W9-DBQ-364

NELSON

TEXTBOOK *of* PEDIATRICS

Richard E. Behrman, MD

Clinical Professor of Pediatrics
Stanford University School of Medicine
University of California, San Francisco,
School of Medicine

Senior Vice President for Medical Affairs
The Lucile Packard Foundation for Children's Health
Palo Alto, California

Robert M. Kliegman, MD

Professor and Chair
Department of Pediatrics
Medical College of Wisconsin
Pediatrician-in-Chief
Children's Hospital of Wisconsin
Milwaukee, Wisconsin

Hal B. Jenson, MD

Professor
Departments of Pediatrics and Microbiology
Chief, Pediatric Infectious Diseases
The University of Texas Health Science
Center at San Antonio
San Antonio, Texas

16TH EDITION

W.B. SAUNDERS COMPANY

A Harcourt Health Sciences Company

Philadelphia London New York St. Louis Sydney Toronto

W.B. SAUNDERS COMPANY
A Harcourt Health Sciences Company

The Curtis Center
Independence Square West
Philadelphia, Pennsylvania 19106

Library of Congress Cataloging-in-Publication Data

Nelson textbook of pediatrics.—16th ed. / [edited by] Richard E. Behrman, Robert M. Kliegman, Hal B. Jenson.

p. cm.

Includes bibliographical references and index.

ISBN 0–7216–7767–3

1. Pediatrics. I. Behrman, Richard E. II. Kliegman, Robert. III. Jenson, Hal B. IV. Title: Textbook of pediatrics.

[DNLM: 1. Pediatrics. WS 100 N432 2000]
RJ45.N4 2000

618.92—dc21

DNLM/DLC 98-50604

NELSON TEXTBOOK OF PEDIATRICS ISBN 0–7216–7767–3

Printed in the United States of America.

Last digit is the print number: 9 8 7 6 5 4 3 2

Dedication

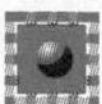

We dedicate this edition to those parents whose love and nurture provide the foundation for the optimal development and good health of their children everywhere.

PREFACE

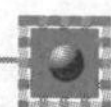

The publication of this 16th Edition of *Nelson Textbook of Pediatrics* coincides with the beginning of the 21st century. The bridging of two centuries creates the opportunity to reflect on past accomplishments, current capabilities, and future hopes. There have been dramatic advances in the prevention and treatment of diseases of childhood. Indeed, many diseases have all but disappeared, and research offers great promise in addressing the new and re-emerging diseases that plague the health of children. Although war, famine, pestilence, poverty, and malfunctioning social systems continue to afflict many of the world's children, ironically the promise of medicine and biologic sciences has never been greater.

From molecular to sociologic levels, knowledge of human development, behavior, and disease is expanding. This has led to greater understanding of health and illness in children and advances in the quality of care that it is possible to provide. Unfortunately, many children worldwide are little affected by these spectacular improvements in medical care, because we have the means but not the political will or wisdom to prevent, to ameliorate, to cure. Not only continually increasing our knowledge but also ensuring that all children are beneficiaries is our challenge for the new century. Good medicine demands ardent advocacy.

In our continuing effort, we address in this edition the full spectrum of problems related to the health and welfare of children and youth that are faced by practitioners, house staff, and medical students. Our goal, as in previous editions, is to be comprehensive, concise, and reader friendly within a single volume. We try to do this in a manner that acknowledges both the science and the art of pediatrics.

The 16th Edition constitutes a major revision and reorganization of the textbook based on a complete review of the field of pediatrics. There are many new chapters as well as substantial modification and expansion of others. Every area of the book has been carefully scrutinized for possible improvement, and, we hope, no chapter has been left unimproved. Although to an ill child and his or her family and physician even the rarest disorder is of vital importance, it is not possible to cover all health problems with the same degree of detail in a general textbook of pediatrics. Thus, leading articles and subspecialty texts are referenced and should be consulted when more information is desired.

A successful textbook is the sum of its expert contributors, and we celebrate ours for their hard work and knowledge as well as their thought and judgment. Our sincere appreciation also goes to Lisette Bralow and Dolores Meloni at W.B. Saunders. We have all worked hard to produce an edition that will be helpful to those who provide care for children and to those wishing to know more about children's health worldwide.

In this edition, we have had informal assistance from faculty and house staff of departments of pediatrics at Stanford University, the Medical College of Wisconsin, the University of California at San Francisco, and the University of Texas Health Science Center at San Antonio. The help of these individuals and numerous practicing pediatricians elsewhere in the United States and around the world who have taken the time to offer thoughtful suggestions is greatly appreciated.

We especially wish to thank Ann Behrman, Sharon Kliegman, and Pauline Jenson for their patience and understanding, without which this textbook would not have been possible.

RICHARD E. BEHRMAN, M.D.

ROBERT M. KLIEGMAN, M.D.

HAL B. JENSON, M.D.

Contributors

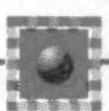

William G. Adams, M.D.
Assistant Professor of Pediatrics, Boston University School of Medicine; Attending Physician, Boston Medical Center, Boston, Massachusetts
Rabies

Raymond D. Adelman, M.D.
Professor of Pediatrics and Associate Dean for Community Affairs, Eastern Virginia Medical School; Director of Community Health and Pediatric Nephrologist, Children's Hospital of the King's Daughters, Norfolk, Virginia
Pathophysiology of Body Fluids and Fluid Therapy

Peter M. Anderson, M.D., Ph.D.
Associate Professor, Mayo Medical School; Consultant, Pediatric Hematology/Oncology, Mayo Clinic, Rochester, Minnesota
Bone Marrow Transplant; Acute Myeloid Leukemia; Neoplasms of the Kidney

Alia Y. Antoon, M.D.
Assistant Clinical Professor of Pediatrics, Harvard Medical School; Chief of Pediatrics, Shriners Hospitals for Children and Shriners Burns Hospital, Boston, Massachusetts
Burn Injuries; Cold Injuries

Ronald L. Ariagno, M.D.
Professor of Pediatrics, Department of Pediatrics, Division of Neonatal and Developmental Medicine, Stanford University School of Medicine; Attending, Packard Children's Hospital at Stanford, Palo Alto, California
Sleep Disorders

Carola A. S. Arndt, M.D.
Associate Professor of Pediatrics and Consultant, Department of Pediatric and Adolescent Medicine, Mayo Medical School and Mayo Clinic and Foundation, Rochester, Minnesota
Acute Myeloid Leukemia; Soft Tissue Sarcomas; Neoplasms of Bone; Benign Tumors

Stephen S. Arnon, M.D.
Senior Investigator and Chief, Infant Botulism Treatment and Prevention Program, California Department of Health Services, Berkeley, California
Botulism; Tetanus

Stephen Aronoff, M.D.
Professor and Chairman, Department of Pediatrics, Temple University School of Medicine; Chief Medical Officer, Temple University Children's Medical Center, Philadelphia, Pennsylvania
Candida; Cryptococcus neoformans; Aspergillus; ***Histoplasmosis*** **(Histoplasma capsulatum);** ***Blastomycosis*** **(Blastomyces dermatitidis); Paracoccidioides brasiliensis;** ***Sporotrichosis*** **(Sporothrix schenckii);** ***Mucormycosis; Primary Amebic Meningoencephalitis; Nonbacterial Food Poisoning***

David M. Asher, M.D.
Chief, Laboratory of Method Development, Office of Vaccine Research and Review, Division of Viral Products, Center for Biologics Evaluation and Research, U.S. Food and Drug Administration, Rockville, Maryland
Transmissible Spongiform Encephalopathies

Jane T. Atkins, M.D.
Assistant Professor, University of Texas–Houston Medical School; Attending, Hermann Children's Hospital, Houston, Texas
Escherichia coli; Aeromonas ***and*** **Plesiomonas**

Marilyn Augustyn, M.D.
Assistant Professor and Director of Training, Division of Developmental and Behavioral Pediatrics, Boston University School of Medicine, Boston, Massachusetts
Impact of Violence on Children

Parvin Azimi, M.D.
Clinical Professor of Pediatrics, University of California, San Francisco; Director of Infectious Diseases, Children's Hospital, Oakland, California
Chancroid **(Haemophilus ducreyi);** ***Syphilis*** **(Treponema pallidum);** ***Nonvenereal Treponemal Infections;*** **Leptospira;** ***Relapsing Fever*** **(Borrelia)**

William F. Balistreri, M.D.
Professor of Pediatrics and Medicine, University of Cincinnati College of Medicine; Director, Division of Pediatric Gastroenterology and Nutrition, Children's Hospital Medical Center, Cincinnati, Ohio
The Liver and Biliary System: Development and Function; Manifestations of Liver Disease; Cholestasis; Metabolic Diseases of the Liver; Liver Abscess; Liver Disease Associated with Systemic Disorders; Reye Syndrome and "Reye-like" Diseases

Robert S. Baltimore, M.D.
Professor of Pediatrics and of Epidemiology and Public Health, Yale University School of Medicine; Associate Hospital Epidemiologist, Yale–New Haven Hospital; Attending Pediatrician, Yale–New Haven Children's Hospital, New Haven, Connecticut
Listeria monocytogenes; Pseudomonas, Burkholderia, ***and*** **Stenotrophomonas**

Lewis A. Barness, M.D.
Professor of Pediatrics, University of South Florida College of Medicine; Staff Pediatrician, The Tampa General Hospital, Tampa, Florida
Nutrition

Fred F. Barrett, M.D.
Professor of Pediatrics, University of Tennessee; Medical Director, Le Bonheur Children's Medical Center, Memphis, Tennessee
Infections Associated with Medical Devices

Dorsey M. Bass, M.D.
Associate Professor of Pediatrics, Stanford University, Stanford; Attending Physician, Lucile Packard Children's Hospital, Palo Alto, California
Rotavirus and Other Agents of Viral Gastroenteritis

Howard Bauchner, M.D.
Professor of Pediatrics and Public Health, Boston University School of Medicine/Boston Medical Center, Boston, Massachusetts
Failure to Thrive

Richard E. Behrman, M.D.
Clinical Professor of Pediatrics, Stanford University School of Medicine and University of California, San Francisco, School of Medicine; Senior Vice President for Medical Affairs, The Lucile Packard Foundation for Children's Health, Palo Alto, California
Overview of Pediatrics; Children at Special Risk

Charles B. Berde, M.D., Ph.D.
Professor of Anaesthesia and Pediatrics, Harvard Medical School; Senior Associate in Anesthesia; Director of Pain Treatment Service, Children's Hospital, Boston, Massachusetts
Anesthesia and Perioperative Care; Pain Management in Children

Jerry M. Bergstein, M.D.
Professor, Department of Pediatrics, Indiana University School of Medicine; Director, Section of Nephrology, James Whitcomb Riley Hospital for Children, Indianapolis, Indiana
Nephrology. Glomerular Disease; Conditions Particularly Associated with Hematuria; Conditions Particularly Associated with Proteinuria; Tubular Function; Renal Tubular Acidosis; Nephrogenic Diabetes Insipidus; Barrter Syndrome; Interstitial Nephritis; Toxic Nephropathy; Cortical Necrosis; Renal Failure

Daniel Bernstein, M.D.
Associate Professor of Pediatrics, Stanford University; Chief, Pediatric Cardiology, Lucile Salter Packard Children's Hospital at Stanford, Stanford, California
The Cardiovascular System

Ronald Blanton, M.D.
Associate Professor of Medicine, Case Western Reserve University School of Medicine, Cleveland, Ohio
Echinococcosis (Echinococcus granulosus *and* E. multilocularis); *Adult Tapeworm Infections; Cysticercosis*

Thomas F. Boat, M.D.
Professor and Chair, Department of Pediatrics, University of Cincinnati College of Medicine; Director, Research Foundation, Physician in Chief, Children's Hospital Medical Center, Cincinnati, Ohio
Chronic or Recurrent Respiratory Symptoms; Cystic Fibrosis

Robert A. Bonomo, M.D.
Assistant Professor of Medicine, Case Western Reserve University School of Medicine; Attending, University Hospitals of Cleveland, Cleveland, Ohio
American Trypanosomiasis (Chagas Disease; Trypanosoma cruzi*); Health Advice for Children Traveling Internationally*

Laurence A. Boxer, M.D.
Professor of Pediatrics, University of Michigan; Director, Pediatric Hematology/Oncology, C.S. Mott Children's Hospital, Ann Arbor, Michigan
The Phagocytic System; Neutrophils; Eosinophils; Disorders of Phagocyte Function; Leukopenia; Leukocytosis

Richard J. Bram, M.D.
Assistant Member, St. Jude Children's Research Hospital, Department of Experimental Oncology, Memphis, Tennessee
Neoplastic Diseases and Tumors: Molecular Pathogenesis

W. Ted Brown, M.D., Ph.D, FACMG
Professor, State University of New York—Health Science Center at Brooklyn; Chairman, Department of Human Genetics, and Director, George A. Jervis Clinic, Institute for Basic Research in Developmental Disabilities, New York State Office of Mental Retardation and Developmental Disabilities, Staten Island, New York
Progeria

Dena R. Brownstein, M.D.
Associate Professor, Department of Pediatrics, University of Washington School of Medicine; Attending Physician, Emergency Services, Children's Hospital and Regional Medical Center, Seattle, Washington
Emergency Medical Services for Children

Rebecca H. Buckley, M.D.
J. Buren Sidbury Professor of Pediatrics and Professor of Immunology, Duke University School of Medicine; Chief, Division of Allergy and Immunology, Duke University Medical Center, Durham, North Carolina
Evaluation of the Immune System; T-, B-, and NK-Cell Systems

Bruce M. Camitta, M.D.
Professor of Pediatrics and Rebecca Jean Slye Professor of Pediatric Oncology, Medical College of Wisconsin; Director, Midwest Children's Cancer Center, Children's Hospital of Wisconsin, Milwaukee, Wisconsin
Polycythemia (Erythrocytosis); The Spleen; The Lymphatic System

James T. Cassidy, M.D.
Professor, Department of Child Health, and Chief, Division of Pediatric Rheumatology, University of Missouri–Columbia School of Medicine, Columbia, Missouri
Treatment of Rheumatic Diseases; Juvenile Rheumatoid Arthritis; Postinfectious Arthritis and Related Conditions

Ellen Gould Chadwick, M.D.
Associate Professor, Northwestern University Medical School; Associate Director, Section of Pediatrics and Maternal HIV Infection, Children's Memorial Hospital, Chicago, Illinois
Acquired Immunodeficiency Syndrome (Human Immunodeficiency Virus)

Yuan-Tsong Chen, M.D., Ph.D.
Professor of Pediatrics and Genetics and Chief, Division of Medical Genetics, Duke University Medical Center, Durham, North Carolina
Defects in Metabolism of Carbohydrates

Russell W. Chesney, M.D.
Le Bonheur Professor and Chair, Department of Pediatrics University of Tennessee College of Medicine, Vice President for Academic Affairs and Co-Director, Center of Excellence in Pediatric Pharmacology and Therapeutics, Le Bonheur Children's Medical Center, Memphis, Tennessee
Hepatic Rickets; Rickets Associated with Anticonvulsant Therapy; Rickets Associated with Renal Tubular Acidosis; Metabolic Bone Disease

Joseph N. Chorley, M.D.
Assistant Professor of Pediatrics, Adolescent Medicine and Sports Medicine Section, Baylor College of Medicine; Team Physician, Texas Southern University, and Assistant Medical Director, Houston Marathon, Texas Children's Hospital, Houston, Texas
Sports Medicine

Robert D. Christensen, M.D.
Professor of Pediatrics, The University of Florida and Shands Teaching Hospital, Gainesville, Florida
Development of the Hematopoietic System

Thomas G. Cleary, M.D.
Professor of Pediatrics, University of Texas–Houston Medical School; Director, Pediatric Infectious Diseases, Hermann Children's Hospital, Houston, Texas
Salmonella; Shigella; Escherichia coli; *Cholera* (Vibrio cholerae); Campylobacter; Yersinia; Aeromonas *and* Plesiomonas

Pinchas Cohen, M.D.
Professor and Director of Research and Training, Division of Pediatric Endocrinology, University of California, Los Angeles, School of Medicine, Los Angeles, California
Hyperpituitarism, Tall Stature, and Overgrowth Syndromes

Harvey R. Colten, M.D.
Dean, Vice President for Medical Affairs and Professor of Pediatrics, Northwestern University Medical School, Chicago, Illinois
Pulmonary Alveolar Proteinosis

Kenneth L. Cox, M.D.
Professor of Pediatrics, Stanford University; Clinical Professor of Pediatrics, University of California, San Francisco; Pediatric Medical Officer, UCSF-Stanford Health Care; Chief, Pediatric Gastroenterology, Lucile Packard Children's Hospitals, Stanford University, Stanford, California
Liver Transplantation

William M. Crist, M.D.
Professor, Mayo Medical School; Chair, Department of Pediatric and Adolescent Medicine, and Consultant, Department of Pediatric and Adolescent Medicine, Mayo Clinic and Foundation, Rochester, Minnesota
Introduction to Pediatric Neoplastic Diseases and Tumors; Epidemiology; Principles of Diagnosis; Principles of Treatment; The Leukemias

John S. Curran, M.D.
Professor of Pediatrics and Vice Dean, University of South Florida College of Medicine; Chief of Pediatrics, The Tampa General Hospital, Tampa, Florida
Nutrition

Richard Dalton, M.D.
Professor of Psychiatry and Pediatrics, Tulane University School of Medicine; Clinical Professor of Psychiatry, Louisiana State University School of Medicine, New Orleans, Louisiana
Psychosocial Problems; Psychiatric Considerations of Central Nervous System Injury; Psychosomatic Illness; Vegetative Disorders; Habit Disorders; Anxiety Disorders; Mood Disorders; Suicide and Attempted Suicide; Disruptive Behavioral Disorders; Sexual Behavior and Its Variations; Pervasive Developmental Disorders and Childhood Psychosis; Psychologic Treatment of Children and Adolescents; Attention Deficit Hyperactivity Disorder; Separation and Death

Alan D. D'Andrea, M.D.
Associate Professor of Pediatrics, Harvard Medical School; Staff, Children's Hospital, Boston, Massachusetts
The Pancytopenias

Gary L. Darmstadt, M.S., M.D.
Assistant Professor of Pediatrics, Division of Dermatology and Division of Infectious Diseases, Department of Pediatrics; Division of Dermatology, Department of Medicine, University of Washington School of Medicine, Seattle, Washington; Adjunct Assistant Professor, Department of International Health, The Johns Hopkins Medical Institutions, Baltimore, Maryland
The Skin

Jorge H. Daruna, Ph.D.
Associate Professor of Psychiatry, Division of Child and Adolescent Psychiatry, Tulane University School of Medicine, New Orleans, Louisiana
The Clinical Interview (History); Attention Deficit Hyperactivity Disorder

Robert S. Daum, M.D., C.M.
Professor, Department of Pediatrics, University of Chicago Pritzker School of Medicine; Chief, Section of Infectious Diseases, University of Chicago Children's Hospital, Chicago, Illinois
Haemophilus influenzae

Dorr G. Dearborn, Ph.D., M.D.
Associate Professor of Pediatrics and Biochemistry, Case Western Reserve University School of Medicine; Physician, Rainbow Babies and Children's Hospital of University Hospitals of Cleveland, Cleveland, Ohio
Pulmonary Hemosiderosis (Pulmonary Hemorrhage)

Melinda T. Derish, M.D.
Assistant Professor, Pediatrics, Stanford University School of Medicine; Associate Director, Pediatric Intensive Care Unit, and Assistant Director, Pulmonary Function Laboratory, Lucile Salter Packard Children's Hospital at Stanford, Stanford, California
Respiratory Distress and Failure; Mechanical Ventilation; Unconventional Forms of Respiratory Support

Robert J. Desnick, Ph.D., M.D.
Professor of Human Genetics and Pediatrics and Chairman, Department of Human Genetics, Mount Sinai School of Medicine, New York, New York
Lipidoses; Mucolipidoses; Disorders of Glycoprotein Degradation and Structure

Joseph V. DiCarlo, M.D.
Assistant Professor of Pediatrics, Stanford University School of Medicine, Stanford, California
Scoring Systems and Predictors of Mortality; Renal Stabilization; Nutritional Stabilization; Neurologic Stabilization; Acute (Adult) Respiratory Distress Syndrome; Continuous Hemofiltration

Angelo M. DiGeorge, M.D.
Professor Emeritus, Department of Pediatrics, Temple University School of Medicine; Member, Section of Endocrinology, Diabetes, and Metabolism, Temple University Children's Medical Center, Philadelphia, Pennsylvania
Disorders of the Parathyroid Glands; Disorders of the Adrenal Glands

Mary K. Donovan, B.S.N., M.S., CPNP
Pediatric Nurse Practitioner/Care Coordinator, Shriners Burn Hospital, Boston, Massachusetts
Pediatric Emergencies and Resuscitation; Burn Injuries; Cold Injuries

Daniel A. Doyle, M.D.
Assistant Professor, Department of Pediatrics, Temple University School of Medicine; Member, Section of Endocrinology, Diabetes, and Metabolism, Temple University Children's Medical Center, Philadelphia, Pennsylvania
Disorders of the Parathyroid Glands

J. Stephen Dumler, M.D.
Associate Professor, The Johns Hopkins University Schools of Medicine and Hygiene and Public Health; Director, Division of Medical Microbiology, Department of Pathology, The Johns Hopkins Hospital, Baltimore, Maryland
Spotted Fever Group Rickettsioses; Scrub Typhus **(Orientia tsutsugamushi)**; *Typhus Group Rickettsioses; Ehrlichioses; Q Fever* **(Coxiella burnetii)**

Paul H. Dworkin, M.D.
Professor and Chair, Department of Pediatrics, University of Connecticut School of Medicine, Farmington; Physician-in-Chief, Connecticut Children's Medical Center and Director and Chair, Department of Pediatrics, St. Francis Hospital and Medical Center, Hartford, Connecticut
Child Care

Jack S. Elder, M.D.
Professor of Urology and Pediatrics, Case Western Reserve University School of Medicine; Director of Pediatric Urology, Rainbow Babies and Children's Hospital, Cleveland, Ohio
Urologic Disorders in Infants and Children

Michele Estabrook, M.D.
Assistant Clinical Professor, University of California, San Francisco, School of Medicine; Clinical Assistant Professor, Stanford University School of Medicine, Stanford, California
Neisseria meningitidis *(Meningococcus)*; Neisseria gonorrhoeae *(Gonococcus)*

Ruth A. Etzel, M.D., Ph.D.
Director, Division of Epidemiology and Risk Assessment, Office of Public Health and Science, Washington, D.C.
Chemical Pollutants

Margaret C. Fisher, M.D.
Professor of Pediatrics, MCP Hahnemann School of Medicine; Member, Section of Infectious Diseases, St. Christopher's Hospital for Children, Philadelphia, Pennsylvania
Pseudomembranous Colitis (Clostridium difficile); *Other Anaerobic Infections; Infection Control and Prophylaxis*

Patricia M. Flynn, M.D.
Associate Professor of Pediatrics, University of Tennessee, Memphis; Associate Member, St. Jude Children's Research Hospital, Memphis, Tennessee
Infections Associated with Medical Devices; Spore-Forming Intestinal Protozoa

Marc A. Forman, M.D.
Emeritus Professor of Psychiatry and Pediatrics, Tulane University School of Medicine, New Orleans, Louisiana; Senior Medical Consultant for Clinical Research, SARAH Network of Hospitals of the Locomotor System, Brasilia, Brazil
Assessment and Interviewing; Psychiatric Considerations of Central Nervous System Injury; Psychosomatic Illness; Mood Disorders; Pervasive Developmental Disorders and Childhood Psychosis; Attention Deficit Hyperactivity Disorder; Separation and Death

Norman Fost, M.D., M.P.H.
Professor, Pediatrics and History of Medicine, and Director, Program in Medical Ethics, University of Wisconsin—Madison; Staff Pediatrician and Director, Child Protection Team, University of Wisconsin Hospital, Madison, Wisconsin
Ethics in Pediatric Care

Kenneth Fox, M.D.
Instructor, Department of Social Medicine, Harvard Medical School; Assistant Professor of Pediatrics, Department of Pediatrics, and Staff Physician, Boston Medical Center, South End Community Health Center, Boston, Massachusetts
Cultural Issues in Pediatric Care

Lorry R. Frankel, M.D.
Associate Professor of Pediatrics, Stanford University School of Medicine; Director, Critical Care Services, Lucile Salter Packard Children's Hospital, Stanford, California
Pediatric Critical Care: An Overview; Interfacility Transfer of the Critically Ill Infant and Child; Effective Communication with Families in the PICU; Monitoring of the Critically Ill Infant and Child; Scoring Systems and Predictors of Mortality; Pediatric Emergencies and Resuscitation; Shock; Respiratory Distress and Failure; Mechanical Ventilation; Neurologic Stabilization; Acute (Adult) Respiratory Distress Syndrome; Transplantation Issues in the PICU; Withdrawal or Withholding of Life Support, Brain Death, and Organ Procurement

James French, M.D.
Major, U.S. Air Force, Keesler Air Force Base, Biloxi, Mississippi
The Spleen

Peter Gal, Pharm.D.
Clinical Professor, School of Pharmacy, University of North Carolina at Chapel Hill; Director, Pharmacy Education and Research, Greensboro Area Health Education Center, Moses Cone Health System, Greensboro, North Carolina
Principles of Drug Therapy; Medications

Luigi Garibaldi, M.D.
Associate Director, Division of Pediatric Endocrinology, Children's Hospital of New Jersey at Newark Beth Israel Medical Center, St. Barnabas Medical Center, and Joslin Center for Diabetes, Livingston, New Jersey
Physiology of Puberty; Disorders of Pubertal Development

Abraham Gedalia, M.D.
Professor of Pediatrics, Louisiana State University Medical Center School of Medicine; Head, Division of Pediatric Rheumatology, Children's Hospital, New Orleans, Louisiana
Behçet's Disease; Sjögren's Syndrome; Familial Mediterranean Fever; Amyloidosis

Fayez K. Ghishan, M.D.
Professor of Pediatrics and Physiology and Head, Department of Pediatrics, University of Arizona Health Sciences Center, Tucson, Arizona
Chronic Diarrhea

Gerald S. Gilchrist, M.D.
Helen C. Levitt Professor, Department of Pediatric and Adolescent Medicine, Mayo Medical School; Consultant in Pediatric Hematology and Oncology, Mayo Clinic, Mayo Eugenio Litta Children's Hospital, Rochester, Minnesota
Lymphoma; Neuroblastoma; Retinoblastoma

Charles M. Ginsburg, M.D.
Professor and Chairman of Pediatrics, Marilyn R. Corrigan Distinguished Chair, University of Texas Southwestern Medical Center; Chief of Staff, Children's Medical Center of Dallas, Dallas, Texas
Animal and Human Bites

Jeffrey L. Goldhagen, M.D., M.P.H.
Associate Clinical Professor of Pediatrics, University of Florida School of Medicine; Director, Duval County Health Department, Jacksonville, Florida
Child Health in the Developing World

Donald A. Goldmann, M.D.
Professor of Pediatrics, Harvard Medical School; Director, Microbiology Laboratories, Hospital Epidemiologist, and Vice Chair for Health Outcomes, Children's Hospital, Boston, Massachusetts
Diagnostic Microbiology

Henry F. Gomez, M.D.
Assistant Professor of Pediatrics, University of Texas, Houston, Medical School, Houston, Texas
Shigella; *Cholera* (Vibrio cholerae)

Collin S. Goto, M.D.
Assistant Professor, Department of Pediatrics, Division of Pediatric Emergency Medicine, University of Texas Southwestern Medical School; Attending Physician, Emergency Department, Children's Medical Center of Dallas, Dallas, Texas
Heavy Metal Intoxication

Samuel P. Gotoff, M.D.
Professor of Pediatrics, Rush Medical College; Chairman of Pediatrics, Rush Children's Hospital and Rush Presbyterian St. Luke's Medical Center, Chicago, Illinois
The Fetus and the Neonatal Infant. Infections of the Neonatal Infant; Group B Streptococcus

Gregory A. Grabowski, M.D.
Professor of Pediatrics, University of Cincinnati College of Medicine; Director, Division and Program in Human Genetics, Children's Hospital Medical Center, Cincinnati, Ohio
Gene Therapy

Christine D. Greco, M.D.
Instructor in Anaesthesia, Harvard Medical School and Children's Hospital, Boston, Massachusetts
Pain Management in Children

David Grossman, M.D., M.P.H.
Associate Professor, Department of Pediatrics, University of Washington School of Medicine; Attending Physician, Harborview Medical Center, Seattle, Washington
Injury Control

Laura T. Gutman, M.D.
Associate Professor of Pediatrics and Pharmacology, Duke University Medical Center, Durham, North Carolina
Papillomaviruses

Gabriel G. Haddad, M.D.
Professor of Pediatrics and of Cellular and Molecular Physiology; Section Chief, Respiratory Medicine, Yale University School of Medicine; Attending Physician, Yale–New Haven Children's Hospital, New Haven, Connecticut
The Respiratory System. Development and Function; Obstructive Sleep Apnea and Hypoventilation in Children; Primary Ciliary Dyskinesia (Immotile Cilia Syndrome)

Judith G. Hall, M.D.
Professor and Head, Department of Pediatrics, University of British Columbia, Vancouver, British Columbia, Canada
Chromosomal Clinical Abnormalities; Genetic Counseling

Scott B. Halstead, M.D.
Senior Scientist, Department of Molecular Microbiology and Immunology, Johns Hopkins School of Public Health, Baltimore, Maryland; Chief Scientist, Division of Medical Science and Technology, Office of Naval Research, Arlington, Virginia
Arboviral Encephalitis in North America; Arboviral Encephalitis Outside North America; Dengue Fever/Dengue Hemorrhagic Fever; Yellow Fever; Other Viral Hemorrhagic Fevers; Hantaviruses

Margaret R. Hammerschlag, M.D.
Professor of Pediatrics and Medicine and Director, Division of Pediatric Infectious Diseases, State University of New York Health Science Center at Brooklyn, Brooklyn, New York
Chlamydia pneumoniae; Chlamydia trachomatis; *Psittacosis* **(Chlamydia psittaci)**

Aaron Hamvas, M.D.
Associate Professor of Pediatrics, Washington University School of Medicine; Staff, St. Louis Children's Hospital, St. Louis, Missouri
Pulmonary Alveolar Proteinosis

H. William Harris, Jr., M.D., Ph.D.
Associate Professor of Pediatrics, Harvard Medical School; Director of Renal Research, Children's Hospital, Boston, Massachusetts
Diabetes Insipidus; Other Abnormalities of Arginine Vasopressin Metabolism and Action

James C. Harris, M.D.
Professor of Psychiatry and Behavioral Sciences and Pediatrics, The Johns Hopkins University School of Medicine; Director, Developmental Neuropsychiatry, The Johns Hopkins Hospital, Baltimore, Maryland
Defects of Purine and Pyrimidine Metabolism

Gary E. Hartman, M.D.
Professor of Surgery and Pediatrics, The George Washington University School of Medicine; Chairman, Department of Pediatric Surgery, Children's National Medical Center, Washington, D.C.
Acute Appendicitis; Diaphragmatic Hernia; Epigastric Hernia

Robert H. A. Haslam, M.D., FAAP, FRCP(C)
Professor of Pediatrics and Medicine (Neurology) and Chairman of Pediatrics Emeritus, University of Toronto; Staff Physician and Child Neurologist, Hospital for Sick Children, Toronto, Ontario, Canada
The Nervous System

Jacqueline T. Hecht, Ph.D.
Professor, Pediatrics, University of Texas Medical School, Houston, Texas
Section 3: The Skeletal Dysplasias

John J. Herbst, M.D.
Professor of Pediatrics, Louisiana State University School of Medicine; Chief, Section of Pediatric Gastroenterology and Nutrition, Louisiana State University Medical Center, Shreveport, Louisiana
The Esophagus; Ulcer Disease

Neil E. Herendeen, M.D.
Clinical Assistant Professor of Pediatrics, University of Rochester School of Medicine and Dentistry; Director of the Pediatric Practice, Children's Hospital at Strong, Rochester, New York
Infections of the Upper Respiratory Tract

Gloria P. Heresi, M.D.
Assistant Professor, Department of Pediatrics, University of Texas Medical School, Houston, Texas
Campylobacter

Albert Hergenroeder, M.D.
Associate Professor of Pediatrics and Section Chief, Adolescent Medicine and Sports Medicine, Baylor College of Medicine; Chief, Sports Medicine Clinic, Texas Children's Hospital, Houston, Texas
Sports Medicine

William H. Hetznecker, M.D.
Clinical Professor of Psychiatry, Temple University Medical School; Inactive Staff, Department of Child Psychiatry, St. Christopher's Hospital for Children, Philadelphia, Pennsylvania
The Clinical Interview (History)

Steve Holve, M.D.
Clinical Instructor of Pediatrics, The Johns Hopkins School of Medicine, Baltimore, Maryland; Chief of Pediatrics, Tuba City Indian Medical Center, Tuba City, Arizona
Envenomations

George R. Honig, M.D., Ph.D.
Professor and Head, Department of Pediatrics, University of Illinois College of Medicine, Chicago, Illinois
Hemoglobin Disorders

William A. Horton, M.D.
Professor, Molecular and Medical Genetics, Oregon Health Sciences University; Director of Research, Shriners Hospital for Children, Portland, Oregon
The Skeletal Dysplasias

Peter J. Hotez, M.D., Ph.D.
Associate Professor of Pediatrics and of Epidemiology and Public Health, Yale University School of Medicine; Associate Physician, Children's Hospital at Yale, New Haven, Connecticut
Hookworms

Walter Hughes, M.D.
Professor of Pediatrics and Preventive Medicine, University of Tennessee College of Medicine; Emeritus Member, Department of Infectious Diseases, St. Jude Children's Research Hospital, Memphis, Tennessee
Infections in Immunocompromised Hosts; Pneumocystis carinii

Carl E. Hunt, M.D.
Professor of Pediatrics, Medical College of Ohio; Staff, St. Vincent Mercy Medical Center, Toledo, Ohio
Sudden Infant Death Syndrome

Jeffrey S. Hyams, M.D.
Professor of Pediatrics, University of Connecticut School of Medicine, Farmington; Head, Division of Digestive Diseases and Nutrition, Connecticut Children's Medical Center, Hartford, Connecticut
Malformations; Ascites; Peritonitis

Richard F. Jacobs, M.D., FAAP
Horace C. Cabe Professor of Pediatrics, University of Arkansas for Medical Sciences; Chief, Pediatric Infectious Diseases, Arkansas Children's Hospital, Little Rock, Arkansas
Actinomycosis; Nocardia; *Tularemia* (Francisella tularensis); Brucella

Renée R. Jenkins, M.D.
Professor and Chairman, Department of Pediatrics, Howard University College of Medicine, Washington, D.C.
Special Health Problems During Adolescence

Hal B. Jenson, M.D.
Professor, Departments of Pediatrics and Microbiology, and Chief, Pediatric Infectious Diseases, The University of Texas Health Science Center at San Antonio, San Antonio, Texas
Epstein-Barr Virus; Lymphocytic Choriomeningitis Virus; Polyomaviruses; Human T-Cell Lymphotropic Viruses Types I and II; Chronic Fatigue Syndrome

David Johnsen, D.D.S.
Dean, College of Dentistry, University of Iowa, Iowa City, Iowa
The Oral Cavity

Charles F. Johnson, M.D.
Professor of Pediatrics, The Ohio State University College of Medicine; Director, Child Abuse Program, Children's Hospital, Columbus, Ohio
Abuse and Neglect of Children

Richard B. Johnston, Jr., M.D.
Professor of Pediatrics, University of Colorado School of Medicine, National Jewish Medical and Research Center, Denver, Colorado
Monocytes and Macrophages; The Complement System

Kenneth Lyons Jones, M.D.
Professor of Pediatrics, University of California, San Diego, School of Medicine, La Jolla; Chief, Division of Dysmorphology, University of California, San Diego, Medical Center, San Diego, California
Dysmorphology

Harry J. Kallas, M.D.
Assistant Professor of Pediatrics, University of California, Davis, School of Medicine; Associate Director, Pediatric Critical Care, University of California, Davis, Medical Center, Sacramento, California
Drowning and Near-Drowning

James W. Kazura, M.D.
Professor of Medicine and International Health, Case Western Reserve University School of Medicine; Chief, Division of Geographic Medicine, University Hospitals of Cleveland, Cleveland, Ohio
Ascariasis (Ascaris lumbricoides); *Enterobiasis (Pinworm,* Enterobius vermicularis*); Toxocariasis (Visceral and Ocular Larva Migrans); Strongyloidiasis* (Strongyloides stercoralis); *Lymphatic Filariasis* (Brugia malayi, Brugia timori, Wuchereria bancrofti); *Infection with Animal Filariae;* Angiostrongylus cantonensis; *Onchocerciasis* (Onchocerca volvulus); *Dracunculiasis (Guinea Worm Infection,* Dracunculus medinensis*); Loiasis* (Loa loa); Gnathostoma spinigerum; *Trichinosis* (Trichinella spiralis); *Trichuriasis* (Trichuris trichiura)

Margaret Kenna, M.D.
Associate Professor, Otology and Laryngology, Harvard Medical School; Associate in Otolaryngology, Children's Hospital, Boston, Massachusetts
Upper Respiratory Tract; The Ear

Charles H. King, M.D.
Associate Professor of Medicine and International Health, Case Western Reserve University School of Medicine; Attending Physician, University Hospitals of Cleveland, Cleveland, Ohio
Schistosomiasis (Schistosoma); Flukes (Liver, Lung, and Intestinal)

Marisa S. Klein-Gitelman, M.D., M.P.H.
Assistant Professor of Pediatrics, Northwestern University Medical School; Attending Physician, Children's Memorial Hospital, Chicago, Illinois
Systemic Lupus Erythematosus

Robert M. Kliegman, M.D.
Professor and Chair, Department of Pediatrics, Medical College of Wisconsin; Pediatrician-in-Chief, Children's Hospital of Wisconsin, Milwaukee, Wisconsin
The Fetus and Neonatal Infant, Noninfectious Disorders

William C. Koch, M.D.
Associate Professor of Pediatrics, Department of Pediatrics, Division of Infectious Diseases, Medical College of Virginia of Virginia Commonwealth University; Attending Physician, Medical College of Virginia Hospitals, Richmond, Virginia
Parvovirus B19

Steve Kohl, M.D.
Professor of Pediatrics, Division of Pediatric Infectious Diseases, University of California, San Francisco; Attending Physician, Moffitt-Long Hospital and San Francisco General Hospital, San Francisco, California
Herpes Simplex Virus

Peter J. Krause, M.D.
Professor, Department of Pediatrics, University of Connecticut School of Medicine, Farmington; Attending Physician, Connecticut Children's Medical Center, Hartford, Connecticut
Malaria (Plasmodium); *Babesiosis* (Babesia)

Danielle J. Laborde, M.P.H., Ph.D.
Visiting Assistant Professor, Clemson University, College of Health, Education, and Human Development, Clemson, South Carolina
Child Care and Communicable Diseases

Stephan Ladisch, M.D.
Professor of Pediatrics and Biochemistry/Molecular Biology, George Washington University School of Medicine; Scientific Director, Children's Research Institute, Children's National Medical Center, Washington, D.C.
Histiocytosis Syndromes of Childhood

Stephen LaFranchi, M.D.
Professor, Department of Pediatrics, and Head, Pediatric Endocrinology, Oregon Health Sciences University; Staff Physician, Doernbecher Children's Hospital, Portland, Oregon
Disorders of the Thyroid Gland

Philip J. Landrigan, M.D., M.Sc.
Ethel H. Wise Professor and Chair, Department of Community and Preventive Medicine, and Professor of Pediatrics, Mount Sinai School of Medicine, New York, New York
Chemical Pollutants

Charles T. Leach, M.D.
Associate Professor of Pediatrics, The University of Texas Health Science Center at San Antonio; Attending Physician, University Hospital and Christus Santa Rosa Children's Hospital, San Antonio, Texas
Roseola (Human Herpesvirus Types 6 and 7); Human Herpesvirus Type 8

Margaret W. Leigh, M.D.
Professor of Pediatrics and Chief, Division of Pulmonary Medicine and Allergy, University of North Carolina at Chapel Hill; Staff Physician, University of North Carolina Hospitals, Chapel Hill, North Carolina
Sarcoidosis

Lenore S. Levine, M.D.
Professor of Pediatrics and Director, Division of Pediatric Endocrinology, College of Physicians and Surgeons, Columbia, University, New York, New York
Disorders of the Adrenal Glands

Melvin D. Levine, M.D.
Professor of Pediatrics and Director, Center for the Study of Development and Learning, University of North Carolina, Chapel Hill, North Carolina
Patterns of Development and Function

Stephen Liben, B.Sc., MDCM
Assistant Professor of Pediatrics, McGill University; Director, Palliative Care Program, and Attending Physician, Pediatric Critical Care Unit, The Montreal Children's Hospital, Montreal, Quebec, Canada
Pediatric Palliative Care: The Care of Children with Life-Limiting Illness

Iris Litt, M.D.
Professor of Pediatrics, Stanford University School of Medicine; Director, Division of Adolescent Medicine, Lucile Packard Children's Hospital at Stanford, Stanford, California
Anorexia Nervosa and Bulimia

Sarah S. Long, M.D.
Professor of Pediatrics, MCP Hahnemann University School of Medicine; Chief, Section of Infectious Diseases, St. Christopher's Hospital for Children, Philadelphia, Pennsylvania
Diphtheria (Corynebacterium diphtheriae); *Pertussis* (Bordetella pertussis *and* B. parapertussis)

Daniel J. Lovell, M.D., M.P.H.
Associate Professor of Pediatrics, University of Cincinnati; Deputy Director, Rowe Division of Rheumatology, Children's Hospital Medical Center, Cincinnati, Ohio
Treatment of Rheumatic Diseases

G. Reid Lyon, Ph.D.
Chief, Child Development and Behavior Branch, National Institute of Child Health and Human Development, National Institutes of Health, Bethesda, Maryland
Specific Reading Disability (Dyslexia)

Adel A. F. Mahmoud, M.D., Ph.D.
President, Merck Vaccines, Whitehouse Station, New Jersey
African Trypanosomiasis (Sleeping Sickness; Trypanosoma brucei*)*

Yvonne Maldonaldo, M.D.
Associate Professor, Department of Pediatrics, Stanford University School of Medicine; Attending Physician, Lucile Salter Packard Children's Hospital at Stanford, Stanford University Hospital, and UCSF-Stanford Healthcare, Stanford, California
Measles; Rubella; Mumps

Joan C. Marini, M.D., Ph.D.
Branch Chief, Heritable Disorders Branch, National Institute of Child Health and Development, National Institutes of Health, Bethesda, Maryland
Osteogenesis Imperfecta

Reuben K. Matalon, M.D., Ph.D.
Professor of Pediatrics and Human Biological Chemistry and Genetics, University of Texas Medical Branch, Galveston, Texas; Adjunct Professor, Department of Human Nutrition and of Pathology, University of Illinois, Chicago, Illinois
Aspartic Acid (Canavan Disease)

Lawrence H. Mathers, Jr., M.D., Ph.D.
Associate Professor of Pediatrics (Critical Care) and Surgery (Human Anatomy) and Chief, Division of Human Anatomy, Stanford University School of Medicine, Stanford, California
Effective Communication with Families in the PICU; Pediatric Emergencies and Resuscitation; Shock; Transplantation Issues in the PICU; Withdrawal or Withholding of Life Support, Brain Death, and Organ Procurement

Nancy J. Matyunas, Pharm.D.
Assistant Clinical Professor of Pediatrics, University of Louisville School of Medicine, Louisville, Kentucky
Poisonings: Drugs, Chemicals, and Plants

Paul L. McCarthy, M.D.
Professor of Pediatrics, Yale University School of Medicine; Head, General Pediatrics, and Medical Director, Pediatric Primary Care, Yale–New Haven Children's Hospital, New Haven, Connecticut
The Well Child; Evaluation of the Sick Child in the Office and Clinic

Margaret M. McGovern, M.D., Ph.D.
Associate Professor of Human Genetics and Pediatrics and Vice Chair, Department of Human Genetics, Mount Sinai School of Medicine, New York, New York
Lipidoses; Mucolipidoses; Disorders of Glycoprotein Degradation and Structure

Kenneth McIntosh, M.D.
Professor of Pediatrics, Harvard Medical School; Chief, Division of Infectious Diseases, Children's Hospital, Boston, Massachusetts
Respiratory Syncytial Virus; Adenoviruses; Rhinoviruses

Rima McLeod, M.D.
Jules and Doris Stein Professor of Research to Prevent Blindness, Visual Sciences Department, University of Chicago Medical School, Chicago, Illinois
Toxoplasmosis (Toxoplasma gondii)

Michael J. McManus, M.D.
Assistant Professor of Pediatrics and Biochemistry/Molecular Biology, Mayo Medical School; Associate Consultant, Pediatric Hematology/Oncology, Mayo Clinic, Rochester, Minnesota
Neoplastic Diseases and Tumors; Molecular Pathogenesis; Neuroblastoma; Neoplasms of the Liver

Peter C. Melby, M.D.
Associate Professor, Departments of Medicine and Microbiology, The University of Texas Health Science Center at San Antonio; Staff Physician, Medical Service, South Texas Veterans Health Care System, Audie L. Murphy VA Hospital, San Antonio, Texas
Leishmania

Fred A. Mettler Jr., M.D., M.P.H.
Professor and Chairman, Department of Radiology, University of New Mexico Health Sciences Center, Albuquerque, New Mexico
Pediatric Radiation Injuries

Michael L. Miller, M.D.
Associate Professor of Pediatrics, Northwestern University Medical School; Director of Clinical Services, Division of Immunology and Rheumatology, Children's Memorial Hospital, Chicago, Illinois
Evaluation of the Patient with Suspected Rheumatic Disease; Treatment of Rheumatic Diseases; Juvenile Rheumatoid Arthritis; Ankylosing Spondylitis and Other Spondyloarthropathies; Postinfectious Arthritis and Related Conditions; Systemic Lupus Erythematosus; Scleroderma; Vasculitis Syndromes; Musculoskeletal Pain Syndromes; Miscellaneous Conditions Associated with Arthritis

Majid Mirmiran, M.D., Ph.D.
Visiting Professor, Department of Pediatrics, Division of Neonatology, Stanford University School of Medicine, Stanford, California; Professor, Netherlands Institute for Brain Research, Amsterdam, The Netherlands
Sleep Disorders

Robert R. Montgomery, M.D.
Professor and Vice Chair for Research, Department of Pediatrics, Medical College of Wisconsin; Senior Investigator, Blood Research Institute; Attending Physician, Children's Hospital of Wisconsin, Milwaukee, Wisconsin
Hemorrhagic and Thrombotic Diseases

Abraham Morag, M.D.
Associate Professor (Clinical Virology), The Hebrew University–Hadassah Medical School; Head, Clinical Virology Unit, Hadassah Medical Center, Jerusalem, Israel
Enteroviruses

Hugo W. Moser, M.D.
Professor of Neurology and Pediatrics, The Johns Hopkins University; Director of Neurogenetics Research, Kennedy Krieger Institute, Baltimore, Maryland
Disorders of Very Long Chain Fatty Acids

Joseph Muenzer, M.D.
Professor, Division of Genetics and Metabolism, Department of Pediatrics, University of North Carolina, Chapel Hill, North Carolina
Mucopolysaccharidoses

Flor Munoz, M.D.
Fellow, Department of Pediatrics, Division of Pediatric Infectious Diseases, Baylor College of Medicine, Houston, Texas
Tuberculosis

James R. Murphy
Professor, Department of Pediatrics, University of Texas–Houston Medical School, Houston, Texas
Campylobacter

Martin G. Myers, M.D.
Professor and Chairman, Department of Pediatrics, Northwestern University Medical School and Children's Memorial Hospital, Chicago, Illinois
Varicella-Zoster Virus

Robert D. Needlman, M.D.
Assistant Professor of Pediatrics, Case Western Reserve University School of Medicine; Attending Physician Rainbow Babies and Children's Hospital, University Hospitals of Cleveland, Cleveland, Ohio
Growth and Development

John D. Nelson, M.D.
Professor Emeritus, Department of Pediatrics, The University of Texas Southwestern Medical Center at Dallas; Honorary Staff Membership, Children's Medical Center and Parkland Memorial Hospital, Dallas, Texas
Osteomyelitis and Suppurative Arthritis

Leonard B. Nelson, M.D.
Professor of Ophthalmology and Pediatrics, Jefferson Medical College of Thomas Jefferson University; Co-Director, Pediatric Ophthalmology, Wills Eye Hospital, Philadelphia, Pennsylvania
Disorders of the Eye

John F. Nicholson, M.D.
Associate Professor of Pediatrics and Pathology, Columbia University College of Physicians and Surgeons; Director, Point-of-Care, New York Presbyterian Hospital at Columbia Presbyterian Medical Center, New York, New York
Laboratory Testing in Infants and Children; Reference Ranges for Laboratory Tests and Procedures

Pearay L. Ogra, M.D.
John Sealy Distinguished Chair and Professor of Pediatrics, University of Texas Medical Branch, Galveston, Texas
Enteroviruses

Robin K. Ohls, M.D.
Associate Professor of Pediatrics, The University of New Mexico, The Childrens Hospital of New Mexico, Albuquerque, New Mexico
Development of the Hematopoietic System

Scott E. Olitsky, M.D.
Assistant Professor of Ophthalmology, State University of New York at Buffalo; Staff, The Children's Hospital of Buffalo, Buffalo, New York
Disorders of the Eye

David M. Orenstein, M.D.
Professor of Pediatrics, School of Medicine; Professor of Health, Physical and Recreation Education and Exercise Physiology, School of Education, University of Pittsburgh School of Medicine; Director, Division of Pediatric Pulmonary and Cystic Fibrosis Center, Children's Hospital of Pittsburgh, Pittsburgh, Pennsylvania
Lower Respiratory Tract; Acute Inflammatory Upper Airway Obstruction; Foreign Bodies in the Larynx, Trachea, and Bronchi; Subglottic Stenosis; Bronchitis; Bronchiolitis; Bronchiolitis Obliterans; Aspiration Pneumonias and Gastroesophageal Reflux–Related Respiratory Disease; Emphysema and Overinflation; Pulmonary Edema; Chronic or Recurrent Respiratory Symptoms; Diseases of the Pleura; Neuromuscular and Skeletal Diseases Affecting Pulmonary Function

Lauren M. Pachman, M.D.
Professor of Pediatrics, Northwestern University Medical School; Chief, Division of Pediatrics, Immunology/Rheumatology, The Children's Memorial Hospital, Chicago, Illinois
Juvenile Dermatomyositis; Vasculitis Syndromes

Regina M. Palazzo, M.D.
Assistant Professor of Pediatrics, Section of Respiratory Medicine, Yale University School of Medicine; Director, Cystic Fibrosis Center; Attending Physician, Yale–New Haven Children's Hospital, New Haven, Connecticut
Diagnostic Approach to Respiratory Disease

Demosthenes Pappagianis, M.D., Ph.D.
Professor, Department of Medical Microbiology and Immunology, School of Medicine, University of California, Davis, Davis, California
Coccidioidomycosis (Coccidioides immitis)

John S. Parks, M.D., Ph.D.
Professor of Pediatrics and Director of Pediatric Endocrinology, Emory University School of Medicine; Director, Pediatric Endocrinology, Egleston Children's Hospital, Atlanta, Georgia
Hormones of the Hypothalamus and Pituitary; Hypopituitarism

Alberto Peña, M.D.
Professor of Surgery, Albert Einstein College of Medicine, The Bronx; Chief, Pediatric Surgery, Schneider Children's Hospital, Long Island Jewish Medical Center, New Hyde Park, New York
Anorectal Malformations; Surgical Conditions of the Anus, Rectum, and Colon

J. Julio Pérez-Fontán, M.D.
Professor of Pediatrics and Anesthesiology, Washington University School of Medicine; Director, Division of Pediatric Critical Care Medicine and Pediatric Intensive Care Unit, Department of Pediatrics, St. Louis Children's Hospital, St. Louis, Missouri
Development of the Respiratory System; Respiratory Pathophysiology; Defense Mechanisms and Metabolic Functions of the Lung

James M. Perrin, M.D.
Associate Professor of Pediatrics, Harvard Medical School; Director, Division of General Pediatrics, Massachusetts General Hospital, Boston, Massachusetts
Developmental Disabilities and Chronic Illness: An Overview; Chronic Illness in Childhood

Michael A. Pesce, Ph.D.
Associate Professor of Clinical Pathology, Columbia University College of Physicians and Surgeons; Director, Specialty Laboratory, New York Presbyterian Hospital at Columbia-Presbyterian Medical Center, New York, New York
Laboratory Testing in Infants and Children; Reference Ranges for Laboratory Tests and Procedures

Georges Peter, M.D.
Professor of Pediatrics, Brown University School of Medicine; Director, Division of Pediatric Infectious Disease, Rhode Island Hospital, Providence, Rhode Island
Immunization Practices

Ross E. Petty, M.D., Ph.D.
Professor and Head, Division of Pediatric Rheumatology, Department of Pediatrics, The University of British Columbia and Children's Hospital, Vancouver, British Columbia, Canada
Ankylosing Spondylitis and Other Spondyloarthropathies

Larry K. Pickering, M.D.
Professor of Pediatrics, Eastern Virginia Medical School of the Medical College of Hampton Roads; Chair in Pediatrics Research and Director, Center for Pediatric Research, Children's Hospital of the King's Daughters, Norfolk, Virginia
Gastroenteritis; Viral Hepatitis; Giardiasis and Balantidiasis; Child Day Care and Communicable Diseases

Sergio Piomelli, M.D.
James A. Wolff Professor of Pediatrics, Columbia University College of Physicians and Surgeons; Director, Pediatric Hematology, Babies and Children's Hospital, New York, New York
Lead Poisoning

Philip A. Pizzo, M.D.
Thomas Margon Rotch Professor and Chair, Department of Pediatrics, Harvard Medical School; Physician-in-Chief and Chair, Department of Medicine, Children's Hospital, Boston, Massachusetts
Infections in Immunocompromised Hosts; The Pancytopenias

Dwight A. Powell, M.D.
Professor of Pediatrics, The Ohio State University College of Medicine and Public Health; Chief, Section of Pediatric Infectious Diseases, Children's Hospital, Columbus, Ohio
Leprosy (Hansen Disease); Atypical Mycobacteria; Mycoplasma pneumoniae; *Genital Mycoplasmas* (Mycoplasma hominis *and* Ureaplasma urealyticum)

Keith R. Powell, M.D.
Professor and Chairman, Department of Pediatrics, Northeastern Ohio Universities College of Medicine, Dr. Noah Miller Chair of Pediatric Medicine, Children's Hospital Medical Center of Akron, Akron, Ohio
Fever; Fever Without a Focus; Sepsis and Shock

Charles G. Prober, M.D.
Professor of Pediatrics, Medicine, Microbiology, and Immunology and Associate Chairman, Department of Pediatrics, Stanford University School of Medicine, Stanford, California
Central Nervous System Infections; Pneumonia

Daniel J. Rader, M.D.
Assistant Professor of Medicine, Pediatrics, Pathology, and Laboratory Medicine, University of Pennsylvania School of Medicine; Director, Preventive Cardiology and Lipid Research Center, University of Pennsylvania Health System, Philadelphia, Pennsylvania
Disorders of Lipoprotein Metabolism and Transport

Robert Rapaport, M.D.
Associate Professor of Pediatrics, University of Medicine and Dentistry of New Jersey, Newark; Director, Pediatric Endocrinology and Metabolism, St. Barnabas Health Care System and Children's Hospital of New Jersey at Newark, Beth Israel Medical Center, Livingston and Newark, New Jersey
Disorders of the Gonads

Michael D. Reed, Pharm.D.
Professor of Pediatrics, Case Western Reserve University, School of Medicine; Director, Pediatric Clinical Pharmacology and Toxicology, Rainbow Babies and Children's Hospital, Cleveland, Ohio
Principles of Drug Therapy; Medications

Jack S. Remington, M.D.
Professor of Medicine, Division of Infectious Diseases and Geographic Medicine, Stanford University School of Medicine; Marcus A. Krupp Research Chair and Chairman, Department of Immunology and Infectious Diseases, Research Institute, Palo Alto Medical Foundation, Palo Alto, California
Toxoplasmosis (Toxoplasma gondii)

Iraj Rezvani, M.D.
Professor of Pediatrics, Department of Pediatrics, Temple University School of Medicine; Chief, Section of Endocrine, Diabetes, and Metabolic Disorders, Temple University Children's Medical Center, Philadelphia, Pennsylvania
An Approach to Inborn Errors; Phenylalanine; Tyrosine; Methionine; Cysteine/Cystine; Tryptophan; Valine, Leucine, Isoleucine, and Related Organic Acidemias; Glycine; Serine; Proline and Hydroxyproline; Glutamic Acid; Urea Cycle and Hyperammonemia; Histidine; Lysine

Frederick P. Rivara, M.D., M.P.H.
George Adkins Professor of Pediatrics, University of Washington School of Medicine; Director, Harborview Injury Prevention and Research Center, Harborview Medical Center, Seattle, Washington
Injury Control; Emergency Medical Services for Children

Dennis M. Robertson, M.D.
Professor of Ophthalmology, Mayo Medical School; Consultant in Ophthalmology, Mayo Clinic and Foundation, Rochester, Minnesota
Retinoblastoma

Kent A. Robertson, M.D., Ph.D.
Associate Professor of Pediatrics and Investigator, Herman B. Wells Center for Pediatric Research, Indiana University School of Medicine; Staff, Riley Hospital for Children, Indianapolis, Indiana
Bone Marrow Transplantation

Luther K. Robinson, M.D.
Associate Professor of Pediatrics, State University of New York at Buffalo, School of Medicine and Biomedical Sciences; Director, Dysmorphology and Clinical Genetics, Kaleida Health—Children's Hospital of Buffalo, Buffalo, New York
Marfan Syndrome

Alice Rock, M.D.
Assistant Professor of Pediatrics, Medical College of Wisconsin and Children's Hospital of Wisconsin, Milwaukee, Wisconsin
The Lymphatic System

George C. Rodgers, Jr., M.D., Ph.D.
Professor of Pediatrics, Pharmacology/Toxicology, and International Pediatrics, University of Louisville School of Medicine; Medical Director, Kentucky Regional Poison Center, Louisville, Kentucky
Poisonings: Drugs, Chemicals, and Plants

Carol L. Rosen, M.D.
Associate Professor of Pediatrics, Section of Respiratory Medicine, Yale University School of Medicine; Medical Director, Children's Sleep Laboratory, Children's Clinical Research Center; Attending Physician, Yale–New Haven Children's Hospital, New Haven, Connecticut
Obstructive Sleep Apnea and Hypoventilation in Children

David S. Rosenblatt, M.D.C.M.
Professor of Pediatrics, Medicine, and Human Genetics, McGill University; Director, Division of Medical Genetics, Department of Medicine, McGill University Health Center, Montreal, Quebec, Canada
An Approach to Inborn Errors; Valine, Leucine, Isoleucine, and Related Organic Acidemias

Anne H. Rowley, M.D.
Associate Professor of Pediatrics and of Microbiology and Immunology, Northwestern University Medical School; Attending Physician, Division of Infectious Diseases, Children's Memorial Hospital, Chicago, Illinois
Kawasaki Disease

Robert A. Salata, M.D.
Professor of Medicine, Case Western Reserve University School of Medicine, Department of Medicine, International Health, Epidemiology, and Biostatistics; Chief, Division of Infectious Diseases, and Hospital Epidemiologist, University Hospitals of Cleveland, Cleveland, Ohio
Amebiasis; Trichomoniasis (Trichomonas vaginalis)*; American Trypanosomiasis (Chagas Disease;* Trypanosoma cruzi*); Health Advice for Children Traveling Internationally*

Joseph S. Sanfilippo, M.D.
Professor and Chairman, Obstetrics and Gynecology, MCP Hahnemann School of Medicine; Allegheny General Hospital, Philadelphia, Pennsylvania
Gynecologic Problems of Childhood

Harvey B. Sarnat, M.D., FRCPC
Professor of Neurology, Pediatrics, and Pathology (Neuropathology), University of Washington School of Medicine; Pediatric Neurologist and Neuropathologist, Children's Hospital and Regional Medical Center, Seattle, Washington
Neuromuscular Disorders

Shigeru Sassa, M.D., Ph.D.
Associate Professor and Head, Laboratory of Biochemical Hematology, The Rockefeller University; Physician, The Rockefeller University Hospital, New York, New York
The Porphyrias

Robert Schechter, M.D., M.Sc.
Clinical Director, Infant Botulism Treatment and Prevention Program, California Department of Health Services, Berkeley; Staff Physician, Children's Hospital, Oakland, California
Botulism

William S. Schechter, M.D., FAAP
Assistant Professor of Anesthesiology and Pediatrics and Director, Pediatric Pain Treatment and Sedation Service, Department of Anesthesiology, Babies and Children's Hospital, New York, New York
Anesthesia and Perioperative Care

Gordon E. Schutze, M.D., FAAP
Associate Professor of Pediatrics and Pathology, University of Arkansas for Medical Sciences; Pediatric Residency Program Director, Pediatric Infectious Diseases, Arkansas Children's Hospital, Little Rock, Arkansas
Actinomycosis; Nocardia; *Tularemia* (Francisella tularensis)*; Brucella*

Elias Schwartz, M.D.
Professor of Pediatrics, Jefferson Medical College of Thomas Jefferson University; Pediatric Hematologist, Cardeza Foundation, Thomas Jefferson University Hospital, Philadelphia, Pennsylvania and Alfred I. duPont Hospital for Children, Wilmington, Delaware
The Anemias; Anemias of Inadequate Production

Peter V. Scoles, M.D.
Professor, Department of Orthopedic Surgery, Case Western Reserve University, Cleveland, Ohio
Bone and Joint Disorders, Orthopedic Problems

Charles Scott, M.D.
Director, Forensic Psychiatry Training, University of California, Davis, Sacramento, California
Vegetative Disorders

J. Paul Scott, M.D.
Professor of Pediatrics, Medical College of Wisconsin; Investigator, Blood Research Institute; Attending Physician, Children's Hospital of Wisconsin, Milwaukee, Wisconsin
Hemorrhagic and Thrombotic Diseases

Theodore C. Sectish, M.D.
Assistant Professor of Pediatrics, Stanford University School of Medicine; Director, Residency Training Program in Pediatrics, Lucile Salter Packard Children's Hospital at Stanford, Palo Alto, California
Preventive Pediatrics

George B. Segel, M.D.
Professor of Pediatrics, Medicine, Genetics, and Oncology; Chief, Pediatric Hematology/Oncology and Genetics; Vice Chair, Department of Pediatrics, University of Rochester Medical Center, Rochester, New York
Diseases of the Blood. Hemolytic Anemias: Definitions and Classification of Hemolytic Anemias; Hereditary Spherocytosis; Hereditary Elliptocytosis; Hereditary Stomatocytosis; Other Membrane Defects; Enzymatic Defects; Hemolytic Anemias Resulting from Extracellular Factors; Hemolytic Anemias Secondary to Other Extracellular Factors

Eugene D. Shapiro, M.D.
Professor of Pediatrics and of Epidemiology and Public Health and the Children's Clinical Research Center, Yale University School of Medicine; Attending Pediatrician, Children's Hospital at Yale–New Haven, New Haven, Connecticut
Lyme Disease (Borrelia burgdorferi)

Larry Shapiro, M.D.
W.H. and Marie Wattis Distinguished Professor and Chairman, Department of Pediatrics, University of California, San Francisco, School of Medicine; Chief of Pediatric Services, UCSF Medical Center, San Francisco, California
Molecular Basis of Genetic Disorders; Molecular Diagnosis of Genetic Diseases; Patterns of Inheritance

William J. Shaughnessy, M.D.
Assistant Professor of Pediatrics, Mayo Medical School; Consultant, Mayo Clinic, Rochester, Minnesota
Benign Tumors

Sally E. Shaywitz, M.D.
Professor of Pediatrics, Director, Learning Disorders Unit, and Co-Director, Center for the Study of Learning and Attention, Yale University School of Medicine, New Haven, Connecticut
Specific Reading Disability (Dyslexia)

Benjamin L. Shneider, M.D.
Associate Professor of Pediatrics, Mount Sinai School of Medicine; Director, Pediatric Liver Program, Mount Sinai Medical Center, New York, New York
Autoimmune (Chronic) Hepatitis

Stephen J. Shochat, M.D.
Professor of Surgery and Pediatrics, University of Tennessee Health Science Center; Surgeon-in-Chief and Chairman, Department of Surgery, St. Jude Children's Research Hospital, Memphis, Tennessee
Inguinal Hernias

Jack P. Shonkoff, M.D.
Samuel F. and Rose B. Gingold Professor of Human Development and Dean of the Heller Graduate School, Brandeis University, Waltham, Massachusetts
Developmental Disabilities and Chronic Illness: An Overview; Mental Retardation

Stanford T. Shulman, M.D.
Professor of Pediatrics and Associate Dean, Northwestern University Medical School; Chief, Division of Infectious Diseases, Children's Memorial Hospital, Chicago, Illinois
Kawasaki Disease

Mark D. Simms, M.D., M.P.H.
Associate Professor of Pediatrics, Medical College of Wisconsin; Medical Director, Child Development Center, Children's Hospital of Wisconsin, Milwaukee, Wisconsin
Adoption; Foster Care

R. Michael Sly, M.D.
Professor of Pediatrics, The George Washington University School of Medicine and Health Sciences; Head, Section of Allergy and Immunology, Children's National Medical Center, Washington, D.C.
Allergic Disorders

William A. Smithson, M.D.
Associate Professor of Pediatric Hematology/Oncology, Mayo Medical School; Consultant, Department of Pediatric and Adolescent Medicine and Head, Section of Pediatric Hematology/Oncology, Mayo Clinic and Foundation, Rochester, Minnesota
The Leukemias; Gonadal and Germ Cell Neoplasms; Gastrointestinal Neoplasms; Carcinomas; Cancer of the Skin

John Snyder, M.D.
Professor of Pediatrics, University of California, San Francisco, San Fransicso, California
Gastroenteritis; Viral Hepatitis

Michael J. Solhaug, M.D.
Professor of Pediatrics and Assistant Professor of Physiology, Eastern Virginia Medical School; Director, Pediatric Nephrology, Children's Hospital of the King's Daughters, Norfolk, Virginia
Pathophysiology of Body Fluids and Fluid Therapy

Mark A. Sperling, M.D.
Vira I. Heinz Professor of Pediatrics and Chair, Department of Pediatrics, University of Pittsburgh School of Medicine; Pediatrician-in-Chief, Children's Hospital of Pittsburgh, Pittsburgh, Pennsylvania
Hypoglycemia; Diabetes Mellitus in Children

Sergio Stagno, M.D.
Professor and Chairman, University of Alabama at Birmingham; Physician-in-Chief, Children's Hospital of Alabama, Birmingham, Alabama
Cytomegalovirus

Lawrence R. Stanberry, M.D., Ph.D.
Albert B. Sabin Professor, Department of Pediatrics, University of Cincinnati College of Medicine; Director, Division of Infectious Diseases, Children's Hospital Medical Center, Cincinnati, Ohio
Varicella-Zoster Virus

Charles A. Stanley, M.D.
Professor of Pediatrics, University of Pennsylvania School of Medicine; Senior Endocrinologist, Endocrine Division, The Children's Hospital of Philadelphia, Philadelphia, Pennsylvania
Disorders of Mitochondrial Fatty Acid Oxidation

Jeffrey R. Starke, M.D.
Associate Professor of Pediatrics, Baylor College of Medicine; Director, Children's Tuberculosis Clinic, and Deputy Chief of Pediatrics, Ben Taub General Hospital, Houston, Texas
Tuberculosis

Barbara W. Stechenberg, M.D.
Professor of Pediatrics, Tufts University School of Medicine, Boston; Vice Chairman and Director of Pediatric Infectious Diseases, Baystate Medical Center Children's Hospital, Springfield, Massachusetts
Bartonella

Robert C. Stern, M.D.
Professor of Pediatrics, Case Western Reserve University School of Medicine; Associate Pediatrician, Rainbow Babies and Children's Hospital, Cleveland, Ohio
The Respiratory System. Lower Respiratory Tract: Congenital Anomalies; Trauma to the Larynx; Neoplasms of the Larynx and Trachea; Silo Filler's Disease; Paraquat Lung; Hypersensitivity to Inhaled Materials; Pulmonary Aspergillosis; Loeffler Syndrome; Pulmonary Involvement in Collagen Diseases; Desquamative Interstitial Pneumonitis

Barbara J. Stoll, M.D.
Professor of Pediatrics, Emory University School of Medicine, Atlanta, Georgia
The Fetus and the Neonatal Infant, Noninfectious Disorders

Ronald G. Strauss, M.D.
Professor, Pathology and Pediatrics, University of Iowa College of Medicine; Medical Director, University of Iowa DeGowin Blood Center, University of Iowa Hospitals and Clinics, Iowa City, Iowa
Blood and Blood Component Transfusions

Frederick J. Suchy, M.D.
Professor and Chair, Department of Pediatrics, Mount Sinai School of Medicine; Pediatrician-in-Chief, Mount Sinai Hospital, New York, New York
Autoimmune (Chronic) Hepatitis; Drug- and Toxin-Induced Liver Injury; Fulminant Hepatic Failure; Cystic Diseases of the Biliary Tract and Liver; Diseases of the Gallbladder; Portal Hypertension and Varices

Peter G. Szilagyi, M.D., M.P.H.
Associate Professor of Pediatrics, Director, Pediatric Ambulatory Services, and Associate Director, Division of General Pediatrics, University of Rochester School of Medicine and Dentistry, Rochester, New York
Infections of the Upper Respiratory Tract

Andrew M. Tershakovec, M.D.
Associate Professor, Department of Pediatrics, University of Pennsylvania School of Medicine; Associate Physician, Division of Gastroenterology and Nutrition, The Children's Hospital of Philadelphia, Philadelphia, Pennsylvania
Disorders of Lipoprotein Metabolism and Transport

George H. Thompson, M.D.
Professor, Orthopaedic Surgery and Pediatrics, Case Western Reserve University; Director, Pediatric Orthopedics, Rainbow Babies and Children's Hospital, Cleveland, Ohio
Bone and Joint Disorders, Orthopedic Problems

Norman Tinanoff, D.D.S.
Professor and Chairman, Department of Pediatric Dentistry, University of Maryland Dental School, Baltimore, Maryland
The Oral Cavity

James K. Todd, M.D.
Professor of Pediatrics, Microbiology, and Preventive Medicine, University of Colorado School of Medicine; Director of Epidemiology and Clinical Microbiology, The Children's Hospital, Denver, Colorado
Staphylococcal Infections; Streptococcus pneumoniae *(Pneumococcus); Group A Streptocococcus; Other Streptococci*

Lucy Tompkins, M.D., Ph.D.
Professor, Department of Medicine (Division of Infectious Diseases and Geographic Medicine) and Microbiology and Immunology, Stanford University School of Medicine; Medical Director, Clinical Microbiology/Virology Laboratory; Medical Director, Hospital Epidemiology and Infection Prevention Department, University of California, San Francisco, and Stanford University Medical Center, Stanford, California
Legionella

Martin Ulshen, M.D.
Professor of Pediatrics, Duke University Medical Center, Durham, North Carolina
Clinical Manifestations of Gastrointestinal Disease; Normal Development, Structure, and Function of Stomach and Intestines; Inflammatory Bowel Disease; Food Allergy; Eosinophilic Gastroenteritis; Malabsorptive Disorders; Recurrent Abdominal Pain of Childhood; Tumors of the Digestive Tract

Rodrigo E. Urizar, M.D.
Professor of Pediatrics and Associate Professor of Medicine, Albany Medical College; Attending Nephrologist, Department of Pediatrics and Medicine; Medical Director, Pediatric Dialysis Services, Albany Medical Center Children's Hospital, Albany, New York
Renal Transplantation

Martin Weisse, M.D.
Associate Professor, Infectious Diseases and General Pediatrics, Department of Pediatrics, West Virginia University Health Science Center, School of Medicine; Director, Pediatrics Residency Program, West Virginia University Hospitals, Morgantown, West Virginia
Candida; Malassezia furfur; *Primary Amebic Meningoencephalitis*

Sharon Weissman, M.D.
Assistant Professor of Medicine, Case Western University Medical School, Department of Medicine, Division of Infectious Disease, and Cleveland Louis Stokes Veterans Affairs Medical Center, Cleveland, Ohio
Amebiasis; Trichomoniasis (Trichomonas vaginalis)

Steven L. Werlin, M.D.
Professor of Pediatrics, Medical College of Wisconsin, Milwaukee, Wisconsin
Exocrine Pancreas

Jeffrey A. Whitsett, M.D.
Professor of Pediatrics, University of Cincinnati; Director, Divisions of Pulmonary Biology and Neonatology, Children's Hospital Medical Center, Cincinnati, Ohio
Gene Therapy

Susan L. Williamson, M.D.
Professor and Chief of Pediatric Radiology, Department of Radiology, University of New Mexico Health Sciences Center, Albuquerque, New Mexico
Pediatric Radiation Injuries

Peter Wright, M.D.
Professor of Pediatrics and Microbiology and Immunology, Head, Department of Pediatric Infectious Diseases, and Director, Center for International Health, Vanderbilt University Medical Center, Nashville, Tennessee
Influenza Viruses; Parainfluenza Viruses

Robert Wyllie, M.D.
Chairman, Department of Pediatric Gastroenterology and Nutrition, Cleveland Clinic Foundation, Cleveland, Ohio
Pyloric Stenosis and Other Congenital Anomalies of the Stomach; Intestinal Atresia, Stenosis, and Malrotation; Intestinal Duplication, Meckel Diverticulum, and Other Remnants of the Omphalomesenteric Duct; Motility Disorders and Hirschsprung Disease; Ileus, Adhesions, Intussusception, and Closed-Loop Obstructions; Foreign Bodies and Bezoars

Ram Yogev, M.D.
Professor of Pediatrics, Northwestern University Medical School; Director, Section of Pediatric and Maternal HIV Infection, Children's Memorial Hospital, Chicago, Illinois
Acquired Immunodeficiency Syndrome (Human Immunodeficiency Virus)

Anita K. M. Zaidi, M.B., S.M.
Instructor in Pediatrics, Harvard Medical School; Assistant in Medicine and Infectious Diseases, Children's Hospital, Boston, Massachusetts
Diagnostic Microbiology

Barry Zuckerman, M.D.
Professor and Chair, Department of Pediatrics, Boston University School of Medicine, Boston, Massachusetts
Impact of Violence on Children

CONTENTS

NOTICE

Pediatrics is an ever-changing field. Standard safety precautions must be followed, but as new research and clinical experience broaden our knowledge, changes in treatment and drug therapy become necessary or appropriate. Readers are advised to check the product information currently provided by the manufacturer of each drug to be administered to verify the recommended dose, the method and duration of administration, and the contraindications. It is the responsibility of the treating physician, relying on experience and knowledge of the patient, to determine dosages and the best treatment for the patient. Neither the Publisher nor the editor assumes any responsibility for any injury and/or damage to persons or property.

THE PUBLISHER

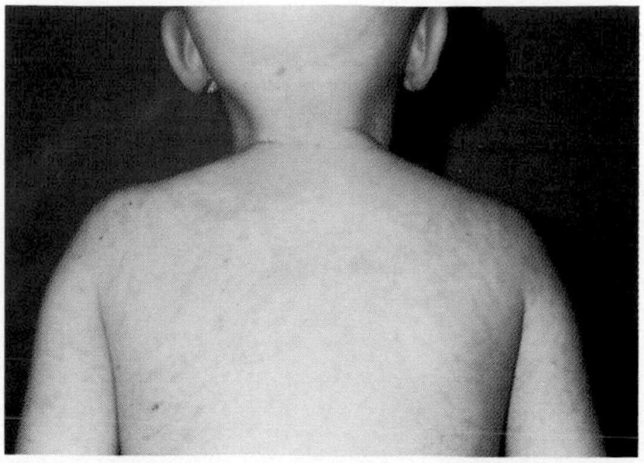

Figure 137–1

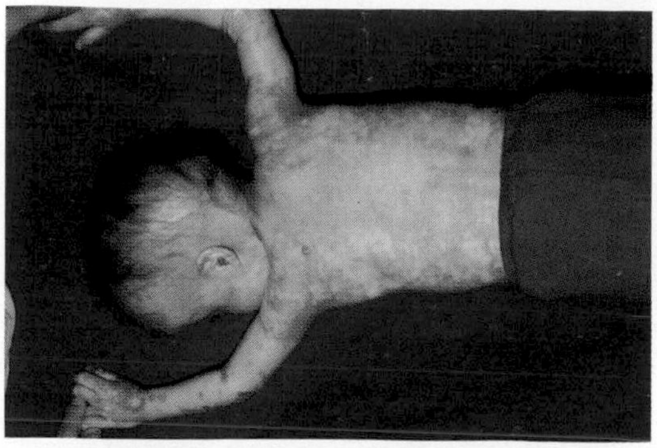

Figure 137–2

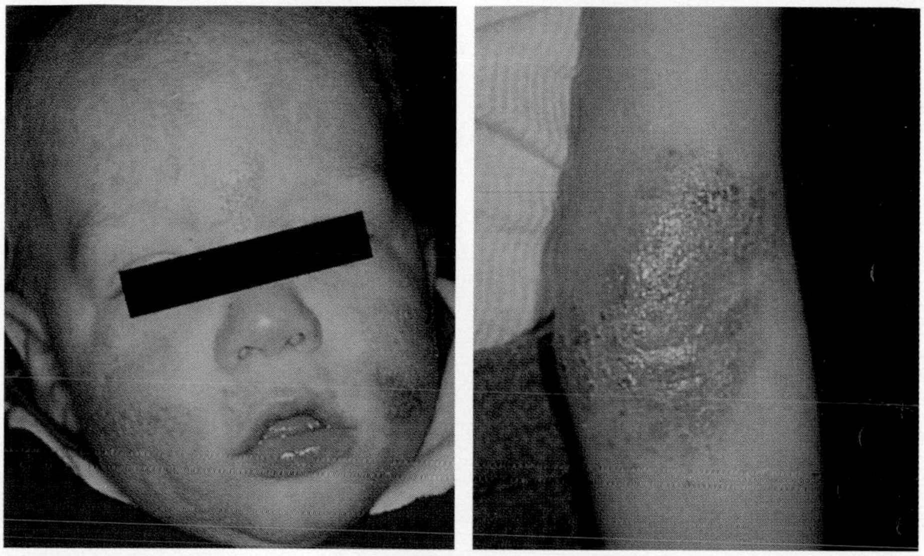

Figure 146–1

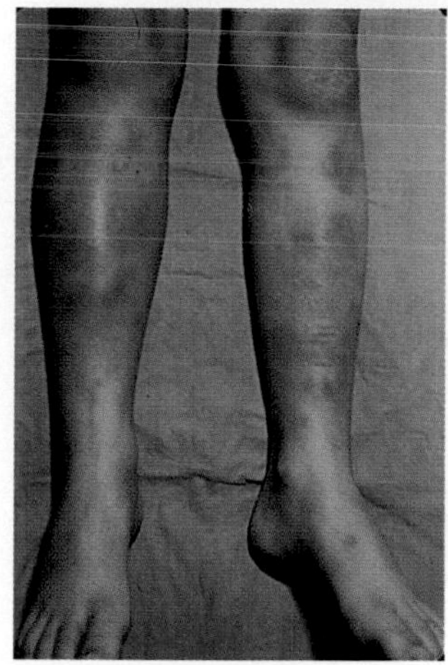

Figure 154–1

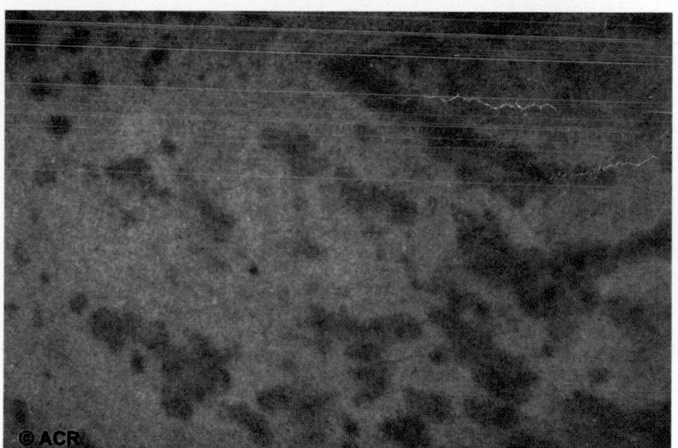

Figure 156–8

Figure 137–1 Acute graft-versus-host disease of the skin with ear, arm, shoulder, and trunk involvement. (Courtesy of Evan Farmer, M.D.)

Figure 137–2 Chronic graft versus host disease of the skin with sclerodermoid changes. (Courtesy of Evan Farmer, M.D.)

Figure 146–1 *A–B,* Infantile atopic dermatitis begins typically as a pruritic, erythematous, papulovesicular eruption over the cheeks but may also involve the wrists and extensor aspects of the extremities or may become generalized, usually sparing the diaper area. By 2 yr of age, involvement of antecubital and popliteal spaces, neck, wrists, and ankles is common with scaling, excoriations, lichenification, and hyperpigmentation. Crusting indicates superimposed infection. (From The Dermatologic Dozen, 1980. Used with permission of Westwood Pharmaceuticals, Inc.)

Figure 154–1 Erythema nodosum: legs. Erythematous nodules and plaques are present over both shins. The skin overlying the lesions is red, smooth, and shiny. The nodules are usually tender. Erythema nodosum is considered a hypersensitivity reaction and can be associated with a variety of diseases, including sarcoidosis, β-hemolytic streptococcal infection, tuberculosis, coccidioidomycosis, and ulcerative colitis.

Figure 156–8 The rash of systemic-onset juvenile rheumatoid arthritis. The rash is salmon colored, macular, and nonpruritic. Individual lesions are transient and occur in crops over the trunk and extremities.

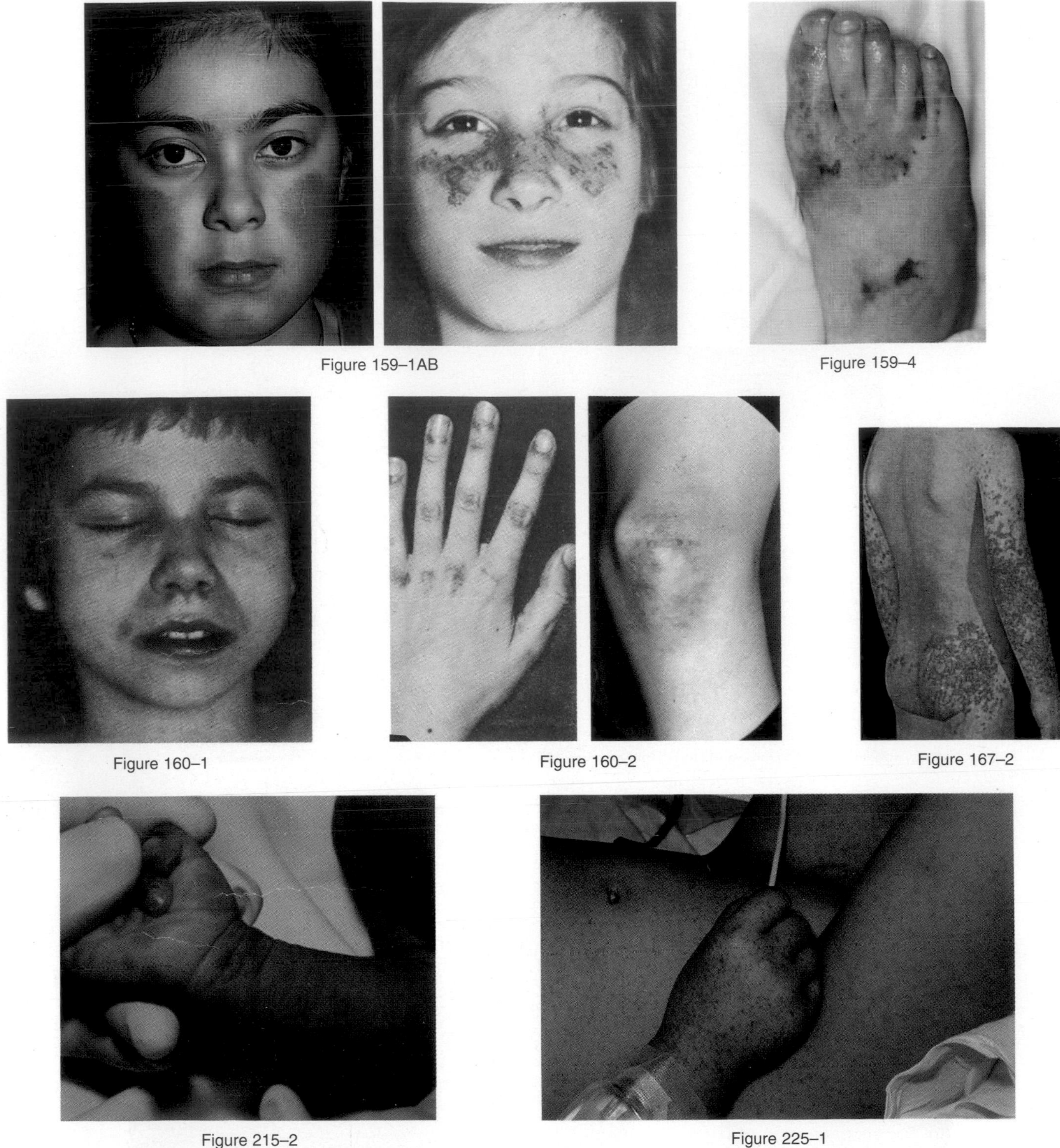

Figure 159–1AB

Figure 159–4

Figure 160–1

Figure 160–2

Figure 167–2

Figure 215–2

Figure 225–1

Figure 159–1 The butterfly rash of systemic lupus erythematosus. The rash can vary from an erythematous blush *(A)* to thickened epidermis to scaly patches *(B).*

Figure 159–4 A 12-yr-old girl with systemic lupus erythematosus and antiphospholipid antibodies with painful cutaneous vasculitis of the right foot. Arterial thrombosis documented by angiography resulted in cyanosis of the large toe. Symptoms resolved with treatment with heparin and corticosteroids.

Figure 160–1 The facial rash of dermatomyositis. Notice the faint erythema over the bridge of the nose and malar areas and the heliotropic discoloration of the upper eyelids.

Figure 160–2 Rash of dermatomyositis. Notice the skin changes over the knuckles *(left)* and over the knee *(right).*

Figure 167–2 Henoch-Schönlein purpura (anaphylactoid purpura). (From Korting GW: Hautkrankheiten bei Kindern und Jugendlichen, 3rd ed. Stuttgart, Germany, FK Schattauer Verlag, 1982.)

Figure 215–2 The mucocutaneous rash of congenital syphilis.

Figure 225–1 Patient with Rocky Mountain spotted fever. Note the predominance of the rash on the extremities. (Courtesy of Debra Karp Klopicki, M.D., Baltimore.)

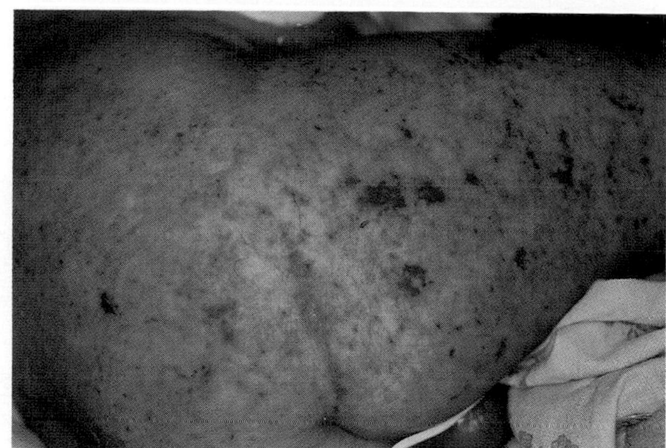

Figure 225–2

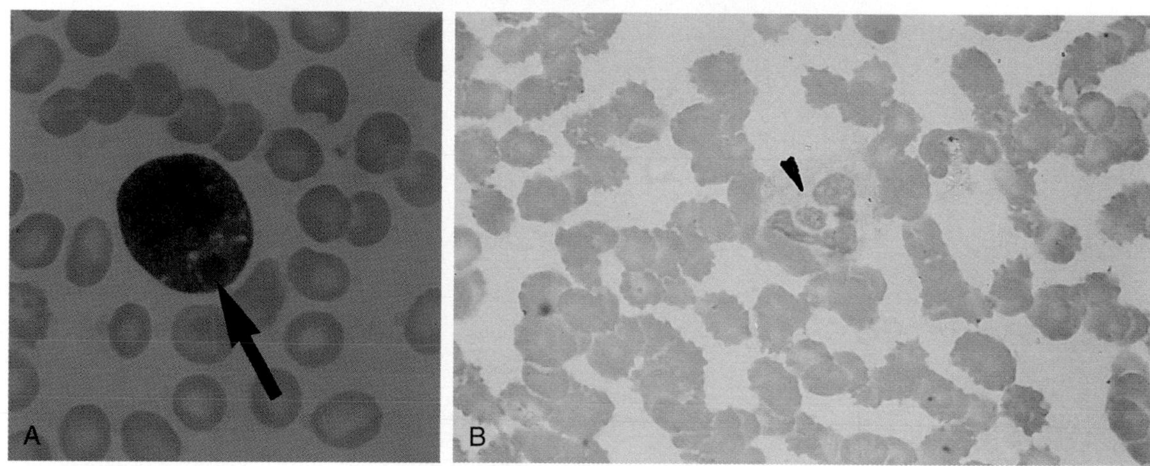

Figure 228–1AB

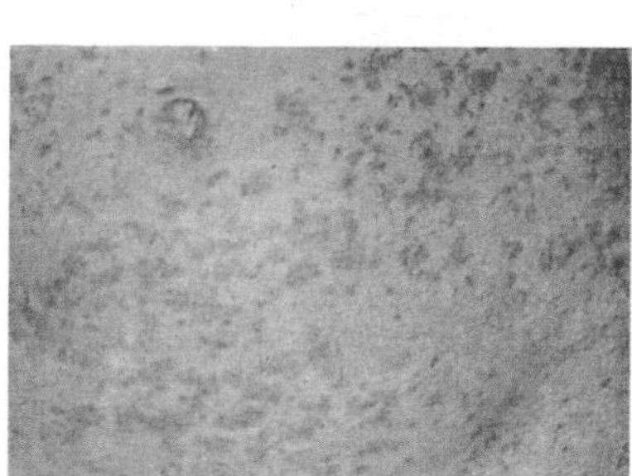

Figure 240–1

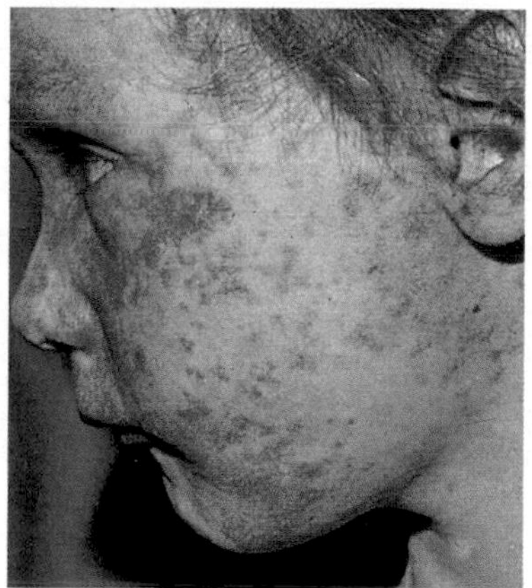

Figure 241–1

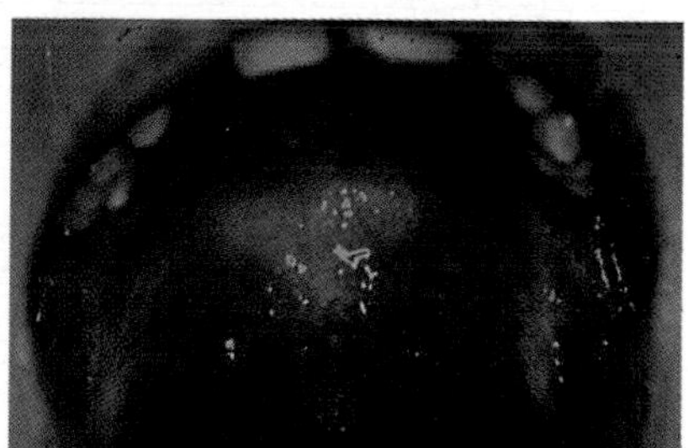

Figure 243–3

Figure 225–2 Later in the course of Rocky Mountain spotted fever the rash may become hemorrhagic or purpuric. (Courtesy of Debra Karp Skopicki, M.D., Baltimore.)

Figure 228–1 *Ehrlichia* morulae in peripheral blood leukocytes: *A,* Morulae *(arrows)* containing *Ehrlichia chaffeensis* in a monocyte. *B, Ehrlichia phagocytophila* group in a neutrophil. (Wright stains, original magnifications × 1,200). *Ehrlichia chaffeensis* and the human granulocytic ehrlichia have similar morphologies but are serologically and genetically distinct.

Figure 240–1 Maculopapular rash of measles. (From Korting GW: Hautkrankheiten bei Kindern und Jugendlichen, 3rd ed. Stuttgart, Germany, FK Schattauer Verlag, 1982.)

Figure 241–1 Rash of rubella (German measles). (From Korting GW: Hautkrankheiten bei Kindern und Jugendlichen, 3rd ed. Stuttgart, Germany, FK Schattauer Verlag, 1982.)

Figure 243–3 Herpangina. This enanthem is predominantly a disease of children and is caused by group A coxsackieviruses. These lesions resemble the ones caused by herpes simplex virus. (From Edmond's Color Atlas of Infectious Diseases. Wolfe Medical Publishers, 1990, p 313.)

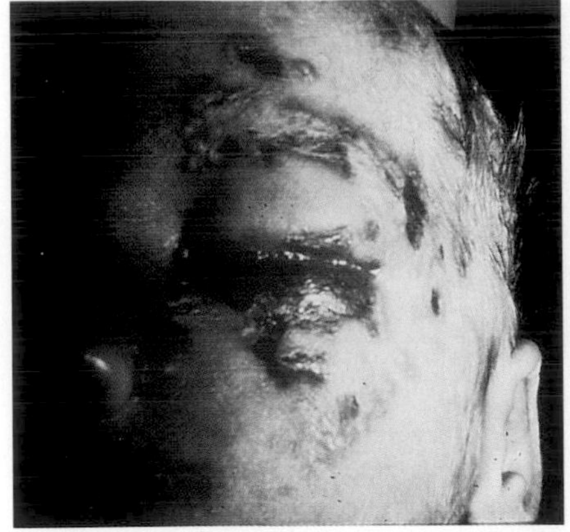

Figure 245–4

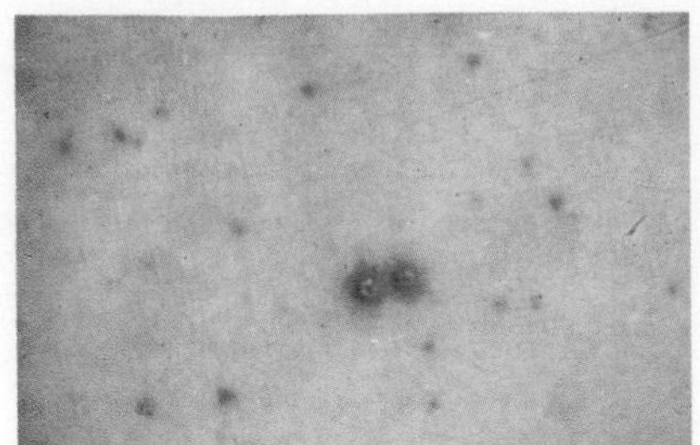

Figure 246–1

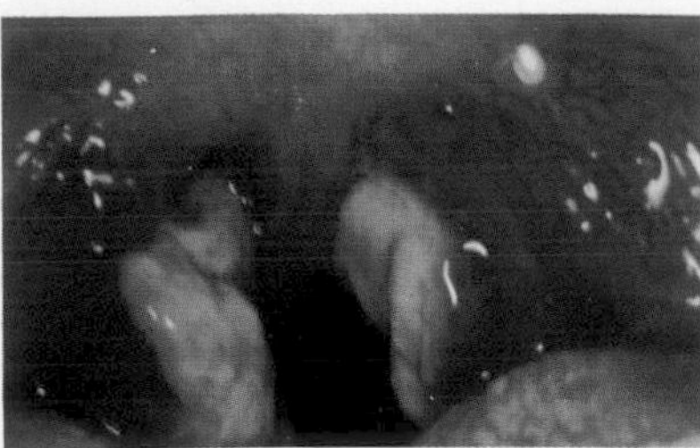

Figure 247–1

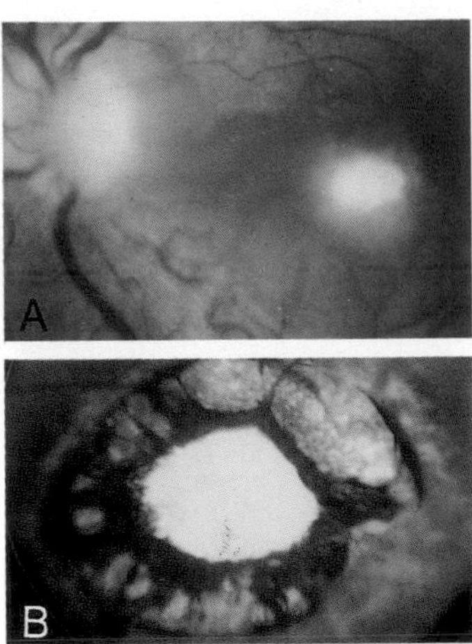

Figure 280–2

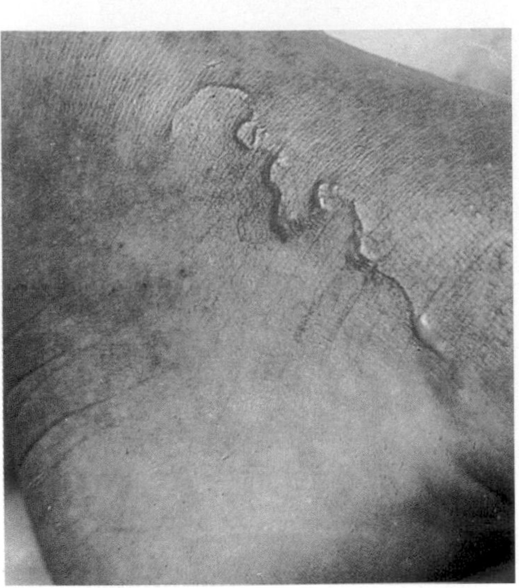

Figure 283–2

Figure 245–4 Vesicular-pustular lesions on the face of an HSV-infected neonate. (From Kohl S: Neonatal herpes simplex virus infection. Clin Perinatol 24:129, 1997.)

Figure 246–1 Skin lesions of chickenpox. Note the varying stages of development (macules, papules, and vesicles) present at the same time. (Courtesy of PF Lucchesi, M.D.)

Figure 247–1 Tonsillitis with membrane formation in infectious mononucleosis. (Courtesy of Alex J. Steigman, M.D.)

Figure 280–2 Toxoplasmic chorioretinitis. *A,* Active acute lesion by indirect ophthalmoscopy. *B,* Old, quiescent lesion. (*B,* adapted from Desmonts G, Remington J: Congenital Toxoplasmosis. *In:* Remington J, Klein J (eds): Infectious Diseases of the Fetus and Newborn Infant, 3rd ed. Philadelphia, WB Saunders, 1991.)

Figure 283–2 Creeping eruption of cutaneous larva migrans. (From Korting GW: Hautkrankheiten bei Kindern und Jugendlichen. Stuttgart, Germany, FK Schattauer Verlag, 1969.)

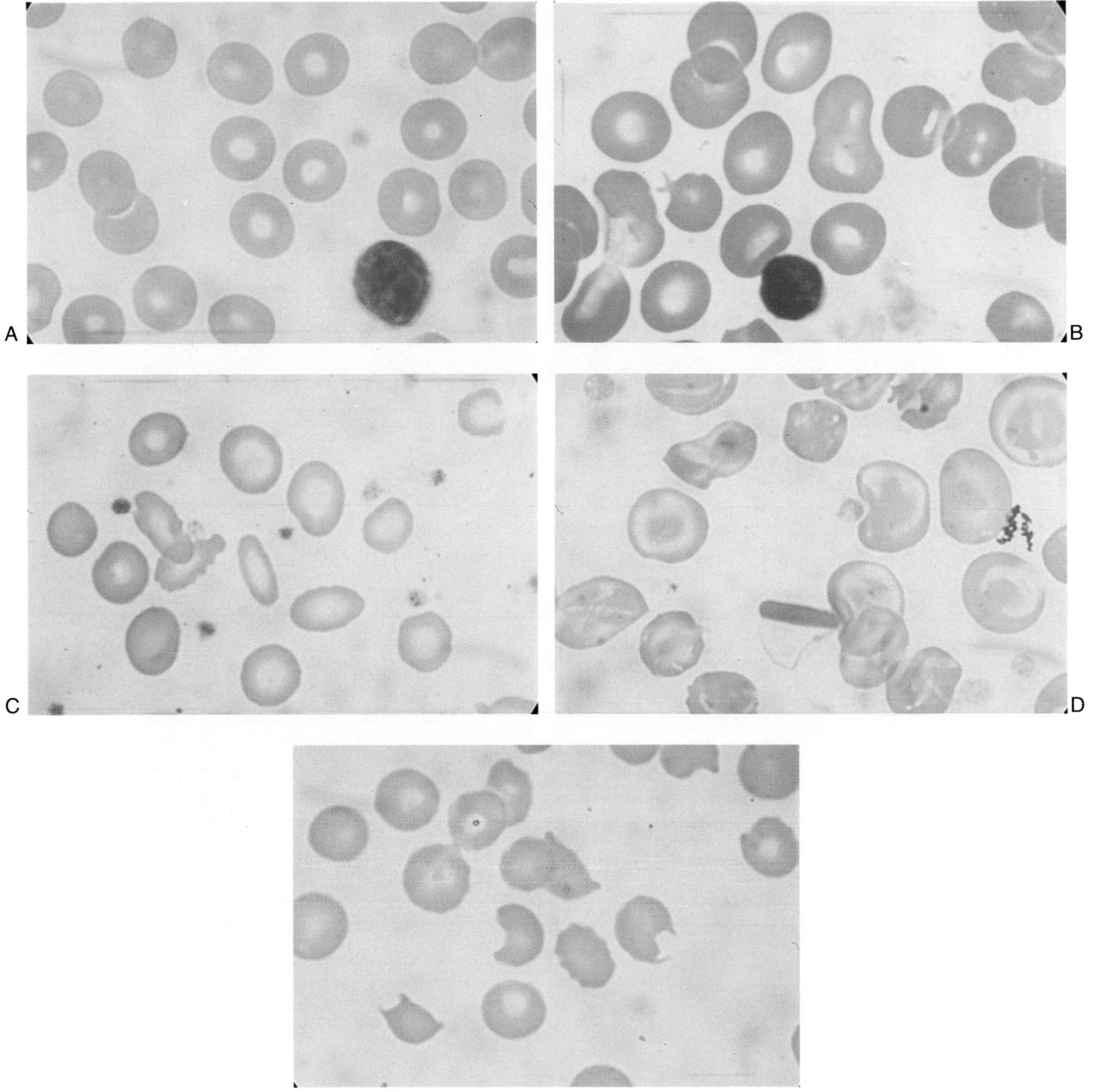

Figure 453–1 Morphologic abnormalities of the red blood cell. *A,* Normal. *B,* Macrocytes (folic acid or vitamin B_{12} deficiency). *C,* Hypochromic microcytes (iron deficiency). *D,* Target cells (Hb CC disease). *E,* Schizocytes (hemolytic-uremic syndrome). (Provided by Dr. E. Schwartz.)

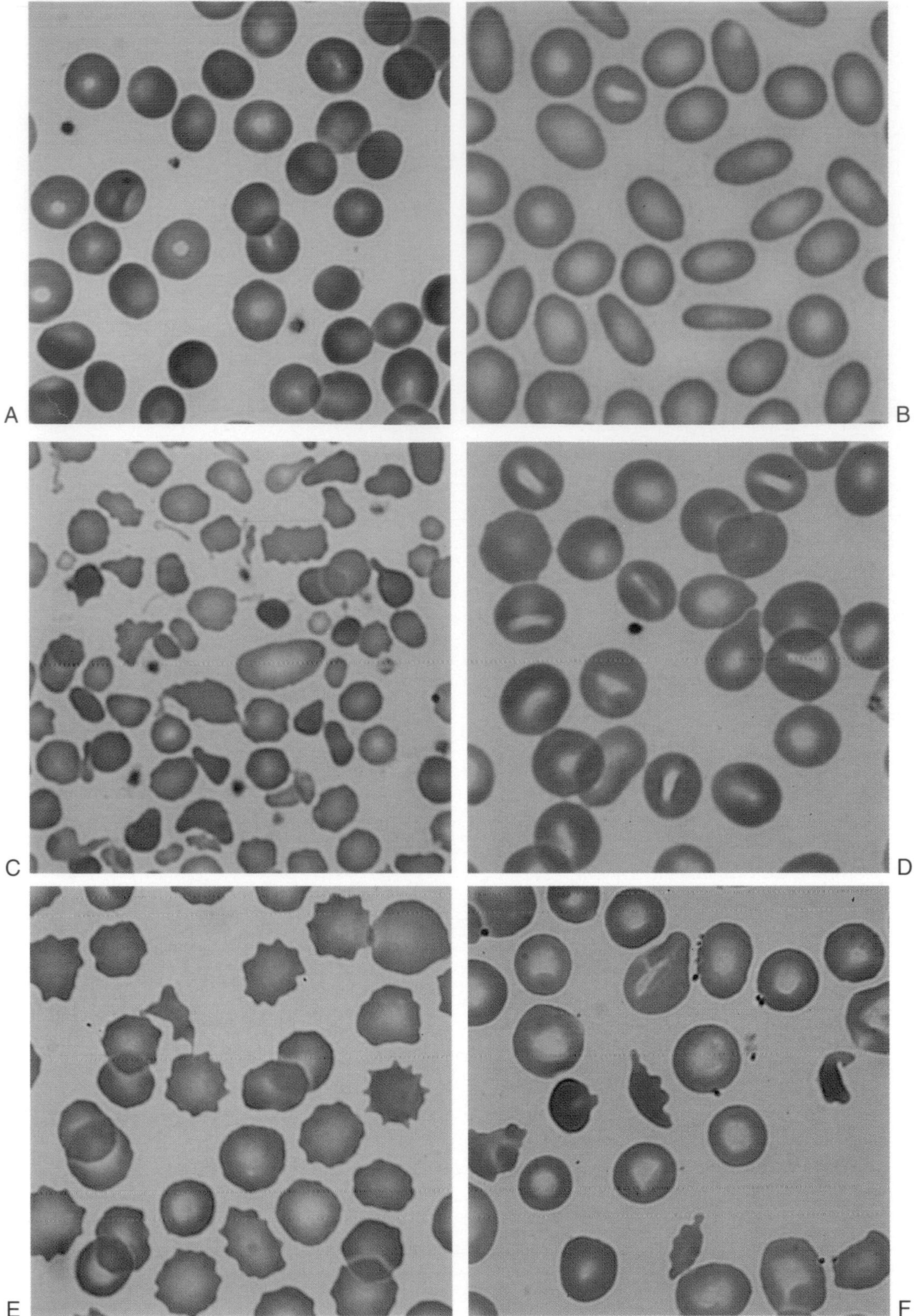

Figure 464–2 Morphology of abnormal red cells. *A,* Hereditary spherocytosis; *B,* hereditary elliptocytosis; *C,* hereditary pyropoikilocytosis; *D,* hereditary stomatocytosis; *E,* acanthocytosis; *F,* fragmentation hemolysis.

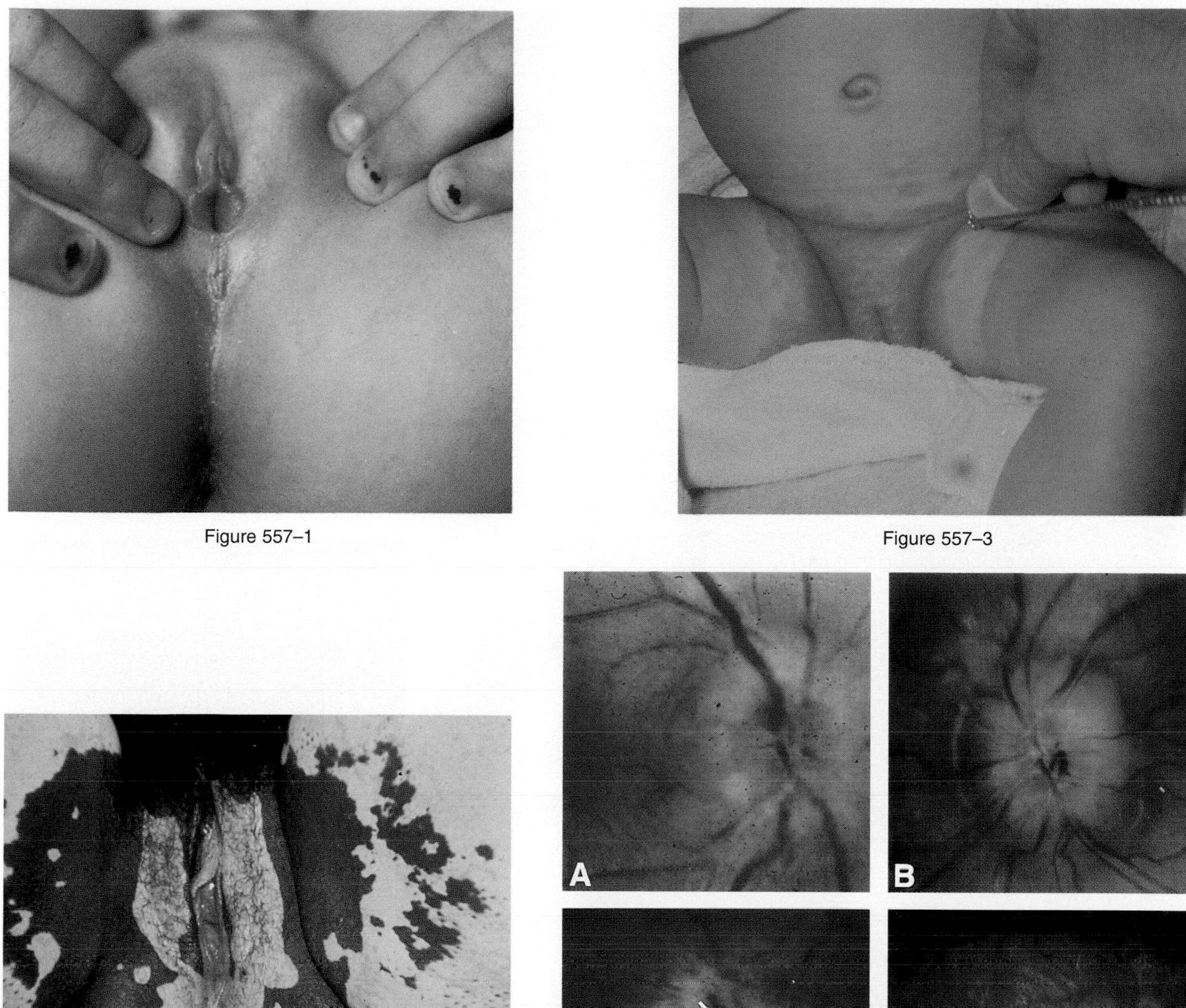

Figure 557–1

Figure 557–3

Figure 557–4

Figure 600–1

Figure 557–1 Labial adhesions.

Figure 557–3 Vulvasoriasi.

Figure 557–4 Vitiligo.

Figure 600–1 *A,* Mild papilledema. Blurred disc margins and venous congestion. *B,* Moderate papilledema. Disc edematous and raised. Vessels buried within substance of nerve tissue. *C,* Severe papilledema. Hemorrhages are evident within disc *(arrow),* and there are microinfarcts (soft exudates) in the nerve fiber layer. *D,* Macular star *(arrow)* with edema residues distributed within the Henle layer of the macula.

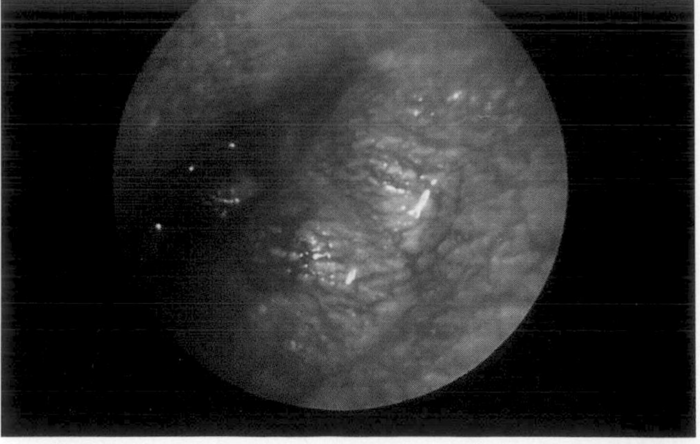

Figure 646–1

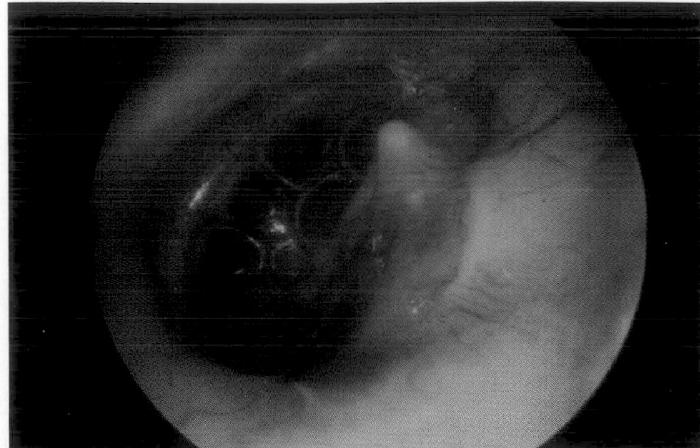

Figure 646–3

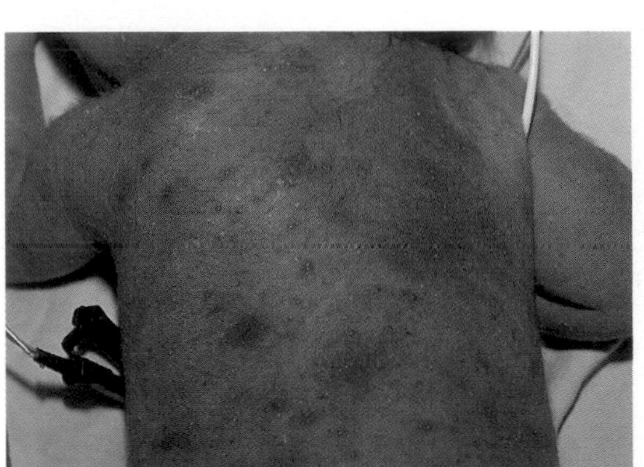

Figure 653–1

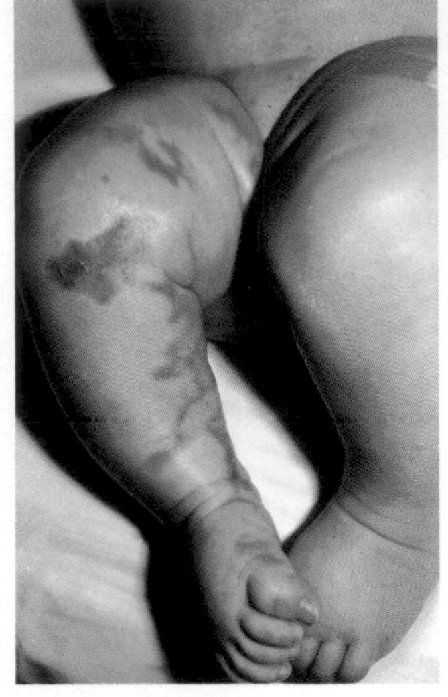

Figure 656–4

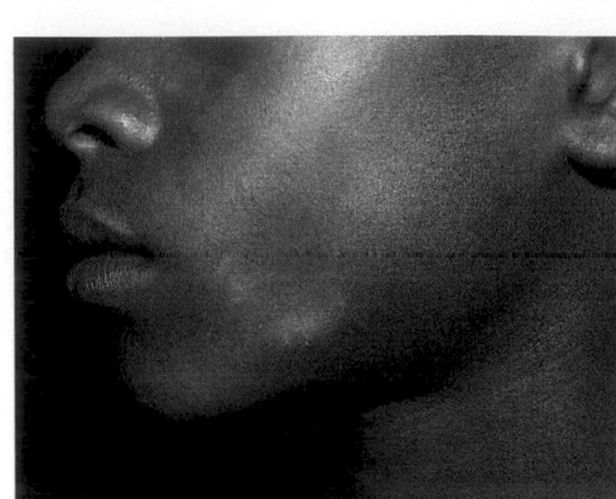

Figure 661–3

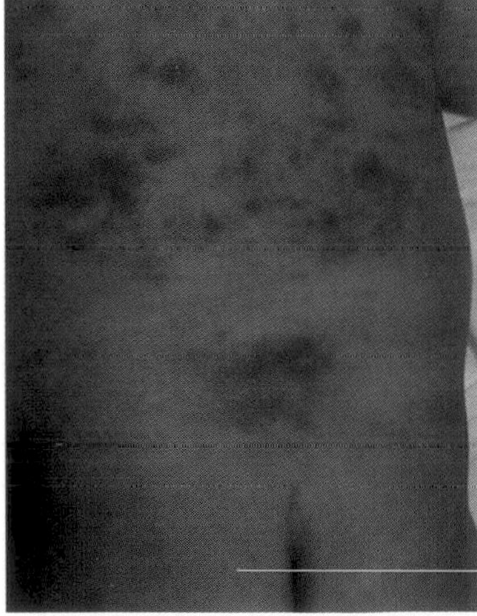

Figure 666–1

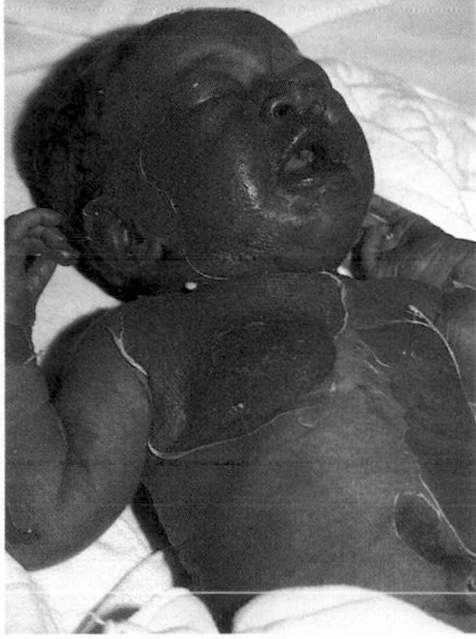

Figure 671–2

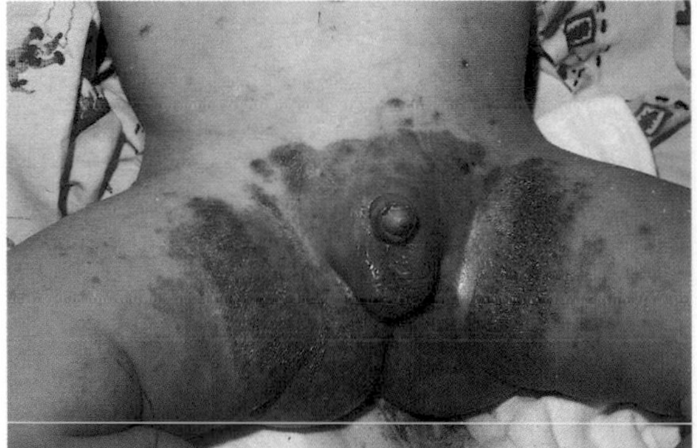

Figure 672–5

Figure 646–1 Acute left otitis media.

Figure 646–3 Otitis media with effusion of left ear. Retracted ear drum, prominent short process of malleus, and air bubbles seen anteriorly through the tympanic membrane.

Figure 653–1 Erythema toxicum on the trunk of a newborn infant.

Figure 656–4 Marbled pattern of cutis marmorata telangiectatica congenita on the right leg.

Figure 661–3 Patchy hypopigmented lesions with diffuse borders characteristic of pityriasis alba.

Figure 666–1 Red-purple nodular infiltration of skin of back caused by subcutaneous fat necrosis.

Figure 671–2 Infant with staphylococcal scalded skin syndrome.

Figure 672–5 Erythematous confluent plaque with satellite pustules caused by candidal infection.

PART I

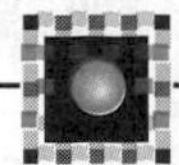

The Field of Pediatrics

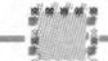

CHAPTER 1
Overview of Pediatrics

Richard E. Behrman

Pediatrics is concerned with the health of infants, children, and adolescents; their growth and development; and their opportunity to achieve full potential as adults. As physicians who assume a responsibility for children's physical, mental, and emotional progress from conception to maturity, pediatricians must be concerned with social and environmental influences, which have a major impact on the health and well-being of children and their families, as well as with particular organ systems and biologic processes. The young are often among the most vulnerable or disadvantaged in society, and thus their needs require special attention.

SCOPE AND HISTORY OF PEDIATRICS AND VITAL STATISTICS

More than a century ago, pediatrics emerged as a medical specialty in response to increasing awareness that the health problems of children differ from those of adults and that a child's response to illness and stress varies with age. The emphasis and scope of pediatrics continue to change, but these basic observations remain valid.

The health problems of children and youth vary widely among the nations of the world depending on a number of factors, which are often interrelated. These factors include (1) the prevalence and ecology of infectious agents and their hosts; (2) climate and geography; (3) agricultural resources and practices; (4) educational, economic, social, and cultural considerations; (5) stage of industrialization and urbanization; and (6), in many instances, the gene frequencies for some disorders.

Not only do problems differ in various parts of the world, but priorities do also, because they must reflect local concerns, resources, and needs. Assessment of the state of health of any community must begin with a description of the incidence of illness and must continue with studies that show the changes that occur with time and in response to programs of prevention, case finding, therapy, and adequate surveillance. As contemporary problems in any community yield to study and to improved management, new problems become the foci of the attention and efforts of pediatric clinicians and research workers. Accordingly, with time, the relative importance of the various causes of childhood morbidity and mortality may undergo major changes.

In the late 19th century in the United States, of every 1,000 children born alive, 200 might be expected to die before the age of 1 yr of conditions such as dysentery, pneumonia, measles, diphtheria, and whooping cough. The efforts of pediatricians, combined with those of scientists and pioneers in public health, have led to such better understanding of the origin and management of many problems of infants that in the past half century the infant mortality rate in the United States has fallen from around 75/1,000 live births in 1925 to approximately 7.2 in 1996. Both neonatal (<1 mo) and postneonatal (1–11 mo) mortality have had major reductions. However, most of the decline in infant mortality since 1970 is attributable to a decrease in the birthweight-specific infant mortality rate related to pediatric care, not to the prevention of low-birthweight births. The majority of deaths of infants under 1 yr of age occur within the first 28 days of life, most of these within the first 7 days; moreover, a large proportion of those within the first 7 days occur within the 1st day. However, an increasing number of severely ill infants born at very low birthweight survive the neonatal period and die later in infancy of neonatal disease, its sequelae, or its complications. Tables 1–1 and 1–2 show the persistent disproportionately high death rate within the 1st yr, compared with the remainder of childhood.

Postneonatal infant mortality for the United States in 1996 was 2.5/1,000 live births (5.0/1,000 for black infants and 2.1/1,000 for white infants). The leading cause of death in this age group was sudden infant death syndrome (SIDS), followed in order by congenital anomalies, perinatal conditions, respiratory system diseases, accidents, and infectious and parasitic diseases. Maternal risk characteristics, such as unmarried status, adolescence, high parity, and less than 12 yr of education, are correlated significantly with increased risk of postneonatal mortality and morbidity and low birthweight.

In developed countries early in the 20th century, efforts at control of infectious disease began to be complemented by better understanding of nutrition. New and continuing discoveries in these areas led to establishment of public well child clinics for low-income families. Along with acute infections and the chronic disturbances associated with deficits of calories, vitamins, minerals, or proteins, the acute nutritional and metabolic disturbances that accompany acute diarrhea received attention.

In the middle years of the 20th century, a profound revolution in child health was brought about by the introduction of antibacterial chemicals and antibiotic agents. With improved control of infectious disease through both prevention and treatment and with other scientific and technical advances, pediatric medicine increasingly turned its attention to conditions affecting relatively small numbers of children. These included both potentially lethal conditions and temporarily or permanently handicapping conditions; among these disorders were leukemia, cystic fibrosis, diseases of the newborn infant, congenital heart disease, mental retardation, genetic defects, rheumatic diseases, renal diseases, and metabolic and endocrine disorders.

The last two decades of this century have been marked by accelerated understanding of and new approaches to the management of many disorders as a consequence of advances in molecular biology, genetics, and immunology. Increasing attention also has been given to behavioral and social aspects of child health, ranging from re-examination of child-rearing

TABLE 1–1 Death Rates* for All Causes, According to Sex, Race, and Age: United States, Selected Years, 1950–1990

	1950		1960		1970		1980		1990	
	White	*Black*	*White*	*Black*	*White*	*Black*	*White*	*Black*	*White*	*Black*
Male										
<1 yr	3,401	1,413	2,694	5,307	2,113	4,299	1,230	2,587	896	2,112
1–4 yr	136		105	209	84	151	66	111	46	86
5–14 yr	67	95	53	75	48	67	35	47	26	41
15–24 yr	152	290	144	212	171	321	167	209	131	252
Female										
<1 yr	2,567	1,139	2,008	4,162	1,615	3,369	963	2,124	690	1,736
1–4 yr	112		85	173	66	129	49	84	36	68
5–14 yr	45	73	35	54	30	44	23	31	18	28
15–24 yr	72	213	55	108	62	112	56	71	46	69

**Death rates per 100,000 population.*
Adapted from Table 119, Statistical Abstract of the United States 1993, 113th ed. Lanham, MD, Berman Press, 1993.

practices to creation of major programs aimed at prevention and management of abuse and neglect of infants and children. Developmental psychologists, child psychiatrists, neuroscientists, sociologists, anthropologists, ethnologists, and others have brought us new insights into human potential, including new views of the importance of the environmental circumstances during pregnancy, surrounding birth, and in the early years of child rearing. However, during these latter years of the 20th century there has also been a resurgence of some of the infectious diseases previously controlled in developed countries, such as tuberculosis and syphilis; the emergence of new infectious pathogens, such as the human immunodeficiency virus (HIV); and the recognition of new disorders related to innovative therapies. In addition, in developing countries, many of the disorders facing children earlier in this century persist, sometimes aggravated by war and famine.

Table 1–3 shows the six leading causes of death in various age groups in 1996. The problems of these children have changed significantly in the United States over a generation. Table 1–3 highlights the impact of violent deaths on mortality in older children, adolescents, and young adults.

Tables 1–1 and 1–2 show that the nonwhite children and other racial and ethnic groups of children in the United States have not fully benefited from the changes in infant mortality in this century owing to various socioeconomic and other disadvantages that have resisted the efforts of many who have struggled to reduce this disparity, including many pediatricians. Similar disparities between races and ethnic groups, occur in several indices of health, such as rates of diseases of the heart and homicides.

In the United States, existing programs for meeting child health problems are not available to all families in need, with gaps between eligibility for public support and parents' ability to pay for services. Needed services are often either nonexistent or fragmented among programs, agencies, or policies. Programs are often poorly coordinated, and the data collection is inadequate. The resources available for maternal and child health care services are also generally inadequate. These findings reflect a need, not just in the United States but in many other parts of the world as well, for continuing re-examination and revision of the system of health care, especially with regard to its impact on the health status of children.

These problems are exacerbated by social and demographic changes in the United States. By 1996, 26.4% of all children under 18 yr of age were living with one parent, about twice

TABLE 1–2 Death Rates* by Age, Sex, Race, and Hispanic Origin, 1996†

	White	Black	Hispanic	Asian/Pacific Islander	American Indian
Male					
< 1 yr	683.4	1697.9	680.8	461.1	899.4
1–4 yr	37.3	72.8	37.8	27.2	74.1
5–14 yr	23.5	38.5	23.7	18.6	39.1
15–24 yr	115.1	234.7	140.3	72.4	176.2
Female					
< 1 yr	557.1	1406.6	527.6	343.8	703.0
1–4 yr	28.3	63.1	27.7	26.8	65.9
5–14 yr	16.4	26.3	17.0	11.3	24.1
15–24 yr	42.8	66.5	38.8	31.1	64.0

**Per 100,000 U.S. Standard Population.*
†Preliminary, National Center for Health Statistics.

TABLE 1–3 Causes of Death at Various Ages

Rank*	Causes	Sub-rank	Rate
	Under 1 Yr: All Causes		875†
1	Perinatal conditions		
	Intrauterine growth retardation/low birthweight	1	
	Respiratory distress syndrome	2	
	Newborn affected by maternal complications of pregnancy	3	
	Newborn affected by complications of placenta, cord, and membranes	4	
	Infections, perinatal	5	
	Intrauterine hypoxia/birth asphyxia	6	
2	Congenital anomalies		
3	Sudden infant death syndrome		
4	Accidents and adverse events		
5	Infections (respiratory)		
	1–4 Yr: All Causes		38†
1	Injuries		
2	Congenital anomalies		
3	Malignant neoplasms		
4	Homicide and legal intervention		
5	Diseases of the heart‡		
6	Respiratory infections		
	5–14 Yr: All Causes		22†
1	Injuries		
2	Malignant neoplasms		
3	Homicide and legal interventions		
4	Congenital anomalies		
5	Diseases of the heart‡		
6	Suicide		
	15–24 Yr: All Causes		90†
1	Injuries		
2	Homicide		
3	Suicide		
4	Malignant neoplasms		
5	Diseases of the heart‡		

**Adapted from Monthly Vital Statistics Report 46:2, 1997. Rates and rankings are for 1996 (Provisional). Source U.S. National Center for Health Statistics.*
†Rate per 100,000 population.
‡Excludes congenital heart anomalies.

the number of such children in 1970. Of these one-parent families, 92% consisted of children living with their mother. There are substantial differences among children: 56.9% of black, 28.6% of Hispanic, 17.9% of white, and 36.5% of Native American children live with one parent. Furthermore, in 1995, 59% of women with children under 3 yr of age, 62% with children under 6, and 77% with children ages 6–17 yr, worked full time or part time outside the home. In 1996, Welfare reform increased incentives for women with low incomes to enter the workforce. The number of children under 5 yr of age in child-care centers or family daycare homes (7.7 million in 1993) is anticipated to increase significantly.

Family income is central to the health and well-being of children. Children living in poor families are much more likely than children living in rich or middle class families to experience material deprivation and poor health, die during childhood, score lower on standardized tests, be retained in grade, drop out of school, have out-of-wedlock births, experience violent crime, end up as poor adults, and suffer other undesirable outcomes. In 1995, 20.8% (14 million) of all children in the United States lived in poverty,* including more than 5 million children under 6 yr of age. One in 3 children spent at least 1 yr in poverty before reaching adulthood; for more than 5% of children, poverty lasts 10 yr or more. Children who live in single-parent families with poorly educated, young, minority (particularly African American), or disabled adults are more likely to be poor and live in poverty longer than those who do not live in such families.

The aforementioned findings have generated three sets of goals. The first set included that all families have access to adequate perinatal, preschool, and family-planning services; that governmental activities be effectively coordinated at national and local levels; that services be so organized that they reach populations at special risk; that there be no insurmountable or inequitable financial barriers to adequate care; that the health care of children have continuity from prenatal through adolescent age periods; and that every family ultimately have access to *all* necessary services, including dental, genetic, and mental health services. A second set of goals addresses the needs for reducing accidents and environmental risks, for meeting nutritional needs, and for health education aimed at fostering health-promoting lifestyles. A third set of goals covers needs for research in biomedical and behavioral science, in fundamentals of bioscience and human biology, and in the particular problems of mothers and children.

The unfinished business in the quest for physical, mental, and social health in the community is illustrated by the disparities with which deaths due to disease, to injuries, and to violence are distributed between white and nonwhite children. Homicide has become a major cause of adolescent deaths and has increased in rate also among the very young, in whom the increase may in part represent the more accurate identification of child abuse (Chapter 35); among adolescents it may reflect unresolved social tensions, the epidemic of substance abuse (especially cocaine and crack), and an unhealthy preoccupation in our society with violence. Some of the issues underlying these problems are discussed in Chapters 24, 34, 39, and Part XII.

PATTERNS OF HEALTH CARE

In 1991, children (0–21 yr) made up 31.9% (80.3 million) of the population of the United States. The number of births has been increasing since 1976 and is expected to continue to increase at 1–2% annually. There were 3,899,589 live births in 1996. Table 1–4 indicates the distribution of children in the population by age. The population of children less than 5 yr of age has been increasing since 1980. The adolescent population (15–19 yr of age) will reach a crest in 2005, reflecting the peak of younger children. The racial, ethnic, and cultural diversity among children is increasing significantly. However, the proportion of children is decreasing relative to the adult population.

TABLE 1–4 Distribution of Children by Age in the United States in 1998 Number (Resident Population in 1000s)

Age (yr)	Total	White	Black	American Indian/ Eskimo/Aleut	Asian/Pacific Islander
< 1	3,795	3,016	558	41	89
1	3,777	3,015	545	40	87
2	3,771	3,005	522	39	86
3	3,824	3,027	581	40	87
4	3,923	3,090	618	42	85
0–4	19,090	15,153	2,855	201	434
5	3,985	3,137	629	43	85
6	4,022	3,175	631	42	85
7	4,087	3,205	643	46	83
8	3,805	3,002	611	47	71
9	3,960	3,105	648	49	77
5–9	19,838	15,624	3,162	226	400
10	3,902	3,079	622	48	74
11	3,794	3,009	589	47	72
12	3,836	3,036	596	48	77
13	3,775	2,994	575	49	78
14	3,783	2,996	579	49	79
10–14	19,090	15,113	2,960	240	380
15	3,910	3,091	608	49	80
16	3,753	2,978	575	46	75
17	4,029	3,197	629	47	77
18	3,754	2,990	86	41	68
19	3,827	3,044	596	41	72
15–19	19,273	15,300	2,994	224	372
20	3,811	3,042	585	39	72
21	3,580	2,859	533	38	74
0–21	84,682	67,091	13,089	968	1,732
22–85+	184,500	155,307	1,141	1,374	8,481
Total	269,182	222,398	34,230	2,342	10,213

U.S. Bureau of Census.

In 1996, there were about 141 million visits to physicians' offices and 15 million visits to hospital outpatient departments by children younger than 15 yr; an additional 59 million and 8 million visits, respectively, were made by children and young adults (15–24 yr). The principal diagnoses accounting for almost 40% of these visits were well child visit (15%), middle-ear infection (12%), and injury (10%). The rate of ambulatory visits by children and youth decreases with increasing age. The opposite occurs with adults. In contrast to the large number of children seen in ambulatory settings, 3,873,000 children younger than 14 yr (excluding newborn births) were hospitalized in the United States in 1995. Nonwhite children are more likely than are white children to use hospital facilities for their ambulatory care, and well child visits are almost 80% higher among white infants than black infants.

Hospitals, particularly in urban areas, are sources of both routine and intensive child care, with medical and surgical services that may range from immunization and developmental counseling to open heart surgery and renal transplantation. Clinical conditions and procedures requiring intensive care are likely to be clustered in university affilitated centers serving as regional resources. The hospitalization rates for children (excluding newborn infants) are less than those of adults under 65 yr of age, except during the first year of life. In 1995, the rates per 1,000 population were: under 1 yr, 205.3; 1–4 yr, 47.2; 5–14 yr, 22.9; 15–19 yr, 67.7 (excluding obstetrics). The rate of hospitalization and lengths of hospital stay have declined significantly for children and adults during the past decade. Children represent less than 8% of the total acute hospital discharges, and in children's hospitals about 70% of admissions are for chronic conditions. Ten to 12%

*Weighted average poverty thresholds in 1995 in the United States were $12,158 for three-person families and $15,569 for four-person families.

of pediatric hospitalizations are related to birth defects and genetic diseases.

PLANNING AND IMPLEMENTING A SYSTEM OF CARE

Physicians caring for children have been increasingly called on to advise in the management of disturbed behavior or in relationships between child and parent, child and school, or child and community and are increasingly concerned with problems of mental, social, and societal health. There is also an increasing concern with disparities in how the benefits of what we know about child health reach various groups of children. Just as in many developing countries, so in the United States the health of children lags far behind what it could be if the means and will to apply current knowledge could be brought to bear. The medical problems of children are often intimately related to problems of mental and social health. The children most at risk are disproportionately represented among ethnic minority groups. Pediatricians have a responsibility to address aggressively problems such as these.

Linked with these views of the broad scope of pediatric concern is the concept that access to at least a basic level of quality services to promote health and treat illness is a right of every person. Among children in the United States, having health insurance is strongly associated with access to primary care. The failure of health services and health benefits to reach all who need them has led to re-examination of the design of health care systems in many countries, but unresolved problems remain in most health care systems, such as the maldistribution of physicians, institutional unresponsiveness to the perceived needs of the individual, failure of medical services to be adapted to the need and convenience of patients, and deficiencies in health education. Efforts to make the delivery of health care more efficient and effective have led imaginative pediatricians to create new categories of health care providers, such as pediatric nurse practitioners, and to participate in new organizations for providing care to children, such as various managed care arrangements.

New insights into the needs of children have reshaped the child health care system in other ways. Growing understanding of the need of infants for certain qualities of stimulation and care has led to restudy and revision of the care of newborn infants (Chapters 9 and 90) and of procedures leading to an adoption or to placement with foster families (Chapters 30 and 31). For handicapped children, the massive centralized institutions of past years are being replaced by community-centered arrangements offering a better opportunity for these children to achieve their maximal potential. Pediatricians have been involved in shaping these and other institutions that provide services to children, and their insights and active contributions will continue to be needed.

COSTS OF HEALTH CARE

The growth of high technology, the redesign of health institutions (particularly with respect to the needs for and the uses of personnel), the public's demand for medical services, and the manner in which the costs of health care are paid have driven the costs of health care in the United States up to a point at which they represent a significant proportion of the gross national product. Although children (0–18 yr) represent about 30% of the population, they account for only about 14% of the personal health care expenditures, or about 60% of adult per capita expenditures. Efforts to contain costs have led to revisions of the way in which physicians and hospitals are paid for services. Limits have been set on the fees for some services, capitated prepayment and various managed care systems flourish, a program of reimbursement (diagnosis-related groups [DRGs]) based on the diagnosis rather than on the particular services rendered to an individual patient has been implemented, and a relative value scale for varying rates of payment among different physician services has been implemented. These and other changes in the system of financing health services raise important ethical issues for pediatricians to address (Chapter 2).

EVALUATION OF HEALTH CARE

The shaping of health care systems to meet the needs of children and their families requires accurate statistical data and difficult decisions in setting priorities. Along with growing concerns about the design and cost of health care systems and the ability to distribute health services equitably has come increasing concern about the quality of health care and about its efficiency and effectiveness. There are large local and regional variations among similar populations of children in the rates of use of procedures and technology and of hospital admissions. These variations require continuing evaluation and explanation in terms of the actual impact of medical and surgical services on health status and the outcome of illness.

GROWTH OF SPECIALIZATION

The amount of information relevant to child health care is rapidly expanding, and no person can become master of it all. Physicians are increasingly dependent on one another for the highest quality of care for their patients; group practices in pediatrics are common in the United States, and although the vast majority of pediatricians are primary care generalists, as many as 25% claim an area of special knowledge and skill.

The growth of specialization within pediatrics has taken a number of different forms: Interests in problems of *age groups* of children have created neonatology and adolescent medicine; interests in *organ systems* have created pediatric cardiology, allergy, hematology, nephrology, gastroenterology, pulmonology, endocrinology, and specialization in metabolism and genetics; interests in the *health care system* have created pediatricians devoted to ambulatory care on the one hand or to intensive care on the other; and finally, multidisciplinary subspecialties have grown up around the problems of *handicapped children,* to which pediatrics, neurology, psychiatry, psychology, nursing, physical and occupational therapy, special education, speech therapy, audiology, and nutrition all make essential contributions. This growth of specialization has been most conspicuous in university-affiliated departments of pediatrics and medical centers for children.

NEED FOR CONTINUING SELF-EDUCATION

The explosion of information has also created a need for continuing education, which was felt much less keenly in earlier years, when the new information in any field of medicine was easily accessible through a relatively small number of journals, texts, or monographs. Now, relevant information is so widely scattered among the many published journals that elaborate electronic data systems are necessary to make it accessible. The Internet has dramatically improved access to information by physicians and patients, but judgment about the quality, clinical significance, and appropriate use of such information is a continuing challenge. New auditory and visual aids to learning abound, as well as postgraduate courses through which participating physicians can be brought up to date on various aspects of child health care. The American Board of Pediatrics and the American Academy of Pediatrics have arranged for close linkage of continuing education of pediatricians to recertification in pediatrics.

There is no touchstone through which physicians can ensure that the process of their own continuing education will keep them abreast of advancing knowledge in the field, but they must find a way to base their decisions on the best available scientific evidence if they are to discharge their responsibility to their patients. An essential element of this process may be for physicians to take an *active* role, such as participating in medical student and resident education. Efforts in continuing self-education will also be fostered, for example, if clinical problems can be made a stimulus for a review of standard literature, alone or in consultation with an appropriate colleague or consultant. This continuing review will do much to identify those inconsistencies or contradictions that will indicate, in the ultimate best interest of patients, that things are not what they seem or have been said to be. Physicians still learn most from their patients, but this will not be the case if they fall into the easy habit of accepting their patients' problems casually or at face value because they appear to be simple.

The tools that physicians must use in dealing with the problems of children and their families fall into three main categories: *cognitive* (up-to-date factual information about diagnostic and therapeutic issues, available on recall or easily found in readily accessible sources, and the ability to relate this information to the pathophysiology of their patients in the context of individual biologic variability); *interpersonal or manual* (e.g., the ability to carry out a productive interview, execute a reliable physical examination, perform a deft venipuncture, or manage cardiac arrest or resuscitation of a depressed newborn infant); and *attitudinal* (the physician's commitment to the fullest possible implementation of knowledge and skills on behalf of children and their families in an atmosphere of empathic sensitivity and concern). With regard to this last category, it is important that children participate with their families in informed decision-making about their own health care in a manner appropriate to their stage of development and the nature of the particular health problem.

The workaday needs of professional persons for knowledge and skills in care of children vary widely. Primary care physicians need depth in developmental concepts and in the ability to organize an effective system for achieving quality and continuity in assessing and planning for health care during the entire period of growth. They may often have little or no need for immediate recall of esoterica. On the other hand, consultants or subspecialists not only need a comfortable grasp of esoterica within their field and perhaps within related fields but also must be able to cope with controversial issues with flexibility that will permit adaptation of various points of view to the best interest of their unique patient.

At whatever level of care (primary, secondary, or tertiary), or in whatever role (as student, as pediatric nurse practitioner, as resident pediatrician, as a practitioner of pediatrics or of family medicine, or as a pediatric or other subspecialist), professional persons dealing with children must be able to identify their roles of the moment and their levels of engagement with a child's problem; each must determine whether his or her experience and other resources at hand are adequate to deal with this problem and must be ready to seek other help when they are not. Among the necessary resources are general textbooks, more detailed monographs in subspecialty areas, selected journals, audiovisual materials, and, above all, colleagues with exceptional or complementary experience and expertise. The intercommunication of all these levels of engagement with medical and health problems of children offers the best hope of bringing us closer to the goal of providing the opportunity for all children to achieve their maximum potential.

Advance Data, Nos. 294 and 295. National Center for Health Statistics, 1997.
The Future of Children: Welfare to work. 7:4–138, 1997.
The Future of Children: Children and poverty. 7:4–157, 1997.
Monthly Vital Statistics Report 46(Suppl 2):1997. National Center for Health Statistics.
Newacheck PW, Stoddard JJ, Hughes DC, et al: Health insurance and access to primary care for children. N Engl J Med 338:513, 1998.
Singh GR, Yu SM: U.S. Mortality, 1950 through 1993: Trends and socioeconomic differentials. Am J Public Health 86:505, 1996.
The State of America's Children. Year Book Medical Publishers, 1997. Children's Defense Fund.
Vital and Health Statistics, Series 13, No. 133, 137. National Center for Health Statistics, 1998.
Yoon PW, Olney RS, Khoury MJ, et al: Contribution of birth defects and genetic diseases to pediatric hospitalizations. Arch Pediatr Adolesc Med 151:1096, 1997.

CHAPTER 2
Ethics in Pediatric Care

Norman Fost

Ethical issues permeate all interactions between physicians and patients: How much information should be disclosed? Is this patient consuming an unfair share of the physician's or society's resources? Should clinical decisions be made by the patient, the parent, or the physician? In pediatrics, these familiar dilemmas are compounded by the variable competence of the patient, the sometimes competing interests of parents and children, and the long-standing tradition of treating children more paternalistically than is acceptable for adult patients.

This chapter reviews the major conceptual principles in medical ethics, identifies the central issues in the common clinical/ethical dilemmas involving children, identifies areas of apparent consensus, and suggests a procedural approach to ethical decision-making.

CONCEPTUAL ISSUES

AUTONOMY. This is a central principle in medical ethics. Its purpose is to allow competent patients to make their own health care decisions based on their own values. In the United States and many other nations, competent patients have almost an absolute right to decide what shall be done to their own bodies. This right is not contingent on the patient's making rational decisions. Thus, a patient may permissibly refuse lifesaving care for religious or other reasons, even though others may believe that he or she is making a foolish or unwise decision. This principle is particularly relevant in adolescence, when a patient's competence begins to resemble that of an adult, but younger children are also sometimes competent to make their own health care decisions.

COMPETENCE. The principle of autonomy is intertwined inextricably with the concept of competence, because only competent patients are granted the right to make their own health care decisions. The most common definition of competence is based on patients' ability to understand the possible consequences of their decision and the available alternatives. Many adolescents meet this standard, creating potential conflicts when they are still under the supervision of their parents.

BENEFICENCE. This refers to the duties to avoid harm as well as to advance the welfare of others. It is at the root of the ancient nostrum "Do no harm"—an obvious oversimplification, because little medical benefit can be gained without the risk of harm. A more complete principle would include some sense of not causing harm without a likelihood of compensating good, but individuals vary in respect to what they consider a harm or a good and how much harm they are willing to risk in exchange for a potential benefit. The primacy of autonomy in the United States has led to a widespread though not unanimous view that competent patients should be allowed to decide for themselves how to balance harms and goods. Interference in these decisions is often based on claims of justified paternalism.

PATERNALISM. This is defined as interfering with the liberty of another person for his or her own benefit. It is generally considered to be a duty of parents, although this assumption has been questioned and is usually considered to be morally unjustified with regard to competent patients, with limited exceptions. Physicians have historically believed that they had a right and duty to be paternalistic, based on the claim that their responsibility is *beneficence*—to promote patients' health, not their autonomy. There is general support for the opinion that paternalism is justified at least when there is a high probability of serious harm, when interference with the patient's liberty is likely to prevent the harm, and when there is a reasonable likelihood that the patient would want to be treated in this manner or will appreciate it later on. This view of paternalism provides the justification for many intrusions for the benefit of children over their apparent objection, such as surgery for suspected appendicitis or immunizations against serious diseases, but it leaves unanswered questions about the appropriateness of intrusions of uncertain effectiveness, particularly if the child objects, or of intrusions for the purpose of preventing uncertain or minimal harms.

TRUTH TELLING. The duty to tell the truth is a requisite for any moral community. It has special importance in the physician-patient relationship, in which trust is essential because of unequal power and because of the serious consequences of medical decisions. Failure to respect this principle occurs by actively lying, which is wrong under almost all circumstances in the health care setting, or by intentional omission of information. Omissions should not be made for the purpose of deception or of manipulating a patient's response.

CONFIDENTIALITY. Patients need to trust their physicians not to disclose private information to others because confidentiality facilitates full disclosure of information relevant for providing effective personal health care, may prevent disorders that threaten others in the community, and possibly reduces the total human and financial cost of illness and related disability through early treatment. There is an implied promise by the physician not to disclose information except with the consent of the patient, or of his or her representative, or when required by law. Exceptions to this principle are generally limited to circumstances carrying a high risk of serious physical harm to others that is most likely to be prevented only by unconsented disclosure (e.g., reporting suspected child abuse on the basis of information obtained from the potential abuser in what was presumed to be a confidential relationship).

CONFLICTS OF INTEREST. Because a child patient is usually represented by someone else, the potential exists for a pediatrician to perceive the best interests of the child differently from the way in which they are perceived by the parent(s) or guardian(s). In addition, a physician's sense of responsibility for the rest of the family may result in conflicts between the interests of the family and the interests of the child patient (e.g., see the following section on "Baby Doe").

WITHHOLDING AND WITHDRAWING LIFE SUPPORT

One of the most important ethical dilemmas that physicians face is whether to withhold or withdraw life support. In pediatrics, these issues arise most commonly in the newborn period, involving infants with limited prospects for survival without significant lifelong morbidity. These cases, however, are only one part of the general question about the justifications for withholding or withdrawing life support from children with various illnesses from birth through adolescence (see also Chapter 38).

A strong ethical consensus in the United States is that competent individuals have an almost absolute right to determine what shall be done with their own bodies. This implies a right to refuse health care, even if the patient has excellent prospects for long-term survival and death is the certain result of refusing treatment. There is a similar tradition in the law. A familiar example is the common occurrence of a Jehovah's Witness's refusing a lifesaving blood transfusion, although religious justifications are not an essential aspect of this ethical or legal principle. Accordingly, adolescent patients who are competent in the sense of understanding the consequences of their decision, including the prospects for survival and the likely quality of life if treatment is accepted and the certainty of death if treatment is withheld, should have a major role in such decisions. The more problematic cases involve younger children at the boundary of competence and disorders with limited prospects for long-term survival.

Most pediatric patients are clearly not competent to make their own decisions with regard to the termination of care. Although parents have traditionally made such decisions on behalf of their children, with little controversy, the limits of such authority are increasingly questioned. This has occurred primarily in decisions involving handicapped or critically ill newborns—the so-called Baby Doe controversy.

"Baby Doe" Dilemma

The "Baby Doe" term arose in a 1982 conflict over an infant who had Down syndrome and esophageal atresia and who was allowed to die at 6 days of age at the parents' request. The case was similar to many others that had occurred during the preceding decade, particularly involving undertreatment of newborns with Down syndrome and spina bifida. Many of these children appeared to have excellent prospects for long, happy lives, suggesting that the decisions were not being made in the interests of the children. Furthermore, in two large surveys, most pediatricians supported parental control of such decisions; some pediatricians stated that they considered their duty was not to serve the interests of their patient but rather to serve the interests of the parents. These problems were compounded by the fact that decisions were often based on erroneous medical assumptions, including inappropriately pessimistic prognoses about quality of life.

As a consequence of concern about this issue in the United States, regulations were eventually promulgated under the authority of the child abuse law that prohibited withholding medically beneficial treatment simply because a child might survive with handicaps, however severe. This rule seemed to disqualify the most common justification for discontinuing life-sustaining care from children—namely, the likelihood that continued biologic existence would not serve the patients' interests precisely because they would be so handicapped that the burdens of treatment would be greater than the benefits. One consequence of this rule was an apparent shift from undertreatment to widespread overtreatment, defined as life-prolonging treatment that, in the opinion of the physician, does not serve the interests of the child.

The effort to find an acceptable middle ground between undertreatment and overtreatment has led to increasing support for a procedural approach to deciding what is in the interests of the child based on the *ideal observer theory.* In this view, a decision is morally acceptable if it could be approved of by an ideal ethical observer with five characteristics: (1) *omniscience*—the decision has included all the readily available and relevant facts; (2) *omnipercipience*—the decision has empathically taken into account the feelings of those involved; (3) *disinterest*—the decision is not based on vested interests; (4) *dispassion*—the decision is not made under conditions in which strong emotions obscure critical thinking; and (5) *consistency*—the hallmark of ethical reasoning, meaning that similar cases are decided similarly. Because no person can attain this ideal, a collaborative process is used to approximate these characteristics, such as a hospital ethics committee. These committees or an appropriate alternative is now required by the Joint Commission on Accreditation of Hospitals. Such committees have a consultative role in cases in which parents and medical staff cannot agree on the proper course of action, but they have acquired considerable influence and are increasingly recognized by state courts as an important factor in decision-making.

Withholding Versus Withdrawing Treatment

It is widely accepted that there is no moral distinction between withholding and withdrawing treatment. Although physicians and nurses historically and psychologically are more reluctant to discontinue a treatment once it has begun, withdrawal of treatment is more justified for two reasons. First, withdrawal of treatment has the benefit of coming after a clinical trial, resulting in more data about the likely outcome than if treatment had been withheld. *Good ethics starts with good facts,* and it is generally preferable to avoid irreversible decisions in the presence of major uncertainty. Second, the traditional prohibition of withdrawing treatment led some physicians to withhold treatment from some infants who had reasonable prospects of benefit, for fear that if the outcome were later shown to be bleak, there would be no recourse other than to keep patients alive as long as technology would allow—for example, very small premature infants allowed to die in the delivery room without the benefit of a clinical trial. No physician in the United States has ever been found liable, civilly or criminally, for withholding or withdrawing any life-sustaining treatment from any patient for any reason.

Active Versus Passive Euthanasia

As the preceding discussion implies, there has been broad support for passive euthanasia allowing a patient to die of some intrinsic disease or defect. Active euthanasia, in comparison, is considered to be more problematic and has long been generally opposed, though opinion is shifting and one state (Oregon) has legalized physician-assisted suicide, a variant of active euthanasia, for competent patients. The reasons for opposition are only partly related to concerns for the interests of patients. If a decision has been made that continued survival is not in a patient's interest, it would seem irrelevant whether he or she died by active or passive means. Indeed, active euthanasia might be preferable because of the opportunity to minimize suffering. The objections are based, in part, on the swiftness and irreversibility of action, precluding the possibility of changing course if it is discovered that the decision was wrong. The greater concern, however, has been for slippery slope effects: the claim that lowering the barrier against killing will make it easier for physicians to kill others, that boundaries will become less distinct, and that patients without a clear interest in dying will be harmed. The accounts of the two countries with the greatest experience in active euthanasia, Germany in the 1930s and contemporary Holland, lend some support to this concern.

SCREENING

Screening is the search for asymptomatic illness in a defined population; it is usually performed for the purpose of treatment but is sometimes done for counseling or research. Several programs, such as screening for inborn errors of metabolism (e.g., phenylketonuria [PKU] and hypothyroidism), are counted among the triumphs of contemporary pediatrics. The success of such programs sometimes obscures serious ethical issues that continue to arise in proposals to screen for other conditions for which the benefits, risks, and costs have not been clearly established. Advances in genetics have led to exponential growth in the number of conditions for which screening tests are available, with insufficient opportunity to study each proposed testing program.

The central ethical principle that should justify screening programs is no different from that which should guide all medical care: *Do no harm without compensating benefit and informed consent.* In the context of drugs and devices, the implementation of this principle means that new treatments are not offered or implemented on a wide scale until benefits and risks have been demonstrated and costs have been found to be acceptable, and then only with the informed consent of patients or their representative. In addition, tests that identify candidates for treatment need to have demonstrated sensitivity, specificity, and high predictive value, lest individuals be falsely labeled and subject to possibly toxic treatments or to psychosocial risks. These safeguards have not always been systematically applied to screening programs, often resulting in serious harm to many children without compensating benefits. Familiar examples include routine fetal monitoring, which contributed to the rising rate of cesarean sections with little benefit for many infants, and screening premature infants for acidosis, resulting in administration of toxic amounts of sodium bicarbonate before its risks were adequately studied.

The growing epidemic of acquired immunodeficiency syndrome (AIDS) infection has stimulated controversy over screening newborns for human immunodeficiency virus (HIV) infection, particularly in high-prevalence areas. Whether such screening will have benefits proportional to the risks remains disputed. As with genetic testing, this carried the added complexity of identifying other affected persons without their consent. In contrast, the value of screening pregnant women for HIV infection has become accepted with the discovery of an intervention that reduces the risk of transmission of the virus to the fetus.

Screening has become such a ubiquitous and accepted component of the health care of healthy and sick patients that its benefits are often assumed and the risk is rarely assessed. Routine pediatric procedures, such as the annual physical examination, urine cultures, and developmental screening before school entry, may be examples of common interventions of uncertain benefit and potential risks, organic and psychosocial. Two ethical principles are important in making judgments about screening: New programs should be considered experimental until the risks and benefits are demonstrated and parents should generally be given the opportunity to exercise informed consent or refusal. Concern is often expressed that seeking informed consent is ethically inappropriate for tests of clear benefit, such as PKU screening, because refusal would constitute neglect, but one study showed that a reasonable attempt at consent could be made on a statewide basis without excessive time or cost and without undue effects on compliance.

ADOLESCENT HEALTH CARE (also see Part XII)

Many adolescents resemble adults more than they do children in their competence to consent to health care. Competence, however, is not a global quality: Teenagers may not be able to support themselves yet may still be competent to consent to health care.

In addition to the role of competence, there are public health reasons, reflected in statutes and court decisions, for allowing adolescents to consent to their own health care with regard to reproductive decisions, such as contraception and abortion, and treatment of sexually transmitted diseases. Strict requirements for parental consent may deter many adolescents from seeking health care, with serious implications for their health and other community interests.

Weighed against these concerns are the legitimate interests of parents in maintaining responsibility and authority for child rearing, including the opportunity to influence the sexual attitudes and practices of one's children. Another claim is that public support for access to such treatment, particularly contraception and abortion, implicitly endorses and encourages sexual activity, aggravating rather than ameliorating the problems. Similar concerns underlie the objection to providing sterile needles for intravenous drug abusers, for the purpose of reducing the risk of acquiring hepatitis or HIV. Critics complain that such programs give children the message that illegal drug use is supported by the state as long as it is done safely, though it is now generally accepted that access to sterile needles results in a decrease in new cases of AIDS. Pediatricians' role and behavior in these disputes will be influenced by their own moral beliefs and by assessments of the competing facts and arguments. Physicians need to consider the possibility that a moralistic position may deter adolescents from seeking health care or counseling (also see Chapter 5).

RESEARCH

The central ethical distinction between research and standard clinical practice is researchers' commitment to future patients, or societal interests, in addition to their responsibility for patients who are the human subjects of the investigation. Research is defined in the federal regulations as the "systematic collection of information for the benefit of others." In *therapeutic research,* an expectation is that the patient/subject may also benefit, but the uncertainty about benefits and risks is typically greater compared with standard treatment. In addition, the need to collect data may be greater than would normally be necessary, thus exposing patients to more discomfort or risk.

In *nontherapeutic research,* there is usually no expected benefit for the subject; therefore, any risk presents a very high risk: benefit ratio. Some argue that children, along with other nonconsenting subjects, should never be used in nontherapeutic research, because of the violation of Kant's dictum that a person should never be used solely as a means to an end. The more widely held opinion is that children may be exposed to at least *minimal risks,* although the reasons for this exception are disputed. Some argue that children have a duty to contribute to the social welfare, although the federal regulations do not allow competent adults to be used as research subjects for this justification without their consent. The federal regulations define minimal risk as risks "similar to those encountered in the course of a routine office visit." Some interpret this to include procedures similar to those done in routine office visits, but others claim that an invasive procedure such as a liver biopsy may be done if the risks, in the hands of a particular investigator, are empirically no higher than those of a routine office visit or if the procedure is routine for a visit to a specialist. Others have argued that the *incremental* risk of the research is the relevant factor, so that risks should be compared with the risk of no treatment or to the risk of standard treatment.

Innovative therapy is defined as a new and unproven intervention done primarily for the benefit of the patient, with no intent to gather new information. Such innovations may be more hazardous and ethically more problematic than research, in part because they are not subject to peer review and because toxicity is not being systematically assessed. This therapy is also subject to abuse because its definition is a matter of intent, difficult for others to disprove.

As with all medical care, *informed consent* of the patient or his or her representative is at the core of protecting subjects. The standard for consent in a research setting is higher because the risks and benefits are typically less clear, the investigator has a conflict of interest, and humans have historically been subjected to unauthorized risks when strict requirements for consent were not respected. Adolescents who are competent may sometimes consent to be research subjects. It is also generally acknowledged that children should be given the opportunity to *dissent,* particularly for nontherapeutic research, when there cannot be a claim that participation is in the child's interest. In the United States, national regulations require that reasonable efforts be made at least to inform children who are capable of understanding that participation is not part of their care and that, therefore, they are free to refuse to participate.

In addition to the protection that informed consent is intended to provide, virtually all research in the United States is reviewed by an institutional review board, required by federal regulations for institutions receiving federal research funds. It is uncertain whether such review is legally required for research that is not federally funded or for research in settings that receive no federal funds, such as private clinics. The principles of ethical decision-making that led to the involvement of ethics committees in clinical decisions argue for similar review of research involving children, regardless of the source of funding.

MATERNAL-FETAL CONFLICTS

In addition to the continuing debate over abortion in the United States, there is increased discussion about the proper balancing of maternal and fetal interests when a pregnant woman's behavior affects the well-being of her fetus. This is usually not limited to maternal-fetal conflicts of interest, because in virtually all cases the concern is also over the well-being of future infants and children.

The most dramatic of these conflicts arise when a pregnant woman refuses standard, effective treatment essential for the benefit of a fetus/infant who is at high risk of death or serious disability, such as refusal of cesarean section for placenta previa in a voluntary pregnancy near term involving a presumably normal fetus/infant. Courts in the United States have sometimes decided that a woman can be required to undergo such a procedure when the benefit to the emergent child is clear. A federal court decided that such an order was inappropriate in a case involving a 26-wk-old fetus and, by implication, other cases in which the benefit of intervention was in doubt. Pediatricians may be required in such cases prenatally to initiate or support court proceedings in the interests of the future child or to consider postnatal sanctions, including reporting of child abuse or neglect.

Child abuse statutes have also been invoked in attempts to modify the behavior of women who ingest alcohol or illicit drugs during pregnancy and expose the fetus/infant to harm. Pediatricians considering reporting such cases must consider the likelihood of benefit from reporting, the harms to the child as well as to the mother if criminal charges or custody changes are sought, and the possible effects that reporting may have in driving pregnant women away from the health care system, particularly from prenatal care.

ACCESS TO HEALTH CARE; RATIONING (DISTRIBUTIVE JUSTICE)

The most serious ethical problem in health care in the United States may be the inequality in access to care. No other major industrial country rations basic health care on the basis of ability to pay. Approximately 10 million children are estimated to lack adequate health insurance, with serious consequences in terms of death, disability, and suffering. The central ethical principle at stake is fair opportunity to participate in the benefits of society; preventable death and disability undermine the claim that the society is one of equal opportunity. Another aspect of the claim of unfairness is that the present system is maintained by those who are already advantaged because of financial or social status, thereby aggravating existing inequalities.

Rationing of health care can be defined as limiting access to wanted and needed services of known benefit. It is increasingly recognized that no society can provide all beneficial services to all its citizens; rationing is therefore unavoidable. The question is not whether to ration health care services but how to do so fairly. Other ways of rationing are based on cost:benefit analysis, age, or likely effects on quality of life.

Beauchamp T, Walters L: Contemporary Issues in Bioethics, 4th ed. Belmont, CA, Wadsworth Publishing, 1994.
Brock D, Daniels N: Ethical foundations of health care reform. JAMA 271:1189, 1994.
Fost N: Genetic diagnosis and treatment: Ethical considerations. Am J Dis Child 147:1190, 1993.
Gaylin W, Macklin R (eds): Who Speaks for the Child?: The Problems of Proxy Consent. New York, Plenum Publishing Corp, 1982.
Holder AR: Legal Issues in Pediatric and Adolescent Medicine, 2nd ed. New Haven, CT, Yale Press, 1985.
Levine R: Ethics and Regulation of Clinical Research, 2nd ed. Baltimore, Urban & Schwarzenberg, 1986.
Menzel PT: Strong Medicine: The Ethical Rationing of Health Care. New York, Oxford University Press, 1990.
O'Neill O, Ruddick W: Having Children: Philosophical and Legal Reflections of Parenthood. New York, Oxford University Press, 1979.
Wall SN, Partridge JC: Death in the intensive care nursery: Physician practice of withdrawing and withholding life support. Pediatrics 99:64, 1997.
Weir R: Selective Nontreatment of Handicapped Newborns: Moral Dilemmas in Neonatal Medicine. New York, Oxford University Press, 1984.

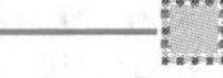

CHAPTER 3
Cultural Issues in Pediatric Care

Kenneth Fox

WHAT ARE CULTURES?

Cultures are dynamic large-scale human social forces that generate structures and meanings of thought and action and enable people to recognize and interpret the meanings of ideas, actions, experiences, places, things, and relationships. Cultures become particularly important for pediatrics as these social forces influence the process of growth and development. Cultural expressions are often unspoken, tacit, and below the level of consciousness. Cultures help structure our understandings about what is natural or common sense and affect what we do and how we do it. In contrast to earlier cognitive notions of cultures as timeless shared ideas or attributes that distill the wisdom of the generations and represent a group's essential life ways, mores, attitudes, and beliefs (including health beliefs), contemporary anthropologists emphasize cultures' situational, historical, and changeable dimensions.

ENCOUNTERING OTHERS IN THE GLOBAL VILLAGE

Today's children grow up in a global village. Conception and birth, health and affliction, growth and development, care and healing, learning and play, life and—sometimes, tragically—death happen for today's children in a busy new human social intersection called the *global economy.* Human cultures exist in a world linked by Internet, phone, and fax and by global media, transportation, and trade networks. These structural features of the global village make encounters between patients and healers from different social, cultural, racial, religious, ethnic, linguistic, national, and class backgrounds a part of everyday life. Cross-cultural experiences are commonplace in many kinds of social settings, including medical ones. However, this time of great cross-cultural contact and economic interdependence is also marked by inequalities in health, wealth, and power.

Encounters with others happen on a grand scale in the flow of goods and services, capital, conflict, ideas, action, images, germs, waste, and labor through busy social intersections. In this global village, we find historically unparalleled movements of large, diverse groups of people. These groups include some 70 million international labor migrants, 20 million refugees, and another 20 million persons displaced within their own national boundaries. Movement and mixing of peoples who draw on diverse identities and resources to make meaning over the life course are fundamental large-scale social forces at work in the global village.

GROUP INEQUALITIES IN THE GLOBAL VILLAGE

Relations of power between different cultural, racial, ethnic, religious, and linguistic groups and the politics of minority/majority group relations have profound implications for health and medical care. A key aspect of the meaning of one's cultural identity is how that identity influences one's position within a social structural framework. In turn, social position shapes health risks and opportunities for care. The United States, for example, is a society with a majority group composed of non-Hispanic whites of European origin and a range of minority "peoples of color" in increasing proportions. Though much has been made of processes like acculturation in the American melting pot, some groups have consistently enjoyed better social structural positions and better health outcomes than others. In patterned, systematic, and enduring ways, United States majority and minority groups are unequally positioned in terms of health, wealth, and power.

At the population level, majority and minority groups have different social statuses, different privileges and burdens, and different health opportunities and risks. For example, minority children in the United States are three times more likely to live below the federal poverty line than non-Hispanic white children. In North American culture, poor health is one of the great burdens of socioeconomic inequality. In New York City, an African American or Latino boy of 15 in the poor borough of Harlem has only a 37% chance of living to age 65. In terms of health, racial and ethnic differences begin early in life. Minority children are disproportionately poor, and poor children have more illnesses, are sicker longer, and have worse health outcomes than nonpoor children (see Chapters 1 and 39). Poor children have higher lead levels, more behavioral and developmental problems, and poorer nutritional, vision, and dental status than more affluent children. They are less likely to be immunized, miss more time from school, and are twice as likely to be restricted from play by chronic health problems than are children from high-income families. Poor children are three times more likely than nonpoor children to die in childhood and have less access to health care than their more privileged peers. However, at any given socioeconomic status level, racial and ethnic disparities in health and health care also may be demonstrated.

Opportunities for human growth, development, and care are similarly unevenly distributed in the global village. Of the world's 5 billion inhabitants, about 1 billion live in abject poverty, on less than a dollar per day. About 1.5 billion have no access to health care facilities at all. Furthermore, demographers predict that the vast majority of the growth of human populations during the next 30 years will happen in Africa, Asia, and Latin America in the world's poorest countries.

Poverty is a key feature of the social contexts in which cultural differences are made to matter. This large-scale social force is the single most important predictor of health outcomes among children all over the world. Cultural, racial, and ethnic differences in the global village are thus suffused with the facts of social structural position.

CULTURE AND RACISM

Racial inequalities in health status are essentially embodiments of social structural inequalities, and racial differences in health often persist even after adjustment for socioeconomic status. Health outcomes are shaped by the cumulative effects of discrimination all along the life course. Whether one explores the most basic elements of primary care (anticipatory guidance, history taking, physical examination, immunization, and so on) or the most sophisticated procedures (e.g., renal transplants), racial inequalities have been demonstrated. These facts are important in pediatrics because competent practice often has the ability to undo or mitigate the health-harming effects of social structural inequalities.

MAKING DIFFERENCES MATTER

Life courses from birth to death are experienced, marked, and managed differently by different cultural and social groups. Identities are shaped by our histories, social institutions, rituals, traditions, concepts of food and nutrition, child rearing, and caretaking practices. Cultures enable us to distinguish self from others according to our sensibilities, values, expectations, and beliefs. One way differences are made to matter is through social processes that generate health risks and opportunities as well as systems of healing and therapy. We express ourselves through distinctive idioms of distress and different explanations about the causes, courses, and threats of illness. Although no one can ever hope to master substantial knowledge about every cultural, racial, or ethnic group encountered, the facts of diversity compel us to incorporate some basic concepts and skills of social analysis into the everyday thought and practice of pediatrics.

DISEASE/ILLNESS; EXPLANATORY MODELS

Medical anthropology is a discipline that explores what people think and do about health and illness across different cultures and different historical periods. *Illness* refers to the uniquely human experience of symptoms and suffering. How a person recognizes, interprets, and responds to symptoms is shaped by his or her social experience and cultural identity. This varies from culture to culture. *Disease* refers to changes, disruptions, or abnormalities of biologic structure or function at the genetic, cellular, tissue, organ/anatomic, or systems levels. For example, a child with asthma has a chronic *disease* caused by reversible hyperactivity of smooth muscle in the airways, airway inflammation, and excessive mucus production. However, the experience of respiratory distress (shortness of breath, wheezing); suffering from a disability that causes restriction from school or play; the family's choices of and access to health care; the child's anxiety and fear of death; the parents' grief over their child's affliction; and the community's outrage over racial/ethnic group disparities in the disease's prevalence, morbidity, and mortality generated by unequal and unjust environmental risk exposures all are aspects of the *illness,* asthma. A healer's capacity and inclination to reframe, translate, and reduce a patient's story to the terms and categories of the biomedical culture are at the heart of traditional standards of clinical competence. However, whether a therapeutic alliance develops between patient and healer depends in large part on the healer's *cultural competence*—his or her ability to hear, interpret, and respond to the illness experience represented by the patient's story (also called the *illness narrative*).

Different cultures have different ways of explaining disease and illness. Every healing system interprets the meanings of symptoms, imagines their course, and responds in characteristic and recognizable ways; they often have distinctive ways of understanding, classifying, and treating illness. Care-seeking and care use behaviors are, in part, shaped by these considerations. Any healing system may be divided for analytic purposes into professional, folk, and popular sectors. In the United States, for example, the professional sector includes physicians, nurses, and ancillary health care providers; the biomedical scientific knowledge base to which they are socialized; and the health care institutions within which they work. The popular sector would include "lay public" ideas, institutions, and practices. The folk sectors would include "folk illnesses" (diagnostic classificatory systems traditionally recognized within a cultural or ethnic group but not usually recognized by categories of biomedical science) and traditional healers. An example of a folk illness is *empacho* among individuals in many Latino ethnic and cultural groups (including Puerto Ricans, Mexicans, Mexican Americans and Guatemalans). *Empacho* is an illness that explains symptoms of nausea, vomiting, diarrhea, cramping, bloating, and anorexia that occur when food or milk gets "stuck" in the stomach as a consequence of dietary indiscretion (e.g., gluttony, inappropriate type or combinations of food, or improper timing of meals). The folk illness may be responsive to different types of intervention: A folk healer *(santiguadora)* may use massage, prayer, or various dietary regimens, which have the effect of "cleaning" the stomach and curing the illness.

The concept of the *explanatory model* (EM) may be helpful in caring for children of various cultures. EMs specify the causes, mechanisms, courses, severity, outcomes, and treatment of symptoms. A physician can begin to explore a patient's EM with some of the following questions: (1) What do you call this problem? Is it an illness? What kind of illness is it? (2) What is the cause of the illness? (3) Why did it start when it did? (4) How does it affect your body? How does it work? (5) What do you expect will happen as consequence of the illness? How severe is it? Will it get better or worse? (6) What do you fear most about the illness? (7) What are the main problems the illness has caused you? (8) What treatment is appropriate? (9) What do you fear about the treatment? The physician then makes explicit his or her own EM. The models are then compared and contrasted. Doctor and patient work to achieve a therapeutic alliance through the process of negotiating an illness narrative and a plan for therapy.

People may make use of more than one healing system at a time. *Cultural pluralism* in medicine refers to systems in which many competing or combining resources are available for people to draw on as they create explanatory models. Explanatory models may be incomplete or contradictory and may change over time in the same individual. Nevertheless, EMs are important because they may help determine pathways of care and amplify the voice of the patient in the medical encounter. In turn, EMs enhance communication and improve patients' satisfaction with and adherence to treatment regimens. Cultural differences between provider and patient may be less significant than differences between professional and lay explanatory models.

Desjarlais R, Eisenberg L, Good B, et al: World Mental Health: Problems and Priorities in Low Income Countries. New York, Oxford University Press, 1995.

Hahn R: Sickness and Healing: An Anthropological Perspective. New Haven, Yale University Press, 1995.

Harwood A (ed): Ethnicity and Medical Care. Cambridge, Harvard University Press, 1981.

Jecker N, Carrese J, Pearlman R: Caring for Patients in Cross-Cultural Settings. Hastings Center Report 25:6–14, 1995.

Kleinman A, Eisenberg L, Good B: Culture illness and care. Clinical lessons from anthropologic and cross cultural research. Ann Intern Med 88:251, 1978.

Krieger N, Rowley D, Herman A, et al: Racism, sexism, and social class: Implications for studies of health disease and well-being. Am J Prev Med 9:82, 1993.

Nichter M: Idioms of distress: Alternatives in the expression of psychosocial distress: A case study from South India. Cult Med Psychiatry 5:379, 1981.

Pachter L: Culture and clinical care: Folk beliefs and behaviors and their implications for health care delivery. JAMA 271:690, 1994.

Pachter L, Dworkin P: Maternal expectations about normal child development in 4 cultural groups. Arch Pediatr Adolesc Med 151:1144, 1997.

Sassen S: The Global City: New York, London, Tokyo. Princeton, NJ, Princeton University Press, 1991.

Williams D, Collins C: US socioeconomic and racial differences in health: Patterns and explanations. Ann Rev Sociol 21:349, 1995.

CHAPTER 4
Child Health in the Developing World

Jeffrey L. Goldhagen

More than 90% of the world's children are born each year in the developing world. Thirty-five thousand of them die each day, most of common and preventable problems. Health and illness for these children are a result of a complex dynamic of environmental, social, political, and economic factors. No single intervention will successfully interrupt the cycles of morbidity and mortality that plague them.

Much has been learned and many successes achieved during the past several decades with regard to the health needs of these children. Eighty per cent of children throughout the world are now being immunized. Polio has been eradicated in the Western hemisphere, and strategies to eliminate measles are being successfully implemented. Oral rehydration therapy (ORT) and community-based protocols dealing with respiratory and other childhood illnesses save millions of children's lives each year. National health policies related to health promotion and disease prevention and treatment are being subjected increasingly to rigorous evidence-based analyses to ensure their effectiveness and cost:benefits.

The relevance of this experience to health services in the United States and other developed countries has gained acceptance. The United States has adopted year-2000 goals patterned after those delineated by the United Nations International Children's Emergency Fund (UNICEF) and the World Health Organization (WHO) in 1978.

PRINCIPLES OF CHILD HEALTH IN DEVELOPING COUNTRIES

Approaches to child health evolved rapidly after World War II. This was because of the efforts of UNICEF and WHO, the emergence of non-government relief and development organizations (NGOs), and changing strategies for international development assistance.

The Thirtieth World Health Assembly (1977) and Alma Ata International Conference on Primary Health Care (1978) defined the contemporary context for international health development. The 1977 World Health Assembly established the main goal of WHO to be the attainment, by all people of the world, of a level of health that would permit them to lead a socially and economically productive life by the year 2000.

The Declaration of Alma Ata asserted primary care to be the key strategy for attaining year-2000 goals. The Declaration has had a profound impact on the structure and function of health systems in all regions of the world. It established 10 precepts for primary care: (1) Health is a state of complete well-being and not merely the absence of disease or infirmity; (2) inequities of health within and between countries are unacceptable and of global concern; (3) economic and social development are reciprocally tied to health development; (4) people have the right to participate in their own health care; (5) individual's health should permit socially and economically productive lives; (6) primary health care is essential for overall social and economic development; (7) components of primary health care include personal health services, nutrition, safe water and sanitation, maternal and child health, immunization, essential drugs, and related sectors including agriculture, housing, public works, and so forth; (8) national policies should support comprehensive intersectoral health systems; (9) all countries should cooperate in a global health strategy; and (10) better use of resources, including diversion of those involved in military pursuits, would facilitate attaining year-2000 goals.

International debate has focused on the balance between two approaches to achieving year-2000 goals. An emphasis on developing comprehensive primary care systems is based on long-term efforts to build equitable systems that address all the health issues of a community. Alternatively, UNICEF, WHO, and developed countries, which contribute most of the world's assistance funds, have argued for more selective programs whose outcomes and cost can be readily measured. Selective strategies for the Child Survival Revolution were implemented after the Alma Ata conference using simple methods of *G*rowth monitoring, *O*ral rehydration, *B*reast-feeding, and *I*mmunization (GOBI). Later, categories of *F*ood, *F*emale education, and *F*amily planning were added (GOBI-FFF). GOBI-FFF has remained the developed world's primary strategy for health development.

Two decades of experience with child survival programs has resulted in numerous innovative approaches to child health initiatives. Networks of indigenous health workers have been established throughout the world, and health professionals trained to manage them. Social marketing strategies, operations and evaluation research, rapid assessment techniques, and so forth have been developed. The importance of the role of women, the household environment, female education, family planning, and birth spacing have been better defined, and related strategies integrated into health programs.

The knowledge and experience accrued in the past several decades provide reasons for optimism. The dramatic decrease in childhood mortality in the developed world before the delivery and use of antibiotics and vaccines is evidence of the importance of basic public health programs and their potential to improve the lives of all children everywhere.

BASIC HEALTH INDICATORS

Despite many successes, great disparity exists among nations in the health status of children. Annual health statistics and related indicators are reported in UNICEF's *The State of the World's Children.* Average infant and under-5-yr mortality rates (U5MR) range from almost 200/1,000 in least-developed countries to less than 9/1,000 in developed countries. Comparing economically poor and wealthy countries reveals (1) more than twice the number of infants born small for gestational age (SGA), (2) a third versus 0% of children under 5 years as moderately to severely malnourished, (3) a fourfold greater average annual population growth rate, and (4) a sevenfold difference in crude birth and fertility rates. With respect to women, (1) the contraceptive prevalence is less than 10% in developing countries and greater than 70% in wealthier nations, (2) maternal mortality rates are 50 times greater in developing than in economically developed countries (approximately 650 vs 12/100,000 live births), and (3) in the developing world less than one third of pregnant women are immunized against tetanus.

Key environmental and education indices related to health outcomes in less developed countries demonstrate similar disparities. Less than one half of the population in these countries has access to safe water and adequate sanitation. Adult literacy rates are 60% and 40% for males and females, respectively. Less than one half of children are enrolled in primary school, and only about one half of these children complete it.

Economic indices reveal increasing inequities between countries and predict potential deterioration in the health status of poorer nations. The per capita gross national product (GNP) (US$) in economically less developed countries is $250–$800 versus $15,000 in developed nations. The per capita average annual income growth rate during the past decade is 0.1% in least-developed countries compared with over 2.4% in developed nations, and the rate of inflation is up to 15-fold greater than that of developed countries. Seventy per cent of the population in the least-developed countries have lived in poverty during the past decade.

Trends in the health indices in developing countries are a cause for both optimism and pessimism. U5MR has fallen by more than 50% during the past 30 years, with the most significant decrease registered in the past decade. Adult literacy and school enrollment rates have more than doubled. Crude birth and death rates have fallen by almost 50%, and life expectancy has increased from 39 to 50 years.

Despite these improvements, increasing disparity in economic indicators is a cause for alarm. In developing nations, the average annual per cent growth rates in per capita GNP have remained stagnant or declined during the past decade relative to the previous 15–20 years. Debt service has risen by 30% (as a percentage of exports of goods and services). Fertility rate reduction has remained virtually unchanged, and average annual population growth rates have actually increased during the past decade. Population growth in combination with deteriorating economic conditions portends increased difficulties for children in affected countries. Child labor, sexual exploitation, environmental poisoning, abandonment, and so on are among the critical child health issues that result from the economic status of poorer countries.

EPIDEMIOLOGY OF ILLNESS AND SPECIFIC INTERVENTION STRATEGIES

Each year, more than 10 million children die. Seven in 10 of these deaths are due to respiratory infections, diarrhea, measles and other vaccine-preventable illnesses, malaria, and/or malnutrition. Although simple and affordable single interventions have had measured success in the past, recognition that morbidity and mortality are most frequently due to a combination of factors has led to the implementation of the WHO Integrated Management of Childhood Illness (IMCI) strategy. The strategy combines improved management of childhood illnesses with combination therapies (e.g., vaccines, antibiotics, ORT, nutritional supplements, contraceptives) and other maternal and child health interventions. Health system modifications required to sustain IMCI include (1) improvement in health personnel case management skills and development of region-specific protocols for IMCI, (2) involvement of families and communities in the implementation of IMCI protocols, and (3) the definition and funding of priority "essential" health services. Overall, more than 65% of child deaths are preventable at low cost.

Pneumonia

Pneumonia causes the majority of child deaths. Pathogens in developing countries are similar to those in economically advanced nations, but the frequency of primary and secondary bacterial infections is much greater. Respiratory viruses, in particular respiratory syncytial virus (RSV), cause the majority of acute lower respiratory tract infections (ALRTI). *Streptococcus pneumoniae, Haemophilus influenzae, Moraxella catarrhalis,* and *Staphylococcus aureus* account for the majority of bacterial infections. Cytomegalovirus, *Chlamydia, Mycoplasma pneumoniae,* and *Mycobacterium tuberculosis* also are common pathogens.

Vitamin A deficiency is clearly associated with increased incidence, morbidity, and mortality of respiratory tract disease (see Chapter 44). Vitamin A stabilizes the structure and function of mucosal surfaces and is involved with immune response (particularly T-cell function) and mucus production. At least a 2-fold increase in the incidence of respiratory disease and a 4- to 12-fold increase in mortality are noted in children with even mild vitamin A deficiency. This explains the association of measles with vitamin A deficiency, xerophthalmia, respiratory and diarrheal diseases, and increased child mortality. Supplementation with as little as a single 200,000 IU vitamin A capsule per year has been shown to decrease childhood mortality by 50%. Treatment of measles with vitamin A supplementation is now recommended by the American Academy of Pediatrics.

Primary malnutrition can result in vitamin A deficiency, which increases a child's susceptibility to respiratory and diarrheal diseases. Viral and bacterial infections can also lead to vitamin A deficiency and further malnutrition. This vicious circle of malnutrition and infection is the principal cause of child deaths in the developing world.

Other simple interventions can decrease mortality due to pneumonia. Breast milk provides the required vitamin A through the first 6 mo of life and most of the requirement until age 2 yr. Prevention of hypothermia through continuous skin-to-skin contact of babies with their parents or surrogates (the kangaroo method) can prevent hypothermia in premature and SGA infants. Oiling the skin can also prevent loss of body heat and moisture.

As an example of a successful low-cost strategy to deal with major childhood illnesses, national acute respiratory infection (ARI) programs have been established in all regions of the world. Millions of mothers have learned to recognize respiratory distress by counting respirations and identifying chest indrawing and fever. Use of antibiotics at home for children identified as having moderately severe ARIs and referral to health care facilities for those with severe disease have reduced mortality and the inappropriate use of antibiotics. National ARI programs train parents, supervise health workers, ensure adequate distribution of essential drugs and access of families to health facilities, monitor and evaluate programs, and provide ongoing surveillance for drug resistance.

Diarrheal Diseases (also see Chapter 176)

The epidemiology of diarrheal disease in developing nations is similar to that in economically advanced countries. Rotavirus and other enteric viruses are the principal pathogens. Bacterial disease is usually caused by *Salmonella* and *Shigella.* Parasitic infections are endemic but generally result in nutritional deficiencies and not acute diarrheal disease. Cholera remains a problem throughout all regions of the developing world.

Oral rehydration solution (ORS) save the lives of millions of children and adults each year. When given in the right proportion, (see Chapter 55), electrolytes and water are absorbed across the intestine despite ongoing diarrhea. Hundreds of millions of ORS packets containing electrolytes and carbohydrates in powder form have been distributed worldwide. The content of oral rehydration solutions has evolved to include indigenous and culturally acceptable sources of carbohydrate as well as homemade recipes that use appropriate finger measurements for locally available containers. UNICEF and WHO's child survival strategy uses ORT (and breast-feeding) as two of its four pillars.

Diarrheal disease programs have significantly reduced mortality. International promotion of breast-feeding has included strict restrictions on advertising and sale of formula, development of baby-friendly hospitals, and extensive social marketing campaigns. Diarrheal disease programs also have had an important impact on the structure and function of national health service delivery systems. Effective, inexpensive, and simple therapies for diarrhea provide an example of how health can be promoted. Networks of indigenous health workers have been developed to teach people about the cause, prevention, and treatment of diarrhea.

These networks have served as the foundation for other health initiatives and have had a profound impact on the culture of many communities. Women, who have traditionally been denied access to important community roles, and traditional healers, who have been generally kept out of mainstream governmental initiatives, have been integrated into health systems. The fundamental role of women and the concept of health as a product generated in the context of a household have been recognized. The importance of birth spacing and female education to efforts to decrease child mortality also has been appreciated.

Immunization-Preventable Diseases (also see Chapter 301)

The six immunization-preventable diseases (measles, polio, diphtheria, pertussis, tetanus, and tuberculosis) kill, blind, cripple, and cause mental damage to some 10 million children each year. Immunization of all the world's children and eradication of a number of diseases are now international priorities. The Expanded Program on Immunization (EPI) is among the joint efforts of WHO, UNICEF, and other governmental and nongovernmental organizations to attain these goals.

Dramatic successes have been achieved. The cold chain, necessary for preservation of heat-intolerant vaccines, reaches virtually everywhere on the globe; effective evaluation and surveillance techniques to ensure vaccine viability have been implemented; new vaccines (HIB, HEP-B) have been introduced in some parts of the world, and others, including vaccines for rotavirus, RSV, malaria, and dengue fever, are under development or already in trials; multiple antigen and new single-dose and heat-resistant vaccines have been introduced or are in final stages of development; new vaccine delivery systems and practices to minimize missed opportunities to vaccinate have been implemented; EPI funding resources and personnel have been expanded; management techniques and strategies for global eradication of diseases are being perfected; communication, computer, and surveillance systems have been introduced; and the commitment of virtually every nation in the world has been secured.

MALNUTRITION (also see Chapter 42)

Malnutrition is a primary cause of morbidity and mortality and a complicating factor for other illnesses. In utero caloric deprivation results in some SGA births. Subsequent protein, calorie, and micronutrient malnutrition results in moderate to severe stunting in 50% of children, with concomitant deficiencies in cognitive development. Susceptibility to infectious diseases is increased. Acute and chronic infections may further exacerbate a child's nutritional deficiencies and often result in a child's death. Anorexia and inaccessible tertiary care make nutritional resuscitation difficult or impossible.

In addition to unavailability of food and chronic parasitic infestation, protein-calorie malnutrition and micronutrient deficiencies sometimes result from cultural food practices. Use of foods with low protein and calorie content as weaning foods, early displacement of infants from the breast (often because of the belief that infants should not be nursed if the mother is pregnant), and failure to initiate breast-feeding or early cessation of it are common causes of primary malnutrition. Female education, family planning, and birth spacing are among the most effective strategies to prevent malnutrition.

OTHER CHILD HEALTH ISSUES

Malaria, schistosomiasis, and dengue fever are examples of other infectious diseases common to children in developing countries. However, the medical, psychologic, and social impact of AIDS and violence is eclipsing all other causes of morbidity and mortality in many regions of the world. In areas of Central Africa, as many as 40% of women are infected with human immunodeficiency virus (HIV). Without access to antiretroviral drugs that can greatly decrease rates of perinatal HIV transmission, approximately 25% of their offspring will be infected with HIV through vertical transmission. Uninfected children are often left orphaned and potentially without the support and nurturing required for normal early childhood development. The personal effect on families is complicated by the economic impact that the death of productive individuals has on whole communities.

War and natural disasters have always had a disproportionate effect on children. Conflicts persist in many regions of the world, exposing children to acts of violence and traumatic stress disorders. The specific targeting of children, health care providers, and hospitals in recent conflicts in Europe and Africa is unique in history and is of particular concern. The susceptibility of children to land mine injuries through normal play has spawned an international movement to limit their distribution and production—a movement that was awarded a 1997 Nobel prize.

Violence directed at children, however, is not limited to war. Street children are routinely tortured and often killed; widespread childhood prostitution and forced labor persist, particularly in Southeast Asia and India; and patterns of abuse continue in all countries. The treatment of detained and incarcerated children is under increased international scrutiny, including the treatment of these children in the United States.

The unique and extensive impact of natural and man-made disasters on the physical and mental health of children has only recently become recognized as an important international child health issue. International efforts are under way to study these impacts, develop intervention strategies, and train personnel to respond.

WORLD SUMMIT FOR CHILDREN AND CONVENTION ON THE RIGHTS OF THE CHILD

In response to the acute needs of children throughout the world, the 1990 United Nations World Summit for Children was convened to establish national programs of action for achieving basic health and social goals. The U.N. Convention on the Rights of Children was presented at the Summit as a legally binding geopolitical contract to extend certain human rights to children. The Convention established standards for survival, protection, and development for all children.

The Convention is being used worldwide as a legal and ethical framework for improving the health and social status of children. To date, only the United States and Somalia have not ratified the Convention, but there is far from full implementation of the Convention among signatories. However, the awareness and dialogue it has engendered have already done much to strengthen the inherent social contract the present adult generation has with their children. The world community's future focus on implementation and monitoring of the Convention will sustain this international commitment to children.

Bertrand W, Walmus B: Maternal knowledge, attitudes and practice as predictors of diarrhoeal disease in young children. Int J Epidemiol 12:205, 1983.

Bloom A, Reid J: Anthropology and primary health care in developing countries. Soc Sci Med 19:183, 1984.

Centers for Disease Control and Prevention: Progress toward global measles control and elimination, 1990–1996. MMWR 46:893, 1997.

Forgie I, O'Neill K, Lloyd-Evans N, et al: Etiology of acute lower respiratory tract infection in Gambian children: II. Acute lower respiratory tract infection in children ages one to nine years presenting at the hospital. Pediatr Infect Dis J 10:42, 1991.

Forgie I, O'Neill K, Lloyd-Evans N, et al: Etiology of acute lower respiratory tract infections in infants presenting at the hospital. Pediatr Infect Dis J 10:33, 1991.

Grant J: The State of the World's Children. Oxford, Oxford University Press, 1996.

Mandl P: A Child Survival and Development Revolution, 2nd ed. Geneva, United Nations Children's Fund, 1983.

Morley D, Lovel H: My Name is Today. London, Macmillan, 1986.

Mulholland K, Weber M: Recognising causes and signs of pneumonia. ARI News 24:2, 1992.

Murray C, Lopez D: Evidence-based health policy-lessons from the Global Burden of Disease Study. Science 274:740, 1996.

Oplatka E: Vitamin A treatment of measles. American Academy of Pediatrics News 9:7, 1993.

Pebley A, Millman S: Birth spacing and child survival. Healthy People 2000. 12:71, 1986.
Sommer A, Katz J, Tarwotjo I: Increased risk of respiratory disease and diarrhea in children with preexisting mild vitamin A deficiency. Am J Clin Nutr 40:1090, 1984.
UNICEF: The Progress of Nations. New York, United Nations Press, 1996.
Werner D, Bower B: Helping Health Workers Learn. Palo Alto, CA, The Hesperian Foundation, 1984.
World Health Organization: The Management of Childhood Illness in Developing Countries: The Rationale for an Integrated Strategy, http://cdrwww/who.ch/.

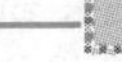

CHAPTER 5
Preventive Pediatrics

Theodore C. Sectish

Prevention in the health care of infants, children, and adolescents is at the core of pediatrics. The outcomes of preventive interventions in childhood are measurable in terms of decades of remaining years of life. Therefore, preventive pediatrics has a substantial impact on our society. During the course of the 20th century, the issues that spawned the development of the field of pediatrics have been largely addressed through advances in biologic science and public health. The threat of mortality and morbidity from infectious disease has been reduced by the development of therapeutic agents and immunizations and by quality improvements in our water system and food supply. Pediatricians have led the way in this and many other scientific, public health, and public policy efforts to address issues that affect the lives of children.

Pediatricians practice preventive pediatrics through their day-to-day clinical activities in health supervision and through their professional activities as educators, advocates, and experts in child health. Their focus should be on the individual patient and on children as a population and should encompass

- Health supervision of healthy infants, children, and adolescents
- Practical approaches to some common issues presenting during health supervision
- Health supervision of children with chronic conditions

HEALTH SUPERVISION OF HEALTHY INFANTS, CHILDREN, AND ADOLESCENTS

ENHANCED HEALTH SUPERVISION GUIDELINES. Pediatricians have the opportunity to improve the lives of children significantly by making effective use of health care supervision visits. New guidelines for supervision have expanded content that addresses continuing and new morbidities facing children and their families, including childhood injuries, educational failure, child abuse and neglect, family violence, teenage pregnancy, environmental health concerns, and risk-taking behaviors such as the use of tobacco, alcohol, and drugs (*Guidelines for Health Supervision III,* developed by the American Academy of Pediatrics, and *Bright Futures,* sponsored by the Maternal and Child Health Bureau). In addition to using the traditional history taking and physical examination, pediatricians must assess cognitive development, social competence, and family life during well child visits in order to address these morbidities. By emphasizing the importance of establishing a therapeutic alliance with the family and promoting a collaborative effort to achieve optimal health, these guidelines suggest the process as well as the content of health supervision visits.

THE THERAPEUTIC ALLIANCE. A *partnership in health supervision* requires an understanding and appreciation of the individual context of each child and his or her family. Children have many unique attributes based on the diversity of their families, culture, ethnicity, language, socioeconomic status, special health needs, and educational backgrounds. Teaming up with families and empowering them with knowledge allow greater opportunity for primary prevention and early detection of disease during the intervals between health supervision visits. Collaboration enables families to participate in the establishment of goals, share responsibility for health care, and develop self-esteem, confidence, and competence.

DOCTOR-PATIENT COMMUNICATION (see Chapter 17.1). Effective physician communication is at the heart of establishing a therapeutic alliance. In health supervision visits, the role of the pediatrician is expanded beyond diagnostician to that of healer, educator, and counselor. Although a complete discussion of communication skills is beyond the scope of this chapter, several key aspects of effective physician-patient communication within health supervision visits should be noted. Pediatricians should

- Demonstrate respect and empathy for patients and families
- Actively listen to the concerns of patients and families
- Use nonjudgmental, open-ended questions to promote a dialogue
- Foster self-esteem and confidence with supportive comments and observations
- Relate to the child separately from the parents
- Consider the family's perspective in formulating a therapeutic plan

PERIODIC HEALTH SUPERVISION VISITS. Pediatricians spend 25–40% of their time performing clinical preventive services throughout infancy, childhood, and adolescence. Although these visits are brief encounters in the life of a child and his or her family, significant relationships are built over time. It is the longitudinal nature of health supervision that helps these brief encounters to have a lasting impact. Eighty per cent of children in the United States receive these preventive services and other acute health care through private practice or a health maintenance organization.

The suggested sequence of health supervision visits is listed in Table 5–1. Beyond the traditional history and physical examination, screening, and immunizations, health supervision visits should include surveillance of developmental milestones, observations of parent-child interaction, counseling, anticipatory guidance, and an opportunity to meet the family's agenda with the use of open-ended or trigger questions. Enhancements to the health supervision visit have been suggested in both *Guidelines for Health Supervision III* and *Bright Futures.* Table 5–2 provides a list of the essential elements in health supervision visits abstracted from these new guidelines.

Because of the large number of potential topics suggested for each periodic health supervision visit and the need for documentation in the medical record, pediatricians should consider using structured encounter forms. Besides improving documentation and efficiency, structured encounter forms may

TABLE 5–1 Suggested Schedule of Health Supervision Visits

Infancy 0–1 yr	Early Childhood 1–4 yr	Middle Childhood 5–10 yr	Adolescence 11–21 yr
Prenatal	15 mo	5 yr	11 yr
Neonatal	18 mo	6 yr	12 yr
First week	2 yr	8 yr	13 yr
1 mo	3 yr	10 yr	14 yr
2 mo	4 yr		15 yr
4 mo			16 yr
6 mo			17 yr
9 mo			18 yr
12 mo			19 yr
			20 yr
			21 yr

TABLE 5–2 Preventive Evaluation at Specific Ages*

Activity	1st week	1 mo	2 mo	4 mo	6 mo	9 mo	12 mo	15 mo	18 mo	2 yr	3 yr	4 yr	5 yr	6 yr	8 yr	10 yr	11–14 yr	15–17 yr	18–21 yr
Interview (for special attention)	√	√	√	√	√	√	√	√	√	√	√	√	√	√	√	√	√	√	√
Family history	√	√								√		√		√	√	√	√	√	√
Pregnancy and delivery	√																		
Neonatal course	√	√																	
Developmental evaluation/ milestones	√	√	√	√	√	√	√	√	√	√	√	√	√	√	√	√	√	√	√
Body systems (for special attention)																			
Hearing/vision	√	√	√	√	√	√	√		√	√	√	√	√		√	√	√	√	
CNS (including sleep)	√	√	√	√	√	√	√		√	√	√	√							
Gastrointestinal/feeding	√	√	√	√	√	√	√		√	√	√	√	√		√	√	√	√	
Urinary	√	√	√							√									
Dental care					√	√	√	√	√	√	√	√	√	√	√	√	√	√	
Drugs, alcohol, tobacco															√	√	√	√	√
Pica						√	√	√	√	√	√	√							
Sexual behavior															√	√	√	√	√
Observations of parent-child interaction	√	√	√	√	√	√	√	√	√	√	√	√	√	√	√	√	√	√	√
Physical Examination (complete) (for special attention)	√	√	√	√	√	√	√	√	√	√	√	√	√	√	√	√	√	√	√
Height and weight	√	√	√	√	√	√	√	√	√	√	√	√	√	√	√	√	√	√	√
Head circumference	√	√	√	√	√	√	√	√											
Blood pressure											√	√	√	√	√	√	√	√	√
Skin	√	√	√	√	√	√	√	√	√	√	√	√	√	√	√	√	√	√	√
Vision																			
Tear ducts	√	√	√	√															
Fixed eyes	√	√																	
Red reflex	√	√	√	√	√	√	√												
Fundi											√	√	√	√	√	√	√	√	√
Strabismus/eye movements	√	√	√	√	√	√				√	√								
Hearing	√	√	√			√	√	√	√	√	√	√	√	√					
Speech		√	√	√	√	√	√	√	√	√	√	√	√	√					
Neurologic problems	√	√	√	√	√	√	√												
Cardiac murmurs	√	√	√	√	√	√	√			√	√	√	√	√	√	√	√	√	√
Abdominal masses	√	√	√	√	√	√	√	√	√	√	√	√	√	√	√	√	√	√	√
External genitalia	√	√	√	√	√	√	√	√	√	√	√	√	√	√	√	√	√	√	√
Hip dysplasia/dislocation	√	√	√	√	√	√	√	√	√	√									
Gait							√	√	√	√	√	√	√	√					
Deformities (metatarsus adductus)	√	√	√	√	√	√	√	√	√										
Sexual development														√	√	√	√	√	
Scoliosis														√	√	√	√	√	√
Evidence of neglect/abuse	√	√	√	√	√	√	√	√	√	√	√	√	√	√	√	√	√	√	
Laboratory testing and screening																			
Hgb/Hct					√ or	√ or	√								√		√	√	
Urinalysis					√ or	√ or	√								√				
Urine culture (girls)					√ or	√ or	√									√	√		
Tuberculin						√ or	√			√		√ or	√ or	√			√ or	√ or	√
Lipids										√	or	√		√		√	√	√	√
Metabolic	√	√																	
Lead					√ or	√ or	√ or	√		√	√		√						
Hearing screening	√ (Prior to 3 mo)												√	√					
Vision screening											√		√	√		√			
STD																	√	√	√
Immunizations (see Chapter 301 for details)	√	√	√	√	√	√	√	√	√			√ or	√				√		
Anticipatory guidance and counseling (for special attention)	√	√	√	√	√	√	√	√	√	√	√	√	√	√	√	√	√	√	√
Parent and child interaction	√	√	√	√	√	√	√	√	√	√	√	√	√	√	√	√	√	√	√
Diet/nutrition	√	√	√	√	√	√	√	√	√	√	√	√	√	√	√	√	√	√	√
Sleep	√	√	√	√	√	√	√	√	√	√	√			√		√	√	√	√
Toilet training								√	√	√	√								
Injury prevention	√	√	√	√	√	√	√	√	√	√	√	√	√	√	√	√	√	√	√
Infant/child care (includes oral health)	√	√	√	√	√	√	√	√	√	√	√	√	√						
School problems											√	√	√	√	√	√	√	√	√
Puberty and sexuality															√	√	√	√	√
Substance abuse															√	√	√	√	√
Family and social relationships	√	√	√	√	√	√	√	√	√	√	√	√	√	√	√	√	√	√	√

**These suggestions or guidelines represent an analysis of recommendations by the American Academy of Pediatrics and Bright Futures. They are not intended to be all inclusive but rather to serve as reminders for some of the important preventive and health promotion activities that should be considered at various ages when physician-patient encounters may occur. The content and timing of visits will need to be altered according to special needs and the presence or absence of risk factors for the child and his or her family.*

improve the delivery of health information and thereby increase parental satisfaction with quality of care. Various preprinted forms are available and should be reviewed to determine which ones are most appropriate for a particular practice setting.

Group well childcare is an effective alternative or complement to the individual well childcare visit. These visits, in which groups of infants and children of similar ages and their families participate in a session (typically 45–60 min) led by a primary care pediatric provider, are designed to facilitate parent education. By allowing ample time for discussion about child-rearing issues, group well child visits promote observations of parent-child interactions and serve as support groups. Pediatricians should consider how to incorporate group visits into their practices and tailor them to the needs of their practice and their patient population. For example, the use of group visits in infancy may improve parental knowledge of parenting and child development; parents of older children may benefit from sessions that address issues of smoking, drinking, or nutrition.

TOPICS OF FREQUENT CONCERN DURING HEALTH SUPERVISION. In the course of well childcare visits, pediatricians provide specific advice in areas of behavior and parenting and educate families about common issues in normal growth and development. By providing information to parents, pediatricians enable parents to feel successful in their roles, become allies in child rearing, and build a therapeutic alliance. In addition to the specific advice offered in the health supervision visit, pediatricians should provide patient education materials (handouts, brochures, references) and train their staff who serve as patient educators on the telephone, in the clinic, and in group visits. As computers become more widespread and families are connected to the Internet, pediatricians should be involved in the development, editing, and updating of patient education information and refer families to useful websites like the American Academy of Pediatrics website, *http://www.aap.org,* which provides access to patient education materials. In the paragraphs that follow, some of the common topics of parenting and childcare, chosen because of their prominence in health supervision visits, are discussed with an emphasis on prevention.

Diaper Dermatitis (see Chapter 653). As the most common skin disorder in infancy and one of the most visible problems in infant care, diaper rash is frequently discussed in well child visits. Diaper dermatitis peaks at age 9–12 mo. Parents need education about its prevalence and an understanding of the pathogenesis. Wearing diapers is the cause of most cases of diaper dermatitis. Diapers provide a warm, dark, moist environment where urine and feces are in contact with skin. Most diaper rashes are self-limited and respond to frequent diaper changes, a period of time without diapers, barrier creams to minimize the contact of urine and feces with skin, and appropriate cleansing of the diaper area with water and a mild, nonperfumed soap. The development of more absorbent diapers has helped to prevent diaper rashes. Diarrheal disease is a major exacerbating factor.

Specific causes such as *Candida albicans* (Chapter 230.1) or underlying skin disorders such as atopic dermatitis, seborrheic dermatitis, or psoriasis may also have a role in the development of diaper dermatitis. Skin infections with bacteria such as *Staphylococcus aureus* occur as secondary infections when the protective barrier of the skin has been compromised. Parents should be alerted to seek additional advice if the diaper rash has been present for more than 5 days; if any exudates, vesicles, or pustules are present; if the rash spreads beyond the diaper area; or if there is cracking or bleeding.

Teething. Most infants have their first teeth erupt at age 6–8 mo (Chapter 307) and may have associated mild symptoms of gingival swelling and sensitivity, increased salivation, and irritability related to gum discomfort. No evidence shows that diarrhea, rhinorrhea, rashes, or fever is related to teething. Parents should be informed about normal behaviors associated with teething and should be given practical advice to help manage its symptoms. Most infants tolerate teething without difficulty if offered a firm object to bite such as teething ring. Rubbing the gums with a cool, wet washcloth can be comforting. If additional pain relief is needed, acetaminophen or ibuprofen may be administered.

Sleep Problems. In the first year, difficulties with transitions to sleep and with night awakening are commonly reported. Parents should be educated about separation anxiety, which develops in the latter half of the first year of life and is related to difficulty with nighttime settling and night awakening. Additionally, parents should be informed about normal sleep requirements to help them understand a child's need for naps, sleep schedules, and bedtimes (see Chapter 10). Older infants and children may experience nightmares or parasomnias such as night terrors, night walking, night talking, or bed-wetting (see Chapter 20.5).

To help a child settle at night, parents should establish a bedtime routine starting with a quiet interaction like reading a bedtime story. Transitional objects, such as blankets and teddy bears, are integral parts of bedtime routines and facilitate falling asleep. It is important to allow infants to settle on their own, so that they are accomplishing a successful independent transition to sleep. If a child protests, parents should use the same consistent approach repeatedly.

When parents experience difficulty with a *child who wakes at night,* the same approach of promoting nighttime settling should be used. It is important to recognize that arousal or awakening from sleep is normal and that hunger does not usually cause night awakening unless the child has been trained to feed at night. Parents should delay their response so that normal arousal states during sleep do not progress to complete awakening. When parents must respond, they should use the same approach as in the bedtime routine.

Nightmares are common and usually involve vivid, scary, or exciting events, which are easily recalled by the child on awakening. *Night terrors* are less common events lasting 10–15 min, during which time the child is not easily aroused and may appear frightened and agitated. On awakening the next morning, a child who experienced a night terror will have amnesia. In advising parents about both nightmares and night terrors, the importance of a calm, soothing approach to facilitate the child's return to sleep should be emphasized.

Bed-wetting is one of the most common sleep problems facing school-age children. By age 7, up to 7% of all children may experience occasional bed-wetting episodes. Parents should be provided information about the prevalence of bed-wetting to foster an understanding of enuresis as a developmental problem and thereby demystify the condition. If a child experiences "dry" nights (nights without bed-wetting) on a weekly basis and is motivated to stop bed-wetting, it may help to involve the child in keeping a record of wet and dry nights on a calendar. The calendar keeps the family and the child focused on the issue and allows for positive reinforcement when dry nights occur. In up to 30% of patients, complete dryness is achieved by this motivational technique. At the time of health supervision visits, it may be helpful to preview the entire range of therapeutic interventions, including conditioning and drug therapies, in the event that the behavioral approach is unsuccessful. The management of enuresis is addressed in greater detail in Chapters 20.3 and 551.

Toilet Training. In the United States, the average age of successful toilet training is 27 mo, with a range of up to 3–4 yr. Early training (before age 2), because of its association with chronic stool retention and encopresis, should be discouraged. The key factor for parents to recognize in successful toilet training is the readiness of the child. Several questions may be used to assess readiness:

"Does your child communicate to you before the passage of urine or stool?"
"Can she 'hold on' for a minute or two before urinating or defecating?"

If these questions are answered affirmatively, the child is ready to train. The process of toilet training involves positive reinforcement by parents who recognize their child's readiness and developmental stage. Minor hurdles in the toilet training process such as fear of sitting on the toilet or accidents when not wearing diapers should be met with a calm and understanding approach.

Temper Tantrums. A child's expression of anger in outbursts of rage is a significant challenge for parents. Parents may blame their ineffective parenting skills, when the problem may be related to a child's personality style or a particular situation. Parents need to understand that temper tantrums are a normal part of child development.

Identifying the type of tantrum may be helpful in offering advice about parental interventions (e.g., frustration or fatigue related, attention seeking or demanding, refusal, disruptive, potentially harmful, or ragelike). If a child is experiencing frustration related to excessive fatigue or hunger, he or she needs support, sleep, or food. Some positive remarks also may help them with their feelings of frustration. For those tantrums in which children are insistent and making unreasonable demands, it is best to ignore them and allow them to regain composure over time. Refusal tantrums related to important issues such as bedtimes or going to school need to be met with firmness and consistency. Parents should be clear in their request for the child to comply and must allow opportunity for compliance. If this approach fails, it may be necessary to move the child physically to bed or into the car. When behavior is so disruptive and out of control or occurs in a public place such as the grocery store, physical removal followed by a time-out is most effective. In advising parents about the length of time-outs, a good rule of thumb is approximately 1 minute per year of age. When significant rage with the potential for physical injury occurs, the best intervention is holding the child to calm and allow him or her to relax in the parent's arms. Even though temper tantrums are a normal part of childhood and parenting, it is important to assess the family and determine if there are any contributing factors such as parental depression or family violence that may require other referrals or interventions.

Discipline. This common subject of well child care is one of the most controversial. Families have little knowledge about the most effective techniques of modifying child behavior, and parents have a tendency to apply the same discipline strategies used by their parents. The strategies suggested by American Academy of Pediatrics include three essential elements: (1) a positive, supportive, loving relationship between parents and children; (2) use of positive reinforcement to increase desired behaviors; and (3) removing reinforcement of undesired behaviors and applying punishment to reduce or eliminate undesired behaviors.

Primary care practitioners should assess the methods of discipline used within families and offer practical advice tailored to the individual family. Well child visits provide opportunities to observe parent-child interaction and to stimulate discussion with trigger questions that address issues of behavior and discipline. The most basic aspect of effective discipline—the positive, supportive, loving relationship—should be evaluated in every well child encounter and serve as a basis for behavioral modification and specific advice for problems. If a pediatrician suspects marital discord, family dysfunction, substance or alcohol abuse, or family violence, a referral for counseling is the most important priority. Parents should be reminded to promote a positive atmosphere within the home and provide clear expectations about desired behaviors. Key factors include positive role modeling, praise, paying attention and listening to children, and devoting special time to build the parent-child relationship. Emphasis should be placed on the need for consistency of parental behavior, open communication within the family, respect for each family member, and ignoring trivial problems to be more selective and effective.

When providing guidance about specific problem behaviors, practitioners need to clarify the distinction between *time-out* or *removal of privileges* and punishment. The former are methods of extinction that are intended to effect a reduction or elimination of undesired behavior. Punishment involves issuing verbal reprimands or inflicting physical pain to reduce or eliminate undesired behaviors. Time-out and removal of privileges require consistency and patience because their effects on behavioral change are more long term than other methods. Parents must provide clear expectations of desired behavior, intervene quickly with time-out or removal of privileges, and communicate to the child about the reason for the consequence. Because a reactive emotional response or tantrum often ensues, parents should remain calm and impassive to avoid prolonging the incident or escalating the child's level of response. These forms of discipline are among the most enduring in changing behavior but require parents to manage their own distress successfully when meting out this form of discipline.

Punishment is a controversial alternative method of discipline. In the United States, surveys have shown that up to 90% of parents use spanking as a regular method of discipline. Behavioral research on corporal punishment is inconclusive and conflicting about the long-term impact of spanking on subsequent behaviors such as antisocial actions and aggression. Clearly, however, some forms of physical punishment may be harsh and abusive. Religious beliefs or influences from other family members may often create inappropriate parental expectations about discipline. Pediatricians must remain empathic, flexible, and committed to working with families so that their role as educators and child advocates may be fulfilled. For example, if a family uses verbal reprimands as a major form of discipline, practitioners should explain how to be most effective. Although verbal reprimands may have some short-term benefit in interrupting or eliminating unwanted behaviors, when verbal reprimands are used during a time-out, they may interfere with the effectiveness of this form of discipline. Verbal reprimands become abusive when the reprimand assaults the character of the child—for example, "Don't wipe your hands on your shirt. You're so sloppy!" Parents can instead comment on the behavior itself—for example, "When you wipe your hands on your shirt, your shirt gets dirty. Please don't do that!"

Building on the therapeutic alliance fostered by primary care, pediatricians have an opportunity to guide and educate families through the challenges of parenting and enable them to be successful in their parental roles. Moreover, as future research in behavioral and social science yields insight into the underpinnings of family violence, child abuse, and violence in our society, the application of this knowledge may be applied to preventive interventions in the context of well child care and appropriate disciplining of children and youth.

HEALTH SUPERVISION OF CHILDREN WITH CHRONIC CONDITIONS (also see Chapter 37)

Several trends within recent decades have influenced the role of primary care pediatricians in the care of children with chronic conditions. Hospital use has decreased, with more care delivered at ambulatory sites. Scientific advances have increased the longevity of children with many chronic conditions; in 1988, 31% of all children were reported by the National Health Interview Survey to have a chronic condition. Changes in health care financing and managed care have placed pediatricians in roles of specialty coordinator, disease manager, and gatekeeper but also may have resulted in disincentives to providing appropriate services for children with chronic conditions.

Most chronic conditions are mild and do not significantly affect the life of a child. For these children, the model of providing health supervision as described in health supervision guidelines is appropriate. For children whose lives are significantly affected by severe chronic conditions, regular health supervision visits must include a special approach to manage the condition, coordinate care, communicate with specialists, and collaborate with family and community resources. The relationship of primary care pediatricians to families and their accessibility suggest that they might provide the majority of health care services to children with these chronic conditions and might work collaboratively with specialists co-managing children with complex conditions. Pediatricians should plan and discuss the frequency of visits needed for management of the condition, thereby avoiding confusion about who should provide certain health care services—the pediatrician or the specialist. Primary care services including health supervision, immunizations, minor illness, or trauma are usually a general pediatrician's domain. However, a joint decision should be made with parents and specialists about who should provide those medical services specific to the condition such as medication checks, interval evaluations, treatment of serious illness, or counseling services. By anticipating these decision points, discussing them with other members of the medical team, and communicating with families and patients, health supervision evolves into chronic condition management and provides patients with a *medical home*.

APPROACH TO PRACTICE. Integration of patients with chronic conditions into a busy clinic or office practice must be adapted to the particular setting and the specific patient. Pediatricians, well trained in the care of childhood *disease*, must also understand the impact of *illness* on patients and families in order to address the needs of these children. They should evaluate a family's ongoing needs for health information, community resources, and social, psychologic, and financial support. Combining chronic condition management and regular health care supervision requires time and commitment.

Several strategies may facilitate the management and improve efficiency in caring for children having a chronic illness within a primary care practice. Orientation of office or clinic staff to the processes of treating patients with chronic conditions is essential. To improve the flow of information and provide appropriate documentation for record keeping and reimbursement, it may be necessary to design special documentation sheets or new medical records systems. Key personnel should be trained and assigned to treat these patients and assist in authorizations, medical record information, and requests from specialists, insurance companies, schools, or agencies. Because visits are more frequent and often more prolonged, special attention should be given to the scheduling. Families need orientation to the procedures involved in providing care such as scheduling, phone calls, medical records, billing, and insurance practices. Pediatricians must also act as advocates for their patients and themselves to negotiate appropriate reimbursement and maintain financial viability in providing the extra care, time, and effort that these children require for counseling and care coordination.

DIRECTIONS FOR PREVENTIVE PEDIATRICS

It is likely that we will have new immunizations to prevent infections, improved screening tests to provide early diagnosis of disease, and enhanced therapeutic agents to manage chronic conditions so that their impact on the lives of children is minimized. The major causes of morbidity and mortality in children, however, will continue to be related to human behavior, our society, and the environment. The challenge for pediatricians in practicing preventive pediatrics is to adopt new practice strategies that address the health concerns of smoking, violence (including spousal as well as child abuse), injuries, drug and alcohol use, teen pregnancy, sexually transmitted diseases, heart-healthy diet, exercise, and sudden infant death syndrome (SIDS). Rather than drugs or immunizations, the effective interventions in these areas will be educational and behavioral, with pediatricians providing information and support. The success of the Back to Sleep Campaign that reduced the incidence of SIDS by promoting the supine sleep position is a powerful example of how an educational intervention can produce significant change in the health of the population.

Preventing nicotine addiction and the health consequences of active and passive smoking is another important area where pediatricians can influence the health of patients and families. Cigarette smoking is the most preventable cause of mortality and morbidity in the United States today. As part of health supervision visits, pediatricians should become active in all aspects of this public health problem. From the time of first meeting a family, especially at the birth of a baby, it is vital to obtain a smoking history and use this information to provide a quit-smoking message. This preventive strategy, directed at the individual family member who smokes, also benefits children who will be exposed to passive smoke. A relatively brief educational message that effectively communicates the relationship of active smoking to lung cancer, ischemic heart disease, and low birthweight can increase rates of smoking cessation. Furthermore, because 80% of people who smoke had their first cigarette before age 18 yr, pediatricians should incorporate smoking prevention as part of the content of health supervision visits.

Pediatricians must also stay abreast of new evidence, technology, and practice guidelines and should shorten the period from the discovery of new knowledge to its application in clinical practice. The continuing commitment to education should not be restricted to the medical literature. The more pediatricians know about their patients, their families, their culture, and their communities, the better able they will be to provide quality primary care, including prevention, to children and their families.

American Academy of Pediatrics: Sleep problems in children: Guidelines for parents. Elk Grove Village, IL, AAP Division of Publications, 1994.

American Academy of Pediatrics: Tobacco, alcohol, and other drugs: The role of the pediatrician in prevention and management of substance abuse. Pediatrics 101:125, 1998.

American Academy of Pediatrics' Committee on Psychosocial Aspects of Child and Family Health: Guidance for Effective Discipline. Pediatrics 101:723, 1998.

Brazelton TB: A child-oriented approach to toilet training. Pediatrics 12:68, 1962.

Cooley WC: Changing care in private practice: Management of chronic conditions in the primary care setting. *In:* Redfern DE (ed): Management of Chronic Illness and Disability in the Primary Care Setting. Report of the 26th Ross Roundtable. Columbus, OH, Ross Products Division, Abbott Laboratories, 1995.

Green M (ed): Bright Futures: Guidelines for Health Supervision of Infants, Children, and Adolescents. Arlington, VA, National Center for Education in Maternal and Child Health, 1994.

Gunnoe ML, Mariner CL: Toward a developmental-contextual model of the effects of parental spanking on children's aggression. Arch Pediatr Adolesc Med 151:768, 1997.

Kessler DA, Natamblut SL, Wilkenfeld JP, et al: Nicotine addiction: A pediatric disease. J Pediatr 103:518, 1997.

Lavin A, Rappo P, Vanchiere CM: CPT Coding and the Medical Home. Elk Grove Village, IL, AAP Division of Publications, 1997.

Moffatt MEK: Nocturnal enuresis: A review of the efficacy of treatments and practical advice for clinicians. J Dev Behav Pediatr 18:49, 1997.

Newacheck PW, Taylor WR: Childhood chronic illness: Prevalence, severity, and impact. Am J Public Health 82:364, 1992.

Schmidt BD: How to deal with temper tantrums. Contemp Pediatr 6:39, 1989.

Singalavanija S, Frieden IJ: Diaper dermatitis. Pediatr Rev 16:142, 1995.

Socolar RRS, Amaya-Jackson L, Eron LD, et al: Research on discipline: The state of the art, deficits, and implications. Arch Pediatr Adolesc Med 151:758, 1997.

Stein MT, Wolraich ML, Aceves J, et al: Guidelines for Health Supervision III. Elk Grove Village, IL, American Academy of Pediatrics, 1997.

Strauss MA, Sugarman DB, Giles-Sims J: Spanking by parents and subsequent antisocial behavior of children. Arch Pediatr Adolesc Med 151:761, 1997.

Taylor JA, Davis RL, Kemper KJ: A randomized controlled trial of group versus

individual well child care for high risk children: Maternal-child interaction and developmental outcomes. Pediatrics. http://www.pediatrics.org/cgi/content/full/99/6/e9.
Wall MA, Severson HH, Andrews JA, et al: Pediatric office-based smoking intervention: Impact on maternal smoking and relapse. Pediatrics 96:622, 1995.
Zenni EA, Robinson TN: Effects of structured encounter forms on pediatric house staff knowledge, parent satisfaction, and quality of care. Arch Pediatr Adolesc Med 150:975, 1996.

CHAPTER 6
The Well Child

Paul L. McCarthy

The most powerful diagnostic maneuver available to pediatricians is the clinical evaluation: the process of observing the child, taking a history, and performing the physical examination. For pediatricians to maximize the benefit of the clinical evaluation, some of the complexities of this process must be appreciated (also see Chapter 5).

UNIQUE CHARACTER OF THE PEDIATRIC CLINICAL EVALUATION. This evaluation involves the physician, the parent(s), and the child. Historical information is often taken from the parents, and it is not until children reach later developmental stages that they can more actively contribute information about symptoms. These considerations change the manner in which pediatricians gather data about symptoms. Rather than asking, for example, if the child has abdominal pain, physicians ask questions that focus on the manner in which abdominal pain would present to an observer. Thus, questions about loss of appetite, sudden episodes of crying and drawing the legs up in a fetal position, or the child's crying when the parent has placed pressure on the abdomen are appropriate. A 24-mo-old child with a sore throat often does not complain of this but rather is observed by the parents to have more difficulty handling oral secretions, to refuse solids, and to have a foul breath odor. Questions are tailored to elicit this information.

As children become older, they may begin to add historical information that expresses symptoms in unique ways. The information provided by a child at times suggests the diagnosis precisely, but at other times a child's information may reflect a less developed sense of cause-and-effect relationships and may be at variance with the data provided by the parents. Thus, a 4-yr-old child with a urinary tract infection may be observed by the parent to be holding his or her abdomen and to have a subtle change in the frequency of urination. The child, on the other hand, may perceive that his or her abdominal complaints are related to a specific food that was ingested just before the onset of symptoms. In this instance, the pediatrician may conclude that the parent's history suggests the correct diagnosis (a urinary tract infection) by eliciting further information about, for example, discomfort when urinating.

PARENTS AND CHILD AS PARTICIPANTS IN THE CLINICAL EVALUATION. It is often left to the judgment of parents whether clinical symptoms should be brought to the attention of a physician. Moreover, children's interpretation of symptoms is intimately related to their developmental stage; this also influences the manner in which they transmit clinical information to a physician. Both parents and children must believe that the pediatrician is interested in their concerns and that interactions with the pediatrician provide them support and enhance the acuity of their clinical perceptions. This process occurs at both well and sick child visits. At well child visits, the parent or child might describe a specific behavior or symptom. The pediatrician demonstrates concern by listening attentively and by asking follow-up questions demonstrating that the behavior or symptom has been understood. These follow-up questions provide an opportunity for the parent or child to explore his or her own interpretation of these behaviors or symptoms, to explore what emotional response they have had, and to learn from the interpretation provided by the physician. For example, parents reporting that their 9-mo-old child cries when being put to bed and has difficulty falling asleep offers an opportunity for the pediatrician to explore their interpretations of this behavior, to discuss their response to it, and to discuss the developmental dimensions of individuation. Based on this discussion and a more precise appreciation of the meaning of that behavior, strategies can evolve as an appropriate response to that behavior.

The same interaction and education process occur during sick child visits (see Chapter 56). Upper respiratory symptoms may concern parents. The pediatrician's discussing the predominance of nasal breathing in younger children, the more prominent symptoms that arise from nasal stuffiness because of this, and the absence of other evidence of serious pulmonary involvement, such as tachypnea, enhances parents' abilities to interpret respiratory symptoms during subsequent upper respiratory infections. Similarly, the pediatrician can explain cause-and-effect relationships between infection and symptoms to an older child. Such encounters, during both well and ill child visits, serve to enhance the confidence of parents and children in their role as participants in the clinical evaluation. Studies have demonstrated the ability of parents to evaluate clinical data reliably and the ability of children, when given developmentally appropriate information, to improve their understanding of clinical causality.

DEVELOPMENTAL DIMENSIONS. The data generated from observation, history (see earlier), and physical examination are greatly influenced by a child's developmental stage. A portion of the observational assessment of a child focuses on signs related to specific organ systems that are intimately related to age. A child of 1 mo has a more rapid respiratory rate (30 breaths/min) than a 3-yr-old child. An infant's respiratory rate is more sensitive to other influences, such as gastric pressure on the diaphragm caused by the recent ingestion of a meal, than that of an older child. Other portions of observational assessment focus on data that are indicators of a child's overall state of well-being or functional status, such as how the child responds visually to the environment. Pediatricians should not only be aware that visual responses undergo developmental change but should also be aware of the manner in which stimuli should be presented to elicit a child's optimal visual response at different developmental stages. A 1-mo-old infant, for example, is more nearsighted and tends to focus on objects held within 1–2 ft of the face; objects presented in the peripheral fields of vision may be ignored. A young infant's ability to maintain attention on a visual stimulus is less developed than that of an older child. Thus, pediatricians must be aware of the developmental dimensions of observing children in order to gather and interpret clinical information accurately.

The data generated during the physical examination are also closely linked to a child's stage of development. Specific findings may be normal in one age group and abnormal in another. For example, a 1-mo-old child normally has a rooting reflex, which facilitates suckling. On the other hand, a rooting reflex found in a 2-yr-old child indicates central nervous system abnormalities. Not only do specific findings differ in different age groups, but the manner in which physical examination findings are elicited varies from one developmental stage to another. An 8-mo-old child, for example, is beginning to develop a sense of individuality and is aware of strangers and frightened by separation. To elicit accurate physical examination data, the child should remain cooperative and not resist the examination, especially during auscultation of the chest and heart. Based on an appreciation of the developmental stage of an 8-mo-old, the examiner should allow the child to remain close to the parent and should approach as unobtrusively as possible. Factors that would lessen the strangeness of a situation, such as the warmth of the room, the stethoscope, and the examiner's voice, help facilitate data gathering. Older children are usually more comfortable with strangers and in separating from the parents; hence, after initial assurances, the physical examination may be done on the examination table.

A pediatric clinical evaluation is a complex interaction because of the manner in which information flows among the participants and because of the influence of developmental trends on gathering and interpreting the observation, history, and physical examination data.

GUIDELINES FOR EVALUATION. During the clinical encounter, it is often difficult to separate each component of the evaluation. As physicians are taking a history from a parent, they are observing the child and observing the interaction with the parent; as physicians perform a physical examination, they are evaluating the child's global responses to the specific maneuver being performed. Nevertheless, certain guidelines can be followed during each part of the evaluation.

Observation is best done with a younger child in a comfortable position, usually on the parent's lap. Upset and anxiety on the parent's part are easily transmitted to the child; thus, the parent and child must be placed at ease with a greeting and reassuring words. The tone of the examiner's voice is important and should convey a willingness to listen and a sensitivity to concerns being expressed. The manner in which an examiner is oriented to the parent and child is also important: If an examiner sits in one corner and regards only the notation page, a sense of unwillingness to communicate is conveyed. Sitting close to the parents and child and facing them directly are more effective. An examiner should observe the manner in which the parent and child are interacting: How are the parents responding to the child's needs, and in turn, how is the child responding to the parents? Pediatricians can modulate the stimuli in this situation to gather important information by observation. The child may initially be clinging to the parent, so the pediatrician should interact with the child, offer the child an object, or attempt some separation of the child and parent to observe the child's response.

A history is best taken with a child in a comfortable position. If the child is quiet and comfortable, the parent can focus better on specific questions. Physicians vary in their amount of note taking during the history. Some prefer to write the history directly to progress notes; others note only key words and, at the end of the examination, transfer the information to the medical record. Whichever technique is used, it is critical that physicians remain responsive to the information being presented. If highly sensitive information is being conveyed and the parent or child is responding emotionally, physicians must convey empathic understanding. This is impossible, however, if note taking continues without interruption. Additional note taking during this critical moment can interfere with important observations about the parent and child and their interaction.

The precision and clarity with which parents and children describe symptoms vary. Ongoing interaction with a family for a time enables pediatricians to learn how clinical information is perceived and transmitted within each family. If, for example, parents perceive their child as vulnerable, minor symptoms may be overemphasized; pediatricians can adjust the assessments accordingly.

The portions of the physical examination that require optimal cooperation are completed initially: the blood pressure measurement, pulmonary and cardiac examinations, and evaluations of the eyes and central nervous system. A younger child may be held by the parent or seated on the parent's lap for these parts of the examination. An older child can be seated on the examination table. The pattern and rate of respirations are evaluated initially. Is there tachypnea? Is there increased work of breathing, as manifested by subcostal, intercostal, and/or supraclavicular retractions? Is there an expiratory grunt indicating that the child is expiring against a closed glottis to keep the small airways open longer? What are the colors of the skin, nails, and mucous membranes? After these assessments have been made, the physician may proceed to palpation, percussion (if indicated), and auscultation. It is not uncommon for a younger child to cry as the stethoscope is placed on the chest, but this can usually be overcome by patience and by increasing the child's comfort, such as offering an infant a bottle. The same sequence may be followed for the cardiac examination. The ophthalmologic examination requires that the child be quietly wakeful; ophthalmoscopy can be done with the child in the parent's lap or as the child is being carried over the parent's shoulder. The other parent can sometimes provide visual stimuli; the retina can be seen more easily as the child focuses on such stimuli. Many portions of the neurologic examination, such as eliciting reflexes, also require cooperation and a state of quiet wakefulness. In an older child, this can be accomplished with the child on the examination table, but it is usually more helpful for a younger child to remain on the parent's lap.

After these portions of the examination, the examiner proceeds to the parts of the examination that are usually more bothersome to a child. Abdominal examination requires that a child be on the examination table. It is helpful to have the parent hold a younger patient's hand and speak reassuringly. Thus, the child does not tense the abdominal musculature unnecessarily, as might occur during crying. After the abdominal examination, the pulses may be palpated, the genitalia examined, and the hips and extremities evaluated for clinical abnormalities. It is at this time that the examiner proceeds to the most intrusive portions of the examination, evaluation of the ear canals and tympanic membranes and examination of the oropharynx. During the ear examination, the parent may hold the child's head to minimize movement against the otoscope. The examiner should recognize that the ear canals are highly sensitive, and the speculum should be introduced gently. The examiner's free hand can be used to put gentle traction on the pinna to straighten the canal. A portion of the hand holding the otoscope, usually the 5th finger, should rest against the head so that the otoscope moves with the head. At times, depending on the amount of cooperation, the ears may be examined with the child in the parent's lap and the head resting against the parent's shoulder. The oropharyngeal examination is performed last, and the tongue blade is introduced gently.

The sequence of performing those portions of the physical examination that require inspection, palpation, percussion, and auscultation (pulmonary, cardiac, and abdominal) varies according to organ system. The most bothersome maneuvers are performed last. For example, during the cardiac examination, inspection can be followed by palpation and percussion and then by auscultation. For the abdominal examination, inspection should be followed by auscultation before percussion and palpation are completed.

With appropriate sensitivity to the child and the parent, an appreciation of the child's developmental stage, and concern for minimizing the discomfort of an examination, pediatricians can almost always obtain accurate clinical information and not cause undue upset to a child.

WELL CHILD EVALUATION. The broad principles of clinical data gathering outlined earlier apply to the clinical evaluation during the well child examination. The recommended schedule of well child visits is outlined in Table 5–1. For children with chronic or intercurrent problems, this sequence may vary. Certain considerations should be addressed at each visit.

Open-Ended Questions. Physicians should ask general questions that allow a parent or child to voice concerns that might not be raised if questions were too specific. Open-ended questions such as "How are you?" or "How is the baby?" transmit an interest in the general well-being of the child and family, as do the behavioral clues that were outlined previously. When such open-ended questions are asked, it is important that physicians explore the leads provided by the parents or child; ending the interaction prematurely, without appropriate follow-up questions, is frustrating to the parents and child and sends a mixed message about the physician's interest and concern.

Development. Each well child visit should determine a child's developmental achievements, such as by the widely used Denver Developmental Screening Test. Questions in the gross motor, personal-social, language, and fine motor adaptive realms can be presented and responses scored. Previous scores serve as a reference point for future visits; the rate of change in specific dimensions, such as language, can be more easily appreciated. As a child matures beyond 5 and 6 yr of age, questions that focus on school performance and talented accomplishments can be substituted for the Denver test. Reviewing developmental milestones provides the parents with a sense of satisfaction in their child's progress and reinforces the efforts they are making to nurture and teach their children. Reviewing an older child's accomplishments is an important demonstration of support for these activities.

Feeding and Diet. Many changes occur in the dietary intake of those in the pediatric age group, and these should be reviewed with the parents and children. During the first 12 mo of life, for example, breast milk or infant formula is the major source of calories and nutrients. The introduction of infant cereals, strained then junior foods, and finally table foods; the change from formula to milk; and the use of vitamins and fluoride are issues of daily concern for parents. In older children, the intake of excessive salt, carbohydrates, or cholesterol can adversely affect health. If the rationale underlying the introduction of certain foods and dietary changes is discussed with parents and children, they can more easily take an active role in this process and feel comfortable with it.

Accident Prevention. At each well child care visit, accident prevention should be reviewed. Potential hazards around the home are emphasized, as well as the importance of car safety measures. Optimal infant sleep position, which is on the back, should be reviewed. Syrup of ipecac is provided at the 6-mo visit, and the phone number of the local poison control center should be given to the parents. For the parents and older children to participate more fully in this process, the developmental aspect of accident prevention should be emphasized. For example, a child's ability to crawl and to grasp and place objects in the mouth make the issue of poison prevention especially critical when these developmental milestones have been reached. The need for having ipecac in the house and for accident-proofing the home then becomes clearer.

Growth. At each well child visit, the height, weight, and head circumference are measured. These are plotted on standard graphs, such as those provided by the National Center for Health Statistics (see Chapter 15). It is important to review growth parameters with parents and children, because these are objective indicators of a child's progress. If abnormalities in the rate of growth are noted, the clinical evaluation can focus on possible causes. When interpreting these data, the pediatrician must focus on what is normal for this child, given the family background. Growth charts rely on normative data from populations with selected growth characteristics; thus, if both parents are slightly below the 3rd percentile for height, these normative data require appropriate interpretation to allay undue concern about this child's growth.

Family and Social Relations. To grow and develop normally, children rely on the support and nurturance provided by their family and the social environment (see Chapter 7). They are sensitive to disturbances in these supports, which can lead to nonoptimal growth, altered development, and adverse behavioral changes. Pediatricians should assess these supports by observation and questions. Observations can include the hygiene of the child and the child's general level of interest and response to people. How do the parents respond to the child's needs? What is the tone of parents' voices as they discuss the child? In what terms do the parents describe the child? If the child begins crying or is disruptive, how do the parents respond? Do the parents face the young child, or do they show lack of interest or concern? Does the child appear depressed or inappropriately anxious? Specific questions from the pediatrician may elucidate other stresses or strengths in the environment. Does the home environment, such as through inclusion of toys and books, nurture the child's developmental potential? Is there an extended network of friends and family that provides support to the children and parents? Is the family under significant stress, such as through illness or loss of a job? A pediatrician's willingness to gather information about these issues and to address them demonstrates a realistic attitude toward what constitutes health or dysfunction for a child and family.

A particular challenge to all who care for children is represented by the special needs of children who live in impoverished environments (see Chapter 39). Empathizing with the difficulties of raising children in these circumstances and recognizing the obstacles that such children often face in realizing their potential are major concerns of pediatric care. Demonstrating a willingness to assist parents and children in overcoming some of these adversities can provide them with a sense of hope and optimism about the future.

Anticipatory Guidance. Based on a developmental orientation, physicians should be aware of issues that might present problems or questions for parents or children between the current and next visits. For example, the rate of growth of a 24-mo-old lessens compared with that of previous months, and a diminished appetite results. Rather than have the parents be unnecessarily concerned about this, it is prudent to preview the child's rate of growth in the next 6 mo and to discuss its impact on food intake. The developmental achievements that the parents might expect in the next several months and the type of activities that facilitate these developments can also be discussed. For example, a 12-mo-old's ability to grasp and bring objects to the mouth makes finger foods an option for a child at this age. In addition, this ability points out the need to remove small objects (e.g., peanuts) from the environment to minimize choking and aspiration hazards. The anticipatory guidance that is provided should also review issues in daily caretaking, such as hygiene and sleep patterns. Again, every effort should be made to integrate these caretaking issues into a wider developmental perspective. See Chapter 5.

Other Concerns. At the initial well child visit, data about the family medical history and the prenatal and perinatal history should be entered into the medical record. At each well child visit, physicians should record and provide a record of immunizations to parents. Notes should be made about any intercurrent illness, such as otitis media or bronchiolitis. At each well child visit, a review of systems is carried out to ascertain whether there have been any symptoms related to specific organ systems, such as the gastrointestinal or neurologic. Finally, a flow sheet of laboratory screening tests, such as hemoglobin level, should be updated.

After the aforementioned considerations have been addressed and the physical examination completed, pediatricians should summarize the child's health status. The parents should be complimented on their strengths as caregivers and children complimented about their achievements and progress. It is also important to recognize problems and to express willingness to work on these together with the family. The pediatrician's availability, if problems arise before the next visit, should be stressed. In this way, the parents and child are reassured about the pediatrician's involvement in ongoing care. Parents and children should again be given an opportunity to ask questions or raise concerns about any aspect of the well child visit.

Committee on Psychosocial Aspects of Child and Family Health. Guidelines for Health Supervision III. Elk Grove Village, IL, American Academy of Pediatrics, 1997.

Green M: Pediatric psychosocial diagnostic interview. *In:* Green M: Pediatric Diagnosis. Philadelphia, WB Saunders, 1998, pp 471–482.

McCarthy PL: Demographic, clinical and psychosocial predictors of the reliability of mothers' clinical judgements. Pediatrics 88:1041, 1991.

PART II

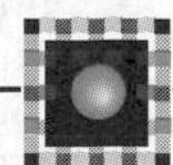

Growth and Development

Robert D. Needlman

CHAPTER 7
Overview and Assessment of Variability

Pediatricians need to understand growth and development in three ways. An understanding of the normative patterns of physical growth and the emergence of motor, cognitive, and emotional competence allows pediatricians to monitor children's progress and to identify delay or deviance. Understanding how biologic and environmental forces interact to shape development allows pediatricians to target factors that increase or decrease risk. Understanding how parents conceptualize development facilitates anticipatory guidance and remedial intervention. The beliefs of parents, like the theoretical models of Freud, Piaget, and Skinner, include implicit or explicit ideas about the nature of children, the characteristics of successful adults, and the processes that control the transformation from one to the other.

By monitoring children and families over time, pediatricians can observe how the processes of growth and development are interrelated: the enlargement of head, trunk, and limbs; the progressive increases in strength and ability to control large and small muscles; the development of social relatedness, thought, and language; and the emergence of personality. At the same time, observation is enhanced by familiarity with developmental theory.

BIOPSYCHOSOCIAL MODELS OF DEVELOPMENT

The debate between nature and nurture is age old. In the nature model, the forces that determine development reside within the child; biology is destiny. In the nurture model, development is determined by forces outside of the individual; the child is infinitely mutable, a blank slate. Biopsychosocial models, now widely accepted, recognize the importance of both intrinsic and extrinsic forces. Height, for example, is a function of a child's genetic endowment (biologic), personal habits of eating (psychologic), and access to nutritious food (social).

Research demonstrating the profound impact of early experience on the development of the brain has further blurred the nature-vs-nurture distinction. The brain comprises 100 billion neurons at birth, developing on average 15,000 synapses per neuron by age 3. Synaptic number under normal circumstances stays roughly constant through the first decade of life, then declines through adolescence. Synaptic pruning, a parallel process, proceeds on a use-it-or-lose-it basis, such that pathways that are frequently used are preserved and those that are less used are not. Thus, early experience has a direct effect on the physical properties of the brain, facilitating or impeding future learning. Early stressful experiences may also have long-standing effects on neurotransmitter and endocrine systems, possibly increasing the risk of mental illness later in life. Biologic, psychologic, and social influences on development are the focus, respectively, of the major theoretical perspectives described next.

BIOLOGIC INFLUENCES. Biologic influences on development include genetics, in utero exposure to teratogens, postpartum illnesses, exposure to hazardous substances, and maturation. Twin studies have established that approximately half of the variance in IQ scores and in various personality characteristics can be accounted for by genetic endowment. The effects on development of prenatal exposure to teratogens such as mercury and alcohol, and of postpartum insults such as meningitis, have been extensively studied. Chronic illness affects growth and development; a particular illness may have specific developmental correlates.

Physical and neurologic maturation propels a child forward and sets lower limits for the emergence of most abilities. The age at which children walk independently is similar around the world, despite great variability in child-rearing practices. Other attainments (e.g., the accomplishment of toilet training or use of two-word sentences) are less tightly bound to a maturational schedule. Maturational changes also create the potential for behavioral problems at predictable times. For example, decrements in growth rate and sleep requirements around 2 yr of age often generate concerns about poor appetite and refusal to nap.

In addition to physical changes in size, body proportions, and strength, maturation is associated with hormonal influences. Sexual differentiation, both somatic and neurologic, begins in utero. Behavioral effects of testosterone may be evident even in young children and continue to be salient throughout life, such as in the association between male gender and aggression.

A biologic influence of particular clinical importance is temperament. Temperament refers to a child's characteristic style of responding. Nine parameters of temperament are proposed (Table 7–1). Temperament, in this model, is intrinsic to a child and relatively resistant to modification by parenting practices. Most temperamental characteristics show only modest stability over time. Active, intense 2-yr-olds, for example, do not necessarily grow into active, intense 22-yr-olds.

Clinically, the concept of temperament is useful in two ways. First, it can help parents understand and accept the characteristics of their children without feeling responsible for having caused them. Second, behavioral and emotional problems tend to occur when the temperamental characteristics of children and parents conflict. Active children may be especially problematic for low-key parents; outgoing parents may pressure a child who is "slow to warm up" and create unnecessary upset; parents who lead highly structured lives may fare poorly with children whose biologic needs occur on a less regular schedule. "Goodness of fit" between the child and parents may be a powerful predictor of outcome.

PSYCHOLOGIC INFLUENCES: ATTACHMENT AND CONTINGENCY. Despite

TABLE 7–1 Temperamental Characteristics: Descriptions and Examples

Characteristic	Description	Example*
Activity level	Amount of gross motor movement	"She ran before she walked." "He would rather sit still than run around."
Rhythmicity	Regularity of biologic cycles	"He is never hungry at the same time each day." "You could set a watch by her nap."
Approach and withdrawal	Typical response to a new stimulus	"She rejects every new food at first." "He loves new people."
Adaptability	How long it takes to adapt to novel stimulus	"Changes upset him." "She adjusts to new people quickly."
Threshold of responsiveness	How intense do stimuli need to be to evoke a response (e.g., feel, sound, light)	"Underwear and socks bother him; he does not like anything touching his skin." "She will eat anything, wear anything, do anything."
Intensity of reaction	How much energy a child expends in emotions and actions	"She shouts when she is happy and wails when she is sad." "He never cries much."
Quality of mood	Usual disposition (e.g., pleasant, glum)	"He does not laugh much." "It seems like she is always happy."
Distractibility	How easily diverted from ongoing activity	"Her mind is always wandering." "He will listen through a whole story."
Attention span and persistence	How long a child pays attention and sticks with difficult tasks	"He goes from toy to toy every minute." "She will keep at a puzzle until she has mastered it."

**Typical statements of parents, reflecting the range for each characteristic from very little to very much.*

the recognized importance of inborn traits, the influence of the child-rearing environment dominates most current models of development. Erik Erikson identified the 1st yr of life as a time when "basic trust" was established, based on a mother's consistent responsiveness to her child's needs. Studies of infants in hospitals and foundling homes documented the devastating effects of maternal deprivation and pointed to the importance of attachment. Attachment refers to a biologically determined tendency of a young child to seek proximity with the parent during times of stress. Children who are securely attached are able to use their parents to re-establish a sense of well-being after a stressful experience, such as a physical examination or immunization. Insecure attachment may signal dysfunction in the parent-child relationship and may be predictive of later behavioral and learning problems.

At all stages of development and across multiple developmental lines, progress is fostered by adult caregivers who observe the child's verbal and nonverbal cues and respond accordingly. In early infancy, such contingent responses of caregivers to signs of overarousal or underarousal help maintain infants in a state of quiet alertness and may foster autonomic self-regulation. Contingent responses to nonverbal gestures create the groundwork for the shared attention and reciprocity critical for later language and social development. At all stages, learning is fostered when new challenges are made contingent on a child's current level of competence, being just slightly harder than what has already been mastered. Such optimal tasks fall within the "zone of proximal development."

SOCIAL FACTORS: FAMILY SYSTEMS AND THE ECOLOGIC MODEL. Contemporary models of child development recognize the critical importance of influences outside of the mother-child dyad. These influences may be conceived of as contributing to a higher or lower level of stress, which then influences the mother-child relationship. An abusive spousal relationship may exacerbate maternal depression, thus impairing the mother's ability to respond appropriately to her child.

Families function as systems, with more or less rigidly defined boundaries, subsystems, roles, and rules for interaction. The impact of these forces on development is often subtle but powerful. In families with rigidly defined parental subsystems, children may be denied any decision-making at all, exacerbating rebelliousness. If the parent-child boundary is overly porous, children may be "parentified," required to take on responsibilities beyond their years or recruited to play a spousal role.

Individuals within systems adopt implicit roles. One child is the "troublemaker," another is the "negotiator," another is "quiet." Changes in an individual's behavior affect every other member of the system; roles change until a new equilibrium is found. After a divorce, an older boy may take on a more parentified role and become the "man of the family," whereas a younger child may take over the role of an irresponsible rebel. The birth of a new child, attainment of developmental milestones such as independent walking, the onset of nighttime fears, and the death of a grandparent all are changes that require renegotiation of roles within the family and have the potential for healthy adaptation or dysfunction.

The family system, in turn, functions within the larger systems of extended family, subculture, culture, and society (see Chapters 3 and 4). The ecologic model depicts these relationships as concentric circles, with the parent-child dyad at the center and the larger society at the periphery. Changes at any level are reflected in the levels above and below. The repeal of Federal Aid to Families with Dependent Children (AFDC, welfare) in favor of time-limited support and workfare is an obvious example of societal change with profound effects on families and children living in poverty.

UNIFYING CONCEPTS: THE TRANSACTIONAL MODEL, RISK, AND RESILIENCE. Current thought has focused on understanding how biology and social interactions influence development. The transactional model proposes that a child's status at any point in time is a function of both biologic and social influences. The influences are bidirectional: Biologic factors such as temperament and health status both affect the child-rearing environment and are affected by it (Fig. 7–1). For example, a premature infant may cry little and sleep for long periods; the infant's depressed parent may welcome this "good" behavior, setting up a cycle that leads to poor nutrition and slow growth. A child's failure to thrive may reinforce the parent's sense of failure as a parent. At a later stage, impulsivity and inattention associated with chronic undernutrition may interact with the parent's depression, leading to a referral for aggressive behav-

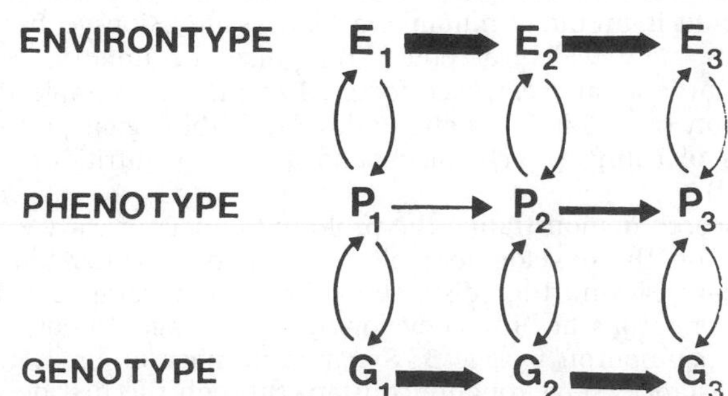

Figure 7–1 Transactional developmental model integrating environmental, genetic, and individual regulating systems. (From Sameroff AJ: *In:* Zeanah C [ed]: Handbook of Infant Mental Health. New York, Guilford Press, 1993, pp 29–41.)

ior. The "cause" of the aggression is not the prematurity, the undernutrition, or the maternal depression but the interaction of all these factors.

Conversely, children with biologic risk factors may nevertheless do well developmentally if the child-rearing environment is supportive. For example, premature infants with electroencephalographic evidence of neurologic immaturity may be at increased risk of cognitive delay. However, this relationship may hold only when the quality of parent-child interaction is poor. When parent-child interactions are optimal, even moderate prematurity carries little risk of developmental disability.

One implication of this model is that developmental assessment at any single point in time has limited ability to predict later outcome because at every stage the developmental trajectory is affected by both past and present conditions. To the extent that certain measures, such as IQ, tend to remain stable over time, this stability may well reflect the continuity of environmental conditions as much as it does the continuity of factors intrinsic to the child. The optimistic interpretation is that change is possible. Such an interpretation conflicts with popular tendencies to see certain early conditions, such as prenatal drug exposure, as "marking" children for life. Children growing up in poverty may be at double jeopardy because they face increased biologic risk factors such as lead poisoning, prematurity, and undernutrition as well as increased social risk factors such as overcrowding, lower maternal education, and exposure to violence (see Chapter 34).

The relative importance of environmental factors can be illustrated by a longitudinal study in which developmental outcome at age 13 yr was directly related to the number of social and family risk factors (Fig. 7–2). As the number of risk factors increases, the percentage of children who developmentally thrive decreases but never reaches zero. Protective factors may make some children resilient though not invulnerable. These factors, like risk factors, may be either biologic (temperamental persistence, athletic talent) or social. The personal histories of children who succeeded despite great risks generally include at least one trusted adult—often a parent, grandparent, or teacher—with whom the child had a close relationship. The clinical assessment should include an enumeration not only of risk factors but of protective strengths as well.

DEVELOPMENTAL DOMAINS AND THEORIES OF EMOTION AND COGNITION. Another approach to child development tracks development within particular domains such as gross motor, fine motor, social, emotional, language, and cognition. Within each of these categories are developmental lines or sequences of changes leading up to particular attainments. One such line, leading from rolling to creeping to independent walking, is widely accepted. Others, such as the line leading to the development of conscience, are less recognized and more controversial.

The concept of a developmental line implies that a child passes though successive stages. The psychoanalytic theories of Sigmund Freud and Erik Erikson and the cognitive theory of Jean Piaget share the idea of stages as qualitatively different epochs in the development of emotion and cognition (Table 7–2). In contrast, the behavioral theory of Skinner relies less on qualitative change and more on gradual modification of behavior or accumulation of knowledge.

Psychoanalytic Theories. At the core of *freudian theory* is the idea of biologically determined drives. The core drive is sexual, broadly defined to include sensations that involve excitation or tension and satisfaction or release. The focus of the sexual drive shifts with maturation, defining discrete stages: oral (1st yr of life), anal (toddlerhood), oedipal (preschool), and genital (puberty and beyond) (see Table 7–2). At each stage, the drive comes into conflict with the social demands of civilization. The emotional health of the child and adult depends on adequate resolution of these conflicts. The phase of latency, corresponding to middle childhood, is relatively free of psychosexual conflict, as the sexual drive is redirected (sublimated) to the achievement of social or external goals.

Controversy remains about many points. Latency may not be as conflict free as once supposed. The nature of aggression is unclear: Is it a primary drive or the result of frustration or feared loss? The consequences of unresolved early conflicts may or may not be lifelong, and progress may or may not require their "working through." Nonetheless, the freudian legacy includes several concepts that are central to an understanding of emotional development: the importance of a child's inner life and sexuality, the normative existence of emotional conflict during childhood, and the possibility of emotional disturbance.

Erikson's chief contribution was to recast Freud's stages in terms of the emerging personality (see Table 7–2). The crisis that establishes a child's internal sense of either autonomy or shame and guilt corresponds with Freud's anal stage; the crisis that establishes a sense of either identity or role diffusion corresponds with Freud's genital stage (puberty). The stages mark the emergence of different issues as salient, although earlier issues remain important. Erikson recognized that these stages arise in the context of Western European societal expectations; in other cultures, the salient issues may be quite different.

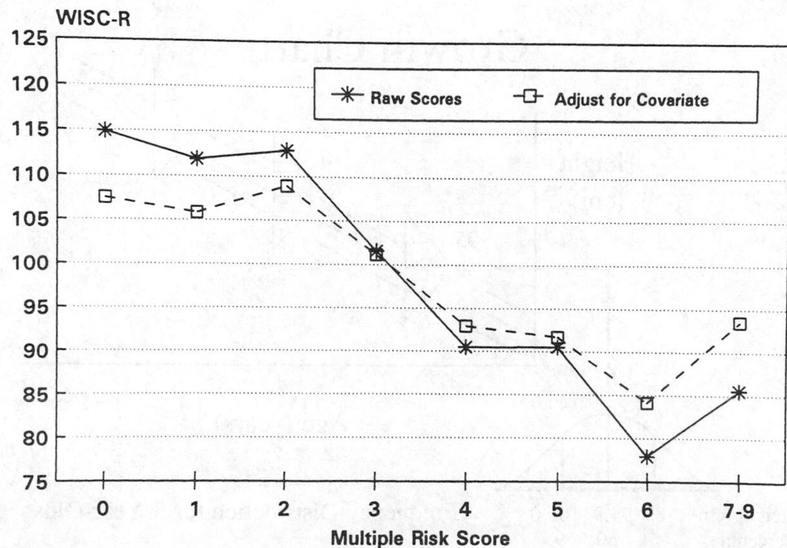

Figure 7–2 Relationship between mean IQ scores at 13 yr (both raw and adjusted for covariation of mother's IQ), as related to the number of risk factors. (From Sameroff AJ, Seifer R, Baldwin A, Baldwin C: Stability of intelligence from preschool to adolescence: The influence of social and family risk factors. Child Dev 64:80, 1993.)

TABLE 7–2 Classic Stage Theories

Theory	Infancy (0–1 yr)	Toddlerhood (2–3 yr)	Preschool (3–6 yr)	School Age (6–12 yr)	Adolescence (12–20 yr)
Freud: psychosexual	Oral	Anal	Oedipal	Latency	Adolescence
Erikson: psychosocial	Basic trust	Autonomy vs shame and doubt	Initiative vs guilt	Industry vs inferiority	Identity vs identity diffusion
Piaget: cognitive	Sensorimotor (stages I–IV)	Sensorimotor (stages V, VI)	Preoperational	Concrete operations	Formal operations

One lasting contribution of Erikson's work is to call attention to the intrapersonal challenges facing children at different ages in a way that facilitates professional intervention. For example, knowing that the salient issue for school-aged children is industry vs inferiority, pediatricians can inquire about a child's experiences of mastery and failure and suggest ways to ensure adequate successes.

Piaget is synonymous with the study of cognitive development. A central tenet of piagetian thought is that cognition is qualitatively different at different stages of development (see Table 7–2). During the sensorimotor stage, thoughts about the nature of objects and their relationships are tied to immediate sensations and a child's ability to manipulate objects. For example, the concept of "in" may be embodied in a child's act of putting a block into a cup. With the arrival of language, the nature of thinking changes dramatically; symbols increasingly take the place of things and actions. Cognitive stages correspond to the major periods of childhood: preoperational (preschool) concrete operations (school age) formal operations (adolescence). Children are not passive recipients of knowledge. Rather, at every stage they actively seek out experiences (assimilation) and use them to build implicit theories about the world. Children periodically reorganize these theories to fit the incoming data better (accommodation). The stages of cognitive reorganization can be mapped by observing children and by asking open-ended questions that make the implicit theories explicit.

Challenges to Piaget have included questions about the timing of various stages, the role of formal teaching, and the extent to which context may affect conclusions about cognitive stage. For example, children's understanding of cause and effect may be considerably more advanced in the context of sibling relationships than in the context of inanimate objects (e.g. various machines); in many children, formal operations appear well before puberty, the age postulated by Piaget. Of undeniable importance are Piaget's focus on cognition as a subject of empirical study, the universality of the progression of cognitive stages (even if details of timing are controversial), and the image of a child as actively and creatively interpreting the world.

Piaget's work is of special importance to pediatricians for three reasons: (1) It helps make sense of many common behaviors of infancy, such as the common exacerbations of sleep problems at 9 and 18 mo of age; (2) piagetian observations often lend themselves to quick replication in the office, with little special equipment; and (3) open-ended questioning, based on Piaget's work, can provide insights into children's understanding of illness and hospitalization.

Behavioral Theory. This major theoretical perspective distinguishes itself by its lack of concern with a child's inner experience. Its sole focus is on observable behaviors and measurable factors that either increase or decrease the frequency with which these behaviors occur. No stages are implied: Children, adults, and indeed animals all respond the same. In its simplest form, the behaviorist orientation asserts that behaviors that are positively reinforced occur more frequently; behaviors that are negatively reinforced or ignored occur less frequently.

The strengths of this position are its simplicity, wide applicability, and conduciveness to scientific verification. A behavioral approach lends itself to readily taught interventions for various common problems such as temper tantrums and nocturnal enuresis. In cognitively limited children, programs designed to reward wanted behaviors and punish or ignore unwanted ones may constitute the therapy of choice. However, in cases in which misbehavior is symptomatic of an underlying emotional, perceptual, or family problem, an exclusive reliance on behavior therapy risks leaving the cause untreated.

STATISTICS USED IN DESCRIBING GROWTH AND DEVELOPMENT (see also Chapters 15 and 16). "Normal" has two potential meanings: that a person or process is healthy or that a measured value falls within the normal range. Anthropometric quantities such as height and weight are normally distributed within a population. Thus, a histogram with the quantity (e.g., height) on the *x*-axis and the frequency (the number of children

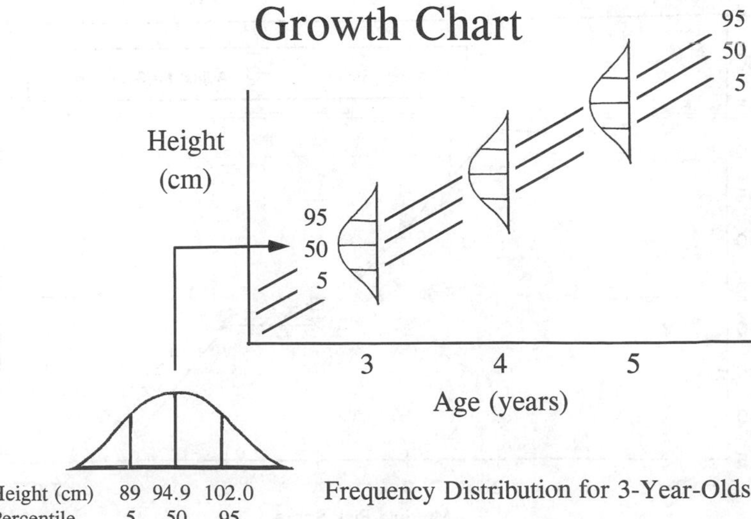

Figure 7–3 Relationship between percentile lines on the growth curve and frequency distributions of height at different ages.

TABLE 7–3 Relationship Between SD and Normal Range for Normally Distributed Quantities

Observations Included in Normal Range		Probability of a "Normal" Measurement Deviating from Mean by This Amount	
SD	*%*	*SD*	*%*
±1	68.3	≥1	16.0
±2	95.4	≥2	2.3
±3	99.7	≥3	0.13

of that height) on the *y*-axis generates a normal (gaussian) distribution, the classic bell-shaped curve. In an ideal bell-shaped curve, the peak of the curve corresponds to the arithmetical mean of the sample, which in turn equals both the median and the mode. The median is the value above and below which 50% of the observations lie; the mode is the value with the highest number of observations. Distributions in which the mean, median, and mode are not equal are termed skewed.

The extent to which observed values cluster near the mean determines the width of the bell and can be described mathematically by the standard deviation (SD). The SD is tied to the concept of the normal range. For quantities that are normally distributed, a range of values extending from 1 SD below the mean to 1 SD above the mean includes approximately 68% of the values; a range encompassing ±2 SD includes 95% of the values, and ±3 SD encompasses 99.7% of the values. For any single measurement, the degree of deviation from the mean, expressed in terms of number of SDs, gives the probability that the individual being measured is truly a member of the same population for which the mean was calculated (Table 7–3). For example, if the population measured is healthy boys and an individual boy's height falls more than 2 SD above the mean, then the probability that this boy belongs to the population of healthy boys is less than 2.3%. He may belong, instead, to the population of "boys with precocious puberty."

Another way of relating an individual to a group uses percentiles. The percentile is the percentage of individuals in the group who have achieved a certain measured quantity (a height of 95 cm) or developmental milestone. For anthropometric data, the percentile cutoffs can be calculated from the mean and SD. The 5th, 10th, and 25th percentiles correspond to −1.65 SD, −1.3 SD, and −0.7 SD, respectively. Figure 7–3 shows how frequency distributions of a particular parameter (height) at different ages translate into percentile lines on the growth curve.

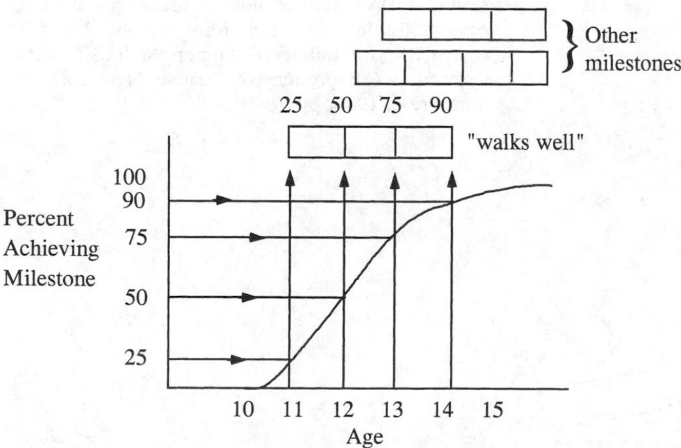

Figure 7–4 Method of presenting percentiles for developmental milestones.

For developmental milestones, the percentiles are often displayed in boxes, derived from graphs plotting age (*x*-axis) against the percentage of subjects achieving the particular milestone (*y*-axis), as shown in Figure 7–4.

Beckwith L, Parmelee A: EEG patterns of preterm infants, home environment, and later IQ. Child Dev 57:777, 1986.
Bronfenbrenner U: The Ecology of Human Development: Experiments by Nature and Design. Cambridge, MA, Harvard University Press, 1979.
Chess S, Thomas A: Temperament in Clinical Practice. New York, Guilford Press, 1986.
Erikson EH: Childhood and Society, 2nd ed. New York, WW Norton & Co, 1963.
Hobson PR: Piaget: On the ways of knowing in childhood. *In:* Rutter M, Hersov L (eds): Child and Adolescent Psychiatry: Modern Approaches. Oxford, England, Blackwell Scientific Publications, 1985, pp 191–203.
Parker S, Greer S, Zuckerman B: Double jeopardy: The impact of poverty on early child development. Pediatr Clin North Am 35:1227, 1988.
Shore R: Rethinking the Brain: New Insights into Early Development. New York, Families and Work Institute, 1997.
Vygotsky LS: Mind in Society: The Development of Higher Psychological Processes. Cambridge, MA, Harvard University Press, 1978.

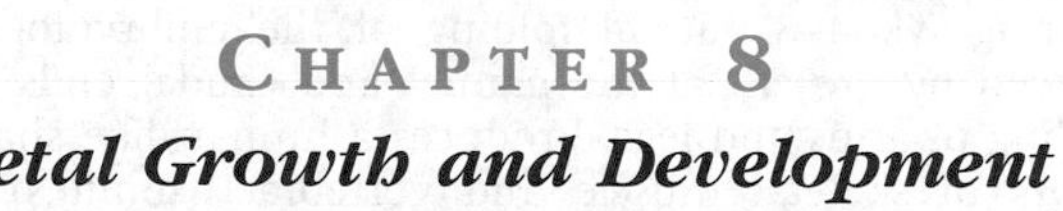

CHAPTER 8
Fetal Growth and Development

The most dramatic events in growth and development occur before birth. These changes are overwhelmingly somatic: the transformation of a single cell into an infant. Behavioral and psychologic developments in the fetus and the parents are also significant. The uterus, although offering a degree of protection, is permeable to social, psychologic, and environmental influences such as maternal drug use. The complex interplay between these forces and the physical transformations occurring in utero shapes infants, as they appear at birth and throughout infancy, and parents.

SOMATIC DEVELOPMENT

Embryonic Period. Milestones of prenatal development are presented in Table 8–1. By 6 days postconceptual age, as implantation begins, the embryo consists of a spherical mass of cells with a central cavity (the blastocyst). By 2 wk, implantation is complete and the uteroplacental circulation has begun; the

TABLE 8–1 Milestones of Prenatal Development

Week	Developmental Events
1	Fertilization and implantation; beginning of embryonic period
2	Endoderm and ectoderm appear (bilaminar embryo)
3	First missed menstrual period; mesoderm appears (trilaminar embryo); somites begin to form
4	Neural folds fuse; folding of embryo into human-like shape; arm and leg buds appear; crown-rump length 4–5 mm
5	Lens placodes, primitive mouth, digital rays on hands
6	Primitive nose, philtrum, primary palate; crown-rump length 21–23 mm
7	Eyelids begin
8	Ovaries and testes distinguishable
9	*Fetal* period begins; crown-rump length 5 cm; weight 8 g
10	External genitals distinguishable
20	Usual lower limit of viability; weight 460 g; length 19 cm
25	Third trimester begins; weight 900 g; length 25 cm
28	Eyes open; fetus turns head down; weight 1,300 g
38	Term

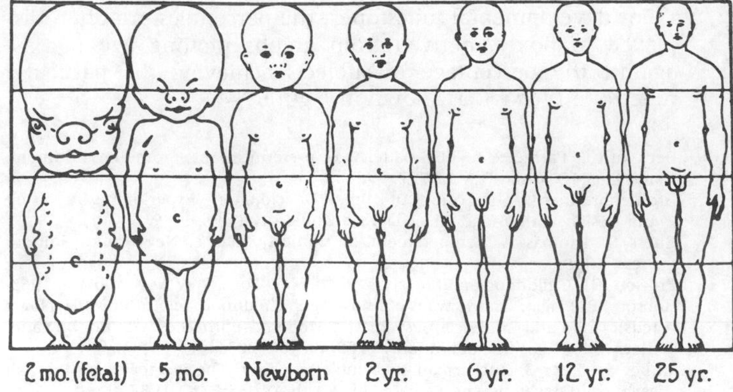

Figure 8–1 Changes in body proportions from the 2nd fetal mo to adulthood. (From Robbins WJ, Brody S, Hogan AG, et al: Growth. New Haven, Yale University Press, 1928.)

embryo has two distinct layers, endoderm and ectoderm, and the amnion has begun to form. By 3 wk, the third primary germ layer (mesoderm) has appeared, along with primitive neural tube and blood vessels. Paired heart tubes have begun to pump.

During wk 4–8, lateral folding of the embryologic plate, followed by growth at the cranial and caudal ends and the budding of arms and legs, produces a human-like shape. Precursors of skeletal muscle and vertebrae (somites) appear, along with the branchial arches that will form the mandible, maxilla, palate, external ear, and other head and neck structures. Lens placodes appear, marking the site of future eyes; the brain grows rapidly. By the end of wk 8, as the embryonic period closes, the rudiments of all major organ systems have developed; the average embryo weighs 9 g and has a crown-rump length of 5 cm.

Fetal Period. From the 9th wk on (the fetal period), fetal somatic changes consist of increases in cell number and size and structural remodeling of several organ systems. Changes in body proportion are depicted in Figure 8–1. By 10 wk, the face is recognizably human. The midgut returns from the umbilical cord into the abdomen, rotating counterclockwise to bring the stomach, small intestine, and large intestine into their normal positions. By 12 wk, the gender of the external genitals becomes clearly distinguishable. Lung development proceeds with the budding of bronchi, bronchioles, and successively smaller divisions. By 20–24 wk, primitive alveoli have formed and surfactant production has begun; before that time, the absence of alveoli renders the lungs useless as organs of gas exchange.

During the 3rd trimester, weight triples and length doubles as body stores of protein, fat, iron, and calcium increase (see Chapter 92). Low birthweight may be due to prematurity, intrauterine growth retardation (small for dates), or both (see Chapter 93).

NEUROLOGIC DEVELOPMENT. During the 3rd wk, a neural plate appears on the ectodermal surface of the trilaminar embryo. Infolding produces a neural tube that will become the central nervous system (CNS) and a neural crest that will become the peripheral nervous system. Neuroectodermal cells differentiate into neurons, astrocytes, oligodendrocytes, and ependymal cells, whereas microglial cells are derived from mesoderm. By the 5th wk, the three main subdivisions of forebrain, midbrain, and hindbrain are evident. The dorsal and ventral horns of the spinal cord have begun to form, along with the peripheral motor and sensory nerves. Myelinization begins at midgestation and continues throughout the 1st 2 yr of life.

By the end of the embryonic period (wk 8), the gross structure of the nervous system has been established. On a cellular level, the growth of axons and dendrites and the elaboration of synaptic connections continue at a rapid pace, making the CNS vulnerable to teratogenic or hypoxic influences throughout gestation. Rates of increase in DNA (a marker of cell number), overall brain weight, and cholesterol (a marker of myelinization) are shown in Figure 8–2. The prenatal and postnatal peaks of DNA probably represent rapid growth of neurons and glia, respectively.

BEHAVIORAL DEVELOPMENT. Muscle contractions first appear around 8 wk, soon followed by lateral flexion movements. By 13–14 wk, breathing and swallowing motions appear and tac-

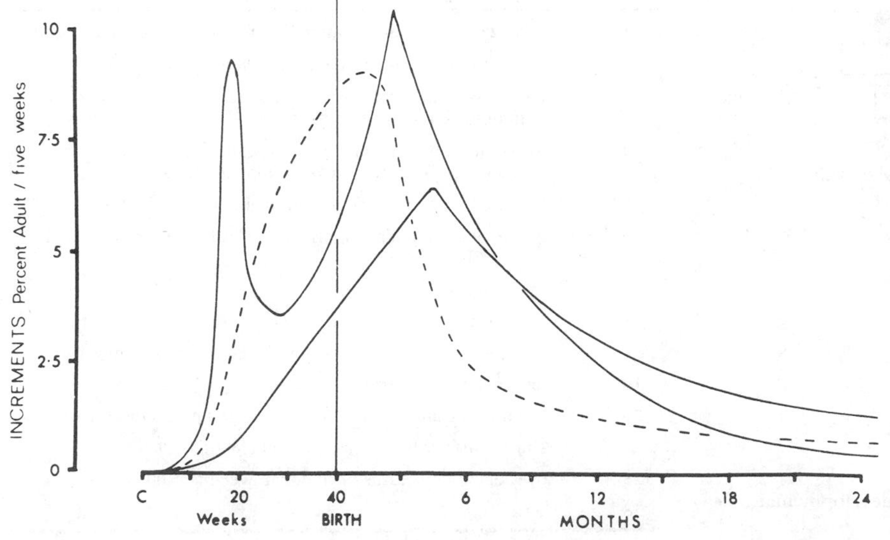

Figure 8–2 Velocity curves of the various components of human brain growth. Solid line with two peaks = DNA; dashed line = brain weight; single peak solid line = cholesterol. (From Brasel JA, Gruen RK. *In:* Falkner F, Tanner JM [eds]: Human Growth: A Comprehensive Treatise. New York, Plenum Press, 1986, pp 78–95.)

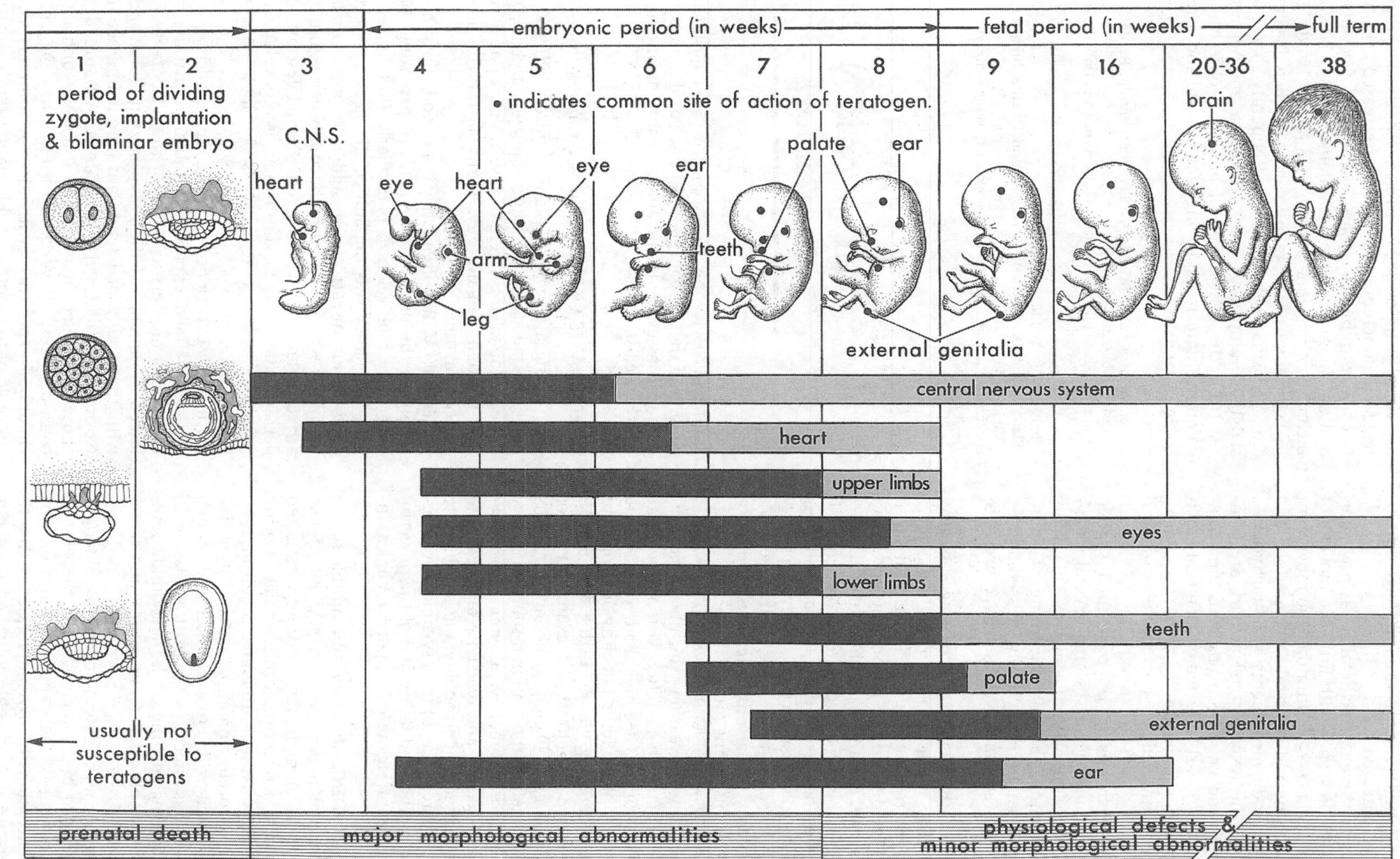

Figure 8–3 Schematic illustration of the sensitive or critical periods in prenatal development. Dark boxes denote highly sensitive periods; light boxes indicate states that are less sensitive to teratogens. (From Moore KL: Before We Are Born: Basic Embryology and Birth Defects, 2nd ed. Philadelphia, WB Saunders, 1977.)

tile stimulation elicits graceful movements. The grasp reflex appears at 17 wk and is well developed by 27 wk. Eye opening occurs around 26 wk. By midgestation, the full range of neonatal movements can be observed.

During the 3rd trimester, three distinct fetal behavioral states have been described: (1) quiescence with little eye movement and little heart rate variability, (2) continuous eye movement with bursts of somatic activity and heart rate accelerations, and (3) continuous eye and body movements with tachycardia. Individual differences in the level of fetal activity are commonly noted by mothers and have been observed ultrasonographically. Fetal behavior is clearly affected by maternal medications and diet, increasing, for example, after ingestion of caffeine, and may be entrained to the mother's diurnal rhythms.

Fetal movement also increases in response to a sudden sound with a specific tone and decreases after several repetitions; a different tone elicits the original response. This ability to habituate to repeated stimuli, a form of learning, is diminished in neurologically impaired or physically stressed fetuses. Similar responses to visual and tactile stimuli have been observed.

PSYCHOLOGIC CHANGES IN THE PARENTS. Three stages of psychologic development may occur in a woman during pregnancy. Stage 1 begins when a woman first learns that she is pregnant. Ambivalent feelings are the norm, whether or not the pregnancy was planned. Elation at the thought of producing a baby and the wish to be the perfect parent compete with fears of inadequacy and of the lifestyle changes that mothering will impose. Old conflicts may resurface as a woman psychologically identifies with her own mother and with herself as a child. The father-to-be faces similar mixed feelings, and problems in the parental relationship may intensify.

Stage 2 begins with awareness of fetal movements, or quickening, at approximately 20 wk or earlier with ultrasonic visualization. This palpable evidence that a fetus exists as a separate being often heightens a woman's feelings, both positive and negative. Parents worry about the fetus's healthy development and mentally rehearse what they will do if the child is malformed. Reassurances based on ultrasound examinations or amniocentesis may not be entirely helpful because the fears arise as much from irrational as from rational sources. During stage 3, toward the end of pregnancy, a woman becomes aware of patterns of fetal activity and reactivity and begins to ascribe to her fetus an individual personality and an ability to survive independently. Appreciation of the psychologic vulnerability of the expectant mother and father and of the powerful contribution of fetal behavior facilitates supportive clinical intervention.

THREATS TO FETAL DEVELOPMENT. Mortality and morbidity are highest during the prenatal period (see Chapter 89). Some 30% of pregnancies end in spontaneous abortion, most often during the 1st trimester as a result of chromosomal or other abnormalities. Major congenital malformations requiring neonatal surgical intervention occur in approximately 2% of live births. Teratogens associated with gross physical and mental abnormalities include various infectious agents (toxoplasmosis, rubella, syphilis), chemical agents (mercury, thalidomide, antiepileptic medications, ethanol), high temperature, and radiation (see Chapters 92 and 718).

For any potential teratogen, the extent and nature of teratogenic effects are determined by characteristics of the host as well as the dose and timing of the exposure. Rates of fetal alcohol syndrome are exceptionally high among Native Americans, for example, because of a possible inherited metabolic vulnerability. Organ systems are most vulnerable during periods of maximum growth and differentiation, generally during the first trimester (organogenesis). Figure 8–3 depicts sensitive periods during gestation for various organ systems.

Teratogenic effects may include not only gross physical malformation but also decreased growth and later cognitive or behavioral deficits. Prenatal exposure to cigarette smoke is associated with lower birthweight, shorter length, and smaller head circumference, as well as decreased IQ and increased rates of learning disabilities. The effects of cocaine on a fetus and an infant may be attributable to associated risk factors including other prenatal exposures (alcohol and cigarettes used in large amounts by many cocaine-addicted women) and to "toxic" postnatal environments frequently characterized by instability, multiple caregivers, and abuse and neglect (see Chapter 102). The wide range of outcomes observed reflects the complex interactions among biologic and social risk and protective factors.

Brazelton TB, Cramer BG: The Earliest Relationship. Reading, MA, Addison-Wesley Publishing Co, 1990.
Hepper PG, Shahidullah S: Habituation in normal and Down's syndrome fetuses. Q J Exp Psychol 44:305, 1992.
Moore KL: Before We Are Born: Basic Embryology and Birth Defects, 2nd ed. Philadelphia, WB Saunders, 1972.
Pillai M, James D: Behavioural states in normal mature human fetuses. Arch Dis Child 65:39, 1990.
Zuckerman B, Frank D: Prenatal cocaine exposure: Nine years later. J Pediatr 124:731, 1994.

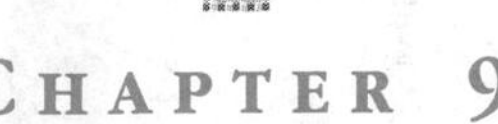

CHAPTER 9
The Newborn

Infants survive physically and psychologically only in the context of their social relationships. For the purposes of developmental assessment and intervention, an infant in isolation does not exist.

DETERMINANTS OF PARENTING (see Chapter 90)

Parenting a newborn infant requires dedication because a newborn's needs are urgent, exhausting, and often unclear. To know what to do, parents must attend to an infant's signals and respond empathically. Many factors influence parents' ability to assume this role.

PRENATAL FACTORS. Pregnancy is a period of psychologic preparation for the profound demands of parenting. Most women experience ambivalence, particularly (but not exclusively) if their pregnancy was unplanned. If financial worries, physical illness, prior miscarriages or stillbirths, or other crises interfere with their working through the ambivalence, the neonate may arrive as an unwelcome guest. For adolescent mothers, the demand that they relinquish their own developmental agenda (e.g., the need for an active social life) may be especially burdensome.

The early experience of being mothered may establish unconsciously held expectations about nurturing relationships that permit mothers to "tune in" to their infants. Research has linked the quality of these expectations (or working models) with the quality of later infant-parent interactions. Mothers whose early childhoods were marked by traumatic separations, abuse, or neglect may find it especially difficult to provide consistent, responsive care. Instead, they may re-enact their childhood experiences with their own infants as if unable to conceive of the mother-child relationship in any other way.

Social support during pregnancy is also important. A supportive relationship with the child's father predicts satisfaction in mothering. At the other extreme, conflict with or abandonment by the father during pregnancy may undermine the mother's ability to become absorbed with her infant. After delivery, anticipation of an early return to work may make committing to the task at hand more difficult. Six months of maternity leave from work may help, although career and financial pressures often force an earlier return.

PERIPARTUM AND POSTPARTUM INFLUENCES. During labor, the continuous presence of a woman trained to offer friendly support and encouragement (a doula) results in shorter labor, fewer obstetric complications, and reduced postpartum hospital stays. Skin-to-skin contact between mothers and infants immediately after birth may correlate with an increased incidence of breast-feeding and longer duration of lactation. An opportunity for increased mother-infant contact over the next several days may result in improved mother-child interactions in the long term and a reduced risk of child abuse. Early separation, although predictably very stressful, does not inevitably impair a mother's ability to bond with her infant. Most new parents value even a brief period of uninterrupted time in which to get to know their new infants. Early discharge home from the maternity ward may undermine bonding in cases in which a new mother is required to resume full responsibility for a busy household.

THE INFANT'S CONTRIBUTION

INTERACTIONAL ABILITIES. Almost immediately after birth, a neonate looks alert and readily suckles if given the opportunity. This first alert-awake period may be adversely modified by some maternal analgesics and anesthetics or fetal hypoxia. Nearsighted, neonates have a fixed focal length of 8–12 in, approximately the distance from the breast to the mother's face, as well as an inborn visual preference for faces. Hearing is well developed, and infants preferentially turn toward a female voice. These innate abilities and predilections ensure that when a mother gazes at her newborn, the gaze is likely to be returned. The initial period of social interaction, usually lasting about 40 min, is followed by a period of somnolence. After that, briefer periods of alertness or excitation alternate with sleep. If a mother misses the first alert-awake period (because she has been anesthetized), she may not experience as long a period of social interaction for several days.

MODULATION OF AROUSAL. Adaptation to extrauterine life requires rapid and profound physiologic changes, including aeration of the lungs, rerouting of the circulation, and activation of the intestinal tract. The necessary behavioral changes are no less profound. To obtain nourishment, to avoid hypothermia or hyperthermia, and to ensure safety, neonates must react appropriately to an expanded range of sensory stimuli. Infants must become aroused in response to stimulation but not so overaroused that behavior becomes random. Underaroused infants are not able to feed and interact; overaroused infants show signs of autonomic instability, including flushing or mottling, perioral pallor, hiccuping, vomiting, uncontrolled limb movements, or inconsolable crying.

BEHAVIORAL STATES. The organization of infant behavior into discrete behavioral states may reflect an infant's inborn ability to regulate arousal. Six states have been described: quiet sleep, active sleep, drowsy, alert, fussy, and crying. In the alert state, infants visually fixate on objects or faces and follow them horizontally and (within a month) vertically; they also reliably turn toward a novel sound, as if searching for its source. When overstimulated, they may calm themselves by looking away, yawning, or sucking on their lips or hands, thereby increasing parasympathetic activity and reducing sympathetic nervous activity. The behavioral state determines an infant's muscle tone, spontaneous movement, electroencephalogram pattern, and response to stimuli. In active sleep, for example, an infant may show progressively less reaction to a repeated heel prick (habituation), whereas in the drowsy state the same stimulus may push a child into fussing or crying.

MUTUAL REGULATION. Parents actively participate in an infant's state regulation, alternately stimulating or soothing to prolong the social interaction. In turn, the parents are regulated by the infant's signals, responding, for example, with a letdown of milk (or with a bottle) in response to cries of hunger. Such interactions constitute a system directed toward furthering the infant's physiologic homeostasis and physical growth. At the same time, they form the basis for the emerging psychologic relationship between parent and child. Infants come to associate the presence of the parent with the pleasurable reduction of tension (as in feeding) and show this preference by calming more quickly for the mother than for a stranger. This response, in turn, strengthens a mother's sense of efficacy and connection with her baby.

CLINICAL IMPLICATIONS: THE PHYSICIAN'S ROLE

Pediatric interventions to support healthy newborn development include (1) promoting optimal medical practices before, during, and after delivery; (2) assessing parent-infant interactions; and (3) teaching parents about their newborn's individual competencies and vulnerabilities.

OPTIMAL PRACTICES. A prenatal pediatric visit allows pediatricians to assess potential problems of bonding (e.g., a tense spousal relationship) and sources of social support and to try to allay unrealistic fears. Supportive hospital policies include use of birthing rooms rather than operating suite/delivery rooms; encouragement for the father or a trusted relative or friend to remain with the mother during labor or provision of a professional support person or doula; the practice of giving the newborn infant to the mother immediately after delivery or after brief stabilization and assessment; and placement of the newborn in the mother's room rather than in a central nursery. After discharge (often within 24 hr of delivery), home visits by nurses and lactation counselors may minimize early feeding problems and allow assessment of medical conditions that arise within the first week. Such family-focused policies may be particularly important for ill infants. For example, infants requiring transport to another hospital should be brought to see the mother first if at all possible. On discharge home, fathers can have an important role in protecting mothers from unnecessary visits and calls and in taking over household duties to allow mothers to get to know their new infants without distractions.

ASSESSING PARENT-INFANT INTERACTIONS. Observation during a feeding or when infants are alert and face to face with parents can be revealing. It is normal for infants and parents to appear absorbed in one another. Infants who become overstimulated by the mother's voice or activity may turn away or appear to fall asleep, leading to a premature termination of the encounter. Alternatively, the infant may be alert and ready to interact, whereas the mother appears preoccupied.

TEACHING ABOUT INDIVIDUAL COMPETENCIES. The Newborn Behavior Assessment Scale (NBAS) provides a formal measure of an infant's neurodevelopmental competencies, including state control, autonomic reactivity, reflexes, habituation, and orientation (the ability to turn toward auditory and visual stimuli). This examination can also be used to demonstrate to parents an infant's capabilities and vulnerabilities. Parents might learn that they need to undress their infant to increase the level of arousal or to swaddle the infant to contain random arm movements and reduce overstimulation. The NBAS can support the development of positive early parent-infant relationships and may prevent early problems that arise from misinterpretation of an infant's behavior. The effects of such early intervention, as with early physical contact, may be long term. Demonstration of the NBAS in the 1st wk of life has been shown to correlate with improvements in the caretaking environment months later.

Brazelton TB: The Neonatal Behavioral Assessment Scale. Philadelphia, JB Lippincott, 1973.

Klaus MH, Kennell JH: Bonding: The Beginnings of Parent-Infant Attachment. St. Louis, CV Mosby, 1983.
Lyons-Ruth K, Zeanah CH: The family context of infant mental health: I. Affective development in the primary caregiving relationship. *In:* Zeanah CH (ed): Handbook of Infant Mental Health. New York, Guilford Press, 1993, pp 14–37.
MacFarlane JA, Smith DM, Garrow DH: The relationship between mother and neonate. *In:* Kitzinger S, Davis JA (eds): The Place of Birth. New York, Oxford University Press, 1978, pp 175–220.
Winnicott DW: The Maturational Processes and the Facilitating Environment. New York, International Universities Press, 1965.

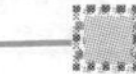

CHAPTER 10
The First Year

During the first year of life, physical growth, maturation, acquisition of competence, and psychologic reorganization occur in rapid, discontinuous bursts. These changes qualitatively change a child's behavior and social relationships. Physical growth during this period is rapid; growth parameters and normal ranges for attainable weight, length, and head circumference can be estimated as noted in Tables 10–1 and 10–2. Table 10–3 presents an overview of milestones in the domains of gross motor, fine motor, and cognitive development. Table 10–4 presents similar information arranged cross-sectionally. Development in each domain affects the others.

AGE 0–2 MO

The biologic and psychologic challenges facing neonates and their parents were described in Chapter 9. These consist of establishing effective feeding and a predictable sleep-wake cycle. The social interactions that occur when parents and infants accomplish these tasks lay the foundation for cognitive and emotional development.

PHYSICAL DEVELOPMENT. A newborn's weight may decrease 10% below birthweight in the 1st wk as a result of excretion of excess extravascular fluid and possibly poor intake. Intake improves as colostrum is replaced by higher-fat milk, as infants learn to latch on and suck more efficiently, and as mothers become more comfortable with feeding techniques. Infants should regain or exceed birthweight by 2 wk of age and should grow at approximately 30 g (1 oz)/day during the 1st mo (Table 10–5). Limb movements consist largely of uncontrolled writhing, with apparently purposeless hand opening and closing. Smiling occurs involuntarily. In contrast, eye gaze, head turning, and sucking are under conscious control and thus can be used to demonstrate infant perception and cognition. For example, an infant's preferential turning toward the mother's voice is evidence of recognition memory.

Six behavioral states have been described (see Chapter 9). Initially, sleep and wakefulness are evenly distributed throughout the 24 hr (Fig. 10–1). Neurologic maturation accounts for the consolidation of sleep periods into longer and longer blocks. Learning has a role as well. Infants whose parents are consistently more interactive and stimulating during the day learn to concentrate their sleeping during the night. By 2 mo of age, most infants are waking briefly two or three times to feed; some sleep 6 hr or more at a stretch. Crying occurs in response to stimuli that may be obvious (a soiled diaper) but are often obscure. Crying normally peaks at about 6 wk of age, when healthy infants cry up to 3 hr/day, then decreases to 1 hr or less by 3 mo.

COGNITIVE DEVELOPMENT. Caretaking activities provide visual, tactile, olfactory, and auditory stimuli; all of these stimuli play an important part in the development of cognition. Studies of habituation and gaze preference provide insights into how infants interpret these stimuli. Infants habituate to the familiar, attending less and less to a stimulus that is repeated several times and then increasing their attention when the stimulus changes. Experiments using habituation and renewed attention as outcomes show that infants can differentiate among similar patterns, colors, and consonants. They can recognize facial expressions (smiles) as similar, even when they appear on different faces. They also can match abstract properties of stimuli, such as contour, intensity, or temporal pattern across sensory modalities. For example, 3-wk-old infants can tell whether a spoken voice corresponds to the movements of the lips on a videotape. Blindfolded and given a bumpy pacifier to

TABLE 10–1 Formulas for Approximate Average Height and Weight of Normal Infants and Children

Weight	Kilograms	(Pounds)
At birth	3.25	(7)
3–12 mo	$\frac{\text{age (mo)} + 9}{2}$	(age [mo] + 11)
1–6 yr	age (yr) × 2 + 8	(age [yr] × 5 + 17)
7–12 yr	$\frac{\text{age (yr)} \times 7 - 5}{2}$	(age [yr] × 7 + 5)
Height	**Centimeters**	**(Inches)**
At birth	50	(20)
At 1 yr	75	(30)
2–12 yr	age (yr) × 6 + 77	(age [yr] × 2½ + 30)

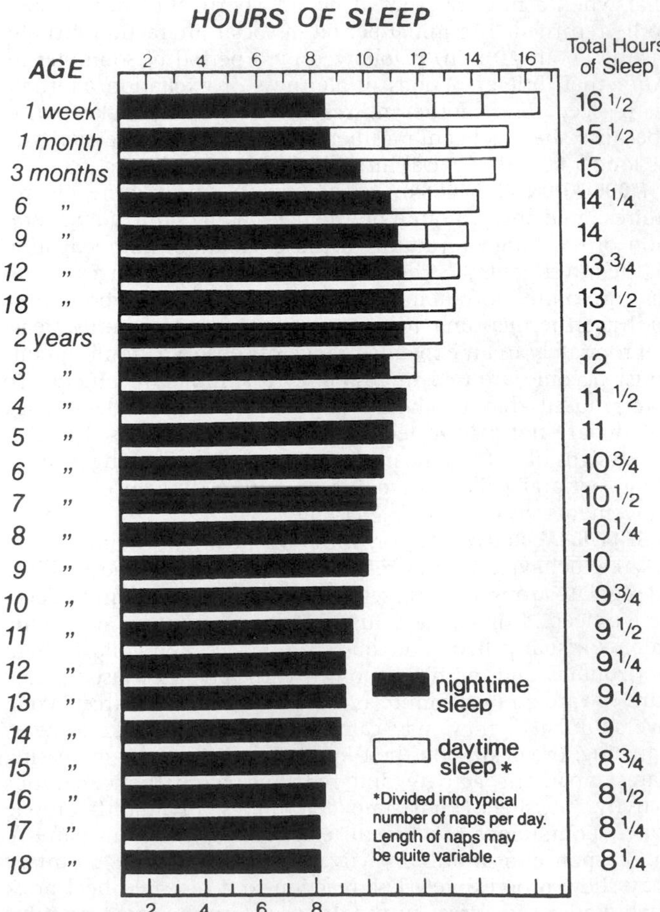

Figure 10–1 Typical sleep requirements in childhood. (From Ferber R: Solve Your Child's Sleep Problems. New York, Simon and Schuster, 1985.)

TABLE 10–2 Length, Weight, and Head Circumference by Age for Boys and Girls: Birth to 36 Mo

	Boys: Percentiles								Girls: Percentiles						
	5th	*10th*	*25th*	*50th*	*75th*	*90th*	*95th*	**Measurement**	*5th*	*10th*	*25th*	*50th*	*75th*	*90th*	*95th*
	46.4	47.5	49.0	50.5	51.8	53.5	54.4	Length, mm	45.4	46.5	48.2	49.9	51.0	52.0	52.9
	(18¼)	(18¾)	(19¼)	(20)	(20½)	(21)	(21½)	(in)	(17¾)	(18¼)	(19)	(19¾)	(20)	(20½)	(20¾)
Birth	2.54	2.78	3.00	3.27	3.64	3.82	4.15	Weight, kg	2.36	2.58	2.93	3.23	3.52	3.64	3.81
	(5½)	(6¼)	(6½)	(7¼)	(8)	(8½)	(9¼)	(lb)	(5¼)	(5¾)	(6½)	(7)	(7¾)	(8)	(8½)
	32.6	33.0	33.9	34.8	35.6	36.6	37.2	Head C, cm	32.1	32.9	33.5	34.3	34.8	35.5	35.9
	(12¾)	(13)	(13¼)	(13¾)	(14)	(14½)	(14¾)	(in)	(12¾)	(13)	(13¼)	(13½)	(13¾)	(14)	(14¼)
	50.4	51.3	53.0	54.6	56.2	57.7	58.6	Length, cm	49.2	50.2	51.9	53.5	54.9	56.1	56.9
	(19¾)	(20¼)	(20¾)	(21½)	(22¼)	(22¾)	(23)	(in)	(19¼)	(19¾)	(20½)	(21)	(21½)	(22)	(22½)
1 mo	3.16	3.43	3.82	4.29	4.75	5.14	5.38	Weight, kg	2.97	3.22	3.59	3.98	4.36	4.65	4.92
	(7)	(7½)	(8½)	(9½)	(10½)	(11¼)	(11¾)	(lb)	(6½)	(7)	(8)	(8¾)	(9½)	(10¼)	(10¾)
	34.9	35.4	36.2	37.2	38.1	39.0	39.6	Head C, cm	34.2	34.8	35.6	36.4	37.1	37.8	38.3
	(13¾)	(14)	(14¼)	(14¾)	(15)	(15¼)	(15½)	(in)	(13½)	(13¾)	(14)	(14¼)	(14½)	(15)	(15)
	56.7	57.7	59.4	61.1	63.0	64.5	65.4	Length, cm	55.4	56.2	57.8	59.5	61.2	62.7	63.4
	(22¼)	(22¾)	(23½)	(24)	(24¾)	(25½)	(25¾)	(in)	(21¾)	(22¼)	(22¾)	(23½)	(24)	(24¾)	(25)
3 mo	4.43	4.78	5.32	5.98	6.56	7.14	7.37	Weight, kg	4.18	4.47	4.88	5.40	5.90	6.39	6.74
	(9¾)	(10½)	(11¾)	(13¼)	(14½)	(15¾)	(16¼)	(lb)	(9¼)	(9¾)	(10¾)	(12)	(13)	(14)	(14¾)
	38.4	38.9	39.7	40.6	41.7	42.5	43.1	Head C, cm	37.3	37.8	38.7	39.5	40.4	41.2	41.7
	(15)	(15¼)	(15¾)	(16)	(16½)	(16¾)	(17)	(in)	(14¾)	(15)	(15¼)	(15½)	(16)	(16¼)	(16½)
	63.4	64.4	66.1	67.8	69.7	71.3	72.3	Length, cm	61.8	62.6	64.2	65.9	67.8	69.4	70.2
	(25)	(25¼)	(26)	(26¾)	(27½)	(28)	(28½)	(in)	(24¼)	(24¾)	(25¼)	(26)	(26¾)	(27¼)	(27¾)
6 mo	6.20	6.61	7.20	7.85	8.49	9.10	9.46	Weight, kg	5.79	6.12	6.60	7.21	7.83	8.38	8.73
	(13¾)	(14½)	(15¾)	(17¼)	(18¾)	(20)	(20¾)	(lb)	(12¾)	(13½)	(14½)	(16)	(17¼)	(18½)	(19¼)
	41.5	42.0	42.8	43.8	44.7	45.6	46.2	Head C, cm	40.3	40.9	41.6	42.4	43.3	44.1	44.6
	(16¼)	(16½)	(16¾)	(17¼)	(17½)	(18)	(18¼)	(in)	(15¾)	(16)	(16½)	(16¾)	(17)	(17¼)	(17½)
	68.0	69.1	70.6	72.3	74.0	75.9	77.1	Length, cm	66.1	67.0	68.7	70.4	72.4	74.0	75.0
	(26¾)	(27¼)	(27¾)	(28½)	(29¼)	(30)	(30¼)	(in)	(26)	(26½)	(27)	(27¾)	(28½)	(29¼)	(29½)
9 mo	7.52	7.95	8.56	9.18	9.88	10.49	10.93	Weight, kg	7.00	7.34	7.89	8.56	9.24	9.83	10.17
	(16½)	(17½)	(18¾)	(20¼)	(21¾)	(23¼)	(24)	(lb)	(15½)	(16¼)	(17½)	(18¾)	(20¼)	(21¾)	(22½)
	43.5	44.0	44.8	45.8	46.6	47.5	48.1	Head C, cm	42.3	42.8	43.5	44.3	45.1	46.0	46.4
	(17¼)	(17¼)	(17¾)	(18)	(18¼)	(18¾)	(19)	(in)	(16¾)	(16¾)	(17¼)	(17½)	(17¾)	(18)	(18¼)
	71.7	72.8	74.3	76.1	77.7	79.8	81.2	Length, cm	69.8	70.8	72.4	74.3	76.3	78.0	79.1
	(28¼)	(28¾)	(29¼)	(30)	(30½)	(31½)	(32)	(in)	(27½)	(27¾)	(28½)	(29¼)	(30)	(30¾)	(31¼)
12 mo	8.43	8.84	9.49	10.15	10.91	11.54	11.99	Weight, kg	7.84	8.19	8.81	9.53	10.23	10.87	11.24
	(18½)	(19½)	(21)	(22½)	(24)	(25½)	(26½)	(lb)	(17¼)	(18)	(19½)	(21)	(22½)	(24)	(24¾)
	44.8	45.3	46.1	47.0	47.9	48.8	49.3	Head C, cm	43.5	44.1	44.8	45.6	46.4	47.2	47.6
	(17¾)	(17¾)	(18¼)	(18½)	(18¾)	(19¼)	(19½)	(in)	(17¼)	(17¼)	(17¾)	(18)	(18¼)	(18½)	(18¾)
	77.5	78.7	80.5	82.4	84.3	86.6	88.1	Length, cm	76.0	77.2	78.8	80.9	83.0	85.0	86.1
	(30½)	(31)	(31¾)	(32½)	(33¼)	(34)	(34¾)	(in)	(30)	(30½)	(31)	(31¾)	(32¾)	(33½)	(34)
18 mo	9.59	9.92	10.67	11.47	12.31	13.05	13.44	Weight, kg	8.92	9.30	10.04	10.82	11.55	12.30	12.76
	(21¼)	(21¾)	(23½)	(25¼)	(27¼)	(28¾)	(29½)	(lb)	(19¾)	(20½)	(22¼)	(23¾)	(25½)	(27)	(28¼)
	46.3	46.7	47.4	48.4	49.3	50.1	50.6	Head C, cm	45.0	45.6	46.3	47.1	47.9	48.6	49.1
	(18¼)	(18½)	(18¾)	(19)	(19½)	(19¾)	(20)	(in)	(17¾)	(18)	(18¼)	(18½)	(18¾)	(19¼)	(19¼)
	82.3	83.5	85.6	87.6	89.9	92.2	93.8	Length, cm	81.3	82.5	84.2	86.5	88.7	90.8	92.0
	(32½)	(32¾)	(33¾)	(34½)	(35½)	(36¼)	(37)	(in)	(32)	(32½)	(33¼)	(34)	(35)	(35¾)	(36¼)
24 mo	10.54	10.85	11.65	12.59	13.44	14.29	14.70	Weight, kg	9.87	10.26	11.10	11.90	12.74	13.57	14.08
	(23¼)	(24)	(25¾)	(27¾)	(29¾)	(31½)	(32½)	(lb)	(21¾)	(22½)	(24½)	(26¼)	(28)	(30)	(31)
	47.3	47.7	48.3	49.2	50.2	51.0	51.4	Head C, cm	46.1	46.5	47.3	48.1	48.8	49.6	50.1
	(18½)	(18¾)	(19)	(19¼)	(19¾)	(20)	(20¼)	(in)	(18¼)	(18¼)	(18½)	(19)	(19¼)	(19½)	(19¾)
	87.0	88.2	90.1	92.3	94.6	97.0	98.7	Length, cm	86.0	87.0	88.9	91.3	93.7	95.6	96.9
	(34¼)	(34¾)	(35½)	(36¼)	(37¼)	(38¼)	(38¾)	(in)	(33¾)	(34¼)	(35)	(36)	(37)	(37¾)	(38¼)
30 mo	11.44	11.80	12.63	13.67	14.51	15.47	15.97	Weight, kg	10.78	11.21	12.11	12.93	13.93	14.81	15.35
	(25¼)	(26)	(27¾)	(30¼)	(32)	(34)	(35¼)	(lb)	(23¾)	(24¾)	(26¾)	(28½)	(30¾)	(32¾)	(33¾)
	48.0	48.4	49.1	49.9	51.0	51.7	52.2	Head C, cm	47.0	47.3	48.0	48.8	49.4	50.3	50.8
	(19)	(19)	(19¼)	(19¾)	(20)	(20¼)	(20½)	(in)	(18½)	(18½)	(19)	(19¼)	(19½)	(19¾)	(20)
	91.2	92.4	94.2	96.5	98.9	101.4	103.1	Length, cm	90.0	91.0	93.1	95.6	98.1	100.0	101.5
	(36)	(36½)	(37)	(38)	(39)	(40)	(40½)	(in)	(35½)	(35¾)	(36¾)	(37¾)	(38½)	(39¼)	(40)
36 mo	12.26	12.69	13.58	14.69	15.59	16.66	17.28	Weight, kg	11.60	12.07	12.99	13.93	15.03	15.97	16.54
	(27)	(28)	(30)	(32½)	(34½)	(36¾)	(38)	(lb)	(25½)	(26½)	(28¾)	(30¾)	(33¼)	(35¼)	(36½)
	48.6	49.0	49.7	50.5	51.5	52.3	52.8	Head C, cm	47.6	47.9	48.5	49.3	50.0	50.8	51.4
	(19¼)	(19¼)	(19½)	(20)	(20¼)	(20½)	(20¾)	(in)	(18¾)	(18¾)	(19)	(19½)	(19¾)	(20)	(20¼)

These data are those of the National Center for Health Statistics (NCHS), Health Resources Administration, Department of Health, Education, and Welfare. They were based on studies of The Fels Research Institute, Yellow Springs, Ohio. Metric data have been smoothed by a least-squares cubic spline technique. For details see Hamill PVV, Drizd TA, Johnson CL, et al: NCHS growth curves for children, birth–18 yr. United States Vital Health Statistics 1977 (Nov 165):1–1V, pp 1–74, 1979.

TABLE 10–3 Developmental Milestones in the First 2 Yr of Life

Milestone	Average Age of Attainment (mo)	Developmental Implications
Gross Motor		
Head steady in sitting	2.0	Allows more visual interaction
Pull to sit, no head lag	3.0	Muscle tone
Hands together in midline	3.0	Self-discovery
Asymmetric tonic neck reflex gone	4.0	Child can inspect hands in midline
Sits without support	6.0	Increasing exploration
Rolls back to stomach	6.5	Truncal flexion, risk of falls
Walks alone	12.0	Exploration, control of proximity to parents
Runs	16.0	Supervision more difficult
Fine Motor		
Grasps rattle	3.5	Object use
Reaches for objects	4.0	Visuomotor coordination
Palmar grasp gone	4.0	Voluntary release
Transfers object hand to hand	5.5	Comparison of objects
Thumb-finger grasp	8.0	Able to explore small objects
Turns pages of book	12.0	Increasing autonomy during book time
Scribbles	13.0	Visuomotor coordination
Builds tower of two cubes	15.0	Uses objects in combination
Builds tower of six cubes	22.0	Requires visual, gross, and fine motor coordination
Communication and Language		
Smiles in response to face, voice	1.5	Child more active social participant
Monosyllabic babble	6.0	Experimentation with sound, tactile sense
Inhibits to "no"	7.0	Response to tone (nonverbal)
Follows one-step command with gesture	7.0	Nonverbal communication
Follows one-step command without gesture (e.g., "Give it to me")	10.0	Verbal receptive language
Speaks first real word	12.0	Beginning of labeling
Speaks 4–6 words	15.0	Acquisition of object and personal names
Speaks 10–15 words	18.0	Acquisition of object and personal names
Speaks two-word sentences (e.g., "Mommy shoe")	19.0	Beginning grammaticization, corresponds with 50+ word vocabulary
Cognitive		
Stares momentarily at spot where object disappeared (e.g., yarn ball dropped)	2.0	Lack of object permanence (out of sight, out of mind)
Stares at own hand	4.0	Self-discovery, cause and effect
Bangs two cubes	8.0	Active comparison of objects
Uncovers toy (after seeing it hidden)	8.0	Object permanence
Egocentric pretend play (e.g., pretends to drink from cup)	12.0	Beginning symbolic thought
Uses stick to reach toy	17.0	Able to link actions to solve problems
Pretend play with doll (gives doll bottle)	17.0	Symbolic thought

suck, they subsequently gaze longer at the bumpy pacifier than at a smooth one when both are presented visually.

Such studies suggest that infants are able to perceive objects and events as coherent, even while noting aspects that are discrepant. These abilities allow infants to sort stimuli into meaningful sets: a set of stimuli that correspond to sucking as well as others that correspond to sucking a bottle, sucking a pacifier, and sucking a finger. Infants appear to seek stimuli actively as though satisfying an innate need to make sense of the world.

EMOTIONAL DEVELOPMENT. Basic trust, the first of Erikson's psychosocial stages, develops as infants learn that their urgent needs are met regularly. The consistent availability of a trusted adult creates the conditions for a secure attachment. Infants who are consistently picked up and held in response to distress cry less at 1 yr and show less aggressive behavior at 2 yr.

The emotional significance of any experience depends on an individual child's temperament as well as the parent's responses. Consider the impact of different feeding schedules. Hunger generates increasing tension; as the urgency peaks, the infant cries, the parent arrives with a bottle or breast, and the tension dissipates. Infants fed "on demand" consistently experience this link between their distress, the arrival of the parent, and the relief from hunger. Most infants fed on a fixed schedule quickly adapt their hunger cycle to the schedule. Those who cannot because they are temperamentally prone to irregular biologic rhythms experience periods of unrelieved hunger as well as unwanted feedings when they already feel full. Similarly, infants fed at the parents' convenience, with neither attention to the infant's hunger cues nor a fixed schedule, may not consistently experience feeding as the pleasurable reduction of tension. These infants often show increased irritability and physiologic instability (spitting, diarrhea, poor weight gain) as well as later behavioral problems.

IMPLICATIONS FOR PARENTS AND PEDIATRICIANS. Success or failure in establishing feeding and sleep cycles determines parents' feelings of efficacy despite the unquestionable importance of infant temperament. When things go well, anxiety, ambivalence, and the exhaustion of the early weeks relent. With physical recovery from delivery and endocrinologic normalization, the mild postpartum depression that affects some 50% of mothers ("baby blues") passes. If sad, overwhelmed, anxious feelings persist, the possibility of true postpartum depression needs to be considered.

AGE 2–6 MO

At about 2 mo, the emergence of voluntary (social) smiles and increasing eye contact mark a change in the parent-child relationship, heightening the parents' sense of being loved back. During the next months, an infant's range of motor and social control and cognitive engagement increases dramatically. Mutual regulation takes the form of complex social interchanges.

PHYSICAL DEVELOPMENT. Between 3 and 4 mo, the rate of growth slows to approximately 20 g/day (see Table 10–5 and

TABLE 10–4 Emerging Patterns of Behavior During the 1st Yr of Life

	Neonatal Period (1st 4 Wk)
Prone:	Lies in flexed attitude; turns head from side to side; head sags on ventral suspension
Supine:	Generally flexed and a little stiff
Visual:	May fixate face or light in line of vision; "doll's-eye" movement of eyes on turning of the body
Reflex:	Moro response active; stepping and placing reflexes; grasp reflex active
Social:	Visual preference for human face
	At 4 Wk
Prone:	Legs more extended; holds chin up; turns head; head lifted momentarily to plane of body on ventral suspension
Supine:	Tonic neck posture predominates; supple and relaxed; head lags on pull to sitting position
Visual:	Watches person; follows moving object
Social:	Body movements in cadence with voice of other in social contact; beginning to smile
	At 8 Wk
Prone:	Raises head slightly farther; head sustained in plane of body on ventral suspension
Supine:	Tonic neck posture predominates; head lags on pull to sitting position
Visual:	Follows moving object 180 degrees
Social:	Smiles on social contact; listens to voice and coos
	At 12 Wk
Prone:	Lifts head and chest, arms extended; head above plane of body on ventral suspension
Supine:	Tonic neck posture predominates; reaches toward and misses objects; waves at toy
Sitting:	Head lag partially compensated on pull to sitting position; early head control with bobbing motion; back rounded
Reflex:	Typical Moro response has not persisted; makes defensive movements or selective withdrawal reactions
Social:	Sustained social contact; listens to music; says "aah, ngah"
	At 16 Wk
Prone:	Lifts head and chest, head in approximately vertical axis; legs extended
Supine:	Symmetric posture predominates, hands in midline; reaches and grasps objects and brings them to mouth
Sitting:	No head lag on pull to sitting position; head steady, tipped forward; enjoys sitting with full truncal support
Standing:	When held erect, pushes with feet
Adaptive:	Sees pellet, but makes no move to it
Social:	Laughs out loud; may show displeasure if social contact is broken; excited at sight of food
	At 28 Wk
Prone:	Rolls over; pivots; crawls or creep-crawls (Knobloch)
Supine:	Lifts head; rolls over; squirming movements
Sitting:	Sits briefly, with support of pelvis; leans forward on hands; back rounded
Standing:	May support most of weight; bounces actively
Adaptive:	Reaches out for and grasps large object; transfers objects from hand to hand; grasp uses radial palm; rakes at pellet
Language:	Polysyllabic vowel sounds formed
Social:	Prefers mother; babbles; enjoys mirror; responds to changes in emotional content of social contact
	At 40 Wk
Sitting:	Sits up alone and indefinitely without support, back straight
Standing:	Pulls to standing position; "cruises" or walks holding on to furniture
Motor:	Creeps or crawls
Adaptive:	Grasps objects with thumb and forefinger; pokes at things with forefinger; picks up pellet with assisted pincer movement; uncovers hidden toy; attempts to retrieve dropped object; releases object grasped by other person
Language:	Repetitive consonant sounds (mama, dada)
Social:	Responds to sound of name; plays peek-a-boo or pat-a-cake; waves bye-bye
	At 52 Wk (1 Yr)
Motor:	Walks with one hand held (48 wk); rises independently, takes several steps (Knobloch)
Adaptive:	Picks up pellet with unassisted pincer movement of forefinger and thumb; releases object to other person on request or gesture
Language:	A few words besides "mama," "dada"
Social:	Plays simple ball game; makes postural adjustment to dressing

Data are derived from those of Gesell (as revised by Knobloch), Shirley, Provence, Wolf, Bailey, and others.

TABLE 10–5 Growth and Caloric Requirements

Age	Approximate Daily Weight Gain (g)	Approximate Monthly Weight Gain	Growth in Length (cm/mo)	Growth in Head Circumference (cm/mo)	Recommended Daily Allowance (kcal/kg/day)
0–3 mo	30	2 lb	3.5	2.00	115
3–6 mo	20	1¼ lb	2.0	1.00	110
6–9 mo	15	1 lb	1.5	0.50	100
9–12 mo	12	13 oz	1.2	0.50	100
1–3 yr	8	8 oz	1.0	0.25	100
4–6 yr	6	6 oz	3 cm/yr	1 cm/yr	90–100

Adapted from National Research Council, Food and Nutrition Board: Recommended Daily Allowances. Washington, DC, National Academy of Sciences, 1989; Frank D, Silva M, Needlman R: Failure to thrive: Myth and method. Contemp Pediatr 10:114, 1993.

Figs. 11–1 and 11–2). Early reflexes that limited voluntary movement recede. Disappearance of the asymmetric tonic neck reflex means that infants can begin to examine objects in the midline and manipulate them with both hands. Waning of the early grasp reflex allows them both to hold objects and voluntarily to let them go. A novel object may elicit purposeful though inefficient reaching. The quality of spontaneous movements also changes, from larger writhing to smaller, circular movements that have been described as "fidgety." Abnormal or absent fidgety movements may constitute a risk factor for later neurologic abnormalities.

Increasing control of truncal flexion makes intentional rolling possible. Infants who routinely sleep on their backs or sides (as recommended to prevent sudden infant death syndrome) may learn to roll somewhat later. Head control improves, allowing infants to gaze across at things rather than merely up and to begin taking food from a spoon. At the same time, maturation of the visual system allows much greater depth of field.

Total sleep requirements are approximately 14–16 hr/24 hr, with about 9–10 hr concentrated at night; about 70% of infants sleep for a 6- to 8-hr stretch by age 6 mo (see Fig. 10–1). By 4–6 mo, the sleep electroencephalogram shows a mature pattern, with demarcation of rapid eye movement (REM) and four stages of non-REM sleep. The sleep cycle remains short, only 50–60 min, compared with the adult cycle, approximately 90 min. As a result, infants arouse to light sleep or wake frequently during the night, setting the stage for behavioral sleep problems.

COGNITIVE DEVELOPMENT. The overall effect of these developments is a qualitative change in an infant. Four-mo-old infants are described as "hatching" socially, becoming interested in a wider world. During feeding, infants no longer focus exclusively on the mother but become distracted. In the mother's arms, the infant may literally turn around, preferring to face outward.

Infants at this age also explore their own bodies, staring intently at their hands, vocalizing, blowing bubbles, and touching their ears, cheeks, and genitals. These explorations represent an early stage in the understanding of cause and effect as infants learn that voluntary muscle movements generate predictable tactile and visual sensations. They also have a role in the emergence of a sense of self. Infants come to associate certain sensations through frequent repetition. For example, the proprioceptive feeling of holding up the hand and wiggling the fingers always accompanies the sight of the fingers moving. Such "self" sensations are consistently linked and reproducible at will. In contrast, sensations that come to be classed as "nonself" occur with less regularity and in varying combinations. The sound, smell, and feel of mother sometimes appears promptly in response to crying but sometimes does not.

EMOTIONAL DEVELOPMENT AND COMMUNICATION. Outward-looking babies interact with increasing sophistication and range. The primary emotions of anger, joy, interest, fear, disgust, and surprise appear in appropriate contexts as distinct facial expressions. Face to face with a trusted adult, the infant and adult match affective expressions about 30% of the time; the intensity of their smiling, eye widening, and lip puckering rises and falls together. Every few seconds, as excitement builds, the infant turns away, settles, and then returns to the interaction. If the parent turns away, the infant leans forward, reaches, or in other ways tries to get the adult involved again; if that fails, the infant cries angrily.

Infants of depressed parents show a different pattern, spending less time in coordinated movement with their parents and making fewer efforts to re-engage. Rather than anger, they show sadness and a loss of energy when the parents continue to be unavailable. Such face-to-face behavior reveals the infant's ability to share emotional states, the first step in the development of communication; it also shows infants' (and parents') developing expectations about social relationships.

IMPLICATIONS FOR PARENTS AND PEDIATRICIANS. Motor and sensory maturation makes infants at 3–6 mo exciting and interactive, at once cuter and more appealing but also more separate than at a younger age. Some parents experience their 4-mo-old's outward turning as a rejection, secretly fearing that their infants no longer love them. For most parents, however, this is a happy period. Most parents excitedly report that they can hold "conversations" with their infants, taking turns vocalizing and listening. Pediatricians share in the enjoyment, as the 4-mo-old flirts and coos. If this visit does not feel joyful and relaxed, causes such as social stress, family dysfunction, parental mental illness, or problems in the infant-parent relationship should be sought.

AGE 6–12 MO

Months 6–12 bring increased mobility and exploration of the inanimate world, advances in cognitive understanding and communicative competence, and new tensions around the themes of attachment and separation. Infants develop will and intentions, characteristics that most parents welcome but still find challenging to manage.

PHYSICAL DEVELOPMENT. Growth slows more (see Table 10–5 and Figs. 11–1 and 11–2). The ability to sit unsupported (about 7 mo) and to pivot while sitting (around 9–10 mo) provides increasing opportunities to manipulate several objects at a time and to experiment with novel combinations of objects. These explorations are aided by the emergence of a pincer grasp (around 9 mo). Many infants begin crawling and pulling to stand around 8 mo and walk before their first birthday either independently or in a walker. Motor achievements correlate with increasing myelinization and cerebellar growth. These ambulatory achievements expand infants' exploratory range and create new physical dangers as well as opportunities for learning. Tooth eruption occurs, usually starting with the mandibular central incisors (Table 10–6). Tooth development also reflects, in part, skeletal maturation and bone age (Table 10–7).

COGNITIVE DEVELOPMENT. At first, everything goes into the mouth; in time, novel objects are picked up, inspected, passed from hand to hand, banged, dropped, and then mouthed. Each action represents a nonverbal idea about what things are for (in piagetian terms, a schema). The complexity of an infant's play, how many different schemata are brought to bear, is a useful index of cognitive development at this age. The pleasure, persistence, and energy with which infants tackle these challenges suggest the existence of an intrinsic drive, or mastery motivation. Mastery behavior occurs when infants feel secure; those with less secure attachments show limited experimentation and less competence.

A major milestone is the achievement (about 9 mo) of object constancy, the understanding that objects continue to exist even when not seen. At 4–7 mo, infants look down for a yarn ball that has been dropped but quickly give up if it is not seen. With object constancy, infants persist in searching, finding objects hidden under a cloth or behind the examiner's back.

EMOTIONAL DEVELOPMENT. The advent of object constancy corresponds with qualitative changes in social and communicative development. Infants looks back and forth between an approaching stranger and a parent, as if to contrast known from unknown, and may cling or cry anxiously. Separations often become more difficult. Infants who have been sleeping through the night for months begin to awaken regularly and cry, as though remembering that parents are in the next room.

At the same time, a new demand for autonomy emerges. Infants no longer consent to be fed but turn away as the spoon approaches or insist on holding it themselves. Self-feeding with finger foods allows infants to exercise newly acquired fine motor skills (the pincer grasp); it may be the only way to

TABLE 10–6 Chronology of Human Dentition of Primary or Deciduous and Secondary or Permanent Teeth

	Calcification		Age at Eruption		Age at Shedding	
Primary Teeth	*Begins at*	*Complete at*	*Maxillary*	*Mandibular*	*Maxillary*	*Mandibular*
Central incisors	5th fetal mo	18–24 mo	6–8 mo	5–7 mo	7–8 yr	6–7 yr
Lateral incisors	5th fetal mo	18–24 mo	8–11 mo	7–10 mo	8–9 yr	7–8 yr
Cuspids (canines)	6th fetal mo	30–36 mo	16–20 mo	16–20 mo	11–12 yr	9–11 yr
First molars	5th fetal mo	24–30 mo	10–16 mo	10–16 mo	10–11 yr	10–12 yr
Second molars	6th fetal mo	36 mo	20–30 mo	20–30 mo	10–12 yr	11–13 yr
Secondary Teeth						
Central incisors	3–4 mo	9–10 yr	7–8 yr	6–7 yr		
Lateral incisors	Max, 10–12 mo Mand, 3–4 mo	10–11 yr	8–9 yr	7–8 yr		
Cuspids (canines)	4–5 mo	12–15 yr	11–12 yr	9–11 yr		
First premolars (bicuspids)	18–21 mo	12–13 yr	10–11 yr	10–12 yr		
Second premolars (bicuspids)	24–30 mo	12–14 yr	10–12 yr	11–13 yr		
First molars	Birth	9–10 yr	6–7 yr	6–7 yr		
Second molars	30–36 mo	14–16 yr	12–13 yr	12–13 yr		
Third molars	Max, 7–9 yr Mand, 8–10 yr	18–25 yr	17–22 yr	17–22 yr		

Max, maxillary; Mand, mandibular.
Adapted from chart prepared by PK Losch, Harvard School of Dental Medicine, who provided the data for this table.

TABLE 10–7 Time of Appearance in Roentgenograms of Centers of Ossification in Infancy and Childhood

Boys—Age at Appearance*	Bones and Epiphyseal Centers	Girls—Age at Appearance*
3 wk	*Humerus, head*	3 wk
	Carpal bones	
2 mo ± 2 mo	Capitate	2 mo ± 2 mo
3 mo ± 2 mo	Hamate	2 mo ± 2 mo
30 mo ± 16 mo	Triangular†	21 mo ± 14 mo
42 mo ± 19 mo	Lunate†	34 mo ± 13 mo
67 mo ± 19 mo	Trapezium†	47 mo ± 14 mo
69 mo ± 15 mo	Trapezoid†	49 mo ± 12 mo
66 mo ± 15 mo	Scaphoid†	51 mo ± 12 mo
No standards available	Pisiform†	No standards available
	Metacarpal bones	
18 mo ± 5 mo	II	12 mo ± 3 mo
20 mo ± 5 mo	III	13 mo ± 3 mo
23 mo ± 6 mo	IV	15 mo ± 4 mo
26 mo ± 7 mo	V	16 mo ± 5 mo
32 mo ± 9 mo	I	18 mo ± 5 mo
	Fingers (epiphyses)	
16 mo ± 4 mo	Proximal phalanx, 3rd finger	10 mo ± 3 mo
16 mo ± 4 mo	Proximal phalanx, 2nd finger	11 mo ± 3 mo
17 mo ± 5 mo	Proximal phalanx, 4th finger	11 mo ± 3 mo
19 mo ± 7 mo	Distal phalanx, 1st finger	12 mo ± 4 mo
21 mo ± 5 mo	Proximal phalanx, 5th finger	14 mo ± 4 mo
24 mo ± 6 mo	Middle phalanx, 3rd finger	15 mo ± 5 mo
24 mo ± 6 mo	Middle phalanx, 4th finger	15 mo ± 5 mo
26 mo ± 6 mo	Middle phalanx, 2nd finger	16 mo ± 5 mo
28 mo ± 6 mo	Distal phalanx, 3rd finger	18 mo ± 4 mo
28 mo ± 6 mo	Distal phalanx, 4th finger	18 mo ± 5 mo
32 mo ± 7 mo	Proximal phalanx, 1st finger	20 mo ± 5 mo
37 mo ± 9 mo	Distal phalanx, 5th finger	23 mo ± 6 mo
37 mo ± 8 mo	Distal phalanx, 2nd finger	23 mo ± 6 mo
39 mo ± 10 mo	Middle phalanx, 5th finger	22 mo ± 7 mo
152 mo ± 18 mo	Sesamoid (adductor pollicis)	121 mo ± 13 mo
	Hip and knee	
Usually present at birth	Femur, distal	Usually present at birth
Usually present at birth	Tibia, proximal	Usually present at birth
4 mo ± 2 mo	Femur, head	4 mo ± 2 mo
46 mo ± 11 mo	Patella	29 mo ± 7 mo
	Foot and ankle‡	

Values represent mean ± standard deviation, when applicable.
**To nearest month.*
†Except for the capitate and hamate bones, the variability of carpal centers is too great to make them very useful clinically.
‡Standards for the foot are available, but normal variation is wide, including some familial variants, so that this area is of little clinical use.
The norms present a composite of published data from the Fels Research Institute, Yellow Springs, OH (Pyle SI, Sontag L: Am J Roentgenol 49:102, 1943), and unpublished data from the Brush Foundation, Case Western Reserve University, Cleveland, OH, and the Harvard School of Public Health, Boston, MA. Compiled by Lieb, Buehl, and Pyle.

get children to eat. Tantrums make their first appearance as the drives for autonomy and mastery come in conflict with parental controls and with infants' still-limited abilities.

COMMUNICATION. Infants at 7 mo are adept at nonverbal communication, expressing a range of emotions and responding to vocal tone and facial expressions. Around 9 mo, infants become aware that emotions can be shared between people; they shows parents toys gleefully, as if to say, "When you see this thing, you'll be happy, too!" Between 8–10 mo, babbling takes on a new complexity, with many syllables ("ba-da-ma") and inflections that mimic the native language. At the same time, infants lose the ability to distinguish between vocal sounds that are undifferentiated in the native language. The first true word—that is, a sound used consistently to refer to a specific object or person—appears in concert with an infant's discovery of object constancy.

At this age, picture books provide an ideal context for verbal language acquisition. With a familiar book as a shared focus of attention, a parent and child engage in repeated cycles of pointing and labeling, with elaboration and feedback by the parent.

IMPLICATIONS FOR PARENTS AND PEDIATRICIANS. With the developmental reorganization around 9 mo, previously resolved issues of feeding and sleeping re-emerge. Pediatricians can prepare parents at the 6-mo visit so that these problems can be understood as the results of developmental progress and not regression. Parental ambivalence about separation can express itself in a delay in introducing finger foods or drinking from a cup (usually before the first birthday) or an intrusive, overly neat approach to meal times. Poor weight gain at this age often reflects a struggle between an infant and parent over control of the infant's eating. Discussions about an infant's drive for autonomy and need for limited choices may avert such problems.

Infants' wariness of strangers often makes the 9-mo examination difficult, particularly if the infant is temperamentally prone to react negatively to unfamiliar situations. Time spent talking with the mother and playing with the child will be rewarded by more cooperation.

Brazelton TB: Touchpoints: The Essential Reference. Reading, MA, Addison-Wesley Publishing Co, 1992.

Cohn JF, Tronick EZ: Three-month-old infants' reactions to simulated maternal deprivation. Child Dev 54:185, 1983.

Lyons-Ruth K, Zeanah CH: The family context of infant mental health: I. Affective development in the primary caregiving relationship. *In:* Zeanah CH (ed): Handbook of Infant Mental Health. New York, Guilford Press, 1993, pp 14–37.

Mahler MS, Pine S, Bergman A: The Psychological Birth of the Infant. London, Hutchinson, 1975.

Needlman R, Zuckerman B: Fight illiteracy: Prescribe a book! Contemp Pediatr 9:41, 1992.

Stern D: The Interpersonal World of the Infant. New York, Basic Books, 1985.

Zuckerman BS, Frank DA: Infancy and toddler years. *In:* Levine MD, Carey WB, Crocker AC (eds): Developmental-Behavioral Pediatrics. Philadelphia, WB Saunders, 1992, pp 27–38.

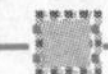

CHAPTER 11
The Second Year

At approximately 18 mo of age, the emergence of symbolic thought causes a reorganization of behavior with implications in many developmental domains.

AGE 12–18 MO

PHYSICAL DEVELOPMENT. The growth rate slows further in the 2nd yr of life (see Table 10–5) and appetite declines. "Baby fat" is burned up by increased mobility; exaggerated lumbar lordosis makes the abdomen protrude. Brain growth continues, with myelinization throughout the 2nd yr (see Fig. 8–2).

Most children begin to walk independently near their first birthday; some do not walk until 15 mo. Highly active, fearless infants tend to walk earlier; less active, more timid infants and those who are preoccupied with exploring objects in detail walk later. Early walking is not associated with advanced development in other domains.

At first, infants toddle with a wide-based gait, knees bent, and arms flexed at the elbow; the entire torso rotates with each stride; the toes may point in or out, and the feet strike the floor flat. Subsequent refinements lead to greater steadiness and energy efficiency. After several months of practice, the center of gravity shifts back and the torso stays more stable, while knees extend and arms swing at the sides for balance. The toes are held in better alignment, and the child is able to stop, pivot, and stoop without toppling over.

COGNITIVE DEVELOPMENT. Object exploration accelerates because reaching, grasping, and releasing are nearly fully mature and walking increases access to interesting things. Toddlers combine objects in novel ways to create interesting effects, such as stacking blocks or putting things into a videocassette recorder slot. Playthings are also more likely to be used for their intended purposes (combs for hair, cups for drinking). Imitation of parents and older children is an important mode of learning. Make-believe play centers on the child's own body (pretending to drink from an empty cup) (Table 11–1; see also Table 10–3).

EMOTIONAL DEVELOPMENT. Infants developmentally approaching the milestone of their first steps may be irritable. Once they start walking, their predominant mood changes markedly. Toddlers are described as "intoxicated" with their new ability and with the power to control the distance between themselves and their parents. Toddlers often orbit around their parents, like planets around the sun, moving away, looking back, moving farther, and then returning for a reassuring touch. In unfamiliar surroundings, with temperamentally timid children, such orbits might be small or nonexistent; in familiar ones, a bold child might orbit out of sight (see Table 11–1).

TABLE 11–1 Emerging Patterns of Behavior from 1 to 5 Yr of Age*

	15 Mo
Motor:	Walks alone; crawls up stairs
Adaptive:	Makes tower of 3 cubes; makes a line with crayon; inserts pellet in bottle
Language:	Jargon; follows simple commands; may name a familiar object (ball)
Social:	Indicates some desires or needs by pointing; hugs parents
	18 Mo
Motor:	Runs stiffly; sits on small chair; walks up stairs with one hand held; explores drawers and wastebaskets
Adaptive:	Makes a tower of 4 cubes; imitates scribbling; imitates vertical stroke; dumps pellet from bottle
Language:	10 words (average); names pictures; identifies one or more parts of body
Social:	Feeds self; seeks help when in trouble; may complain when wet or soiled; kisses parent with pucker
	24 Mo
Motor:	Runs well, walks up and down stairs, one step at a time; opens doors; climbs on furniture; jumps
Adaptive:	Tower of 7 cubes (6 at 21 mo); circular scribbling; imitates horizontal stroke; folds paper once imitatively
Language:	Puts 3 words together (subject, verb, object)
Social:	Handles spoon well; often tells immediate experiences; helps to undress; listens to stories with pictures
	30 Mo
Motor:	Goes up stairs alternating feet
Adaptive:	Tower of 9 cubes; makes vertical and horizontal strokes but generally will not join them to make a cross; imitates circular stroke, forming closed figure
Language:	Refers to self by pronoun "I"; knows full name
Social:	Helps put things away; pretends in play
	36 Mo
Motor:	Rides tricycle; stands momentarily on one foot
Adaptive:	Tower of 10 cubes; imitates construction of "bridge" of 3 cubes; copies a circle; imitates a cross
Language:	Knows age and sex; counts 3 objects correctly; repeats 3 numbers or a sentence of 6 syllables
Social:	Plays simple games (in "parallel" with other children); helps in dressing (unbuttons clothing and puts on shoes); washes hands
	48 Mo
Motor:	Hops on one foot; throws ball overhand; uses scissors to cut out pictures; climbs well
Adaptive:	Copies bridge from model; imitates construction of "gate" of 5 cubes; copies cross and square; draws a man with 2 to 4 parts besides head; names longer of 2 lines
Language:	Counts 4 pennies accurately; tells a story
Social:	Plays with several children with beginning of social interaction and role-playing; goes to toilet alone
	60 Mo
Motor:	Skips
Adaptive:	Draws triangle from copy; names heavier of 2 weights
Language:	Names 4 colors; repeats sentence of 10 syllables; counts 10 pennies correctly
Social:	Dresses and undresses; asks questions about meaning of words; domestic role-playing

**Data are derived from those of Gesell (as revised by Knobloch), Shirley, Provence, Wolf, Bailey, and others. After 5 yr the Stanford-Binet, Wechsler-Bellevue, and other scales offer the most precise estimates of developmental level. In order to have their greatest value, they should be administered only by an experienced and qualified person.*

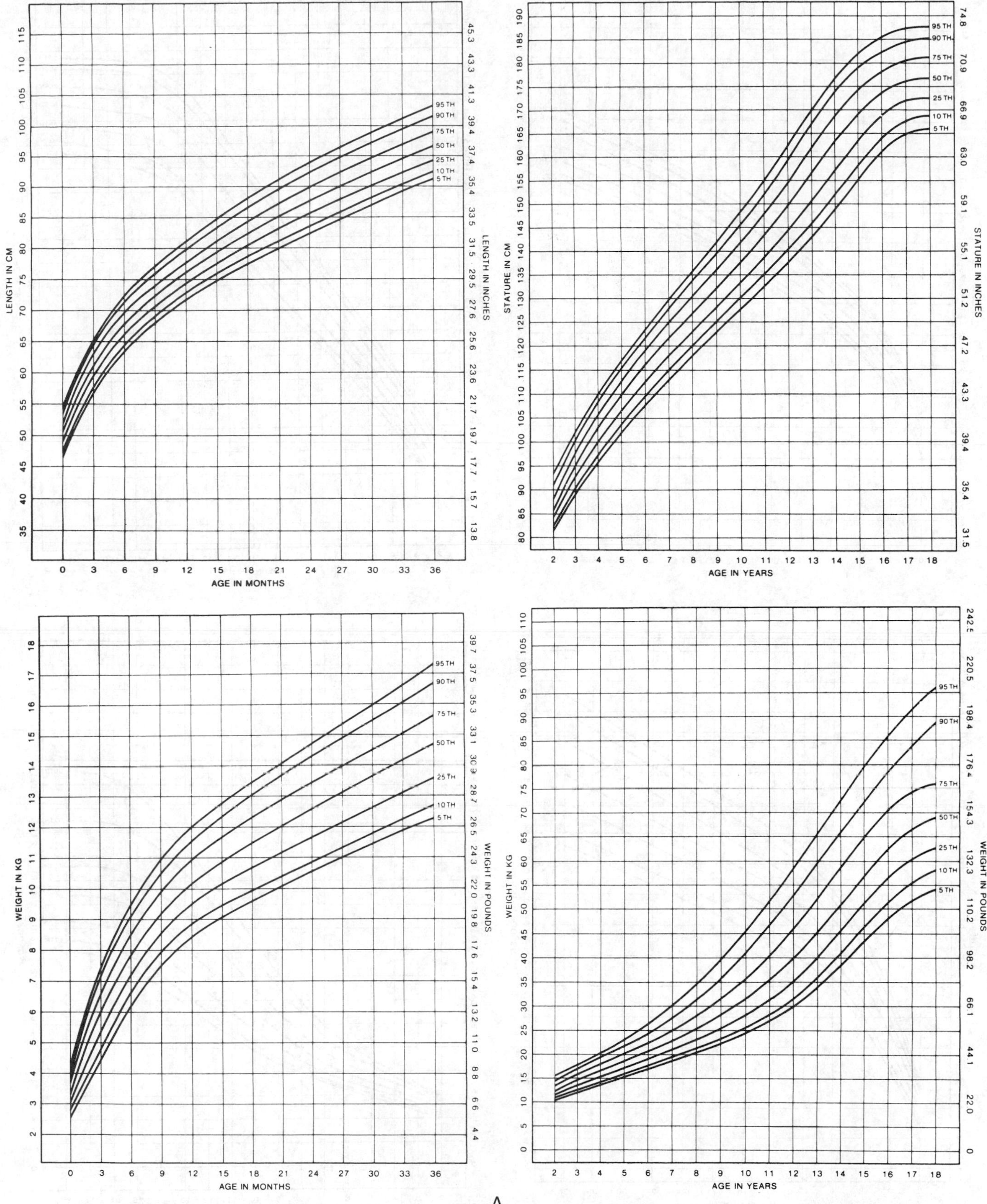

Figure 11–1 *A* and *B*, Charts for BOYS *(A)* and GIRLS *(B)* of length (or stature) by age *(upper curves)* and weight by age *(lower curves)*, each curve corresponding to the indicated percentile level. These charts are based on the data in Tables 10–2 and 12–1. (*A* and *B*, From Hamill PVV, Drizd TA, Johnson CL, et al: Physical growth: National Center for Health Statistics percentiles. Am J Clin Nutr 32:609, 1979.)

Illustration continued on following page

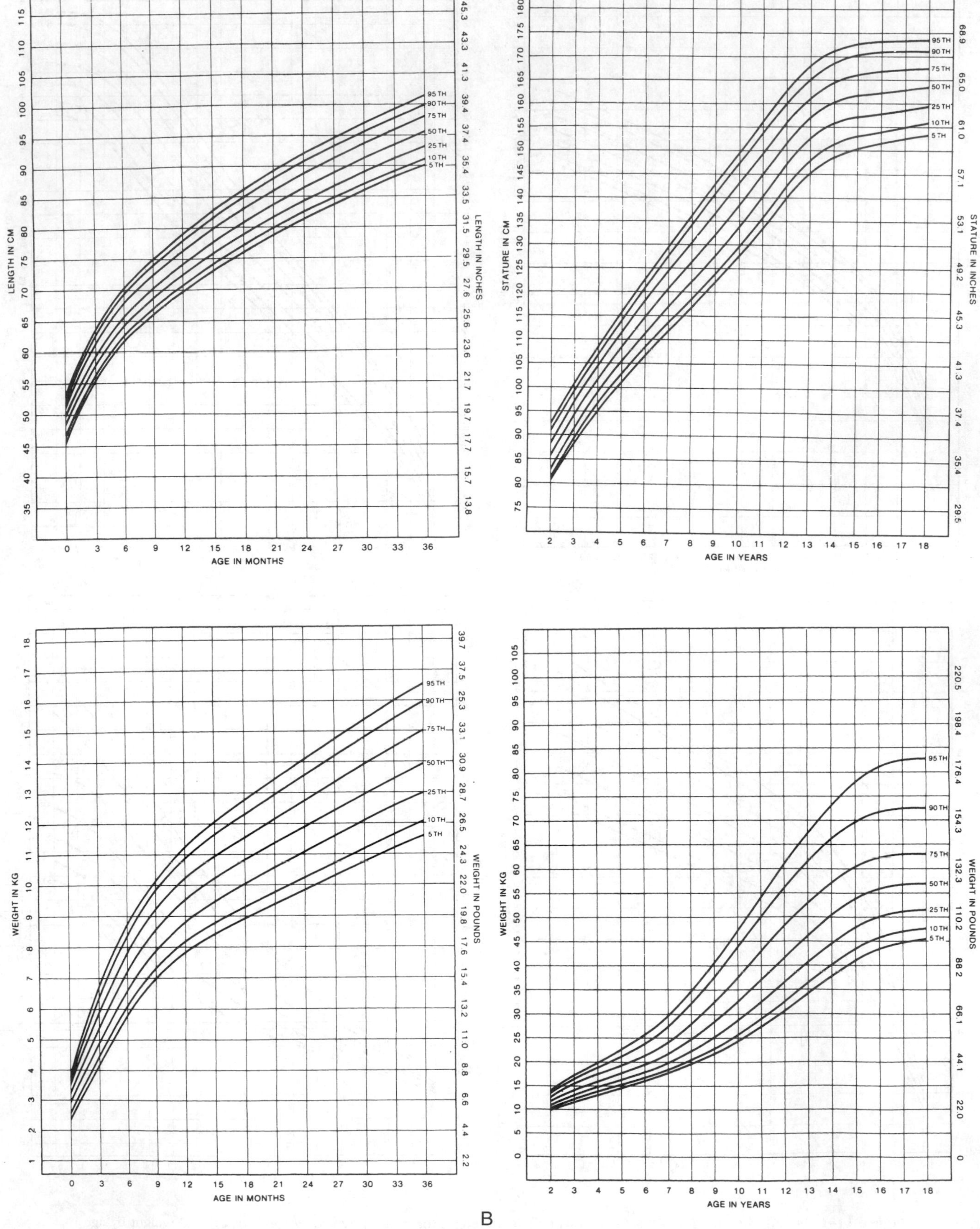

Figure 11–1 *Continued*

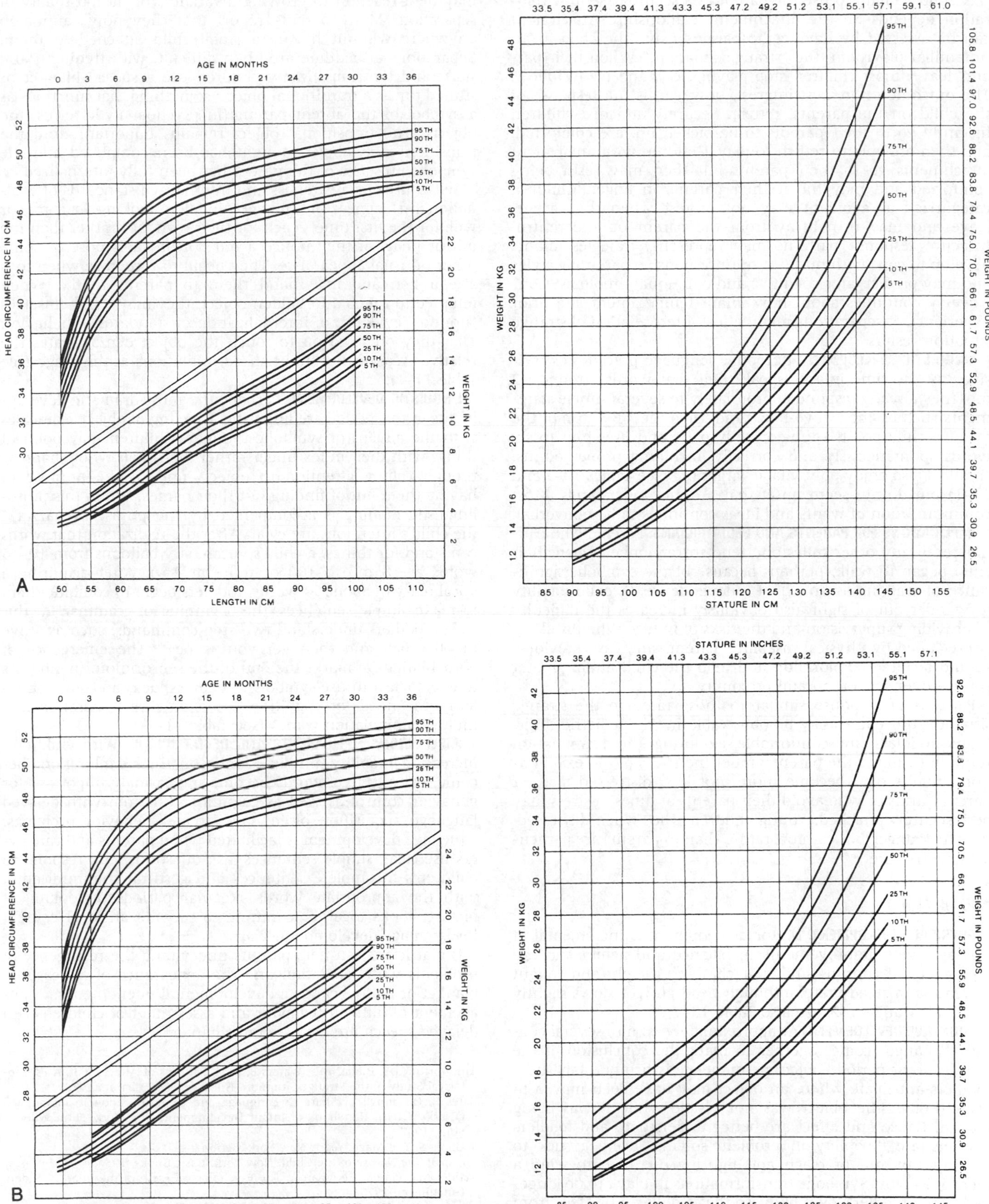

Figure 11–2 Charts for BOYS *(A)* and for GIRLS *(B)* of weight by length (or stature), for infants and young children *(left),* and for older (prepubertal) children *(right).* Head circumference by age is given for infants and young children *(upper left).* These charts are based on the data in Tables 10-2 and 12-1. (*A* and *B,* From Hamill PVV, Drizd TA, Johnson CL, et al: Physical growth: National Center for Health Statistics percentiles. Am J Clin Nutr 32:614, 1979.)

A child's ability to use the parent as a secure base for exploration depends on the attachment relationship. Attachment can be assessed by having the parents leave the child in an unfamiliar playroom, the "strange situation." When their parents leave, most children stop playing, cry, and try to follow. The outcome of greatest interest, however, is the response of the child on the parents' return. Securely attached children instantly go to their parents to be picked up, are comforted, and then are able to return to play. Children with ambivalent attachments go to their parents but then may resist being comforted and may hit at their parents in anger. Children categorized as avoidant may not protest when the parents leave and may turn away from the parent on the return. Insecure response patterns may represent strategies infants develop to cope with punitive or unresponsive parenting styles and may predict later cognitive and emotional problems. Controversy continues about how infant temperament and prior experience of separations might affect interpretation of strange situation results.

LINGUISTIC DEVELOPMENT. Receptive language precedes expressive. By the time infants speak their first words, around 12 mo, they already respond appropriately to several simple statements such as "no," "bye-bye," and "give me." By 15 mo, the average child points to major body parts and uses four to six words spontaneously and correctly, including proper nouns. Toddlers also enjoy polysyllabic jargoning (see Tables 10–3 and 11–1) but do not seem upset that no one understands. Most communication of wants and ideas continues to be nonverbal.

IMPLICATIONS FOR PARENTS AND PEDIATRICIANS. Parents who cannot recall any other milestone tend to remember when their child began to walk, perhaps because of the symbolic significance of walking as an act of independence. A child's ability to wander out of sight also obviously increases the difficulty of providing supervision and the risks of injury. When walking is precluded by physical disability, parents and care providers should facilitate exploration and help the child attain greater control over separation and proximity.

Patterns of response similar to those rated in the strange situation procedure may be observable in the pediatric clinic. Many toddlers are comfortable exploring the examination room but cling to the parents under the stress of the examination. Infants who become more, not less, distressed in their parents' arms or who avoid their parents at times of stress may be insecurely attached. Young children who, when distressed, turn to strangers for comfort rather than to parents are particularly worrisome.

AGE 18–24 MO

PHYSICAL DEVELOPMENT. Motor development is incremental at this age, with improvements in balance and agility and the emergence of running and stair climbing. Height and weight increase at a steady rate, although head growth slows slightly (Figs. 11–1 and 11–2; see also Table 10–5).

COGNITIVE DEVELOPMENT. At approximately 18 mo, several cognitive changes come together to mark the conclusion of the sensorimotor period. Object permanence is firmly established; toddlers anticipate where an object may have been moved to even though the object was not visible while it was being moved. Cause and effect are better understood, and toddlers demonstrate flexibility in problem solving, using a stick to obtain a toy out of reach and figuring out how to wind a mechanical toy. Symbolic transformations in play are no longer tied to the toddler's own body, so that a doll can be "fed" from an empty plate. Like the reorganization at 9 mo, the cognitive changes at 18 mo correlate with important changes in the emotional and linguistic domains (see Table 11–1).

EMOTIONAL DEVELOPMENT. In many children, the relative independence of the preceding period gives way to increased clinginess around 18 mo. This stage, described as *rapprochement,* may be a reaction to growing awareness of the possibility of separation. Many parents report that they now cannot go anywhere without having a small child attached to them. Separations at bedtime are often difficult, with frequent false starts and tantrums. Many children use a special blanket or stuffed toy as a transitional object: something that functions as a symbol of the absent parent (in psychoanalytic terms, the object). The transitional object remains important until the transition to symbolic thought has been completed and the symbolic presence of the parent has been fully internalized.

Self-conscious awareness and internalized standards of evaluation first appear at this age. Toddlers looking in a mirror will, for the first time, reach for their own face rather than the mirror image if they notice a red dot on their nose or some other unusual appearance. They begin to recognize when toys are broken and may hand them to parents to fix. When tempted to touch a forbidden object, they may tell themselves "no, no," evidence of internalization of standards of behavior. That they often go on to touch the object demonstrates the relative weakness of internalized inhibitions at this stage (see Table 11–1).

LINGUISTIC DEVELOPMENT. Perhaps the most dramatic developments in this period are linguistic. Labeling of objects coincides with the advent of symbolic thought. Children may point at things with their index finger rather than their whole hand as though calling attention to objects not for the purpose of having them but of finding out their names. When this protolinguistic naming is accompanied by the phrase "Whazzat?" the child's intentions are clear. After the realization that words can stand for things, a child's vocabulary balloons from 10–15 words at 18 mo to 100 or more at 2 yr. After acquiring a vocabulary of about 50 words, toddlers begin to combine them to make simple sentences, the beginning of grammar. At this stage, toddlers understand two-step commands, such as "Give me the ball and then get your shoes." The emergence of verbal language marks the end of the sensorimotor period. As toddlers learn to use symbols to express ideas and solve problems, the need for cognition based on direct sensation and motor manipulation wanes (see Table 11–1).

IMPLICATIONS FOR PARENTS AND PEDIATRICIANS. With children's increasing mobility, physical limits on their explorations become less effective; words become increasingly important for behavior control as well as cognition. Children with delayed language acquisition often have greater behavior problems. Language development is facilitated when parents and caregivers use clear, simple sentences, ask questions, and respond to children's incomplete sentences and gestural communication with the appropriate words. Regular periods of looking at picture books together continue to provide an ideal context for language development.

Pediatricians can help parents understand the resurgence of problems with separation and the appearance of a treasured blanket or teddy bear as a developmental phenomenon. Management of difficult behavior and assessment of children with delayed speech are discussed in Chapter 12.

Ainsworth MDS, Blehar MC, Waters E, et al: Patterns of Attachment: A Psychological Study of the Strange Situation. Hillsdale, NJ, Erlbaum, 1978.

Bates E, O'Connell B, Share C: Language and communication in infancy. *In:* Osofsky J (ed): Handbook of Infant Development. New York, John Wiley & Sons, 1987.

Fraiberg S: The Magic Years. New York, Scribner's, 1959.

Kagan J: The Nature of the Child. New York, Basic Books, 1984.

Mahler MS, Pine S, Bergman A: The Psychological Birth of the Infant. London, Hutchinson, 1975.

CHAPTER 12
Preschool Years

Between 2 and 5 yr of age, the core issues of attachment and separation are reshaped by the emergence of language and played out in the context of a widening social sphere. As a toddler, a child learned to walk away and come back. As a preschooler, he or she explores emotional separation, alternating between strident opposition and clinging dependence. Increasing time spent in classrooms and playgrounds challenges a child's ability to adapt to new rules and relationships. Tension between a child's growing sense of autonomy and the awareness of internal and external limitations defines the central dynamic of this age. This tension is affected by and in turn affects development in many domains.

PHYSICAL DEVELOPMENT (Tables 12–1 and 12–2)

By the end of the 2nd yr, somatic and brain growth slows, with corresponding decreases in nutritional requirements and in appetite (see Table 10–5). Between the ages of 2 and 5 yr, the average child gains approximately 2 kg in weight and 7 cm in height per year. The toddler's prominent abdomen flattens, and the body becomes leaner. Physical energy peaks, and the need for sleep declines to 11–13 hr/24 hr, usually including one nap (see Fig. 10–1). Visual acuity reaches 20/30 by age 3 yr and 20/20 by age 4. All 20 primary teeth have erupted by 3 yr of age (see Table 10–6).

Gross and fine motor milestones are presented in Table 10–4. Most children walk with a mature gait and run steadily before the end of their 3rd yr. Beyond this basic level, there is wide variation in ability as the range of motor activities expands to include throwing, catching, and kicking balls; riding on bicycles; climbing on playground structures; dancing; and other complex-pattern behaviors. Stylistic features of gross motor activity, such as tempo, intensity, and cautiousness, also vary largely because of inborn predilection. Toe walking, if it persists, may be associated with developmental delays, particularly of speech and language.

The effects of such individual differences on cognitive and emotional development depend in part on the demands of the social environment. Energetic, coordinated children may thrive emotionally with parents who encourage physical activity; lower energy, more cerebral children may thrive with parents who value quiet play.

Handedness is usually established by the 3rd yr. Frustration may result from attempts to change children's hand preference. Variations in fine motor development reflect both individual proclivities and different opportunities for learning. Children who are seldom allowed to use crayons, for example, develop mature pencil grasp later.

Bowel and bladder control emerge during this period (average age 30 mo, with large individual and cultural variation). Daytime bladder control typically precedes bowel control, and girls precede boys. Bed-wetting is normal up to age 4 in girls, 5 in boys (see Chapters 20 and 551). Many children master toileting with ease, particularly once they are able to verbalize their bodily needs. For others, toilet training can involve a protracted power struggle. Refusal to defecate in the toilet or potty is relatively common and can lead to constipation and parental frustration. Defusing the issue by a temporary cessation of training (and return to diapers) often allows toilet mastery to proceed.

IMPLICATIONS FOR PARENTS AND PEDIATRICIANS. The normal decrease in appetite at this age often arouses worry about nutrition. For the most part, parents can be reassured that if growth is normal, the child's intake is adequate. Children normally modulate their food intake to match their somatic needs according to feelings of hunger or satiety. Daily intake fluctuates, at times widely, but intake during the period of a week is relatively stable. Parental attempts to control the child's intake interfere with this self-regulatory mechanism as the child must either accede to or rebel against the pressure. The result may be either overeating or undereating.

Motorically precocious, highly active children face increased risks of injury. Parents of such children benefit from early guidance about the need for childproofing the home, constant supervision, and bicycle helmet use (beginning with the tricycle). Parental concerns about possible hyperactivity may reflect inappropriate expectations, heightened fears, or true overactivity. Children who engage in reckless, uncontrollable activity with no apparent regard for personal safety need a safe environment with close supervision. This pattern of indiscriminate activity is sometimes seen among children who have suffered abuse or neglect.

LANGUAGE, COGNITION, AND PLAY

These three domains all involve the symbolic function, a mode of dealing with the world that emerges during the preschool period.

LANGUAGE. Language development occurs most rapidly between 2 and 5 yr of age. Vocabulary increases from 50–100 words to more than 2,000. Sentence structure advances from telegraphic phrases ("Baby cry") to sentences incorporating all of the major grammatical components. As a rule of thumb, between age 2 and 5, the number of words in a typical sentence equals the child's age (2 by age 2, 3 by age and so on.) By $2\frac{1}{2}$, most children are using possessives ("My ball"), progressives (the "ing" construction, as in "I playing"), questions, and negatives. By 4 they can count to 4 and use the past tense; by 5 they can use the future tense.

An important distinction is between speech, the production of intelligible sounds, and language, the underlying mental act. Language includes both expressive and receptive functions. Receptive language (understanding) varies less in its rate of acquisition than does expressive language and therefore has greater prognostic importance. Language assessment is described more fully in Chapters 16 and 29.

Language acquisition depends critically on environmental input. Key determinants include the amount and variety of speech directed toward children and the frequency with which adults ask questions and encourage verbalization. Striking differences in these parameters between upper- and lower-class parents parallel class-related disparities in preschool language development and later school achievement.

Although experience determines the rate of language development, increasing evidence shows that the basic mechanism for language learning is "hard-wired" in the brain. Children do not simply imitate adult speech. Rather, they abstract the complex rules of grammar from the ambient language, generating implicit hypotheses. Evidence for the existence of such implicit rules comes from analysis of grammatical errors, such as the overgeneralized use of "s" to signify the plural and "ed" to signify the past (e.g., "We seed lots of mouses"). Children have an inborn propensity to create language. For example, deaf orphans raised by nonsigning adults were observed to invent their own sign language, including all of the essential grammar.

Language is a critical barometer of both cognitive and emotional development. Mental retardation may first become apparent with delayed speech at approximately 2 yr. Child abuse and neglect are correlated with delayed language, particularly the ability to convey emotional states. Language plays a critical part in the regulation of behavior through internalized "private

TABLE 12–1 Percentiles of Stature and Weight by Age*

Age (Yr)	5th		10th		25th		50th		75th		90th		95th	
Boys: 2–18 Yr														
2.0†	82.50	(32½)	83.50	(32¾)	85.30	(33½)	86.80	(34¼)	89.20	(35)	92.00	(36¼)	94.40	(37¼)
	10.49	(23¼)	10.96	(24¼)	11.55	(25½)	12.34	(27¼)	13.36	(29½)	14.38	(31¾)	15.50	(34¼)
2.5†	85.40	(33½)	86.50	(34)	88.50	(34¾)	90.40	(35½)	92.90	(36½)	95.60	(37¾)	97.80	(38½)
	11.27	(24¾)	11.77	(26)	12.55	(27¾)	13.52	(29¾)	14.61	(32¼)	15.71	(34¾)	16.61	(36½)
3.0	89.00	(35)	90.30	(35½)	92.60	(36½)	94.90	(37¼)	97.50	(38½)	100.10	(39½)	102.00	(40¼)
	12.05	(26½)	12.58	(27¾)	13.12	(29¾)	14.62	(32¼)	15.78	(34¾)	16.95	(37¼)	17.77	(39¼)
3.5	92.50	(36½)	93.90	(37)	96.40	(38)	99.10	(39)	101.70	(40)	104.30	(41¼)	106.10	(41¾)
	12.84	(28¼)	13.41	(29½)	14.46	(32)	15.68	(34½)	16.90	(37¼)	18.15	(40)	18.98	(41¾)
4.0	95.80	(37¾)	97.30	(38¼)	100.00	(39¼)	102.90	(40½)	105.70	(41½)	108.20	(42½)	109.90	(43¼)
	13.64	(30)	14.24	(31½)	15.39	(34)	16.69	(36¾)	17.99	(39¾)	19.32	(42½)	20.27	(44¾)
4.5	98.90	(39)	100.60	(39½)	103.40	(40¾)	106.60	(42)	109.40	(43)	111.90	(44)	113.50	(44¾)
	14.45	(31¾)	15.10	(33¼)	16.30	(36)	17.69	(39)	19.06	(42)	20.50	(45¼)	21.63	(47¾)
5.0	102.00	(40¼)	103.70	(40¾)	106.50	(42)	109.90	(43¼)	112.80	(44½)	115.40	(45½)	117.00	(46)
	15.27	(33¾)	15.96	(35¾)	17.22	(38)	18.67	(41¼)	20.14	(44½)	21.70	(47¾)	23.09	(51)
5.5	104.90	(41¼)	106.70	(42)	109.60	(43¼)	113.10	(44½)	116.10	(45¾)	118.70	(46¾)	120.30	(47¼)
	16.09	(35½)	16.83	(37)	18.14	(40)	19.67	(43¼)	21.25	(46¾)	22.96	(50½)	24.66	(54¼)
6.0	107.70	(42½)	109.60	(43¼)	112.50	(44¼)	116.10	(45¾)	119.20	(47)	121.90	(48)	123.50	(48½)
	16.93	(37¼)	17.72	(39)	19.07	(42)	20.69	(45½)	22.40	(49½)	24.31	(53½)	26.34	(58)
6.5	110.40	(43½)	112.30	(44¼)	115.30	(45½)	119.00	(46¾)	122.20	(48)	124.90	(49¼)	126.60	(49¾)
	17.78	(39¼)	18.62	(41)	20.02	(44¼)	21.74	(48)	23.62	(52)	25.76	(56¾)	28.16	(62)
7.0	113.00	(44½)	115.00	(45¼)	118.00	(46½)	121.70	(48)	125.00	(49¼)	127.90	(50¼)	129.70	(51)
	18.64	(41)	19.53	(43)	21.00	(46¼)	22.85	(50¼)	24.94	(55)	27.36	(60¼)	30.12	(66½)
7.5	115.60	(45½)	117.60	(46¼)	120.60	(47½)	124.40	(49)	127.80	(50¼)	130.80	(51½)	132.70	(52¼)
	19.52	(43)	20.45	(45)	22.02	(48½)	24.03	(53)	26.36	(58)	29.11	(64¼)	32.73	(72¼)
8.0	118.10	(46½)	120.20	(47¼)	123.20	(48½)	127.00	(50)	130.50	(51½)	133.60	(52½)	135.70	(53½)
	20.40	(45)	21.39	(47¼)	22.09	(51)	25.30	(55¾)	27.91	(61½)	31.06	(68½)	34.51	(76)
8.5	120.50	(47½)	122.70	(48¼)	125.70	(49½)	129.60	(51)	133.20	(52½)	136.50	(53¾)	138.80	(54¾)
	21.31	(47)	22.34	(49¼)	24.21	(53¼)	26.66	(58¾)	29.61	(65¼)	33.22	(73¼)	36.96	(81½)
9.0	122.90	(48½)	125.20	(49¼)	128.20	(50½)	132.20	(52)	136.00	(53½)	139.40	(55)	141.80	(55¾)
	22.25	(49)	23.33	(51½)	25.40	(56)	28.13	(62)	31.46	(69¼)	35.57	(78½)	39.58	(87¾)
9.5	125.30	(49¼)	127.60	(50¼)	130.80	(51½)	134.80	(53)	138.80	(54¾)	142.40	(56)	144.90	(57)
	23.25	(51¼)	24.38	(53¾)	26.88	(58¾)	29.73	(65½)	33.46	(73¾)	38.11	(84)	42.35	(93¼)
10.0	127.70	(50¼)	130.10	(51¼)	133.40	(52½)	137.50	(54¼)	141.60	(55¾)	145.50	(57¼)	148.10	(58¼)
	24.33	(53¾)	25.52	(56¼)	28.07	(62)	31.44	(69¼)	35.61	(78½)	40.80	(90)	45.27	(99¾)
10.5	130.10	(51¼)	132.60	(52¼)	136.00	(53½)	140.30	(55¼)	144.60	(57)	148.70	(58½)	151.50	(59¾)
	25.51	(56¼)	26.78	(59)	29.59	(65¼)	33.30	(73½)	37.92	(83½)	43.63	(96¼)	48.31	(106½)
11.0	132.60	(52¼)	135.10	(53¼)	138.70	(54½)	143.33	(56½)	147.80	(58¼)	152.10	(60)	154.90	(61)
	26.80	(59)	28.17	(62)	31.25	(69)	35.30	(77¾)	40.38	(89)	46.57	(102¾)	51.47	(113½)
11.5	135.00	(53¼)	137.70	(54½)	141.50	(55¾)	146.40	(57¾)	151.10	(59½)	155.60	(61¼)	158.50	(62½)
	28.24	(62¼)	29.72	(65½)	33.08	(73)	37.46	(82½)	43.00	(94¾)	49.61	(109¼)	54.73	(120¾)
12.0	137.60	(54¼)	140.30	(55¼)	144.40	(56¾)	149.70	(59)	154.60	(60¾)	159.40	(62¾)	162.30	(64)
	29.85	(65¾)	31.46	(69¼)	35.09	(77¼)	39.78	(87¾)	45.77	(101)	52.73	(116¼)	58.09	(128)
12.5	140.20	(55¼)	143.00	(56¼)	147.40	(58)	153.00	(60¼)	158.20	(62¼)	163.20	(64¼)	166.10	(65½)
	31.64	(69¾)	33.41	(73¾)	37.31	(82¼)	42.27	(93¼)	48.70	(107¼)	55.91	(123¼)	61.52	(135¾)
13.0	142.90	(56¼)	145.80	(57½)	150.50	(59¼)	156.50	(61½)	161.80	(63¾)	167.00	(65¾)	169.80	(66¾)
	33.64	(74¼)	35.60	(78½)	39.74	(87½)	44.95	(99)	51.79	(114¼)	59.12	(130¼)	65.02	(143¼)
13.5	145.70	(57¼)	148.70	(58½)	153.60	(60½)	159.90	(63)	165.30	(65)	170.50	(67¼)	173.40	(68¼)
	35.85	(79)	38.03	(83¾)	42.40	(93½)	47.81	(105½)	55.02	(121¼)	62.35	(137½)	68.51	(151)
14.0	148.80	(58½)	151.80	(59¾)	156.90	(61¾)	63.10	(64¼)	168.50	(66¼)	173.80	(68½)	176.70	(69½)
	38.22	(84¼)	40.64	(89½)	45.21	(99¾)	50.77	(112)	58.31	(128½)	65.57	(144½)	72.13	(159)
14.5	152.00	(59¾)	155.00	(61)	160.10	(63)	166.20	(65½)	171.50	(67½)	176.60	(69½)	179.50	(70½)
	40.66	(89¾)	43.34	(95½)	48.08	(106)	53.76	(118½)	61.58	(135¾)	68.76	(151½)	75.66	(166¾)
15.0	155.20	(61)	158.20	(62¼)	163.30	(64¼)	169.00	(66½)	174.10	(68½)	178.90	(70½)	181.90	(71½)
	43.11	(95)	46.06	(101½)	50.92	(112¼)	56.71	(125)	64.72	(142¾)	71.91	(158½)	79.12	(174½)

TABLE 12–1 Percentiles of Stature and Weight by Age* *Continued*

Age (Yr)	5th		10th		25th		50th		75th		90th		95th	
15.5	158.30	(62¼)	161.20	(63½)	166.20	(65½)	171.50	(67½)	176.30	(69½)	180.80	(71¼)	183.90	(72½)
	45.50	(100¼)	48.69	(107¼)	53.64	(118¼)	59.51	(131¼)	67.64	(149)	74.98	(165¼)	82.45	(181¾)
16.0	161.10	(63½)	163.90	(64½)	168.70	(66½)	173.50	(68¼)	178.10	(70)	182.40	(71¾)	185.40	(73)
	47.74	(105¼)	51.16	(112¾)	56.16	(123¾)	62.10	(137)	70.26	(155)	77.97	(172)	85.62	(188¾)
16.5	163.40	(64¼)	166.10	(65½)	170.60	(67¼)	175.20	(69)	179.50	(70¾)	183.60	(72¼)	186.60	(73½)
	49.76	(109¾)	53.39	(117¾)	58.38	(128¾)	64.39	(142)	72.46	(159¾)	80.84	(178¼)	88.59	(195¼)
17.0	164.90	(65)	167.70	(66)	171.90	(67¾)	176.20	(69¼)	180.50	(71)	184.40	(72½)	187.30	(73¾)
	51.50	(113½)	55.28	(121¾)	60.22	(132¾)	66.31	(146¼)	74.17	(163½)	83.58	(184¼)	91.31	(201¼)
17.5	165.60	(65¼)	168.50	(66¼)	172.40	(67¾)	176.70	(69½)	181.00	(71¼)	185.00	(72¾)	187.60	(73¾)
	52.89	(116½)	56.78	(125¼)	61.61	(135¾)	67.78	(149½)	75.32	(166)	86.14	(190)	93.73	(206¾)
18.0	165.70	(65¼)	168.70	(66½)	172.30	(67¾)	176.80	(69½)	181.20	(71¼)	185.30	(73)	187.60	(73¾)
	53.97	(119)	57.89	(127½)	62.61	(138)	68.88	(151¾)	76.00	(167¾)	88.41	(195)	95.76	(211)
Girls: 2–18 Yr														
2.0	81.60	(32¼)	82.10	(32¼)	84.00	(33)	86.80	(34¼)	89.30	(35¼)	92.00	(36¼)	93.60	(36¾)
	9.95	(22)	10.32	(22¾)	10.96	(24¼)	11.80	(26)	12.73	(28)	13.58	(30)	14.15	(31¼)
2.5	84.60	(33¼)	85.30	(33½)	87.30	(34½)	90.00	(35½)	92.50	(36½)	95.00	(37½)	96.60	(38)
	10.80	(23¾)	11.35	(25)	12.11	(26¾)	13.03	(28¾)	14.23	(31¼)	15.16	(33½)	15.76	(34¾)
3.0	88.30	(34¾)	89.30	(35¼)	91.40	(36)	94.10	(37)	96.60	(38)	99.00	(39)	100.60	(39½)
	11.61	(25½)	12.26	(27)	13.11	(29)	14.10	(31)	15.50	(34¼)	16.54	(36½)	17.22	(38)
3.5	91.70	(36)	93.00	(36½)	95.20	(37½)	97.90	(38½)	100.50	(39½)	102.80	(40½)	104.50	(41¼)
	12.37	(27¼)	13.08	(28¾)	14.00	(30¾)	15.07	(33¼)	16.59	(36½)	17.77	(39¼)	18.59	(41)
4.0	95.00	(37½)	96.40	(38)	98.80	(39)	101.60	(40)	104.30	(41)	106.60	(42)	108.30	(42¾)
	13.11	(29)	13.84	(30½)	14.80	(32¾)	15.96	(35¼)	17.56	(38¾)	18.93	(41¾)	19.91	(44)
4.5	98.10	(38½)	99.70	(39¼)	102.20	(40¼)	105.00	(41¼)	107.90	(42½)	110.20	(43½)	112.00	(44)
	13.83	(30½)	14.56	(32)	15.55	(34¾)	16.81	(37)	18.48	(40¾)	20.06	(44¼)	21.24	(46¾)
5.0	101.10	(39¾)	102.70	(40½)	105.40	(41½)	108.40	(42¾)	111.40	(43¾)	113.80	(44¾)	115.60	(45½)
	14.55	(32)	15.26	(33¾)	16.29	(36)	17.66	(39)	19.39	(42¾)	21.23	(46¾)	22.62	(49¾)
5.5	103.90	(41)	105.60	(41½)	108.40	(42¾)	111.60	(44)	114.80	(45¼)	117.40	(46¼)	119.20	(47)
	15.29	(33¾)	15.97	(35¼)	17.05	(37½)	18.56	(41)	20.36	(45)	24.48	(49½)	24.11	(53¼)
6.0	106.60	(42)	108.40	(42¾)	111.30	(43¾)	114.60	(45)	118.10	(46½)	120.80	(47½)	122.70	(48¼)
	16.05	(35½)	16.72	(36¾)	17.86	(39¼)	19.52	(43)	21.44	(47¼)	23.89	(52¾)	25.75	(56¾)
6.5	109.20	(43)	111.00	(43¾)	114.10	(45)	117.60	(46¼)	121.30	(47¾)	124.20	(49)	126.10	(49¾)
	16.85	(37¼)	17.51	(38½)	18.76	(41¼)	20.61	(45½)	22.68	(50)	25.50	(56¼)	27.59	(60¾)
7.0	111.80	(44)	113.60	(44¾)	116.80	(46)	120.60	(47½)	124.40	(49)	127.60	(50¼)	129.50	(51)
	17.71	(39)	18.39	(40½)	19.78	(43½)	21.84	(48¼)	24.16	(53¼)	27.39	(60½)	29.68	(65½)
7.5	114.40	(45)	116.20	(45¾)	119.50	(47)	123.50	(48½)	127.50	(50¼)	130.90	(51½)	132.90	(52¼)
	18.62	(41)	19.37	(42¾)	20.95	(46¼)	23.26	(51¼)	25.90	(57)	29.57	(65¼)	32.07	(70¾)
8.0	116.90	(46)	118.70	(46¾)	122.20	(48)	126.40	(49¾)	130.60	(51½)	134.20	(52¾)	136.20	(53½)
	19.62	(43¼)	20.45	(45)	22.26	(49)	24.84	(54¾)	27.88	(61½)	32.04	(70¾)	34.71	(76½)
8.5	119.50	(47)	121.30	(47¾)	124.90	(49¼)	129.30	(51)	133.60	(52½)	137.40	(54)	139.60	(55)
	20.68	(45½)	21.64	(47¾)	23.70	(52¼)	26.58	(58½)	30.08	(66¼)	34.73	(76½)	37.58	(82¾)
9.0	122.10	(48)	123.90	(48¾)	127.70	(50¼)	132.20	(52)	136.70	(53¾)	140.70	(55½)	142.90	(56¼)
	21.82	(48)	22.92	(50½)	25.27	(55¾)	28.46	(62¾)	32.44	(71½)	37.60	(83)	40.64	(89½)
9.5	124.80	(49¼)	126.60	(49¾)	130.60	(51½)	135.20	(53¼)	139.80	(55)	143.90	(56¾)	146.20	(57½)
	23.05	(50¾)	24.29	(53½)	26.94	(59½)	30.45	(67¼)	34.94	(77)	40.61	(89½)	43.85	(96¾)
10.0	127.50	(50¼)	129.50	(51)	133.60	(52½)	138.30	(54½)	142.90	(56¼)	147.20	(58)	149.50	(58¾)
	24.36	(53¾)	25.76	(56¾)	28.71	(63¼)	32.55	(71¾)	37.53	(82¾)	43.70	(96¼)	47.17	(104)
10.5	130.40	(51¼)	132.50	(52¼)	136.70	(53¾)	141.50	(55¾)	146.10	(57½)	150.40	(59¼)	152.80	(60¼)
	25.75	(56¾)	27.32	(60¼)	30.57	(67½)	34.72	(76½)	40.17	(88½)	46.84	(103¼)	50.57	(111½)
11.0	133.50	(52½)	135.60	(53½)	140.00	(55)	144.80	(57)	149.30	(58¾)	153.70	(60½)	56.20	(61½)
	27.24	(60)	28.97	(63¾)	32.49	(71¾)	36.95	(81½)	42.84	(94½)	49.96	(110¼)	54.00	(119)
11.5	136.60	(53¾)	139.00	(54¾)	143.50	(56½)	148.20	(58¼)	152.60	(60)	156.90	(61¾)	159.50	(62¾)
	28.83	(63½)	30.71	(67¾)	34.48	(76)	39.23	(86½)	45.48	(100¼)	53.03	(117)	57.42	(126½)
12.0	139.80	(55)	142.30	(56)	147.00	(57¾)	151.50	(59¾)	155.80	(61¼)	160.00	(63)	162.70	(64)
	30.52	(67¼)	32.53	(71¼)	36.52	(80½)	41.53	(91½)	48.07	(106)	55.99	(123½)	60.81	(134)

Table continued on following page

TABLE 12–1 Percentiles of Stature and Weight by Age* *Continued*

Age (Yr)	5th		10th		25th		50th		75th		90th		95th	
12.5	142.70	(56½)	145.40	(57¼)	150.10	(59)	154.60	(60¾)	158.80	(62½)	162.90	(64½)	165.60	(65¼)
	32.30	(71¾)	34.42	(76)	38.59	(85)	43.84	(96¾)	50.56	(111½)	58.81	(129¾)	64.12	(141¼)
13.0	145.20	(57¼)	148.00	(58¼)	152.80	(60¼)	157.10	(61¾)	161.30	(63½)	165.30	(65)	168.10	(66¼)
	34.14	(75¼)	36.35	(80¼)	40.55	(89½)	46.10	(101¾)	52.91	(116¾)	61.45	(135½)	67.30	(148¼)
13.5	147.20	(58)	150.00	(59)	154.70	(61)	159.00	(62½)	163.20	(64¼)	167.30	(65¾)	170.00	(67)
	35.98	(79¼)	38.26	(84¼)	42.65	(94)	48.26	(106½)	55.11	(121½)	63.87	(140¾)	70.30	(155)
14.0	148.70	(58½)	151.50	(59¾)	155.90	(61½)	160.40	(63¼)	164.60	(64¾)	168.70	(66½)	171.30	(67½)
	37.76	(83¼)	40.11	(88½)	44.54	(98¼)	50.28	(110¾)	57.09	(125¾)	66.04	(145½)	73.08	(161)
14.5	149.70	(59)	152.50	(60)	158.80	(61¾)	161.20	(63½)	165.60	(65¼)	169.80	(66¾)	172.20	(67¾)
	39.45	(87)	41.83	(92¼)	46.28	(102)	52.10	(114¾)	58.84	(129¾)	67.95	(149¾)	75.59	(166¾)
15.0	150.50	(59¼)	153.20	(60¼)	157.20	(62)	161.80	(63¾)	166.30	(65¼)	170.50	(67¼)	172.80	(68)
	40.99	(90¼)	43.38	(95¾)	47.82	(105½)	53.68	(118¼)	60.32	(133)	69.54	(153¼)	77.78	(171½)
15.5	151.10	(59½)	153.60	(60½)	157.50	(62)	162.10	(63¾)	166.70	(65¾)	170.90	(67¼)	173.10	(68¼)
	42.32	(93¼)	44.72	(98½)	49.10	(108¼)	54.96	(121¼)	61.48	(135½)	70.79	(156)	79.59	(176½)
16.0	151.60	(59¾)	154.10	(60¾)	157.80	(62¼)	162.40	(64)	166.90	(65¾)	171.10	(67¼)	173.30	(68¼)
	43.41	(95¾)	45.78	(101)	50.09	(110½)	55.89	(123¼)	62.29	(137¼)	71.68	(158)	80.99	(178½)
16.5	152.20	(60)	154.60	(60¾)	158.20	(62¼)	162.70	(64)	167.10	(65¾)	171.20	(67½)	173.40	(68¼)
	44.20	(97½)	46.54	(102½)	50.75	(112)	56.44	(124½)	62.75	(138¼)	72.18	(159¼)	81.93	(180½)
17.0	152.70	(60)	155.10	(61)	158.70	(62½)	163.10	(64¼)	167.30	(65¾)	171.20	(67½)	173.50	(68¼)
	44.74	(98¾)	47.04	(103¾)	51.14	(112¾)	56.69	(125)	62.91	(138¾)	72.38	(159½)	82.46	(181¾)
17.5	153.20	(60¼)	155.60	(61¼)	159.10	(62¾)	163.40	(64¼)	167.50	(66)	171.10	(67¼)	173.50	(68¼)
	45.08	(99½)	47.33	(104¼)	51.33	(113¼)	56.71	(125)	62.89	(138¾)	72.37	(159½)	82.62	(182¼)
18.0	153.60	(60½)	156.00	(61½)	159.60	(62¾)	163.70	(64½)	167.60	(66)	171.00	(67¼)	173.60	(68¼)
	45.26	(99¾)	47.47	(104¾)	51.39	(113¼)	56.62	(124¾)	62.78	(138½)	72.25	(159¼)	82.47	(181¾)

Stature measured in centimeters (inches); weight measured in kilograms (pounds).

**Data are those of the National Center for Health Statistics, Health Resources Administration, Department of Health, Education, and Welfare, collected in its Health Examination Surveys. Metric data have been smoothed by the least-squares cubic spline technique. For details see footnote to Table 10–2.*

†Stature data for 2.0–3.0 yr include some recumbent length measurements, which make values slightly higher than if all measurements had been of stature.

speech" in which a child repeats adult prohibitions first audibly and then mentally. Language also allows children to express feelings, such as anger or frustration, without acting them out; consequently, language-delayed children show higher rates of tantrums and other externalizing behaviors.

Preschool language development lays the foundation for later success in school. Approximately 35% of children in the United States may enter school lacking the language skills that are the prerequisites of literacy acquisition. Although most children learn to read and write in elementary school, critical foundations for literacy are established during the preschool years. Through repeated early exposure to written words, children learn about the uses of writing (telling stories or sending messages) and about its form (left to right, top to bottom). Early errors in writing, like errors in speaking, reveal that literacy acquisition is an active process involving hypothesis generation and revision. One hypothesis is that words that take longer to say ("big words") have more letters in them regardless of what the letters are. At a later stage, letters may be assigned one to a syllable, such as GNYS to spell "genius."

Picture books have a special role not only in familiarizing young children with the printed word but also in the development of verbal language. Reading aloud with a young child is an interactive process in which a parent focuses the child's attention on a particular picture, requests a response (by asking, "What's that?"), and then gives the child feedback ("Right, it's a dog."). This question-feedback routine is repeated many times in the course of reading a book. As a child's sophistication grows, the parent increases the complexity of the task, requesting descriptions ("What color is the dog?") and later projections ("What's that dog going to do?"). The elements of shared attention, active participation, immediate feedback, repetition, and graduated difficulty make such routines ideal for language learning.

COGNITION. The preschool period corresponds to Piaget's preoperational (prelogical) stage, characterized by magical thinking, egocentrism, and thinking that is dominated by perception (see Table 7–2). Magical thinking includes a confusion of coincidence for causality, animism (attributing motivations to inanimate objects and events), and unrealistic beliefs about the power of wishes. A child might believe that people cause it to rain by carrying umbrellas, that the sun goes down because it's tired, or that feeling resentment toward a sibling can actually make that sibling sick. Egocentrism refers to a child's inability to take another's point of view and does not connote selfishness. A child might try to comfort an upset adult by bringing a favorite stuffed animal.

Piaget demonstrated the dominance of perception over logic by a famous series of conservation experiments. In one, water was poured back and forth from a tall, thin vase to a low, wide dish and children were asked which container had more water. Invariably, they chose the one that looked larger (usually the tall vase), even when the examiner pointed out that no water had been added or taken away. Such misunderstandings reflect young children's developing hypotheses about the nature of the world as well as their difficulty in attending simultaneously to several aspects of a situation.

PLAY. During the preschool period, play is marked by increasing complexity and imagination, from simple scripts replicating common experiences such as shopping and putting baby to bed (age 2 or 3 yr) to more extended scenarios involving singular events such as going to the zoo or going on a trip (age 3 or 4 yr) to creation of scenarios that have only been imagined, such as flying to the moon (age 4 or 5 yr). A similar

TABLE 12–2 Weight by Length*

Recumbent Length	Boys: Weight Percentiles, kg and (lb)							Girls: Weight Percentiles, kg and (lb)						
	5th	*10th*	*25th*	*50th*	*75th*	*90th*	*95th*	*5th*	*10th*	*25th*	*50th*	*75th*	*90th*	*95th*
Boys and Girls Younger Than 4 Years†														
48–50 cm (19–19¾ in)			2.86 (6¼)	3.15 (7)	3.50 (7¾)					3.02 (6¾)	3.29 (7¼)	3.59 (8)		
50–52 cm (19¾–20½ in)			3.16 (7)	3.48 (7¾)	3.86 (8½)					3.25 (7¼)	3.55 (7¾)	3.89 (8½)		
52–54 cm (20½–21¼ in)			3.25 (7¾)	3.88 (8½)	4.28 (9½)					3.56 (7¾)	3.89 (8½)	4.26 (9½)		
54–56 cm (21¼–22 in)	3.49 (7¼)	3.65 (8)	3.95 (8¾)	4.34 (9½)	4.76 (10½)	5.13 (11¼)	5.33 (11¾)	3.54 (7¾)	3.64 (8)	3.93 (8¾)	4.29 (9½)	4.70 (10¼)	5.02 (11)	5.21 (11½)
56–58 cm (22–22¾ in)	3.90 (8½)	4.09 (9)	4.43 (9¾)	4.84 (10¾)	5.29 (11¾)	5.69 (12½)	5.88 (13)	3.93 (8¾)	4.05 (9)	4.37 (9¾)	4.76 (10½)	5.20 (11½)	5.55 (12¼)	5.77 (12¾)
58–60 cm (22¾–23½ in)	4.37 (9¾)	4.58 (10)	4.94 (11)	5.38 (11¾)	5.84 (12¾)	6.28 (13¾)	6.47 (14¼)	4.38 (9¾)	4.50 (10)	4.85 (10¾)	5.27 (11½)	5.73 (12¾)	6.12 (13½)	6.36 (14)
60–62 cm (23½–24½ in)	4.88 (10¾)	5.10 (11¼)	5.49 (12)	5.94 (13)	6.42 (14¼)	6.88 (15¼)	7.08 (15½)	4.85 (10¾)	4.99 (11)	5.37 (11¾)	5.82 (12¾)	6.30 (14)	6.70 (14¾)	6.95 (15¼)
62–64 cm (24½–25¼ in)	5.43 (12)	5.65 (12½)	6.05 (13¼)	6.52 (14¼)	7.02 (15½)	7.50 (16½)	7.72 (17)	5.35 (11¾)	5.50 (12)	5.91 (13)	6.39 (14)	6.89 (15¼)	7.30 (16)	7.55 (16¾)
64–66 cm (25¼–26 in)	5.99 (13¼)	6.20 (13¾)	6.62 (14½)	7.11 (15¾)	7.63 (16¾)	8.13 (18)	8.36 (8½)	5.87 (13)	6.03 (13¼)	6.47 (14¼)	6.97 (15¼)	7.48 (16½)	7.90 (17½)	8.15 (18)
66–68 cm (26–26¾ in)	6.55 (14½)	6.76 (15)	7.19 (15¾)	7.70 (17)	8.23 (18¼)	8.75 (19¼)	8.99 (19¾)	6.38 (14)	6.56 (14½)	7.02 (15½)	7.55 (16¾)	8.07 (17¾)	8.50 (18¾)	8.75 (19¼)
68–70 cm (26¾–27½ in)	7.10 (15¾)	7.31 (16)	7.75 (17)	8.27 (18¼)	8.82 (19½)	9.35 (20½)	9.62 (21¼)	6.89 (15¼)	7.08 (15½)	7.56 (16¾)	8.11 (17¾)	8.64 (19)	9.08 (20)	9.33 (20½)
70–72 cm (27½–28¼ in)	7.63 (16¾)	7.84 (17¼)	8.28 (18¼)	8.82 (19½)	9.39 (20¾)	9.93 (22)	10.21 (22½)	7.37 (16¼)	7.58 (16¾)	8.08 (17¾)	8.64 (19)	9.18 (20¼)	9.63 (21¼)	9.88 (21¾)
72–74 cm (28¼–29¼ in)	8.13 (18)	8.33 (18¼)	8.78 (19¼)	9.33 (20½)	9.92 (21¾)	10.48 (23)	10.77 (23¾)	7.82 (17¼)	8.05 (17¾)	8.56 (18¾)	9.14 (20¼)	9.68 (21¼)	10.15 (22½)	10.41 (23)
74–76 cm (29¼–30 in)	8.58 (19)	8.78 (19¼)	9.24 (20¼)	9.81 (21¾)	10.43 (23)	10.99 (24¼)	11.29 (25)	8.24 (18¼)	8.49 (18¾)	9.00 (19¾)	9.59 (21¼)	10.14 (22¼)	10.63 (23½)	10.91 (24)
76–78 cm (30–30¾ in)	9.00 (19¾)	9.21 (20¼)	9.68 (21¼)	10.27 (22¾)	10.91 (24)	11.48 (25¼)	11.78 (26)	8.62 (19)	8.90 (19½)	9.42 (20¾)	10.02 (22)	10.57 (23¼)	11.08 (24½)	11.39 (25)
78–80 cm (30¾–31½ in)	9.40 (20¾)	9.62 (21¼)	10.09 (22¼)	10.70 (23½)	11.36 (25)	11.94 (26¼)	12.25 (27)	8.99 (19¾)	9.29 (20½)	9.81 (21¾)	10.41 (23)	10.97 (24¼)	11.51 (25¼)	11.85 (26)
80–82 cm (31½–32¼ in)	9.77 (21½)	10.01 (22)	10.49 (23¼)	11.12 (24½)	11.80 (26)	12.39 (27¼)	12.69 (28)	9.34 (20½)	9.67 (21¼)	10.19 (22½)	10.80 (23¾)	11.37 (25)	11.93 (26¼)	12.29 (27)
82–84 cm (32¼–33 in)	10.14 (22¼)	10.39 (23)	10.88 (24)	11.53 (25½)	12.23 (27)	12.83 (28¼)	13.13 (29)	9.68 (21¼)	10.04 (22¼)	10.57 (23¼)	11.18 (24¾)	11.75 (26)	12.35 (27¼)	12.72 (28)
84–86 cm (33–33¾ in)	10.49 (23¼)	10.76 (23¾)	11.27 (24¾)	11.93 (26¼)	12.65 (28)	13.26 (29¼)	13.56 (30)	10.03 (22)	10.41 (23)	10.94 (24)	11.56 (25½)	12.15 (26¾)	12.76 (28¼)	13.15 (29)
86–88 cm (33¾–34¾ in)	10.85 (24)	11.14 (24½)	11.67 (25¾)	12.34 (27¼)	13.07 (28¾)	13.69 (30¼)	14.00 (30¾)	10.39 (23)	10.78 (23¾)	11.33 (25)	11.95 (26¼)	12.55 (27¾)	13.19 (29)	13.57 (30)
88–90 cm (34¾–35½ in)	11.22 (24¾)	11.53 (25½)	12.08 (26¾)	12.76 (28¼)	13.50 (29¾)	14.13 (31¼)	14.44 (31¾)	10.76 (23¾)	11.17 (24½)	11.74 (26)	12.36 (27¼)	12.98 (28½)	13.63 (30)	14.01 (31)
90–92 cm (35½–36¼ in)	11.60 (25½)	11.94 (26¼)	12.52 (27½)	13.20 (29)	13.94 (30¾)	14.58 (32¼)	14.90 (32¾)	11.16 (24½)	11.58 (25½)	12.17 (26¾)	12.80 (28¼)	13.45 (29¾)	14.10 (31)	14.45 (31¾)
92–94 cm (36¼–37 in)	12.00 (26½)	12.37 (27¼)	12.97 (28½)	13.65 (30)	14.40 (31¾)	15.05 (33¼)	15.39 (34)	11.59 (25½)	12.02 (26½)	12.63 (27¾)	13.27 (29¼)	13.95 (30¾)	14.61 (32¼)	14.92 (33)
94–96 cm (37–37¾ in)	12.42 (27½)	12.81 (28¼)	13.45 (29¾)	14.14 (31¼)	14.88 (32¾)	15.54 (34¼)	15.90 (35)	12.05 (26½)	12.48 (27½)	13.12 (29)	13.77 (30¼)	14.48 (32)	15.14 (33½)	15.42 (34)
96–98 cm (37¾–38½ in)	12.88 (28½)	13.28 (29¼)	13.96 (30¾)	14.66 (32¼)	15.39 (34)	16.06 (35½)	16.43 (36¼)	12.55 (27¾)	12.98 (28½)	13.64 (30)	14.31 (31½)	15.04 (33¼)	15.71 (34¾)	15.99 (35¼)
98–100 cm (38½–39¼ in)	13.37 (29½)	13.78 (30½)	14.50 (32)	15.21 (33½)	15.94 (35¼)	16.62 (36¾)	17.00 (37½)	13.10 (29)	13.51 (29¾)	14.19 (31¼)	14.87 (32¾)	15.63 (34½)	16.32 (36)	16.64 (36¾)
100–102 cm (39¼–40¼ in)	13.90 (30¾)	14.30 (31½)	15.06 (33¼)	15.81 (34¾)	16.54 (36½)	17.22 (38)	17.60 (38¾)	13.68 (30¼)	14.08 (31)	14.77 (32½)	15.46 (34)	16.25 (35¾)	16.96 (37½)	17.39 (38¼)
102–104 cm (40¼–41 in)	14.48 (32)	14.85 (32¾)	15.65 (34½)	16.45 (36¼)	17.18 (37¾)	17.87 (39½)	18.24 (40¼)							

Table continued on following page

TABLE 12–2 Weight by Length* *Continued*

Recumbent Length	Boys: Weight Percentiles, kg and (lb)							Girls: Weight Percentiles, kg and (lb)						
	5th	*10th*	*25th*	*50th*	*75th*	*90th*	*95th*	*5th*	*10th*	*25th*	*50th*	*75th*	*90th*	*95th*
Boys and Girls: Prepubescent‡														
90–92 cm (35½–36¼ in)	11.70 (25¾)	11.97 (26½)	12.59 (27¾)	13.41 (29½)	14.35 (31¾)	15.25 (33½)	15.72 (34¾)	11.45 (25¼)	11.67 (25¾)	12.28 (27)	13.14 (29)	14.11 (31)	14.98 (33)	15.74 (34¾)
92–94 cm (36¼–37 in)	12.07 (26½)	12.36 (27¼)	13.03 (28¾)	13.89 (30½)	14.84 (32¾)	15.87 (35)	16.41 (36¼)	11.86 (26¼)	12.10 (26¾)	12.74 (28)	13.63 (30)	14.63 (32¼)	15.57 (34¼)	16.42 (36¼)
94–96 cm (37–37¾ in)	12.46 (27½)	12.77 (28¼)	13.49 (29¾)	14.38 (31¾)	15.34 (33¾)	16.45 (36¼)	17.06 (37½)	12.26 (27)	12.53 (27½)	13.21 (29)	14.12 (31¼)	15.14 (33½)	16.13 (35½)	17.05 (37½)
96–98 cm (37¾–38½ in)	12.87 (28¼)	13.21 (29)	13.98 (30¾)	14.89 (32¾)	15.87 (35)	17.01 (37½)	17.69 (39)	12.66 (28)	12.97 (28½)	13.70 (30¼)	14.62 (32¼)	15.66 (34½)	16.69 (36¾)	17.65 (39)
98–100 cm (38½–39¼ in)	13.31 (29¼)	13.67 (30¼)	14.48 (32)	15.43 (34)	16.41 (36¼)	17.56 (38¾)	18.29 (40¼)	13.06 (28¾)	13.42 (29½)	14.19 (31¼)	15.13 (33¼)	16.19 (35¾)	17.24 (38)	18.23 (40¼)
100–102 cm (39¼–40¼ in)	13.77 (30¼)	14.15 (31¼)	15.00 (33)	15.98 (35¼)	16.98 (37½)	18.11 (40)	18.89 (41¾)	13.48 (29¾)	13.88 (30½)	14.69 (32½)	15.65 (34½)	16.73 (37)	17.80 (39¼)	18.80 (41½)
102–104 cm (40¼–41 in)	14.25 (31½)	14.65 (32¼)	15.54 (34¼)	16.65 (36½)	17.57 (38¾)	18.67 (41¼)	19.50 (43)	13.91 (30¾)	14.36 (31¾)	15.21 (33½)	16.20 (35¾)	17.28 (38)	18.38 (40½)	19.38 (42¾)
104–106 cm (41–41¾ in)	14.76 (32½)	15.18 (33½)	16.10 (35½)	17.13 (37¾)	18.18 (40)	19.25 (42½)	20.12 (44¼)	14.36 (31¾)	14.85 (32¾)	15.75 (34¾)	16.75 (37)	17.86 (39¼)	18.98 (41¾)	19.98 (44)
106–108 cm (41¾–42½ in)	15.30 (33¾)	15.73 (34¾)	16.68 (36¾)	17.74 (39)	18.82 (41½)	19.86 (43¾)	20.76 (45¾)	14.84 (32¾)	15.37 (34)	16.30 (36)	17.33 (38¼)	18.46 (40¾)	19.62 (43¼)	20.61 (45½)
108–110 cm (42½–43¼ in)	15.85 (35)	16.31 (36)	17.28 (38)	18.37 (40½)	19.49 (43)	20.51 (45¼)	21.45 (47¼)	15.35 (33¾)	15.91 (35)	16.87 (37¼)	17.94 (39½)	19.09 (42)	20.30 (44¾)	21.29 (47)
110–112 cm (43¼–44 in)	16.43 (36¼)	16.91 (37¼)	17.90 (39½)	19.02 (42)	20.18 (44½)	21.22 (46¾)	22.18 (49)	15.90 (35)	16.48 (36¼)	17.47 (38½)	18.56 (41)	19.76 (43½)	21.03 (46¼)	22.03 (48½)
112–114 cm (44–45 in)	17.04 (37½)	17.53 (38¾)	18.54 (40¾)	19.70 (43½)	20.91 (46)	21.98 (48½)	22.98 (50¾)	16.48 (36¼)	17.09 (37¾)	18.08 (39¾)	19.22 (42¼)	20.47 (45¼)	21.81 (48)	22.84 (50¼)
114–116 cm (45–45¾ in)	17.66 (39)	18.18 (40)	19.20 (42¼)	20.39 (45)	21.66 (47¾)	22.82 (50¼)	23.85 (52½)	17.11 (37¾)	17.72 (39)	18.72 (41¼)	19.91 (44)	21.23 (46¾)	22.67 (50)	23.73 (52¼)
116–118 cm (45¾–46½ in)	18.32 (40½)	18.85 (41½)	19.89 (43¾)	21.11 (46½)	22.45 (49½)	23.73 (52¼)	24.80 (54¾)	17.77 (39¼)	18.40 (40½)	19.40 (42¾)	20.64 (45½)	22.04 (48½)	23.60 (52)	24.71 (54½)
118–120 cm (46½–47¼ in)	18.99 (41¾)	19.55 (43)	20.60 (45½)	21.85 (48¼)	23.28 (51¼)	24.73 (54½)	25.83 (57)	18.48 (40¾)	19.11 (42¼)	20.11 (44¼)	21.42 (47¼)	22.92 (50½)	24.62 (54¼)	25.81 (57)
120–122 cm (47¼–48 in)	19.70 (43½)	20.28 (44¾)	21.34 (47)	22.63 (50)	24.15 (53¼)	25.80 (57)	26.96 (59½)	19.22 (42¼)	19.85 (43¾)	20.87 (46)	22.25 (49)	23.88 (52¾)	25.73 (56¾)	27.03 (59½)
122–124 cm (48–48¾ in)	20.43 (45)	21.03 (46¼)	22.11 (48¾)	23.45 (51¾)	25.07 (55¼)	26.96 (59½)	28.18 (62¼)	19.99 (44)	20.64 (45½)	21.68 (47¾)	23.13 (51)	24.91 (55)	26.95 (59½)	28.37 (62½)
124–126 cm (48¾–49½ in)	21.20 (46¾)	21.82 (48)	22.92 (50½)	24.32 (53½)	26.05 (57½)	28.18 (62¼)	29.50 (65)	20.80 (45¾)	21.47 (47¼)	22.54 (49¾)	24.09 (53)	26.05 (57½)	28.27 (62¼)	29.87 (65¾)
126–128 cm (49½–50½ in)	21.99 (48½)	22.64 (50)	23.77 (52½)	25.24 (55¾)	27.10 (59¾)	29.48 (65)	30.92 (68¼)	21.65 (47¾)	22.34 (49¼)	23.47 (51¾)	25.11 (55¼)	27.28 (60¼)	29.71 (65½)	31.51 (69½)
128–130 cm (50½–51¾ in)	22.82 (50¼)	23.50 (51¾)	24.67 (54½)	26.22 (57¾)	28.21 (62¼)	30.86 (68)	32.44 (71½)	22.53 (49¾)	23.25 (51¼)	24.46 (54)	26.22 (57¾)	28.63 (63)	31.28 (69)	33.33 (73½)
130–132 cm (51¼–52 in)	23.69 (52¼)	24.59 (53¾)	25.62 (56½)	27.26 (60)	29.41 (64¾)	32.31 (71¼)	34.07 (75)	23.44 (51¾)	24.22 (53½)	25.52 (56¼)	27.40 (60½)	30.09 (66¼)	32.99 (72¾)	35.33 (78)
132–134 cm (52–52¾ in)	24.59 (54¼)	25.32 (55¾)	26.62 (58¾)	28.38 (62½)	30.68 (67¾)	33.82 (74½)	35.81 (79)	24.38 (53¾)	25.22 (55½)	26.66 (58¾)	28.68 (63¼)	31.68 (69¾)	34.84 (76¾)	37.53 (82¾)
134–136 cm (52¾–53½ in)	25.53 (56¼)	26.30 (58)	27.68 (61)	29.58 (65¼)	32.05 (70¾)	35.40 (78)	37.67 (83)	25.35 (56)	26.28 (58)	27.88 (61½)	30.06 (66¼)	33.41 (73¾)	36.84 (81¼)	39.93 (88)
136–138 cm (53½–54¼ in)	26.51 (58½)	27.32 (60¼)	28.80 (63½)	30.86 (68)	33.51 (74)	37.05 (81¾)	39.65 (87½)	26.34 (58)	27.39 (60½)	29.19 (64¼)	31.54 (69½)	35.29 (77¾)	39.01 (86)	42.54 (93¾)
138–140 cm (54¼–55 in)	27.53 (60¾)	28.38 (62½)	29.99 (66)	32.23 (71)	35.08 (77¼)	38.77 (85½)	41.74 (92)							
140–142 cm (55–56 in)	28.59 (63)	29.48 (65)	31.25 (69)	33.70 (74¼)	36.75 (81)	40.55 (89½)	43.97 (97)							
142–144 cm (56–56¾ in)	29.70 (65½)	30.64 (67½)	32.58 (71¾)	35.27 (77¾)	38.54 (85)	42.39 (93½)	46.32 (102)							
144–146 cm (56¾–57½ in)	30.86 (68)	31.85 (70¼)	34.00 (75)	36.95 (81½)	40.45 (89¼)	44.29 (97¾)	48.80 (107½)							

**Data are those of the National Center for Health Statistics (NCHS), Health Resources Administration, Department of Health, Education, and Welfare.*

†Data are based on studies of the Fels Research Institute, Yellow Springs, OH.

‡Data are based on the Health Examination Surveys of the NCHS. For details see footnote to Table 10–2.

progression in socialization moves from minimal social interaction with peers during play (solo or parallel play, age 1 or 2 yr) to cooperative play such as building a tower of blocks together (age 3 or 4 yr) to organized group play with distinct role assignments, as in playing house. Play also becomes increasingly rule governed, from early rules about asking (rather than taking) and sharing (age 2 or 3 yr) to rules that change from moment to moment according to the desires of the players (ages 4 and 5 yr) to the beginning of the recognition of rules as relatively immutable (age 5 yr and beyond).

Play allows children to experience mastery by solving puzzles, practicing adult roles, assuming the aggressor role rather than the victim (spanking a doll), taking on super powers (dinosaur and superhero play), and obtaining things that are denied in real life (a make-believe friend or stuffed pet). Creativity, inherent in all play, is especially visible in drawing, painting, and other artistic activities. The 4-yr-old who chooses to let a big circle with sticks represent a body and limbs knows that real bodies do not actually look like that. The simplicity of the drawing is, at least in part, a matter of choice. Themes and emotions that emerge in a child's drawings often reflect the emotional issues of greatest importance for the child.

Moral thinking mirrors and is constrained by a child's cognitive level. Empathic responses to others' distress arise during the 2nd yr of life, but the ability to cognitively consider another child's point of view remains limited throughout the preschool period. In keeping with a child's inability to focus on more than one aspect of a situation at a time, fairness is taken to mean equal treatment regardless of circumstantial differences. Rules tend to be absolute, with guilt assigned for bad outcomes regardless of intentions.

IMPLICATIONS FOR PARENTS AND PEDIATRICIANS. The significance of language as a target for assessment and intervention cannot be overestimated because of its central role as an indicator of cognitive and emotional development and as a key factor in behavioral regulation and later school success. Detection and assessment of language delays, a critical part of preventive care, is discussed in Chapters 16 and 29. Parents can support emotional development by using words that describe the child's feeling states ("You sound angry right now") and by urging the child to use words to express feelings rather than acting out the feelings.

Parents should have a regular time each day for reading or looking at books with their children. Programs in which pediatricians give out picture books along with appropriate guidance during primary care visits have been effective in increasing reading aloud, particularly in lower income families.

Preoperational thinking constrains how children understand experiences of illness and treatment. Many children perceive needles as huge objects that threaten to puncture them like a balloon. Verbal explanation is often not as reassuring as giving the child an opportunity to administer make-believe shots to a doll and see, repeatedly, that nothing horrible happens. Explanations that involve several contradictory aspects ("This will hurt a little, but it will keep you from getting sick") will be lost on most preoperational children; the immediate presence of a calm parent is more comforting. Children with precocious language development may elicit overly complex explanations from adults who assume incorrectly that their cognitive sophistication matches their verbal skill.

The imaginative intensity that fuels play and the magical, animist thinking characteristic of preoperational cognition can also generate intense fears. More than 80% of parents report at least one fear in their preschool children, and nearly 50% report seven or more fears. Refusal to take baths or to sit on the toilet may arise from the fear of being washed or flushed down, reflecting a child's immature appreciation of relative size. Attempts to demonstrate rationally that there are no monsters in the closet often fail, as the fear arises from prerational thinking. Reassurances that parents will use their "great power" (e.g., monster spray, tape) to guarantee the child's safety may be more effective because they appeal to a child's magical thinking.

EMOTIONAL DEVELOPMENT

Emotional challenges facing preschool children include accepting limits while maintaining a sense of self-direction, reigning in aggressive and sexual impulses, and interacting with a widening circle of adults and peers. At age 2 yr, behavioral limits are predominantly external; by age 5 yr, these controls need to be internalized if a child is to function in a typical classroom. Success in achieving this goal relies on prior emotional development, particularly the ability to use internalized images of trusted adults to provide security in times of stress. Children need to believe themselves worthy of adult approval to be willing to work for it.

Children learn what behaviors are acceptable and how much power they wield vis-à-vis important adults by testing limits. Testing increases when it elicits an exceptional amount of attention, even though that attention is often negative, and when limits are inconsistent. Testing often arouses parental anger or inappropriate solicitude as a child's struggle to separate gives rise to a corresponding challenge for the parents: letting go. Excessively tight limits can undermine a child's sense of initiative, whereas overly loose limits can provoke anxiety in a child who feels that no one is in control.

Control is a central issue. Inability to control some aspect of the external world, such as what to buy or when to leave, often results in a loss of internal control—that is, a *temper tantrum.* Fear, overtiredness, or physical discomfort can also evoke tantrums. When they are reinforced by intermittent rewards, as when a parent occasionally gives in to a child's demands, tantrums can also become an entrenched strategy for exerting control. Tantrums lasting more than 15 min or regularly occurring more than three times a day may reflect underlying medical, emotional, or social problems. Tantrums normally appear toward the end of the 1st yr of life and peak in prevalence between ages 2 and 4 yr. Frequent tantrums after age 5 yr tend to persist throughout childhood.

Preschool children normally experience complicated feelings toward their parents: intense love and jealousy and resentment and fear that angry feelings might lead to abandonment. The swirl of these emotions, most beyond a child's ability to analyze or express, often finds expression in highly labile moods. The resolution of this crisis (a process extending over years) involves a child's unspoken decision to emulate the parents rather than compete with them. Play and language foster the development of emotional controls by allowing children to express emotions and to enjoy gratifications (power or intimacy with parents) that are taboo in real life.

Curiosity about genitals and adult sexual organs is normal, as is *masturbation.* Modesty appears gradually between age 4 and 6 yr, with wide variations among cultures and families. Masturbation that has a compulsive quality or that interferes with a child's normal activities, acting out of sexual intercourse in doll play or with other children, extreme modesty, or mimicry of adult seductive behavior all suggest the possibility of sexual abuse.

IMPLICATIONS FOR PARENTS AND PEDIATRICIANS. Most parents find it difficult to understand their preschool children at least some of the time. Rapid shifts between clinging dependence and defiant independence, between sophisticated-sounding language and infantile helplessness, and between angelic joy and uncontrollable rage can erode parents' self-confidence and patience. Guidance emphasizing appropriate expectations for behavioral and emotional development and acknowledging normal parental feelings of anger, guilt, and confusion can help lessen parents' worries both about their children and about themselves. Many parents fail to raise such concerns during pediatric visits because they feel embarrassed or because they do not think the pediatrician can help. Pediatricians need to let parents know that the child's behavior and the parents' reactions are appropriate topics for discussion.

It may be difficult to decide whether a particular child's behavior is normally challenging or indicative of a true problem. Red flags include parents who do not volunteer any positive statements about their children, evidence of threatening or overtly punitive discipline, and the existence of problems (especially tantrums) in daycare or preschool, where most preschool children manage to maintain self-control. The presence of chronic medical problems, developmental delays, or unusual family stresses signal the need for more detailed assessment. Even apparently normal behavior constitutes a problem if it arouses sufficient parental concern. An extended visit devoted to the issue or referral to a mental health professional is appropriate. Reference to *The Classification of Child and Adolescent Mental Diagnoses in Primary Care: Diagnostic and Statistical Manual for Primary Care (DSM-PC)* will help pediatricians distinguish among normal variations, problems, and disorders that may merit referral.

Corporal punishment is accepted in many traditional cultures but may be inappropriate in the modern context in which most families now live (also see Chapter 5). No evidence shows that spanking per se is harmful, but regular use of corporal punishment may reflect an excessive desire for control, as well as a lack of other parenting techniques. Parents usually claim that they do not like spanking but feel that nothing else works. Pediatricians can point out that the spanking is not working either, or it would not have to be used so often. As children habituate to repeated spanking, parents are forced to spank ever harder to get the desired response, increasing the risk of serious injury. Sufficiently harsh punishment may inhibit undesired behaviors, but at great psychologic cost. Children mimic the corporal punishment they receive, and it is not uncommon for preschool-age children to strike their parents back. Parents may be helped to renounce spanking or at least reserve it for extreme circumstances if they learn more effective discipline techniques including consistent limit setting, clear communication, and frequent approval. Time-out for approximately 1 min per year of age is a form of noncorporal punishment backed by extensive research. Parents may require detailed instruction to use time-out effectively.

Anderson RC, Hiebert EH, Scott JA, et al: Becoming a Nation of Readers: The Report of the Commission on Reading. Washington, DC, The National Institute of Education, 1985.

Faber A, Mazlish E: How to Talk So Kids Will Listen & Listen So Kids Will Talk. New York, Avon, 1980.

Friedman SB, Schonberg SK (eds): The Short- and Long-term Consquences of Corporal Punishment. Supplement to Pediatrics 98:803–858, 1996.

Ginsburg H, Opper S: Piaget's Theory of Intellectual Development. Englewood Cliffs, NJ, Prentice-Hall, 1969.

Satter E: Child of Mine: Feeding with Love and Good Sense. Palo Alto, CA, Bull Publishing, 1986.

Schickedanz JA: More Than the ABCs: The Early Stages of Reading and Writing. Washington, DC, National Association for the Education of Young Children, 1986.

Wolraich ML (ed): The Classification of Child and Adolescent Mental Diagnoses in Primary Care: Diagnostic and Statistical Manual for Primary Care (DSM-PC) Child and Adolescent Version. Elk Grove Village, IL, American Academy of Pediatrics, 1996.

CHAPTER 13
Early School Years

During middle childhood (6–12 yr), children face new challenges. The cognitive power to consider several factors simultaneously confers the ability to evaluate oneself and perceive others' evaluations. As a result, *self-esteem* becomes a central issue. Unlike infants and preschoolers, school-age children are judged according to their ability to produce socially valued outputs, such as good grades or home runs. Accordingly, Erikson identified the central psychosocial issue of this period as the crisis between industry and inferiority. Healthy development requires increasing separation from parents and the ability to find acceptance in the peer group and to negotiate challenges in the outside world.

PHYSICAL DEVELOPMENT. Growth during the period averages 3–3.5 kg (7 lb) and 6 cm (2.5 in) per year (see Figs. 11–1 and 11–2 and Table 12–1). Growth occurs discontinuously, in irregular spurts lasting on average 8 wk, three to six times per year. The head grows only 2–3 cm in circumference throughout the entire period, reflecting slowed brain growth; myelinization is complete by 7 yr of age. Body habitus (endomorphic, mesomorphic, or ectomorphic) tends to remain relatively stable throughout middle childhood.

Growth of the midface and lower face occurs gradually. Loss of deciduous (baby) teeth is a more dramatic sign of maturation, beginning about age 6 yr after eruption of the 1st molars. Replacement with adult teeth occurs at a rate of about four per year. Lymphoid tissues hypertrophy, often giving rise to impressive tonsils and adenoids, which occasionally require surgical treatment.

Muscular strength, coordination, and stamina increase progressively, as does the ability to perform complex movements such as dancing, shooting basketballs, or playing the piano. Such higher order motor skills are a result of both maturation and training; the degree of accomplishment reflects wide variability in innate skill, interest, and opportunity. Epidemiologic studies report a general decline in *physical fitness* among school-age children. Sedentary habits at this age are associated with increased lifetime risk of obesity and cardiovascular disease.

The sexual organs remain physically immature, but interest in gender differences and sexual behavior remains active in many children and increase progressively until puberty. Masturbation is common, if not universal. In more permissive cultures, sexual experimentation often occurs among prepubertal children.

IMPLICATIONS FOR PARENTS AND PEDIATRICIANS. "Normality" encompasses a wide range of physical sizes, shapes, and abilities in school-age children. Just as importantly, children's feelings about their physical attributes range from pride to shame to apparent nonchalance. Fears of being "defective" can lead to avoidance of situations in which physical differences might be revealed, such as gym class or medical examinations. Children with actual physical disabilities may face special stresses because of their difference. The routine physical examination provides an opportunity to elicit concerns and allay fears.

Girls, in particular, often worry that they are overweight, and many engage in unhealthy dieting to achieve an abnormally thin cultural ideal. Shortness, particularly in boys, may be associated with decreased educational attainment and increased risks for behavior problems (although social class remains a more powerful predictor). The availability of recombinant human growth hormone raises the possibility of medical treatment for short children who may not have documentable hormone deficiency. The decision to treat, with its attendant cost and discomfort, needs to be made in view of the meaning of shortness for the individual child (see Chapter 567).

A child's physical appearance may also evoke strong feelings in parents, leading them to undermine the child's self-esteem inadvertently, or, alternatively, to encourage vanity. Pediatricians can help parents distinguish between true health risks and individual variations that should be accepted. Questions about regular physical activities should be part of the medical history for health supervision visits. Participation in organized *sports* can foster skill, teamwork, and fitness, but excessive pressure to compete often has negative effects. Prepubertal children should not engage in high-stress, high-impact sports such as power lifting or football because skeletal immaturity increases the risk of injury.

COGNITIVE AND LANGUAGE DEVELOPMENT. The thinking of young school-aged children differs qualitatively from that of children just 1 or 2 yr younger. In place of magical, egocentric, and perception-bound cognition, school-aged children increasingly apply rules based on observable phenomena, factor in multiple dimensions and points of view, and interpret their perceptions in view of realistic theories about physical laws. This shift from "preoperational" to "concrete logical operations" was documented by Piaget in a series of "conservation" experiments (see Chapter 12). For example, 5-yr-olds who watch a ball of clay being rolled into a snake might insist that the snake has "more" because it is longer. Seven-year-olds typically reply that the ball and snake must weigh the same because nothing has been added or taken away or because the snake is both longer and thinner. This cognitive reorganization occurs at different rates in different contexts. In the context of social interactions with siblings, young children often demonstrate an ability to understand many points of view long before they demonstrate that ability in their thinking about the physical world.

School makes increasing cognitive demands. Mastery of the elementary curriculum requires that a large number of perceptual, cognitive, and language processes work efficiently (Table 13–1). Attention and receptive language affect each other as well as every other aspect of learning. One cannot attend to what one cannot understand or understand without first paying attention. By third grade, children need to be able to sustain attention through a 45-min period.

The first 2 yr of elementary school are devoted to acquiring the fundamentals: reading, writing, and basic mathematics skills. By third or fourth grade, the curriculum requires that children use those fundamentals to learn increasingly complex materials. The goal of reading a paragraph is no longer to decode the words but to understand the content; the goal of writing is no longer spelling or penmanship but composition. The volume of work increases along with the complexity. Children can meet these demands only if they have mastered the basic skills to the point that their execution has become automatic. Children who have to think about how to shape each letter or who have to recalculate basic mathematics facts each time they attempt to solve a word problem fall behind.

Cognitive abilities interact with a wide array of attitudinal and emotional factors in determining classroom performance. A partial list of such factors includes eagerness to please adults, cooperativeness, competitiveness, willingness to work for a delayed reward, belief in one's abilities, and ability to risk trying when success is not ensured. Success predisposes to success, whereas failure undercuts a child's ability to take cognitive-emotional risks in the future.

Children's intellectual activity extends beyond the classroom. Beginning in third or fourth grade, children increasingly enjoy strategy games and word play (puns and insults) that exercise growing cognitive and linguistic mastery. Many become experts on subjects of their own choosing, such as sports trivia or stamps. Others become avid readers.

IMPLICATIONS FOR PARENTS AND PEDIATRICIANS. Children in the cognitive stage of concrete logical operations can understand simple explanations for illnesses and necessary treatments, although they may revert to prelogical thinking under stress (as may adults). A child with pneumonia may be able to explain about white cells fighting the "germs" in the lungs but still secretly harbor the belief that the sickness is a punishment for disobedience.

Academic and classroom behavior problems, like fever, are symptoms that require diagnosis. Among the broad range of possible causes are deficits in specific cognitive, perceptual, or linguistic functions (specific learning disabilities); global cognitive delay (mental retardation); primary attention deficit; and attention deficits secondary to emotional preoccupation, depression, anxiety, or any chronic illness. Commonly, the cause is a combination of several such factors. Assessment of school problems is discussed in Chapters 16 and 29.

Remedial approaches depend on the underlying problem or problems. Children who are inattentive because of receptive language disability will benefit more from language therapy than from stimulant medication. Similarly, psychotherapy is generally less helpful for primary attention deficits than are medication and environmental modifications aimed at increasing structure and decreasing distractions. Simply having a child repeat a failed grade rarely has any beneficial effect and often seriously undercuts the child's self-esteem. See Chapter 29 for a further discussion of learning and behavior problems.

TABLE 13–1 Selected Perceptual, Cognitive, and Language Processes Required for Elementary School Success

Process	Description	Associated Problems
Perceptual		
Visual analysis	Ability to break a complex figure into components and understand their spatial relationships	Persistent letter confusion (e.g., between *b, d,* and *g*); difficulty with basic reading and writing and limited "sight" vocabulary
Proprioception and motor control	Ability to obtain information about body position by feel and unconsciously program complex movements	Poor handwriting, requiring inordinate effort, often with overly tight pencil grasp; special difficulty with timed tasks
Phonologic processing	Ability to perceive differences between similar sounding words and to break down words into constituent sounds	Delayed receptive language skills; attention and behavior problems secondary to not understanding directions; delayed acquisition of letter–sound correlations (phonetics)
Cognitive		
Long-term memory, both storage and recall	Ability to acquire skills that are "automatic" (i.e., accessible without conscious thought)	Delayed mastery of the alphabet (reading and writing letters); slow handwriting; inability to progress beyond basic mathematics
Selective attention	Ability to attend to important stimuli and ignore distractions	Difficulty following multistep instructions, completing assignments, and behaving well; peer interaction problems
Sequencing	Ability to remember things in order; facility with time concepts	Difficulty organizing assignments, planning, spelling, and telling time
Language		
Receptive language	Ability to comprehend complex constructions, function words (e.g., if, when, only, except), nuances of speech, and extended blocks of language (e.g., paragraphs)	Difficulty following directions; wandering attention during lessons and stories; problems with reading comprehension; problems with peer relationships
Expressive language	Ability to recall required words effortlessly (word finding), to control meanings by varying position and word endings, to construct meaningful paragraphs and stories	Difficulty expressing feelings and using words for self-defense, with resulting frustration and physical acting out; struggling during "circle time" and in language-based subjects (e.g., English)

Interventions that allow children to exercise their strengths and experience success have beneficial effects that often spill over into problem areas.

SOCIAL AND EMOTIONAL DEVELOPMENT. In psychoanalytic theory, latency follows the resolution of oedipal conflicts, as sexual energies are channeled away from their original forbidden objects, the parents, and toward the pursuit of socially accepted accomplishments. As part of the resolution, postoedipal children identify with same-sex parents, adopting them as role models. The parents' moral judgments are internalized as the superego. Observations in support of this theory include decreased emotional lability toward parents and an increasing involvement in relationships outside of the home.

Social and emotional development proceeds in three contexts: the home, the school, and the neighborhood. Of these, the home remains the most influential. The parent-child relationship continues to provide a secure base from which children can venture forth. Milestones of a school child's increasing independence include the first sleepover at a friend's house and the first time at overnight camp. Parents should make demands for effort in school and extracurricular activities, celebrate successes, and offer unconditional acceptance when failures occur. Regular chores provide an opportunity for children to contribute to the family in a meaningful way, supporting self-esteem. Siblings have critical roles as competitors, loyal supporters, and role models. Sibling relationships exert lasting effects on personality development, influencing an individual's self-image, approach to conflict resolution, interests, and even career choices.

The beginning of school coincides with a child's further separation from the family and the increasing importance of teacher and peer relationships. In addition to friendships that may persist for months or years, experience with a large number of superficial friendships and antagonisms contributes to a child's growing social competence. Popularity, a central ingredient of self-esteem, may be won through possessions (having the right toys or the right clothes) as well as through personal attractiveness, accomplishments, and actual social skills.

Conformity is rewarded. Some children conform readily and enjoy easy social success; those who adopt individualistic styles or have visible differences may be stigmatized as "weird." Such children may be painfully aware that they are different, or they may be puzzled by their lack of popularity. Children with social skills deficits may go to extreme lengths to win acceptance, only to meet with repeated failure. Attributions conferred by peers, such as funny, stupid, bad, or scary, may become incorporated into a child's self-image.

In the neighborhood, real dangers such as busy streets, bullies, and strangers tax school-aged children's common sense and resourcefulness. Interactions with peers without close adult supervision call on increasing conflict resolution or pugilistic skills. Observation of older children and adults as well as advertisements in store windows and on television expose children to adult materialism, sexuality, and violence. Many of these experiences reinforce children's feeling of powerlessness in the larger world. Compensatory fantasies of being powerful may fuel the fascination with superheroes. Hero worship and adoption of adult-like dress and mannerisms are "dress rehearsals" for adult roles and represent ways of appropriating adult power. A balance between fantasy and appropriate ability to negotiate real world challenges indicates healthy emotional development.

IMPLICATIONS FOR PARENTS AND PEDIATRICIANS. Children need unconditional support as well as realistic demands as they venture into a world that is often frightening. Children who show unusual difficulty in separating from parents and in facing school and neighborhood challenges may be reacting to their parents' difficulty letting them go. Other parents exert excessive pressure on their children to adopt adult behaviors and achieve academic or competitive success. Children often struggle to meet such expectations but may develop behavior problems or somatic symptoms such as headaches or stomachaches as a result (Chapter 19).

Many children face stressors that exceed the normal challenges of separation and "making it" in school and neighborhood. Divorce affects some 40% of children. Violence between parents, parental substance abuse, and other mental health problems may also impair a child's ability to use home as a secure base for refueling emotional energies. In many neighborhoods, the threats of gangs and random violence make the normal development of independence extremely dangerous. Children in late elementary and middle school may join *gangs* as a means of self-protection and a way to appropriate power and belong to a cohesive group. The high prevalence of adjustment disorders among school-aged children attests to the effects of such overwhelming stressors on development.

Pediatricians need to be alert to children's functioning in all contexts (home, school, neighborhood) and consider how each of those environments either supports or overwhelms the child's ability to adapt and grow. Use of the HEADSS mnemonic—*H*ome, *E*ducation and employment, peer *A*ctivities, *D*rugs, *S*exuality, and *S*uicide or depression can help. Originally designed for adolescents, with minor modifications it also works well for school-aged children.

Dunn J: Sisters and Brothers. Cambridge, MA, Harvard University Press, 1985.

Goldenring JM, Cohen E: Getting into adolescent heads. Contemp Pediatr 5:75, 1988.

Lee PDK, Rosenfeld RG: Psychosocial correlates of short stature and delayed puberty. Pediatr Clin North Am 34:851, 1987.

Levine M: Middle childhood. *In:* Levine MD, Carey WB, Crocker AC (eds): Developmental-Behavioral Pediatrics. Philadelphia, WB Saunders, 1992, pp 48–64.

Putnam N: Seven to ten years: Growth and competency. *In:* Dixon SD, Stein MT (eds): Encounters with Children. St. Louis, MO, Mosby–Year Book, 1992, pp 317–326.

Wells RD, Stein MT: Seven to ten years: The world of the elementary school child. *In:* Dixon SD, Stein MT (eds): Encounters with Children. St. Louis, MO, Mosby–Year Book, 1992, pp 329–338.

CHAPTER 14
Adolescence

Also see Part XII.

Between the ages of 10 and 20 yr, children undergo rapid changes in body size, shape, physiology, and psychologic and social functioning. Hormones set the developmental agenda in conjunction with social structures designed to foster the transition from childhood to adulthood.

Adolescence proceeds across three distinct periods—early, middle, and late—each marked by a characteristic set of salient biologic, psychologic, and social issues (Table 14–1). However, individual variation is substantial, both in terms of the timing of somatic changes and the quality of the adolescent's experience. Gender and subculture profoundly affect the developmental course, as do physical and social stressors such as cerebral palsy or parental alcoholism.

EARLY ADOLESCENCE

BIOLOGIC DEVELOPMENT. Adrenal production of androgen (chiefly dehydroepiandrosterone sulfate [DHEAS]) may occur as early as age 6, with development of underarm odor and faint genital hair (adrenarche). Levels of luteinizing hormone (LH) and follicle-stimulating hormone (FSH) rise progressively

TABLE 14–1 Central Issues in Early, Middle, and Late Adolescence

Variable	Early Adolescence	Middle Adolescence	Late Adolescence
Age (yr)	10–13	14–16	17–20 and beyond
SMR*	1–2	3–5	5
Somatic	Secondary sex characteristics; beginning of rapid growth; awkward	Height growth peaks; body shape and composition change; acne and odor; menarche; spermarche	Slower growth
Sexual	Sexual interest usually exceeds sexual activity	Sexual drive surges; experimentation; questions of sexual orientation	Consolidation of sexual identity
Cognitive and moral	Concrete operations; conventional morality	Emergence of abstract thought; questioning mores; self-centered	Idealism; absolutism
Self-concept	Preoccupation with changing body; self-consciousness	Concern with attractiveness, increasing introspection	Relatively stable body image
Family	Bids for increased independence; ambivalence	Continued struggle for acceptance of greater autonomy	Practical independence; family remains secure base
Peers	Same-sex groups; conformity; cliques	Dating; peer groups less important	Intimacy; possibly commitment
Relationship to society	Middle-school adjustment	Gauging skills and opportunities	Career decisions (e.g., drop out, college, work)

**See text and Figures 14–1 and 14–2.*
SMR, sexual maturity rating.

throughout middle childhood without dramatic effect. The rapid changes of puberty begin with increased sensitivity of the pituitary to gonadotropin-releasing hormone (GnRH), pulsatile release of GnRH, LH, and FSH during sleep, and corresponding rises in gonadal androgens and estrogens. The triggers for these changes are incompletely understood. Contemporary children in the United States enter puberty somewhat earlier than the published norms, perhaps related to increased weight and adiposity. The resulting sequence of somatic and physiologic changes gives rise to the sexual maturity rating (SMR) or Tanner stages. Figures 14–1 and 14–2 depict the somatic changes used in the SMR scale; Tables 14–2 and 14–3 describe these changes in words. Table 14–4 lists median ages and normal ranges for key stages of breast, pubic hair, and penile development. Note that the SMR stages are not perfectly synchronized (e.g., SMR2 penis development precedes SMR2 pubic hair by on average 1.5 years). Figures 14–3 and 14–4 depict the typical sequence of pubertal changes in males and females, respectively. The range of normal for progress through the stages of sexual maturity is wide.

In girls, the first visible sign of puberty is the appearance of breast buds, between 8 and 13 yr. Menses typically begin 2–2½ yr later (normal range 9–16 yr), around the peak in height velocity (see Fig. 14–4). Less obvious changes include enlargement of the ovaries, uterus, labia, and clitoris; thickening of endometrium and the vaginal mucosa; and increased vaginal glycogen, predisposing to yeast infections.

In boys, testicular enlargement begins as early as 9½ yr. Peak growth occurs when testis volumes reach approximately 9–10 cm^3. Under the influence of LH and testosterone, the seminiferous tubules, epididymis, seminal vesicles, and prostate enlarge. The left testis normally is lower than the right; the opposite may be true in situs inversus. Some degree of breast hypertrophy occurs in 40–65% of pubertal boys as a result of a relative excess of estrogenic stimulation. Gynecomastia sufficient to cause embarrassment and social disability occurs in fewer than 10%. Breast swelling less than 4 cm in diameter has a 90% chance of spontaneous resolution within 3 yr. For greater degrees of enlargement, hormonal or surgical treatment may be indicated. Obesity may exacerbate gynecomastia and should be addressed through diet and exercise.

For both sexes, growth acceleration begins in early adolescence, but peak growth velocities are not reached until SMR3 or 4. Boys typically peak 2–3 yr later than girls (Fig. 14–5) and continue their linear growth for approximately 2–3 yr after girls have stopped. The growth spurt begins distally, with enlargement of hands and feet followed by the arms and legs and finally by the trunk and chest. This asymmetric growth gives young adolescents a gawky look. Rapid enlargement of the larynx, pharynx, and lungs leads to changes in vocal quality, often heralded by a period of vocal instability (voice cracking) or dysphonation. Adrenal androgens stimulate the sebaceous glands, promoting the development of acne. Elongation

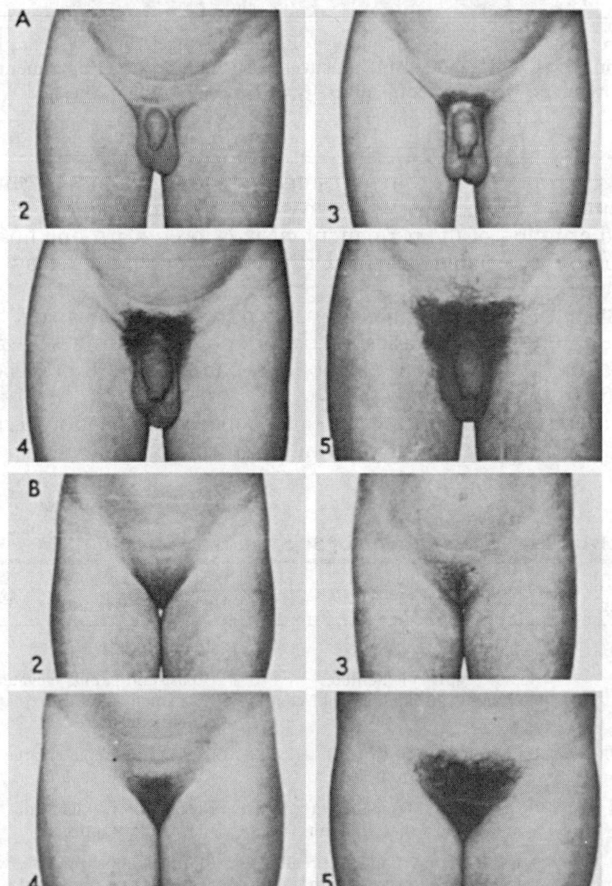

Figure 14–1 Sex maturity ratings of pubic hair changes in adolescent boys and girls. (Courtesy of JM Tanner, M.D., Institute of Child Health, Department of Growth and Development, University of London, London, England.)

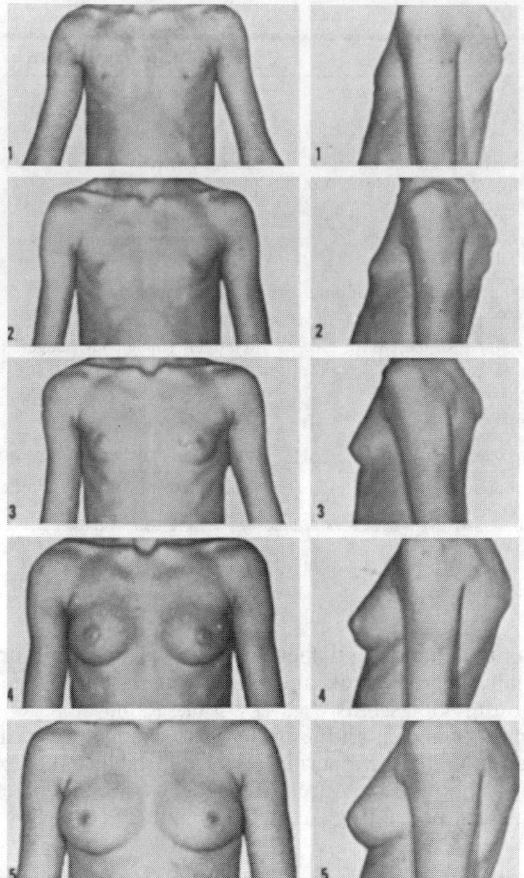

Figure 14–2 Sex maturity ratings of breast changes in adolescent girls. (Courtesy of JM Tanner, M.D., Institute of Child Health, Department of Growth and Development, University of London, London, England.)

of the optic globe often results in nearsightedness. Dental changes include jaw growth, loss of the final deciduous teeth, and eruption of the permanent cuspids, premolars, and finally molars (see Table 10–6). Orthodontic appliances may be needed.

SEXUALITY. Sexuality includes not only sexual behaviors but also interest and fantasies, sexual orientation, attitudes toward sex and its relationship to emotions, and awareness of socially defined roles and mores.

Interest in sex increases in early puberty. Ejaculation occurs for the first time, usually during masturbation and later spontaneously in sleep. Some boys worry that these emissions are signs of infection. Early adolescents sometimes masturbate socially; mutual sexual exploration is not necessarily a sign of homosexuality (Chapter 26). Sexual behavior, other than masturbation, is less common, although 31% of an urban sample reported sexual intercourse before age 14.

The relationship between hormonal changes and sexual interest and activity is controversial; no consistent links between hormones and sexual arousal, age of first intercourse, or frequency of intercourse have been found.

COGNITIVE AND MORAL DEVELOPMENT. In piagetian theory, adolescence marks the transition from the concrete operational thinking characteristic of school-aged children (Chapter 13) to formal logical operations. Formal operations include the ability to manipulate abstractions such as algebraic expressions, to reason from known principles, to weigh many points of view according to varying criteria, and to think about the process of thinking itself. Some early adolescents demonstrate formal

TABLE 14–2 Classification of Sex Maturity Stages in Girls

SMR Stage	Pubic Hair	Breasts
1	Preadolescent	Preadolescent
2	Sparse, lightly pigmented, straight, medial border of labia	Breast and papilla elevated as small mound; areolar diameter increased
3	Darker, beginning to curl, increased amount	Breast and areola enlarged, no contour separation
4	Coarse, curly, abundant but amount less than in adult	Areola and papilla form secondary mound
5	Adult feminine triangle, spread to medial surface of thighs	Mature, nipple projects, areola part of general breast contour

SMR, sexual maturity rating.
From Tanner JM: Growth at Adolescence, 2nd ed. Oxford, England, Blackwell Scientific Publications, 1962.

TABLE 14–3 Classification of Sex Maturity Stages in Boys

SMR Stage	Pubic Hair	Penis	Testes
1	None	Preadolescent	Preadolescent
2	Scanty, long, slightly pigmented	Slight enlargement	Enlarged scrotum, pink, texture altered
3	Darker, starts to curl, small amount	Longer	Larger
4	Resembles adult type but less in quantity; coarse, curly	Larger; glans and breadth increase in size	Larger, scrotum dark
5	Adult distribution, spread to medial surface of thighs	Adult size	Adult size

SMR, sexual maturity rating.
Adapted from Tanner JM: Growth at Adolescence, 2nd ed. Oxford, England, Blackwell Scientific Publications, 1962.

TABLE 14–4 Variability in Timing of Sexual Maturation

SMR	Early (mean − 2 SD Early)	Average (median)	Late (mean + 2 SD Late)
Timing of SMR Stages in Girls			
Pubic Hair			
SMR2	9.0	11.2	13.5
SMR3	9.6	11.9	14.1
SMR4	10.3	12.6	14.8
Breast Development			
SMR2	8.9	10.9	12.9
SMR3	9.8	11.9	13.9
SMR4	10.5	12.9	15.3
Timing of SMR Stages in Boys			
Pubic Hair			
SMR2	9.9	12.0	14.1
SMR3	11.2	13.1	14.9
SMR4	12.0	13.9	15.7
Penis Development			
SMR2	9.2	10.5	13.7
SMR3	10.1	12.4	14.6
SMR4	11.2	13.2	15.4

SMR, sexual maturity rating.
Data from Tanner JM, Davies PSW: Clinical longitudinal standards for height and height velocity for North American children. J Pediatr 107:317, 1985.

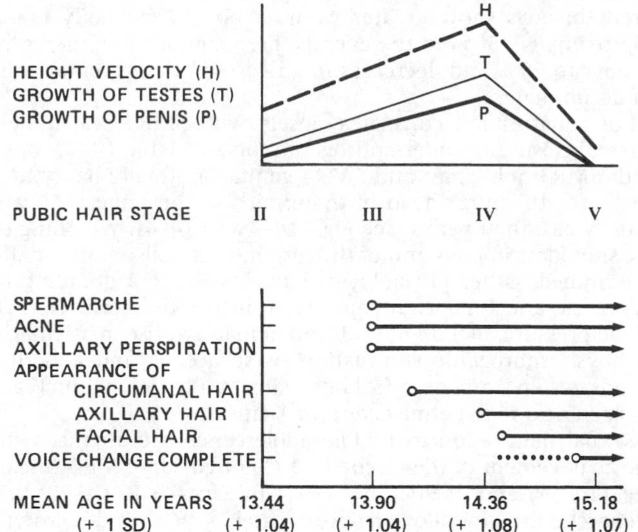

Figure 14–3 Sequence of maturational events in males. (Adapted from Marshall WA, Tanner JM: Variations in the pattern of pubertal changes in boys. Arch Dis Child 45:13, 1970.)

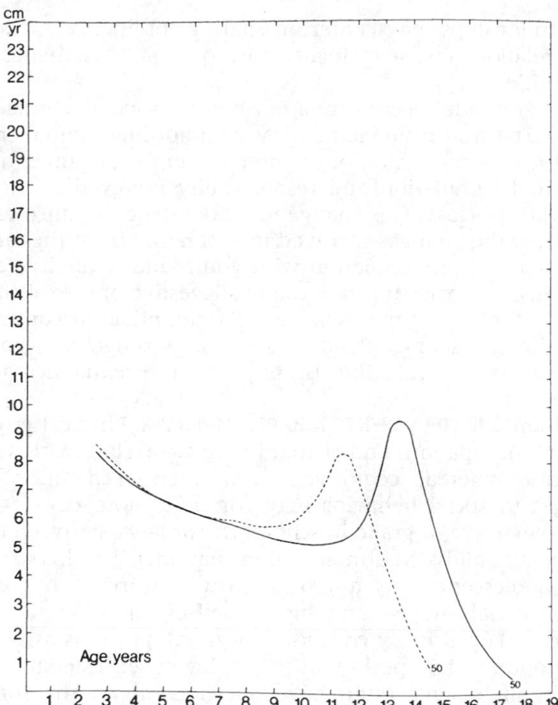

Figure 14–5 Height velocity curves for U.S. boys *(solid line)* and girls *(dashed line)* who have their peak height velocity at the average age (i.e., average growth tempo). (From Tanner JM, Davies PSW: Clinical longitudinal standards for height and height velocity for North American children. J Pediatr 107:317, 1985.)

thinking, others acquire the capability later, and others do not acquire it at all. Young adolescents may be able to apply formal operations to schoolwork but not to personal dilemmas. When the emotional stakes are high, magical thinking, such as the conviction of invulnerability, may interfere with higher order cognition. The ability to treat possibilities as real entities may affect critical decisions, such as whether or not to have unprotected intercourse or engage in other risk-taking behavior.

Some theorists argue that the transition from concrete to formal operations follows from quantitative increases in knowledge, experience, and cognitive efficiency rather than a qualitative reorganization of thinking. Consistent with this view are data showing a steady rise in cognitive processing speed from late childhood through early adulthood, associated with a reduction in synaptic number (pruning of less-used pathways) and progressive maturation of electroencephalographic results. It is unclear whether or not the hormonal changes of puberty directly affect cognitive development.

The development of moral thinking roughly parallels general cognitive development. Most preadolescents perceive right and wrong as absolute and unquestionable. Taking a loaf of bread to feed a starving child is wrong because it is "stealing." Adolescents often question received morality, embracing the behavior standards of the peer group. Group membership may allow them to displace guilt feelings for perceived moral infractions from themselves to the group.

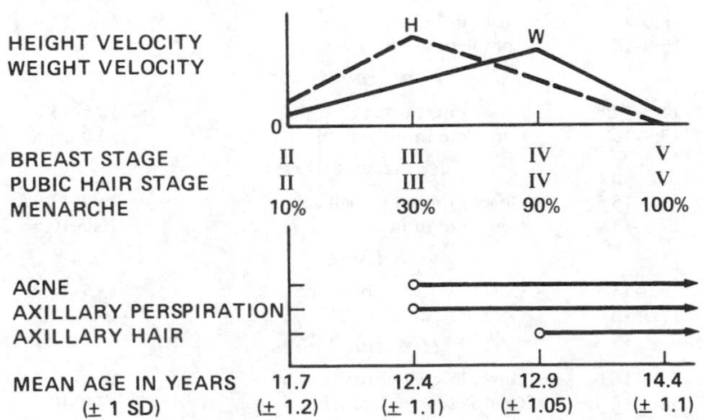

Figure 14–4 Sequence of maturational events in females. (Adapted from Marshall WA, Tanner JM: Variations in pattern of pubertal changes in girls. Arch Dis Child 44:291, 1969.)

SELF-CONCEPT. Self-consciousness increases exponentially in response to the somatic transformations of puberty. Self-awareness at this age tends to center on external characteristics in contrast to the introspection of later adolescence. It is normal for early adolescents to scrutinize their appearance and to feel that everyone else is staring at them too. Girls, in particular, are at risk for viewing themselves as overweight. Dieting behavior is common, and girls who rate themselves as fat/out of shape may be at increased risk of depression (Chapter 23). Severe body image distortions, such as anorexia nervosa, also tend to appear at this age (Chapter 112). There is controversy about whether puberty may increase self-esteem in boys but undermine it in girls as both sexes assume gender roles that incorporate gross inequalities in power and prestige.

RELATIONSHIPS WITH FAMILY, PEERS, AND SOCIETY. In early adolescence, the trend toward separation from family with increasing involvement in peer activities accelerates. A symbolic expression of this shift is the renunciation of family norms of dress and grooming in favor of the peer group "uniform." Such stylistic changes frequently spark conflicts that are truly about power or difficulty accepting separation. Not all adolescents rebel, and not all parents reject such assertions of separateness as signs of insurrection. Most adolescents continue to strive to please their parents even while they disagree on certain issues.

Separation from family often involves selecting adults outside of the family as role models and developing close relationships with particular teachers or the parents of other children. Organizations such as scouting, sports teams, or gangs provide an important sense of extrafamilial belonging.

Early adolescents often socialize in same-sex peer groups. Scatologic jokes, teasing directed against the other gender, and rumor mongering about who likes whom attest to burgeoning sexual interest. Belonging is all important. In one-to-one friendships, boys and girls may differ in important ways. Female friendships may center on sharing confidences, whereas male relationships may focus more on shared activities and competition.

An early adolescent's relationship to society centers on school. The shift from elementary to junior high school entails giving up the protection of the homeroom in exchange for the additional stimulation and responsibility involved in moving from class to class. This change in school structure mirrors and reinforces the changes involved in separating from the family.

The societal preoccupation with youth and sexuality generates constant exposure to sexually suggestive and explicit images. At the same time, reliable information about contraception remains sparse. Ready access to pornography on the Internet may increase the risk of premature sexual activity or exploitation.

IMPLICATIONS FOR PARENTS AND PEDIATRICIANS. Physical growth, body preoccupation, and sexual interest correlate with sexual maturity, whereas cognitive advancement, separation, and changes in social behavior may correlate more closely with chronologic age or grade in school. Discordance between chronologic age and sexual maturation may increase the stress of early adolescence. As a group, early maturing boys enjoy greater social success and higher self-esteem than do later maturers. For girls, by contrast, early maturation is associated with poorer school performance and lower self-esteem.

Early adolescents often have questions about the somatic and sexual changes they are experiencing. In a multicultural sample of rural and urban adolescents, questions may range from sophisticated to poignantly ignorant. During a physical examination, a pediatrician can anticipate concerns and volunteer information that the adolescent may have been too uncomfortable to request. Parents, too, may have concerns that they are hesitant to discuss. If the parent is interviewed alone, it is important that this be done first, before the interview with the child, to avoid undermining the adolescent's trust.

The child's level of cognitive sophistication has implications for the sort of explanations that will be most helpful. Open-ended questions about common dilemmas facing young adolescents (e.g., whether or not to join a clique or gang or to abide by family rules that seem unjustified) can provide information about cognitive level and help assess the likelihood of risky behavior (see Chapters 5 and 17).

Parents and children often need help differentiating between the normal discomforts of the period and truly concerning behaviors. Discomfort with one's body is normal; the conviction that one is overweight and needs to diet despite objective evidence to the contrary is concerning. Bids for autonomy in the form of avoidance of family activities, demands for privacy, and increased argumentativeness are normal; extreme withdrawal or antagonism may be a sign of dysfunction. Interest in sex, sometimes heralded by the appearance of pornographic magazines, is normal; sexual intercourse in early adolescence, though fairly common, is usually a sign of developmental dysfunction. Bewilderment and dysphoria at the start of junior high school are normal; continued failure to adapt several weeks later suggests a more serious problem.

MIDDLE ADOLESCENCE

BIOLOGIC DEVELOPMENT. In middle adolescence, growth accelerates above the prepubertal rate of 6–7 cm (3 in) per year. In the average girl, the growth spurt peaks at 11.5 yr at a top velocity of 8.3 cm (3.8 in) per year and then slows to a stop at 16 yr (see Fig. 14–4). In the average boy, the growth spurt starts later, peaks at 13.5 yr at 9.5 cm (4.3 in) per year, and then slows to a stop at 18 yr. Weight gain parallels linear growth, with a delay of several months, so that adolescents seem first to stretch and then fill out. Pubertal weight gains account for approximately 40% of adult weight. Muscle mass also increases, followed several months later by an increase in strength; boys show greater gains in both. Lean body mass, approximately 80% in the average prepubertal child, increases in boys to 90% and decreases in girls to 75% as subcutaneous fat accumulates.

Bone maturation correlates closely with SMR because epiphyseal closure is under androgenic control (Table 14–5). Boys with SMR3 pubic hair and SMR4 genitals normally have their peak growth spurt ahead of them; girls at the same SMR are usually past their peaks (see Figs. 14–3 and 14–4). Widening of the shoulders in boys and of the hips in girls is also hormonally determined. Other physiologic changes include a doubling in heart size and lung vital capacity from preadolescent norms. Blood pressure, blood volume, and hematocrit rise, particularly in boys. Androgenic stimulation of sebaceous and apocrine glands results in acne and body odor. A physiologic increase in sleepiness may be mistaken for laziness.

Sexual maturation in middle adolescence is dramatic, with the achievement of menarche in 30% of girls by SMR3 (mean age 11.9 yr) and in 90% by SMR4 (mean age 12.6–12.9 yr). Menarche usually follows approximately 1 yr after the growth spurt. The timing of menarche, not completely understood, appears to be determined by genetics as well as such factors as adiposity, chronic illness, and exercise. In developed countries, the average age at menarche has decreased in the past century, perhaps in response to better nutrition and less physical activity. Before menarche, the uterus achieves a mature configuration, vaginal lubrication increases, and a clear vaginal discharge appears, sometimes mistaken for a sign of infection. In boys, spermarche occurs and the penis lengthens and widens.

SEXUALITY. Dating becomes a normative activity during middle adolescence. The degree of sexual activity varies widely. At age 16 yr, approximately 30% of girls and 45% of boys report having sexual intercourse, whereas 17% engage in petting, and some 22% report kissing as the only sexual behavior.

Biologic maturation and social pressures combine to determine sexual activity. High testosterone and low religiosity together may predict which boys become sexually active. Most parents discourage sexual activity, but some actually encourage it in hopes of boosting the child's popularity or of living vicariously through the child's experiences. *Homosexual experimentation* is common and does not necessarily reflect a child's ultimate sexual orientation. Many adolescents worry that they might be homosexual, and dread being found out. As a result, homosexual dating and sexual activity during adolescence are rare. Homosexual adolescents face increased risk of isolation

TABLE 14–5 Modal Age at Onset and Completion of Fusion in Skeletal Areas in Adolescence

Boys: Modal Age Between (yr)	Area	Girls: Modal Age Between (yr)
	Elbow	
13.0–13.5	Onset in humerus	11.0–11.5
15.0–15.5	Complete in ulna	12.5–13.0
	Foot and Ankle	
14.0–14.5	Onset in great toe	12.5–13.0
15.5–16	Complete in tibia, fibula	14.0–14.5
	Hand and Wrist	
15.0–15.5	Onset in distal phalanges	13.0–13.5
17.5–18.0	Complete in radius	16.0–16.5
	Knee	
15.0–15.5	Onset in tibial tuberosity	13.5–14.0
17.5–18.0	Complete in fibula	16.0–16.5
	Hip and Pelvis	
15.5–16.0	Onset in greater trochanter	14.0–14.5
after 18.0	Complete in symphysis	17.5–18.0
	Shoulder and Clavicle	
15.5–16.0	Onset in greater tubercle of humerus	14.0–14.5
after 18.0	Complete in clavicle	17.5–18.0

and depression. Fear of stigmatization may keep them from discussing their concerns with pediatricians or other potentially helpful adults (see Chapter 26).

In addition to sexual orientation, middle adolescents begin to sort out other important aspects of sexual identity, including beliefs about love, honesty, and propriety. Dating relationships are often superficial at this age, emphasizing attractiveness and sexual experimentation rather than intimacy. Adolescents tend to choose one of three sexual paths: celibacy, monogamy, or polygamous experimentation. Most have some knowledge of the risks of pregnancy, acquired immunodeficiency syndrome, and other sexually transmitted diseases, but knowledge does not consistently control behavior. A minority use any contraception at first intercourse, and fewer than 75% consistently use condoms or other effective methods.

COGNITIVE AND MORAL DEVELOPMENT. With the transition to formal operational thought, middle adolescents question and analyze extensively. Questioning of moral conventions fosters the development of personal codes of ethics. Such codes often appear designed to justify the adolescent's sexual appetite: "Anything I want is right." In other cases, adolescents may embrace a code that is more strict than that of their parents, perhaps in response to the anxiety engendered by the weakening of the conventional limits. An adolescent's new flexibility of thought has pervasive effects on relationships with self and others.

SELF-CONCEPT. The peer group exerts less influence over dress, activities, and behavior. Middle adolescents often experiment with different personae, changing styles of dress, groups of friends, and interests from month to month. Many philosophize about the meaning of their lives and wonder, "Who am I?" and "Why am I here?" Intense feelings of inner turmoil and misery are common and may be difficult to differentiate from psychiatric illness. Girls may tend to characterize themselves and their peers according to interpersonal relationships ("I am a girl with close friends"), whereas boys as a group may focus on abilities ("I am good at sports").

RELATIONSHIPS WITH FAMILY, PEERS, AND SOCIETY. Puberty commonly results in strained relationships between adolescents and their parents. As part of separation, adolescents may become distant from parents, redirecting emotional and sexual energies toward peer relationships. Dating can become a lightning rod for parent-child battles, in which the real issue may be the fact of separation rather than the particulars of "with whom" or "how late."

As dating increases, the need to belong to same-sex groups declines. Physical attractiveness and popularity remain critical factors in both peer relationships and self-esteem. Children with visible differences, such as cleft lip, are at risk for problems developing social skills and confidence and may have more difficulty establishing satisfying relationships.

Middle adolescents often begin thinking seriously about what they want to do as adults, a question that formerly had been comfortably hypothetical. The process involves self-assessment and assessment of the opportunities available. The presence or absence of realistic role models, as opposed to the idealized ones of earlier periods, can be crucial.

IMPLICATIONS FOR PARENTS AND PEDIATRICIANS. Physical and sexual maturation, changes in sexual behavior and identity, emotional distance from parents, waning peer group influence, introspection, and growing cognizance of life after childhood all combine to make middle adolescence a time when the opportunity to talk confidentially with a nonjudgmental, informed adult can be particularly appreciated and helpful.

Adolescents vary greatly in their rate of physical and social progress and in the resolution of central conflicts about autonomy and self-esteem. Questions about family and peer relationships can help locate a child along the developmental continuum and facilitate individualized counseling. In asking about dating and sex, it is important not to convey the assumption of heterosexuality because that will reduce the likelihood that concerns about sexual orientation will surface. In talking to a boy, for example, one might observe that some boys are interested sexually in girls, some boys are interested in other boys, and some are interested in both (or neither).

LATE ADOLESCENCE

BIOLOGIC DEVELOPMENT. The somatic changes in this period are modest by comparison. The final stages of breast, penile, and pubic hair development occur by age 17–18 yr in 95% of males and females. Minor changes in hair distribution often continue for several years in males, including the growth of facial and chest hair and the onset of male-pattern baldness in a few.

PSYCHOSOCIAL DEVELOPMENT. Sexual experimentation decreases as adolescents adopt more stable sexual identities. Cognition tends to be less self-centered, with increasing thoughts about concepts such as justice, patriotism, and history. Older adolescents are often idealistic but also may be absolutist and intolerant of opposing views. Religious or political groups that promise answers to complex questions may hold great appeal.

Slowing physical changes permit the emergence of a more stable body image. Intimate relationships are also an important component of identity for many older adolescents. In contrast to the often superficial dating relationships of middle adolescence, these relationships increasingly involve love and commitment. Career decisions become pressing because an adolescent's self-concept is increasingly bound up in the emerging role in society (as student, worker, or parent).

IMPLICATIONS FOR PARENTS AND PEDIATRICIANS. Erikson identified the crucial task of adolescence as that of establishing a stable sense of identity, including separation from family of origin, initiation of intimacy, and realistic planning for economic independence. To achieve these milestones, developmental progress is required of both adolescents and their parents. Continued difficulty in any of these areas may constitute an indication for referral for counseling.

Brown RT, Cromer BA: The pediatrician and the sexually active adolescent: Sexual activity and contraception. Pediatr Clin North Am 44:1379–1390, 1997.

Felice ME: Adolescence. *In:* Levine MD, Carey WB, Crocker AC (eds): Developmental-Behavioral Pediatrics. Philadelphia, WB Saunders, 1992, pp 65–73.

Kohl HW, Hobbs KE: Development of physical activity behaviors among children and adolescents. Pediatrics 101:549, 1998.

Litt IF, Martin JA: Development of sexuality and its problems. *In:* Levine MD, Carey WB, Crocker AC (eds): Developmental-Behavioral Pediatrics. Philadelphia, WB Saunders, 1992, pp 428–442.

Marshall WA, Tanner JM: Variations in the pattern of pubertal change in girls. Arch Dis Child 44:291, 1969.

Marshall WA, Tanner JM: Variations in the pattern of pubertal change in boys. Arch Dis Child 45:13, 1970.

Owens RP: Disorders of puberty. *In:* Kliegman RM (ed): Practical Strategies in Pediatric Diagnosis and Therapy. Philadelphia, WB Saunders, 1996, pp 1008–1020.

Rutter M, Graham P, Chadwick OFD, et al: Adolescent turmoil: Fact or fiction? J Child Psychol Psychiatr 17:35, 1976.

Slap GB: Normal physiological and psychosocial growth in the adolescent. J Adolesc Health Care 7:13S, 1986.

Tanner JM, Davies PSW: Clinical longitudinal standards for height and height velocity for North American children. J Pediatr 107:317, 1985.

CHAPTER 15
Assessment of Growth

Growth assessment is an essential component of pediatric health surveillance because almost any problem within the physiologic, interpersonal, and social domains can adversely affect growth. The most powerful tool in growth assessment is the growth chart (see Figs. 11–1 and 11–2). Combined with an accurate scale, a measuring board, stadiometer, and tape measure, the growth chart provides most of the information needed to assess growth.

GROWTH CHART DERIVATION AND INTERPRETATION

The standard growth charts are based on data collected from 1963 to 1975 by the National Center for Health Statistics (NCHS) and may not reflect normal growth in contemporary U.S. children. New growth charts are scheduled to be released by 1999, based on a nationally representative sample collected from 1988 to 1994 as part of the National Health and Nutrition Examination Survey (NHANES-III). Normative values provided in the present volume (see Tables 12–1 and 12–2) are based on the older NCHS data.

For infants, the measure of linear growth is *length,* taken by two examiners (one to position the child) with the child supine on a measuring board. For older children, the measure is *stature,* taken with a child standing on a stadiometer. This technical difference results in children's appearing to shift down in length as they change from the younger to the older chart. The data are presented in four standard charts: (1) weight for age, (2) height for age, (3) head circumference for age, and (4) weight for height. Separate charts are provided for boys and girls (see Figs. 11–1 and 11–2).

Each chart is composed of seven percentile curves, representing the distribution of weight, length, stature, or head circumference values at each age. The percentile curve indicates the percentage of children at a given age on the *x*-axis whose measured value falls below the corresponding value on the *y*-axis. For example, on the weight chart for boys age 0–36 mo (see Fig. 11–1*A*), the 9-mo age line intersects the 25th percentile curve at 8.5 kg, indicating that 25% of the 9-mo-old boys in the NCHS sample weigh less than 8.5 kg (75% weigh more). Similarly, a 9-mo-old boy weighing more than 11 kg is heavier than 95% of his peers.

By definition, the 50th percentile is the median, the value above (and below) which 50% of the observed values fall. It is also termed the *standard value* in the sense that the standard height for a 7-mo-girl is 120 cm (see Fig. 11–1*B*). The weight-for-height charts (see Fig. 11–2) are constructed in an analogous fashion, with length or stature in place of age on the *x*-axis. According to the chart, the median or standard weight for a girl measuring 125 cm is 24 kg.

It is important to appreciate both the strengths and limitations of these charts. The NCHS data are representative of a population of well-nourished and healthy children in the United States. In the 1963–1975 sample, most of the infants were bottle fed. Although this population is dissimilar to much of the rest of the world, the NCHS charts have been accepted by the World Health Organization as the international standard of growth for the first 5 yr of life. Disparities in growth between developed and developing countries reflect nutritional rather than genetic differences. It is recommended to use the NCHS standards for first-generation American children whose immigrant parents may be short. Such children may have better nutrition and grow taller than their parents.

The NCHS curves are less appropriate for adolescents. Growth during adolescence is linked temporally to the onset of puberty, which varies widely (Chapter 14). The NCHS cross-sectional sample, based solely on chronologic age, lumps together subjects who are at different stages of maturation. The data for 12-yr-old boys include both early-maturing boys who are at the peak of their growth spurts and later-maturing ones who are still growing at their prepubertal rate. The net result is to artifactually level off the growth peak, making it seem as though adolescent children grow more gradually and for a longer period than they do. The NCHS curves may indicate poor or excessive growth when a child is growing normally but happens to be a late or early maturer. Growth charts derived from longitudinal data are recommended for adolescents, when precision is necessary.

The numeric data on which the charts are based are presented in Tables 12–1 and 12–2. The charts are useful because they facilitate assessment of growth over time. Specialized charts have also been developed for U.S. children with various conditions, including Down, Turner, and Klinefelter syndromes and achondroplasia.

ANALYSIS OF GROWTH PATTERNS

Growth is a process rather than a static quality. An infant at the 5th percentile of weight for age may be growing normally, may be failing to grow, or may be recovering from growth failure, depending on the *trajectory* of the growth curve. Typically, infants and children stay within one or two growth channels. This *canalization* attests to the robust control that genes exert over body size.

A normal exception commonly occurs during the 1st 2 yr of life. For full-term infants, size at birth reflects the influence of the uterine environment; size at age 2 yr correlates with mean parental height, reflecting the influence of genes. Between birth and 18 mo, small infants often shift percentiles upward toward their parents' mean percentile. Large neonates with smaller parents often shift downward, with decelerating growth beginning at 3–6 mo and ending as an infant achieves a new growth channel at approximately 13–18 mo.

It is important to correct for various factors in plotting and interpreting growth charts. For premature infants, overdiagnosis of growth failure can be avoided by subtracting the weeks of prematurity from the postnatal age when plotting growth parameters. Very low birthweight (VLBW <1,500 g) infants may continue to show *catch-up growth* through early school age. The presence of neurologic abnormality (e.g., cerebral palsy) in VLBW infants may limit catch-up growth. Special growth charts based on gestational rather than chronologic age have been developed for infants beginning at 26 wk gestational age. These charts are based on a relatively small, possibly nonrepresentative sample, which may limit their general applicability.

For adolescents, normal variations in the timing of the growth spurt can lead to misdiagnosis of growth abnormalities. In general practice, cognizance of the relationship between sexual maturity and growth suffices (see Chapter 14). Special growth charts have been developed for early-, average-, and late-maturing adolescents that can be used when additional precision is needed. For children with particularly tall or short parents, there is a risk of overdiagnosing growth disorders if parental height is not taken into account or, conversely, of underdiagnosing growth disorders if parental height is accepted uncritically as the explanation. Standards have been developed to allow adjustments on the adolescent height curve based on mean parental height. These charts are based on a small, possibly nonrepresentative sample, which limits the generalizability of these standards.

The analysis of growth patterns provides critical information for the diagnosis of *failure to thrive* (FTT) (see Chapter 36). There is no universally agreed-on criterion for FTT or growth failure; most consider the diagnosis if a child's weight is below the 5th percentile or drops down more than two major percentile lines. Calculation of weight gain in grams per day, with comparison with Table 10–5, allows more precise estimation of growth rate.

Weight-for-height below the fifth percentile is the single best growth chart indicator of acute undernutrition. After several months of caloric deprivation, the height-for-age curve drops (stunting), whereas the weight-for-height curve may return toward normal. In infants, chronic, severe undernutrition also depresses head growth, an ominous predictor of later cognitive disability.

TABLE 15–1 Severity of Malnutrition: Stunting and Wasting

Grade of Malnutrition	Weight for Age* (Wasting)	Height for Age† (Stunting)	Weight for Height‡
0, normal	>90	>95	>90
1, mild	75–90	90–95	81–90
2, moderate	60–74	85–89	70–80
3, severe	<60	<85	<70

Values represent percentage of median for age.

**Data from Gomez F, Galvan RR, Frank S, et al: Mortality in second- and third-degree malnutrition. J Trop Pediatr 2:77, 1956.*

†Data from Waterlow JC: Evolution of kwashiorkor and marasmus. Lancet 2:712, 1974.

‡Data from Waterlow JC: Classification and definition of protein-calorie malnutrition. BMJ 3:566, 1972.

When growth parameters fall below the 5th percentile, it becomes necessary to express the values as percentages of the median or standard value. A 12-mo-old girl weighing 7.3 kg is at 75% of the median weight (9.7 kg) for her age. Using the calculated percentage of standard rather than the percentile, growth failure can be graded from mild to severe according to Table 15–1. These designations correlate with risk of mortality in developing countries; their correlation with short- and long-term sequelae of growth failure in the United States is less well documented. Another way to describe extremes of height is the *height age,* the age at which the standard (median) height equals the child's present height. A 30-mo-old child who is as tall as an average 13-mo-old has a height age of 13 mo. The *weight age* is defined analogously.

Nutritional insufficiency must be differentiated from congenital, constitutional, familial, and endocrine causes of decreased linear growth (see also Chapter 42). In the latter cases, the length declines first or at the same time as the weight; weight for height is normal or elevated. In nutritional insufficiency, the weight declines before the length and the weight for height is low (unless there has been chronic stunting). Figure 15–1 depicts typical growth curves for four classes of decreased linear growth. In congenital pathologic short stature, an infant is born small and growth gradually tapers off throughout infancy. Causes include chromosomal abnormalities (Turner syndrome, trisomy 21), infection (TORCH [toxoplasmosis, other infections, rubella, cytomegalovirus infection, and herpes simplex] infections), teratogens (phenytoin [Dilantin], alcohol), and extreme prematurity. In constitutional growth delay, weight and height decrease near the end of infancy, parallel the norm through middle childhood, and accelerate toward the end of adolescence. Adult size is normal. In familial short stature, both the infant and parents are small; growth runs parallel to and just below the normal curves.

Growth charts can confirm an impression of obesity if the weight for height exceeds 120% of the standard (median) weight for height. The *body mass index* (BMI) can be calculated as weight per height^2 when weight is in kilograms and height is in meters (Fig. 15–2). Although widely used as a clinical measure of *obesity,* BMI may not provide an accurate index of adiposity, because it does not differentiate lean tissue and bone from fat. Measurement of triceps and subscapular skinfold thickness can provide an index of adiposity (Fig. 15–3). However, considerable experience is needed for accuracy, and variability in fat distribution may confound the measurement. Dual x-ray absorptiometry provides a more precise estimation of body composition for research purposes.

Accurate measurement of weight and length is of obvious importance. Scales should be calibrated regularly. Supine length should be measured on a board; length measurements using a tape are inaccurate. Stature is best measured using a stadiometer; swing-arm measuring sticks attached to office scales are inaccurate. Head circumference is measured from the supraorbital ridge in front to the farthest point of the occiput in back. Cloth tapes stretch and should be avoided.

OTHER INDICES OF GROWTH

BODY PROPORTIONS. Body proportions follow a sequence of regular changes with development. The head and trunk are relatively large at birth, with progressive lengthening of the limbs throughout development, particularly during puberty (Chapter 14). Proportionality can be assessed by measuring the *lower body segment,* defined as the length from the symphysis pubis to the floor, and the *upper body segment,* defined as the height minus the lower body segment. The ratio of upper body segment divided by lower body segment (U/L ratio) equals approximately 1.7 at birth, 1.3 at 3 yr, and 1.0 after age 7 yr. Higher U/L ratios are characteristic of short-limb dwarfism or bone disorders such as rickets.

SKELETAL MATURATION. Reference standards for bone maturation facilitate estimation of bone age (see Tables 10–7 and 14–5). *Bone age* correlates well with stage of pubertal develop-

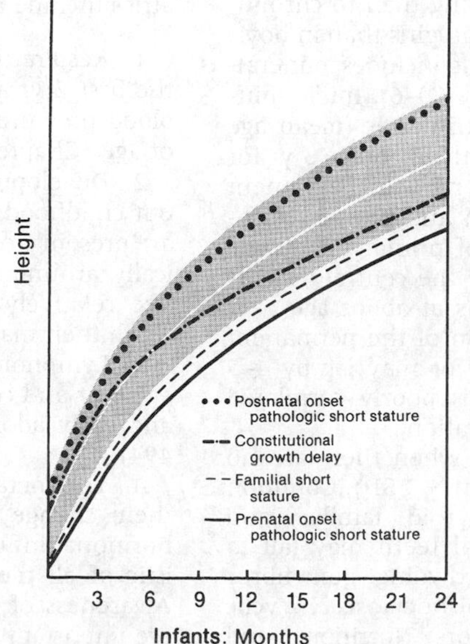

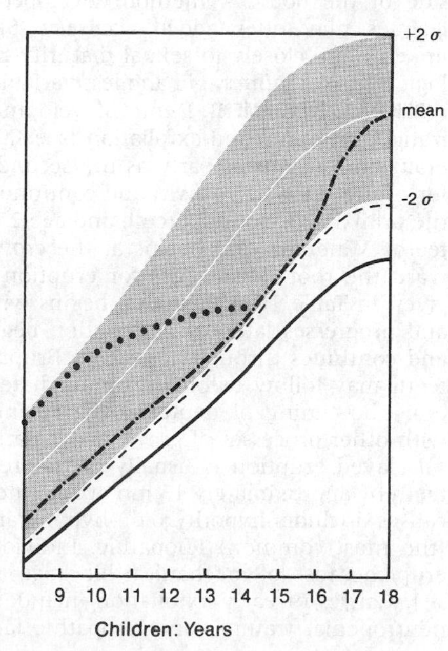

Figure 15–1 Height for age curves of the four general causes of proportional short stature: postnatal onset pathologic short stature, constitutional growth delay, familial short stature, and prenatal onset short stature. (From Mahoney CP: Evaluating the child with short stature. Pediatr Clin North Am 34:825, 1987.)

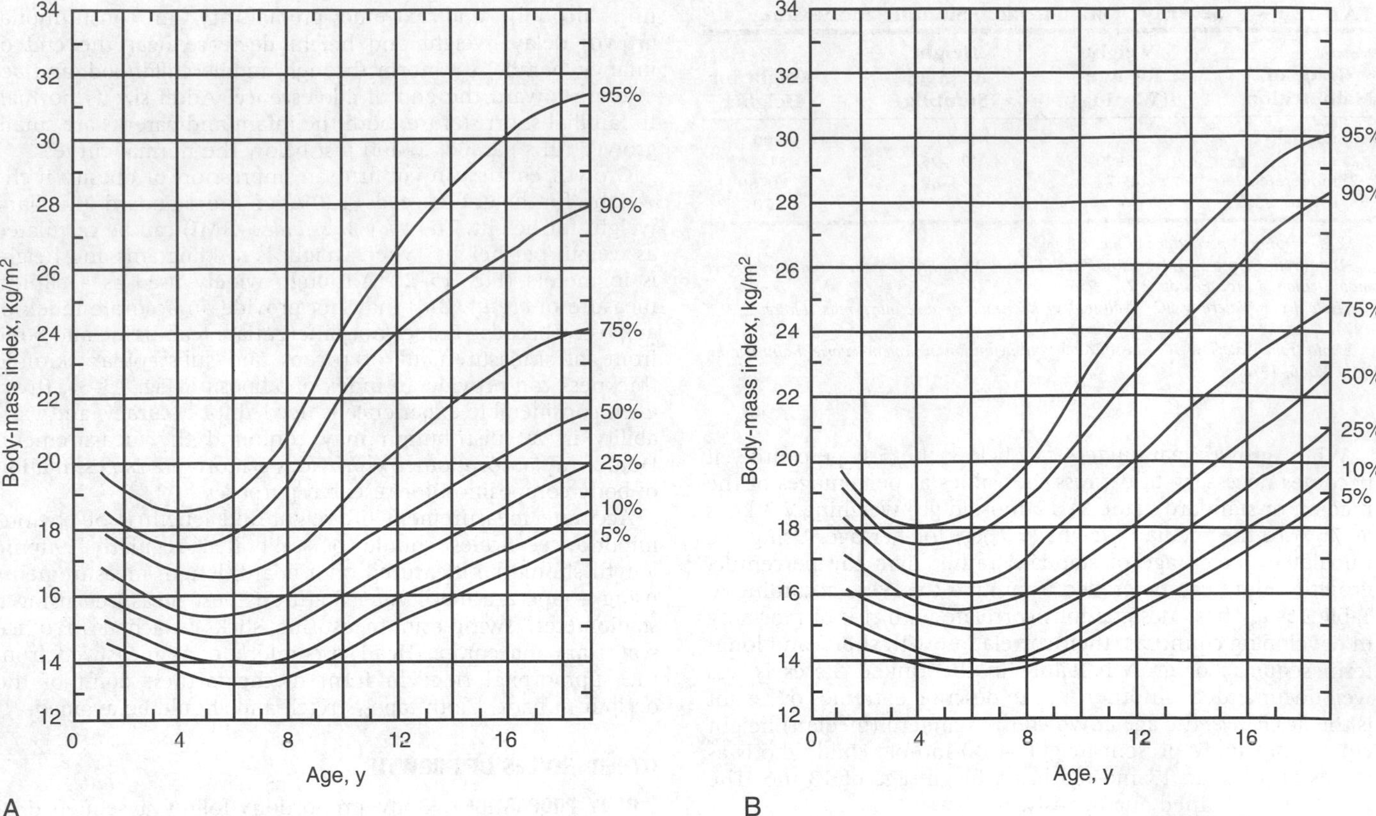

Figure 15–2 Body mass index (BMI) for white females *(A)* and males *(B)* age 1–19 yr. (From Hammer LD, Kraemer HC, Wilson DM, et al: Standardized percentile curves of body-mass index for children and adolescents. Am J Dis Child 145:259, 1991.)

ment and can be helpful in predicting adult height in early- or late-maturing adolescents. In familial short stature, the bone age is normal (comparable to chronologic age). In constitutional delay, endocrinologic short stature, and undernutrition, the bone age is low and comparable to the height age. The most commonly used standards are those of Gruelich and Pyle, which require radiographs of the left hand and wrist; knee films are sometimes added for younger children. Sontag's method requires radiographs of each major joint on the left side of the body. A method developed by Tanner and colleagues may offer added accuracy. Skeletal maturation is linked more closely to sexual maturity rating than to chronologic age. It is more rapid and less variable in girls than in boys.

DENTAL DEVELOPMENT. Dental development includes mineralization, eruption, and exfoliation (see Table 10–6). Initial mineralization begins as early as the second trimester (mean age for central incisors, 14 wk) and continues through age 3 yr for the primary (deciduous) teeth and age 25 yr for the permanent teeth. Mineralization begins at the crown and progresses toward the root. Mean ages for eruption of primary teeth are given in Table 10–6. Eruption begins with the central incisors and progresses laterally. Exfoliation begins at about age 6 yr and continues through age 12 yr. Eruption of the permanent teeth may follow exfoliation immediately or may lag by 4–5 mo. The timing of dental development is poorly correlated with other processes of growth and maturation.

Delayed eruption is usually considered when there are no teeth by approximately 13 mo of age (mean +3 SD). Common causes include hypothyroid, hypoparathyroid, familial, and (the most common) idiopathic. Individual teeth may fail to erupt because of mechanical blockage (crowding, gum fibrosis). Causes of early exfoliation include histiocytosis X, cyclic neutropenia, trauma, and idiopathic factors. Nutritional and metabolic disturbances, prolonged illness, and certain medications (tetracycline) commonly result in discoloration or malformations of the dental enamel. A discrete line of pitting on the enamel suggests a time-limited insult.

PHYSIOLOGIC AND STRUCTURAL GROWTH. Virtually every organ and physiologic process undergoes a predictable sequence of structural or functional changes, or both, during development. Reference values for developmental changes in a wide variety of systems (pituitary and renal function, electroencephalogram, electrocardiogram) have been published. Physiologic and structural changes of particular relevance to general pediatrics include the following:

1. Respiratory rate and pulse rate decrease sharply during the first 2 yr and then more gradually throughout childhood; blood pressure rises steadily beginning at approximately 6 yr of age (Chapters 374 and 429).
2. Development of the paranasal sinuses continues throughout childhood. The ethmoids, maxillary, and sphenoid sinuses are present from birth; the frontal sinuses first appear radiologically around age 6 yr. The ethmoids reach their maximum size relatively early in childhood (age 7–14 yr); the others reach their maximum size after puberty (also see Chapter 373).
3. Lymphoid tissues develop rapidly, reaching adult size by age 6 yr and continuing to hypertrophy throughout childhood and early adolescence before receding to adult size (Chapter 494).
4. The metabolism of medications and a child's response to them change rapidly in the 1st mo of life and again under hormonal influences in puberty. No single pattern is characteristic of all medications, and individual variation is the rule. Awareness of the possibility of changes and close monitoring are important (see Chapter 727).

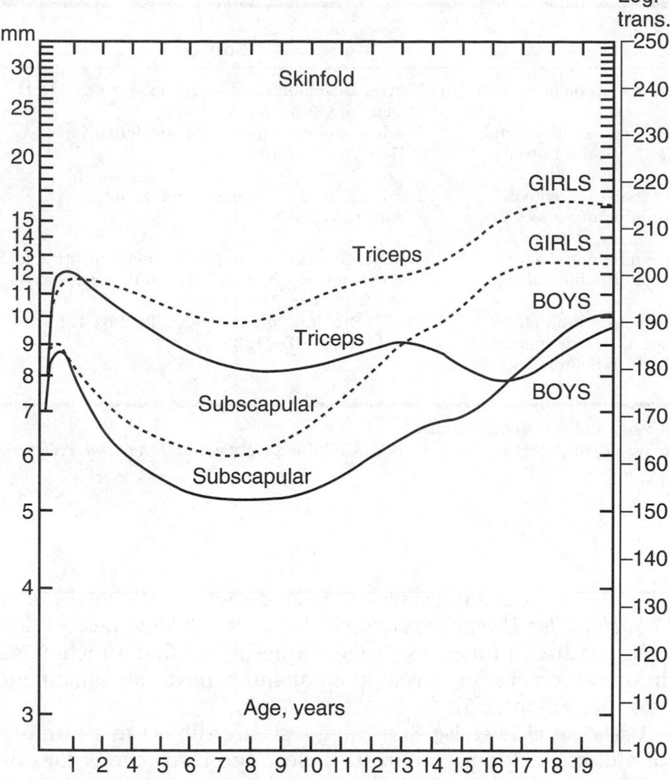

Figure 15–3 Skinfold thickness by age and sex, as measured by Harpenden skinfold calipers over triceps and under scapula. Scale is in millimeters on the left side and logarithmic transformation units on the right side. The lines shown are the 50th percentiles for British children. (From Tanner JM: Fetus into Man: Physical Growth from Conception to Maturity. Cambridge, Harvard University Press, 1978.) The data generating these curves are those of Tanner and Whitehouse (1975).

5. Nutritional needs as well as a wide variety of biochemical and hematologic values undergo marked developmental changes. For example, alkaline phosphatase level increases during periods of rapid bone growth (Chapter 706); hemoglobin has a physiologic nadir at approximately 2 mo of age (see Chapter 459).

Babson SG, Benda GI: Growth graphs for the clinical assessment of infants of varying gestational age. J Pediatr 89:814, 1976.

Bowers DF: Tooth development and abnormalities of appearance. *In:* Johnson TR, Moore WM, Jeffries JE (eds): Children are Different: Developmental Physiology. Columbus, OH, Ross Laboratories, 1978, pp 64–67.

Frank DA, Silva M, Needlman RD: Failure to thrive: Mystery, myth, and method. Contemp Pediatr 10:114, 1993.

Gruelich WW, Pyle SI: Radiographic Atlas of Skeletal Development of the Hand and Wrist. San Francisco, Stanford University Press, 1974.

Hamill PV, Drizd TA, Johnson CL, et al: Physical growth: National Center for Health Statistics percentiles. Am J Clin Nutr 32:607, 1979.

Himes JH, Roche AF, Thissen D, et al: Parent-specific adjustments for evaluation of recumbent length and stature of children. Pediatrics 75:304, 1985.

Smith DW, Truog W, Rogers JE, et al: Shifting linear growth during infancy: Illustration of genetic factors in growth from fetal life through infancy. J Pediatr 89:225, 1976.

Tanner JM, Davies PSW: Clinical longitudinal standards for height and height velocity for North American children. J Pediatr 107:317, 1985.

Tanner JM, Whitehouse RH, Cameron N, et al: Assessment of Skeletal Maturity and Prediction of Adult Height (TW2 Method). London, Academic Press, 1983.

CHAPTER 16
Developmental Assessment

Developmental assessment is the necessary prerequisite to intervention. The 1986 Amendments to the Education for All Handicapped Children Act (PL 99-457) require that every state create a system to identify and treat developmental disabilities in children age 3–5 yr. Most states have opted to extend these entitlements to children beginning at birth and to children deemed at risk for developmental problems as well as those with established delays. Ideally, pediatricians should have a central role in early identification, although in practice this is not always the case (Chapters 29, 37, and 39). In one large multicity study, physicians identified only 23% of emotional problems and 19% of hyperactivity before other professionals did. The mean ages at which physicians detected mental retardation, speech, and hearing problems were 34, 38, and 39 months, respectively; Down syndrome and cerebral palsy were detected earlier, at 0.6 and 10.3 mo.

Developmental assessment is a two-step process: first a screening procedure to pick out children in need of more in-depth assessment; second, developmental diagnosis, the goal of which is to define the developmental problems and their significance in the context of a child's biologic, psychologic, and social strengths and vulnerabilities. This chapter describes common approaches to screening, then discusses developmental diagnosis from infancy through school age.

SCREENING AND SURVEILLANCE. The ideal screening test must be highly sensitive (detect nearly all children with problems) and reasonably specific (not label many children as having problems when they do not in fact have them). It should also measure what it purports to measure (content validity), give similar results on repeat administration and on administration by different examiners (test-retest and inter-rater reliability), and be relatively quick and inexpensive. Table 16–1 lists several of the more common screening tests and their strengths and limitations. The ideal developmental screening test does not exist.

The most widely used and researched test is the Denver-II. The test generates pass-fail ratings in four domains of development—personal-social, fine motor-adaptive, language, and gross motor—for children from birth to 6 yr. It can be administered in 20–30 min without extensive training or expensive equipment. Originally published in 1969 as the Denver Developmental Screening Test (DDST), the name was later changed to "The Denver" in recognition of its limited utility for screening, per se. The test may fail to identify children with subtle delays, and its ability to predict cognitive delays at a later age (predictive validity) is modest. However, the Denver remains of great value, as it offers clinicians 125 well-standardized, easily administered developmental test items, presented in a convenient one-page format.

To increase the efficiency of screening, a series of brief parent questionnaires based on the DDST milestones has been recommended as a prescreen. Agreement with the full DDST is good, although the questionnaires require a high school reading level and may be subject to the same limitations as the Denver itself. The Denver Home Screening Questionnaire for parents provides information on the child-rearing environment, analogous to the well-validated Home Observation for Measurement of the Environment (HOME scale).

Screening for language delays is particularly important because of the strong links between language and cognitive development and later school performance. The Early Language

TABLE 16–1 Instruments and Questionnaires for Brief Developmental Assessment

Instrument	Age Range	Time (min)	Notes	Source
Denver-II	0–6 yr	30–45	Better sensitivity for language delays than older version	Denver Developmental Materials, PO Box 6169, Denver, CO 80206
Early Screening Inventory	3–6 yr	15–20	A quick, multidomain screen with good sensitivity and specificity compared with McCarthy Scales (a well-accepted test)	Teachers College Press, 1234 Amsterdam Ave, New York, NY 10027
ELM	0–3 yr	5–10	Well-normed, quick screen for expressive, receptive, and visual language; very useful in infancy; does not assess other domains	Pro-Ed, 8700 Shoal Creek Boulevard, Austin, TX 78757-6897
CAT/CLAMS	0–3 yr	10–20	CLAMS alone gives quick language quotient; CAT/CLAMS correlates well with Bayley (traditional gold standard)	Contact Dr. AJ Capute, The Kennedy Institute for Handicapped Children, 707 North Broadway St., Baltimore, MD 21205
Ages and Stages Questionnaires (ASQ)	4–48 mo	15–20	Series of self-administered questionnaires; multiple domains; good sensitivity and specificity; designed for ages that fall *between* usual pediatric schedule (e.g., 4, 8, 16 months)	Paul H Brookes Publishing Co., PO Box 10624, Baltimore, MD 21285

ELM, Early Language Milestone Scale; CAT, Clinical Adaptive Test; CLAMS, Clinical Linguistic and Auditory Milestone Scale.
Adapted from Blackman JA: Developmental screening: Infants, toddlers, and preschoolers. In: Levine MD, Carey WB, Crocker AC (eds): Developmental-Behavioral Pediatrics. Philadelphia, WB Saunders, 1992, pp 617–623.

Milestone (ELM) Scale provides pass-fail ratings in expressive, receptive, and visual language, using a format similar to that of the Denver. The scale was normed on a racially mixed sample of middle-class children and has been well validated in both low- and high-risk samples. Administration takes 2–3 min; most items can be completed by parental reporting. Sensitivity for language and cognitive delays is high compared with gold standard diagnostic tests; the test identifies many children even before their parents report being concerned. A modified scoring method can be used to generate a numeric score or age equivalent for diagnostic and research purposes.

Like the ELM, The Clinical Linguistic and Auditory Milestone Scale (CLAMS) is a sequence of language milestones that can be quickly administered, has been validated in infants and toddlers suspected of language delay and in those with known motor delays, and correlates well with standard diagnostic language tests. Paired with a similar series of nonverbal adaptive (problem-solving) milestones, the test correlates well with a gold standard test of mental retardation.

The Ages and Stages Questionnaires (ASQ) are a series of 11 questionnaires designed to be completed at home by parents at several time points from 4 to 48 mo. Validity and reliability are established, with overall agreement with standard developmental tests of 76–91%. However, the ASQ may fail to identify up to 13% of children with developmental delays. Scoring and interpretation are quick, making the ASQ especially suitable for busy practices. The Child Development Inventory is another well-standardized parent-report measure.

An efficient screening strategy relies on eliciting parental concerns verbally, first by asking about concerns in general and then about concerns in specific developmental areas (e.g., learning, talking, and motor development). In a community study of 408 children ages 2–7, parental concerns had sensitivity and specificity roughly comparable to the paper-and-pencil screening tests. Screening efficiency can be further enhanced by using a formal screening test as a second-level screen for any child "flagged" by systematic parent questioning.

Other procedures that can be useful for developmental screening include the draw-a-person test and the kinetic family drawing ("draw your family, with everybody doing something"). Much information can be obtained by asking children about their drawings. Another promising technique combines developmental screening with a modified vision test, the Simultaneous Technique for Acuity and Readiness Testing (START). Behavioral and psychiatric problems are common and often accompany developmental concerns. Screening for behavioral problems using the Pediatric Symptom Checklist (Fig. 16–1) is a simple, well-validated method. *Bright Futures: Guidelines for Health Supervision of Infants, Children and Adolescents* features numerous "trigger questions" that function as informal screens for developmental and behavioral adjustment (also see Chapter 5).

Limitations of Screening. Screening tests are subject to a number of abuses, including failure to follow the instructions for administration and scoring; overinterpretation of the results (essentially confusing screening with diagnosis); focusing on the screening test to the exclusion of other sources of information; screening too infrequently; using tests that are culturally biased; and failing to follow up with further assessments and treatment when indicated.

Concerns have been raised about the utility of community-wide programs of developmental screening. In one study, for example, children flagged by a preschool screening program had the same likelihood of developing later school problems, whether or not their parents were informed of the screening results. Parents who were informed reported worrying more but did not necessarily comply with recommendations for follow-up assessments and intervention.

Developmental Surveillance. Surveillance has been put forward as an antidote to the shortcomings of developmental screening. The transactional nature of development ensures that a child's status at any single point in time can never entirely predict later development. As with physical growth, a series of observations made over time provide much more information than an assessment at a single time point, allowing for estimation of developmental rate. Prediction is more accurate when it makes use of several sources of information, including the medical and social histories. These considerations underlie the concept of developmental surveillance, a process that includes regular elicitation of the developmental history, attention to parental concerns, careful developmental observations, and promotion of development.

Critics of surveillance have pointed out that a pediatrician's judgment is subject to a host of biases that undermine its accuracy. Pediatricians may overestimate IQ in children they know well or in children who are physically attractive or socially adept.

An approach combining ongoing surveillance with periodic use of screening tests may be the most effective and practical solution. A multidomain battery of milestones, such as the Denver, can be used as a framework for regular observations rather than as a stand-alone test. Parent questionnaires can streamline data collection and may encourage parents to voice their questions and concerns. Early identification of develop-

The Pediatric Symptom Checklist[a]

Please mark under the heading that best fits your child:

	Never	Sometimes	Often
1. Complains of aches or pains	____	____	____
2. Spends more time alone	____	____	____
3. Tires easily, little energy	____	____	____
4. Fidgety, unable to sit still	____	____	____
5. Has trouble with a teacher	____	____	____
6. Less interested in school	____	____	____
7. Acts as if driven by a motor	____	____	____
8. Daydreams too much	____	____	____
9. Distracted easily	____	____	____
10. Is afraid of new situations	____	____	____
11. Feels sad, unhappy	____	____	____
12. Is irritable, angry	____	____	____
13. Feels hopeless	____	____	____
14. Has trouble concentrating	____	____	____
15. Less interest in friends	____	____	____
16. Fights with other children	____	____	____
17. Absent from school	____	____	____
18. School grades dropping	____	____	____
19. Is down on him or herself	____	____	____
20. Visits doctor with doctor finding nothing wrong	____	____	____
21. Has trouble sleeping	____	____	____
22. Worries a lot	____	____	____
23. Wants to be with you more than before	____	____	____
24. Feels he or she is bad	____	____	____
25. Takes unnecessary risks	____	____	____
26. Gets hurt frequently	____	____	____
27. Seems to be having less fun	____	____	____
28. Acts younger than children his or her age	____	____	____
29. Does not listen to rules	____	____	____
30. Does not show feelings	____	____	____
31. Does not understand other people's feelings	____	____	____
32. Teases others	____	____	____
33. Blames others for his or her troubles	____	____	____
34. Takes things that do not belong to him or her	____	____	____
35. Refuses to share	____	____	____

[a]School items are in bold. These items were not counted for the 4–5-yr-old sample.

Figure 16–1 The Pediatric Symptom Checklist. (From Little M, Murphy JM, Jellinek MS, et al: Screening 4- and 5-year-old children for psychosocial dysfunction: A preliminary study with the pediatric symptom checklist. J Dev Behav Pediatr 15:191, 1994.)

mental and emotional problems will be maximized by keeping the following five principles in mind:

1. Parents, as a rule, are accurate observers of their children's behaviors; parental concerns about possible developmental delays are often appropriate and need to be taken seriously; conversely, a lack of parental concern should not be relied on as the sole indicator of normal development.
2. No child is too young for formal audiologic testing. In-office audiologic screening cannot rule out clinically significant hearing loss. Hearing-impaired children often use visual cues to "pass" hearing tests. Audiologic testing is indicated by the presence of any of the historic and physical findings listed in Table 16–2.
3. Risk factors are additive. Biologic impairments that may be relatively minor on their own (e.g., recurrent otitis) may have major impacts in the presence of environmental risk factors (e.g., maternal depression). Awareness of problems in one area should trigger increased vigilance in other areas. For example, emotional problems are common causes and consequences of cognitive and language disorders; environmental risk factors, such as maternal depression, frequently coexist with biologic risks, such as prematurity or lead toxicity.
4. Discomfort, fatigue, shyness, and oppositionality may adversely affect a child's performance on developmental testing. Rescreening is appropriate when these factors are suspected but should not be unduly delayed. Caution should be exercised before proclaiming that a child will "grow out of" a problem.
5. Pediatricians and parents may worry about the adverse effects of labeling a child. Screening test results are not diagnoses. Follow-up assessment and intervention are critical. It is a child's progress over time that is important rather than any labels given along the way. In all but the most severe cases, a child's progress cannot be accurately predicted at the outset; an attitude of realistic optimism is appropriate.

TABLE 16–2 Indications for Audiologic Evaluation

- Neonatal intensive care
  - Birth wt <2,500 g: All cases
  - Birth wt >2,500 g: If medical complications (asphyxia, seizures, persistent fetal circulation, intracranial hemorrhage, assisted ventilation, hyperbilirubinemia, ototoxic drugs)
- Proven or suspected intrauterine infection
- Bacterial meningitis
- Anomalies of 1st or 2nd branchial arch (microtia, auricular dysplasia, micrognathia)
- Anomalies of neural crest/ectoderm (widely spaced eyes; pigmentary defects)
- Family history of hereditary or unexplained deafness
- Parental concern about hearing loss
- Delayed speech or language development
- Other developmental disabilities (mental retardation, cerebral palsy, autism, blindness)

From Coplan J: Deafness: Ever heard of it? Delayed recognition of permanent hearing loss. Pediatrics 79:206, 1987.

DIAGNOSTIC ASSESSMENT

Once a child has been identified as having a potential problem, the next step is diagnostic assessment. The form and content of the assessment depend on the age of the child, the nature of the problem, and the available medical and community resources. Pediatricians function as part of a team that may also include psychologists, educators, social workers, and other professionals. Central to a pediatrician's role is medical evaluation of a developmentally disabled child (also see Chapter 37).

MEDICAL EVALUATION OF DEVELOPMENTAL DELAYS. The prevalence of more common developmental disabilities is listed in Table 16–3. The medical evaluation includes history, physical examination, and laboratory testing. Taking a thorough family history, including neurologic, psychiatric, and social difficulties

TABLE 16–3 Prevalence of Developmental Disabilities

Condition	Prevalence per 1,000
Cerebral palsy	2–3
Visual impairment	0.3–0.6
Hearing impairment	0.8–2
Mental retardation	25
Learning disability	75
ADHD	150
Behavioral disorders	6–13%

ADHD, Attention deficit hyperactivity disorder.
Adapted from Levy SE, Hyman SL: Pediatric assessment of the child with developmental delay. Pediatr Clin North Am 40:465, 1993.

(e.g., legal problems), is indispensable. The family history may shed light on the multigenerational origins of family dysfunction and resilience and may illuminate the parents' beliefs about the causes of the child's problem (e.g., "He's just like his uncle") (see Chapter 17).

The prenatal history should include a search for potential teratogenic exposures, including radiation or medications, infectious illnesses, fever, addictive substances, and trauma. The perinatal history includes birthweight, gestational age, Apgar scores, and any medical complications. Postnatal medical factors that are sometimes overlooked include chronic respiratory or allergic illness, recurrent otitis, head trauma, and sleep problems (particularly signs of obstructive sleep apnea [Chapter 383).

In the physical examination, points of particular importance include growth parameters and head circumference, facial and other dysmorphology, eye findings (e.g., cataracts in various inborn errors of metabolism), and signs of neurocutaneous disorders (café au lait spots in neurofibromatosis, hypopigmented macules in tuberous sclerosis).

No single set of laboratory tests is indicated in all cases. Most states screen for phenylketonuria, hypothyroidism, and other metabolic conditions in the neonatal period. Iron deficiency and lead toxicity are common contributors to developmental delays and are easily detected. Electroencephalograms and neuroimaging are not routinely indicated but should be used if there is clinical suspicion of seizure or encephalopathy or in cases of microcephaly or of rapidly expanding head circumference.

The medical evaluation for mental retardation (Chapter 37.2) and autism (Chapter 27.1) should include chromosomal and molecular biologic testing for fragile X, the most commonly identified genetic cause of mental retardation (Chapter 78). Classic physical findings in fragile X such as long facies, large ears, and large testes may be absent in infancy. Milder forms of cognitive and behavioral disturbance have been associated with partial mutations and heterozygosity for fragile X in girls as well as boys. A diagnosis of fragile X does not change therapy but has implications for genetic counseling. Ammonia and organic and amino acids may be included to screen for metabolic disease. With progressive loss of milestones, and particularly if there is associated growth delay, human immunodeficiency virus must be considered (Chapter 268).

DEVELOPMENTAL DIAGNOSIS FOR INFANTS AND PRESCHOOL-AGED CHILDREN. The most widely used newborn behavioral examination is the Brazelton Neonatal Behavioral Assessment Scale (NBAS). The NBAS allows quantitative estimation of an infant's neurologic intactness, adaptation to extrauterine life, primitive reflexes, state organization, self-regulatory ability, and interactive capacities from birth to 1 mo. The examination takes approximately 30–45 min and requires extensive training for an examiner to reach proficiency.

The NBAS is a poor predictor of later development, not surprising given the salience of environmental influences on development. In practice, the assessment functions well as an intervention in its own right (Chapter 9). Demonstrating neonates' behavioral abilities and vulnerabilities to their parents (e.g., their ability to track visually and turn toward sounds and their vulnerability to overstimulation) is consistently associated with improvements in the child-rearing environment months later.

For older infants and preschool-aged children, the diagnostic process may include formal developmental testing, playroom observations, parent and family interviews, home observations, and team meetings. It often involves a multidisciplinary team of educators, psychologists, parents, social workers, therapists, and pediatricians. Pediatricians contribute medical expertise and knowledge of the child and family accumulated over time. Diagnostic and therapeutic services are provided through the federal- and state-mandated early intervention programs and through multidisciplinary child development teams.

For young children, intervention relies on parental participation. The federal Early Intervention law (PL 105-17) mandates family involvement at all stages of the process of assessment, construction of a service plan, and monitoring of a child's progress. Pediatricians can help parents understand their rights and responsibilities under the law, review the process of developmental assessment and service planning to ensure that the parents are comfortable with the plan, and advocate with the early intervention system on behalf of a child.

To monitor a child's progress and advise the parents, a pediatrician needs to have realistic expectations about the effectiveness of early intervention. For children who face predominantly social/environmental risk factors (e.g., poverty), strong evidence shows that early intervention can raise IQ in the short term, as well as rates of school completion, job satisfaction, and social adjustment in the long term. For children at biologic risk because of prematurity, interventions combining direct therapy for a child with family support (home visiting, parent education) have resulted in significant gains in cognitive and emotional development. For children with established disabilities, the findings are more complex and controversial. Gains in IQ are modest overall, with greater gains among less severely affected children. However, improvements in family adjustment and alleviation of parental stress are consistently found. For children with autism-spectrum disorders, intensive language and interpersonal therapy may result in significant gains.

DIAGNOSTIC ASSESSMENT FOR SCHOOL-AGED CHILDREN. Pediatricians are often called on to diagnose specific learning disabilities or attention deficit disorder in school-aged children with academic or behavioral problems or both (Chapter 29.1, 29.2, and 29.3). The medical evaluation includes the factors discussed in the prior chapters. Vision and hearing deficits, although seldom the sole causes of school problems, must be evaluated. The interview should assess functioning in the home, the school, and the neighborhood and with peers (Chapters 13 and 14).

Definitive diagnosis usually requires a team effort. Educational testing is indicated to define areas of academic strength and weakness. Psychologic evaluation is indicated to assess emotional problems, such as depression or anxiety, that may be either causes or consequences of the school problems. Assessment of family functioning is essential. Neuropsychologic testing may be indicated to assess specific functional deficits (short-term memory, verbal processing) that may cause a child to be inattentive (Chapter 13). Pediatricians can facilitate these referrals and synthesize the information for parents and the school. Pediatricians with special interest in assessment of learning problems may also choose to use one of a series of neurodevelopmental tests, such as the Pediatric Early Elementary Examination (PEEX), to obtain a better sense of a child's functioning in various school-related cognitive areas.

Referrals to psychologic and educational specialists may be expensive and may not be covered by insurance. An alternative is assessment in the school. In the United States, under federal law, each child is entitled to comprehensive educational assessment and the establishment of an individualized educational plan (IEP) as part of free public education. The assessment must be completed within approximately 2–3 mo, and parents must approve the IEP before it can be instituted.

In practice, the quality of these educational assessments varies greatly depending on the skills of the school psychologist, the workload, and the educational resources available within the school system. If the assessment is inadequate, the parents have the right to demand an independent evaluation at the school's expense. The following questions can aid pediatricians in the important task of assessing the assessment:

1. Was sufficient time taken for the child to feel comfortable with the examiner and setting? The anxiety of confronting a stranger in a strange room may lower a child's score considerably.
2. Were a psychologic interview and projective testing as well as the more standard educational tests performed? Many school psychologists ignore the emotional aspects of learning, focusing solely on the cognitive.
3. Was IQ testing done? Were individual or group tests done?
4. Did the testing address all major areas of functioning (e.g., receptive and expressive language, visuomotor skills, short- and long-term memory)?
5. Was an attempt made to synthesize the findings in the report, or were the scores simply reported?

AAP Committee on Children with Disabilities: Screening infants and young children for developmental disabilities. Pediatrics 5:863, 1994.

Glascoe FP, Martin ED, Humphrey S: A comparative review of developmental screening tests. Pediatrics 86:547, 1990.

Solomon R: Pediatricians and early intervention: Everything you need to know but are too busy to ask. Infants Young Children 7:31, 1995.

Sturner R, Howard B: Preschool Development 1: Communicative and motor aspects. Pediatr Rev 18:291, 1997.

Zuckerman BS: Family history: A special opportunity for psychosocial intervention. Pediatrics 87:740, 1991.

PART III

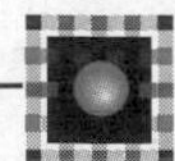

Psychologic Disorders

CHAPTER 17
Assessment and Interviewing

17.1 The Clinical Interview (History)

William H. Hetznecker, Marc A. Forman, and Jorge H. Daruna

The clinical interview is the most common procedure in medicine, but the nature of the process is often poorly defined. The interview is not simply history taking; still less is it a cross-examination of a patient that attempts to fulfill the requirements of a review of systems. It is basically a working alliance between a patient and physician, aimed at the orderly exchange of any and all clinically relevant information between them (see also Chapter 6). The patient is seeking reassurance or help, and the physician possesses knowledge, skills, and the social sanction to be helpful. The most useful perspective in which to view the clinical interview is as a major means of engaging patients and their families in active management of their own care (Chapter 5).

One well-practiced aspect of a clinical interview in most pediatric and general medical settings is the simple collection of those historical medical data that disclose and review the signs and symptoms of a presenting illness, the nature and course of past medical illnesses, the family history, and a review of systems. Other aspects of a patient's life, such as the psychosocial aspects, often get less or scant attention in interviewing. Physicians need to find ways to use clinical interviews to assess the emotional states of their patients, their usual reactions to stress, their self-concept, their systems of values, the nature of their personal relationships, something of their personalities, the quality of their coping abilities, and clues that might point to psychosocial distress or disturbance.

To become an effective interviewer requires motivation, skill, and continuous attentive practice. The skills required develop throughout the course of one's professional life. They are frequently overlooked in medical school, poorly taught, seen as related only to psychiatric patients, or taken for granted once medical school is completed. The development of effective interviewing skills is facilitated when students have the opportunity to practice with simulated patients, to make and watch recordings of their work with simulators or with actual patients, and to have these activities supervised by competent teachers or consultants.

TIME. An interview that attempts comprehensively to explore both psychosocial and biomedical aspects of the condition of a stranger who has just become a new patient needs at least 30–40 min for significant exchange of the most basic relevant information. Physician and patient must have time to become comfortable with each other and to establish the rapport that facilitates exploration of psychologic and social information. When patient and physician have had an adequate earlier initial interview and the physician therefore knows some of the major aspects of the patient's psychosocial status, it is possible to focus on particular issues in periods as brief as 10 min, but an initial interview of 10 min is inadequate, and it may communicate to the family a lack of respect for the sensitivity and importance of material given such casual attention.

SETTING. Privacy is essential, but the need for privacy is most likely to be overlooked with children, who are frequently managed with less respect and sensitivity than are adults. It is difficult to carry on an interview in a relatively unsheltered cubicle in an outpatient department or at bedside, even with curtains drawn to shield the child or family from visual intrusion or distractions. If possible, it is often more productive to seat a hospitalized child in a chair next to the bed rather than to converse with the child while he or she lies in bed. Adverse physical conditions negatively affect the quality and the effectiveness of the clinical interview. Although it may be difficult, it is worth considerable effort to find a private place; in hospitals, this may be a treatment room, an empty conference room, or even an unoccupied office or patient's room. Privacy is more easily arranged in the office of the practicing physician, where closed doors and reasonable comfort are ordinarily routine.

GOALS. The most common deficiency within an interview is the failure of the clinician to define clearly the goals of that particular encounter. No single interview can accomplish everything that needs to be done to complete a clinical assessment. Clinicians must set, define, and state priorities. These will depend on the nature of a patient's condition, whether the interview is an initial visit or a follow-up one, and whether the physician has to elicit sensitive material or to transmit unpleasant or unhappy diagnostic or prognostic information to patient or family. Physicians must become sufficiently familiar with their own styles and learn enough from past experiences to be able to judge accurately what can be accomplished in each interview. For example, if the work of the first interview is to establish a working alliance with a child and family and to identify the primary problems or concerns, then it may be a mistake to attempt a total developmental, family, or school survey on such an occasion.

COMMUNICATION. The major purpose and process of the clinical interview is the exchange of information. When the patients are children, this exchange occurs between parents and physician, between child and parents, and between parents, as well as between child and physician. In any social interaction, communication has two major features: one is the content or message; the other is the process, or the manner in which content is exchanged within the relationship (see also Chapter 5.)

The notion of content refers to the literal meaning of the words exchanged between communicating parties; content is the message or the *what* of communication. The notion of process refers to the relational or nonverbal aspects of communication. The tone of voice, the rate of speech, the inflection of words and phrases, facial expressions, head movements, hand gestures, and body postures and movement all communicate meaning, often more accurately than the words exchanged. The words usually capture the major conscious attention, but the process may frequently determine the success of the venture. The nonverbal features of communication are continually monitored by each sender and receiver, often preconsciously or subconsciously. The nonverbal expression conveys the cognitive, emotional, social, or global state of the sender with respect to what he or she is saying and indicates to the receiver how the content is to be interpreted.

Children attend to and respond to nonverbal communication before they understand the meanings of words. Reciprocal communication of basic feelings and emotions between parent and infant takes place through sounds, gestures, and body contacts long before the infant or the toddler can identify feelings or know what words appropriately express them. Physicians should be aware of how their own facial expressions, tone of voice, or gestures influence children's reactions and determine how messages are interpreted; this knowledge contributes greatly to skill in interviewing. The complementary skill required of a physician is to recognize and interpret a child's emotional state correctly through careful observation of facial expression, tone and inflection of voice, body posture, gestures, and other responses. Children may be unresponsive to questions because they are upset by the loudness of a physician's voice, by the suddenness with which he or she initiates an examination, or even by the closeness of the physician's body. Some children have temperamental characteristics predisposing them to anxiety in new or unfamiliar situations, and the physician has the responsibility for recognizing the signs and knowing how anxiety may be dealt with. Many children are frightened of unfamiliar office or hospital settings, of physical pain, of separation, of uncertainty, of persons or figures to whom they may attribute awesome authority and power, and of all else that goes with the word *doctor.*

Children continually need to know what is happening and what is going to happen to them in the immediate future. Their anxiety will be significantly reduced when physicians take time to explain what they are doing, what they are going to do, and, when they engage the child as an active participant, as much as the clinical situation and good judgment will allow. Making life predictable, within the framework of a short or even a 50-min encounter in the office or hospital, can have a profound effect on the likelihood of obtaining the cooperation of children.

Some children as young as 3–4 yr and most children by the age of 8 yr can participate verbally as well as physically in their own health care. All too frequently, conversation involves only the clinician and a parent, with the interaction between clinician and child being limited to the physical examination and some pleasantries. Children can and will respond relevantly to seriously posed questions about themselves.

By about the age of 13 yr, young persons are to be considered the primary informant and should be dealt with directly in their own right. If parents are at hand, they may be interviewed with the adolescent or separately, but at this age all explanations of diagnostic and treatment procedures should be directed first to the young person rather than to the parents. This procedure does not imply that a patient has veto power over the recommendations of a physician. Patients are still dependent on their parents, and the parents are still the major decision makers. Physical examinations of adolescents should be conducted with their parents not present, unless a patient requests otherwise.

TALKING WITH CHILDREN. Professional conversations with children have certain rules:

1. Don't talk to children in a condescending manner but as a physician talks with any patient.
2. Don't convey to children your thought that their feelings, concerns, or ideas are childish.
3. Don't laugh at what children say unless you are quite sure they intend to be humorous.
4. Don't try always to be funny or amusing to children. Such efforts are best saved for few occasions only and for children you know and who know you very well. Children know the difference between doctors and funny people.
5. Never tease children unless you know them very well and they know that they have permission to tease you in return.
6. Initial or casual encounters with young children are often made easier when introduced in a whisper, which young children may find more personal, private, and reassuring than jollity; they commonly whisper in response.
7. When children are old enough, at 4–5 yr, form the habit of discussing with them their symptoms, diagnoses, and treatments in terms they can understand. The use of drawings to illustrate and explain medical problems can be very useful.
8. Never discuss the illness or treatment of hospitalized children who have acquired receptive language functions in their presence unless you are discussing it with them as well.
9. When children fail to cooperate in their care in office or hospital, the first assumption should be that negativism or struggling means that they are frightened and reacting to fear in a customary personal manner; such behavior is often erroneously perceived as immature and irritating, embarrassing, provocative, or frightening by parents and other adults.

OTHER ASPECTS OF THE INTERVIEW. Certain signs indicate that the progress of an interview or examination should be assessed or reassessed for the effectiveness of communication.

1. When parents do not appear readily reassured by the diagnostic and treatment procedures, look for hidden anxiety due to unanswered questions that they may have difficulty recognizing or stating. Latent anger may have the same result. Physicians should make it comfortable and easy for parents to ask "stupid" questions or to admit "shameful" thoughts or "ungrateful" or angry feelings.
2. When a child is giving evidence of feeling pain, it is a psychologic impossibility that nothing hurts. When parents scold a child with "That doesn't hurt," they must be helped to understand that pain is a purely subjective experience and needs to be respected. Their acceptance of this may help greatly to clear the air.
3. Parents will sometimes be heard denigrating or shaming a child by using such terms as "baby," which is almost as bad as being intentionally cruel or frightening. Such behavior should be dealt with by the physician promptly and its inappropriateness discussed, with as much empathy for the parents' position as possible. "I can see that it's upsetting to you to have your child behaving this way, but I don't think that this approach is going to help us. Let's look at it from her (his) point of view. . . ."
4. Exhortation and other emotional appeals to reason are frequently used by parents and are among the weakest methods of attempting to alter behavior or attitudes. Again, "Let's look at it from the child's point of view. . . ."
5. When only one parent accompanies the child, it is almost always the mother. In many families, including those with working mothers, issues of health care are considered as maternal responsibilities. Physicians should feel increasingly uncomfortable as time passes and they have not yet met the fathers of children for whom they have assumed the responsibility of continuing care. Many fathers will be found eager to see a physician who extends a specific invitation, has clearly stated expectations, and will accommodate his time and schedules.
6. Physicians often, if they adequately explore the matter, find that parents have not complied with recommendations made for the care of their children. Compliance is not simply a matter of hearing, understanding, and doing what the doctor says, nor is noncompliance to be explained simply as ignorance, neglect, or a personality clash. Parents who fail to comply with recommendations may do so for a number of reasons, and these must be accurately identified.

Did the parent really understand what was prescribed or recommended? Does noncompliance express the parent's reservations about the appropriateness of the recommendations, or were the recommendations beyond the capacity of these parents to execute them, for technical, emotional, or financial reasons? Had the parents enough opportunity to ask questions and to discuss the details and ramifications of the child's condition and treatment? Is a noncompliant parent being influenced by information or advice contrary to that of the physician, which may come from the other parent, a grandmother, a friend, a newspaper or magazine article, or television programs?

Does the parent or do the parents have personal or marital problems that so upset and distract them that they cannot be effective, or does the child's illness itself have them so emotionally upset that they cannot accept the initiative and responsibility that has been thrust on them? Depressed mothers can be so psychologically depleted as to be unavailable to the child even though they may consciously want or intend to carry out recommendations. Is the parent expressing anger at the physician through noncompliance? Is the parent of an anxious and resistant child unable to execute a prescribed regimen that may be difficult or uncomfortable because he or she fears that the child may become hurt, resentful, or angry if the required firmness is exercised?

OTHER SOURCES FOR ASSESSMENT

INSTITUTIONS OR AGENCIES. Besides the clinical interview, other data can greatly help in psychosocial assessment. Birth records, for example, may help in questions of injury during pregnancy or at birth. Such records are often deficient, but they may provide the only objective view of events of a patient's birth and early days. Other health records, including those from other physicians or agencies that have cared for the patient, may provide essential information about acute or chronic illness, show a pattern of unusually frequent visits to the physician's office for relatively minor problems, or reveal an obsessive focus on certain areas of the body.

School reports are important to the psychosocial assessment, especially if they include both an academic assessment and a description of the child's relationships with schoolmates and teachers. Requests for school reports should be made only with the written permission of the child's parents or legal guardians.

Reports from child-care agencies may also be helpful, especially in the case of adopted children or children in foster care. Such agencies often have extensive background material and may have reports of earlier psychologic examinations.

PSYCHOLOGIC TESTING. A number of instruments may be administered to parents by trained pediatric staff to assess development, temperament, family stress, and parenting skills. Some examples of such instruments include the Vineland Adaptive Behavior Scales, Denver Developmental Screening Test, Carey Temperament Scales, and Parenting Stress Index. Use of these instruments can facilitate early identification of problems that may necessitate referral to a child psychiatrist or other appropriate specialist. These instruments should not be viewed as providing an adequate assessment by themselves.

Individual psychologic testing should be conducted by trained psychologists. Comprehensive assessments of sensory-motor development, language, and academic achievement may require additional involvement of occupational therapists, speech/language pathologists, or educational consultants. The major tests used in the psychologic assessment of children can be classified into four groups: (1) tests of general intelligence; (2) tests of academic achievement; (3) tests of specific sensory, motor, or cognitive functions; and (4) tests of behavioral or personality characteristics. Tests that are widely used to assess general cognitive proficiency or intelligence for specific age groups (shown in parentheses) include the following: The Bayley Scales of Infant Development (0–42 mo); Stanford-Binet Intelligence Scale, 4th edition (2 yr–adult); McCarthy Scales of Children's Abilities (2.5–8.5 yr); Kaufman Assessment Battery for Children (2.5–12.5 yr); Wechsler Preschool and Primary Intelligence Scale–Revised (3–7 yr); Wechsler Intelligence Scale for Children, 3rd edition (6–16 yr); and Wechsler Adult Intelligence Scale, 3rd edition (16 yr–adult).

Academic achievement tests are designed to measure competence in specific areas of knowledge or skill (e.g., arithmetic, reading) usually acquired through formal education in schools. Some frequently used tests in this category include the Peabody Individual Achievement Test, Revised; the Wide Range Achievement Test, 3rd edition; and the Woodcock-Johnson Psychoeducational Battery, Revised.

Numerous tests have been developed to measure more circumscribed skills such as auditory perception (e.g., Seashore Rhythms test); language (e.g., Boston Naming test); verbal memory (e.g., California Verbal Learning Test); abstract reasoning (e.g., Children's Category Test; Wisconsin Card Sorting Test); constructional ability and nonverbal memory (e.g., Rey's Complex Figure test); motor proficiency (e.g., Finger Tapping Test; Purdue Pegboard Test); and sustained attention (e.g., Continuous Performance tests).

Evaluation of behavioral or personality characteristics often relies on questionnaires completed by parents or teachers (e.g., Conners Rating Scales; Child Behavior Checklist) to rate the frequency with which children show various behaviors (e.g., hyperactivity, aggression). In the case of older children and adolescents, it is also possible to assess self-reported feelings and thoughts using questionnaires such as the Youth Self-Report, Piers-Harris Self-Concept Scale, or Reynolds Child Depression Scale. These scales are useful but do not substitute for carefully conducted clinical interviews. Assessments using projective tests, which require a child to report associations provoked by relatively abstract pictures (e.g., Rorschach inkblot test) or make up stories to pictures depicting specific situations (e.g., Children's Apperception Test; Thematic Apperception Test) are useful in uncovering issues or concerns that preoccupy children as well as distortions or idiosyncrasies that characterize their thought processes.

Neuropsychologic testing is synonymous with extensive testing using various instruments from all of the categories listed earlier. However, it should be noted that more testing is not necessarily better. As often as possible, tests should be chosen to address specific questions that will help make decisions about interventions. In choosing tests, it is essential that they have demonstrable reliability and validity. They should also have norms that are relatively recent and representative of the general population. An ongoing collaborative relationship with a psychologist or other specialist facilitates appropriate use of testing in a pediatric practice.

As a note of caution, psychologic tests should not be used to differentiate between so-called organic and functional causes of behavior. All causes of behavior are organic in the sense that behavior is biologically driven. If a question arises about the type of biologic disturbance that may underlie a behavioral impairment, other forms of assessment should be used, such as brain imaging techniques, neurophysiologic, endocrinologic, immunologic tests, and/or chromosomal-genetic studies.

PSYCHIATRIC CONSULTATION. A psychiatric consultation may be a valuable part of assessment of children in whom physical symptoms may have substantial psychosocial determinants; it often is most acceptable and useful when a child has been hospitalized for study. Other indications include the evaluation of depression in children with major acute or chronic illness, of chronic anxiety problems, of underachievement, and of serious aggressive difficulties. Standardized guidelines for psychiatric assessment of infants, children, and adolescents have been established by the American Academy of Child and Adolescent Psychiatry. Physicians should inform both parent and child that psychiatric consultation is intended to assess how psychosocial factors may contribute to the illness or problem, and they should obtain their consent and prepare them for what to expect.

CORRELATION OF DATA. Physicians must avoid early diagnostic closure even when parents' initial description of their problem gives a reasonably clear idea of what is going on. So long as physicians remain receptive and perceptive listeners, new and important information will emerge, as parents and perhaps patients begin to feel more trusting and as they are educated by a physician's questions. Furthermore, weighing of data must be done in the context of a family's sociocultural pattern (see Chapter 3). It is important that physicians not use their personal value system or style of living as a yardstick against which to measure a family's behavior or their success or failure in coping with their life situation. A family's feelings of anger, frustration, anxiety, failure, or depression are more valid indicators of where they need help.

It is important that the principal item of concern be accurately identified. Parents may present as the prime concern, for example, a problem such as bed-wetting of many years' duration. Why then have they come for help now? It is important to determine whether there may, in fact, be more important hidden issues the parents do not recognize or acknowledge or cannot face. By the same token, it must be understood that parents' assessment of the problem is critical for the child. Physicians, having collected and assessed appropriate data, sometimes can conclude only that children presented by their parents as having a problem are functioning within normal limits. In such a case, it must be determined what personal, familial, social, or cultural considerations compel the parents to see their child's behavior as a major problem. It must then be determined what re-education they may need to feel reassured and not be left with the impression that their anxiety has been casually dismissed.

REFERRAL. When problems have not been internalized by the child, it may be sufficient simply to counsel the parents, school personnel, or both. If this has been done and a maladaptive child or situation continues to present problems, the child and family will probably require more intensive or extensive help and should be referred to a child psychiatrist or psychiatric clinic. It is important that physicians avoid the position that psychiatric referral is a last resort. The need for a psychiatric consultation or referral can perhaps best be expressed in terms of the joint need of the family and physician for help in areas where the psychiatrist has special expertise, with the understanding that the collaboration of physician and family in management of the other health care needs of the child remains intact.

17.2 Psychosocial Problems

Richard Dalton and Marc A. Forman

A psychosocial disorder in a child may be manifested as a disturbance in feelings (e.g., depression, anxiety), in bodily functions (e.g., psychosomatic disorders), in behavior (e.g., conduct disturbances, passive-aggressive behavior), or in performance (e.g., learning problems). Dysfunction may involve any or all of these areas. Psychosocial problems may be produced by such physical or emotional stresses as birth defects, physical injury, inconsistent and contradictory child-rearing practices, marital conflict, child abuse and neglect, overindulgence, chronic illness, and so on. Particular agents do not, however, produce specific symptoms or disorders; rather, children's psychosocial problems are multifactorial in origin, their expression depending on many variables, including temperament, developmental level, the nature and duration of stress, past experiences, and the coping and adaptive abilities of the family. In general, chronic stresses or a series of stressful events are much more difficult for a child and family to manage than a single acute stressful episode. Children may react immediately to traumatic events or may keep their feelings dormant until maladaptive reactions become apparent during later periods of vulnerability.

Anticipatory guidance during periods of stress may considerably help children and their families to achieve more positive outcomes. Parents should be encouraged to prepare their children in advance for potentially traumatic events that can be anticipated (e.g., elective surgery, separation, or divorce). Children should be allowed or encouraged to express their feelings of dismay, fear, or anger rather than being told to be a "good girl" or "brave boy."

Infants and toddlers tend to react to stressful situations with impairment of physiologic functions, such as disturbances of feeding and sleep, with relatively global expressions of anger or fear, as in temper tantrums, or with withdrawal and avoidance behavior. School-aged children demonstrate their difficulties through altered interpersonal relationships with peers and family members, through impairment of school performance, by the development of specific psychologic syndromes, such as phobias or psychosomatic disorders, or by regressing to earlier, more childish modes of functioning.

Parents are frequently concerned whether the particular behaviors of their children are normal or whether they represent problems that require intervention. Some "symptomatic" actions of children may be part of normal development. For example, a temper tantrum may express the normal negativism of a toddler; on the other hand, temper tantrums on slight provocation in a 6-yr-old child may indicate psychosocial disturbance. Whether behavior is judged to be a developmental variation or evidence of a more serious problem depends on the age of the child; on the frequency, intensity, and number of symptoms; and especially on the degree of functional impairment. The decision of parents to seek help is determined, in turn, by the characteristics of their children's behavior; by the amount of distress it causes the children, parents, teachers, and others; and by their past experiences in discussing psychosocial matters with their physicians.

Achenbach TM, Edelbrock CS: Manual for Child Behavior Checklist and Revised Child Behavior Profile. Burlington, VT, University of Vermont, Department of Psychiatry, 1993.

Goodall J: Opening windows into a child's mind. Dev Med Child Neurol 18:173, 1976.

Impara JC, Murphy LJ (eds): Buros Desk References: Psychological Assessment in the Schools. Lincoln, NE, Buros Institute, 1994.

King RA, Work Group on Quality Issues: Practice parameters for the psychiatric assessment of children and adolescents. J Am Acad Child Adolesc Psychiatry 36(Suppl):4S, 1997.

Kestenbaum CJ: The clinical interview of the child. *In:* Wiener JM (ed): Textbook of Child and Adolescent Psychiatry. Washington, DC, American Psychiatric Press, 1991.

Reynolds CR, Kamphaus RW (eds): Handbook of Psychological and Educational Assessment of Children. Vol I. Intelligence and Achievement. Vol II. Personality, Behavior, and Context. New York, Guilford Press, 1990.

Rich J: Interviewing Children and Adolescents. London, Macmillan, 1968.

Thomas JM, Benham AL, Gean M, et al: Practice parameters for the psychiatric assessment of infants and toddlers (0–36 mo). J Am Acad Child Adolesc Psychiatry 36 (Suppl):21S, 1997.

Schowalter JE, King RA: The clinical interview of the adolescent. *In:* Wiener JM (ed): Textbook of Child and Adolescent Psychiatry. Washington, DC, American Psychiatric Press, 1991.

Simmons JE: Psychiatric Examination of Children, 4th ed. Philadelphia, Lea & Febiger, 1987.

Task Force on DSM-IV: Diagnostic and Statistical Manual of Mental Disorders, 4th ed: DSM-IV. Washington, DC, American Psychiatric Association, 1991.

Wood DJ: Talking to young children. Dev Med Child Neurol 24:856, 1982.

CHAPTER 18
Psychiatric Considerations of Central Nervous System Injury

Richard Dalton and Marc A. Forman

Psychiatric difficulties may follow infection; injury; intoxication; or genetic, metabolic, or idiopathic illness involving the central nervous system (CNS). These are not to be confused with the manifestations of "minimal cerebral dysfunction" (also known as minimal brain dysfunction, dysfunctional child, attention deficit disorder, or, in behavioral terms, the hyperactive or hyperkinetic child; for the last condition, see Chapter 29).

Brain injury increases the risk of both intellectual impairment and psychiatric disorder, especially when the injury is severe. Social disinhibition appears to be a specific sequela of brain injury, but no typical psychiatric syndrome is associated. The development of novel psychiatric disorders presenting after brain injury is predicted by the severity of the injury, preinjury family functioning, and preinjury psychiatric history. Psychosis is not a typical result of brain injury or illness in childhood.

Psychiatric disorder accompanies or follows brain injury, illness, or epilepsy in a significant percentage of affected children. The epidemiologic survey of the Isle of Wight found brain-injured or epileptic children 5–15 yr old to have five times the normal risk of psychiatric disorders. Mentally retarded children also are at increased risk of psychiatric disorders.

Prenatal factors have long been suspected of causing brain damage and psychiatric or behavioral disorders. Prematurity and neonatal complications place children at risk for such conditions as hyperactivity, impulsivity, difficulties in socialization, and poor control of emotions, especially anger, and psychiatric disorders in general.

Substance abuse during pregnancy may affect both prenatal and early childhood development. Although placental problems, premature labor, intrauterine growth retardation, and low birthweight are often confounding factors, fetal and infant CNS problems from cocaine include cerebral infarction, microcephaly, developmental delays, and behavioral and learning problems. Although cocaine use during pregnancy is associated with subsequent learning and behavioral deficits in some exposed children, a significant percentage of substance-exposed children are not adversely affected by the prenatal exposure (see Chapter 102).

Children under the age of 3 yr who survive encephalitis or meningitis show more lasting effects on personality and behavior than those who have these illnesses later. This result contradicts the notion that the brain might, in the earlier years, have greater potential for recovery without significant residual dysfunction.

When children with brain damage or injury have problems with impulse or anger control, aggressiveness, hyperactivity, or other emotional reactions, these do not differ in quality from those of children with intact nervous systems who have the same disturbances.

The most significant factor in the child's adjustment to a chronic handicapping organic condition is the capacity of parents to adjust and cope.

In some affected children, stimulant drugs improve the ability to perform in school, smooth out emotional reactivity, and facilitate social interactions with peers and adults. Such medication, taken for extended periods, may produce growth retardation, which must be weighed against possible beneficial effects. Neuroleptics may lessen anxiety and improve emotional control and behavior, but they also tend to produce obtundation and somnolence, which may interfere with learning. In addition, they may have serious side effects (see Chapter 28).

Most children with psychologic disturbances related to CNS injuries, as well as their families, benefit from understanding psychosocial support. A frequently beneficial approach is to help the child to identify his or her ineffective reaction patterns, along with more successful patterns. The approach combines "coaching" and education with an opportunity to discuss depression, isolation, and anger as well as those feelings of being different, rejected, or exploited that so greatly affect self-esteem. The parents have their own needs and will need advice, counseling, and emotional support in dealing with their child's emotional and behavioral problems, both in family matters and in life at school and with friends. Fair, firm discipline is always useful. Behavior modification techniques can help children in whom specific target behaviors can be identified; the technique may be used at home or at school. Both aberrant psychosocial behaviors and learning difficulties may respond to these techniques (see Chapters 28 and 29).

Caplan R, Arbelle S, Guthrie D, et al: Formal thought disorder and psychopathology in pediatric primary generalized and complex partial epilepsy. J Am Acad Child Adolesc Psychiatry 36:1286, 1997.

Cousens P, Waters B, Said J, Stevens M: Cognitive effects of cranial irradiation in leukaemia: A survey and meta-analysis. J Child Psychol Psychiatry 29:839, 1988.

Deonna TH: Annotation: Cognitive and behavioural correlates of epileptic activity in children. J Child Psychol Psychiatry 34:611, 1993.

Gonzales N, Campbell M: Cocaine babies: Does prenatal exposure to cocaine affect development? J Am Acad Child Adolesc Psychiatry 33:16, 1994.

Griffith D, Azuma S, Chasnoff I: Three-year outcome of children exposed prenatally to drugs. J Am Acad Child Adolesc Psychiatry 33:20, 1994.

Kim WJ: Psychiatric aspects of epileptic children and adolescents. J Am Acad Child Adolesc Psychiatry 30:874, 1991.

Max J, Robin D, Lindgren S, et al: Traumatic brain injury in children and adolescents: Psychiatric disorders two years later. J Am Acad Child Adolesc Psychiatry 36:1278, 1997.

Richardson G, Day N: Detrimental effects of prenatal cocaine exposure: Illusion or reality? J Am Acad Child Adolesc Psychiatry 33:28, 1994.

Whitaker A, Van Rossen R, Feldman J, et al: Psychiatric outcomes in low-birthweight children at 6 years: Relation to neonatal cranial ultrasound abnormalities. Arch Gen Psychiatry 54:847, 1997.

CHAPTER 19
Psychosomatic Illness

Richard Dalton and Marc A. Forman

Psychologic conflict that significantly alters somatic function is the hallmark of the psychosomatic disorder. Any kind of emotional distress may be associated with any type of psychosomatic disorder in a child or adolescent; particular types of feeling or conflict do not produce specific kinds of psychosomatic illness. There appear to be both innate constitutional vulnerabilities and environmental factors, neither of which are well understood, that determine why one organ or system, rather than another, becomes dysfunctional.

There are three categories of psychosomatic disorders. The first, consisting of psychologic factors that affect the physical condition (psychophysiologic disorders), occurs when psychologic reactions to either external or internal stimuli affect the development or recurrence of a physical condition with demonstrable pathophysiologic dysfunctions (e.g., diabetes mellitus, rheumatoid arthritis, or asthma). The second, somatoform disorder, presents with somatic complaints and/or dysfunctions that are not under conscious control and for which there is no demonstrable organic cause. These disorders include body dysmorphic disorder, conversion disorder, hypochondriasis, somatization disorder, and somatoform pain disorder. The third, factitious disorder, presents with somatic and psychologic complaints and/or dysfunctions that are consciously controlled and self-induced for the purpose of secondary gain. Munchausen by proxy syndrome is an example of a chronic factitious disorder.

Although there are multiple theories regarding cause, Engel's biopsychosocial approach to development and psychopathology offers the most cogent understanding. Underlying temperamental factors, environmental stress, family issues, and individual psychodynamics all contribute, some more than others, depending on the situation. The notion of specific personality types leading to particular disorders has not been substantiated.

Conversion disorder, the loss or alteration of physical functioning without a demonstrable organic illness, is a type of somatoform disorder that usually presents in adolescence or adulthood. However, numerous childhood cases have occurred. Conversion reactions usually start suddenly, can often be traced to a precipitating environmental event, and end abruptly after a short duration. Voluntary musculature and organs of special sense are the most frequent target sites for the "hysterical" expressions of psychologic conflict. Such reactions may take many forms, including hysterical blindness, paralysis, diplopia, and gait distubances, although pseudoseizures are the most common conversion symptom. Physical examination often fails to reveal objective abnormalities. Histories usually reveal a close relationship with a person who exhibited similar symptoms or a recent episode of actual illness. Deep tendon reflexes can be elicited in a paralyzed leg, and pupillary responses to light are noted in patients with hysterical blindness. Video electroencephalography and postictal increases in serum prolactin can distinguish pseudoseizures from seizures. Although conversion disorder is probably not genetically mediated, two broad patterns of disturbance are found in family members: anxiety and chaotic disorganization. The few follow-up studies that do exist suggest that more than one third of children and adolescents who are initially diagnosed with a conversion disorder ultimately are found to have a not readily apparent organic disorder.

Hypochondriasis, preoccupation with the fear of having a serious illness, and *somatization disorder,* the use of multiple somatic complaints as a means of assuaging inner tension, are also somatoform disorders. As with conversion hysteria, these disorders provide alternative routes and mechanisms for the discharge of physiologic and emotional tension. Community samples show that half of children and adolescents questioned report at least one somatic symptom during the preceding 2 weeks. Recurrent abdominal pain accounts for 2–4% of all pediatric office visits; headaches account from 1–2%. Prevalence studies suggest that 11% of boys and 15% of girls are somatizers.

Munchausen by proxy syndrome is a factitious disorder in which parents induce physical symptoms in their children. It is considered a form of child abuse, sometimes ending in death. Warning observations include (1) a persistent or recurrent illness that cannot be explained; (2) investigation results at variance with the general health of the child; (3) symptoms and signs that lead experienced doctors to say that they have never seen such a case; (4) symptoms that do not occur when the parent is away; (5) a particularly attentive primary caregiver who refuses to leave the child alone in the hospital for even a short time; (6) poorly tolerated treatments; (7) a very rare disorder; (8) a primary caregiver who does not seem as worried as the staff is about the child; and (9) clinical syndromes that do not respond to appropriate treatment.

The signs and symptoms can be varied, including fractures, poisonings, persistent complaints of apnea, and unusual injuries. Therapy includes separation of the child from the abusing parent and further investigation, as in cases of child abuse. The treatment team usually consists of the pediatrician, child psychiatrist, nurse, and social worker. (Also see Chapter 35.3.)

Psychophysiologic disorders have a more insidious onset than somatoform disorders. Chronic anxiety produces functional abnormalities within the autonomic nervous system that lead to structural changes within organ systems. Eczema, bronchial asthma, ulcerative colitis, and peptic ulcer are considered in some children to be psychophysiologic disorders or at least to have significant psychophysiologic components. Although these children have been reported to be obsessive and inhibited, there is no compelling evidence for specific personality characteristics. Vocal cord dysfunction is an often unrecognized disorder in which spasm of the vocal cords leads to narrowing of the glottis, resulting in a dysfunction distinguished from asthma by the absence of nocturnal symptoms, localization of wheezing to the upper chest and throat, normal blood gas values despite extreme symptoms, and significant adduction of the vocal cords when visualized during laryngoscopy.

Reflex sympathetic dystrophy presents with chronic painful swelling in an extremity, decreased skin temperature, cyanosis, delayed capillary refilling, and limitation of function. It often follows injury to the involved limb. The pathophysiology is undetermined but may be related to disregulation of the sympathetic nervous system or inflammation in response to injury.

Several general principles guide the management of children with psychosomatic disorders:

1. The symptoms of affected children are not within their conscious control; they are not acting or malingering, and their pain and their problems are real.
2. It is essential for a psychiatric assessment to be arranged early in the management of these disorders; otherwise, after elaborate and expensive tests have been done, the child and family will often be convinced that the patient has a very serious illness for which a "real" cause exists that cannot be found. Assessment of these disorders is aided by a history of somatization symptoms, a psychiatric history, a model for unexplained symptoms within the child's environment, secondary gain, symptoms that violate anatomic and physiologic boundaries, symptom fluctuation, and placebo response.
3. An explanation of the role of the emotions and the genesis of these disorders must be accepted by the parents before truly effective intervention can be accomplished.
4. Psychotherapy for the child and counseling for the family are often indicated, in addition to pediatric management. The psychiatrist and pediatrician must be in close communication with each other in a therapeutic alliance. Modest amounts of minor tranquilizing medication may be a useful adjunct.
5. Child and family should be helped to live as normally as possible to avoid crippling psychologic invalidism. Stress should be placed on early return to school after acute illness, participation in recreational activities, and normal peer interactions. Parents should know that some children unconsciously use their symptoms to maintain dependency and that firm, gentle insistence on the fullest possible range of activities for the child is indicated.
6. The physician should be alert for indications of psychosomatic or physical illness in parents, with which children may unconsciously identify; successful treatment of parental illness may be necessary to ensure a favorable outcome in the child.

Bools CN, Neale BA, Meadow SR: Follow up of victims of fabricated illness (Munchausen syndrome by proxy). Arch Dis Child 69:625, 1993.

Campo JV, Fritsch SL: Somatization disorder in children and adolescents. J Am Acad Child Adolesc Psychiatry 33:1223, 1994.

Engel G: The clinical application of the biopsychosocial model. Am J Psychiatry 137:535, 1980.

Fritz GK, Fritsch SL, Hagino O: Somatoform disorders in children and adolescents: A review of the past 10 years. J Am Acad Child Adolesc Psychiatry 36:1329, 1997.
Liang S, Boyce WT: The psychobiology of childhood stress. Curr Opin Pediatr 5:545, 1993.
McGrath P, McAlpine LM: Psychological perspectives on pediatric pain. J Pediatr 122:52, 1993.
Mitchell I, Brummett J, DeForest J, Fisher G: Apnea and factitious illness (Munchausen syndrome) by proxy. Pediatrics 92:810, 1993.
Nemzer E: Psychosomatic illnesses in children and adolescents. *In:* Garfinkel B, Carlson G, Weller E (eds): Psychiatric Disorders in Children and Adolescents. Philadelphia, WB Saunders, 1990.
Steinhausen HC, von Aster M, Pfeiffer E, et al: Comparative studies of conversion disorders in childhood and adolescence. J Child Psychol Psychiatry 30:615, 1989.
Taylor DC: Outlandish factitious illness. *In:* David TJ (ed): Recent Advances in Pediatrics No. 10. Edinburgh, Churchill Livingstone, 1992.

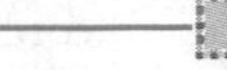

CHAPTER 20
Vegetative Disorders

Charles Scott and Richard Dalton

The five disorders included under this appellation are classified in the *Diagnostic and Statistical Manual of Mental Disorders,* fourth edition, under Eating Disorders (rumination disorder and pica, along with bulimia and anorexia nervosa, which are discussed in Chapter 112), Elimination Disorders (encopresis and enuresis), and Sleep Disorders (dyssomnias and parasomnias of adolescence are also discussed in Chapter 114).

20.1 Rumination Disorder

The hallmark of this disorder is a weight loss or failure to gain at the expected level because of repeated regurgitation of food without nausea or associated gastrointestinal illness. This rare disorder occurs more commonly in males and usually appears between 3 and 14 mo of age. It is potentially fatal; some reports indicate that up to one fourth of affected children die. There are psychogenic and self-stimulating ruminators. The former type occurs in infants with otherwise normal development, although there is often a disturbed parent-child relationship and the child may fail to thrive (Chapter 36). The self-stimulating variety is usually seen in mentally retarded individuals of any age and often occurs even in the presence of nurturing parents. The differential diagnosis should include congenital anomalies that affect the development of the gastrointestinal system and pyloric valve.

Behavioral *treatment* is directed toward positively reinforcing correct eating behavior and negatively reinforcing rumination. Adverse conditioning is often used. Parent counseling and family therapy are often necessary to manage underlying conflicts and to help educate the parents about appropriate approaches to be taken toward the child and the problem.

20.2 Pica

This eating disorder involves repeated or chronic ingestion of non-nutrient substances, which may include plaster, charcoal, clay, wool, ashes, paint, and earth. The age of onset is usually 1–2 yr of age but may be earlier. Pica usually remits in childhood but can continue into adolescence and adulthood. Mental retardation and lack of parental nurturing (psychologic and nutritional) are predisposing factors. Although tasting or mouthing of objects is normal in infants and toddlers, pica after the 2nd yr of life needs investigation. It is often a symptom of family disorganization, poor supervision, and affectional neglect. Pica appears to be more prevalent in the lower socioeconomic classes. Children with pica are at an increased risk for lead poisoning (Chapter 721), iron-deficiency anemia (Chapter 461), and parasitic infections (see Part XVI, Sections 13 and 14). Differential diagnoses include autism, schizophrenia, and certain physical disorders such as Kleine-Levin syndrome.

20.3 Enuresis

(Bedwetting)

Enuresis is defined as the voluntary or involuntary repeated discharge of urine into clothes or bed after a developmental age when bladder control should be established. Most children have obtained bladder control during the day and night by age 5 yr. The diagnosis of enuresis is made when urine is voided twice a week for at least 3 consecutive months or clinically significant distress occurs in areas of the child's life as a result of the wetting. The prevalence of enuresis at age 5 yr is 7% for males and 3% for females. At age 10 yr, it is 3% for males and 2% for females, and at age 18 yr, it is 1% for males and extremely rare in females. Twin studies show that there is a marked familial pattern: a 68% concordance rate in monozygotic twins and a 36% concordance rate in dizygotic twins (see also Chapters 5 and 551).

CLINICAL MANIFESTATIONS. Bed-wetting may be divided into the persistent (primary) type, in which the child has never been dry at night, and the regressive (secondary) type, in which a child who has been continent for at least 1 yr begins to wet the bed again. Primary enuresis represents approximately 90% of all cases. Secondary enuresis most frequently occurs between the ages of 5 and 8 yr and is more common in late school-aged children. Secondary enuresis may occur as a result of stressful environmental events, such as move to a new home, marital conflict, birth of a sibling, or death in the family. Such bed-wetting is typically more transitory and has a better prognosis than primary enuresis. More recent investigations, however, have not identified major psychologic stress differences between nonenuretic children and those with secondary enuresis.

Further classification involves *nocturnal only* enuresis (voiding urine at night), *diurnal only* enuresis (voiding urine while awake), and nocturnal/diurnal, which involves passage of urine while awake and asleep. A strong genetic predisposition is one contributing factor to *nocturnal enuresis.* For example, if both parents have a history of enuresis, the child has a 70% likelihood of having enuresis. A delay in maturational development of the bladder and an underlying medical condition are additional etiologic factors to consider in nocturnal enuresis. Nocturnal enuresis occurs at all stages of sleep and has not been linked to the depth of sleep or arousal patterns. Other proposed but controversial etiologies of nocturnal enuresis include reduced bladder capacity and abnormal secretion patterns of antidiuretic hormone. Currently, there is no substantial evidence that those children with primary nocturnal enuresis continuing until age 10 yr have any increased rate of emotional disorders when compared with nonenuretic children. However, a significant percentage of children with primary nocturnal enuresis that persists past age 10 yr do have symptoms of attention deficit hyperactivity disorder.

Diurnal enuresis (voiding urine during the day) is more common in girls and rarely occurs after the age of 9 yr. The most common cause of daytime enuresis in the preschool child is waiting until the last minute to void urine (micturation deferral). In addition to micturation deferral, etiologic factors to consider in diurnal enuresis include a urinary tract infection, chemical urethritis, associated constipation, diabetes, and giggle or stress incontinence. In both nocturnal and diurnal enuresis, organic pathologic conditions can be found in only a very small number of cases. Physical examination and urinalysis are indicated, but procedures such as urography and cytoscopy should not be pursued unless there is some indication of an organic lesion.

TREATMENT. Management of the child with enuresis depends on an understanding of the possible specific causative factors suggested by an adequate psychosocial evaluation and physical examination. For example, a parent may be helped to establish the proper attitudes and climate for a child's success in toilet training. If the child develops a secondary enuresis as a result of an environmental stressor, the parent should assist the child in coping with this change. Some general suggestions are as follows:

1. It is important to enlist the cooperation of the child to deal with the problem. Rewarding the child for being dry at night is a useful step. The child or parent can chart the dry nights, and, with one or two dry nights, a small reward can be given. More substantial rewards should be given for increasing success.
2. Older children should be expected to launder their own soiled bedclothes and pajamas.
3. The child should void before retiring.
4. Waking the child repeatedly to take him or her to the bathroom is useful in only a few children and may further engender or aggravate anger in child or parents.
5. Punishment or humiliation of the child by parents or others should be strongly discouraged.

The use of conditioning devices (e.g., an alarm that rings when the child wets a special sheet) is usually not necessary and should be reserved for persistent and refractory cases in which the child's self-esteem has been seriously eroded. Consent of the child should be a prerequisite for use of such a device. Such alarm systems have a success rate of approximately 70%, but the relapse rate can be as high as 30%. One study showed that dry bed training (which includes the alarm, night waking, and cleanliness training) has a success rate of 85–100%.

Imipramine (Tofranil) at a maximum dosage of 2.5 mg/kg/24 hr before bedtime has shown a success rate of approximately 50%, with a relapse rate of 30%, similar to that of the alarm system. Desmopressin acetate nasal spray (DDAVP) is typically administered intranasally at bedtime. The fast results of DDAVP suggest a role for special occasions (such as overnights), when rapid control of enuresis is desired. The relapse rate upon discontinuation of desmopressin is very high; rare side effects of hyponatremia and water intoxication with resulting seizures have been noted.

20.4 Encopresis

Encopresis refers to the passage of feces into inappropriate places after a chronological age of 4 yr (or equivalent developmental level). Subtypes include encopresis with constipation and overflow incontinence and encopresis without constipation and overflow incontinence. In children less than 4 yr of age, the male:female ratio for chronic constipation is 1:1. In the schoolage child, encopresis is much more common in males; it affects slightly more than 1% of school-aged children.

CLINICAL MANIFESTATIONS. Chronic soiling may persist from infancy onward (primary) or may appear as a regressive (secondary) phenomenon. It is often associated with chronic constipation, fecal impaction, and overflow incontinence (in about two thirds of cases) and may progress to psychogenic megacolon. Chronic constipation may develop if the child experiences a painful passage of stool and subsequently withholds feces to avoid discomfort. In some children, encopresis may represent unconscious anger and defiance by the child, and the parents may respond with retaliatory, punitive measures. School performance and attendance may be affected as the child becomes the target of scorn and derision from schoolmates because of the offensive odor.

TREATMENT. Management of encopresis should include educating and assisting the parents on how to re-establish normal toileting. For those children less than 2.5 yr of age who are resistant to toilet training, backing off from toilet training attempts should be considered until the child has re-established normal bowel patterns. For older children, relieving constipation and removing impactions can lead to significant improvement in about three fourths of cases. The use of mineral oil and a high-fiber diet helps prevent a recurrence of the constipation. Some children benefit from sitting on the toilet 10–15 min after each meal. Rewards for compliance should be offered. Power and autonomy struggles should be avoided, if possible, and records of the child's elimination should be kept.

Primary encopresis is often more difficult to treat and may require enemas to evacuate the colon. However, chronic use of enemas and laxatives should be avoided. Biofeedback, which is used to train the anal sphincter muscle, has been helpful. The child is encouraged to use the bathroom at specific times and is rewarded accordingly. If the child does not produce a reasonable amount of fecal material, glycerine suppositories may be necessary. A nonhumiliating examination of the child's clothing at the end of the day is necessary. Rewards are offered for nonsoiling, and soiling is met with mild, nonjudgmental consequences. Failure to respond to supportive measures may require psychotherapeutic intervention with the child and family.

American Psychiatric Association: Diagnostic and Statistical Manual of Mental Disorders IV. Washington, DC, 1994.
Bakwin H: The genetics of enuresis. Clin Dev Med 48/49:73, 1973.
Bernstein SA, Williford SL: Intranasal desmopressin-associated hyponatremia: A case report and literature review. J Fam Pract 44:203, 1997.
Fergusson DM, Horwood LJ: Nocturnal enuresis and behavioral problems in adolescence: A 15 year longitudinal study. Pediatrics 94:662, 1994.
Jarvelin MR, Moilanen I, Kangas P, et al: Aetiological and precipitating factors for childhood enuresis. Acta Paediatr Scand 80:361, 1991.
Kales A, Kales JD, Jacobson A, et al: Effects of imipramine on enuretic frequency and sleep stages. Pediatrics 60:431, 1977.
Loening-Baucke V: Constipation in early childhood: Patient characteristics, treatment and long-term follow-up. Am Fam Physician 49:397, 1994
Loening-Baucke V: Encopresis and soiling. Pediatr Clin North Am 43:279, 1996.
Mikkelsen EJ, Rapoport JL: Enuresis: Psychopathology, sleep stage, and drug response. Urol Clin North Am 7:361,1980.
Robson WL, Leung AKC, Bloom DA: Daytime wetting in childhood. Clin Pediatr 35:91, 1996.
Shaffer D, Gardner A, Hedge B: Behavior and bladder disturbance of enuretic children: A rational classification of a common disorder. Dev Med Child Neurol 26:781, 1984.
Sneed TJ, Foxx RM. Dry bed training: Rapid elimination of childhood enuresis. Behav Res Ther 12:147, 1974.
Tietjen DN, Husmann DA: Nocturnal enuresis: A guide to evaluation and treatment. Mayo Clin Proc 71:857, 1996.
Ullom-Minnich M: Diagnosis and management of nocturnal enuresis. Am Fam Physician 54:2259, 1996.

20.5 Sleep Disorders

Ronald L. Ariagno and Majid Mirmiran

A sleep disorder may be characterized by too little or too much sleep than is normal for age (see Chapters 5, 9, and 114); an abnormal type of sleep (e.g., narcolepsy, in which the regulation of sleep and wakefulness is abnormal); abnormal behavior during sleep (e.g., enuresis or sleepwalking); or a pathophysiologic event that occurs during sleep (e.g., obstructive sleep apnea syndrome [OSAS]; see Chapter 383). In evaluating sleep in a child, all daytime naps should be recorded (including brief periods in the car or stroller). The number of naps decreases from 4–6 in the neonate to zero by 2.5–4.5 yr of age. During the same period, daytime sleep decreases from about 8.5 hr to 0. Some sleep disorders identified in adulthood may have started in infancy (e.g., narcolepsy or OSAS). It is important to recognize the possibility of a sleep disorder as early as possible to avoid increased morbidity, e.g., chronic hypoxia and cor pulmonale in case of OSAS or behavioral problems associated with decreased sleep and excessive nighttime awakenings when there is circadian (day/night) desynchronization. Consultation with the pediatric sleep specialist may be helpful in suggesting appropriate tests (Table 20–1).

Nighttime awakenings are common in infancy (Chapter 5). By 1–3 mo of age the longest daily sleep period should be between midnight and early morning. However, by 1 yr of age, 20–30% of infants are still waking at night. Sleeping through the night is an early developmental milestone governed primarily by maturational factors, but parental and environmental factors can influence how early or late the circadian rhythm of sleep is established. A common sleep problem in young children (4–12 yr of age) is normal bedtime resistance; most of these children have both sleep onset delay and awakening problems. The significance of problems in the development of circadian rhythms in infancy and early childhood may be underestimated as a cause of sleep disturbance. Other symptoms of circadian sleep disorders in older children are delayed sleep onset, early morning awakening, or daytime sleepiness.

Infants may respond to biorhythm entrainment by increasing environmental differences (light and sound intensities) between day and nighttime, reducing nighttime feedings, and avoiding mother/infant exposure to light at night. For older children, regular light-dark cycle and regular bedtime/waking time schedules may favor the developing circadian rhythms, whereas environmental disturbances such as irregular/continuous 24-hr lighting regime, irregular bedtime schedule, and co-sleeping with parents may delay them.

Obstructive sleep apnea syndrome (OSAS) and upper airway resistance syndrome (UARS) are breathing-related sleep problems seen in infants, children, and adults. Adenotonsillar hypertrophy is a common cause of OSAS and UARS. Children with small triangular chins, retroposition of the mandible, steep mandibular plane, high hard palate, long oval face, or long soft palate are at high risk for breathing disorders during sleep (also see Chapter 383). **Clinical manifestations** include loud snoring (often continuous), difficulty breathing, marked paradoxical chest and abdominal motion, and retractions during sleep. Owing to sleep deprivation these patients have daytime sleepiness and performance deficits (e.g., behavioral and learning problems). OSAS is characterized by episodes of partial or complete upper airway obstruction that occur during sleep. In the case of large tonsils, OSAS is more likely than UARS. When clinical symptoms such as daytime sleepiness and nighttime sleep disturbances suggest abnormal breathing during sleep, but obstructive sleep apnea is not documented, UARS may be involved.

Polysomnography recording evaluations are important in establishing the **diagnosis** (see Table 20–1). Obstructive apnea is defined by lack of (nasal/mouth) airflow despite continuous respiratory effort. Partial UARS is defined by a breathing pattern with diminished airflow, hyperventilation, and hypercarbia (increase in end-tidal and transcutaneous carbon dioxide); transcutaneous oxygen desaturation; and increase in transpleural esophopharyngeal pressure (Pes). Central apnea is defined by no effort or airflow. Mixed apnea usually starts with a central apnea followed by an obstructive event. Although polysomnography may be useful for identifying breathing-related sleep problems in some infants and young children, periodic breathing (e.g., three or more successive central apneas separated by periods of less than 20 sec of normal breathing) found during both rapid eye movement (REM) and non-REM sleep in preterm and term infants may be normal, unless it is accompanied by oxygen desaturation, hypercarbia, and/or bradycardia.

Adenotonsillectomy is effective **treatment** when adenotonsillar hypertrophy is the cause of OSAS and UARS. Other therapies for functional nonanatomic upper airway obstruction include nasal continuous positive airway pressure (CPAP) and bilevel positive airway pressure (BiPAP) during sleep.

Gastroesophageal reflux (pH <4 in the esophagus, 2 cm above the cardiac sphincter level) associated with sleep apnea may respond to prone sleep positioning and elevation of the head of a crib for infants, pharmacologic therapy, or surgery (see Chapter 323). Apnea of prematurity may evolve into gastroesophageal reflux and reflex apnea with or without chronic pulmonary aspiration and can exacerbate pre-existing chronic lung disease and chronic respiratory failure. Reflux may improve after discontinuing caffeine therapy for apnea.

Craniofacial anomalies such as Pierre Robin syndrome sequence is characterized by abnormalities that can affect upper airway patency (micrognathia, glossoptosis, and cleft palate). Polysomnography shows increased upper airway resistance (increased pressure during the breathing cycle), hypercarbia, and/or decrease in oxygen saturation. Prone position, artificial airway (nasopharyngeal tube), and, in extreme cases, tracheostomy may be necessary.

Narcolepsy is a disorder characterized by excessive daytime sleepiness, cataplexy, sleep paralysis, hypnogogic hallucinations, school academic and athletic failures, irritability, and emotional lability. Onset may be as early as 3–4 yr of age, particularly when there is a strong family history. There is a genetic predisposition. Polysomnography and multiple sleep latency testing (MSLT) are needed for definitive diagnosis. Short REM latency, increased daytime naps, and sleep-onset REM sleep are diagnostic. Stimulants are used to decrease excessive daytime sleep.

Other disorders that may present with sleep disturbances as a prominent clinical feature include insomnia or hypersomnia in depression, daytime sleepiness in Prader-Willi syndrome, OSAS in children with Down syndrome, frequent nighttime arousals in Tourette and Rett syndromes, and sleepiness in Kleine-Levin syndrome. In attention deficit hyperactivity disorder (ADHD), difficulty falling asleep, restless sleep, and early morning awakening are also common (Chapter 29).

TABLE 20–1 Polygraphic Evaluations

Basic Apnea Recording Variables

Respiration effort measured by impedance, inductance, or a strain gauge (e.g., piezoelectrode), and esophageal pressure
Airflow measured by nasal-oral thermistor or carbon dioxide
Heart rate measured by ECG or cardiotachometer*
Oxygenation measured by oxygen saturation via pulse oximetry
Ventilation measured by transcutaneous carbon dioxide or end-tidal carbon dioxide

Gastroesophageal Reflux–Reflex Apnea Recording

Includes basic apnea recording variables plus endoesophageal pH

Sleep Apnea Recording

Includes the above variables with or without pH, plus sleep variables (electroencephalogram C_3/A_2–C_4/A_1;† electro-oculogram; electromyogram, [chin]; and time-lapse video, which makes it possible to determine sleep state)

Respiratory Control or Arousal Recording

Includes sleep apnea recording plus quantitative measures of ventilation response (end-tidal carbon dioxide and pneumotachygraph or plethysmograph to obtain minute ventilation)

*Continuous digitized electrocardiogram may be required for heart rate variability and arrhythmia analysis.

†Clinical multichannel electroencephalogram montage and video recording may be needed to diagnose sleep-related epilepsy.

From Nelson Updates, No. 6. Philadelphia, W.B. Saunders, 1994.

REFERENCES

American Sleep Disorders Association Report: Practice parameters for indications for polysomnography and related procedures. Sleep 20:406, 1997.

American Thoracic Society: Standards and indications for cardiopulmonary sleep studies in children. Am J Respir Crit Care Med 153:866, 1996.

Ariagno RL: Apnea. *In*: Behrman RE (ed): Nelson Updates, No 6. Philadelphia, WB Saunders, 1994, pp 1–12.

Beckerman RC, Brouillette RT, Hunt CE (eds): Respiratory Control Disorders in Infants and Children. Baltimore, Williams & Wilkins, 1992.

Blader JC, Koplewicz HS, Abikoff H, et al: Sleep problems in elementary school children. Arch Pediatr Adolesc Med 151:473, 1997.

Curzi-Dascalova L, Mirmiran M (eds): Manual of Methods for Recording and Analyzing Sleep-Wakefulness States in Preterm and Full Term Infant. Paris, INSERM, 1996.

Ferber R, Kryger M (eds): Principles and Practice of Sleep Medicine in the Child. Philadelphia, WB Saunders, 1995.

Kahn A, Dan B, Groswasser J, et al: Normal sleep architecture in infants and children. J Clin Neurophysiol 13:184, 1996.

Sheldon SH, Spire JP, Levy HB (eds): Pediatric Sleep Medicine. Philadelphia, WB Saunders, 1992.

Wise MS: Childhood narcolepsy. Neurology 50:S37, 1998.

CHAPTER 21
Habit Disorders

Richard Dalton

Habit disorders include tension-discharging phenomena, such as head banging, body rocking, thumb sucking, nail biting, hair pulling (trichotillomania), teeth grinding (bruxism), hitting or biting parts of one's own body, body manipulations, repetitive vocalizations, breath holding, and air swallowing (aerophagia). Tics, which involve the involuntary movement of various muscle groups, are also included. Stuttering is discussed with the habit disorders, although it is not generally regarded as a tension-relieving activity.

All children at various developmental points show repetitive patterns of movement that can be described as habits. Whether they are considered disorders depends on the degree to which they interfere with the child's physical, emotional, or social functioning. Some habit patterns may be learned by imitation of adults. Many begin as a purposeful movement that, for some reason, becomes repetitive, with the habit losing its original significance and becoming a means of discharging tension. For example, a child who has an eye irritation or is attempting not to shed tears might try closing the eyelids several times in rapid succession. This activity may become repetitive and incorporated into the child's behavior as an outlet for tension. Such symptoms are often reinforced by attention from parents or others. Other movements, such as rhythmic head banging and rocking in early life, can persist without parental reinforcement, occurring when the child is put to bed or is alone; these movements seem to provide a kind of sensory solace for the child who is feeling otherwise uncared for or understimulated by human touch or interaction. These movements represent a kind of internal stroking. Such patterns are often seen in the mentally retarded or in children suffering from maternal or emotional deprivation. Equivalent movements are evident in children who twist their hair or touch or play with parts of their bodies in repetitive ways. As involved children become older, they learn to inhibit some of their rhythmic habit patterns, particularly in social situations. The prevalence of habit disorders is not known. The natural course can vary, depending on whether the behavior is part of a chronic problem (e.g., mental retardation) or results from an episodic disorder.

Teeth grinding, or *bruxism,* seems to result from tension that may originate in unexpressed anger or resentment. It may create problems in dental occlusion. Helping the child find ways to express concerns may relieve the problem. Bedtime can be made more enjoyable and relaxed by reading or talking with the child, permitting re-experience and review of some of the fears or angers experienced during the day. Praise and other emotional support are useful at these times.

Thumb sucking is normal in early infancy. It makes the older child appear immature and may interfere with normal alignment of the teeth. Like other rhythmic patterns, it can be seen as a way of securing extra self-nurturance. The best strategy for dealing with thumb sucking is to provide the child with evidence of interest in his or her well-being and other forms of satisfaction. Parents should ignore the symptom, if possible, while giving attention to more positive aspects of the child's behavior. The child who actively tries to restrain thumb sucking should be given praise and encouragement.

Tics involve repetitive movements of muscle groups and represent discharges of tension originating in emotional and physical states that have no apparent useful function. They may have been initially intentional, sometimes becoming nonintentional very quickly. Parts of the body most frequently involved are the muscles of the face, neck, shoulders, trunk, and hands. There may be lip smacking and grimacing, tongue thrusting, eye blinking, throat clearing, and so on. It is very difficult for a person with a tic to inhibit it. Tics can be distinguished from variants of minor seizures in that the child does not experience a transient loss of consciousness or amnesia. They can be distinguished from dyskinetic movements and dystonias by their discontinuation during sleep and by virtue of the conscious control that can be achieved for short periods. Tics usually accompany other psychiatric syndromes or follow encephalitis. In most cases, they seem to have had no physical antecedents and are transient. Undue parental attention can reinforce tics, whereas ignoring them may diminish their occurrence. Electroencephalographic (EEG) findings and cognitive testing do not differentiate patients with tics from control subjects.

Gilles de la Tourette syndrome, which has a lifetime prevalence rate of 0.5/1,000 individuals, is a rare condition in children. It appears prior to 7 yr of age in one half of cases. It is characterized by multiple tics, compulsive barking and grunting, or shouting obscene words. It is more common in the first-degree relatives of patients with Tourette syndrome than in the general population and affects boys three to four times more often than girls. It is more common in whites than in other races. Children with Gilles de la Tourette syndrome often suffer from secondary behavioral, emotional, and academic problems. Children with Tourette syndrome and tic disorder are similar in many ways (psychiatric co-morbidity; impairments in school, neuropsychologic, and psychosocial functioning). However, they are differentiated by the fact that Tourette sufferers have higher rates of oppositional-defiant disorder (OCD) and simple phobia.

Although the etiology is uncertain, the syndrome probably results from an interplay among genetic, neurobiologic, psychologic, and environmental factors. Neuroimaging studies suggest that there is a lack of normal asymmetry within the striatum. Drugs that increase dopaminergic action precipitate or worsen tics and Gilles de la Tourette syndrome. Thus, a dopaminergic theory has been promulgated. In addition, just as with OCD, there is evidence to suggest that a subgroup of children who develop Tourette syndrome suffer with pediatric autoimmune neuropsychiatric disorder (PANDA), in which antibodies to group A streptococcal infections cross react with basal ganglia tissue and subsequently precipitate symptoms. The diagnostic index of suspicion should be raised when symptoms develop de novo after a streptococcal-like illness. A thorough history taking and an ASO titer and other laboratory studies are indicated. Treatment of PANDAs includes acute and prophylactic antibiotic therapy. Lyme disease may also present with clinical manifestations of Tourette syndrome (see Chapter 219). Many environmental precipitants serve as emotional stressors, which also precipitate or increase tics and Gilles de la Tourette syndrome. Laboratory studies are nonspecific; up to 80% of patients with Tourette syndrome have nonspecific abnormal EEG findings. Abnormal amounts of various neurotransmitter metabolites as well as lower scores on verbal subscales of psychometric tests have been reported.

Gilles de la Tourette syndrome can be fairly well managed with haloperidol (Haldol), a dopamine antagonist, or pimozide (Orap), a more powerful dopamine antagonist. Although both reduce the severity of tics by 65%, haloperidol has been viewed as more effective. However, one study suggests that pimozide (3–4 mg/24hr) is significantly more effective than haloperidol in children and young adolescents and that it has far fewer side effects. Clonidine is less frequently associated with side effects but yields only a 25–35% reduction in severity of tics. The disorder usually persists throughout life, but studies have shown a significant diminution in symptoms in one half to two thirds of cases 10–15 yr after the initial evaluation and treatment.

Primary *stuttering* usually begins as an atypical development during the learning of speech. It starts gradually, initially with the repetition of consonants, often followed by a repetition of words and phrases. As the child becomes aware of the dysfluency, anxiety and behavioral responses may occur. As the condition becomes fixed, secondary compulsive and repetitive movements of various muscle systems occur as the child attempts to "force out" the words and release the built-up tension. About 5% of children stutter. Most cases resolve spontaneously, although about 20% continue to suffer the disability in adulthood. A strong family incidence has been noted, and the disorder seems to remit more readily in girls than in boys.

The physician can help parents accept the child's early patterns of dysfluent speech; a decreased emphasis on these early patterns portends a better outcome. The child should be made to feel successful and cared for in other ways. If the pattern persists, a speech therapist should be consulted. Approaches to treatment include breath-control exercises and the use of a miniaturized metronome that "paces" the rhythm of speech.

Chappell P, Leckman J, Riddle M: The pharmacologic treatment of tic disorders. Child Adolesc Psychiatr Clin North Am 4:197, 1995.

Cohen D, Leckman J: Sensory phenomena associated with Gilles de la Tourette syndrome. J Clin Psychiatry 53:319, 1992.

Cohen D, Leckman J: Developmental psychopathology and neurobiology of Tourette's syndrome. J Am Acad Child Adolesc Psychiatry 33:2, 1994.

Lang A: Patient perception of tics and other movement disorders. Neurology 41:223, 1991.

Lehane MC, Swedo SE, Rapoport JL: Rates of obsessive-compulsive disorder in first degree relatives of patients with trichotillomania. J Child Psychol Psychiatry 33:925, 1992.

Sallee FR, Nesbitt L, Jackson C, et al: Relative efficacy of haloperidol and pimozide in children and adolescents with Tourette's disorder. Am J Psychiatry 154:1057, 1997.

Spencer T, Biederman J, Harding M, et al: The relationship between tic disorder and Tourette's syndrome revisited. J Am Acad Child Adolesc Psychiatry 34:1133, 1995.

CHAPTER 22
Anxiety Disorders

Richard Dalton

Anxiety, fearfulness, and worrying are regularly experienced as part of normal development. When they become disattached from specific situations or events or when they become disabling to the point that they negatively affect social interactions and development, they are pathologic and warrant intervention. Separation anxiety disorder, childhood-onset social phobia, generalized anxiety disorder, obsessive-compulsive disorder, phobias, and post-traumatic stress disorder are all defined by the occurrence of either diffuse or specific anxiety related to predictable situations. The Isle of Wight study reported the prevalence of anxiety disorders to be 6.8%. About one third of these children were overanxious, and another third had specific fears or phobias that were disabling.

The antecedents of developmentally normal anxiety initially present at 7–8 mo of age. As infants begin to differentiate from their primary caregivers they often develop wariness and mood changes that previously did not exist when they were in the company of strangers. This *stranger reaction* is to be differentiated from *stranger anxiety*, which is a more intense discomfort that includes obvious psychologic and physiologic distress. Although stranger reaction is typically seen in early development, stranger anxiety often heralds later problems related to attachment and separation. Preschoolers typically develop specific fears related to the dark, to animals, and to imaginary situations. Parental reassurance is usually sufficient to help the child through this period. School-aged children slowly give up imaginary fears and replace them with fears of bodily harm as well as with other potentially real worries. Social anxieties often develop during the teenage years.

There are a number of theories about the origin of fears and phobias. The psychoanalytic view postulates that internal conflict that is not expressed leads to the development of neurotic symptoms. Social learning theory proposes that fears and anxieties are learned within the context of the child's environment. Others think that excessive worrying is related to maternal anxiety. Several studies suggest a genetic cause; 50% of monozygotic twins show concurrent anxiety disorders compared with a much smaller percentage of dizygotic twins. Studies also suggest that anxiety disorders are related genetically to depressive disorders. Finally, research has related persistent childhood anxiety to motor (neurologic) "soft" signs.

Children with *phobias* are anxious only under specific conditions. They try to avoid specific objects or situations that will automatically lead to anxiety. As with other forms of anxiety, phobias become pathologic when they interfere with social, professional, and interpersonal functioning. The parents of phobic children should remain calm in the face of the child's anxiety or panic. If they become upset, the child will conclude that there is, in fact, something to fear. The prevalence of specific phobias in childhood is 0.5–2.0%. Behavioral therapy is indicated, including systematic desensitization, the process of exposing the patient to the fear-inducing situation or object. Anxiety is managed through relaxation techniques. A thorough interpretive session with the parents and child, designed to convey an understanding of what is happening, is important to the development of a trusting therapeutic relationship. Parent training designed to help the family be supportive during stressful periods is also important.

School phobia, a syndrome in which a child will not attend school for various reasons, occurs in about 1–2% of children. The literature has underscored the hostile-dependent nature of the relationship between mother and child that often contributes to this disorder. Bernstein et al. report that over 75% of these patients suffer with either depression plus anxiety or subclinical depression plus anxiety. Management of the disorder involves treatment of the underlying psychiatric problems, family therapy, parent management training, and liaison work with the child's school.

Separation anxiety disorder (SAD) is characterized by unrealistic and persistent worries of possible harm befalling primary caregivers, reluctance to go to school or to sleep without being near the parents, persistent avoidance of being alone, nightmares involving themes of separation, and numerous somatic symptoms and complaints of subjective distress. These are children who come from the middle to lower socioeconomic classes. Often the first clinical sign of this disorder does not appear until third or fourth grade, typically after the Christmas holidays or after a period in which the child has been absent from school because of an illness. Parents frequently encourage the disability in conscious and unconscious ways. The prevalence of SAD in adolescence is 3.6%.

Psychiatric therapy is called for when the usual supportive approaches have failed to return the child to school or to reduce the symptoms. After a thorough assessment, the therapist clearly states to the child the expectations of the family regarding his or her return to school. A program involving the school, the parents, and the child is coordinated by the therapist to minimize the child's use of splitting and manipulation. Parent training as well as family therapy is often necessary to delineate underlying motivations and to teach appropriate ways to help the child fulfill reasonable expectations regarding school attendance. A large percentage of children with SAD develop feelings of panic when they are coerced to separate from their parents. A judicious use of either antidepressant or antianxiety medicines is often necessary to facilitate treatment goals. Initial reports that tricyclic antidepressants significantly ameliorate SAD have not been replicated in subsequent studies. Anecdotal reports support the use of serotonin reuptake blockers (SSRIs), cognitive-behavioral therapy, and operant procedures. Benzodiazepines have shown efficacy in several open trials. Young children with affective symptoms have the best prognosis. SAD with school refusal presenting insidiously in adolescence has a more guarded prognosis.

Childhood-onset social phobia is characterized by an excessive fear of contact with unfamiliar people that leads to social isolation. These children and adolescents maintain the desire for involvement with family and familiar peers. The long-term course is variable. Buspirone, alprazolam, and phenelzine have been shown to be helpful in various types of studies.

Children who suffer from *generalized anxiety disorder (GAD)* have unrealistic worries about future events, the appropriateness of past behavior, and concerns about competence. They frequently present with somatic complaints, are markedly self-conscious, need large amounts of reassurance, and have trouble relaxing. Onset may be gradual or sudden. The prevalence in adolescence is 2.4%. GAD is characteristically seen in middle and upper middle class white children. They are more likely than those with SAD to suffer with other anxiety disorders. Boys and girls are equally affected. Overanxious children are more likely than children with separation anxiety to be diagnosed as having a simple phobia or panic disorder as well. Frequently, GAD does not become manifest until puberty.

Many children present with repetitive thoughts that invade consciousness or repetitive rituals or movements that do not obviously contribute to a high level of adaptation in any given situation—an *obsessive-compulsive disorder (OCD)*. In times of stress (e.g., bedtime, preparing for school), some children touch certain objects, verbalize certain words, or wash their hands continually. The most common *obsessions* are concerned with bodily wastes and secretions, the fear that something calamitous will happen, or the need for sameness. The most common *compulsions* are handwashing, continual checking of locks, and touching. These thoughts and acts occur consciously, often causing great distress in the child. Some children externalize the ritualized behavior, attempting to involve their parents in their compulsions.

These behaviors become part of a disorder when they cause distress, consume time, or interfere with accustomed occupational or social functioning. The National Institute of Mental Health Global Rating Scale and the Yale-Brown Obsessive-Compulsive Scale are useful in distinguishing individuals with OCD from those without the disorder. The lifetime prevalence rate is about 1%. This disorder may be associated with anorexia nervosa, Gilles de la Tourette syndrome, and epilepsy. Positron emission tomography studies have demonstrated increased metabolic activity in the frontal lobes and the basal ganglia in affected children.

Treatment consists of behavioral therapy and pharmacotherapy. Overexposure of the patient to situations that lead to the symptoms and anxiety is a major therapeutic technique, used especially for rituals. Clomipramine (Anafranil), fluoxetine (Prozac), and fluvoxamine have all shown promise in ameliorating OCD symptoms. Because each blocks the neuronal reuptake of serotonin, a major etiologic role for the depletion of serotonin, especially in pathways connecting frontal lobe activity with the basal ganglia, has been hypothesized. Neuroimaging studies support this hypothesis. However, other neurotransmitters, particularly dopamine, are probably involved. A subgroup of children with OCD develop symptoms following a β-hemolytic streptococcal infection. Antineuronal antibodies against group A β-hemolytic streptococcal wall antigens cross react with caudate neural tissue with the consequent initiation of OCD symptoms. What percentage of children with OCD have developed symptoms secondary to these infections is not known. Treatment in these cases includes acute and prophylactic antibiotic therapy along with the usual psychopharmacologic and behavioral therapies used in OCD as well as plasmapheresis and, sometimes, steroids.

POST-TRAUMATIC STRESS DISORDER (PTSD). This anxiety disorder has received considerable attention during the past decade as investigators have explored the long- and short-term effects of trauma on children, adolescents, and adults. Many adolescent and adult psychopathologic conditions such as conduct disorder and various character pathologic findings, which were previously thought to be a product of internal psychologic conflict, have been shown to be related to previous trauma.

Etiology. PTSD results from external traumatic events perceived by the child or adolescent as dangerous. Life-threatening situations that produce considerable stress predispose the child to PTSD. The victim's feelings of helplessness in response to the trauma are important. Witnessing the traumatic death of a family member or close friend also places the child at risk for PTSD. In addition to the trauma itself, predisposing factors include the level of trait anxiety within the individual prior to the trauma. For example, the children with the greatest PTSD reactions after Hurricane Hugo were those with the greatest tendency to experience anxiety or negative emotionality, as measured on the Revised Children's Manifest Anxiety Scale. Younger children and females are also more likely to suffer with PTSD symptoms after significant trauma.

Epidemiology. About 1% of adults suffer with PTSD symptoms sufficient to completely satisfy *Diagnostic and Statistical Manual of Mental Disorders,* 3rd edition, revised criteria for the disorder. In addition, 15% of adults suffer with symptoms and produce behavior indicative of past trauma. Statistics for children and adolescents are not available.

Clinical Manifestations. PTSD is characterized by recurrent and intrusive recollections and dreams of noxious events in addition to intermittently intense psychologic and physiologic distress in situations that symbolize the original trauma. Individuals with this disorder typically try to avoid stimuli associated with the original trauma. Symptoms and behaviors indicative of this disorder include re-experiencing the trauma through intrusive recollections and dreams and re-enactment through play and other behaviors; psychologic numbing by way of amnesia, isolation, avoidance, and reduced interest in activities; and increased states of arousal, as exemplified by sleep problems, agitated emotions, hypervigilance, extreme startle responses, and difficulty concentrating.

Terr suggests that four long-term symptom complexes are

related to childhood traumas. These are visualized or otherwise repeatedly perceived memories of the traumatic event, repetitive behaviors, trauma-specific fears, and changed attitudes about people, life, and the future. Terr further divides childhood trauma into two basic types. Type I trauma is usually a product of an unanticipated single event and includes subsequently developed detailed memories, omens, and misperceptions. Type II is usually the product of long-standing or repeated exposures to extreme external events and is associated with later developing denial and numbing, self-hypnosis, and dissociation, sadness, and rage. Type II is often associated with repetitive physical and sexual abuse. Some overlap exists between these two types.

Treatment. Initial interventions should be directed toward determining the severity of the trauma, the child's vulnerability to the trauma, and the child's reactions to the trauma. Interviews designed to help children explore their understanding of the trauma are very important. This sort of triage helps determine which children require brief vs. extensive treatment and which therapeutic modalities are necessary (e.g., individual vs. group psychotherapy or pharmacotherapy). Treatment goals include the bolstering of ego and reality-testing functions; helping children anticipate, understand, and manage everyday reminders; and assisting the child in making distinctions between current life stresses and past trauma. Both early intervention and psychotherapy provide the child with an opportunity to talk about the trauma and express feelings of sadness, rage, and helplessness, among others. Family therapy and school consultations are often helpful. Pharmacotherapy designed to modify arousal behavior can be an important adjunctive treatment. In one study, propranolol proved effective in reducing PTSD symptoms during the time of its administration. Tricyclic antidepressants are often used effectively with adult PTSD patients (see Chapter 28).

Allen AJ, Leonard H, Swedo J: Current knowledge of medications for the treatment of childhood anxiety disorders. J Am Acad Child Adolesc Psychiatry 34:976, 1995.
American Academy of Child and Adolescent Psychiatry: Practice parameters for the assessment and treatment of anxiety disorders. J Am Acad Child Adolesc Psychiatry 36:695, 1997.
Bernstein GA, Borchardt CM, Perwien AR: Anxiety disorders in children and adolescents: A review of the past 10 years. J Am Acad Child Adolesc Psychiatry 35:1110, 1996.
Famularo R, Fenton T, Kinscherff R: Child maltreatment and the development of post-traumatic stress disorder. Am J Dis Child 147:755, 1993.
Flament MF, Koby E, Rapoport JL, et al: Childhood obsessive-compulsive disorder: A prospective follow-up study. J Child Psychol Psychiatry 31:363, 1990.
Klein RG, Koplewicz HS, Kanner A: Imipramine treatment of children with separation anxiety disorder. J Am Acad Child Adolesc Psychiatry 31:21, 1992.
Leonard HL, Swedo SE, Rapoport JL, et al: Treatment of obsessive-compulsive disorder with clomipramine and desipramine in children and adolescents. Arch Gen Psychiatry 46:1088, 1989.
Lonigan C, Shannon M, Taylor C, et al: Children exposed to disaster: II. Risk factors for the development of post-traumatic symptomatology. J Am Acad Child Adolesc Psychiatry 33:94, 1994.
March JS, Biederman J, Wolkow R, et al: Sertraline in children and adolescents with obsessive-compulsive disorder. JAMA 280:1752, 1998.
Moreau D, Weissman MM: Panic disorder in children and adolescents: A review. Am J Psychiatry 149:1306, 1992.
Pine D, Shaffer D, Schonfeld I: Persistent emotional disorder in children with neurological soft signs. J Am Acad Child Adolesc Psychiatry 32:1229, 1993.
Riddle MA, Scahill L, King RA, et al: Double-blind crossover trial of fluoxetine and placebo in children and adolescents with obsessive-compulsive disorder. J Am Acad Child Adolesc Psychiatry 31:1062, 1992.
Rosenberg D, Keshavan M, O'Hearn K, et al: Frontospatial measurement in treatment-naive children with obsessive-compulsive disorder. Arch Gen Psychiatry 54:824, 1997.
Rutter M, Tizard J, Yule W, et al: Research Report: Isle of Wight studies, 1964–1974. Psychol Med 6:313, 1976.
Shannon M, Lonigan C, Finch A, Taylor C: Children exposed to disaster: I. Epidemiology of post-traumatic symptoms and symptom profiles. J Am Acad Child Adolesc Psychiatry 33:80, 1994.
Simeon JG, Ferguson HG, Knott V, et al: Clinical, cognitive and neurophysiological effects of alprazolam in children and adolescents with overanxious and avoidant disorders. J Am Acad Child Adolesc Psychiatry 31:29, 1992.
Terr LC: Childhood traumas: An outline and overview. Am J Psychiatry 148:1, 1991.
Udwin O: Annotation: Children's reactions to traumatic events. J Child Psychol Psychiatry 34:115, 1993.
Yule W: Post-traumatic stress disorder in children. Curr Opin Pediatr 4:623, 1992.

CHAPTER 23
Mood Disorders

Richard Dalton and Marc A. Forman

Major depressive disorder, dysthymic disorder, and bipolar disorder with alternating mania and depression are the three major types of affective disorder seen in children and adolescents. *Major depression* is characterized by dysphoria and an obvious loss of interest and pleasure in usual activities but also includes a significant weight change secondary to decreased or increased food intake, insomnia or hypersomnia, psychomotor agitation or retardation, fatigue or loss of energy almost every day, feelings of worthlessness and excessive guilt, diminished ability to think and concentrate, and recurrent thoughts of death. In addition, the melancholic subtype of depression includes marked anhedonia and greater feelings of depression in the morning with early morning awakening. *Dysthymic disorder* is a less severe but more protracted syndrome involving depressed mood for at least 1 yr. In addition, poor appetite, sleep problems, decreased energy and self-esteem, and feelings of hopelessness are present. *Bipolar disorder* involves both mania and depression or mania alone.

23.1 Major Depression

Although in the past there was some doubt as to whether prepubertal children experience depression similar to that seen in adults, this view has been dispelled through the use of structured interviews and rating scales.

EPIDEMIOLOGY. The prevalence of depression starting in childhood is 0.4–2.5% and in adolescence, 0.4–8.3%. The lifetime prevalence of depression starting in adolescence is 15–20%. Girls report significantly more depressive symptoms than boys during adolescence but not during the elementary school-aged years.

ETIOLOGY. Although the causes of depression have not been established, there is ample evidence of a genetic basis for major depressive disorders. Genetic factors play a role in 50% of mood disorders. Individuals at high genetic risk appear to be more sensitive to the effects of adverse environmental conditions. Twin studies have shown a 76% concordance for depression among monozygotic twins reared together and 67% for monozygotic twins reared apart compared with 19% for dizygotic twins reared together. Many studies have demonstrated an increased rate of depression (three to six times greater) in first-degree relatives of patients suffering from a major affective disorder. In attempting to assess exactly what it is that is genetically transmitted, researchers have focused on biogenic amines and neurotransmitters. Because of the low urinary levels of 3-methoxyhydroxyphenylglycol and 5-hydroxyindoleacetic acid in depressed patients, low functional levels of norepinephrine and serotonin are thought to be important genetic markers. These views are reinforced by the therapeutic responses to antidepressants that block presynaptic reuptake of these compounds. Cognitive theories have attributed the development of depression to feelings of hopelessness and helplessness secondary to an actual loss or the perception of loss by the individual. Learning theory has postulated that depression is learned within the environment because of a lack of positive reinforcers, e.g, learned helplessness. Others postulate that social skills deficits, problems with self-control, and life stress play a role in the development and maintenance of depression.

CLINICAL MANIFESTATIONS. Depressive symptoms vary according to age and developmental level. Spitz described the *anaclitic depression of infancy.* Bowlby reported that separation from a primary caregiver after 6–7 mo of age leads to protest (crying, searching, panic-like behavior, and hypermotility of both arms and legs). This is followed by the infant's close scrutiny of each approaching adult, looking for the caregiver. The child turns away from everyone else. The final phase involves apathy in which the infant becomes hypotonic and inactive, exhibiting an obviously sad facial expression. These babies cry silently and stare into space. When picked up, they search again for the familiar face; they cling to the stranger and cry but are not consoled.

The clinical picture of depression in children somewhat parallels that of adults, except that children are more likely to present with separation anxiety, phobias, somatic complaints, and behavioral problems. The hallmark of psychotic depression in children is the occurrence of hallucinations; delusions, which require sophisticated cognitive development, are more common in adolescents and adults. Uncomplicated clinical depression in adolescents is similar phenomenologically to depression in adults.

The symptoms of a major depressive episode usually develop over a period of days or weeks. They may develop suddenly, secondary to a severe precipitant. The duration of the symptoms is variable. Untreated, symptoms often persist for 7–9 mo; 6–10% of cases are more protracted. Although the natural history of major depression has not been fully elucidated, several longitudinal studies clearly show that children and adolescents who are depressed are at risk for the development of later episodes of depression. Children who have depression at age 9 yr have been shown to have numerous depressive symptoms at 11–13 yr of age. Other studies have shown that, within 2 yr of the first depressive episode, 40% of children who have had a major depressive disorder experience a relapse. As many as 20–40% of teenagers hospitalized because of major depressive disorders develop a manic episode within 3–4 yr of discharge. Three predictors of such an outcome are (1) a depressive symptom cluster characterized by rapid onset, psychomotor retardation, and mood-congruent psychotic features; (2) a family history of bipolar illness or other affective illness; and (3) induction of hypomania by antidepressant medication. Co-morbidity commonly occurs with major depression: 20–50% have two or more diagnoses, including anxiety disorder (30–80%), behavior disorder (10–80%), dysthymic disorder (30–80%), and substance abuse disorder (20–30%).

DIAGNOSIS. Two measures have been developed that are useful in diagnosing depression: structured interviews or questionnaires and biologic methods that measure physiologic and neuroendocrine dysfunctions. The Children's Depression Inventory, Children's Depression Scale, Depression Self-Rating Scale, and the Center for Epidemiological Studies Depression Scale for Children have all been shown to be useful in diagnosing depression in children and adolescents, although some researchers have questioned the validity of some scales. There are no biologic tests specific for depression. However, during major depressive episodes, some children have been shown to hyposecrete growth hormone in response to insulin-induced hypoglycemia. Some preliminary reports have also suggested that depressed prepubertal children produce higher growth hormone peaks during sleep. Dexamethasone (Decadron) suppression testing (DST) has been shown to be inconclusive in children and adolescents, although it shows some efficacy in diagnosing depressed adults. About one half of depressed children produce a negative DST result. Children with false-negative results are more likely to relapse but are also more likely to respond to pharmacotherapy. Sleep electroencephalographic (EEG) reports in depressed children and adolescents are inconclusive. Although psychologic and biologic tests show promise in their ability to differentiate depression from other psychopathologic syndromes as well as from a normal state, additional research is needed.

TREATMENT. Fluoxetine (Prozac) is significantly more effective than placebo as an antidepressant medication for children and adolescents. Serotonin reuptake inhibitors (SSRIs), of which fluoxetine is one example, reduce depressive symptoms in 70–80% of cases. A less favorable response has been found for tricyclic antidepressanats (TCAs), and their efficacy has yet to be demonstrated in well-controlled studies.

Cognitive behavioral therapy (12–16 wk) is effective in about 70% of cases of adolescent depression. Psychotherapy is especially important for patients with multiple diagnoses.

23.2 Dysthymic Disorder

In this disorder, the dysphoria is generally more intermittent than in a major depression, with periods of normal mood lasting several days to several weeks. The dysphoria is less intense but more chronic, lasting up to several years.

ETIOLOGY. Although the genetic basis of major depression has been demonstrated, it is questionable whether there is also a genetic basis for dysthymic disorder. Dysthymia may be a partial phenotypic expression of an underlying genetic disorder or a different syndrome that has certain symptom clusters in common with major depression.

Prevalence in childhood is 0.6–1.7% and in adolescence, 1.6–8.0%.

CLINICAL MANIFESTATIONS. With the exception of hallucinations and delusions, the symptoms of major depression may be present. Dysthymia frequently is the consequence of a preexisting chronic condition such as anorexia nervosa, somatization disorder, or anxiety disorder. Children who have dysthymia have had frequent disruptions of important relationships, often beginning as early as infancy. There is often a history of depressive illness in both parents. Affected children show more general emotional and social maladjustment. They often present the picture of helpless, passive, clinging, dependent, and lonely children. Others relate in a more hardened, aloof, negativistic manner. They are reluctant to invest emotion or trust in relationships and frequently develop manipulative or expedient approaches to human affairs. These children are less likely than acutely depressed children to show episodes of crying; they attempt to hide their depressed affect. Such children frequently experience problems in school achievement and in their relationships with family and peers. They are at risk for the development of conduct disorders or substance abuse. Untreated dysthymic disorder lasts approximately 4 yr and is associated with increased risk for the subsequent development of major depression (70%), bipolar disorder (13%), and substance abuse disorder (15%). The recovery rate for dysthymic disorder is significantly worse than that for a major affective disorder. The younger the child when dysthymia emerges, the longer it takes to recover.

TREATMENT. Antidepressant pharmacotherapy may be useful in the treatment of dysthymic patients. It is especially helpful for those who display vegetative symptoms of depression. Because dysthymic disorder predisposes the individual to major depression, therapies necessary in the treatment of the latter are often indicated for the treatment of dysthymic disorder. However, when the dysthymic symptoms are a secondary reaction to an underlying disorder (anorexia, somatization disorder, substance abuse disorder, physical illness, personality disorder), the issues causing the underlying disorder should be addressed as well. This often requires a full spectrum of therapies, including alliance building and dynamic psychotherapy, family therapy, parent management training, and liaison work with the child's school.

23.3 Bipolar Disorder

Bipolar illness is characterized by either alternating depression and mania (a typical adult presentation) or a rapid cycling of mood, which is more commonly seen in children and young adolescents. Twenty to 40% of adult bipolar patients report that their bipolar symptoms began in childhood. The lifetime prevalence for the development of bipolar illness is 0.6%. This disorder has been shown to have genetic roots: a concordance rate of 65% in monozygotic twins and less than 20% in dizygotic twins. First-degree relatives of individuals with bipolar disorder are much more likely than the general population to develop various mood disorders. Twenty per cent of adolescents presenting with major depressive symptoms have been shown to develop manic episodes later.

Clinical manifestations include grandiose thoughts, high activity levels (often at bedtime), pressured speech, distractibility, increased pleasurable activities with high levels of danger, overspending, and extreme irritability and emotionality,among others. (See also Chapter 109.)

Lithium carbonate has proved to be very effective in the *treatment* of bipolar illness and manic symptoms. This is administered orally, followed by measurement of blood levels. The ideal therapeutic range for the initial treatment of acute symptoms is 1.0–1.2 mEq/L, and the recommended level for maintenance therapy is 0.5–0.8 mEq/L. During the acute manic phase, neuroleptic medication may also be required because of the psychotic nature of the symptoms. Carbamazepine (Tegretol), a tricyclic compound, and valproate, like carbamazepine an antiseizure medication, have been found to be especially effective in rapid cycling bipolar disorder.

Ambrosini PJ, Bianchi MD, Rabinovich H, et al: Antidepressant treatments in children and adolescents. I. Affective disorders. J Am Acad Child Adolesc Psychiatry 32:1, 1993.

American Academy of Child and Adolescent Psychiatry: Practice parameters for the assessment and treatment of children and adolescents with bipolar disorder. J Am Acad Child Adolesc Psychiatry: 34 (Suppl):157, 1997.

Birmaher B, Ryan ND, Williamson DE, et al: Childhood and adolescent depression: A review of the past 10 years. Part I. J Am Acad Child Adolesc Psychiatry 35:1427, 1996.

Birmaher B, Ryan ND, Williamson DE, et al: Childhood and adolescent depression: A review of the past 10 years. Part II. J Am Acad Child Adolesc Psychiatry 35:1575, 1996.

Bowlby J: Attachment and Loss, Vol 2. Separation. New York, Basic Books, 1973.

Bowring MA, Kovacs M: Difficulties in diagnosing manic disorders among children and adolescents. J Am Acad Child Adolesc Psychiatry 31:611, 1992.

Carlson GA: Child and adolescent mania—diagnostic considerations. J Child Psychol Psychiatry 31:331, 1990.

Geller B, Luby J: Child and adolescent bipolar disorder: A review of the past 10 years. J Am Acad Child Adolesc Psychiatry 36:1178, 1997.

Harrington R: Annotation: The natural history of child and adolescent affective disorders. J Child Psychol Psychiatry 33:1287, 1992.

Jones P, Berney T: Early onset rapid cycling bipolar affective disorder. J Child Psychol Psychiatry 28:731, 1987.

Kafantaris V: Treatment of bipolar disorder in children and adolescents. J Am Acad Child Adolesc Psychiatry 34:732, 1995.

Riddle MA, Geller B, Ryan N: Another sudden death in a child treated with desipramine. J Am Acad Child Adolesc Psychiatry 32:792, 1993.

Riddle MA, Nelson J, Kleinman C, et al: Sudden death in children receiving Norpramin: A review of three reported cases and commentary. J Am Acad Child Adolesc Psychiatry 30:104, 1991.

Schou M: Lithium prophylaxis: Myths and realities. Am J Psychiatry 146:5, 1989.

Spitz R: The First Year of Life. New York, International University Press, 1965.

Steinberg D: The use of lithium carbonate in adolescence. J Child Psychol Psychiatry 21:263, 1980.

CHAPTER 24
Suicide and Attempted Suicide

Richard Dalton

See also Chapter 110.

Adolescents may turn to suicide as a solution to psychologic and environmental problems. It is now the second leading cause of adolescent death. In addition, although few prepubertal children kill themselves, many in this age group consider suicide as a means of handling problems and conflicts.

EPIDEMIOLOGY. Nine to 18% of nonpsychiatrically disturbed preadolescents entertain suicidal ideas, whereas 1.5% actually make suicidal threats. The incidence of suicide in children and youth has been rising since 1950. Furthermore, it is estimated that there are 5 to 45 attempts for each completed act. The suicide rate in males is about threefold that in females, but the opposite sex ratio occurs for attempted suicide. By 1986, suicide was the third leading cause of fatal injuries among those younger than 20 yr; 80% of these suicides (2,151) were males, and firearms were associated with 60% of their deaths. The rate is significantly higher in the 15–19-yr-olds (8.5/100,000 in 1980) than in those younger than 15 yr. In 1991, there were 266 suicides among children younger than 15 yr; the 1990 rate was 0.8/100,000 for this population. The increase in suicide rates has been greater in black than in white youth. Because of undercounting, the rates are estimated to be 1.2 to 3.8 times the reported rates. Brent et al. suggest that this increased incidence of suicide, especially in the 15–19 yr group, is due to increased abuse of alcohol, increased rates of depression and divorce, increased availability of firearms, and an increase in mobility.

The individual and family variables associated with suicidal ideation are different from those associated with suicide. Studies suggest that up to 25% of children and adolescents think about killing themselves. Factors influencing suicidal thoughts include depression, preoccupation with death, and general psychopathologic factors. No particular diagnosis has been associated with suicidal threats. However, a wide range of psychosocial variables were found not to be associated with suicidal ideation: age, sex, social status, race, family size, intelligence, academic achievement, impulse control, reality testing, parental separation and divorce, parental medical and psychiatric problems, and drug or alcohol abuse. Variables associated with completed suicides are different. The preponderance of white, older adolescent males among child and adolescent suicide victims readily points to age, sex, and race as important factors. Alcohol intoxication is a prominent factor in adolescent suicide.

CLINICAL MANIFESTATIONS. Fifteen to 40% of completed suicides are preceded by suicide attempts. Depression and general psychopathologic factors are related to completed suicides. Specific ego functions such as impulsivity, poor reality testing, and ego mechanisms of defense such as projection, regression, and reaction formation are related to suicide attempts. In one third of suicides, a parent, a sibling, or other first-degree relative had previously shown overt suicidal behavior. Just as with suicidal ideation, children and adolescents who kill themselves show an especially prominent preoccupation with death and dying, a wish to die, and feelings of hopelessness or worthlessness prior to the act. In adolescents, the notion of revenge or hostility is particularly prominent, directed either outwardly or against the self; it is present in at least one half of those who succeed in killing themselves. Family studies have shown that fathers of suicidal youngsters have more often been noted to be depressed themselves and to have low self-esteem, whereas mothers have experienced greater anxiety or suicidal ideation. Marital difficulties and child abuse are more likely in families of adolescent suicide victims. Both parents have tended to consume more alcohol than usual. Drug use is a common family problem. Some reports suggest that gender dysphoria is related to adolescent suicide.

Firearms serve as the major method of death in adolescent suicide. Studies suggest that violent suicides by firearms and hanging are increasing and account for the overall increased suicide rate among adolescents. Death from carbon monoxide poisoning and medication overdoses are also prominent. Males are more likely than females to use violent methods. Among preadolescents, jumping from heights is the most common method, followed by self-poisoning, hanging, stabbing, and running into traffic. Episodes of self-poisoning that occur after age 6 yr are less likely to be accidental and should be treated as if the behavior had suicidal potential or as a possible case of child abuse and neglect.

School-aged children in general are surprisingly knowledgeable about the subject of suicide. The major difference between children and adolescents lies in the congruence among knowledge, fantasy, and method. Among adolescents, there is a very high correspondence among knowledge about the kinds of acts that will lead to death, fantasies about what will happen to them if they commit one of these acts, and the particular method chosen for suicide. Prepubertal children, on the other hand, show discrepancies between what they know to be a suicidal act and their fantasies of what will kill and what will not. This may, in part, be why so few prepubertal children kill themselves compared with adolescents.

TREATMENT OF THREATS AND ATTEMPTS AT SUICIDE. Threats of suicide should be seen as acts communicating desperation, and all such threats or attempts should be taken seriously. Physicians, parents, and others must scrupulously avoid sarcasm, kidding, daring, or belittling the individual making such threats. If a suicidal threat is labeled "manipulative," power or control becomes a major issue influencing behavior, and the risk of suicide may increase.

The physician assessing suicidal behavior of a child or adolescent should carefully explore, in detail, the child's life during the 48–72 hr prior to either the threat or the suicide attempt. The precipitating events should be identified. The degree of premeditation or impulsivity should be assessed. It is important to understand whether the patient intended to stop or to be discovered and whether the behavior prior to or subsequent to the attempt promoted or impeded the patient's being discovered before or after the attempt. The physician should judge the margin of error allowed by the patient in terms of the method used or proposed; the closeness or remoteness of available help; whether the patient actually called for help after the attempt if it was not immediately discovered; and whether the patient calculated correctly whether the family would return in time to discover the attempt. The most significant factor in assessing intent is the possibility and probability of rescue, as foreseen by the child or adolescent.

When the patient is able, the physician should investigate the child's frame of mind; the degree of hopelessness, helplessness, or overwhelming shame or guilt; and the presence or absence of anger (directed toward others or toward the self). The degree of depression should be evaluated carefully in terms of both the seriousness of the attempt and whether the patient presents a continuing risk. It is important to determine whether the child acted out a psychotic delusion or paranoid ideation or whether the act was the result of hallucinatory experiences that produce intolerable anxiety or panic. After recovery, it is important to assess the patient's frame of mind, to determine whether the suicide intent persists, and to assess whether there is now a more optimistic sense of being able to solve or to seek help for problems in a constructive manner.

When suicidal patients have been seen in the physician's office, the physician should enter into a no-suicide contract with the patient. The parents should be notified, and a psychiatric consultation should be obtained. Because 50% of suicide attempters do not attend even one outpatient psychiatric session, the physician should procure a specifically arranged appointment within 1 or 2 days. If possible, the patient and family should meet the therapist immediately after the examination by the physician. Suicide attempters who are seen in the emergency room should be admitted to the hospital for 1 day or more so that a more adequate evaluation can be made of the patient's frame of mind and of the circumstances of the family or environment. Such admissions usually require 2–3 days, unless medical needs require a longer stay or a serious psychiatric disorder, such as depression or psychosis, is found. If social service and psychiatric assessments are adequate and arrangements for appropriate follow-up care can be made, disposition can be made fairly rapidly. The physician must give careful attention to how the family and friends have responded to the patient's act. A hostile and angry family, such as is frequently seen, will necessitate a different disposition or resolution than a family that is supportive, sympathetic, and understanding. The latter supports a decision for the patient to return home. Some families may completely deny the seriousness of the behavior; this can be discouraging and provocative to the patient, whose act has been a desperate attempt to compel a different response. The family members should be helped to examine their roles in the interactions that preceded the attempt, without being made to feel overly guilty.

In planning care of patients after suicidal threats or attempts the physician should consider the following factors:

1. Has the patient been restored physiologically? The patient's state of consciousness, orientation, memory, attention, and concentration should be evaluated. Drugs taken during the suicide attempt may produce an acute brain syndrome or delirium that persists after the coma or stupor phase is no longer present. It is important to determine whether the effects of the drugs have cleared the system.
2. Is the patient less depressed, or is the depression masked? This is difficult to determine quickly and may require a pediatric psychiatric consultation. The family can sometimes help determine if or when the patient seems to be returning to his or her usual self.
3. Does the patient appreciate the seriousness of the act, or does he or she still want to die? Answers to these questions are important in deciding about future psychiatric hospitalization as well as in determining the appropriate time to discharge the patient home.
4. Are the precipitating events or other reasons that provoked the suicidal behavior still actively influential? The answer requires assessment of the family and environment by a health care worker.
5. Have the family, friends, teachers, and other persons significant to the patient responded in a relatively positive manner? It is important to determine whether the parents or other significant adults have recovered from their anger or excessive guilt because the child will need their support after discharge. Have the parents and child been able to identify for themselves some changes that they can make to improve things at home, at school, or in the neighborhood?
6. Does the child show evidence of a future orientation after the return home?
7. Have the child's anger, disappointment, shame, guilt, depression, grief, and other strong feelings moderated to the point at which he or she does not feel at the mercy of impulses and feelings? It is particularly important to assess whether hopelessness and helplessness have declined and whether a sense of control over one's life or one's situation has reappeared.

Psychiatric hospitalization is indicated when the individual continues to be actively suicidal, when major psychiatric disorders are found within the attempter, or when major family problems complicate ongoing protection of the attempter.

Brent DA, Kolko DJ, Allan MJ, et al: Suicidality in affectively disordered adolescent inpatients. J Am Acad Child Adolesc Psychiatry 29:586, 1990.
Brent DA, Perper JA, Goldstein CE, et al: Risk factors for adolescent suicide. Arch Gen Psychiatry 45:581, 1988.
Carlson G, Asarnow J, Orbach I: Developmental aspects of suicidal behavior in children. J Am Acad Child Adolesc Psychiatry 26:186, 1987.
Centers for Disease Control: Suicide among black youths—United States, 1980–1995. MMWR 47:193, 1998.
deWilde EJ, Kienhorst ICWM, Diekstra FW, et al: The relationship between adolescent suicidal behavior and life events in childhood and adolescence. Am J Psychiatry 149:45, 1992.
Kaplan S, Pelcovitz D, Salzinger S, et al: Adolescent physical abuse and suicide attempts. J Am Acad Child Adolesc Psychiatry 36:799, 1997.
Ohberg A, Longvist J, Serna S, et al: Violent methods associated with high suicide mortality among the young. J Am Acad Child Adolesc Psychiatry 35: 144, 1996.
Pfeffer CR, Hurt S, Peskin J, et al: Suicidal children grow up: Ego functions associated with suicide attempts. J Am Acad Child Adolesc Psychiatry 34: 1318, 1995.
Pfeffer CR, Normandin L, Kabuma T: Suicidal children grow up: Suicidal behavior and psychiatric disorders among relatives. J Am Acad Child Adolesc Psychiatry 33:1087, 1994.

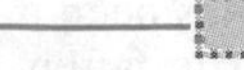

CHAPTER 25
Disruptive Behavioral Disorders

Richard Dalton

Numerous behaviors considered appropriate at certain early developmental levels are obviously pathologic when they present at later ages. Lying, impulsiveness, breath holding, defiance, and temper tantrums are frequently noted around the ages of 2–4 yr, when children begin to need autonomy but do not have the motor and social skills necessary for successful independence. These behaviors are probably the result of frustration and anger. About one half of preschoolers in the United States are brought to the attention of physicians at some time because of destructive and disobedient behaviors. Moreover, some studies suggest that disruptive, antisocial behaviors are intermittently committed by one half of this country's adolescents.

Breath holding is not unusual during the first years of life. It is frequently used by infants and toddlers in an attempt to control their environment and their caregivers. Whereas some children hold their breath until they lose consciousness, sometimes leading to a seizure, there is no increased risk of their later developing a seizure disorder. Parents are best advised to ignore the behavior and leave the room in response. Without sufficient reinforcement, the behavior soon disappears.

Defiance, oppositionalism, and *temper tantrums* are often used by children 18 mo to 3 yr of age, who feel frustrated by their conflicting desires to be in control of their environment on the one hand and, on the other, to be taken care of and pampered in a developmentally regressed way. Parental and caregiver response to this behavior is very important. Caregivers who respond to toddler defiance with punitive anger run the risk of reinforcing the defiance and teaching the child that out-of-control emotions are a reasonable response to frustration. In response to tantrums and oppositionalism, parents are advised to acknowledge verbally to the child that the reasons for frustration are understandable but that the particular response is not acceptable. The child should be given time and space to recover. If the child is unable to give up this behavior but instead presents with escalating oppositionalism, parents should nonemotionally place the child on time-out or a room restriction until he or she is able to adjust more reasonably.

Children are often frightened by the strength and intensity of their own angry feelings as well as by the intensity of the angry feelings they arouse in their parents. It is therefore of prime importance that parents provide models for control of their own anger and aggressive feelings that they wish their children to follow. Many parents who are horrified at their children's loss of control of anger are unable to see that they have often lost control themselves; they are not, therefore, helping their children to internalize controls. Physicians must learn from the parents how they handle anger before making recommendations about how to approach the child's problems. One way to help the toddler develop a sense of autonomy and to feel more in control is to allow him or her to have simple choices of activities that the parents can accept. This helps provide the child with options, thus reducing his or her potential feelings of being powerless, overwhelmed, or engulfed. Such negative, internalized feelings may later have adverse effects on interpersonal relationships, intimacy, and personality development.

Lying is often used by 2–4 yr olds as a method of playing with the language. By observing the reactions of parents and caregivers, preschoolers learn cognitively and affectively about expectations for honesty in communication. In another sense, lying is a form of fantasy for children, who describe things as they wish them to be rather than as they are. For instance, in order to avoid an unpleasant confrontation, a child who has not done something that a parent wanted may say that it has been done to avoid an unpleasant confrontation. The child's sense of time and reason does not permit the realization that this only postpones an even angrier confrontation.

In school-aged children, lying most often represents the child's attempt to avoid the pain of a relative loss of self-esteem. That is, most lying is an effort to cover up something that the child does not want to accept in his or her own behavior. The lie is invented, therefore, to achieve temporary good feeling. Lying can be the result of parental modeling, in which case the child's interpretations of reality are often conflicting, confusing, or unclear. For instance, when mothers and fathers accuse each other frequently of lying, the child may become hopelessly unsure of how the word *lying* is to be interpreted; moreover, a loyalty conflict is added to the already distorted process of reality testing.

Many adolescents lie because they fear that their parents would disapprove of what they are doing. Chronic lying, however, often occurs in combination with several other antisocial behaviors and is a sign of an underlying psychopathologic condition. As with other antisocial behaviors, lying is often used as a method of rebellion.

Regardless of the age or developmental level, when lying becomes a frequent way of managing conflict and anxiety, intervention is warranted. Initially, the parents should confront the child to give a clear message of what is acceptable. Sensitivity and support are necessary for a successful intervention, because children and adolescents are so developmentally vulnerable to shame and embarrassment. If the situation cannot be resolved equitably (i.e., parental understanding of the situation and the child's understanding that lying is not a reasonable alternative), professional intervention is indicated.

Almost all children *steal* something at some point in their lives. It becomes a problem when it happens more than once or twice. Some preschoolers and school-aged children steal as a response to a sense of internal loss. They frequently feel neglected and are, in fact, emotionally deprived. Their stealing is impulsive, but the gratification derived does not satisfy the underlying need. In children and adolescents, stealing can sometimes be an expression of anger or revenge for real or imagined frustrations by the parents. In many instances of children's stealing, there is a strong wish by the child to be caught. Stealing becomes one way in which the child or adolescent can manipulate and attempt to control interactions with parents. Like lying, stealing can be learned from parents. Parents who boast about outwitting tax laws or exceeding speed limits are implicitly condoning stealing as an acceptable behavior.

It is important for parents to help the child undo the theft by returning the stolen articles or by rendering their equivalent either in money that the child can earn or in services. When it is apparent that children are not able to control temptation, money and valuable objects should not be left where they can reach them, to decrease the chances of stealing. It is also important that the act not be overemphasized, lest the behavior or the response to it becomes so exciting that it is reproduced in future periods of discontent.

Unlike the previous behaviors, *truancy* and *run-away behavior* are never developmentally appropriate. Some children skip school because they are afraid of peers or teachers or because of the sense of humiliation secondary to learning difficulties. Others are truant because of separation anxiety symptoms. Most often, truancy represents disorganization within the home or developing personality problems, or both. Whereas younger children often threaten to run away out of frustration or a desire to get back at parents, children who run away with nowhere to go are almost always expressing a serious underlying problem (see Chapter 39). During the latency years, the most common causes are related to abuse and neglect within the home. In adolescence, disagreements with the parents, developing personality problems, and abuse and neglect all must be considered as possible precipitants.

Although the interest in fire is ubiquitous in early childhood, unsupervised *fire setting* is always inappropriate. Early school-aged children tend to set fires because of both curiosity and latent hostility secondary to deprivation within a disorganized and neglectful family. These young children set fires by themselves within their homes. In adolescence, fire setting is a more delinquent sign. Teenagers usually set fires in small groups, seeking revenge upon school and community authorities.

At the very least, fire setting requires intervention by the parents but, most often, also intervention by mental health professionals. A combination of family therapy, alliance-building individual therapy, parent management training, and community involvement is often necessary to effect a reasonable change. The recidivistic young fire setter is very difficult to manage, however. Many adult arsonists were childhood fire setters.

Although there is no totally satisfactory theory about the nature and cause of *antisocial behavior,* risk factors within the individual and family have been identified. Adoption twin studies strongly suggest that both genetic factors and child-rearing practices contribute to later developing aggressive behaviors. In well-controlled studies, adopted children with antisocial biologic fathers presented later in life with more antisocial behaviors than did those with antisocial adoptive fathers. However, children with both biologic and adoptive antisocial fathers were the most antisocial in later life. Sociocultural factors, temperament, some psychiatric conditions, and cognitive limitations can also predispose individuals to antisocial acting out.

Aggression is possibly the most serious of the disorders included in this group. Many theories have attempted to explain human aggression. The drive theory proposes that aggressive responses are biologically programmed within the human species. The phenomenologic approach suggests that everyday life is sufficiently depriving and frustrating that aggression is to be expected. Social learning theory proposes that aggression is learned and successively reinforced throughout young childhood and adolescence. In addition, social theorists suggest that modern crowding, the breakdown of widely shared values, the demise of traditional family patterns of child rearing in kinship systems, and social alienation both in individuals and in large groups are leading to increased aggression in children, adolescents, and adults. Aggression in childhood has also been correlated with family unemployment, discord, criminality, and psychiatric disorders as well as births to teenage or unmarried mothers.

Several factors contribute to aggression. Boys are almost universally reported to be more aggressive than girls. In many animals, administration of male sex hormones to females produces more aggressive behavior. Large children are often more aggressive than smaller ones. More active and intrusive children are perceived as more aggressive. Difficult temperament and later aggressiveness have been shown to be related. Children from larger families are often more aggressive than those from smaller families. Marital discord between parents and aggression within the home certainly contribute to aggression by children.

Clinically, it is important to differentiate the causes and motives for childhood aggression. Many hyperactive, clumsy children are called aggressive because of the accidental results of their behavior. Intentional aggression may be primarily instrumental, to achieve an end, or primarily hostile, to inflict physical or psychologic pain. There is also a relationship between individual aggression and emotional disturbance, school failure, brain damage, overactivity, and character pathologic conditions. Psychopathologic conditions are also associated with conduct-disordered behavior; attention deficit disorder, depression, bipolar disorder, and borderline personality traits have been correlated with aggression. Of particular importance is the relationship between severe reading retardation (as well as cognitive deficits, in general) and the development of symptoms of aggressive conduct disorder, especially in boys.

The child of 2–5 yr may show aggressive outbursts ranging from temper tantrums and screaming to hurting others or destroying toys and furniture. This behavior is frequently the product of particular frustrations and the toddler's inability to manage them. In toddlerhood, aggression is usually directed toward parents; during the preschool years, it is more likely to be directed toward siblings or peers. Verbal aggression increases between 2 and 4 yr, and after 3 yr of age, revenge and retaliation become more prominent as determinants of aggression.

Aggressive behavior in boys is relatively consistent from the preschool period through adolescence; a boy with a high level of aggressive behavior from 3–6 yr of age has a high probability of carrying this behavior into adolescence. On the other hand, girls younger than 6 yr who are aggressive toward peers are less likely to demonstrate that behavior at older ages.

Children exposed to aggressive models on television or in play display more aggressive behavior compared with children not exposed to these models (see Chapter 34). Parents' anger and aggressive or harsh punishment model behavior that children may imitate when they are physically or psychologically hurt. As Lewis has noted, parental abuse may be transmitted to the next generation by several modes: Children imitate aggression that they have witnessed; abuse can cause brain injury (which itself predisposes the child toward violence); and internalized rage more often than not results from abuse.

Passive-aggressive behaviors are common in childhood and adolescence. Prevalence rates of 16–22% have been noted. Children with passive-aggressive behavior express hostility indirectly as procrastination, stubbornness, or resistance. Parents often complain that such children do not hear them and that they fail to respond to repeated requests. Academic underachievement is common. Early histories may reveal excessive negativism during infancy and toddlerhood with feeding disturbances and problems in bladder and bowel training.

Children may unconsciously adopt passive-aggressive strategies for a variety of motives: to gain independence while maintaining dependency; to counter underlying low self-esteem; to maintain control and autonomy when threatened by anxiety; and to get revenge. These children are fearful of direct expression of assertiveness, aggression, and hostility. The child-rearing styles of their parents are often intimidating, critical, and inconsistent or, on the other hand, indulgent and permissive. Both children and parents often find it difficult to deal directly with anger.

Parents should be encouraged to handle passive-aggressive behavior by setting firm limits and expectations for the child. Parents and child should reach agreement on what they consider to be the child's important tasks and responsibilities. The most important issues need to be managed first. Age-appropriate assertiveness and independence should be promoted and rewarded. More refractory cases often require psychiatric intervention.

Conduct disorder is a distinct clinical entity manifested by several different antisocial behaviors: stealing, lying, fire setting, truancy, property destruction, cruelty to animals, rape, use of a weapon while fighting, armed robbery, physical cruelty to others, and repeated attempts to run away from home. A pattern of such behaviors that has existed for at least 6 mo warrants the diagnosis of a conduct disorder. One third to one half of adolescent psychiatric clinic patients present with conduct-disordered behavior. *Oppositional defiant disorder* is defined by less severe behavior than a conduct disorder: temper tantrums, continuous arguing, defiance of rules, continual blaming of others, angry and resentful affect, spiteful and vindictive behavior, and frequent use of obscene language. Studies have significantly differentiated oppositionalism seen in patients with oppositional defiant disorder from delinquent behaviors noted in children with conduct disorder. One third of children and adolescents with psychiatric diagnoses seen in community-based clinics are considered oppositional.

Many argue that conduct disorder is not a unitary illness but instead contains three different syndromes characterized primarily by *aggression, intermittent antisocial behaviors,* and *delinquency.* The latter two types of behavior are differentiated by the number and frequency of antisocial behaviors committed by the child. The antecedents and outcome of patients suffering from each of these subtypes, as they relate specifically to conduct disorder, have not been studied.

The risk factors (from child, parent, and environment) associated with the development of conduct disorders are very similar to those previously mentioned in association with the development of specific antisocial and aggressive behaviors. Specific antisocial symptoms in children have been related to similar behavior in their parents. Aggressive behavior is stable across generations within families. Inconsistent parenting practices as well as overly punitive disciplinary measures have been associated with conduct-disordered children. Parents of conduct-disordered children are less accepting of their children and show less warmth and support for them. However, not all children showing antisocial behavior continue that behavior into adulthood. An early age of onset of disordered behavior, an increased number of episodes and varieties of antisocial behaviors, the seriousness of the behavior as well as the types of symptoms, parental criminality, and marital discord are associated with continuation of antisocial behavior into the adult years.

Many different approaches have been used in the *treatment* of children and adolescents with aggressive behavior, conduct disorder, and oppositional disorder. Individual therapy focusing on alliance building and conflict resolution is sometimes useful in establishing the basic trust necessary for a positive therapeutic outcome; however, this is not especially effective in ameliorating behavioral problems. Group therapy has shown some promise in treating adolescents with behavioral difficulties but has been relatively ineffective with latency-aged children. Anger management therapy has demonstrated some positive results. Training in problem-solving skills involves modeling, role playing, and practicing to help children deal more successfully with interpersonal relations; it is somewhat effective in modifying maladaptive styles of relating and behaving. The most effective results have been obtained with parent management training, in which parents are trained directly to promote prosocial behaviors within the home and to place reasonable limits on unwanted, destructive behaviors. Family therapy designed to improve communication among family members and to elicit underlying conflicts to allow them to be more equitably resolved is also somewhat effective. Pharmacotherapy is, by and large, not indicated for this problem. However, children with underlying biologic vulnerability (intermittent psychotic disorders, attention deficit problems) may benefit from judicious use of appropriate medication. There are no medicines specifically intended for treatment of antisocial behaviors. Lithium, antipsychotics, anticonvulsants such as valproate, and α_2-agonists such as clonidine may be useful in the treatment of violence but have significant side effects. Some children present with such severe behavioral problems that residential treatment and psychiatric hospitalization are necessary for a successful outcome.

American Academy of Child and Adolescent Psychiatry: Practice parameters for the assessment and treatment of children and adolescents with conduct disorder. J Am Acad Child Adolesc Psychiatry 36(Suppl):122, 1997.

Conseur A, Rivara FP, Barnoski R, Emanuel I: Maternal and perinatal risk factors for later delinquency. Pediatrics 99:785, 1997.

Lahey BB, Piacentini JC, McBurnett K, et al: Psychopathology in the parents of children with conduct disorder and hyperactivity. J Am Acad Child Adolesc Psychiatry 27:163, 1988.

Lewis DO: Conduct disorders. *In:* Garfinkel B, Carlson G, Weller E (eds): Psychiatric Disorders in Children and Adolescents. Philadelphia, WB Saunders, 1990.

Marriage K, Fine S, Moretti M, et al: Relationship between depression and conduct disorder in children and adolescents. J Am Acad Child Adolesc Psychiatry 25:687, 1986.

Offord DR, Bennett KJ: Conduct disorder: Long-term outcomes and intervention effectiveness. J Am Acad Child Adolesc Psychiatry 33:1069, 1994.

Rey JM: Oppositional defiant disorder. Am J Psychiatry 150:1769, 1993.

Rutter M: Introduction: Concepts of antisocial behaviour, of cause, and of genetic influences. *In:* Bock CT, Goode J (eds): Genetics of Criminal and Antisocial Behaviour. Chichester, Wiley, 1996, pp 1–20.

Stewart JT, Myers WC, Burket RC, et al: A review of the pharmacotherapy of aggression in children and adolescents. J Am Acad Child Adolesc Psychiatry 29:269, 1990.

Wallander JL: The relationship between attention problems in childhood and antisocial behavior eight years later. J Child Psychol Psychiatry 29:53, 1988.

Webster-Stratton C: Annotation: Strategies for helping families with conduct disordered children. J Child Psychol Psychiatry 32:1047, 1991.

CHAPTER 26
Sexual Behavior and Its Variations

Richard Dalton

See also Chapter 598.

Gender identity refers to the individual's sense of self as a male or a female. *Gender role,* on the other hand, refers to those behaviors within a culture commonly thought to be associated with maleness or femaleness. Thus, one's gender identity is intact when a biologic male identifies himself as a man and a biologic female identifies herself as a woman. If the male performs the sort of behavior associated with being a man within his culture, he is said to fit comfortably within his gender role. However, if a man is uncomfortable with those behaviors identified with men within his culture, the implication is that he has trouble with his gender role. The same is true for women. However, as society has changed, gender roles have changed. In the past, gender roles were shaped by traditionally defined masculine and feminine roles. As the economics of family life have changed—and both sexes have become potentially self-sufficient economically—gender roles, as they relate to job choices and performance, have changed dramatically or, in some cases, have simply disappeared. Fewer behaviors are specific solely to one gender.

Children identify themselves as boys or girls by about 18 mo of age (i.e., establish a gender identity). Between 18 and 30 mo of age, children establish *gender stability,* the concept that boys become men and girls become women. By 30 mo, gender constancy, the immutability of one's gender, is firmly established and resistant to change. Although there are numerous theories suggesting which environmental and biologic factors are most important to the establishment of a firm gender identity, at this point we still do not understand, in a way that has treatment implications, which factors are most important in any given child.

Children are naturally curious about their bodies. The 2-yr-old child ought to be taught the proper names for the parts of the body, including the genitals. Parents should react calmly when their children explore and manipulate their own bodies with enjoyment, although open masturbation by older children suggests poor awareness of social reality or lack of parental censorship. Parents should inform their children that *masturbation* is not a social activity and should be limited to the bedroom when the child is alone. An overly excited or overly punitive reaction will serve only to excite the child. It is important that masturbation be accepted as a normal aspect of the child's sexual life and that guilt be avoided. By puberty, children should be given explanations of its normality. This can be done in conjunction with explanations of ejaculation, orgasm, and menstruation so that children can understand them, too, as normal bodily functions.

It is quite common for preschool children to hug and kiss each other. More explicit sexual behavior, such as oral contact, attempts at simulated intercourse, or anal stimulation, is probably learned through observation or direct involvement with older children or adults. Intervention designed to uncover the source of the child's knowledge followed by appropriate action is indicated in these situations (Chapter 35).

Especially between the ages of 10 and 12 yr, boys and girls typically explore sexual issues with best friends (same-sex friends) as a means of gathering information. This should not be viewed as a prelude for homosexuality but as a developmental stage in most children. At any age, the compulsive need for sex serves as a defense against underlying dependency, separation, and autonomy issues. It is usually during adolescence that gender object interests are realized. The teenager's actual or perceived sexual experiences and their reinforcements are important in shaping ultimate gender role behaviors.

Transsexualism, the conviction by a person biologically of one gender that he or she is a member of the other gender, is the most obvious example of gender identity confusion. Transsexual adolescents feel discomfort and a sense of inappropriateness about their assigned sex. They spend years trying to figure out how to get rid of the primary and secondary sexual characteristics that define them biologically. Gender roles of the opposite biologic sex are usually adopted.

The prevalence of transsexualism is 1/30,000 for males and 1/100,000 for females. Transsexuals usually have a difficult time with social and occupational functioning. Concurrent psychopathologic conditions and depression are part of the reason; societal consternation is the other part. The natural history of transsexualism is not well understood. A preponderance of adult transsexuals had gender identity disorders as children and adolescents. Extreme femininity in boys is a predisposing factor. Some say that they remember being confused about gender identity as early as 2 yr of age. Which particular effeminate boys will later show transsexual behavior cannot be accurately predicted.

Treatment of transsexualism has taken two directions. Many transsexual adults have opted for hormonal and surgical therapies to produce primary and secondary sexual characteristics of the gender with which they identify. Follow-up studies consistently show continued distress after these treatments. Long-term dynamic and behavioral therapies also have been tried. Although there are anecdotal reports of successful re-identification with the given biologic sex, without statistical controls it is impossible to know whether this represents a response to therapy or a spontaneous change that would have occurred without it. Spontaneous remissions have been shown to occur.

Transvestism, cross-dressing, may occur transiently in preschool boys who dress up in their mothers' clothing, or it may occur chronically in preschool and school-aged boys who feel genuinely excited when dressed in women's clothing. Cross-dressing in girls is rarely an identified problem. Chronic cross-dressing might represent underlying transsexualism, although that is generally not the case. Transvestism usually indicates that other gender roles may also be problematic for the individual. Physicians consulted by parents should investigate other areas of gender identification and gender behavior. Does the child verbalize a preference to be of the opposite sex? Does the child deny or disparage his or her own sexual anatomy or assert that opposite anatomic structures will develop? Three to 6% of school-aged boys and 10–12% of school-aged girls often behave like the opposite sex, but less than 2% of boys and 2–4% of girls actually wish to be the opposite sex.

26.1 Gender Identity Disorder

(GID)

Ten or more gender-atypical behaviors (GABs) are exhibited in 22.8% of school-aged boys and 38.6% of girls. Most children exhibit one or more GABs. These behaviors are to be expected in most children and are most often not indicative of GID. However, persistent distress about being a particular gender while being preoccupied with cross-gender roles or repudiation of given anatomic genital structures is the hallmark of GID. It encompasses transsexualism, transvestism, and effeminacy in boys. The etiology of GID is unknown. Some suggest that GID ought not be considered a psychiatric disturbance. Despite the fact that normative studies consistently show that more girls express the wish to be the opposite sex, clinic samples consistently include many more boys than girls (7 to 1).

CLINICAL MANIFESTATIONS. Many GID children develop the disorder prior to 4 yr of age. They are often ostracized by peers and have a difficult social adjustment, sometimes with subsequent depression. One half or more of the boys develop a homosexual orientation during adolescence and adulthood. GID is associated with numerous other childhood and adolescent disorders. Using the Child Behavior Checklist, it has been shown that 84% of feminine boys display behavioral disturbances similar to those seen within a psychiatric clinic population. Sixty per cent endorsed items related to peer difficulties and met the criteria for the diagnosis of separation anxiety disorder. Others have found that GID is unrelated to ethnic background, religion, or educational level. Although the natural history of GID suggests a strong relationship between GID and homosexuality, the fact that many gay men and lesbians do not retrospectively recall a history of cross-gender behavior and the fact that a proportion of individuals with childhood GID (10–30%) later identify as heterosexual indicate that GID is probably not just an early manifestation of homosexuality.

TREATMENT. The relationship between GID and separation anxiety disorder and other disturbances supports the importance of psychotherapy and possibly pharmacotherapy if behaviors satisfy criteria for separation anxiety disorder or other Axis I disorders. Other approaches are often employed and have been shown to be helpful. Parenting techniques that specify which behaviors are appropriate and what is expected of the child regarding gender role behaviors have shown promise in managing a significant percentage of children with GID. In fact, the extent of parental involvement in treatment appears to be correlated with a lessening of cross-gender behaviors. The physician needs to help the parents control their own frustration and disappointment and minimize judgmental, rejecting behavior. Punishment, castigation, or shaming will not support the child's attempts to struggle with whatever intrapsychic, interpersonal, or cultural conflicts exist. Underlying family conflicts and parent-child conflicts need to be managed therapeutically.

26.2 Homosexuality

Homosexuality, the romantic and physical attraction to someone of the same gender, has occurred throughout the ages in about 5% of men and women. Historically, acceptance of homosexuality has waxed and waned within societies. The view is currently held by some that homosexuality is best regarded as an alternative lifestyle. The American Psychiatric Association no longer lists it among mental disorders.

ETIOLOGY. This is uncertain. Many view its development as a normal variant of sexual development; others point to problematic parent-child relationships. Numerous psychologic theories have been proffered to explain homosexual development. They include problems of sexual identification with parents; problematic relationships between either parent and the child; abuse; overly eroticized attachment; and underlying anxiety and affective proclivities in the individual who will later present with homosexual behavior. Although each theory has been accompanied by anecdotal reports and case studies, none has been substantiated in well-controlled studies.

Biologic causes have also been proposed. Focusing on the perceived homology between homosexual behavior in humans and lower animals, researchers have proposed the "dual mating center" theory, stating that there are hypothalamic areas that regulate male and female sexual behavior. It is hypothesized that too little androgen production in males during a critical prenatal period causes the female center to overdevelop; conversely, excessive androgen production in females leads to the overdevelopment of the male center. Proponents point to the fact that some homosexual men demonstrate "estrogen feedback responses," in which, because of decreased androgen levels, administration of estrogen causes increased production of luteinizing hormone. Many other investigators dispute this theory because of the lack of consistent findings (e.g., XY males with testicular feminization syndrome do not exhibit this response).

LeVay's finding that heterosexual and homosexual men have differences in hypothalamic structure and size also suggests a biologic substrate for sexual orientation, although the possibility of AIDS in his post-mortem specimens may have biased these findings. Other researchers have noted that the anterior commissure in homosexual men is significantly larger than that in heterosexual men. This anatomic difference correlates with both sexual orientation and gender; i.e., the anterior commissure is also larger in heterosexual women than in heterosexual men. Furthermore, Hamer et al. discovered a possible genetic marker for male homosexuality in a small group of individuals and are searching for a gene. Many researchers are skeptical of these biologic findings. Some note that the current evidence that postulates biologic factors in the development of sexual orientation is no more compelling than the current evidence linked to psychologic theories.

There are probably multiple mechanisms leading to homosexuality in adolescence and adulthood, just as there are probably multiple mechanisms leading to heterosexuality; many complex factors contribute to sexual development. At this point, it appears probable that cultural, biologic, and psychologic factors contribute to sexual orientation development.

CLINICAL MANIFESTATIONS AND DIAGNOSIS. If a child is found to be engaging in homosexual behavior, parents should not immediately conclude that this means that the child is already homosexual. Sexual behavior during adolescence does not necessarily predict future sexual orientation. It is estimated that 6% of females and 17% of males have had at least one homosexual experience during adolescence. Children sexually explore in the same way that they explore other parts of their environment. The first task of the physician after discovering that a child has engaged in homosexual activity is to help the younger child feel safe and less guilty. Parents should avoid suspicious, scolding, threatening, shaming, or guilt-inducing attitudes or behaviors toward the child. The physician can serve as a model for the parent through his or her own calm, sensitive, careful exploration of feelings and behavior with the child. The physician should expect denials on the part of the child and avoidance of and embarrassment with the subject, but discussion helps the child understand that sexual behavior is comprehensible and that sexual feelings and curiosity are normal. It is important to know whether the child's information and understanding of sexual matters are appropriate for his or her age.

If the same-sex behavior involves another child in the family, he or she should be treated in the same manner. If an older child is the initiator or seducer, he or she should be told clearly and firmly that such behavior will not be tolerated and that he or she will be expected to act with responsibility and control. The older child should talk with a physician or mental health professional; if concerns about emotional and social adjustment become evident, referral for a psychiatric evaluation is indicated. Physicians must not let their own negative feelings aggravate the negative feelings that parents might have for an older child seen as a perpetrator, especially if the older child is not a member of the younger child's family. The physician may need to help the parents of exploited children refrain from ill-considered acts of revenge against the offenders. On the other hand, if there has been physical violence or psychologic coercion, both psychiatric and legal interventions are indicated.

In taking a history of sexual behavior, the pediatrician should not presume exclusively heterosexual behavior. Confidentiality must be maintained, except in sexual abuse cases. Depending on the patient's prior experience, the physical examination should include an assessment of possible sexually transmitted diseases (STDs). The American Academy of Pediatrics recommends that all sexually active males should have appropriate laboratory testing for STDs. Immunization for hepatitis B is recommended and should be provided for all males who anticipate having sex with another male. Human immunodeficiency virus (HIV) testing with the necessary consent is appropriate in these situations. Counseling before and after HIV testing is also necessary. Homosexual activity between adolescent girls is associated with a far lower risk of STDs. However, both HIV infection and other STDs can be transmitted during lesbian sexual activity, especially if one of the partners has also had sex with a man.

When the social opprobrium is considered, it is not surprising that homosexual feelings and wishes create psychologic conflicts in adolescents. Studies suggest that 3–30% of adolescent suicides are attributed to conflicts regarding sexual orientation. In a Minnesota study, 28.1% of gay/bisexual males (grades 7–12) had attempted suicide at least once, compared with 4.2% of heterosexual males of the same age. Although a greater percentage of lesbian adolescents attempted suicide than heterosexual females (20.5% compared with 14.5%), the difference was not statistically significant (see Chapter 24). Troiden's model of homosexual identity development helps elucidate the stages associated with sexual orientation acceptance. These include sensitization, i.e., the awareness of being different because of same-gender attraction; sexual identity confusion, i.e., turmoil often related to trying to reconcile one's feelings with negative societal stigmatization; sexual identity assumption, i.e., acknowledgment of one's own gay identity; and integration and commitment, i.e., incorporation of sexual identity into a positive self-acceptance.

TREATMENT. In spite of some anecdotal reports, very little can be done to change one's sexual orientation. Even in cases in which individuals have expressed the desire to change, significantly less than half of those who have tried have been able to change sexual orientation with various behavioral and dynamic therapies. Often, attempts to change sexual orientation lead only to additional guilt and further stigmatization. Psychotherapy is more appropriately used for concurrent disorders (separation anxiety disorder, conduct disorder, dysthymic disorder, depression) and to help with the conflict that often ensues as one moves toward sexual orientation acceptance. Families usually need assistance in coping with this knowledge and their attendant anger and disappointment. Children need help in understanding how to cope with the reactions of others.

Allen L, Gorski R: Sexual orientation and the size of the anterior commissure in the human brain. Proc Natl Acad Sci USA 89:7199, 1992.

Bailey J, Michael J, Neale M, et al: Heritable factors influencing sexual orientation in women. Arch Gen Psychiatry 50:217, 1993.

Bradley SJ, Zucker KJ: Gender identity disorder: A review of the past 10 years. J Am Acad Child Adolesc Psychiatry 36:872, 1997.

Byrne W, Parsons B: Human sexual orientation: The biologic theories reappraised. Arch Gen Psychiatry 50:228, 1993.

Coates S, Person E: Extreme boyhood femininity: Isolated behavior or pervasive disorder? J Am Acad Child Adolesc Psychiatry 24:702, 1985.

Committee on Adolescence (American Academy of Pediatrics): Homosexuality and adolescence. Pediatrics 92:631, 1993.

DuRant RH, Krowchuk DP, Sinal SH: Victimization, use of violence, and drug use at school among male adolescents who engage in same-sex sexual behavior. J Pediatr 132:13, 1998.

Friedrich WN, Fisher J, Broughton D, et al: Normal sexual behavior in children: A contemporary sample. Pediatrics 101:E9, 1998.

Hamer D, Magnuson V, Pattatucci A: A linkage between DNA markers on the X chromosome and male sexual orientation. Science 261:321, 1993.

LeVay S: The Sexual Brain. Cambridge, MIT Press, 1993.

Sandberg D, Meyer-Bahlburg H, Ehrhardt A, et al: The prevalence of gender-atypical behavior in elementary school children. J Am Acad Child Adolesc Psychiatry 32:306, 1993.

Troiden R: Homosexual identity development. J Adolesc Health Care 9:105, 1989.

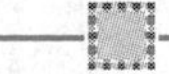

CHAPTER 27

Pervasive Developmental Disorders and Childhood Psychosis

Richard Dalton and Marc A. Forman

Pervasive developmental disorders include autistic disorder, Asperger disorder, childhood disintegrative disorder, and Rett disorder.

27.1 Autistic Disorder

Autism develops before 30 mo of age. It is characterized by a qualitative impairment in verbal and nonverbal communication, in imaginative activity, and in reciprocal social interactions.

CLINICAL MANIFESTATIONS. Among the most notable symptoms and signs are nondeveloped or poorly developed verbal and nonverbal communication skills, abnormalities in speech patterns, impaired ability to sustain a conversation, abnormal social play, lack of empathy, and an inability to make friends. Stereotypical body movements, a marked need for sameness, very narrow interests, and a preoccupation with parts of the body are also frequent. The autistic child is withdrawn and often spends hours in solitary play. Ritualistic behavior prevails, reflecting the child's need to maintain a consistent, predictable environment. Tantrum-like rages may accompany disruptions of routine. Eye contact is minimal or absent. Visual scanning of hand and finger movements, mouthing of objects, and rubbing of surfaces may indicate a heightened awareness and sensitivity to some stimuli, whereas diminished responses to pain and lack of startle responses to sudden loud noises reflect lowered sensitivity to other stimuli. If speech is present, echolalia, pronomial reversal, nonsense rhyming, and other idiosyncratic language forms may predominate.

Intelligence, measured by conventional psychologic testing, usually falls in the functionally retarded range; however, the deficits in language and socialization make it difficult to obtain an accurate estimate of the autistic child's intellectual potential. Some autistic children perform adequately in nonverbal tests, and those with developed speech may demonstrate adequate intellectual capacity. Occasionally, an autistic child may have an isolated, remarkable talent, analogous to that of the adult savant.

Although it was first described as a social illness, most research studies have focused on the communicative and cognitive deficits of autism and, particularly, on the types of cognitive processing deficits most apparent in emotional situations. Deficits in verbal sequencing, abstraction, rote memory, and reciprocal verbal exchange are typical in autistic children. Autistic children also show deficits in their understanding of what the other person might be feeling or thinking, a so-called lack of a "theory of mind." On some psychologic tests, children with autism pay more attention to specific details while overlooking the entire Gestalt of the object, demonstrating a "lack of central coherence."

EPIDEMIOLOGY. The prevalence is 3–4/10,000 children. The disorder is much more common in males than in females (3–4:1). Autism can be associated with other neurologic disorders, particularly tuberous sclerosis, seizure disorders, and to a lesser extent, fragile X syndrome.

ETIOLOGY. The cause of autism is unknown. Genetic factors have been implicated. There is an 80% concordance rate for monozygotic twins and a 20% concordance rate for dizygotic twins. What is actually inherited is not entirely clear; language and cognitive abnormalities are more common in relatives of autistic children than in the general population. Chromosomal abnormalities, especially fragile X syndrome, are also more common in families with autism.

Abnormal neurochemical findings have been associated with autism. Aberrant dopamine functioning has been implicated, and abnormalities have been suggested in a number of catecholamine pathways. Increased levels of serotonin have also been noted.

Theories of causation have also centered on a variety of other possibilities, including brain injury, constitutional vulnerability, developmental aphasia, deficits in the reticular activating system, structural cerebellar changes, forebrain hippocampal lesions, neuroradiologic abnormalities in the prefrontal and temporal lobe areas, and an unfortunate interplay between psychogenic and neurodevelopmental factors. Autistic children have been reported to have increased brain volume in the temporal, parietal, and occipital lobes. Other studies demonstrate anatomic changes in the anterior cingulate gyrus, an area of the brain associated with decision-making and the ascription of feelings and thoughts. Contrary to notions in vogue in the past, autism is not induced by parents.

TREATMENT. Advances have been made in the treatment of autism, especially within the educational, psychosocial, and biologic areas. However, few well-controlled studies have compared the efficacy of individual approaches or of combined treatments. Treatment is most successful when geared toward the individual's particular needs. Therapy with the very young often focuses on speech and language, special education, parent education, training and support, and pharmacotherapy for certain target symptoms. Older children and adolescents with relatively higher intelligence but with poor social skills and psychiatric symptoms (e.g., depression, anxiety, obsessive-compulsive symptoms) may require psychotherapy, behavioral or cognitive therapy, and pharmacotherapy.

Working with families of autistic children is vital to the child's overall care. In general, services have not yet been sufficiently developed to provide support and continuity of care. The most successful educational model at present is the program for the Treatment and Education of Autistic and Related Communication Handicapped Children (TEACCH). The following treatment principles are emphasized: use of objective measures such as the Childhood Autism Rating Scale (CARS); enhancement of skills and acceptance by the environment of autism-related deficits; use of interventions based on cognitive and behavioral theories; use of visual structures for optimal education; and multidisciplinary training for all professionals working with autistic children.

Methods are being developed to help increase spontaneous language usage that maximizes the autistic child's communication. The use of facilitated communication has been disavowed by most professional organizations. Initial findings regarding the use of auditory integration training are hopeful; however, full-scale investigations have not been undertaken.

Behavior modification is a major part of the overall treatment for autism. These procedures include enhancement (i.e., rewards emphasizing appropriate choice) and reduction (extinction, time-out, punishment). Ethical concerns about vigorous aversive therapy approaches have led to specific guidelines. Social skills training is also currently used as a treatment modality.

Because a subgroup of autistic children present with psychiatric symptoms, pharmacotherapy is sometimes used to ameliorate target behaviors. The behaviors include hyperactivity, tantrums, physical aggression, self-injurious behavior, stereotypies, and anxiety symptoms (e.g., obsessive-compulsive behaviors). Among the neuroleptics, haloperidol is the most studied. It is effective in diminishing various generalized behaviors (anger, aggression, uncooperativeness, overactivity). When used on a short-term basis (≤2 mo) in doses ranging from 0.25 mg/24 hr to 4 mg/24 hr, the often seen pernicious side effects (tardive dyskinesia, withdrawal dyskinesia, neuroleptic malignant syndrome) do not usually develop.

Fenfluramine, although once seen as a potentially useful agent, is not helpful. Although naltrexone, an opiate antagonist, was also originally believed to be helpful, its utility has not been proved. Clomipramine, a tricyclic antidepressant with serotonin reuptake inhibition action, is useful in reducing compulsions and stereotypies in autistic children. However, it does lower the seizure threshold and has cardiotoxic and behavior toxicity effects. Other medicines used to treat psychiatric symptoms in autistic children include the stimulants, the SSRIs, and clonidine. Although anecdotal evidence abounds, no scientific evidence substantiates their value.

PROGNOSIS. This is guarded. Some children, especially those with speech, may grow up to live marginal, self-sufficient, albeit isolated, lives in the community, but for some, chronic placement in institutions is the ultimate outcome. The relationship between autism and schizophrenia is uncertain. Cases in which autistic children have later developed schizophrenia have been reported but are not common. A better prognosis is associated with higher intelligence, functional speech, and less bizarre symptoms and behavior. The symptoms often change as children grow older. Seizures and self-injurious behavior become more common with advancing age.

27.2 Asperger Disorder

Children with this disorder have a qualitative impairment in the development of reciprocal social interaction, often demonstrating repetitive behaviors and restricted, obsessional, idiosyncratic interests. They do not, however, have the language impairments that characterize autism. Although somewhat socially aware, these children appear to others to be peculiar or eccentric. Prevalence is estimated to be approximately 3/1,000 children. Asperger disorder may represent a higher functioning form of autism, although this distinction remains controversial.

27.3 Childhood Disintegrative Disorder

This disorder, also known as Heller dementia, is a rare condition of unknown etiology. It is characterized by normal development up to 2–4 yr, followed by severe deterioration of mental and social functioning, with regression to a very impaired "autistic" state. Language, social skills, and imagination are profoundly affected; bowel and bladder control may be lost; and motor stereotypies are often present. While this condition may be the result of an underlying neurologic illness, none has been identified as yet. The outcome appears to be worse than for autistic disorder.

27.4 Rett Disorder

This is an X-linked dominant disorder affecting girls almost exclusively (it is lethal to the male fetus). It has a prevalence of 1–2/ 20,000. Development proceeds normally until approximately 1 yr of age, at which time language and motor development regress and acquired microcephaly becomes apparent. These girls present with midline hand-wringing and unusual sighing. Autistic behaviors are typical. Post-mortem examinations have revealed greatly reduced brain size and weight as well as a reduced number of synapses. No specific etiology or treatment has been identified.

27.5 Childhood Schizophrenia

Psychotic reactions in older children tend to resemble more closely the psychoses of adulthood, and the same diagnostic criteria apply. Affective psychoses, such as bipolar illness, have been described in Chapter 23.

In *childhood schizophrenia,* prominent symptoms include thought disorder, delusions, and hallucinations. The latter two symptoms, in addition to later onset, higher intelligence scores, and fewer perinatal complications, differentiate schizophrenia from autism. As the symptoms imply, schizophrenic children often appear to be chaotic. They may have paranoid delusions, aggressive behavior, hebephrenic silliness, social withdrawal, and alternating moods not apparently related to environmental stimuli, among other possibilities.

The prevalence of adult schizophrenia is 1% of the population. Because the typical age of onset in schizophrenia is late adolescence to early adulthood, a very small percentage of preschool and latency-aged children actually show symptoms that meet the criteria for a diagnosis of schizophrenia. As infants, half of schizophrenic children are said to have had abnormally delayed development and unusual sensory sensitivities. Schizophrenic children show significant premorbid maladjustments. The onset of the disorder is usually insidious. Auditory hallucinations are seen in 80% of schizophrenic children. Delusions and formal thought disorders usually do not present until midadolescence. The prognosis is poor. The symptoms in childhood that most predict psychotic adult psychopathology are affective blunting and disturbed interpersonal relationships, as opposed to delusions and hallucinations.

A multimodal therapeutic approach is necessary to manage this illness. Parent training is necessary to teach effective techniques to modify the schizophrenic child's behavior to a reasonable extent. Individual therapy designed to build a positive alliance is also very important. Neuroleptic therapy is often effective in managing hallucinations and psychotic delusions. School and community liaison work can establish and maintain a day-to-day schedule for the patient.

American Academy of Child and Adolescent Psychiatry: Practice parameters for the assessment and treatment of children and adolescents with schizophrenia. J Am Acad Child Adolesc Psychiatry 36:1775, 1997.

Baron-Cohen S: The autistic child's theory of mind: A case of specific developmental delay. J Child Psychol Psychiatry 30:285, 1989.

Campbell M, Schopler E, Cueva JE, et al: Treatment of autistic disorders. J Am Acad Child Adolesc Psychiatry 35:134, 1996.

Fourbonne E, DuMazaubrun C, Cans C, et al: Autism and associated medical disorders in a French epidemiologic survey. J Am Acad Child Adolesc Psychiatry 36:1561, 1997.

Frith U: Autism: Explaining the Enigma. Oxford, Blackwell, 1989.

Gillberg C: Clinical Child Neuropsychiatry. Cambridge, Cambridge University Press, 1995.

Green WH, Padron-Gayol M, Hardesty AS, et al: Schizophrenia with childhood onset: A phenomenological study of 38 cases. J Am Acad Child Adolesc Psychiatry 31:968, 1992.

Harris JC: Developmental Neuropsychiatry, Vol II: Assessment, Diagnosis, and Treatment Of Developmental Disorders. New York, Oxford University Press, 1995.

Kanner L: Early infantile autism. Am J Orthopsychiatry 19:416, 1949.

Lofgren DP, Bemporad J, King J, et al: A prospective follow-up of so-called borderline children. Am J Psychiatry 148:1541, 1991.

Mars AE, Mauk JE, Dowrick PW: Symptoms of pervasive developmental disorders as observed in prediagnostic home videos of infants and toddlers. J Pediatr 132:500, 1998.

Petti TA, Vela RM: Borderline disorders of childhood: An overview. J Am Acad Child Adolesc Psychiatry 29:327, 1990.

Piven J, Arndt S, Bailey J, et al: Regional brain enlargement in autism: A magnetic resonance imaging study. J Am Acad Child Adolesc Psychiatry 35:530, 1996.

Pomeroy J: Infantile autism and childhood psychosis. *In*: Garfinkel B, Carlson G, Weller E (eds): Psychiatry Disorders in Childhood and Adolescence. Philadelphia, WB Saunders, 1990.

Schopler E, Olley R: Comprehensive educational services for autistic children: The TEACCH model. *In*: Reynolds CR, Gutkin TR (eds): The Handbook of School Psychology. New York, Wiley, 1982.

Schopler E, Reichler RJ, Renner BR: The Childhood Autism Rating Scale (CARS) for Diagnostic Screening and Classification of Autism. New York, Irvington Publishers, 1986.

Treffert DA: The idiot savant: A review of the syndrome. Am J Psychiatry 145:563, 1988.

Ventner A, Lord C, Schopler E: A follow-up study of high-functioning autistic children. J Child Psychol Psychiatry 33:489, 1992.

Volkmar FR: Childhood and adolescent psychosis: A review of the past 10 years. J Am Acad Child Adolesc Psychiatry 35:843, 1996.

Volkmar FR, Cohen DJ: Comorbid association of autism and schizophrenia. Am J Psychiatry 148:1705, 1991.

Wing L: The definition and prevalence of autism: A review. Eur Child Adolesc Psychiatry 2:1, 1993.

CHAPTER 28
Psychologic Treatment of Children and Adolescents

Richard Dalton

28.1 Illness and Death

All clinical phenomena relate to various organizational levels: molecular, anatomic, physiologic, intrapsychic, interpersonal, familial, and social. Accordingly, physicians should focus on patients' discomfort rather than on a categorization of clinical manifestations as either organically or psychologically determined. The psychologic aspects of illness should be evaluated from the outset, and physicians should act as a model for parents and children by showing interest in a child's feelings and demonstrating that it is possible and appropriate to communicate discomfort in verbal, symbolic language.

For *hospitalized children,* potential challenges include coping with separation; adapting to a new environment; adjusting to multiple caregivers; often associating with very sick children; and sometimes experiencing the disorientation of intensive care, anesthesia, and surgery. To help mitigate potential problems, a preadmission visit to the hospital is often important to meet the people who will be offering care and to ask questions about what will happen. For children younger than age 5–6 yr, parents should room with the child if feasible. Creative and active recreational or socialization programs, with liberal visiting hours (including visits from siblings), and chances to act out feared procedures in play with dolls or mannequins all are helpful. Sensitive, sympathetic, and accepting attitudes toward children and parents by the hospital staff are very important. There is often an underlying tension between the hospital caregivers and the parents. Hospital routines and schedules often serve to complicate the relationship between parents and hospital workers. Guilt and anger can result, unnecessarily complicating an already difficult situation.

Ambulatory care in clinics or offices where patients receive discontinuous care from a series of physicians whose intercommunication is often limited may create a problem. Parents often become confused and unable to verbalize major concerns about their children. Recommendations for care may become inappropriate or irrelevant, and compliance with advice or directions becomes poor. At the end of any initial diagnostic or management activity, physicians should habitually inquire whether there are other things parents or children may wish to talk about during this visit. In busy emergency rooms, conflicting expectations between how the professional staff expects the emergency room to be used and what patients actually need can lead to confusion. When these different expectations are critically examined, ways may be found to deal more effectively with the patterns of use of emergency services.

With *chronically or fatally ill children,* every symptom is experienced by patients and parents as a threat to physical integrity and life. The more serious the clinical state, the greater the intensity of the emotions aroused. By age 9 yr, children begin to conceive of death as meaning more than just going away. By adolescence, they think of death in philosophic terms much as adults do, albeit with limited experience (see Chapters 37 and 38).

In dealing with chronic illness that shortens life, such as cystic fibrosis, parents need physicians' early support in developing a relatively guilt-free understanding of the disease and how to manage it. They need guidance to help them comfortably answer their child's questions about the disease. Young children take most cues from their parents. With older children, especially adolescents, parents must be prepared to deal with the anger of their children because of their fate. Children need both the parents' psychologic strengths and resources and the physician's availability and objectivity. The siblings of an ill child require information about the disease and the support and attention of the parents for their own needs.

The role of physicians is difficult. They must stand for hope and for relief of discomfort, ready to help parents and children avoid emotionally crippling psychologic handicaps. For example, parents must be encouraged to meet their own needs, even when this requires temporary and perhaps recurrent separation from their child; at times, this may help a child to learn to tolerate frustration. Parents of critically or fatally ill children may creatively support each other in group meetings under the professional guidance of physicians, psychologists, or social workers.

In potentially *fulminant lethal processes,* the intensity of parental anxiety, guilt, and despair may be greater than it is with more chronic illnesses. With most children older than 9–10 yr, it is most supportive to treat fatal illness factually with a child, so far as diagnosis and prognosis are concerned, but always to offer realistic hope. Children do not usually ask a physician if and when they are going to die, although they may reveal their fears to others in the hospital. Young children primarily want to be reassured that their parents will not desert them and that they are loved. A hospital team approach representing medical, nursing, psychologic, and social work disciplines, among others, should provide support. The primary physician needs to stay involved and close to the child and to the clinical situation.

Organ transplants in children have most often involved the kidney. Dialysis may precede renal transplant for various lengths of time and begins in the hospital, but parents may be expected to learn to carry out this procedure at home. They may be ambivalent about being given control of a life-threatening process. Children receiving dialysis become psychologically dependent and often withdrawn. Bone marrow, heart, lung, and liver transplants also involve many psychologic considerations, such as donor relationships and the stress of isolation and complications (see Chapters 68, 449, and 367).

Family problems multiply with the question of who will donate an organ. If relatives are available as donors, there may be tension about who can and should make such sacrifice. In some cases, guilt may be relieved if the physician arbitrarily (but thoughtfully) makcs this dccision. A medical support team of carefully chosen staff is essential to facilitate decision-making and continuing care. Although the suicide rate among adults undergoing hemodialysis is high, this procedure appears to be less traumatic in children, probably owing to a child's greater capacities for denial and acceptance of a support system. Adolescents are concerned with distortions of body image, which they cannot always express verbally.

After *the death of a child,* the parents need opportunities to talk out their feelings with the physician, one of whose goals should be to help them avoid psychologically encapsulating the lost child in an unmourned state. Many parents can be helped and comforted by being with and holding the dying infant or child or seeing and touching him or her after death. Physicians need the patience to listen (both to the stated and to the implied questions and misconceptions), to answer questions, and to help families with funeral arrangements (see Chapters 38 and 72).

28.2 Psychopharmacology (Table 28–1)

Using drugs to modify children's behavior is controversial. Their effects on behavior are influenced by the maturity of the central nervous system, by intrapsychic and psychosocial factors, by the personality or charisma of the physician prescribing them, by the problem itself, and by the milieu (e.g., patient, parents, time of day given). Although potentially helpful, psychiatric medications can cause very serious side effects. Even though some guidelines are offered in Table 28–1 for their use, only clinicians with appropriate training and experience should prescribe the antipsychotics, mood stabilizers, and tricyclic antidepressants.

Neuroleptics are appropriately used for hallucinations, delusions, thought disorders, and severe agitation. They are primarily indicated for children and adolescents suffering with schizophrenic disorders, mood-congruent and mood-incongruent psychotic reactions secondary to major affective disorders, autism presenting with stereotypic and withdrawal symptoms and self-abuse, and Gilles de la Tourette syndrome. Some advocate the use of haloperidol for aggressive behavior in children and adolescents, but this use remains controversial. Serious questions have been raised about the efficacy of neuroleptics in childhood schizophrenia. This class of medicine is inappropriately used for anxiety, conduct disorder without extreme aggression, and attention deficit disorder.

Neuroleptics can be subdivided into low-potency, midpotency, and high-potency types. Both chlorpromazine and thioridazine are low-potency medicines and usually require a higher dose than the other neuroleptics for symptom remission. Both are rather sedating, producing numerous anticholinergic side effects but causing comparatively fewer extrapyramidal symptoms. Mesoridazine, a midpotency medicine, produces more extrapyramidal symptoms than the low-potency drugs. Thiothixene and haloperidol are high-potency medicines that produce, comparatively, the greatest number of extrapyramidal symptoms. Clozapine, a new atypical neuroleptic, has efficacy in the treatment of negative schizophrenic symptoms. However, threatening side effects include agranulocytosis and seizure development.

The most worrisome side effect of the neuroleptics is the development of *tardive dyskinesia.* This is characterized by choreoathetoid movements of the trunk, limbs, and facial musculature; these movements develop in approximately 20–30% of children treated long-term with neuroleptics. Dyskinesia can occur during the treatment with the drug or after it has been discontinued, in which case it is referred to as *withdrawal dyskinesia.* This latter type of dyskinesia, the symptoms of which can include nausea, vomiting, diaphoresis, ataxia, oral dyskinesia, and various dystonic movements, is reversible in most cases, whereas the dyskinesia developing during drug use may not be reversible. The best instrument for the assessment of abnormal movements is the Abnormal Involuntary Movement Scale (AIMS). It is very helpful with children and adolescents. Treatment of tardive dyskinesia involves decreasing or discontinuing the medication if possible, despite the fact that it has been noted that increasing the neuroleptic causes a temporary diminution of dyskinetic symptoms. Prophylactic measures involving drug-free holidays and periodic discontinuation of neuroleptics are also advisable to help mitigate the development of tardive dyskinesia.

Extrapyramidal symptoms, a Parkinson-like syndrome (akathisia, bradykinesia, torticollis, drooling, and involuntary hand movements, among others), develop in at least one fourth of children treated with neuroleptics. The imbalance created by the dopaminergic blocking action of the antipsychotic medication disrupts a needed balance between the dopaminergic system and the cholinergic system within the basal ganglia. The high-potency neuroleptics, which contain few anticholinergic properties, are the most likely to produce extrapyramidal symptoms. This syndrome can be treated by decreasing the neuroleptic or adding an anticholinergic agent (trihexyphenidyl HCl [Artane], benztropine mesylate [Cogentin]).

Neuroleptic malignant syndrome, a rare side effect of neurolep-

TABLE 28–1 Psychopharmacology

Medication Class		Dosage	Side Effects/ Toxicity/Caution	Pretreatment Work-up
Antipsychotics	***All Classes***	***Low Potency***	***All Classes***	CBC with differential, blood chemistry panel (including hepatic enzymes)
Low Potency/High Dosage Thioridazine (Mellaril) Chlorpromazine (Thorazine) Clozapine (Clozaril) [atypical]	Severe agitation; psychosis; mania; stereotypic symptoms of pervasive developmental disorder and autism; self-abuse, extreme aggressiveness	Initial: 10–30 mg/24 hr in single or divided doses. Maintenance: 100–900 mg/24 hr in divided doses	Sedation, weight gain, anticholinergic effects (dry mouth, blurred vision; constipation); hypersensitivity reactions (hepatic, skin); blood dyscrasias; parkinsonism; neuroleptic malignant syndrome; orthostatic hypotension; agranulocytosis and seizures (especially with clozapine)	
Midpotency/Mid-dosage Mesoridazine (Serentil)		***Midpotency*** 10–75 mg/24 hr in divided doses		
High-potency/Low-dosage Trifluoperazine (Stelazine) Thiothixine (Navane) Haloperidol (Haldol) Risperidone (Risperdal)		***High potency*** Initial: 0.5–1 mg/24 hr in single or divided doses		
Stimulants	***All Drugs***			
(6 yr and older) Methylphenidate (Ritalin) Dextroamphetamine (Dexedrine)	ADHD (with and without behavioral acting out): Narcolepsy (methylphenidate, (dextroamphetamine)	0.3–1.0 mg/kg/24 hr in divided doses. 0.2–0.6 mg/kg/24 hr in divided doses	Lower seizure threshold; insomnia, decreased appetite, possible weight loss; irritability and tearfulness; abdominal pain, headache; elevated systolic blood pressure; development and worsening of tics; possible subnormal height and weight growth. Possible precipitation of hypomania in bipolar patients.	Medical history, heart rate, blood pressure, CBC with differential (with prolonged use)
Pemoline (Cylert)		18.75–112.5 mg/day in divided doses.	Pemoline is associated with hypersensitivity reactions, especially hepatic	Hepatic enzymes with pemoline
Antidepressants **Tricyclics**				
Desipramine (Norpramin)	Major depressive disorder in mid to late adolescence; ADHD (12 yr and older); separation anxiety disorder	For major depression disorder and separation anxiety disorder, 2–3 mg/kg/24 hr in divided doses. (Therapeutic blood level, 100–250 mg/mL)	Possible sudden death in doses >3.5–5 mg/kg; hypertension, orthostatic hypotension, cardiac arrhythmia, lengthening of PR or QRS interval on ECG; overdose leading to death	Thorough individual and family history for cardiologic problems; 12-lead ECG; blood pressure monitoring. Plasma blood levels indicated after therapy has begun only if clinical response is poor
Imipramine (Tofranil)	As above; enuresis	As above. For enuresis usually 25–50 mg qhs (continued for at least 4–6 mo after remission of enuresis)	As above	As above
Clomipramine (Anafranil)	Obsessive-compulsive disorder	Starting dose of 25 mg, which is increased slowly (2–3 wk) to either 100 mg or 3 mg/kg (whichever is smaller) in divided doses. Thereafter, increase to a maximum of 250–300 mg	Seizures; overdose leading to death; ST-T wave changes on ECG, conduction abnormalities; psychiatric changes including mania and confusion; weight gain; hyperthermia; vertigo; constipation	As above
Selective Serotonin Reuptake Inhibitors				
Fluoxetine (Prozac)	Mild-moderate depression, anxiety, OCD	10–20 mg/24 hr (possibly higher for OCD)	Fluoxetine and its principal metabolite have a long half (1–4 days). Can inhibit its own metabolism; thus, an increase in dose may result in a disproportionate increase in side effects. Drug interactions with compounds metabolized by several isoenzymes of the cytochrome P 450 system (especially terfenadine, astemizole, cisapride); gastrointestinal difficulties (nausea, diarrhea, vomiting) CNS effects (agitation, disinhibition, jitteriness, headache, insomnia); tremor; serotonin syndrome (fever, myoclonus, confusion, tachycardia, rigidity. . .) when taken with MAO inhibitors or L-tryptophan; mania; self-injurious behavior and behavioral activation and dyscontrol	

Table continued on following page

TABLE 28–1 Psychopharmacology *Continued*

Medication Class		Dosage	Side Effects/ Toxicity/Caution	Pretreatment Work-up
Paroxetine (Paxil)	As above	20–30 mg/24 hr	As above except shorter half-life (24 hr); withdrawal symptoms if stopped abruptly	
Sertraline (Zoloft)	As above	25 mg/24 hr with meals	Similar to paroxetine; fairly inactive metabolite has longer half-life; exhibits linear relationship between dose and side effects	
Fluvoxamine (Luvox)	OCD	Initial: 50 mg each night. Increase slowly to no more than 300 mg/24 hr in divided doses.	Similar to sertraline; less interference with cytochrome P450 system	
Venlafaxine (Effexor)	Depression	37.5 mg/24 hr increased by no more than 37.5–75 mg/24 hr to a maximum 225 mg/24 hr in divided doses, with meals	As above, except for little interference with cytochrome P450 system	
Aminoketone				
Bupropion (Wellbutrin)	Depression, ADHD	Initial: 75–100 mg/24 hr increased slowly to 200–300 mg/24 hr (bid dosing); total daily dose should not exceed 450 mg	Seizures, restlessness, agitation, weight loss, rashes, nocturia, mania, flulike symptoms	
Mood Stabilizers				
Lithium carbonate	Bipolar cycling typical of older adolescents and adults, some cases of unipolar illness, affective type of aggression	600–1,200 mg/24 hr (therapeutic blood level: 0.6–1.2 mEq/L)	Gastrointestinal disturbance, tremor, ataxia, confusion, coma, death; hypothyroidism. Once discontinued, lithium is often not as effective when restarted. Overdose leading to death	Creatinine clearance, thyroid studies, ECG, electrolytes, calcium, phosphorus
Carbamazepine (Tegretol)	Bipolar cycling including rapid cycling; aggressive behavior in organically impaired patients	Initial: 100–200 mg/24 hr increased to 400–1,000 mg/24 hr (therapeutic blood level: 8–12 μg/mL)	Fever, sore throat, hematologic problems (white cell decrease), dizziness, drowsiness, neuromuscular disturbance, blurred vision; overdose leading to death	Physical examination, medical history, CBC with differential, BUN, hepatic enzymes
Valproic acid (Depakene)	Rapid cycling bipolar disorder, aggression	Initial: 125–250 mg/24 hr or 10–15 mg/kg; increase by 5–10 mg/kg/24 hr up to 60 mg/kg/24 hr in divided doses (therapeutic blood level: 50–100 μg/mL)	Hepatic failure (usually in the first few months of treatment); younger children (under 10 yr, especially under 2 yr), patients with prior hepatic disease history, those on multiple anticonvulsants, those with severe seizure history plus mental retardation, and those with congenital metabolic disorders are especially vulnerable. Obesity, birth defects in pregnancy; possible clotting problems; depression; nausea, vomiting, indigestion (at initiation of therapy), rashes; overdose leading to coma and possibly death	Physical examination, medical history, hepatic enzymes
Antihypertensives				
Clonidine (Catapres)	Hyperactivity; aggression associated with ADHD; secondary use in tic disorder	0.1–0.25 mg/24 hr	Sedating bradycardia, hypotension; withdrawal symptoms; sudden deaths reported when used with stimulants	Physical examination, medical history, blood pressure, ECG
Guanfacine (Tenex)	Aggression associated with ADHD; tic disorder	0.5–1 mg qhs	Sedation, headaches (less hypotension than clonidine)	Blood pressure

ADHD, attention deficit hyperactivity disorder; CBC, complete blood count; ECG, electrocardiogram; OCD, obsessive-compulsive disorder; CNS, central nervous system; MAO, monoamine oxidase; BUN, blood urea nitrogen.

tic use, can be fatal. Its development is heralded by a high fever and a "lead pipe" stiffness of the extremities. Patients' creatinine phosphokinase level is also markedly elevated. Immediate discontinuation of the medicine and supportive care are necessary during the early part of the syndrome.

Stimulant medications are used to treat the signs and symptoms of attention deficit hyperactivity disorder (see Chapter 29.2). Although the mechanism of action is not entirely clear, these medications increase children's ability to attend, improve classroom behavior, and increase social acceptance of affected children in various situations. These stimulants should be used concurrently with individual, family, and community therapy, but this is often not done.

Antidepressants and *mood stabilizers* are useful in the treatment of affective disorders. Antidepressants generally are effective for depression, whereas lithium, carbamazepine, and valproate have shown efficacy with mania. Adult patients with bipolar and unipolar disorders are often treated with long-term pharmacotherapy, and this is becoming more common in childhood and adolescence. Because of the propensity of tricyclic antidepressants to cause heart block, a pretreatment electrocardiogram (ECG) and follow-up ECGs are necessary. This usually takes at least a few weeks. Although deaths in school-aged children taking desipramine have been reported, sudden deaths have not been reported in conjunction with the use of other tricyclics or with other nontricyclic antidepressants. Before prescribing tricyclics in general and desipramine in particular, clinicians must procure a detailed medical history, including examination of a patient's cardiovascular system and ascertainment of any family history of cardiac disease (including unexplained syncope and sudden death). A child with a suspicious history or with abnormal ECG findings should have a pediatric or cardiologic assessment before these medicines are used. The desipramine dose should not exceed 3.5–5.0 mg/kg. A pretreatment lithium evaluation includes thyroid studies, renal function tests, and electrolyte determinations. Lithium blood levels should also be determined while patients are taking the medication. Prolonged use of lithium may cause hypothyroidism.

Serotonin reuptake blockers, especially fluoxetine (Prozac), sertraline (Zoloft), and paroxetine (Paxil), have been shown to be effective in patients with mild depressive symptoms, anxiety, and compulsions. Paroxetine is especially useful because of its relatively short half-life and lack of side effects. Clonidine has been partially successful in treating children with attention deficit hyperactivity disorder and in those who have a personal history of tics (including Gilles de la Tourette syndrome). Pimozide (Orap) reduces vocal and motor tics effectively in both tic disorder and Gilles de la Tourette syndrome.

Carbamazepine, an antiepileptic medicine, is effective in the treatment of mania and episodic dyscontrol syndrome. β-Blocking agents (nadolol [Corgard]) appear to decrease aggressiveness in mentally retarded patients. Opiate antagonists significantly change some behaviors in autistic children and have promise in the treatment of self-injurious behavior in severely and profoundly mentally retarded individuals. Clomipramine (Anafranil) is efficacious in the treatment of obsessive-compulsive disorder. Seizures have been reported secondary to its use, however.

Some parents are adamantly opposed to the use of psychotropic medications. If drugs are used, they should be used for as short a time as possible. As with any clinical disorder, physicians should avoid using several medications and should not shift back and forth from one medication to another when no immediate response occurs. Because psychotropic medications have significant biochemical effects on developing children, it is important for physicians to give an appropriate explanation to parents and children about the rationale for medication. Parents and children must have an opportunity to discuss their feelings and thoughts about psychotropic medication use in general and the specific drug that is ordered. Even with thought disorders, in which pharmacotherapy has a firmly established place, medication is rarely if ever the sole treatment indicated. The complexity of emotional conditions demands an integrated approach involving various therapies: psychodynamic (individual, family, or group), behavioral, milieu, medication, and the use of resources in the family, school, and community. These factors must be knowledgeably selected, judiciously coordinated, and skillfully applied to ensure maximal benefit for a child.

28.3 Psychotherapy

When it has been determined that psychopathology exists in a child or within a family and that it that requires intervention, a pediatrician may develop and implement the therapeutic plan or may refer to a more specialized level of care within the community. The choice of treatment should be left to the consultant, with the referring physician reassuring the family and patient that close communication with the consultant will be maintained. The primary physician should continue to evaluate the child's progress throughout the treatment process and to provide medical care for the patient.

There are many types of individual psychotherapy. Most involve the development of an alliance with patients that provides an opportunity to look at the problems precipitating therapy. Younger children often express their concerns and developmental issues in *play therapy,* a specific modality designed to foster symbolic and metaphoric individual expression. Older children and adolescents are more likely to participate in talking during therapy. *Dynamic therapy* is designed to understand the psychologic motivations for a child's problems and to develop a therapeutic process based on that understanding. *Behavior therapy* and cognitive-behavior therapy are especially useful in treating anxiety, depression, and some behavioral problems.

There are several types of *family therapy:* directive, structural, strategic, and object-relations. In each, the therapist works primarily with the family to impart understanding or to help organize change. A particular directive approach, *parent management training,* is very useful in treating conduct disorder. This approach involves training parents to respond in specific and consistent ways to a child's behavior.

Group therapy is especially useful for children suffering from poorly developed social skills. Group therapy for preadolescents tends to emphasize structured activities through which therapist and children alike can discover how they relate to each other and find ways to change. It is an especially profitable approach for treating the social problems of adolescents.

Barriers to involving the generalist or pediatrician in psychotherapeutic activities with children include a presumed lack of time and lack of adequate conceptual background. Although psychotherapy primarily emphasizes listening and interviewing, two skills important to all fields of medicine, experience is an important and necessary asset for psychotherapists.

28.4 Psychiatric Hospitalization

Psychiatric hospitalization of a disturbed or emotionally ill child in a general, pediatric, or psychiatric hospital is at times helpful or necessary, and it may serve a number of functions. In children with many psychosomatic disorders or in a suicidal or drugged adolescent, indications may be medical as well as psychiatric. If treatment of a child in a psychiatric hospital is thought necessary, consultation with a child psychiatrist is essential for decision-making and planning. The indications for admission include thought, behavior, and affect that are so irrational that they will not respond to less restrictive therapy; complex psychiatric problems that require skilled medical and nursing care; extremely disturbed family interactions that contribute to problematic behavior or interfere with needed care; and dangerous behavior that cannot otherwise be managed. Admission to residential treatment reflects the family's decompensation as often as the child's.

Campbell M, Cueva J: Pharmacology in child and adolescent psychiatry: A review of the past seven years. Part I. J Am Acad Child Adolesc Psychiatry 34:1124, 1995.

Campbell M, Cueva J: Pharmacology in child and adolescent psychiatry: A review of the past seven years. Part II. J Am Acad Child Adolesc Psychiatry 34:1262, 1995.

Dalton R: Psychiatry on the burn unit. *In:* Salisbury R, Dingeldein P, Newman N (eds): A Guide to Burn Unit Therapies. Boston, Little, Brown & Co, 1984.

Dalton R, Forman MA: Psychiatric Hospitalization of School-Age Children. Washington, DC, American Psychiatric Press, 1992.

Gadow KD: Pediatric psychopharmacology: A review of recent research. J Child Psychol Psychiatry 33:153, 1992.

Leonard H, March J, Rickler K, Allen A: Pharmacology of selective serotonin reuptake inhibitors in children and adolescents. J Am Acad Child Adolesc Psychiatry 36:725, 1997.

Schowalter JE: Psychodynamics and medication. J Am Acad Child Adolesc Psychiatry 28:681, 1989.

Special feature: Rating scales and assessment instruments for use in pediatric psychopharmacology research. Psychopharmacol Bull 24:1, 1985.

Spinetta JJ: The dying child's awareness of death. Psychol Bull 81:256, 1974.

Stallard P, Mastroyannopoulou K, Lewis M, et al: The siblings of children with life-threatening conditions. Child Psychol Psychiatr Rev 2:26, 1997.

Van Dongen-Melman JEWM, Sanders-Woudstra JAR: The chronically ill child and his family. *In:* Solnit AJ, Cohen DJ, Schowalter J (eds): Child Psychiatry (Psychiatry, Vol 6). Philadelphia, JB Lippincott, 1986, pp 531–540.
Werry JS, Wollersheim JP: Behavior therapy with children and adolescents: A twenty-year overview. J Am Acad Child Adolesc Psychiatry 28:1, 1989.

CHAPTER 29
Neurodevelopmental Dysfunction in the School-Aged Child

29.1 Patterns of Development and Function

Melvin D. Levine

Neurodevelopmental dysfunctions are central nervous system (CNS)–mediated impairments that are commonly associated with academic underachievement, behavioral difficulties, and problems with social adjustment. It is estimated that 5–15% of school children harbor these so-called low severity–high prevalence handicaps. The prevalence becomes even higher if one includes discrete dysfunctions that lead to a transient self-limited disorder in learning a particular subject area (also see Chapter 29.2.)

ETIOLOGY. Diverse causes underlie these neurodevelopmental dysfunctions. Some reading and spelling disabilities have genetic causes. Many studies have uncovered etiologic associations between disorders of learning or attention and abnormal chromosome patterns, low-level lead intoxication, recurrent otitis media, meningitis, acquired immunodeficiency syndrome, intraventricular hemorrhage, serious head trauma, and low birthweight. Abnormalities of thyroid function have also been documented in a group of children with attentional dysfunction. Environmental and sociocultural deprivation have also been implicated as etiologic factors, or at least potentiators, of neurodevelopmental dysfunction. In individual cases, a definite cause usually cannot be ascertained.

CLINICAL MANIFESTATIONS. School-aged children with neurodevelopmental dysfunctions vary widely with regard to clinical symptoms. Their specific patterns of academic performance and behavior represent final common pathways, the convergence of many forces, including interacting cognitive strengths and deficits, environmental or cultural factors, temperament, educational experience, and intrinsic resiliency. Consequently, a memory dysfunction has different manifestations in a child with strong language skills, well-controlled attention, and a supportive home environment from those evident in an economically deprived youngster whose memory problems are accompanied by weaknesses of attention and difficulties with language. Eight areas of neurodevelopmental function (so-called neurodevelopmental constructs) are especially germane to understanding an academically delayed child.

Attention. Attention subsumes a series of control mechanisms through which the CNS regulates behavior and learning. Children with attentional dysfunction show various patterns of impairment of these controls (also see Chapter 29.2). The resulting symptoms may affect learning, behavior, or social interactions. Located in different parts of the brain, these controls are responsible for regulating the following:

1. CNS arousal, levels of mental energy, and the mobilization and distribution of mental effort: Children with diminished alertness and arousal are likely to exhibit signs of mental fatigue in a classroom. They often yawn, stretch, fidget, and daydream. They sometimes become overactive or hyperkinetic in an effort to attain a higher level of arousal. They may have difficulties falling asleep or awakening on time. They are apt to have difficulty sustaining their concentration, and they may display a reduced ability to mobilize, allocate (to the appropriate functions), and maintain the mental effort required to initiate and complete many academic tasks. Their efforts at work may be erratic and unpredictable. Those affected by this form of weak control may manifest extreme *performance inconsistency.* That is, at certain times or on certain days they are able to use mental energy, but at other times they cannot. Teachers and parents often note such erratic function.
2. The processing of incoming stimuli: These children often show evidence of superficial concentration. As a result, directions and explanations may have to be repeated. Furthermore, such a child is likely to show weaknesses of saliency determination, often focusing on the wrong stimuli at home and in school. Weak saliency determination can make it difficult for a student to take notes, summarize information, or know what to study for a test. More overt forms of weak saliency determination result in various types of distractibility, which may take the form of listening to extraneous noises instead of a teacher, staring out the window, or constantly thinking about the future rather than current salient inputs. In addition, it takes inordinate incoming stimulation to enable many of these children to feel satisfied. They display insatiability and tend to be restless, to feel bored easily, to require constant high levels of stimulation or excitement and to want things or entertainment all the time and not feel satisfied until they receive what they desire.
3. Output or the production of work, behavior, and social activity: These children have a tendency to perform without previewing a likely outcome or thinking through what they are about to do. The consequent *impulsivity* can lead to careless mistakes in academic work and unintended misbehavior. They may show hyperactivity. Such children have difficulty with self-monitoring, not knowing how they are doing during and right after an academic endeavor or a behavior. As a result, they can get into trouble without realizing it. Finally, these children commonly are under-responsive to punishment and reward.

It is important to appreciate that most children with attentional dysfunction also harbor other forms of neurodevelopmental dysfunction. The latter can have a significant impact on the symptoms exhibited by a child. There is also considerable confusion and disagreement about the appropriate terminology to be applied to children with attentional difficulties. The Diagnostic and Statistical Manual of Mental Disorders, fourth edition, uses the *term attention deficit disorder* (ADD) and makes a distinction between individuals who have trouble with inattention and those who exhibit substantial hyperactivity and impulsivity (Chapter 29.2). Through the years, such terms as ADD, hyperactivity, hyperkinetic impulse disorder, and minimal brain dysfunction have been used. In part, the taxonomic flux stems from the marked heterogeneity of groups of affected children. The clinical symptoms summarized earlier are variably present and are of different degrees of severity from case to case. In addition, children with attention deficits show diverse patterns of developmental, academic, or behavioral difficulties. It is likely, therefore, that there are multiple subtypes of attention deficits.

Dysfunctions of Memory. As children proceed through school, demand for the efficient use of memory progressively increases. Students are expected to be selective, systematic, and strategic in entering new procedures and factual data in memory. They must become proficient in their use of both long- and short-term memory to file and retrieve rules, facts, concepts, and skills. By secondary school, rapid and precise recall is heavily emphasized. Not surprisingly, some students experience tremendous frustration when memory dysfunctions prevent them from satisfying academic demands.

Some children have difficulty with the initial *registration of information in short-term memory.* They have trouble keeping pace with the data flow in a classroom. In some cases, children with attentional dysfunction have problems being selective and sufficiently alert to register salient information in memory. Other students have highly specific registration weaknesses. Some may have trouble with registering visual-spatial data in memory, whereas others may be deficient in the registration of language. Verbal instructions and explanations need to repeated several times to become stabilized in memory. Still others have a problem putting *linear chunks* of data in short-term memory; they can enter only small amounts of material that comes arranged in a linear configuration or sequence. Finally, some children can register data in short-term memory, but they cannot do so quickly enough to keep pace with classroom demands.

Many children experience problems with *active working memory.* They are ineffective at temporarily suspending information in memory while they are working on it. Normally active working memory enables a student to keep in mind all of the different components of a task, such as a mathematics problem, while completing it. A student with an active memory dysfunction, for example, might carry a number and then forget what it was that he or she intended to do after carrying that number. Active working memory during reading enables children to remember the beginning of a paragraph when they arrive at the end of it. It lets them remember what they intend to express in writing while they are attempting to remember where to place a comma or how to spell a particular word. Thus, children with active working memory disorders can have trouble performing computations in mathematics, problems with writing, and difficulty in remembering and retelling what they have read.

Other youngsters experience frustration in their efforts at *consolidating information in long-term memory.* They are ineffective when filing data for later access. Ordinarily, consolidation in long-term memory is accomplished in one or more of four ways: (1) pairing two bits of information together (such as a group of letters and the English sound it represents), (2) classifying data in categories (e.g., filing all the insects together in memory), (3) linking new information to established rules (so called rule-based learning), and (4) arranging knowledge in logical chains (such as the months of the year, the alphabet, the steps in a procedure, or the events in a story). Some students struggle unsuccessfully with specific kinds of paired association learning, categories, rules, or chains.

Some children can register and consolidate facts and procedures in memory but seem to have inordinate *difficulty recalling* these items when they need them. Their recall may be painfully slow or imprecise. They are prone to encounter difficulty with *simultaneous recall,* the frequent need to retrieve several facts or procedures at once. This can be especially disabling when writing, a task requiring the simultaneous recall of spelling, punctuation, capitalization, letter formation, ideas, vocabulary, and the directions given for the assignment. Consequently, many children with simultaneous recall problems have their greatest difficulty with written output. When they try to write, they contend with memory overload, often manifested in illegibility (due to a crowding out of memory for letter formation), poor use of punctuation and capitalization, deficient spelling in context, and surprisingly primitive ideation. Some of these children also do poorly in mathematics.

Finally, some students exhibit *delayed automatization.* Not enough of what they have learned in the past is accessible to them instantaneously and with no expenditure of effort. Such skills as letter formation, the mastery of mathematic facts, and word decoding must ultimately become automatic if students are to make good academic progress.

Language. Linguistically proficient children have a distinct advantage in school because much of what is taught is delivered in literate language. All of the basic academic skills are conveyed largely through language. Therefore, it is not surprising that children with language dysfunctions usually have troubled educational careers.

Language disorder has many forms. Some children have particular problems with *phonology* (also see Chapter 29.3). They experience unclear reception of English language sounds and are said to have difficulty with phonologic awareness. They may have trouble discriminating between and forming associations with the sounds of their native language. Commonly, a weak phonologic sense has a negative effect on reading. A student with a poor appreciation of language sounds is likely to form unstable associative linkages between those sounds and visual symbols (i.e., letter combinations). It can be hard for them to conceptualize words as made up of language sound segments (phonemes); thus, their ability to break words down into their constituent sounds and then reblend them into pronounceable words is impeded. They may also have problems manipulating language sounds in their minds. Consequently, while analyzing the last sound in a word, they may forget the first two and thus be unable to blend the sounds to form a word.

Language sounds are most often composed of more than one acoustic signal. For example, in English there are stop consonants, such as "puh" and "kuh." For the brain to process these language sounds, it must accommodate the very rapid transition (about 30 msec in duration) from the sound "k" to the "uh" in "kuh." In some cases, affected students may have trouble processing these acoustic signals within language sounds rapidly enough. A subgroup appears to manifest this difficulty as part of a broader dysfunction involving an inability to process rapidly successive signals of any kind.

Semantic deficits are also common. Affected children have trouble learning and using new words. It is especially hard for them to develop a strong enough sense of how words relate to each other in their meanings. Their grasp of the words they know is likely to be rigid and superficial, lacking shades of meaning. Other common language deficiencies include difficulty with syntax (word order), problems with discourse (paragraphs and passages), an underdeveloped sense of how language works (weak metalinguistics), and trouble with drawing appropriate inferences (i.e., supplying missing information) from language. Many adolescents fail to develop higher language functions. They have problems dealing with abstract and symbolic language, highly technical vocabulary, verbal concepts, densely packed verbal information in textbooks, foreign language learning, and figures of speech (including metaphors and similes).

It is common to distinguish between *receptive language dysfunctions* (those affecting understanding) and *expressive language dysfunctions* (those impeding production or communication). Children with primarily receptive language problems may have serious difficulty following instructions in the classroom, understanding verbal explanations, and interpreting what they have read. Expressive weaknesses include oromotor problems affecting articulation and verbal fluency. Some students experience difficulty with sound sequencing within words. Others find it hard to regulate the rhythm or prosody of their language. Their speech may be dysfluent, hesitant, and somehow inappropriate in its tone.

Problems with *word retrieval* can also thwart expressive language fluency. Despite an adequate vocabulary, affected children have problems in finding exact words when they need them (as in a class discussion). They may reveal marked hesitation and keep subtituting definitions for words (circumlocution). Still others with expressive impediments have trouble formulating sentences, using grammar acceptably, and organizing spoken (and possibly written) narrative. Some children with expressive language problems are hesitant when they speak, so that their verbal communication is unduly laborious.

They may become passive, taciturn, and nonelaborative in communication. Some studies have linked expressive language dysfunction to delinquent behavior. This is especially true when an expressive language disorder occurs in a context of environmental deprivation or turmoil.

Language dysfunctions may be subtle and diagnostically elusive. For example, some children with mild language difficulty function reasonably well in school until they are required to master a second language or become proficient with abstract verbal material (i.e., when the higher language function of secondary school is called for).

Students with strong language strengths may make use of their linguistic facility to overcome other learning problems. For example, it may be possible to verbalize one's way through a mathematics curriculum, thereby circumventing a tendency to be confused by predominantly nonverbal concepts (such as ratio, equation, and diameter).

Visual-Spatial Ordering. Visual processing abilities entail the appreciation of spatial attributes. Shape, position, relative size, foreground and background relationships, and form constancy (the notion that a shape retains its identity regardless of its position in space) are among the constituents of visual-spatial ordering. Children with visual-spatial deficiencies may encounter some initial problems with letter and word recognition. Spelling may emerge as a weakness because these children commonly experience trouble recalling the precise visual configurations of words. In general, however, children who are confused about spatial attributes are unlikely to have long-standing or serious academic problems unless their visual-spatial weaknesses are complicated by additional academically relevant neurodevelopmental dysfunctions. At one time, it was thought that visual-spatial processing dysfunctions were a common cause of chronic reading disabilities; research, for the most part, has refuted this opinion.

Children with visual-spatial dysfunctions may be late in discriminating between left and right. They may show signs of fine or gross motor clumsiness because they may be poor at making use of visual-spatial data to program motor responses.

Temporal-Sequential Ordering. Awareness of time and sequence is an important neurodevelopmental function. Students in school need to be able to manage time, to process and produce multistep explanations and procedures, and to develop memory capacity for extended sequences. The latter includes preservation of serial order in motor procedures, in narrative, and in various mathematical algorithms.

Children who have difficulties with temporal-sequential ordering may be delayed in learning to tell time. They may have great difficulty in following multistep commands, performing acts that necessitate a sequence of steps in the proper order, mastering the months of the year, or organizing narrative. Affected children may also have trouble managing time. They may be frustrated in adhering to schedules, in learning the order of their classes in school, or in meeting deadlines.

Neuromotor Function. There are three distinct yet related forms of neuromotor ability relating to function in school: *graphomotor fluency, gross motor coordination,* and *fine motor dexterity.* Although these competencies ordinarily develop rapidly throughout childhood, some children experience considerable humiliation related to their insufficiently developed motor abilities.

Graphomotor fluency refers to the specific motor aspects of written output. Several subtypes of graphomotor dysfunction significantly impede the writing of certain children. Some of them exhibit signs of *finger agnosia;* they have trouble localizing their fingers while they write. As a result, they need to keep their eyes very close to the page. Ultimately, their writing becomes agonizingly slow and laborious. Others struggle with *graphomotor production deficits.* Such students have trouble planning the highly coordinated motor sequences needed for writing. Although they may understand and be able to visualize what it is they need to write, they have difficulty assigning writing roles to specific muscle groups in their hands. Some of these students also display oromotor production problems, resulting in speech articulation gaps. Some students harbor *weaknesses of visualization* during writing. They have trouble picturing the configurations of letters and words as they write. Their written output tends to be poorly legible, and their problems with visualization frequently also result in poor spelling. These commonly are students who much prefer printing (manuscript) to cursive writing. It is important to emphasize that a child may show excellent fine motor dexterity (as revealed in mechanical or artistic domains) but very poor graphomotor fluency (with labored or poorly legible writing).

Some children exhibit generalized *gross motor delays,* weaknesses, or highly specific deficits with or without fine motor or graphomotor problems. Examples of the latter include problems in using visual-spatial information to guide their gross motor actions; affected children are inept at catching or throwing a ball because they cannot form accurate judgments about trajectories in space. Others are unable to satisfy the motor praxis demands of certain gross motor activities. It is hard for them to recall or plan complex motor procedures (such as those needed for dancing, gymnastics, and swimming). Still others demonstrate diminished *body position sense.* They do not receive or interpret feedback from peripheral joints and muscles. They are likely to be impaired when activities demand balance and the ongoing tracking of body movement.

Children with gross motor problems may suffer a significant loss of self-esteem. They may incur considerable embarrassment in physical education classes. Gross motor weaknesses can lead to social rejection, withdrawal, and generalized feelings of inadequacy.

Problems with *fine motor dexterity* can affect a child's ability to excel in artistic and crafts activities. They may also interfere with learning a musical instrument or mastering a computer keyboard. *Eye-hand incoordination* may be prominent because the child has trouble with the rapid and precise use of visual inputs to govern hand movements.

Higher-Order Cognition. This series of functions consists of various sophisticated thinking skills. Included are the formation of concepts, problem-solving skills, understanding and formulation of rules, critical thinking, brainstorming (and creativity), and metacognition (i.e., the ability to think about thinking).

Children vary considerably in their capacities to understand the *conceptual bases of skills and content areas.* Some of them acquire only a *tenuous grasp of concepts.* As students progress through their education, concepts become increasingly abstract and complex. New concepts are likely to contain previously encountered concepts. Those youngsters who have chronically tenuous grasps of concepts often underachieve. Some of them have a pervasive weak grasp of concepts, whereas others have difficulty only with concepts in highly specific domains (e.g., mathematics, social studies, or science). Some students prefer to conceptualize verbally, whereas others are more comfortable in forming concepts without the interposition of language (perhaps using visual imagery). Many of the best students try to solidify concepts both linguistically and nonverbally.

Problem-solving skills are an important part of mathematics and virtually every other subject in school. Children with good problem-solving skills are good strategists. They are excellent at previewing or estimating answers, coming up with several alternative techniques to meet challenges, selecting the best techniques, and monitoring what they are doing so that they can deploy alternative strategies as needed. Poor problem solvers, on the other hand, tend to be rigid or impulsive. They do not come up with the best strategic approaches. Instead, they become committed irreversibly to a particular technique whether or not it works. They fail to undertake challenges in a stepwise fashion. They may then encounter significant difficulties in course work that requires methodic strategy deployment and flexible problem solving. Many students with attention deficits reveal weak problem-solving skills.

Brainstorming skills are needed to develop a topic for a report, to think about the best way to undertake a project, and to deal with various other open-ended academic challenges. Some students cannot generate original ideas. They prefer to be told exactly what to do. They balk at having to devise a topic, deploy imagination, develop an argument, or think freely and independently.

Critical thinking skills represent another higher cognitive ability acquired during childhood. Successful students often display a keen ability to evaluate statements, products, and people using objective criteria. They are able to tease out their own personal biases and appreciate the viewpoints of others. They are effective in comparing and contrasting their own values and views with those of another. They can think and talk about the qualities of a person. They become adept at assembling qualitative criteria to judge the products they see on television or in stores.

Metacognitive abilities are the capacity to think about thinking. Children with good metacognition are able to observe themselves thinking or studying. They can thereby develop an understanding of thought processes, enabling them to enhance their personal learning strategies and become more efficient and active learners. Those youngsters who lack metacognition tend to perform intellectual tasks the hard way. They are unlikely to appropriate effective techniques to study for a test, to write a report, or to meet other complex academic challenges.

Social Cognition. A student's social abilities are stringently tested throughout the school day and in the neighborhood after school. Increasing evidence shows that social cognition exists as a discrete area of neurodevelopmental function. Some children are extremely adept in social abilities, whereas others exhibit debilitating social skill deficits. There are multiple subskills within social cognition. These include the ability to enter smoothly into new relationships, the capacity to time and stage interactions effectively, the appropriate degree of sensitivity to social feedback cues, the knowledge of how to resolve social conflict without aggression, the adaptive use of language in social contexts *(verbal pragmatics)*, the ability to establish truly reciprocal (sharing) relationships with others (especially peers), and the inclination to overcome one's innate egocentricity to praise or nurture others. In addition to these skills, students need to be conscious of their own image development and to be adept at marketing themselves to peers. Regrettably, some children have no idea of how adversely they are affecting others. As a result, they experience agonizing isolation with little or no insight into the reasons for their rejection.

The plight of a socially unskilled child can be tragic. He or she may sustain verbal abuse, bullying, and outright rejection, with various subtle forms of repudiation. Such students may seek refuge in the company of younger children, animals, a fantasy world, or adults. Social skill deficits can exert an enduring negative effect on behavioral adjustment, mental health, and, ultimately, success in a career.

Academic Effects. Neurodevelopmental dysfunctions are likely to occur in varying clusters within individual children. Combinations of dysfunctions commonly result in academic delays, frequently affecting the acquisition of basic skills and subskills in reading, spelling, writing, and mathematics.

READING. (also see Chapter 29.3). Reading disabilities may stem from many neurodevelopmental factors. Most commonly, subtle or blatant language dysfunctions are present in children with significant reading delays. Initially, such children are likely to reveal *poor phonologic awareness*, as observed in their difficulty appreciating and manipulating language sounds (see above). They may then have debilitating problems in forming associations in memory between English language sounds and combinations of letters. This gap results in deficiencies at the level of decoding individual words. Affected children may be slow to acquire a *sight vocabulary* (a repertoire of words they can identify instantly). When decoding skills are delayed or overly laborious, reading comprehension is subsequently seriously compromised.

Students with visual-spatial dysfunctions may also have trouble learning to read, but this is a relatively rare cause of reading difficulty. Children with weaknesses of temporal-sequential ordering or active working memory may experience difficulty in breaking down words into their component sounds (phonemes) and reblending them into correct sequences. Memory difficulties can cause problems with reading recall and summarization skill, with associative memory for sounds and symbols, and with the acquisition of vocabulary. Some youngsters with higher-order cognitive deficiencies experience trouble in understanding what they read because they lack a strong grasp of the concepts in a text.

Children with reading difficulties commonly avoid reading. Thus, it is not unusual for a child whose reading is deficient to superimpose on this problem a lack of reading practice. Consequently, a delay in reading proficiency becomes increasingly pronounced over time. In particular, language development may stagnate as a result of reading deprivation. Ironically, a language dysfunction may cause a reading disorder, and subsequently, a reading disorder may aggravate an underlying language dysfunction.

SPELLING. Impairments in spelling ability take various forms. Those with language disorders may have difficulty in applying a knowledge of phonology to spelling. They may overuse their visual (configurational) sense of words, and thus their attempts at spelling are phonetically poor approximations yet visually comparable to the actual word (e.g., faght for fight). Other youngsters seem to have the opposite problem, trouble with revisualization or the recall of word configurations. When their phonologic abilities are adequate, their spelling efforts are often phonetically correct but visually far afield (e.g., fite for fight). Some children lack a sense of the *morphology* of language, the sense that certain letter combinations impart certain meanings within words. They may be insensitive to suffixes, prefixes, and word roots. This can be reflected in their spelling patterns. For example, a child may spell the word *played* as *plade*.

Children with certain memory disorders can spell words adequately during a spelling bee or on a spelling list, but they misspell the same words when writing a paragraph. They appear to have a memory problem that leads to difficulty in sustaining several different operations simultaneously. As a result, spelling becomes eclipsed by other task components.

Children who have difficulty preserving *linear chunks* of data tend to omit critical letters in the middle of words. Some students commit *mixed spelling errors*, many of which are orthographically illegal (i.e., they deploy letter combinations never found in English). Such children have the worst prognoses with regard to spelling proficiency. Overall, the analysis of a child's spelling errors can provide valuable insights into the nature of his or her overall neurodevelopmental profile.

WRITING. Writing is an anathema to many youngsters with learning and attention problems. As children proceed through school, demands for large amounts of well-organized written output increase. In many cases, writing is laborious because of an underlying graphomotor dysfunction. In such instances, a child's graphomotor fluency does not keep pace with ideation and language production. The fingers cannot keep pace with the child's thinking. Thoughts may also be forgotten or underdeveloped during writing because the mechanical effort is so taxing.

Just as students with simultaneous memory deficiencies experience difficulty with spelling in paragraphs, they are also prone to serious problems with writing in general. Their written output is often inconsistent in its legibility, ideation, and use of rules (of punctuation, capitalization, and grammar). Children with sequential ordering problems may have difficulty in organizing their ideas effectively when they write. Those with expressive language dysfunctions may not be able to use language effectively on paper. Students with active working memory dysfunctions have difficulty getting the ideas in a paragraph to cohere because they keep forgetting what they wish to express. Finally, students with attentional dysfunction may find it hard to mobilize and sustain the mental effort, the pacing, and the self-monitoring demands of writing. In fact, writing difficulties are the most frequently encountered academic problems among children with weak attention controls.

MATHEMATICS. Delays in mathematical ability can be especially refractory to correction. In one school-based study, it was found that no student who was delayed more than 6 mo in mathematics in 6th grade ever caught up. Thus, significant mathematical weaknesses can become virtually insurmountable, as the subject is so highly cumulative in its structure. Various forms of mathematical disability plague students.

Some children experience mathematics failure because of discrete higher-order cognitive weaknesses. They cannot grasp arithmetical concepts. Good mathematicians are able to deploy both verbal and nonverbal conceptual abilities to understand such concepts as fractions, percentages, equations, and proportion. Impaired student mathematicians may have serious difficulty in moving back and forth from abstract to concrete thinking. It may also be hard for them to apply concepts effectively or be systematic in solving word problems or when confronted with practical situations.

Some youngsters show circumscribed memory weaknesses that compromise mathematical ability. Some have trouble in automatizing mathematical facts (such as the multiplication tables). Others have difficulty in recalling appropriate procedural sequences or *algorithms* (such as the steps involved in solving a long division problem). Still others have weak active working memory; thus, when they focus on one portion of a mathematical problem, they are likely to forget other components of the same problem.

Some students with language dysfunctions have difficulty in mathematics because they have trouble understanding their teachers' verbal explanations of quantitative concepts and operations. Such students are likely to experience frustration in solving word problems and in processing the vast network of technical vocabulary in this subject area.

Many students with attention deficits falter in mathematics classes because they are poor at focusing on fine detail (such as operational signs). They may take an impulsive approach to mathematical problem solving and engage in little or no self-monitoring. Consequently, they commit frequent careless errors.

Mathematics involves a degree of visualization. Children who have difficulty forming and recalling visual imagery to enhance learning may be at a disadvantage in acquiring mathematical skills. It may be hard, for example, for them to picture geometric shapes or to think about fractions.

It is not unusual for individuals with mathematical disabilities to develop superimposed mathematical phobias. Anxiety over mathematics can be especially disheartening and can aggravate an underlying skill delay.

CONTENT AREA SUBJECTS. Children with neurodevelopmental dysfunctions may experience difficulty in a wide range of academic content areas. The sciences may be a special problem, especially because they necessitate the processing of dense verbal material in textbooks and the rapid convergent recall of facts. Social studies courses often entail use of sophisticated language and a mastery of verbal abstract concepts (e.g., democracy, liberalism, and taxation with representation). Students with higher cognitive weaknesses may not grasp such concepts.

Foreign language learning can be a serious problem for students with language disorders or memory gaps. In particular, those with even mild trouble with phonologic awareness, semantics, or syntax in their first language may have serious problems adding a second language. Some adolescents require foreign language waivers to graduate from high school and enter college. Younger children with learning problems often need to postpone foreign language learning until well into their high school years.

Many students with attention deficits can succeed only in content areas that they find romantically attractive. They are likely to exhibit poor performance in courses that contain a great deal of not very exciting detail. They may have trouble distinguishing important data from trivia in a text because their selective attention is too diffuse.

Some students harbor incapacitating *organizational problems* that adversely affect performance in content area subjects. They often lack effective learning strategies. Some are too impulsive to make use of techniques to facilitate studying and work output. Others struggle because they are unable to maintain a systematized notebook, keep track of assignments, get to places on time, meet deadlines, find things, organize a locker, and remember what books to take home from school. Many disorganized students also have trouble studying for tests. They do not seem to know how and what to study and for how long. They frequently lack self-testing skills.

Nonacademic Impacts. Neurodevelopmental dysfunctions commonly exert impacts that extend far beyond school. Some nonacademic impacts are closely related to the dysfunctions themselves, whereas other sequelae are secondary to persistent failure and frustration. The impulsivity and lack of effective self-monitoring of children with attention deficits may lead to unacceptable actions that were unintentional. Children affected by attentional dysfunction may be aggressive or disruptive in the classroom and at home. They may have serious difficulty in accepting behavioral limits, assuming responsibilities, and delaying gratification. Insatiability may lead to highly provocative behaviors, as they perpetually seek intense experience (be it ever so negative). These negative behaviors often subvert the function of an entire family. Adolescents with attentional dysfunction have also been shown to be predisposed to serious automobile accidents.

In some cases, children with neurodevelopmental dysfunctions have excessive performance anxiety or clinical depression. Sadness, self-deprecatory comments, declining self-esteem, chronic fatigue, loss of interests, and even suicidal ideation may ensue. Some children lose motivation. They tend to give up and exhibit *learned helplessness,* a sense that they have no personal control over their destinies. Therefore, they feel no need to exert effort. This perspective ultimately can promote depression, pessimism, and a loss of ambition.

DIAGNOSIS (ASSESSMENT). A child who is functioning poorly during the school years requires a careful multidisciplinary evaluation because of the diverse sources and broad effects of underachievement. An optimal evaluation team should consist of a pediatrician, a psychologist or psychiatrist, and a psychoeducational specialist (sometimes called an educational diagnostician). The latter is a clinician (usually a special educator or educational psychologist) who can undertake a detailed analysis of academic skills and subskills. Other professionals should become involved, as needed, in individual cases, such as a speech and language pathologist, an occupational therapist, a neurologist, and a social worker.

Many children undergo evaluations in school. Such assessments are guaranteed in the United States under Public Law 94-142. In addition, children found to have attentional dysfunction and other disorders may qualify for educational accommodations under Section 501 of the individuals with Disabilities Education Act (IDEA).

Multidisciplinary evaluations conducted in schools are usually very helpful, but they are susceptible to biases and conflicts of interest. For example, if a school does not have a language therapist, that school's evaluation team might tend to be reluctant to recommend language therapy. School budgeting constraints may also affect the quality of evaluations and the extent of recommended services. Because of such limitations, demand for independent evaluations and for second opinions outside of the school setting is growing. Many pediatricians become involved in such outside assessments.

Evaluation of a child with suspected neurodevelopmental dysfunctions should include complete physical, neurologic, and sensory examinations. A physician may also perform an extended neurologic and developmental assessment. Available pediatric neurodevelopmental examination instruments that facilitate direct sampling of various neurodevelopmental functions, such as attention, memory, and so on, include the Pediatric Examination at Three (PEET), the Pediatric Examination of Educational Readiness (PEER), the Pediatric Early Elementary Examination (PEEX II), and the Pediatric Examination of Educational Readiness at Middle Childhood (PEERAMID II). Examinations of this type also include direct behavioral observations and assessment of minor neurologic indicators (sometimes called *soft signs*). The latter include various associated movements and other phenomena frequently associated with neurodevelopmental dysfunction (see also Chapters 37 and 600).

Pediatricians can be helpful in gathering and organizing data relating to a child with neurodevelopmental dysfunctions (also see Chapter 5). They can obtain such data through the use of questionnaires completed by the parents, the school, and (if old enough) the child. These questionnaires can provide up-to-date information about behavioral adjustment, patterns of academic performance, and traits associated with specific developmental dysfunctions. In addition, questionnaires can elicit relevant data about a child's health history, family background, and demographic variables relevant to a child's learning difficulty. The ANSWER System Questionnaires have been developed for this purpose. Standardized behavioral checklists also can aid in evaluation. Among these are the Yale Child Behavioral Inventory, the Connors Questionnaire (for hyperactivity), and the Achenbach Child Behavioral Checklist.

An evaluation commonly includes *intelligence testing*. Although an overall intelligence quotient (IQ) is seldom helpful, testing can be useful in relating specific subtest scores to other diagnostic data. Such comparisons can uncover revealing patterns suggestive of specific neurodevelopmental dysfunctions.

Psychoeducational tests yield relevant data, especially when such assessments include careful analyses that pinpoint where breakdowns are occurring in the processes of reading, spelling, writing, and mathematics. A psychoeducational specialist, making use of input from multiple sources, can help a pediatrician formulate specific recommendations for regular and special educational teachers.

A mental health specialist can be valuable in identifying family-based issues that may be complicating or aggravating neurodevelopmental dysfunctions. Specific psychiatric disorders also may be a part of the clinical picture.

TREATMENT. Treatment of children with neurodevelopmental dysfunctions often also needs to be multidisciplinary. Most children require several of the following forms of intervention.

Demystification. Many children with neurodevelopmental dysfunctions have little or no understanding of the nature or sources of their difficulties. Once an appropriate descriptive assessment has been performed, it is especially important to explain to children the nature of the dysfunction and their strengths. This explanation should be provided in nontechnical, optimistic, and nonaccusatory language. The Concentration Cockpit is an example of a device that can be used to help children understand attentional dysfunction.

Bypass Strategies (Accommodations). Numerous techniques can enable a child to circumvent neurodevelopmental dysfunctions. Such bypass strategies are ordinarily used in the regular classroom; individual forms of intervention in other settings are aimed at strengthening deficient functions. Examples of bypass strategies include using a calculator while solving mathematical problems, writing essays with a word processor, presenting oral instead of written reports, solving fewer mathematical problems, seating a child with attention deficits closer to the teacher to minimize distraction, offering visually presented demonstration models of correctly solved mathematical problems, and granting permission for a student to take scholastic aptitude tests untimed. These bypass strategies do not cure neurodevelopmental dysfunctions but minimize their academic and nonacademic effects.

Remediation of Skills. Tutorial programs are commonly used to bolster deficient academic skills. Reading specialists, mathematical tutors, and other such professionals can make use of diagnostic data to select techniques that make use of a student's neurodevelopmental strengths in an effort to improve decoding skills, writing ability, or mathematical computation. Remediation need not focus exclusively on specific academic areas. Many students need assistance in acquiring study skills, cognitive strategies, and productive organizational habits.

Remediation may take place in a resource room or learning center at school. To qualify for these services in school, students may need to be labeled or classified as learning disabled. To be so designated, testing must document a substantial discrepancy between the child's IQ and his or her academic skill. Unfortunately, some needy students with significant neurodevelopmental dysfunctions do not display such a discrepancy. Fortunately, increasing numbers of schools and regulatory agencies are giving up these arbitrary criteria and providing help to all children who demonstrate a developmental delay.

Students with neurodevelopmental dysfunctions are increasingly being served within regular classrooms. This approach, known as the *inclusionary model*, places an emphasis on bypass strategies and other accommodations rather than resource rooms or other "pullout" services in schools. The success of inclusionary models is highly dependent on the training and orientation of regular classroom teachers.

Developmental Therapies. Considerable controversy exists about the efficacy of treatments to enhance weak developmental functions. It has not been convincingly demonstrated that it is possible to improve substantially a child's fine motor skills, memory, problem-solving proficiency, or temporal-sequential ordering abilities. Nevertheless, some forms of developmental therapy are widely accepted. *Speech and language pathologists* commonly offer intervention for youngsters with various forms of language disability. *Occupational therapists* strive to improve the motor skills of certain students with writing problems or gross motor clumsiness. Considerable interest is being shown in *social skills training*, which usually takes the form of small group sessions in which school children are helped to become more aware of the dynamics of social interaction. *Cognitive-behavioral therapy* is another recently introduced intervention. In this modality of treatment, children learn about their neurodevelopmental dysfunctions and are given specific exercises aimed at enhancing the weak areas. For example, children with attentional dysfunction may be taught about their impulsivity and then provided with exercises that encourage reflection, planning, and a less frenetic tempo.

Curriculum Modifications. Many children with neurodevelopmental dysfunctions require alterations in the school curriculum to succeed. This is particularly true as students progress through secondary school. For example, students with memory weaknesses may need to have their courses selected for them so that they do not have an inordinate cumulative memory load in any one semester. The timing of a foreign language, the selection of a mathematical curriculum, and the choice of science courses are critical issues for many of these struggling adolescents.

Strengthening of Strengths. Affected children need to have their affinities, potentials, and talents identified clearly and exploited widely. It is as important to strengthen strengths as it is to attempt to remedy deficiencies. Athletic skills, artistic inclinations, creative talents, and mechanical aptitudes are among the potential assets of certain students who are underachieving academically. Parents and school personnel need to create opportunities for such students to build on these assets and to achieve respect and praise for their efforts. The strengthening of strengths is essential for sustaining self-esteem and motivation. These well-developed personal assets can ultimately have implications for transitions into young adulthood, including career or college selection.

Individual and Family Counseling. When learning difficulties are complicated by family problems or identifiable psychiatric disorders, psychotherapy may be indicated. Clinical psychologists or child psychiatrists may offer long- or short-term therapy. Such intervention may involve the child alone or the entire family. It is essential, however, that the therapist have a firm understanding of the nature of a child's neurodevelopmental dysfunctions. Both parents and child can become confused if a psychotherapist attributes a child's learning difficulties exclusively to environmental factors, thus ignoring the potent influence of an underlying language disability, attention deficit, or memory problem. Most families do not require a heavily psychoanalytic or psychodynamic approach but instead can benefit from a counseling program that offers them practical advice on behavioral management. Increasingly recognized is the role of short-term problem-oriented counseling (see Chapter 28).

Advocacy. Children with neurodevelopmental dysfunctions require informed advocacy. They need to have their rights upheld in school and in the community. Physicians can be especially helpful in advocating for children in school. Some children, for example, are devastated by being held back in a grade, and the likelihood of benefit is minimal. A physician may need to represent the rights of the child in opposing such grade retention and other sources of public humiliation. A physician may also need to argue strongly for a child to receive services in school or to benefit from modifications in the curriculum. Physicians can also perform advocacy by becoming vocal citizens of their communities. In serving on a school board, for example, a physician can exert a major influence on local policy and on the allocation of resources to school children with special educational needs. Physicians can also be helpful in offering to conduct in-service educational programs for teachers.

Medication. Certain psychopharmacologic agents may be especially helpful in lessening the toll of neurodevelopmental dysfunctions (see Chapter 28.) Most commonly, stimulant medications are used in the treatment of children with attention deficits. They are never a panacea because most youngsters with attention deficits have other associated dysfunctions (such as language disorders, memory problems, motor weaknesses, or social skill deficits). Nevertheless, medications such as methylphenidate (Ritalin), dextroamphetamine (Dexedrine), and pemoline (Cylert) can be important adjuncts to treatment because they seem to help some youngsters focus more selectively and control their impulsivity. Stimulant medication, its indications, administration, and complications are described in Chapter 29.2. When depression or excessive anxiety is a significant component of the clinical picture, antidepressants or antianxiety drugs may be helpful (see Chapters 22 and 23). Other drugs may improve behavioral control (see Chapter 28). Children receiving medication need regular follow-up visits that include a review of current behavioral checklists, a complete physical examination, and appropriate modifications of medication dose, including intervals when they are off the drug so that they can strive to be in control of themselves.

Longitudinal Case Management. All children with neurodevelopmental dysfunctions can benefit from the support and guidance of a case manager or mentor, a professional who can offer advice in a continuing manner and be available to monitor function through the years. Pediatricians may be the ideal professionals to assume this responsibility. With time, new questions inevitably emerge as a child's neurodevelopmental dysfunctions evolve and academic expectations undergo progressive changes. Because children with neurodevelopmental dysfunctions represent an extremely heterogeneous group, no two children require the same management plan, nor is it possible to predict with certainty at age 7 the needs of a youngster when he or she is 14 yr old. Consequently, affected children and their families require vigilant follow-up and individualized objective advice throughout their academic careers.

Barkley RA, Guevremont DC, Anastopoulos AD, et al: Driving-related risks and outcomes of attention deficit hyperactivity disorder in adolescents and young adults: A 3- to 5-year follow-up survey. Pediatrics 92:212, 1993.

Gerber A: Language-Related Learning Disabilities. Baltimore, Paul H. Brookes, 1993.

Hauser P, Zametkin AJ, Martinez P, et al: Attention deficit-hyperactivity disorder in people with generalized resistance to thyroid hormone. N Engl J Med 328:997, 1993.

Levine MD: Attention and memory: Progression and variation during the elementary school years. Pediatr Ann 18:366, 1989.

Levine MD: Keeping a Head in School: A Student's Book About Learning Abilities and Learning Disorders. Cambridge, MA, Educators Publishing Service, 1990.

Levine MD: All Kinds of Minds: A Young Student's Book About Learning Abilities and Learning Disorders. Cambridge, MA, Educators Publishing Service, 1993.

Levine MD: Educational Care. Cambridge, MA, Educators Publishing Service, 1994.

Levine MD: The Pediatric Assessment System for Learning Disorders—Revised. (Questionnaires and Neurodevelopmental Examinations). Cambridge, MA, Educators Publishing Service, 1996.

Levine MD: Developmental Variation and Learning Disorders, 2nd ed. Cambridge, MA, Educators Publishing Service, 1998.

Lyon R (ed): Frames of Reference for the Assessment of Learning Disability. Baltimore, Paul H. Brookes, 1994.

Lyon R, Gray DB, Kavanaugh JF (eds): Better Understanding of Learning Disabilities. Baltimore, Paul H. Brookes, 1993.

29.2 Attention Deficit Hyperactivity Disorder

Jorge H. Daruna, Richard Dalton, and Marc A. Forman

Attention deficit hyperactivity disorder (ADHD) is characterized by poor ability to attend to a task, motoric overactivity, and impulsivity. Oppositional and aggressive behaviors are often seen in conjunction with ADHD. Tic disorders may coexist with ADHD. Many of these children are also afflicted by specific learning disabilities (see also Chapter 29.1). Appropriate management of ADHD requires careful delineation of *all* the problems in need of intervention.

ETIOLOGY. The cause of ADHD is unknown. Genetic factors as well as other factors affecting brain development during prenatal and early postnatal life are most likely responsible. An association of the dopamine receptor D4 gene with a refined phenotype of ADHD has been demonstrated. Growing evidence shows that children with ADHD differ from normal children on neuroimaging measures of brain structure and function. In particular, a prefrontal-striatal-thalamocortical circuit has been implicated. Involvement of the ascending projections of catecholaminergic and serotonergic neurons is likely, given the efficacy of medications (e.g., stimulants) that increase the release of such neurotransmitters. In psychologic terms, ADHD reflects an impairment in the ability to self-regulate arousal and inhibit behavior according to socially acquired rules of conduct.

EPIDEMIOLOGY. The prevalence of ADHD depends on the precise definition adopted, the methods used to evaluate children, and more elusive factors that may ultimately be linked to culture. The *Diagnostic and Statistical Manual* (DSM-IV) estimates the prevalence in school-aged children to be 3–5%. However, estimates have ranged from as low as 1% to as high as 20%. ADHD appears more prevalent in boys; the ratio of boys to girls is approximately 4:1 in epidemiologic surveys and 9:1 in clinic samples. ADHD frequently occurs (65% of cases) in conjunction with at least one other disorder of childhood, particularly oppositional/defiant disorder (50%), conduct disorder (30–50%), anxiety disorders (20–25%), mood disorders (15–20%), and learning disorders (10–25%). In adolescents, substance abuse may be co-morbid with ADHD as well.

CLINICAL MANIFESTATIONS. ADHD-afflicted children display various behaviors indicative of problems with attention, hyperactivity, and impulsivity. According to DSM-IV, inattentiveness is manifested when a child (1) often makes careless mistakes, failing to give close attention; (2) often has difficulty sustaining attention; (3) often does not seem to listen; (4) often does not follow through on tasks; (5) often has difficulty getting organized; (6) often dislikes or avoids sustained mental effort; (7) often loses things; (8) often is easily distracted; and (9) often is forgetful. Hyperactivity is evidenced when a child (1) often fidgets; (2) often is out of his or her seat; (3) runs and climbs excessively; (4) often has difficulty playing quietly; (5) is always on the go as though driven by a motor; and (6) often talks excessively. Impulsivity is reflected in a child who (1) often blurts out answers, (2) often has difficulty awaiting his or her turn, and (3) often interrupts or intrudes on others.

Diagnosis of ADHD requires the presence of at least six manifestations from the inattentiveness cluster, six from the hyperactivity/impulsivity cluster, or both. Children whose symptoms are predominantly from one cluster are said to be primarily inattentive or hyperactive/impulsive. Clinical diagnosis requires that the symptoms be evident before age 7 yr and be constant for at least 6 mo. They must be noted in at least two different settings (e.g., home and school), must exceed what would be expected for the child's developmental level, and must impair the child's functioning (e.g., academic failure; social difficulty).

DIAGNOSIS AND DIFFERENTIAL DIAGNOSES. Initial identification of many children with ADHD commonly occurs when they enter nursery or elementary school. The children are often reported as being disruptive and unresponsive to directions. They often provoke others to anger and do not seem to learn from the negative consequences of their behavior. Some of these same behaviors are commonly noted in children afflicted with other psychiatric disorders, which are primarily characterized by defiance, aggression, overanxiousness, depression, psychosis, or mental retardation. Therefore, it is essential, as part of the diagnostic process, to obtain a detailed description of all problem behaviors exhibited by the child across specific situations and environments. It is common for signs and symptoms of ADHD as well as other disorders to be absent in the clinic setting. Many children with ADHD appear much less affected in novel settings or when they are the focus of attention.

The assessment, aside from obtaining a detailed description of the child's current behavior, should cover events during pregnancy and delivery. Developmental milestones should be ascertained. Description of the child's temperament, reaction to separation from caregivers, and overall activity before the age of 5 should be obtained. Such information can be helpful because many parents of children afflicted with ADHD report pregnancy complications, colicky or temperamentally difficult behavior in infancy, and overactivity from a very early age. Sleep difficulties and feeding problems have also been noted.

Neurologic soft signs (e.g., mixed hand preference, impaired balance, astereognosis, dysdiadochokinesia) or minor physical anomalies (e.g., low-set ears) are not sufficiently specific to assist in diagnosis. This is generally true about laboratory studies. However, such studies can be helpful in ruling out other disorders (e.g., absence seizures) or conditions (e.g., sensory deficits, lead toxicity) that may underlie symptoms of inattentiveness and overactivity. Medical conditions (e.g., thyroid dysfunction) and medicines (e.g., phenobarbital, theophylline) need to be ruled out as causes of any behavioral disturbance.

Psychologic testing provides important data in the process of differential diagnosis. Tests of intelligence (e.g., Wechsler Intelligence Scale for Children, 3rd edition) and educational achievement (i.e., Woodcock-Johnson Psychoeducational Battery, Revised) can serve to rule out intellectual deficits and learning disabilities. Behavior rating scales (e.g., Child Behavior Checklist, Conners Rating Scales, Brown Attention Deficit Disorder Scales) have proved particularly helpful in the assessment of ADHD. Tests of sustained attention (e.g., Continuous Performance tests) can help corroborate the diagnosis of ADHD but are not adequate by themselves. Projective tests (e.g., Rorschach Inkblot Test) can be useful in determining whether disorganization of thought processes may be responsible for behavioral signs of poor concentration and overactivity.

TREATMENT. The approach most likely to be efficacious encompasses both psychosocial interventions and pharmacotherapy. Medications should be used as only part of a comprehensive treatment plan involving the child, parents, and school. Medication should not be used to compensate for an inadequate educational program or parenting deficits without directing therapeutic effort toward those aspects of the child's environment.

A program that gives structure to the child's environment enhances the adaptive function of children afflicted with ADHD. Such children should have a regular daily routine that they are expected to follow promptly and for which they are rewarded with praise. Rules should be simple, clear, and as few as possible. They should be coupled with firm limits, enforced fairly and sympathetically through the use of concrete rewards (e.g., prizes) for adherence and restrictions (loss of privileges) or negative consequences (time-out) for transgressions. Overstimulation and excessive fatigue should be avoided. Time should be set aside for relaxation after play, particularly after vigorous physical activity. The period before bedtime should be quiet, with avoidance of exciting television programs and rough and tumble games.

Children with ADHD should not be expected to respond well to long trips in automobiles or extensive shopping trips. Moreover, the home should be arranged so that valuable, dangerous, or breakable objects are out of the reach of these children. Parents need to be well informed about realistic expectations and should reward with praise and affection even partially successful efforts by the child to maintain appropriate behavior and perform in keeping with parental expectations. Parent training programs or psychoeducational interventions can be helpful in providing parents with needed information and behavior modification techniques (e.g., use of token economies or point systems) useful in creating the needed structure for children with ADHD.

Close communication between the family, the physician, and school personnel is essential. Depending on the level of disability, some children may require placement in special education classes. Federal legislation mandates that appropriate educational services must be provided for children with ADHD. Physicians can act as advocates for children in this regard. Decisions about medication should take into account the views of both parents and teachers. Communication between the teachers and parents should also be built into the daily routine (e.g., daily report cards) in an effort to assist the child to remain on task despite transitions from home to school and back.

Additional forms of treatment are indicated if severe family problems exist or when a child appears to be responding to the disapproval of others with low self-esteem, depression, social withdrawal, school avoidance, or acting-out behavior. Family psychotherapy may be required to help some families overcome interactional problems that hamper the implementation of structure and effective communication in a consistent manner. Child individual psychotherapy, although not efficacious with respect to the core ADHD symptoms, can prove helpful in safeguarding self-esteem and ameliorating social problems secondary to the core ADHD symptoms.

Multimodality therapy brings together many forms of treatment including parent training, social skills training, cognitive therapy, educational interventions, and pharmacotherapy. It is appealing for its comprehensiveness, but it has not lived up to expectations when subjected to empirical evaluation. Nonetheless, it is essential to address *all* problem areas in an efficient and sustained manner. Cessation of treatment can quickly result in the return of the behavioral problems. Coping with the chronic nature of ADHD, in most cases, can be facilitated by referring families to support organizations such as Children with Attention Deficit Disorders (CHADD) or Attention Deficit Disorders Association (ADDA).

A number of alternative treatments for ADHD have gained popularity. The support often is entirely anecdotal or theoretical, and unbiased empirical tests either are lacking or have failed to provide evidence of efficacy. Interventions of this type include the use of megavitamins, electroencephalographic biofeedback, optometric vision training, chiropractic manipulation, and herbal remedies. Dietary management (e.g., restriction of refined sugar or food additives) has been particularly popular even though there is little evidence of clinical effect—except, perhaps, in some very young children. However, when families feel strongly about exploring manipulations of the diet to treat ADHD, they should be allowed to see for themselves as long as other components of treatment are not neglected and the diet is not harmful.

Pharmacotherapy is especially effective in suppressing the core symptoms of ADHD. Stimulants, in particular, and various tricyclic antidepressants have been shown to be effective in reducing overactivity and impulsivity and increasing attention span. As a consequence, they improve the interactions between the child and adults. However, little evidence shows that stimulants improve retention of information or control of anger. Marginal evidence suggests that stimulants significantly enhance academic performance. Peer interaction is not favorably altered with drug treatment. Also, the increased likelihood of developing delinquency during adolescence is unaffected by long-term drug treatment. The long-term benefits of these medicines have not been established.

Methylphenidate is the most commonly used stimulant; it is efficacious in 75–80% of patients when administered in a dose ranging from 0.3–1.0 mg/kg. It generally has an effect for 2–4 hr, although the sustained-release form, available only in 20-mg tablets, lasts considerably longer. Studies of plasma levels suggest that a dose of 0.3 mg/kg helps to improve attention, whereas amelioration of behavioral problems requires 0.7 mg/kg. Methylphenidate should usually be given for at least 2–3 wk so that efficacy can be adequately determined.

Dextroamphetamine is efficacious in approximately 70–75% of patients. Its optimal dose range is 0.2–0.5 mg/kg. It has a longer half-life than methylphenidate, although the therapeutic effect of amphetamine preparations is reported to be no longer than 4 hr. Both dextroamphetamine and methylphenidate should be given about 20–30 min before meals to avoid their deactivation. They should not be given after 4:00 P.M. to avoid insomia, although in some cases their effect on overactivity may facilitate sleep onset. The response to both medications should be noticeable soon after they are started. Children who do not respond show little or no change in behavior with increasing doses.

Magnesium pemoline, a longer-acting stimulant, is effective in 65–70% of children. Its effect develops more slowly, and it may take 2–3 wk to evaluate its efficacy fully. An initial dose of 18.75 mg should be given and increased by one-half tablet per week as needed (see Table 28–1, maximum 112.5 mg/24 hr). About 1–2% of children treated with this medicine may show changes in liver function; accordingly, pretreatment studies and monitoring of liver function are required. Other long-acting stimulant preparations in use include Ritalin-SR, Dexedrine Spansule, Adderall, and Desoxyn Gradumet.

Stimulant drugs can cause complications such as increased nervousness and jitteriness. Major short-term side effects include anorexia, upper abdominal pain, and difficulty sleeping. The abdominal discomfort usually remits spontaneously. Tics have been reported with stimulant use. Alternative medicine should be considered if tics are evident before treatment or if a family history reveals tic disorder. If tics are precipitated by stimulant drugs, it is wise to continue stimulant use only with great caution and close vigilance. Long-term stimulant side effects may include increased heart rate and growth suppression. The effects of increased heart rate are not known. Some think that decreased growth rate is a short-term problem, but others have reported a drop in height of 2% in children who receive an average of 40 mg/24 hr of a stimulant medicine for 2–4 yr. The growth of children receiving stimulants should be monitored, and drug-free periods (weekends, holidays, summer vacations) should be used when practical. Stopping the medication each summer permits the parents and child to reassess the need for continued medication. At the very least, a drug-free period of 2–3 wk/yr should be tried routinely for this purpose.

It is difficult to predict which children will respond most favorably to stimulants. Up to 25% of children with ADHD do not respond positively to stimulant medication for poorly understood reasons. The action of these drugs is the same in children with and without ADHD. Some studies suggest that nonanxious children with the poorest levels of concentration respond best to stimulants.

Tricyclic antidepressants (e.g., imipramine, desipramine) are efficacious in 60–70% of children with ADHD. When they are used for this disorder, it is not necessary to determine blood levels. Unlike stimulants, tricyclic antidepressants have not been found to exacerbate tic disorder or Tourette syndrome. They should be considered for patients with co-morbid tic disorders or significant symptoms of anxiety and depression. However, several cases of sudden death have been associated with desipramine, and families should be informed and given a strong justification for using these drugs. Because of their side effects, these medications should not be used initially. Monoamine oxidase inhibitors have been found effective on the basis of limited data but are impractical owing to dietary restrictions and side effects. Selective serotonin reuptake inhibitors (e.g., Prozac) have not been found effective in reducing the core symptoms of ADHD.

Clonidine (Catapres), an α-noradrenergic agonist, typically used as an antihypertensive, has been shown to be efficacious in treating some ADHD symptoms but may produce hypotension. It is frequently used in conjunction with stimulants, although there have been a few reports of death of children taking this combination. *Guanfacine hydrochloride* (Tenex), a long-acting α_2-noradrenergic agonist, is also useful in treating ADHD and appears to have a side effect profile more favorable than that of clonidine.

Other drugs that have been used in patients with ADHD include bupropion (Wellbutrin) and neuroleptics such as thioridazine. Reduction of seizure threshold and other serious side effects make these drugs much less appropriate. There is little support for the use of fenfluramine, benzodiazepines, lithium, or cabamazepine in the treatment of ADHD.

PROGNOSIS. Prospective follow-up studies of children with ADHD indicate that as many as 50% of these children function well in adulthood. The remaining continue to exhibit symptoms of inattention and impulsivity. Delinquent behavior during adolescence and later antisocial personality disorder may be evident in as many as 50–80% of those who continue to be affected. Alcohol abuse and drug use are also quite prevalent but not related to history of stimulant treatment. Poor outcomes are most common in children who exhibit defiance and aggression toward adults and who have poor peer relationships and below average cognitive function. Research indicates that children who receive sustained comprehensive treatment (i.e., medication, special education, parent counseling, and psychotherapy) are less likely to present with delinquency in adolescence.

Biederman J, Mick E, Faraone SV: Normalized functioning in youths with persistent attention-deficit/hyperactivity disorder. J Pediatr 133:544, 1998.
Castellanos FX: Neuroimaging of attention-deficit hyperactivity disorder. Child Adolesc Psychiatr Clin North Am 6:383–411, 1997.
Elia J, Welsh PA, Gullotta CS, et al: Classroom academic performance: Improvement with both methylphenidate and dextroamphetamine in ADHD boys. J Child Psychol Psychiatry 34:785, 1993.
Fisher M, Barkley R, Fletcher K, et al: The adolescent outcome of hyperactive children: Predictors of psychiatric academic, social and emotional adjustment. J Am Acad Child Adolesc Psychiatry 32:324, 1993.
Goldman LS, Genel M, Bezman R, et al: Diagnosis and treatment of attention-deficit/hyperactivity disorder in children and adolescents. JAMA 279:1100, 1998.
Ialongo NS, Horn WF, Pascoe JM, et al: The effects of a multimodal intervention with attention deficit hyperactivity disorder and tic disorder in children: A 9-month follow-up. J Am Acad Child Adolesc Psychiatry 32:182, 1993.
Practice parameters for the assessment and treatment of children, adolescents and adults with attention deficit hyperactivity disorder. J Am Acad Child Adolesc Psychiatry 36 (Suppl 10):85S–121S, 1997.
Swanson JM, Sergeant JA, Taylor E, et al: Attention-deficit hyperactivity disorder and hyperkinetic disorder. Lancet 351:429, 1998.
Swanson JM, Sunohara GA, Kennedy JL, et al: Association of the dopamine receptor D4 (DRD4) gene with a refined phenotype of attention deficit hyperactivity disorder (ADHD): A family based approach. Mol Psychiatry 3:38, 1998.
Zametkin AJ, Ernst M: Problems in the management of attention-deficit-hyperactivity disorder. N Engl J Med 340:40, 1999.

29.3 Specific Reading Disability (Dyslexia)

G. Reid Lyon and Sally E. Shaywitz

Dyslexia is characterized by an unexpected difficulty in reading in children and adults who otherwise possess the intelligence, motivation, and opportunities to learn considered necessary for accurate and fluent reading. Dyslexia is the most common and most comprehensively studied of the learning disabilities (LD), affecting at least 80% of children identified as manifesting LD. When asked to read aloud, most children and adults with dyslexia display a labored approach to decoding and recognizing single words, an approach characterized by hesitations, mispronunciations, and repeated attempts to sound out unfamiliar words. In contrast to the difficulties they experience in decoding single words, individuals with dyslexia have the vocabulary, syntax, and other higher level abilities involved in comprehension. If asked about the meaning of what has been read, these individuals demonstrate limited comprehension, primarily because the effort and time devoted to decoding and word recognition make retention of the material difficult. If the material is read to the individual, however, comprehension is typically intact. Conversely, hyperlexia, a relatively rare type of reading disability, is diagnosed when word decoding and word reading skills are accurate and fluent but comprehension skills are limited. This subtype of reading disability remains poorly understood.

ETIOLOGY. At a cognitive-linguistic level, dyslexia appears to reflect deficits within a specific component of the language system, the phonologic module, which is engaged in processing the sounds of speech. As predicted by this model, dyslexic individuals have difficulty developing an awareness that words, both spoken and written, can be segmented into smaller units of sound—an essential ability given that reading an alphabetic language (i.e., English) requires that the reader map or link printed symbols to sound. Abundant evidence shows that the linguistic abilities related to learning to read involve phonology, with deficits in phonologic awareness best predicting dyslexia. Theories of dyslexia that implicate the visual system or deficits in the temporal processing of auditory and visual stimuli have not been sufficiently substantiated by research.

Dyslexia is both familial and heritable. Family history is one of the most important risk factors; 23–65% of children who have a parent with dyslexia have the disorder. Studies suggest that there are major genetic loci linked to chromosome 6 for the transmission of phonologic awareness deficits and subsequent reading problems. The specific mechanisms by which genetic factors predispose someone to dyslexia are not clear.

A range of neurobiologic studies using postmortem brain specimens, brain morphometry, functional brain imaging, and electrophysiology suggest differences in the temporoparieto-occipital and inferior frontal brain regions between dyslexic and nonimpaired readers. In functional imaging (fMRI) studies, Shaywitz and associates demonstrated that in comparison with good readers, dyslexic persons displayed relative underactivation in posterior brain regions when attempting to carry out a series of reading tasks ranging from identification of letters to sounding out letters and words. In contrast, during these same reading tasks, a pattern of overactivation (relative to good readers) was observed in the anterior inferior frontal brain region. This pattern of relative under- and overactivation in posterior and anterior regions, respectively, may represent a neural signature for the phonologic difficulties experienced by dyslexic readers. These findings converge with a large literature describing anatomic lesions in posterior brain regions in acquired alexia, specifically in the region of the angular gyrus.

EPIDEMIOLOGY. Dyslexia may be the most common neurobehavioral disorder affecting children, with prevalence rates ranging from 5–10% in clinic- and school-identified samples to 17.5% in unselected population-based samples. Like hypertension and obesity, dyslexia fits a dimensional model in which reading ability and disability occur along a continuum, with dyslexia representing the lower tail of a normal distribution of reading ability. In contrast to traditional assumptions, several converging studies indicate similar numbers of affected males and females. Both prospective and retrospective longitudinal studies indicate dyslexia is a persistent, chronic condition rather than a transient developmental lag. Over time, dyslexic and poor readers maintain their relative positions along the distribution of reading ability. However, approaches using focused, early, and intensive intervention provide promise that these trends can be modified.

CLINICAL MANIFESTATIONS. Difficulties in decoding, word recognition, and reading comprehension may vary according to age and developmental level. However, the cardinal signs of dyslexia observed in school-aged children and adults are an inaccurate and labored approach to decoding, word recognition, and text reading. Listening comprehension is typically robust. In several studies, older children have been found to improve reading accuracy over time, albeit without commensurate gains in reading fluency and comprehension. Difficulties in spelling typically reflect the phonologically based difficulties observed in oral reading. A parental history frequently identifies early subtle language difficulties in dyslexic children. Many children identified as dyslexic during the primary grades displayed difficulties playing rhyming games and learning the names for letters and numbers during the preschool and kindergarten years. Indeed, recent longitudinal studies demonstrate that kindergarten assessments of these language skills are highly predictive of later reading failure. Parents also frequently report that although their child relishes the opportunity to be read to, reading aloud to the parent or reading independently is resisted. Dyslexia may co-occur with attention deficit hyperactivity disorder (ADHD). Although this comorbidity has been documented in both referred samples (40% co-morbidity) and nonreferred samples (15% co-morbidity), the two disorders are distinct and separable.

DIAGNOSIS. Family history, teacher/classroom observation, and tests of language (particularly phonology), reading, spelling, and intellectual ability represent a core assessment for the diagnosis of dyslexia in children; additional tests of mathematics, attention, general memory, and general language skills may be administered as part of a more comprehensive evaluation of cognitive, linguistic, and cognitive function. No single test score is pathognomonic for dyslexia. As with any other medical diagnosis, the diagnosis of dyslexia reflects a thoughtful synthesis of all the clinical data available. In most cases, dyslexic individuals manifest a disparity between average to above average ability to learn as assessed by a measure of general intelligence and scores on measures assessing phonologic, decoding, word recognition, and reading comprehension skills. Dyslexia is distinguished from other disorders that may include reading difficulties by the unique, circumscribed nature of the phonologic deficit. Primary sensory impairments should be ruled out. Some individuals with dyslexia also have ADHD; if inattention may possibly be a problem, the child should also be assessed for specific symptoms of this disorder.

TREATMENT. The causal link between phonologic deficits and dyslexia has provided a strong empirical foundation for treatment intervention studies. No one treatment approach is equally efficacious for all children or adults with dyslexia. Moreover, single modality teaching methods using *either* phonics approaches *or* whole language approaches to developing reading skills are contraindicated for those with dyslexia. Rather, all studies point to the application of combined teaching methods that ensure mastery of phonologic skills, the accurate and fluent applications of these skills when reading text, and direct instruction in reading comprehension strategies. Children with dyslexia do not readily acquire the basic phonologic skills that serve as a linguistic prerequisite to reading; consequently, phonologic awareness must be taught directly and explicitly. In addition to learning that words can be segmented into smaller units of sound (phonologic awareness) and that sounds (phonemes) are linked to specific letters and letter patterns (phonics), children with dyslexia require practice in reading stories, both to allow them to apply their newly acquired decoding skills to reading text and to experience reading for meaning. What is also clear from these and other studies is that early identification and early intensive intervention are critical to improving reading skills among dyslexic individuals. Shaywitz and colleagues report that traditional interventions, which are less intense and less explicit, resulted in limited gains in reading skills for children with dyslexia. The treatment of dyslexia in students in high school, college, and graduate school is typically based on accommodation rather than remediation. College students with a childhood history of dyslexia require extra time in reading and writing assignments as well as examinations. Many adolescent and adult students have been able to improve their reading accuracy, though without commensurate gains in reading speed. Other helpful accommodations include the use of laptop computers with spelling checkers, tape recorders in the classroom, recorded books, access to lecture notes, tutorial services, alternatives to multiple choice tests, and a separate quiet room for taking tests.

Ball EW, Balchman BA: Does phoneme awareness training in kindergarten make a difference in early word recognition and developmental spelling? Read Res Q 26:49, 1991.

Cardon LR, Smith SD, Fulker DW, et al: Quantitative trait locus for reading disability on chromosome 6. Science 266:276, 1994.

Foorman BR, Francis DJ, Fletcher JM, et al: The role of instruction in learning to read: Preventing reading failure in at-risk children. J Educ Psychol 90:1, 1998.

Lyon GR: Toward a definition of dyslexia. Ann Dyslexia 45:3, 1995.

Pennington BF: Genetics of learning disabilities. J Child Neurol 10:S69, 1995.

Shankweiler D, Crain S, Katz L, et al: Cognitive profiles of reading-disabled children: Comparison of language skills in phonology, morphology, and syntax. Psychol Sci 6:149, 1995.

Shaywitz SE: Dyslexia. N Engl J Med 338:307, 1998.

Shaywitz SE, Escobar MD, Shaywitz BA, et al: Evidence that dyslexia may represent the lower tail of the normal distribution of reading ability. N Engl J Med 326:145, 1992.

Shaywitz SE, Shaywitz BA, Pugh K, et al: Functional disruption in the organization of the brain for reading in dyslexia. Proc Natl Acad Sci USA 95:2636, 1998.

Torgesen JK, Morgan S, Davis C: The effects of two types of phonological awareness training on word learning in kindergarten children. J Educ Psychol 84:364, 1992.

PART IV

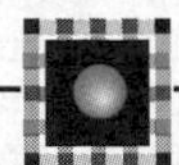

Social Issues

CHAPTER 30
Adoption

Mark D. Simms

Adoption is a social, emotional, and legal process that creates a family for children when the birth family is unable or unwilling to parent. Approximately 1 million children in this country are adopted; 2–4% of all American families have adopted. In 1992, 127,441 children of all races and nationalities were adopted in the United States. Of these, 42% were stepparent or relative adoptions, 15.5% were children in foster care, and 5% were children from other countries adopted by United States families. Approximately one third of adoptions were handled by private agencies or independent practitioners, such as lawyers.

Adoption of children from the foster care system is one of the greatest child welfare policy challenges today. As many as 100,000 children currently in foster care are legally ready for adoption, but the number of finalized adoptions has remained relatively constant at about 18,000 per year over the past decade. Many of these children are considered "special needs" because they are of school age, part of a sibling group, members of ethnic or racial minority groups, or because they have physical, emotional, or developmental needs (including HIV/AIDS infection or prenatal exposure to illicit substances). Federal adoption subsidies, tax credits, special minority recruitment efforts, increased postplacement services, and more open consideration of "nontraditional" families—including single adults and older couples—are aimed at increasing the number of adoption opportunities for these children.

International adoptions have increased 150% in the past decade. In 1996 the primary sending countries for children were China, the Russian Federation, South Korea, and Romania. Most of the children released for adoption overseas have experienced poverty, social hardship, or war. Adoptees may include healthy infants and older children as well as children with "special needs."

ROLE OF PEDIATRICIANS. Pediatricians can help prospective adoptive parents evaluate the health and developmental history of the child and available background information from birth families in order to assess actual and potential problems or risks that children may have. In international adoptions, in particular, prior to traveling abroad, parents should try to learn as much as they can about the child's past experience and current condition. After the child is settled in the new home, pediatricians should encourage adoptive parents to seek comprehensive assessment of the child's health and developmental needs.

Pediatricians can also promote positive adjustment of the child and family by providing guidance and support at all stages in the adoption. Families should be encouraged to speak freely and repeatedly about adoption with the child, beginning in toddler years and continuing through adolescence. Older children may need some encouragement to voice their questions and concerns. Research shows that most adopted children and families adjust well and lead healthy, productive lives. Adoption disruption (of placement) rates vary based on the child's age at placement and are not strongly related to the presence of medical or developmental disabilities; adopted foster children are at greater risk of disruption. Although not required by law, agency placements, particularly for older and "special needs" children, may provide more comprehensive counseling of birth parents, closer attention to resolving birth fathers' rights, more intensive preparation of adoptive parents, greater child development expertise, and the availability of postadoption support and services.

American Academy of Pediatrics, Committee on Early Childhood, Adoption and Dependent Care: Families and adoption: The pediatrician's role in supporting communication. AAP News, February 1992.

American Academy of Pediatrics, Committee on Early Childhood, Adoption and Dependent Care: Initial medical evaluation of an adopted child. Pediatrics 88:642, 1992.

Holloway JS: Outcome in placements for adoption or long-term fostering. Arch Dis Child 76:227, 1997.

Sills Mitchell MA, Jenista JA: Health care of the internationally adopted child. Part 1: Before and at arrival into the adoptive home. J Pediatr Health Care 11:51, 1997.

Sills Mitchell MA, Jenista JA: Health care of the internationally adopted child. Part 2: Chronic care and long-term medical issues. J Pediatr Health Care 11:117, 1997.

CHAPTER 31
Foster Care

Mark D. Simms

Approximately 500,000 children in the United States were living in state-supported foster homes in 1995. Over the past two decades, efforts to reduce the number of children entering foster care have been largely unsuccessful. Developed as a temporary measure to assist families in crisis, the foster care system became overwhelmed in the 1960s and 1970s as placements for child abuse and neglect increased dramatically. By the late 1970s, there was concern that many children were continuing in the system without clear plans for their futures. In 1980, the Child Welfare Reform and Adoption Assistance Act (PL 96-272) changed the emphasis of public policy by requiring states to make "reasonable efforts" to prevent children from entering the foster care system and to eventually reunify with their families children who were placed. The Act advanced the idea of permanency planning to prevent children from remaining in foster care indefinitely. Periodic reviews of the need to maintain placements were required for all children in state custody. Other significant changes in child welfare policy have included increased reliance on relatives to provide care and development of intensive efforts to prevent out-of-home placement of children. However, chronic underfunding of child welfare programs generally, and worsening circumstances for the most disadvantaged segments of society, have continued to plague this fragile system.

Between 1977 and 1994, the number of reported cases of child abuse and neglect (Chapter 35) increased by nearly 450% (from 670,000 to more than 3 million), yet funding for child welfare services that might decrease the need for foster care increased very little. As a result, the focus of child welfare services has narrowed to the point where most children and their families can gain access to help only if the child was abused or significantly neglected. Less serious problems are not considered within the purview of the public agencies. The total number of children who receive child welfare services has decreased by nearly one half (from 1.8 million in 1977 to just under 1 million in 1994). At the same time, the complexity of problems affecting families in which child abuse and neglect occur has grown: parental substance addiction, spousal abuse, inadequate housing or homelessness, lack of parenting skills or employment skills, mental or physical health problems, mental retardation and incarceration. Foster care placement is often the only option available for these children, since services to treat the family's problems are either unavailable or the client's access is severely limited. Thus, while funds for Title IV-B child welfare preventive services increased (in inflation-adjusted dollars) by only 14% between 1977 and 1994, federal expenditures for foster care maintenance payments under Title IV-E increased by more than 900%.

An increasing proportion of children entering foster care are young—nearly half are less than 5 yr old at the time of placement—and from minority groups. Currently, 46% of the children in foster care are African-American, 42% are white, and 12% are Hispanic. Despite a significant decrease in the average duration of placement—from 29 mo in 1977 to 16 mo in 1994—placement rates have continued to rise.

Children who enter foster care have extraordinarily high rates of medical, developmental, and mental health problems. The majority suffer from behavioral and adjustment problems. Nearly 60% of preschoolers are developmentally delayed, and more than half of school-aged children are behind their peers academically. Chronic medical conditions are noted in 35%, physical growth failure in up to 25%, and congenital anomalies in 15%. Children in foster care are high utilizers of all types of care, especially inpatient hospitalization and outpatient mental health services. Similarly, health costs are high for this population. Furthermore, the presence of mental health problems, physical disabilities, and developmental delays in children is associated with a greater chance of being placed in foster care and longer length of placement. Yet when children in foster care receive needed services, significant improvements have been noted in overall health status, stabilization of chronic conditions, and improved growth and development.

In 1988, the Child Welfare League of America, in collaboration with the American Academy of Pediatrics, published *Standards for the Health Care of Children in Out-of-Home Care* to serve as a blueprint for developing effective service delivery structures for children in foster care. These standards have generally not been implemented. Moreover, despite eligibility for comprehensive diagnostic and treatment services under the Medicaid program (EPSDT), the majority of children in foster care do not receive these needed services.

A variety of factors act as "barriers" to care for these children. For example, most public and private agencies caring for foster children have no formal policies or arrangements to provide health services; they rely instead on local physicians and/or health clinics funded by Medicaid. Also, information about children's health prior to placement is often hard to obtain. Frequently, the children have had erratic contact with a number of different health care providers prior to placement, and social workers are not always able to obtain detailed health histories from the biologic parents at the time of removal. Following placement, most decisions as to when and where children receive health care is left to the foster parents. Lacking information about the type and content of services the children receive, social workers cannot oversee the amount or quality of health care delivered. Compounding this is the fact that many of the children have complex problems and require care from a variety of specialists. Lack of coordination between child welfare and health providers, and uncertainty as to who is able to assist in making treatment decisions, further complicates the children's care. This diffusion of responsibility can also result in delay or denial of care while issues of proper authority remain unresolved.

Nearly three quarters of these children experience more than one foster home placement during their time in the foster care system. Changes of residences and caretakers may further disrupt the fragile care network, since the children usually change their health care provider with each move. Similarly, changes in social workers are exceedingly common; as a result, key aspects in planning and coordinating efforts on the child's behalf may be lost.

As America enters the next century, organizing, financing, and delivering health and welfare services to the poor is undergoing fundamental change. The traditional "safety net" of federal and state programs for economically distressed families, formerly represented by the AFDC, SSI, and food stamp programs, is shrinking or being replaced by newer programs with stricter parental work requirements and shorter time limits for eligibility for public assistance. The cumulative impact of these policy and program changes may result in even more foster care placements unless careful attention is paid to meeting the real needs of these vulnerable children and their families.

American Academy of Pediatrics, Committee on Early Childhood, Adoption and Dependent Care: Health care of children in foster care. Pediatrics 93:335, 1994.

Child Welfare League of America: Standards for Health Care Services for Children in Out-of-Home Care. Washington, DC, Child Welfare League of America, 1988.

Simms MD: Foster children and the foster care system, Part I. History and legal structure. Curr Probl Pediatr 21:291, 1991.

Simms MD: Foster children and the foster care system, Part II. Impact on the child. Curr Probl Pediatr 21:345, 1991.

Szilagyi M: The pediatrician and the child in foster care. Pediatr Rev 19:39, 1998.

Takayama JI, Wolfe E, Coulter KP: Relationship between reasons for placement and medical findings among children in foster care. Pediatrics 101:201, 1998.

U.S. Department of Health and Human Services, Children's Bureau: National Study of Protective, Preventive and Reunification Services Delivered to Children and Their Families. Washington, DC, US Government Printing Office, 1997.

U.S. General Accounting Office: Health Needs of Many Young Children Are Unknown and Unmet (GAO/HEHS-95-114). Washington, DC, US General Accounting Office, 1995.

CHAPTER 32
Child Care

Paul H. Dworkin

Profound social and demographic changes have resulted in an increasing number of children receiving a portion of their care from someone other than their parents. In the United States, almost two thirds of mothers with children under 6 yr are working outside the home, including over one half of mothers of infants and toddlers. A high divorce rate and rise in births to single women have contributed to approximately one child in four living within a single-parent household headed by the mother. Women work for the same reasons as men—economic necessity and personal choice. The economic climate and changes in family structure have necessitated the availability of child-care services for working parents.

"Child care" is defined as care provided by an individual outside the nuclear family or in a setting separate from the child's home and is inclusive of such services as baby sitting, daycare, preschool, early childhood program, Head Start, and nursery school. Options for families generally include in-home care, family child care, and center child care. Child care is used for children of all ages. Less than 5% of children of working parents receive in-home care, in which a relative or a nonrelative (such as a nanny, housekeeper, or regular sitter) comes to the child's home to provide care. Approximately 20% of all preschool children who receive supplemental care are in regulated or nonregulated family child care, in which a small group of children, typically six or fewer, receive care in the private home of a caregiver. Nearly one half of employed mothers of 3- and 4-yr-old children report center care as their primary supplemental arrangement. Child-care centers provide care for more than six to ten children at a time and include for-profit centers, which may be independent or operated by large chains, and nonprofit centers, which may be independent or sponsored by the government (e.g., Head Start), religious organizations, public schools, community agencies, or employers. Most child-care centers are licensed, although standards vary from state to state. Different types of child care have advantages and disadvantages, including cost, familiarity of care provider and environment, convenience, availability, flexibility in scheduling, and reliability. From a developmental perspective, the progression from care in the child's own home to care in another home with a few other children to large-group care may be appropriate. Yet for most families, decisions about child care are based largely on considerations of cost, distance from home, and safety.

The effect of child care on children's development depends on a number of inter-related factors, including the quality of the child-care experience, as well as characteristics of the child and family. Although some studies have suggested that infants in child care may be at greater risk of insecure attachments to their mothers, most such infants are securely attached and display no long-term emotional insecurity. In some studies, children with child-care experience have been found to be more sociable, more self-confident, more involved in activities with peers, and less timid. However, such children have also been described as more aggressive (especially boys) and less compliant with adults.

High-quality child care can favorably influence the **cognitive and social development** of children, especially those from disadvantaged populations. Such children perform better on school entry on standardized tests of intelligence, academic achievement, and measures of accomplishment such as grades and teacher ratings. Conversely, poor-quality child care can adversely affect developmental outcomes. Contrary to popular beliefs, middle-class children are not protected from the effects of poor-quality child care.

Good-quality child care has been associated with a low adult-to-child ratio, small group size, and caregiver training in child development. Other important determinants include a caring and supportive staff that is stable and consistent; a developmentally appropriate curriculum that enables children to learn through a variety of fun activities; and a physical setting that affords cleanliness, sanitation, and adequate space for activities and rest as well as protection from environmental hazards. Unfortunately, child care in the United States is often of poor quality. A study of child-care centers in four states found that only 14% of centers gave good-quality care, with the remaining centers rated as mediocre or poor, often endangering the health and safety of young children. A study of family daycare yielded similar findings, with only 12% of regulated family child-care homes found to provide high-quality care. Only 3% of unregulated family child care was considered high quality, as was only 1% of the care provided by relatives in their own homes.

The lack of national standards for child care and uneven regulation from state to state contribute to the variable quality of child care in the United States. The American Academy of Pediatrics and the American Public Health Association have published standards for health and safety in child-care programs. The National Association for the Education of Young Children also has developed criteria for good child-care practice. Yet a national survey of state regulations for center-based infant and toddler care found that no state regulations fulfill the criteria for good practice, and the majority reflect poor or very poor practice. Efforts to upgrade the quality of child care are likely to require the establishment of federal standards that address such characteristics as staff-to-child ratios, group size, caregiver training, and improved salaries for child-care providers. Additional critical policy issues include parental leave, tax credits for child care (currently available), flexible work time, and on-site child care provided by employers.

Pediatric providers may assume a number of important roles in promoting successful child-care experiences. Pediatricians can help parents become informed consumers by discussing the advantages and disadvantages of various child-care options, providing accurate information regarding implications for children's health and development, and directing parents to sources of information about child care in the community. The pediatrician can provide guidance to parents regarding a sick child's participation in child care and serve as health consultant to child-care programs. Pediatric advocacy for the availability of high-quality care for all children includes encouraging the implementation of national child-care standards, paid parental infant care leaves, and improved salaries and training for child-care providers.

Adams GC, Poersch NO: Key Facts About Child Care and Early Education: A Briefing Book. Washington, DC, Government Printing Office, 1994.

American Academy of Pediatrics and American Public Health Association: Caring for Our Children. National Health and Safety Performance Standards: Guidelines for Out-of-Home Child Care Programs. Elk Grove Village, IL, American Academy of Pediatrics, 1993.

Cost, Quality, Child Outcomes Study Team: Cost, Quality and Child Outcomes in Child Care Center: Public Report, 2nd ed. Denver, Department of Economics, University of Colorado, 1995.

Dilks SA: Developmental aspects of child care. Pediatr Clin North Am 38:1529, 1991.

Galinsky E, Howes C, Kontos S, Shinn M: The Study of Children in Family Day Care and Relative Care: Highlights of Findings. New York, Families & Work Institute, 1994.

Saluter AF: Marital Status and Living Arrangements: March 1993. US Bureau of the Census, Current Population Reports, Series P20–478. Washington, DC, Government Printing Office, 1994.

Young KT, Marsland KM, Zigler E: The regulatory status of center-based infant and toddler child care. Am J Orthopsychiatry 67:535, 1997.

Zigler E: School should begin at age 3 years for American children. J Dev Behav Pediatr 19:38, 1998.

CHAPTER 33
Separation and Death

Marc A. Forman and Richard Dalton

Relatively brief separations of children from their parents, such as vacations, usually produce minor transient effects, but more enduring and frequent separations may cause significant sequelae. The potential impact of each event must be considered in the light of the age and stage of development of the child and the particular relationship with the absent person as well as the nature of the separation. For example, it is more frightening for children to be separated from a parent in a hospital than within the familiar surroundings of home. In a marital separation, children are faced with a relative loss of one parent, who may be vilified by the other.

The initial reaction of *young children* to separation may involve crying, either of a tantrum-like, protesting type or of a quieter, sadder type. After a few hours or a day or so of separation, children may appear more subdued, withdrawn, and quiet or irritable, fussy, moody, and resistant to authority. Disturbance of appetite may occur, and there may be special difficulties at bedtime, such as reluctance about going to bed and problems in getting to sleep, with a resurgence of old fears and, in younger children, perhaps such regressive behavior as bed-wetting. Children may repeatedly ask where the absent parent is and when he or she will return home; some children may not refer to parental absence at all. The child may go to the window or door or out into the neighborhood looking for the absent parent; a few may even leave home or their places of temporary placement to try to find where their parents are. This last rather unusual response needs to be considered when a child cannot be found for a while shortly after the separation or departure of a parent.

A child's **response to reunion** may surprise or alarm a parent who is not prepared. A parent who joyfully returns to the family may be met by wary or cautious children, who, after a brief interchange of affection, may move away from the parent and seem indifferent to his or her return. The interpretation of this response depends on the child and his or her style; it may indicate anger at being left and wariness that the event will happen again, or, because children tend to personalize, the child may have felt that he or she caused the parent's departure. For instance, if the mother who frequently says, "Stop it, or you'll give me a headache," is hospitalized, the child may unrealistically feel at fault and guilty. As a result of these feelings, children may seem to be more closely attached to the other parent than to the absent one, or even to the grandparent or baby sitter who cared for them during their parent's absence. Immediately after the reunion or after a few days, some children, particularly younger ones, may become more clinging and dependent than they were before separation, while continuing any regressive behavior that had occurred during separation. Such behavior may engage the returned parent more closely and help to re-establish the bond that the child felt was broken. Such reactions are usually transient; within 1–2 wk, children will have recovered their usual behavior and equilibrium. Recurrent separations may tend to make children more wary and guarded about re-establishing the relationship with the repeatedly absent parent, and these traits may affect other personal relationships. Parents should not try to ameliorate a child's behavior by threatening to leave.

Experiences of loss such as **divorce** or **placement in foster care** can give rise to the same kinds of reactions listed earlier, but they are more intense and possibly more lasting. School-aged children may respond with evident depression, seem indifferent, or be markedly angry. Other children appear to deny or avoid the issue, behaviorally or verbally. Most children may cling to the hope or fantasy that the actual placement or separation is not real. Guilt may be generated by the child's feeling that this loss, separation, or placement represents rejection and perhaps punishment for misbehavior. Children may protect a parent at their own expense, believing and asserting that their own badness caused the parent to depart or to place them with relatives or strangers, rather than that the parent has been bad or irresponsible. Besides having their own feelings of guilt, children cannot blame their parents because they sense it may be fairly risky. Parents who discover that a child harbors resentment might punish further for these thoughts or feelings. Children who feel that their misbehavior caused their parents to separate or become divorced have the fantasy that their own trivial or recurrent behavioral patterns have caused their parents to become angry with each other. Some children develop behavioral or psychosomatic symptoms and unwittingly adopt a "sick" role as a strategy for reuniting their parents.

In response to separation and divorce of parents, *older children and adolescents* commonly show more intense anger. Almost all children cling to the magical belief that their parents will reunite after divorce. Wallerstein and Kelly found that 5 yr after the breakup, about one third of the children studied were "consciously and intensely unhappy and dissatisfied with their life in the post-divorce family." Another third showed clear evidence of a quite satisfactory adjustment, and the remaining third demonstrated "a mixed picture with good achievement in some areas and faltering achievement in others." After 10 yr, 45% were doing well, but 41% were poorly adjusted and had academic, social, and emotional problems. As they entered adulthood, many were reluctant to form intimate relationships, fearful of repeating their parents' experience. A large-scale British study indicates that parental divorce had a moderate long-term negative impact on the adult mental health status of children who had experienced it, even after controlling for changes in economic status and problems before divorce. Good adjustment of children after a divorce is related to ongoing involvement with two psychologically healthy parents who minimize conflict and to the support system offered by siblings and other relatives. Divorcing parents should be encouraged to avoid the adversarial process and to use a trained mediator if they cannot resolve disputes on their own. Joint custody arrangements may reduce ongoing parental conflict, but a study by Steinmann revealed that one third of children in joint custody "felt overburdened by the demands and requirements of maintaining a strong presence in two homes."

Another version of a separation experience occurs when a child's family **moves.** A significant proportion of the population of the United States changes residence each year. The effects of this movement on children and families are frequently overlooked. For children, the move is essentially involuntary; they move because a parent has obtained employment elsewhere, because the birth of a sibling has made a larger home desirable, or for other reasons. When such changes in family structure as divorce or death precipitates moves, children face the stresses created by both the precipitating events and moving itself. When parents are sad because of the circumstances surrounding the move, this unhappiness will be transmitted to their children. Children who move lose their old friends, the comfort of a familiar bedroom and house, and their ties to school and community. They not only must sever old relationships but also are faced with developing new ones in new neighborhoods and new schools. Because movement upward in social standing often accompanies a geographic move, children may enter neighborhoods with new and different customs and values, and because academic standards and curricula vary from community to community, children who have performed well in one school may find themselves struggling in a new one. Frequent moves during the school years are likely to have adverse consequences on social and academic performance.

Migrant children and families present as a special population (see Chapter 39). Migrant children not only need to adjust to a new community, school, and house but also need to adjust to a new culture and, in many cases, to a new language. Because children have faster language acquisition, they may function as translators for the adults in their families. This powerful position may lead to role reversal and potential conflict within the family. Whether or not migrant status per se poses a higher risk to the development of psychopathologic conditions in children is controversial. However, there is agreement that migrant children are more likely to come from families with low socioeconomic status, live in overcrowded conditions, and have poorly educated parents. All of this, plus the previously mentioned factors, can increase the risk for psychopathologic disorders. In the evaluation of migrant children and families, it is also important to ask about the circumstances of the migration; legal status; conflict of loyalties; and moral, ethical, and religious differences.

Parents should prepare children well in advance of any move and allow them to express any unhappy feelings or misgivings. Parents should acknowledge their own mixed feelings and agree that they will miss their old home while looking forward to a new one. Visits to the new home in advance are often useful preludes to the actual move. Transient periods of regressive behavior may be noted in preschool children after moving, and these should be understood and accepted. Parents should assist the entry of their children into the new community, and exchanges of letters with old friends and visits, whenever possible, should be encouraged.

As to the ultimate separation—*death of a parent*—most preadolescent children do not seem to go through a typical mourning process as psychoanalytically defined. A child's mourning may be masked by behavior not typically seen in adults. Among school-aged to adolescent children who had lost a parent through death, Wolfenstein found that immediately after the loss, sad feelings were not markedly evident, nor was there much crying. Children continued in daily activities; the major mechanism in dealing with catastrophe was denial, both overt and unconscious, and maintained by the magical wish and hope for reunion and reappearance. Some children seemed to maintain remarkably good moods; some were more active than usual. Wolfenstein saw these good moods as an effective accompaniment of denial, "If one does not feel bad, then nothing bad has happened." Some children show hostile and angry feelings toward the surviving parent and tend to identify with and idealize the lost parent, sometimes with reunion fantasies accompanying denial. Children may feel guilty, reflecting their egocentric tendency. Alternatively, some children show considerable sorrow at the time of a parent's death or after a delay, when the defense of denial is no longer effective.

Children younger than 5 yr view death as reversible, possibly with belief in the dead coming back to life and in ghosts. In the next stage, up to 8–9 yr, death is personified, for example, as the grim reaper who punishes and avenges. Only after this age do children realistically understand death as a universal and final biologic process.

Physicians can help children and surviving caretakers through a period of separation or adjustment to death of a parent or sibling, first by helping them recognize that the adults themselves are going through a period of grief and mourning. It is not unhealthy for children to see their surviving or remaining parent mourn the loss of a mate or grieve for a divorced or separated spouse. When a parent dies, the child needs the support and reassurance of having the remaining parent or other important caretakers available. Close physical contact and emotional exchange, with verbal explanations and reassurance for those children who can understand, are important aspects of support. Children should not be expected or forced to discuss all their feelings or to put into words their reactions to a parent's death. They should not be expected to interrupt usual social or recreational activities for weeks or months after the death of a parent, either out of respect for that parent or in recognition of the remaining parent's sorrow or grief. Continuance of usual activities should not be interpreted by adults or older children as callousness or indifference but rather as a child's way of dealing, at his or her stage of development, with what is as much a catastrophe for him or her as it is for an adult. Further, children should not be expected to serve as a primary support to the remaining parent or others in their grief.

In most cases, it seems helpful for children to participate appropriately in the rituals that generally surround the death and burial of a parent. Young children can attend a funeral, viewing, or wake so long as there is no morbid preoccupation or demand that they remain a long time or be involved in prolonged religious ceremonies. Keeping young children away from some participation in the burial rituals, whatever they are, is a misguided effort to protect and ultimately will be more confusing and isolating than helpful.

Ash P: Children in divorce litigation. *In:* Alessi NE, Noshpitz JD (eds): Basic Handbook of Child and Adolescent Psychiatry, Vol 4: Varieties of Development. New York, John Wiley & Sons, 1997.

Bolgar R, Zweig-Frank H, Paris J: Childhood antecedents of interpersonal problems in young adult children of divorce. J Am Acad Child Adolesc Psychiatry 34:143, 1995.

Chase-Lansdale PL, Cherlin AJ, Kiernan KE: The long-term effects of parental divorce on the mental health of young adults: A developmental perspective. Child Dev 66:1614, 1995.

Dillon PA, Emery RE: Divorce mediation and resolution of child custody disputes: Long-term effects. Am J Orthopsychiatry 66:131, 1996.

Jensen PS, Lewis RL, Xenakis SN: The military family in review: Context, risk and prevention. J Am Acad Child Adolesc Psychiatry 25:225, 1986.

Monroe-Blum H, Boyle M, Offord D, et al: Immigrant children: Psychiatric disorder, school performance and service utilization. Am J Orthopsychiatry 59:510, 1989.

Nagy M: The child's meaning of death. *In:* Feifel H (ed): The Meaning of Death. New York, McGraw-Hill, 1959.

Puskar KR, Martsolf DS: Adolescent geographic relocation: Theoretical perspective. Issues Mental Health Nursing 15:471, 1994.

Quinn LS, Behrman RE (eds): Children and Divorce. Future Child 4:4, 1994.

Steinmann S: The experience of children in a joint custody arrangement: A report of a study. Am J Orthopsychiatry 53:220, 1981.

Wallerstein JS: The long-term effects of divorce on children: A review. J Am Acad Child Adolesc Psychiatry 30:349, 1991.

Wallerstein JS, Blakeslee S: Second Chances: Men, Women and Children a Decade After Divorce. London, Ticknor & Fields, 1989.

Westermeyer J: Psychiatric Care of Migrants: A Clinical Guide. Washington DC, American Psychiatric Press, 1989.

Wolfenstein M: How is mourning possible? *In:* The Psychoanalytic Study of the Child. New York, International Universities Press, 1966.

CHAPTER 34

Impact of Violence on Children

Marilyn Augustyn and Barry Zuckerman

Violence in the United States is a public health epidemic, affecting victim, witness, and perpetrator. Our focus should not be limited to the traditional care of violence-related injury.

The source of first exposure to violence for children is often *domestic violence*. Occasional wife battering is estimated to exist in 16% of all families, and 3.4% (or 1.8 million women) are beaten regularly by their husbands. One study found that 40% of mothers reported *violence in their families* as a way of "settling disagreements." Family violence is most likely to be perpetrated by those between ages 18 and 30 yr—"the child-rearing years." It is not surprising, then, that the majority of children in these homes have witnessed violence; one study estimated that 3 million children witness domestic violence every year. In a series of 62 domestic incidents, children were **victims** in 15% of domestic violence incidents. Most of the children were injured when they intervened to protect their mother from her partner (see Chapter 35). **Witnessing** violence is only now being recognized as detrimental to children. Because their scars as bystanders are emotional and not physical, the pediatric clinician may not fully appreciate their distress and thereby miss an opportunity to provide needed interventions.

Another source of witnessed violence is *community violence*. More than a third of New Orleans school-aged children had witnessed severe violence, and 40% had seen a dead body. In inner-city Boston, a study of mothers in a pediatric clinic found that 10% of children less than 6 yr had seen a knifing or shooting. In Los Angeles County, the sheriff's office estimates that children witness 20% of all murders. Young children living in high crime and violence areas observe death more frequently and at younger ages than children growing up in more secure surroundings.

The most ubiquitous source of exposure to violence for children in the United States is *television*. The average child 2–5 yr of age watches 20 to 30 hr of television a week, hours that are increasingly filled with scenes of violence. According to a 1994 study by the Center for Media and Public Affairs, scenes of life-threatening violence (assaults with a deadly weapon) increased from 751 per day in 1992 to 1252 per day in 1994. In the same period, TV scenes showing gunplay went from 362 to 526 per day. Although exposure to media violence cannot be equated to exposure to "real-life" violence, many studies confirm that media violence desensitizes children to the meaning and impact of violent behavior. Not all children are affected by television violence. Children most at risk from viewing television violence may be children who are also exposed regularly to real-life violence in their homes and communities.

Real-life violence continues to be a major problem in the United States. About 20,000 people in the country die each year as a result of intentional homicide. The leading cause of death in both black and white teenage males in the United States is gunshot wounds. In 1994 children under age 15 yr represented nearly 13% of all arrests for serious crimes, including murder, forcible rape, robbery, aggravated assault, burglary, motor-vehicle theft, and arson. The Massachusetts Department of Education found in a 1995 survey that one in five public high school students carried a weapon on or off school property in the 30 days prior to the survey. One in 20 had carried a gun.

The violence children experience and witness also has a profound *impact on health and development*. Beyond injuries, violence affects children psychologically and behaviorally; it may influence how they view the world and their place in it. Children can come to see the world as a dangerous and unpredictable place. This fear may thwart their exploration of the environment, which is essential to learning in childhood. Violence, particularly domestic violence, also can teach children especially powerful early lessons about the role of violence in relationships. Children who grow up in violent homes are more likely to be aggressive with their peers. Perhaps the most sobering consequence is that violence may change the way that children view their future—they may believe that they may die at an early age and thus take more risks, such as drinking, abusing drugs, not wearing seatbelts, and not taking prescribed medication.

Infants chronically exposed to violence may have difficulties sleeping and exploring their environment. Toddlers may become more "clingy," finding it hard to separate from caregivers. Young and middle-school children may have difficulty concentrating at school and may be easily distracted or hyperactive. Growth may be slowed in infants, toddlers, and young children. Adolescents may become more easily aroused and "develop a short fuse," quickly resorting to violence to solve conflicts. Finally, some children exposed to severe and/or chronic violence may suffer from post-traumatic stress disorder (PTSD), exhibiting constricted emotions, difficulty concentrating, autonomic disturbances, and re-enactment of the trauma through play or action (see Chapter 22). A particular challenge in treating and diagnosing pediatric PTSD is that a child's caregiver exposed to the same trauma may be suffering from it as well.

The simplest way to recognize if violence has become a problem in a family is to consistently question both patients (when they are old enough) and parents. It is important to assure families that they are not being singled out but that all families are asked about their exposure to violence. For some families a direct approach is useful; e.g., "Violence is a major problem in our world today and one that impacts everyone in our society. Thus I have started asking all my patients and families about violence that they are experiencing in their lives...." In other cases, beginning with general questions and then moving to the specific may be helpful. For example: "Sometimes children may behave differently after watching someone engage in a behavior; have you noticed your children modeling any behaviors that they have seen?" When violence has impacted the child, it is important to gather details about symptoms and behaviors.

Many parents and children who have been exposed to violence can be effectively counseled by the pediatrician. Matters to be covered include gathering the facts and details of the event; gaining access to support services; providing information about the symptoms and behaviors common in children exposed to violence; and helping parents talk to their children about the event. When the symptoms are chronic (more than 6 mo) or not improving, if the violent event involved the death or departure of a parent, if the caregivers are unable to empathize with the child, or if the ongoing safety of the child is a concern, it is important that the family be referred to mental health professionals for additional treatment.

Exposure to violence disrupts the healthy development of a great many children, and pediatricians need to be aware of this threat. Pediatric providers also have a wider responsibility to advocate on local, state, and national levels for safer environments in which all children can grow and thrive.

American Academy of Pediatrics—Committee on Adolescents: Firearms and adolescents. Pediatrics 89:784, 1992.

Augustyn M, Parker S, Groves B, Zuckerman B: Silent victims: Children who witness violence. Contemp Pediatr 12:35, 1995.

Gelles R: Family Violence. Beverly Hills, CA, Sage Publications, 1987.

Groves B: Witness to violence. *In:* Parker S, Zuckerman B (eds): Handbook of Developmental and Behavioral Pediatrics. Boston, Little, Brown & Company, 1995, pp 334–336.

Jaffe PG, Hurley DJ, Wolfe D: Children's observations of violence, part 1 and 2: Critical issues in child development and intervention planning. Can J Psychiatry 35:466, 1990.

Montgomery SM, Bartley MJ, Wilkinson RG: Family conflict and slow growth. Arch Dis Child 77:326, 1997.

Osofsky J: Children Who Witness Violence. SRCD Policy Report, 1997.

Stringham P: Violent youth. *In:* Parker S, Zuckerman B (eds): Handbook of Developmental and Behavioral Pediatrics. Boston, Little, Brown & Company, 1995, pp 329–331.

CHAPTER 35

*Abuse and Neglect of Children**

Charles F. Johnson

Child maltreatment encompasses a spectrum of abusive actions, or acts of commission, and lack of action, or acts of omission, that result in morbidity or death (Fig. 35–1). Acts of omission and commission before birth, such as maternal drug abuse and failure to seek appropriate health care during pregnancy, may also have adverse effects on the child. Physical abuse may be narrowly defined as intentional injuries to a child by a caregiver that result in bruises, burns, fractures, lacerations, punctures, or organ damage. A broader definition would include short- and long-term emotional consequences, which can be more debilitating than the physical effects. Physical neglect, and other acts of omission, may result in failure to

*Some parts adapted from previous sections by B. D. Schmitt and R. D. Krugman.

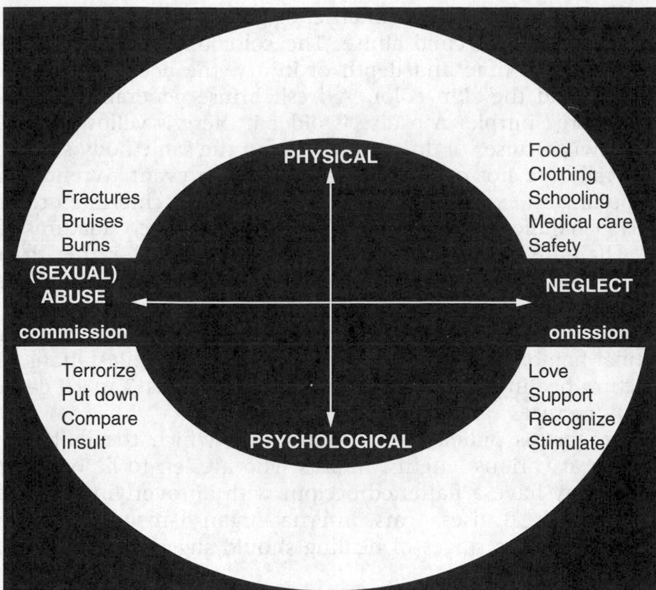

Figure 35–1 The spectrum of child maltreatment. Child maltreatment encompasses acts of commission, or abuse, and acts of omission, or neglect, by a caretaker that adversely affect children. The act can be physical or psychologic. The boundaries between these areas are indistinct and psychologic; physical abuse and neglect overlap and may exist at the same time or various times in the child's life. Sexual abuse may be considered a specific type of physical abuse that has strong emotional components. Physical abuse and neglect invariably have short- and long-term psychologic consequences. Psychologic consequences may persist long after the physical wounds heal.

thrive, develop, and learn. Nutritional neglect is the most common cause of underweight in infancy and may account for more than half the cases of failure to thrive (see Chapter 36). Physicians are most likely to identify medical neglect that results from the failure of a parent to provide appropriate medical care, whereas failure to provide shelter, schooling, adequate clothing, and protection from environmental hazards tends to be observed by neighbors, relatives, teachers, and social workers. Medical neglect of a child with an acute or chronic disease may result in worsening of the condition and death.

Parents may refuse to allow recommended medical treatments because of personal or religious beliefs. The determination of whether this constitutes neglect and, if so, the appropriate action for a physician to take are difficult decisions. Neglect of appropriate precautions by caregivers to ensure a child's safety may also involve difficult matters of judgment. Children may be injured despite a variety of protective actions by well-meaning parents.

Psychologic maltreatment includes intentional verbal or behavioral acts or omissions that result in adverse emotional consequences. A caregiver may intentionally fail to provide nurturing verbal and behavioral actions that are necessary for healthy development. Psychologic maltreatment of a child by a caregiver includes spurning, exploiting/corrupting, withholding emotional responsiveness, isolating, or terrorizing. Psychologic maltreatment may be difficult to document when psychopathology or emotional consequences must be shown to be the direct result of acts or omissions by caregivers. Sexual abuse, or involving a child in any act intended for the sexual gratification of an adult, accounts for the major proportion of the continued increase in abuse reports that are made to agencies. Sexual abuse may be perpetrated by family members (incest), acquaintances, or, least often, strangers.

Medications and toxins may be given to intentionally poison a child. When this or any other deceptive action is undertaken to simulate a disorder, it is referred to as *Munchausen syndrome by proxy.* The induced symptoms and signs may lead to unnecessary medical investigation, hospital admissions, or treatment; death occurs in 10% of these cases.

Legal definitions of what constitutes abuse and neglect vary from state to state. Physicians and other providers of care to children are required by law in all 50 states to report suspected child abuse or neglect. These laws afford protection from lawsuits to mandated reporters who report in good faith; they also allow for clinical and laboratory evaluations and documentation without the parent's or guardian's permission. Failure to report suspected child abuse may result in a penalty. It may also result in a malpractice claim for damages incurred as a result of failure to report and thereby protect the child from further injury.

EPIDEMIOLOGY. The number of reports to children's protective services (CPS) and law enforcement agencies in the county in which the alleged abuse or neglect occurred have steadily increased since mandated reporting began in the 1960s. Reports of all types of abuse increased from 669,000 children in 1976 to 3.0 million in 1995 (1 out of every 25 children). This increase in reports is attributed primarily to improved case finding and reporting. In 1995, 36% (1.0 million) reports were "substantiated" by CPS. It is estimated that 2,000 children die each year of abuse. With the advent of child death review teams, it is expected that more child abuse deaths will be revealed. The prevalence of abuse is unknown. A survey of families with children aged 3–18 yr indicated that 140 of 1,000 (14%) were kicked, bitten, punched, hit with an object, beaten up, or threatened with a knife or gun in 1 yr. A 1995 Gallup telephone survey indicated that 49 of every 1,000 children (5%) may have been physically abused. Approximately 10% of injuries to children younger than 5 yr who are seen in emergency departments are due to abuse; 15% of children admitted for burns and 50% of children less than 1 yr of age with fractures are abused. In 1991, the National Child Abuse and Neglect Data System indicated that 24% of 838,232 reports were for physical abuse; 7% of children were younger than 1 yr; 27% were younger than 4 yr; and 28% were 4–8 yr of age. The rate of reports decreases in older children. Of the 1,229 assessments done in a pediatric hospital during 1991, 223 of 797 reports (28%) were for physical abuse, and the death rate was 6%. The most common perpetrators were the father (21%), mother (21%), boyfriend of the mother (9%), baby sitter (8%), and stepfather (5%). The average age of the abuser was 25 years. In 1997, 233 of 956 hospital reports (24%) were for physical abuse. Nationally, in 1995, neglect, physical abuse, sexual abuse, and emotional abuse constituted 52%, 25%, 13%, and 5%, respectively, of confirmed cases.

Although varying definitions and reporting requirements prevent detailed comparisons, parents who abuse their children have been reported from most ethnic, geographic, religious, educational, occupational, and socioeconomic groups. Groups living in poverty have increased reports of physical abuse because of (1) the increased number of crises in their lives (e.g., unemployment or overcrowding); (2) limited access to economic or social resources for support during times of stress; (3) the increased violence in the communities where they live; (4) an association of poverty with other risk factors, such as teenage and single parenthood and substance abuse; and (5) the possibility of more scrutiny by community agencies and neighbors. An increased incidence of physical abuse also has been noted on military bases. The presence of spouse abuse increases the likelihood of child abuse (see Chapter 34). Substance abuse is a common finding in families with abused children. More than 90% of abusing parents have neither psychotic nor criminal personalities. Rather, they tend to be lonely, unhappy, angry, young, single parents who do not plan their pregnancies, have little or no knowledge of child development, and have unrealistic expectations for child behavior. Mentally retarded children are more at risk for abuse and neglect. Their parents may injure them in anger after being provoked by what they consider a misbehavior that is actually related to the handicap. From 10–40% of abusive parents have experienced physical abuse as children.

Physical abuse is most likely to occur when a high-risk parent is responsible for the care of a high-risk child. High-risk children include premature infants, infants with chronic medical conditions, colicky babies, and children with behavior problems. The child may be normal but misperceived by an inexperienced parent as difficult, unusual, or abnormal. Normal behavior, such as crying, wetting, soiling, and spilling, may cause the parent to lose control and injure a child. The occasion precipitating the abuse may be associated with a family crisis, such as loss of a job or home, marital strife, death of a sibling, physical exhaustion, or development of an acute or chronic physical or mental illness in the parent or child. Risk factors for abuse and neglect should be determined as part of the routine medical history and in all cases of childhood injury. The presence of risk factors should increase the suspicion of abuse; however, when abuse is not documented, significant risk factors may necessitate referral for preventive services.

CLINICAL MANIFESTATIONS. Physical abuse is suspected when an injury is unexplained, unexplainable, or implausible. If an injury is incompatible with the history given or with the child's development, suspected abuse should be reported. It is not necessary to have diagnostic certainty of physical abuse to file a report. It is expected, when children are hurt, that parents will bring them immediately for examination. A delay in seeking medical help should increase suspicion of abuse or neglect. A delay may also be due to a lack of transportation or ignorance about the significance of disease or injury. Before reporting suspected medical neglect, the physician should determine whether the parents have an understanding of disease processes and the intellectual, emotional, and physical resources needed to provide for their children. A report of neglect should bring needed services.

Bruises are the most common manifestation of child abuse and may be found on any body surface. Accidental bruises, from impact trauma, are most likely to be found on leading surfaces overlying superficial bone edges, such as the shins, forearms,and brows. Bruises to the buttocks, genitals, back, and back of the hands are less likely to be due to an accident. Children may be struck, thrown, burned, bitten, lacerated, or punctured. The shape of the injury may suggest the object used. Paddles, belts, hands, and other instruments leave specific marks (Fig. 35–2). The most commonly used "instrument" is the hand. Bilateral, symmetric, or geometric injuries should raise suspicion of child abuse. The color of a bruise is influenced by the time and depth of injury, the body surface involved, and the skin color. A fresh bruise generally appears blue or red-purple. A bruise is older if there is yellow, green, or brown. Bruises of different colors on the same body surface generally are not compatible with a single event. Wrenching or pulling an extremity may result in a corner chip fracture or bucket-handle fracture of the metaphysis. Inflicted fractures of the shaft are more likely to be spiral from twisting rather than transverse from impact. Spiral fractures of the femur before the age of walking are usually inflicted. Cardiopulmonary resuscitation or accidental impact rarely causes rib fractures or retinal hemorrhages in children. The earliest manifestations of fracture healing, manifest as callus formation, is 7 to 10 days. Skull fractures cannot be dated.

Hair that is pulled causes alopecia in which the hairs are broken at various lengths. Infants who are left to lie on their backs may have a flattened occiput with an overlying area of missing hair. Bruises, scars, internal organ damage, and fractures in various stages of healing should suggest the battered child syndrome.

Petechiae of the face and shoulders from intense retching, coughing, or crying may be mistaken for abuse as may a variety of conditions such as mongolian spots, capillary hemangiomas, pigmented nevi, and other congenital, allergic, self-inflicted, and infectious skin conditions. A single 1-cm, round lesion of impetigo may be difficult to differentiate from a fresh cigarette burn. Blood dyscrasias and coagulopathies result in readier bruising. Old and new fractures may be seen in specific chromosomal disorders or rare conditions such as Wilson's disease, Schmid-like metaphyseal chondrodysplasia, and osteogenesis imperfecta. Severe monilia of the diaper area may suggest an immersion burn.

Approximately 10% of cases of physical abuse involve *burns*. The shape or pattern of a burn may be diagnostic when it reflects the pattern of an object or method of injury. Cigarette burns produce circular, punched-out lesions of uniform size (Fig. 35–3). An immersion burn occurs when a child is placed in hot water by accident or as punishment. Extremity immersions result in glove or stocking burn patterns. When a child's body is placed in hot water, the level of burn demarcation is uniform and distinct. Flexion creases may be spared when the child protectively flexes the extremities. Depending on how the child is held when immersed, the hands and feet may be spared and splash burns are not expected. The immersion burn pattern is incompatible with falling into a tub or turning on the hot water while in the bathtub. It is necessary to ascertain

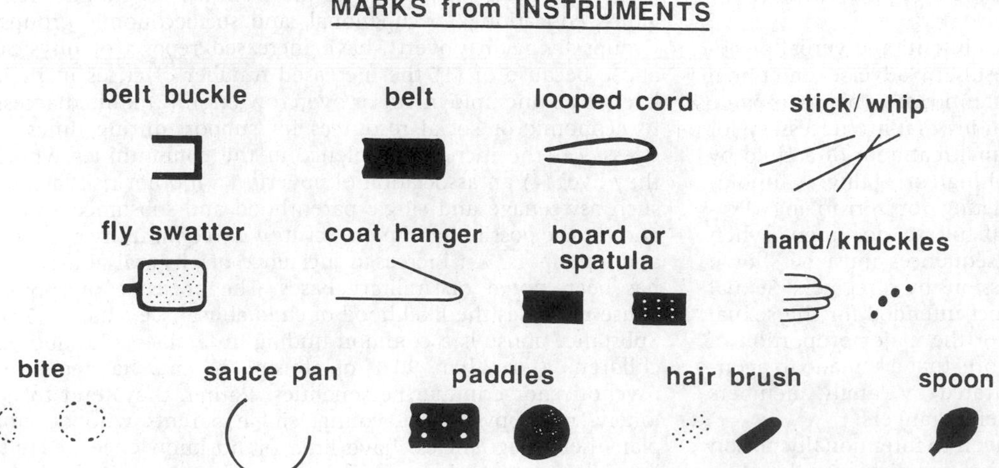

Figure 35–2 A variety of instruments may be used to inflict injury on a child. Often the choice of an instrument is a matter of convenience. Marks tend to silhouette or outline the shape of the instrument. The possiblility of intentional trauma should prompt a high degree of suspicion when injuries to a child are geometric, paired, mirrored, of various ages or types, or on relatively protected parts of the body. Early recognition of intentional trauma is important to provide therapy and prevent escalation to more serious injury.

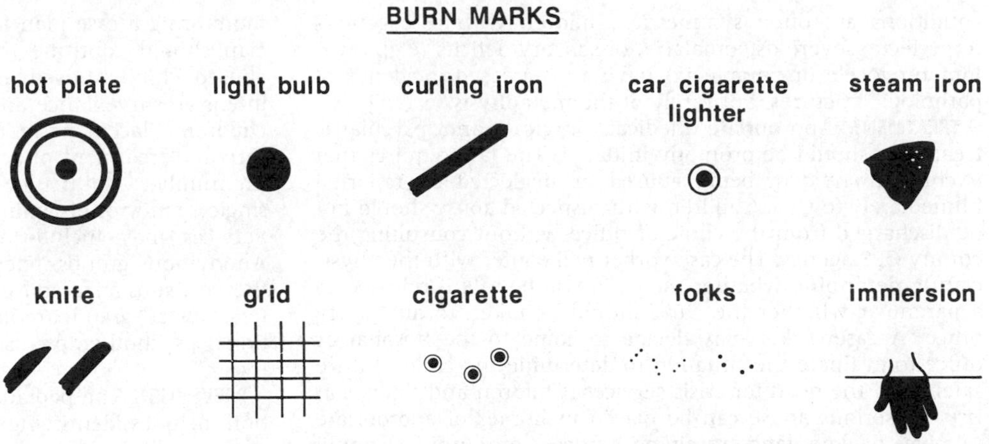

Figure 35–3 Marks from heated objects cause burns in a pattern that duplicates that of the object. Familiarity with the common heated objects that are used to traumatize children facilitates recognition of possible intentional injuries. The location of the burn is important in determining its cause. Children tend to explore surfaces with the palmar surface of the hand and rarely touch a heated object repeatedly.

the developmental skills of the child, water temperature, tub height, and knob type in the investigation of scald burns. Children under 24 mo of age may not be able to enter a tub or turn a rotary knob. Immersion burns are most common in infants.

The most common cause of death from physical abuse is *head trauma.* Twenty-nine per cent of child abuse reports from a children's hospital recorded injuries to the head, face, or cranial contents. More than 95% of serious intracranial injuries during the 1st yr of life are the result of abuse. Injured infants may present with coma, convulsions, apnea, and increased intracranial pressure. A bloody spinal tap may not be iatrogenic, particularly if xanthochromia is present. Subdural hematomas in which there are no scalp marks or skull fractures may result from a blow from a hand. Although grab marks or metaphyseal fractures and rib fractures have been described in association with *shaking* (acceleration-deceleration) and slamming the head against an object, there may be no external marks. Retinal hemorrhages are seen in 85% of infants who are shaken. They also may occur in association with normal birth, coagulopathies, blood dyscrasias, meningitis, endocarditis, and severe hypertension. Retinal hemorrhages rarely result from cardiopulmonary resuscitation or impact trauma.

Intra-abdominal injuries from impacts are the second most common cause of death in battered children. Affected children may present with recurrent vomiting, abdominal distention, absent bowel sounds, localized tenderness, or shock. Because the abdominal wall is flexible, the overlying skin may be free of bruises. If the child is struck with a fist, a row of three to four 1-cm oval bruises in a slight curve may be seen. The blow(s) may result in a ruptured liver or spleen or perforation or laceration of the small intestine at sites of ligamental support, such as the duodenum and proximal jejunum. Intramural hematomas at these sites can lead to temporary obstruction. Chylous ascites and pseudocyst of the pancreas also have been reported.

LABORATORY DATA. Screening tests should be obtained in all cases of bruising to rule out a bleeding diathesis. These tests should include a prothrombin time, partial thromboplastin time, and platelet count. Abnormal results may *follow* intracranial bleeding. Children with a hematologic condition, or any chronic condition, may also be abused.

When physical abuse is suspected in a child younger than 2 yr, a *roentgenologic bone survey* consisting of multiple views of the skull, thorax, long bones, hands, feet, pelvis, and spine is necessary. These films should be repeated in 7 to 10 days to reveal healing of fractures not seen on the initial films. Bone scans may be of value in detecting new fractures of the hands, feet, or ribs. They are not valuable in detecting skull fractures. For children 2–4 yr of age, a bone survey is indicated unless the child is adequately verbal, has very minor injuries, or was in a witnessed and supervised setting (e.g., preschool) when injured. For verbal children older than 4 or 5 yr, roentgenograms need be obtained only if there is bone tenderness or a limited range of motion on physical examination. If films of a tender site are initially negative, they should be repeated in 7 to 10 days to detect any calcification, subperiosteal bleeding, or nondisplaced epiphyseal separations that were initially undetected. Bone trauma is found in 10–20% of physically abused children. Fractures considered highly specific for child abuse include metaphyseal, rib, scapular, outer end of clavicle, vertebral, and finger in preambulating children; fractures of different ages; bilateral fractures; and complex skull fractures. Midclavicular, simple linear, and single diaphyseal fractures have a low specificity for abuse. Despite an absence of CNS abnormalities, a head CT scan and, if indicated, an MRI should be obtained when an infant has been severely injured. Fractures, burns, or bruises may be associated with an old or a new head injury. Liver and pancreatic enzyme studies or an abdominal CT scan may uncover damage to these organs. Urine and stool should be screened for blood if abdominal trauma is suspected.

DIAGNOSIS. Suspicion of physical abuse or neglect is usually based on a history that is not in keeping with physical findings or the child's developmental stage. All information should be legibly recorded. All visible lesions should be photographed with a 35 mm camera. Color charts, patient identification, and measuring scales should be included in the field. An analysis of the circumstances of the injury is critical. For example, the consequences of a fall depend on (1) child variables, such as surface contacted, age, size, motor skills, motor tone, clothing, and momentum; and (2) environmental variables, such as distance and physical qualities (soft, hard, padded, sharp, dull) of contact surfaces. Data from studies of witnessed falls from hospital beds, bunk beds, windows, and schoolyard equipment have been used to estimate the force required to cause brain damage and fractures. A fall from 3 ft may rarely result in a simple linear fracture of the skull or clavicle. Falls from 6 ft may rarely result in concussions, subdural hemorrhages, or lacerations. There are no reports of death or severe brain injury from *witnessed* falls of less than 10 ft.

After separation from caretakers, a child older than age 3 yr may be able to tell a sensitive and skillful interviewer that a particular adult hurt him or her. However, verbal children may not give a history of intentional injury if they are concerned about retribution from the perpetrator or separation from their home, school, siblings, friends, or nonoffending parent.

The differential diagnosis depends on the particular injuries. For example, roentgenograms of bones in scurvy and syphilis and normally growing bone shafts of infants may resemble nonaccidental bone trauma. The bony changes in these conditions are often symmetric. Children with osteogenesis imperfecta, severe osteomalacia, or sensory deficits (e.g., myelomeningocele or paraplegia) have an increased incidence of pathologic fractures, but rarely of the metaphysis.

TREATMENT. Appropriate medical, surgical, and psychiatric treatment should be promptly initiated. The law requires that a child *suspected* of being abused or neglected be reported immediately to CPS. Children with suspected abuse should not be discharged from the clinic or office without consulting the county CPS agency. The caseworker will confer with the physician to determine whether the child will be safe if released to a parent or whether the child should be taken to an agency office. A caseworker may decide to come to the hospital or office to evaluate the situation to determine the child's future safety and the need for crisis services. Children and siblings at risk for serious abuse can be placed in homes of appropriate relatives or emergency receiving homes. Communities should offer intensive services that provide for the immediate and safe return of the child to the home. The CPS should complete its investigation within a reasonable stipulated time. The role of law enforcement is to perform site investigations, to interview suspects, and, if a criminal act has taken place, to contact the prosecutor's office. In most states, 48 hr after the initial report by telephone or fax, a *written* and detailed report is required. The latter is best accomplished using a specialized form.

Hospital admission is indicated for children (1) whose medical or surgical condition requires inpatient management; (2) in whom the diagnosis is unclear; and (3) when no alternative safe place for custody is immediately available. If the safety of the child is in doubt, the physician, agency, and court should err on the side of protecting the child. If the parents refuse hospitalization or treatment, an emergency court order must be obtained. The parents should be told by the physician why an inflicted injury is suspected; that the physician is legally obligated to report the circumstance; that the referral is being made to protect the child; that the family will be provided with services; and that a CPS social worker and law enforcement officer will be involved. Siblings and children baby-sat by suspected abusers should have full examinations within 24 hr of the recognition of child abuse. Approximately 20% of them will be found to have signs of physical abuse.

Professionals should expect anger from abusing or neglectful parents; however, expressing anger toward them damages rapport, increases defensiveness, and makes their cooperation less likely. Repeated interrogations, confrontations, and accusations may be avoided by involving CPS workers and law enforcement early in the investigation. If the child is hospitalized, the supervised parents should be encouraged to visit, and the hospital staff must be counseled to be courteous, helpful, and observant. The primary physician should maintain contact with the parents. An evaluation by hospital social services should be obtained to determine existing problems, needs, and strengths in the family. An agency caseworker and, when needed, a police officer should visit the home. A psychiatric evaluation of the parents may be indicated.

Hospitals caring for children should have a team of professionals who are trained and skilled in child abuse recognition, reporting, and services. This team should include a pediatrician, a hospital social worker, a pediatric nurse, a psychologist or psychiatrist, and a data coordinator. Roles of all team members as well as public agencies involved should be formalized in a community plan and clinical pathways. Legal and medical specialty consultants should be available. When evaluations are completed, the team should meet with the child's primary care physician, ward nurse, the CPS representative, and, as appropriate, a law enforcement officer, prosecutor, or any other community agencies involved with the family in a staffing to share information, clarify medical and social findings, and plan immediate and long-range goals and therapies.

Child welfare agencies are responsible for developing and monitoring a case plan for the child and family. The pediatrician should continue to coordinate the health care of the abused child. Abused and neglected children require more intensive surveillance and well-child care than do nonabused children. Placement in foster care may interrupt preventive care and treatment of acute and chronic illnesses. Because of the number of difficulties experienced by abusive families, no single agency or discipline can provide all the needed services. Services may include parent aides, homemakers, Parents Anonymous groups, telephone hot lines, environmental crisis therapy, substance abuse treatment, Big Brothers and Big Sisters, "foster" grandparents, and child-rearing counseling. Traditional psychotherapy, especially in isolation, may be ineffective.

PREVENTION. The pediatrician's role in primary abuse prevention includes identifying parents at high risk for being unable to accept, love, and properly discipline and care for their offspring. The history obtained from all parents should include information about pregnancy planning and attitudes about the child and child-rearing techniques. Parental risks include a history of family violence or child abuse, drug addiction, depression, lack of support, socioeconomic problems, serious psychiatric illness, mental retardation, young parental age, closely spaced pregnancies, single-parent status of the mother, negative parental comments about the newborn infant, lack of evidence of maternal attachment, infrequent visits to a new infant whose discharge is delayed because of prematurity or illness, inappropriate anger toward or spanking of an infant younger than 18 mo or a handicapped child, and neglect of infant hygiene. The use of an instrument on any part of the body, a bruise from corporal punishment, or striking any part of the body aside from the hands or buttocks may be considered inappropriate and reportable. Child risks include mental or physical handicap, chronic illness, prematurity, being a twin, and learning or behavior problems. Abuse and serious neglect may be prevented when at-risk families receive intensive training and support during pregnancy and after delivery. Prevention efforts should include early and frequent contact between mother and baby in the delivery room, rooming-in, increased parental contact with premature infants, extra help calming the crying or "difficult" infant, more frequent office visits for at-risk infants, ongoing counseling regarding discipline and the use of nonphysical responses to behaviors, public health nurse visits or trained home visitors, parenting classes, stress and anger management classes, close follow-up of acute and chronic illnesses, telephone hot lines, arrangement for child care or preschool, and assistance in family planning.

PROGNOSIS. Early studies of abused children returned to their parents without any intervention indicated that about 5% were killed and that 25% were seriously re-injured. With comprehensive, intensive family treatment, 80–90% of families involved in child maltreatment may be rehabilitated to provide adequate care for their children. Approximately 10–15% of maltreating families, especially those with a history of substance abuse, can only be stabilized and will require an indefinite continuation of supporting services, which may include drug monitoring, until their children are old enough to leave home. Termination of parental rights or continued foster placement is required in 2–3% of cases. If a parent is unable to respond to a treatment plan, this should be documented as soon as possible to afford the child the opportunity to develop in a healthy and permanent home.

Children with injuries to the CNS may develop mental retardation, learning problems, blindness, deafness, motor problems, organic brain syndrome, seizures, hydrocephalus, and ataxia. Common emotional traits of abused children include fearfulness, aggression, hypervigilance, denial, projection, a lack of trust, low self-esteem, juvenile delinquency, substance abuse, and hyperactivity. Unsuccessful treatment may result in children who become juvenile delinquents, violent and antisocial adults, and the next generation of child abusers.

35.1 Sexual Abuse

Sexual abuse includes any activity with a child, before the age of legal consent, that is for the sexual gratification of an adult or a significantly older child. Sexual abuse includes oral-genital, genital-genital, genital-rectal, hand-genital, hand-rectal, or hand-breast contact; exposure of sexual anatomy; forced viewing of sexual anatomy; and showing pornography to a child or using a child in the production of pornography. Sexual intercourse includes vaginal, oral, or rectal penetration. Penetration is entry into an orifice with or without tissue injury. Younger perpetrators tend to have younger victims but are more likely to have intercourse with older victims. Sex acts perpetrated by young children are learned behaviors and are associated with experiencing sexual abuse or exposure to adult sex or pornography. Without detection and intervention, sexual abuse may progress from touching to intercourse. *Sexual play,* on the other hand, may be defined as viewing or touching of the genitals, buttocks, or chest by preadolescent children separated by not more than 4 yr, in which there has been no force or coercion. See Chapter 26 for a discussion of the development of sexual identity and behavior.

Sexual mistreatment of children by family members (incest) and nonrelatives known to the child is the most common type of sexual abuse. The least common offender is a stranger. Intrafamilial sexual abuse is difficult to document and manage, because the child must be protected from additional abuse and coercion to not reveal or to deny the abuse while attempts are made to preserve the family unit. Children also may be coerced to recant accusations of abuse by relatives, or they may decide to recant the abuse for fear of ridicule or teasing, retaliation, attendance in court, or loss of contact with needed or loved relatives and friends.

EPIDEMIOLOGY. Most of the increase in child abuse reports is due to increased reporting of sexual abuse. The rate of sexual abuse, estimated by the American Association for Protecting Children, went from 1.4/10,000 to 17/10,000 children between 1976 and 1984. In a children's hospital, the number of total assessments of sexual abuse increased by a factor of 4 between 1981 and 1991. In 1995, 13% of confirmed reports were of sexual abuse. Surveys of adult women indicate that from 12–38% were sexually abused by 18 yr of age. The results of one study indicated that the likelihood of extrafamilial and intrafamilial sexual abuse being reported were 8% and 2%, respectively. The incidence of sexual abuse of males ranges from 3–9% of the population; males account for up to 20% of reports. Because fixed pedophiles show a predilection for boys, it is theorized that the number of males who are sexually abused is higher. Furthermore, boys may refrain from reporting what they might interpret as a homosexual action or a consequence of their failure to protect themselves from assault.

In 1997, 679 reports (71%) from a children's hospital were for sexual abuse. Of 744 patients referred to a diagnostic clinic for suspected sexual abuse, 230 (31%) were reported. Physical and behavioral findings thought to be due to sexual abuse were responsible for the greater number of diagnoses. A lack of substantiation may be due to a child's young age and inability to give a detailed history or a lack of significant physical or laboratory findings. Caregivers may mistake genital erythema, enuresis, masturbation, or nonspecific behaviors as being due to sexual abuse. Suspicion may be increased during divorce proceedings owing to distrust of the other parent and changes in the child's behavior caused by the divorce process. Approximately one third of sexual abuse victims are less than 6 yr of age; one third are 6–12 yr of age; and one third are 12–18 yr of age. Reported offenders are 97% male. Females are more often perpetrators in child-care settings, including baby sitting. The number of female perpetrators may be higher because younger children may confuse sexual abuse by a female with normal hygiene care, and adolescent males may not be trained to recognize sexual activity with an older female as a form of abuse. Sexual abuse by stepfathers is nearly five times higher than by natural fathers. Incest is described in most cultures and is seen at all socioeconomic levels to a greater degree than are physical abuse and neglect.

ETIOLOGY. The abuse of daughters by fathers and stepfathers is the most common form of reported incest, although brother-sister incest is considered to be the most common type. Studies of incarcerated adult perpetrators indicated that sexual abuse begins with selection of vulnerable and available victims, innocent physical contact, and seduction. The propensity for pedophiles to become sexually involved with children often appears in their adolescence. Pedophiles have indicated that they seek positions and opportunities where they can be in contact with potential victims. The vulnerable children they described include those with mental and physical handicaps, unloved and unwanted children, previously abused children, children in single-parent families, children of drug abusers, and children with low self-esteem and poor achievement. Pornography may be used to initiate sexual activity with a child. Threats and bribes may be used to entice children and keep them from telling. Boys and girls may be told that they are at fault because they did not protect themselves. Obedience and trust of adults, coupled with a need to maintain family unity, are factors associated with incest. A father's need for sexual gratification and a daughter's need for affection and nurturance may lead to incest when the mother is unavailable and there is a desire to maintain the family unit. These incestuous fathers have been described as rigid, patriarchal, and emotionally immature. They are unlikely to engage in extramarital relationships, and there is a high reported incidence of alcoholism. The characteristics of incarcerated perpetrators or perpetrators in therapy, upon which many study results are based, may be different from those of other perpetrators. The mothers have been described as chronically depressed, unavailable to their husbands because of work or illness, and often the victims of childhood sexual abuse. The child victim tends to be pseudomature and to have taken on many of the adult roles, including housekeeping. The tendency for some of these families to be closely knit and socially isolated prevents detection.

Violence is not common in sexual abuse; however, its incidence increases with the age and size of the victim and specific traits in the perpetrator. Violence is more likely to occur in association with a single incident by a stranger. In cases of violent incest, the father has been described as sociopathic, with sexual abuse extending outside the family circle.

CLINICAL MANIFESTATIONS. A child may disclose sexual abuse to the mother and be brought to a physician at that time. If the mother does not believe the child, the child may delay further comment indefinitely or later tell a friend, relative, friend's mother, teacher, or school counselor. Children, given the opportunity, may disclose their abuse to a physician in a private interview or physical examination. The possibility of sexual abuse should be considered as the result of associated physical symptoms, including (1) vaginal, penile, or rectal pain, discharge, or bleeding; (2) chronic dysuria, enuresis, constipation, or encopresis; and (3) rarely, premature puberty in a female. Behaviors more likely to be associated with sexual abuse include sexualized activity with peers, animals, or objects; seductive behavior; and age-inappropriate sexual knowledge and curiosity. Nonspecific behaviors include suicide gestures, fear of an individual or place, nightmares, sleep disorders, regression, aggression, withdrawn behavior, post-traumatic stress disorder (see Chapter 22), low self-esteem, depression, poor school performance, running away, self-mutilation, anxiety, fire setting, multiple personalities, somatization, phobias, trauma, prostitution, drug abuse, eating disorders, dysmenorrhea, and dyspareunia. Because of secrecy, a desire to protect the abuser or family, or threats by the abuser, the cause of symptoms or behaviors may be denied by the child. When the perpetrator is a breadwinner or is violent, it may also be denied by the nonoffending and dependent parent.

Investigating the possibility of sexual abuse requires supportive, sensitive, and detailed *history* taking. Because of variance in the type of abuse, the ages of the victim and perpetrator, and the time since abuse, less than 15% of cases yield physical or laboratory findings. Ideally, the videotaped forensic interview, which uses open-ended, nonleading questions, should be conducted by one or two experienced interviewers in the presence of law enforcement and social service workers who observe behind a one-way mirror. This will obviate the need for repeated interviews and possible further trauma to the child. After an initial interview, children who gain trust and comfort may experience a decrease in guilt and fear of reprisal or loss of love and give more detailed information in subsequent interviews. Interviewing should proceed at the child's pace and level of development. It should begin with discussion of general topics and naming of body parts, including "private" parts, and proceed to details about each incident. The sophistication of the information that can be obtained from the child will vary with the development of the child and the skill of the interviewer. Anatomic pictures or dolls may help clarify the names of body parts and aid in describing the abuse. If a social worker or law enforcement officer has carried out the initial interview, the physician should review this material and decide whether it is necessary to repeat the interview before performing a physical examination. Questions about the abusive actions, including symptoms of trauma, may be asked during the physical examination. Familiarity with the child through participation in the forensic interview, a previous examination, or sick- and well-child care contacts facilitates a cooperative and nontraumatic physical examination. Older female and male victims may prefer that a physician of the same sex examine them; when possible, their desires should be respected.

A thorough physical *examination* should be conducted, with special attention to the neck and mouth. If present, bite marks should be measured, and wax impressions and wiping for saliva should be done to aid in identification of the perpetrator. The abdominal examination should assess the possibility of pregnancy. The mouth should be examined for redness, abrasions, or purpura that may be due to recent trauma. The rectum should be examined for signs of trauma and laxity. The external genitals should be examined for signs of trauma and discharge with the aid of a colposcope or strong light and magnifier. Acute injuries to the hymen occur between the 4 and 8 o'clock positions. In the younger girl, penetration may injure the labia minora, posterior fourchette, or vestibule floor; with deeper penetration, tears of the posterior hymenal ring may occur between the 4 and 8 o'clock positions. With the prepubertal girl in the frog-leg position, separation or traction is applied to the labia with the gloved fingers of the examiner or assistant. The examination should be explained to the girl; anxiety can be reduced by distracting her. She can be asked to blow on a pinwheel, sing, or count. The hymenal walls and orifice are measured. When abnormalities are seen, some physicians repeat the examination with the child in the knee-chest position. The horizontal diameter of the hymen increases with age and lateral traction. If the child is resistant despite preparation, she may be examined while sitting on the parent's lap. Occasionally, the child will be able to separate the labia or buttocks herself. A speculum examination of the vagina with collection of specimens is indicated when the victim is postpubertal or when nonmenstrual vaginal bleeding or major trauma of the external genitals is present. No child should be forced to have an examination. General anesthesia or sedation may be required if there is bleeding from the rectum or vagina. Magnification, using a colposcope or a hand-held magnifier with bright illumination, ensures a detailed examination that can reveal abnormalities in the fourchette and rim of the hymen. The tears from penetration may heal with scarring or a permanent notch. Trauma may cause attenuation or narrowing of the lateral or inferior (dorsal) hymenal rim to less than 0.1 mm.

Drawings of trauma should be supplemented with photographs or video recordings using the colposcope or photos from a hand-held 35-mm camera and macro lens. Normal values for the hymenal opening of non–sexually abused girls of different ages are available and should be referred to in evaluating the hymen; however, owing to normal variations in size and stretching that occurs during examination, hymen size is not considered diagnostic. "Suggestive findings" of sexual abuse also include (1) a hymen with new or healed lacerations and transections, remnants, and attenuations; (2) posterior fourchette lacerations; (3) vaginal wall tears; and (4) perianal lacerations. The presence of sperm and semen is "clear evidence" of sexual abuse. Other suggestive findings include bite marks on the genitals or inner thigh or scarring or tears of the labia minora. Straddle injuries usually result in trauma to the labia and clitoris and do not involve the protected hymen. Accidental penetration of the hymen is rare and is associated with penetration of underclothing and possibly the wall of the vagina.

Abnormal perianal findings even in the face of repeated anal penetration are unusual. If immediate dilation of the anus reveals an anterior-posterior diameter greater than 20 mm, with no stool present in the rectal ampulla, that is a strong marker for possible abuse, warranting further investigation. Scar formation, even following an episode of forceful sodomy, is unusual. However, there are two common, midline, naturally occurring entities that may be confused with scar tissue in the perianal region. The first is a smooth, wedged-shaped area known as diastasis ani. This can be found either anterior or posterior to the anus. The second finding is an extension of the median or perineal raphe that has a taglike appearance on the anterior side of the anus. Anal fissures must be interpreted with caution, since they can be the result of chronic constipation or underlying disease, such as Crohn's disease.

Injuries to the male genitals are usually the result of an accident or physical abuse. A bite mark may be found. The forceful retraction of the foreskin may result in a dehiscence of the tissues. Injury from a sexual assault will most likely cause a nonspecific, transitory redness of the penis.

LABORATORY DATA. Laboratory investigation depends on the history and the time from injury. The body of a victim seen within 72 hr of sexual abuse should be examined under a Wood's lamp for ejaculatory evidence. Suspected areas should be swabbed with a moist cotton applicator. In addition, specimens of possible offender blood and hair and the victim's nail clippings and clothing should be collected. Tests for rectal blood may be indicated. If there is a history of contact with the perpetrator's genitals, gonorrhea and *Chlamydia* cultures should be obtained from the mouth, anus, and genitals. In the vagina, motile sperm can be found for 6 hr; nonmotile sperm exist for longer than 72 hours. Acid phosphatase is present for 24 hr. Sperm and semen may also be recovered from the mouth, rectum, and clothing. Although the presence of semen substantiates the victim's history of vaginal intercourse, the absence of semen does not contradict it. Less than 5% of victims have positive cultures for gonorrhea or *Chlamydia*. Symptomatic victims, those with positive cultures for other venereal diseases, and children with a history of contact with the perpetrator's genitals should also be tested for syphilis, HIV, and hepatitis B. All specimens should be transferred to the forensic laboratory in sealed, signed, and dated envelopes to ensure an official chain of evidence.

DIAGNOSIS. It is most common for the diagnosis of sexual abuse to depend upon the history offered by the victim. False accusations are rare except in unusual cases involving adolescents, emotionally disturbed patients, or patients in custody disputes. Abuse may be revealed during a custody dispute because the child has been separated from an offender and is able to communicate without fear of retaliation or further abuse. The physical or laboratory examination may corroborate a child's history, but normal physical and laboratory examination findings are compatible with sexual abuse. Fondling and oral-genital and labial intercourse may not cause tissue trauma. The genitals and rectum may heal completely after extensive trauma, and minor trauma, such as abrasions, may heal within 3–4 days. In one study of 18 victims whose abusers confessed to vaginal penetration, 7 children had normal genital examination findings. Abnormal physical or laboratory findings should be reported if no history is available.

Laboratory findings of pregnancy, sperm, semen, and *non-pregnancy-* or *delivery-related* syphilis, gonorrhea, *Chlamydia,* herpes type II (genital), and HIV may be considered diagnostic of sexual abuse and reported. Condyloma acuminatum appearing after 3 yr of age and *Trichomonas vaginalis* are considered "probably diagnostic." Herpes type I and nonvenereal warts may be autoinoculated to the genitorectal area or transmitted by a perpetrator's mouth or hand. The significance of bacterial vaginosis and genital *Mycoplasma* infection is uncertain. New techniques, such as DNA typing of blood, semen, sperm, or tissue, may positively identify the perpetrator.

TREATMENT. Sexual abuse is a criminal offense and is investigated by the police. All victims of sexual abuse require psychologic support. Parents, relatives, and siblings may deny the accusation and rebuke or punish the child for reporting the incident. The consequences and appropriate therapy of sexual abuse vary, depending on the type of abuse, the age and other physical and emotional factors in the victim, the frequency of abuse, and the identity of the abuser. Victims of a single nonviolent episode of touching or exposure by a stranger may need only reassurance and a chance to express their feelings about the event in one or two therapy sessions. They may be less distressed by the incident than are their parents. In contrast, a single episode of family-related sexual abuse may cause serious, long-term emotional distress and require prolonged individual and group treatment. The therapist may recommend that the victim of incest be returned home if the perpetrator is out of the home or has confessed and is in therapy. The child victim should be placed in foster care if this is his or her desire; if the nonoffending parent is not protective of the child, does not believe the child's story, or is likely to encourage the child to recant; and if family life is chaotic or collection of evidence is not yet complete. Medication to prevent pregnancy may be given to postmenarchal girls in midcycle who have experienced vaginal intercourse within the previous 72 hr. Treatment with antibiotics is initiated to prevent sexually transmitted disease if the perpetrator is known to be infected, if the victim has signs of infection, or if the likelihood of follow-up is poor. All victims should revisit their primary care physicians within 2 wk to ensure that recommended services have been implemented.

Incest offenders may respond to treatment, but success requires a coordinated, multifaceted, multidisciplinary approach. The offending parent should be referred for psychiatric or psychologic evaluation, and the spouse should be evaluated by a social worker. Offenders should be investigated by the police, and criminal prosecution should be supported. There is evidence, especially in pedophilia, that incarceration may ensure access to, and efficacy of, simultaneous treatment. Incarceration of a breadwinner may have serious adverse consequences for the family. The behavior of chronic sexual offenders may be resistant to a variety of therapies. All juvenile and prejuvenile offenders should receive therapy to prevent recurrences. In one diagnostic center, 17% of offenders were under 17 yr of age.

PREVENTION. The primary prevention of sexual abuse is related, in part, to normal developmental education and sexual behavior (Chapter 26). Teaching children the proper names of all body parts, including the names, function, and significance of "private parts" (nipples, genitals, and rectum) should begin in the home and pediatrician's office and continue in school. Children should be taught to say "no" to inappropriate touches to these latter areas by anyone and to report to a trusted adult any actions that make them uncomfortable. Caregivers, including baby sitters and their companions, should be carefully screened by parents and agencies. Victim therapy should decrease the potential for reactive abuse. Family and classroom discussions of uncomfortable events in the lives of children may reveal unsuspected abuse. To improve diagnostic skills, physicians should appropriately examine the genitals and rectum routinely, record their findings, become familiar with normal rectal and genital anatomy and the consequences of trauma, listen to and seriously consider what children tell them, and be willing to report and testify when abuse is suspected.

PROGNOSIS. With early and adequate intervention, victims may lead normal adult lives. However, even with intervention, certain adolescent victims may run away from home and fall prey to adolescent prostitution, violence, drug addiction, and unprepared parenthood (see Chapter 39). Others who remain at home may manifest a variety of emotional problems, including depression, suicidal gestures, deterioration in school performance, and conversion reactions. As adults, victims may have difficulties with close relationships; enter abusive relationships; have a variety of somatic complaints of the genitourinary, gastrointestinal, and other systems; and need psychiatric help for depression, anxiety, substance abuse, dissociation, and eating disorders. The risk of untoward effects is greatest for incest victims.

35.2 Nonorganic Failure to Thrive (NOFTT)

See Chapter 36 for a full discussion of organic and nonorganic failure to thrive. NOFTT mainly occurs when a child, usually an infant, is not fed adequate calories. The mother may neglect proper feeding because she is involved with external demands and the care of others; is preoccupied with inner problems or depressed; is ignorant about appropriate feeding; is abusing substances; or does not like or understand the infant. Emotional or maternal deprivation is inevitably concurrent with nutritional deprivation. These mothers often feel deprived and unloved themselves and may be acutely or chronically depressed. Multiple and continuing crises, frequently compounded by the physical absence of the father, may overwhelm a mother, who reacts by neglecting her infant. Poverty may also prevent a caregiver from obtaining adequate food for a child. Retarded and emotionally disturbed parents may not have the capacity to provide proper care.

CLINICAL MANIFESTATIONS. The dietary history in infants with nutritional neglect may not be accurate because the parent misinforms the physician that the baby is receiving adequate calories. Depending on severity, the infant with NOFTT may exhibit thin extremities, a narrow face, prominent ribs, and wasted buttocks. Neglect of hygiene is evidenced by diaper rash, unwashed skin, untreated impetigo, uncut and dirty fingernails, or unwashed clothing. A flattened occiput with hair loss may indicate that the child has been lying on his or her back and unattended for prolonged periods. Delays in social and speech development are common. Other findings include an avoidance of eye contact, an expressionless face, and the absence of a cuddling response. The amount of time that the mother spends holding, playing with, and talking to her baby is usually reduced or inappropriate. A rejecting or frustrated mother may feed her baby with anger and unnecessary force. This may result in a torn frenulum and an aversion to feeding.

LABORATORY DATA. Extensive laboratory evaluation should be delayed until dietary management has been attempted for at least 1 wk and has failed. A skeletal survey is indicated in those infants who have a rejecting parent or evidence of associated physical abuse.

DIAGNOSIS. Most children with NOFTT should be hospitalized and given unlimited feedings of a diet appropriate for age for a minimum of 1 wk; this diet usually approaches 150 kcal/kg (ideal weight)/24 hr. Infants with NOFTT usually gain more than 2 oz every 24 hr for 1 wk (approximately 1 lb/wk) or have a gain that is significantly greater than that achieved during a similar period at home. These infants may display a ravenous appetite. A nursing plan should include careful charting of intake, weight, and observations of the mother's feeding style and relationship to the child. Deprivational behaviors may improve or resolve in the hospital setting with attention from the staff. Infants who are difficult to feed owing to neurologic or mechanical problems may gain weight as a result of the intensive efforts by experienced hospital staff.

TREATMENT. All cases of NOFTT caused by underfeeding from maternal neglect should be reported to CPS. After appropriate hospital management, approximately 75% of infants are discharged home with added services for the family; 20% go into temporary foster care while the parents receive therapy; and 5% enter long-term foster care with plans for voluntary relinquishment or termination of parental rights. Exercising this last option should be based mainly on the responsiveness of the mother to treatment. Those infants who are discharged to their natural home require intensive and long-term intervention. The parents should be provided with clear, written dietary instructions at discharge and trained to hold the infant close during feedings and to provide frequent and appropriate stimulation. Families may require a homemaker, public health nurse, health visitor, and other types of outreach services. Weekly medical follow-up is necessary to monitor progress.

PROGNOSIS. Without detection and intervention, a small percentage of infants with nutritional neglect die of starvation. Approximately 5–15% of these infants suffer from physical abuse. Weight loss and understature from malnutrition are reversible, but normal head circumference and brain growth may not be achieved if the infant has suffered from NOFTT beyond 6 mo of age. Emotional and educational problems occur in more than half these children.

35.3 Munchausen Syndrome by Proxy

The term *Munchausen syndrome* was used initially to describe situations in which adults falsified their own symptoms. In Munchausen syndrome by proxy, first described in 1977, a parent, invariably the mother, simulates or causes disease in a child. The parent may (1) fabricate a medical history; (2) cause symptoms by repeatedly exposing the child to a toxin, medication, infectious agent, or physical trauma; or (3) alter laboratory samples or temperature measurements. Depending on the parent's sophistication and secrecy, a variety of convincing, novel, and exotic diseases may be simulated or created. The parent may deny any involvement and, in instances of intentional poisoning, smothering, or trauma, may continue the action while the child is hospitalized. This syndrome is inflicted on children who are either unable or unwilling to identify the true offense and offender. The abusing caregiver gains attention from the relationships formed with health care providers or her own family as a result of the problems created.

CLINICAL MANIFESTATIONS. The child's symptoms, their pattern, or the response to treatment may not be compatible with a recognized disease. They may involve any organ system and suggest a panoply of disease processes. Although generally reported in preverbal children, cases have been recognized in children up to 16 yr of age. There may be an associated actual disease. Symptoms are always associated with the proximity of the mother to the child. The mother may have a background in health care, may be supported by the father who may be unavailable, and may present as a devoted and model parent who forms close relationships with members of the health care team. She may have a history of Munchausen syndrome and seem relatively unconcerned about the child's illness.

Apnea and seizures, two common manifestations, the observation of which may be falsified, may also be created by partial suffocation. Symptoms created by toxins, medications, water, and salts require familiarity with those substances available to families and the wide array of consequences from misuse of these substances. The clinical pattern is variable, depending on the agent. It includes forced ingestion of medications such as ipecac to cause chronic vomiting or laxatives to cause diarrhea, or injection of insulin with consequent seizures. The skin, which is more easily accessible to the perpetrator, may be burned, dyed, tattooed, lacerated, or punctured to simulate acute or chronic skin conditions. Infectious or toxic agents may be administered into any available orifice. Provision of intravenous lines during hospitalization may provide an opportunity for injection of infectious agents from feces, toxins, and pharmacologic agents. Urine and blood samples may be contaminated with foreign blood or stool.

DIAGNOSIS. Investigations should be based on a high index of suspicion of this diagnosis so that unpleasant, dangerous, or unnecessary tests are not undertaken on the child. Specimens should be analyzed for potentially harmful agents and for "foreign" blood. All steps in the diagnosis should be carefully documented. Records from other hospitals for the index child and siblings should be obtained and carefully reviewed. Hospitalized children should be under constant surveillance. This may include hidden television monitoring in coordination with law enforcement. Frequent staff meetings are necessary to ensure that all information is gathered in a planned and forensic manner.

TREATMENT. After all laboratory information is collected and the diagnosis is established, the offending parent should be confronted by a nonaccusatory physician and staff who offer help. Any approach may be met with resistance, denial, and threats. All cases should be reported promptly and with careful documentation to children's services. The consequences of Munchausen syndrome by proxy include persistence of abuse, emotional problems, chronic disability in 8% of cases, and death. Other siblings may be, or may have been, at risk; there is an association of this syndrome with unexplained infant deaths.

General

American Humane Association—Children's Division, 63 Inverness Drive East, Englewood, CA 80112-5117. E-mail http://www.amerhumane.org

American Professional Society Against Child Abuse, 407 South Dearborn, Suite 1300, Chicago, IL 60605. E-mail http://www.apsac.org

Belsey MA: Child abuse: Measuring a global problem. World Health Stat Q 46:69, 1993.

National Clearinghouse on Child Abuse and Neglect. Child maltreatment: Reports from the States to the National Center on Child Abuse and Neglect. P.O. Box 1182, Washington, DC, 20013-1182, 1995. E-mail nccanch@calib.com

Department of Health and Human Services: National Child Abuse and Neglect Data System Working Paper 2, 1991. Summary Data Component. Washington, DC, National Center on Child Abuse and Neglect, 1993.

Jones E, McCurdy K: The links between types of maltreatment and demographic characteristics of children. Child Abuse Negl 16:201, 1992.

Overpeck MD, Brenner RA, Trumble AC, et al: Risk factors for infant homicide in the United States. N Engl J Med 339:1211, 1998.
The Gallup Organization: Disciplining Children in America. A Gallup Poll Report. Princeton, NJ, 1995.
Reece RM: Child Abuse: Medical Diagnosis and Management. Philadelphia, Lea & Febiger, 1994.
Windom MD: Injury prevention and control in children and youth. Elk Grove, IL, American Academy of Pediatrics, 1997.

Physical Abuse

Brewster AL, Nelson JP, Hymel KP, et al: Victim, perpetrator, family and incident characteristics of 32 infant maltreatment deaths in the United States Air Force. Child Abuse Negl 91:101, 1998.
Carty HM: Fractures caused by child abuse. J Bone Joint Surg 75B:849, 1993.
Chadwick DL, Chin S, Salerno C, et al: Deaths from falls in children: How far is fatal? J Trauma 31:1353, 1991.
Duhaime AC, Gennarellia TA, Thibault LE, et al: The shaken baby syndrome: A clinical, pathological, and biomechanical study. J Neurosurg 66:409, 1987.
Duhaime AC, Lewander WJ, Schut L, et al: Head injury in very young children: Mechanisms, injury types, and ophthalmologic findings in 100 hospitalized patients younger than 2 years of age. Pediatrics 9:179, 1992.
Gillham B, Tanner G, Cheyne B, et al: Unemployment rates, single parent density and indices of child poverty: Their relationship to different categories of child abuse and neglect. Child Abuse Negl 22:79, 1998.
Johnson CF: Inflicted injury vs accidental injury: The diagnosis of inflicted injury. Pediatr Clin North Am 37:791, 1990.
Kempe CH: The battered child syndrome. JAMA 181:17, 1962.
Lyons T, Oates RK: Falling out of bed: A relatively benign occurrence. Pediatrics 92:125, 1993.
McClain PW, Sacks JJ, Froehlke RG, et al: Estimates of fatal child abuse and neglect, United States 1979 through 1988. Pediatrics 91:338, 1993.
Nashelsky MB, Dix JD: The time interval between lethal infant shaking and onset of symptoms: A review of the shaken baby syndrome literature. Am J Forensic Med Pathol, 16:154, 1995.
Raiha HK, Soma D: Victims of child abuse and neglect in the U.S. Army. Child Abuse Negl 21:759, 1997.
Schwartz AJ, Ricci LR: How accurately can bruises be aged in abused children? Literature review and synthesis. Pediatrics 97:254, 1966.
Wilkinson WS, Han DP, Rappley MD, et al: Retinal hemorrhage predicts neurologic injury in the shaken baby syndrome. Arch Ophthalmol 107:1472, 1989.
Williams RA: Injuries in infants and small children resulting from witnessed and corroborated free falls. J Trauma 31:1350, 1991.

Sexual Abuse

American Academy of Pediatrics: Guidelines for the evaluation of sexual abuse of children: Subject review. Pediatrics 103:186, 1999.
Adams JA: Significance of medical findings in suspected sexual abuse: Moving toward consensus. J Child Sexual Abuse 1:91, 1993.
Bays J, Chadwick D: Medical diagnosis of the sexually abused child. Child Abuse Negl 17:91, 1993.
Bays J, Jenny C: Genital and anal conditions confused with child sexual abuse. Am J Dis Child 144:1319, 1990.
Holmes WC, Slap GB: Sexual abuse of boys. JAMA 280:1855, 1998.
McCann J, Voris J, Simon M: Genital injuries resulting from sexual abuse: A longitudinal study. Pediatrics 89:307, 1992.
McCann J, Voris J, Simon M, et al: Perianal findings in prepubertal children selected for nonabuse: A descriptive study. Child Abuse Negl 13:179, 1989.
Swanston HY, Tebbutt JS, O'Toole BI, et al: Sexually abused children 5 years after presentation: A case controlled study. Pediatrics 100:600, 1997.

Nonorganic Failure to Thrive

Rosenn DW, Loeb LS, Jura MB: Differentiation of organic from non-organic failure to thrive in infancy. Pediatrics 66:698, 1980.
Schmitt BD, Mauro RD: Nonorganic failure to thrive: An outpatient approach. Child Abuse Negl 13:235, 1989.
Skuse D, Albanese A, Stanhope R, et al: A new stress-related syndrome of growth failure and hyperphagia in children associated with reversibility of growth-hormone insufficiency. Lancet 348:353, 1996.

Munchausen Syndrome by Proxy

Levin AV, Sheridan MS: Munchausen Syndrome by Proxy: Issues in Diagnosis and Treatment. New York, Lexington Books, 1995.
Rosenberg DD: Web of deceit: A literature review of Munchausen syndrome by proxy. Child Abuse Negl 11:547, 1987.
Schreier HA, Libow JA: Munchausen syndrome by proxy: Diagnosis and prevalence. Am J Orthopsychiatry 63:318, 1993.

Other Types of Child Maltreatment

Garbarino J: Psychological child maltreatment—a developmental view. Prim Care 20:6, 1993.
Jaudes PK, Ekwo E, Gosselink CA, et al: Linkage of drug abuse and child abuse. Am J Dis Child 147:482, 1993. [Abstract.]
Johnson CF: Physicians and medical neglect: Variables which affect reporting. Child Abuse Negl 17:605, 1993.

PART V

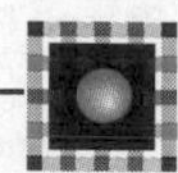

Children with Special Health Needs

CHAPTER 36
Failure to Thrive

Howard Bauchner

Failure to thrive (FTT) is diagnosed in an infant or child whose physical growth is significantly less than that of his or her peers, and it often is associated with poor developmental and socioemotional functioning. Although there is no clear consensus about the definition, FTT usually refers to growth below the 3rd or 5th percentile or a change in growth that has crossed two major growth percentiles (i.e., from above the 75th percentile to below the 25th) in a short time. Traditionally, the diagnosis has been divided into two categories. Organic FTT is marked by an underlying medical condition; nonorganic or psychosocial FTT occurs in a child who is usually younger than age 5 yr and has no known medical condition that causes poor growth (also see Chapter 35.2).

EPIDEMIOLOGY AND ETIOLOGY. The prevalence of FTT depends on the population sampled. From 5–10% of low-birthweight children and children living in poverty may have FTT. Family discord, neonatal problems other than low birthweight, and maternal depression are also associated with FTT. In the United States, psychosocial FTT is far more common than organic FTT.

The causes of organic FTT are numerous (Table 36–1). Every organ system is represented. Psychosocial FTT is most often due to poverty or poor child-parent interaction. It occasionally occurs with severe stress such as child abuse. Organic and nonorganic etiologic factors may also occur together, for example, in children who are victims of abuse and neglect or temperamentally difficult premature infants.

TABLE 36–1 Major Organic Causes of Failure to Thrive

System	Cause
Gastrointestinal	Gastroesophageal reflux, celiac disease, pyloric stenosis, cleft palate/cleft lip, lactose intolerance, Hirschsprung's disease, milk protein intolerance, hepatitis, cirrhosis, pancreatic insufficiency, biliary disease, inflammatory bowel disease, malabsorption
Renal	Urinary tract infection, renal tubular acidosis, diabetes insipidus, chronic renal insufficiency
Cardiopulmonary	Cardiac diseases leading to congestive heart failure, asthma, bronchopulmonary dysplasia, cystic fibrosis, anatomic abnormalities of the upper airway, obstructive sleep apnea
Endocrine	Hypothyroidism, diabetes mellitus, adrenal insufficiency or excess, parathyroid disorders, pituitary disorders, growth hormone deficiency
Neurologic	Mental retardation, cerebral hemorrhages, degenerative disorders
Infectious	Parasitic or bacterial infections of the gastrointestinal tract, tuberculosis, human immunodeficiency virus disease
Metabolic	Inborn errors of metabolism
Congenital	Chromosomal abnormalities, congenital syndromes (fetal alcohol syndrome), perinatal infections
Miscellaneous	Lead poisoning, malignancy, collagen vascular disease, recurrently infected adenoids and tonsils

CLINICAL MANIFESTATIONS. The clinical presentation of FTT ranges from failure to meet expected age norms for height and weight, to alopecia, loss of subcutaneous fat, reduced muscle mass, dermatitis, recurrent infections, marasmus, and kwashiorkor. In developed countries, the most common presentation is poor growth detected in an ambulatory setting; in developing countries, recurrent infections, marasmus, and kwashiorkor are more common presentations.

The degree of FTT is usually measured by calculating each growth parameter (weight, height, and weight/height ratio) as a percentage of the median value for age based on appropriate growth charts. Appropriate growth charts are often not available for children with specific medical problems; serial measurements are especially important for these children. For premature infants, correction must be made for the extent of prematurity. Corrected age, rather than chronologic age, should be used in calculations of their growth percentiles until 1–2 yr of corrected age.

For weight, mild, moderate, and severe FTT is equivalent to 75–90%, 60–74%, and less than 60% of standard, respectively. For height, the corresponding values are 90–95%, 85–89%, and less than 85%. For the weight/height ratio, the values are 81–90%, 70–80%, and less than 70%. The weight for age per cent of the standard value traditionally decreases early in the course of FTT, followed by a decrement of height for age. Children with chronic malnutrition often have a normal weight for height because both their weight and height are reduced.

The laboratory evaluation of children with FTT is often not helpful and, therefore, should be used judiciously. A complete blood count, lead level, urinalysis, and set of electrolyte values represent a reasonable initial screen. Other tests, such as thyroid function studies, tests for gastroesophageal reflux and malabsorption, organic and amino acids, or a sweat test, should be performed if indicated by the history or physical examination.

DIAGNOSIS. The history, physical examination, and observation of the parent-child interaction usually suggest the diagnosis. The latter observation, especially with feeding, is often critical to the diagnosis of psychosocial FTT.

The causes of insufficient growth include (1) failure of a parent to offer adequate calories, (2) failure of the child to take sufficient calories, and (3) failure of the child to retain sufficient calories. Reasons why parents or their substitute may not offer appropriate or sufficient foods include lack of knowledge, parental depression, unusual dietary beliefs, or lack of food. With young infants, it is particularly important to obtain a detailed dietary history, including what the diet consists of, how often the infant is fed, and how the parents respond when the child cries or sleeps for prolonged periods. Children may have difficulty swallowing if they have oral-motor dysfunction, anatomic abnormalities, cardiopulmonary

TABLE 36–2 Approach to Failure to Thrive Based on Age

Age of Onset	Major Diagnostic Consideration
Birth to 3 mo	Psychosocial failure to thrive, perinatal infections, gastroesophageal reflux, inborn errors of metabolism, cystic fibrosis
3–6 mo	Psychosocial failure to thrive, human immunodeficiency virus infection, gastroesophageal reflux, inborn errors of metabolism, milk protein intolerance, cystic fibrosis, renal tubular acidosis
7–12 mo	Psychosocial failure to thrive (autonomy struggles), delayed introduction of solids, gastroesophageal reflux, intestinal parasites, renal tubular acidosis
12+ mo	Psychosocial failure to thrive (coercive feeding, new psychologic stressor), gastroesophageal reflux

Adapted from Frank D, Silva M, Needlman R: Failure to thrive: Mystery, myth and method. Contemp Pediatr 10:114, 1993.

dysfunction, or enlarged and recurrently infected tonsils and adenoids. Vomiting, diarrhea, and malabsorption are general causes of inadequate caloric absorption. It may be helpful to approach the diagnosis in terms of age (Table 36–2) or signs and symptoms (Table 36–3).

A syndrome of growth failure and hyperphagia/polydipsia associated with growth hormone deficiency has also been described. Children age 3–13 yr were affected, many had been abused, and growth hormone levels returned to normal after removal from stressful circumstances.

TREATMENT. The treatment of FTT requires an understanding of all the elements that contribute to a child's growth: a child's health and nutritional status, family issues, and the parent-child interaction. Regardless of cause, an appropriate feeding atmosphere at home is important. Children with severe malnutrition must be refed carefully.

For children with organic FTT, the underlying medical condition should be treated. The type of caloric supplementation must be based on the severity of FTT and the underlying medical condition. For example, in children with renal failure, the amount of protein in the diet must be carefully monitored. The response to caloric supplementation depends on the specific diagnosis, medical treatment, and severity of FTT.

For older infants and young children with psychosocial FTT, mealtimes should be approximately 20–30 min, solid foods should be offered before liquids, environmental distractions should be minimized, and children should eat with other people and not be force fed. The intake of water, juice, and low-calorie beverages should be limited. High-calorie foods, such as peanut butter, whole milk, cheese, and dried fruits, should be emphasized. High-calorie supplementation, such as Polycose, or high-calorie liquids, such as Carnation Instant Breakfast with whole milk, or formulas containing more than 20 calories per ounce (PediaSure, Ensure, and Resource) are

TABLE 36–3 Approach to Failure to Thrive Based on Signs and Symptoms

History/Physical Examination	Diagnostic Consideration
Spitting, vomiting, food refusal	Gastroesophageal reflux
Diarrhea, fatty stools	Malabsorption, intestinal parasite, milk protein intolerance
Snoring, mouth breathing, enlarged tonsils	Adenoid hypertrophy, obstructive sleep apnea
Recurrent wheezing, pulmonary infections	Asthma, aspiration
Recurrent infections	Human immunodeficiency virus disease
Travel to/from developing countries	Parasitic or bacterial infections of the gastrointestinal tract

Adapted from Frank D, Silva M, Needlman R: Failure to thrive: Mystery, myth and method. Contemp Pediatr 10:114, 1993.

sometimes necessary. Weight gain in response to adequate caloric feedings usually establishes the diagnosis of psychosocial FTT.

Indications for hospitalization include severe malnutrition, further diagnostic and laboratory evaluation, lack of catch-up growth, and evaluation of the parent-child feeding interaction. Parents of children with organic FTT should be comfortable with the diagnosis and treatment before discharge. For psychosocial FTT, hospitalization often lasts 10 days to 2 wk. Caloric intake should be monitored, and the parent-child feeding interaction should be observed (Chapter 35.2). The goals of hospitalization are to obtain sustained catch-up growth and educate parents about appropriate foods and feeding styles. For both organic and psychosocial FTT, the approach to feeding in the hospital should mimic the anticipated treatment at home before discharge.

PROGNOSIS. FTT in the 1st yr of life, regardless of cause, is particularly ominous. Maximal postnatal brain growth occurs during the first 6 mo of life. The brain grows as much during the 1st yr of life as during the rest of a child's life. Approximately one third of children with psychosocial FTT are developmentally delayed and have social and emotional problems. The prognosis for children with organic FTT is more variable, depending on the specific diagnosis and severity of FTT. Ongoing assessment and monitoring of cognitive and emotional development, with appropriate intervention, is necessary for all children with FTT.

Berwick DM, Levey JC, Kleinerman R: Failure to thrive: Diagnostic yield of hospitalization. Arch Dis Child 57:347, 1982.
Bithoney WG, Dubowitz H, Egan H: Failure to thrive/growth deficiency. Pediatr Rev 13:453, 1992.
Drotar D, Sturm L: Prediction of intellectual development in young children with early histories of nonorganic failure-to-thrive. J Pediatr Psychol 13:281, 1988.
Fleishe DR: Comprehensive management of infants with gastroesophageal reflux and failure to thrive. Curr Probl Pediatr 25:247, 1995.
Frank D, Silva M, Needlman R: Failure to thrive: Mystery, myth and method. Contemp Pediatr 10:114, 1993.
Kelleher KJ, Casey PH, Bradley RH, et al: Risk factors and outcomes for failure to thrive in low birth weight preterm infants. Pediatrics 91:941, 1993.
Maggion A, Lifshitz F: Nutritional management of failure to thrive. Pediatr Clin North Am 42:791, 1995.
Skuse D, Stanhope R: A new stress-related syndrome of growth failure and hyperphagia in children associated with reversibility of growth hormone insufficiency. Lancet 348:355, 1996.
Wright CM, Waterston A, Aynsley-Green A: Effect of deprivation on weight gain in infancy. Acta Pediatr 83:357, 1994.

CHAPTER 37
Developmental Disabilities and Chronic Illness: An Overview

James M. Perrin and Jack P. Shonkoff

Children with special health care needs constitute a heterogeneous population that includes youngsters with a wide variety of developmental disabilities and chronic illnesses. Although estimates of the size of this population vary greatly (partly because of the wide spectrum of severity of various conditions), data from the 1994–1995 National Health Interview Survey indicate that 15–18% of children and adolescents have some form of chronic condition, including physical conditions, developmental disabilities, disorders of learning, and primary mental health conditions. Adding speech defects, visual and hearing impairments, repeated ear infections, skin allergies, and other common conditions raises the prevalence to over 30%. Approximately 6–7% of all children and adolescents have some limitation of activity due to a chronic health condition, and 1–2% meet the very severe definition of disability used by the federal Supplemental Security Income (SSI) program, which is the main cash support program of the United States for people of all ages with disabling conditions. Within these groups, approximately 40% of children have disorders of development and learning; 35%, chronic physical conditions; and 25%, chronic mental health conditions. With improvements in health care and access to services in the last few decades, almost all these children and adolescents survive to adulthood, although often with major physical or psychologic consequences related to their condition. Although in some cases conditions fall into more than one category, most children's problems fall within a single classification. A core of basic considerations applies to most children with chronic conditions, and these issues will be discussed first.

Early detection of persistent conditions, amelioration of the functional consequences of specific disabilities, and prevention of secondary psychosocial handicaps are central to the provision of care for children with special health needs. Caregivers should recognize the importance of treating the whole child in a family and community context. Health care providers occasionally and inappropriately refer to children with chronic conditions by the name of their condition, such as "asthmatics," "sicklers," "leukemics," or "Down's babies." This tendency to characterize children by their disease or disability adversely influences both parental and professional attitudes as well as objective assessments of the child's current abilities and expectations for the future. In general, parents and professionals should work together on behalf of a child who has a disease rather than allowing the disease to define the child.

Most children receive the majority of their health care from a single provider and are educated in regular school settings that require no modifications to meet special developmental or health concerns. Children with special health needs, on the other hand, may see a variety of health care specialists (e.g., neurologists, orthopedists, cardiologists), interact with multiple professionals (e.g., occupational therapists, respiratory therapists, nutritionists, psychologists), and need major adaptive modifications in their school setting (e.g., barrier-free facilities, special education services, and specialized nursing care). Some of these services, especially those of pediatric subspecialists, are provided in hospital-based programs; others, such as home health care and certain supportive therapies, may be offered in community settings. Thus, the pediatrician needs a working knowledge of community services available to families and should help coordinate the subspecialty services received.

An appreciation of the multiple levels at which prevention or treatment efforts can be implemented requires an understanding of the differences inherent in the concepts of disease, functional limitation, and disability or social impact. Disease refers to a specific health condition affecting a child, such as arthritis or congenital cytomegalovirus (CMV) infection. Functional limitation refers to the problem brought about as a result of the symptoms of the disease, such as a poorly functioning knee or a hearing impairment. Social impact (disability), on the other hand, refers to the social consequences of having the disease or disability, such as the inability to participate competitively in sports or the social isolation that results from difficulty in communicating orally.

Physicians can play a key role in preventing the occurrence of many special health needs and in diminishing their impact on a child's growth and development. Intervention may be targeted at the level of the disease, the functional limitation, or the disability. For the child with arthritis, efforts are directed both toward reducing joint inflammation and toward removing barriers to participation in age-appropriate physical activities. For the child with congenital CMV infection and deafness, successful management focuses on both audiologic habilitation and social integration.

For children under age 3 yr, early intervention (EI) programs provide a mechanism for decreasing the impact of special health or developmental needs on children and their families. EI programs that incorporate the best practices offer individualized services designed to strengthen the inherent adaptiveness of participating children and families. Older children may need special education evaluations and services or special adaptations to maximize their school attendance. Because of their strategic relationship with young children and their parents, physicians have an important responsibility with regard to early identification of children at risk and referral to the appropriate services (see also Chapter 5). This responsibility includes maintaining accurate and updated information on all available resources within a community to ensure that families have access to a full range of needed services. Except in the hospital, a child's family provides most care, at times an extraordinary amount of extra caretaking. Parental health, mental health, and well-being strongly affect child health outcomes in the context of disability. The best predictors of the well-being of children with special health needs include factors that relate to family health and functioning; effective pediatric management should therefore embody a comprehensive approach to the child in the context of the family, addressing the needs of all its members.

Several public programs in the United States assist families of children with special health needs. In addition, parent groups in many communities help parents learn effective techniques for caring for children with chronic conditions and for obtaining the necessary health and educational services. Title V Maternal and Child Health Programs for Children with Special Health Needs provide a variety of coordinating and multidisciplinary clinical services for children who have chronic illnesses and developmental disabilities. The Individuals with Disability Education Act (IDEA) supports state-sponsored early intervention and special education programs and mandates an appropriate education in the least restrictive environment for children with disabilities. The SSI program provides cash benefits for families whose children have severe physical, mental, or developmental disabilities as well as public health insurance coverage (i.e., Medicaid) in almost every state.

Increasingly, whether under private or public insurance, children with special health care needs receive services through managed care organizations. When parents of children with chronic conditions have a choice, they may avoid managed care arrangements. Most states, however, are currently enrolling their Medicaid populations, with and without disability, in managed care plans. Monitoring systems to ensure that children with disabilities have access to enrollment and to appropriate services when enrolled are in development, but most programs currently lack such methods of assessment. Child health professionals should have enough information regarding public programs and public services to refer families appropriately and to provide the clinical information necessary for families to obtain appropriate services. Within managed care arrangements, especially absent effective monitoring systems, pediatricians will need to help assure access to appropriate services.

Despite the variations among conditions and their clinical requirements, families caring for children with any of these long-term conditions typically face key times of transition when additional community and health services may be necessary to improve child and adolescent functioning. This is especially the case at discharge from hospital to home after a long and complex intensive care experience or other management related to the initial diagnosis. Many families initially rely on hospital-based services to provide a wide range of therapies and now must take on responsibilities for home care, including providing services themselves and coordinating services from a variety of therapists in the home setting. Although discharge plans from hospital-based services may work well in the first few months, as nurses and equipment vendors change and as parents increasingly develop their own skills the new arrangement needs ongoing monitoring and help. A second period of difficult transition for families is at entry to school, where the management of the child's health condition—at times specialized services within the school setting—and plans for emergencies or medication use affect the planning for him or her. Clinicians can help ensure both the child's integration into school and the availability of school services and plans appropriate to his or her needs. A third time of transition is at adolescence, when many chronic conditions delay onset of puberty or affect cognitive abilities and make many aspects of adolescent life particularly complex. Chronic conditions may influence the ways of approaching risk-taking behaviors, substance and drug use, or the development of healthy sexuality. Families may need support and advice from clinicians during their child's adolescence. Finally, the transition to adulthood of adolescents with disabilities is made more complex because of difficulties in obtaining health insurance, gaining access to educational and vocational services, shifting from pediatric and adolescent care to adult health services, and achieving personal and economic independence.

37.1 *Chronic Illness in Childhood*

James M. Perrin

EPIDEMIOLOGY, SEVERITY, AND OUTCOME. The *epidemiology* of chronic illness in childhood differs in important ways from that of long-term illness in adults. Adults face a relatively small number of common chronic conditions (e.g., diabetes, osteoarthritis, coronary artery disease) and few rare diseases. Children, in contrast, face a wide variety of mainly quite rare diseases. Only two groups of chronic physical conditions in childhood are common: allergic disorders (mainly asthma, eczema, and hay fever) and neurologic disorders (mainly seizure disorders and neuromuscular conditions such as cerebral palsy). Other conditions often thought to be common, such as childhood diabetes, occur in only about 1 in 1,000 children younger than 16 yr, a much lower rate than is seen in adults. Many of the conditions described in this textbook occur with a frequency of much less than 1/1,000. Table 37–1 indicates prevalence rates for representative childhood conditions.

These epidemiologic distinctions have implications for both physicians and families. The adult pattern means that health care providers for adults have frequent daily experience with the common chronic illnesses of adults, remaining current and knowledgeable about such conditions as hypertension. Similarly, an adult who has been newly diagnosed with high blood pressure probably knows something about the disease and has friends or family members with hypertension. The practicing pediatrician, however, may see a new case of a malignancy only once in a decade and will make the diagnosis of cystic fibrosis or even diabetes infrequently. A family whose child has been newly diagnosed with a rare condition may never even have heard the name of the disease prior to its onset in their child. These epidemiologic facts mean that child health care providers have a difficult task in identifying children with rare conditions and in staying current with applicable technologies.

TABLE 37–1 Estimated Prevalence of Representative Childhood Chronic Conditions, Ages 0–20, United States

Chronic Conditions	Rates/1,000
Asthma (moderate and severe)	15.00
Congenital heart disease	10.00
Seizure disorder	3.00
Arthritis	3.00
Diabetes mellitus	1.40
Cleft lip/palate	1.40
Sickle cell anemia	1.20
Down syndrome	1.00
Cystic fibrosis	0.20
Hemophilia	0.15
Acute lymphocytic leukemia	0.11
Muscular dystrophy	0.06

Adapted from Gortmaker SL, Sappenfield W: Chronic childhood disorders: Prevalence and impact. Pediatr Clin North Am 31:3, 1984; and Newacheck PW, Taylor WR: Childhood chronic illness: Prevalence, severity, and impact. Am J Public Health 82:364, 1992.

The aggregate number of children with all types of chronic health conditions is high, despite the rarity of individual conditions, mainly because the number of different conditions that affect children is very large. Up to 30% of children have some chronic condition, although most are mild, such as acne, hay fever, and other respiratory allergies, or a mild congenital deformity causing a slight limp. Only about 6–7% of children (3–4 million children) have diseases of such physiologic severity that they interfere on a regular basis with a child's daily activities.

Severity is difficult to measure in most chronic illnesses. Although new techniques increasingly define the underlying molecular basis for many conditions, these biologic markers do not commonly correlate well with clinical indicators of severity. Most measures of severity (e.g., asthma rating scales or hemoglobin A_{1C} in diabetes) reflect the interaction of biologic susceptibility, treatment, and other environmental factors. The effect of the condition on the child's development (cognitive, behavioral, and physical) and on functioning with friends or in school is another aspect of severity. Although this chapter focuses on health conditions that physiologically are relatively severe, many of the issues discussed affect children with milder conditions. Further, one type of severity (e.g., physiologic or clinical) may correlate poorly with others (e.g., psychologic or functional).

The percentage of children with severe, long-term illnesses has more than doubled in the past two decades. This change reflects major advances in the technology of medical and surgical care and marked improvements in survival more than increased incidence of chronic conditions. Current estimates are that, even among severely ill children, at least 90% survive to young adulthood. Asthma, the most common chronic condition in childhood, has increased in incidence in the past decade, however. Rates of a few other conditions of much lower prevalence also have increased in recent years, including AIDS, the aftereffects of fetal substance exposure, and major pulmonary or neurologic disease in children leaving neonatal intensive care units. On the other hand, new genetic techniques allow the prenatal and preconception diagnosis of increasing numbers of health conditions, and genetic counseling and other interventions have diminished the incidence of other diseases.

ISSUES COMMON TO DIVERSE CHRONIC CONDITIONS. Health care providers typically view each chronic illness as a distinct and separate entity that has its own etiology, natural history, treatment, complications, and physiologic impact. However, families of children with a variety of long-term illnesses face several issues in common, reflecting chronicity itself rather than aspects of the specific disease.

Many chronic childhood illnesses are *high-cost health conditions*. A small percentage of children with major chronic illnesses utilize a large proportion of the child health dollar; 2–4% of children with severe long-term illnesses account for at least 35% of all child health expenditures. These figures reflect only what is paid by public or private insurance. Families face many other expenses, such as the costs of transportation, long-distance phone calls, and special diets, few of which may be reimbursed. Furthermore, chronic illness in a child makes it more difficult for both parents to work outside the home, thereby diminishing the family's financial resources.

The *daily burden of care rests mainly with the families*, and that burden can be extensive, as with a family with two teenagers with muscular dystrophy, both wheelchair-bound and requiring transportation from place to place, or with a youngster with cystic fibrosis who needs time-consuming pulmonary care prior to leaving for school each day. These daily burdens greatly extend the work of families.

Whereas most children require only a single provider for most of their health care and supervision, *children with long-term health conditions frequently have multiple providers and multiple treatments*. A child with hemophilia may have contact with a hematologist, a pediatrician, a specialized dentist, an orthopedist, a hematology nurse, a physical therapist, a psychologist, and a social worker, among others. The recommendations of any member of this group may vary from those of another, and families must often choose among conflicting advice. Clinically, there usually are trade-offs among the choices, such as the optimal time to do a surgical procedure or the balance between seizure control and alertness. Pediatricians can help families make informed choices.

The comparative rarity of most childhood chronic conditions makes *families feel isolated*. They often wonder why they have been singled out by an unusual condition, and they feel that no other families have had similar experiences. Family programs in specialty centers (e.g., cystic fibrosis or arthritis centers) and parent advocacy programs have worked to break this sense of isolation through groups that help parents learn from each other how to raise children with chronic conditions.

Many of these conditions are unpredictable in their implications, longevity, complications, and developmental impact on the child. The parent whose child has leukemia wonders whether new bleeding signals a relapse that will have a fatal outcome or will be followed by a permanent remission. The parent whose child has mild wheezing at bedtime does not know whether the child will sleep well through the night or awaken severely dyspneic in the middle of the night in need of emergency care. Parents speak frequently of how difficult this unpredictability is for them and how they wish for clear answers to difficult questions, even if the answers may be unfavorable. Many important aspects of chronic disease are unpredictable, both because of great variability in environmental influences and biologic responsiveness to specific conditions and treatments and because little information is available about many rare diseases.

Many chronic conditions and their treatments cause great *pain*, far in excess of that faced by other children. Sickle cell anemia, hemophilia, arthritis, and leukemia are examples of conditions characterized at times by severe pain.

Chronic illness has a *pervasive influence on a child's daily life*. Frequent interactions with the medical care system, occasional hospitalization, and greater dependence on parents and health care providers characterize their lives. A chronic health impairment may create a sense of "differentness," of being unable to do many things that other children can do.

Finally, a chronic illness creates *additional stresses and demands on families and on children* that apparently healthy children do not face. Perhaps as a result, chronically ill children have about twice the frequency of psychologic or behavioral problems found in healthy control subjects; children with significant neurologic handicaps or sensory deficits have as much as a five times greater risk for these problems. The level of severity correlates poorly with psychologic status. Despite this greater risk of psychologic maladjustment, most children with chronic health conditions are psychologically healthy.

DEVELOPMENTAL ASPECTS OF LONG-TERM ILLNESS. Two issues are central to an understanding of the developmental implications of long-term childhood illness: the development of children's understanding of illness mechanisms and the impact of illness at different stages of child development.

Clinicians working with children who have long-term illnesses should understand the *developmental stage of their patients' understanding of illness* in order to explain illness and its mechanisms in age-appropriate terms. Because their understanding follows a typical pattern of growth in cognitive abilities, children need different explanations of their continuing disease as they mature. Young children of preschool or early school age tend to have a concrete and relatively superficial understanding of illness. They view illness as a response to their bad behavior or not following the rules (such as wearing a coat to go outside in the cold). Children at this age believe that getting well occurs by adhering to another set of rules. By about the 4th–6th grade, children begin to differentiate themselves from external events that may cause illness. For this age group, germ theory seems very important; with the notion that germs cause almost all illnesses, illness can be prevented by avoiding germs, and better results will be gained from taking medicines, which are seen as fighting germs. This notion of germs can cause confusion or isolation for children of this age who have conditions such as leukemia or diabetes. By 8th grade or even later, children begin to understand the physiologic mechanisms for illness, appreciating the many interrelated causes and the several symptoms of illness. At this age, children usually begin to understand the interaction of body parts, for example, that lungs and hearts are not only near each other but actually work together to maintain body functions.

Physical illness has different effects on children based on their stage of development (see Chapters 7–16). In infancy, the illness may affect the parameters of growth and development by influencing feeding, sleeping, motor abilities (and therefore exploration of the environment), and sensory functions. Physical deformity or fatigue may affect a child's responsiveness to parents, who may in turn react differently to this child. Frequent hospitalizations may interfere with the normal development of trusting relationships within a family. In later preschool years, when children are developing autonomy, mobility, and self-control, illness may again interfere with these important developmental functions. Early school-aged children may be subject to teasing from classmates; they may need to be absent from school for illness or its treatment and thus miss normal opportunities for early socialization. Middle childhood and adolescence are periods when children expand their areas of competence; responsibility for the care of the child's health condition should shift gradually from the parents to the child. Chronic illness may interfere with this process.

In adolescence, illness may affect the individual's developing independence, greater responsibility for self-care, growing intimacy, and planning for the future. The disease or its treatment may be particularly embarrassing for adolescents and may affect their body image. Adolescence is frequently a time to test the limits of the illness and compliance with recommended therapies. Health conditions that require another person for some care (such as the case of the teenager with cystic fibrosis who needs pulmonary physical therapy before each day of high school) may hinder growth toward independence. With appropriate services, most adolescents with chronic conditions make the transition to adulthood well, with little interference in their finishing education, becoming employed, and entering into significant interpersonal relationships. Sensitivity to the developmental impact of chronic illness will help clinicians provide their patients with appropriate planning and anticipatory guidance and help children and their families find acceptable ways of fulfilling the normal developmental tasks of childhood and adolescence.

Children should take increasing responsibility for the management of their own health condition commensurate with their level of maturity, developmental stage, and understanding of their illness. Areas of responsibility include monitoring the condition, assessing indicators of change and exacerbation, asking for help, and being responsible for self-medication (both at home and at school). Families may need help in learning ways to foster responsibility, and children need education and advice in learning how to become independent in appropriate ways.

INTEGRATING CHILDREN WITH CHRONIC CONDITIONS INTO COMMUNITIES. Changing interests of families, changing notions of the civil rights of people with disabilities, and improved technologies have fostered an increasing emphasis on family-centered services for children with chronic conditions. Parents increasingly take responsibility for monitoring and managing the care of their child, and more care is provided in or near the child's home and less in hospitals. Families want to receive most care in community settings and want to integrate their chronically ill child into community activities, not limiting him or her to services provided mainly for children with special health needs.

Providing services in the community also strengthens early socialization of the child, mainly through participation in child care and, later, social and educational development through participation in school programs. Chronic illness accounts for a sizable number of school absences. Part of that time away from classes reflects the direct effects of illness, such as increased fatigue or necessary hospitalization; however, some represents the need to travel great distances for treatments that are often available only during regular school hours.

Some children with chronic illnesses, especially those with cognitive impairments, need special education services. However, most children with long-term illnesses have no intrinsic cognitive impairment and should be in regular education programs. They may need specialized health services (e.g., access to medicines or planning for emergencies) in order to participate in school, and children who must miss classes frequently need home or hospital instruction to allow them to keep up with their classmates.

Families whose children have long-term health conditions should have access to a wide range of coordinated and comprehensive services. The specific services needed by any one family will vary considerably from those needed by another and will change over time as the child grows and the family changes. The main groups of services that should be available for families include primary and specialized medical and surgical care; nursing services, especially those that will help to strengthen a family's own skills in caring for their child; preventive and therapeutic mental health services; social services; educational planning; and certain special therapies, such as physical therapy, occupational therapy, and nutritional services. Preventive mental health services help diminish the risk of psychologic problems related to the chronicity of the child's condition.

Partly because of the emphasis on specialized medical services and frequent surgeries, hospitalization, or other acute episodes, children with chronic health conditions lack regular pediatric health supervision. They have lower rates of immunization and screening for common health problems and often lack anticipatory guidance in key areas of growth and development, such as behavior and discipline in the preschool years, preparation for entry to school, and preparation for adolescence, with developing sexuality, growth of independence, and opportunity for substance abuse. Lack of adequate primary care has been associated with greater likelihood of hospitalization for children with some chronic conditions such as asthma, in which preventive use of anti-inflammatory drugs can diminish the number and severity of episodes. The primary care provider should help ensure that children receive services aimed at preventing exacerbation of their condition or diminishing its severity (Chapter 5).

PEDIATRIC CARE IN THE COMMUNITY. Community pediatricians have a central role in the care of children with chronic illnesses and in supporting their families. Although the pediatrician's involvement may begin with diagnosis and referral to subspecialty services, he or she should also assume responsibility as a continuing advocate for the child and family. This includes continuing communication with specialty providers and helping families make informed choices, especially when advice is conflicting. Along with ongoing primary care, the pediatrician should work with subspecialty services to coordinate medical care and help with efforts to prevent morbidity. Educating parents and children about the disease process and its management, complications, and developmental implications is a central part of the therapeutic effort. Other responsibilities include continued support for children and family members, helping families locate appropriate community resources, and, especially, collaborating with schools and agencies to integrate the child into the community. Tasks with agencies include referral to early intervention services, when appropriate; providing information that may help determine whether a child needs special or regular education services; and helping the child obtain the school services that enhance school attendance. Needed school services typically include appropriate nursing and related services and access to medications or emergency care, although a few children require more extensive services, including personal attendants.

Communication with families is particularly important. Families want clear information, with details that they can understand and information about both positive and negative aspects of the child's condition. They particularly appreciate receiving information and support from a professional familiar to them who provides compassionate and caring services. The child should also participate in developmentally appropriate ways in information sharing.

American Academy of Pediatrics: Screening infants and young children for developmental disabilities. Pediatrics 93:863, 1994.
American Academy of Pediatrics: Guidelines for home care of infants, children, and adolescents with chronic disease. Pediatrics 96:161, 1995.
American Academy of Pediatrics: Sexuality education of children and adolescents with developmental disabilities. Pediatrics 97:275, 1996.
Goldberg AI, Gardner HG, Gibson LE: Home care: The next frontier of pediatric practice. J Pediatr 125:686, 1994.
Gortmaker SL, Sappenfield W: Chronic childhood disorders: Prevalence and impact. Pediatr Clin North Am 31:3, 1984.
Newacheck PW, Taylor WR: Childhood chronic illness: Prevalence, severity, and impact. Am J Public Health 82:364, 1992.
Perrin EC, Gerrity PS: There's a demon in your belly: Children's understanding of illness. Pediatrics 67:841, 1981.
Perrin EC, Gerrity PS: Development of children with chronic illness. Pediatr Clin North Am 31:19, 1984.
Perrin JM, Shayne MW, Bloom SR: Home and Community Care for Chronically Ill Children. New York, Oxford University Press, 1993.
Pless IB, Power C, Peckham CS: Long-term sequelae of chronic physical disorders in childhood. Pediatrics 91:1131, 1993.
Stein REK (ed): Caring for Children with Chronic Illness. New York, Springer, 1989.
Strauss D, Ashwal S, Shavelle R, et al: Prognosis for survival and improved function in children with severe developmental disabilities. J Pediatr 131:712, 1997.

37.2 *Mental Retardation*

Jack P. Shonkoff

Mental retardation is a condition of both clinical and social importance. It is characterized by limitations in performance that result from significant impairments in measured intelligence and adaptive behavior. It also confers a social status that can be more handicapping than the specific disability itself. Because the boundaries between "normality" and "retardation" frequently are difficult to delineate, the pediatric identification, evaluation, and care of children with cognitive difficulties and their families require a considerable level of both technical sophistication and interpersonal sensitivity.

Dramatic changes in social and political attitudes during the past few decades toward persons with developmental disabilities have revolutionized the pediatric approach to children with mental retardation. Previous practices of withholding life-saving measures from neonates with congenital abnormalities have been modified by legally enforced treatments for children with profound and irreversible disorders. The practice of almost automatically placing young children with disabilities in residential institutions has been replaced by extensive efforts to develop community-based service systems that coordinate resources for both children and their families. The pediatric responsibility has shifted from helping "put the child away" to "normalizing" the life of the child and his or her family.

Concurrent with this shift in sociopolitical values, our theoretical and empirical understanding of the phenomenon of mental retardation has also changed. The expanding knowledge base has led to a rejection of the simplistic debate over "organic" vs "environmental" causes of retardation and to a growing recognition of the interactive contributions of nature and nurture to the development of all children. Consequently, the traditional medical focus on neuropathology has been expanded to an assessment of the interplay among the biologic factors in the child, the adaptive characteristics of the family, and the social context in which they live.

In 1992, the American Association on Mental Retardation revised its official definition to formalize the paradigm shift from viewing mental retardation as an individual trait to thinking of it as an expression of the interaction between a person with limited intellectual functioning and the environment. Consequently, categories of mild, moderate, severe, and profound retardation have been replaced by a classification system that specifies four levels of support systems needed for daily functioning (i.e., intermittent, limited, extensive, and pervasive). Four assumptions were articulated as essential to the appropriate application of the new definition: (1) Valid assessment considers cultural and linguistic diversities; (2) limitations in adaptive skills occur within the context of community environments typical of age peers and indexed to individualized needs for supports; (3) adaptive limitations coexist with strengths; and (4) with appropriate and sustained supports, the life functioning of individuals with mental retardation will generally improve.

ETIOLOGY AND PATHOGENESIS. The determinants of competence in any individual are complex and multifactorial. Regardless of his or her level of performance, each child's abilities are influenced by both the integrity and the maturational status of the nervous system and by the nature and quality of his or her life experience. Some children sustain significant neurologic insults and develop normal skills. Others manifest severe cognitive impairment despite the absence of recognizable focal neurologic findings or historical evidence of significant risk factors for CNS dysfunction. The neurobiologic roots of mental retardation may be found among such diverse factors as structural malformations of the brain, metabolic abnormalities, and CNS deficits related to infection, malnutrition, or hypoxic-ischemic injury. The environmental precursors of retardation may be identified in histories of impaired caregiving related to parental psychopathology, extreme family disorganization, or economic hardship. Children who live in poverty are particularly susceptible to the cumulative burdens of social stress and the greater biologic vulnerability related to a higher prevalence of such risk factors as perinatal complications and nutritional deficiencies.

Table 37–2 lists potential contributing factors in the pathogenesis of mental retardation from preconception through the early childhood years. Few of these etiologic factors, however, provide a complete explanation for the phenomenon of retardation in any single individual. Rather, the evolution of this developmental disability reflects the complex interplay among multiple risk and protective factors.

TABLE 37–2 Potential Contributing Factors in the Pathogenesis of Mental Retardation

Preconceptual Disorders

Single gene abnormalities (e.g., inborn errors of metabolism, neurocutaneous disorders)
Chromosomal abnormalities (e.g., X-linked disorders, translocations, fragile X syndrome)
Mitochondrial abnormalities
Polygenic familial syndromes

Early Embryonic Disruptions

Chromosomal disorders (e.g., trisomies, mosaics)
Infections (e.g., CMV, rubella, toxoplasmosis, HIV)
Teratogens (e.g., alcohol, radiation)
Placental dysfunction
Congenital CNS malformations (idiopathic)

Fetal Brain Insults

Infections (e.g., HIV, toxoplasmosis, CMV, herpes simplex)
Toxins (e.g., alcohol, cocaine, lead, maternal phenylketonuria, maternal tobacco smoking[?])
Placental insufficiency/intrauterine malnutrition

Perinatal Difficulties

Extreme prematurity
Hypoxic-ischemic injury
Intracranial hemorrhage
Metabolic disorders (e.g., hypoglycemia, hyperbilirubinemia)
Infections (e.g., herpes simplex, bacterial meningitis)

Postnatal Brain Insults

Infections (e.g., encephalitis, meningitis)
Trauma (e.g., severe head injury)
Asphyxia (e.g., near-drowning, prolonged apnea, suffocation)
Metabolic disorders (e.g., hypoglycemia, hypernatremia)
Toxins (e.g., lead)
Intracranial hemorrhage
Malnutrition

Postnatal Experiential Disruptions

Poverty and family disorganization
Dysfunctional infant-caregiver interaction
Parental psychopathology
Parental substance abuse

Unknown Influences

EPIDEMIOLOGY. Approximately 3% of the general population has an IQ less than two standard deviations below the mean. It has been estimated that 80–90% of persons with mental retardation function within the mild range, whereas only 5% of the population with mental retardation is severely to profoundly impaired. The prevalence of mild retardation varies inversely with socioeconomic status, whereas moderate to severe disability occurs with equal frequency across all income groups. Because a diagnosis of mental retardation relies on an assessment of adaptive behavior and not solely on IQ, the epidemiology varies with the life cycle. The reported incidence of retardation increases initially with age, the numbers rising sharply in the early school years and then declining in late adolescence as individuals with mild impairments leave the formal education setting and are assimilated into the "normal" adult world. Identification of children with mild retardation in the preschool period is most commonly precipitated by concerns about the development of language.

CLINICAL MANIFESTATIONS. Children with physical findings suggestive of recognizable syndromes that are associated with mental retardation should be identified at birth or during early infancy. Down syndrome, fetal alcohol syndrome, and primary microcephaly are examples of such conditions. These disorders, however, represent a small percentage of the population of youngsters with intellectual impairment. The overwhelming majority are identified because of their failure to meet age-appropriate expectations.

Delayed achievement of developmental milestones is the cardinal symptom of mental retardation. Although youngsters with severe impairment show marked delays in psychomotor skills in the first year of life, children with moderate retardation typically exhibit normal motor development and present with delayed speech and language abilities in the toddler years. Mild retardation, on the other hand, may not be suspected until after entry into school, although participation in an organized preschool or child-care program can highlight discrepancies in the performance of a young child with significantly subaverage abilities.

The natural history of mental retardation is highly variable and influenced by the availability of appropriate educational and therapeutic experiences as well as by neuromaturation and the presence of associated disabilities. Although many youngsters may experience transient "plateau periods" during which measurable progress appears to be minimal, most individuals with mental retardation acquire new skills and continue to learn throughout their lifetimes. The ability to formulate accurate prognoses, except for children who manifest severe to profound retardation, is limited, especially during the preschool years. Generally speaking, children within the relatively mild range of retardation who receive appropriate education can achieve 4th to 6th grade reading levels and may be able to function relatively independently as adults. Individuals with more significant intellectual limitations require greater degrees of supervision, depending on their range of adaptive abilities. Children with histories that suggest a loss of previously acquired skills represent an important subgroup for whom the diagnosis of a progressive rather than a static neurologic disorder must be investigated. In such cases, developmental deterioration is rarely reversible, yet a precise diagnosis is important for genetic counseling and informed family support.

A thorough pediatric history is essential to identify relevant contributing factors as well as to document the evolving pattern of the child's developmental skills over time. The product of the history should be a comprehensive inventory of risk factors (both within the child and within his or her environment) that increase the likelihood of developmental impairment (see Table 37–2) as well as protective factors that may contribute to more adaptive functioning. Important protective factors include good physical health, a normal rate of growth, healthy parent-child attachment, and a cohesive family unit within a supportive social network.

A systematic physical examination may reveal findings that help explain the etiology of the child's disability or that identify particular treatment needs. Table 37–3 lists a number of atypical physical features that have been associated with a higher incidence of mental retardation. In some cases, a specific cluster of phenotypic characteristics may suggest a diagnosable syndrome related to a chromosomal abnormality or known teratogenic effect. It should be emphasized, however, that many of these physical features are found in children without developmental disabilities; some tend to be familial; and several appear with greater prevalence among specific ethnic groups.

TABLE 37–3 Atypical Physical Features That May Be Associated with Increased Incidence of Mental Retardation

Hair	Double whorl Fine, friable, prematurely gray or white locks Sparse or absent hair
Eyes	Microphthalmia Hypertelorism Hypotelorism Upward-and-outward or downward-and-outward slant Inner or outer epicanthal folds Coloboma of iris or retina Brushfield spots Eccentrically placed pupil Nystagmus
Ears	Low-set pinna Simple or abnormal helix formation
Nose	Flattened bridge Small size Upturned nares
Face	Increased length of philtrum Hypoplasia of maxilla or mandible
Mouth	Inverted V-shape of upper lip Wide or high-arched palate
Head	Microcrania Macrocrania
Hands	Short 4th or 5th metacarpals Short, stubby fingers Long, thin, tapered fingers Broad thumbs Clinodactyly Abnormal dermatoglyphics (e.g., distal triradius) Transverse palmar crease Abnormal nails
Feet	Short 4th or 5th metatarsals Overlap of toes Short, stubby toes Broad, large big toes Deep crease leading from angle of 1st and 2nd toes Abnormal dermatoglyphics
Genitals	Ambiguous genitalia Micropenis Large testicles
Skin	Café-au-lait spots Depigmented nevi
Teeth	Evidence of abnormal enamelogenesis Abnormal odontogenesis

DIAGNOSIS. The primary care pediatrician is strategically situated to identify young children with possible mental retardation through routine developmental surveillance in the context of general pediatric care (see Chapter 5). Parental reports of a child's typical skills and behaviors in conjunction with in-office screening procedures are important complementary sources of information. For young children involved in a program outside the home (e.g., child care or preschool), the impressions of the caregiver or teacher are most valuable. Any concern raised by parents, nonparental caregivers, or teachers or by direct observation of the child requires systematic investigation. The extent to which a comprehensive developmental assessment can be performed within the primary care setting depends on the expertise of the physician and the office staff.

Ultimately, the diagnosis of mental retardation requires confirmation of significantly subaverage general intellectual functioning (i.e., an IQ standard score of 70–75 or below) in association with deficits in two or more of the following ten adaptive skill areas: communication, self-care, home living, social skills, community use, self-direction, health and safety, functional academics, leisure, and work. Screening instruments (e.g., the Denver-II) and nonstandardized developmental scales are unacceptable substitutes for validated and reliable diagnostic measures (e.g., the Bayley Scales of Infant Development, the Stanford-Binet Intelligence Scale, or the Wechsler Scales). After the psychometric diagnosis of mental retardation has been confirmed, a comprehensive medical evaluation is necessary to complete the assessment process.

A range of laboratory studies must be considered in the medical evaluation of a youngster with mental retardation. Table 37–4 lists important studies and the indications for their use. Growing appreciation of the frequency of fragile X syndrome has prompted some clinicians to suggest routine karyotypes to rule out this diagnosis in all children with retardation of unknown cause. Furthermore, advances in the technology of chromosome analysis have led some to recommend a repeat study of the karyotype of children with significant retardation who had normal findings several years previously.

TABLE 37–4 Indications for Laboratory Assessment of the Young Child with Mental Retardation

Chromosomal Karyotype with Fragile X Analysis

Unusual number or character of atypical physical features
History of maternal exposure to a teratogen
Major congenital malformations
Abnormal genitalia
Associated autistic features
Family history of unexplained retardation

Serum Amino and Urine Organic Acids

Unexplained seizures in early infancy
Failure to thrive with neurologic regression
Unusual smell of urine or skin
Unusually light-colored hair
Microcephaly
Dermatitis
Unexplained acidosis
Family history

Urine Mucopolysaccharides

Coarse facial features
Kyphosis
Short extremities
Short trunk
Hepatosplenomegaly
Cloudy corneas
Impaired hearing
Short stature
Stiff joints

Urine-Reducing Substances

Cataracts
Hepatomegaly
Seizures

Plasma Ammonia

Episodic vomiting
Metabolic acidosis

Urine Ketoacids

Seizures
Short friable hair

Blood Lead

History of pica
Anemia

Serum Zinc

Acrodermatitis

Serum Copper and Ceruloplasmin

Involuntary movements
Cirrhosis
Kayser-Fleischer rings

White Blood Cell Lysosomal Enzyme Analysis or Skin Biopsy

Loss of motor or cognitive milestones or functions
Optic atrophy
Retinal degeneration
Recurrent cerebellar ataxia
Myoclonus
Hepatosplenomegaly
Coarse loose skin
Seizures
Enlarged head beginning after 1 yr of age

Urine Vanillylmandelic Acid

Episodic vomiting
Poor suck
Symptoms of autonomic dysfunction

Serum Uric Acid

Self-mutilation
Rage attacks
Gout
Choreoathetosis

Plasma Very Long Chain Fatty Acids

Atypical phenotypic features
Hepatomegaly
Early seizures and hypotonia
Hearing loss
Retinal degeneration
Renal cysts
Aberrant bone calcification

Blood Lactate and Pyruvate Plus Special Mitochondrial Studies

Metabolic acidosis
Myoclonic seizures
Progressive weakness
Ataxia
Retinal degeneration
Ophthalmoplegia
Recurrent strokelike episodes

Viral Titers for Congenital Infection

Sensorineural hearing impairment
Neonatal hepatosplenomegaly
Neonatal petechial rash
Chorioretinitis
Microphthalmia
Intracranial calcifications
Microcephaly

Electroencephalogram

Suspected seizure disorder
Severe receptive language impairment

Cranial CT or MRI

Progressive enlargement of head
Suspected tuberous sclerosis or other neurocutaneous syndrome
Suspected gross malformation of brain
Focal seizures
Suspected intracranial mass
Neurologic regression

A comprehensive history, physical examination, and laboratory evaluation often lead to identification of specific factors that contribute to the phenomenon of mental retardation. A thorough diagnostic formulation highlights those contributing factors that are amenable to specific medical treatments (e.g., hypothyroidism or an excessive lead burden), suggests associated problems that require therapeutic intervention or continued surveillance (e.g., a seizure disorder or a sensory impairment), and provides a comprehensive data base that can inform ongoing management decisions. More commonly, however, the results of the medical evaluation are nonspecific and inconclusive. In such cases, when there is no evidence of a specific CNS insult, a family history of disability, or identifiable environmental problems, the retardation is presumed to be secondary to an unknown congenital influence on the development of the brain.

TREATMENT. Management of a child with mental retardation is multidimensional and highly individualized. Although the potential need for a highly specialized multidisciplinary effort should be considered, not all children with mental retardation are served best by a complex array of services and professionals. Wise decisions about resource needs are most likely when they are informed by the development of an individualized family service plan, the goals and objectives of which flow from a careful consideration of the specific risk and protective factors inherent in the child and his or her family.

One of the critical and most demanding roles played by the physician involves the *initial synthesis and presentation of diagnostic findings to the family.* This process involves a highly sensitive interaction, the details of which are often remembered and recounted verbatim by parents for many years thereafter. A skilled clinician provides complete and accurate information on what is known about the nature and possible causes of the child's disability; identifies areas of relative competence and adaptive behaviors; provides emotional support; works with the family to define specific goals and objectives and to formulate a strategy for further management; provides sufficient opportunities for parents to identify their own needs for further information; and responds honestly to unanswerable questions. When managed well, the initial informing interview can provide a strong foundation for ongoing parent-professional collaboration.

Specialized educational and therapeutic services are central elements in the multidisciplinary care of children with mental retardation. During the adolescent years, issues related to sexuality, vocational training, and community living become more prominent. The role of the physician necessarily varies with the needs of the child and family. All children must be assured of routine health maintenance services, including immunizations, monitoring of growth, and prompt treatment of minor illnesses. Specific medical complications that occur with greater frequency among children with developmental disabilities (e.g., seizure disorders, impairments of vision or hearing, and nutritional problems) require accurate diagnosis and prompt management. Ongoing health surveillance should be guided by knowledge of the relative risks of specific associated disorders (e.g., slowly progressive sensorineural hearing impairment in children with congenital CMV infection or the development of hypothyroidism, atlantoaxial instability, conductive hearing loss, or celiac disease in youngsters with Down syndrome). Finally, the physician has an important responsibility to ensure the provision of genetic counseling, regardless of the underlying diagnosis.

Collaboration between the primary care physician and an early intervention service system (and later with the school) is particularly important in the management of children with developmental impairments. In the first years of life, early identification and prompt referral ensure access to individualized therapeutic and educational services for the child in conjunction with flexible support services for the family. Such services are delivered best when they focus on the family as a dynamic system and view child and family adaptation as interdependent and mutually influenced by the environment in which they live. Although significant methodologic limitations (as well as ethical, legal, and practical constraints) compromise the ability to evaluate adequately the full range of effects of early intervention programs through randomized control trials, a substantial body of research demonstrates the capacity to produce positive short-term gains in standardized developmental test scores. The long-term effects of specific early intervention experiences on child social competence and family adaptation remain undocumented.

PREVENTION. Although most pathogenetic mechanisms remain unknown, an increasing number of disorders can be detected through prenatal diagnostic studies such as ultrasound, amniocentesis, or chorionic villus biopsy. The provision of complete information and sensitive medical management are therefore essential to ensure informed family decisions about all available prenatal intervention options, including experimental fetal surgeries (such as the placement in utero of an intracranial shunt) and the elective termination of a pregnancy. When specific early treatments are available for infants with metabolic disorders (such as phenylketonuria) or structural abnormalities (such as hydrocephalus), successful prevention requires prompt diagnosis and sophisticated management. In contrast, identifiable metabolic disorders for which specific therapies are not available must await further advances in molecular biology before effective prevention efforts can be realized. Access to experimental treatments, as they become available, must be handled with care on an individual basis.

The central theme common to all efforts to prevent mental retardation is the promotion of healthy brain development and the provision of a nurturing and growth-promoting environment. Because most individuals with mental retardation are mildly retarded, and because mild retardation is disproportionately prevalent among lower socioeconomic groups, substantial prevention efforts must focus on the biologic well-being and the early life experiences of children living in poverty. In this regard, universal access to prenatal care, regular child health supervision, and selected family support services, such as parenting education, represent major prevention strategies.

American Academy of Pediatrics: Health Supervision for children with Down syndrome. Pediatrics 93:855, 1994.

American Association on Mental Retardation: Mental Retardation—Definition, Classification, and Systems of Supports. Washington, DC, American Association on Mental Retardation, 1992.

Drews CD, Murphy CC, Yeargin-Allsopp M, Decoufle P: The relationship between idiopathic mental retardation and smoking during pregnancy. Pediatrics 97:547, 1996.

Hodapp RM, Burack JA, Zigler E (eds): Issues in the Developmental Approach to Mental Retardation. Cambridge, Cambridge University Press, 1990.

Jones KL: Smith's Recognizable Patterns of Human Malformation. Philadelphia, WB Saunders, 1988.

Shonkoff JP, Meisels SJ (eds): Handbook of Early Childhood Intervention, 2nd ed. New York, Cambridge University Press, 2000.

Shonkoff JP: Biological and social factors contributing to mild mental retardation. *In:* Heller K, Holtzman W, Messick S (eds): Placing Children in Special Education: A Strategy for Equity. Washington, DC, National Academy Press, 1982.

Shonkoff JP, Yatchmink Y: Helping families deal with bad news. *In:* Parker S, Zuckerman B (eds): Developmental and Behavioral Pediatrics: A Handbook for Primary Care. Boston, Little, Brown, 1994.

Smith R (ed): Children with Mental Retardation. A Parent's Guide. Rockville, MD, Woodbine House, 1993.

Strauss D, Kastner T, Ashwal S, et al: Tube feeding and mortality in children with severe disabilities and mental retardation. Pediatrics 99:358, 1997.

Turnbull HR, Turnbull AP: Parents Speak Out? Then and Now, 2nd ed. Columbus, OH, Merrill, 1985.

CHAPTER 38

Pediatric Palliative Care: The Care of Children with Life-Limiting Illness

Stephen Liben

Despite medicine's best efforts to combat illness and the remarkable decline in infant and childhood mortality rates in industrialized nations, children still die. For parents and families the death of a child represents the loss of a lifetime of potential, and it may be the greatest threat to family function and integrity that they will ever have to face. For the physician, a lack of training and experience in the care of the dying child may trigger personal fears about mortality and the meaning of life as well as feelings of professional inadequacy.

Pediatricians assume responsibility for overseeing children's physical, mental, and emotional progress from conception to maturity (Chapter 1). Professionals involved in the care of a child with a life-threatening illness (any illness that may result in death before adulthood) may come to feel that there is nothing left to offer once cure and prolongation of life are no longer possible. Palliative care (also referred to as hospice care) recognizes the importance of quality of life in this setting and has much to offer to patients and families by way of comfort, communication, and healing (also see Chapter 72). To care for children with life-limiting illness and their families the pediatrician requires an active, coordinated, consistent, well-thought-out approach to diagnosis and management. Palliative medicine is directed at the development of a care plan to meet the needs of the child and family, taking into account local resources. The care of the dying child represents a personal and professional challenge to the physician that is never easy, but it also represents a unique and privileged opportunity to guide, comfort, and lay the groundwork for true healing to occur.

SCOPE OF THE PROBLEM: A DIVERSITY OF NEEDS. There are smaller numbers of dying children compared with adults. This means that even professionals specializing in the care of children may only rarely encounter the death of a child. Although childhood mortality rates are low, there are a significant number of children who live with life-limiting illness. In the United Kingdom it is estimated that 1/1000 children/yr have a life-limiting condition. These are children who have a high likelihood of dying before adulthood and who could potentially benefit from a palliative care approach.

Adult palliative care has a large number of patients with cancer. In pediatrics, cancer is an important but less common cause of life-limiting illness and death. In some pediatric hospice/palliative care programs only 10–20% of admitted children have cancer. A diverse group of children with rare diseases, such as inborn errors of metabolism or neurodegenerative disorders, make up the majority receiving palliative care. These are children who may live with a host of physical and intellectual handicaps for years before their death. The time course of these illnesses is varied and often prolonged, and the burden of care taken on by the families is huge. Palliative care for these children may therefore involve some overlap with chronic care, with palliative care becoming more prominent as the child progresses from being chronically ill to being terminally ill.

A working group of the British Pediatric Association has classified life-threatening illness in children into four main groups:

- Cure possible but uncertain (e.g., cancer).
- Chronic course with intermittent intensive treatment; premature death likely (e.g., cystic fibrosis).
- Palliative care from time of diagnosis (e.g., some inborn errors of metabolism).
- Nonprogressive brain injuries; unpredictable course; premature death likely (e.g., severe cerebral palsy).

Children with AIDS are a special group with an ill-defined but increasing life expectancy. Because of the diversity of illness trajectories, there are circumstances in which palliative care may be involved on an unpredictable and intermittent basis, with frequent "crises" followed by return to baseline function.

MODELS OF CARE. Although length of life predictions are frequently inaccurate, it is often possible to recognize that the child either is entering into the final stages of illness or is at high risk for a precipitous death. At this time the child and family should have the opportunity to discuss and coordinate end-of-life care in anticipation of the need for decision-making, symptom control, and advanced care planning. Patients and families may be most comfortable continuing with physicians and other care providers with whom they have an established relationship; in most cases the services of a palliative care specialist or *hospice program* may be consultative to the primary care physician and team. At other times, a transfer of care to a home-care or hospice-care program may be necessary for those patients who prefer to remain at home and who will require intensive home care intervention.

Home care of the dying child requires 24 hr per day accessibility to experts in pediatric palliative care; a team approach with an identified coordinator who will serve as a link between hospitals, the community, and specialists; immediate access to hospital admission as needed; and planned respite care. Provision of *respite services* is of key importance to families caring for children with complex needs for prolonged periods of time. Respite care may involve temporary placement with another family or in an institution such as a hospital or hospice. Many children, when given the choice, prefer to remain at home. Even with comprehensive home support, the child may need to periodically return to the hospital or hospice. It is important to plan a respite admission before the family caring for the child feels overwhelmed. At these times the family should be reassured that they have done well under the most difficult circumstances.

Holistic end-of-life care can be effectively carried out in a hospital setting. In pediatric hospitals the neonatal and pediatric ICUs are the locations where most children die (Chapter 72). Many of the children in ICUs die after discussions that lead to the limitation or withdrawal of therapy. Improving the care of these hospitalized children and their families involves removing the obstacles inherent in intensive care settings, such as routine testing and monitoring of vital signs; liberalizing visiting, including pets; and respecting privacy. The "hospice philosophy" can be successfully implemented in a hospital setting when the focus of care is on comfort and quality of life. All interventions that affect the child and family need to be assessed in relation to these goals. Staff who are comfortable and supportive of this approach need to be carefully chosen. In addition, comprehensive care requires a multidisciplinary approach that may include psychologists, psychiatrists, social workers, pastoral services, child-life specialists, and trained volunteers.

COMMUNICATION ISSUES AND ANTICIPATORY GUIDANCE. "What do I say to my child?" The answer relates to the child's concept of illness and death as well as to the particular circumstances of the child-family relationship. A child's perception of death depends on his or her concepts of universality (the recognition that all things inevitably die), irreversibility (the ability to understand that dead people cannot come back to life), nonfunctionality (the understanding that being dead means that all biologic functions cease with death), and causality (the ability to understand the objective causes of death). Children up to 6 yr of age have difficulty with the concepts of irreversibility and nonfunctionality. They may believe that death is like sleep, and if this belief is reinforced by well-meaning adults they may relate falling asleep with dying. Many young children believe that the dead still eat, drink, and breathe. Children 6–8 yr old begin to understand that not only do others die but they too will die, and they begin to acknowledge the concepts of irreversibility and nonfunctionality. The last concept to become clear is causality. Children in the stage of integrating causality may personify death as a monster that can be avoided or outrun. Children's fears of death are centered on the concrete fear of being separated from parents and other loved ones, rather than on the existential consequences of an afterlife common to adults (see Chapter 33). This fear of separation may be responded to in different ways, with some families giving reassurance that loving relatives will be waiting, and others using religious figures or referring to an eternal spiritual connection ("I will always be there for you"). Adolescents have their own unique issues, including risk-taking behavior that seems to challenge their concept of universality ("I am invincible").

It is also important to recognize that a child's expressed question may have different levels of meaning. A child asking "Am I going to die?" may really be testing the honesty of the person being asked. The child asking "Why is this happening to me?" may be signaling a need to be with someone who is comfortable listening to such unanswerable questions. Many children find nonverbal expression much easier; art, play therapy, and storytelling may bring out more than direct conversation does. Despite the reflex parental instinct to shield the child from "bad things," children cannot be "protected" from the reality of their situation. Bluebond-Langner showed that seriously ill children become aware of their mortality even when there has been a conscious effort at deception (the practice of mutual pretense). Perpetuating the myth that "everything is going to be all right" takes away the chance to explore fears and provide reassurance. For example, many children blame themselves for their illness and the hardships that it causes for their loved ones. Their guilt can be addressed and resolved only by open, honest communication, requiring a sensitive response that takes into account the child's developmental stage and particular circumstances.

Siblings are at special risk both during the course of the illness and after death. Because of the stresses on parents to meet the needs of their ill child, siblings may feel that their needs are not being acknowledged. These feelings of neglect may then trigger guilt about their own good health. Young siblings may react to the stress by becoming seemingly oblivious to the turmoil around them. Parents need to know that this is a normal response, and siblings should be encouraged to maintain the normal routines of daily living. It has been found that siblings who were most involved with their sick brothers or sisters before death adjusted better both at the time of and after the death. Acknowledging their feelings, being honest and open about the situation, and appropriately involving them in the life of their sick sibling offers them the best chance to adapt and adjust.

Parents may blame themselves for their child's illness ("If only I had taken him to the doctor sooner") and may spend considerable energy and resources looking for "miracle cures." The physician should be sensitive to these concerns and realize that parents need an effective listener who is engaged and attentive. Anticipatory guidance involves exploring a variety of options and formulating a care plan. Parents need to know about the availability of home care, respite services, educational books and videotapes, and support groups. It is important to discuss how parents envision their child's death and to address myths surrounding pain control and the benefit of involving siblings. What all parents want to know is that they and their child will not be abandoned and, as the goal of treatment changes from prolongation of life to quality of life, that a skilled team will remain involved in pursuit of the revised diagnostic and therapeutic goals. Regular meetings between caregivers and the family are essential. At these meetings, important issues include finding an appropriate physical setting (not a hospital corridor), reviewing what was previously discussed, listening to concerns and issues as they are revealed, having parents repeat back what was said to ensure clarity, and responding with honest, factual answers in areas of uncertainty.

In communications with the child and family the physician should avoid giving estimates of survival length, even when explicitly asked for. These predictions are invariably inaccurate, as population-based statistics do not predict the course for individual patients. A more honest and effective approach is to say "Nobody really knows how long." At the same time, the physician can ask parents what they might do differently if they knew how long their child would live and then assist them in thinking through the options relating to their specific concerns. It is generally wise to suggest that relatives who wish to visit might do so now to take advantage of whatever time remains. For the child and family the integration of bad news is a process, not an event. The disclosure of the hard realities associated with life-limiting illness should be paced according to the resources of the specific child and family.

Decision-making should remain focused on the goals of therapy, rather than on specific limitations of care; e.g., "This is what we can offer," instead of "This is what we can no longer do." Rather than meeting specifically to discuss a do-not-resuscitate order, a more general discussion centered on the goals of therapy will naturally lead to considering which interventions are in the child's best interests. Unclear terms such as "withholding heroic or extraordinary measures" are best replaced by reference to specific interventions that are then documented in a care plan. Parents should not be left alone in their decision-making. Rather than asking "Do you want us to do CPR?" (placing the full burden of the decision on the parents) it might be better to say "Given what we have discussed, I don't think CPR really makes sense for your child, do you agree?" Once the goals of therapy are agreed upon, the physician can draft a letter that outlines the care plan for the child. The letter should be as detailed as possible, including suggestions for medications and the telephone numbers of caregivers who know the patient best. Such a letter, given to the parents, with copies to involved caregivers and institutions, can be a useful aid in communication, especially in times of crisis.

TABLE 38–1 Pain Treatment Guidelines

Educate patient, parents, and staff. Establish realistic goals.
Always combine pharmacologic with nonpharmacologic strategies.
Titrate analgesics to individual needs: Start with nonopioids (acetaminophen/NSAIDs) and add opioids.
Consider use of adjuvant drugs for specific indications (antidepressants, anticonvulsants for neuropathic pain; neuroleptics for nausea, agitation; sedatives, hypnotics for anxiety or muscle spasm; steroids for tumor effects; stimulants for opioid-induced somnolence).
Consider use of anesthetic blocks for regional pain. Use topical local anesthetics when possible.
Include cognitive (guided imagery, distraction), physical (TENS, physiotherapy, massage), and behavioral (biofeedback, behavior modification) techniques.
Use the least invasive route—by the mouth, when possible.
Use regular (not PRN) medications for ongoing pain.
Frequently reassess effectiveness and modify the treatment plan as needed.

SYMPTOM MANAGEMENT. *Pain control* is of paramount importance in reducing the suffering of the child, family, and caregivers (Chapter 74). Pain is a complex sensation influenced by tissue damage as well as by situational factors, including cognitive, behavioral, emotional, social, and cultural issues that are unique to each person. It is important to form and initiate a pain treatment plan even without a confirmed diagnosis. Many children with life-limiting illness are unable to verbalize their symptoms and will instead communicate their discomfort nonverbally. Presumptive therapy should be initiated promptly, and treatment plans can then be modified based on the response. For the dying child, in whom accurate assessment of the cause of pain may be difficult, it is important to frequently reassess therapy and to be honest in telling parents that it may take several dose adjustments to determine the optimal analgesic requirements of their child. Guidelines for the treatment of pain and the use of opioids are summarized in Tables 38–1 and 38–2.

Dying children have a multitude of symptoms, in addition to pain, for significant periods before their death. *Respiratory symptoms* such as **dyspnea** are common, and many children with chronic life-threatening disease have symptomatic airway secretions. Excessive secretions and salivation due to poor swallowing may be treated with oral glycopyrrolate. As death approaches, a buildup of secretions may result in noisy respiration sometimes referred to as a death rattle. Patients at this stage are usually unconscious, and noisy respirations are often more distressing for others than for the child. Pointing out the child's lack of distress and the use of an anticholinergic drug, such as hyoscine, may be helpful. Pneumonia is a frequent complication in dying children. Dyspnea can be relieved with the use of opioids, and oxygen may be helpful in certain cases to relieve hypoxemia-related headaches. As with all interventions the question must be asked, "Who is being treated?"

TABLE 38–2 Opioid Use Guidelines

Explain the difference between tolerance vs physical dependence vs addiction.
Dispel the myth that strong medications should be saved for last. There is no ceiling dose for potent opioids.
Anticipate and treat/prevent common side effects (constipation, pruritus, nausea, dysphoria, somnolence).
Start with weak opioid for mild pain (e.g., codeine) and use strong opioid (e.g., morphine) for unresponsive or persisting pain. Continue with nonopioids.
Start with short-acting opioid at regular intervals and convert to long-acting when dose requirements have become established. Use short-acting opioid PRN for interdose breakthrough pain.
Consider subcutaneous infusions when oral/rectal routes no longer possible.
Adjust doses depending on age and organ system dysfunction.

(child, parents, or staff). For example, giving the cyanotic child who is quiet and relaxed oxygen by face mask may serve to relieve staff discomfort, not patient distress.

Neurologic symptoms include seizures that are often part of the antecedent illness but that may increase in frequency and severity toward the end of life. Anticonvulsants should be administered, and parents can be taught to use rectal diazepam at home. Increased *irritability* accompanies some neurodegenerative disorders; it may be particularly disruptive because of the resultant break in normal sleep-wake patterns and the difficulty in finding respite facilities for children who have prolonged crying. Judicious use of sedatives in the daytime (benzodiazepines) combined with hypnotics at night (chloral hydrate) may achieve a balance that can dramatically improve the quality of life for both child and caregivers.

Feeding and hydration issues raise ethical questions that include the use of nasogastric and gastrostomy feedings for the child who can no longer feed by mouth (see also Chapter 2). These complex issues require evaluating the risks and benefits of artificial feedings, taking into consideration the child's functional level and prognosis. At times it may be appropriate to initiate a trial of tube feedings with the understanding that they may be discontinued at a later stage of the illness. A commonly held but unsubstantiated belief is that hydration is a "comfort measure," which may result in well-meaning but disruptive and invasive attempts to administer intravenous fluids to a dying child. Studies of dying adults show how the sensation of thirst may be alleviated by careful efforts to keep the mouth moist and clean. There may also be deleterious side effects to artificial hydration in the form of increased secretions, need for frequent urination, and exacerbation of dyspnea.

Nausea demands prompt treatment after a search for common causes (drug effects, constipation, primary disease, metabolic disturbance). Drugs such as metoclopramide, phenothiazines, ondansetron, and steroids may be used depending on the etiology and desired secondary effects (e.g., if sedation is desired, a sedating phenothiazine may be used). *Vomiting* may accompany nausea but may also occur without nausea in the presence of bowel obstruction. *Constipation* is common, and the first step is to assess stool frequency and quantity. Children on regular opioids should routinely be placed on stool softeners (docusate) and may also need the addition of laxative agents (senna derivatives, lactulose). *Diarrhea* may be particularly difficult for the child and family and may be treated with loperamide and opioids. Paradoxical diarrhea, a result of overflow resulting from constipation, must also be ruled out.

Hematologic issues include consideration of transfusions for anemia and thrombocytopenia. Most children in the palliative phase may be managed by intermittent red cell and platelet transfusions for bleeding that interferes with the quality of life. Serious bleeding is disturbing for all concerned, and a plan involving the use of fast-acting sedatives should be prepared in advance.

Skin care issues include the prevention of problems such as **bedsores** by the early use of inexpensive egg-crate type foam mattresses and careful attention to turning the child. **Pruritus** may be secondary to systemic disorders or drug therapy. Treatment includes avoiding excessive use of soap, using moisturizers, trimming fingernails, and wearing loose-fitting clothing, in addition to administering topical or systemic steroids. Oral antihistamines and other specific therapies may also be indicated (e.g., cholestyramine in biliary disease).

When discussing possible therapies or interventions with adolescent patients or with the parents of an ill child, it is important to raise the issue of *complementary* or *alternative medicine*, since it has been shown that many patients use some form of alternative medicine therapy but are reluctant to bring it up with their physician. Although mostly unproven, some therapies are inexpensive and provide subjective relief to individual patients. Other therapies may be expensive, painful, intrusive, and even dangerous. By initiating conversation and inviting discussion in a nonjudgmental way, the physician can offer advice on the safety of different therapies and may help avoid expensive and dangerous interventions.

THE TERMINAL PHASE. As death approaches, the major task of the physician is to help prepare the child and family for expected problems and issues. If the child is cared for at home, arrangements must be made to manage new symptoms as they occur (terminal airway secretions, seizures, irritability, myoclonus, vomiting). Legal issues such as who will perform the declaration of death may be addressed, and the necessary documents can be partially filled out and left in a sealed envelope in the child's home. In the hospital, the care plan should be clear to all involved professionals and should include an understanding of the specific needs and requests of the child and family.

Initiating a discussion of the options for funeral arrangements may be appropriate, as some parents prefer to settle these practical issues before the child's death. Thought to the attendance of young siblings at the funeral should be discussed and sibling participation encouraged. Excluding siblings from the funeral deprives them of an opportunity for closure and may devalue their need to grieve.

In an intensive care setting, where technology can put distance between the child and parent, the physician should discontinue the use of unneeded equipment. Children can be picked up by their parents even while on a ventilator, or they may be removed from the ventilator and placed in their parents' arms. Parents who may not have held their infant since birth may be afraid to ask permission to hold their child but will be relieved to be offered the opportunity when it is presented. Hearing and the ability to sense touch are often present until death. Siblings and family members should be encouraged to talk to and touch the child, even if he or she seems unresponsive. It seems that many children who live with prolonged illness die only after their parents have begun the process of "letting go." Some children appear to wait for "permission to die," and their parents' acceptance of the inevitable may play a role in the timing of their death.

For the family, the moment of death is an event that is recalled in detail for years to come. After death, they should be given the option of remaining with their child for as long as they need to. During this time, physicians and other professionals should avoid trying to "do and say too much." Quietly sitting with the family and gently touching the child transmits the message that it is natural to touch the body. Different ethnic and cultural practices should be taken into consideration and facilitated (Chapter 3). In some traditions it is important to have the family take the child to the place of worship directly, instead of passing through the hospital morgue. Arranging this and other details in advance will help avoid some stress for both family and staff.

The physician should discuss the option of an autopsy, answering questions that parents may be reluctant to ask (e.g., "Will the face be disturbed?"). Parents might also be reminded that they may have questions later on that can be answered by an autopsy. The parents should also be offered genetic counseling, when appropriate.

The physician's decision to attend the funeral is a personal one. It may serve the dual purpose of showing respect as well as helping him or her cope with a personal sense of loss.

Bereavement involves a complex, individualized process that is only partially understood. What is known is that the death of a child is not something to "get over," and intense feelings of sadness may persist for years. The physician should arrange to meet with the family at a set time after the death, to review autopsy results if applicable, and to answer questions that may remain. When the death occurs after a prolonged hospitalization, a hospital memorial service may be held. These services often serve as an opportunity for closure by staff who were involved in care but who may not have been present at the child's death.

The physician can be proactive in preventing the phenomenon of *replacement children*. Physicians have in the past suggested to parents, "Get on with your lives," and "Why not have another child as soon as possible?" Instead, parents should be made aware that nothing can replace the uniqueness of their deceased child and that, although their memories will remain forever, the pain for most does subside with time. Physicians should also be aware that the divorce rate for bereaved couples is not necessarily higher than for the general population. Divorce is therefore not an inevitable result of the grieving process; and couples should be referred for counseling, when appropriate.

Because grieving for a deceased child places parents at risk for psychologic illness, it is recommended that a professional trained in bereavement counseling be consulted following the death of a child. Long-term follow-up should be the norm, including regular phone calls at significant times such as birthdays, anniversaries of the death, and significant holidays. Other interventions that may be helpful include support groups for bereaved parents and siblings, where those who share common experiences can learn from one another. Such support groups include The Compassionate Friends and Candlelighters/Lamplighters.

THE PEDIATRICIAN AND DEATH. The ability to care effectively for dying children and their families is not a skill shared by all. There are situations and times in the professional's own life when the demands of end-of-life care may be difficult to tolerate. At such times the availability of supportive colleagues is invaluable, and it may be appropriate and in the patient's best interest to refer to others. However, for most physicians, the duty to care for their patients through the illness spectrum is a commitment that reaches to the core of their professional identity. Most physicians have had training that emphasized their role as conquerors of disease. This notion, coupled with limited training in psychosocial care, may promote a feeling of personal and professional failure when facing the death of a patient. Effective care of children with life-threatening illness can not only ease the burden of suffering for dying children and their families but also serve as the embodiment of the privileged role that physicians have as healers.

Adams DW, Deveau EJ (eds): Beyond the Innocence of Childhood. Vols 1–3. New York, Baywood Publishing, 1995.

Armstrong-Dailey A, Goltzer SZ (eds): Hospice Care for Children. Oxford, Oxford University Press, 1993.

Association for Children with Life-Threatening or Terminal Conditions and Their Families and the Royal College of Pediatrics and Child Health: A Guide to the Development of Children's Palliative Care Services. Bristol, England, 1997.

Bluebond-Langner M: The Private Worlds of Dying Children. Princeton, Princeton University Press, 1978.

Corr CA, Corr DM (eds): Hospice Approaches to Pediatric Care. New York, Springer, 1985.

Doyle D, Hanks GWC, MacDonald N (eds): Oxford Textbook of Palliative Medicine, 2nd ed. Oxford, Oxford University Press, 1998.

Goldman A (ed): Care of the Dying Child. Oxford, Oxford University Press, 1994.

Roy DJ: When children have to die...pediatric palliative care. J Palliat Care 12:3, 1996.

Sourkes BM: Armfuls of Time: The Psycological Experience of the Child with Life-Threatening Illness. Pittsburgh, University of Pittsburgh Press, 1995.

CHAPTER 39

Children at Special Risk

Richard E. Behrman

In this chapter, the health issues faced by some of the most socioculturally and economically disadvantaged children in the United States are discussed: Native Americans, migrants, immigrants, homeless children, and runaways. Children in foster care are discussed in Chapter 31. The role of poverty in the lives of these and other children has a special significance. The biologic causes of special risk are covered elsewhere. The nonbiologic and biologic causes of special risk often overlap and may confound the risks.

Most children in the United States today grow up loved and supported, although many have problems that disturb their parents and blight their future. However, for a small but significant number of children, their circumstances are so dismal that one wonders how they survive with hope for any quality of future life. Examples of children with even more dismal futures than these also exist elsewhere in the world, such as children growing up in the midst of the Israel-Palestine conflict or in Northern Ireland, Bosnia, or Rwanda. Many of the children growing up in these environments will be damaged and their futures will be compromised, unless effective interventions are mounted. However, in all of these situations, a few children are so resilient that they survive and actually thrive. Werner has characterized these children as "vulnerable but invincible." The fact that a few defy the odds does not absolve society from attempting to help the majority of those who do not, although these resilient ones can teach us what it takes to survive.

The majority of children at special risk need a nurturing environment but have had their futures compromised by actions or policies arising from their families, schools, communities, and nation. The challenge is to improve the environment of these children so that most can achieve their full potential. Many of their problems are due to several causes, and many of these causes are similar, whether the end result is homeless children, runaways, children in foster care, or other disadvantaged groups. From a preventive point of view, the most effective approach involves alleviation of poverty, poor housing, and lack of jobs. From a treatment point of view, optimal care of these children requires specially organized programs, multidiscipline teams, and special financing.

CHILDREN IN POVERTY

Poverty and economic loss diminish the capacity of parents to be supportive, consistent, and involved with their children. Clinicians need to be especially alert to the development and behavior of children whose parents have lost their jobs or who live in permanent poverty. Fathers who become unemployed frequently develop psychosomatic symptoms, and their children often develop similar symptoms. Young children who grew up in the Great Depression and whose parents were subject to acute poverty suffered more than older children, especially if the older ones were able to take on responsibilities for helping the family economically. Such responsibilities during adolescence seem to give purpose and direction to an adolescent's life. But the younger children, faced with parental depression and unable to do anything to help, suffered a higher frequency of illness and a diminished capacity to lead productive lives even as adults. Children who are poor have higher than average rates of death and illness from almost all causes (exceptions being suicide and motor vehicle accidents, which are most common among white, nonpoor children) (Table 39–1). Also see Chapter 1.

Although physicians cannot cure poverty, they have an obligation to ask parents about their economic resources, adverse changes in their financial situation, and the family's attempts to cope. Encouraging concrete methods of coping, suggesting ways to reduce stressful social circumstances while increasing social networks that are supportive, and referring patients and their families to appropriate welfare, job training, and family agencies can significantly improve the health and functioning of children at risk when their families live in poverty. In many cases, special services, especially social services, need to be

TABLE 39–1 Relative Frequency of Health Problems in Low-Income Children Compared with Other Children

Health Problem	Relative Frequency in Low-Income Children
Low birthweight	Double
Delayed immunization	Triple
Asthma	Higher
Bacterial meningitis	Double
Rheumatic fever	Double to triple
Lead poisoning	Triple
Neonatal death	1.5 times
Postneonatal death	Double to triple
Child deaths due to accidents	Double to triple
Child deaths due to disease	Triple to quadruple
Complications of appendicitis	Double to triple
Diabetic ketoacidosis	Double
Complications of bacterial meningitis	Double to triple
Percent with conditions limiting school activity	Double to triple
Lost school days	40% more
Severely impaired vision	Double to triple
Severe iron-deficiency anemia	Double

From Starfield B: Effectiveness of Medical Care: Validating Clinical Wisdom. Baltimore, Johns Hopkins University Press, 1985. In: *Starfield B: Child and adolescent health status measures. Future Child 2:25, 1992.*

added to the traditional medical services, and outreach is required to find and encourage parents to use health services and bring their children into the health care system.

Poverty among children in the United States has increased over 33% since the early 1970s. One in five children lived in poverty in 1995, a higher percentage than in any other developed country. The rates are higher for children (20.8%) than adults (11.3%) and are highest for infants and toddlers. The rates also vary substantially among ethnic groups: white, 16%; black, 41%; Hispanic, 40%; Native American, 41%; and Asian American, 19%. Many factors associated with poverty are responsible for the illnesses seen in these children—crowding, poor hygiene and health care, poor diet, environmental pollution, poor education, and stress.

NATIVE AMERICANS, INCLUDING ALASKAN ESKIMOS AND ALEUTS

Children of Native Americans have higher than average rates of many physical and psychologic disorders. They are one group in the United States for whom a separately organized health service has long been in place, the Indian Health Service. There are approximately 2.1 million Native Americans, 40% of whom are younger than 20 yr, a much higher proportion of children than for the remainder of the United States. More than 50% of Native Americans live in urban areas, not on or near native lands. The unemployment and poverty levels of Native Americans are, respectively, three- and fourfold that of the white population and far fewer Native Americans graduate from high school or go on to college.

The rate of low birthweight is more than the white rate and less than the black rate. The neonatal mortality rate and the postneonatal mortality rate are higher for Native Americans living in urban areas than for urban white Americans. Deaths during the 1st yr of life due to sudden infant death syndrome and pneumonia and influenza are higher than the average in the United States, whereas deaths due to congenital anomalies, respiratory distress syndrome, and disorders relating to short gestation and low birthweight are similar.

Accidental death among Native Americans occurs at twice the rate for other United States populations, whereas deaths due to malignant neoplasms are lower. During adolescence and young adulthood, suicide and homicide are the second and third causes of death in this population and occur at about twice the rates of the rest of the population. There may be significant underreporting of deaths of Native American children.

Recurrent otitis media is an especially frequent problem among Native American children. As many as three quarters of these children have recurrent otitis media and high rates of hearing loss. This results in learning problems for many children. Other infectious disorders, such as tuberculosis and gastroenteritis, which were so much more common among Native Americans in the past, now occur at about the national average.

Psychosocial problems are more prevalent in these populations than in the general population: depression, alcoholism, drug abuse, out-of-wedlock teenage pregnancy, school failure and dropout, and child abuse and neglect. The reasons for these differences are not clear, but the cultural disruption of Native American populations is probably, in part, responsible.

INDIAN HEALTH SERVICE. Since 1954, the Indian Health Service has been the responsibility of the Public Health Service; since the 1975 Indian Self-Determination Act, tribes have been given the option of managing Native American health services in their communities. Thus, today, the Indian Health Service is managed through local administrative units, and some tribes contract outside of the Indian Health Service for health care. The asthma-related hospitalization patterns of Native American children are similar to those in white children despite having socioeconomic characteristics more similar to those of black children. A great deal of emphasis is, however, on adult services: treatment for alcoholism, nutrition and dietetic counseling, and public health nursing services. In addition to programs on Native American reservations, there are currently more than 40 urban programs for Native Americans, with an emphasis on increasing access of this population to existing health services, providing special social services, and developing self-help groups. In an effort to accommodate traditional Western medical, psychologic, and social services to the Native American cultures, such programs increasingly include the "Talking Circle," the "Sweat Lodge," and other interventions based on Native American culture (see Chapter 3). The efficacy of any of these programs, especially those to prevent and treat the sociopsychologic problems peculiar to Native Americans, has not been assessed.

CHILDREN OF MIGRANT FARM WORKERS

There are estimated to be 3–5 million migrant and seasonal farm workers and their families in the United States. The eastern stream of workers winters primarily in Florida, whereas the western stream comes from Texas and the border states, as well as from Mexico. Many children travel with their parents in the migrant streams. The circumstances of migrants often include poor housing, frequent moves, and a socioeconomic system controlled by a crew boss who arranges the jobs, provides transportation, and often, together with the farm owners, provides food, alcohol, and drugs under a "company store" system that leaves migrant families with little money or even in debt at the end of the year. Children often go without schooling because of the moves, and medical care is usually limited.

The medical problems of children of migrant farm workers are similar to those of children of homeless families: increased frequency of infections (including human immunodeficiency virus [HIV] and AIDS), trauma, poor nutrition, poor dental care, low immunization rates, exposures to toxic chemicals, anemia, and developmental delays.

In 1964, the Public Health Service initiated a special program to provide funds for local groups to organize medical care for migrant families. This program has continued to grow. In addition, many migrant health projects, which were staffed initially by part-time providers and were open for only part of the year, have been transformed into community health care centers that provide services not only for migrants but also for other residents in the area. However, health services for migrant farm workers often need to be organized separately from existing primary care programs because the families are migratory. Special record-keeping systems that link the health care provided during winter months in the south with the care provided during the migratory season in the north are difficult to maintain in ordinary group practices or individual physicians' offices. Outreach programs that take medical care to the often remote farm sites are necessary, and specially organized Head Start, early education, and remedial education programs should also be provided. Similar to other groups discussed in this section, children of migrant farm workers require health care that is more extensive than physicians' services; and this sort of health care often requires separate organizations to deliver it.

CHILDREN OF IMMIGRANTS

The United States has always been a country of immigrants, and it is in the midst of a wave of immigration larger than experienced in the early 1900s. There has been a marked increase in immigration from Southeast Asia, South America, and the Soviet Union. About 240,000 children legally immigrate each year, and an estimated 50,000/yr enter the country illegally. During the past decade, about 9 million immigrants attained permanent residency status. There may be 850,000 to 1 million illegal immigrant children currently in residence. Families of different origins obviously bring different health problems and different cultural backgrounds, which influence health practices and use of medical care and need to be understood to provide appropriate services (see Chapter 3). Children from Southeast Asia and South America have growth patterns that are generally below the norms established for children of Western European origin, and high rates of hepatitis, parasitic diseases, and nutritional deficiencies are prevalent, as well as high degrees of psychosocial stress. The high prevalence of hepatitis among women from Southeast Asia makes use of hepatitis B vaccine necessary for newborns in this group.

Although special health care programs have been developed for many of these children (e.g., children of immigrant migrant workers), children of legally immigrant families have usually been more readily incorporated into traditional medical practice in the United States than some of the other groups of children at special risk. However, "linguistically isolated households," in which no one over 14 yr of age speaks English, often present significant obstacles to providing quality health care to children because of difficulties in understanding and communicating basic concerns and instructions and in avoiding compromising privacy and confidentiality interests and obtaining informed consent when using translators.

HOMELESS CHILDREN

Families with children are the fastest growing segment of the homeless population (36–38%), with an estimated 100,000 children living in shelters on a given night and about 500,000 homeless each year. Many homeless are not in shelters, and thus, these figures are low estimates. In addition, an unknown number of thrown-away and runaway children and adolescents are homeless, living in shelters, on the streets, and elsewhere (see later). The population of homeless children has been increasing as a consequence of more families with children living in poverty, fewer available affordable dwellings for these families, decreasing public assistance programs for the nonelderly poor, and the rising prevalence of substance abuse.

Homeless children have an increased frequency of illness, including intestinal infections, anemia, neurologic disorders, seizures, behavior disorders, mental illness, and dental problems, as well as increased frequency of trauma and substance abuse. Homeless children are admitted to hospitals at a much higher rate than the national average. They have higher school failure rates, and the likelihood of their being victims of abuse and neglect is much higher. In one study, 50% of such children were found to have psychosocial problems, such as developmental delays, severe depression, or learning disorders. The increased frequency of maternal psychosocial problems, especially depression, in homeless households has a significant untoward impact on the mental and physical health of these children.

Because families tend to break apart under the strain of poverty and homelessness, many homeless children end up in foster care. And even if their families remain intact, frequent moves make it very difficult for them to receive continuity of medical care. Homeless persons rarely have a family physician, and therefore special programs generally need to be developed to provide health services for this population. Mobile vans, with a team consisting of a physician, nurse, social worker, and welfare worker, have been shown to provide effective comprehensive care, ensure delivery of immunizations, link the children to school health services, and bring the children and their families into a stable relation with the traditional medical system. A special record-keeping system is necessary to enhance continuity and to provide a record of care once the family has moved to a permanent location. Because of the high frequency of developmental delays in this group, linkage of preschool homeless children to Head Start programs is an especially important service. Medical and social services for the parents of homeless children are also essential for preservation of these families.

The basic problem of homeless families cannot be solved by physicians. Provision of adequate housing, job retraining for the parents, and mental health and social services are necessary to prevent homelessness from occurring. Physicians can have an important role in motivating society to adopt the social policies that will prevent homelessness from occurring by pointing out the likelihood that these homeless children will become burdens both to themselves and to society if their special health needs are not met.

RUNAWAY AND THROWN-AWAY CHILDREN

The number of runaway and thrown-away children and youths in 1988 (the most recent national survey) was 577,800, and at least 192,700 of these children had no secure and safe place to stay. Teenagers make up most of both groups. The usual definition of a runaway is a youth less than 18 yr who is gone for at least one night from his or her home without parental permission. Most runaways leave home only once, stay overnight with friends, and have no contact with the police or other agencies. This group is no different from their "healthy" peers in psychologic status. A smaller but unknown number become multiple or permanent "runners" and are significantly different from the one-time runners. Thrown-aways include children directly told to leave the household, children who have been away from home and are not allowed to return, abandoned or deserted children, and children who run away but their caretaker makes no effort to recover them or does not care if they return.

The same constellation of causes common to many of the other special-risk groups is characteristic of permanent runaways. These causes include environmental problems (family dysfunction, abuse, poverty), as well as personal problems of the young person (poor impulse control, psychopathology, substance abuse, or school failure). Thrown-aways experienced more violence and conflicts within their families. The reason why one child enters the group of runaways while another child enters foster care, the juvenile justice system, or mental health systems is not clear.

The minority of runaway youths who become homeless

street people have a high frequency of problem behaviors. Three quarters engage in some type of criminal activity and half engage in prostitution as a means of support. A majority of permanent runaways have serious mental problems; more than one third are the product of families who engage in repeated physical and sexual abuse. These children also have a high frequency of medical problems, including traditional infections, hepatitis, sexually transmitted diseases, and drug abuse. Although runaways usually distrust most social agencies, they will come to and use medical services. Thus, medical care may become the point of re-entry into mainstream society and the path to needed services.

Services for permanent runaways and thrown-aways need to be comprehensive and should include social, psychiatric, foster home, drug detoxification, and more traditional medical services. The only approach that has been successful has been long-term team efforts by people who develop the trust of runaway youths and then can help them to work out a better solution to their problems than by running away, drug use, and prostitution.

Although legal considerations involved in the treatment of homeless minor adolescents may be significant, most states, through their " Good Samaritan" laws and definitions of emancipated minors, authorize treatment of homeless youths. Physician liability is based on the usual malpractice standards. Legal barriers should not be used as an excuse to refuse medical care to runaway or thrown-away youths.

The Runaway Youth Act, Title III of the Juvenile Justice and Delinquency Prevention Act of 1974 (Public Law 93–414), and its amended version (Public Law 95–509) have supported shelters and provide a toll-free 24-hr telephone number (1-800-621-4000) for youths who wish to contact their parents or request help after having run away.

Parents who seek a physician's advice about a runaway child should be asked about the child's history of running away, the presence of family dysfunction, and personal aspects of the child's development. If the youth contacts the physician, he or she should be examined and the youth's health status should be assessed, as well as his or her willingness to return home. If it is not feasible for the youth to return home, foster care, a group home, or an independent living arrangement should be sought by referral to a social worker or a social agency.

INHERENT STRENGTHS IN VULNERABLE CHILDREN AND INTERVENTIONS

By age 20–30 yr, many children who were at special risk will have made moderate successes of their lives. Furstenberg's study of teenage mothers and Werner's study of children in Kauai, most of whom were born prematurely or in poverty, demonstrate that by this age, the majority in each study had defied the odds and made the transition to stable marriages and jobs and were accepted by their communities as responsible citizens.

Certain biologic characteristics are associated with success over the long term, such as being born with an accepting temperament. Avoidance of additional social risks is even more important. Premature infants or preadolescent boys with conduct disorders and poor reading skills, who must also face a broken family, poverty, frequent moves, and family violence, are at much greater risk than children with only one of these handicaps. Perhaps most important are the protective buffers that have been found to enhance children's resilience because these can be aided by an effective health care system and community. Children generally do better if they can gain social support, either from family members or from a nonjudgmental adult outside the family, especially an older mentor or peer. Providers of medical services should develop ways to "prescribe" supportive "other" persons for children who are at risk and isolated. Promotion of self-esteem and self-efficacy seems to be a very central factor in protecting against risks. It is essential to promote competence in some area of these children's lives.

Providers of medical services need the patience to work over a long time frame and the willingness to accept limited improvement. In addition, prediction of the consequences of risk is never 100% accurate. Health professionals as well as families should have hope. However, the confidence that, even without aid, many such children will achieve a good outcome by age 30 yr does not justify ignoring or withholding services from them in early life. It should teach us how to focus our resources on those most in need and provide a basis for hope in individual cases.

Programs that seem to work for high-risk children have a similar group of characteristics. A team is needed, because it is rare for one individual to be able to provide the multiple services needed for high-risk children. At the same time, successful programs are characterized by at least one caring person who can make personal contact with these children and their families. Most successful programs are relatively small (or are large programs divided up into small units) and nonbureaucratic but are intensive, comprehensive, and flexible. They work not only with the individual but also with the family, school, community, and even at broader societal levels. In addition, generally the earlier the programs are started, in terms of the age of the children involved, the better is the chance of success. It is also important for services to be continued over a long period.

General

Lewit EM: Why is poverty increasing among children? Future Child 3:198, 1993.
Starfield B: Effectiveness of Medical Care: Validating Clinical Wisdom. Baltimore, Johns Hopkins University Press, 1985.
Starfield B: Child and adolescent health status measures. Future Child 2:25, 1992.
Children and poverty. Future Child 7:4, 1997.
Children's Defense Fund: The State of America's Children. Mosby–Year Book, 1997.
Werner EE: Vulnerable but Invincible: A Longitudinal Study of Resilient Children and Youth. New York, McGraw-Hill, 1982.
Wilson WJ: The Truly Disadvantaged: The Inner City, the Underclass and Public Policy. Chicago, Chicago University Press, 1987.

Native American, Alaskan Eskimo, and Aleut Children

Epstein M, Moreno R, Bucchetti P: The underreporting of American Indian children in California, 1979 through 1993. Am J Public Health 87:1363, 1997.
Grossman DC, Krieger JW, Sugarman JR, et al: Health status of urban American Indians and Alaska Natives. JAMA 271:845, 1994.
Hismanick JJ, Coddington DA, Gergen PJ: Trends in asthma-related admissions among American Indian and Alaskan Native children from 1979 to 1989. Arch Pediatr Adolesc Med 148:357, 1994.
Potthoff SJ, Bearinger LH, Skay CL, et al: Dimensions of risk behaviors among American Indian youth. Arch Pediatr Adolesc Med 152:157, 1998.
The State of Native American Youth Health. University of Minnesota Health Center, 1994.

Homeless Children

Bassuk EL, Weinreb LF, Buckner JC, et al: The characteristics and needs of sheltered homeless and low-income housed mothers. JAMA 276:640, 1996.
Bassuk EL, Weinreb LF, Dawson R, et al: Determinants of behavior in homeless and low income housed preschool children. Pediatrics 100:92, 1977.
Ensign J, Santelli J: Health status and service use: Comparison of adolescents at a school-based health clinic with homeless adolescents. Arch Pediatr Adolesc Med 152:20, 1998.
Lassauer T, Richman S, Tempia M, et al: Influence of homelessness on acute admissions to hospital. Arch Dis Child 69:423, 1993.
Wood DL, Valdez RB, Hayashi T, et al: Health of homeless children and housed, poor children. Pediatrics 86:858, 1990.
Zima BT, Bussing R, Forness SR, et al: Sheltered homeless children: Their eligibility and unmet need for special education evaluations. Am J Public Health 87:236, 1997.

Children of Migrant Farm Workers and Immigrants

American Academy of Pediatrics: Health care for children of immigrant families. Pediatrics 100:153, 1997.

Dever GEA: Migrant Health Status: Profile of a Population with Complex Health Problems. Monograph Series. Migrant Clinicians Network. National Migrant Resource Program, 1991.

Centers for Disease Control and Prevention: Pregnancy-related behaviors among migrant farm workers—four states, 1989–1993. MMWR 46:283, 1997.

National Commission to Prevent Infant Mortality: HIV/AIDS: A Growing Crisis Among Migrant and Seasonal Farmworker Families, 1993.

Slesinger DP: Health status and needs of migrant farm workers in the United States: A literature review. Res Rev 8:227, 1992.

Runaway and Thrown-Away Children

Finkelhor D, Hotaling G, Sedlak A: Missing, Abducted, Runaway, and Thrown-away Children in America. Washington, DC, Office of Justice Programs. Attorney General U.S., 1990.

Greene JM, Ringwalt CL: Youth and family substance use's associated with suicide attempts among runaway and homeless youth. Subst Use Misuse 31:1058, 1996.

Green JM, Ennett ST, Ringwalt CL: Substance use among runaway and homeless youth in three national samples. Am J Public Health 87:229, 1997.

PART VI

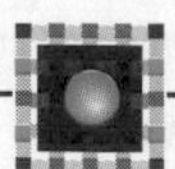

Nutrition

John S. Curran ■ Lewis A. Barness

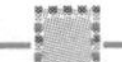

CHAPTER 40
Nutritional Requirements

Individual nutritional requirements vary with genetic and metabolic differences. For infants and children, the basic goals are achievement of satisfactory growth and avoidance of deficiency states. Good nutrition helps to prevent acute and chronic illness, to develop physical and mental potential, and to provide reserves for stress.

The Food and Nutrition Board (NAS-NRC) has identified appropriate dietary allowances for a number of substances that prevent deficiency states in most persons (Table 40–1) and is currently re-examining ranges of requirements. The Food and Nutrition Board (Institute of Medicine, 1997) released new dietary reference intakes (DRIs) for calcium, phosphorus, magnesium, vitamin D, and fluoride. DRIs encompass consideration of the estimated average requirement (EAR), the recommended dietary allowances (RDAs), the adequate intake (AI), and the tolerable upper level (UL). The EAR represents the nutrient intake estimated to meet the requirement of a specified indicator of adequacy in 50% of the individuals at a life stage in a gender group. It is a daily average over time, generally 1 wk. The RDA is the daily dietary intake sufficient to meet the individual nutrient requirements of 97–98% of individuals in the life stage and gender group. If the EAR is available the RDA = +2 SD_{EAR}. In those instances in which there is insufficient scientific evidence to calculate an EAR, the AI is used as an approximation of the average nutrient intake (e.g., for young infants, the AI is based on the daily nutrient intake for healthy full-term infants who are exclusively breastfed). The 1997 report recommends that AIs be used for all nutrients up to 1 yr of age and for calcium, vitamin D, and fluoride for all life stages. Representative values are given in Tables 40–2 and 40–3. It is likely that as further scientific evidence becomes available DRIs will replace RDAs.

Because some essential substances remain unidentifiable, a varied diet may be the only prudent way of providing them after early infancy. Only human milk appears to supply all essentials for a prolonged time. Although some food essentials should be included in the daily diet, others are stored by the body and may be supplied periodically.

Although any diet producing good nutrition varies considerably, mild excesses of nutrients or calories may be as undesirable as mild deficiencies. Because dietary influences on aspects of the aging process (e.g., atherosclerosis and longevity) remain incompletely understood, avoidance of excessive caloric and fat intake appears to be wise at all ages.

40.1 Water

Water (see also Chapter 45) is essential for existence; a lack of it results in death in a matter of days. The water content of infants is relatively higher (75–80% of body weight) than that of adults (55–60%). Although dietary fluids provide the principal source of water, some water is obtained from the oxidation of foods (mixed diets yield about 12 g of H_2O/100 kcal) and, when needed, body tissues.

Human needs for water are related to caloric consumption, to insensible loss, and to the specific gravity of the urine. The infant must consume much larger amounts of water per unit of body weight compared with the adult, but when calculated per unit of caloric intake, the amounts required are almost identical (Tables 40–4 and 40–5). The daily consumption of fluid by the healthy infant is equivalent to 10–15% of body weight compared with 2–4% in the adult. The usual food of infants and children is high in water content; most of the solid food in the child's diet contains 60–70% water, with fruits and vegetables containing 90%.

Water is absorbed throughout the intestinal tract. The quantity of water in the interstitial compartment is readily changed to maintain homeostatic balance between the intracellular and vascular compartments. The interchange of water among these compartments depends on their respective protein and electrolyte concentrations. Depending on the rate of growth, about 0.5–3% of the fluid intake will be retained. Retention of water is in the range of 9–25 mL/24 hr for the "male reference infant" in the first year of life.

Water balance depends on variables, such as the protein and mineral content of diet, that determine solute load presented for renal excretion, metabolic and respiratory rates, and body temperature. Water requirements for low birthweight infants are estimated at 85–170 mL/kg/24 hr. Fecal losses are small (3–10% of intake). Evaporation from lungs and skin accounts for 40–50% of intake (sometimes more) and renal excretion for 40–50% or more. The kidney preserves the fluid and electrolyte equilibrium of the body by varying the osmolar content and volume of urine. Urine usually has a greater osmotic pressure (300–1,000 mOsm/L) than the internal environment (293 mOsm/L); maximum normal urinary concentration is approximately 600–700 mOsm/L.

40.2 Energy

The unit of heat in metabolism is the large calorie, or kilocalorie (1 Cal = 1 kcal); it is used to refer to the energy content of food. A kilocalorie is defined as the amount of heat necessary to raise the temperature of 1 kg of water from 14.5 to 15.5°C. The production of heat varies in the oxidation of different foods, so that measuring the amount of oxygen consumed or measuring the end products of oxidation, carbon dioxide, and water approximates the values obtained by direct calorimetry.

Energy needs of children at different ages and under various conditions (Fig. 40–1) vary greatly. The approximate average expenditures of energy by the child 6–12 yr of age are basal metabolism 50%; growth 12%; physical activity 25%; fecal

TABLE 40–1 Food and Nutrition Board, National Academy of Sciences—National Research Council Recommended Dietary Allowances (Revised 1989)*†

							Fat-Soluble Vitamins			Water-Soluble Vitamins							Minerals			
Category	Age (yr) or Condition	Weight‡ (kg)	Weight‡ (lb)	Height‡ (cm)	Height‡ (in)	Protein (g)	Vitamin A (μg RE)§	Vitamin E (mg α TE)¶	Vitamin K (μg)	Vitamin C (mg)	Thiamine (mg)	Riboflavin (mg)	Niacin (mg NE)**	Vitamin B-6 (mg)	Folate (μg)	Vitamin B-12 (μg)	Iron (mg)	Zinc (mg)	Iodine (μg)	Selenium (μg)
Infants	0.0–0.5	6	13	60	24	13	375	3	5	30	0.3	0.4	5	0.3	25	0.3	6	5	40	10
	0.5–1.0	9	20	71	28	14	375	4	10	35	0.4	0.5	6	0.6	35	0.5	10	5	50	15
Children	1–3	13	29	90	35	16	400	6	15	40	0.7	0.8	9	1.0	50	0.7	10	10	70	20
	4–6	20	44	112	44	24	500	7	20	45	0.9	1.1	12	1.1	75	1.0	10	10	90	20
	7–10	28	62	132	52	28	700	7	30	45	1.0	1.2	13	1.4	100	1.4	10	10	120	30
Males	11–14	45	99	157	62	45	1,000	10	45	50	1.3	1.5	17	1.7	150	2.0	12	15	150	40
	15–18	66	145	176	69	59	1,000	10	65	60	1.5	1.8	20	2.0	200	2.0	12	15	150	50
	19–24	72	160	177	70	58	1,000	10	70	60	1.5	1.7	19	2.0	200	2.0	10	15	150	70
	25–50	79	174	176	70	63	1,000	10	80	60	1.5	1.7	19	2.0	200	2.0	10	15	150	70
	51+	77	170	173	68	63	1,000	10	80	60	1.2	1.4	15	2.0	200	2.0	10	15	150	70
Females	11–14	46	101	157	62	46	800	8	45	50	1.1	1.3	15	1.4	150	2.0	15	12	150	45
	15–18	55	120	163	64	44	800	8	55	60	1.1	1.3	15	1.5	180	2.0	15	12	150	50
	19–24	58	128	164	65	46	800	8	60	60	1.1	1.3	15	1.6	180	2.0	15	12	150	55
	25–50	63	138	163	64	50	800	8	65	60	1.1	1.3	15	1.6	180	2.0	15	12	150	55
	51+	65	143	160	63	50	800	8	65	60	1.0	1.2	13	1.6	180	2.0	10	12	150	55
Pregnant						60	800	10	65	70	1.5	1.6	17	2.2	400	2.2	30	15	175	65
Lactating	1st 6 mo					65	1,300	12	65	95	1.6	1.8	20	2.1	280	2.6	15	19	200	75
	2nd 6 mo					62	1,200	11	65	90	1.6	1.7	20	2.1	260	2.6	15	16	200	75

**The allowances, expressed as average daily intakes over time, are intended to provide for individual variations among most normal persons as they live in the United States under usual environmental stresses. Diets should be based on a variety of common foods in order to provide other nutrients for which human requirements have been less well defined. See text for detailed discussion of allowances and of nutrients not tabulated.*

†Designed for the maintenance of good nutrition of practically all healthy people in the United States.

‡Weights and heights of Reference Adults are actual medians for the population in the United States of the designated age, as reported by National Health and Nutrition Examination Survey (NHANES II). The median weights and heights of those younger than 19 years of age were taken from Hamil H, et al: Physical growth: National Center for Health Statistics percentiles. Am J Clin Nutr 32:607, 1979. The use of these figures does not imply that the height-to-weight ratios are ideal.

§Retinol equivalents. 1 retinol equivalent (RE) = 1 μg retinol or 6 μg β-carotene. See text for calculation of vitamin A activity of diets as retinol equivalents.

¶α-Tocopherol equivalents. 1 mg d-α-tocopherol = 1 mg α-TE. See text for variation in allowances and calculation of vitamin E activity of the diet as α-tocopherol equivalent.

***1 NE (niacin equivalent) is equal to 1 mg of niacin or 60 mg of dietary tryptophan.*

TABLE 40–2 Dietary Reference Intake Values by Life Stage Group

Nutrient	Calcium	Phosphorus			Magnesium						Vitamin D	Fluoride	
					EAR[c] (mg/d)		*RDA*[d] (mg/d)		*AI*[b] (mg/d)			*AI*[b] (mg/d)	
Life Stage Group[a]	*AI*[b] (mg/d)	*EAR*[c] (mg/d)	RDA[d] (mg/d)	AI[b] (mg/d)	Male	Female	Male	Female	Male	Female	*AI*[b,e,f] (μg/d)	Male	Female
0–6 mo	210	-	-	100	-	-	-	-	30	30	5	0.01	0.01
6–12 mo	270	-	-	275	-	-	-	-	75	75	5	0.5	0.5
1–3 y	500	380	460	-	65	65	80	80			5	0.7	0.7
4–8 y	800	405	500	-	110	110	130	130			5	1.1	1.1
9–13 y	1300	1055	1250	-	200	200	240	240			5	2.0	2.0
14–18 y	1300	1055	1250	-	340	300	410	360			5	3.2	2.9
19–30 y	1000	580	700	-	330	255	400	310			5	3.8	3.1
31–50 y	1000	580	700	-	350	265	420	320			5	3.8	3.1
51–70 y	1200	580	700	-	350	265	420	320			10	3.8	3.1
>70 y	1200	580	700	-	350	265	420	320			15	3.8	3.1
Pregnancy													
#18 y	1300	1055	1250	-		335	-	400	-	-	5	-	2.9
19–50 y	1000	580	700	-		290		350	-			-	3.1
31–50 y						300		360					
Lactation													
#18 y	1300	1055	1250	-		300		360	-	-	5	-	2.9
19–50 y	1000	580	700	-		255		310	-	-		-	3.1
31–50 y						265		320					

[a] *All groups except Pregnancy and Lactation are males and females unless separately labeled.*

[b] *AI, Adequate Intake. The observed average or experimentally set intake by a defined population or subgroup that appears to sustain a defined nutritional state, such as growth rate, normal circulating nutrient values, or other functional indicators of health. AI is used if sufficient scientific evidence is not available to derive an EAR. For healthy breast-fed infants, AI is the mean intake. Some seemingly healthy individuals may require higher calcium intakes to minimize risk of osteopenia and some individuals may be at low risk on even lower intakes. The AI is not equivalent to an RDA.*

[c] *EAR, Estimated Average Requirement. The intake that meets the estimated nutrient needs of 50% of the individuals in a group.*

[d] *RDA, Recommended Dietary Allowance. The intake that meets the nutrient need of almost all (97–98%) of individuals in a group.*

[e] *As cholecalciferol. 1 μg cholecalciferol = 40 IU vitamin D.*

[f] *In the absence of adequate exposure to sunlight.*

Adapted from Dietary Reference Intakes for Calcium, Phosphorus, Magnesium, Vitamin D, and Fluoride; Standing Committee on the Scientific Evaluation of Dietary Reference Intakes, Food and Nutrition Board, Institute of Medicine, National Academy of Sciences. Washington, D.C.: National Academy Press, 416 pp., 1997.

TABLE 40–3 Tolerable Upper Intake Levels (UL[a]), by Life Stage Group

Life Stage Group	Calcium (g/d)	Phosphorus (g/d)	Magnesium[b] (mg/d)	Vitamin D (μg/d)[c]	Fluoride (mg/d)
0–6 mo	ND[d]	ND	ND	25	0.7
6–12 mo	ND	ND	ND	25	0.9
1–3 y	2.5	3	65	50	1.3
4–8 y	2.5	3	110	50	2.2
9–18 y	2.5	4	350	50	10
19–70 y	2.5	4	350	50	10
>70 y	2.5	3	350	50	10
Pregnancy					
≤18 y	2.5	3.5	350	50	10
19–50 y	2.5	3.5	350	50	10
Lactation					
≤18 y	2.5	4	350	50	10
19–50 y	2.5	4	350	50	10

[a]*UL, tolerable upper intake level. The maximum level of daily nutrient intake is unlikely to pose risks of adverse effects to members of the general population. Unless specified otherwise, the UL represents total nutrient intake from food, water, and supplements.*

[b]*The UL for magnesium represents intake from a pharmacologic agent only and does not include intake from food and water.*

[c]*As cholecalciferol. 1 μg cholecalciferol = 40 IU vitamin D.*

[d]*ND, not determinable due to lack of data of adverse effects in this age group and concern with regard to lack of ability to handle excess amounts. Source of intake should be from food only in order to prevent high levels of intake.*

Adapted from Dietary Reference Intakes for Calcium, Phosphorus, Magnesium, Vitamin D, and Fluoride; Standing Committee on the Scientific Evaluation of Dietary Reference Intakes, Food and Nutrition Board, Institute of Medicine, National Academy of Sciences. Washington, D.C.: National Academy Press, 416 pp., 1997.

loss about 8%, mainly as unabsorbed fat; and thermic effect of food 5% of the remainder.

Basal metabolism is measured at room temperature (20°C) 10–14 hr after a meal, with the patient physically and emotionally quiet. For each centigrade degree of fever, basal metabolism increases approximately 10%. The basal requirement in infants is about 55 kcal/kg/24 hr; it decreases to 25–30 kcal/kg/24 hr at maturity. The term *thermic effect of food* (TEF) refers to the increase in metabolism over the basal rate by the ingestion and assimilation of food. Protein digestion may increase metabolism as much as 30% above the basal level except when it is being deposited in tissues, whereas fat and carbohydrate, which have a "sparing" effect on the TEF of protein and upon each other, cause increases of only 4 and 6%, respectively. In infants, about 7–8% of the total caloric intake goes to the TEF; in older children on an ordinary mixed diet, it is unlikely to constitute more than about 5% of total intake. The estimated energy necessary to build body tissue (*growth*) is the difference between the calories ingested and those expended for other purposes. The average requirement for *physical activity* is 15–25 kcal/kg/24 hr, with peak utilizations as high as 50–80 kcal/kg/24 hr for short periods. The amount of energy-producing food lost in the stools, except when absorption is impaired, is not more than 10% of the intake.

Although caloric requirements can best be predicted from the surface area rather than from age or weight, the final criteria for evaluating the child's needs depend on the growth pattern, the sense of well-being, and satiety. The daily requirement is approximately 80–120 kcal/kg for the 1st yr of life, with subsequent decreases of about 10 kcal/kg for each succeeding 3 yr period. Periods of rapid growth and development near puberty require increased caloric consumption. The distribution of calories in human milk, in most formulas, and in a well-balanced diet is similar. Approximately 9–15% of the calories are derived from protein; 45–55% are derived from carbohydrate; and 35–45% are derived from fat. In the older child, 10–15% of the calories should be derived from protein, 55–60% from carbohydrate, and about 30% from fat.

Each gram of ingested protein or carbohydrate provides 4 kcal. One gram of short-chain fatty acids provides 5.3 kcal; 1 g of medium-chain fatty acid gives 8.3 kcal; and 1 g of long-chain fatty acids provides 9 kcal. A continued caloric intake greater or less than the body expenditure will increase or decrease body fat. In general, a consistent caloric imbalance of 500 kcal/24 hr changes body weight by about 450 g (1 lb)/wk.

TABLE 40–4 Water Requirements

Urine Specific Gravity	Infant—3 kg 300 Calories* Intake: Water Intake mL	g/100 kcal	g/kg	Adult—70 kg 3,000 Calories* Intake: Water Intake mL	g/100 kcal	g/kg
1.005	650	217	220	6300	210	90
1.015	339	113	116	3180	106	45
1.020	300	100	100	2790	93	40
1.030	264	88	91	2430	81	35

**In this sense Calorie = large calorie = 1 kcal = 1 Cal (see text).*

40.3 Proteins

Protein constitutes about 20% of adult body weight. Its amino acids are essential nutrients in forming cell protoplasm. The kind, number, and arrangement of amino acids in a protein molecule determine its characteristics. Twenty-four amino acids have been identified; nine were found to be essential for infants (threonine, valine, leucine, isoleucine, lysine, tryptophan, phenylalanine, methionine, and histidine). Arginine, cystine, and taurine are essential for low birthweight infants. Nonessential amino acids can be synthesized and need not be

TABLE 40–5 Range of Average Water Requirements of Children at Different Ages Under Ordinary Conditions

Age	Average Body Weight (kg)	Total Water in 24 hr (mL)	Water per Kilogram of Body Weight in 24 hr (mL)
3 days	3.0	250–300	80–100
10 days	3.2	400–500	125–150
3 mo	5.4	750–850	140–160
6 mo	7.3	950–1100	130–155
9 mo	8.6	1,100–1,250	125–145
1 yr	9.5	1,150–1,300	120–135
2 yr	11.8	1,350–1,500	115–125
4 yr	16.2	1,600–1,800	100–110
6 yr	20.0	1,800–2,000	90–100
10 yr	28.7	2,000–2,500	70–85
14 yr	45.0	2,200–2,700	50–60
18 yr	54.0	2,200–2,700	40–50

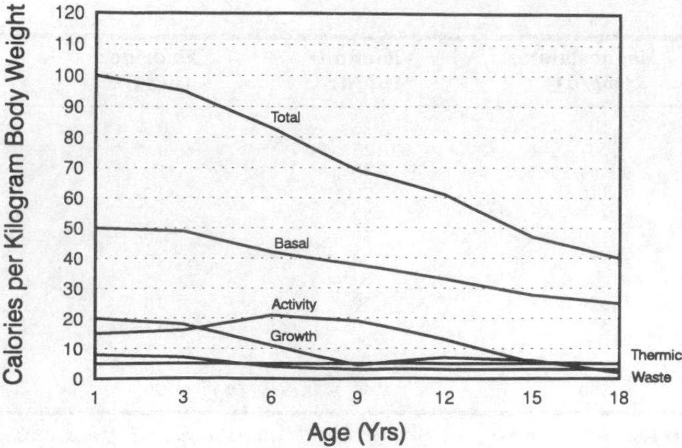

Figure 40–1 Changing energy expenditure with age.

supplied in the diet. New tissue cannot be formed without all the essential amino acids simultaneously present in the diet; the absence or deficiency of only one essential amino acid results in a negative nitrogen balance.

Proteins are broken down in the digestive process to oligopeptides and α-amino acids. The hydrochloric acid of the stomach provides the optimal pH for peptide cleavage by pepsin. Chymosin changes casein of milk to paracasein, which pepsin hydrolyzes along with other proteins. The various proteases show preference for splitting specific peptide linkages; some cleave linkages in the interior of the peptide chain, and others act at more terminal junctures. In the alkaline medium of the intestine, trypsin, chymotrypsin, and carboxypeptidase from the pancreas hydrolyze these proteins and peptones to peptides and to some amino acids; other peptidases from the intestinal juices carry digestion to the amino acid stage.

Minute amounts of certain proteins may be absorbed unchanged, as shown by immunologic reactions, but the hydrolytic products, the amino acids, and some peptides are normally absorbed through the intestinal mucosa. Large oligopeptides may be absorbed in the first few months of life or after episodes of gastroenteritis. The amino acids are carried to the liver by the portal circulation, and from there they are distributed to other tissues. Amino acids are reconstituted to functional human proteins (e.g., albumin, hemoglobin, hormones). Excess amino acids undergo deamination, and the nitrogenous portions are converted to urea in the liver and excreted by the kidneys. The carbon from amino acids is oxidized much like that of carbohydrate or fat; some amino acids are glycogenic; others are ketogenic. Proteins cannot be effectively stored. In protein depletion states, proteins from muscle may be broken down to supply amino acids for more essential sites, such as the brain, and for enzyme synthesis.

Aberrations in the metabolism of protein and the amino acids constitute a significant portion of the disease entities known as inborn errors of metabolism (see Part X).

Protein requirements at various ages are listed in Table 40–1. "Biologic value" of proteins indicates effectiveness of utilization; proteins of high biologic value have the quantity and distribution of essential amino acids appropriate for resynthesis of body tissues and produce little waste, as determined by nitrogen balance studies (Table 40–6). Abundant protein is available for children in the United States, but the supply in many developing countries is limited, and specific disorders of inadequate quality or quantity of protein intake may be encountered.

40.4 Carbohydrates

Carbohydrates, while supplying the necessary bulk of the diet, also supply most of the body's energy needs. In their absence, the body uses proteins and fats for energy. Stored chiefly as glycogen in the liver and muscles, carbohydrates probably constitute no more than 1% of the body weight. Because the size of the infant's liver is 10% that of the adult and the muscle mass is 2%, the infant's glycogen reserve is a fraction (approximately 3.5%) of that of the adult.

Carbohydrates are oxidized as glucose (dextrose) but are consumed in various forms: the monosaccharides (glucose, fructose, galactose), the disaccharides (lactose, sucrose, maltose, isomaltose), and the polysaccharides (starches, dextrins, glycogen, gums, cellulose). Pentoses are poorly absorbed.

Through a series of enzymatic and chemical reactions in the digestive tract, complex carbohydrates are split into simpler structures. Salivary and pancreatic amylases are principally involved in the breakdown of starch to oligosaccharides (dextrins) and disaccharides (primarily maltose). Intestinal amylase may be decreased during the first 4 mo of life. The disaccharides are absorbed intact into the intestinal brush border cells, where disaccharidases in the microvilli complete the hydrolysis to the monosaccharides: one molecule of maltose to two molecules of glucose; sucrose to glucose and fructose; lactose to glucose and galactose. The monosaccharides are absorbed rapidly; glucose and galactose are actively taken up against concentration gradients, whereas fructose absorption is passive. During absorption, phosphoric acid "carrier" radicals combine with hexose sugars in the intestinal mucosa for transport across the cell membrane. Sodium must be present for absorption to continue when the intraintestinal sugar concentration is low. These hexose phosphates separate again into their component parts, permitting the sugar to diffuse into the portal bloodstream.

Some glucose may be oxidized directly, such as in the brain and heart. Most of the absorbed sugar is converted to glycogen in the liver, although glycogenesis also occurs in other tissues. Up to 15% of the weight of the liver and 3% of the muscle may be glycogen; small amounts are also found in practically all other organs. Glycogenolysis in the liver yields glucose as the chief product, whereas glycogen breakdown in the muscle yields lactic acid. The overall oxidation of glucose has two phases, the anaerobic (glycolysis) and the aerobic (tricarboxylic acid cycle). In the former, glucose is broken down to pyruvic acid; in the aerobic cycle, pyruvic acid is completely oxidized to carbon dioxide and water. Insulin and the pituitary and adrenal hormones are involved in these processes, and nicotinic acid, thiamine, riboflavin, and pantothenic acid take part in the enzymatic reactions. Carbohydrate that is not oxidized or stored as glycogen is converted to fat.

The principal carbohydrate metabolic disorders are diabetes mellitus, glycogen storage diseases, galactosemia, fructose intolerance, and glucose intolerance; deficiencies of sugar-splitting enzymes in the intestines (e.g., lactase, sucrase, maltase, isomaltase) are associated with diarrhea and malabsorption resulting from the osmotic effect of the unabsorbed sugar and from fermentation of the carbohydrate by intestinal bacteria.

40.5 Fats

Fats or their metabolic products form an integral part of cellular membranes and are efficient stores of energy. They impart palatability to food and serve as vehicles for fat-soluble vitamins A, D, E, and K. Approximately 98% of natural fats are triglycerides, three fatty acids combined with glycerol. The remaining 2% include free fatty acids, monoglycerides, diglycerides, cholesterol, and phospholipids (including lecithin, cephalin, sphingomyelin, and cerebrosides).

Naturally occurring fats contain straight-chain fatty acids, both saturated and unsaturated, varying in length from 4 to 24 carbon atoms. The degree of absorption generally varies

TABLE 40–6 Functions of Water, Proteins, Carbohydrates, and Fats

Foodstuffs	Functions	Effects of Deficiency	Effects of Excess	Sources
Water	Solvent for cellular changes, medium for ions, transport of nutrients and waste products, regulation of body temperature	Thirst, dryness of tongue, dehydration, anhydremia, high specific gravity of urine, loss of kidney function (acidosis, oliguria, uremia, death)	Abdominal discomfort, headache, cramps (water without salt), intoxication, convulsions, edema, and circulatory failure	Water as such, all foods
Proteins	Supply amino acids for growth and repair of tissue cells, solutions for osmotic equilibrium, buffer. Hemoglobin, nucleoproteins, glycoprotein, and lipoproteins; enzymes, antibodies; protective structures (nails and hair)	Lassitude, abdominal enlargement, edema, depletion of plasma proteins, kwashiorkor (protein malnutrition); marasmus (protein-calorie malnutrition)	Prolonged high protein intake. May aggravate renal insufficiency	Milk, eggs, meat, fish, poultry, cheese, soybeans, peas, beans, cereals, nuts, lentils
Carbohydrates	Readily available source of energy, antiketogenic, structure of cells, antibodies, source of stored calories (glycogen and fat), resynthesis of amino acids, roughage	Ketosis if intake is less than 15% of calories or in starvation; underweight if total calories are low	Overweight if total calories are high. Various syndromes due to inborn errors of sugar metabolism.	Milk, cereals, fruits, sucrose, syrups, starches, vegetables
Fats	Concentrated source of energy; physical protection for vessels, nerves, organs; insulation against changes in temperature; cell membranes and nuclei; vehicle for absorption of vitamins (A, D, E, and K); essential fatty acids, appetite appeal; aid satiety (delay emptying time of stomach)	Lack of satiety (craving for fat), underweight, skin changes with intakes very low in linoleic acid	Overweight, abdominal symptoms in familial hyperlipidemia, high cholesterol intakes may be harmful to selected populations	Milk, butter, egg yolk, lard, bacon, meat, fish, cheese, nuts, vegetable oils. Breast milk usually supplies 4–5% of calories as linoleic acid; vegetable oils vary greatly, with safflower, corn, soy, and others being especially rich

with the melting point, the degree of unsaturation, and the positions of the fatty acids on the glycerol molecule.

Ingested triglycerides are partially hydrolyzed by lingual lipase and emulsified in the stomach. In the duodenum, pancreatic lipase hydrolyzes the triglycerides to monoglycerides and fatty acids and, with bile salts, forms micelles, which increase fat solubility. Unsplit diglycerides and triglycerides are insoluble. Low birthweight infants have decreased amounts of bile and decreased absorption of fat.

Long-chain fatty acids and monoglycerides (those with more than 10 carbon atoms) in micelles are presumably absorbed into the mucosal cell by diffusion. Transport across the cell involves re-esterification of these fatty acids and monoglycerides to triglycerides, which are then "coated" with lipoprotein to form the chylomicron, in which the fat is transported in the lymph system to the venous circulation via the thoracic duct. Transport proteins include very low density, low-density, and high-density lipoproteins synthesized in the liver.

Short- and medium-chain triglycerides are handled differently; they are readily hydrolyzed by pancreatic lipase to free fatty acids, which are transported through the cell. Even when intraluminal hydrolysis is inadequate because of deficiency of pancreatic lipase or of bile salts, these fats will be absorbed and hydrolyzed to free fatty acids within the cell by mucosal lipase. With neither esterification to triglycerides nor subsequent chylomicron formation, these free fatty acids directly enter the intestinal veins and pass to the liver via the portal system. This alternative pathway for short- and medium-chain triglycerides is utilized in nutritional formulations for children with severe absorptive problems.

ESSENTIAL FATTY ACIDS. Humans do not synthesize linoleic or linolenic acid. Both must be supplied in the diet and are, therefore, "essential." Unsaturated fatty acids are named to indicate the position of double bonds. The carbon atom farthest from the carboxyl acid is the omega carbon. Linoleic acid, the precursor of arachidonic acid is an omega-6 acid. Arachidonic acid metabolites are the omega-6 series of prostaglandins and leukotrienes. Linolenic acid, an omega-3 acid, modulates the production of arachidonic acid and is the direct precursor of the omega-3 series of prostaglandins and longer chain fatty acids, such as docosahexaenoic and eicosapentaenoic acids; it affects cerebral nervous structures and neurotransmission. Dietary recommendations indicate that the ratio of linoleic:linolenic acids should be 4–6:1. Essential fatty acids are necessary for growth, skin and hair integrity, regulation of cholesterol metabolism, lipotropic activity, decreased platelet adhesiveness, and reproduction. Diets containing less than 1–2% of the calories as linoleic acid require greater caloric consumption for comparable growth. In children with essential fatty acid deficiency, serum levels of trienoic acid increase relative to tetraenoic acids. Excess unsaturated acids increase peroxidation and may cause membrane destruction. Rapidly growing young infants maintained on diets very low in linoleic acid develop intertrigo and dryness, thickening, and desquamation of the skin.

The relation of dietary fat intake to intimal fat streaking in the major arterial vessels in early life and atheromatous changes in adults remains to be clarified (see Chapter 83.3).

40.6 Minerals

The physiologic roles and dietary sources of the principal minerals with nutritional significance are summarized in Table 40–7. Requirements, except for several of the trace elements, are shown in Tables 40–1 to 40–3.

The ash content of the fetus is about 3% of the body weight at birth. It increases continuously throughout childhood. Adult ash content is 4.35% of body weight; 83% is in the skeleton, and 10% is in the muscle. For each gram of protein retained, 0.3 g of mineral matter is deposited. The principal cations are calcium, magnesium, potassium, and sodium; the comparable anions are phosphorus, sulfur, and chloride. Iron, iodine, and cobalt appear in important organic complexes. The trace elements fluorine, copper, zinc, chromium, manganese, selenium, and molybdenum have known metabolic roles; silicon, boron, nickel, aluminum, arsenic, bromine, and strontium are also present in the diet and in the body.

40.7 Vitamins

The word *vitamin* refers to organic compounds required in minute amounts to catalyze cellular metabolism essential for

TABLE 40–7 Physiology and Sources of Nutritionally Important Minerals

Mineral	Function and Metabolism	Effects of Deficiency	Effects of Excess	Sources
Calcium	Structure of bone and teeth, muscle contraction, nerve irritability, coagulation of blood, cardiac action, production of milk. Absorbed from upper small intestine: aided by vitamin D, ascorbic acid, lactose, acid medium; hindered by excesses of dietary oxalic acid, phytic acid, fat, fiber, phosphate. Deposited in bone trabeculas and maintained in dynamic equilibrium with body tissue through action of parathyroid hormone and thyrocalcitonin. About 70% excreted in feces, 10% in urine, 15–25% retained, depending on growth rate. Serum level 9–11 mg/dL, 60% ionized.	Poor mineralization of bones and teeth; osteomalacia; osteoporosis; tetany; rickets; impairment of growth.	Unknown (dietary) Heart block and renal stones (parenteral).	Milk, cheese, green leafy vegetables, canned salmon, clams, oysters.
Chloride	Osmotic pressure; acid-base balance; HCl in gastric juice. Readily absorbed; about 92% of intake is excreted, mainly in the urine, some in feces and sweat; composes about ⅔ of the blood plasma anions; blood serum level, 99–106 mEq/L; in intracellular and extracellular fluids; parallels sodium intake and output.	Hypochloremic alkalosis may occur with prolonged vomiting or excessive sweating, with parenteral administration of glucose without saline, with excessive ACTH therapy, and with congenital alkalosis.	Unknown	Table salt, meat, milk, eggs.
Chromium	Glycemia regulation and insulin metabolism.	Diabetes in animals	None known	Yeast
Cobalt	Component of vitamin B_{12} (cyanocobalamin) molecule and of erythropoietin.	None known ? Hypothyroidism.	Cardiomyopathy; medicinally, it may be goitrogenic or may produce cardiomyopathy.	Widely distributed
Copper	Essential for production of red blood cells; transferrin, hemoglobin formation; absorption of iron, activities of tyrosinase, catalase, uricase, cytochrome C oxidase, 8-aminolevulinic acid dehydrase, lysyl oxidase. Absorbed with sulfur-rich proteins; transported bound to α-2-globulin as ceruloplasmin; present in erythrocytes in a labile form and the more stable hemocuprein; highest concentration in liver and central nervous system (cerebrocuprein); excreted mainly via the intestinal wall and the bile; deranged metabolism in Wilson disease (hepatolenticular degeneration), and Menkes syndrome.	May be cause of refractory anemia, osteoporosis, neutropenia, depigmentation and delayed bone age, bone infractions, pseudoparalysis, ataxia. Increase of serum cholesterol.	Cirrhosis, gastritis, hemolysis.	Liver, oysters, meats, fish, whole grains, nuts, legumes.
Fluorine	Tooth and bone structure. Retained when intake is above 0.6 mg/day; excreted in urine and sweat; deposited in bones as fluorapatite (dynamic equilibrium).	Tendency to dental caries.	Fluorosis: mottling of teeth with intake of more than 4–8 mg/24 hr.	Water, sea foods, plant and animal foods (dependent on content in soil and water).
Iodine	Constituent of thyroxine (T4) and triiodothyronine (T3). Readily absorbed from intestine; circulates as inorganic and organic iodide; selectively concentrated about 25:1 in the thyroid gland, quickly iodized and incorporated into thyroglobulin; proteolytic enzymes release thyroxine and triiodothyronine into the blood. Excretion mainly in urine. Antithyroid compounds: goitrins and brassicae; certain drugs interfere with iodine metabolism.	Simple goiter, endemic cretinism.	Not harmful (less than 1 mg/24 hr); medicinally, may cause goiter.	Iodized salt, sea food, food grown in nongoitrous areas.
Iron	Structure of hemoglobin and myoglobin for O_2 and CO_2 transport; oxidative enzymes; cytochrome C and catalase. Absorbed in ferrous form according to body need, aided by gastric juice and ascorbic acid; hindered by fiber, phytic acid, steatorrhea. Transported in plasma in ferric state bound to transferrin; stored in liver, spleen, bone marrow, and kidney as ferritin and hemosiderin; conserved and reused; minimal losses in urine and sweat; about 90% of intake excreted in the stool.	Anemia; hypochromic, microcytic, growth failure; hyperactivity (?).	Hemosiderosis in Bantu people of Africa due to low phosphorus and high iron contents of diet. Poisoning by medicinal iron.	Liver, meat, egg yolk, green vegetables, whole grains, legumes, nuts.
Magnesium	Structure of bones and teeth; activation of enzymes in carbohydrate metabolism; muscle and nerve irritability, important intracellular cation, essential to metabolic processes. Principal cation of soft tissue; absorption from small intestine varies with intake; some urinary excretion, but excellent renal conservation; antagonist to calcium action.	Occurs in malabsorption and deficiency states; diabetes, may be expressed clinically as tetany; associated frequently with hypocalcemia; hypokalemia.	None (dietary); toxicity from intravenous medication.	Cereals, legumes, nuts, meat, milk.

TABLE 40–7 Physiology and Sources of Nutritionally Important Minerals *Continued*

Mineral	Function and Metabolism	Effects of Deficiency	Effects of Excess	Sources
Manganese	Enzyme activation, especially superoxide dismutase; normal bone structure, carbohydrate metabolism. Poor absorption from intestine; transported in plasma; particularly high turnover rate in mitochondria; excretion mainly via the intestine in bile; competes with iron.	Not known.	None (dietary); toxicity from chronic inhalation (encephalopathy).	Legumes, nuts, whole grain cereals, green leafy vegetables.
Molybdenum	Component of enzymes; xanthine oxidase for conversion to uric acid and mobilization of ferritin iron in liver, liver aldehyde oxidase, sulfite oxidase. Readily absorbed from intestine; excreted chiefly in urine, some in bile.	Ocular abnormalities, seizures, mental retardation, xanthinuria.	Not established.	Legumes, grains, dark green leafy vegetables, animal organs.
Phosphorus	Constituent of bones and teeth; structure of nucleus and cytoplasm of all cells; acid-base balance; energy transformations and transmission of nerve impulses; metabolism of carbohydrate, protein, and fat. About 70% of intake absorbed as free phosphates; vitamin D and parathormone implicated in intestinal absorption and kidney retention; excreted in urine and feces; occurs in blood as phospholipids, organic esters, and inorganic phosphates; inorganic phosphates in blood serum of infants and children, 4–7 mg/dL; ratio of inorganic to organic phosphates in whole blood is about 1:20.	Rickets may develop in rapidly growing, very low birthweight babies with low intakes of both P and Ca; muscle weakness.	Possibility of tetany during recovery from rickets or in newborn on formula with low Ca:P (1:1) ratio.	Milk, milk products, egg yolk, fresh foods, legumes, nuts, whole grains.
Potassium	Muscle contraction; nerve impulse conduction; intracellular osmotic pressure and fluid balance; heart rhythm. Primarily intracellular; excretion 80% in urine, some in sweat and feces; about 8% retained by growing child; blood serum level 4.0–5.6 mEq/L.	In starvation or in such pathologic conditions as diarrhea, diabetic acidosis, ACTH excess; muscle weakness, anorexia, nausea, abdominal distention, nervous irritability, drowsiness, confusion, tachycardia; deficiency exaggerates effects of sodium.	Heart block at serum levels of 10 mEq/L; important in Addison disease, renal failure, or administration of potassium-containing salts.	All foods.
Selenium	Cofactor of glutathione peroxidase in tissue respiration.	Kashin cardiomyopathy, arthritis (?), Kashin cardiovascular disease, myositis.	Alopecia, nail abnormalities, garlic odor to breath.	Vegetables, meat.
Sodium	Osmotic pressure; acid-base balance; water balance; muscle and nerve irritability. Readily absorbed from intestine; excreted chiefly in urine (98%); parallels chloride intake; renal excretion controlled by ACTH; extracellular cation, but small amount in muscle and cartilage; blood serum level, 135–145 mEq/L.	Nausea; diarrhea, muscle cramps, dehydration, hypotension.	Edema if inadequate excretion or excessive parenteral fluids.	Table salt, fresh foods, milk, eggs, sodium compounds as baking soda and powder, glutamate, seasonings, and preservatives.
Sulfur	Constituent of cellular protein; cocarboxylase; melanin; mucopolysaccharides, vitreous humor, synovial fluid, connective tissues, cartilage, heparin, insulin; metabolism of nerve tissue; detoxification mechanisms; SH group in coenzyme A, cystathionine, and glutathione. Only sources utilized are cystine and methionine; inorganic forms unavailable to body; excreted as inorganic sulfate or ethereal sulfate via urine and bile.	Not known; growth failure from protein deficiency may be due in part to deficiency of sulfur-containing amino acids.	Not harmful, excreted in urine as sulfates.	Protein foods contain about 1%.
Zinc	Constituent of several enzymes; carbonic anhydrase (in erythrocytes) essential for CO_2 exchange; carboxypeptidase of intestine for hydrolysis of protein; dehydrogenase of liver. Found in liver and organs, muscles, bones, red and white blood cells; higher tissue concentration in young subjects; excreted chiefly from intestine, competes with copper.	Dwarfism, iron-deficiency anemia, hepatosplenomegaly, hyperpigmentation and hypogonadism, acrodermatitis enteropathica, depression of immunocompetence, poor wound healing. Functional zinc depletion syndrome. Includes: hepatosplenomegaly, dermatitis, anemia, stunted growth, impaired immune function.	Gastrointestinal upsets (from galvanized iron cooking utensils); copper deficiency; decreased high-density lipoprotein. Hepatosplenomegaly, dermatitis, anemia, stunted growth, impaired immune function.	Meat, grain, nuts, cheese.

TABLE 40–8 Physical and Metabolic Properties and Food Sources of the Vitamins

Names and Synonyms	Characteristics	Biochemical Action	Effects of Deficiency	Effects of Excess	Sources
Vitamin A: retinol (vitamin A1) is an alcohol of high molecular weight; 1 μg of retinol = 3.3 IU vitamin A Provitamin A: the plant pigments α-, β-, and γ-carotenes and cryptoxanthin; ⅙ activity of retinol	Fat soluble; heat stable; destroyed by oxidation, drying, bile necessary for absorption; stored in liver, protected by vitamin E	Component of retinal pigments, rhodopsin and iodopsin, for vision in dim light; bone and tooth development; formation and maturation of epithelia	Nyctalopia, photophobia, xerophthalmia, conjunctivitis, keratomalacia leading to blindness; faulty epiphyseal bone formation; defective tooth enamel; keratinization of mucous membranes and skin; retarded growth; impaired resistance to infection	Anorexia, slow growth, drying and cracking of skin, enlargement of liver and spleen, swelling and pain of long bones, bone fragility, increased intracranial pressure, alopecia, carotenemia	Liver, fish liver oils, whole milk, milk fat products, egg yolk, fortified margarines Carotenoids from plants: green vegetables, yellow fruits and vegetables
Vitamin B Complex: thiamine: vitamin B_1; antiberiberi vitamin; aneurin	Water and alcohol soluble; fat insoluble; stable in slightly acid solution; labile to heat, alkali, sulfites	Component of thiamine pyrophosphate carboxylases, which act in various oxidative decarboxylations, including that of pyruvic acid	Beriberi, fatigue, irritability, anorexia, constipation, headache, insomnia, tachycardia, polyneuritis, cardiac failure, edema, elevated pyruvic acid in the blood, aphonia	None from oral intake	Liver, meat, especially pork, milk, whole grain or enriched cereals, wheat germ, legumes, nuts
Riboflavin: vitamin B_2	Sparingly soluble in water; sensitive to light and alkali; stable to heat, oxidation, acid	Constituent of flavoprotein enzymes important in hydrogen transfer reactions; amino acid, fatty acid, and carbohydrate metabolism and cellular respiration. Retinal pigment for light adaptation	Ariboflavinosis; photophobia, blurred vision, burning and itching of eyes, corneal vascularization, poor growth, cheilosis	Not harmful	Milk, cheese, liver and other organs, meat, eggs, fish, green leafy vegetables, whole or enriched grains
Niacin: nicotinamide; nicotinic acid; antipellagra vitamin	Water and alcohol soluble; stable to acid, alkali, light, heat, oxidation	Constituent of coenzymes I and II. NAD, NADP cofactors in a number of dehydrogenase systems	Pellagra, multiple B-vitamin deficiency syndrome, diarrhea, dementia, dermatitis	Nicotinic acid (not the amide) is vasodilator; skin flushing and itching, hepatopathy	Meat, fish, poultry, liver, whole grain and enriched cereals, green vegetables, peanuts
Folacin: group of related compounds containing pteridine ring, para amino benzoic acid, and glutamic acid. Pteroylglutamic acid (PGA)	Slightly soluble in water: labile to heat, light, acid	Concerned with formation and metabolism of one-carbon units; participates in synthesis of purines, pyrimidines, nucleoproteins, and methyl groups	Megaloblastic anemia (infancy, pregnancy): usually is secondary to malabsorption disease glossitis, pharyngeal ulcers, impaired immunity	Unknown	Liver, green vegetables, nuts, cereals, cheese, fruits, yeast, beans, peas
Cyanocobalamin: vitamin B_{12}	Slightly soluble in water; stable to heat in neutral solution; labile in acid or alkaline ones; destroyed by light. Castle intrinsic factor of the stomach required for absorption	Transfer of one-carbon units in purine and labile methyl group metabolism; essential for maturation of red blood cells in bone marrow; metabolism of nervous tissue; adenosylcobalamin is the coenzyme for methylmalonyl CoA mutase	Juvenile pernicious anemia, due to defect in absorption rather than to dietary lack; also secondary to gastrectomy, celiac disease, inflammatory lesions of small bowel, long-term drug therapy (PAS, neomycin); methylmalonic aciduria; homocystinuria	Unknown	Muscle and organ meats, fish, eggs, milk, cheese
Biotin	Crystallized from yeast; soluble in water	Coenzyme carboxylases; involved in CO_2 transfer	Dermatitis, seborrhea; inactivated by avidin in raw egg white	None known	Yeast, animal products; synthesized in intestine
Vitamin B_6 active forms: pyridoxine, pyridoxal, pyridoxamine	Water soluble; destroyed by ultraviolet light and by heat	Constituent of coenzymes for decarboxylation, transamination, transsulfuration; fatty acid metabolism	Irritability, convulsions, hypochromic anemia; peripheral neuritis in patients receiving isoniazid; oxaluria (see Chapter 44.3)	Sensory neuropathy	Meat, liver, kidney, whole grains, soybeans, nuts, fish, poultry, green vegetables

TABLE 40–8 Physical and Metabolic Properties and Food Sources of the Vitamins *Continued*

Names and Synonyms	Characteristics	Biochemical Action	Effects of Deficiency	Effects of Excess	Sources
Vitamin C: ascorbic acid; vitamin C; antiscorbutic vitamin	Water soluble; easily oxidized, accelerated by heat, light, alkali oxidative enzymes, traces of copper or iron	Integrity and maintenance of intercellular material, facilitates absorption of iron and conversion of folic acid to folinic acid; metabolism of tyrosine and phenylalanine, activity of succinic dehydrogenase and serum phosphatase in infants, not in adults	Scurvy and poor wound healing	Oxaluria (see also Chapter 44.9 and discussion of hyperoxaluria oxalosis)	Citrus fruits, tomatoes, berries, cantaloupe, cabbage, green vegetables. Cooking has destructive effect.
Vitamin D: group of sterols having similar physiologic activity, D_2-calciferol is activated ergosterol. D_3 is activated 7-dehydrocholesterol in skin 1 μg = 40 IU vitamin D	Fat soluble, stable to heat, acid alkali, and oxidation; bile necessary for absorption. Prohormone for 25-OH cholecalciferol	Regulates absorption and deposition of calcium and phosphorus, by affecting permeability of intestinal membrane; regulates level of serum alkaline phosphatase, which is believed to be concerned with calcium phosphate deposition in bones and teeth	Rickets (high serum phosphatase level appears before bone deformities); infantile tetany, poor growth, osteomalacia	Wide variation in tolerance; over 500 μg/24 hr toxic when continued for weeks; prolonged administration of 45 μg/24 hr may be toxic (Chapter 44.12); nausea, diarrhea, weight loss, polyuria, nocturia, calcification of soft tissues, including heart, renal tubules, blood vessels, bronchi, stomach	Vitamin D-fortified milk and margarine, fish liver oils, exposure to sunlight or other ultraviolet sources
Vitamin E: group of related chemical compounds—tocopherols with similar biologic activities	Fat soluble; unstable to ultraviolet light, alkali, readily oxidized by oxygen, iron, rancid fats Antioxidant; bile necessary for absorption	Minimizes oxidation of carotene, vitamin A, and linoleic acid; stabilizes membranes	Requirements related to polyunsaturated fat intake; red blood cell hemolysis in premature infants, loss of neural integrity	Unknown	Germ oils of various seeds, green leafy vegetables, nuts, legumes
Vitamin K: group of naphthoquinones with similar biologic activities; K_1 is phytoquinone	Natural compounds are fat soluble; stable to heat and reducing agents; labile to oxidizing agent, strong acids, alkali, light; bile salts necessary for intestinal absorption	Prothrombin formation, coagulation factors II, VII, IX, and X and osteocalcin are vitamin K dependent, proteins C, S, Z	Hemorrhagic manifestations; bone metabolism	Not established; analogs may produce hyperbilirubinemia in premature infants	Green leafy vegetables, pork, liver. Widely distributed

NAD(P), nicotinamide adenine dinucleotide (phosphate); CoA, coenzyme A; PAS, para-aminosalicylic acid.

growth or maintenance of the organism. Vitamin requirements for infants and children are listed in Tables 40–1 to 40–3. For vitamin functions and disorders, see Table 40–8 and Chapter 44.

40.8 Miscellaneous Factors

FIBER. Recommended dietary intake of fiber is approximately 0.5 g/kg/24 hr to a maximum of 35 g/24 hr. The quantity of undigestible vegetable fiber consumed in acceptable diets may be as much as 170–300 mg/kg/24 hr. Most children who receive well-balanced diets obtain sufficient amounts of fiber. Highly refined foods contain little fiber and may be associated with an increased incidence of constipation, appendicitis, diverticulitis, and other intestinal disorders. High fiber intake may result in decreased absorption of cholesterol as well as zinc and other essential nutrients.

DIGESTIBILITY. The relative amount of a given nutrient available for assimilation is high in most of the common food classes: carbohydrate, 97%; fat, 95%; protein, 92%. Cooking is a factor in digestibility. For example, the boiling of milk reduces the size of the curd and renders it more digestible; on the other hand, heating destroys the activity of vitamin C.

SATIETY. The ingestion of a meal should provide a sense of well-being. Whole milk, cream, eggs, and fatty foods have high satiety values; sugar increases the flow of gastric juice and delays emptying of the stomach, thus increasing satiety. Bread and potatoes have relatively low satiety values, as do lean meat, fish, vegetables, and many fruits.

AVAILABILITY. Poverty, ignorance, and lack of practical education in buying and preparing food are the main causes of malnutrition in children. Diets of lower income families are often deficient in milk, fruits, fresh vegetables, and meats. A suggested method for planning low-cost meals is to divide the money available for food into fifths: one fifth each for vegetables and fruits; for milk and cheese; for meats, fish, and eggs; for bread and cereals; and for fats, sugar, and other food adjuncts.

Geographic location may influence the availability of foods and the development of deficiency disorders, especially among low socioeconomic populations (for example, the relation of dental caries to lack of fluoride in communal water supplies).

BACTERIAL SYNTHESIS OF VITAMINS. Certain vitamins are synthesized in the human gastrointestinal tract; however, the extent to which they can meet the body's needs is uncertain. Once the bacterial flora of the intestinal tract have been established, vitamin K is produced and is available to the body. Pantothenic acid and biotin, essential to human metabolism, can be supplied by bacterial synthesis alone. Thiamine, riboflavin, niacin, vitamin B_6, vitamin B_{12}, and folic acid are synthesized in some

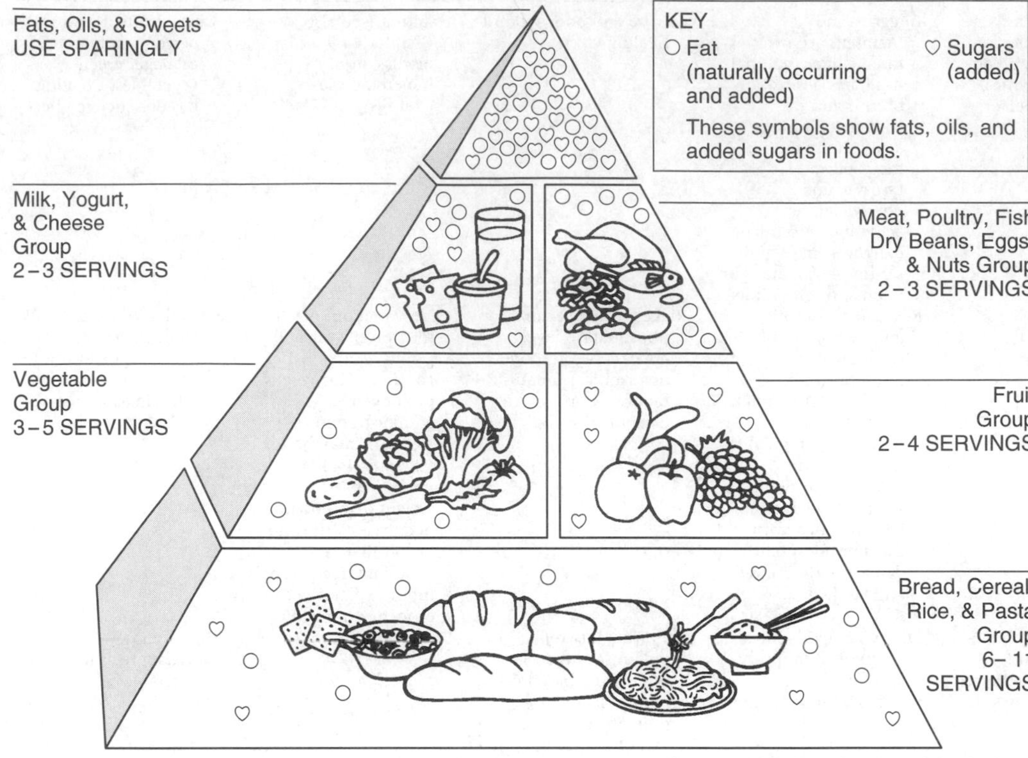

Figure 40–2 Food guide pyramid: a guide to daily food choices.

species, but synthesis is limited or does not exist in humans. The kind of food or the nature of intestinal flora may affect vitamin production or availability. For instance, 3% of the population in Kobe, Japan, harbored intestinal bacteria that split thiamine; evidence of beriberi appeared in these persons.

ANTIMICROBIAL FACTORS. Administration of antimicrobial agents may affect nutritional status. Appetite is sometimes impaired or bacterial flora producing vitamin K are sufficiently altered to precipitate borderline deficiency. Several antibiotics are known to produce steatorrhea. Orally administered broad-spectrum antibiotics decrease nitrogen balance. Isoniazid combines with pyridoxal phosphate and may produce symptoms of vitamin B_6 deficiency. Antimicrobial compounds may be transmitted in breast milk or in foods from animals that are fed these compounds.

ENDOCRINE FACTORS. Antithyroid substances that increase the requirement for iodine (goitrogens) have been found in turnips, rutabagas, cabbage, soybeans, cobalt-containing foods, food additives, and medications. Administering adrenocorticotropic hormone (ACTH) or corticosteroids necessitates an increase in protein and calcium and a decrease in sodium intake. Transient hypoparathyroidism with tetany has been observed in the neonatal period after excessive intake of vitamin D or phosphates.

RADIOACTIVITY. Apparently, little danger results from ^{14}C, because of its low activity. ^{131}I is removed from milk by aeration or storage. ^{137}Cs, which may be found in meat and milk prod-

TABLE 40–9 Recommended Food Intake for Good Nutrition According to Food Groups

Food Group	Serving Size	Servings/d	1 yr	2–3 yr	4+ yr
Bread, cereal, rice, pasta	1 slice 1 oz (cereal)	6–11	1–2	2–4	3–11
Vegetables	½ cup	3–5	1/2	1	3–5
Fruit	1 apple, banana	2–4	1/2	1	2–4
Milk, cheese	1 cup 1½ oz cheese	2–3	1/2	1	1–3
Meat, poultry, etc	2–3 oz	2–3	1/2–1	1/2–1	1–3

After age 2 yr, fats, oils, and sweets should be consumed sparingly.
C = 1 cup or 8 oz or 240 mL.
Tbsp = tablespoon (1 Tbsp = 15 mL = ½ oz).

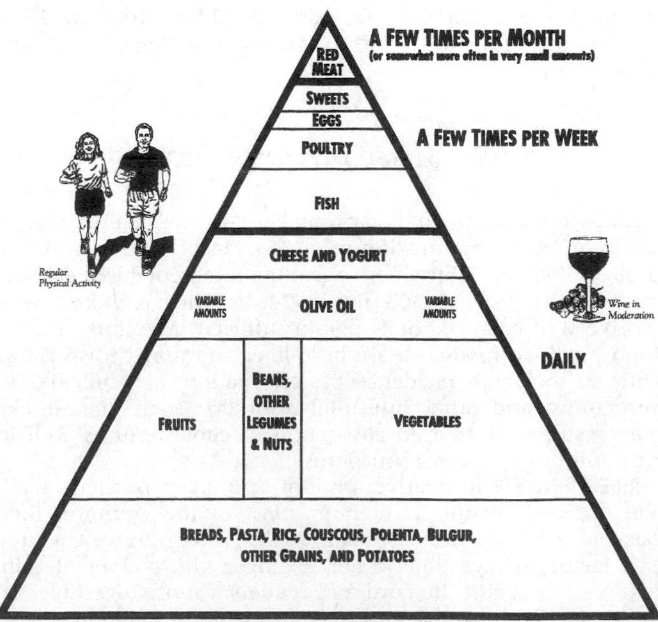

Figure 40–3 Mediterranean diet pyramid.

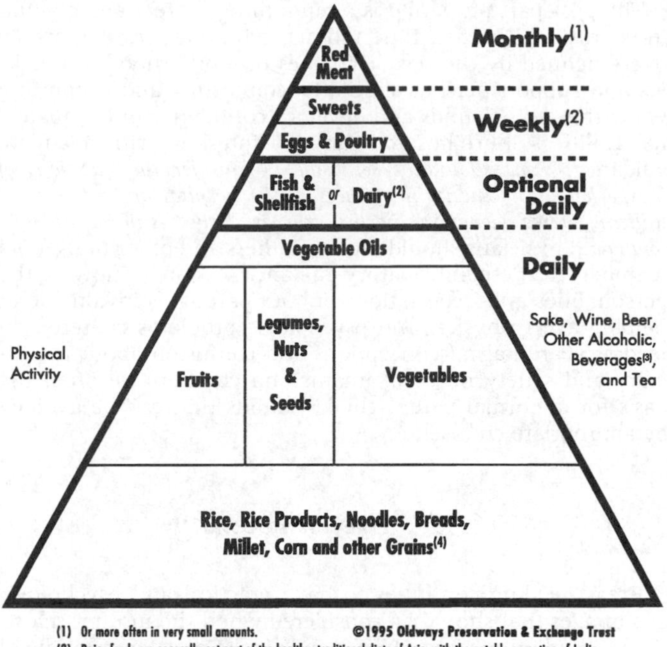

(1) Or more often in very small amounts. ©1995 Oldways Preservation & Exchange Trust
(2) Dairy foods are generally not part of the healthy, traditional diets of Asia, with the notable exception of India. In light of current nutrition research, if dairy foods are consumed on a daily basis, they should be used in low to moderate amounts, and preferably low in fat.
(3) Wine, beer and other alcoholic beverages should be consumed in moderation and primarily with meals,and avoided whenever consumption would put an individual or others at risk.
(4) Minimally refined whenever possible.

Figure 40–4 Asian diet pyramid.

ucts, can be counteracted by a high potassium intake or by acetazolamide. Only 10% of ^{90}Sr ingested by the cow is found in cow's milk. Some foods are irradiated to improve safety and preservation. No adverse effects have been reported from consuming properly irradiated foods.

EMOTIONAL FACTORS. Along with increased knowledge of the significance of various nutrients, excessive parental and professional concern has developed with regard to the food that the individual infant or child cats. For cxamplc, misdirected efforts to control obesity and hypercholesterolemia have led to severe malnutrition in young children.

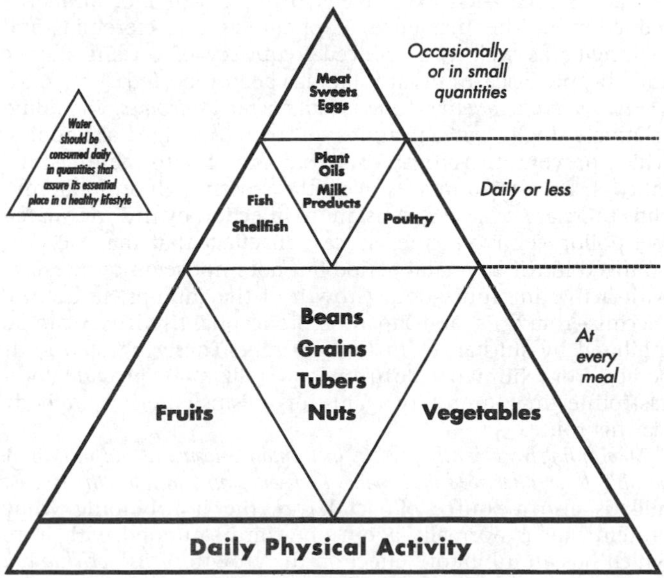

Alcohol may be consumed by adults in moderation and with meals, but consumption should be avoided during pregnancy and whenever it would put the individual or others at risk.

Figure 40–5 Latin American diet pyramid.

40.9 Evaluation of Diet

See Tables 40–9 and Tables 726–11 and 726–12 in Chapter 726 and Figures 40–2 to 40–5.

The recall interview for determining children's food habits is usually satisfactory, but for a more accurate accounting the parent should observe and record the actual food intake and convert to "servings" appropriate to the child's age. It is important to include items that may not be consumed daily.

The 1992–1997 United States Department of Agriculture dietary guide according to food groups provides flexibility (see Fig. 40–2). Similar dietary guides have been prepared for Mediterranean, Asian, and Latin American populations (see Figs. 40–3 to 40–5). A food intake record can indicate possible nutritional imbalances. An excessive intake of foods of one group may result in a high caloric level, producing an overweight child while at the same time leading to a dangerously low intake of some essential nutrients, such as the overconsumption of milk and the underconsumption of other foods with resultant iron-deficiency anemia. When key foods, such as milk, eggs, and citrus fruits, are eliminated for personal or medical reasons, the deficiencies may be compensated for by judicious substitutions.

Dietary Reference Intakes for Calcium, Phosphorus, Magnesium, Vitamin D, and Fluoride; Standing Committee on the Scientific Evaluation of Dietary Reference Intakes, Food and Nutrition Board, Institute of Medicine, National Academy of Sciences. Washington, DC, National Academy Press, 1997.

Hamil H, et al: Physical growth; National Center for Health Statistics Percentiles. Am J Clin Nutr 32:607, 1979.

Sampson B, Kovar IZ, Rauscher A, et al: A case of hyperzincemia with functional zinc depletion: A new disorder? Pediatr Res 42:219, 1997.

CHAPTER 41
The Feeding of Infants and Children

Successful infant feeding requires cooperation between the mother and her baby, beginning with the initial feeding experience and continuing throughout the child's period of dependency. Promptly establishing comfortable, satisfying feeding practices contributes greatly to the infant's and mother's emotional well-being (see Chapter 90). Feeding time should be pleasurable for both mother and child. Because maternal feelings are readily transmitted to the baby and largely determine the emotional setting in which feeding takes place, mothers who are tense, anxious, irritable, easily upset, or emotionally labile are more likely to experience a difficult feeding relationship. They frequently become more comfortable and confident, however, with appropriate guidance and support from an empathetic and experienced relative, friend, lactation consultant, or physician.

As soon after birth as an infant can safely tolerate enteral nutrition, as judged by normal activity, alertness, suck, and cry, feedings should be initiated to maintain normal metabolism and growth during the transition from fetal to extrauterine life; to promote maternal-infant bonding; and to decrease the risks of hypoglycemia, hyperkalemia, hyperbilirubinemia, and azotemia. Mistakes are made by feeding the infant too much or too little. Inadequate fluid intake, particularly in hot environments, may result in "dehydration fever." Most infants may start breast-feeding shortly after birth, and others, within 4–6 hr. When any question about the tolerance of feeding arises because of physical or neurologic status, feeding should be withheld until the newborn is carefully evaluated, and parenteral fluids or other means of enteral feeding may be substituted. Mothers who wish to initiate breast-feeding in the delivery room and continue on a demand basis thereafter should be supported. Subsequent formula or breast feedings are given every 3–4 hr/day and night by the mother. Artificially fed infants should receive sterile water for the first feeding because regurgitation and aspiration of this liquid are less likely to cause significant irritation of the respiratory tract.

The feeding of infants requires practical interpretation of specific nutritional needs and of the widely varying limits of the normal baby's appetite and behavior regarding food. The time that it takes the infant's stomach to empty may vary from 1–4 hr or more; thus, considerable difference in the infant's desire for food is expected at different times of the day. Ideally, the feeding schedule should be based on this reasonable "self-regulation." Variation in the time between feedings and in the amount taken per feeding is to be expected in the first few weeks during the establishment of the self-regulation plan. By the end of the first month, more than 90% of infants will have established a suitable and reasonably regular schedule.

Most healthy, bottle-fed infants will want 6–9 feedings/24 hr by the end of the first week of life. Some will take enough at one feeding to satisfy themselves for approximately 4 hr; others who are smaller or whose gastric emptying time is more rapid will want formula about every 2–3 hr; breast-fed infants often prefer shorter intervals. Most term infants will rapidly increase their intake from 30 mL to 80–90 mL every 3–4 hr at 4–5 days of life. Feeding should be considered as having progressed satisfactorily if the infant is no longer losing weight by 5–7 days and is gaining weight by 12–14 days. Some infants will not awaken for a middle-of-the-night feeding after 3–6 wk of age; some may never want it. Many will not want a late evening feeding between 4 and 8 mo of age and will be satisfied with 3 meals/day by 9–12 mo. However, individual feeding needs are quite variable, and one infant should not be expected to fit the pattern of another infant.

It is important to appreciate that infants cry for reasons other than hunger and *they need not be fed every time they cry.* Some infants are placid; some are unusually active; and some are irritable. Sick infants are often uninterested in food. Infants who awaken and cry consistently at short intervals may not be receiving enough milk at each feeding or may have discomfort from some cause other than hunger, such as too much clothing; colic; soiled, wet, or uncomfortable diapers and clothing; swallowed air ("gas"); uncomfortably hot or cold environment; or illness. Some infants cry to gain sufficient or additional attention, whereas others deprived of adequate mothering become indifferent. Some infants simply need to be held. Those who stop crying when they are picked up or held do not usually need food, but those who continue to cry when held and when food is offered should be carefully evaluated for other causes of distress. The habit of offering frequent, small feedings or of holding and feeding to pacify all crying should not be cultivated.

However, the advantages in satisfying the infant's true hunger needs as they are expressed are several: Physiologic requirements are met promptly; the infant does not learn to associate prolonged crying and discomfort with feeding; and the infant is less likely to develop poor eating practices, such as gulping the feedings or taking small amounts too frequently. Infants soon establish a regular schedule that permits the family to resume normal functioning. If this does not occur, individual feedings or the whole day's schedule can be moved ahead or delayed sufficiently to avoid conflicts with necessary family activities.

Some mothers will not understand the goals of infant "self-regulation"; some will misinterpret the physician's instructions; and others may be unable to adjust themselves to the regimen of the infant. *The orderly, overanxious, and compulsive parent may do better with a more specific outline for the infant's activities.*

The post-partum period is often a time of great anxiety and insecurity for the first-time mother, who may be temporarily overwhelmed by the responsibilities of motherhood. Caretakers and support persons should be comforting and supporting while the mother finds and develops confidence in her maternal abilities. Short hospital stay can interfere with adequate guidance. *Time should be set aside to consider the questions of inexperienced or uncertain mothers at the hospital or in the home utilizing home visitation, particularly as early discharge becomes common.* Physicians should include fathers and other household members in these anticipatory guidance sessions. Knowing the personalities and expectations of both parents is invaluable in helping avert physical and psychologic problems centered on feeding. Parental misconceptions and confusion about the dietary and satiety needs of infants and children are often the basis for abnormal parent-child relations that can be avoided by appropriate counseling.

41.1 Breast-Feeding

Breast-feeding continues to have practical and psychologic advantages that should be considered when the mother selects the method for feeding. Human milk is the most appropriate of all available milks for the human infant because it is uniquely adapted to his or her needs.

ADVANTAGES. *Breast milk is the natural food for full-term infants during the first months of life.* It is always readily available at the proper temperature and needs no time for preparation. The milk is fresh and free of contaminating bacteria, which reduces the chances of gastrointestinal disturbances. Although little if any difference exists in mortality rates in formula-fed and breast-fed infants receiving good care, the potential lifesaving and protective effects of breast milk against enteric pathogens associated with severe diarrhea are most strongly demonstrated in developing countries or where there is not a safe supply of potable water and effective disposal of human waste.

Allergy and intolerance to cow's milk create significant disturbances and feeding difficulties that are not seen in breast-fed infants. The symptoms include diarrhea, intestinal bleeding, and occult melena. "Spitting up," colic, and atopic eczema are less common in infants receiving human milk. A decreased incidence of otitis media in the first year of life has been reported in infants breast-fed exclusively for at least 4 mo. Similarly, reduction in the incidence of pneumonia, bacteremia, and meningitis as well as a reduced frequency of certain allergic and chronic diseases in later life has been reported.

Human milk contains bacterial and viral antibodies, including relatively high concentrations of secretory IgA antibodies, which prevent microorganisms from adhering to the intestinal mucosa. Breast-fed infants of mothers with high antipoliomyelitis titers are relatively resistant to infection by the attenuated live poliomyelitis vaccine viruses, an effect that may be pronounced in the neonatal period but does not seem to interfere with active immunization. Growth of the mumps, influenza, vaccinia, rotavirus, and Japanese B encephalitis viruses can be inhibited by substances in human milk. These ingested antibodies from human colostrum and milk may provide local gastrointestinal immunity against organisms entering the body via this route.

Macrophages normally present in human colostrum and milk may be able to synthesize complement, lysozyme, and lactoferrin. Breast milk is also a source of lactoferrin, the iron-binding whey protein that is normally about one-third saturated with iron, which has an inhibitory effect on the growth of *Escherichia coli* in the intestine. The stool of the breast-fed infant has a pH lower than that of the infant fed cow's milk. The intestinal flora of infants fed human milk may protect them against infections caused by some species of *E. coli.* Bile salt–stimulated lipase kills *Giardia lamblia* and *Entamoeba histolytica*. Transfer of tuberculin responsiveness by breast milk also suggests passive transfer of T-cell immunity.

Milk from the mother whose diet is sufficient and properly balanced *will supply the necessary nutrients*, except, perhaps, fluoride and, after several months, vitamin D. If the water supply is inadequately fluoridated (≤0.3 ppm), the infant should receive 0.25 mg of fluoride daily. If the maternal vitamin D intake is inadequate and the infant's exposure to sunlight is rare (especially in dark-skinned infants), 10 μg of vitamin D is recommended. Iron stores are sufficient for the first 6 mo in term infants. Human milk iron is well absorbed by the infant, but at 4–6 mo of age the diet should be supplemented with the addition of iron-fortified cereals and baby foods or by one of the ferrous iron preparations. Human milk contains sufficient vitamin C for the infant's needs, provided the mother's intake is adequate.

The psychologic advantages of breast-feeding for both mother and infant are well recognized, and successful breast-feeding is a satisfying experience for both. The mother is personally involved in the nurturing of her baby, gaining both a feeling of being essential and a sense of accomplishment. The infant is provided with a close and comfortable physical relationship with the mother. Breast-feeding offers increased opportunity for close sensual contact between the mother and the infant (see Chapter 90.5).

The mother who is unable or does not wish to nurse her infant, however, need have no less sense of accomplishment or of affection for her baby. The quality of attachment and mothering and the degree of security and affection provided can be identical. Women who are less likely to either initiate breast-feeding or be nursing at 6 mo include younger mothers, those enrolled in the Supplemental Food Program for Women, Infants, and Children (WIC), those with a high school education or less, and those with low birthweight infants.

The resumption of *menstruation* should not deter continued nursing, although temporary behavior changes of mother or baby may call for reassurance. *Pregnancy* does not necessitate immediate cessation of nursing, but the combined demands of supplying milk to the infant and nutrients to the fetus are formidable and require special attention to maternal nutrition.

Prematurely born infants weighing 2,000 g (4 1/2 lb) or more usually thrive on breast milk. Infants of lesser birthweights, however, may have such rapid rates of growth that human milk alone may not supply sufficient essential nutrients for normal growth (see Chapter 93). Low birthweight infants too weak to suck or those tiring before ingesting an adequate volume may be given human milk by gavage. Occasionally, breast milk fortifier preparations may be indicated as a supplement to the breast milk feeding of very low birthweight infants (≤1,500 g).

The *low vitamin K content of human milk* may contribute to hemorrhagic disease of the newborn. *Administration of 1 mg of vitamin K_1 parenterally at birth is recommended for all infants, especially for those who will be breast-fed.*

Unconjugated hyperbilirubinemia in breast-fed infants is discussed in Chapter 98.3.

Hemolytic disease of the newborn (erythroblastosis fetalis) is not a contraindication to breast-feeding if the infant's general condition warrants it, because antibodies in the mother's milk are inactivated in the intestinal tract and do not contribute to further hemolysis of the infant's blood cells.

Transmission of HIV by breast-feeding is well documented and contraindicates breast-feeding when there are safe alternatives and there is a low rate of endemic infection. The risk of HIV acquisition by this route is a contraindication to the use of pooled donor milk in the United States and other developed countries. However, in developing countries, breast-feeding may be crucial to infant survival; thus, the risk of HIV transmission must be accepted even though there may be a high endemic infection rate. The World Health Organization currently recommends that, unless safe infant formula is readily available, breast-feeding be continued in areas of high HIV endemicity. Regardless of the risk of transmission of HIV, breast-feeding benefits are significantly greater than the risks of bottle feeding in the developing countries.

Other viruses that have been demonstrated in breast milk include cytomegalovirus (CMV), human T-cell lymphotropic virus type 1, rubella, hepatitis B, and herpes simplex. A study of infants seronegative at birth who were breast-fed by mothers shedding CMV only in their milk demonstrated infection in 63%. Although CMV-specific antibodies may be demonstrated in colostrum and milk, the antibody does not appear to be protective. Transmission to term infants appears to be without symptoms or sequelae; *however*, the risks to preterm infants may be substantially greater, and the use of fresh donor milk is relatively contraindicated unless it is known to be CMV seronegative.

Although hepatitis B has been isolated from maternal milk, the predominant means of transmission appears to be at delivery. Active immunization of the infant within the first 24 hr of life, together with the use of specific high-titer hepatitis B immune globulin and follow-up active vaccination, should permit the mother to nurse, if desired, with minimal risk. If a nursing mother acquires hepatitis B, the infant should receive the accelerated protocol of immunization with doses at birth and at 1 and 2 mo.

Herpes simplex virus has been described in breast milk, with vesicles in the mouth of one infant. Although evidence of breast milk transmission is rare, it appears prudent that women with active lesions who are nursing should observe scrupulous handwashing technique and should avoid nursing if there are active lesions on or near the nipple.

Similarly, rubella virus has been isolated from breast milk, both from maternal acute infection and associated with active immunization of the mother with attenuated virus. Breast-feeding need not be interrupted, because neither virus appears to be associated with significant risk to the infant.

PREPARATION OF THE PROSPECTIVE MOTHER. Most women are physically capable of breast-feeding, provided they receive sufficient encouragement and are protected from discouraging experiences and comments while the secretion of breast milk is becoming established. The physician interested in aiding the prospective mother to breast-feed should discuss its advantages during the midtrimester of pregnancy or whenever the mother begins planning for her baby. Many mothers ambivalent toward breast-feeding will be able to nurse successfully if they are reassured and supported. If the mother rejects the suggestion that she nurse her infant, overpersuasion may be detrimental to mother-infant relationships.

Physical factors conducive to a good breast-feeding experience include establishing and maintaining a state of good health, proper balance of rest and exercise, freedom from worry, early and sufficient treatment of any intercurrent disease, and adequate nutrition.

Retracted nipples usually benefit from daily manual breast-pump traction during the latter weeks of pregnancy; truly *inverted nipples* may be helped by the use of milk cups, starting as early as the 3rd mo of pregnancy.

The mother may be confidently told that she need not gain or lose weight if her diet is adequate. Nursing will help the uterus return to its normal size sooner and may help the mother return to her prepregnancy weight sooner. She should be reassured that breast tone will be preserved by the use of a properly fitted brassiere to support the breasts, especially before delivery and during the nursing period. During the latter part of pregnancy, the mother gains weight and stores fat, which is utilized in lactation. Nutritional requirements for lactation are listed in Table 40–1.

ESTABLISHING AND MAINTAINING THE MILK SUPPLY. The most satisfactory stimulus to the secretion of human milk is regular and complete emptying of the breasts; milk production is reduced when the secreted milk is not drained. Once lactation is well established, mothers are capable of producing more milk than their infants need. There are many reasons for incomplete nursing, but the principal ones are lack of support, weakness of the infant, and failure to initiate the natural hunger cycle. Efforts should be directed toward the early establishment of normal, vigorous nursing by letting the infant empty the breast frequently during the time when only colostrum is being formed. The infant should be allowed to nurse when hungry, whether or not there appears to be any milk.

Breast-feeding should begin as soon after delivery as the condition of the mother and of the baby permits, preferably within the first hours. Infants who cannot be fed on demand should be brought to the mother for feeding about every 3 hr during the day and night. Many infants are hungry within 2 hr of a satisfying nursing episode, and about 75% of the breast's milk has been replenished by this time.

Appropriate care for tender or sore nipples should be instituted before severe pain from abrasions and cracking develops. Exposing the nipples to air; applying pure lanolin; avoiding soap, alcohol, and tincture of benzoin; frequently changing disposable nursing pads lining the brassiere cups; nursing more frequently; manually expressing milk; nursing in different positions; and keeping the breast dry between feedings are recommended. When the tenderness causes the mother apprehension the *milk-ejection reflex* may be delayed, leading to frustration in the infant and to increasingly vigorous nursing, which further injures the nipple and areolar area. Occasionally, nipple shields may be helpful.

The first 2 wk of the neonatal period are crucial for establishing breast-feeding. Daily weight gains may be overly emphasized, and early supplemental bottle feedings given to achieve weight gain may compromise attempts at breast-feeding.

Although the difference between breast and bottle nipples may confuse the infant, this is usually not the case. It may be perfectly satisfactory to have the mother pump her breasts and feed the infant breast milk via a bottle for the 1st wk or 2. She can then attempt breast-feeding one or two times daily when she is relaxed and less anxious, until infant and mother have achieved a successful nursing experience. The additional pumping will usually increase milk production, ensuring an adequate supply. Even after nursing is well established, it may be appropriate for the mother to pump extra milk to store (in a freezer up to 1 mo or refrigerator up to 24 hr) for use when the mother is not available. This will also allow the mother a bit of freedom and afford the father or other caregiver more involvement in the infant's feeding and care.

On the day that the mother is discharged from the hospital, lactation is usually not well established, and the excitement of going home may impede an initially successful nursing experience in the hospital. A wise physician anticipates this possibility and discusses it with the mother. In rare cases, providing her with enough isocaloric formula for one or two complementary feedings may prevent discouragement that might prejudice further nursing.

PSYCHOLOGIC FACTORS. No factor is more important than a happy, relaxed state of mind. Worry and unhappiness are the most effective means for decreasing or abolishing breast secretions.

Mothers may worry that their infants are abnormal when they cry or are drowsy, sneeze, or regurgitate milk. Mothers are upset by any suggestion that their milk may be lacking in quantity or quality. They may be disturbed at the scanty supply of colostrum, at tenderness of the nipples, and at the fullness of the breast on the 4th or 5th day. Many mothers do not feel comfortable when trying to nurse in an open ward or with another person in the room. Mothers may worry about what is going on at home while they are in the hospital or about what is going to happen when they arrive home. An alert physician recognizes and appreciates these worries, particularly if the baby is a first-born, and by tactful reassurance and explanation can help prevent or minimize worry, thus contributing to successful breast-feeding. Attention should be given to social and cultural factors to provide a support plan for the individual mother.

FATIGUE. Avoiding fatigue is important, but the mother should exercise sufficiently to promote her sense of physical well-being.

HYGIENE. Once a day, the breasts should be washed. If soap is drying to the nipple and areolar area, its use should be discontinued. The nipple area should be kept dry. *Boric acid must not be used.* Care should be taken to prevent irritation and infection of the nipples caused by prolonged initial nursing, maceration from wetness of the nipple, or rubbing of clothing.

Some mothers may be more comfortable if they wear a properly fitted brassiere day and night. Plastic liners should be removed. An absorbent pad (commercially available) or a clean cloth or handkerchief may be placed inside the brassiere to absorb any milk that leaks out.

DIET. The diet should contain enough calories to compensate for those secreted in the milk as well as for those required to produce it. The nursing mother needs a varied diet, sufficient to maintain her weight and high in fluid, vitamins, and minerals. She should avoid weight-reducing diets. Milk is important but should not replace other essential foods. If the mother is allergic to or dislikes milk, 1 g of calcium may be added to her daily diet. The fluid intake should approximate 3 qt daily; urinary output is a good measure of the adequacy of fluid in the daily diet.

The idea that substances such as milk, beer, oatmeal, and tea are galactogenic is mistaken. A single food in the mother's diet seldom disturbs the breast-fed infant. Occasionally, however, eating certain berries, tomatoes, onions, members of the cabbage family, chocolate, spices, and condiments may cause gastric distress or loose stools in the infant. No food need be withheld from the mother unless it causes distress to the infant. Whenever possible, nursing mothers should not take drugs, because many preparations are harmful to the neonate and many have not been evaluated (see Table 90–5). Antithyroid medications, lithium, anticancer agents, isoniazid, all recreationally abused drugs, and phenindione are contraindicated. Temporary cessation of nursing is recommended if the mother requires diagnostic radiopharmaceuticals, chloramphenicol, metronidazole, sulfonamides, or anthraquinone-derivative laxatives. Lactating women should not eat sport fish from waters contaminated with polychlorinated biphenyls. It is better to control maternal constipation by inclusion in the diet of raw and cooked fruits and vegetables, whole wheat bread, and an adequate amount of water than by use of laxatives. Smoking cigarettes and drinking alcoholic beverages should be discouraged. Substances such as arsenicals, barbiturates, bromides, iodides, lead, mercurials, salicylates, opium, atropine, most antimicrobial agents, and cascara may be transmitted through the milk and exert an effect on the infant.

TECHNIQUE OF BREAST-FEEDING. The technical aspects of breast-feeding require careful consideration. Breast-feeding sometimes becomes impossible simply because the attending physician fails to recognize that the difficulties are in the feeding technique.

At feeding time, the infant should be hungry, dry, neither too cold nor too warm, and held in a comfortable, semisitting position for his or her enjoyment and for ease of eructation without vomiting. The mother, too, must be comfortable and completely at ease. When she is able to be out of bed, a moderately low chair with an armrest is preferable, and a low stool is advantageous for resting her foot and raising her knee on the nursing side. The baby is supported comfortably with the face held close to the mother's breast by one arm and hand while the other hand supports the breast so that the nipple is easily accessible to the infant's mouth and yet does not obstruct the infant's nasal breathing. The baby's lips should engage considerable areola as well as nipple.

Success in infant feeding depends greatly on the adjustments made during the first few days of life. Difficulties often result from attempts to adapt the infant to a nursing procedure rather than designing a procedure that satisfies the infant's natural desires. Rigidly adhering to clock schedules may make adjustment difficult. Most problems can be avoided by conforming to the infant's spontaneous pattern. If the infant is breast-fed when he or she normally cries in hunger and feeding ends when the baby's appetite is satisfied, the fundamental requirements are met.

At birth, the normal infant is equipped with several reflexes, or behavior patterns, that facilitate breast-feeding. These reflexes are concerned with obtaining food—rooting, sucking, swallowing, and satiety reflexes. The *rooting reflex* is the first to come into play. When infants smell milk, they move their heads around, attempting to find its source. If their cheek is touched by a smooth object (the mother's breast), they will turn toward that object, opening their mouths in anticipation of grasping the nipple (rooting with their mouths for the nipple).

The infant's rooting reflex brings the entire areolar area into the mouth; the contact of the nipple against the palate and posterior tongue elicits sucking or "milking," and the buccal fat pads help keep the nipple in place. This *sucking reflex* is a process of squeezing the sinuses of the areola rather than simply suction on the nipple. The infant's sucking results in afferent impulses to the mother's hypothalamus and then to both anterior and posterior pituitary. Prolactin from the anterior pituitary stimulates milk secretion in the cuboidal cells in the acini or alveoli of the breast. Finally, milk in the infant's mouth triggers the *swallowing reflex.* In contrast, bottle-feeding requires the infant to compress the nipple to avoid choking.

Mothers should know that if the infant is not hungry, he or she will not search for the nipple or suck. Infants are usually sleepy for several days, and most, initially, are not avid suckers. On the 3rd day, when there has been some weight loss, mothers become anxious about infants who seem uninterested in nursing. It reassures them to learn that most healthy babies "wake up" and become good nursers on the 4th day. Infants whose mothers received obstetric sedation during labor suck at lower rates and pressures and consume less milk than comparable infants of mothers given no sedation.

Some infants will empty a breast in 5 min; others nurse more leisurely for 20 min. Most of the milk is obtained early in the feeding: 50% in the first 2 min and 80–90% in the first 4 min. The infant should be permitted to suck until satisfied unless the mother has sore nipples. If the infant does not "unlatch" from the breast, a finger inserted into the corner of the infant's mouth decreases suction and facilitates removal. The infant should not be pulled from the breast. Waking a sleepy infant to nurse by slapping feet, pinching, or shaking is usually unsuccessful and inappropriate.

At the end of the nursing period, the infant should be held erect over the mother's shoulder or on her lap with or without gently rubbing or patting the back to assist in expelling swallowed air; often this "burping" procedure is necessary one or more times during the feeding as well as 5–10 min after the infant has been put into the crib. It is an essential procedure during the early months but should not be overdone. When nursing is completed, the infant should be placed in the crib on the back or on the right side to facilitate emptying of the stomach into the intestines and to reduce the chances of regurgitation or aspiration.

ONE OR BOTH BREASTS PER FEEDING. The infant should empty at least one breast at each feeding; otherwise, it will not be stimulated to refill. Both breasts should be used at each feeding in the early weeks to encourage maximal production of milk. After the milk supply has been established, the breasts may be alternated at successive feedings, and the infant will usually be satisfied with the amount obtained from one. If the secretion of milk becomes too great, both breasts may again be offered at each feeding and incompletely emptied with the intent of securing a partial decrease in lactation.

DETERMINING ADEQUACY OF MILK SUPPLY. If the infant is satisfied after each nursing period, sleeps 2–4 hr, and gains weight adequately, the milk supply is sufficient. Infants who are "light sleepers" require a lot of body contact with the mother during the first months. Mothers of these wakeful and alert infants should not be thought to have a poor milk supply. However, if the infant nurses avidly and completely empties both breasts but appears unsatisfied afterward, does not go to sleep or sleeps fitfully and awakens after 1–2 hr, and fails to gain weight satisfactorily, the milk supply is probably inadequate. The program of La Leche League,* which establishes close relationships between successful nursing mothers and mothers needing assistance, is often helpful in such circumstances.

The "let-down" or *milk-ejection reflex* in the mother is an important sign of successful nursing. Sucking or psychologic stimuli associated with nursing lead to secretion of oxytocin by the posterior pituitary. As a result, the myoepithelial cells surrounding the alveoli deep in the breast contract, squeezing milk into the larger ducts, where it is more easily available to the sucking infant. When this reflex functions well, milk flows from the opposite breast as the infant begins to nurse. This reflex is frequently absent or erratic during periods of pain, fatigue, or emotional distress, and its malfunction is thought to be responsible for milk retention in women unsuccessful in breast-feeding.

In general, a mother's weighing her infant before and after nursing is neither necessary nor desirable in judging adequacy of milk supply. The amount of milk that an infant takes at a time is usually unimportant (the amount ingested at each feeding ranges from one to several ounces throughout a 24-hr period), and the results obtained are readily misinterpreted. Small gains may worry the mother and in turn may diminish her milk supply. She may give the infant a bottle to reassure herself that the infant is getting enough to eat. The better result with the "test bottle" may be so discouraging that subsequent breast-feeding becomes impossible, even when she has an adequate supply of milk. Before assuming that the mother produces insufficient milk, three possibilities should be excluded: (1) errors in feeding technique responsible for the infant's inadequate progress; (2) remediable maternal factors related to diet, rest, or emotional distress; or (3) physical disturbances in the infant that interfere with eating or with weight gain. Infrequently, infants who seem to be nursing well may not thrive because of insufficiency of milk; increased frequency of feeding may be indicated. Nursing more than every 2 hr, however, may inhibit prolactin secretion of the anterior pituitary, decreasing production; this is usually corrected by delaying feedings to 2–2½ hr intervals. Other aids include stimulation of prolactin secretion by administering small doses of chlorpromazine for a few days or by devices such as the LactAid, which supplement the infant's intake.

EXPRESSION OF BREAST MILK. Although manual expression of breast milk is useful to relieve engorgement of the breasts in an emergency, the cost and availability of battery-operated and electric breast pumps usually makes this unnecessary. Pumping can increase milk production and relieve sore nipples for a few feedings because it does not cause the same nipple irritation that suckling may. Again, breast milk can be safely stored in the freezer or refrigerator and used at a later time for the father or caregiver to feed the infant. Although the infant

---

*La Leche League International, 9616 Minneapolis Avenue, Franklin Park, IL 60131, has many local affiliates composed of successfully nursing mothers willing to assist other mothers desiring to nurse.

may balk at anyone else's attempting to feed him or her, perseverance will win out.

SUPPLEMENTARY FEEDINGS. The best-intentioned mother who is returning to work plans on pumping while at work and supplying enough milk to feed her infant in her absence. This is often not possible because of stress and time constraints at work. It is acceptable to feed the infant a commercial formula during the day and to continue nursing in the evening and throughout the night. The breast milk production will gradually decrease so that the mother is not plagued by engorged, leaking breasts. She will usually continue to produce enough milk to supply two or three feedings a day for several months. If formula is to be given after the infant has completed a breast-feeding, the warmed bottle should be available so that it can be offered immediately after the infant has been burped. The holes in the nipples should not be so large that the infant gets this portion of food without any effort, or the infant may quickly abandon any efforts to suck adequately at the mother's breast. Some employers provide child care at the workplace that enables mothers to continue nursing successfully. Such efforts by employers should be commended and encouraged.

WEANING. Most infants gradually reduce the volume and frequency of their demand for breast-feedings at 6–12 mo of age, and they become accustomed to increasing amounts of solid foods and liquids by bottle and cup. As they demand less breast milk, the mother's supply gradually diminishes, causing the mother no discomfort from engorgement. Weaning should be initiated by substituting formula or cow's milk by bottle or cup for part of a breast-feeding and subsequently for all of a breast-feeding. Over several days, one of the breast-feedings is replaced and then subsequently another, and so on, until the infant is weaned completely. Occasionally, the infant takes the cup as readily as the bottle, avoiding the intermediate transfer from breast to bottle to cup. These changes should be made gradually; they should provide a pleasant experience, not a conflict, for the mother and infant. Praise, loving attention, and cuddling are vital to successful weaning.

When cessation of nursing is necessary at an earlier age, a tight breast binder may be used, and ice bags may be applied for a few days to decrease milk production. Restriction of the mother's fluid intake is also helpful. Hormones, such as small doses of estrogen for 1–2 days, also may help decrease milk production at the termination of nursing.

CONTRAINDICATIONS. For the average, healthy, full-term infant there are no disadvantages to breast-feeding, provided that the mother's milk supply is ample and that her diet contains sufficient amounts of protein and vitamins. Infrequently, allergens to which the infant is sensitized may be conveyed in the milk. In such cases, an attempt should be made to find the specific allergen and to remove it from the mother's diet; its presence rarely is a valid reason for weaning the baby.

From the mother's standpoint, there are few contraindications to breast-feeding. Markedly inverted nipples may be troublesome. Fissuring or cracking of the nipples can usually be avoided if engorgement is prevented. Mastitis may be alleviated by continued and frequent nursing on the affected breast to keep it from becoming engorged, by local heat applications, and by antibiotics. Acute infection in the mother may contraindicate breast-feeding if the infant does not have the same infection; otherwise, there is no need to stop nursing unless the condition of either necessitates it. When the infant is unaffected and the mother's condition permits, the breast may be emptied and the milk given to the infant. Septicemia, nephritis, eclampsia, profuse hemorrhage, active tuberculosis, typhoid fever, breast cancer, and malaria are contraindications to nursing, as are chronic poor nutrition, substance abuse, debility, severe neuroses, and post-partum psychoses.

41.2 Formula Feeding

Whole cow's milk or its modified form is the basis for most formulas, although other milks and milk substitutes are available for infants who cannot tolerate it. Sterilization and refrigeration of the formula greatly reduce morbidity and mortality from gastrointestinal infections. Milk processing (ranging from simple home boiling to commercial pasteurization, homogenization, and evaporation) alters the casein so that small and readily digestible curds form in the stomach, eliminating the principal cause for undigestibility of cow's milk protein.

Although breast-feeding is considered superior to formula feeding for normal infants, many infants receive formula from birth. Because they are employed outside the home, many mothers are reluctant to nurse their infants. Others believe that nursing will limit their activities, or they fear failure at nursing. Some regard weight gain and loss of breast tone as unattractive, and some consider breast-feeding socially unacceptable. Whatever the reasons, the present use of artificial feeding was facilitated by prior improvements in the safety and quality of the substitute milks.

Objective nutritional studies of growing infants (e.g., rate of growth in weight and length, normality of various constituents in blood, performance in metabolic studies, body composition) show relatively small differences between infants fed human milk and those fed cow's milk. Although such techniques may not record small but important variations, these investigations attest to the normal infant's ability to thrive by making satisfactory physiologic adjustments to wide ranges of ingested protein, fat, carbohydrate, and minerals.

Conventional formulas of whole and evaporated cow's milk provide approximately 3–4 g of protein/kg/24 hr ("high-protein" intake largely exceeding the basic need), whereas breast milk and many commercially prepared feedings simulating the composition of breast milk supply 1.5–2.5 g/kg/24 hr ("low-protein" intake supplying a smaller degree of excess).

Fomon has calculated the rate of increase in total body protein mass in the "male reference" term infant to average approximately 3.5 g/24 hr in the first 4 mo of life. Assuming 0.5 g/24 hr of nitrogen loss from the skin, total protein need is estimated to be about 4 g/24 hr during the first 4 mo and slightly less during the remainder of the first year.

Commercial formulas are modified from a cow's milk base, and their protein and ash levels are reduced nearer to those of human milk, thus decreasing osmolality and renal excretory load. The saturated fat of cow's milk is replaced with some unsaturated vegetable fatty acids, and vitamins are added. The concentration of lactose is lower in cow's milk than in human milk. Some formulas include higher whey protein and lower casein, such as in breast milk. Low birthweight infants in particular may benefit from the increased cystine of whey proteins. Until more information is available, breast-feeding for all infants appears prudent, but if this is impossible, a formula as compositionally close to breast milk as possible is desirable.

TECHNIQUE OF ARTIFICIAL FEEDING. The setting should be similar to that for breast-feeding, with the caregiver and infant in a comfortable position, unhurried, and free from distractions. The infant should be hungry, fully awake, warm, and dry and be held as though being breast-fed. The bottle should be held so that milk, not air, channels through the nipple. Bottle propping, even with a "safe" holder, should be avoided, because it not only deprives the infant of the physical contact, comfort, and security of being held but may also be dangerous to small infants, who may aspirate if unattended. Otitis media is more common in infants fed with the propped bottle.

The bottle of milk is customarily warmed to body temperature, although no harmful effects have been demonstrated from feedings at room temperature or cooler. The temperature may be tested by dropping milk onto the wrist. The nipple holes should be of a size that milk will drop slowly.

Especially during the first 6–7 mo of life, the eructation of air swallowed during feeding is important for avoiding regurgitation and abdominal discomfort. This technique is similar to that described after breast-feeding. A few infants relieve themselves best after being returned to the crib. All infants will, at times, regurgitate or "spit up" a small amount of milk after feeding, a fact that the mother should know. Spitting up occurs more often in the artificially fed than in the breast-fed infant.

A feeding may last from 5–25 min, depending on the vigor and age of the infant. Because the appetite varies from one feeding to another, each bottle should contain more than the average amount taken per feeding. In no case should the infant be urged to take more than desired, and excess milk should be discarded.

COMPARISON OF HUMAN MILK AND COW'S MILK. Average values for the various constituents of human milk and whole fresh cow's milk are listed in Table 41–1. Both differ during the various stages of lactation and among individuals, although the differences in human milk from women with adequate diets are insignificant. Milk late in pregnancy and early after birth contains more protein, calcium, and other minerals than later during lactation. Cells are also present in colostrum and human milk.

Colostrum. The secretion of the breasts during the latter part of pregnancy and for the 2–4 days after delivery is called colostrum. It has a deep lemon-yellow color; its reaction is alkaline; and its specific gravity is 1.040–1.060, in contrast to the average specific gravity of 1.030 for mature breast milk. The total amount of colostrum secreted daily is 10–40 mL. Human or cow colostrum contains several times the protein of mature breast milk and more minerals but less carbohydrate and fat. Human colostrum also contains some unique immunologic factors. After the first few days of lactation, colostrum is replaced by secretion of a transitional form of milk that gradually assumes the characteristics of mature breast milk by the 3rd or 4th wk.

Water. The relative amounts of water and solids in human and cow's milks are about the same.

TABLE 41–1 Compositions of Human Breast Milk and Cow's Milk

	Breast Milk							
	Mature Milk (15 days–15 mo Postpartum)		***Transitional Milk (6–10 days Postpartum)***		***Colostrum (First 5 days Postpartum)***		**Cow's Milk**	
	Mean	**Experimental Range**	**Mean**	**Experimental Range**	**Mean**	**Experimental Range**	**Mean**	**Experimental Range**
Calories								
(kcal/L)	747	446–1192	735	678–830	671	588–730	701	587–876
(mJ/L)	3.127	1.867–4.989	3.076	2.838–3.474	2.808	2.461–3.055	2.9344	2.457–3.666
Specific gravity	1.031	1.026–1.037	1.035	1.034–1.036	1.034	—	1.031	1.028–1.033
pH	7.01	6.4–7.6	—	—	—	—	6.6	—
Solids, total (g/L)	129	103–175	133	105–156	128	100–167	124	119–142
Ash, total (g/L)	2.02	1.6–2.66	2.67	2.31–3.38	3.08	2.47–3.50	7.15	6.81–7.71
Minerals								
Electropositive elements (mEq/L)	41	—	55	—	68	—	149	—
Sodium (g/L)	0.172	0.064–0.436	0.294	0.192–0.539	0.501	0.265–1.37	0.768	0.392–1.39
	0.189	0.080–0.350	0.536	0.170–1.21	0.956	0.330–2.24	—	—
Potassium (g/L)	0.512	0.373–0.635	0.636	0.528–0.769	0.745	0.658–0.870	1.43	0.38–2.87
	0.553	0.425–0.735	0.692	0.450–0.910	0.581	0.220–0.790	—	—
Calcium (g/L)	0.344	0.173–0.609	0.464	0.23–0.628	0.481	0.242–0.656	1.37	0.56–3.81
	0.271	0.207–0.372	0.320	0.166–0.420	0.261	0.180–0.364	—	—
Magnesium (g/L)	0.035	0.018–0.057	0.035	0.026–0.054	0.042	0.031–0.082	0.13	0.07–0.22
Electronegative elements (mEq/L)	28	—	37	—	40	—	108	—
Phosphorus (g/L)	0.141	0.068–0.268	0.198	0.097–0.317	0.157	0.085–0.251	0.91	0.56–1.12
Sulfur (g/L)	0.14	0.05–0.30	0.20	0.15–0.23	0.23	0.20–0.26	0.30	0.24–0.36
Chlorine (g/L)	0.375	0.088–0.734	0.457	0.305–0.721	0.586	0.435–1.01	1.08	0.93–1.41
Excess electropositive elements (mEq/L)	13	—	18	—	28	—	41	—
Trace elements								
Cobalt (µg/L)	Trace	—	—	—	—	—	0.6	—
Iron (mg/L)	0.50	0.20–0.80	0.59	0.29–1.45	1.0	—	0.45	0.25–0.75
Copper (mg/L)	0.51	—	1.04	—	1.34	—	0.102	—
Manganese (mg/L)	Trace	—	Trace	—	Trace	—	0.02	0.005–0.067
Zinc (mg/L)	1.18	0.17–3.02	3.82	0.39–5.88	5.59	0.72–9.81	3.9	1.7–6.6
Fluorine (mg/L)	0.107	0.0–0.24	—	—	0.131	0.0–0.35	—	0.10–0.28
Iodine (mg/L)	0.061	0.044–0.093	—	—	—	0.045–0.450	0.116	0.036–1.05
Selenium (mg/L)	0.021	—	—	—	—	—	0.04	0.005–0.067
Protein (g/L)								
Total	10.6	7.3–20	15.9	12.7–18.9	22.9	14.6–68.0	32.46	28.16–36.76
	—	—	—	—	55	14–215	—	—
Casein	3.7	1.4–6.8	5.1	4.2–5.9	21	7.3–52	24.9	21.9–28.0
Whey protein	7	4–10	—	—	—	—	7	6–10
Lactalbumin	3.6	1.4–6.0	7.8	6.9–8.6	—	—	2.4	1.4–3.3
Lactoglobulin	—	—	5.0	2.1–13.6	35	4.2–133	1.7	0.7–3.7
Blood-serum albumin	0.32	0.20–0.47	0.37	0.26–0.65	2.5	—	0.4	—
Blood-serum immunoglobulin	0.09	0.02–0.27	0.36	0.01–0.96	1.0	—	0.8	—
Amino acids (g/L)								
Total	12.8	9.0–16.0	9.4	6.0–10.0	12.0	7.0–40.0	33.0	27.0–41.0
Alanine	—	0.36–0.42	—	—	—	—	0.75	—
Arginine	0.43	0.28–0.64	0.63	0.48–0.73	0.74	0.62–0.96	1.4	1.2–1.6
Aspartic acid	—	0.89–0.98	—	—	—	—	1.7	—
Cystine	—	0.23–0.25	—	—	—	—	—	—
Glutamic acid	—	1.89–2.00	—	—	—	—	6.8	—
Glycine	—	0.23–0.24	—	—	—	—	0.11	—
Histidine	0.24	0.12–0.30	0.38	0.29–0.45	0.41	0.35–0.46	1.2	1.1–1.3
Isoleucine	0.61	0.41–0.92	0.97	0.73–1.21	1.01	0.88–1.15	2.5	2.1–2.9
Leucine	0.97	0.65–1.47	1.51	1.13–1.97	1.66	1.33–2.14	3.6	3.2–3.9

Table continued on following page

TABLE 41–1 Compositions of Human Breast Milk and Cow's Milk *Continued*

	Breast Milk							
	Mature Milk (15 days–15 mo Postpartum)		*Transitional Milk (6–10 days Postpartum)*		*Colostrum (First 5 days Postpartum)*		Cow's Milk	
	Mean	Experimental Range	Mean	Experimental Range	Mean	Experimental Range	Mean	Experimental Range
Amino acids (g/L) *Continued*								
Lysine	0.70	0.36–0.93	1.13	0.88–1.48	1.18	0.95–1.41	2.6	2.3–3.1
Methionine	0.12	0.07–0.16	0.24	0.16–0.34	0.25	0.19–0.36	0.8	0.6–0.9
Phenylalanine	0.40	0.24–0.58	0.62	0.48–0.71	0.70	0.60–0.84	1.8	1.5–2.2
Proline	—	0.84–0.94	—	—	—	—	2.5	—
Serine	—	0.47–0.51	—	—	—	—	1.6	—
Threonine	0.52	0.30–0.66	0.78	0.61–0.91	0.85	0.75–1.04	1.7	1.3–2.2
Tryptophan	0.19	0.14–0.26	0.28	0.23–0.32	0.32	0.25–0.42	0.6	0.4–0.8
Tyrosine	—	0.46–0.52	—	—	—	—	—	—
Valine	0.73	0.45–1.14	1.05	0.77–1.36	1.17	0.98–1.49	2.6	2.4–2.8
Nonprotein nitrogen (mg/L)								
Total	324	173–604	479	425–533	910	510–1270	252	181–323
Urea nitrogen	180	127–235	111	—	—	—	132.7	61.3–204
Uric acid nitrogen	22	13–41	—	—	—	—	24.1	11.3–36.9
Creatinine nitrogen	11	8–19	—	—	—	—	7.05	1.9–12.2
Creatine nitrogen	11	2–41	—	—	—	—	40.35	24.5–56.2
Amino acid nitrogen	50	28–113	44	—	—	40–120	6.8	1.7–11.9
Choline nitrogen	10.3	6.2–16.8	—	—	—	—	12	5–19
Enzymes								
Lysozyme (mg/L)	390	30–3000	—	—	460	90–1020	0.13	0.00–2.6
Carbohydrates								
Lactose								
Directly estimated (g/L)	71	49–95	64	61–67	57	11–79	47	45–50
As difference	68	50–92	64	60–68	—	—	—	—
Fucose (g/L)	1.3	—	—	—	—	—	—	—
Glucosamine (g/L)	—	0.7–0.8	—	—	—	1.4–4.3	0	—
Galactosamine (g/L)	—	0.0–0.4	—	—	—	0.04–0.7	0	—
Inositol (g/L)	0.45	0.39–0.56	—	—	—	—	0.08	0.06–0.12
Citric acid (g/L)	—	0.35–1.25	—	—	—	—	2.54	2.15–2.90
Fats, total (g/L)	45.4	13.4–82.9	35.2	27.3–51.8	29.5	24.7–31.8	38.0	34.0–61.0
Cholesterol (mg/L)	139	88–202	241	126–320	280	180–345	110	70–170
Free cholesterol (as percent of total)	76.1	—	76.5	—	79.5	—	—	90–95
Lipid phosphorus (mg/L)	10.5	7–14	15.5	11–20	12	6–17	—	53–70
Vitamins								
Vitamin A (mg/L)	0.61	0.15–2.26	0.88	0.58–1.83	1.61	0.75–3.05	0.27	0.17–0.38
Carotenes (mg/L)	0.25	0.02–0.77	0.38	0.23–0.63	1.37	0.41–3.85	0.37	0.12–0.79
Vitamin D (IU/L)	—	4–100	—	—	—	—	—	5–40
Tocopherol (mg/L)	2.4	1.0–4.8	8.9	4.0–18.5	14.8	2.8–30.0	0.6	0.2–1.0
Thiamine (mg/L)	0.142	0.081–0.227	0.059	0.023–0.105	0.019	0.009–0.034	0.43	0.28–0.90
Riboflavin (mg/L)	0.373	0.198–0.790	0.369	0.275–0.490	0.302	0.120–0.453	1.56	1.16–2.02
Vitamin B_6 (mg/L)	0.18	0.10–0.22	—	—	—	—	0.51	0.40–0.63
Nicotinic acid (mg/L)	1.83	0.66–3.30	1.75	0.60–3.60	0.75	0.50–14.5	0.74	0.50–0.86
Vitamin B_{12} (μg/L)	—	Trace	0.36	0.03–0.70	0.45	0.10–1.5	6.6	3.2–12.4
Folic acid (μg/L)								
(a)	1.4	0.9 1.8	0.2	0.15–0.25	0.5	0.10–1.5	1.3	0.2–4.0
(b)	24.0	7.4–61.0	—	—	—	—	37.7	16.8–63.2
(c)	7.3	2.3–17.6	—	—	—	—	12.6	2.8–43.6
Biotin (μg/L)	2	1–3	—	—	—	—	22	14–29
Pantothenic acid (mg/L)	2.46	0.86–5.84	2.88	1.35–4.12	1.83	0.29–3.02	3.4	2.2–5.5
Ascorbic acid (mg/L)	52	0–112	71	45–90	72	47–104	11	3–23

From Geigy Scientific Tables, 7th ed. Basel, Switzerland, Ciba-Geigy, Ltd.

Calories. The energy value of each milk may vary slightly and is approximately 20 kcal/oz or 0.67 kcal/mL.

Protein. There are quantitative differences between the proteins of the two milks. Human milk contains only 1–1.5% protein compared with approximately 3.3% in cow's milk. The increased protein of cow's milk results almost entirely from its sixfold higher content of casein. Human milk protein consists of approximately 75% whey proteins, largely lactalbumins, and 25% casein; the cow's milk ratio is reversed to 22:78.

Carbohydrate. Human milk contains 6.5–7%, and cow's milk contains about 4.5% lactose. About 10% of the carbohydrate in human milk consists of polysaccharides and glycoproteins.

Fat. The fat content of milks is about 3.5%. In human milk, fat content varies somewhat with maternal diet; during a single nursing, it is higher in the latter portion of the feeding, which may help satiate the infant at the conclusion of nursing.

The milks of different breeds of cattle vary in fat content. Most market milk in urban areas, however, is pooled, and the fat content is adjusted to a standard level, generally from 3.25–4%.

Qualitative differences exist in the fats of human milk and cow's milk. The fats of each consist principally of the triglycerides olein, palmitin, and stearin, but human milk contains twice as much of the more absorbable olein. The volatile fatty acids (butyric, capric, caproic, and caprylic) constitute only about 1.3% of human milk fat but about 9% of cow's milk fat. The small amount of linoleic acid in cow's milk is usually sufficient to prevent deficiency. The premature or debilitated infant may have steatorrhea after ingesting cow's milk fat. For such infants, it is wise to substitute a more readily assimilated vegetable fat or human milk.

Minerals. Cow's milk contains much more of all the minerals except iron and copper than human milk; the total mineral content of cow's milk is 0.7–0.75%; that of human milk is 0.15–0.25%. Cow's milk contains inadequate iron; breast-milk iron, although low, may be sufficient for the infant because it is better absorbed, and during the first 4 mo or so of life iron stored during fetal life compensates for the milk's deficiency. Although the need for calcium and phosphorus is great during periods of rapid growth, adequate balances are maintained on breast milk despite its low content of these minerals.

Vitamins. The vitamin content of each milk varies with the maternal intake. Cow's milk is low in vitamins C and D. Breast milk usually contains adequate vitamin C, if the mother eats appropriate foods, and adequate vitamin D unless she is insufficiently exposed to sunlight or is darkly pigmented. Cow's milk contains more vitamin K than human milk. Both types of milk seem to contain adequate amounts of vitamin A and the B-complex vitamins for the nutritional needs of infants in the first months of life.

Bacterial Content. Although human milk is essentially uncontaminated by bacteria, pathogenic organisms in significant numbers may enter the milk from mastitis. Tubercle and typhoid bacilli and herpes, hepatitis B, rubella, mumps, HIV, and CMV may be found at times in the milk of women infected with these organisms. Cow's milk is regularly contaminated but in most cases by bacteria that are not harmful to humans. Milk, however, is a good culture medium for pathogenic bacteria, and many infections are milk-borne, including streptococcal diseases, diphtheria, typhoid fever, salmonellosis, tuberculosis, and brucellosis. Furthermore, certain bacteria that may not affect older children or adults may cause diarrhea in infants. In most cities, pasteurization of all marketed whole milk is required. In addition, terminal sterilization or boiling the milk immediately before mixing the infant's formula is advisable.

Digestibility. The stomach empties more rapidly after human milk than after whole cow's milk; however, no appreciable difference in gastrointestinal passage time exists between human milk and processed milk formulas during the first 45 days of life. The curd of cow's milk is reduced in size by boiling; it is made considerably less tough and much smaller by the heating required in evaporation, by the addition of acid or alkali, and by homogenization. In contrast, the curd of breast milk is fine and flocculent and is readily broken down in the stomach. The fat of cow's milk is less readily digested than that of breast milk.

MILK USED IN FORMULAS

Raw Milk. This is not advised for infant feeding; it forms large curds in the stomach, is slowly digested, and is easily contaminated with pathogenic organisms. Its sale is forbidden in most urban communities in the United States.

Pasteurized Milk. Pasteurization destroys many pathogenic bacteria and modifies casein so that smaller, less tough curds are produced in the stomach. Raw milk is heated at 63°C (145°F) for 30 min or, more commonly, at 72°C (161°F) for 15 sec, then rapidly cooled. Standards for the bacterial content of pasteurized milk vary in different cities and countries, tolerable counts ranging as high as 50,000 nonpathogenic bacteria/mL; average counts in many cities, however, are as low as 5,000–10,000 bacteria/mL. Pasteurized milk should be boiled when used for infant feeding. If it is allowed to stand in the refrigerator for as long as 48 hr, its bacterial count may increase significantly.

Homogenized Milk. During the process of homogenization, the fat globules are broken into minute particles and remain dispersed. The principal advantage of homogenized milk is the smaller, less tough curd produced in the stomach.

Evaporated Milk. This milk has many advantages, including almost universal availability, especially in regions of the world where breast-feeding is not prevalent and prepared milks are not readily available or acceptable. The unopened can will keep for months without refrigeration. The casein curd produced in the stomach is softer and smaller than that of boiled whole milk; homogenization of the fat also contributes to smaller curd formation. The whey protein or lactoglobulin appears to be less allergenic than that of fresh milk. Evaporated milk can be fed in higher concentrations than whole milk formulas. The standard can contains 13 fluid oz* (384 mL). Each fluid ounce equals about 44 kcal. Vitamin D is usually added in the processing so that each reconstituted quart contains 10 g.

Prepared Milks. Many commercially prepared modified milks (Tables 41–2 and 41–3) are derived from cow's milk, and many are available in powder, concentrated liquid requiring 1:1 dilution with water, and ready-to-feed forms. The composition of the majority simulates breast milk in various ways. All are fortified with vitamin D and other vitamins, and some have added iron. In addition, specially modified preparations for premature infant feeding have been developed (Table 41–4).

These milks are nutritionally adequate for normal infants. They cost more than evaporated milk-water formulas. Recommended ranges of nutrients have been defined (Table 41–5).

Other prepared milks that may have virtue for special circumstances are now available. Milks prepared from hydrolyzed whey or casein may be useful for infants having malabsorption or milk allergy. Special formulas with specific amino acid elimination are useful for infants and children having inborn metabolic errors.

Dried Whole Milk. The fat content of fluid milk is adjusted to 3.5%, and the milk is rapidly evaporated to powder form by spray-, freeze-, or roller-drying. Reconstituted dried milk has most of the advantages of evaporated milk but does not keep well when exposed to air.

Dried Skim Milk. Both nonfat skim milk (fat content 0.5%) and half-skim milk (fat content 1.5%) are available for infants with fat intolerance or for children consuming diets with lowered fat content. Skim milk should not be used in the first 2 yr of life. Its high protein and mineral content in proportion to calories may cause severe dehydration. Many of these products do not contain added vitamin D.

Acid and Fermented Milk. So-called acid milks are prepared by adding acid to previously boiled and cooled cow's milk formulas, or these milks are fermented by adding lactic acid–producing organisms. These milks require less hydrochloric acid for gastric digestion. The casein is altered so that smaller, less tough curds form in the stomach. Acidified milks are now rarely used in infant feedings because they are likely to cause acidosis.

Goat's Milk. In many countries, goat's milk is used extensively for infant feeding; in the United States, its use is limited to managing cow's milk allergies.

Although similar in composition to cow's milk, goat's milk contains less sodium, more potassium and chloride, and more linoleic and arachidonic acids. Its fat may be more digestible and its curd tension lower than that found in cow's milk. It is low in vitamin D, iron, and folic acid; infants fed exclusively on goat's milk are susceptible to megaloblastic anemia due to folate and vitamin B_{12} deficiency. Because the goat is especially susceptible to brucellosis, its milk should be boiled before use. Goat's milk is commercially available in evaporated and powdered forms.

Milk Protein. Powdered protein is used chiefly for increasing protein content of some formulas fed to premature or debilitated infants or to infants with diarrhea. Because of the increased metabolic products and the easy conversion from a balanced to an unbalanced diet, such products should be used carefully and for short durations.

Milk Substitutes and Hypoallergenic Milks. A number of milks and

*One fluid ounce is equivalent to approximately 29.57 mL.

Text continued on page 164

TABLE 41–2 Natural Milks, Prepared Milks, and Milk Substitutes Used in Infant Feeding

	Normal Dilution (kcal/oz)	Approximate Percentage Composition in Normal Dilution (g/dL): Protein	Carbo-hydrate	Fat	PUFA	Minerals	Approximate Electrolyte Composition in Normal Dilution (mEq/L): Na	K	Cl	(mg/L): Ca	P	Fe
Human milk, mature, average	22	1.1	7.0	3.8	0.5–0.55	0.21	6.5	14	12	340	150	1.5
Cow's milk, market, average	20	3.3	4.8	3.7	—	0.72	25	35	29	1.170	920	1.0
Cow's milk, evaporated	22	3.8	5.4	4.0	—	0.80	28	39	32	1.300	1.100	1.0
Prepared formulas, cow's milk based												
AL 110, Nestle	20	1.7	7.5	3.3	0.51	0.35	9.8	20.5	13.9	560	330	4.0
Alfare, Nestle	20	2.3	7.0	3.3	0.40	0.42	17.0	20.6	19.2	540	340	7.8
Alfare, Nestle (22 kcal)	22	2.5	7.8	3.6	0.44	0.47	19.1	23.1	21.1	600	380	8.7
Aptamil Milupa	20	1.5	7.2	3.6	0.43	0.30	7.8	21.2	11.2	580	350	8.0
Bebelac #1, LYEMPF	20	1.5	8.0	3.5	0.55	0.30	9.1	15.9	12.7	550	280	5.5
Dumex Infant Formula, Dumex	20	2.0	7.3	3.2	0.40	0.37	8.6	15.0	13.0	594	396	7.9
Dutch Baby Food, Friesland	20	1.5	7.8	3.3	0.40	0.33	4.6	23.8	14.9	590	400	4.0
Enfamil w/iron, Mead Johnson	20	1.4	7.3	3.6	0.67	0.23	7.9	18.7	12.0	530	360	12.2
Enfamil, Mead Johnson	20	1.4	7.3	3.6	0.67	0.23	7.9	18.7	12.0	530	360	4.7
Follow-Up, Nestle Carnation	20	1.8	8.9	2.8	0.60	0.34	11.5	23.3	17.2	913	609	12.8
Frisolac, Friesland	20	1.4	7.4	3.5	0.48	0.31	4.6	25.4	13.9	560	300	6.2
Gerber Baby Formula	20	1.5	7.2	3.7	0.67	0.37	8.7	18.7	13.2	510	390	3.4
Good Start, Nestle Carnation	20	1.6	7.4	3.4	0.80	0.28	7.0	16.5	11.3	430	240	10.0
Lactofree, Mead Johnson	20	1.4	7.3	3.6	0.50	0.31	8.8	19.1	12.8	550	370	12.2

Lactogen, Nestle	20	1.7	7.4	3.4	0.47	0.36	10.7	20.5	16.1	620	500	8.1
Lactogen FP, Nestle	20	2.9	7.6	2.7	0.39	0.66	17.8	34.8	27.6	1060	880	11.0
Mamex, Dumex	20	1.6	7.3	3.5	0.45	0.26	6.0	14.0	10.0	500	333	7.7
Nan 1 LP, Nestle	20	1.5	7.6	3.4	0.46	0.25	6.9	16.9	12.3	420	210	8.1
Nan 2, Nestle	20	2.2	7.9	2.9	0.44	0.50	14.0	26.9	21.3	810	660	11.0
Nativa, Nestle	20	1.8	6.9	3.6	0.60	0.26	7.4	17.4	13.0	410	210	8.1
Nestac, Nestle	20	3.1	7.4	2.7	0.35	0.69	19.1	37.3	29.4	1120	920	12.0
Nutricia	20	1.8	7.1	3.4	0.28	0.23	8.3	17.2	12.0	600	370	8.0
Promil, Latin America, Wyeth Ayrest	20	2.2	8.2	2.8	0.20	0.30	15	26	16	1150	650	0.8
Pelargon, Nestle	20	1.9	8.0	3.0	0.39	0.43	13.9	23.1	19.4	700	580	8.0
Similac, Ross (also 24 kcal/oz)	20	1.4	7.3	3.7	0.67	0.22	7.0	18.1	12.4	530	280	12.2
Similac, PM 60/40, Ross	20	1.5	6.8	3.8	0.87	0.17	7.0	14.7	11.1	380	190	1.3
S-26, Wyeth Ayerst	20	1.5	7.2	3.6	0.65	0.30	7.0	17.9	12.2	460	333	8.0
Soy Based												
Alsoy, Nestle Carnation	20	1.9	7.5	3.3	0.70	0.35	9.7	20.1	13.5	710	413	12.2
Follow-Up Soy, Nestle Carnation	20	2.1	8.1	3.0	0.70		12.4	20.4	15.1	913	609	12.2
Frisosoy, Friesland	20	1.7	7.1	3.5	0.5	0.29	5.7	28.9	13.9	460	270	7.0
Gerber Soy	20	2.0	6.8	3.6	0.7	0.4	13.9	20.0	16.6	640	500	12.2
Isomil with Iron, Ross	20	1.8	6.8	3.7	0.67	0.27	12.9	18.7	11.8	710	510	12.2
Isomil DF, Ross	20	1.8	6.8	3.7	0.87	0.27	12.9	18.7	11.8	710	510	12.2
Isomil SF, Ross	20	1.8	6.8	3.7	0.67	0.27	12.9	18.7	11.8	710	510	12.2
Nursoy (soy), Wyeth-Ayerst	20	1.8	6.9	3.6	0.65	0.3	8.7	17.9	10.5	600	420	12
ProSobee (soy), Mead Johnson	20	2.0	6.8	3.6	0.67	0.4	10.4	21.0	15.2	710	560	12.2
Soyalac (soy), Loma Linda	20	2.1	6.8	3.7	1.9	0.4	13.0	20.0	13.0	635	370	13

TABLE 41–3 Other Milks, Prepared Milks, and Milk Substitutes Used in Infant Feeding

		Approximate Percentage Composition in Normal Dilution (g/dL)					Approximate Electrolyte Composition in Normal Dilution			
	Normal Dilution (kcal/oz)	*Protein*	*Carbohydrate*	*Fat*	*Notes*	*mOsm/kg water*	*(mEq/L)*		*(mg/L)*	
							Na	*K*	*Ca*	*P*
Specialty Products										
Accupep, Sherwood	30	4.0	19.0	1.0	1	490	30	30	625	625
Advera, Ross	38	6.0	21.6	2.3	—	540	44	65	1080	1080
Alimentum, Ross	20	1.9	6.9	3.7	2	370	13	20	710	510
Alitra Q, Ross	30	5.2	16.5	1.5		575	43	31	733	733
Babelac FL, LYEMPF	20	1.7	7.5	3.7	—	—	9.1	16	550	280
Compleat Pediatric, Novartis	30	3.8	13	3.9	—	380	30	38	1000	1000
Compleat Modified, Novartis	32	4.3	14	3.7	—	300	43	36	670	800
Comply, Sherwood	45	6.0	18.0	6.0	—	410	48	47	1000	1000
Criticare H, Mead Johnson	31	3.8	22.0	0.5	2	650	27	34	530	530
Deliver, Mead Johnson	59	7.5	20	10.2	—	—	35	43	1010	1010
Enfamil Human Milk Fortifier, Mead Johnson	14	0.7	2.7	0.04	—	—	7	15	60	3
Ensure with fiber, Ross	33	4.0	16.2	3.7	—	480	37	43	720	720
Ensure, Ross	31	3.7	16.9	2.6		555	37	40	1270	1270
Ensure High Protein, Ross	28	5.1	13.0	2.5	—	610	53	54	1060	1060
Ensure Plus, Ross	44	5.5	20.0	5.3	—	690	46	50	705	705
Ensure Plus HN, Ross	44	6.3	20.0	5.0	—	650	51	47	1060	1060
Entera, Fresenius	32	4.0	14.6	3.6	—	420	35	34	800	640
Entralife, Corpak	30	3.5	13.6	3.5	—	300	26	25	500	500
Entralife HN30, Corpak	4.2	13.3	3.4	—	—	300	40	32	800	800
FiberSource, Novartis	36	4.3	17	4.1	—	390	48	46	670	670
FiberSource HN, Novartis	36	5.3	16	4.1	—	390	48	46	670	670
Follow-Up Soy, Nestle Carnation	20	2.1	8.1	3.0	—	200	12.4	20.4	913	609
Frisopep 1, Friesland	20	1.5	7.2	3.5	—	—	51	25.4	500	300
Glucerna, Ross	30	4.2	9.6	5.4	—	355	40	40	705	705
Isocal, Mead Johnson	31	4.4	12.4	4.4	—	230	41	41	850	850
Isocal HN, Mead Johnson	31	4.4	12.4	4.4	—	230	41	41	850	850
IsoSource Standard, Novartis	36	4.3	17.0	4.1	5	360	52	43	670	670
IsoSource HN, Novartis	36	5.3	16	4.1	5	330	48	43	670	670
IsoSource 1.5 Cal, Novartis	45	6.8	17	6.5	5	650	57	54	1100	1100
Jevity, Ross	31	4.4	15.2	3.5	—	300	40	40	910	760
Jevity Plus, Ross	36	5.6	17.5	3.9	—	450	59	47	1200	1200
Kindercal	32	3.4	13.6	4.5		275	16	34	850	850
Magnacal, Sherwood	60	7.0	25.0	8.0	—	590	43	32	1000	1000

Meritene, Sandoz	32	6.9	12.0	3.4	—	690	48	32	2200	1900
Mepro, Ross	59	7.0	21.5	9.6	—	635	36	27	1370	690
Neocate, SHS	20	2.0	7.5	2.9	—	340	10	25	790	600
Newtrition, Knight	32	3.6	41.0	4.0	—	450	42	?	600	600
Newtrition Isotonic, Knight	32	3.6	14.8	3.6	—	300	26	26	600	600
Newtrition Isofiber, Knight	36	5.0	16.0	3.7	—	310	36	32	847	847
NextStep Toddler, Mead Johnson	20	1.7	7.4	3.4	—	240	12	22	810	510
NextStep Soy Toddler, Mead Johnson	20	2.0	6.7	3.6	—	210	11	21	710	430
Nutramigen, Mead Johnson	20	1.9	7.4	3.4	2	290	14	19	640	430
Nutrapak, Corpak	32	3.7	14.5	3.7	—	450	37	40	530	530
Nutren 1.0, NCN	30	4.0	12.7	3.8	—	300–350	38.1	32	668	668
Nutren 1.5, NCN	30	6.0	16.9	6.7	—	430–530	50.8	48	1000	1000
Nutren 2.0, NCN	30	8.0	19.6	10.6	—	720	56.6	49.2	1340	1340
Nutren Junior, NCN	30	3.0	12.7	4.2		350	20.0	33.8	1000	800
Nutren, Junior with Fiber, NCN	30	3.0	12.7	4.2		350	20.0	33.8	1000	800
Osmolite, Ross	31	3.7	15.1	3.5	—	300	28	26	530	530
Osmolite HN, Ross	31	4.4	14.4	3.5	—	300	40	40	760	760
Osmolite HN Plus, Ross	36	5.6	15.8	3.9	—	360	62	50	1200	1200
Oxepa, Ross	45	6.3	10.6	9.4	—	493	57	50	1060	1060
Pediasure, Ross	30	3.0	10.9	4.9		345	16	33	970	800
Pediasure with Fiber, Ross	30	3.0	11.4	4.9	—	345	16	33	970	800
Peptamen, NCN	30	4.0	12.7	3.9	1	270–380	24.3	38.5	800	700
Peptamen Junior, NCN	30	3.0	13.7	3.8	1	260–360	20.0	33.8	1000	800
Perative, Ross	38	6.7	17.7	3.7		385	45	44	867	867
Portagen, Mead Johnson	20	2.4	7.8	3.2	—	220	16	22	635	470
Pregestimil PO, Mead Johnson	20	1.9	6.9	3.8	2	290	9	19	640	430
Profiber, Sherwood	30	4.0	14.7	3.5	—	300	32	32	800	800
Promil, Wyeth-Ayerst	20	2.5	8.0	2.8	—	360	14	26	1150	650
Promote, Ross	30	6.3	13.0	2.6	—	340	43	51	1200	1200
Promote with Fiber, Ross	30	6.3	13.9	2.8	—	370	57	51	1200	1200
Pulmocre, Ross	44	6.3	10.5	9.2	—	475	57	44	1060	1060

Table continued on following page

TABLE 41–3 Other Milks, Prepared Milks, and Milk Substitutes Used in Infant Feeding *Continued*

	Normal Dilution (kcal/oz)	Approximate Percentage Composition in Normal Dilution (g/dL) Protein	Carbohydrate	Fat	Notes	mOsm/kg water	Approximate Electrolyte Composition in Normal Dilution (mEq/L) Na	K	(mg/L) Ca	P
RCF, Ross	20	2.0	0	3.6	—	74	13	19	700	500
Resource Standard, Novartis	32	3.8	17	2.5	—	650	41	38	1266	1055
Resource Plus, Novartis	45	5.5	22	4.6	—	870	57	50	1266	1055
Resource Just for Kids, Novartis	30	3.0	11	5.0	—	360	17	31	970	800
S-14, Wyeth-Ayerst	20	1.1	7.1	3.7	—	280	7	12	420	320
S-29, Wyeth-Ayerst	20	1.7	9.8	2.2	—	360	0.4	8	160	190
S-44, Wyeth-Ayerst	20	1.7	9.8	2.2	—	360	0.4	8	160	190
Suplena, Ross	60	3.0	25.5	9.6	—	600	34	29	1385	730
Sustacal, Mead Johnson	30	6.1	14.0	2.3	—	620	41	54	1010	930
Sustacal Plus, Mead Johnson	45	6.1	19.0	5.8	5	520	36	38	850	850
Tolerex, Novartis	30	2.1	23	0.15	3	550	20	31	560	560
Traumacal, Mead Johnson	45	8.3	14.3	6.8	—	440	51	36	750	750
TwoCal HN, Ross	60	8.4	21.7	9.1	—	690	63	63	1050	1050
Vital HN, Ross	30	4.1	18.0	1.1	3, 4, 5	500	25	36	670	670
Vitaneed, Sherwood	30	4.0	13.5	3.5	—	300	27	32	670	670
Vivonex Pediatric, Novartis	24	2.4	13	2.4	3	360	17	31	970	800
Vivonex Ten, Novartis	30	3.8	21	0.28	3	630	20	20	500	500
Vivonex Plus, Novartis	30	4.5	19	0.67	3	650	27	28	560	560

(1) Hydrolyzed whey, (2) hydrolyzed casein, (3) amino acids, (4) partially hydrolyzed whey, and (5) others. Other specialty formulas are available from various manufacturers, low (or free of) carbohydrate, protein, sodium, phenylalanine, branched-chain amino acids, histidine, homocystine, lysine, tyrosine, and methionine.

TABLE 41–4 Natural Milks, Prepared Milks, and Milk Substitutes Used in Premature Infant Feeding

	Normal Dilution (kcal/oz)	Approximate Percentage Composition in Normal Dilution (g/dL) Protein	Carbo-hydrate	Fat	PUFA	Minerals	Approximate Electrolyte Composition in Normal Dilution (mEq/L) Na	K	Cl	(mg/L) Ca	P	Fe
Formulas for Low Birthweight Infants												
Alprem, Prenan, Nestle	24	2.3	8.8	4.2	0.60	0.50	14.6	24.6	14.4	990	544	12.0
Enfamil, Premature Formula, Mead Johnson	24	2.4	8.0	3.4	0.50	0.40	11	19	11.3	700	460	11.0
Similac Natural Care, Ross	24	2.2	8.5	4.4	0.60	0.47	15	27	18	1700	850	3.2
Similac NeoCare, Ross	22	1.9	7.6	4.1	0.60	0.32	11	27	17	780	460	13.3
Similac Special Care with Iron 20, Ross	20	1.8	7.2	3.7	0.50	0.36	13	22	15	1220	610	12.2
Similac Special Care with Iron 24, Ross	24	2.2	8.6	4.4	0.60	0.43	15	27	18	1440	720	14.5
S-26 LBW, Wyeth-Ayerst	24	2.0	8.6	4.4	0.80	0.40	15	22	17	800	425	8

TABLE 41–5 Recommended Ranges of Nutrient Levels in Infant Formulas*

Nutrient (per 100 kcal)	Adequate	Not to Exceed
Protein (g)	1.8†	4.5
Fat (g)	3.3 (30% of kcal)	6 (54% of kcal)
Including essential fatty acid (linoleate) (mg)	300 (2.7% of kcal)	
Vitamins		
A (IU)	250 (75 μg)‡	750 (225 μg)‡
D (μg) cholecalciferol§	1	2.5
K (μg)	4	—
E (tocopherol equivalents)‖	0.5 (at least 0.5/g linoleic acid)	
C (ascorbic acid) (mg)	8	—
B_1 (thiamine) (μg)	40	—
B_2 (riboflavin) (μg)	60	—
B_6 (pyridoxine) (μg)	35 μg/g protein	—
B_{12} (μg)	0.15	
Niacin (μg)	250 (or 0.8 niacin equivalent)	—
Folic acid (μg)	4	—
Pantothenic acid (μg)	300	—
Biotin (μg)	1.4	—
Choline (mg)	7¶	—
Inositol (mg)	4¶	—
Minerals**		
Calcium (mg)	60††	—
Phosphorus (mg)	30††	—
Magnesium (mg)	6	—
Iron (mg)	0.15	2.5‡‡
Iodine (μg)	5	25
Zinc (mg)	0.5	—
Copper (μg)	60	—
Manganese (μg)	5	100
Selenium (μg)	3	—
Sodium (mg)	20 (5.8 mEq/L)	60 (17.5 mEq/L)
Potassium (mg)	80 (13.7 mEq/L)	200 (34.3 mEq/L)
Chloride (mg)	55 (10.4 mEq/L)	150 (28.3 mEq/L)

American Academy of Pediatrics Committee on Nutrition, 1976 recommendations with 1987 modifications.

†*Nutritionally equivalent to casein. For use of other proteins, refer to the commentary on breast feeding and infant formulas, including proposed standards for formulas. Pediatrics 57:278, 1976.*

‡*Retinol equivalents.*

§*1 μg cholecalciferol = 40 IU vitamin D.*

‖*1.49 IU = 1 mg d-α-tocopherol equivalent. The β and γ isomers have less activity.*

¶*Average present in milk-based formulas; should be included in this amount in other formulas.*

***Formula should be made with water low in fluoride and in all cases contain less than 45 μg/100 kcal. For explanation, see statement on fluoride supplementation: revised dosage schedule. American Academy of Pediatrics Committee on Nutrition. Fluoride supplementation: revised dosage schedule. Pediatrics 63:150, 1979.*

††*Calcium to phosphorus ratio should not be less than 1.1 or more than 2.*

‡‡*Prudence indicates there should be an upper limit for iron. If formula is labeled "infant formula with iron," it must not contain less than 1 mg/100 kcal.*

milk substitutes are available for infants allergic to cow's milk. These include evaporated goat's milk, a preparation in which nutrient nitrogen is supplied as an amino acid mixture (casein or whey hydrolysate), and nonmilk foods in which the protein is derived from soybeans. All appear to be nutritionally satisfactory and have a place in the management of infants who cannot tolerate cow's milk; those not containing lactose are useful for infants with galactosemia. Powdered casein and medium-chain triglycerides (MCT oil) are available for special purposes.

Filled and Imitation Milks. Imitation milk products and nondairy "white" beverages in which vegetable fat is substituted for cow (butter) fat are being tested for use in countries where milk and other high-quality protein sources are in short supply. Many of these products lack the full nutritional benefits of fluid milk; they are not intended as formula for infants or as a substitute for breast milk. When they are used for older children, the physician should be aware of the composition and limitations of the product.

Elemental Dietary Substitutes for Milk. A number of specialty products have been developed to meet complicated dietary and nutritional problems in children and adults with malabsorption due to primary disease or extensive surgical resection of the small bowel. These include diets prepared with known quantities of purified chemical elements (free glucose, amino acids, and essential fatty acids). All are low-residue, chemically defined, and nutritionally adequate, at least for short-term use. They have been most useful in treating severely ill infants with intractable diarrhea, in reducing stooling or "resting" the colon in inflammatory bowel disease, in making maximum use of short bowel segments after surgery, and in maintaining very ill patients in positive nitrogen balance while decreasing the bulk and bacterial content of the colon prior to and after major bowel surgery (see inclusion in Table 41–3). Supplements may be necessary and are often used during transitional periods for such patients (Table 41–6).

MILK FORMULAS. The formulas combine milk, sugar, and water, and some modification for a more desirable, smaller curd formation. They should contain about 20 kcal/oz. Recommended ranges of nutrient levels for infant formulas have been described (see Table 41–5).

Caloric Requirements (Chapter 40). The average caloric requirements of full-term infants are about 45–55 kcal/lb or 80–120 kcal/kg during the first few months of life and about 45 kcal/lb or 100 kcal/kg by 1 yr of age; individual variations are significant, and for many infants intakes of this order exceed caloric need.

Fluid Requirements (see Table 40–4). Fluid requirements are high during infancy. During the first 6 mo of life, they range from 2–3 oz/lb/24 hr or 130–190 mL/kg/24 hr and may increase during hot weather. As a rule, the infant regulates his or her own fluid intake, provided adequate amounts are offered. Most of the fluid required is in the formula, but some is supplied in juice and other foods and by water between feedings.

Number of Feedings Daily. The number of feedings required per day decreases throughout the first year; by 1 yr of age, most infants are satisfied with 3 meals/day (Table 41–7). The interval between feedings differs considerably among infants but, in general, ranges from 3–5 hr during the first year of life, averaging 4 hr for full-term, healthy infants. Small or weak infants may prefer feedings at 2- to 3-hr intervals. For the first month or two, feedings are taken throughout the 24-hr period, but thereafter, as the quantity of milk consumed at each feeding increases and the infant adjusts his or her demand to the family pattern of daytime activity, the infant usually sleeps for

TABLE 41–6 Supplements/Substitutes Used in Infant Feeding

	kcal/g	kcal/mL
Carbohydrate Supplements		
LC, Corpak	—	2.5
Moducal, Mead Johnson	3.8	—
PC, Corpak	4.0	—
Polycose powder, Ross	3.8	2.0
Polycose liquid, Ross	—	2.0
Sumacal, Sherwood	3.8	—
Fat Supplements		
Liposyn, Abbott 10%	1.1	1.1
Liposyn, Abbott 20%	2.0	2.0
Intralipid, Cutter 10%	1.1	1.1
Intralipid, Cutter 20%	2.0	2.0
MCT Oil, Mead Johnson	7.7	7.1
MCT Supplement, Corpak	6.1	—
Microlipid, Sherwood	4.5	2.2
Protein Supplements		
Casec, Mead Johnson	3.7	—
Electrodialyzed Whey, Wyeth-Ayerst	1.4	—
Pro-Mix, Corpak	1.4	—
Pro-Mod, Corpak	4.2	—
Propac, Sherwood	4.0	—

TABLE 41–7 Average Daily Number of Feedings

Age	Average No. of Feedings in 24 hr
Birth–1 wk	6–10
1 wk–1 mo	6–8
1–3 mo	5–6
3–7 mo	4–5
4–9 mo	3–4
8–12 mo	3

longer periods at night. As the infant develops psychologically and the loving relationship between the parent and infant evolves, demand feeding should gradually progress to a feeding regimen that accounts for the needs of both the infant and the parents.

Quantity of Formula. The quantity taken at a feeding varies with different infants of the same age and with the same infant at different feedings.

Each infant must be primarily responsible for determining the quantity of intake (Table 41–8). Rarely will an infant want to take more than 7–8 oz of milk at one feeding, if caloric and nutritional needs are adequately supplemented by other foods. The relative requirement for milk is somewhat less in the first 2 wk than in the succeeding 5–6 mo. After this time milk, although still of value, has diminishing importance in meeting total nutritional requirements.

It is rarely necessary to use more than 1 qt of "humanized" formula/24 hr. By the time the infant is taking these quantities, other foods will be added to the diet in increasing amounts. Ingesting more milk has no advantage, but the disadvantage is that other essential foods may be displaced. Some milk may be incorporated in the cereal and in the preparation of other foods. During the first few months, the high quantity of protein and minerals in undiluted cow's milk and insufficient iron content makes unmodified milk unsuitable for infants.

Whereas lactose is the milk sugar of most mammals, other carbohydrates are usually used in home-prepared formulas. Cane sugar, dextrin-maltose preparations, or other easily digestible sugars can be added. Ingested lactose produces a lower pH in the intestine than formulas containing other sugars. The acid pH improves calcium absorption (Table 41–9).

Representative evaporated or whole milk formulas are given in Table 41–10 for those situations in which breast-feeding cannot be sustained or there is lack of availability and/or acceptability of human milk substitutes.

41.3 Other Foods

VITAMINS. Most marketed whole and artificial milks are fortified with 10 g of vitamin D per reconstituted quart; commercially prepared milks vary in the content of other vitamins.

Orange and other citrus fruit juices are natural sources of *vitamin C*, but because many young infants do not seem to tolerate them in amounts large enough to supply an adequate vitamin intake, it is preferable to give 35 mg of ascorbic acid. When at least 2 oz of fresh, frozen, or canned orange juice (or

TABLE 41–8 Average Quantity of Feedings

Age	Average Quantity Taken in Individual Feedings
1st and 2nd wk	2–3 oz (60–90 mL)
3 wk–2 mo	4–5 oz (120–150 mL)
2–3 mo	5–6 oz (150–180 mL)
3–4 mo	6–7 oz (180–210 mL)
5–12 mo	7–8 oz (210–240 mL)

TABLE 41–9 Household Measures of Some Commonly Used Sugars*

	Tablespoonfuls per Ounce
Lactose	3
Sucrose (cane)	2
Dextrin-maltose preparations	
Mead's Dextri-Maltose	4
Karo	2
Cartose	2
Dexin	6
Polycose fluid	2

*Caloric value of each is 120 kcal/oz, except Dexin, 115, and Polycose, 60.

equivalent amount of other sources of vitamin C) is taken daily, the ascorbic acid may be discontinued. Fruit juices should be introduced only when the infant can drink from a cup, in order to diminish nursing-bottle caries. There is a single published report that excessive juice intake may be associated with an increased frequency of obesity in later life.

Vitamin D should be started early in the neonatal period with a daily intake of approximately 10 μg only if the infant is taking a formula that does not contain vitamin D or is receiving an insufficient volume of milk to meet the daily requirement. Low birthweight infants require supplementation (Chapter 93). Vitamin D supplement is not necessary during the first few months of breast-feeding of white infants but may be for black infants and those not exposed to adequate sunlight. Concentrates in water-miscible vehicles are desirable to avoid aspiration of oil.

IRON. Foods rich in iron are less available in the diet of poor families. The most effective way to prevent iron deficiency is to provide iron supplementation in the form of an iron-fortified milk formula or medicinal iron (2 mg/kg up to a total of 15 mg/24 hr) beginning at 6 wk of age. It is doubtful whether iron-supplemented cereals provide sufficient supplementation for infants with reduced iron stores.

"SOLID" FOODS. The caloric contents of the various prepared baby foods differ widely (see Table 726–12). Egg yolk, cereals with added milk, meats, and puddings have greater caloric density than milk, whereas vegetables and fruits have an energy value similar to or lower than that of milk. Without appropriate advice, many mothers select foods with high caloric values that result in obesity. The inclusion of solid foods to the diet before 4–6 mo of age does not contribute significantly to the health of the normal infant nor does it increase the likelihood of the infant's sleeping through the night, providing hunger is avoided with adequate breast-feeding or formula feeding.

Any new food should be initially offered once a day in small amounts (1–2 teaspoonfuls). Any small spoon that easily fits the baby's mouth may be used. New foods are generally best accepted if fairly thin or dilute. Food is frequently pushed out

TABLE 41–10 Representative Formulas*

	1–3 Days	kcal	4–10 Days	kcal	>10 Days	kcal
Evaporated milk	6 oz	240	7 oz	280	13 oz	520
Sugar	1 tbsp	60	1 tbsp	60	3 tbsp	180
Water	14 oz		14 oz		17 oz	
	20 oz	300	21 oz	340	30 oz	700
kcal/oz		14		16		22
kcal/100 mL		47		56		70
Whole milk	12 oz	240	14 oz	280	26 oz	520
Sugar	1 tbsp	60	1 tbsp	60	3 tbsp	180
Water	8 oz		7 oz		6 oz	
	20 oz	300	21 oz	340	32 oz	700

*Total volume is divided into six bottles, and the total intake is regulated by the infant.

by the tongue rather than back, because the baby cannot yet swallow efficiently. This should be mentioned to the mother, who might otherwise interpret the spitting out of new foods as dislike. It is usually wise to offer the same food daily until the baby becomes accustomed to it and not to introduce new foods more often than every 1–2 wk.

The feeding at which these foods are offered is not particularly important. They should be given when the baby's hunger is no longer satisfied by milk alone and when they fit into the daily schedule. There is no reason for persisting with or forcing a particular food that is definitely disliked. The family's dislikes and prejudices for particular foods are contagious and should not be displayed before the infant. The physician should avoid prescribing a definite amount of a given food lest the mother interpret the suggestion too literally. *Many infants are overfed by overzealous parents who mistake acceptance of food for appetite.* The infant's appetite is the best index of the proper amount, and respect for the infant's wishes will avoid many problems.

Cereal. The various precooked cereals on the market provide in a convenient form a variety of grains excellent for infants. Most contain iron and factors of the vitamin B complex.

Fruits. Strained or puréed cooked fruits furnish minerals and some water-soluble vitamins and usually have a mild laxative effect. Raw ripe mashed banana is readily digested and enjoyed by most infants. Many infants who are slow in accepting new foods seem to prefer fruits.

Vegetables. Vegetables are moderately good sources of iron and other minerals and of the B-complex vitamins. They should be freshly cooked and strained or commercially prepared. Vegetables are usually added to the infant's diet by about 7 mo of age.

Meats, Eggs, and Starchy Foods. Eggs and starchy foods are usually introduced during the second 6 mo of life, although some physicians offer egg yolk at an earlier age. The yolk of the egg is used initially and is preferably hard-cooked. As with all new foods, a small amount is offered at first, with gradual increases up to a whole yolk 1–3 times a week. Egg white should be introduced with equal caution to minimize any possible allergic manifestations.

Potatoes, rice, spaghetti, bread, and similar starchy foods have a principally caloric value. As a rule, they are not included in the infant's diet until the more essential foods mentioned earlier are being taken regularly. Zwieback, toast, or graham crackers may be offered to the infant when he or she shows an interest in "gumming" on coarser foods (usually 6–8 mo of age). It is with such foods that infants learn to chew and to feed themselves.

Meat is an excellent source of protein as well as of iron and vitamins. Ground fresh beef or liver or the strained canned meats may be used initially by about 6 mo of age. Meats may be more readily accepted when mixed with another food.

The commercial soups and meat and vegetable mixtures are relatively high in carbohydrate and are not considered optimal sources of iron or protein. Many home-prepared soups are bulky out of proportion to their food value, and much of the vitamin content is lost by overcooking.

Desserts. Pudding, junket, and custard are good foods for older infants, particularly if they temporarily prefer milk in that form. If, however, such foods are given as a bribe or reward or only after other foods have been finished, poor eating habits are likely to be established. Sweet foods should be offered as casually as the rest of the meal and at any point in the meal that the child desires.

SALT INTAKE. To increase their palatability, particularly for the parent, excessive salt used to be added to baby foods. This practice has been discontinued. The significance of large intakes of sodium, which are in the ranges seen in populations with a high incidence of hypertension, is not clear, but the possibility that they might contribute to the development of hypertension later in life cannot be ignored.

FOOD ADDITIVES. Naturally occurring chemicals and food additives, particularly the artificial flavors and colors, have been implicated in health problems. It has been estimated that more than 3,000 flavors are currently being used, and few children are spared exposure to them in their daily diet. Artificial flavors and colors have been associated with respiratory allergic disorders, with urticaria and angioedema, with lesions of the tongue and buccal mucosa, with digestive disturbances, with arthralgia and hydrarthroses, and with headache and behavioral disturbances, including hyperkinesis in childhood.

41.4 First-Year Feeding Problems

UNDERFEEDING. Underfeeding is suggested by restlessness and crying and by failure to gain weight adequately, despite complete emptying of the breast or bottle. Underfeeding may also result from the infant's failure to take a sufficient quantity of food even when offered. In these cases, the frequency of feedings, the mechanics of feeding, the size of the holes in the nipple, the adequacy of eructation of air, the possibility of abnormal mother-infant "bonding," and possible systemic disease in the baby should be investigated (see Chapters 35 and 36).

The extent and duration of underfeeding determine the *clinical manifestations*. Constipation, failure to sleep, irritability, and excessive crying are to be expected. There may be poor gain in weight or an actual loss. In the latter case, the skin becomes dry and wrinkled, subcutaneous tissue disappears, and the infant assumes the appearance of an "old man." Deficiencies of vitamins A, B, C, and D and of iron and protein may be responsible for characteristic clinical manifestations.

Treatment consists of increasing the fluid and caloric intake, correcting deficiencies in vitamin and mineral intake, and instructing the mother in the art of infant feeding. If some underlying systemic disease, child abuse/neglect, or psychologic problem is responsible, specific management of these disorders is necessary.

OVERFEEDING. Overfeeding may be quantitative or qualitative. Regurgitation and vomiting are frequent symptoms of overfeeding. As a rule, infants can be depended on not to take excessive quantities, but occasionally an infant who has postprandial discomfort from eating too much may nonetheless gain weight excessively. Diets too high in fat delay gastric emptying, cause distention and abdominal discomfort, and may cause excessive gain in weight. Diets too high in carbohydrate are likely to cause undue fermentation in the intestine, resulting in distention and flatulence and in too rapid a gain in weight. Such diets may be deficient in essential protein, vitamins, and minerals. Formulas too high in caloric content in the first 1–2 wk of life are likely to result in loose or diarrheal stools. Obesity is undesirable at any time in life; often the excessively fed infant becomes the obese child and adult.

REGURGITATION AND VOMITING. The return of small amounts of swallowed food during or shortly after eating is called regurgitation or spitting up. More complete emptying of the stomach, especially that occurring some time after feeding, is called vomiting. Within limits, regurgitation is a natural occurrence, especially during the first 6 mo or so of life. It can be reduced to a negligible amount, however, by adequate eructation of swallowed air during and after eating, by gentle handling, by avoiding emotional conflicts, and by placing the infant on the right side for a nap immediately after eating. The head should not be lower than the rest of the body during the rest period, because gastroesophageal reflux is common during the first 4–6 mo.

Vomiting, one of the most common symptoms in infancy, may be associated with a variety of disturbances, both trivial and serious. It should be distinguished from rumination; its cause should always be investigated (see Chapters 306, 323, and 329).

LOOSE OR DIARRHEAL STOOLS. Acute infectious diarrhea and chronic diarrheal conditions are discussed in Chapters 176, 306, and 341; only mild disturbances of dietary origin are considered here.

The stool of the breast-fed infant is naturally softer than that of the infant fed cow's milk. From about the 4th to the 6th day of life, the stools go through a transitional stage in which they are rather loose and greenish yellow and contain mucus; within a few days, the typical "milk stool" appears. Subsequently, the use of laxatives or the ingestion of certain foods by the mother may be temporarily responsible for an infant's loose stools. Excessive intake of breast milk may also increase the frequency and the water content of the stool. Actual diarrhea in a breast-fed infant is unusual and should be considered infectious until proved otherwise.

Although the stools of artificially fed infants tend to be firmer than those of breast-fed infants, loose stools may result from artificial feeding. In the first 2 wk or so of life, overfeeding is likely to cause loose, frequent stools. Later, formulas too concentrated or too high in sugar content, especially in lactose, may produce loose, frequent stools. Many temporary diarrheal disturbances in artificially fed infants result from food contaminations that would not disturb an older child and are not serious enough to cause prolonged difficulty for the infant. The ease with which artificially fed infants acquire diarrheal disturbances and their potential seriousness are strong arguments for extreme care in providing food free of pathogenic bacteria.

Mild diarrheal disturbances due to overfeeding respond quickly to temporary decrease or cessation of feeding. Withholding all solid food as well as one or several milk feedings and substituting boiled water or a balanced electrolyte solution are usually all that is required.

CONSTIPATION (see Chapter 306). Constipation is practically unknown in breast-fed infants receiving an adequate amount of milk and is rare in artificially fed infants receiving an adequate diet. The nature of the stool, not its frequency, is the basis for diagnosing. Although most infants have one or more stools daily, an infant will occasionally have a stool of normal consistency only at intervals of 36–48 hr.

Whenever constipation or obstipation is present from birth or shortly thereafter, a rectal examination should be performed. Tight or spastic anal sphincters may occasionally be responsible for obstipation, and correction usually follows finger dilatation. Anal fissures or cracks may also cause constipation. If irritation is alleviated, healing usually occurs quickly. Aganglionic megacolon may be manifested by constipation in early infancy; the absence of stool in the rectum on digital examination suggests this possibility.

Constipation in the artificially fed infant may be caused by an insufficient amount of food or fluid. In other cases, it may result from diets too high in fat or protein or deficient in bulk. Simply increasing the amount of fluid or sugar in the formula may be corrective in the first few months of life. After this age, better results are obtained by adding or increasing the amounts of cereal, vegetables, and fruits. Prune juice (½–1 oz) may be given as a temporary measure, but it is better to add foods with some bulk. Enemas and suppositories should never be more than temporary measures. Milk of magnesia may be given in doses of 1–2 tsp but should be reserved for unresponsive or severe constipation.

COLIC. The term *colic* describes a frequent symptom complex of paroxysmal abdominal pain, presumably of intestinal origin, and of severe crying. It occurs usually in infants younger than 3 mo.

The *clinical manifestations* are characteristic: The attack usually begins suddenly; the cry is loud and more or less continuous; so-called paroxysms may persist for several hours; the face may be flushed, or there may be circumoral pallor; the abdomen is distended and tense; the legs are drawn up on the abdomen, although they may be momentarily extended; the feet are often cold; the hands are clenched. The attack may terminate only when the infant is completely exhausted, but often there is apparent temporary relief with the passage of feces or flatus.

Certain infants seem to be peculiarly susceptible to colic. The *etiology* of recurrent attacks is usually not apparent, although they may be associated with hunger and with swallowed air that has passed into the intestine. Overfeeding may also cause discomfort and distention. Certain foods, especially those of high carbohydrate content, may be responsible for excessive fermentation in the intestines, but a change in diet only occasionally prevents further colic attacks. Crying from intestinal discomfort is seen in infants with intestinal allergy, but colic is not limited to this group. Intestinal obstruction or peritoneal infection may mimic an attack of colic. Recurrent attacks commonly occur late in the afternoon or evening, suggesting that events in the household routine may possibly cause them. Worry, fear, anger, or excitement may cause vomiting in an older child and may cause colic in an infant. No single factor consistently accounts for colic, nor does any treatment consistently provide satisfactory relief. Careful physical examination is important to eliminate the possibility of intussusception, strangulated hernia, hair in the infant's eye, otitis, pyelonephritis, or other disorders.

Holding the baby upright or permitting the baby to lie prone across the lap or on a hot water bottle or heating pad helps occasionally. Passage of flatus or fecal material spontaneously or with expulsion of a suppository or enema sometimes affords relief. Carminatives before feedings are ineffective in preventing the attacks. Sedation is occasionally indicated for a prolonged attack and is sometimes given to the parent or child for a period of time if other measures fail. Temporary hospitalization of the infant, often without more than a change in feeding routine and a period of rest for the mother, may help in extreme cases. Prevention of attacks should be sought by improving feeding techniques, including burping, providing a stable emotional environment, identifying possibly allergenic foods in the infant's or nursing mother's diet, and avoiding underfeeding or overfeeding. Colic rarely persists after 3 mo of age. A supportive, sympathetic physician is important in successfully resolving the problem.

41.5 Feeding During the Second Year of Life

Most infants naturally adapt themselves to a schedule of three meals a day by about the end of the 1st yr of life. Although considerable latitude in the diet of each infant should be permitted to allow for personal idiosyncrasies and family habits, the mother should be given an outline of the daily basic dietary needs (see Table 40–9 and Fig. 40–2). When malnutrition, as either dietary deficiency or excess, or failure to thrive exists despite an apparently satisfactory food intake, the infant or child's family relationships must be evaluated, not only for organic causes but especially for psychosocial ones (see Chapters 35 and 36).

REDUCED CALORIC INTAKE. Toward the end of the 1st yr of life and during the 2nd yr, because of the constantly decelerating rate of growth, there is a gradual reduction in the infant's caloric intake per unit of body weight. In addition, it is not unusual to have temporary periods of lack of interest in certain foods or even in food in general. Failure to recognize these features, especially the decreasing caloric needs, results in attempts to force feed. The child naturally rebels, and feeding problems ensue. Because preventing problems is more effective than correcting them, the changing pattern of the infant's food habits during the 2nd yr of life should be explained to the mother before it appears.

SELF-SELECTION OF DIET. Children's strong likes or dislikes of particular foods should be respected whenever possible and practicable. Spinach is an example of a nonessential food whose virtues have been overemphasized. When consistently rejected foods include basic staples such as milk and cereal, food allergy should be considered.

Children, including infants, tend to select diets that, over several days, assume a balanced nature. Thus, the child may be permitted a wide choice of foods, as long as he or she eats adequately over the longer period. Normally, the child determines the quantity to be eaten of a given food and of the entire meal. At this age, eating habits may be strongly influenced by older children in the family, particularly in respect to food likes and dislikes. Eating patterns and habits developed in the first 2 yr of life usually persist for several years.

SELF-FEEDING BY INFANTS. Before 1 yr of age, the infant should be permitted to participate in the act of feeding. By approximately 6 mo, the infant can hold a bottle; within another 2–3 mo, a cup. Zwieback, graham crackers, or other hand-held foods can be introduced by the age of 7–8 mo. A spoon may be used as soon as it can be held and directed to the mouth, possibly by 10–12 mo of age. Mothers often inhibit this learning process because they object to its messiness.

Acquiring the ability to feed oneself is an important step in developing self-reliance and responsibility. By the end of the 2nd yr of life, infants should be largely responsible for feeding themselves.

Permitting infants and children to go to sleep while sucking intermittently from a bottle of formula, whole milk, sweet fruit juice, or water should be discouraged. Pedodontists emphasize the correlation between this habit and enamel erosion in deciduous teeth, calling it the "baby bottle syndrome."

Although nutritional requirements per unit of body weight constantly decrease with increasing age (110 kcal/kg in infancy; 50 kcal/kg at 15 yr), the need for calories as well as for protein, vitamins, and minerals is relatively greater in children than it is in adults.

DAILY BASIC DIET. Parents should be given a daily basic diet for the child from which the family menu can be prepared. Daily selection from each of the food groups (see Fig. 40–2) provides a balanced diet with sufficient macronutrients and micronutrients. The quantity of intake after the basic requirements have been met can usually be determined by the healthy growing child. The child's history of dietary habits is essential for evaluating the nutritive intake, but such histories are often unreliable unless an accurate dietary diary is kept for several days. From such information, correcting the diet may be more effective.

The older child should learn the content of a basic diet and its importance to proper growth and good health, but this information should never be presented as a threat to enforce rigid feeding practices.

EATING HABITS. Eating habits formed in the 1st yr or 2 of life distinctly affect those of the subsequent years. Feeding difficulties between the ages of 2–5 yr frequently result from excessive parental insistence on eating and subsequent anxiety when the child does not conform to some arbitrary standard. The child's negative reactions naturally result from undue mealtime stress, and correction requires improvement in parent-child relations. Other factors that disturb eating are too much confusion at mealtime, insufficient time for eating on the part of either the adult or the child, food dislikes of other members of the family, and poorly prepared and unattractively served food. A comfortable chair of proper height with a footrest is important for a child's ease at the table. Mealtimes should be happy, and the conversation should be on subjects of interest to the entire family. The child's appetite should be respected; if his or her desire for food is below average at times, there should be no persuasion to eat more. Adults should realize that eating habits are taught better by example than by formal explanation.

SNACKS BETWEEN MEALS. During the 2nd yr and even for several years thereafter, orange juice or other fruit juice or fruit, together with a cracker, may be given in either or both of the between-meal periods. Snacks served in nursery schools and kindergartens should be nutritious. Older children should avoid between-meal snacking if it reduces their appetite for the next meal. After-school snacks, especially of fruit, should be encouraged if they produce greater enthusiasm and energy for play and do not reduce the appetite for the evening meal.

VEGETARIAN DIET. All-vegetable diets supply all necessary nutrients when vegetables are selected from different classes. Vegetables are high in fiber content, vitamins, and minerals. Vegetarians usually have faster gastrointestinal transit time, bulkier stools, and low serum cholesterol levels and are said to have less diverticulitis and appendicitis than meat eaters. Those who consume eggs are ovovegetarians. Those who consume milk are lactovegetarians. Those who consume neither are vegans. Vegans may develop vitamin B_{12} deficiency and, because of high fiber intake, may develop trace mineral deficiency. Nursing vegan mothers must be given added vitamin B_{12} to prevent methylmalonic acidemia in their infants. Vegetarian infants may not grow as rapidly as omnivores in the first 2 yr.

41.6 Later Childhood and Adolescence

As the child reaches age 2 yr, diet is similar to that of the family. All the known nutrients are supplied by a varied diet and should include selections from each of the food groups: cereals, fruits, vegetables, proteins, and dairy. The relative amounts are described by the food pyramid (see Fig. 40–2). Emphasis on cereal, fruits, and vegetables supports the recommendations of the National Cholesterol Education Program. Those recommendations include restriction of total fat in the diet to approximately 30% of the total daily calories, of which 10% is saturated, 7–8% polyunsaturated, and 12–13% monounsaturated fatty acids. Dietary cholesterol should not exceed 100 mg/1,000 calories. This diet, the American Heart Association Step One Diet, is recommended to decrease atherosclerotic heart disease and may also be effective in limiting the development of obesity. The food selections of the pyramid may be made as the infant begins to take supplemental foods, but fat in the diet should not be restricted until the child is past 2 yr of age. Some children given a more restricted diet in infancy fail to thrive.

DIET FOR ATHLETIC ACTIVITIES. Adequate caloric intake is necessary for growth and activity. A varied diet supplies all necessary nutrients. Special food supplements are unnecessary and may be harmful. Water intake should be scheduled regularly before and during athletic events.

SPECIAL NUTRITIONAL SUPPORT PROGRAMS. The Special Supplemental Nutrition Program for Women, Infants, and Children (WIC) is designed to provide specified food items and nutrition education to pregnant and post-partum women, lactating mothers, infants, and children up to 5 yr of age who are assessed as being at nutritional risk and have a family income of less than a specified percent (recently 185%) of the federal poverty level. Programs such as this should be available to women and children as an appropriate public health intervention to facilitate good health.

American Academy of Pediatrics Committee on Nutrition: Pediatric Nutrition Handbook, 4th ed. Elk Grove Village, IL, American Academy of Pediatrics, 1998.

American Academy of Pediatrics Committee on Nutrition: Soy protein–based formulas: Recommendations for use in infant feedings. Pediatrics 101:148, 1998.

Barr RG, Kramer MS, Pless B, et al: Feeding and temperament as determinants of early infant crying/fussing behavior. Pediatrics 84:514, 1989.
Baumgartner TG: Trace elements in clinical nutrition. Nutr Clin Pract 8:251, 1993.
Dennison BA, Rockwell HL, Baker SL: Excess fruit juice consumption by preschool-aged children is associated with short stature and obesity. Pediatrics 99:15, 1997.
Fomon SJ, Ziegler EE: Upper limits of nutrients in infant formulas: Proceedings of a symposium held in Iowa City, IA, Nov 7–8, 1988. Bethesda, American Institute of Nutrition, 1989.
George DR, De Francesca BA: Human milk in comparison to cow milk. *In*: Lebenthal E (ed): Textbook of Gastroenterology and Nutrition in Infancy and Childhood, 2nd ed. New York, Raven Press, 1989, pp 242–243.
La Leche League International: The Womanly Art of Breast Feeding. Franklin Park, IL, La Leche League International, 1976.
Lawrence RA: Breast Feeding, A Guide For the Medical Profession, 4th ed. St. Louis, CV Mosby, 1994.
Lebenthal E (ed): Textbook of Gastroenterology and Nutrition in Infants, 2nd ed. New York, Raven Press, 1989.
Lozoff B: Behavioral alterations in iron deficiency. Adv Pediatr 35:331, 1988.
National Academy of Sciences: Recommended Dietary Allowances, 10th ed. Washington, DC, National Academy Press, 1989.
National Cholesterol Education Program (NCEP): Reports of the Expert Panel on Blood Cholesterol in Children and Adolescents. Pediatrics 89(Suppl):525, 1992.
Oski FA: Iron deficiency in infancy and childhood. N Engl J Med 329:190, 1993.
United States Department of Agriculture: Food Guide Pyramid. A Guide to Daily Food Choices. Home and Garden Bulletin, No. 252. Washington, DC, Human Nutrition Information Services, 1992.
Wright JA, Ashenberg CA, Whitaker RC: Comparison of methods to categorize undernutrition in children. J Pediatr 124:944, 1994.

CHAPTER 42

Malnutrition

Worldwide, malnutrition is one of the leading causes of morbidity and mortality in childhood (see Chapter 4).

Malnutrition may be due to improper or inadequate food intake or may result from inadequate absorption of food. Insufficient food supply, poor dietary habits, food faddism, and emotional factors may limit intake. Certain metabolic abnormalities may also cause malnutrition. Requirements for essential nutrients may be increased during stress and disease and during the administration of antibiotics and of catabolic or anabolic drugs. Malnutrition may be acute or chronic, reversible or irreversible.

Precise evaluation of nutritional status is difficult. Severe disturbances are readily apparent, but mild disturbances may be overlooked, even after careful physical and laboratory examinations. The diagnosis of malnutrition rests on an accurate dietary history; on evaluation of present deviations from average height, weight, head circumference, and past rates of growth; on comparative measurements of midarm circumference and skinfold thickness; and on chemical and other tests. Decreased skinfold thickness suggests protein-calorie malnutrition; excessive thickness indicates obesity. Muscle mass is calculated by subtracting skinfold measurements from arm circumference. For older children and adults, midarm muscle mass circumference (cm) = arm circumference (cm) − (skinfold thickness [cm] × 3.14). Body mass index, BMI, kg/m^2 can be calculated. Lean body mass can be estimated from 24 hr creatinine excretion. Deficiencies of some nutrients may be revealed by finding low blood levels of them or their metabolites, by observing biochemical or clinical effects of administration of the nutrients or their products, or by giving the patient substantial amounts of appropriate nutrients and noting the rate at which they are excreted. Protein reserves are assessed from serum albumin and rapid-turnover proteins. The levels of rapid-turnover proteins, transthyretin with a half-life of 12 hr, prealbumin with a half-life of 1.9 days, and transferrin with a half-life of 8 days, decrease owing to inadequate visceral protein synthesis or depletion of protein stores. Serum levels of essential amino acids may be lower than those of nonessential amino acids. In the severely malnourished child, excretion of hydroxyproline is decreased and excretion of 3-methylhistidine increased, and hair is easily plucked out.

The most acute nutritional disturbances are those that involve water and electrolytes, especially sodium, potassium, chloride, and hydrogen ions (see Part VII). Chronic malnutrition usually involves deficits of more than a single nutrient. Immunologic insufficiency is common in malnutrition and is demonstrated by total lymphocyte counts less than 1,500/mm^3 and anergy to skin test antigens, such as streptokinase-streptodornase, *Candida*, mumps, or tuberculin in exposed persons (see Chapters 36 and 179).

42.1 Marasmus (Infantile Atrophy, Inanition, Athrepsia)

Severe malnutrition in infants is common in areas with insufficient food, inadequate knowledge of feeding techniques, or poor hygiene. The synonyms of marasmus apply to patterns of clinical illness emphasizing one or more features of protein and calorie deficiency.

ETIOLOGY. The clinical picture of marasmus originates from an inadequate caloric intake due to insufficient diet, to improper feeding habits such as those of disturbed parent-child relations, or to metabolic abnormalities or congenital malformations. Severe impairment of any body system may result in malnutrition.

CLINICAL MANIFESTATIONS. Initially there is failure to gain weight, followed by loss of weight until emaciation results, with loss of turgor in skin that becomes wrinkled and loose as subcutaneous fat disappears. Because fat is lost last from the sucking pads of the cheeks, the infant's face may retain a relatively normal appearance for some time before becoming shrunken and wizened. The abdomen may be distended or flat, and the intestinal pattern may be readily visible. Atrophy of muscle occurs, with resultant hypotonia.

The temperature is usually subnormal; the pulse may be slow; and the basal metabolic rate tends to be reduced. At first, the infant may be fretful but later becomes listless, and the appetite diminishes. The infant is usually constipated, but the so-called starvation type of diarrhea may appear, with frequent small stools containing mucus.

42.2 Protein Malnutrition (Protein-Calorie Malnutrition [PCM], Kwashiorkor)

Because they are growing, children must consume enough nitrogenous food to maintain a positive nitrogen balance, whereas adults need only maintain nitrogen equilibrium.

ETIOLOGY. Although deficiencies of calories and other nutrients complicate the clinical and chemical patterns, the principal symptoms of protein malnutrition are due to insufficient intake of protein of good biologic value. There may also be impaired absorption of protein, such as in chronic diarrheal states; abnormal losses of protein in proteinuria (nephrosis), infection, hemorrhage, or burns; and failure of protein synthesis, such as in chronic liver disease.

Kwashiorkor is a clinical syndrome that results from a severe deficiency of protein and an inadequate caloric intake. Either from lack of intake or from excessive losses or increases in metabolic rate caused by chronic infections, secondary vitamin and mineral deficiency may contribute to the signs and symptoms. It is the most serious and prevalent form of malnutrition in the world today, especially in industrially underdeveloped areas. Kwashiorkor means deposed child; that is, the child no longer suckled; the condition may become evident from early infancy to about 5 yr of age, usually after weaning from the breast. Although gains in height and weight are accelerated with treatment, these measurements never equal those of consistently well-nourished children.

CLINICAL MANIFESTATIONS (Fig. 42–1). Early clinical evidence of protein malnutrition is vague but does include lethargy, apathy, or irritability. When well advanced, it results in inadequate growth, lack of stamina, loss of muscular tissue, increased susceptibility to infections, and edema. Secondary immunodeficiency is one of the most serious and constant manifestations. For example, measles, a relatively benign disease of the well nourished, can be devastating and fatal in malnourished children. HIV intercurrent infection rates approximating 25% have been reported in studies from Malawi and may complicate the diagnosis and treatment.

The child may develop anorexia, flabbiness of subcutaneous tissues, and loss of muscle tone. The liver may enlarge early or late; fatty infiltration is common, and hepatic export proteins are reduced. Edema usually develops early; failure to gain weight may be masked by edema, which is often present in internal organs before it can be recognized in the face and limbs. Renal plasma flow, glomerular filtration rate, and renal tubular function are decreased. The heart may be small in the early stages of the disease but is usually enlarged later.

Dermatitis is common. Darkening of the skin appears in irritated areas but not in areas exposed to sunlight, a contrast to the situation in pellagra (see Chapter 44.5). Dyspigmentation may occur in these areas after desquamation, or it may be generalized. The hair is often sparse and thin and loses its elasticity. In dark-haired children, dyspigmentation may result in streaky red or gray hair color (hypochromotrichia). Hair texture becomes coarse in chronic disease.

Infections, both acute and chronic (TB and HIV), and parasitic infestations are common, as are anorexia, vomiting, and continued diarrhea. The muscles are weak, thin, and atrophic, but occasionally there may be an excess of subcutaneous fat. Mental changes, especially irritability and apathy, are common. Stupor, coma, and death may follow with a substantial case fatality rate (~30–40%) even when the disease is diagnosed and appropriately treated.

There are substantial regional and seasonal variations related to diet, intercurrent infectious disease, and other factors in the prevalence of kwashiorkor in different parts of the world.

LABORATORY DATA. Decrease in the concentration of serum albumin is the most characteristic change. Ketonuria is common in the early stage of inanition but frequently disappears in the later stages. Blood glucose values are low, but glucose tolerance curves may be diabetic in type. Urinary excretion of hydroxyproline relative to creatinine may be decreased. Plasma values of essential amino acids may be decreased relative to nonessential ones, and there may be increased aminoaciduria. Potassium and magnesium deficiencies are frequent. Severe hypophosphatemia (<0.32 mmol/L) is associated with increased mortality. The serum cholesterol level is low, but it returns to normal after a few days of treatment. The serum values of amylase, esterase, cholinesterase, transaminase, lipase, and alkaline phosphatase are decreased. There is diminished activity of the pancreatic enzymes and of xanthine oxidase, but these values return to normal shortly after initiation of treatment. Anemia may be normocytic, microcytic, or macrocytic. Signs of vitamin (particularly vitamin A) and mineral

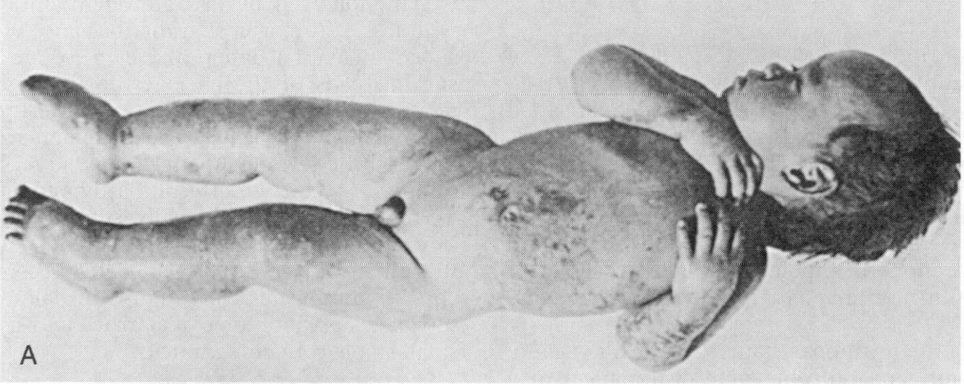

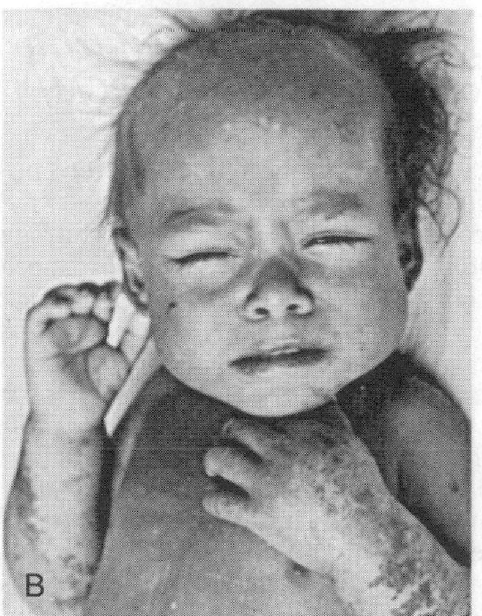

Figure 42–1 *A*, Kwashiorkor in a 2-yr-old boy. Note the generalized edema, the typical skin lesions, and the state of prostration. *B*, Close-up of the same child showing the hair changes and psychic alterations (apathy and misery); the edema of the face and the skin lesions can be seen more clearly. (Photographs made available by the Institute of Nutrition of Central America and Panama, Guatemala, courtesy of Moises Behar, M.D.)

deficiencies are usually evident. Bone growth is usually delayed. Growth hormone secretion may be increased. There is altered intestinal permeability, which correlates with disease severity.

DIFFERENTIAL DIAGNOSIS. Differential diagnosis of protein deprivation includes chronic infections, diseases in which there is an excessive loss of protein through urine or stools, and conditions involving a metabolic inability to synthesize protein.

PREVENTION. This requires a diet containing an adequate quantity of protein of good biologic quality. Because kwashiorkor has not only a serious and often fatal course but often permanent and devastating aftereffects in recovered children and their offspring, adequate dietary instruction and food distribution are urgently needed in endemic areas.

TREATMENT. Immediate management of any acute problems such as those of severe diarrhea, renal failure, and shock (see Chapter 64.2) and, ultimately, the replacement of missing nutrients are essential.

Initial management consists of administration of low-volume, dilute milk feeds with nutrient supplementation (such as Nutriset—a micronutrient supplement with supplemental potassium, calcium, zinc, magnesium, manganese, selenium, iodine, copper, and multivitamins or use of mineral supplements with at least potassium [recommendations range from 4.0–8.0 mmol/kg/24 hr at initiation of therapy rising to 7.7 mmol/kg/24 hr or more in the recovery phase], magnesium, and zinc) advanced incrementally over 2 wk to high-energy milk with supplemention as the patient enters the rapid-growth phase. The routine administration of antibiotics such as co-trimoxazole has also been advocated. Other antimicrobials are used only to treat overt infection because of concerns about emergence of microbial resistance.

Moderate or severe dehydration, manifest or suspected infection, eye signs of severe vitamin A deficiency, severe anemia, hypoglycemia, continuing or recurrent diarrhea, skin and mucous membrane lesions, anorexia, and hypothermia all must be treated. For mild to moderate dehydration, feedings are administered orally or by nasogastric tube, when culturally appropriate, to prevent aspiration (see Chapter 54). A breast-fed infant should be nursed as often as he or she wants.

Intravenous (IV) fluids are necessary for the treatment of severe dehydration (see Chapter 55). If IV fluids cannot be given, an intraosseous (marrow) or intraperitoneal infusion of 70 mL/kg of half-strength Ringer's lactate solution may be lifesaving. Effective antibiotics should be given parenterally for 5–10 days.

When dehydration is corrected, oral or nasogastric feeding starts with small, frequent feeds of dilute milk (66 kcal and 1.0 g protein/100 mL at ~120/mL/kg/24 hr) with nutrient supplementation; strength and volume are gradually increased and frequency decreased over the next 5–7 days. By day 6–8, the child should receive 150 mL/kg/24 hr in ~6 feeds of high-energy milk (114 kcal and 4.1 g protein/100 mL). Cow's milk, or yogurt for the lactose-intolerant child, should be made with 50 g of sugar/L. Special feeds are available from UNICEF.

When high-calorie and high-protein diets are given too early and too rapidly, the liver may become enlarged, the abdomen becomes markedly distended, and the child improves more slowly. Vegetable fat is better absorbed than cow's milk fat. Impaired glucose tolerance may be improved in some affected children by the daily administration of 250 mg of chromium chloride. Vitamins and minerals, especially vitamin A, potassium, and magnesium, are necessary from the outset of treatment. Iron and folic acid usually correct the anemia.

Bacterial infections should be treated concomitantly with the dietary therapy, whereas treatment of parasitic infestations, if they are not severe, may be postponed until recovery is under way. There is not uniform consensus with regard to timing of HIV testing relative to timing of nutritional rehabilitation. Testing should best follow local established practices and take into consideration the availability of specific interventions.

After treatment has been initiated, the patient may lose weight for a few weeks, owing to loss of apparent or inapparent edema. Serum and intestinal enzymes return to normal, and intestinal absorption of fat and protein improves.

If growth and development have been extensively impaired, mental and physical retardation may be permanent. The younger the infant at the time of deprivation, the more devastating are the long-term effects. Deficits in perceptual and abstract abilities are especially long lasting.

Brewster DR, Manary MJ, Graham SM: Case management of kwashiorkor: An intervention project at seven nutrition rehabilitation centers in Malawi. Eur J Clin Nutr 51:139, 1997.

Briend A, Golden MH: Treatment of severe malnutrition in refugee camps. Eur J Clin Nutr: 47:750, 1993.

Manary MJ, Brewster DR: Potassium supplementation in kwashiorkor. J Pediatr Gastroenterol Nutr 24:194, 1997.

Manary MJ, Hart CA, Whyte MP: Severe hypophosphatemia in children with kwashiorkor is associated with increased mortality. J Pediatr 133:789, 1998.

42.3 Malnutrition in Children Beyond Infancy

ETIOLOGY. Malnutrition in children may be a continuation of an undernourished state begun in infancy, or it may arise from factors that become operative during childhood. In general, the causes are the same as those for malnutrition in infants. The problem may be complex. Poor dietary habits may be associated with a generally poor hygienic situation, with chronic disease, with finicky eating habits of other family members, or with disturbed parent-child relations (see Chapter 35).

Poor eating habits in children under the age of 5 or 6 yr can often be traced directly to parental factors, of which overconcern about the quantity or quality of the diet is a common one. In children of all ages, insufficient sleep and too much emotional excitement, such as that associated with movies, computers, video games, and television, are important factors. School-aged children often develop irregular or inappropriate eating habits, especially at breakfast and lunch, because sufficient time is not allotted or because the meals may be inadequate. Some children as young as 5–8 yr eat little because of fear of obesity. These children respond readily to dietary advice and explanation, in contrast to children who have anorexia nervosa. Eating between meals, especially of items such as candy and snack foods, usually reduces the mealtime appetite.

CLINICAL MANIFESTATIONS. Malnutrition does not invariably result in underweight. Fatigue, lassitude, restlessness, and irritability are frequent manifestations. Restlessness and overactivity are frequently misinterpreted by parents as evidences of lack of fatigue. Anorexia, easily induced digestive disturbances, and constipation are common complaints, and even in older children the starvation type of mucoid diarrheal stool may be observed. Malnourished children often have a limited attention span and do poorly in school. They have increased susceptibility to infections. Muscular development is inadequate, and the flabby muscles result in a posture of fatigue, with rounded shoulders, flat chest, and protuberant abdomen. Such children often look tired; the face is pale, the complexion is "muddy," and the eyes lack luster. Hypochromic anemia is common. In protracted cases, there may be delayed epiphyseal development, irregularities in dentition, and delayed puberty.

Evaluation should always include a careful history of dietary habits, psychosocial maladjustments, physical hygiene, and illness, in addition to a thorough physical examination. Laboratory examinations are usually unnecessary.

TREATMENT. Individualized treatment is aimed at correcting underlying psychologic and physical disturbances. An adequate diet (see Chapter 41) should be outlined; vitamin concentrates may be added and continued for a time after the dietary intake has become adequate. When anorexia is a problem, the essential items of the diet should be provided in as concentrated a form as possible, and the fat content should be low. Between-meal snacks need not be prohibited if they do not interfere with the appetite for the next meal; milk or candy should not be given at such times; fruit or fruit juices are appropriate. Re-educating the entire family about eating habits may be necessary.

Committee on Agriculture, House of Representatives: Hunger in America, Its Effects on Children and Families, and Implications for the Future. Committee on Agriculture, House of Representatives: Hearings, Serial No. 102-13, 1991.
Graham GG, Lembeke J, Lancho E, et al: Quality protein maize: Digestibility and utilization by recovering malnourished infants. Pediatrics 83:416, 1989.
Hegsted DM: Protein-calorie malnutrition. Am Sci 66:61, 1978.
Karp RJ (ed): Malnourished Children in the United States. New York, Springer, 1993.
Katz M, Stiehm ER: Host defense in malnutrition. Pediatrics 59:490, 1977.
Robinson H, Picou D: A comparison of fasting plasma insulin and growth hormone concentrations in marasmic, kwashiorkor, marasmic-kwashiorkor and underweight children. Pediatr Res 11:637, 1977.
Select Committee on Hunger, House of Representatives: Hearings, Serial No. 102-28, 36, 38, 1992.
Sleisenger MH, Kim YS: Protein digestion and absorption. N Engl J Med 300:659, 1979.

42.4 Protein Excess

Excessive protein intake, especially in the absence of sufficient water, may lead to signs of dehydration-protein fever. Signs of protein excess are rare, but premature infants fed a high-protein diet may have an increased morbidity. Marasmic infants fed high-protein diets during the recovery phase may develop hyperammonemia; protein intoxication has also been noted in children with other liver disease. Some weight-reducing diets with high protein content may be responsible for protein intoxication.

CHAPTER 43
Obesity

The identification of obesity and overweight in childhood and their management is an important aspect of preventive pediatrics and public health with implications for the promotion of physical, social, and emotional health of children and for significant potential untoward effects in adulthood. The importance of the issue is underlined for children and adolescents by the 30% increase in overweight in the United States observed between the National Health and Nutrition Examination Surveys, NHANES II 1976–1980 and NHANES III (1988–1994). This increased prevalence of body mass in relation to height among children and adolescents in the past 30 yr has also been observed in the United Kingdom and Western Europe.

Obesity in childhood is not a disease but rather a symptom complex having a weak association with adult obesity with its correlates of increased mortality, cardiovascular disease, hypertension, hyperlipidemias, liver disease, cholelithiasis, and adult-onset diabetes. The correlation between body mass index (BMI) in infancy and childhood and the BMI in adults is generally less than 0.5 in subjects reassessed at age 35 to 50 yr. In addition, studies have shown that childhood obesity occurred in a minority (10–30%) of obese adults.

Interpretation of studies assessing the impact and management of childhood obesity has been difficult because there has not been a uniform standard to differentiate obesity (defined as an excess accumulation of body fat) from overweight, in which body size may be increased without increased accumulation of body fat but with increased lean body mass. Excess weight and body fat in adolescents have been associated with increased plasma insulin levels, elevated blood lipid and lipoprotein levels, elevated serum leptin levels, and elevated blood pressure, which are factors known to be associated with obesity-related adult morbidity.

No exact line separates optimal nutrition from overnutrition; practically, the diagnosis is based on a child's appearance rather than an arbitrary weight excess. Stocky children may have relatively large skeletal frames and more than the average amount of muscular tissue so that their weight and height and their "bigness" exceed those of an average child of their age, but they should not be considered obese. Obesity or overnutrition is a generalized and excessive accumulation of fat in subcutaneous and other tissues.

Measures used to differentiate obese and overweight adolescents have included relative weight, weight-stature indices, body circumferences, and skinfold thickness, usually triceps. Weight-for-age percentiles are unsatisfactory because they do not allow for variation in lean body mass. The use of adult reference data such as life tables is inappropriate, as children and adolescents differ greatly in the rate of growth and distribution of weight. BMI is the most useful index used for screening populations of adolescents for obesity because it correlates significantly with both subcutaneous and total body fat in adolescents, particularly those with the greatest proportion of body fat. In addition, BMI elevations correlate with blood pressure, blood lipid levels, and lipoprotein concentrations in adolescence and predict elevated BMI, lipid levels, and blood pressure in young adults. In adults, elevated BMI is predictive of adult obesity-related morbidity and mortality (Figs. 43–1 and 43–2).

ETIOLOGY. Obese children do not eat differently or eat more "junk" food or starch than their peers. The total energy expenditure during exercise of obese children during controlled exercise is increased but, when corrected for increased body mass, is equivalent to that of nonobese children. The resting metabolic rate is also equal when adjusted for metabolically active body mass.

Appetite may be influenced by various factors that include psychologic disturbances; hypothalamic, pituitary, or other brain lesions; and hyperinsulinism. Genetic predisposition to obesity occurs in certain animals as noted and may occur in humans, although environmental effects are thought to be more prominent. Obesity may result from increases in the number or in the size of fat cells, adipocytes. These appear to increase in number when caloric intake is increased, especially in the gestational months and during the 1st yr of life. This stimulus to increase in number continues, although at a reduced rate, throughout puberty. Thus, during periods of adolescent weight reduction, the size but not the number of adipocytes decreases.

Factors related to the occurrence of overweight and obesity are multifactorial in nature with the exception of certain single gene disorders associated with human obesity (Prader-Willi, Bardet-Biedl, Ahlstrom, and Cohen syndromes). A common denominator is the occurrence of a positive energy balance stored as adipose over long periods. Some of the known factors include excessive intake of high-energy foods, inadequate exercise in relation to age and activity and more sedentary lifestyle, low metabolic rate relative to body composition and mass, increased respiratory quotient in the resting state, and increased insulin sensitivity. No specific evidence shows that

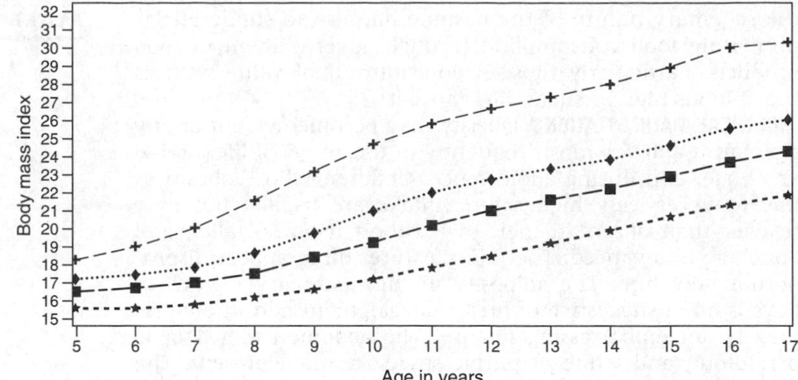

Figure 43–1 Fiftieth, 75th, 85th, and 95th percentile of body mass index for boys 5 to 17 yr of age. Stars denote 50th percentile U.S. weighted values; squares denote 75th percentile U.S. weighted values; diamonds denote 85th percentile U.S. weighted values; crosses denote 95th percentile U.S. weighted values. (From Rosner B, Prineas R, Loggie S, Daniels RD: Percentiles for body mass index in US children 5 to 17 years of age. J Pediatr 132:211, 1998.)

the increased prevalence of overweight is related to a direct increase in caloric intake.

Obese individuals may become resistant to insulin, resulting in an increase in levels of circulating insulin. Insulin decreases lipolysis and increases fat synthesis and uptake. An obese person responds to a carbohydrate meal with increased insulin secretion and a decreased use of free fatty acids. During weight-reduction regimens, an obese person delivers less food to his or her cells than a lean person, owing to decreased mobilization of free fatty acids. In starvation after obesity, fat is mobilized as the serum insulin level decreases. Protein conservation is facilitated as the brain uses ketones for energy. During starvation, serum alanine levels decrease and glycine levels rise. Purified sugars and high-protein diets may cause greater secretion of insulin than do complex carbohydrates.

The repeated and uncritical offering of a bottle as a method of dealing with a fretful or crying infant may establish a habit that leads the infant to expect or seek food whenever experiencing frustration. If obesity is initiated early, it may persist. Excess fruit juice consumption by preschool-age children has been reported to be associated with obesity using a combination of ponderal index greater than 95th percentile and BMI of 75th percentile for age and sex. Similarly, uncritical early introduction of high-calorie solid foods may lead to rapid weight gain and obesity.

In rodents, the protein leptin is essential to the feedback loop related to satiety in the hypothalamic centers; elevated leptin level produces satiety in animal models. Using parallels from animal models of genetic obesity, obese children have been studied with regard to serum leptin levels. Single gene altered rodent models have been extensively studied with regard to leptin deficiency and altered leptin signal transduction. In mice, these alterations are associated with increased food intake and decreased energy expenditure. Studies of obese children show elevated serum leptin concentrations that are highly correlated with BMI. Females had higher leptin levels than males; leptin levels varied with Tanner stage rather than adiposity. Obese children may manifest leptin resistance as a part of normal growth and development, with altered feedback signals to the hypothalamus. Studies in progress are examining specific genes thought to regulate body fatness in humans through metabolic pathways related to energy expenditure in human families, sibling pairs, and specific populations.

EPIDEMIOLOGY. Longitudinal studies in industrialized societies during the past century have shown growth in height and weight compared with previous generations. Individual studies have described a prevalence of childhood overweight of 7–43% (Canada), 7.3% (United Kingdom), and approximately 25% for children and adolescents in the United States. Recent NHANES III data for the United States reports an incidence of BMI greater than 95th percentile for both sexes ages 6 to 11 of 10.6% and for 12 to 17 yr, 10.6%. An additional 14% had a BMI between the 85th and 95th percentiles of the reference population and are considered to be at risk for obesity. (Ranges of the "risk" population were from 10% for non-Hispanic black boys age 6–11 yr to approximately 17% for Mexican-American girls age 6–11 yr and non-Hispanic black and Mexican-American girls age 12–17 yr). The occurrence of overweight does not clearly correlate with parental education, race-ethnicity, or income. In the United States, the highest prevalence is in the Northeast and the incidence decreases in the Midwest, South, and West, respectively. This may relate to decreased seasonal availability of low-caloric density foods or decreased access to facilities for play or exercise in the winter season. Obesity is more prevalent in urban than rural areas.

The incidence of childhood obesity relates strongly to family variables, including parental obesity, small family size, and family patterns of inactivity. Children of parents with high activity levels tend to be leaner than their peers. An increased amount of time spent viewing television, playing video games, or "surfing" the Internet appears to correlate with an increased incidence of childhood obesity and may relate not only to

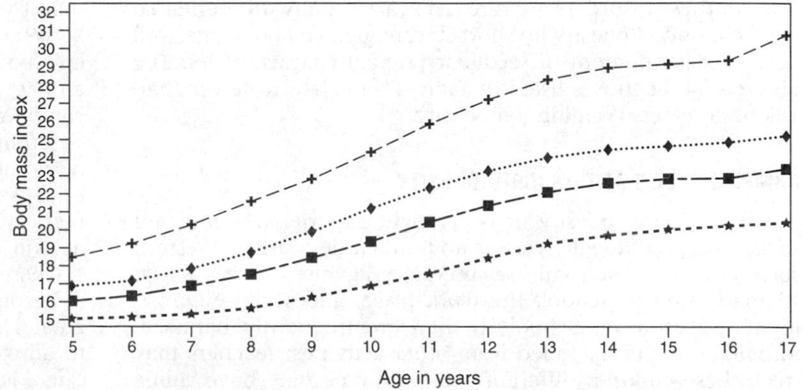

Figure 43–2 Fiftieth, 75th, 85th, and 95th percentile of body mass index for girls 5 to 17 yr of age. Stars denote 50th percentile U.S. weighted values; squares denote 75th percentile U.S. weighted values; diamonds denote 85th percentile U.S. weighted values; crosses denote 95th percentile U.S. weighted values. (From Rosner B, Prineas R, Loggie S, Daniels RD: Percentiles for body mass index in US children 5 to 17 years of age. J Pediatr 132:211, 1998.)

the sedentary nature of the pastime but also to subtle effects promoting food consumption through advertisement of food products, particularly those of low nutritional value such as snack foods high in sugar, fat, and salt.

CLINICAL MANIFESTATIONS. Obesity may become evident at any age, but it appears most frequently in the 1st yr of life, at 5–6 yr of age, and during adolescence. Children whose obesity is due to excessively high caloric intake are usually not only heavier than others in their own cohort but also taller, and bone age is advanced. The facial features often appear disproportionately fine. The adiposity in the mammary regions of boys is often suggestive of breast development and, therefore, may be an embarrassing feature. The abdomen tends to be pendulous, and white or purple striae are often present. The external genitalia of boys appear disproportionately small but actually are most often of average size; the penis is often embedded in the pubic fat. Puberty may occur early, with the result that the ultimate height of obese individuals may be less than that of their slower maturing peers. The development of the external genitalia is normal in most girls, and menarche is usually not delayed and may be advanced. Obesity of the extremities is usually greater in the upper arm and thigh and is sometimes limited to them. The hands may be relatively small and the fingers tapering. Genu valgum is common.

DIAGNOSIS. The BMI is recommended for definition of obesity and overweight populations. Two categories have been defined: (1) adolescents with BMIs at the 95th percentile or more for age and sex or whose BMIs are more than 30 (whichever is smaller) should be considered overweight and should be referred for definitive medical evaluation, and (2) adolescents whose BMIs are at the 85th percentile or more but less than the 95th percentile or equal to 30 (whichever is smaller) should be referred to a second level of screening (see Figs. 43–1 and 43–2). Supplemental consideration of triceps skinfold thickness measurements more than 85th percentile for age and sex may also be helpful.

The proposed second level of screening includes five areas of health risk, as follows: (1) family history (i.e., positive family history of cardiovascular disease, parental elevated total cholesterol level or an unknown history), positive family history of diabetes mellitus or positive family history of parental obesity; (2) blood pressure (i.e., elevated blood pressure using methods and criteria of the Second Task Force on Blood Pressure Control in Children); (3) total cholesterol level (i.e., elevation >5.2 mmol/L or 200 mg/dL); (4) large annual incremental increase in BMI (i.e., an increase over the previous year of two BMI units); and (5) concern about weight (i.e., assessment of personal concerns, emotional or psychologic, related to overweight or the perception of overweight). If any one or more of the five areas are positive, then the patient should receive careful medical evaluation to consider primary medical pathologic conditions as listed under differential diagnosis.

DIFFERENTIAL DIAGNOSIS. Children with obesity defined by elevated BMI should receive careful medical evaluation for disorders that may have a primary medical association with obesity. Most of these disorders are rare. They are usually differentiated from childhood obesity by short stature, delayed bone age, and delayed development of secondary sexual characteristics. The differential diagnoses listed in Table 43–1 relate to fewer than 1% of all cases of childhood obesity.

TABLE 43–1 Differential Diagnosis of Childhood Obesity

Endocrine Causes
Cushing syndrome
Hypothyroidism
Hyperinsulinemia
Growth hormone deficiency
Hypothalamic dysfunction
Prader-Willi syndrome
Stein-Leventhal syndrome (polycystic ovary)
Pseudohypoparathyroidism type I
Genetic Syndromes
Turner syndrome
Laurence-Moon-Biedl syndrome
Alstrom-Hallgren syndrome
Other Syndromes
Cohen syndrome
Carpenter syndrome

Adapted from Dietz WH, Robinson TN: Assessment and treatment of childhood obesity. Pediatr Rev 14:337, 1993.

COMPLICATIONS AND MORBID OBESITY

Children with obesity or overweight experience significant social and psychologic stresses and difficulties. Urban Western society has a strong cultural prejudice against obesity. Social stigmatization in school, the work place, and social environments is common. School children are frequently harassed, intimidated, and excluded from other activities; teachers may treat obese children differently. Sleep apnea may have subtle or unrecognized manifestations and directly diminish participation and academic performance. Negative social attitudes toward obesity have been demonstrated in children as early as age 7 yr. Psychologic disturbances are common in obese children. Even in apparently well-adjusted children, adequate psychologic evaluation often discloses significant underlying emotional problems, which may have initially contributed to the causes of obesity and usually are an additive factor in its maintenance.

Glucose intolerance and non–insulin-dependent diabetes mellitus (NIDDM) occur in obese children and adolescents. Patients have increased basal insulin secretion, stimulated insulin secretion, insulin resistance, and increased visceral body fat as seen on magnetic resonance imaging.

Obese children and adolescents characteristically have elevated serum levels of low-density lipoprotein cholesterol and triglycerides and lowered high-density lipoprotein cholesterol. Long-term consequences in prospective studies have not been assessed.

Children who are overweight have advanced bone age, are taller for age, and usually mature earlier than non-overweight children. Height gain occurs shortly after excessive weight gain and may relate to complex endocrine factors.

Sleep apnea is increasingly identified in obese children and adolescents and may mandate aggressive forms of therapy. It is estimated that sleep apnea occurs in 7% of obese children or in one third of children with BMI exceeding 150th percentile. Because cognitive defects and mortality may occur with sleep apnea, it is essential that children with morbid obesity be so evaluated and a therapeutic regimen be instituted (see Chapter 20.5).

Orthopedic complications of obesity include Blount disease (overgrowth of the proximal medial tibial metaphysis) and slipped capital femoral epiphysis in adolescents. It is estimated that two thirds of patients with Blount disease are obese; between 30 and 50% of patients with slipped capital femoral epiphysis are obese. Each requires specific orthopedic therapy and aggressive weight reduction in order to reduce the risk of complications and recurrence in obese patients.

Although speculative evidence links polycystic ovary disease in women to obesity in adolescence, evidence is insufficient to establish the relationship. An association of obesity, acanthosis nigricans, insulin resistance, and hyperandrogenemia has been described.

Obese infants and children are at moderately increased risk of becoming obese adults. This increased risk is associated with greater severity of childhood obesity, decreased time interval to adult age, and greater number of obese family members. There is an association between childhood obesity and cardiovascular risk factors. In the Muscatine study, obese children had significantly lower high-density lipoprotein cholesterol levels, higher triglyceride levels, and higher systolic blood pressure, although there was no difference from normal ranges for total cholesterol, low-density lipoprotein cholesterol, apolipoprotein A_1, apolipoprotein B, or diastolic blood pressure. Other studies have provided conflicting results and do not prove that childhood obesity increases the risk of cardiovascular disease, nor does evidence at this time show that treatment of childhood obesity decreases the risk of adult coronary artery disease. Table 43–2 provides a list of the complications of obesity described in children, although some of those included have not been firmly established.

The *pickwickian syndrome* (for the fat boy, Joe, in Dickens' Pickwick Papers) is a rare complication of extreme exogenous obesity, in which patients have severe cardiorespiratory distress with alveolar hypoventilation and a decrease in pulmonary, tidal, and expiratory reserve volumes. The manifestations include polycythemia, hypoxemia, cyanosis, cardiac enlargement, congestive cardiac failure, and somnolence. High concentrations of oxygen may be dangerous in treating the cyanosis because respiration may depend solely on the chemoreceptor stimulation of hypoxemia. Weight reduction is extremely important and should be accomplished as rapidly as feasible. Similarly, patients with *Prader-Willi syndrome* have abnormal ventilatory control, which may aggravate those factors directly related to respiratory compromise with morbid obesity. In such patients, aggressive weight loss therapy is essential; in those with concomitant right-sided congestive heart failure, additional benefit may be gained from the use of progesterone to stimulate ventilation through alteration of endogenous P_{CO_2} sensitivity. For patients with obstructive sleep apnea, continuous airway pressure delivered by nasal prongs may be indicated, particularly in those patients at risk for the development of pulmonary hypertension.

PREVENTION AND TREATMENT. Because obesity may be self-perpetuating for psychologic or physiologic reasons, obese children, children of obese parents, or those with obese siblings should be encouraged to adhere to a systematic program of energetic exercise and a balanced diet appropriate to their energy expenditure level. Idealized weight is desirable not only for aesthetic reasons but also potentially to prevent complications of obesity. Untreated overweight infants may remain overweight as adults. Early attempts to modify behavior commencing in the infant period, such as feeding an infant on demand shortly after birth, providing food only at signs of hunger in the 1st yr, avoiding cueing by showing attractive foods or regimenting feeding times by the clock, and by teaching a child to eat only when hungry, may effectively prevent overeating and obesity.

After childhood obesity is established, it is extremely difficult to implement an effective plan for weight reduction and maintenance without active participation and motivation of both the child and the family. Techniques used for fat reduction in adults, including surgery, pharmacotherapy, and gastric balloons, are contraindicated in children. Very low-calorie diets are inappropriate because they may impair growth and development at critical points during childhood. Alternatively, however, maintenance of weight during the growth spurt of adolescence leads to effective weight reduction for age as growth occurs and may be preferable to drastic weight reduction and exercise protocols.

TABLE 43–2 Reported Complications of Childhood Obesity

- Cardiovascular
  - Increased blood pressure
  - Increased total cholesterol
  - Increased serum triglycerides
  - Increased low-density lipoprotein levels
  - Increased very low-density lipoprotein levels
  - Decreased high-density lipoprotein levels
- Hyperinsulinism
- Cholelithiasis
- Blount disease and slipped capital femoral epiphysis
- Pseudotumor cerebri
- Pulmonary
  - Pickwickian syndrome
  - Abnormal results of pulmonary function tests
- Other
  - Sleep apnea

Successful treatment of childhood obesity requires attention to at least the following components: (1) modification of diet and caloric content, (2) definition and use of appropriate exercise programs, (3) behavior modification for the child, and (4) involvement of the family in therapy. Modest success has been gained in behavior modification programs; however, results for individuals have been highly variable. Programs that include simultaneous family therapy seem to be effective in preventing progression to severe obesity as measured by reduction in triceps skinfold thickness during adolescence, if the therapy starts at age 10–11 yr. Such programs also include self-monitoring, stimulus control, reduction in the rate of eating, cognitive restructuring, and increased physical activity. Involvement of the family is most effective if a parent is simultaneously engaged in the therapeutic plan and makes efforts to change the family lifestyle. Although these programs have shown some success, the patients did not reach nonobese status (<20% overweight).

If a decision is made to implement a diet, the basic nutritional needs must be met. At least four practical types of therapeutic approaches may be considered, two of which are contraindicated for children and adolescence at this time:

1. Individual diet counseling and exercise prescription—an individualized program is developed with the family and the patient. This program ensures provision of macronutrients and micronutrients, develops caloric reduction appropriate to maintaining growth of the child, and develops and implements a rigorous plan of exercise acceptable to the child. Goals should include modest reduction of intake and modification of habits to promote a healthy, exercise-oriented lifestyle.

2. Use of a diabetic exchange program with a caloric level sufficient to sustain growth and to promote a goal of 0.5 kg of weight loss per week. A combination of diet and exercise is moderately effective as compared with controls.

3. A "traffic-light" diet program may be implemented; this is a well-planned dietary regimen of 900–1300 kcal/24 hr using the food pyramid (see Chapter 40, Fig. 40–2). Categories include green foods (GO), which may be consumed in unlimited quantities; yellow foods (CAUTION), which have average nutritional value for their food group; and red foods (STOP), or foods that provide less desirable nutrient density because they have high fat or simple carbohydrate content. Long-term obesity changes over 5–10 yr have been observed when this program is combined with exercise, behavioral modification, and family therapy programs. In addition, there is intrinsic shift of preferences to foods of greater nutrient value with this approach.

4. Patients with morbid obesity require aggressive diet therapy with significant restriction. The protein-sparing modified fast (PSMF) diet consists of 600–900 kcal/24 hr, with 1.5–2.5 g/kg/24 hr of high-quality protein provided as lean meat with vitamin and mineral supplementation and assurance of at least 1.5 L of water intake per day. The goal of the PSMF diet is to maximize weight loss, preserve mineral balance, and achieve positive nitrogen balance simultaneously. Duration is restricted to 4–12 wk, and medical supervision is required. This diet generally should not be used by prepubertal children. Short-term goals can be achieved; however, long-term weight loss is not different from less restrictive regimens.

5. Surgical therapy is rarely if ever indicated in children.

The complications of jejunoileal bypass for children with morbid obesity are significant and include encephalopathy, cholelithiasis, nephrolithiasis, renal cortical nephropathy, systemic fatty acid deficiency, hypoproteinemia, multiple nutrient deficiencies, and in 30% reversal of the procedure.

6. Pharmacotherapy is now being prescribed for adult patients. This is rarely if ever indicated for children.

Regardless of the therapeutic plan used, all of the essential dietary needs should be included in a calorically defined diet such as the 1,100–1,300-calorie diet described for children age 10–14 yr for several months (Table 43–3). Some children avoid excessive eating after they have been allowed to return to a free choice of diet. The diet should contain as much bulk as possible. At times, greater cooperation is secured if small portions of the diet are permitted between meals, especially in the afternoon. If adequacy of the daily vitamin intake is in doubt, vitamin concentrates may be prescribed. Vitamin D should be included. Rapid decreases in weight should not be attempted, and medical supervision should be maintained.

Competitive *athletes attempting to achieve rapid weight loss* in order to qualify for specific events can encounter significant hyperthermia and dehydration. Deaths have been reported from such aggressive measures to achieve time-limited weight loss goals. All methods to achieve weight loss should emphasize moderation, and health care professionals should counsel against such methods for athletes engaged in competitive sports.

PROGNOSIS. Results with dietary or exercise modification have been successful only for the short term; follow-up studies of adequate duration show a high rate of relapse at 4–10 yr, with successsful maintenance of reduced (but not normal) weight in only 50% of patients.

A Canadian meta-analysis that evaluated obesity in children, used in the development of practice guidelines, supported the need for sequential weight and height measurements of children principally to rule out failure to thrive, but the analysis was unable to demonstrate sufficient evidence of the success of therapeutic intervention to support screening for childhood obesity. No harm was associated with screening, however. In addition, there was insufficient evidence to either include or exclude counseling about nutrition and exercise for the initial therapy of obese children, although very low-calorie diets should be excluded from the management of preadolescent children. Finally, evidence with regard to the inclusion or exclusion of exercise in the routine treatment of obese children was conflicting. Nevertheless, exercise without diet control or diet without increased exercise almost always results in failure.

Although data do not support massive screening programs for the identification of childhood obesity as a preventive program of pediatrics, it appears prudent for practitioners to initiate, on behalf of the individual motivated patient, judicious dietary and exercise management combined with behavior modification and family therapy. The goal should be to facilitate growth and provide substantial social and psychologic support, even if the direct medical preventive aspects are not well substantiated.

TABLE 43–3 1,100–1,300 Calorie Diet

Breakfast	Dinner
½ cup orange juice	2 oz lean ground beef
¾ cup ready-to-eat cereal	1 oz cheese
6 oz 1% milk	½ tomato
1 tsp sugar	1 cup 1% milk
Lunch	2 taco shells, taco sauce
	1 nectarine
2 oz turkey or lean meat	Lettuce
½ cup noodles or bread	**Snack**
½ cup carrots	
1 tsp margarine	6 Saltines
1 cup 1% milk	1 apple

Total "exchanges" 3 fruit, 2 vegetables, 4 starch, 2¾ milk, 3 medium-fat meat, 2 low-fat meat, 2 fat. Try to incorporate egg, high-fiber sources (e.g., beans, some combination foods).

Andersen R, Crespo C, Bartlett SJ, et al: Relationship of physical activity and television watching with body weight and level of fatness among children. JAMA 279:938, 1998.
Canadian Task Force on the Periodic Health Examination: Periodic health examination, 1994 update: 1. Obesity in childhood. Can Med Assoc J 150:871, 1994.
Dietz WH, Robinson TN: Assessment and treatment of childhood obesity. Pediatr Rev 14:337, 1993.
Dietz WH: Health consequences of obesity in youth: Childhood predictors of adult disease in "The Causes and Health Consequences of Obesity in Children and Adolescents." Pediatr 101 (Suppl):518, 1998.
Editorial: Hyperthermia and dehydration-related deaths associated with rapid weight loss in three collegiate wrestlers—North Carolina, Wisconsin, and Michigan, Nov–Dec 1997. Cited from MMWR 1998:47:105–108. JAMA 279:824–825, 1998.
Epstein LH, Myers MD, Raynor HA, Saelens BE: Treatment of pediatric obesity in "The Causes and Health Consequences of Obesity in Children and Adolescents." Pediatrics 101(Suppl):554, 1998.
Flodmark C, Ohlsson T, Ryden O, et al: Prevention of progression to severe obesity in a group of obese schoolchildren treated with family therapy. Pediatrics 91:880, 1993.
Hassink SG, Sheslow DV, de Lancey E, et al: Serum leptin in children with obesity: Relationship to gender and development. Pediatrics 98:201, 1996.
Himes JH, Dietz WH: Guidelines for overweight in adolescent preventive services: Recommendations from an expert committee. Am J Clin Nutr 59:307, 1994.
Mossberg H: 40-year followup of overweight children. Lancet 2:491, 1989.
Rossner S: Childhood obesity and adult consequences. Acta Pediatr 87:1, 1998.
Schlicker SA, Borra ST, Regan C: The weight and fitness status of United States children. Nutr Rev 52:11, 1994.

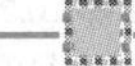

CHAPTER 44
Vitamin Deficiencies and Excesses

Vitamins are essential nutrients that must be supplied exogenously. Functions of vitamins are summarized in Table 40–8, and recommended daily allowances and DRIs in Tables 40–1 to 40–3. Toxicity more commonly results from excesses of the fat-soluble vitamins A and D than with those of the water-soluble vitamins. The vitamin-dependent states are summarized in Table 44–1.

44.1 Vitamin A Deficiency

The term *vitamin A* is a generic label for all β-ionone derivatives other than provitamin A carotenoids. Retinol signifies vitamin A alcohol; retinyl ester, vitamin A ester; retinal, vitamin A aldehyde; and retinoic acid, vitamin A acid.

Provitamin A carotenoids is the generic term for all carotenoids that have the biologic activity of β-carotene. They or their derivatives with vitamin A activity are required in the diets of infants and children.

β-Carotene is partly absorbed by the intestinal lymphatics; the remainder is cleaved into two molecules of retinol. Dietary retinyl ester is hydrolyzed to retinol in the intestine. Retinol is esterified inside mucosal cells with palmitic acid and is stored in the liver as retinyl palmitate; this in turn is hydrolyzed to free retinol for transport to its site of action. Zinc is required for this mobilization. Normal plasma values of retinol in infants are 20–50 μg/dL; in children and adults, 30–225 μg/dL.

Ingested carotenoids are nontoxic and may result in yellow discoloration of the skin but not of the sclera. This disorder, *carotenemia,* is especially likely to occur in children with liver

TABLE 44–1. Vitamin Dependency States

Vitamin	Disease	Untreated State	Daily Dose
A	Darier	Hyperkeratosis follicularis	7,500 μg
B_1	Leigh—pyruvic-lactic acidosis	Ataxia, retardation	600 mg
	Thiamine responsive anemia	Megaloblastic anemia	20 mg
	Maple syrup urine disease	Hypotonia, seizures	10 mg
Riboflavin	Pyruvate kinase deficiency	Hemolysis	10 mg
	Glutaric acidemia (II)	Hypoglycemia	100–300 mg
Niacin	Hartnup	Ataxia, eczema	200 mg
B_6	Cystathioninuria	No symptoms	200 mg
	Homocystinuria	Retardation	200 mg
	B_6-anemia	Hypochromic microcytic anemia	10 mg
	B_6-seizures	Seizures	25 mg
	Xanthurenic aciduria	Retardation	10 mg
	Gyrate atrophy of choroid	Blindness	100 mg
	Oxaluria	Oxalate crystals	100 mg
Folic acid	Formiminotransferase deficiency	Retardation	5 mg
	Folate reductase deficiency	Megaloblastic anemia	5 mg
	Homocystinuria	Retardation	10 mg
B_{12}	Methylmalonic acidemia	Retardation	1 mg
Biotin	Propionic acidemia	Retardation	10 mg
	β-Methylcrotonyl glycinuria	Coma	10 mg
	Biotinidase deficiency	Seizures	5–20 mg
	Holocarboxylase deficiency	Hypotonia	10 mg
C	Chédiak-Higashi	Infections	50 mg
D	Dependence	Rickets	100 μg
	Familial hypophosphatemia	Rickets	2,500 μg

disease, diabetes mellitus, or hypothyroidism and in those who have congenital absence of enzymes that convert provitamin A carotenoids.

ETIOLOGY. At birth, the liver has a low vitamin A content that is rapidly augmented because colostrum and breast milk furnish large amounts of the vitamin. Breast milk and whole cow's milk are satisfactory sources of vitamin A. Other foods (vegetables, fruits, eggs, butter, liver) or vitamin supplements also provide vitamin A. Loss of it in cooking, canning, and freezing of foodstuffs is small; oxidizing agents, however, destroy it.

The risk of vitamin A deficiency is small in healthy children with balanced diets. Deficient diets commonly cause disease by age 2–3 yr. Vitamin A deficiency also results from inadequate intestinal absorption, such as, for example, with chronic intestinal disorders or fat malabsorption. Low intake of dietary fat results in low vitamin A absorption. Vitamin A excretion is increased in cancer, urinary tract disease, and chronic infectious diseases. Low protein intake results in deficient carrier protein and in decreases in plasma concentration of vitamin A.

PATHOLOGY. The human retina contains two distinct photoreceptor systems: The rods are sensitive to light of low intensity, and the cones to colors and to light of high intensity. Retinal is the prosthetic group of the photosensitive pigment in both rods and cones. The major difference between the visual pigments in rods (rhodopsin) and in cones (iodopsin) is the nature of the protein bound to retinal. All-trans retinal isomerizes in the dark to 11-cis form. This combines with opsin to form rhodopsin. Energy from light quanta reconverts 11-cis retinal to the all-trans form; this energy exchange, transmitted via the optic nerves to the brain, results in visual sensation. β-Carotene has been effective in ameliorating photosensitivity in patients with erythropoietic protoporphyria. It has also been suggested that retinitis pigmentosa may be related to a defect in retinol-binding protein.

Retinoids are essential for cell differentiation, in the activation of retinoic acid–responsive genes, and in membrane stability. Both excess and deficiency of vitamin A lead to rupture of lysosomal membranes with release of hydrolases.

Vitamin A has a role in keratinization, cornification, bone metabolism, placental development, growth, spermatogenesis, and mucus formation. Characteristic changes in epithelium include proliferation of basal cells, hyperkeratosis, and the formation of stratified, cornified squamous epithelium. Epithelial changes in the respiratory system may result in bronchiolar obstruction. Squamous metaplasia of the renal pelves, ureters, urinary bladder, enamel organs, and pancreatic and salivary ducts may lead to an increase in infections in these areas.

CLINICAL MANIFESTATIONS. Ocular lesions develop insidiously. The posterior segment of the eye is initially affected, with impairment of dark adaptation resulting in night blindness. Later, drying of the conjunctiva (xerosis conjunctivae) and of the cornea (xerosis corneae) is followed by wrinkling and cloudiness of the cornea (keratomalacia) (Fig. 44–1). Dry, silver-gray plaques may appear on the bulbar conjunctiva (Bitot spots), with follicular hyperkeratosis and photophobia.

Vitamin A deficiency may result in retardation of mental and physical growth and in apathy. Anemia with or without hepatosplenomegaly is usually present.

The skin is dry and scaly, and follicular hyperkeratosis may at times be found on the shoulders, buttocks, and extensor surfaces of the extremities. The vaginal epithelium may become cornified, and epithelial metaplasia of the urinary tract may contribute to pyuria and hematuria. Increased intracranial pressure with wide separation of cranial bones at the sutures may occur. Hydrocephalus, with or without paralyses of the cranial nerves, is an infrequent manifestation.

DIAGNOSIS. Dark adaptation tests may be helpful. Xerosis conjunctivae can be detected by biomicroscopic examination of the conjunctiva. Examination of the scrapings from the eye and vagina is recommended as a diagnostic aid. The plasma carotene concentration falls quickly, but that of vitamin A decreases more slowly.

PREVENTION. Infants should receive at least 500 μg of vitamin A daily; older children and adults, 600–1500 μg of vitamin A or carotene. The average diets of infants and children in the United States supply enough vitamin A to prevent symptoms of deficiency. One microgram of retinol equals 3.3 IU of vitamin A.

For therapeutic reasons, low-fat diets should be supplemented with vitamin A. In disorders with poor absorption of fat or increased excretion of vitamin A, water-miscible preparations should be administered in amounts several times the usual daily requirement. Premature infants, who absorb fats and vitamin A less efficiently than do full-term infants, should also receive water-miscible preparations.

Epidemiologic public health studies in areas of the world where vitamin A deficiency or subclinical deficiency is of high

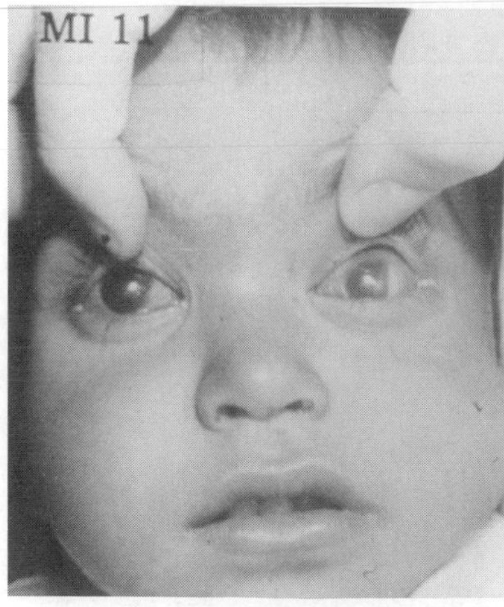

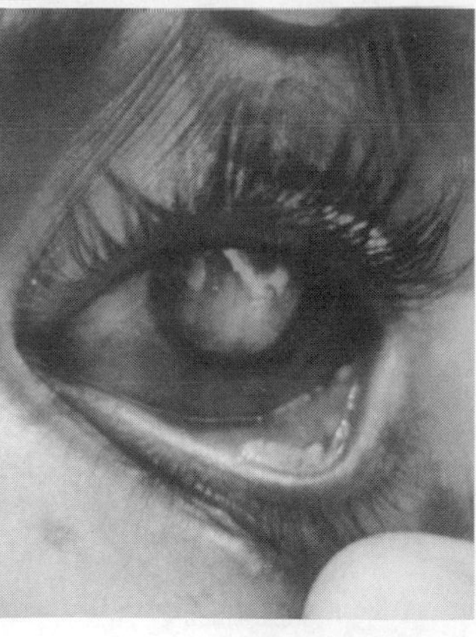

Figure 44–1 Recovery from xerophthalmia, showing permanent eye lesion. (From Bloch CE: Blindness and other diseases arising from deficient nutrition [lack of fat-soluble A factor]. Am J Dis Child 27:139, 1924.)

prevalence because of insufficient dietary intake, seasonal variance, or intercurrent illness have demonstrated that restoration of vitamin A sufficiency is associated with a 20% increase of survival in deficient children. The deficiency is most pronounced in populations with primarily vegetable diets with decreased or absent intake of green leafy vegetables. Effects are not apparent in populations younger than 6 mo; on the other hand, in infants supplemented with 30,000 μg [100,000 IU] of vitamin A (age 6–11 mo) and 60,000 μg [200,000 IU] of vitamin A (age 12 mo–6 yr) given orally in a water-miscible base every 4 mo, mortality associated with severe diarrhea and measles is reduced. There is no consistent effect on the severity or mortality of respiratory disease. The effects may be related to restoration of epithelial integrity and upregulation of immunocompetence in deficient populations. The same dose (30,000 μg [100,000 IU]) should be given postpartum to the mothers of breast-fed infants in these regions. Alternative methods of prevention can include vitamin A fortification of bread, sugar, or margarine.

TREATMENT. In cases of latent vitamin A deficiency, a daily supplement of 1,500 μg of vitamin A is sufficient. For xerophthalmia, 1,500 μg/kg/24 hr is given orally for 5 days and then continued with intramuscular injection of 7,500 μg of vitamin A in oil daily until recovery occurs. Morbidity and mortality rates may decrease in nondeficient children who acquire certain viral infections such as measles when given 1,500–3,000 μg of vitamin A.

HYPERVITAMINOSIS A. Acute hypervitaminosis A may occur in infants after ingesting 100,000 μg or more. The symptoms are nausea, vomiting, drowsiness, and bulging of the fontanel. Diplopia, papilledema, cranial nerve palsies, and other symptoms suggestive of brain tumor (pseudotumor cerebri) may also occur. Toxicity has occurred with supplementation during vaccine administration in developing countries.

Chronic hypervitaminosis A appears after ingestion of excessive doses for several weeks or months. An affected child has anorexia, pruritus, and a lack of weight gain. Also noted are increased irritability, limitation of motion, and tender swelling of the bones. Alopecia, seborrheic cutaneous lesions, fissuring of the corners of the mouth, increased intracranial pressure, and hepatomegaly may develop. Craniotabes and desquamation of the palms and soles are common. Roentgenograms reveal hyperostosis affecting several long bones; it is most notable at the middle of the shafts (Fig. 44–2).

Severe congenital malformations may occur in infants of mothers consuming large amounts of oral retinoids used in treating acne.

A history of excessive ingestion of vitamin A helps to differentiate it from cortical hyperostosis (see Chapter 703). Besides a history of excess, the serum vitamin A level is elevated, and hypercalcemia or liver cirrhosis occurs occasionally.

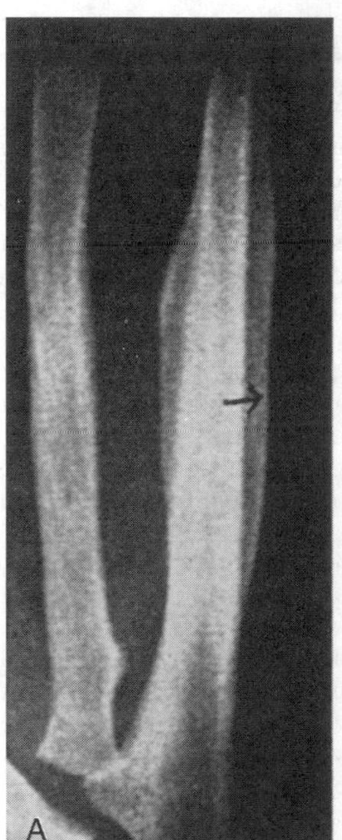

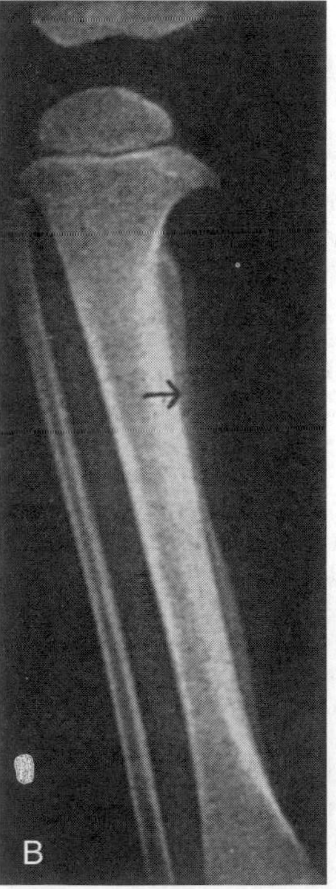

Figure 44–2 Hyperostosis of the ulna and the tibia in an infant 21 mo of age, resulting from vitamin A poisoning. *A*, Long, wavy cortical hyperostosis of the ulna. *B*, Long, wavy cortical hyperostosis of the right tibia; striking absence of metaphyseal changes. (From Caffey J: Pediatric X-ray Diagnosis, 5th ed. Chicago, Year Book, 1967, p 994.)

Caffey J: Pediatric X-Ray Diagnosis, 5th ed. Chicago, Year Book Medical Publishers, 1967, p 994.

de Francisco A, Chakrabory J, Chowdhury HR, et al: Acute toxicity of vitamin A given with vaccines in infancy. Lancet 392:526, 1993.

Fisher KD, Carr CJ, Huff JE, et al: Dark adaptation and night vision. Fed Proc 29:1605, 1970.

Goodman DS: Vitamin A metabolism. Fed Proc 39:2716, 1980.

Hussey GD, Klein M: A randomized controlled trial of vitamin A in children with severe measles. N Engl J Med 323:160, 1990.

Leung AKC: Carotenemia. Adv Pediatr 34:223, 1987.

Mahoney CP, Margolis T, Knauss TA, et al: Chronic vitamin A intoxication in infants fed chicken liver. Pediatrics 65:893, 1980.

McLaren DS, Shirajain E, Tchallian M, et al: Xerophthalmia in Jordan. Am J Clin Nutr 17:117, 1965.

Moon RC: Comparative aspects of carotenoids and retinoids as chemopreventive agents for cancer. J Nutr 119:127, 1989.

Neuzil KM, Gruber WC, Chytil F, et al: Serum vitamin A levels in respiratory syncytial virus infection. J Pediatr 124:433, 1994.

Peck GL: Prolonged remissions of cystic and conglobate acne with 13-cis-retinoic acid. N Engl J Med 300:299, 1979.
Sommer A: Vitamin A prophylaxis. Arch Dis Child 77:191, 1997.

44.2 Vitamin B Complex Deficiency

Vitamin B complex includes several factors whose chemical composition and function vary widely (see Table 40–8). All are important constituents of enzyme systems. Because many of these enzymes are closely related functionally, lack of a single factor can interrupt an entire chain of chemical processes, producing diverse clinical manifestations.

Diets deficient in any one factor of the B complex are frequently poor sources of other B vitamins. Because manifestations of several B deficiencies can usually be found in the same patient, it is generally practical to treat the patient with the entire B complex.

Factors such as pantothenic acid, choline, and inositol are important for normal functioning of the human organism, but at present no specific deficiency syndromes can be ascribed to their lack in the diets of children.

44.3 Thiamine Deficiency (Beriberi)

ETIOLOGY. Vitamin B_1 (thiamine) is water soluble and, as thiamine pyrophosphate or cocarboxylase, functions as a coenzyme in carbohydrate metabolism. Thiamine is required for the synthesis of acetylcholine, and deficiency results in impaired nerve conduction. It is the coenzyme in transketolation and in decarboxylation of α-keto acids. Transketolase participates in the hexose monophosphate shunt that generates nicotinamide adenine dinucleotide phosphate and pentose.

Breast milk or cow's milk, vegetables, cereals, fruits, and eggs are sources of thiamine. Infants whose source of food is the milk of thiamine-deficient mothers may develop beriberi. Older children whose diet contains good sources of thiamine such as meats and legumes do not require thiamine supplements.

Thiamine is easily destroyed by heat in neutral or alkaline media and is readily extracted from foodstuffs by cooking water. An enzyme factor destructive to thiamine is present in some fish. Because the covering of grains of cereals contains most of the vitamin, polishing reduces its availability.

Thiamine absorption decreases with gastrointestinal or liver disease. Requirements increase with fever, surgery, or stress. Thiamine dependence has been described in a child with megaloblastic anemia and in an infant with otherwise typical maple syrup urine disease. The urine of children with Leigh's encephalomyelopathy and of their parents inhibits the formation of thiamine pyrophosphate. Large doses of thiamine improve some of the physical abnormalities associated with the disease.

PATHOLOGY. In fatal cases of beriberi, lesions are located principally in the heart, peripheral nerves, subcutaneous tissue, and serous cavities. The heart is dilated, and fatty degeneration of the myocardium is common. Generalized edema or edema of the legs, serous effusions, and venous engorgement may be present. The peripheral nerves undergo various degrees of degeneration of myelin and axon cylinders, with wallerian degeneration, beginning in the distal locations. The nerves of the lower extremities are affected first. Lesions in the brain include vascular dilatation and hemorrhage.

CLINICAL MANIFESTATIONS. Early manifestations of deficiency include fatigue, apathy, irritability, depression, drowsiness, poor mental concentration, anorexia, nausea, and abdominal discomfort. Signs of progression include peripheral neuritis with tingling, burning, and paresthesias of the toes and feet; decreased tendon reflexes; loss of vibration sense; tenderness and cramping of leg muscles; congestive heart failure; and psychic disturbances. Patients may have ptosis of the eyelids and atrophy of the optic nerve. Hoarseness or aphonia due to paralysis of the laryngeal nerve is a characteristic sign. Muscle atrophy and tenderness of nerve trunks are followed by ataxia, loss of coordination, and loss of deep sensation. Paralytic symptoms are more common in adults than in children. Later, signs of increased intracranial pressure, meningismus, and coma occur.

In dry beriberi, the child may appear plump but is pale, flabby, listless, and dyspneic; the heart rate is rapid, and the liver enlarged. In wet beriberi, the child is undernourished, pale, and edematous and has dyspnea, vomiting, and tachycardia. The skin appears waxy. The urine may contain albumin and casts.

The cardiac signs at first are slight cyanosis and dyspnea. Tachycardia, enlargement of the liver, loss of consciousness, and convulsions may develop rapidly. The heart is enlarged, especially to the right. The electrocardiogram shows increased Q-T interval, inversion of T waves, and low voltage, changes that rapidly revert to normal with treatment. Cardiac failure may lead to death in either chronic or acute beriberi.

Wernicke's Encephalopathy. This is characterized by irritability, somnolence, and ocular signs and less commonly by mental confusion and ataxias; it occurs infrequently in malnourished infants and children. Encephalopathy and beriberi has occurred during total parenteral nutrition, when it is attributable to a shortage of multivitamin infusion. Associated conditions include malignancy, infection, malnutrition gastrointestinal disorders (especially with malabsorption), and premature labor in the parturient.

DIAGNOSIS. Because the early symptoms are encountered in many types of nutritional disturbances besides thiamine deficiency, demonstrations of lowered red blood cell transketolase and high blood or urinary glyoxylate values have been proposed as diagnostic tests. Measurement of excretion after an oral loading dose of thiamine or of its metabolites, thiazole or pyrimidine, may help to identify the deficiency state. Clinical response to administration of thiamine remains the best test for thiamine deficiency.

PREVENTION. A maternal diet containing sufficient amounts of thiamine prevents this deficiency in breast-fed infants (see Table 40–1). Thiamine requirements increase with a high-carbohydrate content of the diet.

TREATMENT. If beriberi occurs in a breast-fed infant, both the mother and child should be treated with thiamine. The daily dose for adults is 50 mg and for children 10 mg or more. Oral administration is effective unless gastrointestinal disturbances prevent absorption. Thiamine should be given intramuscularly or intravenously to children with cardiac failure. Such treatment is followed by dramatic improvement, although complete cure requires several weeks. The heart is not permanently damaged. Because patients with beriberi often have other B complex deficiencies, all other vitamins of the B complex should be administered, in addition to large doses of thiamine chloride.

44.4 Riboflavin Deficiency (Ariboflavinosis)

Riboflavin deficiency without deficiencies of other members of the B complex is rare. Riboflavin, a yellow, fluorescent, water-soluble substance, is stable to heat and acids but is destroyed by light and alkalis. The coenzymes flavin mononucleotide and flavin adenine dinucleotide (FAD) are synthesized from riboflavin, forming the prosthetic groups of several enzymes important in electron transport. Riboflavin is essential for growth and tissue respiration; it may have a role in light adaptation and is required for conversion of pyridoxine to pyridoxal phosphate. Large amounts of riboflavin are found in liver, kidney, brewer's yeast, milk, cheese, eggs, and leafy vegetables; cow's milk contains about five times as much riboflavin as human milk.

Riboflavin deficiency is usually caused by inadequate intake. Faulty absorption may contribute in patients with biliary atresia or hepatitis or in those receiving probenecid, phenothiazine, or oral contraceptives. Phototherapy destroys riboflavin.

CLINICAL MANIFESTATIONS. Evidences of riboflavin deficiency include cheilosis (perlèche), glossitis, keratitis, conjunctivitis, photophobia, lacrimation, marked corneal vascularization, and seborrheic dermatitis. Cheilosis begins with pallor at the angles of the mouth, followed by thinning and maceration of the epithelium. Superficial fissures often covered by yellow crusts develop in the angles of the mouth and extend radially into the skin for distances of 1–2 cm. With glossitis, the tongue is smooth, and loss of papillary structure occurs. A normocytic, normochromic anemia with bone marrow hypoplasia is common.

DIAGNOSIS. Urinary excretion of riboflavin below 30 μg/24 hr is abnormally low. Levels of erythrocyte glutathionine reductase, a flavoprotein requiring FAD, may reflect the stores of riboflavin. A patient with hemolysis due to pyruvate kinase deficiency and reduced erythrocyte glutathionine reductase had both enzyme activities restored to normal on administration of riboflavin.

PREVENTION. Recommended daily allowances are presented in Table 40–1. Riboflavin deficiency is usually prevented by a diet that contains adequate amounts of milk, eggs, leafy vegetables, and lean meats.

TREATMENT. Treatment consists in the oral administration of 3–10 mg of riboflavin daily. If no response occurs within a few days, intramuscular injections of 2 mg of riboflavin in saline solution may be made three times daily. The child should also be given a well-balanced diet and, at least temporarily, more than the usual requirements of the B complex.

44.5 Niacin Deficiency (Pellagra)

ETIOLOGY. Pellagra (pellis, skin; agra, rough), a deficiency disease caused mainly by a lack of niacin (nicotinic acid), affects all tissues of the body. Niacin forms part of two enzymes important in electron transfer and glycolysis: nicotinamide adenine dinucleotide and nicotinamide adenine dinucleotide phosphate. Although dietary tryptophan can partially substitute for niacin, other sources of niacin are necessary. Liver, lean pork, salmon, poultry, and red meat are good sources, but most cereals contain only small amounts of it. Pellagra occurs chiefly in countries where corn (maize), a poor source of tryptophan, is a basic foodstuff. Milk and eggs, which contain little niacin, are good pellagra-preventive foods because of their high content of tryptophan. Because niacin is a stable compound, only small losses occur in cooking.

PATHOLOGY. Histologically, edema and degeneration of the superficial collagen of the dermis occur. The papillary vessels are engorged, and perivascular lymphocytic infiltration is observed in the dermis. The epidermis is hyperkeratotic and later becomes atrophic.

Changes comparable to those in the skin are present in the tongue, buccal mucous membranes, and vagina. These changes may be associated with secondary infection and ulceration. The walls of the colon are thickened and inflamed, with patches of pseudomembrane; the mucosa later atrophies. Changes in the nervous system occur relatively late in the disease and consist of patchy areas of demyelinization and degeneration of ganglion cells; demyelination in the spinal cord may involve the posterior and lateral columns.

CLINICAL MANIFESTATIONS. The early symptoms of pellagra are vague. Anorexia, lassitude, weakness, burning sensations, numbness, and dizziness may be prodromal symptoms. After a long period of niacin deficiency, the characteristic symptoms appear. The classic triad consists of dermatitis, diarrhea, and dementia. Manifestations in children with parasites or chronic disorders may be especially severe.

The most characteristic manifestations are the cutaneous ones, which may develop suddenly or insidiously and may be elicited by irritants, particularly by intense sunlight. They first appear as symmetric erythema of the exposed surfaces that may resemble sunburn and in mild cases may escape recognition. The lesions are usually sharply demarcated from the healthy skin around them, and their distribution may change frequently. The lesions on the hands sometimes have the appearance of a glove (pellagrous glove), and similar demarcations are occasionally seen on the foot and leg (pellagrous boot) or around the neck (Casal necklace) (Fig. 44–3). In some cases, vesicles and bullae develop (wet type), or there may be suppuration beneath the scaly, crusted epidermis; in others, the swelling disappears after a short time and desquamation begins. The healed parts of the skin may remain pigmented.

The cutaneous lesions are sometimes preceded by stomatitis, glossitis, vomiting, or diarrhea. Swelling and redness of the tip of the tongue and its lateral margins may be followed by intense redness of the entire tongue and papillae and even ulceration.

Nervous symptoms include depression, disorientation, insomnia, and delirium.

The classic symptoms of pellagra are usually not well developed in infants and children. Anorexia, irritability, anxiety, and apathy are common in "pellagra families." They may also have sore tongues and lips, and the skin is usually dry and scaly. Diarrhea and constipation may alternate, and a moderate secondary anemia may occur. Children who have pellagra often have evidence of other nutritional deficiency diseases.

DIAGNOSIS. Diagnosis is usually made from the physical signs of glossitis, gastrointestinal symptoms, and a symmetric dermatitis. Rapid clinical response to niacin is an important confirming test. *N*-methylnicotinamide, a normal metabolite of niacin, is almost undetectable in urine during niacin deficiency.

PREVENTION. A well-balanced diet containing meat, vegetables, eggs, and milk meets the recommended daily allowances (see Table 40–1); thus, supplements of niacin are necessary only in breast-fed infants whose mothers have pellagra or in children on restricted diets.

TREATMENT. Children respond rapidly to antipellagral therapy.

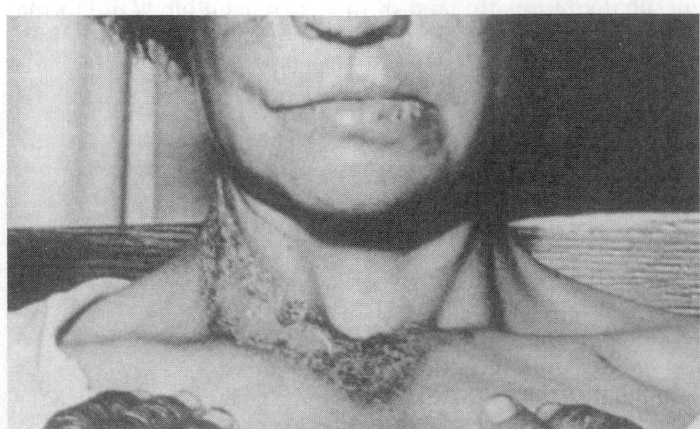

Figure 44–3 Pellagra showing an early lesion on the neck (Casal necklace).

A liberal and well-balanced diet should be supplemented with 50–300 mg/24 hr of niacin; 100 mg may be given intravenously in severe cases or in cases of poor intestinal absorption. Administering large doses of niacin is often followed within a half hour by a sensation of increased local heat and flushing and burning of the skin, unpleasant effects that are not produced by niacinamide. Large doses of niacin may cause cholestatic jaundice or hepatotoxicity.

The diet should also be supplemented with other vitamins, especially with other members of the B complex. Sun exposure should be avoided during the active phase; the skin lesions may be covered with soothing applications. Hypochromic anemia should be treated with iron. The diet of patients cured of pellagra should be supervised continuously to prevent recurrence.

Thiamine Deficiency

Borgna-Pignatti C, Marradi P, Pinelli L, et al: Thiamine-responsive anemia in DIDMOAD syndrome. J Pediatr 114:405, 1989.

Brin M: Erythrocyte as a biopsy tissue for functional evaluation of thiamine adequacy. JAMA 187:762, 1964.

Hahn JS, Benquist W, Alcorn DM, et al: Wernike encephalopathy and beriberi during total parenteral nutrition attributable to multivitamin infusion shortage. Pediatrics 101:1, 1998.

McCandless DW, Schenker S: Neurologic disorders of thiamine deficiency. Nutr Rev 27:213, 1969.

Pihko H, Soarinen U, Paetau A: Wernicke encephalopathy: A preventable cause of death: Report of 2 children with malignant disease. Pediatr Neurol 5:237, 1989.

Vrochota K, Oberg CN, Harris KN: Beriberi in a southeast Asian adolescent. Am J Dis Child 143:270, 1989.

Riboflavin Deficiency

Rillotson JA, Baker EM: An enzymatic measurement of the riboflavin status in man. Am J Clin Nutr 25:425, 1972.

Rivlin RS: Hormones, drugs and riboflavin. Nutr Rev 37:241, 1979.

Staal GEJ, Van Berkel TJC, Nijessen JG, et al: Normalization of red blood cell pyruvate kinase in pyruvate kinase deficiency by riboflavin treatment. Clin Chim Acta 60:323, 1975.

Niacin Deficiency

Darby WJ, McNutt KW, Todhunter EN: Niacin. Nutr Rev 33:289, 1975.

44.6 Pyridoxine (Vitamin B_6) Deficiency

Vitamin B_6 includes pyridoxal, pyridoxine, and pyridoxamine. These are converted to pyridoxal-5-phosphate (or pyridoxamine-5-phosphate), which acts as a coenzyme in decarboxylation and transamination of amino acids, such as in the decarboxylation of 5-hydroxytryptophan in the formation of serotonin and in the metabolism of glycogen and fatty acids. Vitamin B_6 is also essential for the breakdown of kynurenine. When this does not occur, xanthurenic acid appears in the urine. Adequate functioning of the nervous system depends on pyridoxine, deficiency of which leads to seizures and to peripheral neuropathy. Pyridoxal phosphate is the coenzyme for both glutamic decarboxylase and γ-aminobutyric acid transaminase; each is necessary for normal brain metabolism. It participates in active transport of amino acids across cell membranes, in chelation of metals, and in the synthesis of arachidonic acid from linoleic acid. If it is lacking, glycine metabolism may lead to oxaluria. It is excreted largely as 4-pyridoxic acid.

ETIOLOGY. Pyridoxine is adequate in human and cow's milk and in cereals, but prolonged heat processing of the latter two destroys it. Diseases with malabsorption, such as celiac syndrome, may contribute to vitamin B_6 deficiency.

There are several types of *vitamin B_6 dependence syndromes,* presumably a result of errors in enzyme structure or function, in which patients respond to very large amounts of pyridoxine. These syndromes include B_6-dependent convulsions, a B_6-responsive anemia, xanthurenic aciduria, cystathioninuria, and homocystinuria.

Pyridoxine antagonists, such as isoniazid used in the treatment of tuberculosis, increase the requirements for pyridoxine, as do pregnancy and drugs such as penicillamine, hydralazine, and the oral progesterone-estrogen contraceptives.

CLINICAL MANIFESTATIONS. Deficiency symptoms are not as common in children as in adults. Four clinical disturbances caused by vitamin B_6 deficiency have been described in humans: convulsions in infants, peripheral neuritis, dermatitis, and anemia. In adults with elevated serum homocysteine levels, pyridoxine and folic acid decrease the frequency of thrombotic events.

Infants fed a formula deficient in vitamin B_6 for 1–6 mo exhibit irritability and generalized seizures. Gastrointestinal distress and an aggravated startle response are common.

Peripheral neuropathy may occur during treatment of tuberculosis with isonicotinic acid hydrazide (INH). The neuropathy responds to administration of pyridoxine or to a decrease in the dose of the drug. Administration of isonicotinic acid may also be followed by manifestations of pellagra.

Skin lesions include cheilosis, glossitis, and seborrhea around the eyes, nose, and mouth. Microcytic anemia, oxaluria, oxalic acid bladder stones, hyperglycinemia, lymphopenia, decreased antibody formation, and infections also occur.

Convulsions due to B_6 dependence may occur several hours to as long as 6 mo after birth. Seizures are typically myoclonic, with hypsarrhythmic patterns on the electroencephalogram (EEG). In several cases, the mother had received large doses of pyridoxine during pregnancy for control of emesis.

In B_6-dependent anemia, the red blood cells are microcytic and hypochromic. Patients have increased serum iron concentrations, saturation of iron-binding protein, hemosiderin deposits in bone marrow and liver, and failure of iron utilization for hemoglobin synthesis.

Xanthurenic aciduria following tryptophan load tests is an apparently benign occurrence in some families. Xanthurenic acid excretion becomes normal after large doses of vitamin B_6. *Cystathioninuria* is similarly not accompanied by any clear clinical disturbance. Cystathioninase is vitamin B_6 dependent (see Chapter 82.4).

In some patients with homocystinuria, serum levels of homocysteine decline after B_6 administration. Cystathionine synthetase is B_6 dependent (see Chapter 82.4 and 82.5).

LABORATORY DATA. Anemia is not common in affected infants. After administration of 100 mg/kg of tryptophan, large amounts of xanthurenic acid are found in the urine of patients with pyridoxine deficiency; in normal persons, none is detected. The result of this test may be normal in patients with pyridoxine dependence.

DIAGNOSIS. Infants with seizures should be suspected of having vitamin B_6 deficiency or dependence. If more common causes of infantile seizures, such as hypocalcemia, hypoglycemia, and infection, can be eliminated, 100 mg of pyridoxine should be injected. If the seizure stops, B_6 deficiency should be suspected, and a tryptophan loading test is indicated. Similarly, in older children with seizure disorders, 100 mg of pyridoxine may be injected intramuscularly while the EEG is being recorded; a favorable response of the EEG suggests pyridoxine deficiency.

Erythrocyte glutamic pyruvic transaminase is reduced in pyridoxine deficiency; its concentration may be used as an indicator of vitamin B_6 status.

PREVENTION. Balanced diets usually contain enough pyridoxine so that deficiency is rare. Children receiving high-protein diets should have vitamin B_6 added. Infants whose mothers have received large doses of pyridoxine during pregnancy are at increased risk of seizures due to pyridoxine dependence. Any child receiving a pyridoxine antagonist such as isoniazid should be carefully observed for neurologic manifestations. If these develop, either pyridoxine should be administered or the dose of the antagonist decreased. Daily intake of 0.3–0.5 mg of pyridoxine in an infant, 0.5–1.5 mg in a child, or 1.5–2.0 mg in an adult prevents deficiency states.

TREATMENT. For convulsions possibly due to pyridoxine deficiency, 100 mg of the vitamin should be given intramuscularly. One dose should suffice if the diet is adequate. For pyridoxine-dependent children, 2–10 mg intramuscularly or 10–100 mg orally may be necessary daily.

TOXICITY. Excessive intake may cause neuropathy.

Baxter P, Gardner-Medwin D, Kelly T, Griffiths P: Pyridoxine-dependent seizures: Demographic, clinical, MRI and psychometric features, and effect of dose on intelligence quotient. Dev Med Child Neurol 38:998, 1996.

Cinnamon AD, Beaton JR: Biochemical assessment of vitamin B_6 status in man. Am J Clin Nutr 26:96, 1970.

Frimpter GW, Andelman RJ, George WF: Vitamin B_6-dependency syndromes. Am J Clin Nutr 22:794, 1959.

Hansson O, Hagberg B: Effect of pyridoxine treatment in children with epilepsy. Acta Soc Med Upsal 73:35, 1968.

Schaumburg H, Kaplan J, Windebank, A, et al: Sensory neuropathy from pyridoxine abuse. N Engl J Med 309:445, 1983.

Scriver CR: Vitamin B_6 deficiency and dependency in man. Am J Dis Child 113:109, 1967.

44.7 Biotin Deficiency

Biotin deficiency is rare. It is found in those consuming the biotin antagonist avidin, found in raw egg white. Many microorganisms produce biotin.

ETIOLOGY. Biotin is discussed in Chapter 82.6. Avidin ingestion causes symptoms of deficiency. Deficiencies have appeared in those receiving all their nutrition parenterally and occasionally in infants whose mothers are deficient in biotin.

CLINICAL MANIFESTATIONS. Brawny dermatitis, orofacial lesions, alopecia, somnolence, hallucinations, hypotonia, and hyperesthesia with accumulation of organic acids are common. Other neurologic signs and defective immunity may occur. Biotin deficiency has been reported in an infant fed amino acid formula without supplemental biotin and hypoallergenic rice for presumptive cow's milk and soy allergy.

DIAGNOSIS. Biotin deficiency is suggested by organic aciduria, particularly propionic and dicarboxylic acids, with response to clinical and biochemical abnormalities after treatment. Biotinidase can be measured on a filter-paper blood spot in neonatal screening.

PREVENTION AND TREATMENT. Parenteral solutions should contain biotin. Deficient patients respond to oral administration of 10 mg.

Higuchi R, Noda E, Koyama Y, et al: Biotin deficiency in an infant fed with amino acid formula and hypoallergenic rice. Acta Paediatr 85:872, 1996.

44.8 Folate Deficiency

Deficiency of folic acid is best recognized for its hematologic effects (see Chapter 460.1). Folate deficiency in a prepregnant woman results in serious dysmorphologic effects in her fetus and newborn. Consumption of 400 μg/24 hr of folic acid in the periconceptual period decreases the incidence of neurotubular and other anatomic defects and may lower the incidence of premature labor. Food may be fortified with folate as a preventive measure to decrease the incidence of neural tube defect. Doses to achieve intake of 100–200 μg/24 hr have been suggested for fortification of food products.

Thrombotic events related to slightly elevated levels of homocystine may be decreased in adults with consumption of 1 mg/24 hr of folic acid together with 5–100 mg/24 hr pyridoxine. Supplements with betaine and vitamin B_{12} may be required to normalize homocystine levels. These vitamin doses are considerably lower than those given for the inborn error of metabolism homocystinuria (see Chapter 82.3).

Hall JG, Solehdin F: Folate and its various ramifications. Adv Pediatr 45:1, 1998.

VITAMIN B_{12} DEFICIENCY (see Chapter 460.2).

44.9 Vitamin C (Ascorbic Acid) Deficiency (Scurvy)

Ascorbic acid is essential for the formation of normal collagen; the defects in collagen structure arising from deficiency of the vitamin produce many of the metabolic and clinical manifestations of scurvy. Alterations in collagen formation are partly due to failure to incorporate hydroxyproline and proline.

Vitamin C is a potent reducing agent that is easily oxidized and destroyed by heating. The adrenals and lenses have particularly high contents of vitamin C.

Ascorbic acid functions in a number of enzymatic activities (see Table 40–8 and Chapter 82.2). Transient tyrosinemia in the neonatal period, relatively common among low-birthweight infants and occasionally noted in full-term infants fed high-protein diets, is corrected by administering ascorbic acid (see Chapter 93).

Ascorbic acid deficiency may also be a factor in some cases of megaloblastic anemia by interfering in the conversion of folic acid or other conjugates (see Table 40–8 and Chapter 460).

ETIOLOGY. An infant is born with adequate stores of vitamin C if the mother's intake has been adequate; the vitamin C content of cord blood plasma is 2–4 times greater than that of maternal plasma. Under these circumstances, breast milk contains about 4–7 mg/dL of ascorbic acid and is an adequate source of vitamin C. Deficiency of vitamin C in the mother's diet may result in scurvy in her breast-fed infant. Infants fed with evaporated milk formula must receive vitamin C supplements.

The need for vitamin C is increased by febrile illnesses, particularly infectious and diarrheal diseases, and by iron deficiency, cold exposure, protein depletion, or smoking.

PATHOLOGY. During vitamin C deficiency, formation of collagen and of chondroitin sulfate is impaired. The tendency to hemorrhage, defective tooth dentin, and loosening of the teeth are caused by deficient collagen. Because osteoblasts no longer form their normal intercellular substance (osteoid), endochondral bone formation ceases. The bony trabeculae that have been formed become brittle and fracture easily. The periosteum becomes loosened, and subperiosteal hemorrhages occur, especially at the ends of the femur and tibia. Severe scurvy may be marked by degeneration of skeletal muscles, cardiac hypertrophy, bone marrow depression, and adrenal atrophy.

CLINICAL MANIFESTATIONS. Scurvy may occur at any age but is rare in newborn infants. The majority of cases occur in infants age 6–24 mo. Clinical manifestations require time to develop; after a variable period of vitamin C depletion, vague symptoms of irritability, tachypnea, digestive disturbances, and loss of appetite appear. There is evidence of general tenderness, especially noticeable in the legs when the infant is picked up or when the diaper is changed. The pain results in pseudoparalysis, and the legs assume the typical frog position, in which the hips and knees are semiflexed with the feet rotated outward. Edematous swelling along the shafts of the legs may be present. In some cases, a subperiosteal hemorrhage can be palpated at the end of the femur. The facial expression is apprehensive. Changes in the gums, most noticeable when the teeth are erupted, are characterized by bluish purple, spongy swellings of the mucous membrane, usually over the upper incisors. A "rosary" at the costochondral junctions and a depression of the sternum may be noted (Fig. 44–4). The angulation of scorbutic beads is usually sharper than that of a rachitic rosary.

Petechial hemorrhages may occur in the skin and mucous membranes. Hematuria, melena, and orbital or subdural hemorrhages may be found. Low-grade fever is usually present. Anemia may reflect inability to utilize iron or impaired folic acid metabolism (see Chapters 460 and 461). Wound healing is delayed, and apparently healed wounds may break down. Swollen joints and follicular hyperkeratosis may develop, as well as the sicca syndrome of Sjögren, which is usually associated with collagen disorders and includes xerostomia, keratoconjunctivitis sicca, and enlargement of the salivary glands (see Chapter 163).

ROENTGENOGRAPHIC MANIFESTATIONS. The diagnosis of scurvy is usually based on roentgenographic changes in the long bones, especially at their distal ends, greatest in the area of the knee. In the early stages, the appearance resembles that of simple atrophy of bone. The trabeculae of the shaft cannot be discerned, and the bone assumes a ground-glass appearance. The cortex is reduced to pencil-point thinness, and the epiphyseal ends are sharply outlined. The white line of Fraenkel, which represents the zone of well-calcified cartilage, can be discerned as an irregular but thickened white line at the metaphysis. The epiphyseal centers of ossification also have a ground-glass appearance and are surrounded by a white ring (Fig. 44–5).

At this stage, scurvy cannot be diagnosed with certainty from the roentgenogram unless the zone of rarefaction under the white line at the metaphysis becomes apparent. The zone of rarefaction is a linear break in the bone proximal and parallel to the white line and may be seen only in its lateral parts as a triangular defect (see Fig. 44–5*B*). A spur, as a lateral prolongation of the white line, may be present. Epiphyseal separation may occur along the line of destruction, with linear displacement or compression of the epiphysis against the shaft. Subperiosteal hemorrhages are not visible roentgenographically in active scurvy. During healing, however, the elevated periosteum becomes calcified, and the affected bone assumes a dumbbell or club shape.

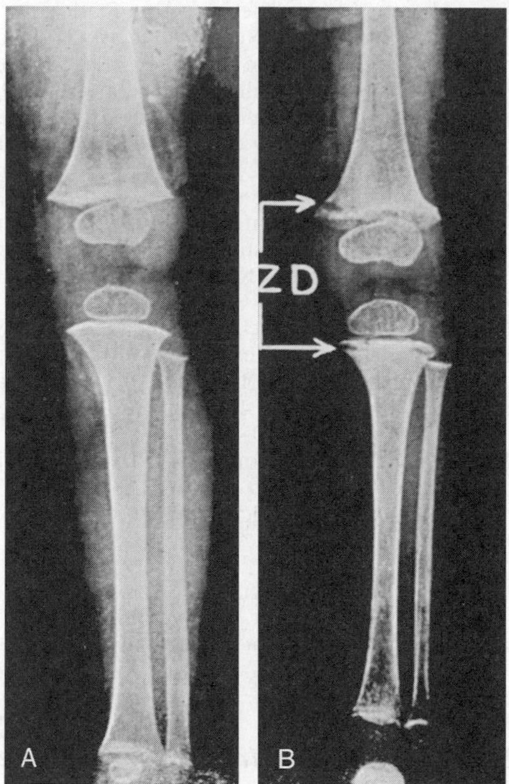

Figure 44–5 Roentgenograms of a leg. *A*, Early scurvy: "white line" is visible on the ends of the shafts of the tibia and fibula; rings around the epiphyses of the femur and tibia. *B*, More advanced scorbutic changes; zones of destruction (ZD) in the femur and tibia.

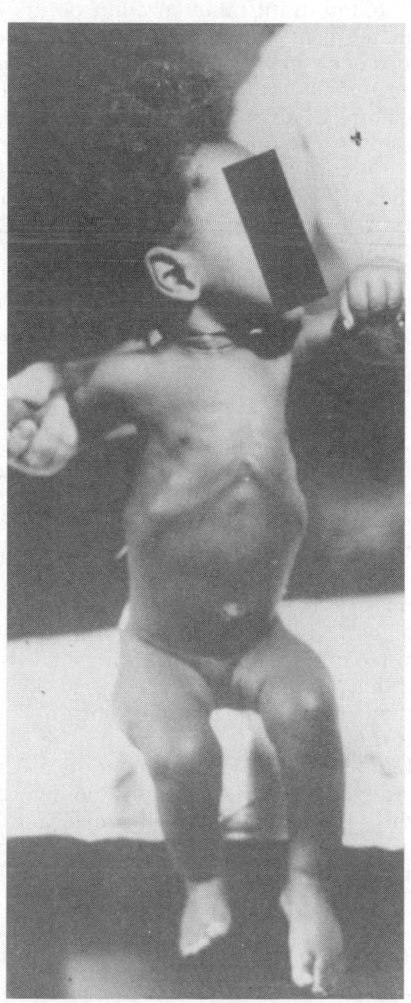

Figure 44–4 Scorbutic rosary and depression of sternum.

DIAGNOSIS. Diagnosis is based mainly on the characteristic clinical picture, the roentgenographic appearance of the long bones, and history of poor intake of vitamin C. A mother may occasionally have been boiling her infant's fruit juices.

Laboratory tests for scurvy are unsatisfactory. A fasting vitamin C level of the blood plasma of over 0.6 mg/dL aids in precluding scurvy, but a lower vitamin C level does not prove its presence. Evidence of vitamin C deficiency is better furnished by the ascorbic acid concentration in the white cell–platelet layer (buffy layer) of centrifuged oxalated blood. A level of zero in this layer indicates latent scurvy, even in the absence of clinical signs of deficiency. Saturation of the tissues with vitamin C can be estimated from the amount of urinary excretion of the vitamin after a test dose of ascorbic acid. During the 3–5 hr after parenteral administration of the test dose, 80% of it can be found in the urine of normal children. A generalized, nonspecific aminoaciduria occurs in scurvy, whereas blood values of amino acids remain normal. After a tyrosine load, scorbutic infants excrete metabolites similar to those of premature infants. Prothrombin time may be greatly increased.

DIFFERENTIAL DIAGNOSIS. The tenderness of the limbs and the pain elicited by movement have often led to a false diagnosis of arthritis or acrodynia. A patient's age aids in differentiating scurvy from rheumatic fever because rheumatic fever is rare in children younger than 2 yr. Suppurative arthritis and osteomyelitis should be considered in the differential diagnosis. The pseudoparalysis of syphilis usually occurs at an earlier age than does that of scurvy and is often accompanied by other signs of syphilis; a roentgenogram may aid in the diagnosis. Henoch-Schönlein purpura, thrombocytopenic purpura, leukemia, meningitis, or nephritis may be suspected.

PROGNOSIS. With proper treatment, recovery occurs rapidly in infants, but the swelling of subperiosteal hemorrhage may require months to disappear. Body growth usually is quickly resumed.

PREVENTION. Scurvy is prevented by a diet adequate in vitamin C; citrus fruits and juices are excellent sources. Formula-fed infants should receive 35 mg of ascorbic acid daily. Lactating mothers should take 100 mg; 45–60 mg/24 hr is needed by children or adults (see Table 40–1).

TREATMENT. Daily administration of 3–4 oz of orange juice or tomato juice quickly produces healing, but ascorbic acid is preferable. The daily therapeutic dose is 100–200 mg or more, orally or parenterally.

Irwin MI, Hutchins BK: A conspectus of research on vitamin C requirements in man. J Nutr 106:823, 1976.

Levine M: New concepts in the biology and biochemistry of ascorbic acid. N Engl J Med 314:892, 1986.

*44.10 Rickets of Vitamin D Deficiency**

Rickets is the term signifying a failure in mineralization of growing bone or osteoid tissue. The characteristic early changes are seen roentgenographically at the ends of long bones; evidence of demineralization also exists in the shafts. Subsequently, if healing is not initiated, clinical manifestations appear (see later). Failure of mature bone to mineralize is called *osteomalacia.*

ETIOLOGY. During the first third of this century, the predominant cause of rickets was nutritional deficiency of vitamin D due either to inadequate direct exposure to ultraviolet rays in sunlight (296–310 nm; these rays do not pass through ordinary window glass) or to inadequate intake of vitamin D, or both. Vitamin D deficiency rickets is rare among infants and children in the industrialized countries. Deficiency may occur in unsupplemented dark-skinned infants or in breast-fed infants of mothers unexposed to sunlight.

In industrialized countries, conditions besides inadequate nutritional prophylaxis with vitamin D collectively produce most of the observed rachitic lesions (see Chapters 366.1, 537.5, and 711–713). These conditions include clinical entities that interfere with the metabolic conversion and activation of vitamin D, such as hepatic and renal lesions, or that disrupt calcium and phosphorus homeostasis in other ways.

Two forms of vitamin D are of practical importance. Vitamin D_2, or calciferol, available as irradiated ergosterol, largely replaced the fish liver oils (cod and percomorph) as a source of dietary and therapeutic vitamin D. Vitamin D_3, available synthetically, is naturally present in human skin in the provitamin stage as 7-dehydrocholesterol. It is activated photochemically to cholecalciferol and transferred to the liver. These irradiated sterols are hydroxylated in the liver to 25-OH-cholecalciferol and, subsequently, in the renal cortical cells to 1, 25-dihydroxycholecalciferol, which functions as a hormone. Receptors of the hormone are found in the kidneys, intestine, osteoblasts of bone, parathyroid, islet cells of the pancreas, cells in the brain, mammary epithelium, and elsewhere. Its antirachitic functions include facilitation of intestinal absorption of calcium and phosphorus and of reabsorption of phosphorus in the kidneys and a direct effect on mineral metabolism of bone (deposition and reabsorption). In conjunction with parathormone and calcitonin, it has a major role in homeostasis of calcium and phosphorus in the body's fluids and tissues.

The diet of infants may contain only small amounts of vitamin D; cow's milk contains only 0.1–1 μg/qt.* Cereals, vegetables, and fruits contain only negligible amounts. Egg yolk contains 3–10 μg/g. Most marketed cow's milk is fortified with vitamin D 10 μg/qt of milk, and most commercially prepared milks for infant formulas are also fortified.

Besides lack of dietary vitamin D and the skin's lack of exposure to ultraviolet irradiation, several factors may predispose to vitamin D deficiency. Rickets or epiphyseal dysplasia is particularly likely to develop during rapid growth, such as in low-birthweight infants and in adolescents. Darkly pigmented children are singularly susceptible to rickets.

Children with disorders such as celiac disease, steatorrhea, or cystic fibrosis may acquire rickets because of deficient absorption of vitamin D or calcium or both. Anticonvulsant therapy, as with the phenytoins or phenobarbital, may interfere in the metabolism of vitamin D. Glucocorticoids appear to be antagonistic to vitamin D in calcium transport.

PATHOLOGY. New bone formation is initiated by osteoblasts, which are responsible for matrix deposition and its subsequent mineralization. Osteoblasts secrete collagen, and changes in polysaccharides, phospholipids, alkaline phosphatase, and pyrophosphatase follow until mineralization occurs in the presence of adequate calcium and phosphorus. Resorption of bone occurs when osteoclasts secrete enzymes on the bone surface, dissolving and removing matrix and mineral. Osteocytes covered by bone both resorb and redeposit bone. Factors affecting bone growth are poorly understood, but phosphorus, calcium, fluoride, and growth hormone all have some influence.

In rickets, defective growth of bone results from retardation or suppression of normal growth of epiphyseal cartilage and of normal calcification. These changes depend on a deficiency in serum of calcium and phosphorus salts for mineralization. Cartilage cells fail to complete their normal cycle of proliferation and degeneration, and subsequent failure of capillary penetration occurs in a patchy manner. The result is a frayed, irregular epiphyseal line at the end of the shaft. Failure of osseous and cartilaginous matrix to mineralize in the zone of preparatory calcification, followed by deposition of newly formed uncalcified osteoid, results in a wide, irregular, frayed zone of nonrigid tissue (the rachitic metaphysis) (Fig. 44–6). This zone, responsible for many of the skeletal deformities, becomes compressed and bulges laterally, producing flaring of the ends of the bones and the rachitic rosary (Fig. 44–7). Mineralization is also lacking in subperiosteal bone; pre-existing cortical bone is resorbed in a normal manner but is replaced by osteoid tissues over the entire shaft, which fails to mineralize. If this process continues, the shaft loses its rigidity, and the resultant softened and rarefied cortical bone is readily distorted by stress; deformities and fractures result.

Healing Rickets. With healing, degeneration of cartilage cells occurs along the metaphyseal-diaphyseal border, capillary penetration of the resultant spaces is resumed, and calcification takes place in the zone of preparatory calcification. This calcification, occurring approximately at the line at which normal calcification would have occurred had the rachitic process not supervened, produces a line clearly demonstrable in roentgenograms (Fig. 44–8*A* and *B*). As healing progresses, the

*For a review of the rachitic lesions, reference should be made to Table 40–8 and Chapters 49 and 51 for calcium and phosphorus metabolism; Chapter 55.9 for hypocalcemic tetany; Part XXV, Section 3, for parathormone, vitamin D, and calcitonin activities; and Chapter 530.1 for additional discussion of vitamin D metabolism and its activities.

*1 μg = 40 IU.

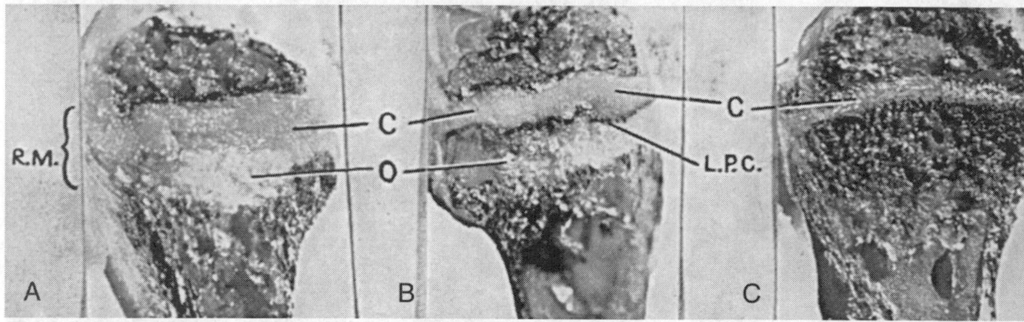

Figure 44–6 Line tests in rats (proximal end of the tibia) (calcified tissue stained with silver appears black). *A*, Active rickets. The light broad zone between the epiphysis and the shaft represents the rachitic metaphysis (R.M.) (C = cartilage; O = osteoid). *B*, Healing rickets. The line of preparatory calcification (L.P.C.) between the zone of cartilage (C) and the osteoid (O). *C*, Healed rickets. Cartilaginous disc (C) between the epiphysis and the normal shaft.

osteoid tissue between this line of preparatory calcification and the diaphysis also becomes mineralized (see Fig. 44–6). Osteoid tissue in the cortex and about the trabeculae in the shaft rapidly becomes mineralized.

Chemical Pathology. Vitamin D–deficient rickets can be conceptualized to be the body's attempt to maintain normal serum calcium levels. In the absence of vitamin D, less calcium is absorbed from the intestine. With slightly lowered serum calcium level, parathormone is secreted, leading to mobilization of calcium and phosphorus from the bone. The serum calcium concentration is thus maintained, but secondary effects occur, including the changes of rickets in bone and the lowered serum phosphorus concentration (because parathormone decreases phosphorus reabsorption in the kidneys) and elevated serum phosphatase levels (due to increased osteoblastic activity).

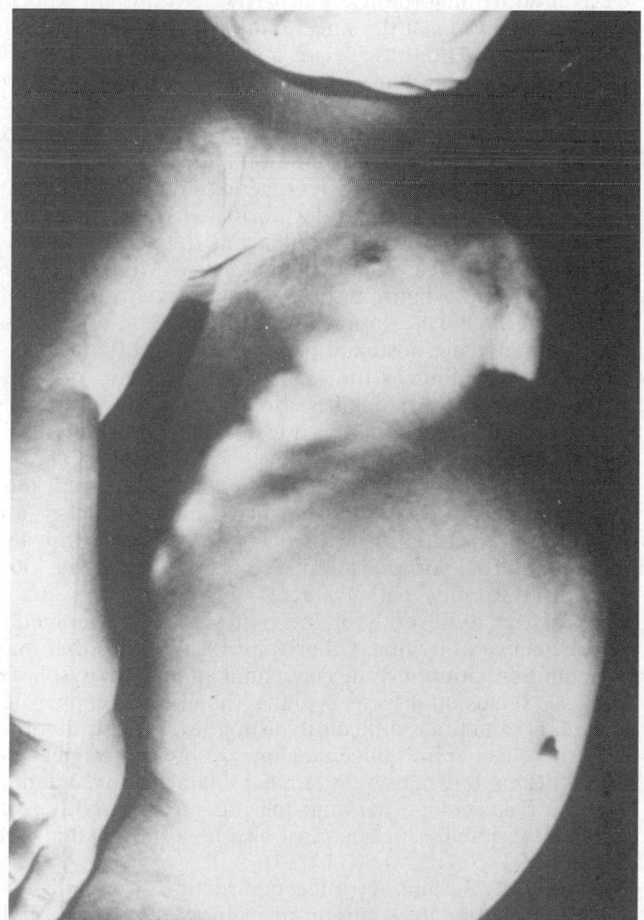

Figure 44–7 Rachitic rosary in a young infant.

The alkaline phosphatase of serum, which in normal children is less than 200 IU/dL, is elevated in mild rickets to more than 500 IU/dL. As rickets heals, the phosphatase value returns slowly to the normal range. Serum alkaline phosphatase levels may be normal in infants who have rickets and who are protein or zinc depleted.

Calcium and phosphorus homeostasis depends on the intestinal absorption of dietary calcium and phosphorus. Maximum calcium absorption occurs in humans when the ratio of calcium to phosphorus in the diet is about 2:1; increase in phosphate decreases absorption of calcium. An increase in calcium absorption occurs with acidity of intestinal contents or when lactose is the dietary sugar. Chelating agents such as ethylenediaminetetraacetic acid or the phytates of cereals may decrease calcium absorption, and dietary iron may decrease absorption of phosphate. High dietary levels of stearic and palmitic acids, which are poorly absorbed, also decrease calcium absorption.

Calcium absorption is facilitated by 1, 25-dihydroxycholecalciferol or similar hydroxylated forms of vitamin D. Calcium deficiency alone rarely leads to the failure of calcification as seen in rickets and osteomalacia; it results in a diminished amount of bone. Alleged dietary calcium deficits have been reported from Nigeria; rickets has been reported from areas of Turkey with elevated soil strontium and a grain cereal diet.

Vitamin D deficiency is also accompanied by generalized aminoaciduria, a decrease of citrate in bone and its increased urinary excretion, decreased ability of the kidneys to make an acid urine, phosphaturia, and, occasionally, mellituria. The parathyroid glands hypertrophy in rickets, and urinary cyclic adenosine monophosphate level is increased.

CLINICAL MANIFESTATIONS. Osseous changes of rickets can be recognized after several months of vitamin D deficiency. In breast-fed infants whose mothers have osteomalacia, rickets may develop within 2 mo. Florid rickets appears toward the end of the 1st and during the 2nd yr of life. Later in childhood, manifest vitamin D–deficient rickets is rare.

One of the early signs of rickets, craniotabes, is due to thinning of the outer table of the skull and detected by pressing firmly over the occiput or posterior parietal bones. A Ping-Pong-ball sensation is felt. Craniotabes near the suture lines is a normal variant. Low-birthweight infants are particularly susceptible to the early development of rickets and to craniotabes. Palpable enlargement of the costochondral junctions (the rachitic rosary) (see Fig. 44–7) and thickening of the wrists and ankles (see Fig. 44–8) are other early evidences of osseous changes. Increased sweating, particularly around the head, may be present.

The softness of the skull may result in flattening and, at times, permanent asymmetry of the head. The anterior fontanel is larger than normal; its closure may be delayed until after

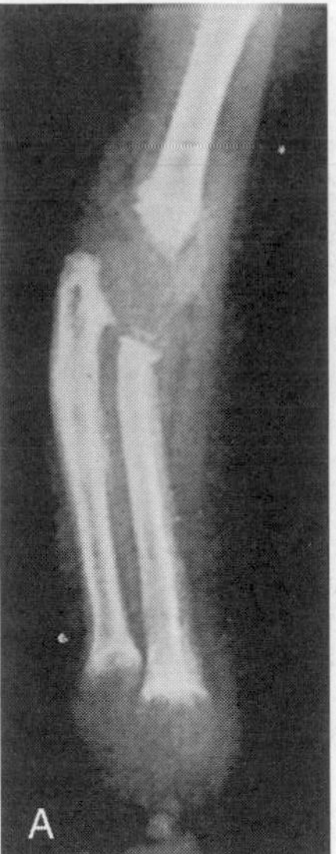

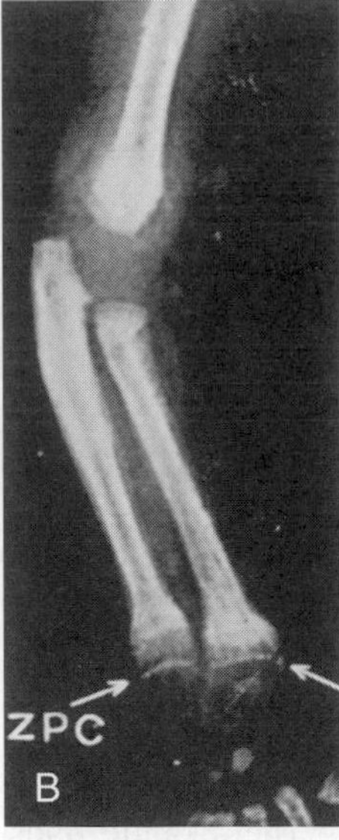

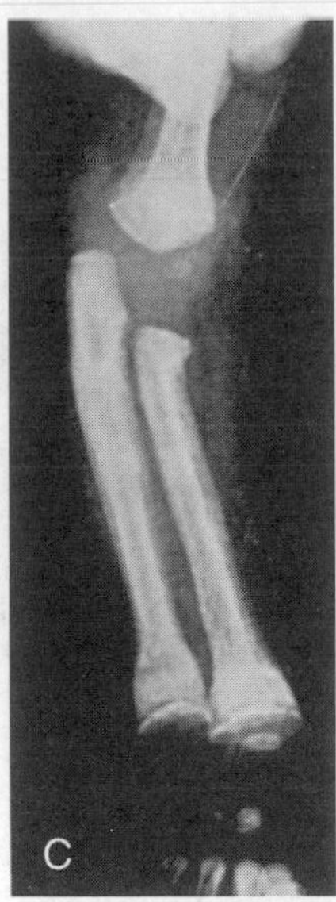

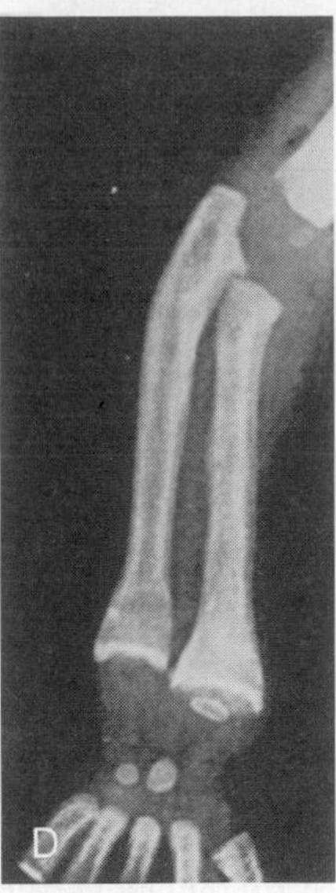

Figure 44–8 *A,* Active rickets; cupping and fraying of the distal ends of the radius and ulna; double contour along the lateral outline of the radius (periosteal osteoid). The two dense zones in the shaft of the ulna are calluses of greenstick fractures. *B,* Healing rickets after 12 days of treatment with vitamin D. Zones of preparatory calcification (ZPC); above them in the rachitic metaphyses there is beginning calcification. *C,* Healing rickets after 18 days of treatment. The zones of preparatory calcification are well defined, and the rachitic metaphyses appear well calcified. The epiphysis of the radius has become visible. *D,* Healing rickets after 29 days of treatment. Zones of preparatory calcification, rachitic metaphyses, and shafts have become united.

the 2nd yr of life. The central parts of the parietal and frontal bones are often thickened, forming prominences or bosses, which give the head a boxlike appearance (caput quadratum). Eruption of the temporary teeth may be delayed, and there may be defects of the enamel and extensive caries. The permanent teeth that are calcifying may also be affected; the permanent incisors, canines, and first molars usually show enamel defects.

Enlargement of the costochondral junctions may become prominent; the beading of the ribs is not only palpable but also visible (see Fig. 44–7). The sternum with its adjacent cartilage appears to be projected forward, producing the so-called pigeon breast deformity. A horizontal depression, Harrison groove (Fig. 44–9), develops along the lower border of the chest.

Affected children frequently have a concomitant deformity of the pelvis, which is also retarded in growth. In girls, these changes, if they become permanent, add to the hazards of childbirth and may necessitate cesarean section.

As the rachitic process continues, the epiphyseal enlargement at the wrists and ankles becomes more noticeable (see Fig. 44–8). Bending of the softened shafts of the femur, tibia, and fibula results in bowlegs or knock-knees. Greenstick fractures occur in the long bones; there often are no clinical symptoms. Deformities of the spine, pelvis, and legs result in reduced stature, rachitic dwarfism. Relaxation of ligaments helps to produce deformities and partly accounts for knock-knees, overextension of the knee joints, weak ankles, kyphosis, and scoliosis. The muscles are poorly developed and lack tone. As a result, children with moderately severe rickets are late in standing and walking (see Fig. 44–9).

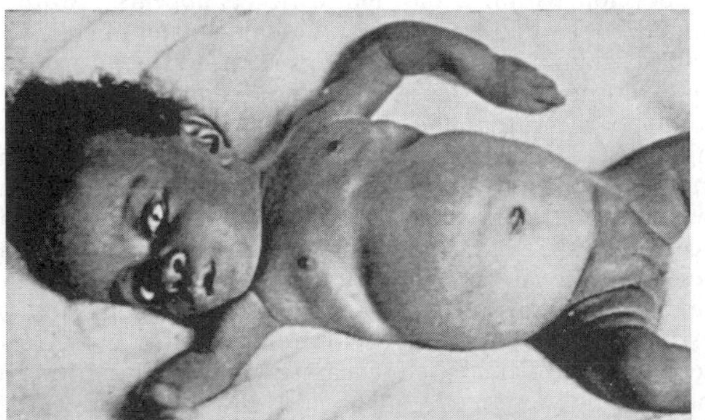

Figure 44–9 Deformities in rickets, showing the curvature of the limbs, potbelly, and Harrison groove.

DIAGNOSIS. The diagnosis of rickets is based on a history of inadequate intake of vitamin D and on clinical observation; it is confirmed chemically and by roentgenographic examination. The serum calcium level may be normal or low, the serum phosphorus level is below 4 mg/dL, and the serum alkaline phosphatase level is elevated. Urinary cyclic AMP level is elevated, and serum 25-hydroxycholecalciferol level is decreased.

DIFFERENTIAL DIAGNOSIS. Nonrachitic craniotabes, at times present in the immediate postnatal period, tends to disappear before rachitic softening of the skull would become manifest (2nd–4th mo of life). Craniotabes also occurs in hydrocephalus and osteogenesis imperfecta, but it is not difficult to differentiate these conditions from rickets.

Enlargement of the costochondral junctions occurs in rickets, scurvy, and chondrodystrophy. The enlargements in rickets are rounded knobs, but in scurvy a ledgelike depression with the chondral or sternal portion is displaced below the osseous ribs. In chondrodystrophy, patients may have irregular, concave outlines of the distal ends of the bones but no roentgenographic evidence of fraying. Other epiphyseal lesions that may require differentiation include congenital epiphyseal dysplasia, cytomegalic inclusion disease, syphilis, rubella, and copper deficiency. It is sometimes difficult to distinguish rachitic deformities of the chest from congenital ones. Bowlegs can be the result of rickets but may be a familial characteristic. Vitamin D–resistant rickets and other metabolic disturbances with osseous lesions resembling rickets must also be differentiated (see Chapters 366.1, 537.5, and 711–713).

COMPLICATIONS. Respiratory infections such as bronchitis and bronchopneumonia are common in rachitic infants, and pulmonary atelectasis is frequently associated with severe deformities of the chest. Anemia due to iron deficiency or accompanying infections often develops in severe rickets.

PROGNOSIS. If sufficient amounts of vitamin D are administered, healing begins within a few days and progresses slowly until the normal bony structure is restored.

Rickets in itself is not a fatal disease, but complications and intercurrent infections such as pneumonia, tuberculosis, and enteritis are more likely to cause death of rachitic children than normal children.

PREVENTION. Rickets can be prevented by exposure to ultraviolet light or by oral administration of vitamin D. Sunlight, as a prophylactic agent, may be effective in the temperate zones only during the summer months in haze-free areas.

The daily requirement of vitamin D is 10 μg or 400 IU. Premature infants or breast-fed infants whose mothers are not exposed to adequate sunlight should receive supplemental vitamin D daily.

Vitamin D should also be administered to pregnant and lactating mothers.

TREATMENT. Natural and artificial light are effective therapeutically, but oral administration of vitamin D is preferred. Daily administration of 50–150 μg of vitamin D_3 or 0.5–2 μg of 1,25-dihydroxycholecalciferol produces healing demonstrable on roentgenograms within 2–4 wk, except in cases of vitamin D refractory rickets.

Administering 15,000 μg of vitamin D in a single dose without further therapy for several months may be advantageous. More rapid healing follows, possibly with earlier differential diagnosis from genetic vitamin D–resistant rickets and less dependence on parents for daily administration of the vitamin. If no healing occurs, the rickets is probably resistant to vitamin D (see Chapters 366.1, 537.5, and 711–713). After healing is complete, the dose of vitamin D should be lowered to 10 μg/24 hr.

Argao EA, Heubi JE: Fat-soluble vitamin deficiency in infants and children. Curr Opin Pediatr 5:562, 1993.

DeLuca HF: New concepts of vitamin D functions. Ann N Y Acad Science 669:59, 1992.

Oginni LM, Worsfold M, Oyelami OA, et al: Etiology of rickets in Nigerian children. J Pediatr 128:692, 1996.

Ozgur S, Sumer H, Kocoglu G: Rickets and soil strontium. Arch Dis Child 75:524, 1996.

Rasmussen H: Cell communication, calcium ion, and cyclic adenosine monophosphate. Science 170:404, 1970.

Reichel H, Koeffler HP, Norman AW: The role of the vitamin D endocrine system in health and disease. N Engl J Med 320:980, 1989.

Root AW, Harrison HE: Recent advances in calcium metabolism. I. Mechanisms of calcium homeostasis. II. Disorders of calcium homeostasis. J Pediatr 88:1, 177, 1976.

Yetgin S, Ozsoylu S, Raucan S, et al: Vitamin D–deficiency rickets and myelofibrosis. J Pediatr 114:213, 1989.

44.11 *Tetany of Vitamin D Deficiency (Infantile Tetany)*

See also Chapter 55.9.

Tetany due to deficiency of vitamin D occasionally accompanies rickets. Relatively common in former times, this type of tetany is rare today owing to widespread prophylactic use of vitamin D. Tetany is occasionally associated with celiac disease, probably as a result of deficient absorption of both vitamin D and calcium. Tetany of vitamin D deficiency occurs most frequently between the ages of 4 mo and 3 yr.

CHEMICAL PATHOLOGY. When the serum ionized calcium concentration falls below 3–4 mg/dL, muscular irritability occurs, apparently owing to the loss of the inhibitory control that calcium exerts on the neuromuscular junctions.

CLINICAL MANIFESTATIONS. The symptoms and signs of tetany are manifested, and rickets usually occurs concurrently. Vitamin D–deficient tetany may exist in either a latent or a clinically manifest stage (see Chapter 55.9).

Latent Tetany. Symptoms are not evident, but they can be elicited by means of the Chvostek, Trousseau, and Erb procedures. The serum calcium level is less than 7–7.5 mg/dL (3–4 mg/dL ionized).

Manifest Tetany. Spontaneous clinical manifestations include carpopedal spasm, laryngospasm, and convulsions. The serum calcium level is often well under 7 mg/dL.

DIAGNOSIS. This is based on the combined presence of rickets, low serum calcium level, and symptoms of tetany. The serum phosphorus level is usually low; the serum alkaline phosphatase level is increased. In the differential diagnosis, causes of tetany such as hypoparathyroidism, hypomagnesemia, and ingestion of phenothiazine must be eliminated.

PROGNOSIS. The prognosis is good unless treatment is delayed. Death rarely occurs, although it may result from laryngospasm and possibly from cardiac dilatation, so-called cardiac tetany.

PREVENTION. Prophylactic treatment is identical to that for rickets.

TREATMENT. Active treatment raises the serum calcium above the tetany level. This level may be attained by administration of calcium chloride in 1–2% solution in milk. For the first 1–2 days, 4–6 g/24 hr may be given in 1-g doses, the initial dose being 2–3 g; smaller doses of 1–3 g/24 hr should then be continued for 1–2 wk. Calcium chloride in more concentrated solution may cause severe gastric ulceration, and large doses may cause acidosis. Calcium lactate may be added to milk in doses of 10–12 g/24 hr for 10 days. When oral medication is impractical, calcium gluconate (5–10 mL of a 10% solution) can be administered intravenously but not subcutaneously or intramuscularly owing to the dangers of local necrosis.

Oxygen inhalation is indicated during convulsive seizures. When intravenously administered calcium gluconate does not quickly control the attacks, sodium phenobarbital may be given intramuscularly. Prolonged attacks of laryngospasm are usually controlled by sedation and by administering calcium salts. Intubation is only occasionally necessary. After the acute manifestations have been controlled, vitamin D in daily doses of 50–100 μg should be started with the oral administration of calcium. When the rickets is healed, the dose of vitamin D should be decreased to the usual prophylactic one.

44.12 *Hypervitaminosis D*

Ingesting excessive amounts of vitamin D results in signs and symptoms similar to those of idiopathic hypercalcemia (see Chapter 708), which may be due to hypersensitivity to vitamin D. Symptoms develop after 1–3 mo of large intakes of vitamin D; they include hypotonia, anorexia, irritability, constipation, polydipsia, polyuria, and pallor. Hypercalcemia and hypercalciuria are notable. Aortic valvular stenosis, vomiting, hypertension, retinopathy, and clouding of the cornea and conjunctiva may occur.

The urine may show proteinuria. With continued excessive intake, renal damage and metastatic calcification occur. Roentgenograms of the long bones reveal metastatic calcification and generalized osteopetrosis.

Excessive intake of vitamin D may result from inadvertently substituting its concentrated form for one more dilute, from the parents' increasing their child's prescribed dose, and from inadequately controlling dosages for children receiving large amounts of vitamin D for chronic hyperphosphatemic states (see Chapter 543.1).

DIFFERENTIAL DIAGNOSIS. Metastatic calcification occurs in chronic nephritis, hyperparathyroidism, and idiopathic hypercalcemia. The latter two are accompanied by hypercalcemia.

PREVENTION. Prevention requires careful evaluation of vitamin D dosage.

TREATMENT. This includes discontinuing vitamin D intake and decreasing intake of calcium. For severely affected infants, aluminum hydroxide by mouth, cortisone, or sodium versenate may be used.

Forbes GB, Cafarelli C, Manning J: Vitamin D and infantile hypercalcemia. Pediatrics 42:203, 1968.

44.13 Vitamin E Deficiency

The effects of vitamin E deficiency vary in different animal species. Vitamin E (α-tocopherol) is a fat-soluble antioxidant that may be involved in nucleic acid metabolism, but its precise biochemical action is unclear. Vitamin E is present in many foods (see Table 40–8).

Deficiency may occur in malabsorption states such as cystic fibrosis and acanthocytosis. Diets high in unsaturated fatty acids increase the vitamin E requirement in premature infants who absorb vitamin E poorly. Excess iron administration exaggerates signs of vitamin E deficiency.

CLINICAL MANIFESTATIONS. Some patients deficient in vitamin E have creatinuria, ceroid deposition in smooth muscle, focal necrosis of striated muscle, and muscle weakness. Some improvement may occur after administration of vitamin E. Vitamin E deficiency has been suggested as a causative factor in the anemia of kwashiorkor. Premature infants may have low serum levels of tocopherol, with development of a hemolytic anemia at age 6–10 wk, correctable by administration of vitamin E. In deficiency states, platelet adhesiveness increases, as do blood platelet levels. The role of vitamin E in retinopathy of prematurity is discussed in Chapters 93.2 and 637. Patients with malabsorption and vitamin E deficiency due to biliary atresia develop a degenerative, potentially reversible, neurologic syndrome consisting of cerebellar ataxia, peripheral neuropathy, and posterior column abnormalities.

DIAGNOSIS. If vitamin E has recently been administered, 3 days should elapse before determination of blood levels because oral vitamin E may circulate for 1–2 days.

PREVENTION. Minimal daily requirements of vitamin E are not known; 0.7 mg/g of unsaturated fat in the diet appears adequate. Children with deficient fat absorption should take more. Premature infants may be given 15–25 IU/24 hr. Large oral or parenteral doses of vitamin E may prevent permanent neurologic abnormalities in children with biliary atresia or abetalipoproteinemia.

Argao EA, Heubi JE: Fat soluble vitamin deficiency in infants and children. Curr Opin Pediatr 5:562, 1993.

Gross S: Hemolytic anemia in premature infants: Relationship to vitamin E, selenium, glutathione peroxidase, and erythrocyte lipids. Semin Hematol 13:187, 1976.

Sokol RJ: Vitamin E and neurologic deficits. Adv Pediatr 37:119, 1990.

44.14 Vitamin K Deficiency

Vitamin K is a naphthoquinone that participates in oxidative phosphorylation. Its absence or its failure to be absorbed from the intestinal tract results in hypoprothrombinemia and decreased hepatic synthesis of proconvertin. Prothrombin (factor II) and proconvertin (factor VII) are important to the second stage of coagulation (see Chapter 483). The second stage of coagulation is studied by the one-stage prothrombin time (Quick). Administering vitamin K to a newborn infant increases concentrations of prothrombin, proconvertin, plasma thromboplastin component (factor IX), and Stuart-Prower factor (factor X). Four vitamin K–dependent proteins contain γ-carboxyglutamate. All require calcium for activity. Factors C and S are anticoagulants. Factors Z and M stimulate platelet activity. Vitamin K–dependent calcium-binding proteins such as osteocalcin promote phospholipid interactions in coagulation and in calcium metabolism.

SOURCES OF VITAMIN K. Naturally occurring vitamin K is fat soluble; it is found in high concentrations of hog's liver, soybeans, and alfalfa and in smaller amounts in some vegetables, such as spinach, tomatoes, and kale. The natural vitamin (2-methyl-3-phytyl-1,4-naphthoquinone) has been labeled vitamin K_1 to distinguish it from vitamin K_2 of bacterial origin and from synthetic naphthoquinones with vitamin K activity.

Suppression of intestinal bacteria by various antibiotics may be responsible for vitamin K deficiency, which results in diminution of prothrombin. Irradiated foods have produced vitamin K deficiency in animals. Cow's milk has more vitamin K than human milk.

CLINICAL MANIFESTATIONS. Deficiency of vitamin K or hypoprothrombinemia should be considered in all patients with a hemorrhagic disturbance. The incidence of hemorrhagic disease of the newborn (see Chapter 99.4) has been sharply decreased by prophylactic administration of vitamin K. In childhood, the deficiency is usually due to factors affecting absorption or utilization of fat or to factors limiting its synthesis in the intestine, such as prolonged use of antibiotics. Diarrhea in infants, particularly breast-fed ones, may cause vitamin K deficiency. Diseases of the liver may lead to hypoprothrombinemia, which usually does not respond to administration of vitamin K.

Hypoprothrombinemia may also result from administering certain drugs. Dicumarol (or bishydroxycoumarin), obtained from spoiled sweet clover, is used specifically for the production of hypoprothrombinemia in the prevention and treatment of venous thrombosis. Dicumarol is thought to prevent the liver from utilizing vitamin K without exerting an effect on prothrombin. Blood prothrombin is continually destroyed in the body; because dicumarol prevents its replacement, a decline in prothrombin occurs. If a dangerously low level results, massive doses of vitamin K_1 may be necessary to restore prothrombin, and whole blood transfusions may also be necessary.

Salicylic acid, a degradation product of dicumarol, produces hypoprothrombinemia by similar action. The reduction in prothrombin resulting from salicylates, however, is mild compared with that of dicumarol. The hemorrhagic manifestations in acute rheumatic fever may be due in some cases to large doses of salicylates; vitamin K is effective in neutralizing this action. Its use in children receiving large doses of salicylates would appear justified.

TREATMENT. Oral administration of vitamin K may correct mild prothrombin deficiency. One to 2 mg/24 hr for an infant usually suffices. If prothrombin deficiency is severe and hemorrhagic manifestations have appeared, 5 mg/24 hr of vitamin K_1 should be given parenterally. Large doses of synthetic vitamin K analogs, but not of vitamin K_1, may result in hyperbilirubinemia and kernicterus in newborns deficient in glucose-6-phosphate dehydrogenase and in premature infants. In hypoprothrombinemia owing to liver damage, vitamin K_1 may be given, but whole blood is usually also necessary.

Corrigan JJ: The vitamin K dependent proteins. Adv Pediatr 28:57, 1981.

Peters C, Casella JF, Marlar RA, et al: Homozygous protein C deficiency. Pediatrics 81:272, 1988.

PART VII

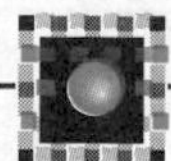

Pathophysiology of Body Fluids and Fluid Therapy*

Raymond D. Adelman ■ Michael J. Solhaug

An understanding of the normal physiology of body fluids is important to managing the abnormalities that alter the normal condition. The discussion of normal body fluid physiology includes the following:

The total amounts of water and solutes in the body as a whole result from carefully regulated balances of intake and output. Many controlling mechanisms, especially for substances having physiologic significance, are extremely complex. Those especially important to the clinician are discussed in some detail.

The distribution of water and the concentration of solutes in the various compartments of the body are critically important because considerable energy is required to maintain steady-state equilibria for most substances. The concentration of solutes depends on the relative amounts of solute and solvent (i.e., water) in that compartment.

The regulation of the fluid compartments that maintain physiologic balance by preventing large changes in solute concentrations, which could disturb function, is addressed in this Part. Alterations of normal body fluid physiology by diseases or other processes are managed best when the expected physiologic responses are known and the physiologic impact of the corrective therapies are fully understood. ■

CHAPTER 45
Water

TOTAL BODY WATER. Water is the most important solvent in the fluid composition of living systems. Total body metabolism of water is maintained by several mechanisms that control water intake and output, but it is balanced principally through excretion of water by the kidney.

Total body water (TBW) as a percentage of body weight changes with age, decreasing rapidly in early life (Fig. 45–1). Prenatally, TBW decreases during gestation. At birth, TBW is 78% of body weight. In the first few months of life, TBW drops dramatically to approximate the adult level of 55–60% of body weight at 1 yr of age. At puberty, a further change in TBW takes place. Because fat has a low water content, TBW as a percentage of body weight is lower in mature women, who have greater amounts of body fat, 55%, than men, 60%. Increased body fat in obese children at any age has a similar effect on TBW. In the nonobese child, a close linear relationship is maintained between TBW and body weight, and TBW can be calculated using body weight alone: TBW (L) = 0.61 × weight (kg) + 0.251.

FLUID COMPARTMENTS. TBW consists of intracellular fluid (ICF) and extracellular fluid (ECF) compartments (Fig. 45–2). In the fetus, the ECF volume is larger than the ICF volume, and the ECF decreases with age. The ECF volume drops precipitously after birth, in large part because of postnatal diuresis. As the ECF volume continues to fall in the 1st yr of life the ICF volume increases, to achieve a ratio of ICF to ECF close to adult levels after 1 yr of age. The relative loss of ECF beyond the immediate postnatal diuresis results from the increasing growth of cellular tissue and the decreasing rate of growth of collagen relative to muscle during the early months of life.

In older children, the ECF volume bears a fairly straight-line relationship to weight and to TBW in normal infants and children (ECF [L] = 0.239 × weight [kg] + 0.325). Under conditions of normal hydration in the older child, exchangeable ECF constitutes 20–25% of body weight and is composed of plasma water (5% of body weight) and interstitial water (15% of body weight) (see Fig. 45–2). At puberty, the ECF volume differs little between males and females. However, because of decreased TBW at this age, girls have a lower ICF volume than boys.

The ICF volume is bounded by the membranes of the cells of the soft tissues. The ICF volume, representing the difference between TBW and extracellular water, is approximately 30–40% of body weight. Although frequently considered a homogeneous fluid, the ICF represents the sum of fluids from the

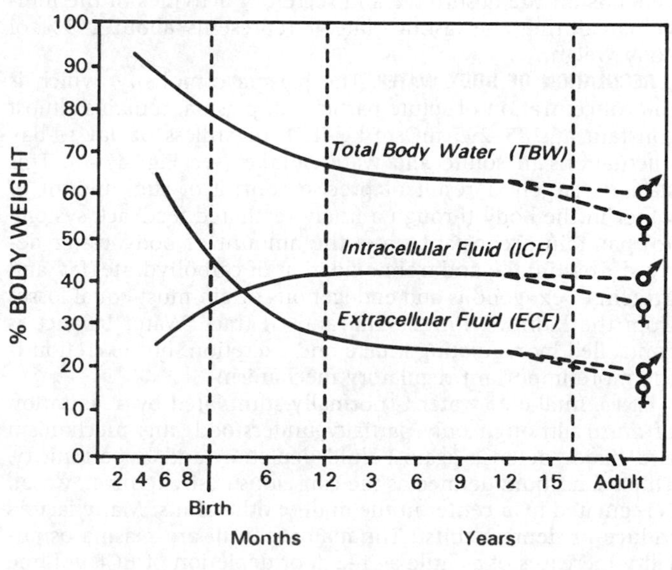

Figure 45–1 Total body water, intracellular fluid, and extracellular fluid as a percentage of body weight and a function of age. (From Winters RW: Water and electrolyte regulation. *In:* Winters RW [ed]: The Body Fluids in Pediatrics. Boston, Little, Brown & Company, 1973.)

*Modified from the 14th edition written by Alan Robson.

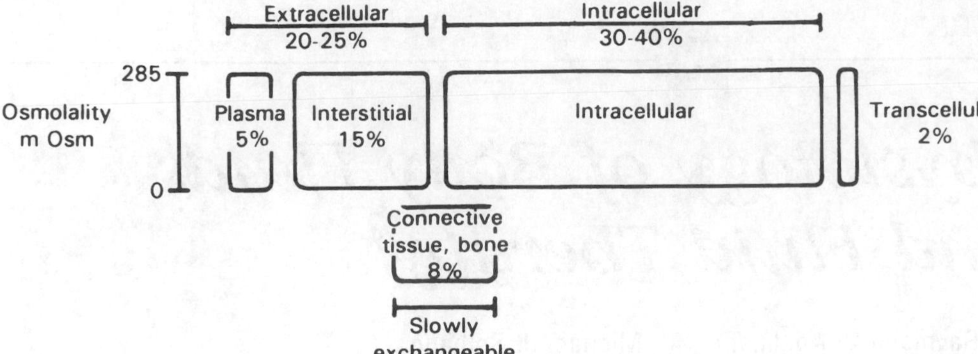

Figure 45–2 Total body water distribution as a percentage of body weight in an older child. (Adapted from Edelman IS, Leibman J: Am J Med 27:256, 1959.)

cells in different locations that have various functions and different intracellular compositions.

The remaining two body water compartments are the transcellular and the slowly exchangeable compartments. Although actually extracellular because of their unique characteristics, these compartments are less important under normal conditions than the ICF and ECF. However, some clinical conditions, especially in the gastrointestinal (GI) tract, render the transcellular compartment an important repository of body water. The *slowly exchangeable fluid compartment,* composing 8–10% of body weight, is contained in bone, dense connective tissue, and cartilage (see Fig. 45–2). Because of its poorly exchangeable nature, this compartment is not accessible to the body fluid regulatory mechanisms. However, fluid infused into the bone compartment can enter the plasma volume, an important physiologic relationship in situations necessitating interosseous fluid resuscitation (see Chapters 58 and 64.2).

The *transcellular water compartment* is influenced by transepithelial transport and, under normal conditions, is more accurately described as extracorporeal. The components of the transcellular fluid compartment are essentially reservoirs of the ECF compartment. The most quantitatively important components of transcellular fluid are the GI tract secretions and the urine in the kidneys and lower urinary tract. Transcellular fluid is also located in cerebrospinal, intraocular, pleural, peritoneal, and synovial fluids. The volume of the transcellular compartment, especially the GI component, varies greatly and depends on the absorptive and secretory activities of the individual; during the fasting state it represents about 1–3% of body weight.

REGULATION OF BODY WATER. The plasma osmolality, which is the concentration of solute particles in plasma, remains almost constant at 285–295 mOsm/kg H_2O, regardless of day-to-day fluctuations in solute and water intake (see Fig. 45–2). This stasis is largely a result of precise control of the amount of water in the body through a finely regulated feedback system. To maintain a constant state, the amount of body water derived from intake and from oxidation of carbohydrate, fat, and protein of exogenous and endogenous origin must equal losses from the kidneys, lungs, skin, and GI tract. Water balance is controlled by regulating intake and excretion, but excretion is the more important regulatory mechanism.

Intake. Intake of water is normally stimulated by a sensation of *thirst;* although only partially understood, this mechanism is a major defense against fluid depletion and hypertonicity. Thirst sensation, defined as the conscious desire to drink water, is regulated by a center in the midhypothalamus. Many factors induce or depress thirst. The major stimuli are plasma osmolality increases of as little as 1–2% or depletion of ECF volume by 10% or more, as occurs with hemorrhage or sodium depletion. The changes in plasma osmolality are monitored by osmoreceptors located in the hypothalamus and possibly located in the pancreas and hepatic portal vein. The mechanisms by which volume depletion induces thirst are less well understood, but depletion may be monitored by baroreceptors in the atria and elsewhere in the vascular bed. Considerable circumstantial evidence suggests that elevated plasma levels of angiotensin II stimulate drinking and may mediate thirst in hypovolemic and hypotensive states.

In clinical situations of conflicting conditions such as decreased plasma osmolality and decreased intravascular volume, the ECF volume changes dominate, and the resultant stimulated thirst causes increased water intake, restoring volume at the expense of tonicity.

The thirst mechanism and the release of antidiuretic hormone (ADH, i.e., arginine vasopressin) may be interrelated. However, at least some of the thirst centers are separated functionally and physically from those involved in release of ADH.

Disorders of the thirst mechanism may be seen in psychologic disorders, diseases of the central nervous system (CNS), potassium deficiency, malnutrition, and alterations in the renin-angiotensin system. These may lead to increased drinking, even though the content of body water is greater than usual and plasma osmolality is decreased, or to a decrease in drinking, as in adipsia.

Excretion. Body water losses can occur from the lungs, skin, GI tract, and kidneys. *Obligatory water losses* represent the minimum volume of fluid a person must ingest every day to maintain fluid balance. After the expenditure of energy, obligatory water losses include *insensible water losses,* which are mainly evaporative water loss from the lungs and skin; *urinary water excretion,* which represents the amount of water necessary to excrete a solute load by the kidneys; and *stool water losses,* which under normal conditions are small but can account for significant water losses during intestinal diseases.

Unlike the excretion of water by the kidneys, which responds to the content of water and solute in the body, *insensible water losses* are regulated by factors generally independent of body water. Because they are evaporative water losses, they are proportionate to the surface area of the body and are influenced by body and environmental temperatures, by the rate of respiration, and by the partial pressure of water vapor in the environment. Evaporative water losses cannot be used to regulate water losses that occur because of changes in the body's water content. The rate of sweating varies with the body temperature and is controlled, in part, by the autonomic nervous system. It may be reduced in heat stress by *severe* deficits in volume of body fluids or in the concentration of electrolytes, but this does not represent a major mechanism for regulating body water. Because of their proportionately high body surface area, premature newborns have much larger evaporative water losses than term newborns and older infants and children. This increased insensible water loss must be taken into account when formulating a fluid management plan for these infants (see Chapter 93).

Urinary water excretion is obligatory, and because an important function of the kidney is to maintain body homeostasis, urinary water excretion closely regulates the composition and volume of ECF. Excess accumulated urea, the end product of protein breakdown, and mineral salts, chiefly dietary sodium, are excreted in the urine daily. The resulting urinary solute load requires a necessary volume of urine for excretion. Alterations in ECF osmolality also require regulation through urinary water excretion. A fall in plasma osmolality, indicating relative excess of water, is corrected by the excretion of an increased volume of dilute urine that has an osmolality below that of plasma. This loss of free water restores plasma osmolality to normal. Conversely, when plasma osmolality rises above normal, the volume of urine falls, and its osmolality rises above that of plasma. This regulation of urine volume and concentration depends principally on the neurohypophyseal-renal axis, the effector of which is ADH. However, because urine volume can be reduced to only that necessary to excrete the solute load, it is also influenced by diet. Other factors that influence urine water output include the glomerular filtration rate (GFR), the state of the renal tubular epithelium, thyroid function, and plasma concentrations of adrenal steroids.

Urinary water excretion is regulated by two complementary mechanisms: the production, storage, and release into the circulation of *ADH;* and the *renal epithelial tubular cell response to ADH,* determined principally by ADH receptor activity of the collecting duct cells and the maintenance of a medullary concentration gradient to provide the passive reabsorption of water. Human ADH, a cyclic octapeptide, is synthesized in the supraoptic nuclei. This neurosecretory substance is transported down axons that descend through the infundibular stem to be stored in the terminal arborizations in the pars nervosa of the posterior pituitary. Release of ADH into the bloodstream occurs by exocytosis in response to stimuli from the hypothalamus. Depletion of ADH in the posterior pituitary occurs in animals deprived of water; storage occurs when water loads are administered (Chapter 55).

Secretion of ADH is regulated by the effective osmotic pressure of the ECF. Pressure is produced by solutes (primarily sodium and chloride) that do not readily penetrate cell membranes. This process is monitored by vesicles in the supraoptic nuclei that act as osmoreceptors. They swell when the osmolality of the ECF is less than that of the ICF and shrink when the osmolality of the ECF exceeds that of the ICF. Administering urea, which readily diffuses across cell membranes to increase the osmolality of the ECF and ICF, produces little shift of water between cells and interstitial fluids and does not evoke consistent antidiuresis. However, intravenous hypertonic saline solution evokes intense antidiuresis; the sodium remains predominantly in the ECF, increasing its osmolality in relation to that of the ICF. Conversely, administering water inhibits the release of ADH.

Normally, the threshold for release of ADH is 280 mOsm/kg of H_2O. Release of vasopressin may be initiated or inhibited with changes in plasma osmolality of as little as 1–2%. The response is graded, permitting the urine volume and the osmolality of the ECF to be continuously regulated, preventing the fluctuations in osmolality that would occur as a consequence of normal variations in intake of fluid and solutes. Levels of ADH also increase significantly after 8% or greater dehydration, and the rise is exponential with more marked dehydration.

The *primary action of ADH* is to increase the permeability of the renal collecting ducts to water. Under conditions of antidiuresis, the interstitium of the renal medulla has an osmolality of as much as 1,200 mOsm/kg H_2O at the level of the papilla. This level of osmolality is achieved by the actions of the countercurrent multiplier (i.e., loops of Henle) and the exchange (i.e., medullary vasa recta blood vessels) systems. ADH activation of specific receptors on the collecting duct cell membrane triggers a series of intracellular events that result in the increase in the cell membrane permeability to water. In the presence of ADH, luminal urine entering the collecting duct has an osmolality of about 285 mOsm/kg H_2O and becomes progressively more concentrated along the course of the collecting duct as water diffuses out of the urine into the hypertonic medullary interstitium by passive osmotic diffusion. By the time the urine enters the calyces, it has achieved the same concentration as the fluid in the hypertonic medullary papillae. Continued reabsorption of sodium in the distal tubule and collecting duct further dilutes the urine. In the absence of ADH, these segments of the nephron are impermeable to water, diffusion into the hypertonic medulla does not occur, and dilute urine is formed.

PATHOPHYSIOLOGIC CONDITIONS. Diabetes insipidus is a specific disease state caused by an inability to effectively conserve urinary water (Chapter 568). The clinical result of excessive urinary water loss is increased concentration of ECF solute (mainly sodium), or hypernatremia. The two types of diabetes insipidus are named according to the site of abnormal function: central and nephrogenic. Central diabetes insipidus occurs if ADH is not released into the circulation. This abnormality is produced by an interruption of the supraoptic-osmoreceptor-hypophyseal axis, preventing the release of ADH in the circulation despite appropriate physiologic stimuli, such as increases in plasma osmolality. In nephrogenic diabetes insipidus, ADH is normally released in response to plasma osmolality changes, but the renal collecting ducts fail to respond to the ADH, often because of a defect in the epithelial cell membrane receptor for ADH.

Factors altering ADH release disrupt the normal mechanisms that regulate it (Chapter 569). ADH release may be stimulated or inhibited by emotional factors. Stressful stimuli such as pain or the mass discharge of peripheral receptors resulting from trauma, burns, or surgery increase ADH output and are important considerations in devising appropriate fluid therapy. Nicotine, prostaglandins, and cholinergic and α-adrenergic drugs are potent stimulators of ADH output. Demerol, morphine, and barbiturates are probably antidiuretic in this way, although their reduction of the GFR may also contribute to their effects in reducing urine flow. Alcohol is a potent inhibitor of ADH release, with a consistent dose-response relationship. Phenytoin and possibly glucocorticoids also inhibit ADH release.

Factors altering the renal response to ADH produce increased urinary excretion of water despite appropriate ADH levels. Anesthesia reduces urinary flow, probably by altering renal hemodynamics. The presence of nonabsorbable, osmotically active solutes in the renal tubular lumen (e.g., glucose in diabetes mellitus) reduces the amount of water than can diffuse into the hypertonic medulla and limits the ability of ADH to conserve water. Intrinsic renal conditions, such as urinary tract obstruction (particularly if it occurs in utero), tubular damage from nephrotoxins or tubular necrosis, and advanced renal disease can reduce renal responsiveness to ADH.

MECHANISMS FOR DISTRIBUTING FLUID WITHIN THE BODY. The distribution of water between the ICF and ECF is determined by physical factors. The *maintenance of the ICF volume* is affected by factors that regulate the concentration of solute within the cell and by the ECF. The ICF volume is maintained relatively constant by osmotic forces operating across cell membranes freely permeable to water. The maintenance of these forces depends on the active transport of potassium into and sodium out of cells by energy-requiring processes, but no evidence exists for active transport or secretion of water. A rise in extracellular osmolality (e.g., with a sodium load) results in a decrease in cell water. Conversely, water intoxication decreases extracellular osmolality and leads to an increase in cell volume. Disturbances in cellular function may also result in an increase in the fluid content of cells.

Maintenance of the ECF volume is critical for the preservation of a normal plasma volume. The amount of fluid in the *plasma volume* (i.e., plasma water) is maintained in a steady state by a balance between renal regulation of solute and water excretion

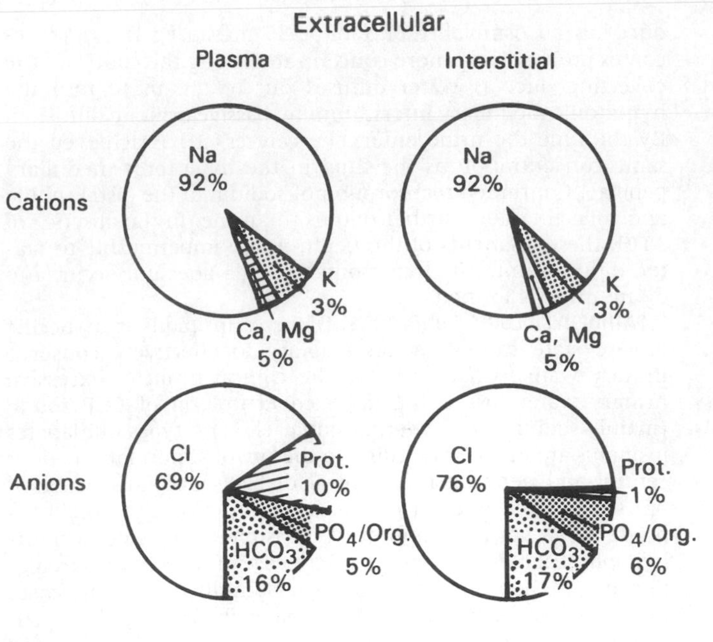

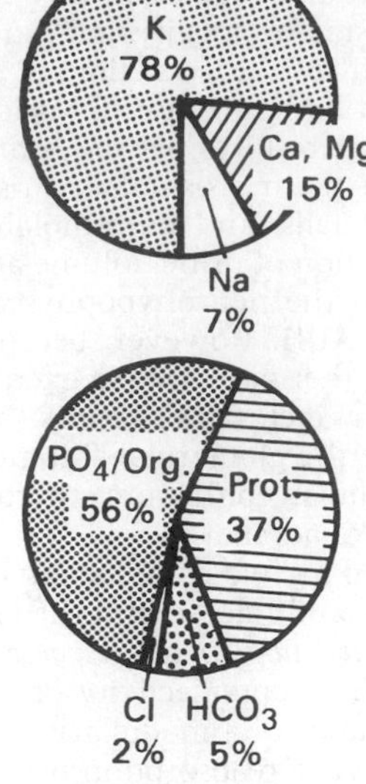

Figure 45–3 The concentrations of the major cations and anions in the extracellular fluid (i.e., plasma and interstitial fluids) and intracellular fluids as a percentage of total electrolyte composition. Na, sodium; K, potassium; Ca, calcium; Mg, magnesium; HCO_3, bicarbonate; PO_4/Org., phosphorus and organ anions; Prot., proteins.

and oncotic forces at the capillary level. Oncotic pressure (i.e., colloid osmotic pressure) represents only a small fraction of the total osmotic pressure,* but its osmotic pressure is exerted by molecules, primarily albumin, that do not readily pass through the capillary pores. The colloid osmotic pressure produces an effective osmotic gradient across capillary walls.

At the arteriolar end of the capillaries, the dominant effect of intracapillary hydrostatic pressure results in a net loss of plasma ultrafiltrate. Normally, at the venous end of the capillary, oncotic pressure causes the net return of a somewhat smaller amount of fluid and electrolytes, with the difference returned to the vascular space through the lymphatic system.

Decreases in protein concentration, as in the nephrotic syndrome, may lead to reductions in plasma volume and equivalent increases in *interstitial volume*. These changes may compromise the intravascular volume enough to reduce the GFR and blood flow to other vital organs. Because the volume of plasma is only one-third that of interstitial fluid, plasma volume reduction achieved by shifting water into the interstitial space may not be observed clinically as *edema*. An increase in capillary permeability to protein, as in angioneurotic edema and diffuse capillary leak syndromes, produces a rise in protein concentration of the interstitial fluid. This rise reduces plasma oncotic pressure, causing a net shift of fluid to the interstitium. The increase may be generalized or localized, appearing as a wheal or urticaria.

Interstitial fluid volume may also be increased by a rise in the hydrostatic pressure at the venous end of the capillary, as occurs with increased venous pressure associated with heart failure or with retention of sodium and resultant hypervolemia in glomerulonephritis.

The *transcellular fluid* space may increase markedly in inflammatory bowel disease, in early severe diarrhea, or in ileus with multiple fluid levels.

OSMOLALITY OF BODY FLUIDS. Individual solute concentrations in the ECF and ICF vary (Fig. 45–3), but the total ionic concentration in the compartments is balanced between cations and anions. The osmolality in the ECF and ICF compartments is balanced as well (see Fig. 45–2). Except for transient changes, the ECF and ICF compartments are in osmotic equilibrium. Because the cell membranes are highly permeable to water, a change in the osmolality of either fluid compartment results in the rapid movement of water to achieve an equilibration of osmolality. Because of its abundance in plasma and interstitial fluids (see Fig. 45–3), sodium is the most important cation contributing to extracellular osmolality. Because sodium and its accompanying anions, chloride and bicarbonate, account for 90% or more of plasma osmolality, a rough estimate of ECF osmolality can be obtained by doubling the plasma sodium concentration. For example, if the normal sodium concentration of plasma is 140 mEq/L, the estimated plasma osmolality is 280 mOsm/L. There are two important exceptions to this rule: hyperglycemia and hyperlipidemia.

Of the nonelectrolytes in plasma, the most important contributor to osmolality is glucose, which does not freely penetrate the cells. At normal plasma glucose concentrations, glucose provides 3–5 mOsm/L to plasma osmolality. However, the high plasma glucose concentrations occurring in diabetic ketoacidosis can increase plasma osmolality, shifting water from the ICF to the ECF compartment. The reduced plasma sodium concentration caused by the influx of water into the ECF volume produces an invalid measure of plasma osmolality. In treating diabetic patients, it is essential to recognize the impact of the changes in plasma glucose concentration on ECF osmolality and on water shifts between the fluid compartments.

The second condition, which does not allow use of plasma sodium to estimate plasma osmolality, occurs with increases in serum solids. For example, when serum solids such as the proteins and lipids are increased, the water content in the serum is markedly decreased (expressed per liter of serum) because of volume displacement of water by lipids. Because electrolytes are dissolved in the aqueous phase of serum, electrolyte concentrations such as that of sodium determined by flame photometry and expressed as milliequivalents per liter of serum appear decreased, even though the concentration per liter of serum water is normal. Treatment of such *pseudohyponatremia* is unnecessary and may be detrimental to the patient. Its occurrence can be recognized by measuring serum osmo-

*The principal colloids in the plasma are the plasma proteins, which exert an osmotic pressure of approximately 28 mm Hg, compared with the 5,100 mm Hg exerted by the plasma's crystalloid solutes. However, the capillary walls are very permeable to the crystalloid solutes, which exert no osmotic force across the capillary walls. Albumin, the most abundant plasma protein and the one having the lowest molecular weight, is the principal solute responsible for colloid osmotic pressure and for regulating net water movement across capillary walls.

lality by freezing point depression, a method that measures solute concentration of the water fraction of serum and more accurately reflects serum sodium concentration. The problem of pseudohyponatremia is avoided by methods measuring sodium concentration with ion-specific electrodes.

CHAPTER 46
Sodium

BODY CONTENT AND DISTRIBUTION OF SODIUM. Sodium, the bulk cation of the extracellular fluid (ECF), is the principal osmotically active solute responsible for the maintenance of intravascular and interstitial volumes. Of the total quantity of sodium in the body, more than 30% is nonexchangeable or only slowly exchangeable, bound in poorly mobilizable tissues (Fig. 46–1). Of total body sodium, 11% is in the plasma sodium pool, 29% is in the interstitial lymph fluid, and 2.5% is in the intracellular fluid (ICF). About 43% of total body sodium is in bone, but only one third of the sodium in bone is exchangeable. Dense connective tissue and cartilage contain 12% of body sodium, of which about two thirds is exchangeable (see Fig. 46–1). The *exchangeable sodium content of the fetus* averages 85 mEq/kg, compared with the adult value of 40 mEq/kg, because the fetus has relatively large amounts of cartilage, connective tissue, and ECF, all of which contain considerable amounts of sodium, and a relatively small mass of muscle cells, which have a low sodium content.

Although cell membranes are relatively permeable to it, sodium is predominantly distributed in the extracellular compartment. Intracellular concentrations are maintained at levels of approximately 10 mEq/L and extracellular concentrations at levels of approximately 140 mEq/L. The low intracellular concentration is achieved by active extrusion of sodium from cells by the sodium-potassium–activated and magnesium-activated ATPase systems. Calcium inhibits ATPase, as do ouabain and related cardiac glycosides.

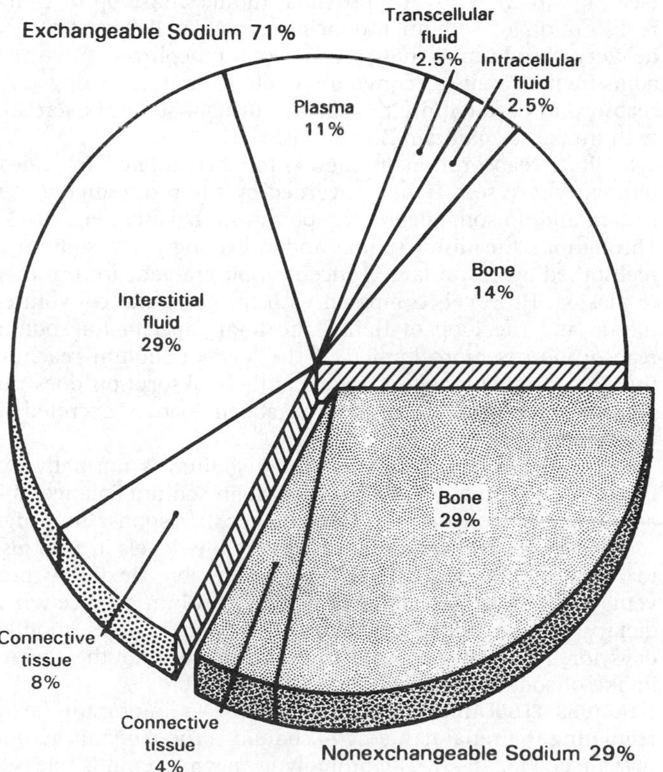

Figure 46–1 Distribution of body sodium as a percentage of the total. Exchangeable sodium (*clear*) and nonexchangeable sodium (*stippled*) are indicated. (From Frohnert pp: Body composition. *In:* Knox FG [ed]: Textbook of Renal Pathophysiology. Hagerstown, MD, Harper & Row, 1978.)

Although intracellular concentrations of sodium are low and represent a small part of total body sodium, they may be critical in modifying certain intracellular enzyme activities. The intracellular sodium content usually remains relatively constant, and changes in total body sodium reflect mostly changes in extracellular sodium. However, redistribution of sodium between the intracellular and extracellular compartments may occur in the absence of significant changes in total body sodium. Such a change (e.g., increased intracellular sodium) may be observed in the severely ill patient, in whom it usually is referred to as the sick cell syndrome. Intracellular sodium may also be increased in some forms of hypertension.

Because of the Donnan distribution of anionic proteins, the concentration of sodium in interstitial fluid is approximately 97% of that of the serum sodium value; changes in concentration of sodium in the serum are reflected by proportional changes in the concentration of sodium in the interstitial fluid. Concentrations of sodium in transcellular fluids vary considerably because such fluids are not in simple diffusion equilibrium with plasma. Unexpected changes in the composition of these fluids may occur and may necessitate changing the therapeutic regimens designed to replace their abnormal loss.

REGULATION OF SODIUM

Intake. The amount of sodium in the body is determined by the balance between intake and excretion. Compared with the thirst mechanism for water, the regulatory mechanism of sodium *intake* is poorly developed but may respond to large changes; for example, salt craving may occur in some patients with salt-wasting syndromes. However, sodium intake normally depends on cultural customs. In the United States, the average adult usually takes in about 170 mEq/24 hr, equivalent to 10 g of salt. Children take in less, proportionate to their smaller food intake but still well in excess of maintenance needs. Infants generally have a relatively high sodium intake because of the high sodium content of cow's milk (21 mEq/L). The sodium content of many infant formulas is also high compared with that of breast milk (7 mEq/L). The sodium dietary intake of older children and adolescents varies but usually is relatively high because of ingestion of fast foods and junk foods.

Absorption. Occurring throughout the gastrointestinal tract, minimally in the stomach and maximally in the jejunum, absorption probably takes place by way of a sodium-potassium–activated adenosine triphosphatase (ATPase) system, which facilitates the movement of sodium by a transport protein that couples sodium with glucose. The intestinal transport mechanism of sodium is augmented by aldosterone or desoxycorticosterone acetate.

Excretion. Sodium excretion occurs through urine, sweat, and feces. The kidney is the principal organ for the facultative regulation of sodium output. Normally, the concentration of sodium in sweat ranges from 5–40 mEq/L. Higher values are seen in cystic fibrosis, which may contribute to body loss of sodium, and Addison's disease; lower values are observed in sodium depletion states and hyperaldosteronism. There is little evidence that changes in the level of sodium in sweat are part of the excretory mechanism for regulating the sodium content of the body under normal circumstances. In the absence of diarrhea, fecal concentrations of sodium are low.

RENAL REGULATION OF SODIUM EXCRETION. Renal regulation of sodium depends on a balance between glomerular filtration and tubular reabsorption. Normally, the amount of sodium filtered daily by the kidneys is more than 100 times that ingested and more than five times the total amount of sodium in the body. However, of the total amount of sodium filtered by the kidneys each day (25,200 mEq/24 hr) less than 1%, or 50 mEq/24 hr, is excreted in the urine; the remaining 99% is reabsorbed along the length of the renal tubule, representing the result of a highly efficient regulatory process.

Glomerular Filtration of Sodium. Under normal conditions, changes in glomerular filtration rate (GFR) do not affect sodium homeostasis. A constant fraction of the filtered load of sodium is reabsorbed in the proximal tubule despite transient, spontaneous variations in the GFR. This balance of filtration and reabsorption, called glomerular-tubular balance, reduces the impact of spontaneous changes in GFR on the amount of renal sodium excretion. Moreover, sodium balance can be achieved when the GFR remains stable even though sodium intake varies. However, the GFR may play a role in sodium excretion during conditions that also stimulate sodium regulatory mechanisms through changes in extracellular volume. The factors that affect the GFR and promote sodium reabsorption in response to a decrease in extracellular volume, such as in hemorrhage or dehydration, are activation of sympathetic renal nervous system and stimulation of the renin-angiotensin system. When extracellular volume expansion occurs, atrial natriuretic peptide (ANP) is released into the circulation from the cardiac atria and causes increased urinary losses of sodium, in part as a response to increased GFR.

Tubular Reabsorption of Sodium. The integrated action of all the nephron segments results in the regulation of renal sodium excretion (Fig. 46–2). Renal sodium handling is characterized by two coordinated tubular processes. First, reabsorption of sodium in the proximal tubule and loop of Henle delivers a constant proportion of the filtered load of sodium to the distal nephron. Second, reabsorption of sodium in the distal tubule and collecting duct is the fine regulator of the final amount of sodium excreted, which closely matches the amount of sodium ingested. Under normal circumstances, approximately two thirds of the filtered sodium is reabsorbed by the proximal convoluted tubule (see Fig. 46–2).

Because the percentages of filtered sodium and water reabsorbed in the proximal tubule are proportional, the fluid remaining at the end of the proximal convoluted tubule has a sodium concentration comparable to that in the plasma. Net movement of sodium out of the proximal tubule represents the balance between sodium reabsorbed from the luminal fluid

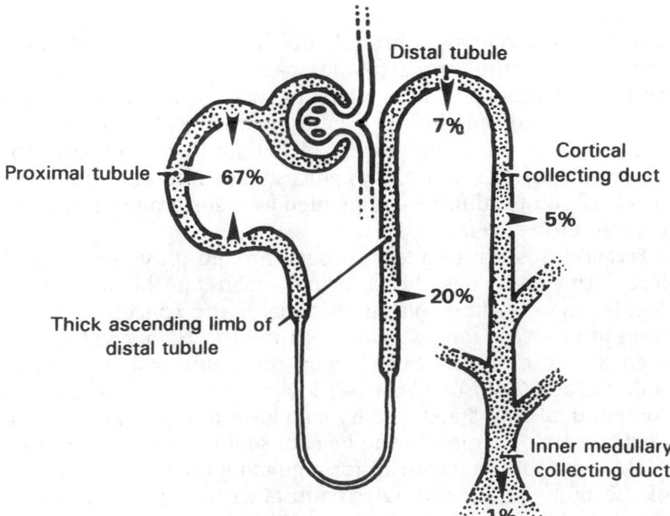

Figure 46–2 Segmental sodium reabsorption along the nephron as a percentage of the filtered load of sodium. (From Koeppen BM, Stanton BA: Renal Physiology. St. Louis, Mosby–Year Book, 1992.)

(i.e., transcellular and paracellular) and that returned through intercellular spaces. The movement of transcellularly reabsorbed sodium across the proximal tubule cell membrane is coupled with the reabsorption of organic solutes and anions, such as glucose and chloride, and facilitated by specific membrane transport proteins. Reabsorbed sodium is actively transported out of the cells across their basolateral membranes, producing an osmotic gradient that causes the movement of an equivalent amount of water. The resulting hydrostatic force in the intercellular spaces and interstitial fluid, as well as the exertion of oncotic pressure by the plasma protein in the peritubular capillary, is responsible for returning the reabsorbed sodium and water into the peritubular capillary and, ultimately, into the systemic circulation.

Significant sodium reabsorption (approximately 20%) occurs in the *loop of Henle* (see Fig. 46–2) and is central to the countercurrent multiplier system essential for water balance and the concentration of urine. Water reabsorption occurs in the descending limb of the loop of Henle, and sodium reabsorption occurs in the ascending limb. Sodium transport at the thick ascending limb is active; it may be secondary to the active transport of chloride, rather than primary, as it is at most other sites. Although the loop of Henle is important in the overall control of sodium reabsorption, no precise regulating mechanism has been delineated, nor has a maximal rate for sodium transport at this site been demonstrated. When the load of sodium delivered to the loop is increased by changes in the GFR or in sodium reabsorption in the proximal tubule, most of the excess load is reabsorbed in the loop, providing a further protective mechanism and limiting the magnitude of changes of sodium delivery to the distal convoluted tubule.

The fine regulation of sodium balance probably occurs throughout the distal nephron in the *distal convoluted tubules* and the *collecting ducts*. The distal convoluted tubule reabsorbs 7% and the collecting duct 5% of the filtered load of sodium (see Fig. 46–2). With the proximal tubule and loop of Henle reabsorption of sodium producing a regulated, proportioned delivery of sodium to these sections of the nephron, only small adjustments in distal convoluted tubule and collecting duct reabsorption are required to balance urinary sodium excretion with intake to maintain homeostasis.

Sodium reabsorption at these sites is regulated by aldosterone, whose secretion is governed by the renin-angiotensin system and, to some degree, by potassium balance (Fig. 46–3). Throughout the distal tubule and collecting duct, sodium is reabsorbed against a large concentration gradient from lumen to plasma. However, compared with the proximal convoluted tubule and the loop of Henle, the total capacity for sodium reabsorption is more limited. If the load of sodium reaching the distal tubule increases significantly, reabsorption does not increase proportionately, and the added load is excreted in the urine.

In health, less than 1% of filtered sodium is normally excreted in the urine. However, to maintain sodium balance, this amount may increase to 10% or higher in response to a high sodium intake and can decrease to very low levels in response to reduced dietary sodium. The considerable flexibility prevents a significantly positive or negative sodium balance when dietary sodium intake fluctuates. However, it takes about 3 days for a new steady state to be achieved after the dietary intake of sodium has been markedly altered.

FACTORS REGULATING SODIUM EXCRETION. An important factor regulating the renal handling of sodium is the *renin-angiotensin system* (see Fig. 46–3). The proteolytic enzyme renin is released from the juxtaglomerular apparatus, which is anatomically composed of the specialized cells in the afferent arteriole and in the segment of the distal tubule that contacts the glomerular vascular pole, the macula densa. Stimuli for the release of renin include decreases in renal perfusion pressure detected

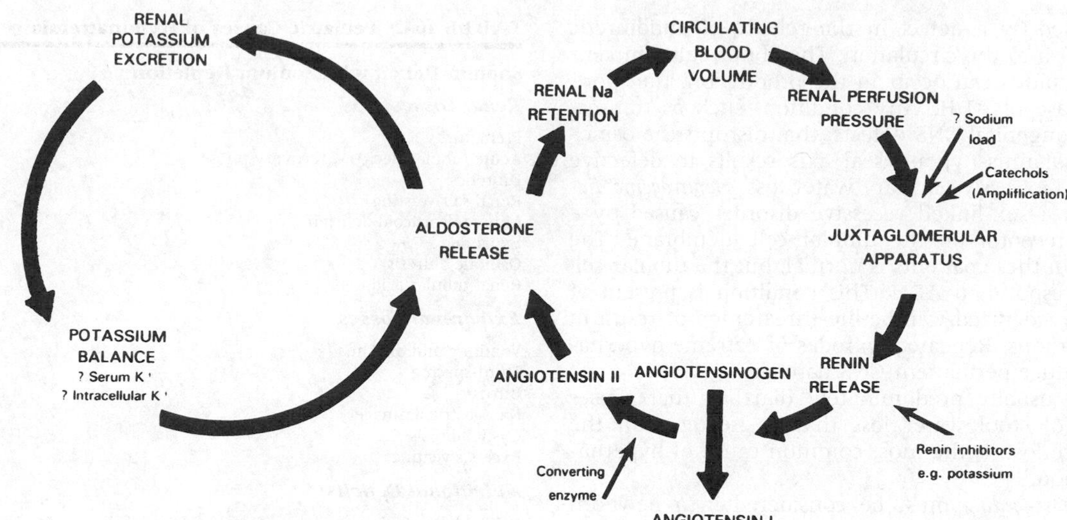

Figure 46–3 Correlations of the volume and potassium feedback loops with aldosterone secretion. Integration of the signals from each loop determines the level of aldosterone secretion. (From Williams GH, Dluhy RG: Aldosterone biosynthesis: Interrelationship of regulating factors. Am J Med 53:595, 1972.)

in the afferent arteriole and a decrease in sodium chloride concentration or delivery to the macula densa.

Angiotensin I is formed by cleavage of the substrate angiotensinogen by renin. Angiotensin I is converted to angiotensin II by a specific converting enzyme. Angiotensin II, by inhibiting renin secretion, acts as a negative-feedback regulator of renin release. The renin-angiotensin system regulates tubular sodium reabsorption by the direct stimulation of sodium reabsorption in the proximal tubule by angiotensin II and by the stimulation of *aldosterone* secretion by angiotensin II. Aldosterone, a mineralocorticoid produced in the adrenal gland, is an important promoter of sodium reabsorption in the late distal convoluted tubule and collecting duct. As it increases sodium reabsorption, aldosterone also increases potassium secretion and the loss of potassium in the urine. In general, activation of the renin-angiotensin system enhances tubular reabsorption of sodium and results in decreased urinary sodium excretion. Under conditions of extracellular volume expansion or plasma sodium excess, the renin-angiotensin system is suppressed and urinary sodium excretion is increased.

Atrial natriuretic peptide (ANP) is a potent natriuretic and diuretic peptide hormone produced and stored in the atrial myocytes. The target organ of ANP is the kidney, in which it increases sodium and water excretion. ANP is released into the circulation from its cardiac location in response to expansion of the ECF volume and the resulting stretch of the cardiac atria. The urinary sodium and water excretory actions of ANP generally antagonize the sodium-retaining mechanisms of the renin-angiotensin system. ANP is an important regulator of acute or short-term changes in ECF volume. However, the role for ANP as a long-term regulator of sodium homeostasis is less certain.

Starling forces in the intercellular space of the proximal tubule cells and the interstitial space between the tubular cells and the peritubular capillaries influence the movement of reabsorbed solute and water into the peritubular capillaries. Normally, the sum of Starling forces favors the movement of solute and water from the intercellular and interstitial spaces into the peritubular capillary. Reabsorbed solute and water are returned to the tubular lumen through paracellular pathways when the normal balance of these forces is altered. Rapid expansion of the ECF volume increases the interstitial hydrostatic pressure, preventing sodium reabsorption and producing increased urinary sodium excretion.

PATHOPHYSIOLOGIC CONDITIONS. Changes in serum sodium concentration in the absence of serum solids excess, such as hyperlipidemia or hyperglycemia, usually result from changes in body water or sodium, or a combination of the two. The serum sodium concentration does not necessarily reflect the status of total body sodium content, as previously described. A particular abnormality of serum sodium concentration must be understood in the context of sodium and water regulation.

Hypernatremia. Hypernatremia (serum sodium >150 mEq/L) is caused by conditions that produce an excessive gain of sodium or result in an excessive loss of body water that is greater than the loss of sodium. Hypernatremia due to an excessive gain of sodium, primary sodium excess (Table 46–1), is usually associated with iatrogenic causes: the substitution of NaCl for glucose in infant formulas prepared on site from basic ingredients, the overuse of saline enemas, inappropriate intravenous administration of hypertonic saline solutions, and NaCl used to induce vomiting. The more commonly encountered causes of hypernatremia are those caused by a primary water deficit (see Table 46–1), in which the loss of total body water exceeds any loss of sodium.

Diabetes insipidus (see Chapter 45) is caused by one of two fundamental defects in renal water regulation. *Central diabetes*

TABLE 46–1 Pediatric Causes of Hypernatremia

Primary Sodium Excess

Improperly mixed formula or rehydration solution
Accidental substitution of NaCl for glucose in infant formulas
Excessive sodium bicarbonate during resuscitation
Hypernatremic enemas
Ingestion of seawater
Hypertonic saline intravenous administration
NaCl used to induce vomiting
Intentional salt poisoning (i.e., Münchausen by proxy)
High breast milk sodium

Primary Water Deficit

Diabetes insipidus
  Central
  Nephrogenic
Diabetes mellitus or other solute diuresis
Gastroenteritis (i.e., water loss greater than solute loss)
Inadequate breast-feeding
Intentional withholding of water intake
Increased insensible water loss (e.g., premature infant)
Adipsia
Inadequate access to free water

insipidus is caused by a defect in the release of antidiuretic hormone (ADH) into the circulation. The abnormality in central diabetes insipidus can occur in the production, transport, storage, or release of ADH. Any condition, such as trauma, neoplasms, or congenital CNS defects, that disrupts the osmoreceptor-hypothalamus-hypophyseal axis results in defective ADH release and excessive urinary water loss. *Nephrogenic diabetes insipidus* is a sex-linked recessive disorder caused by a defective ADH receptor on the tubular cell membrane. The release of ADH in these patients is normal, but the tubular cell is not able to respond to ADH. This condition is present at birth and, if unrecognized, can be life-threatening or result in serious complications. Repeated episodes of extreme hypernatremia may produce permanent CNS damage.

Gastroenteritis, usually predominately diarrhea that causes large amounts of stool water loss that is greater than the amount of solute lost, is the most common cause of hypernatremia in childhood.

Inadequate breast-feeding must be considered in a newborn with hypernatremia. In most of these cases, the breast milk sodium concentration is not elevated, but there have been case reports of hypernatremia associated with elevated breast milk sodium concentration. In an otherwise normal infant, decreased water intake from an inadequate breast milk supply cannot match the obligatory water losses, and hypernatremia ensues.

Withholding of water intake may produce hypernatremia if the water intake is withheld to such a degree that it is exceeded by obligatory water losses. Two groups of children are vulnerable to developing this type of hypernatremia: neurologically compromised individuals who cannot express thirst or obtain water and severely abused children. Lack of access to water also occurs in children who, because of age or a handicapping condition, cannot provide themselves with water intake.

Hyponatremia. Hyponatremia (serum sodium <130 mEq/L) is caused by conditions that create primary sodium deficits resulting in the depletion of sodium; produce a gain in total body water; or combine sodium and water abnormalities (Table 46–2).

TABLE 46–2 Pediatric Causes of Hyponatremia

Sodium Deficit with Sodium Depletion

Renal Losses

Prematurity
Acute tubular necrosis, recovery phase
Diuretics
Renal salt-wasting
Mineralocorticoid deficiency
Expanded ECF
Osmotic diuresis
Renal tubular acidosis

Extrarenal Losses

Vomiting and diarrhea
Third-spacing
Burns
Nasogastric drainage
Cystic fibrosis
Excess sweating

Nutritional Deficits

WIC syndrome (i.e., inadequate oral sodium intake)
Inadequate sodium in parenteral fluids
Cerebrospinal fluid drainage
Burns
Paracentesis

Water Excess with Water Gain

Syndrome of inappropriate ADH secretion
Glucocorticoid deficiency
Hypothyroidism
Drugs
Excess parenteral fluid administration
Psychogenic polydipsia
Tap water enemas

Excess of Sodium and Water

Nephrotic syndrome
Cirrhosis
Cardiac failure
Acute and chronic renal failure

Primary sodium deficits involve a disruption in renal sodium handling. *Renal sodium losses* occur in conditions with intrinsic renal defects in sodium regulation. Premature infants can lose sodium in the urine because of the immaturity of the sodium reabsorptive capacity. *Renal salt wasting* due to congenital urinary tract anomalies, obstruction, hypoplasia, dysplasia, or other congenital renal diseases, such as medullary sponge kidney, produce significant urinary sodium losses despite a low serum sodium. Adrenal insufficiency resulting in *mineralocorticoid deficiency* is most commonly seen in children with congenital adrenal hyperplasia. Renal losses of sodium also occur during the recovery phase of acute tubular necrosis and with the chronic use of diuretics and result from the osmotic diuresis that accompanies diabetes mellitus.

Extrarenal losses of sodium often accompany gastrointestinal fluid losses, through unreplaced nasogastric fluid losses or from gastroenteritis. This type of gastroenteritis, associated with intestinal water losses and significant sodium losses, usually includes vomiting and diarrhea. The hyponatremia produced by the greater loss of sodium than water is exacerbated by the intake of low-solute beverages.

The most common cause of hyponatremia due to decreased *nutritional* sodium intake is the *WIC syndrome*. This form of water intoxication is seen in small infants who receive large amounts of very low sodium–containing fluids, usually to the exclusion of normally concentrated formulas. These infants present with profound hyponatremia and serious CNS symptoms, such as seizures.

Of the disorders resulting in a primary water excess, the most common is the *syndrome of inappropriate ADH secretion (SIADH)*. This disorder, which has many potential causes, is marked by the secretion of ADH in the absence of a physiologic stimulus for its secretion. The increased ADH secretion increases collecting duct water reabsorption and dilutes the ECF, producing hyponatremia. In children, of the many conditions associated with SIADH, the most common is acute meningitis.

The *hyponatremia of water excess* involves the addition of excess water from an exogenous source, such as the use of dilute or sodium-poor intravenous fluids for the treatment of dehydration. Conditions producing hyponatremia combining abnormal retention of sodium and water usually involve the edema-forming diseases of *nephrotic syndrome* and *cirrhosis*. In these conditions, water shifts from plasma to the interstitial spaces, which stimulates thirst and releases ADH, causing water and sodium retention. The resulting water retention is greater than the sodium retention, producing hyponatremia. *Cardiac failure* activates similar water- and sodium-retaining mechanisms, but the plasma oncotic pressure remains normal.

CHAPTER 47
Potassium

BODY CONTENT AND DISTRIBUTION OF POTASSIUM. The body content of potassium, the major intracellular cation, correlates well with the lean body mass. Because potassium is predominantly intracellular (see Fig. 45–3), the change in body potassium content that occurs with growth is an excellent index of cellular mass at different ages. In the adult, 90% of total body potassium is exchangeable. The exchangeable components are intracellular potassium (89.6%) and extracellular potassium:plasma (0.4%) and interstitial lymph (1.0%). The remainder (10%) of total body potassium is nonexchangeable and is contained in dense connective tissue and cartilage (0.4%), bone (7.6%), and as a small amount of intracellular potassium (2%).

Intracellular concentrations of potassium approximate 150 mEq/L of cell water. The extracellular concentration of potassium (4 mEq/L) creates a large concentration difference across the cell membranes. The difference between intracellular and extracellular potassium, sustained by the action of Na^+, K^+-ATPase, is important for maintaining the resting membrane potential difference across the cell membrane. Potassium is critical for the excitability of nerve and muscle cells and for the contractility of cardiac, skeletal, and smooth muscle. Because of its intracellular osmotic contribution, potassium is also important for the maintenance of cell volume.

REGULATION OF POTASSIUM. Potassium exists in remarkably constant quantities in almost all animal and vegetable tissues. A daily intake of 1–2 mEq/kg body weight is recommended, but intakes vary widely. Absorption of potassium is reasonably complete in the upper gastrointestinal tract. More distally, body potassium is exchanged for sodium in the lumen of the lower bowel.

Two sets of mechanisms participate in potassium homeostasis. These mechanisms maintain an intracellular potassium concentration differential and match potassium dietary intake, mainly through regulating renal potassium excretion. Acute potassium loads require well-developed *extrarenal mechanisms* to prevent severe hyperkalemia and to avoid potassium toxicity. In the first 4–6 hr after a potassium load, only one half of the potassium is excreted by the kidneys. Some potassium is secreted into the intestinal tract. More than 40% is translocated into cells, primarily in the liver and muscle. This process is an important protective mechanism and is regulated by insulin and epinephrine, which enhance potassium uptake. The catecholamine effect appears to be mediated through α-receptors. Stimulation of α-adrenergic receptors impairs extrarenal disposal of an acute potassium load.

Aldosterone plays a key role in the renal and extrarenal handling of potassium. Its primary extrarenal site of action may be the gastrointestinal tract, although it also affects muscle transport of potassium. Glucocorticoids may be important in extrarenal potassium homeostasis. Glucagon infusion causes a transient hyperkalemia, but its role in potassium regulation is not clear.

The acid-base balance affects intracellular shifts of potassium. Systemic acidosis results in the movement of potassium out of cells; alkalosis produces the opposite effect. For every 0.1 unit change in blood pH, the plasma potassium concentration changes 0.3–1.3 mEq/L in the opposite direction. The changes depend on numerous factors. For example, the increase in serum potassium accompanying respiratory acidosis is much less than that with metabolic acidosis.

Chronic potassium balance is primarily regulated by the kidneys, which can adjust the amount of potassium excreted over a wide range. Normally, the rate of potassium excretion in the urine approximates 10–15% of that filtered. With the administration of large amounts of potassium, urinary excretion may be more than twice the amount filtered at the glomerulus. Conversely, urinary concentrations can be reduced to very low levels if potassium conservation is required. In the adult, rates of urinary potassium excretion may range from less than 5 mEq to 1,000 mEq/24 hr, depending on the amount of potassium intake.

Potassium is freely filtered in the glomerulus. Its concentration along the length of the proximal convoluted tubule is similar to that of plasma, indicating that reabsorption of potassium in this segment of the nephron is proportionate to that of water, with 60% or more of the filtered potassium absorbed. Concentrations of potassium are increased in the loop of Henle. However, by the time tubular fluid reaches the early distal convoluted tubule, its potassium concentration is below that of plasma, and the amount of potassium delivered to more distal segments of the nephron is less than 10% of the filtered load. The distal tubule and collecting duct have the dual capabilities of potassium reabsorption and secretion.

Under conditions of maximal potassium conservation, continued reabsorption occurs in the distal tubule; when dietary intake is normal or when excretion is increased for other reasons, potassium secretion takes place in the distal tubule and possibly in the collecting duct. The primary mechanism regulating renal control of potassium homeostasis is potassium secretion in these segments of the nephron. The cellular mechanisms of potassium secretion in the distal nephron are regulated by several clinically relevant factors. Increases in plasma potassium stimulate the tubular cell secretion of potassium, and decreases of plasma potassium inhibit tubular secretion.

Aldosterone promotes potassium secretion in the tubule through a series of intracellular events in the tubular cell, including increased luminal membrane permeability to potassium. Aldosterone secretion is stimulated by increased plasma potassium and angiotensin II (see Fig. 46–3). Atrial natriuretic peptide (ANP) and low plasma potassium inhibit aldosterone secretion. Increased tubular flow rate through the potassium-secreting nephron segments due to diuretics or extracellular volume expansion stimulates potassium secretion.

Acid-base status, which affects the cellular potassium concentration, also regulates tubular potassium handling. Alkalosis stimulates and acidosis inhibits secretion. A rise of tubular fluid sodium concentration, such as that produced by diuretics, stimulates potassium secretion. Diuretics can promote renal potassium secretion and urinary potassium loss by increasing tubular fluid flow rate and by increasing tubular sodium concentration. Most of the potassium in the final urine probably results from tubular secretion rather than glomerular filtration.

Potassium is also lost in the feces and in sweat. The exchange of plasma potassium for sodium in the colonic contents contributes to sodium conservation and permits the colon to participate in potassium homeostasis. However, even under conditions of chronic potassium loading, fecal potassium constitutes only a small percentage of the total amount of potassium excreted. The human colon responds to mineralocorticoids by decreasing sodium and increasing the potassium content of the stool. Glucocorticoids have a similar effect.

The potassium content of sweat, normally 10–25 mEq/L, is increased by mineralocorticoids and may be elevated in cases of hyperaldosteronism and in cystic fibrosis. Losses of potassium by this route, however, usually are insignificant, even in disease states.

PATHOPHYSIOLOGIC CONDITIONS

Consequences of Hyperkalemia. The major consequences of hyperkalemia result from its neuromuscular effects. Hyperkalemia reduces transmembrane potential toward threshold levels, producing delayed depolarization, faster repolarization, and a slower conduction velocity. Paresthesias are followed by weakness and eventually by flaccid paralysis if treatment is not instituted. The heart is particularly vulnerable to hyperkalemia. The ECG typically shows peaking of the T waves. Lengthening of the P-R interval and widening of the QRS complex develop later and are particularly ominous, because they often herald the development of ventricular fibrillation. Because the sequence of cardiotoxic events often progresses rapidly, hyperkalemia should be treated as a medical emergency (Chapter 442).

Causes of Hyperkalemia. Hyperkalemia with serum potassium levels of 5.5 mEq/L or greater (normal values of serum potassium vary with age) may result from surprisingly small increases in total body potassium. Acute increases in potassium intake, usually through parenteral administration, may result in hyperkalemia, although it is typically transient. Because the kidney has a large capacity to excrete excess potassium and to prevent hyperkalemia, this electrolyte abnormality is most often seen when renal excretory mechanisms are impaired. It may occur in acute or chronic renal failure, in adrenal insufficiency, in hyporeninemic hypoaldosteronism, and with the use of potassium-sparing diuretics.

Sources of potassium include the potassium salts of penicillin (1.7 mEq/1 million units) and salt substitutes by patients on a salt-restricted diet. Acute tissue breakdown, such as from trauma, major surgery, burns, and cell lysis from chemotherapeutic agents, can release sufficient potassium into the extracellular fluid (ECF) to cause hyperkalemia. An elevated serum potassium may occur with transcellular redistribution of potassium, which is seen typically in metabolic acidosis and shortly before death or in severely ill patients. Certain drugs may increase the serum potassium level by similar mechanisms. Succinylcholine inhibits membrane repolarization, which requires cellular uptake of potassium. Severe digitalis overdose may cause severe hyperkalemia, presumably by inhibiting sodium-potassium exchange by cell membranes.

Because intracellular levels of potassium are 30 times as high as those in the ECF, lysis of red cells during the collection or handling of a blood sample or release of potassium from platelets during clotting may result in pseudohyperkalemia, in which apparent elevations of serum potassium levels are recorded by the laboratory.

Consequences of Hypokalemia. Although it is impossible to predict the degree of potassium loss from the body accurately by measuring serum potassium, a decrease of 1 mEq/L in serum potassium concentration secondary to potassium loss generally corresponds to a loss of approximately 10–30% of body potassium. Many patients tolerate this degree of loss without symptoms. The rate of change in potassium levels and the magnitude of losses probably affect the severity of symptoms.

The relation of extracellular to intracellular potassium concentration is vital to cell function. Membrane depolarization, the process responsible for initiating muscle contraction, requires the abrupt influx of sodium into cells and a comparable efflux of potassium. The process is reversed with repolarization. With hypokalemia, the ratio of intracellular to extracellular potassium concentrations is increased. The transmembrane electrical potential gradient increases so that a wider differential between the resting and excitation potentials exists, which interferes with impulse formation, propagation, and muscle contraction. Hypokalemia produces functional *alterations in skeletal muscle, smooth muscle, and the heart.* The most observable cardiac manifestations of hypokalemia are ECG changes, including a prolonged Q-T interval and flattened T waves.

Hypokalemia also can produce serious *neurologic symptoms,* including autonomic insufficiency, manifested by orthostatic hypotension, tetany, and decreased neuromuscular excitability. The last results in weakness and decreased bowel motility. Weakness is an early manifestation, typically noticed first in limb muscles before trunk and respiratory muscles. Areflexia, paralysis, and death from respiratory muscle failure can develop.

Paralytic ileus and gastric dilatation reflect smooth muscle dysfunction. Hypokalemia affects protein metabolism and diminishes growth hormone release, contributing to the *failure to thrive* of children with chronic hypokalemia, most notable in Bartter's syndrome. *Rhabdomyolysis* is a dramatic complication of hypokalemia.

In the kidney, potassium deficiency may result in vacuolar changes in the tubular epithelium. If sustained for a long time, it leads to *nephrosclerosis* and *interstitial fibrosis,* pathologic lesions indistinguishable from those of chronic pyelonephritis. The kidney has a reduced ability to concentrate or dilute the urine, with polyuria and polydipsia developing. An increase in bicarbonate reabsorption and hydrogen ion secretion results in *systemic alkalosis.* External losses of potassium also result in a shift of potassium from the intracellular to the extracellular fluid. Intracellular potassium is replaced in part by sodium, hydrogen ions, and dibasic amino acids. If these changes become severe, intracellular acidosis in the renal tubular cells may result in excessive exchange of intracellular hydrogen for sodium in the distal tubular fluid, leading to aciduria, with the increased urinary excretion of ammonia, and to systemic alkalosis.

Causes of Hypokalemia. Abnormally low amounts of total body potassium occur in various disease states (such as muscular dystrophy) that are characterized by a decrease in muscle mass. These disorders are not necessarily accompanied by *hypokalemia.* A low serum potassium level may result from a prolonged decreased intake, from increased renal excretion, or from increased extrarenal losses. Renal losses may be increased by the use of diuretics, including osmotic diuretics and carbonic anhydrase inhibitors; by tubular defects, such as renal tubular acidosis; by acid-base disturbances; in endocrinopathies such as Cushing's syndrome, primary aldosteronism, and thyrotoxicosis; and in diabetic ketoacidosis, Bartter's syndrome, and magnesium deficiency.

Extrarenal losses may occur from the bowel (e.g., diarrhea, chronic catharsis, frequent enemas, protracted vomiting, biliary drainage, enterocutaneous fistulas) or from the skin if there is profuse sweating. Movement of potassium into cells during correction of a metabolic acidosis, for example, may also result in hypokalemia, as may *familial hypokalemic periodic paralysis,* a rare disorder in which episodes of paralysis are usually accompanied by an abrupt and marked hypokalemia caused by movement of potassium into an extravascular body compartment (see Chapter 618.1).

When the source of potassium loss is not apparent, measuring urinary potassium may help. A urine concentration of 15 mEq/L or less indicates renal conservation of potassium and suggests that the loss occurred from a nonrenal source.

CHAPTER 48
Chloride

BODY CONTENT AND DISTRIBUTION OF CHLORIDE. Chloride is the major anion of extracellular fluid (ECF) (see Fig. 45–3). Most of total body chloride is extracellular, occurring in plasma chloride (13.6%), interstitial lymph (37.3%), dense connective tissue and cartilage (17%), bone (15.2%), and transcellular fluids (4.5%). Small quantities (12.4%) are present intracellularly. Exchangeable chloride remains relatively constant per unit of body weight at different ages. The low chloride concentration in cells is regulated by two active cell membrane mechanisms. A reciprocal bicarbonate-chloride exchange is sensitive to changes in intracellular pH. When intracellular pH increases, bicarbonate in the cell is exchanged for extracellular chloride, restoring cellular pH to normal. The extrusion of chloride from the cell is mainly accomplished by the large potassium gradient across the cell membrane. The membrane potential, created by the large intracellular potassium concentration, also drives chloride out of the cell passively through anion-selective transport channels or actively by potassium-chloride co-transport.

REGULATION OF CHLORIDE. The intake and output of chloride usually parallel those of sodium, but chloride intake, abnormal extrarenal losses, and renal excretion can occur independently of sodium. The daily turnover of chloride is high, and the renal conservation of chloride is excellent because of efficient renal regulation. In the proximal tubule, a proportional amount (60–70%) of the chloride filtered load is reabsorbed, closely linked to sodium reabsorption (see Fig. 46–2). Chloride reabsorption in the proximal tubule is coupled to sodium, and in the latter portion, chloride is the preferred anion for sodium co-transport. Because of this co-transport mechanism, any change in sodium reabsorption in the proximal tubule influences proximal tubule handling of chloride.

In the thick ascending limb of the loop of Henle, 20–30% of the chloride load is reabsorbed, closely linked to sodium by a special mechanism. Sodium and chloride movement out of the lumen into the tubular cell is driven by active transport. The reabsorption in this segment is mediated by a unique membrane transport symport protein that couples the movement of one sodium, two chlorides, and one potassium ion. Loop diuretics, such as furosemide, inhibit the symport protein, abolishing the reabsorption of sodium and chloride in the thick ascending limb.

Virtually all the remaining filtered load of chloride is reabsorbed in the distal tubule and collecting duct. Chloride plays a special role in the tubular handling of sodium, potassium, and hydrogen ions in these segments, because it is the only anion available for reabsorption under normal conditions. Chloride reabsorption in this portion of the nephron involves a complex combination of sodium-chloride coupling by a symporter protein, an antiporter protein that facilitates chloride-bicarbonate exchange and a significant amount of chloride transcellular transport by mechanisms not completely understood. The clinically relevant feature of chloride handling in the distal tubule and collecting duct involves the requirement that sodium reabsorption be electroneutral, dictating that sodium is exchanged for potassium or hydrogen ions or co-transported with chloride.

The importance of chloride reabsorption in the handling of cations in the distal tubule and collecting duct is demonstrated during conditions of chloride deficiency, which are most commonly caused by diets severely restricted in sodium chloride and extended diuretic use. A lower than normal amount of chloride arrives out of the proximal tubule to the thick ascending limb. Because of the special properties of the co-transport protein, less tubular chloride in this segment results in less reabsorption of sodium. More sodium delivered to the distal tubule and collecting duct enhances sodium reabsorption, which increases the counterexchange of potassium and hydrogen ions. The resulting hypokalemia and hypochloremia produce and perpetuate metabolic alkalosis.

PATHOPHYSIOLOGIC CONDITIONS. Under most clinical circumstances, alterations in chloride concentration in the blood parallel those of sodium. Hypochloremia and hyperchloremia are usually associated with comparable degrees of hyponatremia and hypernatremia, respectively, and are seen most often in patients with dehydration secondary to diarrhea. Occasionally, changes in chloride concentration are not accompanied by equivalent changes in sodium concentration.

Hypochloremia. Hypochloremia is typically seen in metabolic alkalosis. Although chloride is not directly involved in regulating the concentration of free hydrogen ions, it is crucial to the genesis and maintenance of metabolic alkalosis. Chloride depletion as a cause of metabolic alkalosis occurs when chloride is lost from the body in excess of sodium losses. Examples include a loss from the bowel with vomiting or gastric drainage or in chloride diarrhea, a rare congenital disorder in which there is a defect in bowel transport of chloride, and cystic fibrosis. Urinary losses of chloride may exceed those of sodium during the correction of metabolic acidosis and in potassium deficiency.

A decrease in the filtered load of chloride increases bicarbonate reabsorption in the proximal tubule, because it becomes the predominantly available anion for sodium reabsorption. Less chloride available in the thick ascending limb reduces the amount of sodium reabsorbed, and the increased sodium delivered to the distal nephron enhances potassium and hydrogen ion exchange. These same mechanisms allow chloride to maintain a condition of metabolic alkalosis.

Administering chloride is necessary to correct most cases of metabolic alkalosis whether or not it is associated with potassium deficiency. In cases of potassium deficiency, both potassium and chloride must be given before the potassium deficits can be corrected. Treating patients with metabolic alkalosis with potassium or sodium chloride, as appropriate, results in the prompt excretion of bicarbonate into the urine and correction of the alkalosis.

Hypochloremia also results from a protracted, inadequate intake of chloride. Infants fed a chloride-deficient milk formula for several months have developed chronic depletion of body chloride, severe hypochloremia (serum sodium levels usually remained normal), severe hypokalemic metabolic alkalosis, loss of appetite, failure to thrive, muscle weakness, and lethargy. Although adding chloride to the diet quickly reverses the electrolyte abnormalities, long-term sequelae may develop, including disturbed behavioral patterns.

Hyperchloremia. Hyperchloremia may result when chloride is conserved by the kidney in excess of sodium and potassium or when alkaline urine is formed during the renal correction of alkalosis. An increased fractional reabsorption of chloride in the renal proximal tubule in distal renal tubular acidosis also results in hyperchloremia. Early amino acid solutions used in parenteral alimentation contained excessive amounts of chloride, and their administration resulted in hyperchloremic acidosis. Substituting acetate has largely solved this problem. Hyperchloremia also may occur when large amounts of parenteral fluids containing chloride, such as normal saline and lactated Ringer's solution, are administered during acute fluid resuscitation.

Anion Gap. Measurements of the serum chloride level are necessary to determine a patient's *anion gap*. The concentration of the most abundant serum cation (i.e., sodium) is greater than the sum of the two most abundant serum anions (i.e., chloride and bicarbonate). The difference is referred to as the anion gap; *anion gap* $= [Na] - ([HCO_3] + [Cl])$. It is normally about 12 mEq/L (range, 8–16 mEq/L). The anion gap results from the effect of the combined concentrations of the unmeasured anions, such as phosphate, sulfate, proteins, and organic acids, which exceed those of the unmeasured cations, primarily potassium, calcium, and magnesium. Calculating the anion gap permits the detection of an abnormal concentration of an unmeasured anion or cation.

An abnormal condition in which a *normal anion gap* exists is the metabolic acidosis due to renal tubular acidosis or stool losses of bicarbonate. The fractional reabsorption of chloride is increased, because it becomes the predominantly available anion to accompany sodium tubular reabsorption when the plasma bicarbonate concentration is decreased. In the plasma, as bicarbonate falls with this type of acidosis, the chloride rises, and the sum of anions in plasma remains normal.

An *increased anion gap* in renal failure is a result of increased concentrations of phosphate and sulfate; in diabetic ketoacidosis, to β-hydroxybutyrate and acetoacetate; in lactic acidosis, to lactate; in hyperglycemic nonketotic coma, to unidentified organic acids; and in disorders of amino acid metabolism, to various organic acids. Increased anion gap also follows the administration of large amounts of penicillin. After ethylene glycol ingestion, it is caused by glycolate production; after methanol ingestion, by formate production; and after salicylate poisoning, by the salicylate anion and various organic anions secondary to the uncoupling of oxidative phosphorylation.

A *decreased anion gap* occurs less frequently. It may be found in nephrotic syndrome, in which it is caused by a decreased serum concentration of albumin, which is anionic at pH 7.4; after lithium ingestion, with lithium as an unmeasured cation; and in multiple myeloma, because of the presence of cationic proteins.

CHAPTER 49
Calcium

BODY CALCIUM. At all stages of life, 99% of the body's calcium is in bone. Because the bones of infants are less densely mineralized than those of adults, the body contents of calcium in infants and adults are significantly different, about 400 and 950 mEq/kg of body weight, respectively (see Chapters 40, 41, and 44).

Under normal conditions, the extracellular pool of calcium remains remarkably constant despite fairly free exchange with the enormous reservoir in bone. The calcium concentration in serum is also maintained within narrow limits, averaging 2.5 mM/L (10 mg/dL). Approximately 40% is protein bound, and the remaining 60% is ultrafilterable (Table 49–1). Because 1 g of albumin binds 0.8 mg of calcium, but 1 g of globulin binds only 0.16 mg, 80–90% of the bound calcium is bound to albumin, and decreases in serum albumin concentration result in decreases in total serum calcium levels. Of the ultrafilterable calcium, 14% is complexed with anions such as phosphate and citrate, and the remaining 46% (1.2 mM/L or 4.8 mg/dL) is present as free ionic calcium (see Table 49–1).

Ionized calcium exists in equilibrium with the protein-bound form. Changes in hydrogen ion activity in the plasma modify the percentage of calcium that is ionized; for example, a change of 0.1 pH unit alters the concentration of ionized calcium by 10%. Acidosis increases and alkalosis decreases the proportion ionized. The ionized form of calcium is of greatest physiologic importance. The calcium ion plays a major role in many fundamental biologic processes, including bone formation, cell division and growth, coagulation, hormone-response coupling, and electrical stimulus-response coupling in muscle contraction and neurotransmitter release. Although ionized calcium concentrations can be measured, a useful approximation can be made for clinical purposes if the patient's acid-base status is known and by assuming that each 1 g/dL decrease in serum albumin concentration decreases bound and therefore total serum calcium by 1 mg/dL.

REGULATION OF CALCIUM. Overall regulation of calcium homeostasis is provided by a complex system involving intestinal absorption, renal excretion, and hormonal regulation of these processes. Two important variables operate to maintain calcium homeostasis: the total body calcium, mainly determined by the amount of calcium absorbed in the intestinal tract and the amount of calcium excreted by the kidneys, and the distribution of calcium between bone and the extracellular compartment, mainly determined by a balance of hormonal regulation.

Body calcium content is regulated primarily through *intestinal tract absorption of calcium.* The recommended daily dietary intake is 360 mg in the first 6 mo of life, 540 mg in the second 6 mo, 800 mg for 1–10 yr of age, and 1,200 mg for 11–18 yr of age. Dairy products constitute the most important single source. Dietary calcium is absorbed along the small intestine, primarily in the duodenum and early jejunum by an active, carrier-mediated transport mechanism that is stimulated by 1,25-dihydroxyvitamin D_3. It is postulated that hypocalcemia stimulates release of parathyroid hormone (PTH), which increases the renal conversion of 25-hydroxyvitamin D_3 to its more biologically active 1,25 derivative.

The efficiency of intestinal absorption of dietary calcium is increased by low calcium intake in the growing child, in pregnancy, and during depletion of body calcium stores. The mechanisms responsible for this adaptation are unknown. Administering vitamin D and PTH also increases calcium absorption; PTH probably acts by its effect on vitamin D metabolism.

Increases in absorption leading to hypercalcemia occur in sarcoidosis, carcinomatosis, and multiple myeloma. Decreased absorption of calcium results from the presence in the gastrointestinal tract of phytate, oxalate, and citrate, all of which complex the dietary calcium; from increased gastric motility; from reduction of bowel length; and from protein depletion, which may cause a deficiency of the calcium-binding protein in the intestinal mucosa. Some calcium is secreted into the intestinal lumen by the bowel, but this process probably does not represent a regulatory mechanism.

Renal calcium excretion matches the amount of intestinal absorption to maintain the overall calcium balance. Plasma non–protein-bound calcium (i.e., diffusible and ultrafilterable calcium) is filtered at the glomerulus. Normally, about 99% of this filtered calcium is reabsorbed by the tubules, with ionized calcium transported more easily than the complexed form. Reabsorption occurs throughout the nephron. Reabsorption that occurs in the proximal tubule (50–55%) and loop of Henle (20–30%) appears to parallel sodium reabsorption; factors influencing the transport of one of these cations also affect the other. Calcium transport in the distal convoluted tubule (10–15%) and the collecting duct (2–8%) can be dissociated from sodium transport; these sites probably represent the mechanisms that are specifically calciuric. For example, thiazide diuretics decrease tubular sodium reabsorption, producing a natriuresis, but when administered on a chronic basis, they increase calcium reabsorption and reduce urinary calcium excretion. Calcium reabsorption is stimulated specifically by 1,25-dihydroxyvitamin D_3 in the distal tubule.

The most important hormone regulating renal calcium excretion is PTH. PTH dramatically stimulates calcium reabsorption in the thick ascending limb of the loop of Henle and the distal tubule. When PTH is increased, urinary calcium is reduced, and the opposite effect occurs with decreased PTH levels. Contraction of extracellular volume and metabolic alkalosis also stimulate tubular calcium reabsorption and decrease urinary calcium excretion.

Urinary excretion of calcium is also increased by many nonspecific mechanisms. These include expansion of extracellular fluid (ECF) volume; administration of osmotic diuretics, furosemide, growth hormone, thyroid hormone, or glucagon; metabolic acidosis; prolonged fasting; and an increase in the serum phosphate level.

There is a diurnal variation in the excretion of calcium, which peaks at the middle of the day. Alterations in dietary calcium result in only small changes in the urinary excretion of calcium, probably reflecting adaptive changes in the intestinal absorption of calcium. Physical inactivity is associated with

TABLE 49–1 Levels of Plasma, Calcium, Magnesium and Phosphorus

Chemical Status	Calcium	Magnesium	Phosphorus
Ionized (diffusible)	46%	55%	85%*
Complexed (ultrafilterable)	14%	25%	5%
Protein-bound (nondiffusible)	40%	20%	10%

*At pH 7.40 = 68% as HPO_4^{2-}, 17% as HPO_4^{-}.

increased urinary excretion of calcium and, if prolonged, may result in the formation of renal stones.

The balance between deposition and mobilization of calcium in bone largely determines the concentration of ionized calcium in the blood. The *distribution of calcium between bone and the ECF* is determined by *hormonal regulation*. PTH and 1,25-dihydroxyvitamin D_3 act to increase plasma calcium. PTH release is stimulated by hypocalcemia or an increase in plasma phosphorus. PTH increases plasma calcium by stimulating release of calcium from bone and by stimulating the production of 1,25-dihydroxyvitamin D_3, which increases intestinal calcium absorption and stimulates bone release of calcium. PTH also increases renal calcium reabsorption.

Thyrocalcitonin, produced in the parafollicular cells of the thyroid gland, is released in response to hypercalcemia. The major effect of thyrocalcitonin is to lower plasma calcium by inhibiting bone resorption. This hormone also increases urinary calcium excretion.

Plasma pH modifies concentrations of plasma-ionized calcium, as do the amounts of calcium absorbed from the renal tubular fluid and from the bowel, although to a lesser extent. Because the serum concentrations of sodium and potassium may play some role in the balance between deposition and mobilization of bone calcium, treating hypernatremia with fluids low in potassium may result in hypocalcemia.

PATHOPHYSIOLOGIC CONDITIONS. Symptomatic *hypocalcemia* may be caused by a low concentration of ionized calcium resulting from vitamin D deficiency, which is caused by nutritional deficiency, malabsorption, or abnormal metabolism of vitamin D. Hypocalcemia may also be a result of hypoparathyroidism, pseudohypoparathyroidism, hyperphosphatemia, magnesium deficiency, and acute pancreatitis. Because acidosis increases and alkalosis decreases the proportion of calcium that is ionized, symptomatic hypocalcemia may occur during rapid correction or overcorrection of acidosis or with alkalosis.

The neonate is particularly susceptible to hypocalcemia associated with hypoparathyroidism, abnormal vitamin D metabolism, a low calcium intake, or a high phosphate intake (see Chapters 93.2, 102, and 581). Bone mineralization is frequently inadequate in very low birthweight infants during the neonatal period, increasing the incidence of radiologic rickets and fractures. These lesions probably result from an inadequate intake of calcium and phosphorus at the time of rapid postnatal growth and may not respond to vitamin D metabolites.

The causes of *hypercalcemia* include primary or tertiary hyperparathyroidism, hyperthyroidism, vitamin D intoxication, immobilization, malignancies (especially those that metastasize to bone), use of thiazide diuretics, excessive calcium in total parenteral nutrition fluid, milk-alkali syndrome, and sarcoidosis. An idiopathic form may occur in infancy associated with typical elfin facies and supravalvular aortic stenosis; this Williams' syndrome may be caused by hypersensitivity to vitamin D. If their dietary intake of phosphorus is inadequate, low birthweight infants may develop hypercalcemia as a result of resorption of phosphorus and calcium from bone.

Calcium loading increases renal excretion of sodium and potassium and profoundly reduces the ability to concentrate the urine. This effect may explain the polyuria and polydipsia of patients with hypercalcemia resulting from hypervitaminosis D, which may be associated with tubulointerstitial nephropathy. Concentrated calcium solutions should always be administered cautiously, using ECG monitoring, if possible, to minimize cardiac arrhythmias (see Chapter 442).

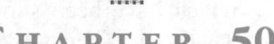

CHAPTER 50
Magnesium

Magnesium is the fourth most abundant cation in the body and the second most common intracellular electrolyte (see Fig. 45–3). Because of its relative intracellular abundance, magnesium plays a major role in cellular enzymatic activity, especially in glycolysis and the stimulation of the ATPases.

BODY CONTENT AND DISTRIBUTION OF MAGNESIUM. Body magnesium concentration is approximately 22 mEq/kg in the infant. In adults the concentration increases to 28 mEq/kg. Bone and muscle cells are the major intracellular pools of magnesium. Sixty per cent of body magnesium is in bone, of which about one third is freely exchangeable. Most of the remaining 40% is intracellular; more than 50% is in muscle and much of the remainder in liver. Only 20–30% of the intracellular magnesium is exchangeable, and the remainder is bound to proteins, RNA, and adenosine triphosphate.

Extracellular magnesium accounts for only 1% of body magnesium. Although freely exchangeable with the large exchangeable pools in bone and cells, extracellular concentrations are maintained at low levels within a relatively narrow normal range. The range of serum magnesium normally is 1.5–1.8 mEq/L, although wider normal ranges have been reported. Approximately 80% is ultrafilterable; this consists of 55% ionized and 25% complexed magnesium. The remaining 20% is protein bound (see Table 49–1).

REGULATION OF MAGNESIUM

Intake. The intake range of magnesium in children is 10–25 mEq/24 hr, depending on age; the highest intakes are required during periods of rapid growth. Green vegetables and many other foods contain high concentrations of magnesium; the intake of most individuals exceeds the minimum requirement of 3.6 mg/kg/24 hr (i.e., 12 mg of magnesium is equivalent to 1 mEq or 0.5 mM). Absorption of dietary magnesium occurs primarily in the upper gastrointestinal tract by mechanisms that are not fully delineated. Vitamin D, parathyroid hormone (PTH), and increased sodium absorption enhance magnesium absorption; calcium, phosphorus, and increased intestinal motility decrease it. Absorption is far from complete; an amount of magnesium equal to about two thirds of intake is excreted in the feces. A small portion of this magnesium is secreted by the bowel.

Renal Excretion. Maintenance of magnesium balance depends primarily on urinary excretion. Normally, less than 5% of the filtered load of magnesium appears in the urine; 20–30% is reabsorbed in the proximal tubule and most of the remainder in the loop of Henle, especially the thick ascending limb, which is the primary site of renal magnesium modification. Under various conditions, magnesium reabsorption parallels that of calcium and sodium. Magnesium competes with calcium for transport. Urinary excretion of magnesium efficiently matches the net intestinal absorption. Renal magnesium reabsorption is inhibited, increasing urinary magnesium, by expansion of the extracellular fluid (ECF) volume; by osmotic, thiazide, mercurial, and loop diuretics; glucagon; by calcium loading; and by decreased PTH levels. Conversely, volume contraction, magnesium deficiency, thyrocalcitonin, and increased PTH levels increase the renal reabsorption of magnesium, decreasing urinary excretion. Acidosis increases urinary excretion of magnesium, but alkalosis decreases urinary magnesium.

The maintenance of magnesium balance and serum magnesium concentrations requires a complex interaction of renal and nonrenal factors. For example, a low-magnesium diet results in reduced urinary magnesium. This reduction may be the consequence of modest reductions in the serum concentration of magnesium, which have been shown to increase the release of PTH. The release of PTH decreases the urinary loss of magnesium and also causes the release of magnesium and calcium into the ECF, increasing the concentrations of both cations. Tubular reabsorption of filtered magnesium can be almost complete. However, the gastrointestinal tract continues to secrete small amounts of magnesium, and depletion may result. The concentration of magnesium in serum depends on intake and output and on the mobilization of magnesium from bone and soft tissue. The serum level is not always a reliable indicator of magnesium balance and may remain normal even with marked magnesium depletion. In severe nutritional deficiency states such as kwashiorkor, serum levels of magnesium may be normal even though the content of magnesium in the muscle is decreased. Conversely, reduced levels may be seen without appreciable losses.

PATHOPHYSIOLOGIC CONDITIONS

Hypomagnesemia. Hypomagnesemia occurs in various clinical states, including malabsorption syndromes, hypoparathyroidism, diuretic therapy, hypercalcemia, renal tubular acidosis, primary aldosteronism, alcoholism, and prolonged intravenous fluid therapy with magnesium-free fluids. At special risk are infants who undergo surgery and receive such fluids for protracted periods. Nephrotoxic agents may produce hypomagnesemia through increased urinary losses. Infants with early or late neonatal tetany also often have hypomagnesemia (see Chapter 55). When associated with early neonatal tetany, hypomagnesemia tends to be mild and transient and may not require treatment with magnesium. In late neonatal tetany, hypocalcemia may fail to respond to treatment until magnesium levels have been returned to normal.

The symptoms of hypomagnesemia are primarily those of increased neuromuscular irritability and include tetany, severe seizures, and tremors. Personality changes, nausea, anorexia, abnormal cardiac rhythms, and ECG changes may also be seen. Symptoms do not always correlate with serum magnesium levels, perhaps because serum levels do not always reflect the body content of magnesium, a predominantly intracellular cation. Alternatively, the symptoms of hypomagnesemia may be minor compared with the symptoms of the primary disease causing the magnesium depletion. A third possibility is that the symptoms may reflect hypomagnesemia complicated by hypocalcemia. Severe hypomagnesemia interferes with the release of PTH and induces skeletal resistance to the action of PTH. Hypomagnesemia and hypocalcemia often coexist.

Hypermagnesemia. Hypermagnesemia, which is an increase in total body magnesium, rarely occurs in the absence of decreased renal function. Normally, the kidney prevents elevations of serum magnesium to dangerous levels even when large magnesium loads are administered. However, hypermagnesemia with serum levels exceeding 5 mEq/L can occur. The usual sources of a magnesium load include magnesium-containing laxatives, enemas, intravenous fluids, and magnesium-containing antacids used as phosphate binders in patients with chronic renal failure. Severe hypermagnesemia may occur in neonates born of mothers who were treated with intramuscular injections of magnesium sulfate for the hypertension of preeclampsia. Neonates born prematurely with asphyxia or hypotonia are at special risk, although it remains to be determined whether the elevated magnesium is the cause or consequence of these abnormalities. Serum magnesium levels tend to spontaneously return to normal within 72 hr. There is also an increased incidence of hypermagnesemia in patients with Addison's disease.

The symptoms of hypermagnesemia occur when magnesium levels exceed 5 mg/dL. Hyporeflexia antedates respiratory depression, drowsiness, and coma. Manifestations are rapidly reversed by intravenous administration of calcium. Coma and death usually occur when the serum magnesium level increases above 15 mg/dL.

CHAPTER 51
Phosphorus

Confusion may exist in understanding the physiology of phosphorus, because the terms *phosphorus* and *phosphate* have frequently and erroneously been used interchangeably. Measurements of phosphate in biologic samples are usually performed as and expressed in terms of total elemental phosphorus concentration. Because the atomic weight of phosphorus is 30.98, a concentration of 3.1 mg/dL (31 mg/L) of phosphorus is equivalent to 1 mM of phosphorus/L. Most of the measured plasma phosphorus exists as monovalent or divalent orthophosphate and behaves as though it has a valence of 1.8 at pH 7.40 (see Table 49–1). Consequently, at pH 7.40, 1 mM of phosphate is equivalent to 1.8 mEq of phosphate (mM × valence = mEq).

BODY CONTENT AND DISTRIBUTION OF PHOSPHORUS. Infants retain phosphorus avidly. A 3 kg infant may retain 40–80 mg/24 hr, which is more than 50% of usual intake. Consequently, total body phosphorus per unit of fat-free body weight (FFBW) increases throughout childhood; it doubles from birth to adulthood, at which time its value is approximately 12 g/kg FFBW. This doubling is primarily the result of an increase in skeletal phosphorus content; more than 80% of body phosphorus is intracellular (see Fig. 45–3), principally in bone, and the remainder is distributed throughout all soft tissues.

In plasma, two thirds of phosphorus occurs as phospholipids. These compounds are insoluble in acid and are not measured in routine plasma phosphorus determinations. The measured portion of plasma phosphorus is acid soluble and is composed of inorganic phosphorus, primarily orthophosphate, 10% of which is bound to protein (see Table 49–1). The remaining 90% is ultrafilterable, 5% of which is complexed as calcium, magnesium, and sodium phosphates, and 85% of which is free phosphate. Of the latter, 80% is the divalent anion (HPO_4^{2-}) and 20% the monovalent anion ($H_2PO_4^-$) (see Table 49–1). Concentrations of phosphorus are low in interstitial fluids.

Cellular phosphorus exists in cell membranes and subcellular organelles as organic phosphoglycerides and sphingolipids. Acid-soluble moieties of intracellular phosphorus include adenosine triphosphate (ATP) and other nucleotides, various glucose-phosphate compounds, creatinine phosphate, and a small amount of cytosolic inorganic phosphate. Intracellular phosphate plays an essential role in forming and releasing energy, as well as in intracellular enzyme activity. Inorganic phosphorus is the principal urinary buffer filtered at the glomerulus and plays a critical function in the regulation of free hydrogen ions (see Chapter 52).

REGULATION OF PHOSPHORUS

Intake and Absorption. The principal sources of *dietary phosphorus* are milk, milk products, and meat. The recommended daily intake is 880 mg/24 hr for children 1–10 yr of age and 1,200 mg for older children. Breast-fed infants ingest 25–30 mg of phosphorus/kg/24 hr. As much as two thirds of the dietary phosphate is absorbed from the bowel, primarily in the jejunum. This absorption is stimulated by vitamin D and its metabolites and by parathyroid hormone (PTH). Absorption is decreased by thyrocalcitonin, by binders such as aluminum hydroxide and carbonate in the bowel, and, at least in animals, by a high dietary calcium intake.

Renal Excretion. Even though phosphate is actively transported across the bowel wall, it is the kidney that plays a major role in regulating body phosphate. Renal handling of phosphate consists of glomerular filtration with facultative reabsorption by the tubule. Ultrafilterable phosphate is freely filtered at the glomerulus, with an average of 90% of this filtered load normally reabsorbed. Eighty per cent of the filtered load reabsorption occurs in the proximal tubule, and the remainder occurs in more distal segments. Under certain circumstances, phosphate may also be secreted by the distal tubules. A maximal rate for tubular reabsorption of phosphorus (T_m) exists in the proximal tubule. Because this transport maximum is only slightly above the normal filtered load, small increases in plasma phosphorus increase the filtered load above the transport maximum and increase urinary phosphorus excretion. Urinary excretion of phosphate shows a circadian rhythm, with the lowest levels in the morning and highest levels in the early evening.

Tubular reabsorption of phosphate is regulated by *PTH,* the effects of which are mediated by the adenylate cyclase system. This hormone reduces tubular reabsorption of phosphorus mainly in the proximal tubule and is associated with phosphaturia. Conversely, large doses of vitamin D stimulate reabsorption of phosphate in the proximal tubule, as does growth hormone. Under many circumstances, renal tubular transport of phosphate parallels that of sodium. Expansion of extracellular fluid (ECF) results in phosphaturia, as does the administration of diuretics, especially those that inhibit carbonic anhydrase. Phosphate transport is also linked to glucose transport and to changes in pH; hyperglycemia therefore results in phosphaturia and a reduced T_m for phosphorus. Conditions that result in an alkaline urine also decrease reabsorption of phosphate.

Plasma Phosphate. In addition to the factors already discussed, plasma phosphate concentration is affected by the continuous exchange of phosphate between the large stores in the bone and those in the ECF. The release of phosphorus from bone stores is stimulated by the same regulating hormones that promote calcium release. Net reabsorption of phosphate from bone is promoted by 1,25-dihydroxyvitamin D_3 and PTH but is opposed by thyrocalcitonin. Phosphate is also readily transported across all cell membranes. Administering glucose or insulin decreases plasma phosphate concentration, probably because of an intracellular flux of phosphate secondary to the phosphorylation of glucose. Hyperventilation, alkalosis, and administration of epinephrine also decrease plasma phosphate concentration. Marked, acute increases in plasma phosphate concentration result in hypocalcemia. Changes in calcium concentration, however, do not necessarily reciprocally alter plasma phosphate concentration.

Plasma phosphorus concentrations are high during infancy and childhood. The range of values at birth is 1.4–2.8 mM/L, which increases progressively in the first week of life to 2.0–3.3 mM/L before declining slowly during childhood. Levels fall to those of the adult (1.0–1.3 mM/L) on completion of growth. Premature infants also have high plasma phosphorus values of 2.5–3.0 mM/L if their intake of phosphorus is adequate.

PATHOPHYSIOLOGIC CONDITIONS

Hyperphosphatemia. Hyperphosphatemia is characteristic of hypoparathyroidism but rarely occurs in the absence of renal insufficiency. Although small changes in the glomerular filtration rate (GFR) have little effect on phosphate excretion in health, *reduction of the GFR* to below 25% of normal leads to an elevation of the serum inorganic phosphate level and to reciprocal changes in the serum calcium level, resulting in secondary hyperparathyroidism. This process begins with small decreases in the GFR but usually does not clinically appear until the GFR has fallen to low levels. *In the young infant,* the GFR is low in relation to active cell mass, and the dietary phosphorus intake is high; consequently, the serum inorganic phosphorus level is high. A reduction in the GFR or relative hypoparathyroidism in infants rapidly leads to very high serum values of phosphate, with consequent depression of the calcium concentration and latent or manifest tetany (see Chapters 44 and 55.9).

Hyperphosphatemia may also result from the excessive administration of phosphate by oral or intravenous routes or of phosphate-containing enemas. Using cytotoxic drugs to treat malignancies, especially lymphomas or leukemias, results in cytolysis, with hyperphosphatemia caused by the release of phosphate into the circulation. The major clinical consequences of hyperphosphatemia are symptoms of the resulting hypocalcemia.

Hypophosphatemia. Hypophosphatemia may result from the phosphate deficiency associated with starvation, protein-calorie malnutrition, and malabsorption syndromes. It may result from intracellular shifts of phosphate, such as those that occur with respiratory or metabolic alkalosis, during the treatment of diabetic ketoacidosis (typically during the first 24 hr), and after the administration of corticosteroids. Increased urinary losses of phosphate may be sufficiently severe to reduce the plasma concentration; this reduction is observed in primary and tertiary hyperparathyroidism, in renal tubular defects, after ECF volume expansion, or after the administration of diuretics. A combination of pathophysiologic mechanisms often is responsible for the hypophosphatemia. Examples include vitamin D–deficient (see Chapter 44) and vitamin D–resistant rickets (see Chapter 711).

The very low birthweight infant requires a high phosphorus intake at the time of rapid postnatal growth. Inadequate intake results in phosphorus depletion and hypophosphatemia. Insufficient phosphorus intake occurs particularly in patients receiving total parenteral nutrition when the physician fails to recognize the need to achieve relatively higher levels of serum phosphorus in premature infants. Bone demineralization, hypercalcemia, and calciuria may occur, probably as a result of mobilization of phosphorus and calcium from the bone.

In most instances, hypophosphatemia is mild or moderate and asymptomatic. Occasionally, plasma phosphate concentrations may fall to very low levels ($\leq$0.3 mM/L [$\leq$1.0 mg/dL]). Such low levels have been observed with the *prolonged use of intravenous alimentation without phosphate supplements* and may produce a very severe, well-defined syndrome. Red cell concentrations of 2,3-diphosphoglycerate and ATP are decreased. The resultant decreased release of oxygen by the red cells produces tissue anoxia. Increased hemolysis may occur, as may leukocyte and platelet dysfunction. Some patients display the symptoms of a metabolic encephalopathy, including irritability, paresthesias, confusion, seizures, and coma; some may develop abnormalities revealed by the electroencephalogram. Hypercalcemia (thought to result from the increased release of calcium from bone), rhabdomyolysis, cardiopathy, and possibly hepatocellular dysfunction also have been reported. Renal tubular defects may occur, and the kidney's ability to excrete hydrogen ions is impaired. Promptly recognizing and treating this syndrome, preferably by oral administration of phosphate salts, is beneficial, but permanent defects may result. Prevention of severe hypophosphatemia should always be the goal.

CHAPTER 52

Hydrogen Ion

(Acid-Base Balance)

TERMINOLOGY. Discussions of acid-base balance have historically been complicated by a confusion about terminology. The current approach emphasizes the hydrogen ion or proton, which is a hydrogen atom with its neutralizing electron removed. The pH is the negative logarithm of the concentration of free hydrogen ions.

An *acid* is a proton (i.e., hydrogen ion) donor. Hydrochloric, sulfuric, phosphoric, and carbonic acids are conventional acids, each dissociating to liberate protons. A strong acid is one that is highly dissociated and therefore produces a high concentration of hydrogen ions; a weak acid is one that is poorly dissociated. A *base* is a hydrogen ion acceptor. Bases bind free hydrogen ions, reducing their concentration. Examples include hydroxyl ions, ammonia, and the anions of weak acids.

A *buffer* is defined as a substance that reduces the change in free hydrogen ion concentration of a solution on the addition of an acid or base. The presence of a buffer in a solution increases the amount of acid or alkali that must be added to cause a change in pH. The addition of a strong acid to any of these buffer systems produces a neutral salt and a weak acid. By generating a poorly dissociated acid, the buffer significantly reduces the increment in free hydrogen ion concentration when the reaction is compared with one that is not buffered.

Aprotes are *cations* such as sodium, potassium, calcium, and magnesium that carry one or more positive charges, depending on valence, or *anions* such as chloride and sulfate that carry negative charges. Because aprotes can neither donate nor accept protons, they are not acids, bases, or buffers.

NORMAL ACID-BASE REGULATION. The number of potential hydrogen ions in the body is huge. Most are buffered and therefore are not in free form. At the usual pH of 7.4, the concentration of free hydrogen ions in the blood is only 0.0000398 mEq/L or 3.98×10^{-8} Eq/L (often expressed as 40 nEq/L; Fig. 52–1):

$$pH = -\log (H^+) = -\log (3.98 \times 10^{-8}) = -(0.60 - 8.0) = 7.4 \quad (1)$$

Normally, the hydrogen ion concentrations of body fluids are maintained in relatively narrow ranges by buffers. Buffers represent the first line of defense against changes in pH, but they cannot maintain the acid-base balance. In disease states or abrupt alterations of hydrogen ion production, buffer systems may not be able to maintain a normal pH for a prolonged period, and their action must be supplemented by compensatory and corrective physiologic changes in the lungs and kidneys.

Compensation of a primary acid-base disorder is a slower process than buffering, but it is more effective in returning the pH to normal. In a primary metabolic disorder, the respiratory system provides the compensating mechanism; the kidneys compensate in a primary respiratory disorder by increasing base or by acid excretion. Compensation reduces pH changes but must be followed by *correction*, which returns all acid-base measurements to normal. This stabilization occurs when the primary disorder is cured. The kidneys correct a metabolic disorder, and the lungs correct a respiratory one. Although discussed separately, the buffering, pulmonary, and renal systems are interdependent and act in concert with one another.

BUFFER SYSTEMS. The principal buffer in the extracellular fluid (ECF) is the bicarbonate-carbonic acid system; intracellular buffers include various proteins and organic phosphates. In the urine, phosphate in its monohydrogen and dihydrogen forms is the major buffer. Only the ECF buffer mechanisms are considered in detail in this chapter.

Hydrogen ions, when added to the plasma, are buffered in large part by bicarbonate, with the generation of a neutral salt and carbonic acid (H_2CO_3):

$$HA + NaHCO_3 \rightarrow NaA + H_2CO_3 \quad (2)$$

H_2CO_3 is a weak acid with a relatively low solubility coefficient and is in equilibrium with dissolved carbon dioxide (CO_2), as follows:

$$[H^+] \cdot [HCO_3^-] \leftrightarrows H_2CO_3 \leftrightarrows CO_2 + H_2O \quad (3)$$

The addition of hydrogen ions drives this equation to the right, generating CO_2 and water. Despite the addition of hydrogen ions, the buffering mechanisms result in relatively little change in free hydrogen ion concentration and in pH. However, buffering is accomplished at the expense of a decrease in bicarbonate concentration, which has been referred to as representing a *base deficit*, and an increase in partial pressure of CO_2 (P_{CO_2}) levels. The Henderson-Hasselbalch equation indicates that these changes must result in some change in pH:

$$pH = pK + \log [A^-]/[HA] \quad (4)$$

In the bicarbonate-H_2CO_3 system, pK (a constant derived from the dissociation of the acid-base pair) is 6.1. Thus,

$$pH = 6.1 + \log [\text{bicarbonate}]/[\text{carbonic acid}] \quad (5)$$

Because H_2CO_3 is in equilibrium with dissolved CO_2, measurement of the P_{CO_2} can be used as a clinical estimate of carbonic acid concentration. By decreasing bicarbonate concentration and increasing P_{CO_2}, the addition of hydrogen ion to the plasma still results in some decrease in pH despite the presence of buffers. However, the changes are of lesser magnitude than would occur in the absence of the buffering mechanism.

CLINICAL ACID-BASE RELATIONSHIPS. The three major compo-

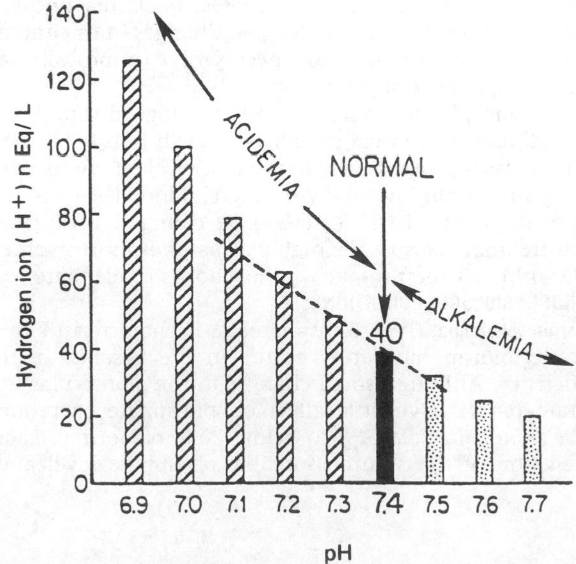

Figure 52–1 Relationship of pH to hydrogen ion concentration. (From Narins RG, Emmett M: Simple and mixed acid-base disorders: A practical approach. Medicine 59:161, 1980.)

nents of clinical acid-base balance are pH, as determined by the hydrogen ion concentration; the partial pressure of CO_2, P_{CO_2}, regulated by pulmonary ventilation; and plasma bicarbonate concentration, HCO_3, initially an extracellular buffer and then regulated primarily and to a much greater degree by the kidneys. The clinically cumbersome Henderson-Hasselbalch equation has been rearranged by Kasirer and Bleich to an equation that has clinical utility for these three components:

$$[H^+] = 24 + P_{CO_2}/HCO_3 \quad (6)$$

This expression emphasizes the important point that hydrogen ion concentration, and therefore pH, is defined by the ratio of P_{CO_2} and plasma bicarbonate, not the absolute values of the individual components. Defining acid-base balance in terms of this important ratio allows a physician to understand how the acid-base balance operates in clinical settings. The interdependence of the three critical acid-base factors—pH, P_{CO_2}, and HCO_3—is vital for understanding the individual effect on acid-base status of primary alterations of P_{CO_2} or HCO_3 produced by clinical abnormalities and for understanding the resultant compensation of the counterbalancing factor, P_{CO_2} or HCO_3, to return the acid-base balance toward normal.

Pulmonary Mechanisms. The aforementioned equation indicates that pH depends not on absolute levels of bicarbonate and P_{CO_2} but on the ratio of the two concentrations. A decrease or increase in concentration of bicarbonate does not modify pH if the P_{CO_2} is lowered or increased in proportion. By altering the rate at which CO_2 is excreted, the lungs can regulate P_{CO_2} and modify pH. Although enormous quantities of CO_2 are produced from normal metabolic activity, little change in pH results because of the unique properties of the bicarbonate-H_2CO_3 buffer system and a highly developed respiratory control mechanism. An increased respiratory rate, stimulated by increased levels of CO_2 increases the excretion of CO_2, decreases P_{CO_2}, and increases pH. Conversely, a decreased respiratory rate increases P_{CO_2} and decreases pH.

Even though the lungs can modify pH by changing the P_{CO_2} and altering the ratio of H_2CO_3 to bicarbonate, this process cannot cause any loss or gain in hydrogen ions. The lungs are incapable of regenerating bicarbonate to replace that lost when the hydrogen ion concentration was buffered. The generation of new bicarbonate and, when required, the excretion of bicarbonate are the responsibilities of the kidneys.

Renal Mechanisms. The kidneys are the most important regulators of acid-base balance on a daily basis under normal conditions. Renal regulation of acid-base balance fulfills two requirements: (1) preventing the loss of bicarbonate in the urine and (2) maintaining plasma bicarbonate levels by excreting an amount of acid equal to the daily production of nonvolatile acids and adding "new" bicarbonate to the blood. Renal regulation to perform these two major requirements is accomplished by two important processes. *Reabsorption of nearly all the filtered bicarbonate* occurs predominately in the proximal tubule (80%) and in the thick ascending limb of the loop of Henle (15%). No net hydrogen ion excretion results, but in adults, this process is responsible for reclaiming up to 5,000 mEq of bicarbonate that is filtered through the glomeruli each day. If this bicarbonate were not reabsorbed, its loss would be equivalent to the retention of an equal amount of hydrogen ions, which would result in severe systemic acidosis. *The excretion of hydrogen ion and the addition of new bicarbonate to the blood* is accomplished by (1) the secretion of fixed hydrogen ion, its combination with buffers, and ultimately excretion in the urine and (2) the excretion of ammonium.

The mechanisms of these steps are highly developed, energy-requiring, active transport processes, in contrast to the pulmonary excretion of CO_2 which results from simple passive diffusion. Both the reabsorption of filtered bicarbonate in the proximal tubule and the net excretion of acid in the proximal and distal tubules are accomplished through the secretion of hydrogen ion from the tubular cell into the tubular lumen (Fig. 52–2). Note in Figure 52–2 that for each hydrogen ion secreted into the tubular lumen, a bicarbonate moves from the cell into the peritubular capillary and the circulation. Increased hydrogen ion secretion increases the movement of bicarbonate into plasma, thereby increasing plasma bicarbonate levels. A decrease in tubular hydrogen ion secretion decreases the amount of bicarbonate entering the plasma.

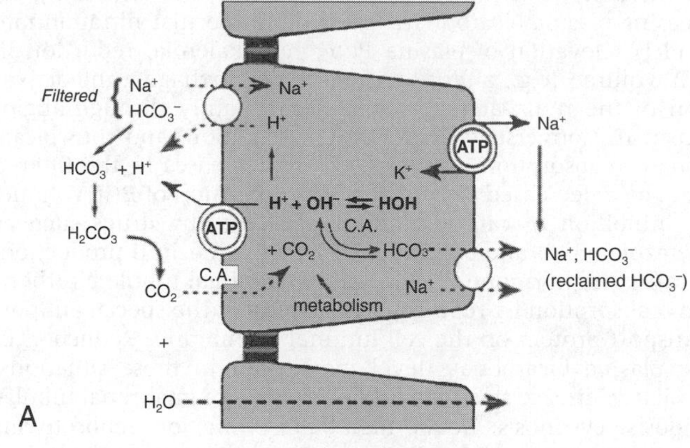

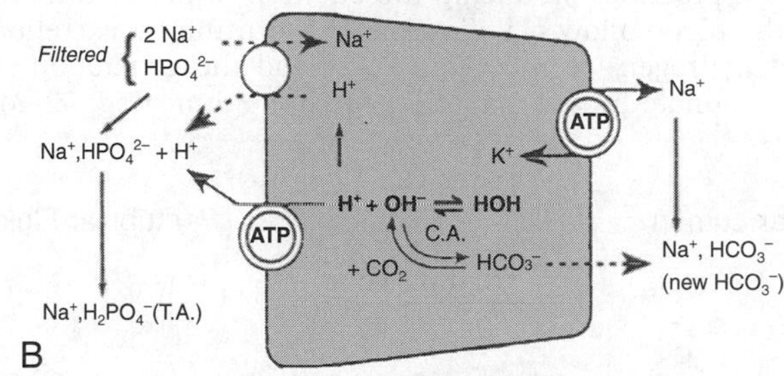

Figure 52–2 *A*, Reabsorption of filtered bicarbonate. *B*, Buffering of secreted hydrogen by phosphate, adding a "new" bicarbonate in the circulation.

As shown in Figure 52–2, reabsorption of bicarbonate centers on the secretion of hydrogen ion from the cell into the tubular lumen in exchange for sodium via an antiporter membrane transport protein. In the proximal tubule cell, hydrogen ion and bicarbonate are produced from H_2CO_3 catalyzed by carbonic anhydrase. As the hydrogen ion is secreted into the tubular lumen, the bicarbonate exits the cell across the basolateral membrane and into the peritubular capillary. Within the tubular lumen, the secreted hydrogen ion combines with filtered bicarbonate to form H_2CO_3. The newly formed H_2CO_3 is rapidly converted to CO_2 and water by the enzyme carbonic anhydrase present on the proximal tubule cell membrane, and exposed to the luminal contents. The H_2CO_3 conversion products, CO_2 and water, rapidly diffuse into the cell, where they are substrate for the reformation of H_2CO_3 within the cell, mediated by intracellular carbonic anhydrase. These mechanisms ensure that virtually no bicarbonate passes to more distal segments of the nephron and that an amount of bicarbonate equal to the amount filtered is returned to the peritubular capillaries. A number of factors cause an increase in the rate of hydrogen ion secretion in the proximal tubules and lead to increased bicarbonate reabsorption with consequent elevation of the serum bicarbonate level. These include an increase in the filtered load of bicarbonate (either by increasing plasma bicarbonate levels or glomerular filtration rate [GFR]), elevation of plasma P_{CO_2}, hypokalemia, reduction in ECF volume (e.g., after vomiting or hemorrhage), and activation of the renin-angiotensin system, mainly through angiotensin II. Conversely, hydrogen ion secretion, and thus bicarbonate reabsorption, is decreased by decreases in the filtered load, by a decreased plasma P_{CO_2}, by expansion of ECF volume, by inhibition of carbonic anhydrase (e.g., by drugs such as acetazolamide), and by inhibition of angiotensin II production. Parathyroid hormone (PTH) inhibits proximal tubule bicarbonate reabsorption by reducing the activity of the special antiport transport protein on the cell luminal membrane. Reduction in the plasma bicarbonate level may occur in these situations. Similarly, disease states such as primary proximal renal tubular acidosis, cystinosis, heavy metal poisoning, or nephrotoxins associated with structural or functional damage to the proximal tubule may limit bicarbonate reabsorption at this site and result in decreased plasma bicarbonate levels, producing systemic acidosis.

The two processes producing the addition of new bicarbonate to the blood allow acidification of the urine by excretion of fixed hydrogen ion (see Fig. 52–2) and the generation of new bicarbonate by the excretion of ammonium (Fig. 52–3).

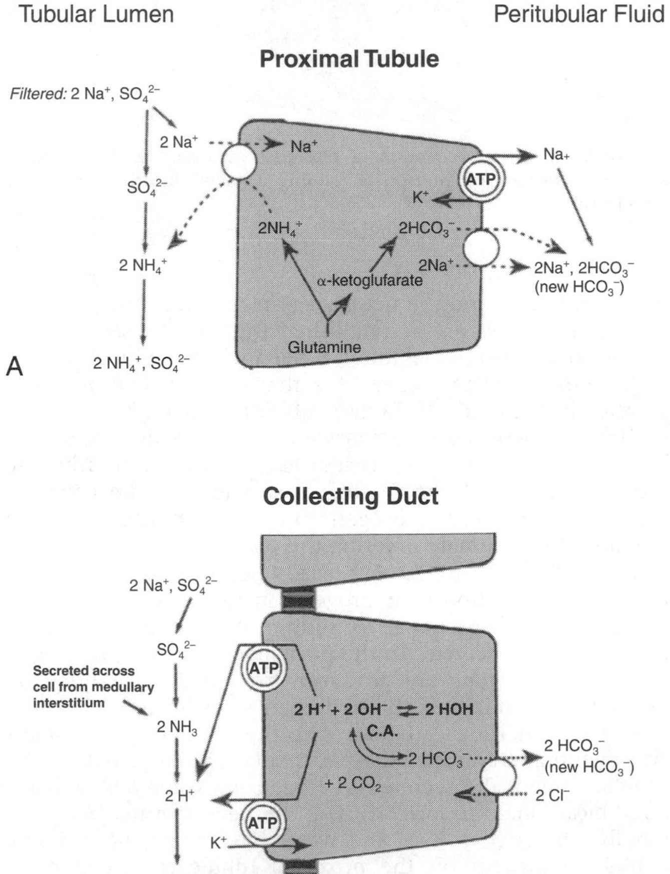

Figure 52–3 Renal excretion of ammonium. *A*, Production of ammonium and "new" bicarbonate by the catabolism of glutamine. Ammonium is secreted into the tubular lumen and excreted. Bicarbonate is delivered to the circulation. *B*, Buffering of secreted hydrogen ion by ammonia and production of "new" bicarbonate.

Excretion of fixed hydrogen ion and addition of new bicarbonate to the blood requires tubular lumen buffering of secreted hydrogen ion, most importantly regulated in the distal convoluted tubule and collecting ducts. Hydrogen ions are generated within these tubular cells by the same process as that described for the proximal tubular cells and secreted into the tubular lumen; in the process, bicarbonate is added to the blood. These nephron segments have a proton-translocating adenosine triphosphatase that actively secretes hydrogen ion under normal conditions. The transport of hydrogen ions at this site appears to be gradient limited, with the distal tubule able to generate a gradient for free hydrogen ion from tubular lumen to tubular cell of up to 1,000:1. Transport is thus facilitated by the presence of buffers in the tubular fluid that decrease the concentration of free hydrogen ion and permit increased movement of hydrogen ion from cells into the tubular fluid. The principal buffers at these sites are phosphate (see Fig. 52–2) and ammonia (see Fig. 52–3).

Once combined with buffers in the tubular fluid, hydrogen ion is excreted, because unlike the proximal tubule, the cell luminal membrane does not have carbonic anhydrase. Filtered, or nonbicarbonate, buffers, principally phosphate, combine with hydrogen ion to excrete titratable acid (see Fig. 52–2), representing the amount of alkali required to bring the urine to a neutral pH. Under most conditions, large amounts of phosphate are present in the distal tubular fluid. In the presence of a high concentration of free hydrogen ions, the phosphate is converted from a monohydrogen to a dihydrogen form, reducing the concentration of free hydrogen ion in the tubular fluid.

The excretion of ammonium accounts for both hydrogen ion buffering and new bicarbonate production. In the proximal tubule cell (see Fig. 52–3), glutamine is hydrolyzed to glutamate and ammonium. Most of the glutamate is then metabolized to α-ketoglutarate, liberating another ammonium. The ammonium is actively secreted into the tubular lumen and excreted. The subsequent metabolism of α-ketoglutarate also yields two bicarbonates, charged cations that cannot readily diffuse back from luminal fluid. The bicarbonate is taken up by the peritubular capillaries, adding new bicarbonate to the blood. Some of the secreted ammonium, NH_4^+, is reabsorbed in the thin loop of Henle and trapped in the medullary interstitium. With changes in interstitial pH, the concentration of ammonia, NH_3^+, increases and then diffuses into the tubular lumen, where it buffers hydrogen ion that has been secreted from the collecting duct (see Fig. 52–3). This allows excretion of hydrogen ion and addition of new bicarbonate similar to the process accomplished by filtered buffers, such as phosphate. These two processes enable an increased rate of transport of hydrogen ions into the distal renal tubule fluid and allow the generation of new bicarbonate, which can enter the plasma and replenish depleted levels of plasma bicarbonate (see Figs. 52–2 and 52–3). The absolute net rate of excretion of hydrogen ions by the kidneys is calculated as the sum of the excretion rates in the urine of titratable acid and ammonium ion minus urine bicarbonate. Living on an average mixed diet, an adult in the United States must excrete about 70 mEq of hydrogen ions each day to maintain balance. Approximately one third is excreted as titratable acid, the remaining two thirds as ammonium.

By stimulating hydrogen ion secretion, aldosterone is a major regulatory factor and, thereby, contributes to the generation of new bicarbonate in the distal nephron. Other factors influencing distal hydrogen ion secretion include the prevailing P_{CO_2} and the amount of sodium delivered to these segments. The distal acidification mechanisms may be impaired by intrinsic defects in the tubule, which cause primary distal renal tubular acidosis, or by various insults such as nephrocalcinosis, vitamin D intoxication, or amphotericin B administration, which produce secondary forms of distal renal tubular acidosis.

NORMAL ACID-BASE BALANCE. Most mixed diets produce a net amount of hydrogen ions; true vegetarians ingest a neutral ash diet. Protein is the largest source of hydrogen ions; its metabolism accounts for approximately 65% of the total, generated primarily from the oxidation of sulfur-containing amino acids to yield sulfuric acid and from the oxidation and hydrolysis of phosphoproteins to yield phosphoric acid. The remainder of the hydrogen ions come from the incomplete catabolism of carbohydrates, fats, and organic acids, such as pyruvic, lactic, acetoacetic, and citric acids. Complete oxidation of these compounds does not produce excess hydrogen ions, because water and CO_2 are the final reaction products; incomplete metabolism results in the formation of organic acids and adds hydrogen ions. Milk and meat diets generate about 70 mEq of hydrogen ions/24 hr in adults and require the kidneys to excrete an equal amount daily to maintain a normal blood pH of 7.35–7.45. Infants and children must excrete proportionally similar amounts of hydrogen ions. As a consequence, the daily turnover of hydrogen ions is large, amounting to more than 50% of the hydrogen ions usually in the body buffers and 10% of the maximum storage capacity of the buffers. This hydrogen ion concentration is initially buffered by the intracellular and ECF buffers and then by respiratory compensation before the kidneys excrete the hydrogen ions to maintain balance.

DISTURBANCES OF ACID-BASE BALANCE

Definitions. Abnormalities in blood pH occur when the hydrogen ion concentration increases above normal, called *acidemia*, or decreases below normal, called *alkalemia* (see Fig. 52–1). The suffix -emia refers to changes in blood pH. The abnormal clinical processes that cause acid or alkali to accumulate are called *acidosis* and *alkalosis*, respectively. The suffix -osis is applied to clinical conditions that may or may not imply that a change in blood pH has occurred. For example, metabolic acidosis need not necessarily be associated with acidemia, because the accumulation of acid might have been handled by the buffer defense mechanisms or respiratory compensation might have occurred to bring the blood pH toward normal.

The simple acid-base disorders are shown in Figure 52–4. The primary alteration refers to the initiating disturbance that produces, at least transiently, a change in the blood pH by altering P_{CO_2} or plasma HCO_3. Acidosis is caused by conditions that result in a primary decrease in plasma HCO_3 or an increase in P_{CO_2} that decreases blood pH below normal (defined as <7.40 in Fig. 52–4) by increasing the hydrogen ion concentration. Alkalosis is caused when the primary disturbance increases plasma HCO_3 or decreases P_{CO_2}, which increases blood pH above normal (>7.40 in Fig. 52–4) by decreasing hydrogen ion concentration.

When a primary acid-base disturbance in plasma HCO_3 or P_{CO_2} occurs, a compensatory response restores blood pH toward normal. Referring to Equation 52–6, acid-base balance (i.e., normal blood pH) is defined as the ratio of P_{CO_2} to plasma HCO_3. The changes of blood pH produced by the primary respiratory and metabolic alterations are determined by the ratio of P_{CO_2} to HCO_3. The offsetting compensatory response necessarily moves in a direction that attempts to restore the ratio, and therefore the blood pH, to normal. Figure 52–4 gives the expected compensation for each primary acid-base disturbance. Primary metabolic disorders elicit respiratory compensation, and primary respiratory disorders elicit metabolic compensation. For example, a primary decrease in the plasma HCO_3 concentration increases blood hydrogen ion concentration, and blood pH falls below normal. This primary metabolic acidosis with a lowered blood pH stimulates the respiratory center to increase alveolar ventilation, which reduces P_{CO_2} and returns the blood pH toward normal. The primary event of metabolic acidosis is a decrease in plasma HCO_3 concentration, lowering blood pH, and the compensatory event is a decrease in P_{CO_2}, accomplished by enhanced ventilation to return the P_{CO_2}/HCO_3 ratio and blood pH toward normal.

A *simple acid-base disorder* is defined as a single primary unidirectional alteration in the respiratory (P_{CO_2}) or metabolic (plasma HCO_3) parameter, with a compensatory response by the remaining parameter. Figure 52–4 provides methods to determine if the expected compensation is appropriate during steady-state conditions. If the actual compensatory response falls outside the expected value, a *mixed acid-base disorder* is likely. Systemic acidosis or alkalosis may result from primary metabolic or respiratory abnormalities. Recovery is unlikely to occur if the blood pH falls below 6.80 or increases above 7.80. The rate of response by the respiratory and renal mechanisms differs. Respiratory responses occur more rapidly: 50% in 6 hr and 100% in 14–16 hr. Renal mechanisms are slower, with renal base excretion more rapid than acid excretion. Renal base excretion is 50% at 8 hr and 100% at 24 hr. Renal acid excretion is 50% at approximately 36 hr and is 100% at 72 hr.

Metabolic Acidosis. This results from an alteration in the balance between production and excretion of acid. Systemic acidosis may result from increased blood hydrogen ion concentration due to accumulation caused by increased intake from an

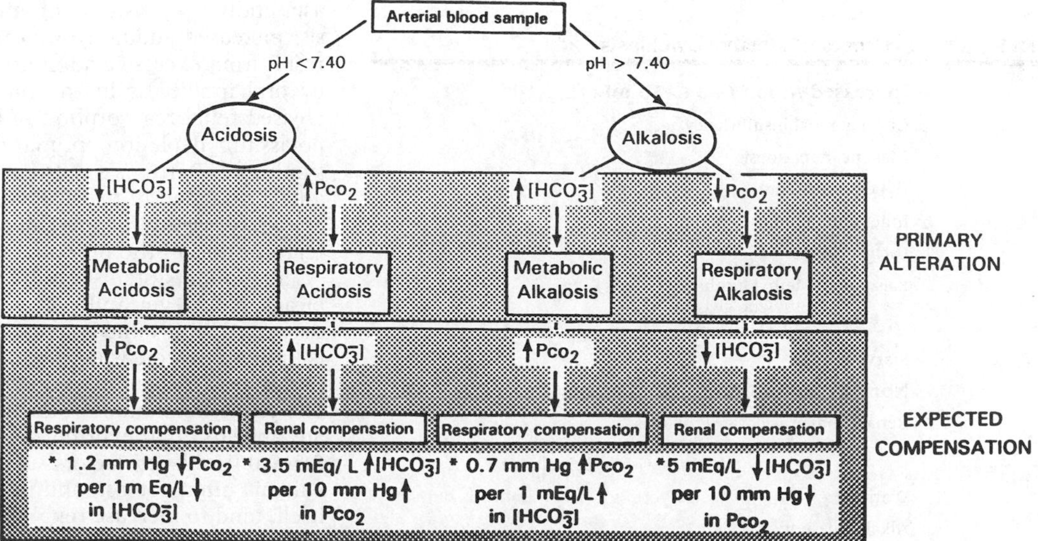

Figure 52–4 Approach for the analysis of simple acid-base disorders. (From Koeppen BM, Stanton BA: Renal Physiology. St. Louis, Mosby-Year Book, 1992.)

exogenous source or increased endogenous production or by inadequate excretion of hydrogen ions or excessive loss of bicarbonate in the urine or stools. Rapid expansion of the ECF space by a bicarbonate-free solution may also produce metabolic acidosis by diluting the bicarbonate in the ECF. The hydrogen ion load is buffered initially by bicarbonate in the ECF and by intracellular buffers such as hemoglobin and phosphate. Bone may be another source of buffer. The serum bicarbonate level and pH fall (to a lesser extent than if no buffering mechanism were available) and Pco_2 rises.

The resulting systemic acidosis and increased Pco_2 stimulate the respiratory center (and possibly peripheral chemoreceptors in the carotid artery and aorta) to increase the respiratory rate, which increases the rate of excretion of CO_2. Plasma Pco_2 and H_2CO_3 levels fall, partially or almost totally correcting the acidosis but at the expense of lowering both plasma bicarbonate and Pco_2. The blood pH is decreased but rarely drops as low as might be predicted from the low level of plasma bicarbonate.

The acidosis also stimulates the kidneys to increase ammonia production and hydrogen ion excretion into the urine. In the distal nephron, the secretion of hydrogen ion is accompanied by the return of a bicarbonate to the circulation (see Fig. 52–2), increasing the generation of bicarbonate and returning the plasma bicarbonate level to normal if the primary disease process has been alleviated. The respiratory rate subsequently decreases, with the Pco_2 returning to normal. At this point, the patient's acid-base status has returned to the normal state that existed before the hydrogen ion load was administered.

The *clinical manifestations* of metabolic acidosis are often nonspecific. The most important physical sign is hyperventilation, the extreme of which is the deep, rapid respirations (i.e., Kussmaul's breathing) needed for respiratory compensation. However, severe acidosis itself may cause a decrease in peripheral vascular resistance and cardiac ventricular function, resulting in hypotension, pulmonary edema, and tissue hypoxia. The laboratory findings are decreased serum pH and decreased levels of HCO_3 and Pco_2 (see Fig. 52–4).

The *anion gap* is an important tool in evaluating metabolic acidosis. As described in Chapter 48, the anion gap represents the unmeasured anions, which along with bicarbonate and chloride counterbalance the positive charge of sodium. The normal anion gap, calculated as [Na] + [K] − ([Cl] + [HCO_3]), is 12 mEq/L, with a range of 8–16 mEq/L. Determining the anion gap in metabolic acidosis is an important clinical clue to narrow the possible causes of the acidosis (Table 52–1). In general, metabolic acidosis associated with an elevated anion gap results from overproduction of endogenous acids, such as keto acids in diabetic ketoacidosis or lactic acidosis; underexcretion of fixed acids with advanced renal failure; or the ingestion of excess exogenous acids, such as salicylates. A normal anion gap (i.e., hyperchloremic) results from the net loss of bicarbonate from the kidneys (e.g., renal tubular acidosis, nephrotoxin related) or the gastrointestinal tract, mainly from diarrhea.

TABLE 52–1 Causes of Metabolic Acidosis

Increased Anion Gap (>16 mEq/L)	
Chronic renal insufficiency	
Diabetic ketoacidosis	
Hyperalimentation	
Inherited aminoacidurias	
Lactic acidosis	
Poisoning:	Methyl alcohol Ethylene glycol Salicylate
Starvation	
Normal Anion Gap (8–16 mEq/L)	
Renal tubular acidosis:	Proximal Distal Distal with hyperkalemia
Diarrhea	
Alkali ingestion	

Renal Causes. The renal causes of metabolic acidosis are numerous. Diseases involving the proximal tubules may limit the ability of this segment of the nephron to secrete hydrogen ions and cause incomplete bicarbonate reabsorption. Increased amounts of bicarbonate are presented to the distal tubular fluid, resulting in the proximal form of *renal tubular acidosis*. In distal renal tubular acidosis, the distal tubule cannot maintain a normal hydrogen ion gradient to promote hydrogen ion secretion into the distal tubular lumen, and the urine pH remains relatively alkaline, rarely falling below 5.5. A reduction of titratable acid, decreased secretion of hydrogen ion, and systemic acidosis result. With *chronic renal insufficiency*, acidification mechanisms work normally or at supranormal rates. However, the reduced tubular mass limits the ability of the kidneys to generate sufficient ammonia and to excrete adequate amounts of hydrogen ions. A *low GFR*, such as in a newborn, also limits the renal capacity to excrete hydrogen ion. The filtered load of phosphate also is reduced, with the bulk reabsorbed in the proximal tubule; little is left for buffering added hydrogen ions in the distal tubule. Hydrogen ion transport is reduced by rapid attainment of a maximal concentration gradient in the absence of buffer. Rarely, *reduction in ammonia synthesis*, as in the cerebro-oculorenal syndrome of Lowe, limits the ability to excrete hydrogens ions.

Other Causes. Metabolic acidosis may also develop in *diabetic ketoacidosis* from incomplete metabolism of body lipids and catabolism of body protein, accompanied by the production of large amounts of acetoacetic, β-hydroxybutyric, phosphoric, and sulfuric acids. In *salicylism*, metabolic acidosis results from hydrogen ions derived from salicylic acid and from the uncoupling of oxidative phosphorylation by salicylate. In *severe diarrhea*, the increased losses of bicarbonate in diarrheal fluid and possibly the formation of organic acids from the incomplete breakdown of carbohydrate in the stools result in metabolic acidosis. Hyperalimentation, lactic acidosis, starvation, and poisoning with either methyl alcohol or ethylene glycol cause systemic acidosis by increasing the production of various strong acids. Metabolic acidosis also occurs in certain inherited aminoacidurias (e.g., methylmalonicaciduria), in hypoxemia, and in shock.

Metabolic Alkalosis. Three basic mechanisms may produce alkalosis: excessive loss of hydrogen ion, as in prolonged gastric aspiration or persistent vomiting associated with pyloric stenosis; increased addition of bicarbonate to the ECF, which may result from excessive administration by the parenteral route or by oral intake, as in the milk-alkali syndrome, or from increased renal reabsorption of bicarbonate caused by profound potassium depletion, primary hyperaldosteronism, Cushing's syndrome, Bartter's syndrome, or excessive intake of licorice; and contraction of the ECF volume, which increases bicarbonate concentration in this fluid space and increases bicarbonate reabsorption in the proximal tubule.

The buffer systems minimize pH change, but the plasma bicarbonate level and pH are increased. Respiration may be depressed with some increase in plasma Pco_2, but this response is limited by increasing hypoxia so that respiratory compensation is always incomplete and never restores the pH to normal. The renal threshold for bicarbonate is exceeded, and bicarbonate appears in the urine, which may have a pH as high as 8.5–9.0. However, factors such as volume depletion and hypokalemia often coexist, and they, along with the increased Pco_2 itself, tend to increase renal reabsorption of bicarbonate, maintaining the metabolic alkalosis. Metabolic alkalosis may be refractory to treatment in the presence of hypokalemia or depletion of ECF volume and often can be treated only after these deficiencies have been corrected.

The diagnosis of metabolic alkalosis should be considered in any patient with an appropriate history; there are no pathognomonic *clinical manifestations* of this electrolyte disturbance. Patients may have cramps or feel weak and may have the signs of tetany if ionized calcium has been reduced by the alkalosis.

Characteristically, the pH, plasma bicarbonate level, and P_{CO_2} of arterial blood are elevated (see Fig. 52–4). Hypochloremia and hypokalemia are usually present, the latter principally resulting from increased urinary losses of potassium. Classically, the urine pH is alkaline, but in the case of severe depletion of potassium, the urinary potassium level is low and *paradoxical aciduria* exists. In patients who have volume depletion and who are responsive to sodium chloride, urine chloride concentrations should be less than 10 mEq/L. Patients who have metabolic alkalosis resulting from excessive mineralocorticoid activity or potassium depletion have a urine chloride level exceeding 20 mEq/L and are resistant to sodium chloride treatment.

Respiratory Acidosis. Inadequate pulmonary excretion of CO_2 in the case of normal production of this gas produces acidosis. It may occur acutely in neuromuscular disorders, such as brain stem injury, Guillain-Barré syndrome, or sedative overdose; in airway obstruction, such as that caused by a foreign body, severe bronchospasm, or laryngeal edema; in vascular diseases, such as massive pulmonary embolism; and in other conditions, such as pneumothorax, pulmonary edema, or severe pneumonia. Chronic respiratory acidosis may accompany the pickwickian syndrome, poliomyelitis, chronic obstructive airway disease, kyphoscoliosis, or chronic administration of sedatives.

In health, increased production of CO_2 stimulates its own respiratory excretion, which maintains a normal P_{CO_2} and acid-base status. In any of the disease states causing respiratory acidosis, the level of P_{CO_2} increases until it is elevated sufficiently to cause pulmonary excretion of CO_2 equal to its production. Although a new steady state is reached, the increase in P_{CO_2} (i.e., hypercapnia) causes a systemic acidosis by increasing serum concentrations of H_2CO_3 and, therefore, of hydrogen ions.

Because CO_2 is a major component of the principal buffer system of the ECF, the rise in P_{CO_2} must be buffered initially by the nonbicarbonate buffers—the proteins in the ECF and phosphate, hemoglobin, other proteins, and lactate in the cells. The acidosis and increased P_{CO_2} stimulate the kidneys to increase hydrogen ion excretion as ammonium and titratable acid and to generate and reabsorb more bicarbonate; the plasma bicarbonate levels may be increased somewhat above normal. At this stage, the increase in the plasma bicarbonate level compensates for the primary increase in P_{CO_2} so that the pH returns toward normal and the respiratory acidosis has been "compensated" by renal mechanisms. The only way to correct the abnormality is to reverse the primary disorder.

The causes of acute respiratory acidosis are often associated with hypoxemia, which usually dominates the *clinical manifestations*, along with the signs of respiratory distress. Hypercapnia results in vasodilatation and increased cerebral blood flow and may be responsible for the headaches and raised intracranial pressure sometimes found in these patients. Severe hypercapnia may be a cerebral depressant; arterial pH is low, P_{CO_2} elevated, and plasma bicarbonate level elevated moderately (see Fig. 52–4).

Respiratory Alkalosis. Excessive pulmonary losses of CO_2, in the presence of normal production result in a fall in P_{CO_2} and produce respiratory alkalosis. This process may be observed with hyperventilation of psychogenic origin, with overventilation from mechanically assisted ventilation, and in the early stages of salicylate overdose as a result of stimulation of the respiratory center by salicylate or of increased sensitivity of the respiratory center to P_{CO_2}. Plasma P_{CO_2} falls, and pH rises. A rapid buffering of this pH change occurs, with hydrogen ions released from body buffers to decrease plasma bicarbonate. Approximately 99% of the hydrogen ions are released from intracellular buffers, with the remaining 1% from extracellular buffers. The renal excretion of bicarbonate, slowly increasing by mechanisms that are incompletely understood, reduces plasma bicarbonate levels and compensates for the excessive loss of CO_2, returning the pH toward normal. However, correction cannot occur until the causative disorder has been removed.

The *clinical manifestations* are usually those of the underlying disease process. However, acute hypercapnia may result in neuromuscular irritability and paresthesias in the extremities and periorally because of a decrease in the concentration of ionized calcium. Arterial pH is elevated, and the P_{CO_2} and plasma bicarbonate levels are decreased (see Fig. 52–4). Despite systemic alkalosis, the urine usually remains acid.

Mixed Disorders. Under certain circumstances, mixed disturbances may occur; in these, more than a single primary cause is responsible for the abnormal acid-base balance. A mixed acid-base disorder should be suspected when the compensatory response falls outside the expected range (see Fig. 52–4 and Fig. 52–5). For example, in respiratory distress syndrome, metabolic and respiratory acidoses often coexist. The respiratory disease prevents the compensatory fall in P_{CO_2}, and the metabolic component limits the ability to increase the plasma bicarbonate level, which would normally buffer a respiratory acidosis. In this situation, the decrease in pH is often profound, of greater magnitude than that of a single disturbance.

Other types of mixed disturbances may be encountered. Patients with congestive heart failure and chronic respiratory acidosis may develop a component of metabolic alkalosis if they use diuretics excessively. The plasma bicarbonate level and pH are higher than in a simple chronic respiratory acidosis. The pH may be normal or even slightly elevated. Patients with hepatic failure may have metabolic acidosis and respiratory alkalosis. The plasma bicarbonate level and P_{CO_2} may be lower

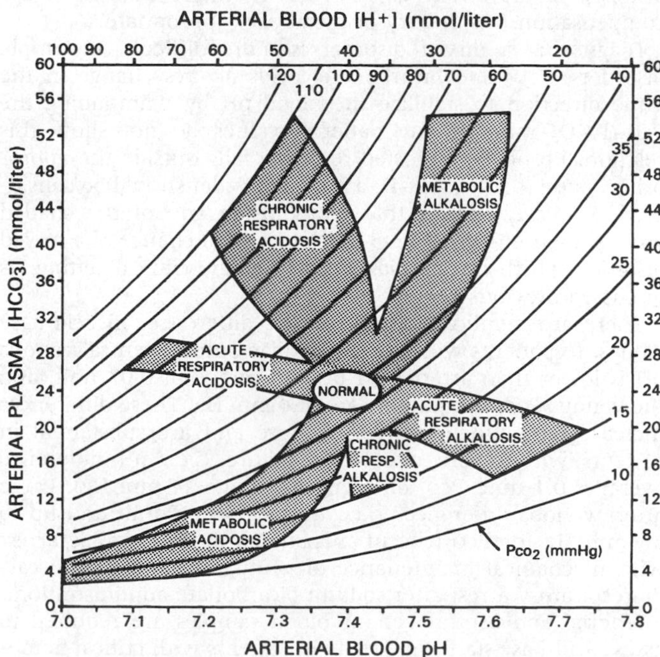

Figure 52–5 The acid-base nomogram shows the 95% confidence limits of metabolic and respiratory compensations for the primary acid-base disturbances. (From Cogan MG, Rector FC: Acid-base disorders. *In*: Brenner BM, Rector FC [eds]: The Kidney. Philadelphia, WB Saunders, 1991.)

than expected with a simple disorder, although the pH may be little changed from normal. Respiratory and metabolic alkaloses also may coexist in some circumstances.

CLINICAL ASSESSMENT OF ACID-BASE DISORDERS. For clinical purposes, acid-base status is determined from serum pH, P_{CO_2}, and bicarbonate levels.

Measurements. Blood pH can be measured accurately in small blood samples; normal values are 7.35–7.45. The concentration of H_2CO_3 in biologic fluids is quantitatively negligible compared with dissolved CO_2. The latter is measured as P_{CO_2} in a gas phase in equilibrium with the biologic fluid; the normal value is approximately 40 mm Hg.

The concentration of bicarbonate ion in plasma can be measured directly, but the precision of this determination is not required for clinical purposes. It is customary to determine total CO_2 concentration of the serum as an estimate of bicarbonate level. This value is 1–2 mEq/L higher than that of true bicarbonate. It is obtained by titration or by generation of CO_2 from serum with a strong acid. The CO_2 is derived principally from bicarbonate but also from dissolved CO_2, H_2CO_3, carbonate ion, and carbamino compounds. The normal value is 25–28 mM/L, except in the first year of life, when values are 20–23 mM/L, probably because of the low renal threshold for bicarbonate.

If only two of these values are known, the third can be derived from one of the nomograms developed for this purpose, or it can be calculated by one of the several methods based on the Henderson-Hasselbalch equation (see Equation 52–6). If all three measurements have been made, the same formulas can be used to check the validity of the values.

Interpretation. It is relatively easy to diagnose a simple acid-base disorder correctly, based on the blood pH, P_{CO_2}, and bicarbonate levels and using an acid-base nomogram such as that shown in Figure 52–5 or the summary of laboratory findings shown in Figure 52–4. Understanding that blood pH is maintained by the ratio of P_{CO_2} to HCO_3, a patient's acid-base status can be readily ascertained. The following steps provide a useful guide for determining an acid-base abnormality. First, is the condition acidosis or alkalosis? Second, is the primary cause metabolic or respiratory? Third, if it is metabolic acidosis, is the anion gap normal or high? Fourth, is the compensation (respiratory or metabolic) appropriate?

Diagnosing a mixed disorder is more difficult. In simple disorders, P_{CO_2} and bicarbonate levels always change in the same direction to stabilize the blood pH by maintaining the P_{CO_2}/HCO_3 ratio. If any patient's values do not show this relationship or the expected response falls outside the appropriate value (see Fig. 52–4), a mixed disorder should be considered. Similarly, results that plot outside any of the shaded areas shown in Figure 52–5 indicate a 95% chance of a mixed disorder, which can be diagnosed from the clinical setting, as discussed previously.

There are significant arteriovenous differences in acid-base values. In patients with normal cardiac output, central venous pH is lower than arterial pH by an average of 0.03 unit, and the venous P_{CO_2} is higher by about 6 mm Hg. These differences increase with moderate heart failure and are substantial in patients with severe circulatory failure (i.e., pH difference averages 0.1 unit; P_{CO_2} differences average 24 mm Hg). Large arteriovenous differences (i.e., up to 0.35 pH unit and up to 56 mm Hg for P_{CO_2}) occur in patients during cardiac arrest with mechanical maintenance of ventilation and during cardiorespiratory arrest after sodium bicarbonate administration.

Arterial and central venous blood samples are required to assess acid-base status optimally in patients with critical hemodynamic compromise. Arterial samples provide information about pulmonary gas exchange, and central venous samples provide more accurate information on the acid-base status of tissues during conditions of severe hypoperfusion.

Intracellular pH. Normal intracellular pH has been estimated to be 6.8; values as low as 6.0 have been obtained using microelectrodes. Mitochondrial pH may be even lower because intracellular pH is probably inhomogeneous.

Because CO_2 diffuses readily across cell membranes, intracellular and extracellular values for P_{CO_2} are similar. The intracellular changes in hydrogen ion concentration may occur as a result of primary respiratory disorders that cause hypocapnia or hypercapnia. With hypocapnia, intracellular alkalosis is proportional to the degree of extracellular alkalosis. With hypercapnia, because intracellular bicarbonate concentrations cannot be adjusted as rapidly as those in the ECF, intracellular acidosis may be proportionally greater than that in the ECF. In contrast to the situation in respiratory acidosis, intracellular pH may be maintained in the presence of severe metabolic acidosis until extracellular pH drops below 7.0.

The effects of extracellular acidosis and alkalosis on cellular functions are not fully understood. A low pH produces a slight change in the Donnan distribution across the capillary membrane, and some decrease in oncotic pressure results in a reduced plasma volume. Low pH also seems to reduce myocardial contractility and impair catecholamine action, and it increases the likelihood of arrhythmia, particularly with hypoxia. Moreover, if the hydrogen ion concentration rises rapidly, it may inhibit further transport of the ion in the kidneys. Metabolic disturbances also alter the exchange of sodium and potassium ions for hydrogen ions; a potassium deficiency may decrease the intracellular pH at the same time that the extracellular pH is elevated.

Changes in intracellular pH probably affect the activities of many enzymes. A decrease in carbohydrate tolerance has been observed in acidosis, and an increase in neuromuscular irritability (i.e., latent or manifest tetany) occurs in alkalosis. Hypocapnia leads to an increase in the blood lactic acid level, with a decrease in the bicarbonate concentration and production of metabolic acidosis.

Cerebrospinal Fluid pH. Bicarbonate and carbonic acid represent virtually all the buffering capacity in cerebrospinal fluid (CSF). CO_2 can diffuse freely between the blood and CSF. Increases or decreases in P_{CO_2} in the blood are reflected by similar changes in the CSF, although the latter value is also modified by the rates of CO_2 production in the brain. In contrast, increases or decreases in the concentration of bicarbonate in blood lead only slowly to small changes in the bicarbonate level in CSF. Consequently, the concentration of hydrogen ions in the CSF does not change instantaneously with changes in extracellular pH; the pHs of these fluids may differ significantly at times, especially if active respiratory compensation of a metabolic acidosis or alkalosis has occurred. Particular problems may develop if a compensated metabolic acidosis is corrected too quickly. Correction results in an increase in P_{CO_2} and bicarbonate levels in the ECF, but only the P_{CO_2} rises in the CSF. The pH of the ECF returns to normal, but that of the CSF falls even further, and continuing neurologic symptoms and abnormalities in respiration may result.

Chan JCM, Gill JR Jr (eds): Kidney Electrolyte Disorders. New York, Churchill Livingstone, 1990.

Cogan MG, Rector FC Jr: Acid-base disorders. *In*: Brenner BM, Rector FC Jr (eds): The Kidney. Philadelphia, WB Saunders, 1991.

Edelman CM Jr (ed): Pediatric Kidney Disease, 2nd ed. Boston, Little, Brown & Co, 1992.

Holliday MA, Barratt TM, Avner ED (eds): Pediatric Nephrology, 3d ed. Baltimore, Williams & Wilkins, 1994.

Koeppen BM, Stanton BA: Renal Physiology. St. Louis, Mosby–Year Book, 1992.

Kokko JP, Tannen RL: Fluids and Electrolytes, 3rd ed. Philadelphia, WB Saunders, 1996.

Narins RG, Emmett M: Simple and mixed acid-base disorders: A practical approach. Medicine 59:161, 1980.

Schrier RW (ed): Renal and Electrolyte Disorders, 5th ed. Philadelphia, Lippincott–Raven, 1997.

Valtin H, Schafer JW: Renal Function, 3rd ed. Boston, Little, Brown & Co, 1995.

CHAPTER 53
Fluid Therapy

Parenteral or oral fluid therapy is employed to maintain or restore the normal volume and composition of body fluids. It should be administered in a safe and efficient manner that maximizes the corrective capability of normal physiologic mechanisms within the body, primarily through the circulatory, respiratory, and renal systems. The goal is to normalize the intracellular and extracellular chemical environments that optimize cell and organ function. Initiated experimentally in the 19th century by Latta, *parenteral fluid therapy* emerged as a scientific and therapeutic entity in the 20th century. This occurred with the development of methods to measure electrolytes such as sodium, potassium, and chloride and to perform balance studies documenting net losses of electrolytes and fluid in children being repleted for diarrheal dehydration. *Oral rehydration,* widely studied since the 1960s, is a simple, safe, and effective way to treat most children with mild to moderate dehydration.

Fluid therapy is an essential component of pediatric medicine throughout the world. In developing countries, 4–5 million youngsters die yearly of dehydration, which is often superimposed on infection and malnutrition. In the United States, about 15–30 million cases of diarrhea in children result annually in 2 billion dollars in health care costs, approximately 10% of admissions to pediatric facilities (roughly 200,000 admissions/yr), and approximately 300 deaths. Dehydration from fluid loss, most commonly vomiting and diarrhea, can be particularly devastating in infants because of limited access to fluids and a turnover of total body water (TBW) of 15–20% per 24 hr, compared with only 5% per 24 hr in adults. Profound diarrheal losses in infants may not be as evident as in adults. In a 3 kg newborn, diarrhea of only 3 tbs every 3 hr results in almost a 50% reduction in extracellular fluid (ECF) volume in a 36 hr period, which is equivalent in an adult to a loss of 8 L of ECF! The problem of diarrheal dehydration is magnified in the malnourished infant, in whom there may be chronic deficits of electrolytes and limited caloric reserves.

DETERMINATION OF REQUIREMENTS. Fluid therapy consists of three categories: maintenance, deficit replacement, and supplemental replacement of ongoing losses. *Maintenance* fluid expenditures are a function of metabolic rate, and maintenance therapy is designed to replace usual body losses of fluid and electrolytes. *Deficit* is described as losses per kg of body weight, and deficit therapy is designed to replace abnormal losses of fluid and electrolytes, usually as a result of an illness. *Supplemental* replacement is based on measured or estimated continuing abnormal losses; supplemental therapy, when indicated, is given in addition to maintenance and deficit fluids.

Each component of therapy can be calculated independently. A fasting preoperatively stable youngster awaiting surgery may need only maintenance fluid and electrolytes before restoration of oral intake postoperatively, but a child with diarrheal dehydration probably needs all components: maintenance, deficit, and supplemental therapy. Although several modified and simple approaches to parenteral therapy have been described (see Chapter 54), it is essential that the physician understand the pathophysiology of body fluids and the specific needs in each of the three areas of fluid therapy. Equally important is the recognition that fluid therapy is based on gross estimates of maintenance requirements, deficit, and ongoing losses. In actual practice, per cent deficit is often overestimated. The patient is always the final common pathway of therapeutic interventions and must be clinically assessed each step of the way.

If the patient is under- or overhydrated after oral or parenteral therapy, the therapy must be readjusted and individualized accordingly. Monitoring is usually easily done at the bedside, with physical examination and assessment of changes in intake, output, and body weight. Serum chemistries may be followed as indicated, but evaluating their results does not replace close bedside monitoring.

MAINTENANCE THERAPY. Maintenance fluid and electrolyte requirements are directly related to metabolic rate. Changes in metabolic rate affect endogenous water production through the oxidation of carbohydrate, fats, and protein; urinary solute excretion, which influences urinary fluid losses; and heat production, 25% of which must be dissipated through the mechanism of insensible water loss. Although several systems have been used to estimate maintenance fluid and electrolyte requirements, the simplified scheme by Holliday and Segar (Table 53–1) that relates caloric expenditure to body weight for a resting, hospitalized patient is easy to use, physiologic, and applicable over the range of pediatric and adult weights. It compares favorably with other approaches and focuses attention on the caloric needs of patients, not just the fluid and electrolyte needs. This is a critical factor in the highly catabolic patient or the child requiring long-term parenteral management. Estimated caloric requirements, if not provided by oral or parenteral intake, are derived through depletion of fat, glycogen, and protein stores.

Maintenance water requirements are determined by water lost from feces and urine and insensible losses. Because fecal water losses are usually negligible, fluid requirements of 100 mL/100 calories primarily address insensible and renal water losses. Approximately one third of this water requirement is for insensible water loss, and two thirds are for renal water loss. **Insensible water loss** occurs through pulmonary and cutaneous routes, with the latter accounting for two thirds and the former for one third of insensible water loss. Conditions that may increase or decrease insensible water loss requirements are associated with changes in caloric expenditure, heat production, and the need for changes in insensible water loss to modulate dissipation of body heat. Insensible water loss increases with increased activity (≥30%), with fever (i.e., 12% increase for each 1°C rise in body temperature), and with reduced vapor tension in the environment. Conversely, insensible water loss decreases with decreased activity, as in comatose states, and with hypothermia, by 12% for every 1°C fall in body temperature. Pulmonary insensible water loss increases with hyperventilation, as in asthma or diabetic ketoacidosis, and decreases with exposure to highly humidified atmospheres or humidified ventilator systems. Cutaneous losses may be especially high in the low birthweight and very low birthweight infant with a large surface area and decreased skin thickness. In this population, insensible water losses of 100–200 mL/kg/24 hr may occur. Insensible water loss is further increased with the use of overhead lights for the treatment of hyperbilirubinemia.

TABLE 53–1 Simplified Method for Calculating Maintenance Fluid Requirements From Body Weight (based on 100 mL for each 100 kcal expended)

Body Weight (kg)	mL/Day*
Up to 10	100 mL/kg
11–20	1,000 mL + 50 mL/kg for each kg above 10 kg
Above 20	1,500 mL + 20 mL/kg for each kg above 20 kg

**Maintenance fluid and electrolytes: 100 mL water (35 mL insensible water loss, 65 mL urinary water loss) and 2–4 mEq of Na and K for every 100 calories expended.*

Urinary water requirements may be increased when renal concentrating ability is diminished by an increased solute load or by diminished secretion of or response to antidiuretic hormone (ADH). The solute load may be increased in diabetes mellitus, after the infusion of mannitol or radiocontrast agents, in electrolyte wasting, or by high-protein diets. ADH deficiency is usually associated with CNS conditions such as craniopharyngioma or other neoplasms, septo-optic dysplasia, head trauma, granulomas, or infections. A diminished response to ADH by the renal tubules occurs in the condition known as nephrogenic diabetes insipidus (NDI). Primary NDI is uncommon and readily diagnosed by family history and clinical presentation. However, secondary NDI may occur in common conditions such as sickle cell disease, chronic pyelonephritis, renal cystic disease, obstructive uropathy, reflux nephropathy, psychogenic polydipsia, hypokalemia and hypercalcemia, as well as in response to certain medications.

Urinary water losses are diminished in conditions associated with oligoanuria such as the syndrome of inappropriate antidiuretic hormone, acute or chronic renal failure, or genitourinary tract obstruction. If urinary water loss is abnormal, maintenance fluid therapy should be adjusted accordingly by replacing insensible water loss plus urinary output on a milliliter for milliliter basis with free water.

Maintenance requirements for sodium and potassium may also be modified for certain patients. Sodium requirements may be higher in patients with increased cutaneous losses from cystic fibrosis; in patients with increased urinary losses from salt-losing nephritis, obstructive uropathy, chronic pyelonephritis, or diuretic therapy; and in patients with increased gastrointestinal losses from fistulas, diversions, nasogastric drainage, or inflammatory bowel disease. Losses from gastric or intestinal drainage are usually replaced by isotonic or half-normal sodium chloride. In some situations, it may be necessary to measure the electrolyte composition of gastrointestinal fluid to aid estimates for electrolyte replacement. Sodium requirements are diminished in edematous states owing to hepatic, cardiac, or renal disease; edema indicates excess body sodium. Patients who have chronic renal failure may require less sodium, especially if they are hypertensive; those with acute anuric renal failure, if euvolemic, should receive no sodium.

Maintenance potassium requirements may also be higher in patients with ongoing abnormal gastrointestinal or genitourinary losses. Potassium-losing states generally parallel sodium-losing states and may occur with chronic renal disease associated with renal medullary injury, with gastric or intestinal drainage, and with chronic laxative or diuretic abuse. Increased renal potassium loss accompanies the alkalosis associated with gastric drainage and loss of hydrochloric acid. In conditions of diminished potassium-excreting ability, such as chronic renal failure and adrenal insufficiency, potassium intake may have to be modified. In cases of acute anuric renal failure, adrenal insufficiency, or severe acidosis with hyperkalemia, no potassium should be administered.

Further maintenance requirements are created by internal shifts of body fluid. In certain clinical situations, **third spacing**, the shift of ECF from the plasma compartment elsewhere, such as interstitial or transcellular spaces, may necessitate changes in the provision of fluid and electrolytes. The volume of third-space fluid is difficult to assess, but the electrolyte composition usually approximates that of ECF. For fluid lost from ECF to another compartment, replacement fluid should be based on clinical assessment, including the impact of third spacing on the effective plasma volume and the resultant effect on circulatory status. Massive increases in ECF from third spacing may necessitate adjustment of drug dosages for medications that are distributed in the ECF compartment.

Maintenance fluid and electrolytes may be given orally or parenterally. Although water, sodium, and potassium needs are easily met by these regimens, the *provision of calories* is insufficient to sustain a positive nitrogen balance. A 5% dextrose solution usually provides enough calories to have some sparing effect on catabolism of protein, but for patients with diminished glycogen and fat storage or those in highly catabolic states, this amount of dextrose may be calorically insufficient. In these patients and in those on parenteral therapy for more than a few days, additional nutrition is provided by parenteral alimentation with 5% or higher dextrose solutions, with or without the addition of amino acids, or by the use of total parenteral nutrition (TPN) delivered through a deep central venous catheter, an arterial line, or an arteriovenous fistula. Such lines are at risk for infection and thrombosis and should be inserted, maintained, or changed only by skilled individuals. Of equal importance is the recognition that TPN represents an important and potentially toxic "medication." The careless use of TPN may result in excess sodium, potassium, magnesium, or osmols given to patients with compromised renal function; inadequate provision of intracellular cations and anions such as potassium, magnesium, and phosphate for highly anabolic patients; or excessive amounts of sodium for patients with renal artery thrombosis or renal failure who are at risk for hypertension. Hyperglycemia, hypophosphatemia, and severe metabolic acidosis may also complicate this therapy and even be life threatening. The ratio of calcium to phosphorus in TPN provided to very low birthweight infants is very important in promoting calcium and phosphorus retention and improving bone mineralization. Inappropriate calcium and phosphorous infusions may lead to hypercalciuria, osteopenia, fractures, and nephrocalcinosis. The physician should pay careful attention on a daily basis to the volume and composition of TPN fluid in terms of the patient's nutrient requirements, which may vary significantly from day to day. Careful attention also should be given to serum electrolytes, calcium, phosphorus, magnesium, glucose, and serum urea nitrogen and to fluid intake, output, and body weight.

DEFICIT THERAPY. Deficits in fluid and electrolytes (Table 53–2) represent the cumulative net impact of oral or parenteral dietary intake, pathologic body losses resulting from disease processes, or physiologic body losses including corrective attempts to modify the volume and composition of losses through normal excretory routes. The net effect produces deficits that are often similar in their magnitude and composition and often, despite different causes, may be treated in a similar fashion. The severity of the deficit reflects the magnitude and rapidity of change, but the type of deficit reflects the relative loss of water and electrolytes, primarily sodium.

Severity of Deficit. The severity of fluid deficit is represented as the percentage of body weight lost (Table 53–3). Acute losses of body weight reflect losses of fluid and electrolytes rather than lean body mass. Although the physician may have a recently recorded baseline weight for the patient, in most clinical situations the percentage of body weight lost is an

TABLE 53–2 Estimated Deficits of Water and Electrolytes in Infants with Moderately Severe Dehydration

Condition	H_2O (mL)	Na (mEq)	K (mEq)†	Cl (mEq)
Fasting and thirsting	100–120*	5–7	1–2	4–6
Diarrhea				
Isonatremic	100–120*	8–10	8–10	8–10
Hypernatremic	100–120*	2–4	0–4	−2 to −6‡
Hyponatremic	100–120*	10–12	8–10	10–12
Pyloric stenosis	100–120*	8–10	10–12	10–12
Diabetic acidosis	100–120*	8–10	5–7	6–8

**All estimated deficits are per kilogram of body weight.*
†Converted for breakdown of tissue cells: − 1 g of N = 3 mEq of K.
‡Negative balance of chloride indicates an excess at the beginning of therapy.

TABLE 53–3 Clinical Assessment of Severity of Dehydration

Signs and Symptoms	Mild Dehydration	Moderate Dehydration	Severe Dehydration
Body weight loss (%)	3–5%	6–9%	10% or more
General appearance and condition; infants and young children	Alert, restless	Thirsty, restless or lethargic, irritable to touch	Lethargic or comatose; limp, cold, sweaty, cyanotic; poor peripheral perfusion
Older children and adults	Thirsty, alert, restless	Thirsty, alert, postural hypotension	Usually conscious; apprehensive; cold, sweaty, cyanotic; wrinkled skin of fingers and toes; muscle cramps
Radial pulse	Normal rate and strength	Rapid and weak	Rapid, feeble, sometimes impalpable
Respiration	Normal	Deep, may be rapid	Deep and rapid
Anterior fontanel	Normal	Sunken	Very sunken
Systolic blood pressure	Normal	Normal or low; orthostatic hypotension	Low, may be unrecordable
Skin elasticity	Pinch retracts immediately	Pinch retracts slowly	Pinch retracts very slowly
Eyes	Normal	Sunken	Grossly sunken
Tears	Present	Absent to reduced	Absent
Mucous membranes	Moist	Dry	Very dry
Urine flow	Normal	Reduced amount and dark	Anuria/severe oliguria
Capillary refill	Normal	±2 sec	>3 sec
Estimated fluid deficit (mL/kg)	30–50	60–90	100 or more

estimate based on the history and physical examination. Infants with a history of fluid loss and no clinical signs of dehydration are considered to have mild dehydration, representing 3–5% of body weight or 30–50 mL/kg of body weight lost. Infants with signs of moderate dehydration are estimated to have 7–10% of body weight lost, and those with marked clinical signs of dehydration have 10–15% of body weight lost or 100–150 mL/kg. In older children and adults, TBW is a smaller percentage of body weight; mild, moderate, and severe dehydration represent 5%, 7%, and 10%, respectively, of body weight lost. The clinical signs of moderate and severe dehydration often overlap and may lead to inaccurate estimates of per cent body weight lost.

The type of dehydration (Table 53–4) is a reflection of the relative net losses of water and electrolytes and is based on serum sodium concentration or plasma osmolality. These types are often used interchangeably, because extracellular osmolality is largely determined by the concentration of sodium, the dominant extracellular cation, and chloride, the dominant extracellular anion that is closely linked to sodium. *Hypotonic* or *hyponatremic dehydration* occurs when serum sodium levels are less than 130 mEq/L; *isonatremic* or *isotonic dehydration* occurs when serum sodium levels are 130–150 mEq/L; and *hypertonic* or *hypernatremic dehydration* occurs when serum sodium levels are greater than 150 mEq/L. Hypertonic dehydration may occur with serum sodium levels less than 150 mEq/L in the presence of other abnormal osmol levels, such as glucose in diabetic ketoacidosis or mannitol. In uremia, increased urea raises extracellular osmolality, but because urea diffuses well across cell membranes into the intracellular space, it has little net effect on extracellular osmolality.

The type of dehydration has important ramifications from the standpoint of pathophysiology, therapy, and prognosis. Intracellular and extracellular osmolality are maintained at equal levels in the body. Changes in the osmolality in one compartment lead to compensatory shifts in water, which is freely diffusible across cell membranes, from one compartment to the other, to restore equality of osmolality between body water compartments. In *isotonic* or *isonatremic* dehydration, no osmotic gradient across cell walls exists, and intracellular fluid (ICF) volume remains unchanged. In *hypotonic* or *hyponatremic* dehydration, the ECF is hypotonic relative to the ICF, and water shifts from the extracellular to the intracellular compartments. Volume depletion through external losses in this form of dehydration is exacerbated by an internal shift of ECF to the intracellular compartment. The resultant marked decrease in extracellular volume may be manifested clinically as profound dehydration leading to circulatory collapse. In patients with *hypertonic* or *hypernatremic* dehydration, the converse occurs; water shifts from the intracellular space to the extracellular space to restore equality of osmolality between compartments. This is the only form of dehydration that significantly decreases intracellular volume. Signs of extracellular depletion are modified because of this compartmental "steal" syndrome.

TABLE 53–4 Dehydration and Serum Sodium Concentration

Type of Dehydration	Electrolyte Status
Hypotonic or hyponatremic	Serum Na <130 mEq/L
Isotonic or isonatremic	Serum Na 130–150 mEq/L
Hypertonic or hypernatremic	Serum Na >150 mEq/L

A careful history can prove provide information for estimating the magnitude and type of deficit. Careful attention must be paid to the types and quantities of fluid intake and output, to any documented changes in body weight or in the frequency and appearance of urine, and to the general appearance and behavior of the child. A child with diarrhea for several days who has ingested adequate water but little sodium may present with hyponatremia. An infant with a high fever for several days and little access to water may have hypernatremia, as may a child with an inaccurately prepared, highly concentrated formula or homemade electrolyte solution. Infants on diuretics or with renal salt-losing conditions may, in the absence of adequate oral intake, develop hyponatremia, but infants with primary or secondary NDI, in the absence of access to free water, are likely to develop hypernatremic dehydration.

Hypernatremic and hyponatremic dehydration each occur in 10–15% of the population, but approximately 70–80% of pediatric dehydration is isotonic, with hypotonic stool losses being replaced, albeit inadequately, with hypotonic oral fluids. Most infants with severe dehydration have a history of lethargy, listlessness, and decreased responsiveness; those with hypernatremic dehydration tend to be irritable and fussy. Decreased urinary frequency and volume is common in severe dehydration, but this sign may be deceptively absent in children with defective renal concentrating ability, who continue to excrete sizable quantities of urine despite severe volume depletion, and in some low birthweight infants.

CLINICAL MANIFESTATIONS. Table 53–3 summarizes the physical findings in children with mild, moderate, and severe dehydration. Children with mild dehydration have a history compatible with dehydration but few physical findings, whereas those with severe dehydration have marked physical signs. Patients with moderate dehydration fall somewhere in between.

The clinical signs of dehydration largely represent the depletion of ECF volume and, therefore, changes in plasma volume, interstitial fluid, and transcellular fluid. Transcellular fluids include fluids of the salivary glands, pancreas, liver, and biliary tracts; mucosal fluids of the respiratory and gastrointestinal tracts; the vitreous humor of the eyes; cerebrospinal fluid; and intraluminal contents of the gastrointestinal tract. Other extracellular-like fluids that may contribute to signs of volume depletion include peritoneal, pleural, and pericardial effusions.

Mild dehydration may be manifested only by thirst and occasionally by changes in behavior. With *moderate to severe dehydration,* the anterior fontanel is sunken, reflecting the depletion in cerebrospinal fluid; mucous membranes are dry from depletion of transcellular fluids; skin demonstrates tenting as a result of decreased interstitial fluid; and eyes are sunken because of the decreased vitreous humor. The appearance of sunken eyes is often obvious to a parent but not necessarily to the physician; it is frequently, however, one of the earliest clinical signs that improves after rehydration. Tenting of the skin, often improperly evaluated, should be tested by pinching and gently twisting the skin of the abdominal or thoracic wall. Tented skin remains in a pinched position rather than springing quickly back to normal. Skin tenting may be difficult to ascertain in the severely malnourished child and in the premature infant. In these patients, dehydration may be overestimated. Tear production may be lacking in severe dehydration, although some tearing still may be observed. With hypovolemia due to contraction of plasma volume, the patient may have hypotension, cool extremities, and activation of the sympathetic nervous system, accompanied by tachycardia and sweating. Postural changes in blood pressure and heart rate occur but are not commonly evaluated. This is unfortunate, because oscillometry and Doppler techniques are usually successful in measuring systolic blood pressure in the infant whose blood pressure may be difficult to obtain by auscultation.

With *very severe dehydration,* circulatory collapse occurs, with cool, cyanotic, sweating extremities; a rapid, thready pulse; mottled skin; and severe lethargy or coma. Delayed capillary refill often occurs in patients with severe dehydration. Capillary refill, measured by compressing the ball of the thumb or large toe and estimating or measuring the time for return of blood flow or a blush, is greater than 3 sec with profound volume depletion. Capillary refill may also be delayed in a cool ambient environment. Although many physical findings may be observed with severe dehydration, the most sensitive and specific appear to be general appearance, decreased capillary refill, dry mucous membranes, and decreased skin turgor. Nonetheless, because many physical findings seen in moderate dehydration are the same as those in severe dehydration, overestimation of severity of dehydration is common, especially among inexperienced physicians.

Different types of dehydration may have different clinical manifestations. Patients with hypotonic dehydration, because of external losses and internal fluid shifts, may present with signs of profound volume depletion and shock. Patients with hypernatremic dehydration tend to have fewer signs of dehydration, even with a similar volume loss. Their skin is warm and has a doughy feel. Patients with hypernatremic dehydration tend to be lethargic, but very irritable when touched, and to be hypertonic and hyperreflexic. Patients with systemic acidosis from diarrhea and excessive stool bicarbonate losses may show Kussmaul breathing; those with hypokalemia may have weakness, abdominal distention, ileus, and cardiac arrhythmias. Patients with hypocalcemia and hypomagnesemia may have associated tetany, muscle twitching, and abnormal ECG findings.

LABORATORY EVALUATION. Laboratory tests can be useful in evaluating the nature and extent of dehydration and in guiding therapy, but they cannot substitute for careful bedside observation of the patient. Management of dehydration requires the clinical skills of the physician. In cases of serious dehydration, therapy should always be initiated promptly, even before receipt of the laboratory test results.

Identifying hemoconcentration, indicated by elevated hemoglobin, hematocrit, and plasma proteins, may help in estimating the severity of dehydration and in monitoring the response to rehydration. However, when hemoglobin and hematocrit appear normal despite severe dehydration, the physician should suspect that hemoconcentration exists and that the patient has an underlying anemia, often due to iron deficiency.

Serum or *plasma electrolyte values* are often helpful. Serum *sodium concentration* defines the type of dehydration and reflects the relative losses of water and electrolytes, not of total body sodium stores. Hypernatremia is not usually caused by sodium excess but is often associated with a mild to moderate deficiency of total body sodium.

Serum potassium values are usually normal or elevated in diarrheal dehydration. Hyperkalemia may be related to acidosis or diminished renal function. Hypokalemia may occur with significant stool losses; with gastric losses associated with alkalosis, as in pyloric stenosis; or with acute intracellular shifts in potassium with the administration of glucose or alkali. Profound depletion of total body potassium usually occurs before extracellular plasma potassium values fall below normal. Hyperkalemia and hypokalemia must be monitored carefully with serial serum sampling and with ECGs or on-line cardiac monitors. Hyperkalemia of whatever cause is a contraindication to parenteral administration of potassium, but hypokalemia is usually addressed with careful and conservative repletion of this cation.

Serum bicarbonate concentrations are helpful in detecting metabolic acidosis or alkalosis. Acidosis is most commonly associated with more severe diarrheal disease because of stool bicarbonate losses and because of retention of anions from tissue catabolism and diminished renal function. Alkalosis occurs in the setting of protracted vomiting or nasogastric drainage. Acute blood gas determinations may be helpful in defining the extent of changes in blood pH and the relative contribution of metabolic and respiratory disorders to the net acid changes.

Because *chloride* values usually parallel those of sodium, hyperchloremia accompanies hypernatremia, and hypochloremia accompanies hyponatremia. The difference in the sum of the measured cations (i.e., sodium and potassium) and anions (i.e., chloride and bicarbonate) is normally about 12 ± 4 mEq/L, the anion gap. The anion gap is elevated in cases of decreased renal function and retention of sulfate, phosphate, and other unmeasured anions and in cases of ketosis and lactic acidosis resulting from tissue breakdown and diminished muscle perfusion. A diminished anion gap may be seen with hypoalbuminemia, but no anion gap often indicates a laboratory error.

Blood urea nitrogen and *serum creatinine levels* may be elevated in severe dehydration because of a decreased glomerular filtration rate (GFR). Increased back-diffusion of urea from the proximal tubule due to decreased urinary flow may produce azotemia in the oliguric child in the absence of elevation in serum creatinine values. Serum urea nitrogen levels may be low in the highly anabolic infant, while actual elevations in serum creatinine values may be overlooked by a physician unaware that normal serum creatinine values in the infant and young child are usually much lower than in the older child and adolescent. A serum creatinine value of 1 mg/dL in an adolescent may represent a normal GFR, but the same value in a 2-mo-old infant could represent a GFR 25% of normal. A child may have severe acute dehydration despite normal values for serum urea nitrogen and creatinine, because accumulation of these waste products due to a decline in renal function occurs over time.

Urinalysis is most helpful in the measurement of urine specific gravity, which is usually elevated in cases of significant dehydration but returns to normal after rehydration. Although infants have a reduced ability to concentrate the urine, even those who are a few weeks of age can show a clear elevation in specific gravity with significant dehydration. A specific gravity less than 1.020 indicates mild or no dehydration or indicates a urinary concentrating defect, as in chronic renal disease or primary or secondary diabetes insipidus. With dehydration, urinalysis may show hyaline and granular casts, a few white cells and red cells, and 30–100 mg/dL of proteinuria. These findings are not usually associated with significant renal pathology, and they remit with therapy.

CHAPTER 54

Principles of Therapy

In the past, fluid and electrolyte therapy emphasized "deficit therapy," that is, repleting fluid and electrolyte losses, primarily sodium and potassium, to restore body composition to normal. This method has been utilized for several decades in the safe and effective management of clinical dehydration; it will be discussed as deficit fluid therapy. Some, however, have proposed a simplified fluid therapy. The proponents argue that deficit therapy is unnecessarily complex, often poorly understood, and consequently seldom followed by practitioners treating children with dehydration. Further, the slow correction over 24 hr of severe extracellular fluid (ECF) depletion, which is the dominant functional change in clinical dehydration, makes little sense, when prompt restoration of ECF will not only restore circulatory status but also set into motion, especially through the kidneys, physiologic corrective changes. Finally, experience with oral rehydration therapy (ORT) has amply demonstrated that one may safely correct, at least orally, all of the deficit in 4–6 hr with excellent results and few complications.

In patients with profound dehydration, intravenous fluid should be administered on an emergent basis, even before a complete evaluation of the patient is undertaken (see Chapter 56). In less urgent situations, before administration of fluids the patient should be evaluated clinically and the type and quantity of fluids calculated. Consideration should be given to the magnitude of water and sodium deficits, the projected changes in body composition resulting from the illness, and the impact on potassium and hydrogen ion balance. Similar therapeutic approaches are often used for patients with dehydration of different causes.

TABLE 54–1 Comparison of Oral Solutions

Solution	Glucose (mmol/L)	Na (mmol/L)	K (mmol/L)	Base (mmol/L)	Osmolality
WHO solution	111	90	20	30	310
Rehydralyte	140	75	20	30	310
Pedialyte	140	45	20	30	250
Pediatric electrolyte	140	45	20	30	250
Infalyte	70	50	25	30	200
Naturalyte	140	45	20	48	265

TABLE 54–2 Composition of External Abnormal Fluid Losses

Fluid	Sodium (mEq/L)	Potassium (mEq/L)	Chloride (mEq/L)	Protein (g/dL)
Gastric	20–80	5–20	100–150	
Pancreatic	120–140	5–15	90–120	
Small intestine	100–140	5–15	90–130	
Bile	120–140	5–15	80–120	
Ileostomy	45–135	3–15	20–115	
Diarrheal	10–90	10–80	10–110	
Sweat*				
Normal	10–30	3–10	10–35	
Cystic fibrosis	50–130	5–25	50–110	
Burns	140	5	110	3–5

Sweat sodium concentrations progressively increase with increasing sweat flow rates.

ORT (Table 54–1) is usually successful in patients with mild to moderate dehydration. Such therapy requires both the close and consistent attention of a caregiver and patient compliance. A variety of oral rehydration solutions varying in sodium and glucose content and in osmolality have been successfully used in both underdeveloped and developed countries in the treatment of the vast majority of children with mild to moderate dehydration. Failure to use ORT in developed countries is a difficult and perplexing cultural issue that reflects primarily the reluctance of many physicians to accept change.

TRADITIONAL FLUID THERAPY. Parenteral therapy is indicated for patients with severe dehydration and those who refuse oral intake or have persistent vomiting. Although the intravenous route is preferable for parenteral therapy, in unusual situations ample fluids may be given intraperitoneally or intraosseously. Parenteral therapy has three phases. *Initial* therapy is designed to expand ECF volume rapidly and improve circulatory and renal function. *Subsequent* therapy is aimed at replacing deficits while providing for maintenance water, electrolyte requirements, and ongoing losses (Table 54–2). During this phase, sodium and water losses are usually almost fully corrected. The *final* phase consists of returning the patient to normal composition, which is usually associated with a return to oral feedings and with the more gradual correction of total body potassium deficits.

Initial Therapy. The goal of initial therapy is to expand ECF volume, especially plasma volume, rapidly to prevent or treat shock (Table 54–3). An isotonic electrolyte solution, similar to plasma in composition, should be used. Isotonic saline (i.e.,

TABLE 54–3 Treatment for 10% Isotonic Dehydration in a 10-kg Infant During the First 24 Hours

Hours	First 8 Hours Water (mL)	First 8 Hours Sodium (mEq/L)	Second 8 Hours Water (mL)	Second 8 Hours Sodium (mEq/L)	Third 8 Hours Water (mL)	Third 8 Hours Sodium (mEq/L)
Deficit	500	†70	250	35	250	35
Isotonic boluses	−250	−35				
Maintenance	333	10	333	10	333	10
Ongoing losses	150	7	150	7	150	7
Total loss	733	52	733	52	733	52
Electrolyte* solution	1,000	70	1,000	70	1,000	70

Approximate electrolyte solution for each 8-hr period is ½ isotonic (after isotonic boluses are given).

0.9%; sodium and chloride, both 154 mEq/L) containing glucose (5 g/dL) is useful, especially in dehydrated patients with metabolic alkalosis. In patients with severe metabolic acidosis, the acidosis may be worsened with the additional chloride load and by dilution of serum bicarbonate levels. In this situation, an isotonic solution in which some chloride is replaced by bicarbonate (e.g., containing 140 mEq/L of sodium, 115 mEq/L of chloride, 25 mEq/L of bicarbonate) may be used. Lactated Ringer's solution provides additional buffer but should be used cautiously in patients with lactic acidosis or impaired ability to convert lactate to bicarbonate.

In the initial phase, 20–40 mL/kg of body weight of isotonic solution should be given by rapid bolus and *repeated* a second or, occasionally, a third time, until the patient is hemodynamically stable. At this time, laboratory values are usually available, and the physician can proceed with a logical and well-planned approach. This initial therapy applies to all forms of dehydration: hypernatremic, hyponatremic, or isotonic. In cases of hypernatremia, some excess in sodium may be provided, but the effect on sodium levels is usually minimal. In hyponatremia, it is not uncommon to require more than one bolus; this reflects the profound intravascular depletion in this condition and the need for additional sodium to restore normal plasma osmolality.

The physician must *never* initially rehydrate a patient with a hypotonic solution. This approach fails to "capture" rehydration fluid within the extracellular compartment; perhaps more seriously, it can cause a rapid fall in serum sodium values in patients with hypernatremia, precipitating cerebral edema, a devastating consequence of inappropriate use of initial solutions that are not isotonic.

Potassium is usually withheld from intravenous fluids unless the patient is hypokalemic or renal function is well established. Ringer's lactate does contain potassium, but the amount is minimal and usually not a concern when it is used as an initial hydrating solution. In desperate situations in which electrolyte solutions are unavailable, pure plasma expansion is needed, and a severe coexisting anemia complicates the patient's clinical condition, blood may be used in the amount of 10 mL/kg. It must be used cautiously, because blood may be associated with potential delays in availability, problems of cross matching, a risk of thrombosis, and the risk of transmission of undetected infectious diseases. A 5% albumin infusion is useful in re-expanding plasma volume but should not replace efforts to restore the total extracellular volume deficit; also, it may offer only temporary benefit in patients with diffuse capillary leak syndrome. Most studies show adequate crystalloid volume expansion to be superior to colloid infusion in hypovolemia.

Subsequent Therapy. The subsequent phase of therapy is devoted to continued replacement of existing deficit, provision of maintenance fluid and electrolytes, and replacement of ongoing losses. It is possible to calculate over 8 hr intervals (see Table 54–3) the water and sodium requirements for deficit, maintenance, and ongoing losses and arrive at a volume and composition of replacement fluid to be used. For example, with 10% isotonic dehydration, the final composition of rehydrating fluid, after the initial boluses have been given, is one-half isotonic. Deficit replacement in this model is over 24 hr but may be shortened to 8–12 hr in patients with isotonic or hypotonic dehydration.

Total body potassium deficits are not fully restored to normal until the patient is on oral feeds or, in cases of protracted parenteral therapy, on total parenteral nutrition. Potassium must move through the ECF compartment to reach the intracellular compartment, in which most potassium is stored. Large amounts of parenterally provided potassium can lead to hyperkalemia, which may have serious cardiac sequelae. Potassium is usually not provided unless the patient has voided and demonstrated acceptable renal function. There are situations, such as patients with prolonged diarrhea, hypokalemic alkalosis (e.g., pyloric stenosis), or diabetic ketoacidosis, in which profound potassium depletion may be assumed and for which repletion should not be delayed.

Provision of dextrose-containing solutions without potassium may worsen hypokalemia and lead to significant or life-threatening complications. In general, solutions are used that contain potassium in the concentration of about 40 mEq/L. Only in exceptional cases, as in patients with profound hypokalemia or substantial ongoing potassium losses (such as those that accompany certain nephrotoxic medications), should higher amounts be used. In these situations, serum levels should be followed carefully, and patients may require ongoing cardiac monitoring.

Correction of Deficits

ISONATREMIC DEHYDRATION. In isonatremic dehydration, the net loss of isotonic fluid from the body produces clinical manifestations resulting predominantly from depletion of ECF compartments such as plasma. Because there is considerable movement of extracellular sodium into cells to compensate for intracellular potassium depletion, it has been argued that only two thirds of the apparent net losses should be replaced. This approach has been validated by balance studies indicating that, in moderately to severely dehydrated children, the net external losses are about 10 mEq of sodium per 100 mL of water. Others have argued that isotonic solutions are indicated for the immediate restoration of ECF volume, because movement of sodium from intracellular spaces is gradual and complete only with full restoration of intracellular potassium levels, a process that may take several days. The net surplus of sodium provided through this approach rarely leads to elevated serum sodium values and, in the presence of normal renal function, is eliminated as sodium shifts from the intracellular compartment.

Table 54–3 indicates both approaches to *treatment* and estimations of the range of sodium deficit in a child with moderate to severe dehydration. Full repletion of deficit is calculated over 24 hr, with one half provided in the first 6–8 hr of therapy. Initial rehydration with fluid boluses is subtracted from the totals for the first 8-hr period. Some experts propose replacement of deficit in 8–12 hr if patients are not hypernatremic. Maintenance requirements exist on an hourly basis and must be met regardless of the deficit and ongoing losses. Certain conditions that may affect insensible water loss, renal water needs, or changes in normal sodium and potassium maintenance requirements can modify these recommendations. For example, a patient with obstructive uropathy and renal salt wasting requires higher amounts of daily sodium as maintenance needs. Similarly, a hyperthermic individual requires provision of more fluid for insensible water loss, and a child with a renal concentrating defect requires more fluid for renal water losses. Ongoing losses represent estimates of continued pathologic losses. In Table 54–3, ongoing stool losses reflect estimates of fluid and electrolyte losses occurring during the first 24 hr of care (see Table 54–2). The patient must be observed carefully, because losses may be less than or more than expected; not recognizing the latter may lead to serious delays in restoration of the ECF volume. If necessary, losses should be measured and replaced more frequently than every 8 hr, as the patient's clinical condition dictates.

HYPONATREMIC DEHYDRATION. Relatively greater losses of sodium than of water produce hyponatremic dehydration. The extra sodium loss can be calculated from the formula

$$\text{Sodium deficit [mEq]} = (\text{Desired } S_{Na} - \text{Actual } S_{Na}) \times \text{total body water [in L]} \ (0.6 \times \text{weight in kg})$$

in which actual S_{Na} represents the measured serum sodium concentration and desired S_{Na} is the targeted serum sodium. Even though sodium is principally an extracellular cation, total body water is used for calculating sodium deficit. This allows for repletion of sodium lost from the ECF, for any expansion of the ECF that occurs with repletion, and for repletion of sodium lost from other pools of exchangeable sodium, such as that in bone (see Chapter 46).

Treatment of hyponatremic dehydration is similar to that for isonatremic dehydration, except that the extra losses of sodium should be taken into account when calculating electrolyte administration. Administering the extra sodium needed to replace losses can be spread over 12–24 hr so that gradual correction of the hyponatremia is accomplished as the volume is expanded. Serum sodium concentrations need not be abruptly elevated by administering hypertonic saline solutions unless symptoms such as convulsions appear. The appearance of symptoms relates as much to the rate of change of serum sodium as to the absolute level and rarely occurs unless serum sodium levels fall below 120 mEq/L. Hyponatremia, with emergent symptoms, such as seizures, is usually treated by intravenous administration of a 3% solution of sodium chloride at a rate of 1 mL/min to a maximum of 12 mL/kg of body weight. Correction of serum sodium by any method must not exceed an increase in serum sodium of 0.5 mmol/hr or 10 mmol/24 hr.

Hypernatremic Dehydration. Fluid therapy for hypernatremic dehydration can be difficult, because severe hyperosmolality may result in cerebral damage with widespread cerebral hemorrhages, thromboses, and subdural effusions. This cerebral injury may result in permanent neurologic deficit. Even in the absence of obvious pathologic lesions, patients with severe hypernatremia are vulnerable to seizures. The diagnosis of cerebral injury secondary to hypernatremia is assisted by finding an elevated protein level in the cerebrospinal fluid. Thrombosis may also occur in other organs, such as in the renal veins.

Frequently, seizures occur during treatment as the serum sodium is returning to normal. During the period of dehydration, in response to increased plasma osmolality, water shifts out of cerebral cells. However, to prevent cellular dehydration, neurons make specialized idiogenic osmoles such as taurine, myo-inositol, glutamine, and glycerophosphorylcholine. With a rapid fall in ECF osmolality due to changes in serum sodium and, occasionally, a fall in the concentration of other osmotically active substances such as glucose, there may be excess movement of water into cerebral cells during rehydration, with the subsequent development of cerebral edema. In some patients, this edema may be irreversible and lethal. This may happen during an overly vigorous correction of hypernatremia or with the use of initial rapid intravenous hydrating solutions that are not isotonic. The incidence of such complications may be reduced by correcting dehydration and hypernatremia slowly over a period of days. Therapy is adjusted to return the serum sodium levels toward normal by not more than 10 mEq/L/24 hr.

Because the sodium deficit in hypernatremic dehydration is relatively small and the ECF volume relatively well maintained, the amounts of sodium and water to be administered in this phase of *treatment* are lower than those in hyponatremic or isonatremic dehydration. A suitable regimen is a 5% dextrose solution containing 25 mEq/L of sodium as a combination of the bicarbonate and chloride. Others have suggested 40 mEq/L of sodium and 40 mEq/L of potassium. Fluids with even higher sodium concentrations have been proposed. Although these fluids result in excess sodium administration to the patient, they may protect against abrupt falls in serum sodium. Most studies indicate that the composition of the rehydration solution is of less importance than careful adherence to a slow and gradual restoration of the deficit over a 48–72 hr period, which is associated with a slow return of serum sodium values to normal.

If seizures occur, they often can be controlled by anticonvulsants, intravenous administration of 3–5 mL/kg of a 3% sodium chloride solution, or measures to reduce increased intracranial pressure, such as mannitol or hyperventilation.

Treatment of hypernatremic dehydration with large amounts of water, with or without salt, frequently results in expansion of the ECF volume before there is any notable excretion of chloride or correction of the acidosis. As a consequence, edema and occasionally cardiac failure may develop. Hypocalcemia occasionally occurs during treatment of hypernatremic dehydration and may require intravenous administration of calcium. Another complication is renal tubular injury with azotemia and loss of concentrating ability.

Although hypernatremic dehydration can be successfully treated, management is difficult and seizures frequently occur, even with the best-designed regimens. It is important to emphasize prevention of neurologic sequelae. The complications of hypernatremic dehydration, especially cerebral edema, are often not the result of hypernatremia per se but of inappropriate and aggressive rehydration.

Supplemental Fluids. Supplemental fluids are mainly needed to replace ongoing losses from diarrhea or from procedures such as nasogastric drainage. In general, replacement fluid should mirror the electrolyte composition of losses (see Table 54–2). For usual diarrhea, one-half normal saline suffices, whereas in patients with cholera, normal saline should be used. Gastric losses are replaced with one-half normal to normal saline with adequate provision of potassium.

Nutritional Deficiencies. Although parenteral fluid therapy results in a caloric intake inadequate to meet the patient's needs, this is rarely a cause for concern because of the short duration of therapy. When the patient can return to a normal diet, any deficits in body fat, glycogen, and protein are soon corrected. If parenteral fluid therapy is required for prolonged periods (e.g., when patients are unable to eat or have intestinal obstruction), increased caloric and nutritional intake is best given by intravenous alimentation, which may be required to prevent the development of malnutrition.

SIMPLIFIED FLUID AND ELECTROLYTE THERAPY

Rapid Rehydration. While rapid intravenous rehydration of diarrheal dehydration is commonly practiced in emergency departments, there are insufficient data in the literature to establish upper limits of safe rapid intravenous rehydration in developed countries with non-cholera dehydration. Most studies have utilized isotonic fluids 20–40 mL/kg given over 1 hr, repeated as necessary to restore circulatory status, followed by oral feeds (preferably ORT) or, if necessary, additional maintenance intravenous fluids. Higher volumes of fluid have been used but primarily in populations with profound dehydration associated with hyponatremia such as cholera. Most balance studies in developed countries indicate that the severity of dehydration tends to be overestimated and that usual deficits for most hospitalized patients range from 4–6%. Hence, isotonic bolus therapy of around 40 mL/kg in actual practice will replete much of the ECF volume loss. Caution must be used if a patient has pre-existing problems such as hypertension, impaired renal function, or impaired myocardial function. Smaller quantities of fluid or a longer rehydration period may be indicated.

ASSESSMENT OF RESPONSE. Many factors modify the amounts and types of fluids to be administered, and the clinician must monitor the response to therapy, which should include frequent clinical observation of the child, including cry, appearance of eyeballs, activity, skin turgor, blood pressure (including orthostatic measurements), and assessment of peripheral perfusion using capillary refill or core:peripheral temperature gap. Frequent and careful measurements of body weight should be made, as well as charting of intake and output of stool and urine, to assess response to therapy. Urinary specific gravity should be measured, because it is a useful gauge of success in the absence of underlying renal disease. Certain circumstances may demand serially following serum and urine electrolyte levels; monitoring osmolality, especially with increased concentrations of nonelectrolyte osmotically active substances such as glucose and mannitol; central venous pressure; and ECGs. In the severely ill child, recording serial determinations on a carefully maintained flow sheet and using them as a guide for adjusting therapy is most important. Unpredicted responses to therapy are not uncommon.

CHAPTER 55
Fluid and Electrolyte Treatment of Specific Disorders

55.1 Acute Diarrhea and Oral Rehydration

Also see Chapters 176 and 306.

Diarrhea continues to be a serious problem in many areas of the world and may be especially lethal when superimposed on malnutrition. It results in large losses of water and electrolytes, especially sodium and potassium (see Table 54–2), and frequently is complicated by severe systemic acidosis. In approximately 70–80% of patients, the losses of water and sodium are proportionate, with *isonatremic dehydration* developing. *Hyponatremic dehydration* is seen in approximately 10–15% of all patients with diarrhea. It occurs when large amounts of electrolytes, especially sodium, are lost in the stool out of proportion to fluid losses. It occurs more frequently with bacillary dysentery or cholera. Hyponatremia may develop or worsen if during diarrhea there is a considerable oral intake of low-electrolyte or electrolyte-free fluids.

Disproportionately large net losses of water compared with losses of electrolytes result in *hypernatremic dehydration.* It is seen in approximately 10–20% of patients with diarrhea and may occur during the course of diarrhea when oral homemade electrolyte solutions with high concentrations of salt are administered or when infants are fed boiled skim milk, which produces a high renal solute load and increased urinary water losses. The potential for hypernatremia also increases with increased evaporative water loss from fever, high environmental temperatures, and hyperventilation and with decreased availability of free water.

The administration of intravenous fluids for treating profound dehydration from severe diarrhea is discussed in Chapter 54. Mild to moderate dehydration from diarrhea of any cause can be treated very effectively in a wide range of age groups using a simple, oral glucose-electrolyte solution (see Table 54–1). Oral rehydration is used in many countries and has significantly reduced the morbidity and mortality from acute diarrhea and lessened diarrhea-associated malnutrition. Oral rehydration is, unfortunately, very underutilized in developed countries but should be attempted for most patients with mild to moderate diarrheal dehydration if adequate supervision is available. Intravenous therapy may still be required for patients with severe dehydration in shock; those with uncontrollable vomiting; those unable to drink because of extreme fatigue, stupor, or coma; or those with gastric or intestinal distention.

The composition of the oral rehydration solution (ORS) recommended by the Diarrhea Disease Control Program of the World Health Organization is shown in Table 54–1. The ingredients should be available in powder form in preweighed packages. Using teaspoons or other household items for measuring the amount of solutes is inaccurate and is not recommended. In the United States, suitable preparations are available commercially. Alternatively, an ORS with similar composition can be prepared from readily available solutions as follows: NaCl (0.9% saline solution), 390 mL; glucose (5% in water), 400 mL; KCl (2 mEq/mL), 10 mL; $NaHCO_3$ (1 mEq/mL), 30 mL; water to 1 L. Glucose is the preferred sugar for use in ORS, because it facilitates the transport of sodium across the bowel wall. Sucrose can be substituted but is slightly less effective, possibly because it has to be hydrolyzed to produce glucose. The concentration of sucrose in grams per liter should be twice that of glucose to obtain the same osmolarity. Solutions containing rice-dextran or rice flour may also be effective.

As a guideline for oral rehydration, 50 mL/kg of the ORS should be given within 4 hr to patients with mild dehydration and 100 mL/kg over 4 hr to those with moderate dehydration. The amounts and rates should be increased if the patient continues to have diarrhea or if rehydration does not appear complete; fluids should be decreased if the patient appears fully hydrated earlier than expected or develops periorbital edema. Breast-feeding should be allowed ad libitum after rehydration in infants who are breast-fed; in other patients, their usual formula, milk, or feeding should be offered after rehydration.

Vomiting may occur during the first 2 hr of administration of ORS, but it usually does not prevent successful oral rehydration if the ORS is given slowly, in small amounts, and at short intervals. If sustained and severe vomiting occurs, intravenous therapy should be instituted. The patient's progress should be assessed frequently and changes in body weight monitored, if possible, to determine the degree of rehydration.

When rehydration is complete, maintenance therapy should be started. Patients with mild diarrhea usually can then be treated at home using 100 mL of ORS/kg/24 hr until the diarrhea stops. Breast-feeding or supplemental water intake should be maintained. Patients with more severe diarrhea require continued supervision. The volume of ORS ingested should equal the volume of stool losses. If stool volume cannot be measured, an intake of 10–15 mL of ORS/kg/hr is appropriate.

This regimen has not been universally accepted. The sodium concentration of ORS (90 mM/L) is two to three times that of other fluids (see Table 54–1) that have traditionally been recommended for oral therapy in patients with diarrhea. Low-sodium solutions were advocated because hypernatremia was seen frequently in the United States when oral electrolyte solutions with sodium concentrations of 50 mEq/L or more were used to treat infantile diarrhea. However, extensive use of ORS in many developing countries has shown hypernatremia to be a rare complication, probably because ORS has been used primarily for rehydration (the major previous role for oral therapy was to prevent dehydration or for maintenance); because large amounts of water are ingested in addition to ORS, often a 2:1 ratio of ORS to H_2O; and because ORS has been administered under close supervision by trained personnel. Oral rehydration has also been effective in treating acute diarrheal illnesses in well-nourished children in developed countries. Hypernatremia did not occur even when solutions containing 90 mEq/L of sodium were used. Several commercially available electrolyte solutions for oral use have been reformulated with a sodium concentration of around 50 mEq/L or higher. All these solutions have been effective in the treatment of mild to moderate dehydration. Reduced osmolality solutions (primarily reduced sodium and glucose) may be associated with reduced stool output.

It has been traditional to omit oral feedings initially when treating infants with severe diarrhea. However, even during acute diarrhea, the small intestine can absorb various nutrients and may absorb up to 60% of the food eaten. Regimens for treating acute diarrhea, including that recommended by the American Academy of Pediatrics, now encourage continued oral intake of nutrients because (1) better weight gain has been documented in infants given a liberal dietary intake during diarrhea compared with others on a more restricted intake; (2) fasting has been shown to further reduce the ability of the small intestine to absorb nutrients; and (3) no physiologic basis exists for giving the bowel a "rest" during acute diarrhea. In patients treated with intravenous therapy, oral feeding of one of the carbohydrate and electrolyte mixtures may be initiated shortly after rehydration if gastric distention and vomiting are absent. As soon as oral feeding is tolerated the caloric intake may be increased gradually by substituting mixtures that also contain fat and protein until the usual dietary intake is attained, usually within 7–8 days. In the young infant with a strong family history of allergy, a hypoallergenic feeding mixture may be used for the recovery phase because permeability of the gastrointestinal tract to whole protein may be increased during this time. The routine use of lactose-free formulas in children with diarrhea is unnecessary; 80% of children with acute diarrhea tolerate full-strength milk well.

In addition to replacing the deficits of water and electrolytes, efforts should be made to obtain an etiologic diagnosis so that specific antimicrobial therapy may be given, if indicated. Such treatment does not modify fluid therapy. Drugs such as opiates, which inhibit peristaltic activity of the bowel; absorbents such as kaolin or pectin; or bismuth subsalicylate, which alters secretion, have little or no effect on the course of infantile diarrhea and are not recommended.

55.2 Diarrhea in Chronically Malnourished Children

Severe malnutrition complicated by diarrheal dehydration is common in tropical and subtropical countries and occurs occasionally in the temperate zones. Therapy should be adapted to meet the specific disturbances in body composition characteristic of the dehydrated *and* malnourished infant, in whom there appears to be an overexpansion of the extracellular space, accompanied by extracellular and presumably intracellular hypo-osmolality. Serum sodium, potassium, and magnesium levels tend to be low, and tetany occasionally may result from a magnesium or calcium deficiency. Serum protein levels are frequently below 3.6 g/dL. The sodium content of muscle is high; potassium and magnesium contents are low. The ECG frequently shows tachycardia, low amplitude, and flat or inverted T waves. Cardiac reserve seems lowered, and heart failure is a common complication.

Despite clinical signs of dehydration and reduced body water, urinary osmolality may be low in the chronically malnourished child. This defect in renal concentration may result from the relative absence of urea to contribute to a hypertonic milieu in the renal papillae, a defect associated with a low dietary protein intake, and resulting in a failure of tubular conservation of water. However, the glomerular filtration rate (GFR) is low, resulting in a smaller loss of water than would otherwise be expected. Renal concentrating ability returns after several days of high-protein feedings. The renal acidifying ability is also limited in patients with malnutrition.

Survival of the malnourished infant with diarrhea is limited by caloric deficit to a greater extent than by water and electrolyte deficit. Reparative calories can be given by slow drip through an indwelling nasogastric tube in conjunction with oral or, when necessary, intravenous rehydration. If appetite is poor and vomiting and gastric distention are absent, feeding is begun early (30–40 cal/kg/24 hr), given by slow intragastric drip. Increases to 50–100 cal/kg/24 hr and 1–2 g of protein/kg/24 hr are made in a few days. Ad libitum intake should be permitted in the succeeding days and weeks, up to 250–300 cal/kg/24 hr, and the diet should include an adequate supply of iron and copper.

Initial parenteral therapy in profound dehydration is designed to improve the circulation and expand extracellular volume. For patients with edema, the quantity of fluid and rate of administration may need to be readjusted from recommended levels to avoid pulmonary edema. Blood should be given if the patient is in shock and severely anemic. Potassium salts can be given early if the urine output is good. Clinical and ECG improvement may be more rapid with magnesium therapy. Seizures occurring during recovery from diarrhea complicating severe malnutrition may respond to magnesium.

55.3 Congenital Alkalosis of Gastrointestinal Origin

Rarely, chronic diarrhea may result from a congenital defect in the transport of chloride in the small and large bowels. The watery stools of these patients have a high content of chloride, and alkalosis results from the ensuing volume depletion. Potassium is lost in the stools and in the urine; the latter losses are a consequence of the alkalosis. Treatment of fluid and electrolyte deficits is similar to that for pyloric stenosis. Long-term therapy must provide an adequate dietary intake of potassium and chloride. Suppression of gastric chloride secretion by a proton pump inhibitor will reduce fecal electrolyte losses. A rare, acute, chloride-losing diarrhea may also occur.

55.4 Pyloric Stenosis

Also see Chapter 329.1.

This condition exemplifies the correction of deficits associated with alkalosis. The therapy differs little from that for other causes of dehydration, except that potassium replacement should begin early, as soon as the child has urinated. In addition, relatively more sodium and potassium should be given as the chloride salt than is usual in treating dehydration; this is partly because of the larger deficit of chloride in pyloric stenosis and partly because this results in some correction of the alkalosis as the volume is expanded. Correction of the hypochloremia and alkalosis by administering ammonium chloride without correcting the potassium deficit is not recommended, because it results in continued dysfunction of renal tubular and other cells.

Severe depletion of intracellular potassium results in the increased exchange of hydrogen ion for sodium in the distal tubules of the kidney. The paradoxical presence of an acid urine with systemic alkalosis should be interpreted as signifying a marked potassium deficit and a need to increase the amount of potassium used for repletion.

It is not uncommon for deficits to be replaced and serum levels of electrolytes returned to normal within 6–12 hr. However, except in the mildly ill infant without signs of dehydration, it is preferable to delay surgery for at least 24–48 hr to achieve optimal readjustment of body functions. During this preparation period, adequate fluid therapy prevents dehydration, and the stomach may be decompressed by gentle suction.

55.5 Fasting and Thirsting

Parenteral fluid therapy is usually required in initially treating the fasting infant or child who has taken little or no water and food for one or more days. Such infants are deficient in water from insensible water loss and in electrolytes, particularly sodium and chloride, that have been excreted in the urine. If fasting and thirsting continue beyond 4–5 days, urinary output falls to such low levels that there is reduced continued loss of electrolytes. Further severe water deficiency associated with continued evaporative losses may result in hypernatremia.

Therapy is begun with an isotonic solution to produce rapid and safe expansion of extracellular volume and to improve renal function. Subsequent therapy is described in Chapter 54. Sodium and water depletion per kilogram of body weight for a given degree of clinical dehydration is generally greater in infants than in children, but potassium deficits are relatively equal in infants, children, and adults. Water, carbohydrate, and electrolytes may be administered orally to the mildly ill patient. Infants with persistent vomiting may require parenteral therapy.

For a detailed discussion of the fluid therapy of children with diabetic ketoacidosis and burns, see Chapters 70 and 599.

55.6 Electrolyte Disturbances Associated with Central Nervous System Disorders

Diseases of the central nervous system are frequently associated with disturbances in sodium concentration. Patients with diverse lesions, such as surgical or traumatic brain injury, encephalitis, brain abscess, brain tumors, Guillain-Barré syndrome, bulbar poliomyelitis, cerebrovascular accidents, tumors of the fourth ventricle, subdural hematomas, and meningitis, may present with hyponatremia. Most hyponatremia in this setting is associated with normal total body sodium, with minimal or no negative sodium balance. A decrease in serum sodium is almost entirely the result of retention of water.

The diagnosis of **syndrome of inappropriate antidiuretic hormone** (SIADH) is considered in the absence of hypovolemia, edema, endocrine dysfunction (including primary and secondary adrenal insufficiency and hypothyroidism), renal failure, and drugs impairing water excretion. Along with CNS causes, such as those mentioned, and neonatal hypoxia or hydrocephalus, this syndrome is also found in patients with pulmonary disorders, including pneumonia, tuberculosis, and asthma, as well as in those on positive-pressure ventilation and with certain carcinomas. The condition represents a defect in osmoregulation of vasopressin; diagnosis is established by measuring inappropriate secretion of ADH under hypotonic conditions. Patients with this syndrome generally have a concentrated urine despite the presence of hyponatremia and a urinary sodium concentration greater than 20 mEq/L. Also see Chapter 569.1.

Treatment of acute symptomatic hyponatremia should be prompt. One may use hypertonic saline in combination with furosemide to enhance free water excretion. Chronic and/or asymptomatic hyponatremia is best managed conservatively by water restriction to allow a gradual increase of serum sodium over 24–48 hr. Rapid normalization of hyponatremia, especially if chronic, should be avoided because of concerns of **myelinolysis**. Occasionally, an individual with a CNS lesion has hyponatremia associated with true salt wasting. In this situation, there are signs of volume depletion including weight loss, signs of dehydration, hypotension, and a diminished GFR with azotemia. Urine output may be excessive, and plasma atrial natriuretic hormone levels are increased. This situation requires the appropriate administration of salt to restore volume status.

Hypernatremia is a consequence of central diabetes insipidus and may be treated by increased oral or parenteral free water, by vasopressin boluses, or by continuous vasopressin infusion at 1.5 to 2.5 mU/kg/hr.

55.7 Perioperative Fluids

Preoperatively, preparing a patient having no pre-existing deficit or in whom the deficit has been repaired consists mainly of supplying adequate carbohydrate for sustenance and protein sparing and the usual maintenance requirements of water and electrolytes. Young infants who are not vomiting should receive carbohydrate and electrolyte mixtures by mouth until 3 hr before the operation. Such fluids are readily absorbed from the gastrointestinal tract. Preparing the newborn involves certain unique hazards. Deficits of water and electrolytes from vomiting or from stasis caused by intestinal obstruction should be replaced prior to the surgery. In cases of intestinal obstruction, conjugated bilirubin may be deglucuronidated by intestinal enzymes; enterohepatic circulation of unconjugated bilirubin can then lead to high serum levels and kernicterus. Hypoprothrombinemia should be prevented by administering 1 mg of vitamin K_1 oxide.

During surgery, blood, plasma, saline, or other volume expanders may be given if blood loss, tissue trauma, third spacing, or excessive evaporative loss occurs. The magnitude of such losses is best judged by the experienced surgeon in the course of the procedure. *The most common error in administering parenteral fluid during and after surgery is excessive administration,* particularly of dextrose in water, rather than use of isotonic solutions. Under most circumstances, little to no potassium need be administered during this time, because extensive tissue trauma or anoxia may result in the release of large amounts of intracellular potassium, with the potential of causing hyperkalemia. If shock occurs, acute renal failure may ensue, impairing the ability to eliminate through the renal route large amounts of released potassium.

Postoperatively, fluid intake should be limited for 24 hr. Thereafter, the usual maintenance therapy is gradually resumed. The water intake should not exceed 85 mL/100 kcal metabolized, because of antidiuresis resulting from trauma, circulatory readjustment, general anesthesia, or narcotic pain relief, unless renal ability to concentrate the urine is limited, as in patients with sickle cell disease, chronic pyelonephritis, or obstructive uropathy. If the intake of water is not limited, whether given parenterally or orally, water intoxication may occur associated with severe hyponatremia and even fatal cerebral edema. This has been reported in post-tonsillectomy patients. Fluid therapy in the postoperative period largely depends on the complex but anticipated response of the body to trauma through modification of water and sodium excretion and the concomitant occurrence of complications from surgery. The patient's clinical condition dictates the final fluid and electrolyte requirements incurred as a result of these processes.

Postoperatively, some children have elevated blood ADH levels due to SIADH or to an appropriate response to fluid restriction and resultant volume contraction. If decreasing urine output after surgery is the result of SIADH, the patient is euvolemic and has a normal circulatory status, stable to slightly increased weight, and an elevated urinary sodium excretion. If a child has oliguria related to third spacing and true depletion of intravascular volume, there is decreased urinary sodium excretion associated with clinical signs of hypovolemia, such as weight loss, tachycardia, changes in skin turgor and peripheral perfusion, and hypotension. Isotonic solutions are indicated in this setting.

55.8 Isolated Disturbances in Blood pH and Concentrations of Electrolytes

ACIDOSIS. Respiratory acidosis, in which the pH may be markedly lowered, primarily owing to retention of carbon dioxide, may be seen with severe respiratory insufficiency as in severe bronchiolitis and asthma, with neonatal respiratory distress syndrome, and in patients receiving assisted ventilation for any reason, who may be inadequately ventilated or have airway blockage. Acute respiratory acidosis may also be a manifestation of child abuse and may be associated with strangulation. Mild metabolic acidosis may coexist because hypoxia leads to the accumulation of lactic and other organic acids in the extracellular fluid (ECF) (see Chapter 52).

Measurements of blood pH and gases should guide the correction of acidosis. The appropriate treatment is to improve ventilation by assisting respiration rather than by administering sodium bicarbonate, which may produce hyperosmolality and cardiac failure.

Metabolic acidosis, which can result from renal tubular acidosis, renal insufficiency, or accumulation of organic acids, may require the administration of alkali, especially if symptoms are evident. In lactic acidosis, in glycogen disorders, or in circulatory insufficiency and hypoxia, sodium lactate may not be adequately metabolized; in these situations, sodium bicarbonate is the preferred agent. The usual initial dose is 1–2 mEq/kg. However, a more precise estimate of the dosage required is given by the general formula

$$(C_d - C_a) \times k \times \text{body weight [in kg]} = \text{mEq required} \quad (1)$$

in which C_d and C_a represent, respectively, the serum bicarbonate concentration desired and the one measured, expressed in units of mEq/L; k represents that fraction of the total body weight in which the administered material is apparently (not actually) distributed. The k for bicarbonate or potential bicarbonate approximates 0.5–0.6. Such calculations indicate that 0.5 mL/kg of a molar solution of sodium bicarbonate would raise the serum bicarbonate concentration approximately 1 mEq/L. However, responses to administered bicarbonate vary widely, because bicarbonate may be sequestered in bone or muscle, lost in urine, or undergoing accelerated systemic consumption.

With renal insufficiency, acidosis should be corrected cautiously, because the sodium administered with bicarbonate may result in further expansion of the ECF volume and lead to hypertension or pulmonary edema. Patients are frequently asymptomatic and have "adjusted" to the acidemic state. Overcorrecting acidosis may lead to tetany if there is an associated hypocalcemia from vitamin D deficiency or phosphate retention. It is rarely necessary to increase serum bicarbonate levels acutely above 15 mEq/L unless the patient is symptomatic. If hyperphosphatemia coexists with acidosis, it should be treated simultaneously with low-phosphate diets and oral calcium carbonate.

Treating acidosis with sodium bicarbonate should always be considered a temporizing measure. Every attempt should be made to treat the underlying cause, such as using glucose and insulin in diabetic ketoacidosis; improving circulation in shock; eliminating salicylates, methanol, or other toxins; and treating underlying sepsis. Severe lactic acidosis due to thiamine deficiency has been seen in patients receiving total parenteral nutrition lacking intravenous multivitamins.

Severe metabolic acidosis is a part of cardiovascular shock of various causes (see Chapter 64.2). Because of differences in pH and P_{CO_2} between arterial and central venous values in this situation, it is often useful to sample from arterial and central venous lines.

ALKALOSIS. Normally, the kidney has an enormous capacity to excrete bicarbonate, and increased amounts of blood bicarbonate are promptly excreted. However, under certain circumstances, *metabolic alkalosis* may develop and be maintained. Typically, it is caused by the administration of excess amounts of alkali, intravenously or orally as in milk alkali syndrome; by the loss of hydrogen ion through emesis from pyloric stenosis or nasogastric drainage; or by acute volume contraction with disproportionate losses of chloride. Severe hypokalemia can result in alkalosis or may perpetuate it (see Chapter 52).

When the plasma bicarbonate level is elevated, respiratory compensation may result in hypoventilation and an increase in P_{CO_2}. Rarely, respiration may be so depressed in infants with severe hypochloremic alkalosis that blood oxygenation is diminished. Severe alkalotic tetany may also occur. In such instances, administering ammonium chloride may effect symptomatic improvement; the dose may be calculated from the general formula (1) presented under metabolic acidosis, with a probable k of 0.2–0.3. Such therapy only relieves symptoms and should not be used in place of correcting the contracted volume of body fluids or administering potassium chloride to repair intracellular deficits.

Metabolic alkalosis associated with volume contraction responds to measures designed to expand volume and replace the chloride and potassium deficits. It occurs in patients with acid-base disorders caused by vomiting, gastric suction, congenital chloride diarrhea, dietary chloride deficiency, or administration of diuretics. In this setting of chloride depletion, urinary chloride concentration is low (≤10 mM/L). A minority of patients are chloride resistant, with urinary chloride concentrations of 15 mM/L or greater because of hyperadrenalism, Bartter's syndrome, severe potassium depletion, or licorice ingestion. Potassium repletion, using potassium chloride, not potassium phosphate, and specific therapy directed to the underlying condition are indicated.

Respiratory alkalosis occurs in salicylate intoxication; in various CNS diseases, such as severe hypoxic insult, trauma, infection, or tumors; with hysterical hyperventilation or fever; with overventilation on a respirator; and in congestive heart failure, hepatic insufficiency, and gram-negative septicemia. Treatment should be directed at removing the underlying cause, although measures designed to return the P_{CO_2} to normal may be indicated. Acidifying agents such as ammonium chloride are not indicated.

HYPONATREMIA. The serum sodium level is usually reduced as a result of true sodium depletion or water intoxication, or a combination of the two (see Table 46–2). In addition, a low serum sodium level, thought to be due to a redistribution of total body sodium, may be associated with severe illnesses or may occur in the terminally ill patient. *Apparent* hyponatremia, an artifact, may be seen in diabetic ketoacidosis and nephrotic syndrome, when the water content of plasma is reduced by the presence of increased quantities of lipids. This error is avoided by laboratory methods that determine sodium activity rather than concentration.

Patients with a serum sodium level below 120 mEq/L are often symptomatic (e.g., convulsions, shock, lethargy), although this depends in part on the rate of change in serum sodium. In infants under 6 mo of age, hyponatremia is a common cause of convulsions. Some patients with serum sodium values below 120 mEq/L, achieved over a period of several months, may be relatively asymptomatic.

The treatment of *asymptomatic hyponatremia* depends on its cause. With water overload, fluid restriction is the appropriate measure; the serum sodium level may return rapidly to normal if there is good renal function, but this may take several days or weeks for patients with SIADH. Adding extra salt to the diet or increasing the sodium concentration of parenterally administered fluid often corrects a sodium deficit.

Measuring urinary sodium concentration helps determine the cause of hyponatremia. Hyponatremic patients with a true deficit in total body sodium due to renal losses from diuretic excess, salt-losing nephritis, metabolic ketoacidosis, osmotic diuresis, or obstructive uropathy or extrarenal losses from vomiting, diarrhea, third spacing, burns, or fistulas generally have clinical signs and symptoms of ECF volume depletion. Urinary sodium concentration is often greater than 20 mmol/L in renal salt-losing conditions and less than 10 mmol/L in other situations. Correction requires administration of isotonic saline. In patients in whom hyponatremia is caused by an excess of total body water (e.g., SIADH, hypothyroidism, pain, use of certain drugs such as morphine, desmopressin, selective serotonin reuptake inhibitors, and street drugs such as ecstasy), urinary sodium concentration usually exceeds 20 mmol/L, and therapy consists of water restriction.

In patients who have excesses of sodium and water, edematous states such as nephrotic syndrome, cirrhosis, or cardiac failure, the urinary sodium level is usually less than 10 mmol/L; however, in edematous patients with acute and chronic renal failure, the urinary sodium level may be in excess of 20 mmol/L. Treatment for hyponatremia associated with edema due to excess water and salt retention is usually water and salt restriction. Inappropriate treatment may not correct an underlying defect and may be detrimental. In some patients, for example, although there is an excess of total body sodium and water, the effective plasma volume is reduced and may be further compromised by aggressive therapy directed toward correction of the edema. In other patients, administering sodium may result in further expansion of ECF volume without correcting the serum sodium level, or, in the patient with renal insufficiency, may produce or exacerbate hypertension.

In the pediatric population, hyponatremia related to sodium deficiency most commonly occurs in conditions with excess gastrointestinal loss from emesis or diarrhea; excess renal loss through salt-losing nephritis, pyelonephritis, obstructive uropathy, and use of diuretics, or excess cutaneous salt losses with cystic fibrosis and burns. Sodium deficiency may also occur in infants receiving inadequate parenteral sodium, such as very low birthweight infants, who may have excessive urinary sodium losses. Perhaps the most common cause of hyponatremia due to insufficient dietary intake of sodium in an otherwise well population in the United States occurs with the **WIC syndrome**, named for the government aid program for poor women, infants, and children. These infants are fed diluted formula or water when eligible parents fail to procure adequate infant formulas (through the WIC food supplementation program) and often present with convulsions. Providing adequate oral salt and water intake corrects this common problem, which should be readily identified by the physician through a careful history. Social service involvement is indicated. Water intoxication conditions not associated with true depletion of total body sodium are most commonly seen with SIADH occurring during CNS infections, asthma, the use of ventilatory machines, and in the postoperative period. Psychogenic polydipsia, reported even in toddlers, can cause hyponatremia.

Treatment of *symptomatic hyponatremia* consists of administering a hypertonic saline solution, calculated according to the formula (1) in the preceding section on acidosis, with k representing serum sodium rather than bicarbonate. Because there is osmotic equilibrium between cells and extracellular water, changes in osmolality are distributed over total body water so that the value for k should be 0.6–0.7 for the child and adolescent and 0.7–0.8 for the newborn or premature infant. A dose of 12 mL/kg of body weight of 3% sodium chloride solution (6 mEq sodium/kg) usually raises the serum sodium level by approximately 10 mEq/L. Rapid correction of hyponatremia may be associated with myelinolysis of the CNS in adults, which presents with disturbed sensorium, spastic quadriparesis, and pseudobulbar palsy. Although there are few data regarding the occurrence and prevalence of this problem in children, it is prudent that the initial rapid therapeutic increase in the serum sodium level should be to a value of only about 125 mEq/L; only the symptomatic individual should be treated; and no more than 10 mEq/L should be used in any 24-hr period. Subsequent elevation of serum sodium concentration should be effected in small increments over several hours. Hypernatremia should be avoided.

HYPERNATREMIA. Hypernatremia (see Table 46–1) may result from faulty preparation of infant formulas, as with the use of condensed instead of evaporated milk or heaped rather than level measures of milk powder. These errors increase the solute load excreted by the kidney relative to the amount of water provided and result in an osmotic diuresis and negative water balance. Hypernatremia can also occur in breast-fed infants, occasionally because of high breast milk sodium content but usually because of inadequate breast milk volume associated with poor weight gain.

Salt poisoning may occur through the accidental ingestion of excessive amounts of sodium chloride (e.g., table salt, seawater) by a child or the ingestion of salt accidentally substituted for sugar. This occurs with sufficient frequency in private homes and institutions to justify the routine use of liquid sugars in infant feeding. Hypernatremia may also result from the intentional salt poisoning of a child or withholding water and may be a manifestation of Munchausen syndrome by proxy (Chapter 35.3).

The excessive intake of sodium is accompanied by increases in total body sodium and in the volume of extracellular water. Severe acidosis results from a shift of organic acids and free hydrogen ions to ECF. With the shift of water from brain cells, distention of cerebral vessels occurs, leading to subdural, subarachnoid, and intracerebral hemorrhage. The complications and residual injury of salt poisoning are similar to, but may be more severe than, those seen with hypernatremic dehydration. Hypernatremia may also be seen in infants with high fever, without access to water, with excessive administration of sodium in parenteral fluids, and with inadequate availability of free water. The latter is not uncommon in the very low birthweight infant with large free water needs because of huge insensible water losses.

Hypernatremia is associated with a high mortality rate, especially if the serum sodium concentration exceeds 158 mEq/L. Treatment is directed toward the rapid removal of excess sodium from the body. Intravenous fluids should consist of glucose in water, potassium acetate, and calcium as needed. In patients with salt poisoning, *peritoneal dialysis* with glucose solutions can remove large quantities of sodium and correct hyperosmolality without the danger of pulmonary edema and heart failure. Approximately 30–45 mL/kg of a commercial dialysis solution containing 4.25% glucose can be injected intraperitoneally for severe hypernatremia (i.e., serum sodium concentration >200 mEq/L) and withdrawn 1 hr later. As the concentration of sodium in the serum falls, subsequent dialysis may be carried out using a solution with 1.5% glucose to prevent removing too much water and dehydrating the patient. Exchange transfusion is not a substitute for dialysis, because enormous quantities of blood are required to effect a change in the osmolality of total body water. Phenobarbital should be administered to prevent or control seizures. Inotropic support may be necessary to treat heart failure.

HYPOKALEMIA. Disturbances in the potassium concentration occurring without changes in volume of body fluids have been described in primary hyperaldosteronism and in Bartter's and Gitelman's syndromes. Large amounts of potassium are lost in the urine, resulting in low serum potassium and high serum bicarbonate concentrations. In congenital alkalosis of gastrointestinal origin, large amounts of potassium and chloride are lost in the stools. Using thiazide and loop diuretics (e.g., ethacrynic acid, furosemide) causes kaliuresis and natriuresis; prolonged use may result in significant potassium loss and hypokalemia. Several drugs, including penicillin, aminoglycosides, amphotericin, and antitumor agents such as cisplatin, have been associated with a significant renal potassium loss and hypokalemia.

Severe hypokalemia may result in weakness of skeletal muscles, decreased peristalsis, ileus, an inability of the kidney to concentrate urine, and excessive thirst. Patients may present with frank paralysis and significant respiratory difficulty (see Chapter 442 for ECG changes). Prolonged hypokalemia results in characteristic pathologic changes in the kidney and decreased function, which may persist even after potassium repletion.

Treatment consists of administration of adequate amounts of potassium (usually up to 3 mEq/kg/24 hr); in Bartter's syndrome or other causes of hypokalemia associated with massive urinary losses, 10 mEq/kg or more may have to be given orally. Indomethacin has proved helpful in Bartter's syndrome. Gitelman's syndrome is treated with $MgCl_2$ alone.

HYPERKALEMIA. Hyperkalemia may be present in renal insufficiency, renal tubular acidosis, Gordon's syndrome, hydronephrosis, severe acidosis, adrenal insufficiency, and tumor lysis syndrome. Marked elevation of the serum potassium level results in ventricular fibrillation and death. Levels above 6.5 mEq/L should be treated promptly, although such levels are often reasonably well tolerated by premature newborns, in whom serum potassium levels tend to be higher because of internal potassium shifts. The presence or absence of ECG changes may be helpful in deciding when to initiate therapy (see Chapter 442). The possibility of oral or parenterally administered excessive amounts of potassium should be considered and all potassium intake discontinued. Occult sources of potassium, such as antibiotics and total parenteral nutrition, may go unrecognized.

Rapid intravenous administration of sodium bicarbonate (1–3 mEq/kg) or glucose and insulin (0.5–1 g of glucose/kg with 1 U crystalline insulin/3 g of glucose) results in the movement of potassium into cells and lowers the serum potassium level. Salbutamol, given intravenously at 5 μg/kg over 15 minutes or by nebulizer at 2.5 to 5.0 mg, is very effective in lowering potassium levels for up to 2 to 4 hr. Intravenous calcium gluconate (up to 0.5 mL of a 10% solution/kg given slowly over several minutes) counters the cardiotoxicity of potassium, but the ECG should be monitored while it is being administered. None of these measures removes significant quantities of potassium from the patient. They are temporizing measures until a negative potassium balance can be established by the use of ion exchange resins, such as Kayexalate (1 g/kg/dose given by oral or rectal routes every 6–12 hr) or by hemodialysis or peritoneal dialysis. Hydrochlorothiazide is effective in lowering potassium in pseudohypoaldosteronism.

HYPOCALCEMIA AND HYPERCALCEMIA. These topics are discussed in Chapters 40, 49, 55, and 102.

HYPOMAGNESEMIA. The importance of magnesium in intravenous therapy is reviewed in Chapters 50 and 55. The only definitive symptom complex associated with hypomagnesemia (i.e., serum magnesium level <1.3 mEq/L) is that of latent or manifest tetany. Convulsions, muscular twitching, disorientation, athetoid movements, carpopedal spasm, and hyperreactivity to mechanical and auditory stimulation have been observed. Lowered serum concentrations and whole body deficits of magnesium are found in cases of chronic diarrhea or vomiting, sprue, celiac disease, prolonged parenteral fluid therapy with low magnesium composition, hyperaldosteronism, familial hypomagnesemia, Gitelman's syndrome, and increased urinary losses of magnesium from nephrotoxic medications such as cisplatin and aminoglycosides. Low serum magnesium levels have been observed in infantile tetany, presumably because of transient hypoparathyroidism.

The intramuscular injection of 0.1 mL of a 24% solution of $MgSO_4 \cdot 7 H_2O$ (0.2 mEq/kg) repeated every 6 hr for three or four doses produces symptomatic and biochemical improvement. Adding 3 mEq/L of magnesium to maintenance fluids for patients requiring long-term therapy may decrease the chance of serious deficiency (see Chapters 50 and 55). *Gitelman's syndrome,* frequently confused with Bartter's syndrome, is seen in older children and young adults. The characteristic features are hypokalemia, occasional tetany, hypomagnesemia, hypocalciuria, and normal growth.

HYPERMAGNESEMIA. Levels of serum magnesium higher than 10 mEq/L are accompanied by drowsiness and occasionally produce coma. Such levels rarely occur in the absence of renal failure. Deep tendon reflexes may be abolished, and respiratory depression may occur at higher concentrations. Disturbances in atrioventricular and intraventricular conduction may be detected at a level of 5 mEq/L. Acute renal failure and Addison's disease are accompanied by significantly elevated serum magnesium levels. Iatrogenic poisoning can result from using magnesium in treating hypertension or toxemia of pregnancy; deaths have been reported from using magnesium sulfate enemas in megacolon and from orally administering it for purging.

Intravenously administering calcium gluconate rapidly reverses the depressant effects of hypermagnesemia and the associated cardiac abnormalities.

AAP Provisional Committee on Quality Improvement, Subcommittee on Acute Gastroenteritis: Practice parameter: The management of acute gastroenteritis in young children. Pediatrics 97:424, 1996.

Brenner BM, Rector FC Jr (eds): The Kidney, 5th ed. Philadelphia, WB Saunders, 1996.

Cooper WO, Atherton HD, Kahana M, et al: Increased incidence of severe breastfeeding malnutrition and hypernatremia in a metropolitan area. Pediatrics 96:957, 1995.

Darrow DC, Pratt EL: Fluid therapy: Relation to tissue composition and expenditure of water and electrolyte. JAMA 154:365, 1950.

European Society of Paediatric Gastroenterology and Nutrition Working Group: Recommendation for composition of oral rehydration for the children of Europe. J Pediatr Gastroenterol Nutr 14:113, 1992.

Finberg L, Kravath R, Hellerstein S, Saenger P (eds): Water and Electrolytes in Pediatrics. Philadelphia, WB Saunders, 1993.

Furth S, Oski FA: Hyponatremia and water intoxication. Am J Dis Child 147:932, 1993.

Gore SM, Fontaine O, Pierce NF: Impact of rice based oral rehydration solution on stool output and duration of diarrhea: Meta-analysis of 13 clinical trials. Br Med J 304:287, 1992.

Hellerstein S: Fluid and electrolytes: Clinical aspects. Pediatr Rev 14:103, 1993.

Holliday M: The evolution of therapy for dehydration: Should deficit therapy still be taught? Pediatrics 98:171, 1996.

Holliday MA, Segar WE: The maintenance need for water in parenteral fluid therapy. Pediatrics 19:823, 1957.

Keating JP, Schears GH, Dodge PR: Oral water intoxication in infants: An American epidemic. Am J Dis Child 145:985, 1991.

Laureno R, Karp BI: Myelinolysis after correction of hyponatremia. Ann Intern Med 126:57, 1997.

Lipschitz CH, Carrazza F: Effect of formula carbohydrate concentration on tolerance and macronutrient absorption in infants with severe chronic diarrhea. J Pediatr 117:378, 1990.

MacKenzie A, Barnes G, Shann F: Clinical signs of dehydration in children. Lancet 2: 605, 1989.

McClure RJ, Prasad VK, Brocklebank JT: Treatment of hyperkalaemia using intravenous and nebulised salbutamol. Arch Dis Child 70:126, 1994.

McRae RG, Wessburg AJ, Chang KW: Iatrogenic hyponatremia: A cause of death following pediatric tonsillectomy. Int J Pediatr Otorhinolaryngol 30:227, 1994.

Meyers A: Fluid and electrolyte therapy for children. Curr Opin Pediatr 6:303, 1994.

Pearce SH, Williamson C, Kifor O, et al: A familial sydrome of hypocalcemia with hypercalciuria due to mutations in the calcium-sensing receptor. N Engl J Med 335:1115, 1996.

Pizarro D, Posada G, Sandi L, et al: Rice-based oral electrolyte solutions for the management of infantile diarrhea. N Engl J Med 324:517, 1991.

Prestridge LL, Schanler RJ, Shulman RJ, et al: Effect of parenteral calcium and phosphorus therapy on mineral retention and bone mineral content in very low birthweight infants. J Pediatr 122:761, 1993.

Rahman O, Bennish M, Alam A, et al: Rapid intravenous rehydration by means of a single polyelectrolyte solution with or without dextrose. J Pediatr 113:654,1988.

Santosham M, Daum RS, Dillman L, et al: Oral rehydration therapy of infantile diarrhea: A controlled study of well-nourished children hospitalized in the United States and Panama. N Engl J Med 306:1070, 1982.

Santosham M, Fayad I, Zikri M, et al: A double-blind clinical trial: Comparing World Health Organization oral rehydration solution with a reduced osmolarity solution containing equal amounts of sodium and glucose. J Pediatr 128:45, 1996.

Sato K, Kondo T, Iwao H, et al: Internal potassium shift in premature infants: Cause of nonoliguric hyperkalemia. J Pediatr 126:109, 1995.

Schrier RW (ed): Renal and Electrolyte Disorders. Boston, Little, Brown & Company, 1992.

Schwab M, Wensel D, Ruder H: Hypernatraemia and cerebral convulsion due to

short term DDAVP therapy for control of enuresis nocturna. Eur J Pediatr 155:46, 1996.
Vesikari T, Isolauri E, Baer M: A comparative trial of rapid oral and intravenous rehydration in acute diarrhoea. Acta Paediatr Scand 76:300, 1987.

55.9 *Tetany*

Tetany, the state of hyperexcitability of the central and peripheral nervous systems, results from abnormal concentrations of ions in the fluid bathing nerve cells. These abnormalities may include decreases of H^+ (alkalosis), Ca^{2+}, or Mg^{2+}. A decrease in H^+ may precipitate tetany when concentrations of Ca^{2+} or Mg^{2+} may otherwise lie above the threshold for manifest tetany. A decreased K^+ can prevent tetany despite low Ca^{2+} concentrations; a rising K^+ can precipitate tetany in a patient with low Ca^{2+}. Hypomagnesemic tetany can occur despite a reduction of K^+ concentration. A range of ionic concentrations exists at which tetany can be latent or manifest.

The serum calcium level, as usually measured, includes ionized calcium (Ca^{2+}) and undissociated calcium proteinate; albumin is the chief serum protein to complex with calcium. Ionized calcium can be measured, but the procedure is not available in all clinical laboratories. At normal concentrations of serum albumin, about 40–50% of the total calcium is ionized (4.0–5.2 mg/dL). When the serum albumin level is reduced, total serum calcium is decreased without necessarily resulting in a decrease in Ca^{2+}; a rule of thumb states that with each decrease of 1 g/dL of albumin, a decrease of 0.8 mg/dL of calcium results. A nephrotic child with a serum albumin level of 1 g/dL may be expected to have a total serum calcium concentration of 7.5–8.0 mg/dL without a reduction of Ca^{2+}.

At physiologic concentrations of H^+ and K^+, tetany may develop at Ca^{2+} concentrations of less than 3.0 mg/dL. Tetany usually is manifested at Ca^{2+} concentrations less than 2.5 mg/dL. At normal concentrations of serum albumin, these levels correspond to total serum calcium concentrations of approximately 7 mg/dL and 5 mg/dL, respectively.

The normal range of magnesium in serum is 1.6–2.6 mg/dL, of which about 75% is Mg^{2+}. Total serum magnesium reduced to less than 1.0 mg/dL may be associated with hyperexcitability of the nervous system.

MANIFEST TETANY. The classic signs of peripheral hyperexcitability of motor nerves are spasms of the muscles of the wrists and ankles (i.e., carpopedal spasm) and of the vocal cords (i.e., laryngospasm). In *carpopedal spasm* the wrists are flexed, the fingers extended, the thumbs adducted over the palms, and the feet extended and adducted. These muscular spasms can be quite painful. *Laryngospasm* causes inspiratory obstruction accompanied by a high-pitched inspiratory crow, which may be confused with asthma or infectious laryngotracheitis; apnea may result. Recurrent croup in an afebrile child without an upper respiratory infection should alert the clinician to the possibility of tetany. The sensory manifestations are *paresthesias,* particularly numbness and tingling of the hands and feet. Motor excitability of the CNS may be manifested by brief but recurrent *convulsions,* which are usually generalized but may be localized to one side of the body. Between seizures, the patient may be apparently conscious, but after a prolonged series of convulsions, a postictal state may result. In young infants, convulsions are frequently the only evidence of hyperexcitability of the nervous system.

LATENT TETANY. This is the condition in which ischemia or mechanical or electrical stimulation of motor nerves is required to produce the motor response characteristic of tetany. Carpopedal spasm may be induced in latent tetany through the production of ischemia of the motor nerves by reducing the arterial blood supply with a tourniquet (i.e., *Trousseau sign*); a blood pressure cuff on the arm is inflated above the systolic blood pressure for 3 min. Motor nerve impulses can be elicited by mechanical tapping, but under normal physiologic conditions, this is not possible. The facial nerve can be stimulated by tapping anterior to the external auditory meatus. Contraction of the orbicularis oris occurs with a twitch of the upper lip or entire mouth (i.e., *Chvostek sign*). The peroneal nerve can be stimulated by tapping the place where it passes over the head of the fibula; a positive *peroneal sign* is dorsiflexion and abduction of the foot.

The motor nerves can also be stimulated electrically. The *Erb sign* is a positive response of motor nerves to electrical stimulation by galvanic currents of amperage less than that required for their stimulation under normal physiologic conditions.

Another manifestation of reduced Ca^{2+} concentration is a prolonged Q-T interval for a given heart rate on the ECG. The normal Q-T interval, calculated as

$$Qt_c = \text{Measured QT (sec)}\sqrt{\text{R-R interval}}\ \text{(sec)}$$

is <0.45 in infants and <0.425 in adolescents. QT_c is the corrected Q-T interval.

ALKALOTIC TETANY. Although rare in infants and young children, alkalotic tetany can be induced through spontaneous overventilation, producing respiratory alkalosis; such hyperventilation is most often of psychogenic origin. The treatment of alkalotic tetany resulting from spontaneous hyperventilation is to have the patient rebreathe into a bag or a balloon to increase the P_{CO_2}. In patients with low Ca^{2+} concentrations, tetany may be precipitated by overventilation or by a metabolic alkalosis after the administration of sodium bicarbonate. The metabolic alkalosis resulting from a loss of gastric juice caused by pyloric obstruction is rarely associated with tetany. Alkalotic tetany has occurred in patients with renal disease who have been protected by concurrent metabolic acidosis or hypokalemia from the consequences of a low Ca^{2+} concentration. Correcting acidosis can cause tetany and convulsions; this may occur accidentally when the noncompliant patient is given in-hospital alkali presumed to be taken at home and well tolerated.

HYPOCALCEMIC TETANY

Disorders of Parathyroid Function. The most common disorder of parathyroid function is *transient physiologic hypoparathyroidism of the newborn infant,* sometimes referred to as *neonatal hypocalcemia.* Clinically, these infants can be separated into two groups: one group with hypocalcemia during the first 72 hr of life, usually before achieving a significant oral intake of milk; and a second group in whom hypocalcemia results from high phosphate load that develops only after ingestion of cow's milk for several days. The onset of symptoms in the second group occurs most commonly during the first 5–10 days of life; clinical manifestations have occasionally appeared as late as 6 wk of age. Both forms presumably result from physiologically underactive parathyroid glands that fail to respond normally to low calcium concentrations. Serum calcium values correlate directly with gestational age, and less mature infants have a greater chance of developing hypocalcemia.

In addition to a relative lack of parathyroid hormone output in the newborn period, a partial refractoriness of the target cells to parathyroid hormone may exist. Moreover, excessive secretion of thyrocalcitonin may be a major contributing factor in persistent hypocalcemia of premature infants, particularly those stressed by anoxia. The low birthweight infant whose mother has had an inadequate intake of vitamin D and little exposure to sunshine also has a low plasma concentration of 25-hydroxyvitamin D, the deficiency of which is associated with relative refractoriness to parathyroid hormone.

The relative hypoparathyroidism of the newborn has been attributed to the increased serum calcium level of the fetus, which reflects a calcium gradient across the placenta. This inhibition of the fetal parathyroids by calcium ions may be augmented by mild maternal hyperparathyroidism. Physiologic hyperparathyroidism, indicated by increased parathyroid hormone levels during pregnancy, may occur more intensely in diabetic women. Occasional cases of infant transient hypoparathyroidism have been associated with asymptomatic maternal clinical hyperparathyroidism and/or hypercalcemia.

Early Hypocalcemia. The infants at greatest risk are low birthweight infants, especially those with intrauterine growth retardation; infants born of diabetic mothers; and infants who have been subjected to prolonged, difficult deliveries (see Chapters 102 and 103). Early hypocalcemia occasionally may be seen in infants of mothers with adenomas or in infants with familial hypoparathyroidism. Calcium intake may be decreased because of the infant's small size or illness, and endogenous phosphate levels may be increased from catabolism. The incidence of hypocalcemia in prematurely born infants is extremely high, particularly in those with respiratory distress and those who have received intravenous sodium bicarbonate. Evaluating the role of hypocalcemia in the morbidity and mortality of such infants is difficult. Although hypocalcemia should be suspected as a possible cause of convulsions, it can be diagnosed only by determining serum concentrations of calcium ions.

Asymptomatic hypocalcemia of premature infants usually resolves spontaneously. However, when possible, oral calcium gluconate should be given, because it usually obviates the subsequent need for intravenous therapy and its attendant complications.

Treatment of clinical manifestations requires the intravenous injection of a 10% solution of calcium gluconate in a dose of about 2 mL/kg (18 mg Ca/kg), which must be given slowly while monitoring the cardiac rate for bradycardia; blood containing excessive calcium concentration that reaches the right atrium may inhibit the rhythmic electrical activity of the sinus node, causing cardiac arrest. Tissue necrosis and calcification may occur if this solution extravasates or is given intramuscularly. Intravenous sites should be carefully watched. The intravenous dose of calcium gluconate can be repeated at 6- to 8-hr intervals until calcium homeostasis becomes stable, or the calcium gluconate (50–75 mg elemental Ca/kg/24 hr) can be added to a constant intravenous infusion. Parenteral calcium should be administered carefully, while monitoring serum ionized calcium levels and urinary calcium levels. Because of decreased protein-bound calcium in hypoalbuminemic infants, parenteral calcium may cause elevations in Ca^{2+} and hypercalciuria associated with nephrocalcinosis.

Administering 1,25-dihydroxyvitamin D_3 during the first day of life to prematurely born infants at risk for hypocalcemia has either successfully prevented or reduced the severity and duration of hypocalcemia, but it is not recommended for routine prevention. When hypomagnesemia occurs with early neonatal tetany, it is usually mild and transient; occasionally, it requires treatment before the hypocalcemia responds to therapy. Calcium gluconate or calcium lactate may be added to the feeding at the same time, as described later. There may be a gradual return to normal calcium levels after 1–3 days. Oral calcium should be continued for about 1 wk.

Late Hypocalcemia. After a feeding of high-phosphate milk, tetany can occur in full-term and prematurely born infants and in infants whose clinical histories have been benign. The intake of a high-phosphate food, such as cow's milk, in a relatively large volume leads to an elevated serum phosphate level because of relatively high tubular reabsorption of phosphate and the physiologically low GFR of the newborn. The elevated serum phosphate level depresses the serum calcium level through deposition of calcium phosphate in bone and possibly in other tissues. The normal physiologic response is an increased output of parathyroid hormone, which increases the solubilization of bone mineral and urine phosphate excretion. This restores the normal serum levels of calcium and phosphate. If the infant's parathyroid glands are not yet able to respond by increasing parathyroid hormone, the level of serum calcium progressively falls, and symptomatic hypocalcemia may result.

Clinical Manifestations. The most important presentation of hypocalcemia in infants is convulsions, usually generalized, short, and without loss of consciousness. Carpopedal spasm is not usually seen, and because the Chvostek sign is common in newborn infants, it cannot be interpreted as a sign of tetany. Laryngospasm with cyanosis and apneic episodes may occur. Irritability, muscular twitching, jitteriness, and tremors are common clinical manifestations in the newborn. In addition to the characteristic signs from increased excitability of the nervous system, nonspecific symptoms clinically suggestive of sepsis may occur, such as poor feeding, vomiting, and lethargy rather than irritability. Serum calcium determinations and other diagnostic studies should be made for infants suspected of having sepsis.

Bradycardia with heart block is rarely noted. A prolonged Q-T interval on the ECG suggests hypocalcemia. A serum calcium concentration below 7 mg/dL establishes the diagnosis; a level below 7.5 mg/dL is suggestive. The serum phosphate level is increased, sometimes to 10–12 mg/dL. The blood urea nitrogen or serum creatinine levels are not elevated, differentiating this condition from the hypocalcemia and hyperphosphatemia seen in severe renal dysfunction. Normal newborns fed cow's milk have serum phosphate concentrations of 6–8 mg/dL; normal premature infants may have concentrations even higher. Hypomagnesemia may also occur.

A favorable response to calcium administration is insufficient in itself to make the diagnosis, because calcium may act nonspecifically during seizures. Symptoms such as irritability and tremors may subside spontaneously, and convulsions resulting from cerebral edema, anoxia, or injury may recur during the neonatal period. Examination of the spinal fluid is indicated because of the possibility of a convulsion caused by infection or hemorrhage in the CNS.

Treatment. Initial treatment of the convulsing infant is intravenous injection of a 10% solution of calcium gluconate (2 mL/kg), with the precautions given previously. The response may be dramatic. After this, specific treatment of late hypocalcemia aims at reducing the serum phosphate level. Because human milk is low in phosphorus, breast-fed infants rarely develop hypocalcemia. Some infant formulas prepared from dialyzed whey of cow's milk are considerably higher in phosphate than human milk.

Phosphate absorption from food can be suppressed by adding a great excess of calcium to the formula, which precipitates as calcium phosphate in the lumen of the intestine (e.g., adding calcium lactate or gluconate to the milk feeding to achieve a calcium to phosphorus ratio of 4:1). Calcium lactate powder is preferred, and its addition to milk produces no significant gastrointestinal disturbances. Because calcium lactate is 13% calcium, 770 mg of this salt provides 100 mg of calcium; calcium gluconate is 9% calcium, and 1,100 mg of it provides 100 mg of calcium. A soluble preparation of calcium gluconate (e.g., syrup of Neo-Calglucon), containing 92 mg Ca/tsp, is a less desirable method of adding calcium, because the required amounts may cause diarrhea. Calcium chloride may cause gastric irritation and hyperchloremic acidosis. Because the salt must dissolve in the milk, calcium lactate tablets should not be used; compressed tablets are insoluble even if fragmented.

As treatment decreases the serum phosphorus level, the serum calcium level returns to normal, possibly even rising to hypercalcemic levels. At this point, the calcium supplement is reduced in steps, not stopped abruptly, because the serum phosphorus level may rise precipitously, and the calcium concentration may fall again to tetanic levels. In most infants, restoration of normal calcium homeostasis and presumably normal parathyroid responsiveness occurs in 1–2 wk. In infants with accompanying hypomagnesemia, plasma magnesium levels usually return to normal.

Occasionally, a more prolonged calcium supplementation period is needed, in which case the treatment must be individualized by serial measurements of calcium and phosphate concentrations. If the infant responds poorly to treatment, the calculations should be checked to determine if sufficient calcium is being added, and the feeding should be examined to see if the calcium lactate or gluconate has been dissolving completely. If no errors are found and the therapeutic response is inadequate, the diagnosis of congenital hypoparathyroidism or, in older infants, of vitamin D deficiency or an absorptive or metabolic abnormality of vitamin D should be entertained.

The *prognosis* for early hypocalcemia with seizures depends on the primary disease; infants with late tetany have an excellent prognosis.

Congenital Absence of the Parathyroids. Absent parathyroid glands can occur in association with aplasia of the thymus (i.e., *DiGeorge syndrome*), in combination with abnormalities of the great vessels of the heart, or as an isolated parathyroid aplasia (see Chapter 125.1). Such patients present with the same symptoms as infants with transient physiologic hypoparathyroidism but respond incompletely to the simple treatment outlined previously and have relapsing hypocalcemia, which requires more definitive treatment.

In total parathyroid deficiency, substituting pharmacologic amounts of vitamin D, vitamin D metabolites, or vitamin D analogs for parathyroid hormone is required. Dihydrotachysterol is more potent than vitamin D in correcting hypocalcemia. It is more rapidly inactivated in the body, not stored, and is not as cumulatively toxic as vitamin D. In the young infant, 0.05–0.1 mg of dihydrotachysterol should be given daily and the dose adjusted by determining serum calcium concentrations, which should be returned to levels of about 9–10 mg/dL. The highly active vitamin D metabolite, 1,25-dihydroxyvitamin D_3, is also available; in doses of 0.25–0.5 μg/24 hr, it is effective in treating hypoparathyroidism. Oral calcium supplements such as calcium gluconate syrup (e.g., Neo-Calglucon) or calcium carbonate tablets (e.g., Tums, Rolaids) are also useful adjunctive therapy. As the child grows, the dosage of either steroid must be increased, as indicated by serum calcium concentrations. Urine calcium to creatinine ratios should be monitored to avoid hypercalciuria (ratio >0.2). Hypoparathyroidism in older children is discussed in Chapter 573.

Hypocalcemia and Tetany Caused by Vitamin D Deficiency or Abnormalities of Vitamin D Metabolism. The onset of vitamin D deficiency tetany usually occurs at 3–6 mo of age, because *depletion of the infant's vitamin D stores* requires this amount of time. However, an infant born of a vitamin D–deficient mother may develop hypocalcemia from vitamin D deficiency within the first wk of life. Tetany and nutritional vitamin D deficiency are now rare, but the latter occasionally develops in a breast-fed infant whose mother, unaware of human milk's vitamin D deficiency, does not provide supplementary vitamin D (see Chapter 44).

Hypocalcemia may also be a result of failure of normal metabolism of vitamin D, which undergoes two hydroxylation steps, first in the liver and then in the kidney, before becoming the metabolically active 1,25-dihydroxyvitamin D_3. Infants with *liver disease,* such as neonatal hepatitis, cytomegalic inclusion disease, or atresia of the bile ducts, may show manifestations of vitamin D deficiency with hypocalcemia because of failure of the liver to metabolize vitamin D. In atresia of the bile ducts, *malabsorption* of vitamin D may complicate the problem. Vitamin D deficiency can also result from steatorrhea caused by pancreatic lipase deficiency or by intrinsic intestinal mucosal disorders. Rickets and osteomalacia are associated with the treatment of convulsive disorders by large doses of combined anticonvulsant *drugs,* principally phenobarbital, phenytoin, and primidone, which alter the liver's metabolism of vitamin D. Phenytoin also inhibits intestinal transport of calcium, and patients may present with hypocalcemia and skeletal changes. *Vitamin D–dependent rickets* type I is caused by a deficiency of 1α-hydroxylase, which converts 25-hydroxyvitamin D to 1,25-dihydroxyvitamin D_3. Levels of the latter are low. Vitamin D–dependent rickets type II is an autosomal recessive condition, in which there is target organ resistance to 1,25-dihydroxyvitamin D_3 and early onset of rickets and hypocalcemia. It is associated with elevated levels of parathyroid hormone and 1,25-dihydroxyvitamin D_3.

Initially, patients with tetany resulting from vitamin D deficiency or failure of normal metabolism of vitamin D can be symptomatically relieved by intravenous injections of 2 mL/kg of a 10% solution of calcium gluconate, with the usual precautionary monitoring of the heart rate to prevent a too-rapid injection. Treatment of vitamin D deficiency is achieved with vitamin D (2,000–4,000 units or 50–100 μg daily). Vitamin D–dependent rickets type I is treated with 2–8 μg/24 hr of 1α-hydroxyvitamin D_3 or 1–4 μg/24 hr of 1,25-dihydroxyvitamin D_3. The daily dosage is halved after radiologic confirmation of healing. Vitamin D–dependent rickets type II responds to high dosages of vitamin D (0.5–5.0 mg/24 hr) or 1α-hydroxyvitamin D_3 or 1,25-dihydroxyvitamin D_3 (5–50 μg/24 hr). An alternative therapy for true vitamin D deficiency is 10,000 units of vitamin D daily for 3 wk or a highly concentrated vitamin D preparation, given in amounts adequate to achieve a rapid physiologic effect (e.g., 600,000 units of vitamin D in a single dose) or divided into several doses over a 24-hr period. Propylene glycol (Drisdol) is unsuitable for this type of therapy, because the large volume of propylene glycol is a depressant. The hypocalcemia of hepatic disorders responds to larger doses of vitamin D; more precise treatment with 25-hydroxyvitamin D_3 or 1,25-dihydroxyvitamin D is possible. Treatment must be individualized and patients closely monitored to avoid vitamin D intoxication (see Chapter 44).

HYPOMAGNESEMIC TETANY. Hypomagnesemia has reportedly caused tetany associated with low or normal serum calcium concentrations. In *transient physiologic hypoparathyroidism* of the newborn, low serum magnesium concentrations may accompany the hyperphosphatemia and hypocalcemia. This hypomagnesemia usually responds to treatment directed at reducing the serum phosphate concentration. Occasionally, newborn infants with hypomagnesemia require specific magnesium therapy: intramuscular injection with 0.2 mL/kg of a 50% solution of $MgSO_4 \cdot 7\ H_2O$ (i.e., 25% solution of $MgSO_4$). This treatment raises serum magnesium concentrations into the normal range within 1 hr and should maintain adequate concentrations for several hours. Often, no further therapy is needed. The mechanism of this transient hypomagnesemia is not understood.

Hypomagnesemic tetany and convulsions beyond the newborn period may result from prolonged parenteral nutrition with magnesium-free solutions or congenital disorders of magnesium transport, causing a failure of absorption of dietary magnesium or failure of tubular reabsorption of magnesium with excessive urinary loss. In Bartter's and Gitelman's syndromes, hypomagnesemia, hypokalemia, and tetany can occur secondary to a renal tubular dysfunction. Intestinal malabsorption of magnesium can result from acquired intestinal injury, such as inflammatory bowel disease or resection of small intestine; rarely, in male infants, it may be caused by a specific malabsorption of magnesium. Renal loss of magnesium may be secondary to nephropathy caused by aminoglycosides or cisplatin. Magnesium depletion, whatever the pathogenesis, can be associated with hypocalcemia, because magnesium is needed for the secretion of parathyroid hormone and responsiveness of target tissues to the hormone. Treatment requires magnesium administered intramuscularly (described earlier), intravenously (2–10 mL/kg of 1% magnesium sulfate solution) by slow infusion, or orally in the form of magnesium salts, such as the chloride, gluconate, or citrate forms (24–48 mg/kg/24 hr; see Chapter 50).

Aarskog D, Harrison H: Disorders of calcium, phosphate, PTH and vitamin D. *In:* Kappy M, Blizzard R, Migeon C (eds): The Diagnosis and Treatment of Endocrine Disorders in Childhood and Adolescence. Springfield, IL, Charles C Thomas, 1994.

Booth BE, Johanson A: Hypomagnesemia due to renal tubular defect in reabsorption of magnesium. J Pediatr 84:350, 1974.

Broner CW, Stidham GL, Westenkirchner DF, et al: A prospective, randomized, double blind comparison of calcium chloride and calcium gluconate therapies for hypocalcemia in critically ill children. J Pediatr 117:986, 1990.

Brown DR, Steranka BH, Taylor FH: Treatment of early-onset neonatal hypocalcemia. Am J Dis Child 135:24, 1981.

Colletti RP, Pan MW, Smith EWP, et al: Detection of hypocalcemia in susceptible neonates. The Q-oTc interval. N Engl J Med 290:931, 1974.

Ezzedeen F, Adelman RD, Ahlfors CE: Renal calcification in preterm infants: Pathophysiology and long-term sequelae. J Pediatr 113:532, 1988.

Fraher LJ, Karmali R, Hinde FRJ, et al: Vitamin D–dependent rickets type II: Extreme end organ resistance to 1,25-dihydroxyvitamin D_3 in a patient without alopecia. Eur J Pediatr 145:389, 1986.

Greig F, Paul E, Dimartino-Nardi J, et al: Transient congenital hypo-parathyroidism: Resolution and recurrence in chromosome 22q11 deletion. J Pediatr 128:563, 1996.

Griffin TA, Hostoffer RW, Tserng KY, et al: Parathyroid hormone resistance and B cell lymphopenia in propionic acidemia. Acta Paediatr 85:875, 1996.

Harrison HE, Harrison HC: Disorders of Calcium and Phosphate Metabolism in Childhood and Adolescence. Philadelphia, WB Saunders, 1979.

Maggioni A, Orzalesi M, Mimouni FB: Intravenous correction of neonatal hypomagnesemia: Effect on ionized magnesium. J Pediatr 132:652, 1998.

Markestad T, Halvorsen S, Halvorsen K, et al: Plasma concentrations of vitamin D metabolites before and during treatment of vitamin D deficiency rickets in children. Acta Paediatr Scand 73:225, 1984.

Marks KH, Kilav R, Naveh-Many T, et al: Calcium, phosphate, vitamin D, and the parathyroid. Pediatr Nephrol 10:364, 1996.

Paunier L, Raddle IC, Kooh SW, et al: Primary hypomagnesemia with secondary hypocalcemia in an infant. Pediatrics 41:385, 1968.

Pearce SH, Williamson C, Kifor O, et al: A familial syndrome of hypocalcemia with hypercalciuria due to mutations in the calcium-sensing receptor. N Engl J Med 335:1115, 1996.

PART VIII

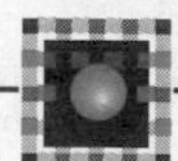

The Acutely Ill Child

CHAPTER 56

Evaluation of the Sick Child in the Office and Clinic

Paul L. McCarthy

Many of the approaches to clinical data gathering presented for the well child evaluation in Chapter 6 are also applicable to the sick child evaluation. There are a number of reasons for a sick child visit, but most visits are made because of acute intercurrent infections, and often the child is febrile.

When evaluating an acutely ill, febrile child, the pediatrician must be aware of statistics about the probable occurrence of serious illness, because one of the major goals of the sick child visit is to identify the seriously ill child, who requires vigorous therapeutic intervention. The risk for, and the cause of, serious illness in children with acute febrile illness vary depending on the child's age. Because of an immature immunologic system, the infant in the first 3 mo of life is more susceptible to sepsis and meningitis caused by group B streptococci and gram-negative organisms. Urinary tract infections are more frequent in male infants; these infants more often have an underlying anatomic abnormality of the urinary tract than do older children with urinary tract infections. As the infant matures beyond 3 mo, the bacterial pathogens that usually cause sepsis and meningitis are *Streptococcus pneumoniae, Haemophilus influenzae* type b (if the child is unimmunized or only partially immunized), and *Neisseria meningitidis*. After infancy, urinary tract infections are seen more often in females. As the child matures, immunity is developed to the bacterial pathogens common during the first 3–4 yr of life. At present, *N. meningitidis* is the leading cause of bacterial meningitis. In children older than 36 mo, pharyngitis caused by group A streptococci is a common bacterial infection. *Mycoplasma pneumoniae* assumes increasing importance as a cause for pulmonary infiltrates in children beyond 5 yr of age. Serious illnesses documented in a series of 996 children in the first 3 yr of life who presented with fever and acute illnesses are shown in Table 56–1. These children were seen in a university hospital and in private practices.

Identifying the acutely ill child with a serious illness is accomplished by careful observation, history taking, physical examination, appreciation of age and body temperature as risk factors, and the judicious use of screening laboratory tests. On the basis of these data, the physician can make informed decisions about the need for more definitive laboratory tests (e.g., urine culture), therapy, and the advisability of hospital admission. Observation, history, and physical examination are discussed separately, but these components are integrated into the sick child evaluation; that is, as the child is being observed, historical data are gathered. History taking and observational assessment often continue as the physical examination is performed. If, for example, abdominal tenderness is found on examination, additional history about blood in the stool, cramping abdominal pain, and vomiting may be sought.

Observation is a key factor in the evaluation of children with acute problems for the possibility of a serious illness. The child should be observed for specific evidence of a serious illness, such as grunting, which might indicate pneumonia or sepsis, or a bulging fontanel, which might indicate bacterial meningitis. *Most observational data that the pediatrician gathers during an acute illness should focus, however, on assessing the child's response to stimuli.* How does the child's crying respond to the parents' comforting? If sleeping, how quickly does the child awaken with a stimulus? Does the child smile when the examiner interacts with him or her? As noted in Chapter 6, assessing responses to stimuli—and often providing those stimuli—require a knowledge of normal responses for different age groups, the manner in which those normal responses are elicited, and to what degree a response might be impaired.

Sometimes the manner in which the child responds to stimuli is readily apparent—for example, the child may vocalize and smile as the examiner enters the room. At other times, more effort and more stimuli are needed to cause the child to act in a normal manner. Often the fussing, irritable child begins to look around and focus on the examiner when held and walked by the parent. This normal visual behavior is an important indicator of well-being. Thus, during observation, the pediatrician must be both clinically and developmentally oriented.

Six observation items and their scales (the Acute Illness Observation Scales) that have reliably and validly identified serious illness in febrile children are shown in Figure 56–1. A normal finding is scored as 1, moderate impairment as 3, and severe impairment as 5. The best possible score is 6 items × 1 = 6; the worst score is 6 items × 5 = 30. The chance of serious illness is 1–2% if the total score is ≤10; if the score is >10, the risk of serious illness increases by at least 10 fold. It is not clear whether these scales can be used in the first 2–3 mo of life, because infants may not have developed the skills required to score some of these items.

The complex nature of history taking has been outlined previously (Chapters 6 and 17.1). Parents must transmit how a younger child has been "feeling." In addition, they should provide information on a specific symptom, such as bloody diarrhea or cyanosis when coughing. The older child's perception of his or her symptoms may reflect a less developmentally

TABLE 56–1 Diagnosis of Serious Illnesses During 996 Episodes of Acute Infectious Illness in Febrile Children Younger Than 36 Mo*

Diagnosis	Cases	
	No.	*%*
Bacterial meningitis	9	0.9
Aseptic meningitis	12	1.2
Pneumonia	30	3.0
Bacteremia	10	1.0
Focal soft tissue infection	10	1.0
Urinary tract infection	8	0.8
Bacterial diarrhea	1	0.1
Abnormal electrolytes, abnormal blood gases	9	0.9
Total	89	8.9

**From McCarthy PL: Acute infectious illness in children. Comp Ther 14:51, 1988.*

6 OBSERVATION ITEMS AND THEIR SCALES

(PLEASE CHECK BOXES THAT DESCRIBE YOUR CHILD'S APPEARANCE AND BEHAVIOR)

OBSERVATION ITEM	NORMAL	MODERATE IMPAIRMENT	SEVERE IMPAIRMENT
1. QUALITY OF CRY	STRONG WITH NORMAL TONE ☐ OR CONTENT AND NOT CRYING ☐	WHIMPERING ☐ OR SOBBING ☐	WEAK ☐ OR MOANING ☐ OR HIGH PITCHED ☐
2. REACTION TO PARENT STIMULATION (Effect on crying when held, patted on back, jiggled on lap, or carried)	CRIES BRIEFLY, THEN STOPS ☐ OR CONTENT AND NOT CRYING ☐	CRIES OFF AND ON ☐	CONTINUAL CRY ☐ OR HARDLY RESPONDS ☐
3. STATE VARIATION (Going from awake to asleep or asleep to awake)	IF AWAKE, THEN STAYS AWAKE ☐ OR IF ASLEEP AND STIMULATED, THEN WAKES UP QUICKLY ☐	EYES CLOSE BRIEFLY, THEN AWAKENS ☐ OR AWAKENS WITH PROLONGED STIMULATION ☐	WILL NOT ROUSE ☐ OR FALLS TO SLEEP ☐
4. COLOR	PINK ☐	PALE HANDS, FEET ☐ OR ACROCYANOSIS (BLUE HANDS AND FEET) ☐	PALE ☐ OR BLUE ☐ OR ASHEN (GRAY) ☐ OR MOTTLED ☐
5. HYDRATION (Moisture in skin, eyes, mouth)	SKIN NORMAL AND EYES, MOUTH MOIST ☐	SKIN, EYES NORMAL AND MOUTH SLIGHTLY DRY ☐	SKIN DOUGHY OR TENTED AND EYES MAY BE SUNKEN AND DRY EYES AND MOUTH ☐
6. RESPONSE TO SOCIAL OVERTURES (Being held, kissed, hugged, touched, talked to, comforted)	SMILES ☐ OR ALERTS ☐ (2 months or less)	BRIEF SMILE ☐ OR ALERTS BRIEFLY ☐ (2 months or less)	NO SMILE, FACE ANXIOUS ☐ OR DULL, EXPRESSIONLESS ☐ OR NO ALERTING ☐ (2 months or less)

Figure 56–1 Acute Illness Observational Scales. Clinical evaluation of the well and sick child. (From McCarthy PL, Sharpe MR, Spiesel SZ, et al: Observation scales to identify serious illness in febrile children. Pediatrics 70:802, 1982. Reproduced by permission of Pediatrics.)

mature understanding of the cause of the illness. The examiner pursues the historical information provided by the parents or child to define the symptoms precisely. For example, if the complaint is blood in the stool, additional questions can be asked about other evidence of bowel inflammation, such as watery stools, mucus in the stools, or increased frequency of stooling. On the other hand, if the historical information indicates crying with defecation and streaks of blood on the outer portion of a hard stool, without other changes in the character or frequency of the stool, a diagnosis of a rectal fissure is tenable.

Questions should focus on those entities that are seen most commonly in acute febrile childhood illnesses. The more serious diagnoses are outlined in Table 56–1. Because most acute illnesses in children are caused by minor viral infections, specific questions about the epidemiology of the illness can offer important insights. Are there other children in the family with similar symptoms? Has the child had other illness exposures? Finally, it is important to be aware of any underlying chronic problems that might predispose the child to recurring infections or a serious acute illness; for example, the child with sickle cell anemia or AIDS is at increased risk for recurrent episodes of bacteremia.

For the sick child, the physical examination follows the same sequence as that outlined for the well child in Chapter 6. The examiner should be aware of illnesses that might be present in the acutely ill child and seek evidence of those illnesses. Initially, it is best to seat the child on the parent's lap; the older child may be seated on the examination table. In addition to the general level of interaction, color, and hydration, as assessed in the Acute Illness Observation Scales (see Fig. 56–1), the child's respiratory status is evaluated. This evaluation includes determining respiratory rate and noting any evidence of inspiratory stridor, expiratory wheezing, grunting, or coughing. Evidence of increased work of breathing—retractions, nasal flaring, and use of abdominal musculature—is sought. Because acute infections in children are most often caused by viral infections, the presence of nasal discharge is noted. It is possible at this time to assess the skin for rashes. Frequently, viral infections cause an exanthematous eruption, and many of these eruptions are diagnostic—for example, the reticulated rash and "slapped-cheek" appearance caused by parvovirus infections or hand-foot-and-mouth disease caused by coxsackievirus. The skin examination may also yield evidence of more serious infections, such as bacterial cellulitis or petechiae associated with bacteremia. When the child is seated and is least perturbed, an assessment of fontanel tension can be completed; it can be determined if the fontanel is depressed, flat, or bulging. It is also important at this time to assess the child's willingness to move and ease of movement. Usually the child with meningitis will hold the neck stiffly and often cry when any attempt is made to move the neck, even during cuddling by the parent. This is termed *paradoxic irritability.* The child with cellulitis, osteomyelitis, or septic arthritis in an extremity will resist movement of that limb. The child with peritoneal inflammation will sit quietly and become irritable during movement. It is reassuring to see the child moving about on the parent's lap with ease and without discomfort.

During this initial portion of the physical examination, when the child is most comfortable, the heart and lungs are auscultated. In the acutely febrile child, because of the relatively frequent occurrence of respiratory illnesses, it is important to assess adequacy of air entry into the lungs, equality of breath sounds, and evidence of adventitial breath sounds, especially wheezes, rales, and rhonchi. The coarse sound of air moving through a congested nasal passage is frequently transmitted to the lungs. The examiner can become attuned to these coarse sounds by placing the stethoscope near the child's nose and then compensating for this sound as the chest is auscultated. The cardiac examination is completed next; findings such as pericardial friction rub, loud murmurs, or distant heart sounds may indicate an infectious process involving the heart. The eyes are examined to identify features that might indicate an infectious process. Often, viral infections result in a watery discharge or redness of the bulbar conjunctivae. Bacterial infection, if superficial, results in purulent drainage; if the infection is more deep-seated, tenderness, swelling, and redness of tissues surrounding the eye are present as well as proptosis, reduced acuity, and altered extraocular movement. The extremities may then be evaluated not only for ease of movement but also for the possibility of swelling, heat, or tenderness; such abnormalities may be indicative of focal infections.

The components of the physical examination that are more bothersome to the child are completed last. This is best done with the patient on the examination table. Initially, the neck is examined to assess for areas of swelling, redness, or tenderness, as may be seen in cervical adenitis. The neck is then flexed to evaluate suppleness; resistance to flexion is indicative of meningeal irritation. Kernig and Brudzinski signs may be sought at this time. In children less than 18 mo, meningeal signs may not always be present with meningitis; if, however, they are present, the diagnostic implications are the same as for the child older than 18 mo. During examination of the abdomen, the diaper is removed. The abdomen is inspected for distention. Auscultation is performed to assess adequacy of bowel sounds, followed by palpation. It is often the case that the child fusses as the abdomen is auscultated and palpated. Every attempt should be made to quiet the child; if this is not possible, increased fussing as the abdomen is palpated may indicate tenderness, especially if this finding is reproducible. In addition to focal tenderness, palpation may elicit involuntary guarding or rebound; these findings indicate peritoneal irritation, as is seen in appendicitis. The inguinal area and genitals are then sequentially examined. In the febrile child, inguinal adenitis or a strangulated hernia may be the cause of fever. The child is then placed in the prone position, and abnormalities of the back are sought. The spine and costovertebral angle (CVA) areas are percussed to elicit any tenderness; such findings may be indicative of osteomyelitis and pyelonephritis, respectively.

The physical examination is completed by examining the ears and throat. These are usually the most bothersome parts of the examination for the child, and parents frequently can be helpful in minimizing head movement. The oropharyngeal examination is important to document the presence of enanthemas; these may be seen in many infectious processes, such as hand-foot-and-mouth disease caused by coxsackievirus. This portion of the examination is also important in documenting inflammation or exudates on the tonsils, which may be viral or bacterial.

At times, repeating portions of observational assessment and the physical examination is indicated. For example, if the child cried continuously during the initial clinical evaluation, the examiner may not be certain if this was due to the high fever or stranger anxiety or is indicative of a serious illness. Continual crying also makes portions of the physical examination, such as auscultation of the chest, more difficult. Before a repeat assessment is performed, maneuvers to make the child as comfortable as possible are indicated. Such maneuvers include reducing the fever with antipyretics and allowing the child to take a bottle. Because most children with fever do not have serious illnesses, repeated assessments are more likely to document normal findings. If, on the other hand, the child is persistently irritable, the possibility of serious illness increases.

The sensitivity of the carefully performed clinical assessment, observation, history, and physical examination for the presence of serious illness is approximately 90%. Careful data gathering is necessary in the observation, history, and physical examination, because each component of the evaluation is as effective as the others in identifying serious illness. Other data, however, should be sought to improve this sensitivity level. In the child with an acute febrile illness, the important supplemental data are age, body temperature, and screening laboratory tests. Febrile children in the first 3 mo of life have yet to achieve immunologic maturity and therefore are more susceptible to severe infections and to infections by unusual organisms. Thus, the febrile infant is at greater risk for serious illness than the child beyond 3 mo of age (see Chapter 172). In febrile children of any age, the higher the fever, the greater the risk for serious illness. The risk of bacteremia increases as the degree of fever increases; at ≥40°C the risk is 7%. The limit of physiologic thermoregulation is 41.1°C; fevers in this range and higher indicate not only bacteremia but also possible central nervous system infection, pneumonia, or pathologic hyperthermia.

Screening laboratory tests can be helpful in identifying the febrile child at increased risk for common serious illnesses. For example, a white blood cell count (WBC) ≥15,000/μL and/or erythrocyte sedimentation rate (ESR) ≥30 mm/hr in children younger than 24 mo with a temperature ≥40°C places those children at five times the risk of bacteremia (15% vs 3%) compared with children in whom the WBC is <15,000/μL and the ESR is <30 mm/hr. A similar association with bacteremia has been found with a WBC ≥15,000/μL, a polymorphonuclear neutrophil count >10,000/μL, and a band count ≥500/μL. The risk of any serious illness in all febrile children is approximately twice as great if the WBC is ≥15,000/μL and/or the ESR is ≥30 mm/hr than if neither of these elevations is present.

DIAGNOSTIC APPROACH (see also Chapters 106 and 172). If the febrile child is older than 3 mo and appears well, if the history or physical examination does not suggest a serious illness, and if no age or temperature risk factors are present, he or she may be followed expectantly. If otitis media is present, it should be treated. This profile applies to most children with acute infectious illnesses. If, on the other hand, the child appears ill or the history or physical examination suggests a serious illness, definitive laboratory tests appropriate for those findings are indicated (e.g., a chest roentgenogram for a child with grunting). The area of greatest controversy is whether laboratory studies are needed on the febrile child who appears well and has no abnormalities on history and physical examination to suggest serious illness but who is less than 3 mo of age or whose temperature is high. Most would agree that a sepsis work-up is indicated in the febrile child <3 mo (see Chapters 105 and 106); obtaining blood cultures in children older than 3 mo with higher grades of fever is gaining acceptance.

If the physician feels comfortable in following the child in whom no specific diagnosis has been established on an outpatient basis, a follow-up examination often yields a diagnosis. During the initial visit, or from one visit to the next during the acute illness, the change in symptoms or in the physical examination over time may provide important diagnostic clues. For the child in whom a diagnosis has already been established and who does not require hospitalization, follow-up by telephone or an office visit should be used to monitor the course of the illness and to further educate and support the parents.

Baker MD, Bell L, Avner J: Outpatient management without antibiotics of fever in selected infants. N Engl J Med 329:1437, 1993.
Baraff LJ, Bass JW, Fleisher GR, et al: Practice guideline for the management of infants and children 0 to 36 months of age with fever without source. Pediatrics 92:1, 1993.
Baskin M, O'Rourke E, Fleisher G: Outpatient treatment of febrile infants 28 to 89 days of age with intramuscular administration of ceftriaxone. J Pediatr 120:22, 1992.
Fleisher G, Rosenberg N, Vinci R, et al: Intramuscular versus oral antibiotic therapy for the prevention of meningitis and other bacterial sequelae in young, febrile children at risk for occult bacteremia. J Pediatr 124:504, 1994.
Kramer MW, Shapiro ED: Management of the young febrile child: A commentary on recent practice guidelines. Pediatrics 100:128, 1997.
Margolis P, Ferkol T, Marsocci S, et al: Accuracy of the clinical examination in detecting hypoxemia in infants with respiratory illness. J Pediatr 124:552, 1994.
McCarthy PL: Fever. Pediatr Rev 19:400, 1998.

CHAPTER 57
Injury Control

Frederick P. Rivara and David Grossman

Injuries are the most common cause of death during childhood beyond the first few months of life and represent one of the most important causes of preventable pediatric morbidity and mortality. Significant advances have been made in understanding the risk factors for injuries as well as in developing successful programs for prevention and control. These principles should be applied daily by the pediatrician, whether in the office, emergency department, hospital, or a community setting.

INJURY CONTROL. The term *accident prevention* has been replaced by *injury control. Accident* implies an event occurring by chance, without pattern or predictability. In fact, most injuries occur under fairly predictable circumstances to high-risk children and families. *Accident* connotes a sense of fatalism—that injuries are an "act of God" and thus cannot be prevented. This fatalistic attitude is a barrier to decreasing mortality and morbidity from injuries. Use of the term *injury* avoids these connotations and focuses attention on the damage to the person.

Reduction in morbidity and mortality from injuries can be accomplished not only through primary prevention (averting the event or injury in the first place) but also through secondary and tertiary prevention. The latter approaches include appropriate emergency medical services for injured children; regionalized trauma care for the multiply injured, severely burned, or head-injured child; and specialized pediatric rehabilitation services that attempt to return children to their prior level of functioning. This broadened scope of prevention is more properly described by the term *injury control.*

This expanded definition encompasses intentional injuries, e.g., assaults and self-inflicted injuries. These injuries are increasingly important among adolescents and young adults, and in some populations they rank first or second as causes of death in these age groups. Many of the same principles of injury control can be applied to these problems, for example, limiting access to firearms.

SCOPE OF THE PROBLEM

Mortality. Injuries cause almost 40% of the deaths among 1- to 4-yr-old children and three times more deaths than the next leading cause, congenital anomalies. For the rest of childhood and adolescence up to the age of 19 yr, nearly 70% of deaths are due to trauma, more than all other causes combined. In 1995, injuries caused 20,269 deaths among individuals 19 yr and younger in the United States (Table 57–1). Injuries result in more years of potential life lost than any other cause.

Motor vehicle injuries lead the list of injury deaths at all ages during childhood and adolescence, even in children under 1 yr of age. Motor vehicle occupant injuries account for the majority of these deaths during childhood as well as in adults. However, among children aged 5–9 yr, pedestrian injuries are the most common cause of death from trauma. During adolescence, occupant injuries are the leading cause of injury death, accounting for more than 50% of the unintentional trauma mortality in this age group.

Drowning ranks second overall as a cause of unintentional trauma deaths, with peaks in the preschool and later teenage years (see Chapter 69). In some areas of the United States, drowning is the leading cause of death from trauma for preschool-aged children. The causes of drowning deaths vary with age and geographic area. In young children, bathtub and swimming pool drownings predominate, whereas in older children and adolescents, drownings occur predominantly in natural bodies of water while swimming or boating.

Fire and burn deaths account for nearly 10% of all trauma deaths and more than 20% in those under 5 yr of age (see Chapter 70). The vast majority of these (85%) are due to house fires, with death due to smoke inhalation and asphyxiation rather than severe burns. Children and the elderly are at greatest risk of these deaths because of difficulty in escaping from burning buildings.

Asphyxiation and choking account for approximately 40% of all unintentional deaths in children under 1 yr of age. The majority of these deaths are due to choking on food items such as hot dogs, candies, grapes, and nuts. Nonfood items include undersized infant pacifiers, small balls, and latex balloons.

Homicide is the leading cause of injury death for infants under 1 yr, the fourth leading cause of injury death for ages 1–14 yr, and the second leading cause of injury death in adolescents (15–19 yr). Homicide among children falls into two patterns: "infantile" and "adolescent." Infantile homicide involves children under the age of 5 yr and represents child abuse (Chapter 35). The perpetrator is usually a caretaker; death is generally due to blunt trauma to the head and/or abdomen. In contrast, the adolescent pattern of homicide involves peers and acquaintances and is due to firearms in more than 80% of cases. The majority of these deaths in-

TABLE 57–1 Number of Fatal Injuries—United States, 1995

Mechanism	No. of Deaths by Age Group				
	0–4	*5–9*	*10–14*	*15–19*	*0–19 Total*
Motor vehicle (overall)	1,004	907	1,150	5,181	8,242
Occupant	487	369	513	3,311	4,680
Pedestrian	245	285	262	308	1,100
Bicycle	8	96	126	62	292
Drowning	631	229	246	461	1,567
Fire and flames	550	248	115	84	997
Unintentional poisoning	38	14	28	178	258
Falls	62	28	36	145	271
Homicide	763	157	404	3,262	4,586
Firearm homicide	82	70	310	2,787	3,249
Suicide	0	7	330	1,890	2,227
Firearm suicide	0	1	183	1,266	1,450
Unintentional firearm injury	20	32	129	259	440
Other	799	55	122	413	1,389
Overall injury	3,875	1,773	2,686	11,935	20,269

From the Naional Center for Health Statistics 1995 mortality data tapes.

volve handguns. Children between these two age groups experience homicides of both types.

Suicide is rare under age 10 yr; only 1% of all suicides occur in children under 15 yr of age. The suicide rate increases markedly after the age of 10 yr, with the result that suicide is now the third leading cause of death for 15- to 19-yr-olds, accounting for more than 100,000 potential years of life lost. Native American teenagers are at the highest risk, followed by white males; black females have the lowest rate of suicide in this age group. Approximately 67% of teenage suicides involve firearms (see Chapters 24 and 110).

Morbidity. Mortality statistics reflect only a small part of the effects of childhood injuries. Approximately 20–25% of children and adolescents receive medical care for an injury each year in hospital emergency departments, and at least an equal number are treated in physician offices. Of these, 2.5% require inpatient care and 55% have at least short-term temporary disability from their injuries.

The distribution of these nonfatal injuries is very different from that of fatal trauma (Fig. 57–1). Falls are the leading causes of both emergency room visits and hospitalizations. Although motor vehicle occupant injuries represent the leading cause of death, falls constitute the leading cause of emergency department visits. Bicycle-related trauma is the most common type of sports and recreational injury, accounting for more than 300,000 emergency department visits annually.

Nonfatal injuries may be associated with severe morbidity. For example, anoxic encephalopathy due to near-drowning, scarring and disfigurement due to burns, and persistent neurologic deficits due to head injury have a great long-term impact on both the injured child and the family.

Trends Over Time. The death rate for childhood injuries has declined throughout the 20th century, with substantial decreases in deaths from unintentional injuries over the last 15 yr. In contrast, rates of intentional injuries have increased. Homicide and suicide are the only leading causes of death to increase from 1950 to 1994. Suicide rates among male teens increased by 50% between 1970 and 1988, largely owing to firearm-related suicides. Since 1988, suicide rates among 15- to 19-yr-olds have decreased. Homicide rates for youth peaked in 1994 and fortunately have decreased since then. Both the increase and the subsequent drop in homicides were firearm-related.

PRINCIPLES OF INJURY CONTROL. For many years, prevention of injuries centered on attempts to pinpoint the innate characteristics of a child that result in greater frequency of injury. Most researchers have now discounted the theory of the "accident-prone child." Although longitudinal studies have demonstrated an association between hyperactivity and impulsivity and increased rates of injuries, the sensitivity and specificity of these traits for risk of injury are extremely low. The concept of "accident proneness" is, in fact, counterproductive in that it shifts attention away from potentially more modifiable factors, such as product design or the environment. It is more productive to examine the physical and social environment of children with frequent rates of injuries than to try to identify particular personality traits or temperaments. At-risk children are likely to be relatively poorly supervised, have disorganized or stressed families, and live in hazardous environments.

Efforts to control injuries include *education or persuasion, changes in product design,* and *modification of the environment,* whether it be the social or physical environment. Efforts to persuade individuals, particularly parents, to change their behaviors have constituted the greater part of injury control efforts. Speaking with parents specifically about using child car seat restraints and bicycle helmets, installing smoke detectors, and checking the tap water temperature is likely to be more successful than well-meaning but too-general advice about supervising the child closely, being careful, and "childproofing" the home. This information should be geared to the developmental stage of the child and presented in moderate doses in the form of anticipatory guidance at well child visits. Important topics to discuss at each developmental stage are shown in Table 57–2.

The most successful injury prevention strategies generally are those involving changes in product design, as shown in Table 57–3. These *passive* interventions protect all individuals in the population, regardless of cooperation or level of skill, and are likely to be more successful than *active* measures, which require repeated behavior change on the part of the parent or child. This must be tempered by the fact that for some types of injuries, effective passive interventions are not available or feasible; we must rely heavily on attempts to change the behavior of individuals. Turning down the water heater temperature, installing smoke detectors, and using child-resistant caps on medicines and household products are examples of effective product modification.

Modification of the environment often requires greater

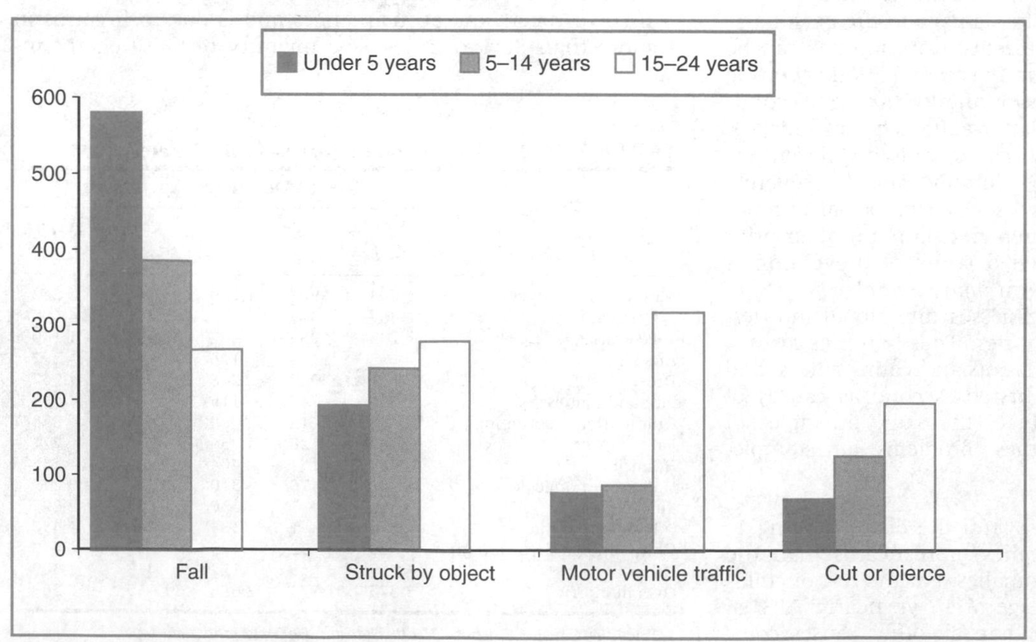

Figure 57–1 Emergency department visit rates for leading first-listed causes of injury by age: United States, 1993–1994. Sources: Centers for Disease Control and Prevention, National Center for Health Statistics, National Hospital Ambulatory Medical Case Survey.

TABLE 57–2 Injury Prevention Topics for Anticipatory Guidance by the Pediatrician

Newborn
- Car seats
- Tap water temperature
- Smoke detectors

Infant
- Car seats
- Tap water temperature
- Bath safety

Toddler and Preschooler
- Car seats
- Pedestrian skills training
- Water safety
- Childproof caps on medicines and household poisons
- Syrup of ipecac

Primary School Child
- Pedestrian skills training
- Water skills training
- Seatbelts
- Bicycle helmets
- Removal of firearms from home

Middle School Child
- Seatbelts
- Removal of firearms from home
- Pedestrian skills

High School and Older Adolescent
- Seatbelts
- Alcohol use, especially while driving, boating, and swimming
- Occupational injuries
- Removal of firearms from home

changes than individual product modification but may be very effective in reducing injuries. The use of smoke detectors, safe roadway design, decreased traffic volume and speed in the neighborhood, and elimination of guns from the environment are examples of such interventions. Included in this concept are changes in the environment through legislation such as mandatory child seat restraint and seatbelt use and mandatory bicycle helmet use.

Campaigns combining two or more of these approaches have been particularly effective in reducing injuries. The classic example is the combination of legislation and education to increase child seat restraint and seatbelt use; other examples are programs to promote bike helmet use among school-aged children and improvements in occupant protection in motor vehicles.

RISK FACTORS FOR CHILDHOOD INJURIES. Factors that increase the risk of injuries to children include age, sex, race, socioeconomic status, and the environment.

Age. Toddlers are at greatest risk for burns, drowning, and falls. As these children acquire mobility and exploratory behavior, poisonings become a risk. Young school-aged children are at greatest risk for pedestrian injuries, bicycle-related injuries (the most serious of which usually involve motor vehicles), motor vehicle occupant injuries, burns, and drowning. During the teenage years, there is a markedly increased risk from motor vehicle occupant trauma, a continued risk from drowning and burns, and the new risk of intentional trauma. Work-related injuries associated with child labor, especially for 14- to 16-yr-olds, are an additional risk.

Injuries occurring at a particular age represent a window of vulnerability during which a child or an adolescent encounters a new task or hazard that he or she may not have the developmental skills to handle successfully. For example, toddlers do not have the judgment to know that medications can be poisonous or that some houseplants are not to be eaten; they do not understand the hazard presented by a swimming pool or an open second-story window. For young children, parents may inadvertently set up this mismatch between the skills of the child and the demands of the task. A walker converts an infant into a mobile toddler and greatly increases contact with hazards. Many parents expect young school-aged children to walk home from school, the playground, or the local candy store, tasks for which most children are not developmentally ready. Likewise, the lack of skills and experience to handle many tasks during the teenage years contributes to an increased risk of injuries, particularly motor vehicle injuries. The high rate of motor vehicle crashes for younger teens is due in part to inexperience but also appears to reflect their level of development and maturity. Alcohol often adds to these limitations.

Age also influences the severity of injury as well as the risk of long-term disability. For example, young school-aged children have an incompletely developed pelvis. In a motor vehicle crash, the seatbelt does not anchor onto the pelvis but rides up onto the abdomen, resulting in the risk of serious abdominal injury. Age interacts with the vehicle characteristics in that most children ride in the rear seat, which in the past was equipped only with lap belts and not lap-shoulder harnesses. Children under the age of 2 yr have much worse outcomes from closed head injuries than do older children and adolescents.

Sex. Beginning at approximately 1–2 yr of age and continuing until the 7th decade of life, males have higher rates of injuries than females. During childhood this does not appear to be due to developmental differences between the sexes, differences in coordination, or differences in muscle strength. Variation in exposure to risk may account for the male predominance in some types of injuries. Although boys in all age groups have higher rates of bicycle-related injuries, adjusting for exposure reduces this excess rate. Boys may have higher rates of injuries because they use bicycles more frequently or for more hours. In contrast, sex differences in rates of pedestrian injuries do not appear to be due to differences in the amount of walking but rather reflect differences in behavior between young girls and boys. Greater risk-taking behavior, combined with greater frequency of alcohol use, may lead to the disproportionately high rate of motor vehicle crashes among teenage males.

Race. There are striking racial variations in childhood and adolescent injury mortality. Blacks have much higher rates of injuries than whites, whereas Asians have lower rates; rates for Hispanics are intermediate between those for blacks and whites. Native Americans have the highest death rate from unintentional injuries. These discrepancies are even more pronounced for some injuries. The homicide rate in black males 18–24 yr was 288 per 100,000 in 1995, compared with 32 per 100,000 for white males. The suicide rate for Native American youth is twice the rate for whites and threefold greater than that for Asians. The rate of fire and burn deaths in black preschool children is more than three times higher than for whites: 12 per 100,000 compared with 3.9 per 100,000, respectively.

These racial differences appear to be primarily related to poverty rather than to race per se. Homicide rates of blacks are nearly equivalent to whites when adjusted for socioeconomic status.

Socioeconomic Status. Poverty is one of the most important risk

TABLE 57–3 Injury Control Interventions: Hierarchy of Effectiveness

Product Modification	>	Environmental Modification	>	Education
Child-resistant caps		Cabinet locks		Anticipatory guidance
Airbags		Roadway design		Public service announcements
Fire-safe cigarettes		Smoke detectors		School safety programs

factors for childhood injury. Mortality from fires, motor vehicle crashes, and drowning is two- to fourfold higher in poor children. Death rates for both blacks and whites have an inverse relationship with income level: the higher the income level, the lower the death rate. Native Americans have especially high rates in low-income areas. Other factors are single-parent families, teenage mothers, and multiple siblings; these are primarily a function of poverty, rather than independent risk factors.

Environment. Poverty increases the risk of injury to children, at least in part through its effect on the environment. Children who are poor are at increased risk of injury because they are exposed to more hazards in their living environments. They may live in poor housing, which is less likely to be protected by smoke detectors. The roads in their neighborhoods are more likely to be major thoroughfares. Their neighborhoods are more likely to be violent, and they are more likely to be victims of assault than are children and adolescents living in middle-class suburbs. The focus on the environment is also important because it directs attention away from relatively immutable factors, such as family dynamics, poverty, and race, and directs efforts toward factors that can be changed through interventions.

MOTOR VEHICLE INJURIES. Motor vehicle injuries are the leading cause of serious and fatal injuries for individuals of all ages. In adolescents, motor vehicle crashes alone account for 40% of *all* deaths, including deaths from natural causes. Large and sustained reductions in motor vehicle crash injuries can be accomplished by approaches already at hand.

Occupants. Injuries to passenger vehicle occupants are the predominant cause of motor vehicle deaths among children and adolescents, with the exception of the 5- to 9-yr group, in whom pedestrian injuries make up the largest proportion. The peak injury and death rate for both males and females occurs between 15 and 19 yr (see Table 57–1).

Much attention has been given to child occupants less than 4 yr of age. Use of child restraint devices can be expected to reduce fatalities by 71% and the risk of serious injuries by 67% in this age group. All 50 states and the District of Columbia have laws mandating their use. Handouts given to parents by physicians emphasizing the positive benefits of child seat restraints have been successful in improving parent acceptance. Pediatricians should point out to parents that toddlers who normally ride restrained behave better during car trips than children who ride unrestrained.

Excellent films are available that discuss the advantages of child seat restraints; these can be shown to parents in waiting rooms or mothers on post-partum hospital floors. Many hospitals and communities have adopted loan programs, renting restraints at low cost. This is especially important for low-income families, who have the lowest rate of restraint use.

A list of acceptable devices is available from the American Academy of Pediatrics. Children under 20 lb may use an infant seat or be placed in a "convertible" infant-toddler child restraint device. Infants under 1 yr or under 20 lb should be placed in the rear seat facing backwards; older toddlers and children can be placed in the back seat in a forward-facing convertible or toddler seat. Emphasis must be given to correct use of these seats, including placing the seat in the right direction, properly routing the belt, and ensuring that the child is correctly buckled into the seat. Children under 13 yr should never be placed in the front seat, especially if an airbag is present. Inflating airbags can be lethal to infants in rear-facing seats and to small children in the front passenger seat.

Older children are often not adequately restrained. Many children ride in the back seat restrained with lap belts only. Unfortunately, the use of lap belts alone has been associated with a marked rise in seatbelt-related injuries, especially fractures of the lumbar spine and hollow-viscus injuries of the abdomen. These flexion-distraction injuries of the spine are usually accompanied by injuries to the abdominal organs; the presence of cutaneous seatbelt contusions in restrained children should alert the clinician. Children should use approved booster seats until large enough to comfortably wear the belt and shoulder harness alone. Shoulder straps placed behind the child or under the arm do not provide adequate crash protection.

Transportation of premature infants presents special problems. The possibility of oxygen desaturation, sometimes associated with bradycardia, among premature infants while in child seat restraints has led the American Academy of Pediatrics to make the following recommendations: monitoring of infants born at less than 37 wk of gestational age in the seat, before discharge and the use of oxygen or alternative restraints for infants who experience desaturation or bradycardia, such as seats that can be reclined and used as a car bed. Monitoring should be done for 60–90 min.

Children riding in the back of pickup trucks are at special risk of injury, because of the possibility of ejection from the truck and serious head injury. Children traveling in the back of covered pickup trucks are at risk for carbon monoxide poisoning from faulty exhaust systems.

Teenage Drivers. Drivers aged 15–17 yr have over twice the rate of collisions per 1,000 registered drivers as motorists 18 yr of age and older. Driver education appears to be ineffective as a primary means of decreasing these collisions. Almost 50% of the fatal crashes involving drivers under age 18 yr occur in the 4 hr before or after midnight. *Restriction on nighttime driving is an effective and surprisingly acceptable strategy* (to teens) to decrease motor vehicle injuries in this age group. In states imposing nighttime driving curfews on teens under 18 yr, there has been a significant decrease in crash involvement and fatalities. Risk of serious injury and mortality is directly related to the speed at the time of the crash and inversely related to the size of the vehicle. Small, fast cars greatly increase the risk of a fatal outcome in the event of a crash, and parents should be counseled accordingly.

Alcohol use is a major cause of motor vehicle trauma among adolescents. The combination of inexperience in driving and inexperience with alcohol is particularly dangerous. Approximately 50% of all deaths from motor vehicle crashes in this age group involve the use of alcohol, with impairment of driving seen at blood alcohol concentrations as low as 0.05 g/dL. All adolescent motor vehicle injury victims should have their blood alcohol concentration measured in the emergency department and be screened for chronic alcohol use with a standard test, such as the CAGE or the Short Michigan Alcohol Screening Test, to identify those with alcohol abuse problems. Individuals who have evidence of alcohol abuse should not leave the emergency department or hospital without plans for appropriate alcohol abuse treatment.

BICYCLE INJURIES. Each year in the United States, approximately 400 children and adolescents die from injuries incurred while riding bicycles; bicycle-related injuries are one of the most common reasons that children with trauma visit emergency rooms. The majority of severe and fatal bicycle injuries involve head trauma. A logical step in the prevention of these head injuries is the use of helmets. Rigorous studies indicate that helmets are very effective, reducing the risk of head injury by 85% and brain injury by 88%. Helmets also protect against injuries to the mid- and upper face. Pediatricians can be effective advocates for the use of bicycle helmets and should incorporate this advice into their anticipatory guidance schedules for parents and children. Appropriate helmets are those with a firm polystyrene liner; they should bear a label indicating that they are approved by either the Snell or American National Standards Institute (ANSI) testing organizations.

Promotion of helmets can and should be extended beyond the office. Community education programs spearheaded by coalitions of physicians, educators, bicycle clubs, and community service organizations have been successful in promoting the wearing of bicycle helmets, resulting in helmet use rates as high as 60% with concomitant reduction in the number of head injuries. Passage of bicycle helmet laws has also led to greatly increased use.

Consideration should also be given to other types of preventive activities, although the evidence supporting their effectiveness is limited. Bicycle paths are a logical method for separating bicycles and motor vehicles. Safe bicycling training for children can be provided in the school and community.

PEDESTRIAN INJURIES. Pedestrian injuries are the single most common cause of traumatic death for 5- to 9-yr-old children in the United States and most industrialized countries. Although case fatality rates are less than 5%, serious nonfatal injuries constitute a much larger problem. Pedestrian injuries are the most important cause of traumatic coma in children and are a frequent cause of serious lower extremity fractures, particularly in the school-aged child.

Most injuries occur during the day, with a peak in the after-school period. Improved lighting or retroreflective clothing would, therefore, be expected to prevent few injuries. Surprisingly, approximately 30% of pedestrian injuries occur while the individual is in a marked crosswalk, perhaps reflecting a false sense of security and decreased vigilance. The risk of pedestrian injury is greater in neighborhoods with high traffic volumes, speeds greater than 40 kph (approximately 25 mph), absence of play space adjacent to the home, household crowding, and low socioeconomic status.

One important risk factor for childhood pedestrian injuries is the developmental level of the child. Children under the age of 5 yr are at risk of being run over in the driveway. Few children under the age of 9 or 10 yr have the developmental skills to successfully negotiate traffic 100% of the time. Young children have poor ability to judge the distance and speed of traffic and are easily distracted by playmates or other factors in the environment. Many parents, however, are not aware of this potential mismatch between the abilities of the young school-aged child and the skills needed to cross streets safely.

Prevention of pedestrian injuries is difficult but should consist of a multifaceted approach. Education of the child in pedestrian safety should be initiated at an early age by the parents and continue into the school-age years. Younger children should be taught never to cross streets when alone; older children should be taught (and practice how) to negotiate quiet streets with little traffic. Major streets should not be crossed alone until the child is 10 yr of age or older.

Pedestrian skills training should constitute part of a more comprehensive pedestrian safety program in a community. Legislation and police enforcement are important components of any campaign to reduce pedestrian injuries. Right-turn-on-red laws increase the hazard to pedestrians. In many cities, few drivers stop for pedestrians in crosswalks, a special hazard for young children. Engineering changes in roadway design are extremely important as passive prevention measures. Most important are measures to slow the speed of traffic and to route traffic away from schools and residential areas. Other modifications include one-way-street networks, proper placement of transit or school bus stops, sidewalks in urban and suburban areas, edge stripping in rural areas to delineate the edge of the road, and curb parking regulations. Comprehensive traffic "calming" schemes employing these strategies have been very successful in reducing child pedestrian injuries in Sweden, the Netherlands, and Germany.

FIRE- AND BURN-RELATED INJURIES (see Chapter 70). Fire- and burn-related injuries are the third most common cause of unintentional injury death in the United States, with about 6,000 burn injury deaths occurring each year. For both injuries and deaths, the first decade of life is the period of highest risk. Burns are second only to motor vehicle crashes in the number of years of life lost *per death,* reflecting the relatively young population involved in serious burn injuries. The likelihood of burn injury is strongly related to low socioeconomic status. Burns are much more frequent among males than females. Among children 10–14 yr of age with burns involving flammable substances, males are burned eight times more frequently than females.

One of the first effective interventions involved flammable fabrics. Flame burns resulting from ignition of clothing were a common, serious burn injury, especially in small children. At least one third of those injuries involved infant sleepwear. Such burns averaged 30% of the body surface, requiring hospitalization for an average of 70 days. In 1967, the Federal Flammable Fabrics Act was passed, *requiring children's sleepwear to be flame retardant.* As a result of this and similar state legislation, clothing ignition burns in small children now account for only a small fraction of burns in children. Despite the withdrawal of tromethamine (*TRIS*)-containing clothing because of potential mutagenicity, federal flammability standards still apply to children's sleepwear. Parents should not circumvent these protective regulations by using cotton T-shirts for infant and child sleepwear.

Another hazard modification resulting in substantial reduction of injury involves *scald burns due to tap water.* Scalds account for 40% of the burn injuries in children requiring hospitalization, and at least 25% of these scald burns involve tap water. Unlike those with flame burns, children with scalds generally do not die; however, many children face long hospitalizations, multiple surgical procedures, and severe disfigurement. The risk of full-thickness burns increases geometrically at water temperatures above 130°F. At 150°F, a full-thickness burn will be produced in adult skin in 2 sec. A simple and effective preventive maneuver is to turn down the water heater temperature to 125°F. At this setting, dishwashers and washing machines operate effectively, but the risk of serious scald injury is greatly reduced. In many cities, the local power company will turn down the temperature without charge. In 1980, Florida became the first state requiring new water heaters to be preset at a temperature of 125°F.

Nearly 70% of all fire deaths in the United States occur in private dwellings. Of these deaths, 60% are caused by smoke asphyxiation and *not* flame burns. *Smoke detectors* are an inexpensive but effective method of preventing the majority of these deaths. Physicians can alter parental behavior and increase smoke detector use by offering information on smoke detectors in their offices.

Cigarettes are estimated to cause 45% of all fires and 22–56% of deaths from house fires. The combination of smoking and alcohol use appears to be particularly lethal. Most cigarettes made in the United States contain additives in both the paper and the tobacco that allow them to burn for as long as 28 min, even if left unattended. If *fire-safe* or *self-extinguishing cigarettes* replaced present types, nearly 2,000 deaths and more than 6,000 burns would be prevented annually.

Other common burn risks include scalds from hot tea, coffee, and foods; fireworks injuries; and burns from cigarette lighters. Scalds from hot foods are the most common reason for a burn admission to the hospital for children under the age of 5 yr. Avoiding the use of electric kettles or frying pans with long cords, not using baby walkers, not drinking hot tea or coffee while holding an infant, and keeping children away from pots cooking on the stove will help to prevent many of these injuries. Community restrictions on certain types of fireworks and adult supervision of use of all fireworks have been effective in decreasing burns, amputations, and ocular injuries due to these devices. Further product modification promises to decrease the hazards associated with certain easy-to-use cigarette lighters commonly found in the home.

Some burns are due to fire setting by children or adolescents. In young children, this usually represents exploratory play. However, such behavior in older children and adolescents may signify a serious conduct disorder and warrants careful psychiatric and family evaluation.

POISONING (see Chapter 722). Deaths by poisoning among children have decreased dramatically over the last two decades, particularly among children less than 5 yr of age. In 1970, 226 poisoning deaths of children under 5 yr occurred, compared with only 38 in 1995. Poisoning prevention represents the effectiveness of passive strategies—*child-resistant packaging* and *dose limits per container*. The Poison Packaging Prevention Act currently includes 16 categories of household products and nearly all prescription drugs. This law has been remarkably effective in reducing poisoning deaths and hospitalizations. However, compliance with the law by pharmacists is only 70–75% at present, indicating that physicians should always specify that prescriptions be dispensed in child-resistant containers. In addition, difficulty using child-resistant containers is an important cause of poisoning in young children today. A survey by the CDC found that 18.5% of households in which poisoning occurred to children less than 5 yr of age had replaced the child-resistant closure and 65% of the ones used did not work properly. Nearly 20% of ingestions occur from drugs owned by grandparents, a group that has difficulty using traditional child-resistant containers. There is a need for better child-resistant closures that do not require manual dexterity or strength greater than the capabilities of older adults.

Other poisoning interventions, such as "Mr. Yuk" stickers, are far less effective. They do not deter young children from ingesting labeled medications and may in fact be attractive to children under 3 yr of age. The most important feature of the Mr. Yuk sticker is the phone number of the local or regional poison control center. Parents of toddlers should also be given a bottle of syrup of ipecac to store in the medicine chest. In the case of an ingestion, they should be instructed to call the poison control center or pediatrician before administering it.

DROWNING (see Chapter 69). In 1995, 1,502 drownings, primarily associated with recreational activities, occurred in children and adolescents in the United States. In young children, drowning ranks second only to motor vehicle injury as a cause of traumatic death. Although no precise data exist on the number of nonfatal water-related injuries, it is estimated that 140,000 occur annually from swimming activities alone. Diving headfirst into water accounts for the most serious aquatic injuries because of spinal cord damage. Of the estimated 700 spinal cord injuries resulting from aquatic activities each year, the majority result in permanent paralysis.

The proportion of drowning deaths that are pool related varies by region of the country. In Los Angeles, half of all drownings take place in residential pools, a rate similar to that in other areas with large numbers of pools. Children under the age of 5 yr do not understand the consequences of falling into deep water and usually do not call for help. A majority of child victims drown during lapses in adult supervision caused by chores, socializing, and phone calls.

Clearly, the most effective way to prevent childhood pool drowning is through *fencing*. To give the greatest protection, these barriers should restrict entry to the pool from the yard and residence, use self-closing and self-latching gates, be at least 5 ft high, and have no vertical openings more than 4 in wide. Ordinances to require appropriate fencing have been demonstrated to be effective. Many people have advocated "water-babies" and other swimming instruction for young children. The efficacy of such techniques is untested. The potential exists for both parent and child to become less vigilant around water, possibly with tragic consequences.

Among adolescents and young adults, alcohol and drug use has been found to be involved in nearly 50% of all drowning deaths. The *restriction of the sale and consumption of alcoholic beverages* in boating, pool, harbor, marina, and beach areas may combat this dangerous combination of activities.

More restrictive licensing of boat owners should also be considered. Coast Guard data show that although only 7% of boats involved in mishaps lacked available personal flotation devices (PFDs), they accounted for 29% of boating fatalities. All children and adolescents should wear a PFD when boating in open water.

The risk of bathtub drowning is markedly increased in children with a seizure disorder, including older children and adolescents. These patients should be instructed to shower instead of using a bathtub.

FIREARM INJURIES. Injuries to children and adolescents involving firearms occur in three different situations: nonintentional injury, suicide attempt, and assault. In each case, the injury induced may be fatal or may result in permanent sequelae.

Among children under the age of 18 yr, firearms are the fifth-ranking cause of death from nonintentional trauma in the United States. More than 700 children and adolescents die each year from nonintentional gunshot wounds. An additional 8,000 children and adolescents are left with permanent sequelae, not including emotional and psychologic problems.

Nonintentional firearm injuries generally occur in a family dwelling; 85% of firearm deaths occur in the home. In gunshot fatalities to children under 16 yr of age, poverty is more closely related to shooting deaths than is race or population density. Urban whites have the lowest death rate, rural whites are intermediate, and urban black children have the highest fatality rate.

Suicide is now the third most common cause of trauma death in teenage males and the fourth for females. During the period from the 1950s to 1982, suicide rates for children and adolescents more than doubled; suicide rates rose by an additional 27% between 1982 and 1991 alone. Firearms have played an important role in this increase and are now the most common means of suicide in males of all ages. The difference in the rate of suicide between males and females is related less to number of attempts than to the method. Women die less often in suicide attempts because they use less lethal means, mainly drugs, and perhaps have a lower degree of intent. The use of firearms in a suicidal act usually converts an attempt into a fatality.

Homicides are second only to motor vehicle crashes among causes of death in teenagers over the age of 15 yr. In 1995, 4,586 children and adolescents were homicide victims; nonwhite teenagers accounted for almost 55% of the total, making homicides the most common cause of death among nonwhite teenagers. At present, almost 80% of homicides among males involve firearms, 75% of which are handguns.

In the United States today, there are an estimated 210 million to 220 million firearms. During the last two decades, over 6 million firearms were sold in the United States each year. Handguns account for approximately 20% of the firearms in use today, yet they are involved in 90% of criminal and other firearm misuse. Home ownership of guns increases the risk of adolescent suicide tenfold and adolescent homicide fourfold. In homes with guns, the risk to the occupants is far greater than the chance the gun will be used against an intruder; for every death occurring in self-defense, there may be 1.3 unintentional deaths, 4.6 homicides, and 37 suicides.

The data seem to indicate that of all firearms, handguns pose the greatest risk to children and adolescents. Access to handguns by adolescents is surprisingly common and is not restricted to those involved in gang or criminal activity. Stricter regulation of handgun access by youth, rather than all firearms, would appear to be the most appropriate focus of efforts to reduce shooting injuries in children and adolescents.

One approach is information and education campaigns in firearm safety. No data exist to support the effectiveness of such programs in decreasing the number of gunshot wounds in children. Safety education is also unlikely to have an effect on the use of firearms in homicides and suicides. Most homicides are between relatives or acquaintances and are acts of rage. Elimination of these weapons from the environment of children and adolescents is the key to reduction in firearm fatalities and injuries. Decreasing access to handguns would certainly not eliminate arguments, but it would decrease the likelihood of a fatal conclusion. In an assault, the chance of death is five times greater with a firearm than with a knife.

Physicians have a responsibility to counsel parents and patients about firearm ownership. This should include information informing them of the risks associated with owning a handgun, the risk of gun injury to all members of the household, and the special risks to adolescent males. Parents should be counseled that the safest approach is to remove the firearm from the household. If the family chooses to keep the gun, parents should be advised to store the gun in a locked container or with a trigger lock, with ammunition stored separately. Further educational information for pediatricians on counseling families and adolescents about guns can be obtained from the American Academy of Pediatrics.

Agran PF, Castillo DN, Winn DG: Comparison of motor vehicle occupant injuries in restrained and unrestrained 4- to 14-year olds. Accid Anal Prev 24:349, 1992.

American Academy of Pediatrics Committee on Injury Prevention and Poison Prevention: Injury Prevention and Control for Children and Youth, 3rd ed. Elk Grove Village, IL, American Academy of Pediatrics, 1997.

Asher KN, Rivara FP, Felix D, et al: Water safety training as a potential means of reducing the risk of young children's drowning. Inj Prev 1:228, 1995.

Baker S, Fowler C, Li G, et al: Head injuries incurred by children and young adults during informal recreation. Am J Public Health 84:649, 1994.

Bergman AB, Rivara FP, Richards DD, et al: Anatomy of a children's bicycle helmet campaign. Am J Dis Child 144:727, 1990.

Braver ER, Ferguson SA, Greene MA, Lund AK: Reduction in deaths in frontal crashes among right front passengers in vehicles equipped with passenger air bags. JAMA 278:1437, 1997.

Chiavello C, Christoph R, Bond G: Infant walker related injuries: A prospective study of severity and incidence. Pediatrics 93:974, 1994.

Colletti RB: Longitudinal evaluation of a statewide network of hospital programs to improve child passenger safety. Pediatrics 7:523, 1986.

Cote TR, Sacks JJ, Lambert-Huber DA, et al: Bicycle helmet use among Maryland children: Effect of legislation and education. Pediatrics 89:1216, 1992.

Cummings P, Grossman DC, Rivara FP, Kopesell TK: State gun safe storage laws and child mortality due to firearms. JAMA 278:1084, 1997.

Davidson L, Durkin M, Kuhn L, et al: The impact of the Safe Kids/Healthy Neighborhood Injury Prevention Project in Harlem, 1988 through 1991. Am J Public Health 84:580, 1994.

Durkin M, Davidson L, Kuhn L, et al: Low income neighborhoods and the risk of severe pediatric injury: A small area analysis in northern Manhattan. Am J Public Health 84:587, 1994.

Evans L, Frick MC: Car size or car mass: Which has greater influence on fatality risk? Am J Public Health 82:1105, 1992.

Fingerhut LA, Cox CS, Warner M: International Comparative Analysis of Injury Mortality. Advance Data. Atlanta, Centers for Disease Control and Prevention, No. 303, October 7, 1998.

Gentilello LM, Donovan DM, Dunn CW, Rivara FP: Alcohol interventions in trauma centers: Current practice and future directions. JAMA 274:1043, 1995

Graham JD, Goldie SJ, Segui-Gomez M, et al: Reducing risks to children in vehicles with passenger airbags. Pediatrics 102:1, 1998. www.Pediatrics.org/cgi/content/full/102/1/@3

Grossman DC, Mang K, Rivara FP: Firearm injury prevention counseling by pediatricians and family physicians: Practices and beliefs. Arch Pediatr Adolesc Med 149:973, 1995.

Johnston C, Rivara F, Soderberg R: Children in car crashes: Analysis of data for injury and use of restraints. Pediatrics 93:960, 1994.

Kassirer JP: Guns in the household. N Engl J Med 329:1117, 1993.

Kellermann AL, Rivara FP, Somes G, et al: Suicide in the home in relation to gun ownership. N Engl J Med 327:467, 1992.

Kellermann AL, Rivara FP, Rushforth NB, et al: Gun ownership as a risk factor for homicide in the home. N Engl J Med 329:1084, 1993.

Laflamme L, Eilert-Petersson E: Injuries to pre-school children in a home setting: Patterns and related products. Acta Paediatr 87:206, 1998.

Mallonee S, Istre GR, Rosenberg M: Surveillance and prevention of residential fire injuries. N Engl J Med 335:27, 1996.

McLoughlin E, McGuire A: The causes, costs and prevention of childhood burn injuries. Am J Dis Child 144:677, 1990.

Quan L, Gore EJ, Wentz K, et al: Ten year study of pediatric drownings and near-drownings in King County, Washington. Lessons in injury prevention. Pediatrics 83:1035, 1989.

Rivara FP, Gurney JG, Ries RK, et al: A descriptive study of trauma, alcohol, and alcoholism in young adults. J Adolesc Health 13:663, 1992.

Rivara FP, Grossman DC: Prevention of traumatic deaths to children in the United States: How far have we come and where do we need to go? Pediatrics 97:791, 1996.

Roberts I, Ashton T, Dunn R, Lee-Joe T: Preventing child pedestrian injury: Pedestrian education or traffic calming? Aust J Public Health 18:209, 1994.

Thompson DC, Nunn ME, Thompson RS, Rivara FP: Effectiveness of bicycle helmets in preventing serious facial injury. JAMA 276:1974, 1996.

Thompson RS, Rivara FP, Thompson DC: A case-control study of the effectiveness of bicycle safety helmets. N Engl J Med 320:1361, 1989.

Wilson M, Baker SP, Teret S, et al: Saving Children: A Guide to Injury Prevention. New York, Oxford University Press, 1991.

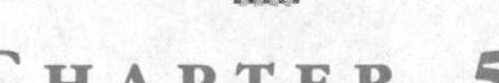

CHAPTER 58
Emergency Medical Services for Children

Dena R. Brownstein and Frederick P. Rivara

Emergency medical services for children (EMS-C) is a concept rather than a distinct entity and represents a continuum of care (Fig. 58–1). Primary care physicians have an important role in the EMS-C system and are responsible for providing parents and children with education on injury prevention and emergency medical services (EMS) access, participating in the pediatric training of EMS providers in the community, and becoming self-educated in appropriate triage and transport of critically ill children. In addition, primary care providers coordinate the care of their sickest patients, from the office to the emergency department (ED), through hospital care to rehabilitation and reintegration into the community.

ANTICIPATORY GUIDANCE. Most injuries are preventable (Chapter 57). Likewise, early recognition and treatment of many illnesses can prevent the need for emergency care. Equally important is education for parents and caregivers on the importance of first aid training, the recognition of signs and symptoms of serious illness or significant injury, and indications for seeking immediate care. The provision of printed handouts and standardized diagnosis-driven discharge instructions, verbal communication during well child or acute care visits, and first aid/cardiopulmonary resuscitation (CPR) classes all are mechanisms for informing parents of emergency care procedures. See Chapter 5.

OFFICE PREPAREDNESS. Although the need for full CPR occurs relatively infrequently in an office setting, most practices see children in need of acute intervention or hospitalization on a regular basis. Despite this, primary care providers and their staffs may find themselves ill equipped to treat patients with impending shock, respiratory failure, or a seizure in an examination room or patients whose condition deteriorates acutely while they are waiting to be seen. Emergency preparedness in the office requires training and continuing education for staff members, policies and procedures for emergency intervention, ready availability of appropriate resuscitation equipment, knowledge of local resources for EMS response and transport, and a working relationship with area EDs to ensure that children are cared for in facilities with expertise in pediatric emergency care.

STAFF TRAINING AND CONTINUING EDUCATION. Initial recognition by an office staff member that a child requires emergency treatment may occur in the course of a telephone call, in the waiting room, or in an examination room. All office personnel, including those seated at the front desk or answering the phone, must be capable of recognizing a child with altered mental status, shock, or respiratory distress/failure and must be aware of an appropriate action plan for rapid intervention.

It is a reasonable expectation that all office staff, including receptionists and medical assistants, be trained in adult and child CPR and first aid and that they maintain their certifica-

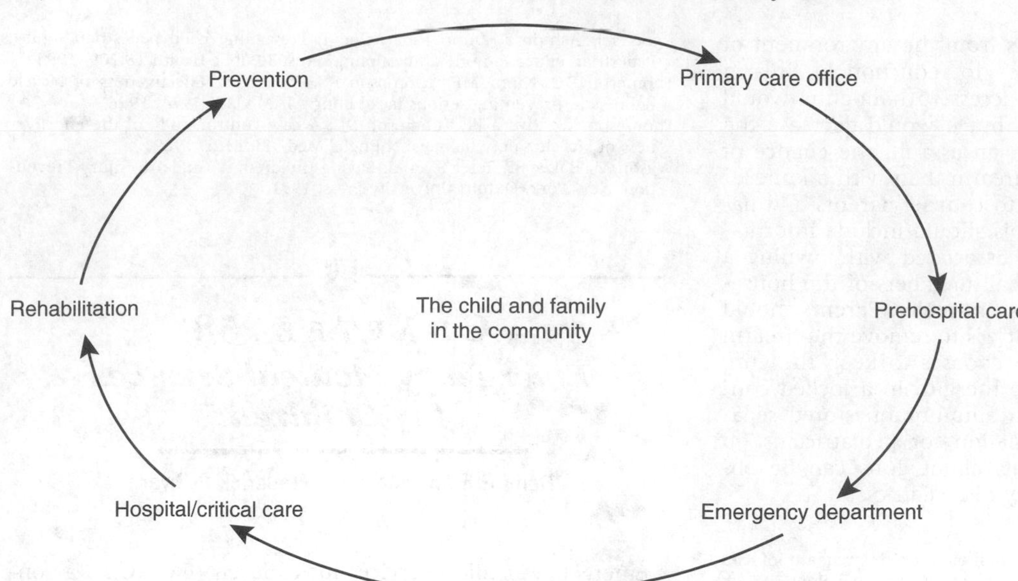

Figure 58–1 The EMS-C continuum of care: Seriously ill and injured children interface with a large number of health care personnel as they move through the EMS-C system. The system both begins and ends in the community.

tion on an annual basis. In addition to these requirements, nurses and physicians should have training in a systematic approach to pediatric medical and trauma resuscitation. Core knowledge may be obtained through standardized courses in pediatric advanced life support (ALS) offered by national medical and nursing associations. Frequent recertification is important for maintaining knowledge and skill. Examples of such curricula include the American Heart Association's Pediatric Advanced Life Support (PALS) course, the Advanced Pediatric Life Support (APLS) course sponsored by the American Academy of Pediatrics and the American College of Emergency Physicians, and the Emergency Nurses Pediatric Course (ENPC) and Pediatric Emergency Nursing self-instruction manual sponsored by the Emergency Nurses Association.

To facilitate emergency response when a child needs rapid intervention in the office, all personnel should have a preassigned role. Organizing a "code team" within the office ensures that necessary equipment is made available to the physician in charge, that an appropriate medical record detailing all interventions and the child's response is generated, and that the call for EMS response or a transport team is made in a timely fashion.

POLICIES AND PROCEDURES. Standardized protocols for telephone triage of seriously ill or injured children are essential, especially if after-hours calls are taken by nonphysician personnel. When a child's status is in question and prehospital care is available, ambulance transport in the care of trained personnel is preferable to transport by private car. This avoids the potentially serious medical consequences of relying on unskilled and worried parents, without the ability to provide even basic life support (BLS) measures, to transport an unstable child to an ED or clinic.

Written policies and procedures for the management of status asthmaticus, upper airway obstruction, seizures, ingestions, shock, sepsis/meningitis, trauma, head injury, anaphylaxis, and cardiopulmonary arrest should be generated and made available to all potentially involved staff members.

RESUSCITATION EQUIPMENT. Availability of necessary equipment is a vital part of a smooth emergency response. Every physician's office should have essential resuscitation equipment and medications packaged in a pediatric resuscitation cart or kit (Table 58–1). This kit should be checked on a routine basis and kept in an accessible location known to all office staff. Outdated medications, a laryngoscope with a failed light source, or an empty oxygen tank represents a catastrophe in a resuscitation setting; these can be easily avoided if an equipment checklist and maintenance schedule are implemented. Responsible staff should receive in-service training on a regular basis on equipment location and use, a task that may best be accomplished by a regular schedule of "mock codes" in which all office staff participate. A pediatric kit that includes posters, laminated cards, or resuscitation tapes specifying emergency drug doses and equipment size by age, weight, or height is invaluable in avoiding critical therapeutic errors during resuscitation.

TRANSPORT. Every office should be prepared to initiate resuscitation on a child with a life-threatening medical problem. This should include, at a minimum, measures to establish adequate oxygenation, ventilation, and perfusion. A decision must be made on how to transport a child to a facility capable of providing definitive care once the child has been stabilized. If a child has required aggressive airway or cardiovascular support, has altered mental status, continues to have unstable vital signs, or has significant potential to deteriorate en route, it is not appropriate to send the child via private car, regardless of proximity to a hospital. Even when an ambulance is called, it is the primary care provider's responsibility to initiate essential life support measures before transport.

In metropolitan centers with numerous public and private ambulance agencies, primary care providers must be knowledgeable about the level of service that is provided by each. The availability of BLS versus ALS services, transport team configuration, and pediatric expertise vary markedly among agencies. It may be appropriate to consider aeromedical transport when definitive or specialized care is not available within a community or when ground transport times are prolonged. In that case, initial transport via ground to a local hospital for interval stabilization may be undertaken pending arrival of the aeromedical team. When a child is to be transported by air or ground ambulance, copies of the child's pertinent medical records as well as any radiologic studies or laboratory results should be sent with the patient (Table 58–2) and a call made to the physicians at the receiving facility to alert them to the referral and any treatments administered. Such prenotification is not merely a courtesy; direct physician-to-physician communication is essential to ensure adequate transmission of patient care information, to allow mobilization of necessary resources in the ED, and to redirect the transport if the emergency physician feels that the child would be better treated at a facility with specialized services.

Not all EDs are equally capable of treating an ill or injured child, and it is the responsibility of the referring physician to

TABLE 58–1 Pediatric Equipment and Medications for Office Emergencies

Respiratory Equipment
- Oxygen cylinder with flowmeter
- Oxygen masks—neonate, infant, child, adult
- Bag-valve-mask resuscitator, with reservoir—child, adult
- Suction machine
- Yankauer suction tip
- Suction catheters—8F, 10F, 14F
- Oral airways—0–5
- Nasal cannulas—infant, child, adult
- Nasogastric tubes—8F, 10F, 14F
- Feeding tubes—5F, 8F
- Intubation equipment*
  - Laryngoscope handle with
    - Straight blade 0, 1, 2
    - Straight or curved blade 2, 3
  - Endotracheal tubes
    - Uncuffed 3.0, 3.5, 4.0, 4.5, 5.0, 5.5 mm ID
    - Cuffed 6.0, 7.0 mm ID
  - Stylets—infant, adult
  - Disposable end-tidal CO_2 detector
- Nebulizer

Fluid Management
- IV catheters, short, over the needle—16, 18, 20, 22, 24 gauge
- Butterfly needles—21, 23, 25 gauge
- IV boards, tape, povidone-iodine and alcohol swabs, tourniquet
- Pediatric infusion set/volume control device
- Intraosseous needles—15–18 gauge
- Isotonic fluids (normal saline or lactated Ringer's solution)

Monitoring
- Blood pressure cuffs—infant, child, adult
- Sphygmomanometer
- Cardiac monitor*
- Pulse oximeter with infant and pediatric probe*
- ECG monitor/defibrillator with pediatric paddles*
- Doppler ultrasound blood pressure monitor*

Cardiac Arrest Board

Medications
- Resuscitation
  - Epinephrine—1:1,000, 1:10,000
  - Atropine
  - Sodium bicarbonate—4.2%, 8.4%
  - Glucose—25% solution
- Anticonvulsants
  - Lorazepam or diazepam
  - Phenobarbital
- Antibiotics, parenteral
- Poisoning
  - Ipecac
  - Activated charcoal
- Respiratory/allergic
  - Albuterol for inhalation
  - Epinephrine—1:1,000
  - Methylprednisolone/prednisolone
  - Diphenhydramine, parenteral
- Miscellaneous
  - Naloxone

**Items are optional.*

be aware of the pediatric capabilities of the hospitals in the area. Critically ill and injured patients may have an improved outcome when cared for in regional referral centers. This is particularly true for neonatal emergencies, major trauma, burns, head injuries, and specific pediatric surgical problems. Thus, although initial stabilization of these patients may take place in a local community hospital, definitive and long-term care may be better delivered in major referral centers especially equipped to provide such care.

PEDIATRIC PREHOSPITAL CARE

Prehospital care refers to emergency assistance rendered by trained emergency medical personnel before a child reaches a fixed medical facility. Although most communities in the United States have a formalized EMS system, the nature of the emergency medical response available depends in large part on local demographics and population base. EMS may be provided by volunteers or paid professionals. A number of key points are important to recognize in considering the interface between the community physician and the local EMS system. These include access to the system, provider capability, response/transport times, and destination.

ACCESS TO THE EMS SYSTEM. Most metropolitan and many rural communities in the United States have a "911" telephone system that provides direct access to a dispatcher who coordinates police, fire, and EMS response. Some communities have an "enhanced 911" system, in which the location of the caller is automatically provided to the dispatcher, permitting emergency response even if the caller, such as a young child, cannot give an address. The extent of medical training for these dispatchers varies between communities, as do the protocols by which they assign an emergency response. In some smaller communities, no coordinated dispatch exists and emergency medical calls are handled by the local law enforcement agency.

In activating the 911 system, it is important for physicians to make it clear to the dispatcher the nature of the medical emergency and the condition of the child. In many communities, dispatchers are trained to ask a series of questions per protocol, allowing them to send out EMS personnel of an appropriate level of training.

PROVIDER CAPABILITY. There are many levels of training for prehospital EMS providers, ranging from individuals capable of providing only first aid to those trained and licensed to provide ALS in the field.

First responders may be law enforcement officers, firefighters, or community volunteers who are dispatched to provide emergency medical assistance. They have approximately 40 hr of training in first aid and CPR. Their role is to provide rapid response and stabilization pending the arrival of more highly trained personnel. In some smaller communities, this represents the only prehospital emergency medical response.

Emergency medical technicians (EMTs) are volunteers or paid professionals who provide the bulk of emergency medical response in the United States. Basic EMTs may staff an ambulance after undergoing an approximately 100-hr training program. They are licensed to provide BLS services but may receive further training to expand their scope of practice to intravenous (IV) placement and fluid administration, endotracheal intubation, and use of an automatic external defibrillator, under the direction of a physician advisor.

Paramedics, or EMT-Ps, represent the highest level of EMT response, with medical training and supervised field experience of approximately 1,000 hr. They provide ALS services in the prehospital setting, functioning out of an ambulance equipped as a mobile intensive care unit. Paramedic skills may include endotracheal intubation; the placement of peripheral, central, or intraosseous lines; IV administration of drugs; ad-

TABLE 58–2 Checklist for Patient Transport

1. Call appropriate transport agency.
2. Copy patient's current and pertinent past medical records, laboratory reports, and radiologic studies.
3. Obtain written permission for transport from parent/guardian.
4. Call receiving physician and document acceptance of transfer in patient's medical record.
5. Stabilize lines and tubes, splint fractures.
6. Give report to transport team, provide copy of records/studies.
7. Provide parent/guardian with patient's destination in writing.

ministration of nebulized aerosols; needle thoracotomy; and cardioversion/defibrillation. Paramedics work under the supervision of a physician advisor.

Aeromedical transport team configuration can vary widely and may include physicians, nurses, respiratory therapists, or paramedics. The amount of pediatric training of team members also varies, and it is important to confirm that an appropriate standard of care can be provided during interfacility transport.

The level of training of the prehospital personnel dispatched to the scene of a medical emergency depends on the condition of the patient, available resources, and local protocols. It is important to realize that attention has only recently been focused on *pediatric* prehospital care. Only about 10% of all EMS calls are for pediatric emergencies. Training and equipment for pediatric emergency care have historically been given inadequate attention in national certification curricula and by EMS agencies primarily geared toward adult patients. In some communities, the standard of pediatric prehospital care may not match that offered to adult patients in similar condition. The EMS-C initiative sponsored by the Maternal and Child Health Bureau, U.S. Department of Health and Human Services, has provided program development grants to improve pediatric emergency services in all 50 states. This has led to increased awareness of the special needs of acutely ill and injured children and to the development of many programs and products to enhance their care.

RESPONSE/TRANSPORT TIMES. Depending on the demographics of a community, the location of the incident, and the nature of the EMS available, EMS response times after a call for assistance may range from a few minutes to longer than an hour. Unfortunately, even in communities with relatively rapid response times, individuals may be a reluctant to call for help because of a misperception that 911 should be activated only for full-blown resuscitations. If a child is physiologically unstable (with marked respiratory distress, cyanosis, signs of early shock, or altered mental status) or has significant potential to deteriorate en route to the ED, or if the parents' ability to comply promptly with recommendations for ED evaluation is in question, an EMS transport should be initiated. Inherent dangers lie in the attitude that a parent can get to the hospital faster by private car. It must be remembered that legal responsibility for patients lies with the referring physician, until responsibility for care is officially transferred to another medical provider.

DESTINATION. The destination to which an EMT transports a pediatric patient may be defined by parental preference, provider preference, or agency protocol. In communities with an organized trauma system or a system of pediatric designation based on objective capabilities of the area hospitals, seriously ill or injured children may be triaged by protocol to the highest-level center reachable within a reasonable time frame. The Pediatric Trauma Score (PTS) (Table 58–3) or Revised Trauma Score (RTS) can be used to assess the severity of injury. Children with a PTS less than 8 or an RTS less than 11 should be treated in a designated trauma center. In communities that do not have a hospital with the equipment and personnel resources to provide definitive inpatient care, interfacility transport of a child to a regional center may be undertaken after initial stabilization. The primary care provider may be involved in this decision-making process and must make a critical assessment of the local hospital's pediatric intensive care capabilities. When interfacility transport is to be undertaken, indications for transfer, parental consent for transfer, and acceptance of the patient by the receiving physician all must be clearly documented in the medical record.

THE PEDIATRIC PATIENT IN THE HOSPITAL EMERGENCY DEPARTMENT: PRIORITIES IN PEDIATRIC RESUSCITATION

The majority of children who require emergency care are evaluated in community hospitals by physicians with variable degrees of pediatric training and experience. Children account for approximately 25% of all ED visits, but only a fraction of them represent true emergencies. Because the volume of critical pediatric cases is low, emergency physicians and nurses often have limited opportunities to reinforce their knowledge and skills in pediatric resuscitation. Pediatricians from the community may be consulted when a seriously ill or injured child presents to the ED and should have a structured approach to initial evaluation and treatment in an unstable child of any age, regardless of the underlying diagnosis. Early recognition of life-threatening abnormalities in oxygenation, ventilation, perfusion, and central nervous system (CNS) function and rapid intervention to correct those abnormalities are key to successful pediatric resuscitation.

Cardiopulmonary arrest in children is rarely the result of a primary cardiac event. Rather, full arrest in children is usually a result of prolonged myocardial ischemia related to untreated hypoxemia or untreated shock. By the time the heart has sustained a sufficient hypoxic insult to result in asystole, the CNS has sustained a severe asphyxial insult as well. This accounts for the poor outcome for children who are brought into the ED with ongoing CPR. Although reported rates of discharge from the hospital for children with prehospital cardiopulmonary arrest range from 0–21%, those with a good neurologic outcome were rapidly resuscitated in the field and arrived in the ED with a perfusing rhythm. In the case of a child who continues to be apneic and pulseless on arrival at the ED, aggressive pharmacologic therapy may re-establish a perfusing cardiac rhythm, but brain death or survival with serious neurologic impairment is the rule.

Whether a child presents with a primary cardiovascular, respiratory, neurologic, infectious, or metabolic disorder, the goal is early recognition of respiratory and circulatory insufficiency. Specific management of these disease states and information about CPR and airway and fluid management are included in Chapter 64. Early intervention is geared toward preventing the progression of hypoxemia and hypoperfusion to full cardiopulmonary arrest, with its attendant poor prognosis. During the primary survey (Table 58–4), *life-threatening conditions* are identified and resuscitation is begun simultaneously. Interventions should be undertaken in a graded progression, from least to most invasive, with careful reassessment after each intervention. A head-to-toe physical assessment, or

TABLE 58–3 Pediatric Trauma Score*

	Score		
Clinical Category	*+2*	*+1*	*−1*
Size	≥20 kg	10–20 kg	<10 kg
Airway	Normal	Maintainable	Unmaintainable
Systolic blood pressure	≤90 mm Hg	50–90 mm Hg	<50 mm Hg
Central nervous system	Awake	Obtunded/loss of consciousness	Coma/decerebrate
Open wound	None	Minor	Major/penetrating
Skeletal	None	Closed fracture	Open/multiple fractures

**From Ford EG: Trauma triage.* In: *Ford EG, Andrassy RJ (eds): Pediatric Trauma Initial Assessment and Management. Philadelphia, WB Saunders, 1994, p 112.*

TABLE 58–4 Pediatric Primary Survey and Resuscitation Measures

A = Airway/Cervical Spine Control

1. Assess airway patency
   If patent and patient conscious—maintain position of comfort
   If compromised—position, suction, ? oral airway
   If unmaintainable—oral endotracheal intubation
2. Maintain cervical spine in neutral position with manual immobilization if head/facial trauma or high-risk injury mechanism

B = Breathing

Assess respiratory rate, color, work of breathing, mental status
  If respiratory effort adequate—administer high-flow supplemental oxygen
  If respiratory effort inadequate—bag-valve-mask ventilation with 100% oxygen, naso/orogastric tube, consider intubation

C = Circulation/Hemorrhage Control

Assess heart rate, pulse quality, color, skin signs, mental status
  If perfusion adequate—apply cardiac monitor, establish IV access, direct pressure to bleeding sites
  If signs of shock—establish vascular access (IV/IO), isotonic fluid bolus, baseline laboratory studies, cardiac monitor, urinary catheter
  If ongoing hemorrhage suspected and continued signs of shock, blood transfusion and surgical consultation

D = Disability (Neurologic Status)

Assess pupillary function, mental status (AVPU)
  If decreased level of consciousness—reassess and optimize oxygenation, ventilation, circulation
  If increased ICP suspected, elevate head of bed, consider mild hyperventilation, neurosurgical consultation

E = Exposure

Remove clothing for complete evaluation. Prevent heat loss with blankets, heat lamps, radiant warmer.

AVPU = alertness, response to voice, response to pain, unresponsive; ICP = intracranial pressure; IO = intraosseous; IV = intravenous.

secondary survey, and definitive care should be undertaken only after the primary survey is complete and appropriate resuscitation is under way. Whether the "code leader" is a pediatrician, surgeon, or emergency physician, clear communication, teamwork, and meticulous documentation are integral to a well-run resuscitation.

A: AIRWAY/SPINAL IMMOBILIZATION. *Airway management* is frequently cited as the key to successful pediatric resuscitation. Because of the anatomic peculiarities of a child's airway, infectious disease susceptibilities, and the vulnerability to foreign body aspiration of orally exploring toddlers, airway emergencies are quite common. In assessing the airway, look for evidence of appropriate chest rise and for signs of increased work of breathing, such as retractions and accessory muscle use. Listen over the trachea for abnormal sounds, such as snoring, gurgling, or stridor, and over the peripheral lung fields for the adequacy of inspiratory effort. Feel for movement of air on expiration and ascertain that the trachea is midline.

If the airway is patent, without evidence of obstruction, allow the child to maintain a position of comfort and administer supplemental oxygen as needed, preferably by mask or nasal prongs. If the child has evidence of partial or complete airway obstruction, reposition the head, placing it in the "sniff" position by using the chin lift or, in trauma patients, jaw thrust, taking care not to hyperextend the neck (see Figs. 64–3 and 64–4). Blood, secretions, or gastric contents should be removed from the mouth with a rigid suction device. If a patent airway cannot be established or maintained with these maneuvers, consideration must be given to placing an oral or nasal airway. These devices are rarely tolerated by a conscious child; placement may lead to gagging, vomiting, and the possibility of aspiration.

Orotracheal intubation (with in-line manual immobilization of the cervical spine in a trauma victim) may be required, if the above-mentioned BLS maneuvers are not successful. Blind nasotracheal intubation is not technically feasible in children, because the glottis is quite anterior and cephalic. The fact that the narrowest part of a child's upper airway lies at the level of the cricoid ring, below the level of the glottic opening, dictates that only uncuffed endotracheal tubes be chosen for children younger than 8 yr. Rapid sequence induction with IV administration of atropine, a neuromuscular blockade agent, and a sedative may be necessary to complete the procedure safely if a child is conscious. In rare situations, when endotracheal intubation cannot be achieved because of severe facial or neck trauma or complete upper airway obstruction, needle cricothyrotomy using a 12- to 14-gauge over-the-needle catheter with jet insufflation of 100% oxygen may be lifesaving.

In managing a child's airway, it is important to remember that adult airway equipment cannot be adapted for use in a pediatric patient. Appropriate-size suction catheters, a full set of oral airways and laryngoscope blades, uncuffed endotracheal tubes of 2.5–5.5 mm ID, and cuffed tubes for older children should be part of the pediatric emergency airway kit.

Spinal immobilization is an integral part of airway management in pediatric trauma patients. The cervical spine must be immobilized in any child who has sustained a high-velocity injury or has evidence of multiple trauma or of significant injury above the level of the clavicles. Optimally, this should be done in the field. If spinal immobilization has not been undertaken in the prehospital setting, it should be achieved immediately on admission to the ED. Although application of an appropriately sized, rigid cervical collar assists in spinal immobilization, it does not prevent movement. A child must therefore be immobilized on a backboard, using towel or blanket rolls to eliminate dead space and 2-in. adhesive tape across the forehead to secure the child's head to the board. Care must be taken to ensure neutral alignment of the head and neck on the backboard. In younger children, this may involve placing a small towel under the shoulders to prevent the child's large occiput from causing cervical spine flexion. Because children are particularly susceptible to spinal cord injury without abnormality on lateral cervical spine films, they should not be removed from the board until a full clinical and radiologic examination is completed. This should include at a minimum anteroposterior, lateral, and open-mouth odontoid views. CT, MRI, or flexion-extension views may need to be obtained if a child's neurologic findings or mechanism of injury is suggestive of a cord injury.

B: BREATHING. Once the patency of a patient's airway is established, the evaluation proceeds to assess the adequacy of the child's minute ventilation, a function of respiratory rate and tidal volume. In a conscious child with spontaneous respiratory effort, look before touching. Observation alone permits evaluation of respiratory rate, skin color, mental status, and work of breathing. Listen over the trachea and over the peripheral lung fields for the adequacy of air entry, symmetry, and abnormal breath sounds such as crackles or wheezing. Placement of a pulse oximetry probe, when available, permits continuous assessment of oxygenation. Tachypnea, in association with increased work of breathing—grunting, nasal flaring, or retractions—may reflect pathology anywhere in the tracheobronchial tree, lung parenchyma, or chest wall. However, effortless tachypnea may represent a compensatory mechanism in the presence of shock and metabolic acidosis, rather than a primary respiratory problem. A respiratory rate too slow for age in a sick child is an ominous sign and may reflect a failure of central respiratory drive—as in closed head injury—or respiratory fatigue. This is a warning sign of imminent respiratory arrest. Cyanosis is a late sign of respiratory failure.

If the airway is patent and minute ventilation appears adequate, high-flow supplemental oxygen should be administered pending objective evaluation of arterial oxygen levels. All seriously ill and injured patients should receive supplemental oxygen. If the airway is patent but spontaneous respiratory effort appears to be inadequate, *positive pressure ventilation* via a bag-valve-mask device with an oxygen reservoir should be initiated. Indications for positive pressure ventilation include but are not limited to poor color or bradycardia unresponsive to supplemental oxygen, gasping, periods of apnea, progressive respiratory distress, and the appearance of respiratory fatigue. Close attention to maintaining a tight mask seal and continual observation of the adequacy of chest rise are imperative. Prolonged positive pressure ventilation in children leads to gastric distention, which impedes diaphragmatic excursion and increases the risk of aspiration of stomach contents. Gastric distention can be minimized by applying cricoid pressure and by placing a nasogastric or orogastric tube to decompress the stomach. If a child fails to respond to positive pressure ventilation with improved color, heart rate, and level of consciousness, equipment and technique should be checked to ensure that the child is being effectively ventilated. If bag-valve-mask ventilation is unsuccessful or prolonged positive pressure ventilation is required, endotracheal intubation must be undertaken.

Pneumothorax must be considered in trauma victims presenting with respiratory failure, especially one who does not improve with supplemental oxygen and positive pressure ventilation. Classically, *tension pneumothorax* produces decreased breath sounds and hyperresonance in the affected hemithorax, mediastinal shift, cyanosis, and distended neck veins, as well as compromised cardiac output caused by decreased venous return to the heart. If the diagnosis is suspected, insert a needle or over-the-needle catheter into the second intercostal space at the midclavicular line, aspirate with a syringe to confirm the presence of free air, and immediately decompress the chest. Definitive treatment involves placing a chest tube in the fifth intercostal space, anterior to the midaxillary line.

C: CIRCULATION. The evaluation of circulation involves assessment of cardiac output and, in cases of trauma, identification and control of exsanguinating hemorrhage. Hypovolemia is the most common cause of shock in children, followed by septic and cardiogenic shock. The early signs and symptoms of shock may be subtle, and tachycardia may be the only objective finding. Cool extremities, mottled or pale skin color, delayed capillary refill time, and effortless tachypnea are relatively early signs of shock, which may be followed by the development of weak or absent peripheral pulses, altered mental status, and hypotension if the shock state is not recognized and treated. Children in shock maintain their blood pressure in the normal range by increasing their heart rate and peripheral vascular resistance. Hypotension is a late sign of shock and does not occur until there has been an acute loss of more than 25% of the blood volume. Shock resuscitation should be initiated long before the blood pressure falls.

Initial priorities in the treatment of shock are directed at restoring adequate perfusion of the vital organs. In trauma victims, shock is almost always due to blood loss. Initial resuscitation efforts should include control of hemorrhage, elevation of the lower extremities, prevention of heat loss, and volume resuscitation. Volume resuscitation is also the cornerstone of therapy in children with hypovolemic shock of medical etiology. The use of pressors should largely be reserved for cases of cardiogenic, septic, or neurogenic shock and is rarely indicated in traumatic shock.

Achieving vascular access in a child in shock may be difficult. The preferred site is the antecubital fossa, using a short, over-the-needle IV catheter. If initial attempts to establish one or, preferably, two large-bore peripheral IV lines are not successful within 2–5 min, alternate methods of vascular access must be undertaken to prevent a dangerous delay in initiating resuscitation. Depending on the experience and expertise of the provider, this might take the form of a surgical venous cutdown, central venous line, or intraosseous (IO) line.

Intraosseous infusion (IOI) is an easily achieved alternative to an IV line when vascular access is imperative and a peripheral IV cannot be rapidly placed in children 6 yr of age and younger. An IOI is established by inserting a 15- to 18-gauge bone marrow needle into the marrow cavity of the proximal tibia (Fig. 58–2). The distal tibia and distal femur are alternate sites of placement. IOI of resuscitation drugs, antibiotics, and anticonvulsants and continuous infusion of crystalloid solutions, blood products, and vasopressors have been successfully used in pediatric resuscitations. Experimental models have demonstrated rapid absorption of resuscitation drugs into the systemic circulation from the tibial marrow space, which serves as a "noncollapsible vein," even in hypotensive subjects or those undergoing CPR.

Although placement of an IO line is easy to learn and rapidly achieved, the technique has some limitations. Flow rates do not approximate those of an IV line of similar caliber and may be inadequate in cases of severe shock or exsanguinating hemorrhage. However, infusion of an initial crystalloid bolus through an IO line may facilitate subsequent placement of IV lines. More rapid infusion rates may be achieved by placing the bag of IV solution in a pressure bag inflated to 300 mm Hg or by "pushing" the bolus with a 60-mL syringe. An IO line cannot be placed in a fractured bone.

Concurrent with IV or IO placement, blood for initial laboratory studies should be drawn and sent. In cases of traumatic shock, this should include a type and cross match for packed red blood cells as well as a baseline hematocrit.

Initial volume resuscitation of patients in shock should be with isotonic crystalloid fluids. Unless a patient has cardiogenic shock, an initial bolus of 20 mL/kg administered as rapidly as possible should be given. Further fluid boluses are administered if reassessment of a patient's response to therapy so warrants, with frequent vital sign checks and attention to signs of end-organ perfusion—skin color and warmth, mental status, and urine output. Placement of an indwelling urinary catheter is helpful in monitoring the effectiveness of shock resuscitation. The production of 1–2 mL/kg/hr of urine is indicative of adequate fluid resuscitation. Transfusion with packed red blood cells may be necessary if an injured child fails to respond to 40 mL/kg of normal saline or lactated Ringer's solution. Early surgical consultation is imperative in any child who remains hemodynamically unstable after an initial fluid bolus, because emergency operative intervention may be necessary.

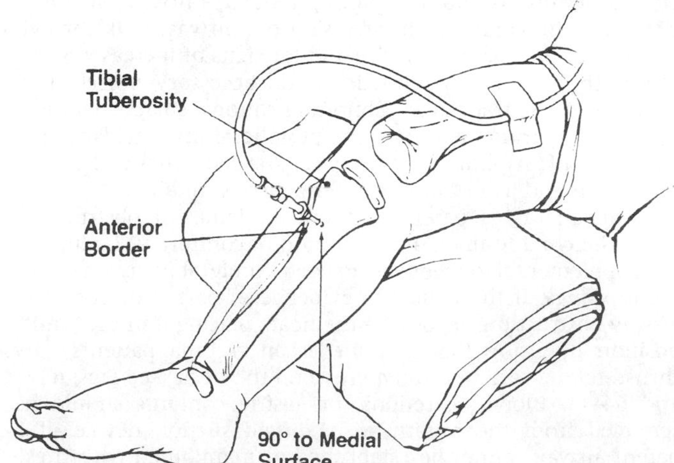

Figure 58–2 Intraosseous cannulation technique. The preferred site for placement of an intraosseous line is approximately one finger breadth below the tibial tuberosity on the flat anteromedial aspect of the bone. Use of a disposable bone marrow needle with stylet prevents plugging with bone. Care should be taken to direct the needle perpendicular to the bone or slightly caudad to avoid the growth plate. (Adapted from Chameides L, Hazinski H [eds]: Pediatric Advanced Life Support. Dallas, TX, American Heart Association, 1997.)

Pneumatic antishock garments have not been demonstrated to be effective in shock therapy for children.

D: DISABILITY. Rapid assessment of both cortical and brain stem function is an important part of the initial assessment of a seriously ill or injured child. Head injury is the most common cause of death due to trauma, accounting for 75% of fatal injuries. The Glasgow Coma Scale or one of the several children's coma scales adapted from that tool may be used to document serial neurologic assessments (see Table 64–7). A more abbreviated initial examination consists of an evaluation of pupillary responses and categorization of mental status based on the acronym AVPU—is the patient **A**lert? Responsive to **V**oice? Responsive to **P**ain? or **U**nresponsive? Frequent reassessment of neurologic status is of utmost importance.

If signs of elevated intracranial pressure (ICP) are identified, immediate stabilizing measures should be undertaken. Adequate oxygenation and ventilation must be ensured. Elevation of the head of the bed and administration of osmotic diuretics may be indicated, depending on the cause of the ICP elevation. The use of hyperventilation to control ICP in the resuscitation setting is a subject of controversy. Again, early surgical consultation is imperative. Attention must also be given to interfacility transport if the hospital does not have CT or neurosurgical capability.

E: EXPOSURE. Undressing and exposing the patient are necessary to perform a thorough examination and to identify all injuries. However, undressed infants and young children are at high risk for excessive heat loss and hypothermia during resuscitation because of their high ratio of surface area to volume. Attention must be paid to preventing heat loss during the emergency evaluation and treatment phase. Blankets, radiant warmers, heat lamps, and warming blankets or chemical heat packs all may have a role in preventing hypothermia.

Once the primary survey has been completed and resuscitation is under way, a thorough head-to-toe physical examination should be performed. A nasogastric or orogastric tube and bladder catheter should be placed unless there are specific contraindications. Radiologic studies, further laboratory evaluation, and consultations with specialists may be undertaken at this time. All seriously injured children need lateral neck, chest, and pelvic radiographs. If equipment or personnel resources for optimal definitive care of a patient are unavailable, consideration should be given to initiating a patient transfer to a facility with greater capability.

PSYCHOSOCIAL/ETHICAL ISSUES IN PEDIATRIC RESUSCITATION

Resuscitation of a child—in particular, failed resuscitation—is an emotionally draining event for all involved. Aggressive efforts must be undertaken whenever there is hope of saving a child's life. However, with the possible exception of children with profound hypothermia, a child brought in apneic and pulseless from a prehospital setting has essentially no chance of neurologically meaningful survival. Extensive resources may be devoted to such futile efforts, with negative consequences for the child and family. The decision not to start resuscitation may be just as difficult as the decision to stop (Chapters 2 and 72).

Parents faced with the sudden unexpected loss of their child may demand that "everything" be done. In reality, when physician-parent communication is good, most families do not insist on unreasonable measures. In dealing with family members faced with the loss of a child, it is important to remember that the spectrum of normal response may range from apparently unnatural calm, to emotional decompensation, to outrage. The anger of family members is often a reflection of their sense of guilt and helplessness.

Parents need to know that everything reasonably possible has been done to save their child—by bystanders, EMTs, or hospital personnel. At the same time, they need to be told clearly but compassionately when there is no hope of survival. By designating one individual to keep the parents informed on the ongoing process of resuscitation, providing them with realistic information as it evolves, and involving them in the decision-making process when the time comes to stop, parents can be given some sense of empowerment at a time of ultimate helplessness. In some situations, allowing the parents to be present in the treatment room to witness the resuscitation may help them come to terms with the gravity of the situation and feel that they were with their child in his or her last moments. If this is to be offered, a staff member must be available to stay with the parents. After resuscitation efforts have stopped, parents and family members should be provided with a private room in which to hold the child and say goodbye.

Death or neurologically poor survival is the rule if asystole persists after administration of two doses of IV epinephrine or after 25 min of CPR. The fact that one can restore a perfusing rhythm with repeated rounds of resuscitation drugs should not be construed as success. We must remember that the goal is survival with good functional neurologic recovery.

At the point at which the code leader wishes to stop CPR and pronounce the child dead, members of the team should be queried to ensure that all personnel involved feel that everything appropriate has been done. An opportunity for staff debriefing should be provided immediately after the code, because emotions tend to run high with the death of a child. Formal code review, looking at process and outcome of each resuscitation, is an important part of the department's quality improvement program.

American Heart Association Emergency Cardiac Care Committee and Subcommittees: Guidelines for cardiopulmonary resuscitation and emergency cardiac care, VI pediatric advanced life support. JAMA 268:2262, 1992.

Baker MD, Ludwig S: Pediatric emergency transport and the private practitioner. Pediatrics 88:691, 1991.

Cales RH: Trauma mortality in Orange County: The effect of implementation of a regional trauma system. Ann Emerg Med 13:1, 1984.

Chameides L, Hazinski H (eds): Pediatric Advanced Life Support. Dallas, TX, American Heart Association, 1997.

Committee on Trauma, American College of Surgeons: Advanced Trauma Life Support. Chicago, American College of Surgeons, 1997.

Day S, McCloskey K, Orr R, et al: Pediatric interhospital critical care transport: Consensus of a national leadership conference. Pediatrics 88:696, 1991.

Doyle CJ, Post H, Burney RE, et al: Family participation during resuscitation: An option. Ann Emerg Med 16:673, 1987.

Durch JS, Lohr KN (eds): Emergency Medical Services for Children. Washington, DC, National Academy Press, 1993.

Eichelberger MR, Gotschall CS, Sacco, et al: A comparison of the Trauma Score, the Revised Trauma Score, and the Pediatric Trauma Score. Ann Emerg Med 18:1053, 1989.

Eisenberg M, Berger L, Hallstrom A: Epidemiology of cardiac arrest and resuscitation in children. Ann Emerg Med 12:672, 1983.

Fiser DH: Intraosseous infusion. N Engl J Med 322:1579, 1990.

Flores G, Weinstock DJ: The preparedness of pediatricians for emergencies in the office. Arch Pediatr Adolesc Med 150:249, 1996.

Gerardi MJ, Sacchetti AD, Cantor RM, et al: Rapid-sequence intubation of the pediatric patient. Ann Emerg Med 28:55, 1996.

Hanson C, Strawser D: Family presence during cardiopulmonary resuscitation: Foote Hospital emergency department's nine-year perspective. J Emerg Nurs 18:104, 1992.

Kaufmann CR, Maier RV, Rivara FP, et al: Evaluation of the Pediatric Trauma Score. JAMA 63:69, 1990.

Lubitz DS, Seidel JS, Chameides L, et al: A rapid method for estimating weight and resuscitation drug dosages from length in the pediatric age group. Ann Emerg Med 17:576, 1988.

Macnab AJ: Optimal escort for interhospital transport of pediatric emergencies. J Trauma 31:205, 1991.

Orlowski JP, Porembka DT, Gallagher JM, et al: Comparison study of intraosseous, central intravenous, and peripheral intravenous infusions of emergency drugs. Am J Dis Child 144:112, 1990.

O'Rourke PP: Outcome of children who are apneic and pulseless in the emergency room. Crit Care Med 14:466, 1986.

Pang D, Wilberger JE: Spinal cord injury without radiographic abnormalities in children. J Neurosurg 57:114, 1982.

Pollack MM, Alexander SR, Clarke N, et al: Improved outcomes from tertiary center pediatric intensive care: A statewide comparison of tertiary and nontertiary care facilities. Crit Care Med 19:150, 1991.

Quan L, Wentz KR, Gore EJ, et al: Outcome and predictors of outcome in pediatric submersion victims receiving prehospital care in King County, Washington. Pediatrics 86:586, 1990.

Schierhout G, Roberts I: Hyperventilation therapy in acute traumatic brain injury. *In:* Alderson P, Fleminger S, Klassen T, et al (eds): Brain and Spinal Cord Injury Module of the Cochrane Database of Systematic Reviews; The Cochrane Library; Issue 4; 1997.

Singer J, Ludwig S (eds): Emergency Medical Services for Children: The Role of the Primary Care Provider. Elk Grove Village, IL, American Academy of Pediatrics, 1992.

Tsai A, Kallsen G: Epidemiology of pediatric prehospital care. Ann Emerg Med 16:284, 1987.

CHAPTER 59

Pediatric Critical Care: An Overview

Lorry R. Frankel

It is important for general pediatricians to understand what constitutes intensive care and to be familiar with some of the nuances of evaluation and stabilization of a child who has an impending life-threatening event or who has recently had a life-threatening event. This knowledge facilitates the management and transfer of the critically ill child to an appropriate facility for care. Pediatric critical care represents a convergence of knowledge, technologies, and approaches to multisystem organ failure from the operating room, neonatal intensive care areas, and adult intensive care units (ICUs). Before the development of specialized areas to care for critically ill or injured pediatric patients, most critically ill children were cared for in either adult intensive care or neonatal intensive care units. This resulted in placement of these children alongside geriatric or neonatal patients, whose medical, nursing, and psychosocial needs were significantly different.

Children having acute neurologic deterioration, respiratory distress, cardiovascular compromise, or life-threatening traumatic injuries constitute the most common admissions to a pediatric intensive care unit (PICU). Unlike pediatric patients who require general care, these patients usually have a disease process that affects more than one organ system, commonly referred to as multiple organ system failure. Successful PICUs use a multidisciplinary approach to care for these patients. Staff are also trained to manage the psychosocial dynamics encountered among the patients, parents and other family members, and the various teams of health care professionals involved in the care of these patients. Communication among the individuals caring for these patients is imperative and involves periodic team conferences with the family, the primary physicians, and the various subspecialists who are caring for these complicated and critically ill patients. The patient population is diverse in age and disease processes. The most active PICUs admit more than 350 patients per year, with a fairly even mix of medical and surgical diseases; the number and distribution vary with the emphasis on various programs.

Patients are admitted to a PICU because they require a very high level of monitoring of vital signs and other body functions not available in other parts of the hospital (see Chapter 62). These patients may need mechanical ventilation, invasive intravascular monitoring, and frequent attention by both the nursing and medical staffs (Table 59–1). The children may be admitted directly from physicians' offices, clinics, the emergency department, or the operating rooms. Most PICUs have active transport programs to facilitate the transfer of critically ill children (Chapter 60). This enables patients to be evaluated and stabilized as well as transported to the appropriate regional PICU. This extension of critical care services to the community and regional areas is essential to provide optimal care to children who have sustained a life-threatening illness or injury.

UNIT ORGANIZATION. PICUs are specially designed and equipped facilities that require nurses, respiratory therapists, pharmacists, and physicians trained to care for critically ill children (see California Children's Services Standards for Pediatric Critical Care Units). The administrative structure for the ICU facilitates the multidisciplinary approach to the care of critically ill patients. It also enables the unit to establish training guidelines for the staff, evaluate equipment, review use of costly resources, and provide objective assessment of the effectiveness of new therapies. A unit director certified in pediatric critical care medicine works closely with nursing leadership and the other physicians to promote integration of critical care and the care provided by other subspecialists who practice in the unit. Assistance from anesthesia is helpful in developing clinical pathways for sedation and pain management and protocols needed to facilitate the transfer of patients from the operating room to the PICU. A surgeon with interests in trauma care is instrumental in developing the appropriate protocols required to care for injured patients. The creation of a critical care committee is also helpful to formulate policies for the ICU, such as those regarding admission and discharge criteria; the

TABLE 59–1 Criteria for PICU Admission and Discharge

	Admission Criteria	Discharge Criteria
PICU	Patients who need *invasive monitoring:* arterial and central venous catheters, pulmonary arterial lines, ICP catheters Patients with evidence of: *respiratory impairment or failure* *cardiovascular compromise:* shock, hypotension, hypertensive crisis *acute neurologic deterioration:* coma, status epilepticus, increased ICP *acute renal failure* requiring dialysis or CVVH *Bleeding disorders* that necessitate massive transfusions	Patient may be discharged from the PICU once the disease process has reversed itself and care can be provided in a less intense environment: Patient no longer requires invasive monitoring Patient can protect his/her airway (cough and gag reflexes) Patient is hemodynamically stable
PIICU	Patients who do *not* require respiratory assistance for acute respiratory failure but may require continuous noninvasive monitoring of vital signs, BP, Sao_2, Tco_2, or $Tcco_2$ Patients who require chronic respiratory support via tracheostomies or noninvasive ventilation Patients who are in early cardiovascular failure and require monitoring of vital signs (noninvasive monitoring) Patients with acute neurologic injury but with a patent airway that they can protect themselves Patients with MSOF who do not need a PICU, but nursing care is not available elsewhere (e.g., trauma victims, DKA)	Patient may be discharged from the PIICU when it has been determined that care can be provided in general care areas

BP = blood pressure; CVVH = continuous venovenous hemofiltration; DKA = diabetic ketoacidosis; ICP = intracranial pressure; MSOF = multisystem organ failure; PICU = pediatric intensive care unit; PIICU = pediatric intermediate intensive care unit; Sao_2 = arterial oxygen saturation; Tco_2 = transcutaneous oxygen; $Tcco_2$ = transcutaneous carbon dioxide.

role of the various attending physicians; credential criteria for physicians and physician extenders who practice in the PICU; the role of the house officers in the care of a critically ill child; transfer agreements with other hospitals to accommodate overflow patients during time of high census; and *quality assurance*. Quality indicators may include mortality, length of ICU stays, adverse neurologic outcomes, reintubation rates for failed extubations, acquired injuries from intubations or other invasive procedures, and unanticipated ICU admissions from various areas within the hospital.

Frankel LR: Pediatric Intensive Care. *In:* Bernstein D, Shelov SP (eds): Pediatrics, Baltimore, Williams & Wilkins, 1996, pp 591–609.
Hyman AI, Arons RR, Milo BJ: Clinical, economic, and political implications of critical care. *In:* Holbrook PR (ed): Textbook of Pediatric Critical Care. Philadelphia, WB Saunders, 1993, pp 1143–1150.
Rabin DS, Wells LA: Admission and Discharge Criteria and Procedures. *In:* Levin DL, Morriss FC (eds): Essentials of Pediatric Intensive Care, 2nd ed. New York, Churchill Livingstone, 1997, pp 1127–1142.
Standards for Pediatric Intensive Care Units; California Children Services: Manual of Procedures. Department of Health Services, State of California, Chapter 3.32, Dec 1998.

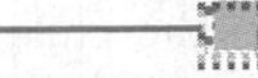

CHAPTER 60

Interfacility Transfer of the Critically Ill Infant and Child

Lorry R. Frankel

As pediatric intensive care units (PICUs) have developed in selected sites, specialized transport programs (interfacility transport) to bring patients from community facilities to the PICU have evolved. Children are usually taken to the local emergency department by the emergency medical services provider or by their parents, where their condition is assessed to determine the extent of injury, severity of illness, and physiologic stability. If the local facility does not have the capabilities to provide comprehensive intensive care, the child must be transported to a PICU. However, unless there is a surgical emergency, the child should be stabilized in the referring hospital while awaiting the arrival of the pediatric transport team. Regional pediatric centers have a responsibility not only to transport patients as rapidly and safely as possible but also to provide community educational programs that enable the providers of health care to develop the necessary skills required for physiologic stabilization until the transport team arrives.

The American Academy of Pediatrics, the Association of Air Medical Services, and the Federal Aviation Administration have developed recommendations for pediatric transport programs. The members of the transport team must have the cognitive and technical skills required for the needs of pediatric patients and should be supervised by an attending physician (medical control physician [MCP]) who has expertise in either pediatric emergency medicine or pediatric critical care. All transport teams should have a team leader able to manage the airway, provide respiratory support, and obtain vascular access and who has basic knowledge of pediatric drug dosing and understands the basic pathophysiology of pediatric disease and the transport environment.

DISPATCH CENTER/TRANSFER CENTER. The regional pediatric center or PICU should provide phone consultation and deploy a team of specialized health care providers to assist in stabilization of patients in order to transport them in a safe mobile environment to the PICU. Once it has been determined that an ill child should be transported, the MCP should be consulted to provide further input into the patient's care while the unseen patient is still at the local facility and to determine the best team composition and vehicle required to transport the patient. The MCP may need to seek additional medical or surgical consultation from other subspecialists.

TEAM COMPOSITION. This is based on a number of factors, including the severity of a patient's illness, the distance to the referring facility, the referring facility's insistence that certain team members be present (e.g., a physician), and the ability of the team members to work together in unfamiliar surroundings. The severity of illness is assessed by the MCP from the information provided by the referring hospital. Many transports can be handled by a nonphysician team leader by phone contact with the MCP. In addition to the team leader, a critical care nurse is helpful to provide nursing care and monitoring and to administer medications. If a child requires airway and respiratory support, a respiratory therapist should be a member of the team.

VEHICLE SELECTION. The selection of the vehicle is made by the MCP in coordination with the referring hospital and those who will participate in transport of the child. Factors taken into consideration are the severity of illness or injury, the distance to the referring hospital, travel time required, weather conditions, vehicle availability, equipment needs, and expense. *Ground ambulance* is used for the majority of transports, which are less than 100 miles. The traffic patterns must be considered in evaluating response time. The major advantages of this mode of transport over the others are the ability to stop en route if the patient's condition worsens and further intervention is required and the ability to take a larger team with more equipment if needed. *Fixed-wing transports* are usually used to reach infants and children who live more than 100–150 miles from the regional PICU. They may be able to fly to areas when the weather or altitude prevents the use of a helicopter. However, the use of fixed-wing aircraft requires several ambulance transfers. In addition, flying at altitude can have serious effects on the partial pressure and volume of gases in various body cavities and closed containers. Thus, patients who have respiratory failure and who require supplemental oxygen or those with a pneumothorax or an ileus require special care to prevent further deterioration. *Helicopters* enable a more rapid response but are expensive; the greatest hazards are poor weather and landing in poorly visualized or nondesignated landing areas. Helicopters are most useful for transports within a 100–200 mile radius and for going directly to the site of an injury.

All vehicles must have the capability of radio or telephone contact with the MCP or the base station. In addition, each vehicle must be able to provide on-board oxygen, electrical power, and suction and must have space for adequate supplies and equipment including oxygen tanks, pharmacy packs, respiratory therapy devices, infusion pumps and solutions, stretchers or Isolettes, and monitors.

COMMUNICATION. This is one of the most crucial components of a regionally based transport system. A critically ill or injured infant or child usually represents an uncommon event for community physicians. Therefore, a referring physician needs to know whom, how, and when to call for assistance in the evaluation, stabilization, and transfer of a child. Telephone contact at all levels is required to ensure that physicians talk to physicians and that nurses talk to nurses. A child's condition often may be changing rapidly; therefore, the ability to obtain information and provide advice needs to be continuing. Using a dispatch center as the patching system to the MCP and others allows the referring physician or hospital to deal with only one phone number.

Once the transport team arrives at the referring facility, the team leader should reassess the patient's condition, review all the pertinent laboratory data and medications, and discuss the situation with the parents and referring physicians. If the patient's condition has changed significantly, the team leader should contact the MCP for additional advice. All medical records including roentgenograms and scans should be copied to take to the accepting facility. Before departing with the child, the MCP should be consulted again and the PICU contacted to finalize preparations to receive the patient.

The referring physician should provide written documentation of the need to transfer the patient to a higher level of care than can be provided at the referring hospital. This should include a statement that the risks, benefits, and alternatives to care for a critically ill patient have been discussed with the parents and their informed consent has been obtained to have their child transferred to another hospital with PICU capacity (see Table 58–2). Medicolegal responsibility is probably shared once communication has begun. It is therefore important to document what has been recommended to the referring facility in order to better stabilize the patient.

It is also important that both the referring facility and the regional PICU have realistic expectations about the transport team's capabilities. If it is determined that a physician with significant critical care skills is required for the transport, then the PICU has an obligation to provide a team leader with this skill level. The referring hospital should not delay lifesaving interventions while awaiting the arrival of the transport team (i.e., intubation of the trachea, initiation of mechanical ventilation or pharmacologic support), especially if this is recommended by the MCP. Federal legislation in the United States requires hospitals to evaluate all patients who arrive with emergent conditions and to stabilize before transfer. It also makes the transferring hospital responsible for selecting a receiving hospital capable of providing appropriate care for the patient's needs. To facilitate the transfer of critically ill pediatric patients, some regional PICUs have developed transfer agreements with referring hospitals to ensure that appropriate and safe transfer of children with life-threatening illness occurs as smoothly and in as safe an environment as possible.

Ackerman N: Aeromedical physiology. *In:* McCloskey KA, Orr RA (eds): Pediatric Transport Medicine, St. Louis, CV Mosby, 1995, pp 143–157.

American Academy of Pediatrics Task Force on Interhospital Transport: Guidelines for Air and Ground Transport of Neonatal and Pediatric Patients. Elk Grove Village, IL, American Academy of Pediatrics, 1993.

Frankel LR: The evaluation, stabilization, and transport of the critically ill child. Int Anesthesiol Clin 25:77, 1987.

Henning R, Farcos F, McNamara V: Difficulties encountered in transport of the critically ill child. Pediatr Emerg Care 7:133, 1991.

Kisson N: Triage and transport of the critically ill child. Crit Care Clin 8:37, 1992.

McCloskey K, Johnston C: Pediatric critical care transport survey: Team composition and training, mobilization time, and mode of transportation. Pediatr Emerg Care 6:1, 1990.

Orr R, Venkataraman S, McCloskey K, et al: Pediatric risk of mortality score (PRISM): A poor predictor in triage of patients for pediatric transport. Crit Care Med 23:224, 1995.

CHAPTER 61

Effective Communication with Families in the PICU

Lawrence H. Mathers and Lorry R. Frankel

THE PEDIATRIC PATIENT IN AN UNFAMILIAR ENVIRONMENT. It is difficult to imagine a situation producing more terror, sadness, fright, and anger in families* than a child's serious illness that requires admission to a pediatric intensive care unit (PICU). Young patients and their families face potentially life-threatening illness or surgery that may result in a permanent disability or death. When families face this frightening experience, they may feel a loss of ability to protect their child from danger, to provide for his or her needs, or to have final determination over which course of treatment should be undertaken. When children are confined to a hospital bed or require restraints to prevent exacerbation of injuries, their natural response is to become more vigorously agitated and to reach out to the parents for relief and reassurance. This behavior, limited visitation, and the presence of medical equipment only heighten the family's feeling of impotence and guilt. Finally, unfamiliar physicians and staff may exacerbate parental distrust and concern.

VISITATION AND PRESENCE IN THE CHILD'S PICU ROOM. Although patients in a PICU may not be fully alert or able to interact normally with those around them, the goal of PICU care should be to allow the maximum amount of time for parents to be with their child and to participate actively in their child's care (*family-centered care*). Limiting the number of visitors at any one time to two may be wise, because most patient areas are crowded with equipment, the child may better benefit from contact with one or two individuals rather than a larger number of visitors, and large crowds may disturb other patients. Siblings and friends should be allowed to visit but should be screened to ensure that they do not have a communicable disease and are psychologically ready to visit a critically ill child. The patient's appearance and the presence of the medical devices may be very frightening to a sibling. Rules for visitation and access to information should be tailored to each particular situation and should maintain patient confidentiality. Visitors may be asked to leave the room during rounds, at change of shift, and when invasive procedures are performed on the child or another when a room is shared. However, it is often desirable for a parent to be present during a procedure to provide comfort to a conscious child. Parents who wish to review their child's chart should be given the opportunity at a convenient time. This provides an occasion to answer questions and explain unfamiliar medical terminology and provides a form of reassurance. Effort should be made to see that the various physicians and nurses caring for a patient take a consistent position on sensitive issues such as reviewing a child's chart.

IDENTIFYING PERSONNEL AND THEIR ROLES. Large medical centers, especially teaching hospitals, are environments in which many physicians, students, nurses, respiratory therapists, social workers, chaplains, and others are involved in the care of a patient in a PICU. A single physician (usually the senior attending physician) should assume primary responsibility for communication with the family. This physician should have sufficient experience to place individual pieces of information about a patient in context and to avoid hasty and incompletely supported conclusions. He or she should communicate at least daily with the family. Nothing frightens and angers families more than to hear significantly different descriptions of their child's condition from physicians, nurses, and others who are involved in the child's care. It is also extremely helpful if early in a child's PICU course parents receive an explanation of the roles played by the different health care providers. Pamphlets containing this information are useful but cannot entirely replace a direct discussion with the family. The family should receive reassurance that those in training may perform independently in certain situations but are always supervised by an attending physician. Expert consultants must exercise diplomacy when they examine a patient in the presence of the parents or family. In general, if patient information is sought by the family from a consultant, it may be best to defer providing it until the attending physician can participate to ensure

*The term "family" or "families" is used here to include parents, grandparents, siblings, friends, and others occupying a traditional family role in the life of a child.

that the consultant's observations and opinions are put in a meaningful context for the family.

THE ROLE OF THE PHYSICIAN. To benefit patients, avoid harm, maintain confidentiality, and respect the dignity of children and their families, an intensivist may assume several roles. This physician may provide information, supporting the family in making the difficult decisions about continuation of support, futility of care, withdrawal of support, organ donation, and so on. The intensivist also may make decisions with minimal or no family input. He or she may convey information, creating a personal relationship with the family and becoming an important participant in the previously mentioned serious decisions with the family. This physician may work together with the family to produce one or more contracts in which real or hypothetical situations are described and actions are agreed on in advance of their occurrence. Each of these models has potential advantages and risks, and an amalgam of these approaches is often used (also see Chapter 2).

INFORMED CONSENT. The goal of informed consent is to provide patients or parents or other adults who are responsible for representing the interests of a child with a full understanding of their choices and the benefits and risks of each potential course of action (Chapter 2). The list of procedures and treatments that require explicit consent grows yearly, and failure to obtain proper consent exposes the caregivers to legal liability. Although informed consent is required only for certain procedures and therapies, the concept should guide virtually all interactions between the physician, the patient, and the patient's family. Caregivers should make efforts to ensure that proper communication occurs despite language barriers or differences in educational or cultural backgrounds (see Chapter 3).

ESTABLISHING A SUPPORTIVE ENVIRONMENT AND RAPPORT. The bedside nurse is the person the family will converse with more often than with any physician involved in the child's care. Families need to be reassured that the nurse providing care to their child is kind, sensitive, and willing to take steps to create a comforting and familiar environment for the sick child. Even when the interior of a child's hospital room is dominated by tubing, cables, monitors, and other machinery used for treatment, parents should be encouraged to decorate areas of the room with pictures, medallions, and cards from friends or other well-wishers.

PROVIDING HEALTH INFORMATION CONSISTENTLY AND ACCURATELY. The goal should be to speak to the family with simple honesty and compassion about the child's condition and prognosis, unless certain circumstances would make such a frank discussion problematic (e.g., psychiatric or other serious illness in a parent). The level of the parents' understanding of medical concepts and terminology should be taken into consideration. Their emotional lability, the need for continued care for other children at home, career and job responsibilities, and so on all guide the physician in choosing the time and circumstances in which to hold a thorough discussion with the parents (see Chapters 38 and 72).

Although informal in-depth discussions among family members and the medical team may be the forum for major decision-making, many family members also need discussions to understand the relative significance of monitor readings, laboratory tests, or an examination. To help with these issues, a *care conference* method is used to exchange information and reach a consensus about children with complex problems or those who have extended PICU stays (>7–10 days). A plenary meeting usually is held with representation from the various the medical and ancillary services involved in a patient's care. Subsequently, the conclusions reached and information are shared with the parents and family at a meeting with the attending physician and, if feasible, the child's primary care physician. This also provides an opportunity to evaluate the parent's concerns, emotional response, and understanding. The primary care physician may be particularly helpful in assisting the family with assimilation of the information.

UNCOOPERATIVE OR HOSTILE FAMILIES. The vast majority of families, despite the stress and anxiety provoked by their child's serious illness, want to work with the medical staff toward the goal of improving their child's health. In all but a handful of cases, an appeal to the importance of the cooperation of parents in treating the child will defuse bad feeling and hostility. However, sometimes families feel that the way to express concern and to maintain parental control over what happens to their child is to challenge the recommendations of the medical staff, resist certain suggestions, and refuse to obey visitation and other PICU regulations. The PICU staff should encourage all families to express their concerns and should indicate a willingness to understand and accommodate their positions whenever possible, but extensive discussion and counseling of these families may be required.

The frustrations, sadness, and anger associated with the illness of a child can lead some family members to become suspicious, aggressive, and occasionally violent. If there is a threat of intimidation or violence against the medical staff, hospital security and the administration should be alerted that a serious conflict has occurred. In such instances, visitation privileges may be limited, allowed only when a security guard is present, and carried out in the company of an appropriate chaperone. The focus is to care for the child, and any conflicts or animosity between family and hospital must not be allowed to detract from that effort.

Gilligan T, Raffin T: Physician virtues and communicating with patients. New Horiz 5:6, 1997.

Paris W, Brawner N, Thompson S, et al: Psychosocial issues in heart transplantation: A review for transplant coordinators. J Transpl Coord 2:88, 1997.

Todres ID: Communication between physician, patient and family in the pediatric intensive care unit. Crit Care Med 21:S383, 1993.

CHAPTER 62

Monitoring of the Critically Ill Infant and Child

Lorry R. Frankel

The ability to provide advanced technologic therapies to critically ill patients makes physiologic monitoring essential. The combination of invasive and noninvasive monitoring is complementary and enables clinicians to understand better the minute-to-minute changes that occur in a critically ill child (Table 62–1). Monitoring device alarms should be set according to age- and disease-specific criteria.

HEMODYNAMIC MONITORING. This is indicated for any patient who is admitted to the intensive care unit and who may be in shock, has respiratory failure or impending respiratory failure, or has sustained an acute neurologic insult. Included in hemodynamic monitoring are heart rate, blood pressure, central venous pressure (CVP), pulmonary capillary wedge pressure (PCWP), and less commonly (e.g., in postoperative cardiovascular patients) left atrial pressure. *Heart rate* is measured with conventional chest electrodes; rhythm strips are usually obtained in lead II, and a 12-lead electrocardiogram (ECG) is indicated if dysrhythmias are suspected.

Blood pressure (BP) can be determined both invasively and noninvasively. Noninvasive BP monitoring provides intermittent readings by a sphygmomanometer or an ultrasonic/Doppler device (see Chapter 429). The cuff should encompass approximately two thirds of the length of the part of the

TABLE 62–1 Monitoring Devices Commonly Used in the PICU

Monitoring Devices	Sites	Measured Variables	Limitations/Concerns
Noninvasive Monitoring			
Cardiorespiratory	Chest leads	Heart rate, rhythm, respiratory rate	Only lead II recording, difficulty with dysrhythmia recognition
Pulse oximetry	Digits, nasal bridge, palms, ear lobe	Continuous Sao_2	Patient must be well perfused; abnormal hemoglobins and nail polish may affect results
Transcutaneous oxygen and carbon dioxide	Usually chest	O_2 and CO_2	Surface electrodes warm skin to 43°C, can cause thermal injury, must be changed every 3–4 hr, useful in young infants
Capnography	End of the endotracheal tube	End-tidal CO_2 using breath-by-breath analysis	Capnographic trace is important to determine actual measurement; it is a true end-tidal representation of alveolar CO_2
Blood pressure	Upper arm, thigh, or calf	Cuff that allows for periodic cycling q 1–15 min	Similar to cuff pressure. Important to have appropriate cuff size
Electroencephalogram	Scalp surface	Provides for continuous monitoring of cranial electrical activity	Requires a specialized technician to place the electrodes and special training in interpreting the waveforms
Invasive Monitoring Techniques			
Arterial	Radial, dorsalis pedis, posterior tibial, femoral, axillary (rarely temporal or brachial)	Continuous determination of blood pressure, ability to measure blood gases and other laboratory tests	Expertise in placement and monitoring needed, may require cutdown technique, may lose distal perfusion
Central venous access for pressure measurement (CVP) and infusion	Femoral, subclavian, internal or external jugular, antecubital, or advanced from the saphenous	Allows for CVP determinations and administration of vasoactive agents and hypertonic solutions (TPN)	Requires expertise in placement, especially in very young patients; attempt to use multilumen catheters; need chest x-ray to determine placement
Pulmonary artery catheter Swan-Ganz catheter	Place through a sheath in the internal or external jugular, femoral, or subclavian	Allows for measurements of cardiac output, Svo_2, pulmonary artery pressure; can calculate SVR and PVR	Less commonly used in pediatrics. May assist in titration of inotropic support, vasodilators, adjustment of PEEP
ICP	Skull, either with a subdural bolt, an epidural fiberoptic device, or an IVC	Measures ICP when CNS pathology is associated with cerebral edema (e.g., head injury, Reye's syndrome, or those with unexplained GCS <8)	Requires a neurosurgeon to insert the device. May be done at the bedside. Increased risk of infection after 5 days. IVC can be used to remove fluid
Jugular bulb catheter	Internal jugular and threaded to the jugular bulb	Measures Svo_2 at the jugular bulb. Cerebral oxygen extraction can be calculated	Technically difficult to insert. Requires training in the utility of the device and the values obtained. May allow modification of therapy

CNS = central nervous system; CVP = central venous pressure; GCS = Glasgow Coma Scale; ICP = intracranial pressure; IVC = intraventricular catheter; PEEP = positive end-expiratory pressure; PVR = pulmonary vascular resistance; Sao_2 = arterial oxygen saturation; Svo_2 = venous oxygen saturation; SVR = systemic vascular resistance; TPN = total parenteral nutrition.

extremity in which it is being measured (upper arm, lower or upper leg). Sites commonly used for invasive arterial monitoring include the radial, ulnar, posterior tibial, and dorsalis pedis arteries; less frequently used sites are the femoral, axillary, brachial, and umbilical arteries. Arterial catheters may be inserted either percutaneously or via cutdown. Before attempting to insert an arterial catheter, collateral circulation should be evaluated if possible by performing an Allen test (Chapter 64.1). Once the catheter is properly inserted, a pressure transducer and pressure tubing are used to connect the catheter to the monitor. A continuous-pressure waveform tracing can then be displayed on the monitor screen along with the simultaneous ECG tracing. The arteral waveform may be helpful in diagnosing hypovolemia (very narrowed and blunted dicrotic notch), determining the severity of cardiac dysrhythmias (pulsus alternans), and evaluating the effects of respirations or high pericardial pressure on BP (pulsus paradoxus). In addition to monitoring BP, arterial lines allow for frequent blood sampling.

Complications from arterial catheterization are infrequent but may be serious. Bleeding and infection are relatively rare. Direct pressure on the insertion site usually reduces bleeding. Cutdowns may require resuturing or placing topical clotting material in the incision. Colonization of the insertion site may produce bacteremia and septicemia. The most serious complication is probably arterial thrombosis. Low cardiac output states (shock), failure to use heparin in the flush solution, and prolonged duration of catheter placement are risk factors. Thrombosis necessitates immediate removal of the catheter, and intravenous heparin or thrombolytic therapy is indicated if the extremity continues to have evidence of poor perfusion. Other complications include vascular spasm, cutaneous mottling, arterial tears, pseudoaneurysms, peripheral nerve damage, and arteriovenous fistula formation. Temporal artery sites have been associated with retrograde flow resulting in a cerebrovascular accident and therefore should be avoided. Finally, decreased flow distal to the catheter insertion may result in serious necrosis of an extremity.

A central venous catheter (CVC) is required to monitor CVP in critically ill children. A CVC is important for evaluating vascular volume. It also facilitates safe infusion of hypertonic solutions and vasoactive agents, which can produce severe peripheral soft tissue damage if they extravasate into the local tissues, and rapid infusion of large volumes of fluids or blood products to treat hypovolemia. These catheters may be inserted at a number of different sites (femoral, subclavian, external jugular, internal jugular, antecubital, and rarely the saphenous veins) with the catheter advanced into the thoracic cavity. The tip of the catheter should be in the inferior or superior vena cava at the atriocaval junction to minimize the risk of cardiac tamponade. Catheters may be inserted percutaneously or via cutdown technique and tunneled under the skin to reduce infectious complications. Ideally, one should attempt to insert a multilumen catheter because it provides several ports for various infusions. Before the procedure, the child should have ECG leads placed for monitoring to detect any dysrhythmias that may occur during the procedure. After insertion of the catheter, its proper position should be confirmed by roentgenogram. Rarely, an intravenous dye contrast study or fluoroscopy is needed to confirm placement of a radiopaque catheter. The catheter is connected via a transducer to the monitor to enable one to evaluate the waveform and obtain a CVP tracing (see Chapter 429). Ultrasonically guided CVC placement may be very helpful in difficult situations.

Complications of CVCs include dysrhythmias, pneumothorax, hydrothorax, hemothorax, air embolism, shearing of the catheter, losing the guide wire, bleeding, or apnea. Infection is associated with longer duration of catheter placement and percutaneous (vs tunneled) catheters. Thrombosis is also associated with longer duration of catheter placement and includes the potential for associated pulmonary embolic events. The most serious and life-threatening complication is cardiac tamponade, usually due to an intra-atrial catheter from a subclavian or internal jugular approach.

Pulmonary artery catheters (PACs) provide the ability to monitor a child's hemodynamic status in situations in which the right- and left-sided filling pressures vary. If a balloon thermodilution catheter is used, monitoring may include core temperature, pulmonary artery pressures (PAP), pulmonary artery occlusion pressure (PaoP), cardiac outputs, and mixed venous oxygen saturations. These data can be used to calculate systemic and pulmonary vascular resistances, oxygen delivery, stroke volume, arteriovenous oxygen content differences, oxygen extraction ratios, and shunt fractions. However, PACs are rarely used in pediatric patients.

The most common indications are cardiogenic shock, severe distributive shock, the use of very high ventilator pressures (to modulate therapy in patients with severe pulmonary hypertension), and perioperative treatment of patients who have undergone complex cardiac or other major surgeries. The limitations to the use of these catheters are predominantly a patient's size and unfamiliarity with these catheters; the smallest multiple-lumen thermodilution catheter is No. 5 French.

Balloon catheters are "floated" into the pulmonary artery and wedged in position, allowing measurement of PaoP or PCWP. These pressures are usually reflective of the left ventricle end-diastolic filling pressure. Once this number is determined, the balloon is deflated and allowed to remain in the pulmonary artery. Complications include pulmonary artery erosion or infarction, dysrhythmias, damage to the pulmonic valve, coiling in the right ventricle, balloon rupture, and infection. These complications are indications for removing a PAC.

PULMONARY MONITORING. Patients receiving respiratory support require monitoring of *blood gases* (see Chapter 52). Arterial blood gas sampling requires techniques similar to inserting an arterial line. Capillary blood sampling requires warming the site to obtain "arteriolized" blood. After the blood is drawn, it is sent to the laboratory to measure the partial pressures of oxygen, as well as carbon dioxide, pH, and bicarbonate. Capillary and venous blood gas sampling has significant limitations. Blood gas sampling provides the most reliable assessment of acid-base and ventilation-oxygenation status in a critically ill child. When a patient requires both continuous BP monitoring and frequent assessments of respiratory status, an indwelling arterial line is indicated.

Noninvasive blood gas devices are frequently used to monitor critically ill infants and children in PICUs. Transcutaneous instruments allow simultaneous or separate determination of carbon dioxide tension and oxygen tension but not pH or bicarbonate levels. Their sensitivity is limited by skin thickness; therefore, transcutaneous monitoring is less useful in larger children. The electrodes must be warmed to 43°C and changed every 3–4 hr to avoid burns. In addition, the electrodes take 20 min to calibrate, and this must be done every 4 hr, which may delay obtaining results. The major advantage of transcutaneous monitoring is the ability to continuously monitor carbon dioxide pressure and therefore to make rapid ventilator adjustments.

Capnography measures the P_{CO_2} in exhaled gas, end-tidal carbon dioxide, using a spectrometric instrument. This technique is used in patients who are intubated and have minimal lung disease without significant intrapulmonary shunting. Capnography is based on the principle that the highest concentration of carbon dioxide sampled in the respiratory circuit represents the alveolar carbon dioxide concentration, which should be very close to the arterial (Pa_{CO_2}) concentration. Gas is constantly monitored from a side port of the connector from the venilator to the endotracheal tube. A small amount of gas is diverted from the respiratory circuit and sent through a spectrophotometric analyzer for P_{CO_2} determination. When interpreting end-tidal carbon dioxide results, it is necessary to evaluate the exhalation capnographic image to ensure that the alveolar plateau and peak are reached. Capnography is helpful to determine that the trachea, not the esophagus, has been intubated in emergent intubations by using an analyzer that changes color on exposure to levels of carbon dioxide; the carbon dioxide concentration in the lungs is markedly higher than in the stomach.

Pulse oximetry is the standard method for noninvasive bedside monitoring of oxygen saturation. An infrared light is directed through tissue and then reflected onto a sensor. The sensor distinguishes between a wavelength that is maximally absorbed by hemoglobin saturated with oxygen and a wavelength maximally absorbed by hemoglobin without oxygen. The ratio of the wavelengths of light indicates the level of oxygen saturation of the hemoglobin. This modality can be used in patients of all ages and does not usually cause tissue damage. Pulse oximetry provides a rapid assessment of oxygenation in critically ill patients. However, the accuracy depends on adequate tissue perfusion, and its utility may be limited in patients with significant vasoconstriction and poor peripheral perfusion. Normal arterial oxygen saturation is 95% or greater (except in patients with cyanotic congenital heart lesions). Pulse oximetry is extremely reliable and relatively inexpensive compared with blood gas analysis.

Continuous or intermittent measurement of blood gases and other substances in blood is also possible via an indwelling arterial catheter that allows blood to flow from the catheter into a *closed-loop system passing electrodes*. These devices are very expensive and require vessels of sufficient size to permit insertion of a large catheter. This point-of-care testing permits the laboratory to come to a patient's bedside and provides almost immediate analysis.

NEUROPHYSIOLOGIC MONITORING. Acute neurologic deterioration (from trauma, tumors, infections, seizures, vascular malformations of the central nervous system, strokes, or various metabolic insults) accounts for a significant number of admissions to a PICU. Frequent clinical observations should include evaluation of the cranial nerves, especially the pupillary reflexes, and use of a modified Glasgow Coma Scale (GCS) for infants and children (see Table 64–7). Most patients with a GCS score less than 12 should be observed in a PICU. Neurophysiologic monitoring involves careful clinical observation accompanied by highly technical noninvasive devices (e.g., electroencephalography, evoked potentials, near-infrared spectroscopy), or invasive catheters (to monitor intracranial pressure [ICP]).

The brain's electrical activity can be monitored by computerized *electroencephalogram* (EEG), which facilitates the diagnosis and treatment of seizures (Chapter 602). EEG artifacts can be caused by the various monitors, ventilators, or other electrical equipment commonly found in a PICU setting. Video-EEG permits correlation of electrical changes associated with a seizure and clinical manifestations.

Evoked potentials are helpful in evaluating various sensory pathways. Visual evoked responses, brain stem auditory evoked potentials, and somatosensory evoked potentials are the most commonly used. They are not affected by the sedative medications that may produce an isoelectric EEG. The brain stem and somatosensory tests are the most commonly performed evoked studies because they may aid in providing prognostic information. However, their utility in diagnosing brain death is not established.

Radionuclide imaging, rarely performed in a PICU, may provide useful information about cerebral blood flow. A portable gamma camera allows tests to be performed at the bedside. These studies estimate cerebral blood flow to injured areas of brain and may provide evidence for brain death (Chapter 72).

Invasive neurologic monitoring includes *ICP monitoring* and *jugular bulb catheterization.* The indications for ICP monitoring include any acute neurologic deterioration in which elevated ICP may produce further injury to the patient. Usually, patients who have experienced acute traumatic events and who have a GCS score of 8 or less have a monitoring device inserted either in the operating room or at the bedside in the PICU. A ventriculostomy tube or intraparenchymal, subdural, or subarachnoid device can be used; except for the intraparenchymal catheter, other devices are connected to a transducer via a fluid-filled tubing device and then to a monitor. The ventriculostomy and the intraparenchymal fiberoptic devices are the most reliable and frequently used, although the intraparenchymal fiberoptic system does not permit the removal of cerebrospinal fluid. A waveform with a numeric value is produced on the monitor. The ICP should be less than 20 cm H_2O. When monitoring ICP, the systemic arterial BP should be determined simultaneously. The difference between the mean arterial pressure and the ICP is the **cerebral perfusion pressure.** This should be greater than 50 cm H_2O in older children and slightly less in younger patients. The complications associated with ICP monitoring include bleeding; infection, especially when the catheter is left in place for more than 5 days; injury to the brain parenchyma (usually only with intraventricular catheters); and leakage of cerebrospinal fluid.

Jugular bulb monitoring provides continuous oxygen saturation measurements using an indwelling fiberoptic catheter placed in the jugular vein and advanced cephalad to the level of the jugular bulb. The values obtained correlate with the jugular Pao_2 content and do not require blood sampling for determination of the oxygen saturation. The jugular bulb, located at the base of the brain just outside of the jugular foramen, is the point of exit of the blood draining most of the cerebral hemispheres. Knowledge of the oxygen saturations in both a systemic artery and the jugular vein permits calculation of the arteriojugular difference for oxygen and estimation of how well the injured brain is using oxygen. This is normally 4–9 vol%. Levels below this may indicate cerebral hyperemia and the need to decrease cerebral blood flow. Levels greater than 10 vol% may indicate ischemia and necessitate further tests to determine the extent of the brain injury.

Deymann A, Moromisato D: Noninvasive respiratory monitoring: Oxygen saturation, transcutaneous oxygen and carbon dioxide, and end-tidal carbon dioxide. *In:* Levin DL, Morriss FC (eds): Essentials of Pediatric Intensive Care, 2nd ed. New York, Churchill Livingstone, 1997, pp 1358–1369.

Ladner E, Javorsky F, Berger J, et al: Respiratory monitoring during postoperative analgesia. J Clin Monit 12:417, 1996.

Levine RL, Fromm RE Jr: Critical Care Monitoring from Pre-Hospital to the ICU. St. Louis, CV Mosby, 1995, pp 210–215.

Lewis SB, Myburgh JA, Reilly PL: Detection of cerebral venous desaturation by continuous jugular bulb oximetry following acute neurotrauma. Anaesth Intens Care 23:307, 1995.

Martin GR, Holley DG: Cardiovascular monitoring and evaluation. *In:* Holbrook PR (ed): Textbook of Pediatric Critical Care. Philadelphia, WB Saunders, 1993, pp 259–278.

Stocchetti N, Paparella A, Bridelli F, et al: Cerebral venous oxygen saturation studied with bilateral samples in the internal jugular veins. Neurosurgery 34:39, 1994.

Takano JS, Howard LA, Toro-Figueroa LO: Advanced hemodynamic monitoring: Pulmonary artery and left atrial catheterization. *In:* Levine DL, Morriss FC (eds): Essentials of Pediatric Intensive Care, 2nd ed. New York, Churchill Livingstone, 1997, pp 1234–1248.

Wahr JA, Tremper KK: Noninvasive oxygen monitoring techniques. Crit Care Clin 11:199, 1995.

CHAPTER 63
Scoring Systems and Predictors of Mortality

Joseph V. DiCarlo and Lorry R. Frankel

Scoring systems are useful for making triage decisions and assessing the performance of an intensive care unit, but they are of limited use in predicting prognosis in individual cases. Various scoring systems are currently used in the pediatric intensive care unit (PICU): (1) *organ specific,* such as the Glasgow Coma Scale (see Chapter 64.1 and Table 64–7) or the croup score (see Chapter 385), (2) *mechanism of injury,* such as the Pediatric Trauma Score (see Table 58–3) or Injury Severity Score, and (3) *pediatric,* such as the Physiologic Stability Index (PSI) or the Pediatric Risk of Mortality (PRISM).

PEDIATRIC RISK OF MORTALITY. This system, a revision of the PSI, assesses the severity of illness in a population of pediatric patients. The PRISM is used to compare and evaluate the performance and resource use among various PICUs. It is based on 17 physiologic variables (Table 63–1). A patient's past medical history is also taken into account, particularly chronic illness and previous PICU days. The PRISM has demonstrated a consistent relationship between the number of malfunctioning organ systems (the score) at 12 and 24 hr and the mortality risk in a given PICU. However, it is of limited predictive value for a single patient. The PRISM is instead most useful in assessing the outcomes for a population of patients in a PICU. A PICU that performs a periodic self-assessment using PRISM can determine whether or not its performance is on a par with a reference population. If performance is below standard, a chart review may reveal the reasons, such as high secondary infection rates, co-morbidity issues, and decisions to withdraw or limit therapy.

PEDIATRIC TRAUMA SCORE (see Table 58–3). This score takes into account a child's size, the accessibility of the airway, the

TABLE 63–1 Physiologic Factors Considered in PRISM Scoring

Vital Signs	Systolic blood pressure Heart rate Stupor/coma (GCS <8) Pupillary reflexes	**Other Factors** Nonoperative disease Chromosomal anomaly Cancer Previous PICU admission Pre-ICU resuscitation (CPR) Postoperative Acute diabetes (e.g., ketoacidosis) Transfer from inpatient unit
Acid-Base Status	pH <7.28 or >7.48 Total CO_2 >34 mmol/L Pao_2 (<50 mm Hg) $Paco_2$ (>50 mm Hg)	
Chemistry	Glucose (>200 mg/dL or >11 nmol/L) Potassium (>6.9 mmol/L) Creatinine increase Blood urea nitrogen increase	
Hematology	White blood cell count (<3,000 cells/mm³) Platelet count (<50,000 or 50,000–200,000/mm³) PT (>22 seconds) or PTT (>57 seconds)	

CPR = cardiopulmonary resuscitation; GCS = Glasgow Coma Scale; ICU = intensive care unit; PICU = pediatric intensive care unit; PT = prothrombin time; PTT = partial thromboplastin time.

systolic blood pressure, the level of consciousness, and the presence or absence of wounds and fractures. Below a certain cutoff, transfer to a dedicated trauma center is recommended (see Chapter 58).

OTHER PHYSIOLOGIC SCORING SYSTEMS. Other scoring systems are less useful in pediatrics. The Acute Physiology and Chronic Health Evaluation (APACHE) system has wide utility in adult intensive care units. However, the refined PRISM III is better suited to the physiology of a child. The PSI is a refinement of APACHE that attempts to make age-related adjustments. The Therapeutic Intervention Scoring System relies on the type and amount of therapy given and therefore may indirectly reflect severity of illness.

Heulitt MJ, Capron C, Fiser DH: Outcome and risk measures. *In:* Levin DL, Morriss FC (eds): Essentials of Pediatric Intensive Care, 2nd ed. New York, Churchill Livingstone, 1997, pp 1138–1142.

Kanter RK, Edge WE, Caldwell CR, et al: Pediatric mortality probability estimated from pre-ICU severity of illness. Pediatrics 99:59, 1997.

Pollack MM, Patel KM, Ruttimann UE: PRISM III: An updated pediatric risk of mortality. Crit Care Med 24:743, 1996.

Pollack MM, Patel KM, Ruttimann UE: The Pediatric Risk of Mortality III—Acute Physiology Score (PRISM-APS): A method of assessing physiologic instability for pediatric intensive care unit patients. J Pediatrics 131:575, 1997.

CHAPTER 64

Stabilization of the Critically Ill Child

64.1 Pediatric Emergencies and Resuscitation

Lawrence H. Mathers and Lorry R. Frankel

Each year in the United States there are over 150,000 emergencies that threaten the lives of children; approximately 10,000 of these children die, and at least 90,000 survive with permanent disability. These emergencies may need immediate treatment in various settings—in the home, hospital, ambulance; en route to the hospital, emergency department (ED); and others. Ideally, those caring for these children will provide immediate resuscitation and support while simultaneously activating the emergency care system and facilitating their transport to the nearest appropriate facility. The growing number of children with increased vulnerability to serious illness, such as surviving premature infants or children with chronic disease, makes knowledge of how to respond to pediatric emergencies ever more important (see Chapter 58).

Pediatric emergencies are of various types—respiratory, cardiac, endocrine, traumatic, and so on. However, most pediatric arrests are respiratory, not cardiac, when injuries and congenital heart diseases are excluded. The proper response to each requires an awareness of the mechanisms of disease and the immediate physiologic threats and their proper treatment. A number of factors contribute to the physiologic instability of infants and young children (Table 64–1). Children prone to suffer from recurring life-threatening illnesses (e.g., seizure disorders, small airways disease, cardiac dysrhythmias) may be able to take precautions to minimize the risk of such threats. Parental vigilance and anticipation of potential dangers in the home, especially for young children, can prevent many injuries and deaths due to these illnesses (see Chapter 57).

TABLE 64–1 Factors Contributing to Infant Physiologic Instability

Temperature	Infants have thin skin (radiating heat) and underdeveloped hypothalmic control. They lack the efficient neural mechanisms for temperature control (e.g., shivering) and are greatly influenced by environmental temperature.
Fluid Requirements	Thin skin allows more evaporation; fluid content in an infant's body is higher than in an adult's (75–80% in newborn); kidneys reabsorb electrolytes inefficiently; infants need proportionately more fluid per unit of weight than adults.
Airway	Airway is small and narrow; resistance to gas flow is inversely proportional to the 4th power of the radius, so small mucous obstructions can seriously threaten air movement; laryngeal and tracheal cartilages are softer than in adults and more easily collapse to obstruct the airway.
Cardiac Output	Heart rate is the major mechanism for varying cardiac output.
Glucose Metabolism	Newborn infants, especially, have only marginal glycogen stores, and hypoglycemia occurs more readily than in adults, because of dependence on exogenous supply of glucose. Glycogenolytic enzymes are not developed in infants.

LIFE-THREATENING EMERGENCIES AND PRE-ARREST STATES IN CHILDREN

The most common life-threatening illnesses in children are those involving respiratory (Table 64–2 and Chapter 64.3), cardiac (Table 64–3 and Chapter 448), or neurologic (Table 64–4 and Chapter 72) failure. Acute failure of the liver (Chapter 363), kidneys (Chapter 543), or adrenals (Chapter 585) also may place pediatric patients in peril and requires early recognition. Pinpointing the cause of all of these various organ failures may take considerable time, but treatment to stabilize a child physiologically should commence immediately.

TABLE 64–2 Respiratory Emergencies

Upper Airway Obstruction	Child usually presents in obvious respiratory distress—with stridor or leaning chin forward and drooling Do not put instruments into the airway unless prepared to intubate immediately. Especially risky in presumed epiglottitis. Lateral neck roentgenogram can show enlarged epiglottis at base of tongue or possibly a foreign body. Major challenge is to avoid irritation of the airway, which can precipitate complete airway obstruction.
Small Airways	Usually an exacerbation of a previously existing condition such as asthma. Patients present with wheezing. Mucus and/or bronchospasm causes air trapping—inspired air more easily enters the alveoli than it leaves them. As a result, the distal airways and alveoli distend with gas and efficient exchange is impaired. In extreme cases, status asthmaticus or bronchiolitis can be fatal. Necessary steps for therapy: oxygen, bronchidilators (aerosols and intravenous), steroids (delayed action), relaxation, and reassurance.
Pneumonia	Impaired gas exchange due to alveolar injury. Usually involves surfactant deficiency, plus fluid in alveoli. Therapy: oxygen, antibiotics, mechanical ventilatory support if serious disease. Parenchymal disease increases the tendency for intrapulmonary shunts, increasing the hypoxia. Pneumonia becomes life threatening only when large portions of the lungs are involved.

TABLE 64–3 Cardiac Emergencies

Bradycardia/Asystole

First priority is to support blood flow and pressure and establish an airway; institute ventilation and compressions as needed. Supply oxygen.
Establish IV or intraosseous access.
Administer atropine (0.1 mg/kg) and epinephrine (0.01 mg/kg of 1:10,000) IV or 0.1 mg/kg of 1:1000 endotracheally (ET).
When ventilation established, administer $NaHCO_3$ (0.5 mEq/kg).
Take steps to normalize temperature.
Perform appropriate blood tests, roentgenograms, and so on.
Treat acidosis and electrolyte disorders as indicated.

Tachycardia

Assess the adequacy of peripheral perfusion—e.g., feel for pulse, assess capillary return time. Supply oxygen.
If HR is rapid but other vital signs are stable, wait—consult with cardiology; consider *less* invasive approaches (e.g., carotid massage, rectal stimulation, fluid support, correction of any electrolyte disorder).
If HR is rapid, patient is acidotic, and other vitals signs are also below acceptable levels, do not delay. DC cardioversion (see Fig. 64–1) should be tried. Mechanical treatments (e.g., carotid massage, rectal stimulation) also should be tried; drug therapies (e.g., digoxin, verapamil, α-agents, propranolol) should be used as well. Mechanical ventilation may be necessary, especially if sedation is used.

Congestive Heart Failure (CHF)

Assess vital signs first. If CHF is severe, lungs may be edematous and oxygen exchange poor. In such cases, intubation, diuresis, and the use of pressors (dopamine, dobutamine, epinephrine) are necessary.
In more stable patients, first step should be to plan minimal necessary fluid input and use diuretics to reduce overall body water, especially lung water. Assess renal function and adjust fluid therapy accordingly.
When the heart is not irreversibly injured and can be expected to recover, then fluid restriction and use of pressors is temporary. Remember that cardiac pressors increase oxygen consumption (especially epinephrine), and the metabolic stress on the heart should be considered.

IV = intravenous; HR = heart rate.

TABLE 64–4 Neurologic Emergencies

Seizures	Observe the patient to see if seizures are (1) focal or generalized and (2) tonic or clonic. Focal seizures are not an emergency; generalized seizures may be an emergency. Prolonged seizures have adverse metabolic effects—acidosis, hypoxia, hypoglycemia. Important risk is the interruption of breathing, either by lack of muscle control or by aspiration. Treatment: Oxygen for generalized seizures; measure glucose, give as needed. Protect airway (tilt head to side, don't instrument mouth). Phenytoin is effective, but cardiac depression is a risk. Phenobarbital is effective but long acting and depresses respiration. Diazepam provides quick action, wears off relatively soon, and often blocks respirations.
Meningitis	Extremely dangerous and often rapidly progressive disease. Causative organisms differ for different ages. Symptoms may be vague and nonspecific: fussiness, anorexia, sleeplessness, weak cry, stiff neck, glassy stare, disorientation, fever, vomiting. Therapy includes restricting fluids, antibiotics (chosen by age group); steroids (debatable) and correcting acidosis or hypoxia. Anticipate shock, respiratory arrest, seizures.
Acute Hydrocephalus	Presents as confusion, stupor, vomiting or headache. If possible, check for papilledema. If patient stable and respiratory status secure, perform CT scan. Consider need for immediate ventriculoperitoneal shunting. Lumbar puncture can be performed to measure pressure and/or rule out meningitis—but controversial, owing to risk of possible high intracranial pressure. Consider dexamethasone, and use diuresis if patient's vital signs stable, Use mannitol, furosemide, ethacrynic acid, acetazolamide. Many patients with acute hydrocephalus have shunts that become infected or obstructed. In such cases, a small fluid sample may be taken from the shunt. Acute hemorrage into the ventricles may cause acute hydrocephalus. Treatment is aimed at relieving intracranial pressure—diuresis, fluid restriction, hyperventilation, alkalosis.

DETECTING AND ASSESSING PHYSIOLOGIC INSTABILITY. A simple and consistent approach is necessary for rapid and efficient evaluation of a pediatric patient who may be in serious distress. *Observation* begins with determination of the alertness of the patient, including response to stimuli, spontaneous vocalization or movement, and muscle tone. This is followed by assessment of the *vital signs* (Table 64–5) and other basic indicators of the physiologic state.

HEART RATE. This varies with age (Table 64–5 and Chapter 429). When a child's heart rate lies outside the physiologic parameters, cardiac output may be affected. A rapid heart rate (e.g., supraventricular tachycardia [SVT]) may be associated with a serious reduction in stroke volume as reflected in poor perfusion, increased fussiness, and poor appetite (Chapter 442.2). Cardiac failure may develop with pulmonary edema (see Chapters 64.2 and 448). Bradycardia also may represent a serious pre-arrest condition (Chapter 442.5). Alternatively, the heart rate change may reflect an appropriate physiologic response and may not necessarily constitute significant pathophysiology.

BLOOD PRESSURE (BP). This is most often measured by auscultation, but automated devices such as the Dinamap can be set to measure BP repeatedly and at very short intervals (see Chapter 429).

ORGAN PERFUSION. This provides a clinical assessment of cardiac output. Skin perfusion is assessed by the temperature of the extremities and capillary refill time. However, the skin temperature may be lowered not only by decreased cardiac output. Low environmental temperature also may cause vasoconstriction. Normal capillary refill time is 2 sec or less. Pulse oximetry may be useful to detect not only inadequate oxygenation but also poor perfusion; a pulsatile signal is not detected. The return of a signal may correlate with the various therapeutic interventions and improvements in perfusion.

CORE TEMPERATURE. The normal temperature range for humans is constant throughout life. Premature infants and small term infants may have difficulty maintaining their appropriate core temperature if they are left uncovered in a cool environment. Also, infants may not be able to generate an elevated temperature in response to infection (Chapter 170).

RESPIRATORY EFFORT. Muscle *retractions* in the chest and neck and *flaring* of the nostrils at inspiration are signs of an abnormally high level of effort required to move air into the lungs. *Grunting* is a moaning noise at expiration, associated with generation of positive pressure to maintain alveolar patancy. A child who is inadequately oxygenated demonstrates *cyanosis*

TABLE 64–5 Vital Signs at Various Ages

Age	Heart Rate (beats/min)	Blood Pressure (mm Hg)	Respiratory Rate (breaths/min)
Premature	120–170*	55–75/35–45†	40–70‡
0–3 mo	100–150*	65–85/45–55	35–55
3–6 mo	90–120	70–90/50–65	30–45
6–12 mo	80–120	80–100/55–65	25–40
1–3 yr	70–110	90–105/55–70	20–30
3–6 yr	65–110	95–110/60–75	20–25
6–12 yr	60–95	100–120/60–75	14–22
12* yr	55–85	110–135/65–85	12–18

**In sleep, infant heart rates may drop significantly lower, but if perfusion is maintained, no intervention is required.*

†A blood pressure cuff should cover approximtely two thirds of the arm; too small a cuff yields spuriously high pressure readings, and too large a cuff yields spuriously low pressure readings.

‡Many premature infants require mechanical ventilatory support, making their spontaneous respiratory rate less relevant.

(a blue or dusky color of the skin and mucous membranes). See Chapters 375 and 377.

GAS EXCHANGE. Although observations of respiratory effort provide useful information about impending respiratory failure, blood gases provide a more quantitative measurement of respiratory gas exchange (see Chapters 52 and 377).

CARDIAC DYSRHYTHMIAS (see Chapter 442). Disturbances in cardiac rate and rhythm are not rare in children, but the majority are fleeting and not pathologic. Life-threatening cardiac emergencies in children are far more likely to involve bradycardia or asystole than they are to involve ventricular fibrillation, which is more common in adults. The overall incidence of rhythm disturbances in children is rising as more children with congenital heart anomalies undergo surgical correction and survive through childhood. Abnormal cardiac rhythms may be manifested as dyspnea, tachypnea, tachycardia, palpitations (the consciousness of skipped or irregular beats), syncope, dizziness, or angina (rarely). Dysrhythmias may not pose any danger to a patient initially, but as they affect the cardiac output they become symptomatic.

The diagnosis and management of specific rhythm disturbances in children are discussed in Chapters 442 and 55.8. However, *asystole* and *bradycardia* present two distinct resuscitative paradigms that require swift recognition and intervention; offices, clinics, and inpatient areas need to be prepared to manage these complicated situations (Figs. 64–1 and 64–2). *Electrolyte imbalances* also may produce life-threatening dysrhythmias. See Chapter 55.8. Children who experience significant fluid loss or who are receiving diuretics or digoxin are especially at risk.

ALTERATIONS OF PULMONARY BLOOD FLOW. In various congenital heart conditions and with some physiologic disturbances, blood flow to the lungs meets with resistance, resulting in pulmonary hypertensive crises. These patients are at risk for serious hypoxic/anoxic events. See Chapter 436.

ASSESSING METABOLIC STATUS. Two of the most important acute destabilizing metabolic disorders are acidosis and hypoglycemia. The causes, consequences, and management of respiratory, metabolic, and mixed *acidosis* are discussed in Chapters 52 and 55. Arterial blood sampling is discussed in Chapter 62. The measurement of the oxygen content of central venous blood (mixed venous O_2 content [Mvo_2]), especially blood from the pulmonary artery (Swan-Ganz) catheter, is also helpful in assessing the adequacy of tissue perfusion and increased anaerobic metabolism. Abnormally low oxygen content of venous blood relative to arterial blood suggests that the delivery of blood to tissues is inadequate, resulting in increased extraction of oxygen and metabolic acidosis. If the venous blood oxygen content is abnormally high, either blood is being delivered too rapidly to the tissues (high cardiac output), so that a lower than normal fraction of oxygen is extracted as blood passes through capillary beds, or there is abnormal mixing of venous and arterial blood near the heart and great vessels or both. Assaying a patient's blood for specific organic acids also may be helpful in diagnosing an underlying metabolic abnormality.

Hypoglycemia is defined as a blood sugar level low enough to threaten destabilization of metabolic activities. See Chapters 88 and 103.2. The brain is particularly dependent on an adequate level of circulating glucose, because the central nervous system (CNS) has no capacity to store glycogen. Hypoglycemia produces weakness and lethargy and then can lead to seizures and coma. Emergency resuscitation should usually include intravenous administration of glucose (250–500 mg/kg, infused over 1–2 min).

ASSESSING CENTRAL NERVOUS SYSTEM FUNCTION. The integrity of the CNS may be assessed through interviewing patients, when feasible, and through various physical examination techniques. Questioning and physical examination techniques should be

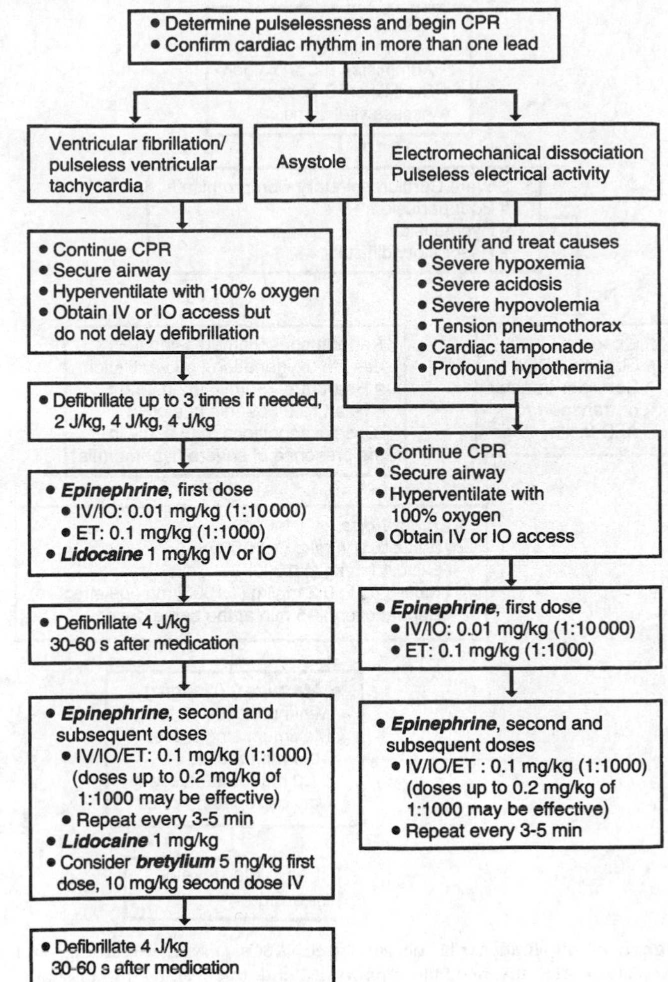

Figure 64–1 Asystole and pulseless arrest decision tree. CPR, cardiopulmonary resuscitation; ET, endotracheal; IO, intraosseous; IV, intravenous. (From Emergency Cardiac Care Committee and Subcommittees, American Heart Association. Pediatric advanced life support, part VI. JAMA 268:2262, 1992.)

age appropriate. See Table 64–6 for an example of encephalopathy staging.

GLASGOW COMA SCALE (GCS). Although this scale has not been validated as a prognostic scoring system for infants and young children, the GCS is commonly used in assessment of pediatric patients with an altered level of consciousness, especially those who have sustained a traumatic head injury (Table 64–7). The GCS provides very rapid assessment of cortical function. Patients with a GCS score of 8 or less may require aggressive management including intracranial pressure monitoring as well as mechanical ventilation.

RESUSCITATION

The goal in pediatric resuscitation is to maintain adequate oxygenation and perfusion of blood throughout the body while steps are taken to stabilize a child and establish long-term homeostasis. An orderly sequence of events similar to those used in adult resuscitation should be instituted, beginning with the ABC principles: airway, breathing, and circulation. (See Chapter 58 and Table 58–4). About 90% of pediatric patients undergoing resuscitation recover to a substantial degree. However, if a patient is asystolic on arrival at the hospital or in the advanced stages of a disease process before he or she receives medical care, then the chances for success decline dramatically.

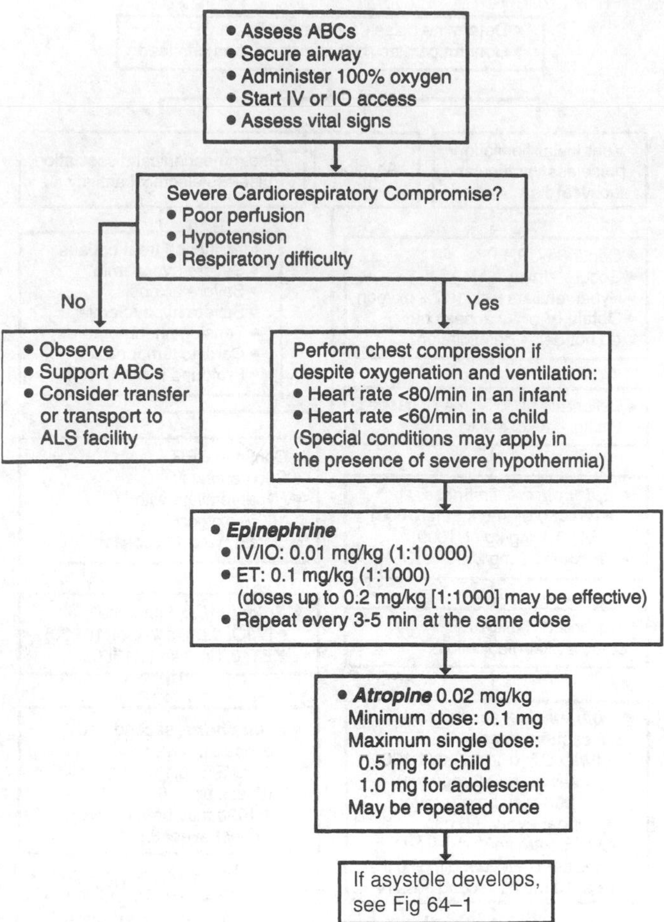

Figure 64–2 Bradycardia decision tree. ABCs, airway, breathing, and circulation; ALS, advanced life support; ET, endotracheal; IO, intraosseous; IV, intravenous. (From Emergency Cardiac Care Committee and Subcommittees, American Heart Association. Pediatric advanced life support, part VI. JAMA 268:2262, 1992.)

RESPIRATORY SUPPORT. If no obstruction by a foreign body is found and if a child has no spontaneous respirations, steps should be immediately taken to breathe for the child. This should be done by *mouth-to-mouth* or *mouth-to-nose* breathing, a mask over patient's nose and mouth and *mouth-to-mask* breathing, or *bag-mask* respirations. If air does not move easily, then head-tilt, chin-lift, and placement of an oral airway or nasal trumpet may be elected (Figs. 64–3 to 64–6). If these measures do not facilitate adequate air entry, then endotracheal intubation is indicated. A simple formula for selecting the appropriate size endotracheal tube is as follows:

$$\frac{\text{Age in years} + 16}{4} = \text{endotracheal tube inner diameter (mm)}$$

The respiratory rate parameters that should be maintained are indicated in Table 64–8.

TABLE 64–7 Glasgow Coma Scale

Eye Opening (total points 4)			
		Spontaneous	4
		To voice	3
		To pain	2
		None	1
Verbal Response (total points 5)			
Older Children		***Infants and Young Children***	
Oriented	5	Appropriate words; smiles, fixes, and follows	5
Confused	4	Consolable crying	4
Inappropriate	3	Persistently irritable	3
Incomprehensible	2	Restless, agitated	2
None	1	None	1
Motor Response (total points 6)			
		Obeys	6
		Localizes pain	5
		Withdraws	4
		Flexion	3
		Extension	2
		None	1

Adapted and modified from Teasdale G, Jennett B: Assessment of coma and impaired consciousness: A practical scale. Lancet 2:81, 1974.

Foreign body aspiration always should be suspected if respiratory distress has had a sudden onset (see Chapter 386) or if the chest does not rise when ventilation is first attempted in an unconscious, apneic infant or child. A conscious child should be permitted to cough spontaneously until coughing is not effective, respiratory distress and stridor increase, or the child becomes unconscious. The airway is then opened with the head-tilt, chin-lift maneuver, and ventilation is attempted. If unsuccessful, the airway is repositioned and ventilation again attempted. If there is still no chest rise, attempts to remove a foreign body are indicated. In the infant younger than 1 yr, a combination of five back blows and five chest thrusts are administered (Fig. 64–7). The foreign body is removed if it is seen. If no foreign body is visualized, ventilation is again attempted. If this is unsuccessful, the head is repositioned and ventilation attempted again. If there is no chest rise, the series of back blows and chest thrusts are repeated.

A conscious child older than 1 yr is administered a series of five abdominal thrusts (the Heimlich maneuver) with the child standing or sitting (Fig. 64–8). If unconscious, this is done with the child lying down (Fig. 64–9). After the abdominal thrusts, the airway is examined for a foreign body, which should be removed if visualized. If no foreign body is seen, the head is repositioned and ventilation attempted. If unsuccessful, repositioning the head and attempted ventilation are repeated. If unsuccessful, the Heimlich sequence is repeated.

CARDIOVASCULAR SUPPORT. As resuscitation proceeds and ventilation is started, support of the *heart rate* also should be provided to sustain adequate blood flow to deliver oxygen to the tissues (Figs. 64–10 and 64–11). The rate and depth of chest compressions vary with age and size (see Table 64–8). Chest compressions in small infants and newborns may be performed by placing two fingers over the midsternum and compressing

TABLE 64–6 Clinical Staging of Encephalopathy

Clinical Stage	1	2	3	4	5
Features	Lethargic Follows commands Pupils reactive Breathing normal *Normal muscle tone	Combative Inconsistent following of commands Pupils sluggish May hyperventilate *Reflexes inconsistent	Comatose Occasional response to commands Eyes may deviate Irregular breathing Decorticate posturing	Comatose Responds only to pain Weak pupillary response Very irregular breathing Decerebrate posturing	Comatose No response to pain No pupillary response Requires mechanical ventilation Absent tendon reflexes—flaccid*

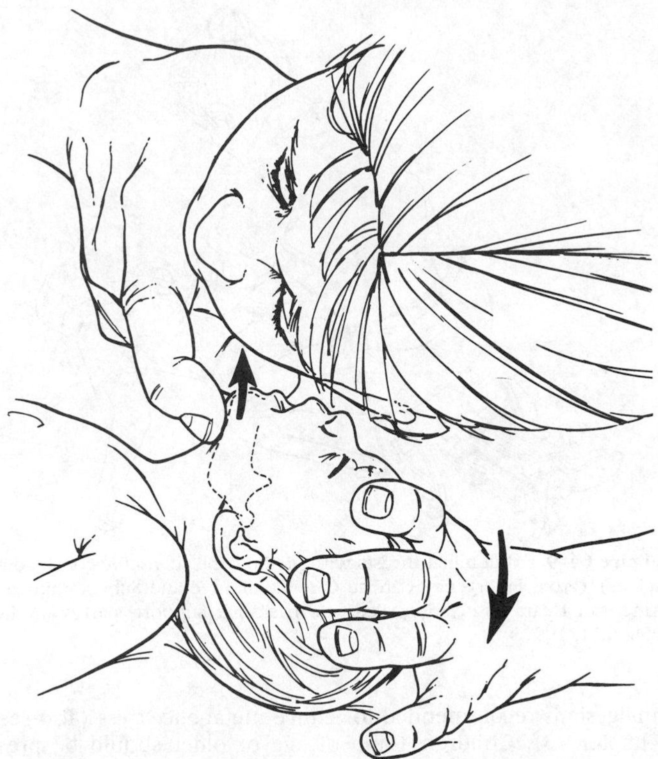

Figure 64–3 Opening the airway with the head tilt–chin lift maneuver. One hand is used to tilt the head, extending the neck. The index finger of the rescuer's other hand lifts the mandible outward by lifting on the chin. Head tilt should not be performed if cervical spine injury is suspected. (From Emergency Cardiac Care Committee and Subcommittees, American Heart Association. Pediatric basic life support, part V. JAMA 268:2251, 1992.)

(See Fig. 64–10) or by holding the child in the supine posture on one's lap, with fingers wrapped around the chest wall to the vertebral column and thumbs positioned over the midportion of the sternum, to perform the compressions. With children, the ratio of chest compressions to breaths should be approximately 5:1. For example, if chest compressions are being performed on a newborn at a rate of 100/min, then after every 5th compression there should be a short pause to deliver a breath (which total 20/min). When feasible, a cardiac resuscitation board should be placed under the child's back, to maximize efficiency of compressions. The resuscitation effort should pause periodically to make an assessment of the possible return of spontaneous heart rate, pulse, and respirations. If the resuscitative efforts do not succeed in re-establishing respiration and heart beat, the medical team must decide whether continued efforts are warranted or if the resuscitation should be stopped. If resuscitation is to continue and spontaneous heart rate and respirations have not returned, then the patient should be intubated, intravenous access established, and administration of inotropic drugs considered.

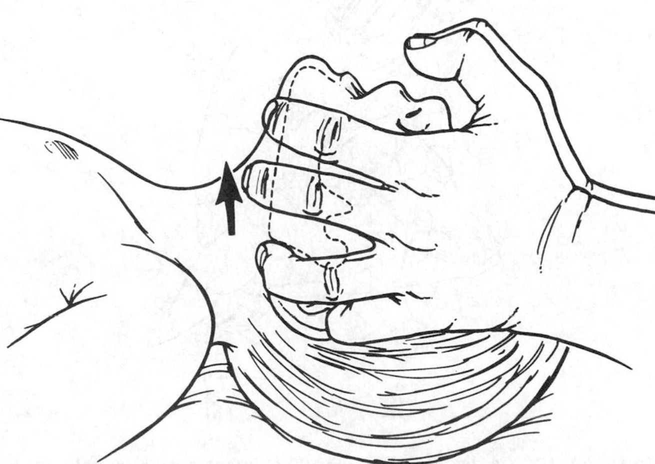

Figure 64–4 Combined jaw thrust–spine stabilization maneuver for the pediatric trauma victim. (From Emergency Cardiac Care Committee and Subcommittees, American Heart Association. Pediatric basic life support, part V. JAMA 268:2251, 1992.)

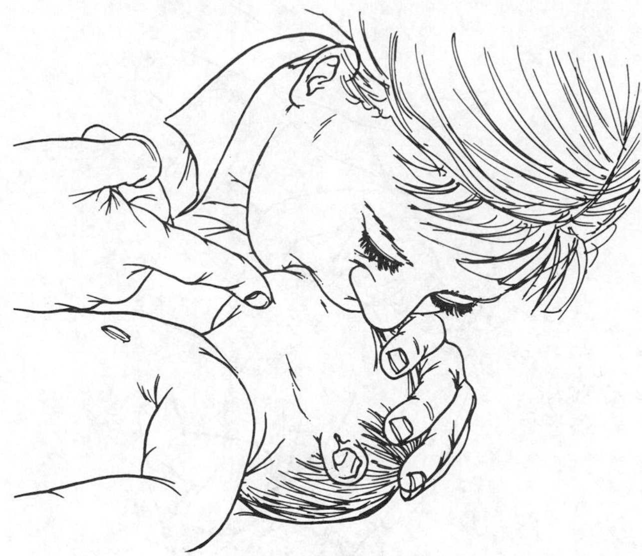

Figure 64–5 Rescue breathing in an infant. The rescuer's mouth covers the infant's nose and mouth, creating a seal. One hand performs head tilt while the other hand lifts the infant's jaw. Avoid head tilt if the infant has sustained head or neck trauma. (From Emergency Cardiac Care Committee and Subcommittees, American Heart Association. Pediatric basic life support, part V. JAMA 268:2251, 1992.)

INTUBATION AND MECHANICAL VENTILATION. Although it is possible to intubate infants without sedation, analgesia, or paralysis,

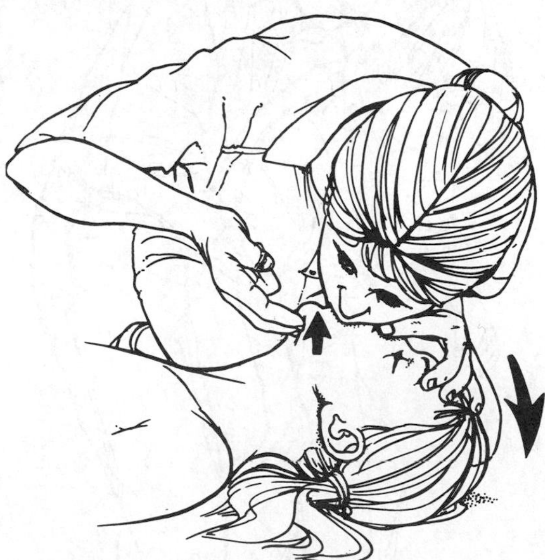

Figure 64–6 Rescue breathing in a child. The rescuer's mouth covers the mouth of the child, creating a mouth-to-mouth seal. One hand maintains the head tilt; the thumb and forefinger of the same hand are used to pinch the child's nose. (From Emergency Cardiac Care Committee and Subcommittees, American Heart Association. Pediatric basic life support, part V. JAMA 268:2251, 1992.)

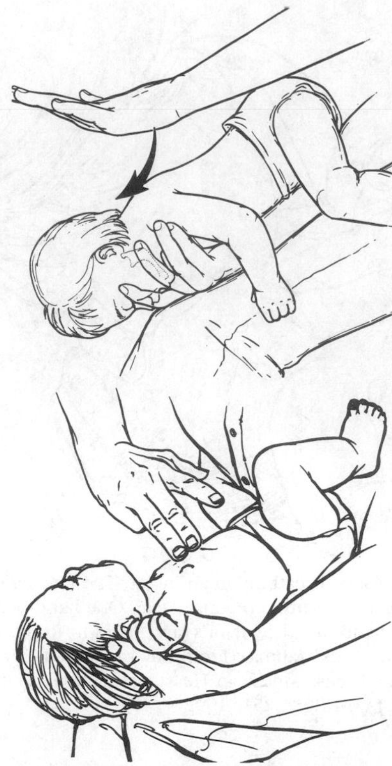

Figure 64–7 Back blows *(top)* and chest thrusts *(bottom)* to relieve foreign-body airway obstruction in the infant. (From Emergency Cardiac Care Committee and Subcommittees, American Heart Association. Pediatric basic life support, part V. JAMA 268:2251, 1992.)

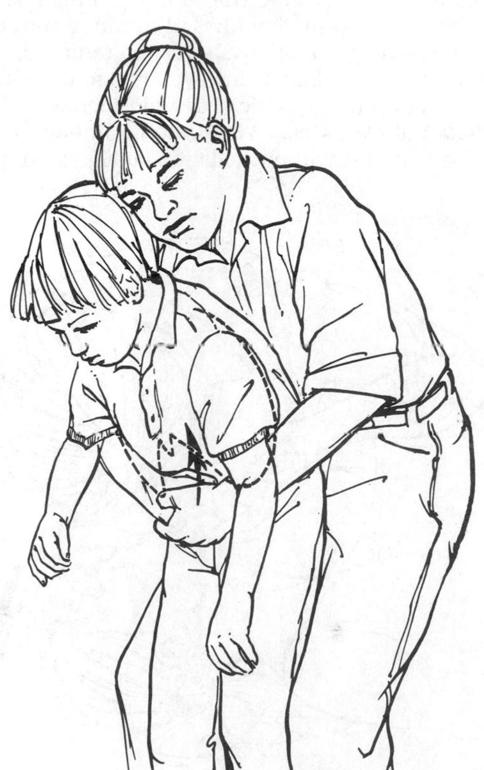

Figure 64–8 Abdominal thrusts with victim standing or sitting (conscious). (From Emergency Cardiac Care Committee and Subcommittees, American Heart Association. Pediatric basic life support, part V. JAMA 268:2251, 1992.)

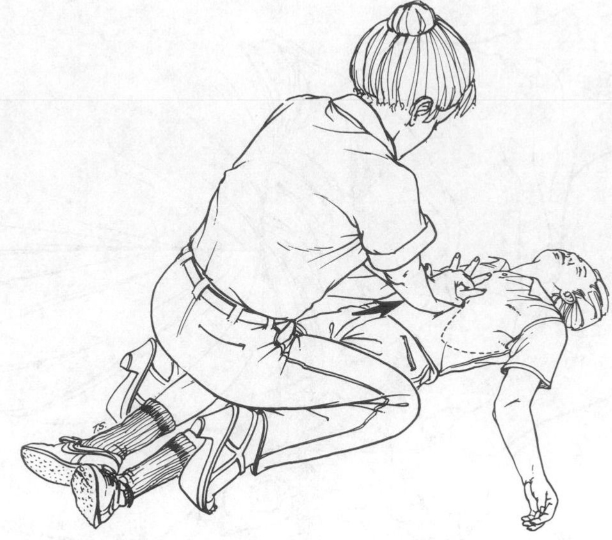

Figure 64–9 Abdominal thrusts with victim lying (conscious or unconscious). (From Emergency Cardiac Care Committee and Subcommittees, American Heart Association. Pediatric basic life support, part V. JAMA 268:2251, 1992.)

analgesia is recommended to reduce metabolic stress (also see Chapter 73). Children 1 mo of age or older should be pretreated with a sedative, an analgesic, and possibly a muscle relaxant unless the situation is an emergency and the adminis-

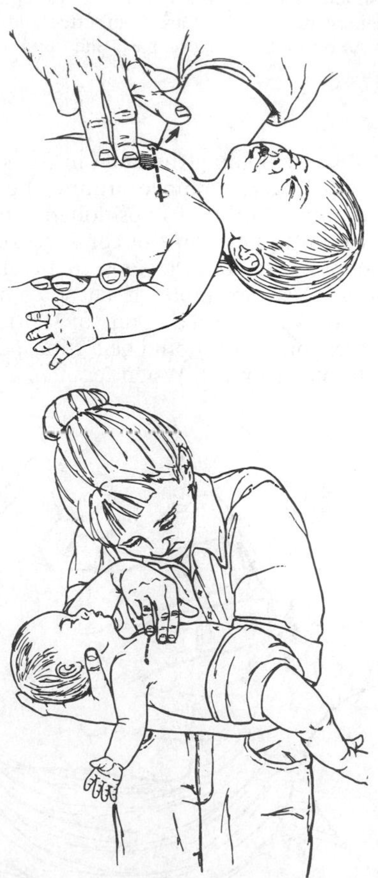

Figure 64–10 Cardiac compressions. *Top*, infant supine on palm of the rescuer's hand. *Bottom*, performing CPR while carrying the infant or small child. Note that the head is kept level with the torso. (From Emergency Cardiac Care Committee and Subcommittees, American Heart Association. Pediatric basic life support, part V. JAMA 268:2251, 1992.)

TABLE 64–8 Parameters for Optimal Cardiorespiratory Resuscitation

Age	Chest Compression Rate	Respiration Rate (breaths/min)	Endotracheal Tube Size
Newborn	100/min; 1 in. deep	20–24	3.5–4.0 mm inner diameter
Child	80/min; 1.5 in. deep	16–20	4.5–6 mm inner diameter
Teen	60/min; 2 in. deep	12–18	6–7.5 mm inner diameter

(From Rogers: Pediatric Intensive Care, 2nd ed. Baltimore, Williams & Wilkins, 1992.)

tration of drugs would cause an unacceptable delay. The intubation technique is shown in Figure 64–12.

In a *controlled intubation,* patients should fast for at least 4 hr or have their stomach emptied by nasogastric tube. The history and physical examination should be reviewed for any allergies or evidence of unusual airway anatomy, and informed consent should be obtained. Equipment necessary for intubation and bag-mask ventilation and an emergency cricothyrotomy tray should be available. After a period of hyperoxygenation, a benzodiazepine (diazepam, midazolam, lorazepam) should be administered, followed by an opiate (fentanyl, remifentanil, morphine), and a paralytic agent (vecuronium, rocuronium).

Because many intubations in critically ill children are emergent, the foregoing steps often cannot be followed, and procedures for *rapid sequence intubation* (RSI) should be initiated (Table 64–9). The goals of RSI are to induce anesthesia and paralysis and complete intubation rapidly. This minimizes elevations of intracranial and blood pressure that may accompany intubation in awake or lightly sedated patients. Because the stomach generally cannot be emptied before RSI, the **Sellick maneuver** (compression of the cricoid cartilage backward, compressing the esophagus against the vertebral column) should be used to prevent aspiration of gastric contents, which is very likely to occur when the laryngoscope and endotracheal tube are inserted into the pharynx and larynx.

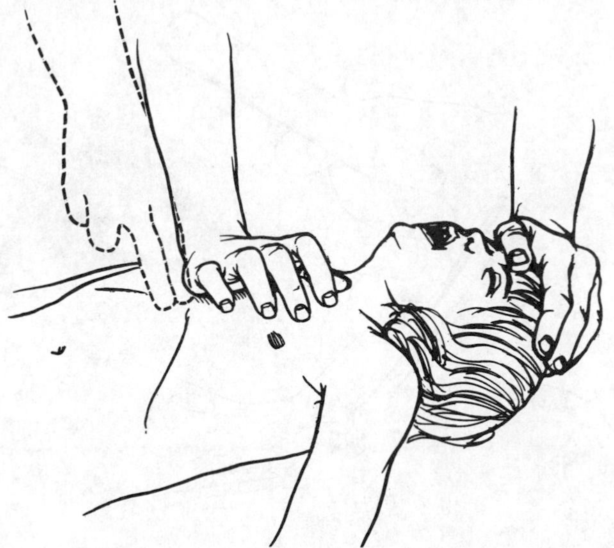

Figure 64–11 Locating hand position for chest compression in a child. Note that the rescuer's other hand is used to maintain head position to facilitate ventilation. (From Emergency Cardiac Care Committee and Subcommittees, American Heart Association. Pediatric basic life support, part V. JAMA 268:2251, 1992.)

Under controlled circumstances, *nasotracheal intubation* may be performed. It is indicated in patients who are going to be lightly sedated or when there is significant oral trauma. A nasotracheal tube causes less noxious sensations than does an *orotracheal tube,* which passes across the tongue and gums, producing a gag reflex in the posterior pharynx. Nasotracheal

TABLE 64–9 Rapid Sequence Intubation

Step	Procedure	Comment-Explanation
1	Brief history and assessment	R/O drug allergies; examine airway anatomy (e.g., micrognathia, cleft palate).
2	Assemble equipment, medications, etc.	See lists below.
3	Preoxygenate patient	With bag/mask, nasal cannula, hood or "blow-by."
4	Premedicate with lidocaine, atropine	Lidocaine minimizes intracranial pressure rise with intubation and can be applied topically to airway mucosa for local anesthesia. Atropine helps blunt the bradycardia associated with upper airway manipulation and reduces airway secretions.
5	Sedation and analgesia induced	Sedatives: *thiopental*—very rapid onset; can cause hypotension. *diazepam*—onset 2–5 min; elimination 30–60 min or more. *ketamine*—onset 1–2 min, elimination in 30–40 min. May cause hallucinations if used alone; causes higher ICP, mucous secretions, increased vital signs, and bronchodilation. Analgesics: *Fentanyl:* 3–10 μg/kg, may repeat 3–4 ×. Rapid administration risks "tight chest" response, with no effective ventilation. Effects wear off in 20–30 min. *Morphine:* 0.05–0.1 mg/kg/dose; may last 30–60 min, may lead to hypotension in hypovolemic patients.
6	Pretreat with nondepolarizing paralytic agent	Small dose of nondepolarizing paralytic agent (see below), with intent of diminishing the depolarizing effect of succinylcholine, which is administered next.
7	Administer muscle relaxants	Succinylcholine dose is 1–2 mg/kg; causes initial contraction of muscles, then relaxation. This depolarization can, however, raise ICP and blood pressure. Onset of paralysis in 30–40 sec; duration 5–10 min. Increased use of pretreatment with a nondepolarizing muscle relaxant, especially rocuronium (1 mg/kg), which has a very quick onset and short duration. Other nondepolarizing agents include vecuronium and pancuronium, both dosed at 0.1 mg/kg.
8	Sellick maneuver	Pressure on cricoid cartilage, to occlude esophagus and prevent regurgitation or aspiration.
9	Endotracheal intubation	Endotracheal tubes: select proper size for age and weight of child. Laryngoscope blades: variety of Miller and Macintosh blades. Patient supine: neck extended moderately to "sniffing" position.
10	Secure tube, verify position with roentgenogram	ET tube secured with tape to cheeks and upper lip or to an adhesive patch applied to the skin near the mouth.
11	Begin mechanical ventilation	Verify tube placement before ventilating with positive pressure; if ET in one bronchus, barotrauma may occur.

ICP = intracranial pressure; ET = endotracheal.

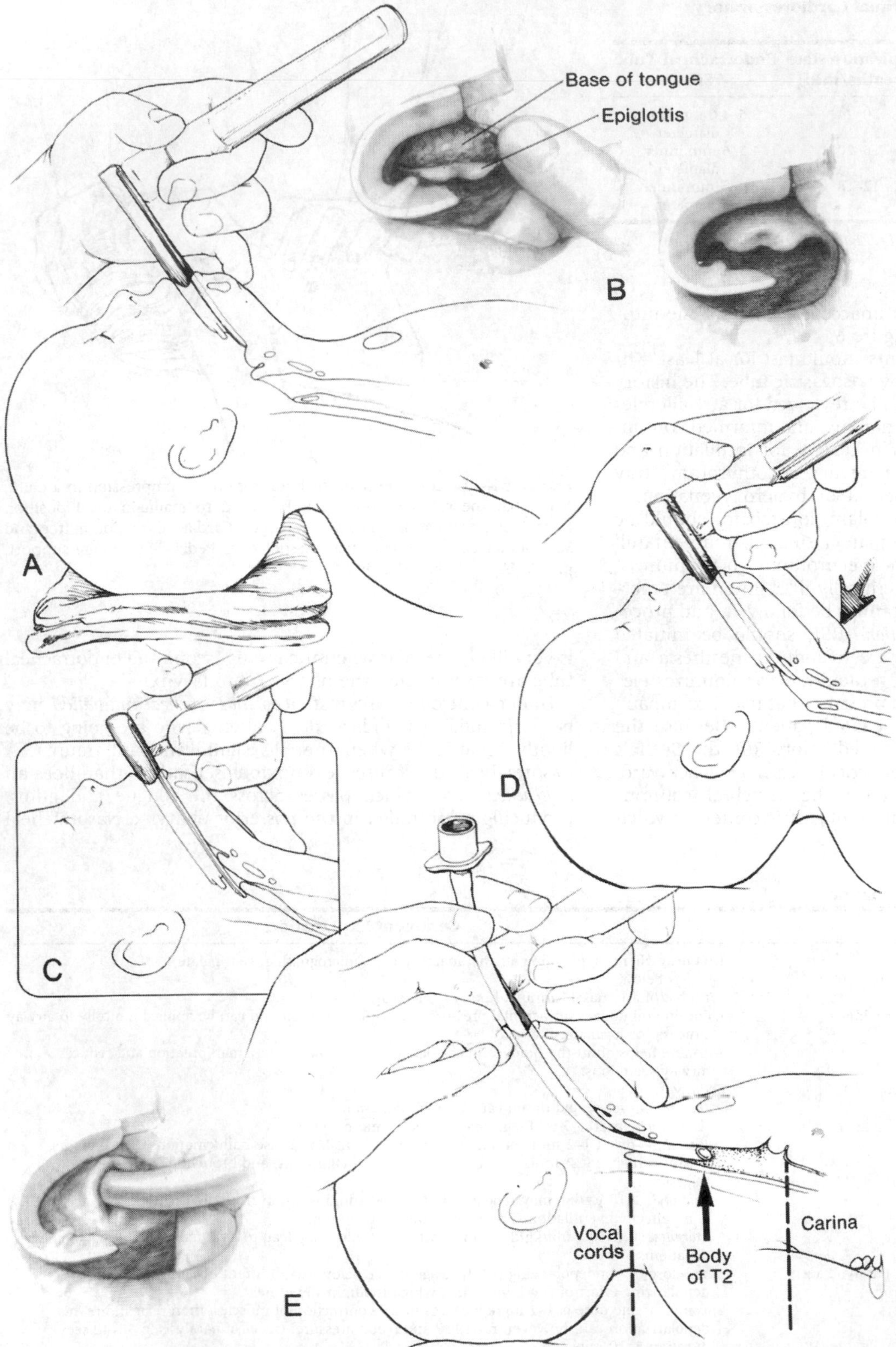

Figure 64–12 Intubation technique. (From Fleisher G, Ludwig S: Textbook of Pediatric Emergency Medicine. Baltimore, Williams & Wilkins, 1983, p 1250.)

tubes do, however, obstruct sinus and eustachian tube drainage, and fever may result.

CRICOTHYROTOMY. When the airway is obstructed and tracheal intubation has not succeeded, *needle cricothyrotomy* is indicated. The patient should be supine with the face looking directly upward. The midpoint of the cricothyroid membrane is palpated, and a 14-gauge intravenous catheter with stylet is advanced slowly through it, inclined inferiorly at about 45 degrees. Quick aspiration of air through a syringe connected to the catheter indicates entry into the trachea. At this point, the metal stylet is removed and the catheter is pushed farther downward into the trachea. Oxygen should be flushed through the catheter at 10–15 L/min. This supports a child, even one with little or no spontaneous respirations, while plans for a more secure airway are made. *Surgical cricothyrotomy* is rarely necessary in children and should always be performed by an experienced surgeon, except in severe emergencies. It involves making a transverse incision in the cricothyroid membrane and advancing a large catheter through the incision downward into the lower trachea. Although similar in principle to a needle cricothyrotomy, the risk of bleeding, upper airway obstruction, and pneumothorax are significantly greater.

INITIATION OF MECHANICAL VENTILATION. Mechanical ventilation is required for patients intubated for airway protection. See Chapters 64.4 and 375.

VENOUS ACCESS. Veins suitable for cannulation are numerous, but there is considerable anatomic variation. The *dorsum of the foot* usually has a large vein in the midline, passing across the ankle joint, but a catheter is difficult to maintain in this vein because dorsiflexion tends to injure it. A second large vein on the *lateral side of the foot,* running in the horizontal plane, usually about 1–2 cm dorsal to the lower margin of the foot, is preferable (Fig. 64–13). The great saphenous vein is accessible in all patients. It is cannulated just anterior to the medial malleolus and may be accessible in the medial leg and thigh in premature infants.

Of the numerous veins on the *dorsum of the hand,* many are suitable for cannulation. The vessels are large, often secured on the flat surface of the dorsum of the hand, and cannulation is well tolerated. There is almost always a large vein lying in the interspace of the 4th and 5th digits, about 1 cm proximal to the metacarpophalangeal joints. The *cephalic vein* is usually cannulated at the wrist, along the forearm, or at the elbow (Fig. 64–14). The *median vein of the forearm* is also suitable because it lies along a flat surface of the forearm. The *basilic vein* is prone to sliding around when attempts are made to cannulate it.

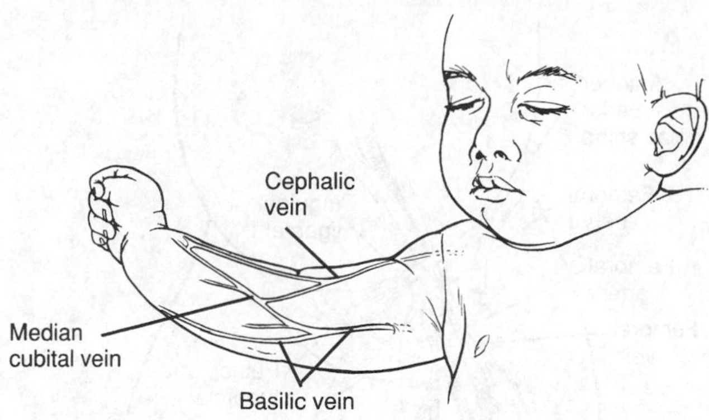

Figure 64–14 Veins of the upper extremity. (From A Textbook of Pediatric Advanced Life Support. Dallas, American Heart Association, 1994.)

Samples of blood may be obtained from the external and internal *jugular veins* or, in neonates, from various *scalp veins.* The two jugular veins are also potential sites for indwelling catheters (Fig. 64–15). The most notable scalp veins are the superficial temporal (just anterior to the ear) and posterior auricular (just behind the ear).

Deeper and larger veins are very valuable because they provide a reliable access for medications, nutritive solutions, and blood sampling. They may be reached by percutaneous cannulation or by surgical exposure. To cannulate the *femoral vein,* after the skin is cleaned, a needle is inserted about 0.5 cm medial to the pulsing femoral artery (or, if no pulse, about two thirds of the way from the anterior superior spine to the pubic tubercle (Fig. 64–16). Slight backward pressure on the plunger of a connected syringe is maintained so that blood flows easily into the syringe once the vessel is punctured. After locating the vessel, a small wire is advanced through the needle into

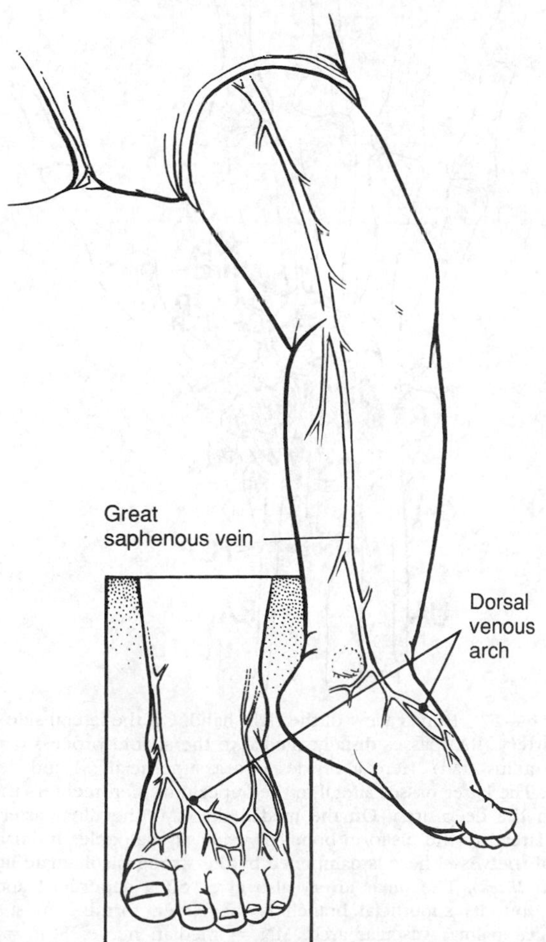

Figure 64–13 Veins of the lower extremity. (From A Textbook of Pediatric Advanced Life Support. Dallas, American Heart Association, 1994.)

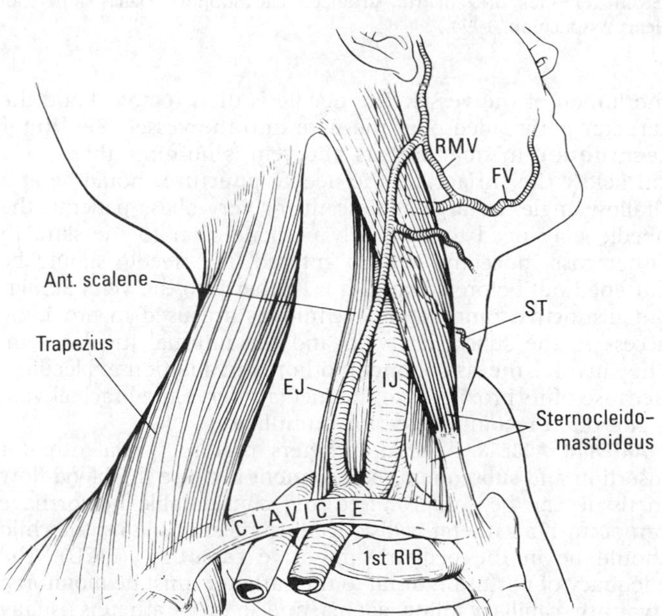

Figure 64–15 The internal and external jugular veins. RMV = retromandibular vein; FV = facial vein; ST = superior thyroid vein; IJ = internal jugular vein; EJ = external jugular vein; SCM = sternocleidomastoid muscle. The two heads of the SCM are indicated by the leader lines connecting that word to the diagram. (From Mathers LW, Smim DW, Frankel L: Anatomic considerations in placement of central venous catheters. Clin Anat 5:89,1992.)

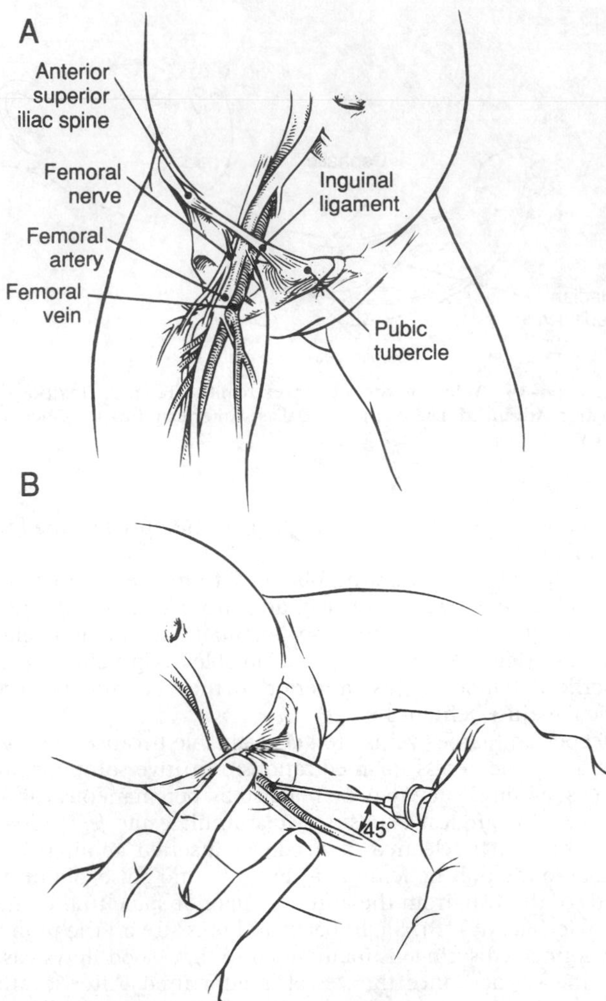

Figure 64–16 Femoral vein (A) anatomy and (B) cannulation technique. (From Textbook of Pediatric Advanced Life Support. Dallas, American Heart Association, 1994.)

the lumen of the vessel. The needle is then removed and the catheter is threaded over the wire into the vessel **(Seldinger technique)**. In small infants, the vein is no more than 0.5–1 cm below the surface, so the needle puncture should be at a shallow angle. In large adolescents or very obese patients, the needle may need to be nearly perpendicular to the skin. In either case, once the vein is entered, the needle should be flattened out before advancing it further into the vein. Similar but distinctive cannulation techniques are used in providing access to the subclavian vein and the internal jugular vein. They involve the risk of pneumothorax in addition to bleeding. Because of its proximity to the median nerve the brachial vein is not often recommended for cannulation.

ARTERIAL ACCESS. Arterial catheters require special care for insertion and subsequent management because the blood flow to tissue can be compromised and considerable hemorrhage can occur if a catheter is dislodged. In most hospitals, the child should be in the pediatric intensive care unit (PICU). The adequacy of perfusion distal to the catheter must be monitored (warmth, capillary filling, edema, and so on). Catheters usually need to be heparinized (1/2–1 unit/mL) to minimize clotting. The *radial artery* lies on the lateral side of the anterior wrist, just medial to the styloid process of the radius. When cannulating this vessel at or beyond the crease of the wrist, the superficial branch of the radial artery is being punctured (Fig. 64–17). *The ulnar artery* is used much less often than the radial. About 2–3 cm above the wrist it becomes superficial, lying just lateral to the tendon of flexor carpi ulnaris. Although it is larger than the radial artery, the ulnar nerve travels side by side with the ulnar artery.

An ulnar or radial artery occasionally may be absent or very small, and cannulation of the normal-sized radial or ulnar vessel may compromise blood flow to the hand. The **Allen test** is used to identify this possibility and consists of simultaneous compression of both the radial and ulnar arteries, instructing patients to clench their fist several times (to blanch the palm of the hand by propelling venous blood upward into the forearm), followed by release of pressure over one of the vessels and observation of how fast and how well the hand regains normal color. The test is then repeated with release of pressure over the other vessel. If, in both cases, the hand quickly becomes pink, it can be adequately perfused with only one of the two main arteries intact, and even if the cannulated artery were to become blocked (a very rare event), the hand would still be adequately perfused.

The *brachial artery* is easily palpable between the brachialis and biceps muscles, on the medial side of the arm, just above the elbow. The median nerve is just medial and may even lie superficial to the artery. Because cannulating this artery may

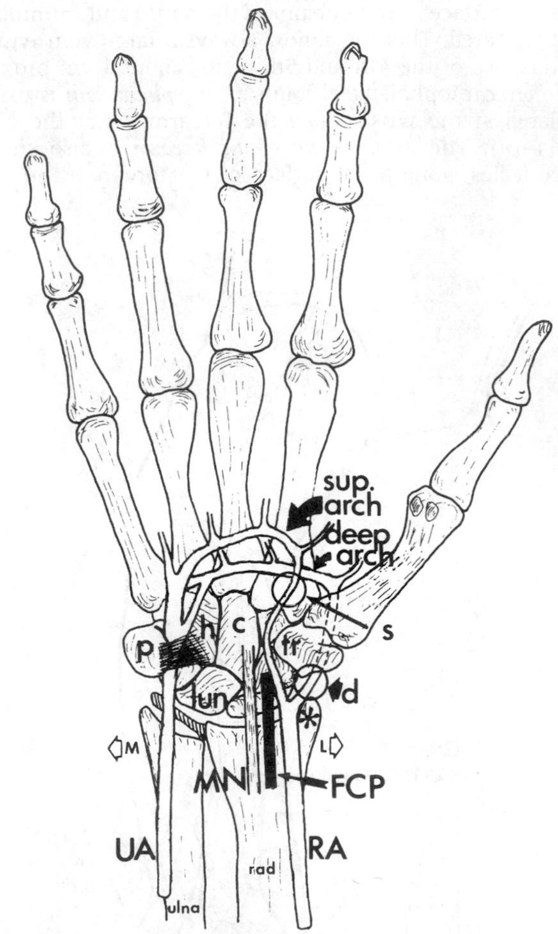

Figure 64–17 Palmar view of the right hand. On the lateral side (L) the radial artery (RA) passes distally, medial to the styloid process (*asterisk*) of the radius (rad). Here it divides into a superficial (s) and deep (d) branch. The latter passes lateral to the trapezium, then reenters the palm to form the deep arch. On the medial side (M) the ulnar artery (UA) passes lateral to the pisiform bone (p), an easily palpable landmark. The pulse of the vessel here is dampened by the strong pisohamate ligament (*dashed lines*). The ulnar artery also gives off a superficial and deep branch, but its superficial branch is the larger, forming most of the superficial palmar vascular arch. MN = median nerve; FCP = flexor carpi radialis; lun = lunate bone; c = capitate bone; h = hamate bone; tr = trapezium bone. (From Mathers LH Jr: Anatomical considerations in obtaining arterial access. J Intensive Care Med 5:110, 1990.)

compromise blood flow distally in the limb, only small catheters should be used (i.e., 22 gauge) and placed distal to the takeoff of the deep brachial artery. Anatomic landmarks and technique for cannulating or sampling from the *femoral artery* are identical to those for the femoral vein (see Fig. 64–16). The *dorsalis pedis artery* lies on the dorsum of the foot between the tendons of tibialis anterior and flexor hallicus longus and is usually palpable. However, cannulation requires immobilization of the foot to minimize the risk of dislodging the catheter with flexion and extension of the ankle. Alternatively, use of the *posterior tibial artery* involves risk to the underlying tibial nerve if profuse bleeding occurs.

INTRAOSSEOUS LINE PLACEMENT. See Chapter 58 and Fig. 58–2. Intraosseous needles have special flanges on the side of the hub for holding the needle and securing it to the patient and an internal stylet that prevents bone fragments from clogging the lumen of the needle. Insertion of the needle too close to the epiphyseal plate may disrupt future bone growth. Further, if the needle is not in the marrow, the infusion of fluids may lead to extravasation into the soft tissues. Osteomyelitis is also a risk, especially because these procedures are often performed hurriedly without adequate sterile precautions.

THORACENTESIS AND CHEST TUBE PLACEMENT. Also see Chapter 377. *Thoracentesis* is the placement of a needle or catheter (chest tube) into the pleural space to evacuate fluid, blood, or air. Most insertions are performed between the 4th and 9th ribs, along the midclavicular line in the anterior chest wall (in adolescents and adults) or in the plane of the midaxillary line. After a skin incision is made, dissection through the chest wall is accomplished in layers, using blunt dissection techniques. The needle (and later chest tube) that enters the pleural space should penetrate the intercostal space by passing over the superior edge of the lower rib, because there are larger vessels along the inferior edge of the rib. The chest tube should lie anterior for air and posterior for fluid accumulation in the pleural space. Final penetration of the intercostal membranes, to enter the pleural space, often takes considerable force, and the instrument (usually a hemostat) inserted into the pleural cavity should be grasped in such a way that there is no risk of uncontrolled deep penetration into the mediastinum, with possible contusion of the lung or heart. After the chest tube is inserted, it should be secured firmly to the chest wall and connected to a source of suction (e.g., Pleurovac) at a pressure of 15–20 cm H_2O. A roentgenogram should be obtained to verify chest tube placement and evacuation of the pleural space.

PERICARDIOCENTESIS. When fluid, blood, or gas accumulates in the pericardial sac, a danger is that the heart will be compressed and will not be able to fill and empty with normal volumes of blood, leading to diminution in cardiac output. The cardinal signs of such a restrictive pericardial effusion are tachycardia, hypotension, and decreasing oxygen saturation. Pericardiocentesis is needle aspiration of the sac performed with or without ultrasound verification of needle placement or attachment of a recording electrode. After proper patient positioning, sterile cleansing of the area around the xiphoid process, and sedation/analgesia, pericardiocentesis begins with a short incision in the skin just below the xiphoid process. The needle should be a 22- or 20-gauge spinal needle, 6.25 cm (2.5 in.) in length. The proximal end of the needle is attached to a stopcock and collection syringe. The needle is inserted through the incision and then positioned so that it points toward the space between the left nipple and the medial end of the clavicle. Once the needle is through the skin, its angle should be flattened considerably with respect to the chest wall so that penetration is not too deep (in larger children or adults, the angle must be steeper). During insertion, the syringe attached to the needle is continuously aspirated with gentle pressure so that when the needle enters the pericardial space there will be a rush of gas or fluid. Once the procedure is concluded, a sterile dressing should be placed over the skin incision and a chest roentgenogram obtained to rule out any complications.

TABLE 64–10 Supplies Needed for Pediatric Intensive Care/Emergency Department

Storage cart for equipment/materials
Defibrillator/portable ECG monitor
Oxygen cylinder
Airway equipment:
- Laryngoscope handle with batteries
- Assortment of blades—Miller 0, 1, 2, 3 and MacIntosh 2, 3
- Large assortment of endotracheal tubes, cuffed and uncuffed, with stylets
- Nasal and oral airways
- Self-inflating resuscitation bags
- Anesthesia bags with oxygen adapter

Suction equipment, including tongue blades, Yankauer suction tip, several catheters
Various nasogastric tubes
Tapes, sponges, IV adapters, T connectors, stopcocks
Masks for bag-mask ventilation, many sizes
Mapleson system with varied bag sizes
Cardiac equipment
- Cardiac arrest board for compressions
- IVs, butterflies, intraosseous needles
- Blood pressure measuring equipment
- Several unit doses of epinephrine, bicarbonate, calcium chloride, lidocaine, naloxone D-25-W

IV fluids and medications
- Various crystalloid and colloid fluids
- Fully equipped IV tray—catheters, alcohol, needles, tape, tourniquets, arm boards
- Cutdown tray
- Umbilical catheter tray
- Tracheostomy tray
- Chest tube tray
- Pleurovac pump
- Cardiac surgery open chest tray (if unit cares for postoperative hearts)
- ICP monitor tray
- General minor surgical procedure tray
- Military antishock trousers (MAST) kit
- Warm packs, sandbags, and so on

Monitoring equipment: pulse oximetry, ECG, end-tidal CO_2, blood pressure

ECG = electrocardiogram; IV = intravenous; ECP = intracranial pressure.

EQUIPMENT AND DRUGS FOR RESUSCITATION. An ED or intensive care unit should have a full supply of resuscitation equipment, frequently checked for both presence and functionality (e.g., available catheters and tubes in appropriate sizes and charged batteries). The supplies needed for a pediatric office or clinic emergency are presented in Chapter 58 and Table 58–1. Those required for a PICU or ED are presented in Table 64–10. See Table 64–11 for drugs that may be urgently required for resuscitation. Some resuscitations involve difficulty in establishing vascular access, and a rapidly deteriorating patient may die without such access if medications are not administered. In such cases, if an airway has been established, certain drugs may be administered via the endotracheal tube (e.g. lidocaine, epinephrine, atropine, and naloxone).

Becker LB, Berg RA, Pepe, et al: A reappraisal of mouth-to-mouth ventilation during bystander-initiated cardiopulmonary resuscitation. A statement for healthcare professionals from the ventilation working group of the basic life support and pediatric life support subcommittees, American Heart Association. Circulation 96(6):2102, 1997.

Brown C, Wiklund L, Bar-Joseph G, et al: Future directions for resuscitation research. IV. Innovative advanced life support pharmacology. Resuscitation 33:163, 1996.

Burns JP, Truog RD: Ethical controversies in pediatric critical care. New Horiz 5:72, 1997.

Carcillo JA, Cunnion RE: Septic shock. Crit Care Clin 13:553, 1997.

Carpenter TC, Stenmark KR: High-dose epinephrine is not superior to standard-dose epinephrine in pediatric in-hospital cardiopulmonary arrest. Pediatrics 99:403, 1997.

Kapklein MJ, Mahadeo R: Pediatric trauma. Mt Sinai J Med 64:302, 1997.

Mathers LH: Anatomical considerations in obtaining arterial access. J Inten Care Med 5:110, 1990.

Mathers LH, Frankel LR, Smith DW: Anatomical considerations in obtaining venous access. Clin Anat 4:1, 1992.

TABLE 64–11 Resuscitation Drugs That May Be Given Urgently

Drug	Indication(s)	Dose	Comments
Epinephrine	Bradycardia/asystole hypotension	10–100 μg/kg; followed by drip of 0.05–2 μg/kg/min	Hepatic excretion; histamine release; bronchospasm
Glucose	Hypoglycemia; stupor, seizures	250–500 mg/kg (1–2 mL/kg of D-25-W)	Too rapid infusion → crenate red blood cells
Atropine	Asystole, bradycardia	10–20 μg/kg	Minimum dose 100 μg; paradoxical bradycardia with very low doses
Calcium chloride	Hypotension, bradycardia; hyperkalemia; overdose of calcium channel blockers	10–20 mg/kg (calcium chloride)	Best in central line, over 2–5 min Clear IV line of drugs that might precipitate (e.g., HCO_3)
Isoproterenol	Bradycardia Vasodilation/hypotension	Continuous infusion 0.1–3.0 μg/kg/min 1,000 ng = 1 μg	Increased risk of dysrhythmias
Prostaglandin E_1	Ductal closure; cyanosis	20–500 ng/kg/min (maximum = 1,000 ng/kg/min)	May cause apnea; hypotension
Naloxone	Opiate overdose	10–25 μg/kg; may repeat × 3; max. single dose = 400 μg	High doses in opiate-dependent patient may cause seizures
Sodium bicarbonate	Metabolic acidosis	0.5–1 mEq/kg	Infuse over 2–5 min; clear IV line if patient not ventilating well, HCO_3 may produce acidosis
Diazoxide	Acute hypertension	1–5 mg/kg; may repeat × 3 over 30 min	Must give IV very rapidly Maximum 15 mg/kg/24 hr
Phenobarbital doses	Seizures	10–20 mg/kg (initial), then 5 mg/kg/24 hr	May depress ventilation in high doses Accelerates liver functions
Phenytoin	Seizures	10–15 mg/kg	Maximum infusion rate 1 mg/kg/min Faster infusion → risk cardiac standstill
Diazepam	Seizures, need sedation	200–400 μg/kg (0.2–0.4 mg/kg)	May be IV, PO, or rectal; has metabolites with long half-lives
Midazolam	Seizures, need sedation	40–100 μg/kg (0.04–0.1 mg/kg)	May be IV, or some give intranasally at dose 3–5× that of IV
Lidocaine	Ventricular dysrhythmias	1 mg/kg loading; then 20–50 μg/kg/min drip	May repeat initial dose 2–3×; should monitor blood levels
Digoxin	Supraventricular tachycardia; congestive heart failure	See Chapter 442.4	Therapeutic range narrow; monitoring levels may help; may cause heart block in high doses
Nitroprusside	Hypertension; poor cardiac output	0.1–2 μg/kg/min	If used >48 h, monitor for cyanide

IV = intravenous; PO = orally.

Schindler MB, Bohn D, Cox PN, et al: Outcome of out-of-hospital cardiac or respiratory arrest in children. N Engl J Med 335:1473, 1996.

Tatman A, Warren A, Williams A, et al: Developments of a modified pediatric coma scale in intensive care practice. Arch Dis Child 77:519, 1997.

Wright R, Reynolds SL, Nachtsheim B: Compartment syndrome secondary to prolonged intrasosseous infusion. Pediatr Emerg Care 10:157, 1994.

Zaritshy A, Nadkarni V, Hazinski MF, et al: Recommended guidelines for uniform reporting of pediatric advanced life support: The pediatric Utstein style. A statement for healthcare professionals from a task force of the American Academy of Pediatrics, the American Heart Association, and the European Resuscitation Council. Pediatrics 96:765, 1995.

64.2 Shock

Lorry R. Frankel and Lawrence H. Mathers

Shock is an acute syndrome characterized by inadequate circulatory perfusion of tissue to meet the metabolic demands of vital organs. Insufficient oxygen is delivered to cells to support aerobic metabolism. There is a shift to less efficient anaerobic metabolism, which produces organic acids resulting in metabolic acidosis (Chapter 52). If inadequate tissue perfusion continues, various metabolic and systemic responses occur as the patient becomes more physiologically unstable (Fig. 64–18). The specific pattern of response and related pathophysiology, clinical manifestations, and treatments varies with the etiology of shock.

EPIDEMIOLOGY. Shock occurs in approximately 2% of all hospitalized children and adults in the United States (300–400,000 cases/yr). The mortality rate is 20–50%. Most patients do not die in the acute hypotensive/hypoxemic phase of shock but as a result of one or more complications associated with the shock state. Multiple organ system failure (MOSF) increases the probability of death (one organ system involved = 25%; 2 organ systems = 60%; 3 or more organ systems = >85%). The mortality rate of shock in pediatric patients has declined as a consequence of educational efforts (pediatric advanced life support [PALS]), which emphasize early recognition and intervention and rapid transfer of critically ill patients to a PICU via a transport service.

PATHOPHYSIOLOGY. Shock may result in tissue injury through a number of pathways (Fig. 64–18) and at various stages in its development (Table 64–12). Production or release of the mediators of injury is triggered by the ischemic or hypoxic insult, which results from inadequate tissue perfusion. However, a separate, highly significant spectrum of injuries occurs during the reperfusion stage of shock when blood flow and oxygen delivery are restored to the previously injured tissues (Table 64–12). Some of the immunity-mediated responses that occur during shock, especially septic episodes, are referred to as the systemic inflammatory response syndrome (SIRS). SIRS may also increase the risk of sepsis and severe shock after bacterial and viral infections.

In the early phases of shock, a number of compensatory physiologic mechanisms act to maintain blood pressure (BP) and preserve tissue perfusion. These responses include increases of heart rate, stroke volume, and vascular smooth muscle tone, regulated through changes in neural and hormonal receptors and substances, to help preserve blood flow to vital organs such as the brain, heart, and kidneys. The respiratory rate is increased to promote the excretion of carbon dioxide and to compensate for the metabolic acidemia. There is also, with time, increased renal excretion of hydrogen ions and retention of bicarbonate, in an effort to maintain normal pH (Chapter 52). Maintenance of vascular volume is facilitated by the renin-angiotensin-atrial natriuretic factor axis (through regulation of sodium), steroid and catecholamine synthesis and secretion, and secretion of antidiuretic hormone. Extracellular fluid also moves into the vascular space as capillary hydrostatic pressure falls.

When the compensatory mechanisms cannot maintain adequate tissue perfusion, shock, tissue injury (Table 64–12), and

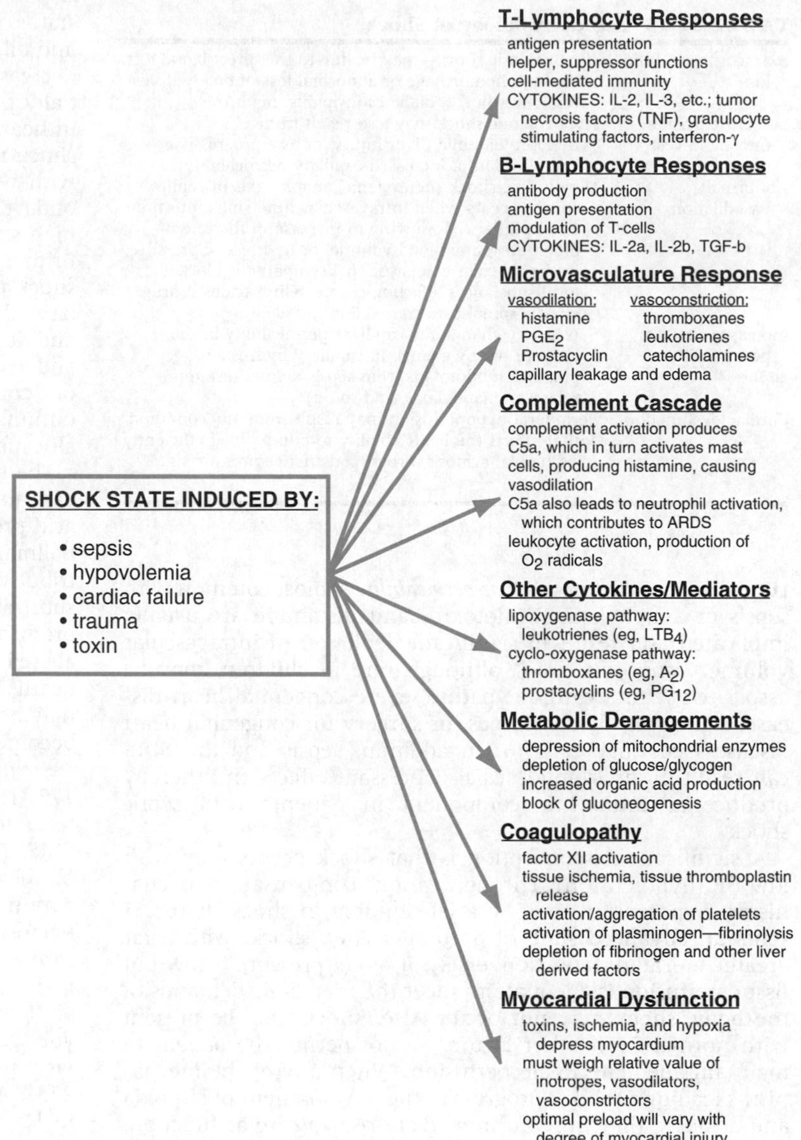

Figure 64–18 Metabolic responses that may occur as a consequence of inadequate perfusion or shock. ARDS = adult respiratory distress syndrome.

cell (and eventually patient) death occur. The major pathophysiologic mechanisms of shock are presented in Table 64–13. It is common for more than one of these processes to occur simultaneously. Extracorporeal fluid loss, commonly accompanying vomiting and diarrhea, trauma, and severe burns, can result in an initial increase in vascular resistance as the body attempts to maintain BP and restore circulating volume, and, subsequently, in hypotension and tissue ischemia from inadequate perfusion. Significant electrolye alterations may also accompany the fluid loss. When there is an associated *lowering of the plasma oncotic pressure,* as occurs with the hypoproteinemia of nephrotic syndrome, hepatic dysfunction, or severe burns, there may be capillary leaking; this may result in greater fluid loss (e.g., edema) and potentially worsening respiratory status. *Abnormal vasodilation* occurs in septic and neurogenic shock and anaphylaxis. The lower systemic vascular resistance (SVR) is usually accompanied by an increase in cardiac output and a redistribution of blood flow, hence the term **distribu-**

TABLE 64–12 Events and Processes Resulting in Tissue Injury from Shock

Inciting Injury	Metabolic Change	Reperfusion Injury	Later Injuries
Blood loss, cardiac arrest, burns, toxic injury	Hypoxia Acidosis Ischemia	Release of free radicals Vasoconstriction	Tissue necrosis Infections Adult respiratory distress syndrome
Underlying Events			
Cells lack oxygen Cells lack adequate perfusion with blood	Organic acids released Increased intracellular water Abnormal ion shifts [Na^+, Ca^{++}] Increase of secondary messengers	Increased oxygen radicals and hydrogen peroxide Increase of secondary messengers Weakened antioxidant defense Release of various cytokines (TNF, interleukins, others) Endothelial cell damage, leading to coagulopathy Activation of leukocytes and macrophages	Increased membrane permeability, causing diffuse edema and depletion of intravascular volume Disseminated coagulopathy Activation of leukocytes and macrophages Irreversible tissue injury and scarring

TABLE 64–13 Pathophysiology of Shock

Extracorporeal fluid loss	Hypovolemic shock—may be due to the direct blood loss through hemorrhage or abnormal loss of bodily fluids (diarrhea, burns, diabetes insipidus, nephrosis)
Lowering plasma oncotic forces	Hypovolemic shock may also result from hypoproteinemia (liver injury, or as a progressive complication of increased capillary permeability).
Abnormal vasodilation	Distributive shock (neurogenic, anaphylaxis or septic shock) occurs when intravascular fluid shifts into the extracellular space owing to increase in the rate of blood flow, and blood volume, or hydrostatic pressure in the vascular compartment (sympathetic blockade, local substances affecting permeability, acidosis, drug effects, spinal cord transection, other).
Increased vascular permeability	Sepsis may change the capillary permeability in the absence of any change in capillary hydrostatic pressure (endotoxins from sepsis, excess histamine relase in anaphylaxis, and so on)
Cardiac dysfunction	Peripheral hypoperfusion may result from any condition that affects the heart's ability to pump blood efficiently (ischemia, acidosis, drugs, constrictive pericarditis, other).

tive shock. *Increased vascular permeability* is most common with sepsis or anaphylaxis. Endotoxins and histamine are usually implicated and result in significant depletion of intravascular volume. *Cardiogenic shock,* although rare in children, may be associated with a cardiomypathy, severe congenital heart disease, significant dysrhythmias, or surgery for congenital heart disease (see Chapter 436). In addition, sepsis and the SIRS can result in direct myocardial depressant effects and thereby produce a cardiogenic component in patients with septic shock.

A significant misconception is that shock occurs only with low BP (hypotension). Through various compensatory mechanisms, hypotension may be a late finding in shock. It represents an advanced state of decompensated shock, with a far greater mortality rate. Conversely, if blood pressure is low but tissue perfusion is adequate to meet the metabolic demands of the body, shock may not occur. Also, shock may be present with normal BP if other factors do not permit the patient to maintain adequate tissue perfusion. When any of the mechanisms leading to shock progress to the development of hypoxia and acidosis, they pose an immediate risk to cardiac function, lessening the strength of contractions and predisposing to dysrhythmias. This results in a cascade of events that, if left undisturbed, result in irreversible shock and death.

CLINICAL MANIFESTATIONS. A classification of shock is presented in Table 64–14. There is significant overlap in these categories, especially between septic and distributive shock. The clinical presentations of shock depend, in part, on the cause; however, if shock is unrecognized and untreated, a very similar untoward progression of clinical signs and pathophysiologic changes occurs (Fig. 64–15). The clinical features of shock may also relate to the stage of the process, e.g., early vs late.

Hypovolemic shock usually presents with changes in mental status, tachypnea, tachycardia, hypotension, cool extremities, and oliguria. See Table 64–15 for clinical signs of a progressive decrease in perfusion. However, hypovolemic shock may initially present with normal or only mild to moderate changes in heart rate and BP and slightly cool distal extremities. Septic shock may initially present as *compensated* or **"warm shock,"** with warm extremities (due to peripheral vasodilatation secondary to low SVR), bounding pulses and tachycardia (due to high stroke volume and cardiac output), tachypnea, adequate urination, and mild metabolic acidosis. In contrast, cardiogenic shock presents with cool extremities, delayed (> 2 sec) capillary filling, hypotension, tachypnea, increasing obtundation, and decreased urination (all due to peripheral vasoconstriction and decreased cardiac output). See Chapter 436. *Uncompensated* or **"cool shock"** (high vascular resistance, decreased cardiac output, oliguria) occurs in the late stage of shock due to almost all causes.

The transition from warm shock to cool shock is not always easy to diagnose. At the cellular level, the increase in lactate acid production, indicating inadequate oxygen delivery, is the hallmark of uncompensated shock. However, in septic or distributive shock, despite excellent cardiac output, appropriate substrate may not be used and lactic acid may accumulate, producing metabolic acidosis. If this process continues unabated, severe shock may become irreversible, resulting in death. In cases of abrupt blood or intravascular fluid loss, there may not be a warm phase of shock, as the patient immediately becomes peripherally vasoconstricted.

Septicemia and septic shock are discussed in Chapters 106 and 173. The associated immune-mediated responses, particularly to endotoxin (see Fig. 173–2), may lead the development of SIRS. The vascular endothelium is one of the principal targets of these inflammatory reactions; these cells in turn release various other mediators such as interleukin I (IL-1) and tumor necrosis factor (TNF-α). SIRS is characterized by fever, tachycardia, tachypnea, and hypotension and hypoperfusion leading to impaired function of multiple organs. Both bacterial and viral infections have been associated with SIRS. Infants younger than 2 mo and having severe respiratory syncytial virus infection may be particularly susceptible to SIRS (Chapter 253). Adult respiratory distress syndrome (ARDS) also occurs in 10–30% of patients having septic shock.

Another unusual form of shock is the *hemorrhagic shock encephalopathy syndrome (HSES)*. This syndrome is similar to heat stoke and is characterized by encephalopathy, fever, shock, watery diarrhea, severe disseminated intravascular coagulation (DIC), and renal and hepatic dysfunction. In addition to the hemodynamic changes associated with poor perfusion and hypotension, patients with HSES may develop seizures and other severe neurologic findings as a result of cerebral edema. These children have an associated rapid onset of abnormal liver function studies and coagulation tests. These abnormalities persist for 3–4 days. Therapy is directed at fluid resuscitation, maintaining adequate cardiac output, supporting the renal and he-

TABLE 64–14 Clinical Classification of Shock. (Also see Table 64-13 for Related Pathophysiologic Processes)

Type of Shock	Septic	Cardiogenic	Distributive	Hypovolemic	Miscellaneous
Characteristics	Infectious organisms release toxins that affect fluid distribution, cardiac output and so on	Primary pump failure produces inadequate tissue perfusion; resultant metabolic acidosis further impairs cardiac function	Neurologic disturbances may cause uneven distribution of fluids, leading to acidosis Overdose of drugs can alter fluid distribution	Reduced fluid volume reduces cardiac output; metabolic acidosis can result from low intravascular volume and poor tissue perfusion; serious electrolyte abnormalities may occur	Various disturbances that lead to fluid loss, pump failure, or maldistribution of fluid
Sample Causes	Bacterial Viral Fungal (all are more likely in immunocompromised)	Ischemic insult Cardiomyopathy Congenital heart disease Tamponade	Neurogenic (disturbance of vasomotor tone) Anaphylaxis Toxic Allergic reactions	Enteritis Hemorrhage Extensive burns Diabetes insipidus Nephrotic syndrome	Major vascular obstruction Hypothermia

TABLE 64–15 Signs of Decreased Perfusion

Organ System	↓ Perfusion	↓ ↓ Perfusion	↓ ↓ ↓ Perfusion
CNS	—	Restless, apathetic	Agitated/confused, stuporous
Respiration	—	↑ Ventilation	↑ ↑ Ventilation
Metabolism	—	Compensated metabolic acidemia	Uncompensated metabolic acidemia
Gut	—	↓ Motility	Ileus
Kidney	↓ Urine volume ↑ Urinary specific gravity	Oliguria	Oliguria/anuria
Skin	Delayed capillary refill	Cool extremities	Mottled, cyanotic, cold extremities
CVS	↑ Heart rate	↑ ↑ Heart rate, ↓ Peripheral pulses	↑ ↑ Heart rate, ↓ blood pressure, central pulses only

CNS, central nervous system; CVS, cardiovascular system; ↑, increased; ↓, decreased.
Adapted with permission from Lister G, Apkon M, Fabry JT: Shock. In: Emmanouilides GC, Riemenschneider TA, Allen HD, Gutgesell HP (eds): Moss & Adam's Heart Disease in Infants, Children and Adolescents: Including the Fetus and Young Adult, 5th ed. Baltimore, Williams & Wilkins, 1994, pp 1725–1746.

patic failure, and ameliorating acute neurologic abnormalities as they arise. Other complications may include myoglobinuria due to rhabdomyolysis. These children have a very high mortality rate, and survivors have a high incidence of neurologic problems.

TREATMENT

Initial Management. In most cases of early shock, a fluid bolus of 20 mL/kg of normal saline or lactated Ringer's, solution should be given rapidly. If it is not possible to insert an intravenous catheter into a peripheral vein within 90 sec or within three attempts, an intraosseus needle should be inserted to administer fluids (Chapters 58 and 64.1). After this infusion, the patient is reassessed to determine if more fluid is required or other forms of therapy should be initiated (i.e., antibiotics, vasoactive agents, or other types of fluids). Children in severe hypovolemic shock may require and tolerate a fluid bolus of 60–80 mL/kg within the first 1–2 hr of presentation. However, the risk of fluid overload must be continually reassessed. If the child's hypovolemia is from loss of blood or protein-rich fluid, replacement with fresh frozen plasma, albumin, whole blood, or red blood cells may be appropriate (administered at 10 mL/kg). The use of limit dextrans may be indicated if there is a need to increase plasma oncotic pressure but blood component therapy cannot be administered. If, after what is considered appropriate fluid resuscitation, the patient continues to demonstrate poor perfusion and shock, vasoactive agents are needed. Also see Chapter 54.

Cardiovascular Management. Also see Chapter 441. Septic, cardiogenic, distributive, and, rarely, hypovolemic shock may require various drugs to stimulate both heart rate (*chronotropic*) and cardiac contractility (*inotropic*). These agents should be infused through a central venous catheter in an intensive care unit. These drugs increase oxygen consumption and the risk of dysrhythmias (Table 64–16). Dopamine is probably the most frequently used agent and is preferred for cardiogenic shock. Epinephrine has many of the same properties as dopamine; however, it is more effective in increasing peripheral vascular tone and has a greater effect on the heart. Epinephrine also causes a greater increase in myocardial oxygen consumption and poses a greater risk of dysrhythmias. Dobutamine has a more selective action than either of these agents in cardiogenic shock and provides afterload reduction. Isoproterenol may decrease coronary perfusion and produce myocardial ischemia. Norepinephrine and phenylephrine are particularly effective in counteracting low SVR. Afterload reduction is seldom indicated in early shock but may be useful in the recovery phase of cardiogenic shock (Table 64–17). Amrinone and milrinone have demonstrated beneficial effects in the advanced treatment of cardiogenic shock because they increase contractility and promote afterload reduction.

OTHER MODES OF SUPPORT IN SHOCK. Coagulation disorders are frequently found in severe shock; DIC is discussed in Chapter 488. Correction of acidosis and hypocalcemia are discussed in Chapters 55.8 and 55.9, respectively.

Rarely, other invasive techniques may be needed to support children in shock who are not responding to fluid, pharmaco-

TABLE 64–16 Cardiovascular Drug Treatment of Shock

Drug	Effect(s)	Dose Range	Comments
Dopamine	Strengthens contractions (throughout dose range) Increases renal blood flow (low/intermediate doses) Vasoconstriction (high doses)	Low dose = 1–5 μg/kg/min Intermediate dose = 5–15 μg/kg/min High dose = 15–25 μg/kg/min	Increasing risk of dysrhythmias at high dose Should be administered in central vein
Epinephrine	Increases heart rate and strength of contractions Potent vasoconstrictor	0.05–3.0 μg/kg/min	May lessen renal perfusion Causes high O_2 consumption in the heart High risk of dysrhythmias
Dobutamine	Increases strength of heart contraction Little effect on heart rate Peripheral vasodilator, especially in vessels to viscera	1–20 μg/kg/min	Has very weak vasoconstriction (high dose) Good for cardiogenic shock; strengthens heart contraction and produces afterload reduction
Isoproterenol	Strong effect on increasing heart rate A potent bronchodilator Virtually no effect on strength of heart contraction	0.05–2.0 μg/kg/min	Increases O_2 consumption Potential for producing dysrhythmias
Norepinephrine	Strong vasoconstrictor Weak effect on strength of heart contraction	0.05–1.5 μg/kg/min	Produces short-run rise in blood pressure (high SVR) Causes increase in O_2 consumption, tendency for dysrhythmias
Phenylephrine	Strong vasoconstrictor Can be used to slow tachycardia through reflex cardiac slowing	0.5–2.0 μg/kg/min	Can cause sudden hypertension Causes increase in O_2 consumption
Amrinone	Potent inotrope Potent chronotrope Peripheral vasodilator	Load with 1.5–5 mg/kg bolus over 20 min, followed by 5–10 μg/kg/min	Phosphodiesterase inhibitor—slows cyclic AMP breakdown

O_2 = oxygen; SVR = systemic vascular resistance.

TABLE 64–17 Vasodilators/Afterload Reducers

Nitroprusside	Vasodilator (mainly arterial)	0.5–1.0 μg/kg/min	Rapid effect Prolonged use (>48 hr risks cyanide toxicity)
Nitroglycerin	Vasodilator (mainly venous)	1.0–20 μg/kg/min	Rapid effect Risk of high intracranial pressure
Prostaglandin E_1	Vasodilator Maintains open ductus arteriosus in newborn	0.05–0.2 μg/kg/min	Can lead to hypotension Risk of apnea when given continuously
Hydralazine	Direct arteriolar smooth muscle dilator	0.1–2.0 mg/kg; may start with low dose and repeat with higher doses to effect	Hypotension and reflex tachycardia Lupus-like effect in chronic use

logic support, or other modes of treatment when the cause of shock is considered treatable and reversible. Extracorporeal membrane oxygenation (ECMO) may be effective in treating young children with septic shock or severe cardiogenic shock and as a bridge to recovery or transplant in patients who have undergone cardiac surgery and who have difficulty in coming off bypass. Left ventricular or biventricular assist devices have also been used to manage severe cardiomyopathy and cardiogenic shock as a bridge to transplantation or until the disease process has reversed itself. Dialysis and hemofiltration have been used to manage fluid overload or pulmonary edema and remove chemical mediators.

American Academy of Pediatrics: Drugs for pediatric emergencies. Pediatrics 101: 1-11, 1998. WWW.Pediatrics.org/cgi/content/full/101/l/e/13.

Ceneviva G, Paschall A, Maffei F, et al: Hemodynamic support in fluid-refractory pediatric septic shock. Pediatrics 102, 1998. WWW.Pediatrics.org/cgi/content/full/102/2/e19.

Cochran Injuries Group Albumin Reviewers. Br Med J 317:235, 1998.

Hayes MA, Timmins AC, Yau EHS, et al: Oxygen transport patterns in patients with sepsis syndrome or septic shock: Influence of treatment and relationship to outcome. Crit Care Med 24:925, 1997.

Hollenberg SM, Cunnion RE: Endothelial and vascular smooth muscle function in sepsis. J Crit Care 9:262, 1994.

Kim KK, Frankel LR: The need for inotropic support in a subgroup of infants with severe life-threatening respiratory syncytial viral infection. J Invest Med 45:1, 1997.

Kumar A, Venkateswarlu T, Dee L, et al: Tumor necrosis factor-α and interleukin-1 β are responsible for in-vitro myocardial cell depression induced by human septic shock serum. J Exp Med 183:949, 1996.

Quirk WF, Sternback G, Jones J: Infection with flesh eating bacteria. J Emerg Med 14:747, 1996.

Teig N, Thomas GN: Haemorrhagic shock encephalopathy syndrome presenting with myglobinuria. Arch Dis Child 74:168, 1996.

Van Lierde S, van Leeuwen WJ, Ceuppens J, et al: Toxic shock syndrome without rash in a young child: Similarity with syndrome of hemorrhagic shock and encephalopathy? J Pediatr 131:130, 1997.

64.3 *Respiratory Distress and Failure*

Melinda T. Derish and Lorry R. Frankel

Respiratory distress/failure is the primary diagnosis in close to 50% of the children admitted to PICUs. There is substantial variability by season, etiology, and severity of illness. The causes of these respiratory problems may be classified by age, anatomic lesions, or abnormalities as involving (1) lung and chest wall mechanics, (2) neuromuscular systems, and (3) CNS control or drive. The presenting clinical findings usually help to determine the type of problem. Increased respiratory rate and effort (tachypnea and dyspnea) suggest mechanical problems of the lung or chest wall. Neuromuscular disease may result in progressively weaker respiratory efforts and eventually fatigue. CNS pathology may present with various respiratory patterns including bradypnea, apnea, and Cheyne-Stokes respirations. The heterogeneous group of pediatric diseases, that can cause respiratory distress and failure requiring mechanical ventilation are discussed in Chapter 377 and Table 64–18.

PATHOGENESIS. Respiratory failure is the inability of the respiratory system to provide exchange of oxygen and carbon dioxide between air and blood, resulting in an impaired supply of oxygen and excretion of carbon dioxide to meet the body's metabolic demands. The normal physiology of respiratory function and gas exchange is discussed in Chapters 373, 374, and 375.1). The oxygen absorption and carbon dioxide excretion that take place at the respiratory membrane occur because these two gases move along their respective concentration gradients, achieving complete equilibrium of pressure for each gas between the blood phase in the end capillary and the gas phase (air) within the alveolus. By the time the inspired air reaches the alveoli, it has changed composition. Inspired atmospheric room air has a PO_2 of approximately 159 mm Hg, and gas inside the alveoli, the *alveolar air,* normally has a PO_2 of 104 mm Hg. Alveolar air has this lower PO_2 because the oxygen in the alveoli is constantly being absorbed into the pulmonary blood. If the atmospheric air is supplemented with a higher concentration of oxygen, then the alveolar PO_2 (PAO_2) will be higher and the increased oxygen gradient between alveolar air and pulmonary blood results in increased absorption of oxygen. Carbon dioxide diffuses through the respiratory membrane so quickly that the mixed venous and alveolar PCO_2 are nearly the same. Atmospheric air has a PCO_2 of approximately zero, and a healthy person's alveolar PCO_2 is about 40 mm Hg.

These relationships are described by the alveolar gas equation:

$$PAO_2 = [FIO_2 (Pb - PH_2O)] - (PaCO_2/R)$$

FIO_2 is the fraction of inspired oxygen—for example, breathing oxygen at room air with a concentration of 21% (an FIO_2 of 0.21). Pb represents barometric pressure (assumed to be 760 mm Hg at sea level), and PH_2O stands for water vapor pressure (which dilutes the dry oxygen content of the atmosphere, about 47 mm Hg). R represents the respiratory quotient (assumed to be 0.8). Thus the PAO_2 of a patient who breathes room air and has a PAO_2 of 40 mm Hg would be predicted as

$$PAO_2 = [0.21 (760 - 47)] - (40/0.8) = 100 \text{ mm Hg}$$

If a patient were breathing a gas mixture with an FIO_2 of 0.5, then the PAO_2 would be 306 mm Hg. The **alveolar-arterial oxygen gradient** is the difference between the predicted PAO_2 and the measured arterial PO_2 (PaO_2). This gradient may be used to assess the severity of impairment of gas exchange. For example, if a patient's blood gas had a PaO_2 of 100 mm Hg and a normal $PaCO_2$, then the alveolar-arterial gradient would be 206 mm Hg. Comparing this with a normal alveolar-arterial gradient of less than 10 mm Hg (for healthy young subjects breathing air at sea level), it is clear that this child's gas exchange is impaired. An alveolar-arterial gradient greater than 300 mm Hg while breathing an FIO_2 of 1.0 signifies a serious oxygenation problem, which may require mechanical ventilation.

Ventilation (V) is the amount of gas delivered to and exhaled from the lungs, and *perfusion (Q)* is the amount of mixed venous blood brought to the pulmonary capillary bed. Gas exchange is determined by both pulmonary ventilation and perfusion, and optimal gas exchange occurs if they are distributed in the same proportion to each other throughout the lungs, the *V/Q ratio*. There is a certain amount of nonuniformity in the distribution of ventilation and perfusion of normal lungs (Chapter 374). Respiratory diseases may cause a spectrum of pathologic derangement from the normal matching of ventilation to perfusion, termed *V/Q mismatch*. Compensatory mechanisms by which the lungs attempt to restore V/Q matching may not be adequate, resulting in ventilated but nonperfused alveoli (V/Q = infinity) and/or perfused but nonventilated alveoli (V/Q = zero).

Dead space ventilation occurs when the inspired gas is delivered to areas with no perfusion. There is an obligatory amount of normal anatomic dead space because inspired gas must traverse the nose, nasopharynx, trachea, and larger conducting airways. However, alveolar dead space occurs when alveoli are ventilated but not perfused. This results from a pathophysiologic process that impedes blood flow through the pulmonary capillary bed, such as pulmonary embolism, pulmonary hypotension, and obstructive lung disease (Chapter 377).

The volume of gas entering and leaving the mouth or nose per breath is the *tidal volume*. Alveolar ventilation, the volume of air entering and leaving the alveoli per minute, is defined by the equation

$$\text{Alveolar ventilation} = (\text{tidal volume} - \text{dead space}) \times \text{frequency}$$

Alveolar ventilation determines the rate of carbon dioxide excretion. Thus, diseases that cause increased dead space result in decreased alveolar ventilation, and unless the tidal volume or frequency of respiration increases enough to compensate, the Pa_{CO_2} will rise.

When alveoli are perfused but not ventilated, the effect is that this portion of the lung acts as an *intrapulmonary shunt*, with mixed venous blood being shunted to the systemic arterial circulation without coming into contact with any inspired gas. The resultant increase in carbon dioxide content of the arterial blood is usually handled by rapid buffering so the effect on $PaCO_2$ is negligible, but the dilution of oxygen content significantly lowers PaO_2. Therefore, diseases that cause increased intrapulmonary shunt cause hypoxemia. The hypoxemia associated with shunt can be severe and is often an indication for mechanical ventilation. Some examples of diseases increasing shunt are ARDS, pneumonia, pulmonary hemorrhage, and pulmonary edema.

Respiratory failure may be classified as due to either lung disease or respiratory pump dysfunction (Table 64–18). Lung diseases involve the airways, alveoli, or pulmonary circulation alone or in combination and result in hypoxemia. When lung disease leads to respiratory failure, patients have dyspnea, increased respiratory drive, and increased alveolar ventilation, which causes respiratory alkalosis unless the patient develops fatigue leading to failure of the respiratory pump as well. The coordinated activities of the CNS and the respiratory muscles act like a respiratory pump; failure can result from CNS, neuromuscular, or muscular dysfunction. Failure of the respiratory pump causes hypoventilation, a decrease in alveolar ventilation, and hypercarbia. Hypoxemia may also occur when the respiratory pump fails; it is treated with supplemental oxygen.

CLINICAL MANIFESTATIONS. Children with impending respiratory failure due to lung disease have respiratory distress characterized by rapid breathing or *tachypnea*; exaggerated use of accessory muscles, *retractions*, which may be much more striking in a child than in an adult because of the increased compliance of a child's chest wall; *nasal flaring*; and *grunting* due to closing of the glottis at the end of expiration to generate positive end-expiratory pressure. Impending respiratory failure caused by respiratory pump dysfunction may be more difficult to recognize because these children may not have any signs of respiratory distress. For example, a patient with a neuromuscular dysfunction such as muscular dystrophy or Werdnig-Hoffman disease may be weak, and the degree of retractions may not be obvious. Other causes of respiratory pump failure, such as a narcotic ingestion or a brain tumor, cause decreased ventilatory drive and hypoventilation. An abnormally low respiratory rate or the shallowness of the breathing may identify these children.

DIAGNOSIS. Severe respiratory distress in children is usually diagnosed by history and physical examination, and very severe distress may need treatment initiated before performing diagnostic procedures or tests. Some of these patients may not tolerate procedures such as an arterial puncture for a blood gas determination or a radiologic study; a change into an uncomfortable position may make it more difficult to breathe. It may be best to leave patients in their position of greatest comfort, provide supplemental oxygen by face mask, and use aerosolized treatments. If these measures are not tolerated and do not result in improvement, then endotracheal intubation is required to secure the airway (see Chapter 64.1).

LABORATORY FINDINGS. Although the clinical presentation may require immediate intubation and mechanical ventilation, for

TABLE 64–18 Anatomic Classification of Respiratory Failure

Lung		Respiratory Pump	
Central airway obstruction	Tracheomalacia	Chest wall deformity	Kyphoscoliosis
	Subglottic stenosis		Diaphragmatic hernia
	Epiglottitis		Flail chest
	Croup		Eventration of diaphragm
	Vocal cord paralysis		Prune-belly syndrome
	Foreign body aspiration		
	Vascular ring		
	Adenotonsillar hypertrophy		
	Near-strangulation		
Peripheral airway obstruction	Bronchiolitis	Brain stem	Sleep apnea
	Asthma		Poisoning
	Aspiration		Trauma
	Cystic fibrosis		Central nervous system infection
	Bronchomalacia		
Diffuse alveolar damage (adult respiratory distress syndrome)	Sepsis	Spinal cord	Trauma
	Pneumonia		Poliomyelitis
	Pulmonary edema		Werdnig-Hoffmann disease
	Near-drowning	Neuromuscular	Postoperative nerve injury
	Pulmonary embolism		Birth trauma
	Lung contusion		Infantile botulism
	Shock		Guillain-Barré syndrome

Adapted from Helfaer M, Nichols D, Rogers M: Developmental physiology of the respiratory system. In: *Rogers MC (ed): Textbook of Pediatric Intensive Care, 2nd ed. Baltimore, Williams & Wilkins, 1992, pp 104–133.*

the majority of children it is possible and helpful to first obtain an arterial blood sample to analyze blood gas tensions (Pa_{O_2} and Pa_{CO_2}) and acid-base status (Chapters 52 and 374) and initiate noninvasive monitoring by pulse oximetry. Hypoxemic respiratory failure is defined as a Pa_{O_2} less than 60 mm Hg with F_{IO_2} greater than 0.6 (in the absence of cyanotic heart disease), and hypercarbic respiratory failure is defined as an acute Pa_{CO_2} greater than 50 mm Hg (see Chapter 416 about chronic hypercapnia). In addition to blood gases obtained at single points in time, the decision to initiate mechanical ventilation should take into account the cause of the respiratory failure, the possibility of reversing the cause of the failure via other interventions, and the overall trend in a patient's clinical status. For example, a patient with respiratory pump failure due to narcotic overdose may have an acute Pa_{CO_2} greater than 50 mm Hg but should respond quickly to administration of a narcotic antagonist and may never require ventilatory support. Conversely, a patient whose lung disease results in hypoxemia and dyspnea that seem adequately treated with supplemental oxygen may have an initially lower than normal Pa_{CO_2} (i.e., respiratory alkalosis). However, if this patient fatigues, an acute rise in the Pa_{CO_2} may indicate impending respiratory failure even if the Pa_{CO_2} is still less than 50 mm Hg.

TREATMENT. Respiratory arrest or repeated apnea requires immediate respiratory support. Severe shock also may require mechanical ventilation, even if arterial blood gases are within acceptable range, because patients need increased oxygen delivery to vital organs. Patients in shock often have respiratory distress due to metabolic acidosis, and the work of breathing and lactic acid production may be ameliorated by ventilatory support. Acute neurologic compromise may require ventilatory support for inadequate or absent ventilation, for loss of protective airway reflexes (cough and gag), or for therapeutic hyperventilation. Intubation and airway management are discussed in Chapters 58 and 64.1. Mechanical ventilation is discussed in Chapter 64.4.

64.4 *Mechanical Ventilation*

(also see Chapter 377)

Melinda T. Derish and Lorry R. Frankel

The complexity and variety of commercially available mechanical ventilators suitable for pediatric use continue to increase. Therefore, a basic understanding of the indications for using this treatment, the basics of management, and terminology (Table 64–19) are presented.

UNDERLYING CONCEPTS AND TERMINOLOGY. Since the 1960s, positive pressure ventilators have been predominately used in adult, pediatric, and neonatal ICUs, and this discussion focuses on these ventilators. During positive pressure mechanical ventilation, the flow of gas during inspiration and exhalation is driven by the airway pressure gradient between the airway opening and the alveoli. Pressure may be administered at the airway opening by a tight-fitting mask connected to a ventilator, mask CPAP (continuous positive airway pressure); to a compressible bag attached to a gas source, bag-mask ventilation; or to both mask BI-PAP (bilevel airway pressure). In a PICU setting, ventilator support is most frequently provided via intubation of the trachea, usually with an endotracheal tube and, on occasion, with a tracheostomy cannula. The endotracheal tube adapter, which attaches to the ventilator tubing, is considered the airway opening. During inspiration, the airway opening pressure is greater than alveolar pressure, thereby driving gas into the lungs and inflating them. Exhalation is usually passive and occurs because, at the end of inspiration, alveolar pressure becomes greater than airway pressure.

TABLE 64–19 Commonly Used Abbreviations for Ventilator Terminology

F_{IO_2}	Fraction of inspired oxygen (% oxygen)
IT	Inspiratory time (I time seconds)
I:E	Inspiratory to expiratory ratio (I:E)
FRC	Functional residual capacity (mL)
PIP	Peak inspiratory pressure (cm H_2O)
PEEP	Positive end-expiratory pressure (cm H_2O)
SIMV	Synchronized intermittent mandatory ventilation
VT	Tidal volume (mL)

TABLE 64–20 Comparison of Pressure-Controlled and Volume-Controlled Ventilation

Pressure-Controlled Ventilation	Volume-Controlled Ventilation
Constant pressure delivered	Constant volume (VT) delivered; less risk of hypoventilation or hyperventilation
Variable volume delivered; reduced risk of barotrauma	Variable pressure (PIP) delivered
Changes in patient's compliance or resistance may lead to alterations in delivered volumes as pressure remains constant	Changes in patient's compliance or resistance leads to potential for dangerously high inflating volume delivered (requires closer monitoring of tidal volume and carbon dioxide, as well as pressure alarms)
Changes in tidal pressures may result in changes in minute ventilation	

Pressures. Peak inspiratory pressure (PIP) occurs during inspiration. Positive end-expiratory pressure (PEEP) helps maintain the end-expiratory resting lung volume. Thus, the maximum pressure gradient is the difference between PIP and PEEP. The mean airway pressure is a measure of the average pressure to which the lungs are exposed during the respiratory cycle. Mean airway pressure can be increased by increasing PEEP, PIP, the ratio of inspiratory time to expiratory time (I:E ratio), or the inspiratory flow. Adjusting the ventilator to increase mean airway pressure is the therapy for hypoxemia that is not responding to an increasing F_{IO_2}. This probably improves oxygenation by decreasing the number of collapsed alveoli or redistributing lung fluid.

Components of the Ventilator Breath. Each complete ventilator breath has an allotted time for inspiration (I time) before the ventilator must cycle into exhalation time (E time). The sum of the I time and E time equals the allotted time per breath. The ventilator delivers a set number of breaths per minute, the ventilator frequency. The frequency determines the length of each breath. For example, a frequency of 20 would result in 3 sec/breath. Most ventilators allow setting either the I time or the I:E ratio. For example, if an I time of 1 sec is ordered and the breath is 3 sec, the I:E ratio will be 1 sec:2 sec. If an I:E ratio of 1:3 is ordered, then the I time would be 0.75 sec, and the E time would be 2.25 sec.

The change in lung volume during the inspiratory period is defined as the tidal volume (VT). It is the volume above the functional residual capacity (FRC)—that is, the volume above the end-expiratory lung volume. By convention, the gas flow is in units of L/sec and the I time is in seconds; however, in pediatrics the VT is usually expressed in mL rather than as fractions of a liter. From the alveolar gas equation, to adjust Pa_{CO_2}, either the VT or the ventilator frequency is changed (Chapter 64.3).

Pressure-Controlled vs Volume-Controlled Ventilation. These are the two primary forms of positive pressure ventilators (Table 64–20). Pressure-controlled ventilators allow a clinician to set the PIP and PEEP. The increase in airway pressure occurs swiftly at the initiation of inspiration to achieve the set PIP. This PIP is then maintained throughout the I time. In pressure-controlled ventilation, the lung volume rises until it reaches its capacity at that PIP or until the ventilator cycles into exhalation. Thus, VT is not set but rather is determined by both the pressure gradient of the ventilator and the pulmonary mechanics of the patient. In volume-controlled ventilation, the VT is preset as a product of setting flow and I time. The airway pressure rises throughout inspiration and reaches its peak when the entire VT has been delivered. Thus, PIP is not set but rather is determined by both the VT and the pulmonary mechanics of the patient.

Ventilator-Patient Interactions. When children are not attempting to breathe spontaneously, the ventilator completely controls the respiratory pattern. For children who can attempt to breathe, the degree to which a ventilator is able to synchronize with the patient's own respiratory efforts may have significant clinical repercussions. Patients whose lung disease is improving and who thus are receiving less sedation in an attempt to wean from ventilator support may find that when they need to, they are unable to draw a breath, thereby experiencing air hunger. Patients also may experience anxiety as gas is pushed into their airway while they are trying to exhale. This dyssynchrony often necessitates pharmacologic interventions with sedation or paralytic agents, which may result in prolonged intubation and ventilation. Patient-ventilator dyssynchrony may also cause barotrauma or pressure injury to the lungs. Advances in mechanical ventilation have attempted to improve patient-ventilator synchronization.

Synchronized Intermittent Mandatory Ventilation (SIMV). SIMV is a ventilator mode that was developed to allow better response by the ventilator to the patient. During SIMV, the ventilator allows the child to trigger a breath by spontaneously attempting to inspire. However, if the patient takes too long to initiate a spontaneous breath, then inspiration is time triggered by the ventilator, a mandatory breath. The determination of how long is too long is a function of the ventilator frequency. Ventilator frequency determines the total time allotted per breath, and some percentage of that time is the window allowed for the patient to initiate inspiration. If the patient does not spontaneously try to breathe during this window of time, then the ventilator initiates inspiration. SIMV may be either volume controlled or pressure controlled. A patient may also breathe spontaneously more often than the set frequency of SIMV, inspiring fresh gas from the circuit, but these breaths are not assisted by the ventilator at the volume or pressure that is ordered for the SIMV breaths.

Despite refinements in triggering based on sensing small changes in pressure or flow, SIMV does not allow for complete spontaneous ventilation. Patients trigger inspiration, but they cannot control when inspiration ends and the ventilator cycles to expiration. Patients cannot control the I time of the ventilator-assisted breaths, even though they can control the I time of the nonassisted breaths in between. The **pressure support mode** allows for spontaneous breathing by patients. The ventilator assists every breath a child initiates by applying a predetermined amount of airway pressure above the set PEEP. A child can control the rate of breathing and the duration of inspiration, so the breathing pattern may truly be called spontaneous. Many ventilators allow both pressure support and SIMV. The pressure support breaths can occur whenever a child attempts to inspire, unless the patient is breathing within that window of time that results in an SIMV breath.

Monitoring and Alarms. What is not controllable is monitored. In pressure-controlled ventilation, the VT is monitored. In volume-controlled ventilation, the airway pressure is monitored; safety precautions include pop-off limits to the peak airway pressure. An oxygen analyzer allows monitoring of FiO_2.

Alarms can be set for a wide array of events. The common alarms are for high or low airway pressure, absence of flow (apnea), loss of electrical power, high or low exhaled VT, and high or low minute volume. When alarms occur, they must then be evaluated to determine if there is a malfunction of the ventilator or a change in the patient. The importance of frequent physical examination cannot be overemphasized; it is the fastest means of diagnosing a variety of ventilator problems, such as patient-ventilator dyssynchrony, endotracheal tube obstruction, and accidental extubation.

APPROACH TO MECHANICAL VENTILATION. The pressure gradient that inflates the lungs must overcome the pulmonary mechanics of the patient's respiratory system. See Chapter 377 for discussion of compliance, resistance, and time constant of the respiratory system. Respiratory diseases result in decreased lung compliance or increased airway resistance or a combination of both. Ventilator strategies are designed to ameliorate physiologic derangements and resulting ventilation-perfusion mismatch.

Diseases of Decreased Compliance. Compliance is decreased in various diseases that affect the lung parenchyma, such as ARDS, atelectasis, pneumonia, pulmonary edema, pulmonary hemorrhage, and RDS. In all of these diseases, FRC is reduced as terminal air spaces are flooded or collapsed, due to the presence of abnormal fluid within the alveoli or atelectasis from the decreased amount of surfactant lining the alveoli. These alveoli are more difficult to inflate. Also, intrapulmonary shunt is increased as blood flows to poorly ventilated lung units. Thus, one goal of mechanical ventilation when lung compliance is decreased is to decrease shunting by improving ventilation to the perfused lung units. The ventilator approach to decreased FRC is to increase mean airway pressure in order to recruit atelectatic areas of lung; this increase is usually achieved by higher PEEPs, although higher PIPs also increase mean airway pressure.

Decreased compliance requires a higher pressure gradient to achieve a given (VT). This means that with volume-controlled ventilation, the PIP will be higher than it would for a patient with normal lungs. If the ventilator is pressure controlled, then a given PIP may result in a VT that will be lower than that of a patient with normal lungs. Diseases that decrease compliance also may respond to higher ventilator rates as the lungs empty and fill more quickly. If neither ventilator pressure nor rate is increased sufficiently to compensate for decreased compliance, then hypercarbia develops.

Diseases of Increased Resistance. Resistance is increased in various diseases that decrease the caliber of the airway lumen by edema, spasm, or obstructing material. Because airways decrease in caliber during exhalation, increased resistance affects expiratory flow more than inspiratory flow. Diseases in which airway resistance is increased include asthma, bronchiolitis, bronchopulmonary dysplasia, and cystic fibrosis.

Diseases of increased resistance are often accompanied by both increased intrapulmonary shunt and dead space ventilation. Shunt occurs if the increased resistance greatly impedes gas flow, decreasing ventilation to alveoli that remain perfused. Dead space ventilation occurs if the increased resistance leads to gas trapping in areas of the lung that contain hyperinflated alveoli. These areas of hyperinflated lung units exert pressure on the surrounding structures, and this results in a reduction of pulmonary capillary blood flow. The increases in both shunt and dead space mean that these diseases produce both significant hypoxemia and hypercarbia. Increased resistance requires that a higher pressure must occur for the flow of gas to reach the terminal air sacs. Therefore, if volume-controlled ventilation is used, an increase in PIP is required to deliver a given VT. If pressure-controlled ventilation is used, tidal volume is lower than in a normal lung at the same pressure.

Increased resistance may result in significant increases in time constant (see Chapters 375 and 377), unless there is a proportional decrease in compliance, which rarely happens in diseases of increased resistance. A longer time constant (time necessary for gas to fill or empty the alveoli) necessitates long I and E times. Therefore, these lung diseases may be adversely affected if the ventilator frequency is too high and the expiratory and inspiratory times are too short. This results in a phenomenon known as gas trapping as the ventilator cycles back into inspiration before the lung has had sufficient time

TABLE 64–21 Guidelines for Initiating Mechanical Ventilation

	Normal Lungs	Decreased Compliance	Increased Resistance
Tidal volume (VT)	8–12 mL/kg (set of volume-controlled and derived if pressure-controlled ventilation)	10–12 mL/kg (may need to use less if the inflating pressures are too high; i.e., risk for volutrauma)	10–12 mL/kg (may need to use less volume if the inflating pressures required are too high; i.e., barotrauma)
Rate (breaths/min)	Physiologic norm for age or lower (depending on the VT used; e.g. infant rate = 30, toddler rate = 20, adolescent rate = 16)	May require higher rates to maintain adequate minute ventilation	Often requires lower rates to allow adequate emptying time
Peak airway pressure PIP (cm H_2O)	Initial PIP = 20–25 cm H_2O; monitor for adequate chest expansion and VT	May require higher PIP to obtain acceptable VT	May require higher PIP to obtain acceptable VT
Positive end-expiratory pressure (PEEP)	2–4 cm H_2O to prevent atelectasis	Frequently requires higher PEEP to achieve oxygenation and improved compliance (e.g., 6–10 cm H_2O) Anticipate decreased venous return and cardiac output	May need to maintain low PEEP to avoid exacerbation of gas trapping and overinflation
Oxygen concentration (FIO_2)	May not need supplemental oxygen; however, one usually begins with FIO_2 of 1.0 and may then quickly wean to an FIO_2 ≤0.5	Begin with an FIO_2 of 1.0 Attempt to wean to ≤0.6 by adjusting mean airway pressure/ PEEP	Begin with an FIO_2 of 1, wean to maintain adequate oxygenation and avoid oxygen toxicity
Inspiratory time (I time)	Normal for age I:E = 1:2, 1:3	Generous I time to allow recruitment of collapsed lung segments (e.g., 1:1.2)	Ensure adequate I time and E time, especially E time, to avoid gas trapping (e.g., I:E of 1:3 or 1:4)

to empty. The ventilator breaths stack on each other as more and more gas is trapped, resulting in an increase in the FRC. This eventually leads to lung hyperinflation and reduction in compliance.

Initial Settings. When initiating mechanical ventilation, there are three approaches: providing support for lungs that function normally, for diseases of decreased compliance, or for diseases of increased resistance (Table 64–21). *For supporting normal lungs,* ventilator frequency may be slightly lower than the normal respiratory rate for age because ventilator VT is usually set higher than a healthy person's VT of 5–7 mL/kg. The customary range for ventilator VT has been 10–15 mL/kg. This larger size of a breath was believed to prevent atelectasis in patients who received ventilator support. This practice may not be suitable for longer-term ventilation or for ventilating diseased lungs; a VT of 8–10 mL/kg is more appropriate. For pressure-controlled ventilation, an initial PIP of 20–25 H_2O is usually sufficient to move an adequate VT, but this must be immediately assessed by observation of chest expansion and measurement of VT.

To initiate *support for diseases of decreased compliance,* mean airway pressures need to be higher. A higher PEEP is often used to achieve this. PEEP is titrated upward in an attempt to provide adequate oxygenation at an FIO_2 less than 0.6. If volume-controlled ventilation is used, the PIP may be much greater than for normal lungs, and clinicians must pay close attention to pressure alarms. If pressure-controlled ventilation is used, the initial PIP may need to exceed 30 cm H_2O. The VT has to be closely monitored. Significant hypoxemia results from these diseases, and it is customary to start with an FIO_2 of 100% and then reduce it as one attempts to avoid oxygen toxicity. The ventilator frequency may be set higher than normal because a decreased time constant permits a faster rate. A common I time is 0.8–1 sec.

Diseases of increased resistance often have very high time constants. Ventilator frequency may need to be set as low as 12–16 breaths/min in severe status asthmaticus to allow adequate I and E times. It is also customary to try to minimize PEEP to 2–3 cm H_2O in these diseases to minimize risk of gas trapping.

Complications. There are many complications of mechanical ventilation, and they may affect organ systems in addition to the pulmonary system. Lung injury may result from positive pressure *(barotrauma), oxygen toxicity,* or excessive volume changes in the lung—volutrauma. Volutrauma may be manifested acutely as pulmonary air leak, such as pneumothoraces, pnemomediastinum, pulmonary interstitial emphysema, and bronchopleural fistula. Volutrauma may also be a cause of chronic repetitive lung injury, exacerbating the primary disease. This may result from subjecting alveolar units to repeated overdistention, such as with excessive VT, or to cyclic collapse and re-expansion, such as with insufficient PEEP to stabilize the resting lung volume. In diseases of decreased compliance, the lung units of higher compliance may receive more of the VT than the less compliant units, leading to volutrauma of the healthier segments of lung. This mechanism may contribute to the chronic lung injury that can develop in ARDS. In diseases of increased resistance, the lung units with higher resistance need more time to fill and empty. This leads to overfilling of the lung units with lower resistance and time constants and to gas trapping and overdistention of the alveoli in the high time constant units with severely obstructed airways.

Positive pressure ventilation also may have effects on the cardiovascular system. Some portion of the mean airway pressure is transmitted through the lungs and raises intrathoracic pressure. This may impede venous return and decrease right ventricular filling. Elevated intrathoracic pressure also may compress the pulmonary circulation and increase the afterload on the right ventricle, which may cause the interventricular septum to shift toward the left ventricle, resulting in a decrease in volume of the left ventricle and a reduction in left ventricular stroke volume. Alternatively, elevations in intrathoracic pressure may cause an afterload reduction for the left ventricle. The net result of these many cardiovascular effects may be beneficial or detrimental, depending on the overall cardiovascular status of the child. In general, high mean airway pressures require close observation for possible hemodynamic compromise and may necessitate support with fluids and inotropic drugs (see Chapter 64.2).

An endotracheal tube may obstruct owing to purulent material or blood or from the child biting on the tube. These are immediately life-threatening complications. An endotracheal tube also may cause injury to the tracheal mucosa, resulting in subglottic stenosis, which is usually not symptomatic until the endotracheal tube is removed. Subglottic stenosis may resolve with time or may ultimately require surgical intervention (Chapter 387).

Prolonged intubation and mechanical ventilation may result in nosocomial infections, often by bacteria with resistance to numerous antibiotics. Nosocomial infection, sepsis, and other organ system failures are the leading cause of death of patients with respiratory failure.

Chatburn RL: A new system for understanding mechanical ventilators. Respir Care 36:1123, 1991.
Ciszek TA, Modanlou HD, Owings D, et al: Mean airway pressure: Significance during mechanical ventilation in neonates. J Pediatr 99:121, 1981.
Fuhrmann BP, Hernan LJ, Papa MC: Conventional mechanical ventilation. *In:* Dieckmann RA, Fiser DH, Selbst SM (eds): Pediatric Emergency and Critical Care Procedures. St. Louis, Mosby–Year Book, 1997, pp 138–147.
Kacmarek RM, Hess D: Basic principles of ventilator machinery. *In:* Tobin MJ (ed): Principles and Practice of Mechanical Ventilation. New York, McGraw-Hill, 1994, pp 65–110.
Lee PC, Helsmoortel CM, Cohn SM, et al: Are low tidal volumes safe? Chest 97:425, 1990.
Levitzky MG (ed): Pulmonary Physiology. New York, McGraw-Hill, 1991, pp 12–104.
Nunn JF (ed): Nunn's Applied Respiratory Physiology, 4th ed. Oxford, Butterworth-Heinemann 1993, pp 156–197.
Parker JC, Hernandez LA, Peevey KJ: Mechanisms of ventilator-induced lung injury. Crit Care Med 21:131, 1993.
Paulson TE, Spear RM, Peterson BM: New concepts in the treatment of children with acute respiratory distress syndrome. J Pediatr 127:163, 1995.

64.5 *Renal Stabilization*

Joseph V. DiCarlo

ETIOLOGY AND EPIDEMIOLOGY. Renal function is often significantly affected by critical illness that does not involve intrinsic renal disease. Renal dysfunction to some degree is frequently encountered but of little consequence, but renal failure in children is most commonly due to shock, sepsis, hypoxia, or nephrotoxic medications. Also see Chapter 543. Severe congenital heart disease is a risk factor for life-threatening renal cortical and medullary necrosis, resulting from renal ischemia. In a series of infants with renal hypoperfusion and ischemic injury, 50% had congenital heart disease, 30% had asphyxial shock or sepsis, and only 1 (of 82) had gastroenteritis and dehydration. There was no association between the renal lesions and the use of radiographic contrast medium. Although renal failure rarely occurs after gastroenteritis and dehydration in children, it can occur as a consequence of hemolytic-uremic syndrome (see Chapter 526). Renal insufficiency or failure associated with hepatic failure or hepatorenal syndrome may also require intensive care. Finally, obstructive uropathy is a potential cause of renal failure necessitating PICU admission.

STRATEGIES TO IMPROVE RENAL FUNCTION. Although oliguria is common in the PICU and may be associated with poor outcomes, often only fluids or low doses of diuretics are needed for correction. In patients with oliguric renal failure, adequate intravascular fluid volumes estimated by the heart rate (within 20% of normal for age) and central venous pressure (at least 4–9 cm H_2O) should be maintained. In addition to treating the underlying cause, loop diuretics may be helpful.

Loop diuretics are commonly used to improve fluid balance in critically ill children. However, tolerance to the effects of the diuretic may require large bolus doses or changing drugs. Some children who demonstrate little effect from furosemide respond to bumetanide. Continuous infusion of loop diuretics may decrease dosage requirements, improve response, and minimize adverse effects. Loop diuretics are often used in the hope of decreasing lung water in children with capillary leak syndrome (e.g., ARDS, septic shock), but the effect is often modest.

Atrial natriuretic factor (ANF), a naturally occurring peptide hormone released in the atria in response to increased atrial filling volumes, has arterial vasodilating effects, especially in the renal vascular bed. Its potential effectiveness in children with fluid overload has not been established.

In the rare instance that renal failure is caused by (or is impending from) a circulating nephrotoxin or substance that might obstruct the renal tubules (e.g., myoglobin), *forced diuresis* may be beneficial. Crystalloid is infused at up to two times the maintenance rate, followed by mannitol (0.5 g/kg) and/or furosemide (0.5 mg/kg) every 4 hr. However, high infusion rates pose the risk of pulmonary edema, and mannitol may cause kidney damage if allowed to crystallize in the interstitium.

VASOACTIVE MEDICATIONS AND RENAL PRESERVATION. Although vasopressor agents can theoretically reduce renal blood flow by causing vasconstriction, renal blood flow and function usually improve when renal perfusion pressure is increased during shock by the infusion of vasopressors. Dopamine at doses of 1–3 μg/kg/min often improves urine output and natriuresis, probably as a result of a direct effect on renal tuules and splanchnic dilatation. However, little evidence shows that dopamine prevents acute renal failure or improves patient outcome.

RENAL REPLACEMENT THERAPIES. See Chapters 543 and 544. Continuous venovenous hemofiltration (CVVH) is the modality of choice for renal replacement therapy in critically ill children. Hemofiltration is usually performed through double-lumen venous catheters, with circulation through the circuit effected by a blood roller-pump fitted with an air trap. Circuit integrity is maintained even during temporary periods of hypotension, which reduces clotting. CVVH is usually more appropriate than conventional hemodialysis in unstable patients because lower blood flows are needed (usually 10 mL/kg/min) and the membranes used may be more biocompatible than the standard hemodialysis membrane. Reasonably high clearances can be obtained during continuous hemodialysis or hemodiafiltration, even in severely catabolic, septic patients. Countercurrent dialysate flow improves clearance rates, and well-designed replacement solutions can correct acidosis and electrolyte imbalances. CVVH may be beneficial in the management of systemic inflammation (e.g., in septic shock or ARDS). The filter removes all substances below a molecular weight of 17,000 that are not protein bound; many proinflammatory substances are of this size or smaller.

Alklgren RL, et al: Anaritide in acute tubular necrosis. N Engl J Med 336:828, 1997.
Bersten AD: Vasoactive drugs and the importance of renal perfusion pressure. New Horiz 3:650, 1995.
Bhimma R: Post-dysenteric hemolytic uremic syndrome in children during an epidemic of Shigella dysentery in Kwazulu/Natal. Pediatr Nephrol 11:560, 1997.
DePriest J: Reversing oliguria in critically ill patients. Postgrad Med 102:245, 1997.
Stewart CL: Acute renal failure in infants, children and adults. Crit Care Clin 13:575, 1997.

64.6 *Nutritional Stabilization*

Joseph V. DiCarlo

Critically ill children need nutritional support to ameliorate negative nitrogen balance resulting from catabolism (Table 64–22). Also see Chapter 42. Carbohydrate (glucose infusion of 3–5 mg/kg/min) also is given to inhibit the breakdown of endogenous protein. Generally, 70% of calories should be derived from carbohydrates and 30% from lipids. It is often difficult to deliver adequate calories to critically ill children because of enteral intolerance or restrictions in fluid volumes, but the caloric goals should be attained within the first week of hospitalization.

TABLE 64–22 Caloric and Protein Requirements in the Critically Ill Child

Critical illness	25–30 kcal/kg/24 hr
Mechanical ventilation	20–25 kcal/kg/24 hr
Receiving growth hormone	15–20 kcal/kg/24 hr as carbohydrate
Burn or trauma	40–45 kcal/kg/24 hr
Protein	1.5–2.5 g/kg/24 hr
Protein (burn >20%)	2.0–3.0 g/kg/24 hr

Amino acids should be provided in reasonable amounts, in any form (1.5 g/kg in older children, 2.0 g/kg in infants). Adequate amounts of glutamine, alanine, and the essential amino acids should be included, but branched-chain amino acids (leucine, cysteine, valine, and lysine) do not confer any special benefit.

Vitamins, particularly water-soluble vitamins B complex and C, are best administered enterally. Vitamin deficiencies, however, can develop even in children receiving parenteral nutrition (e.g. thiamine deficiency leading to Wernicke's encephalopathy and riboflavin deficiency). Essential minerals and trace elements including zinc, magnesium, and selenium should also be provided.

Rarely, growth factors are administered, especially growth hormone. Growth hormone may be beneficial to debilitated children having difficulty in weaning from mechanical ventilation.

ENTERAL FEEDING. Early enteral feeding in critically ill children, particularly those with sepsis, may avert ulcerative complications, preserve the indigenous intestinal flora, avoid overgrowth by pathogens, and prevent atrophy of the mucosa. Normal flora also may be restored, in part, by the administration of *Acidophilus*. If the stomach is relatively atonic, early feeding may be accomplished through a weighted tube passed through the pyloris into the jejunum; fluoroscopic guidance or placement via endoscopy may be necessary. However, septic patients often have ilieus that precludes enteral nutrition and only responds to time (3–7 days).

PARENTERAL NUTRITION. If the gastrointestinal tract cannot be used, parenteral nutrition is necessary. Conversion of maintenance intravenous fluids to parenteral nutrition is often indicated by the 2nd or 3rd day of hospitalization. There is no need to administer amino acids gradually, although protein restriction may be indicated for renal failure.

OVERFEEDING. Excessive intake of carbohydrates is manifested as hyperglycemia, which may result in hyperosmolarity, osmotic diuresis, and dehydration. Subsequently, increased carbon dioxide production and an increase in the respiratory quotient may tax an already compromised respiratory system. Excessive administration of lipids can produce hypertriglyceridemia, fatty liver, and steatorrhea and can make patients prone to infection.

IMMUNOMODULATION THROUGH DIET. Unfed patients, in general, have the highest complication rate. Attempts to enhance immune function through dietary supplementation with glutamine, arginine, omega-3 fatty acids, and nucleotides have failed to demonstrate benefit.

DeBiasse MA, Wilmore DW: What is optimal nutritional support? New Horiz 2:122, 1994.

Sear M: Thiamine, riboflavin, and pyridoxine deficiencies in a population of critically ill children. J Pediatr 121:533, 1992.

Squires RH, Mize CE: Total Enteral Nutrition. *In:* Levin DL, Morriss FC (eds): Essentials of Pediatric Intensive Care, 2nd ed. New York, Churchill Livingstone, 1997, pp 1637–1646.

Squires RH, Mize CE: Total Parenteral Nutrition. *In:* Levin DL, Morriss FC (eds): Essentials of Pediatric Intensive Care, 2nd ed. New York, Churchill Livingstone, 1997, pp 1629–1636.

Wells CL, Erlandsen SL: Bacterial translocation: Association with intestinal epithelial permeability. *In:* Gut Dysfunction in Critical Illness. Rombeau JL, Takala J (eds): New York, Springer-Verlag, 1996, pp 131–149.

64.7 Neurologic Stabilization

Joseph V. DiCarlo and Lorry R. Frankel

Acute neurologic deterioration in children may be a life-threatening event with numerous causes and diverse clinical presentations. Children with an evolving neurologic illness must be quickly stabilized to avoid further injury to the brain. The initial insult produces the "primary injury" to the brain, which gives rise to the various signs and symptoms with which a patient presents. Failure to recognize the intial injury and its clinical manifestations may put a child at significant risk for further secondary injury. The most common causes of global neurologic dysfunction in children are head trauma, hypoxia-ischemia, CNS infection, and encephalopathies due to endogenous metabolites or exogenous toxins. Rarely, idiopathic status epilepticus also can cause a moderate or severe encephalopathy (Chapter 602). Finally, global neurologic dysfunction, coupled with focal signs, may be a late presentation of a CNS tumor (Chapter 611).

Coma, stupor, and lethargy are general findings suggestive of an advancing process that has global CNS implications. Focal findings may reflect a well-defined process localized to one part of the brain. *Coma* is a state in which patients are unable to be aroused or respond to noxious stimuli and are completely unaware of themselves and surroundings. *Stupor* may be confused with normal sleep, but the child can be aroused with painful stimuli. *Lethargy* is subjective and indicates drowsiness or decreased wakefulness; these patients may be confused but are able to communicate.

CLINICAL MANIFESTATIONS

Head Trauma. This diagnosis usually is fairly obvious (Chapter 692). A child occasionally presents with chronic or acute intracranial bleeding due to abuse (Chapter 35). A head CT scan is indicated to identify subdural and epidural hematoma, effusions, punctate intracerebral hemorrhages, skull fractures, atrophy, or hydrocephalus.

Hypoxia-Ischemia. Also see Chapters 95.7 and 607. Encephalopathy due to poor or absent cerebral circulatory perfusion often heralds a poor outcome, especially if the child has experienced a period of asystole and required CPR, as may occur after near drowning episodes, near-miss sudden infant death syndrome, and other life-threatening events. The lack of oxygen supply produces primary neuronal damage. Further, secondary injury may result from mediators that activate a cascade of events through glutamate receptors leading to cell death. As a child's clinical course progresses, imaging studies may be helpful in evaluating the structural brain damage commonly accompanying hypoxic-ischemic encephalopathy. The brain stem is often preserved after this type of injury, but other organ systems (the liver, intestines, and heart) may reflect hypoxic-ischemic injury. The prognosis for children who require significant support of the functions of other organ systems is poor.

Central Nervous System Infection. CNS infections include meningitis, meningoencephalitis, and brain abscess. See Chapters 174.1, 174.2, and 610. Viruses and bacteria are the most common causes, but with immunosuppression the frequency of fungal infections is increasing (Chapter 179). Stupor, coma, or status epilepticus is particularly associated with herpes encephalitis and bacterial abscess with mass effect but may occur with any CNS infection. A CNS infection should be considered with any acute neurologic deterioration associated with fever, signs of meningeal irritation, and an elevated white blood cell count. Complications of acute neurologic infections include vascular infarcts, cerebritis, cranial nerve compression, development of hydrocephalus, and subdural effusion.

Encephalopathies from Endogenous Metabolites or Exogenous Toxins. Profound encephalopathy with obtundation, stupor, or coma may result from metabolic defects (e.g., those that result in hyperammonemia), fulminant hepatic failure (in which NH_3 acts as a marker of other neurodepressant toxins), hypoglycemia (Chapter 88), diabetic katoacidosis (Chapter 599.2), or ingestion of certain drugs or substances (Chapter 722). A child who has an altered level of consciousness without a clear explanation should have a toxicology screen. Other helpful laboratory tests include electrolytes, glucose, blood gases, and serum osmolarity.

Status Epilepticus. Severe status epilepticus may result in stupor or coma and has the potential for permanent cellular damage, if the seizures are prolonged or associated with hypoxia, hypercarbia, and hypotension. Intensive therapies are aimed at halting the seizure activity. See Chapter 602.

Intracranial Hypertension. This often presents first as headache and confusion and then advances to combativeness, somnolence, and coma if not treated. It may occur as a complication of either global or focal encephalopathies. See Chapter 607. An increase in the volume of the cranial contents within the rigid cranial bony cavity produces an increase in intracranial pressure (ICP). As the ICP increases, the effective cerebral perfusion pressure decreases (see Chapter 600). Cerebral perfusion pressure is equal to the mean arterial pressure minus the ICP. Autoregulation of the cerebral vasculature provides the initial protection to maintain cerebral perfusion by increasing BP. However, as the ICP increases, autoregulation may be lost and cerebral blood flow decreased. This may result in significant secondary neuronal injury and even herniation. Intracranial hypertension may initially mimic global encephalopathy with increasing confusion and combativeness that progress to coma and eventual brain stem findings. These are late signs of increased ICP and indicate that herniation of brain structures is occurring, a life-threatening event requiring immediate intervention.

Herniation. Coma may precede herniation of intracranial contents as brain stem herniation proceeds from higher to lower brain centers. Coma is followed by decorticate rigidity, small pupils, and Cheyne-Stokes breathing. As the midbrain and pons become involved, posturing is decerebrate, pupils are midposition and nonreactive, and the breathing pattern is hyperpneic. As the medulla is compromised, the BP and heart rate fluctuate greatly, the patient becomes flaccid, and breathing is irregular and then absent. Uncal herniation may be heralded by ipsilateral anisocoria, loss of pupillary reflexes, and ptosis caused by compression of the third cranial nerve. Later stages of uncal herniation are the same as described earlier. Also see Chapter 611.

Infratentorial Lesions. Lesions in the infratentorial region can cause coma, cranial nerve palsies, and respiratory abnormalities at an early stage of disease. Obstructive hydrocephalus may result from compression of the circulatory and cerebrospinal fluid pathways. This is noted with posterior fossa tumors that may produce brain stem compression without the degree of encephalopathy previously described. The hallmark of infratentorial herniation is early respiratory and autonomic impairment; pupillary responses may be preserved.

TREATMENT OF GLOBAL NEUROLOGIC DYSFUNCTION

Normalize the Circulation and Respiration. The basics of neurologic stabilization include the ABC's and maintenance of adequate oxygenation and perfusion during the various diagnostic tests that must be performed. The decision to intubate and institute mechanical ventilation depends on the need to stabilize respiration and protect the upper airway from aspiration. Although a stuporous child's respiratory drive may be intact, the gag or cough reflex may be absent or upper airway muscle tone lax. Alternatively, if children can protect their airway, spontaneous breathing may not be capable of maintaining adequate gas exchange to avoid hypercarbia and hypoxemia. See Chapter 64.1 for intubation and Chapter 64.4 for mechanical ventilation.

Circulation should be stabilized with the aim of optimizing perfusion to all tissue (Chapter 64.2). If, after appropriate fluid resuscitation, a patient is still without adequate perfusion, inotropic agents may be indicated to enhance cardiac output. Once a patient has been stabilized, modest fluid restriction is beneficial to avoid fluid overload without producing oliguria. Urine output and serum sodium levels should be monitored. The syndrome of inappropriate secretion of antidiuretic hormone (SIADH) is frequently associated with CNS injury or infection; it can also occur with pulmonary disease. See Chapter 569.1. SIADH usually responds to fluid restriction, although it may persist until mechanical ventilation ceases. *Diabetes insipidus,* on the other hand, often heralds a very poor outcome in children with significant brain injury (see Chapter 568). A damaged pituitary or hypothalamus can induce excessive urine output, dehydration, and hypernatremia. The sodium can rise as much as 30 mEq/L in a few hours. Diabetes insipidus is treated with vigorous intravenous fluid resuscitation and vasopressin or desmopressin acetate.

Reduction of Intracranial Hypertension: Positioning and Hyperventilation. The head should be positioned in the midline and elevated about 30 degrees to allow optimal venous drainage. Movement should be minimized with sedation (e.g., intermittent or continuous benzodiazepines and narcotics). Hyperventilation is helpful: cerebral vessels constrict in response to a falling P_{CO_2}. The P_{CO_2} should be maintained between 25 and 30 mm Hg. Lower levels risk severe vasoconstriction and cerebral ischemia. One should consider monitoring jugular venous bulb M_{VO_2} (Chapter 62).

Diuretics and Steroids. Mannitol (0.5 g/kg) promotes a shift of fluid from the intracellular to the intravascular CNS space, from which it can be removed by renal excretion. However, mannitol becomes problematic if the blood-brain barrier is seriously disrupted or if mannitol infusion results in a severe hyperosmolar state that may lead to hemolysis and renal failure. Furosemide is a safer but less effective alternative. The combination is often prescribed. Intravenous corticosteroids are not helpful in the treatment of global cerebral edema but may be of benefit in treating the localized edema surrounding an intracranial mass or a tumor.

Seizures: Benzodiazepines vs Antiepileptics. Both benzodiazepines and antiepileptics reduce cerebral metabolism, but the antiepileptics are more effective at suppressing subsequent seizure activity. Both phenobarbital and phenytoin are effective. If necessary in refractory status epilepticus, phenobarbital can be infused at a very high dose (e.g., to a serum level of 50–200 mg/dL) with very little effect on the cardiovascular system. However, its half-life may be quite long and monitoring of the neurologic status compromised. Phenytoin use is limited by its cardiovascular toxicity. The two are often used in combination in refractory status epilepticus. Also see Chapter 602.

Seizures: Barbiturate-Induced Coma. In the treatment of seizures refractory to the previous agents, a barbiturate-induced coma may be necessary using a shorter-acting agent (usually pentobarbital). Therapy may be titrated to a burst suppression on electroencephalogram, but this is not necessary if the clinical seizures stop. A continuous electroencephalogram should be monitored. Continuous infusions of midazolam have also been used to treat refractory status epilepticus.

Hypothermia. Mild hypothermia (e.g., 32–35°C) results in a decrease in cerebral metabolism but poses risks of superinfection and dysrhythmias and has not been shown to improve outcomes in severe CNS illness. Moderate hypothermia for 24 hr may be beneficial in children with a GCS score of 5–7 after head trauma. See Chapters 69 and 71.

Abramo TJ, Wiebe RA, Scott S, et al: Noninvasive capnometry monitoring for respiratory status during pediatric seizures. Crit Care Med 25:1242, 1997.

Alvarez M, Nav J-M, Rue M, et al: Mortality prediction in head trauma patients: Performance of Glasgow Coma Score and general severity systems. Crit Care Med 26:142, 1998.

Marion DW, Penrod LE, Kelsey SF, et al: Treatment of traumatic brain injury with moderate hypothermia. N Engl J Med 336:540, 1997.

Newell DW, Weber JP, Watson R, et al: Effect of transient moderate hyperventilation on dynamic cerebral autoregulation after severe head injury. Neurosurgery 39:35, 1996.

Skipper P, Seear M, Poskitt K, et al: Effect of hyperventilation on regional cerebral blood flow in head-injured children. Crit Care Med 25:1402, 1997.

CHAPTER 65
Acute (Adult) Respiratory Distress Syndrome

Joseph V. DiCarlo and Lorry R. Frankel

Acute or "adult" respiratory distress syndrome (ARDS) is diagnosed in 2.5–3% of children in the pediatric intensive care unit (PICU); these children account for about 8% of total days spent in the unit and 33% of the deaths. ARDS is more likely to occur in children already compromised by serious illness.

The syndrome consists of (1) hypoxemia ($Pa{O_2}/F{IO_2} \leq 200$), (2) diffuse pulmonary infiltrates on chest roentgenogram, (3) normal pulmonary artery occlusion pressure, and (4) normal cardiac function. The diagnosis is often delayed in children, in part, because pulmonary artery catheters are rarely used in pediatrics and because cardiac function is often not normal, because children with severe pulmonary edema have a combination of leaky capillaries and cardiac dysfunction. The diagnosis can be hastened by a high index of suspicion and an echocardiogram.

EPIDEMIOLOGY AND ETIOLOGY. The mortality rate of ARDS is 40–60%, and as the syndrome progresses with failure of other organ systems, the mortality rate climbs toward 100%. The rate varies for different groups of children, however, from 24% following trauma to 88% following bone marrow transplant. Severe respiratory failure in bone marrow transplant recipients is not always ARDS; diffuse alveolar damage, the histologic hallmark of the ARDS, was found in only 33% of these children. Infectious pneumonia was the most frequent cause of the acute hypoxemic respiratory failure. Nevertheless, ARDS is also associated with viral pneumonia, particularly respiratory syncytial virus, postmeasles pneumonia, and, in immunocompromised children, cytomegalovirus infections. ARDS has also been associated with systemic inflammatory responses that have not begun in the lungs.

PATHOGENESIS. ARDS may be a pulmonary manifestation of a systemic inflammatory process triggered by various events. Three stages can be identified histologically. In the early exudative stage, disruption of the capillary junction allows leakage of protein-rich fluid into the alveoli, with blood and inflammatory cells. This stage either resolves within about 3 days or progresses to the proliferative second stage, in which fibroblasts predominate, leading to the third stage of pulmonary fibrosis at about 3 wk. The lung histology in ARDS is not homogeneous. The predominant alteration in lung function is restrictive, characterized by a decrease in compliance and forced vital capacity.

CLINICAL MANIFESTATIONS. The acute pulmonary deterioration of ARDS may not be appreciated initially. During this latent period, patients may exhibit mild respiratory distress evidenced by tachypnea, dyspnea, and an increased oxygen requirement. Auscultation of the lungs may reveal clear breath sounds or scattered rales. Within a few hours, patients begin to develop more severe hypoxia accompanied by carbon dioxide retention. The onset of ARDS may be quite variable in sepsis, very sudden with pulmonary aspiration, or insidious in acute neurologic injury or shock.

LABORATORY FINDINGS. These patients usually are initially monitored with a pulse oximeter, and when an $F{IO_2}$ greater than 0.5 is required to maintain the arterial oxygen saturation above 92%, the diagnosis of ARDS is considered. An increased alveolar-arterial gradient and a $Pa{O_2}/F{IO_2}$ less than 200 correlates with an intrapulmonary shunt greater than 20%. Radiographic findings are initially nonspecific but may rule out other causes of progressive respiratory failure or cardiomegaly. During the next few hours, the chest radiographs begin to demonstrate interstitial and alveolar pulmonary edema. Positive pressure ventilation may alter the radiographic features of pulmonary edema, but the abnormalities in pulmonary function and blood gases coupled with a worsening respiratory status support the diagnosis. As time passes and the lungs go through the various pathologic stages of ARDS, the chest radiographs correlate with these changes. In addition, barotrauma/volutrauma with air leak may occur. An echocardiogram should not suggest increased pulmonary artery pressure. Although rarely measured, the pulmonary artery occlusion pressure is normal, differentiating cardiogenic pulmonary edema from ARDS.

TREATMENT. The underlying disease (e.g., sepsis, aspiration, shock) should be treated. A minority of patients respond to oxygen therapy and meticulous fluid management. However, most patients progress to severe respiratory failure and require endotracheal intubation and mechanical ventilation in a PICU. The duration of respiratory support may be prolonged, accompanied by numerous complications and a very high mortality rate. Patients with ARDS require invasive monitoring of vital signs, blood gases, and central venous pressure. A pulmonary artery catheter is helpful in titrating ventilator and pharmacologic therapies.

The mainstay of ventilator therapy is positive end-expiratory pressure (PEEP) to improve oxygenation by decreasing intrapulmonary shunting. PEEP is usually titrated in increments of 2–4 cm H_2O with repeated measurement of blood gases to a point where the $F{IO_2}$ is less than 0.6 and the $Pa{O_2}$ is adequate to prevent tissue hypoxia. If the PEEP exceeds 15 cm H_2O, patients may experience significant hemodynamic instability and decreased cardiac output, requiring pharmacologic support (see Table 64–15). Large tidal volume (10–15 mL/kg) and a low ventilation rate, with an inspiratory time approximately 1–1.5 sec, may also be needed to improve the distribution of inhaled gas, decrease $Pa{CO_2}$, and permit more uniform ventilation. It is relatively common for children having severe ARDS to develop air leak syndromes. This risk may be decreased by maintaining the $Pa{CO_2}$ at 55–70 mm Hg, using low-volume pressure-limited ventilation and prone positioning.

High-frequency ventilation may benefit children weighing less than 30 kg by reducing air leak and permitting adequate ventilation to occur with less shear forces on the already injured lung. Although inhaled nitric oxide may increase pulmonary blood flow to poorly perfused lungs, this increase may not occur in all lung units, resulting in more dead space ventilation. Extracorporeal membrane oxygenation (ECMO) has been used to treat children with ARDS refractory to the foregoing modalities. Earlier intervention with ECMO (before 7 days) may be beneficial, but ECMO must still be considered experimental. The effectiveness of liquid ventilation has not been established (Chapter 66).

In addition to treating the underlying disease and respiratory failure, efforts should be taken to prevent nosocomial infections, provide nutritional support, avoid complications, maintain adequate cardiac output, and ensure that patients remain comfortable. Pharmacologic agents that provide appropriate sedation, analgesia, and amnesia should be used to facilitate ventilation and reduce patients' discomfort.

PROGNOSIS. Efficiency of oxygenation is crudely correlated with outcome by the 2nd day after onset of ARDS. An alveolar-arterial oxygen tension difference exceeding 420 is the best early predictor of death. The usual cause of death in ARDS is the failure of multiple organ systems. However, a surviving child can usually expect a return to good function. Follow-up of 14 children approximately 2 yr after PICU discharge showed no limitation of activities, unremarkable findings on physical examinations, room air oxyhemoglobin saturation of greater than 98%, and markedly (but not completely) improved findings on chest radiographs. Four children had normal respiratory function, and the others had evidence of mild restrictive or obstructive disease either at baseline or after challenge tests.

Artigas A, Bernard GR, Carlet J, et al: The American-European Consensus Conference on ARDS: Ventilatory, pharmacologic, supportive therapy, study design strategies, and issues related to recovery and remodeling. Am J Respir Crit Care Med 157:1332, 1998.

Bojko T, Notterman DA, Greenwald BM, et al: Acute hypoxemic respiratory failure in children following bone marrow transplantation: an outcome and pathologic study. Crit Care Med 23:755, 1995.

Davis SL, Furman DP, Costarino AT Jr: Adult respiratory distress syndrome in children: Associated disease, clinical course, and predictors of death. J Pediatr 123:35, 1993.

Meduri GW, Headley AS, Golden E, et al: Effect of Prolonged methylprednisolone therapy in unresolving acute respiratory distress syndrome. JAMA 280:159, 1998.

Newth CJ, Stretton M, Deakers TW, et al: Assessment of pulmonary function in the early phase of ARDS in pediatric patients. Pediatr Pulmonol 23:169, 1997.

Stocker R, Neff T, Stein S, et al: Prone positioning and low-volume pressure-limited ventilation improve survival in patients with severe ARDS. Chest 111:1008, 1997.

Tremblay L, Valenza F, Ribeiro SP, et al: Injurious ventilatory strategies increase cytokine and c-fos m-RNA expression in an isolated rat lung model. J Clin Invst 99:944, 1997.

Weiss I, Ushay HM, DeBruin W, et al: Respiratory and cardiac function in children after acute hypoxemic respiratory failure. Crit Care Med 24:148, 1996.

CHAPTER 66
Special Therapies

66.1 Unconventional Forms of Respiratory Support

Melinda T. Derish

The mortality rate for severe pediatric respiratory failure is 40–60% despite increases in the variety and sophistication of ventilators suitable for pediatric use and the refinements in ventilator strategies. Ventilator-induced iatrogenic lung injury contributes both to this mortality and to the incidence of chronic lung disease (see Chapter 97). Alternatives to conventional ventilation have been developed with the goal of reducing the mortality and the morbidity associated with ventilator-induced lung injury.

INVERSE RATIO VENTILATION (IRV). IRV is rarely used. The ratio of inspiratory to expiratory time is reversed, with inspiration occupying the greater portion of the respiratory cycle of a conventional respirator. Theoretically, prolongation of the inspiratory time results in a higher mean airway pressure and improved oxygenation without an increased peak inspiratory pressure. Prolongation of the inspiratory time may help to recruit collapsed alveoli and re-expand lung units with longer time constants, but the shortened expiratory phase causes gas trapping due to insufficient time to complete exhalation. This results in an increased intrinsic positive end-expiratory pressure (auto-PEEP). No controlled clinical studies indicate that IRV is equal or superior to conventional ventilation in terms of either morbidity or mortality. The main risks of IRV are the potential for gas trapping and elevated intra-alveolar pressures, leading to rupture of the alveolus and air leak. Patients on IRV also generally require deep sedation and often paralytic agents.

HIGH-FREQUENCY VENTILATION (HFV). HFV can be provided in four ways: high-frequency positive-pressure ventilation (HFPPV), high-frequency jet ventilation (HFJV), high-frequency oscillatory ventilation (HFOV), and high-frequency flow interruption (HFFI). All modes of HFV eliminate carbon dioxide by cycling a below normal tidal volume at a supraphysiologic rate. This allows use of relatively high mean airway pressure to improve oxygenation without the superimposition of high peak inspiratory pressures. The delivered tidal volume in HFV is frequently less than the patient's dead space, but carbon dioxide exchange readily occurs. Various mechanisms have been proposed to explain how alveolar ventilation can occur under these circumstances, but the physiologic basis has not been established.

Mean airway pressure is set directly during HFOV and is adjusted by changing end-expiratory pressure for HFPPV, HFJV, and HFFI. Lung volume is usually inferred by frequent chest radiographs, aiming for at least nine ribs of lung expansion, and by assessments of which airway pressure gives the best oxygenation and cardiac output. An optimal lung volume should give the best ventilation-perfusion (V/Q) matching, hence the best oxygenation. HFV can often provide more ventilation for less elevation of intrathoracic pressure than conventional ventilation.

HFV appears to benefit a substantial percentage of children who receive it either as a rescue strategy for air leak syndromes (occurring as a complication of conventional ventilation) or for failure to respond to conventional ventilation (defined as unacceptably low oxygenation or excessive hypercarbia). HFV survivors can be predicted on the basis of a rapid improvement in air leak or a decreased need for high ventilator settings to maintain oxygenation. Controversy persists over the role for HFV as an initial therapeutic mode of ventilation rather than as a rescue strategy for air leak or for respiratory failure unresponsive to conventional ventilation. One study has reported that HFOV resulted in improved oxygenation and decreased lung injury compared with conventional ventilation as the initial therapy for respiratory failure.

HELIUM. Helium, a biologically inert gas, can be combined with oxygen (heliox) and substituted for the usual ventilator gases, which are nitrogen-oxygen mixtures. Heliox has a much lower density than nitrogen and oxygen mixtures. Heliox also has a lower *Reynolds number,* the ratio of kinetic and viscous forces affecting airflow. It is the Reynolds number that determines whether airflow is *turbulent* or *laminar.* The substitution of helium for nitrogen facilitates laminar airflow at lower pressure gradients, lowering airway resistance and decreasing the work of spontaneous breathing. For children receiving mechanical ventilation, heliox allows a lower airway pressure to deliver a given tidal volume. Heliox may reduce partial upper airway obstruction due to causes such as infectious croup, postextubation stridor, tumors, and radiation therapy. More recently, lower airway obstruction has also been treated with heliox. Children hospitalized for status asthmaticus have also shown improvement in their pulmonary function in response to heliox (60–70% helium); however, heliox did not change dyspnea scores or oxygen saturation values. The beneficial effects of helium require a tracheal concentration of at least 40% helium, which limits its use to those patients who can be supported with an FIO_2 less than 0.6.

NITRIC OXIDE (NO). NO is synthesized by many cells in the body, including endothelium, vascular smooth muscle, platelets, hepatocytes, and neurons, and is a chemical messenger in many physiologic systems. It mediates local vasodilatation by activating guanylate cyclase and increasing cyclic guanosine 3′, 5′ -monophosphate. The NO then binds rapidly to hemoglobin and is inactivated. Thus, when NO is delivered as an inhaled drug, it causes selective pulmonary capillary vasodilation with minimal effects on other body systems. Another potent effect is its potential to improve oxygenation by decreasing V/Q mismatch, because the inhaled drug reaches and causes vasodilatation of only those pulmonary capillaries that serve aerated alveoli. See Chapter 97.7 for discussion of NO in the treatment of neonatal persistent pulmonary hypertension. It has also been used to treat severe adult respiratory distress syndrome, and at concentrations ranging from 5–20 ppm it decreased pulmonary artery pressures, improved oxygenation, and did not affect systemic blood pressures. A study of children treated with 20 ppm inhaled NO for severe hypoxemic respiratory failure showed improved oxygenation, lowered pulmonary vascular resistance, and stable systemic arterial pressure. At a similar dose, a randomized controlled trial of neonatal infants with hypoxic respiratory failure demonstrated a reduced need for extracorporeal membrane oxygenation (ECMO) without an effect on the mortality rate. The potential toxicities of inhaled NO relate to the formation of nitrogen dioxide and methemoglobin.

LIQUID VENTILATION. Perfluorochemical (PFC) liquids are being used experimentally to support respiration by a technique known as liquid-assisted ventilation. These inert PFC liquids are substituted for nitrogen as the vehicle for delivering oxygen and removing carbon dioxide. They have low surface tension and viscosity and a high affinity for gases. The liquid fills alveoli, recruiting atelectatic areas to provide an overall greater surface area of gas exchange and better V/Q matching. The lower surface tension of liquid improves pulmonary compliance; hence, PFC liquid can be distributed throughout the lungs at low pressures. Partial liquid ventilation has been used in conjunction with conventional ventilation, HFV, and ECMO. A controlled multicenter trial is in progress.

ECMO (see Chapter 64.2). The ECMO circuit uses a pump to propel a child's mixed venous blood through a membrane oxygenator typically supplying a mixture of 100% oxygen blended with a small amount of carbon dioxide. The membrane takes over the physiologic role of the lung. As blood leaves the oxygenator, it is warmed to body temperature and then returned to either the venous system, in *venovenous* ECMO, or to the arterial system, in *venoarterial* ECMO. While on ECMO support, a patient's lungs are allowed to "rest" on low ventilator settings. For patients with inadequate cardiac function, venoarterial ECMO is used to support perfusion to vital organs while allowing the heart to recover. ECMO requires surgical cannulation of central venous and arterial vessels and systemic heparinization.

The potential complications of ECMO in older children are similar to those in neonatal infants and include bleeding, thromboembolic events, hypoxia and ischemia, and the obligatory exposure to many blood products. The long-term effects of single carotid artery cannulation (and subsequent repair of ligation) in children are not known. Children treated with ECMO have lower survival rates than neonates and tend to require ECMO for longer periods. The overall survival for postneonatal pediatric respiratory failure treated with ECMO is approximately 50% (47–70%). In 1996, a retrospective study by Green and colleagues reported a multicenter (41 pediatric intensive care units) cohort analysis of patients with acute respiratory failure. Patients who received ECMO were matched with patients treated with ECMO for the primary diagnostic etiology of their respiratory failure and for their risk of mortality as predicted by PRISM score (Chapter 63). The ECMO-treated patients had a significantly lower mortality rate.

Abman SH, Griebel JL, Parker DK, et al: Acute effects of inhaled nitric oxide in children with severe hypoxemic respiratory failure. J Pediatr 124:881, 1994.

Arnold JH, Hanson JH, Toro-Figuero LO, et al: Prospective, randomized comparison of high-frequency oscillatory ventilation and conventional mechanical ventilation in pediatric respiratory failure. Crit Care Med 22:1530, 1994.

Carter ER, Webb CR, Moffitt DR: Evaluation of heliox in children hospitalized with acute severe asthma. Chest 109:1256, 1996.

Clarke RH: High-frequency ventilation. J Pediatr 124:661, 1994.

Cueto E, Lopez-Herce J, Sánchez A, et al: Life-threatening effects of discontinuing inhaled nitric oxide in children. Acta Padiatr 86:1337, 1997.

Froese AB, Bruan AC: High-frequency ventilation. Am Rev Respir Dis 135:1363, 1987.

Gluck EH, Onorato DJ, Castriotta R: Helium-oxygen mixtures in intubated patients with status asthmaticus and respiratory acidosis. Chest 98:693, 1990.

Green TP, Timmons OD, Fackler JC, et al: For the Pediatric Critical Care Study Group: The impact of extrcorporeal membrane oxygenation on survival in pediatric patients with acute respiratory failure. Crit Care Med 24:323, 1996.

Marcy TW: Inverse ratio ventilation. *In*: Tobin MJ (ed): Principles and Practice of Mechanical Ventilation. New York, McGraw-Hill, 1994, pp 319–331.

Ring JC, Stidham GL: Novel therapies for acute respiratory failure. Pediatr Clin North Am 41:1325, 1994.

Rossaint R, Falke KJ, Lopez F, et al: Inhaled nitric oxide for the adult respiratory distress syndrome. N Engl J Med 328:399, 1993.

Sarnaik AP, Meert KL, Pappas MD, et al: Predicting outcome in children with severe acute respiratory failure treated with high-frequency ventilation. Crit Care Med 24:1396, 1996.

Shaffer TH, Wolfson MR: Liquid ventilation: An alternative ventilation strategy for management of neonatal respiratory distress. Eur J Pediatr 155(Suppl):S30, 1996.

CHAPTER 67

Continuous Hemofiltration

Joseph V. DiCarlo

Continuous venovenous hemofiltration (CVVH) was designed as a renal replacement therapy for acute renal failure (Chapter 543). It is often used rather than hemodialysis for patients with blood pressure instability; it is generally more efficient than peritoneal dialysis. CVVH is particularly useful in children with multiple organ dysfunction or failure, whose treatment often requires very large amounts of intravenous fluids. A double-lumen dialysis catheter is placed in a large vein (usually femoral vein) and connected to a blood pump and air filter. The hemofilters have an additional port located in the ultrafiltrate compartment, which allows for the countercurrent circulation of an added dialysate solution. This converts CVVH into a hemodialysis system (CVVHD), which augments the clearance of solutes of low molecular weight. To avoid increasing blood viscosity, filtration rate is kept below 25–30%, or replacement intravenous fluids are infused at the proximal (inflow) side of the filter, diluting the blood presented to the filter. Predilution reduces sludging within the filter and may increase filter life, but the efficiency of ultrafiltration is compromised, because the ultrafiltrate now contains a portion of the replacement fluid. Overall efficiency may be enhanced, however, if the ultrafiltration rate is increased. The replacement solution should contain dextrose, sodium, and potassium in physiologic concentrations, and bicarbonate, calcium, magnesium sulfate, chloride, and phosphate.

Goyon JB: Survey on the practice of extrarenal hemofiltration in pediatrics. Arch Pediatr 3:769, 1996.

Heering P: Cytokine removal and cardiovascular hemodynamics in septic patients with continuous venovenous hemofiltration. Intens Care Med 23:288, 1997.

Ronco C: Achievements and new directions in continuous renal replacement therapies. New Horiz 3:708, 1995.

CHAPTER 68

Transplantation Issues in the PICU

Lawrence H. Mathers and Lorry R. Frankel

Children who are in the pediatric intensive care unit (PICU) for post-transplant care or pretransplant evaluation present a series of unique challenges. These problems include sustaining a child with end organ failure while awaiting a suitable donor; complications after transplant such as sepsis, organ rejection, or multiple system organ failure; and various psychologic, emotional, ethical, and social problems. In addition, organ and tissue transplantation is a complex process requiring important decisions involving both the donor and the recipient.

ORGAN AND TISSUE DONATIONS. Donors fall into two broad categories: (1) those who will survive the process of donation (e.g., skin, bone marrow, kidney, and partial liver donors) and (2) those for whom donation can be accomplished only after death. The former group includes both those who donate a dispensable tissue, such as cartilage or bone marrow, and those who donate a part or all of one of their own vital organs (kidney, partial liver, or lung). The latter group requires that there be a determination of a brain death (Chapter 72) and that the vital organs remain perfused and oxygenated.

Certain medical conditions may preclude donation of organs or tissues: severe organ dysfunction, organ injury from trauma, disseminated malignancy, active infection (including HIV), serious vascular disease, diabetes mellitus, and severe hypertension. For some transplants, the size and age of the donor and recipient should be similar.

In most cases, a potential *recipient* of a transplant is identified long in advance of the actual transplant, but in the case of potential *donors* there is often little time to broach the subject of organ donation with the family and secure their support for organ donation. Because of the regionalization of PICUs, it is not unusual that a potential recipient of an organ transplant is in the same hospital or even on the same unit as the potential donor. A family whose child or other family member is being considered as a donor must digest all the factual information about organ donation and come to terms with the idea of their loved one as a donor. The team providing care to the potential donor should introduce the concept of organ donation, beginning with a frank assessment of the degree of injury suffered by the potential donor and the futility of any future care. To avoid even an appearance of conflict of interest, clinicians may wish to obtain consultation from the local organ transplant organization.

Evaluation of potential compatibility between donor and recipient is discussed in Chapters 123 and 136 and in chapters addressing specific organ and tissue transplants. *Hyperacute rejection* may occur within minutes of the transplant in the operating room or in the PICU soon after arriving. It results from the presence of preformed antibodies, and blood flow to the foreign tissue is usually compromised by the acute reaction. The organ must be removed immediately or rested as the body is supported (e.g., extracorporeal membrane oxygenation [ECMO] in postcardiac transplant recipients). Immune responses, immunosuppression, and *acute* and *chronic rejection* are discussed in Chapters 137 and 138. Admission to a PICU is usually not required for bone marrow transplantation unless severe complications develop. In contrast, solid organ transplants that include heart, heart/lung, liver, and kidney require major surgery and result in admission to a PICU, often before and almost always after the transplantation (kidney transplants in older children may be an exception). Many children awaiting solid organ transplantation are in a deteriorating state. Pretransplant treatment of the unstable potential recipient is just as important as postoperative care.

COMPLICATIONS OF BONE MARROW TRANSPLANTATION (BMT). Approximately 10–15% of children having a BMT spend time in a PICU. The most common reasons for PICU admission of these children are life-threatening complications, especially those that occur in the first 20–40 days after transplantation. Patients having significant fluid and electroylyte problems, signs of hemodynamic instability, renal failure, airway obstruction, or progressive respiratory failure are the most frequently admitted. Mortality is particularly high in children requiring mechanical ventilation.

Acute *graft versus host disease* (GVHD) may present with cholestasis, erythematous maculopapular rash, and diarrhea requiring PICU management (Chapter 137). Chronic GVHD often follows acute GVHD. See Chapter 501.4 for treatment.

Veno-occlusive disease (VOD), a thrombotic disorder producing clots in the small venules in the liver, is the third most frequent complication of BMT and occurs most often in patients undergoing BMT for malignancy. These patients may have severe hepatic dysfunction resulting in ascites, respiratory distress, and other evidence of organ failure. They may necessitate aggressive treatment including fluid therapy, anticoagulation, and sometimes thrombolytic agents or procedures.

Infections are of major concern because these children are both immunologically suppressed and neutropenic. Patients should be placed in protective isolation in order to limit infectious exposures. See appropriate chapters on specific infectious agents. Opportunistic infections are discussed in Chapter 179. Seizures, encephalopathy, and psychiatric disturbances associated with infections or drug toxicity require aggressive diagnostic and therapeutic interventions.

Thrombocytopenia may result in bleeding from the respiratory and gastrointestinal tract. Efforts are directed at maintaining platelet counts greater than 50,000 when bleeding is present. Children may require nasal packing for severe nosebleeds. Clotting factors may be required if a coagulopathy is present; this is a high risk in children having VOD. Patients also require red blood cell transfusions for a low hematocrit due to bleeding and the inability to produce red blood cells before engraftment.

Oncologists and intensivists need to confer on all BMT recipients in the PICU, in order to assist the family and the care staff in understanding the realistic prospects for success with continued treatment. The PICU staff, in turn, must understand that BMT recipients can become very ill owing to the immunosuppresive therapy and numerous complications but can still recover. Children with oncologic diseases and their families have typically battled with disease for months or even years and often are prepared for a protracted struggle against complications of their transplants. However, they need to have realistic expectations about the treatment of BMT complications. Frequent conferences, involving oncologists, intensivists, and family, are often necessary to provide optimal care in these complicated cases.

HEART TRANSPLANTATION (See Chapter 449.1). Most pediatric transplant patients transferred to a PICU are receiving chronotropic agents, such as isoproterenol, to maintain the heart rate and ensure adequate cardiac output. Pacing wires from surgery are left in place in the event that direct electrical stimulation of the heart is required during recovery. Early complications include hyperacute rejection, acute rejection, bradycardia, and dysrhythmias. Later, rejection may still occur along with various infections, accelerated coronary artery disease, and lymphoproliferative disorders secondary to immunosuppression. If a child experiences acute or hyperacute rejection, additional vasoactive agents, ECMO or ventricular assist devices, or retransplantation may be necessary. Children having accelerated coronary artery disease can present with severe cardiogenic shock secondary to ischemic myocardial dysfunction.

LUNG TRANSPLANTATION (see Chapter 449.2). Children with cystic fibrosis, pulmonary hypertension, and α_1-antitrypsin deficiency are among the primary candidates. Recipients about to undergo lung transplantation may need to be placed on cardiopulmonary bypass if they cannot sustain adequate ventilation and oxygenation on only one lung. Hyperacute and acute rejection may occur with lung transplants as with other organs. More than half of all recipients experience some degree of rejection in the first 3 mo after transplant. Transbronchial biopsy may confirm the diagnosis. Bronchial and/or tracheal anastomosis dehiscence is also a problem. Infection remains a serious threat, and prophylactic treatment with trimethoprim-sulfa (for *Pneumocystis*), fluconazole (for fungus), and ganciclovir (for cytomegalovirus [CMV]) are used by some centers. **Bronchiolitis obliterans** occurs in 25–50% of survivors and is diagnosed with lung biopsies and treated with pulse steroids and other immunosuppressives (Chapter 392). It may require retransplant.

HEART-LUNG TRANSPLANTATION (see Chapter 449.2). Postoperatively, children require mechanical ventilation with the minimum possible intra-airway pressures, because high pressures increase stress on the tracheal suture lines. Fiberoptic bronchoscopies may be needed to clear potential obstructions. For 2–3 wk the denervated lung is sensitive to exogenous fluid overload and is prone to develop edema. Rejection of the lung also may occur without any evidence of cardiac rejection. This can be assessed with pulmonary function studies that demonstrate alterations in flow patterns, specifically FEF_{25-75}. Bronchoscopy with lavage and biopsies may also be useful in diagnosing rejection. Most deaths are perioperative owing to uncontrollable hemorrhage.

KIDNEY TRANSPLANTATION. (see Chapter 544). The goal in the immediate postoperative period is to encourage graft organ function, and in children this is achieved by maintaining renal perfusion with high levels of preload fluids producing substantial urine output. Even in the youngest children, the goal is to produce several hundred milliliters of urine per hour. Fluid replacement usually consists of normal saline or another physiologic fluid. This not only encourages sufficient urine production but also helps reduce the risk of thrombi at the vascular suture lines. Urine and insensible losses are replaced, and electrolytes are monitored closely. Blood pressure is tolerated at levels 20–30% higher than normal, particularly if a small child has received a transplanted adult kidney. The large fluid infusions when associated with a capillary leak phenomenon can produce significant pulmonary edema and necessitate meticulous respiratory management.

Ultrasound study of the newly transplanted kidney is often performed to confirm proper renal blood flow and to evaluate potential obstructive problems related to the surgery. When oliguria occurs, additional fluid replacement is instituted, assuming that the cause of oliguria is intravascular depletion. If oliguria persists in the presence of adequate intravascular fluid, then a range of problems, from obstruction of the Foley catheter to kinking of the implanted ureter must be considered. If no fluid or mechanical cause can be found, early rejection or acute tubular necrosis may be the problem. Diuretics may be helpful (a continuous furosemide drip is often effective), but if the problem persists, a graft biopsy may be indicated. Postoperative hypertension should not be treated with angiotensin-converting enzyme inhibitors, because their site of action (at the glomerular arterioles) may jeopardize glomerular perfusion. The treatment of rejection is discussed in Chapter 544.

LIVER TRANSPLANTATION (see Chapter 367). The most common indication for liver transplant is biliary atresia. Other indications include various other congenital causes of cirrhosis, several inborn errors of metabolism (tyrosinemia, Wilson disease, others), toxic ingestions (acetaminophen overdose, mushroom poisining), various forms of acute and chronic hepatitis, certain liver malignancies, and liver trauma. Indications for transplantation and immunotherapy are discussed in Chapter 367.

Hepatic failure results in various life-threatening structural changes and metabolic derangements, including acidosis, coagulopathy, hyperammonemia and hepatic coma, hypoalbuminemia and anasarca, and portal hypertension with varices. Hyperammonemic hepatic coma may force consideration of transplant because it produces unconsciousness and apnea as it progresses. Children having fulminant hepatic failure should be transferred to a PICU at a liver transplant center for rapid evaluation for transplantation.

The liver graft is subject to an array of potential problems after transplantation. Hyperacute graft rejection is very rare but may occur within minutes of revascularization of a transplanted organ. The organ must be removed and replaced, if at all possible. Acute rejection can occur within the first 5–7 days after transplant and is manifested by rising levels of liver enzymes, worsening coagulopathy, and hepatic encephalopathy. It can be treated with high-dose steroids, increased doses of cyclosporine, or FK506, and if these fail, antithymocyte antibody preparations. Vascular anastomosis breakdown produces hemorrhage and demands surgical re-exploration. Thrombus formation deprives the liver of blood flow and also requires surgery. Hematobilia may require surgical exploration. Intestinal perforations may occur and can be detected by observation of free air in the abdomen. Various abscesses and other fluid accumulations may need surgical exploration. Nonsurgical problems include hypertension (from fluid overload, steroid treatment, and so on); pulmonary edema secondary to fluid overload; effusions; phrenic nerve injury producing basilar atelectasis; seizures; and coagulopathy. Extensive blood product administration may lead to metabolic alkalosis (from the citrate in blood products). Various electrolyte disturbances are possible and require frequent checks of electrolytes. The kidney may manifest a mild form of acute tubular necrosis due to necessary intraoperative occlusion of the inferior vena cava.

At the time of transplantation, children typically receive corticosteroids and either cyclosporine or FK506 (tacrolimus). In some cases, small doses of antithrombocyte globulin (ATG) or OKT3 are given as well. The early phase of immunosuppression extends for 2–3 wk postoperatively, and most patients continue lifelong small doses of steroids. Patients are also usually treated with antifungal (nystatin, fluconazole), anti-CMV (ganciclovir), and antipneumocystis (trimethoprim-sulfa, pentamidine) prophylactic medications for a limited time after transplant.

MULTIINTESTINAL ORGAN TRANSPLANTATION. Pancreas, small bowel, or various combinations of intestinal viscera transplantation are rarely performed in comparison with other transplants. These are experimental procedures for severe, intractable diseases unresponsive to any other form of therapy. In children, the most common reasons for considering intestinal viscera transplant are necrotizing enterocolitis, gastroschisis, various obstructions, and intestinal atresias, with dependence on total parenteral nutrition.

Whatever intestinal components are transplanted, postoperative risks are common to many transplant operations. In addition, edema of intestinal tissues, and sometimes the inability to close the abdominal wall, may not allow rapid weaning from mechanical ventilation. Maintaining renal perfusion is critically important. Cleansing bowel preparations before surgery are advisable, as is postoperative treatment with enteral amphotericin, gentamicin, and polymixin for several weeks. A short course of ganciclovir (for CMV prophylaxis) is usually also given, and patients may require a prophylactic dose of trimethoprim-sulfa for life. Reintroduction of enteral feeding must be done very gradually, with continuing parenteral nutrition. Bowel transplants also should be assessed carefully for the signs and symptoms of bowel dysfunction—obstruction, abdominal tenderness, emesis, diarrhea, melena, and so on. Endoscopic monitoring of the intestinal mucosa and monitoring fluid losses from ileostomy or colostomy sites are essential.

In the postoperative period, usually at the time of reperfusion of the implanted organs, steroids and FK506 or acyclovir are administerered. Azathioprine may also be added. Prostaglandin E_1 is generally administered for 5–7 days to discourage the formation of clots in the microvasculature of the intestines and to dilate these vascular beds. Graft rejection usually results in fever, pain, distention, emesis, and increased stoma output. Severe rejection can lead to acute ulceration, perforation, and hemorrhage. Any evidence of biliary leakage or obstruction should be pursued vigorously. Vascular problems include microvascular thrombi and breakdown or large clots in vascular anastomoses. The risk of infection is greater than in other solid organ transplants.

POST-TRANSPLANT LYMPHOPROLIFERATIVE DISORDERS (PTLD). PTLD involves the inappropriate growth of lymphoid tissue, which may occur at sites where lymph nodes are ordinarily found or where nodes do not usually occur. The growing tissue may obstruct nearby structures and produce various symptoms. Stridor or wheezing can result from airway obstruction from the proliferation of mediastinal lymph nodes, adenoidal hypertrophy, or hypertrophy of the glottic structures. Dysphagia can occur when the gastric lymph nodes enlarge around the gastroesophageal junction. A bowel obstruction can occur if mesenteric lymph nodes enlarge and compress the bowel. In addition, PTLD may result in perforation of a hollow viscus, resulting in peritonitis and free air within the peritoneum. The diagnosis may require endoscopy or surgical exploration to obtain tissue or relieve an obstruction. Treatment of PTLD involves reduction of immunosuppressive therapy. Rarely, chemotherapeutic agents used in the treatment of lymphomas unassociated with transplantation are required (also see Chapter 503).

Bernstein D, Starnes VA, Baum D: Pediatric heart transplantation. Adv Pediatr 37:413, 1990.
Kocoshis SA: Small bowel transplantation in infants and children. Gastroenterol Clin North Am 23:737, 1994.
Malago M, Rogiers X, Broelsch CE: Liver splitting and liver donor techniques. Br Med Bull 53:860, 1998.
Neumann M: Evaluation of the pediatric renal transplant recipient. ANNA J 24:515, 1997.
Shah V, Friedman AL, Navarro VJ: Immunology of liver transplantation: Clinical management aspects. Gastroenterologist 5:137, 1997.
Spray TL: Transplantation of the heart and lungs in children. Annu Rev Med 45:139, 1994.
Stokes DC: Pulmonary complications of tissue transplantation in children. Curr Opin Pediatr 6:272, 1994.

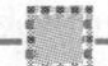

CHAPTER 69
Drowning and Near-Drowning

Harry J. Kallas

Childhood submersion is too commonly a cause of injury and fatality. After submersion in a liquid medium, suffocation and asphyxia may occur, with or without pulmonary aspiration. Irreversible multisystemic injury occurs very rapidly, often leading to death. Death within 24 hr of submersion is termed *drowning,* which may be immediate or may follow resuscitation. Survival of more than 24 hr is termed *near-drowning,* regardless of whether the victim later dies or recovers. Although treatment in the PICU has reduced mortality from the cardiorespiratory consequences of near-drowning, neurologic injury from hypoxemia and ischemia remains the primary cause of mortality and long-term morbidity in survivors.

EPIDEMIOLOGY. Worldwide, approximately 150,000 persons drown each year (approximately 1 person every 3.5 min). Children are particularly at risk for drowning. In the United States, drowning is the fourth leading cause of death for children ≤19 yr old and the single leading cause of injury death for children ≤5 yr of age. There are approximately 8,000 drownings/yr in the United States, but 40% of the victims are ≤4 yr old. Pediatric drowning constitutes 7% of traumatic deaths in children <1 yr of age, 19% of 1- to 4-yr-olds, and 12–14% of older children. From 1986 to 1988, the U.S. drowning rate was 2.53/100,000 for children <19 yr old, but was 5.80/100,000 for 1- to 2-yr-olds.

However, fatality statistics convey only a small part of the greater problem, as there are many more near-drowning than drowning victims, and many near-drowning victims survive with neurologic sequelae. There are an estimated 500,000 significant submersions in the United States each year, and 50,000 of these will require medical intervention. Estimates of cumulative risk for males from birth to 19 yr of age indicate that 1/1,098 will drown, 1/301 will be hospitalized for near-drowning, and 1/75 will be treated or observed in an emergency department (ED) but sent home (comparable risk estimates for females are 1/3,333, 1/913, and 1/228, respectively). Among children <5 yr old, for every 1 pediatric drowning victim, there are 14.6 children hospitalized or seen in the ED with near-drowning. For children <21 yr old in California in 1994, the drowning rate was 1.8/100,000, but 4.7/100,000 were hospitalized for near-drowning; there were 32.8 fatalities for every 100 hospitalized survivors of near-drowning. Of pediatric near-drowning victims treated at a tertiary care facility, 5–12% will survive with profound neurologic damage.

Risk factors for drowning include age, gender, and race. Two age groups are at particular risk: toddlers, who commonly drown in residential swimming pools during brief periods of inadequate supervision; and older adolescent males (15–19 yr old), who often drown in natural bodies of water, frequently in association with risk-taking behavior, alcohol intoxication, or drug use. Young teenagers (10–14 yr old) actually have the lowest drowning rate in the pediatric age group. In California, the near-drowning hospitalization rate is 2.8/100,000, but it is 18.4/100,000 in 1- to 5-yr-olds. Male drowning victims predominate in all age groups, but the male:female ratio increases dramatically from 2:1 in toddlers to 10:1 in teenagers. In the United States, black children have almost double the drowning rate of white children (3.8 vs 2.2/100,000, respectively). In Cape Town, South Africa, black children have triple the drowning rate of white children.

The site of drowning is also a major risk factor in different age groups. The proportion of drowning at various sites is a result of the accessibility to various bodies of water, socioeconomic status, and geographic area. Certainly, any body of water can pose a hazard to the child. However, in most industrialized countries reporting drowning statistics, the swimming pool is the most common drowning site for young children.

Residential swimming pools account for half of all drowning in the United States but are the site of almost 90% of submersion events in children <5 yr old. The U.S. Consumer Product Safety Commission estimated that 3,000 children <5 yr old are seen annually in the ED after submersion in residential pools; 80% of these children are hospitalized for at least 1 day. Most pool submersion events occur at the child's own home, and nearly half occur within the first 6 mo of pool exposure. Brief lapses (<5 min) in supervision account for most submersions. Preschool age swimming pool drowning and near-drowning in California accounts for $5.2 million/yr in acute hospital charges.

Bathtub drowning occurs predominately in infants (1.87/100,000 children <2 yr old), with approximately 86% occurring in children 7–15 mo old. Often, these infants have inadequate supervision and parents who overestimate their child's abilities or coordination. In Japan, half of all drowning occurs in the bathtub, which is the most common drowning site for children <4 yr old.

Hot tubs and spas also pose special hazards, as many have suction devices that can entrap hair, clothing, or body parts, preventing children from surfacing. Again, brief lapses in supervision are noted in most circumstances; however, drowning from entrapment may occur even when the parents are present, directly supervising the child. Children <2 yr old are the most frequent victims.

Children have also been reported to drown in buckets, toilets, washing machines, sinks, and other common areas containing water around the home. Bucket drowning is not uncommon, constituting up to 24% of all toddler drowning in some regions. Children 7–15 mo old account for 88% of these deaths. Children fall headfirst into the bucket and cannot right themselves owing to their relatively cephalic center of gravity and their insufficient body mass to tip it over. Bucket drowning has a high mortality, in part because of substances that buckets contain, such as cleaning fluids and other caustic agents.

In older children and teenagers, as much as 70% of drowning occurs in open bodies of water, such as lakes, ponds, streams, or irrigation ditches, usually when little or no adult supervision exists. One fifth of these drowning events involve boats, and over 50% are associated with alcohol or drug use.

The risk of drowning is increased by the use of alcohol or illicit drugs. Alcohol clouds judgment, increasing the likelihood of injudicious risk-taking behavior, and retards motor coordination. Intoxicated adults are also incapable of providing adequate supervision for younger children near water. In a recent United States survey, 70% of males and 66% of females reported the use of alcohol while participating in aquatic activities during the previous year; the largest group of positive respondents were 16–20 yr old. One third of boaters use alcohol while boating. Adjusted odds ratios for drowning are 4.6 and 31.8 with a blood alcohol level of 10–99 mg/dL and >100 mg/dL, respectively, compared with control subjects at drowning sites.

Concomitant medical conditions may also increase the likelihood of drowning. Children with epilepsy have a 4- to 10-fold increased risk of drowning or near-drowning compared with nonepileptic children. Epileptic children with other associated handicaps are at even greater risk. Epilepsy-associated drowning occurs predominately in bathtubs and swimming pools (86%); the majority of cases are in children >5 yr old. In nonepileptic children, other mental or motor disabilities also increase drowning risk.

Child abuse and homicide by submersion do occur and require a careful history, a high index of suspicion, and an understanding of normal childhood developmental capabilities. Approximately 1 in 30 child homicides are by intentional drowning. Overall, about 1.5 to 8% of all drowning and near-drowning in children <5 yr old is inflicted, most commonly in the bathtub. It is estimated that 5–19% of submersion injuries in children 1–4 yr of age and 10–67% of bathtub submersions may be associated with child abuse or neglect. Eighty-five per cent of intentional bathtub drowning involves children 15–30 mo of age. Compared with unintentional injuries, victims of abuse are less likely to have resuscitation attempted by bystanders and are more likely to die.

PATHOPHYSIOLOGY. Progressively, hypoxemia affects all organs and tissues, with the severity of injury dependent on the duration. If pulmonary aspiration is associated with submersion, hypoxemia and respiratory failure are exacerbated. Additionally, myocardial dysfunction, arrhythmias, or arrest compromise the victim by causing tissue ischemia. The combination of hypoxia and ischemia is a common injury mechanism associated with submersion events. Although severe hypothermia may rarely confer some degree of neurologic protection to individual victims, its pathologic implications are more commonly detrimental if not rapidly corrected.

Anoxic-Ischemic Injury. Following submersion, a conscious animal will initially panic, trying to surface. During this stage, small amounts of water enter the hypopharynx, triggering laryngospasm. Most animals struggle violently and swallow copious amounts of water. They soon lose consciousness from hypoxemia. Vomiting may ensue, accompanied by involuntary aspiration. In about 10% of animals, the initial laryngospasm persists until death without aspiration into the lungs; similarly, aspiration is absent in 10–15% of humans who drown. Profound hypoxemia and medullary depression lead to terminal apnea. Cardiovascular changes include an initial tachycardia followed by severe hypertension with reflex bradycardia, presumably from catecholamine release; arrhythmias may be seen. By 3–4 min, the circulation abruptly fails as myocardial hypoxemia supervenes. The heart may continue to have ineffective contractions or electrical activity for a short time, but there is no effective perfusion. The chance of successful resuscitation quickly becomes impossible as hypoxemia and ischemia cause rapid, progressive, and irreversible injury.

The diving reflex may potentially enhance cerebral and myocardial blood flow when the face is submerged in very cold water (<20°C) and is believed by some authors to contribute to cerebral protection during prolonged submersion. Although this reflex is prominent in many sea mammals, it is relatively weak in humans. The extent of neurologic protection afforded humans by the diving reflex is controversial but is probably minimal.

All organs may be injured from hypoxia and ischemia, but the brain is exquisitely sensitive. With advances in intensive care, the cardiorespiratory consequences of near-drowning have become increasingly manageable and less often the cause of mortality compared with hypoxic-ischemic CNS injury. CNS injury is now the most frequent cause of mortality and long-term morbidity. Although the duration of hypoxemia before irreversible CNS injury occurs is uncertain, it is probably on the order of 3–5 min.

Myriad pathophysiologic biochemical events occur as a result of hypoxemia and ischemia. The brain has minimal energy stores, and adenosine triphosphate (ATP) is depleted after approximately 2 min of anoxia. ATP is necessary to maintain all cellular metabolic functions and ionic gradients, and its depletion likely is a trigger for a number of pathogenic cascades. Blood flow and ongoing nutrient delivery during hypoxic conditions result in anaerobic metabolism, increasing cellular lactate and other intermediary metabolite concentrations. In contrast, total ischemia halts all nutrient delivery, leading to an abrupt cessation of cellular metabolic activity. Secondary injury during reperfusion occurs by various mechanisms. Neuronal injury is exacerbated by the release of glutamate and other "excitatory" amino acids. These excitotoxins activate specific receptors on neural cell membranes, which leads to an influx of calcium. Increased intracellular calcium after hypoxic-ischemic injury is believed to promote irreversible cellular injury. Alteration of calcium homeostasis can perpetuate numerous deleterious responses, including activation of phospholipases, proteases, endonucleases, protein kinases, and nitric oxide synthase and the uncoupling of oxidative phosphorylation. Membrane phospholipid hydrolysis and the release of arachidonic acid metabolites contribute to oxygen free radical generation, the inflammatory response, and cellular damage. Other important pathways leading to oxygen radical formation include cyclooxygenase, lipoxygenase, purine degradation, the electron transport chain, and inflammatory cells. Oxygen radicals produce cellular injury by a variety of mechanisms but most importantly lead to lipid peroxidation; the ensuing chain reaction produces more radicals, affects enzymatic function, and compromises cell membrane integrity. Cellular dysfunction also leads to secondary increases in intracellular sodium and to cytotoxic cerebral edema.

Hyperglycemia has also been implicated in exacerbating CNS injury. After near-drowning, children with initial blood glucose concentrations >300 mg/dL may be more likely to die or survive in a persistent vegetative state (PVS) compared with normoglycemic victims. Although the link between hyperglycemia and neuronal injury is tentative, animal studies suggest a potential mechanism. Hyperglycemic rats have significantly lower CNS levels of adenosine and its metabolites compared with normoglycemic animals. Adenosine, proposed to be an endogenous neuroprotecter, causes cerebral vasodilatation, inhibits the release of neuronal excitotoxins, and affects neutrophil-endothelial interactions. However, control of hyperglycemia with insulin after near-drowning is not recommended in humans at this time. Nevertheless, it is prudent to avoid iatrogenic hyperglycemia. Careful monitoring to avoid hypoglycemia is also imperative to prevent augmenting neuronal injury.

The neurologic consequences of severe hypoxic-ischemic injury culminate in the loss of cerebral autoregulation and blood-brain barrier integrity. Generalized neuronal death often soon follows, resulting in cytotoxic cerebral edema and increased intracranial pressure (ICP). The extent of cerebral edema in near-drowning probably reflects the severity of the initial cytotoxic injury; although severe cerebral edema can elevate ICP, causing further ischemia, its very presence is an ominous sign of extensive neuronal death.

Other organs and tissues may also be injured. In the lung, hypoxia, ischemia, and aspiration can damage pulmonary vascular endothelium, increasing vascular permeability, which can result in noncardiogenic pulmonary edema and the adult respiratory distress syndrome (ARDS) (Chapter 65). Myocardial dysfunction, arrhythmias, and infarction may also occur. Acute tubular necrosis and acute cortical necrosis are common renal complications of significant hypoxic-ischemic events. Vascular endothelial injury, exposing basement membrane, can initiate disseminated intravascular coagulation (DIC) and thrombocytopenia. Factors contributing to gastrointestinal damage include hypoxia, ischemia, hypothermia, the diving reflex, and catecholamine infusions used during resuscitation; a profuse bloody diarrhea with mucosal sloughing may be seen with very severe hypoxic-ischemic events and usually portends a fatal injury. Hepatic transaminases and serum pancreatic enzymes are often acutely elevated. Violation of normal mucosal protective barriers predisposes the victim to bacteremia and sepsis.

Pulmonary Aspiration. Pulmonary aspiration occurs in 85–90% of drowning victims and in 80–90% of the nearly drowned, but, in the great majority of cases, the amount aspirated is small. Nonaspirating victims may still succumb acutely from laryngospasm, hypoxemia, or cardiac arrhythmias. The amount and composition of the aspirated material can affect the patient's clinical course: water salinity, gastric contents, pathogenic organisms, toxic chemicals, and other foreign matter can injure the lung or cause airway obstruction. A few children may have massive aspiration, increasing the likelihood of severe pulmonary dysfunction, fluid shifts, or electrolyte abnormalities.

Although a substantial literature is devoted to the distinction between seawater and freshwater aspiration, clinical management is not significantly different. Seawater is hypertonic (approximately 3% normal saline), establishing an osmotic gradient drawing interstitial and intravascular fluid into the alveoli; furthermore, seawater inactivates surfactant, increasing alveolar surface tension and making the alveolus unstable and prone to atelectasis. On the other hand, hypotonic freshwater aspiration washes out surfactant, also causing alveolar instability and collapse. In either case, hypoxemia and pulmonary insufficiency result from ventilation-perfusion mismatch, increased intrapulmonary shunting, decreased lung compliance, and increased small airway resistance. Profound arterial hypoxemia may result after the aspiration of as little as 2.2 mL/kg.

Pulmonary edema may develop from aspiration of liquid or foreign material, hypoxemic-ischemic injury, severe myocardial dysfunction, or hypothermia. Pulmonary capillary endothelial injury can lead to ARDS. Pulmonary edema in some cases of near-drowning may be neurogenic in origin.

Pulmonary infections, caustic aspirations, and barotrauma are still significant causes of morbidity and mortality. Pneumonia may occur primarily from aspirated contaminated water or emesis or be secondarily associated with endotracheal intubation (ventilator-associated, hospital-acquired pneumonia) or hypothermia. Gastric acid or caustic agent aspiration can directly injure the lung without infection being present. Patients treated with high airway pressures during mechanical ventilation may develop lung injury from barotrauma (pulmonary interstitial emphysema, pneumothorax, pneumomediastinum), ARDS, and possibly multiple organ failure.

Fluid And Electrolyte Alterations. Although submersion victims usually do not aspirate large volumes of fluid, they do swallow copious amounts. Swallowed water, pulmonary aspiration, and intravenous fluids administered during resuscitation can lead to intravascular fluid and electrolyte changes. However, with the exception of pulmonary edema, clinically significant fluid shifts are uncommon in survivors. Only 15% of patients who die in either freshwater or seawater have significant electrolyte changes; children who survive long enough to be seen in the ED rarely have electrolyte aberrations requiring therapy.

Massive seawater ingestion or aspiration can lead to electrolyte changes and fluid shifts because of its high sodium concentration and osmolarity. Hypernatremia may occur. As fluid is osmotically drawn into the lungs and gastrointestinal tract, hemoconcentration from reduced intravascular volume may be observed. However, hypernatremia and hemoconcentration due to hyposmolar diuresis also occurs in diabetes insipidus, usually a sign of profound CNS injury after hypoxic-ischemic events.

Water intoxication can occur in freshwater drowning, causing hyponatremia and hemodilution. Rarely, sudden hypoosmolarity results in red blood cell swelling and hemolysis, leading to hyperkalemia and hemoglobinuria. Hemoglobinuria can cause renal injury; however, plasma-free hemoglobin levels in human near-drowning are usually <500 mg/dL, insufficient to cause significant renal dysfunction from tubular plugging alone. Additionally, free water overload may occur from excess antidiuretic hormone (SIADH), which often accompanies pulmonary or brain injuries (Chapter 569.1). Excess free water can swell cerebral cells, increasing cerebral edema and ICP.

Hypothermia. Core temperature of <35°C after submersion is common (see Chapter 71). Children are at increased risk of developing hypothermia owing to their relatively high body surface area to mass ratio, decreased subcutaneous fat, and limited thermogenic capacity. Hypothermia can develop as a result of surface contact with cold water and potentially after swallowing or aspirating large quantities of fluid. Further drops in body temperature occur after the child is removed from the water as a result of cold air, wet clothes, and transport to hospital. Compensatory mechanisms will usually attempt to restore normothermia at body temperatures above 32°C; below this core temperature, thermoregulation fails and spontaneous rewarming will not occur. Moderate hypothermia (core temperature 32–35°C) increases oxygen consumption owing to shivering thermogenesis and increased sympathetic tone. Below 32°C (severe hypothermia), shivering ceases and the cellular metabolic rate decreases (approximately 7% per °C in the absence of active thermogenesis).

With moderate to severe hypothermia, progressive bradycardia, impaired myocardial contractility, and loss of vasomotor tone contribute to inadequate perfusion, hypotension, and shock. Below 28°C, extreme bradycardia is usually present, and the propensity for spontaneous ventricular fibrillation (VF) or asystole is high. Central respiratory center depression with moderate to severe hypothermia results in hypoventilation and eventual apnea. Deep coma with fixed and dilated pupils and absent reflexes at very low body temperatures (below 25–29°C) may give the false appearance of death.

Depending on the duration and severity of the temperature aberration, other systemic adverse consequences of hypothermia may occur acutely and persist even after rewarming. ARDS secondary to hypothermia can be seen even in the absence of submersion or aspiration. Depressed hepatorenal metabolism and perfusion reduce drug clearance. Either hypoglycemia from glycogen store exhaustion or hyperglycemia due to a hypercholinergic state, altered pancreatic insulin release, and depressed peripheral glucose utilization may be observed. Thrombocytopenia, platelet dysfunction, and DIC also occur. Although hypothermia slows bacterial replication, it also renders the host more susceptible to bacterial and fungal invasion and sepsis by impairing neutrophil and reticuloendothelial function. Hypothermia must be expediently corrected to minimize these adverse consequences.

During initial rewarming efforts, core body temperature may actually drop before increasing. This *afterdrop* may occur secondary to the return of colder blood from the extremities to the relatively warmer central core or by the conduction of heat from the warmer core to cooler surface layers. In patients with severe hypothermia, afterdrop may further compromise cardiac, respiratory, or neurologic function or induce arrhythmias. Afterdrop may be less severe if the extremities are not rewarmed during initial resuscitative efforts in moderately hypothermic victims, focusing rather on core rewarming.

Rewarming shock may be observed following rescue. When subjected to the additional metabolic requirements of increasing body temperature and the vasodilatation accompanying surface rewarming, victims with borderline cardiovascular function cannot respond adequately to meet increased physiologic tissue demands. Hypotension, metabolic acidosis, tissue ischemia, and other consequences of shock may therefore be exacerbated during rewarming (Chapter 64.2).

Controversial Issues Related to Hypothermia. The implications and consequences of hypothermia in near-drowning victims are the subject of significant controversy and confusion. Generally, there is misunderstanding regarding the mechanisms by which hypothermia occurs in submersion victims, the potential for cerebral protection, and changes in resuscitation management in severely hypothermic patients. The last of these issues will be discussed later.

The misconceptions surrounding this issue are fueled by a few case reports of dramatic neurologic recovery after prolonged (10–150 min) icy water submersion. There should be a clear distinction between "cold" and "ice" water. The rare survivor of prolonged submersion typically has been in freezing temperature water (<5°C) and has a core body temperature <28–30°C (usually much lower). Although hypothermia may confer a degree of cerebral protection from hypoxic-ischemic injury in controlled situations and in rare individual victims, hypothermia is most often a poor prognostic sign.

For hypothermia to be protective, core body temperature must fall extremely rapidly, decreasing cellular metabolic rate, before irreversible hypoxic-ischemic injury begins. Hypothermia has been shown to be effective in protecting the brain and other organs from anoxia-ischemia for 75–110 min in controlled circumstances in which core body temperature is first cooled to 18°C and then the heart is stopped. However, once cell death from hypoxia-ischemia has begun (starting at about 5–6 min), hypothermia does not confer a protective effect or improve recovery. The potential hypothetical mechanism for such a rapid drop in body temperature is not well elucidated.

Surface cooling alone is not likely to decrease body temperature fast enough to afford neuroprotection. The cooling rate of the body in nearly drowned victims is difficult to estimate, because, in addition to surface cooling, victims may swallow or aspirate water. However, in the cardiac anesthesia literature, surface cooling of anesthetized naked infants with ice packs and ice water decreases rectal temperature by as little as 2.5°C in the first 10 min; it takes a further 32 min for the temperature to fall to 24–26°C. During surface cooling with flowing ice water (1°C), the nasopharyngeal temperature of a naked infant falls only 1°C every 5 min. Therefore, hypothermia involving surface cooling would seem to require that submersion occur in icy water, as opposed to cold water, and that the victim continue breathing with the head above water as body temperature cools. However, this is not a common event.

The hypothesis that the aspiration of icy water accelerates cooling is also controversial. Most animals and human submersion victims in warm or cold water drowning aspirate very little. Theoretically, for sufficiently rapid neuroprotective-level hypothermia to develop, a very large quantity of icy water would have to be aspirated or swallowed, or the victim would have to rebreathe a smaller quantity of water for a period of time. In human adults and animals, immersion in icy water results in intense involuntary reflex hyperventilation and a decreased breath-holding ability to <10 sec. This response may increase the likelihood of aspiration and rebreathing of icy water in some victims. In Conn's study of ice water–submerged dogs, this rapid and violent hyperventilation lasts about 70 sec. Carotid artery temperatures of lightly anesthetized dogs fell about 8.0°C during the first 2 min in both fresh and salt ice water (4°C) and then relatively slowly during the following 8 min of the experiment. Carotid artery temperature of control animals (same temperature ice water but head kept out of the water) fell only 0.8°C during the same period. Rectal temperature changes lagged behind changes in carotid temperature. Thus, it may be that victims of ice-water submersions are more likely to have involuntary respiration and a greater likelihood of aspiration or fluid rebreathing. In such a case, it may be possible for the brain to cool to a protective level (<30°C) provided that the water aspirated is icy and cardiac output lasts long enough for sufficient heat exchange to occur. Whether this actually occurs in humans is obviously not known.

However, such a mechanism is not likely to benefit cold water near-drowning victims: Hypothermia is most commonly an unfavorable prognostic sign. In a 15-yr series from King County, Washington, where the water is cold but rarely icy, hypothermic protection has not been observed. Ninety-two per cent of survivors with good neurologic outcomes had initial core temperatures >34°C, whereas 61% of those who died or had severe neurologic injury had core temperatures <34°C. Similarly, in a Finland study in which the median water temperature was 16°C, a beneficial effect of hypothermia could not be proved in pediatric submersion victims; submersion duration <10 min had the greatest sensitivity in predicting good outcome.

CLINICAL MANIFESTATIONS AND TREATMENT. A submersion victim's clinical course and outcome are primarily determined by the circumstances of the incident, the duration of submersion, the speed of the rescue, and the effectiveness of resuscitative efforts. Children with brief submersions may arrive at the hospital awake and alert, without obvious clinical injury. Some children may have been apneic (but not pulseless) at the scene, required assisted ventilation, and quickly regained spontaneous respiration. Other victims may develop minimal to severe respiratory insufficiency.

A smaller subset of children arrive at the hospital in more critical condition. These children have had cardiac arrest and prolonged hypoxemia, required more extensive resuscitative efforts, and are at great risk for death or major morbidity. Initial management requires coordinated and experienced prehospital care following the ABCs of emergency resuscitation (Chapter 58). Rapid and high-quality prehospital resuscitation has the greatest probability of improving outcome after submersion has occurred. Subsequent ED and PICU care often involves complex management of multiorgan dysfunction.

Initial Evaluation and Resuscitation (see Chapter 64.1). Once a submersion has occurred, extrication and immediate institution of cardiopulmonary resuscitation (CPR) at the scene potentially have the greatest chance of improving outcome. Children with a good outcome are almost five times as likely to have had immediate scene resuscitation compared with children with a poor outcome, although this is not demonstrated in all series. Waiting for the arrival of paramedical personnel should not delay bystander resuscitative efforts. In a model prehospital system the arrival of paramedics took >10 min in

91% of submersion cases. Prolonged submersion victims are not likely to benefit from any current interventions. In near-drowning victims with cardiac arrest who receive prehospital care, 7–21% will have neurologically intact survival.

The initial out-of-hospital resuscitation of submersion victims must focus on rapidly restoring oxygenation, ventilation, and adequate circulation. The airway should be clear of vomitus or foreign material, which may result in obstruction or aspiration. Abdominal thrusts should not be routinely used for lung fluid removal, as their effectiveness is not established. They may increase the risk of regurgitation, aspiration, and loss of airway control; they may delay or interrupt CPR; and they have the potential to aggravate spinal trauma. Rather, abdominal thrusts or back blows should be reserved for cases in which airway obstruction by a foreign body is suspected.

The cervical spine should be protected in anyone with potential neck injury, such as in child abuse, water sport accidents, and unknown circumstances surrounding the immersion. The neck should be in a neutral position and protected with a well-fitting cervical collar.

If the victim has ineffective respiration or apnea, ventilatory support must be initiated immediately (Chapter 64.3). Mouth-to-mouth or mouth-to-nose breathing by trained bystanders often restores spontaneous ventilation and is preferable to manual methods of artificial respiration. Positive pressure bag-mask ventilation with high inspired oxygen concentration should be substituted as soon as possible in patients with respiratory insufficiency. Supplemental oxygen should be administered uniformly regardless of the patient's condition.

Gastric distention is exacerbated by mouth-to-mouth or bag-mask ventilation. Vomiting is seen in >75% of victims during resuscitation, and nearly 25% aspirate their gastric contents. Cricoid pressure during positive pressure breathing and early nasogastric or orogastric decompression may mitigate further gastric distention, decreasing the risk of vomiting and aspiration (Chapter 64.1).

If apnea, cyanosis, hypoventilation, or labored respiration persists, endotracheal intubation should be performed by trained personnel as soon as possible. Endotracheal intubation is also indicated to protect the airway in patients with depressed mental status or hemodynamic instability. Hypercapnia and hypoxia must be corrected to optimize the chances of recovery.

Concurrent with securing oxygenation, ventilation, and airway control, the child's cardiovascular status must be evaluated. Heart rate and rhythm, blood pressure, temperature, and end-organ perfusion require quick assessment: Slow capillary refill, cool extremities, and altered mental status are potential indicators of shock. ECG monitoring assists with the diagnosis and treatment of arrhythmias. Core temperature must be evaluated, especially in children, because hypothermia can cause arrhythmias, hypotension, and depressed myocardial function. Rough and excessive stimulation should be avoided in the severely hypothermic victim, as this may precipitate asystole or ventricular arrhythmia. Generally, closed-chest cardiac compressions must be instituted immediately in pulseless, bradycardic, or severely hypotensive victims (Chapters 58 and 64.1).

Intravenous fluid administration is often required to improve perfusion. Two large-bore intravenous catheters or a central venous line should be established as soon as possible; intraosseous catheter placement is a potentially lifesaving vascular access technique that avoids the delay often associated with multiple attempts to establish venous access in critically ill children (Chapter 58). Non–dextrose containing, isotonic fluid (lactated Ringer's solution or normal saline) is usually bolused to augment preload. In the hypothermic patient, administered fluids should be warmed (40–43°C), if possible. Although patients with cerebral edema are often fluid restricted, cerebral blood flow cannot be restored if cardiac output is insufficient; thus, establishing effective perfusion takes precedence over measures to minimize cerebral edema.

In children with cardiac arrest after submersion, the first recorded rhythm is asystole in 55%, VF or ventricular tachycardia (VT) in 29%, and bradycardia in 16%. Electrical defibrillation or cardioversion is often urgently necessary for children with VF or VT (Chapter 442). Catecholamine infusions may be required to support myocardial function and blood pressure (Chapter 64.1). In severely hypothermic patients, the restoration of normal sinus rhythm and adequate perfusion is difficult until core body temperature is at least partially corrected. When VF is present in such victims, up to three defibrillation attempts should be delivered. If defibrillation is unsuccessful, CPR should be reinstituted and further defibrillation attempts minimized until the child's core temperature is ≥30°C, at which time successful defibrillation may be possible. The dose of cardioactive medications in hypothermic arrest victims is unchanged, but the frequency of administration may need to be reduced because of decreased drug metabolism and clearance.

Attention to hypothermia in the field is of great importance, both to initiate rewarming measures and to prevent the consequences of deeper hypothermia. A low recording thermometer and a high index of suspicion are required to diagnose hypothermia. Core temperature is best measured at the tympanic membrane; rectal temperature determinations are often inadequate owing to insufficient insertion depth of the thermometer; oral and axillary temperature readings are unreliable. Rewarming efforts should be instituted in the field. All hypothermic victims should have damp clothes removed, the skin dried, warm blankets applied, and a warm environmental temperature provided as soon as possible. If available, both warmed intravenous fluids (40–43°C) and humidified oxygen (42–46°C) should be used. Inhalational rewarming may not significantly contribute to core rewarming in the spontaneously ventilating patient; the potential benefit may be greater in the intubated patient. For victims not in cardiac arrest with core temperatures <34°C, external rewarming measures should be applied only to truncal areas, attempting to avoid afterdrop. In poorly perfused hypothermic victims, the application of warm packs and other external rewarming devices may cause significant skin burns. Patients with severe hypothermia (core temperature <30°C) require active internal warming measures provided as soon as possible.

Rapid assessment of blood glucose should be obtained in the field. If a child is hypoglycemic, 0.5–1.0 mL/kg of 50% dextrose or 2–4 mL/kg of 10% dextrose should be administered. Dextrose-containing solutions should be withheld in children with high blood glucose concentrations, but repeated assessments must be made to avoid unrecognized subsequent hypoglycemia. Insulin is not indicated to correct hyperglycemia after submersion injury.

Controversial Issues in the Resuscitation of Severely Hypothermic Victims with Cardiac Arrest. The cardiorespiratory management of patients with severe hypothermia (core temperature <28°C) is controversial. Ventricular arrhythmias have been temporally associated with endotracheal intubation or chest compressions in occasional reports of severely hypothermic patients. Therefore, some authors advocate withholding artificial ventilation or chest compressions if any respiratory activity or perfusing rhythm is present in order to avoid precipitating VF. However, in a prospective study of 50 severely hypothermic victims, ventricular arrhythmia associated with endotracheal intubation was not observed. Therefore, gentle endotracheal tube placement should be performed in children with hypoxia, apnea, or insufficient respiration.

No prospective studies are available to guide the clinician regarding chest compressions. A few authors would withhold chest compressions if core temperature is <28°C and the ECG shows a perfusing rhythm, regardless of heart rate or hypotension. The logic behind these recommendations follows from observations that effective perfusion often returns with rewarming; rewarming is more effective when any circulation is present; VF or asystole slows rewarming efforts; chest compressions may precipitate VF; and CPR is less effective during severe hypothermia. However, given the lack of data, some practitioners would certainly initiate CPR, attempting to thwart life-threatening compromises of cardiac output. Full CPR with chest compressions is indicated for victims with apparent cardiac arrest if (1) narrow QRS activity is absent on the ECG; or (2) core temperature is unknown or >28°C, no ECG monitor is available, and a pulse cannot be found.

Victims with profound hypothermia may appear clinically dead, but full neurologic recovery is possible, although very rare. Attempts at lifesaving resuscitation should not be withheld based on initial clinical presentation, unless the victim is obviously dead (e.g., dependent lividity or rigor mortis). Body temperature should be taken into account before resuscitative efforts are terminated. Rewarming efforts, in general, should be continued until core temperature is at least 32–34°C; if the victim continues to have no effective cardiac rhythm and remains unresponsive to aggressive CPR, resuscitative efforts may be discontinued.

Complete core rewarming is not indicated for all victims. Some children with severe hypothermia and the appearance of death are really dead. In most situations, discontinuing resuscitative efforts in victims of non–icy water submersions who remain asystolic despite 30–45 min of aggressive advanced CPR is probably warranted. Physicians in hospital settings must use their individual clinical judgment when deciding to stop resuscitative efforts, taking into account the unique circumstances of each incident.

Hospital-Based Evaluation and Treatment. ED and hospital management of the submersion victim includes and extends the aforementioned resuscitative efforts. Excellent prehospital management gives victims the best possible chance for recovery. Hospitalization allows for ongoing and more sophisticated evaluation, diagnostic testing, and therapy.

At a minimum, monitoring of vital signs (especially temperature and respiratory rate), careful examination, chest radiography, and assessment of oxygenation by arterial blood gas or oximetry should be performed on all submersion victims. Even children who initially appear unaffected after a significant submersion need to be carefully observed for at least 8–12 hr. Of initially asymptomatic children, almost half may become symptomatic, usually during the first 4–8 hr postsubmersion. Delayed respiratory symptoms can occur even in children with initially normal chest examination and normal chest radiographs. The great majority of children with minor respiratory symptoms will be asymptomatic by 18 hr after their submersion.

Respiratory Management. The level of respiratory support should be appropriate to the patient's condition. Patients may develop atelectasis, pneumonia, pneumothorax, pneumomediastinum, pulmonary edema, or ARDS. Pulmonary edema in the immediate postinjury period may result from increased capillary permeability, massive fluid overload, aspiration, or myocardial failure. An arterial catheter is often required for reliable and frequent arterial blood gas assessment and continuous blood pressure monitoring in critically ill patients.

Increased inspired oxygen concentration (FIO_2) alone may not resolve hypoxemia in patients with ventilation-perfusion mismatch. Endotracheal intubation, supplemental oxygen, and the application of positive end-expiratory pressure (PEEP) are the most effective means of reversing hypoxemia. The routine use of PEEP in near-drowning has made early death from pulmonary insufficiency uncommon. PEEP increases functional residual capacity, decreases intrapulmonary shunting, improves ventilation-perfusion matching, and may improve pulmonary compliance. The level of PEEP and FIO_2 should restore functional residual capacity and adequate oxygenation, usually to an initial oxygen saturation goal of ≥95%. Excessive PEEP can depress cardiac output. Prolonged use of high FIO_2 (>70–80%) may cause pulmonary oxygen toxicity.

Unintubated children who have mild to moderate hypoxemia despite supplemental oxygen and who are alert and adequately self-ventilating may be candidates for mask continuous positive airway pressure (CPAP). CPAP also restores oxygenation and functional residual capacity, possibly averting endotracheal intubation. A nasogastric tube may be necessary to prevent gastric distention with gas. Ongoing hypoxemia, impaired ventilation, labored respiration, depressed mental status, or other intolerance to CPAP requires endotracheal intubation to secure the airway and breathing.

Hypercapnia should be avoided in potentially brain-injured children. Normal ventilation or mild hyperventilation is usually employed to maintain $PaCO_2$ at 35–40 mm Hg. Excessive hyperventilation is not indicated, and even moderate hyperventilation may lead to cerebral hypoperfusion and worsen ischemic injury.

Children with bronchospasm after near-drowning may benefit from β_2-agonist therapy; however, wheezing may also be caused by pulmonary edema or airway foreign body. Bronchoscopy is indicated if a foreign body is suspected. Diuretics may benefit a few patients with pulmonary edema and stable cardiovascular status, but they are generally not necessary. The routine use of corticosteroids for lung injury after near-drowning is not recommended. Although pneumonia may follow aspiration, prophylactic antibiotics are not generally indicated, except in circumstances in which the aspirate is known to be grossly contaminated.

ARDS is a serious but uncommon complication of near-drowning (Chapter 65). Patients requiring high airway pressures during mechanical ventilation are at increased risk for barotrauma. Sedation and, less often, neuromuscular blockade may be necessary adjuncts to respiratory management, improving thoracic compliance, patient-ventilator synchrony, and gas exchange; however, these medications can obscure neurologic evaluation, making prognostication and decision-making more difficult.

The last decade has seen a plethora of new therapies applied to the treatment of severe respiratory failure after near-drowning. Various modes of high-frequency ventilation have been successfully used in victims failing conventional mechanical ventilation (Chapter 66). In some cases, inhaled nitric oxide may help improve ventilation-perfusion matching and decrease pulmonary hypertension associated with severe lung injury (Chapter 66.1). A few case reports of exogenous surfactant therapy for respiratory failure after near-drowning exist, but indications for its routine use and guidelines for effective delivery in this population do not. Partial liquid ventilation has also been successfully employed in the management of near drowning–associated ARDS (Chapter 66.1). The use of extracorporeal life support for near-drowning victims is extremely controversial; although a few uncontrolled retrospective cases have been reported, the general application of this technology should be limited until good selection criteria and more accurate predictors of neurologic outcome exist (Chapter 64.2). "Defoaming" of pulmonary edema fluid with butyl alcohol vapor has been used in experimental seawater aspiration to improve oxygenation, but this is not currently recommended in children.

Cardiovascular Management. Etiologies contributing to myocardial insufficiency include hypoxic-ischemic injury, ongoing hypoxemia, hypothermia, acidosis, high airway pressures during mechanical ventilation, alterations of intravascular volume, and electrolyte disorders. Heart failure, shock, arrhythmias, or cardiac arrest may occur. Continuous ECG monitoring is mandatory to recognize and treat arrhythmias. In critically ill children, fluid resuscitation and inotropic agents are often necessary to improve myocardial function and restore tissue perfusion. However, overzealous fluid administration, especially in the presence of depressed myocardial function, can worsen pulmonary edema and hypoxemia. Echocardiography, central venous pressure monitoring, or pulmonary artery catheter placement may aid clinical management in patients with severe myocardial dysfunction.

Rewarming Measures. Patients with significant hypothermia, if rapidly rewarmed, may have improved stability and decreased morbidity. Adequate circulation greatly facilitates rewarming. Passive rewarming (e.g., warm room, dry blankets) relies upon the patient's thermogenic ability and is not sufficient for most significantly hypothermic children. Active external rewarming (e.g., warmed blankets, radiant warmers) restores temperature more rapidly (0.8 ± 0.4°C/hr), but decreased surface circulation makes this method less effective. Moderate sources of external heat (e.g., forced-air blanket ≅100 W) may result in skin rewarming and shivering inhibition, but there is little or no rewarming advantage compared with shivering itself. Placing the subject in a forced warm air box (400 W) produces rates of rewarming double that of shivering (6.1 vs 3°C/hr).

Active core rewarming more rapidly improves body temperature and is necessary for moderate to severe hypothermia or for victims with impaired shivering thermogenesis. Simple active core rewarming measures include administration of warmed intravenous fluids (36–40°C), heated humidified inspired oxygen (40–44°C), and warmed gastric, bladder, or peritoneal lavage. More aggressive methods include hemodialysis, extracorporeal rewarming (venovenous or arteriovenous), and cardiopulmonary bypass. Rewarming rates utilizing extracorporeal rewarming (2.1 ± 0.7°C/hr) are significantly faster than external active rewarming methods. For profound hypothermia, especially if circulatory collapse is present, cardiopulmonary bypass may be required and has a very rapid rewarming rate (6.9 ± 1.9°C/hr). The implementation of cardiopulmonary bypass is a difficult decision requiring physician anticipation as well as consultation with, and rapid transfer to, a tertiary care center.

Neurologic Management. Near-drowning victims who present to the hospital awake and alert almost always have normal neurologic outcomes. In comatose victims, CNS injury is a major concern. The most effective neurointensive care in near-drowning is the rapid restoration of adequate oxygenation, ventilation, and perfusion. Otherwise, present neurologic management entails avoiding exacerbation of CNS injury. The primary injury, cell death from hypoxemia and ischemia, is not currently treatable.

Ongoing close monitoring is necessary. Hypoxemia, hypercapnia, and vasodilatory medications can exacerbate ICP elevations and should be avoided. If the child is not hypotensive, mild head elevation may be of hypothetical benefit. Hypoglycemia and hyperglycemia should be avoided. Attempts to control seizures (Chapter 602) and fever are warranted, as they increase cerebral metabolic activity and oxygen utilization. More aggressive neurointensive care measures must be critically scrutinized, given that they have not been shown to improve satisfactory patient outcome.

Head CT scans are not generally helpful in near-drowning, unless there is a suspicion of associated traumatic injury. The great majority of near-drowning victims have normal scans initially. Head CT studies cannot adequately distinguish good outcomes from poor ones. An acutely abnormal CT scan is most frequently associated with death. There is no advantage to head CT scans over neurologic examination in the management of nontrauma near-drowning.

Many neurointensive care measures have been shown not to benefit the usual near-drowning victim. Routine ICP monitoring after near-drowning is not useful. Victims with elevated ICP usually have poor outcomes—either death or severe neurologic sequelae—regardless of ICP management. Children with normal ICP can also have poor outcomes, although less frequently. While ICP monitoring and therapy to reduce increased ICP would seem likely to preserve cerebral perfusion and prevent herniation, in fact, they do not improve outcome for near-drowning victims. ICP monitoring, "therapeutic" hypothermia, and barbiturates combined with more conventional neurointensive care therapies (hyperventilation, osmotic agents, diuretics, fluid restriction, muscle relaxants, and steroids)—measures often used in victims with elevated ICP from different causes—so far have not been shown to benefit the near-drowning victim and should not be routinely utilized. Indeed, these interventions may decrease mortality but at the expense of increasing the number of survivors in PVS. The number of neurologically intact survivors does not increase, nor does neurologic morbidity decrease.

A number of potential therapies directed at hypoxic-ischemic brain injury are now emerging or being re-examined. Potential unproven therapies under investigation include superoxide dismutase and other oxygen radical scavengers; lipid peroxidation inhibitors, such as the 21-aminosteroid tirilazad mesylate (U74006F); calcium channel antagonists, including flunarizine, lidoflazine, and nimodipine; the glutamate antagonists dizocilpine maleate (MK-801) and 2,3-dihydroxy-6-nitro-7-sulfamoylbenzoquinoxaline (NBQX); L-arginine analogs that inhibit nitric oxide synthase; and a re-investigation of barbiturates and "therapeutic" hypothermia.

With optimal management, many initially comatose children can have dramatic neurologic improvement, which usually occurs within the first 24–72 hr. Unfortunately, almost half of deeply comatose children admitted to the PICU will die from their brain injury or survive with severe neurologic damage. Many children become brain dead (Chapter 72). Deeply comatose near-drowning victims who do not show substantial improvement on neurologic examination after 24–72 hr of aggressive cardiorespiratory support and whose altered mental status cannot be otherwise explained should be seriously considered for withdrawal of support (Chapter 72).

Other Management Issues. Some submersion victims may have traumatic injury, especially if they were participating in water sports such as boating, diving, or surfing. A high index of suspicion is required. Spinal precautions should be maintained in victims with altered mental status and suspected traumatic injury. Significant anemia should raise suspicion of trauma and internal hemorrhage.

Hypoxic-ischemic injury can have multiple systemic effects, although clinically significant protracted organ dysfunction is uncommon in the absence of CNS injury. Even after initially severe pulmonary injury, lung function returns to normal in most near-drowning victims. Acute renal failure after hypoxic-ischemic injury can result in albuminuria, hemoglobinuria, oliguria, or anuria. Diuretics, fluid restriction, or dialysis is uncommonly needed to treat fluid overload or electrolyte disturbances; renal function usually normalizes. Profuse bloody diarrhea and mucosal sloughing usually portend a grim prognosis; conservative management includes bowel rest, nasogastric suction, and gastric pH control. Nutritional support for most near-drowning victims is usually not difficult, because the majority of children either die or recover quickly and resume a normal diet within a few days; enteral tube feeding or parenteral nutrition is occasionally indicated. Rhabdomyolysis after cold saltwater drowning has been reported.

One third to one half of near-drowning victims will have a fever during the first 48 hr after their submersion. Fever resolves spontaneously without antibiotics in approximately 80% of patients. Prophylactic antibiotics are not recommended unless the victim has obvious aspiration of contaminated fluid. Pulmonary or disseminated infection, either bacterial or fungal, may be related to aspiration or nosocomial acquisition but results in death uncommonly. Antimicrobial therapy should be considered in victims with persistent fever, worsening pulmonary or general clinical status, or other evidence of infection. Reported causes of near-drowning associated pneumonia include several unusual pathogens, which are frequently specific to the drowning medium and geographic region. Early respiratory and blood cultures should be considered and infectious disease consultation obtained in worrisome cases.

Severe anoxic encephalopathy is seen in 10–30% of PICU survivors after near-drowning. Chronic neurologic sequelae after near-drowning include lowered mentation, cerebral dysfunction, spastic quadriplegia, extrapyramidal syndromes, optic and cerebral atrophy, cortical blindness, peripheral neuromuscular damage, or PVS.

Psychiatric and psychosocial sequelae are also usual, and counseling for the child and family should be considered. Grief, guilt, and anger are common. Divorce rates of up to 80% are reported within a few years of injury, and parents often report difficulties with employment and substance abuse. Friends and families may blame the parents for the event. Professional counseling, pastoral care, or the support of a social worker should be considered for all families.

PROGNOSIS. Approximately 80% of pediatric submersion victims survive, and 92% of survivors make a complete recovery. In those children requiring tertiary intensive care, just over half survive neurologically intact, but approximately 13–35% die and 7–27% survive with severe brain damage.

Accurate neurologic prognostication is important for the child, family, physicians, and society. Victims most likely to have good neurologic outcomes should be offered the most aggressive intensive care measures to prevent death from associated injuries; conversely, children with devastating neurologic injuries can be spared the futility of therapies that will not improve their condition. Early and precise prognostication is important to guide triage decisions, counsel families, reduce unnecessary interventions, guide discussions with families regarding withdrawal of support, and decrease the expenditure of valuable resources on children who will not recover.

Scoring and classification systems as well as individual factors have been used to predict near-drowning outcome. Although many strongly correlate with outcome, to date, none is accurate enough to completely differentiate good from poor outcomes. In many studies, several factors may correlate with outcome, including historical variables, such as submersion duration (SD), intervention at the scene, and water or patient temperature; treatment variables, such as need for CPR in the ED, apnea and pulselessness, swiftness of heartbeat restoration, resuscitation duration (RD), depth of coma and Glasgow Coma Score (GCS), pupillary responsiveness, and neurologic response to therapy; and laboratory values, such as pH, glucose, electroencephalography (EEG), ICP, regional cerebral blood flow reduction, cerebral arteriovenous oxygen difference, and cerebral oxygen consumption.

Prehospital predictors of non–icy water immersion outcomes in King County, Washington, have been comprehensively evaluated (1974–1989). Intact survival or mild neurologic impairment occurred in 91% of children with SD <5 min and in 87% who had successful restoration of cardiovascular function (RD) within 10 min. Children with normal sinus rhythm, reactive pupils, or neurologic responsiveness at the scene virtually always had good outcomes (≥99%). In cases requiring CPR, death or severe neurologic injury occurred in 93% of patients with SD >10 min and in 100% of victims requiring RD >25 min. All victims with SD >25 min died. However, a few other series have noted sporadic intact recovery in non–icy water near-drowning after longer SD and RD than in the King County study, highlighting the difficulty in assigning absolute prognostic classification based on prehospital and ED variables.

Other studies of pediatric non–icy water immersions corroborate these findings. Generally, only a third of victims requiring advanced CPR at the scene survive, but two thirds of survivors have good recoveries. Functional recovery has been reported in 0–24% (average 17%) of patients requiring CPR in ED. However, prolonged CPR after non–icy water submersion almost invariably leads to death or severe neurologic injury. Therefore, the discontinuation of CPR in the hospital is probably warranted for victims of non–icy water submersions who do not respond to aggressive advanced life support within 25–30 min. In a given victim, however, the circumstances surrounding a submersion may not be known, especially during the first 25 min of an ongoing resuscitation; therefore, decisions regarding when to discontinue resuscitative efforts must be individualized, understanding that protracted resuscitation generally is not necessary to salvage survivors who will obviously have good outcomes.

The GCS (see Table 64–7) has some utility in predicting recovery. Children with GCS ≥6 on admission to the hospital generally have good outcomes, whereas those with GCS ≤5 have a higher probability of poor neurologic outcome. Unreactive pupils in the ED or GCS ≤5 on PICU admission have odds ratios of 374 and 51, respectively, for poor outcome. Upward trends in GCS during the first several hours of hospitalization may indicate a better prognosis. Overall, GCS fails to adequately distinguish children who will survive intact from those with major neurologic injury.

Neurologic examination and progression during the first 24–72 hr are currently the best prognosticators of neurologic outcome. Children who awake at the rescue scene or regain consciousness within 72 hr, even after prolonged resuscitation, are unlikely to suffer serious neurologic sequelae. In a small series from Children's Hospital & Medical Center in Seattle, all satisfactory survivors of non–icy water, comatose near-drowning were noted to have spontaneous purposeful movements and normal brain stem function within 24 hr. Good recovery did not occur in any child with abnormal brain stem function and absence of purposeful movements at 24 hr. The highest cortical function at 24 hr seen in victims with eventual poor outcomes was localization to painful stimuli. In another small series of near-drowning victims who remained unconscious >24 hr and survived at least 1 yr, 73% remained in a PVS and the rest had severe neurologic impairment; 45% died after 1 yr but during the follow-up period.

The value of neurologic functional recovery in prognostication was also noted in a larger retrospective series of 274 submersion victims admitted to Loma Linda Children's Hospital (1985–1994). Of patients receiving CPR in the ED (n = 89), 41 survived (8/41 intact and 33/41 PVS). An initial ED GCS of 3 was recorded in 100 patients: 14% survived intact. Of 165 victims with GCS ≥4 in the ED, 2 survived in PVS but the others survived intact. Of 185 intact survivors, 99.5% demonstrated functional recovery (time to first documented purposeful response) within 48 hr. In patients with a first documented purposeful response within 6 hr, all survived intact (n = 168). Conversely, only 5.6% of children who died or survived with PVS had purposeful movement within 48 hr. However, one child with good outcome and one with an intermediate outcome did not have purposeful movement until 1 and 3 mo, respectively.

Because of inexact prognostication in the prehospital setting and the ED, all near-drowning victims should receive appropriate aggressive support initially. Serial neurologic evaluation should be performed over the ensuing 48–72 hr with consideration of withdrawal of support in patients failing to demonstrate neurologic recovery, even though this may occur before absolute prognostic certainty is achieved.

Laboratory and technologic methods to improve prognostication have not proved superior to the neurologic examination. Methods that have been investigated include CT scans, brain stem auditory evoked responses, EEG, somatosensory evoked responses, cerebral spinal fluid creatine kinase and lactate assays, measurements of cerebral blood flow, positron emission tomography, and magnetic resonance spectroscopy.

PREVENTION. The best hope for a "cure" of drowning lies in prevention. These efforts must focus on legislation as well as ongoing education of parents, children, and physicians. Unfortunately, physicians still need more education to be an adequate resource. In a survey of pediatricians in the American Academy of Pediatrics, 85% of respondents believed that it was the responsibility of pediatricians to become involved in community and legislative efforts to prevent childhood drowning; yet only 4.1% were involved in such efforts. Despite the fact that drowning is the second leading cause of injury death in children, only 50.9% of pediatricians gave any anticipatory guidance to children's parents, and only 33.8% gave any guidance to teenagers. Only 17.9% of pediatricians noted having received formal drowning prevention education during their residency training.

The residential swimming pool should be a focus of preventive efforts because of the high drowning rate at this site. In one study of pools where pediatric drowning had occurred, 75% were inadequately fenced; only 18% of submersions were witnessed, even though a supervising adult could be identified 84% of the time. Less than half of households had any member who knew basic CPR, and 42% of children who eventually drowned did not receive CPR until paramedics arrived.

Education (including basic CPR) in addition to appropriate pool fencing could prevent up to 80% of drownings in young children. Fences should be 5 ft high and completely isolate the pool from the house and yard. Gates should be self-closing and self-latching, with the latches mounted near the top of the fence. The relative risk of drowning in a fenced pool is only 0.16 to 0.6 compared with that in an unfenced one. Parents need to supervise children at every moment during swimming. Toys should be removed from the pool area at the end of swim time.

Not all barriers are equally effective. The commonly used 4-ft tall, large chain link (2.5-inch mesh) fence can be scaled by 75% of 2-yr-olds in an average time of 25.6 sec and by 100% of 4-yr-olds in an average 11.5 sec. Increasing the height to 5 ft, narrowing the mesh to 1.25 inch, or retrofitting fences to include additional climbing barriers only minimally decreases the scaling success rate. Obviously, no commonly used barrier is universally insurmountable by young children. However, in one study, the only barrier insurmountable to children ≤4 yr old was a 5 ft ornamental iron fence (vertical bars 3.25 inches apart; horizontal crossbars 45 inches apart; no decorative cutouts on the fence). However, crafty children may be able to climb any fence using aids such as chairs or boxes. Pool covers should be American Society for Testing Materials approved. However, since pool covers are often cumbersome, they are unlikely to be replaced immediately after swim time and therefore are not likely to be an effective barrier. Lightweight covers should be discouraged, because they do not prevent the child from entering the pool and may obscure visualization of the submerged child. Door alarms and automatically closing and locking doors are untested in efficacy. Swimming pool alarms cannot be recommended at this time: In all alarms tested, a significant number of false alarms and failure to alarm were noted.

Parents must be made aware that any body of water, no matter how innocuous, poses a drowning risk, especially in children ≤4 yr of age. Educating parents about the risks of common household fixtures, such as bathtubs, buckets, toilets, and washing machines, should be every pediatrician's task. Parents must be taught to remain with children throughout the entire bath time. Buckets containing water should never be left unattended. Toilet covers and bathroom doors should be closed at all times. Children with epilepsy can enjoy swimming as long as close supervision is maintained; these children should be encouraged to shower in a nonglass cubicle rather than in a bathtub.

Swimming lessons in children ≤4 yr old do not "drown-proof" children and may provide a false sense of security. Swimming lessons for 2- to 4-yr-olds improve water-related skills, but it is unclear whether they have any effect on the risk of submersion injury. School-aged children should be taught to swim but nonetheless prevented from swimming in unsupervised circumstances.

A National Transportation Safety Board review found that only 15% of boaters who drowned wore life vests. Less than one fifth of recreational boaters use life vests, but intensive community boating education efforts have been shown to substantially increase personal flotation device use. Water safety education for children, teenagers, and parents that encourages wearing flotation devices and never swimming alone should be reinforced in the school, community, and physician's office. Teenagers should learn CPR and be counseled about alcohol and drug use, which significantly contribute to submersion and drowning.

Biggart MJ, Bohn DJ: Effect of hypothermia and cardiac arrest on outcome of near-drowning accidents in children. J Pediatr 117:179, 1990.

Bohn DJ, Biggar WD, Smith CR, et al: Influence of hypothermia, barbiturate therapy, and intracranial pressure monitoring on morbidity and mortality after near-drowning. Crit Care Med 14:529, 1986.

Bratton SL, Jardine DS, Morray JP: Serial neurologic examinations after near-drowning and outcome. Arch Pediatr Adolesc Med 148:167, 1994.

Christensen DW, Jansen P, Perkin RM: Outcome and acute care hospital costs after warm water near-drowning in children. Pediatrics 99:715, 1997.

Committee on Injury and Poison Prevention: Drowning in infants, children, and adolescents. Pediatrics 92:292, 1993.

Corneli HM: Accidental hypothermia. J Pediatr 120:671, 1992.

Griest KJ, Zumwalt RE: Child abuse by drowning. Pediatrics 83:41, 1989.

Kallas HJ, O'Rourke PP: Drowning and immersion injuries in children. Curr Opin Pediatr 5:295, 1993.

Kyriacou D, Arcinue E, Peek C, et al: Effect of immediate resuscitation on children with submersion injury. Pediatrics 94:137, 1994.

Modell JH: Drowning. N Engl J Med 328:253, 1993.

Quan L, Kinder D: Pediatric submersions: Pre-hospital predictors of outcome. Pediatrics 90:909, 1992.

Rabinovich BA, Lerner ND, Huey RW: Young children's ability to climb fences. Hum Factors 36:733, 1994.

Wintemute GJ: Childhood drowning and near-drowning in the United States. Am J Dis Child 144:663, 1990.

Zuckerman GB, Gregory PM, Santos-Damiani SM: Predictors of death and neurologic impairment in pediatric submersion injuries. Arch Pediatr Adolesc Med 152:134, 1998.

CHAPTER 70
Burn Injuries

Alia Y. Antoon and Mary K. Donovan

Burns are a leading cause of unintentional death in children, second only to motor vehicular accidents. There has been a significant decline in the national incidence of burn injury necessitating medical care over the last decade. This has coincided with an increased focus on burn treatment and prevention, fire and burn prevention education, availability of regional treatment centers, widespread use of smoke detectors, greater regulation of consumer products and occupational safety, and societal changes such as declines in smoking and alcohol abuse. Although these prophylactic measures have proved effective and should therefore be continued, a significant number of children still suffer fatal burns.

EPIDEMIOLOGY. About 1.2 million people in the United States require medical care for burn injuries each year, with 51,000 requiring hospitalization. Thirty to forty per cent of these patients are under 15 years of age, with an average age of 32 mo. Fire continues to be a major killer of children, accounting for up to 34% of fatal injuries in those younger than 16 yr. Scald burns account for 85% of total injuries and are most prevalent in children under 4 yr of age. Although the incidence of hot water scalding has been reduced by legislation requiring new water heaters to be preset at 130°F, scald injury remains the leading cause of hospitalization for burns. Flame burns account for 13%, the remainder being electrical and chemical burns. Clothing ignition has declined since passage of the Federal Flammable Fabric Act, requiring sleepwear to be flame retardant; however, the Consumer Product Safety Commission voted to relax the existing children's sleepwear flammability standard under the Flammable Fabrics Act. Approximately 18% of burn injuries occur as a result of child abuse, making it important to assess pattern and site of injury and their consistency with history (Chapter 35).

Careful review of the history of injury will usually reveal a common pattern—scald burn to the side of face, neck, and arm if liquid is pulled from a table or stove; a pant leg area burn if clothing ignites; splash areas from cooking; and palm of hand contact with a hot stove. However, "glove or stocking" burns of hands and feet; single-area deep burns on the trunk, buttocks, or back; and small-area, full-thickness burns (cigarette burns) in young children should raise a suspicion of child abuse.

Burn care involves a range of activities: prevention, acute care and resuscitation, wound management, pain relief, reconstruction, rehabilitation, and psychosocial adjustment. Children with massive burns require early and appropriate psychologic and social support as well as resuscitation. Surgical debridement, wound closure, and rehabilitative efforts should be instituted concurrently to promote optimal rehabilitation. Aggressive surgical removal of devitalized tissue, infection control, and judicious use of antibiotics as well as early nutrition and cautious use of intubation and mechanical ventilation are necessary to maximize survival. Children who have sustained burn injuries differ in appearance from their peers, necessitating supportive efforts for re-entry to schooling and social and sporting activities.

PREVENTION. The aim is a continuing reduction in the number of serious burn injuries (Table 70–1). Effective first aid and triage can decrease both the extent (area) and the severity (depth) of injuries. Flame-retardant clothing, smoke detectors, and control of hot water temperature (thermostat settings) within buildings as well as prohibition of cigarette smoking have been partially successful in reducing the incidence of burn injuries. Dedicated burn unit treatment of children with significant burn injuries facilitates medically effective care, improves survival, and leads to greater cost efficiency. Survival of 80% of patients with 90% burns is now usual; overall survival of children with burns of all sizes is 99%. Deaths are more likely in children with irreversible brain injury sustained at the time of the burn.

Pediatricians can play a major role in preventing the most common burns by educating parents and care providers in preventive measures geared to the various stages of child development. Appropriate clothing, smoke detectors, and planned routes for emergency exit from the home are simple, effective, efficient, and cost-effective preventive measures. Child neglect and abuse must be seriously considered when the history of the injury and the distribution of the burn do not match.

TABLE 70–1 Burn Prophylaxis

Prevent Fires

- Smoke detectors
- Control of hot water thermostat—public buildings (maximum water temperature 120° F)
- Learn to use fire-matches-lighter to prevent injury
- Prevent cigarette smoking
- Flame retardant–treated clothing

Prevent Injury

- Roll, not run, if clothing catches fire; wrap in blanket
- Practice escape procedures
- Crawl beneath smoke if indoors
- Use of materials for education*

**National Fire Protection Association pamphlets and videos.*

TABLE 70–2 Indications for Hospitalization for Burns

- Burns greater than 15% body surface area
- High tension-wire electrical burns
- Inhalation injury regardless of the size of body surface area burn
- Inadequate home situation
- Suspected child abuse or neglect
- Burns to hands, feet, genitalia

ACUTE CARE, RESUSCITATION, AND ASSESSMENT

Indications for Admission (Table 70–2). Burns covering greater than 10–15% of total body surface area (BSA), burns associated with smoke inhalation, burns resulting from high-tension electrical injuries, and burns associated with suspected child abuse or neglect should be treated as emergencies and the child hospitalized. Small first- and second-degree burns of the hands, feet, face, perineum, and joint surfaces also require admission if close follow-up care is difficult to provide. Children who have been in enclosed-space fires and those who have face and neck burns should be hospitalized for at least 24 hr of observation.

First Aid Measures. Acute care should include the following:

1. Extinguish flames by rolling on the ground; cover the child with a blanket, coat, or carpet.
2. After determining that the airway is patent, remove smoldering clothing or clothing saturated with hot liquid. Jewelry, particularly rings and bracelets, should be removed or cut away to prevent constriction and vascular compromise during the edema phase in the first 24–72 hr post burn.
3. In cases of chemical injury, brush off any remaining chemical if powdered or solid; then use copious irrigation or wash the affected area with water. Call Poison Control for the neutralizing agent to treat a chemical ingestion.
4. Cover the burned area with clean, dry sheeting and apply cold (not iced) wet compresses to small injuries. Significant large burn surface area injury (>15–20% BSA) decreases body temperature control and contraindicates the use of cold compress dressings.
5. If the burn is caused by hot tar, use mineral oil to remove tar.

Emergency Care (Table 70–3). Life support measures should include the following:

1. Rapidly review the cardiovascular and pulmonary status and document pre-existing or physiologic lesions (asthma, congenital heart disease, renal or hepatic disease).
2. Ensure and maintain an adequate airway and provide humidified oxygen by mask or nasotracheal intubation. The latter may be needed in children who have facial burns or a burn sustained in an enclosed space, before facial or laryngeal edema becomes evident. If hypoxia or carbon monoxide poisoning is suspected, 100% oxygen should be used (see Chapters 58 and 64.1).

TABLE 70–3 Acute Treatment of Burns

- First aid
- Fluid resuscitation
- Supply energy requirements
- Pain control
- Prevention of infection—early excision and grafting
- Control of bacterial wound flora
- Biologic and synthetic dressings to close wound

3. Children with burns greater than 15% of BSA require intravenous fluid resuscitation to maintain adequate perfusion. All inhalation injuries, regardless of the extent of BSA burn, require venous access to control fluid intake. All high-tension and electrical injuries require venous access to ensure forced alkaline diuresis in case of muscle injury and myoglobinuria. Lactated Ringer's solution, 10–20 mL/kg/hr (normal saline may be used if Ringer's lactate is not available), is infused until proper fluid replacement can be calculated. Consultation with a specialized burn unit should be made to coordinate fluid therapy, type of fluid, preferred formula for calculation, and preferences for use of colloid agents, particularly if transfer to a burn center is anticipated.

4. Evaluate the child for associated injuries, which are common in patients with a history of high-tension electrical burn, especially if there has been a fall from a height. Injuries to spine, bones, and thoracic or intra-abdominal organs may occur. The child should be placed on cervical spine precaution until this injury is ruled out. There is a very high risk of cardiac abnormalities, including ventricular tachycardia or ventricular fibrillation, resulting from conductivity of the high electric voltage. Cardiopulmonary resuscitation should be instituted promptly at the scene, and the patient should be placed on a cardiac monitor on arrival at the emergency room (see Chapter 58).

5. Children with burns greater than 15% BSA should not receive oral fluids (initially), as they may develop ileus. These children require insertion of a nasogastric tube in the emergency room to prevent aspiration.

6. A Foley catheter should be inserted to monitor urine output in all children who require intravenous fluid resuscitation.

7. All wounds should be wrapped with sterile towels until a decision is made about whether to treat on an outpatient basis or refer to an appropriate facility for treatment.

Classification of Burns. Proper triage and treatment of burn injury require assessment of the extent and depth of the injury. *First-degree burns* involve only the epidermis and are characterized by swelling, erythema, and pain (similar to a mild sunburn). Tissue damage is usually minimal, and there is no blistering. Pain resolves in 48–72 hr; in a small percentage of patients the damaged epithelium will peel off, leaving no residual scars.

A *second-degree burn* involves injury to the entire epidermis and a variable portion of the dermal layer (vesicle and blister formation are characteristic of second-degree burns). A *superficial* second-degree burn is extremely painful because a large number of remaining viable nerve endings are exposed. Superficial second-degree burns heal in 7–14 days as the epithelium regenerates in the absence of infection. *Midlevel* to *deep* second-degree burns also heal spontaneously if wounds are kept clean and infection free. Pain is less than in more superficial burns, because fewer nerve endings remain viable. Fluid losses and metabolic effects of deep dermal (second-degree) burns are essentially the same as those of third-degree burns.

Full-thickness or *third-degree* burns involve destruction of the entire epidermis and dermis, leaving no residual epidermis cells to repopulate the damaged area. The wound cannot epithelialize and can heal only by wound contraction or skin grafting. The absence of painful sensation and capillary filling demonstrates the loss of nerve and capillary elements.

Estimation of Body Surface Area of Burn. Appropriate burn charts for different childhood age groups should be used to accurately estimate the extent of BSA burned. The volume of fluid needed in resuscitation is calculated from the estimation of the extent and depth of burn surface. Mortality and morbidity also depend on the extent and depth of the burn. The variable growth rate of the head and extremities throughout childhood makes it necessary to use surface area charts, such as that modified by Lund and Brower or the chart used at the Shriners Hospital in Boston (Fig. 70–1). The "rule of nines" used in adults may be used only in children over age 14 yr or as a very rough estimate to institute therapy before transfer to a burn center. In small burns under 10% of BSA, the "rule of palm" may be used, especially in outpatient settings. The area from the wrist crease to finger crease (the palm) in the child equals 1% of the child's BSA.

TREATMENT

Outpatient Management of Minor Burns. First- and second-degree burns less than 10% BSA may be treated on an outpatient basis unless there is inadequate family support or there are issues of child neglect or abuse. These outpatients do not require a tetanus booster or prophylactic penicillin therapy. Children who are not current with immunizations should have their immunizations updated. Blisters should be left intact and dressed with silver sulfadiazine cream (Silvadene). Dressings should be changed twice daily, after the wound is washed with lukewarm water to remove any cream left from the previous application. Very small wounds, especially those on the face, may be treated with bacitracin ointment and left open. Debridement of the devitalized skin is indicated when the blisters rupture. Burns to the palm with large blisters usually heal beneath the blisters, with close follow-up on an outpatient basis. The great majority of superficial burns heal in 10–20 days. Deep second-degree burns take longer to heal. Pain control should be accomplished by using acetaminophen with codeine an hour before dressing changes. Wounds that appear deeper than at initial assessment or that have not healed by 21 days may require a short hospital admission for grafting.

The depth of scald injuries is difficult to assess early; conservative treatment is appropriate to allow maturation and declaration of the depth and area involved before closure is attempted. This obviates the risk of anesthesia and unnecessary grafting and diminishes potential scarring in those patients in whom spontaneous healing is likely to occur.

Fluid Resuscitation. For most children the Parkland formula is an appropriate starting guideline for fluid resuscitation (4 mL Ringer's lactate/kg body weight/% BSA burned). One half of the fluid is given over the first 8 hr calculated from the time of onset of injury. The remaining half is given at an even rate over the next 16 hr. The rate of infusion is adjusted according to the patient's response to therapy. Pulse and blood pressure should return to normal, and an adequate urine output (1 mL/kg body weight/hr) should be accomplished by varying the IV infusion rate. Vital signs, acid-base balance, and mental status reflect the adequacy of the resuscitation. Because of interstitial edema and sequestration of fluid in muscle cells, patients may gain up to 20% over baseline preburn body weight. Patients with burns of 30% BSA require a large venous access (central venous line) to deliver the fluid required over the critical first 24 hr. Patients with burns greater than 60% BSA may require a multilumen central venous catheter; these patients are best cared for in a specialized burn unit.

During the second 24 hr after the burn, patients will begin to reabsorb edema fluid and to diurese. One half of the first day's fluid requirement is infused as lactated Ringer's solution in 5% dextrose. Children under age 5 yr may require the addition of 5% dextrose in the first 24 hrs of resuscitation. Controversy exists as to whether colloid should be provided in the early period of burn resuscitation. One preference is to use colloid replacement concurrently if the burn is greater than 85% total BSA. Colloid is usually instituted 8–24 hr after the burn injury. In children less than 12 mo of age, sodium tolerance is limited; volume and sodium concentration of the resuscitation solution should be decreased if urinary sodium is rising. Adequacy of resuscitation should be constantly assessed using vital signs, blood gases, hematocrit, and protein levels. Some patients require arterial and central venous lines, particularly if undergoing excision and grafting, for monitoring and

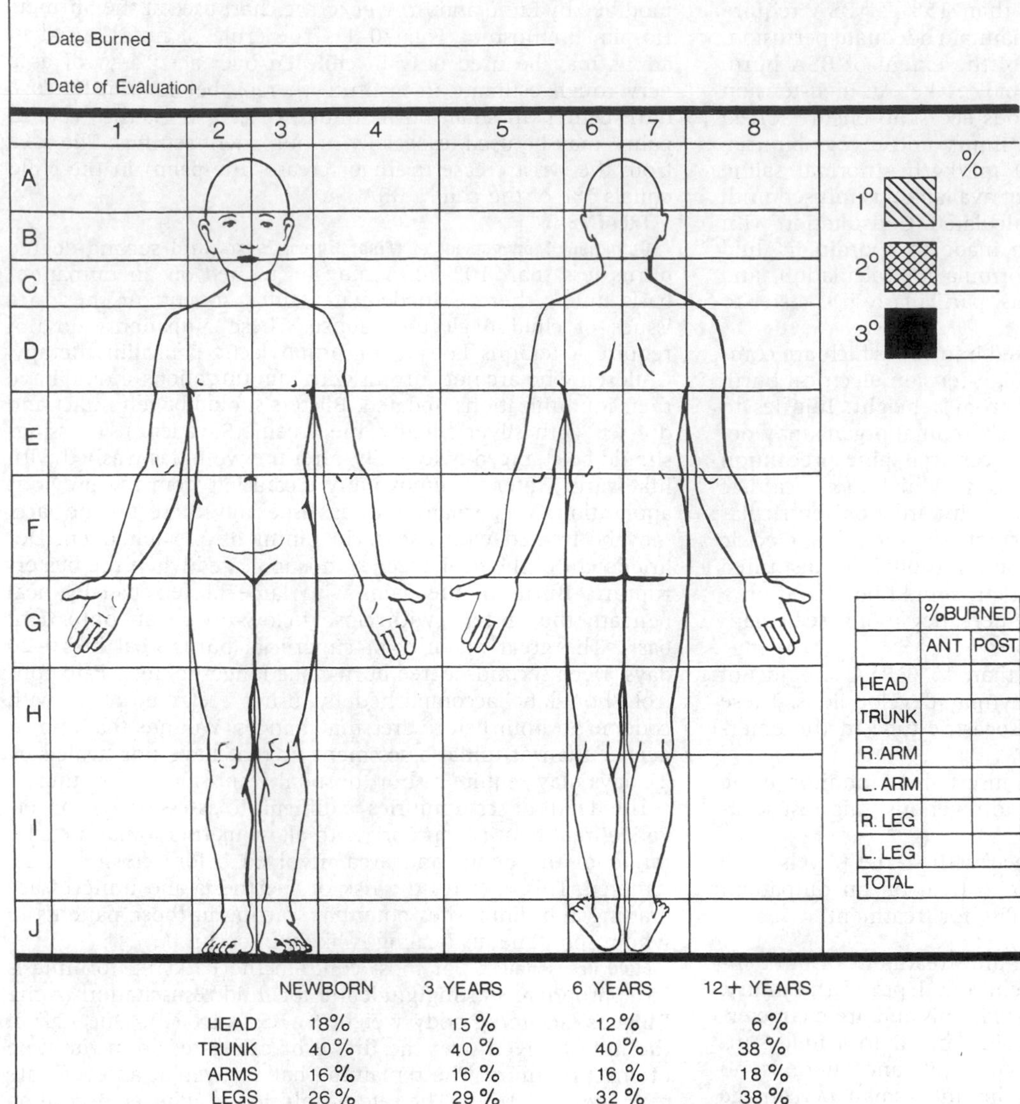

	NEWBORN	3 YEARS	6 YEARS	12 + YEARS
HEAD	18%	15%	12%	6%
TRUNK	40%	40%	40%	38%
ARMS	16%	16%	16%	18%
LEGS	26%	29%	32%	38%

Figure 70–1 Chart to determine developmentally related percent body burn surface area. (Courtesy of Shriners Hospital for Crippled Children, Burn Institute, Boston Unit.)

replacement purposes. Pulmonary artery pressure monitoring may be indicated to assess circulation and urine output in patients with hemodynamic or cardiopulmonary instability.

Oral supplementation may start as early as 48 hr post burn. Milk formula, artificial feedings, homogenized milk, or soy-based products can be given by bolus or constant infusion via a nasogastric or small bowel feeding tube. As oral fluids are tolerated, intravenous fluids are decreased proportionately in an effort to keep the total fluid intake constant, particularly if pulmonary dysfunction is present.

Five per cent albumin infusions may be used to maintain the serum albumin levels at a desired 2 g/dL. The following rates are effective: For total BSA burns of 30–50%, 0.3 mL of 5% albumin/kg body weight/% BSA burn is infused over a 24 hr period; for burns of 50–70% total BSA, 0.4 mL/kg body weight/% BSA burn is infused over 24 hr; and for total BSA burns of 70–100%, 0.5 mL/kg body weight/% BSA burn is infused over 24 hr. Packed red cell infusion is recommended if the hematocrit falls below 24% (hemoglobin ≤8 g/dL). Some recommend treating hematocrits below 30% or hemoglobin under 10 g/dL in patients with systemic infections, hemoglobinopathies, cardiopulmonary disease, or anticipated (or ongoing) blood loss when repeated excision and grafting of full-thickness burns are likely to be needed. Fresh frozen plasma is indicated if clinical and laboratory assessment reveals a deficiency of clotting factors, a prothrombin level above 1.5 times control, or a partial thromboplastin time of greater than 1.2 times control in children who are bleeding or are scheduled for an invasive procedure or a grafting procedure that could result in an estimated blood loss of over half the blood volume. (Fresh frozen plasma is used for volume resuscitation within 72 hr of injury in patients under 2 yr of age with burns over 20% BSA and associated moderate inhalation injury.)

Sodium supplementation may be required for children having burns greater than 20% BSA, if 0.5% silver nitrate solution is used as the topical antibacterial burn dressing. Losses with silver nitrate therapy are regularly as high as 350 mMol sodium/m² burn surface area. Oral sodium chloride supplement of 4 g/m² burn area per 24 hr is usually well tolerated, divided into four to six equal doses to avoid osmotic diarrhea. The aim is to maintain serum sodium levels over 130 mEq/L and urinary sodium concentration over 30 mEq/L. Intravenous potassium supplementation is supplied to maintain serum potassium level over 3 mEq/dL. Potassium losses may be significantly increased when 0.5% silver nitrate solution is used as the topical antibacterial agent or when aminoglycoside, diuretic, or amphotericin therapy is required.

Prevention of Infection. Controversy exists over the prophylactic use of penicillin for all acute hospitalized burn patients and the periodic replacement of central venous catheters. In some units a 5-day course of penicillin therapy is used for all acute burns; standard-dose crystalline penicillin is given orally or intravenously in four divided doses. Erythromycin may be used as an alternative in penicillin-allergic children. Other units have discontinued prophylactic use of penicillin therapy without an increase in the infection rate. Similarly, there is conflicting evidence as to whether relocation of the intravenous catheter every 48–72 hr decreases or increases the incidence of catheter-related sepsis. It is recommended that the central venous catheter be replaced and relocated every 7 days, even if the site is not inflamed and there is no suspicion of catheter-related sepsis.

Mortality related to the burn injury is associated not with the toxic effect of thermally injured skin but with the metabolic and bacterial consequences of a large open wound, reduction of the patient's host resistance, and malnutrition. These abnormalities set the stage for life-threatening bacterial infection originating from the burn wound. Wound treatment and prevention of wound infection also promote early healing and improve esthetic and functional outcomes. *Topical treatment* of the burn wound using 0.5% silver nitrate solution, silver sulfadiazine cream, or Sulfamylon cream aims at prevention of infection (Table 70–4). The latter two agents have tissue-penetrating capacity. Regardless of choice of topical antimicrobial agent, it is essential that all third-degree *burn tissue be fully excised* before bacterial colonization occurs and the area be grafted as early as possible to prevent deep wound sepsis. Children having a BSA burn of over 30% should be housed in a *bacteria-controlled nursing unit* to prevent cross contamination and to provide a temperature- and humidity-controlled environment to minimize hypermetabolism.

Deep second-degree burns greater than 10% BSA benefit from early tangential *excision and grafting*. To improve outcome, sequential excision and grafting of third-degree and deep second-degree burns are required in children with large burns. Prompt excision and immediate wound closure are achieved with autografts, often meshed to increase the efficiency of cover. Alternatives for wound closure, such as allografts, xenografts, and Integra (a bilaminate membrane composed of a porous lattice of cross-linked chondroitin 6-sulfate engineered to induce neovascularization as it is biodegraded), may be important for wound coverage in patients with extensive injury to limit fluid, electrolyte, and protein losses and to reduce pain and minimize temperature loss. Epidermal cultured cells (autologous keratinocytes) are a costly alternative that may be less effective. Early staged or total excision can be safely carried out by an experienced burn team while burn fluid resuscitation continues. Important keys to success include (1) accurate preoperative and intraoperative determination of burn depth, (2) the choice of excision area and appropriate timing, (3) control of intraoperative blood loss, (4) specific instrumentation, (5) choice and use of perioperative antibiotics, and (6) type of wound coverage chosen.

Nutritional Support. Supporting the increased energy requirements of a burn is a high priority. The burn injury produces a hypermetabolic response characterized by both protein and fat catabolism. Children with a 40% total BSA burn require approximately 50% above predicted basal energy expenditure for their age. Early excision and grafting can decrease the energy requirement. Pain, anxiety, and immobilization increase the physiologic demands. Additional energy expenditure is caused by cold stress if environmental humidity and temperature are not controlled; this is especially true in young infants, in whom the largest surface area-to-mass ratio allows proportionately greater heat loss than in adolescents and adults. Calorie demands can be decreased by providing environmental temperatures of 28–33°C, adequate covering during transport, and liberal use of analgesics and anxiolytics. Special units to control ambient temperature and humidity may be necessary for children having large surface area burns. Appropriate sleep intervals are necessary and should be part of the regimen.

TABLE 70–4 Topical Agents for Burns

Agent	Effectiveness	Ease of Use
Silver sulfadiazine (Silvadene cream)	Broad spectrum Good penetration	Closed dressings Changed bid Residue *must* be washed off with each dressing change
Mafenide acetate (Sulfamylon)	Broad spectrum, including *Pseudomonas* Rapid and deep wound penetration	Closed dressings Changed bid Residue *must* be washed off with each dressing change
Povidone-iodine (Betadine 1%)	Broad spectrum, including some fungi	Closed or wet dressings Changed bid

The objective of caloric supplementation programs is to maintain body weight and decrease metabolic demands. This reduces the loss of lean body mass from nitrogenous waste excretion. Calories are provided at 1½ times the basal metabolic rate, 3–4 g/kg body weight of protein per day. Additional calories are necessary for stabilization and growth. Multivitamins, particularly the B vitamin group, vitamin C, vitamin A, and zinc, are also necessary.

Alimentation should be started as soon as is practical, either orally or intravenously, after the resuscitative phase. Patients with greater than 40% total BSA burns need a gastric or small bowel feeding tube to facilitate continuous delivery of calories without the risk of aspiration. In order to decrease the risk of infectious complications, parenteral nutrition is discontinued as soon as is practical after delivery of sufficient enteral calories is established. Growth hormone administration may promote more rapid healing of donor sites, earlier achievement of positive nitrogen balance, and decreased rates of protein breakdown, but the safety of growth hormone admininstration has not been established. Early excision with grafting is the best method to decrease caloric stress.

Topical Therapy. Topical therapy is widely used and is effective against most burn pathogens (see Table 70–4). A number of agents (0.5% silver nitrate, sulfacetamide acetate, silver sulfadiazine cream) are available, and preferences vary among burn units. Each topical agent has advantages and disadvantages in application, comfort, and bacteriostatic spectrum. Sulfacetamide acetate is a very effective broad-spectrum agent with the ability to diffuse through the burn eschar and is thus the treatment of choice in injury to cartilaginous surfaces, such as ears. However, the carbonic anhydrase inhibition activity of sulfacetamide may cause acid-base imbalance if large surface areas are treated, and adverse reactions to the sulfur-containing agents may produce a transient leukopenia.

Inhalational Injury. This injury is serious in the infant and child, particularly if pre-existing pulmonary conditions are present (also see Chapter 64.3). Mortality estimates vary depending upon the criteria for diagnosis but are 45–60% in adults; exact figures are not available in children. Evaluation aims at early identification of inhalational airway injuries. These may occur from (1) direct heat (greater problems occur in steam burns), (2) acute asphyxia, (3) carbon monoxide poisoning, and (4) toxic fumes, including cyanides from combustible plastics. Sulfur and nitrogen oxides and alkalis formed during the combustion of synthetic fabrics produce corrosive chemicals that may erode mucosa and cause significant sloughing. Exposure to smoke may cause degradation of surfactant and decrease its production, resulting in atelectasis. Inhalation injury and burn injury are synergistic, and the combined effect can increase morbidity and mortality.

The pulmonary complications of burns and inhalation can be divided into three syndromes with distinct *clinical manifestations* and temporal patterns: (1) *Early* carbon monoxide poisoning, airway obstruction, and pulmonary edema are major concerns. (2) The acute respiratory distress syndrome (ARDS) usually becomes clinically evident later, at 24–48 hr, although it can occur even later (see Chapter 65). (3) *Late* complications (days to weeks) include pneumonia and pulmonary emboli. Inhalation injury should be assessed by evidence of obvious injury (swelling or carbonaceous material in nasal passages) and laboratory determination of carboxyhemoglobin (HbCO) and arterial blood gases. *Treatment* is initially focused on establishing and maintaining a patent airway through prompt and early nasotracheal intubation and adequate ventilation and oxygenation. Aggressive pulmonary toilet and chest physiotherapy are necessary in prolonged nasotracheal intubation or tracheotomy. The availability of less irritating endotracheal tube materials as well as improved tube and cuff design has allowed progressively longer periods of translaryngeal intubation; wheezing is common, and β-agonist aerosols or inhaled cortisteroids are useful. If tracheotomy has to be performed, it should be delayed until burns at and near the site have healed, and then it should be performed electively with the child under anesthesia and using optimal tracheal positioning and hemostasis. In children having inhalation injury or burns of the face and neck, upper airway obstruction can develop rapidly; endotracheal intubation becomes a lifesaving intervention. An endotracheal tube can be maintained for months without the need for tracheostomy. Extubation should be delayed until the patient meets accepted criteria for maintaining the airway.

Signs of central nervous system injury from hypoxemia due to asphyxia or carbon monoxide poisoning may vary from irritability to depression. Carbon monoxide poisoning may be mild (<20% HbCO), with slight dyspnea and decreased visual acuity and higher cerebral functions; moderate (20–40% HbCO), with irritability, nausea, dimness of vision, impaired judgment, and rapid fatigue; or severe (40–60% HbCO), producing confusion, hallucination, ataxia, collapse, and coma. Direct measurement of HbCO is important for diagnosis and prognosis, because it reflects the degree of tissue hypoxia caused by the combination of carbon monoxide 'and hemoglobin and the change in the shape and position of the oxygen dissociation curve. Pa_{O_2} may be normal and the oxyhemoglobin saturation values misleading because HbCO is not detected by the usual tests of oxygen saturation. Hyberbaric oxygen therapy may need to be delayed in the critically ill burn patient requiring resuscitation and intensive care.

PAIN RELIEF AND PSYCHOLOGIC ADJUSTMENT (see also Chapter 74). It is important to provide adequate analgesia, anxiolytics, and psychologic support to reduce early metabolic stress, decrease the potential for post-traumatic stress syndrome (Chapter 22), and allow future stabilization and rehabilitation. Patients and family require team support to work through a grieving process and accept long-term changes in appearance.

Children having burn injury show frequent and wide fluctuations in pain intensity. Appreciation of pain depends on the depth of the burn, stage of healing, age and stage of emotional development, cognition, experience and efficiency of the treating team, use of analgesics and other drugs, pain threshold, and interpersonal and cultural factors. From the onset of the treatment, pain control during dressing changes is of paramount importance. The use of a variety of nonpharmacologic interventions as well as pharmacologic agents needs to be reviewed throughout the treatment period. Opiate analgesia prescribed in an adequate dose and timed to cover dressing changes is essential to comfort management. A supportive person who is consistently present and "knows" the patient profile can integrate and encourage patient participation in burn care. The problem of undermedication is most prevalent with adolescents, in whom fear of drug dependency may inappropriately influence treatment. A related problem is that the child's specific pain experience may be misinterpreted; for example, for anxious patients, those who are confused and alone, or those with pre-existing emotional disorders, even small wounds may illicit intense pain. Anxiolytic medication added to the analgesic is usually helpful, and it has more than a synergistic effect. Other modalities of pain and anxiety relief, such as relaxation techniques, also can decrease the physiologic stress response. Equal attention is necessary to decrease stress in the intubated patient. Oral morphine sulfate (immediate-release) is recommended on a consistent schedule at a dose of 0.3–0.6 mg/kg body weight q 4–6 hr initially and until wound cover is accomplished. Morphine sulfate intravenous bolus at a dose of 0.05–0.1 mg/kg body weight q 2 hr is administered in older patients using a patient-controlled analgesia (PCA) protocol. Morphine sulfate rectal suppositories may be useful at an added dose of 0.3–0.6 mg/kg body weight q 4 hr. For anxiety, lorazepam (Ativan) is given on a consistent schedule, 0.05–0.1 mg/kg body weight/dose q 8 hr. To control pain during a procedure (dressing changes or debridement), oral morphine at a dose of 0.3–0.6 mg/kg body weight, is given ½ hr prior to the procedure, and this is supplemented by a morphine intravenous bolus at a dose of 0.05–0.1 mg/kg body weight given immediately prior to the procedure. Lorazepam at a dose of 0.04 mg/kg body weight is given orally, or intravenously if necessary, for anxiety prior to the procedure. Midazolam (Versed) is also very useful for control of anxiety and is given at a dose of 0.05–0.1 mg/kg/hr as an infusion or a bolus; it may be repeated in 10 min, with a maximum dose of 0.2 mg/kg. During the process of weaning from analgesics, the dose of oral opiates is reduced by 25% over 1–3 days, sometimes with the addition of acetaminophen as opiates are tapered. Antianxiety medications are tapered by reducing the dose of benzodiazepines at 25–50% per dose daily over 1–3 days.

For ventilated patients, pain control is accomplished by using morphine sulfate intermittently as an intravenous bolus at a dose of 0.05–0.1 mg/kg body weight q 2 hr. Doses may need to be increased gradually, and some children may need continuous infusion; a starting dose of 0.05 mg/kg body weight/hr given as an infusion is increased gradually as the need of the child changes. Naloxone should be immediately available to reverse the effect of morphine, if necessary; if needed for an airway crisis it should be given in a dose of 0.1 mg/kg body weight, either intramuscularly or intravenously. For patients on assisted respiration who require treatment of anxiety, midazolam is used as an intermittent intravenous bolus (dose of 0.04 mg/kg body weight given by a slow push every 4–6 hr) or as a continuous infusion. Intubated patients do not require opiates to be discontinued during the process of weaning from the ventilator. Benzodiazepine should be reduced to about half the dose over 24–72 hr prior to extubation because too rapid weaning from benzodiazepine can lead to seizures.

RECONSTRUCTION AND REHABILITATION. To ensure maximum cosmetic and functional outcome, occupational and physical therapy must begin on the day of admission, continue throughout the hospitalization, and for some patients continue after discharge. Physical rehabilitation involves body and limb positioning, splinting, exercises (active and passive movement), assistance with activities of daily living, and gradual ambulation. These measures maintain adequate joint and muscle activity with as normal a range of movement as possible after healing or reconstruction. Pressure therapy is necessary to reduce hypertrophic scar formation; a variety of prefabricated and custom-made garments are available for use in different body areas for prevention of hypertrophic scarring. These custom-made garments deliver consistent pressure on scarred areas; they shorten the time of scar maturation and decrease the thickness of the scar as well as the redness and associated itching. Continued adjustments to scarred areas (scar release, grafting, rearrangement) and multiple minor cosmetic surgical procedures are necessary to optimize long-term function and to improve appearance. Replacement of areas of alopecia and scarring has been achieved using tissue expander techniques.

School Re-Entry. Social re-entry is as critical for life survival as resuscitation and wound healing. It is best for the child to return to school immediately following discharge. Occasionally, a child may need to attend a few half days (because of rehabilitation needs). However, it is important for the child to return to his or her normal routine of attending school and being with peers. Planning for return to home and school often requires a school re-entry program that is individualized to each child's needs. For a school-aged child, planning for the return to school occurs simultaneously with planning for discharge. The hospital schoolteacher contacts the local school and plans the program with school faculty, nurses, social workers, recreational/child life therapists, and rehabilitation therapists. This team should work with students and staff to ease anxiety, answer questions, and provide information. Burns and scars evoke fears in those who are not familiar with this type of injury and can result in a tendency to withdraw from or reject the burned child. A school re-entry program should be appropriate to a child's development and changing educational needs.

SPECIAL SITUATIONS

Electrical Burns. There are three types of electrical burns. *Minor electrical burns* usually occur as a result of biting on an extension cord. These injuries produce localized burns to the mouth, which usually involve the upper and lower lip that come in contact with the extension cord. The injury may involve or spare the corners of the mouth. Since these are nonconductive injuries (do not extend beyond the site of injury), hospital admission is not necessary and care is focused on the area of the injury visible in the mouth. Treatment with topical antibiotic creams is sufficient until the patient is seen in a burn unit outpatient department or by a plastic surgeon.

A more serious category of electrical burn is the *high-tension electrical wire burn,* for which children need to be admitted for observation regardless of the extent of the surface area burn. Deep muscle injury is usual and cannot be readily assessed initially. These injuries result from high voltage (>1,000 volts) and occur particularly at high-voltage installations, such as electric power stations or railroads; youngsters climb an electric pole and touch an electric box in curiosity or accidentally touch the high-tension electric wire. Such injuries have a mortality rate of 3–15% for children who arrive at the hospital for treatment. Survivors have a high rate of morbidity, including major limb amputations. Points of entry of current through the skin and the exit site show characteristic features consistent with current density and heat. The majority of entrance wounds involve the upper extremity, with small exit wounds in the lower extremity. The electrical path from entrance to exit takes the shortest distance between the two points and may produce injury in any organ or tissue in the path of the current. Multiple exit wounds in some patients attest to the possibility of several electrical pathways in the body, placing virtually any structure in the body at risk. Damage to abdominal viscera, thoracic structures, and the nervous system in areas remote from obvious extremity injury occurs and must be sought, particularly in multiple current pathway injury or injury in which the victim falls from a high pole. Sometimes arcing occurs and results in a concurrent flame burn and clothing fire. Cardiac abnormalities manifested by ventricular fibrillation or cardiac arrest are common; patients with high-tension electrical injury need cardiac monitoring until they are stable and have been fully assessed. Renal damage from deep muscle necrosis and subsequent myoglobinuria is another complication; these patients need a forced alkaline diuresis to minimize renal damage. Aggressive removal of all dead and devitalized tissue, even with risk of functional loss, remains the key to effective management of the electrically damaged extremity. Early debridement will facilitate early closure of the wound. Damaged major vessels must be isolated and buried in a viable muscle to prevent exposure. Survival depends on the immediate intensive care, while functional result depends on long-term care and delayed reconstructive surgery.

Lightning burns occur when high-voltage current directly strikes a person (most dangerous) or when the current strikes the ground or an adjacent (in-contact) object. A step voltage burn is observed when lightning strikes the ground and travels up one leg and down the other leg (the path of least resistance). Lightning burns are dependent on the current path, the type of clothing, the presence of metal, and cutaneous moisture. Entry, exit, and path lesions are possible; the prognosis is poorest for lesions of the head or legs. Internal organ injury along the path is common and does not relate to the severity of the cutaneous burn. Linear burns are in the locations where sweat is present and are usually first or second degree. Feathering or an arborescent pattern is characteristic of lightning injury. Lightning may ignite clothing or produce serious cutaneous burns from heated metal in the clothing. Internal complications of lightning burns include cardiac arrest due to asystole, transient hypertension, premature ventricular contractions, ventricular fibrillation, and myocardial ischemia. Most severe cardiac complications resolve if the patient is supported with CPR (Chapters 58 and 64.1). CNS complications include cerebral edema, CNS bleeds, seizures, mood changes, depression, and lower extremity paralysis. Rhabdomyolysis and myoglobinuria (with possible renal failure) also occur.

Renal Failure in Burn Injury. Also see Chapters 64.5 and 543. Renal failure in burn injury is best classified in relation to the time of onset after the burn injury. Most cases present as a nonoliguric renal failure, making careful fluid and electrolyte monitoring critical. Special considerations of renal failure in a child with burn injury include initial phase capillary leak, making resuscitation difficult; severe catabolic stress with increased risk of hyperkalemia; and rapid development of azotemia. Such children require high caloric and protein intake to prevent catabolic stress and promote wound healing.

Renal failure may occur early or late, after 1–3 wk. *Early* renal failure may occur immediately post burn if late resuscitation with subsequent hypovolemia occurs or if severe pigment nephropathy (hemoglobinuria with burn injury in an enclosed space or myoglobinuria secondary to deep muscle injury or post escharotomy) develops. This is associated with early maximal catabolic stress, and frequently dialysis is necessary to sustain the circulation in the presence of marked capillary leak and to provide sufficient calories and protein to minimize the catabolic stress. *Late* renal failure may result from sepsis or drug toxicity. At this time there is less catabolic stress, and standard indications for dialysis apply.

ABLS Advanced Burn Life Support Course Providers Manual. Lincoln, Nebraska Burn Institute.

Bell SJ, Blackburn GL: Nutritional support of the burn patient. *In:* Martyn JAJ (ed): Acute Management of the Burned Patient. Philadelphia, WB Saunders, 1990, pp 138–158.

Brigham PA, McLoughlin E: Burn incidence and medical care use in the United States: Estimates, trends, and data sources. J Burn Care Rehabil 17:2, 1996.

Flynn AE, Gunter LL: Rehabilitation of the burn patient. *In:* Martyn JAJ (ed): Acute Management of the Burned Patient. Philadelphia, WB Saunders, 1990, pp 320–332.

Goldstein AM, Weber JM, Sheridan RL: Femoral venous access is safe in burned children: An analysis of 224 catheters. J Pediatr 130:3, 1996.

Heimbach D, Luterman A, Burke JF, et al: Artificial dermis for major burns: A multi-center randomized clinical trial. Ann Surg 208:313, 1988.

Herndon DM, Barrow RE, Broemeling LD, et al: Effect of exogenous growth hormone on the rate of donor site healing in pediatric burn patients. Ann Surg 212:424, 1990.

Herrin JT: Management of the pediatric patient with burns. *In:* Ichikawa I (ed): Pediatric Textbook of Fluids and Electrolytes. Baltimore, Williams & Wilkins, 1990, pp 388–401.

Herrin JT: Renal function in burns. *In:* Martyn JAJ (ed): Acute Management of the Burned Patient. Philadelphia, WB Saunders, 1990, pp 239–255.

Milner S, Hodgetts T, Rylah L: The burns calculator: A simple proposed guide for fluid resuscitation. Lancet 342:1089, 1993.

Monafo W: Initial management of burns. N Engl J Med 335:1581, 1996.
Moore P, Blackeney P, Broemeling L, Portman S: Psychologic adjustment after childhood burn injuries as predicted by personality traits. J Burn Care Rehabil 14:80, 1993.
Remensnyder JP: Acute electrical injuries. *In:* Martyn JAJ (ed): Acute Management of the Burned Patient. Philadelphia, WB Saunders, 1990, pp 66–86.
Ryan CM, Schoenfeld DA, Thorpe WP, et al: Objective estimates of probability of death from burn injuries. N Engl J Med 338:362, 1998.
Sheridan RL, Hurford WE, Kacmarek RM, et al: Inhaled nitric oxide in burn patients with respiratory failure. J Trauma 42:629, 1997.
Sheridan RL, Tompkins RG, Burke JF: Management of burn wounds with prompt excision and immediate closure. J Intens Care Med 9:6, 1994.
Strongin J, Hales CA: Pulmonary disorders in the burn patient. *In:* Martyn JAJ (ed): Acute Management of the Burned Patient. Philadelphia, WB Saunders, 1990, pp 25–45.
Volinsky J, Hanson J, Lustig J: Lightning burns. Arch Pediatr Adolesc Med 148:529, 1994.
Walker A: Emergency department management of house fire burns and carbon monoxide poisoning in children. Curr Opin Pediatr 8:239, 1996.
Weber J: Epidemiology of infections and strategies for control. *In:* Carrougher AJ (ed): Burn Care and Therapy. St. Louis, CV Mosby, 1998, pp 185–211.

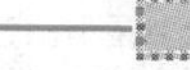

CHAPTER 71
Cold Injuries

Alia Y. Antoon and Mary K. Donovan

The increased involvement of children and youth in snowmobiling, mountain climbing, winter hiking, and skiing has increased the risk of cold injury. Cold injury may produce either local tissue damage, with the injury pattern depending on exposure to damp cold (frostnip, immersion foot or trench foot) dry cold (which leads to local frostbite), or generalized systemic effects (hypothermia).

PATHOPHYSIOLOGY. Ice crystals may form between or within cells, interfering with the sodium pump and leading to rupture of cell membranes. Further damage may result from clumping of red blood cells or platelets, causing microembolism or thrombosis. Blood may be shunted away from an affected area by secondary neurovascular responses to the cold injury; this shunting often further damages an injured part while improving perfusion of other tissues and the whole body. The spectrum of injury ranges from mild to severe and reflects the result of structural and functional disturbance in small blood vessels, nerves, and skin.

ETIOLOGY. In general, body heat may be lost by conduction (wet clothing, contact with metal or other solid conducting objects), convection (wind chill), and radiation. Susceptibility to cold injury may be increased by dehydration, alcohol or drug excess, substance abuse, impaired consciousness, exhaustion, hunger, anemia, impaired circulation due to cardiovascular disease, and sepsis, as well as in very young or aged persons.

Hypothermia occurs when the body can no longer sustain normal temperature. As shivering ceases, the body is unable to warm itself, and when the body core temperature falls below 35°C, the syndrome of hypothermia occurs. Wind chill, wet or inadequate clothing, or other factors both increase local injury and may cause dangerous hypothermia, even in the presence of an ambient temperature that is not lower than 17–20°C (50–60°F).

CLINICAL MANIFESTATIONS

Frostnip. This results in the presence of firm, cold white areas on the face, ears, or extremities. Blistering and peeling may occur over the next 24–72 hr, occasionally leaving mild increased hypersensitivity to cold for some days or weeks. Treatment consists of warming the area with an unaffected hand or warm object before the lesion reaches a stage of stinging or aching and before numbness supervenes.

Immersion Foot (Trench Foot). This occurs in cold weather when the feet remain in damp or wet, poorly ventilated boots. The feet become cold, numb, pale, edematous, and clammy. Tissue maceration and infection are likely, and prolonged autonomic disturbance is common. This autonomic disturbance leads to increased sweating, pain, and hypersensitivity to temperature changes, which may persist for years. The treatment is largely prophylactic and consists of using well-fitting, insulated, waterproof, nonconstricting footwear. Once damage has occurred, patients must choose clothing and footwear that are more appropriate, dry, and well fitting. The disturbance in skin integrity is managed by keeping the affected area dry and well ventilated and preventing or treating infection. Only supportive measures are possible for control of autonomic symptoms.

Frostbite. With frostbite, initial stinging or aching of the skin progresses to cold, hard, white anesthetic and numb areas. On rewarming, the area becomes blotchy, itchy, and often red, swollen, and painful. The injury spectrum can progress to complete normality to extensive tissue damage, even gangrene, if early relief is not obtained.

Treatment consists of warming the damaged area. It is important not to cause further damage by attempting to rub the area with ice or snow; initial warming as in frostnip may be tried. The area may be warmed against an unaffected hand, abdomen, or axilla while in transfer to a facility where more rapid warming with a water bath is possible. If the skin becomes painful and swelling occurs, anti-inflammatory agents are helpful, and an analgesic agent is necessary. Freeze and rethaw cycles are most likely to cause permanent tissue injury, and it may be necessary to delay definitive warming and apply only mild measures if the patient is required to walk on the damaged feet en route to definitive treatment. In the hospital, the affected area should be immersed in warm water (temperature approximately 42°C), being careful not to burn the anesthetized skin. Vasodilating agents, such as prazosin or phenoxybenzamine, may be helpful. Anticoagulants (heparin, dextran) have provided equivocal results; results of chemical and surgical sympathectomy have also been equivocal. Oxygen is of help only at high altitudes. Meticulous local care, prevention of infection, and keeping the rewarmed area dry, open, and sterile provide optimal results. Recovery can be complete, and prolonged observation with conservative therapy is justified before any excision or amputation of tissue is considered. Analgesia and maintenance of good nutrition are necessary throughout the prolonged waiting period.

Hypothermia. Hypothermia may occur in winter sports when injury, equipment failure, or exhaustion decreases the degree of exertion, particularly if sufficient attention is not paid to wind chill. Immersion and wet wind chill rapidly produce hypothermia. As the core temperature of the body falls, an insidious onset of extreme lethargy, fatigue, incoordination, and apathy follows, followed by mental confusion, clumsiness, irritability, hallucinations, and finally bradycardia. A number of medical conditions, such as cardiac disease, diabetes mellitus, hyperinsulinemia, sepsis, and substance abuse, may need to be considered in a differential diagnosis. The decrease in rectal temperature to less than 34°C (93°F) is the most helpful diagnostic feature. Hypothermia associated with near-drowning is discussed in Chapter 69.

Prevention is a high priority. Of extreme importance for those who participate in winter sports is wearing layers of warm clothing, gloves and socks within insulated boots that do not impede circulation, and a warm head covering, as well as applying adequate waterproofing and protecting against the wind. Thirty per cent of heat loss occurs from the head. Ample food and fluid need to be provided during exercise. Those who participate in sports should be alert to the presence of cold or numbing of body parts, particularly the nose, ears, and extremities, and they should review methods to produce local warming and know to seek shelter if they detect symptoms of local cold injury.

Treatment at the scene aims at prevention of further heat loss and early transport to adequate shelter. Dry clothing should be provided as soon as practical, and transport should be undertaken if the victim has a pulse. If no pulse is detected at the initial review, cardiopulmonary resuscitation is indicated (Chapter 58). During transfer, jarring and sudden motion should be avoided, because these may cause ventricular arrhythmia. It is often difficult to attain a normal sinus rhythm during hypothermia.

If the patient is conscious, mild muscle activity should be encouraged and a warm drink offered. If the patient is unconscious, external warming should be initially undertaken using blankets and a sleeping bag, often with snuggling with a warm companion to increase the efficiency of warming. On arrival at a treatment center, inhalation of warm, moist air or oxygen, heating pads, or thermal blankets should be used while a warming bath of 45–48°C (113–118°F) is prepared. Monitoring of serum chemistry values and an electrocardiogram are necessary until the core temperature rises above 35°C and can be stabilized. Control of fluid, pH, blood pressure, and oxygen all are necessary in the early phases of the warming period and resuscitation. In patients with marked abnormalities, warming measures such as gastric or colonic irrigation with warm saline or peritoneal dialysis may be considered, but the effectiveness of these measures to treat hypothermia is unknown. In accidental deep hypothermia (core temperature 28°C) with circulatory arrest, rewarming with cardiopulmonary bypass may be lifesaving for previously healthy young individuals.

Chilblain (Pernio). Chilblain (pernio) is a form of cold injury in which erythematous, vesicular, or ulcerative lesions occur. The lesions are presumed to be of a vascular or vasoconstrictive origin. They are often itchy and may be painful and result in swelling and scabbing. The lesions are most often found at the ears, tips of fingers, and toes and on exposed areas of the legs. The lesions last for approximately 1–2 wk but may persist longer. *Treatment* consists of prophylaxis—avoiding prolonged chilling and protecting potentially susceptible areas with a cap, gloves, and stockings. Prazosin and phenoxybenzamine may be helpful in improving circulation if this is a recurrent problem. For significant itching, local corticosteroid preparations may be helpful.

Cold-Induced Fat Necrosis (Panniculitis). This common, usually benign injury occurs on exposure to cold air, snow, or ice and is manifested in exposed (or, less often, covered) surfaces as red (or, less often, purple to blue) macular, papular, or nodular lesions. *Treatment* is with nonsteroidal anti-inflammatory agents. The lesions may last 10 days to 3 wk. See Chapter 666.

Berkow R (ed): Cold injury. *In:* The Merck Manual of Diagnosis and Therapy. Rahway, NJ, Merck, Sharp, & Dohme, 1992.

Britt LD, Dascombe WH, Rodriguez A: New horizons in management of hypothermia and frostbite injury. Surg Clin North Am 71:345, 1991.

Shepard RJ: Metabolic adaptations to exercise in the cold. Sports Med 16:266, 1993.

Walpoth BH, Walpoth-Aslan BN, Mattle HP, et al: Outcome of survivors of accidental deep hypothermia and circulatory arrest treated with extracorporeal blood warming. N Engl J Med 337:1500, 1997.

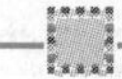

CHAPTER 72

Withdrawal or Withholding of Life Support, Brain Death, and Organ Procurement

Lorry R. Frankel and Lawrence H. Mathers

The major focus of treatment for children with a life-threatening illness is survival with minimal residual injury or cure. However, when a physician realizes that further aggressive treatment is futile and harmful to a patient, the family should be compassionately informed. No decision is more important than the determination that further care is futile and should be discontinued or significantly limited. Such decisions should be based on mutual understanding about quality of life, human dignity, and futility. The practices of a pediatric intensive care unit (PICU) with patients and families facing these tragic circumstances should be consistent and reflect the best in medical practice and community standards (also see Chapter 61). If a patient fulfills brain death criteria, then compassionate medical care should continue during efforts to remove the "brain-dead" patient from life support. Judgments about withholding or withdrawing life support and declaration of brain death should not be influenced by considerations of the potential use of the child's organs or tissues for transplantation or by economic interests.

WITHHOLDING AND WITHDRAWING OF LIFE SUPPORT. Two basically different groups of patients die in a PICU: first, previously healthy children who have recently experienced a catastrophic event (e.g., motor vehicle accident, near drowning, or a serious infection); second, children with severe underlying disease that has become terminal (e.g., cystic fibrosis, severe inborn errors of metabolism, major congenital malformations). For these latter children and their families, it may be possible to provide appropriate terminal care in a more comfortable setting than the hospital, such as the home or hospice (see Chapter 38).

A decision to provide limited or palliative care is difficult and needs to involve the primary and critical care physicians, the child (when appropriate) and parents, social services, and clergy (if appropriate) in order to come to an understanding that further intervention will not improve the outcome. Discussion of this shift from prolongation of life to management of dying should include consideration of resuscitation measures ("code status"), comfort care, and pain management. In the vast majority of cases involving children, families and physicians reach an agreement about limitation of care without involvement of the legal system or ethics committees.

Although not fulfilling the criteria of death, some children may have a very limited quality of continuing life. The most severe form of this state of perpetual debilitation is the *persistent vegetative state* (PVS). This is a state of perpetual unconsciousness, "wakefulness without awareness," in which there may be neurologic responsiveness to external stimuli. PVS exists when there has been lack of neurologic recovery for at least 6 mo, with preservation of only the autonomic nervous system, resulting in the maintenance of vital signs (heart rate, blood pressure, respirations, and temperature). Such patients require significant nursing care, including feeding (usually via gastrostomy), bathing, assistance with bowel and bladder function, skin care to prevent pressure lesions (bed sores), commonly airway access via a tracheotomy, and passive range of motion exercises to minimize joint contractures. These children may be cared for at home or in long-term care nursing

TABLE 72–1 Guidelines for the Determination of Brain Death

Determination of the cause of coma
Preclude toxins, drugs, metabolic disorders, and surgically correctable lesions
Patient must be normotensive and normothermic
Physical examinations performed by at least 2 physicians
Apnea and coma must be present (apnea tests requires monitoring of arterial blood gases or noninvasive determination of carbon dioxide while patient is adequately oxygenated.
Pa_{CO_2} needs to rise to a level ≥60 mm Hg
Absence of brain stem function: no pupillary, corneal, cough, or gag reflexes, as well as absence of spontaneous respirations
Core temperature must be >32°C
Flaccid tone, no spontaneous movements *(spinal cord reflexes may be present)*
Examination findings must be consistent over the duration of observation and testing; observation period is based on age (Table 72–2)
Ancillary tests (optional except in patients <2 mo of age)
Electroencephalogram
Cerebral angiogram
Radionuclide angiogram
Xenon CT scan
Brain stem evoked responses
Doppler sonography
Intracranial pressure monitoring
Endocrinologic studies of function of the brain

facilities. Patients in PVS are susceptible to infections, and death usually occurs as a result of pneumonia, urinary tract infection, or complications of a skin lesion. After months or years of caring for a child in PVS, a family may decide to limit various treatment modalities after careful consideration of the risks and benefits of further interventions for the child.

Withdrawal of support represents cessation of medical treatment and support already being provided to patients. It must be made very clear to a family that as life support is withdrawn from a child who is dependent on this treatment, the outcome is most likely to be death. In practice, withdrawing therapy or care that has already been instituted is more difficult than making the decision not to institute a therapeutic intervention. However, in either case, the decision not to provide a certain level of care is made in the context in which provision of such care would only prolong an inevitable death, perhaps involving additional pain and suffering. Such decisions force families and the medical care team to come to an agreement about the quality of life for the critically ill patient. Although there is little moral distinction between the provision of ventilator support (and other highly technical forms of care) and the provision of artificial hydration and nutrition to critically ill patients, most clinicians find it more difficult to advocate withdrawal of the latter than to recommend that mechanical ventilation or inotropic medicines be withdrawn.

BRAIN DEATH. Criteria to determine brain death for adult and pediatric patients have been established and are accepted by most states (Table 72–1). Death is defined as irreversible cessation of circulatory and respiratory functions or irreversible cessation of all functions of the entire brain, including the brain stem. Guidelines for assessing brain death in children of different ages also have been established because of the judgment that premature or newborn infants require a longer period of observation than older children or adults (Table 72–2).

TABLE 72–2 Age-Specific Criteria for Brain Death

Children 1 wk–2 mo of age: fulfillment of the clinical criteria listed in Table 72–1 in two separate examinations at least 48 hr apart, or one clinical examination followed by an isoelectric EEG at least 48 hr later
Children 2 mo–1 hr: fulfillment of the clinical criteria described in Table 72–1 in two separate examinations, at least 24 hr apart, or one clinical examination followed by an isoelectric EEG or negative results of a cerebral blood flow study at least 24 hr later
Children >1 yr: fulfillment of the clinical criteria described in Table 72–1 in two separate examinations at least 12 hr apart

EEG = electroencephalogram.

The diagnosis of brain death is established once the cause of the coma is determined and the possibility of recovery of any brain function has been ruled out. Brain death results from permanent cessation of all brain function in the absence of any factor or agent that could cloud accurate assessment of brain function. Physical examinations by two physicians must demonstrate loss of brain stem responses and include an apnea test, in which the patient is hyperoxygenated and then removed from the ventilator or placed on continuous positive airway pressure. The Pa_{CO_2} is allowed to rise to a level of 60 mm Hg or greater while maintaining appropriate oxygenation is maintained. Laboratory tests also are required to establish the cause of the coma and to preclude toxic, metabolic, paralytic, or sedative causes. Electroencephalograms, cerebral perfusion studies, and intracranial pressure monitoring may be helpful in convincing the family that their child is brain dead and in facilitating the opportunities for organ donation or discontinuation of life support.

Brain death is equivalent to cardiorespiratory death, and a child should be considered legally dead at the time that the criteria for brain death are fulfilled. This determination is crucial to the process of organ procurement that requires the harvested heart, lung, liver, or bowel to be obtained from a donor whose heart is beating. Despite increasing acceptance of organ donation in the United States, fewer than 20% of eligible donors become organ donors. This results in the death of several thousand potential organ recipients each year while awaiting transplantation.

ORGAN PROCUREMENT (see Chapter 68). In the United States there are more than 250 hospitals offering solid organ transplants and at least 75 regional organizations that monitor organ availability and try to match donors with available organs. Every major metropolitan center has its own such organization or network. If questions arise about organ transplantation, a 24-hr telephone hotline is maintained at 1-800-355-7427. The number of pediatric transplant centers is considerably smaller. Transplant centers often maintain their own transport system and are capable of flying to distant sites to retrieve organs.

Once the diagnosis of brain death has been made and the family wishes to pursue organ donation, a transplant donor network should be contacted to assist in the process. A procurement coordinator generally assumes responsibility for the donation process, including holding family discussions, determining arrangements and logistics, obtaining consent forms, making arrangements for appropriate laboratory tests, contacting various transplant centers to make arrangements for organ retrieval, and checking on recipient lists in order to match the organs to the patient with the highest priority. The coordinator is able to provide the donor's family long-term follow-up about organ placement; many grieving families find this to be very helpful in dealing with their loss. Most donor organizations assume full financial responsibility for the procurement process and the donated organs.

Farrell MM, Levin DL: Brain death in the pediatric patient: Historical, sociological, medical, religious, cultural, legal, and ethical considerations. Crit Care Med 21:1951, 1993.

Holbrook PR: Death. *In:* Holbrook PR (ed): Textbook of Pediatric Critical Care. Philadelphia, WB Saunders, 1993, pp 1131–1133.

Levetown M, Pollack MM, Guerdon TT, et al: Limitations and withdrawal of medical intervention in pediatric critical care. JAMA 272:1271, 1994.

Mjia RE, Pollack MM: Variability in brain death determination practices in children. JAMA 274:7, 1995.

Staworn D, Lewison L, Marks J, et al: Brain death in pediatric intensive care unit patients: Incidence, primary diagnosis, and the clinical occurrence of Turner's triad. Crit Care Med 22:1301, 1994.

Task Force for the Determination of Brain Death in Children: Guidelines for the determination of brain death in children. Pediatrics 80:298, 1987.

CHAPTER 73
Anesthesia and Perioperative Care

Charles B. Berde and William S. Schechter

The prospect of surgery and anesthesia provokes anxiety for most children and their parents. Although pediatricians are generally not called on to direct their patients' perioperative care, they have an essential role in preoperative evaluation and preparation, in counseling patients and families, and in postoperative assessment. Because it is now feasible to provide anesthesia safely for children of all ages, pediatricians should advocate for the rights of infants and children to receive anesthesia and analgesia for both major and minor procedures.

PREOPERATIVE ASSESSMENT

All infants and children scheduled for surgery should be evaluated preoperatively both to screen for conditions that may require specific treatment or optimization of therapy (e.g., evaluation of anemia, adjustment of asthma medications) and to counsel patients and parents about the expected course of anesthesia and surgery. The cornerstone of assessment is a systematic history and detailed physical examination with emphasis on airway anatomy and cardiorespiratory status. A careful history enables the anesthesiologist to plan the management of anesthesia and the postanesthetic period more effectively. The history should include the information listed in Table 73–1.

The physical examination should begin with general observation of the patient and evaluation of vital signs. The airway is assessed for predictors of difficulty with mask ventilation or intubation, including impaired neck mobility, micrognathia, nasal obstruction, adenotonsillar hypertrophy, impaired mouth opening, macroglossia, and various forms of orofacial dysmorphism. The presence of pectus excavatum in a small child may suggest chronic upper airway obstruction. Determination of hydration status is important because most anesthetics are vasodilators or myocardial depressants, and hypovolemia predisposes patients to hypotension after induction. Evidence of cardiac failure, such as tachypnea, tachycardia, or hepatomegaly, may alter the choice of induction agents. The presence of wheezing demands further evaluation before proceeding with an elective operation. Potential sites for venous access must be evaluated with care so that cannulation may proceed rapidly after an inhalation induction. A child's behavior and ability to cooperate can help predict the need for premedication or parental presence at induction.

MATURATION OF ORGAN SYSTEMS: ANESTHETIC IMPLICATIONS. Major anatomic and physiologic differences between a neonate, infant, child, and adult influence anesthetic management. Critical differences for infants are outlined in Table 73–2.

OUTPATIENT SURGERY. More than half of the operations performed on children are performed on an outpatient basis. This has been made possible in part by advances in anesthetic

TABLE 73–1 The Preanesthetic History

Child's Previous Anesthetic and Surgical Procedures

Review anesthetic record for information about mask and endotracheal tube size, type and size of laryngoscope used, difficulties with mask ventilation or intubation

Perinatal Problems (Especially for Infants)

Need for prolonged hospitalization
Need for supplemental oxygen or intubation
History of apnea and bradycardia

Other Major Illnesses and Hospitalizations

Family History of Anesthetic Complications, Malignant Hyperthermia, or Pseudocholinesterase Deficiency

Respiratory Problems

Chronic exposure to environmental tobacco smoke
Obstructive apnea, breathing irregularities, or cyanosis (especially in infants under age 6 mo)
History of snoring or obstructive breathing pattern
Recent upper respiratory tract infection
Recurrent respiratory infections
Previous laryngotracheitis (croup)
Asthma or wheezing during respiratory infections

Cardiac Problems

Murmurs
Dysrhythmia
Exercise intolerance
Syncope
Cyanosis

Gastrointestinal Problems

Reflux and vomiting
Feeding difficulties
Failure to thrive
Liver disease

Exposure to Exanthems or Potentially Infectious Pathogens

Neurologic Problems

Seizures
Developmental delay
Neuromuscular diseases
Increased intracranial pressure

Hematologic Problems

Anemia
Bleeding diathesis
Tumor
Immunocompromise
Prior blood transfusions and reactions

Renal Problems

Renal insufficiency, oliguria, anuria
Fluid and electrolyte abnormalities

Psychosocial Considerations

Post-traumatic stress
Drug abuse, use of cigarettes or alcohol
Physical or sexual abuse
Family dysfunction
Previous traumatic medical and surgical experiences
Psychosis, anxiety, depression

Gynecologic Considerations

Sexual history (sexually transmitted diseases)
Possibility of pregnancy

Current Medications

Prior administration of corticosteroids

Allergies

Drugs
Iodine
Latex products
Surgical tapes
Food allergies (especially soya and egg albumin)

Dental Condition (Loose or Cracked Teeth)

When and What the Child Last Ate (Especially in Emergency Procedures)

TABLE 73–2 Anatomic and Physiologic Features of Infancy: Anesthetic Implications

System/Category	Implications
Airway	
Infant tongue occupies larger proportion of oropharynx	Nasal obstruction may make mask ventilation difficult and require placement of an oral airway; tongue commonly obstructs airway
Cephalic ("anterior") larynx	Difficult visualization of larynx
Infant inlet: C3–C4	Difficult visualization of larynx
Adult inlet: C4–C5	
Omega-shaped epiglottis	
Vocal cords	Difficult visualization of larynx
Angled lower anteriorly than posteriorly in infants	
Small airway diameter	Poiseuille's law Small changes in diameter (e.g., with edema) produce large changes in resistance Greater difficulty with spontaneous ventilation in patient under anesthesia
Cricoid cartilage	Use uncuffed endotreacheal tubes
Narrowest part of pediatric airway	Tubes should have air leak at 20–30 cm H_2O pressure Postanesthetic croup is common in infants
Short tracheal length	Precise endotracheal tube placement required
Lungs	
Rapid desaturation with apnea	High ratio of O_2 consumption to FRC Closing capacity near FRC Rapid induction and emergence from inhalation anesthesia
Rapid induction and emergence from inhalation anesthesia	
Rapid desaturation with apnea	Chest wall compliance high
Atelectasis	
Postoperative apnea	Immature ventilatory reflexes Hypoventilation
Central Nervous System	Reduced anesthetic requirements at birth, increase to a maximum at 6 mo of age, decrease with age thereafter
Autonomic Nervous System	Decreased resting sympathetic tone Increased parasympathetic tone
Cardiac	
Noncompliant ventricles	Relatively fixed stroke volume
Immature sarcoplasmic reticulum	Cardiac output rate dependent
Immature baroreceptors	Greater depression of contractility by inhalation anesthetics Less compensatory tachycardia and vasoconstriction with hypotension
Hepatic	
Immature enzyme systems	Slower metabolism of intravenous anesthetics, some muscle relaxants, and opioids
Renal	
Diminished GFR in the first several weeks of life	Delayed elimination of intravenous anesthetics, some muscle relaxants, and opioid metabolites
Thermal Regulation	Greater temperature fluctuation with environmental changes

FRC = functional residual capacity; GFR = glomerular filtration rate.

techniques that involve more rapid recovery and reduced incidence of nausea.

Advantages of day surgery include (1) less time in a threatening hospital environment, (2) reduced health care costs, and (3) reduced exposure to pathogens. Disadvantages include (1) greater difficulty with follow-up care and observation, (2) greater burden for some families, with potential for increased parental anxiety, (3) less continuity of care, and (4) greater difficulty with management of pain and other symptoms.

Preoperative assessment for "day surgery" patients may vary according to local resources and referral patterns. Patient selection criteria for outpatient surgery are based on three factors: the nature of the operative procedure, parental readiness, and patient status. The most common outpatient procedures are herniorrhaphy, myringotomy, tonsillectomy with or without adenoidectomy, strabismus repair, orchiopexy, and circumcision. In most cases, these procedures cause minor physiologic change and minimal bleeding. Parents must be capable of following specific postoperative instructions. Patients should live close to a hospital or emergency medical care facility should the need arise for medical intervention within the first 24 hr after surgery. Children presenting for outpatient surgery should be in good general health, or if they have chronic illness, they should be optimally prepared. Most outpatients are of American Society of Anesthesiologists (ASA) physical status I and II (Table 73–3), although on occasion patients of ASA status III may be cared for on an outpatient basis. For example, a suitable ASA III patient may be an oncology patient presenting for a diagnostic or therapeutic procedure or for placement of an indwelling catheter.

LABORATORY TESTING. Preoperative laboratory testing for most children should be extremely parsimonious. The predictive value and cost effectiveness of chest radiography and urinalysis in otherwise healthy children are extremely low. In many centers, even preoperative hematocrit determination is no longer required for children who are undergoing minor surgery and who have no specific risk factors for anemia disclosed by history and physical examination. Infants younger than 1 yr are at increased risk of anemia, and most centers currently require a hematocrit or hemogram for infants younger than 6–12 mo. If the sickle cell status is unknown, it should be clarified in susceptible populations. Blood typing and cross matching are recommended for children undergoing surgery for which the potential for significant blood loss is high. Coagulation studies are widely obtained for children undergoing diverse procedures from tonsillectomy to craniotomy. In general, their yield is low in patients without a history of bleeding problems.

There is controversy about the requirement for pregnancy testing in adolescent females. Undisclosed pregnancy rates in adolescent females presenting for elective surgery exceed 1% in some studies. Our practice is to perform urine pregnancy

TABLE 73–3 American Society of Anesthesiologists Physical Status Classification

ASA PS I	Healthy patient
ASA PS II	Mild illness, well controlled
ASA PS III	Serious illness
ASA PS IV	Life-threatening illness
ASA PS V	Moribund

testing on all adolescent females who have begun their menses or have reached the age of 15 yr.

FASTING GUIDELINES (NPO ORDERS). These guidelines are a frequent source of frustration for patients, parents, and health providers. Preoperative fasting is advised because anesthetic induction involves loss of airway reflexes that prevent aspiration of regurgitated gastric contents. Aspiration involves two problems: airway occlusion from particulates in food and gastric acid–induced chemical pneumonitis.

Although a child's stomach should be free of solids before elective anesthesia, it is important not to interrupt fluid intake longer than necessary. Most centers withhold milk or solids for 6–8 hr before elective anesthesia. Several studies have confirmed the safety of preoperative administration of clear liquids (apple juice, glucose-electrolyte solutions) up to 2–4 hr preoperatively in healthy infants and children. Gastric emptying can be delayed in various circumstances, including trauma, gastric outlet obstruction, or severe anxiety. In these circumstances and for most emergency surgery, "full stomach" precautions and a rapid sequence induction of anesthesia may be required. The recommendations in Table 73–4 reflect a review of the evidence and consensus report by a task force of the ASA.

CHILDREN WITH RHINORRHEA OR COUGHING. Anesthesiologists are frequently faced with the prospect of anesthetizing a child with respiratory signs and symptoms. For convenience, we divide common rhinorrhea and cough into three categories: (1) isolated chronic rhinitis, (2) viral upper respiratory tract infection, and (3) lower respiratory tract disease.

Children with *chronic rhinitis* may have chronic purulent sinusitis or a noninfectious condition related to allergy, vasomotor rhinitis, or adenotonsillar hypertrophy. In some of these children, signs and symptoms are persistent. One controlled study found no increased risk of pulmonary complications among children who had chronic rhinitis and were undergoing myringotomy and tube placement. Airway management can sometimes be challenging, because many of these children are mouth breathers and may have significant adenotonsillar hypertrophy.

Acute rhinitis or *pharyngitis* may predispose a child to both intraoperative and postoperative respiratory problems. Because mild airway difficulties are common but serious adverse events are rare in these patients, anesthesiologists may disagree about the safety of proceeding with surgery. The anesthesiologist must judge whether to proceed with an elective anesthetic procedure after the risks and benefits are carefully discussed with the family and surgeon. The presence of fever along with cough, tachypnea, or an abnormality on chest examination suggests lower tract disease and argues against proceeding with elective surgery.

Children who have had *recent viral respiratory tract infection* may demonstrate airway hyperreactivity on pulmonary function tests. These abnormalities may persist for as long as 6–8 wk after resolution of symptoms and are associated with an increased risk of laryngospasm, bronchospasm, and desaturation with anesthesia. After an upper respiratory infection, children who received endotracheal anesthesia may be at an 11 times higher risk of airway problems than those who were treated by mask alone. Postextubation stridor is more common

TABLE 73–4 Fasting Guidelines*

Clear fluids	2 hr
Breast milk	4 hr
Infant formula	6 hr
Solids (light meal)	6 hr
Solids (fatty meal)	8 hr

**These are general guidelines and may not reflect local hospital policies.*
Data from a report of a Task Force on Practice Guidelines of the American Society of Anesthesiologists, 1998. Available from the ASA website at www.asahq.org.

after a respiratory infection. These complications are more severe in infants and toddlers than in older children or adolescents. Household exposure to cigarette smoke has been shown to increase the risk of children's having coughing, laryngospasm, bronchospasm, and desaturation during general anesthesia.

AN ACCEPTABLE HEMATOCRIT. In the past, a hematocrit greater than 30% was widely considered mandatory for patients before elective surgery. The rationale for preferring adequate red blood cell (RBC) mass lies in providing a safety margin for oxygen delivery and anticipated surgical blood loss. With increasing awareness of the infectious and immunologic consequences of transfusion and with greater experience in management of hemodilution under anesthesia, this rule has been relaxed. A hematocrit of 28% lies within the normal range for infants at 3 mo of age. In many patients with chronic renal insufficiency or hematologic disorders, it may be appropriate to administer anesthesia with a substantially lower hematocrit. Causes of anemia should be investigated, and purely elective surgery should be delayed pending such assessment.

SURGICAL TIMING AND EVALUATION OF ANESTHETIC RISK. The proper timing of surgery in infants depends on both anesthetic risks and effects of timing on surgical outcome. For example, prostaglandin infusions to maintain patency of the ductus arteriosus may permit preoperative stabilization before neonatal cardiac surgery and greatly improve the infant's physiologic stability. Conversely, a newborn exsanguinating from a sacrococcygeal teratoma may need immediate surgery to gain control of bleeding. In many other cases, such as repair of cleft lip and palate or craniosynostosis, the timing of the procedure represents a compromise between the benefits of early repair on outcome and the increased risks of anesthesia (or the increased likelihood of needed transfusion) in younger infants.

Parents and older children often ask for assessment of anesthetic risk. It is useful to place these statistics into a context based on a patient's disease, age-related risks, and the type of surgery. It should be noted that anesthetic mishap accounts for only a small percentage (<5%) of perioperative deaths; the majority of perioperative deaths are related to patients' disease-related factors, such as exsanguination after major trauma or inability to separate from cardiopulmonary bypass.

In adults, morbidity and mortality increase as ASA physical status increases; in limited pediatric studies, this trend is less apparent. A study of adverse events in pediatric and adult anesthesia highlights causal differences between pediatric and adult patients. Analyses of critical incidents indicate that two scenarios are most common in infants: (1) inability to manage the airway and deliver oxygen and (2) overdose of inhalation anesthetics with associated myocardial depression. Bradycardia and other dysrhythmias under anesthesia are primarily caused by inadequate ventilation and oxygenation until proved otherwise. A retrospective analysis in one center found statistically reduced mortality among children cared for by pediatric anesthesiologists when compared with those cared for by nonspecialist anesthesiologists. This difference persisted despite controlling for age, illness, and other factors.

The overall risk of anesthetic death is difficult to estimate because a patient's age, pre-existing medical condition, type of surgery, and the surgeon's skill all must be considered. Estimates range from 1/10,000 to 1/185,000. Infants remain at greater risk than older children. Emergency surgery is more risky than elective surgery. Perioperative risk has decreased considerably in the past 30 yr. Factors for this improvement include better intraoperative temperature and fluid management, better monitoring equipment (pulse oximetry, capnography), and better training.

FORMERLY PREMATURE INFANTS. Physiologic immaturity may complicate anesthetic treatment of neonates in general and premature infants in particular. In premature infants, control of airway patency, respiratory drive, temperature, electrolyte balance, and blood pressure is immature. Formerly preterm infants up to perhaps 60 wk after conception are at risk for periodic breathing, apnea, and bradycardia after general anesthesia or sedation. These risks appear diminished with the use of spinal or caudal epidural anesthesia, provided that sedation is avoided. The most common elective procedure in formerly preterm infants is inguinal hernia repair. It is important to emphasize that general anesthesia may be safely administered in this group of patients, if careful monitoring is continued postoperatively and individuals are available to manage respi-

TABLE 73–5 Specific Pediatric Diseases and Their Anesthetic Implications

Disease	Implications
Respiratory System	
Asthma	Intraoperative bronchospasm that may be severe
	Pneumothorax
	Optimal preoperative medical management essential; may require preoperative steroids
Difficult airway	May require special equipment and personnel
	Should be anticipated in children with dysmorphic features or acute airway obstruction as in epiglottitis or laryngotracheobronchitis or with airway foreign body
	Patients with Down syndrome may require evaluation of atlanto-occipital joint
	Patients with storage diseases may be at high risk
Bronchopulmonary dysplasia	Barotrauma with positive pressure ventilation
	Oxygen toxicity, pneumothorax a risk
Cystic fibrosis	Airway reactivity, bronchorrhea
	Risk of pneumothorax, pulmonary hemorrhage
	Atelectasis
	Assess for cor pulmonale
Sleep apnea	Must rule out pulmonary hypertension and cor pulmonale
	Requires careful postoperative observation for obstruction
Cardiac	Need for antibiotic prophylaxis for subacute bacterial endocarditis
	Use of air filters; careful purging of air from intravenous equipment
	Need to understand effects of various anesthetics on the hemodynamics of specific lesions
	Preload optimization and avoidance of hyperviscous states in cyanotic patients
	Possible need for preoperative evaluation of myocardial function and pulmonary vascular resistance
	Provide information about pacemaker function and ventricular device function
Hematologic	
Sickle cell	Possible need for simple or exchange transfusion based on preoperative Hgb and per cent Hgb S
	Importance of avoiding acidosis, hypoxemia, hypothermia, dehydration, and hyperviscosity states
Oncology	Pulmonary evaluation of patients who have received bleomycin, *bis*-chloroethyl-nitrosourea, chloroethyl-cyclohexyl-nitrosourea, methotrexate, or radiation to the chest
	Avoidance of high oxygen concentration
	Cardiac evaluation of patients who have received anthracyclines; risk of severe myocardial depression with volatile agents
	Potential for coagulopathy
Rheumatologic	Limited mobility of temporomandibular joint, cervical spine, arytenoid cartilages
	Requires careful preoperative evaluation
	May be difficult airway
Gastrointestinal	
Esophageal, gastric	Potential for reflux and aspiration
Liver	High overall morbidity and mortality in patients with hepatic dysfunction
	Altered metabolism of some drugs
	Potential for coagulopathy
Renal	Altered electrolyte and acid-base status
	Altered clearance of some drugs
	Need for preoperative dialysis in selected cases
	Succinylcholine to be used with extreme caution and only when serum potassium level is recently shown to be normal
Neurologic	
Seizure disorder	Avoid anesthetics that may lower threshold
	Ensure optimal control preoperatively
	Preoperative anticonvulsant levels
Increased intracranial pressure	Avoid agents that increase cerebral blood flow
	Avoid hypercarbia
Neuromuscular disease	Avoid depolarizing relaxants; at risk for hyperkalemia
	May be at risk for malignant hyperthermia
Developmental delay	May be uncooperative at induction
Psychiatric	Monoamine oxidase inhibitor (or cocaine) may interact with meperidine, resulting in hyperthermia and seizures
	Selective serotonin reuptake inhibitors may induce or inhibit various hepatic enzymes that may alter anesthetic drug clearance
	Illicit drugs may have adverse effects on cardiorespiratory homeostasis and may potentiate the action of anesthetics
Endocrine	
Diabetes	Greatest risk is unrecognized intraoperative hypoglycemia; if insulin is administered, monitor blood glucose level intraoperatively; must provide glucose and insulin with adjustment for fasting condition and surgical stress
Skin	
Burns	Difficult airway
	Risk of rhabdomyolysis and hyperkalemia from succinylcholine
	Fluid shifts
	Bleeding
	Coagulopathy
Immunologic	Retroviral drugs may inhibit benzodiazepine clearance
	Immunodeficiency requires careful infection control practices
	May require cytomegalovirus-negative blood products, irradiation, or leukofiltration
Metabolic	Careful assessment of glucose homeostasis in infants

Hgb = hemoglobin.

ratory problems. Intravenous caffeine administered after induction of general anesthesia stimulates respiration and reduces but does not eliminate the risk of apnea. Other factors may predispose to apnea, including metabolic and electrolyte derangements, sepsis, decreased RBC mass, acidosis, hypocalcemia, and temperature stress. Prudence dictates that nonessential surgery be delayed beyond 60 wk postconceptual age in formerly preterm infants. Postoperative apnea rarely occurs in apparently healthy full-term infants. It is our current practice to recommend overnight observation of term infants if they are under 44 wk postconceptual age.

LATEX ALLERGY. Intraoperative allergic reactions to latex antigens have been described with increasing frequency during the past decade. Latex allergy may present as hypotension, wheezing, hives, or erythema, and these reactions can be life threatening. These reactions were originally described in patients with spina bifida and in patients who had repeated latex exposure from urinary catheterization, but they also occur in otherwise healthy children. When management is guided by history or by risk group, the risk of reactions can be diminished greatly by avoidance of latex antigen contact. In response to this problem, many hospitals have made nonlatex gloves routinely available.

SPECIFIC DISEASES THAT AFFECT ANESTHETIC MANAGEMENT. Table 73–5 outlines a number of disorders that may require anesthetic consultation preoperatively. This listing is not all-inclusive.

PREANESTHETIC PREPARATION AND PREMEDICATION

For most children, the primary purpose of premedication is to diminish the fear and anxiety associated with separation from parents and with other aspects of anesthetic induction, such as fear of the mask. Terrifying experiences may occur during induction of anesthesia or in the immediate postoperative period. These can contribute to psychologic sequelae such as night terrors, enuresis, and temper tantrums. Certain steps can minimize the psychologic trauma. For children older than 3 yr, parents should explain the purpose of the proposed operation in simple terms, telling of the probable sequence of events and discomfort involved. Parents' tension and anxiety are readily transmitted to children. In many locations, preoperative teaching programs are available; the Association for the Care of Children in Hospitals has taken a leadership role in this regard. Teaching films and videotapes are widely available.

Premedication should not substitute for efforts to make the experience of induction as atraumatic as possible. Many healthy children, particularly those older than 4 yr, require no premedication before a mask induction, particularly with a supportive and skilled practitioner. Conversely, it is our impression that many 2-yr-olds are uncooperative unless heavily premedicated. Premedication should be given by a non-noxious route whenever possible. Oral premedications are not intrinsically noxious, but when an uncooperative toddler is forced to drink a bitter-tasting elixir, the result may be heightened distress. An elixir of midazolam is rapidly becoming the most widely used premedication in the United States. Midazolam is a benzodiazepine anxiolytic with inactive metabolites and considerably more rapid clearance than diazepam or lorazepam. Various syrups have been used to mask the bitter taste.

Oral transmucosal fentanyl ("fentanyl lollipop") has the virtue of rapid onset and a pleasant route of administration, but it has a potential for causing significant nausea, chest wall rigidity, and desaturation in preoperative sedation studies. Intranasal medication is commonly disliked by children, although in uncooperative patients, it may on occasion be a feasible route for administration of midazolam, sufentanil, or ketamine.

Intramuscular injections are painful but have a specific limited role for sedation of highly distressed or uncooperative children. In uncooperative children with difficult intravenous access and severe aversion to a mask or oral premedication, a single intramuscular injection of midazolam and ketamine, for example, may ultimately be less distressing than repeated attempts at intravenous cannulation or forced application of a mask. Rectal administration of the barbiturates methohexital or thiamylal or of benzodiazepines such as midazolam usually produces reliable sedation in less than 10 min.

For patients with pain preoperatively (e.g., a child with fractures), it may be helpful to include an opioid as premedication, both to relieve pain and because the risk of dysphoric reactions increases when sedatives are given without analgesics to patients in pain.

Anticholinergics (atropine, scopolamine, glycopyrrolate) were previously routinely given preoperatively, either orally or by intramuscular injection, to patients of all ages to dry secretions, attenuate vagal reflex responses to airway manipulation, and support cardiac output in the presence of myocardial depression and relative bradycardia caused by volatile anesthetics. The drying of secretions produced by anticholinergics is generally regarded as unpleasant in awake children. With currently available anesthetic agents, the need for drying of secretions is diminished, and many pediatric anesthesiologists currently limit their use to specific indications such as (1) prolonged surgery in the prone position, (2) airway surgery, and, (3) ophthalmic surgery to block the oculocardiac reflex. If pancuronium is used for neuromuscular blockade, it generally provides sufficient vagolysis to obviate the need for anticholinergics.

The effect of premedication is variable. Some children are inadequately sedated but others are deeply sedated with premedication. It is therefore essential that the guidelines of the American Academy of Pediatrics be followed with regard to observing patients. In general, patients should be sedated in locations with immediate availability of resuscitation equipment and staff skilled in airway management. Along with respiratory observation, constant attention is needed to keep sedated children from falling or injuring themselves.

ANESTHETIC INDUCTION (Table 73–6)

Before proceeding with an operation, it is important to correct dehydration, decrease excessive fever, correct acid-base balance, and restore a depleted blood volume. Preoperative dehydration can be particularly harmful for children with cyanotic congenital heart disease associated with polycythemia or after Fontan-type procedures. Such patients may at times require that an intravenous catheter be placed preoperatively to avoid the deleterious effects of dehydration.

Choice of anesthetic induction technique is dictated by specific patient risks and disease status in certain circumstances, such as the requirement for an intravenous rapid sequence induction for children at risk of aspiration, but in the majority of cases the primary issue lies in finding a method that is least distressing for the child.

TABLE 73–6 Emotional Responses to Anesthetic Induction

Age	Typical Responses and Implications
0–8 mo	Fewer anticipatory responses Generally calm with strangers Mask induction well tolerated
8 mo–2 yr	Separation anxiety is high Most difficult for mask induction Premedication, preinduction useful
3–7 yr	Separation anxiety still present Mask induction aided by parental presence
7–11 yr	Generally calm with mask induction Fear of needles Fear of loss of control
12–18 yr	Generally prefers intravenous to mask induction

Fear of needles depends on age, developmental factors, and previous experience with noxious procedures. In countries where the local anesthetic lidocaine-prilocaine cream, eutectic mixture of local anesthetics (EMLA), has been used routinely, children are said to approach needle procedures with less apprehension. Conversely, a study of use of EMLA before venous cannulation in American children found that apprehension and distress persisted even though the cannulation site was numb. Adolescents, with some notable exceptions, generally prefer intravenous induction to inhalation induction, in part because of the reduced fear of needles and preference for rapid induction of unconsciousness. Intravenous induction is also generally preferred for most children with indwelling intravenous lines before surgery.

Intravenous induction is medically indicated for most children coming for emergency surgery, who are generally considered at risk for aspiration of gastric contents. The established method to minimize the risk of aspiration is the *rapid sequence induction,* in which (1) the patient inhales 100% oxygen before induction, to prolong the time to arterial desaturation with apnea, (2) anesthesia is induced with a rapid-acting hypnotic along with a muscle relaxant, and (3) cricoid pressure is applied to occlude the esophagus and prevent passive reflux of gastric contents into the pharynx. See Chapter 64.1 and Table 64–9.

Rapid sequence inductions are effective at preventing aspiration in most cases. Nevertheless, they assume certain calculated risks: (1) The ability to intubate the trachea or at least ventilate by mask is assumed but not tested before muscle paralysis; (2) a fixed rather than slowly titrated dose of hypnotic may produce harmful degrees of hypertension or hypotension in susceptible patients; (3) the younger the infant, the shorter the time to hypoxia after preoxygenation and induction; and (4) cricoid pressure does not protect against aspiration of upper airway contents, such as purulent matter from a retropharyngeal abscess.

Awake intubation, or sedated-awake intubation with topical anesthesia, may be safer than rapid sequence induction in certain emergency cases in which there is potential for airway difficulty, such as in children with severe burns and airway swelling or in certain critically ill neonates. A cardinal rule is that *the risk of loss of airway and hypoventilation takes priority over risks related to aspiration.* Various specialized techniques are available to help in intubating children with difficult airways, including fiberoptic bronchoscopes, anterior commissure laryngoscopes, and light wands. The laryngeal mask airway is an alternative method for airway maintenance.

Inhalation induction is well accepted by most children ages 4–10 yr and is the most common induction technique in the United States in this age group. It is aided by (1) calm and quiet surroundings, (2) a confident manner on the part of the anesthesiologist, (3) avoidance of delays, (4) use of flavored aromas for the mask, (5) introduction of nitrous oxide (which is odorless) in oxygen for a few minutes before introducing the more aromatic vapor anesthetics, and (6) gradual introduction of the mask.

Inhalation induction may be medically indicated when preservation of spontaneous breathing is important, such as in cases of airway foreign body. Inhalation induction remains the most widely established technique of induction for children with presumed epiglottitis, although some centers have reported good outcomes with simple intravenous induction. Parental presence at anesthetic induction is increasingly being encouraged in order to diminish the child's distress. Parents should receive specific direction and support from operating room staff.

INTRAOPERATIVE MANAGEMENT (Table 73–7)

Anesthesia can be maintained by either intravenous agents or inhalation anesthetics, or a combination of both. In a critically ill infant or child, particularly one for whom postoperative ventilation is anticipated, high doses of synthetic opioids, such as fentanyl and sufentanil, provide anesthesia with excellent preservation of hemodynamic stability. Blocking the stress of pain perception has beneficial effects on metabolic stability in a newborn or young infant by attenuating the stress response, which is characterized by excessive catecholamine release, hyperglycemia, and protein catabolism. The newer opioid remifentanil has extremely rapid metabolism by plasma esterases and permits the use of "high-dose opioid" or "cardiac-style" anesthesia for cases of virtually any duration, with rapid recovery.

Airway maintenance by mask is useful for many short and elective operations. Tracheal intubation is indicated in the following: (1) operations of the head and neck; (2) thoracic, abdominal, and cranial procedures; (3) operations in the prone position; and (4) most emergency procedures, because there is uncertainty about the contents of the stomach. In younger infants, especially those younger than 6 mo, airway maintenance and adequacy of respiratory effort are more problematic, and tracheal intubation is widely preferred for all but the briefest operations. Controlled ventilation (as opposed to spontaneous ventilation) is preferred for intrathoracic and most intra-abdominal operations.

Although most children prefer to be asleep during surgery, use of regional anesthesia in children is rapidly increasing, both as a supplement to general anesthesia and as the primary form of anesthesia in selected high-risk infants. Peripheral nerve blocks with bupivacaine can provide prolonged analgesia postoperatively and permit rapid, pain-free emergence that can facilitate early discharge, reduced opioid requirements, and reduced nausea and vomiting. Examples include penile block for circumcision and femoral nerve or fascia iliaca block for femur fractures.

Pediatricians should become familiar with *safe dosing guidelines for local anesthetics* in children: 5 mg/kg (7 mg/kg with epinephrine) for lidocaine and 2 mg/kg (2.5 mg/kg with epinephrine) for bupivacaine. Thus, for example, if lidocaine 1% is used to infiltrate for chest tube placement in a 2-kg premature infant, then only 1 mL is permitted. Dose calculation and use of more dilute solutions are especially important for young infants. Mucosal application of lidocaine may also produce toxicity. Excessive dosing can produce seizures, arrhythmias, and myocardial depression.

For major thoracic, abdominal, and pelvic surgery in children, a useful technique involves epidural analgesia combined with a light general anesthetic intraoperatively, followed by epidural analgesia postoperatively. Both epidural opioids and local anesthetics may be used. Case-control studies of children undergoing esophageal repair, fundoplication, and major urologic reconstruction all suggest a reduced requirement for postoperative ventilation and reduced pulmonary complications in patients receiving epidural analgesia.

FLUID THERAPY. For all but the most superficial operations, children should receive intravenous cannulation, both as a port of access for medications and as a means for replacing fluid deficits and providing maintenance requirements. Venous cannulation of chronically hospitalized children may be extremely difficult. These difficulties should be anticipated during preoperative assessment, and in appropriate circumstances, personnel with expertise in pediatric central venous cannulation or venous access via cutdown should be available. When major bleeding is anticipated, venous access with catheters of appropriate gauge is essential. See Chapter 64.1.

Hypoglycemia and hyperglycemia are to be avoided. The clinical signs of hypoglycemia are difficult to interpret in anesthetized patients, and the neurologic consequences may be devastating. Studies indicate that hypoglycemia is very rare in anesthetized older children receiving glucose-free solutions, but it may occur more commonly in fasted infants and in

TABLE 73–7 Selected Drugs Used in Anesthesia

Drug	Uses and Implications
Muscle Relaxants	Used to facilitate endotracheal intubation and maintain muscle relaxation
Succinylcholine (SDC)	A depolarizing neuromuscular blocking agent with rapid onset and offset properties Associated with the development of MH in susceptible patients Degraded by plasma cholinesterase, which may be deficient in some individuals and result in prolonged effect Fasciculations may be associated with immediate increases in intracranial and intraocular pressure as well as postoperative muscle pain
Pancuronium, vecuronium, *cis*-atracurium, D-tubocurarine (curare)	Nondepolarizing neuromuscular blockers Less rapid onset than SDC but longer acting Pancuronium is vagolytic, which may be of benefit in newborns, who have high levels of vagal tone Vecuronium and rocuronium are metabolized by the liver and excreted in bile *Cis*-atracurium is metabolized by plasma cholinesterase and therefore may be of benefit in patients with hepatic or renal disease; curare releases histamine and is long acting
Hypnotics	Used to induce a state of unconsciousness
Thiopental	Rapidly acting hypnotic, but not an analgesic Offset is by redistribution, not by metabolism May cause hypotension because of its myocardial depressant effects and by vasodilation Causes respiratory depression Releases histamine and may be associated with bronchospasm in susceptible individuals Increases seizure threshold
Ketamine	Hypnotic analgesic and amnestic Causes sialorrhea and should be co-administered with an antisialogogue such as atropine or glycopyrrolate May be associated with laryngospasm Causes endogenous catecholamine release, tachycardia, and bronchodilation Increases intracranial and intraocular pressure Decreases seizure threshold
Etomidate	Cardiovascular stability on induction with no increase in intracranial pressure May inhibit corticosteroid synthesis Associated with myoclonus, potential difficulty with assisted ventilation, and pain on injection
Propofol	Rapidly acting hypnotic, amnestic but not analgesic Like pentothal, may cause hypotension Causes respiratory depression May increase seizure threshold Great utility in titrated doses for sedation and with local anesthetic and short-acting opioid for outpatient procedures May suppress nausea
Sedative-Anxiolytics	
Benzodiazepines	May produce sedation, anxiolysis, or hypnosis, depending on dose May produce antegrade but not retrograde amnesia All raise seizure threshold, are metabolized by the liver, and depress respiration, especially when administered with opioids Frequently administered as premedicants Diazepam may be painful on injection and has active metabolites Midazolam can be administered by various routes and has a short half-life Lorazepam has no active metabolites Sedation effected by all benzodiazepines may be reversed by flumazenil, but respiratory depression may not be reliably reversed
Analgesic-Sedatives	
Opioids	Gold standard for providing analgesia May cause respiratory depression Morphine and, to a lesser extent, hydromorphone may cause histamine release The synthetic opioids fentanyl, sufentanil, and short-acting alfentanil may have a greater propensity to cause chest wall rigidity when administered rapidly or in high doses and are also associated with the rapid development of tolerance; these three drugs have particular utility in cardiac surgery because of the hemodynamic stability associated with their use Remifentanil is an ultra–short-acting synthetic opioid that is metabolized by plasma cholinesterase; it may have particular utility when deep sedation and analgesia are required along with the ability to assess neurologic status intermittently
Inhalational Agents	
Nitrous oxide	Amnesia and mild analgesia at low concentrations Danger of hypoxic mixture if oxygen concentration is not monitored and preventive safety mechanisms are not in place
Potent vapors	"Complete anesthetics"—they induce a state of hypnosis, analgesia, and amnesia All are myocardial depressants, and some are vasodilators All are triggers in MH-susceptible individuals Isoflurane and enflurane are fluorinated ethers and isomers Enflurane may lower seizure threshold Halothane has been the gold standard for performing inhalation induction of anesthesia in children, but sevoflurane, a newer drug, is also well tolerated and has more rapid kinetics (onset and offset) because of its low solubility in blood All are bronchodilators at equipotent concentrations Isoflurane, enflurane, and especially desflurane are associated with a higher incidence of laryngospasm, when used for anesthetic induction, than either halothane or sevoflurane Halothane may be associated with an acute fulminant hepatitis, although this is extremely rare in children

MH = malignant hyperthermia.

children with medical conditions that prevent an adequate glycemic response to operative stress. In high-risk circumstances, plasma glucose concentrations should be monitored or patients should receive maintenance glucose infusions. Rapid infusion of glucose-containing solutions should be avoided, because it can produce hyperglycemia.

BLOOD TRANSFUSION (see Chapter 480). Criteria for perioperative transfusion in children have been modified, in part by improved understanding of the safety of mild hemodilution and because of increased concern about blood-borne infections. The decision to transfuse depends not on hematocrit determinations alone (which may not be equilibrated in the setting of ongoing blood loss) but on calculated or estimated blood losses, calculated blood volume, the particular stage of the operation, and patient's risk factors. For example, if an infant loses 30% of his or her blood volume during the initial dissection of a craniotomy or hepatic resection, in which ongoing losses are anticipated and may be rapid, then transfusion should not be delayed. Conversely, if a healthy 45-kg 12-yr-old has lost 30% of his or her blood volume (approximately 1,200 mL) by the end of a hip osteotomy and has stable hemodynamics, excellent urine output, and a hematocrit of 22% after adequate crystalloid replacement, then transfusion can generally be avoided. Children who are iron deficient and who are undergoing elective surgery in which major blood loss is anticipated may sometimes avoid transfusion if the anemia is corrected preoperatively. Blood component therapy is preferable to whole blood transfusion in most circumstances. Complications of rapid transfusion include hyperkalemia and citrate toxicity (ionized hypocalcemia), which may produce arrhythmias and cardiac arrest. Calcium administration may be lifesaving in this setting. For elective surgery with anticipated bleeding in older children and adolescents, predonation of autologous blood should be encouraged. Various techniques are in use to diminish blood loss, including acute hemodilution, controlled hypotension, inhibition of the plasmin system by aprotinin or tranexamic acid, and reinfusion of centrifuged, washed RBCs from the surgical field. Preoperative erythropoietin administration to increase RBC mass, followed by blood donation and autologous transfusion at the time of surgery, is currently under investigation.

THERMOREGULATION. Thermoregulation is impaired during general or major regional anesthesia, and young infants are particularly susceptible to hypothermia or hyperthermia in the operating room. Continuous monitoring of body temperature is essential during general anesthesia. In air-conditioned operating rooms, inadvertent *hypothermia* develops frequently in small infants undergoing laparotomy, thoracotomy, or craniotomy. Deliberate hypothermia is useful for cerebral and myocardial protection in cardiac surgery and other specialized operations. In most other circumstances, hypothermia is to be avoided, because it may detrimentally affect coagulation, ventilatory control, termination of neuromuscular blockade, and metabolic balance. Similarly, hyperthermia increases oxygen consumption and may confuse the differential diagnosis in more serious conditions, such as sepsis and malignant hyperthermia.

Hypothermia can be prevented by the use of overhead radiant heaters, circulating warm water mattresses, and heated humidification of inspired gases, as well as wrapping the child's head and extremities with heat-retaining, nonabrasive materials. Forced-air convective warming is a convenient and highly effective method for treating intraoperative hypothermia.

Malignant hyperpyrexia or *malignant hyperthermia* (MH) is due to a rare life-threatening genetic abnormality of skeletal muscle and is characterized by tachycardia, tachypnea, hypermetabolism, muscle rigidity, hypercarbia, acidosis, and fever following exposure to the vapor inhalation anesthetics (halothane, isoflurane) or the depolarizing muscle relaxant succinylcholine (also see Chapter 618.2). MH is more common among patients with various muscle disorders, including Duchenne muscular dystrophy. Initial management includes (1) cessation of triggering agents, (2) hyperventilation with oxygen, and (3) administration of a specific agent, dantrolene 3 mg/kg, given intravenously mixed in sterile water to a total loading dose of 10 mg/kg if necessary. Along with this, general intensive care measures include (1) treatment of hyperkalemia and acidosis, (2) circulatory support, (3) active cooling measures, and (4) urinary alkalization to prevent tubular injury from myoglobinuria. Nontriggering anesthetics that may be used safely include barbiturates, opioids, propofol, nitrous oxide, local anesthetics, benzodiazepines, butyrophenones, and nondepolarizing muscle relaxants (see Chapter 618.2).

MONITORING (also see Chapter 62). Standard monitors for children in the United States undergoing general or major regional anesthesia include an electrocardiogram, a blood pressure cuff, a precordial or esophageal stethoscope, a temperature probe, an oximeter, a capnograph, and in-line oxygen analyzers. Intra-arterial pressure monitoring is indicated for procedures associated with hemodynamic instability or major blood loss. Other invasive monitoring methods, including central venous or pulmonary artery catheterization and transesophageal echocardiography, may be indicated in specific circumstances.

POSTANESTHETIC RECOVERY

Recovery room facilities and nursing care must be available to provide constant surveillance of airway patency, adequate ventilation, and circulatory stability. Common sequelae of general anesthesia in infants and children include postanesthetic excitement, vomiting, and pain.

Vomiting can be relieved in the majority of cases with butyrophenones (droperidol), phenothiazines (prochlorperazine, perphenazine, trifluoperazine), metoclopramide, or the newer serotonin-3 antagonists, including ondansetron, dolasetron, and gravisetron. Butyrophenones, phenothiazines, and metoclopramide all can have the potential to cause oculogyric or dystonic reactions. These should be treated with immediate administration of intravenous diphenhydramine (Benadryl) 0.5–1 mg/kg. If the patient is not improved, intravenous benztropine (Cogentin) 0.02–0.04 mg/kg should be administered. If intravenous access is not available, both drugs can be given by intramuscular injection. Recognition of extrapyramidal reactions is often delayed or mistaken in postoperative infants and children; these reactions may be erroneously diagnosed and treated as seizures. Other children may react to neuroleptics with a range of other transient but distressing responses, including persistent sedation, difficulty speaking, or dysphoria. Because the serotonin-3 antagonists are associated with a much lower incidence of these adverse reactions, a growing tendency is to prescribe them routinely for postoperative nausea, despite their greater cost.

The recovery period should be of adequate duration to ensure that the child has adequate relief of pain and is not vomiting. It is neither necessary nor desirable to "force fluids" by mouth, because this may exacerbate vomiting, nor is it necessary to delay discharge until the child has voided.

Patients with abnormal upper airways, a history of sleep apnea, or abnormal ventilatory control or patients who have had airway surgery require careful and longer observation.

After tracheal intubation, patients may develop subglottic edema, especially if they have a history of croup or recent upper respiratory tract infection, which can often be relieved by inhaling aerosolized racemic epinephrine. Corticosteroids may be of benefit.

ANESTHESIA AND CONSCIOUS SEDATION AWAY FROM THE OPERATING ROOM (See also Chapter 74)

Common diagnostic and therapeutic procedures include bone marrow aspiration and biopsy, radiologic imaging, radiation therapy, and endoscopic procedures. Sedation and anesthesia in these settings can be of great benefit in reducing children's distress and improving ease of conduct of the procedure. The American Academy of Pediatrics has promoted monitoring standards to reduce the risks of conscious sedation outside the operating room.

The choice of conscious sedation by pediatric subspecialists (oncologists, gastroenterologists, radiologists) versus sedation or anesthesia by anesthesiologists depends on several factors, including (1) the patient's medical or psychologic condition and risk factors; (2) the duration and painfulness of the procedure, as well as the degree of immobility or cooperation required; and (3) resource availability. A wide range of minor procedures can be managed safely using conscious sedation by nonanesthesiologists. Safe practice of conscious sedation requires (1) standardized protocols for monitoring of vital signs; (2) a full-time clinician (nurse, physician, respiratory therapist) who is not occupied with performing the procedure but attends to vital signs, adequacy of airway and breathing efforts, and level of consciousness; and (3) immediate availability of airway equipment, supplemental oxygen, suction, and resuscitative drugs. Consensus should be reached about which procedures are appropriate and maximum doses of sedatives for use by nonanesthesiologists. Pulse oximetry is extremely valuable as a continuous monitor of oxygenation.

There is no perfect combination of medications that provides adequate sedation and cooperation for procedures in all cases with zero risk of respiratory depression. Dosing should be individualized and titrated slowly enough to gauge a patient's response. For many brief procedures that involve noxious stimulation, a useful combination involves midazolam (a short-acting benzodiazepine), to provide anxiolysis and amnesia, along with an opioid (fentanyl), to provide analgesia. This combination of drugs can produce synergistic sedation as well as respiratory depression, and thus titrated dosing and monitoring are essential. It is also advisable to have the reversal agents flumazenil and naloxone, respectively, immediately available in the event of hypoventilation unresponsive to stimulation, for application of supplemental oxygen, or for ventilatory assistance. For painless procedures that require sleep and immobility, such as MRI scans, sedatives without analgesic properties, such as pentobarbital or chloral hydrate, are commonly used. The toxicology of chloral hydrate's metabolites is a subject of unresolved debate.

The management of brief anesthetic procedures in locations remote from the operating suite has been greatly facilitated by the design of ultra–short duration intravenous agents such as propofol that permit very rapid and clear-headed emergence and recovery. Propofol has the additional benefit of antiemetic and antipruritic action.

General References

Badgwell JM (ed): Clinical Pediatric Anesthesia. Philadelphia, Lippincott-Raven, 1997.

Cote CJ, Ryan JF, Todres ID, Goudsouzian N (eds): The Practice of Anesthesia for Infants and Children, 2nd ed. New York, Grune & Stratton, 1993.

Gregory GA (ed): Pediatric Anesthesia, 3rd ed. New York, Churchill Livingstone, 1994.

Motoyama E, Davis P (eds): Smith's Anesthesia for Infants and Children, 5th ed. St. Louis, CV Mosby, 1990.

Steward DJ: Manual of Pediatric Anesthesia, 3rd ed. New York, Churchill Livingstone, 1990.

Preoperative Laboratory Testing

O'Connor ME, Drassner K: Pre-operative laboratory testing of children undergoing elective surgery. Anesth Analg 70:176, 1990.

Patel RI, DeWitt L, Hannallah RS: Preoperative laboratory testing in children undergoing elective surgery: Analysis of current practice. J Clin Anesth 9:569, 1997.

Preoperative Fasting

Moon R: Fasting before surgery. JAMA 273:1171, 1995.

Schriner MS, Treibwasser A, Koen TP: Ingestion of liquids compared to preoperative fasting in pediatric patients. Anesthesiology 72:593, 1990.

Splinter WM, Stewart JA, Muir JG: The effect of pre-operative apple juice on gastric contents, thirst and hunger in children. Can J Anaesth 36:55, 1990.

Warner MA, Caplan RA, Epstein BS, et al: Practice guidelines for preoperative fasting and the use of pharmacologic agents to reduce the risk of pulmonary aspiration. A report by the American Society of Anesthesiologists. Park Ridge, IL, 1998. Available from the ASA website at www.asahq.org.

Postoperative Apnea in Formerly Preterm Infants

Kurth CD, Spitzer AR, Broennle AM, et al: Post-operative apnea in preterm infants. Anesthesiology 66:483, 1987.

Steward DJ: Preterm infants are more prone to complications following minor surgery than are term infants. Anesthesiology 56:304, 1982.

Welborn LG, DeSoto H, Hannallah RS, et al: The use of caffeine in the control of post-anesthetic apnea in former preterm infants. Anesthesiology 68:796, 1988.

Child with Upper Respiratory Infection

Cohen MM, Cameron CB: Should you cancel the operation when a child has an upper respiratory tract infection? Anesth Analg 72:282, 1991.

Desoto H, Patel RI, Soliman IE, et al: Changes in oxygen saturation following general anesthesia in children with upper respiratory infection signs and symptoms undergoing otolaryngological procedures. Anesthesiology 68:276, 1988.

Tait AR, Knight PR: The effects of general anesthesia on upper respiratory tract infections in children. Anesthesiology 67:930, 1987.

Neonatal Anesthesia

Anand KJS, Sippell WG, Aynsley-Green A: Randomized trial of fentanyl anesthesia in preterm babies undergoing surgery. Effects on the stress response. Lancet 1:243, 1987.

Barrington KJ, Byrne PJ: Premedication for neonatal intubation. Am J Perinatol 15:213, 1998.

Berde CB: Anesthesia and analgesia. *In*: Cloherty JP, Stark A (eds): Manual of Neonatal Care, 4th ed. St. Louis, Little, Brown and Co, 1998, pp 667–675.

Cote CJ, Zaslavsky A, Downes JJ, et al: Postoperative apnea in former preterm infants after inguinal herniorrhaphy. A combined analysis. Anesthesiology 82:809, 1995.

Krane EJ, Haberkern CM, Jacobson LE: Postoperative apnea, bradycardia, and oxygen desaturation in formerly premature infants: Prospective comparison of spinal and general anesthesia. Anesth Analg 80:7, 1995.

Lander J, Brady-Fryer B, Metcalfe JB, et al: Comparison of ring block, dorsal penile nerve block, and topical anesthesia for neonatal circumcision: A randomized controlled trial. JAMA 278:2157, 1997.

Sedation

Cote CJ: Sedation for the pediatric patient. A review. Pediatr Clin North Am 41:31, 1994.

Krauss B, Zurakowski D: Sedation patterns in pediatric and general community hospital emergency departments. Pediatr Emerg Care 14:99, 1998.

Marx CM, Stein J, Tyler MK, et al: Ketamine-midazolam versus meperidine-midazolam for painful procedures in pediatric oncology patients. J Clin Oncol 15:94, 1997.

Maxwell LG, Yaster M: The myth of conscious sedation. Arch Pediatr Adolesc Med 150:665, 1996.

Regional Anesthesia and Pain Management

Schechter N, Berde CB, Yaster M: Pain in Infants, Children, and Adolescents. Baltimore, Williams & Wilkins, 1993.

Kain ZN, Berde CB: Pediatric pain management. *In*: Motoyama EK, Davis PJ (eds): Smith's Anesthesia for Infants and Children, 6th ed. St. Louis, CV Mosby, 1995, pp 385–402.

Sethna NF, Berde CB: Pediatric regional anesthesia. *In*: Gregory G (ed): Pediatric Anesthesia, 3rd ed, New York, Churchill Livingstone, 1994, pp 281–317.

Anesthetic Risk

Holtzman R: Morbidity and mortality in pediatric anesthesia. Pediatr Clin North Am 41:239, 1994.

Keenan RL, Boyan CP: Cardiac arrest due to anesthesia. A study of incidence and causes. JAMA 253:2373, 1985.

Morray JP, Geiduschek JM, Caplan RA, et al: A comparison of pediatric and adult anesthesia closed malpractice claims. Anesthesiology 78:461, 1993.

Rosen G, Muckle R, Mahowald M, et al: Postoperative respiratory compromise in children with obstructive sleep apnea syndrome: Can it be anticipated? Pediatrics 93:784, 1994.

Skolnick ET, Vomvolakis MA, Buck KA, et al: Exposure to environmental tobacco smoke and the risk of adverse respiratory events in children receiving general anesthesia. Anesthesiology 38:1144, 1998.

Vichinsky EP, Haberkern C, Neumayr L, et al: Randomized prospective study of conservative versus aggressive transfusion in the management of sickle cell disease. N Engl J Med 333:206, 1995.

Latex Allergy

Holzman RS: Clinical management of latex-allergic children. Anesth Analg 85:529, 1997.

Malignant Hyperthermia

Kaus SJ, Rockoff MA: Malignant hyperthermia. Pediatr Clin North Am 41:221, 1994.

CHAPTER 74
Pain Management in Children

Christine D. Greco and Charles B. Berde

Assessment and treatment of pain are an essential part of pediatric practice. This chapter summarizes (1) the development of pain perception, (2) ways to assess pain in children of different ages, (3) nonpharmacologic methods of relieving pain, and (4) the pharmacology of analgesics in children.

DEVELOPMENT OF PAIN PERCEPTION. Even the smallest neonates can respond to noxious stimulation with signs of stress and distress. Afferent pathways in the human peripheral nervous system and spinal cord connect with peripheral targets during the 2nd trimester, and rostral projections to the thalamus and cortex also develop at this time. The development of pain responses has been studied in infant animals and humans. Reflex withdrawal is evoked by milder stimuli in neonates than in adults. Noxious stimulation in neonatal animals produces more prolonged discharges in spinal neurons than in older animals. Spinal dorsal horn neurons receive inputs from larger portions of the body surface, with greater overlap of cutaneous receptive fields. Spinal descending pain inhibitory pathways, including the dorsal lateral funiculus, become active comparatively later in development. In many respects, neonates can be regarded as hypersensitive to painful stimuli. In general, pain transmission develops before pain modulation.

The long-term consequences of unrelieved pain in infants are a subject of considerable debate. Improved outcomes have been reported among neonates undergoing intensive care when efforts were undertaken to reduce painful experiences. Taddio and coworkers compared responses to immunizations among three groups of infants: those who had undergone circumcision with and without anesthesia and those who had not undergone circumcision. Blinded observers recorded the most distress in the group circumcised without anesthesia and the least distress in the uncircumcised group. These findings could not be attributed to differences in baseline temperament or other demographic variables. Although additional research is needed to clarify these issues, there is reason to conclude that neonates feel pain and that every effort should be made to provide adequate analgesia for noxious procedures.

CLINICAL ASSESSMENT OF PAIN. Whenever feasible, pain is best assessed by asking children about the character, location, quality, and intensity of their pain. For the most part, patients should be believed, and self-report is the most useful guide to assessment. For infants and preverbal children, parents, pediatricians, nurses, and other caregivers are constantly challenged to interpret whether the distressed behaviors of the children represent pain, fear, hunger, or a range of other perceptions or emotions. When behavioral and physiologic responses to pain are unclear, therapeutic trials of comfort measures (cuddling, feeding) and analgesics may be helpful in clarifying the situation.

Behavior and physiologic signs are useful but can be misleading in certain situations. A toddler may scream and grimace during an ear examination because of fear and anxiety rather than from pain; thus, a behavioral scale that scores these distress behaviors over-rates pain in this case. Conversely, children with inadequately relieved persistent pain due to cancer, sickle cell disease, trauma, or surgery often withdraw from their surroundings and appear very quiet, leading observers to conclude falsely that they are comfortable or sedated. In these situations, increased dosing of analgesics may make the child become more, not less, interactive and alert. Similarly, neonates and young infants may close their eyes, furrow their brows, and clench their fists in response to pain. Adequate analgesia is often associated with eye opening and increased involvement in their surroundings.

Investigators have devised a range of behavioral distress scales for infants and younger children, mostly emphasizing facial expressions, crying, and body movement. Facial expression measures appear to be most useful and specific in neonates. Autonomic signs, including tachycardia and hypertension, can indicate pain, but these signs may be nonspecific and may reflect a range of other processes unrelated to pain, including fever, hypoxemia, and cardiac or renal dysfunction.

Children ages 3–7 yr become increasingly articulate in describing intensity, location, and quality of pain. Pain is occasionally referred to adjacent areas; referral of hip pain to the leg or knee is not rare in this age range. Children of these ages generally are unable to use the standard visual analog scales that are well validated in older children and adults. For this reason, several investigators have explored other self-report measures for children ages 3–8 yr, using drawings or pictures of faces or graded color intensity (Table 74–1). Most children age 3 yr and older are able to describe some aspects of the intensity, quality, and location of pain. Children ages 8 yr and older generally can use visual analog pain scales accurately. Several pain intensity scales have been developed for preschool and school-aged children using facial expressions, pictures, and rulers with increasing intensity of red signifying greater pain intensity. Behavioral and physiologic indices of pain can be helpful in children who have severe cognitive and motor disabilities and whose pain is often difficult to assess. Pain is best assessed by correlating verbal reports and behavior and physiologic indices with each other and with the rest of the child's clinical picture. For hospitalized children, particularly those with pain due to cancer, sickle cell disease, or surgery, pain assessment should become a routine part of nursing assessment and documentation.

NONPHARMACOLOGIC APPROACHES TO MANAGEMENT OF PAIN. Various nonpharmacologic methods can be used to relieve pain, fear, and anxiety, including relaxation training, guided imagery, self-hypnosis, and a range of physical therapeutic methods. In general, these approaches have the merit of excellent safety and good effectiveness. For example, studies of management of childhood chronic headaches provide more robust evidence of effectiveness for cognitive and behavioral treatments than for any pharmacologic treatment. These methods are also useful because children can generalize them to new situations. Thus, a child who has cancer and who learns self-hypnosis or guided imagery to reduce distress from lumbar punctures may apply this skill to the management of venipuncture or to remaining immobile and calm while receiving radiation treatments or imaging studies. Conversely, nonpharmacologic techniques may not work for some children and should not be used as an excuse for withholding analgesics when appropriate. Expertise with these techniques requires training and practice. The Society for Behavioral Pediatrics has taken a lead in teaching these hypnosis and related techniques to pediatricians, child psychologists, and other pediatric providers.

Physical approaches to pain include use of aerobic and strength conditioning exercise programs and transcutaneous electrical nerve stimulation (TENS). Many children with chronic musculoskeletal pain become inactive and deconditioned. Exercise appears to have both specific benefits related to muscle functioning and posture and more generalized benefits related to improved body image, body mechanics, sleep, and mood. TENS can be tried for many forms of localized pain. It is quite safe, although evidence of efficacy in several situations is controversial. In newborns and young infants undergoing brief painful procedures, oral sucrose provides some analgesia and excellent safety; sucrose should not be

TABLE 74–1 Pain Measurement Tools

Name	Features	Age Range	Advantages	Limitations
Visual Analog Scale (VAS)	Horizontal 10 cm ruler, subject marks between "no pain" and "worst pain imaginable"	8 yr and older	Good psychometric properties; gold standard	Cannot be used in younger children or those with cognitive limitations
Faces scales (e.g., Wong-Baker, Oucher, Bieri, McGrath scales)	Subjects compare their pain to line drawings of faces or photos of children	4 yr and older	Can use at younger ages than VAS	Choice of anchors affects responses (neutral vs smiling)
Color analog scales	Horizontal or vertical ruler, on which increasing intensity of red signifies more pain	4 yr and older	Can use at younger ages than VAS Converges to VAS at older ages	Cannot be used in toddlers or those with cognitive limitations
Behavioral or combined behavioral-physiologic scales (e.g., CHEOPS, OPS, FACS, NIPS)	Scoring of observed behaviors (e.g., facial expression, limb movement) ± heart rate and blood pressure	Some work for any age; some are specific for age groups	Can be used even for infants and nonverbal children	Overrates fear in toddlers and preschool children Underrates persistent pain Some measures are convenient; others require videotaping and complex processing
Autonomic measures (e.g., heart rate, blood pressure, heart rate spectral analyses)	Scores changes in heart rate, blood pressure, or measures of heart rate variability, e.g., "vagal tone"	All ages	Can be used at all ages Useful for patients receiving mechanical ventilation	Nonspecific; changes can occur unrelated to pain
Hormonal-metabolic measures	Plasma or salivary sampling of hormones, e.g., cortisol, epinephrine	All ages	Can be used at all ages	Nonspecific; changes can occur unrelated to pain Inconvenient, cannot provide "real-time" information

used in lieu of analgesic medications when they are necessary and appropriate. In general, the distress of medical procedures can be diminished by a broad-based approach to make the hospital or office environment a less ominous or terrifying place to children.

DEVELOPMENTAL PHARMACOLOGY. Because the pharmacokinetics and pharmacodynamics of analgesics vary with age, infants and young children respond to drugs differently from older children and adults. The elimination half-life of most analgesics is prolonged in neonates and young children because of their immature hepatic enzyme systems. Clearance of analgesics also may be variable in young infants and children. Renal blood flow, renal plasma flow, glomerular filtration, and tubular secretion increase dramatically in the first weeks and approach adult values by 3–5 mo. Renal clearance of analgesics is often greater in toddlers and preschool children than in adults, whereas premature infants tend to have reduced renal clearance of analgesics. There also are age-related differences in body composition and protein binding, and total body water as a fraction of body weight is greater in neonates. Tissues with greater perfusion such as the brain and heart account for larger proportion of body mass in neonates than do other tissues such as muscle and fat. Because of decreased serum concentrations of albumin and α_1-acid glycoprotein, neonates have reduced protein binding of some drugs, resulting in higher amounts of free, unbound drug.

Analgesic dosing in infants and children is influenced by these differences in metabolism, clearance, and distribution. Because most drug trials have been in adult patients, drug dosing in infants and younger children is often extrapolated from studies in adults and older children using weight-based scaling. Age-specific pharmacologic studies should be useful in determining more appropriate drug dosing for children.

ACETAMINOPHEN, ASPIRIN, AND NONSTEROIDAL ANTI-INFLAMMATORY DRUGS. Acetaminophen and nonsteroidal anti-inflammatory drugs (NSAIDs) have replaced aspirin as the most commonly used antipyretics and oral nonopioid analgesics. Aspirin is indicated for certain rheumatologic conditions and for inhibition of platelet adhesiveness, as in the treatment of Kawasaki disease. Concerns about Reye hepatic encephalopathy have resulted in a substantial decline in pediatric aspirin use during the past 20 yr (Chapter 360).

Acetaminophen is generally a safe nonopioid analgesic and antipyretic that has the advantage of rectal as well as oral routes of administration. In addition, acetaminophen is not associated with the gastrointestinal effects or antiplatelet effects of aspirin and NSAIDs, making it a particularly useful drug in cancer patients. Unlike aspirin and NSAIDs, acetaminophen has little anti-inflammatory action. Plasma concentrations of 10–20 μg/mL are associated with antipyresis and analgesia. Recommended oral dosing is 10–15 mg/kg/q 4 hr. Studies examining the pharmacokinetics of rectally administered acetaminophen show that the rectal route produces delayed and variable uptake. Therapeutic plasma concentrations are achieved with single rectal doses of 35 mg/kg, with peak concentrations occurring at 45–70 min. Because clearance is prolonged with these larger rectal doses, the dosing interval should be extended to at least 6–8 hr in children. Although single doses of 10 mg/kg PO or 20 mg/kg rectally produce safe plasma concentrations in term and preterm neonates, little is known at present about maximum daily dosing for more prolonged use.

Toxicity of acetaminophen can occur from either large single doses or excessive cumulative dosing over days (see Chapter 722.2). Maximum recommended daily oral doses are 90 mg/kg for children and 60 mg/kg for infants. Based on extrapolation from kinetic data, maximum neonatal daily dose recommendations have ranged from 30–40 mg/kg/24 hr, but these numbers should be regarded as provisional. Acetaminophen overdoses have been associated with fulminant hepatic failure in infants and children. Fever and dehydration may be risk factors for hepatic injury.

NSAIDs are used widely for the treatment of pain and fever in children. A study of children with juvenile rheumatoid arthritis found that ibuprofen and aspirin were equally effective, but ibuprofen was associated with fewer side effects and better compliance. The recommended dosing of ibuprofen is 8–10 mg/kg PO every 6 hr. For children undergoing surgery, NSAIDs can provide good analgesia with a low side effect profile. In several studies of major operations, NSAIDs reduced opioid requirements by as much as 35–40% and thereby led to a reduction in side effects such as nausea or sedation. Although NSAIDs can be useful postoperatively, they should not be used as an excuse to withhold opioids from patients with unrelieved pain. **Ketorolac** is a parenterally administered NSAID that is useful in treating moderate to severe acute

TABLE 74–2 Commonly Used Nonopioid Medications

Drug	Dosing Guidelines	Comments
Acetaminophen	10–15 mg/kg PO q 4 h 20–30 mg/kg PR q 4 h Maximum daily dosing: 90 mg/kg/24 hr (children) 60 mg/kg/24 hr (infants) 30–45 mg/kg/24 hr (neonates)	No anti-inflammatory action No antiplatelet or gastric effects Toxic dosing can produce hepatic failure
Aspirin	10–15 mg/kg PO q 4 h Maximum daily dosing: 120 mg/kg/24 hr (children)	Anti-inflammatory effects Prolonged antiplatelet effects Can cause gastritis
Ibuprofen	8–10 mg/kg PO q 6 hr	Anti-inflammatory effects Reversible antiplatelet effects Can cause gastritis Extensive pediatric safety experience
Naprosyn	5–7 mg/kg PO q 8–12 hr	Anti-inflammatory effects Reversible antiplatelet effects Can cause gastritis More prolonged duration than that of ibuprofen
Ketorolac	0.25–0.5 mg/kg IV q 6 hr, to a maximum of 5 days	Anti-inflammatory effects Reversible antiplatelet effects Can cause gastritis Useful for short-term situations when oral dosing is not feasible
Choline magnesium salicylate	10–20 mg/kg PO q 8–12 hr	Weak anti-inflammatory effects Lower risk of bleeding and gastritis than with conventional NSAIDs
Nortriptyline, amitriptyline	Begin at 0.1–0.2 mg/kg PO q 24 hr, advance as needed or tolerated to 1.5 mg/kg/24 hr; some patients require a portion of the dose, e.g., 25%, in the morning, others remain at q hr dosing	Useful for neuropathic pain Rare risk of dysrhythmias; should screen for rhythm disturbances Side effects include dry mouth, sedation, constipation, urinary retention, orthostatic hypotension, palpitations

pain, particularly when patients are unable to swallow oral medications. Recommended dosing is 0.5 mg/kg IV/IM every 6 hr for no longer than 5 days; lower doses may be equally effective. Ketorolac is not unique in its opioid-sparing effect; little evidence suggests any clinically meaningful difference among NSAIDs in their maximum analgesic effects.

Adverse effects of NSAIDs include gastrointestinal bleeding, renal dysfunction, and impaired hemostasis. Although the overall incidence of bleeding is low, NSAIDs should be avoided in children who are at risk for bleeding or when surgical hemostasis is a prominent concern. Gastrointestinal bleeding is extremely rare, with an incidence of 7.2/100,000. Renal injury due to short-term use of ibuprofen in euvolemic children also appears to be quite rare; renal risk is increased by hypovolemia or cardiac dysfunction. The safety of both ibuprofen and acetaminophen for short-term use is well established. Adverse effects are rare with either drug. Table 74–2 lists suggested dosing for NSAIDs and other commonly used analgesics.

NSAIDs and aspirin act via inhibition of cyclooxygenases (COXs), enzymes that catalyze production of prostanoids to form arachidonic acid. COX has two predominant isoenzymes: a constitutively synthesized form, COX-1, found in platelets, gastric mucosa, liver, and kidneys, and an inducible form, COX-2, found in monocytes, peripheral nerve, and spinal cord and induced by injury and inflammation. Inhibition of COX-1 produces side effects, and inhibition of COX-2 produces analgesia. This realization has led to efforts to synthesize COX-2 inhibitors as safer NSAIDs. Clinical trials in adults with several selective COX-2 inhibitors suggest that these agents may provide analgesia similar to that obtained with NSAIDs but with a dramatic reduction in gastric, hemostatic, hepatic, and renal side effects.

OPIOIDS. These are used to treat various types of acute and chronic pain in infants and children. Opioids are most frequently administered for moderate and severe pain, such as acute postoperative pain, sickle cell crisis pain, and cancer pain. Opioids can be administered by a number of routes, including oral, rectal, oral transmucosal, transdermal, intravenous, epidural, subarachnoid, subcutaneous, and intramuscular. Infants and young children have traditionally been underdosed with opioids for fear of significant respiratory side effects. With proper understanding of the pharmacokinetics and pharmacodynamics of opioids, children can receive effective relief of pain and suffering with a good margin of safety. Suggested dosing guidelines for opioids are presented in Tables 74–3 and 74–4.

Opioids act by mimicking actions of endogenous opioid peptides in binding to receptors in the brain, brain stem, spinal cord, and peripheral nervous system. Opioids have dose-dependent respiratory depressant effects and blunt ventilatory responses to hypoxia and hypercarbia. The respiratory depressant effects of opioids can be increased with co-administration of other sedating drugs, such as benzodiazepines and barbiturates.

Although opioids can be used with very good safety, they frequently produce a range of annoying side effects, including constipation, nausea, vomiting, urinary retention, and pruritus. Optimal use of opioids requires proactive and anticipatory management of these side effects. The most common easily treatable side effect is constipation. Stool softeners and stimulant laxatives should be administered to most patients receiving opioids for more than a few days. Constipation often continues to be a problem with long-term opioid administration. Nausea sometimes subsides with long-term dosing but often requires treatment with antiemetics, such as phenothiazines, butyrophenones, antihistamines, and the new serotonin receptor antagonists.

It is important for pediatricians to understand the phenomena of tolerance, dependence, withdrawal, and addiction. *Tolerance* refers to a decreasing effect on continued administration of a drug or a requirement for increased dosing to achieve the same effect. Patients receiving opioids continually, as for cancer pain or for sedation/analgesia during mechanical ventilation, may require increasing doses to achieve analgesia. In general, tolerance to respiratory depression develops in parallel with tolerance to analgesic action. Thus, if patients require larger doses for analgesia, they usually do not develop respiratory depression despite these larger doses. Tolerance is not an insurmountable barrier to effective opioid use; it can be treated in most situations simply by dose escalation. *Dependence* refers to the requirement for continued opioid dosing to prevent a series of symptoms known as the **withdrawal syndrome,** which may include irritability, agitation, autonomic arousal, nasal congestion, piloerection, diarrhea, and so on. In neo-

TABLE 74–3 Practical Aspects of Opioid Prescribing

- Dosing should be titrated and individualized. There is no "right" dose for everyone.
- The right dose is the dose that relieves pain with a good margin of safety.
- Dosing should be more cautious with younger infants, in patients having coexisting diseases that increase risk or impair drug clearance, and with concomitant administration of sedatives.
- Anticipate and treat peripheral side effects, including constipation, nausea, and itching.
- Give doses at sufficient frequency to prevent return of severe pain before the next dose.
- With opioid dosing for more than a week, taper gradually to avoid withdrawal symptoms.
- When converting between parenteral and oral opioid doses, use appropriate potency ratios.

TABLE 74–4 Analgesic Initial Dosage Guidelines*

Drug	Equianalgesic Doses: Parenteral	Equianalgesic Doses: Oral	Usual Starting IV or SC Doses and Intervals: Child <50 kg	Usual Starting IV or SC Doses and Intervals: Child >50 kg	Parenteral/Oral Dose Ratio	Using Starting Oral Doses and Intervals: Child <50 kg	Using Starting Oral Doses and Intervals: Child >50 kg
Codeine	N/R	200 mg	N/R	N/R	1:2	0.5–1 mg/kg q 3–4 hr	30–60 mg q 3–4 hr
Morphine	10 mg	30 mg	Bolus: 0.1 mg/kg q 2–4 hr Infusion: 0.03 mg/kg/hr	Bolus: 5–8 mg q 2–4 hr Infusion: 1.5 mg/hr	1:3	Immediate release: 0.3 mg/kg q 3–4 hr Sustained release: 20–35 kg: 10–15 mg q 8–12 hr 35–50 kg: 15–30 mg q 8–12 hr	Immediate release: 15–20 mg q 3–4 hr Sustained release: 30–45 mg q 8–12 hr
Oxycodone	N/A	30 mg	N/A	N/A	N/A	0.1–0.2 mg q 3–4 hr	5–10 mg q 3–4 hr
Methadone	10 mg	20 mg	0.1 mg/kg q 4–8 hr	5–8 mg q 4–8 hr	1:2	0.2 mg/kg q 4–8 hr	10 mg q 4–8 hr
Methadone requires additional vigilance, because it can accumulate and produce delayed sedation. If sedation occurs, doses should be withheld until sedation resolves. Thereafter, doses should be substantially reduced and/or the dosing interval should be extended to 8–12 hr.							
Fentanyl	100 μg (0.1 mg)	N/A	Bolus: 0.5–1 μg/kg q 1–2 hr Infusion: 0.5–1.5 μg/kg/hr	Bolus: 25–50 μg q 1–2 hr Infusion: 25–75 μg/hr	N/A	N/A	N/A
Hydromorphone	1.5–2 mg	6–8 mg	Bolus: 0.02 mg q 2–4 hr Infusion: 0.006 mg/kg/hr	Bolus: 1 mg q 2–4 hr Infusion: 0.3 mg/hr	1:4	0.04–0.08 mg/kg q 3–4 hr	2–4 mg q 3–4 hr
Meperidine (pethidine)	75 mg	300 mg	Bolus: 0.8–1 mg/kg q 2–3 hr	Bolus: 50–75 mg q 2–3 hr	1:4	2–3 mg/kg q 3–4 hr	100–150 mg q 3–4 hr
Meperidine should generally be avoided if other opioids are available, especially with chronic use, because its metabolite can cause seizures.							

**Doses refer to patients >6 mo of age. In infants <6 mo, initial doses/kg should begin at roughly 25% of the doses/kg recommended here. All doses are approximate and should be adjusted according to clinical circumstances.*

N/A = not applicable; N/R = not recommended.

nates, yawning and jitteriness are common. Dependence can be produced by regular or high-dose opioid administration for as few as 7–10 days, particularly if opioid dosing is abruptly discontinued. In most cases of intermediate-term opioid use, as in postoperative patients, opioid dosing is tapered as pain subsides, so that withdrawal does not occur. In most situations, *withdrawal reactions* can be prevented by gradual tapering of opioid dosing over 7–10 days. In rare circumstances, particularly with very long-term dosing in young infants, slower tapering may be required. Tolerance, dependence, and withdrawal are physiologic responses that should be distinguished from *addiction*, which is defined as a psychologic condition of compulsive drug-seeking behaviors. In general, tolerance and dependence do not imply addiction. Addiction is extremely rare among both children and adults receiving opioids for treatment of pain. There is no basis for the view that opioid underdosing prevents addiction or that generous dosing causes addiction. Evidence suggests the converse: providing adequate relief liberates patients to focus on other concerns, whereas inadequate pain relief heightens patients' concern with obtaining medication to stop the pain.

Continuous opioid infusion is a safe and effective alternative that permits more constant plasma concentrations and clinical effects than intermittent intravenous opioid bolus dosing. Starting morphine infusion rates range from 0.01 mg/kg/hr in younger infants to 0.025 mg/kg/hr for older children. Clinical studies comparing morphine infusions in children vs adults have shown effective analgesia, fewer significant respiratory effects, and more frequent milder side effects, including nausea, pruritus, and ileus. Hypoventilation in infants can be preceded by shallow rather than slow breathing.

Because of the wide individual variation in opioid requirements, a popular approach is to permit patients to titrate their own dosing using a computer-controlled pump, a **patient-controlled analgesia (PCA)** device. Children as young as 5–6 yr can effectively use PCA. When compared with children given intermittent intramuscular morphine, children using PCA reported overall better pain scores and patient satisfaction. PCA has the advantage of adjusting dosing to account for individual pharmacokinetic and pharmacodynamic variation, as well as changing pain intensity in the course of a day. In comparison with continuous infusions titrated by nurses and physicians, PCA affords better pain scores, and in several studies this is achieved with lower overall opioid consumption and fewer side effects. PCA also can help children feel more in control and less helpless. For children too young to use the PCA button, several centers have reported favorable preliminary experience with nurse- or parent-activated PCA, particularly for cancer pain and often in combination with a low-dose continuous infusion. Our practice is to make liberal use of nurse-controlled PCA and to use parent-controlled PCA predominantly in the setting of palliative care (Chapter 38). Overdoses have been reported when well-meaning, inadequately instructed parents pushed the PCA button in medically complicated situations.

Many opioids are used clinically, and differences among them relate in part to differences in relative potency and duration of action. *Morphine* is widely used for infants and children, particularly for acute postoperative pain. Peak analgesic effect occurs in approximately 10 min when this agent is administered intravenously. *Codeine* is a weak opioid; it is often administered in combination with acetaminophen. It has the practical advantage that it can be prescribed over the telephone more readily than other opioids. *Meperidine* is metabolized in the liver into normeperidine, which can cause dysphoria, agitation, and seizures. When compared with meperidine, morphine provides better analgesia with no difference in the incidence of side effects. In general, meperidine use should be discouraged and limited to specific indications, such as in low doses for the treatment of rigors and shivering, particularly in oncology patients receiving amphotericin or blood products. *Hydromorphone* is similar to morphine in most respects and is approximately five times as potent when given intravenously. *Fentanyl* and its analogs are potent analgesics that are usually used for short, painful procedures such as bone marrow aspiration and burn debridement or for brief surgical procedures. Fentanyl is most commonly administered intravenously, although a transdermal patch and transmucosal lozenges are also available. Fentanyl is 70–100 times more potent than morphine and provides rapid onset of intense analgesia with shorter duration of action in smaller doses. With infusions or larger doses, the duration of action can be quite prolonged. With higher doses and rapid administration, fentanyl and its analogs have the additional risk of producing chest wall rigidity, which can make mask ventilation extremely difficult. Chest wall rigidity can sometimes be reversed with naloxone, although in some cases neuromuscular blockade and controlled ventilation are required. Patients receiving fentanyl or its analogs should be carefully monitored, and airway equipment should be readily accessible. *Methadone* is a long-acting opioid that can provide 12–24 hr of analgesia. It can be given either intravenously or orally in an elixir or tablet. Because of its long duration of action, methadone can be especially useful in managing certain types of chronic pain or for patients who are unable to swallow tablets. Methadone requires careful dosing and close observation to avoid accumulation and delayed sedation.

LOCAL ANESTHETICS. Local anesthetics are widely used in children for topical application, cutaneous infiltration, peripheral nerve block, and intraspinal punctures. In general, local anesthetics can be used with excellent safety and effectiveness. Excessive systemic concentrations can cause two major forms of toxicity: in the brain, they produce seizures and central nervous system depression; in the heart, they produce arrhythmia or cardiac depression. Unlike opioids, for which doses can be titrated upward as needed, there is a strict maximum dosing of local anesthetics. Pediatricians need to be aware of the need to calculate these doses and adhere to the guidelines.

Topical local anesthetic preparations have diverse uses in reducing pain, such as for suturing lacerations, intravenous catheter placements, lumbar punctures, and accessing indwelling central ports. Application of tetracaine, epinephrine, and cocaine (**TAC**) results in good anesthesia for suturing wounds. It should not be used on mucous membranes. Cocaine is not essential; combinations of tetracaine with phenylephrine or lidocaine-epinephrine-tetracaine are equally effective. **EMLA** is a topical eutectic mixture of lidocaine and prilocaine that is used to anesthetize intact skin and is commonly applied for venipuncture, lumbar puncture, and other needle procedures. EMLA is safe for use in neonates. When used for newborn circumcision, it partially but not completely suppresses behavioral and autonomic responses. EMLA is more effective than placebo but probably is less effective than ring block of the penis in providing analgesia for circumcision.

Lidocaine is the most commonly used local anesthetic for cutaneous infiltration. Maximum safe doses of lidocaine are 5 mg/kg without epinephrine and 6 mg/kg with epinephrine. Concentrated solutions (e.g., 2%) should be avoided, because solutions as dilute as 0.3% are equally effective as 1–2% solutions, and the dilute solutions permit larger doses. For example, a 5-kg infant receiving infiltration for suturing may safely receive $5 \times 5 = 25$ mg of lidocaine. This maximum dose would be attained with either 1.25 mL of lidocaine 2%, 2.5 mL of lidocaine 1%, or 5 mL of lidocaine 0.5%.

Regional anesthesia is widely used for postoperative pain relief in children after many types of surgery, such as abdominal, orthopedic, and thoracic procedures. It also can reduce the need for systemic opioids in patients with severe lung disease. Epidural analgesia and peripheral nerve blocks provide excellent analgesia and are safe even in term and preterm infants. Spinal anesthesia can be used to avoid the need for general anesthesia and for intubated infants with moderate and severe lung disease undergoing herniorrhaphy or lower extremity procedures.

POSTOPERATIVE PAIN MANAGEMENT. As described in Chapter 73, infants and children can be anesthetized for surgery with excellent safety and physiologic stability. Surgery in neonates receiving inadequate anesthesia evokes an outpouring of stress hormones (e.g., epinephrine, glucagon, cortisol, growth hormone) with resultant consequences including catabolism, immunosuppression, hemodynamic instability, and marked fluctuations in intracranial pressure. Providing adequate anesthesia and analgesia to critically ill neonates may improve outcomes in newborn surgery. Opioids in newborns receiving ventilatory support can blunt stress responses to surgery and intensive care, and the opioids are tolerated with good hemodynamic stability.

Children should receive an age-appropriate explanation of what to expect with anesthesia, surgery, and postoperative care. Depending on the site and severity of surgery, postoperative analgesia may involve combinations of acetaminophen, NSAIDs, opioids, and local anesthetics. In major pediatric centers, multidisciplinary programs for postoperative pain management, such as an acute pain service, have become widely used. These programs help ensure standards for treating postoperative pain, provide immediate pain assessment, monitor responses to analgesics, and provide individualized adjustment of analgesics and management of side effects.

MANAGEMENT OF BRIEF DIAGNOSTIC AND THERAPEUTIC PROCEDURES. Procedures such as endoscopy, bone marrow aspiration and biopsy, or radiologic imaging procedures may require either analgesia to make the procedure more comfortable, anxiolysis to make the procedure less terrifying, or sedation to permit a child to lie motionless for imaging studies or radiation therapy. There is no consensus of a "right way" for all procedures. The term *conscious sedation* refers to a condition in which a patient is sleepy, comfortable, and more cooperative but maintains protective airway and ventilatory reflexes. The term *deep sedation* refers to a state of unarousability to voice and greater suppression of reflex responses. Sedation represents a continuum of responses, and a dose of sedative medication that causes minimal sedation in one subject may produce complete unconsciousness and apnea in another. It is therefore essential that clinicians administer sedatives with an appreciation of these individual differences, that children receive close observation for adequacy of respiration, and that airway equipment and supplemental oxygen delivery sources be immediately available. Conscious sedation for children is often required in various clinical locations, such as in the emergency room, MRI suites, or procedure rooms on pediatric wards. To ensure that patients receive optimal, safe care, it is recommended that hospitals develop conscious sedation guidelines, such as those established by the American Academy of Pediatrics. These guidelines should include recommendations for withholding feeding before procedures, drug dosages (Table 74–5), strategies to achieve patient comfort, necessary monitoring, required resuscitation equipment, and a quality improvement program for tracking outcomes and ensuring efficacy and safety. The guidelines also should specify which subgroups of patients are at increased risk and should have sedation performed by pediatric anesthesiologists.

TREATMENT OF PAIN DUE TO CANCER IN CHILDREN. Children frequently experience pain during cancer treatment, including brief painful diagnostic procedures or surgery, and with mucositis. Children with widespread or terminal disease benefit from a multidimensional approach to supportive care and symptom management that relies not only on medications but also on psychosocial support, nonpharmacologic modalities, and treatment of pain in the context of their emotional distress, grief, and loss (see Chapter 38). In some cases, other symptoms including nausea, itching, dysphoria, myoclonus, or air hunger can be as distressing as pain. The World Health Organization (WHO) proposed a model for analgesic therapy for cancer pain known as the "analgesic ladder" (Fig. 501–2).

TABLE 74–5 Drugs Used for Conscious Sedation in Children

Drug	Suggested Starting Dose(s)	Comments
Midazolam	0.05 mg/kg incremental doses IV q 5–10 min up to 3–5 doses (to a maximum incremental dose of 1 mg) 0.1–0.2 mg/kg IM (maximum dose 10 mg) 0.3–0.6 mg/kg PO (maximum dose 20 mg)	Good anxiolytic Flumazenil is a reversal agent Dose more cautiously when combined with opioids
Fentanyl	0.5 μg/kg increments q 5 min up to 3–5 doses	Rapid infusion of large doses can produce chest wall rigidity Respiratory depression is amplified by co-administration of sedatives
Pentobarbital	1 mg/kg increments IV q 10 min up to 3 doses 2–4 mg/kg IM 4–6 mg/kg PO	Good sedative, no analgesia Used primarily for radiologic procedures Occasionally produces prolonged sedation
Chloral hydrate	25–100 mg/kg PO or PR 30–40 min before the procedure	Higher incidence of failed sedation with 25–50 mg/kg
Ketamine	0.2–0.5 mg/kg increments q 10 min × 3 1–2 mg/kg IM	Co-administration of midazolam or other benzodiazepines is recommended to reduce the risk of dysphoria or bad dreams Use should be restricted to cases managed by physicians with extensive airway expertise

Nonopioid analgesics (e.g., acetaminophen) are used for mild pain. If pain relief is not adequate, a weak opioid (e.g., codeine) is added. If this is not sufficient, then strong opioids (e.g., morphine) are administered for more severe pain. Morphine should be regarded as a first choice in most circumstances. The program emphasizes the oral route of opioid administration whenever feasible, because of its simplicity and demonstrated efficacy. When opioids are used for cancer pain, side effects are frequent, especially constipation, itching, and nausea, and require active management, including the regular use of stimulant laxatives. If sedation becomes a limiting side effect, morning and mid-day dosing of methylphenidate or dextroamphetamine provides increased alertness as well as some analgesia.

Sustained-release oral opioids are convenient for providing prolonged effect. They must be swallowed whole: If sustained-release opioid tablets are crushed, they become immediate-acting. If a prolonged-duration opioid is required for children who cannot swallow tablets, an alternative is oral methadone given as an elixir. When patients who are tolerant to morphine or hydromorphone are switched to methadone, they sometimes show incomplete cross-tolerance and improved efficacy. This incomplete cross-tolerance may be due, in part, to methadone's dual action as a μ-opioid receptor agonist and as an antagonist at the *N*-methyl-D-aspartate (NMDA) class of glutamate receptors.

Although the oral route of opioid administration should be encouraged, some children are unable or unwilling to take oral opioids. Intravenous infusions with a PCA option are commonly used next. Small portable infusion pumps are convenient for home use. If venous access is limited, a useful alternative is to administer opioids (especially morphine or hydromorphone, not methadone or meperidine) via continuous subcutaneous infusion, with or without a bolus option. A small (e.g., 22-gauge) cannula is placed under the skin and secured on the thorax, abdomen, or thigh. Sites may be changed every 3–7 days as needed. Other alternative routes for opioids include transdermal and oral transmucosal.

Collins and colleagues examined the effectiveness of analgesic treatment, patterns of opioid use, and terminal symptoms among 199 children and adolescents dying of cancer. More than 90% could be made comfortable by standard escalation of opioids according to the WHO program. A small subgroup of 12 patients (5%) had enormous opioid dose escalation to more than 100 times standard morphine infusion rates. In all but one of these cases, there was spread of solid tumors to the spinal cord, roots, or plexus, and signs of neuropathic pain were evident. When huge opioid infusion rates are used, myoclonus can occur; it may be treated with clonazepam or other benzodiazepines. In selected cases of intolerable side effects or enormous opioid dose escalation, subarachnoid or epidural infusions of opioids along with local anesthetics can improve pain relief and alertness. In other cases, infusion of sedatives may be required if there is no margin between sedation and unrelieved pain. If continuous sedation is chosen, high-dose opioid infusions should be maintained as well. The choice of extraordinary methods of pain relief, involving either regional anesthesia or sedation, should be made judiciously and with consideration of the individual child's and family's wishes and of the developmental, emotional, and medical situation.

Patients experiencing pain associated with other causes of terminal illnesses, including AIDS, neurodegenerative disorders, and cystic fibrosis, need similar approaches to palliative care that combine emotional support with pharmacologic management of pain and other distressing symptoms. There are some important differences between these conditions and cancer in the progression of illness, hopes, and expectations of children and families and between the particular patterns of pain, air hunger, and other symptoms (see Chapter 38).

CHRONIC AND RECURRENT PAIN IN CHILDREN. It is useful to distinguish between the common recurrent "benign" pains of childhood and the less common forms of chronic persistent pain. A large proportion of otherwise healthy children experience recurrent episodes of nonspecific headache, chest pain, abdominal pain, or limb pains. In general, these problems are characterized by painful episodes alternating with symptom-free periods, and the child appears to be growing and gaining weight and shows no signs suggestive of serious illness. A thorough history and physical examination are the cornerstone of diagnosis, and laboratory testing should be extremely sparse and only as guided by clinical indication. For example, gastrointestinal barium roentgenographic studies in children with recurrent abdominal pains that appear benign from history and physical examination have an extraordinarily low yield. The art of general pediatric practice lies in distinguishing these unpleasant but essentially benign problems from those symptoms that suggest more serious illness. Even when it is concluded that a patient's problem is benign (e.g., "nonspecific recurrent abdominal pain"), it is important not only to avoid overmedicalization but also to maintain an open mind to reassessing the diagnosis if the clinical presentation changes later. Pediatricians must try to reassure children and families that their symptoms are real, that they are believed, but that the symptoms should not keep the child from participating in school and other normal activities. This is sometimes easier said than done.

In evaluating a child with recurrent or persistent pain complaints, along with a thorough medical history and review of systems, a comprehensive psychosocial history is mandatory (see Chapters 17 and 19). It is important in counseling the family to understand how the pain complaint affects social functioning, school attendance, and parental behavior toward the child. Management should emphasize lifestyle interventions, including diet, exercise, and biobehavioral treatment, rather than excessive reliance on medications in isolation. For example for children having recurrent headaches, the evidence for efficacy of relaxation training or hypnosis is more compelling than for that of any medication.

Recurrent headaches are common in children; as many as 5–10% of school-aged children experience them. The most common types of headaches occurring in children are migraine and tension headaches. NSAIDs are widely used and effective for treatment of headaches in children. See Chapter 604.1 for treatment of migraine. *Chronic persistent pains* that occur daily are uncommon in general pediatric practice, although arthritis may produce daily pain (Chapter 154).

Sickle cell anemia is discussed in Chapter 468.1. Both recurrent acute severe pain and chronic persistent pain occur in some affected children. There is a marked variation in the frequency and severity of painful episodes; the majority of people with sickle cell disease come to the hospital only rarely and manage most of their symptoms at home. Children experiencing painful vaso-occlusive episodes deserve generous dosing with opioids and NSAIDs for pain relief without excessive concern about addiction. Several centers that care for these children have reported success with a treatment model that emphasizes (1) self-care and maintenance of normal activities, (2) generous dosing of opioids and NSAIDs at home via the oral route whenever possible, (3) treatment of breakthrough pain in a day-treatment program or clinic rather than in an emergency room and with hospital admission, and (4) teaching of biobehavioral techniques and coping strategies before a cycle develops involving negative experiences with health care personnel. For severe episodes requiring inpatient treatment, intravenous opioid infusions and PCA can be used safely and effectively, although careful dose titration may be needed in many cases. Yaster and colleagues reported favorable effects on pain and respiratory function when continuous epidural infusions were used for children at high risk for acute chest syndrome. This management is not established.

Neuropathic pain is pain due to abnormal excitability in the peripheral or central nervous system that may persist after an injury heals or inflammation subsides. The pain is often described as burning or stabbing and may be associated with cutaneous hypersensitivity (allodynia). Neuropathic pain conditions may be responsible for more than 35% of referrals to chronic pain clinics and commonly include post-traumatic and postsurgical peripheral nerve injuries, phantom pain after amputation, pain after spinal cord injury, and pain due to metabolic neuropathies. In many but not all cases, neuropathic pain may respond poorly to opioids. In adults, evidence suggests the efficacy of several tricyclic antidepressants (e.g., nortriptyline, amitriptyline) and anticonvulsants (e.g., carbamazepine, gabapentin) for treatment of neuropathic pain, and treatment of children is based largely on extrapolation from these adult studies. Antidepressants and anticonvulsants may provide relief for some children, but side effects are common, and a considerable degree of trial and error is involved in this type of pharmacotherapy. Treatment for neuropathic pain should also include a comprehensive approach involving physical therapy and biobehavioral interventions. In many cases, it is important to educate the child and family about the nonprotective character of the pain. It is counterintuitive for most people to move a part of the body that hurts, and many patients with neuropathic pain develop atrophy or contractures of a painful extremity. The notion must be taught that neuropathic pains are "misinformation from nerves" and that movement of the painful area, though unpleasant, does not damage tissues and may diminish pain and dysfunction in the long run. Long-term administration of opioids has a role in a highly selected subgroup of children.

The majority of children with recurrent or chronic pains cope well and maintain school attendance. For a small subgroup of children with chronic pain, school absenteeism should be viewed as a disability syndrome analogous to work absenteeism in adults. In some cases, granting a child long-term home tutoring is analogous to granting an adult a long-term disability claim; it sanctions the disability and maintains the child away from the mainstream social milieu. School avoidance, common among children referred to chronic pain clinics, should not be reinforced.

Berde CB, Lehn B, Yee JD, et al: Patient-controlled analgesia in children and adolescents: A randomized, prospective comparison with intramuscular morphine for postoperative analgesia. J Pediatr 118:460, 1991.

Beyer JE, McGrath PJ, Berde CB: Discordance between self-report and behavioral pain measures in children aged 3–7 years after surgery. J Pain Symptom Manage 5:350, 1990.

Collins JJ, Grier HE, Kinney HC, et al: Control of severe pain in terminal pediatric malignancy. J Pediatr 126:653, 1995.

Grossi E, Borghi C, Cerchiari EL, et al: Analogue chromatic continuous scale (ACCS): A new method for pain assessment. Clin Exp Rheumatol 1:337, 1983.

Himelstein BP, Cnaan A, Blackall CS, et al: Topical application of lidocaine-prilocaine (EMLA) cream reduces the pain of intramuscular infiltration of saline solution. J Pediatr 129:718, 1996.

Houck CS, Wilder RT, McDermott JS, et al: Safety of intravenous ketorolac therapy in children and cost savings with a unit dosing system. J Pediatr 129:292, 1996.

Johnston CC, Strada ME: Acute pain response in infants: A multidimensional description. Pain 24:373, 1986.

Liebelt EL: Current concepts of laceration repair. Curr Opin Pediatr 9:459, 1997.

Maxwell LG, Yaster M: The myth of conscious sedation. Arch Pediatr Adolesc Med 150:665, 1996.

McGrath PA, Seifert CE, Speechley KN, et al: A new analogue scale for assessing children's pain: An initial validation study. Pain 64:435, 1996.

Olness K, Gardner GG: Pediatrics for the clinician: Some guidelines for uses of hypnotherapy in pediatrics. Pediatrics 62:228, 1978.

Parker RI, Mahan RA, Giugliano D, et al: Efficacy and safety of intravenous midazolam and ketamine as sedation for therapeutic and diagnostic procedures for children. Pediatrics 99:427, 1997.

Petrack EM, Christopher NC, Kriwinsky J: Pain management in the emergency department: Patterns of analgesic utilization. Pediatrics 99:711, 1997.

Schechter NF, Berde CB, Yaster MS: Pain in Infants, Children and Adolescents. Baltimore, Williams & Wilkins, 1992.

Smith GA, Strausbaugh SD, Harbeck-Weber C, et al: New non-cocaine-containing topical anesthetics compared with tetracaine-adrenaline-cocaine during repair for lacerations. Pediatrics 100:825, 1997.

Taddio A, Katz J, Lane A, et al: Effect of neonatal circumcision on pain response during subsequent routine vaccination. Lancet 349:599, 1997.

PART IX

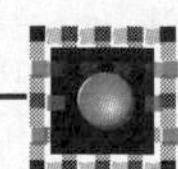

Human Genetics

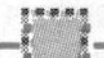

CHAPTER 75
Molecular Basis of Genetic Disorders

Larry Shapiro

Genetic factors influence susceptibility to a variety of human diseases and play a major role in the response of individuals to various environmental events. Appreciation of the importance of inherited components of common diseases, congenital malformations, and cancer has increased substantially as revolutionary developments have occurred in the basic science of genetics. The application of molecular genetics to an understanding of heritable disease has led to extraordinary progress in the practice of medicine, specifically in the approach to diagnosis, genetic counseling, and screening of individuals at risk for genetic disease.

The scope of molecular genetics extends from the structure of genes to the functioning of their products in a cell; this field is dominated by powerful and rapidly changing technology involving the manipulation of DNA, RNA, and protein. A fundamental goal of molecular genetics is to identify a heritable disease at the level of the affected gene and to chemically define the precise mutation. Once the mutation has been identified, efforts are made to understand its impact on the functioning of the cell, on the tissue and organ, and on the organism. The mutation is traced from DNA to the corresponding RNA copies of the gene to the protein translated from the RNA. Such studies also provide novel insights into the biologic design of normal cellular constituents and processes.

With knowledge of the nature of mutations occurring at the DNA level, diagnosis of a mutation may be aimed at direct examination of an individual's DNA. Diagnosis can often be achieved by examination of the DNA from a single cell, and almost any cell from an individual will suffice. Although our diagnostic capacities exceed our therapeutic capabilities, molecular genetics may eventually provide enhanced treatment of disease through direct correction of a mutation at the DNA level. In some cases, a gene can be corrected in a somatic cell by replacement with a normal or modified gene, and, in a few examples, similar replacement of a gene into the germ line of an animal has been accomplished.

This chapter reviews certain essential facts that provide an understanding of how human genetic machinery is organized and discusses applications that have an impact on this study of human disease. There are numerous excellent texts that review the general field of molecular genetics, and the reader is advised to refer to them for a deeper appreciation of the subject.

THE HUMAN GENOME. Each human somatic cell contains two copies of the entire human genetic program, or genome, amounting to 3 billion base pairs (bp) of DNA. DNA is a double-stranded helix, each "step" of the helix comprising a base from one strand connected by hydrogen bonds to a complementary base from the other (a bp either A-T or G-C). Human DNA is portioned into 46 (23 pairs) large fragments, each contained in a specific autosomal chromosome or the X or Y chromosome. The gene is the functional unit of information. Approximately 50,000 genes are thought to be encoded in human DNA. In any one type of cell, only a subset of these genes is actually active and operates to maintain the viability and specialized functions of that cell. The genes within a cell may be expressed at widely varying levels. Some genes are responsible for the specialized function of a cell, such as the globin genes of a red blood cell. Other genes are considered to have a "housekeeping" function; these genes (the products of which are common to most cells) are needed for the maintenance of basic cellular functioning. Some genes are expressed constitutively, and others are expressed in response to a specific stimulus. A major question of modern molecular biology is why certain genes, such as globin in a red blood cell or myosin in a muscle cell, are capable of extraordinary activity in these cells but remain silent in others.

Why genes are located at particular sites in the genome or why they are present on a particular chromosome is unknown. Frequently, however, highly related genes are clustered in a particular region of a chromosome. A well-studied example is the gene for globins on chromosome 11. At this location a cluster of six related globin genes is found. In the case of this globin cluster, one gene is turned on in red blood cells during embryonic life; a different gene is turned on during the later fetal period; and the β-globin gene is turned on around the time of birth, increases in activity, and remains active into adulthood. It is believed that precise developmental regulation of the genes within the globin family depends partly on their physical proximity to each other within the cluster. Also see Chapter 452.

Many proteins consist of different component subunits, which together are needed for complete function. Often, the genes encoding these component proteins are located on different chromosomes, such as the genes for the α- and β-globins, the proteins that assemble into the tetrameric hemoglobin molecule. The genes for α-globin are on chromosome 16, while the gene for the β chain is on chromosome 11. The cell must be able to carefully regulate the relative expression of these physically unconnected genes as well.

Only a small fraction of the DNA that makes up the human genome appears to be represented by functional genes, perhaps about 10% of the total. Most of the human genome consists of DNA sequences without any clear function. Some of this noncoding DNA may be important in the regulation of gene expression or in aspects of chromosome structure and function. Portions of the noncoding DNA are present as single, unique sequences, while other components are repeated hundreds or thousands of times in the genome.

Most, but not all, of the DNA in a human cell is contained in the nucleus. Some genes are also found in the mitochondria. These organelles, which serve energy-producing needs of cells, contain their own genome. The mitochondrial genome consists of a circular double-stranded molecule containing about 16,000 bp of DNA, which has been completely sequenced. Each mitochondrion may harbor several copies of this circular DNA molecule, and, during mitochondrial division, the mitochondrial genome is replicated. A cell may contain different mitochondria with distinctly different genomes. What is remarkable about the mitochondrion is that it is constructed of proteins that are encoded by its own genome as well as proteins that are encoded in genes contained in the cell nucleus. Proteins that are encoded in the mitochondrial genome appear to be synthesized within the mitochondrion, whereas those encoded in the nucleus are made in the cell's cytoplasm and transported into the mitochondrion. The design principle on which the mitochondrion is built affects the patterns of inheritance that are observed for mitochondrial characteristics. On fertilization, the sperm does not carry mitochondria into the oocyte. The fertilized egg, therefore, receives only mitochondria from the maternal gamete. Thus, genes located on the mitochondrial genome are exclusively maternally inherited, and, as a consequence, diseases resulting from mutation of mitochondrial genes exhibit a maternal inheritance pattern.

A collaborative international scientific effort known as the Human Genome Project has the goal of determining the entire DNA sequence of the human genome. As of 1998, there has been remarkable progress in accomplishing this task, with the spatial location of many human genes and DNA segments having been established. This has accelerated the identification and characterization of genes that are important in the pathogenesis of many inherited and acquired human disorders. The diagnostic and therapeutic potential of these efforts may reshape the way in which all medicine is practiced. Access to actual DNA sequence information as well as a host of derivative sources of information can be readily obtained via the internet (Table 75–1).

STRUCTURE OF GENES. A gene is a functional unit of DNA from which RNA is copied *(transcribed)*. Most genes implicated in human disease express a class of RNA that is translated by cellular machinery into protein (messenger RNA [mRNA]). Genes range in length from several hundred bp to more than 2 million bp of DNA. A specialized nuclear enzyme, *RNA polymerase*, recognizes the beginning or start sequence of a gene, attaches to the double-stranded DNA, and proceeds to copy one strand of the gene's DNA sequence into a single strand of RNA as it travels along the length of the gene. The enzyme recognizes another punctuation signal and falls off the gene, releasing the RNA strand. The RNA strand is then processed. The processing reactions involve additions of certain nucleic acids at both ends and removal of certain internal sequences. These processing reactions are necessary for the RNA to be transported from the nucleus to the cytoplasm and to be used effectively by the protein synthetic machinery of the cytoplasm, which must translate this RNA into protein.

TABLE 75–1 Useful Internet Reference Sites

Web Address	Data Base
http://www.ncbi.nlm.nih.gov	General reference maintained by National Library of Medicine
http://www.ncbi.nlm.nih.gov/Omim	Online Mendelian Inheritance in Man (extremely useful for clinicians—over 10,000 entries of genetic traits indexed by gene name, symptoms, and so forth)
http://www.ncbi.nlm.nih.gov/genemap	General reference to current efforts to map the human genome
http://www.ncbi.nlm.nih.gov/Web/Genbank	Searchable repository of all DNA sequence data
http://www.ncbi.nlm.nih.gov/ncicgap	Cancer Genome Anatomy Project (National Cancer Institute)
http://www.nhgri.nih.gov	National Human Genome Research Institute Web Site (useful information about human genetics and ethical issues)
http://www.uwcm.ac.uk/uwcm/mg/hgmd0.html	Human Gene Mutation Database (searchable index of all described mutations in human genes with phenotypes and references)

The most striking processing reaction involves the splicing out of stretches of the RNA, each splicing event taking place at a very precise point in the precursor. In some cases, the total length of RNA removed exceeds the final length of the mature product. Because of this process, mature RNA differs in sequence from the original DNA template. RNA sequences that are retained in mature mRNA are called **exons** of a gene, and those that are excised are called **introns**.

The cellular equipment that splices the RNA precursor accurately is complex and consists of many proteins and small RNA species. The basic principle underlying splicing is that the nuclear splicing machinery somehow recognizes proper splice junctions, cleaves the RNA precisely at these junctions, and rejoins the pieces. The excised piece is destroyed in the nucleus and appears to serve no further function in most cases. Splicing is a very complicated process, fraught with possible opportunities for errors. For example, mutations have been identified that prevent normal splicing by altering critical sequences around the splice junction.

It is unknown why most eukaryotic genes are designed in this manner. However, this splicing mechanism permits a cell to produce different RNA molecules from a single gene by splicing the initial RNA differently. For example, in a muscle cell the initial tropomyosin RNA transcript is spliced in as many as ten different alternative patterns. Each alternatively spliced RNA actually yields a distinctly different final protein product. From a single gene, a family of different proteins, corresponding to RNAs alternatively spliced, can be expressed. This design permits different proteins to be expressed from a single gene. An RNA may be spliced in one way in one cell and in another way in a different cell type, permitting some degree of tissue specificity over the nature of the product expressed from a gene. Splicing permits another level of control and compresses the amount of DNA that we are required to accommodate in our genome.

It is important to understand what causes a particular gene to be expressed in a given cell and how the activity of that gene is regulated. Certain controls exist that can activate a particular battery of genes in a cell (e.g., the genes activated in response to a hormone). Other specialized controls are necessary for activating genes expressing an abundant product in a specific tissue. Another level of control exists to turn on genes at specific times in development. Many of these controls appear to lie within very small DNA sequences residing in the general neighborhood of the expressed sequences. They are commonly found at the front end of the gene (5′-end) before the DNA sequence that is actually copied into RNA. The essential control element of a gene is called a *promoter*, and, in almost every gene, such a group of essential control sequences has been identified. Specific proteins bind to these control sequences and make the gene more accessible to productive transcription by RNA polymerase. The precise mechanism by which proteins accomplish this is not known, but it is thought that they permit RNA polymerase to gain access more easily than when they are absent. For example, it appears that steroid hormone–responsive genes are activated by specific proteins that bind to DNA sequences around responsive genes when associated with a specific hormone.

The other control elements that are needed for tissue-specific activation are called *enhancers*. These enhancers appear to be special sequences that interact with proteins present only in cells of a specific tissue. The presence of this sequence in the vicinity of a gene may be sufficient to lead to its expression in a tissue-specific fashion.

If DNA were fully extended, the total length of the DNA contained in the nucleus of a cell would stretch to about 1 M. Because DNA is condensed into a considerably smaller volume, it is obvious that DNA must be packaged. Packaging is complicated by the fact that genes and other sequences must be accessed. In addition, DNA must be replicated during cellular division. Nuclear DNA is packaged with a set of basic proteins, *histones*, and some additional non-histone chromosomal proteins into a DNA-protein assembly called *chromatin*. The histones themselves organize to form spherical particles around which about 200 bp of DNA are draped. These "beads on a string" are coiled coaxially to form thicker ropes, which are then draped on proteins that constitute the scaffolding of the chromosomes. It is believed that when a gene is active the chromatin assembly containing the gene is less condensed or more "open," and, at certain sequences, histones may be replaced by other specialized proteins or may undergo modification such as acetylation.

After a gene sequence has been copied to an RNA and that RNA has subsequently matured, the RNA is transported to the cytoplasm of a cell. In the cytoplasm, the RNA is translated by ribosomes and associated enzymes into a nascent protein. In some cases, the protein remains in the cytoplasm, where it will ultimately function (e.g., glycolytic enzymes). In other cases, the mRNA directs its protein product into the internal membrane system of a cell, the endoplasmic reticulum, and the newly made protein is shuttled through the internal membrane compartments of a cell. It can be directed from the endoplasmic reticulum to membrane compartments, such as the Golgi network, where chemical modifications, such as the addition of carbohydrate, occur. Proteins may be subsequently delivered into intracellular vesicles, such as lysosomes, or be secreted from the cell, or be delivered to any of the membranes of the cell, such as the plasma membrane. In some cases, proteins synthesized in the cytoplasm are transported into organelles, such as the mitochondrion, the peroxisome, or the nucleus. The precise nature of the signals that specify the particular intracellular compartment in which a protein will ultimately find itself is the subject of intense investigation.

GENETIC ABNORMALITIES. Genetic abnormalities are a common cause of disease, handicap, and death among infants and children. Genetic disease accounts for the primary diagnosis of 11–16% of patients admitted to the pediatric units of teaching hospitals. One per cent of newborn infants have a hereditary malformation, and an additional 0.5% have an inborn error of metabolism or an abnormality of the sex chromosomes.

Many genes have been localized to specific chromosomes. Molecular biology technology now makes gene mapping possible so that gene deletions and point mutations, due to the loss or the substitution of a few bp, can be identified. New methods for staining human chromosomes and identifying subtle duplications and deficiencies of chromosomal material have also enlarged the understanding of human chromosomal abnormalities.

A more complete understanding of the basic defect in many of the genetic diseases has altered clinical classifications. For example, homocystinuria, once considered a single disease, has been shown to be the manifestation of several different metabolic abnormalities. The lethal type of osteogenesis imperfecta, once considered a single disorder, has been shown to be caused by several different alterations of the collagen gene, including internal deletion in the gene's structure, its failure to properly form the collagen triple helix, and failure to secrete the precursors of collagen from cells (see below). Furthermore, although lethal osteogenesis imperfecta was once considered to be due to an autosomal recessive gene, spontaneous and presumably autosomal dominant mutations are now known to be the basis for most affected infants. The study of common genetic disorders has shown that for some, such as cystic fibrosis and phenylketonuria (PKU), most affected individuals have the same mutation, whereas others, such as hemophilia, are due to many different mutations. The identification of genetic markers that are close to mutant genes is making it possible to trace mutant genes in diseases through successive generations.

When clinically appraising and managing the child with an inherited disorder, three phases are critical: (1) recognizing that the condition is inherited, (2) identifying the pattern of inheritance, and (3) clarifying the clinical nature of the disorder, which includes understanding the risk of the disease's occurrence in siblings or other members of the family. Recognition that a condition is hereditary may be difficult when the patient has no affected relatives. The physician should be familiar with the different types of genetic diseases and be able to identify their patterns of inheritance using appropriate references such as *Mendelian Inheritance in Man* by McKusick, which lists conditions caused by single mutant genes. For those with access to the Internet, this resource is available on-line, is heavily annotated, and frequently updated (see Table 75–1).

HUMAN GENETIC MAPS AND THEIR USE TO LOCATE DISEASE GENES. The chromosomal locations of many thousands of human genes are already known. In many cases, data are available on the precise location on a chromosome as well as the relative position between individual genes on the same chromosome. This body of data makes up the human genome map. In some cases, positional information is available about DNA sequences for which there is no known function. These sequences have been mapped to precise locations and help orient us in a particular region of a chromosome, providing us with further guideposts for mapping.

Several approaches have been utilized to map genes and other DNA sequences to specific chromosomes. In the classical approach, genes located on the X chromosome were identified on the basis of sex-linked patterns of inheritance. Other disorders were mapped by virtue of the association of a disease with a visible chromosomal alteration, either a translocation or a deletion (see Chapter 78). It was assumed that segments deleted or disrupted when chromosomes break and rejoin represented the positions of the genes lost or altered and that they were responsible for the disease. By this association, the gene responsible for retinoblastoma was localized to chromosome 13 and that for Wilms tumor was localized to chromosome 11. The precise location of the gene for Duchenne muscular dystrophy (DMD) on the X chromosome was identified by the finding of a deletion encompassing a large enough segment of the X chromosome to be visible by routine cytogenetics.

Another powerful technique for the mapping of genes was the use of human-rodent somatic cell hybrids. By this method, cells of a human and rodent are fused in tissue cultures. Through repeated cell cycle passage, human chromosomes are randomly lost, resulting in a variety of hybrid cells containing one or several human chromosomes. Because the chromosomes of humans and rodents are very distinguishable by karyotype analysis, the human chromosomes persisting in the hybrid can be readily identified. By analyzing each of the cell lines for the presence of specific human enzymes or other biochemical markers, it has been possible to assign the genes expressing specific proteins to individual human chromosomes.

The introduction of molecular genetic techniques has dramatically expanded our ability to localize genes to specific chromosome loci. As mentioned earlier, through application of in situ hybridization, a DNA probe can be physically mapped directly, providing the most powerful and direct approach to this problem.

To construct detailed linkage maps, which relate genes too closely spaced to be visualized as physically distinct on microscopic examination of chromosomes (this amounts to around 1 million bp of DNA), Southern hybridization and related methods are utilized. In this approach, DNA is fragmented, as described previously, into large pieces using restriction endonucleases. To determine if two genes (or DNA sequences) are chromosomal neighbors, one experimentally asks whether or not they lie on the same DNA fragment generated by a restriction nuclease. In addition, once a single gene (or sequence) has been mapped, one can *walk* around the chromosomal region, by cloning segments of DNA that are contiguous with the DNA sequence of interest. By this route, detailed "maps" of many chromosomal loci are assembled.

FINDING A "DISEASE" GENE. The power of modern molecular genetic methodologies is best appreciated in the approach taken to define a gene by positional cloning in contrast to determining the cause of disease by the classic approach. In the latter, the pathophysiology of a disease is determined to a degree of detail that includes identification of the specific protein that is defective. The protein is purified, and the chemical sequence of that purified protein is determined. A comparison between that sequence and the normal sequence determines the nature of the amino acid error. This was how the molecular basis of sickle cell anemia was determined; this condition is now known to result from a valine to glutamic acid substitution in position 6 of the β-globin protein. Subsequently, using molecular genetics, the mRNA for β-globin was isolated, cloned, and sequenced, and the gene was subsequently sequenced. The nature of the mutation was determined at both the RNA and the DNA level. A similar pathway of discovery characterized the elucidation of the defect in Tay-Sachs disease. After discovering that this degenerative disease of the nervous system resulted from expression of a defective enzyme, *hexosaminidase A*, the enzyme was purified. The protein was partially sequenced, and the corresponding mRNA for the enzyme was cloned and sequenced. Molecular genetic methods revealed heterogeneity of the disease. Those of Ashkenazi Jewish origin exhibited the disease as a result of a frameshift mutation in the coding portion of the hexosaminidase A gene, whereas those from other ethnic backgrounds (e.g., French-Canadian kindred) seemed to be missing a segment of the gene.

By the positional cloning approach, it is possible to identify the cause of disease through purely genetic techniques. The defective protein and the biologic processes underlying the disease are studied *after* the gene has been identified by direct genetic analysis. This approach is exemplified by the discovery of the gene that is defective in DMD. It was known for many years that DMD was an X-linked disorder; although pathophysiology was unclear, the defect was profoundly expressed in muscle tissue. After the discovery of a visible deletion on the X-chromosome associated with DMD in a single individual, the chromosomal neighborhood was identified. By use of several techniques, DNA probes were isolated, which mapped to the region identified by the deletion. These probes provided a powerful tool. The probes were used to identify genes in the suspected location that encoded proteins that were expressed in muscle. After one of these genes was identified and characterized, it was shown that the product of that gene was absent from muscle of many patients with DMD. The protein, dystrophin, was subsequently shown to be very large and appeared to be associated with certain membrane functions involved in coupling of electrical activity and muscle contractions.

Another example of this "reverse" genetics is the identification of the gene responsible for cystic fibrosis (CF). Unlike the situation with DMD, no patient was identified with a visible deletion. First, it was shown by family linkage studies that the disease was due to a defective gene on chromosome 7. The precise location of the gene was not evident. To find this gene required precise mapping of the suspect region of chromosome 7, narrowing the boundaries within which the gene had to lie through careful linkage studies at the molecular genetic level by analysis of many different pedigrees. As the region around chromosome 7 linked to CF narrowed, potential candidate genes were surveyed in the region, using probes to determine if any genes were present that expressed RNA in tissues affected in CF. One such candidate gene was identified. After cloning of the RNA product of that gene from the tissues of those with CF and those without, it appeared that a 3 nucleotide deletion occurred in the deduced gene product in about 70% of the mutant alleles. From the nucleic acid sequence of the putative CF gene product, it was possible to deduce a putative structure from the genetic code. The protein sequence was novel but resembled a group of proteins that were implicated in multidrug resistance, proteins that pump out many different classes of drugs that permeate our cells. Although the biochemical basis of CF was unknown, it appeared that epithelial cells from the respiratory mucosa exhibited a defect in the transport of chloride resulting from aberrant chloride channels. Putting these pieces of information together, it was established that the gene that was isolated by positional cloning is in fact a chloride channel or transporter (CFTR). Further study has shown that in addition to the most common mutation in the CFTR gene (a 3 nucleotide deletion), over 400 other discrete alterations of this gene can be found in various patients with CF.

ADVANCES IN UNDERSTANDING MORPHOGENESIS. Approximately 3% of all newborns have recognizable congenital malformations. Lethal malformations account for 25% of all neonatal deaths in the United States and are responsible for 50% of the neonatal mortality when full-term infants are considered alone. In spite of the major importance of malformations, our understanding of their etiology and prevention is inadequate. Both environmental and genetic factors are operative. Experimental work in fruit flies and mice provides reason for cautious optimism in this area. The genome of the mouse is similar to that of the human in its gross architecture; there is a rapidly accumulating data base on mouse genetics. This detailed information can now be combined with some powerful experimental tools to yield profound insights into mammalian development. For example, any desired cloned or modified gene can be introduced into a developing mouse, and, in principle, it is possible to control when and where that introduced gene is expressed. Such methods of transgenic technology can be used to create animal models of human disease. A second set of methodologies can be used to ablate virtually any gene within a developing mouse and to construct so-called knockout animals in the process. Taken together, these protocols are analogous to what physiologists and endocrinologists have enjoyed for more than a century in being able to investigate the function of a gland, for example, by extirpating it, transplanting it, or stimulating its function and examining the impact on an experimental organism.

These techniques of experimental mammalian embryology have been augmented by basic discoveries using simple organisms such as flies and worms. For example, the fruit fly, *Drosophila melanogaster*, is a segmented organism with three head segments, three thoracic segments, and nine abdominal segments. Each segment is destined to give rise to discrete and unique structures. After a finite point in development, the fate of cells in each segment is irreversibly determined; a group of cells will continue to play out this predetermined program, even if transplanted to another location. A variety of mutations have been observed that disrupt this otherwise orderly process. These "homeotic" mutations may result in dramatically aberrant phenotypes such as a fly with legs rather than sensory feelers at the top of the head.

Molecular biologic research has led to a detailed understanding of early events in *Drosophila* development that is relevant to human development. We now understand how the rostral-caudal axis of the *Drosophila* egg is established by gene products contributed by maternal cells that surround the egg (maternal effect genes). Next, a series of stripes across this axis is established via the action of so-called gap and pair rule genes. Then, the anterior and posterior borders of each segment are specified by the action of segment polarity genes. At this point, while all the segments are established, their identities and embryonic potential are equal. The homeobox genes then act in concert to instruct each segment as to whether it is to

TABLE 75–2 Homeobox Mutations Causing Human Disease

Homeobox Gene	Human Disease
HOXA13	Hand-foot-genital syndrome
HOXD13	Polysyndactyly
EMX2	Schizencephaly
PAX6	Aniridia
PAX3	Waardenburg syndrome
MSX1	Hypodontia
MSX2	Craniosynostosis
RIEG	Rieger syndrome
PIT1	Pituitary hormone deficiency
POU3F4	Deafness with fixation of the stapes
HOXA9	Acute myelocytic leukemia
PBX1	Pre–B cell ALL
HOX11	T-cell ALL
PAX3	Rhabdomyosarcoma
PAX7	Rhabdomyosarcoma

become a head segment or an abdominal segment and so on. The homeobox genes are so named because mutations in them cause homeotic transformations in the fate of specific segments, and because each homeobox gene contains a relatively similar region encoding 60 amino acids near one end of the gene. The homeobox genes are thought to act as master switches that can regulate the expression of other genes that act downstream in development. They probably do this by binding to control regions of DNA of these target genes and regulating their transcription. The homeobox genes of *Drosophila* are organized in a specific order on the third chromosome. This order is identical to the spatial order in which they are expressed in the various segments.

The homeobox genes (as well as some other important developmental genes) are highly conserved through evolution; very similar genes can be found in most other organisms, including mice and humans. There are at least 35 human and murine homeobox genes, organized into four clusters, each on a different chromosome. Although the function of most of these genes remains to be clarified, their spatial and temporal expression indicates that they follow a pattern at least grossly reminiscent of that seen in flies. Studies in the mouse using the methods described above are under way, aimed at overexpressing homeobox genes, expressing them in the wrong location, or knocking out their expression in efforts to clarify their function. Early results support the critical role of these genes in development and provide important hints about their role in human malformations. For example, mice in which the Hox 1.6 gene has been knocked out develop defects in neural tube closure. Mice overexpressing Hox 1.1 have vertebral duplications. Mice lacking the Hox 1.5 gene look very similar to human infants with the DiGeorge syndrome. Overexpression of the Hox 1.4 gene produces a phenotype very similar to Hirschsprung disease. More recently, several human disorders that are the direct result of mutations of homeobox genes have been identified (Table 75–2). Understanding of the genes involved in early development may enable us to recognize prenatally (and possibly treat prenatally) a number of human malformations. For those abnormalities that are the product of environmental triggers, we should be able to specify the genes through which these signals act and are transmitted. This may offer a hope of having better screening procedures to recognize environmental teratogens and mitigate their effects.

CHAPTER 76
Molecular Diagnosis of Genetic Diseases

Larry Shapiro

TECHNOLOGY OF MOLECULAR GENETICS. Molecular genetics, as a field, is driven to a large degree by technology; novel methods are frequently introduced that improve and significantly modify approaches to the study of gene structure and function. Both DNA and RNA can be sequenced directly. DNA can be cloned, meaning that a DNA sequence can be amplified to yield unlimited amounts. This procedure involves the insertion of a specific DNA sequence into a *vector* (e.g., a virus or antibiotic-resistant plasmid) that can be propagated indefinitely in bacteria. By simple procedures, the vector, containing an inserted DNA sequence, can be purified, and the inserted DNA sequence can be cleaved out. Other methodologies permit RNA to be transcribed into DNA enzymatically and to be cloned and sequenced. Small stretches of DNA (<100 base pairs [bp]) can be synthesized efficiently by purely chemical methods. DNA can also be manipulated through the use of a variety of enzymes purified from natural sources. Duplex DNA segments can be ligated to each other enzymatically. DNA and RNA can be chemically tagged with radioactive or fluorescent markers. Enzymes (e.g., restriction nucleases, isolated from a variety of microorganisms) cleave specific DNA sequences (between four and eight nucleotides in length) and are used to fragment DNA at specific sites. These tools and others provide an extraordinary ability to manipulate and characterize nucleic acids.

In addition, specific DNA sequences can be detected with high specificity. All methods of detection rely on the double-stranded design of DNA. A single-stranded DNA sequence of sufficient length (a *probe*), corresponding to a segment of DNA in the human genome, will find its complementary sequence when exposed to a preparation of human DNA that has been "melted" into single strands. By several different methods, the formation of such a duplex between a probe, and any DNA preparation to which it has been *hybridized*, can be readily detected.

Molecular hybridization is used in procedures such as Southern blotting and in situ hybridization. In **in situ hybridization**, a chromosome spread is prepared in the same manner as one would prepare a karyotype (Chapter 78). A DNA sequence, corresponding to a sequence within the human genome, is applied to the chromosome spread after the DNA strands have been separated (or denatured). After a period of time, the probe will hybridize to its complementary sequence at a precise location on a specific chromosome. The method of detecting the location of the probe varies. Fluorescent-tagged probes are used most commonly, and their location can be determined by observation of the karyotype under a fluorescent microscope. This is termed fluorescent in situ hybridization, or *FISH*. The precise chromosomal locus can be determined by comparison with karyotypic landmarks.

Another technique utilizing molecular hybridization is called **Southern blotting**. In this procedure, DNA is fragmented with a specific restriction nuclease, which is generally chosen empirically. The digestion of DNA with a specific restriction endonuclease permits a preparation of DNA to be fragmented into discrete pieces at cleavage sites dependent on the particular sequence recognized by the nuclease utilized. Thus, the DNA from every cell is fragmented in the same way, and a uniform population of fragments is generated. In the classic procedure, the fragments are separated on the basis of size by electrophoresis in agarose: they are denatured and then transferred (with their position preserved) onto a nitrocellulose sheet. The sheet bearing the fragments is exposed to a probe, and the position on the sheet bearing the complement is detected. This procedure tells us the presence, and the size, of the fragment bearing the sequence of interest.

RNA can be studied by a similar method called **Northern blotting**. In this procedure, RNA is isolated, analyzed by electrophoresis in agarose, and transferred to a membrane. The presence of a specific RNA as well as its size is detected by hybridization with a probe complementary to the expected RNA sequence.

Southern blotting, along with application of sets of restriction enzymes, permits one to examine the nucleic acid sequence around a gene. Thus, if a sequence necessary for the cutting of a restriction enzyme is missing, that fragment will not be present. A fragment of a different size will result. These differences are called *restriction fragment length polymorphisms* (RFLPs).

Another technique called *polymerase chain reaction* (PCR) has become critically important to molecular genetics. This method permits one to enzymatically amplify a DNA sequence, using short synthetic DNA probes or primers. If a sequence is known, by use of two oligonucleotides (probes) one can specifically amplify the DNA sequence bracketed by the probes. From the DNA contained in a single cell (essentially one or two molecules), enough DNA corresponding to a specific sequence can be generated to sequence it, to detect it by hybridization, or to clone it. This method permits direct examination of mutations and can be applied to situations in which very limited DNA is available. This method is also routinely used in the clinical laboratory to detect and characterize the nucleic acids of bacteria and viruses. One can also use PCR to detect and quantitate the expression of genes by applying it to cellular messenger RNA. By using the enzyme reverse transcriptase, mRNA can be copied into complementary DNA, or cDNA, which can then be further quantitated or sequenced. From a medical geneticist's perspective, the development of PCR technology means that patient DNA from any source (a buccal smear, a blood sample, prenatally obtained amniocytes, and even archived surgical specimens) can be amplified and characterized by hybridization or direct sequencing to identify mutations responsible for heritable disorders.

Finally, there are now extraordinarily powerful tools that can be used to study the function of any given DNA sequence. A gene can be transcribed directly in RNA and translated into protein. The gene can be transferred into a living eukaryotic cell, and expression of the gene can be examined by employing suitable synthetic methods. Any given DNA sequence can be altered at will so that the effect of such changes can be assessed in various systems. The gene can be redesigned and expressed in bacterial or yeast cells and protein products produced in large quantity. In some cases, it is possible to transfer DNA back into the germ line of an animal (e.g., the mouse) and to explore its expression and its effect on development or physiology. The impact of the loss of function of a given DNA sequence can also be studied by using gene targeting or so-called knockout methods.

DIAGNOSIS. The most striking advantage of the diagnosis of genetic disease through the molecular genetic approach is that a gene can be identified through examination of the DNA from almost any cell of a patient. The cell can be obtained at any time in the life of the individual. In the past we often diagnosed a disease by looking for a specific enzymatic defect or for the presence of an abnormal protein. Now, once a disease or a carrier state is suspected, we can make a diagnosis by examination of the individual's DNA. The gene encoding a liver-specific enzyme or red blood cell protein can be examined in any available cell from that individual and from every member of the kindred. Any tissue with chemically intact DNA can be studied. With the advent of PCR, it is possible to perform this study on a single cell's worth of DNA, and it need not even be physically intact. The DNA from a single cell retrieved by biopsy of a human embryo can be defined genetically. Frequently, whole blood is used as a source of DNA, coming from the nucleated cells present in the circulation. Alternatively, buccal epithelial cells, cells shed from the urinary tract, and even a single sperm can serve as a source for DNA to be examined. In prenatal diagnosis, chorionic villus sampling can be used, or amniocytes can be obtained from amniocentesis. Rare fetal cells in the maternal circulation also can be isolated, providing a noninvasive access to fetal DNA. In combination with in vitro fertilization, a cell can be dissected from the cultured human embryo and used for diagnosis before implantation.

Diagnosis of a genetic disorder can be accomplished by either the direct approach or the indirect approach. In the direct approach, we examine a gene for mutations associated with a disease; in the indirect approach, generally applied before a gene has been fully characterized, we follow a "disease" gene within a family by its linkage with defined sequences that are co-inherited with high probability. In general, the direct examination of a gene provides a diagnosis with absolute certainty and represents an essential goal in the advancement of the diagnostic arm of molecular genetics. The linkage approach requires the participation of other relevant family members.

If a disease is associated with a single mutation, we can readily determine whether an individual carries the mutant gene. Thus, the diagnosis of sickle cell anemia or the determination of a carrier state involves positive identification of the specific mutation within the β-globin gene. This can be accomplished by the application of PCR methodology or by hybridization with DNA, with short DNA probes specific for either normal or mutant DNA sequences, permitting direct examination for the presence of a specific sequence at the DNA level associated with expression of the mutant protein. With increasing frequency, direct sequencing with an automated sequencer is used to establish this information. Other techniques on the horizon, such as the DNA or gene chip, may further enhance the acquisition of directly determined gene sequences.

In diseases such as DMD or factor VIII deficiency, in which numerous mutations within the corresponding genes have been identified to result in a disease with a common phenotype, the gene is examined for mutations that are observed with highest frequency. If no previously recognized mutation can be localized, the gene itself can be sequenced directly, and variations from normal that appear to be linked to the disease phenotype can be deduced directly. As data accumulate defining the mutations within a gene responsible for specific diseases, the ability to identify a mutation within a gene directly increases, and catalogues of such data grow more detailed at an extraordinary pace.

In many diseases, however, the responsible defective gene has not been identified. Prenatal diagnosis and carrier status must be determined through linkage analysis. An attempt is made to identify DNA sequences that are co-inherited with the disease phenotype and serve to *mark* the chromosome that has been implicated in carrying the defective allele. In general, these linked sequences lie physically close to the gene and are part of the framework (see under The Nature of Mutations), representing the somewhat polymorphic DNA in which genes are embedded. Molecular genetic methods are used to try to distinguish the DNA neighborhood of the defective gene from the DNA neighborhood or framework surrounding a gene unaffected in a kindred. Sufficient polymorphisms exist in the DNA in which our genes are embedded to distinguish nonidentical chromosomal segments (e.g., alleles deriving from either parent). In practice, considerable investigational effort is mounted to determine highly polymorphic DNA sequences that are linked through patterns of inheritance with a disease. When an individual case is presented for diagnosis, the molecular geneticist must first attempt to identify the chromosome associated with the disease gene in the pedigree. If the disorder is recessive, both chromosomal neighborhoods harboring the defective gene must be "fingerprinted." The fingerprint amounts to a collection of polymorphic sequences that can distinguish a particular chromosomal framework from another. In the case of a recessive disorder, the chromosomes bearing the defective gene must first be identified by examination of the DNA of an affected patient in the pedigree. Then, a determination is made with regard to which of the two maternal and paternal chromosomes is associated with the defective gene. If there is an unaffected sibling, that individual should not have inherited the same set of alleles as the affected individual; he or she provides a control for the molecular genetic analysis. Prenatal diagnosis involves a search for the presence of the set of maternal and paternal chromosomes bearing mutations. If only one is inherited, the patient is a *heterozygote* or *carrier*. If neither chromosome is inherited, the patient will not have inherited the defective gene. Carrier detection within the extended family is based on the same principle that involves tracking of the affected chromosome on which the disease gene is linked.

Prenatal diagnosis or carrier detection through linkage analysis requires an analysis of the DNA of an affected individual. This provides a method of identifying the chromosomes bearing the mutation; DNA from both parents permits characterization of the chromosome that carries the unaffected gene; ideally, DNA of a sibling of the proband who is unaffected provides a "proof" that the chromosomal linkage is correct. The larger the pedigree and the more discriminating the sequence differences characterizing the chromosomal neighborhood in which the gene is embedded, the more accurate the diagnosis. It must be appreciated, however, that diagnosis by linkage analysis can never offer 100% certainty about the inheritance of a defective gene. Because we do not actually examine the defective gene by this method but only track it by association of its immediate chromosomal neighborhood, linkage is never perfect. Significant uncertainty results from a probability that the gene will be separated from the linked DNA sequences during meiosis, and this probability increases as the distance between these linked sequences and the gene increases. In general, however, once the chromosomal neighborhood of a gene has been established, major efforts are directed to characterization of the defective gene itself. If this is accomplished, the diagnosis can be made by direct examination of a gene for the presence of associated mutations.

Diseases expressed in highly specialized tissues (e.g., the liver), appearing late in development, can be determined through direct examination of a gene examined from almost any cell of an individual. When a defective gene responsible for human disease is identified and the mutations associated with it are characterized, it is possible to screen populations for the presence of these mutations. Ethical and societal pressures frequently determine how we apply these techniques in practice.

THE NATURE OF MUTATIONS. Human genetics deals with the variations between individuals. These variations are reflections of differences that exist at the DNA level. Variations that have an impact on the functioning of a gene are usually referred to as mutations. Other variations that do not have an impact on the health or functioning of an organism are called polymorphisms; the dilemma often arises during molecular investigations in deciding whether a newly observed change is a mutation or a harmless polymorphism. Mutations may arise in somatic cells as well as in germ cells, but only those changes present in the germ cells will be heritable. Polymorphisms include single nucleotide substitutions (particularly in introns and extragenic flanking regions of DNA) that may create or abolish a specific restriction enzyme site and thereby lead to length polymorphisms (RFLPs) when restriction endonuclease enzymes are employed to digest or cut DNA. Other neutral variants include a variable number of a tandem repeat (VNTR), the repeating unit consisting of 10 to 60 nucleotides. The human genome also contains short sequence repeats of dinucleotides or trinucleotides. Many of these polymorphisms are useful in genetic analyses and are exploited by the use of either DNA probes and Southern blotting or PCR (see below).

Mutations result from a change of a single bp of DNA (substitution), from the loss or addition of DNA (deletions, insertions, duplications, expansions), and from rearrangements (inversions and translocations). The effects of mutations depend on the alteration in the amount or structure of the protein that is formed and whether the change occurs in domains of the protein crucial for its normal function, such as the catalytic site of enzymes or the transmembrane spanning domain for membrane-associated proteins. These changes in protein structure can occur during translation, during the extensive post-translational modifications (glycosylation and the like) that many proteins undergo, or by causing silencing of transcription or inappropriate gene expression. A mutation in which a base is changed within an exon, resulting in change of a corresponding amino acid in the protein, is called a *missense* mutation.

Such a mutation may result in a dramatic loss of function or of stability or may only mildly affect the protein. An altered protein sequence can also result in mislocalization of the protein within a cell. In some cases, a single base change can add a new stop signal to an RNA molecule, thereby directing the ribosome to prematurely terminate translation (nonsense mutation) and to yield a shortened protein. A classic example of an instructive genotype-phenotype correlation occurs in the dystrophin gene, in which the clinical differences between the allelic conditions of Duchenne muscular dystrophy (DMD) (virtually no dystrophin detectable at the muscle) and the much milder Becker muscular dystrophy (BMD) (variably reduced dystrophin protein) can usually be attributed to whether the deletion disrupts the translational reading frame. In the case of DMD the deletion occurs such that translation of dystrophin occurs out of frame, leading to a severely truncated *(nonsense mutation)* or highly unstable *(missense mutation)* protein. In contrast, BMD mutations usually tend to maintain the translational reading frame and in consequence merely reduce the amount of functional dystrophin protein.

The human genome is a dynamic structure, and rearrangements of DNA sequences can occur as part of a normal mechanism that has evolved to increase the diversity of gene expression. A recently recognized type of mutation involves the expansion of nucleotide triplets repeated in tandem. These trinucleotide repeat arrays are found in normal individuals in certain genes and are capable of occasionally being expanded in size through an increase in trinucleotide repeat number. If the number of repeats exceeds a certain threshold, the repeat array becomes unstable, and additional size increases are likely to occur in succeeding generations. This type of unstable (or dynamic) mutation can result in disease in individuals carrying the expanded repeats. At present these **trinucleotide repeat expansions** fall into three classes, with corresponding classes of phenotypes (Table 76–1). The first class is characterized by large expansions of a CGG trinucleotide, leading to a so-called fragile site in the chromosome. Such a site is so designated because it is associated with chromosome breakage under certain in vitro growth conditions. The prototype for this class is the *fragile X syndrome* (FRAXA), in which an expanded CGG repeat in the 5′ untranslated region of the FMR1 gene leads to underexpression and a clinical phenotype of mental retardation, macro-orchidism, and other somatic changes in affected males. The second class of disorder involves the relatively small expansion of an in-frame CAG repeat in the coding region of

TABLE 76–1 Mutations Showing Triplet Repeat Expansion

Condition	Repeat	Repeat Location	Pathologic Repeat Number
FRAXA	CGG	5′ untranslated	200–1000
FRAXE	CGG		200–1000
FRAXF	CGG		300–500
FRA16A	CGG		1000–2000
Spinal and bulbar muscular atrophy	CAG	Coding region	40–52
Huntington disease	CAG	Coding region	37–86
Spinocerebellar ataxia type I	CAG	Coding region	40–81
Spinocerebellar ataxia type II	CAG	Coding region	35–59
Spinocerebellar ataxia type 6	CAG	Coding region	21–30
Spinocerebellar ataxia type 7	CAG	Coding region	38–130
Dentatorubral-pallidoluysian atrophy	CAG	Coding region	49–75
Myotonic dystrophy	CTG	3′ untranslated	50–2000
Friedreich ataxia	GAA	1st intron	200–900

Adapted from Willems PJ: Dynamic mutations hit double figures. Nat Genet 8:213, 1994.

the respective genes, leading to a polyglutamine stretch in the resulting protein. All the known disorders exhibiting this type of expansion are dominantly inherited, late-onset neurodegenerative diseases, the best known example being *Huntington disease.* The third class of disorder involving triplet repeat expansion is represented by the disorder *myotonic dystrophy.* In this case a CTG repeat in the 3′ untranslated region of the relevant gene is greatly expanded in affected individuals. A commonly observed characteristic of this dominantly inherited disease is an increase in disease severity in successive generations, a clinical phenomenon known as **anticipation.** Anticipation results from the successive increases in repeat expansion; it is observed to a lesser degree in the other classes of disorders.

Another example of the dynamism within the genome that can lead to either harmless (and thus usually unrecognized) polymorphic variation or to a disease is the insertion of repeated sequences of DNA as they are replicated at meiosis into novel sites in the genome. Although only a single case of this type of mutation in humans (a case of hemophilia A) has been attributed to this mechanism, such *retrotransposons* are likely to become recognized more frequently as detailed investigation of disease at the molecular level continues.

For many conditions a variety of different mutations of the same gene account for individual cases of any single disease. Until recently, the analysis of DNA from patients with hemophilia A revealed point mutations, duplications, and deletions of the factor VIII gene as mutational mechanisms but did not explain the molecular basis of many cases of more severe disease. Then, it was recognized that a common inversion brought about by aberrant recombination during sperm production (male meiosis) disrupted the factor VIII gene in these individuals. Similarly, a gene can be disrupted by a translocation, an event that joins a segment of DNA on one chromosome with a segment normally located on another chromosome. In the case of the malignant cells of chronic myelogenous leukemia patients, a balanced translocation between chromosomes 9 and 22 is invariably observed. This translocation brings together two genes (*abl* and *bcr*), allowing expression of an abnormal fusion protein with potent tyrosine kinase activity (acts to transduce external growth promoting stimuli to the nucleus), enabling unregulated clonal expansion to occur.

At the cellular level the effects of mutations in inherited genes responsible for structural proteins can create disease in the heterozygous state and thus be inherited in an autosomal dominant manner. Serious clinical consequences of heterozygous mutations affecting structural proteins is more common than for enzymatic proteins, in which heterozygotes usually show no clinical abnormalities and inheritance of two mutant alleles is required for expression of the disease phenotype (autosomal recessive inheritance). For example, the most common form of *osteogenesis imperfecta* (OI) type I has been associated with a number of mutations in the *Col* α1(I) gene responsible for production of collagen chains of type I procollagen, a triple helical protein composed of α1 and α2 chains that confers tensile and compression strength in those tissues (bone, tendons, skin) that have type I collagen as a major component. The effect of a knockout mutation or inactivation in one allele leads to a half-normal amount of α1(I) protein produced and an alteration in the ratio of α1 to α2 chains from the normal 2:1 to 1:1. Thus, only half the normal amount of type I collagen is produced, and excess fragility of the bones is seen. A related disease mechanism is exemplified by the more severe disorder osteogenesis imperfecta type II, in which mutations in *Col* α1 or *Col* α2 genes, although not quantitative in this condition, qualitatively alter the assembly, function, or degradation of collagen triple helices. The presence of one mutant allele is sufficient to cause this disruption, and this effect is referred to as a dominant negative mutation. This lethal disorder is usually the result of a new dominant mutation in either parent's germline. Comparison of these two OI disease subtypes, due to different types of mutations in the same gene and having their effects on type I collagen, show that reduced amounts of a normal protein may be less deleterious than normal amounts of an aberrant protein.

Mutations can also affect the functioning of a gene by altering the splicing efficiency of the RNA transcribed from the gene. A mutation might lie in an intron and lead to reduced amounts of normally spliced RNA. The classic examples of mutations of this type include several forms of thalassemia.

Mutations can profoundly disturb a cell by altering the normal regulated function of a gene, rather than through disturbing the quality of the actual protein. An example is the expression of the *myc* gene, which encodes a growth-promoting nuclear protein and is translocated into the neighborhood of immunoglobulin heavy-chain genes in certain lymphoid tumors. The *myc* gene, which, when present, is normally regulated in its usual chromosomal setting, is activated when it is translocated beside the immunoglobulin gene, normally active in the plasma cell. The activation of the *myc* gene in this cell, in an unregulated fashion, results in unrestrained growth and a malignant phenotype.

Rearrangements in the human genome occur naturally between generations and are essential for biologic diversity and the evolution of species, including man. This process, termed recombination, occurs during meiosis in germ cells, between maternal and paternal homologues, and appears to be exquisitely precise to allow equal genetic exchange between these homologues. Exchange of DNA even occurs between tiny portions of the short arms of the X and Y chromosomes, the so-called pseudoautosomal regions of the sex chromosomes. On average, there are 52 crossovers per male germ cell examined cytogenetically (obtained by testicular biopsy), between 0 and 2 crossovers per chromosome arm. Since the chromosomes assort independently during meiosis, there are 2^{23} possible combinations of chromosomes in the germ cells from each parent. The process of pairing and recombination can, however, lead to abnormal exchange of genetic material and mutations either by insertion or deletion or by duplication of DNA sequences and can prove deleterious to functional genes. Hereditary sensory and motor neuropathy (Charcot-Marie-Tooth disease) type IA occurs as a result of acquisition of 1.5Mb of DNA including a third copy of the *PMP2* gene acquired by abnormal recombination mediated by a 17kb DNA repeat sequence. This is an example of a *gain of function* mutation. DNA repeat sequences appear to have an important role in the pairing of homologues during meiosis, but this process can go awry, leading to mutation. Aberrant recombination has been among the many mechanisms elucidated as responsible for familial hypercholesterolemia (FH). In one patient, abnormal pairing occurred between two *Alu* repetitive elements found within introns of this gene. Unequal exchange and loss of some exons with duplication of other exons occurred in the LDL receptor gene.

Deletions can vary in their extent and, even when not visible at the cytogenetic level, can involve several genes; these are often termed microdeletions. By a variety of rearrangements, conditions referred to as *contiguous gene syndromes* may be generated. The clinician may be alerted to this possibility by an unusually diverse array of clinical features in any individual or the presence of additional features to a known condition. For example, owing to the close physical proximity of a series of genes, different deletions involving the short arm of the X chromosome can produce individuals with various combinations of the following features: ichthyosis, Kallmann syndrome, ocular albinism, mental retardation, chondrodysplasia punctata, and short stature. The individual features in each case depend on the involvement of these genes and the loss of DNA sequences in the underlying rearrangement. Many other contiguous gene syndromes have been described in humans, including Smith-Magenis, Rubinstein-Taybi, DiGeorge, and Prader-Willi syndromes.

Rearrangements such as translocations also take place in somatic cells. The most well understood are the rearrangements that occur in lymphoid cells. Some rearrangements are required for the formation of functional immunoglobulin in B cells and antigen-recognizing receptors on the T cell. Large segments of DNA, which code for the variable and the constant regions of either immunoglobulin or the T-cell receptor, are physically joined at a specific stage in the development of an immunocompetent lymphocyte. The rearrangements take place during development of the lymphoid cell lineage in humans and result in the extensive diversity of immunoglobulin and T-cell receptor molecules. It is as a result of this post–germ line DNA rearrangement that no two individuals, not even identical twins, are really identical, because mature lymphocytes from each will have undergone random DNA rearrangements at these loci.

During the last decade, as human genes have been cloned and sequenced and variations in particular sequences compared between individuals, certain striking patterns have emerged that characterize DNA variations in humans. Segments of a gene that play a critical functional role, at any level of the pathway of expression of that gene into a functional product, will exhibit very little variation among normal individuals. In contrast, segments of our genome that seem to be less "important" (e.g., regions of DNA between genes) exhibit extensive variation among individuals. Indeed, if these less important areas are examined at the level of nucleic acid sequence, the variation in a specific segment of DNA (e.g., an intron in a globin gene) may amount to a different base in every several hundred. As a result of this pattern of variation, a gene and all the associated sequences that are critical for function may be considered as an island lying in a sea of highly variable DNA. The sequences surrounding this "gene island" can exhibit significant sequence difference when these segments, which tolerate variation, are compared among individuals from different pedigrees, while the genes themselves are strikingly similar. The polymorphic framework that surrounds a gene and a particular framework is called a *haplotype*. The variations that characterize the DNA in which the gene is embedded can be used to identify the particular chromosome from an individual and (if the sequence of the framework is known in sufficient detail and number) would provide a fingerprint, enabling us to distinguish the particular chromosomal region within a population. If a mutation were to arise in the gene of one individual, that mutation could be followed directly (or by tracking variations in the neighborhood of the gene that distinguishes that individual's chromosomes). This linkage concept underlies much of the diagnostic methodology of molecular genetics.

This picture of the genome as consisting of islands of conserved genes embedded in a framework that tolerates considerably more variation also helps us understand the patterns of variation that are observed across evolution. As we compare specific genes among mammals, for example, less variation is noted in the sequences of the genes than in the surrounding genetic environment. When segments of DNA between species are compared by sequence, segments that are conserved in sequence across many species generally mark the presence of genes.

CHAPTER 77
Patterns of Inheritance

Larry Shapiro

Each single mutant gene exhibits one of the four patterns of mendelian inheritance: autosomal recessive, autosomal dominant, X-linked recessive, or dominant. This method of grouping genetic diseases is often helpful in understanding the clinical presentation of a disorder. Concepts such as the basic structure of the DNA molecule and the transmission of genetic information, initially to messenger RNA (mRNA) and then to the formation of a specific polypeptide, help in understanding the basis of diseases such as the various disorders of hemoglobin structure in which the primary abnormalities include amino acid substitutions and deletions, elongated globin chains, and fused or "hybrid" globin chains. Other concepts explaining the mechanisms for the occurrence of genetic abnormalities that are apparent in the study of microorganisms, such as defective function of repressor genes and regulator genes, may also be applicable to understanding human genetic diseases.

In discussing single mutant genes a number of special terms are used. The 23 chromosomes in the sperm combine with the 23 chromosomes in the egg to form a *zygote* with 23 *pairs* of chromosomes. The *gene locus* is the particular location of a specific gene in a specific chromosome. Studies show that the coding portions of a gene are interrupted by *intervening sequences* of DNA of variable lengths. These intervening sequences, *introns*, are not represented in the mature mRNA that corresponds to the gene. Errors in splicing out the introns are the basis for the most common types of β-thalassemia. Each gene has an analog with a similar location in the homologous (other of a pair) chromosome; the identical pair of loci are called *homologous loci*. The genes at the homologous loci are called *alleles*. Allelic genes are analogous (i.e., affect the nature of the same characteristic) but are often not identical; exten-

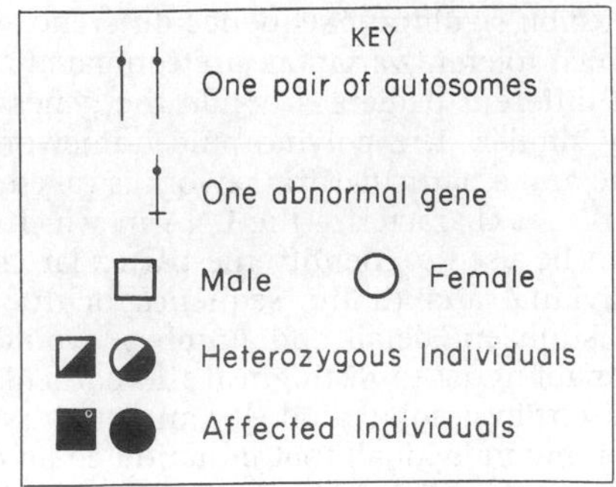

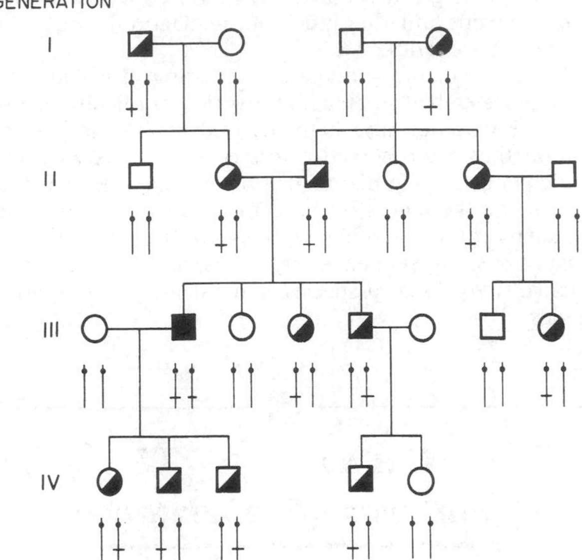

Figure 77–1 Autosomal recessive inheritance.

sive variation may be observed in many of the different types of serum proteins among people of the same as well as of different races. Because of the genetic variation that exists at many gene loci, it is arbitrary to consider some genes as mutant; usually the distinction is that the mutant gene has a major, harmful effect. When a person has a mutant gene at a locus in one chromosome but not at the homologous locus of the other, the person is *heterozygous* for the mutant gene. If the mutant gene does not affect the heterozygous individual, it is called a *recessive gene*. If the mutant gene has an effect in the heterozygous state, it is a *dominant gene*. A person having the same mutant gene at both homologous loci is *homozygous* for that gene. Autosomal recessive genes manifest their clinical effect only in the *homozygote*. The distinctions between recessive and dominant genes become arbitrary when identifying the heterozygote by biochemical testing or when the heterozygote only mildly expresses the disorder. Furthermore, molecular genetic studies have demonstrated that many persons considered homozygous for the same autosomal recessive gene actually have two different mutations.

Each mendelian pattern of inheritance has characteristics that may be useful in establishing a diagnosis or in planning family studies that may be important for a clear explanation to the parents of an affected child.

AUTOSOMAL RECESSIVE INHERITANCE. The pedigree illustrating this pattern of inheritance (Fig. 77–1) shows the following characteristics: The child of two heterozygous parents has a 25% chance of being homozygous (i.e., a 1 in 2 chance of inheriting the mutant gene from each parent: $1/2 \times 1/2 = 1/4$); males and females are affected with equal frequency; the affected individuals are almost always born in only one generation of a family; the children of the affected (homozygous) person are all heterozygotes; and the children of a homozygote can be affected only if the spouse is a heterozygote, which is a rare event because of the low incidence of most adverse recessive genes in the general population.

If the frequency of an autosomal recessive disease is known, the frequency of the heterozygote or carrier state can be calculated from the Hardy-Weinberg formula

$$p^2 + 2pq + q^2 = 1$$

in which p is the frequency of one of a pair of alleles and q is the frequency of the other. For example, if the frequency of cystic fibrosis among white Americans is 1 in 2,500 (p^2), then the frequency of the heterozygote (2 pq) can be calculated: if $p^2 = 1/2{,}500$, then $p = 1/50$ and $q = 49/50$; $2pq = 2 \times 1/50 \times 49/50$ or approximately 1/25 (or 3.92%).

Every human probably has several rare, harmful, recessive genes. Because these mutant genes are frequently not identifiable by laboratory tests, the heterozygous adult usually learns about his or her harmful recessive genes after the birth of a homozygous (and therefore affected) child. Related parents are much more likely to be heterozygous for the same harmful recessive genes because they have a common ancestor. Consanguineous matings are rare in the United States and in many other countries. Therefore, few genetic studies have been carried out to establish the overall risk for healthy but related parents. Based on the information available, the risk for parents who are first cousins of having a child with a birth defect is about double the 2–3% risk faced by healthy unrelated parents.

AUTOSOMAL DOMINANT INHERITANCE. The pedigree in Figure 77–2 shows that both males and females are affected, that transmission occurs from one parent to child, and that the responsible mutant gene can arise by spontaneous mutation of a gene.

X-LINKED RECESSIVE INHERITANCE. The pedigree in Figure 77–3 shows that only males are clinically affected; that affected males are related through carrier females; that all daughters of affected males are carriers of the mutant gene; and that affected males do not have affected sons but may have affected grandsons born to carrier females. The female carrier has a 50% chance of giving her chromosome that bears the mutant gene to each of her children. In other words, each daughter of a carrier has a 50% chance of being a carrier, and each son has a 50% chance of inheriting the mutant gene and having the disease that it causes. Therefore, in each pregnancy the female carrier has a 25% chance of having an affected son.

Initially, both X chromosomes of a female zygote are active. Random inactivation of portions of one X in each cell occurs

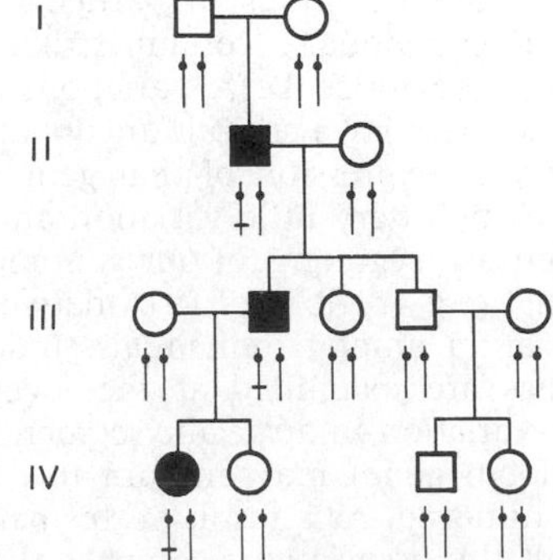

Figure 77–2 Autosomal dominant inheritance. (See Figure 77–1 for key.)

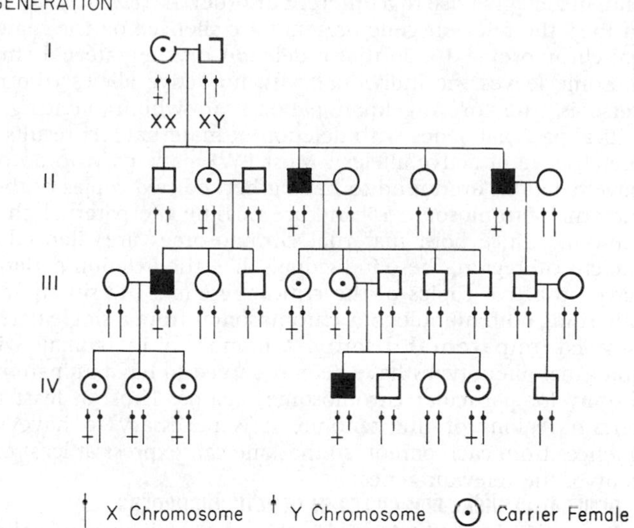

Figure 77–3 X-linked recessive inheritance. (See Figure 77-1 for key.)

early in fetal development. The inactivated X, which replicates later than the active X, is the sex chromatin mass or Barr body, which may be observed in the nucleus of a cell near the nuclear membrane. This random inactivation protects the carrier female from the effect of the X-linked recessive mutant gene, because there is as much chance that the X chromosome that carries the mutant gene will be inactivated as that the other X chromosome will. Therefore, the carrier expresses the effect of the mutant gene in an average of 50% of her cells. For this reason, the female carrier of classic hemophilia will have a reduced level of factor VIII activity but a level not nearly as low as that in her affected son or brother.

X-LINKED DOMINANT INHERITANCE. Very few X-linked dominant genes have been identified in humans. Two examples are vitamin D–resistant rickets and the Melnick-Needles syndrome of multiple malformations. The pedigree in Figure 77–4 shows the essential characteristics: both males and females are affected, but males are often more severely affected; the disorder is transmitted from generation to generation; and all daughters of an affected father will be affected, but none of his sons.

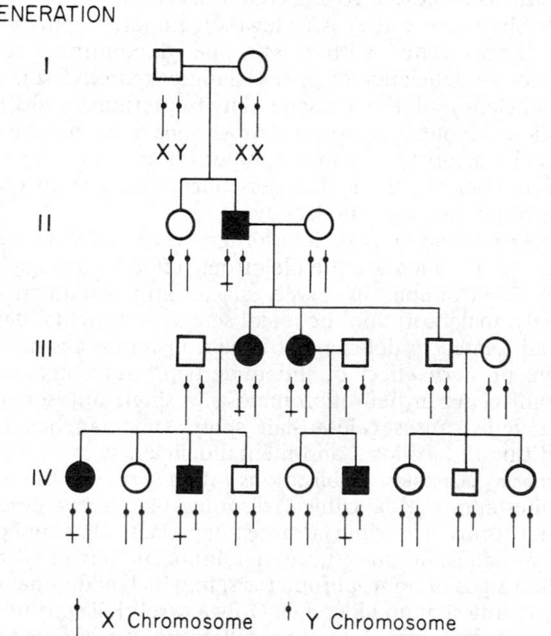

Figure 77–4 X-linked dominant inheritance. (See Figure 77-1 for key.)

MULTIFACTORIAL INHERITANCE. The term *multifactorial inheritance* refers to the process in which either continuously variable (quantitative) traits (such as height or blood pressure) or as disease state is the result of additive and interactive effects of one or more genes plus environmental factors. The estimate of the contribution of genes to such a trait or disorder is termed the *heritability.* These disorders include most of the common malformations (neural tube defects, cleft lip and palate, congenital dislocation of the hip) and common multifactorial diseases of adulthood (schizophrenia, essential hypertension, coronary heart disease, diabetes mellitus) and childhood (allergic diseases, some types of hyperlipidemia). The number of genes involved is often unknown, and either "minor" genes whose harmful impact is the result of cumulative effect (although they individually may not be harmful) or "major" genes with a larger effect (therefore easier to map in genetic studies) are involved. Few of the environmental factors have been identified in humans, but studies of conditions caused by multifactorial inheritance and their environmental triggers in animals emphasize their relevance. Considerable data must be available on many affected persons and their families before the disease or malformation can be attributed to multifactorial inheritance. More accessible data in studies of mice with such disorders make mapping of these genes feasible; by locating the syntenic chromosomal region (those conserved blocks of chromosomes that contain very similar DNA sequences between species) in humans such genes can be identified. This approach has been used in type I diabetes mellitus.

Some features of multifactorial inheritance are similar to mendelian inheritance of single mutant genes (i.e., incidence of a disorder related to racial background persisting after migration), but many of the features of multifactorial inheritance are distinct from mendelian inheritance. A particularly difficult dilemma can occur in distinguishing between a multifactorial etiology and an autosomal dominant disease gene with reduced penetrance (here lowered penetrance refers to the phenomenon of inheriting the mutant gene but not showing the disease phenotype in every instance). Although it may be very difficult to assign multifactorial etiology to a disease in individual instances, most of the features of multifactorial inheritance are quite different and pertinent. Differentiating points are as follows:

1. There is a similar rate of recurrence (typically 2–10%) among all first-degree relatives (parents, siblings, and offspring of the affected child). However, it is unusual to find a substantial increase in risk for relatives related more distantly than second degree to the index case.
2. The risk of recurrence is related to the incidence of the disease.
3. Some disorders have a sex predilection, as indicated by an unequal male:female incidence. Pyloric stenosis is more common in males, whereas congenital dislocation of the hips is more common in females. Where there is an altered sex ratio, the risk is higher for the relatives of an index case in which the sex is less common. For example, the risk to the son of an affected female with infantile pyloric stenosis is 18% compared with the 5% risk for the son of an affected male. The female has passed on a greater genetic susceptibility to her offspring.
4. The likelihood that both identical twins will be affected with the same malformation is less than 100% but much greater than the chance that both members of a nonidentical twin pair will be affected. The frequency of concordance for identical twins ranges from 21% to 63% for the disorders. This distribution contrasts with that of mendelian inheritance, in which identical twins always share a disorder due to a single mutant gene.

5. The risk of recurrence is increased when multiple family members are affected; these instances are often the most problematic for distinguishing a multifactorial from a mendelian etiology. A simple example is that the risk of recurrence for unilateral cleft lip and palate is 4% for a couple with one affected child and increases to 9% with two affected children.

6. The risk of recurrence may be greater when the disorder is more severe. For example, the infant who has long-segment Hirschsprung disease has a greater chance of having an affected sibling than the infant who has short-segment Hirschsprung disease.

ATYPICAL PATTERNS OF INHERITANCE. There is a growing appreciation that genetic disorders are sometimes inherited in ways that do not follow the usual patterns of dominant, recessive, X-linked, or multifactorial inheritance. These atypical patterns of inheritance sometimes involve specific diseases and in other instances can apply to virtually any hereditary disorder. Examples of the latter category are manifested when a de novo mutation occurs at a stage of development of an individual such that the person's gamete population becomes a mixture of normal and mutant alleles. The individual's somatic cells may or may not also constitute a normal/mutant mosaic, but, in general, the person is not recognized to be a carrier of a mutant allele, even upon testing for carrier status. An example would be a mother who does not appear to be a carrier for an X-linked disease such as hemophilia A, even by DNA testing of somatic cells, but who gives birth to more than one affected son. The explanation is that the mother carries multiple mutant gametes in addition to normal ones. This phenomenon is known as **gonadal mosaicism** and is most easily recognized for X-linked and dominant disorders.

Certain diseases display an atypical mode of inheritance because they result from **mutations in mitochondrial DNA.** Mitochondria contain small circular chromosomes that encode as well as ribosomal and transfer RNAs, 13 proteins that function in the respiratory chain of the organelle. Mutations of the mitochondrial genome (which are often deletions) can produce specific diseases. Abnormalities in these disorders are typically seen in one or more specific organs: the brain, eye, and skeletal muscle. Examples of such disorders are *Kearns-Sayre syndrome* and *Leber hereditary optic neuropathy.* Because mitochondria are inherited virtually exclusively from the mother, these conditions are passed from mother to offspring, without regard to sex of the latter (thus differing from X-linked recessive inheritance). Because the mitochondria of an individual constitute a heterogeneous mixture of genotypes both within and between cells, the mitochondrial complement passed in the egg is often not representative of the total mitochondrial population of the mother. Thus, there is a great variability in symptoms within a family, and the observed inheritance may be more complex than a simple maternal pattern. Nonetheless, the finding of a myopathy or neurologic disease that seems to come from the mother's side should alert the clinician to the possibility of a mitochondrial etiology.

Another type of nontraditional inheritance is the result of a phenomenon known as **genomic imprinting** (Chapter 78). This takes place in the germ line and results in certain regions of the genome being inherited differently, depending on the parent of origin. Specifically, genes in the relevant region are functionally inactivated (imprinted) during gamete formation and remain inactive in the resulting zygote. The genes imprinted in the two parental germ lines are mutually exclusive sets; otherwise, the offspring would have no active copies of the pertinent genes. This imprinting phenomenon leads to clinical consequences in the case of *Prader-Willi syndrome* (PWS). About two thirds of these patients have de novo microdeletions of chromosome 15, and the deletions always occur on the paternally derived chromosome. Similar deletions inherited on the maternal chromosome 15 do not result in PWS and, in fact, give rise to a different disorder, *Angelman syndrome.* In PWS the relevant gene or genes are silenced on the maternal chromosome 15, so that a deletion on the paternal chromosome leaves the individual with no active alleles (the reverse is true for Angelman patients, in whom silencing of critical paternal genes with deletion of maternal loci results in the absence of active alleles). Most PWS patients who do not have deletions are found to have inherited two copies of their maternal chromosome 15 and are missing the paternal chromosome. Since both maternal chromosomes are silenced in the critical region, these individuals, like the deletion patients, have no active copies of the critical gene(s). The situation of inheriting both homologous chromosomes from a single parent is called **uniparental disomy**. A number of individuals with abnormal phenotypes have been observed to have uniparental disomy for particular chromosome regions. Thus, at least for certain regions of the genome, it is necessary to have sequences from each parent, so that one can express at least one copy of the relevant genes.

GENERAL CLINICAL PRINCIPLES IN GENETIC DISORDERS.

Negative Family History. A child with a genetic disease or malformation is usually the only known affected member of his or her family. This reflects the fact that the rates of recurrence are very low for common abnormalities of the chromosomes and for conditions attributed to multifactorial inheritance. For example, the recurrence risk for Down syndrome associated with 21-trisomy is 1%; for conditions attributed to multifactorial inheritance it varies from 2% to 10%. The recurrence risk for disorders with a mendelian pattern of inheritance is much higher (e.g., 25% for autosomal recessive disorders), but in small families it is more likely that an autosomal recessive disorder will affect only one of three or four children rather than two. In the case of autosomal dominant disorders, the child may be affected by a spontaneous genetic mutation rather than by inheritance of the mutant gene from an affected parent. Generally speaking, a negative family history may be misleading.

Environmental Factors. Since the family history is usually negative for the disorder under consideration, the parents often blame themselves and look for environmental factors that might have been the cause. The physician should anticipate their feelings of guilt and should carefully discuss the events, including medications taken, to which congenital disorders may be inappropriately attributed by parents.

Genetic Heterogeneity. A single clinical manifestation may have more than one cause. An elevation in serum phenylalanine may be associated with classic phenylketonuria (either the absence or deficiency of phenylalanine hydroxylase); absence or deficiency of the enzyme dihydropteridine reductase; or deficient biopterin synthesis. Arachnodactyly may be an isolated characteristic of a tall, thin person, or it may be a feature of a number of genetic disorders, including Marfan syndrome and contractual arachnodactyly.

Pleiotropism. Some genetic disorders have many different features, all of which are the pleiotropic effect of a single mutant gene. For example, in classic galactosemia, cataracts, hepatomegaly, malabsorption, neonatal sepsis, and mental deficiency are all related to deficiency of the transferase enzyme, which is the primary effect of the underlying autosomal recessive mutant gene. In neurofibromatosis, a single autosomal dominant gene causes café-au-lait spots, subcutaneous nodules, solid tumors, scoliosis, and mental deficiency.

Variable Expression. Publications often present the extreme manifestations of a clinical disorder but rarely describe its milder forms. The clinician must appreciate that two or three café-au-lait spots may be either innocent birthmarks or the earliest signs of neurofibromatosis, in which additional features may manifest at an older age. Only a careful diagnostic evaluation and sometimes long-term follow-up can resolve this diagnostic dilemma. In the case of hereditary disorders without progressive changes, such as the *Treacher Collins syndrome* (mandibulofacial dysostosis), the affected child may have microtia, severe hearing loss, colobomas of the lower eyelids, and marked maxillary hypoplasia, whereas the affected parent may have only mild hearing loss, a downward slant of the palpebral fissures, and a decreased number of lashes on the lower eyelid.

Not Everything Familial is Genetic. Environmental factors, such as infection and teratogens, may simulate genetic conditions; occasionally, two or more children of healthy parents may be affected.

Establishing the Pattern of Inheritance Requires Extensive Data. Data from a small number of families cannot establish a pattern of inheritance. For example, when a presumed genetic disorder has occurred in a son and daughter of healthy parents, it is often concluded that each child is homozygous for an autosomal recessive mutant gene. However, a familial chromosomal abnormality or multifactorial inheritance could also cause the same pattern. Similarly, the pattern of occurrence in families with a disorder due to multifactorial inheritance may simulate mendelian inheritance, for example, the parent and child with a cleft lip and palate mimic autosomal dominant inheritance. With the rate of recurrence among parents and siblings only 4% for Caucasians, almost all children with cleft lip and palate are the only affected members of the family.

American Academy of Pediatrics: General principles in the care of children and adolescents with genetic disorders and other chronic health conditions. Pediatrics 99:643, 1997.

Beaudet AL, Scriner CR, Sly WS, et el: Genetics, biochemistry, and molecular basis of variant human phenotypes. *In*: Scriner CR, Beaudet AL, Sly WS, et al (eds): The Metabolic and Molecular Basis of Inherited Disease. New York, McGraw-Hill, 1995.

Mark M, Chambon P, Rijli FM: Homeobox genes in embryogenesis and pathogenesis. Pediatr Res 42:421, 1997.

Motulsky AG: Screening for genetic disease. N Engl J Med 336:1314, 1997.

Rosenberg RN: DNA-triplet repeats and neurologic disease. N Engl J Med 335:1222, 1996.

Yoon PW, Olney RS, Khoury MJ, et al: Contribution of birth defects and genetic diseases to pediatric hospitalizations. Arch Pediatr Adolesc Med 151:1082, 1997.

CHAPTER 78

Chromosomal Clinical Abnormalities

Judith G. Hall

The chromosomes are made up of DNA and other protein complexes and contain most of the genetic information that is passed from one generation to the next. Chromosomes are normally visualized through the microscope only when they are in a contracted state as they go through cell division. Chromosome studies are important to the pediatrician because abnormal chromosome number (e.g., trisomy 13) and abnormal chromosomal arrangements (e.g., microdeletion 15q) may lead to multiple congenital anomalies. Improved culture and staining techniques have allowed the description of a large number of chromosomal abnormalities associated with specific disorders, and techniques of molecular genetics have facilitated the identification of the specific position of genes as well as their presence or absence along the chromosomes (see Chapters 75 and 76).

In order to report their findings, cytogeneticists arrange chromosomes by size in pairs—the largest being chromosome 1 and the smallest, chromosome 22 (although chromosome 21 has been found to actually be the smallest)—and then the sex chromosomes X and Y. The X chromosome is a large submetacentric chromosome, and the Y chromosome is a small acrocentric chromosome (Fig. 78–1). The position of the centromere in regard to the chromosome arms is another distinguishing feature of each chromosome (Fig. 78–2). The short arm of a chromosome is referred to as p (for petite) and the long arm as q (for the next letter in the alphabet).

NOMENCLATURE. A karyotype is the designation for the visual display of chromosome studies. This display is obtained after the chromosomes are arrested during cell division in prophase and are photographed and arranged in order according to size. The visual display can also be produced by computer. A description of a karyotype consists of three parts: (1) the number of chromosomes, (2) the sex chromosome constitution, and (3) any abnormalities found. The normal karyotype is 46,XX for females and 46,XY for males. If an abnormality is found, it is noted after the sex chromosome constitution. For example, in the case of a female with cri-du-chat syndrome in which a piece of the short arm of the chromosome 5 is missing, the karyotype would be 46,XX,5p–. In a male with Down syndrome in which there is an extra chromosome 21, the karyotype is 47,XY,+21. In the case of translocations, the chromosomes involved are written in brackets preceded by a t, as in 45,XX,t(13q14q), indicating a female carrier of a translocation between the long arms of chromosomes 13 and 14. If the chromosome breaks are along an arm of a chromosome, the band position at which the break occurred is also indicated in the brackets, for example, 45,XY,t(13q2.1–14q1.3), indicating a male carrier of a translocation within the long arms of chromosome 13 and 14.

CELL DIVISION. There are two types of cell division. *Mitosis* is the type of cell division that occurs in most cells of the body. It is during mitosis, specifically the prophase stage of mitosis, that chromosomes are visible and easy to identify for karyotyping. In mitosis, two genetically identical daughter cells are produced from a single parent cell. Prior to cell division, DNA replication has occurred so that there is a doubled amount of DNA and the chromosomes contain two identical sister chromatids. Mitosis is divided into stages. *Prophase* is characterized by spiraling of the chromosome threads into coils to form microscopically identifiable chromosomes; the nuclear membrane and the nucleolus disappear and the mitotic spindle forms. In *metaphase*, the chromosomes condense and are clearly visible as distinct structures. The centromeres of the chromosomes attach to the microtubules of the mitotic spindle and the chromosomes align at the middle of the cell along the spindle. *Anaphase* is characterized by division of the chromosomes along their longitudinal axis to form two daughter chromatids and migration of each chromatid of the pair to opposite poles of the cell. *Telophase*, which completes mitosis, is characterized by reconstitution of the nuclear membrane and nucleolus, duplication of the centriolus, and cytoplasmic cleavage to form the two daughter cells.

Meiosis is the form of cell division that occurs to produce germ cells or gametes (sperm and egg). A diploid cell (with two sets or 46 chromosomes) divides to form haploid cells (with one set or 23 chromosomes). Meiosis is divided into two parts: meiosis I and meiosis II. DNA replication occurs before meiosis I. In male meiosis, the germ cell begins division with two times the normal cellular amount of DNA. In *meiosis I*, each daughter cell gets one of the duplicated chromosomes of each pair. At the beginning of *meiosis II*, each cell contains 23 chromosomes, each with a duplicated pair of chromatids. In meiosis II, the duplicated pair separate and each daughter cell ends up with 1 of each of the 23 chromosomes, that is, there will be four daughter cells, each with a haploid (half the normal number) set of chromosomes. In female meiosis, rather than going through cell divisions, during meiosis I one diploid set of chromosomes condenses and forms a polar body, and during meiosis II one of the haploid sets of chromosomes condenses and forms the 2nd polar body resulting in one egg

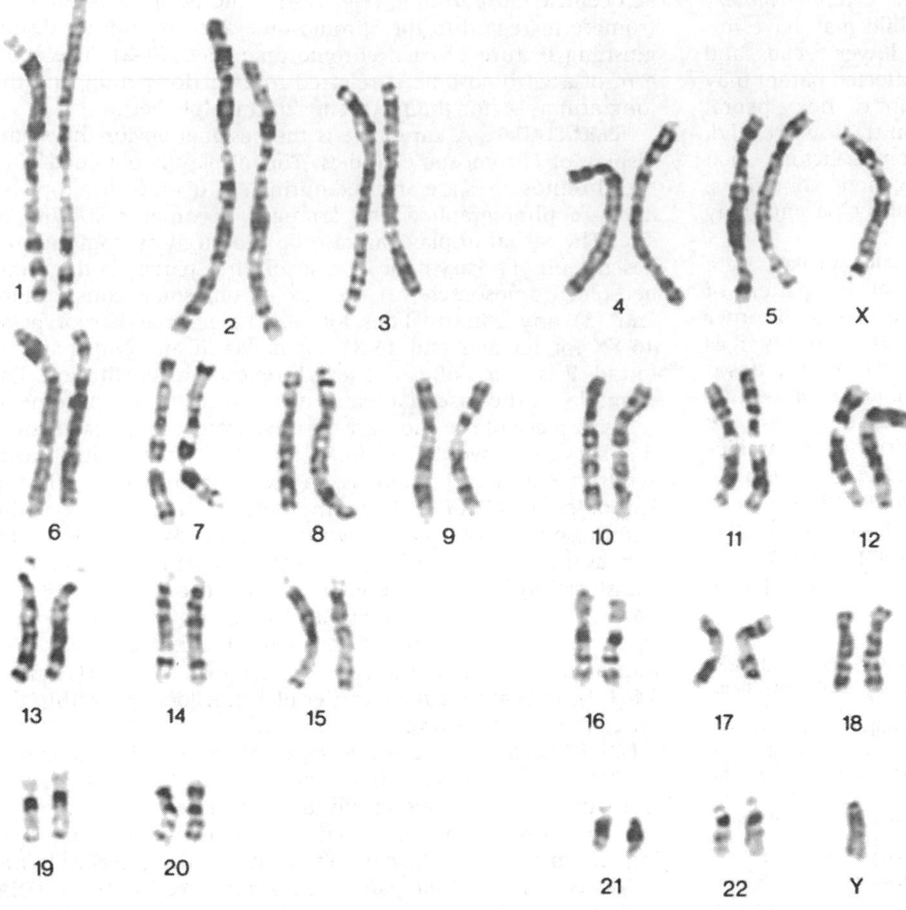

Figure 78–1 Karyotype of normal male with chromosomes in late prophase. The chromosomes are longer, and a greater number of bands are seen than when chromosomes are photographed at metaphase.

with a haploid (half the normal number) set of chromosomes and two polar bodies that contain three sets of chromosomes.

There is exchange between chromosomes (crossing over of chromosome segments) during meiosis, leading to new alignment and combination of genes. Two common errors of cell division occur during meiosis that result in abnormal numbers of chromosomes and chromosomal anomalies. The first is *nondisjunction,* in which two chromosomes fail to separate and migrate together into one of the new cells, producing one cell with two copies of the chromosome and one cell with no copy. The second is *anaphase lag,* in which a chromatid is lost because it fails to move quickly enough during anaphase to become incorporated into one of the new daughter cells (Fig. 78–3).

METHODOLOGY. Chromosome studies can be obtained from any dividing nucleated cell. The techniques for visualization require condensation of chromatin material that occurs at cell division. Because blood is easy to obtain, cytogenetic studies are usually performed on lymphocytes, but cytogenetic studies of fibroblasts must be considered if there is a suspicion of mosaicism. Chromosome studies for prenatal diagnosis are performed with cells obtained from amniotic fluid, chorionic villi tissue, or fetal blood.

Karyotyping refers to the systematic arrangement from a photograph or by a computer of previously stained and banded chromosomes of a single cell by pairs (see Fig. 78–1). The cells are cultured, arrested in mitosis during metaphase, and then fixed and stained. If finer details are necessary, prophase chromosomes may be examined. Because prophase chromosomes are longer and less condensed, they will show 600–1,200 bands, compared with metaphase chromosomes, in which only

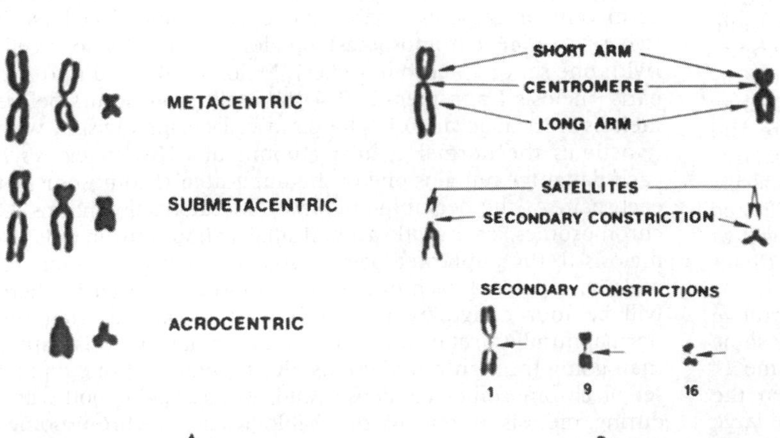

Figure 78–2 *A,* Centromere position determining the three types of chromosomes seen in the normal human karyotype—metacentric, submetacentric, and acrocentric. *B,* Morphologic landmarks useful in chromosome identification.

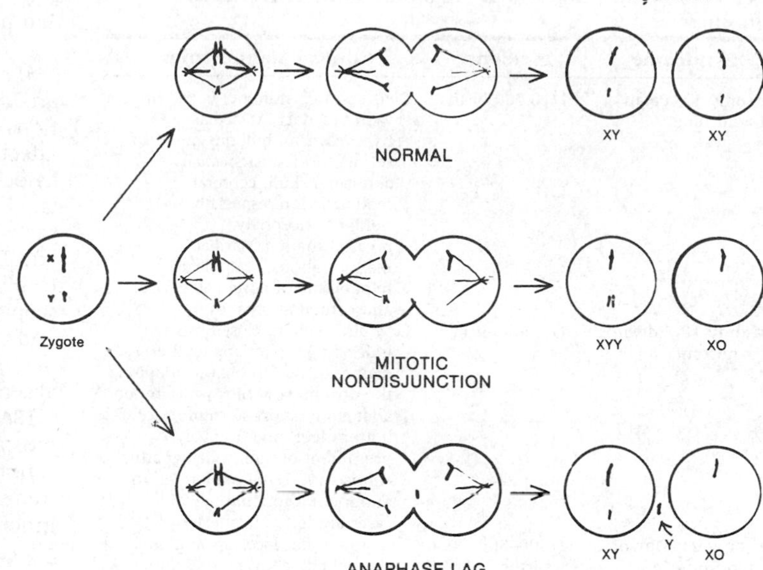

Figure 78–3 The formation of mosaicism. The X and Y chromosomes are used to illustrate two common errors leading to chromosomally abnormal cell populations. In normal mitosis *(top)*, duplicated chromosomes separate and become incorporated into daughter cells. If one replicated chromosome fails to separate, mitotic nondisjunction occurs *(middle)*. Occasionally, normal separation occurs, but one member fails to migrate. This is known as anaphase lag *(bottom)*. (From Wisniewski LP, Hirschhorn K: A Guide to Human Chromosome Defects, 2nd ed. White Plains, NY, March of Dimes Birth Defects Foundation, BD:OAS, 16[6], 1980, with permission from the copyright holder.)

400–600 bands are usually visible. Trypsin-Giemsa staining gives G banding. Quinacrine gives the Q (fluorescent) banding. Special stains are used to demonstrate centromeres.

In situ hybridization is used to identify the presence or absence of specific DNA sequences on a chromosome spread. A molecular probe is used to recognize and attach to homologous DNA sequences on the chromosome spread, identifying a specific chromosome, chromosome segment, or DNA sequence. If fluorescent probes are used, the technique is called *fluorescent in situ hybridization* (FISH) (see Chapters 75 and 76).

CHROMOSOMAL ABNORMALITIES

Chromosomal anomalies occur in 0.4% of live births. They are an important cause of mental retardation and congenital anomalies. Chromosomal anomalies are present in much higher frequencies among spontaneous abortions and still births. The phenotypic anomalies that result from chromosomal aberrations are mainly due to imbalance of genetic information. Chromosomal anomalies include abnormalities of chromosome number and structure.

Abnormalities of Chromosome Number

ANEUPLOIDY AND POLYPLOIDY. When a human cell has 23 chromosomes, it is referred to as a haploid cell (the number of chromosomes in an ova or sperm). Any number of chromosomes that is an exact multiple of the haploid number (e.g., 46, 69, 92 in humans) is referred to as euploid. Euploid cells with more than the normal diploid number of 46 chromosomes are called polyploid cells. Polyploid conceptions are usually not viable. However, they may be present in mosaic (more than one cell line) forms, which allow survival. Cells with three sets of chromosomes are called triploid and are frequently seen in abortus material and occasionally in viable humans, usually in mosaic forms. Cells deviating from the multiples of the haploid number are called *aneuploid* (i.e., not euploid), indicating a missing or extra chromosome.

TRISOMIES. The most common abnormalities of chromosome number are trisomies. These occur when there are three representatives of a particular chromosome instead of the usual two. Trisomies are usually the result of meiotic nondisjunction (failure of a chromosome pair to separate). Trisomy may be present in all cells or may occur in mosaic form. Most individuals with trisomies exhibit a consistent and specific phenotype depending on the chromosome involved (Table 78–1). The most frequent and best known trisomy in humans is *trisomy 21* or Down syndrome (Fig. 78–4). *Trisomies of chromosome 18* (Fig. 78–5) and *chromosome 13* (Fig. 78–6) are also relatively common and are associated with a characteristic set of congenital anomalies and mental retardation.

The incidence of Down syndrome among conceptions is more than twice as high as it is among live births. More than half the trisomy 21 conceptions spontaneously abort early in pregnancy. The occurrence of trisomy 21 as well as other autosomal trisomies increases with advancing maternal age. The increased risk of trisomy 21 in women older than 35 yr is an indication to offer these women amniocentesis or chorionic villus sampling for prenatal diagnosis. Fetal chromosome analysis is a reliable way to detect fetal Down syndrome. In women younger than 35 yr of age, maternal serum testing (triple screen) can be efficacious in prenatal screening for Down syndrome. Low maternal serum α-fetoprotein concentration, low unconjugated estriol, and elevated human chorionic gonadotropin are indicators of Down syndrome.

Translocation Down Syndrome. All individuals with Down syndrome have three copies of chromosome 21. About 95% have three free-standing copies of chromosome 21. Approximately 1% of individuals are mosaic with some normal cells. Approximately 4% of Down syndrome individuals have a translocation involving chromosome 21. Translocations account for 9% of the children with Down syndrome born to mothers younger than 30 yr of age. Half the translocations arise de novo in the affected individual, whereas half are inherited from a translocation carrier parent. Parents who are carriers of a translocation involving chromosome 21 produce three types of viable offspring: normal phenotype and karyotype, a phenotypically normal translocation carrier, and the translocation trisomy 21. The majority of translocations that give rise to Down syndrome are fusions at the centromere between chromosomes 13, 14, 15, or 21 t(21q,21q). The phenotype in translocation Down syndrome is not distinguishable from regular trisomy 21 Down syndrome (see Table 78–1). Chromosome studies must be performed on every Down syndrome individual. If a translocation is identified, parental studies must be performed to identify normal individuals who are translocation carriers with a high recurrence risk for a chromosomally abnormal child and who may also have other family members at risk.

MONOSOMIES. Monosomies occur when only one representative of a chromosome is present. They may be complete or

TABLE 78–1 Chromosomal Trisomies and Their Clinical Findings

Syndrome	Incidence	Clinical Manifestations
Trisomy 13, Patau syndrome	1/10,000 births	Cleft lip often midline; flexed fingers with polydactyly; ocular hypotelorism, bulbous nose; low-set malformed ears; small abnormal skull; cerebral malformation, especially holoprosencephaly; microphthalmia; cardiac malformations; scalp defects; hypoplastic or absent ribs; visceral and genital anomalies
Trisomy 18, Edwards syndrome	1/6,000 births	Low birthweight, closed fists with index finger overlapping the 3rd digit and the 5th digit overlapping the 4th, narrow hips with limited abduction, short sternum, rocker-bottom feet, microcephaly, prominent occiput, micrognathia, cardiac and renal malformations and mental retardation; 95% of cases are lethal in the 1st yr
Trisomy 21, Down syndrome	1/600–800 births	Hypotonia, flat face, upward and slanted palpebral fissures and epicanthic folds, speckled irises (Brushfield spots); varying degrees of mental and growth retardation; dysplasia of the pelvis, cardiac malformations, and simian crease; short, broad hands, hypoplasia of middle phalanx of 5th finger, intestinal atresia, and high arched palate; 5% of patients with Down syndrome are the result of a translocation—t(14q21q), t(15q21q), and t(13q21q)—in which the phenotype is the same as trisomy 21 Down syndrome
Trisomy 8, mosaicism	1/20,000 births	Long face, high prominent forehead, wide upturned nose, thick everted lower lip, microretrognathia, low-set ears, high arched, sometimes cleft palate. Osteoarticular anomalies are common; moderate mental retardation.

partial. Complete monosomies may be the result of nondisjunction or anaphase lag. In nondisjunction during cell division, the two chromosomes in a replicating pair fail to separate; one cell ends up with only one copy (monosomic) and the other with three copies (trisomic) of the specific chromosome. In anaphase lag, a chromosome fails to move into the new daughter cell and is lost. In humans, all complete autosomal monosomies appear to be lethal early in development and only survive in mosaic forms. Partial monosomies are usually the offspring of a translocation carrier.

Abnormalities of Chromosome Structure

DELETIONS. Deletions occur when a piece of a chromosome is missing. They may occur as a simple deletion or as a deletion with duplication of another chromosome segment. The latter is usually caused by a crossover in meiosis in a translocation carrier, resulting in an unbalanced reciprocal chromosomal translocation. Deletions may be located at the chromosome ends or in interstitial segments of the chromosome and are usually associated with mental retardation and malformations. Small telomeric deletions may be relatively common in nonspecific mental retardation with minor anomalies. The most commonly observed deletions in humans are 4p-, 5p-, 9p-, 11p-, 13q-, 18p-, and 18q-, which are associated with well-described phenotypes (Table 78–2). Deletions may be observed in routine chromosome preparations, but microdeletions are detectable only under the microscope with prophase chromosome studies. In submicroscopic deletions, the missing piece can be detected only by using molecular probes or DNA studies.

Microdeletions are defined as small chromosome deletions that are detectable only in high-quality (pro)metaphase preparations. These deletions often involve several genes so that the affected individual may be identified by an unusual phenotype associated with a single gene mutation (e.g., Duchenne muscular dystrophy). Williams, Langer-Giedion, Prader-Willi, Angelman, Rubinstein-Taybi, Smith-Magenis, Miller-Dieker, Alagille and DiGeorge-velocardiofacial syndromes have all been found to be associated with microdeletions (Table 78–3). Submicroscopic deletions are not visible by microscopic examination and are detected only with specific probes for a DNA sequence or DNA studies. The deletion is recognized because of the absence of staining or fluorescence.

TRANSLOCATIONS. Translocations involve the transfer of chromosomal material from one chromosome to another. Translocations may be robertsonian or reciprocal. They occur with a frequency of 1/500 liveborn human infants. They may be inherited from a parent or appear de novo, with no other affected family members.

Robertsonian translocations involve two acrocentric (centromere located at the end) chromosomes that fuse near the centromeric region with subsequent loss of the nonfunctional, very truncated short arms. The translocation chromosome is made up of the long arms of two fused chromosomes, hence the resulting count will be only 45 chromosomes. The loss of the short arms of acrocentric chromosomes has no known deleterious effect. Although carriers of a robertsonian translocation are usually phenotypically normal, they are at increased risk for miscarriages and abnormal offspring. *Reciprocal translocations* are the result of breaks in nonhomologous chromosomes with reciprocal exchange of the broken segments. Carri-

TABLE 78–2 Common Deletions and Their Clinical Manifestations

Deletion	Clinical Abnormalities
4p-	Wolf-Hirschhorn syndrome. The main features are a typical "Greek helmet" facies with ocular hypertelorism, prominent glabella and frontal bossing; microcephaly, dolichocephaly, hypoplasia of the eye socket, ptosis, strabismus, nystagmus, bilateral epicanthic folds, cleft lip and palate, beaked nose with prominent bridge, hypospadias, cardiac malformations, and mental retardation.
5p-	Cri-du-chat syndrome. The main features are hypotonia, short stature, characteristic cry, microcephaly with protruding metopic suture, moonlike face, hypertelorism, bilateral epicanthic folds, high arched palate, wide and flat nasal bridge, and mental retardation.
9p-	The main features are craniofacial dysmorphology with trigonocephaly, slanted palpebral fissures, discrete exophthalmos, arched eyebrows, flat and wide nasal bridge, short neck with pterygium colli, genital anomalies, long fingers and toes, cardiac malformations, and mental retardation.
13q-	The main features are low birthweight, failure to thrive, and severe mental retardation. Facial features include microcephaly, flat wide nasal bridge, hypertelorism, ptosis, micrognathia. Ocular malformations are common. The hands have hypoplastic or absent thumbs and syndactyly.
18p-	A few patients (15%) are severely affected and have cephalic and ocular malformations, cleft lip and palate, and varying degrees of mental retardation. Most (80%) have only minor malformations and mild mental retardation.
18q-	The main features are hypotonia with "froglike" position with the legs flexed, externally rotated, and in hyperabduction. The face is characteristic with depressed midface and apparent protrusion of the mandible, deep-set eyes, short upper lip, everted lower lip ("carplike" mouth); antihelix of the ears is very prominent; varying degrees of mental retardation and belligerent personality.
21q-	The main features are hypertonia, microcephaly, downward-slanting palpebral fissures, high palate, prominent nasal bridge, large low-set ears, micrognathia, and varying degrees of mental retardation. They may have skeletal malformations.

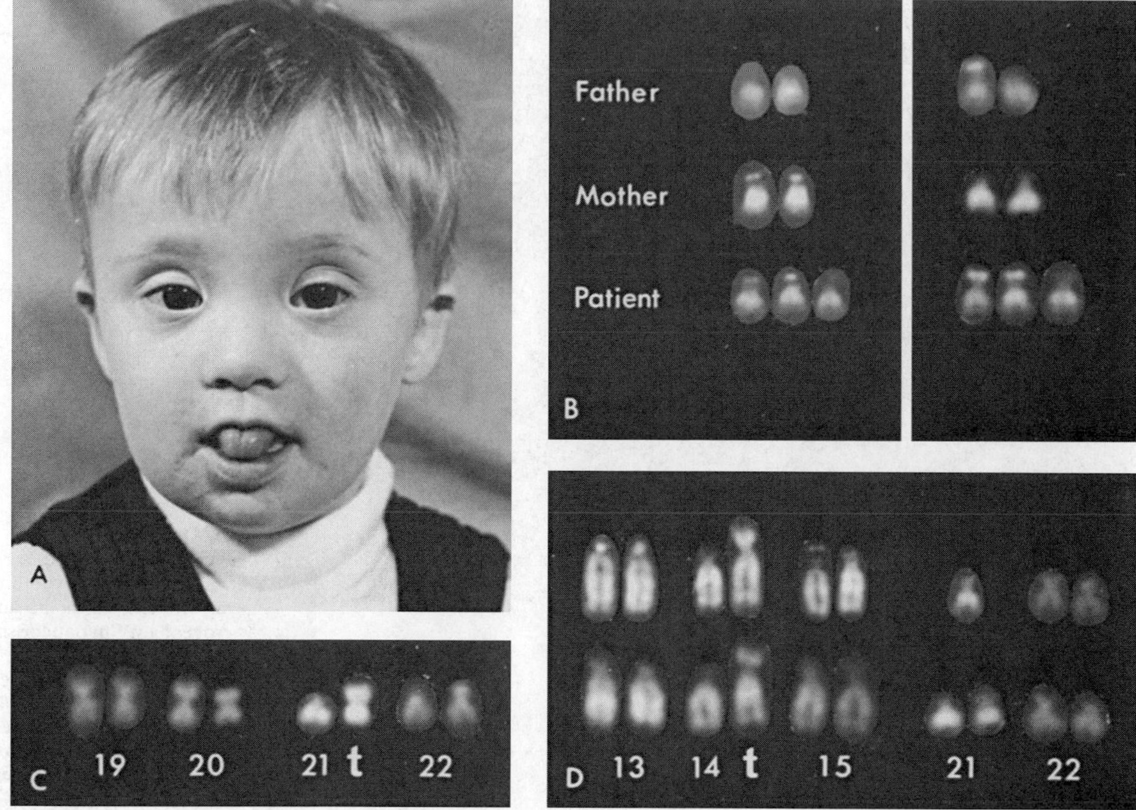

Figure 78–4 Partial karyotypes from patients with Down syndrome. *A,* Patient with trisomy 21. *B,* Chromosome 21 from two patients and their parents. *Left:* Two of a patient's chromosomes with brightly fluorescent satellites were transmitted by the mother. *Right:* Another patient's two chromosomes with bright satellites resulted from paternal nondisjunction at second meiotic division. *C,* 21q21q translocation. *D,* 14q21q translocation in a mother *(above)* and her affected child *(below).*

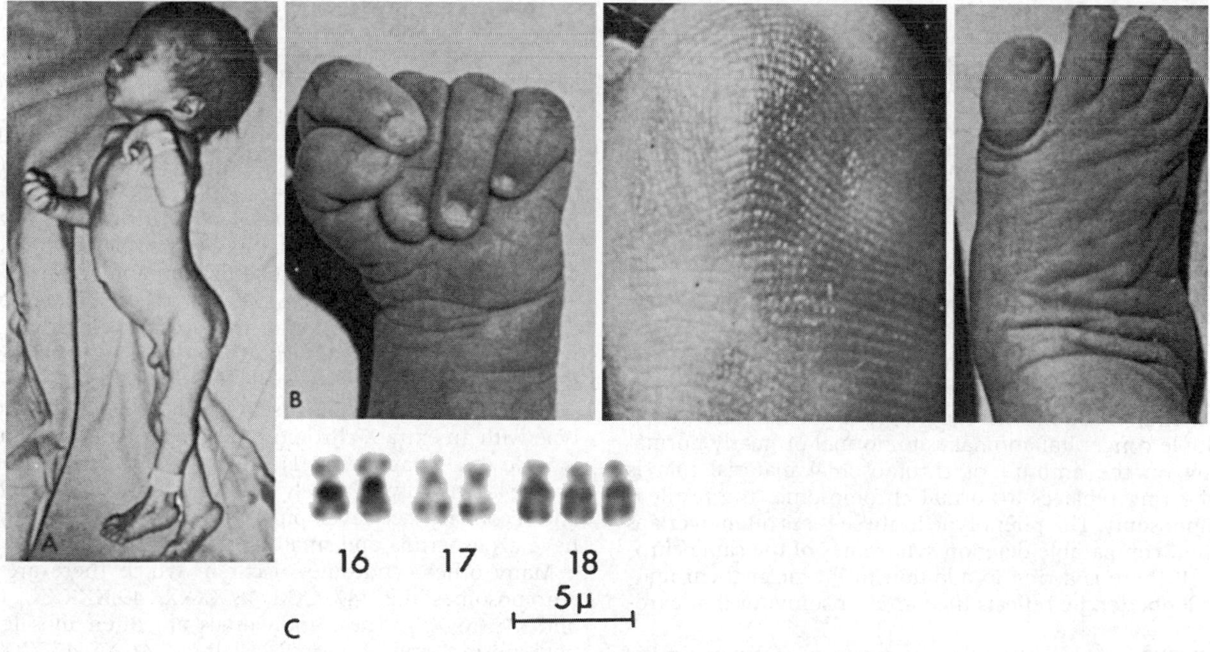

Figure 78–5 *A,* Photograph of male infant with trisomy 18, age 4 days. Note prominent occiput, micrognathia, low-set ears, short sternum, narrow pelvis, prominent calcaneus, and flexion abnormalities of the fingers. (Courtesy of Robert E. Carrel.) *B,* Several of the common anomalies in the 18 trisomy syndrome, including the unusual position of the fingers with hypoplasia of fifth fingernail; the simple arch pattern of the fingerpads; and the dorsiflexed hallux with hypoplasia of toenails. (From Smith DW: Autosomal abnormalities. Am J Obstet Gynecol 90:1055, 1964.) *C,* Partial karyotype of trisomy 18 prepared with modified Giemsa stain.

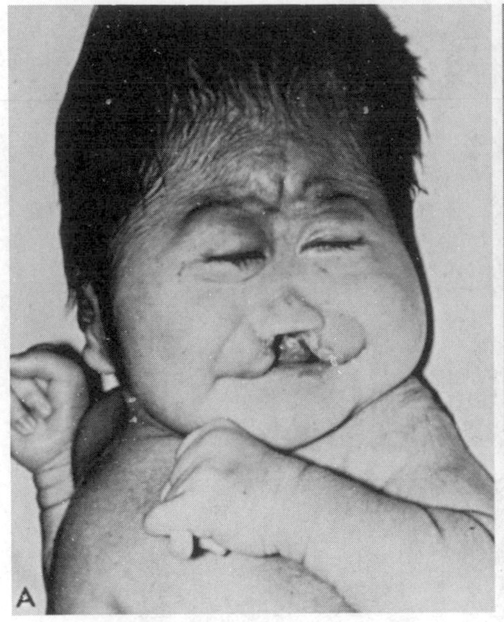

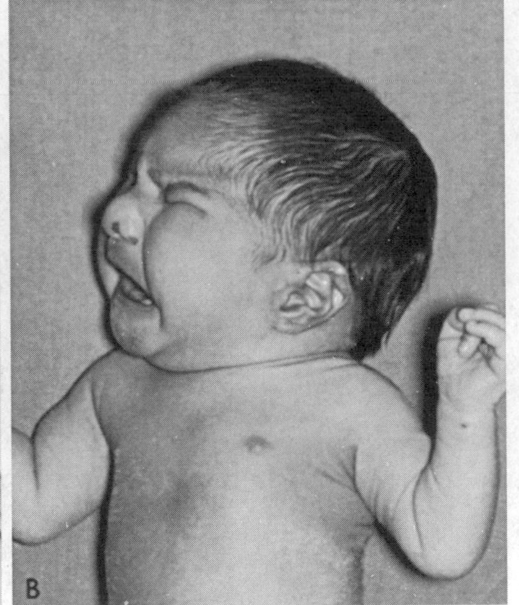

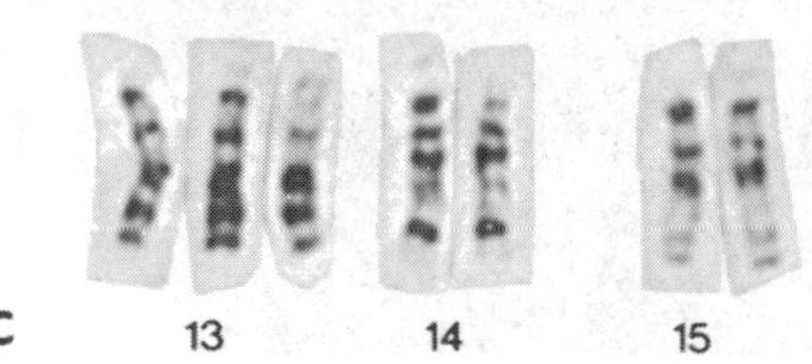

Figure 78–6 *A* and *B*, Female infants with trisomy 13 syndrome. Note the midline cleft of the lip and palate, microcephaly, hypotelorism, microphthalmos, bulbous nose, polydactyly, and overlapping of fingers. Scalp defects (not shown) are also present. (Courtesy of Miriam G. Wilson.) *C*, Partial karyotype showing chromosomes 13, 14, and 15 stained with the trypsin-Giemsa method.

ers of a reciprocal translocation are usually phenotypically normal but also have an increased risk of having chromosomally abnormal offspring and miscarriages because of abnormalities in the segregation of the chromosomes in the germ cells.

INVERSIONS. Inversions require the chromosome to break at two points. The broken piece is then inverted and joined into the same chromosome. Inversions have a frequency of 1/100 liveborns and may be pericentric or paracentric. In *pericentric inversions,* the breaks are in the two opposite arms of the chromosome so that the intervening portion that contains the centromere is reversed. They are usually discovered because they change the position of the centromere. In contrast, *paracentric inversions* involve only chromosomal material from one arm of a chromosome. Carriers of inversions are usually normal, but they may have an increased risk of miscarriages and chromosomally abnormal offspring.

RING CHROMOSOMES. Ring chromosomes are very rare, but they have been found for all human chromosomes. The formation of a ring involves a deletion at each end of the chromosome. The "sticky" ends then join to form the ring. The phenotype of a ring chromosome ranges from mental retardation and multiple congenital anomalies to normal or nearly normal depending on the amount of chromosomal material that is lost. If the ring replaces a normal chromosome, the result is partial monosomy. The phenotype in these cases often overlaps that seen in comparable deletion syndromes of the same chromosome. If there is a ring in addition to the normal chromosomes, the phenotype reflects the partial trisomy for that chromosome.

DUPLICATIONS. A duplication is the presence of extra genetic material from the same chromosome. Duplications may result from the abnormal segregation in carriers of translocations or inversions.

INSERTIONS. Insertions occur when a piece of chromosome breaks at two points and is incorporated into a break in another part of a chromosome. This requires three breakpoints and may occur between two chromosomes or within one.

Sex Chromosome Anomalies

TURNER SYNDROME. This is one of the most common monosomies in liveborn humans (see Chapter 596.1). The chromosomal finding in Turner syndrome is the loss of part or all of one of the sex chromosomes. Half the affected individuals have 45,X in their lymphocyte studies. The other half have a variety of abnormalities of one of their sex chromosomes and may be mosaic. The phenotype in Turner syndrome is female and is characterized by short stature and underdeveloped gonads. The frequency at birth is 0.4/1,000 (i.e., 1/4,000 liveborn females or 1/8,000 livebirths), but it occurs much more frequently with spontaneous abortion.

From 5–10% of individuals with Turner syndrome have some Y chromosome material in all or some cells. These individuals may have some masculinization and are at risk for the development of gonadoblastoma. A careful screening for Y chromosome material should be performed on any individual with Turner syndrome in whom no additional X chromosome (in addition to the one normal X) material has been found.

KLINEFELTER SYNDROME. These individuals have a male karyotype with an extra X chromosome, 47,XXY, and the phenotype is male (see Chapter 593.1). Individuals with Klinefelter syndrome are usually relatively tall. They may have gynecomastia and secondary sex development may be delayed. They usually have azoospermia and small testes and are infertile.

Many other syndromes occur in which there are extra X chromosomes (i.e., 47,XXX, 48,XXXX, 49,XXXXX, 48,XXXY, and 49,XXXXY). These individuals are often mosaic, having both normal and abnormal cell lines (46,XX/47,XXX). In all these syndromes, the number of abnormalities increases with the number of X chromosomes and is specific to each syndrome. Abnormalities of chromosome Y also exist. The most common abnormality is the XYY male.

47,XYY MALE. The frequency of XYY males has been estimated to be 1/1,000 livebirths. Because XYY males do not have any striking phenotypical abnormality, this frequency has been

TABLE 78–3 Microdeletions and Their Clinical Manifestations

Deletion	Syndrome	Clinical Manifestations
7q23-	Williams	Round face with full cheeks and lips, stellate pattern in iris, strabismus, supravalvular aortic stenosis and other cardiac malformations, varying degrees of mental retardation, and a very friendly personality
8q24.1-	Langer-Giedion or tricho-rhino-phalangeal, type II	Sparse hair, multiple cone-shaped epiphyses, multiple cartilaginous exostoses, bulbous nasal tip, thickened alar cartilage, upturned nares, prominent philtrum, large protruding ears, and mild mental retardation
11p13-	WAGR	Hypernephroma (Wilms tumor), aniridia, male genital hypoplasia of varying degrees, gonadoblastoma, long face, upward slanting palpebral fissures, ptosis, beaked nose, low-set poorly formed auricles, and mental retardation
15q11-13 (pat)	Prader-Willi	Severe hypotonia at birth, obesity, short stature (responsive to growth hormone), small hands and feet, hypogonadism, and mental retardation
15q11-13 (mat)	Angelman	Hypotonia, fair hair, midface hypoplasia, prognathism, seizures, jerky ataxic movements, uncontrollable bouts of laughter, and severe mental retardation
16p13-	Rubinstein-Taybi	Microcephaly, ptosis, beaked nose with low-lying philtrum, broad thumbs and large toes, and mental retardation
17p11.2	Smith-Magenis	Brachycephaly, midfacial hypoplasia, prognathism, myopia, cleft palate, short stature, behavioral problems, and mental retardation
17p13.3-	Miller-Dieker	Microcephaly, lissencephaly, pachygyria, narrow forehead, hypoplastic male external genitals, growth retardation, seizures, and profound mental retardation
20p12-	Alagille syndrome	Bile duct paucity with cholestasis, heart defects, particularly pulmonary artery stenosis, ocular abnormalities (posterior embryotoxin), skeletal defects such as butterfly vertebrae, long nose with broad midnose
22q11-	DiGeorge-velocardiofacial CATCH 22	Hypoplasia or agenesis of the thymus and parathyroid glands, hypoplasia of auricle and external auditory canal, conotruncal cardiac anomalies, cleft palate, short stature, behavioral problems

estimated from newborn surveys. XYY males are said to be relatively tall and may have some behavioral problems.

Fragile Sites

Fragile sites are defined as regions of chromosomes that show a tendency to separation, breakage, or attenuation under particular growth conditions. Numerous fragile sites have been identified.

FRAGILE X SYNDROME. The fragile site located on the distal long arm of chromosome X at Xq27.3 has been associated with the fragile X syndrome, which is the most common form of mental retardation in males. This fragile site (FRAXA) becomes visible in chromosome studies only when it is induced under special culture techniques; regular metaphase studies do not demonstrate this fragile site. The fragile site may not always be visible, even with the appropriate chromosome preparation. The diagnosis of fragile X is now usually made by DNA studies, which demonstrate an expanded segment of DNA from the Xq27.3 region. There are two other fragile sites on the X chromosome (FRAXE and FRAXF) also associated with mental retardation and allelic expansion.

The main *clinical manifestations* of fragile X syndrome in affected males are mental retardation; macro-orchidism; large size; characteristic facial features, including long face, prominent jaw, and large prominent ears; and sterotyped behavior and speech. Females affected with fragile X show varying degrees of mental retardation.

The *inheritance of fragile X* is different from the usual single gene inheritance patterns. It involves an area of the gene with CGG/CCG repeats (triplet repeats). Three distinct categories of DNA variation occur at the fragile X locus (normal, up to 50 repeats; premutation, 52 to 200 repeats; and symptomatic, 200–2,000 repeats or greater). A person who carries a small increase of trinucleotide repeats without the phenotypic abnormalities is said to be a carrier of a premutation. When inherited, this premutation is unstable and may expand over a few generations, gradually increasing in size when transmitted by females but usually remaining the same size when transmitted by males. As the mutation is transmitted by a female and increases in size, it may become of a size (usually an additional 600–3,000 base pairs) that is clinically significant and leads to the typical fragile X syndrome phenotype with mental retardation. Also see Chapter 76.

The fragile X syndrome is due to the *allelic expansion*, which interferes with gene function. Allelic expansion refers to the change in the increasing size of a particular DNA sequence. The expansion begins as a small increase in the copy number of trinucleotide repeats. The number of repeats may be unstable and may develop different sizes in different cells or tissues. The number of repeats may increase in size from one generation to the next (and occasionally has been seen to decrease in size). A change in size of the DNA segment between generations or in tissues means that this type of mutation differs from classic mutations in which the change in DNA sequence usually occurs once and is then passed on from generation to generation. Some other disorders associated with allelic expansion are myotonic dystrophy (with CTG repeats), Huntington disease (with CAG repeats), spinobulbar muscular atrophy (with CAG repeats), spinocerebellar ataxia type 1, 2, and 3 (SCA1, SCA2, and SCA3, all with CAG repeats), and dentatorubropallidoluysian atrophy (with CAG repeats).

The number of copies seen in disorders associated with allelic expansion may be related to the age of onset and severity of the disease (Table 78–4). For example, the congenital form of myotonic dystrophy is known to occur with the largest number of repeats but only when it is transmitted by the mother. In Huntington disease, the juvenile onset form of the disease is also associated with the largest number of repeats and occurs primarily when inherited from the father.

Chromosomal Breakage Syndromes

There are a number of recessive disorders that are associated with breakage or rearrangement of chromosomes, or both. The breaks may be spontaneous or they can be induced by a variety of environmental agents and different techniques. Chromatid breaks are found in Fanconi anemia, Nijmegen syndrome, Bloom syndrome, and Werner syndrome. Breaks and nonrandom rearrangements of chromosomes 7 and 14 have been reported in ataxia-telangiectasia. A special cytogenetic study called sister chromatid exchange can be used in some of these disorders for carrier detection and prenatal diagnosis. These disorders have specific phenotypes, but the growth impairment, malformations, and other dysmorphic features have not been directly attributed to the chromosome breaks.

Mosaicism

Mosaicism is the term used to describe an individual who has two different cell lines derived from a single zygote (fertilized

TABLE 78–4 Allelic Expansion

Gene	Location	Normal	Premutation	Affected	Parent of Origin Effect
Huntington disease	4p16.3	11–24 repeats	30–38	42–82	Male transmission usually increases repeat
Myotonic dystrophy	19q13.3	5–37 repeats	37–50	>50	Male may decrease repeat Female usually increases repeat
Fragile X	Xq23.7	6–54 repeats	52–200	>200	Male constant Female may markedly increase repeat

egg) (see Fig. 78–3). Studies of placental tissue from chorionic villus sampling show that at least 2% of all conceptions are mosaic for chromosomal anomalies at or before 10 wk of pregnancy. Compared with complete trisomies, which are usually nonviable for chromosomes other than 13, 18, and 21, the development of a normal cell line may allow a trisomic conception of the other chromosomes to come to term and be viable. If a normal cell line develops, the fetus may survive and the original trisomic cell line may even be lost. Normal disomic cells are found in the placenta of infants who are born alive with trisomies 13 and 18.

Germline mosaicism refers to the presence of mosaicism in the germ cells found in the gonad. This type of mosaicism may be suspected in cases in which there is more than one affected offspring with the same genetic abnormality (usually inherited as a chromosomal or dominant disorder) with phenotypically normal parents. If germline mosaicism is present, there is an increased risk for recurrence of an affected child.

Depending on the point at which the new cell line arises during early embryogenesis, an affected individual may have a variety of clinical presentations. Mosaicism may be present in some tissues and not in others, giving the affected individual a patchy or asymmetric distribution of abnormalities. Cytogenetic studies of fibroblasts must be performed if mosaicism is suspected because blood lymphocyte cells may not tolerate some trisomies, deletions, or chromosomal rearrangements, and thus the finding of normal lymphocyte studies will be misleading.

PALLISTER-KILLIAN SYNDROME. This disorder is characterized by coarse facies, pigmentary skin anomalies, localized alopecia, diaphragmatic hernias, cardiovascular anomalies, supernumerary nipples, and profound mental retardation. The syndrome is due to mosaicism for isochromosome 12p. The presence of the isochromosome 12p in cells gives four copies of 12p in the affected cells. The isochromosome 12p is preferentially cultured from fibroblast and is seldom present in lymphocytes. The abnormalities seen in affected individuals probably reflect the presence of abnormal cells during early embryogenesis.

HYPOMELANOSIS OF ITO. This entity is characterized by unilateral or bilateral macular hypopigmented whorls, streaks, and patches. Abnormalities of the eyes, musculoskeletal system, and central nervous system may also be present. Patients with hypomelanosis of Ito appear to have two genetically distinct cell lines. The mosaic chromosome anomalies that have been observed involve both autosomes and sex chromosomes and have been demonstrated in about 50% of cases. The mosaicism may not be visible in chromosome studies carried out on blood but is more likely to be found when the chromosome studies are obtained from skin fibroblasts. Sometimes the distinct cell lines may not be due to observable chromosomal anomalies but to single gene mutations or other mechanisms.

UNIPARENTAL DISOMY

Uniparental disomy (UPD) is the term used when both chromosomes of a pair of chromosomes in a person with a normal number of chromosomes have been inherited from only one parent. Uniparental isodisomy means that the two chromosomes are identical, whereas uniparental heterodisomy means that the two chromosomes are different members of a pair, both of which were inherited from one parent. The phenotypical result of UPD may vary according to the specific chromosome involved, the parent who contributed the chromosomes, and whether it is isodisomy or heterodisomy. Three types of phenotypic effects are seen in UPD: (1) those related to imprinted genes (see later), that is, the absence of a gene expressed only when inherited from one parent, (2) those related to autosomal recessive disorders, and (3) those related to a vestigial aneuploid. Also see Chapter 77.

In uniparental isodisomy, both chromosomes in a pair are identical; consequently, the genes on both chromosomes will also be identical. This becomes particularly important for the carriers of an autosomal recessive disorder. If the offspring of a carrier parent has isodisomy for a chromosome with an abnormal gene, the abnormal gene will be present in two copies and the phenotype will be that of the autosomal recessive disorder; however, this occurs when only one parent is actually a carrier of the recessive disorder. It is estimated that all human beings carry five to eight abnormal autosomal recessive genes. The autosomal recessive disorders spinal muscular atrophy, cystic fibrosis, cartilage-hair hypoplasia, α- and β-thalassemias, and Bloom syndrome have been reported to have occurred because of uniparental disomy. The possibility of uniparental isodisomy should also be kept in mind when an individual is affected with more than one recessive disorder

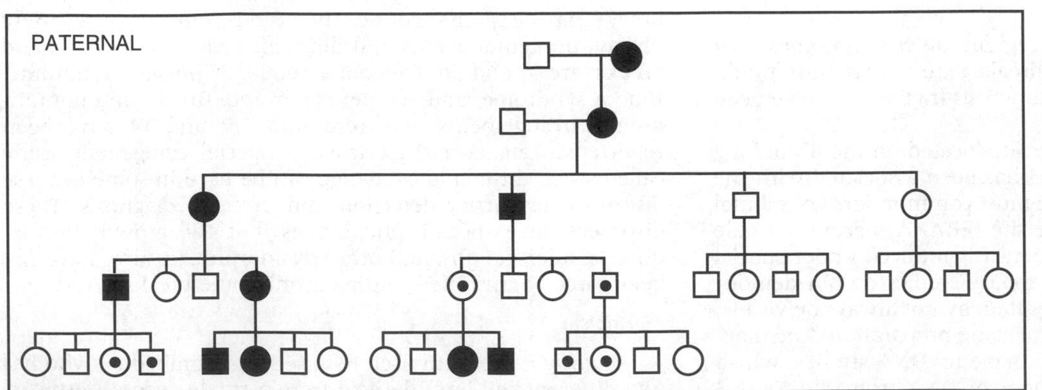

Figure 78–7 In pedigrees suggestive of paternal imprinting, phenotypic effects will occur only when the gene is transmitted from the mother but not when transmitted from the father. There will be an equal number of males and females affected and nonaffected phenotypically in each generation. A nonmanifesting transmitter will give a clue to the sex of the parent who passes the expressed genetic information; in other words, in paternal imprinting there will be "skipped" female nonmanifesting individuals.

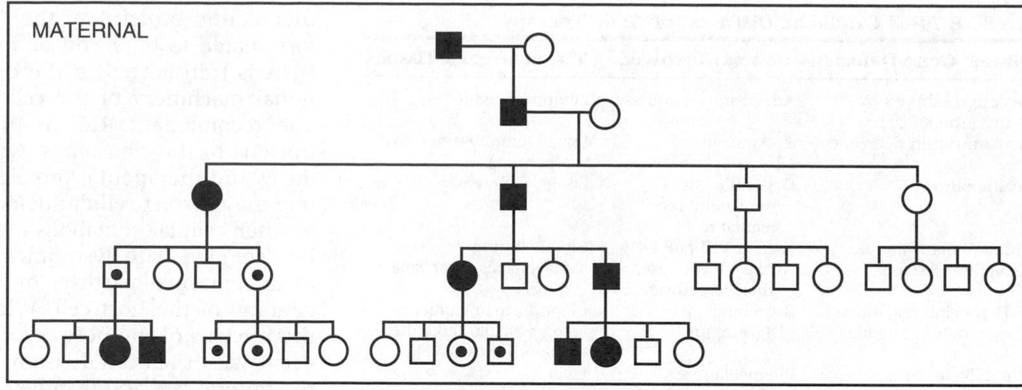

Figure 78–8 In pedigrees suggestive of maternal imprinting, phenotypic effects will occur only when the gene is transmitted from the father but not when transmitted from the mother. There are equal numbers of males and females affected and nonaffected phenotypically in each generation. A nonmanifesting transmitter will give a clue to the sex of the parent who passes the expressed genetic information; in other words, in paternal imprinting there will be "skipped" female nonmanifesting individuals.

because the genes for both disorders could be carried on the same disomic chromosome.

Maternal uniparental disomy involving chromosomes 2, 7, 14, and 15 and paternal uniparental disomy involving chromosomes 6, 11, 15, and 20 are associated with phenotypic abnormalities of growth and behavior. For instance, UPD maternal 7 is associated with a phenotype similar to Russell-Silver syndrome with intrauterine growth retardation. These phenotypic effects are thought to be related to imprinting (see later).

UPD for chromosome 15 has been reported in some cases of Prader-Willi syndrome and Angelman syndrome. In *Prader-Willi syndrome,* about 60% of cases have maternal UPD (i.e., missing the paternal chromosome 15). In a small percentage of individuals with *Angelman syndrome,* paternal UPD of chromosome 15 is observed (i.e., missing the maternal chromosome 15). The phenotype for both Prader-Willi syndrome and Angleman syndrome in cases of UPD is thought to be due to the lack of the functional contribution from a particular parent for chromosome 15. These findings suggest there are differences in function of certain regions of chromosome 15, depending on whether it is inherited from the mother or from the father.

Uniparental disomy most likely arises because a pregnancy starts off as a trisomy. Most trisomies are lethal, and the fetus survives only if a cell line loses one of the extra chromosomes and becomes disomic. One third of the time, the disomic cell line is uniparental. Usually, the viable cell line outgrows the trisomic cell line. When mosaic trisomy is found at prenatal diagnosis, care should be taken to determine whether uniparental disomy has resulted and whether the chromosome involved is one of the disomies known to be associated with phenotypic abnormalities. There must also be concern that some residual cells with trisomy will be present in some tissues, leading to malformations or dysfunction.

IMPRINTING

Genomic imprinting refers to the observation that phenotypic expression depends on the parent of origin for certain genes and chromosome segments. Whether the genetic material is expressed depends on the gender of the parent from whom it was derived. Genomic imprinting is suspected on the basis of a pedigree (Figs. 78–7 and 78–8) with unusual transmission. Imprinting probably occurs in many different parts of the human genome but is thought to be particularly important in gene expression related to development, growth, cancer, evolution, and behavior.

The classic examples of imprinting in humans are the phenotypic differences seen in Prader-Willi and Angelman syndromes, which are associated with deletion and uniparental disomy of the same region of chromosome 15. Thus, in uniparental maternal disomy, there is also lack of the paternal segment of chromosome 15, resulting in Prader-Willi syndrome as well. In Prader-Willi syndrome, the deletion, when it occurs, is always of the paternally derived chromosome 15, suggesting that the phenotype of Prader-Willi is due to a lack of paternally derived genetic information carried on that segment of chromosome 15. In contrast, when there is a deleted chromosome 15 in Angelman syndrome, the deleted chromosome is always maternal in origin, that is, there is lack of maternal information and the UPD is always paternal. There are likely to be many other disorders with this type of parent of origin effect.

Haddow JE, Palomaki GE, Knight GJ, et al: Reducing the need for amniocentesis in women 35 years of age or older with serum markers for screening. N Engl J Med 330:1114, 1994.

Hashimoto T, Mori K, Yoneda Y, et al: Proton magnetic resonance spectroscopy of the brain in patients with Prader-Willi syndrome. Pediatr Neurol 18:30, 1998.

Holm VA, Cassidy SB, Butler MG, et al: Prader-Willi syndrome: Consensus diagnostic criteria. Pediatrics 91:398, 1994.

International System for Human Cytogenetic Nomenclature (ISCN): Published in collaboration with Cytogenetics and Cell Genetics, 1985.

Langlois S, Lopez-Rangel E, Hall JG: New mechanisms for genetic disease and non-traditional modes of inheritance. Adv Pediatr 40:91, 1995.

Lignon AH, Beaudet AL, Shaffer LG: Simultaneous, multilocus FISH analysis for detection of microdeletions in the diagnostic evaluation of development delay and mental retardation. Am J Hum Genet 61:51, 1997.

Lindren AC, Hagenäs L, Müller J, et al: Growth hormone treatment of children with Prader-Willi syndrome affects linear growth and body composition favorably. Acta Pediatr 87:28, 1998.

McCandless SE, Scott JA, Robin NH: Deletion 22q11: A newly recognized cause of behavioral and psychiatric disorders. Arch Pediatr Adolesc Med 152:481, 1998.

Rimoin DL, Connor JM, Pyeritz RE: Emery and Rimoin's Principles and Practice of Medical Genetics, 3rd ed. New York, Churchill Livingston, 1997.

Stevenson RE, Hall JG, Goodman RM: Human Malformations and Related Anomalies. Oxford, Oxford Monographs on Medical Genetics, 1993.

Strachan T, Read AP: Human Molecular Genetics. Oxford, BIOS Scientific Publishers Limited, 1996.

Weinzimer SA, McDonald DM, Driscoll DA, et al: Growth hormone deficiency in patients with a 22q11.2 deletion: Expanding the phenotype. Pediatrics 101:929, 1998.

CHAPTER 79
Gene Therapy

Gregory A. Grabowski and Jeffrey A. Whitsett

The ability to easily manipulate DNA for transfer into cells, wherein transcription of the recombinant gene can be achieved, makes feasible the transfer of corrected or correcting genes for therapy of genetic and gene-influenced diseases. Although continued advances in basic science and technology of gene transfer are required before widespread clinical applications can be achieved, the ultimate importance of these therapeutic approaches and the accelerating progress in the

TABLE 79–1 Candidate Diseases for Gene Therapy

Single Gene Defects	Gene(s) Involved	Target Organs/Tissues
Severe combined immunodeficiency	Adenosine deaminase	Lymphoid tissue
α_1-Antitrypsin deficiency	α_1-Antitrypsin	Lungs (emphysema), liver (cirrhosis)
Cystic fibrosis	Cystic fibrosis transmembrane regulator	Lungs, pancreas
Hemophilia A and B	Factors VIII and IX	Blood clotting
Gaucher's disease	Acid β-glucosidase, glucocerebrosidase	Macrophages; liver, spleen, lungs
β-Hemoglobinopathies	β-Globin	Blood formed elements
Hypercholesterolemia, familial	LDL receptor	Liver; vascular, endothelial; smooth muscle cells
Phenylketonuria	Phenylalanine hydroxylase	Liver
Complex Traits	**Genetic Approach**	**Target Organs/Tissues**
Cancer	Cytokine, HLA genes, thymidine kinase, p53	Various
HIV-1	Antisense constructs, immunoenhancers	Immune system

HIV = human immunodeficiency virus; HLA = human leukocyte antigen; LDL = low-density lipoprotein.

laboratory requires pediatricians to understand how these potential treatments are designed and function.

DEFINITION

Gene therapy is the transfer of recombinant DNA, whether transiently or permanently, into human cells for correction of disease. At present, this involves the transfer of recombinant DNA molecules into somatic cells for correction of a variety of human diseases (Table 79–1; Fig. 79–1). Gene transfer is mediated by vectors, or gene transfer vehicles, that transfer plasmid DNA, RNA, or oligonucleotides to target cells, altering the expression of specific mRNA that directs the synthesis of a

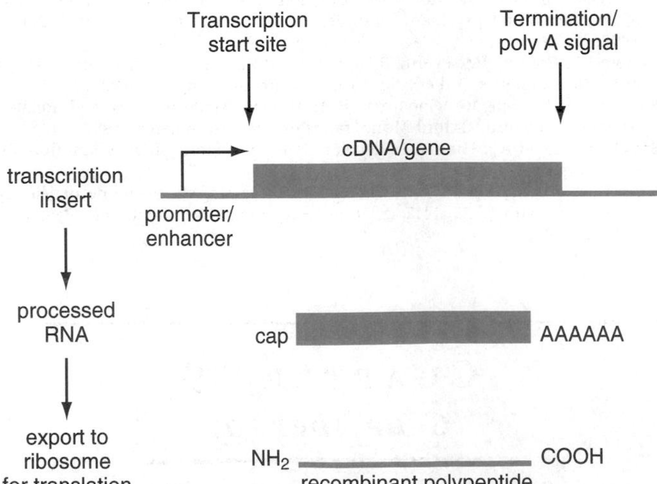

Figure 79–1 Design of a transcriptional unit for expression of recombinant polypeptides. Gene constructs are made using recombinant DNA technology in plasmids. The DNA is engineered to contain promoter enhancer sequences, a transcription start site, cDNA or gene encoding the desired polypeptide, and appropriate termination and polyadenylation signals. After transfer to the target cell, the chimeric gene construct directs synthesis of mRNA. Mature RNA is exported to the ribosomes, where it is translated by cellular machinery into the recombinant polypeptide that can restore physiologic abnormalities in genetically deficient cells or be transferred to distant sites, where therapeutic effects are exerted.

therapeutic protein by the "transfected" cells. The vector is formulated to bind and be internalized by target cells. Vector DNA is transported to the cell nucleus, where the transcriptional machinery of the cell produces a recombinant mRNA. The recombinant RNA is processed and exported from the nucleus to the ribosomes, where translation of the RNA produces the therapeutic protein product. The recombinant protein may correct cellular defects in the target cell or be secreted to alter cellular metabolism at distant sites. Vector DNA may be degraded with lysosomes, maintained within the nucleus as an episomal particle, or integrated permanently into the genome of the host cell. When maintained as an episome in the nucleus of the host cell, loss of the recombinant DNA will occur with each cell division, with expression depending upon the mitotic rate and turnover of the target cells. If recombinant DNA is permanently integrated into the chromosomes of the host progenitor cells that are capable of self-renewal, DNA is permanently transferred to all daughter cells. Transfer and integration of genes into germ cells results in a generationally transmitted trait. Germ line transfer is routinely achieved in a variety of laboratory mammals, that is, transgenic animals. Although it is experimentally feasible to transfer DNA into both human somatic and germ line cells, at present, only transfer to somatic cells is considered ethical. Intense discussions regarding the medical, ethical, social, and economic impact of both somatic cell and germ line gene therapy have accompanied the technical advances that now make gene transfer possible for the treatment of human diseases.

Recombinant DNA technology makes feasible the use of DNA or genes as therapeutic agents or drugs. Detailed understanding of the life cycle of a variety of viruses, including retrovirus, adeno-associated virus, and adenovirus, provides the scientific foundation required to produce delivery vehicles or vectors to transfer the recombinant DNA molecules to a variety of cells and organs. Initially, gene therapy was directed to the transfer of genes to somatic cells to correct single gene disorders, that is, the inborn errors of metabolism, but it is now also directed at treatment of cancers, infectious diseases, and other acquired disorders. Gene therapy (encompassed by the broader term *genetic therapeutics*) also includes treatment with genes that alter a variety of cellular activities or that enhance the properties or activities of existing normal genes, the use of pluripotent stem cells and organoids, the use of both prokaryotes and eukaryotes (both plants and animals) as bioreactors for the production of recombinant molecules of therapeutic interest, and the use of bioengineered proteins and genes for the treatment of inherited and acquired disorders in humans.

SOMATIC CELL VERSUS GERM LINE GENE THERAPY

Two types of gene therapy can be envisioned: (1) the permanent introduction of new or altered genetic material to germ cells, termed germ line gene therapy, which allows generational passage of the genes to offspring; and (2) transfer of DNA to somatic cells that cannot be transmitted to new generations, termed somatic cell gene therapy. The vast majority of diseases currently under consideration for gene therapy result either from single genes or from interactions among multiple genes, and the affected individual is the target of gene therapy. This somatic cell gene therapy to individuals with disease fits the current model of medical care, which treats patients affected by or predisposed to the development of significant life-threatening disease. Since it is not possible, or potentially desirable, to "correct" or alter predisposing genes that might be considered deleterious prior to conception of individuals, germ line gene therapy is outside this model of medicine and is essentially banned worldwide. Therefore, the remainder of this chapter focuses on somatic cell gene therapy: the scientific basis of gene therapy, candidate genes, and some of the current limitations to genetic therapeutics.

Vectors: Delivery Systems for Genes

Transcriptional Unit for Somatic Cell Gene Therapy

Recombinant complementary DNA (cDNA) or genes encoding the therapeutic proteins, like all eukaryotic or prokaryotic genes, must contain all the elements required to direct the transcription of the gene, including a start site and the promoters and enhancers that determine the level and cell-specific regulation of the production of mRNA encoding the therapeutic gene product. Transcriptional control of the introduced gene is directed by the nucleotide sequences (*cis*-acting elements) that are recognized by nuclear proteins (*trans*-acting factors) present in target cells. These *trans*-acting factors direct transcription (the production of RNA from the DNA) of the inserted gene. Transcriptional elements, including enhancers, promoters, silencers, transcriptional start sites, RNA splice-donor sites, and termination and polyadenylation signals, can be incorporated to achieve the desired levels of mRNA, tissue and cell specificity, or the other features of gene regulation required to achieve physiologic correction by the recombinant protein. A typical minimal transcriptional unit is represented by Figure 79–1. More complex constructs containing cell-specific promoter-enhancers or DNA sequences, or both, that control mRNA stability can be engineered into the vectors to confer cell specificity and the ability to control the levels of mRNA produced from the inserted gene. A large repertoire of prokaryotic and eukaryotic promoter-enhancer elements has been developed for achieving appropriate levels of gene expression in specific target cells.

Vector Systems

An idealized vector would be capable of direct in vivo administration through a variety of routes, provide for targeted (tropic) delivery to cells of interest, be safely integrated into the genome in somatic cells, and be transferred to all daughter cells. The site of gene integration would be specific and would include the excision of the defective gene and its replacement by the normal gene. Finally, the vector would be integrated in nononcogenic sites in the genome and require a single administration. Although significant progress has been made in resolving many technical obstacles to the success of gene transfer, current vectors do not satisfy any of these criteria (Table 79–2). Each of these methods has distinct limitations and advantages.

Retroviral, adenoviral, and adeno-associated vectors (AAVs) are currently used in gene therapy protocols in humans. The use of viral vectors for human gene therapy has required substantial modification of the genomes of the wild-type viruses prior to their use to make them nontoxic, monogenic, and nonreplicating. For example, retroviruses are oncoviruses, and expression of their unmodified genomes predisposes the infected organism to malignancy. Adenoviruses can cause severe pulmonary infections and stimulate the host immune system, and they must be administered repeatedly for correction of genetic disorders, since they do not integrate. Although AAV is a nonpathogenic organism in humans, its small capacity for DNA inserts, lack of efficient infection, inefficient production methods, and potential immunogenicity have limited its utility. Because of the need to render the vectors nonreplicating, and therefore nonpathogenic, substantial parts of the viral genomes have been removed, crippling the replication capacity of the virus in vivo. Consequently, cell lines were developed that allow replication and encapsulation of the defective recombinant virus in vitro.

TABLE 79–2 Vectors for Gene Therapy

Vector	Comments
Plasmid DNA	Transient expression
Naked	
Liposomes	
Ligand-DNA complexes	
Retrovirus	Cell division required
RNA virus	Integration into host genome
Adenovirus	Transient expression
DNA virus	Stable virus
	Antigenic
Adeno-associated virus	
DNA parvovirus	

Retroviral Vectors

The retrovirus life cycle is illustrative of the design of packaging cell systems used to produce a noninfectious virus capable of gene transfer. The genomic structure life cycle of a recombinant retrovirus is represented in Figure 79–2. Moloney murine leukemic virus and gibbon leukemic virus have been the most widely used viruses to produce gene transfer vectors. Retroviruses recognize receptors on cell surfaces and are internalized via receptor-mediated endocytosis. The retroviral RNA genome escapes digestion in the endosomes of the transfected cell and is delivered to the nucleus of dividing cells, where preformed viral reverse transcriptase synthesizes a DNA template of the viral genome during mitosis. The viral genome then directs the synthetic processes of the host cell to produce its viral RNA genome and capsid proteins. Following encapsidation, the mature viral particles bud off from the plasma membrane of the packaging cell to produce infective viral particles. The process of incorporation of genomic viral RNA and the use of preformed reverse transcriptase into a complete viral particle is termed *packaging* and requires a specific sequence called the psi (ψ) to signal the packaging events. The ψ sequence is provided in the genome of recombinant viruses used for gene therapy and initiates viral production in the packaging cell lines that complement the genes missing in the disabled retrovirus.

The retroviral genome contains five major elements that include the long terminal repeats, which are powerful promoters; the ψ sequence, which signals packaging events, and three genes called *GAG*, *POL* and *ENV*. These three genes encode encapsidation proteins, reverse transcriptase, and envelope proteins, respectively. Preformed reverse transcriptase that has been carried into the cell with the virus is required for the production of the DNA genome from the viral RNA genome prior to viral replication and production of new viruses. Replication and expression of the viral genes can be separated from the packaging and production of infective viral particles. Consequently, most of the retroviral genome—in particular, the genes that encode for infectivity and oncogenesis *(GAG, POL, ENV)*—can be removed and the therapeutic genes inserted into the regions of the deleted genes. As long as the virus is packaged properly, the genes of the virus are delivered to the appropriate cells and the preformed reverse transcriptase produces the viral DNA for integration into the host genome. Transcription of the therapeutic gene product is directed by gene promoters such as the retroviral LTRs or other promoter-enhancer sequences that can be engineered into the vector.

To achieve the disassociation between pathogenesis and the reproduction of the viral vector carrying the genes of interest, cell lines are produced containing the appropriate retroviral genes for packaging. The retroviral genome is permanently inserted into the chromosomes of the packaging cell line but lacks the ψ sequence. Consequently, a defective retrovirus lacking *GAG*, *POL*, and *ENV*, but containing the promoter, the ψ sequence, and the therapeutic gene, is transfected into the packaging cell line. The latter provides the proteins required for replication and packaging of the recombinant virus. Thus, a recombinant, defective retrovirus uses the packaging and

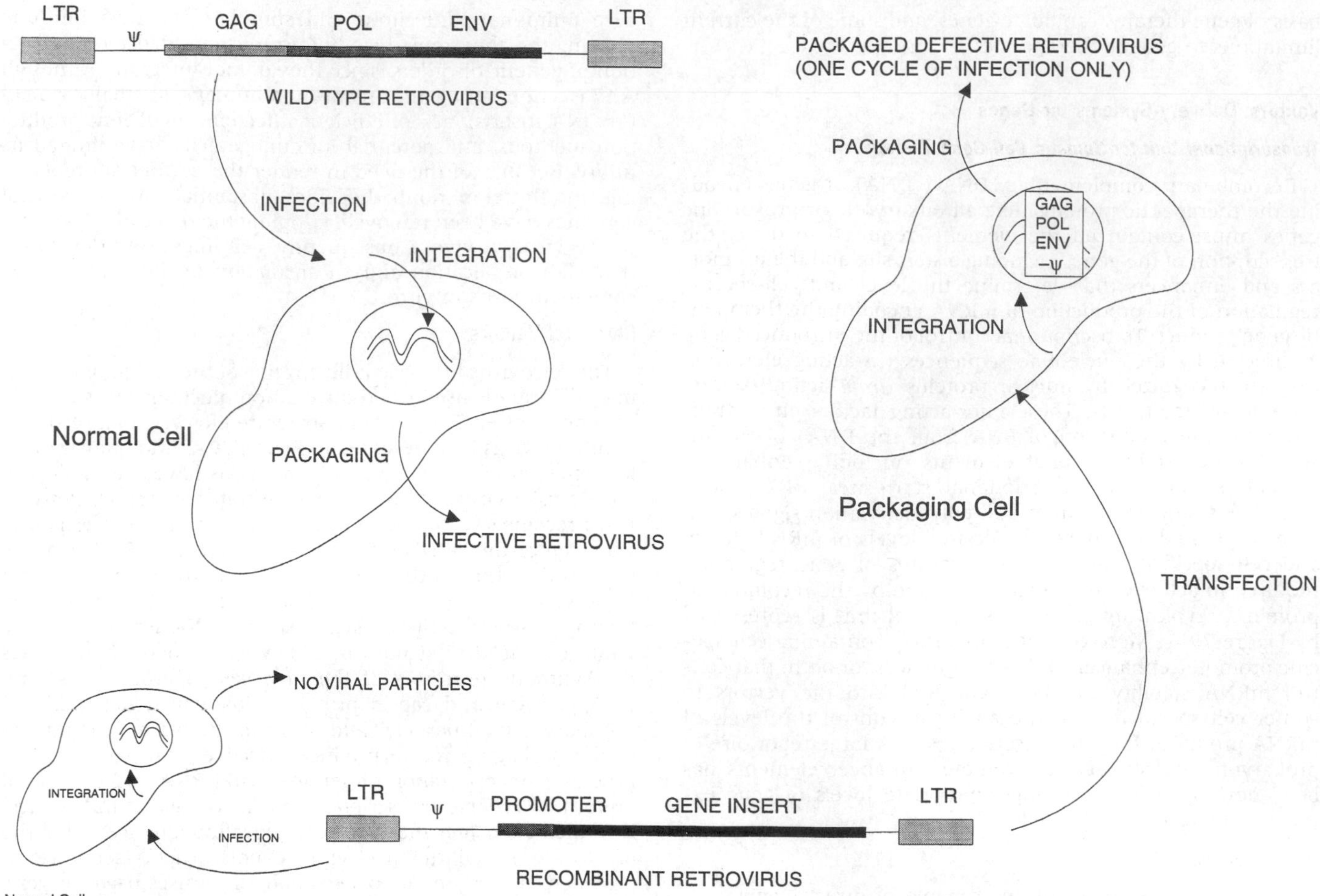

Figure 79–2 Life cycle and organization of wild type and recombinant retrovirus genomes. Retroviruses bind to specific cellular receptors on the target cell surface and are internalized by receptor-mediated endocytosis. Following entry, the retroviral RNA genome is removed from its capsid coat and is reverse transcribed by viral reverse transcriptase into DNA that is transported to the nucleus, where integration into the host genome occurs. In wild type virus, the life cycle is completed by the synthesis of viral proteins and RNA by the host cell, packaging the retroviral particle that is released by budding from the cell surface. Recombinant viruses containing the therapeutic gene or cDNA are replication incompetent, the insert taking the place of the viral genes *GAG, POL,* and *ENV.* "Packaging" lines produce these retroviral gene products in vitro, allowing encapsulation of virus and production of the infectious virions. The "packaged" recombinant virus contains an RNA copy of the therapeutic gene insert that can be used to infect target cells.

encapsidation proteins from the genome of the packaging cell line to make infective viral particles. Resultant viral particles do not contain the genes required for viral pathogenesis and replication but do incorporate the encapsulation proteins and the replication defective recombinant viral RNA genome. High-titer infectious viruses are then obtained by multiple passages through the packaging cell line. The "crippled" recombinant virus is used to transfect the recipient cells of interest, integrating the exogenous genes into the genome of the host cell. Since the genome of the recipient cells does not contain the viral gene sequences for packaging, the crippled retrovirus integrates once and remains in the host cell genome without producing additional viruses. This single integration event does not produce additional viral particles and is termed *transfection* rather than infection. Figure 97–2 shows a typical retroviral vector construct containing the LTRs, the ψ sequence, a promoter, and the gene of interest for incorporation into the target cells.

Since intravenously administered retroviruses are rapidly inactivated, the recombinant retroviruses must be delivered in high titer to the appropriate target cells, by direct local application via physical injection, by organ infusion (i.e., portal vein to the liver), or by ex vivo transfection of stem cells that can be transplanted into the patient. Because of these properties and the clinical importance of hematopoietic disorders, pluripotent bone marrow stem cells have been a primary target for retroviral gene therapy. Although substantial progress has been made in the identification of pluripotent stem cells, they make up a very small percentage of bone marrow cells. The isolation of appropriate quantities of stem cells remains a major limitation of gene therapy. To be transfected, pluripotent stem cells must express receptors for retroviruses and undergo mitosis. Once the pluripotent stem cells are transfected with the retroviral vector, they can be returned to the patient so that the genetic abnormality in bone marrow–derived cells can be corrected. Long-term expression of transgenes has occurred in multiply transplanted mice and in humans receiving autologous bone marrow transplants of genetically marked cells, supporting the ability to transfect bone marrow progenitor cells with retroviruses.

LIMITATIONS OF RETROVIRUSES FOR GENE TRANSFER. Retroviral genomes can incorporate genes of only approximately 4 kb. Most cDNAs for human genes are about 2.5 to 3 kb in length; however, many genes, including hemoglobin, require genomic enhancer sequences on the 5′ and 3′ end to direct their expression. This effectively limits the use of retroviruses in the transfer of relatively small genes or cDNAs that lack desirable regulatory sequences. The ability to permanently integrate exogenous genes into the human genome is a major advantage of retroviruses. Integration is predominantly random, however, making possible the integration into normal genes, which leads to disrupted expression of essential genes. For example, insertion near a tumor suppressor gene could alter its expression and cause tumors. Although "insertional mutagenesis" remains an important theoretical and practical concern, such events appear to be rare. A more serious limitation to the safety of retrovirus for gene therapy is the potential recombination of the therapeutic virus with endogenous retroviruses that can complement the defective virus and allow production of infective retroviral particles. Such recombinations are likely to occur in the packaging cell lines, and major efforts have been directed to ensure the production of "minimal" retroviruses that are incapable of recombination with wild-type retroviruses. Unfortunately, many cell types are not efficiently infected by retrovirus, since this mechanism is perhaps dependent on the presence or absence of specific cell surface receptors on the target cells. Since integration depends on cell division, retroviruses require mitotic cells for integration and expression and are ineffective in transfecting the postmitotic cells present in most adult tissues. Because some retroviruses, including lente virus and foamy virus, do not require cell replication for gene expression, vectors based on these viruses are under investigation.

Adenoviral Vectors

Adenoviruses are DNA viruses that are capable of infecting most cell types; they are being tested for therapy of a variety of human diseases. The life cycle of wild-type adenovirus begins with infection of the host cell by binding to cell surface receptors, followed by endocytosis into the endosomes of the target cell. The adenovirus escapes degradation in the endosomal/lysosomal compartment and is able to efficiently transfer its DNA into the nucleus of the host cells, where it directs replication and reproduction of infective adenoviral particles that are released by cell lysis. The discovery that the *E1* region of the adenoviral genome is critical for the production of infective viral particles led to the design of adenoviruses in which the *E1*, *E3*, or other genes have been deleted, rendering them infective but nonreplicating. Packaging cell lines containing the *E1* genes were developed and used to produce adenovirus containing exogenous cDNAs or genes (Fig. 79–3). The stability of the adenovirus facilitates its production and

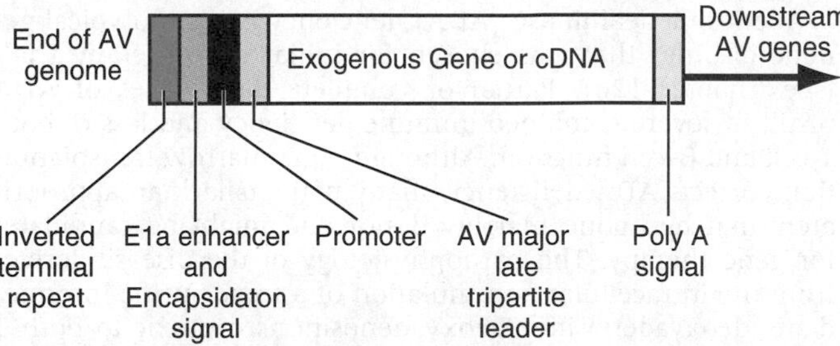

Figure 79–3 Design of *E1*-deleted adenoviral vectors. Adenovirus types 5 and 2, constituting approximately 75 kb, are manipulated using standard recombinant DNA technology in plasmids. The vectors are rendered replication incompetent by deletion of the adenoviral *E1* gene. The exogenous gene or cDNA can be inserted into the adenovirus genome at a variety of sites. For example, deletion of *E3* has been used as a site to insert the exogenous gene. The therapeutic gene is expressed from exogenous promoters or from the LTRs of the adenovirus itself. The replication incompetent adenovirus is propagated in packaging cell lines (293 cells) that provide *E1a* protein in *trans*. The virus is then purified for use as a gene transfer vector. Adenovirus efficiently infects most cell types, directing the synthesis of the exogenous cDNA that directs the synthesis of the therapeutic protein by the target cell.

purification in the laboratory. High-titer, noninfectious adenoviruses have been used to efficiently transfer genes of therapeutic interest to a variety of cell types. Adenoviral DNA is maintained in the cell nucleus in episomal form, directing transient expression of the exogenous therapeutic gene. Episomal DNA is gradually lost by cell replication and DNA degradation, with resultant loss of expression of the transfected gene. Adenoviral vectors do not require cell replication for infectivity or gene expression.

The large genome of adenovirus (75 kb) accommodates gene inserts up to 7 or 8 kb. Highly efficient packaging of cell lines is available and powerful cell selective promoters can be incorporated into the constructs. In contrast to retroviral vectors, which require substantial ex vivo manipulation for infection of pluripotent stem cells, the adenoviral vectors are highly efficient in vivo for delivery of exogenous genes in a variety of cell types. For example, direct instillation of recombinant adenovirus into the respiratory tract is being studied for gene transfer of the cystic fibrosis transmembrane conductance regulator (CFTR) gene for therapy of cystic fibrosis. Administration of adenovirus into the portal vein in experimental animals directs high levels of gene expression in hepatocytes that could be used to transfer α_1-antitryspin or blood clotting factors. Although the transient expression of the adenovirus-delivered genes is a major limitation to permanent gene therapy, adenoviruses are highly efficient and may have advantages in therapy for some diseases. For example, specific antitumor or highly toxic gene sequences could be used to treat malignancies.

Adeno-Associated Viral Vectors

An AAV is a small (4.7 kb) parvovirus whose life cycle requires coinfection with an adenovirus. Interest in the AAV as a gene therapy vector derives from several features of the virus. AAV is nonpathogenic, infects dividing and nondividing cells, integrates into the human genome, and does not express its own genome following transfection of the target cell. Wild-type AAV is capable of site-specific integration on chromosome 19. Similar to retrovirus and adenovirus, production of AAV requires a packaging cell line for replication of recombinant vectors containing the genes of interest. Adenovirus must be added in vitro to achieve viral replication. The need for the adenovirus derives from the life cycle of the AAV. Infective viral particles enter cells via receptor-mediated endocytosis, and their DNA becomes integrated into the genome of cells. During this phase, the virus is nonreplicative and no additional viral particles are produced. Upon exposure of these cells to adenovirus, AAV replication and protein synthesis are activated, and the life cycle of the adenovirus is terminated. The AAV genome contains genes for the entire assembly and production of infective viruses, but their "activation" and release of the integrated virus require the presence of the adenovirus genome and the production of adenoviral proteins *E1*, *E1a*, and *E4*. Following production of capsid and envelope proteins, infective AAV particles are secreted and purified for use in gene transfer. Because the AAV viral cycle includes termination of the adenovirus life cycle, the pathologic consequences of adenoviral infection may be blunted. Similar to other viral vectors, incorporation of specific human genes into AAV requires the removal of the DNA sequences necessary for the life cycle of the AAV. Packaging occurs only in cells that are transfected or infected with adenovirus to produce recombinant AAV virus. Current recombinant AAVs lack the genetic signals that allow selective integration of the AAV genome on human chromosome 19. Like adenovirus, recombinant AAVs used for gene transfer are likely maintained as episomes and do not integrate into the host genome in vivo. The lack of a highly productive packaging cell line, poor efficiency of gene transfer in some tissues, limitations in the size of the DNA that can be inserted into AAV (less than 4–5 kb), and immunologic responses currently limit the use of AAV.

Nonviral Methods of Gene Delivery

A variety of nonviral methods have been developed for gene transfer in vivo and in vitro. These methods use recombinant, plasmid DNA produced in bacteria. Several formulations, including naked DNA and liposomal and protein-DNA conjugates, have been utilized for gene transfer. Incorporation of plasmid DNA into small lipid vesicles or "liposomes," especially when formulated with cationic lipids, markedly enhances the efficiency of DNA delivery to target cells. Altering the composition of the liposomes changes the organ distribution and cellular specificity of the expression of the transferred genes. The lipid-DNA complex binds to the plasma membrane of target cells, perhaps via electrostatic interactions, and is internalized into the endosomes and lysosomes of the target cell. Some DNA escapes degradation in the lysosomes, is released to the cytosol, and is transported to the nucleus. The DNA is maintained as an apisome in the nucleus of the target cells. The DNA is not integrated into the genome and therefore mediates transient gene expression. Thus, repeated administrations of DNA complexes will be required to achieve correction of most genetic disorders. Nevertheless, transient expression may be sufficient for therapeutic effects in a variety of disorders. Plasmid DNA vectors are likely to be applicable for gene therapy of cancer in which toxic genes would be required for relatively short periods of time. The efficiency of gene uptake of plasmid DNA can be further enhanced by linking, covalently or noncovalently, the recombinant plasmid DNA to proteins (ligands) that bind efficiently to cell surface receptors, taking advantage of the high affinity of the ligands for cellular uptake. The DNA-protein complex may be designed to target specific cellular sites expressing receptors recognized by the ligand. Plasmid DNA is readily produced in large quantities in vitro. Furthermore, there are no major limitations in the size of the plasmid DNA that can be transferred into cells. Thus, large cDNAs or genes, including complex regulatory elements, can be incorporated into plasmid-based gene transfer systems. Artificial human chromosomes, which would replicate during cell division, are also being designed for permanent gene transfer.

Host Immunity and Gene Transfer

Host immune responses, both humoral and cellular, are a major obstacle in the application of gene transfer technology for therapy of disease. Immune responses to the vector as well as to the recombinant therapeutic protein result in clearance of cells transfected by the vector. Transfected cells expressing foreign antigens or the recombinant protein can be recognized as non-self and stimulate host immunity. Generation of cytotoxic T cells directed against viral or therapeutic proteins results in the rapid immune cytolysis of transfected cells. Furthermore, neutralizing antibody will block subsequent transfection by the vectors. Thus, vectors must be sought that minimize host immune responses. Antibody produced against the therapeutic protein may be particularly problematic, since it may be recognized as foreign. This occurs with protein replacement therapy in hemophilia and Gaucher's disease; 10% to 15% of treated patients develop antibodies to the administered factor VIII or acid β-glucosidase.

Alternative Strategies

Implantation of genetically altered cells that secrete therapeutic gene products systemically or locally is an alternative approach to in vivo gene therapy. This approach has spawned the field of tissue engineering and the development of *organoids.* Cells that are genetically altered to produce high levels of a secretable gene product are expanded ex vivo. These cells are then transplanted back into the recipient so that the gene product is secreted or delivered locally or systemically to a variety of cell types. Organoids have a variety of advantages for those disorders that can be treated by a secreted protein that functions at distant cellular sites. Examples include expression of factor VIII for hemophilia, β-glucuronidase for correction of mucopolysaccharidosis type VII, and various cytokines for treatment of cancer. The factor VIII cDNA can be permanently transferred to fibroblasts or other cells that are capable of post-translationally modifying and producing factor VIII proenzyme for secretion into the circulation. Transfected ex vivo, the cells are placed subdermally, in blood vessels, or in the peritoneal cavity, or are attached to synthetic membrane supports and transplanted into the recipient. Following vascularization of the graft, factor VIII is secreted into the circulation. Treatment of mucopolysaccharidosis type VII, a β-glucuronidase deficiency, may be possible using organoids capable of attaching a specific ligand—that is, a mannose-6-phosphate—to the β-glucuronidase polypetide. The β-glucuronidase-ligand complex is then delivered to cells expressing mannose-6-phosphate receptors on their surface. The therapeutic enzymes are delivered to the lysosomes of the target cell via endosomal pathways, correcting the β-glucuronidase deficiency in cells bearing this receptor. The pathology of the visceral organs in animal models of mucopolysaccharidosis type VII has been reversed by this approach. Finally, cytokine or cytotoxic genes have been transferred to somatic cells that have been transplanted directly into sites of tumor involvement. The expression of the cytokines, acting as immunoattractants, stimulates an immune response to the tumor cells. Producer cells containing a retrovirus that expresses the herpes thymidine kinase gene have been injected into brain tumors, causing infection of adjacent tumor cells and rendering them susceptible to killing by nucleotide analogs (ganciclovir), which are metabolized to toxic compounds by the viral thymidine kinase but not by the host cell. Systemic administration of ganciclovir to the patient kills tumor cells expressing retroviral-thymidine kinase.

DISEASE TARGETS FOR GENE THERAPY

Genetic diseases that are invariably lethal and without other effective therapies are the appropriate targets for gene therapy. A partial list of such disease candidates for gene therapy is given in Table 79–1.

Adenosine Deaminase Deficiency

Adenosine deaminase (ADA) deficiency is a prototypical genetic disorder that was chosen for initial gene therapy trials (see Chapter 126). Partial or complete deficiencies of ADA result in severe combined immune deficiency and loss of both T-cell and B-cell function. Although bone marrow transplantation corrects ADA deficiency, many patients lack an appropriately matched bone marrow donor and might be candidates for gene therapy. The pathophysiology of the disease derives from the intracellular accumulation of a toxic purine intermediate, deoxyadenosine. Deoxyadenosine is cytotoxic to both T and B cells, resulting in the loss of cellular and humoral immunity and leading to recurrent infections that cause death in childhood. For gene therapy, autologous bone marrow of ADA patients was transfected ex vivo with a recombinant retrovirus containing the ADA cDNA, and these cells were then returned to the patients. Since autologous marrow is used, the therapy represents an isogenic transplant that avoids graft-versus-host reactions. Correction of the recombinant cells results in their selective growth advantage so that the lymphoid cells expressing recombinant ADA live longer than uncorrected cells. Long-term expression of recombinant ADA has been achieved by gene therapy in two patients receiving the retroviral ADA transfected marrow cells.

Currently enzyme replacement therapy with polyethylene glycol–modified bovine ADA (PEG-ADA) infusions is used to treat children who lack the matched donors required for bone marrow transplantation. Although the long-term effects of PEG-ADA treatment have not been assessed and these children still develop serious infections, this therapy leads to partial reconstitution of lymphoid immunity and life saving. Since patients are protected from overwhelming infections by PEG-ADA infusions, the therapeutic effectiveness of gene therapy must be measured during the withdrawal of PEG-ADA or by in vitro methods that are independent of PEG-ADA. Early results suggest a benefit from gene therapy.

Hemoglobinopathies

Hemoglobinopathies and other hematologic disorders are potential candidates for gene therapy (see Table 79–1). Since hematopoietic stem cells can be permanently transfected by retroviral vectors ex vivo and the cells reinserted into the marrow of the patient, diseases like sickle cell anemia, thalassemias, Fanconi's anemia type C, and other disorders of erythropoiesis and myelopoiesis are potentially amenable to gene therapy and are being studied in model laboratory systems.

Lysosomal Storage Diseases

Gaucher disease and mucopolysaccharidosis (MPS) VII are two of the lysosomal storage diseases that are targets for gene therapy (see Chapters 83 and 85). Gaucher disease is caused by mutations in acid β-glucosidase, a protein found in the inner lysosomal membrane of the cell, and MPS VII is caused by a lack of β-glucuronidase, resulting in defective soluble lysosomal protein secreted from cells. Transfection of bone marrow progenitor cells with retrovirus containing the cDNAs encoding these proteins should correct the enzymatic defect in the macrophage/monocyte-derived cells. In contrast, β-glucuronidase is not secreted; thus, correction of Gaucher disease by gene therapy requires transfection of a high percentage of progenitor cells with retrovirus capable of directing the synthesis of the acid β-glucosidase cDNA. Bone marrow ablation or pretreatment with effective enzyme therapy may be required to provide sufficient space for the growth of these transfected bone marrow progenitor cells. Nevertheless, following significant progress in gene therapy in a mouse model of Gaucher disease, human trials using retroviral gene transfer have been initiated.

In MPS VII, the major visceral pathology derives from involvement of bone marrow monocyte/macrophage–derived cell lines and chondrocytes. Central nervous system involvement also occurs in this disease. Gene therapy for MPS VII, with retroviral transfection of bone marrow progenitor cells, should provide functional macrophages that are distributed throughout the body and are capable of secreting the recombinant protein. By expressing high levels of β-glucuronidase, macrophages could also act as organoids, producing the enzyme that will be taken up by macrophages in various organs. In the mouse model of MPS VII, neither enzymes nor transplanted macrophages entered the brain, and pathologic correction was not achieved in the brain, but visceral manifestations of the disease were essentially eradicated by gene transfer. However, Daly et al achieved long-term β-glucuronidase expression and phenotypic reversal, including CNS, in MPS VII mice. These mice received one intravenous dose of AAV containing the β-glucuronidase cDNA during the neonatal period. This suggests the potential of AAV for gene therapy.

Hypercholesterolemia: Low Density Lipoprotein Receptor Defects

Mutations in the low density lipoprotein (LDL) receptor gene (see Chapter 83.3) block LDL uptake in target cells, causing severe, premature atherosclerosis in affected patients. The normal LDL receptor was transferred by retroviral vectors into hepatocytes isolated from the livers of patients with LDL receptor gene defects ex vivo. The transfected cells were grown in culture and reinjected into the patient's portal vein and recolonized the liver. In the two patients who have received this therapy, evidence of decreased serum cholesterol levels was observed. This methodology may be useful for therapy of a variety of metabolic disorders, including phenylketonuria, clotting disorders, and α_1 antitrypsin deficiency.

GENE THERAPY FOR CYSTIC FIBROSIS AND OTHER LUNG DISEASES

Cystic fibrosis is caused by mutations in a membrane protein termed the *cystic fibrosis transmembrane conductance regulator,* or CFTR (see Chapter 416). The CFTR is expressed primarily in epithelial cells and acts as a Cl^- transport protein that enhances Cl^- transport across the epithelial surfaces of numerous organs, including the lungs, gastrointestinal and reproductive tracts, and pancreas. The most common mutation, a deletion of a phenylalanine codon at position 508 of the polypeptide, produces a CFTR protein that is not properly routed to the apical membrane of the affected cells and therefore fails to transport Cl^- following stimulation with cyclic 3′–5′ adenosine monophosphate. Lack of Cl^- and fluid secretion results in the accumulation of mucus in the secretory ducts of many affected organs.

Phase I clinical trials have been initiated with liposomes, adenovirus, and adeno-associated viruses to transfer normal human CFTR cDNA to somatic cells of the epithelium of the lung for correction of the lethal pulmonary complications related to mucous plugging and recurrent infection seen in cystic fibrosis. If the therapy is successful in ameliorating pulmonary disease in these children, it will require repeated administration, since these vectors do not integrate into stem cells of the pulmonary epithelium. The vectors should also not cause untoward toxic or immunologic reactions. Other diseases being studied as targets for gene therapy include lethal hereditary surfactant protein B deficiency, α_1-antitrypsin deficiency, and pulmonary cancer.

RECOMBINANT PROTEIN THERAPIES

The production of recombinant human insulin and human growth hormone in *Escherichia coli* established the value of recombinant DNA technology for production of many medicinal polypeptides and human proteins. However, many potentially therapeutic polypeptides can be produced only in genetically altered eukaryotic cells, such as yeast, insect, and mammalian cells. A variety of support matrices and fibers have been developed to increase production of recombinant proteins from mammalian cell cultures, such as DNAse, tissue plasminogen activator, erythropoietin, and granulocyte-macrophage colony-stimulating factor. The need for mammalian or eukaryotic expression cell systems derives from the specific post-translational processing requirements to produce functional, stable recombinant proteins, including proteolytic processing, oligosaccharide addition and modifications, and polypeptide folding. Transgenic animals and plants also have been developed that use the organism as the bioreactor for the production of human proteins. For example, transgenic goats and cattle have been produced in which the recombinant gene is expressed from promoters that are active only in the mammary gland, the polypeptide being secreted into the milk. Active recombinant proteins are appropriately processed in the mammary gland and can be obtained in large quantities for therapeutic use. Similarly, domesticated plants, such as tobacco, have been used to express human transgenes in leaves.

Protein Modeling and Engineering

Progress in structural biology and the use of site-directed mutagenesis to make mutations in polypeptide sequences that can be expressed by recombinant DNA technology now makes feasible the design and synthesis of novel therapeutic proteins. The alteration of amino acids or groups of amino acids that constitute functional domains in the polypeptide can improve the biologic properties of recombinant polypeptides. For example, polypeptides can be designed to improve synthesis rates, processing, stability, or biologic activity. Likewise, antigenicity of the proteins can be modified to overcome host cell immunity. Not only can novel proteins be designed for administration, but the improved genes themselves could be transferred to direct the synthesis of novel proteins or other gene products that exhibit enhanced biologic activities. By combining the approaches of genetic therapeutics and protein design, it may be possible to overcome some of the limitations related to the lack of efficiency of gene transfer systems. For example, a gene encoding an engineered protein with an increased catalytic rate constant could be incorporated into cells producing a protein with an enhanced therapeutic effect.

ETHICAL AND REGULATORY CONSIDERATIONS

Extensive safeguards have been developed to ensure rigorous scientific assessment of the safety and efficacy of gene therapy trials for both patients and society. A network of review systems has been developed that includes review of protocols by local institutional review boards, supervised by the National Institutes of Health. Once approved, the local institutional protocols are reviewed by the Recombinant DNA Advisory Committee of the National Institutes of Health and, in turn, must then be approved by the Food and Drug Administration. More than 200 individuals have been administered recombinant cells or recombinant vectors for assessment of therapies for lethal diseases under this review process. These important regulatory processes have greatly facilitated the development and widespread acceptance of the scientific validity and ethical appropriateness of gene therapy.

Culver KW: Gene Therapy: A Handbook for Physicians. New York, Mary Ann Liebert, Inc., 1994

Daly TM, Vogler C, Levy B, et al: Neonatal gene transfer leads to widespread correction of pathology in a murine model of lysosomal storage disease. Proc Natl Acad Sci USA 96:2296, 1999.

Davis BD: Germline gene therapy: Evolutionary and moral considerations. Hum Gene Ther 3:336, 1992.

Hoeg JM: Guidelines for trials of gene therapy and somatic gene therapy in cardiovascular disease. Am J Cardiol 81:60F, 1998.

Jane SM, Cunningham JM, Vanin EF: Vector development: A major obstacle in human gene therapy. Ann Med 30:413, 1998.

Suhr ST, Gage FH: Gene therapy in the central nervous system: The use of recombinant retroviruses. Arch Neurol 56:287, 1999.

Wang J, Takabe K, Bidlingmaier SM, et al: Sustained correction of bleeding disorder in hemophilia B mice by gene therapy. Proc Natl Acad Sci USA 96:3906, 1999.

Wang NA, Wilson JM: Methods of gene delivery. Hematol Oncol Clin North Am 12:483, 1998.

CHAPTER 80

Genetic Counseling

Judith G. Hall

When a child is born with multiple congenital anomalies or a family is diagnosed with a genetic disorder, talking with the family is not easy. Giving bad news is always difficult, and the information is often somewhat technical. However, it is important to provide the family with as much information as possible so that they can make informed decisions. Genetic counseling has been defined as "an educational process that seeks to assist affected and/or at risk individuals to understand the nature of a genetic disorder, its transmission and the options available to them in management and family planning."

Although the task of providing information about genetic diseases is often done by a team of highly trained medical geneticists and genetic counselors, the information can also be provided by a family physician, pediatrician, or nurse. Genetic counseling must be done based on an understanding of genetic principles, the ability to recognize and diagnose genetic diseases and rare syndromes, and knowledge of the natural history of the disorder and its recurrence risk. Awareness of prenatal diagnosis and screening programs available in a particular region and access to information about new advances in genetic disorders and medical techniques are also necessary.

TALKING TO FAMILIES

The type of information provided to a family depends on the urgency of the situation, the need to make decisions, and the need to collect additional information. However, there are three general situations in which genetic counseling becomes particularly important.

The first is the prenatal diagnosis of a congenital anomaly or genetic disease. This is a very difficult situation, and the need for information is urgent because a family must often decide whether to continue or to terminate a pregnancy. The second type of situation occurs when a child is born with a congenital anomaly or genetic disease. This also requires urgent information, and decisions must be made immediately with regard to how much support should be provided for the child and whether certain types of therapy should be attempted. The third situation arises later in life when (1) a diagnosis with a genetic implication is made, (2) a couple is planning a family and there is a family history of the problem (e.g., a couple in which one person carries a translocation or is a carrier of cystic fibrosis), or (3) an adolescent or young adult has a family history of an adult-onset genetic disorder (e.g., Huntington's disease or breast cancer). It is often necessary to have several meetings with a family; all of their questions and concerns usually cannot be adequately addressed at one time.

Genetic Counseling

Providing accurate information to families requires (1) taking a careful family history and constructing a pedigree that lists the patient's relatives (including abortions, stillbirths, and deceased individuals) with their sex, age, and state of health; (2) gathering information from hospital records about the affected individual (and in some cases, other family members); (3) documenting the prenatal, pregnancy, and delivery history; (4) reviewing the available information concerning the disorder; (5) careful physical examination of the affected individual (with photographs and measurements) and of apparently unaffected individuals in the family; (6) establishing or confirming the diagnosis by the diagnostic tests available; (7) giving the family information about support groups; and (8) providing new information to the family as it becomes available.

To provide optimal benefits, the counseling session must include certain information.

KNOWLEDGE OF THE DIAGNOSIS OF THE PARTICULAR CONDITION. Although it is not always possible to make an exact diagnosis, having as accurate a diagnosis as possible is important. Estimates of recurrence risk for various family members depend on an accurate diagnosis. When a specific diagnosis cannot be made (as in many cases of multiple congenital anomalies), the various differential diagnoses should be discussed with the family and empirical information provided. If specific diagnostic tests are available, they should be discussed.

NATURAL HISTORY OF THE CONDITION. It is very important to discuss the natural history of the specific genetic disorder in the family. Affected individuals and their families will have questions regarding the prognosis and potential therapy that can be answered only with knowledge of the natural history. If there are other possible differential diagnoses, their natural history may also be discussed. If the disorder is associated with a spectrum of clinical outcomes or complications, the worst and best scenario, as well as treatment and referral to the appropriate specialist, should be addressed.

GENETIC ASPECTS OF THE CONDITION AND RECURRENCE RISK. This is important information for the family because family members need to be aware of their reproductive choices. The genetics of the disorder can be explained with visual aids (e.g., figures of chromosomes). It is important to provide accurate occurrence and recurrence risks for various members of the family, including unaffected individuals, cousins, aunts, and so forth. In cases in which a definite diagnosis cannot be made, it will be necessary to use empirical recurrence risks. Counseling should give the individuals the necessary information to understand the various options and to make their own informed decisions regarding pregnancies, adoption, artificial insemination, prenatal diagnosis, screening, carrier detection, and termination of pregnancy. To complete the educational process, it is often necessary to have more than one counseling session.

PRENATAL DIAGNOSIS AND PREVENTION. Many different methods of prenatal diagnosis are available, depending on the specific genetic disorder. The use of ultrasonography allows prenatal diagnosis of anatomic abnormalities such as neural tube defects. Amniocentesis and chorionic villus sampling are used to obtain fetal tissue for analysis of chromosomal abnormalities, biochemical disorders, and DNA studies. Maternal blood or serum sampling is used for some types of screening.

THERAPIES AND REFERRAL. A number of genetic disorders require the care of a specialist. For example, individuals with Turner's syndrome usually need to be evaluated by an endocrinologist. Prevention of known complications is a priority. The psychologic adjustment of the family may require specific intervention.

SUPPORT GROUPS. Over the last decade, a large number of lay support groups have been formed to provide information and to fund research on specific genetic and nongenetic conditions. An important part of genetic counseling is to give information about these groups to individuals and to suggest a contact person for the families. Many groups have established Web sites with very helpful information.

FOLLOW-UP. Families should be encouraged to continue to ask questions and keep up with new information about the specific disorder. New developments often influence the diagnosis and therapy of specific genetic disorders. Lay groups are a good source of new information.

Alliance of Genetic Support Groups: Directory of National Genetic Voluntary Organizations, 35 Wisconsin Circle, Suite 440, Chevy Chase, Maryland 20815-7015, founded 1995.

Harper PS: Practical Genetic Counselling, 4th ed. Oxford, Butterworth-Heinemann Ltd, 1993.

Hubbard R, Lewontin RC: Pitfalls of genetic testing. N Engl J Med 334:1192, 1996.

OMIM: A guide to the use of OMIM. GBD/OMIM User Support, 2024 East Monument Street, Baltimore, MD 21205 Tel: (410) 955-9705; Fax: (410) 614-0434; e-mail: help@gdb.org.

Stevenson RE, Hall JG, Goodman RM: Human Malformations and Related Anomalies. Oxford, Oxford Monographs on Medical Genetics, 1993.

Task Force on Genetic Testing, National Institutes of Health, Department of Energy Working Group on Ethical, Legal, and Social Implications of Human Genome Research; NA Holtzman, MS Watson (eds): Promoting Safe and Effective Genetic Testing in the United States: Final Report of the Task Force on Genetic Testing. Bethesda, Maryland: The Human Genome Research Institute, 1997.

PART X

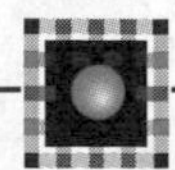

Metabolic Diseases

CHAPTER 81

An Approach to Inborn Errors

Iraj Rezvani and David S. Rosenblatt

Many childhood conditions are caused by gene mutations that encode specific proteins. These mutations can result in the alteration of primary protein structure or the amount of protein synthesized. The functional ability of protein, whether it is an enzyme, receptor, transport vehicle, membrane, or structural element, may be relatively or seriously compromised. These hereditary biochemical disorders were collectively termed *inborn errors of metabolism* by Garrod at the turn of the 20th century.

Most mutations are clinically inconsequential and represent polymorphic differences that set individuals apart *(genetic polymorphism)*. However, some mutations produce disease states that range from very mild to lethal. Most inborn errors of metabolism exhibiting clinical consequences manifest themselves (or can be detected) in the newborn period or shortly thereafter. It is also now possible to screen and detect many of these disorders in utero (see Chapter 92).

Children with inborn errors of metabolism may present with one or more of a large variety of signs and symptoms. These may include metabolic acidosis, persistent vomiting, failure to thrive, developmental delay, elevated blood or urine levels of a particular metabolite (an amino acid or ammonia), a peculiar odor (Table 81–1), or physical changes such as hepatomegaly. Diagnosis is facilitated by considering those presenting in the neonatal period separately from children presenting later in life.

NEONATAL PERIOD. Inborn errors of metabolism causing *clinical manifestations* in the neonatal period are usually severe and are often lethal if proper therapy is not promptly initiated. Clinical findings are usually nonspecific and similar to those seen in infants with sepsis. An inborn error of metabolism should be considered in the differential diagnosis of a severely ill neonatal infant, and special studies should be undertaken if the index of suspicion is high (Fig. 81–1).

TABLE 81–1 Inborn Errors of Amino Acid Metabolism Associated with Abnormal Odor

Inborn Error of Metabolism	Urine Odor
Glutaric acidemia (type II)	Sweaty feet
Hawkinsinuria	Swimming pool
Isovaleric acidemia	Sweaty feet
Maple syrup urine disease	Maple syrup
Hypermethioninemia	Boiled cabbage
Multiple carboxylase deficiency	Tomcat urine
Oasthouse urine disease	Hops-like
Phenylketonuria	Mousy or musty
Trimethylaminuria	Rotting fish
Tyrosinemia	Boiled cabbage

Infants with metabolic disorders are usually normal at birth; however, signs and symptoms such as lethargy, poor feeding, convulsions, and vomiting may develop as early as a few hours after birth. A history of clinical deterioration in a previously normal neonate should suggest an inborn error of metabolism. This clinical course contrasts with many other genetic disorders or perinatal insults, which cause abnormalities from the time of birth. Occasionally, vomiting may be severe enough to suggest the diagnosis of pyloric stenosis, which is usually not present, although it has simultaneously occurred in such infants. Lethargy, poor feeding, convulsions, and coma may also be seen in infants with hypoglycemia (see Chapters 88 and 103.2) or hypocalcemia (see Chapter 55.9). Response to intravenous injection of glucose or calcium usually establishes these diagnoses. Because most inborn errors of metabolism are inherited as autosomal recessive traits, a history of consanguinity and/or death in the neonatal period in the immediate family should increase suspicion of this diagnosis. Some of these disorders have a high incidence in specific population groups. For instance, tyrosinemia type 1 is more common among French-Canadians of Quebec than in the general population. Therefore, the knowledge of ethnic background of the patient may be helpful in diagnosis. *Physical examination* usually reveals nonspecific findings, with most signs related to the central nervous system. Hepatomegaly, however, is a common finding in a variety of inborn errors of metabolism. Occasionally, an unusual odor may offer an invaluable aid to the diagnosis (see Table 81–1). A physician caring for a sick infant should smell the patient and his or her excretions; patients with maple syrup urine disease have the unmistakable odor of maple syrup in their urine and their bodies.

Diagnosis usually requires a variety of specific *laboratory studies*. Measuring serum concentrations of ammonia, bicarbonate, and pH is often very helpful in differentiating major causes of metabolic disorders (see Fig. 81–1). Elevation of blood ammonia is usually due to defects in urea cycle enzymes. These infants with elevated blood ammonia levels commonly have normal serum pH and bicarbonate, and without measurement of blood ammonia they may remain undiagnosed and succumb to their disease. Elevation of serum ammonia, however, has also been observed in some infants with certain organic acidemias. These infants are severely acidotic because of accumulation of organic acids in body fluids.

When blood ammonia, pH, and bicarbonate are normal, other aminoacidopathies (such as hyperglycinemia) or galactosemia should be considered; galactosemic infants may also manifest cataracts, hepatomegaly, ascites, and jaundice.

Most inborn errors of metabolism presenting in the neonatal period are lethal if specific *treatment* is not initiated immediately. Specific diagnosis, even in an infant in whom death seems inevitable, is of great importance for genetic counseling of the family (see Chapter 80). Therefore, every effort should be made to determine the diagnosis while the infant is alive; postmortem examination is usually not helpful.

CHILDREN AFTER THE NEONATAL PERIOD. Most inborn errors of metabolism that cause symptoms in the first few days of life exhibit milder variant forms that have a more insidious onset. These forms may escape detection during the neonatal period, and the diagnosis may be delayed for months or even years.

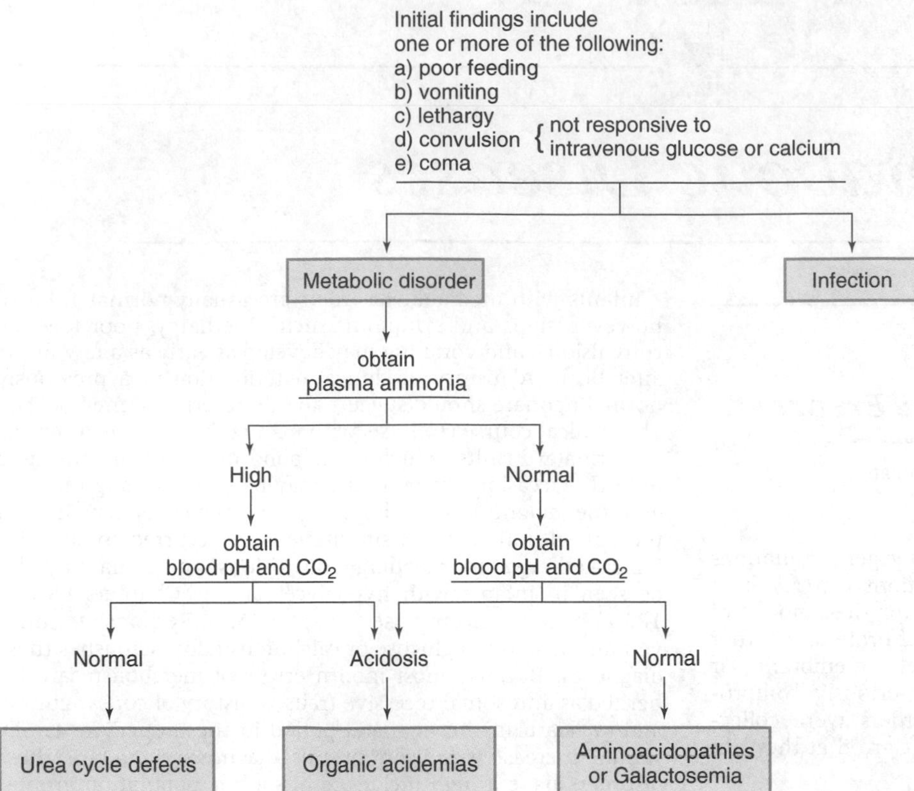

Figure 81–1 Clinical approach to a newborn infant with a suspected metabolic disorder. This schema is a guide to the elucidation of some of the metabolic disorders in newborn infants. Although some exceptions to this schema exist, it is appropriate for most cases.

The early clinical manifestations in children with these forms are commonly nonspecific and may be attributed to perinatal insults. *Clinical manifestations,* such as mental retardation, motor deficits, and convulsions are the most constant findings in these children. There may be an episodic or intermittent pattern with episodes of acute clinical manifestations separated by periods of seemingly disease-free states. The episodes are usually triggered by a stress or a nonspecific insult such as an infection. The child may die during one of these acute attacks. An inborn error of metabolism should be considered in any child with one or more of the following manifestations: (1) unexplained mental retardation, developmental delay, motor deficits, or convulsions; (2) unusual odor, particularly during an acute illness; (3) intermittent episodes of unexplained vomiting, acidosis, mental deterioration, or coma; (4) hepatomegaly; or (5) renal stones.

Inborn errors of metabolism of a given pedigree run true to type. Thus, although symptomatology may vary among siblings, usually if one child in a family, for example, has the neonatal form of a condition, the next affected sibling will have the same form.

CHAPTER 82
Defects in Metabolism of Amino Acids

82.1 Phenylalanine

Iraj Rezvani

Phenylalanine is an essential amino acid. Dietary phenylalanine not utilized for protein synthesis is normally degraded via the tyrosine pathway (Fig. 82–1). Deficiency of the enzyme phenylalanine hydroxylase or of its cofactor tetrahydrobiopterin causes accumulation of phenylalanine in body fluids. Several clinically and biochemically distinct forms of hyperphenylalaninemia exist.

CLASSIC PHENYLKETONURIA (PKU). This form of the disorder is caused by the complete or near-complete deficiency of phenylalanine hydroxylase. Excess phenylalanine is transaminated to phenylpyruvic acid or decarboxylated to phenylethylamine (see Fig. 82–1). These and subsequent metabolites, along with excess phenylalanine, disrupt normal metabolism and cause brain damage.

Clinical Manifestations. The affected infant is normal at birth. Mental retardation may develop gradually and may not be evident for a few months. It has been estimated that an untreated infant loses about 50 points in IQ by the end of the first yr of life (4 IQ points per mo). Mental retardation is usually severe, and most patients require institutional care. Vomiting, sometimes severe enough to be misdiagnosed as pyloric stenosis, may be an early symptom. Older untreated children become hyperactive with purposeless movements, rhythmic rocking, and athetosis.

On physical examination these infants are blonder than unaffected siblings; they have fair skin and blue eyes. Some may have a seborrheic or eczematoid skin rash, which is usually mild and disappears as the child grows older. These children have an unpleasant odor of phenylacetic acid, which has been described as musty or mousey. There are no consistent findings on neurologic examination. However, most infants are hypertonic with hyperactive deep tendon reflexes. About one fourth of children have seizures, and more than 50% have electroencephalographic (EEG) abnormalities. Microcephaly, prominent maxilla with widely spaced teeth, enamel hypoplasia, and growth retardation are other common findings in untreated children. The clinical manifestations of classic PKU are rarely seen in those countries in which neonatal screening programs for the detection of PKU are in effect.

Diagnosis. Infants with PKU are clinically normal at birth, and

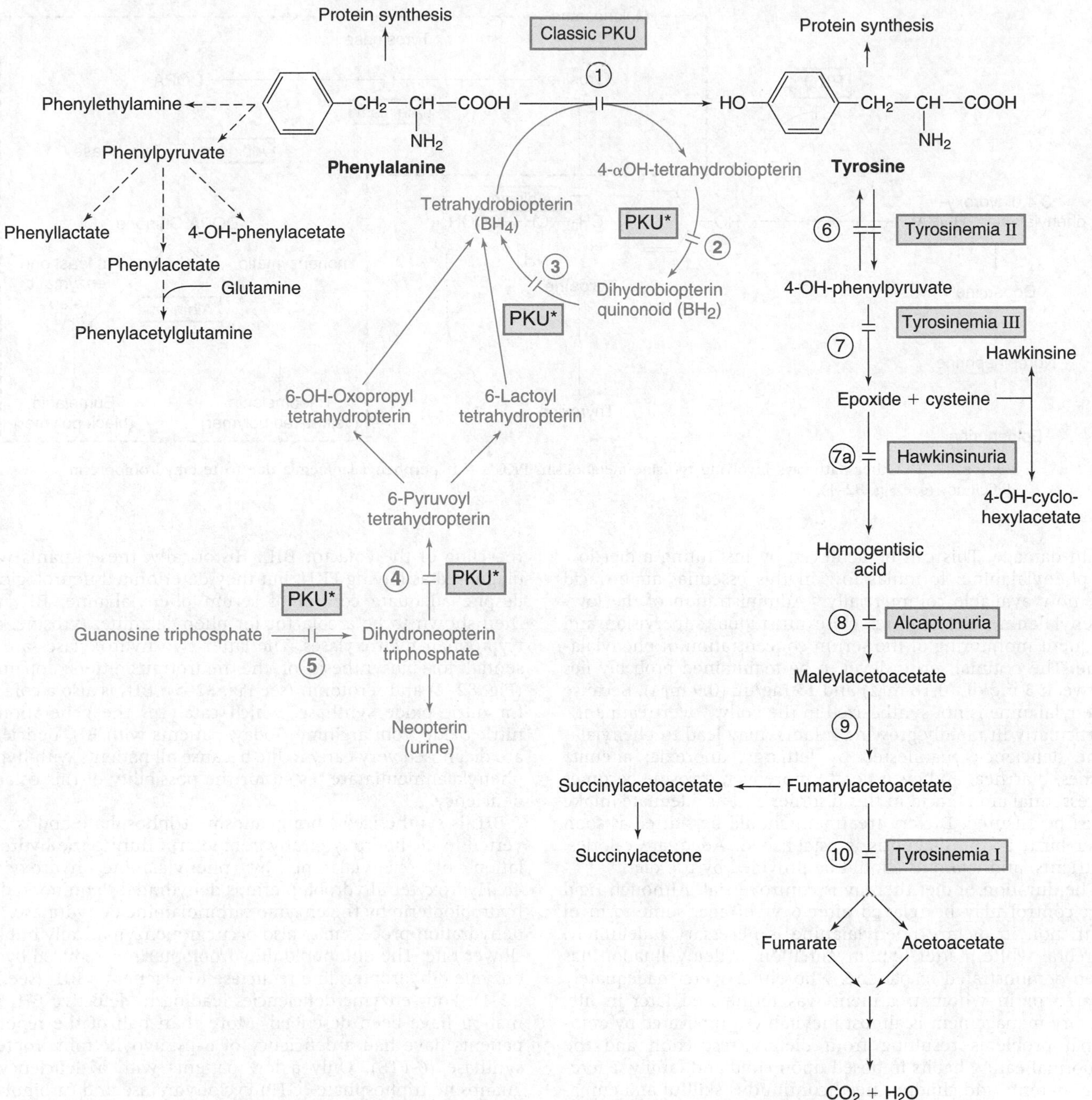

Figure 82–1 Pathways of phenylalanine and tyrosine metabolism. Inborn errors are depicted as bars crossing the reaction arrow(s). Pathways for synthesis of cofactor BH_4 are shown in green. PKU* refers to defects of BH_4 metabolism that affect the phenylalanine, tyrosine, and tryptophan hydroxylases. See Figures 82–2 and 82–4. **Enzymes:** (1) phenylalanine hydroxylase; (2) carbinolamine dehydratase; (3) dihydropteridine reductase; (4) 6-pyruvoyltetrahydropterin synthase; (5) guanosine triphosphate (GTP) cyclohydrolase; (6) tyrosine aminotransferase; (7a) intramolecular rearrangement; (7 + 7a) 4-Hydroxyphenylpyruvate dioxygenase; (8) homogentisic acid dioxygenase; (9) maleylacetoacetate isomerase; (10) fumarylacetoacetate hydroxylase.

tests of their urine for phenylpyruvic acid may be negative in the first few days of life; accordingly, the diagnosis depends on measuring blood levels of phenylalanine. The bacterial inhibition assay method of Guthrie is widely used in the newborn period to screen for PKU. This test requires a few drops of capillary blood, which are placed on a filter paper and mailed to the laboratory for assay. Blood phenylalanine in affected infants may rise to levels necessary to render the Guthrie test positive as early as 4 hr after birth in the absence of any protein feeding. It is recommended, however, that the blood for screening be obtained after 48–72 hr of life and preferably after feeding proteins in order to reduce the possibility of false-negative results. When this test indicates an elevated level of phenylalanine, the phenylalanine and tyrosine concentrations of the plasma should be measured. The criteria for diagnosis of classic PKU are (1) a plasma phenylalanine level above 20 mg/dL (1.2 mM); (2) a normal plasma tyrosine level; (3) increased urinary levels of metabolites of phenylalanine (phenylpyruvic and *o*-hydroxyphenylacetic acids); and (4) a normal concentration of the cofactor tetrahydrobiopterin.

Treatment. The goal of therapy is to reduce phenylalanine and its metabolites in body fluids in order to prevent or minimize

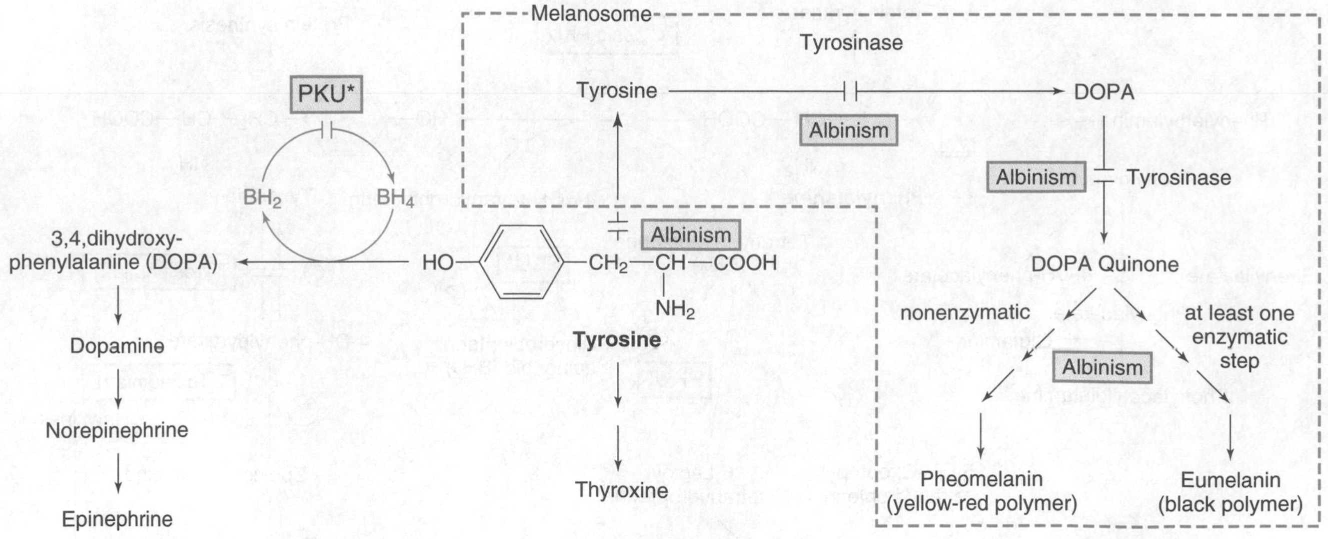

Figure 82–2 Other pathways involving tyrosine metabolism. PKU* = hyperphenylalaninemia due to tetrahydrobiopterin deficiency (see Fig. 82-1).

brain damage. This can be achieved by instituting a diet low in phenylalanine; formulas low in this essential amino acid are now available commercially.* Administration of the low-phenylalanine diet requires close nutritional supervision and frequent monitoring of the serum concentration of phenylalanine. The optimal serum level to be maintained probably lies between 3 mg/dL (0.18 mM) and 15 mg/dL (0.9 mM). Because phenylalanine is not synthesized in the body, "overtreatment," particularly in rapidly growing infants, may lead to phenylalanine deficiency, manifested by lethargy, anorexia, anemia, rashes, diarrhea, and even death; moreover, tyrosine becomes an essential amino acid in this disorder and its adequate intake must be ensured. Dietary treatment should be started as soon after birth as the diagnosis is established. Adequate calories, nutrients, and vitamins should be provided by the diet.

The duration of diet therapy is controversial. Although rigid diet control may be relaxed after 6 yr of age, some form of restriction in dietary phenylalanine is necessary indefinitely. Cerebral white matter hypomyelination or demyelination has been demonstrated in patients who either were inadequately treated or in whom treatment was terminated later in life. Dietary management is almost inevitably complicated by emotional problems resulting from dietary restriction and the abnormal eating habits imposed upon child and family. Therefore, parents and children need continuous skillful and empathetic support and guidance.

Pregnancy in Mothers with PKU (Maternal PKU). Pregnant women with PKU who are not on a low-phenylalanine diet have a higher risk of spontaneous abortion than the general population. Infants born to such mothers are often mentally retarded and may have microcephaly and/or a congenital heart anomaly. Hypoplasia of the corpus callosum is common. These complications are related to high maternal levels of blood phenylalanine during pregnancy. Prospective mothers who have PKU should be started on a low-phenylalanine diet before conception, and every effort should be made to keep blood phenylalanine levels below 10 mg/dL (<600 μM) throughout pregnancy.

HYPERPHENYLALANINEMIA DUE TO DEFICIENCY OF COFACTOR TETRAHYDROBIOPTERIN (BH_4) ("MALIGNANT" HYPERPHENYLALANINEMIA). In about 2% of infants with hyperphenylalaninemia, the defect resides in one of the enzymes necessary for production or recycling of the cofactor BH_4. Historically, these infants were diagnosed as having PKU, but they deteriorated neurologically despite adequate control of serum phenylalanine; BH_4 was then shown to be a cofactor for phenylalanine, tyrosine, and tryptophan hydroxylases. The latter two hydroxylases are essential for biosynthesis of the neurotransmitters dopamine (Fig. 82–2) and serotonin (see Fig. 82–5). BH_4 is also a cofactor for nitric oxide synthase, which catalyzes the generation of nitric oxide from arginine. Today, patients with BH_4 deficiency are diagnosed very early in life because all patients with hyperphenylalaninemia are tested for the possibility of this cofactor deficiency.

BH_4 is synthesized from guanosine triphosphate and is converted to 4α-hydroxytetrahydrobiopterin during the hydroxylation of phenylalanine by phenylalanine hydroxylase. 4α-Hydroxytetrahydrobiopterin is dehydrated to quinonoid dihydrobiopterin by the enzyme carbinolamine dehydratase. The dehydration process may also occur nonenzymatically but at a slower rate. The quinonoid dihydrobiopterin is reduced by the enzyme dihydropteridine reductase to regenerate BH_4 (see Fig. 82–1). Four enzyme deficiencies leading to defective BH_4 formation have been described. More than half of the reported patients have had a deficiency of 6-pyruvoyltetrahydropterin synthase (6-PTS). Only a few patients with a deficiency of guanosine triphosphate (GTP) cyclohydratase and carbinolamine dehydratase have been reported. The remaining patients have had a deficiency of dihydropteridine reductase.

Clinical Manifestations. These signs and symptoms are similar and usually indistinguishable from those of classic PKU. These patients are identified during screening programs for PKU because of evidence of hyperphenylalaninemia, but neurologic manifestations, such as loss of head control, hypertonia, drooling, swallowing difficulties, and myoclonic seizures, develop after 3 mo of age despite adequate dietary therapy. The exception to this malignant course occurs in patients with carbinolamine dehydratase deficiency in whom the clinical manifestations may be none other than mild hyperphenylalaninemia. This is not surprising because BH_2 is formed slowly without the enzyme action. Plasma phenylalanine levels may be as high as those in classic PKU or in the range of benign (persistent) hyperphenylalaninemia (<1.0 mM).

Diagnosis. BH_4 deficiency and the responsible enzyme defect may be established by performing one of the following tests:

1. Measurement of neopterin (oxidative product of dihydroneopterin triphosphate) and biopterin (oxidative product of

*Dietary management with this milk substitute is described in "Phenylketonuria—Low Phenylalanine Dietary Management with Lofenalac," a pamphlet available from Mead Johnson Laboratories, Evansville, IN 47721.

dihydro- and tetrahydrobiopterin) in body fluids (see Fig. 82–1) especially urine. In patients with 6-pyruvoyltetrahydropterin synthase deficiency, there is a marked elevation of neopterin and a concomitant decrease in biopterin exretion (neopterin-biopterin ratio is high). In patients with GTP cyclohydrolase deficiency, urinary excretion of both neopterin and biopterin is very low, and in patients with dihydropteridine reductase deficiency, neopterin is normal, but biopterin is very high (neopterin-biopterin ratio is low). Excretion of biopterin increases in this enzyme deficiency because the quinonoid dihydrobiopterin cannot be recycled into BH_4. Patients with carbinolamine dehydratase deficiency excrete 7-biopterin (an unusual isomer of biopterin) in their urine.

2. BH_4 loading test. An oral or intravenous (more reliable if feasible) dose of BH_4 (7–10 mg/kg) normalizes plasma phenylalanine in patients with BH_4 deficiency within 4–6 hr. This test should be done while the child is receiving normal amounts of phenylalanine in the diet. Some patients with dihydropteridine reductase deficiency may not respond to this loading test.

3. Enzyme assay. The activity of dihydropteridine reductase can be measured in many tissues, including liver, leukocytes, red blood cells, and cultured fibroblasts. 6-Pyruvoyltetrahydropterin synthase can be measured in liver, kidney, and red blood cells. GTP cyclohydrolase can be measured in liver and in phytohemagglutinin-stimulated lymphocytes (the enzyme activity is normally very low in unstimulated lymphocytes). Measurement of the last two enzymes is technically difficult, and assays are not readily available.

4. Gene study. Genes for dihydropteridine reductase and carbinolamine dehydratase have been identified. Identification of mutations in these gene in affected patients and their families is now possible.

Treatment. The long-term efficacy of various therapies is unknown. The various treatment methods include the following:

1. Low-phenylalanine diet. Although phenylalanine does not prevent neurologic damage, such a diet in conjunction with the following therapies is recommended for at least the first 2 yr of life. High levels of phenylalanine inhibit the synthesis of neurotransmitters.

2. Neurotransmitter precursors. Administration of the L-dopa and 5-hydroxytryptophan seems to be the most effective treatment and may prevent neurologic damage if started early in life. Therefore, *all patients with PKU and hyperphenylalaninemia should be tested for BH_4 deficiency as early as possible.* Treatment started after 6 mo of age, although resulting in some improvement, has not reversed existing neurologic damage.

3. BH_4 replacement. Oral administration of the cofactor in small daily doses normalizes serum levels of phenylalanine. This compound, unless given at high doses (20–40 mg/kg/24 hr), does not readily cross the blood-brain barrier, and neurologic damage may continue to progress.

BENIGN HYPERPHENYLALANINEMIA. Infants with hyperphenylalaninemia are occasionally identified as those whose blood levels of phenylalanine are only slightly elevated; these concentrations are not enough (less than 20 mg/dL or 1.2 mM) to result in the excretion of phenylpyruvic acid. Like infants with classic PKU, these patients presumably have a deficiency of the phenylalanine hydroxylase enzyme but with some residual enzyme activity; measured activity has ranged from 1% to 35% of normal, in contrast to the nondetectable enzyme activity found in classic PKU. These infants have been detected by screening tests in the neonatal period; they are asymptomatic and may develop normally without special dietary treatment. They should, however, be tested for the presence of the cofactor tetrahydrobiopterin, and if it is deficient, they should be treated accordingly (see earlier).

For infants who have serum phenylalanine concentrations in the range of 10–20 mg/dL, with normal tyrosine values and no PKU, a simple reduction of dietary protein intake may be sufficient to control serum concentrations of phenylalanine; if this is not effective, specific restriction of dietary phenylalanine is indicated. All infants who are not treated with dietary restriction should be systematically monitored with repeated determinations of plasma phenylalanine and developmental evaluations to establish the safety of continuing partial treatment or nontreatment. Periodic challenges with natural protein may be helpful in determining the need for continuing dietary restriction.

TRANSIENT HYPERPHENYLALANINEMIA. Moderately elevated levels of phenylalanine occur in transient tyrosinemia of the newborn infant (see Chapter 82.2). When the infant's ability to oxidize tyrosine matures, the elevated levels of tyrosine and phenylalanine return to normal.

Absence of or delayed maturation of phenylalanine transaminase can also produce hyperphenylalaninemia if the patient is fed milk with a high protein content. Such infants cannot produce much phenylpyruvic acid, even when their blood levels of phenylalanine approach 30 mg/dL; they have normal blood levels when fed milk products having the protein content of human milk.

GENETICS AND PREVALENCE. All defects causing persistent hyperphenylalaninemia and PKU are inherited as autosomal recessives. They have a collective prevalence of 1:10,000 to 1:20,000 live births, with classic PKU being the most common and GTP cyclohydrolase the rarest. The gene for phenylalanine hydroxylase is located on the long arm of chromosome 12. Over 100 mutations of the gene have been described in different families. Most patients are compound heterozygotes. The genes for carbinolamine dehydratase and dihydropteridine reductase are located on the long arm of chromosome 10 and the short arm of chromosome 4, respectively. Prenatal diagnosis and carrier detection are possible using specific genetic probes in cells obtained from chorionic villus biopsy.

82.2 Tyrosine

Iraj Rezvani

Tyrosine, obtained from ingested protein and synthesized endogenously from phenylalanine, is used for protein synthesis and is a precursor of dopamine, norepinephrine, epinephrine, melanin, and thyroxine. Excess tyrosine is metabolized to carbon dioxide and water (see Fig. 82–1). Hypertyrosinemia is observed with deficiencies of tyrosine aminotransferase, 4-hydroxyphenpyruvate dioxigenase (4-HPPD), or fumarylacetoacetate hydrolase (FAH). The causal relationship of high levels of tyrosine with the diseased state has been established only in deficiency of tyrosine aminotransferase (tyrosinemia type II). The significance of hypertyrosinemia in the pathogenesis of the other two enzyme deficiencies is unclear.

Deficiencies of other enzymes involved in tyrosine degradation cause little or no increase in blood levels of tyrosine. Acquired conditions such as severe hepatocellular dysfunction (liver failure), scurvy (vitamin C is the cofactor of 4-HPPD enzyme), and hyperthyroidism may cause varying degrees of hypertyrosinemia.

TYROSINEMIA TYPE I (Tyrosinosis, Hereditary Tyrosinemia, Hepatorenal Tyrosinemia). In this condition, caused by a deficiency of the enzyme fumarylacetoacetate hydrolase, a moderate elevation of serum tyrosine is associated with severe involvement of the liver, kidney, and central nervous system. These findings are thought to be due to an accumulation of intermediate metabolites of tyrosine in the body, especially succinylacetone. Decreased activities of 4-hydroxyphenylpyruvate dioxygenase and maleylacetoacetate isomerase observed in this condition are presumed to be secondary phenomena (Fig. 82–2).

Clinical Manifestations. The clinical description is based on symptomatology in patients of French-Canadian descent, who have a more severe form of the disease than other ethnic groups.

The affected infant may become symptomatic as early as 2 wk of age or may remain seemingly healthy during the first yr of life. The earlier the presentation, the poorer the prognosis. The 1-yr mortality, which is about 60% in infants who develop symptoms before 2 mo of age, decreases to 4% in infants who become symptomatic after 6 mo.

The major organs affected are the liver, peripheral nerves, and kidneys. An acute *hepatic crisis* commonly heralds the onset of the disease and is precipitated by an intercurrent illness that produces a catabolic state. Fever, irritability, vomiting, hemorrhage (melena, hematemesis, hematuria), hepatomegaly, jaundice, elevated levels of serum transaminases, and hypoglycemia are common. An odor resembling boiled cabbage may be present and may be due to methionine metabolites. Most hepatic crises resolve spontaneously, but progression to liver failure and death may occur. Between the crises, varying degrees of failure to thrive, hepatomegaly, and clotting abnormalities often persist. Cirrhosis of the liver and eventually hepatocellular carcinoma occur in children who survive beyond 2 yr. The incidence of hepatic carcinoma may be as high as 37%.

Episodes of acute *peripheral neuropathy* resembling acute porphyria occur in about 40% of affected children. These crises, often triggered by a minor infection, are characterized by severe pain, often in the legs, associated with hypertonia (causing hyperextension of the trunk and neck), vomiting, paralytic ileus, and, occasionally, self-induced injuries. Marked weakness and paralysis occur in about 30% of the episodes, which may lead to respiratory failure and death. These crises may last 1 to 7 days. Urinary excretion of 5-aminolevulinic acid, which is usually elevated before the crises (see below), is further increased during the episode. Monitoring the urinary excretion of this compound has little diagnostic or predictive value.

Renal involvement is manifested as a Fanconi-like syndrome with metabolic acidosis, hyperphosphaturia, hypophosphatemia, and vitamin D–resistant rickets. Nephromegaly and some degree of nephrocalcinosis are often found by ultrasound examination of the kidneys.

Laboratory Findings. These include normocytic anemia and marked elevations of serum bilirubin (both conjugated and unconjugated), serum transaminases, and α-fetoprotein. An increase in serum levels of α-fetoprotein has been observed in the cord blood of affected infants, indicating intrauterine liver damage. Clotting factors are often markedly decreased. Plasma levels of tyrosine and other amino acids, especially methionine, are moderately increased. Generalized aminoaciduria occurs. Hyperphosphaturia and hypophosphatemia are common. Urinary excretion of 5-aminolevulinic acid (presumably due to inhibition of 5-aminolevulinic hydratase by succinylacetone) may be increased. The presence of succinylacetoacetate and succinylacetone in serum and urine is diagnostic (see Fig. 82–1). Liver histology is usually compatible with chronic active hepatitis and nonspecific cirrhosis. Hyperplasia of pancreatic islet cells is also a common finding.

Diagnosis is established by measurement of fumarylacetoacetate hydrolyase activity in liver biopsy specimens or fibroblast cultured cells. The degree of residual enzyme activity dictates the severity of the disease. This condition should be differentiated from other causes of hepatitis and hepatic failure in infants, including galactosemia, hereditary fructose intolerance, neonatal iron storage disease, and giant cell hepatitis.

Treatment. A diet low in tyrosine, phenylalanine, and methionine may result in some clinical improvement in some patients. However, in most patients the progression of the disease cannot be halted by diet alone. Inhibition of the enzyme 4-hydroxyphenylpyruvate dioxygenase by 2-(nitro-4-trifluoromethylbenzoyl)-1-3-cyclohexanedione (NTBC) has been shown to cause significant improvement in clinical and biochemical findings in five patients with this condition. The long-term effect of this treatment, however, has not yet been determined. Liver transplantation, especially if performed early in the course of the disease, remains the most effective therapy.

Genetics and Prevalence. Tyrosinemia type I is an autosomal recessive trait. The gene for fumarylacetoacetate hydrolase has been mapped to the long arm of chromosome 15. Most reported patients have a French-Canadian or Scandinavian ancestry. The prevalence of the condition is estimated to be 1 in 1,846 newborn infants in the Saguenay–Lac Saint Jean region of the province of Quebec (Canada). The worldwide prevalence is estimated to be 1:100,000 to 1:120,000. Prenatal diagnosis has been achieved by measurement of succinylacetone in amniotic fluid and by the enzyme assay in chorionic villus biopsy. Direct gene analysis is possible in some families.

TYROSINEMIA TYPE II (Richner-Hanhart Syndrome, Oculocutaneous Tyrosinemia). This rare autosomal recessive disorder results in mental retardation, palmar and plantar punctate hyperkeratosis, and herpetiform corneal ulcers. Excessive tearing, redness, pain, and photophobia may occur before skin lesions. Corneal lesions usually occur during the first few months of life and are presumed to be due to tyrosine deposition; skin lesions may develop later in life. Mental retardation, which occurs in less than 50% of patients, is usually mild to moderate and may be associated with self-mutilation.

Significant hypertyrosinemia (20–50 mg/dL) and tyrosinuria are present. The condition is due to the deficiency of the cytosolic fraction of hepatic tyrosine amino transferase (tyrosine transaminase). In contrast to tyrosinemia type I, liver and kidney functions, as well as serum concentrations of other amino acids, are normal.

Treatment with a diet low in tyrosine and phenylalanine has not only corrected the chemical abnormalities but has also resulted in dramatic healing of the skin and eye lesions. Mental retardation may be prevented by early dietary restriction of tyrosine. The gene for tyrosine aminotransferase is located on the long arm of chromosome 16. About half the reported cases are of Italian descent.

Tyrosinemia Type III (Primary Deficiency of 4-Hydroxyphenylpyruvate Dioxygenase, 4-HPPD). Only four cases have been reported. All patients have various neurologic findings but no consistent clinical phenotype. There is doubt as to whether this enzyme deficiency causes any clinical abnormalities. Age of onset has been from 1 to 17 mo. Developmental delay, seizures, intermittent ataxia, and self-destructive behavior have been the main neurologic findings. No liver or renal abnormalities are present.

The diagnosis is established by moderate increases in plasma levels of tyrosine (350–700 μM), the presence of 4-hydroxyphenylpyruvic acid and its metabolites (4-hydroxyphenyllactic and 4-hydroxyphenylacetic acids) in urine, and low activity of 4-HPPD enzyme in liver biopsy.

Diets low in tyrosine and phenylalanine in combination with vitamin C cause a dramatic decrease in plasma tyrosine levels. The beneficial effects of the diet on neurologic abnormalities have not been demonstrated. The mode of inheritance has not yet been established.

TRANSIENT TYROSINEMIA OF THE NEWBORN. In a small number of newborn infants, plasma tyrosine may rise to as high as 60 mg/dL during the first 2 wk of life. Most affected infants are premature and are receiving high-protein diets. The condition is presumably due to delayed maturation of 4-hydroxyphenylpyruvate dioxygenase. Lethargy, poor feeding, and decreased motor activity occur in some of them, but most are asymptomatic and come to medical attention because of a high blood phenylalanine level, rendering the Guthrie test for PKU screening positive. *Laboratory findings* include marked elevation of plasma tyrosine with a moderate increase in plasma phenylalanine. The presence of marked hypertyrosinemia differentiates this condition from phenylketonuria. Four-hydroxyphenylpyruvic acid and its metabolites (4-hydroxyphenyllactic and 4-hydroxyphenylacetic acids) are also present in the urine. Hypertyrosinemia usually resolves spontaneously during the first mo of life. The condition is often corrected promptly by reducing the amount of protein in the diet (to 2 g/kg/24 hr) and by administering vitamin C (200–400 mg/24 hr). Mild intellectual deficits have been reported in some full-term infants with this disorder.

HAWKINSINURIA. This rare condition (named after the first affected family) is due to a deficiency of one of the components of the 4-hydroxyphenylpyruvate dioxygenase enzyme complex. This enzyme oxidizes 4-hydroxyphenylpyruvic acid to form an epoxide intermediate first; the epoxide metabolite undergoes a rearrangement to form the final product, homogentisic acid (see Fig. 82–1). A block in the rearrangement step leads to an accumulation of the epoxide intermediate, which either is reduced to form 4-hydroxycyclohexylacetic acid (4-HCAA) or reacts with glutathione to form the unusual organic acid 2-L-cysteine-S-yl-1-4-dihydroxycyclohex-5-en-1-yl-acetic acid (hawkinsin); secondary glutathionine deficiency may occur.

Individuals with this disorder become symptomatic only during infancy. The symptoms usually appear after weaning from breast-feeding with the introduction of a high-protein diet. Severe metabolic acidosis, ketosis, failure to thrive, mild hepatomegaly, and an unusual odor (of a swimming pool) are common findings. These infants respond well to a diet low in both phenylalanine and tyrosine, and their clinical manifestations resolve spontaneously by 1 yr of age. Adults with this condition are usually asymptomatic despite metabolic abnormalities. Mental development is usually normal.

Affected children and adults excrete 4-hydroxyphenylpyruvic acid and its metabolites 4-hydroxyphenyllactic and 4-hydroxyphenylacetic acids as well as 5-oxoproline (owing to secondary glutathione deficiency) and the two very unusual organic acids 4-HCAA and hawkinsin in their urine. One patient had mild hypertyrosinemia (196 μM).

Treatment consists of a low-protein diet (such as breast milk) or a diet low in phenylalanine and tyrosine. Large doses of vitamin C (up to 1,000 mg/24 hr) are also recommended. No therapy is needed after 1 yr of age. The condition is inherited as an autosomal dominant trait, and all affected patients reported to date have been presumed to be heterozygous for the trait.

ALCAPTONURIA. This rare (incidence 1 in 250,000) autosomal recessive disorder is due to a deficiency of homogentisic acid oxidase, which causes large amounts of homogentisic acid to accumulate in the body and then to be excreted in the urine (see Fig. 82–1). It is most common in the Dominican Republic and Slovakia.

Clinical manifestations of alcaptonuria consist of ochronosis and arthritis. These findings may not become evident until midadult life. The only sign of the disorder in the pediatric age group is a darkening of the urine to almost a black color on standing. This is caused by oxidation and polymerization of the homogentisic acid and is enhanced with an alkaline pH. Therefore, an acid urine may not become dark even after many hours of standing. This is one of the reasons why darkening of the urine may never be noted in an affected person, and the diagnosis may be delayed until adulthood, when arthritis or ochronosis occurs. *Ochronosis,* a term used to describe the darkening of tissue, is due to a slow accumulation of the black polymer of homogentisic acid in cartilage and other mesenchymal tissues. It is manifested clinically as dark, blackened spots in the sclera or as diffuse blackish pigmentation of the conjunctiva, cornea, and ear cartilage. Arthritis is the only disabling effect of this condition, which occurs in almost all affected subjects with advancing age. It involves the large joints (spine, hip, and knee) and is usually more severe in men. The arthritis has the clinical characteristics of rheumatoid arthritis, but the radiologic findings are typical of osteoarthritis. Degenerative changes in the lumbar spine are quite characteristic with narrowing of the joint spaces and fusion of the vertebral bodies. The pathogenesis of arthritic changes remains unclear. High incidences of heart disease (mitral and aortic valvulitis, calcification of the heart valves, and myocardial infarction) have also been noted.

The *diagnosis* is confirmed by measurement of homogentisic acid in urine. Affected subjects may excrete as much as 4–8 g of this compound daily. Homogentisic acid is a strong reducing agent that produces a positive reaction with Fehling or Benedict reagent (but not with glucose oxidase). The dark urine of phenol poisoning and that associated with melanotic tumors do not have these reducing properties. The enzyme is expressed only in the liver and kidneys. The gene for alkaptonuria has been mapped to the long arm of chromosome 3.

There is no effective *treatment* for this disorder. Large doses of vitamin C (1 g/day) may delay the development of arthritic changes.

ALBINISM. Albinism is due to defects in the biosynthesis and distribution of melanin. Melanin is synthesized by melanocytes from tyrosine in a membrane-bound intracellular organelle, the melanosome. Melanocytes originate from the embryonic neural crest and migrate to the skin, eyes (choroid and iris), and hair follicles. The melanin in the eye is not secreted into the adjacent tissues, whereas the pigment in skin and hair follicles is secreted into the epidermis and the hair shaft. The rate of melanogenesis is very low in the eye and very high in the skin and hair. The biosynthetic pathway for melanin synthesis is not completely elucidated. Tyrosine is transported into the melanosome, where it is metabolized to dopa and dopaquinone by a single enzyme, tyrosinase (see Fig. 82–2). This copper-containing enzyme is present only in the melanocytes. Dopaquinone reacts with cysteine to make cysteinyldopa. The latter compound undergoes several poorly understood steps to form a yellow-red pigment called *pheomelanin.* Dopaquinone may alternatively form *eumelanin,* a brown-black pigment, after several enzymatic and nonenzymatic reactions.

Several genes, including at least one on the short arm of the X chromosome, have been found to be involved in melanogenesis (Table 82–1). However, only the product of the tyrosinase gene has been identified to date (tyrosinase enzyme). The products of other genes involved in melanin production are unknown.

Clinical manifestations common in all forms of albinism are hypopigmentation of the skin and hair. Patients with involvement of the eyes may have strabismus, photophobia, decreased visual acuity, and the presence of red reflex. Irides are translucent and pink in infancy and change to light blue or brown with age. Binocular vision is absent because of a decussation defect in which all optic nerve fibers from one eye completely cross to the other side at the chiasma. Blindness and skin cancer are major late sequelae of albinism in its severe forms.

TABLE 82–1 Classification of Albinism

Type	Gene Defect	Chromosome
Oculocutaneous albinism (OCA)		
OCA$_1$ (tyrosinase deficient OCA)	Tyrosinase	11q
OCA$_2$ (normal tyrosinase activity OCA)	p (pink-eyed dilution)	15q
Prader-Willi and Angelman syndrome	p (pink-eyed dilution)	15q
Hermansky-Pudlak syndrome	?	?
Chédiak-Higashi syndrome	?	?
Ocular albinism (OA)		
OA$_1$ (Nettleship-Fallls type)	OA gene	Xq
Localized albinism		
Piebaldism	KIT	4q
Waardenburg syndrome I	PAX3	2q
Waardenburg syndrome II	?	?

Many clinical forms of albinism have been identified. Some of the seemingly distinct clinical forms are caused by different mutations of the same gene. Attempts to differentiate types of albinism based on the mode of inheritance, tyrosinase activity, or the extent of hypopigmentation have failed to yield a comprehensive classification. The following classification is based on the distribution of albinism in the body (see Table 82–1).

Oculocutaneous (Generalized) Albinism (OCA). Lack of pigment is generalized, affecting skin, hair, and eyes. Two genetically distinct forms exist: OCA_1 and OCA_2. The lack of pigmentation is more severe in patients with OCA_1 than in those with OCA_2. Milder forms of OCA_1 may be indistinguishable from OCA_2. Both conditions are inherited as an autosomal recessive trait.

OCA_1 (Tyrosinase-Deficient Albinism). The genetic defect is in the gene encoding for the tyrosinase enzyme, and this gene is on the long arm of chromosome 11. Many mutant alleles have been identified. Most affected individuals are compound heterozygotes. A number of mutations render the enzyme completely inactive (tyrosinase negative or OCA_1A). These individuals have the most severe form of albinism. Lack of pigment in the skin, hair, and eyes is evident at birth and remains unchanged throughout life. Some mutations result in enzymes with some residual activity. These individuals, although completely depigmented at birth, are capable of developing some pigment with age (yellow OCA). There is minimal tyrosinase activity in these patients, as evidenced by the ability of a plucked hair bulb to form minimal amounts of pigments when incubated with tyrosine.

OCA_2 (Tyrosinase-Positive Albinism). This is the most common form of generalized albinism. It is particularly common in African blacks. These individuals demonstrate some pigmentation of the skin and eyes at birth and continue to collect pigment throughout their lives. The hair is yellow at birth and may become darker with age. The tyrosinase activity in the plucked hair bulb is normal. The defect is in the p gene, which is located on the long arm of chromosome 15. This gene produces the p protein, which is involved in the the transport of tyrosine across the melansome membrane. Patients with *Prader-Willi* and *Angelman* syndromes who have deletion of chromosome 15 also have this form of albinism (see Chapter 78).

Hermansky-Pudlak syndrome is a tyrosinase-positive oculocutaneous albinism associated with platelet dysfunction (owing to the absence of platelet-dense bodies) and an accumulation of a ceroid-like material in tissues. The degree of albinism is variable. The condition is most prevalent in Puerto Rico (frequency about 1:2,000). Bleeding tendencies, often manifested as epistaxis, and a prolonged bleeding time are common. The ceroid-like material is histochemically similar to that found in neuronal ceroid-lipofuscinosis. The accumulation of this material in tissues results in restrictive lung disease, inflammatory bowel disease, kidney failure, and cardiomyopathy during the third or fourth decade of life. The basic defect is thought to be a membrane abnormality involving melanosomes, lysosomes, and platelet-dense bodies.

Chédiak-Higashi Syndrome. Patients with this rare autosomal recessive condition have partial albinism and susceptibility to infection with the presence of giant peroxidase-positive lysosomal granules in granulocytes (see Chapter 130.3). These patients have a reduced number of melanosomes, which are abnormally large (macromelanosomes). Patients who survive early childhood may develop a lymphofollicular malignancy.

Ocular Albinism (OA). Albinism is limited to the eyes. All the eye findings of albinism (see above) are present. Skin and hair color are within normal limits but are usually lighter than those in nonaffected siblings. Hair bulb tyrosinase activity is positive. At least three forms of this condition (OA_1, OA_2, and OA_3) have been reported. Only the X-linked recessive form (OA_1) has been segregated as a separate entity. OA_2, which was thought to be an autosomal recessive trait, is now known to be inherited as an X-linked condition and, most probably, is a form of OA_1. OA_3, which has been known as the autosomal recessive ocular albinism, is now known to be a mild variant of type 2 oculocutaneous albinism (OCA_2).

Ocular Albinism 1 (OA_1 Nettleship-Falls Type). In this form only the hemizygote male has the complete manifestation. Some abnormal pigmentation of the retina may be present in heterozygote carriers. The gene for this condition is located on the short arm of the X chromosome. An X-linked ocular albinism with late-onset sensorineural deafness has been reported.

Localized Albinism. This disorder is characterized by localized hypopigmentation of skin and hair, which may be present at birth or develop with time.

Piebaldism. In this autosomal dominant inherited condition, the individual is usually born with a white forelock. The underlying skin is depigmented. In addition, there are usually white macules on the face, trunk, and extremities. The white hair lock and the depigmented underlying skin are devoid of melanocytes. Mutations in KIT gene (tyrosine kinase receptor) have been shown in affected patients.

Waardenburg Syndrome. In this syndrome, lateral displacement of inner canthi, broad nasal bridge, heterochromia of idides and sensorineural deafness are associated with a white forelock. This condition is inherited as an autosomal dominant trait. Two types of this syndrome, types I and II, have been identified. Patients with type I have displacement of inner canthi, while type II patients have normal inner canthi. Mutation in PAX3 gene is the cause of type I Waardenburg syndrome.

82.3 Methionine

Iraj Rezvani

The normal pathway for catabolism of methionine, an essential amino acid, produces *S*-adenosylmethionine, which serves as a methyl group donor for methylation of a variety of compounds in the body, and cysteine, which is formed through a series of reactions called trans-sulfuration (Fig. 82–3).

HOMOCYSTINURIA (Homocystinemia). Most homocysteine, an intermediate compound of methionine degradation, is normally remethylated to methionine. This methionine-sparing reaction is catalyzed by the enzyme methionine synthase, which requires a metabolite of folic acid (5-methyltetrahydrofolate) as a methyl donor and a metabolite of vitamin B_{12} (methylcobalamin) as a cofactor (see Fig. 82–3). Homocysteine (and its dimer homocystine) ordinarily is detectable only in trace amounts in plasma or urine. Three major forms of homocystinemia and homocystinuria have been identified.

Homocystinuria Due to Cystathionine Synthase Deficiency (Homocystinuria Type I, Classic Homocystinuria). This is the most common inborn error of methionine metabolism. About 40% of affected patients respond to high doses of vitamin B_6 and usually have milder clinical manifestations than those who are unresponsive to vitamin B_6 therapy. These patients possess some residual enzyme activity.

Infants with this disorder are normal at birth. *Clinical manifestations* during infancy are nonspecific and may include failure to thrive and developmental delay. The diagnosis is usually made after 3 yr of age, when subluxation of the ocular lens (ectopia lentis) occurs. This causes severe myopia and iridodonesis (quivering of the iris). Astigmatism, glaucoma, staphyloma, cataracts, retinal detachment, and optic atrophy may develop later in life. Progressive mental retardation is common. Normal intelligence, however, has been reported. In an international survey of over 600 patients, IQ scores ranged from 10 to 135. The higher IQ scores were noted in vitamin B_6–responsive patients. Psychiatric and behavioral disorders have been observed in more than 50% of affected patients. Convulsions occur in about 20% of patients. Affected individuals with

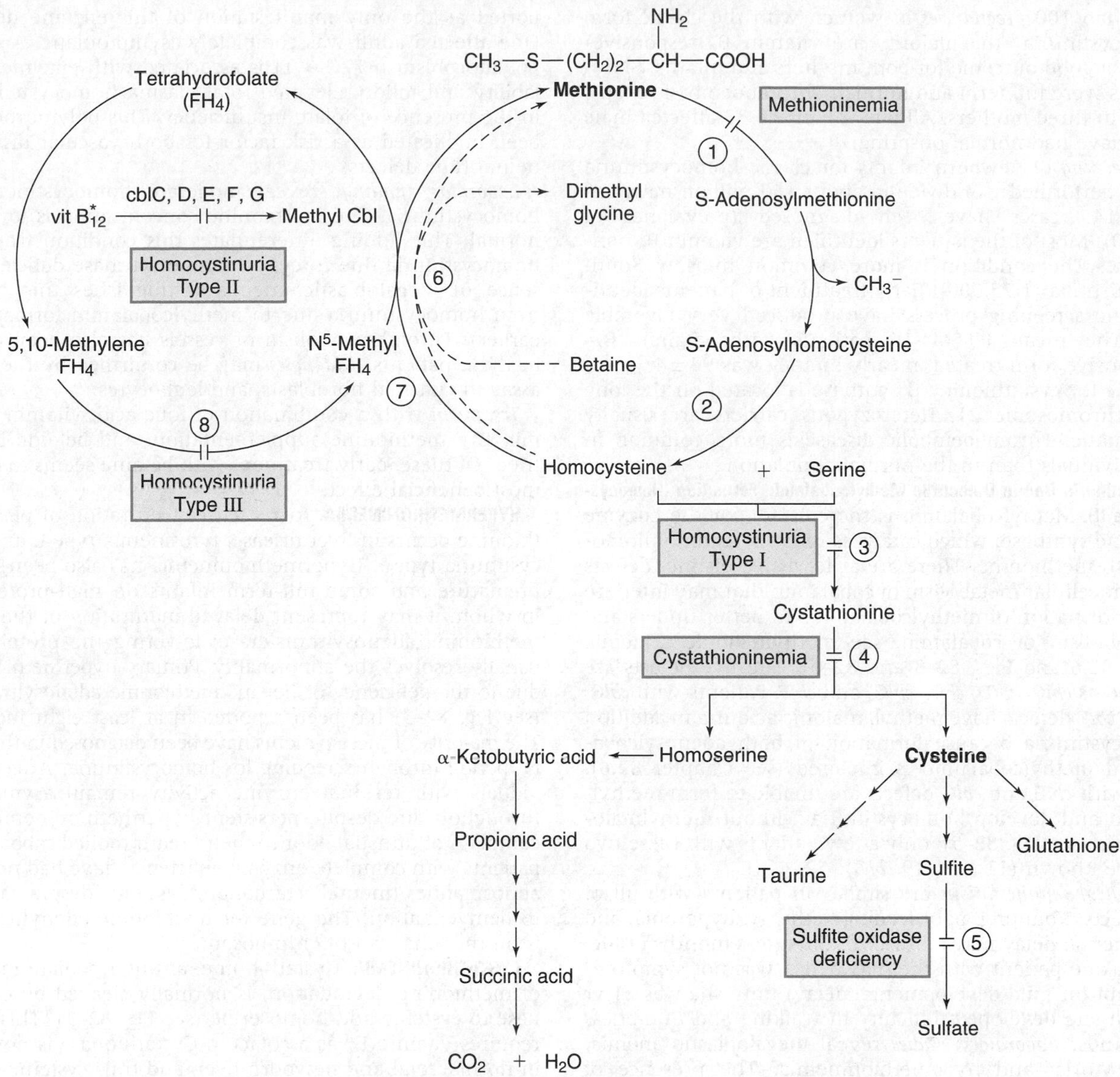

Figure 82–3 Pathways in the metabolism of the sulfur-containing amino acids. **Enzymes:** (1) methionine adenosyltransferase; (2) adenosylhomocysteine hydrolase; (3) cystathionine synthase; (4) cystathionase; (5) sulfite oxidase; (6) betaine homocysteine methyltransferase; (7) methionine synthase; (8) methylene tetrahydrofolate reductase.

homocystinuria manifest skeletal abnormalities resembling those of Marfan syndrome (see Chapter 705); they are usually tall and thin with elongated limbs and arachnodactyly. Scoliosis, pectus excavatum or carinum, genu valgum, pes cavus, high arched palate, and crowding of the teeth are commonly seen. These children usually have fair complexions, blue eyes, and a peculiar malar flush. Generalized osteoporosis is the main roentgenographic finding. Thromboembolic episodes involving both large and small vessels, especially those of the brain, are common and may occur at any age. Optic atrophy, paralysis, seizure disorders, cor pulmonale, and severe hypertension (due to renal infarcts) are among the serious consequences of thromboembolism, which is due to changes in the vascular walls and increased platelet adhesiveness secondary to elevated homocystine levels. The risk of thromboembolism increases following surgical procedures. The incidence of thromboembolic events after surgery is much lower than originally estimated (14 postoperative thromboembolic episodes in 241 major surgical procedures).

Elevations of both methionine and homocystine (or homocysteine) in body fluids are the diagnostic *laboratory findings.* Freshly voided urine should be tested for homocystine, since this compound is unstable and may disappear as the urine is stored. Cystine is low or absent in plasma. The *diagnosis* may be established by assay of the enzyme in liver biopsy specimens, cultured fibroblasts, or phytohemagglutinin-stimulated lymphocytes. Prenatal diagnosis is feasible by performing an enzyme assay of cultured amniotic cells or chorionic villi. An increasing number of mutations have been recognized in different families.

Treatment with high doses of vitamin B_6 (200–1,000 mg/24 hr) causes dramatic improvement in patients who are responsive to this therapy, but some patients may not respond because of folate depletion; therefore, a patient should not be considered unresponsive to vitamin B_6 until folic acid (1–5 mg/24 hr) has been added to the treatment regimen. Restriction of methionine intake in conjunction with cysteine supplementation is recommended for all patients regardless of their response to vitamin B_6. Betaine (trimethylglycine, 6–9 g/24 hr), which also serves as a methyl group donor, lowers homocysteine levels in body fluids by remethylating homocysteine to methionine (Fig. 82–3). This treatment has produced clinical improvement in patients who are unresponsive to vitamin B_6 therapy.

More than 100 *pregnancies* in women with the classic form of homocystinuria (the majority are vitamin B_6 responsive) have had a good outcome for both mothers and infants. Sixty-six infants were full term and normal. Thromboembolic events occurred in three mothers. All but one of the 38 affected male patients have had normal offspring.

The *screening* of newborn infants for classic homocystinuria has been performed worldwide in about 150 million newborn infants; 145 cases have been diagnosed (prevalence of 1:340,000). Most of the patients identified are vitamin B_6 nonresponsive. The condition is more common in New South Wales, Australia (1:75,000). Early treatment of patients identified by the screening process have produced very favorable results. The mean IQ of 16 patients with vitamin B_6–nonresponsive form treated in early infancy was 94 ± 4.

The *gene* for cystathionine β synthase is located on the long arm of chromosome 21. Heterozygous carriers are usually asymptomatic. Thromboembolic disease is more common in these individuals than in the normal population.

Homocystinuria Due to Defects in Methylcobalamin Formation (Homocystinuria Type II). Methylcobalamin is the cofactor for the enzyme methionine synthase, which catalyzes remethylation of homocysteine to methionine. There are at least five distinct defects in the intracellular metabolism of cobalamin that may interfere with the formation of methylcobalamin. To better understand the metabolism of cobalamin, see methylmalonic acidemia (Chapter 82.6 and Figs. 82–3 and 82–5). The five defects are designated as *cbl*C, *cbl*D, *cbl*E, *cbl*G, and *cbl*F. Patients with *cbl*C, *cbl*D, and *cbl*F defects have methylamalonic aciduria in addition to homocystinuria because formation of both adenosylcobalamin and methylcobalamin is impaired (see Chapter 82.6). Patients with *cbl*E and *cbl*G defects are unable to form methylcobalamin and develop homocystinuria without methylmalonic aciduria (see Fig. 82–5); only a few patients with these two defects are known (11 *cbl*E, 19 *cbl*G).

The *clinical manifestations* are similar in patients with all of these defects. Vomiting, poor feeding, lethargy, hypotonia, and developmental delay may occur in the first few months of life. However, one patient with the *cbl*G defect was not symptomatic (except for mild developmental delay) until she was 21 yr old, when she developed difficulty in walking and numbness of the hands. *Laboratory studies* reveal megaloblastic anemia, homocystinuria, and hypomethioninemia. The presence of megaloblastic anemia differentiates these defects from homocystinuria due to methyleneterahydrofolate reductase deficiency. The presence of hypomethioninemia differentiates both of these from cystathionine β synthase deficiency.

Diagnosis is established by complementation studies performed in cultured fibroblasts. Prenatal diagnosis has been accomplished by studies in amniotic cell cultures.

Treatment with vitamin B_{12} in the form of hydroxycobalamin (1–2 mg/24 hr) is used to correct the clinical and biochemical findings. Results vary among both diseases and sibships.

Homocystinuria Due to Deficiency of Methylenetetrahydrofolate Reductase (Homocystinuria Type III). This enzyme reduces 5–10 methylenetetrahydrofolate to form 5-methyltetrahydrofolate, which provides the methyl group needed for remethylation of homocysteine to methionine (see Fig. 82–3). The gene for this enzyme has been located on the short arm of chromosome 1. The condition is transmitted as an autosomal recessive trait and more than 40 cases have been reported.

The severity of the enzyme defect and of the *clinical manifestations* varies considerably in different families. Complete absence of enzyme activity results in neonatal apneic episodes and myoclonic seizures that may lead rapidly to coma and death. Partial deficiency may result in a more chronic clinical picture, manifested by mental retardation, convulsions, microcephaly, and spasticity. One 15-yr-old patient developed schizophrenia and mental deterioration at 11 yr of age. Premature vascular disease or peripheral neuropathy have been reported as the only manifestation of this enzyme deficiency. One affected adult was completely asymptomatic. A common polymorphism (677C→ T) is associated with enzyme thermal lability and mildly elevated total plasma homocysteine levels in the presence of folate insufficiency. This polymorphism has been implicated as a risk factor for both vascular disease and neural tube defects.

Laboratory findings reveal moderate homocystinemia and homocystinuria. The methionine concentration is low or low normal. This finding differentiates this condition from classic homocystinuria due to cystathionine synthase deficiency. Absence of megaloblastic anemia distinguishes this condition from homocystinuria due to methylcobalamin formation (see earlier). Thromboembolism of vessels has also been observed in these patients. *Diagnosis* may be confirmed by the enzyme assay in cultured fibroblasts, and leukocytes.

Treatment with a combination of folic acid, vitamin B_6, vitamin B_{12}, methionine supplementation, and betaine has been tried. Of these, early treatment with betaine seems to have the most beneficial effect.

HYPERMETHIONINEMIA. Increased concentration of plasma methionine occurs in liver disease, tyrosinemia type I, and homocystinuria type I. Hypermethioninemia has also been found in premature and some full-term infants on high-protein diets, in whom it may represent delayed maturation of the enzyme methionine adenosyltransferase; lowering the protein intake usually resolves the abnormality. Primary hypermethioninemia due to the deficiency of hepatic methionine adenosyltransferase (see Fig. 82–3) has been reported in at least eight individuals. The majority of these patients have been diagnosed in the neonatal period through screening for homocystinuria. Affected individuals with residual enzyme activity remain asymptomatic throughout life despite persistent hypermethioninemia. Some complain of unusual odor to their breath (boiled cabbage). Two patients with complete enzyme deficiency have had neurologic abnormalities (mental retardation, dystonia, dyspraxia) related to demyelination. The gene for methionine adenyltransferase is on the long arm of chromosome 10.

CYSTATHIONINEMIA. Cystathionine, an intermediate metabolite of methionine degradation, is normally cleaved by cystathionase to cysteine and homoserine (see Fig. 82–3). This enzyme requires vitamin B_6 as a cofactor. Cystathionase is not present in normal fetal and newborn liver, and thus cysteine becomes an essential amino acid during the newborn period, particularly in the premature infant.

Secondary cystathioninuria occurs in patients with vitamin B_6 or B_{12} deficiency, liver disease (particularly when the liver damage is secondary to galactosemia), thyrotoxicosis, hepatoblastoma, neuroblastoma, ganglioblastoma, or defects in remethylation of homocysteine (homocystinuria types II and III).

Cystathionase deficiency results in massive cystathioninuria and mild to moderate cystathioninemia; cystathionine is not normally detectable in blood. Deficiency of this enzyme is inherited as an autosomal recessive trait. Affected subjects with a wide variety of clinical manifestations have been reported. Lack of a consistent clinical picture and the presence of cystathioninuria in a number of normal persons suggest that cystathionase deficiency perhaps is of no clinical significance. A majority of reported cases are responsive to oral administration of large doses of vitamin B_6 (100 mg or more/24 hr). Once cystathioninuria is discovered in a patient, vitamin B_6 treatment seems indicated, but its beneficial effect has not been established.

82.4 Cysteine/Cystine

Iraj Rezvani

Cysteine is a sulfur-containing nonessential amino acid that is synthesized from methionine (see Fig. 82–3). In the presence of oxygen, two molecules of cysteine are oxidized to form cystine. The most common disorders of cysteine/cystine metabolism, cystinuria (see Chapter 555), and cystinosis (see Chapter 537.3) are discussed elsewhere.

SULFITE OXIDASE DEFICIENCY (Molybdenum Cofactor Deficiency). As the last step in cysteine metabolism, sulfite is oxidized to sulfate by sulfite oxidase, and the sulfate is excreted in the urine (see Fig. 82–3). This enzyme requires a molybdenum-pterin complex named molybdenum cofactor. This cofactor is also necessary for the function of two other enzymes in humans, xanthine dehydrogenase (which oxidizes xanthine and hypoxanthine to uric acid) and aldehyde oxidase. Most patients who were originally diagnosed as having sulfite oxidase deficiency have proved to have molybdenum cofactor deficiency. The condition is inherited as an autosomal recessive trait.

Both deficiencies produce identical *clinical manifestations.* Refusal to feed, vomiting, severe intractable seizures (tonic, clonic, and myoclonic), and severe developmental delay may develop within a few weeks after birth. Bilateral dislocation of ocular lenses is a common finding in patients who survive the neonatal period.

These children excrete large amounts of sulfite, thiosulfate, S-sulfocysteine, xanthine, and hypoxanthine in their urine. Urinary and serum levels of uric acid and urinary concentration of sulfate are diminished. The urine can be screened for the presence of sulfite by a commercially available strip test (Macherey-Nagel strip or Quntofix sulfite test strip). Fresh urine should be used for screening purposes and for quantitative measurements of sulfite, because oxidation at room temperature may produce false-negative results.

Diagnosis is confirmed by measurement of sulfite oxidase and molybdenum cofactor in fibroblasts and liver biopsies, respectively. Prenatal diagnosis is possible by performing an assay of sulfite oxidase activity in cultured amniotic cells or in samples of chorionic villi.

No effective *treatment* is available, and most children die during the first 2 yr of life.

82.5 *Tryptophan*

Iraj Rezvani

Tryptophan is an essential amino acid and a precursor for nicotinic acid and serotonin (Fig. 82–4). Presumed deficiencies of a variety of different enzymes involved in tryptophan metabolism have been reported in isolated cases, but in none of these cases has the enzyme deficiency been documented by direct assay of the enzyme activity. Moreover, because of the paucity of reported patients, the relationship between the symptoms and the putative enzyme deficiency has remained uncertain. Therefore, only disorders of tryptophan metabolism that have been well documented are discussed in this section. The most common disorder involving tryptophan metabolism is Hartnup disorder.

HARTNUP DISORDER. In this autosomal recessive disorder, named after the first reported family, there is a single defect in the transport of monoamino-monocarboxylic amino acids (neutral amino acids) by the intestinal mucosa and renal tubules.

Data from routine urine screening of newborn infants have revealed that most children with Hartnup defect remain asymptomatic. The major *clinical manifestation* in the rare symptomatic patient is cutaneous photosensitivity. The skin becomes rough and red after moderate exposure to the sun, and with greater exposure a pellagra-like rash may develop. The rash may be pruritic, and a chronic eczema may appear. The skin changes have been reported in affected infants as young as 10 days of age. Some patients may have intermittent ataxia with or without the skin rash. Mental deficiency, perhaps an incidental finding in the original kindred, has been reported only in one additional case of a girl who had a severe encephalopathy. Episodic psychologic changes, such as irritability, emotional instability, and suicidal tendencies, have been observed; these changes are usually associated with bouts of ataxia.

Identification of asymptomatic children with Hartnup defect suggests that it can be a benign disorder. The clinical polymorphism may be related to the severity of the defect, especially in the intestinal mucosa. Patients with a severe defect may develop marked amino acid deficiency following minor stress such as diarrhea or a low-protein diet and may then become symptomatic. This theory also explains the episodic nature of the symptoms and the long intervals of spontaneous remission in patients with Hartnup disorder. Hartnup defect, with an overall prevalence of 1 in 24,000 (range 1 in 18,000–42,000) ranks among the most common amino acid disorders in humans. Pregnancy in women with Hartnup disorder has not produced any ill effects in either mother or fetus.

The main *laboratory finding* is aminoaciduria, which is restricted to neutral amino acids (alanine, serine, threonine, valine, leucine, isoleucine, phenylalanine, tyrosine, tryptophan, and histidine). Urinary excretion of proline, hydroxyproline, and arginine remains normal. This is an important

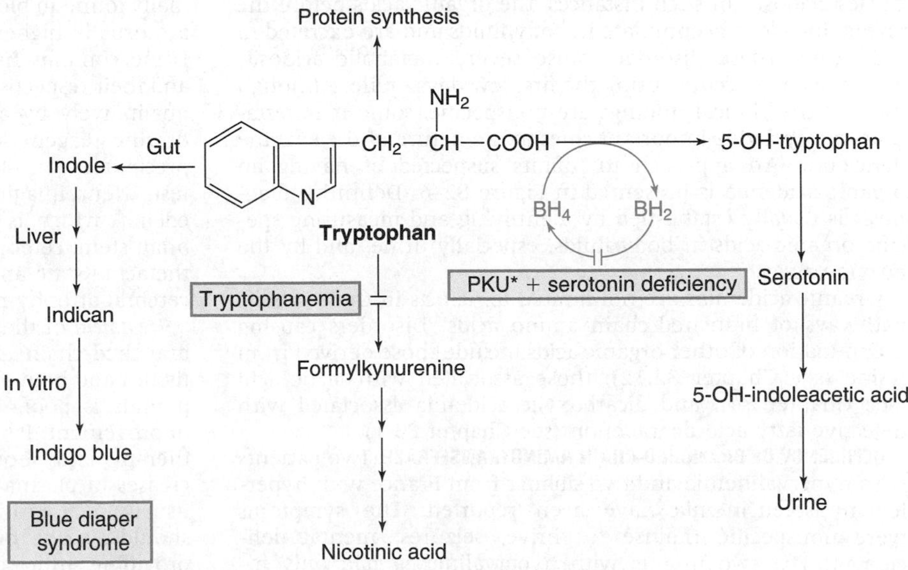

Figure 82–4 Pathways in the metabolism of tryptophan. PKU = hyperphenylalaninemia due to tetrahydrobiopterin deficiency (see Fig. 82–1).

diagnostic finding that differentiates Hartnup disorder from other causes of generalized aminoaciduria such as Fanconi syndrome. Plasma concentrations of neutral amino acids are usually within normal limits. This seemingly unexpected finding is due to absorption of the amino acids as dipeptides because the transport system for small peptides remains intact in Hartnup disorder. The indole derivatives (especially indican) are usually excreted in large amounts in this disorder owing to bacterial breakdown of unabsorbed tryptophan in the intestines.

Treatment with nicotinic acid or nicotinamide (50–300 g/24 hr) and a high-protein diet have resulted in a favorable response in symptomatic patients.

SEROTONIN DEFICIENCY. The first step in serotonin synthesis is the hydroxylation of tryptophan by tryptophan hydroxylase (see Fig. 82–4). This enzyme requires tetrahydrobiopterin as a cofactor. Defects in biopterin metabolism (see Chapter 82.1) cause a deficiency of serotonin in addition to phenylketonuria (PKU). This fact explains why treatment of patients with PKU due to biopterin defects with the usual low-phenylalanine diet alone does not prevent neurologic manifestations.

INDICANURIA (Tryptophan Malabsorption). This condition occurs when tryptophan, poorly absorbed from the gastrointestinal tract, is converted there by bacterial action to indole. Indole is absorbed, oxidized, sulfated, and excreted as an indican (see Fig. 82–4). Indicanuria is commonly observed whenever stasis in the bowels occurs, such as in constipation or in the *blind loop syndrome*; it also occurs in Hartnup disorder, in which tryptophan is poorly absorbed, and in phenylketonuria. The *blue diaper syndrome*, a familial disorder characterized by hypercalcemia, nephrocalcinosis, and indicanuria, derives its name from the fact that indican is oxidized to indigo blue on exposure to air.

82.6 Valine, Leucine, Isoleucine, and Related Organic Acidemias

Iraj Rezvani and David S. Rosenblatt

The early steps in the degradation of these three essential amino acids, the branched-chain amino acids, are similar (see Fig. 82–5). Although valine transaminase may be different from leucine-isoleucine transaminase, only one enzyme system (branched-chain α-ketoacid dehydrogenase) is involved in the decarboxylation of their three ketoacid derivatives. The intermediate metabolites are all organic acids, and deficiency of any of the degradative enzymes, except for the transaminases, causes acidosis; in such instances, the organic acids before the enzymatic block accumulate in body fluids and are excreted in the urine. These disorders cause severe metabolic acidosis, which usually occurs during the first few days of life. Although most of the clinical findings are nonspecific, some manifestations may provide important clues to the nature of the enzyme deficiency. An approach to infants suspected of having an organic acidemia is presented in Figure 82–6. Definitive diagnosis is usually established by identifying and measuring specific organic acids in body fluids, especially urine, and by the enzyme assay.

Organic acidemias are not limited to defects in the catabolic pathways of branched-chain amino acids. Disorders causing accumulation of other organic acids include those derived from lysine (see Chapter 82.12), those associated with lactic acid (see Chapter 84), and dicarboxylic acidemia associated with defective fatty acid degradation (see Chapter 83.1).

DEFICIENCY OF BRANCHED-CHAIN AMINOTRANSFERASE. Two patients with hypervalinemia and two siblings from France with hyperleucine-isoleucinemia have been reported. The symptoms were nonspecific (failure to thrive, seizures, mental deficiency). The two infants with hypervalinemia had only increased concentrations of valine in blood and urine with normal levels of leucine and isoleucine. Impaired transamination of valine was demonstrated in leukocytes. The siblings with hyperleucine-isoleucinemia had elevated plasma concentrations of leucine, isoleucine, and proline with normal levels of valine. Assay of leukocytes revealed no abnormalities of branched-chain ketoacid dehydrogenase or of valine aminotransferase, but there was a 50% reduction in leucine and isoleucine aminotransferase. The urine of these infants neither contained branched-chain ketoacids nor had the odor of maple syrup.

The presence of hypervalinemia and hyperleucine-isoleucinemia as separate entities suggests that the aminotransferase for leucine-isoleucine may be different from that of valine. Two isoforms of the enzyme, cystosolic and mitochondrial, have been identified. Both are equally active for these three amino acids.

MAPLE SYRUP URINE DISEASE (MSUD). Decarboxylation of leucine, isoleucine, and valine is accomplished by a complex enzyme system (branched-chain α-ketoacid dehydrogenase) using thiamine pyrophosphate as a coenzyme. This mitochondrial enzyme consists of four subunits: $E_{1\alpha}$, $E_{1\beta}$, E_2, and E_3. The E_3 subunit is shared with two other dehydrogenases in the body, namely, pyruvate dehydrogenase and α-ketoglutarate dehydrogenase. Deficiency of this enzyme system causes MSUD (see Fig. 82–5), named after the sweet odor of maple syrup found in body fluids, especially urine. Based on clinical and biochemical findings, five phenotypes of MSUD have been identified.

Classic MSUD. This form has the most severe *clinical manifestations*. Affected infants who are normal at birth develop poor feeding and vomiting during the 1st wk of life; lethargy and coma ensue within a few days. Physical examination reveals hypertonicity and muscular rigidity with severe opisthotonos. Periods of hypertonicity may alternate with bouts of flaccidity. Neurologic findings are often mistaken for generalized sepsis and meningitis. Convulsions occur in most infants, and hypoglycemia is common. However, in contrast to most hypoglycemic states, correcting the blood glucose concentration does not improve the clinical condition. Routine laboratory studies are usually unremarkable, except for severe metabolic acidosis. Death usually occurs in untreated patients within the first few weeks or months of life.

Diagnosis is often suspected because of the peculiar odor of maple syrup found in urine, sweat, and cerumen (see Fig. 82–6). It is usually confirmed by amino acid analysis showing marked elevations in plasma levels of leucine, isoleucine, valine, and alloisoleucine (a stereoisomer of isoleucine not normally found in blood) and depression of alanine. Leucine levels are usually higher than those of the other three amino acids. Urine contains high levels of leucine, isoleucine, and valine and their respective ketoacids. These ketoacids may be detected qualitatively by adding a few drops of 2,4-dinitrophenylhydrazine reagent (0.1% in 0.1 N HCl) to the urine; a yellow precipitate of 2–4 diphenylhydrazone is formed in a positive test. Neuroimaging during the acute state shows cerebral edema, which is most prominent in the cerebellum, dorsal brain stem, cerebral peduncle, and internal capsule. Following the acute state and with advancing age, hypomyelination and cerebral atrophy may develop.

Treatment of the acute state is aimed at quick removal of the branched-chain amino acids and their metabolites from the tissues and body fluids. Because renal clearance of these compounds is poor, hydration alone does not produce a rapid improvement. Peritoneal dialysis is the most effective mode of therapy and should be promptly instituted; significant decreases in plasma levels of leucine, isoleucine, and valine are usually seen within 24 hr of institution of treatment. Attempts should also be made to stop the patient's catabolic state by providing sufficient calories intravenously or orally.

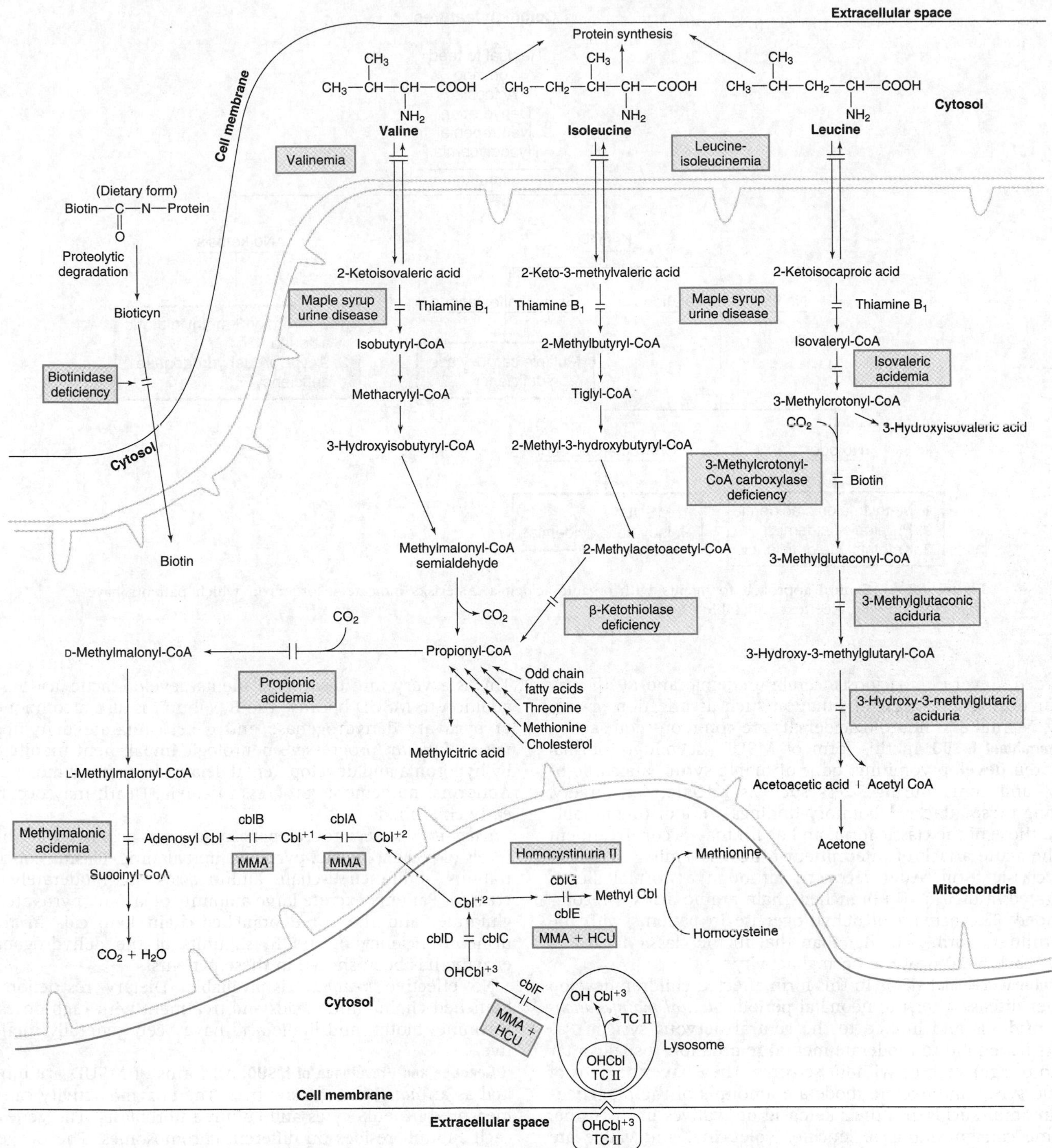

Figure 82–5 Pathways in the metabolism of the branched-chain amino acids, biotin, and vitamin B_{12} (cobalamin). MMA = methylmalonic acidemia; HCU = homocystinuria; Cbl = cobalamin; OHCbl = hydroxycobalamin; cbl = defect in metabolism of cobalamin; TC = transcobalamin.

Treatment after recovery from the acute state requires a low branched-chain amino acid diet. Synthetic formulas devoid of leucine, isoleucine, and valine are now commercially available.* Because these amino acids cannot be synthesized endogenously, small amounts of them should be added to the diet; the amount should be titrated carefully by performing frequent analyses of the plasma amino acids. A clinical condition resembling acrodermatitis enteropathica occurs in affected infants whose plasma isoleucine concentration becomes very low; addition of isoleucine to the diet causes a rapid and complete recovery. Patients with MSUD should remain on the diet for the rest of their lives. Liver transplantation has been performed in two patients with classic MSUD. One patient was a 7½-yr-old with liver failure following fulminant hepatitis A infection. The second patient was a 9-yr-old from the Mennonite community with idiopathic cirrhosis and chronic liver failure. Biochemical abnormalities in one of the children corrected to near-normal values within 12 hr after transplantation. Both children tolerated a normal diet.

The long-term *prognosis* of affected children remains

*MSUD Formula, Mead Johnson Laboratories, Evansville, Indiana.

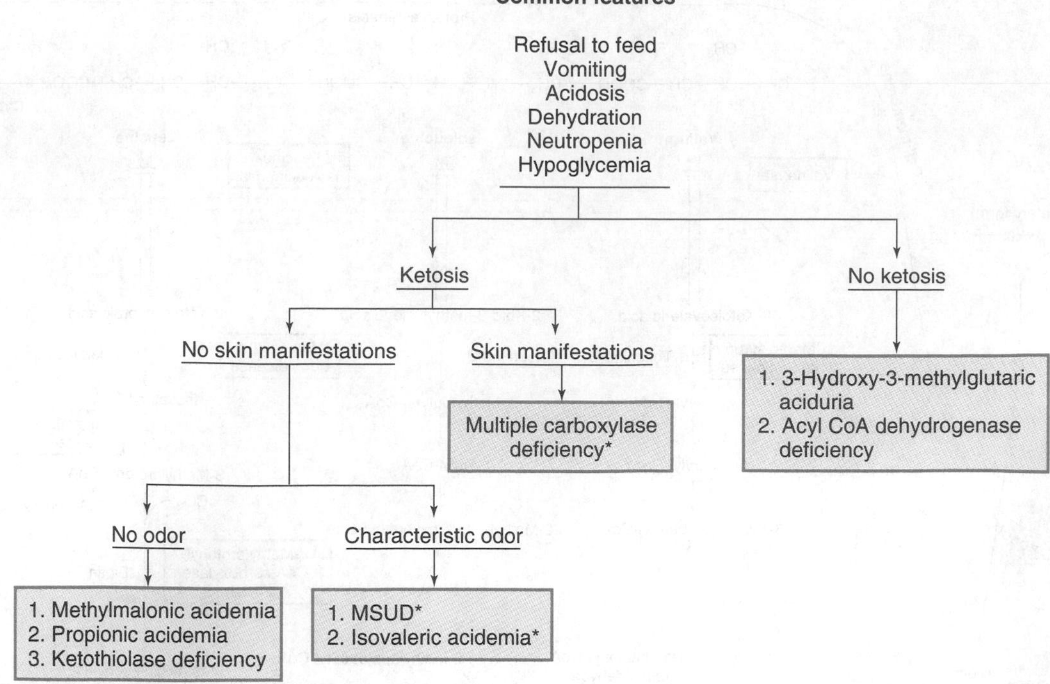

Figure 82–6 Clinical approach to infants with organic acidemia. Asterisks indicate disorders in which patients have a characteristic odor (see text and Table 81-1).

guarded. Severe ketoacidosis, cerebral edema, and death may occur during any stressful situation such as infection or surgery. Mental and neurologic deficits are common sequelae.

Intermittent MSUD. In this form of MSUD, seemingly normal children develop vomiting, odor of maple syrup, ataxia, lethargy, and coma during stress such as infection or surgery. During these attacks, laboratory findings are indistinguishable from those of the classic form, and death may occur. Treatment of the acute attack of intermittent MSUD is similar to that of the classic form. After recovery, although a normal diet is tolerated, a diet low in branched-chain amino acids is recommended. The activity of dehydrogenase in patients with the intermittent form is higher than that in the classic form and may reach 5–20% of the normal activity.

Mild (Intermediate) MSUD. In this form affected children develop milder disease after the neonatal period. *Clinical manifestations* are insidious and limited to the central nervous system. Patients have mild to moderate mental retardation (usually after 5 mo of age) with or without seizures. They have the odor of maple syrup and excrete moderate amounts of the branched-chain amino acids and their ketoacid derivatives in the urine. Plasma concentrations of leucine, isoleucine, and valine are moderately increased. These children are commonly diagnosed during an intercurrent illness when signs and symptoms of classic MSUD occur. The dehydrogenase activity is 15–25% of normal. Since patients with thiamine-responsive MSUD usually have manifestations similar to those seen in the mild form, a trial of thiamine therapy is recommended. Diet therapy similar to that of classic MSUD is needed.

Thiamine-Responsive MSUD. Some children with mild or intermediate forms of MSUD who are treated with high doses of thiamine have dramatic clinical and biochemical improvement. Although some responded to treatment with 10 mg/24 hr thiamine, others require as much as 200 mg/24 hr for at least 3 wk before a favorable response is observed. These patients also require diets deficient in branched-chain amino acids in addition to thiamine supplementation. The enzymatic activity in these patients is 30–40% of normal.

MSUD Due to a Deficiency of E_3 Subunit (Dihydrolipoyl Dehydrogenase). This is a very rare disorder. Patients develop lactic acidosis in addition to MSUD because the E_3 subunit is also a component of pyruvate dehydrogenase and α-ketoglutarate dehydrogenase. *Clinically,* progressive neurologic impairment manifested by hypotonia and developmental delay occur after 2 mo of age. Abnormal movements progress to ataxia. Death may occur in early childhood.

Laboratory studies reveal persistent lactic acidosis with high levels of plasma lactate, pyruvate, and alanine. Plasma concentrations of branched-chain amino acids are moderately increased. Patients excrete large amounts of lactate, pyruvate, α-glutarate, and the three branched-chain ketoacids in their urine. Deficiency of the E_3 subunits of the dehydrogenase enzyme has been shown in these patients.

No effective *treatment* is available. Dietary restriction of branched-chain amino acids and treatment with high doses of thiamine, biotin, and lipoic acid have been generally ineffective.

Genetics and Prevalence of MSUD. All forms of MSUD are inherited as an *autosomal recessive* trait. The enzyme activity can be measured in leukocytes and cultured fibroblasts. The gene for each subunit resides on different chromosomes. The $E_{1\alpha}$ gene is on the long arm of chromosome 19; $E_{1\beta}$ is on the short arm of chromosome 6; E_2 is on the short arm of chromosome 1, and E_3 is on the long arm of chromosome 7. More than 20 different mutations have been identified in patients with different forms of MSUD. A given phenotype is caused by a variety of genotypes. Patients from different pedigrees with the classic form of MSUD have been shown to have mutations in genes for $E_{1\alpha}$, $E_{1\beta}$, or E_2. Most patients are compound heterozygotes inheriting two different mutant alleles.

The *prevalence* of the condition is estimated at 1:185,000. The classic form of MSUD is quite prevalent in the Mennonite population in the United States and is estimated to be 1:176. Affected patients in this population are homozygous for a specific mutation (Try_{393}-to-Asn) in the $E_{1\alpha}$ subunit gene.

Prenatal diagnosis has been accomplished by enzyme assay of the cultured aminocytes, cultured chorionic villi tissue, or direct assay of the chorionic villi samples.

Several successful *pregnancies* have occurred in women with different forms of MSUD. No ill effects have been observed in the offspring of these patients.

ISOVALERIC ACIDEMIA. This rare condition is due to the deficiency of isovaleryl CoA dehydrogenase, which catalyzes the conversion of isovaleric acid to 3-methylcrotonic acid in the leucine degradative pathway (see Fig. 82–5). Isovaleric acidemia is inherited as an autosomal recessive trait. The gene has been mapped to the long arm of chromosome 15. The gene frequency in the general population is not known.

Clinical manifestations in the acute form (about 50% of cases) include vomiting and severe acidosis in the first few days of life. Lethargy, convulsions, and coma ensue, and death may occur if proper therapy is not initiated. The vomiting may be severe enough to suggest pyloric stenosis. The characteristic odor of "sweaty feet" may be present (see Fig. 82–6). A milder form of the disease also exists in which the first clinical manifestation (vomiting, lethargy, acidosis, or coma) may not appear until the infant is a few months or a few years old *(chronic intermittent form)*.

Laboratory findings reveal severe ketoacidosis, neutropenia, thrombocytopenia, and occasionally pancytopenia. Hypocalcemia and moderate to severe hyperammonemia may be present in some patients. Increases in plasma ammonia may suggest a defect in the urea cycle. However, in the latter conditions the infant is not acidotic. Hyperglycemia may be present in some patients.

Diagnosis is established by demonstrating marked elevations of isovaleric acid and its metabolites (isovalerylglycine, 3-hydroxyisovaleric acid) in body fluids, especially urine. Isovaleric acid is volatile and may disappear from the urine if the specimen is not handled properly; however, isovalerylglycine is a stable compound that is more reliable for diagnostic purposes. Measuring the enzyme in cultured skin fibroblasts confirms the diagnosis. Intrauterine diagnosis has been accomplished by measuring isovalerylglycine in amniotic fluid or by enzyme assay in cultured amniocytes.

Treatment of the acute attack is aimed at hydration, correction of metabolic acidosis (by infusing sodium bicarbonate), and removal of the excess isovaleric acid. Because isovalerylglycine has a high urinary clearance, administration of glycine (250 mg/kg/24 hr) is recommended to enhance formation of isovalerylglycine. Carnitine (100 mg/kg/24 hr) also increases removal of isovaleric acid by forming isovalerylcarnitine, which is excreted in the urine. Adequate calories should be provided orally or intravenously to minimize the catabolic state. In patients with significant hyperammonemia (blood ammonia >200 μM), measures that reduce blood ammonia should be employed (Chapter 82.10). Exchange transfusion and peritoneal dialysis may be needed if the above measures fail to induce significant clinical and biochemical improvement. Patients should be kept on a low-protein diet (1.0–1.5 g/kg/24 hr) and should be given glycine and carnitine supplements after recovery from the acute attack. Pancreatitis (acute and recurrent forms) has been reported in survivors. Normal development can be achieved with early and proper treatment. Successful pregnancy with favorable outcome has been reported.

MULTIPLE CARBOXYLASE DEFICIENCY (Defects in Utilization of Biotin). Biotin is a water-soluble vitamin that acts as a cofactor for all four carboxylase enzymes: pyruvate carboxylase, acetyl CoA carboxylase, propionyl CoA carboxylase, and 3-methylcrotonyl CoA carboxylase. The latter two are involved in the metabolic pathways of leucine, isoleucine, and valine (see Fig. 82–5).

Dietary biotin is bound to protein (carboxylases); free biotin is generated in the intestine by the action of digestive enzymes and perhaps biotinidase. The latter enzyme, which is found in serum and most tissues in the body, is also essential for the recycling of biotin in the body by releasing it from a carboxylase (see Fig. 82–5). Free biotin must form a covalent peptide bond with the apoprotein of the above carboxylases in order to render them active. This binding is catalyzed by holocarboxylase synthetase. Deficiencies in this enzyme or in biotinidase result in malfunction of all the carboxylases and in organic acidemia.

Holocarboxylase Synthetase Deficiency (Multiple Carboxylase Deficiency—Infantile or Early Form). Infants with this rare autosomal recessive disorder become symptomatic in the first few weeks of life with breathing difficulties (tachypnea, apnea), hypotonia, seizures, vomiting, and failure to thrive. The urine may have a peculiar odor, which is described as similar to tomcat urine. The clinical finding that may differentiate this disorder from other organic acidemias, especially propionic acidemia, is the skin manifestations, which include generalized erythematous rash with exfoliation and alopecia totalis (see Fig. 82–6).

Laboratory findings include metabolic acidosis, ketosis, and the presence of a variety of organic acids, which include lactic acid, propionic acid, 3-methylcrotonic acid, 3-methylcrotonylglycine, triglylgycine, methylcitrate, and 3-hydroxyisovaleric acid in body fluids. Significant hyperammonemia has occurred in some patients. These infants may also have an immunodeficiency manifested by a decrease in the number of T cells. *Diagnosis* is confirmed by the enzyme assay in lymphocytes or cultured fibroblasts. The mutant enzyme has an increased K_m value for biotin. Thus, the enzyme activity can be restored by the administration of massive doses of biotin.

Treatment with biotin (10 mg/24 hr) results in a dramatic response. Prenatal diagnosis has been accomplished by means of an assay of enzyme activity in cultured amniotic cells and by measurement of intermediate metabolites (3-hydroxyisovalerate and methylcitrate) in amniotic fluid. Prenatal treatment of the mother with biotin has produced normal offspring in two women in whom prenatal diagnosis of holocarboxylase synthetase deficiency was made.

Biotinidase Deficiency (Multiple Carboxylase Deficiency—Juvenile or Late Form). The absence of biotinidase results in biotin deficiency. The prevalence of this autosomal recessive trait is estimated at 1 in 60,000.

Infants with this deficiency may develop *clinical manifestations* similar to those seen in infants with holocarboxylase synthetase deficiency, but, unlike the latter, symptoms may appear later when the child is several months or several years old. The delay is presumably due to the presence of sufficient free biotin derived from the mother or the diet. Atopic or seborrheic dermatitis, alopecia, ataxia, myoclonic seizures, hypotonia, developmental delay, hearing loss, and immunodeficiency may occur. Measurement of biotinidase in 100 Japanese children with intractable seborrheic dermatitis revealed two children with partial (15–30% activity) deficiency of the enzyme; these children were otherwise asymptomatic, and their dermatitis resolved with biotin therapy. Patients with partial deficiency of the enzyme have been identified on neonatal screening and in family members of these infants. Symptoms of biotinidase deficiency were observed only in a few of these individuals. However, the majority of these infants have shown no clinical or biochemical abnormalities.

Laboratory findings and the pattern of organic acids in body fluids resemble those associated with holocarboxylase synthetase deficiency (see earlier). *Diagnosis* can be established by measurement of the enzyme activity in the serum. A simplified method of neonatal screening for biotinidase deficiency is now available that requires a small amount of blood spotted on a filter paper.

Affected children respond dramatically to administration of free biotin (10 mg/24 hr). Treatment with biotin is also suggested for individuals with residual biotinidase activities below 10%.

Multiple Carboxylase Deficiency Due to Dietary Biotin Deficiency. Acquired deficiency of biotin may occur in infants receiving total parenteral nutrition without added biotin, in patients receiving prolonged anticonvulsant drugs, or in children with short gut syndrome or chronic diarrhea who are receiving formulas low in biotin. Excessive ingestion of raw eggs may also cause biotin deficiency because the protein avidin in egg white binds biotin and makes it unavailable for absorption. Infants with biotin deficiency develop dermatitis, alopecia, and moniliasis.

ISOLATED 3-METHYLCROTONYL-CoA CARBOXYLASE DEFICIENCY. This enzyme is one of the four carboxylase enzymes in the body that requires biotin as a cofactor (see Fig. 82–5). An isolated deficiency of this enzyme must be differentiated from disorders of biotin metabolism (multiple carboxylase deficiency), which causes diminished activity of all four carboxylases. Over 12 patients with this disorder have been reported.

Clinically, affected infants who grow and develop normally, have an acute episode of vomiting, hypotonia, lethargy, apnea, and convulsion following a minor infection. The first episode may be as early as 3 mo of age or as late as 5 yr. Death may occur during the acute episode. These episodes may be mistaken for Rye syndrome.

Laboratory studies reveal mild acidosis, ketosis, severe hypoglycemia, hyperammonemia, and elevated levels of liver transaminases. Large amounts of 3-hydroxyisovaleric acid and 3-methylcrotonylglycine are found in the urine. Urinary excretion of 3-methylcrotonic acid is not increased in this condition because the accumulated 3-methylcrotoyl CoA is converted to 3-hydroxyisovaleric acid. Severe secondary carnitine deficiency is common. *Diagnosis* may be confirmed by measurement of the enzyme activity in cultured fibroblasts.

Aggressive *treatment* of acute episodes with hydration, intravenous infusion of glucose, and alkali is recommended. Long-term treatment include a diet restricted in leucine in conjunction with the oral administration of carnitine (75–100 mg/kg/24 hr) and the prevention of catabolic states. Normal growth and development are expected in these patients. The condition is inherited as an autosomal recessive trait.

3-METHYLGLUTACONIC ACIDURIA. At least three inherited conditions are known to be associated with excessive excretion of 3-methylglutaconic acid in the urine. Deficiency of the enzyme 3-methylglutaconyl CoA hydratase (see Fig. 82–5) has been documented only in one condition (type I). In the other two conditions the enzyme activity is normal despite a modest excretion of 3-methylglutaconic aciduria.

3-Methylglutaconic Aciduria Type I (3-Methylglutaconyl CoA Hydratase Deficiency) (Fig. 82–5). This rare condition is manifested by speech retardation, mild psychomotor delay, and the development of metabolic acidosis during a catabolic state. Patients excrete large amounts of 3-methylglutaconic acid and moderate amounts of 3-hydroxyisovaleric and 3-methylglutaric acids. Deficiency of 3-methyltaconyl CoA hydratase has been shown in cultured fibroblasts and lymphoblast. The condition is inherited as an autosomal recessive trait. Treatment with a low protein diet has been suggested. Beneficial effects of this therapy on the clinical course of the disease remain doubtful.

3-Methylglutaconic Aciduria Type II (X-Linked Cardiomyopathy, Neutropenia, Growth Retardation, and 3-Methylglutaconic Aciduria with Normal 3-Methylglutaconyl CoA Hydratase). Over 20 male patients with this condition have been reported. *Clinical manifestations,* which usually occur shortly after birth, include dilated cardiomyopathy (manifested as respiratory distress and heart failure), hypotonia, growth retardation, and neutropenia. If patients survive infancy, relative improvement may occur with advancing age. Cognitive development is usually normal despite delayed motor function.

Laboratory findings reveal mild to moderate increases in urinary excretion of 3-methylglutaconic, 3-methylglutaric, and 2-ethylhydracrylic acids. Neutropenia is a common finding. Lactic acidosis, hypoglycemia, and abnormal mitochondrial ultrastructure have been shown in some patients. Unlike 3-methylglutaconic aciduria type I, urinary excretion of 3-hydroxyoisovaleric acid is not elevated.

The condition is inherited as an X-linked recessive trait. The activity of the enzyme 3-methylglutaconyl CoA hydratase is normal. The reason for the increased excretion of the above organic acids has not been understood. No effective *treatment* is available.

3-Methylglutaconic Aciduria Type III. *Clinical manifestations* in these patients include optic atrophy, choreoathetoid movements, ataxia, and mild developmental delay. All reported patients except one were Iraqi Jews in Israel. These patients excrete moderate amounts of 3-methylglutaconic and 3-methylglutaric acids. As in 3-methyglutaconic aciduria type II, the reason for the increased excretion of these organic acids has not been elucidated. Activity of the enzyme 3-methylglutaconyl CoA hydratase has been normal. About 50% of these patients develop spastic paraplegia during the second decade of life. The condition seems to be inherited as an autosomal recessive trait. No effective *treatment* is available.

β-KETOTHIOLASE DEFICIENCY (Acetoacetyl-CoA Thiolase Deficiency). 2-Methylacetoacetyl CoA thiolase is one of the four existing thiolases in the body. This mitochondrial enzyme cleaves 2-methylacetoacetyl CoA to acetyl CoA and propionyl CoA (see Fig. 82–5). Although deficiencies of the other thiolases have also been reported, the term β-ketothiolase deficiency is traditionally reserved for patients with mitochondrial acetoacetyl-CoA thiolase deficiency. This condition is inherited as an autosomal recessive trait and may be more prevalent than has been appreciated. The gene for this enzyme is located on the long arm of chromosome 11.

The *clinical manifestations* are quite variable, ranging from an asymptomatic course in an adult to severe episodes of acidosis starting in the 1st yr of life. These children have intermittent episodes of severe acidosis, ketosis, and moderate to severe hyperammonemia that may lead to coma and death. These episodes usually occur following an intercurrent infection and respond quickly to intravenous fluids and bicarbonate therapy. The child may be completely asymptomatic between episodes and may tolerate a normal protein diet well. Mental development is normal in most children. The episodes may be misdiagnosed as salicylate poisoning because of the similarity of clinical findings and the interference of elevated blood levels of acetoacetate with the colorimetric assay for salicylate. In an unreported case of our own, the diagnosis was not made until the child was 3½ yr of age, when a third episode of severe acidosis occurred following an upper respiratory infection. The second episode at 14 mo of age was diagnosed as salicylate ingestion. Psychomotor development is normal in affected children.

Laboratory findings during the acute attack include acidosis, ketosis, and hyperammonemia. The urine contains large amounts of 2-methylacetoacetate, and its decarboxylation product butanone, 2-methyl-3-hydroxybutyrate, and tiglylglycine. Mild hyperglycinemia may also be present. The clinical and biochemical findings should be differentiated from those seen with propionic and methylmalonic acidemias (see later). *Diagnosis* may be established by assay of the enzyme in cultured fibroblasts.

Treatment of acute episodes includes hydration and infusion of bicarbonate to correct the acidosis; a 10% glucose solution with the appropriate electrolytes and intravenous lipids may be used to minimize the catabolic state. Hyperammonemia should be treated promptly (see Chapter 82.10). Peritoneal dialysis may be required if the above measures do not produce significant clinical improvement. Restriction of protein intake (1–2 g/kg/24 hr) is recommended for long-term therapy. L-Carnitine (50–100 mg/kg/24 hr) may be used to prevent possible secondary carnitine deficiency. However, secondary deficiency of carnitine has not been documented in this condition.

CYSTOSOLIC ACETOACETYL CoA THIOLASE DEFICIENCY. This enzyme catalyzes the cytosolic production of acetoacetyl CoA from 2 moles of acetyl CoA (see Fig. 82–7). Cytosolic acetoacetyl CoA is the precursor of hepatic cholesterol synthesis. The cytosolic acetoacetyl CoA thiolase is a completely different enzyme from that of mitochondrial thiolase (see Fig. 82–5). Two patients with a deficiency of this enzyme have been reported. *Clinical manifestations* in these patients were similar to those in patients with mavolonic acidemia (see below). Severe progressive developmental delay, hypotonia, and chorioathetoid movements develop in the first few months of life. *Laboratory findings* were nonspecific; one patient had elevated lactate and pyruvate levels in blood and urine with normal acetoacetate and 3-hydroxybutyrate, whereas the other patient had persistent elevations of acetoacetate and 3-hydroxybutyrate. *Diagnosis* was established by demonstrating a deficiency in cytosolic thiolase activity in liver biopsy or in cultured fibroblasts. No effective *treatment* is available.

3-HYDROXY-3-METHYLGLUTARIC (HMG) ACIDURIA. This condition is due to a deficiency of 3-hydroxy-3-methylglutaryl (HMG) CoA lyase (see Fig. 82–5). This enzyme also catalyzes the conversion of 3 HMG CoA to acetoacetate during ketogenesis (Fig. 82–7). *Clinically,* 60% of patients become symptomatic between 3 and 11 mo of age, whereas 30% develop symptoms in the first few days of life. One child remained asymptomatic until 15 yr of age. Episodes of vomiting, severe hypoglycemia, hypotonia, acidosis, and dehydration may rapidly lead to lethargy, ataxia, and coma. These episodes often occur during an intercurrent infection. Hepatomegaly is common. These manifestations may be mistaken for Reye syndrome or medium chain acyl CoA dehydrogenase (MCAD) deficiency. Patients usually have normal development.

Laboratory findings reveal hypoglycemia, moderate to severe hyperammonemia, and acidosis. There is mild or no ketosis because 3-hydroxy-3 methylglutaric CoA, which is an obligatory intermediate metabolite in the formation of ketone bodies, cannot be converted to acetoacetate. Urinary excretion of 3-hydroxy-3-methylglutaric acid and other proximal intermediate metabolites of leucine catabolism (3-methylglutaconic acid and 3-hydroxyisovaleric acid), is markedly increased. These organic acids are excreted in the urine as carnitine conjugates resulting in secondary carnitine deficiency. Glutaric and adipic acids may also be increased in urine during acute attacks. *Diagnosis* may be confirmed by enzyme assay in cultured fibroblasts, leukocytes, or liver specimens. Prenatal diagnosis is possible with an assay of the enzyme in cultured aminocytes or in a chorionic villi biopsy.

Treatment of acute episodes includes hydration, infusion of glucose to control hypoglycemia, and administration of bicarbonate to correct acidosis. Hyperammonemia should be treated promptly (see Chapter 82.10). Exchange transfusion and peritoneal dialysis may be required in patients with severe hyperammonemia. Restriction of protein and fat intake is recommended for long-term management. L-Carnitine (50–100 mg/kg/24 hr, orally) prevents secondary carnitine deficiency. Prolonged fasting should be avoided. One patient died from acute cardiomyopathy at 7 mo of age during a febrile illness. There

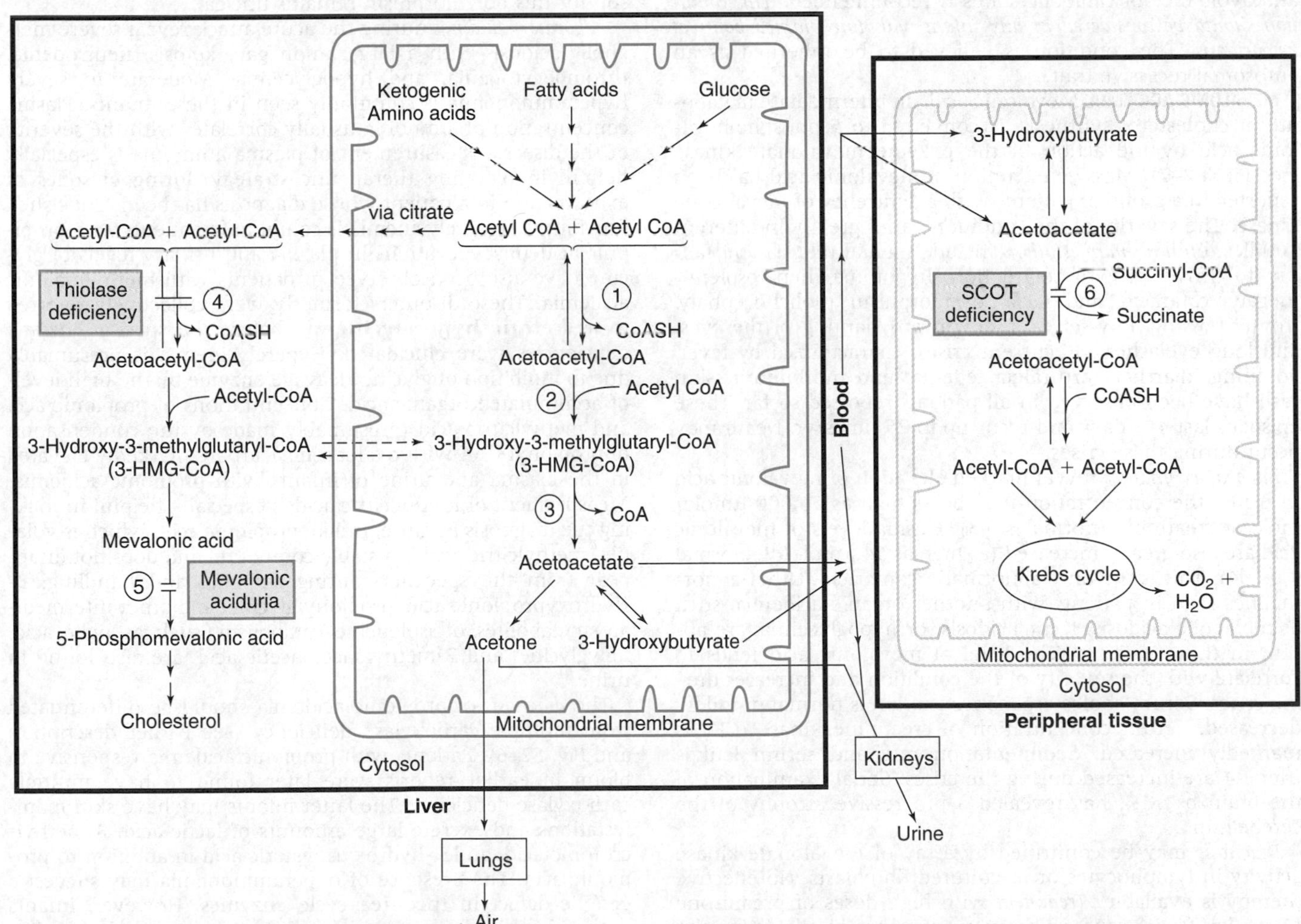

Figure 82–7 Formation (liver) and metabolism (peripheral tissues) of ketone bodies and cholesterol synthesis. **Enzymes:** (1) mitochondrial acetoacetyl-CoA thiolase; (2) HMG-CoA synthase; (3) HMG-CoA lyase; (4) cytosolic acetoacetyl-6A-thiolase; (5) mevalonic kinase; (6) succinyl-CoA: 3-ketoacid CoA transferase (SCOT).

may be a risk in immunization, because one child has died following immunization. The condition is inherited as an autosomal recessive trait. The *gene* for 3HMG CoA lyase resides on the short arm of chromosome 1. The gene defect appears to be more common in the Arabic population.

SUCCINYL CoA: 3-KETOACID CoA TRANSFERASE (SCOT) DEFICIENCY. This enzyme is necessary for the metabolism of ketone bodies (acetoacetate and 3-hydroxybutyrate) in peripheral tissue (see Fig. 82–7). A deficiency of this enzyme results in the underutilization and accumulation of ketone bodies and ketoacidosis. Ten patients with SCOT deficiency have been reported. However, it is believed that the condition is not rare and, in most cases, remains undiagnosed.

The presentation is an acute episode of severe ketoacidosis in an infant who had been growing and developing normally. The acute episode is often precipitated by an intercurrent infection or a catabolic state. Death may occur during these episodes. The first episode may happen as early as 38 hr after birth or as late as 10 mo of age. A chronic subclinical ketosis persists between the attacks. Development is usually normal.

Laboratory findings are nonspecific and include metabolic acidosis and ketonuria with high levels of acetoacetate and 3-hydroxybutyrate in blood and urine. No other organic acids are found in the urine. Plasma amino acids are usually normal. *Diagnosis* can be established by demonstrating a deficiency of enzyme activity in cultured fibroblasts.

Treatment of acute episodes consists of hydration, correction of acidosis, and the provision of a diet adequate in caloric content. Long-term treatment with a high carbohydrate diet and avoidance of catabolic states is recommended. *This condition should be considered in any infant with unexplained bouts of ketoacidosis.* The condition is believed to be inherited as an autosomal recessive trait.

MEVALONIC ACIDEMIA. Mevalonic acid, an intermediate metabolite of cholesterol synthesis, is converted to 5-phosphomevalonic acid by the action of the enzyme mevalonate kinase (see Fig. 82–7). Massive excretion of mevalonic acid has been reported in a group of patients with a deficiency of mevalonate kinase. The severity of the condition varies greatly in different families. *Clinical manifestations* include mental retardation, failure to thrive, growth retardation, hypotonia, hepatosplenomegaly, cataracts, and facial dysmorphism (dolichocephaly, frontal bossing, low-set ears, downward slanting of the eyes, and long eyelashes). Recurrent crises, characterized by fever, vomiting, diarrhea, arthralgia, edema, and morbiliform skin rash have been observed in all patients reported so far. These episodes last 4–5 days and recur up to 25 times/yr. Death may occur during these crises.

Laboratory findings reveal marked elevation of mevalonic acid in urine; the concentration may be as high as 56,000 μmole/mole of creatinine (normal <0.3). Plasma levels of mevalonic acid are also greatly increased (as high as 54 μmole/dL; normal <0.004). This is the only abnormal organic acid. Other abnormalities seen in patients with another organic acidemia, such as metabolic acidosis, lactic acidosis, or hypoglycemia, are absent in these patients. The level of mevalonic acid tends to correlate with the severity of the condition and increases during crises. Serum cholesterol concentration is normal or mildly decreased. Serum concentration of creatinine kinase (CK) is markedly increased. Sedimentation rate and serum leukotriene-4 are increased during the crises. Serial examination of the brain by MRI has revealed a progressive atrophy of the cerebellum.

Diagnosis may be confirmed by assay of mevalonate kinase activity in lymphocytes or in cultured fibroblasts. No effective therapy is available. *Treatment* with high doses of prednisone (2 mg/kg/24 hr) causes a dramatic response in alleviating the acute crises. The condition is inherited as an autosomal recessive trait. *Perinatal diagnosis* is possible by measurement of mevalonic acid in the amniotic fluid or by assay of the enzyme activity in amniocytes or chorionic villi samples. The *gene* for mevalonate kinase is on chromosome 12.

PROPIONIC ACIDEMIA (Propionyl CoA Carboxylase Deficiency). Propionic acid is an intermediate metabolite of isoleucine, valine, threonine, methionine, odd-chain fatty acids, and cholesterol catabolism. It is normally carboxylated to methylmalonic acid by the mitochondrial enzyme propionyl CoA carboxylase, which requires biotin as a cofactor (see Fig. 82–5). The enzyme is composed of two nonidentical subunits, α and β. Biotin is bound to the α subunit.

The prevalence of propionic acidemia, inherited as an autosomal recessive trait, is not known. The gene for the α subunit is located on chromosome 13 and that of the β subunit is mapped to the long arm of chromosome 3.

Clinical findings are nonspecific. The majority of patients develop symptoms in the first few weeks of life. Poor feeding, vomiting, hypotonia, lethargy, dehydration, and clinical signs of acidosis progress rapidly to coma and death. Seizures occur in about 30% of affected infants. If an infant survives the first attack, similar episodes may occur during an intercurrent infection, constipation, or following ingestion of a high-protein diet. Less frequently, the infant may come to medical attention later in life because of mental retardation without acute attacks of ketosis. Some affected children may have episodes of unexplained severe ketoacidosis separated by periods of seemingly normal health. The severity of clinical manifestations may also be variable within a family; in one kindred, a brother was diagnosed at 5 yr of age, whereas his 13-yr-old sister, with the same level of enzyme deficiency, was asymptomatic. The reason for this polymorphism remains unclear.

Laboratory findings during the acute attack reveal severe metabolic acidosis with a large anion gap, ketosis, neutropenia, thrombocytopenia, and hypoglycemia. Moderate to severe hyperammonemia is commonly seen in these infants. Plasma concentration of ammonia usually correlates with the severity of the disease. Measurement of plasma ammonia is especially helpful in planning therapeutic strategy during episodes of exacerbation in a patient whose diagnosis has been established previously. Hyperglycinemia is common in patients with propionic acidemia. Elevations in plasma and urinary levels of glycine have also been observed in patients with methylmalonic acidemia. These disorders formerly were collectively referred to as **ketotic hyperglycinemia** before the specific enzyme deficiencies were elucidated. Hyperglycinemia is presumably due to inhibition of glycine cleavage enzyme by the high levels of accumulated organic acid. Concentrations of propionic acid and methylcitric acid (presumably made by the condensation of propionyl CoA with oxaloacetic acid) are markedly elevated in the plasma and urine of infants with propionic acidemia. Measurement of methylcitric acid is especially helpful in making the diagnosis because, unlike propionic acid, which is volatile, methylcitric acid is a stable compound and does not disappear from the specimen during shipping and handling. 3-Hydroxypropionic acid, propionylglycine, and other intermediate metabolites of isoleucine catabolism, such as tiglic acid, tiglyglycine, and 2-methyloacetoacetic acid, are also found in urine.

The *diagnosis* of propionic acidemia should be differentiated from multiple carboxylase deficiency (see earlier description and Fig. 82–6). Patients with propionic acidemia responsive to biotin in earlier reports were later found to have multiple carboxylase deficiency. The latter infants may have skin manifestations and excrete large amounts of lactic acid, 3-methylcrotonic acid, and 3-hydroxyisovaleric acid in addition to propionic acid. The presence of hyperammonemia may suggest a genetic defect in the urea cycle enzymes. However, infants with defects in the urea cycle are usually not acidotic (see Fig. 81–1). Hyperammonemia is believed to be due to inhibition of carbamylphosphate synthetase (CPS I) by the organic acid. Definitive diagnosis of propionic acidemia can be established by measuring the appropriate enzyme activity in leukocytes or cultured fibroblasts.

Prenatal diagnosis has been accomplished by measuring the enzyme activity in cultured amniotic cells and in samples of uncultured chorionic villi.

Treatment of acute attacks includes rehydration, correction of acidosis, and prevention of the catabolic state by provision of adequate calories through parenteral hyperalimentation. Minimal amounts of protein (0.25 g/kg/24 hr), preferably a protein deficient in propionate precursor, should be provided in the hyperalimentation fluid very early in the course of treatment. To control the possible production of propionic acid by intestinal bacteria, sterilization of the intestinal tract flora by antibiotics (e.g., oral neomycin, metronidazole) should be promptly initiated. Constipation should also be treated. Patients with propionic acidemia may develop carnitine deficiency, presumably as a result of urinary loss of propionylcarnitine formed from the accumulated organic acid. Administration of L-carnitine (50–100 mg/kg/24 hr orally) normalizes fatty acid oxidation and improves acidosis. In patients with concomitant hyperammonemia measures to reduce blood ammonia should be employed (see Chapter 82.10). Very ill patients with severe acidosis and hyperammonemia require peritoneal dialysis or hemodialysis to remove ammonia and other toxic compounds. Although infants with true propionic acidemia are rarely responsive to biotin, this compound should be administered (10 mg/24 hr) to all infants during the initial attack and should be continued until a definitive diagnosis is established.

Long-term treatment consists of a low-protein diet (1.0–1.5 g/kg/24 hr) and administration of L-carnitine (50–100 mg/kg/24 hr orally). Synthetic proteins deficient in propionate precursors* (isoleucine, valine, methionine, and threonine) may be used to increase the amount of dietary protein (to 1.5–2.0 g/kg/24 hr) while causing minimal change in propionate production. However, excessive supplementation with these proteins may cause a deficiency of the essential amino acids. To avoid this problem, natural proteins should comprise most of the dietary protein (50–75%). Some patients may require chronic alkaline therapy to correct low-grade chronic acidosis. The concentration of ammonia in blood usually normalizes between attacks, and chronic treatment of hyperammonemia is rarely needed. Catabolic states that may trigger acute attacks (e.g., infections) should be treated promptly and aggressively. Close monitoring of blood pH, amino acids, urinary content of propionate and its metabolites, and growth parameters is necessary to ensure the proper balance of the diet and the success of therapy.

Long-term *prognosis* is guarded. Death may occur during an acute attack. Normal psychomotor development is possible, but most children manifest some degree of permanent neurodevelopmental deficit such as dystonia, chorea, and pyramidal signs, despite adequate therapy.

METHYLMALONIC ACIDEMIA. Methylmalonic acid, a structural isomer of succinic acid, is normally derived from propionic acid as part of the catabolic pathways of isoleucine, valine, threonine, methionine, cholesterol, and odd-chain fatty acids. Two enzymes are involved in the conversion of D-methylmalonic acid to succinic acid, methylmalonyl CoA racemase (which forms the L-isomer) and methylmalonyl CoA mutase (which converts the L-methylmalonic acid to succinic acid) (see Fig. 82–5). The latter enzyme requires adenosylcobalamin, a metabolite of vitamin B_{12}, as a coenzyme. Deficiency of either the mutase or its coenzyme causes an accumulation of methylmalonic acid and its precursors in body fluids. A deficiency of the racemase has not been confirmed.

At least two forms of mutase apoenzyme deficiency have been identified. These are designated *mut*^{0}, meaning no detectable enzyme activity, and *mut*$^-$, indicating residual, although abnormal, mutase activity. About half of the reported patients with methylmalonic acidemia have a deficiency of the mutase apoenzyme (*mut*^{0} or *mut*$^-$). These patients are not responsive to vitamin B_{12} therapy. The gene for the mutase has been mapped to the short arm of chromosome 6 and about 30 different mutations have been described. In the remaining patients with methylmalonic acidemia, the defect resides in the formation of adenosylcobalamin.

Defects in Metabolism of Vitamin B_{12} (Cobalamin). Dietary vitamin B_{12} requires intrinsic factor, a glycoprotein secreted by the gastric parietal cells, for absorption in the terminal ileum. It is transported in the blood by heptocorrin (TCI) and transcobalamin II (TCII). Genetic disorders involving intrinsic factor and TCII but not TCI result in megaloblastic anemia. The complex of transcobalamin II-cobalamin (TCII-Cbl) is recognized by a specific receptor on the cell membrane and enters the cell by endocytosis. The TCII-Cbl complex is hydrolyzed in the lysosome, and free cobalamin is released into the cytosol (see Fig. 82–5). The cobalt of the molecule is reduced in the cytosol from three valences (cob[III]alamin) to two (cob[II]alamin) before it enters the mitochondria, where further reduction to cob(I)alamin occurs. The latter compound reacts with adenosine to form adenosyl cobalamin (coenzyme for methylmalonyl CoA mutase). The free cobalamin in the cytosol may also undergo a series of poorly understood enzymatic steps to form methylcobalamin (coenzyme for methionine synthase, which catalyzes the remethylation of homocysteine to methionine; see Fig. 82–3).

At least seven different defects in the intracellular metabolism of cobalamin have been identified. These are designated *cbl* A through G (*cbl* stands for a defect in any step of cobalamin metabolism). *cbl*A is probably due to a deficiency of mitochondrial cobalamin reductase; *cbl*B is caused by a deficiency of adenosylcobalamin transferase. Both cause methylmalonic acidemia only. The precise enzymatic deficiencies in the remaining defects are not known. In patients with *cbl*C, *cbl*D, and *cbl*F defects, synthesis of both adenosylcobalamin and methylcobalamin is impaired, causing homocystinuria in addition to methylmalonic acidemia. The *cbl*E defect and the *cbl*G defect involve only the synthesis of methylcobalamin, resulting in homocystinuria without methylmalonic aciduria but usually with megaloblastic anemia. All of the above defects including apoenzyme deficiency (*mut*^{0} and *mut*$^-$) are inherited as autosomal recessive traits and have an overall prevalence of about 1 in 48,000.

Clinical manifestations of patients with *mut*^{0} and *mut*$^-$ and *cbl*A and *cbl*B are similar to those of patients with propionic acidemia (see earlier). However, fulminating neonatal forms causing severe ketosis, acidosis, hyperammonemia, neutropenia, coma, and death are more common in patients with methylmalonic acidemia than in patients with propionic acidemia. If the infant survives the first attack, similar exacerbations may occur during an intercurrent infection or following ingestion of a high-protein diet. The condition may present later in life with failure to thrive, hypotonia, and developmental delay. Some infants with methylmalonic acidemia have characteristic facial features with a triangular mouth and high forehead. Patients with severe clinical manifestations in the first few days of life tend to have mutase deficiency (*mut*^{0} or *mut*$^-$). However, there are wide variations in the clinical presentation regardless of the nature of the enzyme deficiency. Asymptomatic patients with mutase apoenzyme deficiency have been identified through screening of newborn infants. These patients tolerate a normal protein intake and accumulate high levels of methylmalonate in their body fluids.

Laboratory findings include ketosis, acidosis, anemia, neutropenia, thrombocytopenia, hyperglycinemia, hyperammonemia, hypoglycemia, and the presence of large quantities of methylmalonic acid in body fluids (see Fig. 82–6). Propionic acid and its

---

*Milupa OS1. Milupa Corporation, Darien, CT.

metabolites 3-hydroxypropionate and methylcitrate are also found in urine. Hyperammonemia may suggest the presence of genetic defects in the urea cycle enzymes. However, patients with defects in urea cycle enzymes are not acidotic (see Fig. 81–1). The increase in ammonia in patients with methylmalonic acidemia is believed to be due to inhibition of CPS I by the organic acid.

Diagnosis can be confirmed by measuring propionate incorporation or mutase activity and by performing complementation studies in cultured fibroblasts. Prenatal diagnosis has been accomplished by performing an assay of propionate incorporation in cultured amniotic cells.

Treatment of acute attacks is similar to that of attacks in patients with propionic acidemia (see earlier) except that large doses (1–2 mg/24 hr) of vitamin B_{12} are used instead of biotin. Long-term treatment consists of a low-protein diet (1.0–1.5 g/kg/24 hr) and administration of L-carnitine (50–100 mg/kg/24 hr) and vitamin B_{12} (1 mg/24 hr for only those patients with defects in vitamin B_{12} metabolism). The protein composition of the diet is similar to that prescribed for patients with propionic acidemia. Chronic alkaline therapy is usually required to correct low-grade chronic acidosis. Blood levels of ammonia usually normalize between the attacks, and chronic treatment of hyperammonemia is rarely needed. Stressful situations that may trigger acute attacks (such as infection) should be treated promptly. Close monitoring of blood pH, amino acid levels, urinary content of methylmalonate, and growth parameters is necessary to ensure proper balance in the diet and the success of therapy. Glutathione deficiency responsive to high doses of ascorbate was described in a 7-yr-old boy who had been refractory to treatment.

Prognosis depends largely on the type of enzymatic defect that is present. Patients with mutase apoenzyme deficiency (*mut*^{0}, *mut*$^-$) have a worse prognosis. Acute and recurrent pancreatitis have been reported in survivors as young as 13 mo of age. Two of the five children with this complication died during an acute attack of pancreatitis. Unexplained infarcts of basal ganglia and tubulointerstitial nephritis have been observed in some of these patients.

COMBINED METHYLMALONIC ACIDURIA AND HOMOCYSTINURIA (*cbl*C, *cbl*D, and *cbl*F Defects). About 100 patients with methylmalonic acidemia and homocystinuria due to *cbl*C, *cbl*D, and *cbl*F defects (see Figs. 82–3 and 82–5) have been reported. The majority of the patients (about 90) had the *cbl*C defect; only two brothers with *cbl*D and five patients with *cbl*F defects have been identified.

Neurologic findings were prominent in patients with *cbl*C and *cbl*D defects. Most patients with *cbl*D defect came to medical attention in the first few months of life because of failure to thrive, lethargy, poor feeding, mental retardation, and seizures. However, late-onset defects with sudden development of dementia and myelopathy have been reported. Megaloblastic anemia was a common finding in patients with *cbl*C defect. Mild to moderate increases in concentrations of methylmalonic acid and homocysteine were found in body fluids. However, unlike patients with classic homocystinuria, plasma levels of methionine are low to normal in these defects. Neither hyperammonemia nor hyperglycinemia has been observed in these patients. The first two patients with *cbl*F defect were females in whom poor feeding, growth and developmental delay, and persistent stomatitis became manifest in the first 3 wk of life. The first patient did not have megaloblastic anemia and homocystinuria, but both these signs were present in the second infant. Moderate methylmalonic acidemia was present in both infants. One patient was not diagnosed until age 10 yr. He had findings suggestive of rheumatoid arthritis, a pigmented skin abnormality, and became encephalopathic. Vitamin B_{12} malabsorption is seen in patients with *cbl*F defect.

Experience with *treatment* of patients with *cbl*C, *cbl*D, and *cbl*F defects is very limited. Large doses of hydroxycobalamin (1–2 mg/24 hr) in conjunction with betaine (6–9 g/24 hr) seem to produce biochemical improvement with little clinical effect. Unexplained severe hemolytic anemia, hydrocephalus, and congestive heart failure have been major complications in patients with *cbl*C defect.

Patients with *cbl*E and *cbl*G defects do not have methylmalonic acidemia and are discussed further in the section on homocystinuria (see Chapter 82.3).

82.7 *Glycine*

Iraj Rezvani

Glycine is a nonessential amino acid synthesized mainly from serine and threonine. The main catabolic pathway requires the complex glycine cleavage enzyme system to cleave the first carbon of glycine and convert it to carbon dioxide. The second carbon is transferred to tetrahydrofolate (FH_4) to form hydroxymethyltetrahydrofolate, which may either react with another mole of glycine to form serine (Fig. 82–8) or form methyltetrahydrofolate, which serves as a methyl group donor for many reactions in the body (see Fig. 82–3). The glycine cleavage system, a mitochondrial multienzyme system, is composed of four proteins: P protein, H protein, T protein, and L protein.

HYPERGLYCINEMIA. Elevated levels of glycine in body fluids occur in patients having propionic acidemia and methylmalonic acidemia. These disorders have been collectively referred to as *ketotic hyperglycinemia* because episodes of severe acidosis and ketosis occur. The pathogenesis of hyperglycinemia in these disorders is not fully understood, but inhibition of the glycine cleavage enzyme system by the various organic acids has been shown to occur in some of the affected patients. The term *nonketotic hyperglycinemia* is reserved for the clinical condition caused by the genetic deficiency of the glycine cleavage enzyme system (see Fig. 82–8). In this condition hyperglycinemia is present without ketosis.

NONKETOTIC HYPERGLYCINEMIA (NKH). Four forms of NKH have been identified—neonatal, infantile, late onset, and transient.

Neonatal NKH. This is the most common form of NKH. *Clinical manifestations* develop during the first few days of life (between 6 hr to 8 days after birth). Poor feeding, failure to suck, lethargy, and profound hypotonia may progress rapidly to a deep coma, apnea, and death. Convulsions, especially myoclonic seizures and hiccups, are common.

Laboratory findings reveal moderate to severe hyperglycinemia (as high as eight times normal) and hyperglycinuria. The unequivocal elevation of glycine concentration in spinal fluid (15 to 30 times normal) and the high ratio of glycine concentration in spinal fluid to that in plasma (a value greater than 0.08) are diagnostic of NKH. Plasma serine levels are usually low. Serum pH is normal.

About 30% of affected infants die despite supportive therapy. Those who survive develop profound psychomotor retardation and intractable seizure disorders (myoclonic and/or grand mal seizures).

Infantile NKH. These previously normal infants develop *signs and symptoms* of neonatal NKH (see above) after 6 mo of age. Seizures are the common presenting signs. This condition appears to be a milder form; infants usually survive, and mental retardation is not as profound as in the neonatal form.

Laboratory findings in these patients are identical to the neonatal form.

Late Onset NKH. This rare form has been reported only in a few patients. Progressive spastic paraparesis, optic atrophy, and choreoathetotic movements are the main *clinical manifestations*. Age of onset has been between 2 and 33 yr. Mental development is usually normal, but mild retardation has been reported in three patients. Seizures have occurred in only one patient.

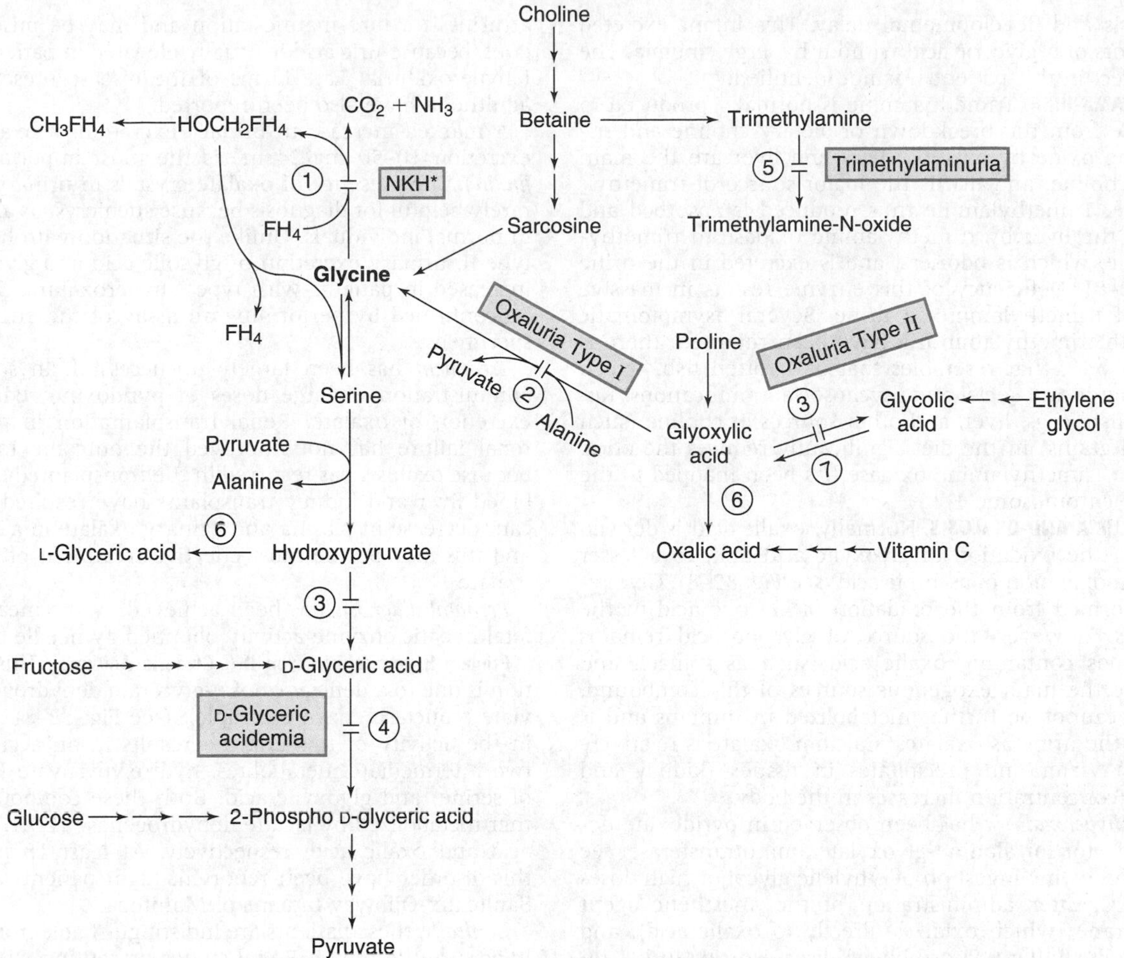

Figure 82–8 Pathways in metabolism of glycine and glyoxylic acid. **Enzymes:** (1) glycine cleavage enzyme; (2) alanine: glyoxylate aminotransferase; (3) D-glyceric acid dehydrogenase; (4) glycerate kinase; (5) trimethylamine oxidase; (6) lactate dehydrogenase; (7) glycolate oxidase; (8) NKH* = nonketotic hyperglycinemia; TH4 = tetrahydrofolate.

Laboratory findings are similar to but not as pronounced as the neonatal form.

Transient NKH. This form has been described in five infants. Clinical and laboratory manifestations are indistinguishable from those of the neonatal form. However, by 2 to 8 wk of age, the elevated glycine levels in plasma and cerebrospinal fluid normalize and a complete clinical recovery occurs. Four of these patients had no neurologic abnormalities, but one had severe mental retardation. The etiology of this condition is not known but it is believed to be due to immaturity of the enzyme system.

All forms of NKH should be differentiated from ketotic hyperglycinemia (see Chapter 82.6), D-glyceric aciduria (see below), and ingestion of valproic acid. This compound causes a moderate increase in blood and urinary glycine concentrations. Repeat assays after discontinuation of the drug should establish the diagnosis.

Diagnosis may be established by assay of the enzyme in liver or brain specimens. Enzyme activity in the neonatal form is close to zero while in the other forms some residual activity is present. In over 80% of patients with the neonatal form, the enzyme defect resides in the P protein. The deficit in the remainder of these patients is in the T protein. The enzyme assay in three patients with the infantile and late-onset forms revealed two patients with the defect in the T protein and one in the H protein.

No effective *treatment* is known. Exchange transfusion, dietary restriction of glycine, and administration of sodium benzoate or folate have not altered the neurologic outcome. Drugs that counteract the effect of glycine on neuronal cells, such as strychnine, diazapam, and dextrometorphan have shown some beneficial effects only in patients with the mild forms of the condition.

NKH is inherited as an autosomal recessive trait. The prevalence is not known but the condition is quite common in northern Finland (1:12,000). The *gene* for P protein is located on the short arm of chromosome 9. *Prenatal diagnosis* has been accomplished by performing an assay of the enzyme activity in chorionic villi biopsy specimens.

SARCOSINEMIA. Increased concentrations of sarcosine (*N*-methylglycine) have been observed in both blood and urine, but no consistent clinical picture can be attributed to this metabolic defect. This is a recessively inherited inborn error involving sarcosine dehydrogenase, the enzyme that converts sarcosine to glycine (see Fig. 82–8).

D-GLYCERIC ACIDURIA. D-Glyceric acid is an intermediate metabolite of serine and fructose metabolism (see Fig. 82–8). At least two forms of this rare condition have been identified. In one form (seen in three patients) clinical manifestations of severe encephalopathy (hypotonia, seizures, and mental and motor deficits) and the laboratory findings of hyperglycinemia and hyperglycinuria were suggestive of nonketotic hyperglycinemia. However, these patients excreted large quantities of D-glyceric acid (this compound is not normally detectable in urine). Enzyme studies indicated a deficiency of glycerate kinase in one patient and decreased activity of D-glyceric dehydrogenase in another.

In the other form, the major findings were persistent metabolic acidosis and developmental delay. This infant excreted large amounts of D-glyceric acid without hyperglycinemia. The enzyme defect in this patient was not identified.

TRIMETHYLAMINURIA. Trimethylamine is normally produced in the intestine from the breakdown of dietary choline and trimethylamine oxide by bacteria. Eggs and liver are the main sources of choline, and fish is the major source of trimethylamine oxide. Trimethylamine thus produced is absorbed and oxidized in the liver by trimethylamine oxidase to trimethylamine oxide, which is odorless, and is excreted in the urine (see Fig. 82–8). Deficiency of this enzyme results in massive excretion of trimethylamine in urine. Several asymptomatic patients with trimethylaminuria have been reported; there is a foul body odor that resembles that of a rotten fish, which may have significant social and psychosocial ramifications. Restriction of fish, eggs, liver, and other sources of choline (such as nuts and grains) in the diet significantly reduces the odor. The gene for trimethylamine oxidase has been mapped to the long arm of chromosome 1.

HYPEROXALURIA AND OXALOSIS. Normally, oxalic acid is derived mostly from the oxidation of glyoxylic acid and, to a lesser degree, from oxidation of ascorbic acid (see Fig. 82–8). Glyoxylic acid is formed from the oxidation of glycolic acid in the preoxisomes. However, the source of glycolic acid remains unclear. Foods containing oxalic acid, such as spinach and rhubarb, are the main exogenous sources of this compound. Oxalic acid cannot be further metabolized in humans and is excreted in the urine as oxalates. Calcium oxalate is relatively insoluble in water and precipitates in tissues (kidney and joints) if its concentration increases in the body.

Secondary hyperoxaluria has been observed in pyridoxine deficiency (cofactor for alanine-glyoxylate aminotransferase, see Fig. 82–8), following ingestion of ethylene glycol or high doses of vitamin C, after administration of the anesthetic agent methoxyflurane (which oxidizes directly to oxalic acid), and in patients with inflammatory bowel disease or extensive resection of bowel *(enteric hyperoxaluria)*. Acute, fatal hyperoxaluria may develop after ingestion of plants with a high oxalic acid content such as sorrel. Intentional ingestion of oxalic acid was a common suicidal agent at the turn of the century when oxalic acid was easily accessible as a common household cleaning agent. Precipitation of calcium oxalate in tissues causes hypocalcemia, liver necrosis, renal failure, cardiac arrhythmia, and death. The lethal dose of oxalic acid is estimated to be between 5 and 30 g.

Primary hyperoxaluria is a rare genetic disorder in which large amounts of oxalates accumulate in the body. Two types of primary hyperoxaluria have been identified. The term *oxalosis* refers to deposition of calcium oxalate in parenchymal tissue.

Primary Hyperoxaluria Type I. This rare condition is the most common form of primary hyperoxaluria. It is due to a deficiency of the peroxisomal enzyme alanine-glyoxylate aminotransferase, which is expressed only in the liver and requires pyridoxine (vitamin B_6) as its cofactor. In the absence of this enzyme, glyoxylic acid, which cannot be converted to glycine, is transferred to the cytosol, where it is oxidized to oxalic acid (see Fig. 82–8). It is inherited as an autosomal recessive trait. The gene for this enzyme resides on the long arm of chromosome 2. Several mutations of the gene have been described in patients with this condition. The most common mutation results in the mistargeting of the enzyme to the mitochondria instead of the proxisomes.

There is a wide variation in the age of presentation. The majority of patients become symptomatic before 5 yr of age. In about 10% of cases symptoms develop before 1 yr of age (neonatal oxaluria). The initial *clinical manifestations* are related to renal stones and nephrocalcinosis. Renal colic and asymptomatic hematuria lead to a gradual deterioration of renal function, manifested by growth retardation and uremia. Most patients die before 20 yr of age from renal failure. Acute arthritis is a rare manifestation and may be misdiagnosed as gout, because uric acid is usually elevated in patients with type I hyperoxaluria. Late forms of the disease presenting during adulthood have also been reported.

A marked increase in urinary excretion of oxalate (normal excretion 10–50 mg/24 hr) is the most important *laboratory finding*. The presence of oxalate crystals in urinary sediment is rarely helpful for diagnosis because such crystals are often seen in normal individuals. Unlike the situation with hyperoxaluria type II, urinary excretion of glycolic acid and glyoxylic acid is increased in patients with type I hyperoxaluria. *Diagnosis* can be confirmed by performing an assay of the enzyme in liver specimens.

Treatment has been largely unsuccessful. In some patients administration of large doses of pyridoxine reduces urinary excretion of oxalate. Renal transplantation in patients with renal failure has not improved the outcome in most cases because oxalosis has recurred in the transplanted kidney. Combined liver and kidney transplants have resulted in a significant decrease in plasma and urinary oxalate in a few patients, and this may be the most effective treatment of this disorder to date.

Prenatal diagnosis has been achieved by the measurement of fetal hepatic enzyme activity obtained by needle biopsy.

Primary Hyperoxaluria Type II (L-Glyceric Aciduria). This rare condition is due to a deficiency of D-glycerate dehydrogenase/glyoxylate reductase enzyme complex (see Fig. 82–8). A deficiency in the activity of this enzyme results in an accumulation of two intermediate metabolites, hydroxypyruvate (the ketoacid of serine) and glyoxylic acid. Both these compounds are further metabolized by lactate dehydrogenase (LDH) to L-glyceric acid and oxalic acid, respectively. At least 18 patients with this disorder have been reported. Eight patients are from the Saulteaux-Ojibway Indians of Manitoba.

Clinically, these patients are indistinguishable from those with hyperoxaluria type I. Renal stones presenting with renal colic and hematuria may develop before age 2 yr. However, renal failure has not been observed in patients with type II oxaluria; the urine contains large amounts of L-glyceric acid in addition to high levels of oxalate (L-glyceric acid is not normally present in urine). Urinary excretion of glycolic acid and glyoxylic acid is not increased. The presence of L-glyceric acid without increased levels of glycolic and glyoxylic acids in urine differentiates this type from type I hyperoxaluria. A similar disease has been recently described in cats.

No effective *therapy* is available.

CREATINE DEFICIENCY (Guanidinoacetate Methyltransferase Deficiency). Creatine is synthesized in the liver and pancreas from arginine and glycine but is not used in these organs (Fig. 82–9). It is transported to muscles and the brain, which contain high activities of creatine kinase. Phosphorylation and dephosphorylation of creatine by this enzyme in conjunction with ADP/ATP provide high-energy phosphate reactions in these organs. Creatine is nonenzymatically metabolized to creatinine at a constant daily rate and is excreted in the urine. A deficiency of guanidinoacetate methyltransferase causing a creatine deficiency state has been reported in two unrelated infants. *Clinical manifestations* were similar in both cases. The first patient was a male infant seen at 22 mo with progressive developmental delay, extrapyramidal movements characterized by dyskinetic-dystonic involuntary movements, and severe hypotonia. The infant had normal growth and development until 5 mo. The second patient, a product of consanguineous Kurdish parents, was first seen at 4 yr. Clinical findings were similar to the index case except that the child also had intractable seizures that developed at 14 mo during a febrile illness. Psychomotor delay was first noted at 6 mo.

Laboratory findings revealed mild hyperammonemia, orotic acidemia, and hyperornithinemia but very low plasma arginine and creatine concentrations. Guanidinoacetate was markedly

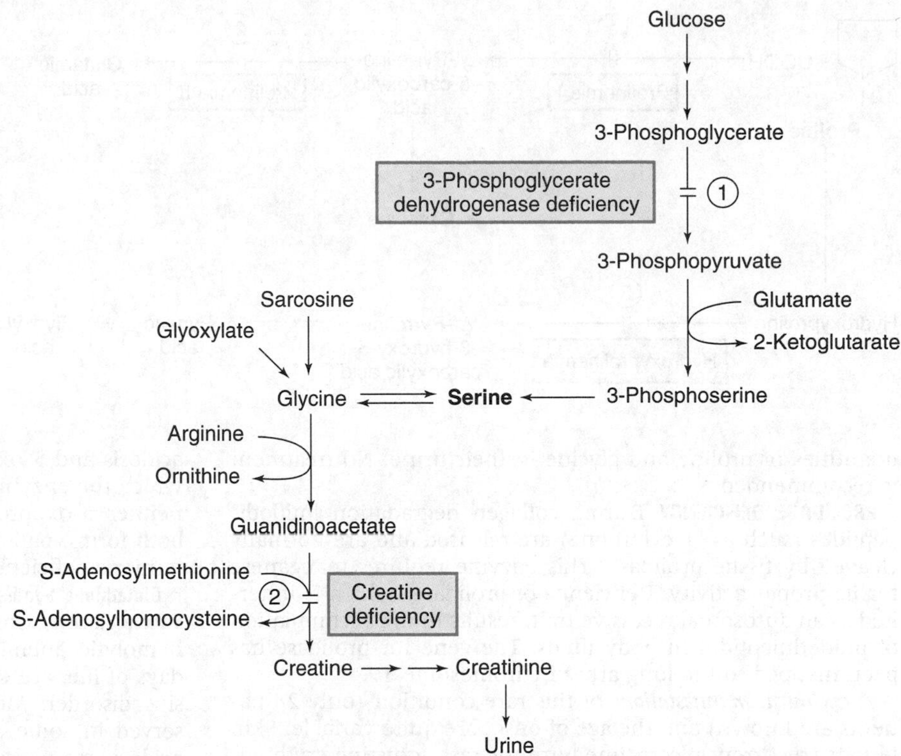

Figure 82–9 Pathways for the synthesis of serine and creatine. **Enzymes:** (1) 3-Phosphoglycerate dehydrogenase; (2) guanidinoacetate methyltransferase.

increased in the urine. Urinary excretion of creatinine was decreased.

Diagnosis was first established by in vivo proton magnetic resonance spectroscopy, which showed a complete deficiency of creatine in the brain. Confirmation of the diagnosis was accomplished by measurement of guanidinoacetate methyltransferase hepatic enzyme activity.

Treatment with supplemental creatine monohydrate (400–500 mg/kg/day) resulted in a dramatic improvement in muscle tone and overall mental status. Extrapyramidal movements abated, but the seizure disorder in the second patient was not alleviated. Significant increases in creatine and creatine phosphate of the brain were noted, and urinary creatinine excretion became normal. The mode of inheritance and the prevalence of the condition is not known at this time. This condition must be considered in any patient with brain and muscle disorders, since treatment can produce a dramatic response.

82.8 Serine

Iraj Rezvani

Serine is a nonessential amino acid synthesized from glucose (through 3-phosphoglycerate) and glycine (see Fig. 82–9).

3-Phosphoglycerate Dehydrogenase Deficiency. Two Turkish brothers born to consanguineous parents developed severe mental retardation, seizures, hypertonia, and microcephaly shortly after birth. One child also had bilateral cataracts.

Laboratory findings revealed low fasting levels of serine and glycine in plasma and very low levels of serine (five times lower than normal) and glycine (two times lower than normal) in cerebrospinal fluid. No abnormal organic acid was found in the urine. Magnetic resonance imaging of the head showed evidence of cortical atrophy and dysmyelination.

Diagnosis was confirmed by measurement of the enzyme activity in cultured fibroblasts.

Treatment with the administration of oral serine (200 mg/kg/24 hr) normalized the serine levels in the blood and in the cerebrospinal fluid. Seizure activity stopped after a wk of treatment. However, the long-term effect of treatment could not be evaluated because of the lack of cooperation of the parents. The mode of inheritance of the disease and its prevalence are not known. The favorable response to a simple treatment makes this diagnosis an important consideration in any child with psychomotor delay, seizure disorder, or other similar findings reported in these patients.

82.9 Proline and Hydroxyproline

Iraj Rezvani

Proline and hydroxyproline are found in high concentrations in collagen. Neither of these amino acids is normally found in urine in the free form except in early infancy. Excretion of "bound" hydroxyproline (dipeptides and tripeptides containing hydroxyproline) reflects collagen turnover and is increased in disorders of accelerated collagen turnover, such as rickets or hyperparathyroidism.

HYPERPROLINEMIA. Two types of this rare autosomal recessive condition have been described. *Type I hyperprolinemia* is due to a deficiency of proline oxidase (dehydrogenase), and *type II* is due to a defect in Δ′-pyrroline-5-carboxylic acid dehydrogenase enzyme (Fig. 82–10). Neither type causes any specific clinical manifestation. Increased blood concentrations of proline (more pronounced in type II) and prolinuria are found in both types. Hydroxyproline and glycine are also excreted in abnormal amounts in the urine because of the saturation of the common tubular reabsorption mechanism by the massive prolinuria. The presence of Δ′-pyrroline-5-carboxylic acid in plasma and urine differentiates type II from type I. No treatment is recommended for the affected individuals.

HYPERHYDROXYPROLINEMIA. This rare autosomal recessive condition is presumably due to a deficiency of hydroxyproline oxidase (see Fig. 82–10). Patients with this disorder are usually asymptomatic. A marked increase in blood concentration of hydroxyproline is diagnostic. These patients also excrete large

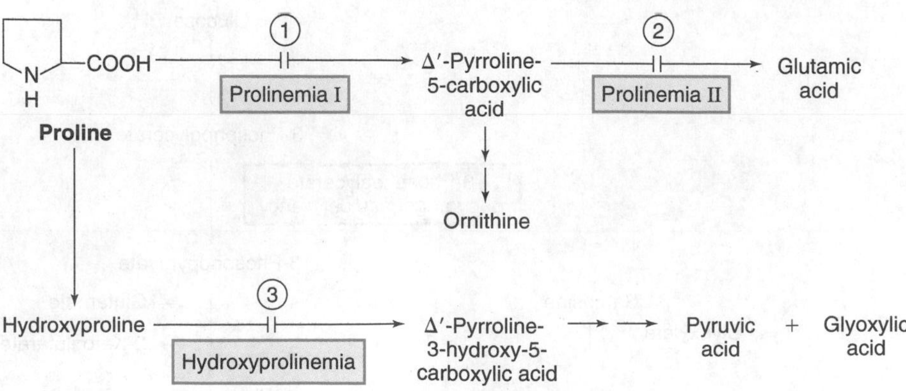

Figure 82–10 Pathways in the metabolism of proline. **Enzymes:** (1) proline oxidase; (2) Δ′-pyrroline-5-carboxylic acid dehydrogenase; (3) hydroxyproline oxidase.

quantities of proline and glycine in their urine. No treatment is recommended.

PROLIDASE DEFICIENCY. During collagen degradation imidodipeptides (such as glycylproline) are released and are normally cleaved by tissue prolidase. This enzyme requires manganese for its proper activity. Deficiency of prolidase, which is inherited as an autosomal recessive trait, results in the accumulation of imidodipeptides in body fluids. The gene for prolidase has been mapped to the long arm of chromosome 19.

The *clinical manifestations* of this rare condition (only 28 patients are known) and the age of onset are quite variable. Skin lesions (recurrent ulcers, fine purpuric rash, crusting erythematous dermatitis), mental and motor deficits, susceptibility to infections, and joint laxity are major findings. Some patients have characteristic craniofacial features with ptosis, ocular proptosis, and prominent cranial sutures. Asymptomatic cases have also been reported. A marked increase in urinary excretion of imidodipeptides is diagnostic. Enzyme assay may be performed in erythrocytes or cultured skin fibroblasts.

Oral supplementation with proline, ascorbic acid, and manganese and the topical use of proline and glycine result in an improvement in leg ulcers.

FAMILIAL IMINOGLYCINURIA. This asymptomatic defect in renal tubular reabsorption of proline is inherited as an autosomal recessive trait. Because proline, hydroxyproline, and glycine are all transported by a common mechanism, patients with familial iminoglycinuria also excrete proline and hydroxyproline in abnormal amounts. The serum concentrations of these amino acids are normal. Many persons so affected also have impaired intestinal transport of proline, and a few may be coincidentally mentally retarded. In a screening program, iminoglycinuria was found in 1 in 15,000 infants. Iminoglycinuria is also seen in patients with hyperprolinemia, hyperhydroxyprolinemia, and Fanconi syndrome.

82.10 Glutamic Acid

Iraj Rezvani

Glutathione (γ-glutamylcysteinylglycine) is the major product of glutamic acid in the body. This ubiquitous tripeptide is synthesized and degraded through a complex cycle called the γ-glutamyl cycle (Fig. 82–11). Because of its free sulfhydryl (-SH) group and its abundance in the cell, glutathione protects other sulfhydryl-containing compounds (such as enzymes and coenzyme A) from oxidation. It is also involved in the detoxification of peroxides, including hydrogen peroxide, and in keeping the cell content in a reduced state. Glutathione may also participate in amino acid transport across the cell membrane through the γ-glutamyl cycle.

GLUTATHIONE SYNTHETASE DEFICIENCY (see Fig. 82–11). Two forms of this condition have been reported. In the *severe form,* which is due to generalized deficiency of the enzyme, severe acidosis and 5-oxoprolinuria are the rule. In the *mild form,* in which the enzyme deficiency is limited to red blood cells only, neither 5-oxoprolinuria nor acidosis has been observed. In both forms, patients have hemolytic anemia secondary to glutathione deficiency.

Glutathione Synthetase Deficiency, Severe Form (Pyroglutamic Acidemia, 5-Oxoprolinuria). Chronic metabolic acidosis and mild to moderate hemolytic anemia, which become manifest in the first few days of life, are cardinal findings in this rare autosomal recessive disorder. Mental and neurologic deficits have been observed in some affected children. Life-threatening metabolic acidosis may occur following a surgical procedure or intercurrent infection. These patients excrete massive amounts (up to 40 g/24 hr) of 5-oxoproline (pyroglutamic acid) in urine. High concentrations of this compound are also found in blood. The glutathione content of erythrocytes is markedly decreased. Increased synthesis of 5-oxoproline in this disorder is believed to be due to the conversion of γ-glutamylcysteine to 5-oxoproline by the enzyme γ-glutamyl cyclotransferase (see Fig. 82–11). γ-Glutamylcysteine production increases greatly because the inhibitory effect of glutathione on the γ-glutamylcysteine synthetase enzyme is removed. A deficiency of glutathione synthetase has been demonstrated in a variety of cells. *Treatment* is mainly directed toward correcting the acidosis, avoiding drugs and oxidants that may cause hemolysis, and preventing stressful states.

Glutathione Synthetase Deficiency, Mild Form. These patients have mild hemolytic anemia and jaundice without 5-oxoprolinuria and acidosis. The enzyme deficiency is limited to the red blood cells.

5-OXOPROLINASE DEFICIENCY. No clear clinical picture has yet been established because only three patients with this disorder have been reported. Two brothers had enterocolitis and renal stones. The other patient had only a low IQ. These findings may be unrelated to the enzyme deficiency. Patients excrete moderate quantities of 5-oxoproline in the urine but, unlike patients with glutathione synthetase deficiency, they are neither acidotic nor have hemolytic anemia. Glutathione and glutamate deficiencies do not occur in this disorder, mainly because glutamic acid is produced from other sources in the body (see Fig. 82–11).

γ-GLUTAMYLCYSTEINE SYNTHETASE DEFICIENCY. Chronic hemolytic anemia, peripheral neuropathy, progressive spinocerebellar degeneration, and generalized aminoaciduria have been reported in two siblings who had very low erythrocytic glutathione levels and a marked deficiency of γ-glutamylcysteine synthetase. Inability to synthesize γ-glutamyl compounds results in impairment of amino acid transport in renal tubules and aminoaciduria (see Fig. 82–11).

GLUTATHIONEMIA (γ-Glutamyl Transpeptidase Deficiency). Mental retardation and severe behavioral problems are the major clinical manifestations of this rare disorder. Patients have glutathionemia, glutathionuria (see Fig. 82–11), and deficient activity

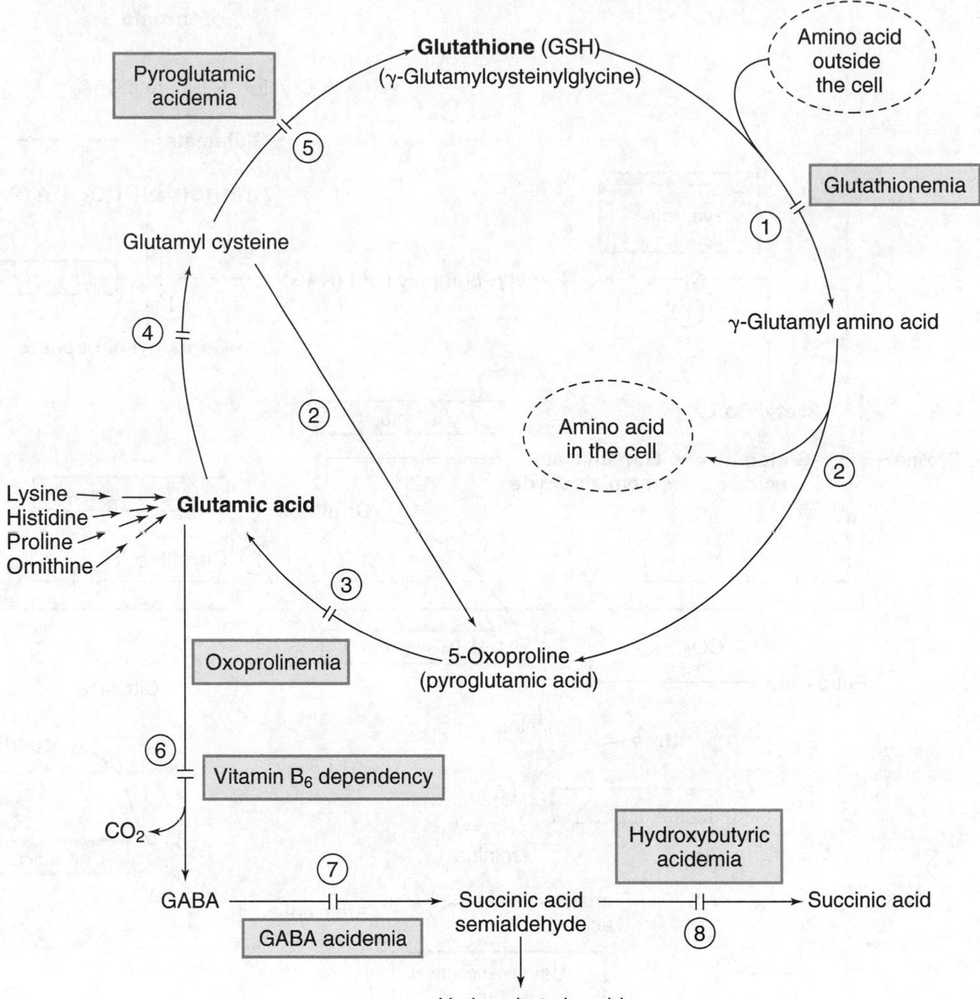

Figure 82–11 The γ-glutamyl cycle. Defects of glutathione synthesis and degradation are noted. **Enzymes:** (1) γ glutamyl transpeptidase; (2) γ glutamyl cyclotransferase; (3) 5-oxoprolinase; (4) γ glutamylcysteine synthetase; (5) glutathione synthetase; (6) glutamic acid decarboxylase; (7) GABA transaminase; (8) succinic semialdehyde dehydrogenase.

of γ-glutamyl transpeptidase in leukocytes and cultured fibroblasts.

INBORN ERRORS OF METABOLISM OF γ-AMINOBUTYRIC ACID (GABA). GABA is synthesized mostly from glutamic acid and, to a lesser degree, from ornithine (see Fig. 82–11). GABA is most abundant in the brain and functions as an inhibitory factor for neurotransmitters.

Vitamin B_6 (Pyridoxine) Dependency. This autosomal recessive condition is due to a deficiency of glutamic acid decarboxylase activity in the brain, which results in decreased production of GABA. This enzyme requires vitamin B_6 as a cofactor (see Fig. 82–11). Diagnosis of pyridoxine dependency should be considered in infants in whom seizures in early life are poorly controlled with conventional anticonvulsant therapy but in whom administration of large doses (10–100 mg/kg) of vitamin B_6 results in dramatic improvement of both seizure activity and EEG abnormalities. Because this defect cannot be detected in fibroblasts, the diagnosis is usually made on the basis of a clinical response to vitamin B_6. Decreased activity of glutamic acid decarboxylase, reversible by the addition of pyridoxine, has been demonstrated in renal tissue but not in the brain. These children require high daily doses of vitamin B_6 indefinitely.

γ-Aminobutyric Acidemia (GABA Transaminase Deficiency). This autosomal recessive condition is manifest as severe psychomotor retardation, hypotonia, and accelerated linear growth. There is a marked elevation of GABA and β-alanine in cerebrospinal fluid and blood (see Fig. 82–11). Increased linear growth occurs, possibly as a result of hypersecretion of growth hormone induced by GABA. GABA transaminase deficiency has been demonstrated in liver biopsy and lymphocytes. Treatment with high doses of vitamin B_6 is ineffective.

γ-Hydroxybutyric Acidemia. A defect in succinic semialdehyde dehydrogenase, inherited as an autosomal recessive disorder, leads to increased production of γ-hydroxybutyric acid, a normal minor metabolite of GABA, which is abundant in the brain (see Fig. 82–11). Ataxia, hypotonia, and neurologic deficits are the main clinical manifestations, which may occur in early infancy. Ataxia improves with advancement of age. Large amounts of γ-hydroxybutyrate and moderate quantities of succinic semialdehyde are found in the urine. Elevated levels of γ-hydroxybutyrate are also detected in the blood and cerebrospinal fluid. These levels may become normal with advancing age. The enzyme deficiency has been demonstrated in lymphocyte lysates. No effective treatment is yet available.

82.11 Urea Cycle and Hyperammonemia

(Arginine, Citrulline, Ornithine)

Iraj Rezvani

Catabolism of amino acids results in the production of free ammonia, which is highly toxic to the central nervous system. Ammonia is detoxified to urea through a series of reactions known as the Krebs-Henseleit or urea cycle (Fig. 82–12). Five enzymes are required for the synthesis of urea: carbamylphosphate synthetase (CPS), ornithine transcarbamylase (OTC), ar-

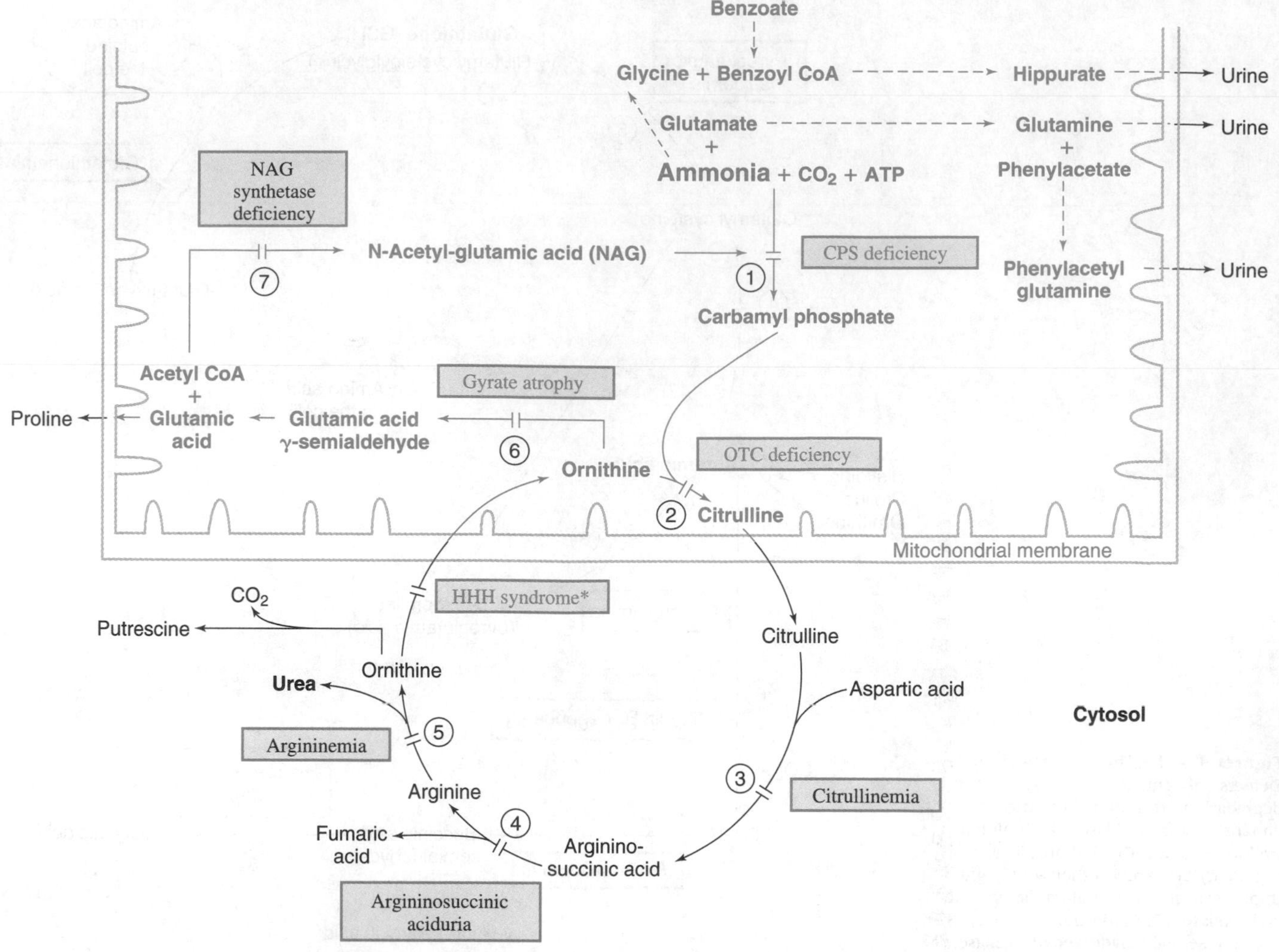

Figure 82–12 Urea Cycle: Pathways for ammonia disposal and ornithine metabolism. Reactions occurring in the mitochondria are depicted in green. Reactions shown with interrupted arrows are the alternate pathways for the disposal of ammonia. **Enzymes:** (1) carbamylphosphate synthetase (CPS); (2) ornithine transcarbamylase (OCT); (3) argininosucccinic acid synthetase; (4) argininosuccinic acid lyase; (5) arginase; (6) ornithine 5-aminotransferase; (7) *N*-acetylglutamate synthetase. *HHH syndrome: Hyperammonemia-Hyperornithinemia-Homocitrullinemia.

gininosuccinate synthetase (AS), argininosuccinate lyase (AL), and arginase. A sixth enzyme, *N*-acetylglutamate synthetase, is also required for synthesis of *N*-acetylglutamate, which is an activator of the CPS enzyme. Individual deficiencies of these enzymes have been observed, and with an overall prevalence of 1 in 30,000 live births, they are the most common genetic causes of hyperammonemia in infants.

GENETIC CAUSES OF HYPERAMMONEMIA. In addition to genetic defects of the urea cycle enzymes, a marked increase in plasma level of ammonia is also observed in other inborn errors of metabolism (Table 82–2). In this section only defects of urea cycle enzymes and transient hyperammonemia of the newborn are discussed.

CLINICAL MANIFESTATIONS OF HYPERAMMONEMIA. In the *neonatal period,* symptoms and signs are mostly related to brain dysfunction and are similar regardless of the cause of the hyperammonemia. In general, the affected infant is normal at birth but becomes symptomatic after a few days of protein feeding. Refusal to eat, vomiting, tachypnea, and lethargy quickly progress to a deep coma. Convulsions are common. Physical examination may reveal hepatomegaly in addition to the neurologic signs of deep coma. In *infants and older children,* acute hyperammonemia is manifested by vomiting and neurologic abnormalities such as ataxia, mental confusion, agitation, irritability, and combativeness. These manifestations may alternate with periods of lethargy and somnolence that may progress to coma.

Routine *laboratory studies* show no specific findings when hyperammonemia is due to defects of the urea cycle enzymes.

TABLE 82–2 Inborn Errors of Metabolism Causing Hyperammonemia

- Deficiencies of the urea cycle enzymes
  - Carbamyl phosphate synthetase (CPS)
  - *N*-acetylglutamate synthetase
  - Ornithine transcarbamylase (OTC)
  - Argininosuccinate synthetase (AS)
  - Argininosuccinate lyase (AL)
  - Arginase
- Organic acidemias
  - Propionic acidemia
  - Methylmalonic acidemia
  - Isovaleric acidemia
  - Ketothiolase deficiency
  - Multiple carboxylase deficiency
  - Fatty acid acyl CoA dehydrogenase deficiency
  - Glutaric acidemia type II
  - 3-Hydroxy-3-methylglutaric acidemia
- Lysinuric protein intolerance
- Hyperammonemia-hyperornithinemia-homocitrullinemia syndrome
- Transient hyperammonemia of the newborn
- Congenital hyperinsulinism with hyperammonemia

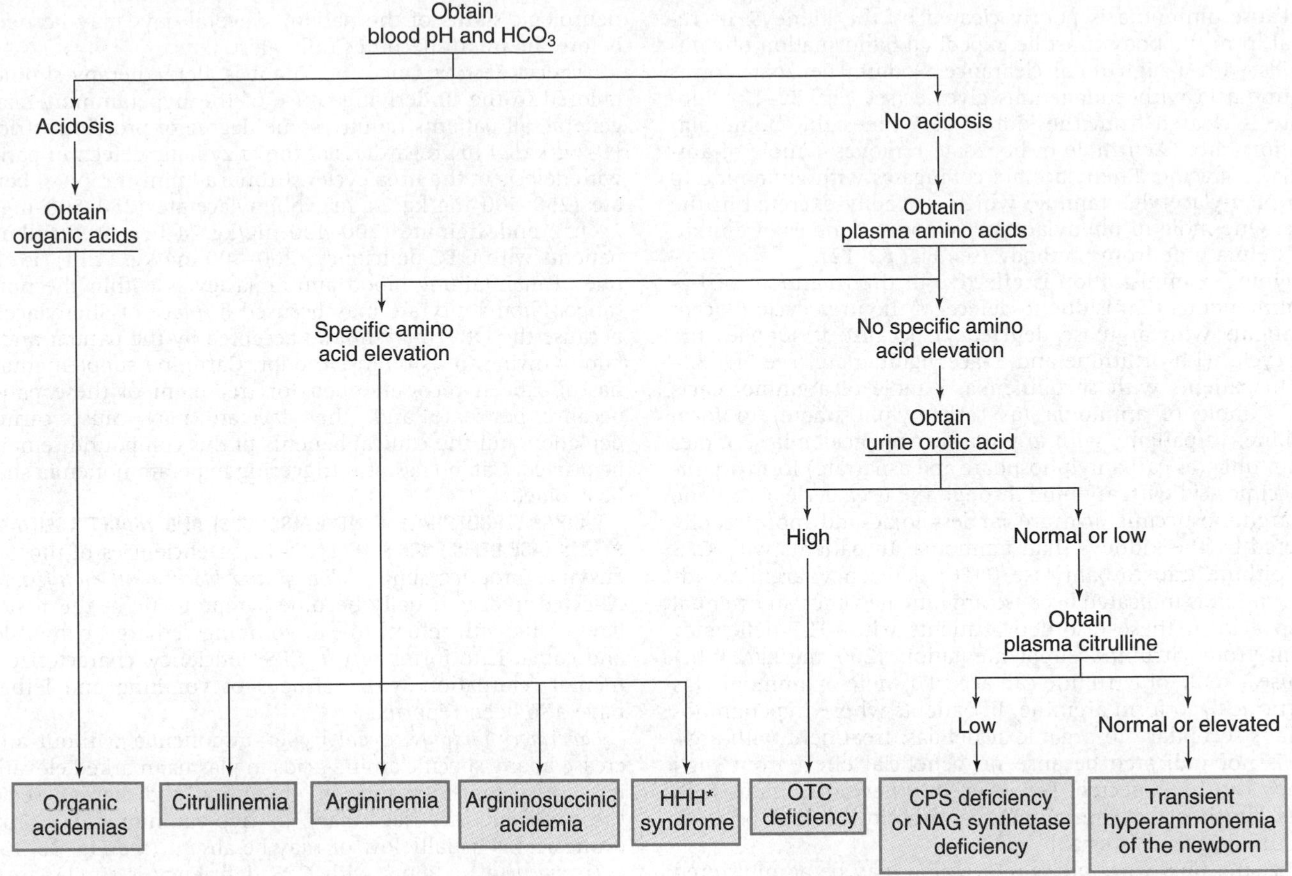

Figure 82–13 Clinical approach to a newborn infant with symptomatic hyperammonemia. HHH syndrome = hyperammonemia-hyperornithinemia-homocitrullinemia.

Blood urea nitrogen is usually very low. In infants with organic acidemias, hyperammonemia is commonly associated with severe acidosis. Newborn infants with hyperammonemia are often misdiagnosed as having a generalized infection, and they may succumb to the disease without a correct diagnosis. Autopsy is usually unremarkable. It is therefore imperative to measure plasma ammonia levels in any ill infant whose clinical manifestations cannot be explained by an obvious infection.

DIAGNOSIS. The main criterion for diagnosis is hyperammonemia. The plasma ammonia concentration in the ill infant is usually above 200 μM (normal values <35 μM). An approach to the differential diagnosis of hyperammonemia in the newborn infant is illustrated in Figure 82–13. Patients with a deficiency of carbamylphosphate synthetase or of ornithine transcarbamylase have no specific abnormalities of plasma amino acids except for increased levels of glutamine, aspartic acid, and alanine secondary to hyperammonemia. A marked increase in urinary orotic acid in patients with ornithine transcarbamylase deficiency differentiates this defect from carbamylphosphate synthetase deficiency. Patients with a deficiency of argininosuccinic acid synthetase, argininosuccinic acid lyase, or arginase have a marked increase in the plasma level of citrulline, argininosuccinic acid, or arginine, respectively. Differentiation between the carbamylphosphate synthetase deficiency and the *N*-acetylglutamate synthetase deficiency may require an assay of the respective enzymes. Clinical improvement occurring after oral administration of carbamylglutamate, however, may suggest *N*-acetylglutamate synthetase deficiency.

TREATMENT OF ACUTE HYPERAMMONEMIA. Acute hyperammonemia should be treated promptly and vigorously. The goal of therapy is to remove ammonia from the body and provide adequate calories and essential amino acids to halt further breakdown of endogenous proteins (Table 82–3). Adequate calories, fluid, and electrolytes should be provided intravenously. Lipids for intravenous use (1 g/kg/24 hr) provide an effective source of calories. Minimal amounts of protein (0.25 g/kg/24 hr), preferably in the form of essential amino acids, should be added to the intravenous fluid to prevent a catabolic state. To supply these essential amino acids without increasing the nitrogen load, ketoacid analogs of essential amino acids have been used by some, but the beneficial effects of these compounds have not been proved clinically. Oral feeding with a low-protein formula (0.5–1.0 g/kg/24 hr) through a nasogastric tube should be started as soon as sufficient improvement in the clinical condition permits it.

TABLE 82–3 Treatment of Acute Hyperammonemia in an Infant

1. Provide adequate calories, fluid, and electrolytes intravenously (10% glucose and intravenous lipids 1 g/kg/24 hr). Add minimal amounts of protein as a mixture of essential amino acids (0.25 g/kg/24 hr) during the first 24 hr of therapy.
2. Give priming doses of the following compounds:
   - Sodium benzoate 250 mg/kg*
   - Sodium phenylacetate 250 mg/kg*
   - Arginine hydrochloride 200–800 mg/kg† as a 10% solution

   } To be added to 20 mL/kg of 10% glucose and infused within 1–2 hr
3. Continue infusion of sodium benzoate* (250–500 mg/kg/24 hr), sodium phenylacetate* (250–500 mg/kg/24 hr), and arginine (200–800 mg/kg/24 hr†) following the above priming doses. These compounds should be added to the daily intravenous fluid.
4. Initiate peritoneal dialysis or hemodialysis if above treatment fails to produce an appreciable decrease in plasma ammonia.

**These compounds are usually prepared as a 1–2% solution for intravenous use. Sodium from these drugs should be included as part of the daily sodium requirement.*

†The higher dose is recommended in the treatment of patients with citrullinemia and argininosuccinic aciduria. Arginine is not recommended in patients with arginase deficiency and in those whose hyperammonemia is secondary to organic acidemia.

Because ammonia is poorly cleared by the kidneys, its removal from the body must be expedited by formation of compounds with a high renal clearance. Sodium benzoate forms hippuric acid with endogenous glycine (see Fig. 82–12); hippurate is cleared from the kidney at 5 times the glomerular filtration rate. Each mole of benzoate removes 1 mole of ammonia as glycine. Phenylacetate conjugates with glutamine to form phenylacetylglutamine, which is readily excreted in the urine. One mole of phenylacetate removes 2 moles of ammonia as glutamine from the body (see Fig. 82–12).

Arginine administration is effective in the treatment of hyperammonemia that is due to defects of the urea cycle (except in patients with arginase deficiency) because it supplies the urea cycle with ornithine and *N*-acetylglutamate (see Fig. 82–12). In patients with citrullinemia, 1 mole of arginine reacts with 1 mole of ammonia (as carbamylphosphate) to form citrulline. In patients with argininosuccinic acidemia, 2 moles of ammonia (as carbamylphosphate and aspartate) form argininosuccinic acid with arginine through the urea cycle. Citrulline and argininosuccinic acid are far less toxic and more readily excreted by the kidneys than ammonia. In patients with CPS or ornithine transcarbamylase (OTC) deficiency, arginine administration is indicated because arginine becomes an essential amino acid in these disorders. Patients with OTC deficiency benefit from citrulline supplementation (200 mg/kg/24 hr) because 1 mole of citrulline can accept 1 mole of ammonia (as aspartic acid) to form arginine. In patients whose hyperammonemia is secondary to organic acidemias, treatment with arginine is not indicated because no beneficial effect from such therapy can be expected. However, in a newborn infant with a first attack of hyperammonemia, arginine should be used until the diagnosis is established.

Benzoate, phenylacetate, and arginine may be administered together for maximal therapeutic effect. A priming dose of these compounds is followed by continuous infusion until recovery from the acute state occurs (see Table 82–3). It should be noted that both benzoate and phenylacetate are supplied as concentrated solutions and should be properly diluted (1–2% solution) for intravenous use. The recommended therapeutic doses of both compounds deliver a substantial amount of sodium to the patient that should be calculated as part of the daily sodium requirement. Benzoate and phenylacetate should be used with caution in newborn infants with hyperbilirubinemia because they may potentiate the risk of hyperbilirubinemia by displacing bilirubin from albumin. In infants at risk, it is advisable to reduce bilirubin to a safe level by exchange transfusion before administering benzoate or phenylacetate.

If the foregoing therapies fail to produce any appreciable change in the blood ammonia level within a few hours, hemodialysis or peritoneal dialysis should be used. Exchange transfusion has little effect on reducing total body ammonia. It should be used only if dialysis cannot be employed promptly or when the patient is a newborn infant with hyperbilirubinemia (see earlier). Hemodialysis, although the most effective measure for removal of ammonia, is technically difficult to perform and may not be readily available in all centers. Peritoneal dialysis, therefore, is the most practical and expeditious method for treatment of patients with severe hyperammonemia; there is usually a dramatic decrease in the plasma ammonia level within a few hours of dialysis, and in most patients the plasma ammonia returns to normal within 48 hr of initiation of peritoneal dialysis. In a patient whose hyperammonemia is due to an organic acidemia, peritoneal dialysis effectively removes both the offending organic acid and ammonia from the body.

To curtail the possible production of ammonia by intestinal bacteria, oral administration of neomycin and lactulose through a nasogastric tube should be initiated very early in the course of therapy. There may be considerable lag between the normalization of ammonia and an improvement in the neurologic status of the patient. Several days may be needed before the infant becomes fully alert.

Long-Term Therapy. Once the infant is alert, therapy should be tailored to the underlying cause of the hyperammonemia. In general, all patients require some degree of protein restriction (1–2 g/kg/24 hr) regardless of the enzymatic defect. In patients with defects in the urea cycle, chronic administration of benzoate (250–500 mg/kg/24 hr), phenylacetate (250–500 mg/kg/24 hr), and arginine (200–400 mg/kg/24 hr), or citrulline in patients with OTC deficiency (200–400 mg/kg/24 hr), is effective in maintaining blood ammonia levels within the normal range. Phenylbutyrate may be used in place of phenylacetate, because the latter may not be accepted by the patient and the family owing to its offensive odor. Carnitine supplementation has also been recommended for treatment of these patients because benzoate and phenylacetate may cause carnitine depletion, but the clinical benefits of this compound remain to be proved. Catabolic states triggering hyperammonemia should be avoided.

CARBAMYLPHOSPHATE SYNTHETASE (CPS) AND *N*-ACETYLGLUTAMATE SYNTHETASE DEFICIENCIES (Fig. 82–12). Deficiencies of these two enzymes produce similar *clinical and biochemical manifestations.* Affected infants usually become symptomatic in the first few days of life with refusal to eat, vomiting, lethargy, convulsions, and coma. Late forms of the CPS deficiency, characterized by mental retardation with episodes of vomiting and lethargy, have also been reported.

Laboratory findings reveal hyperammonemia without an increase in any specific amino acids in plasma; marked elevations in plasma concentrations of glutamine and alanine seen in these patients are secondary to hyperammonemia. Urinary orotic acid is usually low or may be absent (see Fig. 82–13).

Treatment of patients with CPS deficiency is similar to that outlined above for hyperammonemia. Patients with *N*-acetylglutamate synthetase deficiency were shown to benefit from oral administration of carbamylglutamate. It is therefore important to differentiate between these two enzyme deficiencies by assay of the enzyme activities in biopsies obtained from the liver.

CPS deficiency is inherited as an autosomal recessive trait; the enzyme is normally present in liver and intestine. The gene is mapped to the short arm of chromosome 2. *N*-acetylglutamate synthetase has been assayed only in liver specimens obtained at biopsy.

ORNITHINE TRANSCARBAMYLASE (OTC) DEFICIENCY (see Fig. 82–12). In this X-linked dominant disorder the hemizygote males are more severely affected than heterozygote females. More than 20 allelic variants have been documented. The heterozygous female may have either mild disease or no clinical manifestations. This is probably the most common of all the urea cycle disorders.

Clinical manifestations in a male newborn infant are those of severe hyperammonemia (see earlier). Milder forms of the condition are commonly seen in heterozygous females and in some affected males. *Mild* forms characteristically have episodic manifestations. Episodes of hyperammonemia (manifested by vomiting and neurologic abnormalities such as ataxia, mental confusion, agitation, and combativeness) are separated by periods of wellness. Onset may occur in early infancy or early childhood. These episodes usually occur following a high-protein diet or during a situation of stress or infection. Hyperammonemic coma and death may occur during one of these attacks. Some affected children have been diagnosed as having recurrent Reye syndrome. Mental development may proceed normally. However, mild to moderate mental retardation is common. Gallstones have been seen in the survivors; the mechanism remains unclear.

The major *laboratory finding* during the acute attack is hyperammonemia without an increase in any specific amino acid in the blood. As with CPS deficiency, elevation of the plasma concentrations of glutamine and alanine are secondary to hyperammonemia. A marked increase in the urinary excretion of orotic acid differentiates this condition from CPS deficiency (see Fig. 82–13). Orotates may precipitate in urine as gravel or stones. In the mild form, these laboratory abnormalities may revert to normal between attacks. This form should be differentiated from all the episodic conditions of childhood and from poisoning. In particular, lysinuric protein intolerance (Chapter 82.12) mimics the clinical and biochemical characteristics of OTC deficiency. Increased urinary excretion of lysine, ornithine, and arginine and elevated blood concentrations of citrulline, which are salient features of lysinuric protein intolerance, are not seen in patients with OTC deficiency.

The *diagnosis* may be confirmed by performing an assay of enzyme activity that is normally present only in liver. Perinatal diagnosis has been achieved by means of fetal liver biopsy and, more recently, by studying the characteristic DNA polymorphism in chorionic villus samples. Asymptomatic heterozygous female carriers may be identified by using an oral protein load, which increases plasma ammonia and urinary orotic acid levels. A marked increase in urinary excretion of orotidine following an allopurinol loading test has also been used to detect obligate female carriers. Asymptomatic female carriers have mild cerebral dysfunction compared with their unaffected siblings.

Treatment is similar to that given for CPS deficiency except that citrulline may be used in place of arginine. Liver transplantation has been successful as a definite treatment in some patients with OTC deficiency.

ARGININOSUCCINIC ACID SYNTHETASE DEFICIENCY (Citrullinemia) (see Fig. 82–12). Citrullinemia is inherited as an autosomal recessive trait. The gene is located on the long arm of chromosome 9. The severity of the abnormality of the mutant genes inherited from each parent is different in a given patient, indicating that most affected patients are "double or compound" heterozygotes. This disorder shows considerable clinical and biochemical heterogeneity.

The spectrum of *clinical manifestations* ranges from severe forms to asymptomatic ones. The signs and symptoms in the neonatal form are identical to those seen in the severe forms of CPS and OTC deficiencies (see earlier). Mild forms may have a gradual onset with failure to thrive, frequent vomiting, developmental delay, and dry, brittle hair or, like mild forms of OTC deficiency, may appear episodically (see earlier). In some patients symptoms may not appear until 20 yr of age.

Laboratory findings are similar to those found in patients with OTC deficiency except that the plasma citrulline concentration is markedly elevated in patients with citrullinemia (see Fig. 82–13). Urinary secretion of orotic acid is moderately increased in patients with citrullinemia, and crystalluria due to precipitation of orotates may also occur. Patients with argininosuccinic aciduria also show some increase in the plasma concentration of citrulline in addition to elevated levels of argininosuccinic acid. The *diagnosis* is confirmed by performing an assay of the enzyme activity that is normally present in cultured fibroblasts. Prenatal diagnosis is based on an assay of the enzyme activity in cultured amniotic cells.

Treatment is similar to that for other urea cycle disorders (see earlier). Although *prognosis* is very poor for symptomatic neonates, patients with the mild disease usually do well on a protein-restricted diet. Mild to moderate mental deficiency is a common sequela even in a well-treated patient.

ARGININOSUCCINATE LYASE DEFICIENCY (Argininosuccinic Aciduria) (see Fig. 82–12). This deficiency is inherited as an autosomal recessive trait with a prevalence of about 1 in 70,000 live births. The gene is located on the long arm of chromosome 7.

The severity of the *clinical and biochemical manifestations* varies considerably. In the neonatal form severe hyperammonemia develops in the first few days of life, and mortality is usually high. In the subacute or late form the major finding is mental retardation, which is associated with episodic vomiting, failure to thrive, and hepatomegaly. Abnormalities of the hair (characterized by dryness and brittleness) are of special diagnostic value. Microscopically, the hair appears similar to that seen in patients with trichorrhexis nodosa. Less severe hair abnormalities are also seen in patients with citrullinemia. Gallstones have been seen in some of the survivors.

Laboratory findings reveal hyperammonemia, moderate elevation in liver enzymes, nonspecific increases in plasma levels of glutamine and alanine, moderate increase in plasma levels of citrulline (less than that seen in citrullinemia), and marked increase in plasma levels of argininosuccinic acid (see Fig. 82–13). In most amino acid analyzers, argininosuccinic acid appears within the isoleucine or methionine region, which may cause confusion in the diagnosis. Argininosuccinic acid can also be found in large amounts in urine and spinal fluid. The levels in the spinal fluid are usually higher than those in plasma. The enzyme is normally present in erythrocytes, liver, and cultured fibroblasts. Prenatal diagnosis is based on measuring the enzyme activity in cultured amniotic cells. Argininosuccinic acid is also elevated in the amniotic fluid of affected fetuses.

Treatment is similar to that described for citrullinemia.

ARGINASE DEFICIENCY (Hyperargininemia) (see Fig. 82–12). This defect is inherited as an autosomal recessive trait. There are two genetically distinct arginases in humans. One is cystosolic and is expressed in liver and erythrocytes, and the other is found in the renal mitochondria. The cytosolic enzyme, which is the one deficient in patients with arginase deficiency, is mapped to the long arm of chromosome 6.

The *clinical manifestations* of this rare condition are quite different from those of other urea cycle enzyme defects. The onset is insidious; the infant usually remains asymptomatic in the first few months or sometimes years of life. A progressive spastic diplegia with scissoring of the lower extremities, choreoathetotic movements, and loss of developmental milestones in a previously normal infant may suggest a degenerative disease of the central nervous system. Two children were followed for several years with the diagnosis of cerebral palsy before the diagnosis of arginase deficiency was confirmed. Mental retardation is progressive; seizures are common, and episodes of severe hyperammonemia are not usually seen in this disorder. Hepatomegaly may be present.

Laboratory findings reveal marked elevation of arginine in plasma and cerebrospinal fluid (see Fig. 82–13). Urinary orotic acid is moderately increased. Plasma ammonia levels may be normal or mildly elevated. Urinary excretion of arginine, lysine, cystine, and ornithine is usually increased, which may suggest a diagnosis of cystinuria. However, urinary excretion of these amino acids may be normal. Therefore, determination of amino acids in plasma is a critical step before the diagnosis of argininemia can be ruled out. The guanidino compounds (α-keto-guanidinovaleric acid, argininic acid) are markedly increased in urine. The *diagnosis* is confirmed by assaying arginase activity in erythrocytes. Prenatal diagnosis has not yet been achieved.

Treatment consists of a low-protein diet devoid of arginine. Administration of a synthetic protein made of essential amino acids usually results in a dramatic decrease in plasma arginine concentration and an improvement in neurologic abnormalities. The composition of the diet and the daily intake of protein should be monitored by frequent plasma amino acid determinations. Sodium benzoate (250–375 mg/kg/24 hr) is also effective in controlling hyperammonemia. One patient developed type 1 diabetes at age 9 yr while his argininemia was under good control.

TRANSIENT HYPERAMMONEMIA OF THE NEWBORN. Although the plasma levels of ammonia in normal full-term infants are within the normal limits of those seen in older children, a majority of premature infants with low birthweights have a *mild transient hyperammonemia* (40–50 μM), which lasts for about 6–8 wk. These infants are asymptomatic, and follow-up studies up to 18 mo of age have not revealed any significant neurologic deficits.

Severe transient hyperammonemia has been observed in newborn infants. The majority of affected infants have been premature and have had mild respiratory distress syndrome. Hyperammonemic coma may develop within 2–3 days of life, and the infant may succumb to the disease if treatment is not started immediately. Laboratory studies reveal marked hyperammonemia (plasma ammonia as high as 4,000 μM), with moderate increases in plasma levels of glutamine and alanine. Plasma concentrations of urea cycle intermediate amino acids are usually normal except for citrulline, which may be moderately elevated. The cause of the disorder is unknown. Urea cycle enzyme activities are normal. Treatment of hyperammonemia should be initiated promptly and continued vigorously. Recovery without sequelae is common, and hyperammonemia does not recur even with a normal protein diet.

ORNITHINE. Ornithine is one of the intermediate metabolites of the urea cycle that is not incorporated into natural proteins. Rather, it is generated in the cytosol from arginine and must be transported into the mitochondria, where it is used as a substrate for the enzyme OTC to form citrulline. Excess ornithine is catabolized by two enzymes, ornithine 5-aminotransferase, which is a mitochondrial enzyme and converts ornithine to a proline precursor, and ornithine decarboxylase, which resides in the cytosol and converts ornithine to putrescine (see Fig. 82–12). Two genetic disorders result in hyperornithinemia: gyrate atrophy of the retina and hyperammonemia-hyperornithinemia-homocitrullinemia syndrome.

Gyrate Atrophy of the Retina and Choroid. This is an autosomal recessively inherited disorder due to the deficiency of the enzyme ornithine 5-aminotransferase (see Fig. 82–12). About half of the reported cases are from Finland. Clinical manifestations are limited to the eyes and include night blindness, myopia, loss of peripheral vision, and posterior subcapsular cataracts. These eye changes start between 5 and 10 yr of age and progress to complete blindness by the 4th decade of life. Atrophic lesions in the retina resemble cerebral gyri. These patients usually have normal intelligence. There is a 10- to 20-fold increase in plasma levels of ornithine. There is no occurrence of hyperammonemia and no increase in any other amino acids. Plasma levels of glutamate, glutamine, lysine, creatine, and creatinine are moderately decreased. Some patients respond to high doses of pyridoxine (500–1,000 mg/24 hr) and low dietary arginine. In conjunction with supplemental lysine, proline, and creatine. The gene for ornithine 5-aminotransferase is mapped to the long arm of chromosome 10.

Hyperammonemia-Hyperornithinemia-Homocitrullinemia Syndrome (HHH Syndrome). In this autosomal recessively inherited disorder the defect is in the transport system of ornithine from the cytosol into the mitochondria, causing an accumulation of ornithine in the cytosol and a deficiency of ornithine inside the mitochondria. The former causes hyperornithinemia and the latter results in disruption of the urea cycle and hyperammonemia (see Fig. 82–12). Homocitrulline is formed from the reaction of mitochondrial carbamylphosphate with lysine, which occurs because of the intramitochondrial deficiency of ornithine. *Clinical manifestations* of hyperammonemia may develop shortly after birth or may be delayed until adulthood. Acute episodes of hyperammonemia manifest as refusal to feed, vomiting, and lethargy; coma may occur during infancy. Progressive neurologic signs, such as lower limb weakness, increased deep tendon reflexes, spasticity, clonus, seizures, and varying degrees of psychomotor retardation, may develop if the condition remains undiagnosed. No ocular lesions have been observed in these patients.

Laboratory findings reveal marked increases in plasma levels of ornithine and homocitrulline in addition to hyperammonemia. Restriction of protein intake improves hyperammonemia. Ornithine supplementation may produce clinical improvement in some patients. The gene for this disorder is located on the long arm of chromosome 13.

82.12 Histidine

Iraj Rezvani

Histidine is an essential amino acid only during infancy. Its synthetic pathway in older children and adults is poorly understood. Histidine is degraded through the urocanic acid pathway to glutamic acid (Fig. 82–14).

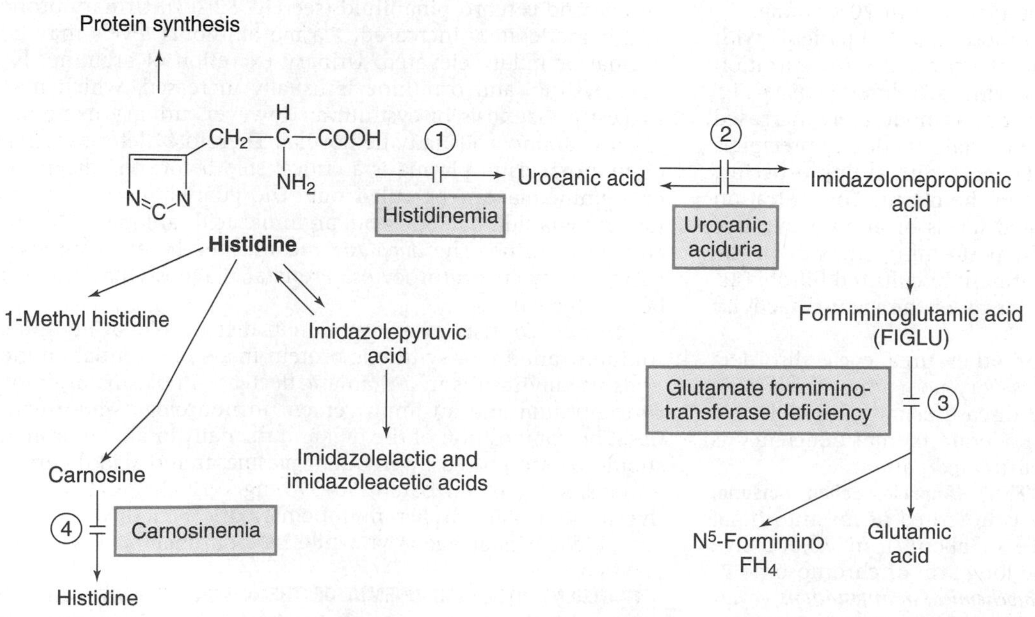

Figure 82–14 Pathways in the metabolism of histidine. FH_4 = tetrahydrofolic acid. **Enzymes:** (1) histidase; (2) urocanase; (3) glutamate formiminotransferase; (4) carnosinase.

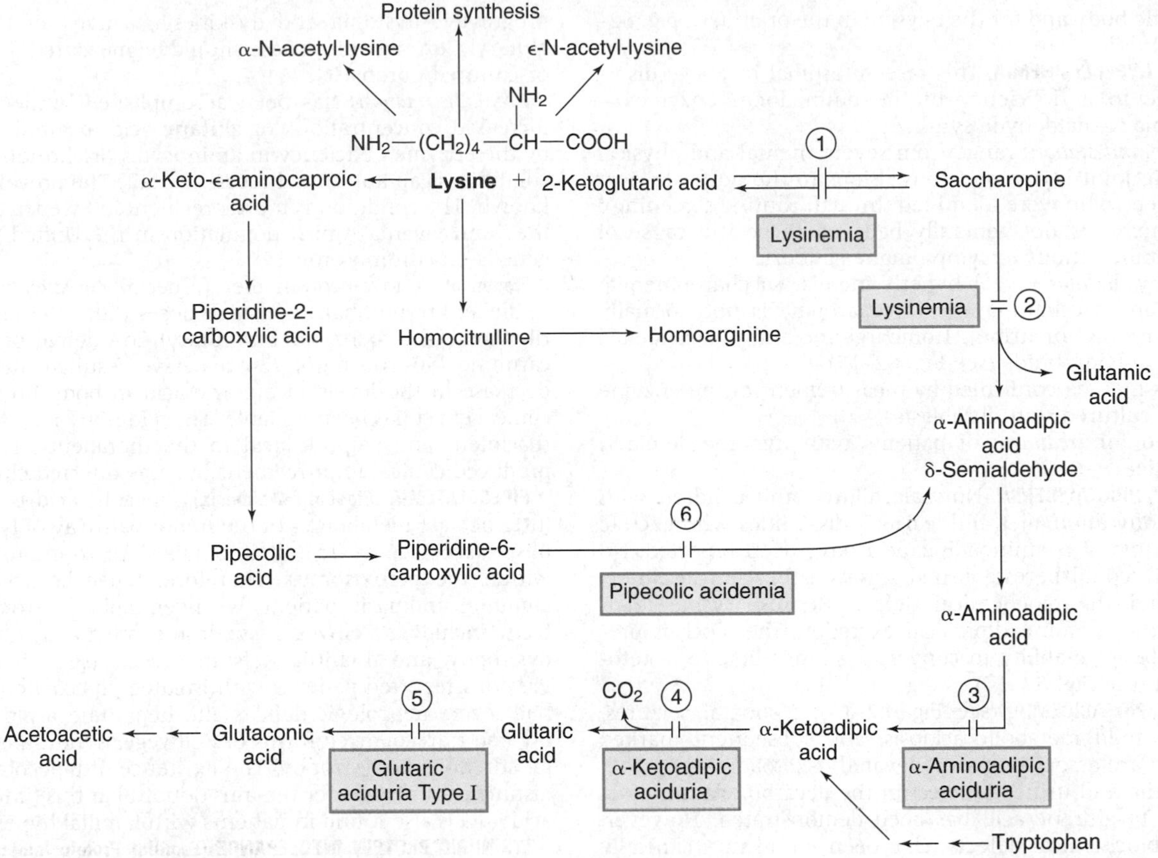

Figure 82–15 Pathways in the metabolism of lysine. **Enzymes:** (1) lysine ketoglutarate reductase; (2) saccharopine dehydrogenase; (3) α-aminoadipic acid transferase; (4) α-ketoadipic acid dehydrogenase; (5) glutaryl CoA dehydrogenase; (6) α-aminoadipic semialdehyde oxidase.

HISTIDINEMIA. This disorder is due to a deficiency of histidase, which normally converts histidine to urocanic acid (see Fig. 82–14). The disorder is inherited as an autosomal recessive trait; its overall prevalence is estimated at 1 in 10,000 worldwide. The gene for histidase is mapped to the long arm of chromosome 12.

Clinical manifestations include impaired speech, growth retardation, or mental retardation. However, the relationship of these findings to histidinemia remains unclear; routine amino acid screening has uncovered a significant number of asymptomatic subjects with histidinemia.

Laboratory findings reveal marked increases in plasma and cerebrospinal fluid concentrations of histidine. There is also an unexplained elevation in the blood level of alanine. Urine contains large amounts of histidine and its transaminated product imidazolepyruvate. The latter compound, like phenylpyruvate, reacts with ferric chloride to produce an intense blue-green color. The *diagnosis* of histidinemia may be confirmed by assay of histidase in liver or skin. Prenatal diagnosis has not yet been achieved because histidase is not present in amniotic cells.

Treatment with a diet low in histidine has produced excellent biochemical control. However, no clinical improvement in symptomatic patients has been observed. Unlike phenylketonuria, maternal histidinemia does not cause any ill effect in the offspring.

UROCANIC ACIDURIA. This disorder is characterized by mental and growth retardation and massive urocanic aciduria (see Fig. 82–14). Urocanase deficiency has been shown in liver biopsies of three of the four reported children. However, the relation of this enzyme deficiency to the clinical findings may be coincidental because normal infants with urocanic aciduria have been identified through routine urine screening of newborns.

GLUTAMATE FORMIMINOTRANSFERASE DEFICIENCY. This disorder is associated with the excretion of formiminoglutamate (FIGLU; see Fig. 82–14). Mildly affected patients have possibly delayed speech. More severely affected patients have mental and physical retardation, abnormal electroencephalogram, and dilatation of the cerebral ventricles with cortical atrophy. Several of the patients had macrocytosis and hyperpigmentation of neutrophils. Only 13 patients have been reported, and the inheritance is autosomal recessive. Although FIGLU excretion may be lowered by folate treatment, it is unclear whether reducing FIGLU excretion is of any value. Glutamate formiminotransferase is not expressed in cultured fibroblasts.

HISTIDINURIA. The urinary excretion of histidine normally increases in pregnant women. Histidinuria also occurs as an overflow phenomenon in patients with histidinemia. Isolated histidinuria without histidinemia due to defective renal tubular reabsorption may occur in children whose parents and siblings have been shown to be heterozygotic for the defect.

82.13 Lysine

Iraj Rezvani

The major pathway in the catabolism of lysine involves its condensation with α-ketoglutaric acid to form saccharopine. Saccahropine is then broken down to α-aminoadipic acid semialdohyde and glutaric acid. These first two steps are catalyzed by α-aminoadipic semialdehyde synthase, which has two activities, lysine-ketoglutarate reductase and saccharopine dehydrogenase (Fig. 82–15). In a minor pathway for lysine degradation, lysine is transmitted first and then condensed to the cyclic form, pipcolic acid. This is the major pathway for D-lysine in the body and for the L-lysine in the brain (see Fig. 82–15).

FAMILIAL HYPERLYSINEMIA. This rare autosomal recessive disorder is due to a deficiency of the bifunctional enzyme α-aminoadipic semialdehyde synthase.

Clinical manifestations range from severe mental and physical retardation, joint laxity, and convulsions to the perfectly normal children (who were identified through routine screening). Hyperlysinemia is not generally believed to be the cause of clinical manifestations in symptomatic patients.

Laboratory findings reveal hyperlysinemia, saccharopinemia, lysinuria, and saccharopinuria (saccharopine is not normally detected in blood or urine). Homoarginine and pipecolic acid are found in body fluids (see Fig. 82–15).

Diagnosis may be confirmed by measurement of the enzyme activity in cultured skin fibroblasts.

The need for *treatment* of patients with hyperlysinemia is controversial.

α-AMINOADIPIC ACIDEMIA. Normal children and children with multiple bony anomalies and learning disabilities who excrete large amounts of α-aminoadipic acid have been reported. No relationship could be established between the clinical abnormalities and the biochemical defect. Because lysine loads increased the α-aminoadipic acid excretion, the block is presumed to be an inability to convert α-aminoadipic to α-ketoadipic acid (see Fig. 82–15).

α-KETOADIPIC ACIDEMIA (see Fig. 82–15). Neonatal seizures, ichthyosis, mild metabolic acidosis, and subsequent marked retardation are associated with elevated α-ketoadipic acid levels in plasma and urine. A defect in the decarboxylation of α-ketoadipic to glutaric acid has been demonstrated. However, the same biochemical defects have been found in a clinically normal sibling of an affected patient, raising doubts about any relationship between the metabolic defect and the mental retardation.

GLUTARIC ACIDURIA TYPE I. Glutaric acid is an intermediate in the degradation of lysine (see Fig. 82–15), hydroxylysine, and tryptophan. Glutaric aciduria type I, a disorder caused by a deficiency of glutaryl CoA dehydrogenase, should be differentiated from glutaric aciduria type II, a distinct clinical and biochemical disorder caused by defects in the electron transport system (see Chapter 83.1).

Clinical Manifestations. Affected patients with glutaric aciduria type I may develop normally up to 2 yr of life. The hallmark of the disease is a progressive dystonia and dyskinesia (choreoathetoic movements). Symptoms of hypotonia, choreoathetosis, seizures, generalized rigidity, opisthotonos, and dystonia may occur suddenly following a minor infection. In other patients, these signs and symptoms may develop gradually during the first few years of life. Hypotonia and choreoathetosis may gradually progress into rigidity and dystonia. Acute episodes of vomiting, ketosis, seizures, and coma with hepatomegaly, hyperammonemia, ketosis, and elevation of serum transaminases, a combination of symptoms that resembles Reye syndrome, may occur during an intercurrent infection or stress. Death usually occurs in the first decade of life during one of these episodes. The intellectual abilities may remain relatively intact in some patients.

Laboratory Findings. During acute episodes mild to moderate metabolic acidosis and ketosis may occur. Hypoglycemia, hyperammonemia, and elevation of serum transaminases have been seen in some patients. High concentrations of glutaric acid are usually found in urine and blood. 3-Hydroxyglutaric acid may also be present in the urine. This finding differentiated glutaric aciduria type I from type II. In glutaric aciduria type II, 2-hydroxyglutaric rather than 3-hydroxyglutaric acid is elevated. Plasma amino acid concentrations are usually within normal limits. Laboratory findings may be unremarkable between attacks. Severely affected children without glutaric aciduria also have been reported. Therefore, in any child with progressive dystonia and dyskinesia, activity of the enzyme glutaryl CoA dehydrogenase should be measured in leukocytes or cultured fibroblasts.

Prenatal diagnosis has been accomplished by demonstrating increased concentrations of glutaric acid in amniotic fluid or by the enzyme deficiency in aminocytes or chorionic villi. The condition is an autosomal recessive trait. The prevalence is not known. The condition is more prevalent in Sweden and among the Pennsylvania Amish population in the United States. The gene is on chromosome 19.

Treatment. A low-protein diet (especially a diet restricted in lysine and tryptophan) and high doses (200–300 mg/24 hr) of riboflavin (the coenzyme for glutaryl CoA dehydrogenase) and carnitine (50–100 mg/kg/24 hr) have resulted in a dramatic decrease in the levels of glutaric acid in body fluids, but the clinical effect has been variable. The addition of a GABA analog (baclofen) and valproic acid to the therapeutic regimen has produced clinical improvement in some affected children.

PIPECOLATEMIA (Pipecolic Acidemia). Pipecolic acid is one of the intermediate metabolites of the minor pathway of lysine catabolism (see Fig. 82–15). It is oxidized to α-aminoadipic acid within the peroxisomes. Therefore, pipecolic acidemia is a common finding in patients with generalized peroxisomal defects, including Zellweger syndrome, neonatal adrenoleukodystrophy, and infantile Refsum disease (see Chapter 83.2). Previous reported patients with isolated pipecolatemia who all had severe neurologic deficits and hepatomegaly most probably had unrecognized forms of Zellweger syndrome or neonatal adrenoleukodystrophy. The existence of pipecolatemia as a distinct clinical disorder remains doubtful at this time. Pipecolic acidemia is also found in patients with familial hyperlysinemia.

LYSINURIC PROTEIN INTOLERANCE (Familial Protein Intolerance). This rare autosomal recessive disorder is due to a defect in the transport of cationic amino acids, lysine, ornithine, and arginine in both kidney and intestine. Unlike patients with cystinuria, urinary excretion of cystine is not increased in these patients. Most reported cases are from Finland, where the prevalence has been estimated to be 1 in 60,000.

Clinical manifestations consist of refusal to feed, nausea, an aversion to protein, vomiting, and mild diarrhea, which may result in failure to thrive, wasting, and hypotonia. Breast-fed infants usually remain asymptomatic until shortly after weaning. This may be due to the low protein content of breast milk. Episodes of hyperammonemia may occur after ingestion of a high-protein diet. Mild to moderate hepatosplenomegaly, sparse brittle hair, thin extremities with moderate centripetal adiposity, and growth retardation are common physical findings in patients when the condition has remained undiagnosed. Mental development is usually normal, but moderate mental retardation has been observed in 20%. Interstitial pneumonitis manifesting as fatigue, cough, and dyspnea occur as an acute episode or as a chronic progressive process. Some patients have remained undiagnosed until the appearance of pulmonary manifestations. Radiographic evidence of pulmonary fibrosis have been observed in up to 65% of patients without clinical manifestations of pulmonary involvement. Acute attacks of pulmonary proteinosis have occurred in older patients. Renal involvement resembling glomerulonephritis has been observed as part of a multisystem disease that may develop as a terminal event.

Laboratory findings may reveal hyperammonemia and elevated concentration of urinary orotic acid, which develop only after protein feeding. Fasting blood ammonia and urinary orotic acid excretion are usually normal. Plasma concentrations of lysine, arginine, and ornithine are usually mildly decreased, but urinary levels of these amino acids, especially lysine, are greatly increased. The exact mechanism producing hyperammonemia is not clear. All enzymes of the urea cycle are normal. Hyperammonemia is thought to be related to a disturbance of the urea cycle secondary to a deficiency of arginine and ornithine. However, in patients with cystinuria, who also have defects in the transport of lysine, arginine, and ornithine in both intestine and kidney, hyperammonemia is not observed. Plasma concentrations of alanine, glutamine, serine, glycine, and citrulline are usually increased. These abnormalities may be secondary to hyperammonemia and are not specific to this disorder.

Mild anemia and increased serum levels of ferritin, lactic dehydrogenase (LDH), and thyroxine-binding globulin also have been observed in these patients. This condition should be differentiated from hyperammonemia due to urea cycle defects (see Chapter 82.10), especially the female heterozygote with OTC deficiency. Increased urinary excretion of lysine, ornithine, and arginine and elevated blood levels of citrulline are not seen in patients with OTC deficiency.

The transport defect in this condition resides in the basolateral (antiluminal) membrane of enterocytes and renal tubular epithelia. This explains the observation that cationic amino acids are unable to cross these cells even when administered as dipeptides. Lysine in the form of dipeptide crosses the luminal membrane of the enterocytes but hydrolyzes to free lysine molecules in the cytoplasm. Free lysine, unable to cross the basolateral membrane of the cells, is diffused back into the lumen.

Treatment with a low-protein diet (1.0–1.5 g/kg/24 hr), supplemented with citrulline (1–4 mmol/kg/24 hr), has produced biochemical and clinical improvement. Episodes of hyperammonemia should be treated promptly (see Chapter 82.10). Supplementation with lysine is not useful because it is poorly absorbed and tends to produce diarrhea and abdominal pain.

Treatment with high doses of prednisone and bronchoalveolar lavage have been effective in the treatment of acute pulmonary complications.

2-HYDROXYGLUTARIC ACIDURIA. Trace amounts of D and L isomers of 2-hydroxyglutaric acid are found in the urine of normal individuals. Pathways for the metabolism of these two isomers have not been elucidated. Two clinically distinct conditions have been identified in which large amounts of either L- or D-2-hydroxyglutaric acids are accumulated in body fluids.

L-2-Hydroxyglutaric Aciduria. In this neurodegenerative condition, patients excrete large amounts of L-2-hydroxyglutaric acid in the urine. The condition has been identified in more than 10 patients, ages 3 to 39 yr.

Clinically, these patients are born normal, but cerebellar signs such as gait instability, ataxia, tremor, hypotonia, dystonia, and other abnormal involuntary movements develop in the first few months of life. Macrocephaly and moderate to severe mental retardation are common findings. Seizures occur in some patients.

Laboratory findings reveal high concentrations of L-2-hydroxyglutaric acid in plasma and to a greater extend in the cerebrospinal fluid. There is a large amount of L-2-hydroxyglutaric acid in the urine. No other organic acid is detected in the urine. An increase of plasma concentration of lysine has been reported in most, but not all, patients. The administration of lysine, glutamate, hydroxylysine, and high-protein or high-lipid diets have not had any effect on the amount of L-2-hydroxyglutaric acid. It is postulated that this compound is derived from the central nervous system. MRI of the brain shows evidence of cerebellar atrophy and subcortical white matter degeneration. Pathologic findings are those of spongiform encephalopathy. These changes are similar to those in Canavan disease. However, patients with Canavan disease have minimal involvement of the cerebellum and excrete large amounts of *N*-acetyl aspartic acid in urine. The condition may be transmitted as an autosomal recessive trait. No effective *therapy* is available.

D-2-Hydroxyglutaric Aciduria. Only five patients with this disorder have been reported. Hypotonia, abnormal involuntary movements, progressive developmental delay, and severe seizures (mainly the myoclonic type) develop shortly after birth. Dysmorphic features such as macrocephaly, prominent cupped ears, hypertelorism, and a flat nasal bridge have been observed in all cases. Dilated cardiomyopathy developed in one patient at 3.5 mo of age. Cortical blindness was noted in two patients. The only *laboratory finding* is the presence of large amounts of D-2-hydroxyglutaric acid in the urine. MRI of the brain showed ventriculomegaly secondary to diminished white matter. No effective *therapy* is known.

82.14 Aspartic Acid

(Canavan Disease)

Reuben K. Matalon

N-Acetylaspartic acid, a derivative of aspartic acid, is synthesized in the brain and is found in a high concentration, similar to that of glutamic acid. Its function is unknown, but excessive amounts of *N* acetylaspartic acid in urine and a deficiency of the enzyme aspartoacylase that cleaves the *N*-acetyl group from *N*-acetylaspartic acid are associated with Canavan disease.

CANAVAN DISEASE. Canavan disease, an autosomal recessive disorder characterized by spongy degeneration of the white matter of the brain, leads to a severe form of leukodystrophy. It is more prevalent in individuals of Ashkenazi Jewish descent than in other ethnic groups.

Etiology and Pathology. The deficiency of the enzyme aspartoacylase leads to the accumulation of *N*-acetylaspartic acid in the brain, especially in white matter, and massive urinary excretion of this compound. Excessive amounts of *N*-acetylaspartic acid are also present in the blood and cerebrospinal fluid. There is striking vacuolization and astrocytic swelling in white matter. Electron microscopy reveals distorted mitochondria. As the disease progresses, the ventricles enlarge, owing to cerebral atrophy.

Clinical Manifestations. The severity of Canavan disease covers a wide spectrum. Infants usually appear normal at birth and may not manifest symptoms of the disease until 3–6 mo of age, when they develop progressive macrocephaly, severe hypotonia, and persistent head lag. As the infant grows older, delayed milestones become evident. These children become hyperreflexic and hypertonic, and joint stiffness may be encountered because of disuse. Seizures and optic atrophy develop as they grow older. Feeding difficulties, poor weight gain, and gastroesophageal reflux may occur in the 1st yr of life; swallowing deteriorates during the 2nd and 3rd yr of life, and nasogastric feeding or permanent gastrostomy may be required. Most patients die in the first decade of life; however, with improved nursing care they may survive through the second decade.

Diagnosis. CT scans and MRI reveal diffuse white matter degeneration, primarily in the cerebral hemispheres, with less involvement in the cerebellum and brain stem (Fig. 82–16). Repeated evaluations may be required. The differential diagnosis of Canavan disease should include Alexander disease, which is another leukodystrophy with macrocephaly. Progression is usually slow in *Alexander disease*; hypotonia is not as pronounced as it is in Canavan disease. Brain biopsy shows spongy degeneration of the myelin fibers, astrocytic swelling, and elongated mitochondria. Definitive diagnosis can be established by finding elevated amounts of *N*-acetylaspartic acid in the urine or blood. A deficiency of aspartoacylase can be found in cultured skin fibroblasts. The biochemical method is the preferred choice for diagnosis. Levels of *N*-acetylaspartic acid in normal urine are only trace amounts (24 ± 16 μmol/mmol creatinine), whereas in patients with Canavan disease they are in the range of 1,440 ± 873 μmol/mmol creatinine. High levels of *N*-acetylaspartic acid in plasma, cerebrospinal fluid, and brain tissue can also be detected. The activity of asparto-

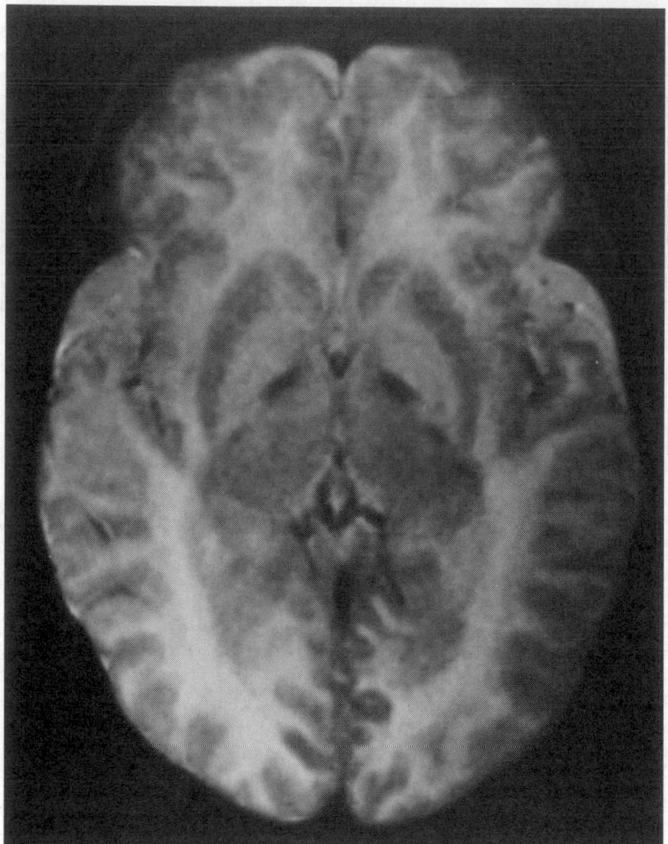

Figure 82–16 Axial T-weighted MRI scan taken of a 2-yr-old patient with Canavan disease. Extensive thickening of the white matter radiation is seen.

acylase in the fibroblasts of obligate carriers is about half or less of the activity found in normal individuals.

The gene for aspartoacylase has been cloned, and mutations leading to Canavan disease have been identified. There are two mutations predominant in the Ashkenazi Jewish population. The first is an amino acid substitution (E285A) in which glutamic acid is substituted to alanine. This mutation is the most frequent and encompasses 83% of 100 mutant alleles examined in Ashkenazi Jewish patients. The second common mutation is a change from tyrosine to a nonsense mutation, leading to a stop in the coding sequence (Y231X). This mutation accounts for 13% of the 100 mutant alleles. In the non-Jewish population more diverse mutations have been observed; the two mutations common in Jewish people are rare. A different mutation (A305E), substitution of alanine for glutamic acid, accounts for 40% of 62 mutant alleles in non-Jewish patients. With the diagnosis of Canavan disease, it is important to obtain a molecular diagnosis because this will lead to accurate counseling and prenatal diagnosis for the family. If the mutations are not known, prenatal diagnosis relies on the level of *N*-acetylaspartic acid in the amniotic fluid. In Ashkenazi Jewish patients the carrier frequency may be as high as 1 in 36, which is close to that of Tay-Sachs disease. Ashkenazi Jewish individuals may need to be screened for Canavan disease.

Treatment and Prevention. No specific treatment is available. Feeding problems and seizures should be treated on an individual basis. Genetic counseling, carrier testing, and prenatal diagnosis are the only methods of prevention. Injection of liposomes with the human aspartoacylase gene was introduced to the ventricles of two children with Canavan disease. The results of this gene therapy have not been encouraging.

Andersson HC, Shapira E: Biochemical and clinical response to hydroxocobalamin versus cyanocobalamin treatment in patients with methylmalonic acidemia and homocystinuria (*cblC*). J Pediatr 132:121, 1998.

Arnold GL, Greene CL, Stout JP, et al: Molybdenum cofactor deficiency. J Pediatr 123:595, 1993.

Baker NS, Sarnat HB, Jack RM, et al: D-2-Hydroxyglutaric aciduria: Hypotonia, cortical blindness, seizures, cardiomyopathy and cylindrical spirals in skeletal muscle. J Clin Neurol 12:31, 1997.

Barth PG: Commentary; L-hydroxyglutaric acidurias. Brain Dev 17:144, 1995.

Burgard P, Rey F, Rupp A, et al: Neuropsychologic functions of early treated patients with phenylketonuria, on and off diet: Results of a cross-national and cross-sectional study. Pediatr Res 41:368, 1997.

Cattaneo M, Martinelli I, Mannucci PM: Hyperhomocysteinemia as a risk factor for deep vein thrombosis. N Engl J Med 335:974, 1996.

Cerone R, Holme E, Schiaffino MC, et al: Tyrosinemia type III: Diagnosis and ten years follow-up. Acta Paediatr 86:1013, 1997.

Chamberlin ME, Ubagai T, Mudd SH, et al: Demyelination of the brain is associated with methionine adenosyltransferase I/III deficiency. J Clin Invest 98:1021, 1996.

Citron BA, Kaufman S, Milstein S, et al: Mutation in the 4α-carbinolamine dehydratase gene leads to mild hyperphenylalaninemia with defective cofactor metabolism. Am J Hum Genet 53:768, 1993.

Committee on Genetics: Newborn screening fact sheets. Pediatrics 98:473, 1996.

Danpure CJ, Jennings PR, Purdue PE, et al: Primary hyperoxaluria type I: Genotypic and phenotypic heterogeneity. J Inherit Metab Dis 17:487, 1994.

Eisensmith RC, Martinez DR, Kuzmin AI, et al: Molecular basis of phenylketonuria and a correlation between genotype and phenotype in a heterogeneous southeastern US population. Pediatrics 97:512, 1996.

Gahl WA, Brantly M, Kaiser-Kupfer MI, et al: Genetic defects and clinical characteristics of patients with a form of oculocutaneous albinism (hermansky-pudlak syndrome). N Engl J Med 338:1258, 1998.

Gibson KM, Cassidy SB, Seaver LH, et al: Fatal cardiomyopathy associated with 3-hydroxy-3-methylglutaryl-CoA lyase deficiency. J Inherit Metab Dis 17:291, 1994.

Gibson KM, Lee CF, Hoffman GF: Screening for defects of branched-chain amino acid metabolism. Eur J Pediatr 153:562, 1994.

Goyette P, Sumner JS, Milos R, et al: Human methylenetetrahydrofolate reductase: Isolation of cDNA, mapping and mutation identification. Nat Genet 7:195, 1994.

Grompe M, St Louis M, Demers SI, et al: A single mutation of the fumarylacetoacetate hydroxylase gene in French-Canadians with hereditary tyrosinemia type I. N Engl J Med 331:353, 1994.

Hoffmann GF, Charpentier C, Mayatepek E, et al: Clinical and biochemical phenotype in 11 patients with mevalonic aciduria. Pediatrics 91:915, 1993.

Hoffman GF, Gibson KM, Trefz FK, et al: Neurologic manifestations of organic acid disorders. Eur J Pediatr 153:594, 1994.

Jaeken J, Detheux M, Van Maldergem L, et al: 3-Phosphoglycerate dehydrogenase deficiency: An inborn error of serine biosynthesis. Arch Dis Child 74:542, 1996.

Janocha S, Wolz W, Srsen S, et al: The human gene for alkaptonuria maps to chromosome 3p. Genomics 19:5, 1994.

Kahler SG, Sherwood G, Woolf D, et al: Pancreatitis in patients with organic acidemias. J Pediatr 124:239, 1994.

Kalayci O, Coskan T, Tokatli A, et al: Infantile spasm as the initial symptoms of biotinidase deficiency. J Pediatr 124:103, 1994.

Kaul R, Gao GP, Aloya M, et al: Canavan disease: Mutations among Jewish and non Jewish patients. Am J Hum Genet 55:27, 1994.

Kerem E, Elpeg ON, Shalev RS, et al: Lysinuria protein intolerance with chronic interstitial lung disease and pulmonary cholesterol granulomas at onset. J Pediatr 123:275, 1993.

Kim SZ, Varvogli L, Waisbren SE, et al: Hydroxyprolinemia: Comparison of a patient and her unaffected twin sister. J Pediatr 130:437, 1997.

Kraus JP: Molecular basis of phenotype expression in homocystinuria. J Inherit Metab Dis 17:383, 1994.

Lee ST, Nicholas RD, Bundey S, et al: Mutations of the p gene in oculocutaneous albinism, ocular albinism and Prader-Willi syndrome plus albinism. N Engl J Med 330:529, 1994.

Levy HL, Lobbregt D, Barnes PD, et al: Maternal phenylketonuria: Magnetic resonance imaging of the brain in offspring. J Pediatr 128:770, 1996.

Linstedt S, Holme E, Lock EA, et al: Treatment of hereditary tyrosinemia type I by inhibition of 4-hydroxyphenylpyruvate dioxygenase. Lancet 340:813, 1992.

Maestri NE, Hauser ER, Bartholomew D, et al: Prospective treatment of urea cycle disorders. J Pediatr 119:923, 1991.

Maestri NE, Brusilow SW, Clissold DB, et al: Long-term treatment of girls with ornithine transcarbamylase deficiency. N Engl J Med 335:855, 1996.

Matalon R, Michaels K, Kaul R: Canavan disease: from spongy degeneration to molecular analysis. J Pediatr 127:511, 1995.

Matalon R, Michaels K: Molecular basis of Canavan disease. Eur J Paediatr Neurol 2:69, 1998.

McKusick V: Mendelian Inheritance in Man, 12th ed. Baltimore, The Johns Hopkins University Press, 1998.

Mater D, Seydewitz HH, Lehnert W, et al: Primary treatment of propionic acidemia complicated by acute thiamine deficiency. J Pediatr 129:758, 1996.

Mehta KC, Zsolway K, Osteroudt, et al: Lessons from the late diagnosis of isovaleric acidemia in a five year old boy. J Pediatr 129:309, 1996.

Morris AAM, Leonard JV: Early recognition of metabolic decompensation. Arch Dis Child 76:555, 1997.

Morton DH, Bennett MJ, Seargeant LE, et al: Glutaric aciduria type I: A common cause of episodic encephalopathy and spastic paralysis in the Amish of Lancaster County, Pennsylvania. Am J Med Genet 41:89, 1991.

Nygard O, Nordrehaug JE, Refsum H, et al: Plasma homocysteine levels and mortality in patients with coronary artery disease. N Engl J Med 337:230, 1997.

Nyhan WL, Rice-Kelts M, Klein J, et al: Treatment of the acute crisis in maple syrup urine disease. Arch Pediatr Adolesc Med 152:593, 1998.

Parenti G, Sebastio G, Strisciuglio A, et al: Lysinuric protein intolerance characterized by bone marrow abnormalities and severe clinical course. J Pediatr 126:246, 1995.

Pearsen KD, Gean-Marton AD, Levy HL, et al: Phenylketonuria: MR imaging of the brain with clinical correlation. Radiology 177:437, 1990.

Peinemann F, Danner DJ: Maple syrup urine disease 1954 to 1993. J Inherit Metab Dis 17:3, 1994.

Peres-Cerda C, Merinero B, Marti M, et al: An unusual late-onset case of propionic acidaemia: Biochemical investigations, neuroradiological findings and mutation analysis. Eur J Pediatr 157:50, 1998.

Pitt DB, Danks DM: The natural history of untreated phenylketonuria. J Pediatr Child Health 27:189, 1991.

Pomponio RJ, Hymes J, Reynolds TR, et al: Mutations in the human biotinidase gene that cause profound biotinidase deficiency in symptomatic children: Molecular, biochemical and clinical analysis. Pediatr Res 42:840, 1997.

Qureshi AA, Crane AM, Matiaszuk NV, et al: Cloning and expression of mutations demonstrating intragenic complementation in *mut*^{0} methylmalonic aciduria. J Clin Invest 93:1812, 1994.

Rabinowitz LG, Williams LR, Anderson CE, et al: Painful keratoderma and photophobia: Hallmarks of tyrosinemia type II. J Pediatr 126:266, 1995.

Riviello J, Rezvani I, DiGeorge A: Cerebral edema causing death in patients with maple syrup urine disease. J Pediatr 119:42, 1991.

Salt A, Barnes ND, Rolles K, et al: Liver transplantation in tyrosinemia type I. The dilemma of timing the operation. Acta Paediatr 81:449, 1992.

Scheuerle AE, McVie R, Beaudet AL, et al: Arginase deficiency presenting as cerebral palsy. Pediatrics 91:995, 1993.

Schulze A, Hess T, Wevers R, et al: Creatine deficiency syndrome caused by guanidinoacetate methyltransferase deficiency. Diagnostic tools for a new inborn error of metabolism. J Pediatr 131:626, 1997.

Seargeant LE, de Groot GW, Dilling LA, et al: Primary oxaluria type 2 (L-glyceric aciduria): A rare cause of nephrolithiasis in children. J Pediatr 118:912, 1991.

Shevell MI, Matiaszuk N, Ledley FD, et al: Varying neurological phenotypes among *mut*^{0} and *mut*$^-$ patients with methylmalomyl CoA mutase deficiency. Am J Med Genet 45:619, 1993.

Smith I, Beasley MG, Ades AE: Intelligence and quality of dietary treatment in phenylketonuria. Arch Dis Child 65:472, 1990.

Snyderman SE and Sansario C: Succinyl-CoA:3-ketoacid CoA transferase deficiency. Pediatrics 101:709, 1998.

Spady DW, Saunders LD, Bamforth F: Who gets missed: coverage in a provincial newborn screening program for metabolic disease. Pediatrics 102 http://www.pediatrics.org/cgi/content/full/102/2/e21, 1998.

Stöckler S, Isbrndt D, Hansfeld F, et al: Guanidinoacetate methyltransferase deficiency: The first inborn error of creatine metabolism in man. Ann J Hum Genet 58:914, 1996.

Stöckler-Ipsiroglu S: Creatine deficiency syndromes: A new perspective on metabolic disorders and a diagnostic challenge. J Pediatr 131:510, 1997.

Treacy E, Arbour L, Chessex P, et al: Glutathione deficiency as a complication of methylmalonic acidemia: Response to high doses of ascorbate. J Pediatr 129:445, 1996.

Topçu M, Erdem G, Saatsi I, et al: Clinical and magnetic resonance imaging features of L-2-hydroxyglutaric aciduria: Report of three cases in comparison with Canavan disease. J Child Neurol 11:373, 1996.

Van Der Meer SB, Poggi F, Spada M, et al: Clinical outcome and long-term management of 17 patients with propionic acidemia. Eur J Pediatr 155:205, 1996.

Van't Hoff WG, Dixon M, Taylor J, et al: Combined liver-kidney transplantation in methylmalonic acidemia. J Pediatr 132:1043, 1998.

Weinzimer SA, Stanley CA, Berry GT, et al: A syndrome of congenital hyperinsulinism and hyperammonemia. J Pediatr 130:661, 1997.

Wolf B, Pomponio RJ, Norrgard KJ: Delayed-onset profound biotinidase deficiency. J Pediatr 132:362, 1998.

Yudkoff M, Daikhin Y, Missim I, et al: In vivo nitrogen metabolism in ornithine transcarbamylase deficiency. J Clin Invest 98:2167, 1996.

Zammarchi E, Ciani F, Pasquini E, et al: Neonatal onset of hyperornithinemia, hyperammonemia, homocitrullinemia syndrome with favorable outcome. J Pediatr 131:440, 1997.

Zeharia A, Elpeleg ON, Mukamel M, et al: 3-Methylglutaconic aciduria. A new variant. Pediatrics 89:1080, 1992.

CHAPTER 83
Defects in Metabolism of Lipids

83.1 Disorders of Mitochondrial Fatty Acid Oxidation

Charles A. Stanley

Mitochondrial oxidation of fatty acids is an essential energy-producing pathway. It becomes especially important during prolonged periods of starvation when the body switches from using predominantly carbohydrates to predominantly fat as its major fuel. Fatty acids are also important fuels for exercising skeletal muscle and are the preferred substrate for the heart. In these tissues, fatty acids are completely oxidized to carbon dioxide and water. However, in the liver, the end products of fatty acid oxidation are the ketones β-hydroxybutyrate and acetoacetate. The ketones cannot be oxidized by the liver but are exported to serve as important fuels in peripheral tissues, particularly the brain.

Genetic defects have been recognized in nearly all the steps in the fatty acid oxidation path. All these disorders are recessively inherited. *Clinical manifestations* are fairly similar among the disorders. The most common presentation is an acute attack of life-threatening coma and hypoglycemia induced by a period of fasting. Other manifestations frequently include chronic cardiomyopathy and muscle weakness or, more rarely, acute rhabdomyolysis. Because the defects can be asymptomatic except during fasting stress, attacks of illness may be misdiagnosed as Reye syndrome or sudden infant death syndrome. Fatty acid oxidation disorders are easily overlooked because the only specific clue to the diagnosis may be the finding of inappropriately low concentrations of urinary ketones in an infant who has hypoglycemia. In a similar manner, genetic defects in ketone utilization may be overlooked because ketosis is an expected finding with fasting hypoglycemia.

Figure 83–1 outlines the steps involved in mitochondrial oxidation of a typical long-chain fatty acid. In the *carnitine cycle,* fatty acids are carried across the barrier of the inner mitochondrial membrane linked to carnitine. Within the mitochondrial matrix, successive turns of the four-step *β-oxidation cycle* convert the fatty acid to acetyl-coenzyme A (CoA) units. Two to four chain-length specific isoenzymes are needed for each of these β-oxidation steps to accommodate the different-sized fatty acids. The *electron transfer pathway* carries electrons generated in the first β-oxidation step to the electron transport chain for adenosine triphosphate production. In the liver, most of the acetyl-CoA generated from β-oxidation flows through the *ketone synthesis pathway* to β-hydroxybutyrate and acetoacetate.

DEFECTS IN THE β-OXIDATION CYCLE

Medium-Chain Acyl-CoA Dehydrogenase Deficiency

Medium-chain acyl-CoA dehydrogenase (MCAD) deficiency is the most common of the fatty acid oxidation disorders. The disorder shows a strong founder effect: Most patients have a northwestern European ancestry, and 85–90% are homozygous for a single common missense mutation, an A to G transition at cDNA position 985.

CLINICAL MANIFESTATIONS. Affected patients usually present in the first 2–3 yr of life with episodes of acute illness triggered by

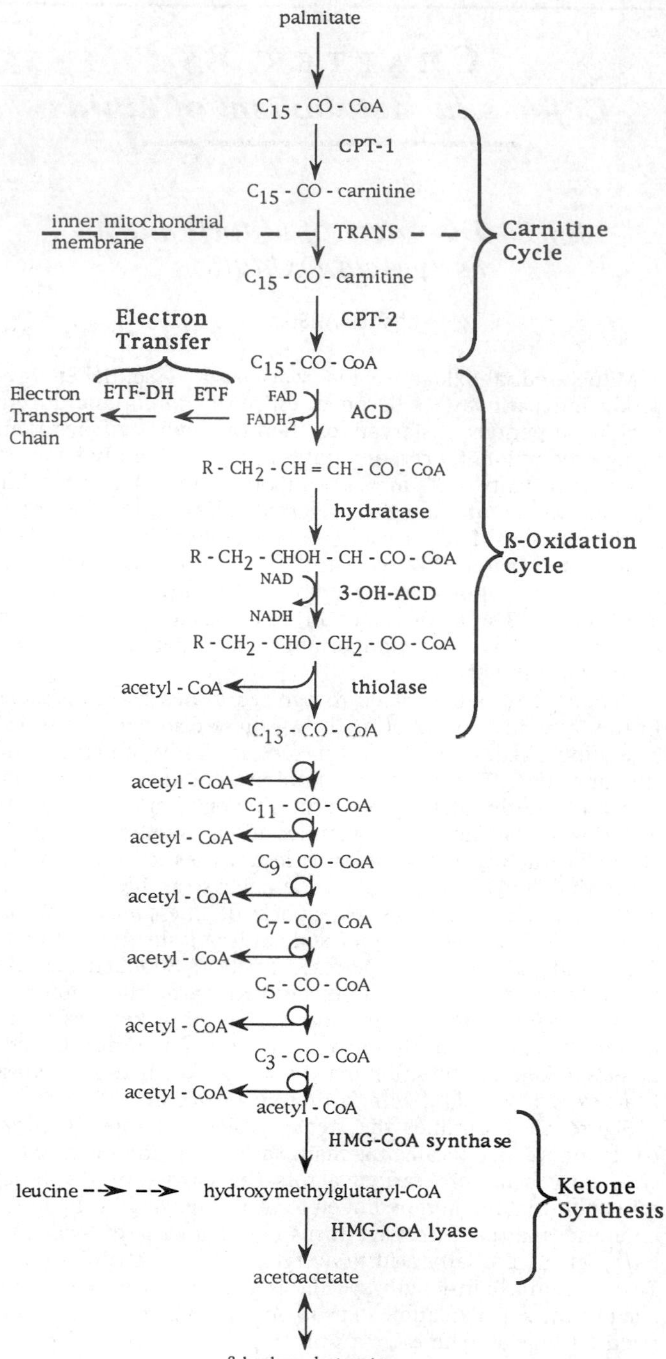

Figure 83–1 Pathway of mitochondrial oxidation of palmitate, a typical 16-carbon long-chain fatty acid. Enzyme steps include carnitine palmitoyltransferase (CPT) 1 and 2, carnitine/acylcarnitine translocase (TRANS), electron transfer flavoprotein (ETF), ETF-dehydrogenase (ETF-DH), acyl-CoA dehydrogenase (ACD), enoyl-CoA hydratase (hydratase), 3-hydroxyacyl-CoA dehydrogenase (3-OH-ACD), β-ketothiolase (thiolase), β-hydroxy-β-methylglutaryl-CoA (HMG-CoA) synthase, and lyase.

prolonged fasting for more than 12–16 hr. Signs and symptoms include vomiting and lethargy, which rapidly progress to coma or seizures and cardiorespiratory collapse. The liver may be slightly enlarged with fat deposition. Attacks are rare until the infant is beyond the first few months of life. Affected infants are at higher risk of illness as they begin to fast through the night or are exposed to fasting stress during intercurrent illnesses. However, presentation in the first days of life has been reported in newborns who were starved inadvertently as they began breast-feeding.

LABORATORY FINDINGS. During acute attacks of illness, hypoglycemia is usually present. Plasma and urinary ketone concentrations are inappropriately low (hypoketotic hypoglycemia). Because of the absence of ketones, there is little or no acidemia. Tests of liver function are abnormal, with elevations of transaminases, urate, urea, ammonia, and prolonged thrombin and partial thromboplastin times. Liver biopsy results at times of acute illness show increased triglyceride deposition in either a micro- or macrovesicular pattern. During fasting stress or at times of acute illness, urinary organic acid profiles by gas chromatography–mass spectrometry show low concentrations of ketones and elevated levels of medium-chain dicarboxylic acids that derive from microsomal and peroxisomal omega oxidation of fatty acids. Plasma and tissue concentrations of total carnitine are reduced to 25–50% of normal, and the fraction of total carnitine esterified is increased. This pattern of *secondary carnitine deficiency* is seen in almost all the fatty acid oxidation defects and reflects competition between increased acylcarnitine levels and free carnitine transport at the plasma membrance. Significant exceptions to this rule are the carnitine transporter, CPT-1 and HMG-CoA synthase deficiencies (see further on). *Diagnosis* can be made by demonstrating abnormal metabolites in plasma (octanoylcarnitine) or urine (glycine conjugates of hexanoate and phenylpropionate) or by showing deficiency of the enzyme in cultured fibroblasts. Expanded mass spectrometry newborn screening programs can diagnose presymptomatic infants based on the detection of octanoylcarnitine in filter paper blood spots. In some cases, the diagnosis can be confirmed by finding the common A985G mutation. A rare mutation G583A is associated with severe MCAD deficiency, hypoglycemia, and sudden neonatal death.

TREATMENT. Acute illnesses should be promptly treated with intravenous fluids containing 10% dextrose in order to suppress lipolysis as rapidly as possible. Chronic therapy consists of ensuring that exposure to starvation stress is eliminated. This usually requires simply adjusting the diet to ensure that overnight fasting periods are limited to less than 10–12 hr. Whether restricting dietary fat or treatment with carnitine is beneficial remains controversial.

PROGNOSIS. Up to 25% of patients may die during their first attack of illness. Some patients may suffer permanent brain injury during an attack. The prognosis for survivors is good because muscle weakness or cardiomyopathy do not occur in MCAD deficiency. With age, fasting tolerance improves and the risk of attacks of illness decreases. It is estimated that as many as 50% of affected patients never have an attack of illness, so testing of siblings of affected patients is important to detect asymptomatic family members.

Long-Chain–Very Long Chain Acyl-CoA Dehydrogenase Deficiency

Long-chain–very long chain acyl-CoA dehydrogenase (LCAD-VLCAD) deficiency was originally termed *LCAD deficiency* before the existence of an additional VLCAD enzyme specific for longer chain fatty acids was known. Some LCAD deficiency patients have been shown to be deficient in the VLCAD enzyme. Patients have usually been more severely affected than those with MCAD deficiency, presenting earlier in infancy and having more chronic problems with muscle weakness or episodes of muscle pain and rhabdomyosis. During acute attacks of fasting illness, evidence of cardiomyopathy may be present. The left ventricle may be hypertrophic or dilatated and show poor contractility on echocardiography. Other physical and routine laboratory features are similar to MCAD deficiency, including secondary carnitine deficiency. The urinary organic acid profile shows a hypoketotic dicarboxylic aciduria. Increased levels of C_{12-14} dicarboxylic acids may be noted in the urine. *Diagnosis* may be suggested by the demonstration of elevated plasma $C_{14:1}$ fatty acid or acylcarnitine, but the specific diagnosis requires assay of enzyme activities of both LCAD and VLCAD in cultured fibroblasts. *Treatment* is avoidance of fasts for more than 10–12 hr. Continuous intragastric feeding has appeared to be useful in some patients.

Short-Chain Acyl-CoA Dehydrogenase Deficiency

The clinical phenotype of short-chain acyl-CoA (SCAD) deficiency remains somewhat unclear. Most patients have not presented with attacks of fasting coma but instead have had chronic acidosis, failure to thrive, muscle weakness, and developmental delay. Some of these features suggest a toxicity syndrome, perhaps due to accumulation of short-chain fatty acid metabolites. One reported patient had normal ketogenesis, implying that there is no impairment of longer chain fatty acid oxidation. Urinary organic acid profile shows elevations of short-chain fatty acid metabolites, including ethylmalonate and butylrylglycine. Secondary carnitine deficiency is present and butyrylcarnitine may be found in urine. *Diagnosis* may be based on the specific metabolite profile in blood and urine, and confirmed by enzyme assay in cultured cells. *Treatment* is limitation of fasting stress and dietary fat.

Long-Chain 3-Hydroxyacyl-CoA Dehydrogenase Deficiency

Long-chain 3-hydroxyacyl-CoA dehydrogenase (LCHAD) deficiency appears to be the second most common of the fatty acid oxidation disorders. The LCHAD enzyme is actually part of a trifunctional protein, which also contains two other steps in β-oxidation, long-chain enoyl-CoA hydratase and β-keto thiolase. In some patients, only LCHAD is affected, whereas others have deficiencies of all three enzymes. *Clinical manifestations* include attacks of acute hypoketotic hypoglycemia similar to MCAD deficiency, but patients often show evidence of more severe disease, including cardiomyopathy, muscle weakness, and abnormal liver function. Some patients have features implying toxic effects of fatty acid metabolites, such as retinopathy, progressive liver failure, peripheral neuropathy, and rhabdomyolysis. A life-threatening illness, acute fatty liver of pregnancy, has been observed in mothers carrying fetuses affected with LCHAD deficiency. Urinary organic acid profile may show increases in levels of 3-hydroxy dicarboxylic acids. Secondary carnitine deficiency is common and plasma 3-hydroxydicarboxylic acid esters of carnitine may be increased. *Treatment* is similar to that for MCAD or LCAD-VLCAD deficiency.

Short-Chain 3-Hydroxyacyl-CoA Dehydrogenase Deficiency

One patient has been reported with attacks of fasting hypoglycemia and myoglobinuria associated with deficiency of short-chain 3-hydroxyacyl-CoA dehydrogenase in muscle but not in cultured fibroblasts. The patient died in adolescence with cardiomyopathy and arrhythmias. Many questions will remain unanswered about this defect until other affected patients are identified.

DEFECTS IN THE CARNITINE CYCLE

Plasma Membrane Carnitine Transport Defect (Primary Carnitine Deficiency)

Primary carnitine deficiency is the only genetic defect in which carnitine deficiency is the cause, rather than the consequence, of impaired fatty acid oxidation. The most common presentation is progressive cardiomyopathy with or without skeletal muscle weakness that begins at 2–4 yr of age. A smaller number of patients may present with fasting hypoketotic hypoglycemia during the 1st yr of life before the cardiomyopathy becomes symptomatic. The underlying defect involves the plasma membrane sodium gradient–dependent carnitine transporter that is present in heart, muscle, and kidney. This transporter is responsible both for maintaining intracellular carnitine concentrations 20- to 50-fold higher than plasma concentrations and for renal conservation of carnitine. *Diagnosis* of the carnitine transporter defect is aided by the fact that patients have extremely reduced carnitine levels in plasma and muscle to 1–2% of normal. Heterozygote parents have plasma carnitine levels approximately 50% of normal. Fasting ketogenesis may be normal because liver carnitine transport is normal, but it may be impaired if dietary carnitine intake is interrupted. The fasting urinary organic acid profile may show a hypoketotic dicarboxylicaciduria pattern if hepatic fatty acid oxidation is impaired, but it is otherwise unremarkable. The defect in carnitine transport can be demonstrated clinically by severe reduction in renal carnitine threshold or in vitro by assay of carnitine uptake using cultured fibroblasts or lymphoblasts. *Treatment* of this disorder with pharmacologic doses of oral carnitine is highly effective in correcting the cardiomyopathy and muscle weakness as well as any impairment in fasting ketogenesis. Muscle total carnitine concentrations remain less than 5% of normal on treatment.

Carnitine Palmitoyltransferase-1 Deficiency

Several infants and children have been described with a deficiency of the liver isozyme of carnitine palmitoyltransferase-1. *Clinical manifestations* include fasting hypoketotic hypoglycemia, occasionally with markedly abnormal liver function tests. The heart and skeletal muscle are not involved because the muscle isozyme is unaffected. Fasting urinary organic acid profile shows a hypoketotic dicarboxylicaciduria but no specific abnormalities. *Diagnosis* is aided by the observation that this is the only fatty acid oxidation disorder in which plasma total carnitine levels are elevated to 150–200% of normal. This may be explained by the fact that the inhibitory effects of long-chain acylcarnitines on the renal tubular carnitine transporter are absent in carnitine palmitoyltransferase-1 deficiency. The enzyme defect can be demonstrated in cultured fibroblasts or lymphoblasts. *Treatment* with diet to avoid fasting is similar to that in MCAD deficiency.

Carnitine–Acylcarnitine Translocase Deficiency

This defect of the inner mitochondrial membrane carrier protein for fatty acylcarnitines blocks the entry of long-chain fatty acids into the mitochondria for oxidation. The few patients identified have had severe and generalized impairment of fatty acid oxidation. All have presented in the newborn period with attacks of fasting-induced hypoglycemia and cardiorespiratory collapse. All have had evidence of cardiomyopathy and muscle weakness. None has survived beyond 2 yr. No distinctive urinary or plasma organic acids were found. Secondary deficiency of carnitine was noted with unusually increased levels of long-chain acylcarnitines. *Diagnosis* can be made using cultured fibroblasts or lymphoblasts. *Treatment* is similar to other fatty acid oxidation disorders.

Carnitine Palmitoyltransferase-2 Deficiency

Two forms of carnitine palmitoyltransferase-2 deficiency have been described. A severe deficiency of enzyme activity is associated with an infantile-onset form. This form shares all the clinical and laboratory features of the carnitine–acylcarnitine translocase deficiency described earlier. A milder defect is associated with an adult presentation of episodic rhabdomyolysis. The first episode usually does not occur until late childhood or early adulthood. Attacks may be precipitated by prolonged exercise. There is aching muscle pain and myoglobinuria that may be severe enough to cause renal shutdown. Serum levels of creatine kinase are elevated to 5,000–10,000 U/L or more. Fasting hypoglycemia has not been described, but fasting may contribute to attacks of myoglobinuria, and ketogenesis may be impaired. Muscle biopsy shows increased deposition of neutral fat. Diagnosis can be made by demonstrating deficient enzyme activity in muscle or other tissues, and in cultured fibroblasts.

DEFECTS IN ELECTRON TRANSFER PATHWAY

Electron Transfer Flavoprotein and Electron Transfer Flavoprotein Dehydrogenase (ETF-DH) Deficiencies (Glutaric Aciduria Type 2, Multiple Acyl-CoA Dehydrogenation Deficiencies)

Electron transfer flavoprotein (ETF) and electron transfer flavoprotein dehydrogenase (ETF-DH) function to transfer electrons into the mitochondrial electron transport chain from dehydrogenation reactions catalyzed by MCAD, SCAD, LCAD, and VLCAD, as well as glutaryl-CoA dehydrogenase and two enzymes involved in branch-chain amino acid oxidation, isovaleryl-CoA dehydrogenase and branch-chain acyl-CoA dehydrogenase. Deficiencies of ETF or ETF-DH, therefore, produce illness that combines the features of impaired fatty acid oxidation and impaired oxidation of several of the amino acids, such as leucine and lysine. Complete deficiencies of either enzyme are associated with severe illness in the newborn period, characterized by acidosis, hypoglycemia, coma, hypotonia, and cardiomyopathy. Some affected neonates have had facial dysmorphia and polycystic kidneys, which suggests that toxic effects of accumulated metabolites may occur in utero. *Diagnosis* can be made from the urinary organic acid profile, which shows abnormalities corresponding to blocks in oxidation of fatty acids (ethylmalonate and dicarboxylic acids), lysine (glutarate), and branched-chain amino acids (isovaleryl-, isobutyryl-, and alpha-methylbutyryl-glycine). Most severely affected infants have not survived the neonatal period.

Partial deficiencies of ETF and ETF-DH produce a disorder that may mimic MCAD deficiency or other milder fatty acid oxidation defects. These patients have attacks of fasting hypoketotic coma. The urinary organic acid profile reveals primarily elevations of dicarboxylic acids and ethylmalonate, derived from short-chain fatty acid intermediates. Secondary carnitine deficiency is present. Some patients with mild forms of ETF–ETF-DH deficiency have been reported to benefit from *treatment* with high doses of riboflavin, the cofactor for these two enzymes as well as for the acyl-CoA dehydrogenases.

DEFECTS IN KETONE SYNTHESIS PATHWAY

β-Hydroxy-β-Methyl Glutaryl-CoA Synthase Deficiency

β-Hydroxy-β-methyl glutaryl-CoA synthase is the rate-limiting step in conversion of acetyl-CoA derived from fatty acid β-oxidation in the liver to ketones. One patient with this defect has been reported, and this may prompt the recognition of other cases. The presentation was one of fasting hypoketotic hypoglycemia without evidence of impaired cardiac or skeletal muscle function. Urinary organic acid profile showed only a hypoketotic dicarboxylic aciduria. Plasma and tissue carnitine levels were normal, in contrast to all the other disorders of fatty acid oxidation. A separate synthase enzyme present in cytosol for cholesterol biosynthesis was not affected. The β-hydroxy-β-methyl glutaryl-CoA synthase defect is expressed only in the liver and cannot be demonstrated in cultured fibroblasts. Treatment with diet to avoid fasting appears to be successful.

β-Hydroxy-β-Methyl Glutaryl-CoA Lyase Deficiency

(See Chapter 82.6)

DEFECTS IN KETONE UTILIZATION

The ketones, β-hydroxybutyrate and acetoacetate, are the end products of hepatic fatty acid oxidation and serve as important metabolic fuels for the brain during late stages of fasting. Two defects in utilization of ketones in brain and other peripheral tissues that present with episodes of "hyperketotic" hypoglycemia have been described.

Succinyl-CoA Acetoacetyl-CoA Transferase Deficiency

Only one patient with succinyl-CoA acetoacetyl-CoA deficiency has been reported. He presented with recurrent episodes of severe ketoacidosis beginning in the newborn period and died at 6 mo of age. Treatment of episodes required infusion of glucose and large amounts of bicarbonate for 3–4 days. The enzyme is responsible for activating acetoacetate in peripheral tissues using succinyl-CoA as a donor to form acetoacetyl-CoA. Deficient activity was demonstrated in brain, muscle, and fibroblasts.

β-Ketothiolase Deficiency (See Chapter 82.6)

Boles RG, Buck EA, Blitzer MG, et al: Retrospective biochemical screening of fatty acid oxidation disorders in postmortem livers of 418 cases of sudden death in the first year of life. J Pediatr 132:924, 1998.

Cederbaum SD: SIDS and disorders of fatty acid oxidation: Where do we go from here? J Pediatr 132:913, 1998.

Chalmers RA, Stanley CA, English N, et al: Mitochondrial carnitine-acylcarnitine translocase deficiency presenting as sudden neonatal death. J Pediatr 131:220, 1997.

Cox GF, Souri M, Aoyama T, et al: Reversal of severe hypertrophic cardiomyopathy and excellent neuropsychologic outcome in very-long-chain acyl-coenzyme A dehydrogenase deficiency. J Pediatr 133:247, 1998.

Demaugre F, Bonnefont J, Mitchell G, et al: Hepatic and muscular presentations of carnitine palmitoyl transferase deficiency: Two distinct entities. Pediatr Res 24:308, 1988.

Frerman FE, Goodman SI: Deficiency of electron transfer flavoprotein or electron transfer flavoprotein:ubiquinone oxidoreductase in glutaric acidemia type II fibroblasts. Proc Natl Acad Sci USA 82:4517, 1985.

Iafolla AK, Thompson RJ, Roe CR: Medium-chain acyl-coenzyme A dehydrogenase deficiency: Clinical course in 120 affected children. J Pediatr 124:409, 1994.

Kamijo T, Indo Y, Souri M, et al: Medium chain 3-ketoacyl-coenzyme A thiolase deficiency: A new disorder of mitochondrial fatty acid β-oxidation. Pediatr Res 42:569, 1997.

Lecoq I, Mallet E, Bonte JB, et al: The A985 to G mutation of the medium-chain acyl-CoA dehydrogenase gene and sudden infant death syndrome in Normandy. Acta Paediatr 85:145, 1996.

Morris AAM, Olpin SE, Brivet M, et al: A patient with carnitine-acylcarnitine translocase deficiency with a mild phenotype. J Pediatr 132:514, 1998.

Pons R, Carrozzo R, Tein I, et al: Deficient muscle carnitine transport in primary carnitine deficiency. Pediatr Res 42:583, 1997.

Rinaldo P, Stanley CA, Hsu BYL, et al: Sudden neonatal death in carnitine transporter deficiency. J Pediatr 131:304, 1997.

Sluysmans T, Tuerlinckx D, Hubinont C, et al: Very long chain acyl-coenzyme A dehydrogenase deficiency in two siblings: Evolution after prenatal diagnosis and prompt management. J Pediatr 131:444, 1997.

Stanley CA: Dissecting the spectrum of fatty acid oxidation disorders. J Pediatr 132:384, 1998.

Stanley CA, Hale DE, Berry GT, et al: A deficiency of carnitine-acylcarnitine translocase in the inner mitochondrial membrane. N Engl J Med 327:19, 1992.

Straussberg R, Harel L, Varsano I, et al: Recurrent myoglobinura as a presenting manifestation of very long chain acyl coenzyme A dehydrogenase deficiency. Pediatrics 99:894, 1997.

Tanaka K, Gregersen N, Ribes A, et al: A survey of the newborn populations in Belgium, Germany, Poland, Czech Republic, Hungary, Bulgaria, Spain, Turkey, and Japan for the G985 variant allele with haplotype analysis at the medium chain acyl-CoA dehydrogenase gene locus: Clinical and evolutionary consideration. Pediatr Res 41:201, 1997.

Thompson GN, Hsu BY, Pitt JJ, et al: Fasting hypoketotic coma in a child with deficiency of mitochondrial 3-hydroxy-3-methylglutaryl-CoA synthase. N Engl J Med 337:1203, 1997.

Treem WR, Rinaldo P, Hale DE, et al: Acute fatty liver of pregnancy and long chain 3-hydroxyacyl-coenzyme A dehydrogenase deficiency. Hepatology 19:339, 1994.

Tyni T, Palotie A, Viinikka L, et al: Long-chain 3-hydroxyacyl-coenzyme A

dehydrogenase deficiency with the G1528C mutation: Clinical presentation of thirteen patients. J Pediatr 130:67, 1997.
Walter JH: L-Carnitine. Arch Dis Child 74:475, 1996.
Yamaguchi S, Indo Y, Coates PM, et al: Identification of very-long-chain acyl CoA dehydrogenase deficiency in three patients previously diagnosed with long-chain acyl-CoA dehydrogenase deficiency. Pediatr Res 34:111, 1993.
Ziadeh R, Hoffman EP, Finegold DM, et al: Medium chain acyl-CoA dehydrogenase deficiency in Pennsylvania: Neonatal screening shows high incidence and unexpected mutation frequencies. Pediatr Res 37:675, 1995.

83.2 Disorders of Very Long Chain Fatty Acids

Hugo W. Moser

PERОXISOMAL DISORDERS

The peroxisomal diseases are genetically determined disorders due to either the failure to form or maintain the peroxisome or a defect in the function of a single enzyme that is normally located in this organelle. These disorders cause serious disability in childhood and occur more frequently and present a wider range of phenotype than has been recognized in the past.

ETIOLOGY. Peroxisomal disorders are subdivided into two major categories (Table 83–1). In Category A (import disorders), the basic defect is the failure to import one or more proteins into the organelle. Category B includes disorders with defects that affect a single peroxisomal protein. The peroxisome is present in all cells except mature erythrocytes and is a subcellular organelle surrounded by a single membrane; 80 peroxisomal enzymes have been identified. Some enzymes are involved in the production and decomposition of hydrogen peroxide; others are concerned with lipid and amino acid metabolism. Most peroxisomal enzymes are first synthesized in their mature form on free polyribosomes and enter the cytoplasm. Proteins that are destined for the peroxisome contain targeting sequences that direct them to the organelle, where they interact with specific receptors. Fifteen additional proteins are required for peroxisome import. The disorders of peroxisome import are due to genetic defects that involve the receptors or one of these other proteins. Currently these proteins are referred to as peroxins and are numbered PEX1 to PEX17.

EPIDEMIOLOGY. Except for X-linked adrenoleukodystrophy (ALD), all the peroxisomal disorders listed in Table 83–1 are inherited as autosomal recessive traits. Their combined incidence is estimated to be between 1/25,000 and 1/50,000. All races are affected.

PATHOLOGY. Absence or reduction in the number of peroxisomes is the pathognomonic feature of disorders of peroxisome biogenesis. In most of these disorders, there are membranous sacs that contain peroxisomal integral membrane proteins, which lack the normal complement of matrix proteins; these are peroxisome "ghosts." Pathologic changes are observed in many organs and include profound and characteristic defects in neuronal migration; micronodular cirrhosis of the liver; renal cysts; chondrodysplasia punctata; corneal clouding, congenital cataracts, glaucoma, and retinopathy; congenital heart disease; and dysmorphic features.

TABLE 83–1 Classification of Peroxisomal Disorders

A: *Disorders of peroxisome import*	B: *Defects of single peroxisomal enzyme*
A1: Zellweger syndrome	B1: X-linked adrenoleukodystrophy
A2: Neonatal adrenoleukodystrophy	B2: Acyl-CoA oxidase deficiency
A3: Infantile Refsum disease	B3: Bifunctional enzyme deficiency
A4: Rhizomelic chondrodysplasia punctata	B4: Peroxisomal thiolase deficiency
	B5: DHAP acyltransferase deficiency
	B6: Alkyl DHAP synthase deficiency
	B7: Classic Refsum disease
	B8: Mevalonic aciduria
	B9: Glutaric aciduria type III
	B10: Hyperoxaluria type I
	B11: Acatalasemia

TABLE 83–2 Abnormal Laboratory Findings Common to Disorders of Peroxisome Biogenesis

Peroxisomes absent or reduced in number
Catalase in cytosol
Deficient synthesis and reduced tissue levels of plasmalogens
Defective oxidation and abnormal accumulation of very long chain fatty acids
Deficient oxidation and age-dependent accumulation of phytanic acid
Defects in certain steps of bile acid formation and accumulation of bile acid intermediates
Defects in oxidation and accumulation of L-pipecolic acid
Increased urinary excretion of dicarboxylic acids

PATHOGENESIS. It is likely that all pathologic changes are secondary to the peroxisome defect. Multiple peroxisomal enzymes fail to function in the group A disorders (Table 83–2). The enzymes that are diminished or absent are synthesized but are degraded abnormally fast because they may be unprotected outside of the peroxisome. It is not clear how defective peroxisome functions lead to the widespread pathologic manifestations.

The disorders of peroxisome import have been subdivided into 11 complementation groups. The phenotype of groups 1–10 is that of the "Zellweger syndrome, neonatal ALD, infantile Refsum disease continuum," whereas group 11 manifests as rhizomelic chondrodysplasia punctata. The molecular defects that underlie seven of these groups are defined. Complementation group 2 is due to a defect in the receptor for peroxisome targeting sequence 1, and rhizomelic chondrodysplasia involves the receptor for targeting sequence 2. The other five disorders involve other peroxins. Approximately 60% of patients with peroxisome import disorders are members of complementation group 1. The defective gene codes for a protein referred to as PEX1 that contains 1,283 amino acids and appears to be required for the stabilization of the receptor for the peroxisome targeting sequence. Mutation analysis has identified a variety of molecular defects in each of these complementation groups. Some of the mutations do not eliminate function completely and are associated with milder phenotypes.

CLINICAL MANIFESTATIONS

Disorders of Peroxisome Biogenesis Group A. Zellweger syndrome, neonatal ALD, and infantile Refsum disease represent a continuum, with the Zellweger syndrome the most severe and infantile Refsum disease the least severe. All three phenotypes have been found in complementation groups 1–10. Rhizomelic chondrodysplasia punctata is distinct and associated only with complementation group 11.

Newborn infants with *Zellweger syndrome* show striking and consistent abnormalities that are easily recognized. Of central diagnostic importance are the typical facial appearance (high forehead, unslanting palpebral fissures, hypoplastic supraorbital ridges, and epicanthal folds [Fig. 83–2]), severe weakness and hypotonia, neonatal seizures, and eye abnormalities (cataracts, glaucoma, corneal clouding, Brushfield spots, pigmentary retinopathy, and optic nerve dysplasia). Because of the hypotonia and "mongoloid" appearance, Down syndrome may be suspected. Infants with Zellweger syndrome rarely live more than a few mo. More than 90% show postnatal growth failure. Table 83–3 lists the main clinical abnormalities.

Patients with *neonatal ALD* show fewer and occasionally no dysmorphic features. Neonatal seizures occur frequently. Some degree of psychomotor development is present; function remains in the severely or profoundly retarded range and may regress after 3–5 yr of age, probably owing to a progressive leukodystrophy. Several patients are now in a stable, albeit disabled, state in the 3rd or 4th decade. Enlarged liver and impaired liver function, pigmentary degeneration of the retina,

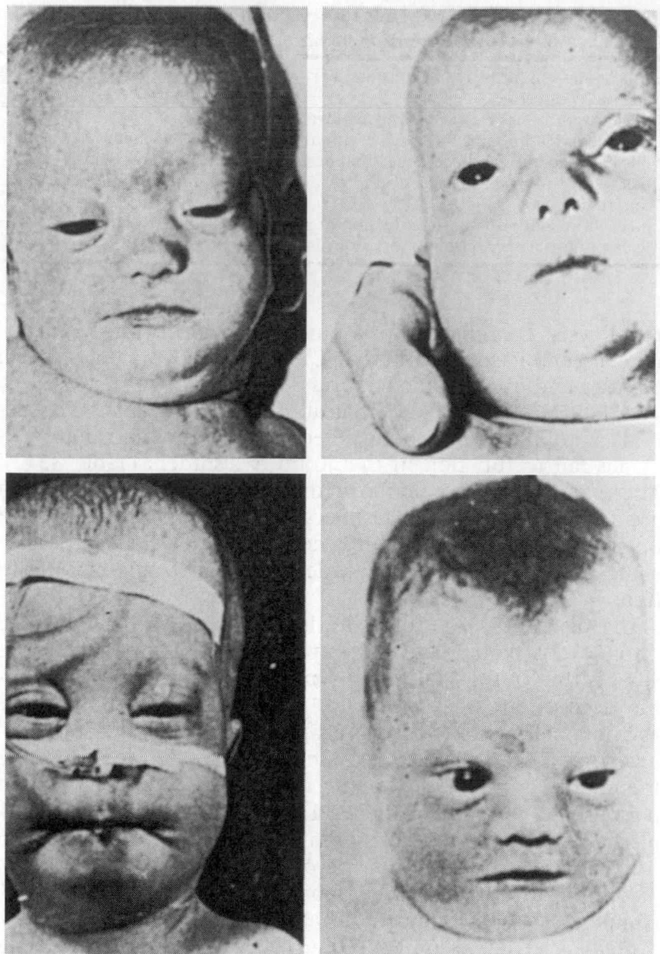

Figure 83–2 Four patients with the Zellweger cerebrohepatorenal syndrome. Note the high forehead, epicanthal folds, and hypoplasia of supraorbital ridges and midface. (Courtesy of Hans Zellweger, M.D. Used by permission.)

and severely impaired hearing are almost always present. Adrenocortical function is usually impaired, but overt Addison disease is rare. Chondrodysplasia punctata and renal cysts are absent.

Patients with *infantile Refsum disease* have survived to the 2nd decade or longer. They are able to walk, although gait may be ataxic and broad-based. Cognitive function is in the severely retarded range. All have sensorineural hearing loss and pigmentary degeneration of the retina. They have moderately dysmorphic features that may include epicanthal folds, a flat bridge of the nose, and low-set ears. Early hypotonia and enlarged liver with impaired function are common. Levels of plasma cholesterol and high- and low-density lipoprotein are often moderately reduced. Chondrodysplasia punctata and renal cortical cysts are absent. Postmortem study in infantile Refsum disease reveals micronodular liver cirrhosis and small hypoplastic adrenals. The brain shows no malformations, except for severe hypoplasia of the cerebellar granule layer and ectopic locations of the Purkinje cells in the molecular layer. Although initial reports indicated a preponderance of males, the mode of inheritance is probably autosomal recessive.

The designation of *hyperpipecolic acidemia* was applied to patients subsequently shown to have diminished or absent peroxisomes, but because of the resemblance of this condition to the Zellweger syndrome or neonatal ALD, this disorder is no longer classified as a separate phenotype.

Rhizomelic Chondrodysplasia Punctata. Rhizomelic chondrodysplasia punctata (RCDP) is characterized by the presence of stippled foci of calcification within the hyaline cartilage and is associated with dwarfing, cataracts (72%), and multiple malformations due to contractures. Vertebral bodies have a coronal cleft filled by cartilage that is a result of an embryonic arrest. Disproportionate short stature affects the proximal parts of the extremities (Fig. 83–3*A*). Radiologic abnormalities consist of shortening of the proximal limb bones, metaphyseal cupping, and disturbed ossification (Fig. 83–3*B*). Height, weight, and head circumference are less than the 3rd percentile, and the children are severely retarded mentally. Skin changes such as those observed in ichthyosiform erythroderma are present in about 25% of patients.

Isolated Defects of Peroxisomal Fatty Acid Oxidation. The disorders labeled B1–B3 (see Table 83–1) each involve one of three enzymes involved in peroxisomal fatty acid oxidation. Their clinical manifestations resemble those of the Zellweger, neonatal ALD, infantile Refsum disease continuum; they can be distinguished from disorders of peroxisome biogenesis by laboratory tests. Defects of bifunctional enzyme are common and are found in approximately 15% of patients with the Zellweger–neonatal ALD–infantile Refsum disease phenotype. Patients with isolated acyl-coenzyme A (CoA) oxidase deficiency have a somewhat milder phenotype that resembles neonatal ALD. Only a single patient with peroxisomal thiolase deficiency has been described. This patient had the Zellweger syndrome phenotype.

Isolated Defects of Plasmalogen Synthesis. Plasmalogens are lipids in which the first carbon of glycerol is linked to an alcohol rather than a fatty acid. They are synthesized through a complex series of reactions, the first two steps of which are catalyzed by the peroxisomal enzymes dihydroxyacetone phosphate alkyl transferase and synthase. Deficiency of either of these enzymes (B4 and B5 in Table 83–1) leads to a phenotype that is clinically indistinguishable from the peroxisomal import disorder rhizomelic chondrodysplasia punctata. This latter dis-

TABLE 83–3 Main Clinical Abnormalities in Zellweger Syndrome

Abnormal Feature	Cases in Which Information About the Feature Was Available		Cases in Which the Feature Was Present	
	No.	*%*	*No.*	*%*
High forehead	60	53	58	97
Flat occiput	16	14	13	81
Large fontanelle(s), wide sutures	57	50	55	96
Shallow orbital ridges	33	29	33	100
Low/broad nasal bridge	23	20	23	100
Epicanthus	36	32	33	92
High arched palate	37	32	35	95
External ear deformity	40	35	39	97
Micrognathia	18	16	18	100
Redundant skin fold of neck	13	11	13	100
Brushfield spots	6	5	5	83
Cataract/cloudy cornea	35	31	30	86
Glaucoma	12	11	7	58
Abnormal retinal pigmentation	15	13	6	40
Optic disk pallor	23	20	17	74
Severe hypotonia	95	83	94	99
Abnormal Moro response	26	23	26	100
Hyporeflexia or areflexia	57	50	56	98
Poor sucking	77	68	74	96
Gavage feeding	26	23	26	100
Epileptic seizures	61	54	56	92
Psychomotor retardation	45	39	45	100
Impaired hearing	21	18	9	40
Nystagmus	37	32	30	81

From Heymans HSA: Cerebro-hepato-renal (Zellweger) syndrome. Clinical and biochemical consequences of peroxisomal dysfunctions. Thesis, University of Amsterdam, 1984.

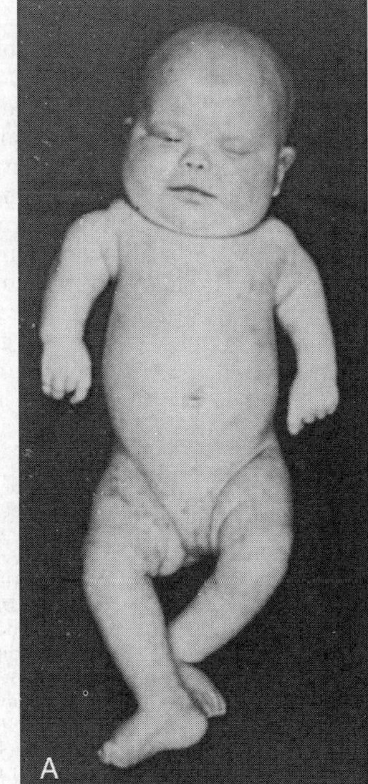

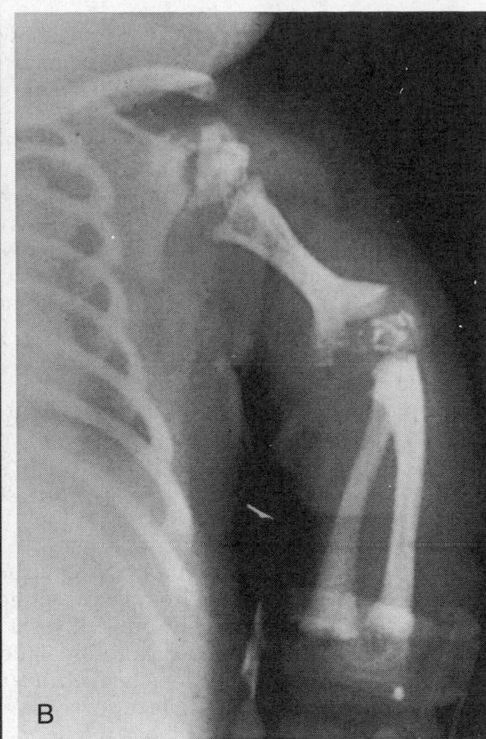

Figure 83–3 *A,* A newborn infant with RCDP. Note the severe shortening of the proximal limbs, the depressed bridge of the nose, hypertelorism, and widespread scaling skin lesions. *B,* Note the marked shortening of the humerus and epiphyseal stippling at the shoulder and the elbow joints. (Courtesy of John P. Dorst, M.D., Johns Hopkins Hospital.)

order is due to a defect in PEX7, the receptor for peroxisome targeting sequence 2. It shares the severe deficiency of plasmalogens with disorders B4 and B5, but in addition has defects of phytanic oxidation. The fact that disorders B4 and B5 are associated with the full phenotype of rhizomelic chondrodysplasia punctata suggests that a deficiency of plasmalogens is sufficient to produce it.

Classic Refsum Disease. The defective enzyme (phytanoyl-CoA oxidase) is localized to the peroxisome. The manifestation of classic Refsum disease includes impaired vision due to retinitis pigmentosa, ichthyosis, peripheral neuropathy, ataxia, and occasionally cardiac arrhythmias. In contrast to infantile Refsum disease, cognitive function is normal, and there are no congenital malformations. Classic Refsum disease often does not become manifested until young adulthood, but visual disturbances, such as night blindness, ichthyosis, and peripheral neuropathy may already be present in childhood and adolescence. Early diagnosis is important because institution of a phytanic acid–restricted diet can reverse the peripheral neuropathy and prevent the progression of the visual and central nervous system manifestations.

LABORATORY FINDINGS. The *group A disorders* display a spectrum of biochemical abnormalities that are secondary to the defect in peroxisome structure (Table 83–4). The pathognomonic feature is the diminished number or absence of peroxisomes combined with defective function of multiple peroxisomal enzymes.

RCDP shows three biochemical abnormalities: (1) an impaired capacity to oxidize phytanic acid, (2) an impaired capacity to synthesize plasmalogens, and (3) a failure to process the peroxisomal thiolase enzyme so that it is present in the precursor rather than the mature form. These three defects are also a feature of the group A disorders. RCDP differs from them in that the peroxisome structure is intact, and the oxidation of very long chain fatty acids and pipecolic acid is unimpaired.

Defects involving the defective function of a single peroxisomal enzyme include lignoceroyl CoA ligase in X-linked ALD; alanine-glyoxylate aminotransferase in hyperoxaluria type 1; catalase in acatalasemia; and acyl-CoA oxidase, bifunctional enzyme, or 3-oxo-acyl-CoA thiolase, respectively, in the three recently described disorders in which a single peroxisomal oxidation enzyme fails to function. In classic Refsum disease, there is a defect in phytanoyl-CoA oxidase.

DIAGNOSIS. There are now several noninvasive laboratory

TABLE 83–4 Peroxisomal Disorders: Biochemical Diagnostic Assays

Disease	Assay	Findings
Disorders of peroxisome biogenesis: Zellweger syndrome, neonatal adrenoleukodystrophy, infantile Refsum disease, hyperpipecolic acidemia	Plasma RBCs Fibroblasts	VLCFAs Pipecolic acid Phytanic acid Bile acids Plasmalogens Plasmalogen synthesis Catalase subcellular localization
X-linked ALD hemizygote	Plasma, RBCs Fibroblasts	VLCFAs VLCFAs
X-linked ALD heterozygotes	Plasma Fibroblasts DNA probe	VLCFAs VLCFAs
Rhizomelic chondrodysplasia punctata	Plasma RBCs Fibroblasts	Phytanic acid Plasmalogens Plasmalogen synthesis Phytanic acid oxidation
Isolated defects of VLCFA degradation	Plasma Fibroblasts	VLCFAs VLCFAs VLCFA oxidation Immunoblot of peroxisomal fatty acid oxidation enzymes
Hyperoxaluria, type 1	Urine Liver	Organic acids Alanine: Glyoxylate amino transferase in percutaneous liver biopsy
Acatalasemia	RBCs	Catalase

VLCFAs = very long chain fatty acids; RBCs = red blood cells; ALD = adrenoleukodystrophy.

tests that permit precise and early diagnosis of peroxisomal disorders (see Table 83–4). For the clinician, the decision is when to order these tests. The challenge in group A disorders is to differentiate them from the large variety of other conditions that can cause hypotonia, seizures, failure to thrive, or dysmorphic features. Experienced clinicians can readily recognize classic Zellweger syndrome by its clinical manifestations. However, group A patients often do not show the full clinical spectrum of disease and may be identifiable only by laboratory assays. Clinical features that may serve as indications for these diagnostic assays include severe psychomotor retardation; weakness and hypotonia; dysmorphic features; neonatal seizures; retinopathy, glaucoma, or cataracts; hearing deficits; enlarged liver and impaired liver function; and chondrodysplasia punctata. The presence of one or more of these abnormalities increases the likelihood of this diagnosis.

Patients with the isolated defects of peroxisomal fatty acid oxidation (group 2) resemble those with group A disorders and can be detected by the demonstration of abnormally high levels of very long chain fatty acids.

Patients with RCDP must be distinguished from patients with other causes of chondrodysplasia punctata. In addition to warfarin embryopathy and the Zellweger syndrome, these disorders include the milder autosomal dominant form of chondrodysplasia punctata *(Conradi-Hünermann syndrome)* which is characterized by longer survival, absence of severe limb shortening, and usually intact intellect; an X-linked dominant form; and an X-linked recessive form associated with a deletion of the terminal portion of the short arm of the X chromosome. RCDP is suspected clinically because of the shortness of limbs, psychomotor retardation, and ichthyosis. The most decisive laboratory test is the demonstration of abnormally low plasmalogen levels in red blood cells and an impaired capacity to synthesize plasmalogens in cultured skin fibroblasts. These biochemical defects are not present in other types of chondrodysplasia punctata.

COMPLICATIONS. Patients with the Zellweger cerebrohepatorenal syndrome have multiple disabilities involving muscle tone, swallowing, cardiac abnormalities, liver disease, and seizures. These conditions are treated symptomatically, but the prognosis is poor, and most patients succumb during the first few months of life.

PREVENTION. See under Genetic Counseling and Chapter 80.

TREATMENT. The most effective therapy is the dietary treatment of classic Refsum disease with a phytanic acid–restricted diet.

For patients with the somewhat milder variants of the peroxisome import disorders, considerable success has been achieved with multidisciplinary early intervention, including physical and occupational therapy, hearing aids, alternative communication, nutrition, and support for the parents. Although most patients continue to function in the profoundly or severely retarded range, some make significant gains in self-help skills, and several are in stable condition in their teens or even early 20s.

Several experimental studies are under way to mitigate some of the secondary biochemical abnormalities. These include the oral administration of docosahexaenoic acid in a dosage of 50–100 mg/24 hr either as the ethyl ester or in the form of a triglyceride in which one of the fatty acids has been replaced by docosahexaenoic acid. This therapy normalizes the plasma and red blood cell levels of this substance, which has important physiologic functions in retina and brain, and the levels of which are reduced greatly in patients with disorders of peroxisome biogenesis because the last step of its synthesis takes place in the peroxisome. There are anecdotal reports of clinical improvement, and double-blind trials to evaluate this therapy are now in progress. Also being studied is the oral administration of cholic acid and chenodeoxycholic in a dosage of 100–250 mg/24 hr, with the aim of reducing the levels of presumably toxic bile acid intermediates.

GENETIC COUNSELING. All the peroxisomal disorders can be diagnosed prenatally in the 1st or 2nd trimester, except for hyperoxaluria type 1. The tests are similar to those described for postnatal diagnosis (see Table 83–4) and use chorionic villus sampling or amniocytes. More than 300 pregnancies have been monitored, and more than 60 affected fetuses have been identified so far without diagnostic error. Because of the 25% recurrence risk, couples who have had an affected child must be advised about the availability of prenatal diagnosis. Heterozygotes can be identified in X-linked adrenoleukodystrophy and in those disorders in which the molecular defect has been identified (see Table 83–4).

Braverman N, Steel G, Obie C, et al: Human PEX7 encodes the peroxisomal PTS2 receptor and is responsible for rhizomelic chondrodysplasia punctata. Nat Genet 15:369, 1997.

Fournier B, Saudubray JM, Benichou B, et al: Large deletion of the peroxisomal acyl-CoA oxidase gene in pseudoneonatal adrenoleukodystrophy. J Clin Invest 94:526, 1994.

Kelley RI, Datta NS, Dobyns WB, et al: Neonatal adrenoleukodystrophy: New cases, biochemical studies, and differentiation from Zellweger and related peroxisomal polydystrophy syndromes. Am J Med Genet 23:869, 1986.

Martinez M, Pineda M, Vidal R, Martin B: Docosahexaenoic acid: A new therapeutic approach to peroxisomal patients. Experience with two cases. Neurology 43:1389, 1993.

Mihalik SJ, Morell SJ, Kim D, et al: Identification of PAHX, a Refsum disease gene. Nat Genet 17:185, 1997.

Moser AB, Rasmussen M, Naidu S, et al: Phenotype of patients with peroxisomal disorders subdivided into 16 complementation groups. J Pediatr 127:13–22, 1995.

Reuber BE, Germain-Lee E, Collins CS, et al: Mutations of *PEX1* are the most common cause of peroxisome biogenesis disorders. Nat Genet 17:445, 1997.

Roels F, DeBie S, Schutgens RBH, Besley GTN: Diagnosis of human peroxisomal disorders, a handbook. J Inherit Metab Dis 18(Suppl):1, 1995.

Setchell KDR, Bragetti P, Zimmer-Nechemias L, et al: Oral bile acid treatment and the patient with Zellweger syndrome. Hepatology 15:198, 1992.

ADRENOLEUKODYSTROPHY (X-LINKED)

X-linked ALD is a genetically determined disorder associated with the accumulation of saturated very long chain fatty acids and a progressive dysfunction of the adrenal cortex and nervous system white matter.

ETIOLOGY. The key biochemical abnormality is the tissue accumulation of saturated very long chain fatty acids. These are unbranched with a carbon chain length of 24 or more. Excess hexacosanoic acid (C26:0) is the most striking and characteristic feature. This accumulation of fatty acids is due to genetically determined deficient degradation of fatty acids, which is a normal peroxisomal function. The key biochemical defect appears to involve the impaired function of peroxisomal lignoceroyl-CoA ligase, which is the enzyme that catalyzes the formation of the CoA derivative of very long chain fatty acids. The gene that is defective codes for a peroxisomal membrane (ALDP) that is thought to be essential for the transport of lignoceroyl-CoA ligase into the peroxisome. More than 100 distinct mutations have been identified, and most families have a mutation that is "private" (unique to that kindred). The gene has been mapped to chromosome Xq28.

EPIDEMIOLOGY. X-linkage has been confirmed by analysis of more than 900 kindreds. All races are affected. Incidence is estimated to be between 1/20,000 and 1/50,000. The various phenotypes often occur in members of the same kindred.

PATHOLOGY. Characteristic lamellar cytoplasmic inclusions can be demonstrated with the electron microscope in adrenocortical cells, testicular Leydig cells, and nervous system macrophages. These inclusions probably consist of cholesterol esterified with very long chain fatty acids. They are most prominent in cells of the zona fasciculata of the adrenal cortex, which at first are distended with lipid and later atrophy.

The nervous system can display two lesions. In the severe childhood cerebral form and in the rapidly progressive adult forms, demyelination is associated with an inflammatory response manifested by the accumulation of perivascular lymphocytes that is most intense in the parieto-occipital region. In the slowly progressive adult form (adrenomyeloneuropathy), the main finding is a distal axonopathy that affects the long tracts in the spinal cord most severely. The inflammatory response is mild or absent.

PATHOGENESIS. The adrenal dysfunction is probably a direct consequence of the accumulation of very long chain fatty acids. The cells in the zona fasciculata are distended with abnormal lipids. Cholesterol esterified with very long chain fatty acids is relatively resistant to adrenocorticotropic hormone (ACTH)-stimulated cholesterol ester hydrolases, and this limits the capacity to convert cholesterol to endocrinologically active steroids. In addition, C26:0 excess increases the viscosity of the plasma membrane and this, in turn, may interfere with receptor and other cellular functions.

There is no correlation between the neurologic phenotype and the nature of the mutation or the severity of the biochemical defect as assessed by levels of very long chain fatty acids or between the degree of adrenal and nervous system involvement. The severity of the illness and the rate of progression correlate with the intensity of the inflammatory response. The inflammatory response may be cytokine-mediated and may involve an autoimmune response triggered in an unknown way by the excess of very long chain fatty acids. Approximately half the patients do not experience the inflammatory response. A modifier gene, which sets the "thermostat" for the inflammatory response, has been postulated.

CLINICAL MANIFESTATIONS. There are seven relatively distinct phenotypes, three of which present in childhood with symptoms and signs. In all the phenotypes, development is usually normal during the first 3–4 yr (see Chapter 83.1).

In the *childhood cerebral* form of ALD, symptoms are first noted most commonly between the ages of 4 and 8 yr and 3 yr at the earliest. The most common initial manifestations are hyperactivity, which is often mistaken for an attention deficit disorder, and worsening school performance in a child who had previously been a good student. Auditory discrimination is often impaired, although tone perception is preserved. This may be evidenced by difficulty in using the telephone and greatly impaired performance on intelligence tests in items that are presented verbally. Spatial orientation is often impaired. Other initial symptoms are disturbances of vision, ataxia, poor handwriting, seizures, and strabismus. Visual disturbances often are due to involvement of the cerebral cortex, which leads to variable and seemingly inconsistent visual capacity. Seizures occur in nearly all patients and may represent the first manifestation of the disease. Some patients present with increased intracranial pressure or with unilateral mass lesions. Impaired cortisol response to ACTH stimulation is present in 85% of patients, and mild hyperpigmentation is noted. However, in most patients with this phenotype, adrenal dysfunction is recognized only after the condition is diagnosed because of the cerebral symptoms. Cerebral childhood ALD tends to progress rapidly with increasing spasticity and paralysis, visual and hearing loss, and loss of ability to speak or swallow. The mean interval between the first neurologic symptom and an apparently vegetative state is 1.9 yr. Patients may continue in this apparently vegetative state for 10 yr or more.

Adolescent ALD designates patients who experience neurologic symptoms between the ages of 10 and 21 yr. The manifestations resemble those of childhood cerebral ALD except that progression is slower.

Adrenomyeloneuropathy first becomes manifested in late adolescence or adulthood as a progressive paraparesis due to long tract degeneration in the spinal cord. Approximately one half of the patients also have involvement of the cerebral white matter.

The "Addison only" phenotype is an important and underdiagnosed condition. Studies in developed countries suggest that as many as 40% of male patients with Addison disease have the biochemical defect of ALD. Many of these patients have intact neurologic systems, whereas others have subtle neurologic signs. Many acquire adrenomyeloneuropathy in adulthood.

The term *presymptomatic ALD* is applied to boys up to 10 yr old who have the biochemical defect of ALD but are free of neurologic or endocrine disturbances. Boys in this category who are 10 yr or older are referred to as asymptomatic. A few persons with the biochemical defect of ALD who are relatives of clinically affected patients with ALD have remained asymptomatic even in the 6th or 7th decade.

Approximately 20–30% of female heterozygotes acquire a syndrome that resembles adrenomyeloneuropathy but is milder and of later onset. Adrenal insufficiency is rare.

LABORATORY FINDINGS. The most specific and important laboratory finding is the demonstration of abnormally high levels of very long chain fatty acids in plasma, red blood cells, or cultured skin fibroblasts. The test should be performed in a laboratory that has experience with this specialized procedure. Positive results are obtained in all male patients with X-linked ALD and in approximately 85% of female carriers of X-linked ALD.

Computed Tomography and Magnetic Resonance Imaging. Patients with childhood cerebral or adolescent ALD show cerebral white matter lesions that are characteristic with respect to location and attenuation patterns on computed tomography (CT) or magnetic resonance imaging (MRI). In 80% of patients, the lesions are symmetric and involve the periventricular white matter in the posterior parietal and occipital lobes. Noncontrast CT scans show bilateral hypodensities in this location. The second characteristic, observed following intravenous injection of contrast material, is the demonstration of a garland of accumulated contrast material adjacent and anterior to the posterior hypodense lesions (Fig. 83–4*A*). This zone corresponds to the zones of intense perivascular lymphocytic infiltration where the blood-brain barrier breaks down. In 12% of patients, the initial lesions are frontal. Unilateral lesions that produce a mass effect suggestive of a brain tumor may occur. MRI provides a clearer delineation of normal and abnormal white matter than does CT and may demonstrate abnormalities missed by CT (see Fig. 83–4*B*).

Impaired Adrenal Function. More than 85% of patients with the childhood form of ALD have elevated levels of ACTH in plasma and a subnormal rise of cortisol levels in plasma following intravenous injection of 250 μg of $ACTH_{1B-4}$ (Cortrosyn).

DIAGNOSIS AND DIFFERENTIAL DIAGNOSIS. The earliest manifestations of childhood cerebral ALD are difficult to distinguish from the more common attention deficit disorders or learning disabilities. Rapid progression, signs of dementia, or difficulty in auditory discrimination suggest ALD. Even in early stages, CT or MRI may show strikingly abnormal changes. Other leukodystrophies or multiple sclerosis may mimic these radiographic findings. Definitive diagnosis depends on demonstration of very long chain fatty acid excess, which occurs only in X-linked ALD and the peroxisomal disorders. The latter may be distinguished from X-linked ALD by their clinical presentation during the neonatal period.

Cerebral forms of ALD may present with increased intracranial pressure and unilateral mass lesions. These have been misdiagnosed as gliomas, even after brain biopsy, and several patients have received radiotherapy before the correct diagnosis was made. Measurement of very long chain fatty acids in plasma or brain biopsy specimens is the most reliable differential test.

Adolescent or adult cerebral ALD can be confused with psychiatric disorders, epilepsy, or dementing disorders. The first clue to the diagnosis of ALD may be the demonstration of

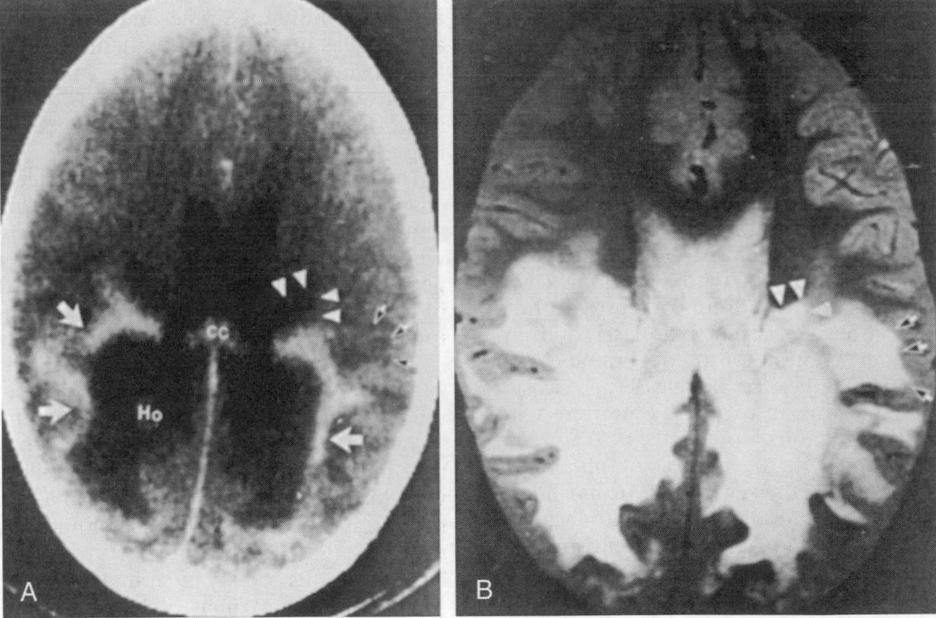

Figure 83–4 *A,* Contrast-enhanced CT abnormalities in ALD with typical parieto-occipital location, showing symmetric bilateral hypodense inactive zones (Ho). The enhancing active periphery zone of hypodensity is demarcated by *arrows.* Compare the anterior zone of hypodensity *(arrowheads)* with the MRI. CC = corpus callosum. (From Kumar et al. 1987, with permission.) *B,* An MRI of the same patient and area shown by CT scanning. MRI-T_2-weighted image shows a high-intensity signal of the abnormally bright parieto-occipital white matter. Subcortical involvement is better identified on MRI. Separation of active zones may be better appreciated by CT scanning, because both inactive and active zones are seen at high-signal areas on MRI. However, it is assumed that such major distinctions afforded by CT will also be demonstrable when IV enhancement (paramagnetic enhancement) becomes readily available. Note the hypodense involvement of CT scanning *(arrowheads* and *arrows* in *A* compared with the well-resolved lesions on MRI in *B.* (From Kumar AJ, Rosenbaum AE, Naidu S, et al: Adrenoleukodystrophy: Correlating MR imaging with CT. Radiology 165:497, 1987.)

white matter lesions by CT or MRI; assays of very long chain fatty acids are confirmatory.

ALD cannot be distinguished clinically from other forms of Addison disease; it is recommended that assays of very long chain fatty acid levels be performed in all male patients with Addison disease. ALD patients usually never have antibodies to adrenal tissue in their plasma.

COMPLICATIONS. An avoidable complication is the occurrence of adrenal insufficiency. The most difficult neurologic problems are those related to bed rest, contracture, coma, and swallowing disturbances. Other complications involve behavioral disturbances and injuries associated with defects of spatial orientation, impaired vision and hearing, and seizures.

TREATMENT. Steroid replacement for adrenal insufficiency or adrenocortical hypofunction is effective (see Chapter 585). Adrenal function should be tested periodically at minimal intervals of 1 yr.

The progressive behavioral and neurologic disturbances associated with the childhood form of ALD are extremely difficult for the family to cope with. ALD patients require the establishment of a comprehensive management program and partnership among the family, physician, visiting nursing staff, school authorities, and counselors. In addition, parent support groups are often helpful.* Communication with school authorities is important because under the provisions of Public Law 94–142 children with ALD qualify for special services as "other health impaired" or "multi-handicapped." Depending on the rate of progression of the disease, special needs might range from relatively low-level resource services within a regular school program to home and hospital-based teaching programs for children who are not mobile.

Management challenges vary with the stage of the illness. The early stages are characterized by subtle changes in affect, behavior, and attention span. Counseling and communication with school authorities are of prime importance. Changes in the sleep-wake cycle can be benefited by the judicious use at night of sedatives such as chloral hydrate (10–50 mg/kg), pentobarbital (5 mg/kg), or diphenhydramine (2–3 mg/kg).

As the leukodystrophy progresses, the modulation of muscle tone and support of bulbar muscular function are major concerns. Baclofen in gradually increasing doses (5 mg twice a day to 25 mg four times a day) is the most effective pharmacologic agent for the treatment of acute episodic painful muscle spasms. Other agents may also be used, care being taken to monitor the occurrence of side effects and drug interactions. As the leukodystrophy progresses, bulbar muscular control is lost. Although initially this can be managed by changing the diet to soft and pureed foods, most patients eventually require a nasogastric tube or a surgical procedure such as gastrostomy or lateral esophagostomy. At least one third of patients have focal or generalized seizures that usually readily respond to standard anticonvulsant medications.

Several specific therapeutic approaches are under investigation. The plasma levels of C26:0 can be normalized within 4 wk by the administration of oils containing certain monounsaturated fatty acids in combination with the dietary restriction of saturated very long chain fatty acids. The most commonly used oil (Lorenzo's oil) is a 4:1 mixture of glyceryl trioleate and glyceryl trierucate. Erucic acid (22:1 n9) is the active component of the latter. These oils appear to act by reducing the rate of endogenous synthesis of the saturated very long chain fatty acids. Although the biochemical effect on plasma C26:0 levels is striking, which led to the hope that this could lead to clinical benefit, the general experience has been that this therapy does not alter the rate of neurologic progression in the childhood cerebral or adrenomyeloneuropathy forms of ALD. There is somewhat encouraging, but not yet proven,

*United Leukodystrophy Foundation, 2304 Highland Drive, Sycamore, IL 60178.

evidence that administration of the oils prior to the development of neurologic symptoms reduces the frequency and severity of later neurologic disability. Although interpretation of the data in asymptomatic patients requires additional study, it is recommended at this time that neurologically asymptomatic ALD patients be placed on this dietary regimen as part of ongoing therapeutic trials. Moderate reductions in platelet counts are observed in 40% of patients on this dietary regimen, and careful medical supervision is required.

Bone marrow transplantation (BMT) is the most effective therapy for X-linked ALD, but its application must be considered with great care. The main indication is in boys with *significant but mild cerebral involvement* for whom a donor with a good HLA match is available. Significant but mild cerebral involvement is judged present if an MRI abnormality characteristic of ALD is combined with moderate deficits in visual or auditory processing or memory-learning that are known to be associated with ALD, or if there is evidence of mild motor, visual, or auditory dysfunction. Under these circumstances, BMT has not only stabilized the course of the disease but in some patients has led to a reversal of the abnormality. It is our impression that severe graft-versus-host disease is not only associated with the expected higher mortality but also jeopardizes the chance of neurologic benefit. Preliminary, but not yet fully confirmed, data suggest that pretransplantation dietary therapy (as described earlier) reduces the risk of transplant-related morbidity and mortality. Because BMT is associated with a 10–20% mortality, even under favorable circumstances, it is not recommended for patients who do not have evidence of cerebral involvement or who have mild cerebral involvement that is nonprogressive (see Chapter 135). Even without therapy, more than half of the patients with the biochemical abnormality of ALD are not "destined" to acquire the severe form of the disease. Although the majority of these patients will acquire adrenomyeloneuropathy in adulthood, and even though this may be a seriously disabling disease, many of these patients have led productive lives, and some have survived to the 8th decade. Furthermore, preliminary experience suggests that dietary therapy administered to neurologically asymptomatic patients reduces the frequency and severity of subsequent neurologic disability, and other forms of therapy are under consideration so that the risk associated with BMT does not appear warranted under these circumstances. BMT is also not recommended for patients with severe cognitive, motor, or visual impairment. The procedure may not be of benefit, and it may accelerate the rate of neurologic progression.

It is our practice to recommend dietary therapy for all persons with the biochemical abnormality of ALD who are asymptomatic or have the "Addison only" phenotype. Neurologic and neuropsychologic examinations and MRI are obtained at 6–12 mo to ensure that the window of opportunity for BMT is not missed.

Studies are in progress to determine whether the rapid rate of progression of childhood cerebral ALD can be modified by pharmacologic agents such as β-interferon, immune globulin, or tumor necrosis factor antagonists such as pentoxifylline or thalidomide. Since the ALD gene has been isolated, efforts toward the development of gene therapy have been initiated.

GENETIC COUNSELING AND PREVENTION. The very long chain fatty acid assay can identify 85% of female carriers, and the accuracy of carrier identification can be increased by use of the DXS52 DNA probe. Prenatal diagnosis of affected male fetuses can be achieved by measurement of very long chain fatty acid levels in cultured amniocytes or chorionic villus cells. Whenever a new patient with X-linked ALD is identified, a detailed pedigree should be constructed, and efforts should be made to identify all at-risk female carriers and affected males. These investigations should be accompanied by careful and sympathetic attention to social, emotional, and ethical issues during counseling.

Aubourg P, Blanche S, Jambaque I, et al: Reversal of early neurologic and neuroradiologic manifestations of X-linked adrenoleukodystrophy by bone marrow transplantation. N Engl J Med 322:1860, 1990.

Dodd A, Rowland SA, Hawkes SLJ, et al: Mutations in the adrenoleukodystrophy gene. Hum Mutat 9:500, 1997.

Krivit W, Lockman LA, Watkins PA, et al: The future for treatment by bone marrow transplantation for adrenoleukodystrophy, metachromatic leukodystrophy, globoid cell leukodystrophy and Hurler syndrome. J Inherit Metab Dis 18:398, 1995.

Malm G, Ringden O, Anvert M, et al: Treatment of adrenoleukodystrophy with bone marrow transplantation. Acta Paediatr 86:484, 1997.

Moser HW: Adrenoleukodystrophy: Phenotype, genetics, pathogenesis and therapy. Brain 120:1485, 1997.

Moser HW, Borel J: Dietary therapy for adrenoleukodystrophy. Annu Rev Nutr 15:379, 1995.

Mosser J, Douar A-M, Sarde C-O, et al: Putative X-linked adrenoleukodystrophy gene shares unexpected homology with ABC transporters. Nature 361:726, 1993.

Van Geel BM, Assies J, Wanders RJA, Barth PG: X-linked adrenoleukodystrophy: Clinical presentation, diagnosis, and therapy. J Neurol Neurosurg Psychiatr 63:4, 1997.

83.3 Disorders of Lipoprotein Metabolism and Transport

Andrew M. Tershakovec and Daniel J. Rader

EPIDEMIOLOGY OF BLOOD LIPIDS AND CARDIOVASCULAR DISEASE

There is an association between fat intake and cholesterol levels and adult coronary heart disease (CHD) mortality. Adult cardiovascular disease has its roots in childhood. American casualties in the Korean and Vietnam wars were found to have a significant prevalence of atherosclerosis, despite their young age. In the Johns Hopkins Precursors Study, cholesterol levels measured in young men in their early 20s were predictive of the risk of CHD developing three to four decades later. The strongest data linking factors in childhood with adult CHD come from the Bogalusa Heart Study and the Pathobiological Determinants of Atherosclerosis in Youth Research Group. These surveys have found significant correlations between early atherosclerotic changes, identified at autopsy of children and young adults, and both total and low-density lipoprotein LDL cholesterol levels.

Although there are no data directly linking cholesterol levels in children with adult heart disease, most of the evidence suggests that such an association exists. Children at risk for the development of premature atherosclerosis in adulthood (those with elevated cholesterol levels) should be identified early in life to try to reduce the associated risk of heart disease. There is a consensus that children with cholesterol levels greater than the 75th percentile should be considered hypercholesterolemic and potentially at risk for adult heart disease. Although many experts agree that hypertriglyceridemia is also a risk factor for premature CHD, the risk is less well defined than the risk associated with hypercholesterolemia.

CLINICAL TRIALS OF CHOLESTEROL REDUCTION. Multiple trials in adults have been performed to assess the impact of cholesterol reduction on a quantitative measure of atherosclerotic disease or on clinical cardiovascular events. A number of trials have been performed to test whether treatment to lower cholesterol would influence the course of angiographic coronary disease. These trials have demonstrated that cholesterol reduction resulted in reduced angiographic progression of coronary disease and even modest regression in some cases. The angiographic differences between treated and control groups has generally been small and by themselves of uncertain clinical significance. However, the reductions in clinical cardiovascular events in the treated groups in many of these studies were surprising and disproportionate to the modest differences in measurable atherosclerosis.

Several secondary prevention trials in adults with clinical

end points have been performed and have confirmed that cholesterol reduction in the setting of established coronary disease is highly effective in reducing cardiovascular events and total mortality. These trials have used a wide variety of interventions, including diet, niacin, bile acid sequestrants, partial ileal bypass surgery, and 3-hydroxy-3-methylglutaryl-coenzyme A (HMG CoA) reductase inhibitors (statins). Two trials with statins enrolled coronary artery disease patients with average cholesterol levels and also demonstrated significant benefit.

Primary prevention of CHD is important, as approximately one quarter to one third of first myocardial infarctions result in death. The issue of drug therapy in primary prevention has been more controversial. The Oslo study, which focused on diet intervention and smoking cessation, demonstrated a 47% decrease in fatal and nonfatal myocardial infarction. Three primary prevention trials using different lipid-lowering drugs (clofibrate, cholestyramine, and gemfibrozil) produced mixed results, generally lowering CHD mortality, but not overall mortality. Subsequently, the West of Scotland Coronary Prevention Trial demonstrated the effectiveness of cholesterol reduction with pravastatin in lowering nonfatal myocardial infarctions, CHD mortality, and overall mortality. This trial clearly established that drug therapy for hypercholesterolemia is safe and effective in relatively high-risk adult men who did not have prior evidence of CHD.

PLASMA LIPOPROTEIN METABOLISM AND TRANSPORT

Cholesterol and triglycerides are transported in the circulation in macromolecular complexes termed *lipoproteins;* the protein components of the complexes are called *apolipoproteins.* Dietary lipoproteins (chylomicrons) are formed in and secreted by the small intestine; other lipoproteins (very low density lipoproteins, VLDL) are synthesized in the liver; still others (high-density lipoproteins, HDL) are secreted as nascent particles by the liver and small intestine, and reach their mature form in the circulation only after exchange of components with other circulating lipoproteins or with tissues.

TRANSPORT OF EXOGENOUS (DIETARY) LIPIDS. After ingestion of a fat-containing meal and hydrolysis of esterified lipids by intestinal and pancreatic lipases, free fatty acids and cholesterol are re-esterified in the intestinal epithelium to form triglycerides and cholesteryl esters, respectively. These lipids are then packaged together with phospholipids, free cholesterol, and the apolipoproteins apoA-I, apo A-IV, and apoB-48 to form chylomicrons (Fig. 83–5). The chylomicrons are then secreted into the intestinal lymph and pass through the thoracic duct into the peripheral circulation. In the circulation, chylomicrons acquire additional apolipoproteins, mainly apoE and several forms of apoC. Triglycerides, which constitute most of the chylomicron mass, are hydrolyzed by lipoprotein lipase at the capillary endothelium; apoC-II is a required cofactor for lipoprotein lipase. The free fatty acid products of this hydrolysis are transferred primarily to adipose tissue for storage as triglycerides or to muscle tissue for β-oxidation. The lipoprotein particles, now smaller and more dense because they have lost much of their triglyceride content, are called *chylomicron remnants.* They have retained most of their cholesteryl ester content, have transferred some of their apolipoproteins (apoCs and apoA-I) to HDL, and have become enriched with respect to their apoE content. These remnants are bound and internalized in part via hepatic membrane receptors specific for apoE on the particles. By this mechanism, dietary cholesterol is delivered to the liver, where it plays a role in the regulation of hepatic cholesterol metabolism. Under normal circumstances, chylomicrons and their remnants are very short-lived in the circulation; following a 12-hr fast, there are no chylomicrons or chylomicron remnants remaining in the plasma.

TRANSPORT OF ENDOGENOUS LIPIDS FROM THE LIVER. The liver secretes a class of lipoproteins called very low density lipoproteins, which contain free and esterified cholesterol, triglycerides, phospholipids, and several apolipoproteins, notably apoB-100, apoCs, and apoE. Like chylomicrons, VLDLs exchange apolipoproteins with other circulating particles and deliver free fatty acids to adipose tissue and muscle after hydrolysis of triglycerides by lipoprotein lipase (Fig. 83–6). In the process, they become smaller and more dense and are termed *VLDL remnants* or *intermediate density lipoproteins* (IDL). Some of these remnant particles are taken up via hepatic receptors specific for apoE, whereas some undergo conversion to LDLs. Conversion of LDL particles requires participation of hepatic lipase, which hydrolyzes the remaining triglycerides, as well as some phospholipids. LDL is almost entirely made up of cholesteryl esters and apoB-100. A specific LDL receptor is present on most cell membranes and recognizes, binds, and internalizes LDL. By this mechanism, LDL particles can deliver cholesterol to extrahepatic tissues for use in membrane or steroid hormone synthesis. LDL receptor expression by the liver is a major regulator of plasma LDL cholesterol levels. LDL particles have a half-life of 3–4 days.

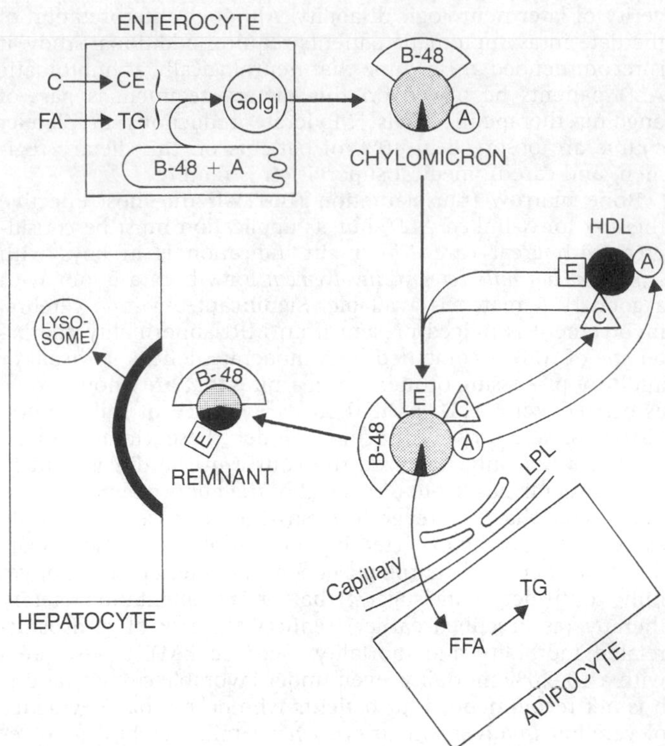

Figure 83–5 Pathway of chylomicron metabolism in human plasma. Fatty acids (FA) and cholesterol (C) are esterified in the intestinal mucosa to form triglycerides (TG) and cholesteryl esters (CE), respectively. They combine with apoA and apoB-48 to form chylomicrons, which are secreted into the circulation: TG *(shaded area)* and CE *(black area).* Chylomicrons undergo lipolysis in the capillary endothelium near adipose tissue and muscle tissue, losing TG via lipoprotein lipase (LPL), gaining apoE from HDL, and losing apoA and apoC to HDL. The resultant chylomicron remnants are taken up by hepatic apoE receptors for degradation by lysosomes. (Adapted from Havel RJ: Approach to the patient with hyperlipidemia. Med Clin North Am 66:319, 1982.)

HIGH-DENSITY LIPOPROTEIN AND REVERSE CHOLESTEROL TRANSPORT. In contrast to chylomicrons and VLDL, which are secreted into the circulation as mature particles, HDL is secreted by the liver and small intestine as nascent discoidal particles composed primarily of phospholipids and apolipoproteins. Nascent HDLs secreted by the small intestine are rich in apoA-I and apoA-IV, whereas those derived from the liver contain predominantly

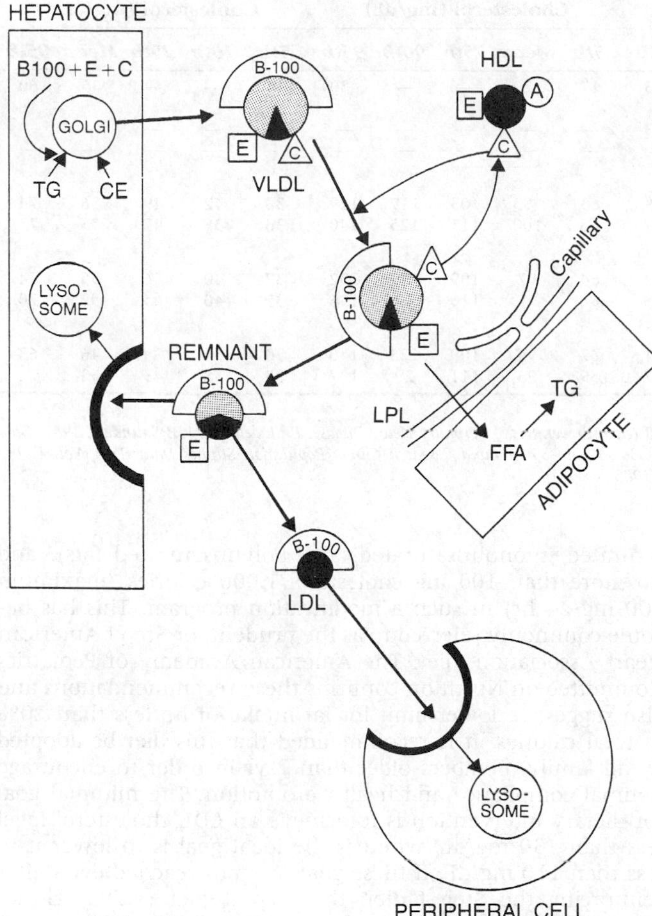

Figure 83–6 Pathways of VLDL and LDL metabolism in human plasma. Triglycerides (TG) and cholesteryl esters (CE) are combined with apoB-100, apoC, and apoE in the liver and then secreted as VLDL, TG *(shaded area),* and CE *(black area).* VLDL undergo lipolysis in the capillary endothelium near adipose tissue and muscle tissue, losing TG via lipoprotein lipase (LPL). The resulting VLDL remnants are either converted to low-density lipoproteins (LDL) for transport to peripheral cells via LDL receptor-mediated uptake or are taken up by hepatic receptors. FFA = free fatty acids. (Adapted from Havel RJ: Approach to the patient with hyperlipidemia. Med Clin North Am 66:319, 1982.)

apoA-I, and apoA-II. HDL particles accept unesterified cholesterol from tissues; this cholesterol is esterified by the enzyme lecithin:cholesterol acyltransferase, which is present on HDL. Cholesteryl esters are either transported in the core of HDL back to the liver or transferred by the cholesteryl ester transfer protein to VLDL and LDL. This process provides a way for returning tissue-derived cholesterol to the liver and has been termed *reverse cholesterol transport.* The liver converts cholesterol to bile acids that are subsequently excreted or directly excretes cholesterol in bile.

PLASMA LIPID AND LIPOPROTEIN LEVELS

Table 83–5 presents normal plasma cholesterol and triglyceride levels from birth through the first 2 decades of life. During the first few months of life, cholesterol levels increase largely because of changes in LDL. Over the next 15–20 yr, in both males and females, there is little change in the total cholesterol level; the mean value fluctuates around 150–165 mg/dL. Mean LDL cholesterol levels remain slightly less than 100 mg/dL in both males and females during this period. HDL cholesterol levels are comparable in males and females early in life; they remain essentially constant in females but decline markedly in males during the 2nd decade to a level that is maintained through adulthood. Plasma triglyceride levels, in contrast, rise transiently in both males and females in the 1st year, fall to a mean of 50–60 mg/dL in the ensuing few years, and then rise to a mean of approximately 75 mg/dL by age 20 yr. In early adulthood, there is a rise in plasma cholesterol that is almost exclusively due to an increase in LDL cholesterol. The rate of increase over the next 30 yr is greater in males than in females. When coupled with their lower HDL cholesterol levels, this puts men at much greater risk than women for atherosclerotic heart disease, at least through menopause. Because of the changes in lipid levels with age, it is more appropriate to use age- and gender-specific percentile figures when comparing levels between individuals and over long periods rather than consider absolute cholesterol levels.

Cholesterol levels track over time. Thus, children with high cholesterol levels tend to have higher levels as young adults, whereas those with low levels as children tend to have lower levels as adults. However, tracking is not perfect. A significant degree of biologic and laboratory variation in cholesterol measurements contributes to this. Lifestyle changes of participants (weight loss, changes in diet) in longitudinal surveys of cholesterol levels in children and young adults may also have contributed to the lower observed degree of tracking. Surveys in adults have described a decline in the prevalence of hypercholesterolemia, presumably related to a decreasing intake of fat in the diet. As similar diet trends have been observed in children, a similar shift in the distribution of cholesterol levels may be occurring among them.

Children may have moderately raised cholesterol levels for a variety of reasons. Some primary genetic defects may be associated with only mild alterations in blood lipid levels. Furthermore, there are secondary causes of hyperlipoproteinemia (HLP) (other disease states) that need to be considered. Finally, inappropriate dietary habits, by themselves or by interacting with any of the preceding factors, can contribute to moderately raised cholesterol levels. Although some children suffer from well-defined familial hyperlipidemia, the majority of individuals with hyperlipidemia do not have such specific syndromes. In addition, although those with hyperlipidemia are at increased risk for heart disease, not all hyperlipidemic individuals acquire clinical heart disease.

SCREENING FOR HYPERCHOLESTEROLEMIA

The Expert Panel on Blood Cholesterol Levels in Children and Adolescents of the National Cholesterol Education Program and the American Academy of Pediatrics Committee on Nutrition have recommended that children with a parental history of elevated total cholesterol levels (>240 mg/dL) should have their total cholesterol level measured. Children with incomplete or unavailable family histories, or those with other risk factors for CHD, should be screened at the discretion of the pediatric care provider. Cholesterol measurements have been shown to be relatively unreliable when undertaken in settings without adequate quality assurance. To avoid inaccurately labeling children as hypercholesterolemic, screening should be completed using only reliable laboratories and methods.

Children with total cholesterol levels less than 170 mg/dL require no intervention other than that recommended for the general population and should be re-evaluated in 5 yr. Children whose total cholesterol level is greater than 200 mg/dL should have a fasting lipid profile performed. Those with borderline levels (170–199 mg/dL) should have another total cholesterol measurement, and the two values should be averaged; if the average total cholesterol level in these two determinations is greater than 170 mg/dL, a lipid profile is recom-

TABLE 83–5 Plasma Cholesterol and Triglyceride Levels in Childhood and Adolescence: Means and Percentiles

	Total Triglyceride (mg/dL)					Total Cholesterol (mg/dL)					Low-Density Lipoprotein Cholesterol (mg/dL)					High-Density Lipoprotein Cholesterol (mg/dL)*				
	5th	*Mean*	*75th*	*90th*	*95th*	*5th*	*Mean*	*75th*	*90th*	*95th*	*5th*	*Mean*	*75th*	*90th*	*95th*	*5th*	*10th*	*25th*	*Mean*	*95th*
Cord	14	34	—	—	84	42	68	—	—	103	17	29	—	—	50	13	—	—	35	60
1–4 yr																				
Male	29	56	68	85	99	114	155	170	190	203	—	—	—	—	—	—	—	—	—	—
Female	34	64	74	95	112	112	156	173	188	200	—	—	—	—	—	—	—	—	—	—
5–9 yr																				
Male	28	52	58	70	85	125	155	168	183	189	63	93	103	117	129	38	42	49	56	74
Female	32	64	74	103	126	131	164	176	190	197	68	100	115	125	140	36	38	47	53	73
10–14 yr																				
Male	33	63	74	94	111	124	160	173	188	202	64	97	109	122	132	37	40	46	55	74
Female	39	72	85	104	120	125	160	171	191	205	68	97	110	126	136	37	40	45	52	70
15–19 yr																				
Male	38	78	88	125	143	118	153	168	183	191	62	94	109	123	130	30	34	39	46	63
Female	36	73	85	112	126	118	159	176	198	207	59	96	111	29	137	35	38	43	52	74

*Note that different percentiles are listed for HDL cholesterol.

Data for cord blood from Strong W: Atherosclerosis: Its pediatric roots. In: *Kaplan N, Stamler J (eds): Prevention of Coronary Heart Disease. Philadelphia, WB Saunders, 1983. Data for children 1–4 yr from Tables 6, 7, 20, and 21, and all other data from Tables 24, 25, 32, 33, 36, and 37 in Lipid Research Clinics Population Studies Data Book, Vol. 1, The prevalence study. NIH Publication No. 80–1527. Washington, DC, National Institutes of Health, 1980.*

mended. The expert panel has likewise recommended that children with a family history of premature coronary heart disease (before the age of 55 yr in a parent or grandparent) should have a lipid profile completed. Lipid profiles of parents and other 1st-degree relatives are necessary to establish whether there is a dominantly inherited defect responsible for the hypercholesterolemia.

A lipid profile (total and HDL cholesterol, triglycerides, calculated LDL cholesterol) is obtained after a 12-hr fast. LDL cholesterol is calculated using the following equation:

$$\text{LDL cholesterol} = \text{total cholesterol} - [\text{HDL cholesterol} + (\text{triglycerides}/5)]$$

Triglycerides must be less than 400 mg/dL to derive an accurate estimate of LDL cholesterol with this method. The average value from two evaluations is recommended because of the biologic and laboratory variability in lipid values. Children with average LDL cholesterol levels greater than 130 mg/dL are considered to have elevated levels, whereas LDL cholesterol levels less than 110 mg/dL are considered acceptable. Levels between 110 and 130 mg/dL are borderline.

These recommendations have been criticized for several reasons. The screening algorithm is complicated to follow for the busy practitioner. Multiple surveys have shown that screening only those with a positive family history misses half or more of the hypercholesterolemic children. This problem is compounded by the fact that many adults do not know their cholesterol levels, as well as the difficulties in obtaining a complete family history. In addition, many parents who may be at risk for CHD are too young to have acquired clinical heart disease while their children are being evaluated; hence their children may not be identified as being at risk.

Those children with *triglyceride* levels greater than the 95th percentile should be scrutinized further. Although elevated triglyceride levels per se may not represent an independent risk factor for premature cardiovascular disease, triglyceride levels greater than the 95th percentile can be a marker of some genetic forms of hyperlipidemia, even if the total cholesterol level is normal.

TREATMENT OF HYPERLIPIDEMIA

DIETARY MANAGEMENT OF HYPERLIPIDEMIA. For hypercholesterolemic children (average LDL cholesterol >110 mg/dL) older than 2 yr, dietary modification is the best initial intervention. Their daily food intake should provide no more than 30% of total calories as fat (approximately equally distributed among saturated, monounsaturated, and polyunsaturated fats), and no more than 100 mg cholesterol/1,000 calories (maximum 300 mg/24 hr) in such a modification program. This has become commonly referred to as the prudent, or Step I American Heart Association, diet. The American Academy of Pediatrics Committee on Nutrition confirms these recommendations and also suggests a lower limit for fat intake of no less than 20% of total calories. It is recommended that this diet be adopted by all family members older than 2 yr in order to encourage optimal compliance and health promotion. The minimal goal for dietary intervention is to achieve an LDL cholesterol level less than 130 mg/dL, whereas the ideal goal is to lower it to less than 110 mg/dL. If these goals are not reached even after reinforcing the Step I diet, the Step II diet (<7% calories as saturated fat and <66 mg cholesterol/1,000 calories to a maximum of 200 mg/24 hr) should be considered.

When recommending dietary intervention, it is important to explain that the response to dietary management is variable and generally does not lower LDL cholesterol levels by more than 10–15%. Individuals commonly have unrealistic expectations about the cholesterol lowering associated with dietary management, which limits their compliance when the response is modest. Even if the initial response to dietary therapy is limited, the potential for adopting a lifelong healthy style of eating should have long-term benefit.

Dietary modification is safe in the treatment of hyperlipidemia in adults and children older than the age of 2 yr. The Dietary Intervention Study for Children demonstrated the safety and efficacy of a low-fat diet for hypercholesterolemic children. However, it must be emphasized that these recommendations are meant only for children older than 2 yr. Children younger than this placed on a similar or more restrictive diet, and older children placed on more restrictive diets by well-meaning caregivers, have demonstrated poor growth. Children younger than 2 yr require a relatively large amount of calories to maintain their rapid growth. Because of the higher caloric density of high-fat food, it is physically difficult for children less than 2 yr to eat enough low-fat food to ensure normal growth. Furthermore, the higher fat intake may be necessary to help ensure an adequate supply of appropriate nutrients for the rapidly developing central nervous system.

There should be proper supervision to ensure the appropriateness of any dietary modification in children. As most pediatricians are unable to provide detailed guidance for such dietary modifications, referral to a trained pediatric dietitian is indicated. Prior to undertaking a screening program, the physician should ensure the availability of such referral for his or her patients. The growth and development of any child undergoing dietary intervention should be monitored, and a specific dietary evaluation should be completed if growth or development is altered. It is also important to explain to the child and family that hypercholesterolemia in childhood is only a risk factor and not an illness. Emphasis should be placed on the positive changes the child and the family can make to minimize the risk.

OTHER DIETARY FACTORS. Dietary fiber, especially soluble fiber, has a modest cholesterol-lowering effect in hypercholesterolemic individuals. However, high-fiber diets must be used with care in children to ensure adequate delivery of calories and nutrients. Monounsaturated fats lower LDL cholesterol levels while maintaining or even raising HDL cholesterol levels, in contrast to the lowering of LDL and HDL cholesterol levels commonly observed with a high polyunsaturated fat diet. Trans-fatty acids (partially hydrogenated vegetable oils), commonly found in processed foods and margarine, seem to raise LDL cholesterol levels. Vegetarian diets have a large and significant cholesterol-lowering effect associated with the substitution of vegetable protein for animal protein and the low fat and cholesterol content of the diet. Although many groups have demonstrated the safety of vegetarian diets for children, care must be taken to ensure the completeness of the diet for the growing child. Although fish oil and antioxidants have little, if any, effect on cholesterol levels, they have been reported to reduce the risk of CHD by other mechanisms. (Fish oil is also used as a treatment for severe hypertriglyceridemia.) However, as these compounds are frequently administered in pharmacologic doses, in the absence of additional experience, their use in children should be discouraged. Dietary modification that increases intake of these nutrients can be considered. For example, encouraging appropriate fruit and vegetable intake will help optimize natural sources of antioxidants.

OTHER FACTORS RELATING TO TREATMENT. Medical management of hypercholesterolemia should be viewed in the context of other lifestyle factors and conditions associated with risk for premature CHD, such as lack of exercise and physical activity and excessive sedentary activity, cigarette smoking, hypertension, obesity, and diabetes. These should be evaluated, controlled, minimized, or eliminated as possible and appropriate. Children already having one risk factor for premature coronary heart disease, such as hyperlipidemia, should be actively treated to minimize any other risk factors. In addition, many of these risk factors are interlinked, and therefore minimizing one may help to ameliorate others (increasing exercise may decrease obesity, which helps to lower blood pressure, LDL cholesterol, and triglyceride levels and, potentially, the risk for non–insulin-dependent diabetes mellitus, while also helping raise HDL cholesterol levels).

DRUG THERAPY. The Expert Panel on Treatment of Hyperlipidemia in Children recommended that drug therapy be considered in children aged 10 yr and older if, after an adequate trial (6 mo–1 yr) of diet therapy:

1. LDL cholesterol remains greater than 190 mg/dL.
2. LDL cholesterol remains greater than 160 mg/dL and
   (a) there is a positive family history of premature CHD (before 55 yr of age), or
   (b) two or more other risk factors are present in the child or adolescent after vigorous attempts have been made to control these risk factors (diabetes, hypertension, smoking, low HDL cholesterol, severe obesity, physical inactivity). It should be noted that the Adult Treatment Panel II of the National Cholesterol Education Program recommended in 1993 that drug therapy could be reasonably deferred in very low risk young adults if the LDL cholesterol level is less than 220 mg/dL. Therefore, it would be reasonable, in the absence of other major risk factors, to defer drug therapy in children unless the LDL cholesterol exceeds 220 mg/dL. This issue is a topic of considerable debate.

Bile acid sequestrants or "resins" (cholestyramine or colestipol) are generally the first-line pediatric drugs for the treatment of hypercholesterolemia in children. Bile acid sequestrants primarily reduce LDL cholesterol and should not be prescribed for patients with triglyceride levels greater than 300 mg/dL because they exacerbate hypertriglyceridemia. These nonabsorbable compounds interrupt the enterohepatic bile acid cycle by the binding of bile acids in the intestine and enhancing their excretion in the stool. This results in shunting of hepatic cholesterol into bile acid synthesis and secondary upregulation of hepatic LDL receptors. As a result, there is increased uptake of LDL from the blood and reduction of LDL cholesterol levels. A 10–32% decrease in LDL cholesterol levels has been reported with cholestyramine therapy in children with familial hypercholesterolemia and familial combined hyperlipidemia (FCHL). However, reported long-term compliance has been poor and related to poor palatability of the medication and gastrointestinal disturbances, including nausea, bloating, and constipation. One packet or scoop contains 4 g of cholestyramine and 5 g of colestipol. The dose is titrated to the severity of hypercholesterolemia and tolerance of the side effects. Generally, resins are started at a dose of one-half packet or scoop twice a day before meals, and the dose is gradually increased over weeks as tolerated and necessary. Doses of three packets or scoops twice a day can be tolerated in some individuals. Colestipol is also available in tablets containing 1 g, but the large size of the tablets may limit their use in children.

The bile acid sequestrants are safe drugs that are not systemically absorbed. However, they are insoluble resins that must be suspended in liquid and are therefore often inconvenient and unpleasant to take. (Colestipol tablets may be preferred by some patients for this reason). In addition, bile acid sequestrants may bind some other drugs (digoxin, warfarin) and interfere with their absorption, creating the need to take other medications 1 hr before or 4 hr after the bile acid sequestrants. Similarly, these resins may interfere with the absorption of fat-soluble vitamins, suggesting the need for multivitamin supplements.

HMG-CoA reductase inhibitors (statins), although not approved for use in children, have been used in children with severe hypercholesterolemia who cannot tolerate or have inadequate response to bile acid sequestrants. HMG-CoA reductase is the rate-limiting step in cholesterol biosynthesis, and inhibition of this enzyme decreases cholesterol synthesis and results in upregulation of hepatic LDL receptors. The Canadian Lovastatin in Children Study demonstrated a 21–36% decrease (dose response–related) in LDL-cholesterol level in boys with familial hypercholesterolemia treated with 10–40 mg/day lovastatin. No serious side effects were noted over the 8-wk follow-up period.

Potential side effects of statins include gastrointestinal upset, headaches, sleep disturbance, fatigue, and muscle or joint pains. Severe myopathy and even rhabdomyolysis have been rarely reported with some HMG-CoA reductase inhibitors in adults. The risk of severe myopathy may be increased in patients taking certain other drugs such as erythromycin, antifungal agents, immunosuppressive agents, and fibric acid derivatives such as gemfibrozil, and niacin. Liver transaminases should be monitored in patients taking statins, but significant (>3 times normal) elevation in transaminase levels is rare in children. However, because the long-term effects of statins remain uncertain, the risk-benefit of using them in children should be carefully considered. They should be used carefully if at all in girls at risk of pregnancy because of the uncertainty of teratogenic defects. Nicotinic acid is also frequently used in adults; however, its side effects (flushing, gastrointestinal upset, hepatic toxicity) may preclude its use in children. The practicing pediatrician should consider referral of all children who may be candidates for drug therapy to a specialized lipid center.

Although drug therapy is used commonly to treat *hypertriglyceridemia* in adults, it is used much less commonly in children. The mainstay of therapy in children with hypertriglyceridemia is diet, exercise, and weight loss. In severe cases of hypertriglyceridemia in children with attendant medical complications, a careful risk-benefit analysis considering the use of medication should be completed by a lipid expert. There are no formal recommendations concerning the treatment of hypertriglyceridemia in children.

Safety Considerations. Dietary intervention must be appropriately supervised to ensure that a complete and balanced diet is provided or available to the affected child. In addition, the potential adverse psychosocial influence of being "labeled" should be considered. Children with heterozygous familial hypercholesterolemia (FH) attending a lipid clinic demonstrated no higher prevalence of psychosocial dysfunction, which could be potentially related to their being labeled "at-risk," than control children. Furthermore, in one cholesterol screening program, the parents of hypercholesterolemic children reported better diets and improved perceptions of the children's health 1 yr after cholesterol screening was completed. This may be an effect of the families' active participation in reducing risk and improving health.

Of some concern are the reports in adults linking low or lowered cholesterol levels with depression, violent tendencies, accidents, and noncardiac illnesses, including some forms of cancer. These reports do not consistently demonstrate the same associations, and other surveys present conflicting data (those reporting an association between high-fat diets and some forms of cancer). In addition, many of the cholesterol-lowering interventions use diet or drugs, or both, and thus negative consequences may be related to the medication. However, the decreased overall mortality reported in recently completed cholesterol lowering trials using HMG-CoA reductase inhibitors support the overall safety and efficacy of lowering cholesterol. Data from other countries, in which mean cholesterol levels are lower than those in the United States, do not support higher overall mortality related to lower cholesterol levels.

SECONDARY HYPERLIPIDEMIAS. Most of the hypertriglyceridemia and hypercholesterolemia seen in clinical practice in children is secondary, at least in part, to exogenous factors or underlying clinical disorders. Obesity, for example, is a major cause of mild elevations of plasma triglycerides, and the hypertriglyceridemia is frequently normalized following a return to desirable weight. Weight loss may also reduce cholesterol levels in overweight individuals.

Pediatric conditions associated with hyperlipidemia include hypothyroidism, diabetes mellitus, nephrotic syndrome, renal failure, storage diseases (glycogen storage disease, Tay-Sachs disease, Niemann-Pick disease [NPD]), congenital biliary atresia and other causes of cholestasis, hepatitis, anorexia nervosa, and systemic lupus erythematosus. Excessive alcohol intake is a well-known cause of hypertriglyceridemia in adults and should be considered in teenagers. Oral contraceptives generally increase triglyceride levels, with varying effects on LDL and HDL cholesterol levels. Other drugs that raise triglyceride levels are 13-*cis*-retinoic acid (isotretinoin or Accutane), thiazide diuretics, and some β-adrenergic blocking agents. Treatment of the underlying condition or removal of the offending drug is usually the first approach to management of the patient with secondary hyperlipidemia. If the elevated lipid levels persist, however, consideration must be given to the possibility that the patient has an underlying primary form of HLP, and therapy appropriate to that condition should be initiated.

PRIMARY (GENETIC) DYSLIPIDEMIAS

One third of patients with their first myocardial infarction before the age of 50 yr in men and 60 yr in women have HLP; about one half of cases are due to an inherited disorder of lipoprotein metabolism. The Frederickson and Levy classification is useful as a guide to accurate diagnosis and effective treatment and is based on the type of lipoprotein that is elevated. For example, in type I, chylomicrons are increased; type IIa implies elevation of LDL; type IV, elevation of VLDL; type IIb, elevation of both LDL and VLDL; type III, elevation of chylomicron and VLDL remnants; and type V, elevation of VLDL and chylomicrons. These descriptive classifications do not imply specific genetic etiology; furthermore, as knowledge about the molecular basis of specific genetic defects in lipoprotein metabolism has grown, the classification has become less useful and may contribute to misunderstanding. Therefore, it seems prudent not to continue its use in most cases; however, because it is still quite prevalent in the literature, physicians need to be aware of the classification.

Disorders Associated with Hypercholesterolemia and Normal Triglycerides (<100 mg/dL)

Elevated cholesterol in the absence of elevated triglycerides generally indicates an elevation in LDL without a concomitant elevation in chylomicrons or VLDL. The LDL receptor plays a major role in regulating the plasma LDL cholesterol levels, and therefore the two major inherited causes of elevated LDL cholesterol both involve the LDL receptor pathway: mutations in the LDL receptor (FH) or in the receptor-binding region of apoB (familial defective apoB).

Familial Hypercholesterolemia. FH is caused by mutations in the LDL receptor, which prevent its synthesis, reduce its appearance on the cell surface, or impair its ability to bind and internalize LDL. Elevated LDL cholesterol levels lead to the major complication of this condition: premature atherosclerotic cardiovascular disease. More than 150 different mutations in the LDL receptor have been described. There are five classes of mutations (null, transport defective, binding defective, internalization defective, and recycling defective) that impair the receptor-mediated uptake of LDL from the circulation (see Fig. 83–6). FH is an autosomal codominant disorder, meaning that heterozygotes have hypercholesterolemia but homozygotes have even more severe hypercholesterolemia. One mutant LDL receptor allele results in the production of only about half of the normal number of LDL receptors, whereas two mutant alleles severely reduce or eliminate functional LDL receptors. Heterozygous and homozygous FH differ clinically in a number of important respects.

Heterozygous Familial Hypercholesterolemia. Heterozygous FH occurs in approximately 1/500 persons worldwide, making it one of the most common single gene disorders. It is characterized by elevated total and LDL cholesterol levels with normal triglycerides and a family history of hypercholesterolemia or premature cardiovascular disease. The finding of tendon xanthomas is virtually diagnostic of FH, although absence of xanthomas does not exclude the diagnosis, especially in children with heterozygous FH in whom xanthomas are rare. Tendon xanthomas are easily recognized on the Achilles tendons, where they cause thickening and irregularity. In fact, any child with suspected Achilles tendon xanthomas should have cholesterol screening to rule out FH. Another common location for tendon xanthomas is the digit extensor tendons on the dorsum of the hands. Premature corneal arcus is frequently seen in adults with heterozygous FH. Secondary causes, especially hypothyroidism and obstructive liver disease, should be excluded. There is currently no definitive diagnostic test for heterozygous FH, which is diagnosed on clinical grounds.

Heterozygous FH is strongly associated with premature atherosclerotic cardiovascular disease, especially CHD. Therefore, children with heterozygous FH should be identified and treated to lower the LDL cholesterol and reduce the long-term risk of atherosclerotic CHD. *Treatment* should be initiated with a Step I diet, and followed by the Step II diet if needed. Dietary therapy can help reduce the LDL cholesterol but rarely normalizes it. Thus most heterozygous FH patients eventually require lipid-lowering drug therapy.

Homozygous Familial Hypercholesterolemia. Homozygous FH is caused by the inheritance of two mutant LDL receptor alleles that result in the production of little or no LDL receptors and a severe defect in the catabolism of LDL. Homozygous FH occurs in approximately 1/1 million persons worldwide and is a much more severe clinical disorder than heterozygous FH. Patients with homozygous FH are often classified into one of two groups based on the LDL cholesterol level and the amount of LDL receptor activity measured in their skin fibroblasts. "Receptor-negative" patients have less than 2% of normal LDL receptor activity and higher LDL cholesterol levels, whereas "receptor-defective" patients have 2–25% of normal LDL receptor activity and not as high LDL cholesterol levels. Receptor-defective patients have a better prognosis than do receptor-negative patients and sometimes have small responses to drug therapy. The clinical heterogeneity among homozygous FH patients is due to the significant genetic heterogeneity of the LDL receptor gene mutations.

Patients with homozygous FH often present in childhood with cutaneous xanthomas on the hands, wrists, elbows, knees, heels, or buttocks. Some patients with homozygous FH do not have cutaneous xanthomas but acquire tuberous or tendon xanthomas on the elbows, knees, or Achilles tendons as older children or adolescents. The absence of xanthomas in children does not exclude the diagnosis. Arcus cornea may be present to some degree. Total cholesterol levels are usually greater than 500 mg/dL and can be as high as 1200 mg/dL. The major complication of homozygous FH is accelerated atherosclerosis, which can result in clinical sequelae even in childhood. Homozygous FH children often have symptoms of vascular disease before puberty, but symptoms can be atypical or go unreported and sudden death is common. Untreated receptor-negative homozygous FH patients rarely survive beyond the 2nd decade; receptor-defective patients have a better prognosis but invariably experience clinical atherosclerotic vascular disease by age 30 and often much sooner.

A child with severe hypercholesterolemia greater than 500 mg/dL with relatively normal triglycerides or with cutaneous or tendon xanthomas, or both, should be suspected of having homozygous FH. The biologic parents and other relatives should be tested for hypercholesterolemia. Obstructive liver disease should be excluded by appropriate tests. The *diagnosis* is made on clinical grounds but can be confirmed in specialized centers by obtaining a skin biopsy specimen and performing an assay of the LDL receptor activity on the skin fibroblasts. Patients with suspected homozygous FH should be referred to a specialized center.

An attempt should be made to try drug therapy using a statin drug plus a bile acid sequestrant. Atorvastatin has been reported to have greater efficacy in homozygous FH than other statins and should be considered. Liver transplantation is effective in decreasing LDL cholesterol levels but is associated with the substantial risks of surgery and long-term immunosuppression. The current *treatment* of choice for homozygous FH is LDL apheresis, which can promote regression of xanthomas and retard progression of atherosclerosis. The age at which LDL apheresis should be initiated is uncertain. Venous access is often problematic in young children, and central catheters are prone to infections, which are especially risky given the frequent aortic valvular and supravalvular flow disturbances. It is generally recommended that initiation of LDL apheresis be delayed until approximately 5 yr of age except when evidence of atherosclerotic vascular disease is present.

Homozygous FH is a model for the development of somatic liver-directed gene therapy because of its serious consequences and poor options for treatment. Five patients with homozygous FH were treated in a gene therapy protocol involving ex vivo gene transfer of the LDL receptor gene into autologous hepatocytes with subsequent reimplantation. At 4 mo, all patients had evidence of LDL receptor transgene expression by liver biopsy. LDL cholesterol levels were decreased in two patients by 17% and 22%, but LDL cholesterol levels in the other three patients were essentially unchanged.

FAMILIAL DEFECTIVE APOLIPOPROTEIN B-100. Familial defective apoB-100 (FDB) is characterized by elevated LDL cholesterol with normal triglycerides, possible tendon xanthomas, and increased risk of premature atherosclerotic cardiovascular disease. Clinically, it resembles heterozygous FH. In contrast to FH, FDB is caused by mutations in the receptor binding region of apoB-100, the ligand for the LDL receptor, which impairs its binding and delays the clearance of LDL from the blood. The most common mutation causing FDB is a substitution of glutamine for arginine at position 3500 in apoB-100. Other mutations have been reported that have a similar effect on apoB binding to the LDL receptor. FDB is a dominantly inherited disorder and occurs in approximately 1/700 persons in Europe and North America. The apoB mutation can be detected in specialized laboratories to make a specific diagnosis. Currently there is no compelling reason to make a specific molecular diagnosis because the clinical management of patients with FDB is similar to that of patients with heterozygous FH.

POLYGENIC HYPERCHOLESTEROLEMIA. Most forms of hypercholesterolemia are not single gene disorders but rather due to a complex interaction of several genetic and environmental factors. For example, genetic differences in cholesterol absorption, cholesterol synthesis, or rates of bile acid synthesis may result in very different cholesterol levels in individuals challenged with a fat-rich diet. Polygenic hypercholesterolemia is characterized by an elevated cholesterol level with triglyceride levels that are usually relatively normal. In polygenic hypercholesterolemia, LDL cholesterol levels usually are not as elevated as they are in heterozygous FH and FDB, and tendon xanthomas are not observed. Only about 7% of 1st-degree relatives of patients with polygenic hypercholesterolemia are hypercholesterolemic, whereas about half of relatives with FCHL, heterozygous FH, and FDB have dyslipidemia. *Treatment* of polygenic hypercholesterolemia follows the same guidelines as the approach to any patient with hypercholesterolemia.

Disorders Associated with Hypercholesterolemia and Moderately Elevated Triglyceride Levels (100–1,000 mg/dL)

The importance of elevated triglyceride levels in the 100–1,000 mg/dL range is primarily related to their potential association with the risk of the development of atherosclerotic CHD because fasting triglyceride levels less than 1,000 mg/dL are not usually associated with risk of acute pancreatitis. The major primary causes of elevated triglycerides in the 100–1,000 mg/dL range are FCHL, familial dysbetalipoproteinemia (type III hyperlipidemia), and familial hypertriglyceridemia. Of the three, FCHL is most likely to present in childhood. It is important to differentiate among them because familial dysbetalipoproteinemia and FCHL are both definitely associated with increased risk of premature atherosclerosis, whereas familial hypertriglyceridemia is often not associated with a substantially increased risk.

FAMILIAL COMBINED HYPERLIPIDEMIA. FCHL is a common primary lipid disorder, occurring in approximately 1/200 adults. It has been estimated that approximately 20% of patients with CHD younger than 60 yr have a form of FCHL. FCHL is characterized by a mixed dyslipidemia usually associated with moderately elevated fasting triglycerides, moderately elevated cholesterol, and reduced HDL cholesterol. In this dominantly inherited syndrome, 1st-degree relatives on one side of the family frequently have hypertriglyceridemia, hypercholesterolemia, or combined elevations of both cholesterol and triglycerides; there is often a family history of premature CHD as well. The hyperlipidemia tends to be modest, and the lipoprotein abnormalities can change from time to time in the same affected individual. Xanthomas are not generally seen in patients with this disorder. Visceral obesity, glucose intolerance, hyperinsulinemia, hypertension, and hyperuricemia are frequently associated with FCHL but are not required for the diagnosis.

FCHL generally presents in adulthood but can be identified in children. In families with FCHL identified through an affected child, half the siblings less than 20 yr of age have hyperlipidemia, compatible with dominant expression of the trait. A correlation between plasma triglyceride level and age and relative weight in affected children has also been observed, which suggests the gradual expression of hyperlipidemia in some children. Experience at our institution suggests that at least 0.5% of all children have hyperlipidemia due to FCHL.

The molecular basis of FCHL is not known. Studies of lipoprotein metabolism in carefully selected individuals have indicated that overproduction of VLDL or LDL, or both, is a common metabolic basis of this condition. It has been suggested that a subset of patients with the FCHL phenotype may be heterozygous for lipoprotein lipase (LPL) deficiency, but LPL mutations are probably not a common cause of FCHL. A variant allele at a locus influencing apoB levels predicts FCHL in a large proportion of families ascertained through affected children; however, the function of this gene is unknown. There is evidence that FCHL is not linked to the apoB structural locus. It is likely that more than one genetic cause of the FCHL phenotype exists.

The *diagnosis* of FCHL is suggested by the presence of a mixed hyperlipidemia with fasting triglyceride and cholesterol levels both greater than the 90th percentile, especially if accompanied by decreased HDL cholesterol levels and in the absence of secondary causes of hyperlipidemia. The formal diagnosis of FCHL requires the presence of dyslipidemia in at least two 1st-degree relatives. Familial dysbetalipoproteinemia should be excluded with appropriate testing. The finding of an elevated apoB level (usually greater than 130 mg/dL or the 90th percentile for age) suggests increased levels of "small dense LDL" and supports the diagnosis of FCHL. *Hyperapobetalipoproteinemia* has been used to describe the syndrome of elevated apoB with normal lipid levels and is probably a subset of FCHL.

The risk of premature heart disease for persons with FCHL is high despite the fact that lipid levels in affected individuals may be only moderately elevated. Children in these families should therefore be identified, and initial dietary *treatment* should be aimed at controlling the hypercholesterolemia and hypertriglyceridemia using the Step I or Step II diet. Dietary modification in children with FCHL has generally demonstrated a 10–15% reduction in the LDL cholesterol level, although fewer than half of the treated children would be expected to have levels less than 130 mg/dL and even fewer would be expected to have levels of less than 110 mg/dL. When dietary modification alone does not achieve desired results, drug therapy may be considered.

FAMILIAL DYSBETALIPOPROTEINEMIA (TYPE III HYPERLIPOPROTEINEMIA). Patients with familial dysbetalipoproteinemia usually present in adulthood with *clinical manifestations* that include distinctive xanthomas, premature atherosclerosis, or asymptomatic hyperlipidemia discovered on routine screening, although children may present with a "strange rash." Two types of xanthomas can be seen in patients with familial dysbetalipoproteinemia. Tuberoeruptive xanthomas begin as clusters of small papules on the elbows, knees, or buttocks and can grow to the size of small grapes. Palmar xanthoma refers to orange-yellow discoloration in the creases of the palms and wrists. The pattern of hyperlipidemia can be a clue to the diagnosis of familial dysbetalipoproteinemia. Patients generally have both hypertriglyceridemia and hypercholesterolemia and, in contrast to most other lipid disorders, the cholesterol and triglyceride are often elevated to a relatively similar degree. In addition, the HDL cholesterol level is often relatively normal, in contrast to most hypertriglyceridemic conditions in which the HDL cholesterol level is usually reduced. The hyperlipidemia can be relatively mild or severe, depending on the presence of other metabolic conditions and unknown factors.

Familial dysbetalipoproteinemia is caused by mutations in the gene for apolipoprotein E (apoE). ApoE is present on chylomicron and VLDL remnants and mediates their removal from the plasma by binding to receptors in the liver. Defective apoE is impaired in its ability to bind to these receptors, resulting in accumulation of chylomicron and VLDL remnants in the plasma. The most common form of familial dysbetalipoproteinemia is related to a common polymorphism of apoE. The "normal" form of apoE is known as apoE3, but another form, apoE2, has an allele frequency of about 7%. The apoE2 protein, which differs from apoE3 by a single amino acid, does not bind to lipoprotein receptors adequately, resulting in defective removal of chylomicron and VLDL remnants. Homozygosity for the E2 allele (the E2/E2 genotype) is the most common cause of familial dysbetalipoproteinemia. However, most individuals with the apoE2/E2 genotype do not have familial dysbetalipoproteinemia; development of this disorder appears to require an additional factor. Some of these factors may include obesity, diabetes mellitus, hypothyroidism, renal disease, and alcohol use; most children with familial dysbetalipoproteinemia have one of these conditions in addition to the apoE2/E2 genotype. However, many adults with familial dysbetalipoproteinemia do not have an obvious predisposing factor in addition to the E2/E2 genotype. There is another common variant of apoE known as apoE4, which has an allele frequency of approximately 14% and is not associated with familial dysbetalipoproteinemia. Other rare mutations in apoE can also cause familial dysbetalipoproteinemia. These mutations generally result in the synthesis of an apoE protein that is severely defective in its ability to bind to lipoprotein receptors and can result in a more severe hyperlipidemia, which may be more likely to present in childhood. Often the inheritance of only one mutant allele is adequate to cause familial dysbetalipoproteinemia, leading to the term *dominant type III HLP.*

The traditional laboratory approach to *diagnosis* is to use lipoprotein electrophoresis, which demonstrates a broad β-band due to the presence of remnant lipoproteins. A second (and preferred) method is often referred to as a "β quantification" in which plasma is subjected to ultracentrifugation to separate lipoproteins; this is available in specialized laboratories. Because this disorder is associated with increased numbers of VLDL remnants that are enriched in cholesterol relative to triglycerides, an elevated ratio of VLDL cholesterol to triglycerides of greater than 0.3 is confirmatory of the diagnosis. Finally, the apoE2/E2 pattern can be determined by using plasma protein methods (apoE phenotype) or DNA-based methods (apoE genotype). The finding of an apoE2/E2 pattern by phenotyping or genotyping in a patient with suspected familial dysbetalipoproteinemia confirms the diagnosis.

Familial dysbetalipoproteinemia is often sensitive to dietary *treatment.* Weight loss to a level appropriate for height, coupled with institution of the Step I diet, can often cause the lipid levels to return to normal. Discontinuance of alcohol can have a major impact on the dyslipidemia. There is little experience with drug treatment of this disorder in children, but adults with familial dysbetalipoproteinemia whose lipid elevations fail to respond to dietary intervention have been treated with fibric acid derivatives, such as gemfibrozil and fenofibrate, and nicotinic acid. HMG-CoA reductase inhibitors have also been used with success in some patients unable to tolerate fibrates or niacin.

FAMILIAL HYPERTRIGLYCERIDEMIA. Familial hypertriglyceridemia (FHTG) is characterized by moderately elevated triglycerides, usually in the absence of significant hypercholesterolemia. FHTG occurs in approximately 1/500 persons and in contrast to FCHL frequently is not associated with premature CHD. Hypertriglyceridemia is often detected by a routine blood test. Triglyceride levels usually range from 250–1,000 mg/dL with normal to mildly increased cholesterol levels and HDL cholesterol levels that are usually decreased. FHTG is inherited as an autosomal dominant trait but is not usually expressed until adulthood. The molecular *etiology* is unknown. The metabolic basis of this disorder is probably heterogeneous but is likely to be related to impaired catabolism of triglyceride-rich lipoproteins in most patients. However, increased production of VLDL by the liver has been observed in some patients with this phenotype. It is possible that VLDL or chylomicron overproduction, or both, may overload the normal catabolic processes and produce hypertriglyceridemia in some patients. It has been proposed that genetic overproduction of apoC-III could cause this syndrome, but this remains to be proved. Increased dietary fat or simple carbohydrates, a sedentary lifestyle, obesity, insulin resistance, alcohol use, and estrogens can all exacerbate the hypertriglyceridemia.

The *diagnosis* is suggested by elevated triglyceride levels (>90th percentile) with normal or mildly increased cholesterol levels (<90th percentile). Hypertriglyceridemia in at least one 1st-degree relative is useful in making the diagnosis. It is important to consider and rule out secondary causes of the hypertriglyceridemia. In the differential diagnosis, both familial dysbetalipoproteinemia (type III HLP) and FCHL should be considered. Relative to the triglyceride level, the total cholesterol level is usually lower in FHTG compared with familial dysbetalipoproteinemia and FCHL.

Children older than 2 yr can usually be *treated* adequately with weight control and use of the Step I diet. Occasionally, further modification of the carbohydrate to fat ratio may be required. Alcohol use should be discouraged. Diabetes mellitus should be aggressively controlled. Lipid-lowering drug therapy is generally not indicated in children, except in extreme cases. In such circumstances, fish oils may be an alternative to drug therapy, although the long-term safety in children is not known.

HEPATIC LIPASE DEFICIENCY. This is a rare autosomal recessive disorder. Hepatic lipase hydrolyzes triglycerides and phospholipids in VLDL remnants and IDL and promotes their conversion to LDL. Genetic deficiency of hepatic lipase impairs the metabolism of VLDL remnants and IDL and is characterized by a mixed hyperlipidemia and the accumulation of lipoprotein remnants in plasma. Hepatic lipase also metabolizes HDL lipids, so levels of HDL cholesterol are often slightly elevated in hepatic lipase deficiency. The *diagnosis* is suggested by a mixed hyperlipidemia with elevation in both triglyceride and cholesterol levels, but an HDL cholesterol level that is normal or elevated rather than low. Familial dysbetalipoproteinemia should be excluded by apoE phenotyping or genotyping. Measurements of hepatic lipase can be made in postheparin plasma by specialized laboratories. The association of hepatic lipase deficiency with atherosclerosis is uncertain, but patients should be *treated* for their hyperlipidemia using an approach similar to that used for familial dysbetalipoproteinemia. Acquired (usually partial) defects in hepatic lipase can be seen in hypothyroidism, chronic renal insufficiency, and chronic liver disease.

Disorders Associated with Hypercholesterolemia and Severely Elevated Triglycerides (>1,000 mg/dL)

Fasting triglycerides greater than 1,000 mg/dL in children reflect severe hyperchylomicronemia and indicates an underlying genetic disorder. In some cases, this genetic factor is exacerbated by another medical condition or a hormonal or environmental factor. The major clinical complication of severe hypertriglyceridemia is acute pancreatitis, and initial treatment is focused on decreasing the triglycerides to less than 1,000 mg/dL to prevent this serious complication. In addition, some patients with severe hypertriglyceridemia are at risk for premature atherosclerotic CHD and require more aggressive therapy even when the triglycerides have been decreased to less than the 1,000 mg/dL threshold.

FAMILIAL CHYLOMICRONEMIA SYNDROME: LIPOPROTEIN LIPASE DEFICIENCY AND APOLIPOPROTEIN C-II DEFICIENCY. The familial chylomicronemia syndrome is characterized by presentation in childhood with acute pancreatitis in the setting of triglyceride levels greater than 1,000 mg/dL. Recurrent abdominal pain is a common historical feature. Rarely, infants present with recurrent "colic." The massive elevation of plasma triglycerides can be clinically silent and is sometimes discovered incidentally due to the lipemic appearance of the blood. On physical examination, eruptive xanthomas (small papular lesions that occur in showers on the buttocks and back) may be seen. Lipemia retinalis (a pale appearance to the retinal veins) is a clue to the existence of severe hypertriglyceridemia; hepatosplenomegaly due to ingestion of chylomicrons by the reticuloendothelial system is often found. Premature atherosclerotic cardiovascular disease is not generally a feature of this disease.

Two different genetic defects can cause the familial chylomicronemia syndrome: LPL deficiency and apoC-II deficiency. The hydrolysis of triglycerides in chylomicrons requires the action of LPL in tissue capillary beds, and apoC-II is a required co-factor for the activation of LPL. Mutations in either the LPL gene or the apoC-II gene result in functional inability to hydrolyze triglycerides in chylomicrons and consequent hyperchylomicronemia. The disorder is autosomal recessive, and both alleles of the LPL or apoC-II gene must be affected. Therefore, the parents of children with this disorder generally have normal or near-normal triglyceride levels, and usually there is no family history of severe hyperlipidemia. Both are rare disorders, but of the two, LPL deficiency is more common (approximately 1/1 million persons) than apoC-II deficiency.

The *diagnosis* of the familial hyperchylomicronemia syndrome is usually made based on the clinical presentation and some key laboratory features. The plasma is lactescent and after overnight refrigeration, a cake of chylomicrons forms on the surface. Triglyceride levels are greater than 1,000 mg/dL and may be as high as 10,000 mg/dL or greater. Total cholesterol levels are also elevated because of the presence of cholesterol in chylomicrons. Lipoprotein electrophoresis demonstrates markedly elevated chylomicrons at the origin but is not essential for making the diagnosis. The diagnosis of LPL and apoC-II deficiency can be confirmed at specialized centers by the quantitation of LPL activity in the plasma after intravenous heparin injection (postheparin lipolytic activity). Patients with suspected familial chylomicronemia syndrome should be referred to a specialized lipid center for diagnosis and management.

The mainstay of *treatment* for familial chylomicronemia syndrome is restriction of total dietary fat. Consultation with a registered dietician familiar with this disorder is essential. Caloric supplementation with medium-chain triglycerides, which are absorbed directly into the portal vein and therefore do not promote chylomicron formation, can be useful. If dietary fat restriction alone is not successful, some patients may respond to a cautious trial of fish oils. For patients with apoC-II deficiency, an attack of acute pancreatitis that fails to resolve can be treated with infusion of fresh frozen plasma to provide an exogenous source of apoC-II in an attempt to clear severe hypertriglyceridemia and promote resolution of the pancreatitis.

TYPE V HYPERLIPOPROTEINEMIA (HLP). Type V HLP is common in adults but rare in children. The *diagnosis* of type V HLP is generally used for a patient with fasting triglyceride levels greater than 1,000 mg/dL (fasting hyperchylomicronemia) who does not have LPL or apoC-II deficiency. Type V HLP is also associated with a risk of acute pancreatitis, which can be the initial presentation of this syndrome and is the major rationale for aggressive treatment. Most but not all patients with type V HLP have a family history of hypertriglyceridemia. Type II diabetes mellitus or glucose intolerance frequently accompanies type V hyperlipidemia, but type V hyperlipidemia also occurs in individuals with normal glucose tolerance. Some patients with nephrotic syndrome can acquire severe hypertriglyceridemia. Estrogen replacement therapy can exacerbate moderate hypertriglyceridemia and lead to a more severe type V hyperlipidemia, as can heavy alcohol use. Finally, treatment with isotretinoin or etretinate sometimes causes severe hypertriglyceridemia.

The *treatment* of type V hyperlipidemia is first targeted to decreasing triglycerides in order to reduce the risk of pancreatitis, followed by further lipid lowering depending on the presence of CHD or other risk factors for cardiovascular disease. Patients taking medications that exacerbate hypertriglyceridemia may need to discontinue them if triglyceride levels are greater than 1,000 mg/dL. Diabetes mellitus should be controlled. Patients should be referred to a registered dietitian for dietary counseling. In general, dietary management includes restriction of total fat as well as simple sugars in the diet. Alcohol should be avoided. Regular aerobic exercise can have a significant impact on triglyceride levels and should be actively encouraged. If the patient is overweight, weight loss can help to decrease triglyceride levels. When fasting triglyceride levels remain greater than 1,000 mg/dL despite institution of appropriate dietary and lifestyle measures and control of secondary causes, drug therapy should be considered in order to decrease the risk of acute pancreatitis. However, none of the agents used in the treatment of hypertriglyceridemia is approved for use in children.

DISORDERS OF HIGH-DENSITY LIPOPROTEIN METABOLISM. HDL cholesterol levels are inversely associated with CHD independent of total and LDL cholesterol levels. Although the National Cholesterol Education Program recommends that all adults older than 20 yr should be screened for total cholesterol and HDL cholesterol levels, it is recommended that only children with a positive family history of premature heart disease have a complete lipid profile including HDL cholesterol. Many causes of low HDL cholesterol are secondary to other factors. Cigarette smoking, obesity, physical inactivity, type II diabetes mellitus, end-stage renal disease, hypertriglyceridemia from any cause and the use of β-blockers, thiazide diuretics, androgens, progestins, and probucol can all reduce HDL cholesterol levels. A low-fat diet can also result in a low level of HDL cholesterol; the low HDL is not considered to be associated with an increased risk of CHD, as persons who eat low-fat diets are at substantially reduced risk of premature CHD. Several rare genetic disorders can also be associated with low HDL cholesterol levels.

FAMILIAL LECITHIN:CHOLESTEROL ACYLTRANSFERASE DEFICIENCY. HDL facilitates the removal of unesterified cholesterol from cells, after which the cholesterol is esterified by the lipoprotein-associated enzyme lecithin:cholesterol acyltransferase (LCAT). Two general types of genetic LCAT deficiency have been described in humans: complete deficiency (classic LCAT deficiency) and partial deficiency (fish-eye disease). Both types are extremely rare. Progressive corneal opacification in young adulthood is characteristic of both types; in addition, complete (classic) LCAT deficiency (but not partial deficiency) is characterized by anemia and progressive proteinuria and renal insufficiency in young adulthood. Both types are characterized by very low plasma levels of HDL cholesterol (usually <10 mg/dL) and variable hypertriglyceridemia. The diagnosis of LCAT deficiency is rarely made in childhood and is suspected when there is corneal opacification, renal insufficiency, or an incidentally discovered very low HDL cholesterol level. The diagnosis can be confirmed in specialized laboratories by quantitation of LCAT and cholesterol esterification activity in the plasma. Remarkably, despite the extremely low levels of HDL cholesterol and apoA-I, there is no apparent increased risk of premature atherosclerotic cardiovascular disease in either complete or partial LCAT deficiency.

TANGIER DISEASE. This is a rare disorder associated with cholesterol accumulation in the reticuloendothelial system resulting in hepatosplenomegaly, intestinal mucosal abnormalities, and pathognomonic enlarged, orange tonsils. Intermittent peripheral neuropathy can also be seen from cholesterol accumulation in Schwann cells. Tangier disease is frequently diagnosed in childhood because of the finding of enlarged orange-colored tonsils. Patients with Tangier disease have HDL cholesterol levels less than 5 mg/dL and extremely low levels of apoA-I due to markedly accelerated HDL catabolism. The genetic etiology of Tangier disease is not known but may be related to a cellular defect in efflux of excess lipid to HDL. Tangier disease is probably associated with some increased risk of premature atherosclerotic disease, but this risk does not seem to be proportional to the markedly decreased HDL cholesterol and apoA-I levels. Tangier disease is an autosomal codominant disease: Obligate heterozygotes have moderately reduced HDL cholesterol levels but no evidence of reticuloendothelial cholesterol accumulation. The risk of premature atherosclerosis in obligate heterozygotes is uncertain but may also be increased.

FAMILIAL APOA-I DEFICIENCY AND STRUCTURAL APOA-I MUTATIONS. Complete genetic deficiency of apoA-I due to deletions of the apoA-I gene or nonsense mutations that prevent the biosynthesis of apoA-I protein result in virtually absent plasma HDL. These extremely rare patients acquire corneal opacities and sometimes cutaneous or planar xanthomas. The risk of premature cardiovascular disease in patients with apoA-I deficiency is increased, but onset of CHD symptoms in these kindreds has varied from the 3rd to the 7th decade. Increased premature cardiovascular disease has not been reported in any kindred with an apoA-I mutation causing low HDL, suggesting that the mechanism causing the low HDL may be an important determinant of the CHD risk associated with low HDL states. Other than corneal opacities, most of these individuals do not appear to have clinical sequelae related to the apoA-I mutations. Interestingly, a few apoA-I mutations have been described in association with systemic amyloidosis, and the mutant apoA-I has been found as a component of the amyloid plaque.

PRIMARY HYPOALPHALIPOPROTEINEMIA. The most common inherited form of low HDL is termed *primary or familial hypoalphalipoproteinemia.* It is defined as an HDL cholesterol level less than the 10th percentile in the setting of relatively normal cholesterol and triglyceride levels, no apparent secondary causes of low HDL, and no clinical signs of LCAT deficiency or Tangier's disease. This syndrome is often referred to as "isolated low HDL." A family history of low HDL cholesterol facilitates the diagnosis of an inherited condition, which usually follows the pattern of an autosomal dominant trait. The genetic etiology of this syndrome is unknown, although the metabolic cause appears to be primarily accelerated catabolism of HDL and its apolipoproteins. The direct relationship of primary hypoalphalipoproteinemia to premature coronary disease is uncertain and may depend on the specific nature of the gene defect or metabolic cause of the low HDL cholesterol level.

CONDITIONS ASSOCIATED WITH LOW CHOLESTEROL LEVELS

ABETALIPOPROTEINEMIA. This is a rare autosomal recessive disease characterized by fat malabsorption, spinocerebellar degeneration, and pigmented retinopathy. The biochemical hallmark of this disease is the strikingly abnormal plasma lipid and lipoprotein profile. Total cholesterol and triglyceride levels are extremely low; there are no detectable plasma chylomicrons, VLDL, or LDL; and apoB is absent from the plasma. This disease is caused by mutations in the gene for the microsomal triglyceride transfer protein, which mediates the intracellular transport of membrane-associated lipids in the intestine and liver and is necessary for the normal formation of chylomicrons in the enterocyte and VLDL in the hepatocyte.

The most prominent and debilitating *clinical manifestations* of abetalipoproteinemia are neurologic and usually begin in the 2nd decade. The first sign of disease is usually the loss of deep tendon reflexes, followed by decreased distal lower extremity vibratory and proprioceptive senses and cerebellar signs such as dysmetria, ataxia, and spastic gait. The clinical outcome is variable, but the result in untreated patients is often severe ataxia and spasticity by the 3rd or 4th decade. These severe effects on the central nervous system are the ultimate cause of death in most patients and often occur by the 5th decade or earlier. Patients with abetalipoproteinemia also acquire a progressive pigmented retinopathy. The presence of both spinocerebellar degeneration and pigmented retinopathy in this disease may result in a misdiagnosis of Friedreich ataxia. The first ophthalmic symptoms are decreased night and color vision. Daytime visual acuity usually deteriorates inexorably to virtual blindness by the 4th decade.

The majority of the clinical symptoms of abetalipoproteinemia are the result of defects in absorption and transport of fat-soluble vitamins, especially vitamin E. Vitamin E is transported from the intestine to the liver, then "repackaged" in the liver and incorporated into the assembling VLDL particle by a specific protein termed the *tocopherol binding protein.* In the circulation, VLDL is converted to LDL, and vitamin E is transported by LDL to peripheral tissues and delivered to cells via the LDL receptor. Patients with abetalipoproteinemia are markedly deficient in vitamin E. Vitamin E metabolism is greatly altered in patients with abetalipoproteinemia because the plasma transport of vitamin E requires hepatic secretion of apoB-containing lipoproteins. Most of the major clinical symptoms, especially those of the nervous system and retina, are primarily due to vitamin E deficiency. This concept is supported by the fact that other diseases involving vitamin E deficiency, such as cholestasis and isolated vitamin E deficiency, are characterized by similar symptoms and pathologic changes. Patients with suspected abetalipoproteinemia should be referred to specialized centers for confirmation of the diagnosis and institution of appropriate therapy.

Obligate heterozygotes (parents of patients with abetalipoproteinemia) have no symptoms and no evidence of reduced plasma lipids. Thus family studies are important in distinguishing abetalipoproteinemia from clinically similar homozygous hypobetalipoproteinemia in which obligate heterozygotes have decreased LDL cholesterol and apoB levels.

FAMILIAL HYPOBETALIPOPROTEINEMIA. Familial hypobetalipoproteinemia, in contrast to abetalipoproteinemia, is autosomal codominant: Heterozygotes have levels of LDL cholesterol and apoB that are approximately one half of normal or less, whereas homozygotes have very low or no plasma apoB. Heterozygous familial hypobetalipoproteinemia is not associated with symptoms, whereas some homozygous patients have symptoms that are similar to those in abetalipoproteinemia patients. The gene defect in this disorder resides in most or all cases within the apoB gene itself. Many are nonsense mutations resulting in a truncated apoB protein; at least 25 such mutations have been described to date. One patient who was initially described as having "normotriglyceridemic abetalipoproteinemia" has subsequently been demonstrated to be homozygous for a truncated apoB and therefore has homozygous hypobetalipoproteinemia.

Clinically, heterozygous hypobetalipoproteinemia is associated with LDL cholesterol levels in the 40–80 mg/dL range, is not associated with clinical sequelae, and requires no specific therapy. However, patients with homozygous hypobetalipoproteinemia have markedly reduced to absent LDL cholesterol and apoB levels and may be at risk for many of the sequelae seen in abetalipoproteinemia. Such patients should therefore be referred to specialized centers for confirmation of the diagnosis and institution of appropriate therapy.

CHYLOMICRON RETENTION DISEASE. Chylomicron retention disease, or Anderson disease, is associated with selective inability to secrete apoB from intestinal enterocytes, resulting in fat malabsorption and sometimes neurologic disease similar to that seen in abetalipoproteinemia and homozygous hypobetalipoproteinemia. In contrast to these two disorders, apoB-100 can be detected in the plasma of patients with chylomicron retention disease, as hepatic VLDL secretion is normal. The molecular defect is unknown but appears to be distinct from both the microsomal triglyceride transfer protein and apoB genes.

SMITH-LEMLI-OPITZ SYNDROME. This syndrome is a recessive genetic disorder characterized by neurologic developmental defects including microcephaly, severe mental retardation, micrognathia, widespread ears, cataracts, and syndactyly. The prevalence of homozygotes is about 1/20,000 births, and the estimated gene carrier frequency is 1–2%. Smith-Lemli-Opitz syndrome is due to defects in the gene encoding the enzyme 7-dehydrocholesterol-δ-7-reductase, which is required to convert 7-dehydrocholesterol to cholesterol. Patients have very low plasma cholesterol levels and the neurologic defects are presumed to be due to limited cholesterol availability within the central nervous system for neural growth. No effective treatment is available.

SELECTED GENETIC DISORDERS OF INTRACELLULAR CHOLESTEROL METABOLISM

Several rare genetic disorders of intracellular cholesterol and lipid metabolism have been described. In some of these diseases, the molecular cause is established, whereas in other cases it remains unknown.

CEREBROTENDINOUS XANTHOMATOSIS. This is an autosomal recessive disorder caused by mutations in the gene for sterol 27-hydroxylase, a mitochondrial enzyme involved in the normal biosynthesis of bile acids in the liver. As a result of the deficiency in sterol 27-hydroxylase, bile acid intermediates are shunted into the synthesis of cholestanol, which then accumulates in multiple tissues. Untreated, patients acquire cataracts, tendon xanthomas, and progressive disease of the central and peripheral nervous system in the 2nd decade of life. Early diagnosis is crucial, as treatment with chenodeoxycholic acid reduces plasma cholestanol levels and prevents the progression of clinical symptoms.

SITOSTEROLEMIA. Sitosterolemia is a rare autosomal recessive disease associated with excess intestinal absorption and tissue accumulation of plant-derived sterols such as sitosterol and cholestanol. The molecular cause of sitosterolemia is unknown. This disease can present with severe hypercholesterolemia, premature atherosclerosis, and tendon xanthomas similar to those seen in patients with homozygous or severe heterozygous FH. Sitosterolemia should be ruled out in patients presenting with this constellation of findings. There is no LDL receptor abnormality in sitosterolemia. Patients with sitosterolemia often benefit from treatment with bile acid sequestrants but do not benefit from HMG-CoA reductase inhibition. Patients suspected of having sitosterolemia should be referred to specialized centers for further evaluation.

CHOLESTEROL ESTER STORAGE DISEASE AND WOLMAN DISEASE. Cholesterol ester storage disease (CESD) or Wolman disease is an autosomal recessive disorder caused by mutations in the gene for lysosomal acid lipase, a lysosomal enzyme required for hydrolysis of cholesteryl esters and triglycerides in the lysosome. See Chapter 83.4.

NIEMANN-PICK C DISEASE. The Niemann-Pick group of diseases are autosomal recessive diseases characterized by accumulation of cholesterol and sphingomyelin in tissues, especially the liver, reticuloendothelial system, and central nervous system. Niemann-Pick A and B are described in Chapters 83.4 and 608.1. Niemann-Pick C disease is a disorder of intracellular cholesterol transport for which the molecular cause has been established. Niemann-Pick C is characterized by hepatosplenomegaly and progressive neurologic disease, often resulting in severe disability and death by the 2nd decade.

American Academy of Pediatrics Committee on Nutrition: Cholesterol in childhood. Pediatrics 101:141, 1998.

Bao W, Srinivasan SR, Valdez R, et al: Longitudinal changes in cardiovascular risk from childhood to young adulthood in offspring of parents with coronary artery disease. The Bogalusa Heart Study. JAMA 278:1749, 1997.

Brunzell JD, Schrott HG, Motulsky AG, et al: Myocardial infarction in the familial forms of hypertriglyceridemia. Metabolism 25:313, 1984.

Clayton PT: Disorders of cholesterol biosynthesis. Arch Dis Child 78:185, 1998.

Connor WE, DeFrancesco C, Connor SL: N-3 fatty acids from fish oil. Effects on plasma lipoproteins and hypertriglyceridemic patients. Ann NY Acad Sci 683:16, 1993.

Cortner JA, Coates PM, Liacouras CA, et al: Familial combined hyperlipidemia in children: Clinical expression, metabolic defects, and management. J Pediatr 123:177, 1993.

Defesche JC, Kastelein JJP: Molecular epidemiology of familial hypercholesterolamia. Lancet 352:1643, 1998.

Dennison BA, Kikuchi DA, Srinavasan SR, et al: Parental history of cardiovascular disease as an indication for screening for lipoprotein abnormalities in children. J Pediatr 115:186, 1989.

Feoli-Fonseca JC, Levy E, Godard M, et al: Familial lipoprotein lipase deficiency in infancy: Clinical, biochemical, and molecular study. J Pediatr 133:417, 1998.

Frerichs RR, Srinavasan SR, Webber LS, et al: Serum cholesterol and triglyceride levels in 3,446 children from a biracial community. The Bogalusa Heart Study. Circulation 54:302, 1976.

Gotto A: Results of recent large cholesterol-lowering trials and implications for clinical management. Am J Cardiol 79:1663, 1997.

Granot E, Deckelbaum RJ: Hypocholesterolemia in childhood. J Pediatr 115:171, 1989.

Grossman M, Rader DJ, Muller DWM, et al: A pilot study of ex vivo gene therapy for homozygous familial hypercholesterolaemia. Nat Med 1:1148, 1995.

Grundy SM, Chait A, Brunzell JD: Familial combined hyperlipidemia workshop. Arteriosclerosis 7:203, 1987.

Johnson MC, Watson MS, Strauss AW: Rational approach to pharmacologic reduction of cholesterol levels in children. J Pediatr 129:4, 1996.

Lambert M, Lupien P-J, Gagne C, et al: Treatment of familial hypercholesterolemia in children and adolescents: Effect of Lovastatin. Pediatrics 97:619, 1996.

Liacouras CA, Coates PM, Gallagher PR, et al: Use of cholestyramine in the treatment of children with familial combined hyperlipidemia. J Pediatr 122:477,1998.

Linton MF, Farese RV Jr, Young SG: Familial hypobetalipoproteinemia. J Lipid Res 34:521, 1993.

Lipid Research Clinics Program: The Lipid Research Clinics Coronary Primary Prevention Trial Results. I and II. JAMA 251:351, 1984.

Mietus-Snyder M, Malloy MJ: Endothelial dysfunction occurs in children with two genetic hyperlipidemias: Improvement with antioxidant vitamin therapy. J Pediatr 133:35, 1998.

National Cholesterol Education Program: Report of the Expert Panel on Blood Cholesterol Levels in Children and Adolescents. Pediatrics 89(Suppl):525, 1992.

Newman WP, Freedman DS, Voors AW, et al: Relation of serum lipoprotein levels and systolic blood pressure to early atherosclerosis. The Bogalusa Heart Study. N Engl J Med 314:138, 1986.

Rader DJ, Brewer HB Jr: Abetalipoproteinemia. New insights into lipoprotein assembly and vitamin E metabolism from a rare genetic disease. JAMA 270:865, 1993.

Rall SC, Mahley RW: The role of apolipopreotein E genetic variants in lipoprotein disorders (review). J Intern Med 231:653, 1992.

Salen G, Shefer S, Nguyen L, et al: Sitosterolemia. J Lipid Res 33:945, 1992.

Shannon BM, Tershakovec AM, Martel JK, et al: Reduction of elevated LDL-cholesterol levels of 4–10 year-old children through home-based dietary education. Pediatrics 94:923, 1994.

Strong WB, Deckelbaum RJ, Gidding SS, et al: Integrated cardiovascular health promotion in childhood. A statement for health professionals from the Subcommittee on Atherosclerosis and Hypertension in Childhood of the Council on Cardiovascular Disease in the Young, American Heart Association. Circulation 85:1638, 1992.

Tershakovec AM, Jawad AF, Stallings VA, et al: Growth of hypercholesterolemic children completing physician-initiated low-fat dietary intervention. J Pediatr 133:26, 1998.

The Writing Group for the DISC Collaborative Research Group: Efficacy and safety of lowering dietary intake of fat and cholesterol in children with elevated low-density lipoprotein cholesterol. JAMA 273:1429, 1995.

Tonstad S, Novik TS, Vandvik IH: Psychosocial function during treatment for familial hypercholesterolemia. Pediatrics 98:249, 1996.

Verschuren WMM, Jacobs DR, Bloemberg BPM, et al: Serum total cholesterol and long-term coronary heart disease mortality in different cultures. Twenty-five-year follow-up of the seven countries study. JAMA 274:131, 1995.

Zwiener RJ, Uany R, Petruska ML, et al: Low density lipoprotein apheresis as a long term treatment for children with homozygous familial hypercholesterolemia. J Pediatr 126:728, 1995.

83.4 Lipidoses

Margaret M. McGovern and Robert J. Desnick

Lipid storage disorders are diverse diseases that are related by their molecular pathology. In each, there is an inherited deficiency of a lysosomal hydrolase leading to the lysosomal accumulation of the enzyme's specific sphingolipid substrate. The lipid substrates share a common structure that includes a ceramide backbone (2-*N*-acyl-sphingosine) from which the various sphingolipids are derived by substitution of hexoses, phosphorylcholine, or one or more sialic acid residues on the terminal hydroxyl group of the ceramide molecule (Fig. 83–7). The pathway of glycosphingolipid metabolism in nervous tissue (Fig. 83–8) and in visceral organs (Fig. 83–9) is known; each catabolic step has a genetically determined metabolic derangement. Since glycosphingolipids are essential components of all cell membranes, the inability to degrade these substances and their subsequent accumulation results in the physiologic and morphologic alterations and characteristic clinical manifestations of the lipid storage disorders. Progressive lysosomal accumulation of glycosphingolipids in the central nervous system leads to neurodegeneration, whereas storage in visceral cells can lead to organomegaly, skeletal abnormalities, pulmonary infiltration, and other manifestations. The storage of a substrate in a specific tissue is dependent on its normal distribution in the body.

The biochemical basis of lipid storage disorders is well characterized, including the determination of each of the enzymatic activities and the various storage products. Diagnostic assays for the identification of affected individuals rely on the measurement of the specific enzymatic activity in isolated leukocytes or cultured fibroblasts. For most disorders, carrier identi-

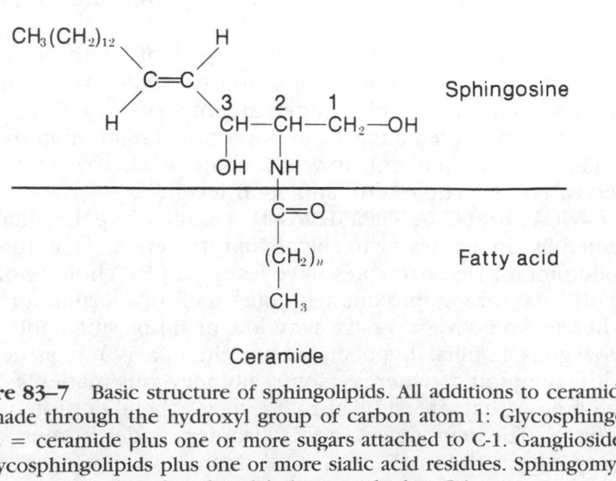

$CH_3(CH_2)_{12}$ H
C=C
Sphingosine
H 3 2 1
CH—CH—CH_2—OH
OH NH
C=O
$(CH_2)_n$
Fatty acid
CH_3
Ceramide

Figure 83–7 Basic structure of sphingolipids. All additions to ceramide are made through the hydroxyl group of carbon atom 1: Glycosphingolipids = ceramide plus one or more sugars attached to C-1. Gangliosides = glycosphingolipids plus one or more sialic acid residues. Sphingomyelin = ceramide plus phosphorylcholine attached to C-1.

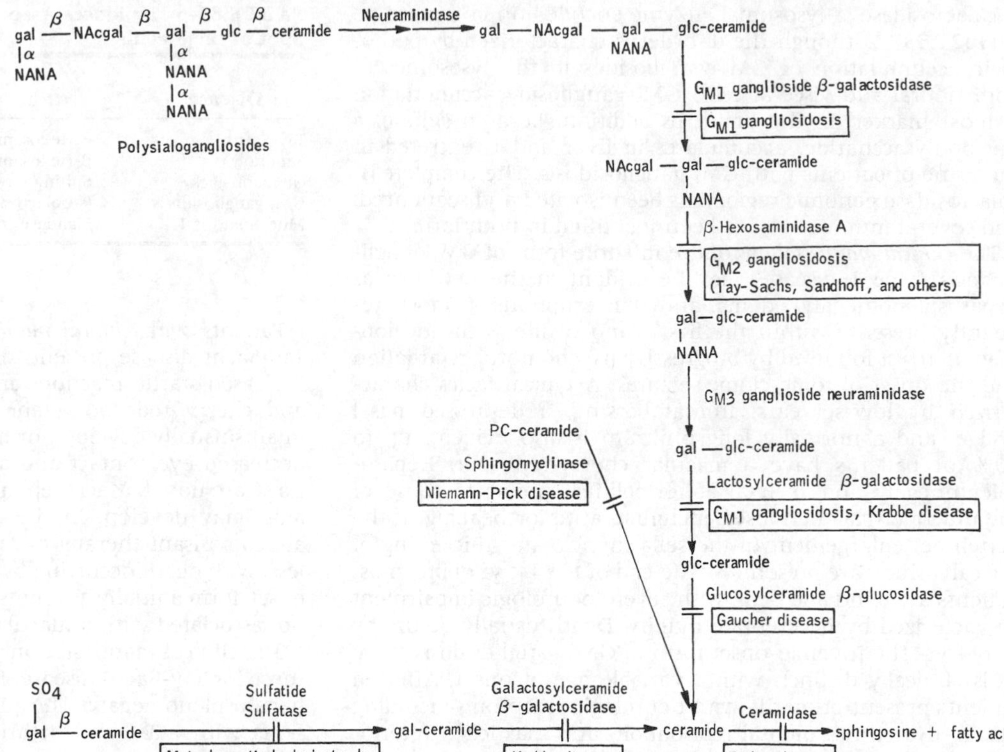

Figure 83–8 Pathways in the metabolism of sphingolipids found in nervous tissues. The name of the enzyme catalyzing each reaction is given with the name of the substrate acted on. Inborn errors are depicted as bars crossing the reaction arrows, and the name of the associated defect or defects is given within the nearest box. The gangliosides are named according to the nomenclature of Svennerholm. Anomeric configurations are given only at the largest starting compound. gal = galactose; glc = glucose; NAcgal = *N*-acetyl-galactosamine; NANA = *N*-acetyl-neuraminic acid; PC = phosphorylcholine.

fication and prenatal diagnosis are available; a specific diagnosis is essential to permit genetic counseling of the family.

The identification of specific disease-causing mutations has led to improved diagnosis, prenatal detection, and carrier identification. For some disorders (Gaucher disease), it has been possible to make genotype-phenotype correlations that predict disease severity and allow more precise genetic counseling. The cloning and characterization of most of the genes that encode the specific enzymes required for sphingolipid metabolism have permitted the development of improved therapeutic options, such as recombinant enzyme replacement therapy, and possibly gene therapy.

GM_1 GANGLIOSIDOSIS. GM_1 gangliosidosis most frequently presents in early infancy (type 1 disease) but has been described in patients with juvenile onset (type 2). Both forms are autosomal recessive traits; each results from the deficient activity of

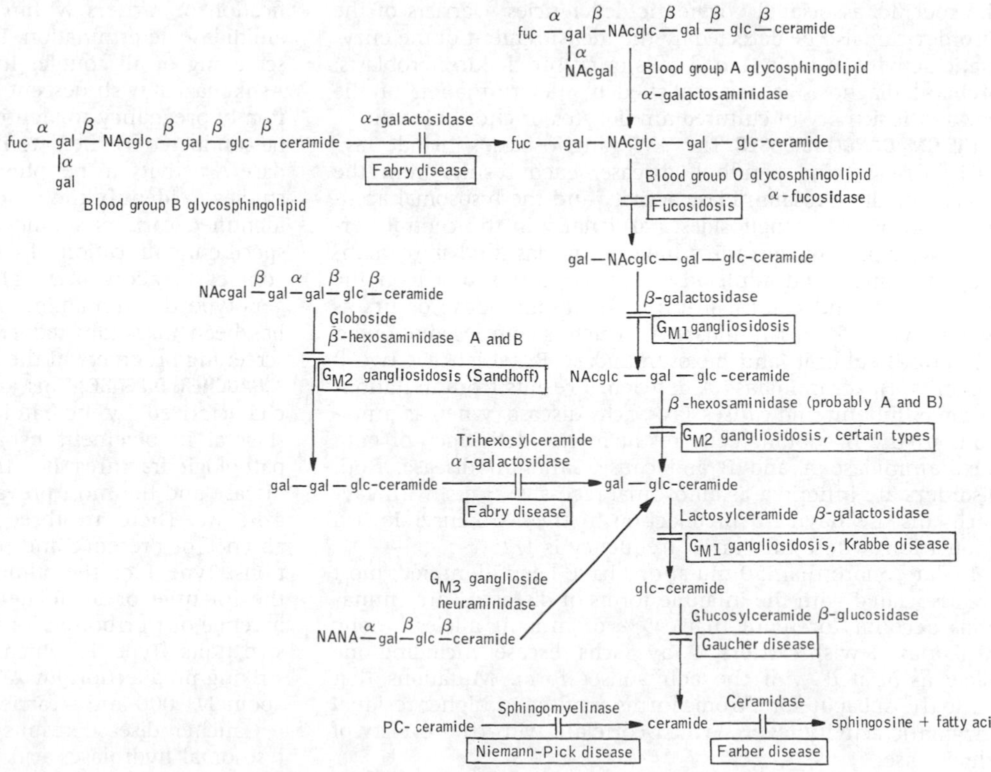

Figure 83–9 Pathways in the degradation of sphingolipids found in visceral organs and red or white blood cells. See also the legend for Figure 83–8. fuc = fucose; NAcglc = *N*-acetylglucosamine.

β-galactosidase, a lysosomal enzyme encoded on chromosome 3 (3p21.33). Although the disorder is characterized by pathologic accumulation of GM_1 gangliosides in the lysosomes of both neural and visceral cells, GM_1 ganglioside accumulation is most marked in the brain. In addition, keratan sulfate, a mucopolysaccharide, accumulates in liver and is excreted in the urine of patients with GM_1 gangliosidosis. The complete β-galactosidase genomic region has been isolated and sequenced, and several mutations have been identified in both forms.

The *clinical manifestations* of the infantile form of GM_1 gangliosidosis (type 1 disease) may be evident in the newborn as hepatosplenomegaly, edema, and skin eruptions. It most frequently presents within the first 6 mo of life with developmental arrest followed by progressive psychomotor retardation and the onset of tonic-clonic seizures. A typical facies characterized by low-set ears, frontal bossing, a depressed nasal bridge, and abnormally long philtrum is also evident; up to 50% of patients have a macular cherry-red spot. Hepatosplenomegaly and skeletal abnormalities similar to those of the mucopolysachharidoses, including anterior beaking of the vertebrae, enlargement of the sella turcica, and thickening of the calvarium, are present. By the end of the 1st yr of life, most patients are blind and deaf, with severe neurologic impairment characterized by decerebrate rigidity. Death usually occurs by 3 to 4 yr. The juvenile-onset form of GM_1 gangliosidosis (type 2) is clinically distinct, with a variable age of onset. Affected patients present primarily with neurologic symptoms including ataxia, dysarthria, mental retardation, and spasticity. Deterioration is slow; patients may survive through the 4th decade of life. These patients lack the visceral involvement, facial abnormalities, and skeletal features seen in type 1 disease. There is no specific *treatment* for either form of GM_1 gangliosidosis.

The *diagnosis* of GM_1 gangliosidosis should be suspected in infants with the clinical features described previously and is confirmed by the demonstration of the deficiency of β-galactosidase activity in peripheral leukocytes or cultured skin fibroblasts. Other disorders that share the features of the GM_1 gangliosidoses include Hurler disease (mucopolysaccharidosis type I), I-cell disease, and Niemann-Pick disease (NPD) type A, which can each be distinguished by the demonstration of the specific, associated enzymatic deficiencies. Carriers of the disorder can also be detected by the measurement of the enzymatic activity in white blood cells or cultured skin fibroblasts; prenatal diagnosis is accomplished by determination of the enzymatic activity in cultured amniocytes or chorionic villi.

THE GM_2 GANGLIOSIDOSES. The GM_2 gangliosidoses include Tay-Sachs disease and Sandhoff disease; each results from the deficiency of hexosaminidase activity and the lysosomal accumulation of GM_2 gangliosides, particularly in the central nervous system. Both disorders have been classified into infantile-, juvenile-, and adult-onset chronic forms based on the age at onset and clinical features. Hexosaminidase occurs as two isozymes, hexosaminidase A, which is composed of one α and one β subunit, and hexosaminidase B, which has two β subunits. Hexosaminidase A deficiency results from mutations in the α subunit and causes Tay-Sachs disease, whereas mutations in the β subunit gene result in the deficiency of both hexosaminidase A and B and cause Sandhoff disease. Both disorders are inherited as autosomal recessive traits, with Tay-Sachs disease having a predilection in the Ashkenazi Jewish population, where the carrier frequency is 1/25.

To date, more than 50 mutations have been identified; most are associated with the infantile forms of disease. Three mutations account for more than 95% of mutant alleles among Ashkenazi Jewish carriers of Tay-Sachs disease, including one allele associated with the adult-onset form. Mutations that cause the subacute or chronic forms resulted in higher residual enzymatic activity levels, which correlate with the severity of the disease.

TABLE 83–6 Lipidoses Associated with Cherry-Red Spot of the Macula

Disease	Enzyme Defect	Visceral Involvement
Tay-Sachs	β-Hexosaminidase A	No organomegaly
Sandhoff	β-Hexosaminidase A and B	Hepatosplenomegaly
Niemann-Pick	Sphingomyelinase	Hepatosplenomegaly
GM_1 gangliosidosis	β-Galactosidase	Hepatosplenomegaly
Mucolipidosis 1	Sialidase (neuraminidase)	Hepatosplenomegaly

Patients with *clinical manifestations* of the infantile form of Tay-Sachs disease present in infancy with loss of motor skills, increased startle reaction, and the presence of macular pallor and cherry red spot (Table 83–6) on retinoscopy. Affected infants usually develop normally until about 5 mo of age when decreased eye contact and an exaggerated startle response to noise are noted. Macrocephaly, not associated with hydrocephalus, may develop. In the 2nd yr of life, seizures requiring anticonvulsant therapy develop. Neurodegeneration is relentless, with death occurring by the age of 4 or 5 yr. The juvenile-onset form initially presents with ataxia and dysarthria; it is not associated with a macular cherry red spot.

The clinical manifestations of Sandhoff disease are similar to those for Tay-Sachs disease. Infants with Sandhoff disease have hepatosplenomegaly. The juvenile form of this disorder presents with ataxia, dysarthria, and mental deterioration, but without visceral enlargement or a macular cherry red spot. There is no *treatment* available for Tay-Sachs disease or Sandhoff disease.

The *diagnosis* of infantile Tay-Sachs disease and Sandhoff disease is usually suspected in an infant with neurologic features and a cherry red spot. Definitive diagnosis is by determination of the level of hexosaminidase in isolated blood leukocytes. The two disorders are distinguished by the enzymatic assay, since in Tay-Sachs disease only the hexosaminidase A isozyme is deficient, whereas in Sandhoff disease both the hexosaminidase A and B isozymes are deficient. Future at-risk pregnancies for both disorders can be monitored by prenatal diagnosis by amniocentesis or chorionic villus sampling. Identification of carriers within families is also possible by hexosaminidase determination. Indeed, for Tay-Sachs disease, carrier screening of all couples in whom at least one member is of Ashkenazi Jewish descent is recommended prior to the initiation of pregnancy to identify couples at risk. These studies can be conducted by the determination of the level of hexosaminidase A activity in peripheral leukocytes or plasma. Molecular studies to identify the exact molecular defect in enzymatically identified carriers should also be performed to permit more specific identification of carriers in the family, and for at-risk couples to allow prenatal diagnosis by both enzymatic and genotype determination. The incidence of Tay-Sachs disease has been markedly reduced since the introduction of carrier screening programs in the Ashkenazi Jewish population.

GAUCHER DISEASE. This disease is a multisystemic lipidosis characterized by hematologic problems, organomegaly, and skeletal involvement usually manifested as bone pain and pathologic fractures. It is the most common lysosomal storage disease and the most prevalent genetic defect among Ashkenazi Jews. There are three clinical subtypes delineated by the absence or presence and progression of neurologic manifestations: Type 1 or the adult, non-neuronopathic form; type 2, the infantile or acute neuronopathic form; and type 3, the juvenile or Norrbotten form. All subtypes are autosomal recessive traits. Type 1, which accounts for 99% of cases, has a striking predilection for Ashkenazi Jews, with an incidence of about 1/1,000 and a carrier frequency of 1/18.

Gaucher disease results from the deficient activity of the lysosomal hydrolase, acid β-glucosidase, which is encoded by a gene on chromosome 1 (q21–q31). The enzymatic defect results in the accumulation of undegraded glycolipid substrates, particularly glucosylceramide, in cells of the reticuloendothelial system. This progressive deposition results in infiltration of the bone marrow, progressive hepatosplenomegaly, and skeletal complications. Four mutations—N370S, L444P, 84insG, and IVS2—account for 90–95% of mutant alleles among Ashkenazi Jewish patients, permitting screening for this disorder in this population. Genotype-phenotype correlations have been noted, providing the molecular basis for the clinical heterogeneity seen in Gaucher disease type 1, which has a wide range of severity and age of onset. Patients who are homozygous for the N370S mutation tend to have later onset with a more indolent course than patients with one copy of N370S and another common allele.

Clinical manifestations of Gaucher disease type 1 have a variable age of onset, from early childhood to late adulthood, with most symptomatic patients presenting by adolescence. At presentation, patients may have easy bruisability due to thrombocytopenia, chronic fatigue secondary to anemia, hepatomegaly with or without elevated liver function test results, splenomegaly, and bone pain. Occasional patients have pulmonary involvement at the time of presentation. Patients presenting in the 1st decade frequently are not Jewish and have growth retardation and a more malignant course. Other patients may be discovered fortuitously during evaluation for other conditions or as part of routine examinations; these patients have a benign course. In symptomatic patients, splenomegaly is progressive and can become massive. Clinically apparent bony involvement, which occurs in more than 20% of patients, can present as bone pain or pathologic fractures. However, more than half of patients have radiologic evidence of skeletal involvement, including an Erlenmeyer flask deformity of the distal femur. In patients with symptomatic bone disease, lytic lesions can develop in the long bones, including the femur, ribs, and pelvis; osteosclerosis may be evident at an early age. Bone crises with severe pain and swelling can occur. Bleeding secondary to thrombocytopenia may manifest as epistaxis and bruising and is frequently overlooked until other symptoms become apparent. With the exception of the severely growth-retarded child, who may experience developmental delays secondary to the effects of chronic disease, development and intelligence are normal.

The pathologic hallmark of Gaucher disease is the Gaucher cell in the reticuloendothelial system, particularly in the bone marrow (Fig. 83–10). These cells, which are 20 to 100 μm in diameter, have a characteristic wrinkled paper appearance resulting from the presence of intracytoplasmic substrate inclusions. The cytoplasm of the Gaucher cell reacts strongly positively with the periodic acid–Schiff stain; the presence of this cell in bone marrow and tissue specimens is highly suggestive of Gaucher disease, although it also may be found in patients with granulocytic leukemia and myeloma.

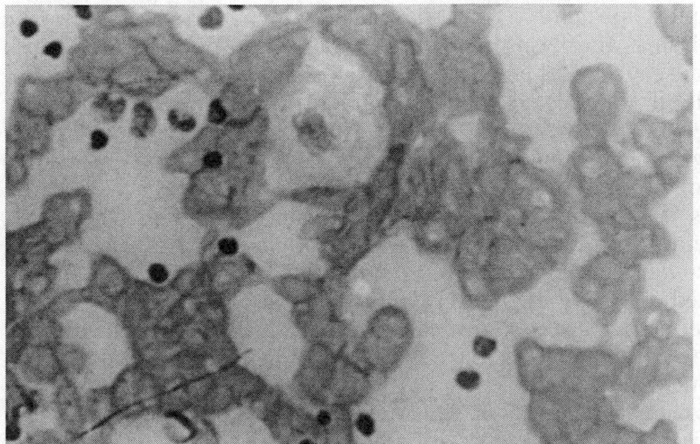

Figure 83–10 Cells from a spleen of a patient with Gaucher disease. A characteristic spleen cell is shown engorged with glucocerebroside.

Gaucher disease type 2 is much less common and does not have a striking ethnic predilection. It is characterized by a rapid neurodegenerative course with extensive visceral involvement and death within the first 2 yr of life. It presents in infancy with increased tone, strabismus, and organomegaly. Failure to thrive and stridor due to laryngospasm are typical. After a several-year period of psychomotor regression, death occurs secondary to respiratory compromise. Gaucher disease type 3 presents with clinical manifestations that are intermediate to those seen in types 1 and 2, with presentation in childhood and death by age 10–15 yr. It has a predilection for the Swedish Norrbottnian population, where the incidence is 1/50,000. Neurologic involvement is present but occurs later and with decreased severity compared wirh type 2. Type 3 is further classified as type 3a and 3b based on the extent of neurologic involvement and whether there is progressive myotonia and dementia (type 3a) or isolated supranuclear gaze palsy (type 3b).

Gaucher disease should be considered in the *differential diagnosis* of patients with unexplained organomegaly, easy bruisability, or bone pain, or a combination of these conditions. Bone marrow examination usually reveals the presence of Gaucher cells; all suspected diagnoses should be confirmed by determination of the acid β-glucosidase activity in isolated leukocytes or cultured fibroblasts. The identification of carriers can be achieved by enzymatic assay, with confirmation of results by molecular testing in most Jewish families. Testing should be offered to all family members, keeping in mind that heterogeneity, even among members of the same kindred, can be so great that nonsymptomatic affected individuals may be diagnosed. Prenatal diagnosis is available by determination of enzyme activity in chorionic villi or cultured amniotic fluid cells.

Treatment of patients with Gaucher disease is primarily symptomatic, including administration of blood transfusions for anemia, partial or total splenectomy for severe mechanical pulmonary compromise or hypersplenism, analgesics for bone pain, and orthopedic procedures for joint replacement in those patients with severe bony involvement. A small number of patients have undergone bone marrow transplantation, which is curative but results in significant morbidity and mortality from the procedure, making the selection of appropriate candidates limited. The safety and efficacy of enzyme replacement with purified placental acid β-glucosidase has been demonstrated in Gaucher disease. Most extraskeletal symptoms are reversed by initial debulking doses of enzyme (30–60 IU/kg) administered by intravenous infusion every other week. The effectiveness of enzyme replacement in reversing and preventing bony manifestations is under study; however, some data indicate that it may also be efficacious. A recombinant form of the enzyme has also been developed and is being studied. The availability of this genetically engineered enzyme provides the potential for unlimited production and the elimination of the risk of transferring human pathogens from the placental purified enzyme.

NIEMANN-PICK DISEASE (NPD). The original description of NPD referred to what is now known as type A NPD, a fatal disorder of infancy characterized by failure to thrive, hepatosplenomegaly, and a rapidly progressive neurodegenerative course that leads to death by 2–3 yr of age. Currently, a total of six subtypes of NPD have been described, including type B, which is a non-neuronopathic form that presents with hepatosplenomegaly, and other, rarer forms that result from cholesterol metabolism defects (see Chapter 83.3). All six subtypes are inherited as autosomal recessive traits and display variable clinical features (see also Chapter 608).

NPD types A and B result from the deficient activity of sphingomyelinase, a lysosomal enzyme encoded by a gene located on chromosome 11 (11p15.1–p15.4). The enzymatic defect results in the pathologic accumulation of sphingomyelin, a ceramide phospholipid, and other lipids in the monocyte-macrophage system, the primary site of pathology. The progressive deposition of sphingomyelin in the central nervous system results in the neurodegenerative course seen in type A and in the systemic disease manifestations of type B, including progressive lung disease in some patients. The complete sphingomyelinase genomic region has been isolated and sequenced, and a number of mutations that cause types A and B NPD have been identified, including single base substitutions and small deletions.

The *clinical manifestations* and course of Type A NPD is uniform and is characterized by a normal appearance at birth (although the newborn period is sometimes complicated by prolonged jaundice). Hepatosplenomegaly, moderate lymphadenopathy, and psychomotor retardation are evident by 6 mo of age, followed by neurodevelopmental regression. With advancing age, the loss of motor function and the deterioration of intellectual capabilities are progressively debilitating and in later stages, spasticity and rigidity are evident; affected infants lose contact with their environment. In contrast to the stereotyped type A phenotype, the clinical presentation and course of patients with type B disease are more variable. Most are diagnosed in infancy or childhood when enlargement of the liver or spleen, or both, is detected during a routine physical examination. At diagnosis, type B NPD patients also have evidence of mild pulmonary involvement, usually detected as a diffuse reticular or finely nodular infiltration on the chest roentenogram. Pulmonary symptoms are not usual until adulthood. In most patients, hepatosplenomegaly is particularly prominent in childhood, but with increasing linear growth, the abdominal protuberance decreases and becomes less conspicuous. In mildly affected patients, the splenomegaly may not be noted until adulthood, and there may be minimal disease manifestations.

In most type B patients, decreased pulmonary diffusion due to alveolar infiltration becomes evident in late childhood and progresses with age. Severely affected individuals may experience significant pulmonary compromise by 15–20 yr of age. Such patients have low Po_2 values and dyspnea on exertion. Life-threatening bronchopneumonias may occur, and cor pulmonale has been described. Severely affected patients may have liver involvement leading to life-threatening cirrhosis, portal hypertension, and ascites. Clinically significant pancytopenia due to secondary hypersplenism may require partial or complete splenectomy; this should be avoided if possible because splenectomy frequently causes progression of pulmonary disease, which can be life-threatening. In general, type B patients do not have neurologic involvement and have a normal IQ. Some patients with type B disease have cherry red maculae or haloes and subtle neurologic symptoms (peripheral neuropathy).

Type C NPD patients often present with prolonged neonatal jaundice, appear normal for 1–2 yr, and then experience a slowly progressive and variable neurodegenerative course. Their hepatosplenomegaly is less severe than that in patients with types A or B NPD, and they may survive into adulthood. The underlying biochemical defect in type C patients is an abnormality in cholesterol transport, leading to the accumulation of sphingomyelin and cholesterol in their lysosomes and a secondary reduction in sphingomyelinase activity (see Chapter 83.3). Type D NPD patients acquire neurologic symptoms later in childhood and have a slower neurodegenerative course than do type C patients. Most individuals with type D disease share a common ancestry traceable to Acadians from Yarmouth county, Nova Scotia. It appears that these patients also have an abnormality in cholesterol metabolism and that the defect may be allelic with type C NPD.

In type B NPD patients, splenomegaly is usually the first manifestation detected. The splenic enlargement is noted in early childhood; however, in very mild disease, the enlargement may be subtle and detection may be delayed until adolescence or adulthood. The presence of the characteristic NPD cells in the bone marrow aspirates supports the diagnosis of type B NPD. However, patients with types C and D NPD also have extensive infiltration of NPD cells in the bone marrow and, thus, all suspected cases should be evaluated enzymatically to confirm the clinical diagnosis by measuring the sphingomyelinase activity level in peripheral leukocytes, cultured fibroblasts, or lymphoblasts, or a combination of these cells. Patients with types A and B NPD have markedly decreased levels (1–10%), whereas patients with types C and D NPD have somewhat decreased sphingomyelinase activities, and patients with Gaucher's disease and other storage disorders presenting with hepatosplenomegaly or neurologic involvement, or both, have normal or near-normal levels of sphingomyelinase activity. The enzymatic identification of NPD carriers is problematic. However, in families in which the specific molecular lesion has been identified, family members can be accurately tested for heterozygote status by DNA analysis. Prenatal diagnosis of NPD can be made reliably by the measurement of sphingomyelinase activity in cultured amniocytes or chorionic villi; molecular analysis of fetal cells can provide the specific diagnosis or serve as a confirmatory test.

Currently, there is no specific *treatment* for NPD. Orthotopic liver transplantation in an infant with type A disease and amniotic cell transplantation in several type B NPD patients have been attempted with little or no success. Bone marrow transplantation in one type B NPD patient was successful in reducing the spleen and liver volumes, the sphingomyelin content in the liver, the number of NPD cells in the marrow, and the radiologic infiltration of the lungs. However, no long-term information is available, as this patient expired 3 mo after transplantation. To date, lung transplantation has not been performed in any severely compromised type B patient.

FABRY DISEASE. This condition is an inborn error of glycosphingolipid metabolism characterized by angiokeratomas (telangiectatic skin lesions), hypohidrosis, corneal and lenticular opacities, acroparesthesias, and vascular disease of the kidney, heart, or brain, or a combination of these organs. The disease is an X-linked recessive trait that is manifested in affected hemizygous males and has an estimated prevalence of 1/40,000. Atypical hemizygous males with residual α-galactosidase A activity may be asymptomatic or have late-onset, mild disease manifestations primarily limited to the heart. Heterozygous females are usually asymptomatic or exhibit mild manifestations.

The disease results from the deficient activity of α-galactosidase A, a lysosomal enzyme encoded by a gene located on the long arm of the X chromosome (Xq22). The enzymatic defect leads to the systemic accumulation of neutral glycosphingolipids, primarily globotriaosylceramide, particularly in the plasma and lysosomes of vascular endothelial and smooth muscle cells. The progressive vascular glycosphingolipid deposition in affected males results in ischemia and infarction, leading to the major disease manifestations. Affected males who have blood group B or AB have a more severe disease course because the blood group B substance also accumulates, as it is normally degraded by α-galactosidase A. The cDNA and genomic sequences encoding α-galactosidase A have been isolated and characterized, and molecular studies have identified a variety of different mutations in the α-galactosidase A gene that are responsible for this lysosomal storage disease, including amino acid substitutions, gene rearrangements, and mRNA splicing defects.

Clinical Manifestations. The angiokeratomas that appear in Fabry disease usually occur in childhood and may lead to early diagnosis. They increase in size and number with age and range from barely visible to several millimeters in diameter.

The lesions are punctate, dark red to blue-black, and flat or slightly raised. They do not blanch with pressure, and the larger ones may show slight hyperkeratosis. Characteristically, the lesions are most dense between the umbilicus and knees, in the "bathing trunk area," but may occur anywhere, including the oral mucosa. The hips, thighs, buttocks, umbilicus, lower abdomen, scrotum, and glans penis are common sites, and there is a tendency toward symmetry. Variants without skin lesions have been described. Sweating is usually decreased or absent. Corneal opacities and characteristic lenticular lesions, observed under slit-lamp examination, are present in affected males as well as in about 70% of asymptomatic heterozygotes. Conjunctival and retinal vascular tortuosity are common and result from the systemic vascular involvement.

Pain is the most debilitating symptom in childhood and adolescence. Fabry crises, lasting from minutes to several days, consist of agonizing, burning pain in the hands and feet and proximal extremities and are usually associated with exercise, fatigue, or fever, or a combination of these factors. These painful acroparesthesias usually become less frequent in the 3rd and 4th decades of life, although in some men they may become more frequent and severe. Attacks of abdominal or flank pain may simulate appendicitis or renal colic.

With increasing age, the major morbid symptoms result from the progressive involvement of the vascular system. Early in the course of the disease, casts, red cells, and lipid inclusions with characteristic birefringent "Maltese crosses" appear in the urinary sediment. Proteinuria, isothenuria, and gradual deterioration of renal function and development of azotemia occur in the 2nd–4th decades. Cardiovascular findings may include hypertension, left ventricular hypertrophy, anginal chest pain, myocardial ischemia or infarction, and heart failure. Mitral insufficiency is the most common valvular lesion. Abnormal electrocardiographic and echocardiographic findings are common. Cerebrovascular manifestations result from multifocal small vessel involvement. Other features may include chronic bronchitis and dyspnea, lymphedema of the legs without hypoproteinemia, episodic diarrhea, osteoporosis, retarded growth, and delayed puberty. Death most often results from uremia or vascular disease of the heart or brain. Prior to hemodialysis or renal transplantation, the mean age of death for affected men was 41 yr. Atypical male variants with residual α-galactosidase A activity who are asymptomatic or mildly affected have been described; several patients with late-onset isolated cardiac or cardiopulmonary disease have been reported without the early classic manifestations. These "cardiac variants" have cardiomegaly, usually involving the left ventricular wall and interventricular septum, and electrocardiographic abnormalities consistent with a cardiomyopathy. Others have had hypertrophic cardiomyopathy or myocardial infarctions, or both.

The *diagnosis* in classically affected males is most readily made from the history of painful acroparesthesias, hypohidrosis, the presence of characteristic skin lesions, and the observation of the characteristic corneal opacities and lenticular lesions. The disorder is often misdiagnosed as rheumatic fever, erythromelalgia, or neurosis. The skin lesions must be differentiated from the benign angiokeratomas of the scrotum (Fordyce disease) or from angiokeratoma circumscriptum. Angiokeratomas identical to those of Fabry disease have been reported in fucosidosis, aspartylglycosaminuria, late-onset GM_1 gangliosidosis, galactosialidosis, α-*N*-acetylgalactosaminidase deficiency, and sialidosis. The diagnosis of the mild cardiac variants should be considered in individuals who present with left ventricular hypertrophy or cardiomyopathy, or both. The diagnosis of classic and variant patients is confirmed biochemically by the demonstration of markedly decreased α-galactosidase A activity in plasma, isolated leukocytes, or cultured fibroblasts or lymphoblasts.

Heterozygous females may have corneal opacities, isolated skin lesions, and intermediate activities of α-galactosidase A in plasma or cell sources. Rare female heterozygotes may have manifestations as severe as those in affected males. However, at-risk females in families affected by Fabry disease who are asymptomatic should be optimally diagnosed by the direct analysis of their family's specific mutation. Prenatal detection of affected males can be accomplished by the demonstration of deficient α-galactosidase A activity or the family's specific gene mutation in chorionic villi obtained in the 1st trimester or in cultured amniocytes obtained by amniocentesis in the 2nd trimester of pregnancy.

Treatment. Phenytoin and carbamazepine have been shown to decrease the frequency and severity of the chronic acroparesthesias and the periodic crises of excruciating pain. Otherwise, treatment of the disease complications is supportive and nonspecific. Renal transplantation and chronic hemodialysis are lifesaving procedures. Replacement therapy using partially purified human enzyme has proved to be biochemically effective in pilot trials. The availability of the cDNA encoding human α galactosidase A has permitted the expression of sufficient quantities of recombinantly produced active enzyme, and trials of enzyme replacement therapy are under way.

FUCOSIDOSIS. Fucosidosis is a rare, autosomal recessive disorder that results from the deficient activity of α-fucosidase and the accumulation of fucose-containing glycosphingolipids, glycoproteins, and oligosaccharides in the lysosomes of the liver, brain, and other organs. The α-fucosidase gene has been localized to chromosome 1 (1p24), and specific mutations have been identified. Although the disorder is panethnic, most affected patients have been from Italy and the United States. There is wide variability in the clinical phenotype, with the most severely affected patients presenting in the 1st yr of life with developmental delay and somatic features similar to those of the mucopolysacharidoses. These features include frontal bossing, hepatosplenomegaly, coarse facial features, and macroglossia. The central nervous system storage results in a relentless neurodegenerative course with death in childhood. Patients with milder disease have angiokeratomata and longer survival. No specific therapy exists for the disorder, which can be diagnosed by the demonstration of deficient α-fucosidase activity in peripheral leukocytes or cultured fibroblasts. Carrier identification studies and prenatal diagnosis are possible by determination of the enzymatic activity.

SCHINDLER DISEASE. This disease is an autosomal recessive neurodegenerative disorder that results from the deficient activity of α-*N*-acetylgalactosaminidase and the accumulation of sialylated and asialoglycopeptides and oligosaccharides. The gene for the enzyme has been cloned and mapped to chromosome 22 (22q13.1–13.2). The disease is clinically heterogeneous, and two major phenotypes have been identified. Type 1 disease is an infantile-onset neuroaxonal dystrophy. Affected infants have normal development for the first 9–15 mo of life followed by a rapid neurodegenerative course that results in severe psychomotor retardation, cortical blindness, and frequent myoclonic seizures. Type II disease is characterized by a variable age of onset, mild retardation, and angiokeratomata. There is no specific therapy for either form of the disorder. The diagnosis is by demonstration of the enzymatic deficiency in white blood cells or cultured skin fibroblasts

METACHROMATIC LEUKODYSTROPHY. Metachromatic leukodystrophy (MLD) is an autosomal recessive white matter disease caused by a deficiency of arylsulfatase A (ASA), which is required for the hydrolysis of sulfated glycosphingolipids (also see Chapter 608). An additional form of MLD is caused by a deficiency of a sphingolipid activator protein (SAP1), a protein required for the formation of substrate enzyme complex. The deficiency of this enzymatic activity results in the white matter storage of sulfated glycosphingolipids, which leads to demyelination and a neurodegenerative course. The ASA gene has been localized to chromosome 22 (22q13.31qter), and specific mutations have been identified that fall into two groups that correlate with disease severity.

Clinical Manifestations. The late infantile form of MLD, which is most common, usually presents between 12 and 18 mo of age with irritability, inability to walk, and hyperextension of the knee causing genu recurvatum. Deep tendon reflexes are diminished or absent. Gradual muscle wasting, weakness, and hypotonia become evident and lead to a debilitated state. As the disease progresses, nystagmus, myoclonic seizures, optic atrophy, and quadriparesis appear, with death in the 1st decade of life. The juvenile form of the disorder has a more indolent course with onset which may occur as late as 20 yr of age. This form of the disease presents with gait disturbances, mental deterioration, urinary incontinence, and emotional difficulties. The adult form, which presents after the 2nd decade, is similar to the juvenile form in its clinical manifestations, although the emotional difficulties and psychosis are more prominent features. Dementia, seizures, diminished reflexes, and optic atrophy also occur in both the juvenile and adult forms. The pathologic hallmark of MLD is the deposition of metachromatic bodies, which stain strongly positive with periodic acid–Schiff and alcian blue, in the white matter of the brain. Neuronal inclusions may be seen in the midbrain, pons, medulla, retina, and spinal cord; demyelination occurs in the peripheral nervous system. Attempts to treat patients with MLD with bone marrow transplantation have resulted in normal enzymatic levels in peripheral blood, but no clear evidence for clinical efficacy in terms of the neurologic course; supportive care remains the primary intervention.

The *diagnosis* of MLD should be suspected in patients with the clinical features of leukodystrophy. Decreased nerve conduction velocities, increased cerebrospinal fluid protein, metachromatic deposits in biopsied segments of sural nerve, and metachromatic granules in urinary sediment are all suggestive of MLD. Confirmation of the diagnosis is based on the demonstration of the reduced activity of ASA in leukocytes or cultured skin fibroblasts. Sphingolipid activator protein deficiency is diagnosed by measuring the concentration of SAP1 in cultured fibroblasts using a specific antibody to the protein. Carrier detection and prenatal diagnosis is available for all forms of the disorder.

MULTIPLE SULFATASE DEFICIENCY. This is an autosomal recessive disorder that results from the deficiency of three enzymatic activities: arylsulfatases A, B, and C. The underlying cause of the disorder remains unknown. Sulfatides, mucopolysaccharides, steroid sulfates, and gangliosides accumulate in the cerebral cortex and visceral tissues, resulting in a clinical phenotype with features of leukodystrophy as well as those of the mucopolysaccharidoses. Severe ichthyosis also may occur. Carrier testing and prenatal diagnosis by measurement of the enzymatic activities can be performed. There is no specific treatment for multiple sulfatase deficiency other than supportive care.

KRABBE DISEASE. This condition, also called *globoid cell leukodystrophy,* is an autosomal recessive fatal disorder of infancy. It results from the deficiency of the enzymatic activity of galactocerebrosidase and the white matter accumulation of galactosylceramide, which is normally found almost exclusively in the myelin sheath. The galactocerebrosidase gene has been localized to chromosome 14 (14q31), and specific disease-causing mutations have been identified. The infantile form of Krabbe disease is rapidly progressive and presents in early infancy with irritability, seizures, and hypertonia. Optic atrophy is evident in the 1st yr of life, and mental development is severely impaired. As the disease progresses, optic atrophy and severe developmental delay become apparent; affected children exhibit opisthotonos and die before 3 yr of age. A second, late infantile form of Krabbe disease also exists and presents after the age of 2 yr. Affected individuals have a disease course similar to that of the early infantile form. Bone marrow transplantation has been attempted in several patients with later onset disease but without significant results. There is no therapy available for this disorder. The diagnosis of Krabbe disease relies on the demonstration of the specific enzymatic deficiency in white blood cells or cultured skin fibroblasts. Carrier identification and prenatal diagnosis are possible.

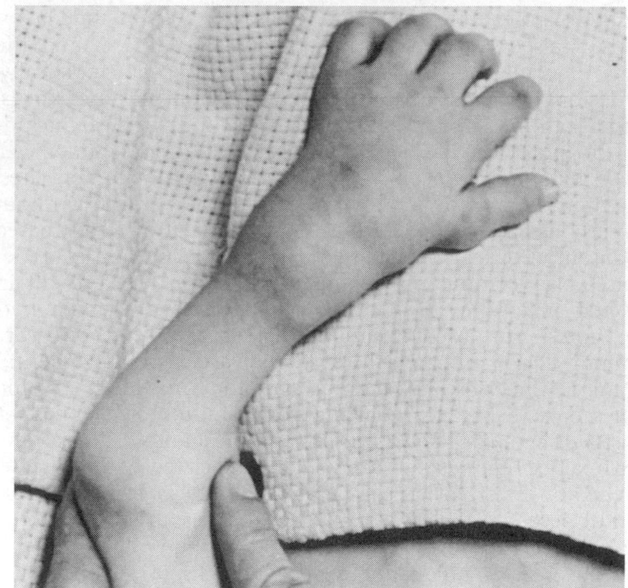

Figure 83–11 A forearm of an 18-mo-old girl with Farber disease. Note the painful joint swelling and the nodule formation. The infant was suspected of having rheumatoid arthritis.

FARBER DISEASE. This is an autosomal recessive disorder that results from the deficiency of the lysosomal enzyme, ceramidase, and the accumulation of ceramide in various tissues, especially the joints. Symptoms can begin as early as the 1st yr of life with painful joint swelling and nodule formation (Fig. 83–11), which is sometimes diagnosed as rheumatoid arthritis. As the disease progresses, nodule or granulomatous formation on the vocal cords can lead to hoarseness and breathing difficulties; failure to thrive is common. In some patients, moderate central nervous system dysfunction is present. Patients may die from recurrent pneumonias in their teens; there is currently no specific therapy. The diagnosis of this disorder should be suspected in patients who have nodule formation over the joints but no other findings of rheumatoid arthritis. In such patients, ceramidase activity should be determined in cultured skin fibroblasts or white blood cells. Carrier detection and prenatal diagnosis are available.

WOLMAN DISEASE AND CHOLESTEROL ESTER DISEASE (CESD). Wolman disease and cholesterol ester storage disease are autosomal recessive lysosomal storage diseases that result from the deficiency of acid lipase and the accumulation of cholesterol esters and triglycerides in histiocytic foam cells of most of the visceral organs. The gene for lysosomal acid lipase has been cloned and mapped to chromosome 10 (10q24q25). Wolman disease is the more severe clinical phenotype and is a fatal disorder of infancy. The clinical features of the disease become apparent in the 1st wk of life and include failure to thrive, relentless vomiting, abdominal distention, steatorrhea, and hepatosplenomegaly. There usually is hyperlipidemia. Hepatic dysfunction and fibrosis may occur. Calcification of the adrenal glands is pathognomonic for the disorder. Death usually occurs within 6 mo. Cholesterol ester storage disease is a less severe disorder that may not be diagnosed until adulthood. Hepatomegaly can be the only detectable abnormality, but affected individuals are at significant risk for premature atherosclerosis. Adrenal calcification is not a feature. Diagnosis and carrier identification are based on measuring acid lipase activity in white blood cells or cultured skin fibroblasts. Prenatal diagnosis depends on measuring decreased enzyme levels in cultured chorionic villi or amniocytes. There is no specific therapy available for either disorder, although the use of pharmacologic agents to suppress cholesterol synthesis in combination with cholestyramine and diet modification have been used in patients with cholesterol ester storage disease (see Chapter 83.3).

Barton NW, Brady RO, Dambrosia JM, et al: Replacement therapy for inherited enzyme deficiency: Macrophage targeted glucocerebrosidase for Gaucher disease. N Engl J Med 324:1464, 1991.
Dawson A, Elias DJ, Rubenson D, et al: Pulmonary hypertension developing after α-glucerase therapy in two patients with type 1 Gaucher disease complicated by hepatopulmonary syndrome. Ann Intern Med 125:901, 1996.
Emery AE, Rimoin DL (eds): Principles and Practice of Medical Genetics, 3rd ed. London, Churchill Livingstone, 1996.
Jan MMS, Camfield PR: Nova Scotia Niemann-Pick disease (type D): Clinical study of 20 cases. J Child Neurol 13:75, 1998.
Johnson WG: The clinical spectrum of hexosaminidase deficiency diseases. Neurology 31:1453, 1981.
NIH Technology Assessment Panel on Gaucher Disease: Gaucher disease: Current issues in diagnosis and treatment. JAMA 275:548, 1996.
Rosenberg RN, Prusiner SB, DiMauro S, et al (eds): The Molecular and Genetic Basis of Neurological Disease. Boston, Butterworth-Heinemann, 1993.
Scriver CR, Beaudet AL, Sly WS, Valle D (eds): The Metabolic Basis of Inherited Disease, 7th ed. New York, McGraw Hill, 1995.
Zimran A, Gross E, West C, et al: Prediction of Gaucher's disease by identification at DNA level. Lancet 2:349, 1989.

83.5 *Mucolipidoses*

Margaret M. McGovern and Robert J. Desnick

I-cell disease (mucolipidosis II, ML-II) and pseudo-Hurler polydystrophy (mucolipidosis III, ML-III) are biochemically related, rare autosomal recessive disorders that share some clinical features with Hurler syndrome. Both diseases result from the abnormal transport of newly synthesized lysosomal enzymes that are normally targeted to the lysosome by the presence of mannose-6-phosphate residues and are recognized by specific lysosomal membrane receptors. These mannose-6-phosphate recognition markers are synthesized in a two-step reaction that occurs in the Golgi apparatus and is mediated by two enzymatic activities. The enzyme that catalyzes the first step, UDP-*N*-acetylglucosamine:lysosomal enzymes *N*-acetylglucosamine-1-phosphotransferase, is defective in both ML-II and ML-III. This enzyme deficiency results in abnormal targeting of the lysosomal enzymes, which are then secreted into the extracellular matrix. Because the lysosomal enzymes require the acidic medium of the lysosome to function, patients with this defect accumulate a variety of different substrates due to the cellular deficiency of all lysosomal enzymes. The diagnosis of ML-II and ML-III can be made by the determination of the serum lysosomal enzymatic activities, which are elevated, or by the demonstration of reduced enzymatic levels in cultured skin fibroblasts. Direct measurement of the phosphotransferase activity is possible. Prenatal diagnosis and carrier identification studies are available for both disorders by measurement of lysosomal enzymatic activities in cultured cells.

I-CELL DISEASE. I-cell disease shares many of the *clinical manifestations* of Hurler syndrome, although there is no mucopolysachariduria and the presentation is earlier. Some patients have clinical features evident at birth, including coarse facial features, craniofacial abnormalities, restricted joint movement, and hypotonia. Nonimmune hydrops may be present in the fetus. The remainder of patients present in the 1st yr with severe psychomotor retardation, coarse facial features, and skeletal manifestations that include kyphoscoliosis and a lumbar gibbus. Patients also may have congenital dislocation of the hips, inguinal hernias, and gingival hypertrophy. Progressive, severe psychomotor retardation leads to death in early childhood. There is no *treatment* available.

PSEUDO-HURLER POLYDYSTROPHY. Pseudo-Hurler polydystrophy is a less severe disorder, with later onset and survival to adulthood reported. Affected children may present around the age of 4 or 5 yr with joint stiffness and short stature. Progressive destruction of the hip joints and moderate dysostosis multiplex are evident. Radiographic evidence of low iliac wings, flattening of the proximal femoral epiphyses with valgus deformity of the femoral head, and hypoplasia of the anterior third of the lumbar vertebrae are characteristic findings. Ophthalmic findings include corneal clouding, retinopathy, and astigmatism; visual complaints are uncommon. Some patients have learning disabilities or mental retardation. Treatment, which should include orthopedic care, is symptomatic.

Matsuda I, Arashuma S, Mitsuyama T, et al: Prenatal diagnosis of I-cell disease. Hun Genet 30:69, 1975.
Scriver CR, Beaudet AL, Sly WS, Valle D (eds): The Metabolic Basis of Inherited Disease, 7th ed. New York, McGraw Hill, 1995.
Varki A, Reitman ML, Vannier A, et al: Demonstration of the heterozygous state for I-cell disease and pseudo-Hurler polydystrophy by assay of N-acetylglucosaminylphosphotransferase in white blood cells and fibroblasts. Am J Hum Genet 34:719, 1982.

CHAPTER 84
Defects in Metabolism of Carbohydrates

Yuan-Tsong Chen

Carbohydrate synthesis and degradation provide the energy required for most metabolic processes. The important carbohydrates include three monosaccharides—glucose, galactose, and fructose—and a polysaccharide, glycogen. The relevant biochemical pathways of these carbohydrates are shown in Figure 84–1. Glucose is the principal substrate of energy metabolism in humans. A continuous source of glucose from dietary intake, gluconeogenesis, and degradation of glycogen maintains normal blood glucose levels. Metabolism of glucose generates adenosine triphosphage (ATP) via glycolysis (conversion of glucose or glycogen to pyruvate) or mitochondria oxidative phosphorylation (conversion of pyruvate to carbon dioxide and water), or both. Dietary sources of glucose come from ingesting polysaccharides, primarily starch, and disaccharides, including lactose, maltose, and sucrose. Oral intake of glucose is intermittent and unreliable. Glucose made de novo (gluconeogenesis) contributes to maintaining the euglycemic state, but this process requires time to be active. The breakdown of hepatic glycogen provides the rapid release of glucose, which maintains a constant blood glucose concentration. Glycogen is also the primary stored energy source in muscle, providing glucose for muscle activity during exercise. Galactose and fructose are monosaccharides that provide fuel for cellular metabolism; their role is much less significant than that of glucose. Galactose is derived from lactose (galactose + glucose), which is found in milk and milk products. Galactose may be incorporated into glycogen and becomes a source of glucose. Galactose is also an important component for certain glycolipids, glycoproteins, and glycosaminoglycans. The two dietary sources of fructose are sucrose (fructose + glucose) and fructose itself, which is found in fruits, vegetables, and honey.

Defects in glycogen metabolism typically cause an accumulation of glycogen in the tissues; hence, the name *glycogen storage disease* (Table 84–1). Defects in gluconeogenesis or the glyco-

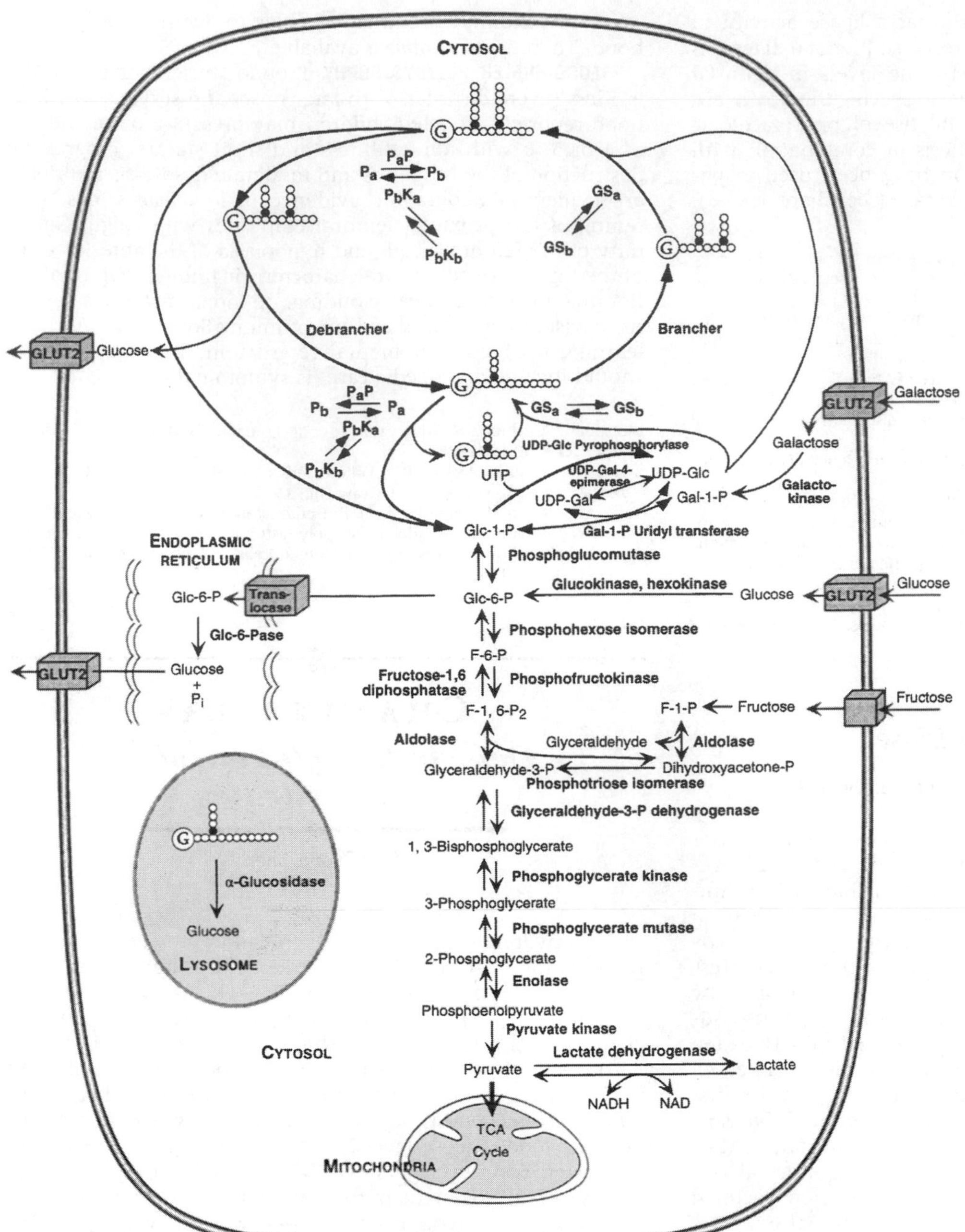

Figure 84–1 Pathway related to glycogen storage diseases and galactose and fructose disorders. Nonstandard abbreviation are as follows: GS_a, active glycogen synthetase; GS_b, inactive glycogen synthetase; P_a, active phosphorylase; P_b, inactive phosphorylase; P_aP, phosphorylase a phosphatase; P_bK_a, active phosphorylase b kinase; P_bK_b, inactive phosphorylase b kinase; G, glycogenin, the primer protein for glycogen synthesis. (Modified from AR Beaudet: Glycogen storage disease. *In:* Isselbacher KJ et al (eds): Harrison's Principles of Internal Medicine, 13th ed. New York, McGraw-Hill, 1994.)

lytic pathway, including galactose and fructose metabolism, do not result in an accumulation of glycogen (see Table 84–1). The defects in pyruvate metabolism in the pathway of the conversion of pyruvate to carbon dioxide and water via mitochondrial oxidative phosphorylation are often associated with lactic acidosis and tissue glycogen accumulation.

Clinical manifestations of disorders of carbohydrate metabolism differ markedly. The symptoms range from harmless to lethal. Dietary therapy has been effective in many of the carbohydrate disorders. Almost all the genes responsible for the inherited defects of carbohydrate metabolism have been cloned and mutations identified.

84.1 Glycogen Storage Diseases

Glycogen storage diseases are inherited disorders affecting glycogen metabolism. Virtually all enzymes involved in the synthesis or degradation of glycogen and its regulation cause some type of glycogen storage disease (see Fig. 84–1). The glycogen found in these disorders is abnormal in either quantity or quality, or in both. The different forms of glycogen storage disease have been categorized by numeric type in accordance with the chronologic order in which these enzymatic defects were identified. This numeric classification is still widely used, at least up to number VII. The glycogen storage diseases can also be classified by organ involvement and clinical manifestations into liver and muscle glycogenoses (Table 84–1).

More than 12 forms of glycogenoses are known at present. Glucose-6-phosphatase deficiency (type I), lysosomal acid α-glucosidase deficiency (type II), debrancher deficiency (type III), and liver phosphorylase kinase deficiency are the most common forms that present in early childhood; myophorphorylase deficiency (type V, McArdle disease) is the most common in adults. The frequency of all forms of glycogen storage disease is approximately 1/20,000 live births.

TABLE 84–1 Features of the Disorders of Carbohydrate Metabolism

Disorders	Basic Defects	Clinical Presentation	Comments
Liver Glycogenoses			
Type/Common Name			
Ia/Von Gierke	Glucose-6-phosphatase	Growth retardation, hepatomegaly, hypoglycemia; elevated blood lactate, cholesterol, triglyceride, and uric acid levels	Common, severe hypoglycemia
Ib	Glucose-6-phosphate translocase	Same as type Ia, with additional findings of neutropenia and impaired neutrophil function	10% of type Ia
II/Pompe			
Infantile	Acid maltase (acid α-glucosidase)	Cardiomegaly, hypotonia, hepatomegaly; onset: birth–6 mo	Common, cardiorespiratory failure leading to death by age 2 yr
Juvenile	Acid maltase (acid α-glucosidase)	Myopathy, variable cardiomyopathy; onset: childhood	Residual enzyme activity
Adult	Acid maltase (acid α-glucosidase)	Myopathy, respiratory insufficiency; onset: adulthood	Residual enzyme activity
IIIa/Cori or Forbes	Liver and muscle debrancher deficiency (amylo, 1,6 glucosidase)	Childhood: hepatomegaly, growth retardation, muscle weakness, hypoglycemia, hyperlipidemia, elevated transaminase levels; liver symptoms improve with age	Common, intermediate severity of hypoglycemia
IIIb	Liver debrancher deficiency; normal muscle enzyme activity	Liver symptoms same as in type IIIa; no muscle symptoms	15% of type III
IV/Andersen	Branching enzyme	Failure to thrive, hypotonia, hepatomegaly, splenomegaly, progressive cirrhosis (death usually before 5th yr), elevated transaminase levels	Rare neuromuscular variants exist
VI/Hers	Liver phosphorylase	Hepatomegaly, mild hypoglycemia, hyperlipidemia, and ketosis	Rare, benign glycogenosis
Phosphorylase kinase deficiency	Phosphorylase kinase	Hepatomegaly, mild hypoglycemia, hyperlipidemia, and ketosis	Common, benign glycogenosis
Glycogen synthetase deficiency	Glycogen synthetase	Early morning drowsiness and fatigue, fasting hypoglycemia, and ketosis	Decreased liver glycogen store
Fanconi-Bickel syndrome	Glucose transporter-2 (GLUT-2)	Failure to thrive, rickets, hepatorenomegaly, proximal renal tubular dysfunction, impaired glucose and galactose utilization	GLUT-2 expressed in liver, kidney, pancreas, and intestine
Muscle Glycogenoses			
Type/Common Name			
V/McArdle	Myophosphorylase	Exercise intolerance, muscle cramps, increased fatigability	Common, male predominance
VII/Tarui	Phosphofructokinase	Exercise intolerance, muscle cramps, hemolytic anemia, myoglobinuria	Prevalent in Japanese and Ashkenazi Jews
Phosphoglycerate kinase deficiency	Phosphoglycerate kinase	As with type V	Rare, X-linked
Phosphoglycerate mutase deficiency	M subunit of phosphoglycerate mutase	As with type V	Rare, majority of patients are African-American
Lactate dehydrogenase deficiency	M subunit of lactate dehydrogenase	As with type V	Rare
Galactose Disorders			
Galactosemia with transferase deficiency	Galactose-1-phosphate uridyltransferase	Vomiting, hepatomegaly, cataracts, amino aciduria, failure to thrive	African-American patients tend to have milder symptoms
Galactokinase deficiency	Galactokinase	Cataracts	Benign
Generalized uridine diphosphate galactose 4-epimerase deficiency	Uridine diphosphate galactose 4-epimerase	Similar to transferase deficiency with additional findings of hypotonia and nerve deafness	A benign variant exists
Fructose Disorders			
Essential fructosuria	Fructokinase	Urine reducing substance	Benign
Hereditary fructose intolerance	Fructose 1-phosphate aldolase	Acute: vomiting, sweating, lethargy Chronic: failure to thrive, hepatic failure	Prognosis good with fructose restriction
Disorders of Gluconeogenesis			
Fructose 1,6-diphosphatase deficiency	Fructose 1,6-disphosphatase	Episodic hypoglycemia, apnea, acidosis	Good prognosis, avoid fasting
Phosphoenolpyruvate carboxykinase deficiency	Phosphoenolpyruvate carboxykinase	Hypoglycemia, hepatomegaly, hypotonia, failure to thrive	Rare

Table continued on following page

TABLE 84–1 Features of the Disorders of Carbohydrate Metabolism *Continued*

Disorders	Basic Defects	Clinical Presentation	Comments
Disorders of Pyruvate Metabolism			
Pyruvate dehydrogenase complex defect	Pyruvate dehydrogenase	Severe fatal neonatal to mild late onset, lactic acidosis, psychomotor retardation, and failure to thrive	Most commonly due to E1 α-subunit defect X-linked
Pyruvate carboxylase deficiency	Pyruvate carboxylase	Same as above	Rare, autosomal recessive
Respiratory chain defects (oxidative phosphorylation disease)	Complex I to V, many mitochondrial DNA mutations	Heterogeneous with multisystem involvement	Mitochondrial inheritance
Other Carbohydrate Disorders			
Pentosuria	L-Xylulose reductase	Urine reducing substance	Benign

Liver Glycogenoses

The glycogen storage diseases that principally affect the liver include glucose-6-phosphatase deficiency (type I), debranching enzyme deficiency (type III), branching enzyme deficiency (type IV), liver phosphorylase deficiency (type VI), phosphorylase kinase deficiency (formerly type VIa or IX), glycogen synthetase deficiency, and glucose transporter-2 defect. Because carbohydrate metabolism in the liver is responsible for plasma glucose homeostasis, this group of disorders typically cause fasting hypoglycemia and hepatomegaly. Some (type III, type IV) are also associated with hepatic cirrhosis. Other organs besides the liver may also be involved, for example, renal dysfunction in type I and myopathy in types III and IV as well as in some rare forms of phosphorylase kinase deficiency.

TYPE I GLYCOGEN STORAGE DISEASE (GLUCOSE-6-PHOSPHATASE OR TRANSLOCASE DEFICIENCY, VON GIERKE DISEASE)

Type I glycogen storage disease is due to the absence or deficiency of glucose-6-phosphatase activity in the liver, kidney, and intestinal mucosa. It can be divided into two subtypes: type Ia, in which the glucose 6-phosphatase enzyme is defective, and type Ib, in which a translocase that transports glucose-6-phosphate across the microsomal membrane is defective. The defects in both type Ia and type Ib lead to inadequate hepatic conversion of glucose-6-phosphate to glucose and thus make affected individuals susceptible to fasting hypoglycemia.

Type I glycogen storage disease is an autosomal recessive disorder. The structure gene for glucose-6-phosphatase is on chromosome 17 and the gene for translocase is on chromosome 11q23. Common mutations responsible for the disease have been identified. Carrier detection and prenatal diagnosis are possible with the DNA-based diagnosis.

CLINICAL MANIFESTATIONS. Patients with type I glycogen storage disease may present in the neonatal period with hypoglycemia and lactic acidosis; however, they more commonly present at 3–4 mo of age with hepatomegaly or hypoglycemic seizures, or both. These children often have doll-like faces with fat cheeks, relatively thin extremities, short stature, and a protuberant abdomen that is due to massive hepatomegaly; the kidneys are also enlarged, whereas the spleen and heart are normal.

The hallmarks of the disease are hypoglycemia, lactic acidosis, hyperuricemia, and hyperlipidemia. Hypoglycemia and lactic acidosis can develop after a short fast. Hyperuricemia is present in young children; gout rarely develops before puberty. Despite marked hepatomegaly, the liver transaminase levels are usually normal or only slightly elevated. Intermittent diarrhea may occur (the mechanism is unknown). Easy bruising and epistaxis are common and are associated with a prolonged bleeding time as a result of impaired platelet aggregation and adhesion.

The plasma may be "milky" in appearance as a result of a striking elevation of triglyceride levels. Cholesterol and phospholipids are also elevated, but less prominently. The lipid abnormality resembles type IV hyperlipidemia and is characterized by increased levels of very low density lipoprotein, low-density lipoprotein, and a unique apolipoprotein profile consisting of increased levels of apo B, C, and E, with relatively normal or reduced levels of apo A and D. The histologic appearance of the liver is characterized by a universal distention of hepatocytes by glycogen and fat. The lipid vacuoles are particularly large and prominent. There is little associated fibrosis.

All these findings apply to both type Ia and type Ib glycogen storage disease, but type Ib has additional features of recurrent bacterial infections due to neutropenia and impaired neutrophil function. Oral and intestinal mucosa ulceration is common, and inflammatory bowel disease may occur.

Although type I glycogen storage disease affects mainly the liver, multiple organ systems are involved. Symptoms of gout usually start around puberty owing to the long-term hyperuricemia. Puberty is often delayed, but fertility appears to be normal. Hypertriglyceridemia causes an increased risk of pancreatitis, but premature atherosclerosis has not been documented. Impaired platelet aggregation may function as a protective mechanism to help reduce the risk of atherosclerosis.

By the 2nd or 3rd decade of life, most patients with type I glycogen storage disease exhibit hepatic adenomas that can hemorrhage and in rare cases may become malignant. Other complications include pulmonary hypertension and osteoporosis.

Renal disease is a late complication, and most patients with type I glycogen storage disease older than age 20 yr have proteinuria. Many also have hypertension, renal stones, nephrocalcinosis, and altered creatinine clearance. Glomerular hyperfiltration, increased renal plasma flow, and microalbuminuria are often found in the early stages of renal dysfunction and can occur before the onset of proteinuria. In younger patients, hyperfiltration and hyperperfusion may be the only signs of renal abnormalities. With the advancement of renal disease, focal segmental glomerulosclerosis and interstitial fibrosis become evident. In some patients, renal function has deteriorated and progressed to failure, requiring dialysis and transplantation. Other renal abnormalities include amyloidosis, a Fanconi-like syndrome, and a distal renal tubular acidification defect.

DIAGNOSIS. The diagnosis of type I glycogen storage disease can be suspected on the basis of clinical presentation and abnormal lactate and lipid values. Administration of glucagon or epinephrine results in little or no rise in blood glucose, but the lactate level rises significantly. A definitive diagnosis requires a liver biopsy to demonstrate either a deficiency of glucose-6-phosphatase activity or of translocase. Identification of the mutations for glucose-6-phosphatase or the translocase gene allows a noninvasive diagnostic method for a majority of patients with type I glycogen storage disease.

TREATMENT. This is designed to maintain normal blood glucose levels and is achieved by continuous nasogastric infusion of glucose or oral administration of uncooked cornstarch. Nasogastric drip feeding can be introduced in early infancy from the time of diagnosis. It may consist of an elemental enteral formula, or it may contain only glucose or glucose polymer to provide sufficient glucose to maintain normoglycemia during the night. Frequent feedings with high carbohydrate content are given during the day.

Uncooked cornstarch acts as a slow-release form of glucose and can be introduced at a dose of 1.6 g/kg every 4 hr for infants younger than 2 yr of age. The response of young infants is variable. As the child grows older, the cornstarch regimen can be changed to every 6 hr at a dose of 1.75 to 2.5 g/kg of body weight. Because fructose and galactose cannot be converted directly to glucose, their dietary intake should be restricted, and dietary supplements of multivitamins and calcium are required. Allopurinol is given to lower the levels of uric acid. In patients with type Ib glycogen storage disease, granulocyte and granulocyte-macrophage colony-stimulating factors are successful in correcting the neutropenia, decreasing the number and severity of bacterial infections, and improving the chronic inflammatory bowel disease.

Prior to surgery, the bleeding status should be evaluated, and good metabolic control should be established. Prolonged bleeding times can be normalized by the use of intensive intravenous glucose infusion for 24–48 hr prior to surgery. Use of 1-deamino-8-D-arginine vasopressin can reduce bleeding complications. Lactated Ringer's solution should be avoided because it contains lactate and no glucose. Glucose levels should be maintained in the normal range throughout surgery with the use of 10% dextrose.

PROGNOSIS. Previously, patients with type I glycogen storage disease died, and the prognosis was guarded for those who survived. The long-term complications discussed previously occur mostly in adults whose disease was not adequately treated during childhood. Early diagnosis and effective treatment have improved the outcome; it remains unknown if all long-term complications can be avoided through good metabolic control.

TYPE III GLYCOGEN STORAGE DISEASE (DEBRANCHER DEFICIENCY, LIMIT DEXTRINOSIS)

Type III glycogen storage disease is caused by a deficiency of glycogen debranching enzyme activity. Debranching enzymes together with phosphorylase are responsible for complete degradation of glycogen; when debranching enzyme is defective, glycogen breakdown is incomplete, and an abnormal glycogen with short outer branch chains and resembling limit dextrin accumulates.

Type III glycogenosis is an autosomal recessive disease that has been reported in many different ethnic groups; the frequency is relatively high in non-Ashkenazic Jews of North African extraction. The gene for debranching enzyme is located on chromosome 1p21. Carrier detection and prenatal diagnosis are possible using DNA-based linkage or mutation analysis.

Deficiency of glycogen debranching enzyme causes hepatomegaly, hypoglycemia, short stature, variable skeletal myopathy, and cardiomyopathy. The disorder usually involves both liver and muscle and is termed *type IIIa glycogen storage disease.* However, in about 15% of patients, the disease appears to involve only liver and is classified as type IIIb (Fig. 84–2).

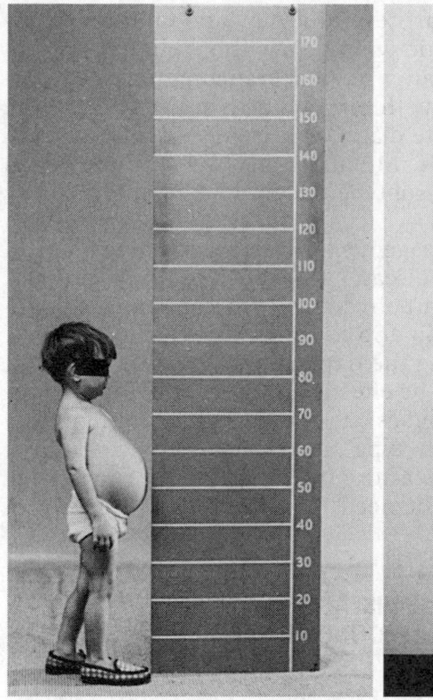

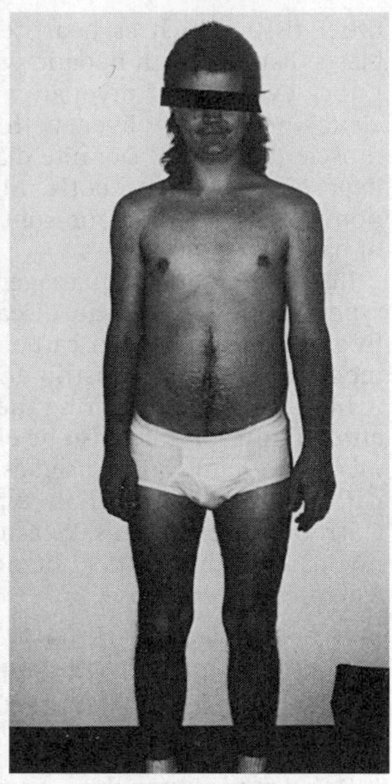

Figure 84–2 Growth and development in a patient with type IIIb glycogen storage disease. The patient has debrancher deficiency in liver but normal activity in muscle. As a child he had hepatomegaly, hypoglycemia, and growth retardation. After puberty, he no longer had hepatomegaly or hypoglycemia, and his final adult height is normal. He has no muscle weakness or atrophy; this is in contrast to type IIIa patients, in whom a progressive myopathy is seen in adulthood.

CLINICAL MANIFESTATIONS. During infancy and childhood, the disease may be indistinguishable from type I glycogen storage disease, as hepatomegaly, hypoglycemia, hyperlipidemia, and growth retardation are common features. Splenomegaly may be present, but the kidney is not enlarged in type III. Remarkably, hepatomegaly and hepatic symptoms in most type III glycogen storage disease improve with age and usually disappear after puberty. Overt liver cirrhosis may occur, especially in Japanese patients. In patients with muscular involvement (type IIIa), muscle weakness is usually minimal during childhood but can become severe after the 3rd or 4th decade as evidenced by slowly progressive weakness and muscle wasting. Electromyography changes are consistent with a widespread myopathy; nerve conduction studies may be abnormal. Ventricular hypertrophy is frequent, but overt cardiac dysfunction is rare. Hepatic symptoms in some patients may be so mild that the diagnosis is not made until adulthood, when the patients show symptoms and signs of neuromuscular disease.

Hypoglycemia and hyperlipidemia are common. In contrast to type I glycogen storage disease, elevation of liver transaminase levels and fasting ketosis are prominent, but blood lactate and uric acid concentrations are usually normal. The administration of glucagon 2 hr after a carbohydrate meal provokes a normal rise of blood glucose, but after an overnight fast, glucagon may provoke no change in blood glucose. Serum creatine kinase levels may be useful to identify patients with muscle involvement, but normal levels do not rule out muscle enzyme deficiency.

DIAGNOSIS. The histologic appearance of the liver is characterized by a universal distention of hepatocytes by glycogen and the presence of fibrous septa. The fibrosis and the paucity of fat distinguish type III glycogenosis from type I. The fibrosis, which ranges from minimal periportal fibrosis to micronodular cirrhosis, in most cases appears to be nonprogressive.

Patients with myopathy and liver symptoms have a generalized enzyme defect (type IIIa). The deficient enzyme activity can be demonstrated not only in liver and muscle but also in other tissues such as heart, erythrocytes, and cultured fibroblasts. Patients with hepatic symptoms without clinical or laboratory evidence of myopathy have debranching enzyme deficiency only in the liver, with enzyme activity retained in the muscle (type IIIb). Definite diagnosis requires enzyme assay in liver or muscle, or both. Mutation analysis can provide a noninvasive method for subtype assignment in the majority of patients.

TREATMENT. Dietary management is less demanding than in type I glycogen storage disease. If hypoglycemia is present, frequent meals high in carbohydrates with cornstarch supplements or nocturnal gastric drip feedings are usually effective. A high-protein diet during the daytime plus overnight protein enteral infusion may also be effective in preventing hypoglycemia, as protein can be used as substrate for gluconeogenesis, a pathway that is intact in type III glycogen storage disease. Currently, there is no satisfactory treatment for the progressive myopathy. Patients do not need to restrict dietary intake of fructose and galactose.

TYPE IV GLYCOGEN STORAGE DISEASE (BRANCHING ENZYME DEFICIENCY AMYLOPECTINOSIS OR ANDERSEN DISEASE)

Deficiency of branching enzyme activity results in accumulation of an abnormal glycogen with poor solubility. The disease is referred to as type IV glycogen storage disease or amylopectinosis because the abnormal glycogen has fewer branch points, more α1–4 linked glucose units, and longer outer chains, resulting in a structure resembling amylopectin.

Type IV glycogen storage disease is an autosomal recessive disorder. The glycogen branching enzyme gene is located on chromosome 3p14. Mutations responsible for type IV glycogen storage disease have been identified, and their characterization in individual patients may be useful in predicting the clinical outcome.

CLINICAL MANIFESTATIONS. This disorder is clinically variable. The most common and classic form is characterized by progressive cirrhosis of the liver and is manifested in the first 18 mo of life as hepatosplenomegaly and failure to thrive. The cirrhosis progresses to portal hypertension, ascites, esophageal varices, and liver failure that leads to death by 5 yr of age. Rare patients survive without progression of liver disease.

A neuromuscular form of the disease has been reported. These patients may (1) present at birth with severe hypotonia, muscle atrophy, and neuronal involvement with death in the neonatal period; (2) present in late childhood with myopathy or cardiomyopathy; or (3) present as adults with diffuse central and peripheral nervous system dysfunction accompanied by accumulation of polyglucosan body disease in the nervous system (so-called adult polyglucosan body disease). For adult polyglucosan disease, leukocyte or nerve biopsy is needed to establish the diagnosis, as the branching enzyme deficiency is limited to those tissues.

DIAGNOSIS. Tissue disposition of amylopectin-like materials can be demonstrated in liver, heart, muscle, skin, intestine, brain, spinal cord, and peripheral nerve. The hepatic histologic findings are characterized by micronodular cirrhosis and faintly stained basophilic inclusions in the hepatocytes. The inclusions consist of coarsely clumped, stored material that is periodic acid–Schiff–positive and partially resistant to diastase digestion. Electron microscopy shows, in addition to the conventional α and β glycogen particles, accumulation of the fibrillar aggregations that are typical of amylopectin. The distinct staining properties of the cytoplasmic inclusions, as well as electron microscopic findings, could be diagnostic. However, polysaccharidoses with histologic features reminiscent of type IV disease, but without enzymatic correlation, have been observed. The definitive diagnosis rests on the demonstration of the deficient branching enzyme activity in liver, muscle, cultured skin fibroblasts, or leukocytes. Prenatal diagnosis is possible by measuring the enzyme activity in cultured amniocytes or chorionic villi.

TREATMENT. There is no specific treatment for type IV glycogen storage disease. For progressive hepatic failure, liver transplantation has been performed, but because it is a multisystem disorder involving many organ systems, the long-term success of liver transplantation is unknown.

TYPE VI GLYCOGEN STORAGE DISEASE (LIVER PHOSPHORYLASE DEFICIENCY, HERS DISEASE)

The number of patients with documented liver phosphorylase deficiency is small. It appears that patients with liver phosphorylase deficiency have a benign course. These patients present with hepatomegaly and growth retardation early in childhood. Hypoglycemia, hyperlipidemia, and hyperketosis are usually mild if present. Lactic acid and uric acid are normal. The heart and skeletal muscles are not involved. The hepatomegaly and growth retardation improve with age and usually disappear around puberty. Treatment is symptomatic. A high-carbohydrate diet and frequent feeding are effective in preventing hypoglycemia; most patients require no specific treatment. The liver phosphorylase gene is located on chromosome 14.

TYPE IX GLYCOGEN STORAGE DISEASE (PHOSPHORYLASE KINASE DEFICIENCY)

Glycogen storage disease due to a deficient phosphorylase kinase represents a heterogeneous group of glycogenoses. Phosphorylase, the rate-limiting enzyme of glycogenolysis, is activated by a cascade of enzymatic reactions involving adenylate cyclase, cyclic adenosine monophophate–dependent protein kinase (protein kinase A), and phosphorylase kinase. The latter enzyme is further complicated by the presence of four subunits, each encoded by different genes on different chromosomes and differentially expressed in various tissues. This cascade of reactions is stimulated primarily by glucagon. Theoretically, the glycogenosis can be the result of any enzyme deficiency along this pathway, but the most common one is the deficiency of phosphorylase kinase.

The numeric classification of phosphorylase kinase deficiency is confusing, ranging from type VIa, to VIII, to IX. It is advisable to refrain from such a designation and to classify the various disorders according to organ involvement and mode of inheritance.

X-LINKED LIVER PHOSPHORYLASE KINASE DEFICIENCY. This is a common form of liver glycogenoses. Enzyme activity may also be deficient in erythrocytes and leukocytes; it is normal in muscle. Typically a 1–5 yr old presents with growth retardation and an incidental finding of hepatomegaly. Cholesterol, triglycerides, and liver enzymes are mildly elevated. Ketosis may occur after fasting. Lactate and uric acid levels are normal. Hypoglycemia is mild, if present. The response in blood glucose to glucagon is normal. Hepatomegaly and abnormal blood chemistries gradually become normal with age. Most adults achieve a normal final height and are practically asymptomatic despite a persistent phosphorylase kinase deficiency. Liver histologic appearance shows glycogen-distended hepatocytes. The accumulated glycogen (α particles, rosette form) has a frayed or burst appearance and is less compact that the glycogen seen in type I or type III glycogen storage disease. Fibrous septal formation and low-grade inflammatory changes may be present.

The structural gene for the liver isoform of the phosphorylase kinase α subunit is located on chromosome Xp22; mutations of this gene have been characterized.

AUTOSOMAL LIVER AND MUSCLE PHOSPHORYLASE KINASE DEFICIENCY. Several patients have been reported with phosphorylase kinase deficiency in liver and blood cells and an autosomal model of inheritance. As with the X-linked form, hepatomegaly and growth retardation apparent in early childhood are the predominant symptoms. Some also exhibited muscle hypotonia. When measured in a few cases, reduced activity of the enzyme has been demonstrated in muscle. Mutations causing autosomally transmitted phosphorylase kinase deficiency are found in the autosomal genes of the subunits β and γ.

MUSCLE-SPECIFIC PHOSPHORYLASE KINASE DEFICIENCY. A few cases of phosphorylase kinase deficiency restricted to muscle have been reported. Several patients, both male and female, presented either with muscle cramps and myoglobinuria with exercise or with progressive muscle weakness and atrophy. Phosphorylase kinase activity was decreased in muscle but normal in liver and blood cells. There was no hepatomegaly or cardiomegaly. Mutation in the structure gene of muscle isoform of the α subunit is located on chromosome Xq12; mutation of this gene has been found in male patients with this disorder.

PHOSPHORYLASE KINASE DEFICIENCY LIMITED TO HEART. These patients present with cardiomyopathy in infancy and rapidly progress to heart failure and death. Phosphorylase kinase deficiency is demonstrated in heart with normal enzyme activity in skeletal muscle and liver.

DIAGNOSIS. Definitive diagnosis of phosphorylase kinase deficiency requires demonstration of the enzymatic defect in affected tissues. Phosphorylase kinase can be measured in leukocytes and erythrocytes, but because the enzyme has many isozymes, the diagnosis can be missed without studies of liver, muscle, or heart.

TREATMENT. The treatment for liver phosphorylase kinase deficiency is symptomatic. A high-carbohydrate diet and frequent feedings are effective in preventing hypoglycemia; most patients require no specific treatment. Prognosis is good. There is currently no treatment for the fatal form of isolated cardiac phosphorylase kinase deficiency other than heart transplantation.

GLYCOGEN SYNTHETASE DEFICIENCY

Deficiency of hepatic glycogen synthetase leads to a decrease of glycogen stored in the liver (less than 1.5%). The patients present in infancy with early-morning drowsiness and fatigue and sometimes convulsions associated with hypoglycemia and hyperketonemia. Blood lactate and alanine levels are low, and there is no hyperlipidemia or hepatomegaly. Prolonged hyperglycemia and elevation of lactate with normal insulin levels after administration of glucose suggest a possible diagnosis of deficiency of glycogen synthetase. Definitive *diagnosis* requires a liver biopsy to measure the enzyme activity. *Treatment* consists of frequent meals, rich protein, and nighttime supplementation with uncooked cornstarch. The liver glycogen synthetase gene is located on chromosome 12p12.2.

HEPATIC GLYCOGENOSIS WITH RENAL FANCONI SYNDROME (FANCONI-BICKEL SYNDROME)

This rare autosomal recessive disorder is caused by defects in the facilitative glucose transporter 2 (GLUT-2) that transports glucose in and out of hepatocytes, pancreatic β cells, and the basolateral membranes of intestinal and renal epithelial cells. The disease is characterized by proximal renal tubular dysfunction, impaired glucose and galactose utilization, and accumulation of glycogen in liver and kidney.

The affected child presents *clinical manifestations* in the 1st yr of life with failure to thrive, rickets, and a protuberant abdomen due to hepato- and renomegaly. Laboratory findings include glucosuria, phosphaturia, generalized amnioaciduria, bicarbonate wasting, hypophosphatemia, increased serum alkaline phosphatase levels, and a radiologic finding of rickets. Mild fasting hypoglycemia and hyperlipidemia may be present. Liver transaminase, plasma lactate, and uric acid levels are usually normal. Oral galactose or glucose tolerance tests show intolerance, which could be explained by the functional loss of GLUT-2 preventing liver uptake of these sugars.

Tissue biopsy results show marked accumulation of glycogen in hepatocytes and proximal renal tubular cells, presumably due to the altered glucose transport out of these organs.

There is no specific *treatment*. Growth retardation persists through adulthood. Symptomatic replacement of water, electrolytes, and vitamin D; restriction of galactose intake; and a diet similar to that used for diabetes mellitus, presented in frequent and small meals with an adequate caloric intake may improve growth.

Muscle Glycogenoses

The role of glycogen in muscle is to provide substrates for the generation of ATP for muscle contraction. The muscle glycogen storage diseases can be divided into two groups. The first group is characterized by progressive skeletal muscle weakness and atrophy or cardiomyopathy, or both, and is represented by a lysosomal glycogen degrading enzyme deficiency, acid α-glucosidase (type II glycogen storage disease). The second group is a muscle energy disorder characterized by muscle pain, exercise intolerance, myoglobinuria, and susceptibility to fatigue. This group includes myophosphorylase deficiency (McArdle disease, type V) and deficiencies of phosphofructokinase (type VII), phosphoglycerate kinase, phosphoglycerate mutase, or lactate dehydrogenase. Some of these latter enzyme deficiencies may also be associated with a compensated hemolysis, suggesting a more generalized defect in glucose metabolism.

TYPE II (LYSOSOMAL ACID α1,4-GLUCOSIDASE DEFICIENCY, POMPE DISEASE)

Type II glycogen storage disease is caused by a deficient activity of lysosomal acid α1,4 glucosidase (acid maltase), an enzyme responsible for the degradation of glycogen in lysosome. The disease is characterized by accumulation of glycogen in lysosome as opposed to its accumulation in cytoplasm in the other glycogenoses.

Pompe disease is an autosomal recessive disorder with an incidence of 1/50,000 live births with no ethnic predilection. The gene for acid α-glucosidase is on chromosome 17q23. A splice site mutation (IVS1-13T→G), commonly seen in adult-onset patients, may be helpful in delineating the phenotypes.

CLINICAL MANIFESTATIONS. The disorder encompasses a range of phenotypes, each including myopathy but differing in age of onset, organ involvement, and clinical severity. The most severe is the *infantile-onset disease*, with prominent cardiomegaly, hypotonia, and death prior to 2 yr of age. Infants appear normal at birth but soon experience generalized muscle weakness with "floppy baby appearance," feeding difficulties, macroglossia, hepatomegaly, and heart failure due to a progressively hypertrophic cardiomyopathy. Electrocardiographic findings include a high-voltage QRS complex and a shortened P-R interval. Death usually results from cardiorespiratory failure or aspiration pneumonia.

The *juvenile form* presents as delayed motor milestones (if age of onset is early enough) or difficult walking in childhood and is followed by swallowing difficulties, proximal muscle weakness, and respiratory muscle involvement. Death from respiratory failure may occur before the end of the 2nd decade. Cardiomegaly is variable, but overt cardiac failure is not seen.

An *adult form* of type II disease presents as a slowly progressive myopathy without cardiac involvement and has its onset between the 2nd and 7th decades. The clinical picture is dominated by slowly progressive proximal muscle weakness with truncal involvement and greater involvement of the lower limbs than the upper limbs. The pelvic girdle, paraspinal muscle, and diaphragm are the muscle groups most seriously affected. The initial symptoms in some patients may be respiratory insufficiency manifested by somnolence, morning headache, orthopnea, and exertional dyspnea.

LABORATORY FINDINGS. These include elevated levels of serum creatine kinase, aspartate aminotransferase, and lactate dehydrogenase. Muscle biopsy shows the presence of vacuoles that stain positively for glycogen; acid phosphatase is increased, presumably from a compensatory increase of lysosomal enzymes. Electron microscopy reveals the glycogen accumulation within the membranous sac and in the cytoplasm. Electromyography reveals myopathic features with excessive electrical irritability of muscle fibers and pseudomyotonic discharges. Serum creatine kinase is not always elevated in adult patients; depending on the muscle biopsied or tested, the muscle histologic appearance on electromyography may not be abnormal. It is prudent to examine the affected muscle.

DIAGNOSIS. This can be established by demonstration of the absence of or reduced levels of acid α-glucosidase activity in muscle or cultured skin fibroblast. Deficiency is usually more severe in the infantile form than in the juvenile and adult forms. Prenatal diagnosis using amniocytes or chorionic villi is available in the fatal infantile form.

TREATMENT. No effective treatment for the infantile form is currently available. A high-protein diet may be useful for the juvenile and adult forms. Nocturnal ventilatory support in adult patients may improve the quality of life and is beneficial during a period of respiratory decompensation.

TYPE V (MUSCLE PHOSPHORYLASE DEFICIENCY, McARDLE DISEASE)

Deficiency of muscle phosphorylase is the prototype of muscle energy disorder. Lack of this enzyme limits muscle ATP generation by glycogenolysis and results in glycogen accumulation.

CLINICAL MANIFESTATIONS. Symptoms usually develop first in late childhood or as an adult and are characterized by exercise intolerance with muscle cramps. Two types of activity tend to cause symptoms: (1) brief exercise of great intensity, such as sprinting or carrying heavy loads and (2) less intense but sustained activity, such as climbing stairs or walking uphill. Moderate exercise, such as walking on level ground, can be performed by most patients for long periods. Many patients experience a characteristic "second wind" phenomenon. If they slow down or pause briefly at the first appearance of muscle pain, they can resume exercise with more ease.

About half report burgundy-colored urine after exercise, the consequence of myoglobinuria secondary to rhabdomyolysis. Intense myoglobinuria after vigorous exercise may cause acute renal failure. In rare cases, electromyographic findings may suggest an inflammatory myopathy, and the diagnosis can be confused with polymyositis.

The level of serum creatine kinase is usually elevated at rest and increases more after exercise. Exercise also increases the levels of blood ammonia, inosine, hypoxanthine, and uric acid. The latter abnormalities are attributed to accelerated recycling of muscle purine nucleotides in the face of insufficient ATP production.

Clinical heterogeneity is uncommon in type V glycogen storage disease, but late-onset disease with no symptoms as late as the 8th decade and an early-onset, fatal form with hypotonia, generalized muscle weakness, and progressive respiratory insufficiency have been described.

DIAGNOSIS. An ischemic exercise test offers rapid diagnostic screening for metabolic myopathy. Lack of an increase in blood lactate and exaggerated blood ammonia elevations are indicative of muscle glycogenosis and suggest a defect in the conversion of glycogen or glucose to lactate. The abnormal ischemic exercise response is not limited to type V glycogen storage disease. Other muscle defects along the pathways of glycogenolysis or glycolysis can produce similar results: deficiencies of muscle phosphofructokinase, phosphoglycerate kinase, phosphoglycerate mutase, or lactate dehydrogenase.

Phosphorus magnetic resonance imaging (^{31}P MRI) allows for the noninvasive evaluation of muscle metabolism. Patients with type V glycogen storage disease have no decrease in intracellular pH and have excessive reduction in phosphocreatine in response to exercise. The diagnosis should be confirmed by enzymatic evaluation of muscle.

Type V glycogen storage disease is an autosomal recessive disorder. The gene for muscle phosphorylase is located on chromosome 11q13-qter. A nonsense mutation changing arginine to a stop at codon 49 (R49X) and a deletion of a single codon (F708) are prevalent in white and Japanese patients, respectively. This allows DNA-based diagnosis and carrier detection for the two populations.

TREATMENT. Exercise tolerance can be augmented by oral administration of glucose or fructose or by injection of glucagon. A high-protein diet may increase muscle endurance in some patients. In general, avoidance of strenuous exercise prevents the symptoms, and there is no need for a specific therapy. Longevity does not appear to be affected.

TYPE VII GLYCOGEN STORAGE DISEASE (MUSCLE PHOSPHOFRUCTOKINASE DEFICIENCY, TARUI DISEASE)

Type VII glycogen storage disease is caused by a deficiency of muscle phosphofructokinase, which catalyzes the ATP-dependent conversion of fructose-6-phosphate to fructose 1,6-diphosphate and is a key regulatory enzyme of glycolysis. Phosphofructokinase is composed of three isoenzyme subunits (M [muscle], L [liver], and P [platelet]) that are encoded by different genes and differentially expressed in tissues. Skeletal muscle contains only the M subunit, and red blood cells contain a hybrid of L and M forms. Type VII disease is due to a defective M isoenzyme, which causes a complete enzyme defect in muscle and a partial defect in red blood cells.

Type VII glycogen storage disease is an autosomal recessive disorder. The disease appears to be prevalent among Japanese and Ashkenazi Jews. The gene for muscle phosphofructokinase is located on chromosome 1cen-1q32. A splicing defect and a nucleotide deletion in the muscle phosphofructokinase gene account for 95% of mutant alleles in Ashkenazi Jews. The molecular diagnosis is possible in this population.

CLINICAL MANIFESTATIONS. The clinical features are similar to those in type V disease. Five features of type VII are distinctive: (1) Exercise intolerance, usually evident in childhood, is more severe than in type V disease, and may be associated with nausea and vomiting. Vigorous exercise causes severe muscle cramps and myoglobinuria. (2) A compensated hemolysis occurs as evidenced by an increased level of serum bilirubin and an elevated reticulocyte count. (3) Hyperuricemia is common and exaggerated by muscle exercise to a more severe degree than that observed in type V or III glycogen storage disease. (4) An abnormal glycogen resembling amylopectin is present in muscle fibers; it is periodic acid–Schiff–positive but resistant to diastase digestion. (5) Exercise intolerance is particularly acute following meals that are rich in carbohydrates because glucose cannot be utilized in muscle and because glucose inhibits lipolysis and thus deprives muscle of fatty acid and ketone substrates. In contrast, patients with type V disease can metabolize blood-borne glucose derived from either liver glycogenolysis or exogenous glucose. Indeed, glucose infusion improves exercise tolerance in type V patients.

Two rare type VII patients have been reported. One variant

presents in infancy with hypotonia and limb weakness and proceeds to a rapidly progressive myopathy that leads to death by 4 yr of age. The other variant presents in adults and is characterized by a slowly progressive, fixed muscle weakness rather than cramps and myoglobinuria.

DIAGNOSIS. To establish a diagnosis, a biochemical or histochemical demonstration of the enzymatic defect in the muscle is required. The absence of the M isoenzyme of phosphofructokinase can also be demonstrated in blood cells and fibroblasts.

TREATMENT. There is no specific treatment for this condition. Avoidance of strenuous exercise is advisable to prevent acute attacks of muscle cramps and myoglobinuria.

OTHER MUSCLE GLYCOGENOSES WITH MUSCLE ENERGY IMPAIRMENT

Three additional enzyme defects—phosphoglycerate kinase, phosphoglycerate mutase, and lactate dehydrogenase in the pathway of the terminal glycolysis—cause symptoms and signs of muscle energy impairment similar to those of types V and VII glycogen storage disease. The failure of blood lactate to increase in response to exercise is a useful diagnostic test and can be used to differentiate muscle glycogenoses from disorders of lipid metabolism, such as carnitine palmitoyl transferase II deficiency and very long chain acyl-CoA dehydrogenase deficiency, which also cause muscle cramps and myoglobinuria. Muscle glycogen levels may be normal in the disorders affecting terminal glycolysis, and definite diagnosis is made by assaying the muscle enzyme activity. There is no specific treatment. Avoidance of strenuous exercise prevents acute attacks of muscle cramps and myoglobinuria.

84.2 Defects in Galactose Metabolism

Milk and dairy products contain lactose, the major dietary source of galactose. The metabolism of galactose produces fuel for cellular metabolism through its conversion to glucose-1-phosphate (see Fig. 84–1). Galactose also plays an important role in the formation of galactosides, which include glycoproteins, glycolipids, and glycosaminoglycans. Galactosemia denotes the elevated level of galactose in the blood and is found in three distinct disorders of galactose metabolism defective in one of the following enzymes: galactose-1-phosphate uridyl transferase, galactokinase, and uridine diphosphate galactose-4-epimerase. The term *galactosemia,* although adequate for the deficiencies for any of these three disorders, generally designates the transferase deficiency.

GALACTOSE-1-PHOSPHATE URIDYL TRANSFERASE DEFICIENCY GALACTOSEMIA

"Classic" galactosemia is a serious disease with early onset of symptoms; the incidence is 1/60,000. The newborn infant normally receives up to 20% of caloric intake as lactose, which consists of glucose and galactose. Without the transferase enzyme, the infant is unable to metabolize galactose-1-phosphate, the accumulation of which results in injury to parenchymal cells of the kidney, liver, and brain. This injury may begin prenatally in the affected fetus by transplacental galactose derived from the diet of the heterozygous mother or by endogenous production of galactose in the fetus.

CLINICAL MANIFESTATIONS. The diagnosis of uridyl transferase deficiency should be considered in newborn or older infants and children with any of the following features: jaundice, hepatomegaly, vomiting, hypoglycemia, convulsions, lethargy, irritability, feeding difficulties, poor weight gain, aminoaciduria, cataracts, vitreous hemorrhage, hepatic cirrhosis, ascites, splenomegaly, or mental retardation. Patients with galactosemia are at increased risk for *Escherichia coli* neonatal sepsis; the onset of sepsis often precedes the diagnosis of galactosemia. When the diagnosis is not made at birth, damage to the liver (cirrhosis) and brain (mental retardation) becomes increasingly severe and irreversible. Therefore, galactosemia should be considered for the newborn or young infant who is not thriving or who has any of the preceding findings.

DIAGNOSIS. Because galactose is injurious to persons with galactosemia, diagnostic tests dependent on administering galactose orally or intravenously should not be used. Galactose administration would result in high concentrations of intracellular galactose-1-phosphate, which can function as a competitive inhibitor of phosphoglucomutase. This inhibition transiently impairs the conversion of glycogen to glucose and produces hypoglycemia. Light and electron microscopy of hepatic tissue reveals fatty infiltration, the formation of pseudoacini, and eventual macronodular cirrhosis. These changes are consistent with a metabolic disease but do not indicate the precise enzymatic defect.

The preliminary diagnosis of galactosemia is made by demonstrating a reducing substance in several urine specimens collected while the patient is receiving human milk, cow's milk, or another formula containing lactose. The reducing substance found in urine by Clinitest can be identified by chromatography or by an enzymatic test specific for galactose. Clinistix or Tes-Tape urine test results are negative because the test materials rely on the action of glucose oxidase, which is specific for glucose and is nonreactive with galactose. Deficient activity of galactose-1-phosphate uridyl transferase is demonstrable in hemolysates of erythrocytes, which also exhibit increased concentrations of galactose-1-phosphate.

GENETICS. Transferase deficiency galactosemia is an autosomal recessive trait. There are several enzymatic variants of galactosemia. The Duarte variant has diminished red cell enzyme activity but usually no clinical significance. Some African-American patients have milder symptoms despite the absence of measurable transferase activity in erythrocytes; these patients retain 10% enzyme activity in liver and intestinal mucosa, whereas most white patients have no detectable activity in any of these tissues. In African-Americans, 48% of alleles are represented by the S135L mutation, a mutation that may be responsible for the milder disease. In the white population, 70% of alleles are represented by the Q188R missense mutation. Carrier testing and prenatal diagnosis can be performed by direct enzyme analysis of amniocytes or chorionic villi; testing can be DNA-based.

TREATMENT AND PROGNOSIS. Because of widespread newborn screening for galactosemia, patients are being identified and treated early. Elimination of galactose from diet reverses growth failure and renal and hepatic dysfunctions. Cataracts regress, and most patients have no impairment of eyesight. Early diagnosis and treatment have improved the prognosis of galactosemia; however, on long-term follow-up, patients still manifest ovarian failure with primary or secondary amenorrhea, developmental delay, and learning disabilities, that increase in severity with age. Most manifest speech disorders, whereas a smaller number demonstrate poor growth and impaired motor function and balance (with or without overt ataxia). The relative control of galactose-1-phosphate levels does not always correlate with long-term outcome, leading to the belief that other factors, such as uridine diphosphate galactose (UDP-galactose) deficiency (a donor for galactolipids and proteins), may be responsible.

GALACTOKINASE DEFICIENCY

The deficient enzyme is galactokinase, which normally catalyzes the phosphorylation of galactose. The principal metabolites accumulated are galactose and galactitol. Mutations leading to galactokinase deficiency have been identified. The gene coding for galactokinase is located on chromosome 17q21–22. In contrast to the multiple organs that are affected in transferase deficiency galactosemia, cataracts are usually the sole manifestation of galactokinase deficiency. The affected infant is otherwise asymptomatic. These patients have an increased concentration of blood galactose levels with normal transferase activity and an absence of galactokinase activity in erythrocytes. Treatment is dietary restriction of galactose intake.

URIDINE DIPHOSPHATE GALACTOSE 4–EPIMERASE DEFICIENCY

The abnormally accumulated metabolites are similar to those in transferase deficiency; however, there is also an increase in cellular UDP-galactose. There are two distinct forms of epimerase deficiency. A benign form was discovered incidentally through a neonatal screening program. Affected persons are healthy and without problems; the enzyme deficiency is limited to leukocytes and erythrocytes. No treatment is required. The second form of epimerase deficiency is severe, and clinical manifestations resemble transferase deficiency with the additional symptoms of hypotonia and nerve deafness. The enzyme deficiency is generalized, and clinical symptoms respond to restriction of dietary galactose. Although this form of galactosemia is rare, it must be considered in a symptomatic patient who has normal transferase activity.

Patients with epimerase deficiency cannot make galactose. Because it is an essential component of many nervous system structural proteins, patients are placed on a galactose-restricted diet rather than a galactose-free diet.

The gene for UDP-galactose 4–epimerase is located on chromosome 1 at 1p32-1pter. Carrier detection is possible by measurement of epimerase activity in the erythrocytes. Prenatal diagnosis for the severe form of epimerase deficiency, using an enzyme assay of cultured amniotic fluid cells, has been achieved.

84.3 Defects in Fructose Metabolism

DEFICIENCY OF FRUCTOKINASE (BENIGN FRUCTOSURIA)

Deficiency of fructokinase is not associated with any clinical manifestations. It is an accidental finding usually made because the asymptomatic patient's urine contains a reducing substance. No treatment is necessary. Inheritance is autosomal recessive with an incidence of 1/120,000. The gene encoding fructokinase is located on chromosome 2p23.3.

Fructokinase catalyzes the first step of metabolism of dietary fructose, conversion of fructose to fructose 1-phosphate (see Fig. 84–1). Without this enzyme, ingested fructose is not metabolized. Its level is increased in the blood, and it is excreted in urine because there is practically no renal threshold for fructose. Both positive and negative Clinitest results reveal the urinary-reducing substance to be something other than glucose. It can be identified as fructose by chromatography.

DEFICIENCY OF FRUCTOSE 1,6-BISPHOSPHATE ALDOLASE (ALDOLASE B) (HEREDITARY FRUCTOSE INTOLERANCE)

Deficiency of fructose 1,6-bisphosphate aldolase is a severe condition of infants that appears with the ingestion of fructose-containing food and is caused by deficiency of fructose 1-phosphate aldolase B activity in the liver, kidney, and intestine. The enzyme catalyzes the hydrolysis of fructose 1-phosphate into triose phosphate and glyceraldehyde. Deficiency of this enzyme activity causes a rapid accumulation of fructose 1-phosphate and initiates severe toxic symptoms when exposed to fructose.

EPIDEMIOLOGY AND GENETICS. The true incidence of hereditary fructose intolerance is unknown but may be as high as 1/23,000. The gene for aldolase B is on chromosome 9q13–32. Several mutations causing heredity fructose intolerance have been identified. A single missense mutation, a G to C transversion in exon 5, which results in the normal alanine at position 149 being replaced by a proline, is the most common mutation identified in northern Europeans. This mutation, plus two other point mutations, account for approximately 80–85% of hereditary fructose intolerance in Europe and the United States. Diagnosis of hereditary fructose intolerance can thus be made by direct DNA analysis. Prenatal diagnosis should be possible by both amniocentesis and chorionic villi, using DNA mutational or linkage analysis.

CLINICAL MANIFESTATIONS. Patients with fructose intolerance are perfectly healthy and asymptomatic until fructose or sucrose (table sugar) is ingested (usually from fruit, fruit juice, or sweetened cereal). Symptoms may occur early in life—soon after birth if foods or formulas containing these sugars are introduced into the diet. Early clinical manifestations resemble galactosemia and include jaundice, hepatomegaly, vomiting, lethargy, irritability, and convulsions. Laboratory findings include prolonged clotting time, hypoalbuminuria, elevation of bilirubin and transaminase levels, and proximal tubular dysfunction. Acute fructose ingestion produces symptomatic hypoglycemia; chronic ingestion results in failure to thrive and hepatic disease. If the intake of the fructose persists, hypoglycemic episodes recur, and liver and kidney failure progress, eventually leading to death.

DIAGNOSIS. Suspicion of the enzyme deficiency is fostered by the presence of a reducing substance in the urine during an episode. The diagnosis could be supported by an intravenous fructose tolerance test, which will cause a rapid fall, first of serum phosphate and then of blood glucose, and a subsequent rise of uric acid and magnesium. An oral tolerance test should not be performed, as patients may become acutely ill. Definitive diagnosis is made by assay of fructaldolase B activity in the liver.

TREATMENT. This consists of the complete elimination of all sources of sucrose, fructose, and sorbitol from the diet. This may be difficult because these sugars are a widely used additive, found even in most medicinal preparations. With treatment, liver and kidney dysfunction improves, and catch-up in growth is common. Intellectual development is usually unimpaired. As the patient matures, symptoms become milder even after fructose ingestion; the long-term prognosis is good. Owing to voluntary dietary avoidance of sucrose, affected patients have few dental caries.

84.4 Defects in Intermediary Carbohydrate Metabolism Associated with Lactic Acidosis

Lactic acidosis occurs with defects of carbohydrate metabolism that interfere with the conversion of pyruvate to glucose via the pathway of gluconeogenesis or to carbon dioxide and water via the mitochondrial enzymes of the citric acid cycle. Figure 84–3 depicts the relevant metabolic pathways. Type I glycogen storage disease, fructose 1,6 diphosphatase deficiency, and phosphoenolpyruvate carboxylase deficiency are disorders of gluconeogenesis associated with lactic acidosis. Pyruvate dehydrogenase complex deficiency, respiratory chain defects, and pyruvate carboxylase deficiency are disorders in the pathway of pyruvate metabolism causing lactic acidosis. Lactic acidosis can also occur in defects of fatty acid oxidation, organic acidurias (see Chapters 82.6, 82.10, and 83.1), or biotin utilization diseases. These disorders are easily distinguishable by the presence of abnormal acylcarnitine profiles in the blood and

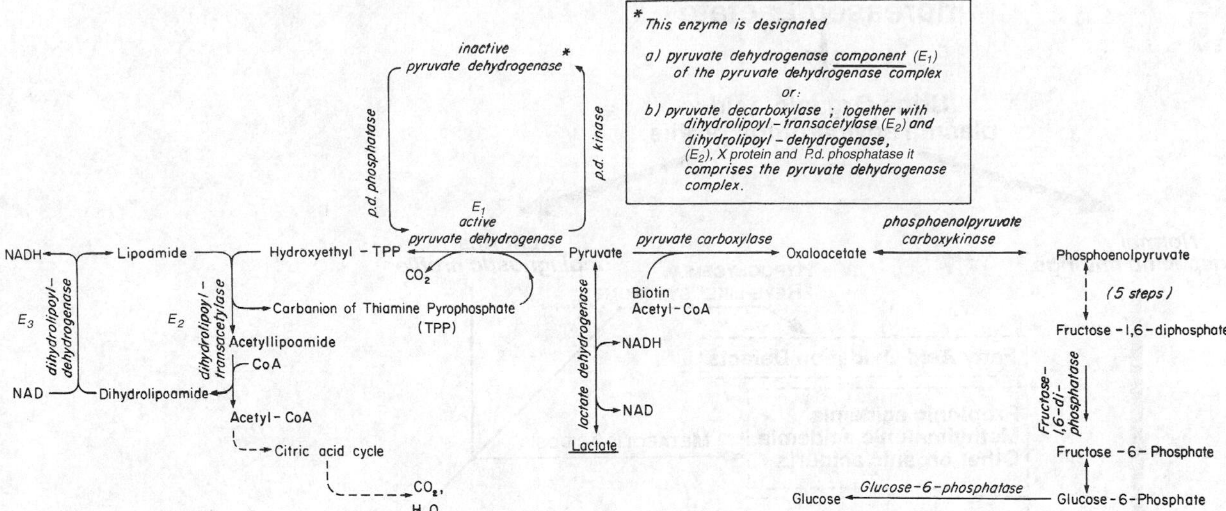

Figure 84–3 Enzymatic reactions of carbohydrate metabolism, deficiencies of which may give rise to lactic acidosis, pyruvate elevations, or hypoglycemia. The pyruvate dehydrogenase complex comprises, in addition to E_1, E_2, and E_3, an extra lipoate-containing protein (not shown), called protein X, and pyruvate dehydrogenase phosphatase.

unusual organic acids in the urine. Therefore, blood lactate and acylcarnitine profiles and the presence of these unusual urine organic acids should be determined in infants and children with unexplained acidosis, especially if there is an increase of anion gap (see Chapter 52).

Lactic acidosis unrelated to an enzymatic defect occurs in hypoxemia. In this case, as well as in defects in the respiratory chain, the serum pyruvate concentration may remain normal (<1.0 mg/dL with an increased lactate:pyruvate ratio), whereas pyruvate is usually increased when lactic acidosis results from an enzymatic defect in gluconeogenesis or pyruvate dehydrogenase complex (both lactate and pyruvate are increased and the ratio is normal). It is useful, therefore, to measure lactate and pyruvate in the same blood specimen and on multiple blood specimens obtained when the patient is symptomatic because dramatic and ultimately fatal lactic acidosis may be intermittent. A algorithm for the differential diagnosis of lactic acidosis is shown in Figure 84–4.

Disorders of Gluconeogenesis

DEFICIENCY OF GLUCOSE-6-PHOSPHATASE (TYPE I GLYCOGEN STORAGE DISEASE)

Type I glycogen storage disease is the only glycogenosis associated with significant lactic acidosis. The chronic metabolic acidosis predisposes these patients to osteopenia, and in an acute setting after prolonged fasting, the acidosis associated with hypoglycemia is a life-threatening condition. This disease is discussed further in Chapter 84.1.

FRUCTOSE 1,6-DIPHOSPHATASE DEFICIENCY

Fructose 1,6-diphosphatase deficiency is not a defect in the fructose pathway; rather, it is a defect involved in gluconeogenesis. The *clinical manifestations* are characterized by life-threatening episodes of acidosis, hypoglycemia, hyperventilation, convulsions, and coma. Half of the patients have an onset in the 1st week of life. In infants and small children, episodes are triggered by febrile infections and gastroenteritis when oral food intake decreases. *Laboratory findings* include low blood glucose and high lactate and uric acid levels and metabolic acidosis. In contrast to hereditary fructose intolerance, there is usually no aversion to sweets, and renal tubular and liver functions are normal.

The *diagnosis* is established by demonstrating an enzyme deficiency in either a liver or intestinal biopsy specimen. The enzyme defect may also be demonstrated in leukocytes in some cases. The gene coding for fructose 1,6-diphosphatase is located on chromosome 9q22. Since mutations are being characterized, carrier detection and prenatal diagnosis should be possible using the DNA-based test.

Treatment of acute attacks consists of correction of hypoglycemia and acidosis by intravenous infusion; the response is usually rapid. Avoidance of fasting and elimination of fructose and sucrose from the diet prevent further episodes. For long-term prevention of hypoglycemia, a slowly released carbohydrate such as cornstarch is useful. Patients who survive childhood seem to develop normally.

PHOSPHOENOLPYRUVATE CARBOXYKINASE DEFICIENCY

Phosphoenolpyruvate carboxykinase (PEPCK) is a key enzyme in gluconeogenesis. It catalyzes the conversion of oxaloacetate to phosphoenolpyruvate (see Fig. 84–3). PEPCK deficiency has been described both as a mitochondrial enzyme deficiency and as a cytosolic enzyme deficiency.

The disease has been reported in only six cases. The clinical features are heterogeneous, with hypoglycemia, lactic acidemia, hepatomegaly, hypotonia, developmental delay, and failure to thrive as the major manifestations. Hepatic and renal dysfunction may be present. The diagnosis is based on the reduced activity of PEPCK in liver, fibroblasts, or lymphocytes. Fibroblasts and lymphocytes are not suitable for diagnosing the cytosolic form of PEPCK deficiency because these tissues possess only mitochondrial PEPCK.

Disorders of Pyruvate Metabolism

Pyruvate is metabolized through four main enzyme systems: lactate dehydrogenase, alanine aminotransferase, pyruvate carboxylase, and pyruvate dehydrogenase complex. Deficiency of the M subunit of lactate dehydrogenase causes exercise

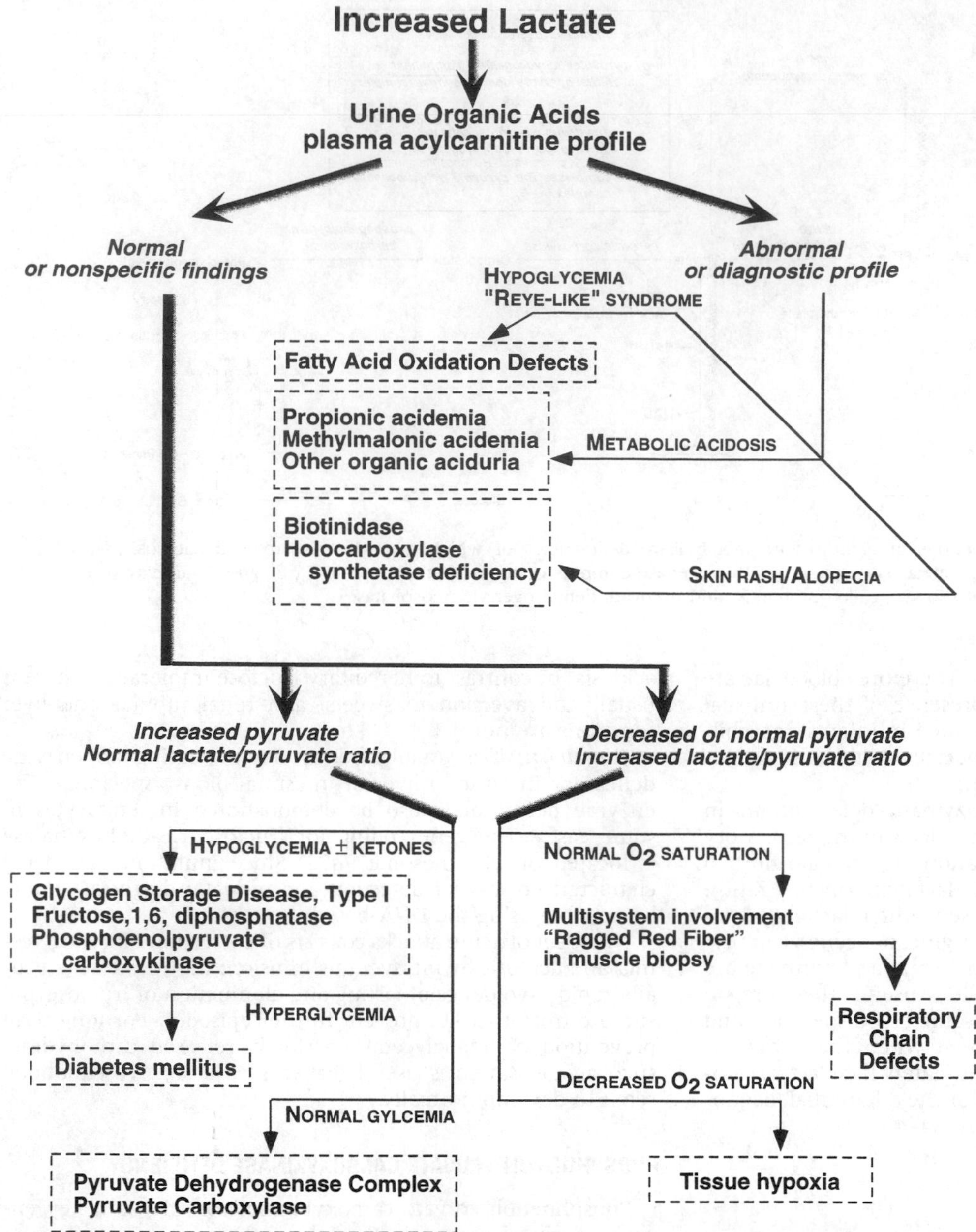

Figure 84–4 Algorithm of the differential diagnosis of lactic acidosis.

intolerance and myoglobinuria (see Chapter 84.1). Genetic deficiency of alanine aminotransferase has not been reported in humans.

DISORDERS OF PYRUVATE DEHYDROGENASE COMPLEX DEFICIENCY

The pyruvate dehydrogenase complex (PDHC) catalyzes the oxidation of pyruvate to acetyl CoA, which enters the tricarboxylic acid cycle for ATP production. The complex comprises five components: E_1, an α ketoacid decarboxylase; E_2, a dihydrolipoyl transacylase; E_3, a dihydrolipoyl dehydrogenase; protein X, an extra lipoate-containing protein; and pyruvate dehydrogenase phosphatase (see Fig. 84–3).

Deficiency of any of these components is associated with lactic acidosis and central nervous system dysfunction. The central nervous system dysfunction is because the brain obtains its energy primarily from oxidation of glucose.

The E_1 defects are caused by mutations in the gene coding for E_1 α subunit, which is X-linked.

CLINICAL MANIFESTATIONS. The disease has a wide spectrum of presentations from the most severe neonatal presentation to a mild late-onset form. The neonatal onset is associated with lethal lactic acidosis, white matter cystic lesions, agenesis of the corpus callosum, and the most severe enzyme deficiency. Infantile onset may be lethal or associated with psychomotor retardation and chronic lactic acidosis, cystic lesions in the brain stem, and basal ganglia pathologic features resembling Leigh disease. Older children, usually boys, may have less acidosis, greater enzyme activity, and manifest ataxia with high-carbohydrate diets. Intelligence may be normal. Patients of all ages may have facial dysmorphologic features similar to those of fetal alcohol syndrome.

The E_2 and protein X-lipoate defects are rare and result in severe psychomotor retardation. The E_3 lipoyl dehydrogenase defect leads to deficient activity not only in the pyruvate dehydrogenase complex but also in the α ketoglutarate and branched-chain ketoacid dehydrogenase complexes. Pyruvate dehydrogenase phosphatase deficiency has also been reported. These other PDHC defects have clinical manifestations within the variable spectrum associated with PDHC deficiency due to E_1 deficiency.

TREATMENT. The general prognosis for these disorders is poor except in rare cases in which mutation is associated with altered affinity for thiamine pyrophosphate, which may respond to thiamine supplementation. Since carbohydrates may aggravate lactic acidosis, a ketogenic diet seems a rational approach. The diet has lowered the blood lactate level, but limited or no long-term benefit is seen. A potential treatment strategy is to maintain any residual PDHC in its active form by dichloroacetate, an inhibitor of E_1 kinase. Beneficial effects in some patients have been shown, but a multicenter, controlled clinical trial has not been performed. Patients usually respond to a daily dose of 25–100 mg/kg by oral or intravenous (50 mg/kg $\times$ 1 may produce a response within 24 hr) routes.

DEFICIENCY OF PYRUVATE CARBOXYLASE

Pyruvate carboxylase catalyzes the conversion of pyruvate to oxaloacetate as the first step for gluconeogenesis. Clinical manifestations of this deficiency have varied from neonatal severe lactic acidosis accompanied by hyperammonemia, citrullinemia, and hyperlysinemia (type B) to late-onset mild to moderate lactic acidosis and developmental delay (type A). In both types, patients who survived usually had severe psychomotor retardation with seizures, spasticity, and microcephaly. Some patients have pathologic changes in the brain stem and basal ganglia that resemble Leigh disease. The clinical severity appears to correlate with the level of the residual enzyme activity. Laboratory findings are characterized by elevated levels of blood lactate, pyruvate, and alanine; in the case of type B, blood ammonia, citrulline, and lysine levels are also elevated, which might suggest a primary defect of the urea cycle. The mechanism is likely due to depletion of oxaloacetate, which leads to reduced levels of aspartate, which is a substrate for argininosuccinate synthetase in the urea cycle (see Chapter 82.10). Diagnosis is made by the measurement of enzyme activity in liver or cultured skin fibroblasts. There is no effective treatment for the disease.

DEFICIENCY OF PYRUVATE CARBOXYLASE SECONDARY TO DEFICIENCY OF HOLOCARBOXYLASE SYNTHETASE OR BIOTINIDASE (See also Chapter 82.6)

Deficiency of either holocarboxylase synthetase or biotinidase, which are enzymes of biotin metabolism, results in a secondary deficiency of pyruvate carboxylase (and other biotin-requiring carboxylases and metabolic reactions) and in *clinical manifestations* associated with the respective deficiencies, as well as skin rash, lactic acidosis, and alopecia. The course of holocarboxylase synthetase or biotinidase deficiency can be protracted, with intermittent exacerbation of chronic lactic acidosis, failure to thrive, seizures, and hypotonia leading to spasticity, lethargy, coma, and death. *Laboratory findings* include metabolic acidosis and abnormal organic acids in the urine. *Diagnosis* can be made in skin fibroblasts or lymphocytes by assay for holocarboxylase synthetase activity and in the case of biotinidase in the serum by screening blood spot. *Treatment* consists of biotin supplementation, 5–20 mg/day and is generally effective if treatment is started before the development of brain damage. Patients identified through newborn screening have been treated with biotin and have remained asymptomatic.

Both enzyme deficiencies are autosomal recessive traits. Holocarboxylase synthetase and biotinidase are located on chromosome 21q22 and 3p25, respectively. Two common mutations (del7/ins3 and A538C) in the biotinidase gene account for 52% of all mutant alleles in patients with biotinidase deficiency.

MITOCHONDRIAL RESPIRATORY CHAIN DEFECTS (OXIDATIVE PHOSPHORYLATION DISEASE)

The mitochondrial respiratory chain catalyzes the oxidation of fuel molecules and transfers the electrons to molecular oxygen with concomitant energy transduction into ATP—so-called oxidative phosphorylation. The respiratory chain produces ATP from NADH or $FADH_2$ and includes five specific complexes (I: nicotinamide-adenine dinucleotide [NADH]–coenzyme Q reductase; II: succinate–coenzyme Q reductase; III: coenzyme QH_2 cytochrome C reductase; IV: cytochrome C oxidase; V: ATP synthase). Each complex is composed of 9–25 individual proteins, encoded by nuclear or mitochondrial DNA (inherited only from the mother by mitochondrial inheritance). Defects in any of these complexes produce chronic lactic acidosis presumably due to a change of redox state with increased concentration of NADH. In contrast to PDHC or pyruvate carboxylase deficiency, skeletal muscle and heart are usually involved in the respiratory chain disorders, and in muscle biopsy "ragged red fiber" (indicating mitochondrial proliferation) is often seen (see Fig. 84–4). Because of the ubiquitous nature of oxidative phosphorylation, a defect of the mitochondrial respiratory chain accounts for a vast array of clinical manifestations and should be considered in patients in all age groups presenting with multisystem involvement. Some deficiencies resemble Leigh disease, whereas others cause infantile myopathies such as MELAS (mitochondrial encephalopathy, myopathy, lactic acidosis, and strokelike episodes), MERRF (myoclonus epilepsy, with ragged-red fibers), and Kearns-Sayre syndrome (external ophthalmoplegia, acidosis, retinal degeneration, heart block, myopathy, high cerebrospinal fluid protein) (see also Chapter 618). Diagnosis requires measurement of enzyme activities in tissues or analysis of mitochondrial DNA mutation, or both. Treatment remains largely symptomatic and does not significantly alter the outcome of disease. However, some patients appear to respond to cofactor supplements such as coenzyme Q_{10}.

LEIGH DISEASE (SUBACUTE NECROTIZING ENCEPHALOPATHY)

Leigh disease remains a neuropathologic description characterized by demylination, gliosis, necrosis, relative neuronal sparing, and capillary proliferation in specific brain regions. In decreasing order of severity, the affected areas are the basal ganglia, brain stem cerebellum, and cerebral cortex (also see Chapter 607). Patients with Leigh disease have been reported to have defects in several enzyme complexes. Dysfunction in cytochrome C oxidase (complex IV) is the most commonly reported defect, followed by NADH–coenzyme Q reductase (complex I), PDHC, and pyruvate carboxylase.

84.5 *Deficiency of Xylulose Dehydrogenase (Essential Benign Pentosuria)*

Essential benign pentosuria is characterized by a reducing substance in the urine in an otherwise healthy individual. Care should be taken not to mistake the reducing substance for glucose. The pentose in the urine reacts with Clinitest but not with glucose oxidase test papers such as Tes-Tape or Clinistix dipsticks.

L-Xylulose dehydrogenase converts L-xylulose (which can arise from D-glucuronate) to xylitol. Xylitol is converted to D-xylulose, which becomes D-xylulose-5-phosphate and enters the pentose phosphate shunt. Deficiency of this enzyme leads to increased concentration of L-xylulose in blood and urine. This rare defect is most common in Jews. No therapy is required.

Pentosuria can be observed in normal individuals if the dietary pentose intake is increased, as with the excessive ingestion of fruit containing pentose. Under these circumstances, there may be urinary excretion of xylose and arabinose up to 200 mg/24 hr in normal individuals.

Bao Y, Kishnani P, Wu JY: Hepatic and neuromuscular forms of glycogen storage disease type IV caused by mutation in the same glycogen branching enzyme gene. J Clin Invest 97:941, 1996.

Bonthron DT, Brady N, Donaldson IA, et al: Molecular basis of essential fructosuria: Molecular cloning and mutational analysis of human ketohexokinase (fructokinase). Hum Mol Genet 3:1627, 1994.

Chen Y-T, Burchell A: Glycogen storage diseases. *In:* Scriver CR, Beaudet AL, Sly WS, Valle D (eds): The Metabolic and Molecular Bases of Inherited Disease, 7th ed. New York, McGraw-Hill, 1995, pp 935–965.

Chen Y-T, Bazzarre CH, Lee MM, et al: Type I glycogen storage disease: Nine years of management with cornstarch. Eur J Pediatr 152:S56, 1993.

Chen Y-T, Cornblath M, Sidbury JB: Cornstarch therapy in type I glycogen storage disease. N Engl J Med 310:171, 1984.

Cormier-Daire V, Chretien D, Rustin P, et al: Neonatal and delayed-onset liver involvement in disorders of oxidative phosphorylation. J Pediatr 130:817, 1997.

el-Schahawi M, Tsujino S, Shanske S, et al: Diagnosis of McArdle's disease by molecular genetic analysis of blood. Neurology 47:579, 1996.

Gerin I, Veiga-da-Cunha M, Achouri Y, et al: Sequence of a putative glucose 6-phosphate translocase, mutated in glycogen storage disease type Ib. FEBS Lett 419:235, 1997.

Gitzelmann R, Spycher MA, Feil G, et al: Liver glycogen synthase deficiency: A rarely diagnosed entity. Eur J Pediatr 155:561, 1996.

Gitzelmann R, Steinmann B, Van Den Berghe G: Disorders of fructose metabolism. *In:* Scriver CR, Beaudet AL, Sly WS, et al (eds): The Metabolic and Molecular Bases of Inherited Disease, 7th ed. New York, McGraw-Hill, 1995, pp 905–934.

Hendricks J, Dams E, Coucke P, et al: X-linked liver glycogenosis type II (XLG II) is caused by mutations in PHKA2, the gene encoding the liver alpha subunit of phosphorylase kinase. Hum Mol Genet 5:649, 1996.

Hirschhorn R: Glycogen storage disease type II: Acid α-glucosidase (acid maltase deficiency). *In:* Scriver CR, Beaudet AL, Sly WS, Valle D (eds): The Metabolic and Molecular Bases of Inherited Disease, 7th ed, Vol 2. New York, McGraw-Hill, 1995, pp 2443–2464.

Holton JB, Leonard JV: Clouds still gathering over galactosemia. Lancet 344:1242, 1994.

James CL, Rellos P, Ali M, et al: Neonatal screening for hereditary fructose intolerance: Frequency of the most common mutant aldolase B allele (A149) in the British population. J Med Genet 33:837, 1996.

Keller KM, Schütz M, Podskarbi T, et al: A new mutation of the glucose-6-phosphatase gene in a 4-year-old girl oligosymptomatic glycogen storage disease type 1a. J Pediatr 132:360, 1998.

Kikawa Y, Inuzuka M, Jin BY, et al: Identification of a genetic mutation in a family with fructose 1, 6-bisphosphatase deficiency. Biochem Biophys Res Commun 210:797, 1995.

Kroos MA, Van der Kraan M, Van Diggelen OP, et al: Glycogen storage disease type II: Frequency of three common mutant alleles and their associated clinical phenotypes studied in 121 patients. J Med Genet 32:836 1995.

Kuroda Y, Ito M, Naito E, et al: Concomitant administration of sodium dichloroacetate and vitamin B_1 for lactic acidemia in children with MELAS syndrome. J Pediatr 131:450, 1997.

Lai K, Langley SD, Singh RH, et al: A prevalent mutation for galactosemia among black Americans. J Pediatr 128:89, 1996.

Lin H-C, Kirby LT, Ng WG, et al: On the molecular nature of the Duarte variant of galactose-1-phosphate uridyl transferase (GALT). Hum Genet 93:167, 1994.

Maichele AJ, Burwinkel B, Maire I, et al: Mutations in the testis/liver isoform of the phosphorylase kinase γ subunit (PHKG2) cause autosomal liver glycogenosis in the gsd rat and in humans. Nat Genet 14:337, 1996.

McConkie-Rosell A, Wilson C, Piccoli DA, et al: Clinical and laboratory findings in four patients with the non-progressive hepatic form of type IV glycogen storage disease. J Inherit Metab Dis 9:51, 1996.

Moses SW: Muscle glycogenosis. J Inherit Metab Dis 13:452, 1990.

Ratner-Kaufman F, Reichardt JKV, Ng WG, et al: Correlation of cognitive, neurologic, and ovarian outcome with the Q188R mutation of the galactose-1-phosphate uridyltransferase gene. J Pediatr 125:225, 1994.

Santer R, Schneppenheim R, Dombrowski A, et al: Mutations in *GLUT2,* the gene for the liver-type glucose transporter, in patients with Fanconi-Bickel syndrome. Nat Genet 17:324, 1997.

Segal S, Berry GT: Disorders of galactose metabolism. *In:* Scriver CR, Beaudet AL, Sly WS, et al (eds): The Metabolic and Molecular Bases of Inherited Disease, 7th ed. New York, McGraw-Hill, 1995, pp 967–1000.

Shen J-J, Bao Y, Liu H-M, et al: Mutations in exon 3 of the glycogen debranching enzyme gene are associated with glycogen storage disease type III that is differentially expressed in liver and muscle. J Clin Invest 98:352, 1996.

Sherman JB, Raben N, Nicastri C, et al: Common mutations in the phosphofructokinase-M gene in Ashkenazi Jewish patients with glycogenesis VII—and their population frequency. Am J Hum Genet 55:305 1994.

Shoffner JM: Maternal inheritance and the evaluation of oxidative phosphorylation diseases. Lancet 348:1283, 1996.

Sokol RJ: Expanding spectrum of mitochondrial disorders. J Pediatr 128:597, 1996.

Stacpoole PW, Barnes CL, Hurbanis MD, et al: Treatment of congenital lactic acidosis with dischloroacetate. Arch Dis Child 77:535, 1997.

Tolan DR, Brooks CC: Molecular analysis of common aldolase B alleles for hereditary fructose intolerance in North Americans. Biochem Med Metab Biol 48:19 1996.

Touati G, Rigal O, Lombs A, et al: In vivo functional investigations of lactic acid in patients with respiratory chain disorders. Arch Dis Child 76:16, 1997.

Van den Berg IET, Van Beurden EACM, Malingre HEM, et al: X-linked liver phosphorylase kinase deficiency is associated with mutations in the human liver phosphorylase kinase α subunit. Hum Mol Genet 3:1983 1994.

Waggoner DD, Buist NRM, Donnell GN: Long-term prognosis in galactosaemia: Results of a survey of 350 cases. J Inherit Metab Dis 13:802, 1990.

Willems PJ, Gerver WJM, Berger R, et al: The natural history of liver glycogenosis due to phosphorylase kinase deficiency: A longitudinal study of 41 patients. Eur J Pediatr 149:268, 1990.

Wolfsdorf JI, Ehrlich S, Landy HS, et al: Optimal daytime feeding regimen to prevent postprandial hypoglycemia in type 1 glycogen storage disease. Am J Clin Nutr 56:587, 1992.

84.6 Disorders of Glycoprotein Degradation and Structure

Margaret M. McGovern and Robert J. Desnick

The disorders of glycoprotein degradation and structure include several lysosomal storage diseases that result from defects in glycoprotein degradation and the carbohydrate-deficient glycoprotein syndrome, which is pathophysiologically unrelated. Glycoproteins are macromolecules that are composed of oligosaccharide chains linked to a peptide backbone. They are synthesized by two pathways, the glycosyltransferase pathway, which synthesizes oligosaccharides linked *O*-glycosidically to serine or threonine residues, and the dolichol, lipid-linked pathway, which synthesizes oligosaccharides linked *N*-glycosidically to asparagine.

Glycoprotein lysosomal storage diseases result from the deficiency of the enzymes that normally participate in the degradation of oligosaccharides and include sialidosis, galactosialidosis, aspartylglucosaminuria and α-mannosidosis. In some instances, the underlying abnormality that leads to glycoprotein accumulation also results in abnormal degradation of other classes of macromolecules that contain similar oligosaccharide linkages, such as certain glycolipids and proteoglycans (Table 84–2). In these instances, the underlying enzymatic deficiency results in the accumulation of both glycoproteins and glycolipids. The classification of these types of disorders as lipidoses or glycoproteinoses is dependent on the nature of the predominantly stored substance. Glycoprotein disorders are characterized by autosomal recessive inheritance and a progressive disease course with clinical features that resemble those seen in the mucopolysaccharidoses.

SIALIDOSIS AND GALACTOSIALIDOSIS

Sialidosis and galactosialidosis are autosomal recessive disorders that result from the deficiency of neuraminidase, and neuraminidase and β-galactosidase, respectively. Neuraminidase normally cleaves terminal sialyl linkages of several oligosaccharides and glycoproteins. Its deficiency results in the accumulation of oligosaccharides and the urinary excretion of sialic acid terminal oligosaccharides and sialylglycopeptides. Examination of tissues from affected individuals reveals pathologic storage of substrate in many tissues, including liver, bone marrow, and brain. Molecular studies have provided evidence that two different genes may be involved in the expression of the glycoprotein-specific neuraminidase that is deficient in sialidosis patients. The neuraminidase deficiency in one sialidosis patient was due to a mutation in a structural gene on chromosome 10, whereas the neuraminidase deficiency in a galactosialidosis patient was caused by a mutation in a gene located on chromosome 20.

CLINICAL MANIFESTATIONS. The clinical phenotype associated with neuraminidase deficiency is variable and includes type I sialidosis, which usually presents in the 2nd decade of life with

TABLE 84–2 Carbohydrate-Deficient Glycoprotein Syndromes: Types and Defects

Transferrin Isoelectric Focus Electrophoresis Pattern	Carbohydrates Deficient Glycoprotein Syndrome	Defect	Glycosylation Pathways Likely to Be Affected	Clinical Features
I	Ia (80%)	PMM (PMM2) (Man-6-P ↔ Man-1-P)	*N*-linked glycophospholipid *O*-mannose (?)	Hypotonia, failure to thrive, inverted nipples, unusual fat deposits, mental and psychomotor retardation, elevated liver function test results, coagulopathy, hepatomegaly, strokelike episodes, seizures, retinitis pigmentosa
	Ib (15%)	PMI (PMI1) (Fru-6-P ↔ Man-6-P)	*N*-linked glycophospholipid *O*-mannose (?)	Hypoglycemia, protein-losing enteropathy, failure to thrive, vomiting, diarrhea, congenital hepatic fibrosis
	—	Glucosylation of LLO	*N*-linked	Moderate CDSG type 1a symptoms and less pronounced neurologic involvement
	—	Normal PMM and PMI	?	Severe fetal-neonatal onset type I; ? lethal, thrombocytopenia, elevated MSAFP
II	IIa	GlcNAc transferase II (MGAT2)	*N*-linked	Severe developmental delay; hypotonia without peripheral neuropathy or cerebellar hypoplasia; generalized dysmyelination
III	III	?	?	Perinatal floppiness without polyneuropathy or cerebellar hypoplasia, generalized dysmyelination
IV	IV	?	?	Essentially no psychomotor development, reduced responsiveness, severe epileptic seizures, hypotonia, gothic palate, microcephaly, optic atrophy

From Freeze HH: Disorders in protein glycosylation and potential therapy: Tip of an iceberg. J Pediatr 133:593, 1998.
CDGS = carbohydrate deficient glycoprotein syndrome; PMI = phosphomannose isomerase; PMM = phosphomannomutase; LLO = lipid-linked oligosaccharide; Man-6-P = mannose 6 phosphate; Man-1-P = mannose 1 phosphate; MGATZ = 2 N-acetylglucosamine transferase II; MSAFP = maternal serum α-fetoprotein.

myoclonus and the presence of a cherry red spot. These patients typically come to attention because of gait disturbances, myoclonus, or visual complaints. In contrast, type II sialidosis occurs as congenital, infantile, and juvenile forms. The congenital and infantile forms result from isolated neuraminidase deficiency, whereas the juvenile form results from both neuraminidase and β-galactosidase deficiency. The congenital type II disease is characterized by hydrops fetalis, neonatal ascites, hepatosplenomegaly, stippling of the epiphyses, periosteal cloaking, and stillbirth or death during infancy. The type II infantile form presents in the 1st yr of life with dysostosis multiplex, moderate mental retardation, visceromegaly, corneal clouding, cherry-red spot, and seizures. The juvenile type II form of sialidosis, which is sometimes designated galactosialidosis, has a variable age of onset ranging from infancy to adulthood. In infancy, the phenotype is similar to that of GM_1 gangliosidosis with edema, ascites, skeletal dysplasia, and a cherry-red spot. Patients with disease of later onset have dysostosis multiplex, visceromegaly, mental retardation, dysmorphism, corneal clouding, progressive neurologic deterioration, and bilateral cherry-red spots.

The *diagnosis* of sialidosis and galactosialidosis is achieved by the demonstration of the specific enzymatic deficiency. Prenatal diagnosis using cultured amniotic cells is also possible.

No specific *treatment* exists for any form of the disease.

ASPARTYLGLUCOSAMINURIA

Aspartylglucosaminuria is a rare autosomal recessive lysosomal storage disorder, except in Finland where the carrier frequency is estimated to be 1/36. The disorder results from the deficient activity of aspartylglucosaminidase and the subsequent accumulation of aspartylglucosamine, particularly in the liver, spleen, and thyroid. The gene for the enzyme has been localized to the long arm of chromosome 4. In the Finnish population, a single mutation in the gene (C163S) accounts for most mutant alleles, whereas outside of Finland a large number of private mutations are present. Affected individuals with aspartylglucosaminuria typically present in the 1st yr of life with recurrent infections, diarrhea, and hernias. Coarsening of the facies and short stature usually develop later. Other features include joint laxity, macroglossia, hoarse voice, crystal-like lens opacities, hypotonia, and spasticity. Psychomotor development is usually near normal until the age of 5 yr when a decline is noted. Behavioral abnormalities are typical, and the IQ in affected adults is less than 40. Survival to adulthood is common, with most early deaths attributable to pneumonia or other pulmonary causes. Definitive diagnosis requires measurement of the enzyme in peripheral blood leukocytes. Molecular diagnosis by analysis of DNA for the C163S mutation is possible for Finnish patients. Prenatal diagnosis by the determination of the level of aspartylglucosaminidase in cultured amniocytes or chorionic villi has been reported. No specific treatment is available, and care is supportive.

α-MANNOSIDOSIS

α-Mannosidosis is an autosomal recessive disorder that results from the deficient activity of α-mannosidase and the accumulation of mannose-rich compounds. The gene encoding the enzyme has been localized to chromosome 19p13.2–q12. Affected patients with this disorder display clinical heterogeneity. There is a severe infantile form, or type I disease, and a milder juvenile variant, type II disease. All patients have psychomotor retardation, facial coarsening, and dysostosis multiplex. However, the infantile form of the disorder is characterized by more rapid mental deterioration, with death occurring between the ages of 3 and 10 yr. Patients with the infantile form also have more severe skeletal involvement and hepatosplenomegaly. The juvenile disorder is characterized by onset of symptoms during early childhood or adolescence with milder somatic features and survival to adulthood. Hearing loss, destructive synovitis, pancytopenia, and spastic paraplegia have all been reported in type II patients. The diagnosis is made by the demonstration of the deficiency of α-mannosidase activity in white blood cells or cultured fibroblasts, and prenatal diagnosis also has been achieved. No specific therapy exists for the disorder.

CARBOHYDRATE-DEFICIENT GLYCOPROTEIN SYNDROME

The carbohydrate-deficient glycoprotein syndrome is a heterogeneous autosomal recessive disorder that results from defects in the processing and synthesis of the carbohydrate moiety of glycoproteins (see Table 84–2). A distinctive biochemical marker of the disorder is the presence of carbohydrate-deficient transferrin in serum and cerebrospinal fluid as determined by isoelectric focusing electrophoresis.

The most consistent *clinical manifestations* of the disorder include psychomotor retardation, which varies in severity, and facial dysmorphic features that include a prominent jaw and ears, and inverted nipples. Frequent neurologic findings in infancy include hypotonia, weakness, hyperreflexia, and strokelike episodes (see Table 84–2). In childhood, ataxia, muscle atrophy, decreased deep tendon reflexes, toe walking, and continued strokelike episodes are observed. The latter events may be related to reduced factor XI, protein C, and antithrombin III. Strabismus is a consistent finding, and retinitis pigmentosa is common. Growth failure, liver dysfunction, retinal degeneration, and skeletal abnormalities have been described. The skeletal features may include contractures, kyphoscoliosis, and pectus carinatum, all of which may be secondary to the neurologic effects of the disorder. Pericardial effusion in older patients and hypertrophic obstructive cardiomyopathy in the infant may occur. Transferrin studies have revealed that infantile olivopontinecerebellar atrophy is a severe form of the carbohydrate-deficient glycoprotein syndrome. Lipodystrophy with prominent fat pads on the buttocks and suprapubic area are distinctive features. The disorder should be considered in patients with mental retardation, cerebellar hypoplasia, hepatic dysfunction, and episodic strokelike episodes. The *diagnosis* can be confirmed by analysis of the transferrin pattern by isoelectric focusing. Although prenatal diagnosis by analysis of transferrin has been attempted, it has not proved reliable.

Treatment of the disorder is symptomatic. Oral mannose has been effective in patients with type Ib CDGS.

Acarregui MJ, George TN, Rhead WJ: Carbohydrate-deficient glycoprotein syndrome type 1 with profound thrombocytopenia and normal phosphomannomutase and phosphomannose issomerase activities. J Pediatr 133:697:1998

Freeze HH: Disorders in protein glycosylation and potential therapy: Tip of an iceberg? J Pediatr 133:593, 1998.

Jaeken J, Stibler H, Hagberg B: The carbohydrate deficient glycoprotein syndrome: A new inherited multisystemic disease with severe nervous system involvement. Acta Pediatr Scand Suppl 375:1, 1991.

CHAPTER 85
Mucopolysaccharidoses

Joseph Muenzer

Mucopolysaccharidoses (MPSs) are inheritable disorders caused by a deficiency of lysosomal enzymes needed for the degradation of glycosaminoglycans (GAGs, also known by the older term *mucopolysaccharides)*. These storage diseases compose a heterogeneous group of disorders characterized by the intralysosomal accumulation of GAGs, excessive urinary excretion of GAGs, progressive mental and physical deterioration and, in severe forms, premature death. Each type has a specific lysosomal enzyme deficiency with a characteristic degree of organ involvement and rate of deterioration (Table 85–1). Depending on the enzyme deficiency, the metabolism of dermatan sulfate, heparan sulfate, or keratan sulfate may be blocked alone or in combination. Lysosomal accumulation of the GAGs eventually results in cell, tissue, and organ dysfunction. The MPS disorders share many clinical features, although in variable degrees. These include a chronic and progressive course, multisystem involvement, organomegaly, dysostosis multiplex, and abnormal facial features. Vision, hearing, airway and cardiovascular function, and joint mobility may be affected. Mental retardation is a common feature of the severe forms. There is clinical similarity among different enzyme deficiencies and conversely a wide spectrum of clinical severity within any enzyme deficiency. MPSs are characterized by autosomal recessive traits except for MPS II, which is an X-linked recessive condition.

CLINICAL MANIFESTATIONS

MUCOPOLYSACCHARIDOSIS I. Deficiency of iduronidase can result in a wide range of clinical involvement from the most severe form, Hurler syndrome, to the mildest form, Scheie syndrome. These represent two ends of a broad clinical spectrum. Hurler syndrome has been the prototype for describing MPSs, but this is misleading because it is not representative of all MPSs but only the most severe end of a spectrum.

Hurler Syndrome. This form of MPS I is a severe progressive disorder with multiple organ and tissue involvement that leads to premature death, usually by 10 yr of age. An infant with Hurler syndrome appears normal at birth. Diagnosis is made between 6 and 24 mo with evidence of hepatosplenomegaly, skeletal deformity, coarse facial features, corneal clouding, large tongue, prominent forehead, joint stiffness, and short stature. Acute cardiomyopathy may be a feature in some infants less than 1 yr of age. Most children with Hurler syndrome acquire only limited language skills because of developmental delay, chronic hearing loss, and an enlarged tongue. Hearing loss is common and is due to a combination of conductive and neurosensory problems. Most patients have recurrent upper respiratory tract and ear infections, noisy breathing, and persistent copious nasal discharge. Progressive ventricular enlargement with increased intracranial pressure caused by communicating hydrocephalus also occurs. Corneal clouding, glaucoma, and retinal degeneration are commonly seen. Obstructive airway disease develops in many patients, necessitating tracheostomy. Obstructive airway disease, respiratory infection, and cardiac complications are the common causes of death.

Radiographic changes seen in Hurler syndrome typify the constellation of skeletal abnormalities in the MPSs and are known as *dysostosis multiplex*. The skull is large, with thickened calvarium, premature closure of lambdoid and sagittal sutures, shallow orbits, enlarged J-shaped sella, and abnormal spacing of teeth with dentigerous cysts. Anterior hypoplasia of the lumbar vertebrae with kyphosis is seen early. The diaphyses of the long bones are enlarged with an irregular appearance of the metaphyses; the epiphyseal centers are not well developed. The pelvis is usually poorly formed with small femoral heads and coxa valga. The clavicles are short, thickened, and irregular. The ribs have been described as oar-shaped—narrowed at the vertebral ends and flat and broad at their sternal ends. The phalanges are short and trapezoid with widening of the diaphyses.

Hurler-Scheie Syndrome. This classification is used to describe a clinical phenotype that is intermediate between Hurler and Scheie syndromes. It is characterized by progressive somatic involvement, including dysostosis multiplex with little or no intellectual dysfunction. The onset of symptoms is usually observed between 3 and 8 yr; survival to adulthood is common. Cardiac involvement and upper airway obstruction contribute to clinical mortality.

Scheie Syndrome. This mild form of MPS I is characterized by joint stiffness, aortic valve disease, corneal clouding, and few other somatic features. Onset of significant symptoms is usually after the age of 5 yr, with diagnosis made between 10 and 20 yr. Patients with Scheie syndrome have normal intelligence and stature but have significant joint and ocular involvement. Ophthalmic features include severe corneal clouding, glaucoma, and retinal degeneration. Obstructive airway disease, causing sleep apnea, develops in some patients, necessitating

TABLE 85–1 Classification of the Mucopolysaccharidoses

Number	Eponym	Enzyme Deficiency	Stored Glycosaminoglycan	Major Clinical Manifestations
MPS I H	Hurler	α-L-Iduronidase	Dermatan sulfate, heparan sulfate	Mental retardation, heart disease, corneal clouding, dysostosis multiplex, organomegaly, death before 10 yr of age
MPS I S	Scheie	α-L-Iduronidase	Dermatan sulfate, heparan sulfate	Normal intelligence and life span, with corneal clouding, stiff joints, and heart disease
MPS I H/S	Hurler-Scheie	α-L-Iduronidase	Dermatan sulfate, heparan sulfate	Phenotype intermediate between Hurler and Scheie syndromes
MPS II	Hunter	Iduronate sulfatase	Dermatan sulfate, heparan sulfate	Wide spectrum of severity, mild to severe; dysostosis multiplex, mental retardation, organomegaly, death before 15 yr in severe form; normal intelligence with variable severity of somatic features in the milder form
MPS III A	Sanfillippo A	Heparan-*N*-sulfatase (sulfamidase)	Heparan sulfate	Hyperactivity, mild somatic features, profound mental deterioration; death usually in 2nd decade
MPS III B	Sanfillippo B	α-*N*-Acetyl-glucosaminidase	Heparan sulfate	Phenotype similar to Sanfillippo A
MPS III C	Sanfillippo C	Acetyl CoA:α-glucosaminidase acetyltransferase	Heparan sulfate	Phenotype similar to Sanfillippo A and B
MPS III D	Sanfillippo D	*N*-Acetylglucosamine 6-sulfatase	Heparan sulfate	Phenotype similar to Sanfillippo A and B
MPS IV A	Morquio A	Galactose-6-sulfatase	Keratan sulfate	Unique skeletal abnormalities, odontoid hypoplasia, short stature, normal intelligence; milder forms exist
MPS IV B	Morquio B	β-Galactosidase	Keratan sulfate	Wild spectrum of clinical severity similar to Morquio A
MPS V	No longer used			
MPS VI	Maroteaux-Lamy	*N*-Acetylgalactosamine-4-sulfatase	Dermatan sulfate	Normal intelligence, dysostosis multiplex, organomegaly, joint stiffness, corneal clouding; milder forms exist
MPS VII	Sly	β-Glucuronidase	Dermatan sulfate, heparan sulfate	Mental retardation, heart disease, corneal clouding, dysostosis multiplex, organomegaly; wide spectrum of clinical severity with fetal and neonatal form
MPS VIII	No longer used			
MPS IX		Hyaluronidase	Hyaluronan	Periarticular soft tissue masses, short stature

tracheostomy. Aortic valve disease is common and has required valve replacement in some patients.

MUCOPOLYSACCHARIDOSIS II. Hunter syndrome (MPS II) comprises two recognized clinical entities, severe and mild, that represent two ends of a wide spectrum of clinical severity. The severe and mild forms of Hunter syndrome can be separated only on clinical grounds because neither has detectable iduronate sulfatase (IDS) activity. The severe form of Hunter syndrome has features similar to Hurler syndrome except for the lack of corneal clouding and the slower progression of somatic and central nervous system deterioration. The mild form is somewhat analogous to Scheie syndrome, with a prolonged life span, minimal central nervous system involvement, and slow progression of somatic deterioration. The severe form of Hunter syndrome is characterized by coarse facial features, short stature, skeletal deformities, joint stiffness, and mental retardation with onset of disease usually between 2 and 4 yr of age. Communicating hydrocephalus is a common feature of the severe form, which can be difficult to detect because of the concurrent central nervous system deterioration. Extensive, slowly progressive neurologic involvement similar to the late stages of Sanfilippo syndrome usually precedes death, which usually occurs between 10 and 15 yr.

A milder form of MPS II has been recognized, with preservation of intelligence in adult life but with obvious clinical features of somatic involvement. Somatic features are similar to the severe form of MPS II but occur at a greatly reduced rate of progression. Airway involvement, hearing impairment, carpal tunnel syndrome, and joint stiffness are common and can result in significant loss of function in both the mild and severe forms.

MUCOPOLYSACCHARIDOSIS III. The Sanfilippo syndrome makes up a biochemically diverse but clinically similar group of four recognized types. Each type is due to a different enzyme deficiency (see Table 85–1). Phenotypical variations exist in MPS III patients but to a lesser degree than other MPS disorders, possibly because a very mild form of MPS III would be difficult to recognize. Patients with Sanfilippo syndrome are characterized by slowly progressive, severe central nervous system involvement but have only mild somatic disease. Such disproportionate involvement of the central nervous system is unique to MPS III. Onset of clinical features usually occurs between 2 and 6 yr in a child who previously appeared normal. Presenting features can include delayed development, hyperactivity with aggressive behavior, coarse hair, hirsutism, sleep disorders, and mild hepatosplenomegaly. Delays in diagnosis of MPS III are common secondary to the mild physical features, hyperactivity, and slowly progressive neurologic disease. Severe neurologic deterioration occurs in most patients by 6–10 yr, accompanied by rapid deterioration of social and adaptive skills. Severe behavior problems, including sleep disturbance, uncontrolled hyperactivity, temper tantrums, destructive behavior, and physical aggression, are common. Profound mental retardation and behavior problems often occur in patients with normal physical strength, making management particularly difficult.

MUCOPOLYSACCHARIDOSIS IV. Morquio syndrome (MPS IV) is caused by defective degradation of keratan sulfate. Two enzyme deficiencies resulting in Morquio syndrome are now recognized, each with a wide spectrum of clinical manifestations. Both types of Morquio syndrome are characterized by short-trunk dwarfism, fine corneal deposits, a skeletal dysplasia that is distinct from other mucopolysaccharidoses, and preservation of intelligence. The predominant clinical features of Morquio syndrome are those related to the skeleton and its effects on the central nervous system. Instability of the odontoid process and ligamentus laxity can result in life-threatening atlantoaxial subluxation. Surgery to stabilize the upper cervical spine, usually by posterior spinal fusion, prior to the development of cervical myelopathy can be lifesaving. The appearance of genu valgus, kyphosis, growth retardation with short trunk and neck, and waddling gait with a tendency to fall are early symptoms of MPS IV. Extraskeletal manifestations may include mild corneal clouding, hepatomegaly, cardiac valvular lesions, and small teeth with abnormally thin enamel and frequent caries formation. Patients with mild forms of MPS IV have been reported with almost normal stature, mild skeletal anomalies with dysplastic hips, corneal clouding, and absent keratosulfaturia.

MUCOPOLYSACCHARIDOSIS VI. Maroteaux-Lamy syndrome, due to deficiency of *N*-acetylgalactosamine-4-sulfatase, is characterized by preservation of intelligence but with severe to mild somatic involvement as seen in MPS I. The somatic involvement of the severe form of MPS IV is characterized by corneal clouding, coarse facial features, joint stiffness, valvular heart disease, communicating hydrocephalus, and dysostosis multiplex. In the severe form, growth can be normal for the first few years of life but seems to virtually stop after the age of 6–8 yr. The mild to intermediate forms of Maroteaux-Lamy syndrome can be easily confused with Scheie syndrome. Spinal cord compression from thickening of the dura in the upper cervical canal with resultant myelopathy is a frequent occurrence in patients with the milder form of MPS VI.

MUCOPOLYSACCHARIDOSIS VII. Sly syndrome (MPS VII), resulting from a deficiency of β-glucuronidase, is the rarest of all forms of MPS but also has the widest range of clinical involvement from a neonatal form to mild disease in adults. A severe neonatal form is characterized by hydrops fetalis, dysostosis multiplex, and clinical and pathologic findings of a lysosomal storage disease. The severe neonatal form of β-glucuronidase deficiency is one of the few lysosomal storage diseases that has been recognized in utero or is present at birth. The clinical involvement in MPS VII is similar to that seen in MPS I, with coarse facial features, hepatosplenomegaly, umbilical hernias, gibbus, and dysostosis multiplex, with varying degrees of clinical severity and mental retardation.

MUCOPOLYSACCHARIDOSIS IX. Major clinical findings in one reported case are bilateral nodular soft tissue periarticular masses, lysosomal storage of GAGs, mildly dysmorphic craniofacial features, short stature, and normal joint movement and intelligence. The clinical findings are presumably the consequences of the inability to degrade the hyaluronan (formerly called hyaluronic acid) that is normally found in cartilage and synovial fluid.

DIAGNOSIS

Analysis of urinary GAGs was the first method available for the diagnosis of MPSs and remains useful as an initial diagnostic test. Spot tests are quick, inexpensive, and useful for initial evaluation but are subject to both false-positive and false-negative results, with reliability largely dependent on the testing laboratory. Many methods are available for urinary GAG analysis, ranging from the semiquantitative spot test to more precise qualitative and quantitative analyses. Any individual who is suspected of an MPS disorder based on clinical features, radiographic results, or urinary mucopolysaccharide screening tests should have a definitive diagnosis established by enzyme assay. Serum, leukocytes, or cultured fibroblasts are generally used as the tissue source for measuring lysosomal enzymes. The choice of tissue used depends on the particular enzyme and the preference of the testing laboratory. Prenatal diagnosis is available for all MPSs and is routinely carried out on cultured cells from amniotic fluid or chorionic villus biopsy. Measurement of GAGs in amniotic fluid is generally unreliable. Carrier testing is difficult to perform by enzyme analysis. Carrier testing by enzyme analysis in Hunter syndrome, an X-linked disorder, is problematic and is not recommended. Molecular diagnosis is the preferred method of carrier testing provided that the mutation in the family under consideration is known.

GENETICS

For most of the MPSs, the lysosomal enzyme has been isolated, the cDNA cloned, and the gene structures characterized. With the isolation of the gene for each MPS, numerous mutations have been idenified in each disorder. However, many patients are compound heterozygotes for rare alleles. Mutation analysis has been beneficial in establishing genotype-phenotype correlation in Hurler syndrome and the severe form of MPS II, but for most mutations, the clinical phenotype cannot be predicted.

MUCOPOLYSACCHARIDOSIS I. The gene encoding α-liduronidase has been localized to chromosome 4p16.3 and spans 19 kilobases and includes 14 exons. Mutation analysis has revealed two major alleles, W402X and Q70X, and a minor allele, P533R, that account for more than half the MPS I alleles in the white population. None of these alleles produce functional enzyme (null alleles), and in homozygosity or compound heterozygosity with each other give rise to Hurler syndrome, the severe form of MPS I. There are numerous mutations that occur in only one or a few individuals.

MUCOPOLYSACCHARIDOSIS II. Hunter syndrome is an X-linked disorder. The gene encoding IDS contains nine exons that span 24 kilobases and has been mapped to Xq28. About 20% of patients with the severe form of MPS II have major deletions or rearrangements of the IDS gene. MPS II patients with an unusually severe phenotype have a very large deletion of the IDS locus, including adjoining genes, resulting in a contiguous gene syndrome. Most MPS II mutations are point mutations, small deletions or insertions, and many occur in only a single family.

MUCOPOLYSACCHARIDOSIS III. The gene encoding heparan *N*-sulfatase (MPS III A [Sanfillipo A]) spans 11 kilobases and is localized to chromosome 17q25.3. The gene encoding α-*N*-acetylglucosaminidase (MPS III B [Sanfillipo B]) spans 8.5 kilobases, comprises six exons, and is localized on chromosome 17q21. Mutations have been found for all the MPS III disorders for which the genes have been isolated. Most MPS III mutations are uncommon, consisting of the missense type, with a few premature terminations and small deletions.

MUCOPOLYSACCHARIDOSIS IV. The gene encoding *N*-acetylgalactosamine-6-sulfatase (MPS IV A [Morquio A) spans about 50 kilobases, contains 14 exons, and has been localized to chromosome 16q24.3. About 100 MPS IV A mutations have been identified, consisting of missense or small deletions. Two mutations are recurring in patients from Northern Ireland and Australia and may explain the relatively high incidence (founder effect) of MPS IV in Northern Ireland. Several missense mutations have been described in the β-galactosidase gene that causes MPS IV B, a rare form of Morquio syndrome.

MUCOPOLYSACCHARIDOSIS VI. The gene encoding *N*-acetylgalactosamine-4-sulfatase (arylsulfatase B) is composed of eight exons and has been localized to chromosome 5q13q14. More than 30 mutations have been identified, most of which have been found in single families. Mutations found in MPS VI have included frameshift, nonsense, and missense mutations.

MUCOPOLYSACCHARIDOSIS VII. The gene encoding β-glucuronidase spans 21 kilobases, contains 12 exons, and has been localized to chromosome 7q21.1. More than 35 mutations have been identified, mostly missense, but also nonsense, frameshift, and splice site.

TREATMENT

Although correction of MPS cultured fibroblasts by "corrective factors" has been possible for at least 3 decades in the laboratory, no definitive therapy is available for patients with an MPS disorder. The corrective factors are the missing lysosomal enzymes that have a mannose-6-phosphate recognition marker for efficient receptor-mediated endocytosis into fibroblasts. Early clinical trials of enzyme replacement by the administration of plasma or leukocytes, fibroblast transplantation, or amnion membrane implantation have failed to make any lasting improvement in the clinical disease. In contrast, bone marrow transplantation has resulted in significant clinical improvement of somatic disease in MPS I and increased long-term survival. Resolution or improvements have been noted in hepatosplenomegaly, joint stiffness, facial appearance, obstructive sleep apnea, heart disease, communicating hydrocephalus, and hearing loss.

In contrast, after bone marrow transplantation, the skeletal and ocular anomalies are not corrected. Orthopedic procedures, including femoral osteotomies, acetabular reconstruction, and posterior spinal fusion, have been necessary for most patients with Hurler syndrome after bone marrow transplantation in an attempt to maintain function and gait. The neuropsychologic outcomes of MPS have varied widely after bone marrow transplantation. Hurler syndrome patients who have undergone transplantation before 24 mo of age and with a baseline mental development index greater than 70 have improved long-term outcome. The microglia cells in the central nervous system, which are of bone marrow origin, are thought to be the source of the enzyme in the brain after bone marrow transplantation. Preservation of intelligence has not occurred in patients with severe MPS II or MPS III. At present, it is not possible to recommend bone marrow transplantation for any MPS disorders except Hurler syndrome in patients who are less than 24 mo of age and have no significant neurologic disease at the time of transplantation. Although bone marrow transplantation has significantly modified the natural history of the disease and improved survival in some patients, the procedure is not curative. Somatic disease has generally improved, except for the skeleton and eyes, but neurologic outcomes have varied.

Enzyme replacement using recombinant enzyme produced in cultured mammalian cells is a potential method to treat the somatic features of MPSs. Experience gained with enzyme replacement in dogs with MPS I has supported an ongoing clinical trial of recombinant α-L-iduronidase for MPS I patients. Early results demonstrate normalization of urinary GAG excretion, decreased liver and spleen size, improved joint range of motion, and activity. Enzyme replacement therapy trials using recombinant enzyme should be initiated in other MPS disorders once adequate quantities of recombinant enzyme are produced. Recombinant enzyme administered peripherally is not expected to cross the blood-brain barrier and improve or stabilize the central nervous system disease.

Since most patients are not candidates for specific therapies at this time, supportive management, with particular attention to respiratory and cardiovascular complications, hearing loss, carpal tunnel syndrome, spinal cord compression, and hydrocephalus, can greatly improve the quality of life for patients and their families. The progressive nature of clinical involvement in MPS patients dictates the need for evaluation of their clinical status on a regular basis.

Cleary MA, Wraith JE: Management of mucopolysaccharidosis type III. Arch Dis Child 69:403, 1993.

Danos O, Heard JM: Mucopolysaccharidosis. Mol Cell Biol Hum Dis 5:350, 1995.

Guffon N, Souillet G, Maire I, et al: Follow-up of nine patients with Hurler syndrome after bone marrow transplantation. J Pediatr 133:119, 1998.

Hopwood JJ, Moris CP: The mucopolysaccharidoses: Diagnosis, molecular genetics and treatment. Mol Biol Med 7:381, 1990.

Hopwood JJ, Bunge S, Morris CP, et al: Molecular basis of mucopolysaccharidosis type II: Mutations in the iduronate-2-sulphatase gene. Hum Mutat 2:435, 1993.

Mikles M, Stanton RP: A review of Morquio syndrome. Am J Orthop 26:533,1997.

Neufeld EF, Muenzer J: The mucopolysaccharidoses. *In*: Scriver CR, Beaudet AL, Sly WS, Valle D (eds): The Metabolic Basis of Inherited Disease, 7th ed, Vol II. New York, McGraw-Hill, 1995, p 2465.

Northover H, Cowie RA, Wraith JE: Mucopolysaccharidosis type IV A (Morquio syndrome): A clinical review. J Inherit Metab Dis 19:357, 1996.

Peters C, Shapiro EG, Anderson J, et al: Hurler syndrome: II. Outcome of HLA-genotypically identical sibling and HLA-haploidentical related donor bone marrow transplantation in fifty-four children. Blood 91:2601, 1998.

Peters C, Shapiro EG, Krivit W: Hurler syndrome: Past, present, and future. J Pediatr 133:79, 1998.

Sands MS, Wolfe JH, Birkenmeier EH, et al: Gene therapy for murine mucopolysaccharidosis type VII. Neuromuscul Disord 7:352, 1997.

Schmidtchen A, Greenberg D, Zhao HG, et al: NAGLU mutations underlying Sanfilippo syndrome type B. Am J Hum Genet 62:64, 1998.

Scott HS, Bunge S, Gal A, et al: Molecular genetics of mucopolysaccharidosis type I: Diagnostic, clinical, and biological implications. Hum Mutat 6:288, 1995.

Shapiro EG, Lockman LA, Balthazor M, et al: Neuropsychological outcomes of several storage diseases with and without bone marrow transplantation. J Inherit Metab Dis 18:413, 1995.

Stone JE: Urine analysis in the diagnosis of mucopolysaccharide disorders. Ann Clin Biochem 35:207, 1998.

Suzuki K, Proia RL, Suzuki K: Mouse models of human lysosomal diseases. Brain Pathol 8:195, 1998.

Tandon V, Williamson JB, Cowie RA, et al: Spinal problems in mucopolysaccharidosis I (Hurler syndrome). J Bone Joint Surg 78:938, 1996.

Van Heest AE, House J, Krivit W, et al: Surgical treatment of carpal tunnel syndrome and trigger digits in children with mucopolysaccharide storage disorders. J Hand Surg 23:236, 1998.

Whitley CB, Belani KG, Chang P, et al: Long- term outcome of Hurler syndrome following bone marrow transplantation. Am J Hum Genet 46:209, 1993.

Wraith JE: The mucopolysaccharidoses: A clinical review and guide to management. Arch Dis Child 72:263, 1995.

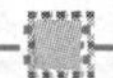

CHAPTER 86
Disorders of Purine and Pyrimidine Metabolism

J. C. Harris

Purines are involved in all biologic processes; all cells require a balanced supply of purines for growth and survival. They provide the primary source of cellular energy through adenosine triphosphate (ATP) and, together with pyrimidines, provide the source for the RNA and DNA that stores, transcribes, and translates genetic information. Purines provide the basic coenzymes (NAD, NADH) for metabolic regulation and play a major role in signal transduction and translation (GTP, cAMP, cGMP). Metabolically active nucleotides are formed from heterocyclic nitrogen-containing purine bases (guanine and adenine) and pyrimidine bases (cytosine, uridine, and thymine). The early steps in the biosynthesis of the purine ring are shown in Figure 86–1. Purines are primarily produced from endogenous sources, and in the usual circumstances dietary purines have a small role. The end product of purine metabolism in human beings is uric acid (2,6,8-trioxypurine).

The inherited disorders of purine and pyrimidine metabolism cover a broad spectrum of illnesses with various presentations. These include hyperuricemia, acute renal failure, gout, unexplained neurologic deficits (seizures, muscle weakness, choreoathetoid and dystonic movements), developmental disability, mental retardation, compulsive self-injury and aggression, autistic-like behavior, unexplained anemia, failure to thrive, susceptibility to recurrent infection (immune deficiency), and deafness.

Although uric acid is not a specific disease marker, increased serum levels in children lead to the investigation of the cause of its elevation. The level of uric acid present at any time depends on the size of the purine nucleotide pool derived from de novo purine synthesis, catabolism of tissue nucleic acids, and increased turnover of preformed purines. Uric acid is

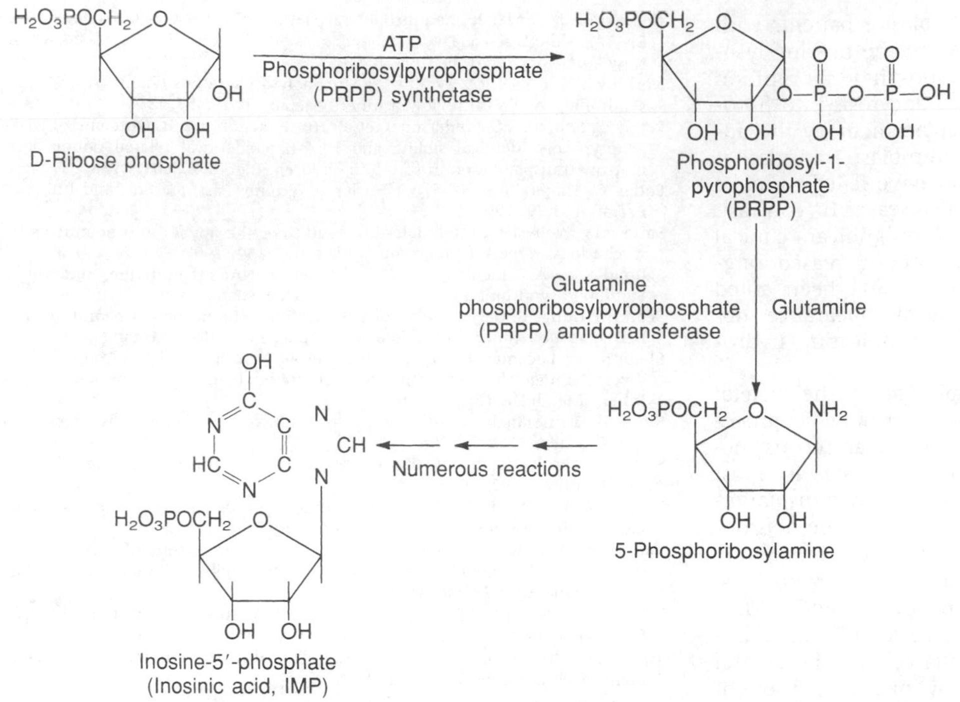

Figure 86–1 Early steps in the biosynthesis of the purine ring.

poorly soluble and must be excreted continuously to avoid toxic accumulations in the body. Its renal excretion involves the following components: (1) glomerular filtration, (2) reabsorption in the proximal convoluted tubule, (3) secretion near the terminus of the proximal tubule, and (4) limited reabsorption near these secretory sites. Thus, renal loss of uric acid is a result of renal tube excretion and is a function of serum uric acid concentration and a homeostatic mechanism to avoid hyperuricemia. Because renal tubule excretion is greater in children than in adults, serum uric acid levels are a less reliable indicator of uric acid production in children than in adults, and consequently measurement of the level in urine may be required to determine excessive production in children. Clearance of a smaller portion of uric acid is via the gastrointestinal tract (biliary and intestinal secretion). Owing to poor solubility of uric acid under normal circumstances, uric acid is near the maximal tolerable limits, and small alterations in production or solubility or changes in secretion may result in high serum levels. In renal insufficiency, urate excretion is increased by residual nephrons and by the gastrointestinal tract. Increased production of uric acid is found in malignancy, Reye syndrome, Down syndrome, psoriasis, sickle cell anemia, cyanotic congenital heart disease, pancreatic enzyme replacement, glycogen storage disease types I, III, IV, and V, hereditary fructose intolerence, acyl-coenzyme A dehydrogenase deficiency, and gout.

The *metabolism* of both purines and pyrimidines can be divided into two biosynthetic pathways and a catabolic pathway. The first involves a multistep biosynthesis from precursors through the de novo pathway that leads to the production of purine and pyrimidine nucleotides from ribose-5-phosphate or carbamyl phosphate, respectively. The second is a single-step salvage pathway that recovers purine and pyrimidine bases derived from either dietary intake or the catabolic pathway (see Figs. 86–1 and 86–3). In the de novo pathway, the nucleosides guanosine, adenosine, cytidine, uridine, and thymidine are formed by the addition of ribose-1-phosphate to the purine bases guanine or adenine, and to the pyrimidine bases cytosine, uracil, and thymine. The phosphorylation of these nucleosides produces monophosphate, diphosphate, and triphosphate nucleotides.

Under usual circumstances, the salvage pathway predominates over the biosynthetic pathway. Synthesis is most active in tissues with high rates of cellular turnover, such as gut epithelium, skin, and bone marrow. The third pathway is catabolism. The end product of the catabolic pathway of the purines is uric acid, whereas catabolism of pyrimidines produces citric acid cycle intermediates. Only a small fraction of the purines turned over each day are degraded and excreted.

Inborn errors in the *synthesis* of purine nucleotides include (1) phosphoribosylpyrophosphate synthetase superactivity and (2) adenylosuccinase deficiency. Disorders resulting from abnormalities in purine *catabolism* include (3) muscle adenosine monophosphate (AMP) deaminase deficiency, (4) adenosine deaminase deficiency, (5) purine nucleoside phosphorylase deficiency, and (6) xanthine oxidase deficiency. Disorders resulting from the purine *salvage* pathway include (7) hypoxanthine-guanine phosphoribosyltransferase (HPRT) deficiency and (8) adenine phosphoribosyltransferase (APRT) deficiency.

Inborn errors of pyrimidine metabolism include (1) hereditary orotic aciduria (uridine monophosphate synthase deficiency), (2) dihydropyrimidine dehydrogenase deficiency, (3) dihydropyrimidinase deficiency, and (4) pyrimidine 5′-nucleotidase deficiency.

GOUT

Gout presents with hyperuricemia, uric acid nephrolithiasis, and arthritis. Gouty arthritis is due to monosodium urate crystal deposits that result in inflammation in joints and surrounding tissues. The presentation is most commonly monoarticular, typically in the metatarsophalangeal joint of the big toe. Tophi, deposits of monosodium urate crystals, may occur over points of insertion of tendons at the elbows, knees, and feet or over the helix of the ears. *Primary gout,* ordinarily occurring in middle-aged men, results from the overproduction, decreased renal excretion, or both, of uric acid. Its biochemical etiology is unknown for most of those affected, and it is considered to be a polygenic trait. When hyperuricemia and gout occur in childhood, it is most often *secondary gout,* the result of another disorder in which there is rapid tissue breakdown or cellular turnover leading to increased production or decreased excretion of uric acid. Gout occurs in any condition that leads to reduced clearance of uric acid: during therapy for malignancy or with dehydration, lactic acidosis, ketoacidosis, starvation, diuretic therapy, and renal shutdown. Excessive purine, alcohol, or carbohydrate ingestion may increase uric acid levels.

Gout is associated with hereditary disorders in three different enzyme disorders that result in hyperuricemia. These include the severe form of HPRT deficiency (Lesch-Nyhan syndrome), partial HPRT deficiency, superactivity of PP-ribose-P synthetase, and glycogen storage disease, type I (glucose-6-phosphatase deficiency) (Chapter 84.1). In the first two, the basis of hyperuricemia is purine nucleotide and uric acid overproduction, whereas in the third it is both excessive uric acid production and impaired uric acid secretion. Glycogen storage disease types III, V, and VII are associated with exercise-induced hyperuricemia, the consequence of rapid ATP utilization and failure to regenerate it effectively during exercise (Chapter 84.1). Finally, *familial juvenile gout* or familial juvenile hyperuricemic nephropathy is associated with severe renal hypoexcretion of uric acid. Although it most commonly presents from puberty up to the 3rd decade, it has been reported in infancy. Familial juvenile hyperuricemic nephropathy is an autosomal dominant disorder, unlike the three inherited purine disorders that are X-linked and the recessively inherited glycogen storage disease. It occurs in both males and females and is frequently associated with a rapid decline in renal function that may lead to death unless diagnosed and treated early.

Treatment of hyperuricemia involves the combination of allopurinal (a xanthine oxidase inhibitor) to decrease uric acid production, probenecid to increase uric acid clearance in those with normal renal function, alkalinization of the urine to increase the solubility of uric acid, and increased fluid intake to reduce the concentration of uric acid. A low purine diet, weight reduction, and reduced alcohol intake are recommended.

ABNORMALITIES IN PURINE SALVAGE

Lesch-Nyhan Syndrome

Lesch-Nyhan syndrome is a rare X-linked disorder of purine metabolism that results from HPRT deficiency. This enzyme is normally present in each cell in the body, but its highest concentration is in the brain, especially in the basal ganglia. *Clinical manifestations* include hyperuricemia, mental retardation, cerebral palsy with early choreoathetosis and later spasticity and dystonia, dysarthric speech, and compulsive self-biting, usually beginning with the eruption of teeth.

There are several clinical presentations of HPRT deficiency. HPRT levels are related to the extent of motor symptoms, to the presence or absence of self-injury, and possibly to the level of cognitive function. The majority of individuals with classic Lesch-Nyhan syndrome have low or undetectable levels of the HPRT enzyme. Partial deficiency in HPRT (Kelley-Seegmiller syndrome) with more than 1.5–2.0% enzyme is associated with hyperuricemia and variable neurologic dysfunction (neurologic HPRT deficiency). HPRT deficiency with levels over 8% leads to a severe form of gout, with apparently normal cerebral functioning (HPRT-related hyperuricemia), although cognitive deficits may occur in some cases.

GENETICS. The *HPRT* gene has been localized to the long arm of the X chromosome (q26-q27). The complete amino acid sequence for *HPRT* is known (approximately 44 kb; 9 exons). The disorder appears in males; occurrence in females is extremely rare and ascribed to nonrandom inactivation of the X chromosome. Absence of *HPRT* prevents the normal metabolism of hypoxanthine, resulting in excessive uric acid production and manifestations of gout, necessitating specific drug treatment (allopurinol). Because of the enzyme deficiency, hypoxanthine accumulates in the cerebrospinal fluid, but uric acid does not; uric acid is not produced in the brain and does not cross the blood-brain barrier. The behavior disorder is not caused by hyperuricemia or excess hypoxanthine because patients with partial HPRT variants with hyperuricemia do not self-injure and infants having isolated hyperuricemia from birth do not develop self-injurious behavior.

The prevalence of the classic Lesch-Nyhan syndrome has been estimated at 1 in 100,000 to 1 in 380,000 based on the number of known cases in the United States. The incidence of partial variants is not known. Those with the classic syndrome rarely survive the 3rd decade because of renal or respiratory compromise. The life span may be normal for patients with partial variants without severe renal involvement.

PATHOLOGY. No brain abnormality is documented after detailed histopathology and electron microscopy of affected brain regions. Magnetic resonance imaging has documented reductions in the volume of basal ganglia nuclei. Abnormalities in neurotransmitter metabolism have been identified in three autopsied cases. All three patients had very low HPRT levels (less than 1% in striatal tissue and 1–2% of control in thalamus cortex). There was a functional loss of 65–90% of the nigrostriatal and mesolimbic dopamine terminals, although the cells of origin in the substantia nigra did not show dopamine reduction. The brain regions primarily involved were the caudate nucleus, putamen, and nucleus accumbens. It is proposed that the neurochemical changes may be linked to functional abnormalities, possibly resulting from a diminution of arborization or branching dendrites rather than cell loss. A neurotransmitter abnormality is suggested by changes in cerebral spinal fluid neurotransmitters and their metabolites, which have been confirmed by positron emission tomography scans. Reductions in vivo in the presynaptic dopamine transporter were documented in the caudate and putamen of six individuals.

The mechanism whereby HPRT leads to the neurologic and behavioral symptoms is unknown. However, guanine triphosphate (GTP) and adenosine have substantial effects on neural tissues. There is a functional link between purine nucleotides and the dopamine system that involves guanine, the precursor of GTP. Dopamine binding to its receptor results in either an activation (D_1 receptor) or an inhibition (D_2 receptor) of adenylcyclase. Both receptor effects are mediated by G proteins (GTP-binding proteins) dependent on guanine diphosphate (GDP) in the GDP/GTP exchange for cellular activation. Dopamine and adenosine systems are also linked through the role of adenosine as a neuroprotective agent in preventing neurotoxicity. Adenosine agonists mimic the biochemical and behavioral actions of dopamine antagonists, whereas adenosine receptor antagonists act as functional dopamine agonists. Two HPRT-deficient strains of mice have been produced.

CLINICAL MANIFESTATIONS. At birth, infants with Lesch-Nyhan syndrome have no apparent neurologic dysfunction. After several months, developmental retardation and neurologic signs become apparent. Before the age of 4 mo, hypotonia, recurrent vomiting, and difficulty with secretions may be noted. By approximately 8–12 mo, extrapyramidal signs appear, including chorea and dystonia. By around 12 mo, in a significant number of cases, pyramidal tract signs may become evident with hyperreflexia, sustained ankle clonus, positive Babinski's sign, and scissoring. Spasticity may become apparent at this time or, in some instances, later in life.

Cognitive function is usually reported to be in the mild-to-moderate range of mental retardation, although some individuals test in the low normal range. Because test scores may be influenced by difficulty in testing the subjects owing to their movement disorder and dysarthric speech, overall intelligence may be underestimated.

The age of onset of self-injury may be as early as 1 yr and occasionally as late as the teens. Self-injury occurs, although all sensory modalities, including pain, are intact. The self-injurious behavior usually begins with self-biting, although other patterns of self-injurious behavior emerge with time. Most characteristically, the fingers, mouth, and buccal mucosa are mutilated. Self-biting is intense and causes tissue damage and may result in the amputation of fingers and substantial loss of tissue around the lips. Extraction of primary teeth may be required. The biting pattern can be asymmetric, with preferential mutilation of the left or right side of the body. The type of behavior is different from that seen in other mental retardation syndromes involving self-injury. Self-hitting and head-banging are the most common initial presentations in other syndromes. The intensity of the self-injurious behavior generally requires that the patient be restrained. When restraints are removed, the individual with Lesch-Nyhan syndrome may appear terrified, and stereotypically place a finger in the mouth. The patient may ask for restraints to prevent elbow movement; when the restraints are placed or replaced, he may appear relaxed and more good humored. Dysarthric speech may cause interpersonal communication problems; however, the higher-functioning children can express themselves fully and participate in verbal therapy.

The self-mutilation presents as a compulsive behavior that the child tries to control but frequently is unable to resist. Older individuals may enlist the help of others and notify them when they are comfortable enough to have restraints removed. In some instances, the behavior may lead to deliberate self-harm. The individual with Lesch-Nyhan syndrome may also show compulsive aggression and inflict injury to others through pinching, grabbing, or hitting or by using verbal forms of aggression. Afterwards he may apologize, stating that this behavior was out of his control. Other maladaptive behaviors include head- or limb-banging, eye-poking, and psychogenic vomiting.

DIAGNOSIS. The presence of dystonia along with self-mutilation of the mouth and fingers suggests Lesch-Nyhan syndrome. With partial HPRT deficiency, recognition is linked to hyperuricemia and a dystonic movement disorder. Serum levels of uric acid that exceed 4–5 mg uric acid/dL and a urine uric acid:creatinine ratio of 3:4 or more are highly suggestive of HPRT deficiency, particularly when associated with neurologic symptoms. The definitive diagnosis requires an analysis of the HPRT enzyme. This is assayed in an erythrocyte lysate. Individuals with classic Lesch-Nyhan syndrome have near 0% enzyme activity and those with partial variants show values between 1.5% and 60%. The enzyme activity in those with partial variants with enzyme levels over 10% shows little correlation with the clinical phenotype. The intact cell HPRT assay in skin fibroblasts offers a good correlation between enzyme activity and the severity of the disease. Molecular techniques are used for gene sequencing and the identification of carriers.

Differential diagnosis includes other causes of infantile hypotonia and dystonia. Children with Lesch-Nyhan syndrome are often initially incorrectly diagnosed as having athetoid cerebral palsy. When a diagnosis of cerebral palsy is suspected in an infant with a normal prenatal, perinatal, and postnatal course, the Lesch-Nyhan syndrome should be considered. Partial HPRT deficiency may be associated with acute renal failure in infancy. An understanding of the molecular disorder has led to effective drug treatment for uric acid accumulation and arthritic tophi, renal stones, and neuropathy. However, reduction in uric acid alone does not influence the neurologic and behavioral aspects of Lesch-Nyhan syndrome. Despite treatment from birth for uric acid elevation, behavioral and neurologic symptoms are unaffected. The most significant complications of Lesch-Nyhan syndrome are renal failure and self-mutilation.

TREATMENT. Medical management of this disorder focuses on the prevention of renal failure by pharmacologic treatment of hyperuricemia with allopurinol, efforts to reduce self-mutilation through behavior management, and the use of restraints or removal of teeth or both. Pharmacologic approaches to decrease anxiety and spasticity with medication have mixed results. Drug therapy focuses on symptomatic management of anticipatory anxiety and on mood stabilization. Although there is no standard drug treatment, diazepam may be helpful for anxiety symptoms, risperidol for aggressive behavior, and carbamazepine for mood stabilization. Each of these medications may alleviate self-injurious behavior by helping to reduce anxiety and stabilize mood.

Bone marrow transplantation, based on the possibility that the central nervous system damage is produced by a circulating toxin, has been done in several patients. Several infant patients have died of complications of bone marrow transplantation. In one adult case in which the transplantation was successful, there was no change in neurologic symptoms or in behavior. In this case, dopamine receptors measured by positron emission tomography before and after the bone marrow transplantation showed no changes in receptor density following the transplantation. To date, there is no evidence that bone marrow transplantation is a beneficial treatment approach; it remains an experimental and potentially dangerous therapy. Two patients received partial exchange transfusions every 2 mo for 3 to 4 yr. Erythrocyte hypoxanthine-guanine phosphoribosyltransferase activity was 10% to 70% of normal during this period, but no reduction of neurologic or behavioral symptoms was apparent.

Both the motivation for self-injury and its biologic basis must be addressed in treatment programs. Yet behavioral techniques alone, using operant conditioning approaches, have not proved to be an adequate general treatment and have limited effectiveness. Although behavioral procedures have had some selective success in reducing self-injury, generalization outside the experimental setting limits this approach because patients under stress may revert to their previous self-injurious behavior. Behavioral approaches may also focus on reducing the self-injurious behavior through the treatment of phobic anxiety associated with being unrestrained. The most common techniques are systematic desensitization, extinction, and differential reinforcement of other (competing) behavior. Stress management has been recommended to assist patients to develop more effective coping mechanisms. Individuals with Lesch-Nyhan syndrome do not respond to contingent electric shock or similar aversive behavioral measures. An increase in self-injury may be observed when aversive methods are utilized.

Restraint (day and night) and dental procedures are common means to prevent self-injury. The time in restraints is linked to the age of onset of self-injury in that the older the patient is at the onset of self-injury, the less time is needed for restraint. Patients who are never restrained at night have a significantly later onset of self-injury. Children with Lesch-Nyhan disease can participate in making decisions regarding restraints and the type of restraints. The time in restraints may potentially be reduced with systematic behavior treatment programs. Many patients have teeth extracted to prevent self-injury. Others use a protective mouth guard designed by a dentist. Most parents suggest that stress reduction and awareness of the patient's needs are the most effective in reducing self-injury. Families reported that they deal with self-injury by attending to physical comfort and adjusting restraints, talking to the child, and finding something more interesting to do. Positive behavioral techniques of reinforcing appropriate behavior are rated effective by almost half of the families.

Adenine Phosphoribosyltransferase Deficiency

Adenine phosphoribosyltransferase deficiency may be present at birth, becoming apparent as early as the first 2 yr of life and as late as the 4th decade. *Clinical manifestations* include urinary calculus formation with crystalluria, urinary tract infections, hematuria, renal colic, and renal failure. The renal calculi, composed of 2,8-dihydroxyadenine, are radiolucent, soft, and easily crushed. These stones are not distinguishable from uric acid stones by routine tests.

The enzyme deficiency causes suppression of the salvage of adenine from nutritional sources and the polyamine pathway, with adenine being oxidized by xanthine dehydrogenase into 2,8-dihydroxyadenine. Urinary levels of adenine, 8-hydroxyadenine, and 2,8-dihydroxyadenine are elevated while plasma uric acid is normal. The deficiency may be complete or partial; the partial deficiency is reported in Japan. The disorder is an autosomal recessive trait with considerable clinical heterogeneity. The *APRT* gene is located on chromosome 16q (16q4) and has been cloned and sequenced. Because identification of 2,8-dihydroxyadenine is complex, the most common diagnostic test is the measurement of APRT activity in red blood cells.

Treatment includes high fluid intake, dietary purine restriction, and allopurinol, which inhibits the conversion of adenine to its metabolites. Alkalinization of the urine is not advised, because, unlike that of uric acid, the solubility of 2,8-dihydroxyadenine does not increase up to pH 9. The prognosis depends on renal function at the time of diagnosis. Early treatment is critical in the prevention of stones because severe renal insufficiency may accompany late recognition.

DISORDERS LINKED TO PURINE NUCLEOTIDE SYNTHESIS

Phosphoribosylpyrophosphate Synthetase Superactivity

Phosphoribosylpyrophosphate (PRPP) synthetase superactivity is a disorder seen primarily in young adult males who present with uric acid stones, gouty arthritis. or both. Blood uric acid may be two to three times normal values, and the urinary excretion of uric acid is increased. In some patients, clinical signs of uric acid overproduction are apparent in infancy and accompanied by neurologic abnormalities, primarily sensorineural deafness, particularly for high frequencies. In addition, hypotonia, delays in motor milestones, ataxia, and autistic-like behavior have been described. The various types of this disorder are sex-linked traits. In those cases in which there is sensorineural hearing loss, heterozygous females have also been found with gout and hearing impairments.

This enzyme produces PRPP from ribose-5-phosphate and ATP, as shown in Figures 86–1 and 86–2. PRPP is the first intermediary compound in the de novo synthesis of purine nucleotides that lead to the formation of inosine monophosphate. Superactivity of the enzyme results in an increased generation of PRPP. Because PRPP amidotransferase, the first enzyme of the de novo pathway, is not physiologically saturated by PRPP, the synthesis of purine nucleotides increases, and, consequently, the production of uric acid is increased. PRPP synthetase superactivity is one of the few hereditary disorders of an enzyme that leads to enhanced activity. A mechanism for the neurologic symptoms is unknown. The diagnosis requires kinetic studies of the enzyme performed in erythrocytes and cultured fibroblasts. This disorder must be differentiated from partial HPRT deficiency involving the salvage pathway, which also results in neurologic HPRT deficiency or hyperuricemia without neurologic features.

Treatment is with allopurinol, which inhibits xanthine dehydrogenase, the last enzyme of the purine catabolic pathway. Uric acid production is reduced and is replaced by hypoxanthine, which is more soluble, and xanthine, which is slightly

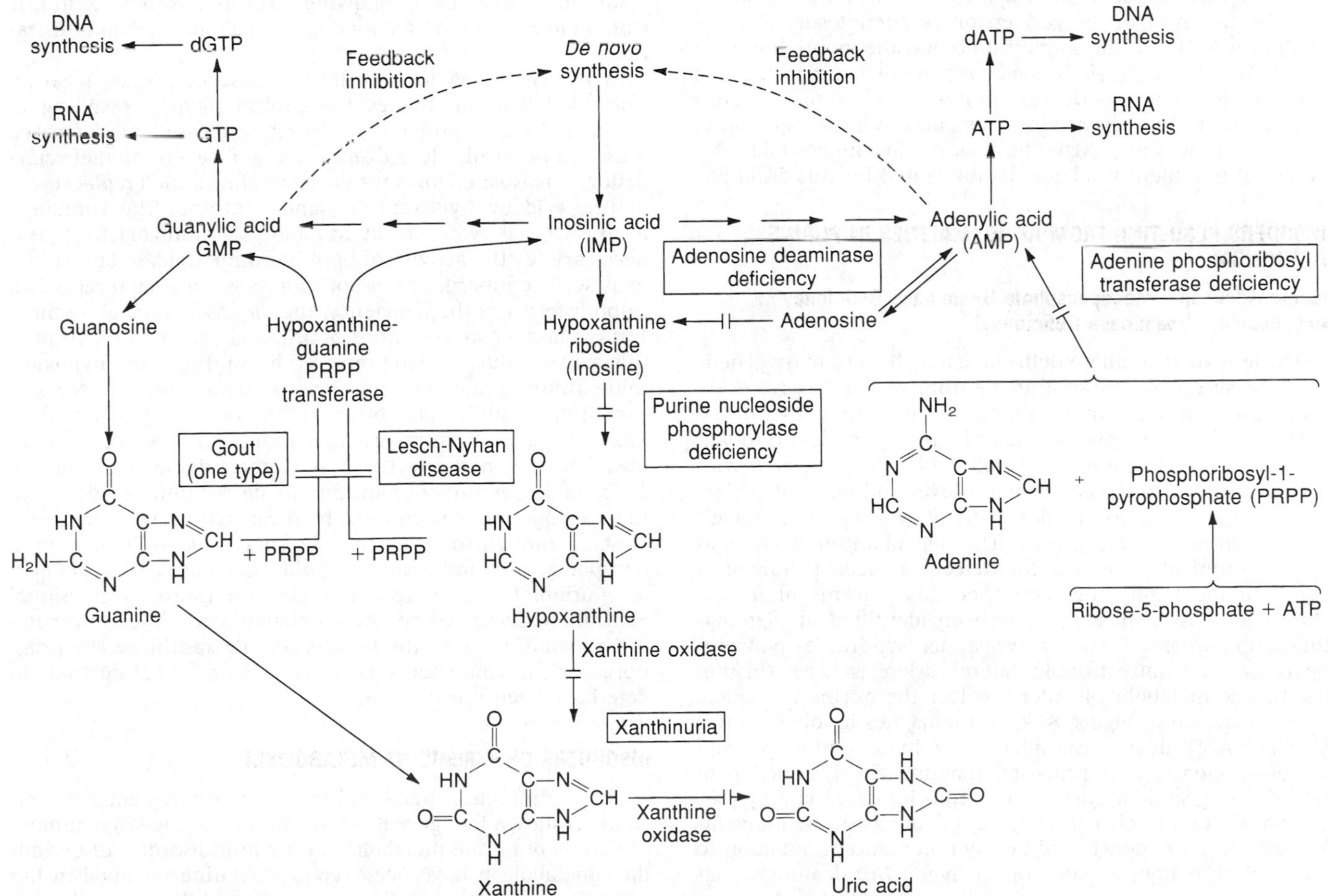

Figure 86–2 Pathways in purine metabolism and salvage.

more soluble than uric acid. The initial dose of allopurinol is 10–20 mg/kg/24 hr in children and is adjusted to maintain normal uric acid levels in plasma. Occasionally, xanthine calculi may form. Consequently, a low purine diet (one free of organ meats, dried beans, and sardines), high fluid intake, and alkalinization of the urine to establish a urinary pH of 6.0–6.5 is necessary. These measures control the hyperuricemia and urate neuropathy but do not affect the neurologic symptoms.

Adenylosuccinase Deficiency

Affected children with adenylosuccinase deficiency show severe psychomotor retardation; the majority have a seizure disorder. Autistic-like behaviors, consisting of failure to make eye contact and repetitive behaviors, are seen in about half of patients. Others demonstrate growth retardation associated with muscle wasting. Fundoscopy, auditory somatosensory and visual-evoked responses, nerve conduction velocities, and electromyelographic findings are normal. Computed tomography and magnetic resonance imaging of the brain may show hypotrophy or hypoplasia of the cerebellum, particularly the vermis. One reported case, a girl, tested in the mild range of mental retardation. The form with profound mental retardation is type I; the variant case is type II. Other patients have an intermediate clinical symptom pattern with moderately delayed psychomotor development, seizures, stereotypies, and agitation. The disease is an autosomal recessive one; the gene is localized on chromosome 22. It is proposed that rather than being caused by purine nucleotide deficiency, the symptoms are due to the toxic effects of accumulating succinyl purines.

Adenylosuccinase catalyzes two reactions in purine metabolism. These are the conversion of succinylaminoimidazole carboxamide (SAICA) riboside into aminoimidazole carboxamide (AICA) ribotide in the de novo synthesis of purine nucleotides. It is also involved in the conversion of adenylosuccinate (S-AMP) into AMP and the conversion of inosine monophosphate into AMP. The *diagnosis* is made when SAICA riboside and succinyl adenosine (S-ADO) are found in body fluids. Diagnosis is based on the presence in urine and cerebrospinal fluid of SAICA riboside and S-ADO, both normally undetectable. No successful treatment has been demonstrated for this disorder.

DISORDERS RESULTING FROM ABNORMALITIES IN PURINE CATABOLISM

Muscle Adenosine Monophosphate Deaminase Deficiency (Myoadenylate Deaminase Deficiency)

Muscle AMP deaminase deficiency may be a primary genetic defect or secondary to another neuromuscular disease. AMP deaminase deficiency most commonly presents with isolated muscle weakness, fatigue, myalgias following moderate-to-vigorous exercise, or cramps. Myalgias may be associated with an increased serum creatine kinase level and detectable electromyelographic abnormalities. Muscle wasting or histologic changes on biopsy are absent. The age of onset may be as early 8 mo of life. The enzyme defect has been identified in asymptomatic family members. Secondary forms of muscle AMP deaminase deficiency have been identified in Werdnig-Hoffmann disease, Kugelberg-Welander syndrome, polyneuropathies, and amyotrophic lateral sclerosis (see Chapter 619.2). The metabolic disorder involves the purine nucleotide cycle. As shown in Figure 86–2, the enzymes involved in this cycle are AMP deaminase, adenylosuccinate synthetase, and adenylosuccinase. It is proposed that muscle dysfunction in AMP deaminase deficiency results from impaired energy production during muscle contraction. It is unclear how individuals may carry the deficit and be asymptomatic. In addition to muscle dysfunction, a mutation of liver AMP deaminase has been proposed as a cause of primary gout, leading to overproduction of uric acid.

This disorder is thought to be an autosomal recessive one. *AMP-D1*, the gene responsible for encoding muscle AMP deaminase, is located on chromosome 1. Population studies reveal that this mutant allele is found at high frequency in white populations. The disorder may be screened for by perfoming an exercise test. The normal elevation of venous plasma ammonia following exercise that is seen in normal subjects is absent in AMP deaminase deficiency. The final diagnosis is made by histochemical or biochemical assays of a muscle biopsy. The primary form is distinguished by the finding of enzyme levels below 2% with little or no immunoprecipitable enzyme. Affected individuals are advised to exercise with caution to prevent rhabdomyolysis and myoglobinuria. A *treatment* administering ribose (2–60 g/24 hr orally, in divided doses) has been reported to improve endurance and muscle strength.

Adenosine Deaminase Deficiency

See Chapter 126.1.

Purine Nucleoside Phosphorylase Deficiency

See Chapter 126.2.

Xanthine Oxidase Deficiency

Xanthine, the immediate precursor of uric acid, is less soluble than uric acid in urine. There are two types of xanthine oxidase (or dehydrogenase) deficiency, namely, the isolated form and a combined xanthine oxidase and sulfite oxidase deficiency. Patients with the isolated form may be asymptomatic; however, renal stones, often not visible on radiography, may appear at any age. Crystalline xanthine deposits may result in muscle pain following exertion. Rarely, xanthine stones have been reported as a result of allopurinol administration.

In the combined form, sulfite oxidase deficiency (also an isolated deficit) dominates the clinical picture, resulting in neonatal feeding problems, seizures, increased or decreased muscle tone, ocular lens dislocation, and severe mental retardation. The isolated form results in an almost total replacement of uric acid by hypoxanthine and xanthine. The combined form is caused by deficiency in a molybdenum cofactor that is necessary for the activity of both xanthine oxidase and sulfite oxidase. The inheritance of both forms is autosomal recessive. In both forms of the deficiency, the *diagnosis* is made by measuring plasma concentrations of uric acid (<1 mg/dL). Urinary uric acid is reduced, being replaced by xanthine and hypoxanthine. In the combined form, there is, in addition, an excessive excretion of sulfite and other sulfur-containing metabolites. Enzyme diagnostic measurement requires jejunal or liver biopsy because these are the only human tissues that contain appreciable amounts of xanthine oxidase. Sulfite oxidase and the molybdenum cofactor can be measured in liver and fibroblasts. Although the isolated deficiency is generally benign, a low purine diet and increased fluid intake are recommended. Allopurinol has been recommended for those with residual xanthine oxidase activity. It completely blocks the conversion of hypoxanthine into the far less soluble xanthine. The prognosis for the combined type is very poor, and drug trials to date have been unsuccessful.

DISORDERS OF PYRIMIDINE METABOLISM

The pyrimidines, uracil and thymine, are degraded in four steps, as shown in Figure 86–3. In contrast to the large number of defects of purine metabolism, only four disorders of pyrimidine metabolism have been reported. Purine metabolism has an easily measurable end point in uric acid; however, there is no equivalent compound in pyrimidine metabolism. The first

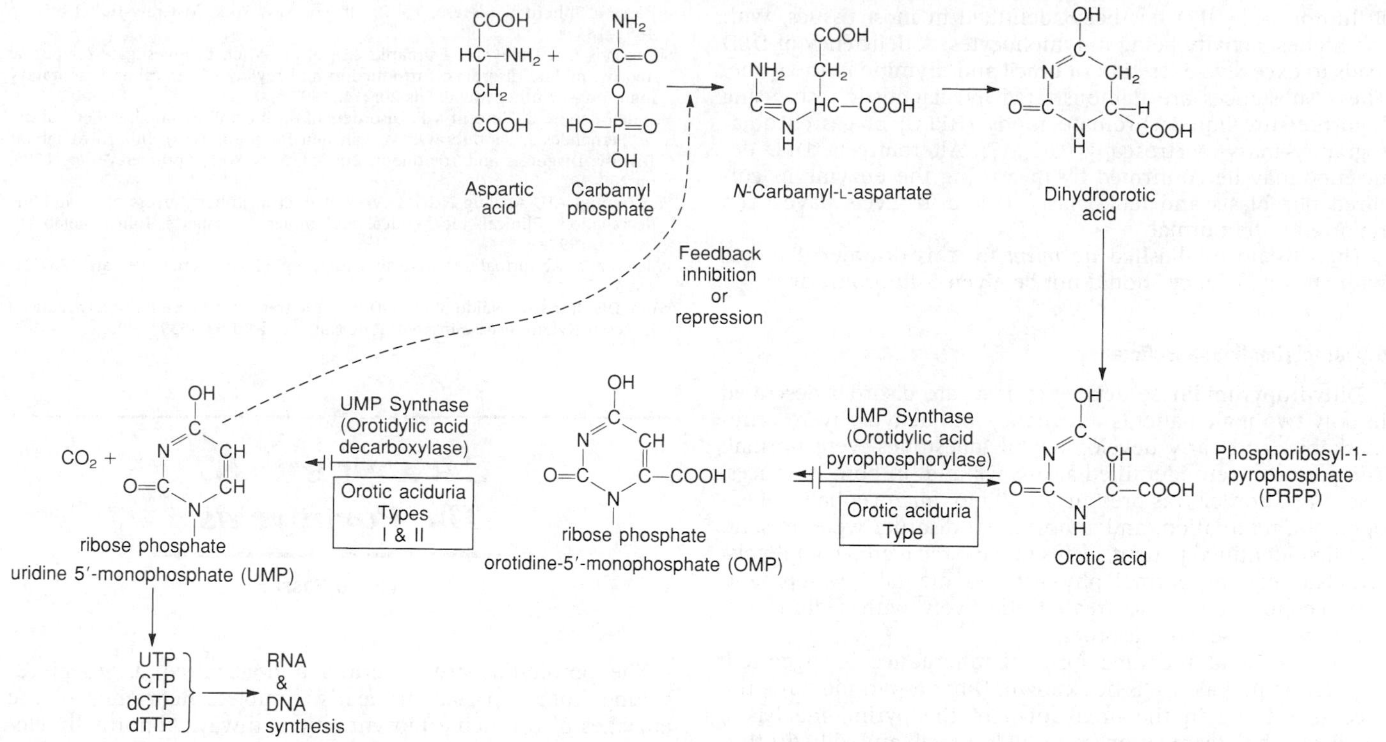

Figure 86–3 Pathways in pyrimidine biosynthesis.

defect, hereditary orotic aciduria, is in the de novo synthetic pathway, whereas the other disorders involve defects in the pyrimidine degradation pathway. The first three steps of the degradation pathways for thymine and uracil, respectively, make use of the same enzymes (DPD, DPH, and UP). These three steps result in the conversion into β-alanine from uracil. Reduced production of the neurotransmitter function of β-alanine is hypothesized to produce clinical symptoms. Clinically, these rare disorders may be overlooked because symptoms are not highly specific; however, they should be considered as possible causes of anemia and neurologic disease and are a contraindication for treatment of cancer patients with certain pyrimidine analogs.

Hereditary Orotic Aciduria (Uridine Monophosphate Synthase Deficiency)

The small number of patients with hereditary orotic aciduria have a macrocytic hypochromic megablastic anemia that is unresponsive to the usual forms of therapy (iron, folic acid, and B_{12}) and sometimes leukopenia. Untreated, this disorder can lead to developmental retardation, failure to thrive, cardiac disease, strabismus, and crystalluria. Renal function is generally normal. Heterozygotes may have mild orotic aciduria but are not otherwise affected.

This disorder is an autosomal recessive one. The gene for uridine monophosphate synthase is located on the long arm of chromosome 3 (3q13). Hereditary orotic aciduria is associated with deficient activity of the last two enzymes of the de novo pyrimidine synthetic pathway (orotic acid phosphoribosyltransferase, orotidine-5′-monophosphate decarboxylase). These two enzymes are contained in a bifunctional protein, uridine monophosphate (UMP) synthase, and catalyze the conversion of orotic acid to UMP. Hereditary orotic aciduria (UMP synthase) deficiency results in the excessive accumulation of orotic acid. The clinical features are thought to be related to pyrimidine nucleotide depletion. Metabolities derived from several pharmacologic agents (5-azauridine, allopurinol) produce secondary orotic aciduria and orotidinuria by specifically inhibiting orotidine-5′-monophosphate decarboxylase. Genetic metabolic defects that involve four of the six enzymes associated with the urea cycle may result in orotic aciduria secondary to PP-ribose-P depletion resulting from a substantial increased flux through the de novo pathway. Orotic aciduria may also occur in association with parenteral nutrition, essential amino acid deficiency, and Reye's syndrome. The enzymatic defect may be demonstrated in liver, lymphoblasts, erythrocytes, leukocytes, and cultured skin fibroblasts. A carrier detection test is available, as is prenatal diagnosis.

The administration of uridine has been effective *treatment* in most cases and leads to clinical improvement and reduction in orotic acid excretion. Lifelong treatment is required. Uracil is ineffective because, unlike purines, pyrimidine salvage occurs at the nucleoside level. The long-term *prognosis* in uncomplicated cases is good; however, congenital malformations and other associated features may adversely affect outcome.

Dihydropyrimidine Dehydrogenase Deficiency

Dihydropyrimidine dehydrogenase (DPD) deficiency has been described in both children and adults. Two clinical forms are described. The *clinical manifestations* in children may vary from seizure disorder, autistic-like behavior, and normal intelligence to severe mental retardation with generalized hypertonia and hyperreflexia. Although there is not one characteristic clinical feature, the more severe form involves developmental retardation with microcephaly, seizure disorder, and muscular hypotonia. In most cases, there is an initial period of normal psychomotor development, followed by subsequent developmental delays. In adult patients, neurotoxicity linked to pyrimidinemia following 5-fluorouracil treatment for breast cancer has been reported in previously healthy individuals.

An autosomal recessive mode of inheritance has been demonstrated in two kindreds. The molecular defect is not known. Prenatal *diagnosis* has been reported. The enzyme, DPD, catalyzes the first metabolic step in the degradation cycle, producing dihydro derivatives of uracil and thymine. This enzyme is also responsible for the breakdown of the antineoplastic agent

5-fluorouracil. DPD has been identified in most tissues, with the highest activity being in lymphocytes. A deficiency of DPD leads to excessive excretion of uracil and thymine in the urine. These substances are demonstrated by diagnostic tests using high-pressure liquid chromatography (HPLC) or gas chromatography–mass spectroscopy (GC-MS). Alternatively, DPD deficiency may be confirmed by measuring the enzyme in cultured fibroblasts and leukoblasts. Uric acid levels have been reported to be normal.

There is no established *treatment* for this disorder. Patients with DPD deficiency should not be given 5-fluorouracil.

Dihydropyrimidinase Deficiency

Dihydropyrimidinase deficiency is a rare disorder described in only two male patients. Pregnancy and delivery were unremarkable, and early developmental milestones were normal. The patients were identified at 6–8 wk and, in both instances, a seizure disorder was present. At 30 mo, microcephaly, developmental retardation, and a movement disorder were present. The first identified patient seems to have recovered completely, with subsequent normal physical and mental development. The second patient was treated effectively with sodium valproate for the seizure disorder.

An autosomal recessive form of inheritance is suggested. Population prevalence is not known. Dihydropyrimidinase, the second enzyme in the breakdown of the pyrimidine bases, catalyzes the degradation of dihydrouracil and dihydrothymine, leading to increased urinary excretion. Organic acid screening by GC-MS may identify increased amounts of these compounds in urine. Oral loading tests with uracil, dihydrouracil, thymine, and dihydrothymine have been used to differentiate this disorder from DPD deficiency.

Pyrimidine 5′-Nucleotidase Deficiency (Uridine Monophosphate Hydrolase Deficiency)

Homozygote patients affected with pyrimidine 5′-nucleotidase deficiency present with a defect restricted to erythrocytes and characterized by nonspherocytic hemolytic anemia with basophilic stippling. Other characteristic features include splenomegaly, increased indirect bilirubin, and hemoglobinuria. This is an autosomal recessive disorder. Pyrimidine 5′-nucleotidase is the first degradative enzyme of the pyrimidine salvage cycle and catalyzes the hydrolysis of pyrimidine 5′-nucleotides. Enzyme deficiency results in high levels of pyrimidine nucleotides in the erythrocytes of those affected. Diagnosis involves the demonstration of a complete deficiency of the major isoenzyme uridine monophosphate hydrolase-1. The enzyme defect should be suspected in patients with nonspherocytic hemolytic anemia. The anemia is usually moderate, and transfusions are rarely necessary. Splenectomy has not proved to be an effective treatment.

Anderson L, Ernst M: Self-injury in Lesch-Nyhan disease. J Aut Dev Disord 24:67, 1994.

Breese GR, Baumeister AA, McCown TJ, et al: Neonatal-6-hydroxydopamine treatment: Model of susceptibility for self-mutilation in Lesch-Nyhan syndrome. Pharmacol Biochem Behav 21:459, 1984.

Cameron JS, Moro F, Simmons HA: Gout, uric acid and purine metabolism in pediatric nephrology. Pediatr Nephrol 7:105, 1993.

Duran M, Dorland L, Meuleman EEE, et al: Inherited defects of purine and pyrimidine metabolism: Laboratory methods for diagnosis. J Inher Metab Dis 20:227, 1997.

Ernst M, Zametkin AJ, Matochik JA, et al: Presynaptic dopaminergic deficits in Lesch-Nyhan disease. N Engl J Med 334:1568, 1996.

Jinnah HA, Wojcik BE, Hunt M, et al: Dopamine deficiency in a genetic mouse model of Lesch-Nyhan disease. J Neurosci 14(3 Pt 1):1164, 1994.

Nyhan WL: The recognition of Lesch-Nyhan syndrome as an inborn error of metabolism. J Inher Metab Dis 20:1718, 1997.

Page T, Yu A, Fontanes J, et al: Developmental disorder associated with increased cellular nucleotidase activity. Proc Natl Acad Sci 94:11601, 1997.

Scriver CR, Beaudet AL, Sly WS, Valle D (eds): The Metabolic and Molecular Bases of Inherited Disease, Vol 2, 7th ed. New York, McGraw-Hill, 1995, pp 1655–1837.

Simmonds HA, Duley JA, Fairbanks LD, et al: When to investigate for purine and pyrimidine disorders: Introduction and review of clinical and laboratory indications. J Inher Metab Dis 20:214, 1997.

Van den Berghe G, Vincent MF: Disorders of purine and pyrimidine metabolism. *In:* Fernandes J, Saudubray J-M, van den Berghe G (eds): Inborn Metabolic Disease: Diagnosis and Treatment, 2nd ed. New York, Springer-Verlag, 1995, pp 289–302.

Van Gennip AH, Abeling NGGM, Vrekan P, et al: Inborn errors of pyrimidine degradation: Clinical, biochemical and molecular aspects. Inher Metab Dis 20:203, 1997.

Wilcox WD: Abnormal serum uric acid levels in children. J Pediatr 128:731, 1996.

Wong DF, Harris JC, Naidu S, et al: Dopamine transporters are markedly reduced in Lesch-Nyhan disease in vivo. Proc Natl Acad Sci 93:5539, 1996.

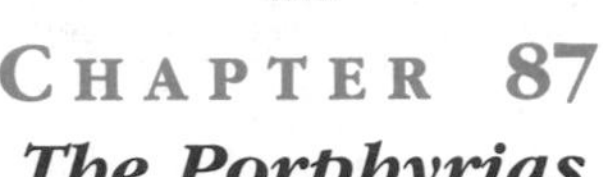

CHAPTER 87
The Porphyrias

Shigeru Sassa

The porphyrias are inherited and acquired disorders resulting from a partial or nearly complete deficiency of the enzymes of the heme biosynthetic pathway. Abnormally elevated levels of porphyrins or their precursors, or both, are produced, accumulate in tissues, and are excreted in urine and stool. Heme is composed of ferrous iron and protoporphyrin IX (Fig. 87–1) and is an essential molecule of heme proteins, such as hemoglobin, myoglobin, mitochondrial and microsomal cytochromes, catalase, peroxidases, and tryptophan pyrrolase. Patients with porphyrias have either cutaneous photosensitivity due to accumulation of porphyrins in the skin or neurologic disturbances due to accumulation of their precursors, or both.

HEME BIOSYNTHETIC PATHWAY

The first step and the last three steps of heme biosynthesis occur in mitochondria; the intermediate steps take place in the cytosol (Fig. 87–2). The two major organs that are active in heme synthesis are the liver and the erythroid bone marrow; inherited enzymatic defects in the porphyrias are mainly ex-

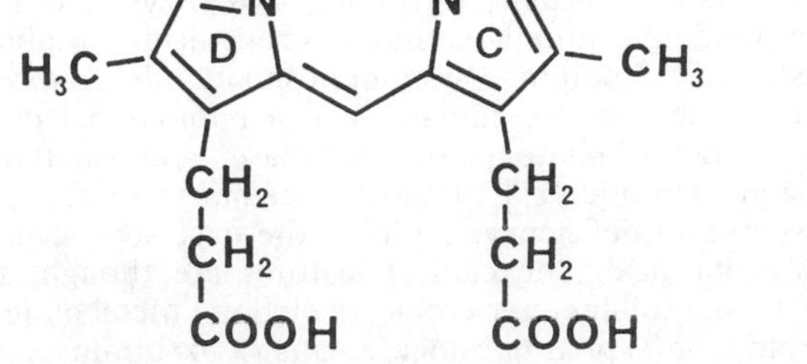

Figure 87–1 Structure of heme.

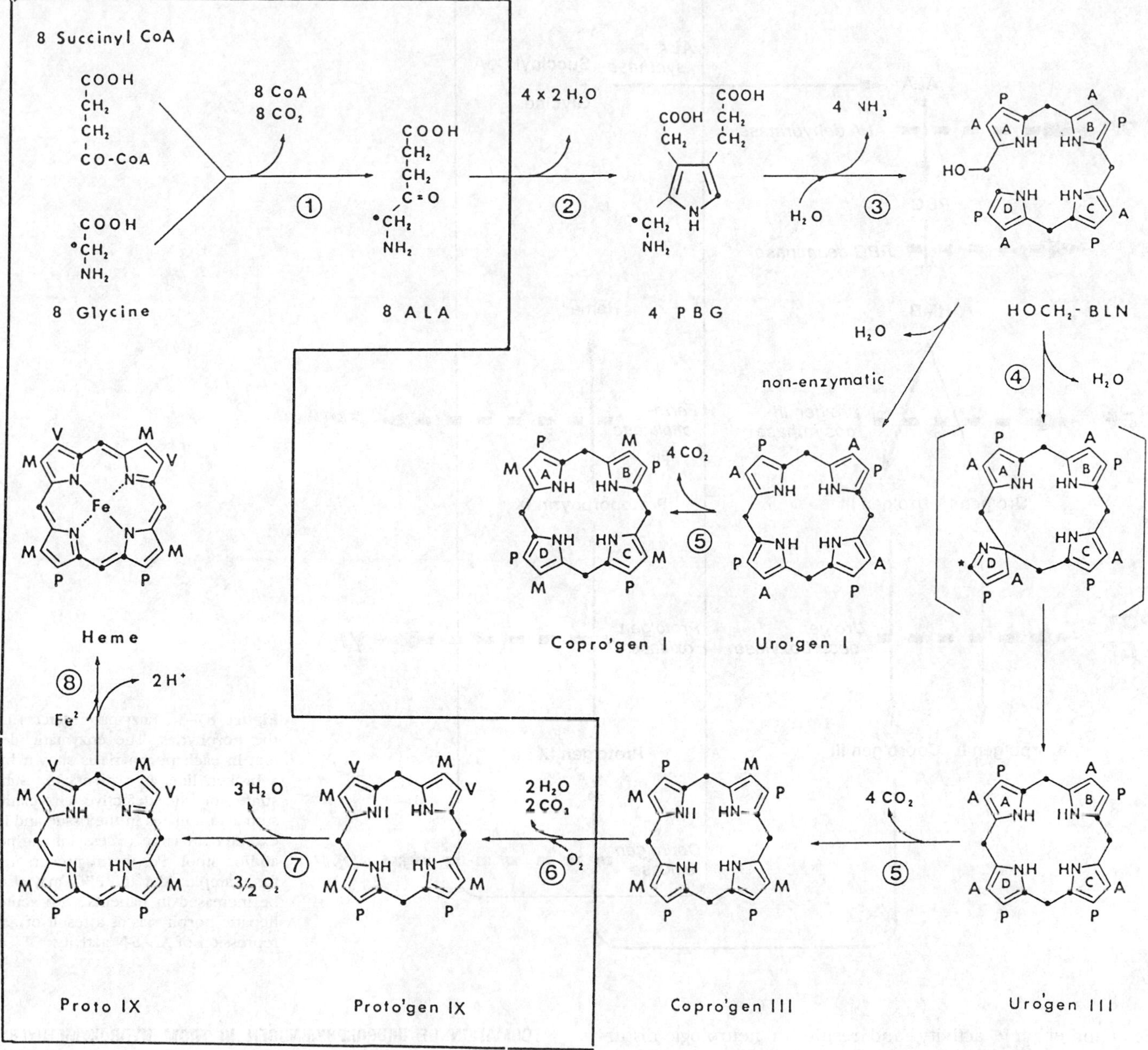

Figure 87–2 The heme biosynthetic pathway. A, -CH_2-COOH; P, -CH_2-CH_2-COOH; M, -CH_3; V, -CH=CH_2; ●, carbon atom derived from the α-carbon of glycine; *, location of the α-carbon atom from glycine in the pyrrole ring that undergoes reversion; [ ], a presumed intermediate. (Modified from Hayashi N: The synthesis of heme and its regulation. Protein, Nucleic Acid Enzyme [Tokyo] 32:797, 1987.)

pressed in these tissues. In erythroid cells, hemoglobin is made in erythroblasts or reticulocytes, which still contain mitochondria, whereas circulating erythrocytes lack the ability to form heme.

FORMATION OF δ-AMINOLEVULINIC ACID. *δ-Aminolevulinate synthase* (ALAS), the first enzyme of the heme biosynthetic pathway, catalyzes the condensation of glycine and succinyl CoA (Fig. 87–2, step 1). The enzyme is localized in the inner membrane of mitochondria and requires pyridoxal 5′-phosphate as a cofactor. ALAS activity is low and rate-limiting for heme formation. Hepatic (or nonspecific) and erythroid ALAS are isozymes that are encoded by two distinct nuclear genes, that is, ALAS-N and ALAS-E. The gene locus for the human ALAS-N is at chromosome 3p21, and that for the ALAS-E is at the Xp11.21. Inherited deficiency of ALAS-E is associated with *X-linked sideroblastic anemia* (see Chapter 349).

FORMATION OF PORPHOBILINOGEN FROM δ-AMINOLEVULINIC ACID. Two molecules of δ-aminolevulinic acid (ALA) are converted by a cytosolic enzyme, *δ-aminolevulinate dehydratase* (ALAD), to a monopyrrole, porphobilinogen (PBG), with the removal of two molecules of water (Fig. 87–2, step 2). ALAD deficiency porphyria (ADP) is due to an almost complete lack of enzyme activity (Fig. 87–3). The human ALAD gene is localized at chromosome 9q34. The enzyme requires an intact sulfhydryl group and a zinc atom per subunit for full activity. Lead inhibits ALAD by displacing zinc from the enzyme, the essential

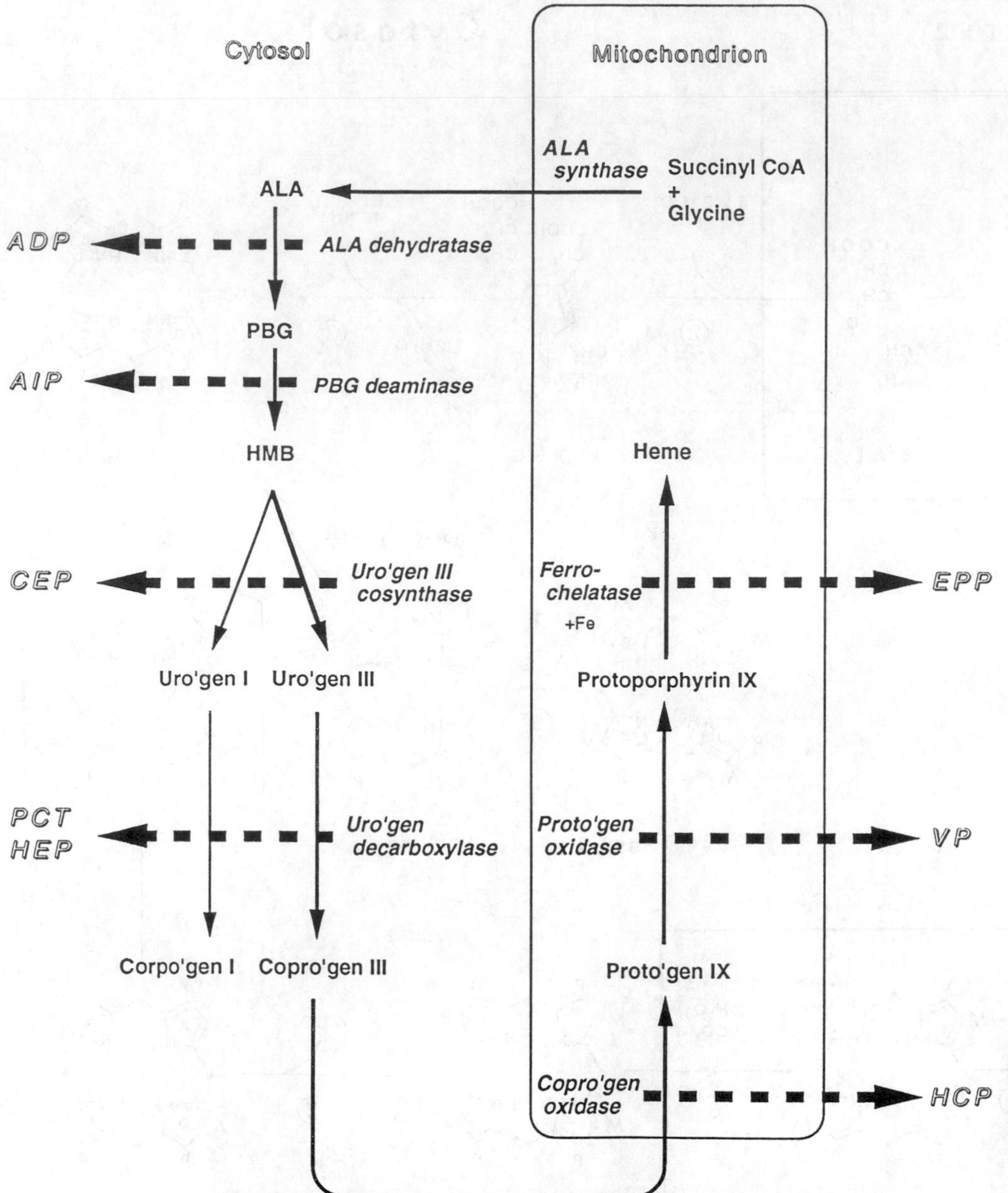

Figure 87–3 Enzymatic defects in the porphyrias. The enzymatic defect in each porphyria is shown by a broken line. In patients the substrate for the defective enzymatic step accumulates in the tissue and is excreted in large excess into urine and/or stool. Porphyrin precursors, for example, ALA and PBG, may also be increased in patients with acute hepatic porphyrias as a result of derepression of ALAS-N activity.

metal for enzyme activity, and results in neurologic disturbances, some of which resemble those of ADP. The most potent inhibitor of the enzyme is succinylacetone, a structural analog of ALA, which is found in urine and blood of patients with hereditary tyrosinemia, who often acquire a condition similar to ADP (see Chapter 82.2).

FORMATION OF HYDROXYMETHYLBILANE FROM PORPHOBILINOGEN. *Porphobilinogen deaminase* (PBGD) catalyzes the condensation of four molecules of PBG to yield a linear tetrapyrrole, hydroxymethylbilane (HMB). In the absence of the subsequent enzyme, uroporphyrinogen III cosynthase (Uro'CoS), the bilane is spontaneously cyclized into the first tetrapyrrole, Uro' I. In the presence of the CoS enzyme, Uro' III is formed, which has an inverted D-ring pyrrole (Fig. 87–2, step 3). The gene locus for human PBGD is at chromosome 11q23→11qter. There are two isozymes of PBGD, that is, erythroid-specific and -nonspecific. The two isoforms of PBGD are produced by distinct mRNAs that are transcribed from a single gene by alternate transcription and splicing of its mRNA. A partial (or heterozygous) deficiency of PBGD is associated with *acute intermittent porphyria* (AIP) (see Fig. 87–3).

FORMATION OF UROPORPHYRINOGEN III FROM HYDROXYMETHYLBILANE. Uro'CoS catalyzes the formation of Uro' III from HMB. This involves an intramolecular rearrangement that affects only ring D of the Uro' (see Fig. 87–2, step 4). Homozygous deficiency of Uro'CoS is associated with *congenital erythropoietic porphyria* (CEP) (see Fig. 87–3).

FORMATION OF COPROPORPHYRINOGEN FROM UROPORPHYRINOGEN. A cytosolic enzyme, *uroporphyrinogen decarboxylase* (Uro'D), catalyzes the sequential removal of the four carboxylic groups of the carboxymethyl side chains in Uro' to yield Copro' (Fig. 87–2, step 5). The gene for Uro'D has been localized to chromosome 1pter→p21. *Porphyria cutanea tarda* (PCT) is due to a partial (or heterozygous) deficiency of Uro'D, whereas *hepatoerythropoietic porphyria* (HEP) is due to a homozygous deficiency of the enzyme (see Fig. 87–3).

FORMATION OF PROTOPORPHYRINOGEN FROM COPROPORPHYRINOGEN. *Coproporphyrinogen oxidase* (Copro'Ox) is a mitochondrial enzyme that catalyzes the removal of the carboxyl group and two hydrogens from the propionic groups of pyrrole rings A and B of Copro' to form vinyl groups at these positions (see Fig. 87–2, step 6). The gene for human Copro'Ox is localized to chromosome 9. *Hereditary coproporphyria* (HCP) is due to a partial (or heterozygous) deficiency of Copro'Ox (see Fig. 87–3).

FORMATION OF PROTOPORPHYRIN FROM PROTOPORPHYRINOGEN. The oxidation of protoporphyrinogen (Proto') to protoporphyrin is mediated by *protoporphyrinogen oxidase* (Proto'Ox), which catalyzes the removal of six hydrogen atoms from the porphyrinogen nucleus (see Fig. 87–2, step 7). *Variegate porphyria* (VP) is due to a partial (or heterozygous) deficiency of Proto'Ox (see Fig. 87–3).

FORMATION OF HEME FROM PROTOPORPHYRIN. The final step of heme biosynthesis is the insertion of iron into protoporphyrin (see Fig. 87–2, step 8). This reaction is catalyzed by the enzyme *ferrochelatase* (FeC). Unlike other steps in the heme biosynthetic pathway, this enzyme uses protoporphyrin IX as a substrate, rather than its reduced form. The enzyme specifically requires ferrous, not ferric, iron. The gene for human FeC has been assigned to chromosome 18q21.3. *Erythropoietic protoporphyria* (EPP) is due to a partial (or heterozygous) FeC deficiency (see Fig. 87–3).

REGULATION OF HEME SYNTHESIS

Hepatic biosynthesis of heme is controlled by the rate of formation of ALAS, that is, ALAS-N. The enzyme activity in normal liver cells is low, whereas its level increases dramatically when the liver needs to make more heme in response to various chemical treatments. The synthesis of the enzyme is also regulated in a feedback fashion by heme (the end product of the biosynthetic pathway). At higher heme concentrations than those that repress the synthesis of ALAS-N, heme induces microsomal heme oxygenase, resulting in enhancement of its own catabolism. Thus heme concentration is maintained by a balance between the synthesis of ALAS-N and heme oxygenase, both of which are under the regulatory influence of heme. In contrast, erythroid ALAS-E synthesis is either refractory to heme treatment or often stimulated by such treatment.

PATHOPHYSIOLOGIC CONSEQUENCES OF PORPHYRINS AND THEIR PRECURSORS

PHOTOSENSITIVITY. Free porphyrins occur in only small amounts in normal tissues, but their levels may become markedly elevated in porphyrias. On illumination at wavelengths greater than 400 nm (Soret band) and in the presence of oxygen, porphyrins cause photodynamic damage to tissues, cells, subcellular elements, and biomolecules via the formation of singlet oxygen.

NEUROLOGIC DISTURBANCES. *Acute hepatic porphyrias*—that is, ADP, AIP, HCP, and VP—are characterized by neurologic disturbances. Most common symptoms are abdominal pain, disturbances in intestinal motility (diarrhea, constipation), dysesthesia, muscular paralysis, and respiratory failure, which can often be fatal. The cause of the neurologic disturbances in the porphyrias remains unclear; it may involve excessive porphyrin precursors, deficient heme synthesis, or increased tryptophan in the central nervous system resulting from decreased hepatic tryptophan pyrrolase activity.

MOLECULAR GENETICS OF THE PORPHYRIAS

Genetic analysis has elucidated the complex nature of molecular defects in the porphyrias and possible consequences of their gene defects on cellular function. The following general conclusions can be drawn from the molecular genetic studies in the porphyrias.

1. In every porphyria, the molecular defect of the enzyme is heterogeneous. There is more than one mutation resulting clinically in a single porphyria disease. There are more than 100 mutations found in the PBGD gene in patients with AIP. There are few founder effect mutations, whereas a pedigree-specific mutation of the enzyme gene is common.
2. The nature of molecular defects is also highly heterogeneous, including promoter mutations, splicing mutations, consensus sequence mutations, mutations producing nonfunctional mRNAs, mutations resulting in unstable proteins, gene deletions, and so on.
3. Even among the dominant form of porphyrias, a homozygous form of the disease can be found in a few patients. The homozygous form appears to be due to mutations with lesser pathophysiologic effects than those found in the heterozygous form of the disease. A subset of homozygous diseases among commonly autosomal dominant diseases has been observed in AIP, HCP, VP, and EPP.
4. Clinically homozygous mutations can be due to a *homoallelic* or a *heteroallelic* mutation. However, a *heteroallelic* mutation, that is, *compound heterozygosity* for two separate mutations, is far more common than a *homoallelic* mutation.
5. Tissue-specific regulation of heme pathway enzymes may be the basis for the tissue-specific expression of different porphyrias.
6. In the case of PBGD, a mutation affecting the splicing of the first intron results in an abnormal enzyme in nonerythroid cells, whereas the same mutation has no effect on the erythroid-specific PBGD, since the transcription of the erythroid PBGD mRNA uses a second AUG, which is located approximately 3 kb downstream of the mutated site. Thus, even in a single form of acute hepatic porphyria, there may be distinct tissue-specific expression of the disease, depending on the type of mutation.
7. Most of the acute hepatic porphyrias, such as AIP, HCP, and VP, require an additional factor or factors for their clinical expression. Such a factor can be either genetic or environmental. Thus porphyrias are not only inborn errors of metabolism but also diseases in which environmental factors have an immense impact on their gene expression.
8. Some hepatic porphyria-like symptoms can be elicited by environmental chemicals that strongly inhibit heme pathway enzymes. For example, PCT may be caused by Uro'D inhibition due to hexachlorobenzene ingestion in normal individuals.

CLASSIFICATION OF PORPHYRIAS

Each porphyria is described according to the order of the enzymes in the heme biosynthetic sequence (see Fig. 87–3). There are eight enzymes of heme synthesis, and with the exception of the first enzyme (ALAS), an enzymatic defect at each step is associated with a form of porphyria (see Fig. 87–3 and Table 87–1). Porphyrias are classified as either hepatic or erythropoietic, depending on the principal site of expression of the specific enzymatic defect (see Table 87–1). They can also be classified as acute hepatic or cutaneous porphyrias. Acute hepatic porphyrias are characterized by acute episodes of neurologic disturbances and by an overproduction of porphyrin precursors, whereas cutaneous porphyrias are characterized by cutaneous photosensitivity and by an excessive production of porphyrins (Table 87–2).

ALAD Deficiency Porphyria

ADP is an autosomal recessive disorder resulting from a homozygous ALAD deficiency (see Fig. 87–3 and Table 87–1). This is the rarest porphyria; only four cases have been reported to date. The symptomatology is similar to that seen in AIP.

CLINICAL MANIFESTATIONS. Patients with ADP have vomiting, pain in the arms and legs, and neuropathy, which is exacerbated following stress, alcohol use, or decreased food intake. A rare infant with ADP has been reported who had a clinical

TABLE 87–1 The Porphyrias and Their Enzymatic Defects

Enzyme Deficiency	Porphyria	Principal Site of Expression	Mode of Transmission	Remarks
ALAD	ADP	Liver	Recessive	
PBGD	AIP			
	Type I	Liver	Dominant	CRIM (−)
	Type II	Liver	Dominant	Normal erythrocyte PBGD
	Type III	Liver	Dominant	CRIM (+)
Uro'CoS	CEP	Bone marrow	Recessive	
Uro'D	PCT			
	Type I	Liver	—	Acquired
	Type II	Liver	Dominant	
	Type III	Liver	Dominant	
	HEP	Liver and bone marrow	Recessive	
Copro'Ox	HCP	Liver	Dominant	
Proto'Ox	VP	Liver	Dominant	
FeC	EPP	Bone marrow	Dominant	

From Sassa S, Kappas A: The porphyrias. In: *Nathan DG, Oski FA (eds): Hematology in Infancy and Childhood, 4th ed. Philadelphia, WB Saunders, 1993, pp 451–471.*
ALAD = δ-aminolevulinate dehydratase; ADP = ALAD deficiency porphyria; PBGD = porphobilinogen deaminase; AIP = acute intermittent porphyria; CRIM = cross-reactive immunologic material; Uro'CoS = uroporphyrinogen III cosynthase; CEP = congenital erythropoietic porphyria; Uro'D = uroporphyrinogen decarboxylase; PCT = porphyria cutanea tarda; HEP = hepatoerythropoietic porphyria; Copro'Ox = coproporphyrinogen oxidase; HCP = hereditary coproporphyria; Proto'Ox = protoporphyrinogen oxidase; VP = variegate porphyria; FeC = ferrochelatase; EPP = erythropoietic protoporphyria.

course from birth onward, including general muscle hypotonia and respiratory insufficiency.

LABORATORY FINDINGS. Urinary ALA excretion is markedly elevated, whereas urinary PBG excretion is normal. Urinary and erythrocyte porphyrins are also markedly elevated (100-fold); no satisfactory explanation has been advanced to account for this observation. Fecal porphyrin excretion is normal or marginally elevated. Patients with ADP display markedly decreased activities of ALAD in erythrocytes, as well as in nonerythroid cells (~2% of normal), whereas their parents show approximately 50% enzyme activity.

DIAGNOSIS. Definitive diagnosis is dependent on the demonstration of impaired ALAD activity and deficiency of enzyme protein in erythrocytes. Supporting evidence includes massive elevations in urinary ALA, substantial elevations of porphyrins in urine and erythrocytes, and perhaps modest elevations in fecal porphyrins. Clinical symptoms of ADP occur only in homozygous patients, whereas heterozygous subjects (parents and certain siblings) remain clinically unaffected.

TREATMENT. The similarities in symptoms between ADP and AIP suggest that prudent management of ADP should probably be the same as that for AIP.

Acute Intermittent Porphyria

AIP, which may also be termed *Swedish porphyria, pyrroloporphyria,* or *intermittent acute porphyria,* is an autosomal dominant disorder resulting from a partial PBGD deficiency (see Fig. 87–3 and Table 87–1). The deficient enzyme activity (~50% of normal) is found in all tissues, including erythrocytes, in the majority of patients (~85%). This is consistent with the heterozygous state of affected individuals. However, a subset of patients (~15%) show deficient enzyme activity only in nonerythroid cells. The majority (~90%) of individuals with PBGD

TABLE 87–2 Clinical and Laboratory Features of the Porphyrias

Porphyria	Clinical Features	Laboratory Features: *Erythrocytes*	*Plasma*	*Urine*	*Stool*
ADP	Neurologic (as in AIP)	ZnPP	—	ALA	—
AIP	Neurologic: nausea, vomiting, abdominal pain, diarrhea, constipation, ileus, dysuria, muscle hypotonia, respiratory failure, sensory neuropathy, seizures	—	—	ALA, PBG	—
CEP	Photosensitivity: bullae, crusts, scar formation, sclerodermoid change, hyper- and hypopigmentation, hypertrichosis, erythrodontia, hemolytic anemia, splenomegaly	Uro'I, Copro'I	Uro'I, Copro'I	Uro'I, Copro'I	—
PCT	Photosensitivity: skin fragility, bullae, crusts, scar formation, sclerodermoid change, hyper- and hypopigmentation, hypertrichosis	—	Uro'I, 7-carboxyl III	Uro'I, 7-carboxyl III	Uro', 7-carboxyl, Isocopro'
HEP	Photosensitivity (as in CEP)	ZnPP	Uro'I, 7-carboxyl III	Uro'I, 7-carboxyl III	Uro, 7-carboxyl, Isocopro'
HCP	Neurologic (as in ADP, AIP, and VP) and photosensitive (as in VP)	—	Copro'	Copro', ALA, PBG	Copro'
VP	Neurologic (as in ADP, AIP, and HCP) and photosensitive (as in HCP)	—	Proto'	ALA, PBG	Proto'
EPP	Photosensitivity: burning sensation, edema, erythema, itching, scarring vesicles	Proto'	Proto'	—	Proto'

ADP = ALAD deficiency porphyria; AIP = acute intermittent porphyria; ALA = δ-aminolevulinic acid; PBG = porphobilinogen; CEP = congenital erythropoietic porphyria; Uro'I = uroporphyrinogen I; Copro'I = coproporphyrinogen I; PCT = porphyria cutanea tarda; Isocopro' = isocoprophyrinogen; HEP = hepatoerythropoietic porphyria; HCP = hereditary coproporphyria; VP = variegate porphyria; EPP = erythropoietic protoporphyria; Proto' = protoporphyrinogen.

deficiency remain biochemically and clinically normal. Clinical expression of the disease is usually linked to environmental or acquired factors (nutritional status, drugs, steroids, other chemicals of endogenous or exogenous origin, and so on). The cardinal pathobiologic feature of the disease is a neurologic dysfunction that may affect the peripheral, autonomic, or central nervous system (see Table 87–2).

EPIDEMIOLOGY. AIP is probably the most common genetic porphyria. The highest incidence occurs in Lapland, Scandinavia and the United Kingdom, although it has been reported in many population groups. The prevalence of AIP was estimated to be 1–2/100,000 in Europe and 2.4/100,000 in Finland. The frequency of low PBGD activity, which includes both patients with AIP and latent gene carriers, is as high as 1/500 in Finland. The disorder is expressed clinically after puberty and more commonly in women than in men.

CLINICAL MANIFESTATIONS. Abdominal pain (generalized or localized) is the most common symptom and is often the initial sign of an acute attack. Other gastroenterologic features may include nausea, vomiting, constipation or diarrhea, abdominal distention, and ileus. Urinary retention, incontinence, and dysuria are observed. In severe cases, the urine develops a port-wine color due to a high content of porphobilin, an auto-oxidation product of PBG. Tachycardia and hypertension, and less frequently fever, sweating, restlessness, and tremor, are observed. In up to 40% of patients, hypertension may become sustained between acute attacks.

Neuropathy is a common feature of AIP. Muscle weakness often begins proximally in the legs but may involve the arms or the distal extremities. Motor neuropathy may also involve the cranial nerves and lead to bulbar paralysis, respiratory deficiency, and death. Sensory patchy neuropathy may occur. Acute attacks of AIP may be accompanied by seizures, especially in patients with hyponatremia due to vomiting, inappropriate fluid therapy, or the syndrome of inappropriate antidiuretic hormone release. The course of an acute attack of AIP is highly variable, both in individuals and among patients, with attacks lasting from a few days to several months. There are no cutaneous manifestations associated with this enzyme deficiency.

Asymptomatic heterozygotes (~90% of subjects with documented PBGD deficiency) may display neither abnormalities in concentrations of porphyrin precursors nor clinical symptoms. An acute attack may be precipitated by endogenous or exogenous environmental factors in individuals with both latent and previously clinically expressed AIP. There are at least five different classes of *precipitating factors* in this disease. (1) *ALAS-N inducers:* Most precipitating factors can be related to an associated increase in the activity of ALAS-N in the liver. An overproduction of ALA then makes the partially deficient PBGD activity rate-limiting. (2) *Endocrine factors:* The clinical disease is more common in women, especially at the time of menses. The disease also rarely is manifested before puberty. (3) *Calorie intake:* Reduced calorie intake often leads to exacerbations of AIP. Additional calories in a diet may reduce PBG excretion and suppress clinical symptoms. (4) *Drugs and foreign chemicals:* Many chemicals—for example, barbiturates, sex steroids, and other foreign chemicals—that exacerbate porphyria have the potential to induce cytochrome P450. The resultant enhanced demand for heme synthesis may lead to induction of hepatic ALAS-N. (5) *Stress:* Stress is known to upregulate the heme oxygenase gene and leads to exacerbation of AIP. Similarly, other forms of stress, including intercurrent illnesses, infections, alcoholic excess, and surgery, all contribute to an acute attack.

LABORATORY FINDINGS. Patients with clinically expressed AIP, as well as a few individuals with latent AIP, excrete variably increased amounts of ALA and PBG in the urine between attacks. In the majority of cases, the onset of an acute attack is accompanied by further increases in excretion of these precursors. Acute attacks may also be associated with elevations in the serum concentrations of ALA, PBG, and porphyrins, which are normally undetectable. Stool porphyrins are usually normal or only slightly elevated in this disorder. The Watson-Schwartz test is widely used as a screening test for urinary PBG. Although this test is highly sensitive, it is neither specific nor quantitative, and its results need to be confirmed and quantified by the column chromatographic method of Mauzerall and Granick. Hemoglobin and bilirubin production is normal in AIP.

GENETICS. Patients with AIP can be classified into three subsets (see Table 87–1). Patients with *type I* mutations are characterized by cross-reactive immunologic material–negative PBGD mutation; they exhibit both intermediately reduced enzyme activity and protein content (~50% of normal). *Type II* mutations are observed in less than 15% of all AIP cases and are characterized by a decreased PBGD activity in nonerythroid cells, but with normal erythroid PBGD activity. Patients with *type III* mutations are characterized by cross-reactive immunologic material–positive mutations, that is, decreased enzyme activity with the presence of structurally abnormal enzyme protein. Various mutations of the human PBGD gene are summarized in Table 87–2. Mutations found in type I AIP are single base substitutions or deletions that result in a single amino acid change or in truncated proteins. The mutations found in type II AIP are single base substitutions that occur in the exon-intron boundary of exon 1, resulting in a splicing defect that affects only the nonspecific form of PBGD, not the erythroid-specific PBGD, because the transcription of the gene in erythroid cells starts downstream of the site of mutation. Mutations characterizing type III AIP are observed in the region that is thought to be essential for catalytic activity.

DIAGNOSIS. Diagnosis of types I and III AIP can be made by demonstrating decreased PBGD activity in erythrocytes in the majority of patients (~85%), whereas the distinction between carrier or latent status and clinically expressed AIP requires demonstration of elevated urinary excretion of PBG and ALA. Elevated levels of both ALA and PBG may also be seen in HCP and VP; measurement of urinary and stool porphyrins usually differentiates these conditions from AIP. The diagnosis of type II AIP requires either the demonstration of PBGD deficiency in nonerythroid cells or DNA hybridization using allele-specific oligonucleotide specific for the mutation.

TREATMENT. The treatment of AIP is essentially identical to that of ADP, HCP, and VP. Treatment between attacks comprises adequate nutritional intake, avoidance of drugs known to exacerbate porphyria, and prompt treatment of other intercurrent diseases or infections. Unresponsive severe cases should be treated with intravenous administration of dextrose to provide a minimum of 300 g of carbohydrate/24 hr. Intravenous hematin (4 mg/kg, every 12 hr) is also effective in reducing ALA and PBG excretion as well as in curtailing acute attacks. Nasal or subcutaneous administration of long-acting agonistic analogs of luteinizing hormone–releasing hormone has been shown to inhibit ovulation and greatly reduce the incidence of perimenstrual attacks of AIP in some women with cyclic exacerbations of the disease. Synthetic heme analogs—for example, Sn-mesoporphyrin—which inhibit heme oxygenase activity have also been shown to diminish the output of ALA, PBG, or porphyrins, or all three, in AIP and VP patients, presumably because of an effective blockade of heme catabolism.

Congenital Erythropoietic Porphyria

CEP, which may also be referred to as Günther disease, is an autosomal recessive disorder (see Fig. 87–3 and Table 87–1). The primary abnormality is decreased Uro'CoS activity, which results in accumulation and hyperexcretion of predominantly type I porphyrins (see Table 87–2). Clinically, this enzymatic defect is expressed in utero as brownish amniotic fluid resulting from excessive amounts of porphyrins and results in cutaneous photosensitivity, hemolysis, and a decreased life expectancy after birth.

EPIDEMIOLOGY. Fewer than 200 cases have been reported and some of these patients may have had PCT or HEP. There is no clear racial or sexual predominance.

CLINICAL MANIFESTATIONS. The diagnosis of CEP is suggested at birth by pink to dark brown staining of the diapers in infants resulting from large amounts of porphyrins in urine. Early onset of cutaneous photosensitivity is characteristic and is exacerbated by exposure to sunlight. Subepidermal bullous lesions progress to crusted erosions, which heal with scarring and either hyperpigmentation or, less commonly, hypopigmentation. Hypertrichosis and alopecia are frequent, and erythrodontia (with red fluorescence under ultraviolet light) is virtually pathognomonic of CEP. Patients may display hemolytic anemia with splenomegaly and porphyrin-rich gallstones. Bone marrow shows erythroid hyperplasia, which may result in pathologic fractures or vertebral compression-collapse and shortness of stature. Although the onset of symptoms of CEP is most often observed in early infancy, a few patients may present as adults.

PATHOGENESIS. The primary site of expression of the enzymatic defect is the bone marrow; fluorescence secondary to porphyrin accumulation is variably distributed but invariably present. Most marrow normoblasts display fluorescence, principally localized in the nuclei of the cells. Massive elevations of systemic porphyrins in CEP are derived from porphyrin-laden erythrocytes, which accounts for the multiple pathologic features of the integument.

LABORATORY FINDINGS. Urinary porphyrins are always elevated (20–60-fold) to greater than normal levels. Uroporphyrin and coproporphyrin are mostly type I isomers. Occasionally anemia may be severe and require transfusion.

DIAGNOSIS. Pink urine or the onset of severe cutaneous photosensitivity, or both, in infancy (or rarely in adults) suggests the diagnosis of CEP. Demonstration of elevated urinary, fecal, and erythrocyte porphyrins, with elevated type I isomers of uro- and coproporphyrin, establishes the diagnosis. Demonstration of a deficiency of Uro'CoS activity is definitive.

TREATMENT. The avoidance of sunlight, trauma to the skin, and infections is the most important preventive measure in CEP. Topical sunscreens may be of some help, as may oral treatment with β-carotene. Transfusions with packed erythrocytes transiently decrease hemolysis and its attendant drive to increased erythropoiesis and also decrease porphyrin excretion. Splenectomy has been used fairly frequently and has produced short-term reductions in hemolysis, porphyrin excretion, and skin manifestations, but not all patients respond. Treatment with charcoal in a man with CEP was reported to have lowered porphyrin levels and induced complete clinical remission during therapy. Bone-marrow transplantation may also be successful.

Porphyria Cutanea Tarda and Hepatoerythropoietic Porphyria

PCT is due to a heterozygous deficiency, and HEP is due to a homozygous deficiency, of Uro'D, respectively (see Fig. 87–3 and Table 87–1).

Porphyria Cutanea Tarda

PCT refers to a heterogeneous group of cutaneous porphyria diseases caused by Uro'D deficiency, which may be either inherited or, more commonly, acquired. Both forms of the disease display reductions in hepatic Uro'D activity, but erythrocyte Uro'D activity may or may not be decreased, depending on the type of PCT. *Type I* PCT is an acquired disease that typically presents in adults, with decreased hepatic but not erythrocyte Uro'D activity. The disease may occur spontaneously but more commonly occurs in conjunction with precipitating environmental factors such as alcohol, estrogen, or drug use, or in association with other disorders. *Type II* PCT is, in contrast, inherited in an autosomal dominant fashion and is associated with decreased Uro'D activity in all tissues. *Type III* PCT is also inherited, but the defect is confined to the liver, and erythrocyte Uro'D activity is normal.

EPIDEMIOLOGY. PCT is probably the most common of all the porphyrias, but its exact incidence is not clear. The disease is recognized worldwide, and there is no racial predilection except among the Bantus in South Africa, secondary to their high incidence of hemosiderosis. Type I PCT is generally more common than type II PCT in Europe, South Africa, and South America, although the trend may be less obvious in North America. PCT was once thought to be more common in men, perhaps secondary to their higher alcohol intake; the incidence in females has increased to the level seen in males, perhaps because of increased use of contraceptive steroids, postmenopausal estrogens, and alcohol.

CLINICAL MANIFESTATIONS. The pathognomonic clinical feature of PCT is the formation of vesicles on sun-exposed areas of the skin, particularly the dorsa of the hands. The vesicles are superseded by crusting, superficial scar, or milia formation, and residual pigmentation. Facial hypertrichosis may be present and is conspicuous in women. Hypopigmented indurated plaques of skin may develop and resemble those seen in scleroderma. Photo-onycholysis is occasionally present. Neurologic dysfunction does not occur.

PATHOGENESIS. Phototoxic porphyrins in the skin are derived from the liver and, to some extent, formed locally in the skin. Activation of the complement system after irradiation has been demonstrated in PCT patients and is presumed to result from the generation of reactive oxygen species. Bullous fluid is known to contain prostaglandin E_2, and photoactivation of uroporphyrin damages lysosomes. The liver in patients with PCT almost invariably displays siderosis with fatty changes, necrosis, chronic inflammatory changes, and granuloma formation. Iron, estrogens, alcohol, and chlorinated hydrocarbons, which are all potential hepatotoxins, may aggravate PCT. The incidence of hepatitis B and C infection may also be higher than normal. The incidence of hepatocellular carcinoma in PCT is greater than in the general population. A significant association of human immunodeficiency virus–infected patients with PCT has been reported.

LABORATORY FINDINGS. Increased concentrations of uroporphyrin (mainly isomer I) and 7-carboxylic porphyrins (isomer III) are found in the urine in PCT, with lesser increases of coproporphyrin and 5- and 6-carboxylic porphyrins. Small quantities of isocoproporphyrin may be detected in serum or in urine, but in feces this is often the dominant porphyrin excreted and represents the most important diagnostic criterion for PCT. Total daily fecal porphyrin excretion exceeds total urinary porphyrin excretion. Skin porphyrins are increased, especially in areas that are protected from photoactivation. Serum iron and ferritin concentrations are frequently elevated.

DIAGNOSIS. The clinical picture in PCT is fairly specific but can be confused with other photosensitive porphyric (VP) and nonporphyric (systemic lupus erythematosus, scleroderma) diseases. Urinary fluorescence under ultraviolet light illumination and quantification of porphyrins and separation and identification of porphyrins by thin-layer chromatography and high-pressure liquid chromatography assist the diagnosis. Plasma porphyrins are elevated in PCT and in other photosensitizing porphyrias. Fecal porphyrins are often elevated; isocoproporphyrin, or an isocoproporphyrin:coproporphyrin ratio greater than or equal to 0.1, is virtually diagnostic of PCT.

TREATMENT. In type I PCT, the identification and avoidance of precipitating factors is the first line of treatment. The clinical response to cessation of alcohol ingestion is highly variable; nonetheless, abstinence should be recommended because the majority of patients have an associated heavy history of alcohol ingestion. Phlebotomy is usually effective in reducing urinary porphyrin concentrations and in induction of clinical remissions. There is strong evidence that the beneficial effects of phlebotomy result from a diminution in the stores of body iron. If phlebotomy is ineffective or contraindicated because of the presence of other diseases such as anemia, low-dose chloroquine therapy may be considered. The efficacy of chloroquine therapy and that of phlebotomy are probably similar, and a combined approach may diminish the incidence of side effects. The mechanism of action of chloroquine therapy is thought to be related to its ability to chelate porphyrins in a water-soluble and hence more easily excretable form.

Hepatoerythropoietic Porphyria

HEP is a rare form of porphyria probably resulting from a homozygous defect of Uro'D. Clinically, HEP is characterized by the childhood onset of severe photosensitivity and skin fragility and is indistinguishable from CEP. Some 20 cases have been reported.

CLINICAL MANIFESTATIONS. These findings are similar to those seen in CEP. Pink urine, severe photosensitivity leading to scarring and mutilation of sun-exposed areas of skin, sclerodermoid changes, hypertrichosis, erythrodontia, anemia (often hemolytic), and hepatosplenomegaly characterize HEP. Onset is usually in early infancy or childhood, but adult onset has also been described. In contrast to PCT, serum iron concentrations are usually normal, and phlebotomy has no beneficial effects in HEP patients.

LABORATORY FINDINGS. Elevations in urinary porphyrins, predominantly uroporphyrin of isomer type I with lesser quantities of 7-carboxylic porphyrins, mainly type III, are commonly found. Isocoproporphyrin concentrations equal to or greater than coproporphyrin levels are also found in urine and feces. Elevated erythrocyte Zn-protoporphyrin is commonly observed (see Table 87–2). Anemia and biochemical evidence of impaired hepatic function are highly variable.

DIAGNOSIS. The diagnosis must be suspected in patients with severe photosensitivity and especially considered in the differential diagnosis of CEP. Diagnostic criteria include elevated levels of fecal or urinary isocoproporphyrin and erythrocyte Zn-protoporphyrin. The differential diagnosis of HEP includes EPP, in which erythrocyte protoporphyrin is also elevated but in which, in contrast to HEP, urinary porphyrins are normal. EPP is also clinically milder than HEP. Measurement of erythrocyte or fibroblast Uro'D activities typically shows reductions to 2–10% of normal control values, with intermediate reductions of Uro'D activities in family members.

TREATMENT. Avoidance of the sun and the use of topical sunscreens are all that can be offered to these patients. The response to phlebotomy has not been observed, although this is perhaps not surprising, as serum iron levels, in contrast to those in PCT patients, are invariably normal.

Hereditary Coproporphyria

HCP is caused by a heterozygous deficiency of Copro'Ox activity, which is an autosomal dominant disorder (see Fig. 87–3 and Table 87–1). Clinically, the disease is similar to ADP or AIP, although it is often milder; HCP may be associated with photosensitivity. Expression of the disease is variable and is influenced by precipitating factors that are similar to those responsible for the exacerbation of AIP. Very rarely, homozygous deficiency of this enzyme may occur and is associated with a more severe form.

EPIDEMIOLOGY. Clinically expressed HCP is much less common than is clinically expressed AIP but, as with the latter disease, latent HCP or HCP gene carriers are found with greater frequency.

CLINICAL MANIFESTATIONS. Neurovisceral symptomatology is indistinguishable from that of ADP or AIP. Abdominal pain, vomiting, constipation, neuropathies, and psychiatric manifestations are common. Cutaneous photosensitivity is a feature in about 30% of cases. Attacks can be precipitated by pregnancy, the menstrual cycle, and contraceptive steroids, but the most common precipitating factor is drug administration, most notably phenobarbital.

LABORATORY FINDINGS. The biochemical hallmark of HCP is hyperexcretion of coproporphyrin (predominantly type III) into the urine and feces. Fecal coproporphyrin may be chelated with copper, and fecal protoporphyrin may be modestly elevated. Hyperexcretion of ALA, PBG, and uroporphyrin into the urine may accompany exacerbation of the disease but, in contrast to AIP, these findings generally normalize between attacks. Copro'Ox activity is typically reduced by about 50% in heterozygotes and by about 90–98% in homozygotes.

DIAGNOSIS. The diagnosis of HCP should be suspected in patients with the signs, symptoms, and clinical course characteristic of the acute hepatic porphyrias (ADP, AIP, HCP, and VP) but in whom PBGD activity is normal. Urinary excretion of heme precursors is similar in HCP and VP, but the predominant or exclusive presence of fecal coproporphyrin is highly suggestive of HCP. Fecal or urinary predominance of harderoporphyrin, with greatly reduced Copro'Ox activity, was reported in a case of harderoporphyria, a variant form of HCP.

TREATMENT. The identification and avoidance of precipitating factors are essential. Treatment of acute attacks is similar to that in the treatment of AIP.

Variegate Porphyria

VP (also termed *porphyria variegata, protocoproporphyria, South African genetic porphyria,* or *Royal malady)* is caused by a heterozygous deficiency in Proto'Ox activity and is an autosomal dominant disease (see Fig. 87–3 and Table 87–1). Patients may show neurovisceral symptoms or photosensitivity, or both (see Table 87–2). Very rare forms of VP are seen with homozygous deficiencies in Proto'Ox activity.

EPIDEMIOLOGY. The incidence of VP of 3/1,000 in South Africa is substantially higher than elsewhere. Affected individuals in South Africa may all be descendants of a single union between two Dutch settlers in 1680. However, the disease is recognized worldwide and, with the exception of South Africa, there is probably no racial or geographic predilection. Outside of South Africa, VP is probably less common than AIP.

CLINICAL MANIFESTATIONS. The neurovisceral symptomatology is identical to that observed in ADP, AIP, and HCP. Photosensitivity is more common, and the resulting lesions tend to be more chronic in VP than in HCP. Cutaneous manifestations comprise vesicles, bullae, hyperpigmentation, milia, hypertrichosis, and increased skin fragility. Lesions are clinically and histologically indistinguishable from PCT. Skin manifestations are less frequently observed in cold climates than in hot climates. The same spectrum of factors that leads to activation of ADP, AIP, and HCP may also exacerbate VP. Thus, barbiturates, dapsone, lead from "moonshine" whiskey, contraceptive steroids, pregnancy, and decreased carbohydrate intake have all been reported to induce or exacerbate VP.

PATHOGENESIS. Proto'Ox activity in most patients with VP is decreased 50%. In very rare cases of homozygous VP, however, there is a virtual absence of Proto'Ox activity. Symptoms consisted of severe photosensitivity, growth and mental retardation, and marked neurologic abnormalities in some cases; the onset of homozygous VP is in childhood.

LABORATORY FINDINGS. The biochemical hallmark of VP is elevated fecal porphyrin, usually with protoporphyrin IX exceeding coproporphyrin (mostly isomer III). Fecal X-porphyrins (ether-acetic acid–insoluble, extracted with urea-Triton), a heterogeneous group of porphyrin-peptide conjugates, are elevated in VP more than in any other type of porphyria.

Urinary coproporphyrin (type III), ALA, and PBG are often normal between attacks but may become markedly elevated during acute attacks. Plasma invariably shows a fluorescence emission that probably represents a protoporphyrin-peptide conjugate.

DIAGNOSIS. VP should be considered in the differential diagnosis of acute porphyria, especially if PBGD activity is normal. Characteristic plasma porphyrin fluorescence, having a different fluorescence emission maximum from PCT, is seen in VP. The differentiation of VP from HCP is usually possible following fecal porphyrin analysis and in patients with only cutaneous manifestations. The demonstration of urinary 8- and 7-carboxylic porphyrins and isocoproporphyrin in PCT is usually sufficient for differentiation from VP. Proto'Ox deficiency can be demonstrated in fibroblasts or lymphocytes.

TREATMENT. Identification and avoidance of precipitating factors are essential. Photosensitivity can be minimized by protective clothing, and Canthaxanthin (a β-carotene analog) may be of some help. The treatment of neurovisceral symptoms is identical to that described for AIP.

Erythropoietic Protoporphyria

EPP (also referred to as *protoporphyria* or *erythrohepatic protoporphyria)* is associated with a partial deficiency of FeC and is inherited in an autosomal dominant fashion (see Fig. 87–3 and Table 87–1). Biochemically, this defect results in massive accumulations of protoporphyrin in erythrocytes, plasma, and feces. Clinically, the disease is characterized by the childhood onset of cutaneous photosensitivity in light-exposed areas, but skin lesions are milder and less disfiguring than those seen in CEP.

EPIDEMIOLOGY. EPP is the most common form of erythropoietic porphyria. There is no racial or sexual predilection, and onset is typically in childhood.

CLINICAL MANIFESTATIONS. Cutaneous photosensitivity of EPP is different from that seen in CEP or PCT. Stinging or painful burning sensations in the skin occur within 1 hr of exposure to the sun and are followed several hours later by erythema and edema. Some patients experience burning sensations in the absence of such objective signs of cutaneous phototoxicity, resulting in the erroneous diagnosis of a psychiatric illness. Petechiae or, more rarely, purpura, vesicles, and crusting may develop and persist for several days after sun exposure. Artificial lights may also cause photosensitivity, especially when the patient is operated on under surgical room lights. Symptoms are usually worse during spring and summer and occur on light-exposed areas, especially the face and hands. Intense and repeated exposure to the sun may result in onycholysis, leathery hyperkeratotic skin over the dorsa of the hands, and mild scarring. Gallstones, sometimes presenting at an unusually early age, are fairly common, and hepatic disease, although unusual, may be severe and associated with significant morbidity. Anemia is uncommon. There are no known precipitating factors and no neurovisceral manifestations.

PATHOGENESIS. The peak light absorption range for porphyrins corresponds well to the wavelength of light (400 nm) known to trigger photosensitivity reactions in the skin of EPP patients. Light-excited porphyrins generate free radicals. Thus, such radicals, notably singlet oxygen, may lead to peroxidation of lipids and cross linking of membrane proteins, which, in erythrocytes, may result in reduced deformability and thus hemolysis. Interestingly, protoporphyrin, but not Zn-protoporphyrin, is released from erythrocytes following irradiation, which may explain why EPP is associated with photosensitivity, whereas lead intoxication and iron deficiency are not. Forearm irradiation in EPP patients leads to complement activation and polymorphonuclear chemotaxis.

LABORATORY FINDINGS. The biochemical hallmark of EPP is excessive concentrations of free protoporphyrin in erythrocytes, plasma, bile, and feces; this is due to its poor solubility in water, not in urine. The bone marrow and the newly released erythrocytes appear to be the major source of elevated protoporphyrin concentrations, although the liver may contribute in certain cases.

DIAGNOSIS. Photosensitivity, which is distinct from that seen in CEP or PCT, should suggest the diagnosis, which can be confirmed by the demonstration of elevated concentrations of free protoporphyrin in erythrocytes, plasma, and stools, with normal urinary porphyrins. The presence of protoporphyrin in both plasma and erythrocytes is specific for EPP. Fluorescent reticulocytes on examination of a peripheral blood smear may also suggest the diagnosis.

TREATMENT. Avoidance of the sun and the use of topical sunscreen agents may be helpful. Oral administration of β-carotene may afford systemic photoprotection, resulting in improved, although highly variable, tolerance to the sun. The recommended serum β-carotene level of 600–800 μg/dL is usually achieved with oral doses of 120–180 mg daily, and beneficial effects are typically seen 1–3 mo after the onset of therapy. The mechanism probably involves quenching of activated oxygen radicals.

Bishop DF, Astrin KH, Ioannou YA: Human δ-aminolevulinate synthase: Isolation, characterization, and mapping of house-keeping and erythroid-specific genes. Am J Hum Genet 45:A176, 1989.

Blauvelt A, Harris HR, Hogan DJ, et al: Porphyria cutanea tarda and human immunodeficiency virus infection. Int J Dermatol 31:474, 1992.

Brenner DA, Didier JM, Frasier F, et al: A molecular defect in human protoporphyria. Am J Hum Genet 50:1203, 1992.

Cotter PD, Baumann M, Bishop DF: Enzymatic defect in "X-linked" sideroblastic anemia: Molecular evidence for erythroid δ-aminolevulinate synthase deficiency. Proc Natl Acad Sci 89:4028, 1992.

Deybach JC, de Verneuil H, Boulechfar S, et al: Point mutations in the uroporphyrinogen III synthase gene in congenital erythropoietic porphyria (Gunther's disease). Blood 75:1763, 1990.

Eales L, Day RS, Blekkenhorst GH: The clinical and biochemical features of variegate porphyria: An analysis of 300 cases studied at Groote Schuur Hospital, Cape Town. Int J Biochem 12:837, 1980.

Elder GH, Hift RJ, Meissner PN: The acute porphyrias. Lancet 349:1613, 1997.

Fujita H, Kondo M, Takatani S, et al: Characterization of cDNA encoding coproporphyrinogen oxidase from a patient with hereditary coproporphyria. Hum Mol Genet 3:1807, 1994.

Held JL, Sassa S, Kappas A, et al: Erythrocyte uroporphyrinogen decarboxylase activity in porphyria cutanea tarda: A study of 40 consecutive patients. J Invest Dermatol 93:332, 1989.

Herrero C, Vicente A, Bruguera M, et al: Is hepatitis C virus infection a trigger of porphyria cutanea tarda? Lancet 341:788, 1993.

Ishida N, Fujita H, Fukuda Y, et al: Cloning and expression of the defective genes from a patient with δ-aminolevulinate dehydratase porphyria. J Clin Invest 89:1431, 1992.

Mantasek P, Nordmann Y, Grandchamp B: Homozygous hereditary coproporphyria caused by an arginine to tryptophan substitution in coproporphyrinogen oxidase and common introgenic polymorphisms. Hum Mol Genet 3:477, 1994.

Mathews-Roth MM, Pathak MA, Fitzpatrick TB, et al: Beta carotene therapy for erythropoietic protoporphyria and other photosensitivity diseases. Arch Dermatol 113:1229, 1977.

Meguro K, Fujita H, Ishida N, et al: Molecular defects of uroporphyrinogen decarboxylase in a patient with mild hepatoerythropoietic porphyria. J Invest Dermatol 98:128, 1994.

Mustajoki P, Kauppinen R, Lannfelt L, et al: Frequency of low porphobilinogen deaminase activity in Finland. J Intern Med 231:389, 1992.

Mustajoki P, Tenhunen R, Niemi KM, et al: Homozygous variegate porphyria. A severe skin disease of infancy. Clin Genet 32:300, 1987.

Mustajoki P, Tenhunen R, Pierach C, et al: Heme in the treatment of porphyrias and hematological disorders. Semin Hematol 26:1, 1989.

Nakahashi Y, Fujita H, Taketani S, et al: The molecular defect of ferrochelatase in a patient with erythropoietic protoporphyria. Proc Natl Acad Sci USA 89:281, 1992.

Nakahashi Y, Miyazaki H, Kadota Y, et al: Molecular defect in human erythropoietic protoporphyria with fatal liver failure. Hum Genet 91:303, 1993.

Pimstone NR, Gandhi SN, Mukerji SK: Therapeutic efficacy of oral charcoal in congenital erythropoietic porphyria. N Engl J Med 316:390, 1987.

Plewinska M, Thunell S, Holmberg L, et al: δ-Aminolevulinate dehydratase deficient porphyria: Identification of the molecular lesions in a severely affected homozygote. Am J Hum Genet 49:167, 1991.

Sassa S, Furuyama K: How genetic defects are identified in the porphyrias. Clin Dermatol 16:235, 1998.

Sassa S, Kappas A: Hereditary tyrosinemia and the heme biosynthetic pathway. Profound inhibition of δ-aminolevulinic acid dehydratase activity by succinylacetone. J Clin Invest 71:625, 1983.

Taketani S, Kohno H, Furukawa T, et al: Molecular cloning, sequencing and expression of cDNA encoding human coproporphyrinogen oxidase. Biochim Biophys Acta 1183:547, 1994.

Thomas C, Ged C, Nordmann Y, et al: Correction of congenital erythropoietic porphyria by bone marrow transplantation. J Pediatr 29:453, 1996.

Thunell S, Holmberg L, Lundgreen J: Aminolevulinate dehydratase porphyria in infancy. A clinical and biochemical study. J Clin Chem Clin Biochem 25:5, 1987.

Toback AC, Sassa S, Poh Fitzpatrick MB, et al: Hepatoerythropoietic porphyria: Clinical, biochemical, and enzymatic studies in a three-generation family lineage. N Engl J Med 316:645, 1987.

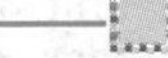

CHAPTER 88
Hypoglycemia

Mark A. Sperling

Glucose has a central role in fuel economy and is a source of energy storage in the form of glycogen, fat, and protein (see Chapter 84). Glucose, an immediate source of energy, provides 38 mol of adenosine triphosphate (ATP)/mol of glucose oxidized. It is important for cerebral energy metabolism because it is usually the preferred substrate and its utilization accounts for nearly all the oxygen consumption in brain. Cerebral glucose uptake occurs through a glucose transporter molecule or molecules that are not regulated by insulin. Cerebral transport of glucose is a carrier-mediated, facilitated diffusion process that is dependent on blood glucose concentration. Deficiency of brain glucose transporters can result in seizures because of low cerebral glucose concentration while blood glucose is normal. To maintain the blood glucose concentration and prevent it from precipitously falling to levels that impair brain function, an elaborate regulatory system has evolved.

The defense against hypoglycemia is integrated by the autonomic nervous system and by hormones that act in concert to enhance glucose production through enzymatic modulation of glycogenolysis and gluconeogenesis while simultaneously limiting peripheral glucose utilization. Hypoglycemia represents a defect in one or several of the complex interactions that normally integrate glucose homeostasis during feeding and fasting. This process is particularly important for neonates, in whom there is an abrupt transition from intrauterine life, characterized by dependence on transplacental glucose supply, to extrauterine life, characterized ultimately by the autonomous ability to maintain euglycemia. Because prematurity or placental insufficiency may limit tissue nutrient deposits, and genetic abnormalities in enzymes or hormones may become evident in the neonate, hypoglycemia is common in the neonatal period.

DEFINITION

In neonates, there is not always an obvious correlation between blood glucose concentration and the classic clinical manifestations of hypoglycemia. The absence of symptoms does not indicate that glucose concentration is normal and has not fallen to less than some optimal level for maintaining brain metabolism. There is evidence that hypoxemia and ischemia may potentiate the role of hypoglycemia in causing permanent brain damage. Consequently, the lower limit of accepted normality of the blood glucose level in newborn infants with associated illness that already impairs cerebral metabolism has not been determined (see Chapter 103.2). Out of concern for possible neurologic, intellectual, or psychologic sequelae in later life, many authorities now urge that any value of blood glucose less than 40 mg/dL in neonates be viewed with suspicion and vigorously treated. This is particularly applicable after the initial 2–3 hr of life, when glucose normally has reached its nadir; subsequently, blood glucose levels begin to rise and achieve values of 50 mg/dL or higher after 12–24 hr. In older infants and children, a blood glucose concentration of less than 40 mg/dL (10–15% higher for serum or plasma) represents hypoglycemia.

SIGNIFICANCE AND SEQUELAE

Metabolism by the adult brain accounts for some 80% of total basal glucose turnover. The brain in infants and children can utilize glucose at a rate in excess of 4–5 mg/100 g of brain weight/min. Thus, the brain of a full-term neonate, weighing about 420 g in a 3.5-kg infant, would require glucose at a rate of approximately 20 mg/min, representing glucose production of 5–7 mg/kg body weight/min. Measurements of the endogenous glucose production rate in infants and children demonstrate values of 5–8 mg/kg/min. Thus, most of the endogenous glucose production in infants and young children can be accounted for by brain metabolism. Furthermore, there is a correlation between glucose production and estimated brain weight at all ages.

Because the brain grows most rapidly during the 1st yr of life and because the larger proportion of glucose turnover is used for brain metabolism, sustained or repetitive hypoglycemia in infants and children can retard brain development and function. In the rapidly growing brain, glucose may also be a source of membrane lipids and protein synthesis; structural proteins and myelination are important for normal brain maturation. Under conditions of severe and sustained hypoglycemia, these cerebral structural substrates may be degraded to energy-usable intermediates such as lactate, pyruvate, amino acids, and ketoacids, which can support brain metabolism at the expense of brain growth. The capacity of the newborn brain to take up and oxidize ketone bodies is about fivefold greater than that in the adult brain. However, the liver's capacity to produce ketone bodies may be limited in the newborn period, especially in the presence of hyperinsulinemia, which acutely inhibits hepatic glucose output, lipolysis, and ketogenesis, thereby depriving the brain of alternate fuel sources. The deprivation of the brain's major energy source during hypoglycemia and the limited availability of alternate fuel sources during hyperinsulinemia have predictable adverse consequences on brain metabolism and growth: decreased brain oxygen consumption and increased breakdown of endogenous structural components with destruction of functional membrane integrity. Hypoglycemia may thus lead to permanent impairment of brain growth and function. The potentiating effects of hypoxia may exacerbate brain damage or indeed be responsible for it when blood glucose values are not in the classic hypoglycemic range.

The major long-term sequelae of severe, prolonged hypoglycemia are mental retardation or recurrent seizure activity, or both. Subtle effects on personality are also possible but have not been clearly defined. Permanent neurologic sequelae are present in more than half of patients with severe recurrent hypoglycemia who are younger than 6 mo of age, the period of most rapid brain growth. These sequelae are reflected in pathologic changes characterized by atrophic gyri, reduced myelination in cerebral white matter, and atrophy in the cerebral cortex. Infarcts are absent if hypoxia-ischemia did not contribute to cerebral manifestations, and the cerebellum is spared if hypoglycemia was the sole insult. These sequelae are more likely when alternative fuel sources are limited as occurs with hyperinsulinemia, when the episodes of hypoglycemia are repetitive or prolonged, or when they are compounded by hypoxia. There is no precise knowledge relating the duration or severity of hypoglycemia to subsequent neurologic development of children in a predictable manner. Although less common, hypoglycemia in older children may also produce long-term neurologic defects through neuronal death mediated, in part, by cerebral excitotoxins released during hypoglycemia.

SUBSTRATE, ENZYME, AND HORMONAL INTEGRATION OF GLUCOSE HOMEOSTASIS

IN THE NEWBORN (see also Chapter 103). Under nonstressed conditions, fetal glucose is derived entirely from the mother through placental transfer. Therefore, fetal glucose concentration usually reflects maternal glucose levels. Catecholamine release, which occurs with fetal stress such as hypoxia, mobilizes fetal glucose and free fatty acids through β-adrenergic mechanisms, reflecting β-adrenergic activity in fetal liver and adipose tissue. Catecholamines may also inhibit fetal insulin and stimulate glucagon release.

The acute interruption of maternal glucose transfer to the fetus at delivery imposes an immediate need to mobilize endogenous glucose. Three related events facilitate this transition: changes in hormones, changes in their receptors, and changes in key enzyme activity. There is a three- to fivefold abrupt increase in glucagon concentration within minutes to hours of birth. Insulin usually falls initially and remains in the basal range for several days without demonstrating the usual brisk response to physiologic stimuli such as glucose. A dramatic surge in spontaneous catecholamine secretion also is characteristic. Epinephrine can also augment growth hormone secretion by α-adrenergic mechanisms; growth hormone levels are elevated at birth. Acting in unison, these hormonal changes at birth mobilize glucose via glycogenolysis and gluconeogenesis, activate lipolysis, and promote ketogenesis. As a result of this process, plasma glucose concentration stabilizes after a transient decrease immediately after birth, liver glycogen stores become rapidly depleted within hours of birth, and gluconeogenesis from alanine, a major gluconeogenic amino acid, can account for approximately 10% of glucose turnover in the human newborn infant by several hours of age. Free fatty acid concentrations also rise sharply in concert with the surges in glucagon and epinephrine and are followed by rises in ketone bodies. Glucose is thus spared for brain utilization while free fatty acids and ketones provide alternative fuel sources for muscle as well as essential gluconeogenic factors such as acetyl-coenzyme A (CoA) and the reduced form of nicotinamide-adenine dinucleotide (NADH) from hepatic fatty acid oxidation, which is required to drive gluconeogenesis.

In the early postnatal period, responses of the endocrine pancreas favor glucagon secretion at the relative expense of insulin secretion so that blood glucose concentration can be maintained. These adaptive changes in hormone secretion are paralleled by similarly striking adaptive changes in hormone receptors. Key enzymes involved in glucose production also change dramatically in the perinatal period. Thus, there is a rapid fall in glycogen synthase activity and a sharp rise in phosphorylase after delivery. Similarly, the rate-limiting enzyme for gluconeogenesis, phosphoenol pyruvate carboxykinase, rises dramatically after birth, activated in part by the surge in glucagon and the fall in insulin. This framework can explain several causes of neonatal hypoglycemia based on inappropriate changes in hormone secretion and unavailability of adequate reserves of substrates in the form of hepatic glycogen, muscle as a source of amino acids for gluconeogenesis, and lipid stores for the release of fatty acids. In addition, appropriate activities of key enzymes governing glucose homeostasis as outlined in Figure 84–2 are required.

IN OLDER INFANTS AND CHILDREN. Hypoglycemia in older infants and children is analogous to that of adults, in whom glucose homeostasis is maintained by glycogenolysis in the immediate postfeeding period and by gluconeogenesis several hours after meals. The liver of a 10-kg child contains 20–25 g of glycogen, which is sufficient to meet glucose requirements of 4–6 mg/kg/min for only 6–12 hr. Beyond this period, hepatic gluconeogenesis must be activated. Both glycogenolysis and gluconeogenesis depend on the metabolic pathway summarized in Figures 84–1 and 84–3. Defects in gluconeogenesis may not become manifested in infants until the frequent feeding of 3- to 4-hr intervals ceases and infants sleep through the night, a situation usually present by 3–6 mo of age. The source of gluconeogenic precursors is derived primarily from muscle protein. The muscle bulk of infants and small children is substantially smaller relative to body mass than that of adults, whereas glucose requirements/unit of body mass are greater in children, so the ability to compensate for glucose deprivation by gluconeogenesis is more limited in infants and children, as is the ability to withstand fasting for prolonged periods. The ability of muscle to generate alanine, the principal gluconeogenic amino acid, may also be limited. Thus, in young children, the blood glucose level falls after 24 hr of fasting, insulin concentrations fall appropriately to levels of less than 5–10 μU/mL, lipolysis and ketogenesis are activated, and ketones may appear in the urine.

The switch from glycogen synthesis during and immediately after meals to glycogen breakdown and later gluconeogenesis is governed by hormones, of which insulin is of central importance (see Chapter 84). Plasma insulin concentrations increase to peak levels of 50–100 μU/mL after meals, which serves to lower blood glucose through the activation of glycogen synthesis, enhancement of peripheral glucose uptake, and inhibition of glucose production. In addition, lipogenesis is stimulated, whereas lipolysis and ketogenesis are curtailed. During fasting, plasma insulin concentrations fall to 5–10 μU/mL and, together with other hormonal changes, this fall results in activation of gluconeogenic pathways (see Fig. 84–1). Fasting glucose concentrations are maintained through the activation of glycogenolysis and gluconeogenesis, inhibition of glycogen synthesis, and activation of lipolysis and ketogenesis. It should be emphasized that a plasma insulin concentration of greater than 10 μU/mL, in association with a blood glucose concentration of 40 mg/dL (2.2 mM) or less, is abnormal, indicating a hyperinsulinemic state and failure of the mechanisms that normally result in suppression of insulin secretion during fasting or hypoglycemia.

The hypoglycemic effects of insulin are opposed by the actions of several hormones whose concentration in plasma increases as blood glucose falls. These counterregulatory hormones are glucagon, growth hormone, cortisol, and epinephrine. Acting in concert, they increase blood glucose concentration by activating glycogenolytic enzymes (glucagon, epinephrine); inducing gluconeogenic enzymes (glucagon, cortisol); inhibiting glucose uptake by muscle (epinephrine, growth hormone, cortisol); mobilizing amino acids from muscle for gluconeogenesis (cortisol); activating lipolysis, providing glycerol for gluconeogenesis and fatty acids for ketogenesis (epinephrine, cortisol, growth hormone, glucagon); and inhibiting insulin release and promotion of growth hormone and glucagon secretion (epinephrine).

Congenital or acquired deficiencies in these hormones may result in hypoglycemia, which occurs when endogenous glucose production cannot be mobilized to meet energy needs in the postabsorptive state, that is, 8–12 hr after meals or during fasting. Concurrent deficiency of several hormones (hypopituitarism) may result in hypoglycemia that is more severe or appears earlier than that seen with isolated hormone deficiencies.

CLINICAL MANIFESTATIONS (see also Chapter 103)

Clinical features generally fall into two categories. The first includes symptoms associated with the activation of the autonomic nervous system and epinephrine release, usually seen

TABLE 88–1 Manifestations of Hypoglycemia in Childhood

Features Associated with Activation of Autonomic Nervous System and Epinephrine Release*	Features Associated with Cerebral Glucopenia
Anxiety†	Headache†
Perspiration†	Mental confusion†
Palpitation (tachycardia)†	Visual disturbances (↓ acuity, diplopia)†
Pallor	Organic personality changes†
Tremulousness	Inability to concentrate†
Weakness	Dysarthria
Hunger	Staring
Nausea	Seizures
Emesis	Ataxia, incoordination
Angina (with normal coronary arteries)	Somnolence, lethargy
	Coma
	Stroke, hemiplegia, aphasia
	Paresthesias
	Dizziness
	Amnesia
	Decerebrate or decorticate posture

**Some of these features will be attenuated if the patient is receiving β-adrenergic blocking agents.*

†Common.

with a rapid decline in blood glucose (Table 88–1). The second category includes symptoms due to decreased cerebral glucose utilization, usually associated with a slow decline in blood glucose or prolonged hypoglycemia (see Table 88–1). Although these classic symptoms occur in older children, the symptoms of hypoglycemia in infants may be more subtle and include cyanosis, apnea, hypothermia, hypotonia, poor feeding, lethargy, and seizures. Some of these symptoms may be so mild that they are missed. Occasionally, hypoglycemia may be asymptomatic in the immediate newborn period. In childhood, hypoglycemia may present as behavior problems, inattention, ravenous appetite, or seizures. It may be misdiagnosed as epilepsy, inebriation, personality disorders, hysteria, and retardation. A blood glucose determination should always be performed in sick neonates, who should be vigorously treated if concentrations are less than 40 mg/dL. At any age level, hypoglycemia should be considered a cause of an initial episode of convulsions or a sudden deterioration in psychobehavioral functioning.

CLASSIFICATION OF HYPOGLYCEMIA IN INFANTS AND CHILDREN

Classification is based on a knowledge of the control of glucose homeostasis in infants and children (Table 88–2).

NEONATAL, TRANSIENT, SMALL FOR GESTATIONAL AGE, AND PREMATURE INFANTS (see Chapter 103). The overall incidence of symptomatic hypoglycemia in newborns varies between 1.3 and 3.0/1,000 live births. This incidence is increased severalfold in certain high-risk neonatal groups (see Table 88–2). The premature and small for gestational age (SGA) infants are vulnerable to the development of hypoglycemia. The factors responsible for the high frequency of hypoglycemia in this group, as well as in other groups outlined in Table 88–2, are related to the inadequate stores of liver glycogen, muscle protein, and body fat needed to sustain the substrates required to meet energy needs. These infants are small by virtue of prematurity or impaired placental transfer of nutrients. Their enzyme systems for gluconeogenesis may not be fully developed.

In contrast to deficiency of substrates or enzymes, the hormonal system appears to be functioning normally at birth in most low-risk neonates. Despite hypoglycemia, plasma concentrations of alanine, lactate, and pyruvate are higher, implying their diminished rate of utilization as substrates for gluconeogenesis. Infusion of alanine elicits further glucagon secretion but causes no significant rise in glucose. During the initial 24 hr of life, plasma concentrations of acetoacetate and β-hydroxybutyrate are lower in SGA infants than in full-term infants, implying diminished lipid stores, diminished fatty acid mobilization, or impaired ketogenesis, or a combination of these conditions. Diminished lipid stores are most likely because triglyceride feeding of newborns results in a rise in the plasma levels of glucose, free fatty acids (FFAs), and ketones. In addition, infants with perinatal asphyxia and some SGA newborns may have transient hyperinsulinemia, which promotes hypoglycemia and diminishes FFAs.

The role of FFAs and their oxidation in stimulating neonatal gluconeogenesis is essential. The provision of FFAs as triglyceride feedings together with gluconeogenic precursors may prevent the hypoglycemia that usually ensues after fasting. For these and other reasons, milk feedings are introduced early (at birth or within 4–6 hr) after delivery. In the hospital setting, when feeding is precluded by virtue of respiratory distress or when feedings alone cannot maintain blood glucose concentrations at levels greater than 40 mg/dL, intravenous glucose at a rate that supplies approximately 4–8 mg/kg/min should be started. Infants can usually maintain the blood glucose level spontaneously after 3–5 days of life.

INFANTS BORN TO DIABETIC MOTHERS (see Chapter 103.1). Of the transient hyperinsulinemic states, infants born to diabetic mothers is the most common. Gestational diabetes affects some 2% of pregnant women, and approximately 1/1,000 pregnant women has insulin-dependent diabetes. At birth, infants born to these mothers may be large and plethoric, and their body stores of glycogen, protein, and fat are replete.

Hypoglycemia in infants of diabetic mothers is mostly related to hyperinsulinemia and partly related to diminished glucagon secretion. Hypertrophy and hyperplasia of the islets is present, as is a brisk, biphasic, and typically adult insulin response to glucose; this insulin response is absent in normal infants. Infants born to diabetic mothers also have a subnormal surge in plasma glucagon immediately after birth, subnormal glucagon secretion in response to stimuli and, initially, excessive sympathetic activity that may lead to adrenomedullary exhaustion as reflected in urinary excretion of epinephrine, which is diminished. The normal plasma hormonal pattern of low insulin, high glucagon, and high catecholamines is reversed to a pattern of high insulin, low glucagon, and low epinephrine. As a consequence of this abnormal hormonal profile, the endogenous glucose production is significantly inhibited compared with that in normal infants, thus predisposing them to hypoglycemia.

Infants born with *erythroblastosis fetalis* also have hyperinsulinemia and share many physical features, such as large body size, with infants born to diabetic mothers. The cause of the hyperinsulinemia in infants with erythroblastosis is not entirely clear but may be related to compensatory hypersecretion as a result of the hemolysis that provides increased glutathione, which splits the disulfide bonds of insulin.

Mothers whose diabetes has been well controlled during pregnancy generally have babies near normal size who are less likely to acquire neonatal hypoglycemia and other complications formerly considered typical of such infants (see Chapter 103.1). In supplying glucose to these infants, it is important to avoid hyperglycemia that evokes prompt insulin release, which may result in rebound hypoglycemia. When needed, glucose should be provided at rates of 4–8 mg/kg/min, but the appropriate dose for each patient should be individually adjusted. During labor and delivery, maternal hyperglycemia should be avoided because it results in fetal hyperglycemia, which predisposes to hypoglycemia when the glucose supply is interrupted at birth. Hypoglycemia persisting or occurring after 1 wk of life requires an evaluation for the causes listed in Table 88–2.

TABLE 88–2 Classification of Hypoglycemia in Infants and Children

Neonatal—Transient Hypoglycemia	Other Etiologies
Associated with inadequate substrate or enzyme function	Poisoning—drugs
Prematurity	Salicylates
Small for gestational age (SGA)	Alcohol
Smaller of twins	Oral hypoglycemic agents
Infants with severe respiratory distress	Insulin
Infant of toxemic mother	Propranolol
Associated with hyperinsulinemia	Pentamidine
Infants of diabetic mothers	Quinine
Infants with erythroblastosis fetalis	Disopyramide
Perinatal asphyxia—SGA	Ackee fruit (unripe)—hypoglycin
Neonatal—Infantile or Childhood Persistent Hypoglycemia	Vacor (rat poison)
	Trimethoprim-sulfamethoxazole (with renal failure)
Hyperinsulinemic states	Liver disease
PHHI	Reye syndrome
Autosomal recessive (SUR and $K_{IR}6.2$ mutations)*	Hepatitis
Autosomal dominant	Cirrhosis
Glucokinase activating mutation	Hepatoma
Glutamate dehydrogenase activating mutation	Amino acid and organic acid disorders
Sporadic	Maple syrup urine disease
β-cell hyperplasia	Propionic acidemia
β-cell adenoma	Methylmalonic acidemia
Beckwith-Wiedemann syndrome	Tyrosinosis
Leucine sensitivity	Glutaric aciduria
Falciparum malaria	3-Hydroxy-3-methylglutaric aciduria
Hormone deficiency	Systemic disorders
Panhypopituitarism	Sepsis
Isolated growth hormone deficiency	Carcinoma/sarcoma (secreting—insulin-like growth factor II)
ACTH deficiency	Heart failure
Addison disease	Malnutrition
Glucagon deficiency	Malabsorption
Epinephrine deficiency	Anti-insulin receptor antibodies
Substrate limited	Anti-insulin antibodies
Ketotic hypoglycemia	Neonatal hyperviscosity
Branched-chain ketonuria (maple syrup urine disease)	Renal failure
Glycogen storage disease	Diarrhea
Glucose-6-phosphatase deficiency	Burns
Amylo-1,6-glucosidase deficiency	Shock
Liver phosphorylase deficiency	Postsurgical
Glycogen synthetase deficiency	Pseudohypoglycemia (leukocytosis, polycythemia)
Disorders of gluconeogenesis	Excessive insulin therapy of insulin-dependent diabetes mellitus
Acute alcohol intoxication	Factitious
Hyperglycinemia, carnitine deficiency	
Salicylate intoxication	
Fructose-1,6-diphosphatase deficiency	
Pyruvate carboxylase deficiency	
Phosphoenol pyruvate carboxykinase (PEPCK deficiency)	
Other enzyme defects	
Galactosemia: galactose-1-phosphate uridyl transferase deficiency	
Fructose intolerance: fructose-1-phosphate aldolase deficiency	
Disorders of fat (alternate fuel) metabolism	
Primary carnitine deficiency	
Secondary carnitine deficiency	
Carnitine palmitoyl transferase deficiency	
Long-, medium-, short-chain fatty acid acyl-CoA dehydrogenase deficiency	

Adapted from Sperling M, Chernausek S: Nelson's Essentials of Pediatrics. Philadelphia, WB Saunders, 1990, p 617.
PHHI = persistent hyperinsulinemic hypoglycemia of infancy.
**Sur = sulfonylurea receptor; $K_{IR}6.2$ = inward rectifying potassium channel (See Fig. 88–1 and text for details).*

PERSISTENT OR RECURRENT HYPOGLYCEMIA IN INFANTS AND CHILDREN

Hyperinsulinism

Most children with hyperinsulinism that causes hypoglycemia present in infancy; hyperinsulinism is the most common cause of persistent hypoglycemia in early infancy. Hyperinsulinemic infants may be macrosomic at birth, reflecting the anabolic effects of insulin in utero. There is, however, no history and no biochemical evidence of maternal diabetes. The onset is from birth to 18 mo of age. Insulin concentrations are inappropriately elevated at the time of documented hypoglyce-

TABLE 88–3 Hypoglycemia in Infants and Children: Clinical and Laboratory Features

Group	Age at Diagnosis (mo)	Glucose (mg/dL)	Insulin (μU/mL)	Fasting Time to Hypoglycemia (hr)
Hyperinsulinemia (n = 12)				
Mean	7.4	23.1	22.4	2.1
SEM	2.0	2.7	3.2	0.6
Nonhyperinsulinemia (n = 16)				
Mean	41.8	36.1	5.8	18.2
SEM	7.3	2.4	0.9	2.9

Adapted from Antunes JD, Geffner ME, Lippe BM, et al: J Pediatr 116:105–108, 1990.

TABLE 88–4 Persistent Hyperinsulinemic Hypoglycemia of Infancy

Age at Onset	Severity of Hypoglycemia	Associated Clinical or Biochemical Features	Response to Medical Management	Molecular Basis	Inheritance
Day 1 or 2 of life up to 3 mo of life	Severe	Macrosomia at birth Diffuse pancreatic β cell hyperplasia Focal adenomatous pancreatic lesions	Poor	SUR/K_{IR}6.2	Autosomal recessive
First wk of life	Severe	Macrosomia Macroglossia Exophthalmos Distinct ear lobe groove Hemihypertrophy	Fair	Gene deletion chromosome 11p	Sporadic Beckwith-Wiedemann syndrome
Later than 6 mo, average 12 mo (may present at older ages)	Moderate	Rarely large at birth	Good	Activated glucokinase or unknown	Autosomal dominant or spontaneous mutation
3 mo to 10 yr	Mild or moderate	Hyperammonemia	Good	Activated glutamate dehydrogenase	Autosomal dominant or spontaneous mutation

mia; with nonhyperinsulinemic hypoglycemia, plasma insulin concentrations should be less than 5 μU/mL and no higher than 10 μU/mL. In affected infants, however, plasma insulin concentrations at the time of hypoglycemia are commonly greater than 5–10 μU/mL. The insulin (μU/mL):glucose (mg/dL) ratio is commonly 0.4 or greater; plasma ketones and FFA levels are low. Macrosomic infants may present with hypoglycemia from the 1st days of life. Infants with lesser degrees of hyperinsulinemia, however, may manifest hypoglycemia after the 1st few wk to mo, when the frequency of feedings has been decreased to permit the infant to sleep through the night and hyperinsulinemia prevents the mobilization of endogenous glucose. Increasing appetite and demands for feeding, wilting spells, jitteriness, and frank seizures are the most common presenting features. Additional clues include the rapid development of fasting hypoglycemia within 4–8 hr of food deprivation compared with other causes of hypoglycemia (Tables 88–3, 88–4); the need for high rates of exogenous glucose infusion to prevent hypoglycemia, often at rates greater than 10–15 mg/kg/min; absence of ketonemia or acidosis; and elevated C-peptide or proinsulin levels at the time of hypoglycemia. The latter insulin-related products are absent in factitious hypoglycemia from exogenous administration of insulin. Provocative tests with tolbutamide or leucine are not necessary in infants; hypoglycemia is invariably provoked by withholding feedings for several hours, permitting simultaneous measurement of glucose, insulin, ketones, and FFAs in the same sample at the time of clinically manifested hypoglycemia. The glycemic response to glucagon at the time of hypoglycemia reveals a brisk rise in glucose of at least 40 mg/dL and implies that glucose mobilization has been restrained by insulin but that glycogenolytic mechanisms are intact (Table 88–5).

The measurement of serum insulin-like growth factor binding protein-1 (IGFBP-1) concentration is a useful test. The secretion of IGFBP-1 is acutely inhibited by insulin; IGFBP-1 concentrations are low during hyperinsulinism-induced hypoglycemia. In infants and children with spontaneous or fasting-induced hypoglycemia with a low insulin level (ketotic hypoglycemia, normal fasting), IGFBP-1 concentrations are significantly higher.

Once endogenous hyperinsulinism has been established through these concurrent measurements taken at the time of spontaneous or fasting-induced hypoglycemia, the differential diagnosis includes *familial and nonfamilial hyperinsulinism of infancy,* β*-cell hyperplasia,* and β*-cell adenoma*. These entities cannot be distinguished by the plasma levels of insulin alone. They represent diffuse genetic defects or localized abnormalities in the endocrine pancreas, characterized by autonomous insulin secretion that is not appropriately reduced when blood glucose declines spontaneously or in response to provocative maneuvers such as fasting (see Table 88–4). Clinical, biochemical, and molecular genetic approaches permit classification of congenital hyperinsulinism, formerly termed *nesidioblastosis,* into at least three entities. One form of persistent hyperinsulinemic hypoglycemia of infancy (PHHI) is inherited in an autosomal recessive pattern, is severe, and is caused by mutations in the regulation of the potassium channel intimately involved in insulin secretion by the pancreatic β-cell (Fig. 88–1). Normally, glucose entry into the β-cell is enabled by the non–insulin responsive glucose transporter, GLUT-2. On entry, glucose is phosphorylated to glucose-6-phosphate by the enzyme glucokinase, enabling glucose metabolism to generate ATP. The rise in the molar ratio of ATP relative to adenosine diphosphate (ADP) closes the ATP-sensitive potassium channel in the cell membrane (K_{ATP} channel). This channel is composed of two subunits, the K_{IR}6.2 channel, part of the family of inward-rectifier potassium channels, and a regulatory component in intimate association with K_{IR}6.2 known as the sulfonylurea receptor (SUR). Together, K_{IR}6.2 and SUR constitute the potassium-sensitive ATP channel, K_{ATP}. Normally, the K_{ATP} is open, but with the rise in ATP and closure of the channel, potassium accumulates intracellularly causing depolarization of the membrane, opening of voltage-gated calcium channels, influx of calcium into the cytoplasm, and secretion of insulin via exocytosis. The genes for both SUR and K_{IR}6.2 are located close together on the short arm of chromosome 11, the site of the insulin gene. Inactivating mutations in the gene for SUR

TABLE 88–5 Analysis of Blood Sample Before and 30 Minutes After Glucagon*

Substrates	Hormones
Glucose	Insulin
Free fatty acids	Cortisol
Ketones	Growth hormone
Lactate	T_4, TSH†
Uric acid	
Ammonia	

**Glucagon 30 μg/kg IV or IM.*

†Measure once only before or after glucagon administration. Rise in glucose of ≥40 mg/dL after glucagon given at the time of hypoglycemia strongly suggests a hyperinsulinemic state with adequate hepatic glycogen stores and intact glycogenolytic enzymes. If ammonia is elevated to 100–200 μM, consider activating mutation of glutamate dehydrogenase.

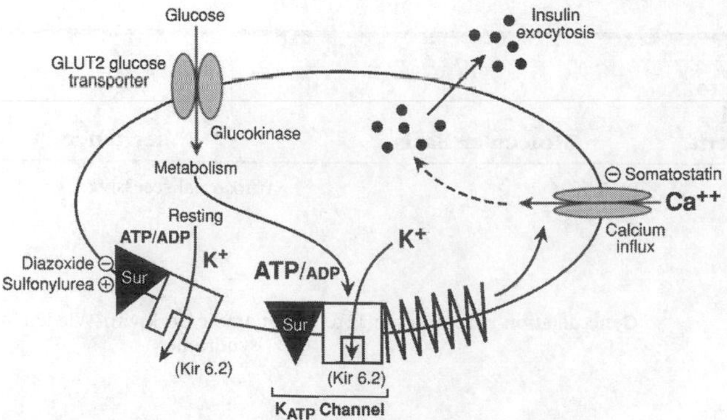

Figure 88–1 Schematic representation of the pancreatic β cell with some important steps in insulin secretion. The membrane-spanning, adenosine triphosphate (ATP)–sensitive potassium (K^+) channel (K_{ATP}) consists of two subunits: the sulfonylurea receptor (SUR) and the inward rectifying K channel ($K_{IR}6.2$). In the resting state, the ratio of ATP to adenosine diphosphate (ADP) maintains K_{ATP} in an open state, permitting efflux of intracellular K^+. When blood glucose concentration rises, its entry into the β cell is facilitated by the GLUT-2 glucose transporter, a process not regulated by insulin. Within the β cell, glucose is converted to glucose-6-phosphate by the enzyme glucokinase and then undergoes metabolism to generate energy. The resultant increase in ATP relative to ADP closes K_{ATP}, preventing efflux of K^+, and the rise of intracellular K^+ depolarizes the cell membrane and opens a calcium (Ca^{2+}) channel. The intracellular rise in Ca^{2+} triggers insulin secretion via exocytosis. Sulfonylureas trigger insulin secretion by reacting with their receptor (SUR) to close K_{ATP}; diazoxide inhibits this process, whereas somatostatin, or its analog octreotide, inhibits insulin secretion by interfering with calcium influx. Genetic mutations in SUR or $K_{IR}6.2$ that prevent K_{ATP} from being open are responsible for autosomal recessive forms of persistent hyperinsulinemic hypoglycemia of infancy (PHHI). One form of autosomal dominant PHHI is due to an activating mutation in glucokinase. The amino acid leucine also triggers insulin secretion by closure of K_{ATP}. Metabolism of leucine is facilitated by the enzyme glutamate dehydrogenase (GDH) and overactivity of this enzyme in the pancreas leads to hyperinsulinemia with hypoglycemia, associated with hyperammonemia from overactivity of GDH in the liver.

or $K_{IR}6.2$ prevent the potassium channel from opening; it remains essentially closed with constant depolarization and, therefore, constant inward flux of calcium; insulin secretion is constant. Likewise, an activating mutation in glucokinase results in closure of the potassium channel through overproduction of ATP and hyperinsulinism. Inactivating mutations of the glucokinase gene are responsible for inadequate insulin secretion and form the basis of type 2 maturity-onset diabetes of youth (see Chapter 599).

The familial forms of PHHI are more common in certain populations, notably Arabic and Ashkenazi Jewish communities where it may reach an incidence of about 1/2,500, compared with the sporadic rates in the general population of approximately 1/50,000. These *autosomal recessive forms* of PHHI typically present in the immediate newborn period in macrosomic newborns with a weight in excess of 4.0 kg and severe recurrent or persistent hypoglycemia manifesting in the 1st hr or days of life. Glucose infusions of as much as 15–20 mg/kg/min and frequent feedings fail to maintain euglycemia. Diazoxide, which functions by opening K_{ATP} channels (see Fig. 88–1), also fails to control hypoglycemia adequately. Somatostatin, which also opens K_{ATP} and inhibits calcium flux, may be partially effective in about 50% of patients (see Fig. 88–1). When affected patients are unresponsive to these measures, pancreatectomy is strongly recommended to avoid the long-term neurologic sequelae of hypoglycemia. If surgery is undertaken, preoperative computed tomography or magnetic resonance imaging may rarely reveal an adenoma, permitting local resection. Also, intraoperative ultrasonography may identify a small impalpable adenoma, permitting local resection. Distinguishing between focal and diffuse cases of hyperinsulinism has been reported with the use of a combination of transhepatic portal venous catheterization and intraoperative histologic techniques. It is claimed that diffuse hyperinsulinism is characterized by large β cells with abnormally large nuclei, whereas focal adenomatous lesions display small and normal β cell nuclei. Although Sur1 mutations are present in both types, the focal lesions arise by a random loss of a maternally imprinted growth-inhibitory gene on maternal chromosome 11p in association with paternal transmission of a mutated Sur1 or $K_{IR}6.2$ paternal chromosome 11p. Local excision of focal adenomatous islet-cell hyperplasia results in a cure with little or no recurrence. If local resection is not possible, near-total resection of 85–90% of the pancreas is recommended. In contrast, the near-total pancreatectomy required for the diffuse hyperplastic lesions is often associated with persistent hypoglycemia and later development of hyperglycemia or frank, insulin-requiring diabetes mellitus.

Further resection of the remaining pancreas may occasionally be necessary if hypoglycemia recurs and cannot be controlled by medical measures, such as the use of somatostatin or diazoxide with cortisone. Surgery should be performed by experienced pediatric surgeons in medical centers equipped to provide the necessary preoperative and postoperative care, diagnostic evaluation, and management.

If hypoglycemia first becomes manifested between 3 and 6 mo of age or later, a therapeutic trial using medical approaches with somatostatin, diazoxide, steroids, and frequent feedings can be attempted for up to 2–4 wk. Failure to maintain euglycemia without undesirable side effects from the drugs prompts the need for surgery. Some success in suppressing insulin release and correcting hypoglycemia in patients with PHHI has been reported with the use of the long-acting somatostatin analog octreotide. Most cases of neonatal PHHI are sporadic; familial forms permit genetic counseling on the basis of anticipated autosomal recessive inheritance. However, infants manifesting hypoglycemia at 3–6 mo of age are likely to have other forms of PHHI.

A second form of familial PHHI suggests *autosomal dominant inheritance*. The clinical features tend to be less severe and onset of hypoglycemia is most likely, but not exclusively, to occur beyond the immediate newborn period and usually beyond the period of weaning at an average age of onset of about 1 yr. At birth, macrosomia is rarely observed, and response to diazoxide is almost uniform. The initial presentation may be delayed and occur as late as 30 yr unless provoked by fasting. The genetic basis for this autosomal dominant form has not been delineated; it is not linked to $K_{IR}6.2$/SUR, although the activating mutation in glucokinase is transmitted in an autosomal dominant manner. If a family history is present, genetic counseling for a 50% recurrence rate can be given for future offspring.

A third form of persistent PHHI is associated with *mild hyperammonemia,* usually as a sporadic occurrence although dominant inheritance occurs. Presentation is more like the autosomal dominant form rather than the autosomal recessive form. Diet and diazoxide control symptoms, but pancreatectomy may be necessary in some cases. The association of hyperinsulinism and hyperammonemia is caused by an inherited or de novo gain-of-function mutation in the enzyme glutamate dehydrogenase. The resulting increase in glutamate oxidation in the pancreatic β cell raises the ATP concentration and, hence, the ratio of ATP:ADP, which closes K_{ATP}, leading to membrane depolarization, calcium influx, and insulin secretion (see Fig. 88–1). In the liver, the excessive oxidation of glutamate to β-ketoglutarate also generates ammonia and diverts glutamate from being processed to *N*-acetylglutamate, an essential cofactor for removal of ammonia through the urea cycle via activation of the enzyme carbamoyl phosphate synthetase. The hyperammonemia is mild, with concentrations of about 100–200 μM/L but without the central nervous system symptoms or consequences of other hyperammonemic states. Leucine, a potent amino acid for stimulating insulin secretion and implicated in leucine-sensitive hypoglycemia, acts by allosterically stimulating glutamate dehydrogenase. Thus, *leucine-sensitive hypoglycemia* may be a form of the hyperinsulinemia-hyperammonemia syndrome or a potentiation of mild disorders of the K_{ATP} channel.

Hypoglycemia associated with hyperinsulinemia is also seen in approximately 50% of patients with the *Beckwith-Wiedemann syndrome* (see Chapter 103). This syndrome is characterized by exophthalmos, gigantism, macroglossia, microcephaly, and visceromegaly. Distinctive lateral earlobe fissures are present, and hemihypertrophy occurs in many of these infants. Diffuse islet cell hyperplasia occurs in infants with hypoglycemia. The diagnostic and therapeutic approaches are the same as those discussed previously, although microcephaly and retarded brain development may occur independently of hypoglycemia. Patients with the Beckwith-Wiedemann syndrome may acquire tumors, including Wilms tumor, hepatoblastoma, adrenal carcinoma, and rhabdomyosarcoma. This overgrowth syndrome is caused by mutations in the chromosome 11p15.5 region close to the genes for insulin SUR, $K_{IR}6.2$, and IGF-2. Duplications in this region and genetic imprinting from a defective or absent copy of the maternally derived gene are involved in the variable features and patterns of transmission.

After the first 12 mo of life, hyperinsulinemic states are uncommon until islet cell adenomas reappear as a cause after the patient is several years of age. Hyperinsulinemia due to *islet cell adenoma* should be considered in any child 5 yr or older presenting with hypoglycemia. The diagnostic approach is outlined in Tables 88–6 and 88–7. Fasting for 24–36 hr usually provokes hypoglycemia; coexisting hyperinsulinemia confirms the diagnosis provided that factitious administration of insulin by the parents, a form of *Munchausen syndrome by proxy,* has been excluded. Occasionally, provocative tests may be required. Exogenously administered insulin can be distinguished from endogenous insulin by simultaneous measurement of C-peptide concentration. If C-peptide levels are elevated, endogenous insulin secretion is responsible for the hypoglycemia; if C-peptide levels are low but insulin values are high, exogenous insulin has been administered, perhaps as a form of child abuse. Islet cell adenomas at this age are treated by surgical excision; familial multiple endocrine adenomatosis type I (Wermer syndrome) should be considered in the differential diagnosis. Antibodies to insulin or the insulin receptor (insulinomimetic action) are also rarely associated with hypoglycemia. Some tumors are reported to produce insulin-like growth factors, thereby provoking hypoglycemia by interacting with the insulin receptor.

Endocrine Deficiency

Hypoglycemia associated with endocrine deficiency is usually due to adrenal insufficiency with or without associated growth hormone deficiency (see Chapters 567 and 585). In patients with panhypopituitarism, isolated adrenocorticotropic hormone (ACTH) or growth hormone deficiency, or combined ACTH deficiency plus growth hormone deficiency, the incidence of hypoglycemia is as high as 20%. In the newborn period, hypoglycemia may be the presenting feature of hypopituitarism; in males, a microphallus may provide a clue to a coexistent deficiency of gonadotropin. Newborns with hypopituitarism often have a form of "hepatitis" and the syndrome of *septo-optic dysplasia.* When adrenal disease is severe, as in congenital adrenal hyperplasia due to cortisol synthetic enzyme defects, adrenal hemorrhage, or congenital absence of the adrenal glands, disturbances in serum electrolytes with hyponatremia and hyperkalemia or ambiguous genitals may provide diagnostic clues (see Chapter 586). In older children, failure of growth should suggest growth hormone deficiency. Hyperpigmentation may provide the clue to Addison disease with increased ACTH levels or adrenal unresponsiveness to ACTH due to a defect in the adrenal receptor for ACTH. The frequent association of Addison disease in childhood with hypoparathyroidism (hypocalcemia), chronic mucocutaneous candidiasis, and other endocrinopathies should be considered. Adrenoleukodystrophy should also be considered in the differential diagnosis of primary Addison disease in older children (see Chapter 83.2).

The cause of hypoglycemia in cortisol–growth hormone deficiency may be due to decreased gluconeogenic enzymes with cortisol deficiency, increased glucose utilization due to a lack of the antagonistic effects of growth hormone on insulin action, or failure to supply endogenous gluconeogenic substrate in the form of alanine and lactate with compensatory breakdown of fat and generation of ketones. Deficiency of these hormones results in reduced gluconeogenic substrate, which resembles the syndrome of ketotic hypoglycemia. Investigation of a child with hypoglycemia, therefore, requires exclusion of ACTH-cortisol or growth hormone deficiency, and if diagnosed, its appropriate replacement with cortisol or growth hormone.

Epinephrine deficiency could theoretically be responsible for hypoglycemia. Urinary excretion of epinephrine has been diminished in some patients with spontaneous or insulin-induced hypoglycemia in whom absence of pallor and tachycardia was also noted, suggesting that failure of catecholamine release, due to a defect anywhere along the hypothalamic-autonomic-adrenomedullary axis, might be responsible for the hypoglycemia. This possibility has been challenged owing to the rarity of hypoglycemia in patients with bilateral adrenalectomy provided that they receive adequate glucocorticoid replacement and because diminished epinephrine excretion is found in normal patients with repeated insulin-induced hypoglycemia. Many of the patients described as having hypoglycemia with failure of epinephrine excretion fit the criteria for ketotic hypoglycemia.

Glucagon deficiency in infants or children may rarely be associated with hypoglycemia.

Substrate Limited

KETOTIC HYPOGLYCEMIA. This is the most common form of childhood hypoglycemia. This condition usually presents between the ages of 18 mo and 5 yr and remits spontaneously by the age of 8–9 yr. Hypoglycemic episodes typically occur during periods of intercurrent illness when food intake is limited. The classic history is of a child who eats poorly or completely avoids the evening meal, is difficult to arouse from sleep the following morning, and may have a seizure or be comatose by midmorning. Another common presentation occurs when parents sleep late and the affected child is unable to eat breakfast, thus prolonging the overnight fast.

At the time of documented hypoglycemia, there is associated ketonuria and ketonemia; plasma insulin concentrations are appropriately low, 5–10 μU/mL or less, thus excluding hyperinsulinemia. A ketogenic provocative diet, formerly used as a diagnostic test, is not essential to establish the diagnosis because fasting alone provokes a hypoglycemic episode with ketonemia and ketonuria within 12–18 hr in susceptible individuals. Normal children of similar age can withstand fasting without hypoglycemia developing during the same period, although even normal children may acquire these features by 36 hr of fasting.

Children with ketotic hypoglycemia have plasma alanine concentrations that are markedly reduced in the basal state after an overnight fast and decline even further with prolonged fasting. Alanine, produced in muscle, is a major gluconeogenic precursor. Alanine is the only amino acid that is significantly lower in these children, and infusions of alanine (250 mg/

kg) produce a rapid rise in plasma glucose without causing significant changes in blood lactate or pyruvate levels, indicating that the entire gluconeogenic pathway from the level of pyruvate is intact but that there is a deficiency of substrate. Glycogenolytic pathways are also intact because glucagon induces a normal glycemic response in affected children during the fed state. The levels of hormones that counter hypoglycemia are appropriately elevated, and insulin is appropriately low.

The *etiology* of ketotic hypoglycemia may be a defect in any of the complex steps involved in protein catabolism, oxidative deamination of amino acids, transamination, alanine synthesis, or alanine efflux from muscle. Children with ketotic hypoglycemia are frequently smaller than age-matched controls and often have a history of transient neonatal hypoglycemia. Any decrease in muscle mass may compromise the supply of gluconeogenic substrate at a time when glucose demands per unit of body weight are already relatively high, thus predisposing the patient to the rapid development of hypoglycemia, with ketosis representing the attempt to switch to an alternative fuel supply. Children with ketotic hypoglycemia may represent the low end of the spectrum of children's capacity to tolerate fasting. Similar relative intolerance to fasting is present in normal children, who cannot maintain blood glucose after 30–36 hr of fasting, compared with the adult's capacity for prolonged fasting. Although the defect may be present at birth, it may not become manifested until the child is stressed by more prolonged periods of calorie restriction. Moreover, the spontaneous remission observed in children at age 8–9 yr might be explained by the increase in muscle bulk with its resultant increase in supply of endogenous substrate and the relative decrease in glucose requirement per unit of body mass with increasing age. There is also some evidence to support the contention that impaired epinephrine secretion due to immaturity of autonomic innervation contributes to ketotic hypoglycemia. Rarely, inborn errors of fatty acid metabolism present as ketotic hypoglycemia, although typically, fatty acid oxidation defects produce hypoketotic hypoglycemia.

In anticipation of spontaneous resolution of this syndrome, *treatment* of ketotic hypoglycemia consists of frequent feedings of a high-protein, high-carbohydrate diet. During intercurrent illnesses, parents should test the child's urine for the presence of ketones, the appearance of which precedes hypoglycemia by several hours. In the presence of ketonuria, liquids of high carbohydrate content should be offered to the child. If these cannot be tolerated, the child should be offered a short course of steroids or admitted to the hospital for intravenous glucose administration.

BRANCHED-CHAIN KETONURIA (MAPLE SYRUP URINE DISEASE) (see Chapter 82.6). The hypoglycemic episodes were once attributed to high levels of leucine, but evidence indicates that interference with the production of alanine and its availability as a gluconeogenic substrate during calorie deprivation is responsible for hypoglycemia.

Glycogen Storage Disease See Chapter 84.1.

GLUCOSE-6-PHOSPHATASE DEFICIENCY (TYPE I GLYCOGEN STORAGE DISEASE). Typically, affected children display a remarkable tolerance to their chronic hypoglycemia; blood glucose values in the range of 20–50 mg/dL are not associated with the classic symptoms of hypoglycemia, possibly reflecting the adaptation of the central nervous system to ketone bodies as an alternative fuel.

Affected untreated children manifest growth failure, mental retardation, and a shortened life span unless they are treated. Continuous intragastric feeding or total parenteral nutrition improves the metabolic and clinical findings by reducing the frequency and severity of hypoglycemia, thereby avoiding the secondary hormonal changes that appear to be responsible for the metabolic derangements. Continuous intragastric feeding at night, combined with frequent daytime feedings, produces equally effective amelioration of the biochemical disturbances and avoids the inconvenience of 24-hr continuous gastric feeding and the problems associated with long-term parenteral nutrition. The daytime feedings are given every 3–4 hr: 60–70% of the calories as carbohydrate low in fructose and galactose, 12–15% of the calories as protein, and 15–25% of the calories as fat. At night, a small nasogastric tube is passed by the patient (or a parent for younger children), and approximately one third of the daily caloric requirements is continuously infused over 8–12 hr using a small continuous infusion pump. One commercially available formula for nocturnal infusion contains 89% of the calories as glucose and glucose oligosaccharides, 1.8% as safflower oil, and 9.2% as crystalline amino acids.* Nocturnal cornstarch therapy also has been used successfully. Transient nocturnal hypoglycemia is not completely prevented and renal glomerular dysfunction plus formation of hepatic adenoma remain serious complications. Liver transplantation offers promise of long-term cure.

Amylo-1,6-Glucosidase Deficiency (Debrancher Enzyme Deficiency; Type III Glycogen Storage Disease). See Chapter 84.

Liver Phosphorylase Deficiency (Type VI Glycogen Storage Disease). (see also Chapter 84). Low hepatic phosphorylase activity may result from a defect in any of the steps of activation; a variety of defects have been described. Hepatomegaly, excessive deposition of glycogen in liver, growth retardation, and occasional symptomatic hypoglycemia occur. A diet high in protein and reduced in carbohydrate usually prevents hypoglycemia.

Glycogen Synthetase Deficiency. (see also Chapter 84). The inability to synthesize glycogen is extremely rare. There is fasting hypoglycemia and hyperketonemia; hyperglycemia occurs with glucosuria after meals. During fasting hypoglycemia, levels of the counterregulatory hormones, including catecholamines, are appropriately elevated or normal, and insulin levels are appropriately low. The liver is not enlarged. Protein-rich feedings at frequent intervals result in dramatic clinical improvement, including growth velocity. This condition mimics the syndrome of ketotic hypoglycemia and should be considered in the differential diagnosis of that syndrome.

Disorders of Gluconeogenesis

ACUTE ALCOHOL INTOXICATION. The liver metabolizes alcohol as a preferred fuel, and generation of reducing equivalents during the oxidation of ethanol alters the NADH:NAD ratio, which is essential for certain gluconeogenic steps. As a result, gluconeogenesis is impaired, and hypoglycemia may ensue if glycogen stores are depleted by starvation or by pre-existing abnormalities in glycogen metabolism. In toddlers who have been unfed for some time, even the consumption of small quantities of alcohol can precipitate these events. The hypoglycemia promptly responds to intravenous glucose, which should always be given to a child who presents initially with coma or seizure, after taking a blood sample to determine glucose concentration. The possibility of the child's ingesting alcoholic drinks must also be considered if there was a preceding adult evening party. A careful history allows the diagnosis to be made and may avoid needless and expensive hospitalization and investigation.

DEFECTS IN FATTY ACID OXIDATION (see also Chapter 83.1). The important role of fatty acid oxidation in maintaining gluconeogenesis is underscored by examples of congenital or drug-induced defects in fatty acid metabolism that may be associated with fasting hypoglycemia.

Various congenital enzymatic deficiencies causing defective carnitine or fatty acid metabolism also occur. A severe and relatively common form of fasting hypoglycemia with hepatomegaly, cardiomyopathy, and hypotonia occurs with long- and medium-chain fatty acid coenzyme-A dehydrogenase defi-

*Vivonex, Eaton Laboratories

ciency (LCAD and MCAD). Plasma carnitine levels are low, ketones are not present in urine, but dicarboxylic aciduria is present. Clinically, patients with *acyl CoA dehydrogenase deficiency* present with a Reye-like syndrome, recurrent episodes of severe fasting hypoglycemic coma, and cardiorespiratory arrest (sudden infant death syndrome–like events). Severe hypoglycemia and metabolic acidosis without ketosis also occur in patients with multiple acyl-CoA dehydrogenase disorders. Hypotonia, seizures, and acrid odor are other clinical clues. Survival depends on whether the defects are severe or mild; diagnosis is established from studies of enzyme activity in liver biopsy tissue or in cultured fibroblasts from affected patients. Tandem mass spectrometry can be employed for blood samples, even those on filter paper, for screening of congenital inborn errors. The frequency of this disorder, about 1/10,000–15,000 births, suggests that screening for medium-chain acyl-CoA dehydrogenase deficiency is indicated; molecular diagnostic methods are being developed. Avoidance of fasting and supplementation with carnitine may be lifesaving in these patients who generally present in infancy.

Interference with fatty acid metabolism also underlies the fasting hypoglycemia associated with Jamaican vomiting sickness, with atractyloside, and with the drug valproate. In *Jamaican vomiting sickness,* the unripe ackee fruit contains a water-soluble toxin, hypoglycin, which produces vomiting, central nervous system depression, and severe hypoglycemia. The hypoglycemic activity of hypoglycin derives from its inhibition of gluconeogenesis secondary to its interference with the acyl-CoA and carnitine metabolism essential for the oxidation of long-chain fatty acids. The disease is almost totally confined to Jamaica, where ackee forms a staple of the diet for the poor. The ripe ackee fruit no longer contains this toxic principle. *Atractyloside* is a reagent that inhibits oxidative phosphorylation in mitochondria by preventing the translocation of adenine nucleotides, such as ATP, across the mitochondrial membrane. Atractyloside is a perhydrophenanthrenic glycoside derived from *Atractylis gummifera.* This plant is found in the Mediterranean basin; ingestion of this "thistle" is associated with hypoglycemia and a syndrome similar to Jamaican vomiting sickness. More commonly, the anticonvulsant drug *valproate* is associated with side effects, predominantly in young infants, which include a Reye-like syndrome, low serum carnitine levels, and the potential for fasting hypoglycemia. In all these conditions, hypoglycemia *is not associated with ketonuria.*

SALICYLATE INTOXICATION (see also Chapter 722.5). Both hyperglycemia and hypoglycemia occur in children with salicylate intoxication. Accelerated utilization of glucose, due to augmentation of insulin secretion by salicylates, and possible interference with gluconeogenesis may contribute to hypoglycemia. Infants are more susceptible than are older children. Monitoring of blood glucose levels with appropriate glucose infusion in the event of hypoglycemia should form part of the therapeutic approach to salicylate intoxication in childhood. Ketosis may occur.

FRUCTOSE-1,6-DIPHOSPHATASE DEFICIENCY (see Chapter 84.3). A deficiency of this enzyme results in a block of gluconeogenesis from all possible precursors below the level of fructose-1,6-diphosphate. Infusion of these gluconeogenic precursors results in lactic acidosis without a rise in glucose, and acute hypoglycemia may be provoked by inhibition of glycogenolysis. Normally, glycogenolysis remains intact, and glucagon elicits a normal glycemic response in the fed, but not in the fasted, state. Accordingly, affected individuals have hypoglycemia only during caloric deprivation, as in fasting, or during intercurrent illness. Although glycogen stores remain normal, hypoglycemia does not develop. In affected families, there may be a history of siblings with known hepatomegaly who died in infancy with unexplained metabolic acidosis.

Clinical features simulate those of type I glycogen storage disease. Hepatomegaly in individuals with fructose-1,6-diphosphatase deficiency is due to lipid storage rather than glycogen storage. Lactic acidosis, ketosis, hyperlipidemia, and hyperuricemia occur; their pathogenesis is related to the severity and duration of hypoglycemia and the resultant low levels of insulin and high levels of counterregulatory hormones. Therapy for these infants, consisting of a diet high in carbohydrates (56%, excluding fructose, which cannot be utilized), low in protein (12%), and normal in fat composition (32%), has permitted normal growth and development. Continuous nocturnal provision of calories through the intragastric infusion system described earlier for type I glycogen storage disease is also applicable to children with fructose-1,6-diphosphatase deficiency. During intercurrent illnesses with vomiting, intravenous glucose infusion is necessary to prevent severe hypoglycemia.

PYRUVATE CARBOXYLASE DEFICIENCY (see Chapter 84). This is predominantly a disease of the central nervous system characterized by a subacute necrotizing encephalomyelopathy and high levels of blood lactate and pyruvate. Hypoglycemia is not a prominent feature of this syndrome, presumably because gluconeogenesis from precursors other than alanine remains intact, and these precursors bypass the pyruvate carboxylase step. The utilization of alanine as well as lactate through pyruvate cannot proceed, however, so these substrates accumulate in blood, and modest hypoglycemia may result during fasting. Affected patients usually die of progressive central nervous system disease.

PHOSPHOENOL PYRUVATE CARBOXYKINASE DEFICIENCY. Deficiency of this rate-limiting gluconeogenic enzyme is associated with severe fasting hypoglycemia and variable onset after birth. Hypoglycemia may occur within 24 hr after birth, and defective gluconeogenesis from alanine can be documented in vivo. At postmortem examination, liver, kidney, and myocardium demonstrate fatty infiltration, and atrophy of the optic nerve and visual cortex may occur. Extensive fatty deposition in liver, kidney, and other tissues also occurs in phosphoenol pyruvate carboxykinase deficiency. Hypoglycemia may be profound. Lactate and pyruvate levels in plasma have been normal, but a mild metabolic acidosis may be present. The fatty infiltration of various organs is due to increased formation of acetyl CoA, which becomes available for fatty acid synthesis. Diagnosis of this rare entity can be made with certainty only through appropriate enzymatic determinations in liver biopsy material. Avoidance of periods of fasting through frequent feedings rich in carbohydrate should be helpful because glycogen synthesis and breakdown are intact.

Other Enzyme Defects

GALACTOSEMIA (GALACTOSE-1-PHOSPHATE URIDYL TRANSFERASE DEFICIENCY). See Chapter 84.

FRUCTOSE INTOLERANCE (FRUCTOSE-1-PHOSPHATE ALDOLASE DEFICIENCY) (see Chapter 84). Acute hypoglycemia is due to the inhibition by fructose-1-phosphate of glycogenolysis via the phosphorylase system and of gluconeogenesis at the level of fructose-1,6-diphosphate aldolase. Affected individuals usually learn to eliminate fructose from their diet spontaneously.

DIAGNOSIS AND DIFFERENTIAL DIAGNOSIS

Table 88–6 lists the pertinent clinical and biochemical findings in the common childhood disorders associated with hypoglycemia. A careful and detailed history is essential in every suspected or documented case of hypoglycemia (Table 88–7). Specific points to be noted include age of onset, temporal relation to meals or caloric deprivation, and a family history of prior infants known to have had hypoglycemia or of unexplained infant deaths. In the 1st wk of life, the majority of infants have the transient form of neonatal hypoglycemia either as a result of prematurity–intrauterine growth retardation

TABLE 88–6 Clinical Manifestations and Differential Diagnosis in Childhood Hypoglycemia

Condition	Hypoglycemia	Urinary Ketones (K) or Reducing Sugars	Hepato-megaly	Serum		Effect of 24–36-hr Fast on Plasma					Glycemic Response to Glucagon		Glycemic Response to Infusion of	
				Lipids	*Uric Acid*	*Glucose*	*Insulin*	*Ketones*	*Alanine*	*Lactate*	*Fed*	*Fasted*	*Alanine*	*Glycerol*
Normal	0	0	0	Normal	Normal	↓	↓	↑	↓	Normal	↑	↓	↑	↑
Hyperinsulinemia	Recurrent severe	0	0	Normal or ↑	Normal	↓↓	↑↑	↓↓	Normal	Normal	↑	↑	↑	↑
Ketotic hypoglycemia	Severe with missed meals	Ketonuria + + +	0	Normal	Normal	↓↓	↓	↑↑	↓↓	Normal	↑	↓↓	↑	↑
Fatty acid oxidation disorder	Severe with missed meals	Absent	0 to + Abnormal liver function test results	Abnormal	↑			Contraindicated			↑	↓	Not indicated	
Hypopituitarism	Moderate with missed meals	Ketonuria + +	0	Normal	Normal	↓↓	↓	↑↑	↓↓	Normal	↑	↓↓	↑	↑
Adrenal insufficiency	Severe with missed meals	Ketonuria + +	0	Normal	Normal	↓↓	↓	↑↑	↓↓	Normal	↑	↓↓	↑	↑
Enzyme deficiencies														
Glucose-6-phosphatase	Severe–constant	Ketonuria + + +	+ + +	↑↑	↑↑	↓↓	↓	↑↑	↑↑	↑↑	0	0–↓↓	0	0
Debrancher	Moderate with fasting	Ketonuria + +	+ +	Normal	Normal	↓↓	↓	↑↑	↓↓	Normal	↑	0–↓↓	↑	↑
Phosphorylase	Mild–moderate	Ketonuria + +	+	Normal	Normal	↓	↓	↑↑	↓↓	Normal	0–↑	0–↓↓	↑	↑
Fructose-1,6-diphosphatase	Severe with fasting	Ketonuria + + +	+ + +	↑↑	↑↑	↓↓	↓	↑↑	↑↑	↑↑	↑	0–↓↓	↓	↓
Galactosemia	After milk or milk products	0 Ketones;(s) +	+ + +	Normal	Normal	↓	↓	↑	↓	Normal	↑	0–↓↓	↑	↑
Fructose intolerance	After fructose	0 Ketones;(s) +	+ + +	Normal	Normal	↓	↓	↑	↓	Normal	↑	0–↓↓	↑	↑

0 = absence; ↑ or ↓ indicates respectively small increase or decrease; ↑↑ or ↓↓ indicates respectively large increase or decrease.
Details of each condition are discussed in the text.

TABLE 88–7 Diagnosis of Acute Hypoglycemia in Infants and Children

Acute Symptoms Present	History Suggestive: Acute Symptoms Not Present
1. Obtain blood sample before and 30 min after glucagon administration 2. Obtain urine as soon as possible. Examine for ketones; if not present and hypoglycemia confirmed, suspect hyperinsulinemia or fatty acid oxidation defect; if present, suspect ketotic, hormone deficiency, inborn error of glycogen metabolism, or gluconeogenesis 3. Measure glucose in the original blood sample. If hypoglycemia is confirmed, proceed with substrate-hormone measurement as in Table 88–5 4. If glycemic increment after glucagon exceeds 40 mg/dL above basal, suspect hyperinsulinemia 5. If insulin level at time of confirmed hypoglycemia is greater than 10 μU/mL, suspect endogenous hyperinsulinemia; if greater than 100 μU/mL, suspect factitious hyperinsulinemia (exogenous insulin injection). Admit to hospital for provocative testing 6. If cortisol less than 10 μg/dL or growth hormone less than 5 ng/mL, or both, suspect adrenal insufficiency or pituitary disease, or both. Admit to hospital for provocative testing	1. Careful history for relation of symptoms to time and type of food intake, bearing in mind age of patient (see Table 88–2). Exclude possibility of alcohol or drug ingestion. Assess possibility of insulin injection, salt craving, growth velocity, intracranial pathology 2. Careful examination for hepatomegaly (glycogen storage disease; defect in gluconeogenesis); pigmentation (adrenal failure); stature and neurologic status (pituitary disease) 3. Admit to hospital for provocative testing: a. 24-hr fast under careful observation; when symptoms provoked proceed with steps 1–4 as when acute symptoms present b. Pituitary-adrenal function using arginine-insulin stimulation test if indicated 4. Liver biopsy for histologic and enzyme determinations if indicated 5. Oral glucose tolerance test (1.75 g/kg; max 75 g) if reactive hypoglycemia suspected in an adolescent

or by virtue of being born to diabetic mothers. The absence of a history of maternal diabetes, macrosomia, or the characteristic large plethoric appearance of an "infant of a diabetic mother" should arouse suspicion of hyperinsulinemic hypoglycemia of infancy probably due to a K_{ATP} channel defect that is familial (autosomal recessive) or sporadic; plasma insulin concentrations greater than 10 μU/mL in the presence of documented hypoglycemia confirm this diagnosis. The presence of hepatomegaly should arouse suspicion of an enzyme deficiency; if nonglucose-reducing sugar is present in the urine, galactosemia is most likely. In males, the presence of a microphallus suggests the possibility of hypopituitarism, which may be also associated with jaundice in both sexes.

Past the newborn period, clues to the cause of persistent or recurrent hypoglycemia can be obtained through a careful history, physical examination, and initial laboratory findings. The temporal relation of the hypoglycemia to food intake may suggest that the defect is one of gluconeogenesis, if symptoms occur 6 hr or more after meals. If hypoglycemia occurs shortly after meals, galactosemia or fructose intolerance is most likely, and the presence of reducing substances in the urine rapidly distinguishes these possibilities. The autosomal dominant forms of hyperinsulinemic hypoglycemia need to be considered, with measurement of glucose, insulin, ammonia, and careful history for other affected family members of any age. Measurement of IGFBP-1 may be useful; it is low in hyperinsulinemia states and high in other forms of hypoglycemia. The presence of hepatomegaly suggests one of the enzyme deficiencies in glycogen synthesis or breakdown or in gluconeogenesis, as outlined in Table 88–6. The absence of ketonemia or ketonuria at the time of initial presentation strongly suggests hyperinsulinemia or a defect in fatty acid oxidation. In most other causes of hypoglycemia, with the exception of galactosemia and fructose intolerance, ketonemia and ketonuria are present at the time of fasting hypoglycemia. At the time of the hypoglycemia, serum should be obtained for determination of hormones and substrates, followed by repeated measurement after an intramuscular or intravenous injection of glucagon as outlined in Table 88–7. Interpretation of the findings is summarized in Table 88–6. Hypoglycemia with ketonuria in children between the ages of 18 mo and 5 yr is most likely to be ketotic hypoglycemia, especially if hepatomegaly is absent. The ingestion of a toxin, including alcohol or salicylate, can usually be excluded rapidly by the history.

When the history is suggestive but acute symptoms are not present, a 24- to 36-hr fast can usually provoke hypoglycemia and resolve the question of hyperinsulinemia or other conditions (see Table 88–6). Such a fast is contraindicated if a fatty acid oxidation defect is suspected; other approaches such as mass tandem spectrometry or molecular diagnosis, or both, should be considered. Because adrenal insufficiency may mimic ketotic hypoglycemia, plasma cortisol levels should be determined at the time of documented hypoglycemia; increased buccal or skin pigmentation may provide the clue to primary adrenal insufficiency with elevated ACTH (melanocyte-stimulating hormone) activity. Short stature or a decrease in the growth rate may provide the clue to pituitary insufficiency involving growth hormone as well as ACTH. Definitive tests of pituitary-adrenal function such as the arginine-insulin stimulation test for growth hormone IGF-1, IGFPB-3, and cortisol release may be necessary.

In the presence of hepatomegaly and hypoglycemia, a presumptive diagnosis of the enzyme defect can often be made through the clinical manifestations, presence of hyperlipidemia, acidosis, hyperuricemia, response to glucagon in the fed and fasted states, and the response to infusion of various appropriate precursors (see Tables 88–6 and 88–7). These clinical findings and investigative approaches are summarized in Table 88–6. Definitive diagnosis of the glycogen storage disease may require an open liver biopsy (see Chapter 81). Occasional patients with all the manifestations of glycogen storage disease are found to have normal enzyme activity. These definitive studies require special expertise available only in certain institutions.

TREATMENT

The prevention of hypoglycemia and its resultant effects on central nervous system development are important in the newborn period. For neonates with hyperinsulinemia not associated with maternal diabetes, subtotal pancreatectomy may be needed, unless hypoglycemia can be readily controlled with somatostatin analogs or diazoxide. The therapeutic approach to specific causes is discussed with the description of each condition.

Treatment of acute neonatal or infant hypoglycemia includes intravenous administration of 2 mL/kg of $D_{10}W$, followed by a continuous infusion of glucose at 6–8 mg/kg/min, adjusting the rate to maintain blood glucose levels in the normal range.

The management of persistent neonatal or infantile hypoglycemia includes increasing the rate of intravenous glucose infusion to 8–15 mg/kg/min or more, if needed. This may require a central venous catheter to administer a hypertonic 15–20% glucose solution. In addition, intramuscular or intravenous hydrocortisone, 5 mg/kg/24 hr given in divided doses every 8 hr, or oral prednisone, 1–2 mg/kg/24 hr given in divided doses every 6–12 hr, and intramuscular growth hormone, 1 mg/24 hr, may be added if hypoglycemia is unresponsive to intravenous glucose.

Oral diazoxide, 10–25 mg/kg/24 hr given in divided doses every 6 hr, may reverse hyperinsulinemic hypoglycemia but also may produce hirsutism, edema, nausea, hyperuricemia, electrolyte disturbances, advanced bone age, IgG deficiency and, rarely, hypertension with prolonged use. A long-acting somatostatin analog (octreotide, formerly SMS 201–995) has been effective in controlling hyperinsulinemic hypoglycemia in a number of patients with islet cell disorders not caused by genetic mutations in K_{ATP} channel and islet cell adenoma. Octreotide is administered subcutaneously every 6–12 hr in doses of 20–50 μg in neonates and young infants. Potential but unusual complications include poor growth due to inhibition of growth hormone release, pain at the injection site, vomiting, diarrhea, and hepatic dysfunction (hepatitis, cholelithiasis). Octreotide is usually employed as a temporizing agent for various periods prior to subtotal pancreatectomy for K_{ATP} channel disorders. It may be particularly useful for the treatment of refractory hypoglycemia despite subtotal pancreatectomy. Total pancreatectomy is not optimal therapy owing to the risks of surgery, permanent diabetes mellitus, and exocrine pancreatic insufficiency.

Antunes JD, Geffner ME, Lippe BM, et al: Childhood hypoglycemia: Differentiating hyperinsulinemic from nonhyperinsulinemic causes. J Pediatr 116:105, 1990.

Apak RA, Yurdakok M, Oran O, et al: Preoperative use of octreotide in a newborn with persistent hyperinsulinemic hypoglycemia of infancy. J Pediatr Endocrinol Metab 11:143, 1998.

Auer RN, Hugh J, Cosgrove E, Curry B: Neuropathologic findings in three cases of profound hypoglycemia. Clin Neuropathol 8:63, 1989.

Aynsley-Green A, Polak JM, Bloom SR, et al: Nesidioblastosis of the pancreas: Definition of the syndrome and the management of the severe neonatal hyperinsulinemic hypoglycemia. Arch Dis Child 56:496, 1981.

Bennett MJ, Weinberger MJ, Kobori JA, et al: Mitochondrial short-chain L-3-hydroxyacyl-coenzyme A dehydrogenase deficiency: A new defect of fatty acid oxidation. Pediatr Res 39:185, 1996.

Bennish M, Kalam Azad A, Rahman O, et al: Hypoglycemia during diarrhea in childhood. Prevalence, pathophysiology and outcome. N Engl J Med 322:1357, 1990.

Burchell A, Bell JE, Busuttil A: Hepatic microsomal glucose-6-phosphatase system and sudden infant death syndrome. Lancet 2:291, 1989.

Chalmers RA, Stanley CA, English N, Wigglesworth JS: Mitochondrial carnitine-acylcarnitine translocase deficiency presenting as sudden neonatal death. J Pediatr 131:220, 1997.

Chaussain JL, Georges P, Olive G, Job JC: Glycemic response to 24-hour fast in normal children and children with ketotic hypoglycemia: II. Hormonal and metabolic changes. J Pediatr 85:776, 1974.

Cornblath M, Schwartz R: Disorders of Carbohydrate Metabolism in Infancy, 3rd ed. Boston, Blackwell, 1991.

Dacou-Voutetakis C, Psychou F, Maniati-Christidis M: Persistent hyperinsulinemic hypoglycemia of infancy: Long term results. J Pediatr Endocrinol Metab 11:131, 1998.

de Lonlay-Debeney P, Poggi-Travert F, Fournet J-C, et al: Clinical features of 52 neonates with hyperinsulinism. N Engl J Med 340:1169, 1999.

DeVivo DC, Trifiletti RR, Jacobson RI, et al: Defective glucose transport across the blood-brain barrier as a cause of persistent hypoglycorrhachia, seizures, and developmental delay. N Engl J Med 325:703, 1991.

Dunne MJ, Kane C, Shepherd RM, et al: Familial persistent hyperinsulinemic hypoglycemia of infancy and mutations in the sulfonylurea receptor. N Engl J Med 336:703, 1997.

Elliott M, Maher ER: Beckwith-Wiedemann syndrome. J Med Genet 31:560, 1994.

Freckmann ML, Thorburn DR, Kirby DM, et al: Mitochondrial electron transport chain defect presenting as hypoglycemia. J Pediatr 130:431, 1997.

Glaser B, Chiu KC, Anker R, et al: Familial hyperinsulinism maps to chromosome 11p14–15.1, 30 cM centromeric to the insulin gene. Nat Genet 7:185, 1994.

Glaser B, Kesavan P, Heyman M, et al: Familial hyperinsulinism caused by an activating glucokinase mutation. N Engl J Med 338:226, 1998.

Gottschalk ME, Geffner ME, Yasuda PM, et al: Reversal of microcephaly and developmental delay after cure of hyperinsulinemic hypoglycemia. J Pediatr 117:432, 1990.

Hatada I, Ohashi H, Fukushima Y, et al: An imprinted gene p57(KIP2) is mutated in Beckwith-Wiedemann syndrome. Nat Genet 14:171, 1996.

Kane C, Lindley KJ, Johnson PRV, et al: Therapy for persistent hyperinsulinemic hypoglycemia of infancy. J Clin Invest 100:1888, 1997.

Kane C, Shepherd RM, Squires PE, et al: Loss of functional K_{atp} channels in pancreatic β cells causes persistent hyperinsulinemic hypoglycemia of infancy. Nat Med 2:1344, 1996.

Kaufman FR, Costin G, Thomas DW, et al: Neonatal cholestasis and hypopituitarism. Arch Dis Child 59:787, 1984.

Kelly RI: The role of carnitine supplementation in valproic acid therapy. Pediatrics 97:892, 1994.

Koh TH, Aynsley-Green A, Tarbit M, et al: Neural dysfunction during hypoglycemia. Arch Dis Child 63:1353, 1988.

Lamberts SWJ, Van Der Lely AJ, De Herder WW, et al: Octreotide. N Engl J Med 334:246, 1996.

Lei KJ, Shelly LL, Pan CJ, et al: Mutations in the glucose-6-phosphatase gene that cause glycogen storage disease type 1a. Science 262:580, 1993.

Levitt-Katz LE, Satin-Smith MS, Collett-Solberg P, et al: Insulin-like growth factor binding protein-1 levels in the diagnosis of hypoglycemia caused by hyperinsulinism. J Pediatr 131:193, 1997.

Lucas A, Morley R, Cole TJ: Adverse neurodevelopmental outcome of moderate neonatal hypoglycemia. Br Med J 297:1304, 1988.

Maaswinkel-Mooij PD, Van den Bogert C, Scholte HR, et al: Depletion of mitochondrial DNA in the liver of a patient with lactic acidemia and hypoketotic hypoglycemia. J Pediatr 128:679, 1996.

Martin LW, Rychman FC, Sheldon CA: Experience with 95 percent pancreatectomy and splenic salvage for neonatal nesidioblastosis. Ann Surg 200:355, 1984.

Mayefsky JH, Sarnaik AP, Postellon DC: Factitious hypoglycemia. Pediatrics 69:804, 1982.

Nestorowicz A, Inagaki N, Gonoi T, et al: A nonsense mutation in the inward rectifier potassium channel gene, *Kir* 6.2, is associated with familial hyperinsulinism. Diabetes 46:1743, 1997.

Phillip M, Bashan N, Smith CPA, et al: An algorithmic approach to diagnosis of hypoglycemia. J Pediatr 110:387, 1987.

Pollack ES, Pollack CV Jr: Ketotic hypoglycemia: A case report. J Emerg Med 11:531, 1993.

Rinaldo P, Stanley CA, Hsu BY, et al: Sudden neonatal death in carnitine transporter deficiency. J Pediatr 131:304, 1997.

Schwenk WF, Haymond MW: Optimal rate of enteral glucose administration in children with glycogen storage disease type I. N Engl J Med 314:682, 1986.

Stanley CA: Hyperinsulinism in infants and children. Pediatr Clin North Am 44:363, 1997.

Stanley CA: Dissecting the spectrum of fatty acid oxidation disorders. J Pediatr 132:384, 1998.

Stanley CA, Baker L: The causes of neonatal hypoglycemia (letter). N Engl J Med 340:1200, 1999.

Stanley CA, Lieu YK, Hsu BYL, et al: Hyperinsulinism and hyperammonemia in infants with regulatory mutations of the glutamate dehydrogenase gene. N Engl J Med 338:1352, 1998.

Taylor SI, Barbetti F, Accili D, et al: Syndromes of autoimmunity and hypoglycemia: Autoantibodies directed against insulin and its receptor. Endocrinol Metab Clin North Am 18:123, 1989.

Thompson GN, Hsu BY, Pitt JJ, et al: Fasting hypoketotic coma in a child with deficiency of mitochondrial 3 hydroxy-3-methylglutaryl-CoA synthase. N Engl J Med 337:1203, 1997.

Thornton PS, Alter CA, Katz LE, et al: Short and long-term use of octreotide in the treatment of congenital hyperinsulinism. J Pediatr 123:637, 1993.

Thornton PS, Satin-Smith MS, Herold K, et al: Familial hyperinsulinism with apparent autosomal dominant inheritance: Clinical and genetic differences from the autosomal recessive variant. J Pediatr 132:9, 1998.

Tyrala EE, Chen X, Boden G: Glucose metabolism in the infant weighing less than 1100 grams. J Pediatr 125:283, 1994.

Vidnes J, Oyasaeter S: Glucagon deficiency causing severe neonatal hypoglycemia in a patient with normal insulin secretion. Pediatr Res 11:943, 1977.

White NJ, Marsh K, Turner RC, et al: Hypoglycemia in African children with severe malaria. Lancet 1:708, 1987.

Wolfsdorf JI: Hyperinsulinemic hypoglycemia of infancy. J Pediatr 132:1, 1998.

Wolfsdorf JI, Keller RJ, Landy H, et al: Glucose therapy for glycogenosis type 1 in infants: Comparison of intermittent uncooked cornstarch and continuous overnight glucose feedings. J Pediatr 117:384, 1990.

Ziadeh R, Hoffman EP, Finegold DN, et al: Medium chain acyl-CoA dehydrogenase deficiency in Pennsylvania: Neonatal screening shows high incidence and unexpected mutation frequencies. Pediatr Res 37:675, 1995.

PART XI

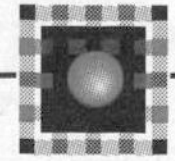

The Fetus and the Neonatal Infant

SECTION 1

Noninfectious Disorders

Barbara J. Stoll ▪ Robert M. Kliegman

CHAPTER 89

Overview of Mortality and Morbidity

Although the neonatal period* is considered to be the first 4 wk of life after birth, both fetal and extrauterine life form a continuum during which human growth and development are affected by genetic, socioeconomic, and environmental factors. For example, maternal toxemia may decrease the rate of fetal growth and cause an increased incidence of neonatal hypoglycemia. Low economic status is frequently associated with prematurity, which is correlated with high rates of morbidity and mortality, not only in the neonatal period but also throughout infancy. In the United States, the significantly higher black neonatal and infant mortality rates over that of white infants (Fig. 89–1) reflect cultural and socioeconomic factors. Although social influences, such as physician shortages in poor underserved areas, affect the availability of medical care for those most needing it, the failure of many mothers in these areas to use available prenatal and preventive medical care effectively also contributes to fetal and infant morbidity and mortality. Their failure results in part from inadequate public health education, lack of money to pay for the care, and limited access to health facilities and providers. Social factors leading to pregnancies among unwed women and cultural practices, such as the use of illicit drugs, also increase the incidence of fetal and neonatal disease.

Neonatal mortality has progressively decreased; it is highest during the first 24 hr of life and overall accounts for about 65% of deaths before age 1 yr. Further reduction of mortality and related morbidity depends primarily on preventing the birth of low-birthweight (LBW) infants, prenatal diagnosis, and early treatment of diseases that result from factors acting during gestation and at delivery (Table 89–1 and Figs. 89–2 and 89–3). *Perinatal mortality* designates fetal and neonatal deaths influenced by prenatal conditions and circumstances surrounding delivery. It is often defined as deaths of fetuses and infants from the 20th wk of gestational life through the 28th day after birth; additional definitions include the period from the 28th wk of gestation to the 7th day of life or the 20th wk of gestation to the 7th day of life.

In the United States each year there are approximately 6 million pregnancies, 4 million live births, and 28,000 infant deaths within the first 12 mo of life. Thirteen per cent of births are to women between 15 and 19 yr, and 32% are to unmarried women. Fetal deaths are associated with intrauterine growth retardation and conditions such as placental insufficiency that predispose the fetus to asphyxia. Neonatal deaths are due to diseases associated with LBW and to lethal congenital anomalies (see Table 89–1).

Infant mortality rates (deaths occurring from birth–12 mo/1,000 live births) vary by country; in 1996, they were lowest in Singapore and Japan (3.8/1,000 births); moderate in the United States (7.3/1,000); and highest in developing countries (30–150/1,000). Although socioeconomic, cultural, and perhaps geographic factors influence perinatal mortality, preventive variables such as health education, prenatal care, nutrition, social support, risk identification, and obstetric care can effectively reduce perinatal mortality. The number of LBW infants is a major determinant of both the neonatal and infant mortality rates and, together with lethal congenital anomalies (e.g., cardiac, central nervous system, and respiratory), contribute significantly to childhood morbidity. The LBW rate is directly related to the variance of infant mortality rates among different countries.

The *LBW rate* (infants weighing 2,500 g or less at birth each year) in the United States increased from 6.6% to 7.5%

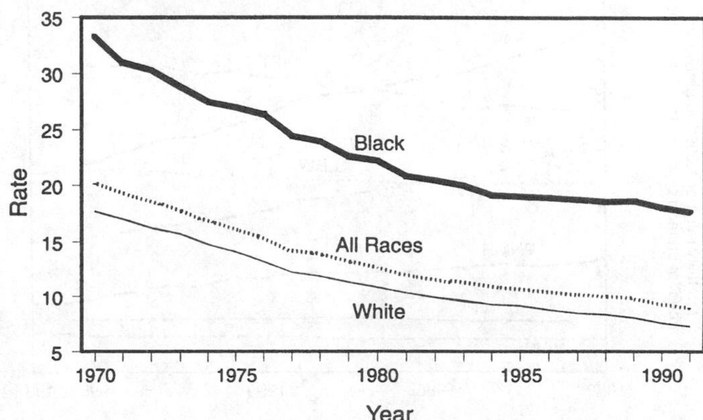

Figure 89–1 Infant mortality rates by race of mother. Deaths at <1 yr of age per 1,000 live births in specified group. Includes Hispanic and non-Hispanic infants; rates are presented only for black and white infants because the Linked Birth/Infant Death Data Set (used to more accurately estimate infant mortality rates for other racial groups) was not available for 1990 and 1991. (From Infant mortality—United States, 1991. MMWR 42:926, 1993.)

*The neonatal period may be further subdivided: period I—birth to <24 hr, period II—24 hr to <7 d, period III—7 d to <28 d.

TABLE 89–1 Major Causes of Perinatal Mortality

Fetal	Preterm	Full Term
Placental insufficiency	Severe immaturity	Congenital abnormalities
Intrauterine infection	Respiratory distress syndrome	Birth asphyxia, trauma
Severe congenital malformations	Intraventricular hemorrhage	Infection
Umbilical cord accident	Congenital anomalies	Meconium aspiration pneumonia
Abruptio placentae	Infection	Persistent pulmonary hypertension (PPHN)
Hydrops fetalis	Necrotizing enterocolitis	
	Chronic lung disease (CLD)	

between 1981 and 1997, while the very low birthweight (VLBW) rate (infants weighing 1,500 g or less at birth) has been 1.1–1.4% of all births. The LBW and VLBW rates and the infant mortality rates are 2 times higher in black infants than in whites. Infants born in the United States to African-born black women have birthweight distributions similar to those born to white women and higher than infants born to black women born in the United States. Despite advances in perinatal care, these data suggest a major need for preventive programs.

The predominant cause of LBW infants in the United States is premature birth, whereas in developing countries and those nations with higher LBW rates the cause is often intrauterine growth retardation. VLBW infants are most often premature (<37 wk of gestation), although intrauterine growth retardation may also complicate their early delivery. VLBW infants represent a larger proportion of infant deaths and infants with neurodevelopmental handicaps. The causes of premature birth include chorioamnionitis, bacterial vaginosis with genitourinary tract bacteria (*Chlamydia trachomatis, Ureaplasma ureolyticum, Mycoplasma hominis,* group B streptococcus, *Gardnerella vaginalis*), premature rupture of the membranes, uterine abnormalities, placental bleeding (abruptio, previa), multifetal gestation, drug misuse, maternal chronic illnesses, fetal distress, and maternal pyelonephritis. Nonetheless, in many cases the cause of preterm delivery is unknown.

Although 99% of births occur in hospitals, only 82% of pregnant women receive *prenatal care* in the 1st trimester. Many women who receive inadequate prenatal care are at risk for perinatal complications. The content of prenatal care is critical, as women receiving health behavior advice have a

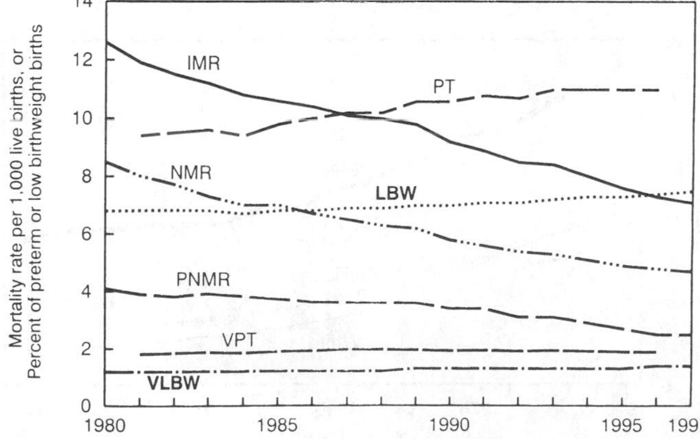

Figure 89–2 Infant, neonatal, and postnatal mortality, LBW and VLBW, and preterm and very preterm delivery, United States, 1980–1997. IMR = infant mortality rate per 1,000 live births; LBW = per cent low birthweight rate (<2,500 g); VLBW = per cent very low birthweight rate (<1,500 g); PT = per cent preterm (>37 wk of gestation); VPT = per cent very preterm (<32 wk of gestation). (From Guyer B, MacDorman MF, Martin JA, et al: Annual Summary of Vital Statistics. Pediatrics 102:1139, 1998.)

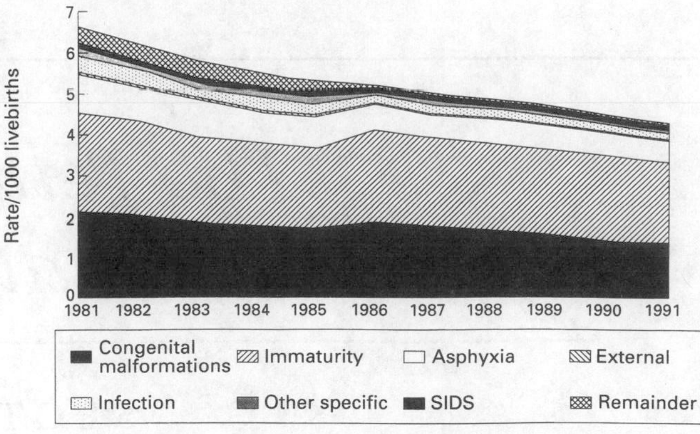

Figure 89–3 Trends in cause groups of neonatal deaths in England and Wales, 1981-1991. External refers to malnutrition, aspiration, pneumonia, hypothermia, injury, or poisoning. (From Alberman E, Botting B, Blatchley N, et al: A new hierarchical classification of causes of infant deaths in England and Wales. Arch Dis Child 70:403, 1994.)

lower incidence of LBW births. Barriers to prenatal care include absent or insufficient money or insurance to pay for care, poor coordination of services, and inadequate effective education about the importance of prenatal care. Successful and adequate provision of high-quality prenatal and perinatal care requires competent health care professionals and coordination of services among physicians' offices, clinics, community hospitals, special regionalized programs for high-risk mothers and infants, and tertiary care centers. Regional peri-

TABLE 89–2 Levels of In-Hospital Perinatal Care

Maternal	Neonate
Basic	
Monitor and care for low-risk patients	Well neonatal care
Triage for high risk for transfer	Resuscitation
Detection and care of unanticipated labor problems	Stabilization
Emergency cesarean delivery within 30 min	Transfer protocols
Blood bank, anesthesia, radiology, ultrasound, and laboratory support	Nursery care
Care of postpartum problems	Back (reverse) transfer
Obstetrician, nurse, midwife staff	Visitation
	General pediatrician staff (capable of neonatal resuscitation)
Special Care	
Basic services plus	*Basic services plus*
Care of high-risk pregnancies	Care of high-risk neonate with short-term problems
Triage, transfer of high-risk pregnancies (<32 weeks, IUGR, preeclampsia, severe anomalies, chorioamnionitis, severe maternal medical illness)	Stabilization before transfer (<1500 g, <32 wk, critically ill)
	Accept convalescing back (reverse) transfers
Subspeciality Care	
Basic plus speciality care plus	*Basic plus speciality care plus*
Experienced perinatologist (24-hr coverage)	Experienced neonatologist (24-hr coverage)
Evaluation of high-risk therapies	Inborn plus transferred patients
Care for severe maternal medical or obstetric illnesses	Evaluation of high-risk therapies
High-risk fetal care (Rh disease, nonimmune hydrops, life-threatening anomalies)	All pediatric medical, radiologic, and surgical subspecialties
Outcomes research	NICU with operating room capabilities
Community education	High-risk follow-up
	Outcomes research
	Community education

From Guidelines for Perinatal Care, 4th ed. AAP, ACOG 1997.
IUGR, intrauterine growth retardation; NICU, neonatal intensive care unit.

TABLE 89–3 Morbidities and Sequelae of Perinatal and Neonatal Illness

Morbidities	Examples
Central Nervous System	
Spastic diplegic-quadriplegic cerebral palsy	Hypoxic-ischemic encephalopathy, periventricular leukomalacia, undetermined antenatal factors
Choreoathetotic cerebral palsy	Bilirubin encephalopathy (kernicterus)
Microcephaly	Hypoxic-ischemic encephalopathy, intrauterine infection (rubella, CMV)
Communicating hydrocephalus	Intraventricular hemorrhage, meningitis
Seizures	Hypoxic-ischemic encephalopathy, hypoglycemia
Encephalopathy	Congenital infections (rubella, CMV, human immunodeficiency virus, toxoplasmosis)
Educational failure	Immaturity, hypoxia, low socioeconomic status
Mental retardation	Hypoxia, hypoglycemia, cerebral palsy, intraventricular hemorrhage
Sensation-Peripheral Nerves	
Reduced visual acuity (blindness)	Retinopathy of prematurity (ROP)
Strabismus	Undetermined
Hearing impairment (deafness)	Drug toxicity (furosemide, aminoglycosides), bilirubin encephalopathy, hypoxia ± hyperventilation
Poor speech	Immaturity, chronic illness, hypoxia, prolonged endotracheal intubation, hearing deficit
Paralysis-paresis	Birth trauma—brachial plexus, phrenic nerve, spinal cord
Respiratory	
Chronic lung disease (CLD)	Oxygen toxicity, barotrauma
Subglottic stenosis	Endotracheal tube injury
Sudden infant death syndrome	Prematurity, BPD, infant of illicit drug user
Choanal stenosis, nasal septum destruction	Nasotracheal intubation
Cardiovascular	
Cyanosis	Precorrective palliative care of congenital cyanotic heart disease, cor pulmonale from BPD, reactive airway disease
Heart failure	Precorrective palliative care of complex congenital heart disease, BPD, ventricular septal defect
Gastrointestinal	
Short gut syndrome	Nectrotizing enterocolitis, gastroschisis, malrotation-volvulus, cystic fibrosis, intestinal atresias
Cholestatic liver disease (cirrhosis, hepatic failure)	Hyperalimentation toxicity, sepsis, short gut syndrome
Failure to thrive	Short gut syndrome, cholestasis, BPD, cerebral palsy, severe congenital heart disease
Inguinal hernia	Unknown
Miscellaneous	
Cutaneous scars	Chest tube, IV placement; hyperalimentation subcutaneous infiltration; fetal puncture; intrauterine varicella; cutis aplasia
Absent radial artery pulse	Frequent arterial punctures
Hypertension	Renal thrombi; repair of coarctation of aorta

BPD = bronchopulmonary dysplasia; CMV = cytomegalovirus.

natal programs should provide continuing education and consultation in both the community and the referral center and transportation for pregnant women and newborn infants to appropriate hospitals; they should also include a regional hospital with facilities, equipment, and personnel for obstetric and neonatal intensive care (Table 89–2).

Fetal deaths slightly exceed neonatal deaths in their contribution to perinatal mortality. Obstetricians have a central role in reducing perinatal mortality and morbidity. Recently, intrapartum fetal deaths have declined more than antepartum fetal deaths, and this decline may reflect an increase in the use of fetal monitoring during labor and a more liberal use of cesarean section for fetal distress and other obstetric complications. It also emphasizes the need to be able to predict the maturity and functional reserve of a fetus before labor. In order to identify as early as possible those fetuses and infants at greatest risk, the obstetrician and pediatrician must effectively interact to anticipate perinatal problems and to take prompt preventive and therapeutic measures.

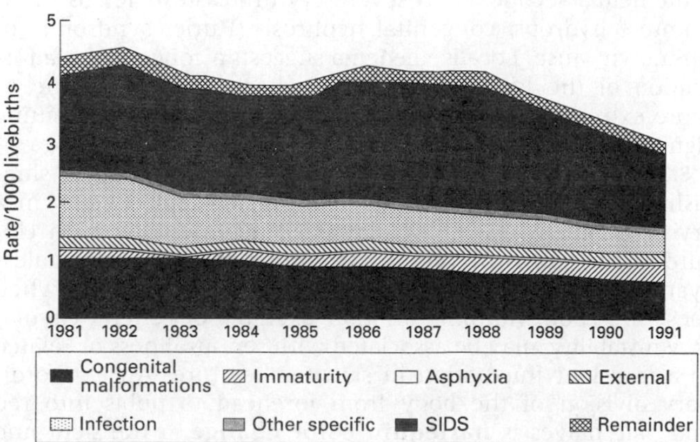

Figure 89–4 Trends in cause groups of postneonatal deaths in England and Wales, 1981–1991. External refers to malnutrition, aspiration, pneumonia, hypothermia, injury, or poisoning. (From Alberman E, Botting B, Blatchley N, et al: A new hierarchical classification of causes of infant deaths in England and Wales. Arch Dis Child 70:403, 1994.)

Postneonatal mortality refers to deaths between 28 days and 1 yr of life. Historically, these infant deaths were due to causes outside the neonatal period, such as sudden infant death syndrome (SIDS), infections (respiratory, enteric), and trauma. With the advent of modern neonatal care, many VLBW infants who would have died in the 1st mo of life now survive the neonatal period only to succumb to the sequelae noted in Table 89–3 and Figure 89–4. This delayed neonatal mortality is an important contributor to postneonatal mortality.

Along with the need to lower perinatal mortality rates is the need to reduce the incidence of handicaps among high-risk infants (see Table 89–3). Because both mortality and permanent neurologic sequelae are largely caused by the same or similar disturbances, research and public health measures directed at reducing perinatal mortality should also reduce the conditions contributing to the incidence of handicaps.

Alexander GR: Annotation: The accurate measurement of gestational age—a critical step toward improving fetal death reporting and perinatal health. Am J Public Health 87:1278, 1997.

Cogswell ME, Yip R: The influence of fetal and maternal factors on the distribution of birthweight. Semin Perinatol 19:222, 1995.

David RJ, Collins JW: Differing birth weight among infants of U.S.-born blacks, African-born blacks, and U.S.-born blacks. N Engl J Med 337:1209, 1997.

Guyer B, MacDorman MF, Martin JA, et al: Annual summary of vital statistics—1997. Pediatrics 102:1333, 1998.

Lumley J: How important is social class a factor in preterm birth? Lancet 349:1040, 1997.

Phibbs CS, Bronstein JM, Buxton E, et al: The effects of patient volume and level of care at the hospital of birth on neonatal mortality. JAMA 276:1054, 1996.

Ray WA, Gigante J, Mitchel EF, et al: Perinatal outcomes following implementation of Tenncare. JAMA 279:314, 1998.
Schoendorf KC, Kiely JL: Birth weight and age-specific analysis of the 1990 US infant mortality drop. Arch Pediatr Adolesc Med 151:129, 1997.

CHAPTER 90
The Newborn Infant

See also Chapter 9.

The neonatal period is a highly vulnerable time for an infant, who is completing many of the physiologic adjustments required for extrauterine existence. The high neonatal morbidity and mortality rates attest to the fragility of life during this period; in the United States, of all deaths occurring in the 1st yr, two thirds are in the neonatal period. Deaths during the 1st yr mark an annual rate unequaled until the 7th decade.

An infant's intrauterine to extrauterine transition requires many biochemical and physiologic changes. No longer dependent on maternal circulation via the placenta, a newborn's pulmonary function is activated for self-sufficient respiratory exchange of oxygen and carbon dioxide. Newborn infants also become dependent on gastrointestinal tract function for absorbing food, renal function for excreting wastes and maintaining chemical homeostasis, hepatic function for neutralizing and excreting toxic substances, and the function of the immunologic system for protecting against infection. Unsupported by the maternal placental system, the neonatal cardiovascular and endocrine systems also adapt for self-sufficient functioning. Many of a newborn's special problems are related to poor adaptation due to asphyxia, premature birth, life-threatening congenital anomalies, or adverse effects of delivery.

90.1 History in Neonatal Pediatrics

The neonatal history should (1) identify disabling diseases that are amenable to prompt preventive action or treatment (e.g., respiratory distress syndrome); (2) anticipate conditions that may be of later importance (e.g., gonococcal conjunctivitis); and (3) uncover possible causative factors that may explain pathologic conditions regardless of their immediate or future significance (e.g., screening for inborn errors of metabolism). The perinatal history should include demographic and social data (socioeconomic status, age, race), past medical illnesses in the family (cardiopulmonary disorders, infectious diseases, genetic disorders, diabetes mellitus), prior maternal reproductive problems (stillbirth, prematurity, blood group sensitization), events occurring in the present pregnancy (vaginal bleeding, medications, acute illness, duration of rupture of membranes), and a description of the labor (duration, fetal presentation, fetal distress, fever) and delivery (cesarean section, anesthesia or sedation, use of forceps, Apgar score, need for resuscitation).

90.2 Physical Examination of the Newborn Infant

Many physical and behavioral characteristics of a normal newborn infant are described in Chapter 9, which should be reviewed before reading this section.

The initial examination of a newborn infant should be performed as soon as possible after delivery to detect abnormalities and to establish a baseline for subsequent examinations. Infants should have temperature, pulse, respiratory rate, color, type of respiration, tone, activity, and level of consciousness monitored every 30 min after birth for 2 hr or until stabilized. For high-risk deliveries, this examination should take place in the delivery room and focus on congenital anomalies and pathophysiologic problems that may interfere with normal cardiopulmonary and metabolic adaptation to extrauterine life. Congenital anomalies may be present in 3–5% of infants. After a stable delivery room course, a second and more detailed examination should be performed within 24 hr of birth. If an infant remains in the hospital >48 hr, a discharge examination should be performed within 24 hr of discharge. With a healthy infant, the mother should be present during this examination; even minor, seemingly insignificant anatomic variations may worry a family and should be explained. The explanation must be careful and skillful so that otherwise unworried families are not unduly alarmed. No infant should be discharged from the hospital without a final examination, because certain abnormalities, particularly heart murmurs, often appear or disappear in the immediate neonatal period, or there may be evidence of disease that has just been acquired. Pulse (normal 120–160 beats/min), respiratory rate (normal 30–60 breaths/min), temperature, weight, length, head circumference, and dimensions of any visible or palpable structural abnormality should be recorded. Blood pressure is determined if a neonate appears ill.

Examining a newborn requires patience, gentleness, and procedural flexibility. Thus, if the infant is quiet and relaxed at the beginning of the examination, palpation of the abdomen or auscultation of the heart should be performed first before other, more disturbing manipulations are done.

GENERAL APPEARANCE. Physical activity may be absent during the relaxation of normal sleep, or it may be decreased by the effects of illness or drugs; an infant may be either lying with extremities motionless, to conserve energy for the effort of difficult breathing, or vigorously crying with accompanying activity of arms and legs. Both active and passive muscle tone and any unusual posture should be recorded. Coarse, tremulous movements with ankle or jaw myoclonus are more common and less significant in newborn infants than at any other age. Such movements tend to occur when an infant is active, whereas convulsive twitching usually occurs in a quiet state. Edema may produce a superficial appearance of good nutrition. Pitting after applied pressure may or may not be noted, but the skin of the fingers and toes lacks the normal fine wrinkles when puffed with fluid. Edema of the eyelids commonly results from irritation caused by administration of silver nitrate. Generalized edema may occur with prematurity, hypoproteinemia secondary to severe erythroblastosis fetalis, nonimmune hydrops, congenital nephrosis, Hurler syndrome, or unknown cause. Localized edema suggests a congenital malformation of the lymphatic system; when confined to one or more extremities of a female infant, it may be the presenting sign of Turner syndrome (Chapters 78 and 596.1).

SKIN. Vasomotor instability and peripheral circulatory sluggishness are revealed by deep redness or purple lividity in a crying infant, whose color may darken profoundly with closure of the glottis preceding a vigorous cry, and by harmless cyanosis (acrocyanosis) of the hands and feet, especially when these are cool. Mottling, another example of general circulatory instability, may be associated with serious illness or related to a transient fluctuation in skin temperature. An extraordinary division of the body from forehead to pubis into red and pale halves is **harlequin color change,** a transient and harmless condition. Significant *cyanosis* may be masked by the pallor of circulatory failure or anemia; alternatively, the relatively high hemoglobin content of the first few days and the thin skin may combine to produce an appearance of cyanosis at a higher Pa_{O_2} than in older children. Localized cyanosis is differentiated from ecchymosis by the momentary blanching pallor (with cyanosis) that occurs following pressure. The same maneuver also helps in demonstrating *icterus*, possibly significant but unnoticed if the skin is suffused with blood. *Pallor* may represent asphyxia, anemia, shock, or edema. Early recognition of anemia may lead to a diagnosis of erythroblastosis fetalis, subcapsular hematoma of the liver or spleen, subdural hemorrhage, or fetal-maternal or twin-twin transfusion. Without being anemic, postmature infants tend to have paler and thicker skin than do term or premature infants. The ruddy red appearance of *plethora* is seen with polycythemia.

The vernix and common transitory macular capillary hemangiomas of the eyelids and neck are described in Chapter 653. Cavernous hemangiomas are deeper, blue masses, which, if large, may trap platelets and produce disseminated intravascular coagulation or may interfere with local organ function. Scattered petechiae may be present in the scalp or face after a difficult delivery. Slate blue, well-demarcated areas of pigmentation are seen over the buttocks, back, and sometimes other parts of the body in more than 50% of black, Native American, or Asian infants and occasionally in white ones. These have no known anthropologic significance despite their name, **mongolian spots**; they tend to disappear within the first year. The vernix, skin, and especially the cord may be stained brownish yellow if the amniotic fluid has been colored by passage of meconium during or before birth, often because of intrauterine anoxia.

The skin of premature infants is thin and delicate and tends to be deep red; in extremely premature infants, the skin appears almost gelatinous and bleeds and bruises easily. Fine, soft, immature hair—**lanugo**—frequently covers the scalp and brow and may also cover the face of premature infants. Lanugo has usually been lost or replaced by vellus hair in term infants. Tufts of hair over the lumbosacral spine suggest an underlying abnormality such as occult spina bifida, sinus tract, or tumor. The nails are rudimentary in very premature infants, but they may protrude beyond the fingertips in infants born past term. Post-term infants may have a peeling, parchment-like skin (Fig. 90–1), a severe degree of which suggests ichthyosis congenita (Chapter 664).

Many neonates develop small, white, occasionally vesiculopustular papules on an erythematous base 1–3 days after birth. This benign rash, *erythema toxicum*, persists for as long as 1 wk, contains eosinophils, and is usually distributed on the face, trunk, and extremities (Chapter 653). *Pustular melanosis*, a benign lesion seen predominantly in black neonates, contains neutrophils and is present at birth as a vesiculopustular eruption around the chin, neck, back, extremities, and palms or soles; it lasts 2–3 days. Both lesions need to be distinguished from more dangerous vesicular eruptions such as herpes simplex (Chapter 245) and staphylococcal disease of the skin (Chapter 182).

Amniotic bands may disrupt the skin, extremities (amputation, ring constriction, syndactyly), face (clefts), or trunk (abdominal or thoracic wall defects). Their cause is uncertain but may be related to amniotic membrane rupture or vascular compromise with fibrous band formation. Excessive skin fragility and extensibility with joint hypermobility suggest Ehlers-Danlos syndrome, Marfan's syndrome, congenital contractural arachnodactyly, or other disorders of collagen synthesis.

SKULL. All infants should have their head circumference noted in the chart. The skull may be molded, particularly if the infant is the first-born and if the head has been engaged for a considerable time. The parietal bones tend to override the occipital and frontal bones. The head of an infant born by cesarean section or from a breech presentation is characterized by its roundness. The suture lines and the size and tension of the anterior and posterior fontanels should be determined digitally. Premature fusion of sutures (cranial synostosis) demonstrates a hard nonmovable ridge over the suture and an abnormally shaped skull. Great variation in the size of the fontanels exists at birth; if small, the anterior fontanel usually tends to enlarge during the first few months of life. Persistence of excessively large anterior (normal: 20 ± 10 mm) and posterior fontanels has been associated with several disorders (Table 90–1). Persistently small fontanels suggest microcephaly, craniosynostosis, congenital hyperthyroidism, or wormian bones; a 3rd fontanel suggests trisomy 21 but is seen in preterm infants. Soft areas (**craniotabes**) are occasionally found in the parietal bones at the vertex near the sagittal suture; they are more common in premature infants and in infants who have been exposed to uterine compression. Although usually insignificant, their possible pathologic cause should be investigated if they persist. Soft areas in the occipital region suggest the irregular calcification and wormian bone formation associated with osteogenesis imperfecta, cleidocranial dysostosis, lacunar skull, cretinism, and occasionally Down syndrome. Transillumination of an abnormal skull in a dark room or examination by ultrasound or computed tomography scan rules out hy-

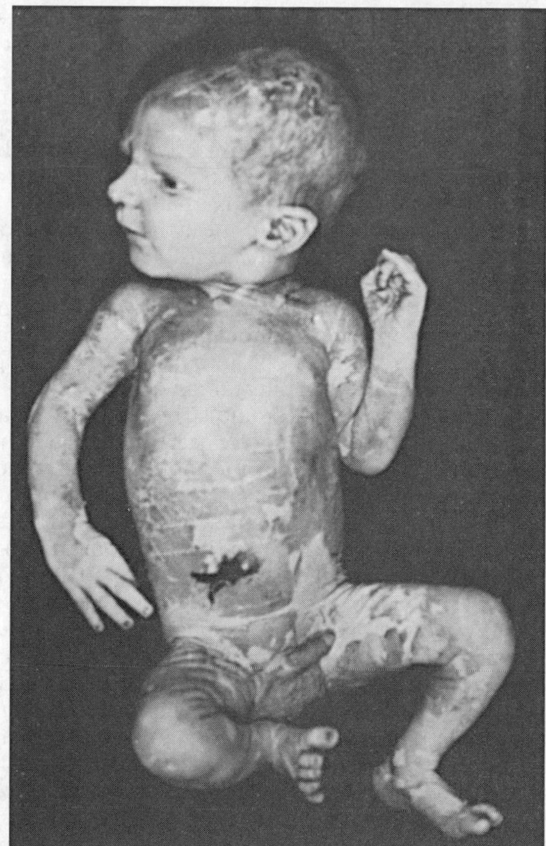

Figure 90–1 Infant with intrauterine growth retardation due to placental insufficiency. Note the long, thin appearance with peeling parchment-like dry skin, alert expression, meconium staining of the skin, and long nails. (From Clifford S: Advances in Pediatrics, Vol 9. Chicago, Year Book Medical Publishers, 1962.)

TABLE 90–1 Disorders Associated with a Large Anterior Fontanel

Achondroplasia	Intrauterine growth retardation
Apert syndrome	Kenny syndrome
Athyrotic hypothyroidism	Osteogenesis imperfecta
Cleidocranial dysostosis	Prematurity
Congenital rubella syndrome	Pyknodysostosis
Hallermann-Streiff syndrome	Russell-Silver syndrome
Hydrocephaly	13-, 18-, 21-trisomies
Hypophosphatasia	Vitamin D deficiency rickets

dranencephaly or hydrocephaly (Chapter 601). An excessively large head (megalencephaly) suggests hydrocephaly, storage disease, achondroplasia, cerebral gigantism, neurocutaneous syndromes, or inborn errors of metabolism, or it may be familial. The skull of a premature infant may suggest hydrocephaly because of the relatively larger brain growth compared with that of other organs. Depression of the skull (indentation, fracture, Ping-Pong-ball deformity) is usually of prenatal onset from prolonged focal pressure of the bony pelvis. Atrophic-alopecia scalp areas may be *aplasia cutis congenita,* which may be sporadic or autosomal dominant or associated with trisomy 13, chromosome 4 deletion, or Johanson-Blizzard syndrome.

FACE. The general appearance should be noted with regard to dysmorphic features, such as epicanthal folds, widely spaced eyes, microphthalmia, long philtrum, and low-set ears, often associated with congenital syndromes. The face may be asymmetric as a result of a 7th nerve palsy, hypoplasia of the depressor muscle at the angle of the mouth, or an abnormal fetal posture (Chapter 104); when the jaw has been held against a shoulder or an extremity during the intrauterine period, the mandible may deviate strikingly from the midline. Symmetric facial palsy suggests absence or hypoplasia of the 7th nerve nucleus (Möbius syndrome).

EYES. The eyes often open spontaneously if the infant is held up and tipped gently forward and backward. This maneuver, a result of labyrinthine and neck reflexes, is more successful for inspecting the eyes than forcing the lids apart. *Conjunctival and retinal hemorrhages* are usually benign. The pupillary reflexes are present after 28–30 wk of gestation. The iris should be inspected for colobomas and heterochromia. A cornea greater than 1 cm in diameter in a term infant suggests congenital glaucoma and requires prompt ophthalmologic consultation. The presence of bilateral *red reflexes* suggests the absence of cataracts or of intraocular pathology (Chapters 629, 634–639). Leukokoria (white pupillary reflex) suggests cataracts, tumor, chorioretinitis, retinopathy of prematurity, or a persistent hyperplastic primary vitreous and warrants an immediate ophthalmologic consultation.

EARS. Deformities of the pinnae are occasionally seen. Unilateral or bilateral preauricular skin tags occur frequently; if pedunculated, they can be ligated tightly at the base; dry gangrene and slough result. The tympanic membrane, easily seen otoscopically through the short, straight external auditory canal, normally appears dull gray.

NOSE. The nose may be slightly obstructed by mucus accumulated in the narrow nostrils. The nares should be symmetric and patent. The nasal cartilage may be dislocated from the vomerian groove, resulting in asymmetric nares.

MOUTH. A normal mouth rarely shows precocious dentition, with natal (present at birth) or neonatal (erupt after birth) *teeth* in the lower incisor position or aberrantly placed; these teeth are shed before the deciduous ones erupt. Alternatively, such teeth occur in Ellis-van Creveld, Hallermann-Streiff, and other syndromes. Extraction is usually not indicated. Premature eruption of deciduous teeth is even more unusual. The **soft** and **hard palate** should be inspected for a complete or submucosal cleft, and the contour noted if the arch is excessively high or the uvula bifid. On the hard palate on either side of the raphe may be temporary accumulations of epithelial cells called **Epstein pearls.** Retention cysts of similar appearance may also be seen on the gums. Both disappear spontaneously, usually within a few weeks of birth. Clusters of small white or yellow follicles or ulcers on an erythematous base may be found on the anterior tonsillar pillars, most frequently on the 2nd–3rd day of life. Of unknown cause, they clear without treatment in 2–4 days.

There is no active salivation. The **tongue** appears relatively large; the **frenulum** may be short, but rarely, if ever, is this a reason for cutting it. The sublingual mucous membrane occasionally forms a prominent fold. The **cheeks** have a fullness on both the buccal and the external aspects owing to the accumulation of fat making up the **sucking pads.** These pads, as well as the labial tubercle on the upper lip (sucking callus), disappear when suckling ceases. A marble-sized buccal mass is usually due to benign idiopathic fat necrosis.

The **throat** of a newborn infant is hard to see because of the low arch of the palate; however, it should be clearly viewed because it is easily possible to miss posterior palatal or uvular clefts. The tonsils are small.

NECK. The neck appears relatively short. Abnormalities are not common; they include goiter, cystic hygroma, branchial cleft rests, teratoma, hemangioma, and lesions of the sternocleidomastoid muscle that are presumably traumatic or are due to fixed positioning in utero that produces either a hematoma or fibrosis, respectively. *Congenital torticollis* causes the head to turn toward and the face to turn away from the affected side. Plagiocephaly, facial asymmetry, and hemihypoplasia may develop if it is untreated (see Chapter 686.1). Redundant skin or webbing in a female infant suggests intrauterine lymphedema, and Turner syndrome (Chapter 596.1). Both clavicles should be palpated for fractures.

CHEST. Breast hypertrophy is common, and milk may be present (but should not be expressed). Asymmetry, erythema, induration, and tenderness should suggest a breast abscess. Look for supernumerary nipples or widely spaced nipples with a shield-shaped chest; the latter suggests Turner syndrome.

LUNGS. Much can be learned by observing breathing. Variations in rate and rhythm are characteristic, fluctuating according to physical activity, state of wakefulness, or presence of crying. Because fluctuations are rapid, the respiratory rate should be counted for a full minute with the infant in the resting state, preferably asleep. Under these circumstances, the usual rate for normal term infants is 30–40/min; for premature infants the rate is higher and fluctuates more widely. A rate consistently over 60/min during periods of regular breathing usually indicates pulmonary, cardiac, or metabolic disease. Premature infants may breathe with a Cheyne-Stokes rhythm, known as periodic respiration, or with complete irregularity. Irregular gasping, sometimes accompanied by spasmodic movements of the mouth and chin, strongly indicates serious impairment of respiratory centers.

The breathing of newborn infants is almost entirely diaphragmatic, so that during inspiration the soft front of the thorax usually is drawn inward while the abdomen protrudes. If the baby is quiet, relaxed, and of good color, this "paradoxic movement" does not necessarily signify insufficient ventilation. On the other hand, labored respiration is important evidence of respiratory distress syndrome, pneumonia, anomalies, or mechanical disturbance of the lungs. A weak persistent or intermittent groaning, whining cry or **grunting** during expiration signifies potentially serious cardiopulmonary disease. Flaring of the alae nasi and retractions of the intercostal muscles and sternum are common signs of pulmonary pathology.

Normally, the breath sounds are bronchovesicular. Suspected pulmonary pathology due to diminished breath sounds, rales, or percussion dullness should always be followed up with a chest roentgenogram.

HEART. The size is difficult to estimate owing to normal variations in the size and shape of the chest. The location of the heart should be determined to detect dextrocardia. There may be transitory murmurs. Congenital heart disease may not initially produce the murmur that will be present later; only a 1:12 chance exists that a murmur heard at birth represents congenital heart disease. Evaluating the heart by roentgenography, echocardiography, and electrocardiography is essential when the possibility of a significant lesion exists. The pulse may vary normally from 90/min in relaxed sleep to 180/min during activity. The still higher rate of supraventricular tachycardia may be counted better on a cardiac monitor or electrocardiogram than by ear. Premature infants, whose resting heart rate is usually 140–150/min, may have a sudden onset of **sinus bradycardia.** Pulses should be palpated in the upper and lower extremities to detect coarctation of the aorta on both admission and discharge from the nursery.

Blood pressure measurements may be a valuable diagnostic aid in ill infants (Chapter 429). The *oscillometric method* is the easiest and most accurate noninvasive method available. Continuous or intermittent direct measurement of blood pressure using an umbilical artery catheter may be indicated in special circumstances for infants who are under close observation in an intensive care unit (Fig. 90–2).

ABDOMEN. The liver is usually palpable, sometimes as much as 2 cm below the rib margin. Less commonly, the spleen tip may be felt. The approximate size and location of each kidney can usually be determined on deep palpation. At no other period of life does the amount of air in the gastrointestinal tract vary so greatly, nor is it usually so great under normal circumstances. Gas should normally be present in the rectum on roentgenogram by 24 hr of age. The abdominal wall is normally weak (especially in premature infants), and **diastasis recti** and umbilical hernias are common, particularly among black infants.

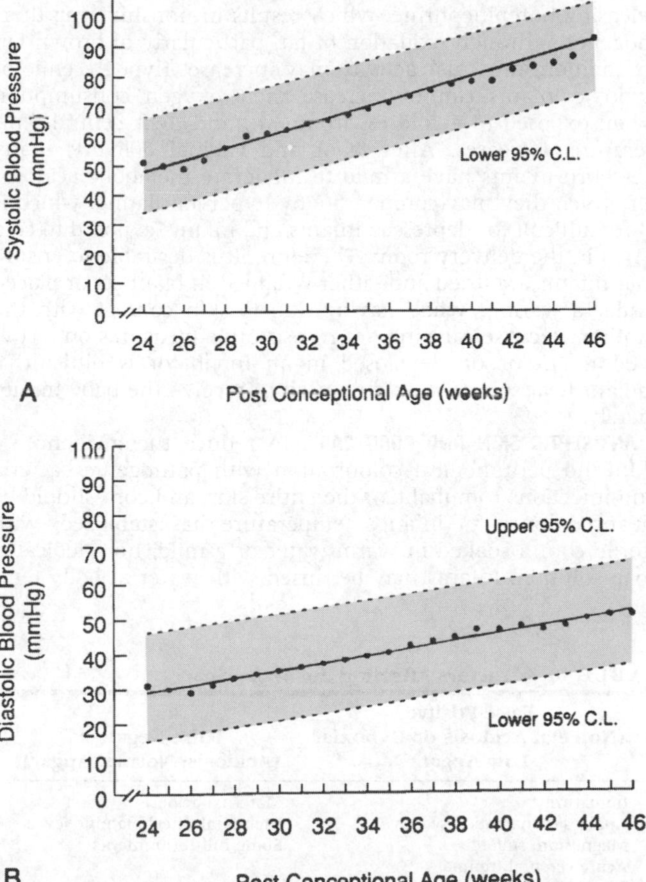

Figure 90–2 Postconceptional age (gestational age in weeks + weeks after delivery) is computed daily for each infant (8,566 daily records) and regressed against mean SBP *(A)* and DBP *(B)* for that day. Regression lines and equations are presented in terms of postconceptional weeks, which is more useful clinically. Regression equations are SBP = (0.255 • postconceptional age in weeks • 7) + 6.34, r = 0.61, $p < 0.0001$ and DBP = (0.151 • postconceptional age in weeks • 7) + 3.32, r = 0.46, $p < 0.0001$. Observed means of SBP and DBP for each postconceptional week are also plotted. C.L., Confidence limits. (From Zubrow AB, Hulman S, Kushner H, et al: Determinants of blood pressure in infants admitted to neonatal intensive care units: A prospective multicenter study. J Perinatol 15:470, 1995.)

Unusual masses should be investigated immediately by ultrasonography. Renal pathology is the cause of 55% of neonatal abdominal masses. Cystic abdominal masses include hydronephrosis, multicystic-dysplastic kidneys, adrenal hemorrhage, hydrometrocolpos, intestinal duplication, and choledochal, ovarian, omental, or pancreatic cysts. Solid masses include neuroblastoma, congenital mesoblastic nephroma, hepatoblastoma, and teratoma. A solid flank mass may be due to renal vein thrombosis, which becomes apparent with hematuria, hypertension, and thrombocytopenia. Renal vein thrombosis in infants is associated with polycythemia, dehydration, diabetic mothers, asphyxia, sepsis, and coagulopathies such as antithrombin III or protein C deficiencies.

Abdominal distention at birth or shortly afterward suggests either obstruction or perforation of the gastrointestinal tract, often due to meconium ileus; later distention suggests lower bowel obstruction, sepsis, or peritonitis. A scaphoid abdomen in a newborn suggests diaphragmatic hernia. **Abdominal wall defects** produce an omphalocele (Chapter 101) when they occur through the umbilicus and a gastroschisis when they occur lateral to the midline. Omphaloceles are associated with other anomalies and syndromes such as Beckwith-Wiedemann syndrome, conjoined twins, 18-trisomy, meningomyelocele, and imperforate anus. **Omphalitis** is an acute inflammation of the periumbilical tissue that may extend into the portal vein, producing acute pyophlebitis and later chronic portal hypertension.

GENITALIA. The **genitalia** and **mammary glands** normally respond to transplacentally obtained maternal hormones to produce enlargement and secretion of the breasts in both sexes and prominence of the female genitalia, often with considerable nonpurulent discharge. These transitory manifestations require observation but no interference.

Imperforate hymen may result in **hydrometrocolpos** and a lower abdominal mass. The normal scrotum is relatively large; its size may be increased by the trauma of breech delivery or by a **transitory hydrocele,** which is distinguished from a hernia by palpation and transillumination. The testes should be in the scrotum or palpable in the canals. Black male infants usually have dark pigmentation of the scrotum before the rest of the skin assumes its permanent color.

The **prepuce** of a newborn infant is normally tight and adherent. Severe hypospadias or epispadias should always lead one to suspect either that abnormal sex chromosomes are present (Chapter 78) or that the infant is actually a masculinized female with an enlarged clitoris, because this may be the first evidence of the adrenogenital syndrome (Chapter 586). Erection of the penis is common and has no significance. Urine is usually passed during or immediately after birth; a period without voiding may normally follow. However, most void by 12 hr, and about 95% of preterm and term infants void within 24 hr.

ANUS. Some passage of **meconium** usually occurs within the first 12 hr after birth; 99% of term infants and 95% of premature infants pass meconium within 48 hr of birth. **Imperforate anus** is not always visible and may require evidence obtained by gentle insertion of the little finger or a rectal tube. Roentgenographic study is required. The dimple or irregularity of skinfold often normally present in the sacrococcygeal midline may be mistaken for an actual or potential neurocutaneous sinus.

EXTREMITIES. In examining the extremities, the effects of fetal posture (Chapter 678) should be noted so that their cause and usual transitory nature can be explained to the mother. This is particularly important after breech presentations. The suspicion of a fracture or nerve injury associated with delivery is more commonly aroused by observing the extremities in spontaneous or stimulated activity than by any other means.

TABLE 90–2 Apgar Evaluation of the Newborn Infant

Sign	0	1	2
Heart rate	Absent	Below 100	Over 100
Respiratory effort	Absent	Slow, irregular	Good, crying
Muscle tone	Limp	Some flexion of extremities	Active motion
Response to catheter in nostril (tested after oropharynx is clear)	No response	Grimace	Cough or sneeze
Color	Blue, pale	Body pink, extremities blue	Completely pink

Sixty sec after the complete birth of the infant (disregarding the cord and placenta), the 5 objective signs above are evaluated, and each is given a score of 0, 1, or 2. A total score of 10 indicates an infant in the best possible condition. An infant with a score of 0–3 requires immediate resuscitation.
Modified from Apgar V: Res Anesth Analg 32:260, 1953.

The hands and feet should be examined for polydactyly, syndactyly, and abnormal dermatoglyphic patterns such as a simian crease.

The hips of all infants should be examined to rule out congenital dislocation (Chapter 684.1).

NEUROLOGIC EXAMINATION. See Chapters 6 and 600. In utero neuromuscular diseases associated with limited fetal motion produce a constellation of signs and symptoms that are independent of the specific disease. Severe positional deformation and contractures produce arthrogryposis. Other manifestations of fetal neuromuscular disease include breech presentation, failure to breathe at birth, pulmonary hypoplasia, dislocated hips, undescended testes, thin ribs, and clubfoot.

90.3 Routine Delivery Room Care

Low-risk infants should be placed head downward immediately after delivery in order to clear the mouth, pharynx, and nose of fluid, mucus, blood, and amniotic debris by gravity; gentle suction with a bulb syringe or soft rubber catheter may also be helpful in removing this material. Wiping the palate and pharynx with gauze may lead to abrasions and the development of thrush, pterygoid ulcers (Bednar aphthae), or, rarely, tooth bud infection with maxillary osteomyelitis and retrobulbar abscess formation. The stomachs of infants delivered by cesarean section may contain more fluid than those of infants delivered vaginally. Their stomachs should be emptied by gastric tube to prevent aspiration of gastric contents. If infants appear to be in satisfactory condition, they may be given directly to their mothers for immediate bonding and nursing. If there is any concern about respiratory distress, they should be placed under a warmer, with the head dependent.

The **Apgar score** is a practical method of systematically assessing newborn infants immediately after birth to help identify infants requiring resuscitation (Table 90–2). A low score does not necessarily signify fetal hypoxia-acidosis; additional factors may reduce the score (Table 90–3). The Apgar score also does not predict neonatal mortality or subsequent cerebral palsy. Indeed, the score is normal in most patients who subsequently develop cerebral palsy, and the incidence of cerebral palsy is very low among infants with Apgar scores of 0–3 at 5 min. The 1-min Apgar score may signal the need for immediate resuscitation, and the 5-, 10-, 15-, and 20-min scores may indicate the probability of successfully resuscitating an infant. Apgar scores of 0–3 at 20 min predict high mortality and morbidity.

Infants who fail to initiate respiration should receive prompt resuscitation and close observation subsequently (Chapter 96).

MAINTENANCE OF BODY HEAT. Relative to body weight, the body surface of an newborn infant is approximately 3 times that of an adult, and in low-birthweight infants the insulating layer of subcutaneous fat is thinner. The estimated rate of heat loss in a newborn is approximately 4 times that of an adult. Under the usual delivery room conditions (20–25°C), an infant's skin temperature falls approximately 0.3°C/min, and the deep body temperature approximately 0.1°C/min during the period immediately after delivery, resulting usually in a cumulative loss of 2–3°C in deep body temperature (corresponding to a heat loss of approximately 200 kcal/kg). The heat loss occurs by *convection* of heat energy to the cooler surrounding air, by *conduction* of heat to colder materials on which the infant is resting, by heat *radiation* from the infant to other nearby solid objects, and by *evaporation* from moist skin and lungs (a function of alveolar ventilation).

Term infants exposed to cold after birth may develop metabolic acidosis, hypoxemia, hypoglycemia, and increased renal excretion of water and solutes owing to their efforts to compensate for heat loss. They augment heat production by increasing the metabolic rate and oxygen consumption and by releasing norepinephrine, which results in nonshivering thermogenesis through oxidation of fat, particularly of brown fat. In addition, muscular activity may increase. Hypoglycemic or hypoxic infants cannot increase their oxygen consumption when exposed to a cold environment, and their central temperature decreases. After labor and vaginal delivery, many newborn infants have a mild to moderate metabolic acidosis, for which they may compensate by hyperventilating, which is more difficult for depressed infants and infants exposed to cold stress in the delivery room. Therefore, it is desirable to ensure that infants are dried and either wrapped in blankets or placed under a warmer while having skin-to-skin contact with the mother. Because carrying out resuscitative measures on a covered infant or one enclosed in an incubator is difficult, a radiant heat source should be used to receive the baby immediately.

ANTISEPTIC SKIN AND CORD CARE. To reduce the incidence of skin and periumbilical colonization with pathogenic bacteria and infections (omphalitis), the entire skin and cord should be cleansed, once an infant's temperature has stabilized, with sterile cotton soaked in warm water or a mild, nonmedicated soap solution. Infants may be rinsed with water at body tem-

TABLE 90–3 Factors Affecting the Apgar Score

False-Positve (No Fetal Acidosis or Hypoxia; Low Apgar)	False-Negative (Acidosis; Normal Apgar)
Immaturity	Maternal acidosis
Analgesics, narcotics, sedatives	High fetal catecholamine levels
Magnesium sulfate	Some full-term infants
Acute cerebral trauma	
Precipitous delivery	
Congenital myopathy	
Congenital neuropathy	
Spinal cord trauma	
Central nervous system anomaly	
Lung anomaly (diaphragmatic hernia)	
Airway obstruction (choanal atresia)	
Congenital pneumonia and sepsis	
Prior episodes of fetal asphyxia (recovered)	
Hemorrhage-hypovolemia	

Regardless of the etiology, a low Apgar score due to fetal asphyxia, immaturity, central nervous depression, or airway obstruction identifies an infant needing immediate resuscitation.

perature if care is taken to avoid chilling. They are then dried and wrapped in sterile blankets and taken to the nursery. To lessen the chance of carrying pathogenic organisms into the nursery, the outer blanket can be discarded at the nursery door. To reduce colonization with *Staphylococcus aureus* and other pathogenic bacteria, the umbilical cord may be treated daily with triple dye, a bactericidal agent, or bacitracin. Alternatively, chlorhexidine washing or, on rare occasions during *S. aureus* epidemics, a single hexachlorophene bath may be used. Repeated total body exposure to hexachlorophene may be neurotoxic, particularly in low-birthweight infants, and is contraindicated. Nursery personnel should use chlorhexidine or iodophor-containing antiseptic soaps for routine handwashing before caring for each infant. Rigidly enforcing hand-to-elbow washing for 2 min in the initial wash and 15–30 sec in the second wash is essential for staff and visitors entering the nursery. Shorter but equally thorough washes between handling infants should also be required.

OTHER MEASURES. The **eyes** of all infants must be protected against gonococcal infection by instilling 1% *silver nitrate* drops, the best-proven therapy; erythromycin (0.5%) and tetracycline (1.0%) sterile ophthalmic ointments are alternative measures. Povidone-iodine (2.5% solution) may also be effective as a one-time prophylactic agent. This procedure may be delayed during the initial short alert period after birth to promote bonding, but once applied, drops should not be rinsed out. Also see Chapters 192 and 223.

Although hemorrhage in newborn infants can be due to factors other than *vitamin K deficiency*, an intramuscular injection of 1 mg of water-soluble vitamin K_1 (phytonadione) is recommended for all infants immediately after birth to prevent hemorrhagic disease of the newborn (see Chapter 99.4). Higher dose, repeated administration of oral vitamin K may also be useful, but this treatment is not yet established. Larger intravenous doses predispose to the development of hyperbilirubinemia and kernicterus and should be avoided. Administration of vitamin K to the mother during labor is not recommended owing to unpredictable placental transfer.

Neonatal screening is available for various genetic, metabolic, hematologic, and endocrine diseases. All states have neonatal screening programs, although specific tests required vary. Laboratory tests performed on infant heel puncture blood samples include those for hypothyroidism, phenylketonuria, galactosemia, maple syrup urine disease, homocystinuria, biotinidase deficiency, adrenal hyperplasia, hemoglobinopathy, cystic fibrosis, tyrosinemia, and other organic or amino acidopathies. To be effective in the timely identification and prompt therapy of treatable diseases, screening programs must include not only high-quality laboratory tests but also follow-up of infants with abnormal test results; education, counseling, and psychologic support for families; and prompt referral of the neonate for accurate diagnosis and therapy. There is no need to routinely screen the hematocrit or blood glucose in the absence of risk factors. *Hearing impairment,* a serious morbidity that affects speech and language development, may be severe in 2:1,000 and overall affects 5:1,000 births. All infants should be screened with otoacoustic emission hearing testing.

90.4 Nursery Care

Non–high-risk healthy infants may be taken to the "regular" newborn nursery or placed in the mother's room if the hospital has rooming-in.

The bassinet, preferably of clear plastic to allow for easy visibility and care, should be cleaned frequently. All professional care should be given in the bassinet, including the physical examination, clothing changes, temperature taking, skin cleansing, and other procedures that, if performed elsewhere, would establish a common contact point and possibly provide a channel for cross-infection. The clothing and bedding should be minimal, only those needed for an infant's comfort; the nursery temperature should be kept at approximately 24°C (75°F). The infant's temperature should be taken by axillary measurement; although the interval between temperature taking depends on many circumstances, it need not be shorter than 4 hr during the first 2–3 days and 8 hr thereafter. Axillary temperatures of 36.4 37.0°C (97.0–98.5°F) are within normal limits. Weighing at birth and daily thereafter is sufficient. Healthy infants should be placed supine to reduce the risk of sudden infant death syndrome.

Vernix is spontaneously shed within 2–3 days, much of it adhering to the clothing, which should be completely changed daily. The diaper should be checked before and after feeding and when the baby cries; it should be changed when wet or soiled. Meconium or feces should be cleansed from the buttocks with sterile cotton moistened with sterile water. The foreskin of the male infant should not be retracted. Circumcision is an elective procedure.

Early discharge (<48 hr) or very early discharge (<24 hr) may increase the risk of rehospitalization for hyperbilirubinemia, sepsis, failure to thrive, dehydration, and missed congenital anomalies. Early discharge requires careful ambulatory follow-up at home (visiting nurse) or in the office within 48 hr. Additional criteria for the early discharge of term neonates have been developed by the American Academy of Pediatrics and American College of Obstetrics and Gynecology (Table 90–4).

TABLE 90–4 Recommendations for Early Discharge from the Normal Newborn Nursery (It is not likely that all of these criteria will be met before 48 hr of age)

- Uncomplicated antepartum, intrapartum, postpartum courses
- Vaginal delivery
- Singleton at 38–42 wk: appropriate for gestational age
- Normal vital signs including respiratory rate <60 breaths/min; axillary temperature 36.1–37° C (97.0–98.6° F) in open crib
- Physical examination reveals no abnormalities requiring immediate attention
- Urination; stool X1
- At least two uneventful, successful feedings
- No excessive bleeding after (2 hr) circumcision
- No jaundice within 24 hr of birth
- Evidence of parental knowledge, ability, and confidence to care for the baby at home
  - Feeding
  - Cord, skin, genital care
  - Recognition of illness (jaundice, poor feeding, lethargy, fever, etc.)
  - Infant safety (car seat, supine sleep position, etc.)
- Availability of family and physician support (physician follow-up)
- Laboratory evaluation
  - Venereal Disease Research Laboratories (VDRL)
  - Hepatitis B surface antigen and vaccination or appointment for vaccination
  - State screening (e.g., phenyketonuria, thyroid, galactosemia, sickle cell, etc.)
  - Coombs test
- No social risks
  - Substance abuse
  - History of child abuse
  - Domestic violence
  - Mental illness
  - Teen mother
  - Homeless

Adapted from Guidelines for Perinatal Care, 4th ed, AAP ACOG, 1997.

90.5 Parent-Infant Bonding

See also Chapter 9.

Normal infant development depends partly on a series of affectionate responses exchanged between a mother and her newborn infant, binding them together psychologically and physiologically. This bonding is facilitated and reinforced by

TABLE 90–5 Drugs and Breast-Feeding

Contraindicated	Avoid or Give with Great Caution	Probably Safe But Give with Caution
Antineoplastic agents	Amiodarone	Acetaminophen
Amphetamines	Anthroquinones (laxatives)	Acyclovir
Bromocriptine	Aspirin (salicylates)	Aldomet
Clemastine	Atropine	Anesthetics
Cimetidine	Birth control pills	Antibiotics (not tetracycline)
Chloramphenicol	Bromides	Antithyroid (not methimazole)
Cocaine	Calciferol	Antiepileptics
Cyclophosphamide	Cascara	Antihistamines*
Cyclosporine	Danthron	Antihypertensive/cardiovascular
Diethylstilbestrol	Dihydrotachysterol	Bishydroxycoumarin
Doxorubicin	Estrogens	Chlorpromazine*
Ergots	Ethanol	Codine*
Gold salts	Metoclopramide	Digoxin
Heroin	Metronidazole	Dilantin
Immunosuppressants	Narcotics	Diuretics
Iodides	Phenobarbital*	Fluoxetine
Lithium	Primidone	Furosemide
Meprobamate	Psychotropic drugs	Haloperidol*
Methimazole	Reserpine	Hydralazine
Methylamphetamine	Salicylazosulfapyridine (sulfasalazine)	Indomethacin, other nonsteroidal anti-inflammatory drugs
Nicotine (smoking)		Methadone*
Phencyclidine (PCP)		Muscle relaxants
Phenindione		Prednisone
Radiopharmaceuticals		Propranolol
Tetracycline		Propylthiouracil
Thiouracil		Quinolones
		Sedatives*
		Theophylline
		Vitamins
		Warfarin

**Watch for sedation.*

the emotional support of a loving husband and family. The attachment process may be important in enabling some mothers to provide loving care during the neonatal period and subsequently during childhood. It is initiated before birth with the planning and confirmation of the pregnancy and with the growing acceptance of the fetus as an individual. After delivery and during the ensuing weeks, visual and physical contact between mother and baby triggers various mutually rewarding and pleasurable interactions such as the mother's touching the infant's extremities and face with her fingertips and encompassing and gently massaging the infant's trunk with her hands. Touching an infant's cheek elicits responsive turning toward the mother's face or toward the breast with nuzzling and licking of the nipple, a powerful stimulus for prolactin secretion. An infant's initial quiet alert state provides the opportunity for eye-to-eye contact, which is particularly important in stimulating the loving and possessive feelings of many parents for their babies. An infant's crying elicits the maternal response of touching the infant and speaking in a soft, soothing, higher-toned voice. Initial contact between mother and infant should take place in the delivery room, and opportunities for extended intimate contact should be provided within the first hours after birth. Delayed or abnormal maternal-infant bonding, occurring because of prematurity, infant or maternal illness, birth defects, or family stress, may harm infant development and maternal caretaking ability. Hospital routines should be designed to encourage parent-infant contact.

NURSERIES AND BREAST-FEEDING. See Chapter 41 for full discussions of breast- and formula feeding. Many hospital practices contribute to difficulties in breast-feeding by enforcing 4-hr feeding schedules, limiting nursing time, using only one breast at a feeding, washing nipples with substances other than water, delaying the first feeding, providing formula supplements, and using heavy intrapartum sedation.

Hospital practices that encourage successful breast-feeding include immediate postpartum mother-infant contact with suckling, rooming-in, demand feeding, inclusion of fathers in prenatal breast-feeding education, and support from experienced women. Nursing at least 5 min at each breast is reasonable and allows a baby to obtain most of the available breast contents and to provide effective stimulation for increasing milk supply. Nursing episodes should then be extended according to the comfort and desire of the mother and infant. A confident and relaxed mother, supported by an encouraging home and hospital environment, is likely to nurse well.

DRUGS AND BREAST-FEEDING. Maternal medications may affect the production and safety of breast milk (Table 90–5). Most commonly used medications, such as antihypertensive agents, are safe, but each should be investigated if used during breast-feeding. Maternal sedatives may result in the infant's sedation. Maternal drugs that are weak acids, composed of large molecules, plasma bound, or poorly absorbed from the maternal or neonatal intestine are less likely to affect a neonate. When fresh breast milk is fed by tube or bottle, bacteriologic evaluation of stored milk should be performed within 24 hr.

Medical contraindications to breast-feeding include infection with HIV (except in developing nations), primary cytomegalovirus, and hepatitis B virus (until an infant receives hepatitis immune globulin and vaccine) (see Table 90–5).

American Academy of Pediatrics, American College of Obstetricians and Gynecologists: Guidelines for Perinatal Care, 4th ed. Elk Grove Village, IL, American Academy of Pediatrics, 1997.

Committee on Drugs: The transfer of drugs and other chemicals into human milk. Pediatrics 93:137, 1994.

Committee on Fetus and Newborn: Use and abuse of the Apgar score. Pediatrics 78:1148, 1986.

Committee on Genetics: Newborn screening fact sheets. Pediatrics 98:473, 1996.

Cooper WO, Kotagal UR, Atherton HD, et al: Use of health care services by inner-city infants in an early discharge program. Pediatrics 98:686, 1996.

Hegyi T, Carbone T, Anwar M, et al: The Apgar score and its components in the preterm infant. Pediatrics 101:77, 1998.

Kennell JH, Klaus MH: Bonding: Recent observations that alter perinatal care. Pediatr Rev 19:4, 1998.

Kugelman A, Hadad B, Ben-David J, et al: Preauricular tags and pits in the newborn: The role of hearing tests. Acta Paediatr 86:170, 1997.

Lawrence R: A review of the medical benefits and contraindications of breast-feeding in the United States. Maternal and Child Health Technical Information Bulletin, HRSA, 1997.

Liu LL, Clemens CJ, Shay DK, et al: The safety of newborn early discharge. JAMA 278:293, 1997.

Margolis LH, Kotelchuck M, Chang HY: Factors associated with early maternal postpartum discharge from the hospital. Arch Pediatr Adolesc Med 151:466, 1997.

Mehl AL, Thomson V: Newborn hearing screening: The great omission. Pediatrics 101:http://www.pediatrics.org/cgi/content/full/101/1/e4, 1998.

CHAPTER 91
High-Risk Pregnancies

Pregnancies in which factors exist that increase the likelihood of abortion, fetal death, premature delivery, intrauterine growth retardation, fetal or neonatal disease, congenital malformations, mental retardation, or other handicaps are called high-risk pregnancies (Table 91–1; see also Chapter 92). Some factors, such as ingestion of a teratogenic drug in the 1st trimester, are causally related to the risk; others, such as hydramnios, are associations that alert a physician to the existence of the risk or risks. Based on their history, 10–20% of pregnant patients can be identified as high risk; less than half of all perinatal mortality and morbidity is associated with these

TABLE 91–1 Factors Associated with High-Risk Pregnancy

Economic	Reproductive
Poverty	Prior cesarean section
Unemployment	Prior infertility
Uninsured, underinsured health insurance	Prolonged gestation
Poor access to prenatal care	Prolonged labor
Cultural-Behavioral	Prior infant with cerebral palsy, mental retardation, birth trauma, congenital anomalies
Low educational status	Abnormal lie (breech)
Poor health care attitudes	Multiple gestation
No care or inadequate prenatal care	Premature rupture of membranes
Cigarette, alcohol, drug abuse	Infections (systemic, amniotic, extra-amniotic, cervical)
Age less than 16 or over 35 yr	Pre-eclampsia or eclampsia
Unmarried	Uterine bleeding (abruptio placentae, placenta previa)
Short interpregnancy interval	Parity (0 or more than 5)
Lack of support group (husband, family, religion)	Uterine or cervical anomalies
Stress (physical, psychologic)	Fetal disease
Black race	Abnormal fetal growth
Biologic-Genetic	Idiopathic premature labor
	Iatrogenic prematurity
Previous low-birthweight infant	High or low levels of maternal serum α-fetoprotein
Low maternal weight at her birth	**Medical**
Low weight for height	Diabetes mellitus
Poor weight gain during pregnancy	Hypertension
Short stature	Congenital heart disease
Poor nutrition	Autoimmune disease
Inbreeding (autosomal recessive?)	Sickle cell anemia
Intergenerational effects	TORCH infection
Hereditary diseases (inborn error of metabolism)	Intercurrent surgery or trauma
	Sexually transmitted diseases
	Maternal hypercoaguable states

pregnancies. Although assessing antepartum risk is important in reducing perinatal mortality and morbidity, some women become at high risk only during labor and delivery; therefore, careful monitoring is critical throughout the intrapartum course.

Identifying high-risk pregnancies is important not only because it is the first step toward prevention but also because therapeutic steps may often be taken to reduce the risks to the fetus or neonate if the physician knows of the potential for difficulty.

GENETIC FACTORS. The occurrence of chromosomal abnormalities, congenital anomalies, inborn errors of metabolism, mental retardation, or any familial disease in blood relatives increases the risk of the same condition in the infant. Because many parents recognize only obvious clinical manifestations of genetically determined diseases, specific inquiry should be made about any disease affecting one or more blood relative(s).

MATERNAL FACTORS. The lowest neonatal mortality rate occurs in infants of mothers who receive adequate prenatal care and who are age 20–30 yr. Both teenage pregnancies and those among women older than 40 yr, particularly primiparous women, carry an increased risk for intrauterine growth retardation, fetal distress, and intrauterine death.

Maternal illness (Table 91–2); multiple pregnancies, particularly those involving monochorionic twinning; infections (Table 91–3), and certain drugs (Chapter 92) increase the risk for the fetus.

Preterm birth is common among high-risk pregnancies (Chapter 93). Factors associated with prematurity are noted in Table 91–1 and include biologic markers such as cervical shortening, genital infection, fetal fibronectin in the cervicovaginal secretions, and preterm premature rupture of the membranes. The latter occurs in 1% of pregnancies but is noted in 30–40% of preterm deliveries, and it is a leading identifiable cause of prematurity.

Polyhydramnios and *oligohydramnios* indicate high-risk pregnancies. Although there is a rapid turnover rate, during normal pregnancy the amniotic fluid volume gradually increases at a rate of less than 10 mL/day until about the 34th wk of pregnancy, after which it slowly diminishes. The volumes vary widely in normal pregnancy; term volume may be 500–2000 mL. A volume estimated at greater than 2,000 mL in the 3rd trimester constitutes polyhydramnios, and a volume estimated at less than 500 mL indicates oligohydramnios. Polyhydramnios complicates 1–3% and oligohydramnios complicates 1–5% of pregnancies. The ultrasonographic criteria for these diagnoses are based on the *amniotic fluid index,* which is determined by measuring the vertical diameter of amniotic fluid pockets in 4 quadrants; an index greater than 24 cm suggests polyhydramnios, while one less than 5 cm suggests oligohydramnios.

Acute polyhydramnios is rare and is usually associated with premature labor and delivery before 28 wk. Chronic polyhydramnios is diagnosed in the 3rd trimester by the discrepancy between uterine size and gestational age; it occasionally goes undiagnosed until the patient has dysfunctional labor or an abnormally large amount of amniotic fluid is noted during delivery. Polyhydramnios is associated with premature labor, abruptio placentae, and fetal neuromuscular dysfunction or obstruction of the gastrointestinal tract that interferes with reabsorption of amniotic fluid swallowed by the fetus (Table 91–4). Increased fetal urination or edema formation is also associated with excessive amniotic fluid volume. Ultrasound demonstrates the increased amniotic fluid surrounding the fetus and detects associated fetal anomalies, hydrops, pleural effusions, or ascites. In 60% of patients, no cause is identified. Polyhydramnios may be managed by serial amniocentesis or maternal administration of indomethacin if due to excessive fetal urination; treatment is indicated for acute maternal respiratory distress, threatened preterm labor, or to provide time for administered steroid to act.

Oligohydramnios is associated with congenital anomalies, intrauterine growth retardation, severe renal anomalies, and drugs that interfere with fetal urination (see Table 91–4). This becomes most evident after 20 wk of gestation, when fetal urination is the major source of amniotic fluid. Rupture of the membranes must be ruled out when oligohydramnios is suspected, especially if a normal-sized bladder is seen with fetal ultrasonography. Oligohydramnios causes fetal compression abnormalities such as clubfoot, spadelike hands, and a flattened nasal bridge. The most serious complication of chronic oligohydramnios is pulmonary hypoplasia. The risk of umbilical cord compression during labor and delivery is increased in pregnancies complicated by oligohydramnios and may be alleviated by saline amnioinfusion. Ultrasonography may reveal small (1–2 cm) pockets of fluid in addition to the associated growth retardation or anomalies. Oligohydramnios in combination with an elevated α-fetoprotein level, uterine bleeding, or intrauterine growth retardation carries an increased risk of intrauterine fetal demise.

Second-trimester screening (15–18 wk) of maternal serum α-fetoprotein (MSAFP) levels helps identify high-risk pregnancies. *Elevated MSAFP* is associated with multifetal gestation, more advanced dates than expected, open neural tube defects, threatened abortion, hydrops with ascites, cystic hygroma, gastroschisis, omphalocele, congenital nephrosis, polycystic renal disease, epidermolysis bullosum, amniotic bands, ectopia cordis, placental hemangioma, retroplacental hemorrhage, Kell or Rh sensitization, and maternal diseases such as liver cancer, yolk sac tumors, viral hepatitis, and lupus anticoagulant; elevated levels may occasionally be normal. *Low MSAFP* is associated with incorrect gestational age estimate, trisomy 18 or 21, and intrauterine growth retardation. A combination of low MSAFP, reduced maternal serum unconjugated estriol, and elevated pregnancy-associated protein A, inhibin, and maternal human chorionic gonadotropin levels between 11–15 wk gestation is highly suggestive of trisomy 21. Fetal ultrasonogra-

TABLE 91–2 Maternal Disease Affecting the Fetus or Neonate

Disorder	Effects	Mechanism
Cholestasis	Preterm delivery	Unknown; possible hepatitis E
Cyanotic heart disease	Intrauterine growth retardation	Low fetal oxygen delivery
Diabetes mellitus		
Mild	Large for gestational age, hypoglycemia	Fetal hyperglycemia—produces hyperinsulinemia; insulin promotes growth
Severe	Growth retardation	Vascular disease, placental insufficiency
Drug addiction	Intrauterine growth retardation, neonatal withdrawal	Direct drug effect, plus poor diet
Endemic goiter	Hypothyroidism	Iodine deficiency
Graves disease	Transient neonatal thyrotoxicosis	Placental immunoglobin passage of thyroid-stimulating antibody
Herpes gestationalis	Bullous rash	Unknown
Hyperparathyroidism	Neonatal hypocalcemia	Maternal calcium crosses to fetus and suppresses fetal parathyroid gland
Hypertension	Intrauterine growth retardation, intrauterine fetal demise	Placental insufficiency, fetal hypoxia
Idiopathic thrombocytopenic purpura	Thrombocytopenia	Nonspecific maternal platelet antibodies cross placenta
Isoimmune neutropenia or thrombocytopenia	Neutropenia or thrombocytopenia	Specific antifetal neutrophil or platelet antibody crosses placenta after sensitization of mother
Malignant melanoma	Placental or fetal tumor	Metastasis
Myasthenia gravis	Transient neonatal myasthenia	Immunoglobin to acetylcholine receptor crosses placenta
Myotonic dystrophy	Neonatal myotonic dystrophy, congenital contractures, respiratory insufficiency	Genetic anticipation
Obesity	Macrosomia, hypoglycemia	Unknown
Phenylketonuria	Microcephaly, retardation	Elevated fetal phenylalanine levels
Pre-eclampsia, eclampsia	Intrauterine growth retardation, thrombocytopenia, neutropenia, fetal demise	Uteroplacental insufficiency, fetal hypoxia, vasoconstriction
Renal transplant	Intrauterine growth retardation	Uteroplacental insufficiency
Rhesus or other blood group sensitization	Fetal anemia, hypoalbuminemia, hydrops, neonatal jaundice	Antibody crosses placenta directed to fetal cells with antigen
Sickle cell anemia	Preterm birth, intrauterine growth retardation	Maternal sickling producing fetal hypoxia
Systemic lupus erythematosus	Congenital heart block, rash, anemia, thrombocytopenia, neutropenia	Antibody directed to fetal heart, red and white blood cells, and platelets
Thrombophilia (familial)	Stillborn, growth retardation	Thrombosis of uteroplacental circulation

TABLE 91–3 Maternal Infections Affecting the Fetus or Newborn

Infection	Mode of Transmission	Outcome
Bacteria		
Group B streptococcus	Ascending cervical	Sepsis, pneumonia
Escherichia coli	Ascending cervical	Sepsis, pneumonia
Listeria monocytogenes	Transplacental	Sepsis, pneumonia
Ureaplasma urealyticum	Ascending cervical	Pneumonia, meningitis
Mycoplasma hominis	Ascending cervical	Pneumonia
Chlamydia trachomatis	Vaginal passage	Conjunctivitis, pneumonia
Syphilis	Transplacental, vaginal passage	Congenital syphilis
Borrelia burgdorferi	Transplacental	Prematurity, fetal demise
Neisseria gonorrhoeae	Vaginal passage	Ophthalmia (conjunctivitis), sepsis, meningitis
Mycobacterium tuberculosis	Transplacental	Prematurity, fetal demise, congenital tuberculosis
Granulocytic ehrlichiosis	Transplacental	Sepsis
Virus		
Rubella	Transplacental	Congenital rubella
Cytomegalovirus	Transplacental, breast milk (rare)	Congenital cytomegalovirus or asymptomatic
Human immunodeficiency virus	Transplacental, vaginal passage, breast milk	Congenital acquired immunodeficiency syndrome
Hepatitis B	Vaginal passage, transplacental, breast milk	Neonatal hepatitis, chronic HBsAg carrier
Hepatitis C	Transplacental	Uncommon but neonatal hepatitis, chronic carrier possible
Lymphocytic choriomeningitis	Transplacental	Fetal, neonatal death; hydrocephalus, chorioretinitis
Herpes simplex II	Transplacental	Congenital herpes simplex virus
	Vaginal passage, ascending	Neonatal encephalitis, disseminated viremia
Varicella-zoster	Transplacental, early	Congenital anomalies
	Transplacental, late	Neonatal varicella
Parvovirus	Transplacental	Fetal anemia, hydrops
Coxsackie virus B	Fecal-oral	Myocarditis, meningitis, hepatitis
Poliomyelitis	Transplacental	Congenital poliomyelitis
Epstein-Barr	Transplacental	Anomalies (?)
Rubeola	Transplacental	Abortion, fetal measles
Parasites		
Toxoplasmosis	Transplacental	Congenital toxoplasmosis or asymptomatic
Malaria	Transplacental	Abortion, prematurity, intrauterine growth retardation
Trypanosomiasis	Transplacental	Congenital Chagas' disease
Fungi		
Candida	Ascending, cervical	Sepsis, pneumonia, rash
Prion		
Creutzfeld-Jakob disease	Transplacental, colostrum	Hypothetical route, no long-term data

TABLE 91–4 Conditions Associated With Disorders of Amniotic Fluid Volume

Oligohydramnios	Polyhydramnios
Intrauterine growth retardation Fetal anomalies Twin-twin transfusion (donor) Amniotic fluid leak Renal agenesis (Potter syndrome) Urethral atresia Prune-belly syndrome Pulmonary hypoplasia Amnion nodosum Indomethacin Angiotensin-converting enzyme inhibitors Intestinal pseudo-obstruction	*Congenital anomalies:* Anencephaly, hydrocephaly, tracheoesophageal fistula, duodenal atresia, spina bifida, cleft lip or palate, cystic adenomatoid lung malformation, diaphragmatic hernia *Syndromes:* Achondroplasia, Klippel-Feil, 18-, 21-trisomy, TORCH, hydrops fetalis, multiple congenital anomalad *Other:* Diabetes mellitus, twin-twin transfusion (recipient), fetal anemia, fetal heart failure, polyuric renal disease, neuromuscular diseases, nonimmune hydrops, chylothorax, teratoma *Idiopathic*

phy may demonstrate nuchal fluid accumulations (translucency), a short femur, and congenital heart disease; chromosome analysis on cells from an amniocentesis confirms the diagnosis.

Obstetric conditions are understandably important because fetuses weighing more than 2,500 g make up a very high proportion of total fetal deaths, and neonatal mortality is greatest during the first 24 hr after delivery. A pregnancy should be considered high risk when the uterus is inappropriately large or small. A uterus large for the estimated stage of gestation suggests the presence of multiple fetuses, hydramnios, or an excessively large infant; an inappropriately small one suggests oligohydramnios or retardation of intrauterine growth. Premature rupture of membranes (PROM) earlier than 24 hr before delivery carries a risk of fetal infection. PROM also increases the risk of premature birth. PROM at term usually results in the onset of labor within 48 hr but has the risk of chorioamnionitis and umbilical cord compression. PROM before 37 wk has a longer latency until labor starts and has the added risks of cord prolapse, oligohydramnios, abruptio placentae, fetal malposition, and, if present for more than 7 days, for pulmonary hypoplasia, uterine-induced deformations, and contractures. Prolonged and difficult labors increase the risks of mechanical and hypoxic damage. A tumultuous short labor, with a precipitous delivery, increases the risk of birth asphyxia, and intracranial hemorrhage. Placental separation at any time before delivery and abnormal implantation or compression of the cord increase the possibility of brain damage due to fetal anoxia; brown or muddy amniotic fluid suggests that meconium has been passed, possibly during an episode of fetal anoxia.

Although the safety of any type of delivery depends on the skill of the obstetrician, additional hazards accompany particular methods and result from the circumstances that dictated them. Neonatal deaths following deliveries by mid and high forceps, breech extraction, and version are likely to be related to traumatic intracranial injury.

Infants born by *cesarean section* present problems possibly related to the unfavorable obstetric circumstance that necessitated the operation or to prolonged maternal anesthesia. In normal term pregnancies, when there is no indication of fetal distress, delivery through the abdomen carries a greater risk than delivery through the birth canal. However, controversy exists regarding the safest type of delivery for a nondistressed viable immature fetus, especially in a breech presentation; cesarean section may involve less risk than the "stress" of labor and the potentially anoxic effects of uterine contractions during vaginal delivery. A small percentage of mature infants delivered by cesarean section have some degree of respiratory difficulty for 1–2 days. Although transient tachypnea is the most frequently associated problem, hyaline membrane disease may develop, particularly in infants born to women not in labor, those with uncertain dates or pulmonary maturity, and those born to diabetic mothers or following asphyxia.

Anesthesia and analgesia affect the fetus as well as the mother; mild maternal hypoxemia due to hypoventilation, or hypotension due to epidural anesthesia, may result in severe fetal hypoxia and shock. Skilled use of medication avoids severe fetal narcosis while securing the benefits of gentle and unhurried delivery. Even skilled administration may result in a mildly depressed infant whose crying and breathing may be delayed 1–2 min and who may be somewhat inactive for several hours. When anesthesia and analgesia are carelessly used or when their milder effects are added to already unfavorable fetal circumstances such as prematurity, anoxia, or trauma, the result may be catastrophic.

Cheng M, Hannah M: Breech delivery at term: A critical review of the literature. Obstet Gynecol 82:605, 1993.

Epstein FH: Premature rupture of the fetal membranes. N Engl J Med 338:663, 1998.

Haddow J, Palomaki G, Knight G, et al: Screening of maternal serum for fetal Down's syndrome in the first trimester. N Engl J Med 338:955, 1998.

Hook B, Kiwi R, Amini SB, et al: Neonatal morbidity after elective repeat cesarean section and trial of labor. Pediatrics 100:348, 1997.

McCurdy CM, Seeds JW: Oligohydramnios: Problems and treatment. Semin Perinatol 17:183, 1993.

Moise KJ: Polyhydramnios: Problems and treatment. Semin Perinatol 17:197, 1993.

Vergani P, Ceruti P, Strobelt N, et al: Transabdominal aminoinfusion in oligohydramnios at term before induction of labor with intact membranes: A randomized clinical trial. Am J Obstet Gynecol 175:465, 1996.

Whittle M: Ultrasonographic "soft markers" of fetal chromosomal defects. Br Med J 314:918, 1997.

CHAPTER 92

The Fetus

Genetic and environmental influences may affect an embryo and fetus at any time during development; the fetal genome itself has a role in development and fetal survival.

The major emphases in fetal medicine are (1) assessing fetal growth and maturity, (2) evaluating fetal well-being or distress, (3) assessing the effects of maternal disease on the fetus, (4) evaluating the fetal effects of drugs administered to the mother, and (5) identifying and treating fetal disease or anomalies. Increasing knowledge of fetal physiology has paved the way for effective fetal therapy, intervention during fetal distress, and improved adaptation of a newborn infant, particularly of a premature one, to extrauterine life. Some aspects of human fetal growth and development are summarized in Chapter 8.

92.1 Fetal Growth and Maturity

Ultrasonography of the fetus, a common obstetric procedure, is both safe and accurate. Indications for antenatal ultrasonography include estimation of gestational age (unknown dates, discrepancy between uterine size and dates or suspected growth retardation, multiple gestation, and abnormalities of amniotic fluid volume), location of the placenta, determination of the number and position of fetuses, and identification of congenital anomalies.

Fetal growth can be assessed by ultrasonography as early as 6 to 8 wk. The most accurate assessment of gestational age is by a first trimester ultrasound measurement of crown-rump

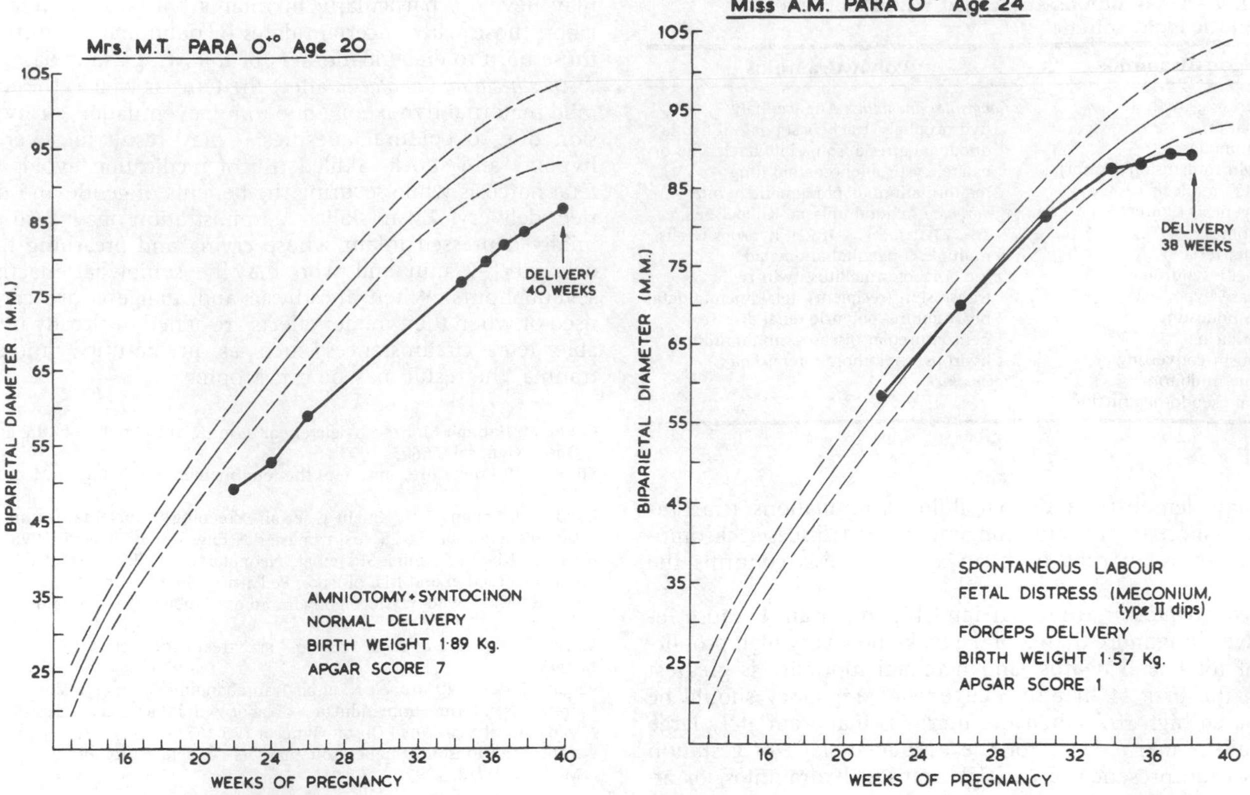

Figure 92–1 *A,* Example of "low profile" growth retardation pattern. Uneventful pregnancy and labor. Baby cried at 1 min and did not develop hypoglycemia. Birth weight was below the 5th percentile weight for gestational age. *B,* Example of "late flattening" growth retardation pattern. Typical history of preeclampsia, intrapartum fetal distress, low Apgar score, and postnatal hypoglycemia. Birthweight was below the 5th percentile weight for gestational age. (From Campbell S: Clin Obstet Gynecol 1:41, 1974.)

length. The biparietal diameter (BPD) is used to assess gestational age beginning in the second trimester. Through 34 wk the BPD accurately estimates gestation to within plus or minus 10 days. Later in gestation, the accuracy falls to plus or minus 3 wk. Methods used to assess gestational age at term include measurement of abdominal circumference and femur length. An estimate of gestational age by dating of the last menstrual period should also be obtained. If a single ultrasound examination is performed, the most information can be obtained with a scan at 18 to 20 wk, when both gestational age and fetal anatomy can be evaluated. Serial scans may be useful in assessing fetal growth. Two patterns of fetal growth retardation have been identified: continuous fetal growth 2 standard deviations below the mean for gestational age and a normal fetal growth curve that abruptly slows or flattens later in gestation (Fig. 92–1).

Fetal maturity is usually assessed by accurate ultrasonographic dating of gestational age but may also be estimated by determining the amniotic fluid surfactant content (Chapters 92.5 and 97). Determination of the extent of calcification by ultrasound (placental maturity index), detection of the first audible fetal heart tones (16–18 wk), and observation of the initial fetal movements (18–20 wk) may also aid in evaluating the maturity of a fetus.

92.2 Fetal Distress

Fetal compromise may occur during the antepartum or intrapartum periods. Fetal compromise may be asymptomatic in the antenatal period. Antepartum fetal surveillance is warranted for women at increased risk for fetal distress, including those with a history of stillbirth, intrauterine growth retardation (IUGR) oligohydramnios or polyhydramnios, multiple gestation, rhesus sensitization, hypertensive disorders, diabetes mellitus or other chronic maternal disease, decreased fetal movement, and post-term pregnancy. The predominant cause of antepartum fetal distress is uteroplacental insufficiency. Fetal distress may be manifested as IUGR, fetal hypoxia, increased vascular resistance in fetal blood vessels (Figs. 92–2 and 92–3), and, when severe, mixed respiratory and metabolic (lactic) acidosis. The goals of antepartum fetal surveillance are to prevent intrauterine fetal demise, to prevent hypoxic brain injury, and to prolong gestation in women at risk for preterm delivery, when this is safe, or to deliver a fetus when it is in jeopardy. The most commonly used tests are the *nonstress test* (NST), the *contraction stress test* (CST), and the *biophysical profile* (BPP). Methods for assessing fetal well-being are listed in Table 92–1.

The NST monitors the presence of fetal heart rate accelerations that follow fetal movement. A reactive (normal) NST result demonstrates 2 fetal heart rate accelerations of at least 15 beats/min lasting 15 sec. A nonreactive NST result suggests fetal compromise and requires further assessment with a CST or the BPP. A CST observes the fetal heart rate response to spontaneous, nipple-, or oxytocin-stimulated uterine contractions. Fetal compromise is suggested when 3 contractions in 10 min are followed by late decelerations. CST is contraindicated in women having preterm premature rupture of membranes or a prior uterine scar from a classic C-section and in those with multiple gestations, an incompetent cervix, or placenta previa. The goals of fetal monitoring are to prevent intrauterine fetal demise and hypoxic brain injury. Although the CST and NST have low false-negative rates, both have high false-positive rates. The BPP assesses fetal breathing, body

TABLE 92–1 Fetal Diagnosis and Assessment

Method	Comment and Indications
Imaging	
Ultrasound (real-time)	Biometry (growth), anomaly (morphology) detection. Biophysical profile. Amniotic fluid volume, hydrops, determine gestational age and IUGR
Ultrasound (Doppler)	Velocimetry (blood flow velocity). Detection of increased vascular resistance secondary to fetal hypoxia, IUGR
Embryoscopy	Early diagnosis of limb anomaly
Fetoscopy	Detection of facial, limb, cutaneous anomalies
Fluid Analysis	
Amniocentesis	Fetal maturity (L/S ratio), karyotype (cytogenetics), biochemical enzyme analysis, molecular genetic DNA diagnosis, bilirubin, or α-fetoprotein determination. Bacterial culture, pathogen antigen or genome detection
Fetal urine	Prognosis of obstructive uropathy?
Cordocentesis (Percutaneous Umbilical Blood Sampling [PUBS])	Detection of blood type, anemia, hemoglobinopathies, thrombocytopenia, acidosis, hypoxia, polycythemia, IgM antibody response to infection. Rapid karyotyping and molecular DNA genetic diagnosis. Fetal therapy (see Table 92–6)
Fetal Tissue Analysis	
Chorionic villus biopsy	Karyotype, molecular DNA genetic analysis, enzyme assays
Skin biopsy	Hereditary skin disease*
Liver biopsy	Enzyme assay*
Circulating fetal cells in maternal blood	Molecular DNA genetic analysis
Maternal Serum α-Fetoprotein	
Elevated	Twins, neural tube defects (anencephaly, spina bifida), intestinal atresia, hepatitis, nephrosis, fetal demise, incorrect gestational age
Reduced	Trisomies, aneuploidy
Maternal Cervix	
Fetal fibronectin	Indicates risk of preterm birth
Bacterial culture	Identifies risk of fetal infection (group B streptococcus, *N. gonorrhoeae*)
Fluid	Determination of premature rupture of the membranes
Antepartum Biophysical Monitoring	
Nonstress test	Fetal distress; hypoxia
Contraction stress test	Fetal distress; hypoxia
Biophysical profile	Fetal distress; hypoxia
Intrapartum Fetal Heart Rate Monitoring	See Fig. 92–4

**DNA genetic analysis on chorionic villus samples, amniocytes from amniocentesis, or fetal cells recovered from the maternal circulation may obviate the need for direct fetal tissue biopsy if the gene or genetic marker is available (e.g., the gene for Duchenne's muscular dystrophy).*
IUGR = intrauterine growth retardation.

movement, tone, and heart rate and amniotic fluid volume, and it is used to improve the accurate and safe identification of fetal compromise (Table 92–2). A score of 2 is given for each observation present. A total score of 8–10 is reassuring; a score of 6 is equivocal, and retesting should be done in 12–24 hr; a score of 4 or less warrants immediate evaluation and possible delivery. Signs of compromise seen on Doppler ultrasonography include a reduced, absent, or reversed diastolic waveform velocity in the fetal aorta or umbilical artery (see Fig. 92–3 and Table 92–1). High-risk fetuses often demonstrate combinations of abnormalities such as oligohydramnios, reversed diastolic Doppler umbilical artery blood flow velocity, and a low BPP.

Fetal distress during labor may be detected by monitoring

TABLE 92–2 Biophysical Profile Scoring: Technique and Interpretation

Biophysical Variable	Normal Score (2)	Abnormal (Score = 0)
Fetal breathing movements	At least 1 episode of FBM of at least 30 sec duration in 30 min observation	Absent FBM or no episode of ≥30 sec in 30 min
Gross body movement	At least 3 discrete body/limb movements in 30 min (episodes of active continuous movement considered as single movement)	2 or fewer episodes of body/limb movements in 30 min
Fetal tone	At least 1 episode of active extension with return to flexion of fetal limb(s) or trunk. Opening and closing of hand considered normal tone	Either slow extension with return to partial flexion or movement of limb in full extension or absent fetal movement with fetal hand held in complete or partial deflection
Reactive FHR	At least 2 episodes of FHR acceleration of ≥15 beats/min and of at least 15 sec duration associated with fetal movement in 30 min	Less than 2 episodes of acceleration of FHR or acceleration of <15 beats/min in 30 min
Qualitative AFV*	At least 1 pocket of AF that measures at least 2 cm in 2 perpendicular planes	Either no AF pockets or a pocket <2 cm in two perpendicular planes

**Modification of the criteria for reduced amniotic fluid from <1 cm to <2 cm would seem reasonable. Fetal biophysical assessment by ultrasound. (From Creasy RK, Resnik R [eds]: Maternal-Fetal Medicine: Principles and Practice, 3rd ed. Philadelphia, WB Saunders, 1994.)*
FBM = fetal breathing movement; FHR = fetal heart rate; AFV = amniotic fluid volume; AF = amniotic fluid.

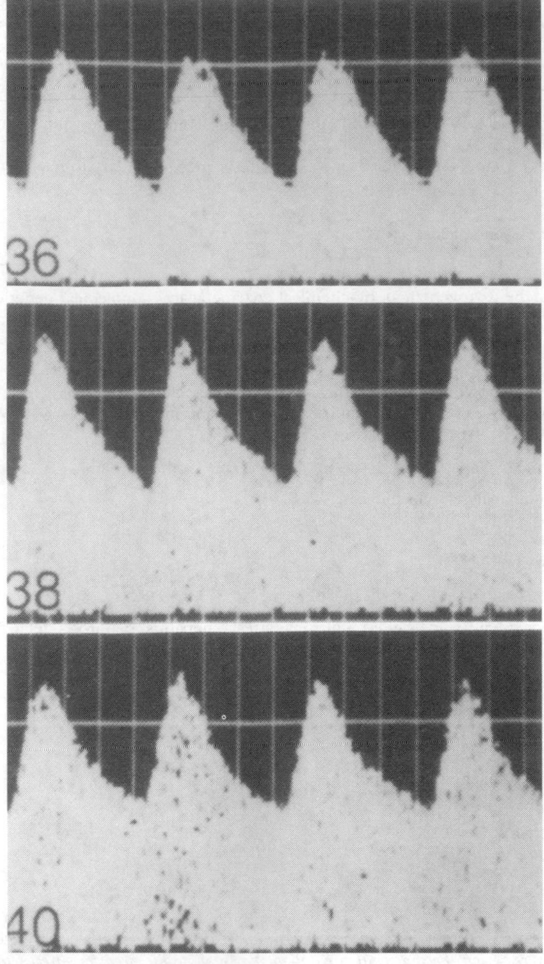

Figure 92–2 Normal Doppler velocimetry. Sequential Doppler studies, from one normal pregnancy, of fetal umbilical artery flow velocity waveforms. Note systolic peak flow with lower but constant flow during diastole. The systolic diastolic ratio can be determined and in normal pregnancies is <3 after the 30th wk of gestation. The numbers indicate the week of gestation. (From Trudinger B: Doppler ultrasound assessment of blood flow. *In:* Creasy RK, Resnik R [eds]: Maternal-Fetal Medicine: Principles and Practice, 3rd ed. Philadelphia, WB Saunders, 1994.)

fetal heart rate, uterine pressure, and fetal scalp blood pH (Fig. 92–4).

Continuous fetal heart rate monitoring detects abnormal cardiac patterns by instruments that compute the beat-to-beat fetal heart rate from a fetal electrocardiographic signal. Signals are derived from an electrode attached to the fetal presenting part; from an ultrasonic transducer placed on the maternal abdominal wall to detect continuous ultrasonic waves reflected from the contractions of the heart; or from a phonotransducer placed on the mother's abdomen. Uterine contractions are simultaneously recorded from an amniotic fluid catheter and pressure transducer or from a tocotransducer applied to the maternal abdominal wall overlying the uterus.

Fetal heart rate patterns show various characteristics, some of which suggest fetal distress. Baseline fetal heart rate is the average rate between uterine contractions, which gradually decreases from about 155 beats/min in early pregnancy to about 135 beats/min at term; the normal range at term is 120–160 beats/min. **Tachycardia** (>160 beats/min) is associated with early fetal hypoxia, maternal fever, maternal hyperthyroidism, maternal β-sympathomimetic or atropine therapy, fetal anemia, and some fetal arrhythmias. The latter do not generally occur with congenital heart disease and tend to resolve spontaneously at birth. **Fetal bradycardia** (<120 beats/min) occurs with fetal hypoxia, placental transfer of local anesthetic agents and β-adrenergic blocking agents, and, occasionally, heart block with or without congenital heart disease.

Normally, the baseline fetal heart rate is variable, with long-term changes of 3–6 cycles/min as well as short-term beat-to-beat variation. This variability may be decreased or lost with fetal hypoxemia or the placental transfer of drugs such as atropine, diazepam, promethazine, magnesium sulfate, and most sedative and narcotic agents. Prematurity, sleep state, and fetal tachycardia may also diminish beat-to-beat variability.

Periodic accelerations or decelerations of fetal heart rate in response to uterine contractions may also be monitored (see Fig. 92–4). **Early deceleration** (type I dips), associated with head compression, is a repetitive pattern of slowing, synchronous with and proportional to the amplitude of the uterine contraction. **Variable deceleration** (associated with cord compression) is characterized by variable shape, abrupt onset and occurrence with consecutive contractions, and return to baseline at or after the conclusion of the contraction. **Late deceleration** (type II dips), associated with fetal hypoxemia, occurs repetitively after a uterine contraction is well established, is proportional to its amplitude, and persists into the interval following contractions. The late deceleration pattern is usually associated with maternal hypotension or excessive uterine activity but may be a response to any maternal, placental, umbilical cord, or fetal factor that limits effective oxygenation of the fetus. Reflex late decelerations with normal beat-to-beat variability are associated with chronic compensated fetal hypoxia and occur during uterine contractions that temporarily impede oxygen transport to the heart. Nonreflex late decelerations are more ominous and indicate severe hypoxic depression of myocardial function. The latter, together with decreased beat-to-beat variability or spontaneous decelerations in the absence of uterine contractions, either warrants further assessment by fetal blood sampling or is an indication for delivery.

Fetal scalp blood sampling during labor through a slightly dilated cervix may aid in confirming fetal distress suspected on the basis of variations in fetal heart rate or the presence of meconium in the amniotic fluid. The proper use of this technique may result in earlier delivery of depressed infants who thus have a better chance of successful resuscitation, increased survival, and less morbidity. Alternatively, when continuous fetal heart rate monitoring or general clinical evaluation suggests that a fetus is at risk, a normal fetal scalp blood sample may help avert obstetric intervention.

Fetal scalp blood pH in normal labor decreases from about 7.33 early in labor to approximately 7.25 at the time of vaginal

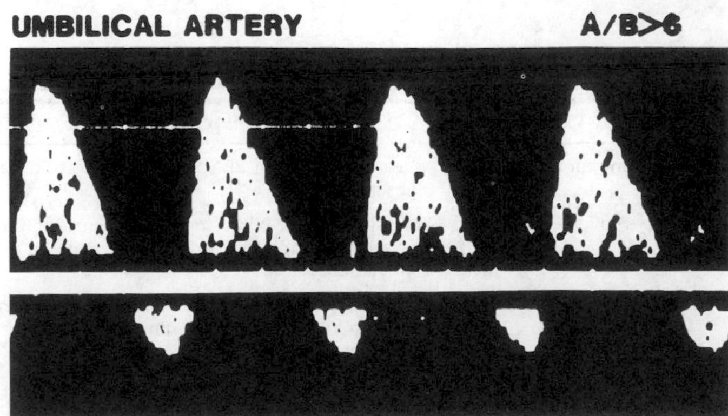

Figure 92–3 Abnormal Doppler velocimetry. An umbilical artery Doppler flow velocity waveform in which umbilical placental impedance is so high that the diastolic component shows flow in a reverse direction. This is an indication of severe intrauterine hypoxia and intrauterine growth retardation. (From Trudinger B: Doppler ultrasound assessment of blood flow. *In:* Creasy RK, Resnik R [eds]: Maternal-Fetal Medicine: Principles and Practice, 3rd ed. Philadelphia, WB Saunders, 1994.)

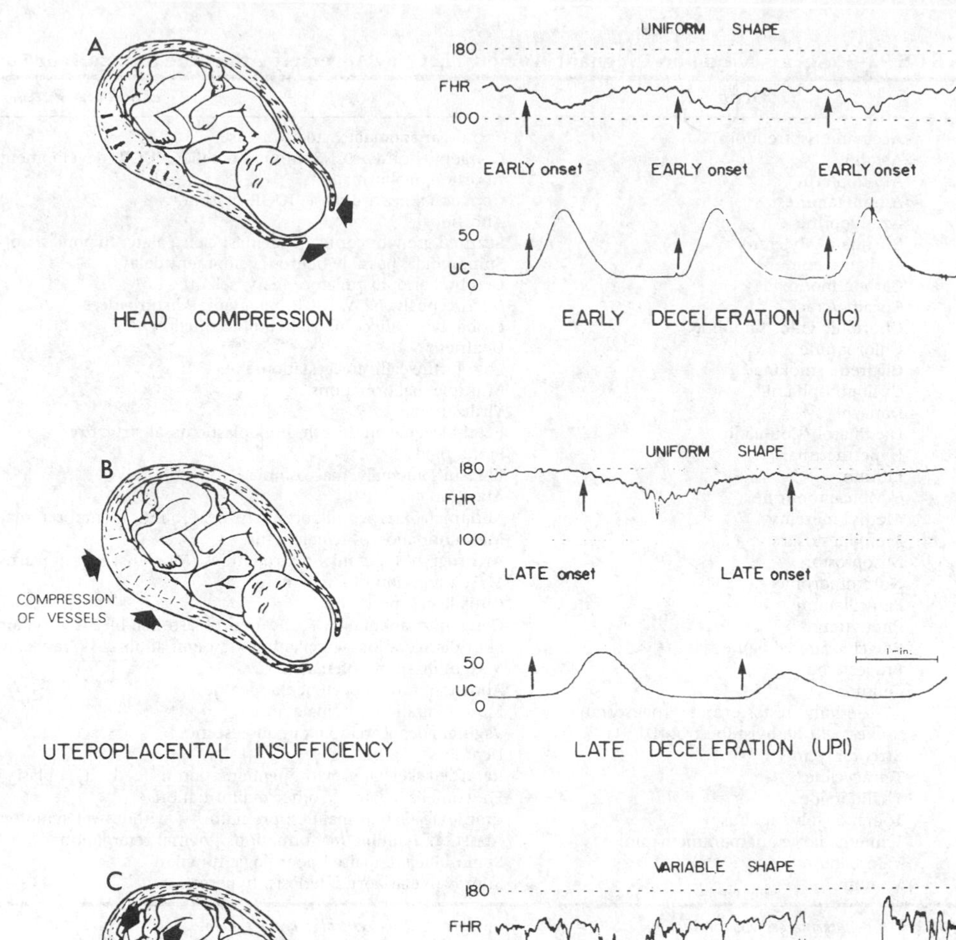

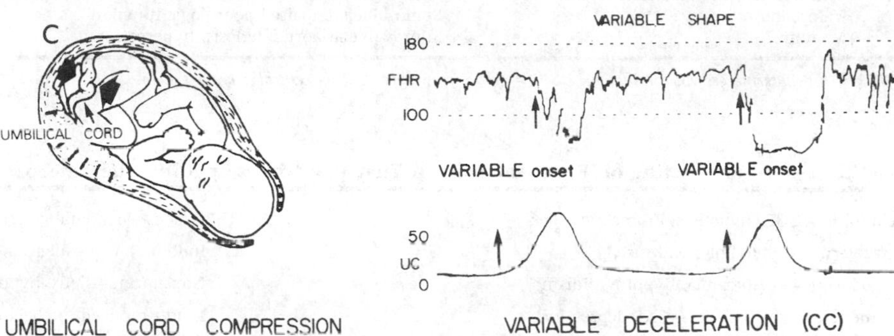

Figure 92–4 Patterns of periodic fetal heart rate decelerations. Tracing in *A* shows early deceleration that occurs during the peak of uterine contractions and is due to pressure on the fetal head. *B*, Late deceleration due to uteroplacental insufficiency. *C*, Variable deceleration due to umbilical cord compression. Arrows denote time relation between the onset of FHR changes and uterine contractions. (From Hon EH: An Atlas of Fetal Heart Rate Patterns, New Haven, CT, Harty Press, 1968.)

delivery; the base deficit is about 4–6 mEq/L. Changes in the buffer base may be particularly helpful in assessing fetal status, because they correspond to fetal lactic acid accumulation. A pH of less than 7.25 strongly suggests fetal distress, and a pH of less than 7.20 is an indication for further assessment and intervention.

Complications of fetal scalp sampling and internal monitoring devices are relatively uncommon but include bleeding (usually due to an underlying coagulation defect), puncture of the fontanel, and scalp abscesses with or without adjacent osteomyelitis. Abscesses may be due to *Staphylococcus aureus* or gram-negative rods; more often they are sterile.

Umbilical cord blood samples obtained at the time of delivery are useful to document fetal acid-base status. Although the exact cord blood pH value that defines significant fetal acidemia is unknown, an umbilical artery pH of less than 7.0 has been associated with greater need for resuscitation and a higher incidence of respiratory, gastrointestinal, cardiovascular, and neurologic complications. However, when a low pH is measured, many newborns will be neurologically normal.

92.3 Maternal Disease and the Fetus

INFECTIOUS DISEASES (see Table 91–3). Almost any maternal infection with severe systemic manifestations may result in miscarriage, stillbirth, or premature labor. Whether these results are due to infection of the fetus or are secondary to stress is not always clear. Maternal hyperthermia during infections may be associated with an increased incidence of congenital anomalies. Regardless of the severity of the maternal infection, certain agents frequently infect a fetus, with serious sequelae. Such fetuses are frequently small for gestational age. Some infections, such as rubella, may also produce congenital malformations if they occur during the period of organogenesis.

NONINFECTIOUS DISEASES (see Table 91–2). *Maternal diabetes* may result in organomegaly, hypertrophy and hyperplasia of the β cells of the fetal pancreas, and metabolic derangements in the neonate (Chapter 103.1). A high incidence of intrauterine death occurs after the 36th wk of gestation in unmonitored and poorly controlled mothers. *Eclampsia–pre-eclampsia* of pregnancy, chronic hypertension, and renal disease result in small fetal size for gestational age, prematurity, and intrauterine death, all probably due to diminished uteroplacental perfusion. Uncontrolled maternal *hypothyroidism* or *hyperthyroidism* is responsible for relative infertility, a tendency to abort, premature labor, and fetal death. Maternal *immunologic diseases,* such as idiopathic thrombocytopenic purpura, systemic lupus, myasthenia gravis, and Graves disease, all of which are mediated by IgG autoantibodies that can cross the placenta, frequently result in a transient illness in the newborn. Untreated maternal

TABLE 92–3 Agents Acting on Pregnant Women That May Adversely Affect the Structure or Function of the Fetus and Newborn

Drug	Effect on Fetus
Accutane (isotretinoin)	Facial-ear anomalies, heart disease
Alcohol	Congenital cardiac CNS, limb anomalies, IUGR, developmental delay, attention deficits, autism
Aminopterin	Abortion, malformations
Amphetamines	Congenital heart disease, IUGR, withdrawal
Azathioprine	Abortion
Busulfan (Myleran)	Stunted growth; corneal opacities; cleft palate; hypoplasia of ovaries, thyroid, and parathyroids
Carbamazepine	Spina bifida, possible neurodevelopment delay
Carbon monoxide	Cerebral atrophy, microcephaly, seizures
Cocaine/crack	Microcephaly, LBW, IUGR, behavioral disturbances
Chorionic villus sampling	Probably no effect, possibly limb reduction
Chloroquine	Deafness
Cigarette smoking	Low birthweight for gestational age
Cyclophosphamide	Multiple malformations
Danazol	Virilization
Dicumarol (Coumadin)	Fetal bleeding and death, hypoplastic nasal structures
Hyperthermia	Spina bifida
Lithium	Ebstein's anomaly, macrosomia
6-Mercaptopurine	Abortion
Methyl mercury	Minamata disease, microcephaly, deaf, blind, mental retardation
Methyltestoserone	Masculinization of female fetus
Misoprostol	Arthrogryposis, cranial neuropathies (Moebius), equinovarus
Norethindrome	Masculinization of female fetus
Penicillamine	Cutis laxa syndrome
Phenytonin	Congenital anomalies, IUGR, neuroblastoma, bleeding (vitamin K deficiency)
Polychlorinated biphenyls	Skin discoloration—thickening, desquamation, LBW, acne, developmental delay
Progesterone	Masculinization of female fetus
Quinine	Abortion, thrombocytopenia, deafness
17-α-ethinyl testosterone (Progestoral)	Masculinization of female fetus
Stilbestrol (diethylstilbestrol [DES])	Vaginal adenocarcinoma in adolescence
Streptomycin	Deafness
Tetracycline	Retarded skeletal growth, pigmentation of teeth, hypoplasia of enamel, cataract, limb malformations
Thalidomide	Phocomelia, deafness, other malformations
Toluene (solvent abuse)	Craniofacial abnormalities, prematurity, withdrawal symptoms, hypertonia
Trimethadione and paramethadione	Abortion, multiple malformations, mental retardation
Valproate	Spina bifida, impaired neurologic function
Vitamin D	Supravalvular aortic stenosis, hypercalcemia

IUGR = intrauterine growth retardation; LBW = low birthweight; CNS = central nervous system.

TABLE 92–4 Agents Acting on Pregnant Women That May Adversely Affect the Newborn Infant

Acebutolol—IUGR, hypotension, bradycardia

Acetazolamide—metabolic acidosis

Aminodarone—bradycardia, hypothyroidism

Anesthetic agents (volatile)—CNS depression

Adrenal corticosteroids—adrenocortical failure (rare)

Ammonium chloride—acidosis (clinically inapparent)

Aspirin—neonatal bleeding, prolonged gestation

Atenolol—IUGR, hypoglycemia

Blue cohosh herbal tea—neonatal heart failure

Bromides—rash, CNS depression, IUGR

Captopril, enalopril—transient anuric renal failure, oligohydramnios

Caudal—paracervical anesthesia with mepivacaine (accidental introduction of anesthetic into scalp of baby)—bradypnea, apnea, bradycardia, convulsions

Cholinergic agents (edrophonium, pyridostigmine)—transient muscle weakness

CNS depressants (narcotics, barbiturates, benzodiazepams) during labor—CNS depression, hypotonia

Cephalothin—positive direct Coombs' test reaction

Fluoxetine—possible transient neonatal withdrawal, hypertonicity, minor anomalies

Haloperidol—withdrawal

Hexamethonium bromide—paralytic ileus

Ibuprofen—oligohydramnios

Imipramine—withdrawal

Intravenous fluids during labor (e.g., salt-free solutions)—electrolyte disturbances, hyponatremia, hypoglycemia

Iodide (radioactive)—goiter

Iodides—neonatal goiter

Indomethacin—oliguria, oligohydramnios, intestinal perforation

Isoxsuprine—ileus, hypocalcemia, hypoglycemia, hypotension

Lead—reduced intellectual function

Magnesium sulfate—respiratory depression, meconium plug, hypotonia

Methimazole—goiter, hypothyroidism

Morphine and its derivatives (addiction)—withdrawal symptoms (poor feeding, vomiting, diarrhea, restlessness, yawning and stretching, dyspnea and cyanosis, fever and sweating, pallor, tremors, convulsions)

Naphthalene—hemolytic anemia (in G6PD-deficient infants)

Nitrofurantoin—hemolytic anemia (in G6PD-deficient infants)

Oxytocin—hyperbilirubinemia, hyponatremia

Phenobarbital—bleeding diathesis (vitamin K deficiency), possible long-term reduction in IQ, sedation

Primaquine—hemolytic anemia (in G6PD-deficient infants)

Propranolol—hypoglycemia, bradycardia, apnea

Propylthiouracil (PTU)—goiter, hypothyroidism

Pyridoxine—seizures

Reserpine—drowsiness, nasal congestion, poor temperature stability

Silicone breast implants—possible esophageal dysmotility in breast-fed infants

Sulfonamides—interfere with protein binding of bilirubin; kernicterus at low levels of serum bilirubin, hemolysis with G6PD deficiency

Sulfonylurea—refractory hypoglycemia

Sympathomimetic (tocolytic-β agonist) agents—tachycardia

Thiazides—neonatal thrombocytopenia (rare)

IUGR = intrauterine growth retardation; CNS = central nervous system; G6PD = glucose-6-phosphate dehydrogenase.

phenylketonuria results in miscarriage, congenital malformations, and injury to the brain of the nonphenylketonuric fetus.

92.4 Maternal Medication and the Fetus

The effects of drugs taken by the mother vary considerably, especially in relation to the time in pregnancy when they are taken. Miscarriage or congenital malformations result from maternal ingestion of teratogenic drugs during the period of organogenesis. Maternal medications taken later, particularly during the last few weeks of gestation or during labor, tend to affect the function of specific organs or enzyme systems, adversely affecting the neonate rather than the fetus (Tables 92–3 and 92–4). Individual genetic makeup may determine susceptibility to some drugs. For example, phenytoin teratogenesis may be mediated by enzymatic production of epoxide metabolites determined by inheritance. In addition, the effects of drugs may be evident immediately in the delivery room or may be delayed, such as with the development of vaginal adenocarcinoma and genital lesions in adolescent female offspring of women exposed to diethylstilbestrol during pregnancy or childhood tumors following fetal alcohol or phenytoin exposure. Consumption of medications in pregnancy is frequent; surveys indicate that 90% of pregnant patients have taken at least one drug. The average mother has taken four drugs other than vitamins or iron during pregnancy; 4% have taken 10 drugs or more. Many are exposed to environmental agents such as solvents, pesticides, or hair products. In view of the limits of current knowledge of the fetal effects of maternal medication, no drugs should be prescribed during pregnancy without weighing the maternal need against the risk of fetal damage. All women should be specifically counseled to abstain from the use of alcohol, tobacco, or illicit drugs during pregnancy.

92.5 Identification of Fetal Disease

(Intrauterine Diagnosis) (see Table 92–1)

See 92.2 for a discussion of fetal distress.

Diagnostic procedures are used to identify fetal diseases when abortion is being considered, when direct fetal treatment is possible, or when a decision is made to deliver a viable but premature infant to avoid intrauterine fetal demise. Fetal assessment is also indicated in a broader context when the family, medical, or reproductive history of the mother suggests the presence of a high-risk pregnancy or a high-risk fetus (Chapters 91 and 92.3).

Various methods are used for identifying fetal disease (see Table 92–1). Fetal ultrasonographic imaging may detect fetal growth abnormalities (by biometric measurements of BPD, femur length, or head or abdominal circumference) or fetal malformations (Fig. 92–5). Although 95% of fetuses whose BPD is 9.5 cm or more are at least 37 wk of gestation, the lungs of these fetuses may not be mature. Serial determination

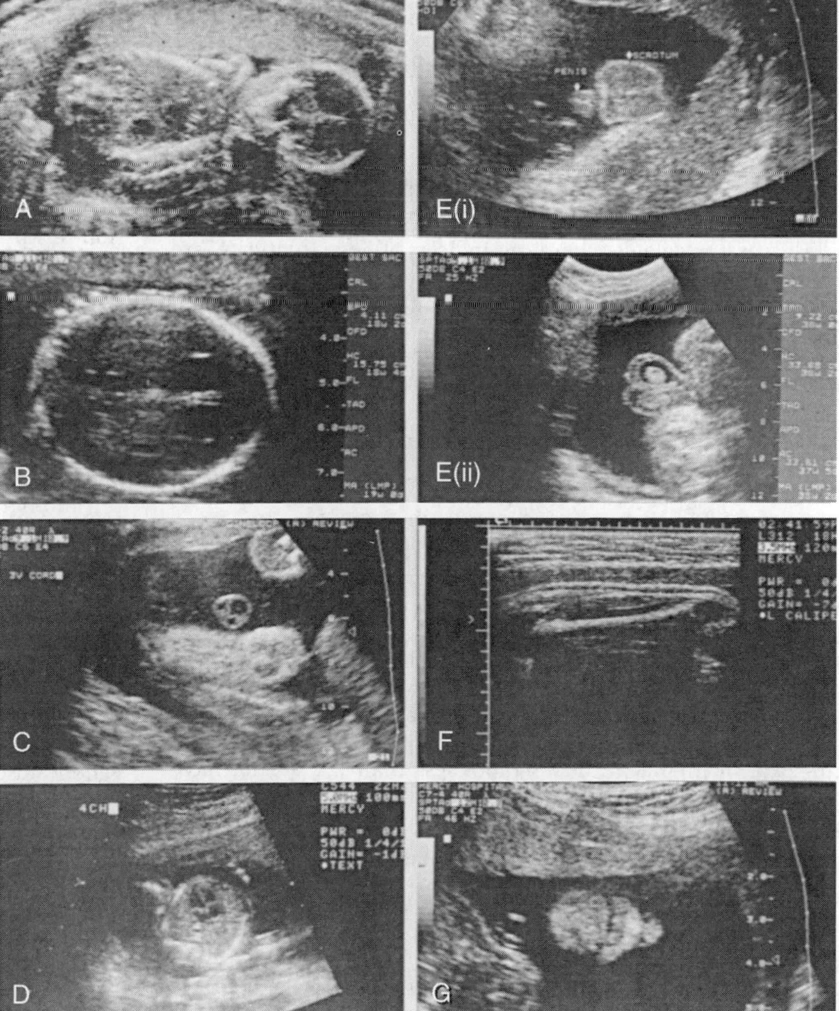

Figure 92–5 Assessment of fetal anatomy. *A,* Overall view of uterus at 24 wk showing a longitudinal section of the fetus and an anterior placenta. *B,* Transverse section at the level of the lateral ventricle at 18 wk showing *(right)* prominent anterior horns of the lateral ventricles on either side of the midline echo of the falx. *C,* Cross section of the umbilical cord showing that the lumen of the umbilical vein is much wider than those of the two umbilical arteries. *D,* Four-chambered view of the heart at 18 wk with equal-sized ventricles shown above equal-sized atria. *E,* (i) Normal male genitalia near term; (ii) hydrocele outlining testicle within scrotum projecting into a normal-sized pocket of amniotic fluid at 38 wk. Approximately 2% of male infants after birth have clinical evidence of a hydrocele that is often bilateral, not to be confused with subcutaneous edema occurring during vaginal breech birth. *F,* Section of thigh near term showing thick subcutaneous tissue (4.6 mm between markers) above the femur of a fetus with macrosomia. *G,* Fetal face viewed from below showing (from right to left) the nose, alveolar margin, and chin at 20 wk. (From Special investigative procedures. *In* Beischer NA, Mackay EV, Colditz PB (eds): Obstetrics and the Newborn, 3rd ed. Philadelphia, WB Saunders, 1997.)

of growth velocity and the head-to-abdominal circumference ratio enhances the ability to detect IUGR. Real-time ultrasonography may identify placental abnormalities (abruptio placentae, placenta previa) and fetal anomalies such as hydrocephalus, anencephalus, spina bifida, duodenal atresia, diaphragmatic hernia, renal agenesis, bladder outlet obstruction, congenital heart disease, limb abnormalities, sacrococcygeal teratoma, cystic hygroma, omphalocele, gastroschisis, and hydrops (Table 92–5).

Real-time ultrasonography also facilitates performance of *cordocentesis* and the BPP by imaging fetal breathing, body movements, tone, and amniotic fluid volume (see Table 92–2). *Doppler velocimetry* assesses fetal arterial blood flow (vascular resistance) (see Figs. 92–2 and 92–3). Roentgenographic examination of the fetus has been replaced by real-time ultrasonography and fetoscopy.

Amniocentesis, the transabdominal withdrawal of amniotic fluid during pregnancy for diagnostic purposes (see Table 92–1), is frequently done to determine the timing of the delivery of fetuses with erythroblastosis fetalis or the need for a fetal transfusion. It is also done for genetic indications, usually between the 15th and 16th gestational weeks, with results available within 1–2 wk. The most common indication for genetic amniocentesis is advanced maternal age (risk for chromosome abnormality at age 21 is 1/526 vs at age 49, 1/8). The amniotic fluid may be directly analyzed for amino acids, enzymes, hormones, and abnormal metabolic products; and amniotic fluid cells may be cultivated to permit detailed cytologic analysis for prenatal detection of chromosomal abnormalities and DNA-gene or enzymatic analysis for the detection of inborn metabolic errors. Analysis of amniotic fluid may also help in identifying neural tube defects (elevation of α-fetoprotein), adrenogenital syndrome (elevation of 17-ketosteroids and pregnanetriol), and thyroid dysfunction. Chorionic villus biopsy (transvaginal or transabdominal) performed in the 1st trimester also provides fetal cells but may pose a slightly increased risk for fetal loss or limb reduction defects. Cell sorting methods plus polymerase chain reaction techniques on fetal cells in a mother's circulation may eliminate the need for amniocentesis or chorionic villus biopsy.

The best available chemical indices of fetal maturity are provided by determinations of amniotic fluid creatinine and lecithin, which reflect the maturity of the fetal kidneys and lungs, respectively. Lecithin (L) is produced in the lungs by type II alveolar cells and eventually reaches the amniotic fluid via the effluent from the trachea. Until the middle of the 3rd trimester, its concentration nearly equals that of sphingomyelin (S); thereafter, S remains constant in amniotic fluid while L increases. By 35 wk, on the average, the L/S ratio is about 2:1, indicating lung maturity.

Earlier lung maturation may occur when there is severe premature separation of the placenta, premature rupture of the fetal membranes, narcotic addiction, or maternal hypertensive and renal vascular disease. A delay in pulmonary maturation may be associated with hydrops fetalis or maternal diabetes without vascular disease. The likelihood of hyaline membrane disease is greatly reduced with L/S ratios of 2:1 or more, although hypoxia, acidosis, and hypothermia may increase the risk despite this "mature" L/S ratio. However, 20–25% of infants with L/S ratios less than 2:1 do not have hyaline membrane disease. Maternal and fetal blood have an L/S ratio of about 1:4; thus, contamination will not alter the significance of a ratio of 2:1 or more. Meconium contamination, storage, and centrifugation all may reduce the reliability of the L/S ratio.

A determination of saturated phosphatidylcholine (L) or phosphatidylglycerol (PG) concentrations in amniotic fluid may be more specific and sensitive predictors of pulmonary maturity, especially in high-risk pregnancies such as those occurring in women with diabetes (see Chapters 97 and 103).

Although amniocentesis can be carried out with little discomfort to the mother, there is, even in experienced hands, a small risk of direct damage to the fetus, of placental puncture and bleeding with secondary damage to the fetus, of stimulating uterine contraction and premature labor, of amnionitis, and of maternal sensitization to fetal blood. The earlier in gestation amniotic puncture is done, the greater the risk to the fetus. The risks can be reduced by using ultrasound for placental and fetal localization. The procedure should be limited to those cases in which the potential benefits of the findings will outweigh the risk.

Cordocentesis, or percutaneous umbilical blood sampling (PUBS), is used to diagnose fetal hematologic abnormalities, genetic disorders, infections, and fetal acidosis (see Table 92–1). Under direct ultrasonographic visualization, a long needle is passed into the umbilical vein at its entrance to the placenta or fetal abdominal wall. Blood may be withdrawn to determine fetal hemoglobin, platelet concentration, lymphocyte DNA, or $Pa{O_2}$, pH, $P{CO_2}$, and lactate levels. Transfusion or administration of drugs can be given through the umbilical vein (Table 92–6).

92.6 Treatment and Prevention of Fetal Disease

Management of fetal diseases continues to depend on coordinated advances in accuracy of diagnosis and knowledge of the disease's natural history; understanding of fetal nutrition, pharmacology, immunology, and pathophysiology; availability of antimicrobial and antiviral drugs; and therapeutic procedures. Progress in providing specific treatments for accurately diagnosed diseases has improved with the advent of real-time ultrasonography and cordocentesis (see Tables 92–1 and 92–6).

The incidence of sensitization of Rh negative women by Rh-positive fetuses has been reduced by prophylactic administration of Rh(D) immunoglobulin to mothers early in pregnancy and after each delivery or abortion, thus reducing the frequency of hemolytic disease in their subsequent offspring. Fetal erythroblastosis (Chapter 99) may now be accurately diagnosed by amniotic fluid analysis and treated with intrauterine intraperitoneal or intravenous transfusions of packed Rh-negative blood cells to maintain the fetus until it is mature enough to have a reasonable chance of survival.

Fetal hypoxia or distress may now be diagnosed with moderate success. Treatment, however, remains limited to supplying the mother with high concentrations of oxygen, positioning the uterus to avoid vascular compression, and initiating operative delivery before severe fetal injury occurs.

Pharmacologic approaches to fetal immaturity (e.g., administration of steroids to the mother to accelerate fetal lung maturation and to decrease the incidence of respiratory distress syndrome [Chapter 97] in prematurely delivered infants) are successful. Inhibiting labor with β-sympathomimetic tocolytic agents is unfortunately not successful in most patients with premature labor. Management of definitively diagnosed fetal genetic disease or congenital anomalies consists of parental counseling or abortion; rarely, high-dose vitamin therapy for a responsive inborn error of metabolism (e.g., biotin-dependent disorders) or fetal transfusion (with red blood cells or platelets) may be indicated. Fetal surgery (see Table 92–6) remains an experimental approach to therapy and is available only in a few highly specialized perinatal centers. The nature of the defect and its consequences, as well as the ethical implications for the fetus and the parents, must be considered.

TABLE 92–5 Significance of Fetal Ultrasonographic Anatomic Findings

Prenatal Observation	Definition	Differential Diagnosis	Significance	Postnatal Evaluation
Dilated cerebral ventricles	Ventriculomegaly ≥ 10 mm	Hydrocephalus Hydrancephalus Dandy-Walker cyst Agenesis of corpus callosum	Transient isolated ventriculomegaly common and benign. Persistent or progressive more worrisome. Identify associated cranial and extracranial anomalies	Serial head US or CT. Evaluate for extracranial anomalies
Choroid plexus cysts	1–3% incidence Size ~ 10 mm: unilateral or bilateral	Abnormal karyotype (trisomy 18, 21). Aneuploidy risk 1 : 100 if isolated. ↑ risk (1 : 3) with other anomalies. Risk ↑ if large, complex, or bilateral cysts or advanced maternal age	Often isolated, benign; resolves by 24–28 wk. Examine for other organ anomalies then amniocentesis for karyotype	Head US or CT. Examine for extracranial anomalies; karyotype if indicated
Nuchal pad thickening	≥ 6 mm at 15–20 wk; cystic hygroma	Trisomy 21, 18 Turner's syndrome (XO) Nonchromosomal syndromes Normal (~25%)	~50% have chromosome abnormalities Amniocentesis for karyotype	Evaluate for multiple organ malformations; karyotype if indicated
Dilated renal pelvis	Pyelectasis ≥ 5 to 10 mm 0.6–1% incidence	UPJ obstruction Vesicoureteral reflux Posterior ureteral valves Etopic ureterocele Large-volume nonobstruction	Often "physiologic" and transient. Reflux is common. If > 10 mm or with caliectasis, consider pathologic cause. Large bladder consider posterior urethral valves, megacystic syndrome.	Repeat US; VCUG, prophylactic antibiotics
Echogenic bowel	0.6% incidence	Cystic fibrosis; meconium peritonitis; trisomy 21 or 18; other chromosomal abnormalities CMV, toxoplasmosis. GI obstruction	Often normal (65%) 10% have CF 1.5% have aneuploidy	Sweat chloride and DNA testing Karyotype Surgery for obstruction TORCH evaluation
Stomach appearance	Small or absent, or double bubble	Upper GI obstruction (esophageal atresia) Double bubble signifies duodenal atresia Abnormal karyotype Polyhydramnios Stomach in chest signifies diaphragmatic hernia	Must also consider neurologic disorders that reduce swallowing. >30% with double bubble have trisomy 21	Chromosomes, KUB if indicated, upper GI, neurologic evaluation

UPJ = ureteropelvic junction; CMV = cytomegalovirus; GI = gastrointestinal; CF = cystic fibrosis; US = ultrasonography; CT = computed tomography; VCUG = voiding cystourethrogram; TORCH = toxoplasmosis, other, rubella, CMV, herpes simplex; KUB = kidney, ureter, and bladder.

TABLE 92–6 Fetal Therapy

Disorder	Possible Treatment
Hematology	
Anemia with hydrops (erythroblastosis fetalis)	Umbilical vein packed red blood cell transfusion
Thalassemia	Fetal stem cell transplantation
Thrombocytopenia	
Isoimmune	Umbilical vein platelet transfusion, maternal intravenous immunoglobulin
Autoimmune (ITP)	Maternal steroids and intravenous immunoglobulin
Chronic granulomatous disease	Fetal stem cell transplantation
Metabolic-Endocrine	
Maternal PKU	Phenylalanine restriction
Fetal galactosemia	Galactose-free diet (?)
Multiple carboxylase deficiency	Biotin if responsive
Methylmalonic acidemia	Vitamin B_{12} if responsive
21-Hydroxylase deficiency	Dexamethasone
Maternal diabetes mellitus	Tight insulin control during pregnancy, labor, and delivery
Fetal goiter	Maternal hyperthyroidism—maternal propylthiouracil Fetal hypothyroidism—intra-amniotic T_4
Fetal Distress	
Hypoxia	Maternal oxygen, position
Intrauterine growth retardation	Maternal oxygen, position, improve nutrition if deficient
Oligohydramnios, premature rupture of membranes with variable deceleration	Amnioinfusion (antepartum and intrapartum)
Polyhydramnios	Amnioreduction (serial), indomethacin (if due to ↑ urine output) if indicated
Supraventricular tachycardia	Maternal digoxin,* flecainide, procainamide, amiodarone, quinidine
Lupus anticoagulant	Maternal aspirin, prednisone
Meconium stained fluid	Amnioinfusion
Congenital heart block	Dexamethasone, pacemaker (with hydrops)
Premature labor	Sympathomimetics, magnesium sulfate, antibiotics
Respiratory	
Pulmonary immaturity	Dexamethasone
Bilateral chylothorax—pleural effusions	Thoracentesis, pleuroamniotic shunt
***Congenital Abnormalities*†**	
Neural tube defects	Folate, vitamins (prevention)
Diaphragmatic hernia	Surgery (correction or plug therapy) (?)
Obstructive uropathy (with oligohydramnios without renal dysplasia)	> 24 wk < 32 wk, vesicoamniotic shunt plus amniofusion
Cystic adenomatoid malformation (with hydrops)	Pleuroamniotic shunt or resection
Infectious Disease	
Group B streptococcus	Ampicillin, penicillin (prevention)
Chorioamnionitis	Antibiotics
Toxoplasmosis	Spiramycin, pyrimethamine, sulfadiazine, and folic acid
Syphilis	Penicillin
Tuberculosis	Antituberculosis drugs
Lyme disease	Penicillin, ceftriaxone
Parvovirus	Intrauterine red blood cell transfusion for hydrops, severe anemia
Chlamydia trachomatis	Erythromycin
HIV-AIDS	Zidovudine (AZT) plus protease inhibitors
Cytomegalovirus	Ganciclovir by umbilical vein
Other	
Nonimmune hydrops (anemia)	Umbilical vein packed red blood cell transfusion
Narcotic abstinence (withdrawal)	Maternal low-dose methadone
Severe combined immunodeficiency disease	Fetal stem cell transplantation
Sacrococcygeal teratoma (with hydrops)	In utero resection, or vessel obliteration
Twin-twin transfusion syndrome	Repeated amniocentesis, YAG-laser photocoagulation of shared vessels
Twin reversed arterial perfusion syndrome (TRAP)	Digoxin, indomethacin, cord occlusion
Multifetal gestation	Selective reduction

(?) Denotes possible but not proved efficacy.

**Drug of choice (may require percutaneous umbilical cord sampling and umbilical vein administration if hydrops is present). Most drug therapy is given to the mother, with subsequent placental passage to the fetus.*

†Detail fetal ultrasonography is needed to detect other anomalies; karyotype is also indicated.

Aronson M, Hagberg B, Gillberg C: Attention deficits and autistic spectrum problems in children exposed to alcohol during gestation: A follow-up study. Dev Med Child Neurol 39:583, 1997.

Arduini D, Rizzo G, Romanini C: The development of abnormal heart rate patterns after absent end-diastolic velocity in umbilical artery: Analysis of risk factors. Am J Obstet Gynecol 168:43, 1993.

Caritis S, Sibai B, Hauth J, et al: Low-dose aspirin to prevent preclampsia in women at high risk. N Engl J Med 338:701, 1998.

Committee on Genetics: Folic acid for the prevention of neural tube defects. Pediatrics 92:493, 1993.

Crombleholme TM: Invasive fetal therapy: Current status and future directions. Semin Perinatol 18:385, 1994.

D'Alton ME: Prenatal diagnostic procedures. Semin Perinatol 18:140, 1994.

Dudley JA, Haworth JM, McGraw ME, et al: Clinical relevance and implications of antenatal hydronephrosis. Arch Dis Child 76:F31, 1997.

Elias S, Emerson DS, Simpson JL, et al: Ultrasound-guided fetal skin sampling for prenatal diagnosis of genodermatoses. Obstet Gynecol 83:337, 1994.

Ewigman BG, Crane JP, Frigoletto FD, et al: Effect of prenatal ultrasound screening on perinatal outcome. N Engl J Med 329:821, 1993.

Flake AW, Zanjani ED: In utero hematopoietic stem cell transplantation. JAMA 278:932, 1997.

Kimber C, Spitz L, Cuschieri A: Current state of antenatal in utero surgical interventions. Arch Dis Child 76:F134, 1997.

Linder N, Davidovitch N, Reichman B, et al: Topical iodine-containing antiseptics and subclinical hypothyroidism in preterm infants. J Pediatr 131:434, 1997.

Lockwood CJ, Wein R, Lapinski R, et al: The presence of cervical and vaginal fetal fibronectin predicts preterm delivery in an inner-city obstetric population. Am J Obstet Gynecol 169:798, 1993.

Lynch A, Marlar R, Murphy J, et al: Antiphospholipid antibodies in predicting adverse pregnancy outcome. A prospective study. Ann Intern Med 120:470, 1994.

MacDonald W, Newnham J, Gurrin L, et al: Effect of frequent prenatal ultrasound on birthweight: Follow-up at 1 year of age. Lancet 348:482, 1996.
Machover Reinisch J, Sanders SA, Mortensen EK, et al: In utero exposure to phenobarbital and intelligence deficits in adult men. JAMA 274:1518, 1995.
Manning FA, Snijders R, Harman CR, et al: Fetal biophysical profile score. VI. Correlation with antepartum umbilical venous fetal pH. Am J Obstet Gynecol 169:755, 1993.
McDonnell M, Serra-Serra V, Gaffney G, et al: Neonatal outcome after pregnancy complicated by abnormal velocity waveforms in the umbilical artery. Arch Dis Child 70:F84, 1994.
Mercer BM, Miodovnik M, Thurnau GR, et al: Antibiotic therapy for reduction of infant morbidity after preterm premature rupture of the membranes. JAMA 278:989, 1997.
Neilson JP: Assessment of fetal nuchal translucency test for Down's syndrome. Lancet 350:754, 1997.
Nulman I, Rovet J, Stewart DE, et al: Neurodevelopment of children exposed in utero to antidepressant drugs. N Engl J Med 336:258, 1997.
Pearson MA, Hoyme HE, Seaver LH, et al: Toluene embryopathy: Delineation of the phenotype and comparison with fetal alcohol syndrome. Pediatrics 93:211, 1994.
Pleet H, Graham J, Smith D: Central nervous system and facial defects associated with maternal hyperthermia at 4–14 wk gestation. Pediatrics 67:785, 1981.
Quintero RA, Johnson MP, Romero R, et al: In-utero percutaneous cystoscopy in the management of fetal lower obstructive uropathy. Lancet 346:537, 1995.
Schwartz LB: Understanding human parturition. Lancet 350:1792, 1997.
Simpson JL, Elias S: Isolating fetal cells from maternal blood. Advances in prenatal diagnosis through molecular technology. JAMA 270:2357, 1993.
Tejani N, Maran LI, Bhakthavathsalan A, et al: Correlation of fetal heart rate–uterine contraction patterns with fetal scalp blood pH. Obstet Gynecol 46:392, 1975.
Theion ATA, Soothill P: Antenatal invasive therapy. Eur J Pediatr 157:52, 1998.
van Wijk IJ, van Vugt JMG, Mulders MAM, et al: Enrichment of fetal trophoblast cells from the maternal peripheral blood followed by detection of fetal deoxyribonucleic acid with a nested X/Y polymerase chain reaction. Am J Obstet Gynecol 174:871, 1996.
Weiner CP, Williamson RA: Evaluation of severe growth retardation using cordocentesis-hematologic and metabolic alterations by etiology. Obstet Gynecol 73:225, 1989.

92.7 Teratogens

When an infant or child is malformed or mentally retarded, the parents often wrongly blame themselves and attribute the child's problems to events that occurred during pregnancy. Because infections occur and several drugs are often taken during many pregnancies, the pediatrician must evaluate the presumed viral infections and the drugs ingested to help parents understand their child's birth defect. The causes of approximately 40% of congenital malformations are unknown. Although only a relatively few agents teratogenic in humans are recognized (see Tables 91–2, 91–3, 92–3, and 92–4), new agents continue to be identified. Overall, only 10% of anomalies are due to recognizable teratogens. The time of exposure is usually less than 60 days of gestation during organogenesis. Specific agents produce predictable lesions. For some there is a dose or threshold effect; below the threshold, no alterations of growth, function, or structure occur. The agent's effects may be species specific. Genetic variables such as the presence of specific enzymes may metabolize a benign agent into a more toxic-teratogenic form (phenytoin conversion to its epoxide). In many circumstances, the same agent and dose may not consistently produce the lesion.

Reduced enzyme activity of the folate methylation pathway, particularly the formation of 5-methyltetrahydrofolate, may be responsible for neural tube or other birth defects. The common thermolabile mutation of 5,10-methylene tetrahydrofolate reductase may be one of the responsible enzymes. Folate supplementation for all pregnant women (by direct fortification of cereal grains—mandatory in the United States) during organogenesis may overcome this genetic enzyme defect, thus reducing the incidence of neural tube defects.

Mechanisms of teratogenesis include cell death without reparative regeneration; mitotic delay; delayed differentiation; physical or vascular constraining; reduced histogenesis secondary to cell depletion, necrosis, calcification, or scarring; inhibited cellular migration; and inflammation. Many mechanisms occur secondary to chromosomal or DNA damage and poor molecular repair.

The Food and Drug Administration classifies drugs in five pregnancy risk categories: *Category A* suggests no risk based on evidence from controlled human trials. *Category B* suggests either no risk shown in animal studies but no adequate studies of humans or some risk in animal studies that are not confirmed by human studies. *Category C* is either definite risk shown in animal studies but no adequate human studies or no available data for animals or humans. *Category D* includes drugs with some risk but with a benefit that may exceed that risk for the treated life-threatening condition, such as streptomycin for tuberculosis. *Category X* is for drugs that are contraindicated in pregnancy on the basis of animal and human evidence and whose risk exceeds the benefits.

The specific mechanism of action is known or postulated for very few teratogens. Warfarin, an anticoagulant because it is a vitamin K antagonist, prevents carboxylation of γ-carboxyglutamic acid, which is a component of osteocalcin and other vitamin K–dependent bone proteins. The teratogenic effect on developing cartilage, especially nasal cartilage, appears to be avoided if the pregnant woman's treatment between weeks 6 and 12 of gestation is switched from warfarin to heparin. Hypothyroidism in the fetus may be caused by maternal ingestion of an excessive amount of iodides or of propylthiouracil; each interferes with the conversion of inorganic to organic iodides. Phenytoin may be teratogenic because of the accumulation of a metabolite as a result of deficiency of epoxide hydrolase.

Recognition of teratogens offers the opportunity for prevention of related birth defects. For example, if a pregnant woman is informed of the potentially harmful effects of alcohol on her unborn infant, she may be motivated to control this problem during pregnancy. A woman with insulin-dependent diabetes mellitus may significantly decrease her risk for having a child with birth defects by achieving good control of her disease *before* conception.

Ardinger HH, Atkin JF, Blackston RD, et al: Verification of the fetal valproate syndrome phenotype. Am J Med Genet 29:171, 1988.
Beckman DA, Brent RL: Mechanism of known environmental teratogens: Drugs and chemicals. Clin Perinatol 13:649, 1986.
Czeizel AE, Elek C, Gundy S, et al: Environmental trichlorfon and cluster of congenital abnormalities. Lancet 341:539, 1993.
Gonzalez C, Marquez-Dias M, Kim C, et al: Congenital abnormalities in Brazilian children associated with misoprostol misuse in the first trimester of pregnancy. Lancet 351:1624, 1998.
Jacobson SJ, Jones K, Johnson K, et al: Prospective multicentre study of pregnancy outcome after lithium exposure during first trimester. Lancet 339:530, 1992.
Jones KJ, Lacro RV, Johnson KA, et al: Pattern of malformations in the children of women treated with carbamazepine during pregnancy. N Engl J Med 320:1661, 1989.
Koch S, Jäger-Roman E, Lösche G, et al: Antiepileptic drug treatment in pregnancy: Drug side effects in the neonate and neurological outcome. Acta Paediatr 84:739, 1996.
Koren G, Pastuszak A, Ito S: Drugs in pregnancy. N Engl J Med 338:1128, 1998.
Kulin NA, Pastuszak A, Sage SR, et al: Pregnancy outcome following maternal use of the new selective serotonin reuptake inhibitors. JAMA 279:609, 1998.
Lammer EJ, Chen CT, Hoar RM, et al: Retinoic acid embryopathy. N Engl J Med 313:837, 1985.
Litsey SE, Noonan JA, O'Connor WN, et al: Maternal connective tissue disease and congenital heart block. N Engl J Med 312:98, 1985.
Molloy AM, Daly S, Mills JL, et al: Thermolabile variant of 5,10-methylenetetrahydrofolate reductase associated with low red cell folates: Implications for folate intake recommendations. Lancet 349:1591, 1997.
Newman CGH: The thalidomide syndrome: Risks of exposure and spectrum of malformations. Clin Perinatol 13:555, 1986.
Pauli RM, Lian JB, Mosher DF, et al: Association of congenital deficiency of multiple vitamin K-dependent coagulation factors and the phenotype of the warfarin embryopathy: Clues to the mechanism of teratogenicity of coumarin derivatives. Am J Hum Genet 41:566, 1987.
Stickler SM, Dansky LV, Miller MA, et al: Genetic predisposition to phenytoin-induced birth defects. Lancet ii:746, 1985.
US Department of Health and Human Services, Food and Drug Administration: Food standards: Amendment of the standards of identity for enriched grain products to require addition of folic acid. Federal Register 61:8781, 1996.
van der Put NM, van den Heuvel LP, Steegers-Theunissen RP, et al: Decreased

methylene tetrahydrofolate reductase activity due to the 677C T mutation in families with spina bifida offspring. J Mol Med 74:691, 1996.

92.8 Radiation (also see Chapter 718)

Accidental exposure of pregnant women to radiation is a common cause for anxiety among women, their families, and their physicians, usually about whether the fetus will have birth defects or genetic abnormalities. It is unlikely that exposure to diagnostic radiation will cause gene mutations; no increase in genetic abnormalities has been identified in the offspring exposed as unborn fetuses to the atomic bomb explosions in Japan in 1945.

A more realistic concern is whether the exposed human fetus will show birth defects or a higher incidence of malignancy. The recommended occupational limit of maternal exposure to radiation from all sources is 500 millirads (mrad) for the entire 40 wk of a pregnancy. See Chapter 718 for discussion of the gonadal exposure for the mother and the whole body exposure of the fetus. The limited data on human fetuses show that large doses of radiation (20,000–50,000 mrad) are harmful to the central nervous system, as evidenced by microcephaly, mental retardation, and IUGR.

Therapeutic abortion is often recommended when exposure exceeds 10,000 mrad. It is more likely that a human fetus will be exposed to 1,000–3,000 mrad, an amount not shown to cause malformations. Whether this level of fetal exposure is associated with an increased risk of developing childhood cancer or leukemia is controversial.

Brent R: The effects of embryonic and fetal exposure to x-ray, microwaves and ultrasound. Clin Perinatol 13:615, 1986.
The Effects on Populations of Exposure to Low Levels of Ionizing Radiation (BEIR Report). Washington, DC, National Academy of Sciences. National Research Council, November, 1972.
Griem ML, Meier P, Dobben GD: Analysis of the morbidity and mortality of children irradiated in fetal life. Radiology 88:347, 1967.

CHAPTER 93
The High-Risk Infant

Infants particularly at risk during the neonatal period should be identified as early as possible in order to decrease neonatal morbidity and mortality (see also Chapter 89). The term *high-risk infant* designates an infant who should be under close observation by experienced physicians and nurses. Approximately 9% of all births require special or neonatal intensive care. Usually needed for only a few days, such observations may last from a few hours to several months. Some institutions find it advantageous to provide a special or transitional care nursery for high-risk infants, often within the labor and delivery suite. This facility should be equipped and staffed similarly to a neonatal intensive care area, where well but high-risk term infants can be observed and cared for immediately after birth without being separated from their mothers. Infants in the high-risk category are listed in Table 93–1.

Examination of a fresh *placenta, cord,* and *membranes* may alert the physician to newborn infants at high risk. Fetal blood loss may be indicated by placental pallor, **retroplacental hematoma,** and tears of a velamentous cord or of chorionic blood vessels supplying succenturiate lobes. **Placental edema** and subsequent deficiency of immunoglobulin G in newborns may be associated with fetofetal transfusion syndrome, hydrops fetalis, congenital nephrosis, or hepatic disease. **Amnion nodosum** (granules on the amnion) and **oligohydramnios** are associated with pulmonary hypoplasia and renal agenesis, whereas small whitish **nodules** on the cord suggest a candidal infection. **Short cords** and noncoiled cords occur with chromosome abnormalities and omphalocele. **Chorioangiomas** are associated with prematurity, abruptio, polyhydramnios, and intrauterine growth retardation (IUGR). **Meconium staining** suggests asphyxia and the risk of pneumonia, and opacity of the fetal placental surface suggests infection. **Single umbilical arteries** are associated with an increased incidence of congenital abnormalities.

Many high-risk infants are born prematurely, are breech deliveries, have small weight for gestational age (SGA), have significant perinatal asphyxia, or are born with life-threatening

TABLE 93–1 High-Risk Infants

Demographic Social Factors
Maternal age <16 or >40 yr
Illicit drug, alcohol, cigarette use
Poverty
Unmarried
Emotional or physical stress
Past Medical History
Genetic disorders
Diabetes mellitus
Hypertension
Asymptomatic bacteriuria
Rheumatologic illness (SLE)
Long-term medication (see Tables 92–3 and 92–4)
Prior Pregnancy
Intrauterine fetal demise
Neonatal death
Prematurity
Intrauterine growth retardation
Congenital malformation
Incompetent cervix
Blood group sensitization, neonatal jaundice
Neonatal thrombocytopenia
Hydrops
Inborn errors of metabolism
Present Pregnancy
Vaginal bleeding (abruptio placentae, placenta previa)
Sexually transmitted diseases (colonization: herpes simplex, group B streptococcus), chlamydia, syphilis, hepatitis B
Multiple gestation
Preeclampsia
Premature rupture of membranes
Short interpregnancy time
Poly-oligohydramnios
Acute medical or surgical illness
Inadequate prenatal care
Familial or acquired hypercoagulable states
Labor and Delivery
Premature labor (<37 wk)
Postdates (>42 wk)
Fetal distress
Immature L/S ratio: absent phosphatidylglycerol
Breech presentation
Meconium-stained fluid
Nuchal cord
Cesarean section
Forceps delivery
Apgar score < 4 at 1 min
Neonate
Birthweight <2,500 or >4,000 g
Birth before 37 or after 42 wk of gestation
SGA, LGA growth status
Tachypnea, cyanosis
Congenital malformation
Pallor, plethora, petechiae

SLE = Systemic lupus erythematosus; SGA = small for gestational age; LGA = large for gestational age.

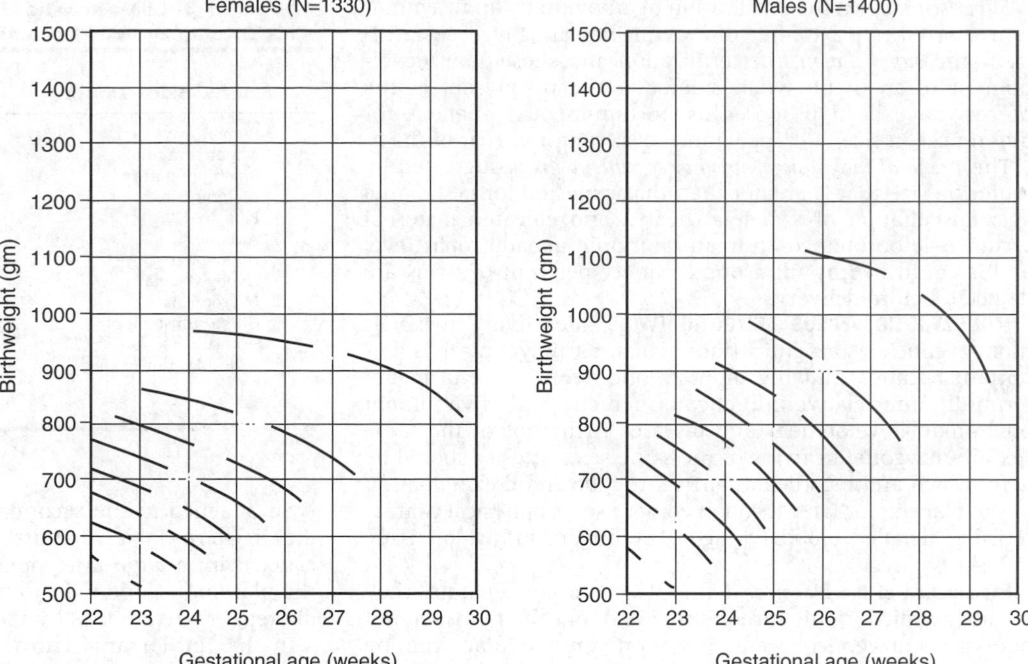

Figure 93–1 Estimated mortality by birthweight, gestational age, and gender. (From Fanaroff AA, Wright LL, Stevenson DK, et al: Very-low-birth-weight outcomes of the National Institute of Child Health and Human Development Neonatal Research Network, May 1991 through December 1992. Am J Obstet Gynecol 173:1423, 1995.)

congenital anomalies without exhibiting previously identified risk factors. Generally speaking, for any given duration of gestation, the lower the birthweight, the higher the neonatal mortality, and for any given weight, the shorter the gestational duration, the higher the neonatal mortality (Fig. 93–1). The highest risk of neonatal mortality occurs among infants who weigh less than 1,000 g at birth and whose gestation was less than 30 wk. The lowest risk of neonatal mortality occurs among infants with birthweights of 3,000–4,000 g whose gestational age was 38–42 wk. As birthweight increases from 500 to 3,000 g, a logarithmic decrease in neonatal mortality occurs; for every week increase in gestational age from the 25th to 37th wk, the neonatal mortality rate decreases by approximately one half. Nevertheless, approximately 40% of all *perinatal deaths* occur after 37 wk of gestation in infants weighing 2,500 g or more; many of these deaths occur in the period immediately before birth and are more readily preventable than those of smaller and more immature infants. In addition, neonatal mortality rates rise sharply for infants weighing over 4,000 g at birth and for those whose gestational period is 42 wk or longer. Because neonatal mortality largely depends on birthweight and gestational age, Figure 93–1 helps to identify high-risk infants quickly. However, this analysis is based on total live births and therefore describes the mortality risk only *at birth.* Because most neonatal mortality occurs within the first hours and days after birth, the outlook improves dramatically with increasing postnatal survival.

Amini SB, Catalano PM, Hirsch V, et al: An analysis of birth weight by gestational age using a computerized perinatal data base, 1975–1992. Obstet Gynecol 83:342, 1994.

Bateman DA, O'Bryan L, Nicholas SW, et al: Outcome of unattended out-of-hospital births in Harlem. Arch Pediatr Adolesc Med 148:147, 1994.

Brett KM, Schoendorf KC, Kiely JL: Differences between black and white women in the use of prenatal care technologies. Am J Obstet Gynecol 170:41, 1994.

Howell EM, Vert P: Neonatal intensive care and birth weight–specific perinatal mortality in Michigan and Lorraine. Pediatrics 91:464, 1993.

Strong TH, Finberg HJ, Mattox JH: Antepartum diagnosis of noncoiled umbilical cords. Am J Obstet Gynecol 170:1729, 1994.

Wigton TR, Tamura RK, Wickstrom E, et al: Neonatal morbidity after preterm delivery in the presence of documented lung maturity. Am J Obstet Gynecol 169:951, 1993.

Wolf EJ, Vintzileos AM, Rosenkrantz TS, et al: Do survival and morbidity of very-low-birth-weight infants vary according to the primary pregnancy complication that results in preterm delivery? Am J Obstet Gynecol 169:1233, 1993.

93.1 Multiple Pregnancies

INCIDENCE. The reported incidence of spontaneous twinning is highest among blacks and East Indians, followed by Northern European whites, and is lowest among the Asian races. Specific rates include Belgium, 1:56; American blacks, 1:70; Italy, 1:86; American whites, 1:88; Greece, 1:130; Japan, 1:150; and China, 1:300. Differences in the incidence of twins mainly involve fraternal (polyovular) dizygotic twins. Triplets are estimated to occur in 1 of 86^2 pregnancies and quadruplets in 1 of 86^3 pregnancies in the United States. The incidence of monozygotic twins is unaffected by racial or familial factors (3–5:1,000). The incidence of twins detected by ultrasonography at 12 wk of gestation (3–5%) is much higher than that occurring later in pregnancy; the vanishing twin syndrome results in a singleton fetus. Although the incidence of spontaneous multifetal gestation is stable, the overall incidence is increasing owing to the treatment of infertility with ovarian stimulants (clomiphene, gonadotropins) and in vitro fertilization. Twins represent about 2.5% of births but 20% of very low birthweight (VLBW) infants.

ETIOLOGY. The occurrence of monovular twins appears to be independent of genetic influences. Polyovular pregnancies are more frequent beyond the second pregnancy, in older women, and in families with a history of polyovular twins. They may result from simultaneous maturation of multiple ovarian follicles, but follicles containing two ova have been described as a genetic trait leading to twin pregnancies. Twin-prone women have higher levels of gonadotropins. Polyovular pregnancies occur in many women treated for infertility.

Conjoined twins (Siamese twins—incidence 1:50,000) probably result from relatively late monovular separation, as does the presence of two separate embryos in one amniotic sac. The latter condition has a high fatality rate that is due to obstruction of the circulation secondary to intertwining of the umbilical cords. The prognosis for conjoined twins depends on the possibility of surgical separation, which depends on the degree of sharing of vital organs. The site of connections varies: thoracoomphalopagus (28% of conjoined twins), thoracopagus (18%), omphalopagus (10%), craniopagus (6%), incomplete duplication (10%). Most conjoined twins are female.

Superfecundation, the fertilization of an ovum by an insemination that takes place after one ovum has already been fertilized, and *superfetation,* the fertilization and subsequent development of an ovum when a fetus is already present in the uterus, have been proposed as uncommon explanations for differences in size and appearance of certain twins at birth.

The *prenatal diagnosis of pregnancy with twins* is suggested by a uterine size that is greater than that expected for gestational age, auscultation of two fetal hearts, and elevated maternal serum α-fetoprotein or human chorionic gonadotropin level and is confirmed by ultrasound. Ninety per cent of twins are detected before delivery.

MONOZYGOTIC VERSUS DIZYGOTIC TWINS. Identifying twins as monozygotic or dizygotic (monovular or polyovular) is important because studying monozygotic twins is useful in determining the relative influence of heredity and environment on human development and disease. Twins not of the same sex are dizygotic. In twins of the same sex, zygosity should be determined and recorded at birth through careful examination of the placenta or later through comparison of physical characteristics, detailed blood typing, DNA fingerprinting, or tissue (HL-A) typing.

Examination of the Placenta. If the placentas are separate, they are always dichorionic (present in 75%), but the twins are not necessarily dizygotic, because initiation of monovular twinning at the first cell division or during the morula stage may result in two amnions, two chorions, and even two placentas. One third of monozygotic twins are dichorionic and diamniotic.

An apparently single placenta may be present with either monovular or polyovular twins, yet inspecting a polyovular placenta usually reveals that each twin has a separate chorion that crosses the placenta between the attachments of the cords and two amnions. Separate or fused dichorionic placentas may be disproportionate in size. The fetus attached to the smaller placenta or portion of placenta is usually smaller than its twin or is malformed. Monochorionic twins may be presumed to be monovular. They are usually diamnionic, and almost invariably, the placenta is a single mass.

Problems of twin gestation include polyhydramnios, hyperemesis gravidarum, preeclampsia, prolonged rupture of membranes, vasa previa, velamentous insertion of the umbilical cord, abnormal presentations (breech), and premature labor. Compared with the first-born twin, the second or B twin is at increased risk for respiratory distress syndrome and asphyxia. Twins are at risk for IUGR, twin-twin transfusion, and congenital anomalies that occur predominantly in monozygotic twins. Anomalies are due to uterine compression deformations from crowding (hip dislocation); vascular communication with embolization (ileal atresia, porencephaly, cutis aplasia) or without embolization (acardiac twin); and unknown factors that cause twinning (conjoined twins, anencephaly, meningomyelocele).

Placental vascular anastomoses occur with high frequency only in monochorionic twins. In monochorionic placentas, the fetal vasculature is usually joined, sometimes in a very complex manner. The vascular anastomoses in monochorionic placentas may be artery to artery, vein to vein, or artery to vein. They are usually well enough balanced so that neither twin suffers. Artery-to-artery communications cross over placental veins, and when anastomoses are present, blood can readily be stroked from one fetal vascular bed to the other. Vein-to-vein communications are similarly recognized and are less common. A combination of artery-to-artery and vein-to-vein anastomoses is associated with the lethal *acardiac fetus.* This rare lethal anomaly (1:35,000) is secondary to the TRAP sequence—twin reversed arterial perfusion. Neodymium:yttrium-aluminum-garnet (Nd:YAG) laser ablation of the anastomosis or cord occlusion in utero can treat heart failure of the surviving twin. In rare cases, one umbilical cord may arise from the other after leaving the placenta. In such cases, the twin attached to the secondary cord is usually malformed or dies in utero. Table 93–2 lists the more frequent changes associated with a large uncompensated arteriovenous shunt from the placenta of one twin to that of the other; twins of widely discrepant size are usually monochorionic.

TABLE 93–2 Characteristic Changes in Monochorionic Twins with Uncompensated Placental Arteriovenous Shunts

Twin on	
Arterial Side—Donor	**Venous Side—Recipient**
Prematurity	Prematurity
Oligohydramnios	Polyhydramnios
Small premature	Hydrops
Malnourished	Large premature
Pale	Well nourished
Anemic	Plethoric
Hypovolemia	Polycythemic
Hypoglycemia	Hypervolemic
Microcardia	Cardiac hypertrophy
Glomeruli small or normal	Myocardial dysfunction
	Tricuspid valve regurgitation
Arterioles thin walled	Right ventricle outflow obstruction
	Glomeruli large
	Arterioles thick walled

In the **fetal transfusion syndrome,** an artery from one twin acutely or chronically delivers blood that is drained into the vein of the other. The latter becomes plethoric and large, and the former is anemic and small. Generally, with chronicity there is a 5 g/dL hemoglobin and 20% body weight difference in this syndrome. Maternal hydramnios in a twin pregnancy suggests the fetal transfusion syndrome. Anticipating this possibility by preparing to transfuse the donor twin or to bleed the recipient twin may be lifesaving. Death of the donor twin in utero may result in generalized fibrin thrombi in the smaller arterioles of the recipient twin, possibly as the result of transfusion of thromboplastin-rich blood from the macerating donor fetus. The surviving twin may develop disseminated intravascular coagulation. Treatment of this highly lethal problem includes maternal digoxin, reductive amniocentesis for polyhydramnios, selective twin termination, or Nd:YAG laser or fetoscopic ablation of the anastomosis.

Postnatal Identification. *Physical criteria* for determining monovular twins are as follows: (1) Both must be of the same sex; (2) their features, including ears and teeth, must be obviously alike (but they need not resemble each other more than the lateral halves of one individual); (3) their hair must be identical in color, texture, natural curl, and distribution; (4) their eyes must be of the same color and shade; (5) their skin must be of the same texture and color (nevi may be differently apportioned and distributed); (6) their hands and feet must be of the same conformation and of similar size; and (7) their anthropometric values must show close agreement.

PROGNOSIS. Most twins are born prematurely, and maternal complications of pregnancy are more common than with single pregnancies. Although there is a significant increase in perinatal mortality among monochorionic twins, there is no significant difference between the neonatal mortality rates of twin and single births in comparable weight groups. Because most twins are premature by weight, their overall mortality is higher than that of single births. The perinatal mortality of twins is about four times that of singletons. Monoamniotic twins have an increased likelihood of entangling their cords, which may lead to asphyxia. Theoretically, the second twin is more subject to anoxia than the first because the placenta may separate after the birth of the first twin and before the birth of the second. In addition, the delivery of the second twin may be difficult because it may be in an abnormal presentation (breech, entangled), uterine tone may be decreased, or the cervix may begin to close after the first twin's birth. A growth-retarded twin is at high risk for hypoglycemia. Notable differences in size at birth of monovular twins usually disappear by the time the infants are age 6 mo. The mortality for multiple gestations with four or more fetuses is excessively high for each fetus. Because of this poor prognosis, selective fetal reduction (with transabdominal intrathoracic injection of KCl) to two to three fetuses has been offered as a treatment option.

TREATMENT. Prenatal diagnosis enables the obstetrician and the pediatrician to anticipate the birth of infants who are at high risk because of twinning. Close observation is indicated during labor and in the immediate neonatal period so that prompt treatment of asphyxia or fetal transfusion syndrome can be initiated. The decision to perform an immediate blood transfusion in a severely anemic "donor twin" or to perform a partial exchange transfusion of a "recipient twin" must be based on clinical judgment.

Albrecht JL, Tomich PG: The maternal and neonatal outcome of triplet gestations. Am J Obstet Gynecol 174:1551, 1996.

Cragan JD, Martin ML, Waters GD, et al: Increased risk of small intestinal atresia among twins in the United States. Arch Pediatr Adolesc Med 148:733, 1994.

D'Alton ME, Simpson LL: Syndromes in twins. Semin Perinatol 19:375, 1995.

Evans MI, Dommergues M, Wapner RJ, et al: Efficacy of transabdominal multifetal pregnancy reduction: Collaborative experience among the world's largest centers. Obstet Gynecol 82:61, 1993.

Lopriore E, Vandenbussche FPHA, Tiersma ESM, et al: Twin-to-twin transfusion syndrome: New perspectives. J Pediatr 127:675, 1995.

Luke B: The changing pattern of multiple births in the United States: Maternal and infant characteristics, 1973 and 1990. Obstet Gynecol 84:101, 1994.

93.2 Prematurity and Intrauterine Growth Retardation

DEFINITIONS. Liveborn* infants delivered before 37 wk from the first day of the last menstrual period are termed *premature* by the World Health Organization. *Premature* is also often used to denote immaturity. Infants of extremely low birthweight (ELBW) are less than 1,000 g. Historically, prematurity was defined by a birthweight of 2,500 g or less, but today infants who weigh 2,500 g or less at birth, *low birthweight* (LBW) *infants*, are considered to be premature with a shortened gestational period, to have IUGR for their gestational age (also referred to as *small for gestational age* [SGA]), or both. Prematurity and IUGR are associated with increased neonatal morbidity and mortality. Ideally, the definitions of low birthweight for individual populations should be based on data that are as genetically and environmentally homogeneous as possible. Figure 93–1 presents variations in neonatal mortality based on birthweight.

INCIDENCE. During 1997, 7.5% of liveborn neonates in the United States weighed less than 2,500 g; the rate for blacks was more than twice that for whites. Since 1981, the LBW rate has increased primarily because of an increased number of preterm births. Approximately 30% of LBW infants in the United States have IUGR and are born after 37 wk. At LBW rates greater than 10%, the contribution of IUGR increases and that of prematurity decreases. In developing countries, approximately 70% of LBW infants have IUGR. Infants with IUGR have a greater morbidity and mortality than appropriately grown gestational age-matched infants (see Fig. 93–1).

VERY LOW BIRTHWEIGHT INFANTS. VLBW infants weigh less than 1,500 g and are predominantly premature. In the United States in 1997, the VLBW rate was approximately 1.4%, 3.0% among blacks and 1.1% among whites. The VLBW rate is an accurate predictor of the infant mortality rate (relative risk of 93). VLBW infants account for over 50% of neonatal deaths and 50% of handicapped infants; their survival is directly related to birthweight, with approximately 20% of those between 500 and 600 g and 85–90% of those between 1,250 and 1,500 g surviving. The VLBW rate has remained unchanged for black Americans but has increased in whites, perhaps because of a rise in multiple births in whites. Perinatal care has improved the rate of survival of LBW infants. Compared with term infants, VLBW neonates have a higher incidence of rehospitalization during the 1st yr of life for sequelae of prematurity, infections, neurologic sequelae, and psychosocial disorders (see later discussion in this section on prognosis).

FACTORS RELATED TO PREMATURE BIRTH AND LOW BIRTHWEIGHT. It is difficult to completely separate factors associated with prematurity from those associated with IUGR (see also Chapters 90 and 91). A strong positive correlation exists between both premature birth and IUGR and low socioeconomic status. Families of low socioeconomic status have relatively high incidences of maternal undernutrition, anemia, and illness; inadequate prenatal care; drug addiction; obstetric complications; and maternal histories of reproductive inefficiency (relative infertility, abortions, stillbirths, premature or LBW infants). Other associated factors such as single-parent families, teenage pregnancies, close spacing of pregnancies, and mothers who have borne more than four previous children are also encountered more frequently. Systematic differences in fetal growth have also been described in association with maternal size, birth order, sibling weight, social class, maternal smoking habit, and other factors. The degree to which the variance in birthweights among various populations is due to environmental (extrafetal) rather than to genetic differences in growth potential is difficult to determine.

Premature birth of infants whose LBW is appropriate for their preterm gestational age is associated with medical conditions in which there is inability of the uterus to retain the fetus, interference with the course of the pregnancy, premature separation of the placenta, or an undetermined stimulus to effective uterine contractions before term (Table 93–3).

Overt or symptomatic (group B streptococci, *Listeria monocytogenes, Ureaplasma ureolyticum, Mycoplasma hominis, Chlamydia, Gardnerella vaginalis, Bacteroides* spp.) bacterial infection of the amniotic fluid and membranes (chorioamnionitis) may initiate

TABLE 93–3 Identifiable Causes of Preterm Birth

Fetal
- Fetal distress
- Multiple gestation
- Erythroblastosis
- Nonimmune hydrops

Placental
- Placental dysfunction
- Placenta previa
- Abruptio placentae

Uterine
- Bicornate uterus
- Incompetent cervix (premature dilation)

Maternal
- Preeclampsia
- Chronic medical illness (e.g., cyanotic heart disease, renal disease)
- Infection (e.g., *Listeria monocytogenes*, group B streptococcus, urinary tract infection, bacterial vaginosis, chorioamnionitis)
- Drug abuse (e.g., cocaine)

Other
- Premature rupture of membranes
- Polyhydramnios
- Iatrogenic

*Live birth is defined by the World Health Assembly (1950) as "the complete expulsion or extraction from its mother of a product of conception . . . which, after such separation, breathes or shows any other evidence of life such as beating of the heart, pulsation of the umbilical cord, or definite movement of the voluntary muscles, whether or not the umbilical cord has been cut or the placenta is attached." This definition is approved by the American Public Health Association.

TABLE 93–4 Factors Often Associated with Intrauterine Growth Retardation

Fetal

Chromosomal disorders (e.g., autosomal trisomies)
Chronic fetal infections (e.g., cytomegalic inclusion disease, congenital rubella, syphilis)
Congenital anomalies—syndrome complexes
Radiation
Multiple gestation
Pancreatic aplasia
Insulin deficiency
Insulin-like growth factor I deficiency

Placental

Decreased placental weight or cellularity or both
Decrease in surface area
Villous placentitis (bacterial, viral, parasitic)
Infarction
Tumor (chorioangioma, hydatidiform mole)
Placental separation
Twin transfusion syndrome

Maternal

Toxemia
Hypertension or renal disease or both
Hypoxemia (high altitude, cyanotic cardiac or pulmonary disease)
Malnutrition or chronic illness
Sickle cell anemia
Drugs (narcotics, alcohol, cigarettes, cocaine, antimetabolites)

TABLE 93–5 Problems of IUGR (SGA) Infants

Problem	Pathogenesis
Intrauterine fetal demise	Hypoxia, acidosis, infection, lethal anomaly
Perinatal asphyxia	↓ Uteroplacental perfusion during labor ± chronic fetal hypoxia-acidosis; meconium aspiration syndrome
Hypoglycemia	↓ Tissue glycogen stores, ↓ gluconeogenesis, hyperinsulinism, ↑ glucose needs of hypoxia, hypothermia, large brain
Polycythemia-hyperviscosity	Fetal hypoxia with ↑ erythropoietin production
Reduced oxygen consumption/hypothermia	Hypoxia, hypoglycemia, starvation affect, poor subcutaneous fat stores
Dysmorphology	Syndrome anomalads, chromosomal-genetic disorders, oligohydramnios-induced deformations, TORCH infection

Other problems include pulmonary hemorrhage and those common to the gestational age–related risks of prematurity if born <37 wk (see Table 93–6).
IUGR = intrauterine growth retardation; SGA = small for gestational age.

preterm labor. Bacterial products may stimulate local cytokine production (interleukin 6, prostaglandins), which may induce premature uterine contractions or a local inflammatory response with focal membrane rupture. Appropriate antibiotic therapy reduces the risk of fetal infection and may prolong gestation. The use of β-sympathomimetic receptor agonists (ritodrine, terbutaline) has not prevented premature birth. Other agents (indomethacin) have significant neonatal complications (necrotizing enterocolitis).

IUGR is associated with medical conditions that interfere with the circulation and efficiency of the placenta, with the development or growth of the fetus, or with the general health and nutrition of the mother (Table 93–4). Many factors are common to both prematurely born and LBW infants with IUGR.

IUGR may be a normal fetal response to nutritional or oxygen deprivation. Therefore, the issue is not the IUGR but rather the ongoing risk of malnutrition or hypoxia. Similarly, some preterm births signify a need for early delivery from a potentially disadvantageous intrauterine environment. IUGR is often classified as reduced growth that is symmetric (head circumference, length, and weight equally affected) or asymmetric (with relative head growth sparing) (see Fig. 92–1). Symmetric IUGR often has an earlier onset and is associated with diseases that seriously affect fetal cell number, such as conditions with chromosomal, genetic, malformation, teratogenic, infectious, or severe maternal hypertensive etiologies. Asymmetric IUGR is often of late onset, demonstrates preser-

Physical maturity	−1	0	1	2	3	4	5
Skin	Sticky, friable, transparent	Gelatinous, red, translucent	Smooth, pink, visible veins	Superficial peeling &/or rash, few veins	Cracking, pale areas, rare veins	Parchment, deep cracking, no vessels	Leathery, cracked, wrinkled
Lanugo	None	Sparse	Abundant	Thinning	Bald areas	Mostly bald	
Plantar surface	Heel–toe 40–50 mm:-1 <40 mm:-2	<50 mm, no crease	Faint red marks	Anterior transverse crease only	Creases on ant. 2/3	Creases over entire sole	
Breast	Imperceptible	Barely perceptible	Flat areola–no bud	Stripped areola, 1–2 mm bud	Raised areola, 3–4 mm bud	Full areola, 5–10 mm bud	
Eye/ear	Lids fused loosely (-1), tightly (-2)	Lids open, pinna flat, stays folded	Slightly curved pinna; soft; slow recoil	Well-curved pinna, soft but ready recoil	Formed & firm, instant recoil	Thick cartilage, ear stiff	
Genitals male	Scrotum flat, smooth	Scrotum empty, faint rugae	Testes in upper canal, rare rugae	Testes descending, few rugae	Testes down, good rugae	Testes pendulous, deep rugae	
Genitals female	Clitoris prominent, labia flat	Prominent clitoris, small labia minora	Prominent clitoris, enlarging minora	Majora & minora equally prominent	Majora large, minora small	Majora cover clitoris & minora	

Figure 93–2 Physical criteria for maturity. Expanded New Ballard Score (NBS) includes extremely premature infants and has been refined to improve accuracy in more mature infants. (From Ballard JL, Khoury JC, Wedig K, et al: New Ballard Score, expanded to include extremely premature infants. J Pediatr 119:417, 1991.)

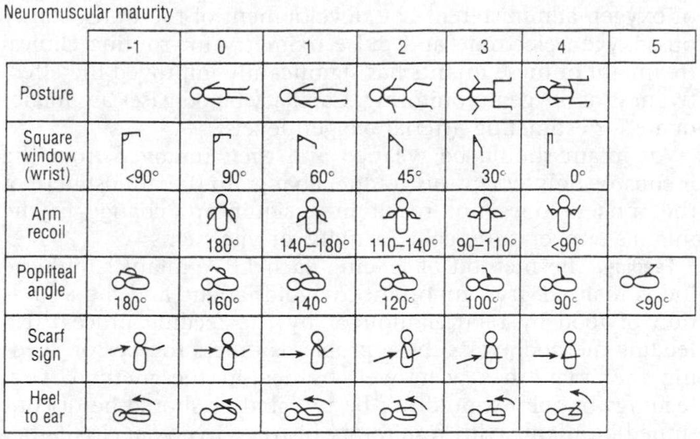

Neuromuscular maturity

	-1	0	1	2	3	4	5
Posture							
Square window (wrist)	<90°	90°	60°	45°	30°	0°	
Arm recoil		180°	140–180°	110–140°	90–110°	<90°	
Popliteal angle	180°	160°	140°	120°	100°	90°	<90°
Scarf sign							
Heel to ear							

Figure 93–3 Neuromuscular criteria for maturity. Expanded NBS includes extremely premature infants and has been refined to improve accuracy in more mature infants. (From Ballard JL, Khoury JC, Wedig K, et al: New Ballard Score, expanded to include extremely premature infants. J Pediatr 119:417, 1991.)

vation of Doppler waveform velocity to the carotid vessels, and is associated with poor maternal nutrition or late onset or exacerbation of maternal vascular disease (preeclampsia, chronic hypertension). Problems of infants with IUGR are noted in Table 93–5.

ASSESSMENT OF GESTATIONAL AGE AT BIRTH. Compared with a premature infant of appropriate weight, an infant with IUGR has a reduced birthweight and may appear to have a *disproportionately larger head relative to body size;* infants in both groups lack subcutaneous fat. In general, neurologic maturity (e.g., nerve conduction velocity) correlates with gestational age despite reduced fetal weight.

Maturity rating

Score	Weeks
-10	20
-5	22
0	24
5	26
10	28
15	30
20	32
25	34
30	36
35	38
40	40
45	42
50	44

Figure 93–4 Maturity rating as calculated by adding the physical and neurologic score, thus calculating the gestational age. (From Ballard JL, Khoury JC, Wedig K, et al: New Ballard Score, expanded to include extremely premature infants. J Pediatr 119:417, 1991.)

Physical signs may be useful in estimating gestational age at birth. Commonly used, the Ballard scoring system is accurate to ±2 wk (Figs. 93–2 to 93–4). An infant should be presumed to be at high risk of mortality or morbidity if a discrepancy exists between the estimation of gestational age by physical examination, the mother's estimated date of last menstrual period, and fetal ultrasonic evaluation.

SPECTRUM OF DISEASE IN LOW BIRTHWEIGHT INFANTS. Immaturity tends to increase the severity but reduce the distinctiveness of the clinical manifestations of most neonatal diseases. Immature organ function, complications of therapy, and the specific disorders that caused the premature onset of labor contribute to neonatal morbidity and mortality associated with premature, LBW infants (Table 93–6). Among VLBW infants, morbidity is inversely related to birthweight; respiratory distress syndrome

TABLE 93–6 Neonatal Problems Associated with Premature Infants

Respiratory

Respiratory distress syndrome—RDS (hyaline membrane disease—HMD)*
Chronic lung disease (bronchopulmonary dysplasia—BPD)*
Pneumothorax, pneumomediastinum; interstitial emphysema
Congenital pneumonia
Pulmonary hypoplasia
Pulmonary hemorrhage
Apnea*

Cardiovascular

Patent ductus arteriosus—PDA*
Hypotension
Hypertension
Bradycardia (with apnea)*
Congenital malformations

Hematologic

Anemia (early or late onset)
Hyperbilirubinemia—indirect*
Subcutaneous, organ (liver, adrenal) hemorrhage*
Disseminated intravascular coagulopathy
Vitamin K deficiency
Hydrops—immune or nonimmune

Gastrointestinal

Poor gastrointestinal function—poor motility*
Necrotizing enterocolitis
Hyperbilirubinemia—direct
Congenital anomalies producing polyhydramnios

Metabolic-Endocrine

Hypocalcemia*
Hypoglycemia*
Hyperglycemia*
Late metabolic acidosis
Hypothermia*
Euthyroid but low T_4 status

Central Nervous System

Intraventricular hemorrhage*
Periventricular leukomalacia
Hypoxic-ischemic encephalopathy
Seizures
Retinopathy of prematurity
Deafness
Hypotonia*
Congenital malformations
Kernicterus (bilirubin encephalopathy)
Drug (narcotic) withdrawal

Renal

Hyponatremia*
Hypernatremia*
Hyperkalemia*
Renal tubular acidosis
Renal glycosuria
Edema

Other

Infections* (congenital, perinatal, nosocomial: bacterial, viral, fungal, protozoal)

**Common.*

is noted in 90% of infants less than 750 g, 80% less than 1,000 g, 60% between 1,000 and 1,250 g, and 40% between 1,250 and 1,500 g; severe intraventricular hemorrhage (IVH) is noted in 25% less than 750 g, 16% between 750 and 1,000 g, 11% between 1,000 and 1,250 g, and 3% between 1,250 and 1,500 g. Overall, the risk of late sepsis (25%), chronic lung disease (18%), severe IVH (11%), necrotizing enterocolitis (5%), and prolonged hospitalization (45–125 days) is high in VLBW infants. Problems associated with IUGR LBW infants are noted in Table 93–5; those added problems are often superimposed on those noted in Table 93–6 if an infant with IUGR is also premature.

NURSERY CARE. At birth, the measures needed for clearing the airway, initiating breathing, caring for the cord and eyes, and administering vitamin K are the same in immature infants as in those of normal weight and maturity (Chapter 90). Special care is required to maintain a patent airway and avoid potential aspiration of gastric contents. Additional considerations are the need for (1) incubator care and heart rate and respiration monitoring, (2) oxygen therapy, and (3) special attention to the details of feeding. Safeguards against infection can never be relaxed. Everyone involved must be aware that routine procedures that disturb these infants may result in hypoxia. Finally, the need for regular and active participation by the parents in the infant's care in the nursery, the need to instruct the mother in at-home care of her infant, and the question of prognosis for later growth and development require special consideration.

Incubator Care. Modern incubators conserve body heat through provision of a warm atmospheric environment and standard conditions of humidity. They also may reduce atmospheric contamination if they are scrupulously cleaned. The survival of LBW and sick infants is greater when they are cared for at or near their *neutral thermal environment.* This is a set of thermal conditions, including air and radiating surface temperatures, relative humidity, and airflow, at which heat production (measured as oxygen consumption) is minimal and the infant's core temperature is within the normal range. It is a function of the size and postnatal age of an infant; larger, older infants require lower environmental temperatures than smaller, younger infants. The optimal incubator temperature for minimal heat loss and oxygen consumption for an unclothed infant is that which maintains the infant's core temperature at 36.5–37.0°C. This depends on an infant's size and maturity; the smaller and more immature the infant, the higher the environmental temperature required. A Plexiglas heat shield or head caps and body clothing may be required when incubator care alone is insufficient to keep a small premature infant warm. Radiant warmers are alternatives to incubators, especially for seriously ill neonates.

Maintaining a relative *humidity* of 40–60% aids in stabilizing body temperature by reducing heat loss at lower environmental temperatures; by preventing drying and irritation of the lining of respiratory passages, especially during administration of oxygen and following or during endotracheal intubation (usually 100% humidity); and by thinning viscid secretions and reducing insensible water loss from the lungs.

Administering *oxygen* to reduce the risk of injury from hypoxia and circulatory insufficiency must be balanced against the risks of hyperoxia to the eyes (retinopathy of prematurity) and oxygen injury to the lungs. Oxygen should be administered by a head hood, nasal cannula, continuous positive airway pressure apparatus, or endotracheal tube to maintain stable and safe inspired oxygen concentration. Although cyanosis, tachypnea, and apnea are definite clinical indications whose treatment should include only the amount of oxygen needed to eliminate these signs, the potential harm resulting from hypoxia or hyperoxia cannot be minimized without monitoring the oxygen tension of arterial blood (Pa_{O_2}) and, based on laboratory analysis, continuously readjusting the concentration of oxygen administered. The development of the transcutaneous oxygen electrode and pulse oximetry for routine clinical treatment of these infants has significantly improved the effectiveness of oxygen monitoring. Capillary blood gases are inadequate for estimating arterial oxygen levels.

An infant should be weaned and then removed from the incubator only when the gradual change to the atmosphere of the nursery does not result in a significant change in the infant's temperature, color, activity, or vital signs.

Feeding. The method of feeding each LBW infant should be individualized. It is important to avoid fatigue and the aspiration of food by regurgitation or by the feeding process. No feeding method averts these problems unless the person feeding the infant has been well trained in the method. Oral feedings (nipple) should not be initiated or should be discontinued in infants with respiratory distress, hypoxia, circulatory insufficiency, excessive secretions, gagging, sepsis, central nervous system depression, immaturity, or signs of serious illness. These infants require parenteral or gavage feedings to supply calories, fluid, and electrolytes.

Large premature infants can often be fed by bottle or at the breast. Because the effort of sucking is usually the limiting factor, breast-feeding is less likely to succeed until the infant matures. Bottle-feeding of expressed breast milk may be a temporary alternative. In *bottle-feeding,* effort may be reduced by use of special small, soft nipples with large holes. The process of oral alimentation requires, in addition to a strong suck, the coordination of swallowing, epiglottal and uvular closure of the larynx and nasal passages, and normal esophageal motility, a synchronized process that is usually absent before 34 wk gestation.

Smaller or less vigorous infants should be fed by *gavage*: A soft plastic tube of No. 5 French external and approximately 0.05 cm internal diameters with a rounded atraumatic tip and two holes on alternate sides is preferable. The tube is passed through the nose until approximately 2.5 cm (1 in) of the lower end is in the stomach. The free end of the tube has an adapter into which the tip of a syringe is fitted, and the measured amount of feeding is allowed to flow in slowly by gravity. Such tubes may be left in place for 3–7 days before being replaced by a similar tube through the alternate nostril. An infant occasionally has enough local irritation from an indwelling tube that he or she may gag or troublesome secretions may gather around it in the nasopharynx. In such cases, a catheter may be passed through the mouth by a skilled person and removed at the end of each feeding. Change to bottle- or breast-feeding may be instituted gradually as soon as an infant displays general vigor adequate for oral feeding without fatigue.

Continuous nasogastric and nasojejunal feedings have also been used successfully in LBW infants who are unable to ingest adequate calories by bottle or intermittent gavage owing to poor suck, uncoordinated swallowing, and delayed gastric emptying. Intestinal perforation has occurred during nasojejunal feedings.

Gastrostomy feeding is usually not indicated in premature infants because of an associated increase in mortality, except as an adjunct to surgical management of specific gastrointestinal conditions or in neurologically injured patients unable to feed. Partial or total *intravenous alimentation* for premature infants should not be used routinely as a substitute for oral or gavage feedings but only for situations in which the latter are contraindicated by an infant's condition.

INITIATION OF FEEDING. The main principle in feeding premature infants is to proceed cautiously and gradually. Careful early feeding of glucose or formula tends to reduce the risk of hypoglycemia, dehydration, and hyperbilirubinemia without the additional risk of aspiration, provided the presence of respiratory distress or other disorders does not present an indication for withholding oral feedings and administering electrolytes, fluids, and calories intravenously.

If an infant is well, is making sucking movements, and is in no distress, oral feeding may be attempted, although most infants weighing less than 1,500 g require tube feeding because they are unable to coordinate breathing, sucking, and swallowing. Intestinal tract readiness for feedings may be determined by active bowel sounds, passage of meconium, absence of abdominal distention or signs of peritonitis, and no bilious aspirates or emesis. For infants under 1,000 g, the initial feedings are either half- or full-strength breast milk or preterm formula at 10 mL/kg/24 hr as a continuous nasogastric tube drip (or given by intermittent gavage every 2–3 hr). If the initial feeding is tolerated, the volume is increased by 10–15 mL/kg/24 hr. The daily milk volume increment should not exceed 20 mL/kg/24 hr. Once a volume of 150 mL/kg/24 hr has been achieved, the caloric content may be increased to 24 or 27 kcal/oz. With high caloric density, infants are at risk for dehydration, edema, lactose intolerance, diarrhea, flatus, and delayed gastric emptying with emesis. Intravenous fluids are needed until feeds provide approximately 120 mL/kg/24 hr. The feeding protocol for premature infants weighing over 1,500 g is initiated at a volume of 20–25 mL/kg/24 hr of full-strength breast milk or preterm formula given as bolus feeds every 3 hr. Thereafter, total daily formula volume increments should not exceed 20 mL/kg/24 hr. The expected weight increments for premature infants of various birthweights are projected from Figure 93–5. Infants with IUGR may not demonstrate the initial weight loss noted in premature infants.

Regurgitation, vomiting, abdominal distention, or gastric residuals from prior feedings should arouse suspicion of sepsis, necrotizing enterocolitis, or intestinal obstruction; these are indications to drop back in the schedule and increase subsequent feedings slowly or to change to intravenous alimentation and to evaluate for more serious problems (Chapter 98.2). Weight gain may not be achieved for 10–12 days, and a daily intake of 130–150 mL/kg or more may be necessary for some infants. Alternatively, in vigorous infants whose feeding schedule is advanced successfully in calories or volume, weight gain may appear within a few days.

When tube feeding is used, the contents of the stomach should be aspirated before each feeding. If only air or small amounts of mucus are obtained, the feeding is given as planned. If all or a substantial part of the previous feeding is obtained, it is advisable to reduce the amount of the feeding and to proceed more gradually with subsequent increases.

The digestive enzyme systems of infants greater than 28 wk gestation are mature enough to permit adequate digestion and absorption of protein and carbohydrate. Fat is less well absorbed owing primarily to inadequate amounts of bile salt; unsaturated fats and the fat of human milk are absorbed better than those of cow's milk. Weight gain of infants weighing under 2,000 g at birth should be adequate when human milk or "humanized" milk (40% casein and 60% whey) with a protein intake of 2.25–2.75 g/kg/24 hr is fed. These two alternatives should provide all amino acids essential for premature infants, including tyrosine, cystine, and histidine. Higher protein intakes may be well tolerated and are generally safe, especially for older, rapidly growing infants. However, protein intake as high as 4.5 g/kg/24 hr may be hazardous: Although linear growth may be promoted, high-protein formulas may cause abnormal plasma aminograms; elevations in blood urea nitrogen, ammonia, and sodium concentrations; metabolic acidosis (cow's milk formulas); and untoward effects on neurologic development. Furthermore, the high protein and mineral contents of balanced cow's milk formulas of high caloric content constitute a large solute load for the kidneys, a fact important in maintaining water balance, especially in infants with diarrhea or fever.

Breast milk from the infant's mother is the preferred milk for all infants, including VLBW infants. Once a premature infant takes 120 mL/kg/24 hr, breast milk fortifiers may supplement breast milk with protein, calcium, and phosphorus, or if breast milk is unavailable, specialized premature formulas may be used. Premature formula should not be continued at the time of discharge or at approximately 34–36 wk gestational

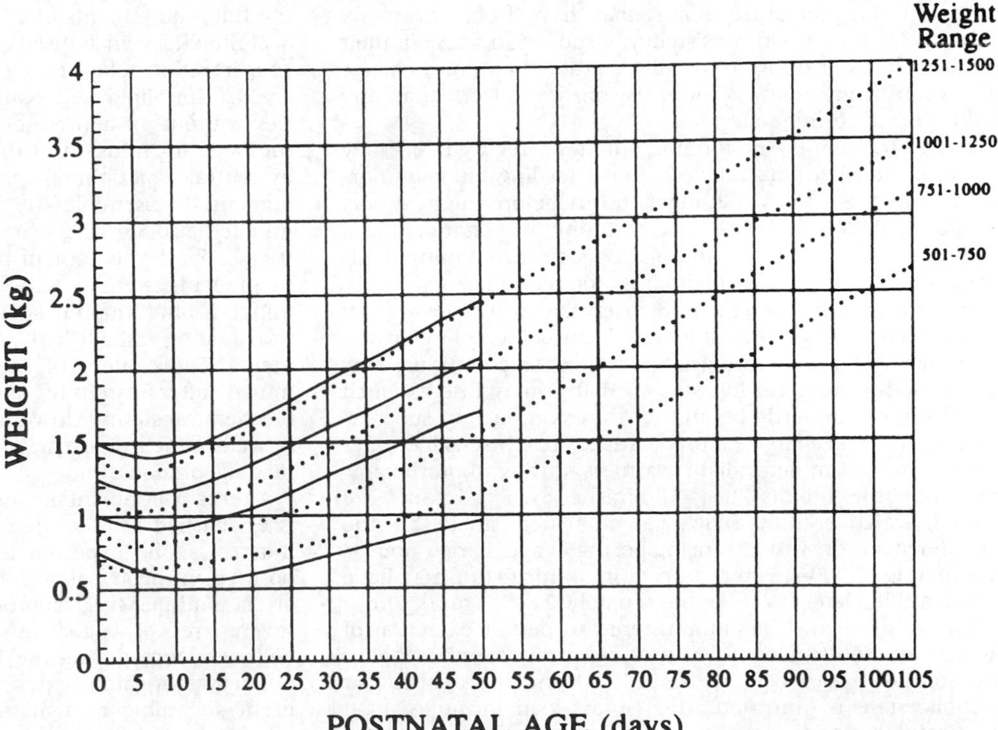

Figure 93–5 Average daily weight (grams) vs postnatal age (days) for infants with birthweight ranges 501–750 g, 751–1,000 g, 1,001–1,250 g, and 1,251–1,500 g *(dotted lines)*, plotted with the curves of Dancis et al. for infants with birthweights 750 g, 1,000 g, 1,250 g, and 1,500 g *(solid lines)*. (From Wright K, Dawson JP, Fallis D, et al: New postnatal growth grids for very low birth weight infants. Pediatrics 91:922, 1993.)

age (unless metabolic bone disease is present—see Chapter 102) because hypercalcemia may develop as a result of the formula's higher calcium and vitamin D levels.

Although formula in amounts necessary for adequate growth probably contains sufficient amounts of all vitamins, the volume of milk sufficient to satisfy requirements may not be ingested for several weeks. Therefore, LBW infants should be given supplemental vitamins. Because requirements for these infants have not been precisely established, the recommended daily allowances for term infants should be given (see Chapter 40). Furthermore, these infants may have a special need for certain vitamins. Intermediary metabolism of phenylalanine and tyrosine depends, in part, on vitamin C. Decreased fat absorption with increased fecal fat loss may be associated with decreased absorption of *vitamin D*, other fat-soluble vitamins, and calcium in premature infants. VLBW infants are particularly prone to develop rickets, but their total intake of vitamin D should not exceed 1,500 IU/24 hr. *Folic acid* is essential for the formation of DNA and production of new cells; serum and erythrocyte levels decrease in preterm infants during the first few weeks of life and remain low for 2–3 mo. Therefore, supplementation is recommended, though it does not result in improved growth or increased hemoglobin concentration. Deficiency of vitamin E is uncommon but is associated with increased hemolysis and, if severe, with anemia in premature infants. Vitamin E functions as an antioxidant to prevent peroxidation of excessive polyunsaturated fatty acids in red blood cell membranes; its need may increase because of the increased membrane content of these fatty acids from older formulas with high polyunsaturated fatty acids. Vitamin K deficiency is discussed in Chapter 99.4.

In LBW infants, physiologic anemia due to postnatal suppression of erythropoiesis is exacerbated by smaller fetal iron stores and greater expansion of blood volume resulting from a more rapid growth compared with that of term infants; therefore, the anemia develops earlier and reaches a lower ultimate level. Fetal or neonatal blood loss accentuates this problem. Iron stores, even in VLBW neonates, are usually adequate until an infant's birthweight has doubled or if an infant is treated with erythropoietin (Chapter 99); iron supplementation (2 mg/kg/24 hr) should then be started. Iron supplements should be started whenever an infant receives erythropoietin.

Properly fed premature infants may have from one to six daily stools of semisolid consistency; a sudden increase in their number, the appearance of occult or gross blood, or a change to a watery consistency is more reason for concern than any arbitrarily stated frequency.

Premature infants should not vomit or regurgitate. They should be satisfied and relaxed after a feeding but may normally show the activity of hunger shortly before the next one.

FLUID REQUIREMENTS. These vary according to gestational age, environmental conditions, and disease states. Assuming minimal water losses in stool of infants not receiving oral fluids, their water needs are equal to insensible water loss, renal solute excretion, growth, and any unusual ongoing losses. Insensible water loss is indirectly related to gestational age; very immature preterm infants (<1,000 g) may lose as much as 2–3 mL/kg/hr, partly because of thin skin, lack of subcutaneous tissue, and a large exposed surface area. Insensible water loss is increased under radiant warmers, during phototherapy, and in febrile infants. It is diminished when infants are clothed, are covered by a Plexiglas inner heat shield, breathe humidified air, or with advancing postnatal age. Larger premature infants (2,000–2,500 g) nursed in an incubator may have an insensible water loss of approximately 0.6–0.7 mL/kg/hr.

Fluids also need to be administered to permit excretion of the urinary solute load (e.g., urea, electrolytes, phosphate). The amount varies with dietary intake and the anabolic or catabolic state of nutrition. High-solute-load formulas, high protein intake, and catabolism increase the end products that require urinary excretion and thus increase the requirement for water. Renal solute loads may vary between 7.5 and 30 mOsm/kg. Newborn infants, especially those with VLBW, also are less able to concentrate urine; thus, their fluid intake required to excrete solutes increases.

Water intake in term infants is usually begun at 60–70 mL/kg on day 1 and increased to 100–120 mL/kg by days 2–3. Smaller, more premature infants may need to be started with 70–100 mL/kg on day 1 and advanced to 150 mL/kg or more by days 3–4. Fluid volumes should be titrated individually, although it is unusual to exceed 150 mL/kg/24 hr. Infants weighing less than 750 g in the first wk of life have immature skin and a large surface area, leading to a high rate of transepidermal fluid loss, at times requiring high rates of intravenous fluids (150–250 mL/kg/24 hr). Daily weights, urine output and specific gravity, and serum urea nitrogen with electrolytes should be monitored carefully to detect abnormal states of hydration, because clinical observations and physical examinations are poor indicators of the state of hydration of premature infants. Conditions that increase fluid losses, such as glycosuria, the polyuric phase of acute tubular necrosis, and diarrhea, may place additional strain on kidneys that have not yet developed their maximum capacity to conserve water and electrolytes, the results of which may be severe dehydration. Alternatively, fluid overload may lead to edema, heart failure, a patent ductus arteriosus, and chronic lung disease.

TOTAL PARENTERAL NUTRITION. When oral feeding is impossible for prolonged periods, total intravenous alimentation may provide sufficient fluid, calories, amino acids, electrolytes, and vitamins to sustain growth of LBW infants. This technique has been lifesaving for infants who have had intractable diarrheal syndromes or extensive bowel resection. Infusions may be administered through an indwelling central vein catheter or through a peripheral vein.

The goal of parenteral alimentation is to deliver enough nonprotein calories to allow an infant to use most of the protein for growth. The infusate should contain synthetic amino acids of 2.5–3 g/dL and hypertonic glucose in the range of 10–25 g/dL in addition to appropriate quantities of electrolytes, trace minerals, and vitamins. The initial daily infusion should deliver 10–15 g/kg/24 hr of glucose and increase gradually to 25–30 g/kg/24 hr when glucose alone is used to meet the full requirements of 100–120 nonprotein kcal/kg/24 hr. If a peripheral vein is used, it is advisable to keep the glucose concentration below 12.5 g/dL. Intravenous fat emulsions such as 20% Intralipid (2.2 kcal/mL) may be used to provide calories without an appreciable osmotic load, thereby decreasing the need for infusion of the higher concentrations of glucose by central or peripheral vein and usually preventing the development of essential fatty acid deficiency. Intralipid may be initiated at 0.5 g/kg/24 hr and advanced to 3–4 g/kg/24 hr, if triglyceride levels remain normal; 0.5 g/kg/24 hr is sufficient to prevent essential fatty acid deficiency. Electrolytes, trace minerals, and vitamin additives are included in amounts approximating established intravenous maintenance requirements. The content of each day's infusate should be determined after carefully assessing the infant's clinical and biochemical status. Slow and continuous infusion is advisable. A well-trained pharmacist using a laminar flow hood should mix all solutions.

After a caloric intake of greater than 100 kcal/kg/24 hr is established by total parenteral intravenous nutrition, LBW infants can be expected to gain about 15 g/kg/24 hr, with positive nitrogen balances of 150–200 mg/kg/24 hr, if there are no multiple surgical procedures, episodes of sepsis, or other severe stress. This goal usually can be achieved and the catabolic tendency during the 1st wk of life reversed with subsequent weight gains by peripheral vein infusions of 2.5 g/kg/24 hr of an amino acid mixture, 10 g/dL of glucose, and 2–3 g/kg/24 hr of Intralipid.

The complications of intravenous alimentation are related to both the catheter and the metabolism of the infusate. **Sepsis** is the most important problem of central vein infusions and can be minimized only by meticulous catheter care and aseptic preparation of the infusate. *Staphylococcus aureus, S. epidermidis,* and *Candida albicans* are the common infecting organisms. Treatment includes appropriate antibiotics. If an infection persists, the line must be removed. Thrombosis, extravasation of fluid, and accidental dislodgement of catheters have also occurred. Sepsis is rarely attributable to peripheral vein infusions, but phlebitis, cutaneous sloughs, and superficial infection occasionally occur. The **metabolic complications** include hyperglycemia from the high glucose concentration of the infusate, which may lead to an osmotic diuresis and dehydration; azotemia; possible increased risk of nephrocalcinosis; hypoglycemia from a sudden accidental cessation of the infusate; hyperlipidemia and possibly hypoxemia from intravenous lipid infusions; tissue accumulation of aluminum (a contaminant); and hyperammonemia, which may be due to high levels of certain amino acids. Cholestatic jaundice has also been noted. Hyperchloremic acidosis occurs in infants receiving synthetic amino acids unless there is an appropriate balance between cationic and anionic amino acids and salts. Abnormal elevations of blood amino acid levels are an additional potential hazard. If intravenous fat emulsions are not used, essential fatty acid deficiency may also occur. When the infusion is given through a peripheral vein, the osmolality of the solution may limit the length of time an infusion site can be used; at the same time, it may require greater volumes of fluid than can be tolerated. Continuous chemical and physiologic monitoring of infants receiving intravenous alimentation is indicated because of the frequency and seriousness of complications.

Intravenous Supplementation of Tolerated Oral Feedings. A combination of intravenous and gavage alimentation is the usual method of feeding preterm infants. Once an infant is stable (2nd–3rd day of life), small nasogastric milk feedings are supplemented with peripheral alimentation solutions. Initiation of enteric feeding is possible in the presence of an endotracheal tube and an umbilical artery catheter. Glucose, amino acid mixtures, and lipid emulsions may be infused into peripheral veins when sufficient calories cannot be provided to LBW infants by oral feeding alone. Increases in weight, length, and head circumference approaching those expected in utero have been achieved with mixtures of amino acids, glucose, and lipids. Although the complications of both techniques may occur, the combination of nutrient delivery methods allows smaller volumes of enteral feedings, thus decreasing the risk of aspiration. Provision of enteral calories reduces the incidence of cholestatic jaundice and rickets of prematurity.

PREVENTION OF INFECTION. Premature infants have an increased susceptibility to infection, which requires nursery personnel to wash rigorously hand to elbow before and after handling each infant, take measures to reduce contamination of food and objects coming in contact with the infant, prevent air contamination, avoid overcrowding, and limit direct and indirect contacts with themselves and other infants. No one with an infection should be permitted into the nursery. However, the risks of infection must be balanced against the disadvantages of limiting the infant's contacts with the family, which may be detrimental to the infant's ultimate development; early and frequent participation by parents in the nursery care of their infant does not significantly increase the risk when preventive precautions are maintained. Routine immunizations should be given on the regular schedule at standard doses (Chapter 301).

Preventing transmission of infection from infant to infant is difficult because often neither term nor premature newborn infants manifest clear clinical evidence of an infection early in its course. Universal precautions require gloves to be worn whenever blood or body fluids are handled. When epidemics occur within a nursery, cohort nursing and isolation rooms should be used in addition to routine antiseptic care.

IMMATURITY OF DRUG METABOLISM. Renal clearances for almost all substances excreted in the urine are diminished in newborn infants, but more so in premature ones. Intervals between doses may, therefore, need to be extended when administering drugs excreted chiefly by the kidneys. For instance, highly satisfactory levels of penicillin, gentamicin, and kanamycin are maintained on doses given at 12-hr intervals. Drugs detoxified in the liver or requiring chemical conjugation before renal excretion should also be given with caution and in doses smaller than usual. When possible, blood levels should be obtained for potentially toxic drugs, especially if renal or hepatic dysfunction is present. Decisions about the choice and dose of antibacterial agents and route of administration should be made on an individual basis rather than routinely, owing to the dangers of (1) development of infections with organisms resistant to antibacterial agents, (2) destruction or inhibition of intestinal bacteria that manufacture significant amounts of essential vitamins (e.g., vitamin K and thiamine), and (3) harmful interference in important metabolic processes.

Many drugs apparently safe for adults on the basis of toxicity studies may be harmful to newborn infants, especially premature ones. Oxygen and a number of drugs have proved toxic to premature infants in amounts not harmful to term infants (Table 93–7). Thus, administering any drug, particularly in large doses, without pharmacologic testing in premature infants, should be carefully undertaken after weighing risk against benefit.

PROGNOSIS. There is now a 95% or greater chance of survival for infants born weighing 1,501–2,500 g, but those weighing less still have a significantly higher mortality (see Fig. 93–1). Intensive care has extended the period during which a VLBW infant is likely to die of complications of perinatal disease, such as chronic lung disease, necrotizing enterocolitis, or secondary

TABLE 93–7 Potential Adverse Reactions to Drugs Administered to Premature Infants

Drug	Reaction
Oxygen	Retinopathy of prematurity, chronic lung disease
Sulfisoxazole	Kernicterus
Chloramphenicol	Gray baby—shock, bone marrow suppression
Vitamin K analogs	Jaundice
Novobiocin	Jaundice
Hexachlorophene	Encephalopathy
Benzyl alcohol	Acidosis, collapse, intraventricular bleeding
Intravenous vitamin E	Ascites, shock
Phenolic detergents	Jaundice
$NaHCO_3$	Intraventricular hemorrhage
Amphotericin	Anuric renal failure, hypokalemia, hypomagnesemia
Reserpine	Nasal stuffiness
Indomethacin	Oliguria, hyponatremia, intestinal perforation
Cisapride	Prolonged QTc interval
Tetracycline	Enamel hypoplasia
Tolazoline	Hypotension, gastrointestinal bleeding
Calcium salts	Subcutaneous necrosis
Aminoglycosides	Deafness, renal toxicity
Enteric gentamicin	Resistant bacteria
Prostaglandins	Seizures, diarrhea, apnea, hyperostosis, pyloric stenosis
Phenobarbital	Altered state, drowsiness
Morphine	Hypotension, urine retention, withdrawal
Pancuronium/vecuronium	Edema, hypovolemia, hypotension, tachycardia, contractions, prolonged hypotonia
Iodine antiseptics	Hypothyroidism, goiter
Fentanyl	Seizures, chest wall rigidity, withdrawal
Dexamethasone	Gastrointestinal bleeding, hypertension, infection, hyperglycemia, cardiomyopathy, reduced growth
Lasix	Deafness, hyponatremia, hypokalemia, hypochloremia, nephrocalcinosis, biliary stones
Heparin (not low-dose prophylactic use)	Bleeding, intraventricular hemorrhage, thrombocytopenia

TABLE 93–8 Sequelae of Low Birthweight

Immediate	Late
Hypoxia, ischemia	Mental retardation, spastic diplegia, microcephaly, seizures, poor school performance
Intraventricular hemorrhage	Mental retardation, spasticity, seizures, hydrocephalus
Sensorineural injury	Hearing, visual impairment, retinopathy of prematurity, strabismus, myopia
Respiratory failure	Chronic lung disease, cor pulmonale, bronchospasm, malnutrition, subglottic stenosis, iatrogenic cleft palate, recurrent pneumonia
Necrotizing enterocolitis	Short bowel syndrome, malabsorption, malnutrition, infectious diarrhea
Cholestatic liver disease	Cirrhosis, hepatic failure, carcinoma, malnutrition
Nutrient deficiency	Osteopenia, fractures, anemia, vitamin E, growth failure
Social stress	Child abuse or neglect, failure to thrive, divorce
Other	Sudden infant death syndrome, infections, inguinal hernia, cutaneous scars (chest tube, patent ductus arteriosus ligation, intravenous infiltration), gastroesophageal reflux, hypertension, craniosynostosis, cholelithiasis, nephrocalcinosis, cutaneous hemangiomas

infection (Table 93–8). The mortality rate of LBW infants who survive to be discharged from the hospital is higher than that of term infants during the first 2 yr of life. Because many of these deaths are attributable to infection, they are at least theoretically preventable. There is also an increased incidence of failure to thrive, sudden infant death syndrome, child abuse, and inadequate maternal-infant bonding among premature infants. Biologic risks from poor cardiorespiratory regulation due to immaturity or to complications of underlying perinatal disease and social risks associated with poverty also contribute to the high mortality and morbidity of these infants. Congenital anomalies are present in approximately 3–7% of LBW infants.

In the absence of congenital abnormalities, central nervous system injury, VLBW or marked IUGR, physical growth of LBW infants tends to approximate that of term infants by the 2nd yr; this occurs earlier in premature infants of larger birth size. VLBW infants may not catch up, especially if they have severe chronic sequelae (see Table 93–8), insufficient nutritional intake, or an inadequate caretaking environment. Premature birth in itself may prejudice later development. In general, the greater the immaturity and the lower the birthweight, the greater the likelihood of intellectual and neurologic deficit; as many as 50% of 500–750 g infants have a significant neurodevelopmental handicap (blindness, deafness, mental retardation, cerebral palsy). Small head circumference at birth may be similarly related to poor neurobehavioral prognosis. Many surviving LBW infants have hypotonia before 8 mo corrected age, which improves by the time they are 8 mo–1 yr old. This transient hypotonia is not a poor prognostic sign. The overall incidence of neurologic and developmental handicap in VLBW infants ranges from 10–20%, including cerebral palsy (3–6%) and moderate to severe hearing and visual defects (1–4%). Mean global IQ is 90–97. Thirty to 50% of VLBW children have poor school performance at age 7 yr (repeat grades, special classes, learning disorders, poor speech and language), despite normal IQ. Risks for poor academic performance include grade IV IVH, periventricular leukomalacia, birthweight less than 750 g, low socioeconomic status, chronic lung disease, cerebral atrophy, posthemorrhagic hydrocephalus, IUGR, and, possibly, low thyroxine levels. Adolescents who were VLBW report satisfactory health; 94% are integrated in regular classes despite neurosensory disabilities (hearing, vision, cerebral palsy, cognition) in 24%.

PREDICTING NEONATAL MORTALITY. Birthweight has traditionally been used as a strong indicator for the risk of neonatal death. Indeed, survival at 22 wk of gestation is close to 0%; survival increases with increasing gestational age to approximately 15% at 23 wk, 56% at 24 wk, and 79% at 25 wk. In addition, birthweight-specific neonatal diseases, such as grade IV IVH, severe group B streptococcal pneumonia, and pulmonary hypoplasia, also contribute to a poor outcome. Scoring systems that have been developed take into consideration physiologic abnormalities (hypo-hypertension, acidosis, hypoxia, hypercarbia, anemia, neutropenia) in the Score for Neonatal Acute Physiology (SNAP) or clinical parameters (gestational age, birthweight, anomalies, acidosis, FIO_2) in the Clinical Risk Index for Babies (CRIB). CRIB includes 6 parameters collected in the first 12 hr after birth, and SNAP has 26 variables collected in the first 24 hr. Although these risk scoring systems may provide prognostic information for mortality, they may not be useful for predicting morbidity among survivors. Furthermore, when compared with the clinical judgment of experienced neonatologists (based on birthweight, illness severity, low Apgar score, IUGR, therapeutic requirements), objective risk scores provide similar predictability. Combining a physician's judgment and an objective score may produce a more accurate assessment of the mortality risk.

DISCHARGE FROM HOSPITAL. Before discharge, a premature infant should be taking all nutrition by nipple, either bottle or breast (Table 93–9). Growth should be occurring at steady increments of approximately 10–30 g/24 hr. Temperature should be stabilized in an open crib. There should have been no recent apnea or bradycardia, and parenteral drug administration should have been discontinued or converted to oral dosing. Stable infants recovering from chronic lung disease may be discharged on oxygen given by nasal cannula as long as careful follow-up is arranged with frequent pulse oximetry monitoring and outpatient visits. Infants previously treated

TABLE 93–9 Recommendations for the Discharge of High-Risk LBW Infants

- Resolution of acute life-threatening illnesses
- Ongoing follow-up for chronic but stable problems
  - Chronic lung disease
  - Intraventricular hemorrhage
  - Necrotizing enterocolitis
  - Ventricular septal defect; other cardiac lesions
  - Anemia
  - Retinopathy of prematurity
  - Hearing
  - Apnea
  - Cholestasis
- Stable temperature regulation
- Gaining weight on oral feedings
  - Breast-feeding
  - Bottle-feeding
  - Gastric tube
- Free of significant apnea; home monitoring for apnea if needed
- Appropriate immunizations
- Hearing screenings
- Ophthalmologic examination < 27 wk or < 1,250 g at birth
- Mother's knowledge, skill, confidence documented in
  - Administration of medications (diuretics, methylxanthines, aerosols, etc.)
  - Use of oxygen; apnea monitors; oximeters
  - Nutritional support
    - Timing
    - Volume
    - Mixing concentrated formulas
  - Recognition of illness and deterioration
  - Basic cardiopulmonary resuscitation
  - Infant safety (see Table 93–1)
- Scheduling of referrals
  - Primary care provider
  - Neonatal follow-up clinic
  - Occupational therapy/physical therapy
  - Imaging (head ultrasound)
- Assessment of and solution to social risks (see Table 93–1)

Adapted from Guidelines for Perinatal Care, 4th ed, AAP, ACOG, 1997.

with oxygen should have an eye examination to determine the presence, stage, or absence of retinopathy of prematurity. All LBW infants should have a hearing test. Those who had indwelling umbilical arterial catheters should have their blood pressure measured to check for renal vascular hypertension. Hemoglobin level or hematocrit should be determined to evaluate possible anemia. If all major medical problems have resolved and the home setting is adequate, premature infants may then be discharged when their weight approaches 1,800–2,100 g; close follow-up and easy access to health care providers are essential for early discharge protocols. Alternatively, if the medical or social environment is not ideal, high-risk neonates transported to neonatal intensive care units whose major illness has resolved may be returned to their hospital of birth for an additional period of hospitalization. Standard vaccinations with full doses should commence after discharge or if in the hospital, with vaccines that do not contain live viruses. For RSV prophylaxis and rotovirus vaccine, see Chapters 253, 256, and 301.

HOME CARE. While the infant is in the hospital, the mother should be instructed in how to care for the baby after discharge. This program should include at least one visit to her home by someone capable of evaluating domestic arrangements and advising about any needed improvements.

93.3 Post-Term Infants

Post-term infants are those born after 42 wk of gestation, calculated from the mother's last menstrual period, regardless of weight at birth. This designation is often used synonymously with the term "postmature" for infants whose gestation exceeds the normal 280 days by 7 days or more. Approximately 25% of all pregnancies end on or after the 287th day of gestation, 12% on or after the 294th day, and 5% on or after the 301st day. The cause of post-term birth or postmaturity is unknown. Large size of the infant correlates poorly with late delivery but does correlate with large size of either parent, multigravidity, or a prediabetic or diabetic state in the mother.

CLINICAL MANIFESTATIONS. Post-term infants may be clinically indistinguishable from term infants, but some have received the designation postmature because their appearance and behavior suggest those of an infant 1–3 wk of age. These post-term, postmature infants are often of increased birthweight and characterized by the absence of lanugo, decreased or absent vernix caseosa, long nails, abundant scalp hair, white parchment-like or desquamating skin, and increased alertness. If *placental insufficiency* occurs, the amniotic fluid and fetus may be meconium stained, and abnormal fetal heart rates may be observed; the infant may have growth retardation. Although this syndrome is frequently confused with postmaturity, *only about 20% of infants with placental insufficiency syndrome are post term.* The majority of those affected are term and preterm infants, particularly those SGA who are infants of toxemic mothers, older primigravidas, and women with chronic hypertension. The placentas are often small or poorly attached. This syndrome has been postulated to result from degenerative changes in the placenta that progressively reduce oxygen and nourishment to the fetus.

Those infants born post term in association with presumed placental insufficiency may have various physical signs; desquamation, long nails, abundant hair, pale skin, alert faces, and loose skin, especially around the thighs and buttocks, giving them the appearance of having recently lost weight; meconium-stained nails, skin, vernix, umbilical cord, and placental membranes (see Fig. 90–1).

PROGNOSIS. When delivery is delayed 3 wk or more beyond term, there is a significant increase in mortality, which in some series has approximated 3 times that of a control group of infants born at term. Mortality has been lowered markedly through improved obstetric management.

TREATMENT. Careful obstetric monitoring, including nonstress testing, biophysical profile, or Doppler velocimetry, usually provides a rational basis for choosing a course of nonintervention, induction of labor, or cesarean section. Induction of labor or cesarean section may be indicated in older primigravidas who go more than 2–4 wk beyond term, particularly if there is evidence of fetal distress. Meconium aspiration pneumonia or hypoxic encephalopathy is treated symptomatically.

93.4 Large for Gestational Age

See also Chapter 103.

Neonatal mortality rates decrease with increasing birth weight until approximately 4,000 g, after which mortality increases. These oversized infants are usually born at term, but preterm infants with weights high for gestational age also have a significantly higher mortality than infants of the same size born at term; maternal diabetes and obesity are predisposing factors. Infants who are very large, regardless of their gestational age, have a higher incidence of birth injuries, such as cervical and brachial plexus injuries, phrenic nerve damage with paralysis of the diaphragm, fractured clavicles, cephalhematomas, subdural hematomas, and ecchymoses of the head and face. The incidence of congenital anomalies, particularly congenital heart disease, is also higher than in term infants of normal weight. Intellectual and developmental retardation is statistically more common in high-birthweight term and preterm infants than in babies of appropriate weight for gestational age.

93.5 Infant Transport

With the advent of regionalized care of high-risk neonates, increasing numbers of sick infants are being transported to neonatal intensive care units in hospitals at which they were not born. Ideally, high-risk mothers should be transported to and delivered at centers where these specialized units are located. Neonatal transport should include consultation about the infant's problem and care before transport, ease of access to the transport team, and transport and stabilization by the team before moving the infant. Securing an airway, providing oxygen, assisting with infant ventilation, providing antimicrobial therapy, maintaining the circulation, providing a warmed environment, and placing intravenous or arterial lines or chest tubes all should be initiated, if indicated, before transport. Infant and maternal records, laboratory reports, and a tube of clotted maternal blood should also be provided. Before departing, the mother should be briefly reassured and allowed to see her stabilized infant, if practical; the father should follow the transport vehicle to the unit. The transport officer or nurse should also call ahead to inform the receiving unit about the nature of the patient's illness.

The transport vehicle should be equipped with appropriate medicines, fluids, oxygen tanks, catheters, chest tubes, endotracheal tubes, laryngoscopes, and an infant warming device. It should be well illuminated and have ample room for emergency procedures and monitoring equipment. With efficient transport and appropriately educated nursing and medical staff at the referring hospitals, the mortality of "outborn" neonates should be no higher than that of those born within the tertiary care center.

Akintorin SM, Kamat M, Pildes RS, et al: A prospective randomized trial of feeding methods in very low birth weight infants. Pediatrics 100: http://www.pediatrics.org/cgi/content/full/100/4/e4, 1997.
American Academy of Pediatrics: Hospital Care of Newborn Infants. Evanston IL, The Academy, 1997.
Anonymous: Breast not necessarily the best. Lancet 1:624, 1988.
Asuncion M, Silvestre A, Morbach CA, et al: A prospective randomized trial comparing continuous versus intermittent feeding methods in very low birth weight neonates. J Pediatr 128:748, 1996.
Bardin C, Zelkowitz P, Papageorgiou A: Outcome of small-for-gestational-age and appropriate-for-gestational age infants born before 27 weeks of gestation. Pediatrics 100:http://www.pediatrics.org/cgi/content/full/1001/2/e4, 1997.
Blaymore Bier J, Ferguson AE, Morales Y, et al: Breastfeeding infants who were extremely low birth weight. Pediatrics 100:http://www.pediatrics.org/cgi/content/full/100/6/e3, 1997.
Dammann O, Alfred EN, Veelken N: Increased risk of spastic diplegia among very low birth weight children after preterm labor or prelabor rupture of membranes. J Pediatr 132:531, 1998.
Davey AM, Wagner CL, Cox C, et al: Feeding premature infants while low umbilical artery catheters are in place: A prospective, randomized trial. J Pediatr 124:795, 1994.
Dunn L, Hulman S, Weiner J, et al: Beneficial effects of early hypocaloric enteral feeding on neonatal gastrointestinal function: Preliminary report of a randomized trial. J Pediatr 112:622, 1988.
Fanaroff AA, Wright LL, Stevenson DK, et al: Very-low-birth-weight outcomes of the National Institute of Child Health and Human Development Neonatal Research Network, May 1991 through December 1992. Am J Obstet Gynecol 173:1423, 1995.
Hegyi T, Carbone T, Anwar M, et al: The Apgar score and its components in the preterm infant. Pediatrics 101:77, 1998.
Heird WC, Gomez MR: Total parenteral nutrition in necrotizing enterocolitis. Clin Perinatol 21:389, 1994.
Higby K, Xenakis EM-J, Pauerstein CJ: Do tocolytic agents stop preterm labor? A critical and comprehensive review of efficacy and safety. Am J Obstet Gynecol 168:1247, 1993.
Hutton JL, Pharoah POD, Cooke RWI, et al: Differential effects of preterm birth and small gestational age on cognitive and motor development. Arch Dis Child 76:F75, 1997.
Kalhoff H, Diekmann L, Hettrich B, et al: Modified cow's milk formula with reduced renal acid load preventing incipient late metabolic acidosis in premature infants. J Pediatr 25:46, 1997.
La Gamma EF, Browne LE: Feeding practices for infants weighing less than 1500 g at birth and the pathogenesis of necrotizing enterocolitis. Clin Perinatol 21:271, 1994.
Lau C, Sheena HR, Shulman RJ, et al: Oral feeding in low birth weight infants. J Pediatr 130:561, 1997.
Lorenz JM, Kleinman LI, Ahmed G, et al: Phases of fluid and electrolyte homeostasis in the extremely low birth weight infant. Pediatrics 96:484, 1995.
Lucas A, Morley R, Cole TJ, et al: A randomised multicentre study of human milk versus formula and later development in preterm infants. Arch Dis Child 70:F141, 1994.
Major CA, Lewis DF, Harding JA, et al: Tocolysis with indomethacin increases the incidence of necrotizing enterocolitis in the low-birth-weight neonate. Am J Obstet Gynecol 170:102, 1994.
Modi N. Sodium intake and preterm babies: Arch Dis Child 69:87, 1993.
Moreno A, Dominguez C, Ballabriga A: Aluminum in the neonate related to parenteral nutrition. Acta Paediatr 83:25, 1994.
O'Shea TM, Klinepeter KL, Goldstein DJ, et al: Survival and developmental disability in infants with birth weights of 501 to 800 grams, born between 1979 and 1994. Pediatrics 100:982, 1997.
O'Shea TM, Prilisser JS, Klinepeter KL, et al: Trends in mortality and cerebral palsy in a geographically based cohort of very low birth weight neonates born between 1982 to 1994. Pediatrics 101:642, 1998.
Perez-Escamilla R, Pollitt E, Lonnerdal B, et al: Infant feeding policies in maternity wards and their effect on breast-feeding success: An analytical overview. Am J Public Health 84:89, 1994.
Prestridge LL, Schanler RJ, Shulman RJ, et al: Effect of parenteral calcium and phosphorus therapy on mineral retention and bone mineral content in very low birth weight infants. J Pediatr 122:761, 1993.
Rautonen J, Makela A, Boyd H, et al: CRIB and SNAP: Assessing the risk of death for preterm neonates. Lancet 343:1272, 1994.
Romero R, Sibai B, Caritis S, et al: Antibiotic treatment of preterm labor with intact membranes: A multicenter, randomized, double-blinded, placebo-controlled trial. Am J Obstet Gynecol 169:764, 1993.
Saigal S, Feeny D, Rosenbaum P, et al: Self-perceived health status and health-related quality of life of extremely low-birth-weight infants at adolescence. JAMA 276:453, 1996.
Sauer P, Visser M: The neutral temperature of very low birth weight infants. Pediatrics 74:788, 1984.
Sauve RS, Robertson C, Etches P, et al: Before viability: A geographical based outcome study of infants weighing 500 grams or less at birth. Pediatrics 101:438, 1998.
Schaap AHP, Wolf H, Bruinse HW, et al: Influence of obstetric management on outcome of extremely preterm growth retarded infants. Arch Dis Child 77:F95, 1997.
Singer L, Yamashita T, Lilien L, et al: A longitudinal study of developmental outcomes of infants with bronchopulmonary dysplasia and very low birth weight. Pediatrics 100:987, 1997.
Sommerfelt K: Long-term outcome for non-handicapped low birth weight infants—is the fog clearing? Eur J Pediatr 157:1, 1998.
Stevens SM, Richardson DK, Gray JE, et al: Estimating neonatal mortality risk: An analysis of clinicians' judgments. Pediatrics 93:945, 1994.
Strauss RS, Dietz WH: Effects of intrauterine growth retardation in premature infants on early childhood growth. J Pediatr 130:95, 1997.
Van Wassenaer AG, Kok JH, De Vijlder JJM, et al: Effects of thyroxine supplementation on neurologic development on infants born at less than 30 weeks' gestation. N Engl J Med 336:21, 1997.
The Victorian Infant Collaborative Study Group: Improved outcome into the 1990s for infants weighing 500–999 g at birth. Arch Dis Child 77:F91, 1997.
Wariyar U, Tin W, Hey E: Gestational assessment assessed. Arch Dis Child 77:F216, 1997.
Whitaker AH, Feldman JF, Van Rossem R, et al: Neonatal cranial ultrasound abnormalities in low birth weight infants: Relation to cognitive outcomes at six years of age. Pediatrics 98:719, 1996.
Whitaker AH, Van Rossem R, Feldman J, et al: Psychiatric outcomes in low-birth-weight children at age 6: Relation to neonatal cranial ultrasound abnormalities. Arch Gen Psychiatry 54:847, 1997.
Whitfield MF, Eckstein Grunau RV, Holsti L: Extremely premature (≤ 800 g) schoolchildren: Multiple areas of hidden disability. Arch Dis Child 77:F85, 1997.
Wilson DC, Cairns P, Halliday HL, et al: Randomised controlled trial of an aggressive nutritional regimen in sick very low birthweight infants. Arch Dis Child 77:F4, 1997.
Woods KA, Camacho-Hübner C, Savage MO, et al: Intrauterine growth retardation and postnatal growth failure associated with deletion of the insulin-like growth factor I gene. N Engl J Med 335:1363, 1996.

CHAPTER 94

Clinical Manifestations of Diseases in the Newborn Period

An infant's physician should appreciate the wide variety of disorders that may originate in utero, during birth, or in the immediate postnatal period. The disorders may represent genetic mutations, chromosomal aberrations, or acquired diseases and injuries. Recognizing disease in newborn infants depends on knowledge about the disorder and evaluation of a limited number of relatively nonspecific clinical signs and symptoms.

Central cyanosis has respiratory, cardiac, central nervous system (CNS), hematologic, or metabolic causes (Table 94–1). Respiratory insufficiency may be due to pulmonary conditions or may be secondary to CNS depression due to drugs, intracranial hemorrhage, or anoxia. If it is caused by the former, respirations tend to be rapid and may be accompanied by retraction of the thoracic cage. If it is due to the latter, respirations tend to be irregular and weak and are often slow. Cyanosis persisting for several days, unaccompanied by obvious signs of respiratory difficulty, suggests cyanotic congenital heart disease or methemoglobinemia. Cyanosis resulting from congenital heart disease may, however, be difficult to distinguish clinically from cyanosis caused by respiratory disease. Episodes of cyanosis also may be the presenting sign of hypoglycemia, bacteremia, meningitis, shock, or pulmonary hypertension. Peripheral acrocyanosis is common and usually does not warrant concern.

Pallor, in addition to anemia or acute hemorrhage, should suggest hypoxia, asphyxia, hypoglycemia, sepsis, shock, or adrenal failure.

Hypotension in term infants suggests shock due to hypovolemia (hemorrhage, dehydration), the systemic inflammatory response syndrome (SIRS due to sepsis, TORCH), cardiac dysfunction (left heart obstructive lesions—hypoplastic left heart syndrome, myocarditis, asphyxia-induced myocardial stun, anomalous coronary artery), pneumothorax, pneumopericardium, pericardial effusion, or metabolic disorders (hypoglycemia, adrenal insufficiency—salt-losing adrenogenital syndrome).

TABLE 94–1 Differential Diagnosis of Cyanosis in the Newborn

Central or peripheral nervous system hypoventilation
- Birth asphyxia
- Intracranial hypertension, hemorrhage
- Oversedation (direct or through maternal route)
- Diaphragm palsy
- Neuromuscular diseases
- Seizures

Respiratory disease
- Upper airway
  - Choanal atresia/stenosis
  - Pierre Robin syndrome
  - Intrinsic airway obstruction (laryngeal/bronchial/tracheal stenosis)
  - Extrinsic airway obstruction (bronchogenic cyst, duplication cyst, vascular compression)
- Lower airway
  - Respiratory distress syndrome
  - Transient tachypnea
  - Meconium aspiration
  - Pneumonia (sepsis)
  - Pneumothorax
  - Congenital diaphragmatic hernia
  - Pulmonary hypoplasia
  - Persistent fetal circulation (persistent pulmonary hypertension of newborn)

Cardiac right-to-left shunt
- Abnormal connections (pulmonary blood flow normal or increased)
  - Transposition of the great vessels
  - Total anomalous pulmonary venous return
  - Truncus arteriosus
  - Hypoplastic left heart syndrome
  - Single ventricle or tricuspid atresia with large ventricular septal defect without pulmonic stenosis
- Obstructed pulmonary blood flow (pulmonary blood flow decreased)
  - Pulmonic atresia with intact ventricular septum
  - Tetralogy of Fallot
  - Critical pulmonic stenosis with patent foramen ovale or atrial septal defect
  - Tricuspid atresia
  - Single ventricle with pulmonic stenosis
  - Ebstein malformation of the tricuspid valve
  - Persistent fetal circulation (persistent pulmonary hypertension of newborn)

Methemoglobinemia
- Congenital (hemoglobin M, methemoglobin reductase deficiency)
- Acquired (e.g., nitrates, nitrites)

Inadequate ambient O_2 or less O_2 delivered than expected (rare)
- Disconnection of O_2 supply to nasal cannula, head hood
- Connection of air, rather than O_2, to a mechanical ventilator

Spurious/artifactual
- Oximeter artifact (poor contact between probe and skin, poor pulse searching)
- Arterial blood gas artifact (contamination with venous blood)

Other
- Hypoglycemia
- Adrenogenital syndrome
- Polycythemia
- Blood loss

From Smith F: Cyanosis. In: *Kliegman R, Nieder M, Super D (eds): Practical Strategies in Pediatric Diagnosis and Therapy. Philadelphia, WB Saunders, 1996.*

Hypotension is a common problem in sick infants with very low birthweight (VLBW) and may be due to any of the problems noted in a term infant. Infants with severe respiratory distress syndrome (RDS) may develop hypotension that responds to fluids (normal saline equally as effective as 5% albumin) or dopamine (5–20 μg/kg/min). Some infants weighing less than 1,000 g do not respond to fluids or inotropic agents but may respond to therapy with hydrocortisone (2.5 mg/kg q 4–6 hr). Sudden onset of hypotension in VLBW infants suggests a pneumothorax, intraventricular hemorrhage, or subcapsular hepatic hematoma.

Convulsions (Chapter 602.5) usually point to a disorder of the CNS and suggest hypoxic-ischemic encephalopathy resulting from asphyxia, intracranial hemorrhage, cerebral anomaly, subdural effusion, meningitis, hypocalcemia, hypoglycemia, infarction, benign familial seizures, and, rarely, pyridoxine dependence, hyponatremia, hypernatremia, inborn errors of metabolism, or drug withdrawal. Seizures beginning in the delivery room or shortly thereafter may be due to unintentional injection of maternal local anesthetic into the fetus. Convulsions may also result from administration of large amounts of hypotonic fluids to the mother shortly before and during delivery, leading to subsequent hyponatremia and water intoxication in the infant.

Convulsions should be distinguished from the jitteriness that may be present in normal newborns, in infants of diabetic mothers, in those who experienced birth asphyxia or drug withdrawal, and in polycythemic neonates. Jitteriness resembling simple tremors may be stopped by holding the infant's extremity; it often depends on sensory stimuli and is not associated with abnormal eye movements. Seizures in premature infants are often subtle and associated with abnormal eye (fluttering, deviation, stare) or facial (chewing, tongue thrusting) movements; the motor component is often that of tonic extension of the limbs, neck, and trunk. Term infants may have focal or multifocal, clonic or myoclonic movements but may also show more subtle seizure activity. *Apnea* may be the first manifestation of seizure activity, particularly in a premature infant.

After severe birth asphyxia, infants may have *motor automatisms* characterized by oral-buccal-lingual movements, rotary limb activities (rowing, pedaling, swimming), tonic posturing, or myoclonus. These motor seizures are not usually accompanied by time-synchronized electroencephalographic discharges, may not signify cortical epileptic activity, respond poorly to anticonvulsant therapy, and are associated with a poor prognosis. Such automatisms may represent cortical depression that produces a brain stem release phenomenon or subcortical seizures.

Lethargy may be a manifestation of infection, asphyxia, hypoglycemia, hypercarbia, sedation from maternal analgesia or anesthesia, cerebral defect, and, indeed, of almost any severe disease including inborn errors of metabolism. Lethargy appearing after the 2nd day should, in particular, suggest infection. Lethargy with emesis suggests increased intracranial pressure or an inborn error of metabolism.

Irritability may be a sign of discomfort accompanying intra-abdominal conditions, meningeal irritation, drug withdrawal, infections, congenital glaucoma, or any condition producing pain. As in later infancy, the eardrums should always be examined as a possible source of pain.

Pain and discomfort are potentially avoidable problems during the treatment of VLBW infants. In the absence of adequate pain control, VLBW infants develop hypotension, metabolic acidosis, and prolonged recovery from surgical procedures. Relief from nociceptive stimuli (painful procedures, intubation, mechanical ventilation) must be provided with analgesic drugs with or without anxiolytic agents. Pre-emptive narcotics (morphine, fentanyl) and/or benzodiazepines (midazolam, lorazepam, diazepam) should be used before pain or anxiety develops. Some painful procedures on well neonates have also been managed with oral concentrated (25–50%) sucrose solutions.

Hyperactivity, especially of the premature infant, may be a sign of hypoxia, pneumothorax, emphysema, hypoglycemia, hypocalcemia, central nervous system damage, drug withdrawal, thyrotoxicosis, bronchospasm, esophageal reflux, or discomfort due to a cold environment.

Failure to feed well is seen in most sick newborn infants and should always occasion a careful search for infection, central or peripheral nervous system disorder, intestinal obstruction, and other abnormal conditions.

Fever may be the result of too high an environmental temperature due to weather, overheated nurseries or incubators, or too many clothes or bedclothes. It is also noted in "dehydration fever" of newborn infants. If these causes of fever can be eliminated, then serious infection (pneumonia, bacteremia, meningitis, and viral infections, particularly herpes simplex or enteroviruses) must be considered, although such infections often occur without provoking a febrile response in newborn infants (see Chapters 105 and 106). An unexplained *fall in*

TABLE 94–2 Common Life-Threatening Congenital Anomalies

Name	Manifestations
Choanal atresia	Respiratory distress in delivery room, apnea, unable to pass nasogastric tube through nares. Suspect CHARGE syndrome
Pierre Robin syndrome	Migrognathia, cleft palate, airway obstruction
Diaphragmatic hernia	Scaphoid abdomen, bowel sounds present in chest, respiratory distress
Tracheoesophageal fistula	Polyhydramnios, aspiration pneumonia, excessive salivation, unable to place nasogastric tube in stomach. Suspect VATER syndrome
Intestinal obstruction: volvulus, duodenal atresia, ileal atresia	Polyhydramnios, bile-stained emesis, abdominal distention. Suspect 21-trisomy, cystic fibrosis, cocaine
Gastroschisis, omphalocele	Polyhydramnios, intestinal obstruction
Renal agenesis, Potter syndrome	Oligohydramnios, anuria, pulmonary hypoplasia, pneumothorax
Neural tube defects: anencephalus, meningomyelocele	Polyhydramnios, elevated α-fetoprotein, decreased fetal activity
Ductal dependent congenital heart disease	Cyanosis, hypotension, murmur

body temperature may accompany infection or other serious disturbances of the circulation or CNS. A sudden servo-controlled increase in incubator temperature to maintain body temperature is often associated with sepsis.

Periods of *apnea*, particularly in premature infants, may be associated with various disturbances (see Chapter 97.2). When apneas recur or when the intervals are longer than 20 sec or are associated with cyanosis or bradycardia, they warrant an immediate diagnostic evaluation.

Jaundice during the first 24 hr of life should be considered to be due to erythroblastosis fetalis until proved otherwise. Septicemia and intrauterine infections such as syphilis, cytomegalovirus, and toxoplasmosis should also be considered, especially if there is an increase in plasma direct-reacting bilirubin.

Jaundice after the first 24 hr may be "physiologic" or may be due to septicemia, hemolytic anemia, galactosemia, hepatitis, congenital atresia of the bile ducts, inspissated bile syndrome following erythroblastosis fetalis, syphilis, herpes simplex, or congenital infections (see Chapter 98.3).

Vomiting during the 1st day of life suggests obstruction in the upper digestive tract or increased intracranial pressure. Roentgenographic studies are indicated when obstruction is suspected. Vomiting also may be a nonspecific symptom of an illness such as septicemia. It is a common manifestation of overfeeding or inexperienced feeding technique, pyloric stenosis, milk allergy, duodenal ulcer, stress ulcer, or adrenal insufficiency. Infants placed in body casts for orthopedic treatment often vomit transiently. Vomitus containing dark blood is usually a sign of a serious illness; the benign possibility of swallowed maternal blood should also be considered. Bile-stained vomitus strongly suggests obstruction below the ampulla of Vater and warrants contrast radiography.

Diarrhea may be a symptom of overfeeding (especially high-caloric-density formula), acute gastroenteritis, or malabsorption or a nonspecific symptom of infection. It may occur in conditions accompanied by compromised circulation of part of the intestinal or genital tract, such as mesenteric thrombosis, necrotizing enterocolitis, strangulated hernia, intussusception, and torsion of the ovary or testis.

Abdominal distention, usually a sign of intestinal obstruction or an intra-abdominal mass, may also be seen in infants with enteritis, necrotizing enterocolitis, ileus accompanying sepsis, respiratory distress, ascites, or hypokalemia.

Failure to move an extremity (pseudoparalysis) or part of it suggests fracture, dislocation, or nerve injury. It is also seen in osteomyelitis and other infections that cause pain on movement of the affected part.

CONGENITAL ANOMALIES

Congenital anomalies are a major cause of stillbirths and neonatal deaths but are perhaps even more important as causes of physical defects and metabolic disorders. (Anomalies are discussed in general in Chapters 78 and 104 and specifically in the chapters on the various systems of the body.) Early recognition of anomalies is important for planning care; for some, such as tracheoesophageal fistula, diaphragmatic hernia, choanal atresia, and intestinal obstruction, immediate medical and surgical therapy is essential for survival (Table 94–2). Parents are likely to feel anxious and guilty on learning of the existence of a congenital anomaly and require sensitive counseling.

CHAPTER 95
Birth Injury

The term *birth injury* is used to denote avoidable and unavoidable mechanical and hypoxic-ischemic injury incurred by an infant during labor and delivery. These injuries may result from inappropriate or deficient medical skill or attention, or they may occur, despite skilled and competent obstetric care, independently of any acts or omissions. To avoid later misunderstandings, recriminations, or parental guilt, it is important to counsel parents who have a child with a residuum from birth trauma or hypoxic-ischemic injury about this broad use of the term *birth injury.* The definition does not include injury from amniocentesis, intrauterine transfusion, scalp blood sampling, or resuscitation procedures, all of which are discussed elsewhere.

The incidence of birth injuries has been estimated at 2–7/1,000 live births. Predisposing factors include macrosomia, prematurity, cephalopelvic disproportion, dystocia, prolonged labor, and breech presentation. Overall, 5–8/100,000 infants die of birth trauma, and 25/100,000 die of anoxic injuries; such injuries represent 2–3% of infant deaths. Even transient injuries readily apparent to the parents result in anxiety and questioning that require supportive and informative counseling. Some injuries may be latent initially but later result in severe illness or sequelae.

95.1 Cranial Injuries

Caput succedaneum is a diffuse, sometimes ecchymotic, edematous swelling of the soft tissues of the scalp involving the portion presenting during vertex delivery. It may extend across the midline and across suture lines. The edema disappears within the first few days of life. Analogous swelling, discoloration, and distortion of the face are seen in face presentations. No specific treatment is needed, but if there are extensive ecchymoses, phototherapy for hyperbilirubinemia may be indicated. *Molding* of the head and overriding of the parietal bones are frequently associated with caput succedaneum and become more evident after the caput has receded but disappear during the first weeks of life. Rarely, a hemorrhagic caput may result in shock and require blood transfusion.

Erythema, abrasions, ecchymoses, and *subcutaneous fat necrosis* of facial or scalp soft tissues may be seen after forceps or vacuum-assisted deliveries. Their location depends on the area of application of the forceps. Ecchymoses may be seen after manipulative deliveries and occasionally in premature infants for no discernible reason.

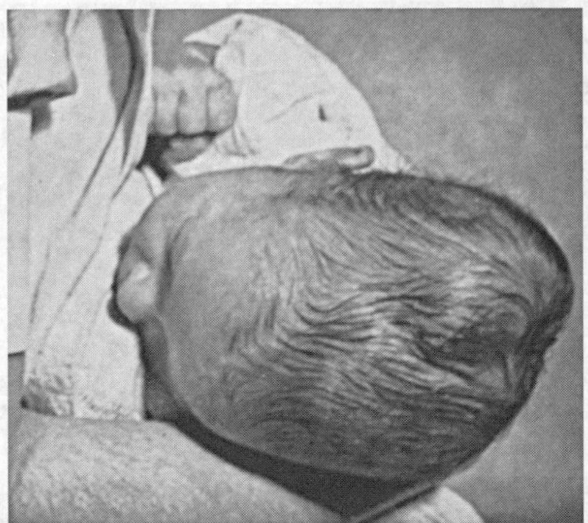

Figure 95–1 Cephalohematoma of the right parietal bone.

Subconjunctival and retinal hemorrhages are frequent, and *petechiae* of the skin of the head and neck are common. All are probably secondary to a sudden increase in intrathoracic pressure during passage of the chest through the birth canal. Parents should be assured that they are temporary and the result of *normal* hazards of delivery.

Cephalohematoma (Fig. 95–1) is a subperiosteal hemorrhage, hence always limited to the surface of one cranial bone. There is no discoloration of the overlying scalp, and swelling is usually not visible until several hours after birth, because subperiosteal bleeding is a slow process. An underlying skull fracture, usually linear and not depressed, is occasionally associated with cephalohematoma. Cranial meningocele may be differentiated from cephalohematoma by pulsation, increased pressure on crying, and the roentgenographic evidence of bony defect. Most cephalohematomas are resorbed within 2 wk–3 mo, depending on their size. They may begin to calcify by the end of the 2nd wk. A sensation of central depression suggesting but not indicative of an underlying fracture or bony defect is usually encountered on palpation of the organized rim of a cephalohematoma. A few remain for years as bony protuberances and are detectable roentgenographically as widening of the diploic space; cystlike defects may persist for months or years. Despite these residuals, cephalohematomas require no treatment, although phototherapy may be necessary to ameliorate hyperbilirubinemia. Incision and drainage are contraindicated because of the risk of introducing infection in a benign condition. A massive cephalohematoma may rarely result in blood loss severe enough to require transfusion. It may also be associated with a skull fracture, coagulopathy, and intracranial hemorrhage.

Fractures of the skull may occur as a result of pressure from forceps or from the maternal symphysis pubis, sacral promontory, or ischial spines. Linear fractures, the most common, cause no symptoms and require no treatment. Depressed fractures are usually indentations of the calvarium similar to a dent in a Ping-Pong ball; they usually are a complication of forceps delivery or fetal compression. Affected infants may be asymptomatic unless there is associated intracranial injury; it is advisable to elevate severe depressions to prevent cortical injury from sustained pressure. Fracture of the occipital bone with separation of the basal and squamous portions almost invariably causes fatal hemorrhage owing to disruption of the underlying vascular sinuses. It may result during breech deliveries from traction on the hyperextended spine of the infant with the head fixed in the maternal pelvis.

95.2 Intracranial-Intraventricular Hemorrhage

ETIOLOGY AND EPIDEMIOLOGY. Intracranial hemorrhage may result from trauma or asphyxia and, rarely, from a primary hemorrhagic disturbance or congenital vascular anomaly. Traumatic epidural, subdural, or subarachnoid hemorrhage is especially likely when the fetal head is large in proportion to the size of the mother's pelvic outlet; when for other reasons the labor is prolonged; in breech or precipitate deliveries; or as a result of mechanical assistance with delivery. Massive subdural hemorrhages, often associated with tears in the tentorium cerebelli or, less frequently, in the falx cerebri, are rare but are encountered more often in full-term than in premature infants. Primary hemorrhagic disturbances and vascular malformations are rare and usually give rise to subarachnoid or intracerebral hemorrhage. Intracranial bleeding may be associated with disseminated intravascular coagulopathy, isoimmune thrombocytopenia, and neonatal vitamin K deficiency (especially in infants born to mothers receiving phenobarbital or phenytoin). Intracranial hemorrhages often involve the ventricles (**intraventricular hemorrhage** [IVH]) of premature infants delivered spontaneously without apparent trauma.

PATHOGENESIS OF INTRAVENTRICULAR HEMORRHAGE. IVH in premature infants occurs in the gelatinous subependymal germinal matrix. This periventricular area is the site of embryonal neurons and fetal glial cells, which migrate to the cortex. Immature blood vessels in this highly vascular area may be subjected to various forces that, together with poor tissue vascular support, predispose premature infants to IVH. By term, the germinal matrix has become attenuated and the tissue's vascular support has strengthened. *Predisposing factors or events* for IVH include prematurity, respiratory distress syndrome (RDS), hypoxic-ischemic or hypotensive injury, reperfusion of damaged vessels, increased or decreased cerebral blood flow, reduced vascular integrity, increased venous pressure, pneumothorax, hypervolemia, and hypertension. These factors result in rupture of the germinal matrix blood vessels. Similar injurious factors (hypoxic-ischemic-hypotensive) or venous obstruction from an IVH may produce periventricular hemorrhage/necrosis (echodensities) due to hemorrhagic infarction. Periventricular leukomalacia (PVL), a common associated cystic finding, may be due to prenatal or neonatal ischemic or reperfusion injury. PVL with or without severe IVH is the result of necrosis of the periventricular white matter and damage to the corticospinal fibers in the internal capsule.

CLINICAL MANIFESTATIONS. The incidence of IVH increases with decreasing birthweight: 60–70% of 500- to 750-g infants and 10–20% of 1,000- to 1,500-g infants. IVH is rarely present at birth; however, 80–90% of cases occur between birth and the 3rd day of life, 50% occur on the 1st day. Twenty to forty per cent of cases progress during the 1st wk of life. Delayed hemorrhage may occur in 10–15% of patients after the 1st wk of life. New-onset IVH is rare after the 1st mo of life regardless of birthweight. The most common symptoms are diminished or absent Moro reflex, poor muscle tone, lethargy, apnea, and somnolence. Premature infants with IVH often have a precipitous deterioration on the 2nd or 3rd day of life. Periods of apnea, pallor, or cyanosis; failure to suck well; abnormal eye signs; a high-pitched, shrill cry; muscular twitchings, convulsions, decreased muscle tone, or paralyses; metabolic acidosis; shock, and a decreased hematocrit or its failure to increase after transfusion may be the first indications. The fontanel *may* be tense and bulging. Severe neurologic depression progresses to coma after more severe IVH, with associated hemorrhage in the cerebral cortex and ventricular dilation. A saltatory pattern demonstrates symptomatic episodes with intervening asymptomatic periods. In some cases (grade I, II) there may be no clinical manifestations.

PVL is usually asymptomatic until the neurologic sequelae of white matter necrosis become apparent in later infancy as spastic diplegia. As a result of symmetric, nonhemorrhagic ischemic injury, PVL often coexists with IVH. PVL may be present at birth but usually occurs later as an early echodense phase (3–10 days of life) followed by the typical echolucent (cystic) phase (14–20 days of life).

DIAGNOSIS. Intracranial hemorrhage is diagnosed on the basis of the history, clinical manifestations, transfontanel cranial ultrasonography or computed tomography (CT), and knowledge of the birthweight-specific risks of the type of hemorrhage. The diagnosis of *subdural hemorrhage* in a LGA term infant with cephalopelvic disproportion may be delayed 1 mo until the chronic subdural fluid volume expands, producing megalocephaly, frontal bossing, a bulging fontanel, seizures, and anemia. Alternatively, a well neonate with a seizure of short duration may have a benign *subarachnoid hemorrhage*.

Although preterm infants with IVH manifest rapid shock, mottling, anemia, coma, or a bulging fontanel, many signs of IVH are nonspecific or absent. Therefore, it is recommended that the premature infant be evaluated with real-time *cerebral ultrasonography* through the anterior fontanel to detect IVH. Infants weighing under 1,500 g are at high risk for IVH and should be examined within the first 3–5 days of life and again the following week. Ultrasound examination also detects the precystic and cystic symmetric lesions of PVL and the asymmetric intraparenchymal echogenic lesions of cortical hemorrhagic infarction. Furthermore, the delayed development of cortical atrophy, or porencephaly, and the severity, progression, or regression of posthemorrhagic hydrocephalus can be determined with ultrasonography.

Three levels of increasing severity of IVH are defined by ultrasound for LBW infants: Grade I is bleeding confined to the germinal matrix–subependymal region or to less than 10% of the ventricle (~ 35% of IVH); grade II is intraventricular bleeding with 10–50% filling of the ventricle (~ 40% of IVH); grade III is more than 50% involvement with dilated ventricles (Fig. 95–2). Another classification includes a grade IV IVH, which is similar to grade III plus intraparenchymal hemorrhage. Periventricular echodensities are intraparenchymal lesions that are not a direct extension of the IVH but represent an asymmetric infarct. Severe IVH is independently associated with immaturity and the severity of RDS. Immature infants without RDS are at risk for IVH, whereas infants with severe RDS are at greater risk than those with mild or no RDS at the same gestational age.

CT or magnetic resonance imaging (MRI) is indicated for term infants in whom the diagnosis is suspected, because ultrasound may not reveal intraparenchymal hemorrhage or infarction. Lumbar puncture is indicated in the presence of signs of increased intracranial pressure or deteriorating clinical condition to identify gross subarachnoid hemorrhage or to rule out the possibility of bacterial meningitis; the cerebrospinal fluid usually has elevated protein levels with many red blood cells. Not infrequently there is hypoglycorrhachia and a mild lymphocytosis. Because a small amount of bleeding into the cerebrospinal fluid often occurs in the course of normal and even cesarean deliveries, small numbers of red blood cells or slight xanthochromia in subarachnoid fluid does not necessarily indicate significant intracranial hemorrhage. Conversely, the subarachnoid fluid may be absolutely clear in the presence of severe subdural or intracerebral hemorrhage when there is no communication with the subarachnoid space.

PROGNOSIS. Patients with massive hemorrhage associated with tears of the tentorium or falx cerebri rapidly deteriorate and may die after birth. In utero hemorrhage associated with maternal idiopathic or, more often, fetal alloimmune thrombocytopenia may occur as severe cerebral hemorrhage or a porencephalic cyst after resolution of a fetal cortical hemorrhage.

Most infants with IVH and acute ventricular distention do not develop *posthemorrhagic hydrocephalus*. Ten to 15% of LBW neonates with IVH have hydrocephalus, which initially may be present without clinical signs such as enlarging head circumference, apnea, bradycardia, lethargy, bulging fontanel, or widely split sutures. In infants who develop symptomatic hydrocephalus, clinical signs may be delayed 2–4 wk despite progressive ventricular distention and compression (thinning) of the cerebral cortex. Posthemorrhagic hydrocephalus is arrested or regresses in 65% of affected infants.

Progressive hydrocephalus requiring ventricular-peritoneal shunting, gestational age of less than 30 wk, prolonged mechanical ventilation (>28 days), intraparenchymal hemorrhage, and extensive PVL are associated with a poor prognosis. Because PVL and intraparenchymal bleeding represent hypoxic-ischemic injury, they are independent risk factors for spastic diplegia and other motor deficits. IVH with intraparenchymal echodensities greater than 1 cm are associated with a

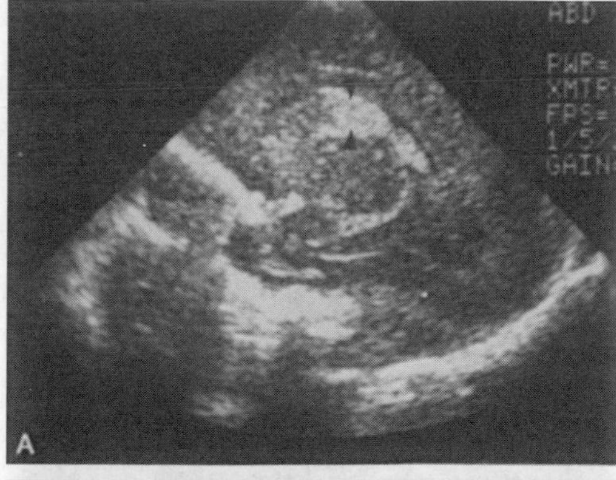

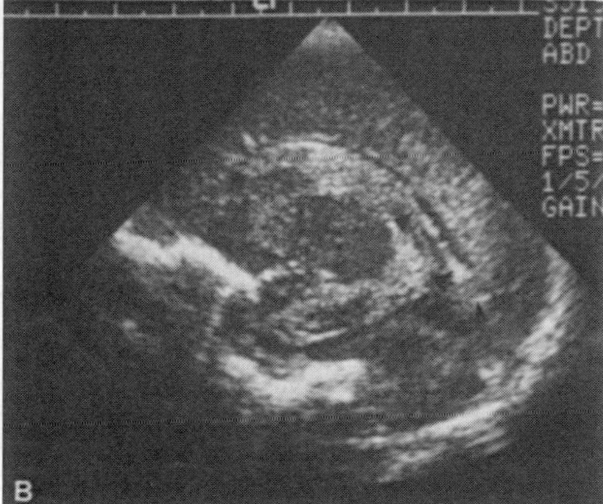

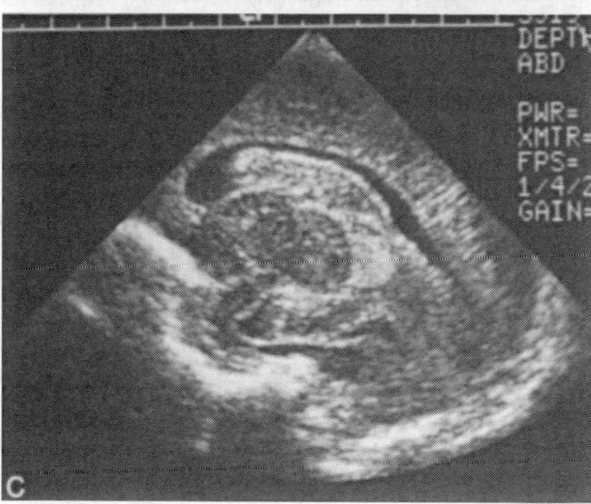

Figure 95–2 Grading the severity of germinal matrix–intraventricular hemorrhage with parasagittal ultrasound scans. *A*, Grade I. Note echogenic blood in germinal matrix *(arrowheads)* just anterior to the anterior tip of the choroid plexus, which (normally) also is echogenic. *B*, Grade II. Note echogenic blood *(arrowheads)* filling <50% of the ventricular area. *C*, Grade III. Note large blood clot nearly completely filling and distending the entire lateral ventricle. (From intracranial hemorrhage: Germinal matrix–intraventricular hemorrhage of the premature infant. *In* Volpe JJ [ed]: Neurology of the Newborn, 3rd ed. Philadelphia, WB Saunders, 1995.)

high mortality and a high incidence of motor and cognitive deficits. Grade I–II IVH may be due to factors other than severe hypoxia-ischemia, and in such a case has a lower risk of long-term neurologic sequelae if it is unassociated with PVL or intraparenchymal hemorrhage.

PREVENTION. The incidence of traumatic intracranial hemorrhage may be reduced by judicious management of cephalopelvic disproportion and operative (forceps, cesarean section) delivery. Fetal or neonatal hemorrhage due to maternal idiopathic thrombocytopenic purpura (ITP) or alloimmune thrombocytopenia may be prevented by maternal treatment with steroids, intravenous immunoglobulin, or fetal platelet transfusion. The incidence of IVH may be reduced by antenatal steroids and by postnatal administration of low-dose indomethacin. Wide fluctuations of blood pressure should be avoided. Vitamin K should be given before delivery to all women receiving phenobarbital or phenytoin during the pregnancy.

TREATMENT. IVH associated with hypoxic-ischemic encephalopathy is frequently associated with multiple organ system dysfunction. Seizures are treated with anticonvulsant drugs, anemia-shock requires transfusion with packed red blood cells or fresh frozen plasma, and acidosis is treated with judicious and slow administration of 1–2 mEq/kg sodium bicarbonate. Serial lumbar punctures have no role during the acute hemorrhage; however, repeated lumbar punctures may reduce the symptoms of posthemorrhagic hydrocephalus. Repeat lumbar punctures may increase the risk of nosocomial meningitis. Neurosurgical placement of an external ventriculostomy catheter may be needed in the early stage of uncontrolled symptomatic hydrocephalus. When the VLBW infant is large enough, a permanent ventricular-peritoneal shunt is put in place.

Symptomatic subdural hemorrhage in large term infants should be treated by removing the subdural fluid collection by means of a spinal needle placed through the lateral margin of the anterior fontanel. In addition to birth trauma, child abuse should be suspected in all infants with subdural effusions.

95.3 Spine and Spinal Cord

Strong traction exerted when the spine is hyperextended or when the direction of pull is lateral, or forceful longitudinal traction on the trunk while the head is still firmly engaged in the pelvis, especially when combined with flexion and torsion of the vertical axis, may produce fracture and separation of the vertebrae. Such injuries, rarely diagnosed clinically, are most likely to occur when difficulty is encountered in delivering the shoulders in cephalic presentations and the head in breech presentations. The injury occurs most commonly at the level of the 4th cervical vertebra with cephalic presentations and the lower cervical–upper thoracic vertebrae with breech presentations. Transection of the cord may occur with or without vertebral fractures; hemorrhage and edema may produce neurologic signs that are indistinguishable from those of transection except that they may not be permanent. Areflexia, loss of sensation, and complete paralysis of voluntary motion occur below the level of injury, although the persistence of a withdrawal reflex mediated through spinal centers distal to the area of injury is frequently misinterpreted as representing voluntary motion. If the injury is severe, the infant, who from birth may be in poor condition owing to respiratory depression, shock, or hypothermia, may deteriorate rapidly to death within several hours before neurologic signs are obvious. Alternatively, the course may be protracted, with symptoms and signs appearing at birth or later in the 1st wk; immobility, flaccidity, and associated brachial plexus injuries may not be recognized for several days. Constipation may also be present. Some infants survive for prolonged periods, their initial flaccidity, immobility, and areflexia being replaced after several weeks or months by rigid flexion of extremities, increased muscle tone, and spasms. Apnea on day 1 and poor motor recovery by 3 mo are poor prognostic signs.

The differential diagnosis includes amyotonia congenita and myelodysplasia associated with spina bifida occulta. The diagnosis is confirmed by ultrasonography or MRI. Treatment of the survivors is supportive, including home ventilation; patients often remain permanently injured. When there is compression from a fracture or dislocation, the prognosis is related to the time elapsing before the compression is relieved.

95.4 Peripheral Nerve Injuries

BRACHIAL PALSY. Injury to the brachial plexus may cause paralysis of the upper arm with or without paralysis of the forearm or hand or, more commonly, paralysis of the entire arm. These injuries occur in macrosomic infants and when lateral traction is exerted on the head and neck during delivery of the shoulder in a vertex presentation, when the arms are extended over the head in a breech presentation, or when excessive traction is placed on the shoulders. Approximately 45% are associated with shoulder dystocia.

In **Erb-Duchenne paralysis,** the injury is limited to the 5th and 6th cervical nerves. The infant loses the power to abduct the arm from the shoulder, to rotate the arm externally, and to supinate the forearm. The characteristic position consists of adduction and internal rotation of the arm with pronation of the forearm. The power of extension of the forearm is retained, but the biceps reflex is absent; the Moro reflex is absent on the affected side (Fig. 95–3). There may be some sensory impairment on the outer aspect of the arm. The power in the forearm and the hand grasp are preserved unless the lower part of the plexus is also injured; the presence of the hand grasp is a favorable prognostic sign. When the injury includes the phrenic nerve, alteration of the diaphragmatic excursion may be observed fluoroscopically.

Klumpke's paralysis is a rarer form of brachial palsy; in-

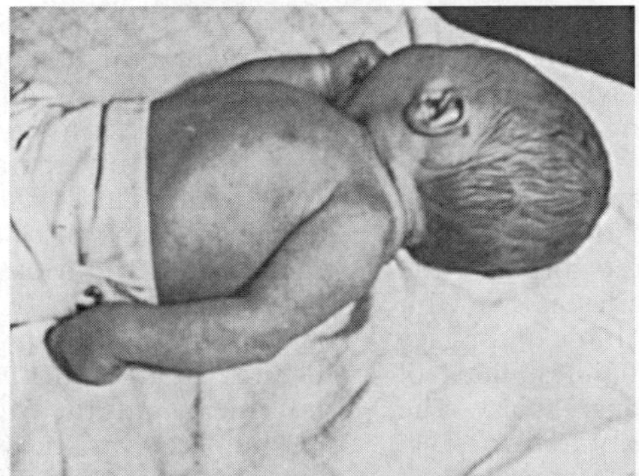
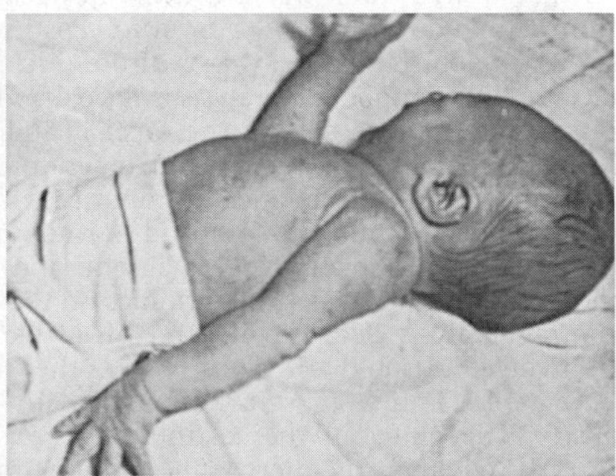

Figure 95–3 Brachial palsy of the left arm (asymmetric Moro reflex).

jury to the 7th and 8th cervical nerves and the 1st thoracic nerve produces a paralyzed hand, and ipsilateral ptosis and miosis (Horner syndrome) if the sympathetic fibers of the 1st thoracic root are also injured.

The mild cases may not be detected immediately after birth. Differentiation must be made from cerebral injury; from fracture, dislocation, or epiphyseal separation of the humerus; and from fracture of the clavicle. MRI demonstrates nerve root rupture or avulsion.

The *prognosis* depends on whether the nerve was merely injured or was lacerated. If the paralysis was due to edema and hemorrhage about the nerve fibers, function should return within a few months; if due to laceration, permanent damage may result. Involvement of the deltoid is usually the most serious problem and may result in a shoulder drop secondary to muscle atrophy. In general, paralysis of the upper arm has a better prognosis than paralysis of the lower arm.

Treatment consists of partial immobilization and appropriate positioning to prevent development of contractures. In upper arm paralysis, the arm should be abducted 90 degrees, with external rotation at the shoulder and with full supination of the forearm and slight extension at the wrist with the palm turned toward the face. This may be done with a brace or splint during the first 1–2 wk. Immobilization should be intermittent through the day while the infant is asleep and between feedings. In lower arm or hand paralysis, the wrist should be splinted in a neutral position and padding placed in the fist. When the entire arm is paralyzed, the same treatment principles should be followed. Gentle massage and range of motion exercises may be started by 7–10 days of age. Infants should be closely monitored with active and passive corrective exercises. If the paralysis persists without improvement for 3–6 mo, neuroplasty, neurolysis, end-to-end anastomosis, or nerve grafting offers hope for partial recovery.

PHRENIC NERVE PARALYSIS. Phrenic nerve injury (3rd, 4th, 5th cervical nerves) with diaphragmatic paralysis must be considered when cyanosis and irregular and labored respirations develop. Such injuries, usually unilateral, are associated with ipsilateral upper brachial palsy. Because breathing is thoracic in type, the abdomen does not bulge with inspiration. Breath sounds are diminished on the affected side. The thrust of the diaphragm, which often may be felt just under the costal margin on the normal side, is absent on the affected side. The *diagnosis* is established by ultrasonography or fluoroscopic examination, which reveals elevation of the diaphragm on the paralyzed side and seesaw movements of the two sides of the diaphragm during respiration.

There is no specific *treatment*; infants should be placed on the involved side and given oxygen if necessary. Initially, intravenous feedings may be needed; later, progressive gavage or oral feedings may be started, depending on an infant's condition. Pulmonary infections are a serious complication. Recovery usually occurs spontaneously by 1–3 mo; rarely, surgical plication of the diaphragm may be indicated.

FACIAL NERVE PALSY. Facial palsy usually is a peripheral paralysis that results from pressure over the facial nerve in utero, from efforts during labor, or from forceps use during delivery. Rarely nonobstetric, it may result from nuclear agenesis of the facial nerve. Peripheral paralysis is flaccid and, when complete, involves the entire side of the face, including the forehead. When the infant cries, there is movement only on the nonparalyzed side of the face, and the mouth is drawn to that side. On the affected side the forehead is smooth, the eye cannot be closed, the nasolabial fold is absent, and the corner of the mouth droops. The forehead wrinkles on the affected side with central paralysis, because only the lower two thirds of the face is involved. Usually there are also other manifestations of intracranial injury, most commonly a 6th nerve palsy. The *prognosis* depends on whether the nerve was injured by pressure or whether the nerve fibers were torn. Improvement occurs within a few weeks in the former instance. Care of the exposed eye is essential. Neuroplasty may be indicated when the paralysis is persistent. Facial palsy may be confused with the absence of the depressor muscles of the mouth, which is a benign problem.

Other peripheral nerves are seldom injured in utero or at birth except when they are involved in fractures or hemorrhages.

95.5 Viscera

The **liver** is the only internal organ other than the brain that is injured with any frequency during birth. The damage usually results from pressure on the liver during delivery of the head in breech presentations. Large infant size, intrauterine asphyxia, coagulation disorders, extreme prematurity, and hepatomegaly are contributing factors. Incorrect cardiac massage is a less frequent cause. Hepatic rupture may result in the formation of a subcapsular hematoma, which may tamponade further bleeding. Infants usually appear normal for the first 1–3 days. Nonspecific signs related to loss of blood into the hematoma may appear early and include poor feeding, listlessness, pallor, jaundice, tachypnea, and tachycardia. A mass may be palpable in the right upper quadrant; the abdomen may appear blue. The hematoma may be large enough to cause anemia. Shock and death may occur if the hematoma breaks through the capsule into the peritoneal cavity, reducing pressure and allowing fresh hemorrhage. Early suspicion by means of ultrasonographic diagnosis and prompt supportive therapy can decrease the mortality of this disorder. Surgical repair of a laceration may be required.

Rupture of the spleen may occur alone or in association with rupture of the liver. The causes, complications, treatment, and prevention are similar.

Although **adrenal hemorrhage** occurs with some frequency, especially after breech delivery in LGA infants or infants of diabetic mothers, its cause is undetermined; it may be due to trauma, anoxia, or severe stress, as in overwhelming infections. Ninety per cent are unilateral; 75% are right sided. Calcified central hematomas of the adrenal have been identified roentgenographically or at autopsy in older infants and children, suggesting that not all adrenal hemorrhages are immediately fatal. In severe cases, the diagnosis is usually made at postmortem examination. The symptoms are profound shock and cyanosis. There may be a mass in the flank, with overlying skin discoloration; jaundice may also develop. If adrenal hemorrhage is suspected, abdominal ultrasonography may be helpful, and treatment for acute adrenal failure may be indicated (Chapter 585).

95.6 Fractures

CLAVICLE. This bone is fractured during labor and delivery more frequently than any other bone; it is particularly vulnerable when there is difficulty in delivery of the shoulder in vertex presentations and of the extended arms in breech deliveries. The infant characteristically does not move the arm freely on the affected side; crepitus and bony irregularity may be palpated, and discoloration is occasionally visible over the fracture site. The Moro reflex is absent on the affected side, and there is spasm of the sternocleidomastoid muscle with obliteration of the supraclavicular depression at the site of the fracture. In greenstick fractures there may be no limitation of movement, and the Moro reflex may be present. Fracture of the humerus or brachial palsy may also be responsible for limitation of movement of an arm and absence of a Moro reflex on the affected side. The *prognosis* is excellent. *Treatment,* if any, consists of immobilization of the arm and shoulder on the affected side. A remarkable degree of callus develops at the site within a week and may be the first evidence of the fracture.

EXTREMITIES

In fractures of the long bones, spontaneous movement of the extremity is usually absent. The Moro reflex is also absent from the involved extremity. There may be associated nerve involvement. Satisfactory results of treatment for a fractured humerus are obtained with 2–4 wk of immobilization during which the arm is strapped to the chest, a triangular splint and a Velpeau bandage are applied, or a cast is applied. For fracture of the femur, good results are obtained with traction-suspension of both lower extremities, even if the fracture is unilateral; the legs, immobilized in a spica cast, are attached to an overhead frame. Splints are effective for treatment of fractures of the forearm or leg. Healing is usually accompanied by excess callus formation. The *prognosis* is excellent for fractures of the extremities. Fractures in preterm infants may be related to osteopenia (Chapter 102).

Dislocations and **epiphyseal separations** rarely result from birth trauma. The upper femoral epiphysis may be separated by forcible manipulation of the infant's leg, as, for example, in breech extraction or after version. The affected leg shows swelling, slight shortening, limitation of active motion, painful passive motion, and external rotation. The diagnosis is established roentgenographically. The prognosis is good for the milder injuries, but coxa vara frequently results from extensive displacement.

NOSE. The most prevalent injury of the nose is a dislocation of the cartilaginous portion of the septum from the vomerine groove and the columella. The infant may have difficulty in nursing and some impairment in nasal respiration. On physical examination, the nares appear asymmetric and the nose flattened. An oral airway rarely is needed, and surgical consultation should be obtained for definitive treatment.

95.7 Hypoxia-Ischemia

Anoxia is a term used to indicate the consequences of a complete lack of oxygen due to a number of primary causes. *Hypoxia* refers to an arterial concentration of oxygen that is less than normal, and *ischemia* refers to blood flow to cells or organs that is insufficient to maintain their normal function. *Hypoxic-ischemic encephalopathy* is an important cause of permanent damage to central nervous system cells, which may result in neonatal death or which may be manifested later as cerebral palsy or mental deficiency. Fifteen to 20% of infants with hypoxic-ischemic encephalopathy die in the neonatal period; 25–30% of survivors develop permanent neurodevelopmental abnormalities (cerebral palsy, mental retardation). Its prevention and treatment are those of the basic conditions that cause it; death and disability may sometimes be prevented through symptomatic treatment with oxygen or artificial respiration and the correction of associated multiorgan system dysfunction (Table 95–1). *Asphyxia* is considered in the presence of fetal acidosis (pH <7.0), a 5-min Apgar score of 0–3, hypoxic-ischemic encephalopathy (altered tone, depressed level of consciousness, seizures), and other multiple organ system signs (Table 95–1).

ETIOLOGY. Fetal hypoxia may result from (1) inadequate oxygenation of maternal blood as a result of hypoventilation during anesthesia, cyanotic heart disease, respiratory failure, or carbon monoxide poisoning; (2) low maternal blood pressure as a result of the hypotension that may complicate spinal anesthesia or that may result from compression of the vena cava and aorta by the gravid uterus; (3) inadequate relaxation of the uterus to permit placental filling as a result of uterine tetany caused by excessive administration of oxytocin; (4) premature separation of the placenta; (5) impedance to the circulation of blood through the umbilical cord as a result of compression or knotting of the cord; (6) uterine vessel vasoconstriction by cocaine; and (7) placental insufficiency from numerous causes, including toxemia and postmaturity.

TABLE 95–1 Effects of Asphyxia

System	Effect
Central nervous system	Hypoxic-ischemic encephalopathy, infarction, intracranial hemorrhage, seizures, cerebral edema, hypotonia, hypertonia
Cardiovascular	Myocardial ischemia, poor contractility, cardiac stun, tricuspid insufficiency, hypotension
Pulmonary	Pulmonary hypertension, pulmonary hemorrhage, respiratory distress syndrome
Renal	Acute tubular or cortical necrosis
Adrenal	Adrenal hemorrhage
Gastrointestinal	Perforation, ulceration with hemorrhage, necrosis
Metabolic	Inappropriate secretion of antidiuretic hormone, hyponatremia, hypoglycemia, hypocalcemia, myoglobinuria
Integument	Subcutaneous fat necrosis
Hematology	Disseminated intravascular coagulation

Placental insufficiency often remains undetected on clinical assessment. Chronically hypoxic fetuses may develop intrauterine growth retardation without traditional signs of fetal distress (e.g., bradycardia). Doppler umbilical waveform velocimetry (demonstrating increased fetal vascular resistance, Fig. 92–3) and cordocentesis (demonstrating fetal hypoxia) identify the chronically hypoxic infant. Uterine contractions further reduce umbilical oxygenation, depressing the fetal cardiovascular and central nervous systems and resulting in low Apgar scores and postnatal hypoxia in the delivery room.

After birth, hypoxia may result from (1) anemia severe enough to lower the oxygen content of the blood to a critical level owing to severe hemorrhage or hemolytic disease; (2) shock severe enough to interfere with the transport of oxygen to vital cells from overwhelming infection, massive blood loss, and intracranial or adrenal hemorrhage; (3) a deficit in arterial oxygen saturation resulting from failure to breathe adequately postnatally owing to a cerebral defect, narcosis, or injury; and (4) failure of oxygenation of an adequate amount of blood resulting from severe forms of cyanotic congenital heart disease or pulmonary disease.

PATHOPHYSIOLOGY AND PATHOLOGY. Within minutes of the onset of total fetal hypoxia, bradycardia, hypotension, decreased cardiac output, and severe metabolic as well as respiratory acidosis occur. The initial circulatory response of a fetus is increased shunting through the ductus venosus, ductus arteriosus, and foramen ovale, with transient maintenance of perfusion of the brain, heart, and adrenals in preference to the lungs (owing to pulmonary vasoconstriction), liver, kidneys, and intestine.

The pathology of hypoxia-ischemia is dependent on the affected organ and the severity of the insult. Early congestion, fluid leak from increased capillary permeability, and endothelial cell swelling may then lead to signs of coagulation necrosis and cell death. Congestion and petechiae are seen in the pericardium, pleura, thymus, heart, adrenals, and meninges. Prolonged intrauterine hypoxia may result in PVL and pulmonary arteriole smooth muscle hyperplasia, which predisposes the infant to pulmonary hypertension (Chapter 97.7). If fetal distress produces gasping, amniotic fluid contents (meconium, squames, lanugo) are aspirated into the trachea or lungs.

The combination of chronic fetal hypoxia and acute hypoxic-ischemic injury after birth results in gestational age-specific neuropathology. Term infants demonstrate neuronal necrosis of the cortex (later cortical atrophy) and parasagittal ischemic injury. Preterm infants demonstrate PVL (later spastic diplegia), status marmoratus of the basal ganglia, and IVH. Term, more often than preterm, infants demonstrate focal or multifocal cortical infarcts that produce focal seizures and hemiplegia. Infarctions are best visualized with CT scanning or MRI. In addition to focal lesions, CT scanning may demonstrate diffuse decreases of tissue attenuation. Cerebral edema with resultant increased intracranial pressure occurs in some infants who have severe hypoxic-ischemic encephalopathy. Excitatory amino acids may have an important role in the pathogenesis of asphyxial brain injury.

CLINICAL MANIFESTATIONS. The signs of hypoxia in a *fetus* are usually noted a few minutes to a few days before delivery. Intrauterine growth retardation with increased vascular resistance may be the first indication of fetal hypoxia. The fetal heart rate slows, and the beat-to-beat variability declines. Continuous heart rate recording may reveal a variable or late (type II dips) deceleration pattern (see Fig. 92–4), and fetal scalp blood analysis may show a pH less than 7.20. The acidosis is made up of various degrees of metabolic or respiratory components. Particularly in infants near term, these signs should lead to administration of high concentrations of oxygen to the mother and immediate delivery to avoid fetal death or central nervous system damage.

At *delivery,* the presence of yellow, meconium-stained amniotic fluid is evidence that fetal distress has occurred. At birth, these infants are frequently depressed and fail to breathe spontaneously. During the ensuing hours, they may remain hypotonic or change from hypotonia to extreme hypertonia, or their tone may appear normal (Table 95–2). Pallor, cyanosis, apnea, slow heart rate, and unresponsiveness to stimulation also are signs of hypoxic-ischemic encephalopathy. Cerebral edema may develop during the next 24 hr and result in profound brain stem depression. During this time, seizure activity may occur, and it may be severe and refractory to the usual doses of anticonvulsants. Phenobartital, the drug of choice, is given with an intravenous loading dose (20 mg/kg); additional doses of 10 mg/kg (up to 40–50 mg/kg total) may be needed. Phenytoin (20 mg/kg loading dose) or lorazepam (0.1 mg/kg) may be needed for refractory seizures. Phenobarbital levels should be monitored 24 hr after the loading dose and maintenance therapy (5 mg/kg/24 hr) are begun. Therapeutic phenobarbital levels are 20–40 μg/mL. Although most often a result of the hypoxic-ischemic encephalopathy, seizures in asphyxiated newborns may also be due to hypocalcemia and hypoglycemia.

In addition to central nervous system dysfunction, congestive heart failure and cardiogenic shock, persistent pulmonary hypertension (persistent fetal circulation), respiratory distress syndrome, gastrointestinal perforation, hematuria, and acute tubular necrosis are associated with perinatal asphyxia (see Table 95–1).

After delivery, hypoxia is due to respiratory failure and circulatory insufficiency (Chapter 97).

TREATMENT. Therapy is supportive and directed at the organ system manifestations. There is no established effective treatment for the brain tissue injury, although many drugs (phenobarbital, allopurinol, calcium channel blockers) and procedures (local cranial hypothermia, hyperglycemia) are under study.

PROGNOSIS. The outcome of perinatal asphyxia depends on whether its metabolic and cardiopulmonary complications (hypoxia, hypoglycemia, shock) can be treated, on the infant's gestational age (outcome is poorest if the infant is preterm), and on the severity of the hypoxic-ischemic encephalopathy. Severe encephalopathy (stage 3, see Table 95–2), characterized by flaccid coma, apnea, absent oculocephalic reflexes, refractory seizures, and a marked decrease of cortical attenuation on CT, is associated with a poor prognosis. A low Apgar score at 20 min, absence of spontaneous respirations at 20 min age, and persistence of abnormal neurologic signs at age 2 wk also predict death or severe cognitive and motor deficits.

Brain death following neonatal hypoxic-ischemic encephalopathy is diagnosed by the clinical findings of coma that is unresponsive to pain, auditory, or visual stimulation; apnea with P_{CO_2} rising from 40 to over 60 mm Hg; and absent brain stem reflexes (pupil, oculocephalic, oculovestibular, corneal, gag, sucking). These must occur in the absence of hypothermia, hypotension, and elevated levels of depressant drugs (e.g., phenobarbital). The absence of cerebral blood flow on radionuclide scan and electrical activity on EEG (electrocerebral silence) is inconsistently observed in clinically brain dead neonatal infants. Persistence of the clinical criteria for 2 days in term and 3 days in preterm infants predicts brain death in most asphyxiated newborns. Nonetheless, there is no universal agreement about the definition of neonatal brain death. Consideration of withdrawal of life support should include discussions with the family, the health care team, and, if there is disagreement, an ethics committee. The best interest of the infant involves judgments about the benefits and harm of continuing therapy and of avoiding continuing futile therapy.

TABLE 95–2 Hypoxic-Ischemic Encephalopathy in Term Infants

Signs	Stage 1	Stage 2	Stage 3
Level of consciousness	Hyperalert	Lethargic	Stuporous, coma
Muscle tone	Normal	Hypotonic	Flaccid
Posture	Normal	Flexion	Decerebrate
Tendon reflexes/ clonus	Hyperactive	Hyperactive	Absent
Myoclonus	Present	Present	Absent
Moro reflex	Strong	Weak	Absent
Pupils	Mydriasis	Miosis	Unequal, poor light reflex
Seizures	None	Common	Decerebration
Electroencephalographic	Normal	Low voltage changing to seizure activity	Burst suppression to isoelectric
Duration	<24 hr if progresses; otherwise, may remain normal	24 hr to 14 days	Days to weeks
Outcome	Good	Variable	Death, severe deficits

Modified from Sarnat H, Sarnat M: Neonatal encephalopathy following fetal distress: A clinical and electroencephalographic study. Arch Neurol 33:696, 1976. Copyright 1976, American Medical Association.

Bager B: Perinatally acquired brachial plexus palsy—a persisting challenge. Acta Paediatr 86:1214, 1997.
Cordes I, Roland EH, Lupton BA, et al: Early prediction of the development of microcephaly after hypoxic-ischemic encephalopathy in the full-term newborn. Pediatrics 93:703, 1994.
de Vries LS, Eken P, Groenendaal F, et al: Antenatal onset of haemorrhagic and/or ischaemic lesions in preterm infants: Prevalence and associated obstetric variables. Arch Dis Child 78:F51, 1998.
Ekert P, Perlman M, Steinlin M, et al: Predicting the outcome of postasphyxial hypoxic-ischemic encephalopathy within 4 hours of birth. J Pediatr 131:613, 1997.
Evans D, Levene M: Neonatal seizures. Arch Dis Child 78:F70, 1998.
Hall RT, Hall FK, Daily DK: High-dose phenobarbital therapy in term newborn infants with severe perinatal asphyxia: A randomized, prospective study with three-year follow-up. J Pediatr 132:345, 1998.
MacKinnon JA, Perlman M, Kirpalani H, et al: Spinal cord injury at birth: Diagnostic and prognostic data in twenty-two patients. J Pediatr 122:431, 1993.
Martin-Ancel A, García-Alix A, Gayá F, et al: Multiple organ involvement in perinatal asphyxia. J Pediatr 127:786, 1995.
Nocon JJ, McKenzie DK, Thomas LJ, et al: Shoulder dystocia: An analysis of risks and obstetric maneuvers. Am J Obstet Gynecol 168:1732, 1993.
Perlman JM, Risser R, Broyles RS: Bilateral cystic periventricular leukomalacia in the premature infant: Associated risk factors. Pediatrics 97:822, 1996.
Rehan VK, Seshia MMK: Spinal cord birth injury—diagnostic difficulties. Arch Dis Child 69:92, 1993.
Rogers B, Msall M, Owens T, et al: Cystic periventricular leukomalacia and type of cerebral palsy in preterm infants. J Pediatr 125:S1, 1994.

Schullinger JN: Birth trauma. Pediatr Clin North Am 40:1351, 1993.

Van Bel F, Shadid M, Morson RMW, et al: Effect of allopurinol on postasphyxial free radical formation, cerebral hemodynamics, and electrical brain activity. Pediatrics 101:185, 1998.

Vannucci RC, Perlman JM: Interventions for perinatal hypoxic-ischemic encephalopathy. Pediatrics 100:1004, 1997.

Ventriculomegaly Trial Group: Randomised trial of early tapping in neonatal posthaemorrhagic ventricular dilatation: Results at 30 months. Arch Dis Child 70:F129, 1994.

Wiswell TE, Graziani LJ, Kornhauser MS, et al: Effects of hypocarbia on the development of cystic periventricular leukomalacia in premature infants treated with high-frequency jet ventilation. Pediatrics 98:918, 1996.

CHAPTER 96
Delivery Room Emergencies

The most common and important emergency related to newborn infants in the delivery room is the failure to initiate and maintain respirations. Less frequent but of major importance are shock (Chapter 94), severe anemia (Chapter 99.1), plethora (Chapter 99.3), convulsions (Chapter 602.5), and management of life-threatening congenital malformations (Chapter 94).

RESPIRATORY DISTRESS AND FAILURE. Disorders of respiration in newborn infants can be categorized as either *central nervous system* (CNS) *failure,* representing depression or failure of the respiratory center, or *peripheral respiratory difficulty,* indicating interference with the alveolar exchange of oxygen and carbon dioxide. Cyanosis occurs in both groups (see Table 94–1). The respiratory problems encountered in the delivery room are most frequently those of airway obstruction and of depression of the CNS (maternal medications, asphyxia), with the absence of adequate respiratory effort.

Respiratory distress in the presence of good respiratory effort should lead to an immediate consideration of peripheral causes; *it is an indication for a roentgenographic examination of the chest,* if this is at all possible.

If respiratory movements are made with the mouth closed but the infant fails to move air in and out of the lungs, bilateral **choanal atresia** (Chapter 378) or other obstruction of the upper respiratory tract should be suspected. The mouth should be opened, and the mouth and posterior pharynx cleared of secretions by gentle suction. An oropharyngeal airway should be inserted, and the source of the obstruction sought immediately. If effective respiratory flow is not produced by opening the infant's mouth and clearing the airway, laryngoscopy is indicated. With obstructive malformations of the mandible, epiglottis, larynx, or trachea, an endotracheal tube should be inserted; prolonged endotracheal intubation or tracheostomy may be required. Respiratory failure due to depression or injury of the CNS may require continuous artificial ventilation with a face mask and bag or through an endotracheal tube.

Hypoplasia of the mandible (Pierre Robin, DiGeorge's, and other syndromes) (Chapter 311) with posterior displacement of the tongue may result in symptoms similar to those of choanal atresia, which may be temporarily relieved by pulling the tongue forward. A scaphoid abdomen suggests a **diaphragmatic hernia** or **eventration,** as does asymmetry of contour or movement of the chest or shift of the apical impulse of the heart; these latter manifestations are also compatible with tension pneumothorax. A pneumothorax in the 1st day of life suggests pulmonary hypoplasia, renal malformations, or both.

Causes of peripheral respiratory difficulty are discussed in Chapter 97.

FAILURE TO INITIATE OR SUSTAIN RESPIRATION. This usually originates in the CNS as a result of asphyxia; immaturity in itself is seldom a causative factor except in infants weighing less than 1,000 g. Intrapulmonary problems, such as the pulmonary hypoplasia associated with Potter syndrome, bilateral pleural effusions (hydrops fetalis), and severe organized intrauterine pneumonia, may at times result in poorly sustained ventilation. The lungs in these infants are very noncompliant, and efforts to begin respirations may be inadequate to start sufficient ventilation.

Narcosis results from heavy doses of morphine, meperidine (Demerol), fentanyl, barbiturates, or tranquilizers administered to the mother shortly before delivery or from maternal anesthesia, given during the second stage of labor. Infants are cyanotic and hypotonic at birth and slow to cry or breathe; when respiration is established, it is extremely slow.

Narcosis should be avoided by using appropriate analgesic and anesthetic practices. Treatment includes initial physical stimulation and securing a patent airway. If effective ventilation is not initiated, artificial breathing with a mask and bag must be instituted. At the same time, if depression is due to morphine or its derivatives, naloxone hydrochloride (Narcan), 0.1 mg/kg, should be given by intravenous, subcutaneous, intratracheal, or intramuscular routes and repeated two to three times if needed. Narcan is contraindicated with maternal opiate addiction because it precipitates acute neonatal withdrawal with severe seizures. Ventilation is essential before and during administration of this antidote. If depression is due to other anesthetics or analgesics, artificial respiration should be continued until the infant is able to sustain ventilation. CNS stimulant drugs should not be used because they are ineffective and may be harmful.

Prenatal or **perinatal hypoxia** of whatever cause, if sufficiently severe, produces brain stem depression and secondary apnea, which is unresponsive to sensory stimulation. Death due to apnea may be prevented by resuscitation, provided the basic cause of the hypoxia can be eliminated within a reasonable time while artificial respiration, if necessary, is being carried out. External cardiac massage, correction of acidosis, and circulatory support with drugs may be important adjuncts to ventilation.

RESUSCITATION. The *goals* of neonatal resuscitation are to prevent the morbidity and mortality associated with hypoxic-ischemic tissue (brain, heart, kidney) injury and to re-establish adequate spontaneous respiration and cardiac output. High-risk situations should be anticipated by the history of the pregnancy, labor, and delivery and by identification of the signs of fetal distress. Although the Apgar score is helpful in evaluating patients in need of attention, infants who are born limp, cyanotic, apneic, or pulseless require immediate resuscitation before assignment of the 1-min Apgar score. Rapid and appropriate resuscitative efforts improve the likelihood of preventing brain damage and achieving a successful outcome.

Immediately after birth, an asphyxiated infant should be placed under a radiant heater (to avoid hypothermia), dried, positioned head down and slightly extended, the airway cleared by suctioning, and gentle tactile stimulation provided (slapping the foot, rubbing the back). Simultaneously, the infant's color, heart rate, and respiratory effort should be assessed.

The steps in neonatal resuscitation follow the ABCs: **A,** *a*nticipate and establish a patent *a*irway by suctioning and, if necessary, perform endotracheal intubation; **B,** initiate *b*reathing using tactile stimulation or positive pressure ventilation with a bag and mask or through an endotracheal tube; **C,** maintain the *c*irculation with chest compression and medications, if needed.

If there are no respirations or if the heart rate is below 100/min, *positive pressure ventilation* with 100% oxygen is given through a tightly fitted face mask and bag for 15–30 sec. Although the first breath may require pressures as low as

15–20 cm H_2O, pressures as high as 30–40 cm H_2O may be needed. Subsequent breaths are given at a rate of 40–60/min, with pressures of 15–20 cm H_2O. Noncompliant stiff lungs due to hyaline membrane disease, congenital pneumonia, or meconium aspiration need higher pressures (20–40 cm H_2O). Successful ventilation is determined by good chest rise, symmetric breath sounds, improved pink color, heart rate greater than 100/min, spontaneous respirations, and improved tone.

If the mother has a history of analgesic narcotic drug administration, Narcan is given while adequate ventilation is maintained. Breathing for the depressed infant should be maintained until a response to Narcan is noted. Continuous observation of the infant is important because repeated doses of Narcan may be needed.

If the heart rate does not improve after 15–30 sec with bag and mask (or endotracheal) ventilation and remains below 60/min or if the rate is less than 80/min and not rising, ventilation is continued and *chest compression* with two fingers is initiated over the lower third of the sternum at a rate of 120/min. The ratio of compressions to ventilation is 3:1. Bradycardia in neonatal infants is usually due to hypoxia resulting from respiratory arrest and often responds to ventilation with 100% oxygen. Persistent bradycardia despite ventilation with 100% oxygen suggests more severe cardiac compromise or inadequate ventilation techniques. Poor response to ventilation may be due to a loosely fitted mask, poor positioning of the airway, intraesophageal intubation, airway obstruction, insufficient pressure, pleural effusions, pneumothorax, excessive air in the stomach, asystole, hypovolemia, diaphragmatic hernia, or prolonged intrauterine asphyxia.

Endotracheal intubation should be performed by an experienced person for any infant who does not respond to initial bag and mask ventilation or who was born apneic, pulseless, cyanotic, and limp.

Medications should be administered when the heart rate is less than 80/min after 30 sec of combined ventilation and chest compressions or during asystole. The umbilical vein usually can be readily cannulated and should be used for immediate administration of medications, glucose, and volume expanders during neonatal resuscitation. Epinephrine (0.1–0.3 mL/kg of a 1:10,000 solution, intravenous or intratracheal) is given for asystole or for failure to respond to 30 sec of combined resuscitation. The dose may be repeated every 5 min. If there is no response, some authorities recommend using 5 to 10 times the standard dose of epinephrine. Ten to 20 mL/kg of volume expanders (normal saline, blood, Ringer's lactate, 5% albumin) should be given for hypovolemia, pallor, electrical-mechanical dissociation (weak pulses with normal heart rate), history of blood loss, suspicion of septic shock, hypotension, or poor response to resuscitation. Sodium bicarbonate (1–2 mEq/kg, 0.5 mEq/mL of a 4.2% solution) should be given slowly (1 mEq/kg/min) if there is a documented metabolic acidosis and the resuscitation is prolonged. Sodium bicarbonate should be given after effective ventilation has been established because such therapy may increase blood CO_2, producing a respiratory acidosis. Restoration of oxygenation and tissue perfusion is the main treatment for the metabolic acidosis associated with asphyxia.

Severe asphyxia also may depress myocardial function, causing cardiogenic shock despite recovery of heart and respiratory rates. Dopamine or dobutamine administered as a continuous infusion (5–20 μg/kg/min) and volume expanders should be started after the initial resuscitation effort to improve cardiac output in an infant with poor peripheral perfusion, weak pulses, hypotension, tachycardia, and poor urine output. Epinephrine (0.1–1.0 μg/kg/min) may be indicated for infants in severe shock who do not respond to dopamine or dobutamine.

Less severe degrees of asphyxia can usually be managed by brief periods of bag and mask ventilation of 100% oxygen. Chest compression and medications are not needed for most neonates who have mild to moderate birth depression. Regardless of the severity of asphyxia or the response to resuscitation, asphyxiated infants should be monitored closely for signs of multiorgan hypoxic-ischemic tissue injury (see Table 95–1).

SHOCK. Circulatory insufficiency may present at birth as a result of severe asphyxia or of internal hemorrhage; fetal bleeding during gestation, labor, or delivery (e.g., fetofetal or fetomaternal transfusion syndrome); bleeding from the fetal circulation secondary to a placental tear during amniocentesis; excessive bleeding from a severed or torn umbilical cord; or severe hemolytic anemia. Clinical manifestations include signs of respiratory distress, cyanosis, pallor, flaccidity, cold mottled skin, tachycardia or bradycardia, hepatosplenomegaly, and, rarely, convulsions. **Edema** and hepatosplenomegaly also may suggest hydrops fetalis or heart failure without shock. Shock from overwhelming infection may also be present after birth.

Supportive treatment with type O Rh negative blood or electrolyte solutions is indicated for hemorrhage or hypovolemia, respectively. Oxygen should be administered and metabolic acidosis corrected with sodium bicarbonate, β-sympathomimetic agents, such as dopamine or dobutamine, may be needed to support cardiac output and blood pressure. The diagnosis and treatment of erythroblastosis fetalis are discussed in Chapter 99.2. If infection is present, appropriate antibiotics must be started as soon as possible.

After supportive measures have stabilized the infant's condition, a specific diagnosis should be established and appropriate continuing treatment instituted.

Blair E, Stanley FJ: Intrapartum asphyxia: A rare cause of cerebral palsy. J Pediatr 112:515, 1988.
Carrasco M, Martell M, Estol PC: Oronasopharyngeal suction at birth: Effects on arterial oxygen saturation. J Pediatr 130:832, 1997.
Davis DJ: How aggressive should delivery room cardiopulmonary resuscitation be for extremely low birth weight neonates? Pediatrics 92:447, 1993.
Emergency Cardiac Care Committee and Subcommittees, American Heart Association: Guidelines for cardiopulmonary resuscitation and emergency cardiac care. Neonatal resuscitation. JAMA 268:2276, 1992.
Lees M, King D: Cyanosis in the newborn. Pediatr Rev 9:36, 1987.
Marrin M, Paes BA: Birth asphyxia: Does the Apgar score have diagnostic value? Obstet Gynecol 72:120, 1988.
Perlman JM, Risser R: Cardiopulmonary resuscitation in the delivery room. Arch Pediatr Adolesc Med 149:20, 1995.
Perlman JM, Tack ED, Martin T, et al: Acute systemic organ injury in term infants after asphyxia. Am J Dis Child 143:617, 1989.
Wimmer JE: Neonatal resuscitation. Pediatr Rev 15:255, 1994.

CHAPTER 97
Respiratory Tract Disorders

Disturbances of respiration in the immediate postnatal period may have originated in utero, in the delivery room, or in the nursery. A wide variety of pathologic lesions may be responsible for one or more of the signs of respiratory distress (see Tables 94–1 and 94–2); cyanosis is common, and if respiratory embarrassment is severe, pallor may also be present. It is occasionally difficult to distinguish cardiovascular from respiratory disturbances on the basis of clinical signs alone. Signs of respiratory distress in newborn infants may suggest hyaline membrane disease (HMD; respiratory distress syndrome [RDS]), aspiration syndrome, pneumonia, sepsis, congenital heart disease, heart failure, pulmonary hypertension, choanal atresia, hypoglycemia, hypoplasia of the mandible with posterior displacement of the tongue, macroglossia, malformation of the epiglottis, malformation or injury of the larynx, cysts or neoplasms of the larynx or chest, pneumothorax, lobar emphysema, pulmonary agenesis or hypoplasia, congenital pulmonary lymphangiectasis, tracheoesophageal fistula, avulsion of the phrenic nerve, hernia or eventration of the diaphragm, intracranial lesions, neuromuscular disorders, and metabolic disturbances. *Any sign of postnatal respiratory distress is an indication for a roentgenogram of the chest.*

97.1 Transition to Pulmonary Respiration

Successful establishment of adequate lung function at birth is dependent on unobstructed anatomy and maturity of respiratory control. Fluid filling the fetal lungs must be removed, gas-containing functional residual capacity (FRC) established and maintained, and a ventilation-perfusion relationship developed that will provide optimal exchange of oxygen and carbon dioxide between alveoli and blood (Chapters 373–376).

THE FIRST BREATH. During vaginal delivery, intermittent compression of the thorax facilitates removal of lung fluid. Surfactant lining the alveoli enhances aeration of gas-free lungs by reducing surface tension, thereby lowering the pressure required to open alveoli. Nevertheless, the opening pressures required to inflate the airless lungs are higher than those needed at any other period of life; they range from 10–50 cm (usually 10–20 cm) H_2O for 0.5- to 1.0-sec intervals compared with about 4 cm for normal breathing in term infants and adults. Higher pressures necessary to initiate respiration are required to overcome the opposing forces of surface tension (particularly in small airways) and the viscosity of liquid remaining in the airways as well as to introduce about 50 mL of air into the lungs, 20–30 mL of which remains after the first breath to establish the FRC. Most of the liquid in the lungs is removed by the pulmonary circulation, which increases many fold at birth because all of the right ventricular output now perfuses the pulmonary vascular bed. The remainder of the fluid is removed by the pulmonary lymphatics, expelled by the infant, swallowed, or aspirated from the oropharynx; removal may be impaired after cesarean section or as a result of endothelial cell damage, hypoalbuminemia, high pulmonary venous pressure, or neonatal sedation.

The stimuli responsible for the first breath are numerous, and their relative importance is uncertain. They include a decline in Po_2 and pH and a rise in Pco_2 due to the interruption of the placental circulation, a redistribution of cardiac output after the umbilical cord is clamped, a decrease in body temperature, and various tactile stimuli.

Compared with term infants, low birthweight (LBW) infants who have a very compliant chest wall may be at a disadvantage in accomplishing the first breath. The FRC is least in the most immature infants, reflecting the presence of atelectasis. Abnormalities in the ventilation-perfusion ratio are greater and persist for longer periods, as does gas trapping. There may be a low Pao_2 (50–60 mm Hg) and elevated $Paco_2$, reflecting atelectasis, intrapulmonary shunting, and hypoventilation. The smallest immature infants have the most profound disturbances, which may resemble RDS.

BREATHING PATTERNS IN NEWBORNS. During sleep in the first months of life, normal full-term infants may have infrequent episodes when regular breathing is interrupted with short pauses. This **periodic breathing** pattern, shifting from a regular rhythmicity to cyclic brief episodes of intermittent apnea, is more common in premature infants, who may have apneic pauses of 5–10 sec followed by a burst of rapid respirations at a rate of 50–60/min for 10–15 sec. They rarely have an associated change in color or heart rate, and it often stops without apparent reason. Periodic breathing persists intermittently, usually until premature infants are about 36 wk of gestational age. If an infant is hypoxic, an increase in inspired oxygen concentration often converts periodic to regular breathing. There is no prognostic significance to periodic breathing, a normal characteristic of neonatal respiration.

97.2 Apnea

Periodic breathing must be distinguished from prolonged apneic pauses, because the latter may be associated with serious illnesses. Apnea is due to many primary diseases that affect neonates (Table 97–1). Such disorders produce direct depression of the central nervous system's control of respiration (e.g., hypoglycemia, meningitis, drugs, hemorrhage, seizures), disturbances of oxygen delivery by perfusion (shock, sepsis, anemia), or ventilation defects (pneumonia, HMD, persistent pulmonary hypertension [PPHN], muscle weakness).

Idiopathic apnea of prematurity occurs in the absence of identifiable predisposing diseases. Apnea is a disorder of respiratory control and may be obstructive, central, or mixed. In obstructive apnea (pharyngeal instability, neck flexion, nasal occlusion) there is absent airflow but persistent chest wall motion. Pharyngeal collapse may follow negative airway pressures generated during inspiration, or it may result from incoordination of the tongue and other upper airway muscles involved in maintaining airway patency. Central apnea, due to decreased central nervous system (CNS) stimuli to respiratory muscles, has simultaneously no airflow or chest wall motion. Gestational age is the most important determinant of respiratory control; the frequency of apnea is inversely related to gestational age. The immaturity of the brain stem respiratory centers is manifested by an attenuated response to carbon dioxide and a paradoxical response to hypoxia, resulting in apnea rather than hyperventilation. The most common pattern of idiopathic apnea among preterm neonates has a mixed etiology (50–75%), with obstructive apnea preceding (usually) or following central apnea. Short apneas are usually central, whereas prolonged apneas are often mixed.

Apnea is sleep state dependent; the frequency increases during active (rapid-eye-movement) sleep. Paradoxical chest wall movement (inspiratory abdominal expansion and inward chest wall movement) is common during active sleep and may cause a fall in Pao_2 due to ventilation-perfusion defects. Furthermore, increased negative pressure during paradoxical breathing and inhibition of pharyngeal muscle tone during active sleep may contribute to upper airway collapse and obstructive apnea.

CLINICAL MANIFESTATIONS. The incidence of idiopathic apnea of prematurity varies inversely with gestational age. In preterm infants, it is rare on the 1st day of life; apnea immediately after birth signifies another illness. The onset of idiopathic

TABLE 97–1 Potential Causes of Neonatal Apnea and Bradycardia

Central nervous system	Intraventricular hemorrhage, drugs, seizures, hypoxic injury, herniation, neuromuscular disorders, Leigh syndrome, brain stem infarction or anomalies (e.g., olivopontocerebellar atrophy), following general anesthesia
Respiratory	Pneumonia, obstructive airway lesions, upper airway collapse, atelectasis, extreme prematurity (<1,000 g), laryngeal reflex, phrenic nerve paralysis, severe hyaline membrane disease, pneumothorax, hypoxia
Infectious	Sepsis, necrotizing enterocolitis, meningitis (bacterial, fungal, viral), respiratory syncytial virus
Gastrointestinal	Oral feeding, bowel movement, gastroesophageal reflux, esophagitis, intestinal perforation
Metabolic	↓ Glucose, ↓ calcium, ↓ ↑ sodium, ↑ ammonia, ↑ organic acids, ↑ ambient temperature, hypothermia
Cardiovascular	Hypotension, hypertension, heart failure, anemia, hypovolemia, vagal tone
Other	Immaturity of respiratory center, sleep state

apnea occurs on the 2nd–7th day of life. The onset of apnea in a previously well premature neonate after the 2nd wk of life or in a term infant at any time is a critical event that warrants immediate investigation. In preterm infants, serious apnea is defined as cessation of breathing for longer than 20 sec or any duration if accompanied by cyanosis and sinus bradycardia. The incidence of associated bradycardia increases with the length of the preceding apnea and correlates with the severity of hypoxia. Short apneas (10 sec) are rarely associated with bradycardia, whereas longer apneas (>20 sec) have a higher incidence of bradycardia. Bradycardia follows the apnea by 1–2 sec in more than 95% of cases; vagal responses and, rarely, heart block are causes of bradycardia without apnea.

TREATMENT. Infants at risk for apnea should be monitored with apnea monitors. Gentle *cutaneous stimulation* is often adequate therapy for neonatal infants having mild and intermittent episodes. Infants having recurrent and prolonged apnea require immediate *bag and mask ventilation. Oxygen* should be administered to treat hypoxia. Apnea of prematurity not due to a precipitating identifiable cause should be treated with *theophylline* or *caffeine.* Methylxanthines enhance ventilation through a central mechanism or by improving diaphragmatic strength. Loading doses of 5 mg/kg of theophylline (PO) or aminophylline (IV) should be followed by doses of 1–2 mg/kg given every 6–8 hr using oral or intravenous routes. Loading doses of 10 mg/kg of caffeine are followed 24 hr later by maintenance doses of 2.5 mg/kg/24 hr qd. PO. These doses should be monitored by observation of vital signs, clinical response, and serum drug levels (therapeutic levels: theophylline, 6–10 μg/mL; caffeine, 8–20 μg/mL). *Transfusion of packed red blood cells* also may reduce the incidence of idiopathic apnea among severely anemic infants.

Nasal continuous positive airway pressure (CPAP, 3–5 cm H_2O) is effective therapy for mixed or obstructive apneas. CPAP may splint the upper airway, preventing obstruction. When apnea is due to a precipitating illness, airway stability and oxygenation must be maintained in addition to the therapy of the underlying disease.

PROGNOSIS. Unless severe, recurrent, and refractory to therapy, apnea of prematurity does not alter an infant's prognosis. Associated problems of intraventricular hemorrhage, chronic lung disease (CLD), and retinopathy of prematurity are critical in determining the prognosis for apneic infants. Apnea of prematurity usually resolves by 36 wk postconceptional age (gestational age at birth plus postnatal age) and does not predict future episodes of sudden infant death syndrome.

Darnall RA, Kattwinkel J, Nattie C, et al: Margin of safety for discharge after apnea in preterm infants. Pediatrics 100:795, 1997.
Eichenwald EC, Aina A, Stark AR: Apnea frequently persists beyond term gestation in infants delivered at 24 to 28 weeks. Pediatrics 100:354, 1997.
Gerhardt T, Bancalari E: Apnea of prematurity. 1: Lung function and regulation of breathing. Pediatrics 74:58, 1984.
Gerhardt T, Bancalari E: Apnea of prematurity. 2: Respiratory reflexes. Pediatrics 74:63, 1984.
Martin RJ, Miller MJ, Carlo WA: Pathogenesis of apnea in preterm infants. J Pediatr 109:733, 1986.
Miller MJ, Carlo WA, Martin RJ: Continuous positive airway pressure selectively reduces obstructive apnea in preterm infants. J Pediatr 106:91, 1985.
Southall DP, Richards JM, Rhoden KJ: Prolonged apnea and cardiac arrhythmias in infants discharged from neonatal intensive care units: Failure to predict an increased risk for SIDS. Pediatrics 70:844, 1982.
Upton CJ, Milner AD, Stokes GM: Upper airway patency during apnoea of prematurity. Arch Dis Child 67:419, 1992.

97.3 Hyaline Membrane Disease

(Respiratory Distress Syndrome)

INCIDENCE. HMD occurs primarily in premature infants; incidence is inversely proportional to the gestational age and birthweight. It occurs in 60–80% of infants less than 28 wk of gestational age, in 15–30% of those between 32 and 36 wk, in about 5% beyond 37 wk, and rarely at term. An increased frequency is associated with infants of diabetic mothers, delivery before 37 wk gestation, multifetal pregnancies, cesarean section delivery, precipitous delivery, asphyxia, cold stress, and a history of prior affected infants. The incidence is highest among preterm male or white infants. The risk of HMD is reduced in pregnancies with chronic or pregnancy-associated hypertension, maternal opiate addiction, prolonged rupture of the membranes, and antenatal corticosteroid use.

ETIOLOGY AND PATHOPHYSIOLOGY. Surfactant deficiency (decreased production and secretion) is the primary cause of HMD. The failure to develop an FRC and the tendency of affected lungs to become atelectatic correlate with high surface tensions and the absence of pulmonary surfactant. The major constituents of surfactant are dipalmitoylphosphatidylcholine (lecithin), phosphatidylglycerol, apoproteins (surfactant proteins SP-A, B, C, D), and cholesterol (Fig. 97–1). With progressive gestational age, increasing amounts of phospholipids are synthesized and stored in type II alveolar cells (Fig. 97–2). These surface-active agents are released into the alveoli, reducing the surface tension and helping to maintain alveolar stability by preventing the collapse of small air spaces at end-expiration. However, the amounts produced or released may be insufficient to meet postnatal demands because of immaturity. Surfactant is present in high concentrations in fetal lung homogenates by 20 wk of gestation but does not reach the surface of the lungs until later. It appears in the amniotic fluid between 28 and 32 wk. Mature levels of pulmonary surfactant are usually present after 35 wk.

Surfactant synthesis depends in part on normal pH, temperature, and perfusion. Asphyxia, hypoxemia, and pulmonary ischemia, particularly in association with hypovolemia, hypotension, and cold stress, may suppress surfactant synthesis. The epithelial lining of the lungs may also be injured by high oxygen concentrations and the effects of respirator management, resulting in further reduction in surfactant.

Alveolar atelectasis, hyaline membrane formation, and interstitial edema make the lungs less compliant, requiring greater pressure to expand the small alveoli and airways. In affected infants, the lower chest wall is pulled in as the diaphragm descends and the intrathoracic pressure becomes negative, thus limiting the amount of intrathoracic pressure that can be produced; the result is a tendency to develop atelectasis. The highly compliant chest wall of preterm infants offers less resistance than that of mature infants against the natural tendency

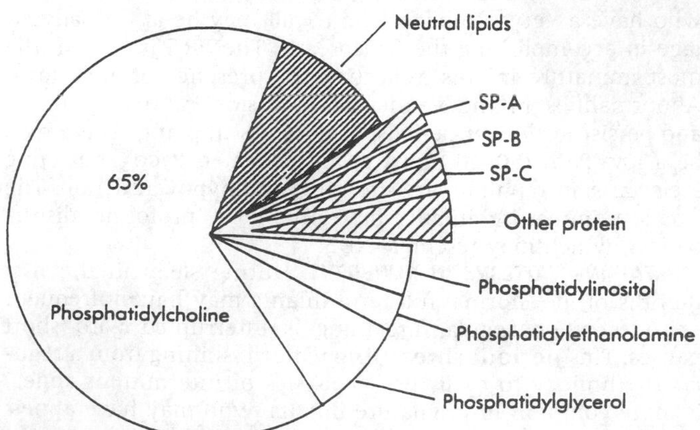

Figure 97–1 Composition of surfactant recovered by alveolar wash. The quantities of the different components are similar for surfactant from mature lungs of mammals. (From Jobe AH: Fetal lung development, tests for maturation, induction of maturation, and treatment. *In:* Creasy RK, Resnik R [eds]: Maternal-Fetal Medicine: Principles and Practice, 3rd ed. Philadelphia, WB Saunders, 1994.)

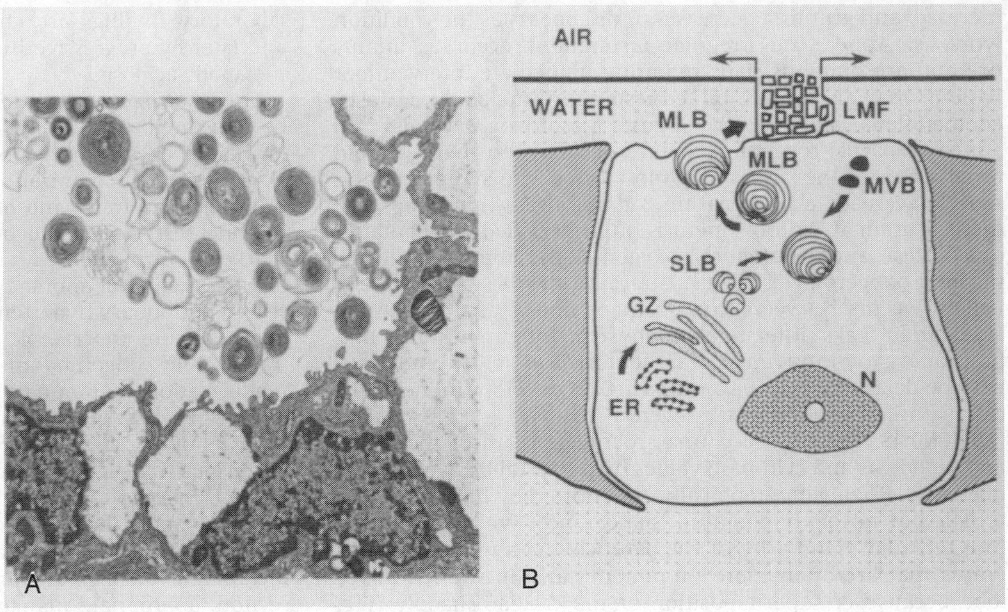

Figure 97–2 *A,* Fetal rat lung (low magnification), day 20 (term day 22), showing developing type II cells, stored glycogen *(pale areas),* secreted lamellar bodies, and tubular myelin. (Courtesy of Mary Williams, M.D., University of California, San Francisco.) *B,* Possible pathway for transport, secretion, and reuptake of surfactant. N, nucleus; ER, endoplasmic reticulum; GZ, Golgi zone; SLB, small lamellar body; MLB, mature lamellar body; LMF, lattice (tubular) myelin figure; MVB, multivesicular body. (From Hansen T, Corbet A: Lung development and function. *In:* Taeusch HW, Ballard RA, Avery MA [eds]: Schaffer and Avery's Diseases of the Newborn, 6th ed. Philadelphia, WB Saunders, 1991.)

of the lungs to collapse. Thus, at end-expiration, the volume of the thorax and lungs tends to approach the residual volume, leading to atelectasis.

Deficient synthesis or release of surfactant, together with small respiratory units and compliant chest wall, produces atelectasis, resulting in perfused but not ventilated alveoli, which causes hypoxia. Decreased lung compliance, small tidal volumes, increased physiologic dead space, increased work of breathing, and insufficient alveolar ventilation eventually result in hypercarbia. The combination of hypercarbia, hypoxia, and acidosis produces pulmonary arterial vasoconstriction with increased right-to-left shunting through the foramen ovale and ductus arteriosus and within the lung itself. Pulmonary blood flow is reduced, and ischemic injury to the cells producing surfactant and to the vascular bed results in an effusion of proteinaceous material into the alveolar spaces (Fig. 97–3).

PATHOLOGY. The lungs appear deep purplish red and are liver-like in consistency. Microscopically there is extensive atelectasis with engorgement of the interalveolar capillaries and lymphatics. A number of the alveolar ducts, alveoli, and respiratory bronchioles are lined with acidophilic, homogeneous, or granular membranes. Amniotic debris, intra-alveolar hemorrhage, and interstitial emphysema are additional but inconstant findings; interstitial emphysema may be marked when an infant has been ventilated with positive end-expiratory pressure (PEEP). The characteristic hyaline membranes are rarely seen in infants dying earlier than 6–8 hr after birth.

CLINICAL MANIFESTATIONS. Signs of HMD usually appear within minutes of birth, although they may not be recognized for several hours in larger premature infants until rapid, shallow respirations have increased to 60/min or greater. The late onset of tachypnea should suggest other conditions. Some patients require resuscitation at birth because of intrapartum asphyxia or initial severe respiratory distress (especially if birthweight is <1,000 g). Characteristically, tachypnea, prominent (often audible) grunting, intercostal and subcostal retractions, nasal flaring, and duskiness are noted. Cyanosis increases and is often relatively unresponsive to oxygen administration. Breath sounds may be normal or diminished, with a harsh tubular quality, and on deep inspiration, fine rales may be heard, especially over the lung bases posteriorly. The natural course is characterized by progressive worsening of cyanosis and dyspnea. If the condition is inadequately treated, blood pressure and body temperature may fall; fatigue, cyanosis, and pallor

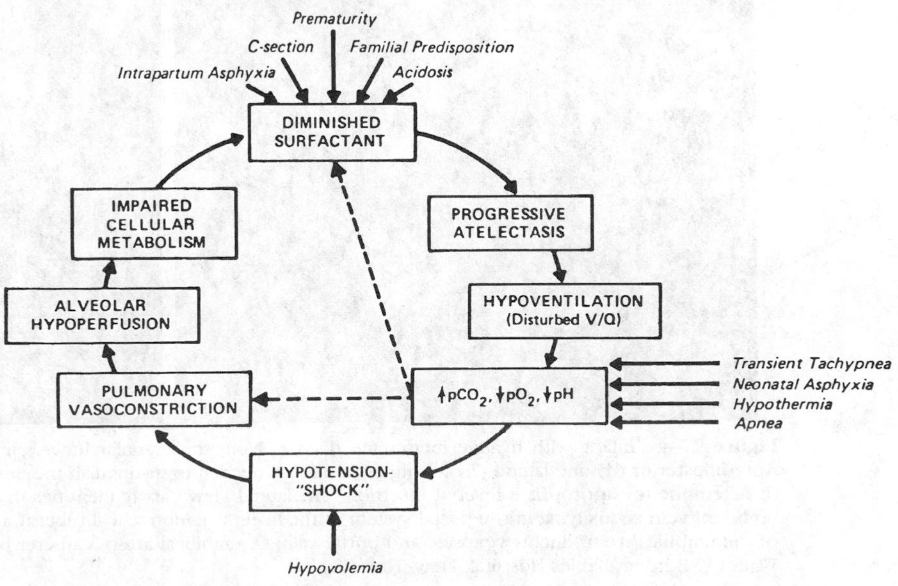

Figure 97–3 Contributing factors in the pathogenesis of hyaline membrane disease. Potential "vicious circle" perpetuating hypoxia and pulmonary insufficiency. (From Farrell P, Zachman R. *In:* Quilligan EJ, Kretchmer N [eds]: Fetal and Maternal Medicine. © 1980. Reprinted by permission of John Wiley & Sons, Inc.)

increase, and grunting decreases or disappears as the condition worsens. Apnea and irregular respirations occur as infants tire and are ominous signs requiring immediate intervention. Patients may also have a mixed respiratory-metabolic acidosis, edema, ileus, and oliguria. Signs of asphyxia secondary to apnea or partial respiratory failure occur when there is rapid progression of the disease. In most cases, the symptoms and signs may reach a peak within 3 days, after which improvement is gradual. Improvement is often heralded by spontaneous diuresis and the ability to oxygenate the infant with lower inspired oxygen levels. Death is rare on the 1st day of illness, usually occurs between days 2 and 7, and is associated with alveolar air leaks (interstitial emphysema, pneumothorax) and pulmonary or intraventricular hemorrhage (IVH). Mortality may be delayed weeks or months if CLD develops in mechanically ventilated infants with severe HMD.

DIAGNOSIS. The clinical course, roentgenogram of the chest, and blood gas and acid-base values help to establish the clinical diagnosis. Roentgenographically, the lungs may have a characteristic but not pathognomonic appearance, which includes a fine reticular granularity of the parenchyma and air bronchograms that are often more prominent early in the left lower lobe because of superimposition of the cardiac shadow (Fig. 97–4). The initial roentgenogram occasionally is normal, only to develop the typical pattern at 6–12 hr. Considerable variation among films may be seen, depending on the phase of respiration and the use of CPAP, often resulting in poor correlation between the roentgenograms and clinical course. The laboratory findings are characterized initially by hypoxemia and later by progressive hypoxemia, hypercarbia, and variable metabolic acidosis.

In the *differential diagnosis,* group B streptococcal sepsis may be indistinguishable from HMD. In pneumonia presenting at birth, the chest roentgenogram may be identical to that for HMD; maternal colonization, gram-positive cocci in the gastric or tracheal aspirates and buffy coat smear, a positive result of a urine test for streptococcal antigen, and the presence of marked neutropenia may suggest this diagnosis. Cyanotic heart disease (e.g., total anomalous pulmonary venous return), persistent pulmonary hypertension, aspiration syndromes, spontaneous pneumothorax, pleural effusions, diaphragmatic eventration, and congenital anomalies such as cystic adenomatoid malformation, pulmonary lymphangiectasia, diaphragmatic hernia, or lobar emphysema must be considered and require roentgenographic evaluation. Transient tachypnea may be distinguished by its short and mild clinical course. *Congenital alveolar proteinosis* is a rare familial disease that often presents as severe and lethal RDS (see Chapter 403).

PREVENTION. Most important is prevention of prematurity, including avoidance of unnecessary or poorly timed cesarean section, appropriate management of high-risk pregnancy and labor, and prediction and possible in utero acceleration of pulmonary immaturity (Chapter 92). In timing cesarean section or inducing labor, estimation of the fetal head circumference by ultrasonography and determination of the lecithin concentration in the amniotic fluid by the lecithin-sphingomy-

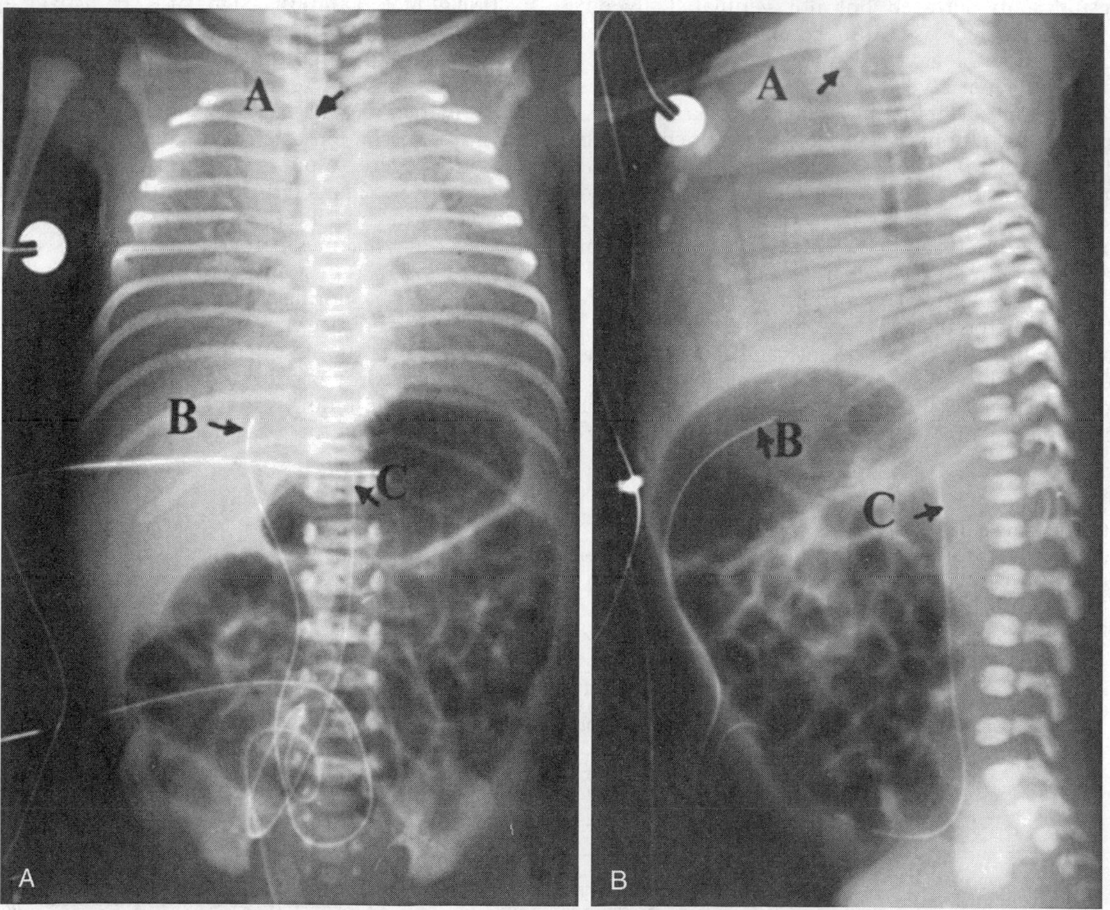

Figure 97–4 Infant with hyaline membrane disease. Note the granular lungs, air bronchogram, and air-filled esophagus. Anteroposterior *(A)* and lateral *(B)* roentgenograms are needed to distinguish the umbilical artery from the vein catheter and to determine the appropriate level of insertion. The lateral view clearly identifies that the catheter has been inserted into an umbilical vein and is lying in the portal system of the liver. A, Endotracheal tube; B, umbilical venous catheter at the junction of the umbilical vein, ductus venosus, and portal vein; C, umbilical artery catheter passed up the aorta to T-12. (Courtesy of Walter E. Berdon, Babies Hospital, New York City.)

elin (L/S) ratio (particularly useful with phosphatidylglycerol in diabetic pregnancies) decrease the likelihood of delivering a premature infant. Intrauterine antenatal and intrapartum monitoring may similarly decrease the risk of fetal asphyxia, which is associated with an increased incidence and severity of HMD.

Administration of *dexamethasone* or *betamethasone* to women 48 hr before delivery of fetuses between 24 and 34 wk of gestation significantly reduces the incidence and the mortality and morbidity of HMD. It is appropriate to administer these corticosteroids intramuscularly to all pregnant women who are likely to deliver in 1 wk between 24 and 34 wk. Prenatal glucocorticoid therapy decreases the severity of RDS and reduces the incidence of other complications of prematurity, such as IVH, patent ductus arteriosus (PDA), pneumothorax, and necrotizing enterocolitis (NEC), without affecting neonatal growth, development, lung mechanics or growth, or the incidence of infection. Prenatal glucocorticoids may act synergistically with postnatal exogenous surfactant therapy.

Administration of a first dose of *surfactant* into the trachea of symptomatic premature infants immediately after birth or during the first 24 hr of life reduces the mortality from HMD but does not alter the incidence of CLD.

TREATMENT. The basic defect requiring treatment is inadequate pulmonary exchange of oxygen and carbon dioxide; metabolic acidosis and circulatory insufficiency are secondary manifestations. Early supportive care of LBW infants, especially in the treatment of acidosis, hypoxia, hypotension (see Chapter 94), and hypothermia, appears to lessen the severity of HMD. Therapy requires careful and frequent monitoring of heart and respiratory rates, arterial Po_2, Pco_2, pH, bicarbonate, electrolytes, blood glucose, hematocrit, blood pressure, and temperature. Arterial catheterization is frequently necessary. Because most cases of HMD are self-limiting, the goal of treatment is to minimize abnormal physiologic variations and superimposed iatrogenic problems. Treatment of these infants is best carried out in a specially staffed and equipped hospital unit, the neonatal intensive care unit (NICU).

The general principles for supportive care of any LBW infant should be adhered to, including gentle handling and minimal disturbance consistent with management. To avoid chilling and to minimize oxygen consumption, infants should be placed in an Isolette and core temperature maintained between 36.5 and 37°C (Chapter 93). Calories and fluids should be provided intravenously. For the first 24 hr, 10% glucose and water should be infused through a peripheral vein at a rate of 65–75 mL/kg/24 hr. Subsequently, electrolytes should be added and fluid volumes increased gradually to 120–150 mL/kg/24 hr. Excessive fluids contribute to the development of a PDA. Chest physiotherapy may be associated with brain damage in extremely premature infants.

Warm humidified oxygen should be provided at a concentration sufficient initially to keep arterial levels between 55 and 70 mm Hg (>90% saturation), with stable vital signs to maintain normal tissue oxygenation while minimizing the risk of oxygen toxicity. If the Pao_2 cannot be maintained above 50 mm Hg at inspired oxygen concentrations of 60% or greater, applying CPAP at a pressure of 6–10 cm H_2O by nasal prongs is indicated; this usually produces a sharp rise in Pao_2. The amount of pressure required usually decreases abruptly at about 72 hr of age, and infants can be weaned from CPAP shortly thereafter. If an infant on CPAP cannot maintain an arterial oxygen tension above 50 mm Hg while breathing 70–100% oxygen, assisted ventilation is required.

Infants with severe HMD or those who develop complications resulting in persistent apnea require *assisted mechanical ventilation*. Reasonable indications for its use are (1) arterial blood pH of less than 7.20; (2) arterial blood Pco_2 of 60 mm Hg or more; (3) arterial blood Po_2 of 50 mm Hg or less at oxygen concentrations of 70–100% and CPAP of 8–10 cm H_2O; or (4) persistent apnea. Assisted ventilation by pressure- or flow-limited conventional respirators through an endotracheal tube should include PEEP. (See Chapter 64.3.)

The goals of mechanical ventilation are to improve oxygenation and carbon dioxide elimination without causing excessive pulmonary barotrauma or oxygen toxicity. Acceptable ranges of blood gas values, balancing the risks of hypoxia and acidosis against those of mechanical ventilation, are Pao_2 of 55–70 mm Hg; Pco_2 of 45–55 mm Hg; and pH of 7.25–7.45. During mechanical ventilation, oxygenation is improved by increasing the Fio_2 or the mean airway pressure. The latter can be increased by increasing the peak inspiratory pressure, gas flow, inspiratory to expiratory ratio, or PEEP. Excessive PEEP may cause pneumothorax or impede venous return, reducing cardiac output despite improvement of Pao_2 and thus decreasing oxygen delivery. PEEPs of 4–6 cm H_2O are usually safe and effective. Carbon dioxide elimination is achieved by increasing the peak inspiratory pressure (tidal volume) or the rate of the ventilator.

The rate ranges of conventional ventilators are 10–80 breaths/min; of high-frequency jet ventilation (HFJV), 150–600/min; and of oscillators, 300–1,800/min. HFJV and oscillators may improve carbon dioxide elimination, lower mean airway pressure, and improve oxygenation in patients who do not respond to conventional ventilators and who have HMD, interstitial emphysema, many pneumothoraces, or meconium aspiration pneumonia. HFJV may cause necrotizing tracheal damage, especially in the presence of hypotension or poor humidification, and oscillator therapy has been associated with an increased risk of air leaks, intraventricular hemorrhage, and periventricular leukomalacia. Both methods may cause gas trapping. Strategies of high-frequency oscillation that promote lung recruitment, combined with surfactant therapy, may reduce the risk of CLD without increasing the risks of IVH or periventricular leukomalacia. Complications of endotracheal intubation (plugging of tube, extubation, subglottic granuloma, and stenosis) and mechanical ventilation (pneumothorax, interstitial emphysema, reduced cardiac output) may be minimized by the interventions of specially trained physicians, nurses, and respiratory therapists in an NICU.

Multidose endotracheal instillation of *exogenous surfactant* to LBW infants requiring 30% oxygen and mechanical ventilation for the treatment (*rescue therapy*) of RDS has dramatically improved survival and reduced the incidence of pulmonary air leaks but has not consistently reduced the incidence of CLD. The immediate effects include improved alveolar-arterial oxygen gradients, reduced ventilator mean airway pressure, increased pulmonary compliance, and improved appearance of the chest roentgenogram. Survanta is an exogenous surfactant prepared from minced bovine lung with lipid extraction and enriched with phosphatidylcholine, palmitic acid, and triglycerides. Survanta contains SP-B and SP-C but no SP-A. Exosurf is a synthetic surfactant containing dipalmitoylphosphatidylcholine, hexadecanol, and tyloxapol. The latter two organic compounds improve spreading of the surfactant along the alveoli, because dipalmitoylphosphatidylcholine alone has poor surface-active properties. Additional surfactants undergoing testing include Curosurf and Infasurf (both natural) and ALEC (artificial lung expanding compound; 7:3 mixture of dipalmitoylphosphatidylcholine and phosphatidylglycerol).

Treatment (rescue) is initiated as soon as possible in the first 24 hr of life; therapy is given via the endotracheal tube every 6–12 hr for a total of 2–4 doses, depending on the preparation. Exogenous surfactant should be given by a physician who is qualified in neonatal resuscitation and respiratory management and who is able to care for the infant beyond the 1st hr of stabilization. Additional on-site required staff support includes nurses and respiratory therapists who are experienced in ventilatory management of LBW infants. In addition, appropriate monitoring equipment must be available (radiology, blood gas laboratory, and pulse oximetry). Furthermore, each institution should have an approved protocol for administration of surfactant. Complications of surfactant therapy include transient hypoxia and hypotension, blockage of the endotracheal tube, and pulmonary hemorrhage.

Partial liquid ventilation with oxygen-carrying perflubron, administered into the endotracheal tube, has resulted in improvement in oxygenation. *Inhaled nitric oxide* has also acutely improved oxygenation but may not improve overall outcome of HMD. These are both experimental therapies.

Respiratory acidosis may require short-term or prolonged assisted ventilation. In severe respiratory acidosis and hypoxia, treatment with sodium bicarbonate may exacerbate hypercarbia.

Metabolic acidosis in HMD may be a result of perinatal asphyxia and hypotension and is often encountered when an infant has required resuscitation (Chapter 96). Sodium bicarbonate, 1–2 mEq/kg, may be administered for treatment over a 10- to 15-min period through a peripheral vein with the acid-base determination repeated within 30 min, or it may be administered over several hours. Often, sodium bicarbonate is administered on an emergency basis through an umbilical venous catheter. Alkali therapy may result in skin sloughs due to infiltration, increased serum osmolarity, hypernatremia, hypocalcemia, hypokalemia, and liver injury when concentrated solutions are administered rapidly through an umbilical vein.

Monitoring of *aortic blood pressure* through an umbilical or peripheral arterial catheter or by oscillometric technique may be useful in managing the shocklike state that may occur during the 1st hour or so after premature birth of an infant who has been asphyxiated or who has developed severe respiratory distress (see Fig. 90–2). Hypotension has been associated with an increased risk of intraventricular hemorrhage and should be treated with dopamine, crystalloid or colloid fluids, or, less often, dobutamine. Occasionally hypotension may be glucocorticoid responsive (see Chapter 94). Radiopaque umbilical catheters should have their position checked roentgenographically after insertion (see Fig. 97–4). The tip of an umbilical artery catheter should lie just above the bifurcation of the aorta (L3–L5) or above the celiac axis (T6–T10). The preferred sites for peripheral catheters are the radial or posterior tibial arteries. Placement and supervision should be done by skilled and experienced personnel. Catheters should be removed as soon as there is no indication for their continued use—usually when PaO_2 is stable and the FIO_2 is less than 40%.

Periodic monitoring of PaO_2 and $PaCO_2$ and of pH is an important part of the management; if assisted ventilation is being used, it is essential. Blood should be obtained from the umbilical or peripheral artery. Tissue PO_2 may also be estimated continuously from transcutaneous electrodes or pulse oximetry (oxygen saturation). Capillary blood samples are of limited value for determining PO_2 but may be useful for evaluating PCO_2 and pH.

Owing to the difficulty of distinguishing group B streptococcal or other infections from HMD, routinely administering antibacterial agents is indicated until the results of blood cultures are available. Penicillin or ampicillin with kanamycin or gentamicin is suggested, depending on the recent pattern of bacterial sensitivities in the hospital where the infant is being treated (Chapters 105 and 106).

COMPLICATIONS OF HMD AND INTENSIVE CARE. The most serious complications of **tracheal intubation** are asphyxia from obstruction of the tube, cardiac arrest during intubation or suctioning, and subsequent development of subglottic stenosis. Other complications include bleeding due to trauma during intubation, posterior pharyngeal pseudodiverticula, difficult extubation requiring tracheostomy, ulceration of the nares due to pressure from the tube, permanent narrowing of the nostril due to tissue damage and scarring from irritation or infection around the tube, erosion of the palate, avulsion of a vocal cord, laryngeal ulcer, papilloma of a vocal cord, and persistent hoarseness, stridor, or edema of the larynx.

Measures to reduce the incidence of these complications include skillfully securing the tube; using polyvinyl endotracheal tubes that do not contain tin, which is toxic to cells; using a tube of the smallest practicable size to reduce local ischemia and pressure necrosis; avoiding frequent changes of the tube; avoiding motion of the tube in situ; avoiding too frequent or vigorous suctioning; and avoiding infection through meticulous cleanliness and frequent sterilization of all apparatus attached to or passed through the tube. The personnel inserting and caring for the endotracheal tube should be experienced and skilled.

The risks of **umbilical arterial catheterization** include vascular embolization, thrombosis, spasm, and perforation; ischemic or chemical necrosis of abdominal viscera; infection; accidental hemorrhage; and impaired circulation to a leg, with subsequent gangrene. Although at necropsy the reported incidence of thrombotic complications varies from 1–23%, aortography has demonstrated that clots form in or about the tips of 95% of catheters placed in an umbilical artery. Aortic ultrasonography can also be used to investigate the presence of thrombosis. The risk of a serious clinical complication resulting from umbilical catheterization is probably between 2 and 5%.

Transient blanching of the leg may occur during catheterization of the umbilical artery. It is usually due to reflex arterial spasm, the incidence of which is lessened by using the smallest available catheters, particularly in very small infants. The catheter should be removed immediately; catheterization of the other artery may then be attempted. Persistent spasm after removal of the catheter may be relieved by topical nitroglycerin applied over the femoral artery or, rarely, by warming the opposite leg. Blood sampling from a radial artery may similarly result in spasm or thrombosis, and the same treatment is indicated. Intermittent severe spasm or unrelieved spasm may respond to the cautious use of topical nitroglycerin or local infusion of tolazoline (Priscoline), 1–2 mg injected intra-arterially over 5 min. Accidentally lodging the catheter in a smaller artery, either blocking it completely or causing unrecognized local vascular spasm, may result in gangrene of the organ or area supplied by the vessel. To prevent this complication, the catheter should be removed promptly if blood cannot be obtained through it.

Serious hemorrhage on removal of the catheter is rare. Thrombi may form in the artery or in the catheter; their incidence is lowered by using a smooth-tipped catheter with a hole only at its end, by rinsing the catheter with a small amount of saline solution containing heparin, or by continuously infusing a solution containing 1–5 U/mL of heparin. The risks of thrombus formation with potential vascular occlusion can also be reduced by removing the catheter when there are early signs of thrombosis, such as narrowing of pulse pressure and disappearance of the dicrotic notch. Some prefer to use the umbilical artery for blood sampling only, leaving the catheter filled with heparinized saline between samplings. *Renovascular hypertension* may occur days to weeks after umbilical arterial catheterization in a small number of neonates.

Umbilical vein catheterization is associated with many of the same risks as artery catheterization. An additional risk is cardiac perforation and pericardial tamponade if the catheter is placed in the right atrium and there is an association with subsequent portal hypertension from portal vein thrombosis.

Extrapulmonary extravasation of air is another frequent complication of the management of HMD (Chapter 97.8).

There may be clinically significant shunting through a **PDA** in some neonates with HMD, the delayed closure being due to associated hypoxia, acidosis, increased pulmonary pressure secondary to vasoconstriction, systemic hypotension, immaturity, and local release of prostaglandins, which dilate the ductus. This shunting may be bidirectional or right to left through the ductus arteriosus. As HMD resolves, pulmonary vascular resistance decreases, and there may be left-to-right shunting leading to left ventricular volume overload and pulmonary edema. The manifestations of PDA may include (1) persistent apnea for unexplained reasons in an infant recovering from HMD; (2) an active heaving precordium, bounding peripheral pulses, wide pulse pressure, and a systolic or to-and-fro murmur; (3) carbon dioxide retention; (4) increasing oxygen dependence; (5) roentgenographic evidence of cardiomegaly and increased pulmonary vascular markings; and (6) hepatomegaly. The diagnosis is confirmed by echocardiographic visualization of a PDA with Doppler flow evidence of left-to-right shunting. Most infants respond to general supportive measures, including diuretics and fluid restriction. In patients in whom spontaneous closure does not occur and in whom there is progressive deterioration despite supportive and cardiotonic treatment, intravenous indomethacin, 0.2 mg/kg at 12- to 24-hr intervals for 3 doses, may induce pharmacologic closure by inhibiting prostaglandin synthesis; repeated courses may be needed. Some physicians use indomethacin prophylactically to reduce the incidence of IVH and PDA. Contraindications to indomethacin include thrombocytopenia (<50,000/mm³), bleeding disorders, oliguria (<1 mL/kg/hr), NEC, and elevated plasma creatinine level (>1.8 mg/dL). Ibuprofen (0.2 mg/kg q 12 hr × 3), unlike indomethacin, does not reduce cerebral blood flow and may be equally effective in closing a PDA. Indications for surgical closure are failure to close the ductus after one to two courses of indomethacin therapy with persistent heart failure and ventilator dependence.

Chronic lung disease, previously called bronchopulmonary dysplasia (BPD), is a result of lung injury in infants requiring mechanical ventilation and supplemental oxygen. CLD is present if the neonate is oxygen dependent at 36 wk after conception. The occurrence of CLD is inversely related to gestational age. Instead of showing improvement on the 3rd–4th day, consistent with the natural course of RDS, some infants who have been on intermittent positive-pressure breathing using increased concentrations of oxygen roentgenographically show a worsening of their pulmonary condition (Fig. 97–5*A*). Respiratory distress persists and is characterized by hypoxia, hypercarbia, oxygen dependence, and, in severe cases, the development of right-sided heart failure. The chest roentgenogram is described as gradually changing from a picture of almost complete opacification with air bronchogram and interstitial emphysema to one of small, round, lucent areas alternating with areas of irregular density resembling a sponge (Fig. 97–5*B*). Histologic study at this stage (10–20 days after beginning oxygen therapy) shows less evidence of hyaline membrane formation, progressive alveolar coalescence with atelectasis of surrounding alveoli, interstitial edema, coarse focal thickening of the basement membrane, and widespread bronchial and bronchiolar mucosal metaplasia and hyperplasia. These findings correspond to a severe maldistribution of ventilation.

Most surviving neonates with persistent roentgenographic changes recover by 6–12 mo, but some require prolonged

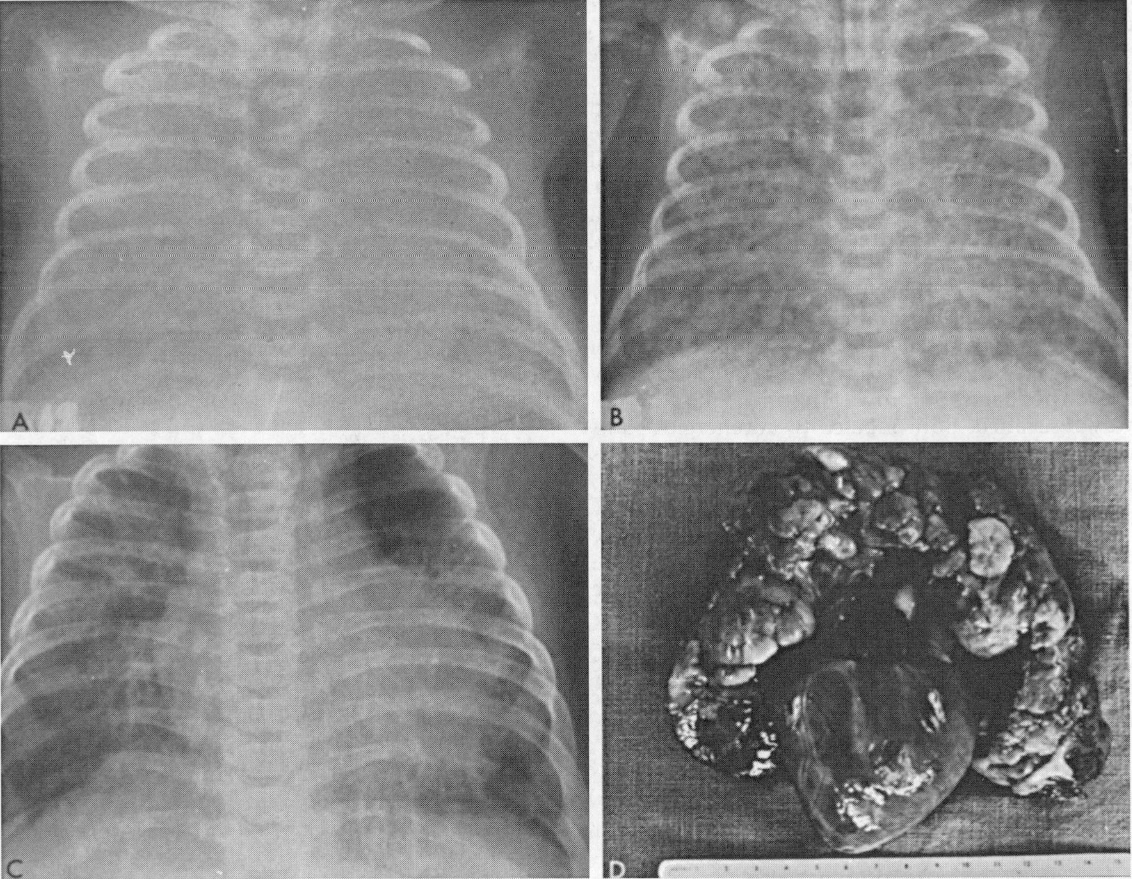

Figure 97–5 Pulmonary changes in infants who were treated in the immediate postnatal period for the clinical syndrome of hyaline membrane disease with prolonged, intermittent positive-pressure breathing with air containing 80–100% oxygen. *A,* A 5-day-old infant with nearly complete opacification of lungs. *B,* A 13-day-old infant with "bubbly lungs" simulating the roentgenographic appearance of the Wilson-Mikity syndrome. *C,* A 7-mo-old infant with irregular, dense strands in both lungs, hyperinflation, and cardiomegaly suggestive of chronic lung disease. *D,* Large right ventricle and cobbly irregularly aerated lung of an infant who died at 11 mo of age. This infant also had a patent ductus arteriosus. (From Northway WH Jr, Rosan RC, Porter DY: N Engl J Med 276:357, 1967.)

hospitalization and may have respiratory symptoms persisting through childhood (bronchospasm). Right-sided heart failure and viral necrotizing bronchiolitis are major causes of death in infancy. Pathology reveals cardiac enlargement and pulmonary changes consisting of focal areas of emphysematous alveoli with hypertrophy of the peribronchial smooth muscle of the tributary bronchioles, some perimucosal fibrosis and widespread metaplasia of the bronchiolar mucosa, thickening of basement membranes, and separation of the capillaries from the alveolar epithelial cells.

Infants at risk for CLD usually have severe respiratory distress requiring prolonged periods of mechanical ventilation and oxygen therapy. Additional associations include the presence of pulmonary interstitial emphysema, lower gestational age, male sex, low Pco_2 at 48 hr, patent ductus arteriosus, high peak inspiratory pressure, increased airway resistance in the 1st wk of life, increased pulmonary artery pressure, and possibly a family history of asthma. Some very low birthweight (VLBW) infants without HMD who require mechanical ventilation for apnea develop CLD that does not follow the classic pattern for CLD.

Severe CLD requires continued mechanical ventilation until weaning from the respirator becomes possible. Acceptable blood gas concentrations for a patient with CLD include Pco_2 of 50–70 mm Hg (if pH > 7.30) and Pao_2 of 55–60 mm Hg with oxygen saturation of $\geq 95\%$. Lower levels of Pao_2 may exacerbate pulmonary hypertension, produce cor pulmonale, and inhibit growth. Airway obstruction in CLD may be due to mucus and edema production, bronchospasm, and collapse of acquired tracheomalacia. These events may contribute to "blue spells." Alternatively, blue spells may be due to acute cor pulmonale or myocardial ischemia.

The *treatment* of CLD includes nutritional support, fluid restriction, drug therapy, maintenance of adequate oxygenation, and prompt treatment of infection. Growth must be monitored because recovery is dependent on the growth of lung tissue and remodeling of the pulmonary vascular bed. Nutritional supplementation to provide added calories (24–30 cal/30 mL formula) and protein (3–3.5 g/kg/24 hr) is needed for growth. Diuretic therapy results in a short-term improvement in lung mechanics and may result in decreased oxygen and ventilatory requirements. Furosemide (1 mg/kg/dose IV bid or 2 mg/kg/dose PO bid) given daily or every other day and hydrochlorothiazide (20 mg/kg/dose bid) alone or in combination with potassium chloride, if needed, or spironolactone are commonly used drugs. Bronchodilators improve lung mechanics by decreasing airway resistance. Both inhaled β_2-adrenergic agents and systemic aminophylline or theophylline (at serum levels of 12–15 mg/L) are used. The use of dexamethasone reduces the duration of mechanical ventilation. Therapy is usually initiated at 4 wk of age at a dose of 0.25 mg/kg bid; the dose is tapered over 1–2 wk. The optimal dose, time of initiation, and duration of steroid use are unknown. Because of side effects of dexamethasone (hypertension, hyperglycemia, gastrointestinal bleeding, adrenal suppression, sepsis, cardiomyopathy, reduced growth), the lowest effective dose for the shortest duration is used. Infants who fail to respond within 1 wk of therapy are unlikely to improve with longer courses. Some infants who respond initially rebound with worsening respiratory status when dexamethasone is discontinued. Earlier use of corticosteroids may prevent CLD (days 1–7). Adequate oxygenation (pulse oximeter $\geq 95\%$) is essential to prevent or treat cor pulmonale and to promote optimal growth and neurodevelopmental outcome. Mortality in infants with CLD ranges from 10–25% and is highest in infants who remain ventilator dependent for over 6 mo. Cardiorespiratory failure (associated with cor pulmonale) and infection (respiratory syncytial virus) are common causes of death.

Complications of CLD include growth failure, psychomotor retardation, and parental stress as well as sequelae of therapy such as nephrolithiasis (due to diuretics and total intravenous alimentation), osteopenia, and subglottic stenosis, which may require tracheotomy or an anterior cricoid split procedure to relieve upper airway obstruction.

Patients with CLD often go home on oxygen, diuretics, and bronchodilator therapy. Prevention of sleep-associated hypoxia improves growth, as does hypercaloric formula. The long-term *prognosis* is good for infants who have been weaned off oxygen before discharge from the NICU. Prolonged ventilation, IVH, pulmonary hypertension, cor pulmonale, and oxygen dependence beyond 1 yr of life are poor prognostic signs. Airway obstruction and hyperactivity and hyperinflation may be demonstrated in some adolescents.

PROGNOSIS. Early provision of intensive observation and care of high-risk newborn infants can significantly reduce morbidity and mortality due to HMD and other acute neonatal illnesses. Antenatal steroids, postnatal surfactant use, improved modes of ventilation, and supportive NICUs have resulted in a low mortality from HMD (~10%). Mortality increases with decreasing gestational age. Good results depend on the availability of experienced and skilled personnel, specially designed and organized regional hospital units, proper equipment, and lack of complications such as severe asphyxia, intracranial hemorrhage, or irremediable congenital malformation. Surfactant therapy has reduced mortality from HMD approximately 40%; CLD incidence has not been measurably affected.

Overall mortality for LBW infants referred to intensive care centers is steadily declining (see Chapter 93.2). Although 85–90% of all infants surviving HMD after requiring ventilatory support with respirators are normal, the outlook is much better for those weighing above 1,500 g; about 80% of those under 1,500 g have no neurologic or mental sequelae. The long-term prognosis for normal pulmonary function in most infants surviving HMD is excellent. However, survivors of severe neonatal respiratory failure may have significant pulmonary and neurodevelopmental impairment.

Bloom BT, Kattwinkel J, Hall RT, et al: Comparison of Infasurf (calf lung surfactant extract) to Survanta (beractant) in the treatment and prevention of respiratory distress syndrome. Pediatrics 100:31, 1997.

Clyman RI: Recommendations for the postnatal use of indomethacin: An analysis of four separate treatment strategies. J Pediatr 128:601, 1996.

Egberts J, Brand R, Walti H, et al: Mortality, severe respiratory distress syndrome, and chronic lung disease of the newborn are reduced more after prophylactic than after therapeutic administration of the surfactant Curosurf. Pediatrics 100:http://www.pediatrics.org/cgi/content/full/100/1/e4, 1997.

Ford LR, Willi SM, Hollis BW, et al: Suppression and recovery of the neonatal hypothalamic-pituitary-adrenal axis after prolonged dexamethasone therapy. J Pediatr 131:722, 1997.

Giacoia GP, Venkataraman PS, West-Wilson KI, et al: Follow-up of school-age children with bronchopulmonary dysplasia. J Pediatr 130:400, 1997.

Hamvas A, Nogee LM, Mallory GB Jr, et al: Lung transplantation for treatment of infants with surfactant protein B deficiency. J Pediatr 130:231, 1997.

Harding JE, Miles FKI, Becroft DMO, et al: Chest physiotherapy may be associated with brain damage in extremely premature infants. J Pediatr 132:440, 1998.

Hawgood S: Surfactant protein genes and human disease: The plot thickens. J Pediatr 132:198, 1998.

Iles R, Edmunds AT: Assessment of pulmonary function in resolving chronic lung disease of prematurity. Arch Dis Child 76:F113, 1997.

Jobe AH: Too many unvalidated new therapies to prevent chronic lung disease in preterm infants. J Pediatr 132:200, 1998.

Keszler M, Modanlou HD, Brudno S, et al: Multicenter controlled clinical trial of high-frequency jet ventilation in preterm infants with uncomplicated respiratory distress syndrome. Pediatrics 100:593, 1997.

Klein JM, Thompson MW, Snyder JM, et al: Transient surfactant protein B deficiency in a term infant with severe respiratory failure. J Pediatr 132:244, 1998.

Leach C, Greenspan JS, Rubenstein SD, et al: Partial liquid ventilation with perflubron in premature infants with severe respiratory distress syndrome. N Engl J Med 335:761, 1996.

Marlow N: High frequency ventilation and respiratory distress syndrome: Do we have an answer? Arch Dis Child 78:F1, 1998.

McEvoy C, Mendoza ME, Bowling S, et al: Prone positioning decreases episodes of hypoxemia in extremely low birth weight infants (1000 grams or less) with chronic lung disease. J Pediatr 130:305, 1997.

Mosca F, Bray M, Lattanzio M, et al: Comparative evaluation of the effects of

indomethacin and ibuprofen on cerebral perfusion and oxygenation in preterm infants with patent ductus arteriosus. J Pediatr 131:549, 1997.
Moyer-Mileur LJ, Nielson DW, Pfeffer KD, et al: Eliminating sleep-associated hypoxemia improves growth in infants with bronchopulmonary dysplasia. Pediatrics 98:779, 1996.
Nagourney BA, Kramer MS, Klebanoff MA, et al: Recurrent respiratory distress syndrome in successive preterm pregnancies. J Pediatr 129:591, 1996.
Palta M, Sadek M, Barnet JH, et al: Evaluation of criteria for chronic lung disease in surviving very low birth weight infants. J Pediatr 132:57, 1998.
Papile L, Tyson JE, Stoll BJ, et al: A multicenter trial of two dexamethasone regimens in ventilator-dependent premature infants. N Engl J Med 338:1112, 1998.
Rettwitz-Volk W, Veldman A, Roth B, et al: A prospective, randomized, multicenter trial of high-frequency oscillatory ventilation compared with conventional ventilation in preterm infants with respiratory distress syndrome receiving surfactant. J Pediatr 132:249, 1998.
Singer L, Yamashita T, Lilien L, et al: A longitudinal study of developmental outcome of infants with bronchopulmonary dysplasia and very low birth weight. Pediatrics 100:987, 1997.
Skimming JW, Bender KA, Hutchinson AA, et al: Nitric oxide inhalation in infants with respiratory distress syndrome. J Pediatr 130:225, 1997.
Skinner J: The effects of surfactant on haemodynamics in hyaline membrane disease. Arch Dis Child 76:F67, 1997.
Subhedar NV, Hamdan AH, Ryan SW, et al: Pulmonary artery pressure: Early predictor of chronic lung disease in preterm infants. Arch Dis Child 78:F20, 1998.
Subhedar NV, Shaw NJ: Changes in oxygenation and pulmonary haemodynamics in preterm infants treated with inhaled nitric oxide. Arch Dis Child 77:F191, 1997.
Tapia JL, Ramirez R, Cifuentes J, et al: The effect of early dexamethasone administration on bronchopulmonary dysplasia in preterm infants with respiratory distress syndrome. J Pediatr 132:48, 1998.
Van Overmeire B, Follens I, Hartmann S, et al: Treatment of patent ductus arteriosus with ibuprofen. Arch Dis Child 76:F179, 1997.
Vyas J, Kotecha S: Effects of antenatal and postnatal corticosteroids on the preterm lung. Arch Dis Child 77:F147, 1997.
Yanowitz TD, Yao AC, Werner JC, et al: Effects of prophylactic low-dose indomethacin on hemodynamics in very low birth weight infants. J Pediatr 132:28, 1998.
Yeh TF, Lin YJ, Hsieh WS, et al: Early postnatal dexamethasone therapy for the prevention of chronic lung disease in preterm infants with respiratory distress syndrome: A multicenter clinical trial. Pediatrics 101:http://www.pediatrics.org/cgi/content/full/100/4/e3, 1997.

97.4 Transient Tachypnea of the Newborn

Transient tachypnea, occasionally called **respiratory distress syndrome type II,** usually follows uneventful normal preterm or term vaginal delivery or cesarean delivery. It may be characterized by the early onset of tachypnea, sometimes with retractions, or expiratory grunting and, occasionally, cyanosis that is relieved by minimal oxygen (<40%). Patients usually recover rapidly within 3 days, although they may rarely appear severely ill and have a more protracted course. The lungs are usually clear without rales or rhonchi, and the chest roentgenogram shows prominent pulmonary vascular markings, fluid lines in the fissures, overaeration, flat diaphragms, and, occasionally, pleural fluid. Hypoxemia, hypercapnia, and acidosis are uncommon. Distinguishing the disease from HMD may be very difficult; the distinctive features of transient tachypnea are the infant's sudden recovery and the absence of a roentgenographic reticulogranular pattern or air bronchograms. The syndrome is believed to be secondary to slow absorption of fetal lung fluid resulting in decreased pulmonary compliance and tidal volume and increased dead space.

Avery ME, Gatewood OB, Brumley G: Transient tachypnea of newborn. Possible delayed reabsorption of fluid at birth. Am J Dis Child 111:380, 1966.
Gross TL, Sokol RJ, Kwong MS, et al: Transient tachypnea of the newborn: The relationship to preterm delivery and significant neonatal morbidity. Am J Obstet Gynecol 146:236, 1983.
Sundell H, Garrott J, Blankenship WJ, et al: Studies on infants with type II respiratory distress syndrome. J Pediatr 78:754, 1971.

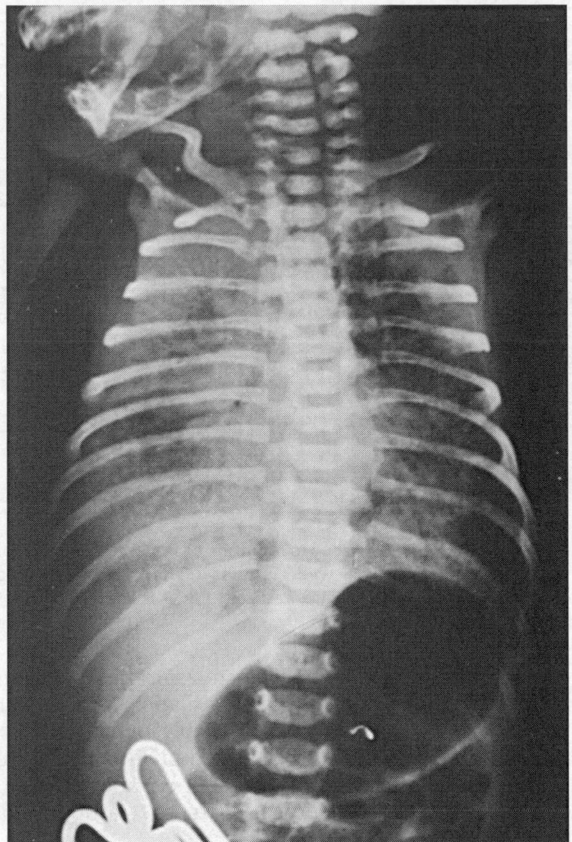

Figure 97–6 Fetal aspiration syndrome (aspiration pneumonia). Note the coarsely granular pattern with irregular aeration typical of fetal distress from aspiration of material, such as vernix caseosa, epithelial cells, and meconium contained in amniotic fluid.

97.5 Aspiration of Foreign Material

(Fetal Aspiration Syndrome: Aspiration Pneumonia)

During prolonged labors and difficult deliveries, infants often initiate vigorous respiratory movements in utero because of interference with the supply of oxygen through the placenta. Under such circumstances, the infant may aspirate amniotic fluid containing vernix caseosa, epithelial cells, meconium, or material from the birth canal, which may block the smallest airways and interfere with alveolar exchange of oxygen and carbon dioxide. Pathogenic bacteria may accompany the aspirated material, and pneumonia may ensue, but even in the noninfected cases respiratory distress accompanied by roentgenographic evidences of aspiration is seen (Fig. 97–6).

Pulmonary aspiration may also occur in newborn infants because of tracheoesophageal fistula, esophageal and duodenal obstructions, gastroesophageal reflux, improper feeding practices, and administration of depressant medicines.

The contents of the stomach should be aspirated through a soft catheter just before operation or other procedures that require anesthesia or significantly disturb an infant. Once aspiration has occurred, treatment consists of general and respiratory support and treatment of pneumonia (Chapters 97.3 and 175).

Goodwin SR, Graves SA, Haberkern CM: Aspiration in intubated premature infants. Pediatrics 75:85, 1985.

97.6 Meconium Aspiration

Meconium-stained amniotic fluid is found in 5–15% of births and usually occurs in term or post-term infants. Five per

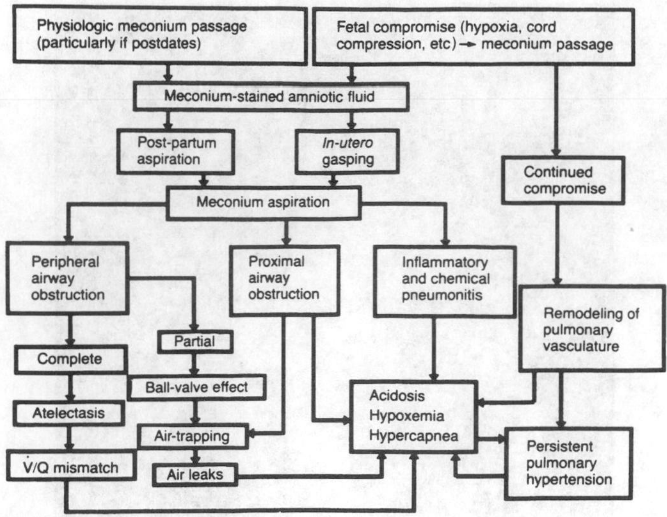

Figure 97–7 Pathophysiology of meconium passage and the meconium aspiration syndrome. (From Wiswell TE, Bent RC: Meconium staining and the meconium aspiration syndrome. Pediatr Clin North Am 40:955, 1993.)

cent of such infants develop meconium aspiration pneumonia; 30% of these require mechanical ventilation, and less than 5–10% expire. Usually but not invariably, fetal distress and hypoxia occur with passage of meconium into the amniotic fluid. These infants are meconium stained and may be depressed and require resuscitation at birth. The pathophysiology is noted in Figure 97–7.

CLINICAL MANIFESTATIONS. Either in utero or more often with the first breath, thick, particulate meconium is aspirated into the lungs. The resulting small airway obstruction may produce respiratory distress within the first hours, with tachypnea, retraction, grunting, and cyanosis in severely affected infants. Partial obstruction of some airways may lead to pneumothorax or pneumomediastinum, or both. Prompt treatment may delay the onset of respiratory distress, which may consist only of tachypnea without retractions. Overdistention of the chest may be prominent. The condition usually improves within 72 hr, but when its course requires assisted ventilation, it may be severe and its potential for mortality high. Tachypnea may persist for many days or even several weeks. The typical chest roentgenogram is characterized by patchy infiltrates, coarse streaking of both lung fields, increased anteroposterior diameter, and flattening of the diaphragm. A normal chest roentgenogram in an infant with severe hypoxia and no cardiac malformation suggests the diagnosis of pulmonary hypertension (Chapter 97.7). Arterial Po_2 may be low in either disease, and if hypoxia has occurred, metabolic acidosis is usually present.

PREVENTION. The risk of meconium aspiration may be decreased by paying careful attention to fetal distress and initiating prompt delivery in the presence of fetal acidosis, late decelerations, or poor beat-to-beat variability. Amnio-infusion and DeLee suctioning of the oropharynx after the head is delivered reduce the incidence of meconium aspiration.

TREATMENT. In the absence of fetal distress, a vigorous infant (Apgar score of 8 or more) can be born through thin meconium and may not require treatment. Depressed infants (those with hypotonia, bradycardia, fetal acidosis, or apnea) and possibly those delivered through thick particulate (pea soup) meconium-stained fluid (particularly those who did not undergo DeLee suctioning) should undergo endotracheal intubation, and suction should be applied directly to the endotracheal tube to remove meconium from the airway. The risks of laryngoscopy and endotracheal intubation (bradycardia, laryngospasm, hypoxia, posterior pharyngeal laceration with pseudodiverticulum formation) are less than the risks of meconium aspiration syndrome in these severe circumstances.

Treatment of meconium aspiration pneumonia includes supportive care and standard management for respiratory distress. The oxygenation benefit of PEEP must be weighed against the risk of pneumothorax. Severe meconium aspiration may be complicated by persistent pulmonary hypertension and requires similar treatment. Patients who are refractory to conventional mechanical or high-frequency ventilation benefit from surfactant therapy (regardless of gestational age), inhaled nitric oxide, or extracorporeal membrane oxygenation (ECMO) (see Chapter 97.7).

PROGNOSIS. The mortality of meconium-stained infants is considerably higher than that of nonstained infants, and meconium aspiration used to account for a significant proportion of neonatal deaths. Residual lung problems are rare but include symptomatic cough, wheezing, and persistent hyperinflation for up to 5–10 yr. Ultimate prognosis depends on the extent of CNS injury from asphyxia and the presence of associated problems such as pulmonary hypertension.

Cialone PR, Sherer DM, Ryan RM, et al: Amnioinfusion during labor complicated by particulate meconium-stained amniotic fluid decreases neonatal morbidity. Am J Obstet Gynecol 170:842, 1994.

Cunningham A, Lawson E, Martin R, et al: Tracheal suction and meconium: A proposed standard of care. J Pediatr 116:153, 1990.

Findlay RD, Taeusch HW, Walther FJ: Surfactant replacement therapy for meconium aspiration syndrome. Pediatrics 97:48, 1996.

Gregory GA, Gooding CA, Phibbs RH, et al: Meconium aspiration infants; a prospective study. J Pediatr 85:848, 1974.

Ramin KD, Leveno KJ, Kelly MA, et al: Amniotic fluid meconium: A fetal environmental hazard. Obstet Gynecol 87:181, 1996.

Sunno C, Kosasa TS, Hale RW: Meconium aspiration syndrome without evidence of fetal distress in early labor before elective cesarean delivery. Obstet Gynecol 73:707, 1989.

Wiswell TE, Bent RC: Meconium staining and the meconium aspiration syndrome. Pediatr Clin North Am 40:955, 1993.

Yoder BA: Meconium-stained amniotic fluid and respiratory complications: Impact of selective tracheal suction. Obstet Gynecol 83:77, 1994.

97.7 Persistent Pulmonary Hypertension of the Newborn (PPHN)

Persistent Fetal Circulation (PFC)

PPHN occurs in term and post-term infants after birth asphyxia, meconium aspiration pneumonia, group B streptococcal sepsis, HMD, hypoglycemia, polycythemia, and pulmonary hypoplasia due to diaphragmatic hernia, amniotic fluid leak, oligohydramnios, or pleural effusions. PPHN is often idiopathic. The incidence is 1:500 to 1:700 live births.

PATHOPHYSIOLOGY. Persistence of the fetal circulatory pattern of right-to-left shunting through the PDA and foramen ovale after birth is due to excessively high pulmonary vascular resistance. Fetal pulmonary vascular resistance is usually elevated relative to fetal systemic or postnatal pulmonary pressure. This fetal state permits shunting of oxygenated umbilical venous blood to the left atrium (and brain) through the foramen ovale and bypasses the lungs through the ductus arteriosus to the descending aorta. After birth, pulmonary vascular resistance normally declines rapidly as a consequence of vasodilation due to gas filling the lungs, a rise in postnatal Pao_2, a reduction in Pco_2, increased pH, and release of vasoactive substances. Increased neonatal pulmonary vascular resistance may be (1) maladaptive from an acute injury (e.g., not demonstrating normal vasodilation in response to increased oxygen and other changes after birth); (2) the result of increased pulmonary artery medial muscle thickness and extension of smooth muscle layers into the usually nonmuscular, more peripheral pulmonary arterioles in response to chronic fetal hypoxia; (3) due to pulmonary hypoplasia (diaphragmatic hernia, Potter syndrome); (4) obstructive owing to polycythemia or total anomalous pulmonary venous return; or (5) due to alveolar capillary dysplasia, a lethal, possibly familial disorder with thickened alveolar septum and reduced numbers of small pulmonary arteries and capillaries. Apart from the etiology, profound hypoxia from right-to-left shunting and normal or elevated P_{CO_2} are present.

CLINICAL MANIFESTATIONS. Infants become ill in the delivery room or within the first 12 hr of life. PPHN due to polycythemia, idiopathic causes, hypoglycemia, or asphyxia may result in severe cyanosis with tachypnea, although there may initially be minimal signs of respiratory distress. Infants who have PPHN associated with meconium aspiration, group B streptococcal pneumonia, diaphragmatic hernia, or pulmonary hypoplasia usually have cyanosis, grunting, flaring, retractions, tachycardia, and shock. Multiorgan involvement may be present (see Table 95–1). Myocardial ischemia, papillary muscle dysfunction with mitral and tricuspid regurgitation, and cardiac stun produce cardiogenic shock with decreased pulmonary blood flow, tissue perfusion, and oxygen delivery. *Hypoxia is quite labile and often out of proportion to the findings on chest roentgenograms.*

DIAGNOSIS. PPHN should be suspected in all term infants with cyanosis with or without fetal distress, intrauterine growth retardation, meconium-stained amniotic fluid, hypoglycemia, polycythemia, diaphragmatic hernia, pleural effusions, and birth asphyxia. Hypoxia is universal and is unresponsive to 100% oxygen given by oxygen hood but may respond transiently to hyperoxic hyperventilation administered after endotracheal intubation or application of a bag and mask. A Pa_{O_2} gradient between a preductal (right radial artery) and a postductal (umbilical artery) site of blood sampling greater than 20 mm Hg suggests right-to-left shunting through the ductus arteriosus. Real-time echocardiography combined with Doppler flow studies demonstrates right-to-left shunting across a patent foramen ovale and a ductus arteriosus. Deviation of the intra-atrial septum into the left atrium is seen in severe PPHN. Tricuspid or mitral insufficiency may be noted on auscultation as a holosystolic murmur and visualized echocardiographically together with poor contractility when PPHN is associated with myocardial ischemia. The degree of tricuspid regurgitation can estimate the pulmonary artery pressure. The second heart sound is accentuated and is not split. In asphyxia-associated and idiopathic PPHN, the chest roentgenogram is normal, whereas in PPHN associated with pneumonia and diaphragmatic hernia it shows the specific lesions of parenchymal opacification and bowel in the chest, respectively. The *differential diagnosis* of PPHN includes cyanotic heart disease (especially total anomalous pulmonary venous return) and the associated etiologic entities that predispose to PPHN (e.g., hypoglycemia, polycythemia, sepsis).

TREATMENT. Therapy is directed toward correcting any predisposing disease (hypoglycemia, polycythemia) and improving poor tissue oxygenation. The response to therapy is often unpredictable, transient, and complicated by adverse effects of drugs or mechanical ventilation. Initial management includes oxygen administration and correction of acidosis, hypotension, and hypercarbia. Persistent hypoxia should be managed with intubation and mechanical ventilation.

One approach to treatment of severe PPHN consists of instituting mechanical ventilation with or without pancuronium paralysis; ventilator settings are initially selected to achieve a Pa_{O_2} of 50–70 mm Hg and a P_{CO_2} of 50–55 mm Hg. Tolazoline (1 mg/kg), a nonselective α-adrenergic antagonist, is sometimes used as an adjunct to nonselectively vasodilate the pulmonary arterial system but also results in systemic hypotension, which is treated with volume expansion and dopamine. In another approach to treating severe PPHN, hyperventilation is used to reduce pulmonary vasoconstriction by lowering P_{CO_2} (~25 mm Hg) and increasing pH (7.50–7.55). This requires high peak inspiratory pressures and rapid respiratory rates, often necessitating the use of pancuronium paralysis to control ventilation in order to achieve a Pa_{O_2} between 90 and 100 mm Hg. Complications of hyperventilation include hyperinflation with reduced carbon dioxide elimination, reduced cardiac output, barotrauma, pneumothorax, decreased cerebral blood flow, increased fluid requirements, and edema resulting from paralysis. Alkalination with sodium bicarbonate also has been used to elevate the plasma pH to induce pulmonary arterial vasodilation. Both methods of mechanical ventilation may be successful, and specific indications for one or the other have not been defined. Patients not responding to conventional ventilation may later respond to hyperventilation or high-frequency ventilation. Cardiogenic shock should be treated with inotropic agents such as dopamine and dobutamine.

Exogenous surfactant therapy has been beneficial in some patients. Inhaled nitric oxide (iNO), a potent and selective pulmonary vasodilator (equivalent to endothelium-derived relaxation factor), when given in 10–20 ppm (occasionally 60–80), has improved oxygenation in patients with PPHN and reduced the need for ECMO. Four responses to iNO include: no improvement; initial improvement but not sustained, requiring ECMO; initial and sustained, usually weaned by the 5th day of therapy; and initial response but prolonged dependency, possibly due to pulmonary hypoplasia or alveolar capillary dysplasia. Methemoglobinemia is a possible complication of iNO.

Extracorporeal Membrane Oxygenation. In 5–10% of patients with PPHN (approximately 1:4,000 births) there is a poor response to 100% oxygen, mechanical ventilation, and drugs. In such patients, the alveolar-arterial oxygen gradient (roughly at sea level [760 − 47] − Pa_{CO_2} − Pa_{O_2}) or the oxygenation index, OI,

$$(\text{mean airway pressure} \times F_{IO_2} \times 100) \div \text{postductal } Pa_{O_2}$$

has been used to predict a greater than 80% mortality. PA_{O_2} − Pa_{O_2} gradients of greater than 620 for 8–12 hr and an OI of more than 40 that are unresponsive to nitric oxide inhalation predict a high mortality and are indications for ECMO. ECMO has also been used to treat carefully selected severely ill infants who have HMD, meconium aspiration pneumonia, or group B streptococcal sepsis. ECMO is indicated in hypoxic patients with diaphragmatic hernia, especially when the ventilation index (rate × mean airway pressure) exceeds 1,000 and the P_{CO_2} exceeds 40 mm Hg.

ECMO is a form of cardiopulmonary bypass that augments systemic perfusion and provides gas exchange. Most experience has been with venoarterial bypass, which requires placement of large catheters in the right internal jugular vein and carotid artery and may necessitate carotid artery ligation. (Venovenous bypass avoids this ligation and provides gas exchange but does not support cardiac output.) Blood is initially pumped through the ECMO circuit at a rate that approximates 80% of the estimated cardiac output of 150–200 mL/kg/min. Venous return passes through a membrane oxygenator, is warmed, and returns into the aortic arch. Venous oxygen saturations are used to monitor tissue oxygen delivery and subsequent extraction. The rate of ECMO flow is adjusted to achieve satisfactory venous oxygen saturation (>65%) and cardiovascular stability. When an infant is started on ECMO, the existing ventilator support is weaned to room air at a low rate and pressure to reduce the risk of oxygen toxicity and barotrauma, thus permitting time for the lungs to rest and heal.

Because ECMO requires complete heparinization to prevent clotting in the circuit, patients with or at risk for IVH (weight <2 kg, age <35 wk gestation) are not candidates for this therapy. In addition, infants for whom ECMO is being considered should have reversible lung disease, no signs of systemic bleeding, and an absence of severe asphyxia or lethal malformations, and they should have been ventilated for less than

7–10 days. Complications of ECMO include thromboembolism, air embolization, bleeding, stroke, seizures, atelectasis, cholestatic jaundice, thrombocytopenia, neutropenia, hemolysis, infectious complications of blood transfusions, edema formation, and systemic hypertension.

PROGNOSIS. The outcome for infants with PPHN is related to the associated hypoxic-ischemic encephalopathy and the ability to reduce pulmonary vascular resistance. The long-term prognosis for infants who have PPHN and who survive after treatment with hyperventilation is comparable to that for infants who have underlying illnesses of equivalent severity (e.g., birth asphyxia, hypoglycemia, polycythemia). The outcome for infants who have PPHN treated with ECMO is also favorable; 85–90% survive, and 70–75% of survivors appear normal at 1 yr of age. Infants who have diaphragmatic hernia associated with severe PPHN fare poorly if the presurgery and postsurgery P_{CO_2} exceeds 40 mm Hg despite mechanical ventilation. Such patients may respond to ECMO; rarely, it is not possible to wean them from bypass, or they expire after ECMO has been discontinued. Lung transplantation may benefit these infants.

Barrington KJ, Finer NN: Care of near term infants with respiratory failure. Br Med J 315:1215, 1997.
Chelliah BP, Brown D, Cohen M, et al: Alveolar capillary dysplasia—a cause of persistent pulmonary hypertension unresponsive to a second course of extracorporeal membrane oxygenation. Pediatrics 96:1159, 1995.
Davidson D, Barefield ES, Kattwinkel J: Inhaled nitric oxide for the early treatment of persistent pulmonary hypertension of the term newborn: A randomized, double-masked, placebo-controlled, dose-response, multicenter study. Pediatrics 101:325, 1998.
Goldman AP, Tasker RC, Haworth SG, et al: Four patterns of response to inhaled nitric oxide for persistent pulmonary hypertension of the newborn. Pediatrics 98:706, 1996.
Hoffman GM, Ross GA, Day SE, et al: Inhaled nitric oxide reduces the utilization of extracorporeal membrane oxygenation in persistent pulmonary hypertension of the newborn. Crit Care Med 25:352, 1997.
Kinsella JP, Truog WE, Walsh WF, et al: Randomized, multicenter trial of inhaled nitric oxide and high-frequency oscillatory ventilation in severe, persistent pulmonary hypertension of the newborn. J Pediatr 131:55, 1997.
Lotze A, Mitchell BR, Bulas DI, et al: Multicenter study of surfactant (beractant) use in the treatment of term infants with severe respiratory failure. Pediatrics 132:40, 1998.
Nakajima W, Ishida A, Arai H, et al: Methaemoglobinaemia after inhalation of nitric oxide in infants with pulmonary hypertension. Lancet 350:1002, 1997.
The Neonatal Inhaled Nitric Oxide Study Group: Inhaled nitric oxide in full-term and nearly full-term infants with hypoxic respiratory failure. N Engl J Med 336:597, 1997.
Steinhorn RH, Cox PN, Fineman JR, et al: Inhaled nitric oxide enhances oxygenation but not survival in infants with alveolar capillary dysplasia. J Pediatr 130:417, 1997.
UK Collaborative ECMO Trial Group: UK collaborative randomised trial of neonatal extracorporeal membrane oxygenation. Lancet 348:75, 1996.

97.8 Extrapulmonary Extravasation of Air

(Pneumothorax, Pneumomediastinum, and Pulmonary Interstitial Emphysema)

Asymptomatic pneumothorax, usually unilateral, is estimated to occur in 1–2% of all newborn infants; symptomatic pneumothorax and pneumomediastinum are less common. Pneumothorax is more common in males than in females and in term and post-term infants than in premature ones. The incidence is increased among infants with lung disease, such as meconium aspiration and HMD; in those who have had vigorous resuscitation or are receiving assisted ventilation, especially if high inspiratory pressure or a continuous elevation of end-expiratory pressure is used; and in infants with urinary tract anomalies.

ETIOLOGY AND PATHOPHYSIOLOGY. The most common cause of pneumothorax is overinflation resulting in alveolar rupture. It may be "spontaneous" or idiopathic or secondary to underlying pulmonary disease, such as lobar emphysema or rupture of a congenital or pneumonic cyst; to trauma; or to a "ball-valve" type of bronchial or bronchiolar obstruction resulting from aspiration. Air leaks occur during the first 24–36 hr in infants with meconium aspiration, pneumonia, and HMD when lung compliance is reduced and later during the recovery phase of HMD if inspiratory pressure and PEEP are not reduced simultaneously with improved respiratory function.

Pneumothorax associated with pulmonary hypoplasia is common, occurs in the first day of life, and is due to reduced alveolar surface area and poorly compliant lungs. It is associated with disorders of decreased amniotic fluid volume (Potter syndrome; renal agenesis, renal dysplasia, chronic amniotic fluid leak), decreased fetal breathing movement (oligohydramnios, neuromuscular disease), pulmonary space-occupying lesions (diaphragmatic hernia, pleural effusion, chylothorax), and thoracic abnormalities (asphyxiating thoracic dystrophies).

Air from a ruptured alveolus escapes into the interstitial spaces of the lung, where it may cause *interstitial emphysema* or may dissect along the peribronchial and perivascular connective tissue sheaths to the root of the lung. If the volume of escaped air is great enough, it may follow the vascular sheaths to cause mediastinal emphysema or a rupture with subsequent pneumomediastinum, pneumothorax, and subcutaneous emphysema. Rarely, increased mediastinal pressure may compress pulmonary veins at the hilum, interfering with venous return to the heart and cardiac output. On occasion, air may embolize into the circulation, producing cutaneous blanching, air in intravascular catheters, an air-filled heart on chest roentgenograms, and death.

Tension pneumothorax occurs if an accumulation of air within the pleural space is sufficient to elevate intrapleural pressure above atmospheric pressure. A unilateral tension pneumothorax results in impaired ventilation not only in the collapsed lung but also in the normal lung by a mediastinal shift to the other side. Compression of the vena cava and torsion of the great vessels may interfere with venous return.

CLINICAL MANIFESTATIONS. The physical findings of *asymptomatic pneumothorax* are hyperresonance and diminished breath sounds over the involved side of the chest with or without tachypnea.

Symptomatic pneumothorax is characterized by respiratory distress, which varies from only an increased respiratory rate to severe dyspnea, tachypnea, and cyanosis. Irritability and restlessness or apnea may be the earliest signs. The onset is usually sudden but may be gradual; an infant may rapidly become critically ill. The chest may appear asymmetric with increased anteroposterior diameter and bulging of the intercostal spaces on the affected side, and there may be hyperresonance and diminished or absent breath sounds. The heart is displaced toward the unaffected side, and the diaphragm is displaced downward, as is the liver with right-sided pneumothorax. Because both sides are affected in approximately 10% of patients, symmetry of findings does not rule out pneumothorax. In tension pneumothorax there may be signs of shock, and the apex of the heart is pushed away from the affected side.

Pneumomediastinum occurs in at least 25% of patients with pneumothorax and is usually asymptomatic. The degree of respiratory distress depends on the amount of trapped air. If it is great, there is bulging of the midthoracic area, the neck veins are distended, and the blood pressure is low. The last two findings are a result of blockage of the circulation by compression of the systemic and pulmonary veins. Although few clinical signs may exist, subcutaneous emphysema in newborn infants is almost pathognomonic of pneumomediastinum.

Pulmonary interstitial emphysema (PIE) may precede the development of a pneumothorax or may occur independently, resulting in increasing respiratory distress due to decreased compliance, hypercarbia, and hypoxia. The latter is due to an increased alveolar-arterial oxygen gradient and in-

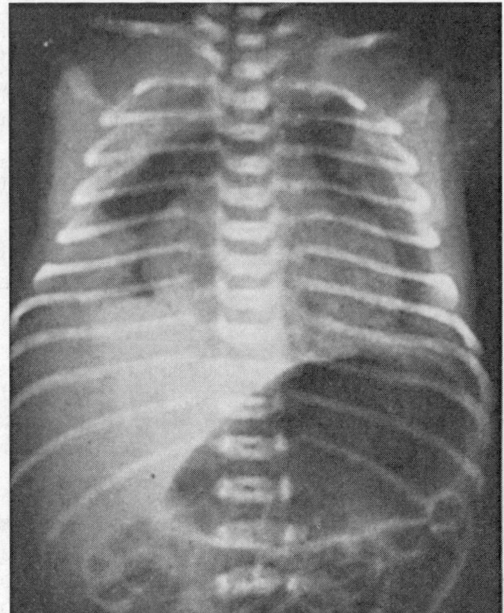
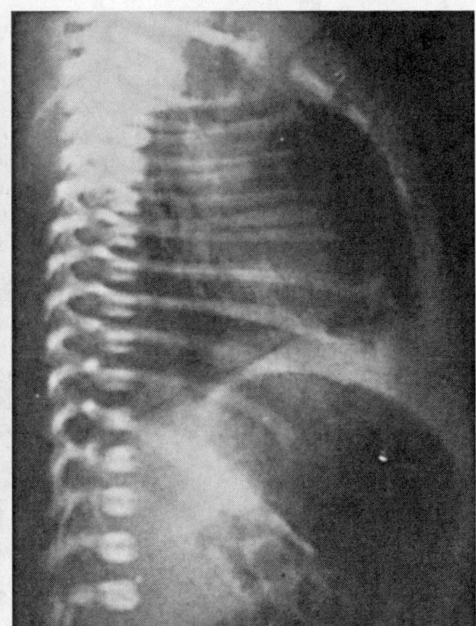

Figure 97–8 Pneumomediastinum in a newborn infant. Anteroposterior view demonstrates compression of lungs and the lateral view shows bulging of the sternum, each resulting from distention of the mediastinum by trapped air.

trapulmonary shunting. Progressive enlargement of blebs or air may result in cystic dilatations and respiratory deterioration resembling pneumothorax. In severe cases, PIE precedes the development of CLD. Avoidance of high inspiratory or mean ventilatory pressures may prevent the development of PIE. Treatment may include bronchoscopy if there is evidence of mucus plugging, selective intubation and ventilation of the uninvolved bronchus, oxygen, general respiratory care, and high-frequency ventilation.

DIAGNOSIS. Pneumothorax and pneumomediastinum should be suspected in any newborn infant who shows signs of respiratory distress or who displays restlessness or irritability, or has a sudden change in condition. The diagnosis is established roentgenographically, with the edge of the collapsed lung standing out in relief against the pneumothorax (see Fig. 419–1), and in pneumomediastinum with hyperlucency around the heart border and between the sternum and the heart border (Fig. 97–8). Transillumination of the thorax is often helpful in the emergency diagnosis of pneumothorax; the affected side transmits excessive light. Associated renal anomalies are identified by ultrasonography. Pulmonary hypoplasia is suggested by signs of uterine compression (extremity contractures), a small thorax on chest roentgenogram, severe hypoxia with hypercarbia, and signs of the primary disease (hypotonia, diaphragmatic hernia, Potter syndrome).

Pneumopericardium may be asymptomatic, requiring only general supportive treatment, but usually presents as sudden shock with tachycardia, muffled heart sounds, and poor pulses suggesting tamponade, which requires prompt evacuation of entrapped air. **Pneumoperitoneum** from air dissecting through the diaphragmatic apertures during mechanical ventilation may also be confused with perforation of an abdominal organ.

TREATMENT. Without a continued air leak, asymptomatic and mildly symptomatic small pneumothoraces require only close observation. Frequent small feedings may prevent gastric dilatation and minimize crying, which can further compromise ventilation and worsen the pneumothorax. Breathing 100% oxygen accelerates the resorption of free pleural air into the blood by reducing the nitrogen tension in blood, producing a resultant nitrogen pressure gradient from the trapped air into the blood, but the benefit must be weighed against the risks of oxygen toxicity. With severe respiratory or circulatory embarrassment, emergency needle aspiration is indicated. Either immediately or after needle aspiration, a chest tube should be inserted and attached to underwater-seal drainage. Severe localized interstitial emphysema may respond to selective bronchial intubation. Judicious use of Pavulon in infants fighting the ventilator may reduce the incidence of pneumothorax. Surfactant therapy for RDS reduces the incidence of pneumothorax.

Gonzalez F, Harris T, Black P, et al: Decreased gas flow through pneumothoraces in neonates receiving high-frequency jet versus conventional ventilation. J Pediatr 110:464, 1987.

Hall RT, Rhodes PG: Pneumothorax and pneumomediastinum in infants with idiopathic respiratory distress syndrome receiving CPAP. Pediatrics 55:493, 1975.

Primhak RA: Factors associated with pulmonary air leak in premature infants receiving mechanical ventilation. J Pediatr 102:764, 1983.

Ryan CA, Barrington KJ, Phillips HJ, et al: Contralateral pneumothoraces in the newborn: Incidence and predisposing factors. Pediatrics 79:417, 1987.

97.9 Interstitial Pulmonary Fibrosis

(Wilson-Mikity Syndrome; Pulmonary Insufficiency of the Premature)

Wilson and Mikity described a pulmonary syndrome of premature infants, usually of less than 32 wk gestation and birthweights below 1,500 g, and without a history of HMD. It was characterized by insidious onset of dyspnea, tachypnea, retractions, and cyanosis during the 1st mo of life. Rare cases have been reported in full-term infants, usually those having a history of meconium aspiration or oxygen administration. Viral infections also have been implicated.

Cough, wheezing, and rales may develop, but fever occurs only with concomitant infection. There may be collapse of a lobe or lung; other complications are right-sided heart failure, osteoporosis, and rib fractures. The symptoms usually increase over 2–6 wk, with increasing oxygen dependence persisting for several months, followed by gradual resolution or progressive respiratory and cardiac failure. Infants who recover from the severe form may have an increased number of lower respiratory tract infections in the 1st yr of life. The most characteristic features of this syndrome are roentgenographic. Early, they include bilateral coarse reticular streaky infiltrates and, often, overexpansion of the lungs with small areas of emphysema that develop into multicystic lesions. Subsequently, the cysts enlarge and coalesce to give a hyperlucent, bubbly appearance (see Fig. 97–5*B*). The roentgenograms tend to clear gradually over months to several years. The roentgenographic changes in Wilson-Mikity syndrome may be indistinguishable from those of CLD.

The syndrome must be differentiated from pneumonia due to cytomegalovirus, *Pneumocystis carinii, Ureaplasma urealyticum*, or *Chlamydia* and from cystic fibrosis. *Chronic pulmonary insufficiency of prematurity* is progressive lung disease developing in VLBW infants requiring mechanical ventilation due to failure to maintain adequate spontaneous ventilation. Usually a VLBW infant without respiratory distress syndrome develops apnea on day 2–5. Atelectasis and a reduced functional residual capacity follow, requiring treatment with CPAP or mechanical ventilation. With prolonged ventilation, CLD develops.

Treatment consists of supportive measures: oxygen for cyanosis, bronchodilators, diuretics for cardiac failure, acid-base correction, correction of anemia with transfusion or erythropoietin, and assisted ventilation when indicated.

Hudak BB, Allen MC, Hudal ML, et al: Home oxygen therapy for chronic lung disease in extremely low-birth-weight infants. Am J Dis Child 143:357, 1989.
Kao LC, Durand DJ, McCrea RC, et al: Randomized trial of long-term diuretic therapy for infants with oxygen-dependent bronchopulmonary dysplasia. J Pediatr 124:772, 1994.
Wilson MG, Mikity VG: A new form of respiratory distress in premature infants. Am J Dis Child 99:489, 1960.
Zimmerman JJ, Farrell PM: Advances and issues in bronchopulmonary dysplasia. Curr Probl Pediatr 24:159, 1994.

97.10 Pulmonary Hemorrhage

Massive pulmonary hemorrhage is present in 15% of neonates who come to autopsy in the first 2 wk of life. The reported incidence at autopsy varies from 1–4/1,000 live births. About three fourths of the patients weigh less than 2,500 g at birth.

Most infants in whom pulmonary hemorrhage is demonstrated at autopsy have had symptoms of respiratory distress that are indistinguishable from those of HMD. The onset may occur at birth or may be delayed several days. One fourth to one half of affected infants cough up or regurgitate material containing old or fresh blood from the nose, mouth, or endotracheal tube. In severe cases there may be cardiovascular collapse, poor lung compliance, profound cyanosis, and hypercarbia. Roentgenographic findings are varied and nonspecific, ranging from minor streaking or patchy infiltrates to massive consolidation.

The cause of massive pulmonary hemorrhage is usually not identified; the incidence is increased in association with acute pulmonary infection, severe asphyxia, HMD, surfactant therapy, assisted ventilation, congenital heart disease, erythroblastosis fetalis, hemorrhagic disease of the newborn, kernicterus, inborn errors of ammonia metabolism, and cold injury. Although in the majority of instances bleeding into other organs is observed at autopsy, bleeding other than through the nostrils and mouth and intraventricular bleeding are relatively rare during life and should suggest the possibility of an additional bleeding diathesis such as disseminated intravascular coagulation. Bleeding is predominantly alveolar in about two thirds of cases and interstitial in the rest. In some infants, the pulmonary hemorrhage represents hemorrhagic pulmonary edema due to severe left-sided heart failure resulting from hypoxia.

The little available information that describes the prognosis of infants who bleed through the mouth or nostrils suggests that it is extremely poor. Death occurs in the first 48 hr of life in two thirds of the infants who come to autopsy. Treatment includes blood replacement, positive end-expiratory pressure, suctioning to clear the airway, and intratracheal administration of epinephrine.

Acute pulmonary hemorrhage may also rarely occur in postneonatal full-term infants. The cause is unknown. These infants have acute respiratory distress with bilateral alveolar infiltrates and usually respond to intensive supportive treatment (see Chapter 402).

Cole VA, Norman ICS, Reynolds EOR, et al: Pathogenesis of hemorrhagic pulmonary edema and massive pulmonary hemorrhage in the newborn. Pediatrics 51:175, 1973.
CDC: Acute pulmonary hemorrhage among infants. MMWR 44:67, 1995.
Pappin A, Shenker N, Hack M, et al: Extensive intraalveolar pulmonary hemorrhage in infants dying after surfactant therapy. J Pediatr 124:621, 1994.

CHAPTER 98
Digestive System Disorders

VOMITING. Infants may vomit mucus, occasionally blood-streaked, in the first few hours after birth. This vomiting rarely persists after the first few feedings; it may be due to irritation of the gastric mucosa by material swallowed during delivery. If the vomiting is protracted, gastric lavage with physiologic saline solution may relieve it.

Vomiting is a relatively frequent symptom during the neonatal period. In the majority of instances, it is simply regurgitation from overfeeding or from failure to permit the infant to eructate swallowed air. (See Chapter 323 for discussion of gastric emptying and gastroesophageal reflux.) When vomiting occurs shortly after birth and is persistent, the possibilities of intestinal obstruction and increased intracranial pressure must be considered. A history of maternal hydramnios suggests upper gastrointestinal (esophageal, duodenal, ileal) atresia.

Bile-stained emesis suggests intestinal obstruction beyond the duodenum, but it may also be idiopathic. Abdominal roentgenograms (kidney-ureter-bladder [KUB] and cross-table lateral views) should be performed in neonates with persistent emesis and in all infants with bile-stained emesis to detect air-fluid levels, distended bowel loops, characteristic patterns of obstruction (double bubble: duodenal atresia), and pneumoperitoneum (intestinal perforation). A barium swallow roentgenogram with small bowel follow-through is indicated in the presence of bilious emesis.

Obstructive lesions of the digestive tract occur most frequently in the esophagus and intestines (see Chapters 319, 329, and 330). Vomiting from esophageal obstruction occurs with the first feeding. The diagnosis of esophageal atresia can be suspected if there is unusual drooling from the mouth and if resistance is encountered in an attempt to pass a catheter into the stomach. Diagnosis should be made before the infant chokes on oral feedings and risks aspiration pneumonia. Infantile achalasia (cardiospasm), a rare cause of vomiting in newborn infants, is demonstrable roentgenographically by obstruction at the cardiac end of the esophagus, without organic stenosis. Regurgitation of feedings due to continuous relaxation of the esophageal-gastric sphincter, chalasia, is a cause of vomiting. It can be controlled by keeping the infant in a semi-upright position, thickening the feeding, or administering prokinetic drugs.

Vomiting due to *obstruction of the small intestine* usually begins on the 1st day of life and is frequent, persistent, usually nonprojectile, copious, and, unless the obstruction is above the ampulla of Vater, bile-stained; it is associated with abdominal distention, visible deep peristaltic waves, and reduced or absent bowel movements. Malrotation with obstruction from midgut volvulus is an acute emergency that must be considered. Upright roentgenographic films of the abdomen show the distribution of air in the intestine and often aid in locating the site of the obstruction; malrotation may be identified by contrast studies. Normally, air can be demonstrated roentgenographically in the jejunum by 15–60 min, in the ileum by 2–3 hr, and in the colon by 3 hr after birth. Absence of rectal gas at 24 hr is abnormal. Persistent vomiting may occur with congenital hernia of the diaphragm. The vomiting of pyloric stenosis may begin any time after birth but does not assume its characteristic pattern before the 2nd–3rd wk. Vomiting with obstipation is a sign of Hirschsprung disease. Vomiting may occur with many other disturbances that do not obstruct the digestive tract, such as milk allergy, adrenal hyperplasia of the salt-losing variety, galactosemia, hyperammonemias, organic acidemias, increased intracranial pressure, septicemia, meningitis, and urinary tract infections.

THRUSH (ORAL CANDIDOSIS). Thrush of the mouth occurs in healthy infants; later, it is rare except in debilitated infants, in those receiving antibiotic or immunosuppressive therapy, and in those with acquired immunodeficiency syndrome (AIDS). Infants with AIDS also manifest failure to thrive, psychomotor retardation, hepatosplenomegaly, diarrhea, lymphadenopathy, and hypergammaglobulinemia (see Chapter 268).

Transmission of the infection from maternal vaginal moniliasis to the infant's oral mucosa is the primary means of infection in healthy newborns. Secondary cases develop in the hospital nursery, presumably owing to contact with infected infants and contaminated supplies or caretakers.

Oral thrush in an otherwise healthy infant is usually a self-limited infection, but treatment is advised, especially in the presence of candidal diaper rash (Chapter 230).

DIARRHEA. See Chapters 55.1, 55.2, 176, and 337–341.

CONSTIPATION. More than 90% of full-term newborn infants pass meconium within the first 24 hr, and most of the remainder do so within 36 hr; the possibility of intestinal obstruction should be considered in any infant who does not. Intestinal atresia or stenosis, congenital aganglionic megacolon, milk bolus obstruction, meconium ileus, or meconium plugs may present as constipation. About 20% of very low birthweight (VLBW) infants do not pass meconium within the first 24 hr. Constipation not present from birth but appearing during the 1st mo of life suggests short-segment congenital aganglionic megacolon, hypothyroidism, or anal stenosis. It must be kept in mind that infrequent bowel movements do not necessarily mean constipation. A breast-fed infant usually has frequent bowel movements, whereas a formula-fed infant may have one to two movements a day or every other day.

MECONIUM PLUGS. Lower colonic or anorectal plugs (Fig. 98–1) with a lower than normal water content may cause intestinal obstruction. Rarely, a firm mass of meconium may form elsewhere in the intestine and cause intrauterine intestinal obstruction and meconium peritonitis unrelated to cystic fibrosis (CF). Anorectal plugs may also cause intestinal ulceration and perforation. Meconium plugs are associated with small left colon syndrome in the infant of a diabetic mother, CF, rectal aganglionosis, maternal drug abuse, and magnesium sulfate therapy for preeclampsia. The plug may be evacuated by irrigating it with isotonic sodium chloride solution. Enemas with the iodinated contrast medium Gastrografin usually cause passage of the plug, presumably because the high osmolarity (1,900 mOsm/L) of the medium draws fluid rapidly into the intestinal lumen and loosens inspissated material. Because this rapid loss of fluid into the bowel may result in acute dehydration and shock, it is advisable to dilute the contrast material with an equal amount of water, to correct any existing dehydration and to provide intravenous fluids during and for several hours after the procedure. *After removal of a meconium plug, the infant should be observed closely for the possible presence of congenital aganglionic megacolon.*

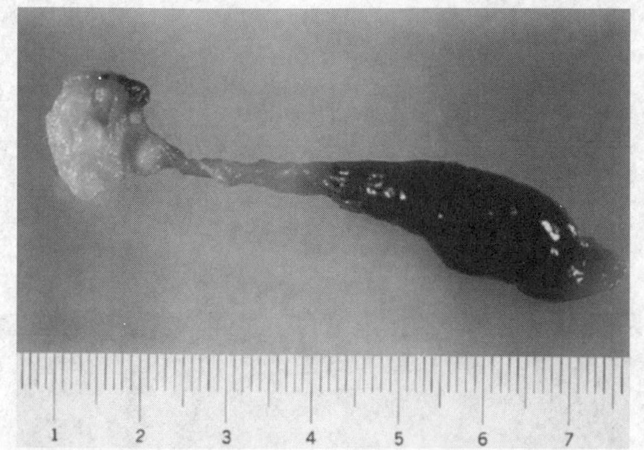

Figure 98–1 This plug of meconium and mucus (scale in cm) caused bowel obstruction in a premature infant. X-ray showed marked gaseous distention and multiple fluid levels at 30 hr of age. Dramatic improvement occurred when the plug was passed following an enema. (From The abnormal fetus. *In:* Beischer NA, Mackay EV, Colditz PB [eds]: Obstetrics and the Newborn, 3rd ed. Philadelphia, WB Saunders, 1997.)

98.1 Meconium Ileus in Cystic Fibrosis

In a newborn infant, impaction of meconium causes intestinal obstructions often associated with CF. The absence of fetal pancreatic enzymes limits normal digestive activities in the intestine, and meconium is left in a viscid, mucilaginous state. It clings to the intestinal wall and is moved with difficulty. The inspissated and impacted meconium fills the intestinal canal but is most concentrated in the lower ileum.

Clinically, the pattern is that of congenital intestinal obstruction with or without intestinal perforation. Abdominal distention is prominent, and persistent vomiting soon occurs. Infrequently, one or more inspissated meconium stools may be passed shortly after birth.

The *differential diagnosis* involves other causes of intestinal obstruction, including intestinal pseudo-obstruction and pancreatic insufficiency; an exact diagnosis cannot be made except at laparotomy. A presumptive diagnosis can be made on the basis of a history of CF in a sibling, by palpation of doughy or cordlike masses of intestines through the abdominal wall, and by the roentgenographic appearance. Roentgenographically, in contrast to the generally evenly distended intestinal loops above an atresia, the loops may vary in width and are not as evenly filled with gas. At points of heaviest meconium concentration, the infiltrated gas may create a bubbly granular appearance (Figs. 98–2 and 98–3). A negative sweat test result in the neonatal period may not rule out CF. Genetic testing confirms the diagnosis of CF.

Most infants survive the neonatal period; their subsequent prognosis depends on the basic disturbance, CF (Chapter 416).

Treatment is high Gastrografin enemas as described under Meconium Plugs (see earlier). If they are unsuccessful or if there is reason to suspect a perforation of the bowel wall, laparotomy is performed and the ileum opened at the point of greatest diameter of the impaction. Approximately 50% of infants have associated intestinal atresia, stenosis, or volvulus that does not respond to contrast enema and requires surgery. The inspissated meconium is removed by gentle and patient irrigation with warm isotonic sodium chloride or acetylcysteine (Mucomyst) solution introduced through a fine catheter, which may be passed between the impaction and the bowel wall.

MECONIUM PERITONITIS. Perforation of the intestine may occur in utero or shortly after birth. Either the tear may be sealed by natural processes relatively quickly with only a small amount of meconium escaping, or the meconial contents may largely be emptied into the peritoneal cavity. Such perforations

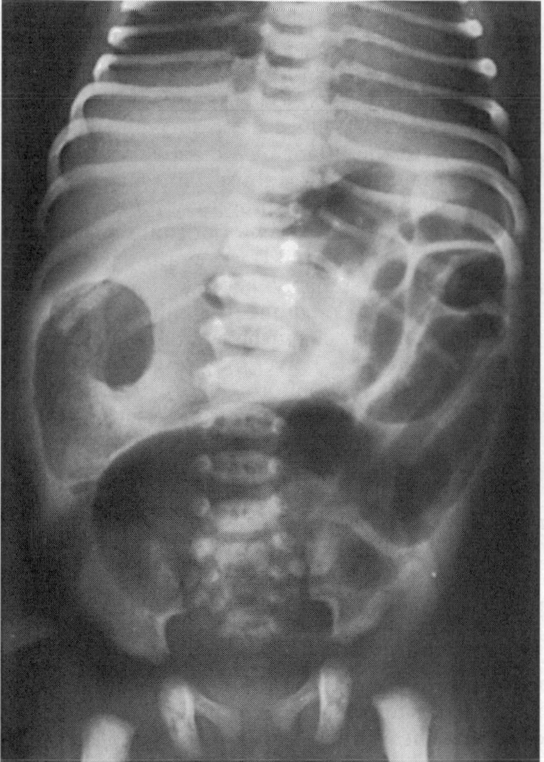

Figure 98–2 Meconium ileus. Impacted meconium with small amounts of air interspersed throughout it in loops of intestine on the right side of abdomen. Intestinal loops above this impaction are greatly distended.

occur most often as a complication of meconium ileus in infants with CF, but the perforation occasionally is due to a meconium plug or intestinal obstruction of another cause.

When the intestinal perforation is spontaneously sealed and only a small amount of meconium has escaped, the event may never be detected, except when meconium becomes calcified and is later fortuitously discovered on roentgenograms of the abdomen. Alternatively, the clinical picture may be dominated by the signs of intestinal obstruction (as in meconium ileus) or peritonitis. Characteristically noted are abdominal distention, vomiting, and absence of stools. Treatment consists primarily of elimination of the intestinal obstruction and drainage of the peritoneal cavity.

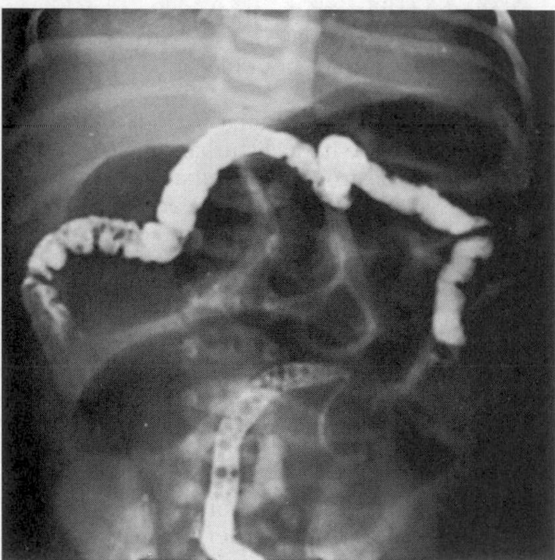

Figure 98–3 Meconium ileus. The colon, outlined by contrast material, is small because meconium has not reached it.

98.2 Neonatal Necrotizing Enterocolitis (NEC)

This serious disease of the newborn is of unknown cause and is characterized by various degrees of mucosal or transmural necrosis of the intestine. Incidence ranges from 1–5% of admissions to neonatal intensive care units. Because very small, ill preterm infants are particularly susceptible to NEC, a rising incidence may reflect improved survival of this high-risk group of patients. The disease rarely occurs in term infants.

PATHOLOGY AND PATHOGENESIS. Many factors may contribute to the development of a necrotic segment of intestine, the gas accumulation in the submucosa of the bowel wall (pneumatosis intestinalis), and progression of the necrosis leading to perforation, sepsis, and death. The distal ileum and proximal colon are involved most frequently; fatal cases have gangrene from the stomach to the rectum. Various factors such as polycythemia, hypertonic milk or oral medicines, or too rapid feeding protocols may contribute to mucosal injury and subsequent infection leading to bowel necrosis. NEC also occurs in premature infants without stress, particularly during epidemics. The clustering of cases suggests a primary role for an infectious agent; *Clostridium perfringens, Escherichia coli, Staphylococcus epidermidis,* and rotavirus have been recovered from cultures. Nonetheless, in most situations no pathogen is identified.

CLINICAL MANIFESTATIONS. Onset usually occurs in the first 2 wk but can be as late as 3 mo of age in VLBW infants. Age of onset is inversely related to gestational age. The first signs are abdominal distention with gastric retention. Manifestations usually develop after the onset of enteric feedings. Obvious bloody stools are seen in 25% of patients. The onset is often insidious, and sepsis may be suspected before an intestinal lesion is noted. There is a wide spectrum of illness from mild with only guaiac-positive stools to severe with peritonitis, bowel perforation, systemic inflammatory response syndrome,

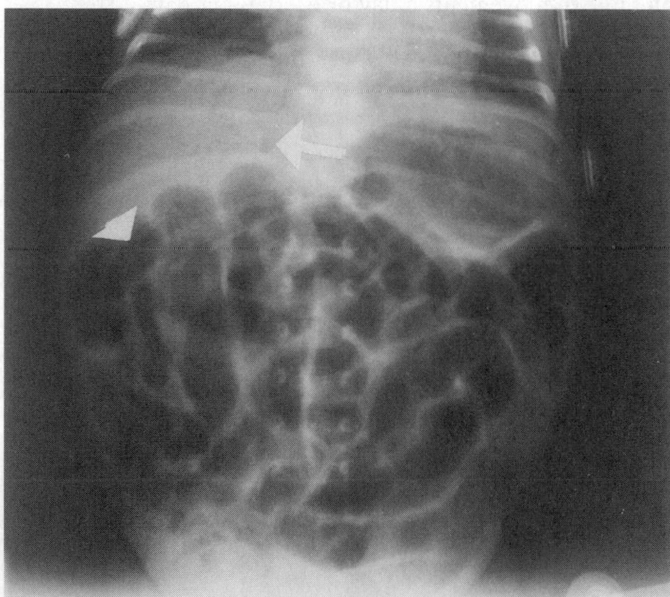

Figure 98–4 Necrotizing enterocolitis. KUB demonstrates abdominal distention, hepatic portal venous gas *(arrow)*, and bubbly appearance of pneumatosis intestinalis *(arrowhead; right lower quadrant)*. The latter two signs are felt to be pathognomonic for neonatal necrotizing enterocolitis.

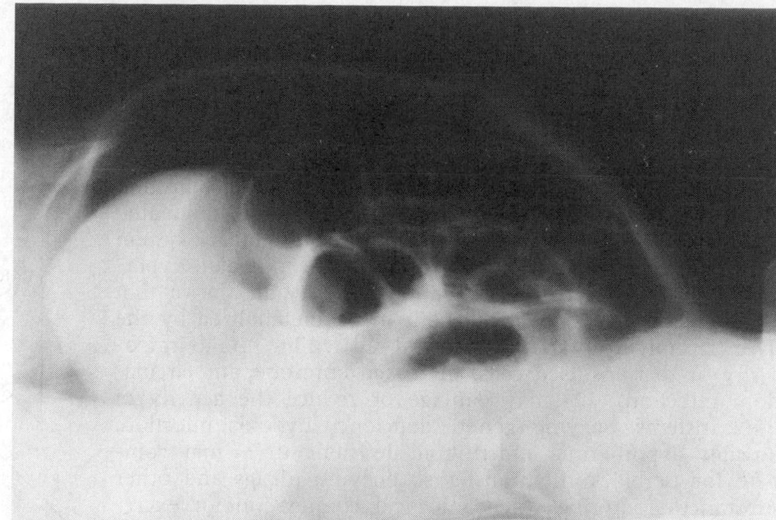

Figure 98–5 Intestinal perforation. Cross-table abdominal roentgenogram in a patient with neonatal necrotizing enterocolitis demonstrating marked distention and massive pneumoperitoneum as evidenced by the free air below the anterior abdominal wall.

shock, and death. Progression may be rapid, but it is unusual for the disease to progress from mild to severe after 72 hr.

DIAGNOSIS. A very high index of suspicion in treating infants at risk is essential. Plain abdominal roentgenograms may demonstrate pneumatosis intestinalis, a finding that is diagnostic of NEC in a newborn infant; 50–75% of patients have pneumatosis when treatment is started (Fig. 98–4). Portal vein gas is a sign of severe disease, and pneumoperitoneum indicates a perforation (Figs. 98–4 and 98–5).

The *differential diagnosis* of NEC includes specific infections (systemic or intestinal), obstruction, and volvulus. Indomethacin may produce focal intestinal perforation, which may also be idiopathic. Such patients manifest pneumoperitoneum but usually are less ill than those with NEC. Cultures and roentgenograms may be diagnostic. Gastrografin enema may demonstrate pneumatosis intestinalis and should be used if congenital obstruction or midgut volvulus is a possible diagnosis; hepatic ultrasonography may detect portal venous gas despite normal abdominal roentgenograms.

TREATMENT. Intensive therapy is advisable for suspected as well as diagnosed cases. Cessation of feeding, nasogastric decompression, and intravenous fluids with careful attention to respiratory status, coagulation profile, and acid-base and electrolyte balance are very important. Once blood cultures are taken, systemic antibiotics (usually ampicillin or an antipseudomonas penicillin [e.g., ticarcillin] with an aminoglycoside [e.g., gentamicin]) should be started. When present, umbilical catheters should be removed, and ventilation should be assisted if distention is contributing to hypoxia and hypercapnia. If hypotension develops, resuscitation with crystalloid, blood, plasma, and dopamine is essential.

The patient's course should be monitored by frequent cross-table lateral abdominal roentgenograms in search of perforation and by hematocrit, platelet, electrolyte, and acid-base determinations. Gown and glove isolation and grouping infants at similar increased risk into cohorts separate from other infants should be instituted to contain an epidemic.

A surgeon should be consulted early in the course of treatment. Evidence of perforation is usually an indication for resection of necrotic bowel. Pneumoperitoneum and brown paracentesis fluid suggest perforation. Failure to respond to medical management, a single fixed bowel loop, erythema of the abdominal wall, and a palpable mass are additional indications for exploratory laparotomy, resection of necrotic bowel, and external ostomy diversion. Peritoneal drainage may be helpful for patients in extremis with peritonitis who are unable to withstand bowel resection.

PROGNOSIS. Medical management fails in about 20% of patients with pneumatosis intestinalis at diagnosis; of these, 9–25% die. Strictures develop at the site of the necrotizing lesion in about 10% of patients. Resection of the obstructing stricture is curative. Complications of NEC following massive intestinal resection include short bowel syndrome (malabsorption, growth failure, malnutrition), complications of total parenteral alimentation due to central venous catheters (sepsis, thrombosis), and cholestatic jaundice. *Prevention* may be possible with judicious feeding protocols (slow advancement of no more than 15–20 mL/kg/24 hr) and the use of breast milk or formula with egg phospholipids.

Carlson S, Montalto M, Ponder D, et al: Lower incidence of necrotizing enterocolitis in infants fed a preterm formula with egg phospholipids. Pediatr Res 44:491, 1998.

Grosfeld JL, Molinari F, Chaet M, et al: Gastrointestinal perforation and peritonitis in infants and children: Experience with 179 cases over ten years. Surgery 120:650, 1996.

Holman R, Stoll B, Clarke M, et al: The epidemiology of necrotizing enterocolitis infant mortality in the United States. Am J Public Health 87:2026, 1997.

Kanto WP, Hunter JE, Stoll BJ: Recognition and medical management of necrotizing enterocolitis. Clin Perinatol 21:335, 1994.

Kliegman RM, Walker WA, Yolken RH: Necrotizing enterocolitis: Research agenda for a disease of unknown etiology and pathogenesis. Clin Perinatol 21:437, 1994.

Rovin J, Rodgers B, Burns C, et al: The role of peritoneal drainage for intestinal perforation in infants with and without necrotizing enterocolitis. J Pediatr Surg 34:143, 1999.

Wilcox DT, Borowitz DS, Stovroff MC, et al: Chronic intestinal pseudo-obstruction with meconium ileus at onset. J Pediatr 123:751, 1993.

98.3 Jaundice and Hyperbilirubinemia in the Newborn

Hyperbilirubinemia is a common and in most cases benign problem in neonates. Nonetheless, untreated severe, indirect hyperbilirubinemia is potentially neurotoxic, and conjugated-direct hyperbilirubinemia often signifies a serious illness. Jaundice is observed during the 1st wk of life in approximately 60% of term infants and 80% of preterm infants. The color usually results from accumulation in the skin of unconjugated, nonpolar, lipid-soluble bilirubin pigment (indirect-reacting) formed from hemoglobin by the action of heme oxygenase, biliverdin reductase, and nonenzymatic reducing agents in the reticuloendothelial cells; it may also be due in part to deposition of the pigment after it has been converted in the liver cell microsome by the enzyme uridine diphosphoglucuronic acid glucuronyl transferase to the polar, water-soluble ester glucuronide of bilirubin (direct-reacting). The unconjugated form is neurotoxic for infants at certain concentrations and under various conditions. Conjugated bilirubin is not neurotoxic but indicates a potentially serious disorder. Mild elevations of bilirubin may have antioxidant properties.

ETIOLOGY. A newborn infant's metabolism of bilirubin is in transition from the fetal stage, during which the placenta is the principal route of elimination of the lipid-soluble bilirubin, to the adult stage, during which the water-soluble conjugated form is excreted from the hepatic cells into the biliary system and then into the gastrointestinal tract. Unconjugated hyperbilirubinemia may be caused or increased by any factor that (1) increases the load of bilirubin to be metabolized by the liver (hemolytic anemias, shortened red cell life due to immaturity or to transfused cells, increased enterohepatic circulation, infection); (2) may damage or reduce the activity of the transferase enzyme (genetic deficiency, hypoxia, infection, possibly hypothermia and thyroid deficiency); (3) may compete for or block the transferase enzyme (drugs and other substances requiring glucuronic acid conjugation for excretion); or (4) leads to an absence of or decreased amounts of the enzyme or to reduction of bilirubin uptake by the liver cells (genetic defect, prematurity). The toxic effects from elevated levels of unconjugated bilirubin in serum are increased by factors that reduce the retention of bilirubin in the circulation (hypoproteinemia, displacement of bilirubin from its binding sites on albumin by competitive binding of drugs such as sulfisoxazole and moxalactam, Chuen-Lin herbal tea, acidosis, increased free fatty acid concentration secondary to hypoglycemia, starvation, or hypothermia), or by factors that increase the permeability of the blood-brain barrier or nerve cell membranes to bilirubin or the susceptibility of brain cells to its toxicity such as asphyxia, prematurity, hyperosmolality, and infection. Early feeding decreases, whereas breast-feeding and dehydration increase the serum levels of bilirubin. Meconium has 1 mg bilirubin/dL and may contribute to jaundice by the enterohepatic circulation after deconjugation by intestinal glucuronidase (Fig. 98–6). Drugs such as oxytocin and chemicals used in the nursery such as phenolic detergents may also produce unconjugated hyperbilirubinemia.

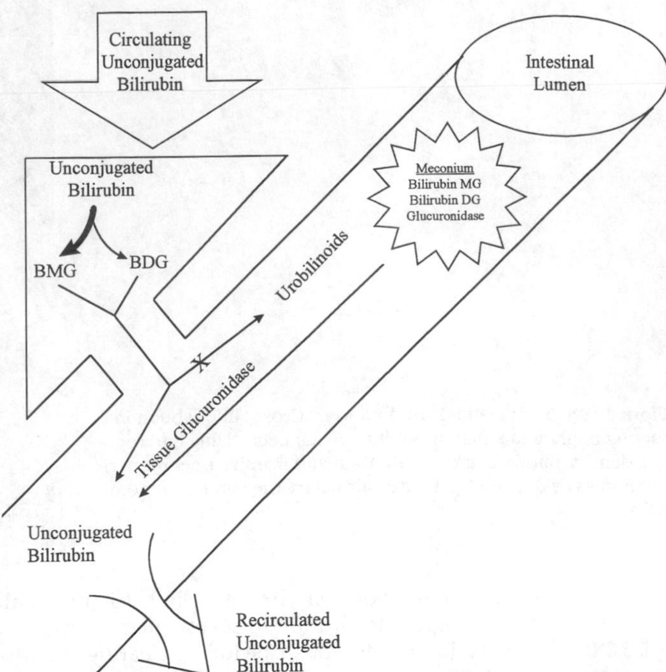

Figure 98–6 The neonatal production rate of bilirubin is 6–8 mg/kg/24 hr (contrast to 3–4 mg/kg/24 hr in adults). Water-insoluble bilirubin is bound to albumin. At the plasma hepatocyte interface, a liver membrane carrier (bilitranslocase) transports bilirubin to a cytosolic binding protein (ligandin or Y protein, now known to be glutathione S-transferase), which prevents back-absorption to plasma. Bilirubin is converted to bilirubin mono (BMG) or diglucuronide (BDG) by several classes of the enzyme bilirubin glucuronyltransferase. The neonate excretes more BMG than adults. In the fetus, conjugated lipid-insoluble BMG and BDG must be deconjugated by tissue β-glucuronidases to facilitate placental transfer of lipid-soluble unconjugated bilirubin across the placental lipid membranes. After birth, intestinal or milk-containing glucuronidases contribute to the enterohepatic recirculation of bilirubin and possibly to the development of hyperbilirubinemia.

CLINICAL MANIFESTATIONS. Jaundice may be present at birth or may appear at any time during the neonatal period, depending on the cause. Jaundice usually begins on the face and, as the serum level increases, progresses to the abdomen and then the feet. Dermal pressure may reveal the anatomic progression of jaundice (face ~ 5 mg/dL, midabdomen ~ 15 mg/dL, soles ~ 20 mg/dL) but cannot be depended on to estimate blood levels. Jaundice to the midabdomen, signs or symptoms, high-risk factors that suggest nonphysiologic jaundice, or hemolysis must be evaluated further. An icterometer or transcutaneous jaundice meter may be used to screen infants, but a serum bilirubin level is indicated for those patients with progressing jaundice, symptoms, or a risk for hemolysis or sepsis. Jaundice resulting from deposition of indirect bilirubin in the skin tends to appear bright yellow or orange; jaundice of the obstructive type (direct bilirubin), a greenish or muddy yellow. This difference is usually apparent only in severe jaundice. Affected infants may be lethargic and may feed poorly. Signs of kernicterus rarely appear on the first day of jaundice (Chapter 98.4).

DIFFERENTIAL DIAGNOSIS. Jaundice, consisting of indirect or direct bilirubin, that is present at birth or appears within the first 24 hr of life requires immediate attention and may be due to erythroblastosis fetalis, concealed hemorrhage, sepsis, cytomegalic inclusion disease, rubella, or congenital toxoplasmosis. Hemolysis is suggested by a rapid rise of serum bilirubin (>0.5 mg/dL/hr), anemia, pallor, reticulocytosis, hepatosplenomegaly, and a positive family history. Jaundice in infants who have received intrauterine transfusions may be characterized by an unusually high proportion of direct-reacting bilirubin. Jaundice that first appears on the 2nd or 3rd day is usually "physiologic" but may represent a more severe form. Familial nonhemolytic icterus (Crigler-Najjar syndrome) and early onset breast-feeding jaundice are seen initially on the 2nd or 3rd day. *Jaundice appearing after the 3rd day and within the 1st wk should suggest bacterial sepsis or urinary tract infections*; it may be due to other infections, notably syphilis, toxoplasmosis, cytomegalovirus, or enterovirus. Jaundice secondary to extensive ecchymosis or hematoma may occur during the 1st day or later, especially in premature infants. Polycythemia may lead to early jaundice.

Jaundice that is noted initially after the 1st wk of life suggests breast milk jaundice, septicemia, congenital atresia of the bile ducts, hepatitis, galactosemia, hypothyroidism, CF, paucity of bile ducts, congenital hemolytic anemia (spherocytosis), or possibly the crises of other hemolytic anemias (such as pyruvate kinase and other glycolytic enzyme deficiencies or hereditary nonspherocytic anemia), or hemolytic anemia due to drugs (as in congenital deficiencies of the enzymes glucose-6-phosphate dehydrogenase [G6PD], glutathione synthetase, reductase, or peroxidase) (Fig. 98–7).

Persistent jaundice during the 1st mo of life suggests the inspissated bile syndrome (which may follow hemolytic disease of the newborn), hyperalimentation-associated cholestasis, hepatitis, cytomegalic inclusion disease, syphilis, toxoplasmosis, familial nonhemolytic icterus, congenital atresia of the bile ducts, or galactosemia. Rarely, physiologic jaundice may be prolonged for several weeks, as in infants with hypothyroidism or pyloric stenosis.

Low-risk jaundiced infants who are full term and asymptomatic may be evaluated by monitoring serum total bilirubin

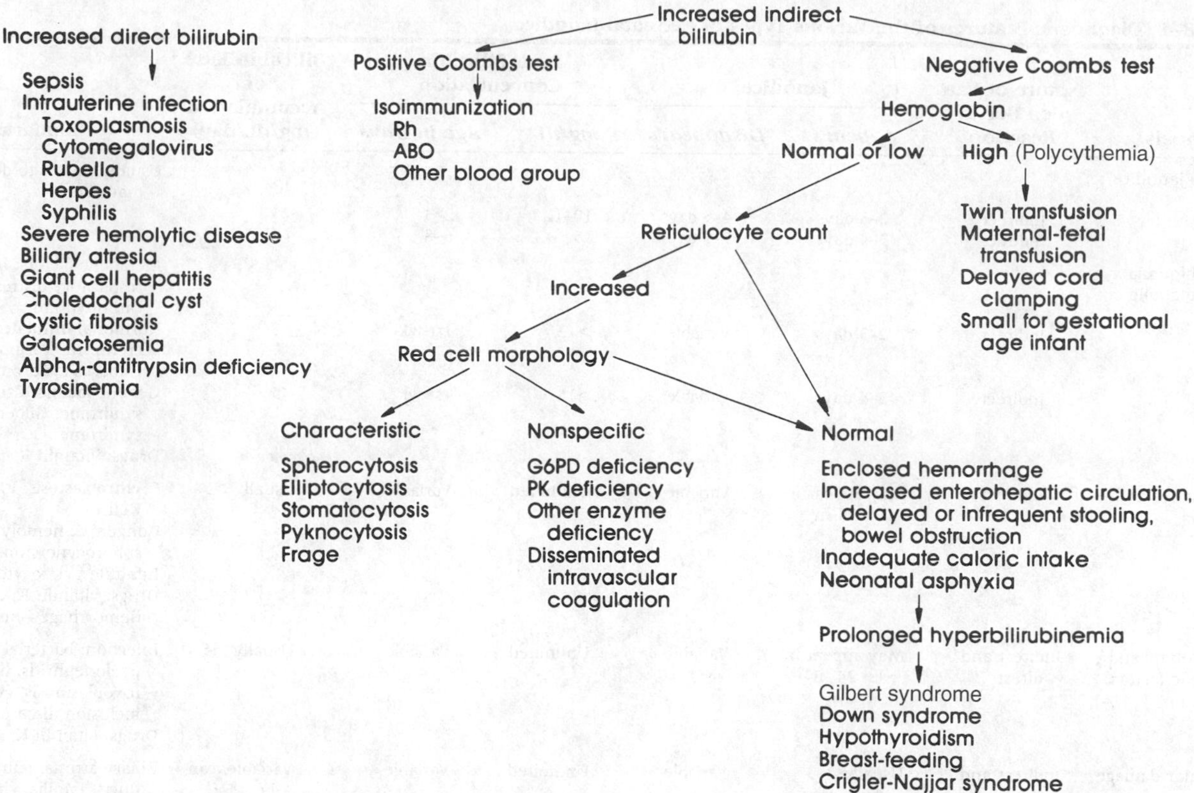

Figure 98–7 Schematic approach to the diagnosis of neonatal jaundice. (From Oski FA: Differential diagnosis of jaundice. *In:* Taeusch HW, Ballard RA, Avery MA [eds]: Schaffer and Avery's Diseases of the Newborn, 6th ed. Philadelphia, WB Saunders, 1991.)

levels. Regardless of the gestational age or time of appearance of jaundice, significant hyperbilirubinemia and all patients with symptoms or signs require a complete diagnostic evaluation, which should include determination of the direct and indirect bilirubin fractions, hemoglobin, reticulocyte count, blood type, Coombs' test, and an examination of the peripheral blood smear (Table 98–1). Indirect-reacting bilirubinemia, reticulocytosis, and a smear demonstrating evidence of red blood cell destruction suggest hemolysis; in the absence of blood group incompatibility, nonimmunologically induced hemolysis should be considered. If there is direct-reacting hyperbilirubinemia, hepatitis, cholestasis, inborn errors of metabolism, cystic fibrosis, and sepsis are diagnostic possibilities. If the reticulocyte count, Coombs test, and direct bilirubin are normal, physiologic or pathologic indirect hyperbilirubinemia may be present (Fig. 98–7).

PHYSIOLOGIC JAUNDICE (ICTERUS NEONATORUM). Under normal circumstances, the level of indirect-reacting bilirubin in umbilical cord serum is 1–3 mg/dL and rises at a rate of less than 5 mg/dL/24 hr; thus, jaundice becomes visible on the 2nd–3rd day, usually peaking between the 2nd and 4th days at 5–6 mg/dL and decreasing to below 2 mg/dL between the 5th and 7th days of life. Jaundice associated with these changes is designated "physiologic" and is believed to be the result of increased bilirubin production following breakdown of fetal red blood cells combined with transient limitation in the conjugation of bilirubin by the liver.

Overall, 6–7% of full-term infants have indirect bilirubin levels greater than 12.9 mg/dL and less than 3% have levels greater than 15 mg/dL. Risk factors for indirect hyperbilirubinemia include maternal diabetes, race (Chinese, Japanese, Korean, and Native American), prematurity, drugs (vitamin K_3, novobiocin), altitude, polycythemia, male sex, 21-trisomy, cutaneous bruising, cephalohematoma, oxytocin induction, breast-feeding, weight loss (dehydration or caloric deprivation), delayed bowel movement, and a sibling who had physiologic jaundice. Infants without these variables rarely develop indirect bilirubin levels above 12 mg/dL, whereas infants with several risks are more likely to have higher bilirubin levels. Indirect bilirubin levels in full-term infants decline to adult levels (1 mg/dL) by 10–14 days of life.

The ability to predict which neonatal infants are at risk for exaggerated physiologic jaundice can be based on hour-specific bilirubin levels in the first 24–72 hr of life (Fig. 98–8).

Persistent indirect hyperbilirubinemia beyond 2 wk suggests hemolysis, hereditary glucuronyl transferase deficiency, breast milk jaundice, hypothyroidism, or intestinal obstruction. Jaundice associated with pyloric stenosis may be due to caloric deprivation, deficiency of hepatic UDP-glucuronyl transferase, or ileus-induced increased enterohepatic circulation of bilirubin.

Among premature infants, the rise in serum bilirubin tends to be the same or a little slower than that in term infants but is of longer duration, which generally results in higher levels, the peak being reached between the 4th and 7th days; the pattern depends on the time required for the preterm infant to achieve mature mechanisms for the metabolism and excretion of bilirubin. Peak levels of 8–12 mg/dL usually are not reached until the 5th–7th day, and jaundice is infrequently observed after the 10th day.

The diagnosis of physiologic jaundice in term or preterm infants can be established only by precluding known causes of jaundice on the basis of the history and clinical and laboratory findings (see Table 98–1). In general, a search to determine the cause of jaundice should be made if (1) it appears in the first 24–36 hr of life; (2) serum bilirubin is rising at a rate greater than 5 mg/dL/24 hr; (3) serum bilirubin is greater than 12 mg/dL in full-term (especially in the absence of risk factors) or 10–14 mg/dL in preterm infants; (4) jaundice persists after 10–14 days of life; or (5) direct-reacting bilirubin is greater

TABLE 98–1 Diagnostic Features of the Various Types of Neonatal Jaundice

Diagnosis	Nature of Van den Bergh Reaction	Jaundice		Peak Bilirubin Concentration		Bilirubin Rate of Accumulation (mg/dL/day)	Remarks
		Appears	*Disappears*	*mg/dL*	*Age in Days*		
"Physiologic jaundice":							Usually relates to degree of maturity
Full-term	Indirect	2–3 days	4–5 days	10–12	2–3	<5	
Premature	Indirect	3–4 days	7–9 days	15	6–8	<5	
Hyperbilirubinemia due to metabolic factors							Metabolic factors: hypoxia, respiratory distress, lack of carbohydrate
Full-term	Indirect	2–3 days	Variable	>12	1st wk	<5	Hormonal influences: cretinism, hormones, Gilbert's syndrome
Premature	Indirect	3–4 days	Variable	>15	1st wk	<5	Genetic factors: Crigler-Najjar syndrome, Gilbert's syndrome Drugs: vitamin K, novobiocin
Hemolytic states and hematoma	Indirect	May appear in 1st 24 hr	Variable	Unlimited	Variable	Usually >5	Erythroblastosis: Rh, ABO, Kell Congenital hemolytic states: spherocytic, nonspherocytic Infantile pyknocytosis Drugs: vitamin K. Enclosed hemorrhage—hematoma
Mixed hemolytic and hepatotoxic factors	Indirect and direct	May appear in 1st 24 hr	Variable	Unlimited	Variable	Usually >5	Infection: bacterial sepsis, pyelonephritis, hepatitis, toxoplasmosis, cytomegalic inclusion disease, rubella Drugs: vitamin K
Hepatocellular damage	Indirect and direct	Usually 2–3 days, may appear by 2nd wk	Variable	Unlimited	Variable	Variable, can be >5	Biliary atresia; paucity of bile ducts, familial cholestasis, galactosemia; hepatitis and infection

From Brown AK: Pediatr Clin North Am 9:589, 1962.

than 2 mg/dL at any time. Among other factors suggesting a nonphysiologic cause of jaundice are family history of hemolytic disease, pallor, hepatomegaly, splenomegaly, failure of phototherapy to lower bilirubin, vomiting, lethargy, poor feeding, excessive weight loss, apnea, bradycardia, abnormal vital signs including hypothermia, light-colored stools, dark urine positive for bilirubin, and signs of kernicterus (Chapter 98.4).

PATHOLOGIC HYPERBILIRUBINEMIA. Jaundice and its underlying hyperbilirubinemia are considered pathologic if their time of appearance, duration, or pattern of serially determined serum

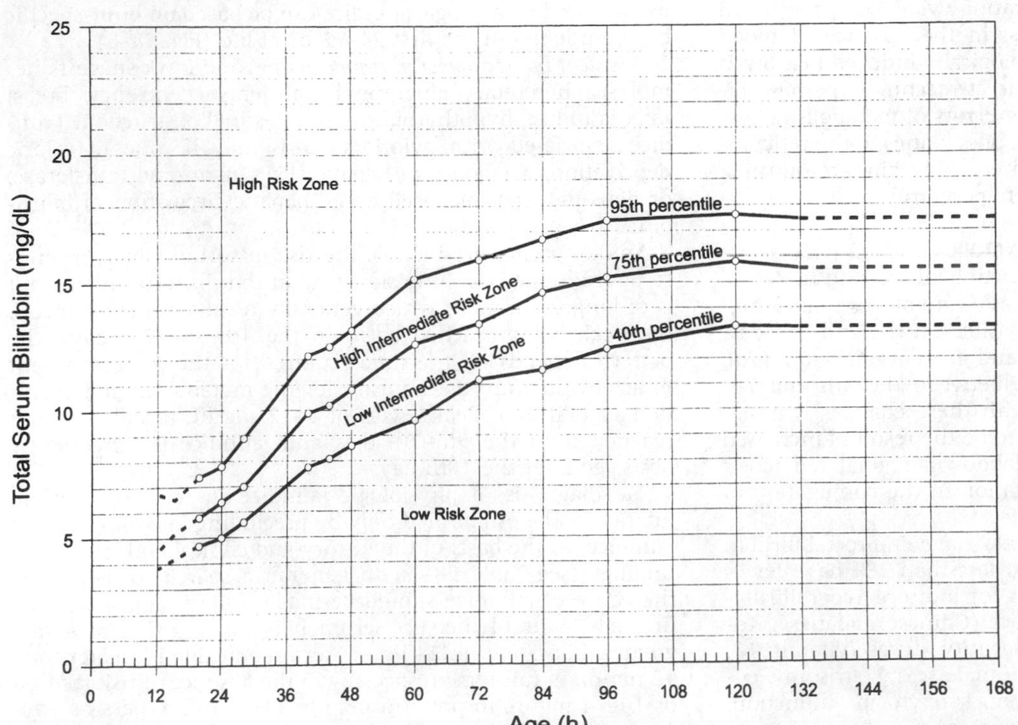

Figure 98–8 Risk designation of term and near-term well newborns based on their hour-specific serum bilirubin values. The high-risk zone is designated by the 95th percentile track. The intermediate-risk zone is subdivided into upper and lower risk zones by the 75th percentile track. The low-risk zone has been electively and statistically defined by the 40th percentile track. (Dotted extensions are based on <300 total serum bilirubin values/epoch). (From Bhutani VK, Johnson L, Sivieri EM: Predictive ability of a predischarge hour-specific serum bilirubin for subsequent significant hyperbilirubinemia in healthy term and near-term newborns. Pediatrics 103:9, 1999).

bilirubin concentrations varies significantly from that of physiologic jaundice; or if the course is compatible with physiologic jaundice but other reasons exist to suspect that the infant is at special risk from the neurotoxicity of unconjugated bilirubin. It may not be possible to determine precisely the cause of an abnormal elevation of unconjugated bilirubin. Many of these infants have an associated risk factor such as Asian race, prematurity, breast-feeding, or weight loss; hence the terms exaggerated physiologic jaundice and hyperbilirubinemia of the newborn are used for those infants whose primary problem is probably a deficiency or inactivity of bilirubin glucuronyl transferase (e.g., Gilbert syndrome) rather than an excessive load of bilirubin for excretion. The combination of G6PD deficiency and a mutation of the promoter region of UDP-glucuronyl transferase 1 produces an indirect hyperbilirubinemia in the absence of signs of hemolysis.

The risk of hyperbilirubinemia is related to the development of kernicterus (bilirubin encephalopathy) at high indirect serum bilirubin levels (Chapter 98.4). The level of serum bilirubin associated with kernicterus is dependent in part on the cause of the jaundice. Kernicterus develops at lower bilirubin levels in preterm infants and in the presence of asphyxia, intraventricular hemorrhage, hemolysis, or drugs that displace bilirubin from albumin. Kernicterus is unusual in patients with breast milk jaundice.

JAUNDICE ASSOCIATED WITH BREAST-FEEDING. An estimated 2% of breast-fed term infants develop significant elevations in unconjugated bilirubin (breast milk jaundice) after the 7th day of life, reaching maximum concentrations as high as 10–30 mg/dL during the 2nd–3rd wk. If breast-feeding is continued, the hyperbilirubinemia gradually decreases and then may persist for 3–10 wk at lower levels. If nursing is discontinued, the serum bilirubin level falls rapidly, usually reaching normal levels within a few days. Cessation of breast-feeding for 1–2 days and substitution of formula for breast milk results in a rapid decline in serum bilirubin, after which nursing can be resumed without a return of the hyperbilirubinemia to its previously high levels. If indicated, phototherapy may be of benefit (Chapter 98.4). These infants have no other sign of illness; nonetheless, kernicterus has been reported. The cause is unclear, but in some the milk contains a glucuronidase that may be responsible for jaundice.

This syndrome should be distinguished from an early onset accentuated unconjugated hyperbilirubinemia (breast-feeding jaundice) in the 1st wk of life, when breast-fed infants have higher bilirubin levels than formula-fed infants (Fig. 98–9). Thirteen per cent of breast-fed infants develop hyperbilirubinemia (>12 mg/dL) in the 1st wk of life. This observation may be due to decreased milk intake with dehydration or reduced caloric intake. Giving supplements of glucose water to breast-fed infants is associated with higher bilirubin levels owing in part to reduced intake of the higher caloric density breast milk. Frequent breast feedings (>10/24 hr), rooming-in with night feedings, and discouraging 5% dextrose or water supplementation may reduce the incidence of early breast-feeding jaundice.

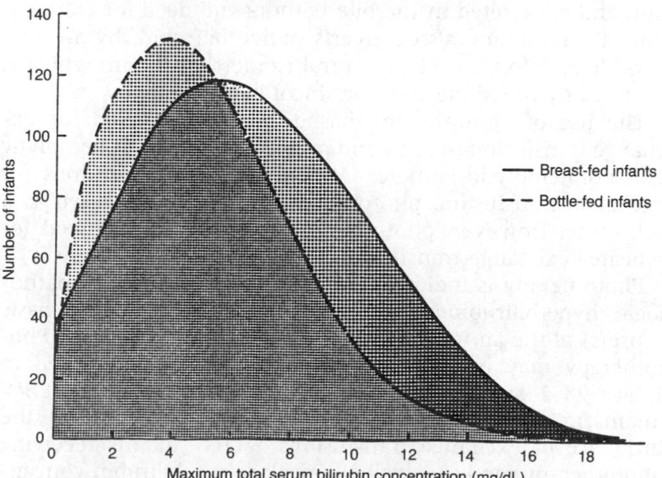

Figure 98–9 Distribution of maximum bilirubin levels during the 1st wk of life in breast-fed and formula-fed white infants >2,500 g. (From Maisels J, Gifford K: Normal serum bilirubin levels in the newborn and the effect of breast-feeding. Pediatrics 78:837, 1986.)

NEONATAL HEPATITIS. See Chapter 356.1.

CONGENITAL ATRESIA OF THE BILE DUCTS. See Chapter 356.1. Jaundice persisting for more than 2 wk or associated with acholic stools and dark urine suggests biliary atresia. All such infants should have a direct bilirubin determination.

INSPISSATED BILE SYNDROME. See Late Complications in Chapter 99.

98.4 Kernicterus

Kernicterus is a neurologic syndrome resulting from the deposition of unconjugated bilirubin in brain cells. The risk in infants with erythroblastosis fetalis is directly related to serum bilirubin levels; the relationship between serum bilirubin level and kernicterus among *healthy term infants* is uncertain. Lipid-soluble indirect bilirubin may cross the blood-brain barrier and enter the brain by diffusion if the bilirubin-binding capacity of albumin and other plasma proteins is exceeded and plasma free bilirubin levels increase. Alternatively, bilirubin may enter the brain after damage to the blood-brain barrier by asphyxia or hyperosmolality.

The precise blood level above which indirect-reacting bilirubin or free bilirubin will be toxic for an individual infant is unpredictable, but kernicterus is rare in healthy term infants and in the absence of hemolysis if the serum level is under 25 mg/dL. The duration of exposure necessary to produce toxic effects is also unknown. Little evidence suggests that the level of indirect bilirubin less than 25 mg/dL affects the IQ of healthy term infants without hemolytic disease. *Nonetheless the less mature the infant, the greater the susceptibility to kernicterus.* Factors that potentiate the movement of bilirubin into brain cells and its adverse effects on them are discussed in Chapter 98.3. In exceptional circumstances, kernicterus in VLBW infants with serum bilirubin concentrations as low as 8–12 mg/dL has been associated with an apparently cumulative effect of a number of these factors.

CLINICAL MANIFESTATIONS. Signs and symptoms of kernicterus usually appear 2–5 days after birth in term infants and as late as the 7th day in premature ones, but hyperbilirubinemia may lead to the syndrome at any time during the neonatal period. The early signs may be subtle and indistinguishable from those of sepsis, asphyxia, hypoglycemia, intracranial hemorrhage, and other acute systemic illnesses in a neonatal infant. Lethargy, poor feeding, and loss of the Moro reflex are common initial signs. Subsequently, the infant may appear gravely ill and prostrated, with diminished tendon reflexes and respiratory distress. Opisthotonos, with a bulging fontanel, twitching of face or limbs, and a shrill high-pitched cry may follow. In advanced cases, convulsions and spasm occur, with the infant stiffly extending his or her arms in inward rotation with fists clenched. Rigidity is rare at this late stage.

Many infants who progress to these severe neurologic signs die; the survivors are usually seriously damaged but may appear to recover and for 2–3 mo show few abnormalities. Later in the 1st yr of life, opisthotonos, muscle rigidity, irregular movements, and convulsions tend to recur. In the 2nd yr, opisthotonos and seizures abate but irregular, involuntary movements, muscle rigidity, or, in some infants, hypotonia increases steadily. By age 3 yr, the complete neurologic syndrome is often apparent, consisting of bilateral choreoathetosis with involuntary muscle spasm, extrapyramidal signs, seizures, mental deficiency, dysarthric speech, high-frequency hearing loss, squinting, and defective upward movement of the eyes. Pyramidal signs, hypotonia, and ataxia occur in a few infants. In mildly affected infants, the syndrome may be characterized only by mild to moderate neuromuscular incoordination, partial deafness, or "minimal brain dysfunction," occurring singly or in combination; these problems may be inapparent until the child enters school.

PATHOLOGY. The surface of the brain is usually pale yellow. On cutting, certain regions are characteristically stained yellow by unconjugated bilirubin, particularly the corpus subthalamicum, hippocampus and adjacent olfactory areas, striate bodies, thalamus, globus pallidus, putamen, inferior clivus, cerebellar nuclei, and cranial nerve nuclei. Nonpigmented areas may also be damaged. Loss of neurons, reactive gliosis, and atrophy of involved fiber systems are found in late disease. The pattern of injury has been related to the development of oxidative enzyme systems in various regions of the brain and overlaps with that found in hypoxic brain damage. Evidence favors the hypothesis that bilirubin interferes with oxygen utilization by cerebral tissue, possibly by injuring the cell membrane; antecedent hypoxic injury increases the susceptibility of brain cells to injury. Gross bilirubin staining without the specific microscopic changes of kernicterus may not be the same entity.

INCIDENCE AND PROGNOSIS. Using pathologic criteria, one third of infants (all gestational ages) with untreated *hemolytic disease* and bilirubin levels in excess of 25–30 mg/dL will develop kernicterus. The incidence at autopsy in hyperbilirubinemic premature infants is 2–16% and is related to the risk factors discussed in Chapter 98.3. Reliable estimates of the frequency of the clinical syndrome are not available because of the wide spectrum of manifestations. Overt neurologic signs have a grave prognosis; 75% or more of such infants die, and 80% of affected survivors have bilateral choreoathetosis with involuntary muscle spasm. Mental retardation, deafness, and spastic quadriplegia are common. Infants at risk should have screening hearing tests.

TREATMENT OF HYPERBILIRUBINEMIA. Regardless of cause, the goal of therapy is to prevent the concentration of indirect-reacting bilirubin in the blood from reaching levels at which neurotoxicity may occur; it is recommended that phototherapy and, if unsuccessful, exchange transfusion be used to keep the maximum total serum bilirubin below the levels indicated in Tables 98–2 (for preterm) and 98–3 (for healthy term infants without hemolysis). The risk of injury to the central nervous system from bilirubin must be balanced against the risk inherent in the treatment for each infant. The criteria for initiating phototherapy are not generally agreed on. Because phototherapy may require 6–12 hr to have a measurable effect, it must be started at bilirubin levels below those indicated for exchange transfusion. When identified, the underlying cause of the icterus should be treated—for example, antibiotics for septicemia. Physiologic factors that increase the risk of neurologic damage should also be treated (e.g., correction of acidosis).

TABLE 98–2 Suggested Maximum Indirect Serum Bilirubin Concentrations (mg/dL) in Preterm Infants

Birthweight (g)	Uncomplicated	Complicated*
<1,000	12–13	10–12
1,000–1,250	12–14	10–12
1,251–1,499	14–16	12–14
1,500–1,999	16–20	15–17
2,000–2,500	20–22	18–20

**Complications include perinatal asphyxia, acidosis, hypoxia, hypothermia, hypoalbuminemia, meningitis, intraventricular hemorrhage, hemolysis, hypoglycemia, or signs of kernicterus.*

Phototherapy is usually started at 50–70% of the maximum indirect level. If values greatly exceed this level, if phototherapy is unsuccessful in reducing the maximum bilirubin level, or if there are signs of kernicterus, exchange transfusion is indicated.

TABLE 98–3 Approach to Indirect Hyperbilirubinemia in Healthy Term Infants Without Hemolysis¶

Age (hr)	Treatment Strategies: Phototherapy	Intensive Phototherapy and Preparation for Exchange Transfusion*	Exchange Transfusion if Phototherapy Fails§
<24	†	†	†
24–48‖	≥15–18	≥25	≥20
49–72	≥18–20	≥30	≥25
>72	≥20	≥30	≥25
>2 wk	‡	‡	‡

**If the initial bilirubin on presentation is high, intense phototherapy should be initiated and preparation made for exchange transfusion. If the phototherapy fails to reduce the bilirubin level to the levels noted on the column to the right, initiate exchange transfusion.*

†Jaundice in the 1st 24 hr of life is not seen in "healthy" infants (see Chapter 98.3).

‡Jaundice suddenly appearing in the 2nd wk of life or continuing beyond the 2nd wk of life with significant hyperbilirubinemia levels to warrant therapy should be investigated in detail, as it most probably is due to a serious underlying cause such as biliary atresia, galactosemia, hypothyroidism, or neonatal hepatitis.

§Intensive phototherapy should be initiated for bilirubin levels in this column and usually reduces serum bilirubin levels 1–2 mg/dL in 4–6 hr; this is often associated with administration of intravenous fluids at 1–1.5 times maintenance; oral alimentation should also continue.

‖Hyperbilirubinemia of this degree within 48 hr of birth is unusual and should suggest hemolysis, concealed hemorrhage, or causes of conjugated (direct) hyperbilirubinemia.

¶With hemolysis, exchange transfusion is initiated with an indirect bilirubin of ≥20, at any age.

The precise level of unconjugated bilirubin among healthy breast-fed term infants that requires therapy is unknown. Treatment options include continued breast-feeding and initiation of phototherapy, or interrupted breast-feeding (use formula as substitute) with or without phototherapy.

If there are any signs of kernicterus during the evaluation or treatment as suggested anywhere in the table or at any level of bilirubin, an emergent exchange transfusion must be performed.

Phototherapy. Clinical jaundice and indirect hyperbilirubinemia are reduced on exposure to a high intensity of light in the visible spectrum. Bilirubin absorbs light maximally in the blue range (from 420–470 nm). Nonetheless, broad-spectrum white, blue, special narrow-spectrum (super) blue, and, less often, green lights have been effective in reducing bilirubin levels. Bilirubin in the skin absorbs light energy, which by photoisomerization converts the toxic native unconjugated 4Z,15Z-bilirubin into the unconjugated configurational isomer, 4Z,15E-bilirubin. The latter is the product of a reversible reaction and is excreted in the bile without the need for conjugation. Phototherapy also converts native bilirubin, by an irreversible reaction, to the structural isomer lumirubin, which is excreted by the kidneys in the unconjugated state.

The use of phototherapy has decreased the need for exchange transfusion in term and preterm infants with hemolytic and nonhemolytic jaundice. When there are indications for exchange transfusion, phototherapy should not be used as a substitute. However, phototherapy may reduce the need for repeated exchange transfusions in infants with hemolysis.

Phototherapy is indicated only after the presence of pathologic hyperbilirubinemia has been established. The basic cause(s) of the jaundice should be treated concomitantly. Phototherapy may be initiated at the bilirubin levels noted in Tables 98–2 and 98–3. Prophylactic phototherapy in VLBW infants may prevent hyperbilirubinemia and may reduce the incidence of exchange transfusions. VLBW infants receiving phototherapy for 1–3 days have peak serum bilirubin concentrations about one-half those of untreated infants. In premature infants without significant hemolysis, serum bilirubin usually declines 1–3 mg/dL after 12–24 hr of conventional phototherapy, and peak levels attained may be decreased by

3–6 mg/dL. The therapeutic effect depends on the light energy emitted in the effective range of wavelengths, the distance between the lights and the infant, and the amount of skin exposed, as well as on the rate of hemolysis and in vivo metabolism and excretion of bilirubin. Available commercial phototherapy units vary considerably in the spectral output and intensity of radiation emitted; therefore, the dose can be accurately measured only at the skin surface. Dark skin does not reduce the efficacy of phototherapy.

Maximum-intensive phototherapy should be used when indirect bilirubin levels approach those noted in Tables 98–2 and 98–3. Such therapy includes "special blue" fluorescent tubes, placing the lamps within 15–20 cm of the infant, and using a fiberoptic phototherapy blanket placed under the infant's back, thus increasing the exposed surface area.

Conventional phototherapy is applied continuously, and the infant is turned frequently for maximal skin exposure. It should be discontinued as soon as the indirect bilirubin concentration has been reduced to levels considered safe in view of the infant's age and condition. Serum bilirubin levels and hematocrit should be monitored every 4–8 hr in infants with hemolytic disease or those with bilirubin levels near the range considered toxic for the individual infant. Others, particularly older infants, may be monitored at 12–24 hr intervals. Monitoring should continue for at least 24 hr after cessation of phototherapy in patients with hemolytic disease, because unexpected rises of serum bilirubin sometimes occur and require further treatment. Skin color cannot be relied on for evaluating the effectiveness of phototherapy; the skin of babies exposed to light may appear almost without jaundice in the presence of marked hyperbilirubinemia. The infant's eyes should be closed and adequately covered to prevent exposure to light. (Excessive pressure from an eye bandage may injure the closed eyes, or the corneas may be excoriated if the infant can open his or her eyes under the bandage.) Body temperature should be monitored, and the infant should be shielded from bulb breakage. If feasible, irradiance should be measured directly, and details of the exposure should be recorded (type and age of bulbs, duration of exposure, distance from light source to infant, and so forth). *In infants with hemolytic disease, care must be taken not to overlook developing anemia, which may require transfusion.*

Complications of phototherapy include loose stools, erythematous macular rashes, a purpuric rash associated with transient porphyrinemia, overheating and dehydration (increased insensible water loss, diarrhea), chilling from exposure of the infant, and bronze baby syndrome. Phototherapy is contraindicated in the presence of porphyria. Eye injury or nasal occlusion from the bandages is uncommon.

The term *bronze baby syndrome* refers to a dark grayish-brown discoloration of the skin sometimes noted in infants undergoing phototherapy. Almost all infants observed with this syndrome have had a mixed type of hyperbilirubinemia with significant elevation of direct-reacting bilirubin and often with other evidence of obstructive liver disease. The discoloration may be due to photoinduced modification of porphyrins, which are often present during cholestatic jaundice and may last for many months.

Wide clinical experience suggests that long-term adverse biologic effects of phototherapy are absent, minimal, or unrecognized. However, those using phototherapy should remain alert to these possibilities and avoid its unnecessary use, because untoward effects on DNA have been demonstrated in vitro.

Exchange Transfusion. This widely accepted treatment should be repeated as frequently as necessary to keep indirect bilirubin levels in the serum under those noted in Tables 98–2 and 98–3. (See Exchange Transfusion in Chapter 99.) Various factors may alter this criterion in either direction in an individual patient. Appearance of clinical signs suggesting kernicterus is an indication for exchange transfusion at any level of serum bilirubin. A healthy full-term infant with physiologic or breast milk jaundice may tolerate a concentration slightly higher than 25 mg/dL with no apparent ill effect, whereas a sick premature infant may develop kernicterus at a significantly lower level. A level approaching that considered critical for the individual infant may be an indication for exchange transfusion during the 1st day or two of life when a further rise is anticipated but not on the 4th day in term infants or on the 7th day in premature infants, when an imminent fall may be anticipated as the hepatic conjugating mechanism becomes more effective.

Tin (Sn)-protoporphyrin (or tin-mesoporphyrin) administration has also been proposed for reduction of bilirubin levels. It may inhibit the conversion of biliverdin to bilirubin by heme oxygenase. A single intramuscular dose on the 1st day of life may reduce the need for phototherapy. In patients with hyperbilirubinemia, bilirubin levels may decline, but the effect is no greater than that achieved with phototherapy. Complications include transient erythema if the infant is receiving phototherapy. More data are needed about its efficacy and toxicity before these compounds can be recommended as therapy for hyperbilirubinemia.

Bhutani V, Johnson L, Sivier E: Predictive ability of a predischarge hour specific serum bilirubin for subsequent significant hyperbilirubinemia in healthy term and near-term newborns. Pediatrics 103:6, 1999.

Gourley G: Bilirubin metabolism and kernicterus. Adv Pediatr 44:173, 1997.

Jackson JC: Adverse events associated with exchange transfusion in healthy and ill newborns. Pediatrics 99:http://www.pediatrics.org/cgi/content/full/99/5/e7, 1997.

Kaplan M, Hammerman C: Severe neonatal hyperbilirubinemia: A potential complication of glucose-6-phosphate dehydrogenase deficiency. Clin Perinatol 25:575, 1998.

Madlon-Kay DJ: Recognition of the presence and severity of newborn jaundice by parents, nurses, physicians, and icterometer. Pediatrics 100:http://www.pediatrics.org/cgi/content/full/100/3/e3, 1997.

Maisels MJ, Newman TB: Kernicterus in otherwise healthy, breast-fed term newborns. Pediatrics 96:730, 1995.

Martinez J, Garcia H, Otheguy L, et al: Control of hyperbilirubinemia in full term newborns with the inhibitor of bilirubin production SN-mesoporphyrin. Pediatrics 103:1, 1999.

Monaghan G, Ryan M, Seddon R, et al: Genetic variation in bilirubin UDP-glucuronosyltransferase gene promoter and Gilbert's syndrome. Lancet 347:578, 1996.

Rubaltelli FF, Da Riol R, D'Amore ESG, et al: The bronze baby syndrome: Evidence of increased tissue concentration of copper porphyrins. Acta Paediatr 85:381, 1996.

Yokochi K: Magnetic resonance imaging in children with kernicterus. Acta Paediatr 84:937, 1995.

CHAPTER 99
Blood Disorders

99.1 Anemia in the Newborn Infant

Hemoglobin increases with advancing gestational age: at term, cord blood hemoglobin is 16.8 g/dL (14–20 g/dL); hemoglobin levels in very low birthweight (VLBW) infants are 1–2 g/dL below those at term (Fig. 99–1). Determinations of less than the normal range for birthweight and postnatal age are defined as anemia (see Table 453–1). A "physiologic" decrease in hemoglobin content is noticed at 8–12 wk in term infants (hemoglobin 11 g/dL) and at about 6 wk in premature infants (7–10 g/dL).

Anemia at birth is manifested by pallor, heart failure, or shock (Fig. 99–2). It may be due to acute or chronic blood loss, hemolysis, or underproduction of erythrocytes. It is usually caused by hemolytic disease of the newborn but may also be a result of tearing or cutting of the umbilical cord during

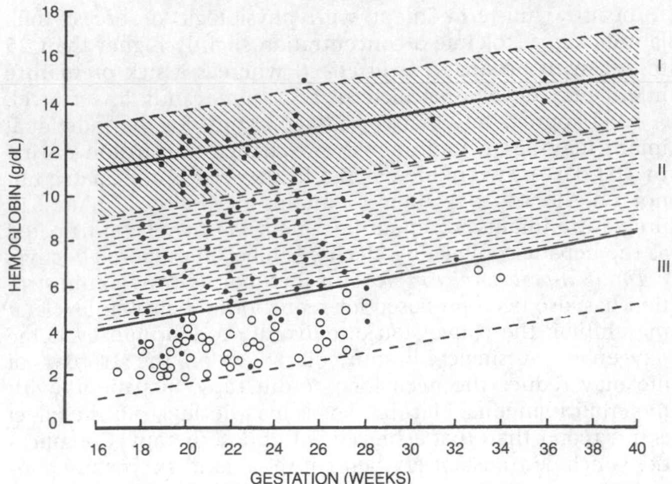

Figure 99–1 Range (mean and 95% confidence limits) of hemoglobin concentration from 16–40 wk of gestational age from normal (zone I) fetuses obtained by cordocentesis (percutaneous umbilical blood sample. Solid circles (●) depict maternal red blood cell isoimmunization; open circles (○) indicate hemoglobin levels in fetus with ultrasonographic evidence of hydrops (zone III). (From Soothill P: Cordocentesis: Role in assessment of fetal condition. Clin Perinatol 16:755, 1989.)

delivery, abnormal cord insertions, communicating placental vessels, placenta previa or abruptio, nuchal cord, incision into the placenta, internal hemorrhage (liver, spleen, or intracranial), α-thalassemia, congenital parvovirus infection or hypoplastic anemias, and twin-twin transfusion in monozygotic twins with arteriovenous placental connections (Chapter 93).

Transplacental hemorrhage, with bleeding from the fetal into the maternal circulation, is probably more common than is generally recognized and, unless severe, is usually not sufficient to cause clinically apparent anemia at birth. The cause of transplacental hemorrhage is not clear, but its occurrence has been proved by demonstrating significant amounts of fetal hemoglobin and red blood cells (RBCs) in the maternal blood on the day of delivery by the Kleihauer-Betke test.

Acute blood loss usually results in severe distress at birth, initially with a normal hemoglobin level, no hepatosplenomegaly, and early onset of shock. In contrast, chronic blood loss in utero produces marked pallor, less distress, low hemoglobin level with microcytic indices, and, if severe, heart failure.

Anemia appearing in the first few days after birth is also most frequently a result of hemolytic disease of the newborn. Other causes are hemorrhagic disease of the newborn, bleeding from an improperly tied or clamped umbilical cord, large cephalohematoma, intracranial hemorrhage, or subcapsular bleeding from rupture of the liver, spleen, adrenals, or kidneys. Rapid decreases in hemoglobin or hematocrit values during the first few days of life may be the initial clue to these conditions.

Later in the neonatal period, delayed anemia from hemolytic disease of the newborn, with or without exchange transfusion or phototherapy, may be seen. Vitamin K (as Synkayvite) in large doses may cause anemia in premature infants, which is characterized by inclusion bodies (Heinz bodies) in the erythrocytes. Congenital hemolytic anemia (spherocytosis) occasionally appears during the 1st mo of life, and hereditary nonspherocytic hemolytic anemia has been described during the neonatal period secondary to deficiency of such enzymes as glucose-6-phosphate dehydrogenase (G6PD) and pyruvate kinase. Bleeding from hemangiomas of the upper gastrointestinal tract or from ulcers caused by aberrant gastric mucosa in a Meckel diverticulum or duplication is a rare source of anemia in newborns. Repeated blood sampling of infants requiring frequent monitoring of blood gases and chemistries is a common cause of anemia. Deficiency of minerals such as copper may cause anemia in infants on total parenteral nutrition.

Anemia of prematurity occurs in low birthweight (LBW) infants 1–3 mo after birth, is associated with hemoglobin levels below 7–10 g/dL, and presents with clinical manifestations such as pallor, apnea, poor weight gain, decreased activity, tachypnea, tachycardia, and feeding problems. Repeated phlebotomy for blood tests, shortened red blood cell (RBC) survival, rapid growth, and the physiologic effects of the transition from fetal (low Pa_{O_2} and hemoglobin saturation) to neonatal

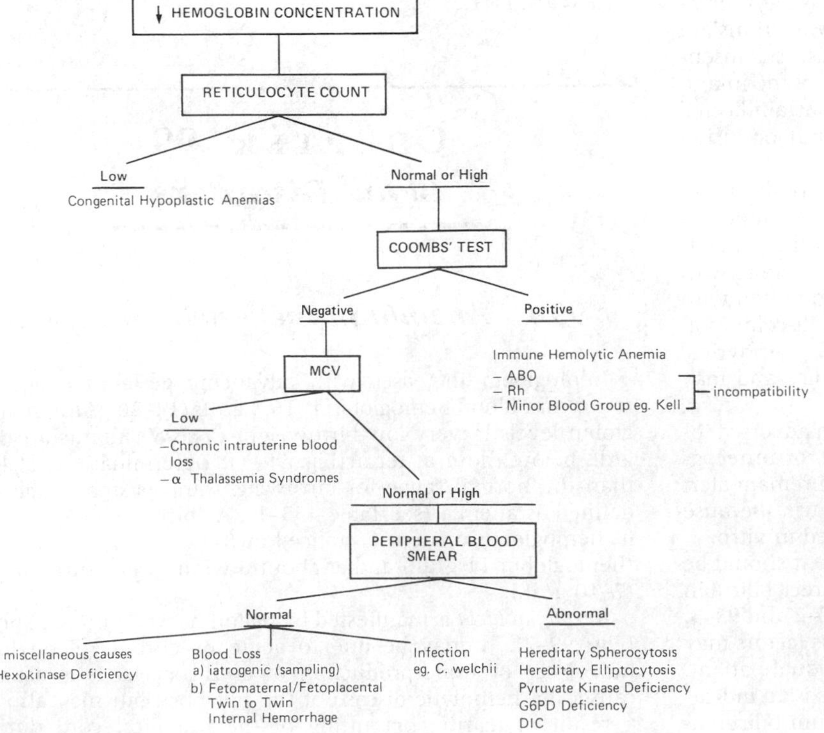

Figure 99–2 Diagnostic approach to anemia in the newborn infant. (From Blanchette V, Zipursky A: Assessment of anemia in newborn infants. Clin Perinatol 11:489, 1984.)

life (high Pa_{O_2} and hemoglobin saturation) contribute to anemia of prematurity. The oxygen available to neonatal tissue is lower than that in adults, but a neonate's erythropoietin response is attenuated for the degree of anemia, resulting in low hemoglobin levels with reticulocytopenia.

Treatment of neonatal anemia by blood transfusion depends on the severity of symptoms, the hemoglobin level, and the presence of co-morbid diseases (chronic lung disease, cyanotic congenital heart disease, hyaline membrane disease) that interfere with oxygen delivery. Treatment with blood should be balanced by concern about transfusion-acquired infection (cytomegalovirus [CMV], human immunodeficiency virus [HIV], hepatitis B and C). The risk of CMV infection can be almost eliminated by the use of CMV antibody-negative or irradiated white-blood-cell poor blood, and that for HIV and hepatitis B and C viruses is reduced but not eliminated by antibody screening of donated blood. Blood banking techniques that limit multiple donor exposures should be encouraged.

Asymptomatic full-term infants with a hemoglobin level of 10 g/dL may be observed, whereas symptomatic neonates born after an abruptio placentae or with severe hemolytic disease of the newborn warrant immediate transfusion. Preterm infants who have repeated episodes of apnea and bradycardia despite theophylline therapy and a hemoglobin level of less than 10 g/dL may benefit from RBC transfusion. In addition, infants with hyaline membrane disease or severe chronic lung disease may need hemoglobin levels of 12–14 g/dL to improve oxygen delivery. No transfusion is needed to replace blood removed for testing or for asymptomatic anemia. Neonatal infants with reticulocytopenia and hemoglobin levels less than 6.5 g/dL may require transfusion; if a transfusion is not provided, close observation is essential. Packed RBC transfusion (10–15 mL/kg) is given at a rate of 2–3 mL/kg/hr to raise the hemoglobin concentration; 2 mL/kg raises the hemoglobin level 0.5–1 g/dL. Hemorrhage should be treated with whole blood if available; alternatively, fluid resuscitation is initiated and followed by packed RBC transfusion.

Recombinant human erythropoietin (rHuEpo) has been used to prevent or treat chronic anemia associated with prematurity, chronic lung disease, and the hyporegenerative anemia of erythroblastosis fetalis. The anemia of prematurity is associated with abnormally low endogenous levels of serum erythropoietin but with rHuEpo-responsive erythrocyte progenitor cells. Therapy with rHuEpo is given by intravenous or subcutaneous routes and must be supplemented with oral iron and possibly vitamin E. Doses and regimens vary from 100–200 U/kg/dose 5 days/wk to 400 U/kg/dose 3 days/wk to 150–200 U/kg/dose q 3 days.

99.2 *Hemolytic Disease of the Newborn*

(Erythroblastosis Fetalis)

Erythroblastosis fetalis results from transplacental passage of maternal antibody active against RBC antigens of the infant, leading to an increased rate of RBC destruction. It continues to be an important cause of anemia and jaundice in newborn infants despite the development of a method of prevention of maternal isoimmunization by Rh antigens. Although more than 60 different RBC antigens capable of eliciting an antibody response in a suitable recipient have been identified, significant disease is associated primarily with the D antigen of the Rh group and with incompatibility of ABO factors. Rarely, hemolytic disease may be caused by C or E antigens or by other RBC antigens, such as C^w, C^x, D^u, K(Kell), M, Duffy, S, P, MNS, Xg, Lutheran, Diego, and Kidd. Anti-Lewis antibodies do not cause disease.

HEMOLYTIC DISEASE OF THE NEWBORN DUE TO RH INCOMPATIBILITY

The Rh antigenic determinants are genetically transmitted from each parent and determine the Rh type and direct the production of a number of blood group factors (C, c, D, d, E, and e). Each factor can elicit a specific antibody response under suitable conditions; 90% are due to D antigen, the remainder to C or E.

PATHOGENESIS. Isoimmune hemolytic disease from D antigen is approximately three times more frequent in white persons than in blacks. When Rh positive blood is infused into an Rh negative woman through error or when small quantities (usually more than 1 mL) of Rh positive fetal blood containing D antigen inherited from an Rh positive father enter the maternal circulation during pregnancy, with spontaneous or induced abortion, or at delivery, antibody formation against D may be induced in the unsensitized Rh negative recipient mother. Once immunization has occurred, considerably smaller doses of antigen can stimulate an increase in antibody titer. Initially, a rise of antibody in the 19S gamma globulin fraction occurs, which later is replaced by 7S (IgG) antibody; the latter readily crosses the placenta, causing hemolytic manifestations.

Hemolytic disease rarely occurs during a first pregnancy, because transfusions of Rh positive fetal blood into an Rh negative mother tend to occur near the time of delivery, too late for the mother to become sensitized and transmit antibody to her infant before delivery. The fact that 55% of Rh positive fathers are heterozygous (D/d) and may have Rh negative offspring and that only 50% of pregnancies have fetal-to-maternal transfusions reduces the chance of sensitization, as does small family size, in which the opportunities for its occurrence are fewer. Finally, the capacity of Rh negative women to form antibodies is variable, some producing low titers even after adequate antigenic challenge. Thus, the overall incidence of isoimmunization of Rh negative mothers at risk is low, with antibody to D detected in less than 10% of those studied, even after five or more pregnancies; only about 5% ever have babies with hemolytic disease.

When mother and fetus are also incompatible with respect to group A or B, the mother is partially protected against sensitization by the rapid removal of Rh positive cells from her circulation by her anti-A or anti-B, which are IgM antibodies and do not cross the placenta. Once a mother has been sensitized, her infant is likely to have hemolytic disease. There is a tendency for the severity of Rh illness to worsen with successive pregnancies. The possibility that the first affected infant after sensitization may represent the end of the mother's childbearing potential for Rh positive infants argues urgently for the prevention of sensitization when this is possible. Such prevention consists of injection into the mother of anti-D gamma globulin (RhoGAM) immediately after the delivery of each Rh positive infant (see later).

CLINICAL MANIFESTATIONS. A wide spectrum of hemolytic disease occurs in affected infants born to sensitized mothers, depending on the nature of the individual immune response. The severity of the disease may range from only laboratory evidence of mild hemolysis (15% of cases) to severe anemia with compensatory hyperplasia of erythropoietic tissue, leading to massive enlargement of the liver and spleen. When the compensatory capacity of the hematopoietic system is exceeded, profound anemia results in pallor, signs of cardiac decompensation (cardiomegaly, respiratory distress), massive anasarca, and circulatory collapse. This clinical picture of excessive abnormal fluid in two or more fetal compartments (skin, pleura, pericardium, placenta, peritoneum, amniotic fluid), termed *hydrops fetalis,* frequently results in death in utero or shortly after birth. With the use of RhoGAM to prevent Rh sensitization, nonimmune-nonhemolytic condi-

TABLE 99–1 Etiology of Hydrops Fetalis*

Category	Disorders
Anemia	Immune (Rh, Kell) hemolysis
	α-thalassemia
	Red blood cell enzyme deficiencies (G6PD)
	Fetomaternal hemorrhage
	Donor in twin-to-twin transfusion
Cardiac dysrhythmias	Supraventricular tachycardia
	Atrial flutter
	Congenital heart block
Structural heart lesions	Premature closure of foramen ovale
	Tricuspid insufficiency
	Hypoplastic left heart
	Endocardial cushion defect
	Cardiomyopathy
	Endocardial fibroelastosis
	Tuberous sclerosis with cardiac rhabdomyoma
	Pericardial teratoma
Vascular	Chorioangioma of placenta, chorionic vessels, or umbilical vessels
	Umbilical artery aneurysm
	Angiomyxoma of umbilical cord
	True knot of umbilical cord
	Hepatic hemangioma
	Cerebral arteriovenous malformation (aneurysm of vein of Galen)
	Angiosteohypertrophy (Klippel-Trenaunay syndrome)
	Thrombosis of renal or umbilical vein or inferior vena cava
	Recipient in twin-to-twin transfusion
Lymphatic	Lymphangiectasia
	Cystic hygroma
	Chylothorax, chylous ascites
	Noonan's syndrome
	Multiple pterygium syndrome
Central nervous system	Absent corpus callosum
	Encephalocele
	Intracranial hemorrhage
	Holoprosencephaly
Thoracic lesions	Cystic adenomatoid malformation of lung
	Mediastinal teratoma
	Diaphragmatic hernia
	Sequestered lung
Teratomas	Choriocarcinoma
	Sacrococcygeal teratoma
Tumors and storage diseases	Neuroblastoma
	Hepatoblastoma
	Gaucher disease
	Niemann-Pick disease
	Mucolipidosis
	GM_1 gangliosidosis
	Mucopolysaccharidosis
Chromosome abnormalities	Trisomy 13, 15, 16, 18, 21
	XX/XY, 45XO
	Partial duplication chromosome 11, 15, 17, 18
	Partial deletion chromosome 13, 18
	Triploidy
	Tetraploidy
Bone diseases	Osteogenesis imperfecta
	Asphyxiating thoracic dystrophy
	Skeletal dysplasias
Congenital infections	Cytomegalovirus
	Parvovirus
	Rubella
	Toxoplasmosis
	Syphilis
	Leptospirosis
	Chagas' disease
Others	Bowel obstruction with perforation and meconium peritonitis, volvulus
	Hepatic fibrosis
	Beckwith-Wiedemann syndrome
	Prune-belly syndrome
	Congenital nephrosis
	Infant of a diabetic mother
	Myotonic dystrophy
	Neu-Laxova syndrome
	Maternal therapy with indomethacin
	Multiple congenital anomaly syndromes
Idiopathic	

**The incidence of nonimmune (nonhemolytic) hydrops fetalis is 1:2,000–1:3,500 births.*
Modified from Phibbs R: In: *Polin N, Fox W: Fetal and Neonatal Physiology, 2nd ed. Philadelphia, WB Saunders, 1998.*

tions are more frequent causes of hydrops (Table 99–1). The severity of hydrops is related to the level of anemia and the degree of reduction in serum albumin (oncotic pressure), which is due in part to hepatic dysfunction. Alternatively, heart failure may increase right heart pressures, with the development of edema and ascites. Failure to initiate spontaneous effective ventilation because of pulmonary edema or bilateral pleural effusions results in birth asphyxia; after successful resuscitation, severe respiratory distress may develop. Petechiae, purpura, and thrombocytopenia may also be present in severe cases, reflecting decreased platelet production or the presence of concurrent disseminated intravascular coagulation.

Jaundice may be absent at birth because of placental clearance of lipid-soluble unconjugated bilirubin, but in severe cases bilirubin pigments stain the amniotic fluid, cord, and vernix caseosa yellow. Icterus is generally evident on the 1st day of life because the infant's bilirubin-conjugating and excretory systems are unable to cope with the load resulting from massive hemolysis. Indirect-reacting bilirubin therefore accumulates postnatally and may rapidly reach extremely high levels, which represent a significant risk of bilirubin encephalopathy. There is a greater risk of developing kernicterus from hemolytic disease than from comparable nonhemolytic hyperbilirubinemia, although the risk in an individual patient may be a function only of the severity of illness (e.g., anoxia, acidosis). Hypoglycemia occurs frequently in infants with severe isoimmune hemolytic disease and may be related to hyperinsulinism and hypertrophy of the pancreatic islet cells in these infants.

Infants born after intrauterine transfusion for prenatally diagnosed erythroblastosis may be severely affected, because the indications for the transfusion are evidence of already severe disease in utero (e.g., hydrops, fetal anemia). Such infants usually have very high (but extremely variable) cord levels of bilirubin, which reflects the severity of hemolysis and its effects on hepatic function. Infants treated with intraumbilical vein transfusions in utero may also have a benign postnatal course, if anemia and hydrops resolve before birth. Anemia from continuing hemolysis may be masked by the prior intrauterine transfusion, and the clinical manifestations of erythroblastosis may be superimposed on various degrees of immaturity resulting from spontaneous or induced premature delivery.

LABORATORY DATA. Before treatment, the direct Coombs test result is usually positive. Anemia is usual. The cord blood hemoglobin varies, usually proportionally to the severity of the disease; with hydrops fetalis it may be as low as 3–4 g/dL (30–40 g/L). Alternatively, despite hemolysis, it may be within the normal range owing to compensatory bone marrow and extramedullary hematopoiesis. The blood smear usually shows polychromasia and a marked increase in nucleated RBCs. The reticulocyte count is increased. The white blood cell count is usually normal but may be elevated; there may be thrombocytopenia in severe cases. The cord bilirubin is usually between 3 and 5 mg/dL (51–86 μmol/L); there may be a substantial elevation of direct-reacting (conjugated) bilirubin. The indirect-reacting bilirubin rises rapidly to high levels in the first 6 hr of life.

After intrauterine transfusions, the cord blood may show a

normal hemoglobin concentration, negative direct Coombs test results, predominantly type O Rh negative adult RBCs, and a relatively normal smear. Marked elevation of both indirect- and direct-reacting bilirubin levels has been reported in these infants.

DIAGNOSIS. The definitive diagnosis of erythroblastosis fetalis requires demonstration of blood group incompatibility and of corresponding antibody bound to the infant's RBCs.

Antenatal Diagnosis. In Rh negative women, a history of previous transfusions, abortion, or pregnancy should suggest the possibility of sensitization. Expectant parents' blood types should be tested for potential incompatibility, and the maternal titer of IgG antibodies to D should be assayed at 12–16, 28–32, and 36 wk. The fetal Rh status may be determined by isolating fetal cells or fetal DNA (plasma) from the maternal circulation or by amniocentesis and polymerase chain reaction with primers to the Rh gene. The presence of measurable antibody titer at the beginning of pregnancy, a rapid rise in titer, or a titer of 1:64 or greater suggests significant hemolytic disease, although the exact titer correlates poorly with the severity of disease. If a mother is found to have antibody against D at a titer of 1:16 or greater at any time during a subsequent pregnancy, the severity of fetal disease should be monitored by amniocentesis, percutaneous umbilical blood sampling (PUBS), and ultrasonography. If there is a history of a previously affected infant or a stillbirth, an Rh positive infant is usually equally or more severely affected than the previous infant, and the severity of disease in the fetus should be followed.

Assessment of the fetus may require information obtained from ultrasonography, amniocentesis, and PUBS. Real-time ultrasonography is used to detect the progression of disease with hydrops defined as skin or scalp edema, pleural or pericardial effusions, and ascites. Early ultrasonographic signs of hydrops include organomegaly (liver, spleen, heart), double bowel wall sign (bowel edema), and placental thickening. Progression to polyhydramnios, ascites, pleural or pericardial effusions, and skin or scalp edema may then follow. If pleural effusions precede ascites and hydrops by a significant time, causes other than fetal anemia should be suspected (see Table 99–1). Extramedullary hematopoiesis and, less so, hepatic congestion compress the intrahepatic vessels, producing venous stasis with portal hypertension, hepatocellular dysfunction, and decreased albumin synthesis.

Hydrops is present when fetal hemoglobin is less than 5 g/dL, frequent when under 7 g/dL, and variable between 7 and 9 g/dL. Real-time ultrasonography predicts fetal well-being by the biophysical profile (see Table 92–2), whereas Doppler ultrasonography assesses fetal distress by demonstrating increased vascular resistance. If there is ultrasonographic evidence of hemolysis (hepatosplenomegaly), early or late hydrops, or fetal distress, amniocentesis or PUBS should be performed.

Amniocentesis is used to assess fetal hemolysis. Hemolysis of fetal RBCs produces hyperbilirubinemia before the onset of severe anemia. Bilirubin is cleared by the placenta, but a significant proportion enters the amniotic fluid and can be measured by spectrophotometry. Amniocentesis is performed if there is evidence of maternal sensitization (titer ≥ 1:16), if the father is Rh positive, or if there are ultrasonographic signs of hemolysis, hydrops, or distress. Ultrasonographically guided transabdominal aspiration of amniotic fluid may be performed as early as 18–20 wk of gestation. Spectrophotometric scanning of amniotic fluid wavelengths demonstrates a positive optical density (OD) deviation of absorption for bilirubin from normal at 450 nm (Fig. 99–3). The OD 450 is a reflection of fetal bilirubin levels, and thus hemolysis, and indicates the severity of anemia and the risk of intrauterine death. With maturity, the level of amniotic fluid bilirubin normally declines; thus the fetal risk assessed during gestation in terms of three relative but declining zones of OD 450, with zone III representing the highest risk. However, some fetuses in zone III do not have life-threatening fetal anemia and thus do not require intrauterine transfusion. If the OD 450 is in zone III or if hydrops or other signs suggesting fetal anemia are present, PUBS should be performed to determine fetal hemoglobin levels, and packed RBCs should be transfused if serious anemia (hematocrit of 25–30%) exists.

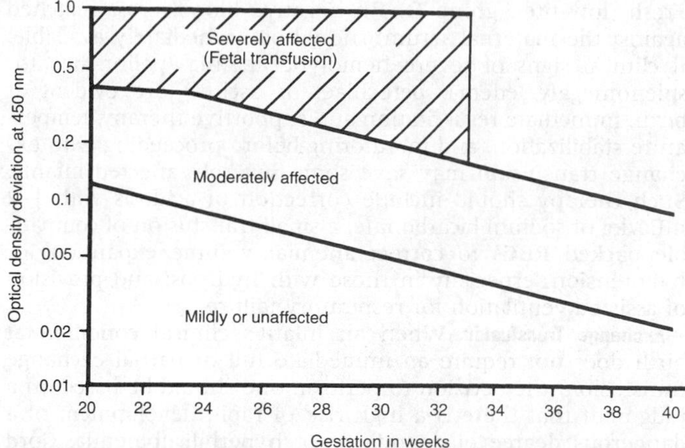

Figure 99–3 Optical density of amniotic fluid plotted against weeks of gestation. Severely affected infants are managed by intrauterine transfusion before 32-33 wk and delivery thereafter. A moderately affected fetus warrants repeated amniocentesis, monitoring by cardiotocography, with delivery at 34-37 wk. A mildly affected fetus warrants delivery at 37–40 wk. (From Blood group incompatibility. *In:* Beischer NA, Mackay EV, Colditz PB [eds]: Obstetrics and the Newborn, 3rd ed. Philadelphia, WB Saunders, 1997.)

Postnatal Diagnosis. Immediately after the birth of any infant to an Rh negative woman, blood from the umbilical cord or from the infant should be examined for ABO blood group, Rh type, hematocrit and hemoglobin, and reaction of the direct Coombs' test. If the Coombs' test result is positive, baseline serum bilirubin level should be measured, and a commercially available RBC panel should be used to identify RBC antibodies that are present in the mother's serum, both tests being done not only to establish the diagnosis but also to ensure the selection of the most compatible blood for exchange transfusion should it be necessary. The direct Coombs test result is usually strongly positive in clinically affected infants and may remain so for a few days up to several months.

TREATMENT. The main goals of therapy are (1) to prevent intrauterine or extrauterine death from severe anemia and hypoxia and (2) to avoid neurotoxicity from hyperbilirubinemia.

Treatment of the Unborn Infant. Survival of a severely affected fetus has been improved by the use of ultrasonographic and amniotic fluid analysis to identify the need for in utero transfusion. Intrauterine transfusion into the fetal peritoneal cavity is being replaced by direct intravascular transfusion of packed RBCs. Hydrops or fetal anemia (hematocrit <30%) is an indication for umbilical vein transfusion in infants with pulmonary immaturity (see Fig. 99–1). Intravascular transfusion is facilitated by maternal and hence fetal sedation with diazepam and by fetal paralysis with pancuronium. Packed RBCs are given by slow-push infusion after cross matching with the mother's serum. The cells should be obtained from a CMV-negative donor and irradiated to kill lymphocytes in order to avoid graft versus host disease. Transfusions should achieve a post-transfusion hematocrit of 45–55% and can be repeated every 3–5 wk. Indications for delivery include pulmonary maturity, fetal distress, complications of PUBS, or 35–37 wk of gestation.

Treatment of the Liveborn Infant. The birth should be attended by the physician who will care for the affected infant afterward.

Fresh, low-titer, group O, Rh negative blood, cross matched against the maternal serum, should be immediately available. If clinical signs of severe hemolytic anemia (pallor, hepatosplenomegaly, edema, petechiae, or ascites) are evident at birth, immediate resuscitation and supportive therapy, temperature stabilization, and monitoring before proceeding with exchange transfusion may save some severely affected infants. Such therapy should include correction of acidosis with 1–2 mEq/kg of sodium bicarbonate; a small transfusion of compatible packed RBCs to correct anemia; volume expansion for hypotension, especially in those with hydrops; and provision of assisted ventilation for respiratory failure.

Exchange Transfusion. When an infant's clinical condition at birth does not require an immediate full or partial exchange transfusion, the decision to perform one should be based on a judgment that there is a high risk of rapid development of a dangerous degree of anemia or of hyperbilirubinemia. Cord hemoglobin of 10 g/dL or less and bilirubin of 5 mg/dL or more suggest severe hemolysis but inconsistently predict the need for immediate exchange transfusion. Some physicians consider previous kernicterus or severe erythroblastosis in a sibling, reticulocyte counts greater than 15%, and prematurity to be further factors supporting a decision for early exchange transfusion. Intrauterine, intravascular transfusions have decreased the need for exchange transfusion.

The hemoglobin, hematocrit, and serum bilirubin levels should be measured at 4- to 6-hr intervals at first, with extension to longer intervals if and as the rate of change diminishes. The decision to perform an exchange transfusion is based on the likelihood that the trend of bilirubin levels plotted against hours of age indicates that the serum bilirubin will reach the level indicated in Table 98–2 and in term infants with levels ≥20 mg/dL, above which there is an increased risk of kernicterus. Ordinary transfusions of compatible Rh-negative RBCs may be necessary to correct anemia at any stage of the disease up to 6–8 wk of age, when the infant's own blood-forming mechanism may be expected to take over. Weekly determinations of hemoglobin or hematocrit should be done until a spontaneous rise has been demonstrated.

Careful monitoring of the serum bilirubin level is essential until a falling trend has been demonstrated in the absence of phototherapy (Chapter 98.4). Even then, an occasional infant, particularly if premature, may experience an unpredicted significant rise in serum bilirubin as late as the 7th day of life. Attempts to predict the attainment of dangerously high levels of serum bilirubin, based on observed levels exceeding 6 mg/dL in the first 6 hr or 10 mg/dL in the second 6 hr of life or on rates of rise exceeding 0.5–1.0 mg/dL/hr, can be unreliable. Indices of free bilirubin and bilirubin binding have not been shown to be routinely reliable aids in evaluating the risk associated with hyperbilirubinemia.

Blood for exchange transfusion should be as fresh as possible. Heparin or adenosine-citrate-phosphate-dextrose may be used as an anticoagulant. If the blood is obtained before delivery, it should be taken from a type O, Rh negative donor with a low titer of anti-A and anti-B and should be compatible with the mother's serum by indirect Coombs' test. After delivery, blood should be obtained from an Rh negative donor whose cells are compatible with both the infant's and the mother's serum; when possible, type O donor cells are usually used, but cells of the infant's ABO blood type may be used when the mother has the same type. A complete cross match, including indirect Coombs' test, should be performed before the second and subsequent transfusions. Blood should be gradually warmed to and maintained at a temperature between 35° and 37°C throughout the exchange transfusion. It should be kept well mixed by gentle squeezing or agitation of the bag to avoid sedimentation; otherwise, the use of supernatant serum with a low RBC count at the end of the exchange will leave the infant anemic. Whole blood or packed RBCs reconstituted with fresh frozen plasma to a hematocrit of 40% should be used. The infant's stomach should be emptied before transfusion to prevent aspiration, and body temperature should be maintained and vital signs monitored. A competent assistant should be present to help monitor, tally the volume of blood exchanged, and perform emergency procedures.

Using strict aseptic technique, the umbilical vein is cannulated with a polyvinyl catheter to a distance no greater than 7 cm in a full-term infant. When free flow of blood is obtained, the catheter is usually in a large hepatic vein or the inferior vena cava. Alternatively, the exchange may be performed through placement of peripheral arterial (drawn out) and venous (infused in) lines. Exchange should be carried out over a 45- to 60-min period, alternating aspirations of 20 mL of infant blood and infusions of 20 mL of donor blood. Smaller aliquots (5–10 mL) may be indicated for sick and premature infants. The goal should be an isovolumetric exchange of approximately two blood volumes of the infant (2×85 mL/kg).

Infants with acidosis and hypoxia from respiratory distress, sepsis, or shock may be further compromised by the significant acute acid load contained in citrated blood, which usually has a pH between 7 and 7.2. The subsequent metabolism of citrate may result in a later metabolic alkalosis if citrated blood is used. Fresh heparinized blood avoids this problem. During the exchange, the blood pH and Pa_{O_2} should be serially monitored, because infants often become acidotic and hypoxic during exchange transfusions. Symptomatic hypoglycemia may occur before or during exchange transfusion in moderately to severely affected infants; it may also occur 1–3 hr after exchange. Acute complications, noted in 5–10% of infants, include transient bradycardia with or without calcium infusion, cyanosis, transient vasospasm, thrombosis, apnea with bradycardia requiring resuscitation, and death. Infectious risks include CMV, HIV, and hepatitis. Necrotizing enterocolitis is a rare complication of exchange transfusion.

The risk of death from exchange transfusion performed by experienced physicians is 0.3/100 procedures. However, with the decreasing use of this procedure as a result of the prevalent use of phototherapy and because sensitization is being prevented, the general level of physician competence is decreasing. Thus, it is best to concentrate this mode of treatment in neonatal referral centers.

After exchange transfusion, the bilirubin level must be determined at frequent intervals (every 4–8 hr), as bilirubin may rebound 40–50% within hours. Repeated exchange transfusions should be carried out to keep the indirect fraction from exceeding the levels indicated in Table 98–2 and in term infants with levels 20 mg/dL. Symptoms suggestive of kernicterus are mandatory indications for exchange transfusion at any time.

Late Complications. Infants who have hemolytic disease or who have had an exchange or an intrauterine transfusion must be observed carefully for the development of anemia and cholestasis. Late anemia may be hemolytic or hyporegenerative. Treatment with supplemental iron, erythropoietin, or blood transfusion may be indicated. A mild graft versus host reaction may be manifested as diarrhea, rash, hepatitis, and eosinophilia.

Inspissated bile syndrome refers to the rare occurrence of persistent icterus in association with significant elevations of direct as well as indirect bilirubin in infants with hemolytic disease. The cause is unclear, but the jaundice clears spontaneously within a few weeks or months.

Portal vein thrombosis and *portal hypertension* may occur among children who have been subjected to exchange transfusion as newborn infants. It is probably associated with prolonged, traumatic, or septic umbilical vein catheterization.

Prevention of Rh Sensitization. The risk of initial sensitization of Rh negative mothers has been reduced from between 10 and 20% to less than 1% by intramuscular injection of 300 μg of human anti-D globulin (1 mL of RhoGAM) within 72 hr of delivery of an ectopic pregnancy, abdominal trauma in pregnancy, amniocentesis, chorionic villus biopsy, or abortion. This quantity is sufficient to eliminate approximately 10 mL of potentially antigenic fetal cells from the maternal circulation. Large fetal-to-maternal transfers of blood may require proportionately more RhoGAM. RhoGAM administered at 28–32 wk and again at birth (40 wk) is more effective than a single dose. The use of this technique, combined with improved methods of detecting maternal sensitization and measuring the extent of the fetal-to-maternal transfusion, plus the use of fewer obstetric procedures that increase the risk of such fetal-to-maternal bleeding (versions, manual separation of the placenta, and so on), should further reduce the incidence of erythroblastosis fetalis.

HEMOLYTIC DISEASE OF THE NEWBORN DUE TO A AND B INCOMPATIBILITY

Major blood group incompatibility between mother and fetus usually results in milder disease than does Rh incompatibility. Maternal antibody may be formed against B cells if the mother is type A or against A cells if the mother is type B. However, usually the mother is type O and the infant is type A or B. Although ABO incompatibility occurs in 20–25% of pregnancies, hemolytic disease develops in only 10% of such offspring, and usually the infants are of type A_1, which is more antigenic than A_2. Low antigenicity of the ABO factors in the fetus and newborn infant may account for the low incidence of severe ABO hemolytic disease relative to the incidence of incompatibility between the blood groups of mother and child. Although antibodies against A and B factors occur without prior immunization ("natural" antibodies), these are ordinarily present in the 19S (IgM) fraction of gamma globulin, which does not cross the placenta. However, univalent, incomplete (albumin active) antibodies to A antigen may be present in the 7S (IgG) fraction, which does cross the placenta, so that A-O isoimmune hemolytic disease may be found in first-born infants. Mothers who have become immunized against A or B factors from a previous incompatible pregnancy also exhibit antibody in the 7S gamma globulin fraction. These "immune" antibodies are the primary mediators in ABO isoimmune disease.

CLINICAL MANIFESTATIONS. Most cases are mild, with jaundice as the only clinical manifestation. The infant is not generally affected at birth; pallor is not present, and hydrops fetalis is extremely rare. The liver and spleen are not greatly enlarged, if at all. Jaundice usually appears during the first 24 hr. Rarely, it may become severe, and symptoms and signs of kernicterus develop rapidly.

DIAGNOSIS. A presumptive diagnosis is based on the presence of ABO incompatibility, a weakly to moderately positive direct Coombs test result, and spherocytes in the blood smear, which may at times suggest the presence of hereditary spherocytosis. Hyperbilirubinemia is often the only other laboratory abnormality. The hemoglobin level is usually normal but may be as low as 10–12 g/dL (100–120 g/L). Reticulocytes may be increased to 10–15%, with extensive polychromasia and increased numbers of nucleated RBCs. In 10–20% of affected infants, the unconjugated serum bilirubin level may reach 20 mg/dL or more unless phototherapy is used.

TREATMENT. Phototherapy may be effective in lowering serum bilirubin levels (Chapter 98.4). Otherwise, treatment is directed at correcting dangerous degrees of anemia or hyperbilirubinemia by exchange transfusions with type O blood of the same Rh type as the infant. The indications for this procedure are similar to those previously described for hemolytic disease due to Rh incompatibility.

OTHER FORMS OF HEMOLYTIC DISEASE

Blood group incompatibilities other than Rh or ABO (c, E, Kell [K], and so on) account for less than 5% of hemolytic disease of the newborn. The direct Coombs test is invariably positive, and exchange transfusion may be indicated for hyperbilirubinemia and anemia. Hemolytic disease, anemia, and hydrops fetalis due to anti-Kell antibodies are not predictable from the previous obstetric history, amniotic fluid OD_{450} bilirubin determinants, or the maternal antibody titer. Erythroid suppression may contribute to the anemia; PUBS is beneficial in actually measuring the fetal hematocrit.

Congenital infections, such as cytomegalic inclusion disease, toxoplasmosis, rubella, and syphilis, may present with hemolytic anemia, jaundice, hepatosplenomegaly, and thrombocytopenia, but the direct Coombs test result is negative and there are usually other distinguishing clinical findings. Homozygous α-thalassemia may present with severe hemolytic anemia and a clinical picture resembling hydrops fetalis; it can be distinguished by a negative direct Coombs test result and characteristic clinical and laboratory findings (Chapter 468.9). Anemia and jaundice may occur in infancy from hereditary spherocytosis (Chapter 464) and, if untreated, can result in kernicterus. Hemolytic anemia producing jaundice in the 1st wk of life may also be secondary to congenital deficiencies in RBC enzymes, such as pyruvate kinase or G6PD.

99.3 *Plethora in the Newborn Infant*

(Polycythemia)

See Chapters 472 and 473.

Plethora, a ruddy, deep red-purple appearance associated with a high hematocrit, is often due to polycythemia, defined as a central hematocrit of 65% or higher. Peripheral (heelstick) hematocrit values are higher than central values, whereas Coulter counter results are lower than hematocrit values determined by microcentrifugation. The incidence of neonatal polycythemia is increased at high altitude (Denver 5% vs Texas 1.6%), in postmature (3%) vs term (1–2%) infants, in small-for-gestational-age (SGA) (8%) vs large-for-gestational-age (LGA) (3%) vs average-for-gestational-age (1–2%) infants, during the 1st day of life (peak 2–3 hr), in the recipient infant of a twin-twin transfusion, after delayed clamping of the umbilical cord, in infants of diabetic mothers, in 13-, 18-, or 21-trisomy, in adrenogenital syndrome, in neonatal Graves' disease, in hypothyroidism, and in Beckwith-Wiedemann syndrome. Infants of diabetic mothers and those with growth retardation may have been exposed to chronic fetal hypoxia, which stimulates erythropoietin production and increases RBC production.

Clinical manifestations include anorexia, lethargy, tachypnea, respiratory distress, feeding disturbances, hyperbilirubinemia, hypoglycemia, and thrombocytopenia. Severe complications include seizures, pulmonary hypertension, necrotizing enterocolitis, and renal failure. Many affected infants are asymptomatic. Hyperviscosity is present in most infants with central hematocrit values of 65% or more and accounts for the symptoms of polycythemia. Hyperviscosity determined at constant shear rates (e.g., 11.5 sec^{-1}) is present when whole blood viscosity is above 18 cycles/sec (18 cps). Hyperviscosity is accentuated because neonatal RBCs have decreased deformability and filterability, predisposing to stasis in the microcirculation.

The *treatment* of symptomatic plethora of newborns is phlebotomy and replacement with saline or, less often, albumin. A partial exchange transfusion to reduce the hematocrit to 50% is a technically simpler and therapeutically more effective approach. The volume exchanged is calculated from the following formula:

$$\text{Volume of exchange (mL)} = \text{Blood volume} \times \frac{\text{Observed} - \text{desired hematocrit}}{\text{Observed hematocrit}}$$

The long-term *prognosis* of polycythemic infants is unclear. Reported adverse outcomes include speech deficits, abnormal fine motor control, reduced IQ, and other neurologic abnormalities. Partial exchange transfusion may reduce the risk of neurologic problems, poor school performance, and fine motor deficit but is associated with feeding disturbances and, if performed through an umbilical vein, may increase the risk of necrotizing enterocolitis.

99.4 Hemorrhage in the Newborn Infant

HEMORRHAGIC DISEASE OF THE NEWBORN. A moderate decrease of factors II, VII, IX, and X normally occurs in all newborn infants by 48–72 hr after birth, with a gradual return to birth levels by 7–10 days of age. This transient deficiency of vitamin K–dependent factors probably is due to lack of free vitamin K in the mother and absence of bacterial intestinal flora normally responsible for synthesis of vitamin K. Rarely, among term infants and more frequently among premature infants there is an accentuation and prolongation of this deficiency between the 2nd and 7th days of life, resulting in spontaneous and prolonged bleeding. Breast milk is a poor source of vitamin K, and hemorrhagic complications have appeared more commonly in breast-fed than in formula-fed infants. This classic form of hemorrhagic disease of the newborn, which is responsive to vitamin K therapy, must be distinguished from disseminated intravascular coagulopathy and from rarer congenital deficiencies of one or more of the other factors that are unresponsive to vitamin K (Chapter 482). Early-onset life-threatening vitamin K deficiency induced bleeding (onset birth–24 hr) also occurs if the mother has been treated with drugs (phenobarbital, phenytoin) that interfere with vitamin K function. Late onset (>1 wk) is often associated with vitamin K malabsorption as noted in neonatal hepatitis or biliary atresia (Table 99–2).

Hemorrhagic disease of the newborn resulting from severe transient deficiencies of vitamin K–dependent factors is characterized by bleeding that tends to be gastrointestinal, nasal, subgaleal, intracranial, or a result of circumcision. Prodromal or warning signs (mild bleeding) may occur before serious intracranial hemorrhage. The prothrombin time, blood coagulation time, and partial thromboplastin time are prolonged, and the levels of prothrombin (II) and factors VII, IX, and X are significantly decreased. Vitamin K facilitates post-transcriptional carboxylation of factors II, VII, IX, and X. In the absence of carboxylation, such factors form PIVKA (protein induced in vitamin K absence), which is a sensitive marker for vitamin K status. Bleeding time, fibrinogen, factors V and VIII, platelets, capillary fragility, and clot retraction are normal for maturity.

Administering 1 mg of natural oil-soluble vitamin K intramuscularly (phylloquinone) at the time of birth prevents the fall in vitamin K–dependent factors in full-term infants but is not uniformly effective in the prophylaxis of hemorrhagic disease of the newborn in premature infants. The disease may be effectively treated with a slow intravenous infusion of 1–5 mg of vitamin K_1, with improvement of coagulation defects and cessation of bleeding within a few hours. However, serious bleeding, particularly in premature infants or those with liver disease, may require a transfusion of fresh frozen plasma or whole blood. The mortality rate is low among treated patients.

A particularly severe form of deficiency of vitamin K–dependent coagulation factors has been reported in infants born to mothers receiving anticonvulsive medications (phenobarbital and phenytoin) during pregnancy. They may suffer severe bleeding, with onset within the first 24 hr of life; this is usually corrected by vitamin K_1, although in some the response is poor or delayed. A prothrombin time (PT) should be obtained on cord blood and the infant given 1–2 mg of vitamin K intravenously. If the PT is greatly prolonged and fails to improve, 10 mL/kg of fresh frozen plasma should be given.

The recommended drug and dose of vitamin K (IM) for prophylaxis in the United States has been safe and is not associated with an increased risk of cancer. Although oral vitamin K (birth, discharge, 3–4 wk: 1–2 mg) has been suggested as an alternative, the oral route is not universally accepted and the IM route remains the method of choice.

Other forms of bleeding may be clinically indistinguishable from hemorrhagic disease of the newborn responsive to vitamin K but are neither prevented nor successfully treated with it. A clinical pattern identical to that of hemorrhagic disease of the newborn may also result from any of the congenital defects in blood coagulation (Chapters 482, 483, and 488). Hematomas, melena, and postcircumcision and umbilical cord bleeding may be present; only 5–35% of factors VIII and IX deficiencies become clinically apparent in the newborn period. Treatment of the rare congenital deficiencies of coagulation factors requires fresh frozen plasma or specific factor replacement.

Disseminated intravascular coagulopathy in newborn infants results in consumption of coagulation factors and bleeding. Affected infants are often premature; the clinical course is frequently characterized by hypoxia, acidosis, shock, hemangiomas, or infection. Treatment is directed at correcting the primary clinical problem, such as infection, and at interrupting consumption and replacing clotting factors (Chapter 489).

Infants with central nervous system or other bleeding constituting an *immediate threat to life* should receive fresh frozen plasma, vitamin K, and blood if needed as soon as possible after blood has been drawn for coagulation studies, which should include determination of the number of platelets.

The so-called swallowed blood syndrome, in which blood or

TABLE 99–2 Hemorrhagic Disease of the Newborn

	Early Onset	Classic Disease	Late Onset
Age	0–24 hours	2–7 days	1–6 months
Site of hemorrhage	Cephalohematoma Subgaleal Intracranial Gastrointestinal Umbilicus Intra-abdominal	Gastrointestinal Ear-nose-throat–mucosal Intracranial Circumcision Cutaneous Gastrointestinal Injection sites	Intracranial Gastrointestinal Cutaneous Ear-nose-throat–mucosal Injection sites Thoracic
Etiology/risks	Maternal drugs (phenobarbital, phenytoin, warfarin, rifampin, isoniazid) that interfere with vitamin K Inherited coagulopathy	Vitamin K deficiency Breast-feeding	Cholestasis—malabsorption of vitamin K (biliary atresia, cystic fibrosis, hepatitis) Abetalipoprotein deficiency Idiopathic in Asian breast-fed infants Warfarin ingestion
Prevention	Possible vitamin K at birth or to mother (20 mg) before birth Avoid high-risk medications	Prevented by parental vitamin K at birth. Oral vitamin K regimens require repeated dosing over time	Prevented by parental and high-dose oral vitamin K during periods of malabsorption or cholestasis
Incidence	Very rare	~2% if not given vitamin K	Dependent on primary disease

bloody stools are passed, usually on the 2nd or 3rd day of life, may be confused with hemorrhage from the GI tract. The blood may be swallowed during delivery or from a fissure in the mother's nipple. Differentiation from GI hemorrhage is based on the fact that the infant's blood contains mostly fetal hemoglobin, which is alkali resistant, whereas swallowed blood from a maternal source contains adult hemoglobin, which is promptly changed to alkaline hematin on the addition of alkali. Apt devised the following test for this differentiation:

> (1) Rinse a bloodstained diaper or some grossly bloody stool with a suitable amount of water to obtain a distinctly pink supernatant hemoglobin solution. (2) Centrifuge the mixture. Decant the supernatant solution. (3) To 5 parts of the supernatant fluid add 1 part of 0.25 normal (1%) sodium hydroxide. Within 1–2 min a color reaction takes place: a yellow-brown color indicates that the blood is maternal in origin; a persistent pink, that it is from the infant. A control test with known adult or infant blood, or both, is advisable.

Widespread subcutaneous ecchymoses in premature infants at or immediately after birth are apparently a result of fragile superficial blood vessels rather than of a coagulation defect. Administering vitamin K_1 to the mother during labor has no effect on their incidence. Occasionally, an infant is born with petechiae or a generalized bluish suffusion limited to the face, head, and neck; this is probably a result of venous obstruction caused by a nuchal cord or sudden increases in intrathoracic pressure during delivery. It may take 2–3 wk for such suffusions to disappear.

NEONATAL THROMBOCYTOPENIC PURPURA. See Chapter 490.9.

Delaney-Black V, Camp BW, Lubchenco LO, et al: Neonatal hyperviscosity association with lower achievement and IQ scores at school age. Pediatrics 83:662, 1989.
Desjardins L, Blaychman M, Chintu C, et al: The spectrum of ABO hemolytic disease of the newborn infant. J Pediatr 95:447, 1979.
de Almeida V, Bowman JM: Massive fetomaternal hemorrhage: Manitoba experience. Obstet Gynecol 83:323, 1994.
Draper G, McNinch A: Vitamin K for neonates: The controversy. A definitive conclusion is still not possible. Br Med J 308:867, 1994.
Howard H, Martlew V, McFadyen I, et al: Consequences for fetus and neonate of maternal red cell allo-immunisation. Arch Dis Child 78:F62, 1998.
Janssens HM, de Haan MJJ, van Kamp IL, et al: Outcome for children treated with fetal intravascular transfusions because of severe blood group antagonism. J Pediatr 131:373, 1997.
Liu EA, Mannino FL, Lane TA: Prospective, randomized trial of the safety and efficacy of a limited donor exposure transfusion program for premature neonates. J Pediatr 125:92, 1994.
Lo D, Hjelm N, Fidler C, et al: Prenatal diagnosis of fetal RhD status by molecular analysis of maternal plasma. N Engl J Med 339:1734, 1998.
Nørgaard Hansen K, Ebbesen F: Neonatal vitamin K prophylaxis in Denmark: Three years' experience with oral administration during the first three months of life compared with one oral administration at birth. Acta Paediatr 85:1137, 1996.
Ohls RK, Harcum J, Schibler KR, et al: The effect of erythropoietin on the transfusion requirements of preterm infants weighing 750 grams or less: A randomized, double-blind, placebo-controlled study. J Pediatr 131:661, 1997.
Ringer SA, Richardson DK, Sacher RA, et al: Variations in transfusion practice in neonatal intensive care. Pediatrics 101:194, 1998.
Robson SC, Lee D, Urbanik S: Anti-D immunoglobulin in RhD prophylaxis. Br J Obstet Gynaecol 105:129, 1998.
Sekizawa A, Watanabe A, Kimura T, et al: Prenatal diagnosis of the fetal RhD blood type using a single fetal nucleated erythrocyte from maternal blood. Obstet Gynecol 87:501, 1996.
Stephenson T, Zuccollo J, Mohajer M: Diagnosis and management of nonimmune hydrops in the newborn. Arch Dis Child 70:F151, 1994.
van Dijk B: Preventing RhD haemolytic disease of the newborn. Br Med J 315:1480, 1997.
Vaughan JI, Manning M, Warwick RM, et al: Inhibition of erythroid progenitor cells by anti-Kell antibodies in fetal alloimmune anemia. N Engl J Med 338:798, 1998.
Wang-Rodriguez J, Mannino FL, Liu E, et al: A novel strategy to limit blood donor exposure and blood waste in multiply transfused premature infants. Transfusion 36:64, 1996.
Wong W, Fok TF, Lee CH, et al: Randomised controlled trial: Comparison of colloid or crystalloid for partial exchange transfusion for treatment of neonatal polycythaemia. Arch Dis Child 77:F115, 1997.
Zipursky A: Vitamin K at birth. Br Med J 313:179, 1996.

CHAPTER 100
Genitourinary System

See also Part XXIII.

Urinary tract anomalies (hydronephrosis, dysplasia, solitary kidney) are frequently identified by prenatal ultrasonography (see Table 92–5). After birth, all such anomalies need to be confirmed and followed with detailed evaluation.

One or both kidneys are often easily palpable in a newborn infant. When both are palpable and similar, there is usually no particular diagnostic problem, but when only one kidney can be felt, a frequent impression is that it is larger than normal or is displaced by an intrinsic or extrinsic mass. Fetal lobulation may contribute to this impression. The problem usually resolves itself as the kidney becomes progressively less easily palpable during the early months of life. Because palpable enlargement or displacement of a kidney in a newborn may be due to hydronephrosis, neuroblastoma, mesoblastic nephroma, adrenal hemorrhage, or a cystic malformation, ultrasound examination is indicated.

THROMBOSIS OF THE RENAL VEIN. See Chapter 103.

CIRCUMCISION. (See Chapter 552.) Circumcision is the most common elective surgical procedure performed on newborn boys in the United States. The benefits relate to cultural beliefs and, possibly, to a reduced incidence of balanitis, penile cancer, sexually transmitted diseases (including HIV), and urinary tract infections (in infant males). The risks are low (local infection, bleeding), but as with any surgical procedure, pain relief must be provided. Analgesia may include concentrated oral sucrose, dorsal penile nerve block, or topical lidocaine-prilocaine cream.

Howard C, Howard F, Garfunkel L, et al: Neonatal circumcision and pain relief: Current training practices. Pediatrics 101:423, 1998.
Task Force on Circumcision, AAP: Circumcision policy statement. Pediatrics 103:686, 1999.

CHAPTER 101
The Umbilicus

UMBILICAL CORD. The cord contains the two umbilical arteries, the vein, the rudimentary allantois, the remnant of the omphalomesenteric duct, and a gelatinous substance called Wharton's jelly. The sheath of the umbilical cord is derived from the amnion. The muscular umbilical arteries contract readily, but the vein does not. The vein retains a fairly large lumen after birth. Abnormally short cords are associated with fetal hypotonia; long cords are at risk for true knots or wrapping around fetal parts (neck, arm); and straight untwisted cords are associated with fetal distress, anomalies, and intrauterine fetal demise.

When the cord sloughs after birth, portions of these structures remain in the base. The blood vessels are functionally closed but are patent anatomically for 10–20 days. The arteries become the lateral umbilical ligaments; the vein, the ligamentum teres; and the ductus venosus, the ligamentum venosum. During this interval, the umbilical vessels are potential portals of entry for infection. The umbilical cord usually sloughs within 2 wk. *Delayed separation of the cord,* after more than than 1 mo, has been associated with neutrophil chemotactic defects and overwhelming bacterial infection (Chapter 130.2).

A **single umbilical artery** is present in about 5–10/1,000 births; the frequency is about 35–70/1,000 twin births. Approximately one third of infants with a single umbilical artery have congenital abnormalities, usually more than one, and many such infants are stillborn or die shortly after birth. 18-Trisomy is one of the more frequent abnormalities. Because many abnormalities are not apparent on gross physical examination, it is important that at every delivery the cut cord and the maternal and fetal surfaces of the placenta be inspected. The number of arteries present should be recorded as an aid to the early suspicion and identification of abnormalities in such infants. Renal ultrasonography is recommended by some for infants with a single umbilical artery.

Patency of the omphalomesenteric (vitelline) *duct* may be responsible for an intestinal fistula, prolapse of the bowel, polyp (cyst), or a Meckel diverticulum (Chapter 331.2).

A *persistent urachus* (urachal cyst) is due to failure of closure of the allantoic duct and is associated with bladder outlet obstruction. Patency should be suspected if there is a clear, light yellow, urine-like discharge from the umbilicus.

CONGENITAL OMPHALOCELE. An omphalocele is a herniation or protrusion of abdominal contents into the base of the umbilical cord. In contrast to the more common umbilical hernia, the sac is covered with peritoneum without overlying skin. The size of the sac that lies outside the abdominal cavity depends on its contents. Herniation of intestines into the cord occurs in about 1/5,000 births, and of liver and intestines in 1/10,000 births. The abdominal cavity is proportionately small because the impetus to grow and develop is deficient. Immediate surgical repair, before infection has taken place and before the tissues have been damaged by drying (saline-soaked sterile dressings should be applied immediately) or by rupture of the sac, is essential for survival. Mersilene or similar synthetic material may be used to cover the viscera if the sac has ruptured or if excessive mobilization of the skin would be necessary to cover the mass and its intact sac. Omphalocele, macrosomia, and hypoglycemia suggest Beckwith's syndrome (Chapter 103).

TUMORS. Tumors of the umbilicus are rare; they include angioma, enteroteratoma, dermoid cyst, myxosarcoma, and cysts of urachal or omphalomesenteric duct remnants.

HEMORRHAGE. Hemorrhage from the umbilical cord may be due to trauma, inadequate ligation of the cord, or failure of normal thrombus formation. It may also indicate hemorrhagic disease of the newborn or other coagulopathies (factor XIII deficiency), septicemia, or local infection. The infant should be observed frequently during the first few days of life so that if hemorrhage does occur, it will be detected promptly.

GRANULOMA. The umbilical cord usually dries and separates within 6–8 days after birth. The raw surface becomes covered by a thin layer of skin, scar tissue forms, and the wound is usually healed within 12–15 days. The presence of saprophytic organisms delays separation of the cord and increases the possibility of invasion by pathogenic organisms. Mild infection may result in a moist granulating area at the base of the cord with a slight mucoid or mucopurulent discharge. Good results are usually obtained by cleansing with alcohol several times daily.

Persistence of exuberant granulation tissue at the base of the umbilicus is common. The tissue is soft, vascular and granular, and dull red or pink, and it may have a seropurulent secretion. The *treatment* is cauterization with silver nitrate; it should be repeated at intervals of several days until the base is dry.

Umbilical granuloma must be differentiated from **umbilical polyp,** a rare anomaly resulting from persistence of all or part of the omphalomesenteric duct or of the urachus. The tissue of the polyp is firm and resistant, is bright red, and has a mucoid secretion. If there is a communication with the ileum or bladder, small amounts of fecal material or urine may be discharged intermittently. Histologically, the polyp consists of intestinal or urinary tract mucosa. Treatment is surgical excision of the *entire* omphalomesenteric or urachal remnant.

INFECTIONS. Inflammation in the umbilical region, which may be caused by any of the pyogenic bacteria, is especially serious because of the danger of hematogenous spread or extension to the liver or peritoneum. Portal vein phlebitis may develop, resulting in later onset of extrahepatic portal hypertension. The general manifestations may be minimal (periumbilical erythema) even when septicemia or hepatitis has resulted. Daily baths or daily application of triple dye to the umbilical stump and surrounding skin may reduce the incidence of umbilical infection. *Treatment* includes prompt antibacterial therapy and, if there is abscess formation, surgical incision and drainage.

UMBILICAL HERNIA. Often associated with diastasis recti, umbilical hernia is due to an imperfect closure or weakness of the umbilical ring. Common especially in low birthweight, female, and black infants, it appears as a soft swelling covered by skin that protrudes during crying, coughing, or straining and can be reduced easily through the fibrous ring at the umbilicus. The hernia consists of omentum or portions of the small intestine. The size of the defect varies from less than 1 cm in diameter to as much as 5 cm, but large ones are rare.

Treatment. Most umbilical hernias that appear before the age of 6 mo disappear spontaneously by 1 yr of age. Even large hernias (5–6 cm in all dimensions) have been known to disappear spontaneously by 5–6 yr of age. Strangulation is extremely rare. There is considerable agreement that "strapping" is ineffective. Surgery is not advised unless the hernia persists to the age of 3–4 yr, causes symptoms, becomes strangulated, or becomes progressively larger after the age of 1–2 yr. Defects exceeding 2 cm are less likely to close spontaneously.

CHAPTER 102
Metabolic Disturbances

HYPERTHERMIA IN THE NEWBORN

(Transitory Fever of the Newborn; Dehydration Fever)

Elevations of temperature (38–39°C or 100–103°F) are occasionally noted on the 2nd–3rd day of life in infants whose clinical course has been otherwise satisfactory. This disturbance is especially likely to occur in breast-fed infants whose intake of fluid has been particularly low or in infants exposed to high environmental temperatures, either in an incubator or in a bassinet near a radiator or in the sun.

The infant may lose weight. There may not be a consistent relationship between the fever and the extent of weight loss or inadequacy of fluid intake. The urinary output and frequency of voiding diminish. The fontanel may be depressed. The infant takes fluids avidly. The apparent vigor of the infant contrasts with the usual appearance of "being sick" in the presence of infection. The rise in temperature may be associated with an increase in serum levels of protein, sodium, and hematocrit. The possibility of local or systemic infection should be evaluated. Administering oral or parenteral fluids or lowering the environmental temperature leads to prompt reduction of the fever and alleviation of symptoms.

A *more severe form of neonatal hyperthermia* occurs among both newborn and older infants when they are warmly dressed for outdoor low temperatures that do not exist in their immediate indoor environment. The diminished sweating capacity of newborn infants is a contributing factor. Warmly dressed infants left near stoves or radiators, traveling in well-heated automobiles, or left with bright sunlight shining directly on them through the windows of a closed room or automobile are likely victims. Overclothing in hot weather, especially when the infant is left in the sun, is a less common cause. Body temperature is often as high as 41–44°C (106–111°F). The skin is hot and dry, and initially the infant usually appears flushed and apathetic. There may be tachypnea and irritability. This stage may be followed by stupor, grayish pallor, coma, and convulsions. Hypernatremia may contribute to the convulsions. The mortality and morbidity rates (brain damage) are high. Hyperthermia has been associated with sudden infant death and the hemorrhagic shock and encephalopathy syndrome (Chapter 64.2). The condition is prevented by dressing infants in clothing suitable for the temperature of the *immediate* environment. In newborn infants, exposure of the body to usual room temperature or immersion in tepid water usually suffices to bring the temperature back to normal levels. Older infants may require cooling for a longer time by repeated immersions or by use of a water-cooled mattress or other apparatus for induction of hypothermia. Attention to possible fluid and electrolyte disturbance is essential.

NEONATAL COLD INJURY

Neonatal cold injury usually occurs among infants in inadequately heated homes during damp cold spells when the outside temperature is in the freezing range. The presenting features are apathy, refusal of food, oliguria, and coldness to touch. The body temperature is usually between 29.5 and 35°C (85–95°F), and immobility, edema, and redness of the extremities, especially of the hands, feet, and face, are observed. Bradycardia and apnea may also occur. The facial erythema frequently gives a false impression of health, delaying recognition that the infant is ill. Local hardening over areas of edema may lead to confusion with scleredema. Rhinitis is common, as are serious metabolic disturbances, particularly hypoglycemia and acidosis. Hemorrhagic manifestations are frequent; massive pulmonary hemorrhage is a common finding at autopsy. Treatment consists of warming and paying scrupulous attention to recognizing and correcting hypotension and metabolic imbalances, particularly hypoglycemia. Prevention consists of providing adequate environmental heat. The mortality rate is about 10%; about 10% of the survivors have evidence of brain damage.

EDEMA

Generalized edema occurs in association with hydrops fetalis and in the offspring of diabetic mothers. In premature infants, edema is often a consequence of a decreased ability to excrete water or sodium, although some have considerable edema without identifiable reason. Infants with hyaline membrane disease may become edematous without heart failure. Edema of the face and scalp may result from pressure from the umbilical cord around the neck, and transient localized swellings of the hands or feet may similarly be due to intrauterine pressures. Edema may be present with heart failure due to congenital cardiac lesions; a lag in renal excretion of electrolytes and water may result in edema when there has been a sudden large increase in intake of electrolytes, particularly with feeding of concentrated cow's milk formulas. High-protein formulas also may cause edema owing to the excessive solute load, particularly in premature infants. It is difficult to show a relationship between low serum protein or low hemoglobin levels and the occurrence of edema in older premature infants. Edema also occurs in association with anemia and vitamin E deficiency in premature infants. Rarely, *idiopathic hypoproteinemia* with edema lasting weeks or months is observed in term infants. The cause is unclear, and the disturbance is benign. Persistent edema of one or more extremities may represent congenital lymphedema (Milroy's disease) or, in females, *Turner's syndrome.* Generalized edema with hypoproteinemia may be seen in the neonatal period with congenital nephrosis and rarely with Hurler's syndrome or after feeding hypoallergenic formulas to infants with cystic fibrosis of the pancreas. *Sclerema* is described in Chapter 653.

HYPOCALCEMIA

(Tetany)

See Chapters 44.11 and 55.9.

OSTEOPENIA OF PREMATURITY. Very small premature infants with chronic illnesses often develop a rickets-like syndrome with pathologic fractures and demineralized bones. There may be associated cholestasis and vitamin D or calcium malabsorption; urine calcium loss due to diuretics; and poor calcium, phosphorus, or vitamin D intake, or aluminum toxicity. The treatment of fractures requires immobilization and administration of calcium and, if needed, phosphorus (for hypophosphatemia) and vitamin D (not more than 1,000 IU/day unless severe cholestasis or vitamin D resistance). Appropriate formulas for premature infants should provide a more optimal intake of calcium, phosphorus, and vitamin D and promote bone mineralization. See also Chapters 49, 55.9, 580, and 712.

HYPOMAGNESEMIA

Rarely, hypomagnesemia of unknown cause may occur in newborn infants, usually in association with hypocalcemia. It may also be associated with insufficient stores of skeletal magnesium secondary to deficient placental transfer, decreased intestinal absorption, neonatal hypoparathyroidism, hyperphosphatemia, renal loss (primary or drugs—e.g., amphotericin B), a defect in magnesium and calcium homeostasis, or an iatrogenic deficiency due to loss incurred during exchange transfusion or insufficient replacement during total intravenous alimentation. Infants of diabetic mothers may have serum magnesium levels that are lower than normal. The clinical manifestations of hypomagnesemia are indistinguishable from those of hypocalcemia and tetany and may, in fact, contribute to the accompanying hypocalcemia.

Hypomagnesemia occurs when serum magnesium levels fall below 1.5 mg/dL (0.62 mmol/L), although clinical signs usually do not develop until serum magnesium levels fall below 1.2 mg/dL. During exchange transfusion with citrated blood, which is low in magnesium because of binding by citrate, the serum magnesium drops about 0.5 mg/dL (0.2 mmol/L); approximately 10 days are required for a return to normal. In noniatrogenic hypomagnesemia, the serum magnesium level may be less than 0.5 mg/dL. The serum calcium in either instance is usually at levels noted in hypocalcemia tetany, but the serum phosphorus value is normal or high. Because the hypocalcemia accompanying hypomagnesemia is inadequately corrected by administering calcium alone, hypomagnesemia should also be suspected in any patient with tetany not responding to calcium therapy.

Immediate *treatment* consists of intramuscular injection of magnesium sulfate. For newborn infants, 0.25 mL/kg of a 50% solution daily usually suffices. The accompanying hypocalcemia usually corrects itself as the hypomagnesemia is relieved. The same daily dose can be given for oral maintenance therapy. Four to five times higher doses may be required in malabsorptive states. In most cases, the metabolic defect is transient, and treatment can be discontinued after 1–2 wk. A few patients appear to have a permanent form of the disease that requires continuous oral supplementation with magnesium to prevent recurrence of hypomagnesemia. No residual damage to the central nervous system is evident after prompt treatment.

HYPERMAGNESEMIA

Hypermagnesemia may occur in newborn infants of mothers treated with magnesium sulfate for eclampsia. At high serum levels the central nervous system is depressed and totally paralyzed so that artificial respiration is required. Lower levels may result in hypoventilation, hypotension, lethargy, flaccidity, and hyporeflexia. The upper limit of normal magnesium is 2.8 mg/dL (1.15 mmol/L), but serious symptoms occur at levels above 5 mg/dL (2.1 mmol/L). Hypermagnesemia may be associated with failure to pass meconium (meconium plug syndrome). Exchange transfusion has been used as a means of rapid removal of magnesium ion from the blood. Calcium salts and diuresis have also been used. Recovery appears to be complete.

OTHER METABOLIC DISEASES

A number of inborn errors of metabolism may be manifested during the neonatal period; these include phenylketonuria, galactosemia, the urea cycle defects, methylmalonic acidemia, and maple syrup urine disease (see Chapters 82 and 84). Pyridoxine deficiency and dependence are considered in Chapter 44.

SUBSTANCE ABUSE AND WITHDRAWALS

Physiologic addiction to narcotics or toxic effects occur in most infants born to actively addicted mothers, because opiates cross the placenta. Withdrawal may be manifested even before birth by increased activity of the fetus when the mother feels the need for the drug or develops withdrawal symptoms. Heroin and methadone are the drugs most frequently associated with withdrawal syndromes, but these syndromes may also occur with alcohol, phenobarbital, pentazocine, codeine, propoxyphene, hydroxyzine, amphetamines, neuroleptics, antidepressants, and benzodiazepines.

Pregnancy in women who use illegal drugs or alcohol is, by definition, a high risk. Prenatal care is usually inadequate, and there is a higher incidence of sexually transmitted diseases including syphilis, AIDS, and hepatitis; toxemia; premature rupture of the membranes; breech presentations; prolapsed cords; preterm and small for gestational age infants; and perinatal morbidity and mortality. More than one drug frequently is being abused in these pregnancies.

Heroin addiction results in a 50% incidence of low birthweight infants, half of whom are small for gestational age; infections, maternal undernutrition, and a direct fetal growth inhibiting effect are possible causes. The rate of stillbirths is increased, but not the incidence of congenital anomalies. *Clinical manifestations* of withdrawal occur in 50–75% of infants, usually beginning within the first 48 hr, depending on the daily maternal dose (<6 mg/24 hr is associated with no or mild symptoms); duration of addiction (>1 yr has a >70% incidence of withdrawal); and time of last maternal dose (there is a higher incidence if the last dose was taken within 24 hr of birth). Symptoms rarely appear as late as 4–6 wk of age. The incidence of hyaline membrane disease and hyperbilirubinemia may be decreased in low birthweight infants of heroin addicts; hyperventilation leading to respiratory alkalosis or accelerated production of surfactant may explain the former, and enzyme induction of glucuronyl transferase the latter.

Tremors and hyperirritability are the most prominent symptoms. The tremors may be fine or jittery and indistinguishable from those of hypoglycemia but are more often coarse, "flapping," and bilateral; the limbs are often rigid, hyperreflexic, and resistant to flexion and extension. Irritability and hyperactivity are generally marked and may lead to skin abrasions. Other signs include wakefulness, hyperacusis, hypertonicity, tachypnea, diarrhea, vomiting, high-pitched cry, fist sucking, poor feeding (disorganized sucking), and fever. Sneezing, yawning, hiccups, myoclonic jerks, convulsions, abnormal sleep cycles, nasal stuffiness, apnea, flushing alternating rapidly with pallor, and lacrimation are less common. The *diagnosis* is generally established by the history and clinical presentation. Examining the urine for opiates may reveal only low levels during withdrawal, but quinine, which is often mixed with heroin, may be present in higher concentrations. Hypoglycemia and hypocalcemia should be excluded.

Methadone addiction is associated with severe withdrawal symptoms, the incidence varying from 20–90%. In general, mothers taking methadone have better prenatal care than those taking heroin; however, there is a high incidence of polysubstance abuse, including alcohol, barbiturates, and tranquilizers, and these mothers are often heavy smokers. There is no increased incidence of congenital anomalies. The average birthweight of infants of mothers taking methadone is higher than that of infants of heroin-addicted mothers; the *clinical manifestations* are similar except that the former group has a higher incidence of seizures (10–20%) and of late onset (2–6 wk of age) of symptoms and signs.

Alcohol withdrawal is uncommon. The infants of women who have been drinking immediately before delivery may have alcohol on their breath for several hours, because it rapidly crosses the placenta, and blood levels in the infant are similar to those in the mother. Hypoglycemia and acidosis may be present. Infants who develop withdrawal symptoms often become agitated and hyperactive, with marked tremors lasting for 72 hr, followed by about 48 hr of lethargy before return to normal activity. Seizures may develop.

Phenobarbital withdrawal usually occurs in full-term, appropriate for gestational age infants of addicted mothers. Symptoms begin at a median age of 7 days (range 2–14 days). There may be a brief acute stage consisting of irritability, constant crying, sleeplessness, hiccups, and mouthing movements, followed by a subacute stage that may last 2–4 mo and consisting of voracious appetite, frequent regurgitation and gagging, episodic irritability, hyperacusis, sweating, and a disturbed sleep pattern.

Cocaine abuse among pregnant women is common, but withdrawal in their infants is unusual; pregnancy may be complicated by premature labor, abruptio placentae, and fetal asphyxia. Infants may have intrauterine growth retardation, microcephaly, intracranial hemorrhage, possible anomalies of the gastrointestinal and renal tracts, sudden infant death syndrome (SIDS), and neurobehavioral deficits characterized by rigidity, impaired state regulation, developmental delay, and learning disabilities. Family disorganization, child abuse, neglect, and AIDS are common in these families.

Treatment of heroin and methadone withdrawals has been successful using various combinations of narcotics, sedatives, and hypnotics. Therapy is indicated for seizures, for diarrhea, or for such irritability that normal sleep and feeding patterns are disturbed and weight gain is poor. Methadone withdrawal may require larger amounts of medication for longer periods than does heroin withdrawal to control clinical manifestations. Phenobarbital, 5–10 mg/kg/24 hr in 3–4 divided doses, can effectively reduce irritability and prevent seizures. Paregoric at a beginning dose of 0.05–0.1 mL/kg is given every 3–4 hr and increased by 0.05 mL every 4 hr if necessary, depending on the size and response of the infant. Paregoric abolishes most withdrawal symptoms, especially diarrhea. Tincture of opium (10 mg/mL), diluted 25-fold results in the same morphine equivalency as paregoric. The recommended dose of diluted tincture of opium is 0.1 mL/kg (~2 drops/kg) with feedings every 4 hr. The dose may be increased by 2 drops every 4 hr if needed. The dose and duration of therapy may be adjusted according to the clinical response. Parenteral administration of fluids may be necessary to prevent aspiration or dehydration until the symptoms are brought under control. Narcotic and phenobarbital withdrawal also requires swaddling, frequent feedings, and protection from noxious external stimuli.

Current mortality from withdrawal is not over 5% and with early recognition and treatment may be negligible. *Prognosis* for normal development is affected by the adverse circumstances of high-risk pregnancy and delivery and by the environment to which the infant is returned after recovery, as well as by the effects of the particular drug on fetal and subsequent neonatal development.

FETAL ALCOHOL SYNDROME. High levels of alcohol ingestion during pregnancy can be damaging to embryonic and fetal development. A specific pattern of malformation identified as the *fetal alcohol syndrome* has been documented, and major and minor components of the syndrome are expressed in 1–2 infants/1,000 live births. Both moderate and high levels of alcohol intake during early pregnancy may result in alterations in growth and morphogenesis of the fetus; the greater the intake, the more severe the signs. Infants born to heavy drinkers have twice the risk of abnormality compared with those born to moderate drinkers; 32% of infants born to heavy drinkers demonstrated congenital anomalies, compared with 9% in the abstinent and 14% in the moderate group.

The characteristics of the fetal alcohol syndrome include (1) prenatal onset and persistence of growth deficiency for length, weight, and head circumference; (2) facial abnormalities, including short palpebral fissures, epicanthal folds, maxillary hypoplasia, micrognathia, and thin upper lip; (3) cardiac defects, primarily septal defects; (4) minor joint and limb abnormalities, including some restriction of movement and altered palmar crease patterns; and (5) delayed development and mental deficiency varying from borderline to severe. Fetal alcohol syndrome is a common cause of mental retardation. The severity of dysmorphogenesis may range from severely affected infants with full manifestations of the fetal alcohol syndrome to those mildly affected with only a few manifestations.

The detrimental effects may be due to the alcohol itself or to one of its breakdown products. Some evidence suggests that alcohol may impair placental transfer of essential amino acids and zinc, both necessary for protein synthesis, which accounts for the intrauterine growth retardation.

Treatment of these infants may be difficult, because no specific therapy exists. These infants may remain hypotonic and tremulous despite sedation, and the prognosis is poor. Counseling with regard to recurrence is important. *Prevention* is achieved by eliminating alcohol intake after conception.

LATE METABOLIC ACIDOSIS

Between 5 and 10% of preterm low birthweight infants develop a metabolic acidosis during the 2nd or 3rd wk of life. Usually there is no history of asphyxia, respiratory distress, or other problems, and the infants are vigorous. However, they often have received cow's milk formulas of high protein and casein content shortly after birth and have had a delayed start of postnatal weight gain. Blood base deficit values range from −10 to −16 mEq/L, the anion gap is elevated, and P_{CO_2} values are usually less than 40 mm Hg. The condition probably represents an abnormally high rate of endogenous acid formation. Treatment includes administering $NaHCO_3$ and changing to a formula of lower protein content with a whey:casein ratio of 60:40. Renal tubular acidosis may produce a nonanionic gap acidosis in premature infants.

Committee on Drugs, AAP: Neonatal drug withdrawal. Pediatrics 101:1079, 1998.
Davis Eyler F, Behnke M, Conlon M, et al: Birth outcome from a prospective, matched study of prenatal crack/cocaine use: I. interactive and dose effects on health and growth. Pediatrics 101:229, 1998.
Doberczak TM, Kandall SR, Friedmann P: Relationships between maternal methadone dosage, maternal-neonatal methadone levels, and neonatal withdrawal. Obstet Gynecol 81:936, 1993.
Forsyth BWC, Leventhal JM, Qi K, et al: Health care and hospitalizations of young children born to cocaine-using women. Arch Pediatr Adolesc Med 152:177, 1998.
Horsman A, Ryan SW, Congdon PJ, et al: Osteopenia in extremely low birthweight infants. Arch Dis Child 64:485, 1989.
Hurt H, Malmud E, Betancourt L, et al: Children with in utero cocaine exposure do not differ from control subjects on intelligence testing. Arch Pediatr Adolesc Med 151:1237, 1997.
Kildeberg P: Late metabolic acidosis of premature infants. *In:* Winters RW (ed): The Body Fluids in Pediatrics. Boston, Little, Brown & Co, 1973.
Mattson SN, Riley EP, Gramling L, et al: Heavy prenatal alcohol exposure with or without physical features of fetal alcohol syndrome leads to IQ deficits. J Pediatr 131:718, 1997.
Nervez CT, Shott RJ, Bergstrom WH, et al: Prophylaxis against hypocalcemia in low birth weight infants receiving bicarbonate infusion. J Pediatr 87:439, 1975.
Neuman L, Cohen S: The neonatal narcotic withdrawal syndrome. Clin Perinatol 2:99, 1975.
Ostrea EM Jr, Ostrea AR, Simpson PM: Mortality within the first 2 years in infants exposed to cocaine, opiate, or cannabinoid during gestation. Pediatrics 100:79, 1997.
Ryan S: Nutritional aspects of metabolic bone disease in the newborn. Arch Dis Child 74:F145, 1996.

CHAPTER 103
The Endocrine System

The endocrinopathies are discussed in Part XXV. The purpose of this section is to call attention to those endocrine disturbances that may be identified at birth or during the first month of life.

Pituitary dwarfism is usually not apparent at birth, although panhypopituitary male infants may present with neonatal hypoglycemia and micropenis. Conversely, constitutional dwarfs usually demonstrate length and weight consistent with prematurity when born after a normal gestational period; otherwise, their physical appearance is normal.

Primary hypothyroidism occurs in approximately 1/4,000 births. Because most of these infants are asymptomatic at birth, all states screen for this serious and treatable disease. *Thyroid deficiency* may also be apparent at birth in genetically determined **cretinism** or in infants of mothers treated with thiouracil or its derivatives during pregnancy. Constipation, prolonged jaundice, goiter, lethargy, or poor peripheral circulation as shown by persistently mottled skin or cold extremities should suggest cretinism. Early diagnosis and treatment of congenital deficiency of thyroid hormone improves intellectual outcome and is facilitated by screening all newborn infants for this deficiency. Transient hypothyroxinemia of prematurity is most common in ill infants of very low birthweight. Because the relationship between the low thyroid levels and neurodevelopmental outcome is unclear, it remains uncertain if premature infants with this transient problem should be treated with thyroid hormone.

Temporary *hyperthyroidism* may occur at birth in the infants of mothers with hyperthyroidism or of those who have been receiving thyroid medication.

Transient *hypoparathyroidism* may be manifested as tetany of the newborn.

The *adrenal glands* are subject to numerous disturbances, which may become apparent and require lifesaving treatment during the neonatal period. Acute adrenal *hemorrhage* and failure may occur after breech or other traumatic deliveries or in association with overwhelming infection. *Adrenocortical hyperplasia* is suggested by vomiting, diarrhea, dehydration, hyperkalemia, hyponatremia, shock, or clitoral enlargement. Because the condition is genetically determined, newborn siblings of patients with the salt-losing variety of adrenocortical hyperplasia should be closely observed for manifestations of adrenal insufficiency. Screening is also possible for this disorder.

Congenitally hypoplastic adrenal glands may also give rise to adrenal insufficiency during the first few weeks of life.

Female infants with webbing of the neck, lymphangiectatic edema, hypoplasia of the nipples, cutis laxa, low hairline at the nape of the neck, low-set ears, high-arched palate, deformities of the nails, cubitus valgus, and other anomalies should be suspected of having *gonadal dysgenesis.*

Transient *diabetes mellitus* (Chapter 599) is rare and is encountered only in newborns. It usually presents as dehydration, loss of weight, or acidosis in small for gestational age infants.

103.1 *Infants of Diabetic Mothers*

Control of diabetes mellitus with insulin has led to improved outcome for diabetic women who bear children. Their infants and the infants of women who later develop diabetes share certain distinctive morphologic characteristics, macrosomia, and high morbidity risks. Diabetic mothers have a high incidence of polyhydramnios, preeclampsia, pyelonephritis, preterm labor, and chronic hypertension; their fetal mortality rate, which is high at all gestational ages, especially after 32 wk, is greater than that of nondiabetic mothers. Fetal loss throughout pregnancy is associated with poorly controlled maternal diabetes (especially ketoacidosis) and congenital anomalies. Diabetic mothers produce an excess of high birthweight infants at all gestational ages and, if complicated with vascular disease, of low birthweight infants at 37- to 40-wk gestations. The neonatal mortality rate is over five times that of infants of nondiabetic mothers and is higher at all gestational ages and in every birthweight for gestational age category.

PATHOPHYSIOLOGY. The probable pathogenic sequence is that maternal hyperglycemia causes fetal hyperglycemia, and the fetal pancreatic response leads to fetal hyperinsulinemia; fetal hyperinsulinemia and hyperglycemia then cause increased hepatic glucose uptake and glycogen synthesis, accelerated lipogenesis, and augmented protein synthesis. Related pathologic findings are hypertrophy and hyperplasia of the pancreatic islets with a disproportionate increase in the number of β cells; increased weight of the placenta and infant organs except for the brain; myocardial hypertrophy; increased amounts of cytoplasm in liver cells; and extramedullary hematopoiesis. Hyperinsulinism and hyperglycemia produce fetal acidosis, which may result in an increased rate of stillbirth. Separation of the placenta at birth suddenly interrupts glucose infusion into the neonate without a proportional effect on the hyperinsulinism, resulting in hypoglycemia and attenuated lipolysis during the first hours after birth.

Hyperinsulinemia has been documented in infants of gestational diabetic mothers and in those of insulin-dependent diabetic mothers without insulin antibodies. The former group also have significantly higher fasting plasma insulin levels than normal newborns despite similar glucose levels; they respond to glucose with an abnormally prompt elevation of plasma insulin and assimilate a glucose load more rapidly. After arginine administration, they also have an enhanced insulin response and increased disappearance rates of glucose, compared with normal infants. In contrast, fasting glucose utilization rates are diminished. The lower free fatty acid levels in infants of insulin-dependent diabetic mothers probably also reflect their hyperinsulinemia. With good prenatal diabetic control, the incidences of macrosomia and hypoglycemia have decreased.

Although hyperinsulinism is probably the main cause of

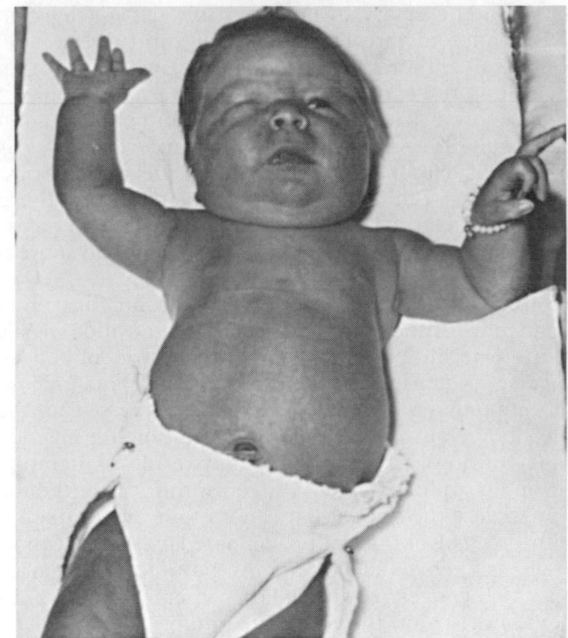

Figure 103–1 Large, plump, plethoric infant of a gestational diabetic mother. Baby was born at 38 wk of gestation but weighed 9 lb 11 oz (4,408 g). Mild respiratory distress was the only symptom other than appearance.

hypoglycemia, the diminished epinephrine and glucagon responses that occur may be contributing factors. Cortisol and human growth hormone levels are normal. Congenital anomalies correlate with poor metabolic control during the periconception and organogenesis periods and may be due to hyperglycemia-induced teratogenesis.

CLINICAL MANIFESTATIONS. The infants of diabetic and gestational diabetic mothers often bear a surprising resemblance to each other (Fig. 103–1). They tend to be large and plump as a result of increased body fat and enlarged viscera, with puffy, plethoric facies resembling those of patients who have been receiving a corticosteroid. These infants may, however, also be of normal or low birthweight, particularly if they are delivered before term or if there is associated maternal vascular disease.

The infants tend to be jumpy, tremulous, and hyperexcitable during the first 3 days of life, although hypotonia, lethargy, and poor sucking also may occur. They may have any of the diverse manifestations of hypoglycemia. Early appearance of these signs is more likely to be related to hypoglycemia, and later appearance related to hypocalcemia; these abnormalities also may occur together. Perinatal asphyxia or hyperbilirubinemia may produce similar signs. Hypomagnesemia may be associated with the hypocalcemia.

About 25–50% of infants of diabetic mothers and 15–25% of infants of mothers with gestational diabetes develop hypoglycemia, but only a small percentage of these infants become symptomatic. The probability of an infant's developing hypoglycemia increases and the glucose levels are likely to be lower at higher cord or maternal fasting blood glucose levels. The nadir in an infant's blood glucose concentration is usually reached between 1 and 3 hr; spontaneous recovery may begin by 4–6 hr.

Many infants of diabetic mothers develop tachypnea during the first 5 days of life, which may be a transient manifestation of hypoglycemia, hypothermia, polycythemia, cardiac failure, transient tachypnea, or cerebral edema due to birth trauma or asphyxia. A greater incidence of respiratory distress syndrome appears in infants of diabetic mothers than in infants of normal mothers born at comparable gestational age; the greater incidence is possibly related to an antagonistic effect between cortisol and insulin on surfactant synthesis.

Cardiomegaly is common (30%), and heart failure occurs in 5–10% of infants of diabetic mothers. Asymmetric septal hypertrophy may occur, becoming manifested similarly to idiopathic hypertrophic subaortic stenosis. Birth trauma is also common owing to fetal macrosomia.

Neurologic development and ossification centers tend to be immature and correlate with the brain size (which is not increased) and gestational age rather than with total body weight. There is also an increased incidence of hyperbilirubinemia, polycythemia, and renal vein thrombosis; the latter should be suspected in the presence of a flank mass, hematuria, and thrombocytopenia.

The incidence of congenital anomalies is increased threefold in infants of diabetic mothers; cardiac malformations (ventricular or atrial septal defect, transposition of the great vessels, truncus arteriosus, double-outlet right ventricle, coarctation of the aorta) and lumbosacral agenesis are most common. Additional anomalies include neural tube defects, hydronephrosis, renal agenesis and dysplasia, duodenal or anorectal atresia, situs inversus, double ureter, and holoprosencephaly. These infants may also develop abdominal distention caused by a transient delay in the development of the left side of the colon, the *small left colon syndrome.* The incidence of Down syndrome may also be increased.

PROGNOSIS. The subsequent incidence of diabetes mellitus in infants of diabetic mothers is increased compared with that of the general population. Physical development is normal, but oversized infants may be predisposed to childhood obesity that may extend into adult life. Disagreement persists about whether or not a slightly increased risk of impaired intellectual development exists unrelated to hypoglycemia; symptomatic hypoglycemia increases the risk, as does maternal ketonuria.

TREATMENT. Treatment of these infants should be initiated before birth by frequent prenatal evaluation of all pregnant women with overt or gestational diabetes, by evaluation of fetal maturity, by biophysical profile, by Doppler velocimetry, and by planning delivery of these infants in hospitals where expert obstetric and pediatric care is continuously available. Periconception glucose control reduces the risk of anomalies, and glucose control during labor reduces the incidence of neonatal hypoglycemia. Regardless of size, all infants of diabetic mothers should initially receive intensive observation and care. Asymptomatic infants should have a blood glucose determination within 1 hr of birth and then every hour for the next 6–8 hr; if clinically well and normoglycemic oral or gavage feedings with breast milk or formula should be started as soon as possible and continued at 3-hr intervals. If any question arises about an infant's ability to tolerate oral feeding, the feeding should be discontinued and glucose given by peripheral intravenous infusion at a rate of 4–8 mg/kg/min. Hypoglycemia should be treated, even in asymptomatic infants, with intravenous infusions of glucose sufficient to keep the blood levels well above this level. Bolus injections of hypertonic glucose should be avoided because they may cause further hyperinsulinemia and potentially produce rebound hypoglycemia. Managing hypoglycemia in sick or symptomatic infants is discussed in the following section. For treatment of *hypocalcemia* and *hypomagnesemia,* see Chapter 102; for *hyaline membrane disease* treatment, see Chapter 97.3; for treatment of *polycythemia,* see Chapter 99.3.

103.2 Hypoglycemia

See also Chapter 88.

Hypoglycemia is present when serum glucose levels are significantly lower than the range among postnatal age-matched

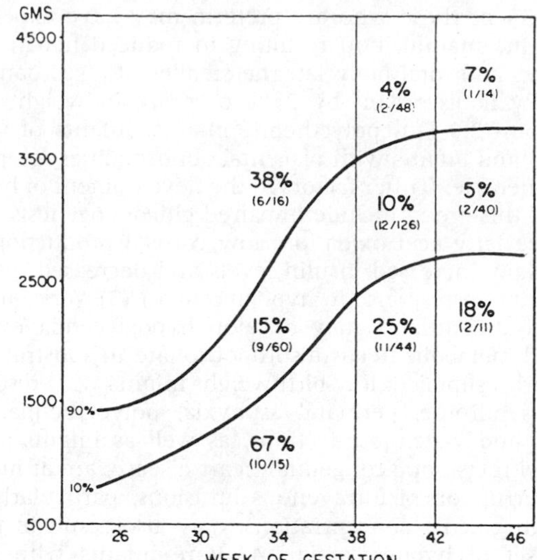

Figure 103–2 Incidence of hypoglycemia by birthweight, gestational age, and intrauterine growth. (From Lubchenco LO [ed]: Incidence of hypoglycemia in newborn infants classified by birth weight and gestational age. Pediatrics 47:832, 1971.)

normal infants. Although hypoglycemia may also be defined as the presence of neurologic (lethargy, coma, apnea, seizures) or sympathomimetic (pallor, palpitations, diaphoresis) manifestations that respond to glucose, many neonates with low serum glucose levels are asymptomatic, whereas normoglycemic infants may have nonspecific signs of hypoglycemia.

The *incidence of hypoglycemia* varies with the definition, population, method and timing of feeding, and type of glucose assay (serum levels are higher than whole blood values) (Fig. 103–2). Early feeding decreases the incidence, whereas prematurity, hypothermia, hypoxia, maternal diabetes, maternal glucose infusion in labor, and intrauterine growth retardation (IUGR) increase the incidence of hypoglycemia. Serum glucose levels decline after birth until 1–3 hr of age, when levels spontaneously increase in normal infants. In healthy term infants, serum glucose values are rarely less than 35 mg/dL (1.9 mmol/L) between 1 and 3 hr of life, less than 40 mg/dL (2.2 mmol/L) from 3–24 hr, and less than 45 mg/dL (2.5 mmol/L) after 24 hr. Although previous studies, performed when premature infants were fasted in the 1st day of life, suggested that premature infants have statistically lower glucose levels than term infants and that preterm infants may be unaffected by low glucose values, evidence does not support these conclusions. Both premature and full-term infants are at risk for serious neurodevelopmental deficits from equally low glucose levels. This risk is related to the depth and duration of the hypoglycemia.

Four pathophysiologic groups of *neonatal infants are at high risk of developing hypoglycemia*: (1) Infants of mothers with diabetes mellitus or gestational diabetes, infants with severe erythroblastosis fetalis, insulinomas, leucine sensitivity with hyperammonemia, familial or sporadic hyperinsulinemia, Beckwith's syndrome (see later), and panhypopituitarism have hyperinsulinism. *Familial hyperinsulinemic hypoglycemia* (nesidioblastosis) may be an autosomal recessive disease characterized by excessive fetal growth and severe neonatal hypoglycemia, often unresponsive to medical management. This severe form is due to defects in either of the two components of the islet β-cell K_{ATP} channel (either the sulfonylurea receptor or the Kir6.2 inward rectifier K^+ channel). A milder autosomal dominant form with delayed onset has an unknown cause. Familial or sporadic hyperammonemic hyperinsulinemia is due to a mutation of the glutamate dehydrogenase gene (increased glutamate oxidation in the β cell releases insulin). (2) Infants with IUGR or those who are preterm may have experienced intrauterine malnutrition resulting in reduced hepatic glycogen stores and total body fat; the smaller of discordant twins (especially if discordant by 25% or more in weight with a weight of <2.0 kg), polycthemic infants, infants of toxemic mothers, and infants with placental abnormalities are particularly vulnerable. (Other factors in the development of hypoglycemia in this group include impaired gluconeogenesis, diminished free fatty acid oxidation, low cortisol production rates, and possibly increased insulin levels and decreased output of epinephrine in response to hypoglycemia.) (3) Very immature or severely ill infants may develop hypoglycemia owing to increased metabolic needs disproportionate to substrate stores and calories supplied; low birthweight infants with respiratory distress syndrome, perinatal asphyxia, polycythemia, hypothermia, and systemic infections, as well as infants in heart failure with cyanotic congenital heart disease, are at increased risk. Interruption of intravenous infusions, particularly those with high glucose concentrations, may also result in precipitous onset of hypoglycemia. (4) Rare infants with genetic or primary metabolic defects, such as galactosemia, glycogen storage disease, fructose intolerance, propionic acidemia, methylmalonic acidemia, tyrosinemia, maple syrup urine disease, and long- or medium-chain acyl-CoA dehydrogenase deficiency are also susceptible.

CLINICAL MANIFESTATIONS. In contrast to the frequency of chemical hypoglycemia, the incidence of symptomatic hypoglycemia is highest in small for gestational age infants (see Fig. 103–2). These infants usually fall into category two or three of the earlier pathophysiologic groupings, and some are referred to as having *transient symptomatic idiopathic neonatal hypoglycemia*. Because many of the symptoms also occur together with other conditions such as infections—especially sepsis and meningitis; central nervous system anomalies, hemorrhage, or edema; hypocalcemia and hypomagnesemia; asphyxia; drug withdrawal; apnea of prematurity; congenital heart disease; or polycythemia—and because some may be seen in normoglycemic well infants, the exact incidence of symptomatic hypoglycemia has been difficult to establish. It probably varies between 1 and 3 per 1,000 live births and affects about 5–15% of growth-retarded infants.

The onset of symptoms varies from a few hours to a week after birth. In approximate order of frequency there are jitteriness or tremors, apathy, episodes of cyanosis, convulsions, intermittent apneic spells or tachypnea, weak or high-pitched cry, limpness or lethargy, difficulty in feeding, and eye rolling. Episodes of sweating, sudden pallor, hypothermia, and cardiac arrest and failure also occur. There is frequently a clustering of episodic symptoms. Because these clinical manifestations may result from various causes, it is critical to measure serum glucose levels and to determine whether they disappear with the administration of sufficient glucose to raise the blood sugar to normal levels; if they do not, other diagnoses must be considered.

TREATMENT. When symptoms other than seizures are present, an intravenous bolus of 200 mg/kg (2 mL/kg) of 10% glucose is effective in elevating the blood glucose concentration. In the presence of convulsions, 4 mL/kg of 10% glucose as a bolus injection is indicated.

After initial therapy, a glucose infusion should be given at 8 mg/kg/min. If hypoglycemia recurs, the infusion rate should be increased until 15–20% glucose is used. If intravenous infusions of 20% glucose are inadequate to eliminate symptoms and maintain constant normal serum glucose concentrations, hyperinsulinemia is probably present and diazoxide should be administered. If this is unsuccessful, octreotide could be added; ultimately, many infants with persistent hyperinsulinemic hypoglycemia undergo subtotal pancreatectomy. Serum glucose level should be measured every 2 hr after initiating therapy until several determinations are above 40 mg/dL. Subsequently, levels should be obtained every 4–6 hr and the treatment gradually reduced and finally discontinued when the serum glucose value has been in the normal range and the baby asymptomatic for 24–48 hr. Treatment is usually necessary for a few days to a week, rarely for several weeks.

Infants who are at increased risk of developing hypoglycemia should have their serum glucose measured within 1 hr of birth and subsequently every 1–2 hr for the first 6–8 hr, then every 4–6 hr until 24 hr of life. Normoglycemic high-risk infants should receive oral or gavage feedings with human milk or formula started at 1–3 hr of age and continued at 2- to 3-hr intervals for 24–48 hr. An intravenous infusion of glucose at 4 mg/kg/min should be provided if oral feedings are poorly tolerated or if *asymptomatic transient neonatal hypoglycemia* develops.

PROGNOSIS. Prognosis is good in asymptomatic patients with hypoglycemia of short duration. Hypoglycemia recurs in 10–15% of infants after adequate treatment. Recurrences are more common if intravenous fluids are extravasated or are too rapidly discontinued before oral feedings are well tolerated. Children who later develop ketotic hypoglycemia have an increased incidence of neonatal hypoglycemia. Prognosis for normal intellectual function must be guarded, because prolonged and severe symptomatic hypoglycemia may be associated with neurologic sequelae. Symptomatic infants with hypoglycemia, particularly low birthweight infants, those with persistent hyperinsulinemic hypoglycemia, and infants of diabetic mothers, have a poorer prognosis for subsequent normal intellectual development than do asymptomatic infants.

HYPOGLYCEMIA WITH MACROGLOSSIA

(Beckwith's Syndrome)

Beckwith described a syndrome of intractable neonatal hypoglycemia occurring in infants with macroglossia, large size, visceromegaly, mild microcephaly, omphalocele, facial nevus flammeus, a characteristic earlobe crease, increased risk of tumors (Wilms', hepatoblastoma, gonadoblastoma) and renal medullary dysplasia. The visceromegaly involves chiefly the liver and the kidneys, in which there is a noncystic hyperplasia. Some infants are also polycythemic. Hyperinsulinemia has been demonstrated. Some infants with Beckwith's syndrome have a partial duplication of chromosome llp, a region that encodes the insulin-like growth factor II gene. Although usually sporadic, familial inheritance has been noted. Treatment is that of hyperinsulinemic hypoglycemia; in this syndrome, hypoglycemia may be severe and may persist for several months. The prognosis is poor.

Severe hypoglycemia has also been demonstrated in extremely high birthweight infants who do not have the anomalies present in Beckwith's syndrome. These *infant giants* weigh from 3.8–5.3 kg, and, in some, pancreatic hyperplasia has been described.

Buchanan TA, Kitzmiller JL: Metabolic interactions of diabetes and pregnancy. Annu Rev Med 45:245, 1994.

Casey BM, Lucas MJ, McIntire DD, et al: Pregnancy outcomes in women with gestational diabetes compared with the general obstetric population. Obstet Gynecol 90:869, 1997.

Cordero L, Treuer SH, Landon MB, et al: Management of infants of diabetic mothers. Arch Pediatr Adolesc Med 152:249, 1998.

Kukuvitis A, Deal C, Arbour L, et al: An autosomal dominant form of familial persistent hyperinsulinemic hypoglycemia of infancy, not linked to the sulfonylurea receptor locus. J Clin Endocrinol Metab 82:1192, 1997.

Langer O, Rodriguez DA, Xenakis EMJ, et al: Intensified versus conventional management of gestational diabetes. Am J Obstet Gynecol 170:1036, 1994.

Lilien L, Pildes R, Srinivasan G, et al: Treatment of neonatal hypoglycemia with minibolus and intravenous glucose infusion. J Pediatr 97:295, 1980.

Lucas A, Morley R, Cole TJ: Adverse neurodevelopmental outcome of moderate neonatal hypoglycaemia. Br Med J 297:1304, 1989.

Mehta A: Prevention and management of neonatal hypoglycaemia. Arch Dis Child 70:F54, 1994.

Nanchi H, Kulaylat: High incidence of Down's syndrome in infants of diabetic mothers. Arch Dis Child 77:242, 1997.

Nestorowicz A, Inagaki N, Gonoi T, et al: A nonsense mutation in the inward

rectifier potassium channel gene, Kir6.2, is associated with familial hyperinsulinism. Diabetes 46:1743, 1997.
Sells CJ, Robinson NM, Brown Z, et al: Long-term developmental follow-up of infants of diabetic mothers. J Pediatr 125:S9, 1994.
Seppänen MP, Ojanperä OS, Kääpä PO, et al: Delayed postnatal adaptation of pulmonary hemodynamics in infants of diabetic mothers. J Pediatr 131:545, 1997.
Simmons D: Persistently poor pregnancy outcomes in women with insulin dependent diabetes. Br Med J 315:263, 1997.
Weinzimer SA, Stanley CA, Berry GT, et al: A syndrome of congenital hyperinsulinism and hyperammonemia. J Pediatr 130:661, 1997.
Wilcken B, Carpenter KH, Hammond J: Neonatal symptoms in medium chain acyl coenzyme A dehydrogenase deficiency. Arch Dis Child 69:292, 1993.
Wolfsdorf JI: Hyperinsulinemic hypoglycemia of infancy. J Pediatr 132:1, 1998.
Zammarchi E, Filippi L, Novembre E, et al: Biochemical evaluation of a patient with a familial form of leucine-sensitive hypoglycemic and concomitant hyperammonemia. Metabolism 45:957, 1996.

CHAPTER 104
Dysmorphology

Kenneth Lyons Jones

The field of dysmorphology has expanded dramatically as the number of recognizable patterns of malformation has more than tripled during the last 25 years. New insights have been gained into the pathogenesis of various structural defects; the potential prenatal effect of various drugs, chemicals, and environmental agents has been better appreciated; and the number of defects in which prenatal detection is possible has increased. Because of their vast number, a listing of all known recognizable patterns of malformation will not be presented. Rather, this chapter provides an approach to the child with the prenatal onset of structural defects. The approach is predicated on the concept that the nature of the structural defects represents a clue to the time of onset, mechanism of injury, and possible etiology of the problem, all of which determine the necessary evaluation. This permits a systematic narrowing of the diagnostic possibilities so that other sections of this textbook or one of the basic compendiums on dysmorphology can be used to make a specific diagnosis.

Structural defects of prenatal onset can be separated into those that represent a single primary defect in development and those that represent a multiple malformation syndrome. In most cases of a single primary defect, the defect involves only a single structure, the child being otherwise completely normal. The seven most common single primary defects in development are congenital hip dislocation (Chapter 684.1), talipes equinovarus (Chapter 680.3), cleft lip with or without cleft palate (Chapter 310), cleft palate alone (Chapter 310), cardiac septal defects (Chapters 433 and 434), pyloric stenosis (Chapter 329), and defects in neural tube closure (Chapter 601). For most, the etiology is unknown, and counseling as to recurrence risk is difficult. However, many of the more common single primary defects are explained on the basis of multifactorial inheritance (Chapter 77), which carries a recurrence risk of between 2% and 5% for the next child of unaffected parents with one affected child. The multifactorial threshold model was developed to explain the empirical 3–5% risk for recurrence in siblings for common single primary defects. Although this figure remains the basis for recurrence risk counseling, the model may not be completely accurate. As the genetic basis for common malformations is elucidated, genetic heterogeneity becomes apparent. For some defects, a few major genes rather than many genes may determine genetic susceptibility. For others, a monogenetic etiology may be apparent. For example, a study of the offspring of adults with major heart defects indicates that atrioventricular septal defect is most likely a single gene defect, whereas tetralogy of Fallot is most likely a polygenic defect with a small number of interacting genes.

The extent to which multifactorial inheritance contributes to the etiology of some of the less common single defects in development is unclear. The fact that single primary defects are etiologically heterogeneous implies that some have an environmental etiology and others result from dominantly or recessively inherited single altered genes. Craniosynostosis (Chapter 601.12) secondary to in utero constraint is an example of the former, whereas postaxial polydactyly (Chapter 687.7) illustrates the latter. Before multifactorial risk figures are used for counseling when a single primary defect is recognized, references should be consulted to determine whether other risk figures are available.

In contrast to the concept of the single primary defect in development, the designation *multiple malformation syndrome* is used when several observed structural defects all have the same known or presumed etiology. The defects usually include a number of anatomically unrelated errors in morphogenesis. Multiple malformation syndromes are caused by chromosomal abnormalities, by teratogens, and by single gene defects inherited in mendelian patterns. Risks of recurrence range from zero, in cases that represent fresh gene mutations or are caused by teratogens, to 100%, in the case of a child with Down syndrome in which the mother is a balanced 21/21 translocation carrier (Chapter 78).

SINGLE PRIMARY DEFECTS IN DEVELOPMENT. These defects are subcategorized according to the nature of the error in morphogenesis that has produced the observed structural defect: malformation, deformation, disruption, or dysplasia of a developing structure. A *malformation* is a primary structural defect arising from a localized error in morphogenesis. A *deformation* is an alteration in shape or structure of a part that has differentiated normally. The term *disruption* is used for a structural defect resulting from destruction of a previously normally formed part. The term *dysplasia* refers to an abnormal organization of cells and the structural consequences.

Malformations. Most children with a localized malformation, such as cardiac septal defect or pyloric stenosis, are otherwise completely normal. After surgical correction, the prognosis is excellent. When neither dominant nor recessive inheritance is established, multifactorial recurrence risk factors (2–5%) apply to unaffected parents.

Deformations. Most deformations involve the musculoskeletal system and are probably caused by intrauterine molding. The pressure producing such molding may be intrinsic, the result of neuromuscular imbalance within the fetus, or extrinsic, secondary to fetal crowding. In either case, the impaired ability of the fetus to kick results in decreased fetal movement, an important factor in development of the normal musculoskeletal system, particularly with respect to normal joint development. In addition, marked positional deformation of any body part can occur when the fetus is unable to change position and thus alter the direction along which potentially deforming forces are being directed.

Intrinsically derived positional deformation of prenatal onset occurs in disorders involving muscle degeneration, such as the Steinert myotonic dystrophy syndrome, and disorders involving motor neurons, such as Werdnig-Hoffmann disease (Chapter 619.2). Early defects in development of the central nervous system (CNS) are more common causes of positional deformations and should be seriously considered whenever a structural defect is thought to be intrinsically derived.

Fetal crowding, the common cause of an extrinsically derived deformation of prenatal onset, is usually due to a decreased volume of amniotic fluid, a situation that occurs normally during the later weeks of gestation, when the fetus is undergoing extremely rapid growth. However, it also occurs abnormally with diminished fetal urinary output and chronic leakage of amniotic fluid.

Other extrinsic factors associated with the development of deformations include breech presentation and the shape of the amniotic cavity. When a fetus is in the breech position, the legs may be trapped between the body and the uterine wall. In that position, the fetus is unable to kick optimally, resulting in a 10-fold increase in the incidence of deformations. The shape of the amniotic cavity, which has profound influence on the shape of the fetus that lies within it, is influenced by many factors, including uterine shape; volume of amniotic fluid; size and shape of the fetus; presence of more than one fetus; site of placental implantation; presence of uterine tumors; shape of the abdominal cavity, which is influenced by the pelvis, sacral promontory, and neighboring abdominal organs; and tightness of abdominal musculature.

Various forms of talipes and congenital hip dislocation are the most frequently observed congenital postural deformities. Most children with these deformations are otherwise completely normal, and their prognosis is excellent. Correction usually occurs spontaneously. However, recognizing that a structural defect represents a deformation does not always imply "normal" fetal crowding and should lead to careful consideration of other etiologic possibilities that might have far greater significance to the child. For example, because decreased fetal movement can be secondary to serious neurologic abnormalities, multiple joint contractures should alert the physician to the possibility of a malformation in CNS development. Although congenital hip dislocations and talipes have a 2–5% recurrence risk, most deformations are the result of physiologic crowding and have a lower recurrence risk. Deformations that are due to pathologic crowding (e.g., uterine tumors or malformation) have a much higher recurrence risk, unless the factors leading to crowding are altered prior to subsequent pregnancies. Deformations that are the result of an underlying malformation (e.g., renal agenesis) have a recurrence risk similar to that of the underlying malformation.

Disruption. These defects occur when there is destruction of a previously normally formed part. At least two basic mechanisms are known to produce disruption. One involves entanglement followed by the tearing apart or amputation of a normally developed structure, usually a digit, arm, or leg, by strands of amnion floating within amniotic fluid (i.e., amniotic bands) (Chapter 92). The second involves the interruption of blood supply to a developing part, leading to infarction, necrosis, and/or resorption of structures distal to the insult. If interruption of blood supply occurs early in gestation, the disruptive defect that is seen at term usually involves atresia or absence of a particular part. If the infarction occurs later, necrosis is more likely to be present. Examples of disruptive single primary defects for which infarctive mechanisms have been implicated include nonduodenal intestinal atresia, gastroschisis (Chapter 368), porencephaly (Chapter 601), and terminal transverse limb reduction defects. The extent to which disruption of a developing structure plays a role in dysmorphogenesis is unknown.

Genetic factors play a minor role in the pathogenesis of disruptions; most are sporadic events in otherwise normal families. The prognosis for a disruptive defect is determined entirely by the extent and location of the tissue loss. Thus, a child with a limb amputation has an excellent prognosis for normal function, whereas a child with porencephaly does not.

Dysplasia. Dysplasias may be localized or generalized. Localized dysplasias are usually single primary defects in development (e.g., hemangiomas). However, generalized dysplasias, such as connective tissue disorders, usually present as multiple malformation syndromes in that a wide variety of structures are involved because of the widespread distribution of the dysplastic tissue.

The causes of the vast majority of localized dysplasias are unknown. Since many generalized dysplasias are the result of abnormal genes, it is possible that localized dysplasias will reflect somatic mutation in specific tissues. The hypothesis is consistent with the observation that empirical recurrence risk for localized dysplasias is low. The process of dysplasia appears to involve deregulation of growth; hence, most dysplasias change over time. For example, capillary hemangiomas become involuted, and bathing trunk nevi carry a risk for malignant transformation. Knowledge of the natural history of a lesion is critical in the long-term follow-up of children with localized dysplasias.

Sequence. The pattern of multiple anomalies that occurs when a single primary defect in early morphogenesis produces multiple abnormalities through a cascading process of secondary and tertiary errors in morphogenesis is called a sequence. When evaluating a child with multiple anomalies, the physician must differentiate between multiple anomalies secondary to a single localized error in morphogenesis (a sequence) and a multiple malformation syndrome. In the former, recurrence risk counseling for the multiple anomalies depends entirely on the recurrence risk for the single localized malformation.

The terms *malformation, deformation,* and *disruption sequence* are used to describe only the initiating error in morphogenesis of a sequence if it is known. For example, the Robin malformation sequence (Chapter 311) is a pattern of multiple anomalies, all of which are produced by a single prenatal onset defect in development, mandibular hypoplasia. Because the tongue is relatively small for the oral cavity, it drops back (glossoptosis), blocking closure of the posterior palatal shelves and causing a U-shaped cleft palate. Recognizing that all the observed defects are due to a single localized error permits recurrence risk counseling based on the single defect.

The patient shown in Figure 104–1 has bathrocephaly, torticollis, facial asymmetry, a dislocated hip, and valgus anomalies of both feet, resulting from compression of developing fetal parts. This pattern is the *breech deformation sequence.* Intrauterine crowding occurred because the large-sized infant was delivered from a breech position to a small, primigravida mother; recurrence risk is therefore negligible. Recognizing the defor-

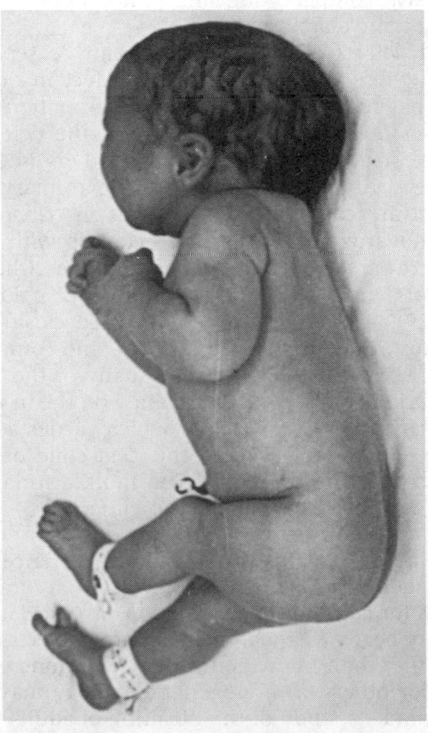

Figure 104–1 Breech deformation sequence.

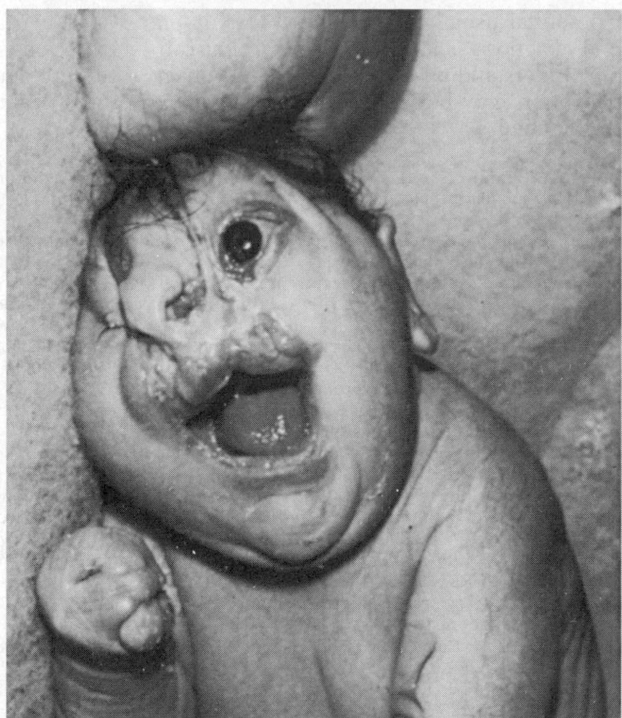

Figure 104–2 Amniotic band disruption sequence.

mational nature of the abnormalities is helpful with respect to prognosis. All the problems should resolve spontaneously or with postural therapy.

In the *amniotic band disruption sequence,* all the craniofacial and limb defects are secondary to constrictions caused by entanglement in multiple fibrous strands of amnion extending from the placental insertion of the umbilical cord to the surface of the amnion-denuded chorion or floating freely within the chorionic sac (Fig. 104–2). These strands of amnion, which result from disruption of the normally formed membrane, can cause secondary defects through several mechanisms. Malformations occur if a strand of amnion interferes with the normal sequence of development; for example, a strand of amnion may interrupt fusion of the facial processes so that a cleft lip results. Disruptions occur secondary to tearing apart of structures that have previously developed normally; for example, an amniotic band might cleave areas in the developing craniofacies along lines not conforming to the normal planes of facial closure.

Deformations due to fetal compression occur secondary to *oligohydramnios* or *tethering of a fetal part.* The former may result from rupture of both amnion and chorion, leading to chronic leakage of amniotic fluid. Tethering occurs when the fetus or one of its parts becomes immobilized by the constraining effect of an amniotic band so that it is unable to change position and thus alter the direction along which potentially deforming forces are being directed. The recurrence risk is based upon the recurrence risk for amnion rupture; unaffected parents have not been reported to have given birth to more than one child affected with this disorder.

MULTIPLE MALFORMATION SYNDROMES. This category includes patients in whom one or more developmental anomalies of two or more systems have occurred, all of which are thought to be due to common etiology. Other than Down syndrome, with an incidence of 1:660, and XXY syndromes (1:500 males), none of these disorders occurs more frequently than 1/3,000 live births.

Multiple malformation syndromes may be caused by chromosomal and genetic abnormalities and by teratogens. A number of these are associated with chromosome abnormalities (Chapter 78).

Disorders that are due to single mutant genes (dominant or X-linked in males) or to pairs of mutant genes (autosomal recessive) also cause a number of recognizable multiple malformation syndromes of prenatal onset. Their correct diagnosis depends on clinical recognition, since in most cases there is no laboratory test to confirm the diagnosis. A family history of a similarly affected individual is extremely helpful. However, in many patients with multiple malformation syndromes of genetic etiology, the occurrence is sporadic and thus represents fresh gene mutations. In such situations, all family members are normal, and the diagnosis depends entirely on the evaluation of the patient's phenotype.

Disorders caused by teratogens include multiple malformation syndromes due to the effect of specific infections or of pharmacologic or chemical agents with which the embryo or fetus has come in contact during gestation. These conditions may be prevented before conception, particularly in the case of drugs and chemicals, if the mother is aware that the agent in question can affect her baby. It is difficult, on the other hand, for a pregnant woman to avoid contact with all infectious agents.

A careful history of drug intake (Chapter 90.1) and chemical exposure (Chapters 719 and 720) should be obtained from the parents of all children with multiple malformation syndromes, especially when the etiology of the disorder is unknown. *A Catalog of Teratogenic Agents,* by T. H. Shepard, and *Drugs in Pregnancy and Lactation,* by Briggs, Freeman, and Yaffe are excellent references for determining whether the agent that the mother has been exposed to is a known teratogen.

Specific and easily distinguishable phenotypes do not exist for each of the infectious diseases commonly associated with altered fetal development, but intrauterine infection can frequently be suspected if there is an overall pattern of malformation (Chapters 105 and 106). Any patient should be suspected of having had an intrauterine infection if he or she is small for gestational age or developmentally delayed; in addition, the infant may be affected by microcephaly or hydrocephalus; by ocular defects, including microphthalmia, chorioretinitis, cataracts, or glaucoma; and by hepatosplenomegaly and thrombocytopenia. Intrauterine infections have a wide spectrum of clinical manifestations, from the severely affected newborn with multiple malformations to the child with no malformations who first manifests learning disabilities at school age.

There are also some well-recognized multiple malformation syndromes in which virtually all cases have been sporadic in otherwise normal families. It is now possible through the newer molecular techniques to determine the etiology of some of these disorders. For example, studies utilizing fluorescent in situ hybridization indicate that the *Williams syndrome* is due to a deletion of one elastin allele located within chromosome subunit 7q 11.23, while the *Rubinstein-Taybi syndrome* is due to a microdeletion in 16p 13.3 (see Chapter 78). For *Prader-Willi syndrome,* another common sporadic disorder, the presence of the phenotype is dependent on whether the gene has been inherited from the mother or the father, a mechanism known as genetic imprinting. Greater than 50% of children with Prader-Willi syndrome have a chromosomal deletion involving band q11.2 of the long arm of chromosome 15. In all cases, the deleted chromosome is paternally derived (see Chapters 77 and 78). Although the gene for *Brachmann–de Lange syndrome* has not been localized, most cases are believed to be due to a single gene transmitted as an autosomal dominant. The low recurrence risk most likely represents the inability of more severely affected individuals to reproduce. Experience with many children having each of these disorders has provided a vast amount of information that can be extremely helpful to parents in understanding their child's behavior and to educators in planning an appropriate curriculum. For example, a specific behavioral phenotype has been delineated for the de Lange syndrome; the parents' awareness that the child's aberrant behavior is "normal" for the de Lange syndrome rather than being "their fault" can be extremely helpful in relieving their anxiety and guilt. For the *Williams syndrome*, a different but equally characteristic behavioral phenotype has been documented and includes the following: multiple developmental motor disabilities affecting strength, balance, coordination, and motor planning; sensory integration dysfunction relating primarily to hypersensitivity to sound; hyperactivity; delayed expressive and receptive language skills with simultaneous age-appropriate grammar and articulation; better reading than mathematics ability; and cognitive dysfunction ranging from learning disabilities to mental retardation. This knowledge of a child's particular strengths and weaknesses may allow educators to develop a curriculum that will give affected children a better chance to reach their potential.

Finally, there are certain nonrandom associations of malformations for which it has not been determined whether the pattern is a sequence or a syndrome. These are designated **associations**. One important clinical example is the *VATER association*, which includes vertebral defects, anal atresia, tracheoesophageal fistula with atresia, radial upper limb hypoplasia, and renal defects. Single umbilical artery and cardiac and genital anomalies are also seen in this association. These defects are likely to occur together in almost any combination of two or more and usually represent a sporadic occurrence in an otherwise normal family.

The ultimate goal in evaluating a child with structural defects is making a specific overall diagnosis. When this is achieved, appropriate recurrence risk counseling for the parents, accurate prognostication about the child's future development, and an appropriate plan to help the child reach his or her potential usually are possible (see Chapter 37). When an overall diagnosis is lacking, the most that can be expected is a better understanding of the nature and onset of the problem, which often may be helpful to parents and to others dealing with the child.

Breuning MH, Dauwerse HG, Fugazza G, et al: Rubinstein-Taybi syndrome caused by submicroscopic deletions within 16p 13.3. Am J Hum Genet 52:249, 1993.

Briggs GG, Freeman RK, Yaffe SJ: Drugs in Pregnancy and Lactation, 4th ed. Baltimore, Williams & Wilkins, 1994.

Burn J, Brennan P, Little J, et al: Recurrence risks in offspring of adults with major heart defects: Results from first cohort of British collaborative study. Lancet 351:311, 1998.

Dilts CV, Morris CA, Leonard CO: Hypothesis for development of a behavioral phenotype in Williams syndrome. Am J Med Genet (Suppl)6:126, 1990.

Dunn PM: Congenital postural deformities. Br Med Bull 32:71, 1976.

Ewart AK, Morris CA, Atkinson D, et al: Hemizygosity at the elastin locus in a developmental disorder, Williams syndrome. Nat Genet 5:11, 1993.

Gorlin RJ, Cohen MM, Levin LS: Syndromes of the Head and Neck, 3rd ed. New York, Oxford University Press, 1990.

Higginbottom MC, Jones KL, Hall BD, et al: The amniotic band disruption complex. Timing of amniotic rupture and variable spectra of consequent defects. J Pediatr 95:544, 1979.

Johnson HG, Ekman P, Frieseu W, et al: A behavioral phenotype in the de Lange syndrome. Pediatr Res 10:843, 1976.

Jones KL: Smith's Recognizable Patterns of Human Malformation, 5th ed. Philadelphia, WB Saunders, 1997.

Kalter H, Warkany J: Congenital malformation, etiologic factors and their role in prevention. N Engl J Med 308:424, 1983.

Kausseff BG, Newkirk P, Root AW: Brachmann-de Lange syndrome. 1994 update. Arch Pediatr Adolesc Med 148:749, 1994.

Kazazian HH Jr: The nature of mutation. Hosp Pract 20:55, 1985.

Lie RT, Wilcox AJ, Skjaervcn R: A population-based study of the risk of recurrence of birth defects. N Engl J Med 331:1, 1994.

McKusick VA: Mendelian Inheritance in Man. Catalog of Autosomal Dominant, Autosomal Recessive and X-linked Phenotypes, 10th ed. Baltimore, The Johns Hopkins University Press, 1992.

Shepard TH: A Catalog of Teratogenic Agents, 7th ed. Baltimore, The Johns Hopkins University Press, 1992.

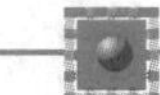

SECTION 2

Infections of the Neonatal Infant

Samuel P. Gotoff

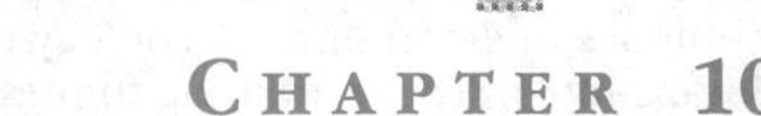

CHAPTER 105
Pathogenesis and Epidemiology

Infections are a frequent and important cause of morbidity and mortality in the neonatal period (see Chapter 89). As many as 2% of fetuses are infected in utero, and up to 10% of infants are infected in the first month of life. The uniqueness of neonatal infections is a result of a number of factors. (1) There are diverse modes of transmission of infectious agents from mother to fetus or newborn infant. Transplacental hematogenous spread may occur at different times during gestation, with manifestations present at birth or delayed for months or years. Vertical transmission of infection from mother to infant may take place in utero, just before delivery, or during the process of delivery. After birth, neonates may be exposed to infectious diseases in the nursery or in the community. With the increasing complexity of neonatal intensive care, gestationally younger and lower birthweight newborns are surviving and remaining for a longer time in an environment with a high risk of infection. (2) Newborn infants may be less capable of responding to infection due to one or more immunologic deficiencies involving the reticuloendothelial system, complement, polymorphonuclear leukocytes, cytokines, antibody, or cell-mediated immunity. (3) Coexisting diseases of newborns often complicate the diagnosis and management of neonatal infections. Respiratory disorders such as hyaline membrane disease may coexist with bacterial pneumonia. Acidosis impairs functions of polymorphonuclear leukocytes. (4) The extremely variable manifestations of infectious diseases in newborn infants include subclinical infection, congenital malformations resulting from infection in the first trimester present at birth or appearing later in life, and mild to severe manifestations of focal or systemic infection. The timing of exposure in utero, inoculum size, immune status, and the etiologic agent influence the expression of disease in a fetus or newborn infant. Etiologic agents include a wide variety of bacteria, viruses, fungi, protozoa, and mycoplasma. Maternal infection that is the source of transplacental fetal infection may be clinical, often with nonspecific symptoms and signs, or subclinical, identified retrospectively by serologic methods, as part of the evaluation of suspected neonatal infection.

105.1 Immunity

Many studies have compared immunologic function of newborn infants with that in adults. Diminished concentrations of immunologic factors and decreased function are often demonstrated. Despite these defects in immunity in premature and full-term infants, the rate of invasive infectious diseases is low in the absence of obstetric and neonatal risk factors. It is important to maintain this perspective when evaluating immunologic prophylactic measures such as the use of intravenous immunoglobulin in newborns. The immunologic system is discussed in Part XIII. This section contrasts the immunologic function of newborns with that of older children and adults. Other maternal factors that influence the exposure of pregnant women to potential pathogens include socioeconomic status, sexual promiscuity, and adolescent age.

IMMUNOGLOBULINS. Active transport of immunoglobulin G (IgG) occurs across the placenta, with concentrations in a full-term infant comparable to those of the mother. The specificity of IgG antibody in cord blood is dependent on the mother's antigenic experience and immunologic response. Other classes of Igs are not transferred, although a fetus can synthesize IgA and IgM in response to intrauterine infection. In premature infants, cord IgG levels are directly proportional to gestational age. Studies of type-specific IgG antibodies to group B streptococci (GBS) have shown that the ratio of cord to maternal serum concentrations is 1.0, 0.5, and 0.3 at term, 32 wk, and 28 wk of gestation, respectively. Infants with birthweights less than 1,500 g become significantly hypogammaglobulinemic, with mean plasma IgG concentrations in the range of 200–300 mg/dL in the 1st wk of life.

The presence of specific IgG antibody in adequate concentrations provides neonates with protection against those infections in which protection is mediated by antibody (e.g., tetanus antitoxin and antibody to encapsulated bacteria such as GBS). Specific bactericidal and opsonic antibodies against enteric bacilli are predominantly in the IgM class. In general, newborn infants lack antibody-mediated protection against *Escherichia coli* and other Enterobacteriaceae.

COMPLEMENT. Complement mediates bactericidal activity against certain organisms such as *E. coli* and functions as an opsonin with antibody in optimal phagocytosis of bacteria such as GBS. There is essentially no transfer of complement from the maternal circulation. A fetus begins to synthesize complement components as early as the 1st trimester. Full-term newborn infants have slightly diminished classic pathway complement activity and moderately diminished alternative pathway activity. There is considerable variability in both concentration of complement components and activity. The alternative pathway components (B and P) are usually 35–60% of normal. Premature infants have lower levels of complement components and less complement activity than full-term newborns. These deficiencies contribute to diminished complement-derived chemotactic activity and to diminished ability to opsonize certain organisms in the absence of antibody. Many studies have been performed with different strains of microorganisms and different conditions, examining both classic and alternative pathways. In general, opsonization of *Staphylococcus aureus* is normal in neonatal sera, but various degrees of impairment have been noted with GBS and *E. coli*.

NEUTROPHILS. Chemotaxis of neonatal neutrophils is diminished, and adherence, aggregation, and deformability are decreased, all of which may delay the response to infection. With adequate opsonization, phagocytosis and killing by neutrophils from healthy newborn infants are comparable to those in adults. However, in infants with respiratory distress, hypoglycemia, hyperbilirubinemia, and sepsis, microbicidal activity is impaired.

The number of circulating neutrophils is elevated after birth in both full-term and premature infants, with a peak at 12 hr, returning to normal by 22 hr. Band neutrophils constitute less than 15% in normal newborns and may increase in newborns with infection and other stress responses such as asphyxia.

The neutrophil storage pool in newborn infants is 20–30% of that in adults. Neutrophils are much more likely to be depleted in neonatal infections; this depletion is the major host factor contributing to poor outcome in bacterial sepsis.

MONOCYTE-MACROPHAGE SYSTEM. The monocyte-macrophage system consists of circulating monocytes and tissue macrophages of the reticuloendothelial system (RES), particularly in the spleen and liver. The number of circulating monocytes in neonatal blood is normal, but the mass or function of the macrophages in the RES apparently is diminished in newborns and particularly in premature infants, as estimated by the relative increase in the number of damaged erythrocytes (pocked cells) in the circulation. In both term and premature infants, chemotaxis of monocytes is impaired; this impairment affects the inflammatory response in tissues and the results of delayed hypersensitivity skin tests. Monocytes from neonates ingest and kill microorganisms as well as monocytes from adults.

NATURAL KILLER (NK) CELLS. NK cells are a subgroup of lymphocytes that are cytolytic against cells infected with viruses. NK cells also lyse cells coated with antibody in a process called antibody-dependent cell-mediated cytotoxicity (ADCC). They are present in cord blood in numbers equivalent to those in adults.

Neonatal NK cells have decreased cytotoxic activity and ADCC compared with adult cells. The diminished cytotoxicity against herpes simplex virus (HSV)–infected cells may predispose to disseminated HSV infection in newborns (see Chapter 245).

CYTOKINES. Interferon (INF)-α and -β are normal, but INF-γ synthesis is diminished. TNF-α levels are elevated in infants with neonatal sepsis, but the response may be less consistent than in adults. Interleukin (IL)-2 activity in cord blood from full-term and premature infants was reported to be higher than in adults, but messenger RNA (mRNA) for the IL-2 receptor could not be detected in cells from premature infants. In full-term infants, the level of mRNA for IL-2R was comparable to that in adults.

IL-6 levels are increased in serum of newborns with neonatal sepsis and necrotizing enterocolitis (NEC). This response appears to be the most consistent of the cytokine responses in newborns.

105.2 Etiology

A number of agents may infect newborns in utero, intrapartum, or post partum (Tables 105–1 and 105–2). Prenatal infections that are known to be transmitted transplacentally include syphilis, *Borrelia burgdorferi*, rubella, cytomegalovirus (CMV), parvovirus B19, hepatitis B virus, HSV, HIV, varicella-zoster, *Listeria monocytogenes*, toxoplasmosis, tuberculosis, and *Trypanosoma cruzi*.

Any microorganism inhabiting the vagina or lower gastrointestinal tract may cause intrapartum and postpartum infection. The most common bacteria are GBS, enteric organisms, gonococci, and chlamydiae. The more common viruses include HSV and enteroviruses. Community-acquired pathogens, such as *Streptococcus pneumoniae*, may also cause infection in newborn infants after discharge from the hospital.

The list of organisms causing nosocomial infections is long. The common causes are coagulase-negative staphylococci, gram-negative bacilli *(Klebsiella pneumoniae, E. coli, Salmonella, Campylobacter, Enterobacter, Citrobacter, Pseudomonas aeruginosa, Serratia)*, enterococci, *S. aureus*, and *Candida*. Viruses contribut-

TABLE 105–1 Bacterial Causes of Systemic Neonatal Infections

Bacteria	Early Onset	Late Onset, Maternal Origin	Late Onset, Nosocomial	Late Onset, Community
Gram-positive				
Clostridia	+		+	*
Enterococci	+		++	
Group B streptococcus	+++	+	+	+
Listeria monocytogenes	+	+		
Other streptococci	++			+
Staphylococcus aureus	+		++	+
Staphylococcus, coagulase negative	+		+++	
Streptococcus pneumoniae	+			++
Streptococcus viridans	+		++	
Gram-negative				
Bacteroides	+		+	
Campylobacter	+			
Citrobacter			+	+
Enterobacter			+	
Escherichia coli	+++		+	++
Haemophilus influenzae	+			+
Klebsiella			+	
Neisseria gonorrhoeae	+			
Neisseria meningitidis	+		+	
Proteus			+	
Pseudomonas			+	
Salmonella		+		+
Serratia			+	
Others				
Treponema pallidum	+	+		
Mycobacterium tuberculosis		+		

*C. tetani *in some developing countries.*
+ = *Relative frequency.*

ing to nosocomial neonatal infections include enteroviruses, CMV, hepatitis A, adenoviruses, influenza, respiratory syncytial virus, rhinovirus, parainfluenza, HSV, and rotavirus.

Congenital pneumonia may be caused by CMV, rubella virus, and *Treponema pallidum* and less commonly by the other agents producing transplacental infection (Table 105–3). Microorganisms causing **pneumonia acquired in the perinatal period** include GBS, gram-negative enteric aerobes, *Listeria monocytogenes*, genital *Mycoplasma, Chlamydia trachomatis*, CMV, herpes simplex virus, and *Candida* species.

Bacteria responsible for most cases of **nosocomial pneumonia** typically include staphylococcal species, gram-negative enteric aerobes, and occasionally *Pseudomonas*. Fungi are responsible for an increasing number of systemic infections acquired during prolonged hospitalization of neonates, although their etiologic role in nosocomial pneumonia may be difficult to document. Finally, respiratory viruses cause isolated cases and outbreaks of nosocomial pneumonia. These viruses, usually endemic during the winter months and acquired from infected hospital staff or visitors to the nursery, include respiratory syncytial virus, parainfluenza virus, influenza viruses, enteroviruses, and adenovirus. Respiratory viruses are the single most important cause of community-acquired pneumonitis and are usually contracted from infected siblings or parents.

The most common bacterial causes of neonatal **meningitis** are GBS, *E. coli* K1, and *Listeria. S. pneumoniae*, other streptococci, nontypable *Haemophilus influenzae*, both coagulase-positive and coagulase-negative staphylococci, *Klebsiella, Enterobacter, Pseudomonas, T. pallidum*, and *Mycobacterium tuberculosis* may also produce meningitis. *Citrobacter diversus* is an important cause of brain abscess. Additional pathogens include *Mycoplasma hominis, Ureaplasma urealyticum, Candida albicans* and other fungi, *Toxoplasma gondii*, and viruses (enteroviruses, HSV type 2 more often than type 1, rubella, CMV, and HIV).

Bacteria, viruses, fungi, and rarely protozoa may produce neonatal **sepsis** (see Table 106–4). The most common causes of early-onset sepsis are GBS and enteric bacteria acquired from the maternal genital tract. Late-onset sepsis may be due to GBS, HSV, enteroviruses, and *E. coli* K1 and other enteric organisms. In very low birthweight infants, *Candida* and coagulase-negative staphylococci (CONS) are the most common pathogens in late-onset sepsis.

TABLE 105–2 Nonbacterial Causes of Systemic Neonatal Infections

Viruses	Mycoplasma
Adenovirus	*M. hominis*
Cytomegalovirus	*Ureaplasma urealyticum*
Enteroviruses	**Fungi**
Herpes simplex virus	*Candida* species
Human immunodeficiency virus	*Malassezia* species
Parvovirus	**Parasites**
Rubella virus	Plasmodia
Varicella-zoster virus	*Toxoplasma gondii*
	Trypanosoma cruzi

TABLE 105–3 Etiologic Agents of Neonatal Pneumonia According to Timing of Acquisition

Transplacental	Perinatal	Postnatal
Cytomegalovirus	Anaerobic bacteria	Adenovirus
Herpes simplex virus	*Chlamydia*	**Candida* species
Mycobacterium tuberculosis	Cytomegalovirus	Coagulase-negative staphylococci
Rubella virus	Enteric bacteria	Cytomegalovirus
Treponema pallidum	Group B streptococci	Echoviruses
Varicella-zoster virus	*Haemophilus influenzae*	*Enteric bacteria
	Herpes simplex virus	Influenza viruses A, B
	Listeria monocytogenes	Parainfluenza
	Mycoplasma	**Pseudomonas*
		Respiratory syncytial virus
		Staphylococcus aureus

**More likely in infants on mechanical ventilation, with indwelling catheters, or after abdominal surgery.*

TABLE 105–4 Frequency of Major Neonatal Infections

Agent	Attack Rate/1,000 Live Births
Cytomegalovirus*	
Congenital	6–24
Perinatal	20–60
Postnatal	140–210
Enteroviruses	2–38
Group B streptococci	1–3
Hepatitis B*	0–61
Herpes simplex virus	0.1–0.6
Toxoplasma gondii	0.1–10
Treponema pallidum	0.3

**Most infections are asymptomatic.*

105.3 Epidemiology

The *frequency of neonatal infections* in the United States is presented in Table 105–4. The most common congenital infection in the United States is due to CMV, with an attack rate of 6–24/1,000 live births. However, perinatal and postnatal transmission of CMV may increase the frequency of neonatal CMV infection 10-fold. Congenital rubella is now rare in countries using rubella vaccine. Certain infections, such as hepatitis B, tetanus, malaria, and HIV, are endemic in some developing countries. Up to 50% of women in sub-Saharan Africa are infected with HIV.

The attack rates of *neonatal bacterial infections* also vary geographically, depending on the prevalence of organisms in the community. GBS and gram-negative enteric bacilli are common colonizers of the gastrointestinal tract and vagina, whereas *L. monocytogenes* is uncommon and usually related to food-borne epidemics. Exposure to *T. gondii* in uncooked meat varies according to dietary practices. Epidemic disease in the community, such as enteroviral infections, has a seasonal variability.

A number of factors in addition to geographic region influence the rates of neonatal infection. Socioeconomic status, maternal age, race, and sexual practices influence the prevalence of a number of maternal infections. The status of a woman's immunity, for example, to rubella, determines whether maternal infection occurs during pregnancy. Hospital-to-hospital variability in incidence may be related to rates of prematurity, prenatal care, conduct of labor, and environmental conditions in nurseries.

The *incidence of neonatal sepsis* varies according to definition, from 1–4/1,000 live births in developed countries with considerable fluctuation over time and with geographic location. Males have an approximately twofold higher incidence of sepsis than females, suggesting the possibility of a sex-linked factor in host susceptibility. Attack rates of neonatal sepsis increase significantly in low birthweight infants, in the presence of maternal chorioamnionitis, congenital immune defects, asplenia, galactosemia *(E. coli)*, and malformation leading to high inocula of bacteria (obstructive uropathy).

The *incidence of meningitis* in newborn infants is 0.2–0.4/1,000 live births and is higher in preterm infants. Bacterial meningitis may be associated with sepsis or may present as a focal infection. Meningitis currently occurs in fewer than 20% of newborn infants with early-onset invasive bacterial infections. Surveillance in 22 counties in the United States revealed an incidence of neonatal meningitis of 125, 39, and 15.7 cases per 100,000 for GBS, *L. monocytogenes*, and *S. pneumoniae*, respectively.

PREMATURITY. The most important neonatal factor predisposing to infection is prematurity or low birthweight; these infants have a 3- to 10-fold higher incidence of infection and sepsis than do full-term, normal birthweight infants. There are a number of possible explanations for increased incidence of infection in premature infants. (1) Maternal genital tract infection is considered to be a significant cause of premature labor, with an increased risk of vertical transmission to the newborn. However, culture-positive intra-amniotic infection may not be associated with clinical chorioamnionitis, and there is a higher frequency of intra-amniotic infection in patients with preterm labor and intact membranes and in patients with preterm premature rupture of membranes. (2) Premature infants have less well-developed immune systems. (3) Premature infants are more likely to have diseases such as hyaline membrane disease and necrotizing enterocolitis, which are often complicated by infection. (4) Premature infants may require intravenous access or endotracheal tubes, which provide a portal of entry or impair clearance mechanisms.

CHORIOAMNIONITIS. Attack rates of neonatal infection increase significantly in the presence of chorioamnionitis, diagnosed by amniotic fluid analysis or histologically. Clinical signs of chorioamnionitis include intrapartum fever (>38°C), maternal leukocytosis (WBC >18,000), and uterine tenderness. By 24 hr of membrane rupture, there is histologic evidence of chorioamnionitis, and prolonged rupture of membranes greater than 18 hr increases the risk of GBS infections.

EARLY-ONSET AND LATE-ONSET INFECTIONS. Neonatal infections are those presenting during the first 28 days of life; however, similar infections may occur in older infants, particularly premature infants, during the first 6 mo of life (Table 105–5). These are referred to as late, late-onset infections. The terms early-onset and late-onset infections refer to the age of onset of infection in the neonatal period. Originally divided arbitrarily by 1 wk of age, those infections are more usefully separated according to peripartum pathogenesis (i.e., acquisition of the agent before or during delivery as early onset). Late-onset infections are usually acquired in the normal newborn nursery or neonatal intensive care unit (NICU) or in the community. The age of onset depends on the latent period of the infection, with pyogenic infections such as GBS usually presenting clinical manifestations within a 24-hr incubation period. Although some infections in which the organism is acquired at delivery may not present clinically until after 72 hr or a week of life, separation of early- and late-onset infections has been useful in developing and evaluating interventional strategies.

NOSOCOMIAL NURSERY INFECTION. (See also Chapter 302.) Neonatal infections acquired in the hospital are nosocomial. The organisms may be acquired in the delivery room (e.g., from contaminated equipment), in the normal newborn nursery, or in the NICU. Maternally acquired infections usually appear within the first 48 hr of life. Thus, presentation 48 hr after admission to the nursery is generally used as a criterion for nosocomial infection in a newborn. Nosocomial infections may be sporadic or occur as epidemics, and they may occur while

TABLE 105–5 Neonatal Infection by Age of Onset

Feature	Early Onset	Late Onset	Late, Late Onset
Age	Birth–1 wk, usually <72 hr	8–28 days	1–6 mo
Risk factors	Prematurity, amnionitis, maternal infection or colonization	Prematurity	Prematurity
Site	Normal newborn nursery, community	NICU, community	NICU, community

NICU = neonatal intensive care unit.

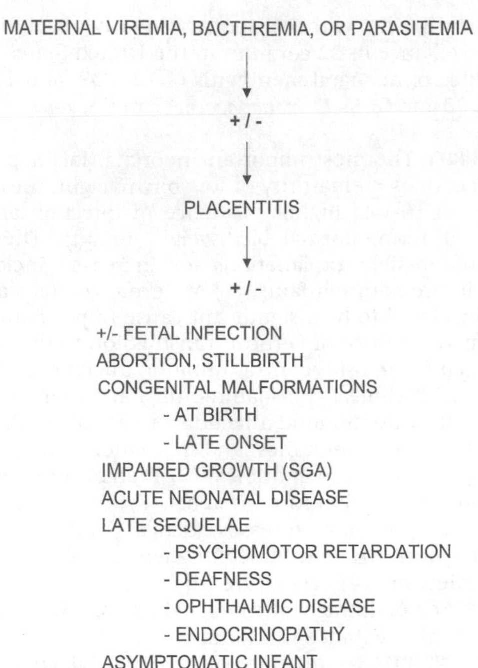

Figure 105–1 Intrauterine (transplacental) infections.

in the hospital or after discharge. Rarely, late-onset infections are due to organisms acquired from the mother's genital tract (e.g., some GBS infections).

Nosocomial infections are relatively uncommon in normal full-term infants; the rate ranges from 0.5–1.7% of term infants. They usually involve the skin and are caused by *S. aureus* or *Candida* (see Chapters 182 and 230). Conjunctivitis, an exception, is relatively common in these infants. In contrast, the rates of nosocomial infections among low birthweight infants in NICUs are higher than in any other site in the hospital and range from 20–33%; the incidence increases with the duration of hospitalization and lower gestational ages. The most common infection is **bacteremia**, usually associated with umbilical or central intravenous catheters, followed by **pneumonia**.

Various organisms may colonize infants, hospital personnel, or visiting families in the NICU and can be transmitted by direct contact or indirect contact through contaminated vehicles (intravenous fluids, medications, disinfectants, respiratory equipment, stool, breast milk, and blood). Colonization of an infant's skin, umbilicus, nasopharynx, and gastrointestinal tract by pathogenic bacteria or fungi is a common prerequisite for subsequent nosocomial infection. Antibiotics interfere with colonization by the normal flora and facilitate colonization by pathogens. Crowding and inadequate infection control techniques (handwashing between patient examinations) may also contribute to the problem.

Multiple risk factors influence the probability of nosocomial infection in the NICU. These include low birthweight, length of stay, invasive procedures, indwelling vascular catheters, ventricular shunts, endotracheal tubes, alterations in the skin and mucous membrane barriers, and frequent use of broad-spectrum antibiotics. In infants weighing less than 1,500 g, the use of intravenous lipid emulsions was the major determinant of coagulase-negative bacteremias in one nursery. Frequent use of antibiotics has led to methicillin-resistant *S. aureus*, gentamicin-resistant *E. coli*, and vancomycin-resistant enterococci.

Transmission of CMV via breast milk and blood transfusion is a significant risk for systemic infection with sequelae, particularly in infants with birthweights less than 1,500 g.

Surveillance for nosocomial infection is based on the ongoing review of nursery infections and data from the microbiology laboratory; routine surveillance to detect colonization is not indicated. Cultures should indicate the bacterial isolate and the antimicrobial sensitivity pattern. Assessment of other microbial markers (biotype, serotype, plasmid, DNA fingerprint) may be helpful in epidemics. During epidemics, investigation of possible reservoirs of infection, modes of transmission, and risk factors is necessary. Identification of colonized infants and nursery personnel may be helpful.

Those infections acquired after discharge from the nursery are called community-acquired infections. They have the same epidemiologic considerations as other community-acquired infections in infants and children, except for protection provided by maternal antibody.

105.4 Pathogenesis

Newborns may be infected at different times via three different routes (Figs. 105–1 and 105–2): in utero (transplacental), intrapartum (ascending), and post partum (nosocomial or community). In most cases, intrauterine infection is a result of clinical or subclinical maternal infection with transplacental transmission to the fetus. Infection acquired in utero may result in resorption of the embryo, abortion, stillbirth, congenital malformation, intrauterine growth retardation, premature birth, acute disease in the neonatal period, or asymptomatic

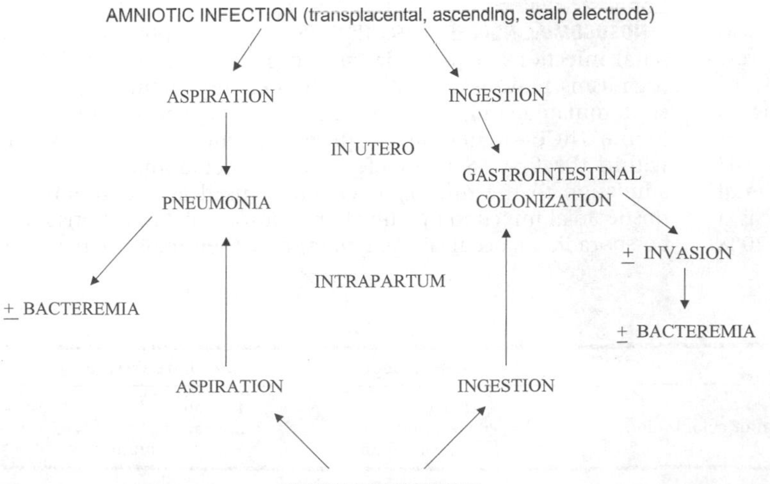

Figure 105–2 Pathways of ascending or intrapartum infections.

TABLE 105–6 The Effect of Maternal Antibody on Immunity to Transplacental and Perinatal Infections

Infection	Antibody Protective	Prevalence of Antibody	Laboratory Availability	Comment
Adenovirus	?	Moderate	Research	Many serotypes
Candida	No	High	Research	Low virulence
Chlamydia	No	Moderate	Research	Many strains
Coxsackievirus	Yes	Low	Hospital	Many strains
Cytomegalovirus	No	High	Hospital	Many strains; antibody reduces risk and severity of disease
Echovirus	Yes	Low	Research	Many strains
Epstein-Barr virus	No	High	Hospital	
Gonorrhea	No	Moderate	Research	
Group B streptococci	Yes	Low	Research	Many types; protection may be overcome by large inoculum
Hepatitis B virus	Yes	Low	Hospital	Except when HBsAg and/or HBeAg is present
Herpes simplex virus	No	Moderate	Hospital	Antibody reduces incidence and severity
HIV	No	Low	Hospital	
Measles	Yes	High	Hospital	
Mumps	Yes	High	Hospital	
Mycoplasmas	?	?	Research	Low virulence
Parvovirus	Yes	Low	Research	
Poliovirus	Yes	High	Hospital	
Rubella	Yes	High	Hospital	
Syphilis	No	Low	Hospital	
Toxoplasmosis	Yes	Moderate	Hospital	Except immunocompromised women
Varicella	Yes	High	Hospital	
Western equine encephalitis	Yes	Low	Research	

persistent infection with neurologic sequelae later in life. In some cases, there are no apparent effects on the newborn infant. The timing of infection during gestation affects outcome. First-trimester infection usually alters embryogenesis, with resulting congenital malformations. Third-trimester infection often results in active infection at the time of delivery. However, late gestational infections may lead to a delay in clinical manifestations until some time after birth (e.g., syphilis). In addition to transplacental transmission, a fetus may be infected by organisms from the vagina, invading the amniotic fluid through the cervix, with or without intact membranes.

Maternal infection is a necessary prerequisite for transplacental infections. For some etiologic agents, maternal immunity is solid and antibody is protective in the woman and her fetus (Table 105–6). For other agents, maternal antibody may ameliorate the outcome of infection or have no effect. Even without maternal antibody, transplacental transmission of infection to a fetus is variable, and the placenta often functions as an effective barrier.

Perinatal infections are acquired just before or during delivery, with vertical transmission of the microorganism from mother to newborn infant. The **amniotic infection syndrome** refers to microbial invasion of amniotic fluid, usually as a result of prolonged rupture of the chorioamniotic membrane. On occasion, amniotic infection occurs with apparently intact membranes or with a relatively brief duration of rupture. Amniotic infection may complicate fetal monitoring. Amniotic fluid infection may be asymptomatic or may produce maternal fever, with or without local or systemic signs of chorioamnionitis. The duration of membrane rupture is directly correlated with the presence of chorioamnionitis. For many years, longer than 24 hr was considered prolonged rupture of membranes, because microscopic evidence of inflammation of membranes is uniformly present when the duration of rupture exceeds 24 hr. However, at 18 hr of membrane rupture, there is a significant increase in the incidence of early-onset GBS disease. Therefore, longer than 18 hr is currently the cutoff point for increased risk of neonatal infection. Difficult or traumatic delivery and premature delivery are also associated with an increased frequency of neonatal infections.

Exposure to and aspiration of bacteria in amniotic fluid lead to congenital pneumonia or systemic infection, with manifestations becoming apparent before delivery (fetal distress, tachycardia), at delivery (perinatal asphyxia), or after a latent period of a few hours (respiratory distress, shock). Aspiration of bacteria during the birth process may lead to infection after an interval of 1–2 days.

Resuscitation at birth, particularly if it involves endotracheal intubation, insertion of an umbilical vessel catheter, or both, is associated with an increased risk of bacterial infection, possibly because of prematurity, the presence of infection at the time of birth, or impairment of normal respiratory tract clearance mechanisms.

Postnatal infections may be transmitted by direct contact from various human sources, such as the mother, family contacts, and hospital personnel; from breast milk (HIV, CMV); or from inanimate sources, such as contaminated equipment.

Most cases of **meningitis** result from hematogenous dissemination. Less often, meningitis results from contiguous spread as a result of contamination of neural tube defects, congenital sinus tracts, or penetrating wounds from fetal scalp sampling or internal fetal electrocardiographic monitors.

Cerebritis and septic infarcts are common in bacterial meningitis. Abscess formation, ventriculitis, hydrocephalus, and subdural effusions occur more often in newborn infants than in older children.

SEPSIS. The physiologic manifestations of the inflammatory response are mediated by various proinflammatory cytokines, principally tumor necrosis factor (TNF), IL-1 and IL-6, and by-products of activation of the complement and coagulation systems (see Chapter 173). Studies of newborn infants are limited, but it appears that some cytokine production may be diminished; this observation is consistent with an impaired inflammatory response. However, elevated levels of IL-6, TNF, and platelet-activating factor have been reported in newborn infants with neonatal sepsis and NEC. IL-6 appears to be the cytokine most often elevated in neonatal sepsis.

CHAPTER 106
Clinical Syndromes

106.1 Clinical Manifestations of Neonatal Infections

Infection in newborn infants may be limited to a single organ or may involve many organs (focal or systemic). Asymptomatic bacteremia occurs in infants born to women with chorioamnionitis. The infection may be mild, moderate, or severe and acute, subacute, or chronic; or it may be asymptomatic. The absence of clinical signs at the time of the initial physical examination does not preclude infection. Some infections may be asymptomatic and remain asymptomatic, (e.g., cytomegalovirus [CMV]). Others may involve an organ system and thus may require a special examination (e.g., roentgenographic changes in rubella or syphilis). Early manifestations of infection may be subtle and nonspecific, such as inability to tolerate feeding, irritability, or lethargy. Many organs and tissues alone or in combination may become infected from hematogenous spread. Nonspecific clinical manifestations of neonatal infections are listed in Table 106–1. Table 106–2 lists the signs of transplacental infections, and the manifestations of neonatal bacterial infections are found in Table 106–3.

FEVER. Only about 50% of infected newborn infants have a temperature greater than 37.8°C (axillary), and fever in newborn infants does not always signify infection. Fever may be caused by increased ambient temperature, dehydration, central nervous system (CNS) disorders, hyperthyroidism, familial dysautonomia, or ectodermal dysplasia. A single temperature elevation is infrequently associated with infection; fever sustained over 1 hr is more likely to be due to infection. Most febrile infected infants have additional signs compatible with infection, although a focus of infection may not be apparent. In premature infants, the normal body temperature is lower, and hypothermia or temperature instability is more likely to accompany infection, but some degree of temperature instability is not unusual in low birthweight infants. Acute febrile illnesses without localization later in the neonatal period may be caused by many agents including enteroviruses, respiratory syncytial virus (RSV), and herpesvirus 6.

TABLE 106–1 Presenting Signs and Symptoms of Infection in Newborn Infants

General	**Cardiovascular System**
Fever, temperature instability	Pallor; mottling; cold, clammy skin
"Not doing well"	Tachycardia
Poor feeding	Hypotension
Edema	Bradycardia
Gastrointestinal System	**Central Nervous System**
Abdominal distention	Irritability, lethargy
Vomiting	Tremors, seizures
Diarrhea	Hyporeflexia, hypotonia
Hepatomegaly	Abnormal Moro reflex
Respiratory System	Irregular respirations
Apnea, dyspnea	Full fontanel
Tachypnea, retraction	High-pitched cry
Flaring, grunting	**Hematologic System**
Cyanosis	Jaundice
Renal System	Splenomegaly
Oliguria	Pallor
	Petechiae, purpura
	Bleeding

RASH. Cutaneous manifestations of infection include impetigo, cellulitis, mastitis, omphalitis, and subcutaneous abscesses. **Ecthyma gangrenosum** is indicative of pseudomonal infection. The presence of small salmon-pink papules suggests *Listeria monocytogenes* infection. A vesicular rash is consistent with herpesvirus infection. The mucocutaneous lesions of *Candida albicans* are discussed elsewhere (Chapter 230). Petechiae and purpura may have an infectious cause. Purple papulonodular lesions are referred to as "blueberry-muffin" rash and represent **dermal erythropoiesis**. The causes include congenital viral infections (CMV, rubella, and *Parvovirus*), congenital neoplastic disease, and Rh hemolytic disease.

OMPHALITIS. Omphalitis is a unique neonatal infection resulting from inadequate care of the umbilical cord. The umbilical stump is colonized by bacteria from the maternal genital tract and the environment. Omphalitis may spread to the abdominal wall, leading to fasciitis or to the umbilical or portal vessels, the liver and peritoneum, often resulting in sepsis.

TETANUS (see Chapter 209). Neonatal tetanus is a major cause of death in Southeast Asia, Africa, and the eastern Mediterranean region; it usually results from unhygienic birth and management of the umbilical cord. In developed countries, infants are usually protected by transplacental tetanus antitoxin. The onset is usually at 3–14 days, marked by poor sucking and irritability. With the more specific signs of trismus, difficulty swallowing, spasms, and opisthotonos, diagnosis is relatively simple. Bronchopneumonia, presumably due to aspiration, is a common complication.

Treatment includes neutralization of toxin with human tetanus immunoglobulin, omphalectomy to remove the site of production of toxin, antimicrobial therapy, and management of seizures and respirations. Because penicillin may act as an agonist to tetanospasmin, metronidazole is the treatment of choice in many centers.

PNEUMONIA. Early signs and symptoms of pneumonia often are nonspecific, including poor feeding, lethargy, irritability, poor color, alteration in temperature, abdominal distention, and the overall impression that the infant is doing less well than previously. Cough indicates an abnormality, often infection, of the lower respiratory tract. As the degree of respiratory compromise increases, tachypnea, tachycardia, flaring of alae nasi, grunting, retractions, cyanosis, apnea, and progressive respiratory failure may ensue. If the infant is premature, these signs of progressive respiratory distress may be superimposed on hyaline membrane disease (HMD) or bronchopulmonary dysplasia (BPD). If an infant is being ventilated at the time of infection, the most prominent change may be the need for an increasing amount of ventilatory support.

The physical signs of pneumonia, such as dullness to percussion, change in breath sounds, and the presence of rales or rhonchi, are very difficult to appreciate in a neonate. Roentgenograms of the chest may reveal new infiltrates or an effusion, but if the neonate has underlying HMD or BPD, it usually is not possible to determine whether the radiographic changes represent a new process or worsening of the underlying process.

The progression of neonatal pneumonia can be variable. Fulminant infection is most commonly associated with group B streptococcal (GBS) septicemia in term or premature infants (see Chapter 185). Onset may be during the first hours or days of life, with the infant often manifesting rapidly progressive circulatory collapse and respiratory failure. The clinical course and radiographs of the chest may be indistinguishable from severe HMD, although with infection, systemic symptoms tend to be more severe, progression is more rapid, and less mechanical pressure is needed to provide effective ventilation.

In contrast to the rapid progression of pneumonitis caused by pyogenic organisms, older infants with community-acquired infection often have an indolent course. Onset usually is preceded by upper respiratory tract symptoms or conjunctivitis. A

TABLE 106–2 Clinical Manifestations of Transplacental Infections

Manifestation	Pathogen
Small for Gestational Age	CMV, rubella, toxoplasmosis, *Treponema pallidum, Trypanosoma cruzi,* VZV
Congenital Anatomic Defects	
Cataracts	Rubella
Heart defects	Rubella
Hydrocephalus	HSV, lymphocytic choriomeningitis virus, rubella, toxoplasmosis
Intracranial calcification	CMV, HIV, toxoplasmosis, *T. cruzi*
Limb hypoplasia	VZV
Microcephaly	CMV, HSV, rubella, toxoplasmosis
Microphthalmia	CMV, rubella, toxoplasmosis
Neonatal Organ Involvement	
Anemia	CMV, *Parvovirus, Plasmodium,* rubella, toxoplasmosis, *T. cruzi, T. pallidum*
Carditis	Coxsackieviruses, rubella, *T. cruzi*
Encephalitis	CMV, enteroviruses, HSV, rubella, toxoplasmosis, *T. cruzi, T. pallidum*
Hepatitis	CMV, enteroviruses, HSV
Hepatosplenomegaly	CMV, enteroviruses, HIV, HSV, *Plasmodium,* rubella, *T. cruzi, T. pallidum*
Hydrops	*Parvovirus, T. pallidum,* toxoplasmosis
Lymphadenopathy	CMV, HIV, rubella, toxoplasmosis, *T. pallidum*
Osteitis	Rubella, *T. pallidum*
Petechiae, purpura	CMV, enteroviruses, rubella, *T. cruzi*
Pneumonitis	CMV, enteroviruses, HSV, measles, rubella, toxoplasmosis, *T. pallidum,* VZV
Retinitis	CMV, HSV, lymphocytic choriomeningitis virus, rubella, toxoplasmosis, *T. pallidum*
Rhinitis	Enteroviruses, *T. pallidum*
Skin lesions	Entroviruses, HSV, measles, rubella, *T. pallidum,* VZV
Thrombocytopenia	CMV, enteroviruses, HIV, HSV, rubella, toxoplasmosis, *T. pallidum*
Late Sequelae	
Convulsions	CMV, enteroviruses, rubella, toxoplasmosis
Deafness	CMV, rubella, toxoplasmosis
Dental/skeletal	Rubella, *T. pallidum*
Endocrinopathies	Rubella, toxoplasmosis
Eye pathology	HSV, rubella, toxoplasmosis, *T. cruzi, T. pallidum,* VZV
Hepatitis	Hepatitis B
Mental retardation	CMV, HIV, HSV, rubella, toxoplasmosis, *T. cruzi,* VZV
Nephrotic syndrome	*Plasmodium, T. pallidum*

CMV = cytomegalovirus; VZV = varicella-zoster virus; HSV = herpes simplex virus.

nonproductive cough ensues, and the degree of respiratory compromise is variable. Fever usually is absent, and radiographic examination of the chest shows focal or diffuse interstitial pneumonitis. This infection has been called the "afebrile pneumonia syndrome" and usually is caused by *Chlamydia trachomatis,* CMV, *Ureaplasma urealyticum,* or one of the respiratory viruses. Although *Pneumocystis carinii* was implicated in the original description of this syndrome, its etiologic role now is in doubt, except in newborns infected with HIV.

SEPSIS. Neonatal sepsis, sepsis neonatorum, and neonatal septicemia are terms that have been used to describe the systemic response to infection in newborn infants. There is little agreement on the proper use of the term—that is, whether it should be restricted to bacterial infections, positive blood cultures, or severity of illness. There has been an explosion of information on the pathogenesis of sepsis and the availability of new potentially therapeutic agents, such as monoclonal antibodies to endotoxin and tumor necrosis factor (TNF), which can alter the lethal outcome of sepsis in animal experiments. However, to evaluate and use these new therapeutic modalities in children, "sepsis" requires a more rigorous definition. On adult inpatient services, particularly intensive care units, the term *systemic inflammatory response syndrome* (SIRS) is used to describe a clinical syndrome characterized by two or more of the following: (1) fever or hypothermia, (2) tachycardia, (3) tachypnea, and (4) abnormal white blood cells (WBCs) or increase in immature forms. SIRS may be a result of trauma, hemorrhagic shock, other causes of ischemia, pancreatitis, or immunologic injury. When it is a result of infection, it is termed *sepsis.* These criteria are probably not applicable to unselected infants and children and are unlikely to be applicable to newborn infants. Nevertheless, the concept of sepsis as a syndrome caused by metabolic and hemodynamic consequences of infection is logical and important. In the future, the definition of sepsis in newborn infants and in children will become more precise. At this time, criteria for neonatal sepsis should include documentation of infection in a newborn infant with a serious systemic illness in which noninfectious explanations for the abnormal pathophysiologic state are excluded or unlikely.

In patients with multisystem involvement or when the cardiorespiratory signs are consistent with severe illness, **sepsis** should be considered. Sepsis may be manifested by the signs listed in Table 106–4. The initial presentation may be limited to only one system, such as apnea, tachypnea with retractions, or tachycardia, but a full clinical and laboratory evaluation usually reveals other abnormalities (Table 106–5). Infants with suspected sepsis should be evaluated for multiorgan system disease. Metabolic acidosis is common. Hypoxemia and carbon dioxide retention may be associated with adult and congenital respiratory distress syndrome (RDS) or pneumonia.

Many newborn infants with infections do not have serious systemic physiologic abnormalities. Many infants with pneumonia and infants with stage II necrotizing enterocolitis (NEC) (see Chapter 98.2) do not have sepsis. In contrast, stage III NEC is usually accompanied by the systemic manifestations of sepsis, and urinary tract infections (UTIs) secondary to obstructive uropathy may have hematologic and hepatic abnormalities consistent with sepsis (urosepsis). Each infant should be reevaluated over time to determine whether physiologic changes secondary to infection have reached a moderate to severe level of severity that is consistent with sepsis.

Late manifestations of sepsis include signs of cerebral edema or thromboses; respiratory failure as a result of acute respiratory distress syndrome (ARDS); pulmonary hypertension; cardiac failure; renal failure; hepatocellular disease with hyperbili-

TABLE 106–3 Manifestations of Neonatal Bacterial Infections

	Time		Occurrence	
	Early Onset	*Late Onset*	*Common*	*Uncommon*
Abdomen				
Peritonitis	+	+	+	
Hepatitis	+	+		+
Adrenal abscess	+	+		+
Gallbladder hydrops	+	+		+
Brain				
Meningitis	+	+	+	
Abscess		+	+	
Subdural empyema		+	+	
Cerebritis	+	+	+	
Ventriculitis		+	+	
Cardiovascular				
Endovascular infection		+	+	
Enocarditis	+	+		+
Pericarditis	+	+		+
Myocarditis	+	+		+
Ocular				
Conjunctivitis	+	+	+	
Endophthalmitis	+	+		+
Chorioretinitis		+		+
Osteoarticular				
Arthritis	+	+		+
Osteomyelitis		+		+
Dactylitis		+		+
Respiratory Tract				
Pneumonia	+	+	+	
Ethmoiditis	+	+		+
Otitis media		+		+
Mastoiditis		+		+
Salivary glands		+		+
Retropharyngeal cellulitis		+		+
Empyema	+	+	+	
Skin, Soft Tissue				
Breast abscess	+	+	+	
Facial cellulitis	+	+		+
Adenitis		+		+
Fasciitis	+	+		+
Impetigo		+	+	
Purpura fulminans	+	+		+
Omphalitis		+		+
Scalp abscess	+	+		+
Abscess of cystic hygroma		+		+
Urinary tract infection	+	+	+	
No focus				
Bacteremia	+	+	+	
Sepsis	+	+	+	

rubinemia and elevated enzymes, prolonged prothrombin time (PT) and partial thromboplastin time (PTT); septic shock; adrenal hemorrhage with adrenal insufficiency; bone marrow failure (thrombocytopenia, neutropenia, anemia); and disseminated intravascular coagulation (DIC).

106.2 Diagnosis

The differential diagnosis in symptomatic newborn infants with primary respiratory disorders, cardiac disease, CNS injury, anemia, and metabolic abnormalities usually includes infection. The newborn infant may have been exposed to a central or peripheral intravenous line, umbilical or Foley catheter, endotracheal tube, peritoneal dialysis, or surgical procedure.

The maternal history may provide important information about maternal infection, exposure to infection in a sexual partner, maternal immunity (natural or acquired), maternal colonization, and obstetric risk factors (prematurity, prolonged ruptured membranes, maternal chorioamnionitis) (Table 106–5). Serologic screening tests may have been performed for *Treponema pallidum*, rubella, and hepatitis B virus. Maternal cultures may have been taken for *Neisseria gonorrhoeae*, GBS, herpes simplex, or *Chlamydia*.

In most cases of suspected *fetal infection*, concern is not raised until the pregnant woman has been ill for several weeks or, in retrospect, at parturition. At this time, the maternal immune response to the suspected pathogen may no longer reflect an acute infection—that is, the specific immunoglobulin (Ig) M response is no longer detectable and the IgG response has already reached a plateau. Also, many of the pathogen-specific IgM serologic assays require considerable skill to perform and tend to be less reliable than the more common IgG assays. For this reason, the results of the IgM assays can be either falsely negative or falsely positive.

If there is a high likelihood of maternal infection with a known teratogenic agent, fetal ultrasound examination is strongly recommended. If the examination demonstrates either delayed growth for gestational age or a physical abnormality, examination of a fetal blood sample may be warranted. Cordocentesis can provide a sufficient sample for both total and pathogen-specific IgM assays. The total IgM value is important because the normal fetal IgM level is less than 5 mg/dL. Any elevation in total IgM may indicate an underlying fetal infection that has stimulated the fetal immune system. Specific IgM antibody tests are available for CMV, *T. pallidum*, and toxoplasmosis. However, IgM tests are useful only when the results are strongly positive. A negative pathogen-specific IgM finding does not necessarily rule out that pathogen as a cause of fetopathy.

If the serologic studies of the mother point to a specific pathogen, it is sometimes possible to culture the organism from amniotic fluid. Amniocentesis can be performed and the fluid sent for viral culture. The presence of CMV in the amniotic fluid indicates that the fetus is infected and at high risk

TABLE 106–4 Serious Systemic Illness in Newborns (Differential Diagnosis of Neonatal Sepsis)

Infection (Sepsis)	
Bacteria:	Group B streptococci, *Escherichia coli*, *Listeria*, coagulase-negative staphylococcus, *Treponema pallidum*
Viruses:	Herpes simplex, enterovirus, adenovirus
Fungi:	*Candida*, *Malassezia*
Protozoa:	Malaria
Perinatal Asphyxia	
Respiratory	
Aspiration pneumonia:	Amniotic fluid, meconium, or gastric contents
Cardiac	
Congenital:	Hypoplastic left heart syndrome, persistent pulmonary hypertension
Acquired:	Myocarditis
Metabolic	
Hypoglycemia	
Adrenal insufficiency (congenital adrenal hyperplasia)	
Organic acidoses	
Urea cycle disorders	
Salicylate toxicity	
Neurologic	
Intracranial hemorrhage	
Hematologic	
Neonatal purpura fulminans	
Severe anemia	
Malignancies (congenital leukemia)	

TABLE 106–5 Evaluation of a Newborn for Infection or Sepsis

History (Specific Risk Factors)

Maternal infection during gestation or at parturition (type and duration of antimicrobial therapy)
- Urinary tract infection
- Chorioamnionitis

Maternal colonization with GBS, *Neisseria gonorrhoeae*, herpes simplex
Gestational age/birthweight
Multiple birth
Duration of membrane rupture
Complicated delivery
Fetal tachycardia (distress)
Age at onset (in utero, birth, early postnatal, late)
Location at onset (hospital, community)
Medical intervention
- Vascular access
- Endotracheal intubation
- Parenteral nutrition
- Surgery

Evidence for Other Diseases*

Congenital malformations (heart disease, neural tube defect)
Respiratory tract disease (HMD, aspiration)
Necrotizing enterocolitis
Metabolic disease, e.g., galactosemia

Evidence for Focal or Systemic Disease

General appearance, neurologic status
Abnormal vital signs
Organ system disease
Feeding, stools, urine output

Laboratory Studies

Evidence for Infection

Culture from a normally sterile site (blood, CSF, other)
Demonstration of a microorganism in tissue or fluid
Antigen detection (urine, CSF)
Maternal or neonatal serology (syphilis, toxoplasmosis)
Autopsy

Evidence for Inflammation

Leukocytosis, increased immature/total neutrophil count ratio
Acute-phase reactants: CRP, ESR
Cytokines: interleukin-6
Pleocytosis in CSF, synovial, or pleural fluid
Disseminated intravascular coagulation: fibrin split proucts

Evidence for Multiorgan System Disease

Metabolic acidosis: pH, Pco_2
Pulmonary function: Po_2, Pco_2
Renal function: BUN, creatinine
Hepatic injury/function: bilirubin, SGPT, SGOT, ammonia, PT, PTT
Bone marrow function: neutropenia, anemia, thrombocytopenia

**Diseases that increase the risk of infection or may overlap with signs of sepsis.*
GBS = group B streptococci; HMD = hyaline membrane disease; CSF = cerebrospinal fluid; CRP = C-reactive protein; ESR = erythrocyte sedimentation rate; Pco_2 = partial pressure of carbon dioxide; Po_2 = partial pressure of oxygen; BUN = blood urea nitrogen; SGPT = serum glutamic pyruvic transaminase; SGOT = serum glutamic oxaloacetic transaminase; PT = prothrombin time; PTT = partial thromboplastin time.

but does not always mean that the fetus will have severe sequelae. *Toxoplasma* also can be grown from amniotic fluid samples. In contrast, herpes simplex virus (HSV) and varicella-zoster virus (VZV) are rarely isolated from amniotic fluid samples. Both CMV and *Toxoplasma* also can be isolated from cordocentesis sampling. Chorionic villus sampling to obtain tissue for virus culture is usually contraindicated because of its associated high risks.

Parvovirus does not grow in the cell cultures commonly available in the virology laboratory. Furthermore, an IgM response is not always detectable in women with primary infections. When a fetus is infected with parvovirus, large quantities of viral particles are usually present in fetal serum, effusions, or amniotic fluid. The likelihood of viral visualization by electron microscopy can be increased by aggregating the viral particles with parvovirus-specific antiserum before placing the sample on a grid for examination by electron microscopy.

Polymerase chain reaction (PCR) is particularly helpful to diagnose HIV infection in cordocentesis samples and in blood samples taken from the newborn infant (see Chapter 268). PCR may also be used for diagnosis of toxoplasmosis, CMV, HSV, *Parvovirus*, rubella, and syphilis.

Neonatal infections due to toxoplasmosis, rubella, CMV, HSV, and syphilis present a diagnostic dilemma because (1) their clinical features overlap and may initially be indistinguishable, (2) disease may be inapparent, (3) maternal infection is often asymptomatic, (4) special laboratory studies may be needed, and (5) specific treatment for toxoplasmosis, syphilis, and HSV is predicated on an accurate diagnosis and may reduce significant long-term morbidity. Common shared features that should suggest the diagnosis of an intrauterine infection include prematurity, intrauterine growth retardation, and hematologic involvement (anemia, neutropenia, thrombocytopenia, petechiae, purpura), ocular signs (chorioretinitis, cataracts, keratoconjunctivitis, glaucoma, microphthalmia), CNS signs (microcephaly, hydrocephaly, intracranial calcifications), and other organ system involvement (pneumonia, myocarditis, nephritis, hepatitis with hepatosplenomegaly, jaundice), or nonimmune hydrops.

Physical examination shortly after birth can identify a **congenital infection**, either acute or chronic. Chronic signs include microcephaly, hydrocephaly, intracranial calcification, retinitis, hepatomegaly, lymphadenopathy and splenomegaly, implicating infection via the transplacental route (see Table 106–2). Acute congenital infection usually presents as a serious illness in an infant with low Apgar scores, CNS depression, and respiratory insufficiency.

Late-onset infection with *Candida* species should be considered in very low birthweight infants who develop abnormal blood glucose values and leukocytosis. Risk factors include intravenous alimentation and exposure to antimicrobial therapy.

Diagnostic studies in newborns with suspected chronic intrauterine infection should specifically test each diagnostic consideration.

When the clinical presentation suggests an acute infection and the focus is unclear, additional studies should be performed. These include, in addition to blood cultures, a lumbar puncture, urine examination and culture, gastric aspirate for Gram stain and culture, and a chest roentgenogram. Urine should be collected by catheterization or suprapubic aspiration; urine culture for bacteria can be omitted in systemic early-onset infections because hematogenous spread to the urinary tract is rare at this time. Examination of the buffy coat with Gram or methylene blue stain may demonstrate intracellular pathogens. Demonstration of bacteria and inflammatory cells in Gram-stained gastric aspirates on the 1st day of life may reflect maternal amnionitis, which is a risk factor for early-onset infection. Stains of endotracheal secretions in infants with early-onset pneumonia may demonstrate intracellular bacteria, and cultures may reveal either pathogens or upper respiratory tract flora. Careful examination of the placenta should be helpful in diagnosis of both chronic and acute intrauterine infections.

Diagnostic evaluations may be indicated for **asymptomatic infants** because of maternal chorioamnionitis. The probability of neonatal infection and subsequent neonatal sepsis correlates with the degree of prematurity and bacterial contamination of amniotic fluid. In an asymptomatic term infant whose mother has chorioamnionitis, two blood cultures should be obtained and a gastric aspirate should be examined to confirm the maternal diagnosis and identify presumptively the organisms by Gram stain. Presumptive treatment should be initiated. A lumbar puncture is not necessary because infants with bacterial meningitis are almost always symptomatic. If the blood culture result is positive or if the infant becomes symptomatic, lumbar puncture should then be performed. If the mother has been treated with antibiotics for chorioamnionitis, the newborn's blood culture result is usually negative, and the clinician must rely on observation and other laboratory tests.

The diagnosis of **pneumonia** in a neonate usually is presumptive; microbiologic proof of infection generally is lacking because lung tissue is not easily cultured. Although some rely on the results of bacteriologic culture of material obtained from the trachea as "proof" of cause, the interpretation of such cultures is fraught with pitfalls. These cultures often simply reflect upper respiratory tract commensal organisms, and they have no etiologic significance. Even cultures obtained by bronchoalveolar lavage in a neonate are unreliable because the tiny bronchoscopes used in neonates cannot be protected from contamination as they are introduced into the distal airways. Short of tissue obtained by lung biopsy, the only reliable bacteriologic cultures are those obtained from blood or pleural fluid. Unfortunately, blood culture results usually are negative, and sufficient pleural fluid for culture rarely is present. Interpretation of fungal cultures is associated with the same problems as for bacterial cultures. Cultures of respiratory secretions for *U. urealyticum* and other genital *Mycoplasma* are of little value because normal neonates often are colonized with these agents as a result of contamination with secretions from the maternal genital tract. Cultures for respiratory viruses and *C. trachomatis* may be valuable; they are never indigenous flora, and their isolation therefore suggests an etiologic role.

Serologic tests may be helpful in evaluating neonates with suspected pneumonia. Although there are no useful serologic tests for bacteria or fungi, reliable tests for respiratory viruses and *C. trachomatis* are available. Serologic tests for *U. urealyticum* are complicated and technically demanding and therefore are not clinically useful at this time.

Other tests of potential value in evaluating neonates with possible infectious pneumonitis are discussed under diagnosis of infections (see Chapter 175).

The differential diagnosis of pneumonitis in neonates is broad and includes HMD, meconium aspiration syndrome, transient tachypnea of the newborn, diaphragmatic hernia, congenital heart disease, persistent fetal circulation, and BPD.

The diagnosis of **meningitis** is confirmed by examination of the cerebrospinal fluid (CSF) and identification of a bacterium, virus, or fungus by culture or antigen detection. Blood culture and complete blood count are part of the initial evaluation because 70–85% of neonates with meningitis have positive results of a blood culture. The incidence of positive blood cultures is highest with early-onset sepsis and meningitis. Infants with bacteremia should have a CSF examination and culture.

Lumbar puncture may be deferred in a severely ill infant if the lumbar puncture would further compromise respiratory status. In these situations, blood culture and antigen detection assays should be performed and treatment initiated for presumed meningitis until a lumbar puncture can be safely performed.

Normal, uninfected infants from 0–4 wk may have elevated CSF protein levels = 84 ± 45 mg/dL, glucose = 46 ± 10, and elevated CSF leukocyte counts = 11 ± 10 with the 90th percentile = 22. The percent of polymorphonuclear leukocytes = 2.2 ± 3.8, with 90th percentile = 6. The upper limit of absolute neutrophil count (ANC) = 3/mm^3. Preterm infants may develop elevated CSF protein levels and leukocyte counts and hypoglycorrhachia after intraventricular hemorrhage. Many nonpyogenic congenital infections also can produce asymptomatic alterations of CSF protein and leukocytes (toxoplasmosis, CMV, syphilis, HIV).

The Gram stain of CSF yields a positive result in the majority of patients with bacterial meningitis. The leukocyte count is usually elevated, with a predominance of neutrophils (>70–90%); the number is often greater than 1,000 but may be less than 100 in infants with neutropenia or early in the disease. Microorganisms are recovered from most patients who have not been pretreated with antibiotics. Bacteria have also been isolated from CSF that did not have an abnormal number of cells (<25) or an abnormal protein level (<200 mg/dL). This is more typical of GBS meningitis but emphasizes the importance of performing a culture and Gram stain on all CSF specimens. Contamination of CSF by bacteremia in a traumatic lumbar puncture is another consideration. Culture-negative meningitis may occur with antibiotic pretreatment, infection with *Mycobacterium hominis, U. urealyticum*, or *Bacteroides fragilis*, a brain abscess, enterovirus infection, or HSV.

Head ultrasonography or CT scan with contrast enhancement may be helpful in diagnosing ventriculitis and brain abscess. Neonatal HSV meningitis may be confirmed by isolation of the virus from the CSF or other site (skin, eye, mouth) or by HSV antigen or DNA detection.

Documentation of infection is the first diagnostic criterion that must be met for **sepsis** (see Table 106–5). It is important to note that patients with bacterial sepsis may have negative results of blood cultures, and thus other approaches to identification of infection should be taken. The total neutrophil count and the ratio of immature to total neutrophils provide some diagnostic information but have limitations in sensitivity and specificity. Neutropenia is more common than neutrophilia in severe neonatal sepsis, but it also occurs in association with maternal hypertension, neonatal sensitization, periventricular hemorrhage, seizures, surgery, and possibly hemolysis. A ratio of immature neutrophils to total neutrophils of 0.16 or greater suggests bacterial infection. Thrombocytopenia is a nonspecific indicator of infection. Tests to demonstrate an inflammatory response include erythrocyte sedimentation rate (ESR), C-reactive protein (CRP), haptoglobin, fibrinogen, nitroblue tetrazolium dye, interleukin-6 (IL-6), and leukocyte alkaline phosphatase. Procalcitonin and IL-6 appear to have some promise for identification of sepsis, particularly in determining which infants require a complete course of therapy in the absence of positive culture results.

Serious systemic illness in newborn infants (see Table 106–4) may be caused by perinatal asphyxia or by respiratory tract, cardiac, metabolic, neurologic, or hematologic diseases. Sepsis occurs in a small proportion of all neonatal infections. Results of blood cultures may be negative, increasing the difficulty in establishing infection etiologically. Finally, infection with or without sepsis may be present concurrently with a noninfectious illness in newborn infants, children, or adults.

Criteria for the magnitude of physiologic change in newborn infants with sepsis are not currently defined but should be consistent with the systemic effect of endogenous mediators on one or more organ systems. For example, the effect of sepsis from pneumonia on respiratory function may be due to ARDS as well as the local inflammatory response in the lung. Thus, a work-up for sepsis should include the laboratory studies listed in Table 106–5.

106.3 Laboratory Findings

The acronym *TORCH* refers to *t*oxoplasmosis, *o*ther agents, *r*ubella, *C*MV, and *H*SV. It was modified to *STORCH* to include syphilis. Although the term may be helpful in remembering some of the etiologic agents of neonatal infections, the TORCH battery of serologic tests has a poor diagnostic yield, and the appropriate diagnostic studies should be selected for each etiologic agent under consideration. CMV and HSV require cultural methods.

Neonatal *IgG antibody titers* are often difficult to interpret because IgG is acquired from the mother by transplacental passage and neonatal *IgM titers* to specific pathogens are technically difficult to perform and are not universally available. IgM titers to specific pathogens have high specificity but only moderate sensitivity; they should not be used to preclude infection. Paired maternal and fetal-neonatal IgG titers with higher newborn IgG levels or rising IgG titers during infancy may be used to diagnose some congenital infections. Total cord blood IgM, IgA (both are not actively transported across the placenta to the fetus), or the presence of *IgM-rheumatoid factor* in neonatal serum has been used as a screening tool to identify infants at risk for any intrauterine infection. Measurement of total IgM has a high rate of both false-positive and false-negative results.

Identification of a bacterial or fungal infection may be made by isolating the etiologic agent from a body fluid that is normally sterile (blood, CSF, urine, joint fluid), by demonstrating endotoxin or bacterial antigen in a body fluid (CSF, urine, or serum), or by demonstrating infection in the placenta or at autopsy. It is preferable to obtain two specimens for **blood culture** by venipuncture from different sites to avoid confusion caused by skin contamination. Samples should be obtained from an umbilical catheter only at the time of initial insertion. A peripheral venous sample should also be obtained when samples for cultures are drawn from central venous catheters. Blood cultures performed by radiometric methods may demonstrate growth within 24–72 hr. Although blood cultures are usually the basis for a diagnosis of bacterial infection, the bacteremic phase of the illness may be missed by poor timing or blood sample size. Low-level bacteremia (<10 colony-forming units/mL) has been observed in a majority of infants from birth to 2 mo with positive cultures. More cases of bacteremia were detected with greater than 2 mL of blood inoculated into two or more culture devices. Both conventional broth culture and new systems (BACTEC, ISOLATOR) may be used. Although anaerobes account for about 2% of isolates from infected newborns, anaerobic cultures might be limited to infants with risk factors for anaerobic infection such as mothers with cerclage, early-onset disease (maternal vaginal source), omphalitis, and NEC. Avoiding cultures from heelsticks, umbilical vessels, and other intravascular catheters minimizes questions of contaminated cultures. Depending on the acuteness and severity of infection, performing more than one blood culture may increase the likelihood of detection and reduce the confusion over interpretation when coagulase-negative staphylococci or other commensal organisms are cultured. Focal infections that produce systemic manifestations such as meningitis, arthritis, and UTIs may be diagnosed by positive culture results from specific, normally sterile sites in the absence of positive blood culture results. Bacterial pneumonia has been reported at autopsy in infants with negative results of blood cultures before antimicrobial therapy.

Interpretation of *tests for bacterial antigen* may also be difficult. Latex particle agglutination and counterimmunoelectrophoresis are used for identification of GBS and *E. coli* K1 capsular polysaccharides in biologic fluids. The commercially available antigen detection kits are not as sensitive as blood cultures, and false-positive results may occur, particularly errors due to contamination of urine collected in bags. Because urine is an excellent fluid for use in antigen detection, this test should be confirmed with specimens collected by suprapubic aspiration or catheterization. Antigen detection is most useful in the presence of prior antimicrobial therapy.

DNA probes are currently under investigation for the diagnosis of rubella, CMV, HSV, enteroviruses, HIV, parvovirus B19, syphilis, and toxoplasmosis using amniotic fluid samples and other biologic fluids.

The *total WBC count and differential* and the *ratio of immature to total neutrophils* provide immediately predictive information when compared with age standards. Neutropenia is more common than neutrophilia in severe neonatal sepsis, but neutropenia also occurs in association with maternal hypertension, preeclampsia, intrauterine growth retardation, neonatal sensitization, NEC, periventricular hemorrhage, seizures, surgery, and possibly hemolysis. An immature neutrophil–total ratio of 0.16 or greater suggests bacterial infection. Systemic infections with CMV, HSV, and enteroviruses frequently involve the liver. If these infections are suspected, biochemical studies should be performed.

106.4 Treatment

Treatment of suspected neonatal infection is determined by the pattern of disease and the organisms that are common for the age of the infant and the flora of the nursery. Once *bacterial infection* has been suspected and appropriate cultures have been obtained, intravenous or intramuscular antibiotic therapy should be instituted immediately. **Initial empirical treatment** of early-onset and late-onset community-acquired bacterial infections should consist of ampicillin and an aminoglycoside (usually gentamicin). Nosocomial infections acquired in a neonatal intensive care unit (NICU) are more likely to be caused by staphylococci, various Enterobacteriaceae, *Pseudomonas*, or *Candida*. Thus, an antistaphylococcal drug, nafcillin for *S. aureus* or vancomycin for coagulase-negative staphylococci (CONS), should be substituted for ampicillin. A history of recent antimicrobial therapy or the presence of antibiotic-resistant infections in the NICU suggests the need for a different aminoglycoside agent (amikacin), and vancomycin is used for methicillin-resistant staphylococci. When the history or the presence of necrotic skin lesions suggests *Pseudomonas* infection, initial therapy should be ticarcillin or carbenicillin and gentamicin. Doses of the commonly used antibiotics are provided in Table 106–6. Peak and trough levels of gentamicin (peak 15–20 mg/mL; trough <2 mg/mL) and vancomycin (peak 15–30 mg/mL; trough <10 mg/mL) are useful to ensure therapeutic levels and minimize toxicity if administered for more than 2–3 days. The increasing use of vancomycin to treat CONS must be balanced against the risk of developing vancomycin-resistant enterococci.

Once the pathogen has been identified and the antibiotic sensitivities determined, the most appropriate drug(s) should be selected. For most of the gram-negative enteric bacteria, ampicillin and an aminoglycoside, or a third-generation cephalosporin (cefotaxime or ceftazidime) should be used. Enterococci should be treated with both a penicillin (ampicillin or piperacillin) and an aminoglycoside, because synergism has been demonstrated with this combination of antibiotics in many strains. Ampicillin alone is adequate for *L. monocytogenes*, and penicillin suffices for GBS. Clindamycin or metronidazole is appropriate for anaerobic infections.

Third-generation cephalosporins such as cefotaxime are valuable additions for treating documented neonatal sepsis and meningitis because (1) the minimal inhibitory concentrations needed for treatment of gram-negative enteric bacilli are much lower than those for the aminoglycosides; (2) excellent penetration into the CSF occurs in the presence of inflamed meninges; and (3) much higher doses can be given. The end result is much higher bactericidal titers in serum and CSF than are achievable with ampicillin-aminoglycoside combinations. However, cephalosporins should not be used alone as empirical therapy or indiscriminantly because they have only modest activity against *S. aureus* and *L. monocytogenes* and enterococci are uniformly resistant. Moreover, rapid emergence of resistant organisms is possible with frequent use in a NICU.

Therapy for most infections should be continued for a total of 7–10 days or for at least 5–7 days after a clinical response has occurred. The course of treatment for meningitis caused by GBS is usually for 14 days and for a minimum of 14 days after sterilization of the CSF in gram-negative meningitis. A blood culture taken 24–48 hr after initiation of therapy should yield negative results. If the culture results are positive, the possibility of an infected indwelling catheter, endocarditis, an

TABLE 106–6 Dosages of Antibiotics Commonly Prescribed for Newborns*

		Dosages (mg/kg) and Intervals of Administration				
		Weight <1,200 g	*Weight 1,200–2,000 g*		*Weight >2,000 g*	
Antibiotics	**Routes**	**Age 0–4 wk**	**Age 0–7 days**	**>7 days**	**Age 0–7 days**	**>7 days**
Amikacin†	IV, IM	7.5 q18–24hr	7.5 q12–18hr	7.5 q8–12hr	10 q12hr	10 q8hr
Ampicillin	IV, IM					
Meningitis		50 q12hr	50 q12hr	50 q8hr	50 q8hr	50 q6hr
Other diseases		25 q12hr	25 q12hr	25 q8hr	25 q8hr	25 q6hr
Aztreonam	IV, IM	30 q12hr	30 q12hr	30 q8hr	30 q8hr	30 q6hr
Cefazolin	IV, IM	20 q12hr	20 q12hr	20 q12hr	20 q12hr	20 q8hr
Cefotaxime	IV, IM	50 q12hr	50 q12hr	50 q8hr	50 q12hr	50 q8hr
Ceftazidime	IV, IM	50 q12hr	50 q12hr	50 q8hr	50 q8hr	50 q8hr
Ceftriaxone	IV, IM	50 q24hr	50 q24hr	50 q24hr	50 q24hr	75 q24hr
Cephalothin	IV	20 q12hr	20 q12h	20 q8hr	20 q8hr	20 q6hr
Chloramphenicol‡	IV, PO	25 q24hr	25 q24hr	25 q24hr	25 q24hr	25 q12hr
Clindamycin	IV, IM, PO	5 q12hr	5 q12hr	5 q8hr	5 q8hr	5 q6hr
Erythromycin	PO	10 q12hr	10 q12hr	10 q8hr	10 q12hr	10 q8hr
Gentamicin	IV, IM	2.5 q18–24hr	2.5 q12–18hr	2.5 q8hr	2.5 q12hr	2.5 q8hr
Imipenem	IV, IM	20 q18–24hr	20 q12hr	20 q12hr	20 q12hr	20 q8hr
Kanamycin	IV, IM	7.5 q18–24hr	7.5 q12–18hr	7.5 q8–12hr	10 q12h	10 q8hr
Methicillin	IV, IM					
Meningitis		50 q12hr	50 q12hr	50 q8hr	50 q8hr	50 q6hr
Other diseases		25 q12hr	25 q12hr	25 q8hr	25 q8hr	25 q6hr
Metronidazole	IV, PO	7.5 q48hr	7.5 q12hr	7.5 q12hr	7.5 q12hr	15 q12hr
Mezlocillin	IV, IM	75 q12hr	75 q12hr	75 q8hr	75 q12hr	75 q8hr
Nafcillin	IV	25 q12hr	25 q12hr	25 q8hr	25 q8hr	25 q6hr
Netilmicin§	IV, IM	2.5 q18–24hr	2.5 q12–18hr	2.5 q8–12hr	2.5 q12hr	2.5 q8hr
Oxacillin	IV, IM	25 q12hr	25 q12hr	30 q8hr	25 q8hr	25 q6hr
Penicillin G	IV					
Meningitis		50,000 U q12hr	50,000 U q12hr	75,000 U q8hr	50,000 U q8hr	50,000 U q6hr
Other diseases		25,000 U q12hr	25,000 U q12hr	25,000 U q8hr	25,000 U q8hr	25,000 U q6hr
Penicillin G	IM					
Benzathine			50,000 U (one dose)	50,000 U (one dose)	50,000 U (one dose)	50,000 U (one dose)
Procaine			50,000 U q24hr	50,000 U q24hr	50,000 U q24hr	50,000 U q24hr
Ticarcillin	IV, IM	75 q12hr	75 q12hr	75 q8hr	75 q8hr	75 q6hr
Tobramycin†	IV, IM	2.5 q18–24hr	2.5 q12–18hr	2.5 q8–12hr	2.5 q12hr	2.5 q8hr
Vancomycin‖	IV	15 q24hr	10 q12–18hr	15 q8–12hr	15 q12hr	15 q8hr

Recommendations for infants weighing <1,000 g based on Prober et al: Pediatr Infect Dis J 9:111, 1990.
**Adapted from Nelson JD: Pocketbook of Pediatric Antimicrobial Therapy, 12th ed. Baltimore, Williams & Wilkins, 1997.*
†Aminoglycoside levels should be monitored if therapy continues >3 days. Optimal peak levels 6–8 μg/mL, trough < 2 μg/mL.
‡Serum levels are highly variable. Chloramphenicol should be given to newborns only if serum levels can be monitored.
§0.5 mg/kg/24 hr can increase to 1 mg/kg/24 hr if needed or give every other day. Treat for cumulative dose of 10–30 mg/kg.
‖Because of variable pharmacokinetics, vancomycin levels should be monitored if therapy continues >3 days. Optimal peak levels 20–30 μg/mL, trough < 10 μg/mL.

infected thrombus, an occult abscess, subtherapeutic antibiotic levels, or resistant organisms should be considered. A change in antibiotics, longer duration of therapy, or removal of the catheter may be indicated.

Antimicrobial therapy is often begun presumptively on the basis of nonspecific clinical findings, and cultures are subsequently sterile. The use of antifungal therapy should be considered in very low birthweight infants who have mucosal colonization with *C. albicans* and who are at high risk for invasive disease.

Because a negative blood culture result does not preclude bacterial infection, the clinician must decide whether an infection is likely and antibiotics should be continued. With another explanation for the clinical findings and normal laboratory data (neutrophils, ESR, CRP, IL-6), infection is unlikely and antibiotics may be discontinued.

Treatment of newborn infants whose mothers received antibiotics during labor should be individualized. If in utero infection is likely, then treatment of the infant should be continued until there is evidence that there was no infection (the infant remains asymptomatic for 24–72 hr) or there is clinical and laboratory evidence of recovery. Antigen detection tests may be helpful in symptomatic infants but are not indicated in asymptomatic infants. The size of the bacterial inoculum needed to produce a positive test result in urine should lead to signs of infection.

For **pneumonia** presenting in the first 7–10 days of life a combination of ampicillin and an aminoglycoside or cefotaxime is appropriate. Nosocomial pneumonia, generally manifested after this time, can be treated empirically with methicillin or vancomycin and a third-generation cephalosporin. *Pseudomonas* pneumonia should be treated with an aminoglycoside combined with ticarcillin or ceftazidime. Pneumonia caused by *C. trachomatis* is treated with either erythromycin or trimethoprim-sulfamethoxazole; *U. urealyticum* infection is treated with erythromycin. Viral pneumonia caused by respiratory syncytial virus may respond to treatment with aerosolized ribavirin, and influenzavirus infection can be treated with amantadine.

In addition to antimicrobial therapy, oxygen or ventilator support may be necessary if hypoxia or apnea ensue. For the most desperately ill neonates with pneumonitis, extracorporeal membrane oxygenation may be valuable. Empyema is usually managed with closed chest drainage.

Presumptive antimicrobial therapy of **bacterial meningitis** should include ampicillin in maximum doses and cefotaxime or ampicillin and gentamicin unless staphylococci are likely, which are an indication for vancomycin. Susceptibility testing of gram-negative enteric organisms is important because resistance to cephalosporins and aminoglycosides occurs. Most aminoglycosides administered by parenteral routes do not achieve sufficiently high antibiotic levels in the lumbar CSF or ventricles to inhibit growth of gram-negative bacilli. Although intraventricular administration of aminoglycosides has been proposed as therapy for gram-negative meningitis and ventriculitis, many authorities recommend a combination of intravenous ampicillin and a third-generation cephalosporin for the treatment of neonatal gram-negative meningitis. Cephalosporins should not be used as empirical monotherapy because *L. monocytogenes* is resistant to all cephalosporins.

Meningitis due to GBS usually responds within 24–48 hr and should be treated for 14–21 days. Gram-negative bacilli may continue to grow from repeated CSF samples for 72–96 hr after therapy despite the use of appropriate antibiotics. Treatment of gram-negative meningitis should be continued for 21 days or for at least 14 days after sterilization of the CSF, whichever is longer. Meningitis due to *Pseudomonas aeruginosa* infection should be treated with ceftazidime. Metronidazole is the treatment of choice for infection caused by *B. fragilis.* Prolonged antibiotic administration, with or without needle drainage for treatment and diagnosis, is indicated for neonatal cerebral abscesses. CT scans are indicated for patients with suspected ventriculitis, hydrocephalus, or cerebral abscess (initial and follow-up assessments) and for those with an unexpectedly complicated course (prolonged coma, focal neurologic deficits, persistent or recurrent fever). Neonatal herpes meningoencephalitis should be treated with acyclovir, and empirical therapy should be considered in symptomatic infants with a CSF mononuclear pleocytosis. Although no definitive studies have been conducted, some clinicians use intravenous immunoglobulin (IVIG) to treat enteroviral meningoencephalitis. Treatment of candidal meningitis is discussed in Chapter 230.

Supportive care includes anticonvulsants for seizures and management of cerebral edema, inappropriate antidiuretic hormone secretion, and hydrocephalus. Although monitoring of gentamicin and vancomycin drug levels is currently recommended, modification of these guidelines is likely.

Treatment of **sepsis** may be divided into antimicrobial therapy for the suspected or known pathogen and supportive care. Fluids, electrolytes, and glucose levels should be monitored carefully with correction of hypovolemia, hyponatremia, hypocalcemia, and hypoglycemia and limitation of fluids if there is inappropriate antidiuretic hormone secretion. Shock, hypoxia, and metabolic acidosis should be identified and managed with inotropic agents, fluid resuscitation, and mechanical ventilation. Corticosteroids should be administered for adrenal insufficiency. Adequate oxygenation of tissues should be maintained; ventilatory support is frequently necessary for respiratory failure caused by congenital pneumonia, persistent fetal circulation, or ARDS (shock lung). ARDS should be treated with surfactant (see Chapter 65). Refractory hypoxia and shock may require extracorporeal membrane oxygenation, which has reduced mortality rates in full-term infants with septic shock and primary pulmonary hypertension. Hyperbilirubinemia should be monitored and treated with exchange transfusion because the risk of kernicterus increases in the presence of sepsis and meningitis. Parenteral nutrition should be considered for infants who cannot sustain enteral feedings.

DIC may complicate neonatal septicemia. Platelet counts, hemoglobin, PT, PTT, and fibrin split products should be monitored. DIC may be treated by management of the primary sepsis, but if bleeding occurs, DIC may be treated with fresh frozen plasma, platelet transfusions, or whole blood.

Because neutrophil storage pool depletion has been associated with a poor prognosis, a number of clinical trials of polymorphonuclear replacement therapy have been conducted, with variable results. Sepsis that is unresponsive to antibiotics with persistent neutropenia may be an indication for granulocyte transfusion, but this therapy poses logistical problems and potential side effects. The use of granulocyte-macrophage colony-stimulating factor (GM-CSF) has not been effective but is still under investigation. IVIG may be considered as adjunctive therapy but has not been demonstrated to be effective. Selected IVIG containing specific antibodies and monoclonal antibodies is being studied.

It is important to remember that nonbacterial infectious agents can produce the syndrome of neonatal sepsis. HSV infection requires specific treatment (Chapter 245), as does systemic candidal infection (Chapter 230).

106.5 Complications and Prognosis

The sequelae of intrauterine infections due to specific pathogens are described in their respective chapters. In general, complications of neonatal infections may be divided into those related to the inflammatory process per se and those that complicate concomitant neonatal problems such as respiratory function and fluid and electrolyte management.

Complications of bacteremic infections include endocarditis, septic emboli, abscess formation, septic joints with residual disability, and osteomyelitis and bone destruction. Recurrent bacteremia may occur in fewer than 5% of patients. Candidemia may lead to vasculitis, endocarditis, and endophthalmitis as well as abscesses in the kidneys, liver, lungs, and brain.

Mortality rates from the sepsis syndrome depend on the definition of sepsis. In adults, the mortality rate approaches 50%, and the rate in newborn infants is probably at least that high. However, reported mortality rates in neonatal sepsis are as low as 20% because all bacteremic infections are included in the definition. Sequelae of sepsis may result from septic shock, DIC, or organ failure.

The case fatality rate for neonatal bacterial meningitis is between 20 and 25%. Many of these cases have associated sepsis. Immediate complications of meningitis include ventriculitis, cerebritis, and brain abscess. Late complications of meningitis occur in 40–50% of survivors. These include hearing loss, abnormal behavior, developmental delay, cerebral palsy, focal motor disability, seizure disorders, and hydrocephalus. CT has demonstrated cerebritis, brain abscess, infarct, subdural effusions, cortical atrophy, and diffuse encephalomalacia in newborns surviving meningitis. A number of these sequelae may be encountered in infants with sepsis without meningitis as a result of cerebritis or septic shock.

106.6 Prevention

A number of intrauterine infections are preventable through maternal immunization. These include hepatitis B, polio, rubella, tetanus, and VZV. CMV vaccines are under study. Toxoplasmosis is preventable with appropriate diet and avoidance of exposure to cat feces. Malaria during pregnancy can be minimized with chemoprophylaxis.

Neonatal tetanus is also preventable with proper care of the umbilical cord. Vertical transmission of GBS (Chapter 185) and *Chlamydia* (Chapter 222) may be interrupted by intrapartum chemoprophylaxis. Transmission of HIV may be diminished with maternal treatment (Chapter 268).

Aggressive management of suspected maternal chorioamnionitis with antibiotics before delivery, rapid delivery of the infant, and selective intrapartum chemoprophylaxis appears to have decreased the morbidity and mortality rates of ampicillin-sensitive neonatal bacterial infections, primarily group B streptococcal infections (see Chapter 185).

Prevention of neonatal nosocomial infection is complex and includes a 2-min scrub before entering the nursery, 15-sec washing between patients, scrub suits for nurses and residents, adequate nursing staff, avoidance of overcrowding, and specific isolation precautions (see Chapters 105 and 302). Control of outbreaks depends on the pathogen and epidemiology (see Chapter 105). Commonly used measures include investigation of the extent of colonization in infants and caretakers, a search for a common source or reservoir, cohorting of infants and caretakers, changes in handwashing solutions and protocols, and antimicrobial prophylaxis. Cord care, equipment sterilization, and handwashing are essential, but gowns have not been consistently demonstrated to be effective.

Three of four multicenter studies of IVIG in prevention of

late-onset infections in low birthweight infants have shown no significant effect. When single and multicenter studies were included in a meta-analysis, a modest significant benefit was noted. However, none of the large trials have shown a difference in mortality or duration of hospitalization, and a National Institutes of Health Consensus Statement concluded that IVIG should not be routinely given to low birthweight infants.

Ahmed A, Hickey SM, Ehrett S, et al: Cerebrospinal fluid values in the term neonate. Pediatr Infect Dis J 15:298, 1996.

Chang HJ, Miller HL, Watkins N, et al: An epidemic of *Malassezia pachydermatis* in an intensive care nursery associated with colonization of health care workers' pet dogs. N Engl J Med 338:706, 1998.

Davies PA, Rudd PT: Neonatal meningitis. Clin Dev Med 1994.

Engle WD, Rosenfeld CR, Mouzinho A, et al: Circulating neutrophils in septic preterm neonates: Comparison of two reference ranges. Pediatrics 99:10, 1997.

Gaynes RP, Edwards JR, Jarvis WR, et al: Nosocomial infections among neonates in high-risk nurseries in the United States. Pediatrics 98:357, 1996.

Horowitz HW, Kilchevsky E, Haber S, et al: Perinatal transmission of the agent of human granulocyte ehrlichiosis. N Engl J Med 339:375, 1998.

Huskins WC, Goldman DA: Nosocomial infections. *In*: Feigin RD, Cherry JD (eds): Textbook of Pediatric Infectious Diseases, 4th ed. Philadelphia, WB Saunders, 1998, pp 2545–2584.

Kellogg JA, Ferrentino FL, Goodstein MH, et al: Frequency of low level bacteremia in infants from birth to two months of age. Pediatr Infect Dis J 16:381, 1997.

Klein JO, Remington JS: Current concepts of infections of the fetus and newborn infant. *In*: Remington JS, Klein JO (eds): Infectious Diseases of the Fetus and Newborn Infant, 4th ed. Philadelphia, WB Saunders, 1995, pp 1–19.

Lewis DB, Wilson CB: Developmental immunology and role of host defenses in neonatal susceptibility to infection. *In*: Remington JS, Klein JO (eds): Infectious Diseases of the Fetus and Newborn Infant, 4th ed. Philadelphia, WB Saunders, 1995, pp 20–98.

Litwin CM, Hill H: Serologic and DNA-based testing for congenital and perinatal infections. Pediatr Infect Dis J 16:1166, 1997.

Ortego-Barria E: *Trypansoma* species (trypanosomiasis) *In*: Long SS, Pickering LK, Prober CG (eds): Principles and Practice of Pediatric Infectious Diseases. New York, Churchill Livingstone, 1997, pp 1451–1458.

Panero A, Pacifico L, Rossi N, et al: Interleukin 6 in neonates with early and late onset infection. Pediatr Infect Dis J 16:370, 1997.

Powell KR, Marcy SM: Laboratory aids for diagnosis of neonatal sepsis. *In*: Remington JS, Klein JO (eds). Infectious Diseases of the Fetus and Newborn Infant, 4th ed. Philadelphia, WB Saunders, 1995, p 1223.

Prober CG: Clinical approach to the infected neonate. *In*: Long SS, Pickering LK, Prober CG (eds): Principles and Practice of Pediatric Infectious Diseases. New York, Churchill Livingstone, 1997, pp 603–605.

Sáez-Llorens X, McCracken GH Jr: Clinical pharmacology of antibacterial agents. *In*: Remington JS, Klein JO (eds). Infectious Diseases of the Fetus and Newborn Infant, 4th ed. Philadelphia, WB Saunders, 1995, pp 1287–1386.

Schuchat A, Robinson K, Wenger JD: Bacterial meningitis in the United States in 1995. N Engl J Med 337:970, 1997.

Shackelford PG: Immunologic development and susceptibility to infection. *In*: Long SS, Pickering LK, Prober CG (eds): Principles and Practice of Pediatric Infectious Diseases. New York, Churchill Livingstone, 1997, pp 596–602.

Silver MM, Hellmann J, Zielenska M, et al: Anemia, blueberry-muffin rash, and hepatomegaly in a newborn infant. J Pediatr 128:579, 1996.

Stiehm ER: Human intravenous immunoglobulin in primary and secondary antibody deficiencies. Pediatr Infect Dis J 16:696, 1997.

Stoll BJ: The global impact of neonatal infection. Clin Perinatol 24:1, 1997.

Stoll BJ, Gordon T, Korones SB, et al: Early-onset sepsis in very low birth weight neonates: A report from the National Institute of Child Health and Human Development Neonatal Research Network. J Pediatr 129:72, 1996.

Stoll BJ, Gordon T, Korones SB, et al: Late-onset sepsis in very low birth weight neonates: A report from the National Institute of Child Health and Human Development Neonatal Research Network. J Pediatr 129:63, 1996.

PART XII

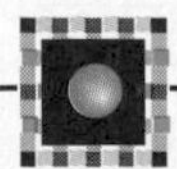

Special Health Problems During Adolescence

Renée R. Jenkins

CHAPTER 107

The Epidemiology of Adolescent Disease

Behavioral and psychosocial risks, including injuries, account for a substantial proportion of both the utilization of health care services by adolescents and the causes of morbidity and mortality. Adolescents make fewer visits to physicians for ambulatory care than does any other age group, yet school-age children and adolescents are more likely than younger children to have unmet health needs and delayed medical care because of cost. Adolescents and young adults are less likely to be insured than all other age groups, and uninsured adolescents are less likely to have visited a physician in the previous 2 yr than are insured adolescents.

Most ambulatory visits for all age groups occur in physician offices, as compared with outpatient or emergency departments. However, in 1996, 15–24 yr olds received more of their care in emergency rooms than did any other age group. In a 1994 survey of emergency room visits in the United States, 11–21 yr olds, males, and older adolescents were the highest utilization subgroups, although half the visits for all groups were for nonurgent causes. Injuries were the leading diagnostic category overall, but females presented most often with complaints related to abdominal pain and sore throat. In the general ambulatory setting, health supervision (10%), and normal pregnancy (9.9%) lead the lists of diagnoses for 10–14 yr olds and 15–24 yr olds, respectively. Acne or diseases of the sebaceous glands and inflammation of the pharynx or sinus complete the list of the most common diagnoses. Children with disabilities, as a group, access health care services more frequently than do nondisabled children, and adolescents represent the largest proportion of children who are disabled, 84.3 cases/1,000 (ages 12–17 yr) compared with 33.2 cases/1,000 for children less than 6 yr of age. Overall, impairments of speech, special senses, and intelligence (primarily mental retardation) as well as respiratory disease (primarily asthma) make up the largest categories of disability diagnoses.

The leading causes of hospitalization in adolescents parallel the diagnoses of adolescents seen in the ambulatory setting, with the exception of mental disorders. Hospitalizations for mental disorders composed 13% of the top five discharge diagnoses in 1996 for 10–21 yr olds, with pregnancy and childbirth (56%), injuries (11%), diseases of the digestive system (9.5%), and respiratory tract diseases (8%) completing the list. The overall hospitalization rates have declined, with rates for 15–19 yr and 20–24 yr dropping 29% and 27%, respectively, for the years 1986 to 1996.

The health conditions having the greatest impact on the status of adolescent health are early unintended pregnancy, sexually transmitted diseases, mental disorders, injuries, and substance use and abuse. The trends in the frequency vary over time relative to prevention programs, legislative actions, and other societal factors. Teen births, at 54.7 births/1,000, have declined steadily since 1991 (Fig. 118–1) but have yet to reach the nadir of the early to mid-1980s of 50–53/1,000. Reportable sexually transmitted diseases such as gonorrhea and syphilis have the highest prevalence in 15–24 yr olds; rates for both diseases declined in 1996, compared with 1993 and 1990. Less comprehensive survey data are available to identify trends for chlamydia, pelvic inflammatory disease, human papillomavirus, and human immunodeficiency virus infection.

Health destructive behavior, such as cigarette and marijuana smoking and the abuse of alcohol and recreational drugs (often in combination with driving), continues to present a serious problem for adolescents. Unlike the trends in morbidity related to sexuality, survey data demonstrate modest increases in marijuana and alcohol use from 1996–1997 (2.7% and 2.3%, respectively).

Automobile and motorcycle accidents are the leading causes of adolescent morbidity and mortality (see Chapter 57). Sixteen- to 19-yr-olds compose 5% of licensed drivers and account for 15% of vehicular fatalities. Alcohol is a factor in approximately one third of the fatal accidents involving adolescents. In addition, other drugs, such as marijuana, are involved in 10–15% of accidents. About 100 nonfatal injuries occur for every adolescent killed in a motor vehicle accident. These injuries are the leading cause of disability from head and spinal cord injuries for adolescents. Graduated licensing systems, more vigorously enforced drinking age laws, and nighttime driving restrictions have demonstrated successful preventive outcomes in some states.

Violent deaths and injuries have a significant impact on adolescents. Homicides are the second leading cause of death for all adolescents and the most common cause of death for black males. Firearm deaths and injuries are a major contributor to these events. Although reliable national firearm injury data are not available, estimates range as high as 100 nonfatal violent assaults resulting in injury for each firearm death. The trend in the death rate has declined since 1980, reaching its nadir in 1985 (Fig. 107–1). From 1983 to 1993, the firearm homicide rate more than tripled from 5 to 18/100,000. Since 1993, the rates of fatal and nonfatal firearm injuries have declined.

Certain chronic diseases affecting adults have their origins during adolescence. Heart disease, diabetes, and respiratory conditions related to smoking are most common. Obesity is a major risk factor for cardiovascular diseases in adulthood but

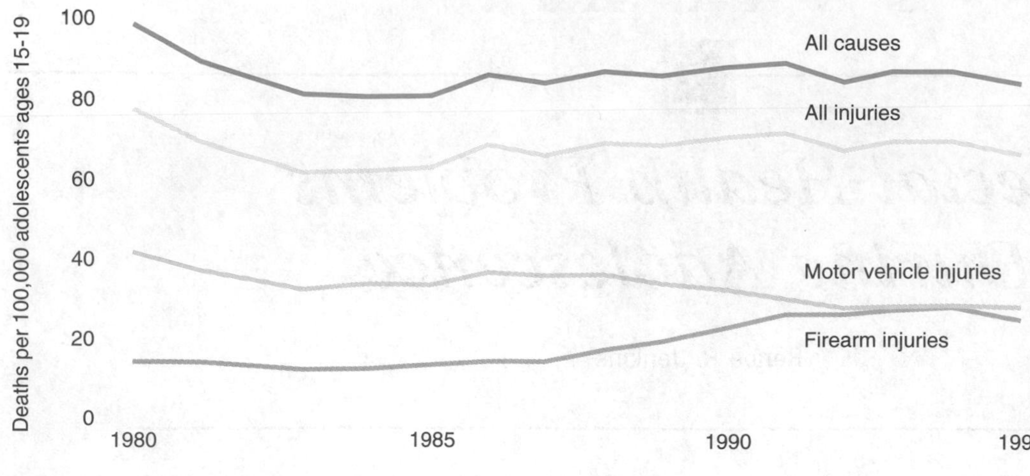

Figure 107–1 Mortality rate among adolescents ages 15-19 yr by cause of death, 1980-1995. (From Federal Interagency Forum on Child and Family Statistics: America's Children: Key National Indicators of Well-Being. Washington, DC, US Government Printing Office, 1998.)

is also independently correlated with hypertension, hypercholesterolemia, diabetes mellitus, gallbladder disease, arthritis, and gout. Poor nutritional habits, such as increased consumption of high-fat foods are correlated with low socioeconomic status in females. As many as 26% of white females and 25% of black females are classified as obese by skinfold thickness. Additional risks for chronic diseases, such as cigarette smoking, sedentary lifestyle, and episodic heavy drinking, are also health behavior risks with significant prevalence in adolescence and are related to low socioeconomic status. Human immunodeficiency virus infection rises in its ranking as a cause of mortality from school-age children through adulthood; by age 25–44 yr it represents the most common cause of death for Hispanics and blacks and the 3rd most common cause of death for whites. According to the natural history of the disease, many of these infections were transmitted during adolescence or young adulthood.

American Medical Association. AMA guidelines for Adolescent Preventive Services: Recommendations and Rationale. Baltimore, Williams & Wilkins, 1994.

Anderson RN, Kochanek MA, Murphy SL: Report of Final Mortality Statistics, 1995. Monthly Vital Statistics Report; Vol 45, No 11, Suppl 2. Hyattsville MD, National Center for Health Statistics, 1997.

Committee on Injury Poison Prevention and Committee on Adolescence: The teenage driver. Pediatrics 98:987, 1996.

Fingerhut LA, Ingram DD, Feldman JJ: Homicide rates amoung US teenagers and young adults. JAMA 280:423, 1998.

Lowry R, Kann L, Collins JL, Kolbe LJ: The effect of socioeconomic status on chronic disease risk behaviors among US adolescents. JAMA 276:792, 1996.

National Center for Health Statistics, unpublished data, September 1998.

Newacheck PW, Halfon N: Prevalence and impact of disabling chronic conditions in childhood. Am J Public Health 88:610, 1998.

Ozer EM, Brindis CD, Millstein SG, et al: America's Adolescents—Are they Healthy? San Francisco, University of California, San Francisco, National Adolescent Health Information Center, 1998.

Ziv A, Boulet JR, Slap GB: Emergency deprtment utilization by adolescents in the United States. Pediatrics 101:987, 1998.

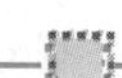

CHAPTER 108
Delivery of Health Care to Adolescents

The leading causes of death and disability among adolescents are preventable, suggesting that society has failed to address the health needs of this age group adequately. Further, teenagers who require medical treatment may not receive the care they need. Although one may concede that the greatest proportion of health problems in adolescents are behaviorally related and less amenable to prevention and treatment by traditional medical services, there is still much that can be done to improve the effectiveness of their health care. Access, confidentiality, and the delivery of age-appropriate care are the primary issues for this age group. The Society for Adolescent Medicine identified seven criteria critical to access to care for adolescents: availability, visibility, quality, confidentiality, affordability, flexibility, and coordination.

Availability addresses age-appropriate services at the community level and includes the creation and dissemination of and provider education about adolescent preventive health guidelines. The ease of recognition or expectation that an adolescent's needs can be addressed in a setting relates to the *visibility* criterion. The *quality* of care should be kept at a guaranteed standard that is satisfactory to the patient as well. *Confidentiality* and access to care that requires consent by the adolescent should be available, while family involvement should be encouraged. Poor *affordability* is an obvious deterrent to access. Adolescents have the lowest annual rate of visits to office-based physicians than do all other age groups (Fig. 108–1). For all age groups, including adolescents, individuals without insurance receive less health care, and insurance coverage is worsening for adolescents: In 1988, 13.7% of 12–17 yr olds had no health insurance, a figure that increased to 19.9% by 1992. In 1993, older adolescents and young adults were the least likely to be insured, at 25.2%; the uninsured level decreased with decreasing age, 19.9% of 15–18 yr olds and 14% of 10–14 yr olds. Service providers who are *flexible* and adaptable recognize and respond to the cultural, ethnic, and social diversity issues of adolescents. Teens with multiple concerns and a broad range of health-related issues require *coordination* of medical, mental health, social, and other services.

The complexity and interaction of physical, cognitive, and psychosocial developmental processes during adolescence require sensitivity and skill on the part of the pediatrician and a greater number of contacts than is currently appreciated or financed. Health education and promotion as well as disease prevention should be the focus of every visit with a teenager. To ensure that this is carried out comprehensively and systematically, guidelines have been promulgated from three major sources: the American Academy of Pediatrics' Health Supervision III, the American Medical Association's Guidelines for Adolescent Preventive Services (GAPS), and the Maternal and Child Health Bureau's Bright Futures (BF) Guidelines. The criteria for establishing the guidelines varied according to the organization. The GAPS guidelines represent the most stringent or evidence-based criteria, whereas the other guidelines used expert consensus (also see Chapter 5).

A comparative analysis of the three sets of guidelines reveals more similarity than differences (Table 108–1). The GAPS guidelines, having been designed exclusively for adolescents,

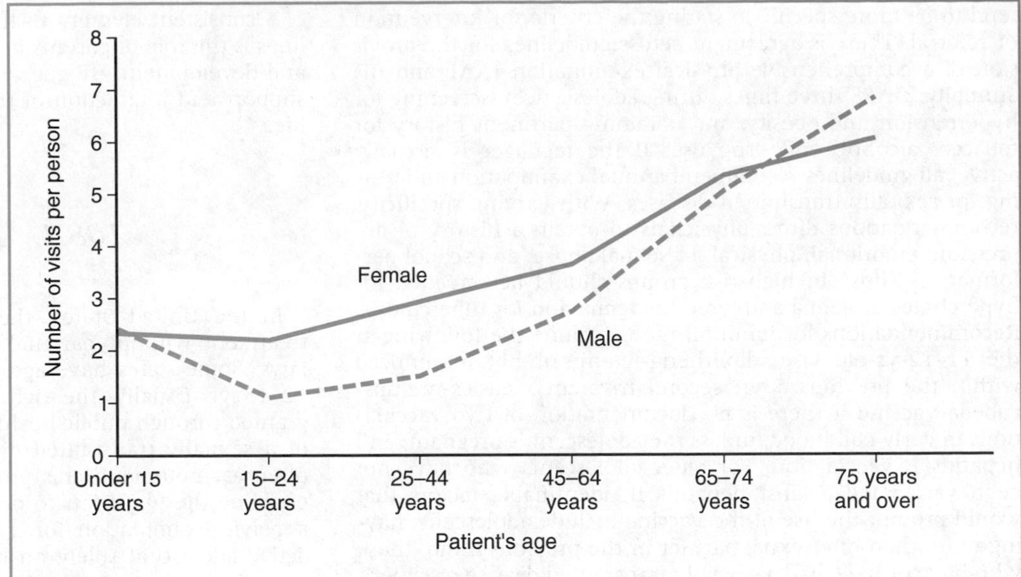

Figure 108–1 Annual rate of visits to office-based physicians by patient's age and sex: United States, 1996. (From Woodwell DA: National Ambulatory Medical Care Survey. Hyattsville, MD, National Center for Health Statistics, 1996.)

TABLE 108–1 Comparison of Supervision Guidelines

Source	AAP	GAPS	Bright Futures
Periodicity	***Annually***	***Annually***	***Annually***
Anticipatory Guidance			
Parenting	X	X	X
Adolescent development	X	X	X
Safety practices	X	X	X
Diet and fitness	X	X	X
Healthy lifestyles	X	X	X
Oral health	X		X
Screening			
History			
Tobacco use	X	X	X
Alcohol and drug use	X	X	X
Sexual behavior	X	X	X
School performance	X	X	X
Depression/suicide risk	X	X	X
Eating disorders	X	X	
Learning problems		X	X
Abuse	X	X	X
Physical Assessment with Specific Recommendations			
Hypertension	X[1]	X	
Obesity	X[1]	X	X
Breast cancer (self-examination)	X		X
Comprehensive examination	X	X	X
Scoliosis	X		X
Tests			
Hyperlipidemia	X	X	X
Tuberculin	X[2]	X[2]	X[3]
Vision	X		X
Anemia	X		X
GC, chlamydia, syphilis[4]	X	X	X
Genital warts (HPV)[4]		X	
HIV infection	X	X	X
Cervical cancer[5]	X	X	X
Immunizations			
MMR	X	X	X
dT	X	X	X
Hepatitis B	X	X	X

[1]*Recommends obtaining and plotting measures only.*
[2]*Under specific conditions.*
[3]*At least one during adolescence (14–16 year old).*
[4]*For adolescents who are sexually active.*
[5]*For adolescent girls who are sexually active or ≥18 yr old.*

tend to be more specific in stating the criteria for intervention or referral. There is agreement across guidelines for the provision of a comprehensive physical examination (AAP and BF, annually; GAPS three times during adolescence), screening for hypertension and obesity, and obtaining pertinent history for tobacco, alcohol, and drug use. If the teenager is sexually active, all guidelines recommend annual examination and testing for sexually transmitted diseases. With varying specificity, recommendations direct physicians to obtain a history of depression; emotional, physical, or sexual abuse; and school performance. Those in high-risk groups should be screened for hypercholesterolemia and hyperlipidemia and for tuberculosis. Recommendations for immunizations include the following at the 11–12-yr-old visit: diphtheria-tetanus if not immunized within the previous 5 yr; second trivalent measles-mumps-rubella vaccine if there is no documentation of two vaccinations in early childhood, unless the adolescent is pregnant; and hepatitis B vaccination. For older adolescents who have not been vaccinated against hepatitis B, identifiable factors that would prompt the use of the vaccine include adolescents having more than one sexual partner in the previous 6 mo, those who have or have had a sexually transmitted disease or experienced a pregnancy, and those living in areas where parenteral drug use is prevalent or if the adolescent uses intravenous drugs. A companion document to the GAPS guidelines provides algorithms for each of the major preventive directives. Figure 108–2 provides a sample using the algorithm for sexuality (also see Chapter 14).

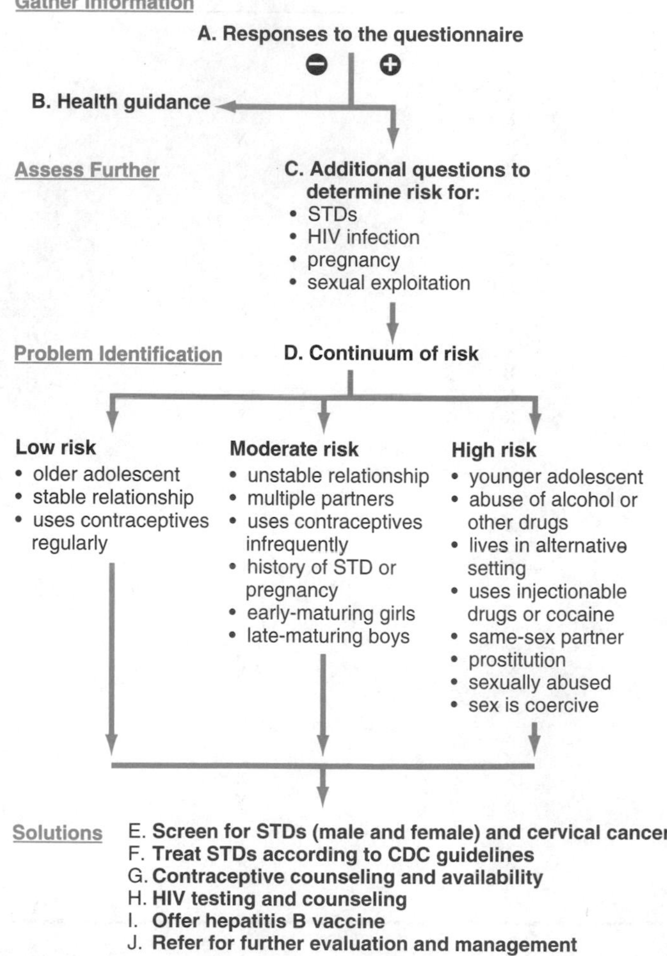

Figure 108–2 Sexuality algorithm. (From Levenberg PB, Elster AB: Guidelines for Adolescent Preventive Services. Clinical Evaluation and Management Handbook. Chicago, American Medical Association, 1995.)

A consistent element to the approach of each of the guidelines is the role of parents in support of the adolescent's health and development. BF goes even further in recommending the support and interaction of the community in the adolescent's life.

108.1 Legal Issues

In the United States, the right of a minor to *consent* to treatment without parental knowledge is governed by state laws. Some states have age limitations, generally around age 12–15 yr. Usually, the right to self-consent for treatment is granted through public health statutes when there is suspicion of a sexually transmitted disease. Because such diseases are often asymptomatic, this provision is generally interpreted as enabling the physician to perform an examination (including a pelvic examination for a young woman) in any sexually active adolescent solely on his or her own consent. In many states, adolescents may consent to receive care for drug abuse or mental health problems. The minor's right to *contraceptives* has not been reviewed by the Supreme Court, although the right to privacy has been upheld (except in a decision allowing searches in schools without due process) and accordingly, most states permit the provision of contraceptives to teenagers on their own consent. Although attempts at restricting Title X–funded programs to provision of contraception only after parents have been informed has not been legislated, the publicity received by the proposal has left many teenagers with the mistaken notion that their parents will be informed if they seek birth control from any physician. The right of an adolescent to obtain an *abortion* without parental consent or over parental objection varies by state.

Minors are also exempt from the requirement of parental consent for medical treatment under the following circumstances:

1. *Emancipated minors*. These are children who live away from home, are no longer subject to parental control, are economically self-supporting, are married, or are members of the military.
2. *Emergencies*. In a medical emergency, a minor may be treated without consent of parents if, in the physician's judgment, the delay resulting from attempts to contact parents would jeopardize the life or health of the minor.
3. *Mature minor rule*. An emerging trend in the law is the recognition that many minors are sufficiently mature to understand the nature of their illness and the potential risks and benefits of proposed therapy and, therefore, should receive such treatment on their own consent. This is particularly the case when the care is low risk, will benefit the minor, and is within established medical practice standards. In these cases, the physician should document that the adolescent has acted in a responsible manner.

Legal policies regarding the confidentiality of information are less consistent than those governing consent. In general, the right to self-consent for health care carries with it the right to confidentiality about that information. Exceptions exist when there are mandatory reporting requirements, as in abuse cases, some legal provision requiring parental disclosure, or a self-imposed danger to the minor. When exceptions exists, this should be divulged to the adolescent and an opportunity for assent or agreement provided.

A chaperone should be present whenever an adolescent female patient is examined by a male physician. The necessity for chaperones in the situation of a female physician examining a male adolescent patient has not yet become an issue.

108.2 Screening Procedures

INTERVIEWING THE ADOLESCENT (Also see Chapters 5 and 17). The preparation for a successful interview with an adolescent patient varies based on the prior history of the relationship with the patient. Patients, who are going from preadolescence to adolescence while seeing the same provider, and their parents should be guided through the transition. Although the rules for confidentiality are the same for new and continuing patients, the change in the physician-patient relationship, allowing more privacy during the visit and more autonomy in the health process, may be threatening for the parent as well as the adolescent. For new patients, the initial phases of the interview are more challenging given the need to establish rapport rapidly with the patient in order to meet the goals of the encounter. Issues of confidentiality and privacy should be explicitly stated along with the conditions under which that confidentiality may need to be altered, that is, in life- or safety-threatening situations. For new patients, the parents should be interviewed with the adolescent or before the adolescent to ensure that the adolescent does not perceive a breech of confidentiality. The physician who takes time to listen, avoids judgmental statements and the use of street jargon, and shows respect for the adolescent's emerging maturity will have an easier time communicating with him or her. The use of open-ended questions, rather than closed-ended questions, will further facilitate history-taking (e.g., the close-ended question, "Do you get along with your father?" leading to the answer, "Yes" compared with the question, "What would you like to change in your relationship with your father?" which may lead to an answer such as "I would like to stop him from always putting me down, especially in front of my friends").

The goals of the interview or clinical encounter are to establish an information base, identify problems and issues from the patient's perspective, and identify problems and issues from the perspective of the provider based on knowledge of the health and other issues relevant to the adolescent age group. The adolescent should be given an opportunity to express concerns and the reasons for seeking medical attention. The adolescent as well as the parent should also be given an opportunity to express the strengths and successes of the adolescent, in addition to the risk assessment.

Barriers to an effective interview occur when the interviewer is distracted by other events or individuals in the office, when there are extreme time limitations obvious to either party, or when there is expressible discomfort with either the patient or the interviewer. The need for an interpreter when a patient is hearing impaired or if the patient and interviewer are not language-compatible provides a challenge but not necessarily a barrier under most circumstances. Observations during the interview can be useful to the overall assessment of the patient's maturity, presence or absence of depression, and the parent-adolescent relationship. Given the key role of a successful interview in the screening process, adequate training and experience should be sought by physicians wishing to give comprehensive care to adolescent patients.

PSYCHOSOCIAL ASSESSMENT. A few questions should be asked to detect the adolescent who is having difficulty with peer relationships (e.g., "Do you have a best friend with whom you can share even the most personal secret?"); self-image (e.g., "Is there anything you would like to change about yourself?" or "What do you consider to be your best features?"); with depression (e.g., "What do you see yourself doing 5 yr from now?" or "Are you ever so sad that you think of dying?"); school (e.g., "How are your grades this year compared with last year?" and "How many days have you been absent from school this year compared with last year?"); personal decisions (e.g., "Are you feeling pressured to engage in any behavior for which you do not feel you are ready?" or "Is there anything you would like to change in your relationship with your boyfriend, your father, and so on?"); and an eating disorder (e.g., "Do you ever feel that food controls you rather than vice versa?"). The GAPS material provides questions and algorithms to structure these assessments. Based on those algorithms, appropriate counseling or referrals are recommended for more thorough probing or for in-depth interviewing.

PHYSICAL EXAMINATION

Audiometry. Highly amplified music of the kind enjoyed by many adolescents may result in hearing loss (see Chapter 643). Therefore, a hearing screening is recommended by the BF guidelines for adolescents who are exposed to loud noises regularly, have had recurring ear infections, or report problems.

Vision Testing. The pubertal growth spurt may involve the optic globe, resulting in its elongation and myopia in genetically predisposed individuals. Vision testing should, therefore, be performed in order to detect this problem before it affects school performance.

Blood Pressure Determination. Criteria for a diagnosis of hypertension are based on age-specific norms that increase with pubertal maturation (see Chapter 451). An individual whose blood pressure exceeds the 95th percentile for his or her age is suspect for having hypertension, regardless of the absolute reading. Those adolescents with blood pressure between the 90th and 95th percentiles should receive appropriate counseling relative to weight and have a follow-up examination in 6 mo. Those with blood pressure below the 90th percentile should have their blood pressure measured on three separate occasions to determine the stability of the elevation before moving forward with an intervention stategy. The technique is important; false-positive results may be obtained if the cuff covers less than two thirds of the upper arm. The patient should be seated, and an average should be taken of the 2nd and 3rd consecutive readings, using the change rather than the disappearance as the diastolic pressure. Most adolescents with elevations of blood pressure have labile hypertension (see Chapter 451). If the blood pressure is below 2 standard deviations for age, anorexia nervosa and Addison disease should be considered.

Scoliosis (Also see Chapter 685.1). Approximately 5% of male and 10–14% of female adolescents have a mild curvature of the spine. This is two to four times the rate in younger children. Scoliosis is typically manifested during the peak of the height velocity curve, at approximately 12 yr in females and 14 yr in males. Curves measuring greater than 10 degrees should be monitored by an orthopedist until growth is complete.

Breast Examination. Examination of the female adolescent's breasts is performed to detect masses (see Chapters 556 and 559), evaluate progression of sexual maturation, provide reassurance about development, and teach the technique of self-examination with the hope that this practice will continue into the higher risk later years. Although self-examination is promoted in two of the three guidelines, there is disagreement on the justification for promoting this routinely, given the rare instances of malignant breast masses in this age group.

Scrotum Examination. The peak incidence of germ cell tumors of the testes is in late adolescence and early adulthood. For that reason, palpation of the testes may have an immediate yield and should serve as a model for instruction of self-examination. Because varicoceles often appear during puberty, the examination also provides an opportunity to explain and reassure the patient about this entity (see Chapter 553).

Pelvic Examination. Refer to Chapter 556.

LABORATORY TESTING. During early adolescence, a screening *urinalysis and culture* are indicated for the female. Polymorphonuclear leukocytes in the urinary sediment suggest the possibility of either cervicitis, vaginitis, urethritis, or an asymptomatic infection of the urinary tract; the last is a common finding in adolescent females. The increased incidence of iron-deficiency anemia after menarche also mandates the performance of a *hematocrit* annually in young women with moderate to heavy menses. The reference standard for this test changes with progression of puberty, as estrogen suppresses erythropoietin (see Chapter 452). Populations with nutritional risk should also have the hematocrit monitored. Androgens have the opposite effect, causing the hematocrit to rise during male puberty; Sex Maturity Rating 1 males have an average hematocrit of 39%, whereas those who have completed puberty (Sexual Maturation Rating 5) have an average value of 43%. *Tuberculosis testing* on an annual basis is important in adolescents with risk factors related to socioeconomic circumstances and area of residence because puberty has been shown to activate this disease in those not previously treated. Sexually active adolescents should undergo screening for *sexually transmitted diseases,* regardless of symptoms (see Chapter 119). *HIV testing* should be included for those at increased risk, that is, a history of sexually transmitted diseases, more than one sex partner in the last 6 mo, bisexual and homosexual males, sexual partners of at-risk individuals, and intravenous drug users. *Papanicolaou smears* are also indicated in sexually active females, regardless of age, because 5–35/1,000 have early neoplastic changes. Technique is important; the practice of obtaining two successive cervical scrapes increases the yield by 26% over that obtained by a single cervical specimen. Although not included in any of the guidelines, screening tests for *genetic defect carrier states,* such as sickle cell anemia, are commonly performed in affected populations. Age-appropriate counseling should be immediately available to ensure an opportunity to have questions answered and to have unspoken fears allayed. The use of *spirometry* screening for adolescents who smoke may, over time, serve as a deterrent if deterioration of respiratory status can be demonstrated.

108.3 Health Enhancement

The health status of adolescents may be enhanced by application of principles of prevention and anticipatory guidance. Prevention of infectious disease should include immunization and counseling. Prevention of sexually transmitted diseases and pregnancy is an important issue to be addressed in sexually active adolescents of both sexes. Prevention of the use of harmful illicit drugs and alcohol and the potential for related injuries should be reviewed. Prevention of automotive accidents and interpersonal conflicts ending violently, the leading killer of adolescents, and of smoking, the leading killer of adults, should also be discussed. Facilitating an optimal health outcome for the adolescent patient also includes supporting him or her in successfully negotiating adolescence through school, job, and personal and family relations.

American Medical Association: Guidelines for Adolescent Preventive Services, Recommendations Monograph, 3rd ed. Chicago, American Medical Association, 1996.

Committee on Psychosocial Aspects of Child and Family Health 1995–1996: Guidelines for Health Supervision III. Elk Grove Village, IL, American Academy of Pediatrics, 1997.

Elston AB: Comparison of recommendations for adolescent clinical preventive services developed by national organizations. Arch Pediatr Adolesc Med 152:193, 1998.

Green M (ed): Bright Futures: Guidelines for Health Supervision of Infants, Children, and Adolescents. Arlington, VA, National Center for Education in Maternal and Child Health, 1994.

Society for Adolescent Medicine: Access to health care for adolescents: A position paper of the Society for Adolescent Medicine. J Adolesc Health 13:162, 1992.

Strasburger VC, Brown RT: Acne: What every pediatrician should know about treatment. Pediatr Clin North Am 44:1505, 1997.

Woodwell DA: National Ambulatory Medical Care Survey: 1996 Summary. Advance data from vital and health statistics; No. 295. Hyattsville, MD, National Center for Health Statistics, 1997.

CHAPTER 109
Depression

Changes in mood are part of the normative developmental "adjustment" to changes in body, roles, and relationships in adolescence (also see Chapter 23). The challenge for a pediatrician is to distinguish between these normative variations and disorders requiring mental health intervention. The widespread belief that major depression in children and adolescents is rare or self-limited has led to underdiagnosis and delayed treatment for approximately two thirds of adolescents with clinical depression.

EPIDEMIOLOGY. The rate of depression in girls and boys changes significantly as a function of puberty. Gender variations are not characteristic of childhood depression, but depression is two to three times higher in postpubertal girls than in postpubertal boys. The lifetime prevalence of major depression is similar to adults and ranges between 15 and 20%. The co-occurrence of depression and another mental health disorder is reported from 40–70% of the time and is common in the adolescent age group. The most frequent co-morbid disorders are anxiety disorders, substance abuse, attention deficit disorder, and disruptive behavior disorders.

ETIOLOGY. There appears to be an interactive effect of genetics and environment in major depressive disorders, with studies in adults suggesting individuals with a high genetic risk may be more vulnerable to adverse environmental stressors when compared with those with low genetic risk. A family history of depressed parents increases the adolescent's risk of lifetime major depression threefold. Other parenting factors such as marital conflict, inadequate parenting, or death of a parent are also associated with depression. Controversy exists about the temporal relationship of symptoms such as low-self esteem, high self-criticism, hopelessness, and social skill deficits to their role as risk factors or as a prodrome of depression.

CLINICAL MANIFESTATIONS. An adolescent who presents with school failure or another behavioral disorder may have an underlying depressive issue. The *Diagnostic and Statistical Manual for Primary Care, Child and Adolescent Version,* provides the clinical presentation of the range of "sadness" symptoms in young persons from the developmental variation, associated with bereavement or other stressors, through a sadness problem, and onto the full-blown disorder such as major depression. The characteristics of a sadness problem encompass (1) depressed or irritable mood, (2) diminished interest or pleasure, (3) weight loss or gain or failure to make expected weight gains, (4) insomnia or hypersomnia, (5) psychomotor agitation or retardation, (6) fatigue or energy loss, (7) feelings of worthlessness or excessive or inappropriate guilt, and (8) diminished ability to think or concentrate. The quality of these symptoms is less intense with a sadness problem, as compared with major depression, and the impact on the adolescent's functioning is mild. When these symptoms occur daily for a period of 2 wk or longer, with or without recurrent thoughts of death and suicidal ideation, the diagnosis falls into the realm of a major depressive disorder. When these symptoms occur within 3 mo of an identifiable stressor, the presentation is considered an adjustment disorder with depressed mood.

DIFFERENTIAL DIAGNOSIS. Physical and metabolic disturbances should be ruled out during the assessment of an adolescent with depressive symptoms. Hypothyroidism, nutritional deficiencies, a chronic infection such as mononucleosis, or a chronic systemic disease such as systemic lupus erythematosus should be ruled out. Substance abuse can mask the depression symptoms as well as imitate depression. A chronic learning disability leading to low self-esteem can also present with depressive-like symptoms.

OFFICE SCREENING FOR DEPRESSION. The screening for depressive symptoms is recommended as a component of the routine health maintenance assessment for an adolescent. Although the diagnosis of the full depressive disorder is based on interviewing the adolescent and obtaining observational data from parents or primary caretakers, alertness during a medical evaluation can raise suspicion early in the course of the disorder. One strategy recommended by the American Medical Association's Guidelines for Adolescent Preventive Services guidelines is to pose a series of screening questions to determine whether depressive symptoms at the level of mild, moderate to severe, or high risk exist. General questions such as, "Have you had fun during the past 2 weeks?" or "In general, are you happy with the way things are going for you these days?" alert the clinician to the need to ask more probing follow-up questions to elicit the presence or absence of diagnostic symptom criteria for depression. Another strategy is to use a depressive screening questionnaire such as the 21-question Beck Depression Inventory to confirm the clinical suspicion of depression.

TREATMENT. There are several therapeutic modalities for the treatment of depression, including individual and group therapy, family intervention, and others along with, or independent of, psychopharmacologic treatment. The role of the pediatrician relative to the timing of a referral to a mental health professional is determined by his or her training and experience in managing mental health problems. The education of parents and patients about depressive disorders and the success of intervention is important, as is the removal of the cultural stigma that may be associated with mental health therapy. The significance of timely intervention should be stressed, including the potential for a depressive disorder to disrupt the normal adolescent developmental process. An extended disruption can lead to impaired functioning even after recovery from the depressive episode. The importance of following early identification with prompt treatment cannot be overemphasized.

PROGNOSIS AND OUTCOME. In one survey of adolescents and young adults, more than one fifth of those with major depression reported ever attempting suicide, the most adverse outcome of a depressive disorder. An untreated major depressive episode can last up to 7–9 months, with about 40% of cases recurring within 2 yr and 70% within 5 yr. The earlier the onset of depression, the more severe and recurrent the course. Outcomes of untreated major depression persist into adulthood and are manifested as impaired psychologic, social, and academic functioning. (See Chapter 28.2 for a discussion of pharmacotherapy.)

Beasley PJ, Beardslee WR: Depression in the adolescent patient. Adolesc Med: State of Art Rev 9:351, 1998.

Kessler RC, Walters EE: Epidemiology of DSM-III-R major depression and minor depression among adolescents and young adults in the national comorbidity survey. Depress Anxiety 7:3, 1998.

Levenberg PB, Elster AB: Guidelines for Adolescent Preventive Services (GAPS), Clinical Evaluation and Management Handbook. Chicago, American Medical Association, 1995.

Wolraich ML, Felice ME, Drotar D (eds): The Classification of Child and Adolescent Mental Diagnoses in Primary Care: Diagnostic and Statistical Manual for Primary Care (DSM-PC) Child and Adolescent Version. Elk Grove Village, IL, American Academy of Pediatrics, 1996.

CHAPTER 110
Suicide

The recognition of risk factors for suicidal behavior is an important aspect in the prevention efforts directed toward adolescents, particularly those with mood disorders (see also Chapter 24).

EPIDEMIOLOGY. Suicide is the third leading cause of death for all adolescents and young adults 15–24 yr old; it is the second leading cause of death for white males. Higher rates of suicide have also been reported in Alaskan, Asian-American, and Native American youth. From 1980 to 1995, the suicide rate for black males aged 15–19 yr increased 146%, compared with a 22% increase in white males during the same period. The chronically ill adolescent is also at increased risk for suicide exacerbated by interpersonal difficulties and increased access to medications that can be used in a suicide attempt. Finland and Norway are among the European countries with the highest suicide rates in this age group. Although data on the rate of suicide attempts in the United States are not available, estimates range from 50 to 200 attempts per successful suicide. Males more frequently complete suicides and females attempt suicide more often. More violent methods, such as hanging, shooting, or wrist slashing, are used most often by males. Guns and firearms are the most prevalent method used to complete suicide among children and youth.

ETIOLOGY. There are at least three proposed contexts to account for an increased risk of suicidal behavior in adolescents. The traditional psychiatric model of risk factors focuses on interpersonal and family factors such as having a psychiatric disorder, family clustering of suicidal behavior, substance use and abuse, sexual abuse, and serotonin abnormalities. Substance abuse is less often a risk factor in prepubertal adolescents; parent-child conflict is identified as a common risk factor. Gay and bisexual youth plagued with gender identity issues also represent a population at increased risk. The "injury" model for increased suicide risk takes additional community risk factors into account such as local suicide and violence exposure rates, the availability or nonavailability of supportive social networks and suicide prevention programs in the community, and the availability of lethal means such as firearms. A third approach that is more developmentally driven looks at suicidal risk in the context of other age-related problem behaviors, noting the high correlation between suicide attempts and lack of seatbelt use, carrying a gun in the 30 days prior to the suicide attempt, physical fights in the prior 12 mo, recent tobacco use, and intravenous drug use. The complex set of factors represented in these three approaches has a direct impact on the strategies taken in suicide prevention programs.

CLINICAL MANIFESTATIONS. Suicidal ideation alone is not necessarily a risk factor for suicidal behavior. As many as 12–25% of older children and adolescents express some form of suicidal ideation. The risk should be taken much more seriously when the ideation is accompanied by a specific plan. Psychologic autopsies following successful suicides have also uncovered the frequent occurrence of a stressful event, such as a disciplinary crisis, disappointment, or rejection, immediately preceding the suicide. When a suicide attempt is made, it is often difficult to assess the seriousness of the intent by the actual potency of the method. Beck and associates found medical lethality of methods to correlate poorly with seriousness of intent. There was, however, good correlation between the latter and the patient's expectation of lethality, which was often inaccurate. Although most adolescents who attempt suicide do not become successful, increased risk exists for later morbidity, mortality, depression, behavioral disturbances, and impaired social and academic skills.

TREATMENT. Consultation with a skilled psychiatrist is essential in the assessment of every teenager who attempts suicide. The evaluation may result in an outpatient referral or hospitalization. When the three most serious risk factors—prior suicide attempt, mood disorder, and substance abuse—are present, there is no proof that hospitalization prevents repeated attempts and the ultimate completion of suicide. However, a hospitalization may assist in resolution of an existing conflict and provide a secure setting in which the patient can have underlying problems addressed. Outpatient management is poorly complied with in this population, with a higher frequency of failure to make an initial visit and a higher rate of termination of treatment observed in adolescents who attempt suicide compared with adolescents who do not attempt suicide.

PREVENTION. A Centers for Disease Control and Prevention review of youth suicide prevention programs categorizes them as school gatekeeper programs, community gatekeeper programs, peer support programs, crisis center and hotlines, restriction of access to lethal means, and intervention after suicide. The review concluded that the lack of rigorous evaluation of these programs limited the evidence for their effectiveness. The complexity of the risk factors noted substantiates the immense challenge of addressing suicide prevention in the most comprehensive fashion, including an adequately designed evaluation. Given the significance of the problem in the United States, efforts should be vigorously pursued to address reducing suicide death in children, adolescents, and young adults.

Beck A, Steer R, Kovacs M, et al: Hopelessness and eventual suicide: A 10-year propsective study of patients hospitalized with suicidal ideation. Am J Psychiatry 142:559, 1985.

Gessner BD: Temporal trends and geographic patterns of teen suicide in Alaska, 1979–1993. Suicide Life Threat Behav 27:264, 1997.

Greenhill LL, Waslick B: Management of suicidal behavior in children and adolescents. Psychiatr Clin North Am 20:641, 1997.

Hawton K, Arensman E, Wasserman D, et al: Relations between attempted suicide and suicide rates among young people in Europe. J Epidemiol Community Health 52:191, 1998.

Suicide among black youths—United States, 1980–1995. JAMA 279:1431, 1998.

Woods ER, Lin YG, Middleman A, et al: The association of suicide attempts in adolescents. Pediatrics 99:791, 1997.

CHAPTER 111
Violent Behavior

Interpersonal and community violence, physical abuse, and domestic violence lead to significant rates of injury and death for specific age, gender, and racial sectors of the population in the United States (also see Chapter 34). Youth and minority populations are disproportionately affected. Violent behavior permeates the youth culture, whether by media or personal experiences in the family, community, or school. For surveillance and research purposes, the Centers for Disease Control and Prevention has accepted a definition of a violent injury as "a threatened or actual use of physical force against a person or group that either results or is likely to result in injury or death." Youth are perpetrators of violence, victims of violence, or observers of violence with varying severity of impact on the individual. Violent acts may result in, or are contributed to by, mental health problems or disorders. Pediatricians are challenged to screen for these disorders and counsel or refer adolescents with serious disorders to mental health professionals. The public health and educational communities have launched a variety of violence prevention interventions to increase youth prosocial behavior and reduce violence as a societal problem.

EPIDEMIOLOGY. In 1993–1994, the United States led the industrialized world in the number of youth deaths due to firearms, both homicide and unintentional firearm deaths (Figs. 111–1 and 111–2). From 1983–1993, the firearm homicide rate more than tripled from 5 to 18/100,000. Since 1993, the rates of fatal and nonfatal firearm injuries have declined. However, from 1993–1995, the estimated case fatality rate increased among males aged 15–24 yr, suggesting that the use of higher powered, semiautomatic handguns has increased the lethality of firearm injuries. Males are much more likely to be victims than are females in fatal and nonfatal injuries; however, 15–24 yr old women have the highest proportion of injuries compared with women in other age groups. Black males, aged 15–19 yr, are twice as likely as Hispanic males to be killed by a firearm and more than six times as likely as non-Hispanic males.

The Youth Risk Behavior Surveillance System reported that in 1995, 20% of students (31% male and 8% female) carried a weapon such as a gun, knife, or club within the 30 days preceding the survey. However, compared with the baseline survey of 1991, weapon carrying had decreased. Thirty-nine per cent of students also reported being in a fight in the prior year, and this too has declined from 137/100 students/12 mo in 1993 to 128/100 students/12 mo in 1995.

Adolescents are more likely to be victims of violence than are any other age group. In 1994, the victimization rate was 115/1,000 for 12–15 yr olds and 122/1,000 for 6–19 yr olds. Although adolescents are infrequently the age group that comes to mind when considering child abuse, adolescents make up almost one quarter of the child abuse and neglect cases in the United States. Adolescents and children less than 5 yr of age are the most likely victims of physical abuse that causes injury.

ETIOLOGY. The theories emerging to address violence come from the perspective of varying disciplines. The development psychopathology theoretical model of Mofitt identifies two types of antisocial youth: one that is life course–persistent and one that is life course limited. Adolescent-limited offenders have no childhood aberrant behaviors and are more likely to commit status offenses such as vandalism, running away, and other behaviors symbolic of their struggle for autonomy from parents. Life course–persistent offenders, in contrast, exhibit aberrant behavior in childhood, such as problems with temperament, behavioral development, and cognition, and as adolescents participate in more victim-oriented crimes. The public health model emphasizes the environment and other external influences. It focuses primarily on preventive strategies that view violence as amenable to systematic, science-based, multidisciplinary, and sustained interventions (Table 111–1). A third theoretical model examines violent behaviors across the spectrum occurring within and outside the family and is referred to as the cycle of violence. This hypothesis proposes that precursors such as child abuse and neglect, a child witnessing violence, adolescent sexual and physical abuse, and adolescent exposure to violence and violent assaults predispose youth to outcomes of violent behavior, violent crime, delinquency, violent assaults, suicide, or premature death. An additional common paradigm for high-risk violence behavior poses a balance of risk and protective factors at the individual, family, and community level. None of these theories successfully explains violent behavior.

CLINICAL MANIFESTATIONS. There are several clinical entities directly associated with violent behavior that require recognition and intervention. The most common behavioral diagnoses associated with aggressive behavior in adolescents are mental retardation, learning disabilities, moderately severe language disorders, and mental disorders such as attention deficit hyperactivity, mood, anxiety, and personality disorders. Inability to

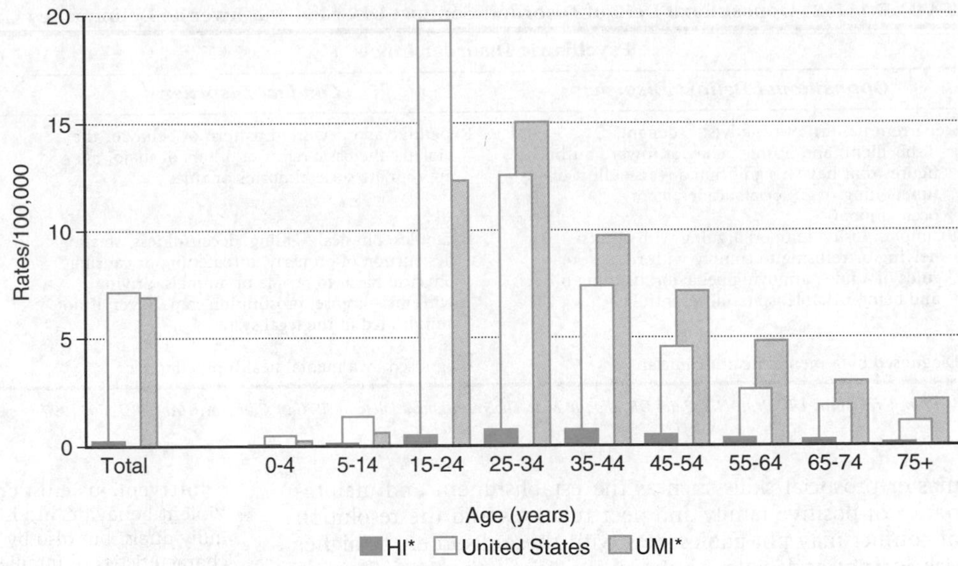

Figure 111–1 Firearm-related homicide rates by age; 36 high- and upper middle-income countries by income group. (From Krug EG, Powell KE, Dahlberg LL: Firearm-related deaths in the United States and 35 other high- and upper-middle income countries. Int J Epidemiol 27:214, 1998.)

TABLE 111–1 Public Health Approach to Youth Violence Prevention Model with Examples

	Victim (Host)	Perpetrator (Vector)	Firearm (Agent)	Social Environment	Physical Environment
Primary prevention	Conflict resolution Violence anticipatory guidance	Substance abuse treatment Home visiting programs for new and single parents	Handgun and assault weapons ban Firearm registration	Job opportunities Adult-supervised activities	Better lighting Zoning-enforced limits in liquor licenses
Secondary prevention	Medical services Psychologic services	Job training Psychosocial rehabilitation	Handgun locks Public education on risks of ownership	School incident debriefing Safe havens	Increased police presence Graffiti removal
Tertiary prevention	Physical rehabilitation Psychosocial services	Incarceration Educational-psychosocial rehabilitation	Firearm surveillance	Foster care Alternative schools	Urban planning, e.g., decrease population density in public housing and mixture of income levels

From Calhoun AD, Clark-Jones F: Theoretical frameworks: Developmental psychopathology, the public health approach to violence, and the cycle of violence. Pediatr Clin North Am 45:287, 1998.

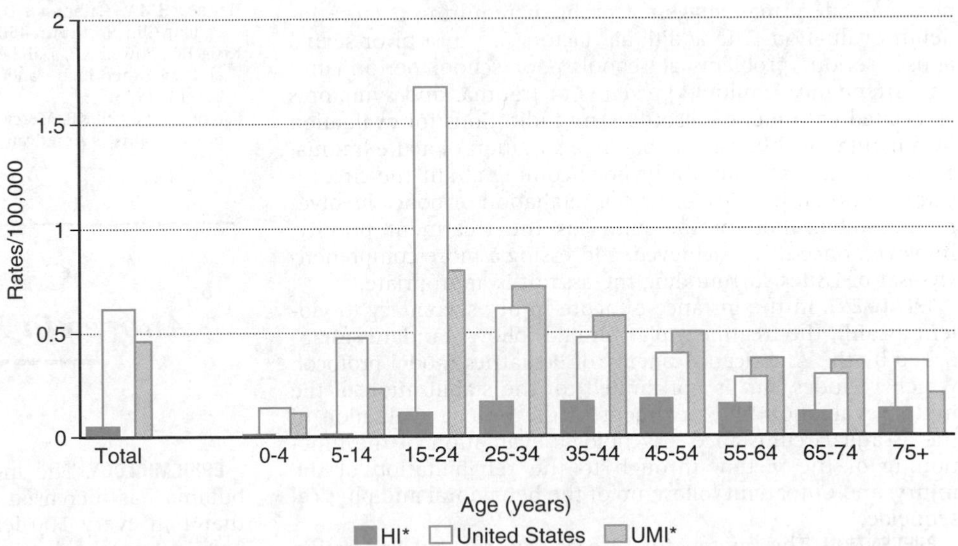

Figure 111–2 Unintentional firearm-related death rates by age; 36 high- and upper middle-income countries by income group. (From Krug EG, Powell KE, Dahlberg LL: Firearm-related deaths in the United States and 35 other high- and upper-middle income countries. Int J Epidemiol 27:214, 1998.)

TABLE 111–2 Oppositional Defiant Disorder, Conduct Disorder, and Juvenile Delinquency

Psychiatric Disorder Labels		Legal Label
Oppositional Defiant Disorder	***Conduct Disorder***	***Juvenile Delinquency***
Recurrent pattern of negativistic, defiant, disobedient, and hostile behavior toward authority figures that have a significant adverse effect on functioning (e.g., social, academic, or occupational)	Repetitive and persistent pattern of behavior that violates the basic rights of others or major age-appropriate societal norms or rules	Offenses that are illegal because of age; illegal acts
Examples: losing temper; arguing with adults; defying or refusing to comply with request or rules of adults; annoying behavior; blaming others; and being irritable, spiteful, resentful	Examples: physical fighting, deceitfulness, stealing, destruction of property, threatening or causing physical harm to people or animals, driving without a license, prostitution, rape (even if not adjudicated in the legal system)	Examples: single or multiple instances of being arrested or adjudicated for any of the following: stealing, destruction of property, threatening or causing physical harm to people or animals, driving without a license, prostitution, rape
Diagnosed by a mental health clinician	Diagnosed by a mental health practitioner	Adjudicated in the legal system

From Greydanus DE, Pratt HD, Patel DR, Sloane MA: The rebellious adolescent. Pediatr Clin North Am 44:1460, 1997.

master prosocial skills such as the establishment and maintenance of positive family and peer relations and the resolution of conflict may put adolescents with these disorders at higher risk for physical violence and other risky behaviors. Conduct disorder and oppositional defiant disorder are specific psychiatric diagnoses whose definitions are associated with violent behavior (Table 111–2). They occur co-morbidly with other disorders such as attention deficit hyperactivity disorder and increase an adolescent's vulnerability for juvenile delinquency, substance use or abuse, sexual promiscuity, adult criminal behavior, incarceration, and antisocial personality disorder.

In an emergency or urgent care setting, one is highly likely to encounter victims of assault. Rather than treat the physical injury in isolation, the American Academy of Pediatrics has established a model protocol for assault victims. The guidelines recommend psychologic evaluation and support, social service evaluation of the circumstance surrounding the assault, and a treatment plan on discharge that is designed to protect the adolescent from subsequent injury episodes and minimize the development of psychologic disability.

Victims as well as witnesses of violence are at risk for post-traumatic stress disorder (see Chapter 22).

DIAGNOSIS. The assessment of an adolescent at risk for, or with a history of, violent behavior should be a part of the health maintenance visit of all adolescents. The answers to questions about recent history of involvement in a physical fight, carrying a weapon, or firearms in the household, as well as concerns that the adolescent may have about his or her personal safety may suggest a problem requiring a more in-depth evaluation. The additional factors of physical or sexual abuse, serious problems at school, poor school performance and attendance, multiple incidents of trauma, and symptoms associated with mental disorders are indications for evaluation by a mental health professional. In a situation of acute trauma, assault victims are not always forthcoming about the circumstances of their injuries for fear of retaliation or police involvement. Stabilization of the injury is the treatment priority; however, once this is achieved, addressing a more comprehensive set of issues surrounding the assault is appropriate.

TREATMENT. In the instance of acute injury secondary to violent assault, the treatment plan should follow standards established by the American Academy of Pediatrics model protocol, which includes, but is not limited to, the stabilization of the injury, evaluation and treatment of the injury, evaluation of the assault circumstance, psychologic evaluation of the functioning of the victim, through to the rehabilitation of the injury, and outpatient follow-up of the behavioral and physical sequelae.

PREVENTION. The Centers for Disease Control and Prevention is the lead federal agency in health for the funding of violence prevention programs. The strategy for selecting potentially successful interventions is:

> Interventions must encompass individual and social factors. Violent behaviors are influenced not only by characteristics of individuals, but also by—moving out from the individual—characteristics of families, such as cohesion and parent practices; characteristics of peers, such as delinquent behaviors; characteristics of schools, such as teacher practices and school atmosphere; characteristics of community organization, such as the frequency and type of youth activities; and characteristics of the larger society, such as economic opportunity, misuse of firearms, or media exposure. Violence-prevention efforts to date have emphasized individually oriented strategies, directed toward students in school or patients in clinical setting. These approaches should be continued, but need to be complemented by activities designed to modify exposures at the family, peer, community, and society level. (Am J Preventive Medicine, v–vi)

American Academy of Pediatrics, Task Force on Adolescent Assault Victim Needs: Adolescent assault victim needs: A review of issues and a model protocol. Pediatrics 98:991, 1996.

Anglin TM: The medical clinician's roles in preventing adolescent involvement in violence. Adolesc Med: State of the Art Rev 8:501, 1997.

Cherry D, Annest JL, Mercy JA, et al: Trends in nonfatal and fatal firearm-related injury rates in the U.S., 1985–95. Ann Emerg Med 32:51, 1998.

Federal Interagency Forum on Child and Family Statistics: America's children: Key National Indicators of Well-Being, 1998. Federal Interagency Forum on Child and Family Statistics, Washington, DC, US Government Printing Office, 1998.

Greydanus DE, Pratt HD, Patel DR, Sloane MA: The rebellious adolescent: Evaluation and management of oppositional and conduct disorders. Pediatr Clin North Am 44:1457, 1997.

Harrington D, Dubowitz H: Family violence and development during adolescence. Adolesc Med: State of Art Rev 6:199, 1995.

Hennes HMA, Calhoun AD (eds): Violence among children and adolescents. Pediatr Clin North Am 45:269, 1998.

Krug EG, Powell KE, Dahlberg LL: Firearm-related deaths in the United States and 35 other high- and upper-middle-income countries. Int J Epidemiol 27:214, 1998.

Satcher D, Powell KE, Mercy JA, Rosenberg ML: Opening commentary: Violence prevention is as American as apple pie. Am J Prev Med 12(Suppl):v, 1996.

CHAPTER 112
Anorexia Nervosa and Bulimia

Iris F. Litt

EPIDEMIOLOGY. The incidence of anorexia nervosa (AN) and bulimia has increased over the last 2 decades. It is estimated that 1 in every 100 females, 16–18 yr old, has anorexia nervosa. A bimodal distribution occurs, with one peak at 14.5 and the other at 18 yr; 25% may be younger than the age of 13. The increased incidence has been documented in all Western countries, with sporadic reports from other nations. Affected females outnumber males 10:1. Initially reported only in middle and upper socioeconomic groups, AN is now occurring in those from the lower socioeconomic levels. It is being diagnosed in a variety of ethnic and racial groups. Bulimia is more common than AN. An increased incidence of eating disorders among primary relatives of those with AN and bulimia suggests a familial basis.

DIAGNOSIS. The *Diagnostic and Statistical Manual of Mental Disorders (DSM-IV)* criteria for the diagnosis of AN include (1) intense fear of becoming obese, which does not diminish as weight loss progresses; (2) disturbance in the way in which one's body weight, size, or shape is experienced (e.g., claiming to "feel fat" even when one is emaciated or believing that one area of the body is "too fat" even when obviously underweight); (3) refusal to maintain body weight over a minimal normal weight for age and height (e.g., weight loss leading to maintenance of body weight 15% below expected, failure to make expected weight gain during period of growth leading to body weight 15% less than that expected); and (4) in females, absence of at least three consecutive menstrual cycles when otherwise expected to occur (primary or secondary amenorrhea).

AN is characterized further by excessive physical activity in the face of apparent inanition; denial of hunger; preoccupation with food preparation, frequently accompanied by bizarre eating behaviors; and often studiousness and academic success. Most youth are described as having been "model children" before the onset of the illness. Patients who have AN are subdivided into the *restrictor* and *bulimia* subgroups, according to their method of caloric reduction. Restrictors severely limit their intake of carbohydrate and fat-containing foods, whereas bulimics tend to eat in binges and then to purge themselves of food by self-induced vomiting or the use of cathartics. Excoriations on the dorsum of the hand from self-induced vomiting may suggest the diagnosis.

DSM-IV separates *bulimia* from AN as a diagnostic entity, defining bulimia as (1) recurrent episodes of binge eating (rapid consumption of a large amount of food in a discrete period of time, usually less than 2 hr); (2) during the eating binges, a fear of not being able to stop eating, (3) regularly engaging in self-induced vomiting, use of laxatives, or rigorous dieting or fasting in order to counteract the effects of binge eating; (4) a minimum average of two binge eating episodes per week for at least 3 mo; and (5) self-evaluation is unduly influenced by body weight and shape, but the disturbance does not occur exclusively during episodes of AN. The binge-purge pattern may occur in youngsters who have normal weight or are slightly obese.

ETIOLOGY AND PSYCHODYNAMICS. Eating disorders commonly begin as innocent dieting behavior, not unlike that seen in many other adolescent women, but those with AN gradually progress to profound weight loss with emaciation. Premorbid psychiatric characteristics of patients with AN may include excessive dependency, developmental immaturity, and isolation. Their families have been described as having difficulty with problem solving and as being intrusive and overprotective. The onset of these conditions at the time of puberty has prompted psychoanalysts to regard them as defenses against emerging sexuality, an opinion that dominated thinking until the 1950s, when Bruch conceptualized AN as a problem in identity development. Others consider that AN may represent a disorder of mood accompanied by manic or depressive symptoms. Patients with AN have also been subcategorized on the basis of psychologic characteristics in order to demonstrate that different subgroups are dynamically and prognostically different. Biogenic amine neurotransmitter abnormalities are found in some patients with AN. Their etiologic significance is unclear.

CLINICAL MANIFESTATIONS. AN and bulimia are associated with disturbances in almost every organ system, although it is uncertain which may be primary and which is the result of severe malnutrition. The death rate in AN is approximately 10% and is usually caused by severe electrolyte disturbance, cardiac arrhythmia, or congestive heart failure in the recovery phase. *Bradycardia* and *postural hypotension* are common, with pulse rates as low as 20 beat/min. Both improve with nutritional therapy. A variety of electrocardiographic abnormalities is common, including low voltage, T-wave inversion and flattening, and ST depression, as well as supraventricular and ventricular dysrhythmias, some preceded by a prolonged QT_c interval. Death from congestive heart failure is a late event and may result from unduly rapid rehydration and refeeding. On a regimen achieving a daily weight gain limited to 0.2–0.4 kg, none of our patients has experienced this complication.

Sleep disturbances occur in some anorexics and include a short rapid eye movement latency time, similar to that often found in depressed patients. Problems of thermal regulation, particularly hypothermia, are common (15% of our patients had temperatures recorded below 35°C). Hypothermia also occurs in some bulimics of normal weight.

Disorders of the hypothalamic-pituitary-ovarian axis are manifested as amenorrhea associated with immature patterns of secretion of luteinizing hormone. These findings may represent a primary hypothalamic defect rather than being secondary to weight loss (which also causes amenorrhea), in as much as amenorrhea antedates weight loss in one third to one half of patients with AN, and a similar proportion fail to resume menses when normal weight is restored. One quarter of patients may be amenorrheic 8 yr later, despite weight rehabilitation. Evidence for hypothalamic-pituitary-adrenal axis dysfunction includes increased secretion of cortisol, loss of diurnal variation in its secretion, and failure of dexamethasone to suppress it. The last may also be found in starvation; however, in 44% of our patients with AN, abnormal results of dexamethasone suppression tests have persisted after weight rehabilitation. Growth hormone secretion is abnormally high in these patients, and somatomedin-C is low. Thyroid-stimulating hormone levels are normal, thyroxine and triiodothyronine are low, and reverse triiodothyronine is elevated, presumably in adaptation to a lowered basal metabolic rate as a result of malnutrition and carbohydrate deprivation. In some patients, peripheral edema in the absence of congestive heart failure or hypoproteinemia has been attributed to inappropriate secretion of antidiuretic hormone.

Elevations of blood urea nitrogen may occur, reflecting dehydration and decreased glomerular filtration rate, but normal levels may be found under these same conditions because of low protein intake even in the dehydrated patient. Mild proteinuria, hematuria, and pyuria, with negative urine cultures, generally resolve with proper rehydration. Pseudoproteinuria is often found because the alkalinity of the urine gives a false-positive reaction to albumin on the dipstick.

Neuropsychologic effects of AN include impairment of concentration and problem solving, as well as attentional-perceptual motor function. Structural changes occur in the brain, such as deficits in volume of white and gray matter, the latter persisting after weight rehabilitation. Persistence of elevated cerebrospinal fluid volume has also been reported.

Bone marrow hypoplasia is common in AN, with leukopenia, anemia, and (rarely) thrombocytopenia. Low erythrocyte sedimentation rates are common, perhaps reflecting low fibrinogen production secondary to malnutrition.

Constipation is a common complication of motility problems in AN, as is esophagitis in those who vomit. Decreased gastrointestinal tract motility may be a cause of perforation, which has been reported to occur when a nasogastric tube has been inserted in patients who refuse to eat. Elevations in amylase levels may be associated with bilateral parotid swelling or with pancreatitis.

Electrolyte imbalance results from vomiting, "waterloading" (a practice of surreptitiously drinking large amounts of water in order to achieve an agreed-upon weight gain), or abuse of diuretics or laxatives. Potassium depletion, associated with a hypochloremic alkalosis, is common. Abnormalities of calcium, magnesium, and phosphorus metabolism may result from laxative abuse, either secondary to malabsorption or resulting from the use of preparations containing phosphate.

Patients with AN appear to be remarkably resistant to infection, and the few studies of their immunologic status support this view. The fact that protein intake is relatively good in these otherwise malnourished persons may contribute to this finding. Bone density may be abnormally low, but this osteopenia appears to improve with weight gain. A number of possible mechanisms have been suggested to explain this finding, including low levels of estrogen and calcium and elevated cortisol levels. The skin of patients with AN is dry, and lanugo hair is often seen. Hair loss often occurs in the refeeding phase.

TREATMENT. Systematic, controlled studies of treatment in these disorders are not available. Most of the regimens in current use combine psychotherapy (individual and family), behavior modification techniques, and nutritional rehabilitation. Pharmacologic therapy (primarily with antidepressant medications) appears to be helpful for that subset of depressed patients with eating disorders. The success rate in short-term follow-up studies is about 70%. The frequent occurrence of medical complications and the possibility of death during the acute or rehabilitation phase require the inclusion of a medically and physiologically oriented physician in the management team.

Fisher M, Golden NH, Katzman DK, et al: Eating disorders in adolescents: A background paper. J Adolesc Health 16:420, 1995.

Katzman DK, Zipursky RB, Lambe EK, Mikulis DJ: A longitudinal magnetic resonance imaging study of brain changes in adolescents with anorexia nervosa. Arch Pediatr Adolesc Med 151:793, 1997.

CHAPTER 113
Substance Abuse

Cultural and societal norms frame acceptable standards for substance use. These standards also have a historical context. The nonacceptance of alcohol use during prohibition and the acceptance of marijuana use during the 1970s are examples of the cultural and historical context in the United States. Adolescents are influenced by these factors and by adult role models and environmental messages related to substances. In the context of the 1990s, occasional or situational use of certain substances such as alcohol, marijuana, and cigarettes may be viewed as "normative" given the proportion of youth who report some experience with these substances. Some studies suggest that otherwise normal, healthy, adolescents who "experiment" with drugs may be better adjusted than those who lack that experience. Others view the potential for adverse outcomes even with occasional use in immature adolescents, such as motor vehicle accidents and other injuries, sufficient justification to consider any drug use in younger adolescents a considerable risk.

The developmental considerations are probably the most important for this age group. Substance use for most teenagers is not an issue of psychopathology but of the influence on normal functioning. Drug use in younger, less experienced adolescents can act as a substitute for developing age-appropriate coping strategies and enhance vulnerability to poor decision-making. When drug use begins to negatively alter functioning in older adolescents at school and in the family, and risk-taking behavior is seen, intervention is warranted. Serious drug use is not an isolated phenomenon. It is a part of a complex set of family and individual issues that should be addressed in a comprehensive fashion. The challenge to the clinician is to determine which type of behavior one is observing and to take the necessary action. The challenge to the community and society is to create norms that decrease the likelihood of adverse health outcomes for adolescents and promote and facilitate opportunities for adolescents to choose healthier and safer options for experimentation.

ETIOLOGY. The determinants of adolescent substance use and abuse have been explained using a number of theoretical models. Most of the models include factors at the individual level, the level of significant relationships with others, and the level of the setting, that is, community or other environment. Models have also begun to include a balance of risk and protective or coping factors that tend to account for individual differences among adolescents with similar risk factors who in fact escape adverse outcomes. Duncan and Petrosa also argue for differentiating the risk factors for adolescent use compared with adolescent abuse. Adolescent use is more commonly related to social and peer factors, whereas abuse is more a function of psychologic and biologic factors. The likelihood that an otherwise normal adolescent would experiment with drugs may be dependent on the availability of the drug to the adolescent, the perceived positive or otherwise functional value to the adolescent, and the presence of absence of restraints as determined by the adolescent's cultural or other important value system. An abusing adolescent, in contrast, may have operative genetic or biologic factors coexisting with dependence on a particular drug for coping with day-to-day activities. In addition, such an adolescent may adopt the identification with the addicted role, specifically with a fear of the consequences of withdrawal.

Specific historical questions can assist in determining the severity of the drug problem through a rating system as depicted in Table 113–1. The type of drug used (e.g., marijuana versus heroin), the circumstances of use (e.g., alone or in a group setting), the frequency and timing of use (e.g., daily before school versus rarely on a weekend), the premorbid personality (depressed versus happy), as well as the teenager's general functional status should all be considered in evaluating any youngster found to be abusing a drug. In addition, certain protective factors are acknowledged to play a part in buffering the risk factors as well as assisting in anticipating the long-term outcome of experimentation. Emotionally supportive parents with open communication styles, involvement in organized school activities, and recognition of the importance of academic achievement are a few of the most commonly recognized protective factors. Involvement in organized sports activ-

TABLE 113–1 Assessing the Seriousness of Adolescent Drug Abuse

Variable	0	+1	+2
Age (yr)	>15 yr	<15 yr	
Sex	Male	Female	
Family history of drug abuse		Yes	
Setting of drug use	In group		Alone
Affect before drug use	Happy	Always poor	Sad
School performance	Good, improving		Recently poor
Use before driving	None		Yes
History of accidents	None		Yes
Time of week	Weekend	Weekdays	
Time of day		After school	Before school
Type of drug	Marijuana, beer, wine	Hallucinogens, amphetamines	Whiskey, opiates, cocaine, barbiturates

Total score: 0–3 less worrisome, 3–8 serious, 8–18 very serious.

ities is usually protective, but it may be a risk factor in regard to the use of anabolic steroids. Any use of a psychoactive drug in the context of the use of machinery or a motor vehicle or in a potentially volatile interpersonal interaction can add an increased health risk, regardless of the extent of any prior use.

EPIDEMIOLOGY. Surveys on adolescent substance use have a variety of limitations due to sampling and questionnaire differences. The National Household Survey on Drug Abuse and the Youth Risk Behavior Surveillance System (Centers for Disease Control) also may reflect refusal to report use within a household. School-based surveys (Monitoring the Future study of middle and high school students) do not capture school dropouts, school absenteeism, and high rates of refusal. The rates of drug use in the Monitoring the Future survey are higher than in the household survey. However, certain observations are consistent across surveys. Alcohol and cigarettes are the most prevalent drugs (Table 113–2). Marijuana tends to be the most commonly reported illicit drug ever used, with the exception of inhalants in younger teenagers (8th grade). The prevalence of substance use varies by age, gender, geographic region, race, and other demographic factors. Younger teenagers tend to report less use of most drugs than do older teenagers, with the exception of inhalants (21% in 8th grade, 18.3% in 10th grade, and 16.1% in 12th grade, 1997). Males strongly predominate in the lifetime prevalence reports for smokeless tobacco and anabolic steroids compared with females (50.3% male, 12.8% female; 3.8% male, 0.8% female, respectively). Forty-two per cent of students in the Northeast report ever using an illicit drug, whereas 36% of students in the South report such use. Marijuana use is reported more frequently in large metropolitan areas, whereas less urbanized areas report more binge drinking and daily cigarette use. In school surveys, Hispanics report more experience with cocaine, whereas white students report high rates of smokeless tobacco and daily cigarette smoking. By 12th grade, blacks report less use of drugs across all categories, with similar low rates of reports in 8th and 10th grade, challenging the assumption that the low rates are a reflection of dropout rates in senior high.

Students reporting marijuana use over the prior year in 8th, 10th, and 12th grades were 22.6%, 42.3%, and 49.6%, respectively. For students who have ever used alcohol, reporting shows 53.8%, 72.0%, and 65.4%, with nicotine at 47.3%, 60.2% and 65.4%, respectively for 8th, 10th, and 12th grades. Trend data for 12th grade students are available from 1975, and 8th and 10th grade data are available from 1991. Eighth graders on the whole show a modest annual decrease across all substances. Patterns of use in 10th graders varies significantly by the type of substance. The nadir of illicit drug use in 12th graders occurred in 1992, and since that time it has been gradually rising. Marijuana use shows the largest annual increase from 1996–1997, 2.7%. Annual alcohol use also increased at the rate of 2.3% for the same year.

PATHOGENESIS. The process of physical growth and development that characterizes puberty may be affected adversely by the use of drugs. For example, one third of adolescent females who use *heroin* have secondary amenorrhea, even in the absence of weight loss. The higher incidence of menstrual abnormalities in the adolescent heroin user probably results from a greater vulnerability of the hypothalamic-pituitary-ovarian axis in the maturing individual. Experiments with naloxone, the opiate antagonist, suggest that endogenous opiates block the release of gonadotropin-releasing hormone. *Amphetamines* interfere with stage 4 sleep and may impair the intimate relationship between sleep and augmentation of secretion of gonadotropin during early adolescence. To derive calories mainly from *ethanol* during the peak of the pubertal growth spurt deprives the body of the protein necessary for normal muscle growth.

TABLE 113–2 Lifetime Use of Cigarettes, Alcohol, Marijuana in 8th, 10th, and 12th Grade Students

	8th Grade	10th Grade	12th Grade
Cigarettes	47%	60.2%	65.4%
Alcohol	53.8%	72.0%	81.7%
Marijuana	22.6%	42.3%	49.6%

From Johnston LD, O'Malley PM, Bachman JG: Drug abuse among American teens show some signs of leveling after a long rise. Ann Arbor, University of Michigan News and Information Services, December 18, 1997.

The metabolism of certain prescribed drugs may be affected by coincident abuse of illicit drugs or alcohol. Induction of hepatic smooth endoplasmic reticulum by barbiturates or alcohol may accelerate the metabolism and enhance the excretion of substances requiring glucuronidation. As a result of this mechanism, estrogen-containing oral contraceptives taken by an abuser of these substances may result in a vulnerability to pregnancy. Conversely, the use of estrogens increases the risk of intoxication from alcohol as a result of decreased ethanol metabolism. The potentiating interaction of alcohol and barbiturates must also be considered when prescribing anticonvulsant medications. Abdominal pain and vomiting occur when metronidazole is ingested by an alcohol-abusing adolescent because of the antagonistic effect of alcohol on acetaldehyde.

CLINICAL MANIFESTATIONS. Although manifestations vary by the specific substance of use, adolescents who use drugs often present in an office setting with no obvious physical findings. Drug use is more frequently detected in adolescents who are victims of motor vehicle accidents or intentional injuries. Eliciting appropriate historical information regarding substance use followed by a urine drug screen is recommended in emergency settings. In addition, an adolescent presenting to an emergency setting with an impaired sensorium as part of a toxic syndrome should be evaluated for substance use as a part of the differential diagnosis, again accompanied by appropriate screening and physical examination (Table 113–3). Certain psychiatric and behavioral diagnoses are frequently associated with substance use and should be considered once such use is detected. Conversely, screening for substance use is recommended for patients with psychiatric and behavioral diagnoses. Diagnoses that are commonly considered range from conduct disorders, with or without attention deficit disorder, to personality disorders. Other clinical manifestations of substance use are associated with the route of use, that is, intravenous drug use is associated with venous "tracks" and needle marks, and nasal mucosal injuries are associated with nasal insufflation of drugs. Seizures can be a direct effect of drugs such as cocaine and amphetamines or an effect of drug withdrawal in the case of barbiturates or tranquilizers. Additional specific clinical manifestations are described in the following sections on each substance.

SCREENING FOR SUBSTANCE ABUSE AND USE. The annual health maintenance examination provides an opportunity for identifying adolescents with substance use or abuse issues (see Chapter 108.2). The direct questions as well as the assessment of school, family relations, and peer activities may necessitate a more in-depth interview if there are suggestions of difficulties in those areas. Several self-report screening questionnaires are available with varying degrees of standardization, length, and reliability. The use of urine screening is recommended in select circumstances, most of which are constructed to provide for the confidentiality and informed choice of the adolescent. Such indications include (1) psychiatric symptoms, to rule out comorbidity or dual diagnoses; (2) significant changes in school performance or other daily behaviors; (3) frequently occurring accidents; (4) frequently occurring episodes or respiratory problems; (5) evaluation of serious motor vehicular or other injuries; and (6) as a monitoring procedure for a recovery program. Table 113–4 demonstrates the types of test com-

TABLE 113–3 The Most Common Toxic Syndromes

Anticholinergic Syndromes	
Common signs	Delirium with mumbling speech, tachycardia, dry, flushed skin, dilated pupils, myoclonus, slightly elevated temperature, urinary retention, and decreased bowel sounds. Seizures and dysrhythmias may occur in severe cases.
Common causes	Antihistamines, antiparkinsonian medication, atropine, scopolamine, amantadine, antipsychotic agents, antidepressant agents, antispasmodic agents, mydriatic agents, skeletal muscle relaxants, and many plants (notably jimson weed and *Amanita muscaria*).
Sympathomimetic Syndromes	
Common signs	Delusions, paranoia, tachycardia (or bradycardia if the drug is a pure α-adrenergic agonist), hypertension, hyperpyrexia, diaphoresis, piloerection, mydriasis, and hyperreflexia. Seizures, hypotension, and dysrhythmias may occur in severe cases.
Common causes	Cocaine, amphetamine, methamphetamine (and its derivatives 3,4-methylenedioxyamphetamine, 3,4-methylenedioxymethamphetamine, 3,4-methylenedioxyethamphetamine, and 2,5-dimethoxy-4-bromoamphetamine), and over-the-counter decongestants (phenylpropanolamine, ephedrine, and pseudoephedrine). In caffeine and theophylline overdoses, similar findings, except for the organic psychiatric signs, result from catecholamine release.
Opiate, Sedative, or Ethanol Intoxication	
Common signs	Coma, respiratory depression, miosis, hypotension, bradycardia, hypothermia, pulmonary edema, decreased bowel sounds, hyporeflexia, and needle marks. Seizures may occur after overdoses of some narcotics, notably propoxyphene.
Common causes	Narcotics, barbiturates, benzodiazepines, ethchlorvynol, glutethimide, methyprylon, methaqualone, meprobamate, ethanol, clonidine, and guanabenz.
Cholinergic Syndromes	
Common signs	Confusion, central nervous system depression, weakness, salivation, lacrimation, urinary and fecal incontinence, gastrointestinal cramping, emesis, diaphoresis, muscle fasciculations, pulmonary edema, miosis, bradycardia or tachycardia, and seizures.
Common causes	Organophosphate and carbamate insecticides, physostigmine, edrophonium, and some mushrooms.

From Kulig K: Initial management of ingestions of toxic substances. N Engl J Med 326:1678, 1992.

monly used for detection by substance, along with the approximate retention time between the use and the identification of the substance in the urine. Most initial screening uses an immunoassay method such as the enzyme-multiplied immunoassay technique followed by a confirmatory test using the highly sensitive, highly specific gas chromatography-mass spectrometry. The substances that can cause false-positive results should be considered, especially when there is a discrepancy between the physical findings and the urine drug screen result.

DIAGNOSIS. Diagnostic criteria that classify the severity of substance use-abuse ranges from substance use variation, through the diagnosis of a substance abuse problem, to the definition of a substance abuse disorder. Substance abuse variation refers to the experimentation that commonly occurs in this age group. An adolescent is considered to have a diagnosis of a substance abuse problem if the use occurs more than on a one-time basis and involves impaired memory or other motor function deficits. A substance abuse disorder carries with it the observation of impaired functioning in key settings such as in school, at home, and with peers. The criteria for a disorder encompasses the issues of tolerance, frequency or volume of drug taken, period of time of use, inability to stop the use, and amount of time consumed by drug activities relative to normal activities. Specific diagnostic codes are assigned to substance abuse, substance intoxication, and substance withdrawal.

COMPLICATIONS. Substance use in adolescence has psychologic as well as physical risks. Youth may engage in robbery, bur-

TABLE 113–4 Urine Screening for Drugs Commonly Abused by Adolescents

Drug	Major Metabolite	Initial	First Confirmation	Second Confirmation	Approximate Retention Time
Alcohol (blood)	Acetaldehyde	GC	IA		7–10 hr
Alcohol (urine)	Acetaldehyde	GC	IA		10–13 hr
Amphetamines		TLC	IA	GC,GC/MS	48 hr
Barbiturates		IA	TLC	GC,GC/MS	Short-acting (24 hr); long-acting (2–3 wk)
Benzodiazepines		IA	TLC	GC,GC/MS	3 days
Cannabinoids	Carboxy- and hydroxymetabolites	IA	TLC	GC/MS	3–10 days (occasional user); 1–2 mo (chronic user)
Cocaine	Benzoyl ecgonine	IA	TLC	GC/MS	2–4 days
Methaqualone	Hydroxylated metabolites	TLC	IA	GC/MS	2 wk
Opiates					
Heroin	Morphine Glucuronide	IA	TLC	GC,GC/MS	2 days
Morphine	Morphine Glucuronide	IA	TLC	GC,GC/MS	2 days
Codeine	Morphine Glucuronide	IA	TLC	GC,GC/MS	2 days
Phencyclidine		TLC	IA	GC,GC/MS	8 days

Modified from Drugs of abuse—Urine screening [Physician information sheet]. Los Angeles: Pacific Toxicology.
GC = gas chromatography; IA = immunoassay; TLC = thin-layer chromatography; MS = mass spectrometry.
From MacKenzie RG, Kipke MD: Substance use and abuse. In: Friedman SB, Fisher M, Schonberg SK (eds): Comprehensive Adolescent Health Care. St. Louis, Quality Medical Publishing, Inc., 1992, p 783.

glary, drug dealing, or prostitution for the purpose of acquiring the money necessary to buy drugs or alcohol. Regular use of any drug eventually diminishes judgment and is associated with unprotected sexual activity with its consequences of pregnancy and sexually transmitted diseases, including human immunodeficiency virus (HIV), as well as physical violence and trauma. Several studies of adolescent trauma victims have identified cannabinoids and cocaine in blood and urine samples in significant proportions, in addition to the more common identification of alcohol. Drug and alcohol use are closely associated with trauma in the adolescent population. Any use of injected substances involves the risk of hepatitis and HIV.

PREVENTION. The model of prevention relevant to the problem of adolescent drug or alcohol use is one that anticipates experimentation with some agent at some point in the normal development of the adolescent and that attempts to delay that event as long as possible, to make its use as limited in amount and setting as possible, and to prevent entirely any use while operating a motor vehicle or any other machinery. Educational efforts based on scare techniques have not been successful, whereas those that present unemotional, factual information about medical complications of drug use combined with skills training to resist drug use have had some impact. The effect of intervention programs vary according to the type of substance most influenced by the intervention (see specific drugs).

TREATMENT. Acute management is discussed in the following sections on specific agents. A variety of chronic treatment programs are available in inpatient and ambulatory settings. In general, these programs have not been adequately evaluated. Important features of successful long-term management of these adolescents include continuing medical evaluation after detoxification and the provision of developmentally appropriate psychosocial support systems.

PROGNOSIS. For adolescent substance abusers who have been referred to a drug treatment program, outcomes are directly related to regular attendance in post-treatment groups. For males with learning problems, these outcomes were worse than were those of their peers. Peer use patterns and parental use have a major influence on outcome for males. For females, factors such as self-esteem and anxiety are more important influences on outcomes. The chronicity of a substance abuse disorder makes relapse an issue that must always be kept in mind when managing patients after treatment, and appropriate assistance from a health professional qualified in substance abuse management should be obtained.

113.1 Alcohol

Alcohol use among adolescents has increased during the past decade and poses a threat to the normal functioning of the teenager as well as to the lives of those potentially jeopardized by drunken drivers. The usual progression is from beer to wine to hard liquor, although regional differences may alter this pattern. Four ounces of hard liquor (86 proof) consumed on an empty stomach produces a plasma ethanol level of approximately 65 mg/dL in an adult male of average weight and 80 mg/dL in a premenstrual female of adult weight. The legal definition of intoxication in most statutes is a blood ethanol level of 100 mg/dL (0.08% or 0.10%).

Alcohol is noted as a contributing factor in 8,000 adolescent deaths and 45,000 injuries each year. Approximately 40% of the 10,000 annual nonautomotive accidental deaths, such as drowning and falls, are also associated with alcohol use. The estimates for involvement in suicide and homicide reach about 5,000/diagnosis/year. For a legal drug, alcohol contributes to more deaths in young individuals than all the illicit drugs combined. Therefore, pediatricians should not underestimate the need to recognize alcohol use and abuse in this age group.

PHARMACOLOGY AND PATHOPHYSIOLOGY. Alcohol (ethyl alcohol or ethanol) is rapidly absorbed in the stomach and is transported to the liver and metabolized by two pathways. The primary pathway involves removal of two hydrogen atoms to form acetaldehyde, a reaction catalyzed by alcohol dehydrogenase through reduction of a cofactor nicotinamide-adenine dinucleotide. The removed hydrogen atoms supply energy (7.1 kcal/g of alcohol) and contribute to the excess synthesis of triglycerides, a phenomenon that is responsible for producing a fatty liver, even in those who are well nourished. Engorgement of hepatocytes with fat causes necrosis, triggering an inflammatory process (alcoholic hepatitis), which is followed by fibrosis, the hallmark of cirrhosis. Early hepatic involvement may result in elevation in γ-glutamyl transpeptidase and serum glutamic-pyruvic transaminase. The 2nd metabolic pathway, which is utilized at high serum alcohol levels, involves the microsomal system of the liver, in which the cofactor is reduced nicotinamide-adenine dinucleotide phosphate. The net effect of activation of this pathway is to decrease metabolism of drugs that share this system and to allow for their accumulation, enhanced effect, and possible toxicity (e.g., drinking alcohol and ingesting tranquilizers results in the potentiation of each.

CLINICAL MANIFESTATIONS. Alcohol acts primarily as a central nervous system (CNS) depressant. It produces euphoria, grogginess, talkativeness, and impaired short-term memory, and it increases the pain threshold. Alcohol's ability to produce vasodilation and hypothermia is also centrally mediated. At very high serum levels, respiratory depression occurs. Its inhibitory effect on pituitary antidiuretic hormone release is responsible for its diuretic effect. The gastrointestinal complications of alcohol use can occur from a single large ingestion. The most common is acute erosive gastritis, which is manifested by epigastric pain, anorexia, vomiting, and guaiac-positive stools. Less commonly, vomiting and midabdominal pain may be caused by acute alcoholic pancreatitis; diagnosis is confirmed by the finding of elevated serum amylase and lipase activities.

Only a small number of adolescents become young alcoholics; however, problem drinking during adolescence requiring a therapeutic intervention is not uncommon. Adolescents who report having been drunk six or more times in the past year; having problems with school authorities, friends, or the police; having been criticized by dates for drinking habits; or having driven after drinking are considered problem drinkers.

DIAGNOSIS. In addition to the general risk factors noted for substance use, a positive family history of alcohol abuse is significant. The genetic influences for the predisposition to alcoholism is supported by family, twin, and adoption studies. Children of alcoholic parents demonstrate a three- to fourfold increase in the risk for alcoholism. The *alcohol overdose syndrome* should be suspected in any teenager who appears disoriented, lethargic, or comatose. Although the distinctive aroma of alcohol may assist in diagnosis, confirmation by analysis of blood is recommended. There is a high correlation between results obtained by serum and breath analyses so that the latter method may be reliably used. At levels greater than 200 mg/dL, the adolescent is at risk of death, and levels greater than 500 mg/dL (median lethal dose) are usually associated with a fatal outcome. When the level of depression appears excessive for the reported blood level, head trauma or ingestion of other drugs should be considered as possible confounding factors.

TREATMENT. The usual mechanism of death from the alcohol overdose syndrome is respiratory depression, and artificial ventilatory support must be provided until the liver can eliminate sufficient amounts of alcohol from the body. In a patient without alcoholism, it generally takes 20 hr to reduce the blood level of alcohol from 400 mg/dL to zero. Dialysis should be considered when the blood level is higher than 400 mg/dL.

113.2 Marijuana

Marijuana and alcohol, the most popular substances of abuse among adolescents, share a number of psychopharmacologic qualities. Both decrease short-term memory and fine coordination, prolong reaction time, and produce "mental clouding." About 300 mg of cannabis is equivalent to 70 g of alcohol.

PHARMACOLOGY. Marijuana (THC, "pot," "weed," "hash," "grass") is synthesized from the resin of the *Cannabis sativa* plant, which flourishes in temperate and hot, dry climates. The tetrahydrocannabinol (THC) fraction of the resin is responsible for its hallucinogenic properties and has been synthesized (δ-9-THC). THC is absorbed rapidly by the nasal or oral routes, producing a peak of subjective effect at 10 min and 1 hr, respectively. Marijuana is generally consumed as a "reefer" or "joint," made by rolling the crushed plant material in paper. Although there is much variation in content, each cigarette contains approximately 1 g of marijuana or 20 mg of δ-9-THC. Another popular form that is smoked, a "blunt," is a hollowed-out small cigar refilled with marijuana.

CLINICAL MANIFESTATIONS. In addition to the "desired" effects of elation and euphoria, marijuana may cause impairment of short-term memory, poor performance of tasks requiring divided attention (e.g., those involved in driving), loss of critical judgment, and distortion of time perception. Visual hallucinations and perceived body distortions occur rarely, but there may be "flashbacks" or recall of frightening hallucinations experienced under marijuana's influence that usually occur during stress or with fever.

Temperature may be lowered. Tachycardia is apparent within 20 min of smoking marijuana and is followed 1/2 hr later by transient systolic and diastolic hypertension, which disappears by 3 hr. Tachypnea is observed only in the experienced user. In placebo-controlled studies of experienced users, smoking marijuana caused hypercapnic ventilation and a decrease in forced expired volume, maximal midexpiratory flow rate, airway conductance, and diffusing capacity. Reduction in bronchospasm has also been demonstrated. Both δ-9-THC and marijuana (smoking a single joint) cause a significant fall in intraocular pressure, lasting up to 5 hr in normal persons as well as in patients with glaucoma.

Kolodny demonstrated dose-related suppression of plasma testosterone levels and spermatogenesis as a result of smoking marijuana for a minimum of 4 days/wk for 6 mo, prompting concern about the potential deleterious effect of smoking marijuana before completion of pubertal growth and development. Smoking marijuana for 1 wk also decreases glucose tolerance. There is an antiemetic effect of oral THC or smoked marijuana, often followed by appetite stimulation, which is the basis of the drug's use in patients receiving cancer chemotherapy. Although the possibility of teratogenicity and carcinogenesis has been raised because of findings in animals, there is no evidence for such effects in humans. Although an "amotivational" syndrome has been described in chronic marijuana users who lose interest in age-appropriate behavior, there is no proof of physiologic dependency. Certain drugs may interact with marijuana to potentiate sedation (i.e., alcohol, diazepam), potentiate stimulation (i.e., cocaine, amphetamines), or be antagonistic (i.e., propranolol, phenytoin).

113.3 Tobacco

CIGARETTES

In 1997, 24.6% of 12th graders, 18% of 10th graders, and 9% of 8th graders reported smoking on a daily basis. These figures represent a 2.6% annual increase for 12th graders, but a small decline for the other two grades. However, most alarming is the compelling evidence of the addictive nature of cigarette smoking, with the natural course of the addiction beginning during the childhood and adolescent years. Compared with all other substances and firearms, tobacco kills more individuals in the United States each year than all these other factors combined. The severity of atherosclerosis may be correlated with the duration of smoking, increasing its risk among those who begin smoking during adolescence. Eighty-five per cent of all current cigarette smokers began smoking before 21 yr of age.

PHARMACOLOGY. Human and animal studies confirm the addictive effect of nicotine, the primary active ingredient in cigarettes. It produces a syndrome of dependence as well as withdrawal. Nicotine is absorbed by multiple sites in the body, including lungs, skin, gastrointestinal tract, and buccal and nasal mucosa. The average nicotine content of one cigarette is 10 mg and the average nicotine intake per cigarette ranges from 1.0 mg to 3 mg. Nicotine, as delivered in cigarette smoke, has a half-life of 10–20 min, with an elimination half-life of 2–3 hr. Nicotine's effect on the brain takes less than 20 sec. The action of nicotine is mediated through nicotinic acetylcholine receptors. These receptors are located on noncholinergic presynaptic and postsynaptic sites in the brain. Cotinine is the major metabolite of nicotine via C-oxidation. It has a biologic half-life of 19–24 hr and can be detected in urine, serum, and saliva.

CLINICAL MANIFESTATIONS. Adverse health effects of smoking may occur during adolescence. These adverse effects include an increased prevalence of chronic cough, phlegm production, and wheezing. Smoking during pregnancy is associated with an average decrease in fetal weight of 200 g; this, added to the already smaller size of infants born to teenagers, increases perinatal morbidity and mortality. Smoking in combination with the use of estrogen-containing oral contraceptives is associated with an increased risk of myocardial infarction. Tobacco smoke induces hepatic smooth endoplasmic reticulum and, as a result, may also influence metabolism of drugs and of endogenously produced hormones. Phenacetin, theophylline, and imipramine are examples of drugs affected in this manner. In addition, laboratory test results may be affected by smoking, for example, white blood cell count, hemoglobin, hematocrit, mean corpuscular volume, and platelet aggregation are increased and serum creatinine, albumin, globulin (in females), and uric acid (in males) are decreased (see Chapter 725).

TREATMENT. The approach to smoking cessation in adolescents is primarily anecdotal; however, clinicians are encouraged to adapt adult programs to adolescents who express a desire to quit. Clinical practice guidelines are available for practical office-based counseling strategies. Recommendations for the use of nicotine replacement therapy vary with the type of product. There is little empirical evidence on the efficacy and safety of such products. Although there are no contraindications for use of the patch or gum, nicotine nasal spray is not recommended for use by adolescents. Over-the-counter products cannot be purchased by persons under 18 yr of age. Consequently, health supervision and supportive counseling are necessary components to smoking cessation management in adolescents.

SMOKELESS TOBACCO

Surveys in the late 1980s and 1990s indicating the increased use of smokeless tobacco (ST) prompted the National Cancer Institute to lead the United States' federal government effort to prevent ST use, especially in adolescents. Surveys now indicate that since the early to mid-1990s, lifetime prevalence of ST use has declined in 8th, 10th, and 12 graders. Regular users of ST risk physical dependence on nicotine. Chewing tobacco may result in lesions, primarily in the mandibular mucobuccal fold. With chronic use, these lesions may become malignant.

113.4 Volatile Substances

The practice of inhalation of a variety of euphoriants has enjoyed popularity among adolescents for centuries. The first well-described documentation of this phenomenon related to an "epidemic" of ether sniffing by Irish teenagers in the 19th century. Young adolescents are attracted to these substances because of their rapid action, easy availability, and low cost. The most popular inhalants among adolescent are glue, gasoline, and volatile nitrites. The 1980 restrictions placed on the use of fluorocarbons in aerosols reduced the prevalence of its use.

CLINICAL MANIFESTATIONS. The major effects of inhalants are psychoactive. Toluene, the main ingredient in airplane glue and some rubber cements, causes relaxation and pleasant hallucinations for up to 2 hr. Tolerance and physical dependence may occur. Gasoline, a popular substance among rural adolescents and Native American youth, contains a complex mixture of organic solvents. Euphoria is followed by violent excitement, and coma may result from prolonged or rapid inhalation. Volatile nitrites, such as amyl nitrite, butyl nitrite, and related compounds marketed as room deodorizers, are used as euphoriants, enhancers of musical appreciation, and aphrodisiacs among older adolescents and young adults. They may result in headaches, syncope, and lightheadedness; profound hypotension and cutaneous flushing followed by vasoconstriction and tachycardia; transiently inverted T waves and depressed ST segments on electrocardiography; methemoglobinemia; increased bronchial irritation; and increased intraocular pressure.

COMPLICATIONS. Airplane glue has been responsible for a wide range of complications, relating to chemical toxicity, to the method of administration (e.g., in plastic bags, with resultant suffocation), and to the often dangerous setting in which the inhalation occurs (e.g., inner-city roof tops). Gasoline toxicity is acute as well as chronic. Death in the acute phase may result from cerebral or pulmonary edema or myocardial involvement. Chronic use may cause pulmonary hypertension, restrictive lung defects or reduced diffusion capacity, peripheral neuropathy, acute rhabdomyolysis, hematuria, tubular acidosis, and possibly cerebral and cerebellar atrophy. Other behavioral disturbances such as inattentiveness, lack of coordination, and general disorientation have been linked to chronic solvent abuse.

DIAGNOSIS. The brief effect of the inhalants makes it unlikely to diagnose unless there is a complication or death from use. In extreme intoxication, a user may manifest symptoms of restlessness, general muscle weakness, dysarthria, nystagmus, disruptive behavior, and occasionally hallucinations, placing inhalant use in the differential diagnoses for acute intoxication of an adolescent. Toluene is excreted rapidly in the urine as hippuric acid, with the residual detectable in the serum by gas chromatography.

TREATMENT. Treatment is generally supportive and directed toward control of arrhythmia and stabilization of respirations and circulation. Withdrawal symptoms do not usually occur.

113.5 Hallucinogens

Several naturally occurring and synthetic substances have been used by adolescents for their hallucinogenic properties. Lysergic acid diethylamide (LSD), methylenedioxymethamphetamine (MDMA) or ecstasy, and phencyclidine (PCP) are the most commonly reported hallucinogens in high school. Among high school seniors in 1997, 15.1% reported ever using a hallucinogen, with 13.6% reporting the use of LSD, 6.9% reporting the use of MDMA, and 3.9% reporting the use of PCP. These reports reflect an increasing trend in use from 1991 to 1997. National household survey rates for all hallucinogens report lifetime use for 12–17 yr olds at 5.6%, with use in the prior year at 4.3%. Illicit drugs sold on the street are not labeled and are frequency misrepresented. In one survey, 11% of the confiscated drugs submitted as LSD to the Los Angeles County Street Drug Identification Program contained no identifiable LSD. The reported experiences with these drugs still represent a significant level of experimentation with dangerous chemicals.

LYSERGIC ACID DIETHYLAMIDE

LSD (acid, big "D," blotters) is one of the constituents found in rye fungus. Morning glory seeds contain lysergic acid derivatives, although the commercially packaged varieties have often been treated with toxic chemicals such as insecticides and fungicides. Although the specific mechanisms of action of LSD are still under study, it is proposed to alter neurotransmitters mediated by serotonin. LSD is a very potent hallucinogen with doses as low as 20 μg causing effects in some individuals. Its high potency allows effective doses to be applied to objects as small as postage stamps and paper blotters. It is rapidly absorbed from the gastrointestinal tract. The onset of action can be between 30 and 60 min, and it peaks between 2 and 4 hr. By 10–12 hours, an individual returns to the predrug state.

CLINICAL MANIFESTATIONS. The effects of LSD can be divided into three categories: somatic (physical effects), perceptual (altered changes in vision and hearing), and psychic effects (changes in sensorium). The common somatic symptoms are dizziness, dilatated pupils, nausea, flushing, elevated temperature, and tachycardia. The sensation of synesthesia or "seeing" smells and "hearing" colors has been reported with LSD use. Delusional ideation, body distortion, and suspiciousness to the point of toxic psychosis are the more serious of the psychic symptoms.

TREATMENT. An individual is considered to have a "bad trip" when the setting causes the user to become terrified or panicked. These episodes should be treated by removing the individual from the aggravating situation or setting and attempting to re establish contact with reality through calm verbal interaction. Any physical complications such as hyperthermia, seizure, or hypertension should be treated supportively. "Flashbacks" or LSD-induced states after the drug has worn off and tolerance to the effects of the drug are additional complications of its use. LSD use has not been associated with a withdrawal syndrome.

METHYLENEDIOXYMETHAMPHETAMINE

MDMA ("X," ecstasy), a phenylisopropylamine hallucinogen, is a synthetic compound similar to mescaline, commonly referred to as a "designer drug." Like other hallucinogens, this drug is proposed to interact with serotoninergic neurons in the CNS.

CLINICAL MANIFESTATIONS. Euphoria, a heightened sensual awareness, and increased psychic and emotional energy are the observed acute effects of MDMA. Compared with other hallucinogens, MDMA is less likely to produce emotional lability, depersonalization, and disturbances of thought. Adverse effects can be physical as well as psychic. Nausea, jaw clenching, teeth grinding, and blurred vision are somatic symptoms, whereas anxiety, panic attacks, and psychosis are the adverse psychic outcomes. A few deaths have been reported after ingestion of the drug. There are no specific treatment regimens recommended for acute toxicity.

PHENCYCLIDINE

PCP (sternyl, angel dust, "hog," "peace pill," "sheets") is an arylcyclohexalamine whose popularity is related, in part, to its ease of synthesis in home laboratories. One of the by-products of home synthesis causes cramps, diarrhea, and hematemesis. The drug is thought to potentiate adrenergic effects by inhibiting neuronal reuptake of catecholamines. PCP is available as a tablet, liquid, or powder, which may be used alone or sprinkled on cigarettes ("joints"). The powders and tablets generally contain 2–6 mg of PCP, whereas joints average 1 mg for every 150 mg of tobacco leaves, or approximately 30–50 mg per joint.

CLINICAL MANIFESTATIONS. The clinical manifestations are dose-related. Euphoria, nystagmus, ataxia, and emotional lability occur within 2–3 min after smoking 1–5 mg and last for hours. Hallucination may involve bizarre distortions of body image that often precipitate panic reactions. With doses of 5–15 mg, a toxic psychosis may occur, with disorientation, hypersalivation, and abusive language lasting for more than 1 hr. After oral ingestion of 15 mg or more, the patient usually becomes comatose within 30–60 min, with alternating periods of wakefulness, with dystonic posturing, muscular rigidity, or myoclonic jerks. Hypotension, generalized seizures, and cardiac arrhythmias commonly occur with plasma concentrations from 40–200 mg/dL. Death has been reported during psychotic delirium, from hypertension, hypotension, hypothermia, seizures, and trauma. The coma of PCP may be distinguished from that of the opiates by the absence of respiratory depression; the presence of muscle rigidity, hyperreflexia, and nystagmus; and lack of response to naloxone. PCP psychosis may be difficult to distinguish from schizophrenia. In the absence of history of use, analysis of urine must be depended on for diagnosis.

TREATMENT. Management of the PCP-intoxicated patient includes placement in a darkened, quiet room on a floor pad, safe from injury. Diazepam, in a dose of 10–20 mg orally or 10 mg intramuscularly every 4 hr, may be helpful if the patient is agitated and not comatose. Supportive therapy of the comatose patient is indicated with particular attention to hydration, which may be compromised by PCP-induced diuresis.

113.6 Cocaine

Crack cocaine, the highly addictive smokable form of cocaine, has increased availability and severity of cocaine use in the face of a decrease in use in the overall population. From 1985 to 1990, the number of cocaine users (prior 30 days) in the United States dropped from 5.8 million to 1.6 million. Lifetime or "ever use" in high school seniors dropped from a level of 17.3% in 1985 to 9.4% in 1990. However, since a low of 5.9% in 1994, the 1997 rate was back to 8.7% Use of crack cocaine represents almost half the total cocaine use.

Cocaine, an alkaloid extracted from the leaves of the South American *Erythroxylon coca,* is supplied as the hydrochloride salt in crystalline form. It is rapidly absorbed from the nasal mucosa, detoxified by the liver, and excreted in the urine as benzoyl ecgonine. Its half-life is slightly more than 1 hr. The perceived effect of "snorting" cocaine may be influenced by some of the many diluents now being added to or actually substituted for the drug (heroin, amphetamines, PCP, or fillers such as mannitol or quinine). Smoking the cocaine alkaloid ("freebasing") in pipes or cigarettes, mixed with tobacco, marijuana, parsley, or as a paste, has become a popular method of use. Accidental burns are potential complications of this practice. With crack cocaine, the smoker feels "high" in less than 10 sec. The technique for extracting crack cocaine does not involve ether and is a safer and simpler technique compared with making freebase cocaine. The risk of addiction with this method is higher and more rapidly progressive than from snorting cocaine. Tolerance develops and the user must increase the dose or change the route of administration, or both, to achieve the same effect.

CLINICAL MANIFESTATIONS. Cocaine produces euphoria, increased motor activity, decreased fatigability, and occasionally paranoid ideation. Its sympathomimetic properties are responsible for pupillary dilatation, tachycardia, hypertension, and hyperthermia. Binge patterns of use are common. Neurologic effects such as dizziness, paresthesias, and seizures can occur. Use in group settings has been associated with sexual promiscuity and increased risks of sexually transmitted infections. Lethal effects are possible, especially when cocaine is used in combination with other drugs, such as heroin, in an injectable form known as a "speedball." Although addiction and tolerance develop in the chronic user, withdrawal symptoms on its discontinuation have not been reported, suggesting that physical dependency does not occur. Pregnant adolescents who use cocaine place their fetus at risk for premature delivery, complications of low birthweight, and possibly congenital malformations and developmental disorders.

TREATMENT. Intensive supportive therapy is directed at the clinical manifestations of acute intoxication.

113.7 Amphetamines

Stimulants, particularly amphetamines, are among the most frequently reported illicit drugs used by high school seniors other than marijuana. They are also one of the few drugs in which prevalence in the 10th grade exceeded that of high school seniors in 1997 (17% vs 16.5%). Methamphetamine, commonly known as "ice," accounted for more than 25% of stimulant use. Methamphetamine is particularly popular among adolescents and young adults because of its potency and ease of absorption. It can be used by snorting, smoking, ingesting by mouth, or absorption across mucous membranes, such as vaginal mucosa. Its use is especially common in the western and southwestern regions of the United States. Amphetamines have multiple CNS effects, among them the release of neurotramsmitters and an indirect catecholamine agonist effect. In high doses, they may also affect serotonergic receptors.

CLINICAL MANIFESTATIONS. The effects of amphetamines can be dose-related. High doses produce slowing of cardiac conduction in the face of ventricular irritability. Hypertensive and hyperpyrexic episodes can occur as can seizures. Binge effects result in the development of psychotic ideation with the potential for sudden violence. Cerebrovascular damage and psychosis can result from chronic use. There is a withdrawal syndrome associated with amphetamine use, with early, intermediate, and late phases. The early phase is characterized as a "crash" phase with depression, agitation, anergia, and desire for more of the drug. Loss of physical and mental energy, limited interest in the environment, and anhedonia mark the intermediate phase. In the final phase, drug craving returns, often triggered by particular situations or objects.

TREATMENT. Agitation and delusional behaviors can be treated with haloperidol or droperidol. Phenothiazines are contraindicated and may cause a rapid drop in blood pressure or seizure activity. Other supportive treatment consists of a cooling blanket for hyperthermia and treatment of the hypertension and arrhythmias, which may respond to sedation with lorazepam (Ativan) or diazepam (Valium).

113.8 Opiates

Opiate abuse by adolescents decreased considerably during the 1980s, but the magnitude and variety of its medical sequelae warrant continued attention. Although it has been one of the least frequently reported drugs of use since 1991, the proportion of seniors reporting having ever used it increased from 0.9% in 1991 to 2.1% in 1997. Johnston and colleagues link this increase to a change in the route of administration, with more students snorting and smoking rather than injecting. Moreover, a resurgence of its use in conjunction with "crack" cocaine has occurred. Heroin produces euphoria and analgesia. Heroin is hydrolyzed to morphine, which undergoes hepatic conjugation with glucuronic acid before excretion, usually within 24 hr of administration. It can be detected in urine by thin-layer chromatography up to 48 hr after administration. The route of administration influences the timing of the onset of action. When the drug is inhaled ("snorting"), it requires almost 30 min before the desired effect is achieved. By the subcutaneous route ("skin-popping"), the effect is achieved within minutes; when injected intravenously ("mainlining"), it has an immediate effect. A larger dose can be administered intravenously. Tolerance develops to the euphoric effect and only rarely to the inhibitory effect on smooth muscle, which causes both constipation and miosis.

CLINICAL MANIFESTATIONS. The clinical manifestations are determined by the pharmacologic effects of heroin or its adulterants, combined with the conditions and the route of administration. The cerebral effects include euphoria, diminution in pain, and pinpoint pupils. An effect on the hypothalamus is suggested by the lowering of body temperature. Vasodilation is a major cardiovascular manifestation related to the method of administration of the drug. Respiratory depression is mediated centrally and is characterized by alveolar underventilation. Pulmonary edema is common in death from the overdose syndrome, but it may also be seen as an incidental roentgenologic finding in an otherwise asymptomatic adolescent heroin abuser. The most common dermatologic lesions are the "tracks," the hypertrophic linear scars that follow the course of large veins. Smaller, discrete peripheral scars, resembling healed insect bites, may be easily overlooked. The adolescent who injects heroin subcutaneously may have fat necrosis, lipodystrophy, and atrophy over portions of the extremities. Attempts at concealment of these stigmata may include amateur tattoos in unusual sites. Abscesses secondary to unsterile techniques of drug administration are commonly found. There is a loss of libido; the mechanism is unknown. The female heroin user may resort to prostitution to support the habit, thus increasing the risk of sexually transmitted disease (including HIV), pregnancy, and other hazards. Constipation results from decreased smooth muscle propulsive contractions and increased anal sphincter tone. The practice of concealment of heroin in a swallowed condom or balloon may cause intestinal obstruction or sudden (often fatal) overdosage if the container breaks. Hepatic enzyme activities are frequently elevated in heroin users, the majority of whom have serologic evidence suggesting viral infection with hepatitis B. The absence of sterile technique in injection may lead to cerebral microabscesses or endocarditis, usually caused by *Staphylococcus aureus*. Infection with HIV is another complication of needle use. Abnormal serologic reactions are also common, including false-positive Venereal Disease Research Laboratory (VDRL) and latex fixation tests. Depression of lymphocyte response to stimulation by mitogens in culture has been reported but may be due to coincident acquired immunodeficiency syndrome in parenteral drug users.

Withdrawal. After a period of 8 hr or more without heroin, the addicted individual undergoes, during a period of 24–36 hr, a series of physiologic disturbances referred to collectively as "withdrawal" or the *abstinence syndrome*. The earliest sign is yawning, followed by lacrimation, mydriasis, insomnia, "goose flesh," cramping of the voluntary musculature, hyperactive bowel sounds and diarrhea, tachycardia, and systolic hypertension. The occurrence of grand mal seizures is rare in adolescent addicts. A short course of diazepam is effective and safe treatment for heroin detoxification. An alternative for detoxification is *treatment* with methadone. This synthetic opiate is effective by the oral route and is pharmacologically similar to heroin, with the exception of its lack of euphoric effect. Neither the safety nor the dosage of methadone has been established for children or adolescents.

Overdose Syndrome. The overdose syndrome is an acute reaction after the administration of an opiate. It is the leading cause of death among drug users. The rapidity of onset, the finding of eosinophilia after recovery, and the fact that it occurs only in those who have used the drug previously suggest a hypersensitivity mechanism. The clinical signs include stupor or coma, seizures, miotic pupils (unless severe anoxia has occurred), respiratory depression, cyanosis, and pulmonary edema. The differential diagnosis includes CNS trauma, diabetic coma, hepatic (and other) encephalopathy, Reye's syndrome, as well as overdose of alcohol, barbiturates, PCP, or methadone. Diagnosis of opiate toxicity is facilitated by intravenous administration of the opiate antagonist naloxone, 0.01 mg/kg (a vial of 0.4 mg usually suffices for an adolescent), which causes dilation of pupils constricted by the opiate. Diagnosis is confirmed by the finding of morphine in the serum.

Treatment consists of maintaining adequate oxygenation and continued administration of naloxone every 5 min, when necessary, to improve and maintain adequate ventilation. Naloxone may have to be continued for 24 hr if methadone, rather than shorter-acting heroin, has been taken.

113.9 Anabolic Steroids

The quest for enhanced athletic performance has led to the abuse of anabolic steroids by competitive athletes of both sexes. As with other substances, prevalence data varies across surveys. Reports of anabolic steroids having ever been used range from 0.7–3.7%, usually with male use predominating. However, two of three surveys show significant increases in females who had ever used anabolic steroids in the 1990s. Although the percentages are low, population estimates based on 1995 data suggest that about 375,000 males and 175,000 females of high school age have ever used anabolic steroids for performance enhancement. The evidence for increased muscle mass and strength are controversial but are supported by objective data. The effects appear to be related to the myotrophic action at androgen receptors as well as competitive antagonism at catabolism-mediating corticosteroid receptors. Erythropoietic and psychologic effects may also contribute to their enhancement effects. The most common forms of anabolic steroids used are the oral 17-α-methyl derivatives of testosterone and the injectable esters of testosterone and 19-nortestosterone.

CLINICAL MANIFESTATIONS. Some of the adverse side effects of these drugs are reversible; others are not. The most immediate effects for all users is increasing acneiform lesions. Other dermatologic manifestations include linear keloids, stria, oily hair, and hirsutism. These findings may be the first recognizable effects. Males can experience gynecomastia, breast pain, testicular atrophy, and azoospermia. Women experience more irreversible side effects such as breast atrophy, clitoral enlargement, and menstrual abnormalities. Serious psychologic effects also have been reported from the use of high doses of these agents (often 100 times the therapeutic doses), including uncontrollable rage, depression, mania, mood fluctuations, and alterations in libido. Users choosing the injectable route increase the risk of HIV if injection equipment is shared with others.

Abnormalities of the liver can be acute, such as hepatitis and hepatomegaly, or more long-term, such as the increased risk of hepatocellular carcinoma, particularly with the 17-α-alkylated forms. Fluid retention is a common side effect that prompts users to take diuretics. In addition to these effects, which occur in individuals of all ages, the early adolescent is at risk for growth retardation because of the possibility of accelerating epiphyseal closure.

DIAGNOSIS AND TREATMENT. The clinical signs noted, coupled with a complete history, provide a diagnosis in most instances. Although urine testing is available and performed at the Olympic and collegiate competitive levels, few laboratories perform these tests and they are very expensive. Therefore, the secondary school approach primarily has been limited to education and prevention.

American Academy of Child and Adolescent Psychiatry Work Group on Quality Issues: Practice parameters for the assessment and treatment of children and adolescents with substance use disorders. J Am Acad Child Adolesc Psychiatry 36:140S, 1997.
Blum RW: Adolescent substance use and abuse. Arch Pediatr Adolesc Med 151:805, 1997.
Duncan D, Petrosa R: Social and community factors associated with drug use and abuse among adolescents. *In:* Gullotta T, Adams GR (eds): Substance Misuse in Adolescence. Thousand Oaks, CA, Sage Publication, 1994.
Heyman RB: Tobacco: Prevention and cessation strategies. Adolesc Health Update 9:(3), 1997.
Johnston LD, O'Malley PM, Bachman JG: National Survey Results on Drug Abuse from The Monitoring the Future Study, 1975–1995, Vol I secondary School Students, NIDA, U.S. Department of Health and Human Services, 1996.
Johnston LD, O'Malley PM, Bachman JG: Drug abuse among American teens shows some signs of leveling after a long rise. Ann Arbor, University of Michigan News and Information Services, December 18, 1997.
Kahn L, Warren CW, Harris WA, et al: Youth risk behavior surveillance—United States, 1995. J School Health 66:365, 1996.
Kokotailo P: Physical health problems associated with adolescent substance abuse. *In:* Rahdert ER, Czechowicz D (eds): Adolescent Drug Abuse: Clinical Assessment and Therapeutic Interventions. Rockville, MD, National Institute on Drug Abuse, 1995.
Lowinson JH, Ruiz P, Millman RB, et al: Substance Abuse: A Comprehensive Textbook, 3rd ed. Baltimore, Williams & Wilkins, 1997.
Neinstein LS, Pinsky D, Heischober BS: Drug Use and Abuse. *In:* Neinstein LS (ed): Adolescent Health Care: A Practical Guide, 3rd ed. Baltimore, Williams & Wilkins, 1996.
Neumark YD, Delva J, Anthony JC: The epidemiology of adolescent inhalant drug involvement. Arch Pediatr Adolesc Med 152:781, 1998.
Rogers PD, Werner MJ: Substance abuse. Pediatr Clin North Am 42:241, 1995.
Substance Abuse and Mental Health Services Administration, National Household Survey on Drug Abuse: Population Estimates 1996. Washington, D.C., U.S. Department of Health and Human Services, July 1997.
Yesalis CE, Barsukiewicz MS, Kopstein AN, et al: Trends in anabolic-androgenic steroid use among adolescents. Arch Pediatr Adolesc Med 151:1197, 1997.

CHAPTER 114
*Sleep Disorders**

The maturational changes in sleep patterns during adolescence indicate that between sex maturation stages 3 and 4 there is an increase in daytime sleepiness and a decrease in slow wave sleep, the deepest level of non–rapid eye movement (REM) sleep. There is also a secretory spurt of gonadotropins and growth hormone with each completed sleep cycle during early puberty, a pattern not found at any other time of life.

Sleep disturbances or disorders (see also Chapter 20.5) are divided into patterns of excessive daytime sleepiness, sleeplessness, and nocturnal arousals. *Narcolepsy,* a neurologically based disorder, often first becomes symptomatic during adolescence. The syndrome includes (1) attacks of rapid eye movement sleep during wakefulness, with excessive daytime sleepiness; (2) hypnagogic hallucinations and frightening and recurring visual hallucinations; (3) *cataplexy,* the sudden inhibition of tone of a muscle group, the effects being dependent on the muscle group involved; and (4) sleep paralysis, a paralysis of voluntary musculature while falling asleep. **Kleine-Levin syndrome** is a unique and rare disorder of recurrent hypersomnia, primarily in adolescent males, and often associated with binge eating, hypersexuality, irritability, and aggression. It can occur in either gender, at any age, and is usually self-limited and treated symptomatically. The *obstructive sleep apnea syndrome* also may first become symptomatic during adolescence and consists of increased daytime sleepiness after multiple episodes of brief nighttime waking after each of the apneic spells, which results from airway obstruction (see Chapter 383). Other medical conditions that may interfere with sleep onset, fragment nighttime sleep, and disturb the circadian rhythm sufficiently to cause daytime sleepiness include encephalitis, meningitis, seizure, traumatic or metabolic brain injury, structural central nervous system disturbance, blindness, pain (acute and chronic), and infection.

Insomnia affects 10–20% of adolescents. The cause may be depression or the delayed sleep phase syndrome in which the difficulty lies in falling asleep rather than awakening once sleep has begun. According to Anders, "adolescents may be particularly susceptible to this syndrome, because the changing social demands, which result in later bedtimes, interact with the changing neuroendocrine secretion patterns of puberty, which affect sleep state relationships."

Nocturnal arousal disorders, or parasomnia can occur in adolescents secondary to post-traumatic stress or attention deficit disorders. The most common substances associated with sleep fragmentation are stimulants (such as methylphenidate), asthma medication, caffeine, alcohol, and cocaine.

Anders TF, Keener MA: Sleep-wake state. Development and disorders of sleep in infants, children, and adolescents. *In:* Levine MD, Carey WB, Crocker AC, et al (eds): Developmental-Behavioral Pediatrics. Philadelphia, WB Saunders, 1983.
Stores G: Practitioner review: Assessment and treatment of sleep disorders in children and adolescents. J Child Psychol Psychiatry 37:907, 1996.
Wolraich ML, Felice ME, Drotar D (eds): The Classification of Child and Adolescent Mental Diagnoses in Primary Care: Diagnostic and Statistical Manual for Primary Care (DSM-PC) Child and Adolescent Version. Elk Grove Village, IL, American Academy of Pediatrics, 1996.

*Adapted from Chapter 106 by I. Litt in 15th edition.

CHAPTER 115
The Breast

Breast development is one of the first obvious signs of puberty, but it is often the focus of attention and a cause of anxiety in an adolescent, whether the issue is normal progression, some variation in progression, or a definable disorder. Normal breast development during puberty is described using a Sex Maturity Rating scale of 1–5, as the breast becomes more mature (see Chapter 14).

NORMAL VARIANTS. Minor breast asymmetry is common in adult females and sexually mature adolescent females. Other conditions that rarely occur but should be ruled out include **Poland syndrome** and unilateral breast aplasia, hypoplasia, or hypertrophy. Poland syndrome is marked by a hypoplastic breast nipple and areola with hypoplastic ipsilateral chest wall structures. Unilateral or bilateral juvenile (virginal) hypertrophy occurs with specific histopathologic changes but without any known cause. The enlargement may be mild and cause back pain and postural problems or severe enough to be associated with tissue and skin necrosis. Accessory breast tissue can also occur in males and females. This lesion can consist of a supernumerary nipple or breast tissue, or both, and usually occurs along both milk lines of the thorax and the abdomen.

Reconstructive surgical repair is indicated in severe breast asymmetry but is recommended after sex maturity rating 5 has been reached.

FEMALE DISORDERS (also see Chapter 559).

Masses. The most common adolescent breast disorder is a mass, the majority of which are benign cysts or fibroadenomas. *Cysts* vary in size over the course of a menstrual cycle, so a patient should be re-examined 2 wk after the initial examination. Persistence of the mass or its enlargement over three menstrual cycles is an indication for surgical consultation. Aspiration is usually attempted under local anesthesia, often resulting in curative drainage if it proves to be a cyst. If no fluid is obtained, an excisional biopsy is indicated. When multiple small masses are palpable, associated with pain or tenderness and varying with the stage of the menstrual cycle, they are most often *fibrocystic lesions.* The use of combination oral contraceptives of low progesterone potency may be beneficial. A biopsy is rarely indicated with this presentation. Most fibroadenomas are benign, mobile, well-defined rubbery feeling masses. Multiple fibroadenomas occur in 10–20% of patients. The *fibroadenoma* tends not to vary in size during the menstrual cycle, often distinguishing it from a cyst. *Cystosarcoma phylloides* is a rare variant of a fibroadenoma distinguished by having a more cellular stroma. It is typically larger than a fibroadenoma and can, rarely, be malignant. In one biopsy series of adolescent breast masses, 71% were found to be fibroadenomas, 11% were abscesses, and 2% were cystosarcoma phylloides. *Carcinoma* of the breast in the adolescent is rare. The efficacy and possible sequelae of mammography in managing adolescent breast masses are unknown. The dense breast tissue of the adolescent obstructs the visualization of a palpable mass, thus mammography is not advised for this age group. Ultrasonography is useful is distinguishing cystic from solid masses.

Nipple Discharge. Nipple discharge in adolescents is usually due to local stimulation; use of medications, including oral contraceptives; and pregnancy. Rarely, it results from a pituitary or breast neoplasm or infection. Examination of the discharge assists in diagnosis: Benign conditions are associated with a milky, sticky, thick discharge; infection is associated with a purulent discharge; and intraductal papilloma and cancer are associated with a serous, serosanguineous or bloody discharge. Elevation of the serum prolactin level may occur in the **amenorrhea-galactorrhea syndromes,** associated with the use of certain antihypertensive medications, oral contraceptives, or tranquilizers, or secondary to a pituitary adenoma. The latter is assciated with central nervous system signs and is evaluated with a computed tomography scan or magnetic resonance imaging of the head. The possibility of a breast neoplasm is an indication for cytologic examination of the discharge and surgical consultation. Infection in the non–breast-feeding adolescent is rare and may be secondary to a human bite or the initial symptom of diabetes mellitus. Culture of the discharge, followed by appropriate antibiotic therapy (usually directed against *Staphylococcus aureus*) is indicated; surgical drainage is rarely necessary.

MALE DISORDERS. Gynecomastia occurs in approximately one third of normal males during early to midpuberty and often causes concern that may not be openly voiced. The response should be factual information and reassurance of its usually transient nature. Rarely is it of such magnitude or persistence as to warrant surgery. Nonpubertal gynecomastia with hypogonadism is associated with Klinefelter syndrome and places a patient at a higher risk for breast cancer (see Chapter 593). Other conditions associated with nonpubertal gynecomastia are secondary to endocrine disorders, neoplasms, chronic disease, trauma, and myriad medication as well as drugs of abuse (Table 115–1).

TABLE 115–1 Drugs Associated with Gynecomastia

Hormones	**Antibiotics**
Estrogens	Isoniazid
Aromatizable androgens	Ketoconazole
Anabolic steroids	Metronidazole
Gonadotropins	**Cytotoxic Drugs**
Psychoactive Drugs	Cyclophosphamide
Tricyclic antidepressants	Methotrexate
Phenothiazines	Vincristine
Benzodiazepines	**Other**
Cardiovascular Drugs	Auranofin
Calcium channel blockers	Ergotamine
Angiotensin-converting enzyme Inhibitors	Etretinate
Digoxin	Metoclopramide
Diuretics	Minoxidil
Spironolactone	Penicillamine
Thiazides	Sulindac
Gastric Acid Inhibitors	Theophylline
Cimetidine	**Drugs of Abuse**
Omeprazole	Alcohol
	Marijuana
	Heroin
	Methadone
	Amphetamines

From Davis AJ, Kulig JW: Adolescent breast disorders. Adolescent Health Update 9:7, 1996.

CHAPTER 116
Menstrual Problems

Some variety of menstrual dysfunction occurs in about 50% of adolescent females. Most of the problems are minor; however, severe dysmenorrhea or prolonged menstrual bleeding can be debilitating to a teenager. Adolescents with mild dysfunction that does not require medical intervention should have their condition explained to them and should be reassured about their reproductive normalcy.

NORMAL MENSTRUATION. The age of normal menarche varies according to the characteristics of the population. In a large office-based study in the United States, 35% of white girls and 62% of African-American girls had initiated menses between ages 12 and 13 yr. The age of menarche in Tanner's English series ranges from ages 9–16 yr, with a mean age of 13.46 yr. The age of menarche is closely related to other parameters of pubertal maturation and correlated closely with bone age. The onset and continuation of normal menstrual cycling depends on the functional and anatomic integrity of (1) the hypothalamus together with higher centers, including possibly the pineal gland; (2) the anterior pituitary; (3) the ovary; and (4) the uterus. The percentage of body fat is also a factor in the onset of menarche, with a minimal fatness of 17% of body weight being necessary for the onset of menstrual cycles and a minimum of 22% fatness necessary to maintain regular ovulatory cycles. Menarche usually occurs about 2.3 yr after the initiation of puberty, with a range of 1–3 yr, and becomes regular after 2–2.5 yr. The length of the menstrual cycle from the first day of menses of one cycle to the first day of the next cycle can range from 21–45 days, although the average is about 28 days. The length of blood flow ranges from 2–7 days, with an average of 3–5 days. Anovulatory cycles are generally longer. The average blood flow usually results in about 40 mL of blood loss with a range of 25–70 mL. The later the age of menarche, the longer until the establishment of ovulatory cycles.

Menstrual cycle irregularities are described according to variation in frequency of menses, amount, and both frequency and amount (Table 116–1). A complete history for evaluating

TABLE 116–1 Terms for Menstrual Cycle Irregularities

Variations in frequency
- Polymenorrhea: frequent regular or irregular bleeding at <21-day intervals
- Oligomenorrhea: infrequent irregular bleeding at >45-day intervals
- Primary amenorrhea: no menstrual flow by age 16 yr
- Secondary amenorrhea: absence of vaginal bleeding for >3 mo
- Irregular menses: bleeding at varying intervals, ≥21-day intervals but <45-day intervals

Variations in amount
- Hypomenorrhea: decreased menstrual flow at regular intervals
- Hypermenorrhea: profuse menstrual flow of normal duration at regular intervals

Variations in amount and duration
- Metrorrhagia: intermenstrual irregular bleeding between regular periods
- Menorrhagia: excessive amount and increased duration of uterine bleeding occurring regularly
- Menometrorrhagia: frequent irregular, excessive, and prolonged episodes of uterine bleeding
- Dysfunctional uterine bleeding: prolonged excessive menstrual bleeding associated with irregular periods: usually due to immaturity of reproductive axis in adolescence if within first 2 yr of menarche

From Blythe MI: Common menstrual problems of adolescence. Adoles Med State of the Art Rev 8:87, 1997.

a patient with menstrual dysfunction should include questions specifically related to puberty and menstrual patterns, a family history of gynecologic problems, and a past medical history noting hospitalizations, chronic illness, medication or substance use, and infections. The related association of weight change, nutrition, exercise, and sports participation can be critically important in considering a differential diagnosis. Regardless of the age of the adolescent, an appropriate history of any type of sexual activity should be elicited, and the pediatrician should be cognizant of the need to rule out sexual abuse as an issue in young adolescents when other findings suggest sexual activity.

In addition to the basic growth parameters of weight, height, blood pressure, heart rate, and body mass index, signs of virilization should be assessed, such as hirsutism and clitoromegaly. A careful external and internal pelvic examination is a key to ruling out anatomic defects and accumulating additional specimens for the evaluation. In the young adolescent, this examination should be performed by someone with expertise in this age group and with the proper-sized equipment.

ETIOLOGY OF MENSTRUAL IRREGULARITIES. The distinction among menstrual irregularities is somewhat artificial given that the causes of the entities are often similar, that is, many of the problems of pubertal delay, such as Turner's mosaic syndrome, may present as primary amenorrhea or secondary amenorrhea. Thyroid disorders can be the source of secondary amenorrhea or abnormal vaginal bleeding. The common cause of all of these disorders is a disturbance of the hypothalamic-pituitary-ovarian axis. The amenorrheic disorders are categorized on the basis of follicle-stimulating hormone (FSH) levels into hypergonadotrophic hypogonadism (ovarian failure) and hypogonadotrophic hypogonadism (hypothalamic or pituitary dysfunction). FSH–luteininzing hormone (LH) patterns in perimenarchaeal girls with anovulatory bleeding also suggests the prevalence of a maturational defect for normal negative feedback cyclicity. The rising levels of estrogen do not cause a fall in FSH and the subsequent suppression of estrogen secretion, and consequently the endometrium becomes thickened, promoting irregular and heavier blood flow with shedding.

Psychogenic factors have been implicated in amenorrhea. It is often difficult to separate psychologic from nutritional factors because weight loss is a common confounding variable in many of these situations, for example, depression, anorexia nervosa, or stress.

CLINICAL MANIFESTATIONS. Amenorrhea, or absence of menses, may be primary or secondary. The diagnosis of primary amenorrhea assumes that the patient has passed the age at which menarche normally occurs, from 10–16 yr. Accordingly, the determination of primary amenorrhea should first be based on an assessment of the patient's stage of pubertal development; 10% of girls have menarche at Sex Maturity Rating (SMSR) 2, 20% reach menarche at SMR 3, 60% reach it at SMR 4, and 10% reach menarche at SMR 5. If the patient has not entered puberty by the expected time or if pubertal development is completed without the onset of menses, she should be thoroughly evaluated, even if her chronologic age is within the normal range. Similarly, the close concordance of the age of menarche between daughters and mothers and among siblings should suggest this diagnosis when the patient is more than 1 yr older than were the mother or sisters when their menarche occurred. The distinguishing characteristic of the clinical presentation of amenorrhea is the presence or absence of virilization. Clinical features such as clitoromegaly, hirsutism, or excessive acne are associated with adrenal or ovarian disease. Other clinical presentations such as slender or obese body habitus or short stature also are characteristic of syndromes associated with amenorrhea.

The first consideration in the adolescent who presents with secondary amenorrhea is pregnancy. This possibility also exists, albeit rarely, as a cause of primary amenorrhea, if fertilization of the first released ovum occurred before menses. A history of sexual intercourse, nausea, and breast tenderness and physical findings of increased pigmentation of nipples and linea alba, cyanosis and softening of the cervix, and an enlarged uterus form the classic picture. In the clinical presentation of abnormal vaginal bleeding, mild to moderate bleeding may present without any specific clinical findings; however, severe bleeding is accompanied by the abnormal vital signs associated with hypovolemia. Very severe bleeding may progress to syncope and death, making this one of the few gynecologic emergencies of adolescence.

Laboratory evaluations should be directed toward the differential diagnosis of the specific pattern of menstrual irregularity.

116.1 Amenorrhea

DIFFERENTIAL DIAGNOSIS. In *primary amenorrhea,* chromosomal or congenital abnormalities, such as gonadal dysgenesis, the triple X syndrome, isochromosomal abnormalities, testicular feminization syndrome and, rarely, true hermaphroditism, should be considered in addition to the conditions that cause secondary amenorrhea. Elevated levels of FSH and LH suggest primary gonadal failure, and chromosome analysis elucidates its cause. When primary amenorrhea occurs with advanced pubertal development, a structural anomaly of the müllerian duct system should be suspected. **Imperforate hymen** is most common and is associated with recurrent (monthly) abdominal pain and, after some time has passed, a midline lower abdominal mass, the blood-filled vagina, or **hematocolpos.** Diagnosis is made by inspection of the introitus, revealing a bulging hymen with bluish discoloration. If the obstruction is at the level of the cervix, the blood-filled uterus **(hematometrium)** is apparent on bimanual examination or ultrasonography. Agenesis of the cervix or uterus is rare but occurs in association with sacral agenesis.

Primary or *secondary* amenorrhea may also be caused by chronic illness, particularly that associated with malnutrition or tissue hypoxia, such as diabetes mellitus, inflammatory bowel disease, cystic fibrosis, or cyanotic congenital heart disease. In most cases, the illness has not been diagnosed previously but, occasionally, the amenorrhea is its first manifestation. A central nervous system (CNS) tumor, most commonly a craniopharyngioma, may present with amenorrhea. Prolactinomas, although rare, are the most common pituitary tumor in adolescence. Abnormalities of the thyroid gland, typically hyperthyroidism, may first be suspected by delayed sexual maturation or amenorrhea, even in the absence of other signs and symptoms. Hypothyroidism may cause precocious puberty but may also be associated with delayed puberty or abnormal uterine bleeding. Anorexia nervosa, which may present with either primary or secondary amenorrhea, is occasionally confused with hyperthyroidism because of weight loss, hyperactivity, and personality changes seen in both entities. Ingestion of drugs, both legal and illegal, may cause amenorrhea and, in the case of phenothiazines, even a false-positive urine pregnancy test. Some drugs, including phenothiazines and certain antihypertensive agents, may cause galactorrhea, further mimicking pregnancy. A thorough drug history is, therefore, necessary.

LABORATORY FINDINGS. The approach to the clinical evaluation of delayed menarche (Fig. 116–1) suggests a stepwise progression initiated by the history and physical examination. The pregnancy test, preferably a qualitative serum β-subunit human chorionic gonadotropin (hCG), is the key laboratory test to perform in the evaluation of secondary amenorrhea (Fig. 116–2) regardless of the history or sexual activity given by the patient or signs of virilization. The next step for laboratory determinations follows the scheme and is performed according to the individual's response to an initial progesterone challenge or after the findings of the vaginal smear for estrogen. The direct correlation of bone age to menstrual age enhances the value of a radiograph before proceeding with an extensive work-up. The measurement of FSH is critical in determining whether chromosomal abnormalities (with FSH elevation >25 mIU/mL) or other endocrinopathies or CNS tumors (with normal or low FSH <5 mIU/mL) are present. Prolonged amenorrhea (>6 mo) and persistent oligomenorrhea without an explanation should prompt the measurement of thyroid-stimulating hormone, FSH, LH, and prolactin levels, even in the face of a normal progesterone challenge. Elevated LH and normal FSH levels require the measurement of androgen excess even in the absence of obvious virilization. An LH:FSH ratio greater than 3 and an elevated free testosterone level is common in adolescents with polycystic ovary (PCO). Although abnormalities of insulin and an increased risk of diabetes mellitus is one of the features of PCO, the measurement of insulin is not currently part of the evaluation (see Chapter 560). An elevated prolactin level or other clinical features suggesting a CNS tumor should be followed up with cranial computed tomography scan or, preferably, magnetic resonance imaging.

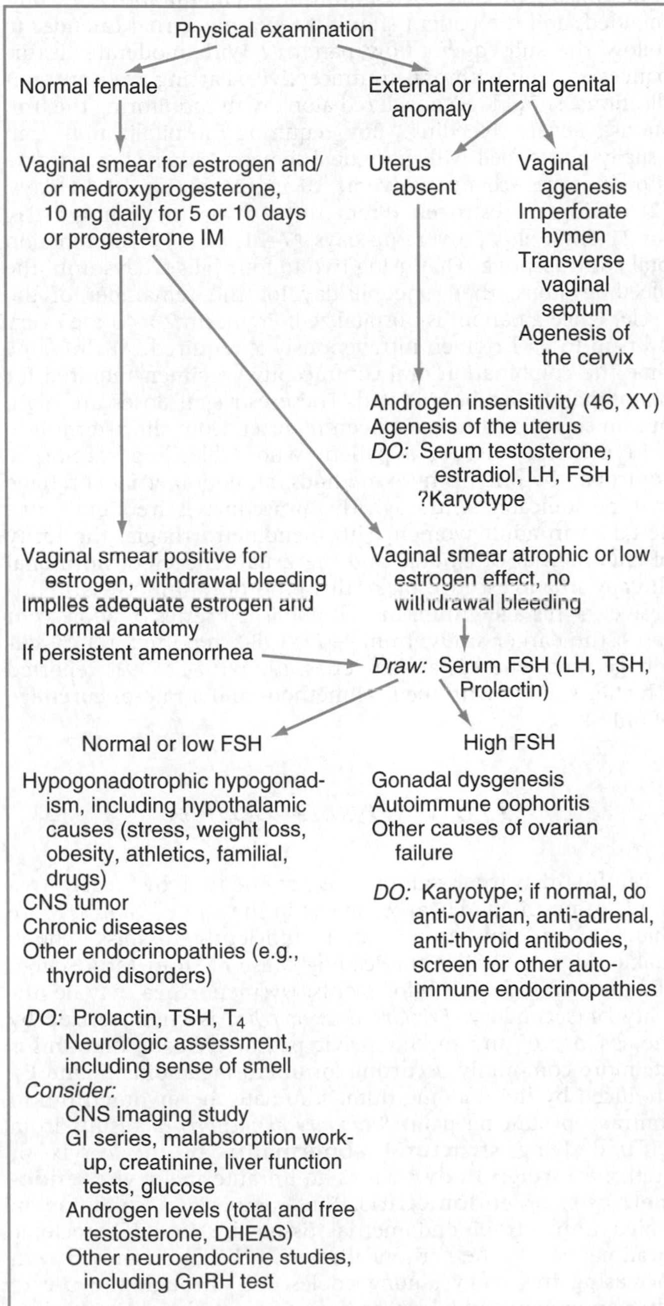

Figure 116–1 Delayed menarche. (From Emans SJH, Laufer MR, Goldstein DP [eds]: Pediatric and Adolescent Gynecology, 4th ed. Philadelphia, Lippincott-Raven, 1998.)

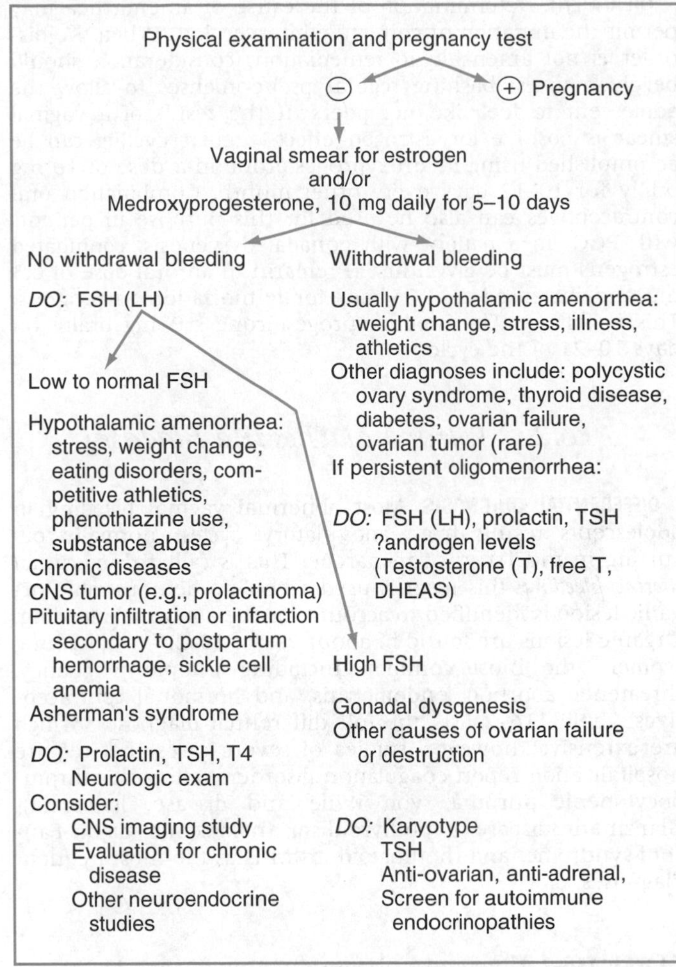

Figure 116–2 Evaluation of secondary amenorrhea. (From Emans SJH, Laufer MR, Goldstein DP [eds]: Pediatric and Adolescent Gynecology, 4th ed. Philadelphia, Lippincott-Raven, 1998.)

TREATMENT. Determination of the cause of amenorrhea may permit the initiation of corrective intervention. When the disorder is not amenable to remediation, consideration should be given to establishing regular pseudomenses to allow the adolescent to feel like her peers. If the result of a vaginal smear is positive for estrogen effect, regular cycling can be accomplished using medroxyprogesterone in a dose of 10 mg orally for 10–12 days every other month. Combination oral contraceptives can also be used for this purpose in patients with PCO. In a patient with gonadal dysgenesis, conjugated estrogens must be given first (Premarin in an oral dose of 0.3 mg and increased to 1.25 mg) for feminization to progress. This is followed by medroxyprogesterone, 10 mg orally on days 10–21 of the cycle.

116.2 Abnormal Uterine Bleeding

DIFFERENTIAL DIAGNOSIS. Most abnormal vaginal bleeding in adolescents results from anovulatory cycles, normally occurring in the 1st yr of menarche. This is called *dysfunctional uterine bleeding;* this term is used when no demonstrable organic lesion is identified to account for the abnormal bleeding. Organic lesions are found in about 9% of 10–20-yr-old young women, the most common including ectopic pregnancy, threatened abortion, endometritis, and hormonal contraceptives. Table 116–2 lists the full differential diagnoses, which are extensive; however, studies of severe cases that require hospitalization report coagulation disorders (idiopathic thrombocytopenic purpura, von Willebrand disease, leukemia), Glanzmann disease, hypothyroidism, thalassemia major, Fanconi syndrome, and rheumatoid arthritis as the most frequent diagnoses.

TABLE 116–2 Differential Diagnosis of Abnormal Vaginal Bleeding in the Adolescent Girl

Anovulatory Uterine Bleeding

Pregnancy-Related Complications
- Threatened abortion
- Spontaneous, incomplete, or missed abortion
- Ectopic pregnancy
- Gestational trophoblastic disease
- Complications of termination procedures

Infection
- Pelvic inflammatory disease
- Endometritis
- Cervicitis
- Vaginitis

Blood Dyscrasias
- Thrombocytopenia (e.g., idiopathic thrombocytopenic purpura, leukemia, aplastic anemia, hypersplenism, chemotherapy)
- Clotting disorders (e.g., von Willebrand disease, other disorders of platelet function, liver dysfunction)

Endocrine Disorders
- Hypo- or hyperthyroidism
- Adrenal disease
- Hyperprolactinemia
- Polycystic ovary syndrome
- Ovarian failure

Vaginal Abnormalities
- Carcinoma
- Laceration

Cervical Problems
- Cervicitis
- Polyp
- Hemangioma
- Carcinoma

Uterine Problems
- Submucous myoma
- Congenital anomalies
- Polyp
- Carcinoma
- Use of intrauterine device
- Breakthrough bleeding associated with oral contraceptives or other hormonal contraceptives
- Ovulation bleeding

Ovarian Problems
- Cyst
- Tumor (benign, malignant)

Endometriosis

Trauma

Foreign Body (e.g., retained tampon)

Systemic Diseases
- Diabetes mellitus
- Renal disease
- Systemic lupus erythematosus

Medications
- Hormonal contraceptives
- Anticoagulants
- Platelet inhibitors
- Androgens
- Spironolactone

From Emans SJH, Laufer MR, Goldstein DP: Pediatric and Adolescent Gynecology, 4th ed. Philadelphia, Lippincott-Raven, 1998, p 239.

LABORATORY FINDINGS. The hemoglobin and hematocrit from a complete blood count are the most important elements in the initial evaluation. They establish the severity of the bleeding, with levels less than a hemoglobin of 9 g/dL or a hematocrit of 27% considered severe, 9–11 g/dL and 27–33% considered moderate, and greater than 11 g/dL and greater than 33% considered mild. Hospitalization is generally recommended for adolescents with a hemoglobin less than 7 gm/dL or a hemoglobin less than 10 gm/dL with significant postural blood pressure changes or excessive heavy bleeding. For sexually active teenagers, tests for gonorrhea and chlamydia and a pregnancy test are also performed. The secondary evaluation should include liver and thyroid function studies, prothrombin time, partial thromboplastin time, and bleeding time. If these studies are not performed at the first visit, they must be performed before any estrogen therapy is initiated that might interfere with interpreting the results.

TREATMENT. In mild cases, iron supplementation is recommended, and the patient should keep a menstrual calendar to follow the subsequent flow patterns. With moderate disturbances, cycling with oral contraceptives, barring any contraindications, should be considered along with monitoring the iron status. Severe bleeding, not requiring hospitalization, can usually be stopped with hormonal therapy, either (1) medroxyprogesterone acetate (Provera) 10 mg/24 hr for 10–14 days; (2) conjugated estrogen (Premarin) 2.5 mg four times a day for 21 days, plus Provera on days 17–21; or (3) a combination oral contraceptive (OC) using two to four pills a days until the bleeding stops, then one pill/day for the remainder of the cycle. Once a patient is hospitalized, Premarin 20–40 mg every 4 hr up to 24 hr given intravenously is required. At the same time the combination oral contraceptive regimen required for maintenance can be initiated. These estrogen doses are high, but no complications have been reported from short-term use.

In the rare case of a patient whose bleeding cannot be controlled by one of these methods, an endometrial curettage may be indicated. Although this procedure is frequently undertaken in adult women with menometrorrhagia, the rarity of endometrial carcinoma and the usual efficacy of hormonal therapy in adolescence make this procedure unnecessarily invasive in this age group. In two published series of adolescent cases, the earlier study, from 1971–1980, reported a 34% curettage rate, whereas a later series, from 1981–1991, reported a higher success with medical methods and a rate of curettage of only 8%.

116.3 Dysmenorrhea

Painful menstrual cramps are experienced by nearly two thirds of postmenarcheal teenagers in the United States. More than 10% of this group suffer sufficiently to miss school, making dysmenorrhea the leading cause of short-term school absenteeism in female adolescents. Dysmenorrhea may be primary or secondary. *Primary dysmenorrhea* is characterized by the absence of any specific pelvic pathologic condition and is the more commonly occurring form. Prostaglandins F_2 and E_2, produced by the endometrium, stimulate the myometrium to contract, producing pain. *Secondary dysmenorrhea* results from an underlying **structural abnormality** of the cervix or uterus, a **foreign body** such as an intrauterine device, **endometriosis**, or **endometritis.** Endometriosis, a condition in which implants of endometrial tissue are found at ectopic locations within the peritoneal cavity, is being diagnosed with increasing frequency among adolescents through the use of ultrasonography and laparoscopy. Characteristically, there is severe pain at the time of menses; its specific location depends on the site of the implants.

A pelvic examination must be performed to exclude the

causes of secondary dysmenorrhea, and if none is found, a diagnosis of *primary dysmenorrhea* should be considered. Adolescents suffering from dysmenorrhea have high levels of prostaglandins F_2 and E_2 and experience symptomatic relief when prostaglandin synthetase inhibitors are administered. If given before a menstrual period (or shortly after it begins), administration of a rapidly absorbed prostaglandin synthetase inhibitor, such as naproxen sodium, is effective in destroying the prostaglandins before they produce pain (e.g., two tablets of 275 mg each taken with the onset of menses and one tablet taken every 6–8 hr after that for the 1st 24 hr). Medication is rarely needed beyond the 1st day. For the teenager with dysmenorrhea who requires contraception, oral contraceptive therapy may be indicated. It is not certain whether the beneficial effect of such use derives from the ability of oral contraceptives to inhibit ovulation and thus eliminate progesterone production from the corpus luteum or from their ability to limit endometrial proliferation and therefore the production of prostaglandins.

In adolescent patients with endometriosis, danazol, an antigonadotrophin, is rarely prescribed because of the unacceptable side effects of weight gain, edema, irregular menses, acne, oily skin, hirsutism, and a deep voice change. The use of gonadotropin–releasing hormone (GnRH) agonists such as nafarelin and leuprolide are more commonly used with the goal of the creation of an acyclic, low-estrogen environment. This prevents bleeding at the site of the implants and further seeding of the pelvis during retrograde menstruation. To reduce the risk of decreased bone density, a long-term side effect of gonadotropin–releasing hormone analog therapy, prescriptions for courses of therapy lasting longer than 6 consecutive mo are not recommended.

116.4 Premenstrual Syndrome

Premenstrual syndrome, or the late luteal phase syndrome, is a complex of physical signs and behavioral symptoms occurring during the second half of the menstrual cycle, which may resolve with the onset of menses. Clinical manifestations may include breast fullness and tenderness; bloating; fatigue; headache; increased appetite, especially for sweets and salty foods; irritability and mood swings; and depression, inability to concentrate, tearfulness, and violent tendencies. About one third of women in the reproductive age group may have premenstrual syndrome, but the absence of objective findings makes this difficult to corroborate. It is not common among adolescents, and it does not relate to the presence of dysmenorrhea, which is much more common in this age group. The popular use of vitamin B_6 and progesterone supplementation is not based on evidence of their effectiveness, nor is there a theoretical basis for their use. Use of a gonadotropin-releasing hormone agonist on a short-term basis is supported by carefully controlled studies, but long-term effects, such as osteoporosis and potential complications have not yet been evaluated, making its use in adolescents premature.

CHAPTER 117
Contraception

Adolescents bear a disproportionate risk for the adverse consequences of sexual activity, sexually transmitted diseases, and early unintended pregnancy. They should be encouraged to postpone sexual involvement; however, contraceptive counseling and services should be offered to adolescents who are sexually active.

EPIDEMIOLOGY. The National Survey of Family Growth (1995) reported a decline in sexual activity from 1988–1995, with intercourse in young women aged 15–19 yr dropping from 55 to 50% and percentages in young men dropping from 60 to 55%. However, the Centers for Disease Control and Prevention's Youth Risk Behavior Survey notes that 66.4% of high school seniors report having ever had intercourse, with 49.7% currently active sexually, which was defined as having had intercourse during the 3 mo preceding the survey. In 9th grade, 36.9% reported ever having had sex, with 23.6% being sexually active. Differential patterns of activity were reported by gender and ethnicity, with boys being more sexually active than girls, and black students with higher rates of sexual activity than Hispanic and white students. Many other factors are associated with early sexual activity and may account for differential effects, including but not limited to lower expectations for education, poor perception of life options, low school grades, and involvement in other high-risk behaviors.

There is some variability in the reporting of the percentage of teenagers who use contraception depending on the study and the way in which the question was worded. Overall contraceptive use among adolescents aged 15–19 yr, according to the National Survey of Family Growth, increased significantly from 1982–1988 (24.2–32.1%); however, more recent data demonstrate a decline between 1988 and 1995 (29.8%). Contraceptive use at first intercourse, and condom use in general, have increased during this same period. The type of method selected also varies by ethnicity, with nonwhite teens more likely to select pills, and black teens using pills as the first choice, but being two times more likely than whites to use an injectable method (Table 117–1). Sexually active adolescent women delay going to a clinic or a doctor for a medical contraceptive for an average of 6 mo after initiating intercourse. A higher likelihood of contraceptive use is associated with older age at sexual initiation, aspirations for higher academic achievement, acceptance of one's own sexuality, and a positive attitude toward contraception.

CONTRACEPTIVE COUNSELING. The health screening interview during the adolescent preventive visit offers the opportunity

TABLE 117–1 Percentage Distribution of Non-Hispanic White and Non-Hispanic Black Contraceptive Users Aged 15–19 Years by Current Method, 1982–1995

Race-Ethnicity and Method	1982	1988	1995
Non-Hispanic White			
Female sterilization	0	2	0
Male sterilization	0	0	0
Pill	62	56	49
Implant	NA	NA	1
Injectable	NA	NA	8
IUD	0	0	0
Diaphragm	7	1	0
Male condom	23	34	36
Other methods	7	7	7
Non-Hispanic Black			
Female sterilization	0	2	0
Male sterilization	0	0	0
Pill	70	75	32
Implant	NA	NA	5
Injectable	NA	NA	19
IUD	5	0	0
Diaphragm	2	0	0
Male condom	13	21	38
Other methods	10	2	5
TOTAL	100	100	100

IUD = intrauterine device; NA = not available.

Adapted from Piccinino LJ, Mosher WD: Trends in contraceptive use in the United States: 1982–1995. Family Planning Perspect 30:4, 46, 1998.

to support the adolescent who is abstinent to continue to be so and also presents an opportunity to identify the sexually active adolescent who has unsafe sexual practices (see Chapter 108). Adolescents with chronic diseases are particularly vulnerable to having these issues omitted from the health maintenance visit. There may be particular cautions related to concurrent medication to be noted for these chronically ill teenagers; however, sexuality and contraceptive issues need to be addressed. The goals of a counseling intervention with the adolescent are to understand the adolescent's perceptions and misperceptions about contraceptives, help him or her put the risk of unprotected intercourse in a personal perspective, and educate the adolescent regarding the real risk and contraindications for the various methods available. The adolescent should also be made aware of the "perfect" use failure rates vs the "typical" failure rates based on patient compliance (Table 117–2). Once an adolescent chooses a method, recognition of the common side effects, with clear plans on management, communication with the provider about the realistic expectation for failure, and a contingency plan for that possibility between the adolescent and the provider give closure to the counseling session and provide strategies for close follow-up. The pelvic examination as a requirement to obtain medical contraception creates a barrier for some teenagers; consequently, clinicians have commonly delayed the examination for 3–6 mo for adolescents who might otherwise postpone the acceptance of a contraceptive device. Confidentiality and consent issues related to contraceptive management are discussed in Chapter 108.

117.1 Barrier Methods

CONDOMS. This method prevents sperm from being deposited in the vagina. There are no major side effects associated with the use of a condom. Its effectiveness in preventing pregnancy is low, however, with 15 pregnancies occurring/100 woman-years of use by adult women in the United States. No comparative figures are available for adolescents, but acceptance of this method in the past has been low in teenagers. A 1979 study found that only 23% of 15- to 19-yr-old girls reported that their partner ever used a condom. The acquired immunodeficiency syndrome scare appears to have increased the use of condoms among adolescents, with 33% of young women reporting partner condom use in 1988 and 37% in 1995. Condoms used in the United States are thicker than those marketed in other countries where they enjoy widespread use. The main advantages of condoms are their low price, availability without prescription, little need for advance planning, and, most important for this age group, their effectiveness in preventing transmission of sexually transmitted diseases, including human immunodeficiency virus. Condoms are recommended as protection against sexually transmitted diseases (STDs), to be used along with all nonbarrier medical methods for adolescents. A female condom is now available over the counter in single size disposable units. It is a second choice over the male latex condom because of the complexity of properly using the device, its low typical efficacy rate, and the lack of evidence demonstrating its effectiveness against STDs. Most adolescents would require intensive education and hands-on practice to use it effectively.

DIAPHRAGM AND CERVICAL CAP. These methods have few side effects but are much less likely to be used by teenagers. Adolescents tend to object to the messiness of the jelly or to the fact that the insertion of a diaphragm may interrupt the spontaneity of sex, or they may express discomfort about touching their genitals.

TABLE 117–2 First-Year Failure Rates by Contraceptive Method

	Women Experiencing Pregnancy (%)	
	Typical Use	*Perfect Use*
Implant	0.09	0.09
Injectable	0.3	0.3
IUD		
Copper T380A	0.7	0.6
Progesterone T	2.0	1.5
Oral contraceptive		
Combined	2.5–6.0	0.1
Progestin-only	3.0–10.0	0.5
Male condom	12.0	3.0
Diaphragm with spermicide	16.0–18.0	6.0
Cervical cap	17.4	6.0
Withdrawal	19.0	4.0
Periodic abstinence	20.0	
Calendar "rhythm"		9.0
Cervical mucus		3.0
Symptothermal		2.0
Spermicides	21.0	6.0
Female condom	21.0–26.0	5.0
No method	85.0	85.0

FDA labeled rates noted are adapted from Hatcher RA, Trussell J, Stewart F, et al: Contraceptive Technology, 16th revised ed. New York, Irvington Publishers, 1994 and Jones EF, Forrest JD: Contraceptive failure rates based on 1988 NSFG. Fam Plann Perspect 24:12, 1992.

117.2 Spermicides

A variety of agents containing the spermicide nonoxynol-9 are available as foams, jellies, creams, films, or effervescent vaginal suppositories. They must be placed in the vaginal cavity shortly before intercourse and reinserted before each subsequent ejaculation in order to be effective. Rare side effects consist of contact vaginitis. Effectiveness is in the range of the barrier methods (approximately 85%), and the finding that nonoxynol-9 is gonococcocidal and spirocheticidal enhances the attractiveness of these agents for adolescents because of the disproportionately high risk for sexually transmitted diseases in adolescents.

117.3 Combination Methods

The conjoint use of the condom by the male and spermicidal foam by the female adolescent is extremely effective; the failure rate is 2% (perfect use), without any of the potential side effects and complications associated with the use of other forms of contraception having comparable efficacy. This combination also prevents STDs, including human immunodeficiency virus.

117.4 Hormonal Methods

Hormonal methods currently employ either an estrogenic substance in combination with a progestin or a progestin alone. The action of the estrogen-progestin combination is to prevent the surge of luteinizing hormone and, as a result, to inhibit ovulation. Progestin may prevent ovulation, but this is not reliable. It does, however, affect fallopian tube transport and the composition of cervical mucus in such a way as to make fertilization or implantation less likely.

COMBINATION ORAL CONTRACEPTIVES. Oral contraceptives (OCs) are commonly referred to as "the pill" and currently contain either 50, 35, 30, or 20 μg of estrogenic substance, typically either mestranol or ethinyl estradiol, and a progestin. The pill is one of the most reliable contraceptive methods available, with a perfect-use pregnancy rate in the range of 0.1%/yr. Typical-use failure rates in 15–19 yr old women have ranged up to 18.1%. Thrombophlebitis, hepatic adenomas, myocardial infarction, and carbohydrate intolerance are some of the more serious potential complications of exogenous estrogen use. These disorders are, however, exceedingly rare in adolescents. Even though teenaged smokers who use OCs have a relative risk of more than 2.0 for myocardial infarction, the likelihood of its occurrence is much smaller, and thus insignificant, than the risk of dying from pregnancy-related complications. Some long-range beneficial effects of estrogen use include decreased risks of benign breast disease, ovarian disease, and anemia.

The short-term adverse effects of OCs, such as nausea and weight gain, often interfere with compliance in adolescent patients. These effects are usually transient and may be overshadowed by the beneficial effects of a shortened menses and the relief of dysmenorrhea. The inhibition of ovulation or the suppressant effect of estrogens on prostaglandin production by the endometrium make oral contraceptives effective in preventing dysmenorrhea (see Chapter 116). An initial concern for younger adolescents regarding the potentially untoward effect of estrogens on epiphyseal growth has diminished. This does not occur, either because the amount of estrogen in oral contraceptives is small or because they are taken at a time when most growth has been completed. Amenorrhea occurring after cessation of OC use is seen with greater frequency in adolescents than in adults. It may persist for up to 18 mo after the discontinuation of the pill. The increased risk may not be due to age alone but may reflect oligomenorrhea or low body weight (<47 kg) before the initiation of use of the pill. Acne may be worsened by some and improved by other oral contraceptive preparations. The newer pills with nonandrogenic progestins are particularly effective in reducing acne and hirsutism as side effects. An additional beneficial cardiovascular effect occurs for adolescents taking estrogen-containing oral contraceptives; these young women have higher levels of cardioprotective high-density lipoproteins than seen in controls.

Major and minor contraindications to the use of estrogen-containing oral contraceptives include hepatocellular disease, migraine headaches, breast disease, any condition in which hypercoagulability may be a problem (e.g., replaced cardiac valve, thrombophlebitis, sickle cell anemia) because of the increased levels of factor VIII and decreased production of antithrombin III, and known or suspected pregnancy. The risks of pregnancy must be balanced against the benefits of reliable contraception in patients with chronic diseases such as diabetes, epilepsy, and sickle cell disease. The initial history taken before prescribing OCs should specifically address these risks. Table 117–3 also presents the potential alterations of various laboratory tests that can occur in patients taking OCs.

ALL-PROGESTIN CONTRACEPTIVES. Progestin-only contraceptives are available for the adolescent in whom the use of estrogen is potentially deleterious, for example, those with liver disease, replaced cardiac valves, or hypercoagulable states. These agents ("mini-pills") are less reliable in inhibiting ovulation and are associated with a 0.5%/yr pregnancy rate (perfect use). Acceptance by adolescents is limited by the necessity of taking the pill daily, the higher incidence of amenorrhea, and increased bleeding.

An **injectable progestin,** medroxyprogesterone (Depo-Provera, DMPA), is highly effective in birth control, with failure rates typically at 0.3–0.4%. This substance needs to be administered only once every 3 mo and is completely reversible in its anovulatory action; furthermore, the cessation of menses is conterminous with its use. The most common side effect of DMPA is menstrual disturbance, either amenorrhea or abnormal vaginal bleeding. Weight gain and lowered bone density have been observed in women taking DMPA; however,

TABLE 117–3 Laboratory Tests and Potential Alteration

Group	Increased	Decreased
Carbohydrate metabolism	Fasting blood sugar and 2-hr pp Insulin	Glucose tolerance
Hematologic and coagulation	Coagulation factors II, VII, XIII, IX, X, XII Fibrinogen Leukocyte count PTT, PT Plasminogen Platelet count, platelet aggregation, platelet adhesiveness	Antithrombin III Hematocrit PT
Lipid metabolism	Cholesterol, lipoproteins HDL increased by estrogen Triglycerides	 HDL decreased by progestins
Liver function and gastrointestinal tests	Alkaline phosphatase Bilirubin, SGOT, SGPT, GGT Protoporphyrin, coproporphyrin excretion (urine)	 Haptoglobin Urobilinogen excretion (urine)
Metals	Copper and ceruloplasmin Iron, iron-binding capacity, and transferrin	Magnesium Zinc
Thyroid function	Thyroid-binding globulin Thyroxine	Free thyroxine
Vitamins	Vitamin A	Folate Vitamins B_6, B_{12} Vitamin C
Other hormones and enzymes	Aldosterone Angiotensinogen Angiotensin I and II Cortisol Growth hormone Testosterone	Estradiol FSH, LH 17-hydroxycorticosteroids Renin
Miscellaneous	α_1-Antitrypsin Antinuclear antibody Lactate Sodium	Albumin Calcium Immunoglobulins A, G, M

FSH = follicle-stimulating hormone; GGT = γ-glutamyltransferase; HDL = high-density lipoprotein; LH = luteinizing hormone; PP = postprandial; PT = prothrombin time; PTT = partial thromboplastin time; SGOT = serum glutamic-oxaloacetic transaminase, SGPT = serum glutamic-pyruvic transaminase.

From Neinstein LS: Adolescent Health Care, 3rd ed. Baltimore, Williams & Wilkins, 1996.

the data confirming the agent as the sole cause of these changes are still under study. Issues relative to bone density are of particular concern during adolescence, the developmental period in which the accumulation of bone density is at its greatest. Studies thus far indicate that the effect is reversible on discontinuation of the drug. DMPA is particularly attractive for adolescents who have difficulty with compliance, mentally retarded teenagers, and teenagers with chronic illnesses who have a relative contraindication to estrogen use. Continuation rates when compared with oral contraceptives are somewhat disappointing and are primarily related to the length of action rather than to the contraceptive behavior of the adolescent.

A *long-acting progestational agent*, levonorgestrel (Norplant), is contained in six small Silastic tubes that are implanted subcutaneously. The contraceptive potency remains for 5 yr. This method is the most effective of all reversible birth control methods available, with a typical 1st-yr failure rate for all women at 0.09% and 5-yr failure rates at 0.9–1.1%. Failure rates specifically calculated for adolescent women are not available. Implants have been used primarily in postpartum adolescents with good tolerance and acceptability. When compared with oral contraceptive use in this population, implant users have better continuation rates and fewer pregnancies over a 1–2 yr period. Requests for early removal of this device have led to its diminished use in adolescent women. Norplant II has been approved in Finland and China as a device with two Silastic rods to be implanted for 3 yr. Other biodegradable implants are also in research and development.

117.5 Emergency Contraception

Unprotected intercourse at midcycle carries a pregnancy risk of 20–30%. At any other time during the cycle, the risk drops to 2–4%. The risk may be reduced or eliminated by intervention within 72 hr after unprotected intercourse. Outside the United States, several agents are used for emergency contraception: oral high-dose estrogens, high-dose combination estrogen-progestins, high-dose progestins, danazol, mifepristone, and the postcoital insertion of a copper intrauterine device (IUD). The Yuzpe method is most commonly used in the United States, consisting of combination pills totaling 200 μg of ethinyl estradiol and 2.0 mg of norgestrel or 1.0 mg levonorgestrel (Table 117–4). The high-dose combination OCs disrupt the luteal phase hormone pattern, creating an unstable and unsuitable uterine lining for implantation. If used midcycle, when ovulation is about to occur, the high-dose estrogen and progestin blunt the luteinizing hormone surge and impair ovulation. This method is effective in reducing the risk of pregnancy by 75%. The most common side effect is nausea (50%) and vomiting (20%), prompting some clinicians to prescribe or recommend antiemetics along with the OCs. In most health care facilities, a urine pregnancy test is required prior to dispensing the pills to rule out an existing pregnancy. There is some controversy about the need to do this, since there is no evidence to suggest that OCs used in this manner affect early fetal development and the dose as prescribed would not disrupt a previously undetected pregnancy. A 2-wk follow-up appointment is recommended to determine the effectiveness of treatment and to diagnose a possible early pregnancy. The visit also provides an opportunity to counsel the adolescent, explore the situation leading up to the unprotected intercourse, test for STDs, and initiate continuing contraception when appropriate.

TABLE 117–4 Emergency Contraceptive Pill Regimens

Brand Name	Instructions	Total Estrogen and Progesterone
Ovral	2 tablets orally, then 2 tablets in 12 hr	200 μg ethinyl estradiol plus 2.0 mg norgestrel
Lo-Ovral	4 tablets orally, then 4 tablets in 12 hr	240 μg ethinyl estradiol plus 2.4 mg norgestrel
Nordette, or Levlen	4 tablets orally, then 4 tablets in 12 hr	240 μg ethinyl estradiol plus 1.2 mg levonorgestrel
Triphasil, or Tri-Levlen	4 tablets orally, then 4† tablets in 12 hr	240 μg ethinyl estradiol plus 1.0 mg levonorgestrel
Ovrette*	20 tablets, then 20 tablets in 12 hr	3.0 mg levonorgestrel

**Must start within 48 hr of unprotected intercourse.*
†Yellow tablets only.
From Gold MA: Emergency contraception: A second chance at preventing adolescent unintended pregnancy. Curr Opin Pediatr 9:300, 1997.

117.6 Intrauterine Devices

IUDs are small, flexible, plastic objects introduced into the uterine cavity through the cervix. They differ in size, shape, and the presence or absence of pharmacologically active substances (e.g., copper or progesterone). The mechanism of action of IUDs is uncertain, although they render the endometrium unsuitable for implantation by inducing a local polymorphonuclear leukocyte response, production of prostaglandins E_2 and F_2, and stimulation of uterine contractility. They are effective in preventing pregnancy in 97–99% of women. Young patients and those with multiple sexual partners are at increased risk of infection, and the prescription of an IUD to teenagers who require passive contraception should be limited to the method of last resort.

CHAPTER 118
Pregnancy

Sexual activity at an early age coupled with nonuse or improper use of contraceptives contributes to a disproportionately high rate of teenage pregnancy in the United States when compared with other industrialized nations. By virtue of the trajectory of early sexual activity to early unintended pregnancy, the risk and protective factors are similar. Factors associated with childbearing as the outcome for teenage pregnancy, however, are strongly linked to poverty and the absence of opportunity for other life choices.

EPIDEMIOLOGY. The estimated number of pregnancies in adolescent women fell to approximately 800,000 in 1994. This decline has been under way since 1991 but still fails to approach the historical low of the late 1980s (Fig. 118–1). However, when considered in the context of the number of sexually active adolescents, the decline is impressive. Most of the pregnancies are unintended, and a significant proportion of young women voluntarily terminate the pregnancy. Forty-eight per cent of girls younger than 15 yrs of age, and 35.3% of 15–19 yr olds elected abortion in 1994, although the overall rates of abortion are also down. Internationally, the United States leads all other industrialized countries in the number of births to 15–19 yr olds, which was 14% in 1996. Overall, the proportion of women who have their first child by age 20 yr is declining worldwide and is largely attributed to increases in women's educational level (Fig. 118–2).

ETIOLOGY. As with early initiation of intercourse, the factors associated with pregnancy are multifactorial at the individual,

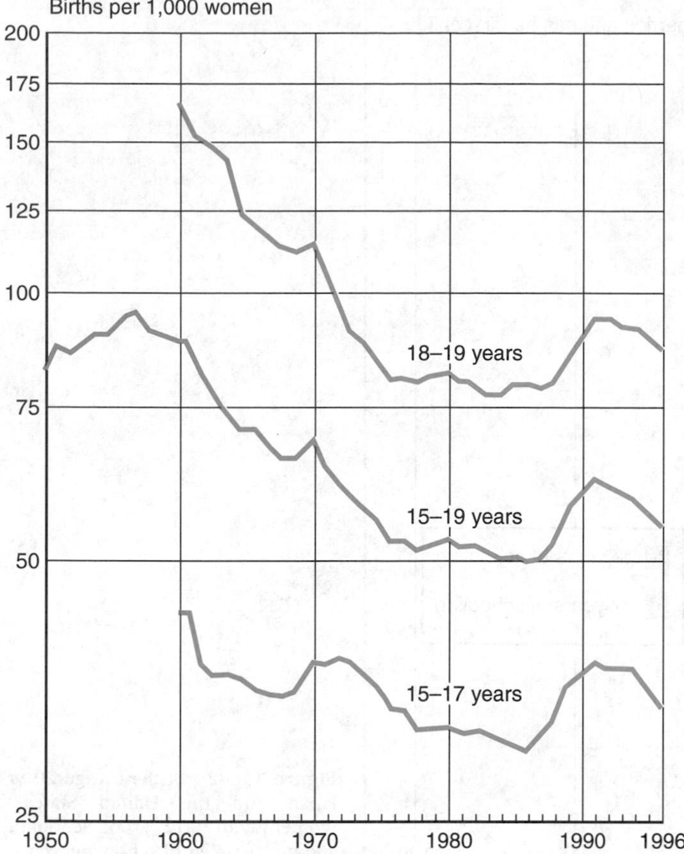

Figure 118–1 Birth rates for teenagers by age: United States, 1950–1996. (From Ventura SJ, Curtin SC, Mathews TJ: Teenage births in the United States: National and state trends 1950–1996. Hyattsville, MD, National Center for Health Statistics, 1998.)

family, and environmental levels (Chapter 107). The sexually active female teenager's success in avoiding unintended pregnancy is determined by her ability to use an effective contraceptive method consistently. Young teenagers are likely to be less deliberative and logical about their sexual decisions than are adults, and their sexual activity is likely to be sporadic and coercive, factors contributing to inconsistent contraceptive use and greater risk of pregnancy. Once the pregnancy has occurred, the decision to bear a child, keep or place the child for adoption, or terminate the pregnancy is influenced again by multiple issues. Parents, most often mothers, have a tremendous influence on what the adolescent decides to do. Friends and sexual partners play a lesser role. Better employment prospects as well as other lifestyle benefits are associated with lowered probability of childbearing. A young woman's attitude toward abortion is the strongest factor associated with that choice. Access to abortion services and individual factors such as high self-esteem and aspirations for further education play a role. Adoption appears to be an option less often considered currently and is associated with younger age, expectations of fewer children and, less often, receiving welfare support prior to pregnancy. Marriage following a first teenager birth is least likely to occur in young teenagers and teenagers with less than a high school education and more likely to occur in some cultural groups, such as Hispanic teens. Overall, adoption and marriage are choices less often selected by pregnant adolescents.

CLINICAL MANIFESTATIONS. Adolescents may experience the traditional symptoms of pregnancy, that is, morning sickness, swollen tender breasts, weight gain, and amenorrhea; however, the presentation is often more vague. Headache, fatigue, abdominal pain, and scanty or irregular menses are common presenting symptoms.

Denial of sexual activity and menstrual irregularity should not preclude the diagnosis in face of other clinical or historical information. An unanticipated request for a complete checkup or a visit for contraception may uncover a suspected pregnancy in some cases. Pregnancy is still the most common diagnosis when an adolescent presents with secondary amenorrhea.

DIAGNOSIS. On physical examination, the findings of an enlarged uterus, cervical cyanosis (Chadwick sign), or a soft cervix (Goodell sign) are highly suggestive of an intrauterine pregnancy. A confirmatory pregnancy test is always recommended. The most commonly used method is a qualitative measurement of the beta subunit for human chorionic gonadotropin (hCG) by blood or urine. The results are positive in 98% of women within 7 days after implantation. The most sensitive test is a quantitative β-hCG radioimmunoassay in which results are reliable within 7 days after fertilization. This test is more expensive and less likely to be used under routine circumstances. Evaluation for a possible ectopic pregnancy, a retained placenta following an abortion, or a molar pregnancy are some of its more common uses. Slide tests are less reliable in diagnosing an early pregnancy but can be useful in confirming a pregnancy after 6–16 wk of gestation. These tests have cross reactions and are less specific for the beta subunit of hCG.

TREATMENT. Confidentiality and privacy are key components of counseling the adolescent in whom pregnancy is suspected. The younger the adolescent, the greater should be the concern that the sexual activity may have been coercive. Special sensitivity is required to explore this issue with the adolescent as is knowledge of proper procedures for enlisting help for the adolescent and reporting suspected abuse. If the adolescent's pregnancy test result is negative, it is prudent to repeat the test in 2 wk. If the repeat test result is negative, the opportunity to counsel the adolescent and provide the appropriate intervention should be seized. If the adolescent is pregnant, the options available to manage the pregnancy should be presented and discussed in the context of her family, as well as individual, situation. Adolescents should be encouraged to include parents fully in the discussion of their options. When parents are not available or the adolescent is resistant to their initial involvement, the adolescent is urged to involve a trusted adult—for example, a relative or counselor—in the decision-making process. Follow-up is necessary to ensure this involvement, given the possibility that denial, fear, and indecisiveness may delay the adolescent's seeking adult support.

RISKS AND CONSEQUENCES OF TEENAGE CHILDBEARING. Adverse outcomes for pregnant teenagers are reduced significantly by early prenatal care. Twenty per cent of teenagers younger than age 15 yr, and 12% of all teenagers are likely to receive third trimester care or no care at all prior to delivery. Adolescent parenting has implications for the adolescent mother, father, and child. When adolescent mothers are compared with their peers, they are less likely to complete high school and have steady employment and are more likely to be on public assistance at some point in their lives and to be in unstable marriages. Infants born to adolescent mothers less than 15 yr old are at greater risk for low birthweight. The children of adolescents experience more problems in school, showing difficulties with cognitive functioning, and have an increased risk of experiencing an accident within the home and of being hospitalized before 5 yr of age. Men who father the children of adolescent mothers are usually 2–3 yr older than the mother and often not teenagers themselves. However, fathers who are adolescents often suffer the same social and economic risks of the teenage mother, with many fewer resources and programs to

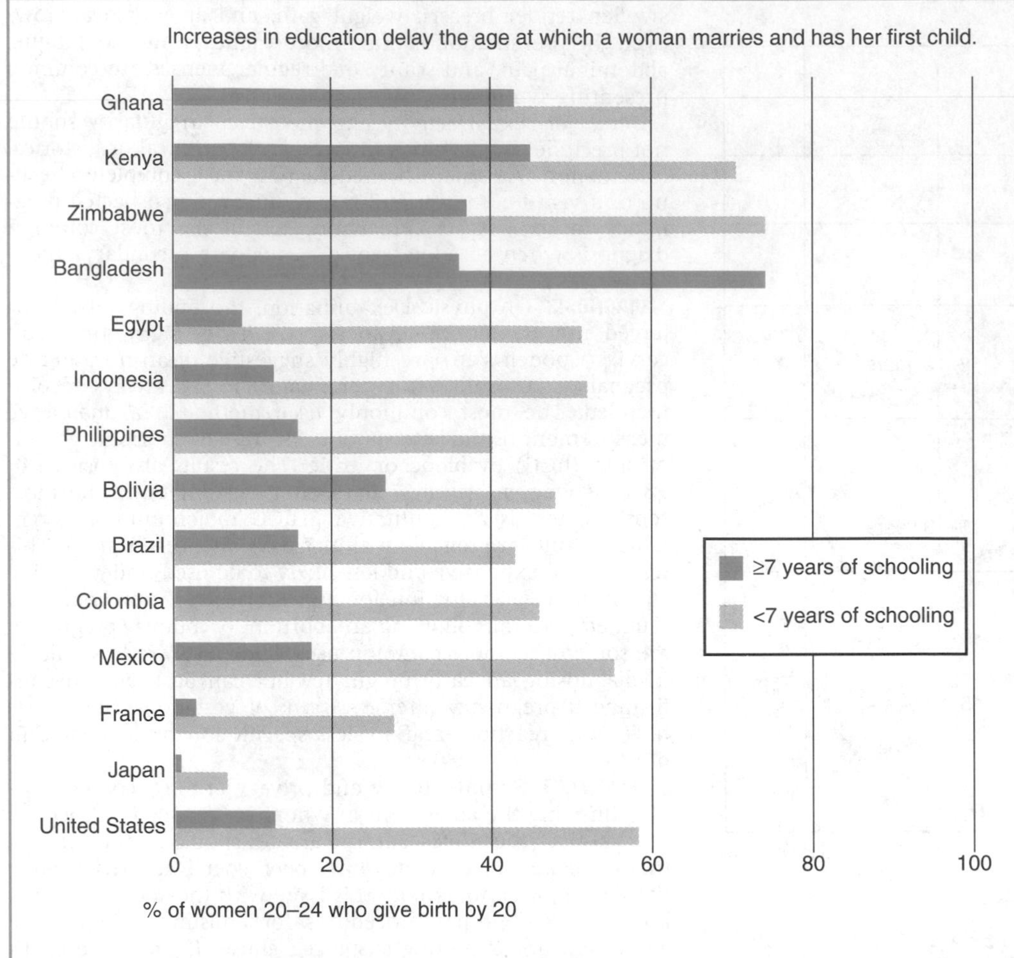

Figure 118–2 Births by age 20 yr, Japan and the United States—women with ≤12 yr of schooling and with ≥12 yr of schooling. (From The Alan Guttmacher Institute: Risks and Realities of Early Childbearing Worldwide: Issues in Brief, New York, AGI, 1996.)

assist them. Some controversy exists as to whether the social and economic outcomes are a function of maternal age or maternal and family poverty.

PREVENTION. The reductions in teenage pregnancy rates, although limited, have been attributed to an increase in contraceptive use at first intercourse and a decrease in sexual activity. Although researchers are still actively seeking successful teenage pregnancy interventions, the multifactorial nature of the issue suggests a multilevel approach. On the individual level, postponing sexual involvement until psychosocial maturity guides a more responsible preventive behavior and is the principle underlying a number of successful programs. The pediatrician contributes to this strategy through anticipatory guidance. The next level is to provide birth control counseling to adolescents who are sexually active to protect against pregnancy and sexually transmitted disease. On the community level, one looks to improved access to protective medical measures with attention to age-appropriate health care delivery models and the removal of financial barriers to these services. At a societal level, corroborated by the international experience, improved economic opportunities and the enhancement of life options for young women and young men play a pivotal role in the positive outcomes related to teenage sexual behavior and the risk of pregnancy and parenthood.

Allan Guttmacher Institute: Issues in Brief. Risks and Realities of Early Childbearing Worldwide, February, 1997.

American Academy of Pediatrics, Committee on Adolescents: Counseling the adolesecent about pregnancy options. Pediatrics 101:938, 1998.

Blythe J: Common menstrual problems of adolescence. Adolesc Med: State of Art Rev 8:87, 1997.

Delbanco SF, Parker ML, McIntosh M, et al: Missed opportunities. Arch Pediatr Adolesc Med 152:727, 1998.

Emans SJH, Laufer MR, Goldstein DP: Pediatric and Adolescent Gynecology, 4th ed. Philadelphia, Lippincott-Raven, 1998.

Gold MA: Emergency contraception: A second chance at preventing adolescent unintended pregnancy. Curr Opin Pediatr 9:300, 1997.

Gold MA: Emergency contraception. Adolesc Med: State of the Art Rev 8:455, 1997.

Henshaw SK: Unintended pregnancy in the United States. Fam Plan Perspect 30:24, 46, 1998.

Litt IF: Pregnancy in adolescence [editorial, comment]. JAMA 275:1030, 1996.

Moore KA, Miller BC, Sugland BW, et al: Beginning Too Soon: Adolescent Sexual Behavior, Pregnancy and Parenthood. Washington, DC, Child Trends, Inc., June, 1995.

Neinstein LS: Adolescent Health Care: A Practical Guide, 3rd ed. Baltimore, Williams & Wilkins, 1996.

O'Connell BJ: The pediatrician and the sexually active adolescent: Treatment of common menstrual disorders. Pediatr Clin North Am 44:1391, 1997.

Ozer EM, Brindis CD, Millstein SG, et al: America's Adolescents—Are They Healthy? San Francisco, University of California at San Francisco, National Adolescent Health Information Center, 1998.

Piccinino LJ, Mosher WD: Trends in contraceptive use in the United States: 1982–1995. Fam Plan Perspect 30:4, 46, 1998.

Polaneczky M, Slap G, Forke C, et al: The use of levonorgestrel implants (Norplant) for contraception in adolescent mothers. N Engl J Med 331:1201, 1994.

Saenger P: Turner's syndrome. N Engl J Med 335:1749, 1996.

CHAPTER 119
Sexually Transmitted Diseases

The behavioral and physiologic characteristics of adolescence predispose sexually active adolescents to the increased acquisition and adverse consequences of sexually transmitted diseases (STDs). When controlled for sexual activity, age-specific rates of many STDs are highest among sexually experienced adolescents. For STD pathogens, intimate sexual contact is the common mode of transmission; however, the clinical expression can be listed according to STD syndromes based on a constellation of clinical signs and symptoms. Different microorganisms are responsible for similar symptoms. Almost all STD pathogens can also infect an adolescent without manifesting any clinical symptoms. The approach to prevention and control of these diseases lies in education, screening, and early diagnosis and treatment. (See Chapters discussing specific microorganisms in Part XVI.)

ETIOLOGY. The risk of contracting an STD exists in any adolescent who has had sexual intercourse. The risk is increased for specific STDs when certain factors exist. The younger the adolescent at the time of initiation of sexual activity, the higher the risk. Inadequate time to develop decision-making and cognitive skills as well as biologic status contribute to this susceptibility. The use of drugs and alcohol removes inhibitions and contributes to unplanned and unprotected sexual activity. Intravenous drug use, sex with homosexual or bisexual males, and a history of exchanging sex for food, shelter, money, or drugs are all associated with increasing risk for human immunodeficiency virus (HIV) and other serious STDs. Exposure to uncommon sexual pathogens is increased with anal sex. Sex with more than one partner in 6 mo and failure to use condoms consistently are behaviors for which educational interventions may have some impact. Adolescents who are victims of sexual abuse or rape may not consider themselves "sexually active," given the context of the encounter and need reassurance, protection, and appropriate intervention when these risk factors are uncovered.

EPIDEMIOLOGY. Although adolescents and young adults younger than 25 yr of age have the highest reported prevalence of gonorrhea and chlamydial infection, the rates have been declining in recent years. Rates for gonorrhea in the United States are highest for 15–19 yr old females and 20–24 yr old males. They have dropped from 851.6/100,000 to 756.8/100,000 for females and 729.9/100,000 to 522/100,000 for males for 1996 as compared with 1993. Although national data are not reported for chlamydial infection, regional data show that adolescent women less than 17 yr have the highest prevalence of reported infection. The proportion of teenagers testing positive dropped from 12% to less than 6% from 1988 to 1996. After peaking in 1990, the rates for primary and secondary syphilis are declining for all ages, with adolescents age 15–19 yr having the 3rd highest reported prevalence for females and the 2nd lowest prevalence for males. Pelvic inflammatory disease (PID) rates are reported to be highest in females age 15–25 yr old when compared with older women. Thirty-three per cent of those infections are in females younger than age 19 yr. In some surveys, 15–20% of adolescents and young adults seeking routine gynecologic care have HIV infection detected. Acquired immunodeficiency syndrome, but not HIV, is reportable in the United States, giving a somewhat skewed perception of a lower rate of infection in adolescents. The lengthy incubation period coupled with a range of smaller seroprevalence studies underscore the serious risk of HIV disease for this population.

PATHOGENESIS. During puberty, increasing levels of estrogen cause the vaginal epithelium to thicken and cornify and the cellular glycogen content to rise, the latter causing vaginal pH to fall. These changes increase the resistance of the vaginal epithelium to penetration by certain organisms (including *Gonococcus*) and increase the susceptibility to others (e.g., *Candida albicans* and *Trichomonas*). The transformation of the vaginal cells leaves columnar cells on the ectocervix, forming a border of the two cell types on the ectocervix, known as the squamocolumnar junction. The appearance is referred to as *ectopy.* With maturation, this tissue involutes. Prior to involution, it represents a unique vulnerability to infection for adolescent females. As a result of these physiologic changes, gonococcal infection becomes primarily cervical, and susceptibility to ascending infection is greatest during menses, when the pH is 6.8–7.0. Menstruation in an adolescent with an endocervical colonization presents a risk factor for the development of PID.

CLINICAL MANIFESTATIONS. STD syndromes are generally characterized by the location of the manifestation (vaginitis) or the type of lesion (genital ulcer). In addition, certain constellations of presenting symptoms suggest the inclusion of a possible STD in the differential diagnosis. The syndromes and the conditions suggestive of STDs are listed in Table 119–1.

Urethritis. Urethritis is an inflammation of the urethra classically presenting as a urethral discharge or dysuria, or both. Urgency, frequency of urination, erythema of the urethral meatus, and scrotal pain are less common clinical presentations. Asymptomatic or minimally symptomatic presentations are common in males. Adolescent males, in particular, are likely to ignore symptoms that improve spontaneously or sometimes ignore obvious physical signs. Consequently, the genital examination should be thorough, including retraction of the foreskin in uncircumcised males, regardless of the denial of symptoms by the adolescent. Examining a patient prior to a urinary void is an important factor in observing a minimally symptomatic discharge. *C. trachomatis* and *Neisseria gonorrhoeae* are the most common pathogens. *Ureaplasma urealyticum* and *Mycoplasma genitalium* are still considered potential pathogens in nongonococcal urethritis, when *Chlamydia* cannot be confirmed. Diagnostic tests for these pathogens are not readily available. *T. vaginalis* and herpes simplex virus (HSV) are considered in the differential diagnosis when nongonococcal urethritis is resistant to treatment. There are classic descriptions of discharges, associating pathogens with color and consistency, that is, yellow-green purulent discharge for gonococci and white mucopurulent discharge for chlamydia; however, co-infection and other factors can alter the appearance of discharges. Co-infection with gonococcal and chlamydial ure-

TABLE 119–1 Sexually Transmitted Disease Clinical Syndromes

Sexually Transmitted Disease Syndromes
Urethritis
Epididymitis
Vaginitis (vulvitis)
Cervicitis
Pelvic inflammatory disease
Genital ulcer disease
Genital lesions and ectoparasites
Conditions Suggestive of Sexually Transmitted Disease
Lower abdominal pain (female)
Scrotal swelling and pain
Arthritis
Exanthem, alopecia
Pharyngitis
Conjunctivitis
Hepatitis, perihepatitis
Local and generalized lymphadenitis
Proctitis

From Morse SA, Moreland AA, Holmes KK: Atlas of Sexually Transmitted Diseases and AIDS, 2nd ed. London, Mosby-Wolfe, 1996.

thritis is reported in more than 25% of men with urethritis. Consequently, laboratory evaluation is key to determining the involved pathogens.

Epididymitis. The inflammation of the epididymis in adolescent males, unlike that in adult males, is most often associated with an STD. The same pathogens associated with urethritis are prevalent. The presentation of scrotal swelling and tenderness, associated with the history of a spontaneously resolving urethral discharge, constitute the presumptive diagnosis of epididymitis. A urethral discharge may still be present at the time of examination. Males who practice insertive anal intercourse are also vulnerable to *Escherichia coli* infection.

Vaginitis (Vulvitis). Vaginitis is a superficial infection of the vaginal mucosa frequently presenting as a vaginal discharge, with or without vulvar involvement (see Chapter 557). Pruritus and the presence of an odor help differentiate the cause of the infection. Colonization without infection, as in bacterial vaginosis, can also present as a vaginal discharge. No longer categorized strictly as an STD, sexual activity is associated with increased frequency of vaginosis. Trichomoniasis and candidiasis, together with bacterial vaginosis, are the predominant diseases associated with vaginal discharge. The clinical observations of the color, consistency (frothy, floccular, homogeneous), odor, extent of vulvar involvement, and cervical changes lead one to a presumptive diagnosis. However, laboratory confirmation is recommended in determining the presence of one or more infections that may present in an uncharacteristic manner. The differential diagnosis for vaginitis with the classic presentations is presented in Figure 119–1.

Cervicitis. The inflammatory process in cervicitis involves the deeper structures in the mucous membrane of the cervix uteri. Vaginal discharge can be a manifestation of cervicitis, if the cervical discharge is profuse. Less subtle clinical manifestations of cervicitis are irregular or postcoital bleeding, mucopurulent discharge from the os, and a friable cervix. The cervical changes associated with cervicitis must be distinguished from cervical ectopy in the younger adolescent to avoid the overdiagnosis of inflammation. The pathogens associated most commonly with cervicitis are *C. trachomatis* and *N. gonorrhoeae,* which are responsible for about 50–60% of cases. HSV is a less common pathogen associated with ulcerative and necrotic lesions on the cervix.

Pelvic Inflammatory Disease. A spectrum of inflammatory disorders of the upper genital tract in females is encompassed under the diagnosis of PID. The spectrum includes endometritis, salpingitis, tubo-ovarian abscess, and pelvic peritonitis, usually in combination rather than as separate entities. *N. gonorrhoeae* and *C. trachomatis* predominate as the involved pathogenic organisms in younger adolescents; maturation and recurrent disease increase the appearance of other anaerobic and aerobic bacteria such as *Mycoplasma hominis,* group B streptococci, streptococci, *Peptostreptococcus* spp., *Gardnerella vaginalis, E. coli,* and various *Bacteroides* spp.

The clinical diagnosis of PID is based on the minimal criteria of lower abdominal tenderness, adnexal tenderness, and cervical motion tenderness in a sexually active female adolescent with no other causes for illness. Although embarrassment may preclude an adolescent's honest answer regarding prior sexual activity, this history should not preclude gathering of evidence for this possible diagnosis. The presence of a recent increase in dysmenorrhea, onset of symptoms following menses, fever, urinary symptoms, abnormal vaginal bleeding, and abnormal vaginal discharge add support to the clinical diagnosis.

Genital Ulcer Syndromes. An ulcerative lesion in a mucosal area exposed to sexual contact is the unifying characteristic of diseases associated with these syndromes. These lesions are most commonly seen on the penis and vulva, but also occur on oral and rectal mucosa depending on the sexual practices of the adolescent. HSV, *Treponema pallidum* (syphilis), and *Haemophilus ducreyi* (chancroid) are the organisms associated with geni-

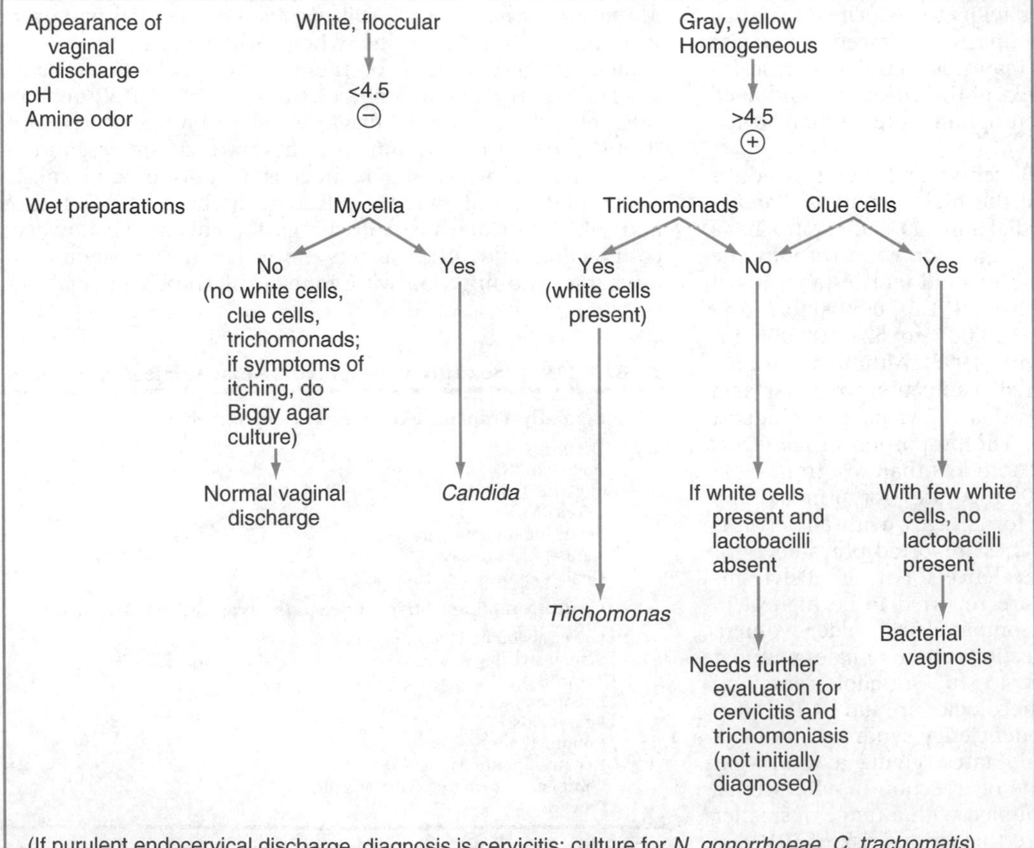

Figure 119–1 Differential diagnosis of vaginitis. (From Emans SJH, Laufer MR, Goldstein DP [eds]: Pediatric and Adolescent Gynecology, 4th ed. Philadelphia, Lippincott-Raven, 1998, p 427.)

tal ulcer syndromes. Although the initial herpetic lesion is a vesicle, by the time the patient presents clinically, the vesicle most often has ruptured spontaneously, leaving a shallow, painful ulcer. Of these syndromes, syphilis and chancroid are less common in adolescents than in adults. HSV-2 predominates as the pathogen in this age group, with an increasing incidence of HSV-1 recovered in genital lesions, especially in women. Clinical characteristics differentiating the lesions are presented in Table 119–2, along with the required laboratory diagnosis to identify the causative agent accurately.

Genital Lesions and Ectoparasites. Lesions that present as outgrowths on the surface of the epithelium and other limited epidermal lesions are included under this categorization of syndromes. Human papillomavirus with its association to cervical cancer causes the most concern for the long-term outcome for individuals infected during adolescence (see Chapter 257). Molluscum contagiosum, and condyloma lata associated with secondary syphilis complete this classification of syndromes.

Human Immunodeficiency Virus Disease and Hepatitis B. HIV disease presents as an asymptomatic, unexpected occurrence in most infected adolescents. Risk factors identified in the history are much more likely to result in suspicion of disease, leading to the appropriate laboratory screening, than are clinical manifestations in this age group.

DIAGNOSIS

Asymptomatic Patients. Health screening guidelines (see Chapter 108) recommend testing for STDs in asymptomatic patients on an annual basis. Asymptomatic infections with viral pathogens, such as HIV, HSV, and hepatitis B, are the most common presentations for these diseases, whereas asymptomatic infections for chlamydial infection and gonorrhea range from 17–56% and 2–33%, respectively. Adolescent males are more likely to be asymptomatic with *Chlamydia,* whereas adolescent females have a higher rate of asymptomatic gonococcal infections. Based on the preceding observations, the recommendations for screening sexually active adolescents are listed in Table 108–1.

Symptomatic Patients. Based on the clinical presentation, further evaluations may be needed to identify the causative agent of the syndrome accurately. For urethritis, a Gram stain when a urethral discharge is present confirms the diagnosis of gonorrhea at the time of the presenting symptom. The wet mount is useful in determining the possible pathogen causing a vaginal discharge (see Fig. 119–1). The definitive diagnosis of PID is difficult based on clinical findings alone. In addition to an elevated temperature (>101°F or >38.3°C) and an abnormal cervical or vaginal discharge, the finding of an elevated erythrocyte sedimentation rate or an elevated C-reactive protein level in combination with confirmative laboratory documentation of *N. gonorrhoeae* or *C. trachomatis* is recommended to avoid incorrect diagnosis and inappropriate management. Imaging techniques demonstrating thickened fluid-filled tubes with or without free pelvic fluid or a tubo-ovarian complex are definite criteria. Direct visualization through the laparoscopic technique with cultures from the fallopian tube, while infrequently performed in the United States, is the gold standard for definitive diagnosis. The HSV direct fluorescent antibody test or the herpes culture is readily available in most clinical settings to help determine the pathogen in genital ulcer syndromes. Darkfield microscopy and fluorescent antibody tests to confirm syphilis are less frequently available, with most clinicians relying on serologic confirmation. Tests to confirm the diagnosis of human papillomavirus are discussed in Chapter 257, although Papanicolaou's smear often reveals the first evidence of vaginal or cervical involvement in adolescents.

Differential Diagnoses. The differential diagnoses are particular to each of the clinical syndromes. Reiter syndrome is considered an autoimmune response to an STD or enteric pathogen and is characterized by arthritis, nonbacterial urethritis or cervicitis, conjunctivitis, and mucocutaneous lesions. The urinary symptoms associated with urethritis mimic a urinary tract infection, a condition much less common than an STD in adolescent males. Testicular torsion, the main differential diagnosis to consider in scrotal pain constitutes a surgical emergency, although trauma is a more common occurrence, especially in adolescent males involved in contact sports (see Chapters 554 and 696). Vaginitis and vulvar irritation can result from a foreign body or chemical irritant, for example, bubble bath or spermicide.

The differential diagnosis for PID, presenting as acute lower abdominal pain, is extensive, involving the gastrointestinal, reproductive, and urinary systems. The most emergent differential diagnosis in a sexually active adolescent is to distinguish PID from appendicitis or an ectopic pregnancy, which both require surgical intervention. Given the complexity of the management approach, clinical practice guidelines are extremely useful in moving swiftly and logically to the correct diagnosis (Table 119–3). Most of the conditions in the differential diagnosis of genital ulcerative lesions rarely occur in teenagers in the United States (i.e., lymphogranuloma venereum,

TABLE 119–2 Signs, Symptoms, and Presumptive and Definitive Diagnoses of Genital Ulcers

Signs/Symptoms	Herpes Simplex Virus	Syphilis Primary	Chancroid
Ulcers	Vesicles rupture to form shallow ulcers	Ulcer with well-demarcated indurated borders and a clean base (chancre)	Unindurated and undermined borders and a purulent base
Painful	Painful	Painless*	Painful
Number of lesions	Usually multiple	Usually single	Multiple
Inguinal lymphadenopathy	First-time infections may cause constitutional symptoms and lymphadenopathy	Usually mild and minimally tender	Unilateral or bilateral painful adenopathy in >50% Inguinal bubo formation and rupture may occur
Presumptive diagnosis	Typical lesions plus any of the following: a previously known outbreak, a positive Tzanck smear of lesion scraping, exclusion of other causes of ulcers, or a fourfold increase in acute and convalescent antibody titers (in a first-time infection)	Early syphilis: a typical chancre plus a reactive nontreponemal test (RPR, VDRL) and no history of syphilis or a fourfold increase in a quantitative nontreponemal test in a person with a history of syphilis	Exclusion of other causes of ulcers in the presence of (1) typical ulcers and lymphadenopathy, (2) a typical Gram stain and a history of contact with a high-risk individual (prostitute) or living in an endemic area
Definitive diagnosis	Detection of HSV by culture or nonculture methods (DFA) from ulcer scraping or aspiration of vesicle fluid	Identification *T. pallidum,* from a chancre or lymph node aspirate, on darkfield microscopy or by DFA	Detection of *H. ducreyi* by culture

**Primary syphilitic ulcers may be painful if they become co-infected with bacteria or one of the other organisms responsible for genital ulcers.*
DFA = direct fluorescent antibody; RPR = rapid plasma reagin; VDRL = Venereal Disease Research Laboratory; HSV = herpes simplex virus.
Data from Centers for Disease Control and Prevention Sexually Transmitted Disease Clinical Practice Guidelines, May 1991; Centers for Disease Control and Prevention 1993 Sexually Transmitted Disease Treatment Guidelines; and Hoffman I, Schmitz J: Genital ulcers management in the HIV era. Post Grad Med 98:67, 1995.
From Lappa S, Moscicki A: The pediatrician and the sexually active adolescent: A primer for sexually transmitted diseases. Pediatr Clin North Am 44:1430, 1997.

TABLE 119–3 Uncomplicated Pelvic Inflammatory Disease Clinical Practice Guideline Inclusion Checklist

Patient MUST meet *all* of the following criteria, in the absence of another established cause:
- ☐ lower abdominal pain
- ☐ cervical motion tenderness
- ☐ adnexal tenderness

Patients MUST meet *at least one* of the following criteria:
- ☐ oral temp. >38.3°C
- ☐ WBC ≥13,000 K/mm³
- ☐ abnormal cervical or vaginal discharge
- ☐ ESR >20 mm/hr
- ☐ laboratory documentation of cervical infection with *N. gonorrheae* or *C. trachomatis*

All patients should have the following as part of the initial evaluation:
- ☐ pelvic examination
- ☐ endocervical culture for *gonorrheae*
- ☐ endocervical EIA or culture for chlamydia
- ☐ CBC with differential
- ☐ ESR or C-reactive protein
- ☐ RPR
- ☐ urine βhCG
- ☐ urine dipstick
- ☐ urine culture

The following should be considered:
- ☐ serum βhCG if urine βhCG is negative and suspect ectopic
- ☐ U/S if mass or difficult examination
- ☐ GYN consult immediately if pregnant or if needs U/S
- ☐ surgical consult if suspect appendicitis or other surgical problem

DIFFERENTIAL DIAGNOSIS (partial list):

GI—appendicitis, constipation, diverticulitis, gastroenteritis, IBD, irritable bowel syndrome

GYN—rupture or torsion of ovarian cyst, endometriosis, dysmenorrhea, ectopic pregnancy, mittelschmerz, ruptured follicle, septic or threatened abortion, tubo-ovarian abscess

Urinary tract—cystitis, pyelonephritis, urethritis, nephrolithiasis

☐ Check box if patient was placed on the PID clinical practice guideline.

ESR = erythrocyte sedimentation rate; EIA = enzyme immunoassay; CBC = complete blood count; RPR = rapid plasma reagin; BhCG = human chorionic gonadotropin; U/S = ultrasonography; GYN = gynecologic; GI = gastrointestinal.

From Emans SJH, Laufer MR, Goldstein DP: Pediatric and Adolescent Gynecology, 4th ed. Philadelphia, Lippincott-Raven, 1998, p 480.

granuloma inguinale); however, trauma is a common cause that can be detected with a careful history.

TREATMENT. The Centers for Disease Control and Prevention guidelines offer treatment options for uncomplicated urethritis, cervicitis, and vaginal discharges that reduce patient noncompliance, single-dose oral medications (see Part XVI for chapters on the treatment of specific microorganisms). Treatment regimens with over-the-counter products as in *Candida* vaginitis, genital warts, and pediculosis reduce financial and access barriers to rapid treatment for adolescents, but there are potential risks for inappropriate self-treatment and complications from untreated more serious infections that must be considered before using this approach. Minimizing noncompliance with treatment, finding and treating the sexual partner, addressing prevention and contraceptive issues, and making every effort to preserve fertility are additional responsibilities. The latter often requires intensive parenteral therapy for PID.

Diagnosis and therapy are often necessarily carried out within the context of a confidential relationship between the physician and the patient. Therefore, the need to report certain sexually transmitted diseases to health department authorities should be clarified at the outset. Most health departments will not violate confidentiality, if assured that treatment and case finding have been accomplished and that the patient can be expected to follow through in a responsible, mature manner.

PREVENTION. The prevention messages to be communicated to adolescents regarding the avoidance of STDs are in direct contrast to the known risk factors for contracting the disease: (1) maintaining a healthier sexual behavior, (2) using barrier methods, (3) adopting healthy medical care–seeking behavior, (4) complying with management instruction, and (5) ensuring examination of sexual partners. The elements of maintaining a healthier sexual behavior include postponing sexual behavior until *at least* 2–3 yr after menarche, limiting the number of sexual partners, eliciting information about a partner's STD status, inspecting the genitals of sexual partners, and abstaining from sex if STD symptoms develop. The upsurge in sexuality education as a result of the HIV epidemic may have played some role in the increased use of condoms in adolescents. The 1995 National Youth Risk Behavior Survey reports 54.4% of students responding that either they or their partner used a condom during last sexual intercourse.

Centers for Disease Control and Prevention: 1998 Guidelines for treatment of sexually transmitted diseases. MMWR 47:1, 1998.

Emans SJ, Laufer MR, Goldstein DP: Pediatric and Adolescent Gynecology, 4th ed. Philadelphia, Lippincott-Raven, 1998.

Kann L, Warren CW, Harris WA, et al: Youth Risk Behavior Surveillance—U.S., 1995. Centers for Disease Control and Prevention. CDC Surveillance Summaries, September 27, 1996. MMWR 45:1, 1996.

Neinstein LS: Adolescent Health Care: A Practical Guide, 3rd ed. Baltimore, Williams & Wilkins, 1996.

Saxena SB, Jenkins RR: Sexually transmitted diseases in adolescents: Screening and treatment. Compr Ther 23:108, 1997.

Strasburger VC, Brown RT: What every pediatrician should know about infectious mononucleosis in adolescents. Pediatr Clin North Am 44:1541, 1997.

CHAPTER 120
Skin Problems

Androgenic stimulation early in puberty induces the increased sebaceous gland activity contributing to acne. The pathogenesis, clinical picture, and management of acne are discussed in Chapter 675. As adolescents become preoccupied with their appearance, acne assumes great importance. For that reason, offering treatment even to the youngster whose acne is mild may enhance self-image and is appropriate. An adolescent anxious to be free of acne should be counseled about the expected time (several weeks) for obvious improvement of lesions and the potential irritability that can be caused by overuse of some products. Special considerations in the treatment of acne in adolescent girls include the need to be sure that the patient is not pregnant and is using a reliable contraceptive method if sexually active before instituting therapy with either tetracycline or *cis*-retinoic acid. She should also be informed about the possibility that chronic tetracycline therapy may cause vaginal infection with *Candida* and appreciate that acne may be worsened or improved by oral contraceptives, depending on the type of estrogen or progestin. Tricyclen was in fact approved by the United States Food and Drug Administration in 1997, specifically for the treatment of acne.

The skin of the adolescent is influenced not only by the hormones of puberty but also by psychosocial factors occurring at this time. For example, sexual experimentation may result in a sexually transmitted disease with dermatologic manifestations (Chapter 119); stress may be manifested by trichotillomania; contact sports, most notably wrestling, may be associated with herpes simplex infection; and drug abuse may cause skin lesions (Chapter 113). Certain other conditions not related to adolescent behavior, such as tinea versicolor, have their peak incidence in the adolescent–young adult age group.

Strasburger V: Acne: What every pediatrician should know about treatment. PCNA 44:1505, 1997.

CHAPTER 121
Orthopedic Problems

Puberty is associated with rapid growth of long bones, open epiphyses, and increased traction at sites of insertion of muscles, all of which contribute to the increased rate and unique types of orthopedic problems in this age group (see Chapters 14 and 678). The timing of the growth spurt (Sex Maturity Rating 2 in girls, Sex Maturity Rating 4 in boys) is a particularly vulnerable period associated with the occurrence or worsening of several conditions. The diagnoses common in this period include idiopathic adolescent scoliosis, slipped capital femoral epiphysis, Osgood-Schlatter disease, Tilleaux fracture, spondylolisthesis, and osteosarcoma. Conditions that are also common in this period but with a less clearly defined association are Freiberg disease and Ewing sarcoma. Adolescents who are involved in sports are disproportionately affected with patellofemoral syndrome, Osgood-Schlatter disease, and acute and repetitive overuse injuries. A history of a prior injury and failure to rehabilitate should exclude a youth from further sports participation subject to an updated evaluation.

The most common presentation for most of the previously mentioned conditions is pain. Pain can be due to a benign self-limiting condition such as costochrondritis (Tietze syndrome) or Osgood-Schlatter disease or, less commonly, can be associated with more serious diagnoses such as slipped capital femoral epiphysis, osteosarcoma, or Ewing sarcoma. Other presentations like limp, limited range of motion, palpation of a mass in a bony area, or discomfort following physical activity suggests other musculoskeletal disorders. With arthralgias and arthritis as a part of a more systemic presentation in this age group, disseminated gonococcal disease, collagen vascular disorders, and viral infections, such as infectious mononucleosis and rubella, should be considered in the differential diagnosis.

Tolo VT, Wood B: Pediatric Orthopaedics in Primary Care. Baltimore, Williams & Wilkins, 1993.

PART XIII

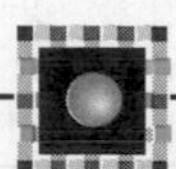

The Immunologic System and Disorders

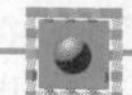

SECTION 1

Evaluation of the Immune System

Rebecca H. Buckley

CHAPTER 122

The Child with Suspected Immunodeficiency

Children with recurrent infections are among the most frequent types of patients seen by primary care physicians. However, despite an exponential rise in the number of patients with HIV infections during the past 18 years, the number of pediatric patients suspected of having primary or secondary immunodeficiency far exceeds the number with either of these two types of diseases. Most patients with recurrent infections do not have an identifiable immunodeficiency disorder. One major cause of recurrent infections is excessive exposure of infants or children to infectious agents in child-care or other group settings. Excessive use of antibiotics by physicians has, however, masked the classic presentation of many of the primary immunodeficiency diseases.

Primary care physicians must have a high index of suspicion if defects of the immune system are to be diagnosed early enough that appropriate treatment can be instituted before irreversible damage is done. Evaluations of immune function should be initiated for children with clinical manifestations of a specific immune disorder or with unusual, chronic, or recurrent infections such as (1) two or more systemic bacterial infections (e.g., sepsis, osteomyelitis or meningitis), (2) three or more serious respiratory or documented bacterial infections (e.g., cellulitis, draining otitis media, or lymphadenitis within 1 yr), (3) infections occurring at unusual sites (e.g., the liver or a brain abscess), (4) infections with unusual pathogens (e.g., *Aspergillus* spp, *Serratia marcescens, Nocardia* spp, or *Pseudomonas cepacia*), and (5) infections with common childhood pathogens but of unusual severity.

It is important that the screening tests selected for immunologic evaluation be broadly informative, reliable, and cost effective. Familiarity with certain clinical guidelines aids in the initial selection of tests. Patients with deficiencies of antibodies, phagocytic cells, or complement have recurrent infections with encapsulated bacteria. Thus, patients with only repeated viral infections (with the exception of persistent enterovirus infections) are not as likely to have any of these disorders. Children with defects in these components of the immune system may grow and develop normally, despite their recurring infections, unless they develop bronchiectasis from repeated lower respiratory tract bacterial infections or persistent enteroviral infections of the central nervous system. By contrast, patients with deficiencies in T-cell function usually develop opportunistic infections early in life and fail to thrive.

The initial evaluation of immunocompetence includes a thorough history, physical examination, and family history. Most immunologic defects can be excluded at minimal cost with the proper choice of screening tests (Table 122–1). A complete blood count (CBC) and erythrocyte sedimentation rate (ESR) are among the most cost-effective screening tests. If the ESR is normal, chronic bacterial or fungal infection is unlikely. If an infant's neutrophil count is persistently elevated, even in the absence of any signs of infection, a leukocyte adhesion deficiency should be suspected. If the absolute neutrophil count is normal, congenital and acquired neutropenia and severe chemotactic defects are eliminated. If the absolute lymphocyte count is normal, the patient is not likely to have a severe T-cell defect. Normal lymphocyte counts are higher in infancy and early childhood than later in life. For example, at

TABLE 122–1 Initial Immunologic Testing of the Child with Recurrent Infections

Complete Blood Count, Manual Differential, and Erythrocyte Sedimentation Rate

Absolute lymphocyte count (normal result [Chapter 726] makes T-cell defect unlikely)
Absolute neutrophil count (normal result [Chapter 726] precludes congenital or acquired neutropenia and (usually) both forms of leukocyte adhesion deficiency, in which elevated counts are present even between infections)
Platelet count (normal result excludes Wiskott-Aldrich syndrome)
Howell-Jolly bodies (absence rules against asplenia)
Erythrocyte sedimentation rate (normal result indicates chronic bacterial or fungal infection unlikely)

Screening Tests for B-Cell Defects

IgA measurement; if abnormal, IgG and IgM measurement
Isohemagglutinins
Antibody titers to tetanus, diphtheria, *Haemophilus influenzae,* and pneumococci

Screening Tests for T-Cell Defects

Absolute lymphocyte count (normal result indicates T-cell defect unlikely)
Candida albicans intradermal skin test: 0.1 mL of a 1 : 1,000 dilution for patients older than 6 yr, 0.1 mL of a 1 : 100 dilution for patients younger than 6 yr

Screening Tests for Phagocytic Cell Defects

Absolute neutrophil count
Respiratory burst assay

Screening Test for Complement Deficiency

CH_{50}

9 mo of age—an age when infants affected with severe T-cell immunodeficiency are likely to present—the lower limit of normal is 4,500 lymphocytes/mm³ (Chapter 726). Examination of red cells for Howell-Jolly bodies helps exclude congenital asplenia. If the platelet count is normal, Wiskott-Aldrich syndrome is ruled out. If a CBC and a manual differential were performed on the cord blood of all infants, severe combined immunodeficiency (SCID) could be detected at birth, and lifesaving immunologic reconstitution could then be given all such infants.

Patients found to have abnormalities on any screening tests should be characterized as fully as possible before any type of immunologic treatment is begun, unless there is a life-threatening illness. Some "abnormalities" may prove to be laboratory artifacts, and conversely, what may appear to be a straightforward diagnosis may prove to be a much more complex disorder. If results of the initial screening including the CBC, immunoglobulin levels, and complement levels are normal, evaluations of T-cell and phagocytic cell functions may be indicated for patients with recurrent or unusual bacterial infections.

B-CELLS. A simple screening test is used to determine the presence and titer of antibodies to type A and B red blood cell polysaccharide antigens (isohemagglutinins). As assayed in most blood banks, this test measures predominantly IgM antibodies. However, isohemagglutinins may be normally absent in the first 2 yr of life and are always absent if the patient is blood type AB. Because most infants and children have received diphtheria-tetanus-pertussis (DTP) and *Haemophilus influenzae* type b (Hib) immunizations, it is informative to test for antibodies to diphtheria, tetanus, and *H. influenzae* polyribose phosphate antigens. If the titers are low, measurement of antibodies to diphtheria or tetanus toxoids before and 2 wk after a pediatric DT booster is helpful in assessing the capacity to form IgG antibodies to protein antigens. These antibody studies can be performed in several different laboratories, but it is important to choose a reliable laboratory and to use the same laboratory to study the child before and after a booster. To evaluate a patient's ability to respond to polysaccharide antigens, antipneumococcal antibodies can be measured before and 3 wk after immunization with a pneumococcal vaccine in patients older than 2–3 yr. Antibodies detected in these tests are of the IgG isotype. Patients with significant or permanent B-cell defects do not produce either IgM or IgG antibodies normally. However, the finding of normal IgM and IgG antibody levels does not preclude IgA deficiency, transient hypogammaglobulinemia of infancy, or protein-losing states. Selective IgA deficiency, the most common B-cell defect, can be ruled out by measuring serum IgA (Chapter 124). If the IgA concentration is normal, most of the permanent types of hypogammaglobulinemia are also excluded, as IgA is usually very low or absent in those conditions as well. If IgA is low, IgG and IgM should also be measured (Chapter 726). Patients who are receiving corticosteroids often have low IgG concentrations but make antibodies normally. Very high serum concentrations of one or more immunoglobulin classes suggest HIV infection or chronic granulomatous disease.

IgG subclass measurements are seldom helpful in assessing immune function in children with recurrent infections. It is difficult to know the biologic significance of the various mild to moderate deficiencies of IgG subclasses, particularly when completely asymptomatic individuals have been described as totally lacking IgG1, IgG2, IgG4, and/or IgA1 owing to immunoglobulin heavy chain gene deletions. Moreover, a number of healthy children have been described as having low levels of IgG2 but normal responses to polysaccharide antigens when immunized. When children with low IgG2 subclass levels and histories of frequent infections were studied in depth, they were found to have broader immunologic dysfunction, including poor responses to protein antigens as well, suggesting that their condition may have been in the process of developing into common variable immunodeficiency (CVID). Only when antibody deficiencies are detected despite normal levels of immunoglobulins are IgG subclass measurements occasionally helpful. Children who lack IgG2 are usually unable to make antibodies to polysaccharide antigens; however, this can be true even in those with normal IgG2. Thus, antibody measurements are far more cost effective than IgG subclass determinations.

Patients found to be agammaglobulinemic should have their blood B cells enumerated by flow cytometry using dye-conjugated monoclonal antibodies to B-cell–specific CD antigens (usually CD19 or CD20). Normally, approximately 10% of circulating lymphocytes are B cells. In X-linked agammaglobulinemia (XLA), such cells are missing, whereas in CVID, B cells are usually present. This distinction is important because children with these two different types of hypogammaglobulinemia can have different clinical problems, and the two defects clearly have different inheritance patterns. Patients with XLA have a heightened susceptibility to persistent enteroviral infections, whereas those with CVID have more problems with autoimmune diseases and lymphoid hyperplasia. Specific molecular diagnostic tests for XLA (Chapter 124.1) are necessary in cases in which there is no family history to aid genetic counseling. T-cell numbers and function should also be evaluated in patients with agammaglobulinemia, because some patients with CVID have T-cell abnormalities.

The capacity of blood B lymphocytes to differentiate into plasma cells that synthesize and secrete immunoglobulin can be assessed in in vitro cultures to which pokeweed mitogen (PWM) or anti-CD40 plus cytokines are added as differentiating agents. If results of all of these tests prove to be normal and the immunoglobulins remain low, trace label studies of serum proteins should be carried out to make certain that the immunoglobulins are not being lost through the urinary or gastrointestinal tracts, such as occurs in the nephrotic syndrome, protein-losing enteropathies, or intestinal lymphangiectasia.

T CELLS. The *Candida* skin test is the most cost-effective test of T-cell function. Adults and children older than 6 yr should be tested intradermally with 0.1 mL of a 1:1,000 dilution of a known potent *Candida albicans* extract. If the test result is negative at 24, 48, and 72 hr, a 1:100 dilution should be tested. The latter concentration can be used in the initial testing of children under 6 yr. If the test result is positive, as defined by erythema and induration of 10 mm or more at 48 hr, virtually all primary T-cell defects are precluded, and this obviates the need for more expensive in vitro tests, such as lymphocyte phenotyping or assessments of responses to mitogens.

T cells and T-cell subpopulations can be enumerated by flow cytometry using dye-conjugated monoclonal antibodies recognizing CD antigens present on T cells (i.e., CD2, CD3, CD4, and CD8). This is a particularly important test to perform on any infant who is lymphopenic, because SCID is a pediatric emergency that can be successfully treated by bone marrow transplantation in more than 90% of cases if diagnosed before untreatable infections develop. CD3+ T cells usually make up 70% of peripheral lymphocytes. Normally there are roughly twice as many CD4+ (helper) T cells as there are CD8+ (cytotoxic) T cells. Because there are examples of severe immunodeficiency in which phenotypically normal T cells are present, tests of T-cell function are far more informative and cost effective than determination of T-cell subpopulations alone. T cells are normally stimulated through their T-cell receptors (TCRs) by antigen present in the groove of major histocompatibility complex (MHC) molecules; however, the TCR can also be stimulated directly with mitogens such as phytohemagglutinin (PHA), concanavalin A (Con A), or PWM. After a 3–5-day period of incubation with the mitogen, the proliferation of T cells is measured by the incorporation of radiolabeled thymidine into DNA. Other stimulants that can be used to assess T-cell function in the same type of assay include antigens (for example, *Candida* or tetanus toxoid) and allogeneic cells. Additional assays of T-cell function include determining the ability of allogeneic cells to stimulate the generation of cytotoxic T cells and the measurement of cytokine production by T lymphocytes stimulated with any of the previously mentioned agents (see Table 123–2).

PHAGOCYTIC CELLS. Killing defects of phagocytic cells, which should be suspected if a patient has recurrent staphylococcal abscesses or gram-negative infections, can be evaluated by screening tests measuring the neutrophil respiratory burst after phorbol ester stimulation. The most reliable and useful test of this type is a flow cytometric assessment of the respiratory burst using rhodamine dye; this test has replaced the previously used nitroblue tetrazolium (NBT) dye test, which had technical problems with reproducibility. Leukocyte adhesion deficiencies can be easily diagnosed by flow cytometric assays of blood lymphocytes or neutrophils, using monoclonal antibodies to CD18 or CD11 (LAD1) or to CD15 (LAD2).

NK cells can be enumerated by flow cytometry using monoclonal antibodies to NK-specific CD antigens, usually CD16 or CD56. NK function is assessed by a radiolabeled chromium-release assay, using a cell line called K562, which is readily killed by NK cells.

Phagocytic cell defects can be further defined according to their molecular cause. Mutations in the genes encoding four different components of the electron transport chain have been discovered in various patients with chronic granulomatous disease (CGD). It is important to identify which molecular type of CGD a patient has for genetic counseling (one type is X linked, and the other three types are autosomal recessive), prenatal diagnosis, and the eventual prospect of gene therapy. New flow cytometric methods for identifying the defective molecules have been developed but are currently available only in research laboratories. In the case of the leukocyte adhesion deficiencies, early diagnosis is of crucial importance because bone marrow transplantation can be lifesaving. A confirmatory test for LAD1 (if flow cytometry suggests that defect) is NK cell function, because the lack of adhesion molecules prevents the NK cells of such patients from attaching to the target cells.

COMPLEMENT. Complement defects can be most effectively screened for by a CH_{50} assay, which measures the intactness of the entire complement pathway. Genetic deficiencies in the complement system are usually characterized by extremely low CH_{50} values. The CH_{50} is a bioassay that yields abnormal results if complement has been consumed from the specimen for any reason. The most common cause of an abnormal CH_{50} result is a delay in or improper transport of the specimen to the laboratory. Specific immunoassays for C3 and C4 are commercially available, but further identification of other complement component deficiencies is usually possible only in research laboratories. However, it is extremely important to identify which component is missing, because there are different disease susceptibilities depending on whether there are deficiencies of early or late components. Knowing the mode of inheritance is also important for genetic counseling. Properdin deficiency is X linked, but all of the other complement deficiencies are autosomal. Measurement of C4 can be helpful in assessing suspected hereditary angioedema.

Johnston RB: Recurrent bacterial infections in children. N Engl J Med 310:1237, 1984.
Lopez M, Fleisher T, deShazo RD: Use and interpretation of diagnostic immunologic laboratory tests. JAMA 268:2970, 1992.
Shannon DC, Johnson G, Rosen FS, et al: Cellular reactivity to *Candida albicans* antigen. N Engl J Med 275:690, 1966.
Wheeler JG, Steiner D: Evaluation of humoral responsiveness in children. Pediatr Infect Dis J 11:304, 1992.

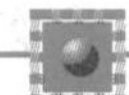

SECTION 2

T-, B-, and NK-Cell Systems

Rebecca H. Buckley

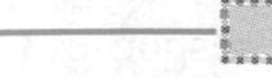

CHAPTER 123
T, B, and NK Cells

Bodily defense against infectious agents is secured through a combination of physical barriers, including the skin, mucous membranes, mucous blanket, and ciliated epithelial cells, and the various components of the immune system. The immune system consists of T lymphocytes, B lymphocytes, natural killer (NK) cells, dendritic and phagocytic cells, and complement proteins. The immune system also serves to protect against autoimmune diseases and malignancy.

LYMPHOPOIESIS IN THE FETUS

SOURCE OF LYMPHOID CELLS AND THE PROCESS OF ORGANOGENESIS. The human immune system arises in the embryo from gut-associated tissue. Pluripotential hematopoietic stem cells first appear in the yolk sac at 2.5–3 wk of gestational age and migrate to the fetal liver at 5 wk of gestation; they later reside in the bone marrow, where they remain throughout life (Fig. 123–1). Lymphoid stem cells develop from such precursor cells and differentiate into T, B, or NK cells, depending on the organs or tissues to which the stem cells traffic. Primary lymphoid organ (thymus, bone marrow) development begins during the middle of the first trimester of gestation and proceeds rapidly; secondary lymphoid organ (spleen, lymph nodes, tonsils, Peyer's patches, lamina propria) development soon follows. These organs continue to serve as sites of differentiation of T, B, and NK lymphocytes from stem cells throughout life. Both the initial organogenesis and the continued cell differentiation occur as a consequence of the interaction of a vast array of lymphocytic and microenvironmental cell surface molecules and proteins secreted by the involved cells. The complexity and number of such cell surface molecules led to the development of an international nomenclature and classification of these differentiation antigens, which are now referred to as *clusters of differentiation* (CD) (Table 123–1).

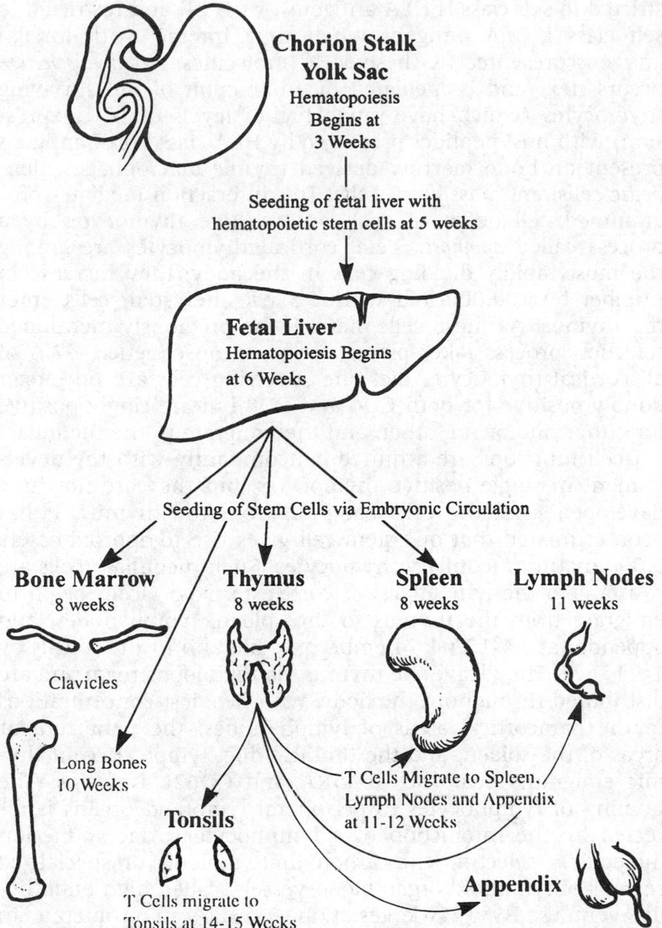

Figure 123–1 Migration patterns of hematopoietic stem cells and mature lymphocytes during human fetal development. (From Haynes BF, Denning SM: Lymphopoiesis. *In:* Stamatoyannopoulis G, Nienhuis A, Majerus P, Varmus H [eds]: Molecular Basis of Blood Diseases, 2nd ed. Philadelphia, WB Saunders, 1994.)

T and B lymphocytes are the only components of the immune system that have antigen-specific recognition capabilities; they are responsible for adaptive immunity. NK cells are lymphocytes that are also derived from hematopoietic stem cells; they are thought to have a role in host defense against viral infections, in tumor surveillance, and in immune regulation. The proteins synthesized and secreted by T, B, and NK cells, and by the cells with which they interact, are referred to as *cytokines.* Several such proteins have been given an official nomenclature as *interleukins* (ILs) (Table 123–2). Cytokines have the ability to act in an autocrine, paracrine, or endocrine manner to promote and facilitate differentiation and proliferation of the cells of the immune system.

T-CELL DEVELOPMENT AND DIFFERENTIATION. The primitive thymic rudiment is formed from the ectoderm of the third branchial cleft and endoderm of the third branchial pouch at 4 wk gestation. Beginning at 7–8 wk, the right and left rudiments move caudally and fuse in the midline. Blood-borne T-cell precursors from the fetal liver then begin to colonize the perithymic mesenchyme at 8 wk gestation. These precursor (pro-T) cells are identified by surface proteins designated as CD7 and CD34. At 8–8.5 wk gestation, CD7+ cells are found intrathymically, and some cells also coexpress CD4, a protein present on the surfaces of mature T-helper (TH) cells, and CD8, a protein found on both mature cytotoxic cells and NK cells. In addition, some cells bear single T-cell receptor (TCR) chains (β, δ, or γ) but none bear complete TCRs.

The mature TCR is a heterodimer of two chains, either α and β or γ and δ; it is coexpressed on the cell surface with CD3, a complex of five polypeptide chains (γ, δ, ϵ, ζ, η). TCR gene rearrangement occurs by a process in which large, noncontiguous blocks of DNA are spliced together. These segments, known as V (variable), D (diversity), and J (joining), each have a number of variants. VDJ segments are joined to a constant region of the α gene, and VJ segments are joined to the β gene to complete the receptor polypeptide genes. Random combinations of the segments account for much of the enormous diversity of TCRs that enables humans to recognize millions of different antigens. TCR gene rearrangement requires the presence of recombinase activating genes, referred to as RAG-1 and RAG-2, as well as other recombinase components. This process is flawed in mice with severe combined immunodeficiency (SCID) and in some humans with SCID. Rearrangement of TCR genes signifies commitment of pro-T cells to T-lineage development—that is, to become pre-T cells. TCR gene rearrangement begins shortly after colonization of the thymus with stem cells, and the establishment of the T-cell repertoire begins at 8–10 wk of gestation. By 9.5–10 wk, more than 95% of thymocytes are CD7+, CD2+, CD4+, CD8+, and c(cytoplasmic)CD3+, and approximately 30% bear the CD1 inner cortical thymocyte antigen. By 10 wk, 25% of thymocytes bear αβ TCRs. Ti αβ+ cells gradually

TABLE 123–1 CD Classification of Some Lymphocyte Surface Molecules

CD Number	Other Names	Tissue/Lineage	Function
CD1	T6	Cortical thymocytes; Langerhans cells	Antigen presentation to TCRγ/δ cells
CD2	SRBC receptor	T and NK cells	Binds LFA-3 (CD58); alternative pathway of T-cell activation
CD3	T3, Leu 4	T cells	TCR-associated; transduces signals from TCR
CD4	T4, Leu3a	Helper T-cell subset	Receptor for HLA class II antigens; associated with p56 *lck* tyrosine kinase
CD7	3A1, Leu 9	T and NK cells and their precursors	Co-mitogenic for T lymphocytes
CD8	T8, Leu2a	Cytotoxic T-cell subset; also on 30% of NK cells	Receptor for HLA class I antigens; associated with p56 *lck* tyrosine kinase
CD10	cALLA	B-cell progenitors	Peptide cleavage
CD11a	LFA-1a α chain	T, B, and NK cells	With CD18, ligand for ICAM 1, 2, and 3
CD11b, c	MAC-1, CR3; CR4	NK cells	With CD18, receptors for C3bi
CD16	FcRγIII	NK cells	FcR for IgG
CD19	B4	B cells	Regulates B-cell activation
CD20	B1	B cells	Mediates B-cell activation
CD21	B2, CR2	B cells	Receptor for EBV and C3d (complement)
CD34	My10	Precursor cells	Unknown
CD45	Leukocyte common antigen, T200	All leukocytes	Tyrosine phosphatase that regulates lymphocyte activation; CD45RO isoform on memory T cells, CD45RA isoform on naive T cells
CD56	N-CAM; NKH-1	NK cells	Mediates NK homotypic adhesion
CD154	CD40 ligand; gp39	Activated CD4+ T cells	Ligates CD40 on B cells and initiates isotype switching

TABLE 123–2 Functional Classification of Cytokines*

Cytokines Involved in Natural Immune Responses

Type I interferons—IFN-α and IFN-β—inhibit viral replication, inhibit cell proliferation, activate NK cells, upregulate class I MHC molecule expression
TNF-α—mediates host response to gram-negative bacteria and other infectious agents
IL-1α and -β—mediate host inflammatory response to infectious agents
IL-1Ra—a natural antagonist of IL-1, blocks signals delivered by IL-1
IL-6—mediates and regulates inflammatory responses
Chemokines (IL-8, monocyte chemotactic protein-1 [MCP-1], RANTES, and others)—mediate leukocyte chemotaxis and activation

Lymphocyte Regulatory Cytokines

Immunostimulatory or Growth Promoting

IL-1—co-stimulates activation of T cells
IL-2—growth factor for T, B, NK cells; activates effector cells
IL-4—T- and B-cell growth factor; stimulates IgE production; upregulates classes I and II MHC molecule and FcRεII expression on macrophages; expansion of TH2 subset
IL-5—B cell growth and activation
IL-6—growth factor for B cells
IL-7—stromal cell factor; growth factor for precursor B and T cells
IL-9—growth factor for T cells
IL-10—growth and differentiation factor for B cells
IL-12—expansion of TH1 subset; powerful stimulator of IFN-γ production by T cells and NK cells
IL-13—growth and differentiating factor for B cells; stimulates IgE production; upregulates classes I and II MHC molecule and FcRεII expression on macrophages
TNF-β—stimulates effector cell function
IFN-γ—activates macrophages, NK cells; upregulates classes I and II MHC molecule expression; inhibits IL-4 or IL-13–induced IgE production

Immunosuppressive

IL-1Ra—regulates IL-1 activities
TGF-β—antagonizes lymphocyte responses
IL-10—inhibits activities of TH1 cells

Hematopoiesis-Regulating Cytokines

GM-CSF, G-CSF, M-CSF—colony-stimulating factors
Erythropoietin (EPO)—differentiation of erythroid precursors
IL-3, SCR, *c-kit* receptor—regulate stem cell development
IL-4—mast cell development
IL-5—eosinophil differentiation and proliferation
IL-6—differentiation of B cells
IL-7—differentiation of B and T cells

Proinflammatory Cytokines

IL-1, TNF-α, IL-6—participate in the acute-phase response and synergize to mediate inflammation, shock, and death

Anti-Inflammatory Cytokines

IL-4—reduces endotoxin-induced TNF and IL-1 production
IL-6—inhibits TNF production
IL-10—suppresses lymphocyte functions and downregulates production of proinflammatory cytokines
IL-13—downregulates functions of macrophages; suppresses production of proinflammatory cytokines
TGF-β—has immunosuppressive effects, inhibits IL-1 and TNF gene expression
IL-1Ra—competes with the binding of IL-1 to its cell surface receptors and blocks IL-1 effects
TNFsR—soluble TNF receptors; by binding TNF, block interaction of TNF with the target cell

**This is not an exhaustive list.*
MHC = major histocompatibility complex; NK = natural killer; TNF = tumor necrosis factor; IL = interleukin.
Modified from Whiteside TL: Cytokine measurements and interpretation of cytokine assays in human disease. J Clin Immunol 14:329, 1994.

increase in number during embryonic life and represent more than 95% of thymocytes postnatally.

As immature cortical thymocytes begin to express TCRs, the processes of positive and negative selection take place. *Positive selection* occurs through the interaction of immature thymocytes (which express low levels of TCR) with major histocompatibility complex (MHC) antigens present on cortical thymic epithelial cells. As a result, thymocytes with TCR capable of interacting with foreign antigens presented on self MHC antigens are activated and develop to maturity. Mature thymocytes that survive the selection process are either CD4+ and restricted to self class II HLA antigens or CD8+ and restricted to self class I HLA antigens when they interact with foreign antigens presented by these MHC molecules. *Negative selection* occurs next and is mediated by interaction of the surviving thymocytes (which have much higher levels of TCR expression) with host peptides presented by HLA class I or II antigens present on bone marrow–derived thymic macrophages, dendritic cells, and possibly B cells. This interaction mediates programmed cell death of such autoreactive thymocytes by a process called *apoptosis.* Fetal cortical thymocytes are among the most rapidly dividing cells in the body; they increase in number by 100,000-fold within 2 wk after stem cells enter the thymus. As these cells mature, the previously mentioned selection process takes place, and as a consequence, 97% of all cortical thymocytes die. The surviving cells are no longer doubly positive for both CD4 and CD8 but are singly positive for either one or the other, and they migrate to the medulla.

T-cell functions are acquired concomitantly with the development of single-positive thymocytes, but they are not fully developed until the cells emigrate from the thymus. It has been estimated that one stem cell gives rise to approximately 3,000 mature medullary thymocytes. Such medullary cells are resistant to the lytic effects of corticosteroids. T cells begin to emigrate from the thymus to the spleen, lymph nodes, and appendix at 11–12 wk of embryonic life and to the tonsils by 14–15 wk. They leave the thymus via the bloodstream and are distributed throughout the body, with heaviest concentrations in the paracortical areas of lymph nodes, the periarteriolar areas of the spleen, and the thoracic duct lymph. Recent thymic emigrants bear the CD45RA and CD62L isoforms. The homing of lymphocytes to peripheral lymphoid organs is directed by the interaction of a lymphocyte surface adhesion molecule, L-selectin, with carbohydrate moieties on specialized regions of lymphoid organ blood vessels, called high endothelial venules. By 12 wk gestation, T cells can proliferate in response to plant lectins (phytohemagglutinin [PHA] and concanavalin A [Con A]) and to allogeneic cells; antigen-binding T cells have been found by 20 wk gestation. Hassall's bodies (swirls of terminally differentiated medullary epithelial cells) are first seen in the thymic medulla at 16–18 wk of embryonic life.

B-CELL DEVELOPMENT AND DIFFERENTIATION. In parallel with T-cell differentiation, B-cell development begins in the fetal liver before 7 wk gestation. Fetal liver CD34+ stem cells are seeded to the bone marrow of the clavicles by 8 wk of embryonic life and to that of the long bones by 10 wk (see Fig. 123–1). *Antigen-independent* stages of B-cell development have been defined according to immunoglobulin gene rearrangement patterns and the surface proteins the cells bear. The *pro-B cell* is the first descendent of the pluripotential stem cell committed to B-lineage development and is detected by the presence of both CD34 and CD10 on its surface; in it the immunoglobulin genes remain germ line (Fig. 123–2). The next stage is the *pre-pre–B-cell* stage, during which immunoglobulin genes are rearranged, but there is no cytoplasmic expression of μ heavy chains or surface IgM (sIgM); these cells are further characterized by the coexpression of membrane CD34, CD10, CD19, and CD40, and (somewhat later) by the additional presence of CD73, CD22, CD24, and CD38. The *pre–B-cell* stage is next; these cells are distinguished by the expression of cytoplasmic μ heavy chains but no sIgM, because no immunoglobulin light chains are produced yet. They also continue to express all CD antigens seen at the pre-pre–B-cell stage except CD34 and CD10 (which are lost); in addition, they express CD21. Next is the *immature B-cell* stage, during which sIgM is expressed (because light-chain genes have now been rearranged) but not sIgD; CD38 is lost, but all other *pre–B-cell* CD antigens persist. The last stage of antigen-independent B-cell development is the *mature* or *virgin B cell,* which coexpresses both sIgM and sIgD; CD23 is also acquired at this stage, and all of the other

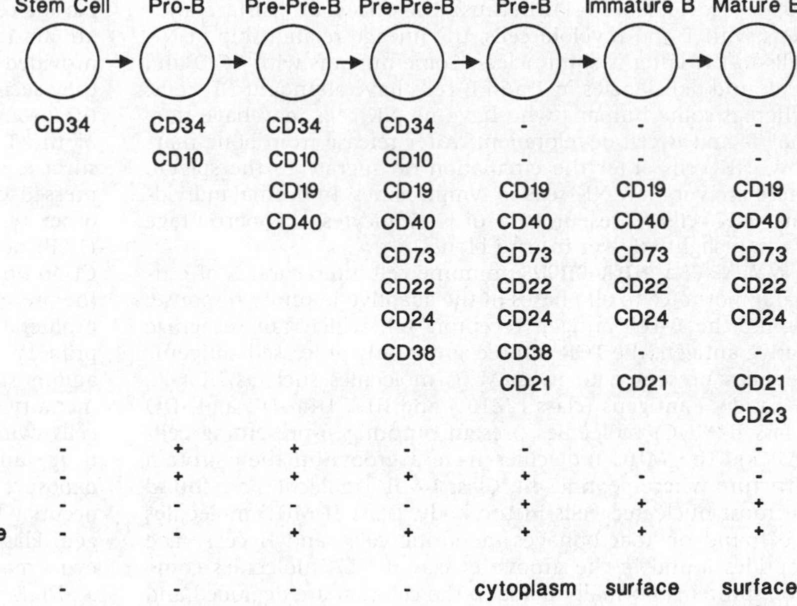

Figure 123–2 Antigen-independent human B-cell development. (From Haynes BF, Denning SM: Lymphopoiesis. *In:* Stamatoyannopoulis G, Nienhuis A, Majerus P, Varmus H [eds]: Molecular Basis of Blood Diseases, 2nd ed. Philadelphia, WB Saunders, 1994.)

CD antigens present on immature B cells persist. Pre-B cells can be found in fetal liver at 7 wk gestation, sIgM+ and sIgG+ B cells at between 7 and 11 wk, and sIgD+ and sIgA+ B cells by 12–13 wk. By 14 wk of embryonic life, the percentage of circulating lymphocytes bearing sIgM and sIgD is the same as in cord blood and slightly higher than in the blood of adults. *Antigen-dependent* stages of B-cell development are those that develop after the mature or virgin B cell is stimulated by antigen through its antigen receptor (sIg); the outcome is the differentiation of the cell and its progeny into sIg+ memory B cells (for that particular antigen) and plasma cells, which synthesize and secrete antigen specific immunoglobulin—that is, antibody. There are five immunoglobulin *isotypes* (defined by unique heavy-chain antigens present on each): IgM, IgG, IgA, IgD, and IgE. IgG and IgM, the only complement-fixing isotypes, are the most important immunoglobulins in the blood and other internal body fluids for protection against infectious agents; IgM is confined primarily to the intravascular compartment because of its large size, whereas IgG is present in all internal body fluids. IgA is the major protective immunoglobulin of external secretions—that is, those of the gastrointestinal, respiratory, and urogenital tracts—but it is also present in the circulation. IgE, present in both internal and external body fluids, has a major role in host defense against parasites. However, because of high-affinity IgE receptors on basophils and mast cells, IgE is the principal if not sole mediator of allergic reactions of the immediate type. The significance of IgD is still not clear. There are also immunoglobulin subclasses (again defined by unique heavy-chain antigens present on each, in addition to their class-specific heavy-chain antigen), including four subclasses of IgG—IgG1, IgG2, IgG3, and IgG4—and two subclasses of IgA—IgA1 and IgA2. These subclasses each have different biologic roles; for example, antipolysaccharide antibody activity is found predominantly in the IgG2 subclass. Secreted IgM and IgE have been found in abortuses as young as 10 wk, and IgG as early as 11–12 wk. Even though these B-cell developmental stages have been described in the context of B-cell ontogeny, it is important to recognize that the process of B-cell development from pluripotential stem cells goes on throughout postnatal life.

Despite the capacity of fetal B lymphocytes to differentiate into immunoglobulin-synthesizing and -secreting cells, plasma cells are not usually found in lymphoid tissues of a fetus until about 20 wk gestation, then only rarely, because of the sterile environment of the uterus. Peyer's patches have been found in significant numbers by the 5th intrauterine month, and plasma cells have been seen in the lamina propria by 25 wk gestation. Before birth there may be primary follicles in lymph nodes, but secondary follicles are usually not present.

A human fetus begins to receive significant quantities of maternal IgG transplacentally at around 12 wk gestation, and the quantity steadily increases until at birth cord serum contains a concentration of IgG comparable to or greater than that of maternal serum. IgG is the only class to cross the placenta to any significant degree; all four subclasses do this, but IgG2 does so least well. A small amount of IgM (10% of adult levels) and a few nanograms of IgA, IgD, and IgE are normally found in cord serum; because none of these proteins cross the placenta, they are presumed to be of fetal origin. These observations raise the possibility that certain antigenic stimuli normally cross the placenta to provoke responses, even in noninfected fetuses. Some atopic infants occasionally have reaginic antibodies to antigens (such as egg white) to which they have had no known exposure during postnatal life, suggesting that synthesis of these IgE antibodies could have been induced in the fetus by antigens ingested by the mother.

NATURAL KILLER (NK)–CELL DEVELOPMENT. NK-cell activity has been found in human fetal liver cells at 8–11 wk of gestation. NK lymphocytes are also derived from bone marrow precursors. Thymic processing is not necessary for NK-cell development, although NK cells have been found in the thymus. They are defined by their functional capacity to mediate non–(classic) MHC-restricted cytotoxicity. However, NK cells do have killer inhibitory receptors (KIRS) that recognize other MHC antigens and inhibit the killing of normal allogeneic cells in four specific patterns of reactivity. The genetic locus controlling these patterns is different from conventional MHC alloantigenic loci, although it has been mapped to chromosome 6 in the region of the MHC class I genes. Unlike T and B cells, NK cells do not rearrange antigen receptor genes during their development. Virtually all NK cells express CD56, and more than 90% bear CD16 (FcγRIII) molecules on their cell surface. Other CD antigens found on NK cells include CD57 (on 50–60%), CD7 and CD2 (70–90%), and CD8 (30–40%) (see Table 123–1). Because NK cells share surface antigens with T and myeloid cells, the lineage relationship of NK cells to the latter is still unclear. Some humans with SCID and profound deficiencies in T and B cells have abundant NK cells, whereas some humans who have no NK cells may have normal T- and B-cell development. After release from bone marrow, NK cells enter the circulation or migrate to the spleen; there are very few NK cells in lymph nodes. In normal individuals, NK cells represent 10% of lymphocytes; this percentage is often slightly lower in cord blood.

IMMUNE CELL INTERACTIONS. Immune cell interaction is of crucial importance to all phases of the adaptive immune response. Unlike the B-cell antigen receptor (Ig), which can recognize native antigen, the TCR can recognize only processed antigenic peptides presented to it by MHC molecules such as HLA-A, -B, and -C antigens (class I MHC) and HLA-DR, -DP, and -DQ (class II MHC) molecules present on antigen-presenting cells (APCs). The MHC molecules have a groove in their protein structure where peptides fit. Class I MHC molecules are found on most nucleated cells in the body. Class II MHC molecules are found on macrophages, dendritic cells, and B cells. The peptides found in the groove of class I HLA molecules come from proteins normally made in the cell that are degraded and inserted into the groove. The peptides include viral peptides if the cell is infected with a virus. The peptides present in the groove of class II molecules come from exogenous native antigens such as vaccine and bacterial proteins. These proteins are taken up by APCs (macrophages, dendritic cells and B cells), degraded, and expressed on the cell surface in the groove of class II HLA molecules. The TCR then interacts with the peptide-bearing HLA molecule and, through its functional and physical link to the CD3 complex of signal-transducing molecules, sends a signal to the T cell to produce cytokines that ultimately result in T-cell activation and proliferation.

Two of the main functions of T cells are (1) to signal B cells to make antibody by producing cytokines and membrane molecules that can serve as ligands for B-cell surface molecules and (2) to kill virally infected cells or tumor cells. For a T cell to carry out either of these functions, it first must bind to an APC or to a target cell. For high-affinity binding of T cells to APCs or target cells, several molecules on T cells, in addition to TCRs, bind to molecules on APCs or target cells. For example, the CD4 molecule present on TH cells binds directly to MHC class II molecules on APCs. CD8 on killer T cells binds the MHC class I molecule on the target cell. Both CD4 and CD8 molecules are directly involved in the regulation of T-cell activation and are physically linked intracellularly to the p56-lck protein tyrosine kinase. The cytoplasmic tail of CD45 is a tyrosine phosphatase capable of regulating T-cell signal-transduction events by virtue of the fact that p56-lck has been shown to be a substrate for CD45 phosphatase activity. Depending on which isoform of CD45 is present on the T cell (CD45RO on memory T cells, CD45RA on naive T cells), mechanisms by which CD45 could upregulate or downregulate T-cell triggering have been proposed. LFA-1 on the T cell binds a protein called ICAM-1 (intracellular adhesion molecule 1), now designated CD54, on APCs. CD2 on T cells binds LFA-3 (CD58) on the APCs. With the adhesion of T cells to antigen-presenting cells, TH cells are stimulated to make interleukins and cell surface molecules, such as the CD40 ligand (CD154), that provide help for B cells, and cytotoxic T cells are stimulated to kill their targets.

In the *primary antibody response,* native antigen is carried to a lymph node draining the site, taken up by specialized cells called follicular dendritic cells (FDCs), and expressed on their surfaces. Virgin B cells bearing sIg specific for that antigen then bind to the antigen on the surfaces of the FDCs. If the affinity of the B-cell sIg antibody for the antigen present on the FDCs is high enough, and if other signals are provided by activated T-helper cells, the B cell develops into an antibody-producing plasma cell. If the affinity is not high enough or if T-cell signals are not received, the B cell dies through apoptosis. The signals provided by activated TH cells include those from cytokines they secrete (IL-4, IL-5, IL-6, and IL-13; see Table 123–2) and that from a surface T-cell molecule, CD154, which, on contact of the T cell with the B cell, binds to CD40 on the B-cell surface. CD40 is a type I integral membrane glycoprotein expressed on B cells, monocytes, some carcinomas, and a few other types of cells. It belongs to the tumor necrosis factor (TNF)/nerve growth factor receptor family. Cross linking of CD40 on B cells by allowing CD40 to interact with CD154 in the presence of certain cytokines causes the B cells to undergo proliferation and to initiate immunoglobulin synthesis. In the primary immune response, only IgM antibody is usually made, and most of it is of relatively low affinity. Some B cells become memory B cells during the primary immune response. These cells switch their immunoglobulin genes so that IgG, IgA, and/or IgE antibodies of higher affinity are formed on a secondary exposure to the same antigen. The *secondary immune response* occurs when these memory B cells again encounter that antigen. Plasma cells form, just as in the primary response; however, many more cells are rapidly generated, and IgG, IgA, and IgE antibodies are made. In addition, genetic changes in immunoglobulin genes (somatic mutation) lead to increased affinity of those antibodies. The exact pattern of isotype response to antigen varies, depending on the type of antigen and the cytokines present in the microenvironment.

For NK-mediated lysis, binding to the target is of crucial importance. This is best exemplified by humans with mutations in CD18, or the β chain of three different adhesion molecules, who also lack NK function. Thus, binding of NK cells to their targets is facilitated by LFA-1-ICAM interactions. CD56 or NCAM (neural cell adhesion molecule) also mediates homotypic adhesion of NK cells. FcγRIII, or the low-affinity IgG receptor, has a higher affinity for IgG when it is present on NK cells than when it is on neutrophils; it permits NK cells also to mediate antibody-dependent cellular cytotoxicity (ADCC). In this reaction, antibody is bound through its Fc region to the FcγRIII. The antibody-combining portion of the IgG attaches to the target. The NK cell, now attached to the target by antibody, kills the target cell.

POSTNATAL LYMPHOPOIESIS

T CELLS AND T-CELL SUBSETS. Although the percentage of CD3+ T cells in cord blood is somewhat less than in the peripheral blood of children and adults, T cells are actually present in higher number because of a higher absolute lymphocyte count in all normal infants. An additional distinction is that the ratio of CD4+ to CD8+ T cells is usually higher (3.5–4:1) in cord blood than in blood of children and adults (1.5–2:1). Virtually all T cells in cord blood bear the CD45RA (naive) isoform, and a dominance of CD45RA+ over CD45RO+ T cells persists during the first 2–3 yr of life, after which time the numbers of cells bearing these two isoforms gradually equalize. TH cells can be further subdivided according to the cytokines they produce when activated. TH1 cells produce IL-2 and IFN-γ, thereby promoting cytotoxic T-cell or delayed hypersensitivity types of responses, whereas TH2 cells produce IL-4, IL-5, IL-6, and IL-13 (Table 123–2), which promote B-cell responses and allergic sensitization. Cord blood T cells have the capacity to respond normally to the two T-cell mitogens, PHA and Con A, and they are capable of mounting a normal mixed leukocyte response. Normal newborn infants also have the capacity to develop antigen-specific T cell responses at birth, as evidenced by vigorous tuberculin reactivity a few weeks after BCG vaccination on day 1 of life. Because patients in the first few months of life may have unrecognized severe T-cell defects, most hospitals now routinely irradiate all blood products given young infants.

B CELLS AND IMMUNOGLOBULINS. Newborn infants are quite susceptible to infections with gram-negative organisms, because they have not received IgM antibodies (i.e., heat-stable opsonins) to these organisms from the mother. Quantities of the heat-labile opsonin, C3b, are also lower in newborn serum than in adults. These factors probably account for the finding of impaired phagocytosis of some organisms by newborn polymorphonuclear cells. Maternally transmitted IgG antibodies serve quite adequately as heat-stable opsonins for most gram-positive bacteria, and IgG antibodies to viruses afford adequate protection against those agents. However, because there is a relative deficiency of the IgG2 subclass, antibodies to capsular polysaccharide antigens may be deficient. Because premature infants have received less maternal IgG by the time of birth than full-term infants, their serum opsonic activity is low for all types of organisms.

B lymphocytes are present in cord blood in slightly higher percentages but considerably higher numbers than in the blood of children and adults because of higher absolute lymphocyte counts in all normal infants. However, cord blood B cells do not synthesize the range of immunoglobulin isotypes made by B cells from children and adults when stimulated with either pokeweed mitogen (PWM) or anti-CD40 plus IL-4 or IL-10, producing primarily IgM and at a much reduced quantity.

Neonates begin to synthesize antibodies of the IgM class at an increased rate very soon after birth in response to the immense antigenic stimulation of their new environment. Premature infants appear to be as capable of doing this as do full-term infants. At about 6 days after birth, the serum concentration of IgM rises sharply. This rise continues until adult levels are achieved by approximately 1 yr of age. Cord serum from noninfected normal newborns does not contain detectable IgA. Serum IgA is normally first detected at around the 13th day of postnatal life; the level gradually increases during early childhood until adult levels are achieved and preserved between the 6th and 7th yr of life. Cord serum contains an IgG concentration comparable to or greater than that of maternal serum. Maternal IgG gradually disappears during the first 6–8 mo of life, while the rate of infant IgG synthesis increases (IgG1 and IgG3 faster than IgG2 and IgG4 during the 1st year) until adult concentrations of total IgG are reached and maintained by 7–8 yr of age. However, IgG1 and IgG4 reach adult levels first, followed by IgG3 at 10 yr and IgG2 at 12 yr of age. The total immunoglobulin level in infants usually reaches a low point at approximately 4–5 mo of postnatal life. The rate of development of IgE has generally been found to follow that of IgA. After adult concentrations of each of the three major immunoglobulins are reached, these levels remain remarkably constant for a normal individual. The capacity to produce specific antibodies to protein antigens is intact at the time of birth. However, normal infants cannot produce antibodies to polysaccharide antigens until usually after age 2 yr unless the polysaccharide is conjugated to a protein carrier, as is the case for the conjugate *Haemophilus influenzae* type b (Hib) vaccines.

NK CELLS. The percentage of NK cells in cord blood is usually lower than in the blood of children and adults, but the absolute number of NK cells is approximately the same owing to the higher lymphocyte count. The capacity of cord blood NK cells to mediate target lysis in either NK-cell assays or ADCC assays is roughly two-thirds that of adults.

LYMPHOID ORGAN DEVELOPMENT. Lymphoid tissue is proportionally small but rather well developed at birth and matures rapidly in the postnatal period. The thymus is largest relative to body size during fetal life and at birth is ordinarily two thirds of its mature weight, which it attains during the 1st year of life. It reaches its peak mass, however, just before puberty, then gradually involutes thereafter. By 1 yr of age, all lymphoid structures are mature histologically. Absolute lymphocyte counts in the peripheral blood also reach a peak during the 1st yr of life. Peripheral lymphoid tissue increases rapidly in mass during infancy and early childhood. It reaches adult size by approximately 6 yr of age, exceeds those dimensions during the prepubertal years, and then undergoes involution coincident with puberty. The spleen, however, gradually accrues its mass during maturation and does not reach full weight until adulthood. The mean number of Peyer's patches at birth is one half the adult number and gradually increases until the adult mean number is exceeded during adolescent years.

INHERITANCE OF ABNORMALITIES IN T-, B-, AND NK-CELL DEVELOPMENT

More than 70 immunodeficiency syndromes have been described. Until recently, there was little insight into the fundamental problems underlying most of these conditions. However, specific molecular defects have been identified in a growing number of primary immunodeficiency diseases. Most are recessive traits, some of which are caused by mutations in genes on the X chromosome and others by mutations on autosomal chromosomes. Examples of the latter include (1) combined immunodeficiencies due to abnormalities of purine salvage pathway enzymes, either adenosine deaminase (ADA, encoded by a gene on chromosome 20q13-ter) or purine nucleoside phosphorylase (PNP, encoded by a gene on chromosome 14q13.1); (2) mutations in the gene encoding ZAP-70 (localized to chromosome 2q12), a non-src family protein tyrosine kinase important in T-cell signaling; and (3) mutations in the gene encoding Janus kinase 3 (Jak3), the primary signal transducer from the common cytokine receptor γ chain (γ). The molecular bases of five X-linked immunodeficiency disorders affecting T, B, and/or NK cells have been reported: X-linked immunodeficiency with hyper IgM, X-linked lymphoproliferative syndrome, X-linked agammaglobulinemia, X-linked SCID, and the Wiskott-Aldrich syndrome (Chapters 124–126). The identification and cloning of the genes for these immunodeficiency diseases have obvious implications for potential future somatic cell gene therapy for these patients.

PRENATAL DIAGNOSIS AND CARRIER DETECTION

Intrauterine diagnosis of ADA and PNP deficiencies can be made by enzyme analyses on amnion cells (fresh or cultured) obtained before 20 wk gestation. Diagnosis of several X-linked defects can be made by direct mutation analysis or by restriction fragment length polymorphism (RFLP) studies of the X chromosome of cells obtained by chorionic villus sampling or by amniocentesis from male infants whose mothers have been identified as carriers and who are heterozygous for informative DNA polymorphisms. Diagnosis of enzyme-normal SCID or other severe T-cell deficiencies, MHC class I and/or II antigen deficiencies, chronic granulomatous disease (CGD), or Wiskott-Aldrich syndrome (by platelet size) can be made by appropriate tests of phenotype or function on small samples of blood obtained by fetoscopy at 18–22 wk of gestation, but this procedure carries significant risk. Carriers of ADA and PNP deficiency can be detected by quantitative enzyme analyses of blood samples. Carriers of X-linked agammaglobulinemia, X-linked SCID, or the Wiskott-Aldrich syndrome can be identified by techniques designed to detect nonrandom X-chromosome inactivation in one or more blood cell lineages or by direct mutation analysis if the family's mutation is known.

Buckley RH: Breakthroughs in the understanding and therapy of primary immunodeficiency. Pediatr Clin North Am 41:665, 1994.

Burke F, Naylor MS, Davies B, et al: The cytokine wall chart. Immunol Today 14:165, 1993.

Comans-Bitter WM, de Groot R, van den Beemd R, et al: Immunophenotyping of blood lymphocytes in childhood. J Pediatr 130:388, 1997.
Haynes BF, Denning SM: Lymphopoiesis. *In:* Stamatoyannopoulis G, Nienhuis A, Majerus P, Varmus H (eds): Molecular Basis of Blood Diseases, 2nd ed. Philadelphia, WB Saunders, 1994, pp 425–462.
Noelle RJ, Roy M, Shepherd DM, et al: A 39-kDa protein on activated helper T cells binds CD40 and transduces the signal for cognate activation of B cells. Proc Natl Acad Sci U S A 89:6550, 1992.
Puck JM: Molecular and genetic basis of X-linked immunodeficiency disorders. J Clin Immunol 14:81, 1994.
Schlossman SF, Boumsell L, Gilks W, et al (eds): Leucocyte Typing V: White Cell Differentiation Antigens. Oxford, Oxford University Press, 1995.
WHO Scientific Group: Primary immunodeficiency diseases: Report of a WHO scientific group. Clin Exp Immunol 99:1, 1997.

CHAPTER 124
Primary B-Cell Diseases

Of all of the primary immunodeficiency diseases, those affecting B-cell function are most frequent. Selective absence of serum and secretory IgA is the most common defect, with rates ranging from 1/333 persons to 1/16,000 among different races. By contrast, it has been estimated that agammaglobulinemia occurs with a frequency of only 1/50,000 persons. Patients with antibody deficiency are usually recognized because they have recurrent infections with encapsulated bacteria or a history of failure responding to antibiotic treatment, but some individuals with selective IgA deficiency or infants with transient hypogammaglobulinemia may have few or no infections. The defective gene products for many primary B-cell diseases have been identified (Table 124–1).

124.1 X-Linked (XLA or Bruton) Agammaglobulinemia (XLA)

Patients with this primary immunodeficiency disease have profound defects in B lymphocyte numbers and function, resulting in severe hypogammaglobulinemia.

GENETICS AND PATHOPHYSIOLOGY. The abnormal gene in XLA was mapped to q22 on the long arm of the X chromosome and was found to encode for a B-cell protein tyrosine kinase, named *Btk* (Bruton tyrosine kinase). *Btk* is a member of the src-related tyrosine kinase family, which includes *Lck, Fyn,* and *Lyn,* and which is thought to be involved in signal transduction in many hematopoietic cells. *Btk* is expressed at high levels in all B-lineage cells, including pre-B cells; it is not detected in any cells of T lineage but is found in myeloid cells. *Btk* is hypothesized to have a role in B-cell differentiation at all stages. Some pre-B cells are found in the bone marrow; however, peripheral blood B lymphocytes are absent or present in very low numbers. Thus far, all males with XLA (by family history) have had low to undetectable *Btk* mRNA and kinase activity. Mutations in the *Btk* gene also occur in some agammaglobulinemic boys with no family history. More than 250 different mutations in the human *Btk* gene have been recognized (Fig. 124–1). Carriers are detected by finding nonrandom X-chromosome inactivation in B cells or by direct mutation analysis. Prenatal diagnosis of affected male fetuses is possible by direct mutation analysis or by using closely linked probes and restriction fragment length polymorphism (RFLP) analysis.

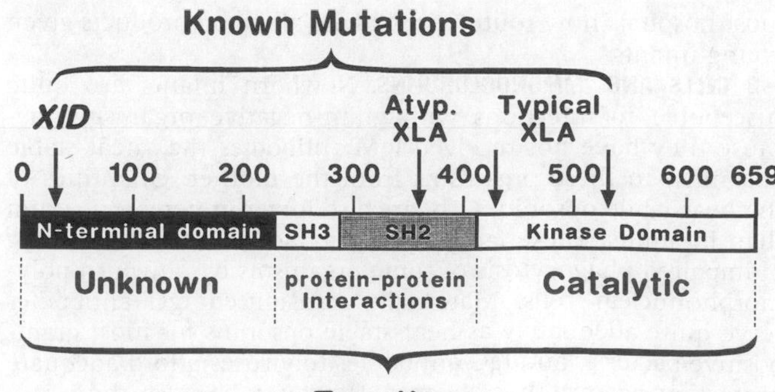

Figure 124–1 Location of mutations in the functional domains of the *Btk* protein. Deletion and point mutations in *Btk* identified to date in many boys with classic XLA are in the kinase domain, whereas CBA/N xid mice with a less severe B-cell defect have a point mutation causing an amino acid substitution at position 28 in the N-terminal domain. A male with a less severe B-cell defect than in classic XLA has had a point mutation at position 361 in the SH2 domain. More recently, however, boys with classic XLA are also reported to have mutations at the xid mutation site and in the SH2 domain. (From Buckley RH: Breakthroughs in the understanding and therapy of primary immunodeficiency. Pediatr Clin North Am 41:665, 1994.)

Polymorphonuclear functions are usually normal, but intermittent neutropenia is observed. The fact that *Btk* is also expressed in cells of myeloid lineage is of interest, because boys with XLA often have neutropenia at the height of an acute infection. It is conceivable that *Btk* is only one of the signaling molecules participating in myeloid maturation and that neutropenia is observed in XLA only when rapid production of such cells is needed. In most patients, the percentage of T cells is increased, ratios of T-cell subsets are normal, and T-cell function is intact. The thymus was morphologically normal in patients who underwent autopsy. An absence of circulating B cells that resembles XLA phenotypically and functionally is also found in girls. This autosomal recessive defect has been shown to be due to mutations in the μ heavy chain gene. XLA is reported in association with growth hormone deficiency.

TABLE 124–1 Primary B-Cell Immunodeficiency Diseases

Chromosome and Region	Gene Product	Disorder	Functional Deficiencies
2p11	Kappa chain*	Kappa chain deficiency	Absence of immunoglobulins bearing kappa chains
6p21.3	Unknown	IgA deficiency; CVID	Low or absent serum IgA; low concentrations of all immunoglobulins in CVID
14q32.3	Immunoglobulin heavy chains*	B-cell negative agammaglobulinemia (μ) or selective deficiencies of other isotypes	Absence of antibody production and lack of B cells in μ chain mutations; subclasses missing but B cells present in others
Xq22	Bruton tyrosine kinase (*Btk*)*	X-linked (Bruton) agammaglobulinemia	Absence of antibody production, lack of B cells
Xq25	SLAM-associated protein (SAP)	X-linked lymphoproliferative (XLP) syndrome	Lack of anti-EBNA and long-lived T-cell immunity to EBV; low immunoglobulins

**Gene cloned and sequenced, gene product known.*
CVID = common variable immunodeficiency; EBV = Epstein-Barr virus.

CLINICAL MANIFESTATIONS. Most boys afflicted with XLA remain well during the first 6–9 mo of life by virtue of maternally transmitted IgG antibodies. Thereafter, they acquire infections with extracellular pyogenic organisms such as *Streptococcus pneumoniae* and *Haemophilus influenzae* unless given prophylactic antibiotics or immunoglobulin therapy. Chronic fungal infections are not usually present, and *Pneumocystis carinii* pneumonia rarely occurs unless there is an associated neutropenia. Viral infections are also usually handled normally, with the exceptions of hepatitis viruses and enteroviruses. Several examples of paralysis after polio vaccine administration have occurred, and chronic, eventually fatal central nervous system infections with various echoviruses have occurred in more than 40 patients. These observations suggest a primary role for antibody, particularly secretory IgA, in host defense against enteroviruses, because normal T-cell function has been present in X-linked agammaglobulinemic patients with such persistent infections. Infections with *Mycoplasma* are also particularly problematic for these patients.

The diagnosis of XLA is suspected if serum concentrations of IgG, IgA, IgM, and IgE are far below the 95% confidence limits for appropriate age- and race-matched controls (i.e., usually <100 mg/dL total immunoglobulin) and circulating B cells are absent. Tests for natural antibodies to blood group substances and for antibodies to antigens given during standard courses of immunization are useful in distinguishing this disorder from transient hypogammaglobulinemia of infancy. Hypoplasia of adenoids, tonsils, and peripheral lymph nodes is the rule; germinal centers are not found, and plasma cells are rare.

124.2 Common Variable Immunodeficiency (CVID)

CVID, also known as "acquired" hypogammaglobulinemia, is similar clinically to XLA. The bacterial pathogens and types of infections that occur are generally the same for the two defects, although echovirus meningoencephalitis is rare in patients with CVID. In contrast to XLA, the sex distribution in CVID is almost equal, the age of onset is later, and infections are less severe.

GENETICS AND PATHOPHYSIOLOGY. Because this disorder occurs in first-degree relatives of patients with selective IgA deficiency, and some patients with IgA deficiency later become panhypogammaglobulinemic, these diseases may have a common genetic basis. The high incidences of abnormal immunoglobulin concentrations, autoantibodies, autoimmune disease, and malignancy in families of both types of patients also suggest a shared hereditary influence. This concept is supported by the discovery of a high incidence of C4-A gene deletions and C2 rare gene alleles in the class III major histocompatibility complex (MHC) region in individuals with either IgA deficiency or CVID, suggesting that the susceptibility genes are in this region on chromosome 6. A small number of HLA haplotypes are shared by individuals affected with IgA deficiency and CVID, with at least one of two particular haplotypes being present in 77% of those affected. In one large family with 13 members, two had IgA deficiency and three had CVID. All of the immunodeficient patients in the family had at least one copy of an MHC haplotype that is abnormally frequent in IgA deficiency and CVID: HLA-DQB1 *0201, HLA-DR3, C4B-Sf, C4A-deleted, G11-15, Bf-0.4, C2a, HSP70-7.5, TNFa-5, HLA-B8, and HLA-A1. However, four immunologically normal members of the pedigree also possessed this haplotype, indicating that its presence is not sufficient for expression of the defects. Environmental factors, particularly drugs such as phenytoin, D-penicillamine, gold, and sulfasalazine, are suspected to be triggers for disease expression in individuals with the permissive genetic background.

The serum immunoglobulin and antibody deficiencies in CVID may be as profound as in XLA. Despite normal numbers of circulating immunoglobulin-bearing B lymphocytes and the presence of lymphoid cortical follicles, blood B lymphocytes from CVID patients do not differentiate normally into immunoglobulin-producing cells when stimulated with pokeweed mitogen (PWM) in vitro, even when co-cultured with normal T cells. However, studies have shown that CVID B cells can be stimulated both to switch isotype and to synthesize and secrete immunoglobulin when stimulated with anti-CD40 and IL-4 or IL-10. T cells and T-cell subsets are usually present in normal percentages, although T-cell function is depressed in some patients. Mitogen-activated T cells from some CVID patients are deficient in expression of genes for several lymphokines while retaining a normal capacity to proliferate. Some patients with CVID have significantly depressed (but not absent) expression of CD154 mRNA and surface protein in activated T lymphocytes, suggesting that inefficient signaling by poorly expressed CD154 on T cells could account for failure of B cells to differentiate. CVID is reported to resolve transiently or permanently in patients who acquire HIV infection.

CLINICAL MANIFESTATIONS. Patients with CVID often have autoantibody formation and normal-sized or enlarged tonsils and lymph nodes, and approximately 25% of patients have splenomegaly. CVID has also been associated with a spruelike syndrome, with or without nodular follicular lymphoid hyperplasia of the intestine; thymoma; alopecia areata; hemolytic anemia; gastric atrophy; achlorhydria; and pernicious anemia. Lymphoid interstitial pneumonia, pseudolymphoma, B-cell lymphomas, amyloidosis, and noncaseating sarcoid-like granulomas of the lungs, spleen, skin, and liver also occur. There is a 438-fold increase in lymphomas among affected women in the 5th and 6th decades of life.

124.3 Selective IgA Deficiency

An isolated absence or near absence (i.e., <10 mg/dL) of serum and secretory IgA is the most common well-defined immunodeficiency disorder, with a frequency of 1/333 reported among some apparently healthy blood donors. However, this condition is also commonly associated with ill health.

GENETICS AND PATHOPHYSIOLOGY. As is the case for CVID, the basic defect leading to IgA deficiency is unknown. Phenotypically normal blood B cells are present in both conditions. IgA deficiency occasionally remits after discontinuation of phenytoin (Dilantin) therapy or spontaneously. The occurrence of IgA deficiency in both males and females and in members of successive generations within families suggests autosomal dominant inheritance with variable expressivity. This defect also commonly occurs in pedigrees containing individuals with CVID. Indeed, IgA deficiency has been noted to evolve into CVID, and the finding of rare alleles and deletions of MHC class III genes in both conditions suggests that the susceptibility genes for these two defects may reside in the MHC class III region on chromosome 6. IgA deficiency is noted in patients treated with the same drugs associated with producing CVID, suggesting that environmental factors may also lead to expression of this defect.

CLINICAL MANIFESTATIONS. Infections occur predominantly in the respiratory, gastrointestinal, and urogenital tracts. Bacterial agents responsible are the same as in other antibody deficiency syndromes. No clear evidence shows that patients with this disorder have an undue susceptibility to viral agents. Children with IgA deficiency vaccinated with killed poliovirus intranasally produce local IgM and IgG antibodies. Serum concentrations of other immunoglobulins are usually normal in patients with selective IgA deficiency, although IgG2 (and other) subclass deficiency is reported, and IgM (usually elevated) may be monomeric.

Patients with IgA deficiency often have IgG antibodies against cow's milk and ruminant serum proteins. These antiruminant antibodies may cause false-positive results in immunoassays for IgA that use goat (but not rabbit) antisera. A sprue-like syndrome occurs in adults with this defect, which may or may not respond to a gluten-free diet. High incidences of autoantibodies and autoimmune diseases are noted, and the incidence of malignancy is increased. Serum antibodies to IgA are reported in as many as 44% of patients with selective IgA deficiency. If of the IgE isotype, these antibodies can cause severe or fatal anaphylactic reactions after intravenous administration of blood products containing IgA. For this reason, only five times washed (in 200 mL volumes) normal donor erythrocytes or blood products from other IgA absent individuals should be administered to these patients. Intravenous immunoglobulin (IVIG), which is greater than 99% IgG, is not indicated because most IgA-deficient patients make IgG antibodies normally. Moreover, many IVIG preparations contain sufficient IgA to cause anaphylactic reactions.

124.4 Transient Hypogammaglobulinemia of Infancy (THI)

After birth, the levels of serum antibodies in an infant diminish with the decline of maternally derived antibodies, reaching a nadir at 3–4 mo of age, and then rise as an infant's own IgG production gradually increases. Extension of hypogammaglobulinemia beyond 6 mo of age is termed THI. B and T lymphocytes are present in normal numbers, and T lymphocyte function is normal. Unlike patients with XLA or CVID, patients with THI synthesize antibodies to human type A and B erythrocytes and to diphtheria and tetanus toxoids normally, usually by 6–11 mo of age, and well before immunoglobulin concentrations become normal. This condition likely represents the extremes of normal variability of the immune system. THI patients may have an increased frequency of otitis media and sinusitis, but infections are not life threatening and respond to appropriate antimicrobial therapy. IVIG therapy is not indicated in this condition.

124.5 IgG Subclass Deficiencies

Some patients have deficiencies of one or more subclasses of IgG, despite normal or elevated total IgG serum concentrations. Most patients with absent or very low concentrations of IgG2 have IgA deficiency. Other patients with IgG2 deficiency have an evolving pattern of immunodeficiency (such as CVID), suggesting that the presence of IgG subclass deficiency may be a marker for more general immune dysfunction. The biologic significance of the numerous moderate deficiencies of IgG subclasses reported is difficult to assess, particularly because commercial laboratory measurement of IgG subclasses is problematic. The more relevant issue is a patient's capacity to make specific antibodies to protein and polysaccharide antigens, because profound deficiencies of antipolysaccharide antibodies are noted even in the presence of normal concentrations of IgG2. IVIG should not be given to IgG subclass–deficient patients unless they are shown to have a deficiency of antibodies to a broad array of antigens.

124.6 Immunoglobulin Heavy- and Light-Chain Deletions

Some completely asymptomatic individuals have a total absence of IgG1, IgG2, IgG4, and/or IgA1 due to gene deletions. These abnormalities were discovered fortuitously in 16 individuals, 15 of whom had no history of undue susceptibility to infection. They produced antibodies of all other isotypes in normal quantity. These patients illustrate the importance of assessing specific antibody formation before deciding to initiate IVIG therapy.

124.7 X-Linked Lymphoproliferative Disease (XLP)

XLP, also referred to as Duncan's disease (after the original kindred in which it was described), is an X-linked recessive trait characterized by an inadequate immune response to infection with Epstein-Barr virus (EBV). The defective gene has been localized to Xq25, cloned, and sequenced. The gene product is known as SAP (SLAM-associated protein). SLAM stands for signaling lymphocyte activation molecule, which is upregulated on both T and B cells with infection or other stimulation. SAP inhibits the upregulation of SLAM, preventing uncontrolled lymphoproliferation in EBV infection in normal hosts. Affected males are healthy until they acquire EBV infection. It is possible to identify affected males of affected kindreds through mutation or RFLP analysis before they develop primary EBV infection. Immunologic studies demonstrated elevated IgA or IgM or variable deficiency of IgG, IgG1, and IgG3 in 13/13 RFLP-positive but in none of 14 RFLP-negative, EBV-negative males.

The mean age of presentation is less than 5 yr. The most common form of presentation (75%) is severe EBV infection with 80% mortality, primarily due to extensive liver necrosis caused by polyclonally activated alloreactive cytotoxic T cells that recognize EBV-infected autologous B cells. Most patients surviving the primary infection develop global cellular immune defects involving T, B, and natural killer (NK) cells; lymphomas; or hypogammaglobulinemia. There is a marked impairment in production of antibodies to the EBV nuclear antigen (EBNA), whereas titers of antibodies to the viral capsid antigen have ranged from zero to markedly elevated. Antibody-dependent cell-mediated cytotoxicity (ADCC) against EBV-infected cells is low in many patients, and NK function is also depressed. There is also a deficiency in memory T-cell immunity to EBV. The percentage of CD8+ T cells is often elevated. Immunoglobulin synthesis in response to PWM stimulation in vitro is markedly depressed.

124.8 Treatment of B-Cell Defects

Judicious use of antibiotics and regular administration of antibodies are the only effective treatments for B-cell disorders. The most common form of replacement therapy is with IVIG. Broad antibody deficiency should be carefully documented before such therapy is initiated. The rationale for the use of these preparations is to provide missing antibodies, not to raise the serum IgG concentration. The development of safe and effective IVIG is a major advance in the treatment of patients with severe antibody deficiencies, although it is expensive. Almost all commercial preparations are isolated from normal plasma by the Cohn's alcohol fractionation method or a modification of it. Cohn's fraction II is then further treated to remove aggregated IgG. Additional stabilizing agents, such as sugars, glycine, and albumin, are added to prevent reaggregation and protect the IgG molecule during lyophilization. HIV is inactivated by the ethanol used in preparation of ISG and IVIG; a solvent/detergent is also added to eliminate hepatitis viruses. Most commercial lots are produced from plasma pooled from more than 60,000 donors and therefore contain a broad spectrum of antibodies. Each pool must contain adequate levels of antibody to antigens in various vaccines, such as tetanus and measles. However, there is no standardization based on titers of antibodies to more clinically relevant organisms, such as *Streptococcus pneumoniae* or *Haemophilus influenzae.*

The IVIG preparations available in the United States have similar efficacy and safety. There has been rare transmission of hepatitis C virus but no documented transmission of HIV by any of these preparations. The potential transmission of hepatitis C virus has been resolved by additional treatment with an organic solvent/detergent mixture. IVIG, 400 mg/kg/mo, achieves trough IgG levels close to the normal range. Systemic reactions to IVIG may occur, but rarely are these true anaphylactic reactions. Anaphylactic reactions caused by a patient's IgE antibodies to IgA in the IVIG preparation may, however, occur in patients with CVID or IgA deficiency. All patients with newly diagnosed cases of CVID should be screened for anti-IgA antibodies through the American Red Cross before undergoing IVIG therapy. If antibodies are detected, IVIG therapy may still be possible by use of the one available IVIG preparation containing almost no IgA (Gammagard S/D, Baxter); carefully screened lots of it can be used safely in patients who have antibodies to IgA.

Buckley RH: Breakthroughs in the understanding and therapy of primary immunodeficiency. Pediatr Clin North Am 41:665, 1994.

Buckley RH, Schiff RI: The use of intravenous immunoglobulin in immunodeficiency diseases. N Engl J Med 325:110, 1991.

Coffey AJ, Brooksbank RA, Brandau O, et al: Host response to EBV infection in X-linked lymphoproliferative disease results from mutations in an SH2-domain encoding gene. Nat Genet 20:129, 1998.

Cunningham-Rundles C: Clinical and immunologic analyses of 103 patients with common variable immunodeficiency. J Clin Immunol 9:22, 1989.

Dalal I, Reid B, Nisbet-Brown E, et al: The outcome of patients with hypogammaglobulinemia in infancy and early childhood. J Pediatr 133:144, 1998.

Nonoyama S, Farrington M, Ochs HM: Activated B cells from patients with common variable immunodeficiency proliferate and synthesize immunoglobulin. J Clin Invest 92:1281, 1993.

North ME, Webster ADB, Farrant J: Primary defect in CD8+ lymphocytes in the antibody deficiency disease (common variable immunodeficiency): Abnormalities in intracellular production of interferon-gamma (IFN-γ) in CD28+ ('cytotoxic') and CD28− ('suppressor') CD8+ subsets. Clin Exp Immunol 111:70, 1998.

Puck JM: Molecular and genetic basis of X-linked immunodeficiency disorders. J Clin Immunol 14:81, 1994.

Sayos J, Wu C, Morra M, et al: The X-linked lymphoproliferative-disease gene product SAP regulates signals induced through the co-receptor SLAM. Nature 395:462, 1998.

Schroeder HW, Zhu Z, March RE, et al: Susceptibility locus for IgA deficiency and common variable immunodeficiency in the HLA-DR3, -B8, -A1 haplotypes. Mol Med 4:72, 1998.

Spickett GP, Webster ADB, Farrant J: Cellular abnormalities in common variable immunodeficiency. Immunodefic Rev 2:199, 1990.

Tsukada S, Saffran DC, Rawlings DJ, et al: Deficient expression of a B cell cytoplasmic tyrosine kinase in human X-linked agammaglobulinemia. Cell 72:279, 1993.

Vetrie D, Vorechovsky I, Sideras P, et al: The gene involved in X-linked agammaglobulinaemia is a member of the src family of protein-tyrosine kinases. Nature 361:226, 1993.

CHAPTER 125
Primary T-Cell Diseases

In general, patients with defects in T-cell function have infections or other clinical problems that are more severe than in patients with antibody deficiency disorders. These individuals rarely survive beyond infancy or childhood. However, exceptions are being recognized as newer primary T-cell defects are identified, such as X-linked immunodeficiency with hyper-IgM and CD3 deficiency. The defective gene products for many primary T-cell diseases have been identified (Table 125–1).

125.1 Thymic Hypoplasia (DiGeorge Syndrome)

Thymic hypoplasia results from dysmorphogenesis of the 3rd and 4th pharyngeal pouches during early embryogenesis, leading to hypoplasia or aplasia of the thymus and parathyroid glands. Other structures forming at the same age are also frequently affected, resulting in anomalies of the great vessels (right-sided aortic arch), esophageal atresia, bifid uvula, congenital heart disease (atrial and ventricular septal defects), a short philtrum, hypertelorism, an antimongoloid slant to the eyes, mandibular hypoplasia, and low-set, often notched ears. The diagnosis is often first suggested by hypocalcemic seizures during the neonatal period. Similar facial features and conotruncal heart lesions are seen in the fetal alcohol syndrome.

GENETICS. DiGeorge syndrome occurs in both males and females. Because familial occurrence is rare, the defect was thought unlikely to be heritable. However, microdeletions of specific DNA sequences from chromosome 22q11.2 (the DiGeorge chromosomal region [DGCR]) have been found in more than 95% of cases. Several candidate genes have been identified in this region. There appears to be an excess of 22q11.2 deletions of maternal origin. Polymerase chain reaction (PCR)–based genotyping using microsatellite DNA markers located within the commonly deleted region permits rapid detection of such microdeletions. Similarities are observed between the DiGeorge syndrome, the velocardiofacial syndrome (VCFS), and the conotruncal anomaly face syndrome (CTAFS), as all three have conotruncal heart defects and 22q deletions. The CATCH 22 syndrome (*C*ardiac, *A*bnormal facies, *T*hymic Hypoplasia, *C*left palate, *H*ypocalcemia) includes the broad clinical spectrum of conditions with 22q11.2 deletions. Other deletions associated with DiGeorge and velocardiofacial syndromes have been identified on chromosome 10p13 (also see Chapters 76 and 77).

TABLE 125–1 Primary T-Cell Immunodeficiency Diseases

Chromosome and Region	Gene Product	Disorder	Functional Deficiencies
2q12	ZAP70*	CD8 lymphocytopenia	Failure of CD4+ T cells to respond to usual signals
10p13	Unknown	Thymic hypoplasia (DiGeorge syndrome)/velocardiofacial syndrome	Low numbers of T cells and impaired T-cell function
11	CD3 γ* or ε*	CD3 deficiency	Poor T-cell responses to mitogens; lack of cytotoxic T cells; IgG subclass deficiency
22q11.2	Unknown	Thymic hypoplasia (DiGeorge syndrome)/velocardiofacial syndrome	Low numbers of T cells and impaired T-cell function
Xq26	CD154 (CD40 ligand)*	X-linked hyper-IgM syndrome	Failure to produce IgG, IgA, and IgE antibodies

**Gene cloned and sequenced, gene product known.*

CLINICAL MANIFESTATIONS. A variable degree of hypoplasia of the thymus and parathyroid glands is more frequent than total aplasia. Children with variable hypoplasia are referred to as having partial DiGeorge syndrome; they may have little trouble with infections and grow normally. Patients with complete DiGeorge syndrome resemble patients with severe combined immunodeficiency (SCID) in their susceptibility to infections with low-grade or opportunistic pathogens, including fungi, viruses, and *Pneumocystis carinii,* and to graft versus host disease (GVHD) from nonirradiated blood transfusions. Concentrations of serum immunoglobulins are usually normal, but IgA may be diminished and IgE elevated. Absolute lymphocyte counts are usually only moderately low for age. The CD3+ T-cell counts are variably decreased in number, corresponding to the degree of thymic hypoplasia, and as a result the percentage of B cells is increased. The proportion of CD4+ and CD8+ T cells is usually normal (2:1). Lymphocyte responses to mitogen stimulation are absent, reduced, or normal, depending on the degrees of thymic deficiency. Thymic tissue, when found, contains Hassall corpuscles and a normal density of thymocytes; corticomedullary distinction is present. Lymphoid follicles are usually present, but lymph node paracortical areas and thymus-dependent regions of the spleen show variable degrees of depletion.

TREATMENT. The immune deficiency in the complete DiGeorge syndrome has been corrected by thymic tissue transplants and by unfractionated HLA-identical bone marrow transplantation.

125.2 X-Linked Immunodeficiency with Hyper-IgM (Hyper IgM)

X-linked immunodeficiency with hyper-IgM, or hyper-IgM syndrome, is characterized by very low serum concentrations of IgG and IgA with a normal or, more frequently, a markedly elevated concentration of polyclonal IgM. It was formerly classified as a B-cell defect.

GENETICS. B cells from boys with the X-linked form of this defect are capable of synthesizing not only IgM but also IgA and IgG when co-cultured with a "switch" T-cell line, indicating that the defect is in the T-cell lineage. The abnormal gene is localized to Xq26, and the gene product, CD154, is the ligand for CD40 on B cells; it is upregulated on activated T cells. Mutations in CD154 on activated T cells from males with X-linked hyper-IgM result in an inability to signal B cells to undergo isotype switching, and thus they produce only IgM. Defective T-cell function may explain the occurrence of *P. carinii* pneumonia and extensive verruca vulgaris lesions in some patients with this condition. A growing number of mutations in the CD154 gene have been reported, all but one of which are clustered in the tumor necrosis factor (TNF) homology domain located in the C-terminus region. A highly polymorphic microsatellite dinucleotide (CA) repeat region has been identified in the 3′ untranslated end of the CD154 gene. Approximately 80% of women are heterozygous for this polymorphism, consisting of eight alleles. This marker can be used to detect carriers of X-linked hyper-IgM, and it can be used to make a prenatal diagnosis of this condition. However, mutations in CD154 are not the only cause of the hyper-IgM syndrome. A number of male and female patients with hyper-IgM have been identified as having normal T-cell CD154, but they appear to have intrinsic B-cell defects that prevent isotype switching. The molecular defects in these patients remain unknown.

CLINICAL MANIFESTATIONS. Like patients with X-linked agammaglobulinemia (XLA), affected boys become symptomatic during the 1st or 2nd year of life with recurrent pyogenic infections, including otitis media, sinusitis, pneumonia, and tonsillitis. In contrast to patients with XLA, the frequent presence of lymphoid hyperplasia often leads away from a diagnosis of immunodeficiency. Thymic-dependent lymphoid tissues and T-cell functions are usually normal, but some affected males have decreased T-cell function. High titers of IgM antibodies to blood group substances and to salmonella O antigen are found in some patients, but very low titers or no IgM antibody is noted in others. The frequency of autoimmune disorders is even higher than it is with other antibody-deficiency syndromes. Hemolytic anemia and thrombocytopenia may occur, and transient, persistent, or cyclic neutropenia is a common feature. Normal numbers of B lymphocytes are found in the blood of these patients.

125.3 Defective Expression of the T-Cell Receptor-CD3 Complex (Ti-CD3)

The first type of this disorder was found in two brothers in a Spanish family. The proband presented with severe infections and died at 31 mo of age with autoimmune hemolytic anemia and viral pneumonia. His lymphocytes had responded poorly to mitogens and to anti-CD3 in vitro and could not be stimulated to develop cytotoxic T cells. However, his antibody responses to protein antigens had been normal, indicating normal T-helper cell function. His 12-yr-old brother was healthy but had almost no CD3-bearing T cells and had IgG2 deficiency similar to his sibling. The defect in this family is due to mutations in the CD3γ chain. The second type of this disorder was diagnosed in a 4-yr-old French boy who had recurrent *Haemophilus influenzae* pneumonia and otitis media in early life but is now healthy. He has a partial defect in expression of Ti-CD3, and thus the percentage of CD3+ cells is about half-normal but the level of expression is markedly decreased. His T cells do not proliferate in response to anti-CD3 or anti-CD2, nor do they express the IL-2 receptor or have normal calcium influx after these treatments. However, they do respond normally to stimulation with anti-CD28 or antigens, such as tetanus toxoid. The defect was shown to be due to two independent CD3ϵ gene mutations, leading to defective CD3ϵ chain synthesis and preventing normal association and membrane expression of the TCR/CD3 complex.

125.4 Defective Cytokine Production

Two main defects of cytokine production are known. The first is a selective inability to produce IL-2. In the two reported cases, patients had severe recurrent infections in infancy. The IL-2 gene was present in both, but no IL-2 message or protein was produced. Other T-cell cytokines were produced normally. The second type was found in a single patient who also presented during infancy with severe recurrent infections and failure to thrive. She had defective transcription of several lymphokine genes, including IL-2, IL-3, IL-4, and IL-5, possibly as a result of abnormal binding of nuclear factor of activated T cells (NFAT-1) to response elements in IL-2 and IL-4 enhancers. She was treated with recombinant IL-2 with some clinical improvement.

125.5 T-Cell Activation Defects

These conditions are characterized by the presence of normal or elevated numbers of blood T cells that appear phenotypically normal but that fail to proliferate or produce cytokines in response to stimulation with mitogens, antigens, or other signals delivered to the T-cell antigen receptor (TCR), owing to defective signal transduction from the TCR to intracellular metabolic pathways. These patients have problems similar to those of other T-cell–deficient individuals, and some with severe T-cell activation defects may resemble SCID patients clinically.

125.6 CD8$^+$ Lymphocytopenia

Patients with this T-cell activation defect present during infancy with severe, recurrent, often fatal infections. A majority of reported cases occur in Mennonites. They have normal or elevated numbers of blood B cells and low to elevated serum immunoglobulin concentrations. Their blood lymphocytes exhibit normal expression of the T-cell surface antigens CD3 and CD4, but CD8+ cells are almost totally absent. These cells fail to respond to mitogens or to allogeneic cells in vitro or to generate cytotoxic T lymphocytes. By contrast, natural killer (NK) activity is normal. The thymus of one patient exhibited normal architecture with normal numbers of CD4:CD8 double-positive thymocytes but an absence of CD8 single-positive thymocytes. This condition is due to mutations in the gene encoding ZAP-70, a non-src family protein tyrosine kinase important in T-cell signaling. The gene is localized to chromosome 2q12. The hypothesis about why there are normal numbers of CD4:CD8 double-positive T cells is that thymocytes can use the other member of the same tyrosine kinase family, Syk, to facilitate positive selection. Syk is present at fourfold higher levels in thymocytes than in peripheral T cells, possibly accounting for the lack of normal responses by the CD4+ blood T cells.

Allen RC, Armitage RJ, Conley ME, et al: CD40 ligand gene defects responsible for X-linked hyper IgM syndrome. Science 259:990, 1993.
Arnaiz-Villena A, Timon M, Corell A, et al: Brief report: Primary immunodeficiency caused by mutations in the gene encoding the CD3-γ subunit of the T lymphocyte receptor. N Engl J Med 327:529, 1992.
Arpaia E, Shahar M, Dadi H, et al: Defective T cell receptor signaling and CD8+ thymic selection in humans lacking zap-70 kinase. Cell 76:947, 1994.
Callard RE, Armitage RJ, Fanslow WC, et al: CD40 ligand and its role in X-linked hyper IgM syndrome. Immunol Today 14:559, 1993.
Chatila T, Wong R, Young M, et al: An immunodeficiency characterized by defective signal transduction in T lymphocytes. N Engl J Med 320:696, 1989.
Disanto JP, Keever CA, Small TN, et al: Absence of interleukin 2 production in a severe combined immunodeficiency disease syndrome with T cells. J Exp Med 171:1697, 1990.
Disanto JP, Markiewicz S, Gauchat J, et al: Brief report: Prenatal diagnosis of X-linked hyper IgM syndrome. N Engl J Med 330:969, 1994.
Driscoll DA, Budarf ML, Emanuel BS: A genetic etiology for DiGeorge syndrome: Consistent deletions and microdeletions of 22q11. Am J Hum Genet 50:924, 1992.
Elder ME, Lin D, Clever J, et al: Human severe combined immunodeficiency due to a defect in ZAP-70, a T cell tyrosine kinase. Science 264:1596, 1994.
Mayer L, Swan SP, Thompson C: Evidence for a defect in "switch" T cells in patients with immunodeficiency and hyperimmunoglobulinemia M. N Engl J Med 314:409, 1986.
Rijkers GT, Scharenberg JGM, VanDongen JJM, et al: Abnormal signal transduction in a patient with severe combined immunodeficiency disease. Pediatr Res 29:306, 1991.
Weinberg K, Parkman R: Severe combined immunodeficiency due to a specific defect in the production of interleukin-2. N Engl J Med 322:1718, 1990.

CHAPTER 126
Combined B- and T-Cell Diseases

Patients with combined B- and T-cell defects have severe, frequently opportunistic infections that lead to death in infancy or childhood without bone marrow transplantation early in life. These are rare defects; for example, severe combined immunodeficiency (SCID) has been estimated to occur in 1/100,000 live births. The defective gene products for many combined B- and T-cell diseases have been identified (Table 126–1).

126.1 Combined Immunodeficiency (CID)

Combined immunodeficiency (CID) is distinguished from SCID by low but not absent T-cell function. Like SCID, however, it is a syndrome of diverse genetic causes. Patients with CID have recurrent or chronic pulmonary infections, failure to

TABLE 126–1 Combined B- and T-Cell Diseases

Chromosome and Region	Gene Product	Disorder	Functional Deficiencies
1q	RFX5	MHC class II antigen deficiency	Low immunoglobulins, lack of T-cell responses to antigens, CD4+ deficiency
5p13	IL-7Rα*	T−B+NK+ SCID	Absence of T- and B-cell functions
6p21.3	TAP	MHC class I antigen deficiency	Marked deficiency of CD8+ cells; combined B- and T-cell defects
6q22–q23	IFN-γ R1*	Disseminated mycobacterial infections	Failure of macrophages and other cells to produce TNF-α in response to IFN-γ
9p21–p13	Unknown	Cartilage-hair hypoplasia	Combined T- and B-cell defects of varying severity
10p14–15	IL-2Rα*	Lymphoproliferative syndrome	Poor T-cell responses; impaired apoptosis; increased bcl-2; autoimmunity
11p13	RAG1 or RAG2*	T−B−NK+SCID	Absence of T- and B-cell functions
11q22.3	DNA-dependent kinase*	Ataxia-telangiectasia	Selective IgA deficiency; T-cell deficiency
13q	RFXAP*	MHC class II antigen deficiency	Low immunoglobulins, lack of T-cell responses to antigens, CD4+ deficiency
14q13.1	Purine nucleosidase*	PNP deficiency	Severe T-cell deficiency; may have immunoglobulins
16p13	CIITA*	MHC class II antigen deficiency	Low immunoglobulins, lack of T-cell responses to antigens, CD4+ deficiency
19p13.1	Jak3*	T−B+NK−SCID	Absence of T-, B-, and NK-cell functions
20q13.11	ADA*	T−B−NK−SCID	Absence of T- and B-cell functions
Xp11.23	WASP*	Wiskott-Aldrich syndrome	Thrombocytopenia; poor antipolysaccharide antibody production; T-cell deficiency
Xq13.1	Common γ chain (γc)*	T−B+NK−SCID	Absence of T-, B-, and NK-cell functions

**Gene cloned and sequenced, gene product known.*
WASP = Wiskott-Aldrich syndrome protein; TH1 = T-helper cell type 1; TH2 = T-helper cell type 2; PNP = purine nucleoside phosphorylase; IL2Rα = interleukin 2 receptor α chain; ADA = adenosine deaminase; Jak3 = Janus kinase 3; IL7Rα = interleukin 7 receptor α chain; RAG1 and RAG2 = recombinase activating genes 1 and 2; IFN-γR1 = interferon γ receptor chain 1; IL-12Rβ1 = interleukin-12β1 chain; MHC = major histocompatibility complex; SCID = severe combined immunodeficiency; TAP = transporter of antigenic peptide; CIITA = class II transactivator.

thrive, oral or cutaneous candidiasis, chronic diarrhea, recurrent skin infections, gram-negative sepsis, urinary tract infections, or severe varicella in infancy. Although they usually survive longer than infants with SCID, they fail to thrive and die early in life. Neutropenia and eosinophilia are common. Serum immunoglobulins may be normal or elevated for all classes, but selective IgA deficiency, marked elevation of IgE, and elevated IgD levels occur in some cases. Although antibody-forming capacity is impaired in most patients, it is not absent. Moreover, plasma cells are usually abundant in the lamina propria and lymph nodes.

Studies of cellular immune function show lymphopenia, profound deficiencies of T cells, and extremely low but not absent lymphocyte proliferative responses to mitogens, antigens, and allogeneic cells in vitro. Peripheral lymphoid tissues demonstrate paracortical lymphocyte depletion. The thymus is very small with a paucity of thymocytes and usually no Hassall corpuscles. An autosomal recessive pattern of inheritance is common.

126.2 Purine Nucleoside Phosphorylase (PNP) Deficiency

More than 40 patients with CID have been found to have PNP deficiency. Point mutations identified in the PNP gene on chromosome 14q13.1 account for these deficiencies. In contrast to adenosine deaminase (ADA) deficiency, in this condition, serum and urinary uric acid are usually markedly deficient and no characteristic physical or skeletal abnormalities have been noted. Deaths result from generalized vaccinia, varicella, lymphosarcoma, and graft versus host disease (GVHD) mediated by allogeneic T cells in nonirradiated blood or bone marrow. Two thirds of patients have neurologic abnormalities, and one third have autoimmune diseases. Lymphopenia is striking, primarily because of a marked deficiency of T cells; T-cell function is decreased to various degrees. Natural killer (NK) cells are increased. Prenatal diagnosis is possible. Gene therapy is a possibility for the future, but thus far bone marrow transplantation has been the only successful form of therapy.

126.3 Cartilage Hair Hypoplasia (CHH)

This unusual form of short-limbed dwarfism with frequent and severe infections occurs among the Pennsylvania Amish; non-Amish patients have been described. Features include short, pudgy hands; redundant skin; hyperextensible joints of hands and feet but an inability to extend the elbows completely; and fine, sparse, light hair and eyebrows. Radiographically, the bones show scalloping and sclerotic or cystic changes in the metaphyses and flaring of the costochondral junctions of the ribs. Severe and often fatal varicella infections, progressive vaccinia, and vaccine-associated poliomyelitis have been observed.

The severity of the immunodeficiency varies; in one series, 11 of 77 patients died before age 20 yr but two were still alive at age 76. Three patterns of immune dysfunction have emerged: defective antibody-mediated immunity, CID (most common), and SCID. In vitro studies have shown decreased numbers of T cells and defective T-cell proliferation due to an intrinsic defect related to the G1 phase, resulting in a longer cell cycle for individual cells. However, NK cells are increased in number and function. CHH is an autosomal recessive condition, and the defective gene has been mapped to chromosome 9p21–p13 in Amish and Finnish families but has not been identified.

126.4 Interleukin 2 Receptor α Chain (IL-2R α [CD25]) Mutation

An infant boy born of a consanguineous union developed cytomegalovirus (CMV) pneumonia, persistent candidiasis, adenoviral gastroenteritis, failure to thrive, lymphadenopathy, hepatosplenomegaly, and chronic inflammation of his lungs and mandible. Biopsies revealed extensive lymphocytic infiltration of his lung, liver, intestines, and bone. Serum IgA level was low. He had T-cell lymphocytopenia, and the T cells responded poorly to anti-CD3, phytohemagglutinin (PHA) and other mitogens, and to IL-2. He was found to have a mutation of the gene encoding the IL-2 receptor α chain (IL-2Rα [CD25]), leading to truncation of the protein. He had no CD1 in his thymus and an elevation of the anti-apoptotic protein bcl-2. This defect reveals that some components of cytokine receptors normally serve a negative regulatory role. Mutations in those components can result in unchecked lymphoproliferation and autoimmunity in addition to immunodeficiency.

126.5 Severe Combined Immunodeficiency

The syndromes of SCID are caused by diverse genetic mutations that lead to absence of all adaptive immune function and, in many cases, in a lack of NK cells (Table 126–1). Patients with this group of disorders have the most severe of all of the recognized immunodeficiencies.

CLINICAL MANIFESTATIONS. Affected infants present within the first few months of life with diarrhea, pneumonia, otitis, sepsis, and cutaneous infections. Growth may appear normal initially, but extreme wasting usually ensues after diarrhea and infections begin. Persistent infections with opportunistic organisms such as *Candida albicans, Pneumocystis carinii,* varicella, measles, parainfluenza 3, CMV, Epstein-Barr virus (EBV), and bacillus Calmette-Guérin (BCG) lead to death. Affected infants also lack the ability to reject foreign tissue and are therefore at risk for GVHD from maternal immunocompetent T cells crossing the placenta or from T lymphocytes in nonirradiated blood products or allogeneic bone marrow.

Infants with SCID have lymphopenia. This is present at birth, indicating that the condition could be diagnosed in all affected infants if routine white blood counts and manual differential counts were done on all cord bloods. They also have an absence of lymphocyte proliferative responses to mitogens, antigens, and allogeneic cells in vitro; and delayed cutaneous anergy. Patients with ADA deficiency have the lowest absolute lymphocyte counts, usually less than 500/mm^3. Serum immunoglobulin concentrations are diminished to absent, and no antibody formation occurs after immunization. Analyses of lymphocyte populations and subpopulations demonstrate distinctive phenotypes for the various genetic forms of SCID. T cells are extremely low or absent in all types; when present, they are in most cases transplacentally derived maternal T cells.

PATHOLOGY. Typically, patients with SCID have very small thymuses (<1 g) that usually fail to descend from the neck, contain few thymocytes, and lack corticomedullary distinction and Hassall corpuscles. The thymic epithelium appears histologically normal. Both the follicular and paracortical areas of the spleen are depleted of lymphocytes; lymph nodes, tonsils, adenoids, and Peyer's patches are absent or extremely underdeveloped.

TREATMENT. This is a true pediatric emergency: Unless immunologic reconstitution is achieved through bone marrow transplantation, death usually occurs in the 1st year of life and almost invariably before the end of the 2nd yr. If diagnosed at birth or within the first 3 mo of life, 95% of cases can be treated successfully with HLA-identical or T-cell–depleted haploidentical bone marrow stem cells without the need for pretransplant chemoablation or post-transplant GVHD prophylaxis.

126.6 X-Linked Severe Combined Immunodeficiency (XSCID)

X-linked SCID (XSCID) is the most common form of SCID in the United States, accounting for approximately 47% of cases. Clinically, immunologically, and histopathologically, affected individuals appear similar to those with other forms of SCID except for having uniformly low percentages of T and NK cells and an elevated percentage of B cells (T−, B+, NK−), a characteristic feature they share only with Janus kinase 3 (Jak3)–deficient patients with SCID. The abnormal gene in XSCID was mapped to Xq13, cloned, and found to encode the common γ (γ_c) chain for several cytokine receptors, including IL-2, IL-4, IL-7, IL-9, and IL-15. The shared γ_c chain functions both to increase the affinity of the receptor for the respective cytokine and to enable the receptors to mediate intracellular signaling. Incapacitation of the receptors for all of these developmentally crucial cytokines by genetic mutations in the common γ chain provides an explanation for the severity of the immunodeficiency in XSCID. In the first 136 patients studied, 95 distinct mutations spanning all 8 IL2RG exons were identified, most of them consisting of small changes at the level of one to a few nucleotides. These mutations resulted in abnormal γ_c chains in two thirds of the cases and absent γ_c protein in the remainder. Carriers can be detected by demonstrating nonrandom X-chromosome inactivation or the deleterious mutation in their T, B, or NK lymphocytes. Unless donor B or NK cells develop, patients with SCID have very poor B- and NK-cell function after nonablated bone marrow cell transplantation because of the many cytokine receptor defects, despite excellent reconstitution of T-cell function by donor-derived T cells.

126.7 Autosomal Recessive SCID

This pattern of inheritance of SCID is less common in the United States than in Europe. Mutated genes on autosomal chromosomes have been identified in four forms of SCID: ADA deficiency, Jak3 deficiency, IL-7 receptor α chain (IL-7Rα) deficiency, and RAG1 or RAG2 deficiency; other causes are likely to be discovered.

ADA DEFICIENCY. An absence of the enzyme ADA is observed in approximately 15% of patients with SCID, resulting from various point and deletion mutations in the ADA gene (on chromosome 20q13-ter). Marked accumulations of adenosine, 2′-deoxyadenosine, and 2′-*O*-methyladenosine lead directly or indirectly to T-cell apoptosis, which causes the immunodeficiency. ADA-deficient patients usually have a much more profound lymphopenia than do infants with other types of SCID, with mean absolute lymphocyte counts of less than 500/mm^3; they rarely have elevated percentages of B or NK cells. They do have normal NK function, and after T-cell function is conferred by bone marrow transplantation without pretransplant chemotherapy, they generally have excellent B-cell function. This is because ADA deficiency affects primarily T-cell function. Milder forms of this condition have been reported as leading to delayed diagnosis of immunodeficiency, even to adulthood. Other distinguishing features of ADA-deficient SCID include the presence of rib cage abnormalities similar to a rachitic rosary and numerous skeletal abnormalities of chondro-osseous dysplasia, which occur predominantly at the costochondral junctions, at the apophyses of the iliac bones, and in the vertebral bodies.

As with other types of SCID, ADA deficiency can be cured by HLA-identical or haploidentical T-cell–depleted bone marrow transplantation without the need for pre- or post-transplant chemotherapy; this remains the treatment of choice. Enzyme replacement therapy should not be initiated if bone marrow transplantation is possible, because it confers graft-rejection capability. Gene therapy has been attempted but has thus far been unsuccessful. A spontaneous in vivo reversion to normal of a mutation in the ADA gene has been reported.

JAK3 DEFICIENCY. Patients with this recently discovered autosomal recessive defect resemble all other types of SCID patients clinically. However, they have a lymphocyte phenotype similar only to that of patients with XSCID—that is, an elevated percentage of B cells and very low or no T and NK cells. Because Jak3 is the only signaling molecule known to be associated with γ_c, it was a candidate gene for mutations leading to autosomal recessive SCID not due to ADA deficiency. It accounts for approximately 7% of SCID cases. Even after successful T-cell reconstitution by transplantation of haploidentical stem cells, patients with Jak3-deficient SCID fail to develop NK cells or normal B-cell function owing to the defective function of the many types of cytokine receptors that share γ_c.

RAG1 OR RAG2 DEFICIENCIES. Infants with this cause of SCID have a different lymphocyte phenotype from those of patients with SCID due to γ_c, Jak3, or ADA deficiencies in that they lack both B and T lymphocytes (so-called T− B− SCID) and have primarily NK cells in their circulation. This suggested a problem with their antigen receptor genes that led to the discovery of mutations in recombinase activating genes, RAG1 or RAG2. Such mutations result in a functional inability to form antigen receptors through genetic recombination.

IL-7Rα DEFICIENCY. Patients with SCID and this defect also have a distinctive lymphocyte phenotype in that they have normal or elevated numbers of both B and NK cells. The prevalence of this form of SCID is yet unknown. In contrast to patients with γ_c and Jak3-deficient SCID, the immunologic defect in these patients is completely correctable even by T-cell–depleted haploidentical bone marrow stem cell transplantation.

126.8 Reticular Dysgenesis

This condition was first described in identical twin boys who exhibited a total lack of both lymphocytes and granulocytes in their peripheral blood and bone marrow. Seven of eight infants with this defect died between 3 and 119 days of age as a result of overwhelming infections; 7 infants have been cured by bone marrow transplantation. The thymus glands have all weighed less than 1 g, no Hassall corpuscles have been found, and few or no thymocytes have been seen. Reticular dysgenesis is considered a variant of SCID. The molecular basis of this autosomal recessive disorder is unknown.

126.9 Defective Expression of Major Histocompatibility Complex (MHC) Antigens

The two main forms of immunodeficiency and abnormalities of expression of the MHC are MHC class I (HLA-A, -B, and -C) antigen deficiency (bare lymphocyte syndrome) and MHC class II (HLA-DR, -DQ, and -DP) antigen deficiency.

MHC CLASS I ANTIGEN DEFICIENCY. An isolated deficiency of MHC class I antigens is rare, and the resulting immunodeficiency is much milder than in SCID, contributing to a later age of presentation. Sera from affected children contain normal quantities of MHC class I antigens and β_2-microglobulin, but MHC class I antigens are not detected on any cells in the body. A deficiency of CD8+ but not CD4+ T cells is noted. A nonsense mutation was found in *TAP2*, one of two genes (*TAP1* and *TAP2*) within the MHC locus on chromosome 6 that encode the protein TAP. TAP functions to transport antigenic peptides from the cytoplasm across the Golgi apparatus membrane to join the α chain of MHC class 1 antigens and β_2-microglobulin. All these are then assembled into a MHC class I complex that can then move to the cell surface. If the assembly of the complex cannot be completed because there is no antigenic peptide, the MHC class I complex is destroyed in the cytoplasm.

MHC CLASS II ANTIGEN DEFICIENCY. Many affected with this autosomal recessive syndrome are of North African descent. Patients present in early infancy with persistent diarrhea that is often associated with cryptosporidiosis and enteroviral infections (poliovirus, coxsackievirus). They also have an increased frequency of infections with herpesviruses and other viruses, oral candidiasis, bacterial pneumonia, *P. carinii* pneumonia, and septicemia. The immunodeficiency is not as severe as in SCID, as evidenced by their failure to develop disseminated infection after BCG vaccination or GVHD from nonirradiated blood transfusions.

MHC class II–deficient patients have a very low number of CD4+ T cells but normal or elevated numbers of CD8+ T cells. Lymphopenia is only moderate. The MHC class II antigens HLA-DP, DQ, and DR are undetectable on blood B cells and monocytes, even though B cells are present in normal number. Patients are hypogammaglobulinemic owing to impaired antigen-specific responses caused by the absence of these antigen-presenting molecules. In addition, MHC antigen-deficient B cells fail to stimulate allogeneic cells in mixed leukocyte culture. Lymphocyte proliferation studies show normal responses to mitogens but no response to antigens. The thymus and other lymphoid organs are severely hypoplastic, and the lack of class II molecules results in abnormal thymic selection. The latter results in circulating CD4+ T cells that have altered CDR3 profiles. The associated defects of both B- and T-cell immunity and of HLA expression emphasize the important biologic role for HLA determinants in effective immune cell cooperation. Three different molecular defects have been defined. These include mutations in (1) the gene for RFX5, a promoter protein encoded on chromosome 1q that binds to the MHC class II gene promoter region X-box; (2) the gene for RFXAP, a similar factor encoded on chromosome 13q; and (3) a gene on chromosome 16p13 that encodes a novel MHC class II transactivator (CIITA) that coordinates the binding of proteins to the MHC class II gene promoter region.

126.10 Omenn Syndrome

Omenn syndrome of CID with hypereosinophilia is an autosomal recessively inherited, fatal condition characterized by profound susceptibility to infection, with T-cell infiltration of skin, intestines, liver, and spleen, leading to an exfoliative erythroderma, lymphadenopathy, hepatosplenomegaly, and intractable diarrhea. Infants so affected have a persistent leukocytosis with marked eosinophilia; elevated serum IgE; low IgG, IgA, and IgM; low or absent blood B cells; and elevated numbers of T cells but impaired T-cell function due to restricted heterogeneity of the host T-cell repertoire. A TH2-like cell dominance is suggested. Mutations in the recombinase activating genes, RAG1 and RAG2, have been found in several patients with this condition.

126.11 Immunodeficiency with Thrombocytopenia and Eczema (Wiskott-Aldrich Syndrome)

Wiskott-Aldrich syndrome, an X-linked recessive syndrome, is characterized by atopic dermatitis, thrombocytopenic purpura with normal-appearing megakaryocytes but small defective platelets, and undue susceptibility to infection.

GENETICS. The abnormal gene, on the proximal arm of the X chromosome at Xp11.22–11.23 near the centromere, encodes a 501 amino acid proline-rich cytoplasmic protein restricted in its expression to lymphocytic and megakaryocytic cell lineages. This protein, now referred to as the Wiskott-Aldrich syndrome protein (WASP), has been shown to bind CDC42H2 and rac, members of the Rho family of guanosine triphosphatases. WASP appears to control the assembly of actin filaments required for microvesicle formation downstream of protein kinase C and tyrosine kinase signaling. Carriers can be detected by nonrandom X-chromosome inactivation in several hematopoietic cell lineages or by demonstration of the deleterious mutation.

CLINICAL MANIFESTATIONS. Patients often have prolonged bleeding from the circumcision site or bloody diarrhea during infancy. The thrombocytopenia is not initially due to antiplatelet antibodies. Atopic dermatitis and recurrent infections usually develop during the 1st year of life. Infections are caused by pneumococci and other bacteria having polysaccharide capsules, resulting in otitis media, pneumonia, meningitis, or sepsis. Later, infections with agents such as *P. carinii* and the herpesviruses become more frequent. Survival beyond the teens is rare; infections, bleeding, and EBV-induced malignancy are major causes of death.

Patients with this defect uniformly have an impaired humoral immune response to polysaccharide antigens, as evidenced by absent or markedly diminished isohemagglutinins, and poor or absent antibody responses after immunization with polysaccharide vaccines. Anamnestic responses to antibody are poor or absent. There is an accelerated rate of synthesis as well as hypercatabolism of albumin, IgG, IgA, and IgM, resulting in highly variable concentrations of different immunoglobulins, even within the same patient. The predominant immunoglobulin pattern is a low serum level of IgM, elevated IgA and IgE, and a normal or slightly low IgG concentration. IgG2 subclass concentrations, surprisingly, are normal. Percentages of T cells are moderately reduced, and lymphocyte responses to mitogens are variably depressed.

126.12 Ataxia-Telangiectasia

Ataxia-telangiectasia is a complex syndrome with neurologic, immunologic, endocrinologic, hepatic, and cutaneous abnormalities.

GENETICS AND PATHOGENESIS. The mutated gene (ATM) responsible for this defect was mapped to the long arm of chromosome 11 (11q22–23) and has been cloned. The gene product is a DNA-dependent protein kinase localized predominantly to the nucleus. It is involved in mitogenic signal transduction, meiotic recombination, and cell cycle control.

Cells from patients as well as those of heterozygous carriers have increased sensitivity to ionizing radiation, defective DNA repair, and frequent chromosomal abnormalities. The malignancies reported in this condition are usually of the lymphoreticular type, but adenocarcinomas are also found, and unaffected relatives have an increased incidence of malignancy.

CLINICAL MANIFESTATIONS. The most prominent clinical features are progressive cerebellar ataxia, oculocutaneous telangiectasias, chronic sinopulmonary disease, a high incidence of malignancy, and variable humoral and cellular immunodeficiency. Ataxia typically becomes evident soon after children begin to walk and progresses until they are confined to a wheelchair, usually by the age of 10–12 yr. The telangiectasias develop between 3 and 6 yr of age. Recurrent sinopulmonary infections occur in approximately 80% of these patients. Although common viral infections have not usually resulted in untoward sequelae, fatal varicella has occurred.

DIAGNOSIS. The most frequent humoral immunologic abnormality is the selective absence of IgA, found in 50–80% of these patients; hypercatabolism of IgA also occurs. IgE concentrations are usually low, and the IgM may be of the low molecular weight variety. IgG2 or total IgG levels may be decreased. Specific antibody titers may be decreased or normal. In vitro tests of lymphocyte function have generally shown moderately depressed proliferative responses to T- and B-cell mitogens. Percentages of CD3+ and CD4+ T cells are moderately reduced, with normal or increased percentages of CD8+ and elevated numbers of Tig/δ+ T cells. Studies of immunoglobulin synthesis have shown both helper T-cell and intrinsic B-cell defects. The thymus is very hypoplastic, exhibits poor organization, and lacks Hassall corpuscles.

126.13 Interferon-γ Receptor 1 and IL-12 Receptor β1 Mutations

Disseminated BCG infections occur in patients with severe T-cell defects. However, in approximately half of cases, no specific host defect is found. There are other possible explanations for this predilection. The first was found in a 2.5-mo-old Tunisian girl who had fatal idiopathic disseminated BCG infection and in four children from Malta who had disseminated atypical mycobacterial infection in the absence of a recognized immunodeficiency. There was consanguinity in all, and each had a functional defect in the upregulation of tumor necrosis factor α (TNF-α) production by their blood macrophages in response to stimulation with interferon-γ (IFN-γ). Each was also found to have a mutation in the gene on chromosome 6q22–q23 that encodes the IFN-γ receptor 1 (IFN-γR1). A second type of defect was found in other patients who had disseminated mycobacterial infections and who were found to have mutations in the β1 chain of the IL-12 receptor (IL-12Rβ1). IL-12 is a powerful inducer of IFN-γ production by T and NK cells. The mutated receptor chain resulted in unresponsiveness of these patients' cells to IL-12 and inadequate IFN-γ production. Interestingly, both the IFN-γR1 and IL-12Rβ1–deficient children appeared not to be susceptible to infection with many agents other than mycobacteria. TH1 responses appeared to be normal in these patients. The susceptibility of these patients to mycobacterial infections thus apparently results from an intrinsic impairment of the IFN-γ pathway response to these particular intracellular pathogens, showing that IFN-γ is obligatory for efficient macrophage antimycobacterial activity.

126.14 Hyperimmunoglobulinemia E (Hyper-IgE) Syndrome

The hyper-IgE syndrome is a relatively rare primary immunodeficiency syndrome characterized by recurrent severe staphylococcal abscesses and markedly elevated levels of serum IgE. More than 200 patients with the condition have been reported. The inheritance pattern is as a single locus autosomal dominant trait with variable expression.

CLINICAL MANIFESTATIONS. These patients have histories from infancy of staphylococcal abscesses involving the skin, lungs, joints, and other sites; persistent pneumatoceles develop as a result of their recurrent pneumonias. The pruritic dermatitis that occurs is not typical atopic eczema, and it does not always persist; respiratory allergic symptoms are usually absent. In older children, delay in shedding primary teeth, recurrent fractures, hyperextensible joints, and scoliosis occur.

Laboratory features include exceptionally high serum IgE concentrations; elevated serum IgD concentrations; usually normal concentrations of IgG, IgA, and IgM; pronounced blood and sputum eosinophilia; abnormally low anamnestic antibody responses; and poor antibody and cell-mediated responses to neoantigens. In vitro studies have shown normal percentages of blood T, B, and NK lymphocytes, except that there is a decreased percentage of T cells with the memory (CD45RO) phenotype. Paradoxically, B cells from these patients demonstrate very low levels of IL-4–stimulated IgE synthesis in vitro, suggesting that they have already been maximally stimulated by a high level of endogenous IL-4. The molecular basis of this disorder remains unknown. Most patients have normal T-lymphocyte proliferative responses to mitogens but very low or absent responses to antigens or allogeneic cells from family members. Blood, sputum, and histologic sections of lymph nodes, spleen, and lung cysts show striking eosinophilia. Hassall corpuscles and thymic architecture are normal. Phagocytic cell ingestion, metabolism and killing, and total hemolytic complement activity are normal in all patients. Results of chemotaxis studies have been mostly normal; thus, defective chemotaxis is not the basic problem in this syndrome.

TREATMENT. The most effective therapy is long-term administration of therapeutic doses of a penicillinase-resistant antibiotic, adding other agents as required for specific infections. Intravenous immunoglobulin (IVIG) should be administered to antibody-deficient patients, and appropriate thoracic surgery should be provided for superinfected pneumatoceles or those persisting beyond 6 mo.

126.15 Treatment of Cellular Immunodeficiency

Transplantation of MHC-compatible or haploidentical (half-matched) parental bone marrow is the treatment of choice for patients with fatal T-cell or combined T- and B-cell defects. The major risk to the recipient from transplants of bone marrow is that of GVHD. The development of techniques to deplete all post-thymic T cells from donor marrow permits safe and successful use of haploidentical bone marrow stem cells for the correction of SCID and other fatal immunodeficiency syndromes. Patients with less severe forms of cellular immunodeficiency, such as some with CID, Wiskott-Aldrich syndrome, cytokine deficiency, or MHC antigen deficiency, reject even HLA-identical marrow grafts unless they are given chemoablative treatment before transplantation. Several patients with these conditions have been treated successfully with HLA-identical bone marrow transplantation after conditioning.

From 1968–1977, only 14 (or 29%) of 48 infants with SCID worldwide were long-term survivors after successful HLA class II compatible bone marrow transplantation. Possibly because of earlier diagnosis before untreatable opportunistic infections develop, the results of bone marrow transplantation have improved considerably during the past two decades. A more recent worldwide survey revealed that 224 of 285, or 79%, of patients with primary immunodeficiency transplanted with HLA-identical marrow over the past 30 yr survive. Most encouraging are the results of T-cell–depleted haploidentical marrow transplants in patients with primary immunodeficiency; 605 patients have had such transplants performed in the past 17 yr, and of these, 332 (or 55%) survive. The significance is even more impressive when it is realized that most of the 605 recipients would have died had not the T-cell depletion techniques been developed. The greatest success has been in patients with SCID, who do not require pretransplant conditioning or GVHD prophylaxis; 82% of 92 patients with SCID treated by the author during the past 17 years survive, and all but 12 received T-cell–depleted parental marrow. Until somatic cell gene therapy is more fully developed, bone marrow transplantation remains the most important and effective therapy for these inborn errors of the immune system.

Altare F, Durandy A, Lammas D, et al: Impairment of mycobacterial immunity in human interleukin-12 receptor deficiency. Science 280:1432, 1998.
Buckley RH, Schiff SE, Schiff RI, et al: Hematopoietic stem-cell transplantation for the treatment of severe combined immunodeficiency. N Engl J Med 340:508, 1999.
Buckley RH, Schiff RI, Schiff SE, et al: Human severe combined immunodeficiency (SCID): Genetic, phenotypic and functional diversity in 108 infants. J Pediatr 130:378, 1997.
Buckley RH, Wray BB, Belmaker EZ: Extreme hyperimmunoglobulinemia E and undue susceptibility to infection. Pediatrics 49:59, 1972.
de Jong R, Altare F, Haagen I, et al: Severe mycobacterial and *Salmonella* infections in interleukin-12 receptor-deficient patients. Science 280:1435, 1998.
Derry JMJ, Ochs HD, Francke U: Isolation of a novel gene mutated in Wiskott-Aldrich syndrome. Cell 78:635, 1994.
Fischer A, Malissen B: Natural and engineered disorders of lymphocyte development. Science 280:237, 1998.
Gilad S, Chessa L, Khosravi R, et al: Genotype-phenotype relationships in ataxia telangiectasia and variants. Am J Hum Genet 62:551, 1998.
Grimbacher B, Holland SM, Gallin JI, et al: Hyper-IgE syndrome with recurrent infections—an autosomal dominant multisystem disorder. N Engl J Med 340:692, 1999.
Klein C, Lisowska-Grospierre B, LeDeist F, et al: Major histocompatibility complex class II deficiency: Clinical manifestations, immunologic features, and outcome. J Pediatr 123:921, 1993.
Markert ML: Purine nucleoside phosphorylase deficiency. Immunodefic Rev 3:45, 1991.
Newport MJ, Huxley CM, Huston S, et al: A mutation in the interferon-gamma-receptor gene and susceptibility to mycobacterial infection. N Engl J Med 335:1941, 1996.
Puck JM, Pepper AE, Henthorn PS, et al: Mutation analysis of IL2RG in human X-linked severe combined immunodeficiency. Blood 89:1968, 1997.
Puel A, Ziegler SF, Buckley RH, et al: Defective IL7R expression in T(−)B(+)NK(+) severe combined immunodeficiency. Nat Genet 20:394, 1998.
Sharfe N, Dadi HK, Shahar M, et al: Human immune disorder arising from mutation of the alpha chain of the interleukin-2 receptor. Proc Natl Acad Sci U S A 94:3168, 1997.

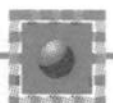

SECTION 3

The Phagocytic System

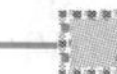

CHAPTER 127
Neutrophils

Laurence A. Boxer

THE PHAGOCYTIC INFLAMMATORY RESPONSE. Neutrophils and mononuclear phagocytes share primary functions including the unusual ability to ingest large particles. Neutrophils, however, are of only one type, but many varieties of mononuclear phagocytes exist (Chapter 128).

Neutrophils, monocytes, and eosinophils are derived from stem cell progenitors in the bone marrow. The hematopoietic progenitor system can be envisioned as a continuum of functional compartments (Table 127–1). The most primitive compartment is composed of very rare cells known as pluripotential stem cells, which have high self-renewal capacity. Pluripotential stem cells give rise to more mature stem cells, including cells that are committed to either lymphoid or myeloid development. Lymphoid stem cells give rise to T- and B-cell precursors and their mature progeny (Chapter 123). Trilineage myeloid stem cells, called CFU-S for the spleen colony-forming unit described in mice, eventually give rise to committed single-lineage progenitors of the recognizable precursors through a random process of lineage restriction in a stepwise process (Fig. 127–1). The lineage restriction arises from cell-surface expression of lineage-specific growth factor receptors. Single-lineage progenitors, including erythroid burst-forming units (BFU-E), erythroid colony-forming units (CFU-E), megakaryocyte colony-forming units (CFU-Meg), and basophil, granulocyte, monocyte, and eosinophil colony-forming units (CFU-Baso, CFU-G, CFU-M, and CFU-Eo, respectively) proliferate and differentiate into their respective precursors in response to the growth factors that bind to their unique receptors. The capacity of lineage-specific committed progenitors to proliferate and differentiate in response to demand constitutes the most important buffer of the hematopoietic system against increased requirement for mature blood cell production.

HEMATOPOIETIC GROWTH FACTORS. The proliferation, differentiation, and survival of immature hematopoietic progenitor cells are governed by a family of glycoproteins, the hematopoietic growth factors (HGFs; Table 127–2). Besides regulating proliferation and differentiation of progenitors, these factors influence the survival and function of mature blood cells. The HGFs include the interleukins and the colony-stimulating factors (CSFs), which have been named on their ability to stimulate progenitor cells to form colonies of recognizable mature cells in vitro. The majority of lineage-specific progenitors require the presence of additional growth factors such as interleukin 3 (IL-3) or granulocyte-macrophage (GM–CSF) in addition to a lineage-specific HGF to generate the colonies for which they are programmed. Hence, immature committed progenitors

TABLE 127–1 Neutrophil and Monocyte Kinetics

Neutrophils	
Average time in mitosis (myeloblast to myelocyte)	7–9 days
Average time in postmitosis and storage (metamyelocyte to neutrophil)	3–7 days
Average half-life in the circulation	6 hours
Average total body pool	6.5×10^8 cells/kg
Average circulating pool	3.2×10^8 cells/kg
Average marginating pool	3.3×10^8 cells/kg
Average daily turnover rate	1.8×10^{10} cells/kg
Mononuclear Phagocytes	
Average time in mitosis	30–48 hours
Average half-life in the circulation	36–104 hours
Average circulating pool (monocytes)	1.8×10^7 cells/kg
Average daily turnover rate	1.8×10^9 cells/kg
Average survival in tissues (macrophages)	Months

From Boxer LA: Function of neutrophils and mononuclear phagocytes. In: *Bennett JC, Plum F (eds): Cecil Textbook of Internal Medicine, 20th ed. Philadelphia, WB Saunders, 1996.*

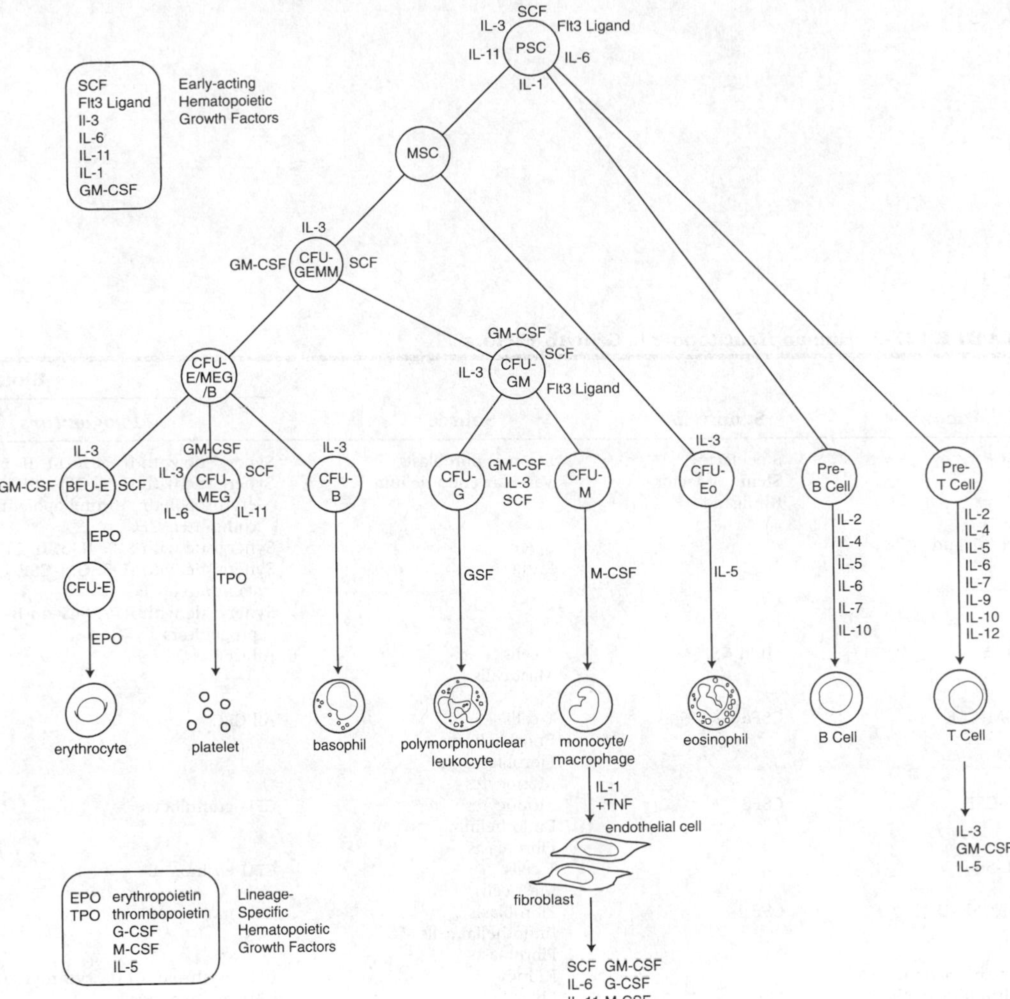

Figure 127–1 Major cytokine sources and actions. Cells of the bone marrow microenvironment such as macrophages (ma), endothelial cells (ec), and reticular fibroblastoid cells (fb) produce macrophage colony-stimulating factor (M-CSF), granulocyte-macrophage colony-stimulating factor (GM-CSF), granulocyte colony-stimulating factor (G-CSF), interleukin (IL-6), and probably stem cell factor (SCF; cellular sources not yet precisely determined) after induction with endotoxin (ma) or IL-1/TNF (ec, fb). T cells produce IL-3, GM-CSF and IL-5 in response to antigenic and IL-1 stimulation. These cytokines have overlapping actions during hematopoietic differentiation, as indicated, and for all lineages optimal development requires a combination of early- and late acting factors. PSC = pluripotent stem cells; MSC = myeloid stem cells; TNF = tumor necrosis factor. (Modified from Sieff CA, Nathan DG, Clark SC: The anatomy and physiology of hematopoiesis. *In:* Nathan DG and Orkin SH [eds]: Hematology of Infancy and Childhood, 5th ed. Philadelphia, WB Saunders, 1997.)

bear receptors for IL-3, stem cell factor (SCF), GM-CSF, and IL-6 (Fig. 127–2). These committed progenitors differ from one another with respect to their lineage-specific receptors; this allows the lineage-specific HGF to produce the colonies for which they are programmed. During granulopoiesis and monopoiesis, several cytokines regulate progenitor cells or mature effector cells at each stage of maturation and differentiation from the primitive pluripotent stem cells to nondividing terminally differentiated cells (monocytes, neutrophils, eosinophils, and basophils). The actions of these growth factors are mediated through lineage-specific receptors. As cells mature, they lose receptors for most cytokines, especially those that influence early cell development, such as SCF. Once the cells have matured, however, they express receptors for chemokines, which help direct the cells to sites of inflammation.

NEUTROPHIL MATURATION AND KINETICS. The bone marrow microenvironment supporting the progenitors and precursors must provide for the normal steady-state rates of renewal of the cellular elements of blood. Normally, the production rates precisely equal destruction rates. Granulocytes survive intravascularly for 6–12 hr. To maintain a level of circulating granulocytes of $5 \times 10^3/\mu L$ requires a daily production of $2 \times 10^4/\mu L$ of blood. In contrast, lymphocytes that can exhibit lifetimes measured in months or years require daily renewal of certain lymphocyte progenitors at rates substantially lower than the other hematopoietic progenitors.

The process of intramedullary granulocyte maturation involves changes in nuclear configuration and accumulation of specific intracytoplasmic granules (Table 127–2). The relatively small peripheral blood pool is compartmentalized into circulating and marginating pools. The peripheral blood pool provides entrance into the tissue and is buffered by an immense marrow reserve of identifiable precursors, some of which are undergoing mitosis and some of which are maturing into bands and neutrophils. Proliferation of myeloid cells consisting of approximately five divisions takes place only during the first three stages of neutrophil development (myeloblast, promyelocyte, and myelocyte). After the myelocyte stage, the cells terminally differentiate into metamyelocytes, bands, and neutrophils. Neutrophil maturation is associated with changes in the nucleus and with the production of azurophilic primary granules and specific or secondary granules. A myeloblast is a relatively undifferentiated cell with a large oval nucleus, a sizeable nucleoli, and a deficiency of granules. Promyelocytes acquire peroxidase-positive azurophilic granules, and myelocytes acquire specific granules. Chromatin condensation, loss of nucleoli, and the shape changes of the nucleus result in the morphometric characteristic of the segmented neutrophil.

NEUTROPHIL FUNCTION. Neutrophil responses are initiated as circulating neutrophils flowing through the postcapillary venules detect low levels of chemokines and other chemotactic substances released from a site of infection. These soluble effectors of inflammation trigger subtle changes in the array and activity of surface molecules on both endothelial cells and neutrophils. The initial associations are low affinity, reversible, and mediated primarily by cell-selectin-carbohydrate interactions. This leads to the phenomenon known as leukocyte "rolling," in which loose adhesions are made and broken, causing

TABLE 127–2 Human Hematopoietic Growth Factors

Factor	Synonym	Source	Biologic Activities	
			Progenitors	***Mature Cells***
SCF	Steel factor Stem cell factor Kit ligand	Stromal fibroblasts Vascular endothelium	Synergistic with IL-3, IL-11, IL-6 on blast CFC Synergistic with IL-3, GM-CSF, G-CSF, erythropoietin, thrombopoietin on committed CFC	Mast cell growth
Flt_3 ligand		Spleen Lung	Synergistic with SCF, IL-3, IL-11 on blast CFC Synergistic with IL-3, GM-CSF, G-CSF on committed CFC Synergistic with IL-7, SCF on B-cell progenitors	
IL-3	Multi CSF	T cells Mast cells	All CFC	Eosinophils B cells Monocytes
GM-CSF	CSFα	T cells Endothelium Fibroblasts Monocytes	All CFC	Neutrophils Monocytes Eosinophils
G-CSF	CSFβ	Monocytes Endothelium Fibroblasts	CFU-granulocyte	Neutrophils
IL-5		T cells Mast cells	CFU-eosinophil	Eosinophils
M-CSF	CSF-1	Fibroblasts Endothelial cells Fibroblasts	CFU-monocyte	Monocytes
Erythropoietin		Kidney	BFU-erythroid, CFU-erythroid	Erythroblasts
Thrombopoietin		Liver Kidney Fibroblasts Endothelium	CFU-megakaryocyte	Megakaryocyte
IL-1α		Monocytes Fibroblasts Endothelium	Synergistic with SCF, IL-3 on blast CFU	Activates cytokine production
IL-1β		Monocytes Fibroblasts Endothelium Kupffer cells Smooth muscle		
IL-6		Monocytes T cells B cells Fibroblasts Endothelium Kupffer cells	Synergistic: SCF, IL-3, on blast CFU	
IL-11		Stromal fibroblasts	Synergistic with SCF, IL-3 on blast CFC Synergistic with IL-3, SCF on CFU-megakaryocyte	Megakaryocytes

SCF = stem cell factor; CFC = colony-forming cell; CFU = colony-forming unit; BFU-E = erythroid burst-forming unit; IL = interleukin; GM-CSF = granulocyte-macrophage colony-stimulating factor; G-CSF = granulocyte colony-stimulating factor; M-CSF = monocyte colony-stimulating factor.

Modified from Sieff CA, Nathan DG, Clark SC: The anatomy and physiology of hematopoiesis. In: *Nathan DG, Orkin SH (eds): Hematology of Infancy and Childhood, 5th ed. Philadelphia, WB Saunders, 1997.*

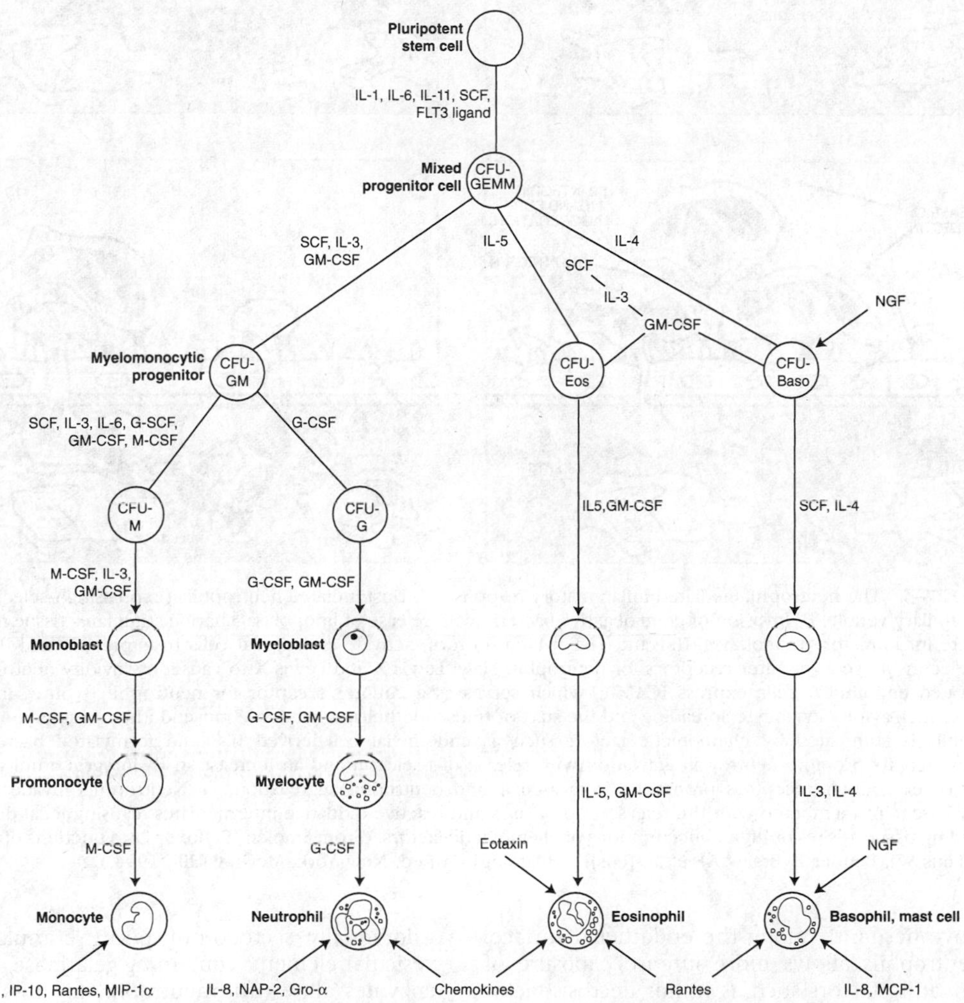

Figure 127–2 Various cytokines and chemokines that act at different levels of granulopoiesis and monocytopoiesis. Multiple cytokines regulate progenitor cells or mature effector cells at each stage of maturation/differentiation from the primitive pluripotent stem cell to nondividing terminally differentiated precursors (monocytes, neutrophils, eosinophils, and basophil/mast cells). The cytokines and chemokines also have varying degrees of specificity; some, such as M-CSF and IL-5, act predominantly on the monocytic and eosinophilic pathways, respectively, while others, such as CSF-GM, act on multiple granulocytic-monocytic (erythroid not shown) cell types. (Modified from Abboud CN, Liesveld JL: Granulopoiesis and monocytopoiesis. *In:* Hoffman R, Benz EB, Shattil SJ, et al [eds]: Hematology: Basic Principles and Practice, 2nd ed. New York, Churchill Livingstone, 1995.)

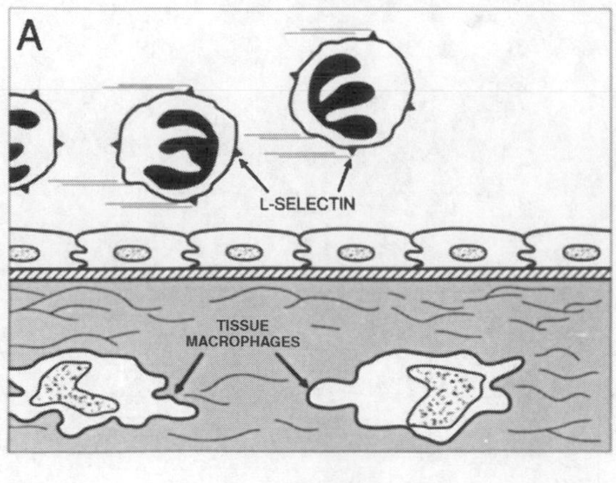

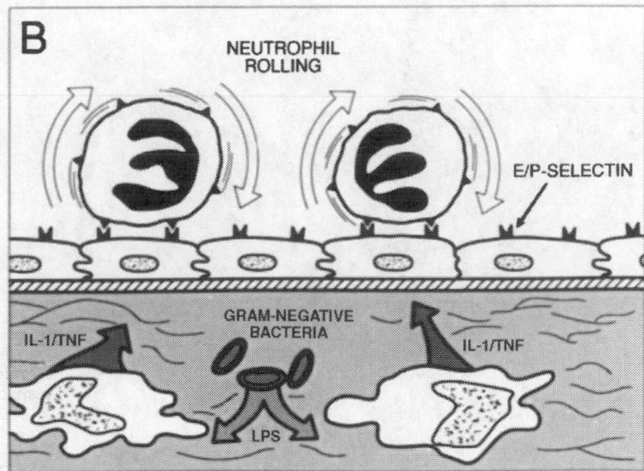

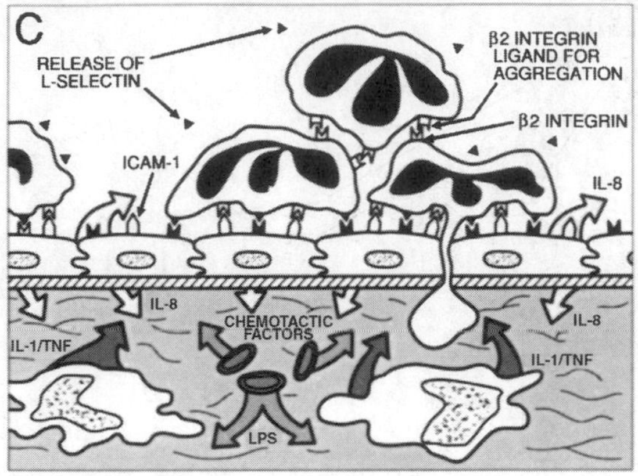

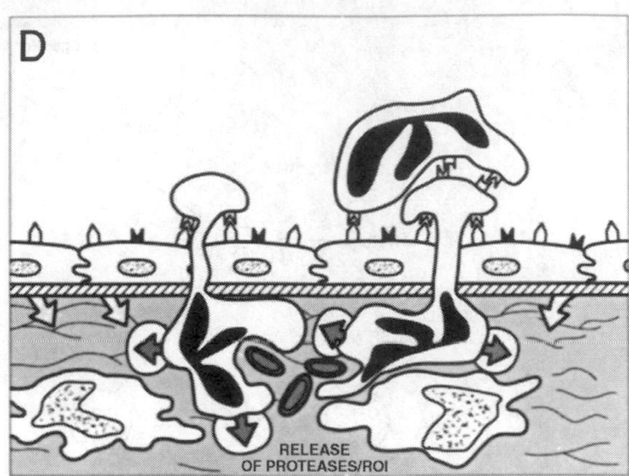

Figure 127–3 The neutrophil-mediated inflammatory response. *A*, Unstimulated neutrophils (expressing L-selectin) entering a post capillary venule. *B*, Invasion of gram-negative bacteria with release of lipopolysaccharide stimulates tissue macrophages to secrete inflammatory monokines, IL-1 and TNF, which, in turn, activate endothelial cells to express E- and P-selectins. E- and P-selectins serve as counter receptors for neutrophils sialyl Lewis X and Lewis X to cause low avidity neutrophil rolling. *C*, Activated endothelial cells express ICAM-1, which serves as a counter receptor for neutrophil β_2 integrin molecules, leading to high-avidity leukocyte spreading and the start of transendothelial migration. Transendothelial migration of activated neutrophils is stimulated by chemotactic factors such as endothelial cell-derived IL-8 and formylated bacterial factors. Chemoattractants promote neutrophil activation with release of L-selectin and an increase in β_2 integrin affinity for ICAM-1 and for other counter receptors promoting intravascular and neutrophil aggregation. *D*, Neutrophils invade through the vascular basement membrane with the release of proteases and reactive oxidative intermediates, causing local destruction of surrounding tissue at sites of high concentrations of chemotactic factors. (From Smolen JE, Boxer LA: Functions of neutrophils. *In:* Williams WJ, Beutler E, Erslev AJ, et al. [eds]: Hematology, 5th ed. New York, McGraw-Hill, 1994.)

neutrophils to move hesitantly along the endothelial surface. The rolling of neutrophils allows more intense exposure of neutrophils to activating factors such as tumor necrosis factor (TNF) or IL-1 (Fig. 127–3). This leads to induction of qualitative and quantitative changes in the family of β2 integrin adhesion receptors on the neutrophils (the CD11/CD18 group of surface molecules). The activated integrin receptors mediate tight heterotypic adhesion between neutrophils and endothelial cells and hemotypic adhesion of neutrophils with each other. The net result of these interdependent intercellular interactions is that neutrophils flatten onto the endothelial cells, while neutrophil/neutrophil and neutrophil/platelet aggregates partially occlude the venule and reduce blood flow.

The next phase involves loosening of the integrin adhesion through the process of mobilizing integrin receptors to the trailing pseudopod of the neutrophil. The neutrophil is able to displace its integrin receptors and undergo conformational changes allowing it to migrate between endothelial cell junctions into the extravascular tissue. Once through the endothelium, the neutrophil senses the gradient of chemokines or other chemoattractants and migrates to sites of infection. Neutrophil migration is a complex process involving rounds of receptor engagement, signal transduction, and remodeling of the actin-microfilaments composing in part the cytoskeleton. Additionally, secretion of specific granules or related secretory vesicular elements containing gelatinase, heparinase, and other enzymes allows the neutrophil to cross the basement membrane and transit through connective tissues. When the neutrophil reaches the site of infection, it recognizes pathogens by means of Fc immunoglobulin and complement receptors, fibronectin receptors, and other adhesion molecules.

The neutrophil ingests microbes that are opsonized (prepared for ingestion) by heat-soluble and heat-labeled factors in human serum that include immunoglobulin G (IgG) and C3, respectively. These opsonins facilitate phagocytosis of microbes, in which the pathogens are engulfed into a closed vacuole called a phagosome (Fig. 127–4).

As phagocytosis proceeds, two cellular responses essential for optimal microbicidal activity occur concomitantly, degranulation and activation of nicotinamide-adenine dinucleotide phosphate (NADPH)–dependent oxidase. Fusion of neutrophil granule membranes with the phagosome membrane occurs, resulting in the delivery of potent antimicrobial proteins into the phagosome. In coordinated succession, the contents of the specific granules and then contents of the azurophil granules are secreted into the phagosome. Occurring concomitantly are assembly and activation of NADPH oxidase at the phagosome membrane (Fig. 127–5). This enzyme generates large amounts

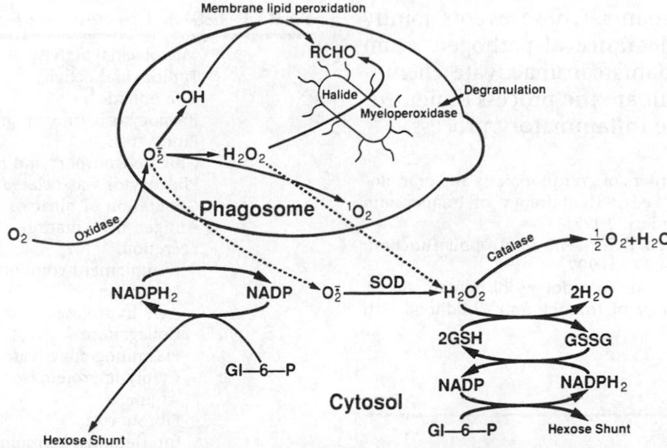

Figure 127–4 The mechanisms for the production, action, and detoxification of peroxides in neutrophils. Oxygen is reduced to superoxide (O_2^-) by an oxidase. NADPH is regenerated from NADPH by the hexose monophosphate shunt. Superoxide may spontaneously decompose to hydrogen peroxide in singlet oxygen ($^1O_2$). Hydrogen peroxide can react with superoxide to form hydroxyl radicals and generate bactericidal aldehydes (RCHO) by oxidizing bacterial constituents in the presence of halide ions and myeloperoxidase that were delivered to the phagosome by degranulation. Hydroxyl radicals (·OH) can peroxidize unsaturated fatty acids of the phagosomal membrane and thus yield the potentially bactericidal aldehydes. Hydrogen peroxide in the presence of myeloperoxidase and chloride ion can create hypochlorous acid (HOCl) in the phagosome. Superoxide leaking out of the phagosome may be converted rapidly to hydrogen peroxide by superoxide dismutase (SOD). Hydrogen peroxide in the cytosol is destroyed by catalase or reduced glutathione (GSH). Glutathione is regenerated by coupled reactions that stimulate the flow of glucose-6-phosphate (G-6-P) into the hexose monophosphate shunt. (Modified from Stossel TP, Boxer LA: Functions of neutrophils. *In:* William WJ, Beutler E, Erslev AJ, Lichtman MA [eds]: Hematology, 3rd ed. New York, McGraw-Hill, 1972.)

of superoxide (O_2^-) from molecular oxygen that in turn decomposes to produce hydrogen peroxide (H_2O_2) and singlet oxygen. H_2O_2 can react with O_2^- to form hydroxyl radicals. In the presence of myeloperoxidase (a major azurophil granule component), a reaction is catalyzed and uses H_2O_2 and ubiquitously present chloride ion to create hypochlorous acid (HOCl) in the phagosome. Although H_2O_2 and HOCl are microbicidal, evidence shows that these agents modulate host defense. First, these oxidants can denature proteins, making them more susceptible to proteolysis. Additionally, some of the neutrophil

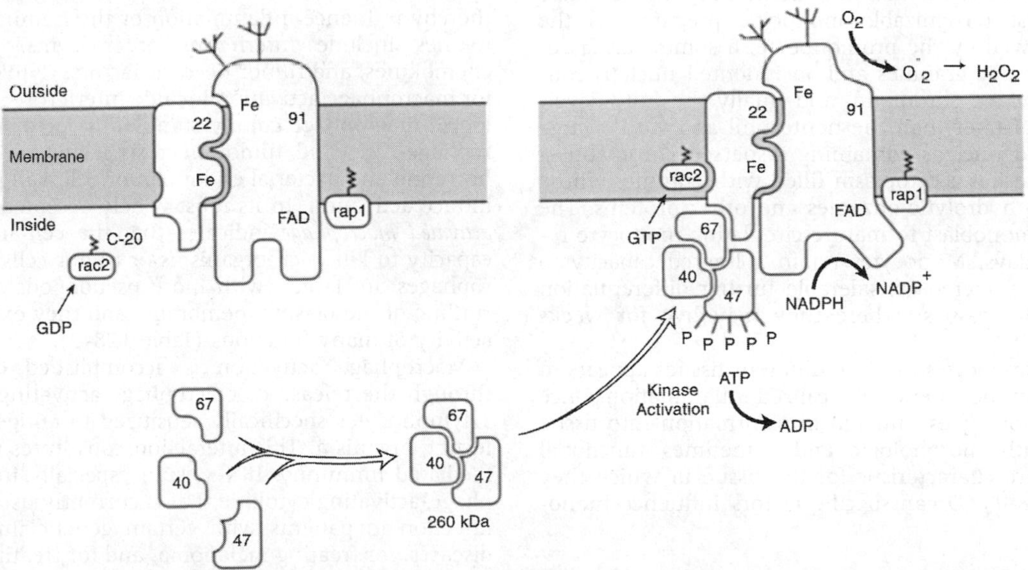

Figure 127–5 This is a modification of a hypothetical model of NADPH oxidase activation. Current knowledge suggests that the oxidase in its dormant state *(left)* is composed of both membrane-bound and cytosolic components. The former includes the gp91^{phox} and p22^{phox} subunits of cytochrome-b (and possibly Rap-1A). The flavin and heme groups (Fe) that mediate the transfer of electrons from NADPH to molecular oxygen are localized in the cytochrome. The cytosolic components p47^{phox} and p67^{phox} may exist as a preformed complex of 260 kDa, which may also include a third protein, possibly p40^{phox}. The small GTPase Rac2 is present in the cytosol in its inactive guanosine. Following phagocyte activation, the cytosolic complex translocates to the membrane, which may be under the control of the active guanosine triphosphate (GTP)-bound form of Rac2 and further regulated by phosphorylation of p47^{phox}. (Modified from Curnutte J, Orkin S, Dinauer M: Genetic disorders of phagocyte function. *In:* Stamatopyannopoulous G. [ed]: The Molecular Basis of Blood Diseases, 2nd ed. Philadelphia, WB Saunders, 1994.)

proteases are activated by the oxidants. These events jointly serve to enhance breakdown or clearance of pathogens from the site of infection. Also, the oxidants can inactivate chemotactic factors and may serve to terminate the process of neutrophil influx, thereby attenuating the inflammatory process.

Dinauer MC: The phagocyte system and disorders of granulopoiesis and granulocyte function. *In:* Nathan DG, Orkin SH (eds): Hematology of Infancy and Childhood, 5th ed. Philadelphia, WB Saunders, 1997.
Malech HL, Nauseef WM: Primary inherited defects in neutrophil function: Etiology and treatment. Semin Hematol 34:279, 1997.
Sieff CA, Nathan DG, Clark SC: The anatomy and physiology of hematopoiesis. *In:* Nathan DG, Orkin SH (eds): Hematology of Infancy and Childhood, 5th ed. Philadelphia, WB Saunders, 1997.

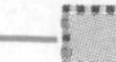

CHAPTER 128
Monocytes and Macrophages

Richard B. Johnston, Jr.

Mononuclear phagocytes (monocytes and macrophages) have a central and essential role in the immune response, in host defense against infection, and in tissue repair and remodeling. No human has been identified as having congenital absence of this cell line, probably because macrophages are required to remove primitive tissues during fetal development as new tissues develop to replace them. Monocytes and tissue macrophages in their various forms (Table 128–1) make up the *mononuclear phagocyte system.* These cells are a system because of their common origin, similar morphology, and common functions, particularly efficient phagocytosis.

DEVELOPMENT. Monocytes, the circulating precursors of tissue macrophages, develop more rapidly in the bone marrow and remain longer in the circulation than do neutrophils (see Table 127–1). The first recognizable monocyte precursor is the monoblast, followed by the promonocyte, a somewhat larger cell with cytoplasmic granules and an indented nucleus containing finely divided chromatin, and finally the fully developed monocyte. Larger than the neutrophil and with a large horseshoe-shaped nucleus containing dispersed chromatin, a mature monocyte has a cytoplasm filled with granules whose contents include hydrolytic enzymes and other proteins. The transition from monoblast to mature circulating monocyte requires about 6 days. Monocytes retain a limited capacity to divide, and they undergo considerable further differentiation after entering the tissues, where they may live for weeks to months.

Migration of monocytes into the different tissues appears to occur randomly in the absence of localized inflammation. Once in the tissues, monocytes undergo transformation into tissue macrophages with morphologic and sometimes functional properties that are characteristic for the tissue in which they reside (Table 128–1). Organ-specific factors influence monocyte differentiation and endow each tissue macrophage with particular metabolic and structural features. Monocytes in the liver become Kupffer cells that bridge the sinusoids separating adjacent plates of hepatocytes. Those in the lungs become large ellipsoid alveolar macrophages. All macrophages have at least three major functions in common: presentation of antigens, phagocytosis, and immunomodulation through release of various interleukins, interferons, growth factors, and cytokines. At sites of inflammation, monocytes and macrophages can fuse to form multinucleated giant cells, the terminal stage of development in the mononuclear phagocyte line.

TABLE 128–1 Principal Sites of Macrophages in Tissues

Liver (Kupffer cells)
Lung (interstitial and alveolar macrophages)
Connective tissue
Serous cavities (pleural and peritoneal macrophages)
Bone (osteoclasts)
Brain (reactive microglial cells)
Spleen, lymph node, bone marrow
Intestinal wall
Breast milk
Placenta
Granuloma (multinucleated giant cells)

TABLE 128–2 Upregulated Functions in Activated Macrophages

Microbicidal activity
Tumoricidal activity
Chemotaxis
Phagocytosis (most particles)
Pinocytosis
Glucose transport and metabolism
Phagocytosis-associated respiratory burst (O_2^-, H_2O_2)
Generation of nitric oxide
Antigen presentation
Secretion
Complement components
Lysozyme
Acid hydrolases
Collagenase
Plasminogen activator
Cytolytic proteinase
Arginase
Fibronectin
Interleukins, including IL-1, -10, -12, and -15
Tumor necrosis factor-α
Interferon-α and -β
Angiogenesis factor

O_2^- = superoxide anion; H_2O_2 = hydrogen peroxide.

ACTIVATION. The most important step in the functional maturation of macrophages is the conversion from a resting to an activated macrophage. Activation is driven primarily by certain cytokines, proteins that mediate signaling between cells and thereby influence inflammation or the immune response. Cytokines include interferons, interleukins, growth factors, chemokines, and tumor necrosis factors. Cytokines responsible for macrophage activation include interferon-γ (IFN-γ); granulocyte-macrophage colony-stimulating factor (GM-CSF); macrophage-CSF; and tumor necrosis factor-α (TNF-α). Growth hormone and bacterial endotoxin or cell wall proteins also can induce activation. In its most widely accepted sense, the term *activated macrophage* indicates that the cell has an enhanced capacity to kill microorganisms or tumor cells. Activated macrophages are larger, with more pseudopods and pronounced ruffling of the plasma membrane, and they exhibit accelerated activity of many functions (Table 128–2).

Macrophage activation is accomplished during infection through the release of macrophage-activating cytokines from T lymphocytes specifically sensitized to antigens from the infecting organism. This interaction constitutes the basis of cell-mediated immunity. IFN-γ is an especially important macrophage-activating cytokine that is currently used for preventing infection in patients with certain genetic immunodeficiency diseases, for treating melanoma, and for treating the decreased bone resorption of congenital osteopetrosis, which is caused by decreased function of osteoclasts (bone macrophages).

Macrophages exposed to endotoxin or other inflammatory mediators release TNF-α, which itself can activate macrophages. As macrophages become activated, they express greater numbers of receptors for TNF-α. Thus, macrophages at sites of inflammation have the potential to activate themselves and thereby achieve enhanced function more rapidly than through the classic cell-mediated immune response, which requires accumulation of a population of memory T lymphocytes. Conversely, macrophages, as well as helper T cells, secrete interleukin-10 (IL-10), which inhibits the production of IFN-γ and serves to suppress the potentially damaging effects of uncontrolled macrophage activation.

FUNCTIONAL ACTIVITIES. The principal functions of mononuclear phagocytes in host defense and the changes that take place in these functions when the macrophage is activated are summarized in Table 128–2. Obviously important are the ingestion and killing of such intracellular pathogens as *Mycobacterium tuberculosis, Listeria, Leishmania, Toxoplasma,* and some fungi, but macrophages also clear from the bloodstream and eliminate such extracellular pathogens as pneumococci. Killing of the ingested organisms depends heavily on products of the respiratory burst (e.g., hydrogen peroxide) and on nitric oxide, and release of these toxic metabolites is enhanced in activated macrophages.

The activity of mononuclear phagocytes against cancers in humans is less well understood. This activity may not involve the phagocytic process. Rather, macrophages may kill tumor cells by means of secreted products, including lysosomal enzymes, nitric oxide, oxygen metabolites, cytolytic proteinases, and TNF-α. Proteolytic enzymes and cytocidal factors present on the surface membrane of monocytes may have a role in tumor rejection.

Essential to the monocyte's protective function is its capacity to undergo diapedesis across the endothelial wall of blood vessels and to migrate to sites of microbial invasion in tissues. Chemotactic factors for monocytes include complement products and chemoattractants (chemokines) derived from neutrophils, lymphocytes, and other cell types. Phagocytosis of the invading organisms or cells can then occur, influenced by the presence or absence of opsonins for the invader (antibody, complement, mannose-binding and surfactant proteins), the inherent surface properties of the microorganism or tumor, and the state of activation of the macrophage.

Another important function of macrophages is disposal of cells that are damaged or dying. Macrophages lining the sinusoids of the spleen are particularly important in ingesting aged erythrocytes, which they differentiate from young ones through a special receptor. Macrophages are also involved in removing tissue debris and repairing wounds. Macrophages are phylogenetically primitive and can be identified early in fetal development, where they function to remove debris as one maturing embryonic tissue replaces another. They are also important in removing inorganic particles, such as elements of cigarette smoke or dust that enter the alveoli.

Macrophages are integrally involved in the induction and expression of specific immune responses, including antibody formation and cell-mediated immunity. This involvement depends on their capacity to break down foreign material in phagocytic and pinocytic vesicles and then present individual antigens on their surface as peptides or polysaccharides bound to class II major histocompatibility complex (MHC) molecules. B lymphocytes and, especially, dendritic cells can also present antigen and serve as "accessory cells" for the specific immune response. Expression of MHC class II molecules is increased in activated macrophages, and antigen presentation is more effective.

The heightened capacity of activated macrophages to synthesize and release various hydrolytic enzymes and potentially microbicidal materials (Table 128–2) probably plays a part in their increased killing capacity, although not every macrophage product is secreted in increased amounts when the cell is activated. The macrophage is an extraordinarily active secretory cell; approximately 100 distinct substances have been identified as being secreted by it, placing this cell in a class with the hepatocyte. Because of the profound effect of some of these secretory products on other cells, the large number of macrophages, and their widespread distribution, the mononuclear phagocyte system can be viewed as an important endocrine organ. IL-1 illustrates this point well. Microbes and microbial products, burns, ischemia-reperfusion, and other causes of inflammation or tissue damage stimulate the release of IL-1, mainly by monocytes and macrophages. In turn, IL-1 elicits fever, sleep, and release of IL-6, which induces production of acute phase proteins.

ABNORMALITIES OF MONOCYTE-MACROPHAGE FUNCTION. Mononuclear phagocytes, as well as neutrophils, from patients with *chronic granulomatous disease* exhibit a profound defect of phagocytic killing (Chapter 130). The inability of affected macrophages to kill ingested organisms leads to abscess formation and characteristic granulomas at sites of macrophage accumulation in the liver, lungs, spleen, and lymph nodes. Genetic deficiency of the CD11–CD18 complex of membrane adherence glycoproteins *(leukocyte adhesion defect),* which includes a receptor for opsonic complement component 3, results in impaired phagocytosis by monocytes (Chapter 130).

The monocyte-macrophage system is prominently involved in several *lipid-storage diseases* (sphingolipidoses; Chapter 83.3). In these conditions, the expression in macrophages of a systemic enzymatic defect permits the accumulation of cell debris that is normally cleared by macrophages. Resistance to infection can be impaired, at least partly because of impairment in macrophage function. *Gaucher disease* is the prototype for these disorders. In this condition, the enzyme glucocerebrosidase functions abnormally, thus allowing accumulation of glucosylceramide (glucocerebroside) from cell membranes in Gaucher cells throughout the body. In all locations, the Gaucher cell is an altered macrophage.

The cytokine IL-12 is a powerful inducer of IFN-γ production by T cells and natural killer cells. Individuals with inherited *deficiency in macrophage receptors for IFN-γ or lymphocyte receptors for IL-12* suffer a severe, profound, and selective susceptibility to infection by nontuberculous mycobacteria such as *Mycobacterium avium* or bacillus Calmette-Guérin (BCG).

Monocyte-macrophage function has been shown to be abnormal in various other clinical conditions. In most of these, however, the abnormality is partial and a suspected, though not a proven, cause of increased infection. For example, cultured mononuclear phagocytes of newborns are more readily infected than adult cells by human HIV-1 and measles virus. Macrophages from newborns release less G-CSF and IL-6, in culture, and this deficiency is accentuated in cells from preterm infants. This finding supports the observations that levels of G-CSF are significantly decreased in blood from term and preterm infants, and that the bone marrow granulocyte storage pool is diminished in infants, particularly those born before term. Macrophages from newborns are poorly activated by IFN-γ, which could weaken resistance to infection by intracellular pathogens.

The term *histiocyte* was originally used to describe cells thought to be macrophages in fixed tissue preparations. Since the discovery of dendritic cells in the late 1970s, it has become clear that histiocytosis X represents a malignancy-like overgrowth of Langerhans-type dendritic cells, not macrophages (Chapter 515). Thus, the term *Langerhans cell histiocytoses* is preferred for these disorders because *histiocyte* is a histologic term and not cell specific.

Borish L, Rosenwasser LJ: Update on cytokines. J Allergy Clin Immunol 97:719, 1996.

Johnston RB Jr: Function and cell biology of neutrophils and mononuclear phagocytes in the newborn infant. Vaccine 16:1363, 1998.

CHAPTER 129
Eosinophils

Laurence A. Boxer

Eosinophils are distinguished from other leukocytes by their morphology, constituent products, and association with specific diseases. Eosinophils are nondividing fully differentiated cells with a diameter of approximately 8 μm and a bilobed nucleus. They differentiate from stem cell precursors in the bone marrow under the control of T-cell–derived interleukin 3 (IL-3), IL-5, and granulocyte-macrophage colony-stimulating factor (GM-CSF). Their characteristic membrane-bound specific granules stain reddish brown with eosin and consist of a crystalline core made up of major basic protein (MBP) surrounded by matrix containing the eosinophil cationic protein (ECP), eosinophil peroxidase (EPO), and eosinophil-derived neurotoxin (EDN). These basic proteins are cytotoxic for the larval stages of helminthic parasites such as *Schistosoma mansoni*. They are also thought to contribute to much of the inflammation associated with asthma, causing sloughing of epithelial cells and contributing to clinical dysfunction (Chapter 145). Both eosinophil MBP and ECP are also present in large quantities in the airways of patients who have died of asthma and are thought to inflict epithelial cell damage that contributes to airway hyperresponsiveness. MBP has the potential to activate other proinflammatory cells including mast cells, basophils, neutrophils, and platelets. Eosinophils have the capacity to generate large amounts of the lipid mediators, platelet-activating factor (PAF) and leukotriene-C4, both of which can cause vasoconstriction and mucus hypersecretion. Eosinophils are a source of a number of proinflammatory cytokines including IL-1, IL-3, IL-5, and GM-CSF. Thus, eosinophils have a potent armory of mediators whose potential to initiate and sustain an inflammatory response is considerable.

Eosinophil migration from the vasculature into the extracellular tissue is mediated by the binding of leukocyte adhesion receptors to their ligands or counterstructures on the postcapillary endothelium. Similar to neutrophils, transmigration begins as the eosinophil selectin receptor binds to the endothelial carbohydrate ligand in loose association, which promotes eosinophils rolling along the endothelial surface until they encounter a priming stimulus such as a chemotactic mediator. Eosinophils then establish a high-affinity bond between integrin receptors and their corresponding immunoglobulin-like ligand. Unlike neutrophils, which become flattened before transmigrating between the tight junctions of the endothelial cells, eosinophils can use unique integrins, known as VLA-4, to bind to vascular cell adhesion molecule (VCAM)-1, which enhances eosinophil adhesion and transmigration through endothelium. These unique pathways account for selective accumulation of eosinophils in allergic inflammation. Eosinophils normally dwell primarily in tissues, especially tissues with an epithelial interface with the environment, including the respiratory, gastrointestinal, and lower genitourinary tracts. The life span of eosinophils may extend for weeks within tissues.

In addition to selectively enhancing eosinophil production as well as adhesion to endothelial cells, IL-5 also has a number of important effects on eosinophil function. Considerable evidence shows that IL-5 has a pivotal role in promoting eosinophil accumulation. It is the predominant cytokine in allergen-induced pulmonary late-phase reaction, and antibodies against IL-5 block eosinophil infiltration into the lungs in animal models associated with airway hyperresponsiveness following allergen challenge. Eosinophils also bear unique receptors for several chemokines. These include RANTES, eotaxin, monocyte chemotactic protein (MCP)–3, and MCP-4. These chemokines appear to be key mediators in the induction of tissue eosinophilia.

Blood eosinophil numbers do not always reflect the extent of eosinophil involvement in disease-affected tissues. Eosinophils usually number fewer than 450 cells/μL in the blood and vary diurnally, being more abundant in the early morning and diminishing as endogenous glucocorticoid levels rise. Eosinopenia occurs after corticosteroid administration and with active bacterial and viral infections.

DISEASES ASSOCIATED WITH EOSINOPHILIA. Many diseases are associated with eosinophilia (Table 129–1). The genesis of sustained eosinophilia in some patients remains unclear. Patients with sustained blood eosinophilia may develop organ damage, especially cardiac damage as found in the idiopathic hypereosinophilic syndrome, and should be monitored for evidence of cardiac disease.

Allergic Diseases. Allergy is the most common cause of eosinophilia in children in the United States. Acute allergic reactions may cause leukemoid eosinophilic responses with absolute eosinophil counts exceeding 20,000 cells/μL; chronic allergy is rarely associated with eosinophil counts of more than 2,000 cells/μL. Hypersensitivity drug reactions can elicit eosinophilia often not accompanied by drug fever or organ dysfunction. Various skin diseases have also been associated with eosinophilia, including atopic dermatitis, eczema, pemphigus, urticaria, and toxic epidermal necrolysis.

Infectious Diseases. Eosinophilia is often associated with infection with multicellular helminthic parasites. The level of eosin-

TABLE 129–1 Causes of Eosinophilia

Allergic disorders
- Allergic rhinitis
- Asthma
- Acute urticaria
- Hypersensitivity drug reactions

Infectious diseases
- Tissue-invasive helminth infection
  - Trichinosis
  - Toxocariasis
  - Strongyloidosis
  - Ascaris
  - Filariasis
  - Schistosomiasis
  - Echinococcosis
- *Pneumocystis carinii*
- Toxoplasmosis
- Amebiasis
- Malaria
- Bronchopulmonary aspergillosis
- Coccidioidomycosis
- Scabies

Malignant disorders
- Brain tumors
- Hodgkin disease and T-cell lymphomas
- Myeloproliferative disorders
- Acute myelogenous leukemia

Gastrointestinal disorders
- Inflammatory bowel disease
- Peritoneal dialysis
- Eosinophilic gastroenteritis
- Milk precipitin disease

Immunodeficiency disease
- Hyper-IgE syndrome
- Wiskott-Aldrich syndrome
- Graft vs host reaction

Pulmonary disease
- Loeffler's syndrome
- Eosinophilic leukemia
- Hypersensitivity pneumonias

Miscellaneous
- Thrombocytopenia with absent radii
- Vasculitis
- Postirradiation of abdomen
- Histiocytosis with cutaneous involvement

ophilia tends to parallel the magnitude and extent of tissue invasion, especially by larvae. Eosinophilia often does not occur in established parasitic infections that are well contained within tissues or are solely intraluminal in the gastrointestinal tract, such as *Giardia lamblia* and *Enterobius vermicularis*.

In evaluating patients with unexplained eosinophilia, the dietary history and geographic or travel history may indicate potential exposures to helminthic parasites. It is necessary to examine the stool for ova and larvae at least three times. Additionally, for many of the helminthic parasites that cause eosinophilia, the diagnostic parasite stages never appear in feces. Thus, normal results of stool examinations do not absolutely preclude a helminthic cause of eosinophilia, and diagnostic blood tests or tissue biopsy may be needed.

Two fungal diseases may be associated with eosinophilia: aspergillosis in the form of allergic bronchopulmonary aspergillosis (Chapter 233.1) and coccidioidomycosis (Chapter 236) following primary infection, especially in conjunction with erythema nodosum.

Hypereosinophilic Syndrome. The idiopathic hypereosinophilic syndrome is a leukoproliferative disease characterized by sustained overproduction of eosinophils. The three diagnostic criteria for this disorder are (1) eosinophilia of at least 1,500 cells/μL persisting for longer than 6 mo, (2) lack of another diagnosis to explain the eosinophilia, and (3) signs and symptoms of organ involvement. The clinical signs and symptoms of hypereosinophilic syndrome can be heterogeneous because of the diversity of potential organ involvement. One of the most serious and life-threatening complications is cardiac disease due to endomyocardial thrombosis and fibrosis. Other organ systems that can be involved can include the skin, liver, spleen, gastrointestinal tract, brain, and lungs. Therapy is aimed at suppressing eosinophilia and is initiated with corticosteroids. Hydroxyurea may be beneficial in patients unresponsive to corticosteroids. The underlying causes of hypereosinophilic syndrome remain unknown. For patients with prominent organ involvement and those who fail to respond to therapy, the mortality is approximately 75% after 3 years.

Miscellaneous Diseases. Eosinophilia is observed in many patients with primary immunodeficiency syndromes, especially hyper-IgE syndrome and Wiskott-Aldrich syndrome. Eosinophilia is also frequently present in syndromes of thrombocytopenia with absent radii and in familial reticuloendotheliosis with eosinophilia. Mild eosinophilia is found in 20% of patients with Hodgkin's disease and in gastrointestinal disorders including ulcerative colitis, Crohn's disease during symptomatic phases, gastroenteritis that is associated with milk precipitins, and chronic hepatitis.

Walsh GM: Human eosinophils: Their accumulation, activation, and fate. Br J Haematol 97:701, 1997.
Weller PF, Bubley GJ: The idiopathic hypereosinophilic syndrome. Blood 83:2759, 1994.

CHAPTER 130
Disorders of Phagocyte Function

Laurence A. Boxer

Neutrophils are particularly important in protecting the skin, mucous membranes, and lining of the respiratory and gastrointestinal tracts as part of the first line of defense against microbial invasion. During the critical 2–4 hr-period after microbial invasion, phagocytic cells must arrive at the site of inflammation if the infection is to be contained. If not, the resulting infection leads to a larger local lesion or disseminates throughout the host.

Immunologic evaluation of patients presenting with recurrent or unusual bacterial infections is formidable (Table 130–1). The differential diagnosis of diseases can be complicated by similar presentations of neutrophil defects or antibody or complement deficiency.

A thorough clinical history and physical examination, along with laboratory testing, are necessary to evaluate immune function (Chapter 122). Disorders of phagocyte function should be considered if results of initial screening tests (see Table 122–1) are normal and the patient has had recurrent or unusual bacterial infections (Fig. 130–1). Despite the rarity of the inherited phagocyte disorders, the understanding gleaned from evaluating the molecular mechanisms underlying the inherited disorders has contributed immensely to our knowledge of normal neutrophil function.

130.1 Chemotaxis

Direct migration of cells into sites of infection, chemotaxis, involves a complex series of events (Chapter 127). Studies of defective in vitro chemotaxis of neutrophils obtained from children having various clinical conditions have not established whether the increased number of infections arises from a chemotactic abnormality or secondary to medical complications of the underlying disorder (Table 130–1). The hyperimmunoglobulin E (hyper-IgE) syndrome is characterized by reduced neutrophil motility accompanied by markedly elevated levels of IgE leading to chronic dermatitis and recurrent sinopulmonary infections (Chapter 126).

130.2 Leukocyte Adhesion Deficiency

Leukocyte adhesion deficiency-1 (LAD-1) and -2 (LAD-2) are rare autosomal recessive disorders of leukocyte function (Table 130–1). LAD-1 affects about 1/10^6 individuals and is characterized by recurrent bacterial and fungal infections and depressed inflammatory responses despite striking blood neutrophilia.

PATHOGENESIS. *LAD-1* results from mutations of the gene on chromosome 21q22.3 encoding CD18, the 95-kd β_2 leukocyte integrin subunit. Normal neutrophils express three heterodimeric adhesion molecules known as LFA-1 (CD11a/CD18), Mac-1 (CD11b/CD18 (also known as CR3 or iC3b receptor), and p150, 95 (CD11c/CD18). These three transmembrane adhesion molecules are composed of unique α_1 subunits of 185, 190, and 150 kd, respectively, encoded on chromosome 16 and sharing a common β_2 subunit. This group of leukocyte integrins is responsible for the tight adhesion of neutrophils to the endothelial cell surface, their egress from the circulation, and their adhesion to iC3b-coated microorganisms, which promotes phagocytosis and particulate activation of the nicotinamide-adenine dinucleotide phosphate (NADPH) oxidase.

Mutations in the CD18 gene either impair or prevent mRNA production or affect the structure of the synthesized CD18 peptide, leading to abnormal post-translational processing and loss of the abnormal CD11/CD18. The CD11α_1 subunits are not stable as polymers, resulting in deficiency of LAD-1 neutrophils in the three CD11α_1 subunits. Some mutations of CD11/CD18 allow a low level of assembly and functional active integrin molecules. These children retain some neutrophil integrin adhesion function and have a moderate phenotype. In contrast, failure of neutrophils to bear the β_2 integrins leads to inability to migrate to sites of inflammation outside of the lung because of their inability to adhere firmly to surfaces

TABLE 130–1 Disorders of Phagocyte Dysfunction

Disorder	Etiology	Impaired Function	Clinical Consequences
Degranulation Abnormalities			
Chédiak-Higashi syndrome	Autosomal recessive; disordered coalescence of lysosomal granules	Decreased neutrophil chemotaxis, degranulation, bactericidal activity; platelet storage pool defect; impaired NK function, failure to disperse melanosomes	Neutropenia; recurrent pyogenic infections; propensity to develop marked hepatosplenomegaly in the accelerated phase; pigment dilution in skin and fundus
Specific granule deficiency	Autosomal recessive; abnormal regulation of expression of various myeloid granule genes by a transacting factor	Impaired chemotaxis and bactericidal activity; bilobed nuclei in neutrophils; reduced content of neutrophil defensins, gelatinase, collagenase, vitamin B_{12} binding protein, lactoferrin	Recurrent deep-seated skin abscesses
Adhesion Abnormalities			
Leukocyte adhesion deficiency 1 (LAD-1)	Absence of CD11/CD18 surface adhesive glycoprotein (β_2 integrins) on leukocyte membranes arising from failure to express CD18 mRNA	Decreased binding of complement to C3bi and endothelial ICAM-1 and ICAM-2	Neutrophilia, recurrent bacterial infections without pus
Leukocyte adhesion deficiency 2 (LAD-2)	Absence of sialyl-Lewis X	Decreased adhesion to inflamed endothelium	Neutrophilia, recurrent bacterial infections without pus
Neutrophil actin dysfunction	Impaired polymerization of neutrophil cytoplasmic actin perhaps arising from the presence of an inhibitor to F-actin formation	Impaired neutrophil chemotaxis, adhesion, and bacterial killing	Neutrophilia, recurrent bacterial infections without pus
Disorders of Chemotaxis			
Defects in the generation of chemotactic signals	IgG deficiencies, C3 deficiency, and properdin deficiency can arise from genetic or acquired abnormalities	Deficiency of serum chemotaxis and opsonic activities	Recurrent pyogenic infections
Intrinsic defects of the neutrophil such as in the newborn	Diminished ability to express neutrophil β_2 integrin function	Diminished chemotaxis	Mild propensity to develop pyogenic infections
Direct inhibition of neutrophil mobility by drugs	Ethanol, glucocorticoids, cyclic AMP	Impaired locomotion and ingestion, impaired adherence	Possible cause for frequent infections, neutrophilia seen with epinephrine is the result of cyclic AMP release from endothelium
Immune complexes	Bind to Fc receptors on neutrophils in patients with rheumatoid arthritis, systemic lupus erythematosus, other inflammatory states	Impaired chemotaxis	Recurrent pyogenic infections
Hyperimmunoglobulin E syndrome	Autosomal dominant; variable expression of a soluble inhibitor from mononuclear cells affecting neutrophil chemotaxis; high levels of antistaphylococcal IgE	Impaired chemotaxis at times, impaired IgG opsonization of *Staphylococcus aureus*	Recurrent skin and sinopulmonary infections
Defects of Microbicidal Activity			
Chronic granulomatous disease	Failure to express functional gp91^{phox} in the membrane in X-linked CGD; failure to express functional protein in the membrane in p22^{phox} (AR), other AR CGD arises from failure to express protein p47^{phox} or p67^{phox}	Failure to activate neutrophil respiratory burst, leading to failure to kill catalase-positive microbes	Recurrent pyogenic infections with catalase-positive microorganisms
G6PD deficiency	Less than 5% of normal activity of G6PD	Failure to activate NADPH-dependent oxidase	Infections with catalase-positive microorganisms
Myeloperoxidase deficiency	Failure to process post-translationally modified precursor protein due to a missense mutation	H_2O_2-dependent antimicrobial activity not potentiated by myeloperoxidase	None
Deficiencies of glutathione reductase and glutathione synthetase	Failure to detoxify H_2O_2	Excessive formation of H_2O_2	Minimal problems with recurrent pyogenic infections
Impaired Spleen Function			
Splenic absence or splenic dysfunction	Congenital absence of spleen, removal of spleen, vascular occlusion of spleen	Removal or impaired function of splenic macrophages	Propensity to infection with encapsulated bacteria

X = X-linked; AR = autosomal recessive; G6PD = glucose-6-phosphate dehydrogenase; CGD = chronic granulomatous disease; ICAM = intracellular adhesion molecule; NK = natural killer; C = complement; m = messenger; H_2O_2 = hydrogen peroxide; NADPH = nicotinamide-adenine dinucleotide phosphate; AMP = adenosine monophosphate.

Modified from Boxer LA: Qualitative abnormalities of granulocytes. In: *Williams WJ, Beutler E, Erslev AJ, Lichtman MA (eds): Hematology, 5th ed. New York, McGraw-Hill, 1994.*

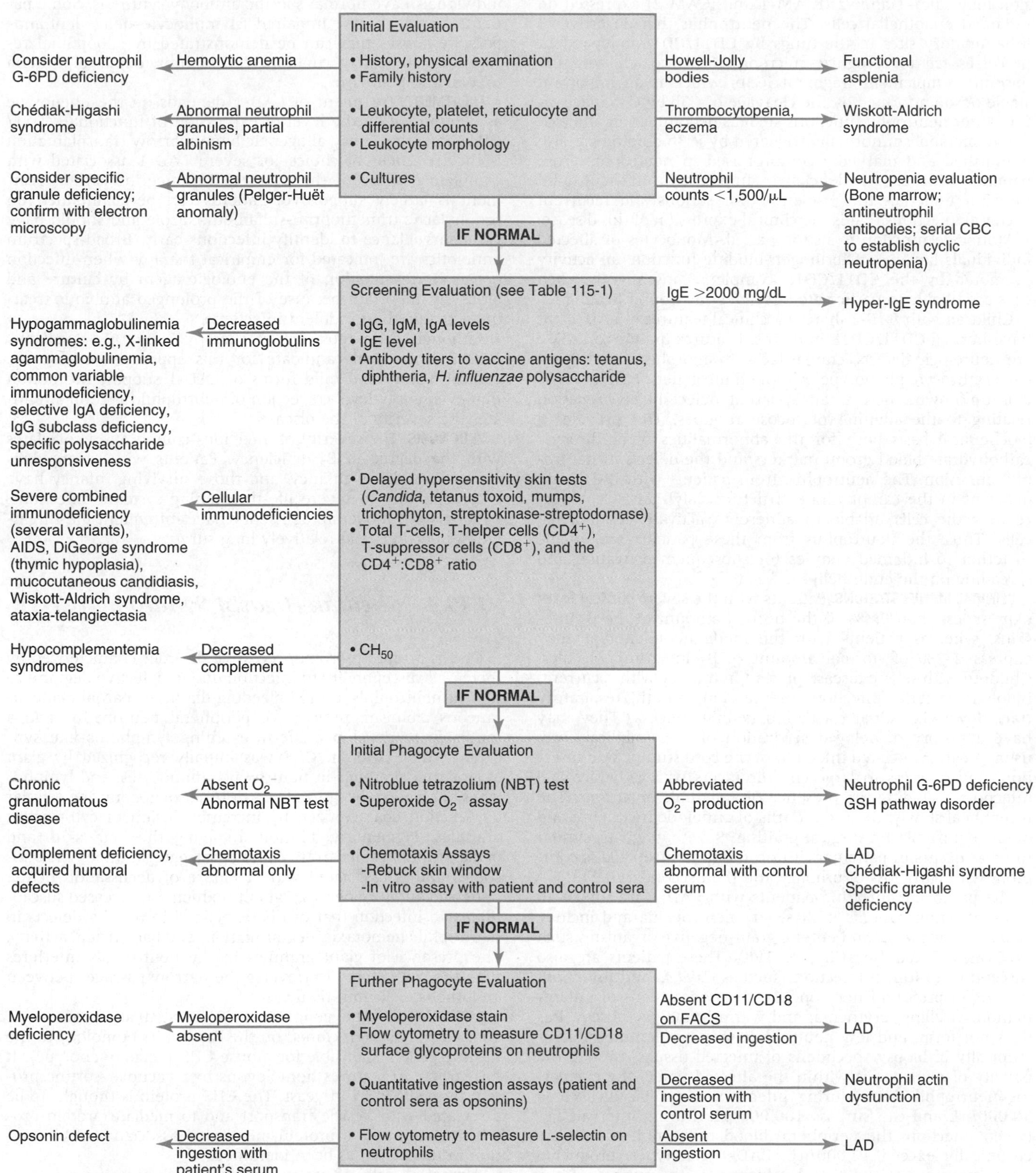

Figure 130–1 Algorithm for the evaluation of the patient with recurrent infections. CBC = Complete blood count; Ig = immunoglobulin; G-6-PD = glucose-6-phosphate dehydrogenase; LAD = leukocyte adhesion deficiency. (Modified from Curnutte JT: Chronic granulomatous disease: Clinical and genetic aspects. Ann Intern Med 109:138, 1988.)

and undergo transendothelial migration. Failure of the CD11/CD18-deficient neutrophils to undergo transendothelial migration occurs because the β_2 integrins bind to intracellular adhesion molecules–1 and -2 (ICAM-1 and ICAM-2) expressed on inflamed endothelial cells. The neutrophils that do arrive at inflammatory sites in the lungs by CD11/CD18-independent processes fail to recognize microorganisms coated with the opsonin complement fragment iC3b, which is an important stable opsonin formed by the cleavage of C3b by C3b inactivator. Other neutrophil functions such as degranulation and oxidative metabolism normally triggered by iC3b binding are also diminished and markedly compromised in neutrophils from patients with LAD-1 deficiency. Impairment in neutrophil function underlies the propensity for serious and recurrent bacterial infections that is the clinical expression of this disease.

Monocyte function is also impaired. Monocytes of affected individuals have poor fibrinogen-binding function, an activity promoted by the CD11/CD18 complex; consequently, such cells are unable to participate effectively in wound healing.

Children with *LAD-2* share the clinical features of LAD-1 but have normal CD11/CD18 integrins. Features unique to LAD-2 are neurologic defects, cranial facial dysmorphism, and Bombay erythrocyte phenotype. Although the genetic basis of LAD-2 is unknown, there is an apparent defect in glycosylation relating to the addition of fucose residues. This provides a biochemical basis both for the abnormalities of erythrocyte carbohydrate blood group markers and the defects in neutrophil adhesion. The neutrophils from patients with LAD-2 are deficient in the carbohydrate structure sialyl-Lewis X, which renders the cells unable to adhere to activated endothelial cells. Thus, the neutrophils from these patients are unable to tether to inflamed venules for subsequent activation and spreading on the endothelium.

CLINICAL MANIFESTATIONS. Patients with the severe clinical form express less than 0.3% of the normal amount of the β_2 integrins, whereas patients with the moderate phenotype may express 2–7% of normal amount of β_2 integrin molecules. Children with severe disease present in infancy with recurrent, indolent bacterial infections of the skin, mouth, respiratory tract, lower intestinal tract, and genital mucosa. They may have a history of delayed separation of the umbilical cord, usually with associated infection of the cord stump. Skin infection may progress to large chronic ulcers with polymicrobial infection, including the presence of anaerobic organisms. The ulcers heal slowly, require months of antibiotic treatment, and often require plastic surgical grafting. Severe gingivitis similar to what occurs in patients with profound neutropenia is common, with early loss of primary and then secondary teeth.

The pathogens infecting patients with LAD-1 are similar to those affecting patients with severe neutropenia and include *Staphylococcus aureus* and enteric gram-negative organisms such as *Escherichia coli* (see Chapter 198). These patients are also susceptible to fungal infections such as *Candida* and *Aspergillus* spp. As in profound neutropenia, the typical signs of inflammation, swelling, erythema, and warmth, may be absent. Pus does not form, and few neutrophils may be identified microscopically in biopsy specimens of infected tissues. Despite the paucity of neutrophils within the affected tissue, the circulating neutrophil count during infection may typically exceed 30,000/μL and can surpass 100,000/μL. During intervals between infection, the peripheral blood neutrophil count may chronically exceed 12,000/μL. LAD-1 genotypes, producing small amounts of functional integrins at the surface of the neutrophil, significantly reduce the severity and frequency of infections compared with children with the severe form.

LABORATORY FINDINGS. The diagnosis of LAD-1 is made most readily by flow cytometric measurements of surface CD11b in stimulated and unstimulated neutrophils using monoclonal antibodies directed against CD11b. Assessment of neutrophil and monocyte adherence, aggregation, chemotaxis, and iC3b-mediated phagocytosis generally demonstrates striking abnormalities that directly correspond to the molecular deficiency. Delayed-type hypersensitivity reactions are normal, and most individuals have normal specific antibody synthesis. Some patients, however, have impaired T-lymphocyte–dependent antibody responses that can be demonstrated by suboptimal responses to repeat vaccination with tetanus toxoid, diphtheria toxoid, and poliovirus.

TREATMENT. Treatment of LAD-1 depends on the phenotype as determined by the level of expression of functional CD11/CD18 integrins. Early allogeneic bone marrow transplantation is the treatment of choice for severe LAD-1 associated with complete absence of the CD11/CD18 integrins. Other treatment is largely supportive. Patients can be maintained on prophylactic trimethoprim-sulfamethoxazole and should have close surveillance to identify infections early. Broad-spectrum antibiotics are indicated for empirical therapy when infection occurs. Determination of the etiologic agent by culture and biopsy is important because of the prolonged antibiotic treatment required for indolent infections.

Although gene replacement therapy is not yet available, LAD-1 is an ideal candidate for this approach because the clinical history and mild forms of LAD-1 support the notion that even a low-level correction of neutrophil function attenuates the severity of the disease.

PROGNOSIS. The severity of infectious complication correlates with the degree of β_2 deficiency. Patients with severe deficiency may die in infancy, and those surviving infancy have a susceptibility to severe life-threatening systemic infections. Patients with moderate deficiency have infrequent life-threatening infections and relatively long survival.

130.3 Chédiak-Higashi Syndrome (CHS)

CHS is a rare autosomal recessive disorder characterized by increased susceptibility to infection due to defective degranulation of neutrophils, a mild bleeding diathesis, partial oculocutaneous albinism, progressive peripheral neuropathy, and a tendency to develop a life-threatening lymphoma-like syndrome (Table 130–1). CHS was initially recognized by giant cytoplasmic granules in neutrophils, monocytes, and lymphocytes but is now recognized as a disorder of generalized cellular dysfunction characterized by increased fusion of cytoplasmic granules. Pigmentary dilution involving the hair, skin, and ocular fundi results from pathologic aggregation of melanosomes and is associated with a failure of decussation of the optic and auditory nerves. Patients exhibit an increased susceptibility to infection that can be explained in part by defects in neutrophil chemotaxis, degranulation, and bactericidal activity. The presence of giant granules in the neutrophils interferes with the cell's ability to traverse the narrow passages between endothelial cells into tissue.

PATHOGENESIS. The gene for CHS, located at chromosome 1q42–q44, has been cloned on the basis of its homology to the murine gene responsible for mouse CHS (beige phenotype). It has structural features homologous to a vacuolar sorting protein termed VPS15 in yeast. The CHS protein is thought to be associated with vesicle transport and to mediate protein-protein interaction and protein-membrane associations. A mutation in this gene has been identified.

Almost all cells of patients with CHS show some aspect of the oversized and dysmorphic lysosomes, storage granules, or related vesicular structures. Melanosomes or melanocytes are oversized, and delivery to the keratinocytes and hair follicles is compromised because of the failure to properly disperse the giant melanosomes, resulting in hair shafts devoid of pigment granules. This leads to the macroscopic impression of hair and skin that is lighter than expected from parental coloration. The same abnormality in melanocytes leads to the partial ocular albinism associated with light sensitivity.

Beginning early in neutrophil development there is spontaneous fusion of giant primary granules with each other or with cytoplasmic membrane components, resulting in huge secondary lysosomes that contain reduced content of hydrolytic enzymes including proteinases, elastase, and cathepsin G. In turn, the deficiency of proteolytic enzymes may be responsible for the impaired killing of microorganisms by CHS neutrophils. Because the CHS blood cell membranes are more fluid than cells of normal individuals, it is possible that the altered membrane structure could lead to defective regulation of membrane activation. Changes in membrane fluidity may conceivably affect cell function by altering expression of membrane receptors. This could result in the elevated levels of intracellular cyclic adenosine monophosphate, disordered assembly of microtubules, and defective interaction of microtubules with lysosome membranes. The latter have been reported in this disorder.

CLINICAL MANIFESTATIONS. Patients with CHS have light skin and silvery hair. They frequently complain of solar sensitivity and photophobia. Other signs and symptoms vary considerably, but frequent infections and neuropathy are common. The infections involve mucous membranes, skin, and respiratory tract. Affected children are susceptible to gram-positive and gram-negative bacteria and fungi, with *S. aureus* being the most common offending organism. The neuropathy may be sensory or motor in type, and ataxia may be a prominent feature. Neuropathy often begins in the teenage years and becomes the most prominent problem.

Patients with CHS have prolonged bleeding times with normal platelet counts, resulting in impaired platelet aggregation associated with a deficiency of the dense granules containing adenosine diphosphate and serotonin. Natural killer cell function is also impaired.

The most life-threatening complication of CHS is the development of an accelerated phase of a lymphoma-like syndrome characterized by pancytopenia, high fever, and lymphohistiocytic infiltration of liver, spleen, and lymph nodes. The accelerated phase may occur at any age. The onset of this accelerated phase may be related to the inability of these patients to contain and control Epstein-Barr virus infection, which leads to features simulating virus-mediated hemophagocytic syndrome. The lymphocytic proliferation is associated with recurrent bacterial and viral infections and usually results in death. At autopsy, the lymphohistiocytic infiltrates in the liver, spleen, and lymph nodes are extensive but are not neoplastic by histopathologic criteria.

LABORATORY FINDINGS. The diagnosis of CHS is established by finding large inclusions in all nucleated blood cells. These can be seen on Wright-stained blood films but are accentuated by a peroxidase stain.

TREATMENT. High-dose ascorbic acid (200 mg/24hr for infants, 2,000 mg/24 hr for adults) improves the clinical status of some children in the stable phase. Although controversy surrounds the efficacy of ascorbic acid, given the safety of the vitamin, it is reasonable to administer ascorbic acid to all patients.

The only curative therapy for the accelerated phase is bone marrow transplantation from an HLA-compatible donor or an unrelated donor compatible at the D locus. Marrow transplantation reconstitutes normal hematopoietic and immunologic function and corrects the natural killer cell deficiency in patients entering the accelerated phase. However, bone marrow transplantation does not correct or prevent the peripheral neuropathy.

130.4 Myeloperoxidase Deficiency

Myeloperoxidase (MPO) deficiency is a disorder of oxidative metabolism (Table 130–1) and is one of the most common inherited disorders of phagocytes, occurring at a frequency approaching 1/4,000 individuals. MPO is a green heme protein located in the azurophilic lysosomes of neutrophils and monocytes and is the basis for the greenish tinge to pus accumulated at a site of infection. Most individuals with the trait do not have an increased rate of infection or other clinical manifestations of disease.

PATHOGENESIS. Mutations in the MPO gene causing this defect have been defined and provide insight into the post-translational processing of this granule protein. MPO mRNA is transcribed exclusively during the promyelocytic stage of granulopoiesis. The primary translation product of the MPO gene is a single-chain peptide of 80kd that undergoes co-translational glycosylation followed by a series of modifications of the oligosaccharides. MPO deficiency is caused by a missense mutation in the MPO gene that replaces an arginine with tryptophan and results in an MPO precursor that does not incorporate heme. Although this mutation is the most common cause of MPO deficiency, many patients are compound heterozygotes with one allele bearing the common mutation and the other being normal or possessing a mutation not yet identified. A partial deficiency results if only one allele is normal.

Partial or complete MPO deficiency leads to diminished production of hypochlorous acid (HOCl) and HOCl-derived chloramines. The deficiency in HOCl leads to early depression of gram-positive and gram-negative bacterial rates of killing in vitro that normalizes after 1 hr incubation. These data indicate that deficient cells use an MPO-independent microbicidal system that is slower to kill pathogens than the MPO-H_2O_2-halide system used by normal neutrophils.

CLINICAL MANIFESTATIONS. MPO deficiency usually is clinically silent. Rarely, patients may have disseminated candidiasis, usually in conjunction with diabetes.

Acquired partial MPO deficiency can be seen in acute myelogenous leukemia and in myelodysplastic syndromes.

LABORATORY FINDINGS. Deficiency of neutrophil and monocyte MPO can be identified by histochemical analysis.

TREATMENT. There is no specific therapy. The prognosis is usually excellent. Aggressive treatment with antifungal agents should be used in patients with candidal infections.

130.5 Chronic Granulomatous Disease

Chronic granulomatous disease (CGD) is characterized by the ability of neutrophils and monocytes to ingest but their inability to kill catalase-positive microorganisms because of a defect in the generation of microbial oxygen metabolites (Table 130–1). CGD is a rare disease with an incidence of 4–5 per million, caused by genes affecting one X-linked and three autosomal recessive chromosomes.

PATHOGENESIS. Activation of NADPH oxidase requires stimulation of the neutrophils and involves assembly from cytoplasmic and integral membrane subunits. Oxidase activation initially arises from phosphorylation of a cationic cytoplasmic protein, $p47^{phox}$ (47kd "phagocyte oxidase" protein). Phosphorylated $p47^{phox}$ together with two other cytoplasmic components of the oxidase, $p67^{phox}$ and a low molecular weight guanine triphosphatase (Rac-2), translocates to the membrane where they interact with the cytoplasmic domains of the transmembrane flavocytochrome b_{558} to form the active oxidase (see Fig. 127–5). The flavocytochrome is a heterodimer of two peptides $p22^{phox}$ and highly glycosylated $gp91^{phox}$. Current models are consistent with three transmembrane domains within the N-terminus of the flavocytochrome that contain the histidines that coordinate heme binding. The role of $p22^{phox}$ peptide is required for stability of $gp91^{phox}$ and for oxidase activity. The role of $p40^{phox}$ in oxidase activation remains unclear. The $gp91^{phox}$ peptide is required for electron transport through use of a NADPH-binding domain, a flavin-binding domain, and a heme-binding domain. In turn, the gp91^{phox} is stabilized by p22^{phox}. Furthermore, p22^{phox} provides a docking site for the cytoplasmic subunits. The cytoplasmic p47^{phox}, p67^{phox}, and Rac-2 appear to serve as regulatory elements for activation of cytochrome b_{558}.

Approximately two thirds of patients with CGD are males who inherit their disorder as a result of mutations in the X-chromosome gene encoding gp91^{phox}. About one third of patients inherit CGD in an autosomal recessive fashion resulting from mutations in the gene encoding p47^{phox} on chromosome 7. Defects in the genes encoding p67^{phox} (chromosome 1) or p22^{phox} (chromosome 16) also occur; these are inherited in an autosomal recessive manner and account for about 5% of cases of CGD.

Effective neutrophil phagocytosis requires activation of NADPH-dependent oxidase (Chapter 127). After activation of neutrophils, electrons are passed from NADPH to flavin and then to the heme prosthetic group on cytochrome b_{558} and finally to molecular oxygen to form O_2^- mutations in the gene for cytochrome b_{558}. Alternatively, the cytosolic factor renders the electron transport system ineffective in generating O_2^-.

The metabolic deficiency of the CGD neutrophil predisposes the host to infection; the CGD phagocytic vacuoles remain acidic, and the bacteria are not digested properly (Fig. 130–2). Hematoxylin-eosin–stained sections from patients' macrophages may contain a golden pigment that reflects this abnormal accumulation of ingested material and contributes to the diffuse granulomas that give CGD its descriptive name.

CLINICAL MANIFESTATIONS. Although the clinical presentation is variable, several features suggest the diagnosis of CGD. Any patient with recurrent or unusual lymphadenitis, hepatic abscesses, osteomyelitis at multiple sites, a family history of recurrent infections, or unusual infections with catalase-positive organisms (e.g., *S. aureus*) require clinical evaluation for this disorder.

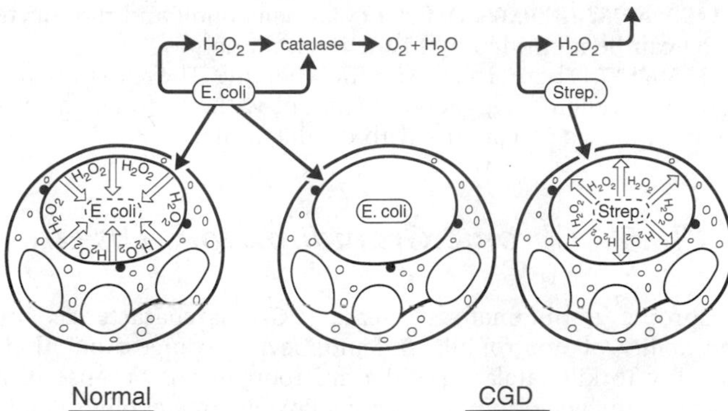

Figure 130–2 The pathogenesis of chronic granulomatous disease (CGD). The manner in which the metabolic deficiency of the CGD neutrophil predisposes the host to infection is shown schematically. Normal neutrophils stimulate hydrogen peroxide in the phagosome containing ingested *Escherichia coli*. Myeloperoxidase is delivered to the phagosome by degranulation, as indicated by the closed circles. In this setting, hydrogen peroxide acts as a substrate for myeloperoxidase to oxidize halide to hypochlorous acid in chloramines that kill the microbes. The quantity of hydrogen peroxide produced by the normal neutrophil is sufficient to exceed the capacity of catalase, a hydrogen peroxide-catabolizing enzyme of many aerobic microorganisms, including most gram-negative enteric bacteria, *Staphylococcus aureus, Candida albicans,* and *Aspergillus* spp. When organisms such as *E. coli* gain entry into CGD neutrophils, they are not exposed to hydrogen peroxide because the neutrophils do not produce it, and the hydrogen peroxide generated by microorganisms themselves is destroyed by their own catalase. When CGD neutrophils ingest streptococci or pneumococci, these organisms, which lack catalase, generate enough hydrogen peroxide to result in a microbicidal effect. As indicated *(middle)*, catalase-positive microbes such as *E. coli* can survive within the phagosome of the CGD neutrophil. (From Boxer LA: Neutrophil disorders: Qualitative abnormalities of the neutrophil. *In:* Williams WJ, Beutler E, Erslev AJ, et al [eds]: Hematology, 5th ed. New York, McGraw-Hill, 1994.)

The onset of clinical signs and symptoms may occur from early infancy to young adulthood. The attack rate and severity of infections are exceedingly variable. The most common pathogen is *S. aureus,* although any catalase-positive microorganisms may be involved. Infections with *Serratia marcescens, Pseudomonas cepacia, Aspergillus* spp, *Candida albicans,* and *Mycobacterium tuberculosis* occur most frequently. Pneumonias, lymphadenitis, and skin infections are the most common infections encountered. Patients may suffer from the sequelae of chronic infection, including the anemia of chronic disease, lymphadenopathy, hepatosplenomegaly, chronic purulent dermatitis, restrictive lung disease, gingivitis, hydronephrosis, and gastroenteral narrowing. Perirectal abscesses and recurrent skin infections, including folliculitis, cutaneous granulomas, and discoid lupus erythematosus also suggest the possibility of CGD.

LABORATORY FINDINGS. For screening of CGD, the nitroblue tetrazolium (NBT) dye test is still widely used, but it is rapidly being replaced by the more accurate flow cytometry test using dihydrorhodamine 123 fluorescence (DHR test). DHR detects oxidant production because it increases fluorescence when oxidized by H_2O_2.

Neutrophils from patients with CGD have normal glucose-6-phosphate dehydrogenase (G6PD) activity. However, a few individuals with apparent CGD have been described as having neutrophils deficient in G6PD activity. The erythrocytes of these patients also lack the enzyme, and the patients have chronic hemolysis. CGD and G6PD deficiency can be distinguished by the hemolytic anemia associated with G6PD deficiency and by the normal erythrocyte G6PD activity in CGD compared with the markedly reduced activity in G6PD deficiency.

Granuloma formation and inflammatory processes are a hallmark of CGD and may be the presenting symptoms that prompt testing for CGD. Examples are pyloric outlet obstruction, bladder outlet obstruction, and rectal fistula simulating Crohn's disease.

TREATMENT. Marrow transplantation is the only known cure for CGD. Vigorous supportive care along with recombinant interferon-γ is used before transplantation. As part of supportive care, patients with CGD should be given daily oral trimethoprim-sulfamethoxazole for infection prophylaxis. Cultures must be obtained as soon as infection is suspected. Most abscesses require surgical drainage for therapeutic and diagnostic purposes. Prolonged use of antibiotics is often required. If fever occurs without an obvious focus, it is advisable to consider the use of roentgenograms of the chest and skeleton as well as CT scans of the liver to determine if pneumonia, osteomyelitis, or liver abscesses are present. The cause of fever cannot always be established, and enteric empirical treatment with broad-spectrum parental antibiotics is often required. The erythrocyte sedimentation rate may be used to help determine the duration of antibiotic treatment.

Aspergillus spp infection requires treatment with amphotericin B. Corticosteroids may also be useful for the treatment of children with antral and urethral obstruction. Granulomas may be sensitive to low doses of prednisone (0.5 mg/24hr); treatment should be tapered over several weeks.

Interferon-γ (50 μg/m^2, three times per week) can reduce the number of serious infections. The mechanism of action of interferon-γ therapy in CGD is unknown. In the future, somatic gene therapy may be used to correct defective phagocyte oxidase function in selected patients with CGD.

Genetic Counseling. Identifying a patient's specific genetic subgroup is useful primarily for genetic counseling and prenatal diagnosis. In cases of suspected X-linked CGD, further analysis is not necessary if the fetus is initially demonstrated to be a 46,XX female. Fetal blood sampling and NBT slide test analysis of fetal neutrophils can be used for prenatal diagnosis of CGD. DNA analysis of amniotic fluid cells or chorionic villus biopsy is an option for early prenatal diagnosis of CGD. Restriction fragment polymorphisms have been identified for gp91^{phox} and p67^{phox} and have proved useful for diagnosis. In families in which the specific mutation is known, prenatal diagnosis is made by analysis of fetal DNA for the presence of mutant alleles using the polymerase chain reaction.

PROGNOSIS. The overall mortality rate for CGD is about two patient deaths/year/100 cases followed. The mortality rate is highest in young children. The long-term prognosis for patients with CGD has greatly improved during the past 20 yr. This can be attributed to an increased understanding of the biology of CGD, the development of effective infection prophylactic regimens, close surveillance for signs of infections, and aggressive surgical and medical interventions.

Boxer LA: Neutrophil disorders: Qualitative abnormalities of the neutrophil. *In:* Williams WJ, Beutler, E, Erslev AJ, et al (eds): Hematology, 5th ed. New York, McGraw-Hill, 1994.

Malech HL, Nauseef WA: Primary inherited defects in neutrophil function: Etiology and treatment. Semin Hematol 34:279, 1997.

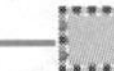

CHAPTER 131
Leukopenia

Laurence A. Boxer

Marked developmental changes in normal values for the white blood cell (WBC) count occur during childhood (Chapter 726). The mean WBC count at birth is high, followed by a rapid fall beginning at 12 hr until the end of the first week. Thereafter, values are stable until 1 yr of age. A slow, steady decline in the WBC count subsequently continues throughout childhood until the value characteristic of an adult is reached in adolescence. Leukopenia in adults is defined as a total WBC count less than 4,000/μL. Evaluation of patients with leukopenia, neutropenia, or lymphopenia begins with a through history, physical examination, family history, and screening laboratory tests (Fig. 131–1).

131.1 Neutropenia

Neutropenia is an absolute neutrophil count (ANC = total WBC count/μL × per cent of neutrophils and bands) more than two standard deviations below the normal mean. Normal neutrophil counts must be stratified for age and race. For whites, the lower limit of normal for the neutrophil count is 1,500/μL; for blacks, the lower limit of normal is 1,200/μL. The relatively low counts in blacks probably reflect a relative decrease in neutrophils in the storage compartment of the bone marrow.

Acute neutropenia evolving over a few days often occurs when neutrophil use is rapid and production is compromised. Chronic neutropenia lasting months or years usually arises from reduced production or excessive splenic sequestration of neutrophils. Neutropenia may be classified by whether it arises secondary to factors extrinsic to marrow myeloid cells (Table 131–1), which is common, or whether an intrinsic defect, which is rare, affects the myeloid progenitors (Table 131–2).

Neutropenia may be characterized as mild, with cell counts of 1,000–1,500/μL; moderate, with counts of 500–1,000/μL; or severe, with counts below 500/μL. This stratification aids in predicting the risk of pyogenic infection because only patients with severe neutropenia have significantly increased susceptibility to life-threatening infections.

INFECTIOUS CAUSES. Transient neutropenia often accompanies viral infections. Neutropenia associated with common childhood viral disease occurs during the first 1–2 days of illness and may persist for 3–8 days. It usually corresponds to a period of acute viremia and is related to virus-induced redistribution of neutrophils from the circulating to the marginal pool. Neutrophil sequestration possibly occurs after virus-induced tissue damage. Moderate to severe neutropenia may also be associated with a wide variety of other infectious causes (Table 131–3). Bacterial sepsis is a particularly serious cause of neutropenia.

Chronic neutropenia often accompanies infection with HIV-1, associated with AIDS. The neutropenia associated with AIDS probably arises from a combination of impaired neutrophil production and the accelerated destruction of neutrophils by antibodies.

DRUG-INDUCED NEUTROPENIA. Drug use remains one of the most common causes of neutropenia (Table 131–4). The incidence of drug-induced neutropenia increases precipitously with age; only 10% of cases occur in children and young adults, whereas more than 50% of cases occur in adults. Drug-induced neutropenia has several underlying mechanisms (i.e., immune-mediated, toxic, idiosyncratic, or hypersensitivity reactions) and should be differentiated from the severe neutropenia that predictably occurs after large doses of cytoreductive cancer drugs or radiotherapy (Table 131–4). Cytotoxic chemotherapy induces neutropenia because of the high proliferative rate of neutrophil precursors and the rapid turnover of blood neutrophils.

Immune-mediated neutropenia usually lasts for 1 wk and is thought to arise from effects of drugs, such as propylthiouracil or penicillin, that act as haptens to stimulate antibody formation. Other drugs, including the antipsychotic drugs such as the phenothiazines, can cause neutropenia when given in toxic amounts. In contrast, idiosyncratic reactions, such as to chloramphenicol, are unpredictable with regard to dose or duration of use. Hypersensitivity reactions are rare and occasionally may involve arene oxide metabolites of aromatic anticonvulsants. Fever, rash, lymphadenopathy, hepatitis, nephritis, pneumonitis, or aplastic anemia may often be associated with hypersensitivity-induced neutropenia. Acute hypersensitivity reactions such as those caused by phenytoin or phenobarbital may last for only a few days if the offending drug is discontinued. Chronic hypersensitivity may last for months to years. Drug-induced neutropenia may occasionally be asymptomatic despite severely reduced numbers of neutrophils and is noted only because of regular monitoring of WBC counts during drug therapy.

Neutropenia accompanying the use of anticancer drugs or radiation therapy (especially therapy directed at the pelvis or sternum) is a common cause of neutropenia, secondary to the effects of the cytotoxicity on replicating cells. A decline in the WBC count typically occurs 7–10 days after administration of the anticancer drug and may persist for 2–3 wk. The neutropenia accompanying both malignancy and the use of cancer chemotherapy is frequently associated with compromised cellular immunity, thereby predisposing patients to a much greater risk of infection than those disorders associated with isolated neutropenia (Chapter 179).

BONE MARROW REPLACEMENT. Various acquired disorders may lead to neutropenia accompanied by anemia and thrombocytopenia. The most important among these are hematologic malignancies including leukemia and lymphoma, and metastatic solid tumors such as neuroblastoma, rhabdomyosarcoma, and Ewing's sarcoma that infiltrate the bone marrow and lead to

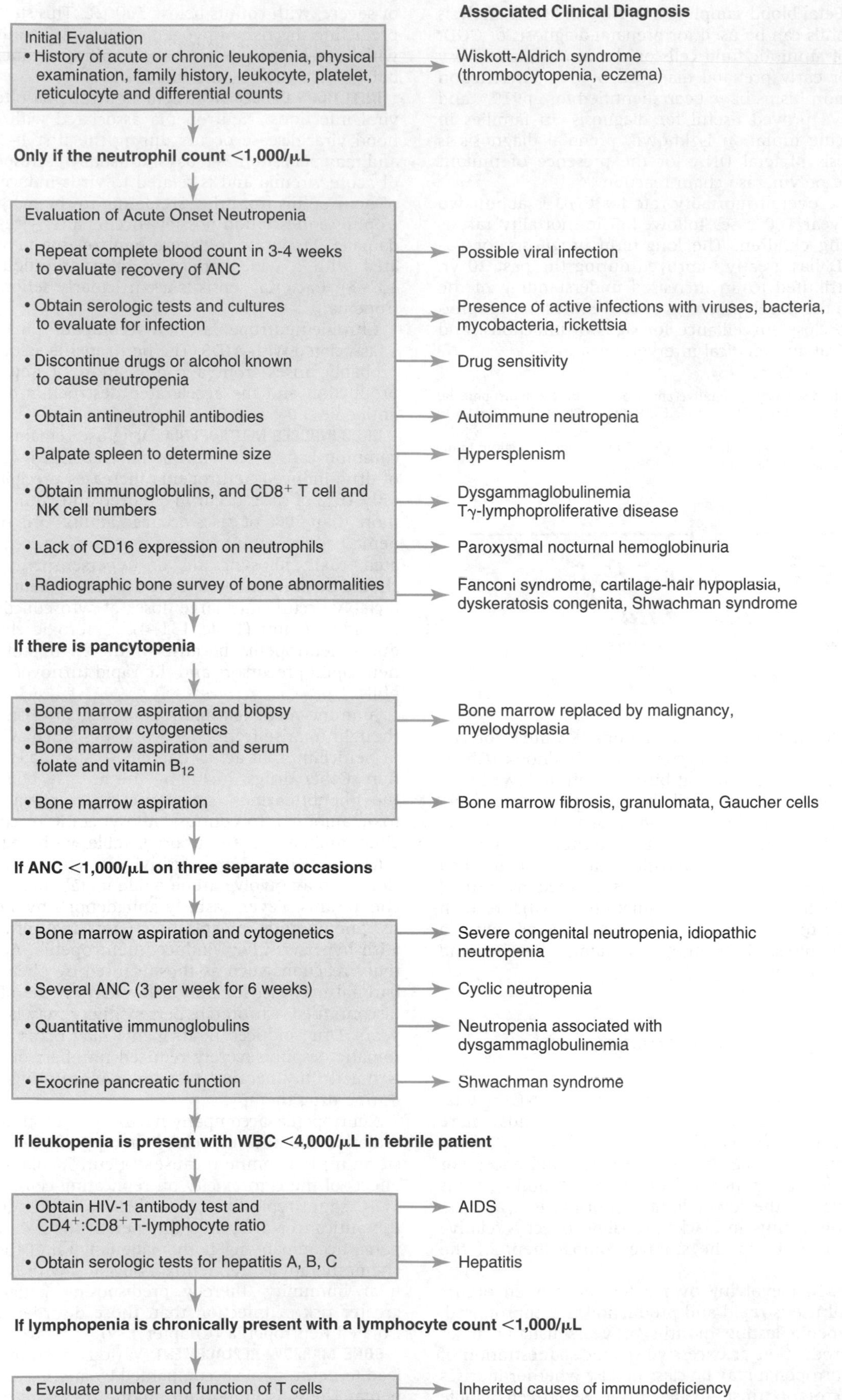

Figure 131–1 Algorithm for the evaluation of the patient with leukopenia or recurrent or unusual bacterial infections.

TABLE 131–1 Causes of Neutropenia Extrinsic to Bone Marrow Myeloid Cells

Cause	Etiologic Factors/Agents	Associated Findings
Infection	Viral, bacterial, protozoal, rickettsial, fungal	Redistribution from circulating to marginating pools, impaired production, accelerated destruction
Drug induced	Phenothiazines, sulfonamides, anticonvulsants, penicillins, aminopyrines	Hypersensitivity reaction (fever, lymphadenopathy, rash, hepatitis, nephritis, pneumonitis, aplastic anemia), antineutrophil antibodies
Immune neutropenia	Isoimmune; autoimmune	Variable arrest from metamyelocyte to segmented neutrophils in bone marrow
Reticuloendothelial sequestration	Hypersplenism	Anemia, thrombocytopenia
Bone marrow replacement	Malignancy (leukemia, lymphoma, metastatic solid tumors), Gaucher disease, granuloma, fibrosis	Anemia, thrombocytopenia, presence of immature myeloid and erythroid precursor in peripheral blood
Cancer chemotherapy or radiation therapy to bone marrow	Suppression of myeloid cell production	Bone marrow hypoplasia, anemia, thrombocytopenia
Ineffective myelopoiesis	Malnutrition (marasmus, anorexia nervosa), vitamin B_{12} or folate deficiency	Megaloblastic anemia, hypersegmented neutrophils

Modified from Boxer LA, Blackwood RA: Leukocyte disorders: Quantitative and qualitative disorders of the neutrophil, part 1. Pediatr Rev 17:19, 1996.

suppression of myelopoiesis. Neutropenia may also accompany myelodysplastic disorders or preleukemic syndromes, which typically are characterized by peripheral cytopenias and macrocytic blood cells associated with impaired production of myeloid precursors.

RETICULOENDOTHELIAL SEQUESTRATION. Splenic enlargement resulting from intrinsic splenic disease, portal hypertension, or other causes of splenic hyperplasia can lead to neutropenia. The neutropenia often is mild to moderate and accompanied by a corresponding degree of thrombocytopenia and anemia, and it may be corrected by successfully treating the underlying disease. The reduced neutrophil survival corresponds to the size of the spleen, and the extent of the neutropenia is proportional to bone marrow compensatory mechanisms. In selected cases, splenectomy may be necessary to restore the neutrophil count to normal, but this predisposes patients to infections by encapsulated bacterial organisms.

IMMUNE NEUTROPENIA. Immune neutropenias are associated with the presence of circulating antineutrophil antibodies. The antibodies may mediate neutrophil destruction by complement-mediated lysis or splenic phagocytosis of opsonized neutrophils.

Alloimmune Neonatal Neutropenia (ANN). This form of neonatal neutropenia occurs after transplacental transfer of maternal alloantibodies directed against antigens on the infant's neutrophils, analogous to Rh hemolytic disease. Prenatal sensitization induces maternal IgG antibodies to neutrophil antigens on fetal cells. The antibodies are usually complement-activating and are frequently directed to neutrophil-specific antigens. The pathogenesis of ANN usually involves phagocytosis of antibody-coated neutrophils by splenic macrophages. Symptomatic infants may present with delayed separation of the umbilical cord, mild skin infections, fever, and pneumonia within the first 2 weeks of life; these resolve with antibiotic therapy. The neutropenia is often severe and associated with fever and infections due to the usual microbes that cause neonatal disease. By 7 wk of age, the infant's neutrophil count usually returns to normal; this change reflects the duration of survival of maternal antibody in the infant's circulation. Treatment consists of supportive care and appropriate antibiotics for clinical infections.

Autoimmune Neutropenia. Autoimmune neutropenia is analogous to autoimmune hemolytic anemia and thrombocytopenia. Antibodies causing neutropenia have been detected in patients

TABLE 131–2 Intrinsic Disorders Associated with Neutropenia

Disorder	Mode of Inheritance	Associated Findings	Bone Marrow Findings
Cyclic neutropenia	AD	Periodic oscillation in ANC	Hypoplasia or myeloid maturation arrest, increased number of eosinophils
Severe congenital neutropenia (Kostmann syndrome)	Sporadic occurrence	Profound neutropenia, monocytosis, eosinophila	Arrest in myeloid maturation at promyelocyte stage
Chronic idiopathic neutropenia	?	Acquired	Variable pattern, arrest in maturation between promyelocyte and band
Chronic benign neutropenia	AD, AR, sporadic	Mild neutropenia	Variable pattern, including normal-appearing marrow
Shwachman-Diamond syndrome	AR	Pancreatic insufficiency with fatty replacement and atrophy, anemia, thrombocytopenia, metaphyseal dysostosis	Hypocellularity associated with leukemic transformation
Cartilage hair hypoplasia	AR	Short-limb dwarfism, fine hair, moderate neutropenia, impaired cellular immunity	Myeloid hypoplasia
Dyskeratosis congenita	X	Nail dystrophy, leukoplakia, reticulated hyperpigmentation of the skin	Marrow hypoplasia
Glycogen storage disease type Ib	AR	Hepatic enlargement, growth retardation, impaired neutrophil motility	Myeloid hypoplasia
Chédiak-Higashi syndrome	AR	Partial albinism, giant granules in myeloid cells, platelet storage pool defect, natural killer cell function impaired, ineffective myelopoiesis	Myeloid hypoplasia
Myelokathexis	AR	Neutrophils have cytoplasmic vacuoles and abnormal nuclei with thin filaments connecting the nuclear lobes	Myeloid hyperplasia
Preleukemia syndromes	?	Often associated with an acquired marrow cytogenetic abnormality, e.g., of monosomy 7	Marrow hypoplasia

AD = autosomal dominant; AR = autosomal recessive; X = X-linked recessive; ANC = absolute neutrophil count.
Modified from Boxer LA, Blackwood RA: Leukocyte disorders: Quantitative and qualitative disorders of the neutrophil, part 1. Pediatr Rev 17:19, 1996.

TABLE 131–3 Infections Associated with Neutropenia

Viral	Fungal
Respiratory syncytial virus	Histoplasmosis (disseminated)
Dengue fever	**Protozoal**
Colorado tick fever	Malaria
Mumps	Leishmaniasis (kala-azar)
Viral hepatitis	**Rickettsial**
Infectious mononucleosis	Rocky Mountain spotted fever
Influenza	Typhus fever
Measles	Rickettsialpox
Rubella	
Roseola	
Varicella	
Cytomegalovirus	
HIV-1	
Sandfly fever	
Bacterial	
Pertussis	
Typhoid fever	
Paratyphoid fever	
Tuberculosis (disseminated)	
Brucellosis	
Tularemia	
Gram-negative sepsis	
Psittacosis	

From Boxer LA, Blackwood RA: Leukocyte disorders: Quantitative and quantitative disorders of the neutrophils, part 1. Pediatr Rev 17:19, 1996.

who have no other signs of autoimmune disease, in patients who have additional antibodies against red blood cells and/or platelets, and in patients who have a connective tissue disorder. Autoimmune neutropenia is distinguished from other forms of neutropenia only by the demonstration of antineutrophil antibodies rather than by abnormal bone marrow histology. Autoimmune neutropenia frequently occurs in children with congenital and acquired forms of immune deficiencies, including dysgammaglobulinemia.

Autoimmune Neutropenia of Infancy (ANI). This benign condition has been diagnosed more frequently as reliable techniques for detection of antineutrophil antibodies have become more widely available. The exact incidence of ANI remains unknown, but because of its benign nature, the disorder may be more common than is suggested by the literature. In one study, ANI occurred with an annual incidence of approximately 1/100,000 among children between the ages of infancy and 10 yr. All patients recognized as having ANI have severe neutropenia on presentation, with an ANC usually less than 500/μL, but the total WBC count is always within normal limits. Monocytosis or eosinophilia may occur but does not seem to affect the rate of infection. The median age at diagnosis is 8 mo (range, 3–30 mo), with a female:male ratio of 6:4. None of the affected children have evidence of other autoimmune diseases. Children with ANI present with minor infections such as otitis media, gingivitis, respiratory tract infections, gastroenteritis, or cellulitis. The diagnosis often is considered only after the blood count reveals neutropenia. Occasionally, children may present with more severe infections including pneumonia, sepsis, or abscesses. Longitudinal studies of infants with ANI demonstrate a median duration of disease of approximately 30 mo (range, 6–60 mo), but 95% of children recover by 4 yr of age.

Neonatal Autoimmune Neutropenia. Mothers with autoimmune disease may give birth to infants who develop transient neutropenia. The duration of the neutropenia depends on the time that it takes for the infant to clear the maternally transferred circulating IgG antibody, and in most cases it persists for a few weeks to a few months. Neonates almost always remains asymptomatic.

INEFFECTIVE MYELOPOIESIS. Ineffective myelopoiesis may be acquired as a result of deficiency of vitamin B_{12} or folic acid. Megaloblastic pancytopenia also can result from extended use of antibiotics such as trimethoprim-sulfamethoxazole that inhibit folic acid metabolism and from the use of phenytoin, which may impair absorption of folate in the small intestine. Neutropenia also occurs with starvation and such conditions as marasmus in infants and anorexia nervosa, and it occasionally affects patients receiving prolonged parenteral feedings. Vitamin B_{12} deficiency may also result from resection of the distal ileum.

INTRINSIC DISORDERS OF PROLIFERATION AND MATURATION OF MYELOID STEM CELLS. The isolated disorders of proliferation and maturation of myeloid stem cells are rare. These patients frequently benefit from recombinant human granulocyte colony-stimulating factor (rhG-CSF) therapy. Congenital disorders that have severe neutropenia as a clinical feature include the severe combined immunodeficiency syndromes, hyperimmunoglobulin M syndrome, and common variable immune deficiencies (Chapter 126).

Cyclic Neutropenia. Cyclic neutropenia, a congenital granulopoietic disorder, is inherited in an autosomal dominant manner in some patients. It is characterized by regular, periodic oscillation in the number of peripheral neutrophils from normal to neutropenic values. The mean oscillatory period is 21 ± 3 days. During the neutropenic phase, most patients suffer from oral ulcers, fever, stomatitis, or pharyngitis, occasionally associated with lymph node enlargement. Serious infections occur occasionally and may lead to pneumonia, recurrent ulcerations of the oral, vaginal, and rectal mucosa, and death. Pneumonias and chronic periodontitis often occur, and sepsis may arise from *Clostridium perfringens* infection. Cyclic neutropenia arises from a regulatory abnormality involving early hematopoietic precursor cells, but the exact nature of the defect remains obscure. Many patients live for a considerable number of years, some actually experiencing abatement of symptoms as they age. The cycles tend to become less noticeable in older patients, and the hematologic picture often begins to resemble that of chronic neutropenia.

Severe Congenital Neutropenia. Severe congenital neutropenia, Kostmann disease, is characterized by an arrest in myeloid maturation at the promyelocyte stage of the bone marrow, resulting in an ANC of less than 200/μL. This disorder occurs sporadically or as an autosomal recessive disorder. Patients

TABLE 131–4 Immune-Mediated, Toxic, and Hypersensitivity-Mediated Neutropenia

Characteristic	Immunologic Form	Toxic Form	Hypersensitivity Form
Paradigm drugs	Aminopyrine, propylthiouracil, penicillin	Phenothiazine	Phenytoin, phenobarbital
Time to onset	Days to weeks	Weeks to months	Weeks to months
Clinical appearance	Acute, often explosive symptoms	Often asymptomatic or insidious onset	May be associated with fever, rash, nephritis, pneumonitis, or aplastic anemia
Rechallenge	Prompt recurrence with small test dose	Latent period; high doses required	Latent period; high doses required
Laboratory findings	Antibody test results positive	Evidence of direct toxicity to cells	Evidence of metabolite-mediated damage to cells

From Boxer LA: Approach to the patient with leukopenia. In: *Kelley WN (ed): Textbook of Internal Medicine, 3rd ed. Philadelphia, Lippincott-Raven, 1996.*

typically show monocytosis and eosinophilia and suffer from recurrent, severe pyogenic infections especially of the skin, mouth, and rectum. Patients often have the anemia associated with chronic inflammatory disease. Before the use of rhG-CSF, two thirds of these patients died of fatal infections before reaching adolescence. A few patients have developed acute myelogenous leukemia or myelodysplasia associated with monosomy 7.

Shwachman-Diamond Syndrome. Shwachman-Diamond syndrome is an autosomal recessive disorder characterized by digestive abnormalities and abnormally low WBC counts. The initial symptoms of this syndrome are usually diarrhea and failure to thrive because of insufficient absorption of nutrients. Almost all infants develop malabsorption by 4 mo of age. Growth failure and metaphyseal chondrodysplasia associated with dwarfism are especially prominent during the 1st or 2nd yr of life. Puberty is often delayed. Some patients have respiratory problems with pneumonia and frequent otitis media, as well as eczema. Virtually all patients with Shwachman-Diamond syndrome have neutropenia, with the ANC periodically falling below 1,000/μL. Some children have been reported to have a chemotactic defect that may contribute to the increased susceptibility to pyogenic infection. The illness may progress to bone marrow hypoplasia leading to moderate thrombocytopenia and anemia. Myelodysplasia and acute myelogenous leukemia associated with monosomy 7 have also been reported in this syndrome.

Cartilage-Hair Hypoplasia. Cartilage-hair hypoplasia is a multisystem autosomal recessive disorder characterized by short limbs and short stature resulting from abnormal development of long bone cartilage (Chapter 126.3). The major symptoms include abnormalities of the spine, hypermobile fingers, and very fine, thin hair on the head, eyebrows, and eyelashes. Decreased cell-mediated immunity, neutropenia, macrocytic anemia, and increased rates of malignancy have been described. Bone marrow transplantation has restored cellular immunity and corrected the neutropenia in two patients.

Glycogen Storage Disease Type Ib. Recurrent infections with neutropenia are a distinctive feature of glycogen storage disease (GSD) type Ib. Both classic von Gierke glycogen storage disease (GSDIa) and GSDIb cause massive enlargement of liver and severe growth retardation. In contrast to GSDIa, glucose-6-phosphatase activity is present on in vitro assays but glucose is not liberated from glucose-6-phosphate in vivo in GSDIb. In the liver, glucose-6-phosphatase requires two microsomal membrane components: a specific transfer system, glucose-6-phosphatase translocase, that shuttles glucose-6-phosphate from the cytoplasm to the lumen of the endoplasmic reticulum and another enzyme bound to the luminal surface of the membrane, glucose-6-phosphate phosphohydrolase. Neutrophils also appear to have a defective transport system. A defect of neutrophil motility is associated with the neutropenia. When the neutropenia is severe, these patients are predisposed to recurrent bacterial infections.

Severe Chronic Neutropenia. Some patients have acquired, idiopathic chronic symptomatic neutropenia. The onset of neutropenia typically occurs after the age of 2 yr, and the disorder more frequently afflicts adults. It is characterized by neutrophil counts that occasionally fall below 500/μL. Patients who consistently maintain an ANC less than 500/μL are afflicted with recurrent pyogenic infections involving the skin, mucous membranes, lungs, and lymph nodes. Bone marrow examination reveals variable patterns of myeloid formation with arrest generally occurring between the myelocyte and band forms.

Some forms of chronic neutropenia, such as myelokathexis, arise from an impaired release of neutrophils from the bone marrow into the peripheral blood. Children with myelokathexis have morphologic abnormalities of the neutrophils, with the cells showing cytoplasmic vacuoles of thin strands connecting the nuclear lobes. In some cases, these patients also have cellular immune defects and are predisposed to recurrent bacterial infections.

Chronic Benign Neutropenia. In contrast to severe congenital neutropenia, chronic benign neutropenia of childhood represents a common group of disorders characterized by mild to moderate neutropenia that does not lead to an increased risk of pyogenic infections. Spontaneous remissions have often been reported, although these may represent misdiagnosis of autoimmune neutropenia of infancy, in which remissions occur commonly during childhood. Chronic benign neutropenia may be inherited in either a dominant or recessive form. An autosomal recessive form of benign neutropenia is encountered in Yemenite Jews. Because of the relatively low risk of serious infection, patients should be not subjected to the potential toxic effects of prolonged administration of corticosteroids, splenectomy, or cytotoxic therapy.

CLINICAL MANIFESTATIONS. Individuals with neutrophil counts below 500/μL are at substantial risk for developing infections, primarily from their endogenous flora as well as from nosocomial organisms. Some patients with isolated chronic neutropenia with ANC less than 200/μL may not experience many serious infections, probably because the remainder of the immune system remains intact. In contrast, children whose neutropenia is secondary to acquired disorders of production such as with cytotoxic therapy, immunosuppressive drugs, or radiation therapy, particularly in conjunction with malignancies, are likely to develop serious bacterial infections because many arms of the immune system are markedly compromised.

Leukopenia associated with neutropenia, in addition to monocytopenia and lymphocytopenia, is often more serious than neutropenia alone. The integrity of skin and mucous membranes, the vascular supply to tissues, and the nutritional status of patients influence the risk of infection.

The clinical presentation in most patients with profound neutropenia is temperature exceeding 101°F, cellulitis, and furunculosis. Stomatitis, gingivitis, perirectal inflammation, colitis, sinusitis, and otitis media are frequent accompaniments of profound neutropenia in children. Other clinical manifestations of profound neutropenia may include hepatic abscesses, recurrent pneumonias, and septicemia. In contrast, isolated neutropenia does not heighten a patient's susceptibility to fungal, parasitic, or viral infections or to bacterial meningitis.

The most common pathogens isolated from neutropenic patients are *Staphylococcus aureus* and gram-negative bacteria. The usual signs and symptoms of local infection and inflammation such as exudate, fluctuance, and regional lymphadenopathy are generally less prominent in neutropenic patients than in non-neutropenic patients because of the neutropenic patients' inability to form pus. However, neutropenic patients can experience pain at sites of inflammation.

LABORATORY FINDINGS. Isolated absolute neutropenia has a limited number of causes (Tables 131–1 and 131–2). The duration and severity of the neutropenia greatly influence the extent of laboratory evaluation. Patients with chronic neutropenia since infancy and a history of recurrent fevers and chronic gingivitis should have WBC counts and differential counts determined three times weekly for 6 wk to evaluate the periodicity suggestive of cyclic neutropenia. Bone marrow aspiration and biopsy should be performed on selected patients to assess cellularity. Additional marrow studies such as cytogenetic analysis and special stains for detecting leukemia and other malignant disorders should be obtained for patients with suspected intrinsic defects in the myeloid cells or the progenitors and for patients with suspected malignancy. Selection of further laboratory tests is determined by the duration and severity of the neutropenia and by findings on physical examination (Fig. 131–1).

TREATMENT. The management of acquired transient neutropenia associated with malignancies, myelosuppressive chemotherapy, or immunosuppressive chemotherapy differs from that of congenital or chronic forms of neutropenia. In the former situation, infections sometimes are heralded only by fever, and sepsis is a major cause of death. Early recognition and treatment of infections may be lifesaving (Chapter 179).

Therapy of severe chronic neutropenia is dictated by the clinical manifestations. Patients with benign neutropenia and no evidence of repeated bacterial infections or chronic gingivitis require no specific therapy. Superficial infections in children with mild to moderate neutropenia may be treated with appropriate oral antibiotics. However, in patients who have life-threatening infections, broad-spectrum intravenous antibiotics should be started promptly.

Effective treatment of severe chronic neutropenia including severe congenital neutropenia, chronic symptomatic idiopathic neutropenia, and cyclic neutropenia is now possible. A randomized controlled trial involving these patients and using subcutaneously administered rhG-CSF at doses ranging from 3.4–11.50 μg/kg/24 hr led to dramatic increases in neutrophil counts, resulting in marked attenuation of infection and inflammation. rhG-CSF has also been successfully administered to some patients with drug-induced neutropenia whose neutrophil count failed to increase after cessation of the offending drug. The long-term effects of rhG-CSF therapy are unknown but include a propensity for the development of moderate splenomegaly, thrombocytopenia, and, occasionally, vasculitis. Autoimmune neutropenia may be responsive to intermittent corticosteroids, especially if it is part of an underlying disease process such as systemic lupus erythematosus. Although this remains unproved by controlled studies, use of rhG-CSF has benefited some patients who have immune neutropenias.

Those patients with severe congenital neutropenia or Shwachman-Diamond syndrome who develop myelodysplasia or acute myelogenous leukemia respond only to allogeneic bone marrow transplantation. Chemotherapy is ineffective.

131.2 Lymphopenia

Lymphocytes account for about 30% of the circulating WBCs in a newborn. The proportion of lymphocytes then increases rapidly within the 1st mo, reaching an average of 60% by 2 yr of age. The normal lymphocyte count in children younger than 2 yr is 3,000–9,500/μL and in adults is 1,000–4,8000/μL. At 6 yr of age, the lower limit of normal is 1,500/μL.

Almost 65% of blood T lymphocytes are $CD4^+$ (helper) T lymphocytes. Most patients with lymphocytopenia have a reduction in the absolute number of T lymphocytes, particularly in the number of $CD4^+$ T lymphocytes. The average number of $CD4^+$ T lymphocytes in adult blood is 1,100/μL (range, 300–1,300/μL), and the average number of $CD8^+$ (suppressor) T lymphocytes is 600/μL (range, 100–900/μL).

Lymphocytopenia per se usually causes no symptoms and is often detected in the evaluation of other illnesses, particularly recurrent viral, fungal, and parasitic infections. Lymphocyte subpopulations can be measured by multiparameter flow cytometry, which uses the pattern of antigen expression to classify and characterize these cells.

Inherited Causes of Lymphocytopenia. Inherited immunodeficiency disorders may have a quantitative or qualitative stem cell abnormality resulting in ineffective lymphocytopoiesis (Table 131–5). Other disorders such as Wiskott-Aldrich syndrome may have associated lymphocytopenia arising from accelerated destruction of T cells. A similar mechanism is present in patients with adenosine deaminase deficiency and purine nucleoside phosphorylase deficiency.

TABLE 131–5 Causes of Lymphocytopenia

Acquired Causes

- Infectious diseases
  - AIDS
  - Viral hepatitis
  - Influenza
  - Tuberculosis
  - Typhoid fever
  - Sepsis
- Iatrogenic
  - Immunosuppressive therapy
  - Corticosteroids
  - High-dose PUVA therapy
  - Cytotoxic chemotherapy
  - Radiation
  - Thoracic duct drainage
- Systemic and other diseases
  - Systemic lupus erythematosus
  - Myasthenia gravis
  - Hodgkin's disease
  - Protein-losing enteropathy
  - Renal failure
  - Sarcoidosis
  - Thermal injury
  - Aplastic anemia
- Dietary deficiency
  - Dietary deficiency associated with ethanol abuse
  - Zinc deficiency

Inherited Causes

- Aplasia of lymphopoietic stem cells
- Severe combined immunodeficiency associated with defect in IL-2 receptor γ-chain, deficiency of ADA or PNP, or unknown
- Ataxia-telangiectasia
- Wiskott-Aldrich syndrome
- Immunodeficiency with thymoma
- Cartilage-hair hypoplasia
- Idiopathic $CD4^+$ T lymphocytopenia

ADA = adenosine deaminase; PNP = purine nucleoside phosphorylase; IL-2 = interleukin-2; PUVA = psoralen and ultraviolet A irradiation.

From Boxer LA: Approach to the patient with leukopenia. In: *Kelley WN (ed): Textbook of Internal Medicine, 3rd ed. Philadelphia, Lippincott-Raven, 1996.*

Acquired Lymphocytopenia. Acquired lymphocytopenia is the result of depletion of blood lymphocytes that is not secondary to inherited diseases. AIDS is the most common infectious disease associated with lymphocytopenia, which results from destruction of $CD4^+$ T cells infected with HIV-1 or HIV-2. Other viral and bacterial diseases may be associated with lymphocytopenia. In some instances of acute viremia with other viral infections, lymphocytes may undergo accelerated destruction from intracellular viral replication, may be trapped in the spleen or nodes, or may migrate to the respiratory tract.

Iatrogenic lymphocytopenia is caused by cytotoxic chemotherapy, radiation therapy, or long-term administration of antilymphocyte globulin. Long-term treatment of psoriasis using psoralen and ultraviolet irradiation may destroy T lymphocytes. Corticosteroids can cause lymphopenia through increased cell destruction. Systemic autoimmune diseases such as systemic lupus erythematosus are associated with lymphocytopenia. Other conditions such as protein-losing enteropathy and aberrant or surgical drainage of the thoracic duct are associated with lymphocyte depletion causing lymphocytopenia.

Boxer LA: Approach to the patient with leukopenia. *In:* Kelley WN (ed): Textbook of Internal Medicine, 3rd ed. Philadelphia, Lippincott-Raven, 1996.

Boxer LA, Blackwood RA: Leukocyte disorders: Quantitative and qualitative disorders of the neutrophils, part 1. Pediatr Rev 17:19, 1996.

CHAPTER 132
Leukocytosis

Laurence A. Boxer

Leukocytosis is an elevation in the total white blood cell (WBC) count that is two standard deviations above the mean count for a particular age (Chapter 726). The various causes of leukocytosis are categorized by the class of WBCs that is elevated and whether the leukocytosis is acute, chronic, or lifelong.

A WBC count exceeding 50,000/μL is termed a *leukemoid reaction* because of the simulation of the features of leukemia. Leukemoid reactions are usually neutrophilic and are most frequently associated with septicemia and severe bacterial infections including shigellosis, salmonellosis, and meningococcemia. Infection in children with WBC adhesion defects results in WBC counts approaching or exceeding 100,000/μL.

A significant proportion of greater than 5% of immature to mature neutrophil cells is termed a *shift to the left* and indicates rapid release of cells from the bone marrow. This may result in increased circulating band forms, which usually constitute 1–5% of circulating neutrophilic cells, or metamyelocytes and myelocytes, which are not usually found in the peripheral circulation. Higher degrees of shift to the left with more immature neutrophil precursors are indicative of serious bacterial infections but may also be encountered with trauma, burns, surgery, and acute hemolysis or hemorrhage.

NEUTROPHILIA. Neutrophilia is an increase in the total number of blood neutrophils in excess of 8,000/μL for adults. During the first day of life, the upper limit of the normal neutrophil count ranges from 7,000–12,000/μL. Thereafter, in the 1st mo of life the neutrophil count is 1,800–5,400/μL. By 1 yr of age, the range of the neutrophil count is 1,500–8,500/μL.

An increase in circulating neutrophils is a result of a disturbance of the normal equilibrium involving neutrophil bone marrow production, movement out of the marrow compartments into the circulation, and neutrophil destruction. Neutrophilia may arise either alone or in combination with enhanced mobilization into the circulating pool from either the bone marrow storage compartment or the peripheral blood marginating pool, by impaired neutrophil egress into tissues, or after expansion of the circulating neutrophil pool secondary to increased progenitor cell proliferation and terminal differentiation through the myeloid series.

Acute Acquired Neutrophilia. Neutrophilia is usually an acquired disorder and is a common finding with inflammation, infection, injury, or stress. Acute or chronic bacterial infections, trauma, and surgery are among the most common causes encountered in clinical practice. Neutrophilia is often associated with sickle cell disease, some chronic hemolytic anemias, heatstroke, burns, and diabetic ketoacidosis. Drugs commonly associated with neutrophilia include epinephrine, corticosteroids, and recombinant growth factors such as recombinant human granulocyte colony-stimulating factor (rhG-CSF) and recombinant human granulocyte-macrophage colony stimulating factor (rhGM-CSF). Epinephrine causes release into the circulation of a sequestered pool of neutrophils that normally marginate along the vascular endothelium. Corticosteroids accelerate the release of neutrophils and bands from a large storage pool within the bone marrow and impair the migration of neutrophils from the circulation into tissues. The hematopoietic growth factors stimulate myeloid production.

Chronic Acquired Neutrophilia. Chronic neutrophilia is usually associated with continued stimulation of neutrophil production resulting from persistent inflammatory reactions or infections such as those occurring with tuberculosis, vasculitis, postsplenectomy states, Hodgkin's disease, chronic myelogenous leukemia, chronic blood loss, and the prolonged administration of corticosteroids.

Lifelong Neutrophilia. Congenital asplenia is associated with chronic neutrophilia. Uncommon genetic disorders that present with neutrophilia include WBC adhesion deficiency, familial myeloproliferative disease, and Down syndrome. In an autosomal dominant form of hereditary neutrophilia, patients maintain an absolute neutrophil count between 1,400 and 150,000/μL that is associated with hepatosplenomegaly, an increased alkaline phosphatase level, and Gaucher-type histiocytes in the bone marrow.

Evaluation of persistent neutrophilia requires a careful history, physical examination, and laboratory studies to search for infectious, inflammatory, and neoplastic conditions. The leukocyte alkaline phosphatase cytochemical stain of circulating WBCs may be used to differentiate chronic myelogenous leukemia, in which the count is uniformly near zero, from reactive or secondary neutrophilias, in which normal to elevated levels are found.

MONOCYTOSIS. The average absolute blood monocyte count varies with age and must be considered in the assessment of monocytosis. Given the role of monocytes in antigen presentation and cytokine secretion and as effectors of ingestion of invading organisms, it is not surprising that many clinical disorders give rise to monocytosis (Table 132–1). Monocytosis is often a sign of an acute bacterial, viral, protozoal, or rickettsial infection. Chronic inflammatory conditions can stimulate sustained monocytosis. Monocytosis can be observed in malignant disorders such as preleukemia, acute myelogenous leukemia, chronic myelogenous leukemia, and lymphomas. It is found in some patients with Hodgkin disease. Monocytosis also occurs in some forms of chronic neutropenia and postsplenectomy states. Most commonly, monocytosis occurs in patients recovering from myelosuppressive chemotherapy and is a harbinger of the return of the neutrophil count to normal.

LYMPHOCYTOSIS. Chronic bacterial infections such as tuberculosis and brucellosis may lead to a sustained lymphocytosis.

TABLE 132–1 Causes of Monocytosis

- Infections
  - Bacterial infections
    - Tuberculosis
    - Brucellosis
    - Syphilis
    - Typhoid fever
    - Infective endocarditis
  - Nonbacterial infections
    - Fungal infections
    - Rocky Mountain spotted fever
    - Kala-azar
    - Typhus
- Hematologic and oncologic disorders
  - Hodgkin's disease
  - Chronic myelomonocytic leukemia
  - Preleukemia
  - Congenital and acquired neutropenias
  - Postsplenectomy states
  - Hemolytic anemias
  - Juvenile chronic myelogenous leukemia
- Collagen vascular diseases
  - Systemic lupus erythematosus
  - Rheumatoid arthritis
  - Polyarteritis nodosa
- Gastrointestinal disorders
  - Ulcerative colitis
  - Granulomatous colitis
  - Cirrhosis
- Miscellaneous
  - Drug reactions
  - Sarcoidosis
  - Recovery from marrow suppression induced by chemotherapy

Pertussis is accompanied by lymphocytosis in approximately 25% of infants infected before 6 mo of age. The viral diseases classically associated with lymphocytosis are infectious mononucleosis, cytomegalovirus infection, and viral hepatitis. Thyrotoxicosis and Addison disease are endocrine disorders associated with lymphocytosis. Acute lymphocytic leukemia should be considered especially with persistent or profound lymphocytosis.

Lymphocytosis is a normal response to most viral infections, because the majority of circulating lymphocytes are T cells. Thus, the most common cause of lymphocytosis is an acute viral illness. In infectious mononucleosis, the B cells are infected with the Epstein-Barr virus and the T cells react to the viral antigens present in the B cells, resulting in T-cell lymphocytosis with the typical large, vacuolated morphology.

Calhoun DA, Kirk JF, Christensen RD: Incidence, significance, and kinetic mechanism responsible for leukemoid reactions in patients in the neonatal intensive care unit: A prospective evaluation. J Pediatr 129:403, 1996.

Christensen RD: Neutrophil kinetics in the fetus and neonate. Am J Pediatr Hematol Oncol 11:215, 1989.

Peterson L, Hrisinko MA: Benign lymphocytosis and reactive neutrophilia. Laboratory features provide diagnostic clues. Clin Lab Med 13:863, 1993.

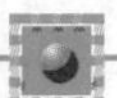

SECTION 4

The Complement System

Richard B. Johnston, Jr.

CHAPTER 133
The Complement System

Complement was originally defined through the study of bacteriolysis, which requires both specific antibody and a nonspecific, heat-labile complementary principle, now termed *complement.* By the 1960s, nine complement components were known, one of which had three subcomponents. By the early 1970s, a second major pathway of activation of complement, the *alternative pathway,* had been described. The latter system contains two unique factors. In addition, at least seven (perhaps 10) regulators that control activity of either or both pathways exist in serum, and at least five such regulatory proteins exist on the surface of cells. The original system of four components, C1423, is now referred to as the classical pathway. The term *complement system,* as broadly conceptualized now, refers to both pathways, which interact and depend on each other for their full activity; the *membrane attack complex* (C5b6789), formed from activity of either pathway; the seven serum and five membrane regulatory proteins; a serosal regulatory protein; and eight cell membrane receptors that bind complement components or fragments (Table 133–1). All of the 20 serum components and regulators are proteins. Together they make up about 10% of the globulin fraction of serum. The normal concentrations of serum complement components in children are given in Reference Ranges for Laboratory Tests, Chapter 726.

NOMENCLATURE. The terminology applied to complement is cryptic but logical and consists of only a few rules. The components have been assigned numbers in the order of their discovery and are preceded by the letter C. Unfortunately, the first four components do not interact in the sequence in which they were discovered but rather in the order C1423. The remaining components react in the appropriate numeric order, C56789. C1 has three subcomponents, C1q, C1r, and C1s. Fragments of components resulting from cleavage by other components acting as enzymes are assigned lowercase letters (a, b, c, d, or e); with the exception of C2 fragments, the smaller piece that is released into surrounding fluids is assigned the lowercase letter a, and the major part of the molecule, bound to other components or to some part of the immune complex, is assigned b—for example, C3a and C3b. When a component is activated (becomes an active enzyme), a bar is placed above the number, for example, C$\overline{1}$.

Components of the alternative pathway, B and D, have been assigned uppercase letters, as have the control proteins I and H, which downregulate both pathways. Factor B has an active form denoted $\overline{\text{Bb}}$. C3 (in particular, its major fragment, C3b) is a component of both the classical and alternative pathways.

GENERAL CONCEPTS. Complement is a *system* of interacting proteins. The biologic functions of the system depend on the interactions of individual components, which occur in sequential fashion. This has been referred to as a *cascade,* in analogy to the clotting system of blood; activation of each component (except the 1st) depends on activation of the prior component or components in the sequence.

TABLE 133–1 Constituents of the Complement System

Serum Components	Membrane Regulatory Proteins
Classical Pathway	CR1
C1q	Membrane cofactor protein
C1r	Decay-accelerating factor (DAF)
C1s	Membrane inhibitor of reactive lysis (CD59)
C4	C8-binding protein (C8bp)
C2	**Serosal Regulatory Protein**
C3	C5a/IL-8 inactivator
Alternative Pathway	**Membrane Receptors**
Factor B	CR1
Factor D	CR2 (CD21)
Membrane Attack Complex	CR3
C5	CR4
C6	C4a/C3a receptor
C7	C5a receptor
C8	C1q receptors (cC1qR, gC1qR)
C9	
Control Protein, Enhancing	
Properdin	
Control Proteins, Downregulating	
C1 inhibitor (C1 INH)	
C4-binding protein (C4-bp)	
Factor H	
Factor I	
S protein (vitronectin)	
Anaphylatoxin inactivator	

CR = complement receptor; IL = interleukin.

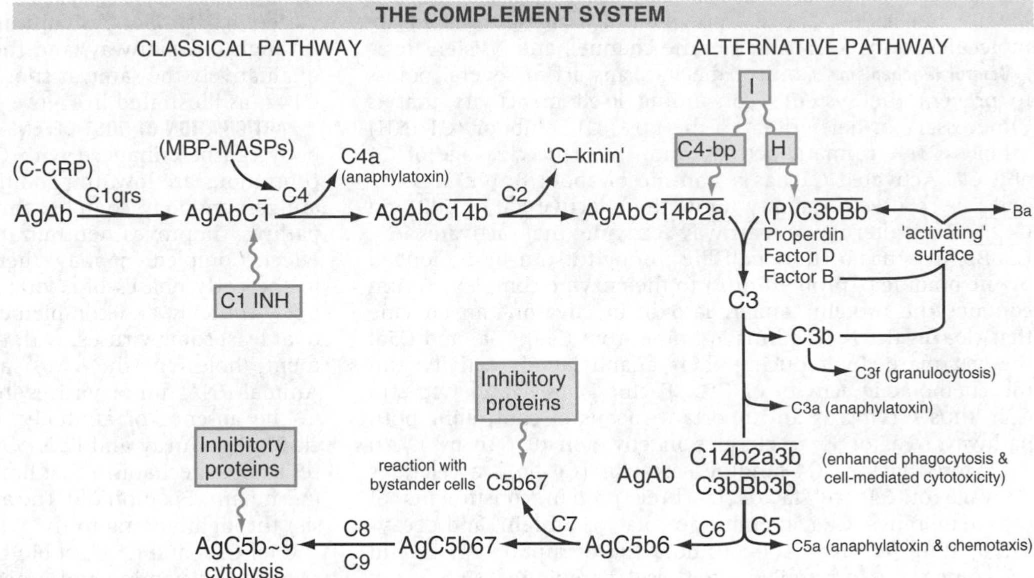

Figure 133–1 Sequence of activation of the components of the classical pathway of complement and interaction with the alternative pathway. (Ag = antigen [bacterium, virus, tumor cell, or erythrocyte]; Ab = antibody [IgG or IgM class only]; C-CRP = C carbohydrate–C-reactive protein; C1 INH = C1 inhibitor; C3f = C3 fragment; I = factor I; C4-bp = C4-binding protein; H = factor H; MBP = mannose-binding protein; MASPs = MBP-associated serine proteases.) Inhibitory regulator proteins are enclosed in a box. S protein is the best defined of the "inhibitory proteins" that act on the membrane attack complex (C5b6789).

Interaction occurs along two pathways (Fig. 133–1): the classical pathway, in the order antigen-antibody-C142356789; and the alternative pathway, in the order activator-(antibody)-C3bBD-C356789. Antibody accelerates the rate of activation of the alternative pathway, but activation can occur on appropriate surfaces in the absence of antibody. The classical and the alternative pathways interact with each other through the ability of both to activate C3.

The interaction of the early-acting components of complement (C1423) results in the generation of a series of active enzymes, $C\bar{1}$, $C\overline{42}$, and $C\overline{423}$. Thus, *activation* refers to transformation of the component into part of an active enzyme. In contrast, the interaction among C5b, C6, C7, C8, and C9 is nonenzymatic. In the case of C1, activation is a result of its interaction with antibody. Activation of C4, C2, C3, and C5, as well as factor B of the alternative pathway, is secondary to cleavage by a preceding activated component. Thus, activation of early components generates enzymes that fix to the antigen-antibody complex and catalyze a reaction on the next component, whereas later-acting components (C6–C9) adsorb to the complex or the underlying cell by an interaction that depends on a change in their configuration.

Classical Pathway. The sequence begins with fixation of C1, by way of C1q, to the Fc non–antigen-binding part of the antibody molecule after antigen-antibody interaction. The C1 tricomplex changes configuration, and the C1s subcomponent becomes an active enzyme, $C\bar{1}$ esterase.

C-reactive protein (CRP), which reacts with C carbohydrate from microorganisms and is increased in certain inflammatory states, can substitute for antibody in the fixation of C1q and initiate reaction of the entire sequence in the absence of antibody. Other agents that can activate C1 directly, without a requirement for antibody, include certain bacteria, *Mycoplasma*, RNA viruses, uric acid crystals, the lipid A component of bacterial endotoxin, and the membranes of certain intracellular organelles.

Mannose-binding protein (MBP) is a member of the "collectin" family of carbohydrate-binding proteins that are believed to play an important part in innate, nonspecific immunity. MBP in association with MBP-associated serine proteases (MASPs) can function like C1s to cleave C4 and C2 and activate the complement cascade. In the next two steps of the classical pathway, polypeptide fragments are split from C4 and C2 during their activation and fixation by the enzymatic action of C1. One of these, a kinin-like peptide split from C2, can induce vascular permeability and edema through direct action on postcapillary venules. The peptide C4a has anaphylatoxin activity; it reacts with mast cells to release the chemical mediators of immediate hypersensitivity, including histamine. Fixation of C4b to the complex permits it to adhere to various mammalian cells, including neutrophils, monocytes, and erythrocytes.

Cleavage of C3 and generation of C3b is the next step in the sequence and the most crucial in terms of biologic activity. Cleavage of C3 can be achieved through $C\overline{142}$, the C3 convertase of the classical pathway, or through the C3 convertase of the alternative pathway, $C\overline{3bBb}$ (see later). Once fixed to the complex, C3b permits adherence of the antigen-antibody complex to cells with receptors for C3b (complement receptor 1, CR1), including B lymphocytes, erythrocytes, and phagocytic cells (neutrophils, monocytes, and macrophages), leading, in the last case, to phagocytosis. Without C3 bound to them, phagocytosis of most microorganisms in vitro, especially by neutrophils, is very inefficient. The severe pyogenic infections that commonly occur in C3-deficient patients indicate that without C3, phagocytosis is also inefficient in vivo. The biologic activity of C3b is controlled by cleavage by factor I (C3b inactivator) to iC3b, which is further degraded by factor I and serum or tissue enzymes to C3c, which is released, and to C3dg and C3d, which stay bound. iC3b promotes phagocytosis on binding to the iC3b receptor (CR3) on phagocytes. Receptors for C3dg and C3d exist on B lymphocytes (CR2) and phagocytes (CR4). Further cleavage of C3c creates a fragment that induces release of granulocytes from bone marrow.

The peptide C3a, generated when C3 is acted on by either pathway, has anaphylatoxin activity. The action of $C\overline{423}$ or of the alternative pathway C5 convertase on C5 releases C5a, a powerful anaphylatoxin that can react with neutrophils, macrophages, mast cells, smooth muscle cells, and certain T cells to induce release of various mediators of inflammation. This same peptide serves as a potent chemical attractant for phagocytic cells.

Membrane Attack Complex. This sequence leading to cytolysis begins with the attachment of C5b to the C5-activating enzyme from the classical pathway, $C\overline{4b2a3b}$, or from the alternative pathway, $C\overline{3bBb3b}$. C6 is bound to C5b without being cleaved, stabilizing the activated C5b fragment. The C5b6 complex then dissociates from $C\overline{423}$ and reacts with C7. C5b67 complexes must attach to the cell membrane promptly or lose their activity and remain in the fluid phase. Next, C8 binds, and the C5b678 complex then promotes the addition of multiple C9 molecules. The C9 polymer of at least three to six molecules forms a transmembrane channel, and lysis ensues.

Control Mechanisms. Control mechanisms act at several points to prevent the system's consuming itself in activity that is unnecessary or deleterious to the host. C1 inhibitor (C1 INH) inhibits $\overline{\text{C1s}}$ enzymatic activity and, thus, the cleavage of C4 and C2. Activated C2 has a half-life of about 8 min at 37°C, and this relative instability limits the effective life of $\overline{\text{C42}}$ and $\overline{\text{C423}}$. The alternative pathway enzyme that activates C3, C3bBb, also has a short half-life, though it can be prolonged by the binding of properdin (P) to the enzyme complex. Serum contains the protein "anaphylatoxin inactivator," an enzyme that cleaves the N-terminus arginine from C4a, C3a, and C5a, thereby markedly reducing their anaphylatoxic activity and the chemotactic activity of C5a. Factor I inactivates C4b and C3b, thus serving as an important means of controlling both pathways. Factor H accelerates inactivation of C3b by I. An analogous factor, C4-binding protein (C4-bp), accelerates cleavage of C4b by factor I. Three protein constituents of cell membranes, CR1, membrane cofactor protein, and decay-accelerating factor (DAF), promote the disruption of C3 and C5 convertases assembled on those membranes. Other cell membrane–associated proteins (C8-binding protein and CD59) can bind C8 or both C8 and C9, thereby interfering with insertion of the membrane attack complex (C5b6789). Certain serum proteins (S protein, or vitronectin, being the best studied) can inhibit attachment of the C5b67 complex to cell membranes, bind C8 or C9 in a full membrane attack complex, or otherwise interfere with the formation or insertion of this complex.

ALTERNATIVE PATHWAY. The alternative pathway can be activated by C3b generated through classical pathway activity, through leukocyte proteases released by degranulation, or perhaps through activation of thrombin or plasmin during blood coagulation. It can also be activated by a form of C3 created by low-grade, spontaneous reaction of native C3 with a molecule of water, which occurs constantly in plasma. Once formed, C3b or this hydrolyzed C3 can bind to any nearby cell or to factor B. Factor B attached to C3b in the plasma or on the surface of a particle can be cleaved to Bb by D, which exists as an active proteolytic enzyme. The complex $\overline{\text{C3bBb}}$ becomes an efficient C3 convertase, which generates more C3b through an "amplification loop" (see Fig. 133–1). P can bind to $\overline{\text{C3bBb}}$, increasing stability of the enzyme and protecting it from inactivation by factors I and H, which serve to modulate the loop. Cleavage of B releases Ba, which has weak chemotactic activity.

Certain materials promote alternative pathway activation if C3b is fixed to their surface—for example, teichoic acid from bacterial cell wall, endotoxic lipopolysaccharide, or immunoglobulin aggregates, especially of the IgA class. This activation depends on the ability of the $\overline{\text{C3bBb}}$ enzyme complex to escape the efficient control otherwise exercised by factors I and H. The surface of rabbit red blood cells also protects $\overline{\text{C3bBb}}$ from inactivation. This phenomenon serves as the basis for an assay of serum alternative pathway activity. Endotoxin may alter normally "nonactivating" cell surfaces in vivo so that $\overline{\text{C3bBb}}$ is relatively protected from inactivation, which may partially explain the activation of the alternative pathway in patients with gram-negative bacteremia. Sialic acid on the surface of microorganisms or cells prevents formation of an effective alternative pathway C3 convertase by promoting activity of I and H.

Although $\overline{\text{C3bBb}}$ can activate C3 efficiently on only a limited variety of surfaces, significant activation of C3 can occur through this pathway, and the resultant biologic activities are qualitatively the same as those achieved through activation by $\overline{\text{C142}}$, as illustrated in Figure 133–1.

PARTICIPATION IN HOST DEFENSE. Neutralization of virus by antibody can be enhanced with C1 and C4. When antibody concentrations are low, the additional fixation of C3b to the viral antigen-antibody complex through the classical or alternative pathway improves neutralization; C5 and C6 add little to the effect. Complement may, therefore, be particularly important in the early phases of a viral infection when antibody is limited. Antibody and complement can also eliminate infectivity of at least some viruses, with the production of typical complement "holes" in the virus, as seen by electron microscopy. Animal RNA tumor viruses interact directly with human C1q in the absence of antibody, with resulting activation of the classical pathway and lysis of the virus. This may be a natural resistance mechanism that limits the infectivity of these viruses in humans. Fixation of C1q can opsonize (promote phagocytosis) through binding to the C1q receptor.

C4a, C3a, and C5a can bind to mast cells and thereby trigger release of histamine and other mediators, leading to vasodilatation and to the swelling and redness of inflammation. C5a can induce monocytes to release the cytokines tumor necrosis factor and interleukin 1, which amplify the inflammatory response. C5a is a major chemical stimulus for the influx into inflammatory sites of neutrophils, monocytes, and eosinophils, which can efficiently phagocytize microorganisms coated (opsonized) with C3b or cleaved C3b (iC3b). Further inactivation of cell-bound C3b by cleavage to C3d removes its opsonizing activity. Fixation of C3b to a target cell can enhance its lysis by cytolytic cells.

Insoluble immune complexes can be solubilized if they bind C3b, apparently because C3b disrupts the orderly antigen-antibody lattice. Binding C3b to a complex also allows it to adhere to C3 receptors (CR1) on red blood cells, which then transport the complexes to fixed macrophages for removal. These findings offer the best explanation for the immune complex disease found in patients who lack C1, C4, C2, or C3.

The complement system may be involved in certain aspects of B- and T-lymphocyte–mediated specific immunity. C3b- and C3d-coated particles can bind to B lymphocytes, which appears to activate them and to enhance the primary antibody response. C3a may suppress antibody formation, whereas C5a and C1q appear to enhance this response. A cleavage product generated during the inactivation of C3 induces an increase in circulating granulocytes.

Neutralization of endotoxin in vitro and protection from its lethal effects in experimental animals require later-acting components of complement, at least through C6. Finally, activation of the entire complement sequence can result in lysis of virus-infected cells, tumor cells, and most types of microorganisms. Bactericidal activity of complement has not appeared to be important to host defense, except for the occurrence of infections with *Neisseria meningitidis* in patients lacking later-acting components of complement (Chapter 191).

Berger M, Frank MM: The serum complement system. *In:* Stiehm ER (ed): Immunologic Disorders in Infants and Children, 4th ed. Philadelphia, WB Saunders, 1996, p 133.

Carroll MC, Fischer MB: Complement and the immune response. Curr Opin Immunol 9:64, 1997.

Johnston RB Jr: The complement system in host defense and inflammation: The cutting edges of a double edged sword. Pediatr Infect Dis J 12:933, 1993.

Whaley K, Schwaeble W: Complement and complement deficiencies. Semin Liver Dis 17:297, 1997.

CHAPTER 134
Disorders of the Complement System

134.1 Evaluation of the Complement System

Testing for total hemolytic complement activity (CH_{50}) is a useful screening procedure for most of the diseases of the complement system. A normal result in this assay depends on the ability of all 11 component proteins of the classical pathway and membrane attack complex to interact and lyse antibody-coated erythrocytes. The dilution of serum that lyses 50% of the cells determines the end-point. In congenital deficiencies of C1 through C8, the CH_{50} value is about 0; in C9 deficiency, the value is approximately half-normal. Values in the acquired deficiencies vary with the severity of the underlying disorder. This assay does not detect deficiencies of the alternative pathway component B or D, or of properdin. Deficiency of factor I or H permits consumption of C3, with partial reduction in the CH_{50} value.

In *hereditary angioedema,* depression of C4 and C2 during an attack significantly reduces the CH_{50}. Serum concentrations of C4 and C3 can be determined by radial immunodiffusion. In hereditary angioedema, C4 is characteristically low and C3 normal. Concentrations of C1 inhibitor can be determined with antibody, but a normal result can be anticipated in about 15% of cases. Because C1 acts as an esterase, the specific diagnosis can be made by showing increased capacity of patients' sera to hydrolyze synthetic esters.

Decreased serum concentrations of both C4 and C3 suggest activation of the classical pathway by immune complexes. In contrast, decreased C3 and normal C4 levels suggest activation of the alternative pathway. This difference is particularly useful in distinguishing nephritis secondary to complex deposition from that due to NeF (nephritic factor). In the latter condition and in deficiency of factor I or H, factor B is consumed, and its serum concentration is low as measured by radial immunodiffusion. Alternative pathway activity can be measured with a relatively simple and reproducible hemolytic assay that depends on the capacity of rabbit erythroctyes to serve as both an "activating" (permissive) surface and a target of alternative pathway activity.

A defect of complement function should be suspected in any patient with collagen vascular disease or chronic nephritis or with recurrent pyogenic infections or *Neisseria meningitidis* or disseminated gonococcal infections, angioedema, partial lipodystrophy, or a second episode of septicemia at any age.

134.2 Primary Deficiencies of Complement Components

Congenital deficiencies of all 11 proteins of the classical and membrane attack pathway and of factors D and B of the alternative pathway have been described (Table 134–1).

Most patients with primary **deficiency of C1q** have had systemic lupus erythematosus (SLE), an SLE-like syndrome without typical SLE serology, a chronic rash that has shown an underlying vasculitis on biopsy, or membranoproliferative glomerulonephritis (MPGN). Three C1q-deficient children suffered from serious infections; two of these died of meningitis-septicemia. **C1r deficiency** can occur as an isolated defect or in association with C1s deficiency.

Like individuals with C1q deficiency, patients with **C1r, C1r/C1s, C4, C2,** and **C3 deficiencies** have had a high incidence of vasculitis syndromes (see Table 134–1), especially SLE or an SLE-like syndrome in which antinuclear antibody level is not elevated. A few patients with **C5, C6, C7,** or **C8 deficiency** have had such a disorder, but recurrent neisserial infections are much more likely to be the major problem in this group. The reason for the concurrence of deficiencies of components of complement and these "autoimmune" diseases is not entirely clear, but deposition of C3 on autoimmune complexes facilitates their removal from the circulation through binding to complement receptor 1 (CR1) on erythrocytes and transport to the spleen and liver. Inefficiency of this process best explains the particular predisposition to collagen vascular disease in individuals with a defect in the classical pathway.

Several patients with **C2 deficiency** have had repeated life-threatening septicemic illnesses, most commonly due to pneumococci. Most have not had problems with increased susceptibility to infection, presumably because of the protective function of the alternative pathway. The genes for C2, factor B, and C4 are situated close to each other on chromosome 6, and a depression of factor B levels can occur in conjunction with C2 deficiency. Persons with a deficiency of both proteins may be at particular risk.

Because C3 can be activated by C142 or by the alternative pathway, a defect in the function of either pathway can be compensated, at least to some extent. Without C3, however, the chemotactic fragment from C5 (C5a) is not generated, and opsonization of bacteria is inefficient. Some organisms must be well opsonized in order to be cleared, and **genetic deficiency of C3** has been associated with recurrent, severe pyogenic infections due to pneumococci and meningococci. Some C3-deficient patients have had sluggish neutrophilic responses to infection, in agreement with reports that a cleavage factor of C3 elicits an increase in blood neutrophils.

More than half of the individuals reported to have congenital **C5, C6, C7,** or **C8 deficiency** have had meningococcal meningitis or extragenital gonococcal infection. A few have had a collagen vascular disease. In seven studies of patients with systemic meningococcal disease, about 15% had a genetic deficiency of C5, C6, C7, C8, or C9. It is not clear why patients with a deficiency of one of the late-acting components suffer a particular predisposition to neisserial infections; it may be that serum bacteriolysis is uniquely important in defense against this organism. Some persons with such a deficiency have had no significant illness. Patients with C9 deficiency retain about half-normal hemolytic complement titers; a third of these patients have had neisserial disease.

A few individuals have had **deficiency of factor D** or **factor B** of the alternative pathway. All have had recurrent infections. Hemolytic complement activity in their serum was normal, but alternative pathway activity was markedly deficient or absent.

Deficiencies of C1r, C1rs, C4, C2, C3, C5, C6, C7, C8, and C9 are transmitted as autosomal recessive traits, of the autosomal co-dominant variety; that is, each parent transmits a gene that codes for synthesis of half the serum level of the component. The mode of transmission of deficiency of C1q and factors D, B, H, and I is probably also autosomal recessive. Properdin deficiency is transmitted as an X-linked trait. A rare form of C4 deficiency may be inherited as an autosomal dominant trait.

134.3 Deficiencies of Plasma, Membrane, or Serosal Complement Control Proteins

Congenital deficiencies of five plasma complement control proteins have been described (see Table 134–1). **Factor I de-**

TABLE 134–1 Genetic Deficiencies of Plasma Complement Components and Associated Clinical Findings

Deficient Component	Infection*			Collagen Vascular Disease*		
	Common	*Less Common*	*Occasional*	*Common*	*Less Common*	*Occasional*
Classical Pathway						
C1q			Pneumococcal B/M, other pyogenic	SLE	GN	DV/DLE
C1r		Other pyogenic	Pneumococcal B/M, DGI	SLE		GN
C1rs		Other pyogenic		SLE		
C4		Other pyogenic		SLE	Other CVD	GN
C2		Other pyogenic, pneumococcal B/M, meningococcal M			SLE, GN, DV/DLE, other CVD	
C3	Other pyogenic	Pneumococcal B/M, meningococcal M			GN, DV/DLE	SLE, other CVD
C5	Meningococcal M	DGI	Other pyogenic			SLE, GN
C6	Meningococcal M	DGI	Other pyogenic			SLE, GN, other CVD
C7	Meningococcal M		DGI, other pyogenic		SLE, other CVD	
C8	Meningococcal M	DGI	Other pyogenic			SLE, GN
C9		Meningococcal M				
Alternative Pathway						
Factor D			DGI, meningococcal M			
Factor B	Meningococcal M					
Control Proteins						
C1 INH	Hereditary angioedema†					
Factor I	Other pyogenic, meningococcal M	Pneumococcal B/M				
Factor H		Meningococcal B/M	Other pyogenic		GN	SLE
Properdin		Meningococcal M	Pneumococcal B/M, other pyogenic		DV/DLE	
C4-binding protein						Other CVD

**A finding was reported as "common" if it occurred in 50% or more of reported cases, "less common" if reported in about 5–50% of cases, and "occasional" if present in one or two cases or <5% of the more frequent deficiencies.*

†Hereditary angioedema is a specific entity not associated with infection or CVD.

B/M = Bacteremia or meningitis; DGI = disseminated gonococcal infection; DV/DLE = dermal vasculitis or typical discoid lupus erythematosus; GN = glomerulonephritis in various forms, often membranoproliferative; M = meningitis; other CVD = other collagen vascular diseases (almost all possible diagnoses have been reported); other pyogenic = serious deep or systemic infection due to, or typically caused by, a pyogenic bacterium (abscess, osteomyelitis, pneumonia, bacteremia other than pneumococcal, meningitis other than meningococcal or pneumococcal, cellulitis, myopericarditis, and peritonitis); SLE = typical systemic lupus erythematosus or an SLE-like syndrome without characteristic serologic findings.

Data from Figueroa JE, Densen P: Infectious diseases associated with complement deficiencies. Clin Microbiol Rev 4:359, 1991; and from Ross SC, Densen P: Complement deficiency states and infection: Epidemiology, pathogenesis and consequences of neisserial and other infections in an immune deficiency. Medicine 63:243, 1984; table modified from Johnston RB Jr: Disorders of the complement system. In: *Stiehem ER (ed): Immunologic Disorders in Infants and Children, 4th ed. Philadelphia, WB Saunders, 1996.*

ficiency was originally reported as a deficiency of C3 owing to its hypercatabolism. The first patient described had suffered a series of severe pyogenic infections similar to those seen with agammaglobulinemia or congenital deficiency of C3. Further studies indicated that the primary deficiency was that of factor I, an essential regulator of both pathways. This deficiency permits prolonged existence of C3b in the C3 convertase of the alternative pathway, C3bBb, resulting in constant activation of the alternative pathway and cleavage of more C3 to C3b, in circular fashion. Intravenous infusion of plasma or purified factor I induced a prompt rise in serum C3 concentration in the patient and a return to normal of in vitro C3-dependent functions such as opsonization.

The effects of **factor H deficiency** are like those of factor I deficiency because factor H assists in dismantling the alternative pathway C3 convertase. Levels of C3, factor B, total hemolytic activity, and alternative pathway activity have been low or undetectable in all patients tested. Patients have sustained systemic infections due to pyogenic bacteria, particularly meningococci, and glomerulonephritis has occurred in almost half the cases. The three patients thus far reported as having **deficiency of C4-binding protein** have had about 25% of the normal levels of the protein and no typical disease presentation.

Persons with **properdin deficiency** have had a predisposition to meningococcal meningitis. All reported patients have been male, and their families have had a striking history of male deaths due to meningitis. The predisposition to infection in these patients indicates a requirement for the alternative pathway in host defense against bacterial infection. Serum hemolytic complement activity is normal in these patients, and the presence of specific antibody should avoid the need for the alternative pathway and properdin. Several patients have had dermal vasculitis or discoid lupus.

Hereditary angioedema occurs in persons born without the ability to synthesize normally functioning C1 inhibitor (C1 INH). In 85% of affected families, the affected members have markedly reduced concentrations of inhibitor (5–30% of normal); in the other 15%, normal or elevated concentrations of an immunologically cross-reacting but nonfunctional protein occur. Both forms of the disease are transmitted as an autosomal dominant trait.

In the absence of C1 INH functions, activation of C1 leads to uncontrolled C1 activity, with breakdown of C4 and C2 and release of a vasoactive peptide (kinin) from C2. Episodic, localized, nonpitting edema results from the vasodilatory effects of the kinin on the postcapillary venule. The mechanism by which C1 is activated in these patients is not clear.

Swelling of the affected part progresses rapidly, without urticaria, itching, discoloration, or redness, and often without severe pain. Swelling of the intestinal wall, however, can lead to intense abdominal cramping, sometimes with vomiting or diarrhea; concurrent subcutaneous edema is often absent, and patients have undergone abdominal surgery or psychiatric examination before the true diagnosis was made. Laryngeal edema can be fatal. Attacks last 2–3 days and then gradually abate. They may occur at sites of trauma, after vigorous exercise, with menses, or with emotional stress. Attacks can begin in the first 2 yr of life but are usually not severe until late childhood or adolescence. **Acquired C1 INH deficiency** can occur in association with B-cell cancer or autoantibody to C1 INH. SLE and glomerulonephritis have been reported in patients with the congenital disease.

Three of the membrane complement control proteins, CR1, membrane cofactor protein, and decay-accelerating factor (DAF), prevent the formation of the full C3-cleaving enzyme, C3bBb, that is triggered by C3b deposition. The other two, membrane inhibitor of reactive lysis (CD59) and C8-binding protein (C8-bp), prevent the full development of the membrane attack complex that creates the "hole." **Paroxysmal nocturnal hemoglobinuria** (PNH) is a hemolytic anemia that occurs when DAF, CD59, and C8-bp are not expressed on the erythrocyte surface. The condition is acquired as a somatic mutation in a hematopoietic stem cell of the PIG-A gene on the X chromosome. The product of this gene is required for normal synthesis of a glycosyl-phosphatidylinositol molecule that anchors about 20 proteins to cell membranes, including DAF, CD59, and C8-bp. One patient with **genetic isolated CD59 deficiency** had a mild PNH-like disease in spite of normal expression of membrane DAF. In contrast, **genetic isolated DAF deficiency** has not resulted in hemolytic anemia.

Patients with SLE and their asymptomatic family members have a partial **deficiency of CR1**, which is possibly inherited. This deficiency could increase the risk of developing immune complex disease, thereby contributing to the pathogenesis of SLE.

Strong evidence indicates that serosal fluids contain yet another complement control protein, a protease that normally destroys the chemotactic activity of C5a and interleukin 8 (IL-8), important chemotactic factors for neutrophils. A defect in this protease in peritoneal and synovial fluids occurs in **familial Mediterranean fever** (FMF). Missense mutations in a gene encoding a transcription factor termed *pyrin* may represent the basic defect. Patients with FMF suffer recurrent episodes of fever in association with painful inflammation of joints and pleural and peritoneal cavities (Chapter 164). Thus, it appears that C5a or IL-8 or both are generated at serosal surfaces under normal conditions and that serosal fluids contain an inhibitor of these chemotactic agents that serves to prevent the inflammatory response that would otherwise ensue.

134.4 Secondary Disorders of Complement

Partial deficiency of C1q has occurred in patients with *severe combined immunodeficiency disease* or *hypogammaglobulinemia*, apparently secondary to the deficiency of IgG, which normally binds reversibly to C1q and prevents its rapid catabolism.

Serum from patients with *chronic membranoproliferative glomerulonephritis* (MPGN) contains a protein termed *nephritic factor* (NeF) that promotes activation of the alternative pathway. NeF is an IgG antibody to the C3-cleaving enzyme of the alternative pathway, C3bBb, that protects the enzyme from inactivation. The result is increased consumption of C3. Serum C3 concentrations vary widely from patient to patient, however. Pyogenic infections, including meningitis, may occur if the serum C3 level drops below about 10% of normal. This disorder has been found in children and adults with *partial lipodystrophy*. Adipocytes can synthesize C3, factor D, and factor B; exposure to NeF induces their lysis. An IgG nephritic factor that binds to and protects C42, the classical pathway C3 convertase, has been described in *acute postinfectious nephritis* and in SLE. The consumption of C3 that characterizes poststreptococcal nephritis and SLE could be due to this factor, to activation of complement by immune complexes, or to both. A related disorder illustrates the importance of factor H in restraining the uncontrolled conversion of C3. A patient has been described as having had a circulating inhibitor of factor H and hypocomplementemic MPGN.

Newborn infants are known to have mild to moderate deficiencies of all plasma components of the complement system. Opsonization and generation of chemotactic activity in serum from full-term newborns can be markedly deficient through either the classical or the alternative pathway. Complement activity is even lower in preterm infants than in full-term babies. Patients with *malnutrition* or *anorexia nervosa* may also have significant depletion of components and functional activity of complement. Although synthesis of components is depressed in these conditions, serum from some patients with malnutrition also appears to contain immune complexes that could accelerate depletion. Severe chronic *cirrhosis of the liver* and *hepatic failure* may also result in decreased synthesis of C3.

Patients with *sickle cell disease* have normal activity of the classical pathway, but some have defective function of the alternative pathway in opsonization of pneumococci, in bacteriolysis and opsonization of salmonellae, and in lysis of rabbit erythrocytes. Deoxygenation of erythrocytes from patients with sickle cell disease alters their membranes to increase exposure of phospholipids that can activate the alternative pathway and consume its components. An alternative pathway defect has been described in about 10% of individuals who have undergone *splenectomy* and in some patients with *β-thalassemia major.* The underlying mechanism for this defect in these last two conditions has not been defined. Children with *nephrotic syndrome* may have subnormal serum opsonizing activity in association with decreased serum levels of factor B; factor D levels also may be low.

Immune complexes, including those initiated by microorganisms or their by-products, may induce consumption of components of complement. Activation occurs primarily through fixation of C1 to antibody, thereby initiating the classic pathway. In *SLE*, immune complexes activate the classical pathway and C3 is deposited at sites of tissue damage, including kidneys and skin; depressed synthesis of C3 is also noted. Formation of immune complexes and consumption of complement have been demonstrated in *lepromatous leprosy, subacute bacterial endocarditis, infected ventriculojugular shunts, malaria, infectious mononucleosis, dengue, hemorrhagic fever,* and *acute hepatitis B*. Nephritis or arthritis may develop as a result of deposition of immune complexes and activation of complement in these infections. The syndrome of *recurrent urticaria, angioedema, eosinophilia,* and *hypocomplementemia* secondary to activation of the classical pathway may be due to circulating immune complexes. Circulating immune complexes and decreased C3 have been reported in some patients with *dermatitis herpetiformis, celiac disease, primary biliary cirrhosis,* and *Reye syndrome.*

In patients with *bacteremic shock*, bacterial products appear to initiate direct activation of the alternative pathway. *Intravenous injection of iodinated roentgenographic contrast medium* can induce a rapid and significant activation of the alternative pathway, which may explain at least some of the occasional reactions that occur in patients undergoing this procedure.

Burns can induce massive activation of the complement system, especially the alternative pathway, within a few hours after injury. Generation of C3a and C5a occurs, which stimulates neutrophils and induces their sequestration in the lungs. These events may play an important part in the development of shock lung after burn injury. Cardiopulmonary bypass, plasma exchange, or hemodialysis using cellophane membranes may be associated with a similar syndrome due to activation of plasma complement, with release of C3a and C5a. In patients with *erythropoietic protoporphyria* or *porphyria cutanea tarda,* exposure of the skin to light of certain wavelengths activates complement, generating chemotactic activity. Phototoxicity is associated histologically with lysis of capillary endothelial cells, mast cell degranulation, and the appearance of neutrophils in the dermis.

134.5 Treatment of Disorders of the Complement System

No specific therapy is available at present for genetic deficiencies of the complement system except hereditary angioedema, but much can be done to protect patients with any of these disorders from serious complications. Management of *hereditary angioedema* starts with avoidance of precipitating factors, usually trauma. Infusion of vapor-heated C1 INH concentrate aborts acute attacks and is safe and effective in long-term prophylaxis or in preparation for surgery or dental procedures. Adults with hereditary angioedema respond to danazol, a synthetic androgen with weak virilizing and mild anabolic potential. The drug, given orally, increases the level of C1 INH severalfold and prevents attacks. It has not been recommended for use in children.

Only supportive management is available for other primary diseases of the complement system. It should be emphasized, however, that identification of a specific defect in the complement system may have an important impact on a patient's health. Concern for the associated complications (collagen vascular disease and infection) should encourage vigorous diagnostic efforts and earlier institution of therapy. With the onset of unexplained fever, cultures should be obtained and antibiotic therapy instituted more quickly and with less stringent indications than in a normal child. The parent or patient should be given letters describing any predisposition to systemic bacterial infection associated with the patient's deficiency, along with the recommended approach to management, for possible use by school, camp, or emergency room physicians. The patient and close household contacts should be immunized with vaccines for pneumococci, *Haemophilus influenzae,* and *N. meningitidis.* High titers of specific antibody might opsonize effectively without the full complement system, and immunization of household members could reduce the risk of exposing patients to these particularly threatening pathogens.

Babior BM, Matzner Y: The familial Mediterranean fever gene—cloned at last. N Engl J Med 337:1548, 1997.

Colten HR, Rosen FS: Complement deficiencies. Annu Rev Immunol 10:809, 1992.

Eichenfield LF, Johnston RB Jr: Secondary disorders of the complement system. Am J Dis Child 143:595, 1989.

Figueroa JE, Densen P: Infectious disease associated with complement deficiencies. Clin Microbiol Rev 4:359, 1991.

Johnston RB Jr: Disorders of the complement system. *In:* Stiehm ER (ed): Immunologic Disorders in Infants and Children, 4th ed. Philadelphia, WB Saunders, 1996, p 490.

Johnston RB Jr: Complement disorders. *In:* Burg FD, Ingelfinger JR, Wald ER, Polin RA (eds): Gellis & Kagan's Current Pediatric Therapy 16. Philadelphia, WB Saunders, 1999, p 1077.

Ross SC, Densen P: Complement deficiency states and infection: Epidemiology, pathogenesis and consequences of neisserial and other infections in an immune deficiency. Medicine 63:243, 1984.

Rosse WF: Paroxysmal nocturnal hemoglobinuria as a molecular disease. Medicine (Baltimore) 76:63, 1997.

Walport MJ, Davies KA, Morley BJ, et al: Complement deficiency and autoimmunity. Ann NY Acad Sci 815:267, 1997.

Wang RH, Phillips G Jr, Medof ME, et al: Activation of the alternative complement pathway by exposure of phosphatidylethanolamine and phosphatidylserine on erythrocytes from sickle cell disease patients. J Clin Invest 92:1326, 1993.

Waytes AT, Rosen FS, Frank MM: Treatment of hereditary angioedema with a vapor-heated C1 inhibitor concentrate. N Engl J Med 334:1630, 1996.

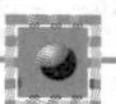

SECTION 5

Bone Marrow Transplantation

Kent A. Robertson

Bone marrow transplantation (BMT) involves treatment with marrow-ablative chemoradiotherapy followed by an infusion of either the patient's own marrow (autologous BMT) or marrow from a donor (allogeneic BMT) or some other source of marrow stem cells (cord blood, peripheral blood stem cells, fetal liver). BMT is the treatment of choice for some malignant diseases, such as chronic myelogenous leukemia, and for acquired and inherited nonmalignant disorders, such as aplastic anemia and Fanconi anemia. It may also be used for some malignancies that are unresponsive to conventional therapy. The process of stem cell transplantation also encompasses replacing an absent or defective gene with a normal gene in the patient's own cells (gene therapy). Although the use of BMT for malignancies is common, disease relapses continue to be a problem. Because only 25% of patients have human leukocyte antigen (HLA)–matched sibling donors, the use of mismatched related donor marrow and unrelated donor marrow or umbilical cord blood provides an alternate source of stem cells but at the cost of increased graft rejection and graft versus host disease (GVHD). As the use of BMT becomes widespread, pediatricians are more often called on to take an important role in the evaluation and consideration of patients for possible transplant and the long-term follow-up of patients who have undergone BMT. ■

CHAPTER 135 *Clinical Indications*

ACQUIRED DISEASES

APLASTIC ANEMIA. Aplastic anemia, a disorder of unknown cause, results in pancytopenia and bone marrow hypoplasia, and, if severe (platelet count <20,000/mm³; absolute neutrophil count <500/mm³ ; or reticulocyte count <1% when anemia is present), often results in death within the first 6 mo due to infection or bleeding. See Chapter 453. The marrow dysfunction may result from inherited disorders (Fanconi anemia or paroxysmal nocturnal hemoglobinuria), autoimmunity, or dysregulated cytokine production and is occasionally associated with exposure to chemicals (benzene or chloramphenicol) and non-A, non-B, non-C hepatitis. Transfusion should be avoided if possible, because sensitization to blood products increases the likelihood of graft rejection should BMT be needed. BMT is the treatment of choice in patients who have severe aplastic anemia and who have an HLA-matched family donor; the survival rate at 2 yr is 69%, based on data from the International Bone Marrow Transplant Registry. The 15-yr survival rate was 100% among children younger than 6 yr (n=12) and 78% for children 6–19 yr old (n=63) who received HLA-matched sibling BMT for aplastic anemia in Seattle. Patients receiving transplants for aplastic anemia exhibit a higher incidence of graft rejection than that seen with other kinds of HLA-matched sibling transplants, but the addition of antithymocyte globulin to cyclophosphamide for the preparative regimen decreases rejection significantly. Since the institution of this preparative regimen, an actuarial 3-yr survival rate of 92% has been achieved (Fig. 135–1). Transplantation using family donors who are more disparate or matched unrelated donors usually requires more immunosuppressive therapy with the addition of radiation and or chemotherapy, which increases the incidence of secondary cancers from 3.8% to 14%. This risk increases to 42% if the underlying diagnosis is Fanconi's anemia. For patients without donors, immunosuppressive regimens have been effective, with survivals after 5 yr of 50–75%.

ACUTE MYELOGENOUS LEUKEMIA. Acute myelogenous leukemia (AML) is a heterogeneous group of leukemias derived from myeloid progenitor cells (Chapter 502.2). BMT is the accepted therapy for AML in first remission. Disease-free survival rates range from 55% to 83% for matched sibling marrow transplant in patients in first complete remission. In a randomized trial of matched sibling BMT, high-dose chemotherapy alone, and autologous BMT, the 3-yr disease-free survival rates were 70%, 55%, and 40% respectively.

BMT also improves survival of children with acute megakaryocytic (M7) leukemia (Chapter 502.3) and secondary AML resulting from prior cancer therapy because both respond poorly to chemotherapy. BMT is indicated for patients who have AML that does not enter remission, using marrow from an HLA-identical family donor, mismatched family donors, or matched unrelated donors. In patients who achieve a first remission, BMT is indicated if they have an HLA-identical family donor. One exception to this strategy is M3, or promyelocytic leukemia, which is quite responsive to all-*trans*-retinoic acid and consolidation chemotherapy (Chapter 501). Patients who relapse or are in second remission should be considered for BMT using HLA-matched family members, unrelated donors, or previously stored autologous marrow. Patients with numerous relapses, resistant disease, or secondary AML are candidates for two to three antigen-mismatched donor transplants.

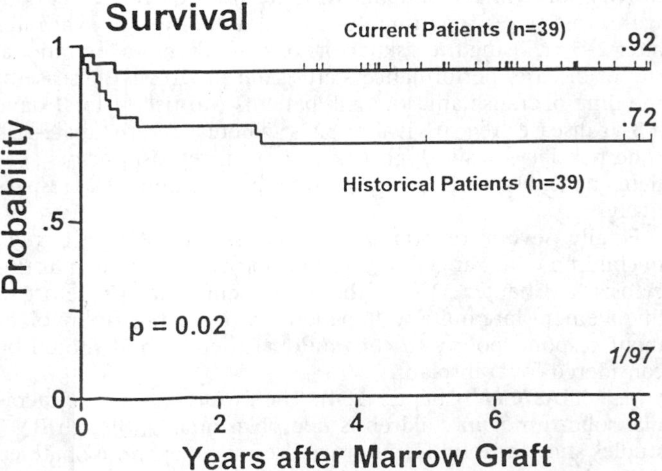

Figure 135–1 Marrow grafts for aplastic anemia (AA). Kaplan-Meier estimates of survival in 78 patients with aplastic anemia given HLA-identical marrow transplants. Thirty-nine were conditioned with cyclophosphamide/ATG (current patients), and thirty-nine received cyclophosphamide alone (historical patients). Tick marks indicate surviving patients. (From Storb R, Leisenering W, Anasetti C, et al: Long-term follow-up of allogeneic marrow transplants in patients with aplastic anemia conditioned by cyclophosphamide combined with antithymocyte globulin. Blood 89:3890, 1997.)

TABLE 135–1 High-Risk Acute Lymphoblastic Leukemia

Congenital or infant (<1 yr) ALL
Chromosomal translocations: t(4,11), t(9,22)-Philadelphia, t(8,14)
Fab L-3 morphology (Burkitt)
White blood cell count ≥100,000
More than 1 mo to achieve remission
Failure to achieve remission
Relapse while on chemotherapy
Second and subsequent remissions (when first remission <30 mo)
More than one extramedullary site of relapse without a marrow relapse
Secondary ALL resulting from prior cancer therapy

ALL = acute lymphoblastic leukemia.

ACUTE LYMPHOBLASTIC LEUKEMIA. Acute lymphoblastic leukemia (ALL) is the most common malignancy of childhood, and approximately 70% of cases are cured by conventional chemotherapy (Chapter 502.1). A subgroup of these patients have a high risk (75–100%) for relapse with conventional therapy and should be considered for BMT using various marrow-purging techniques and preparative regimens (Table 135–1). Disease-free survival rates range from 15% to 65% in general, with relapse rates of 30–70%.

Patients who have HLA-matched donors may be eligible for allogeneic BMT for high-risk ALL. Children receiving HLA-matched sibling marrow transplants for high-risk ALL in first complete remission have disease-free survival rates of 70–80%, with low relapse rates of 0–10%, although the numbers are small and some high-risk groups such as patients with Philadelphia chromosome–positive ALL have lower survival rates of 30–50%. Patients who do not have high-risk features at the time of diagnosis but who later suffer relapse and have an HLA-identical family donor also benefit from transplantation, with disease-free survivals of 40–60%. Patients have a better outcome if they undergo transplantation in remission, and patients in whom remission occurs earlier have a higher disease-free survival rate. Total body irradiation given before chemotherapy may be advantageous. Patients without a family donor may benefit from unrelated donor BMT, with disease-free survival rates of 30–40%.

Comparisons of allogeneic and autologous BMT or chemotherapy for ALL relapse support the recommendation that these children should be offered BMT when possible. A review of 376 children receiving HLA-identical sibling marrow transplants compared with 540 children receiving chemotherapy for ALL in second remission revealed disease-free survival rates of 40% and 17%, with relapse rates of 45% and 80%, respectively. Other studies comparing allogeneic and autologous BMT for relapsed ALL have shown disease-free survival rates of 33–61% for allografts and 21–47% for autografts, illustrating the advantage of allogeneic BMT over autologous transplants despite increased toxicity.

The lower incidence of relapse in allogeneic BMT is related to GVHD/graft versus leukemia (GVL) effect. The probability of relapse is 25 ± 6%, 22 ± 5%, 10 ± 7%, 7 ± 3%, 46 ± 15%, and 41 ± 8% for allogeneic grafts without GVHD, acute GVHD only, chronic GVHD only, acute and chronic GVHD, syngeneic grafts, and allogeneic T-cell–depleted grafts, respectively. These results are the same for the individual diseases (ALL, AML, chronic myelogenous leukemia [CML]), emphasizing and the importance of the immune system in eliminating residual leukemia cells.

Infant leukemia (Chapter 502.4) occurring within the first 12 mo of life is rare and carries a very poor prognosis, with survival rates of 20–30% after 5 yr with conventional chemotherapy. Infants with a normal 11q23 locus have a very good response to conventional chemotherapy, with a disease-free survival of 80% at a median follow-up of 46 mo, whereas those with a rearranged 11q23 have a very poor response, with a 15% disease-free survival. A total of 29 patients with infant leukemia have received BMT for ALL or AML; disease-free survival occurs in 40–50% of patients receiving BMT while in remission, compared with 10–20% if BMT is performed after relapse, using various sources of marrow. Cases of acute leukemia with chromosomal rearrangements involving 11q23 diagnosed within the first year of life are best treated with intense induction chemotherapy followed by BMT if a suitable donor is available.

MYELODYSPLASTIC AND MYELOPROLIFERATIVE DISORDERS. *Myelodysplastic syndrome* (MDS) includes a group of disorders with a defect in hematopoietic cell development close to the level of the marrow stem cell, which eventually progresses from a picture of dysplastic ineffective hematopoiesis to aggressive overt myeloid leukemia (Chapter 502.2). These are classified as refractory anemia, refractory anemia with ringed sideroblasts, refractory anemia with excess blasts, refractory anemia with excess blasts in transformation, and chronic myelomonocytic leukemia. Because of the close relationship to AML, patients with MDS are treated according to AML protocols. The transplant outcome in patients with MDS is similar to that in patients with AML. In one series of 23 pediatric patients, the disease-free survival at 5 yr was 64% using HLA-matched family donors, and for 15 pediatric patients receiving HLA-matched unrelated donor BMTs the disease-free survival was 53%. Transplant should be considered early after diagnosis because patients in whom the disease has progressed with increasing blasts have a much poorer outcome and a higher rate of relapse. Conventional chemotherapy and other nontransplant forms of treatment have not made a significant impact on the natural progression of the disease.

The *myeloproliferative disorders* are characterized by a single-lineage myeloid proliferation that can progress to an AML-like leukemia. These diseases include CML, essential thrombocythemia (ET), polycythemia vera, agnogenic myeloid metaplasia (AMM), and juvenile myelomonocytic leukemia (JMML). BMT is the treatment of choice for CML (Chapter 502.5). HLA-identical sibling transplantation results in an 80% long-term disease-free survival, compared with 45–74% for matched unrelated donor BMT. Transplantation is recommended within 1 yr from diagnosis, because delay results in a significant decrease in the disease-free survival to 40–60%. Patients receiving BMT in accelerated phase or blast crisis have disease-free survival rates of 35–40% and 10–20%, respectively, and a 60% chance of relapse compared with a 10–20% chance of relapse in patients receiving BMT in the chronic phase.

Successful BMT has also been performed for some of the more uncommon myeloproliferative disorders. BMT should be considered in those patients who fail to respond to conservative management or whose disease progresses to an AML-like leukemic condition. BMT is a possible approach for childhood *polycythemia vera.* BMT has been attempted for ET in a few patients without success. AMM, or idiopathic myelofibrosis, is characterized by splenomegaly and progressive fibrosis of the marrow compartment, resulting in anemia. The mean survival for patients with AMM is 5 yr, and the only known curative therapy is BMT; 7 of 12 patients receiving BMT for AMM survived.

JMML, formerly known as *juvenile chronic myelogenous leukemia* (Chapter 502.3), is an aggressive clonal proliferation of immature myeloid precursors associated with neurofibromatosis type 1 and monosomy 7. The clinical course is rapid, with resistance to conventional chemotherapy and death at an average of 9 mo from the time of diagnosis. BMT is curative in these patients and should be pursued aggressively once the diagnosis is confirmed. Among the 43 children receiving BMT by the European group from matched sibling donors (n = 25) or from mismatched family members/matched unrelated donors (n = 18), the disease-free survivals were 38% and 22%, respectively, with follow-up of 9–65 mo. The Milwaukee transplant group reported six patients with JMML given T-cell–depleted matched unrelated donor BMT; three of the six were alive at 6 mo–6 yr. Some patients with JMML have been found to respond to 13-*cis*-retinoic acid with temporary remissions, which may provide the time needed to identify potential marrow donors for these patients.

LYMPHOMAS. Non-Hodgkin lymphoma (NHL) and Hodgkin disease (HD) are malignant, usually clonal proliferations arising from the lymphoreticular system (Chapters 503.2 and 503.1). Childhood lymphomas are quite responsive to conventional chemoradiotherapy, but a subset of these patients have high-risk disease and relapse, requiring more intensive therapy to achieve a cure. BMT can cure some patients with NHL and HD and should be offered early after relapse, while the disease is still sensitive to therapy, there is little bulky disease, and there is a greater likelihood of being able to tolerate a transplant regimen. Pretransplant salvage chemotherapy may be of some benefit to reduce the tumor burden. If an HLA-identical sibling is available, allogeneic transplant should be offered to take advantage of the GVL effect, which has reduced the relapse rate by as much as 25–30% in some series. Finally, early results using peripheral blood stem cells for transplantation appear to be as good as or better than those with autologous transplantation. A European Lymphoma Registry study described autologous BMT for children with poor-risk B-cell or Burkitt lymphoma including those with relapsed or resistant disease. The 5-yr disease-free survival was 39.4% in these children with otherwise incurable disease. In a report from 6 Spanish centers, 46 pediatric patients received BMT for NHL including lymphoblastic lymphoma, Burkitt lymphoma, and large cell lymphoma, with a 3-yr disease-free survival of 58%. A separate but distinct clincopathologic entity is the CD30- or Ki-1–positive peripheral T-cell lymphomas including anaplastic large cell lymphomas associated with chromosomal translocation t (2;5). These tumors are aggressive and tend to relapse but have responded well to BMT, with an 80% 5-yr disease-free survival.

Hematopoietic stem cell transplantation has resulted in improved survival for patients with relapsed or refractory HD, with most series reporting 40–60% disease-free survival rates after 2–5 yr. Using the risk factors of more than one extranodal site of disease, performance status, and progressive disease at the time of transplant, low-risk patients (no risk factors) have a 3-yr disease-free survival of 82%, whereas intermediate-risk (one risk factor) and high-risk (two to three risk factors) patients have disease-free survival rates of 56% and 19%, respectively.

Finally, several reports describe successful BMTs performed in children with Langerhans' cell histiocytosis, including histiocytosis X (Chapter 515). Although patients with single-organ involvement fare quite well, patients with multiorgan involvement respond poorly to conventional therapy and should be considered for transplant.

NEUROBLASTOMA (Chapter 504). The most common extracranial solid tumor in children is neuroblastoma. Although BMT studies show a trend for improved results over those obtained with chemotherapy, randomized trials to compare the two approaches are ongoing. Disease-free (3-yr) survival rates for patients receiving BMT after progression of disease are 7–25%, compared with 25–55% for those receiving BMT before progression of disease. Certain high-risk groups have significant improvement with BMT, including those with N-*myc* amplification, age of 2 yr or older, a partial remission to induction therapy, and bone/bone marrow metastasis. Protocols use various combinations of sequential cycles of chemotherapy with peripheral blood stem cell support and radiation to localized disease, followed by transplantation of autologous T cell–purged marrow.

BRAIN TUMORS. Tumors of the central nervous system (CNS) are the most common solid tumors in children, accounting for 20% of childhood malignancies (Chapter 611). Phase I–II trials are helping to define the role of BMT in treating brain tumors. The Italian group treated 11 children with recurrent medulloblastoma (3), glioblastoma multiforme (2), supratentorial primitive neuroectodermal tumor (PNET) (2), ependymoma (2), anaplastic astrocytoma (1), and anaplastic oligodendroglioma (1) using a conditioning regimen of etoposide (VP-16) and *bis*-chlorethylnitrosourea (BCNU) or thiotepa followed by autologous marrow infusion; five who had no measurable disease at the time of transplant are alive without evidence of disease after a median follow-up period of 20 mo. A Children's Cancer Group study used carboplatin, thiotepa, and etoposide as a preparative regimen for 23 patients with recurrent medulloblastoma, resulting in a 34% disease-free survival after 3 yr. Another study focused on using a similar chemotherapy-only transplant regimen after standard induction therapy (vincristine, cisplatin, cyclophosphamide, and etoposide) for young children with newly diagnosed brain tumors (malignant glioma, 9; ependymoma, 10; brain stem glioma, 6; medulloblastoma, 13; PNET, 14; other, 10) in an effort to avoid the toxicity of cranial irradiation; of 62 children enrolled, 37 had no disease progression with induction therapy and went on to autologous BMT with a disease-free survival of 41% (27% for all 62 enrolled) after 2 yr.

SOLID TUMORS. Many solid tumors are quite responsive to conventional chemoradiotherapy; however, a subset of these are associated with a very poor prognosis (Chapters 504 to 513). These tumors are high risk by virtue of their histology (alveolar rhabdomyosarcomas, anaplastic Wilms tumor), location (pelvic, trunk, or proximal extremity Ewing sarcoma, axial skeletal osteogenic sarcoma), or widespread metastatic presentation. Phase I–II trials are exploring the use of dose intensification of chemotherapy with or without total body irradiation, followed by autologous marrow rescue. The European Bone Marrow Transplantation Solid Tumor Registry described 25 children who received autologous BMT for refractory or relapsed *Wilms tumor* (Chapter 505.1). Eight of 17 children who received BMT after remission reinduction are disease free 14–90 mo after BMT; one of eight children receiving BMT in relapse survives disease free after 3 yr. The Memorial Sloan Kettering group treated 26 patients with high-risk rhabdomyosarcoma (n = 21), undifferentiated sarcoma (n = 3), or extraosseous Ewing sarcoma (n = 2) using the strategy of induction chemotherapy followed by split-course hyperfractionated radiotherapy. Those with a complete or partial remission received consolidation therapy with high-dose melphalan/etoposide and autologous BMT, which resulted in a 2-yr progression-free survival of 53%. Patients with primary refractory or relapsed rhabdomyosarcoma respond less well to BMT, with disease-free survival rates of 24%. In another study, patients with various solid tumors were treated with escalating doses of cyclophosphamide in addition to carboplatin, etoposide, and melphalan as a preparative regimen for autologous BMT. Four of six patients with metastatic Ewing sarcoma who received BMT in first complete remission remain disease free after 3 yr. One series of 24 children received BMT for relapsed osteosarcoma; after a follow-up of only 6 mo, half were disease-free survivors.

GENETIC DISEASES

IMMUNODEFICIENCY DISORDERS (Chapters 124 to 126). BMT is the treatment of choice for some forms of severe combined immunodeficiency (SCID). See Chapter 126.1. BMT has been performed in other forms of immunodeficiency, including Wiskott-Aldrich syndrome, DiGeorge syndrome, Kostmann neutropenia, leukocyte adherence deficiency, chronic granulomatous disease, Chédiak-Higashi syndrome, familial erythrophagocytic lymphohistiocytosis, Duncan syndrome, and neutrophil actin deficiencies. Survival rates are 68% when matched sibling donors are used and 35% when mismatched donors are used. The presentation of DiGeorge syndrome can be variable; however, those patients with initial profoundly depressed T-cell function do not recover over time and are candidates for BMT. If other forms of therapy are available, such as interferon-gamma for chronic granulomatous disease or granulocyte colony-stimulating factor for Kostmann neutropenia, BMT should be reserved for patients who are unresponsive.

FANCONI ANEMIA (Chapter 474). The characteristic sensitivity to DNA cross-linking agents makes children who have Fanconi anemia (FA) quite sensitive to conventional BMT conditioning regimens, requiring dose reduction to avoid excessive toxicity. Transplant-related toxicities include severe oral mucositis, hemorrhagic cystitis, erythroderma, and GVHD. Disease-free survival rates are 25–75%, depending on the source of stem cells. Patients receiving reduced conditioning regimens and matched sibling donor BMT have the best outcomes, although mismatched and unrelated donor BMTs have been successful. Patients with FA and an HLA-identical family member who has a negative result on FA screening should be offered BMT at the first sign of pancytopenia. Alternative donor transplants including cord blood should be considered in the absence of a matched family member, given the poor outlook for these patients once leukemic transformation occurs.

STORAGE DISEASES. The metabolic storage diseases are a heterogeneous group of disorders resulting from single gene mutations producing enzyme defects and the subsequent toxic accumulation of metabolites. The end result is progressive neurologic deterioration or visceral infiltration, which is usually fatal. Some disorders, such as adrenoleukodystrophy, respond to dietary measures, whereas others, such as Gaucher disease types I and III, respond to enzyme supplementation. In most cases, however, no successful supplementation therapy is available. BMT provides a source of enzyme through the bone marrow–derived monocyte/phagocytic cell system, which includes the liver (Kupffer cells), brain (microglial cells), skin (Langerhans cells), marrow (osteoclasts), lung (pulmonary macrophages), and lymph nodes (histiocytes). The results of transplant in several storage disorders are variable, with some patients showing a good response (with adrenoleukodystrophy, metachromatic leukodystrophy, globoid cell leukodystrophy, Hurler syndrome), whereas other results have been more dismal (Sanfilippo and Hunter syndromes). The risk of transplant-related mortality is about 10% for matched sibling donors and 37% for mismatched and unrelated donors. Transplant before the disease progresses to extensive end-organ damage is necessary. Efforts should be directed toward early diagnosis and BMT before significant neurologic damage occurs.

THALASSEMIA (Chapter 468.9). Three risk factors that influence the outcome of BMT for thalassemia include hepatomegaly, portal fibrosis, and a history of inconsistent iron chelation before transplant. Other factors, such as the number of transfusions, ferritin level, degree of hemosiderosis, hepatic iron concentration, and splenomegaly, have no effect. More than 500 children (≤16 yr) in Italy have received HLA-identical family member donor BMTs (Fig. 135–2). Disease-free survival rates of up to 90% are obtained in children receiving BMT before the development of hepatomegaly or portal fibrosis. Hepatic hemosiderosis and portal fibrosis may improve after BMT if the damage is not too extensive. In the United States, 17/27 children (63%) who received HLA-matched family donor BMTs survived disease free; one required a second BMT. Another five patients survived after graft rejections and lived with

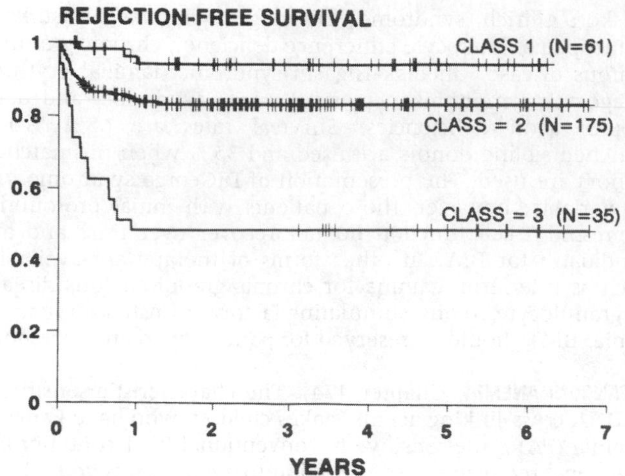

Figure 135–2 The probabilities of rejection-free survival for 271 patients younger than 17 yr with thalassemia who received marrow transplants from human leukocyte antigen identical family members after conditioning with busulfan and cyclophosphamide. (From Forman SJ, Blume KG, Thomas ED: Bone Marrow Transplantation. Boston, Blackwell, 1994.)

recurrent thalassemia, for an overall survival rate of 81%. If an HLA-identical family member is available, BMT should be performed before the patient develops advanced disease.

SICKLE CELL DISEASE (Chapter 468.1). With supportive care, more than 90% of children with sickle cell (SS) disease live into their 3rd and 4th decades and 60% survive to 50 yr. Disease severity varies among patients with homozygous hemoglobin S (HbS) disease; 5–20% suffer significant morbidity from vaso-occlusive crises and pulmonary, renal, and CNS damage. New approaches include antisickling agents, gene therapy, and induction of increased hemoglobin F by drugs such as hydroxyurea, but BMT is the only curative treatment for sickle cell anemia.

In the United States, 34 patients (ages 3–15 yr) have received BMTs using HLA-identical sibling donors; two donors had the sickle trait. The indications for BMT included history of strokes, recurrent acute chest syndrome, and recurrent vaso-occlusive crises. Thirty-two survived (93%), with four patients (14%) experiencing graft rejection or recurrence of SS disease for a disease-free survival of 79% at a median follow-up of 26 mo. Forty-five patients (ages 1–23 yr) received HLA-identical family member donor BMT for SS disease in Belgium and France. After follow-up of 1–75 mo, 95% survive, with a disease-free survival rate of 86%. No vaso-occlusive events have occurred among the 38 patients with successful engraftment, and some have recovered splenic function. Although BMT can cure homozygous HbS disease, selecting appropriate candidates for BMT is difficult. Patients with SS disease may survive for decades, but some patients have a poor quality of life, with repeated hospitalizations for painful vaso-occlusive crises and CNS infarcts. Patients with SS disease, such as those with the Central African Republic haplotype, can be predicted to have serious complications. BMT should be considered in young patients who have recurrent severe vaso-occlusive crises, evidence of developing end-organ damage, CNS infarcts, or a history of strokes and who have an HLA-identical family member donor.

OTHER CONGENITAL ANEMIAS. BMT is successful in some other congenital anemias. *Diamond-Blackfan syndrome,* or congenital pure red blood cell aplasia, is characterized by normochromic-macrocytic anemia with a normocellular marrow (Chapter 454). Patients who fail to respond to initial therapies may benefit from BMT using an HLA-identical sibling donor. Twenty-four of 35 patients who were given BMT for Diamond-Blackfan anemia are alive disease free at 6 mo–10 yr after transplant, including three cord blood transplants. *Congenital sideroblastic anemia* results from a mitochondrial abnormality in erythroblasts (Chapter 458). One 34-mo-old child received a BMT from a phenotypically identical cousin and has some persistent liver enlargement after 3 yr but remains transfusion independent, with normal serum iron and ferritin levels.

General References

Forman SJ, Blume KG, Thomas ED (eds): Hematopoietic Cell Transplantation, 2nd ed. Boston, Blackwell Scientific Publications, 1998.
Robertson KA: Pediatric bone marrow transplantation. Curr Opin Pediatr 5:103, 1993.
Sanders JE: Bone marrow transplantation for pediatric malignancies. Pediatr Clin North Am 44:1005, 1997.

Aplastic Anemia

Doney K, Leisenring W, Storb R, et al: Primary treatment of acquired aplastic anemia: Outcomes with bone marrow transplantation and immunosuppressive therapy. Ann Intern Med 126:107, 1997.
Gillio AP, Boulad F, Small T, et al: Comparison of long-term outcome of children with severe aplastic anemia treated with immunosuppression versus bone marrow transplantation. Biol Blood Marrow Transplant 3:18, 1997.
Locatelli F, Ports F, Zecca M, et al: Successful bone marrow transplantation in children with severe aplastic anemia using HLA-partially matched family donors. Am J Hematol 42:328, 1993.

Acute Myelogenous Leukemia

Appelbaum FR: Indications for bone marrow transplantation in the treatment of acute myeloid leukemia. Leukemia 7:1081, 1993.
Hongeng S, Krance RA, Bowman LC, et al: Outcomes of transplantation with matched-sibling and unrelated bone marrow in children with leukemia. Lancet 350:767, 1997.
Vormoor J, Boos J, Stahnke K, et al: Therapy of childhood acute myelogenous leukemias. Ann Hematol 73:11, 1996.
Woods WG, Neudorf S, Gold S, et al: Aggressive post-remission chemotherapy is better than autologous bone marrow transplantation and allogeneic BMT is superior to both in children with acute myeloid leukemia. Proc Am Soc Clin Oncol/J Clin Oncol 15:368, 1996.

Acute Lymphoblastic Leukemia

Borgmann A, Baumgarten E, Schmid H, et al: Allogeneic bone marrow transplantation for a subset of children with acute lymphoblastic leukemia in third remission: A conceivable alternative? Bone Marrow Transplant 20:939, 1997.
Davies SM, Wagner JE, Shu XO, et al: Unrelated donor bone marrow transplantation for children with acute leukemia. J Clin Oncol 15:557, 1997.
Emminger W, Emminger-Schmidmeier W, Haas OA, et al: Treatment of infant leukemia with busulfan, cyclophosphamide + etoposide and bone marrow transplantation. Bone Marrow Transplant 9:313, 1992.
Feig SA, Harris RE, Sather, HN: Bone marrow transplantation versus chemotherapy for maintenance of second remission of childhood acute lymphoblastic leukemia: A study of the Children's Cancer Group (CCG-1884). Med Pediatr Oncol 29:534, 1997.
Marks DI, Bird JM, Cornish JM, et al: Unrelated donor bone marrow transplantation for children and adolescents with Philadelphia-positive acute lymphoblastic leukemia. J Clin Oncol 16:931, 1998.
Saarinen UM, Mellander L, Nysom K, et al: Allogeneic bone marrow transplantation in first remission for children with very high-risk acute lymphoblastic leukemia: A retrospective case controlled study in the Nordic countries. Bone Marrow Transplant 17:357, 1996.
Weisdorf DJ, Billet AL, Hanan P, et al: Autologous versus unrelated donor allogeneic marrow transplantation for acute lymphoblastic leukemia. Blood 90:2962, 1997.

Myelodysplastic and Myeloproliferative Syndromes

Anderson J, Appelbaum FR, Storb R: An update on allogeneic marrow transplantation for myelodysplastic syndrome. Leuk Lymphoma 17:95, 1995.
Dini G, Rondelli R, Miano M, et al: Unrelated-donor bone marrow transplantation for Philadelphia chromosome-positive chronic myelogenous leukemia in children: Experience of eight European countries. Bone Marrow Transplant 18(Suppl 2):80, 1996.
Locatelli F, Niemeyer C, Angelucci E, et al: Allogeneic bone marrow transplantation for chronic myelomonocytic leukemia in childhood: A report from the European Working Group on Myelodysplastic Syndrome in Childhood. J Clin Oncol 15:566, 1997.

Lymphomas

Bureo E, Ortega JJ, MuZoz A, et al: Bone marrow transplantation in 46 pediatric with non-Hodgkin's lymphoma. Bone Marrow Transplant 15:353, 1995.
Landenstein R, Pearce R, Hartmann O, et al: High-dose chemotherapy with autologous bone marrow rescue in children with poor-risk Burkitt's lym-

phoma: A report from the European Lymphoma Bone Marrow Transplantation Registry. Blood 90:2921, 1997.

Schiffman K, Buckner CD, Maziarz R, et al: High-dose busulfan, melphalan, and thiotepa followed by autologous peripheral blood stem cell transplantation in patients with aggressive lymphoma or relapsed Hodgkin's disease. Biol Blood Marrow Transplant 3:261, 1997.

Wheeler C, Eickhoff C, Elias A, et al: High-dose cyclophosphamide, carmustine, and etoposide with autologous transplantation in Hodgkin's disease: A prognostic model for treatment outcomes. Biol Blood Marrow Transplant 3:98, 1997.

Neuroblastoma

Kletzel M, Abella EM, Sandler E, et al: Thiotepa and cyclophosphamide with stem cell rescue for consolidation therapy for children with high-risk neuroblastoma: A phase I/II study of the Pediatric Blood and Marrow Transplant Consortium. J Pediatr Hematol Oncol 20:49, 1998.

Landenstein R, Philip T, Lasset C, et al: Multivariate analysis of risk factors in stage 4 neuroblastoma patients over the age of one year treated with megatherapy and stem-cell transplantation: A report from the European Bone Marrow Transplantation Solid Tumor Registry. J Clin Oncol 16:953, 1998.

Matthay KK: Impact of myeloablative therapy with bone marrow transplantation in advanced neuroblastoma. Bone Marrow Transplant 18(Suppl 3):21, 1996.

Brain Tumors

Busca A, Miniero R., Besenzon L, et al: Etoposide-containing regimens with autologous bone marrow transplantation in children with malignant brain tumors. Childs Nerv Syst 13:572, 1997.

Dunkel IJ, Bayett JM, Yates A, et al: High-dose carboplatin, thiotepa, and etoposide with autologous stem-cell rescue for patients with recurrent medulloblastoma. J Clin Oncol 16:222, 1998.

Mason WP, Grovas A, Halpern S, et al: Intensive chemotherapy and bone marrow rescue for young children with newly diagnosed malignant brain tumors. J Clin Oncol 16:210, 1998.

Solid Tumors

Boulad F, Kernan NA, LaQuaglia MP, et al: Hig-dose induction chemoradiotherapy followed by autologous bone marrow transplantation as consolidation therapy in rhabdomyosarcoma, extraosseous Ewing's sarcoma, and undifferentiated sarcoma. J Clin Oncol 16:1697, 1998.

Garaventa A, Hartmann O, Bernard JL, et al: Autologous bone marrow transplantation for pediatric Wilm's tumor: The experience of the European Bone Marrow Transplantation Solid Tumor Registry. Med Pediatr Oncol 22:11, 1994.

Ozkaynak MF, Matthay KK, Cairo M, et al: Double alkylator non-total-body irradiation regimen with autologous hematopoietic stem-cell transplantation in pediatric solid tumors. J Clin Oncol 16:937, 1998.

Immune Deficiency Syndromes

Blanche S, Caniglia M, Girault D, et al: Treatment of hemophagocytic lymphohistiocytosis with chemotherapy and bone marrow transplantation: A single center study of 22 cases. Blood 78:51, 1991.

Jabado N, Le Deist F, Cant A, et al: Bone marrow transplantation from genetically HLA-nonidentical donors in children with fatal inherited disorders excluding severe combined immunodeficiencies. Pediatrics 98:420, 1996.

Onodera M, Ariga T, Kawamura N et al: Successful periphera; T-lymphocyte–directed gene transfer for a patient with severe combined immune deficiency caused by adenosine deaminase deficiency. Blood 91:30, 1998.

Smart BA and Ochs HD: The molecular basis and treatment of primary immunodeficiency disorders. Curr Opin Pediatr 9:570, 1997.

Fanconi Anemia

Flowers MED, Zanis J, Pasquini R, et al: Marrow transplantation for Fanconi anemia with reduced doses of cyclophosphamide without radiation. Br J Hematol 92:699, 1996.

Gluckman E: Allogeneic bone marrow transplantation in Fanconi anemia. Bone Marrow Transplant 18(Suppl 3):S33, 1996.

Metabolic Storage Diseases

Hoogerbrugge PM, Brouwer OF, Bordigoni P, et al: Allogenic bone marrow transplantation for lysosomal storage diseases. The European Group for Bone Marrow Transplantation. Lancet 345:1398, 1995.

Krivit W, Lockman LA, Watkins PA, et al: The future for treatment by bone marrow transplantation for adrenoleukodystrophy, metachromatic leukodystrophy, globoid cell leukodystrophy and Hurler syndrome. J Inherit Metab Dis 18:398, 1995.

Thalassemia

Lucarelli G, Giardini C, Angelucci E: Bone marrow transplantation in thalassemia. Cancer Treat Res 77:305, 1997.

Walters MC, Thomas ED: Bone marrow transplantation for thalassemia, the USA experience. Am J Pediatr Hematol Oncol 16:11, 1994.

Sickle Cell Anemia

Vermylen C, Cornu G, Ferster A, et al: Sickle cell disease and haematopoietic stem cell transplantation in Belgium. Bone Marrow Transplant 19(Suppl 2):99, 1997.

Walters MC, Patience M, Leisenring W, et al: Collaborative multicenter investigation of marrow transplantation for sickle cell disease: Current results and future directions. Biol Blood Marrow Transplant 3:310, 1997.

CHAPTER 136

Matching and Rejection

(also see Chapter 501)

The immunologic goal of bone marrow transplantation (BMT) is a graft that can respond to foreign antigens without reacting to the host and that is not rejected. The most important factor determining tolerance is the histocompatibility between donor and host. The genes defining histocompatibility are encoded in the major histocompatibility complex (MHC) on the short arm of chromosome 6. The MHC spans approximately 4,000 kb of DNA and contains the genes for a series of cell surface glycoproteins termed the *human leukocyte antigens* (HLAs). The HLA genes are tightly linked and can be divided into class I glycoproteins that dimerize with β_2-microglobulin and class II glycoproteins with α and β peptides that form heterodimers. Although there are more than 35 HLA class I and II genes and over 684 alleles, HLA-A, HLA-B (class I), and HLA-DRB1 (class II) genes are used as the primary determinants for histocompatibility of donors and recipients for BMT. The HLA genes on a single chromosome 6 make up a haplotype that, along with the HLA genes on the other copy of chromosome 6, constitute the genotype. Class I genes are determined by serotyping, isoelectric focusing gel electrophoresis, and DNA sequence analysis, whereas class II genes are identified primarily by DNA typing. Several potential combinations of donor/recipient may be identified, including syngeneic (twins), genotypically matched siblings, phenotypically matched family members or unrelated donors, and various degrees of mismatch (one-antigen, two-antigen, or three-antigen mismatch = haploidentical). Minor mismatches as well as partial matches based on graft versus host disease (GVHD) and rejection vectors may also be identified. Because only 25–30% of patients have an HLA-identical sibling, identification of phenotypically matched unrelated donors is most feasible using large unrelated donor registries. In the United States, the National Marrow Donor Program has typed more than 3 million volunteer donors and uses 118 donor centers and over 57 transplant centers to add 40,000 potential new donors each month. The chance of identifying an unrelated donor for a given individual is about 20–67%, depending on the ethnic/HLA background. Transplants using one-antigen mismatched, unrelated donors may be possible if the mismatch is with cross-reactive or very closely related HLA antigens.

Graft failure and graft rejection are influenced by several factors (Table 136–1); HLA disparity is the most important variable. Failure to engraft may occur in autologous as well as allogeneic BMT and may result from an inadequate stem cell

TABLE 136–1 Factors Influencing Engraftment and Graft Rejection

HLA disparity
Pretransplant alloimmunization by transfusions
Conditioning regimen
Transplanted marrow cell dose
Marrow stroma/microenvironment
Post-transplant/immunosuppression
Donor T cells
Drug toxicity
Viral infections

dose or from marrow stromal damage by prior therapy in conjunction with the transplant preparative regimen. Graft rejection may occur immediately, without an increase in cell counts, or may follow a brief period of engraftment. Rejection is usually mediated by residual host T cells, cytotoxic antibodies, or lymphokines and is manifested by a fall in donor cell counts with a persistence of host lymphocytes. BMT using marrow from HLA-disparate donors significantly increases the risk for graft rejection/failure. For example, the risk of graft failure in HLA-identical sibling donor BMT is 1–2%, whereas in haploidentical donor BMT the risk is 3–15%. Alloimmunization by exposure to numerous transfusions before BMT may sensitize a patient to HLA antigens, increasing the potential for graft rejection; this is observed most often with aplastic anemia. Because adequate immunosuppression of the host before marrow infusion is required to ensure engraftment and prevent rejection, the incidence of rejection depends in part on the conditioning regimen. With matched sibling donor BMT for aplastic anemia, there is a 24% incidence of graft rejection when cyclophosphamide is used alone as a preparative regimen, compared with 3% when antithymocyte globulin is added. Post-transplant immunosuppression is useful to prevent GVHD and to minimize the likelihood of graft rejection. One effective approach to GVHD is to eliminate T cells from the donor marrow before infusion, but elimination of T cells allows the persistence of host lymphocytes, which are capable of mediating graft rejection in about 10% of cases. Graft rejection may be difficult to differentiate from the effects of drugs or viral infections on the graft.

Quinones RR: Hematopoietic engraftment and graft failure after bone marrow transplantation. Am J Pediatr Hematol Oncol 15:3, 1993.

CHAPTER 137
Graft Versus Host Disease (GVHD)

Engraftment by donor lymphocytes in an immunologically compromised host (congenital or radiation- or chemotherapy-induced immune defects) can result in donor T-cell activation against host major histocompatibility complex (MHC) antigens, with resultant GVHD. Cell death results from cell-mediated cytotoxic activity (e.g., by natural killer cells) and a complex cascade of lymphokines released by activated lymphocytes (e.g., tumor necrosis factor [TNF]). For this reaction to occur, the graft must contain immunocompetent cells, the host must be immunocompromised and unable to reject or mount a response to the graft, and there must be histocompatibility differences between the graft and the host. GVHD is classified as acute, occurring within the first 100 days after bone marrow transplant, or chronic, occurring after the first 100 days. As discussed in Chapter 135, GVHD may have some benefit by producing a graft versus leukemia (GVL) effect and a lower relapse rate in patients receiving a transplant for leukemia. The process of GVHD represents a loss of "tolerance" normally maintained by thymic elimination of alloreactive lymphocytes; modulation of the T-cell receptor, rendering alloreactive cells anergic; and active suppressor cells that hold activated T cells in check. Attempts at generating GVHD/GVL effects in patients with autologous BMT have been based on altering these tolerance factors with immunodulatory agents such as cyclosporine.

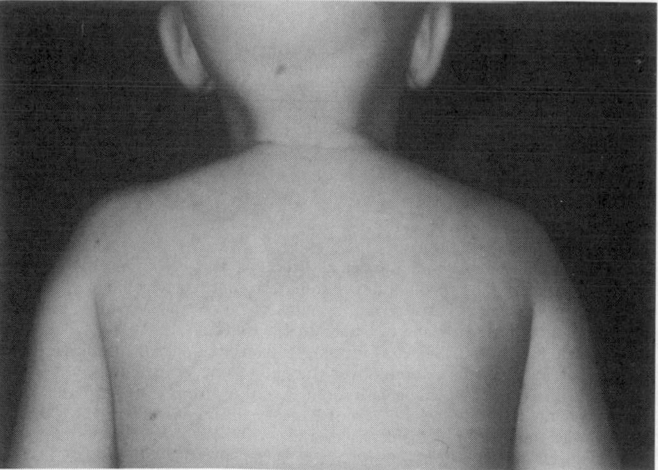

Figure 137–1 Acute graft versus host disease of the skin with ear, arm, shoulder, and trunk involvement. (Courtesy of Evan Farmer, M.D.) See also color section.

ACUTE GVHD. The acute form of GVHD (aGVHD) is characterized by erythroderma, cholestatic hepatitis, and enteritis (Table 137–1). Typically, aGVHD presents about day 19 (median), when patients are starting to engraft. It usually starts with a pruritic macular/papular rash on the ears, palms, and soles and may progress to involve the trunk (Fig. 137–1) and extremities, potentially becoming a more confluent erythroderma with bulla formation and exfoliation. Fever may or may not be present. Differential diagnostic considerations include

TABLE 137–1 Clinical Staging and Grading of Graft Versus Host Disease

Stage	Skin	Liver	Intestinal Tract
+	Maculopapular rash <25% of body surface	Bilirubin 2–3 mg/100 mL	>500 mL diarrhea/day
++	Maculopapular rash <25–50% of body surface	Bilirubin 3–6 mg/100 mL	>1,000 mL diarrhea/day
+++	Generalized erythroderma	Bilirubin 6–15 mg/100 mL	>1,500 mL diarrhea/day
++++	Generalized erythroderma with bullous formation and desquamation	Bilirubin >15 mg/100 mL	Severe abdominal pain with or without ileus

GVHD Grade	Skin Stage	Liver Stage	Intestinal Tract Stage	Decrease in Clinical Performance
I	+ to ++	0	0	None
II	+ to +++	+	+	Mild
III	++ to +++	++ to ++++	++ to +++	Marked
IV	++ to ++++	++ to ++++	++ to ++++	Extreme

Adapted from Thomas ED, Storb R, Clift RA, et al: Bone marrow transplantation. N Engl J Med 292:832, 895, 1975.

toxicity from the immunosuppressive regimen, drug rash, and viral or other infectious exanthems. Hepatic manifestations include cholestatic jaundice with elevated values on liver function testing. The differential diagnosis includes hepatitis, venoocclusive disease, or drug effect. The intestinal symptoms of aGVHD include crampy abdominal pain and watery diarrhea, often with blood. The conditioning regimen and infectious agents may produce similar symptoms. Eosinophilia, lymphocytosis, protein-losing enteropathy, bone marrow aplasia (neutropenia, thrombocytopenia, anemia), peripheral edema, and secondary infections may ensue. Factors related to the development of aGVHD include histocompatibility differences between donor and patient, gender mismatching, donor parity, age, active or relapsed malignancy at the time of transplantation, and increasing doses of radiation. Prevention and treatment of GVHD require various immunosuppressive agents (see Chapter 138).

CHRONIC GVHD. Maturation of the graft may include the development of chronic GVHD (cGVHD), usually after day 100 but as early as day 60–70. cGVHD resembles a multisystem autoimmune process manifesting as Sjögren's (sicca) syndrome, systemic lupus erythematosus, and scleroderma (Fig. 137–2), lichen planus, and primary biliary cirrhosis. Recurrent infections (sepsis, sinusitis, pneumonia) with encapsulated bacteria and fungal and viral organisms are common and contribute significantly to transplant-related morbidity and mortality. Prophylaxis with trimethoprim-sulfamethoxazole reduces the incidence of *Pneumocystis carinii* pneumonia. Risks for chronic GVHD include increasing age (donor or host), prior acute GVHD, buffy coat transfusions, and high level of parity of a female donor. Therapy for cGVHD consists of additional immunosuppression with agents (prednisone and cyclosporine are front-line drugs) as described in Chapter 138, again with the disadvantage of putting patients at risk for infectious complications.

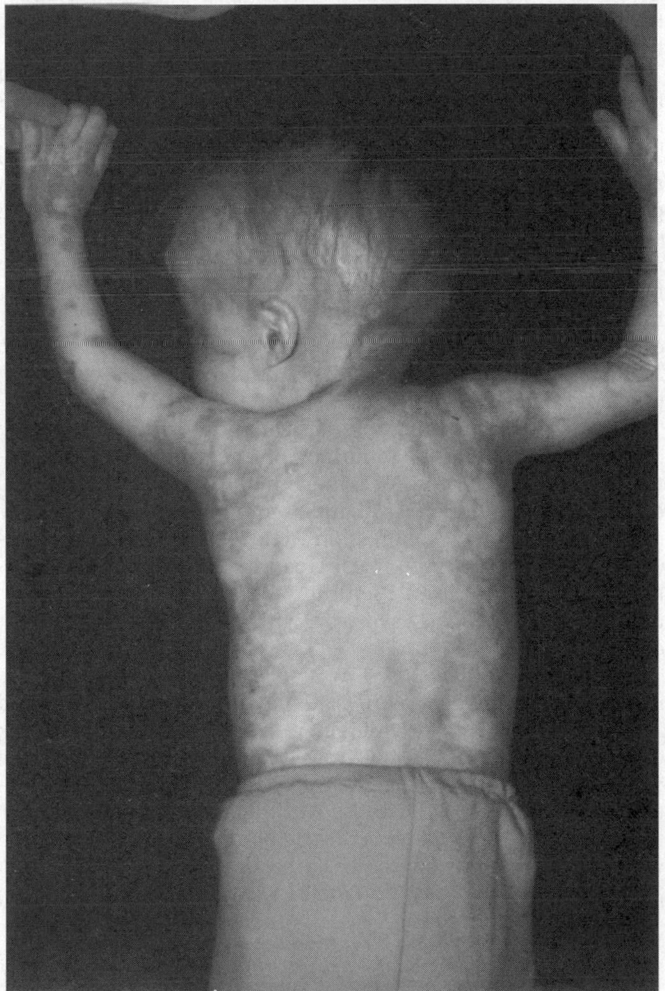

Figure 137–2 Chronic graft versus host disease of the skin with sclerodermoid changes. (Courtesy of Evan Farmer, M.D.) See also color section.

Klingebiel T, Schlegel PG: GVHD: Overview on pathophysiology, incidence, clinical and biological features. Bone Marrow Transplant 21(Suppl 2):S45, 1998.
Parkman R: Chronic graft-versus-host disease. Curr Opin Hematol 5:22, 1998.

CHAPTER 138
Principles of Immunosuppression

Immunosuppressive agents are used to prevent and treat allograft rejection and graft versus host disease (GVHD). Because differences in major or minor histocompatibility antigens induce recipient T-lymphocyte activation and subsequent donor allograft rejection, immunosuppression is needed for all tissue transplantation, except from identical twins and in certain stem cell transplants for severe immunodeficiencies. Solid organ transplantation requires lifelong immunosuppression to prevent graft rejection (see Chapters 367, 449, and 544), whereas BMT recipients are treated for 6–12 mo until a state of tolerance is attained. Transplant strategies using selected stem and T cells to enhance engraftment but avoid GVHD and more potent immunosuppressive agents permit successful bone marrow transplantation (BMT) across greater degrees of mismatched HLA antigens. The ideal immunosuppressive agent inhibits the host lymphocyte subsets that mediate rejection and inhibits donor lymphocytes that mediate GVHD without altering immunity against infection or malignancy (graft versus leukemia [GVL]).

PREPARATIVE REGIMEN. Different preparative regimens are used for BMT for different diseases. Most agents have antineoplastic as well as immunosuppressant activity. Cyclophosphamide is a nitrogen mustard derivative that requires metabolic activation to generate a bifunctional alkylating metabolite and is the most widely used immunosuppressant in BMT-preparative regimens. Total body irradiation (TBI) is also an important therapeutic agent, with excellent antineoplastic activity and immunosuppressive qualities that can effectively treat all parts of the body. Other chemotherapeutic agents that have greater antitumor effects than immunosuppression have been used in combination with TBI and cyclophosphamide and include busulfan, etoposide (VP-16), melphalan, carmustine (BCNU), cytosine arabinoside (ara-C), thiotepa, ifosfamide, and carboplatin. The combinations are designed to achieve adequate immunosuppression allowing rapid engraftment without excessive toxicity and with the capacity to eliminate a malignant clone.

T-CELL DEPLETION. Prevention of graft rejection and GVHD along with treatment of GVHD in the peritransplant period involves several different strategies. Because donor T cells are responsible for GVHD, donor marrows have been depleted of T cells using monoclonal antibodies or physical separation techniques such as soy lectin agglutination. Depletion results in a dramatic reduction in GVHD but can cause graft rejection and relapse. Donor T cells have an important role in eliminating residual host T cells as well as in mediating a GVL effect. Alternatives to T-cell depletion are being explored, including adding back-selected T cells that may help engraftment and retain antitumor activity but without GVHD activity.

METHOTREXATE. This competitive inhibitor of dihydrofolate reductase is an excellent immunosuppressive agent, in addition to being a cancer chemotherapeutic drug. A regimen of methotrexate given on days 1, 3, 6, and 11 is effective at preventing GVHD, with additional improvement if the drug is given weekly for the first 100 days. Methotrexate may aggravate mucositis resulting from the conditioning regimen and may require rescue with leucovorin if a patient has renal impairment or a fluid collection, such as a pleural effusion. Trimetrexate is an antifolate drug with structural similarity to methotrexate, but it is eliminated by the liver and may be an alternative for patients who have significant renal impairment.

CYCLOSPORINE. This lipophilic (hydrophobic), cyclic, 11-amino-acid peptide is a potent and specific immunosuppressive agent that selectively inhibits the translation of interleukin (IL)–2 mRNA by helper T cells. Cyclosporine may also inhibit IL-1, IL-3, and γ-interferon synthesis. T-cell activation is attenuated in the absence of IL-2. Cyclosporine inhibits IL-2 receptor formation at higher doses. Cyclosporine has no myelosuppressive or anti-inflammatory effects, but it is very useful for preventing graft rejection. Cyclosporine is metabolized by the hepatic cytochrome P450 enzyme system and can be involved in a number of drug interactions. Cyclosporine levels increase in the presence of ketoconazole, erythromycin, methylprednisolone, warfarin, verapamil, ethanol, imipenem-cilastatin, metoclopramide, and fluconazole; cyclosporine levels decrease in the presence of phenytoin, phenobarbital, carbamazepine, valproate, nafcillin, and rifampin.

Cyclosporine has significant nonimmunosuppressant toxic effects, including neurotoxicity (tremors, paresthesias, headache, confusion, somnolence, seizures, coma), hypertrichosis, gingival hyperplasia, anorexia, nausea, vomiting, hepatotoxicity (cholestasis, cholelithiasis, hemorrhagic necrosis), endocrinopathies (ketosis, hyperprolactinemia, hypertestosteronemia, gynecomastia, impaired spermatogenesis), metabolic disorders (hypomagnesemia, hyperuricemia, hyperglycemia, hyperkalemia, hypocholesterolemia), vascular derangements (hypertension, increased sympathetic nervous system activation, vasculitic-hemolytic-uremic syndrome–like illness, atherogenesis), and nephrotoxicity. Renal toxicity is a significant limitation of cyclosporine use and is manifested as an increased creatinine level, oliguria, hypertension, fluid retention, vasoconstriction of the afferent glomerular filtration rate, renal tubular damage, and hemolytic-uremic syndrome–like lesions. Chronic nephrotoxicity (interstitial fibrosis, tubular atrophy) may require a reduction of the cyclosporine dose or a change to other immunosuppressant drugs. Nephrotoxicity may be exacerbated by aminoglycosides, amphotericin B, acyclovir, digoxin, furosemide, indomethacin, or trimethoprim. The renal toxicity may be reduced by adjusting dosing based on blood cyclosporine levels. Levels may also be influenced by clinical conditions affecting absorption, including diarrhea, intestinal disorders (due to GVHD, viral infections, or therapy), and altered hepatic function. Although the drug is lipophilic, obesity does not influence the distribution of the drug, and dosing should be based on ideal body weight. Cyclosporine is as effective as methotrexate for post-BMT immunosuppression, and the combination of cyclosporine with methotrexate is better than either drug alone.

TACROLIMUS. This macrolide immunosuppressive drug, produced by the fungus *Streptomyces tsukubaensis*, is chemically distinct from cyclosporine but has similar effects on the immune system. Although it binds specific proteins, it has the same effects on the expression of IL-2 and the IL-2 receptor as cyclosporine. Tacrolimus has little advantage over cyclosporine, except possibly in the treatment of GVHD of the liver because it is concentrated in the liver. The toxicities and drug interactions are similar to those of cyclosporine. The combination of these drugs causes synergistic toxicity.

CORTICOSTEROIDS. Prednisone, usually in combination with other immunosuppressive agents, is often used to treat or prevent GVHD and to prevent rejection. Corticosteroids may interfere with T-lymphocyte proliferation by directly blocking activation of the genes for IL-1 and IL-6. Because IL-2 secretion depends in part on IL-1 and IL-6 release, steroids block IL-2 action indirectly. Corticosteroids also produce a more rapid anti-inflammatory response by inducing the production of lipocortin, an inhibitor of phopholipase A_2, which reduces the synthesis of inflammatory prostaglandins. They may also lyse small populations of activated lymphocytes and reduce the migration of monocytes to sites of inflammation. Nonspecific and pronounced immunosuppressant effects of corticosteroids (and other immunosuppressants) place patients at risk for serious opportunistic infections. Other long-term complications of steroid use include growth failure, cushingoid appearance, hypertension, cataracts, gastrointestinal bleeding, pancreatitis, psychosis, hyperglycemia, osteoporosis, aseptic necrosis of the femoral head, and suppression of the pituitary-adrenal axis.

ANTITHYMOCYTE GLOBULIN. Heterologous antibodies against human thymocytes have been generated from horses, rabbits, and other sources. These antibody preparations are potent immunosuppressants and have been useful in preparative regimens as well as for treatment of resistant GVHD. Toxicities include fever, hypotension, rash-urticaria, tachycardia, dyspnea, chills, myalgias, serum sickness, and potential anaphylaxis. Diphenhydramine, acetaminophen, and hydrocortisone help to minimize side effects.

OKT3. This is a murine monoclonal antibody directed against the T3 (CD3) surface glycoprotein on T cells. Although OKT3 eliminates T cells by binding to CD3 and inducing clearance by the reticuloendothelial system, it also activates T cells, with resultant toxicity that includes fever, chills, dyspnea, chest pain, wheezing, nausea, and vomiting. Modified antibodies such as BC3 have been developed; these bind CD3 but are unable to interact with the Fc receptors on monocytes and do not activate T cells. These newer antibodies are more effective for treating GVHD and have fewer side effects. Another strategy is to conjugate antibodies to cytologic toxins such as ricin A. Ricin A linked to an anti-CD5 antibody (XomaZyme) that binds T cells and some B cells mediates cytospecific toxicity.

AZATHIOPRINE. This imidazole derivative of 6-mercaptopurine blocks DNA synthesis by inhibiting purine synthesis. Both azathioprine and 6-mercaptopurine inhibit T-cell activation and decrease the number of migrating mononuclear cells. Toxic effects include myelosuppression (neutropenia), hepatic veno-occlusive disease, hepatitis, pancreatitis, and secondary malignancies. It has not been useful for acute GVHD because of its toxicities but has been used with variable benefit for resistant chronic GVHD (cGVHD).

THALIDOMIDE. Initially used as a sedative but found to have immunosuppressive properties, thalidomide has been studied in phase I–II trials for treating cGVHD. Patients with high-risk or refractory cGVHD treated with thalidomide have shown a 59% response rate, with a 76% survival for those with refractory cGVHD and 48% for those with high-risk cGVHD. Studies to determine the relative efficacy of thalidomide compared with other regimens for cGVHD are in progress.

Lazarus HM, Vogelsang, GB, Rowe JM: Prevention and treatment of acute graft-versus-host disease: The old and the new. A report from the Eastern Cooperative Oncology Group. Bone Marrow Transplant 19:577, 1997.

Vogelsang GB, Farmer E, Hess A, et al: Thalidomide for the treatment of chronic graft-versus-host disease. N Engl J Med 326:1055, 1992.

CHAPTER 139
Late Effects of Bone Marrow Transplantation

As more children are undergoing bone marrow transplantation (BMT) for a widening spectrum of indications and an increasing number of these children become long-term survivors, late effects of the transplant process have a lasting impact on the health and well-being of the individual. Pediatricians should be aware of possible delayed complications, including effects on growth and development, neuroendocrine dysfunction, fertility, second tumors, chronic graft versus host disease (GVHD), cataracts, leukoencephalopathy, and immune dysfunction.

NEUROLOGIC FUNCTION. Infections, metabolic encephalopathy (resulting from hepatic dysfunction), and drug/radiation therapy all may contribute to neurologic sequelae. Cyclosporine may produce headache (most responsive to propranolol), tremor, confusion, visual disturbance, seizures, and frank encephalopathy. Most of these effects are reversible with discontinuation of the drug. The incidence of cataracts is approximately 80% in patients receiving single-dose total body irradiation (TBI), 20–50% with fractionated TBI, and 20% after chemotherapy-only regimens. A dry eye syndrome is often related to chronic GVHD and is treated with artificial tears and lubricants. *Leukoencephalopathy* is a clinical syndrome characterized by lethargy, slurred speech, ataxia, seizures, confusion, dysphagia, and decerebrate posturing. It may present with minimal symptoms or can result in coma or death in its most severe form. MRI and CT scans reveal multifocal areas of white matter degeneration with necrosis. Leukoencephalopathy is observed almost exclusively in patients who have received extensive intrathecal chemotherapy or cranial irradiation before transplant, with an overall incidence of 7% in patients at risk.

SECONDARY MALIGNANCIES. The overall risk of developing a secondary form of cancer is about six to eight times that in the general population, with the greatest risk being within the 1st yr. Approximately half of the secondary tumors are non-Hodgkin lymphomas, and two thirds of these are Epstein-Barr virus (EBV) positive. Other malignancies observed tend to occur later (1–30 yr) and include leukemia/myelodysplastic syndrome, brain tumors, melanomas, and various carcinomas of the skin, liver, lung, and thyroid. Risk factors that are associated with second malignancies include the diagnosis of immunodeficiency, use of antithymocyte globulin (ATG), T-cell depletion of the donor marrow, and TBI in the preparative regimen. EBV-related B-cell lymphomas, which are aggressive and resistant to most therapeutic interventions, have been successfully treated with infusions of donor T cells.

GROWTH AND DEVELOPMENT. Long-term follow-up studies of patients who have received TBI-containing regimens reveal significant growth depression and growth hormone deficiency. After 5 yr, TBI-treated patients were more than two standard deviations below the mean height for age and dropped to three to four standard deviations below the mean by 8 yr after transplant. This decrease in growth velocity is similar for boys and girls and does not vary with the use of cranial irradiation or different regimens of radiation (single vs fractionated). Children receiving radiation-containing regimens also have no pubertal growth spurt. The pubertal growth spurt depends on the presence of adequate growth hormone and gonadal hormones, both of which may be low after transplant. A major determinant of final height is the amount of growth before puberty. Children receiving BMT before the age of 11 have a final height below the 10th percentile, whereas those after age 11 attain a height close to the average. Chronic GVHD and its treatment with corticosteroids may also contribute to growth impairment after transplant. In an attempt to avoid TBI-related growth effects in children, chemotherapy-only regimens such as busulfan/cyclophosphamide have been used. Early results of growth studies suggest that busulfan has much less of an impact on growth. Preparative regimens using only cyclophosphamide for aplastic anemia have little effect on normal growth and development. Irradiation of the long bones and vertebral bodies for neuroblastoma also contributes to decreased growth velocity. Therapy with recombinant growth hormone after age 12 yr prevents a further decrease in growth velocity, but little or no catch-up growth is achieved.

Annual growth hormone evaluation is essential in all children after transplant. Current studies are aimed at identifying children with growth hormone deficiencies at an earlier age and administering supplemental growth hormone to achieve a normal pubertal growth spurt. Gonadal hormones are essential for normal pubertal growth as well as development of secondary sexual characteristics. About three quarters of patients receiving TBI-containing regimens show delayed development of secondary sexual characteristics, resulting from primary ovarian or testicular failure. Laboratory evaluation reveals elevated follicle-stimulating hormone (FSH) and luteinizing hormone (LH) levels with depressed estradiol and testosterone. These patients require careful follow-up with annual Tanner scores and endocrine evaluation. Supplementation of gonadal hormones is useful for primary gonadal failure and is given along with growth hormone to promote normal pubertal growth.

THYROID FUNCTION. The use of TBI with or without additional conventional radiation involving the thyroid gland may result in hypothyroidism. Some children who have received single-dose TBI develop compensated (28–56%) or overt (9–13%) hypothyroidism. The use of fractionated TBI has significantly reduced the incidence of compensated (10–14%) and overt (<5%) hypothyroidism. Risk factors for the development of hypothyroidism appear to be related only to the use of radiation, with no influence of age, sex, or GVHD. The site of injury by radiation is at the level of the thyroid gland rather than at the pituitary or hypothalamus. Therapy with thyroxine is very effective for overt hypothyroidism, but treatment of compensated hypothyroidism is more controversial. Despite treatment of hypothyroidism, there remains a risk for thyroid carcinomas. Because the risk of hypothyroidism continues for many years, annual thyroid function studies are important. Chemotherapy-only preparative regimens have far fewer effects on normal thyroid function.

IMMUNE RECONSTITUTION. Chemoradiotherapy for BMT results in complete eradication of host B- and T-cell immunity. After infusion of donor marrow, recovery of the normal immune functions takes many months or years. The ability of newly engrafting B cells to respond to mitogenic stimulation is intact by 2–3 mo. Because the production of antibodies requires B- and T-cell interaction, normal IgM levels are not observed until 4–6 mo after transplant; IgG levels take 7–9 mo to normalize, and it may take 2 yr before normal IgA levels are achieved. T-cell recovery also takes many months. $CD8^+$ T cells recover by about 4 mo, but $CD4^+$ T cells do not increase until 6–9 mo, resulting in an inverted $CD4^+/CD8^+$ ratio for the first 6–9 mo after transplant. Factors that prolong this interval include T-cell depletion of the marrow, post-transplant immunosuppression, and chronic GVHD. Patients with chronic GVHD have a continued decrease in the number of cytotoxic T lymphocytes and helper T cells, along with increased suppressor T cells. Live virus vaccines *should be avoided* in immunocompromised patients. *Reimmunization* of an individual will be successful only after adequate recovery of immune function. For patients without chronic GVHD, diphtheria and tetanus toxoid series, pertussis (in children <7 yr old), inactivated (Salk) polio series, hepatitis B series, pneumococcal, and *Haemophilus influenzae* type b series immunizations may be given 12 mo after transplant, and measles-mumps-rubella after 2 yr. Influenza vaccines should be given every fall. If chronic GVHD is present, reimmunization should be postponed and IgG supplemented until it resolves.

Boulad F, Bromley M, Black P, et al: Thyroid dysfunction following bone marrow transplantation using hyperfractionated radiation. Bone Marrow Transplant 15:71, 1995.

Deeg HJ, Socié G: Malignancies after hematopoietic stem cell transplantation: Many questions, some answers. Blood 91:1833, 1998.

Giorgiani G, Bozzola M, Locatelli F, et al: Role of busulfan and total body irradiation on growth of prepubertal children receiving bone marrow transplantation and results of treatment with recombinant human growth hormone. Blood 86:825, 1995.

Sanders JE: Pubertal development of children treated with marrow transplantation before puberty. J Pediatr 130:174, 1997.

Thompson CB, Sanders JE, Flournoy N, et al: The risks of central nervous system relapse and leukoencephalopathy in patients receiving marrow transplants for acute leukemia. Blood 67:195, 1986.

Chapter 140 *Umbilical Cord Blood Transplantation (CBT)*

Although allogeneic stem cell transplantation has been successful during the past 30 yr, not all candidates for transplantation have a suitable family member donor. Alternate sources of stem cells have been developed, the most recognized source being unrelated donor marrow, using donor registries such as the National Marrow Donor Program. In the past decade, human umbilical cord blood has become an additional source of stem cells for hematopoietic cell transplantation. An estimated 600 CBTs have been performed. After delivery of an infant and clamping of the cord, 40–200 mL of umbilical cord blood is collected aseptically and stored. In the numerous cord blood banks both public and private that have been established around the world, cord blood can be donated or stored for potential personal use. Cord blood has been successfully used in transplants for virtually every indication for which marrow has been used, demonstrating the utility of cord blood as a stem cell product. The time to myeloid engraftment is 8–56 days. The incidence of grade III–IV acute graft versus host disease (GVHD) in early studies appears to be less than in marrow transplants, with rates of 3–10% in matched sibling CBTs and 10–20% in unrelated donor CBTs. The overall survival has been 30–65% for both related donor and unrelated donor CBT. Numerous adults have had successful transplants using cord blood stem cells, although size restrictions and cell dose requirements are still being defined. Immune reconstitution appears to be complete, with normal natural killer cell function, immunoglobulin production, and B- and T-cell repertoires. Current studies are addressing engraftment and GVHD issues in a large multi-institutional trial by the National Heart, Lung, and Blood Institute. Other investigations are targeted at ex vivo expansion of cord blood cells to accelerate engraftment and gene therapy applications. The early success of CBTs, along with the ease of collection and availability, makes cord blood a valuable resource for future transplants.

Cairo MS, Wagner JE: Placental and/or umbilical cord blood: An alternative source of hematopoietic stem cells for transplantation. Blood 90:4665, 1997.

Gluckman E, Rocha V, Boyer-Chammard A, et al: Outcome of cord-blood transplantation from related and unrelated donors. N Engl J Med 337:373, 1997.

Kurtzburg J, Laughlin M, Graham ML, et al: Placental blood as a source of hematopoietic stem cells for transplantation into unrelated recipients. N Engl J Med 335:157, 1996.

PART XIV

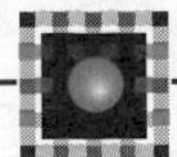

Allergic Disorders

Michael Sly

Chapter 141

Allergy and the Immunologic Basis of Atopic Disease

Allergy is a specific, acquired change in host reactivity mediated by an immunologic mechanism and causing an untoward physiologic response. This definition precludes the use of the term *allergy* for disorders in which immunologic mechanisms have not been demonstrated. For example, some adverse reactions after food or drug ingestion may resemble typical allergic reactions without an immunologic basis. Sometimes there is a biochemical basis for the reaction, as in diarrhea after milk ingestion in people with disaccharidase deficiency. When there is no reason to suspect that allergy is responsible for signs or symptoms, the use of immunologic methods in diagnosis or treatment is irrational.

The terms *antigen* and *allergen* are often used interchangeably, but not all antigens are good allergens and vice versa. For example, tetanus and diphtheria toxoids are highly antigenic but are only rarely responsible for allergic reactions. Conversely, ragweed pollen protein, one of the most potent allergens, is not a particularly potent antigen by immunologic criteria. Most naturally occurring allergens share several common characteristics. They are protein in part, are acidic with isoelectric points of 2–5.5, and have molecular weights of 10,000–70,000 d. Molecules smaller than 10,000 d would be unable to bridge the gap between adjacent immunoglobulin E (IgE) antibody molecules on the surface of mast cells, a requirement for release of the mediators of the allergic reaction (Fig. 141–1). Molecules larger than 70,000 d would not easily pass through mucosal surfaces to reach IgE-forming plasma cells.

The use of the term *atopy* or *atopic* in designating an allergic reaction implies a hereditary factor expressed as susceptibility to hay fever, asthma, and eczematoid dermatitis in the families of affected individuals. Twin studies suggest that 75% of the variance in asthma is due to genetic factors. Atopic susceptibility genes may be involved in the regulation of specific IgE antibody production or in mediating the effector functions of IgE. Although no single "atopic gene" has been discovered, atopy has been linked to certain human leukocyte antigen (HLA) histocompatability types as well as to various chromosome loci (11q, 14, and 5q). Chromosome 5q31-33 has multiple candidate genes linked to atopy that would regulate IgE synthesis (interleukins 4, 5, 13 [IL-4, IL-5, IL-13]) or modify response to therapy (greater downregulation of the β_2 receptor). Polymorphisms of the β_2 receptor have been associated with some types of asthma. Furthermore, altered signal transduction secondary to an allele of the IL-4 receptor is associated with atopy. In contrast to classic mendelian recessive or dominant traits, it is possible that multiple major and minor genes involved in the inflammatory pathway (enhancers, modifiers, inhibitors) are responsible for atopy in individual families. There may be one specific gene involved in each affected family, or a combination of different genes may produce atopy.

The formation of IgE antibodies is revealed in atopic persons by "wheal and flare" reactions on skin testing with allergenic extracts. However, the capacity to form IgE antibody is not limited to atopic individuals because IgE is found in the sera and on mast cells of most normal individuals. Under intense allergen exposure, as in certain occupations, or in response to particular allergens, such as ascaris, nonatopic individuals may form large quantities of allergen-specific IgE antibodies. Atopic persons, however, form IgE antibodies on exposure to common environmental substances such as pollens and mites in house dust, thus distinguishing them from nonatopic individuals. Among patients with asthma, hay fever, or atopic dermatitis, we can identify "highly atopic" persons and others with lesser atopic tendencies.

It is useful to characterize immunologic reactions by the reactants involved in order to understand the mechanism by which injury occurs. Immunologically mediated tissue injury may occur as a result of the interaction of humoral antibody with antigen or the interaction of antigen with lymphocytes (cell-mediated or delayed-type hypersensitivity). There are three forms of humoral antibody-antigen reactions, two of which occur on the surface of cells and the third in the extracellular fluids.

Of the two reactions occurring on the surface of the cells, *type I hypersensitivity, mediated by IgE* (immediate type or anaphylactic hypersensitivity) is of greatest interest to the allergist. In this circumstance, circulating basophils and tissue mast cells, the latter strategically located around blood vessels, become "sensitized" through the binding of IgE antibodies to their surface receptors. This is the initial event in the production of immune tissue injury following allergen interaction with cell-bound IgE antibody molecules; the ultimate outcome of the reaction depends on a broad spectrum of secondary events involving various types of lymphoid cells, inflammatory cells, mediator-producing cells, and the soluble products derived not only from all these cells but also from other tissues (platelets, endothelial cells) at the site of the reaction. For example, in particularly intense allergen-induced immediate reactions in the skin, the initial wheal and flare does not entirely disappear but is replaced by an inflammatory lesion that reaches its maximal size at 6–12 hr and disappears in 24–72 hr. This late cutaneous response depends on recruitment of inflammatory cells (polymorphonuclear leukocytes, eosinophils, and mononuclear cells) by chemotactic factors released in the early response. Late-phase reactions also occur in the lung and nose.

The terms *reaginic IgE, IgE reagins,* and *homocytotropic antibodies* refer to molecules with activities against specific allergens, such as ragweed pollen, whereas "nonspecific" IgE molecules are found in the sera and tissues of all normal individuals. The

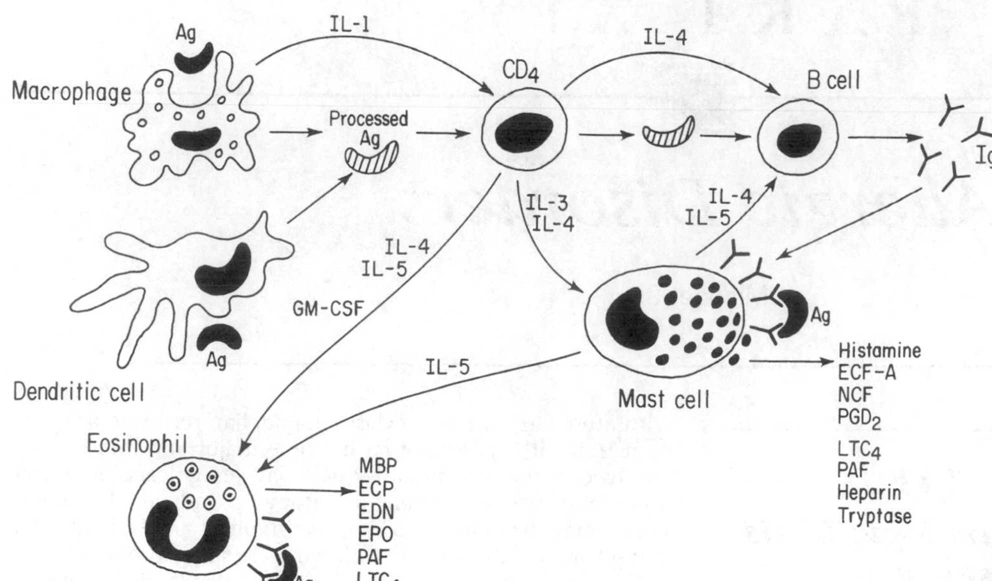

Figure 141–1 Sequential events that lead to allergic sensitization and subsequent allergic reactions after exposure to allergen. (Ag = antigen; IL = interleukin; GM-CSF = granulocyte-macrophage colony-stimulating factor; ECF-A = eosinophil chemotactic factor of anaphylaxis; NCF = neutrophil chemotactic factor; PGD_2 = prostaglandin D_2; LTC_4 = leukotriene C_4; PAF = platelet-activating factor; MBP = major basic protein; ECP = eosinophil cationic protein; IgE = immunoglobulin E; EDN = eosinophil-derived neurotoxin; EPO = eosinophil peroxidase.)

"normal" role of IgE antibody appears to be to defend the host against tissue-invasive parasites. In humans, the ability to induce antigen-specific release of mediators from mast cells and basophils is principally confined to antibodies of the IgE class.

IgE antibodies, like IgA antibodies, are synthesized by plasma cells located predominantly under mucosal surfaces and particularly in the respiratory and gastrointestinal tracts. IgE-forming plasma cells arise following antigen-stimulated differentiation of B cells or their precursors.

Chemical modifications of antigens used in immunotherapy of allergic diseases suppress IgE responses. The association of IgE responses with HLA-linked immune response (IR) genes has been shown for several allergens (ragweed antigen Ra3 and HLA-A2, ragweed antigen Ra5 and HLA-B7, rye grass antigen I and HLA-B8). IgE synthesis in general, and specifically hypersensitivity, is genetically determined by immune cells, probably the specific helper T cells. Bone marrow transplantation from an atopic donor to a nonatopic recipient transfers the allergic diathesis to the recipient. Macrophages and dendritic cells process antigen for presentation to CD4 (helper T) cells, which are activated by IL-1. As a result, these T cells differentiate into TH2 cells, which after activation by processed antigen can synthesize IL-3, IL-4, IL-5, and granulocyte-macrophage colony-stimulating factor as well as other cytokines (see Fig. 141–1). IL-4 plays an important role in isotype switching of B cells from synthesis of IgM and IgG to synthesis of IgE. For optimal IgE synthesis, IL-5 (a nonisotype B cell growth factor) and IL-6 (a nonisotype B cell differentiation factor) are also needed. IL-5 and granulocyte-macrophage colony-stimulating factor also induce eosinophil differentiation. IL-3 and IL-4 are mast cell growth factors. Interferon-γ produced by another subset of T lymphocytes can inhibit IL-4–dependent IgE synthesis and IL-4–induced expression of low-affinity IgE receptors (CD23) on B cells. TH1 cells, characterized by production of IL-2, interferon-γ, and tumor necrosis factor-β, are important mediators of cellular immune responses rather than allergy or other humoral immune responses. Interferon-γ antagonizes B cell isotype switching to production of IgE (mediated by IL-4), whereas IL-4 and IL-10, produced by TH2 cells, inhibit production of interferon-γ.

Once formed, IgE antibody becomes reversibly bound or "fixed" to surface receptors of mast cells and basophils. The binding of IgE to its receptor (F_ER) involves the C4 and C3 domains of the Fc portion of the immunoglobulin molecule. In nonatopic individuals, only 20–50% of the receptors are occupied by IgE molecules. In atopic individuals with high serum IgE concentrations, a larger percentage, up to almost 100%, of their basophil and mast cell receptors is occupied by IgE. Once binding of IgE occurs, the basophils and mast cells are "sensitized." On subsequent contact with this specific allergen, and if cell-bound IgE molecules are sufficiently numerous, allergen may bridge adjacent IgE molecules, causing an interaction between the IgE receptors. This causes a series of biochemical reactions (activation of methyltransferases, phospholipid methylation, Ca^{2+} influx, and activation of the phospholipid diacylglycerol cycle). This results in fusion of the mast cell granules with the mast cell plasma membrane, causing release of pharmacologically active substances (such as histamine), known as chemical mediators. The released mediators act on other cellular receptors to cause symptoms. The reaction is largely reversible; the mast cells and basophils participating in the reaction are not lysed, and the effects of mediators are only temporary. Although aggregated IgE can fix late components of the complement system through an alternative pathway, participation of the complement system in IgE-mediated hypersensitivity disorders has not been shown. Newly synthesized chemical mediators are released by the mast cell 6–8 hr after antigenic stimulation. Thus, the late-phase reaction may last 12–48 hr.

Interactions of cytokines with endothelial cells are important in localization of eosinophils at the site of the allergic reaction. Activation of endothelial cells by IL-1 causes upregulation of endothelial adhesion molecules, including E-selectin (endothelial leukocyte adhesion molecule-1), intercellular adhesion molecule-1 (ICAM-1), and vascular cell adhesion molecule-1 (VCAM-1). Endothelial activation by IL-4 results in upregulation of VCAM-1. Lectin-binding regions of selectins interact with ligands on leukocytes, causing rolling of leukocytes over endothelial cells. Interactions with the integrins ICAM-1 and VCAM-1 then arrest the leukocytes, facilitating movement out of the vasculature at the site of the allergic reaction. The ligand for VCAM-1 is late activation antigen-4; it is found on eosinophils but not on neutrophils.

The usual tests for inhalant or food sensitivity make use of the reaction that occurs on the surface of mast cells between antigen and IgE antibody. Small amounts of extracts of pollens, molds, danders, and foods are introduced into the patient's skin by scratch, puncture, or intradermal techniques. If IgE antibody specific for the test antigen is bound to the subject's mast cells, the interaction of injected antigen with cell-bound IgE releases histamine, a potent vasoactive agent that causes increased capillary permeability and dilatation and axon reflex stimulation, leading to the familiar wheal and flare reaction. The prototypic *anaphylactic* or *IgE-mediated* disease is ragweed hay fever. Others include anaphylactic reactions to insect venom, food-induced urticaria, and allergic conjunctivitis or rhinitis.

In *type II hypersensitivity (cytotoxic) interactions* between antigen and antibody at cell surfaces, IgG or IgM immunoglobulins react with antigenic determinants* that either are integral parts of the cell membrane or have become adsorbed to or incorporated into the membrane. In contrast to the IgE or anaphylactic type of reaction, this second kind of reaction activates the complement system in most instances, and the involved cell is destroyed. An example of this type of immunologic injury occurs after transfusion of incompatible red cells. The recipient's isohemagglutinins (antibodies directed against determinants on the surface of the red cells) react with the incompatible cells, the complement system is activated, and sequential action of complement proteins leads to lysis of the cell. Analogous immune injury may involve platelets or leukocytes. In the case of drug-induced immune hemolytic anemias, various other mechanisms are also involved ("innocent bystander," drug adsorption).

The *type III immunopathologic mechanism* (Arthus or immune complex) of tissue injury involving humoral antibody and antigen occurs in the extracellular spaces. At certain ratios of antigen to antibody, antigen-antibody complexes are formed that are "toxic" to tissues in which they are deposited. For example, complexes may lodge in the filtering organs of the body (such as the kidney or lung) or infiltrate the walls of small blood vessels, activating the complement cascade. There is release of biologically active substances, including factors that are chemotactic for polymorphonuclear leukocytes, which are attracted to the site. With phagocytosis of the complexes, the polymorphonuclear leukocytes are lysed, and basic proteins and proteolytic enzymes are released that damage tissue. Immune complex disease is responsible for poststreptococcal glomerulonephritis.

Toxic complex injury involves cooperation among different antibodies in the production of tissue injury. The deposition of immune complexes containing IgG_1, IgG_2, IgG_3, and IgM in small blood vessels in the kidney in experimental serum sickness in animals depends on an increase in the permeability of these vessels. This is brought about by histamine liberated in the course of a simultaneous interaction of IgE antibody and antigen, which leads to "leakiness" of the capillaries and prepares them to receive the toxic complexes. Such deposition can be largely prevented by pretreatment with antihistamine drugs in the animal model. Examples of *type III reactions* include serum sickness and immune complex pericarditis or arthritis following meningococcal or *Haemophilus influenzae* infection.

In *type IV cell-mediated or delayed-type hypersensitivity,* pathologic changes follow interaction of antigen with specifically sensitized, thymus-derived T lymphocytes. The basis for the tissue injury in classic cell-mediated immune reactions is not completely understood, but it is clear that macrophages and cytotoxic cells play major roles. Contact allergy (poison ivy, chemical-induced contact dermatitis) is the prototype of allergic disease mediated by delayed-type hypersensitivity. Drug reactions with involvement of liver, lung, and kidney may be further examples of T cell–mediated disease. Cell-mediated immunity is involved in certain infiltrative hypersensitivity lung diseases in which granuloma formation is a pathologic feature. Tuberculin reactivity, graft-versus-host disease, and tissue transplant reaction are additional type IV hypersensitivity reactions.

*An antigenic determinant or epitope is a restricted portion of an antigen molecule that determines the specificity of an antigen-antibody reaction. Antigenic determinants may consist of only four or five amino acid residues. In complex antigens found in nature, such as pollens, there may be several hundred determinants on the surface of an antigen molecule, each capable of initiating immune responses and reacting with specific antibody.

141.1 Chemical Mediators of Allergic Reactions and Mechanisms of Release

Mast cells play the central role in immediate hypersensitivity responses. Considerable heterogeneity probably exists among populations of mast cells and basophils in humans; differences among these metachromatically staining cells can be measured by morphologic, immunologic, biochemical, and functional criteria. Mast cells and basophils are involved not only in IgE-mediated reactions but also in other chronic inflammatory disorders, for example, inflammatory bowel disease, rheumatoid arthritis, and parasitic infections.

The critical triggering event in mast cell degranulation and release of chemical mediators of allergic injury is the cross-linking of receptor-bound IgE antibodies (which may be viewed as an extension of the receptor) by multivalent specific antigen. Although antigen is usually the principal factor in causing the approximation of IgE receptors, this can be accomplished in the absence of antigen or even IgE antibody, for example, by the action of purified antibody to the IgE receptor itself. Other stimuli can also cause mast cell activation without involving antigen and cell-bound IgE. These stimuli include products of activation of the complement system (C3a, C5a), kinins, neutrophil-derived lysosomal basic proteins, and lymphokines.

Whatever the nature of the mast cell surface signal that acts as the degranulation stimulus, a series of biochemical reactions takes place that results in granule discharge. Activation of a serine esterase, utilization of intracellular energy stores, calcium influx or remobilization of intracellular calcium, and changes in the mast cell cytoskeleton such as polymerization of microtubules occur during mediator release. Changes in membrane phospholipid metabolism also occur, including methylation and activation of phospholipases and generation of phospholipid by-products, which participate in the fusion of the mast cell granules with the cell membrane, leading to extrusion of the granules. Once discharged from the mast cell, the granules, which are relatively water insoluble, may remain intact for hours. The preformed mediators, such as histamine, eosinophil chemotactic factor, and other chemotactic factors, are rapidly eluted from the granule matrix and act immediately on local tissues—smooth muscles and endothelial cells in blood vessels. Another set of mediators, which are preformed but granule associated (e.g., heparin, arylsulfatase B, enzymes such as trypsin and chymotrypsin, and inflammatory factors) may be involved in the immediate and late-phase reactions; these mediators express their activity either while they are still part of the intact granule or only after the granule begins to dissolve.

Bridging of adjacent, cell-bound IgE molecules also causes liberation of arachidonic acid from membrane phospholipids, either directly by action of phospholipase A_2 or indirectly by sequential actions of phospholipase C and diglyceride lipase. A cofactor in the nuclear membrane, 5-lipoxygenase–activating protein, can present arachidonate to the enzyme 5-lipoxygenase. Metabolism of arachidonic acid by the lipoxygenase pathway leads to the new formation of 5-hydroxyeicosatetraenoic acid and the leukotrienes B_4, C_4, D_4, and E_4. Metabolism of arachidonic acid by the cyclo-oxygenase pathway results in new formation of the various prostaglandins and thromboxanes. Prostaglandin D_2 is the chief prostaglandin product of mast cells. Other cells also generate prostaglandins and leukotrienes, which have various actions (Table 141–1).

Increases in intracellular concentrations of cyclic adenosine

TABLE 141–1 Chemical Mediators of Allergic Reactions

Mediator	Structural Characteristics	Actions
Histamine (preformed)	5-β-Imidazolylethylamine MW 111	H_1 receptors: Increase in venular permeability Contraction of smooth muscle Increase in cGMP levels Generation of prostaglandins Increase in nasal mucus production Positive chemokinetic effect on neutrophils and eosinophils* Positive chemotactic effect on neutrophils and eosinophils Bronchial irritant receptor stimulation Pruritus H_2 receptors: Increase in vascular permeability Increase in gastric acid secretion Positive chemokinetic effect on neutrophils and eosinophils Negative chemotactic effect on neutrophils and eosinophils Inhibition of T-cell responses Inhibition of basophil (not mast cell) mediator response Augmentation of gastric acid secretion Stimulation of airway mucus secretion Increase in AMP Increase in chronotropic and inotropic effects on heart
ECF-A tetrapeptides (preformed)	Val/Ala-Gly-Ser-Glu MW 400–500	Chemotactic attraction and deactivation of eosinophils Increase in eosinophil complement receptors
ECF-oligopeptides (preformed)	Peptides MW 1,500–3,000	Chemotactic attraction and deactivation of eosinophils and mononuclear leukocytes
HMW-NCF (preformed)	Neutral protein MW 600,000	Chemotactic attraction and deactivation of neutrophils
PAF (newly formed)	AGEPC MW 551 (hexadecyl), MW 523 (octadecyl)	Aggregation of platelets and secretion of amines Neutrophil aggregation and enzyme release Production of prostaglandins and thromboxanes by platelets Increase in vascular permeability Mimics physiologic and intravascular sequelae of IgE-mediated human systemic anaphylaxis Potent chemotactic attraction and activation of eosinophils Prolonged increase in bronchial hyperresponsiveness
Heparin (preformed)	Acidic proteoglycan MW 60,000 (human)	Anticoagulation (antithrombin III binding activity) Anticomplementary activity (at several sites) Augments inactivation of histamine
Arachidonic acid (newly formed) Cyclo-oxygenase products: PGD_2 (newly formed)	20-carbon fatty acid	Contraction of smooth muscle Bronchoconstriction Vasodilation (skin) Chemokinesis of granulocytes Chronotropic effect on heart Increase in vascular permeability Sneezing Rhinorrhea
PGE_2 (newly formed)		Relaxation of smooth muscle Bronchodilation Vasodilation
$PGF_{2\alpha}$ (newly formed)		Bronchoconstriction Constriction of microvasculature and pulmonary vasculature
PGI_2 (newly formed)		Relaxation of smooth muscle Pulmonary vasodilation
TXA_2 (newly formed)		Bronchoconstriction Constriction of microvasculature Platelet aggregation
Lipoxygenase products: LTC_4, LTD_4, LTE_4 (newly formed)	MW 400–600	Smooth muscle contraction and bronchoconstriction, especially of peripheral airway Airway mucus secretion Dilatation and increased permeability of microvasculature Constriction of coronary and cerebral arteries Depression of myocardial contractility
LTB_4 (newly formed)	MW 400	Chemotactic and chemokinetic for neutrophils and eosinophils Increased leukocyte adherence to endothelium Leukocyte activation Suppression of T-lymphocyte function
HETEs (newly formed)		Chemotaxis and chemokinesis of eosinophils and neutrophils

**Chemotactic migration requires a concentration gradient from the stimulus side. Movement in the absence of a gradient of the stimulus is termed* positive chemokinesis.

GMP = guanosine monophosphate; cGMP = cyclic GMP; AMP = adenosine monophosphate; cAMP = cyclic AMP; ECF = eosinophil chemotactic factor; A = anaphylaxis; HMW = high molecular weight; NCF = neutrophil chemotactic factor; PAF = platelet-activating factor; PG = prostaglandin; TXA_2 = thromboxane A_2; MW = molecular weight; Ig = immunoglobulin; HETEs = hydroxyeicosatetraenoic acids; AGEPC = acetyl-glyceryl-ether-phosphorylcholine.

monophosphate (cAMP) are associated with inhibition of release of mediators from mast cells. Prostaglandins of the E series and β-adrenergic agonists can cause increases in cAMP.

FACTORS NOT DERIVED FROM MAST CELLS THAT PARTICIPATE IN IMMEDIATE-TYPE HYPERSENSITIVITY DISEASES

Eosinophil-derived molecules of potent biologic activity may contribute to tissue injury in IgE-mediated and other diseases. *Eosinophil major basic protein* (MBP) causes dose-dependent epithelial damage in guinea pig trachea and in human bronchial epithelium. Immunofluorescent staining discloses extracellular deposition of MBP in areas of airway epithelial destruction in patients who have died of status asthmatics. If MBP causes destruction of airway epithelium, it may play a role in the bronchial hyperresponsiveness characteristic of asthma. Deposition of MBP is also demonstrable in lesions of atopic dermatitis and often in those of chronic urticaria. MBP also stimulates histamine release from human basophils and causes a wheal and flare reaction when injected into human skin. In a variety of in vitro systems (bacteria, parasites, tumor cells), *eosinophil peroxidase* causes injury. Both eosinophil-derived neurotoxin and eosinophil cationic protein cause damage to myelinated cells in animals.

Kinins are another system of proteins activated in inflammatory processes that have amplifier and effector properties. Their activities include chemotaxis, increased vascular permeability, and smooth muscle contraction. Bradykinin, a nonapeptide, is the most important product of the kinin system. The kinin, complement, and clotting systems are interrelated. Activation of Hageman factor (factor XII) is the initial step in kinin generation and amplification, with positive feedback loops resembling those in the complement pathway. Hageman factor (HF) is activated by tissue injury from a number of agents, including IgG aggregates and immune complexes. HF and complexes of high molecular weight kininogen and prekallikrein and high molecular weight kininogen and factor XI are bound together. HF appears to autoactivate to form activated HF (HFa), which converts prekallikrein to kallikrein. Kallikrein digests high molecular weight kininogen to liberate the vasoactive peptide bradykinin. Bradykinin has potent contractile effects on smooth muscle, causes increased vascular permeability, and dilates peripheral arterioles. It also stimulates pain receptors. At least two other plasma kinins have biologic activities similar to those of bradykinin. The role of bradykinin in allergic disease is uncertain. Several patients with cold urticaria have had increased concentrations of bradykinin in plasma.

Platelet-activating factor (PAF), a phospholipid, is synthesized by a variety of cells, including vascular endothelial cells, monocytes, macrophages, neutrophils, and especially eosinophils, as well as platelets. It is a potent inducer of increased vascular permeability. Its inhalation causes acute transient bronchoconstriction in both normal and asthmatic subjects. Bronchial hyperresponsiveness follows and may persist for weeks in normal individuals but may not occur in patients with asthma, possibly because of hyperresponsiveness already induced by endogenous PAF. Mediators released or formed in response to bridging of cell-bound IgE molecules, such as eosinophil chemotactic factors and LTB_4, may attract eosinophils and other cells that synthesize PAF, which, in turn, may cause a late-phase reaction several hours after the initial antigen-antibody reaction occurred.

Type I hypersensitivity reactions involve early-phase (10–30 min) and late-phase (4–8 hr) reactions. Early reactions after antigenic stimulation include vasodilation, edema formation from increased vascular permeability, smooth muscle constriction (bronchoconstriction), and mucus production. This response is due to the release of preformed and newly synthesized mast cell mediators and may be treated with antihistamines and mast cell membrane stabilizers such as cromolyn sodium. The late-phase reaction perpetuates the early changes of vascular permeability but includes the recruitment of inflammatory cell types in addition to mast cells. These recruited cells (eosinophils, neutrophils, lymphocytes) are located in the perivascular space. Erythema, edema, and induration are present, as is airway hyperirritability to rechallenge with allergens. This late, chronic inflammatory reaction probably contributes to the hyperresponsiveness found in allergic children with asthma, rhinitis, and atopic dermatitis. Late-phase reactions respond poorly to antihistamines or bronchodilator therapy but may respond to corticosteroids.

Serotonin (5-hydroxytryptamine) is a vasoactive amine that, in experimental animals, induces contraction of smooth muscle and increases vascular permeability. Ninety per cent of the body's stores of serotonin are found in the gastrointestinal tract, with the remainder divided between the central nervous system and platelets. Human mast cells lack serotonin. Serotonin has been reported to induce bronchoconstriction in asthmatics but not in normal persons, but it has no significant role in immediate hypersensitivity reactions in humans. It is associated distinctively with diarrhea in the carcinoid syndrome.

Although not mediators in the same sense as products released from mast cells or basophils, certain components of the *complement system* have activities that may contribute to allergic reactions.

1. Aggregated IgE can initiate complement system activity in vitro through the alternative pathway; this probably does not occur in vivo because of the large quantities of IgE required.
2. Certain "split" or "cleavage" products of the complement cascade, C3a and C5a, can induce mediator (histamine) release from basophils and from mast cells in the skin, producing wheal and flare reactions. C3a and C5a have been termed *anaphylatoxins* because they release histamine and resemble components of serum capable of causing guinea pig anaphylaxis. C5a and, to a much lesser extent, C3a are chemotactic for various leukocytes. Neutrophils attracted to the site of complement activation by C5a may degranulate, releasing basic lysosomal proteins that trigger mediator liberation from mast cells. The result in the skin is urticaria mimicking an antigen-IgE reaction. Small *N*-formylated peptides, derived from bacterial products, also possess potent granulocyte chemotactic activity and may operate in a manner similar to that of C5a to cause urticaria.
3. A kinin-like peptide derived from C2 as a result of reduced functional activity of the inhibitor of C1-esterase is thought to mediate the angioedema observed in hereditary angioedema.

From the foregoing considerations it is evident that the signs and symptoms of typical, immediate-type allergic reactions such as anaphylaxis, although most often involving the IgE mechanism, may result from non-IgE immunologic mechanisms or from nonimmunologic mechanisms.

Jarvis D, Burney P: The epidemiology of allergic disease. Br Med J 316:607, 1998.

Jirapongsananuruk O, Leung DYM: Clinical applications of cytokines: New directions in the therapy of atopic disease. Ann Allergy Asthma Immunol 79:5, 1997.

Holgate ST: Asthma: Past, present and future. Eur Respir J 6:1507, 1993.

Leung DYM: Immunologic basis of chronic allergic diseases: Clinical messages from the laboratory bench. Pediatr Res 42:559, 1997.

Luster AD: Chemokines—chemotactic cytokines that mediate inflammation. N Engl J Med 338:434, 1998.

CHAPTER 142
Diagnosis

GENERAL AND SPECIFIC METHODS OF DIAGNOSIS

ALLERGY HISTORY. The allergy history includes a detailed history of "exposure" to potential allergens. The frequency, duration, intensity, location, and progression of symptoms are relevant to a determination of their possible causes and to decisions about the types of therapy that may be effective. Seasonal symptoms may correlate with exposure to seasonal allergens such as pollens. Exposure to the highest concentrations of house dust mites, the chief source of allergens in house dust, often occurs at the end of the summer because high humidity favors mite proliferation. Allergy to house dust mites, however, usually causes perennial symptoms. Allergy to pet dogs or cats that have access to the house also usually causes perennial symptoms. Patients may deny an association between exposure to the animal and their symptoms because they fail to recognize that contamination of the house and its furnishings with animal dander results in continual exposure to allergen despite only intermittent exposure to the animal itself. Onset or worsening of symptoms shortly after acquisition of an animal or relief when the child is away from the house should arouse suspicion.

A relationship between symptoms and where they occur may suggest a cause. Exposure to pollens is often more intense outdoors than indoors, especially when windows are closed and air conditioners are operating. Onset of symptoms shortly after moving to a different dwelling should suggest an environmental cause. Changes in symptoms during trips away from home may provide helpful clues to the cause. Worsening of symptoms in a damp, musty basement should suggest allergy to fungi. An increase in symptoms at night may suggest increased exposure to allergen in the bedroom, but asthma commonly worsens at night even without exposure to allergens. Weekend remissions suggest a source of allergen at school or the workplace.

An association between symptoms and certain activities may be diagnostically helpful. Respiratory symptoms that follow exposure to freshly cut grass suggest allergy to pollen or fungi. Symptoms provoked by dusting or carpet cleaning are often due to allergy to house dust mites. Coughing or wheezing following strenous exercise may occur in children who have asthma. Provocation of coughing by laughter, crying, or exposure to smoke or specific odors also suggests the bronchial hyperresponsiveness characteristic of asthma.

The nature of the symptoms is important. An intermittent, recurrent, dry cough or a cough productive of clear mucus is consistent with asthma, but a chronic persistent cough productive of purulent sputum suggests bronchiectasis or cystic fibrosis. Aspiration of a foreign body often causes a sudden onset of coughing with choking followed by wheezing. Coughing associated with aphonia or dysphonia may be due to a hypopharyngeal or laryngeal foreign body or laryngeal papilloma. Glottic or subglottic obstruction can cause a harsh, barking cough. Paroxysmal coughing suggests pertussis or a bronchial foreign body.

Allergic rhinitis is the most common cause of a chronic or recurrent clear nasal discharge, especially when associated with sneezing or conjunctival itching and injection with excessive tearing. A purulent nasal discharge suggests infection. A postnasal drip caused by allergic rhinitis or sinusitis may cause frequent clearing of the throat, hoarseness, and nocturnal coughing. Intense conjunctival itching associated with photophobia and a viscid, white conjunctival discharge suggest vernal conjunctivitis.

A history of any beneficial or adverse effects of previous treatment may be helpful in establishing the diagnosis as well as guiding further therapy. Improvement of rhinitis in response to an antihistamine suggests allergy rather than infection. Antihistamines often relieve coughing as a result of postnasal drainage associated with allergic rhinitis, but relief of coughing by a bronchodilator suggests asthma.

The immediate family history is relevant. Atopic allergy manifested by allergic rhinitis, asthma, atopic dermatitis, or urticaria, and the specific manifestations of these disorders tend to be familial. Asthma may be familial whether or not it is due to allergy. Nonetheless, any of these conditions can also occur without a positive family history.

PHYSICAL EXAMINATION. Results of the physical examination depend upon the duration and severity of the allergic disorder. *Height and weight* should be compared with normal values for age. Both severe asthma and treatment with adrenal corticosteroids can suppress growth. Poor weight gain may suggest cystic fibrosis, a consideration in the differential diagnosis of asthma.

Pulsus paradoxus, the difference in systemic arterial blood pressure during inspiration and expiration, normally does not exceed 10 mm Hg. During acute asthma it is often increased, and the extent to which it exceeds 10 mm Hg is an index of the severity of the airway obstruction. An increase to more than 20 mm Hg indicates moderate or severe airway obstruction. Other possible causes of increased pulsus paradoxus include cystic fibrosis, heart failure, and cardiac tamponade.

Cyanosis resulting from airway obstruction may be evident if arterial oxygen saturation is less than 85%. The need for a marked reduction in intrapleural (high negative) pressure to initiate inspiration through obstructed airways may cause *supraclavicular and intercostal retractions.* Air trapping during expiration may cause bulging of the intercostal spaces during acute asthma. *Flaring of the alae nasi* may be evident. Bobbing of the head with each inspiration indicates *dyspnea* in infants lying supine.

Mouth breathing and a dark discoloration beneath the lower eyelids *(allergic shiners)* indicate nasal obstruction, usually caused by allergic rhinitis. Frequent wrinkling of the nose and the *allergic salute* (habitual wiping of the running nose) also suggest allergic rhinitis. Frequently repeated salutes for months or years elevate the tip of the nose, causing a transverse nasal crease at the junction of the cartilaginous and bony bridge of the nose. A familial transverse nasal groove, inherited as a mendelian dominant trait, is unrelated to rhinitis. *Dennie lines* (Dennie-Morgan folds), wrinkles beneath the lower eyelids, are associated with allergic rhinitis, asthma, and atopic dermatitis.

Digital clubbing is extremely rare in patients with uncomplicated asthma. Its presence suggests a complication such as bronchiectasis or another disease (Table 142–1). Comparison of the depth of the index finger at the base of the nail with its depth at the distal interphalangeal joint is the best method of recognizing digital clubbing. The depth at the base of the nail is normally smaller. A depth at the base of the nail equal to that at the distal interphalangeal joint is 2.5 standard deviations above normal, indicating mild clubbing.

Inspection of the skin may disclose evidence of *atopic dermatitis*—an erythematous, maculopapular eruption; fine scaling; or weeping and oozing with excoriations caused by frequent scratching (see also Chapters 146 and 671). Crusting may be evident if there is superimposed infection. The dermatitis may be generalized, but in infancy there is usually a predilection for the cheeks and extensor surfaces of the extremities. In older children, involvement of the antecubital spaces, popliteal spaces, and neck is most frequent and licheni-

TABLE 142–1 Diseases Associated with Acquired Digital Clubbing

Cardiac	Gastrointestinal
Cyanotic congenital heart disease	Celiac disease
Bacterial endocarditis	Chronic dysentery
Pulmonary	Ulcerative colitis
Abscess	Crohn's disease
Bronchiectasis	Multiple polyposis
Chronic pneumonia	Hepatic
Cystic fibrosis	Biliary cirrhosis
Empyema	Chronic active hepatitis
Malignant neoplasms	Other
Tuberculosis	Hodgkin's disease
Pleural	Thyrotoxicosis
Mesothelioma	Congenital methemoglobinemia
	Familial

fication and either hyperpigmentation or hypopigmentation may be evident.

Urticarial lesions may vary in appearance from multiple, 1- to 3-mm wheals with flares typical of cholinergic urticaria to giant wheals that may be associated with angioedema. Wheals are often evanescent, resolving in minutes or hours, only to appear elsewhere. There is often associated *dermographism. Contact dermatitis* is manifested by an erythematous or papulovesicular eruption in the area exposed to the contactant.

Examination of the eyes may disclose the conjunctival injection, excessive tearing, and periorbital edema of *allergic conjunctivitis.* A tenacious, ropy, mucoid conjunctival discharge associated with giant papillae on the upper palpebral conjunctiva, pseudoptosis, and photophobia should suggest *vernal conjunctivitis.*

The *nasal mucosa* may be pale, blue, or pink in children with allergic rhinitis. A profuse, clear nasal discharge is typical. Nasal turbinates are usually edematous. Hypertrophy of tonsils and adenoids is a common complication of allergic rhinitis.

Examination of the chest may disclose an increase in the *anteroposterior diameter* associated with asthma. Comparison of the depth with the width of the chest, measured with chest or obstetric calipers, permits objective evaluation of the chest configuration. The chest of the normal newborn infant is almost circular in cross-section. With growth, the width increases more than the depth (anteroposterior diameter). By the time the child's height reaches 95 cm at approximately 3 yr of age, the depth-width ratio has decreased to 0.75 and remains between 0.70 and 0.75 thereafter. Abnormal increases in the depth-width ratio occur during acute asthma but return toward normal after response to bronchodilator treatment. A persistent increase in this ratio may occur in children with frequently recurrent or continual asthma episodes but is more characteristic of chronic conditions associated with persistent airway obstruction, such as cystic fibrosis.

In patients with asthma, auscultation of the lungs may disclose *wheezing,* more pronounced on expiration, and prolongation of the expiratory phase of respiration. Wheezing is usually generalized, but there may be minor differences in intensity from segment to segment as a result of segmental atelectasis.

IN VITRO TESTS. A white cell count and a differential count are useful in establishing whether *eosinophilia* is present. The total eosinophil count is more accurate than estimates from blood smears. Eosinophils are subject to a diurnal rhythm, their numbers being highest in the early morning. Because eosinophilia may be intermittent, two or three normal results should be obtained before concluding that there is no eosinophilia. Eosinophil counts in children usually approximate 250 cells/mm^3, but as many as 700/mm^3 may be normal. Eosinophilia of respiratory tract secretions in a patient with rhinorrhea or cough is important. A smear of nasal secretions or bronchial mucus should be stained on a microscope slide with an eosin-methylene blue stain (Hansel's stain). A finding of more than 5–10% eosinophils in nasal secretions supports the diagnosis of allergic rhinitis. Eosinophils in bronchial mucus strongly suggest asthma. Blood eosinophilia in allergic conditions does not generally exceed 15–20% but may rarely be as high as 35% in allergic children in the absence of other disorders known to cause eosinophilia. Eosinophilia is also noted in drug hypersensitivity, rheumatologic disorders (periarteritis nodosa, rheumatoid arthritis), pemphigus, dermatitis herpetiformis, inherited eosinophilia, allergic bronchopulmonary aspergillosis, various malignancies (leukemias, lymphomas, Hodgkin's disease), eosinophilic fasciitis, toxic oil syndrome, and eosinophilic-myalgia syndrome (associated with L-tryptophan). High eosinophil counts are also noted in parasitic infections with tissue-invading helminths *(Toxocara,* trichinosis, *Echinococcus, Ascaris)* or malaria and in hypereosinophilic syndrome (Löffler's syndrome, pulmonary infiltrates, cardiomyopathy). Corticosteroids cause eosinopenia for up to 6 hr following a dose; the timing of collection of a blood specimen should be appropriately adjusted.

A number of in vitro immunologic tests are of value in allergy diagnosis, such as measurement of the *total and specific immunoglobulin (Ig) content of serum* and determination of the sensitivity of the patient's leukocytes for antigen-induced histamine release. Table 142–2 shows the serum concentrations of IgE in normal Swedish subjects of different ages. Normal values vary in different populations. Mean concentrations of IgE in atopic individuals are often higher than normal, although a significant number of allergic individuals have normal or low IgE concentrations. Indeed, low levels of serum IgE may be more useful in excluding atopic disease than elevated levels are in confirming this diagnosis, although patients with low IgE levels can have atopy. In patients with active atopic dermatitis, however, serum IgE levels are usually greatly elevated. Increased total IgE levels during infancy suggest the likelihood of subsequent development of atopic diseases. Table 142–3 shows some nonatopic disorders associated with increased concentrations of serum IgE.

The *radioallergosorbent test* (RAST) determines antigen-specific IgE concentrations in serum (Fig. 142–1). The correlation among RAST results and medical histories, provocation tests, or leukocyte histamine release tests is good. Correlation with allergy skin testing is also good, but RAST is somewhat less sensitive than skin testing. There has been considerable interlaboratory and intralaboratory variability in RAST results on the same specimen. Selection of a reliable laboratory is essen-

TABLE 142–2 Levels of Serum Imunoglobulin E of Normal Subjects at Different Ages*

Age	Range (IU/mL)	Geometric Mean (±2 SD) (IU/mL)
0 days	<0.1–1.5	0.22 (0.04–1.28)
6 wk	<0.1–2.8	0.69 (0.08–6.12)
3 mo	0.3–3.1	0.82 (0.18–3.76)
6 mo	0.9–28.0	2.68 (0.44–16.26)
9 mo	0.7–8.1	2.36 (0.76–7.31)
1 yr	1.1–10.2	3.49 (0.80–15.22)
2 yr	1.1–49.0	3.03 (0.31–29.48)
3 yr	0.5–7.7	1.80 (0.19–16.86)
4 yr	2.4–34.8	8.58 (1.07–68.86)
7 yr	1.6–60.0	12.89 (1.03–161.32)
10 yr	0.3–215	23.66 (0.98–570.61)
14 yr	1.9–159	20.07 (2.06–195.18)
18–83 yr	1–178	21.20 (Modal values 10–20 IU/ml)†

**Data on ages 0–14 yr adapted from Kjellman N-IM, Johansson SGO, Roth A: Clin Allergy 6:51, 1976; data on ages 18–83 yr adapted from Nye L, Merrett TG, Landon J, et al: Clin Allergy 1:13, 1975, The method used was a double antibody assay. To convert IU/mL to μg/L, multiply by 2.4.*

†*Modal values—the most common values observed.*

TABLE 142–3 Nonallergic Diseases Associated with Increased Serum IgE Concentrations

Parasitic infestations	Neoplastic diseases
Ascariasis	Hodgkin's disease
Capillariasis	IgE myeloma
Echinococcosis	Other diseases and disorders
Fascioliasis	Burns
Filariasis	Cystic fibrosis
Hookworm	Dermatitis, chronic acral
Onchocerciasis	Erythema nodosum, streptococcal
Paragonimiasis	Guillain-Barré syndrome
Schistosomiasis	Hemosiderosis, primary pulmonary
Strongyloidiasis	Intestinal nephritis, drug-induced
Trichinosis	Kawaski's disease
Visceral larva migrans	Liver disease
Infections	Pemphigoid, bullous
Allergic bronchopulmonary aspergillosis	Polyarteritis nodosa, infantile
Candidiasis, systemic	Rheumatoid arthritis
Coccidioidomycosis	
Cytomegalovirus mononucleosis	
Infectious mononucleosis (Epstein-Barr virus)	
Leprosy	
Immunodeficiency	
Hyperimmunoglobulinemia E syndrome	
IgA deficiency, selective	
Nezelof's syndrome	
Thymic hypoplasia (DiGeorge's anomaly)	
Wiskott-Aldrich syndrome	

Ig = immunoglobulin.

tial. More recent modifications of in vitro methods for determining specific IgE incorporate different types of solid supports for binding allergen and different labels for antihuman IgE antibody, resulting in colored, luminescent, or fluorescent detectable products.

In vitro methods of determining specific IgE to several allergens simultaneously have been marketed as screening tests for allergy. The few published data evaluating such methods indicate that they are relatively insensitive and may fail to identify more than 30% of children with allergy.

Whatever the method for determining specific IgE, results must be correlated with the patient's medical history to establish clinical relevance. In vitro determination of specific IgE has both advantages and disadvantages compared with allergy skin testing (Table 142–4). For experienced clinicians, allergy skin testing remains the method of choice for most patients.

IN VIVO TESTS. Determination of allergic reactivity through direct *skin testing* of the patient is an important tool in the diagnosis of IgE-mediated sensitivity. A small quantity of allergenic extract is introduced into the skin by prick or puncture (epidermal or epicutaneous method) or by intradermal technique. If the patient's mast cells have IgE antibodies specific for the allergen on their surfaces, an allergen-IgE interaction triggers biochemical events that culminate in release of histamine and other mediators from the mast cell. The histamine acts on histamine receptors in small vessels, causing increased permeability and dilatation and axon reflex stimulation, which cause a wheal and flare reaction. A positive intradermal reaction is a wheal of at least 5 mm of induration, plus surrounding erythema, occurring 15 min after injection of antigen. The immediate wheal and flare reaction usually peaks within 15–30 min and then resolves. In some patients, however, when the wheal has exceeded 10 mm in diameter, a late-phase reaction may follow. The wheal becomes less distinct, but edema and erythema persist, peak at 6–8 hr, and often resolve by 24 hr. Late-phase reactions are associated with burning, pruritus, and warmth and may become more than double the size of the antecedent immediate reaction. Histologic examination of this late-phase reaction discloses a mixed cellular infiltrate including mononuclear cells, eosinophils, and neutrophils.

The immediate wheal and flare reaction in skin indicates that specific IgE antibody is also present on the mast cells in the tissue of the clinically affected organ. *It does not indicate that the patient will necessarily have clinical symptoms on exposure to the allergen.* Some atopic individuals have no symptoms following natural exposure to allergens that elicit positive wheal and flare reactions on skin testing. As a general rule, the larger the size of the wheal and flare reaction, the more likely is the test antigen to be clinically relevant. However, one must be cautious not to overinterpret skin test results.

Positive skin test results obtained by the puncture technique correlate better than the more sensitive intradermal tests with measurements of specific IgE antibody and with the appearance of clinical symptoms on exposure to the allergen. With the intradermal technique, only those positive test results ob-

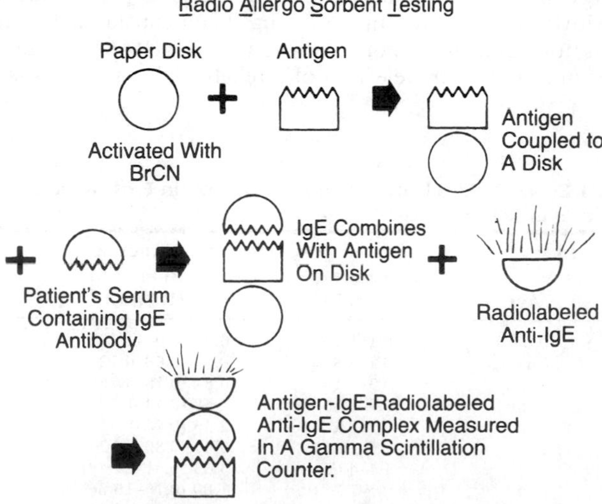

Figure 142–1 The principle of the radioallergosorbent test (RAST). After activation of some form of cellulose (e.g., a paper disk) by cyanogen bromide (BrCN), antigen is coupled covalently to the disk to render the antigen insoluble. Incubation with the patient's serum permits any specific antibodies to bind to the antigen. These antibodies remain bound to antigen after washing. Addition of radiolabeled antihuman immunoglobulin E (IgE) results in labeling of the antigen-IgE complex. The complex is then counted in a gamma scintillation counter. The number of disintegrations per minute is proportional to the amount of specific IgE in the serum sample.

TABLE 142–4 Determination of Specific IgE by Radioallergosorbent Test* and Skin Testing

Variable	Skin Test	Radioallergosorbent Test
Risk of allergic reaction	Yes	No
Sensitive†	Very	Less
Affected by antihistamines	Yes	No
Affected by corticosteroids	Usually not	No
Affected by extensive dermatitis or dermographism	Yes	No
Convenience, less patient anxiety	No	Yes
Broad selection of antigens	Yes	No
Immediate results	Yes	No
Expensive	No	Yes
Semiquantitative	No	Yes
Lability of allergens	Yes	No
Results evident to patient	Yes	No

*Radioallergosorbent test as example of other in vitro tests.

†Because skin tests are more sensitive, they are more reliable than RAST in confirming life-threatening anaphylactic conditions if maximal sensitivity is required (e.g., penicillin, Hymenoptera hypersensitivity).

tained with high dilutions (weak concentrations) of extract have as high correlations. If only concentrated solutions of allergenic extract (e.g., 1–100 or 1–10 weight/volume) elicit positive intracutaneous test results, the results will more often than not be of little clinical significance. A histamine control should also be used for comparison. Overinterpretation of such reactions has led to overuse of allergenic extracts in immunotherapy.

Various drugs, extracts that contain irritant materials or substances that are too concentrated, and improper technique can induce nonimmunologic histamine release from tissue mast cells. The resulting wheal and flare reaction cannot be differentiated from that following IgE-allergen interaction, and IgE sensitivity may be mistakenly inferred. Other drugs may inhibit full expression of clinically relevant positive skin test results. Among these are certain adrenergic drugs such as epinephrine and ephedrine and the antihistamines. These drugs should be withheld prior to skin testing (ephedrine for at least 12 hr and most antihistamines for at least 72 hr, hydroxyzine for 5 days, and astemizole for at least 2 mo). To make sure that the skin is capable of reacting to endogenously released histamine, a positive histamine control (histamine phosphate, 1%) should always be used. Corticosteroids administered for only a few days have no appreciable inhibitory effects on IgE-mediated wheal and flare reactions and need not be withheld before skin testing, but administration of systemic corticosteroids daily or on alternate days for as long as 1 yr can suppress cutaneous reactivity to codeine (but not to histamine), suggesting suppression of histamine release from mast cells.

Because the appearance of symptoms on natural exposure may not correlate well with results of skin testing, *provocation testing* by direct exposure of the mucous membrane of the affected organ to the suspected allergen (usually in the form of an extract or aerosol of the material) has received considerable attention. Mucous membrane (bronchial) provocation testing has been used mostly in patients with asthma. As commonly performed, the test requires that increasing concentrations of extracts of various allergens be inhaled by the patient after nebulization with a suitable device. A positive response is manifested by an increase in airway obstruction as monitored with pulmonary function testing. The patient's degree of sensitivity should be determined by skin tests before provocation testing to permit appropriate initial concentrations of allergenic extract to be used. With reasonable precautions, the method is safe, and the results of provocation testing correlate well with clinical data. It is time-consuming, however, and is not suitable for general use in the office or clinic. Bronchial challenge testing may be most useful in patients who have many positive skin test results, in whom it can guide selection of those allergens that may be most clinically significant for inclusion in an immunotherapy extract mixture. Selection in this way permits a greater concentration of the more clinically significant allergens in the mixture than would be possible if all the allergens possibly implicated by skin testing were to be included. Studies have shown excellent correlations in the results of provocative bronchial challenge testing, RAST, and quantitative intradermal skin tests (end-point dilution method); accordingly, bronchial challenge testing is principally reserved for research purposes. Conversely, bronchial provocative testing with methacholine or histamine is valuable when the degree of airway reactivity in asthma must be determined and when the diagnosis of asthma is uncertain. Methacholine bronchial challenge testing produces marked bronchoconstriction in patients with asthma compared with normal controls. Atopic children without asthma also have increased hyperresponsiveness to methacholine provocation, suggesting a predisposition to nonspecific bronchial hyperactivity.

Oral provocation should be performed in a facility equipped for cardiopulmonary resuscitation and is contraindicated if anaphylactic reactions have occurred. Provocation testing with foods has been used to diagnose IgE-mediated food allergy and food-induced atopic dermatitis. Following an elimination diet, food antigens are introduced in a double-blind provocation trial. Skin testing may help to identify the offending food, especially in the presence of an association between ingestion and IgE-mediated events (anaphylaxis, urticaria, angioedema, eczema, abdominal cramps). Oral provocation is indicated if the history is equivocal and symptoms improve during an elimination diet. The specific food is given in gelatin capsules, and the child is evaluated for the immediate recurrence of symptoms or signs. Manifestations of allergy appear within 10–90 min and include pruritus, erythematous macular morbilliform rash, wheezing, sneezing, cough, abdominal pain, nausea, emesis, and increased serum histamine levels.

Aberg N, Engstrom I: Natural history of allergic diseases in children. Acta Pediatr Scand 79:206, 1990.

American College of Physicians: Allergy testing. Ann Intern Med 110:317, 1989.

Bierman CW, Pearlman DS (eds): Allergic Diseases from Infancy to Adulthood, 2nd ed. Philadelphia, WB Saunders, 1988.

Broadbent JB, Sampson H: Food hypersensitivity and atopic dermatitis. Pediatr Clin North Am 35:1115, 1988.

deShazo R, Smith D: Primer on allergic and immunologic diseases. JAMA 268:2785, 1992.

Ownby DR: Allergy testing: In vivo versus in vitro. Pediatr Clin North Am 35:995, 1988.

Pacheco S, Shearer W: Laboratory aspects of immunology. Pediatr Clin North Am 41:623, 1994.

Van Arsdel PP, Larson E: Diagnostic tests for patients with suspected allergic disease: Utility and limitations. Ann Intern Med 110:304, 1989.

CHAPTER 143
Principles of Treatment

Successful management of allergic disorders is based on avoidance of allergens or irritants, pharmacologic therapy, immunotherapy (hyposensitization or desensitization), and prophylaxis.

When clinically relevant allergens are identified by history and judicious use of allergy skin tests, their elimination or *avoidance* is all that is needed in many cases of IgE-mediated disease. If the history and skin testing indicate reactivity to house dust mites or molds, or if dog or cat allergen is contributing to the patient's symptoms, these allergens should be eliminated from the home to the greatest extent possible. The recommendation that a family pet be removed from a home is frequently difficult to implement. When the allergic disorder is a serious one, such as asthma, and when the child has a positive skin test result to the dog or cat allergen, parents can generally be persuaded to remove the animal. When skin test results to danders are negative, the problem may be more difficult; most allergists believe that elimination of potentially sensitizing pets from the household of the allergic child is desirable for prophylaxis.

Allergy to **house dust mites** requires precautions to minimize exposure to mite allergens. Avoidance in the bedroom is often sufficient because children spend more time there than in other rooms of the house. Mattresses, box springs, and pillows should be encased in airtight, allergen-proof covers.* Vacuuming the covered mattress at least weekly is necessary to remove mites. Bedding should be washed at least weekly in hot water (>70°C); cool water does not kill the mites. There

---

*Allergy Control Products, 96 Danbury Road, PO Box 793, Ridgefield, CT 06877-0793.

should be no carpet or rug in the bedroom because either may be a rich source of mites. A small cotton throw rug may be acceptable if it is washed at least weekly in hot water. There should be no upholstered furniture and no stuffed toys in the bedroom. When removal of carpet from a bedroom is impossible, treatment of the carpet with a solution of tannic acid inactivates mite allergens.* Repeated treatments of the carpet at intervals of 2–3 mo are necessary because the solution does not kill the mites. Benzyl benzoate (Acarosan) kills mites; carpet treatment every few months is necessary to control mite populations. Use of tannic acid or benzyl benzoate is of less value than elimination of carpet.

Household humidity should be kept at less than 50% to inhibit survival of mites. It is prudent to avoid use of vaporizers. Dehumidifiers may be necessary in damp basements. Air conditioning helps to control humidity and also reduces exposure to atmospheric pollens and molds. If elimination of a cat from a home is impossible, other measures that can reduce allergen exposure include exclusion of the animal from the house, washing the cat more often than weekly, removal of carpets and upholstered furniture, and improvement of ventilation. Cat allergen is ubiquitous in public places and homes without cats.

Avoidance of irritants is important in the control and prevention of asthma. Potential sources of irritants include kerosene heaters and wood-burning stoves. Smoking should not be permitted indoors, and patients with asthma should avoid public facilities where exposure to cigarette smoke is likely.

Pharmacologic therapy is a major element in the management of allergic diseases (see Chapter 143.1). The drugs used have specific roles in the interruption of pathways leading to tissue damage as a consequence of antigen-antibody interaction. Certain drugs, for example, modulate the antigen-induced release of mediators (histamine, leukotrienes) or block their actions; others affect the tension of smooth muscle and still others prevent the migration to the site of an allergic reaction of inflammatory cells having the potential for producing tissue injury. Drug therapy may be effective whether or not an allergic mechanism is involved. Patients with nonimmunologic or nonallergic asthma may respond to drug treatment as well as do those in whom allergy plays a major role.

Immunotherapy is appropriate for the treatment of allergic rhinitis or asthma mediated by IgE antibody-antigen interactions caused by unavoidable inhalant allergens (see Chapter 143.2).

A predisposition to form IgE antibodies to substances of "high" allergenic potential is an important characteristic of the atopic state. Therefore, prevention of exposure of infants and children at risk has a rational basis. It is appropriate to recommend breast-feeding for infants born into families with strong histories of hay fever, asthma, or atopic dermatitis and to delay for at least 6 mo the introduction of solid foods into the diet of such infants, especially foods of highly allergenic potential, such as eggs, cow milk, wheat, fish, citrus fruit, and peanut butter. The nursing mother should avoid highly allergenic foods in her diet because there is evidence that the breast-fed infant can become sensitized to food antigens that are transmitted in breast milk. It is not definitively established whether postponing cow milk feedings in an atopic infant can prevent the development of cow milk allergy, of allergic diseases in general, or of atopic dermatitis in particular, although there is some evidence of such effects.

Environmental exposure to high concentrations of house dust mite allergen is a risk factor for subsequent sensitization and asthma. There are no prospective studies that indicate convincingly that avoidance of environmental exposure of atopic infants and children to other inhalant allergens such as dog and cat allergen lessens the likelihood of their sensitization, although such a result seems reasonable. Cord blood IgE levels greater than 1.3 IU/mL, elevated serum IgE levels, eosinophilia during infancy, and a family history of atopic dermatitis, asthma, or allergic rhinitis may predict a child at risk for future atopic disorders who might benefit from allergenic avoidance.

*Allergy Control Products, 96 Danbury Road, PO Box 793, Ridgefield, CT 06877-0793.

143.1 Pharmacologic Therapy

ADRENERGICS. These agents combine with α- and β-receptors on the surfaces of cells. With several exceptions, drugs that affect α-receptors cause physiologic responses that are excitatory (vasoconstriction), whereas drugs that influence β-receptors produce inhibitory responses (bronchodilation). In a given tissue the response to a drug depends both on the relative numbers of α- and β-receptors and on whether the drug stimulates predominantly α-receptors or β-receptors, or both.

Variations in the sensitivity of β-receptors of different organs to β-agonists (stimulants) and differences in the response to β-blocking drugs of diverse chemical structure have led to separation of β-receptors into two subclasses, β_1 and β_2; β_1-receptors have approximately equal affinity for epinephrine and norepinephrine, whereas β_2-receptors have an approximately 10-fold higher affinity for epinephrine than for norepinephrine. Agents with greater β_2-selective activity (isoetharine, metaproterenol, terbutaline, albuterol, fenoterol, bitolterol, pirbuterol, salmeterol) provide effective bronchodilation in asthma with less of the increase in heart rate that may occur with isoproterenol or epinephrine because the latter drugs stimulate both bronchial β_2-receptors and cardiac β_1-receptors, causing tachycardia. Selectivity for β_2-receptors is relative, however, and some patients experience tachycardia after administration of putative β_2-selective agents. Selective β_2 drugs have essentially no α-adrenergic activity and thus no pressor effect. These agents stimulate skeletal muscle and may induce tremors. They also stimulate glycogenolysis and may produce hypokalemia. Accordingly, such drugs do not cause the pallor that may follow epinephrine administration. The function of β_3-adrenergic receptors is uncertain.

Alpha-adrenergic receptors have been subclassified into α_1 and α_2 subtypes; these have wide distribution and mediate different effects. Stimulation of α_1-receptors contracts vascular and airway smooth muscle. Additional subtypes of α_1- and α_2-adrenergic receptors have distinctive patterns of distribution.

Although experiments in vitro with human tissues have shown that adrenergic drugs can inhibit allergen-induced mediator release from mast cells and basophils, their use in allergic disorders depends principally on their effects on smooth muscle in blood vessels and in the bronchial airways. For example, stimulation of α-adrenergic receptors reduces edema of nasal mucous membranes through vasoconstriction and decreases the permeability of venules and capillaries, whereas β-adrenergic stimulation causes smooth muscle relaxation, which relieves at least one component of obstruction of the airway in asthma.

Adrenergic drugs include catecholamines (epinephrine, isoetharine, isoproterenol, and bitolterol) and noncatecholamines (ephedrine, albuterol, metaproterenol, salmeterol, terbutaline, pirbuterol, procaterol, and fenoterol). Those of the former group are rapidly inactivated by enzymes found in the gastrointestinal tract and liver; accordingly, the use of epinephrine and isoproterenol is limited largely to injection, inhalation, and topical application to mucous membranes. Ephedrine, the oldest of the noncatecholamine sympathomimetics, has relatively weak β-stimulant activity and frequently causes adverse side effects, including increased activity, insomnia, irritability, and headache. Newer noncatecholamine adrenergic agents (metaproterenol, terbutaline, and albuterol), which may also be given orally, have a somewhat longer duration of action (up to 6 hr) than ephedrine (4 hr) and have relatively selective activity on the β_2-receptors in the airways, with less of the cardiovascular effects of isoproterenol and epinephrine, especially when delivered by inhalation. Salmeterol is a long-acting derivative of albuterol; its long action is due to a long lipophilic side chain that interacts with a binding site near the β_2-receptor, permitting the phenylethanolamine head of the molecule to interact repeatedly with the β_2-receptor. Inhalation of a single dose of salmeterol can elicit bronchodilation for at least 12 hr, inhibit both immediate and late-phase reactions to inhaled allergen, and inhibit allergen-induced bronchial hyperresponsiveness for 24 hr. Because severalfold lower doses of adrenergic drugs are effective when the agents are given by the inhalational rather than the oral route, aerosol administration is preferred wherever possible to minimize adverse side effects.

Autoantibodies against β_2-adrenergic receptors have been identified in small proportions of patients with asthma, a few patients with cystic fibrosis, and a few normal controls. The presence of these autoantibodies has been associated with β-adrenergic hyporesponsiveness. Such autoantibodies may account for some of the abnormalities in autonomic function in some patients with asthma. Tolerance or desensitization to adrenergic agents may occur, but if such agents are used as prescribed, the small decrease in the duration or intensity of drug effect usually has no serious therapeutic implications. Desensitization is related to genetic polymorphisms of the β_2-receptor gene.

Adverse side effects of adrenergic drugs may include skeletal muscle tremor, cardiac stimulation, worsening of hypoxemia, increased airway obstruction, headache, insomnia, irritability, nausea, vomiting, epigastric pain, flushing, hyperglycemia, hypokalemia, and tolerance (subsensitivity, refractoriness). Benzalkonium chloride, the preservative in most albuterol and metaproterenol nebulization solutions, can occasionally cause bronchoconstriction in asthmatic patients, which may limit the response to the bronchodilator; medications delivered from metered-dose inhalers contain no benzalkonium chloride. Metabisulfite, used as a stabilizing agent in solution for nebulization, may exacerbate bronchoconstriction because of hypersensitivity to this agent. Over-reliance on metered-dose adrenergic agents or home-aerosolized sympathomimetic drugs may be responsible for delay in seeking medical attention, increasing the risk of morbidity and even mortality.

THEOPHYLLINE. This is a therapeutic agent for the treatment of both acute and chronic asthma. Its mode of action is uncertain. It is no longer held that it inhibits cyclic adenosine monophosphate (cAMP) phosphodiesterase because the concentrations necessary to demonstrate this effect are toxic in vivo. Moreover, other potent phosphodiesterase inhibitors (e.g., papaverine) are ineffective in asthma. Other possible modes of action include adenosine antagonism, an effect on calcium flux across cell membranes, prostaglandin antagonism, release of or synergistic interactions with β-adrenergic agonists, and enhancement of binding of cAMP to a cAMP-binding protein. Theophylline causes bronchodilation by relaxing bronchial smooth muscle, increases concentrations of endogenous catecholamines in the circulation, and enhances the contractility of the fatigued diaphragm. It can inhibit both immediate and late-phase asthmatic responses to allergenic challenge and sometimes reduces bronchial hyperresponsiveness.

Both the therapeutic and toxic effects of theophylline are related to the serum concentration. The incidence of toxic effects increases as the serum levels rise progressively to greater than 20 μg/mL. *Measurement of serum theophylline concentration* is an important element in effective and safe use of the drug. Methods for theophylline analysis are specific, sensitive, and rapid and require only a small serum sample; they should be available in all hospitals. A 15-min method that requires no instrument for determination of theophylline level in finger prick blood (AccuLevel) gives excellent results.

Pharmacokinetics. Both the rapidly absorbed and most (but not all) slow-release (SR) formulations of theophylline are completely bioavailable. Rapidly absorbed preparations may be given with food without significant effect on rate or extent of absorption, but absorption characteristics of SR products may be altered when they are administered with a meal, being either accelerated or delayed, depending on the product. Administration of TheoDur tablets or Slo-bid Gyrocaps with a meal can delay attainment of peak serum concentrations by 1–2 hr usually with little or no effect on bioavailability. Conversely, administration of Uniphyl with a meal can almost double the amount of drug absorbed. Unless the physician wishes to take advantage of the fact that food delays absorption of a specific SR product (e.g., Theolair-SR), SR products other than TheoDur tablets and Slo-bid Gyrocaps are best given 60 min before meals. The ultraslow-release formulations may be incompletely bioavailable when given to patients with rapid gastrointestinal transit times (especially young children). The absorption from an SR product can vary from time to time, even in the same patient, leading to confused interpretation of serum concentration data. Occasionally, a "trough" theophylline level will be higher than that in a specimen drawn at a time thought to represent a "peak" level. Peak serum concentrations usually occur 4–8 hr after administration of most SR products (6–10 hr after TheoDur or Uniphyl).

The marketed SR products differ in theophylline-release characteristics, and care must be exercised in switching from one product to another. Substitution of a generic for a proprietary preparation without the physician's or patient's knowledge is a potential source of problems. Such unauthorized substitution by the pharmacist is legal in most states unless it is specifically forbidden on the prescription.

Despite these limitations, SR formulations of theophylline represent an advance in dealing with the fluctuations in serum concentrations seen with rapidly absorbed products, particularly in young patients who metabolize the drug rapidly. Even with the SR products, patients who metabolize theophylline rapidly may have unacceptable fluctuations in the serum theophylline level if the drug is given at 12-hr intervals rather than 8-hr intervals. Theophylline absorption is slower during night-time hours; accordingly, administration every 12 hr may produce early morning levels that are higher than those later in the day. Theophylline salts such as aminophylline (theophylline ethylenediamine) do not improve efficacy and may cause adverse effects because of the development of ethylenediamine hypersensitivity.

After its absorption, about 60% of theophylline is bound to protein (somewhat less in premature infants). Free theophylline is distributed rapidly into body fluids, equilibration between serum and tissues being complete within 1 hr following intravenous injection. Salivary concentrations are about 60% of those in serum. Estimates of serum theophylline concentration derived from analysis of *appropriately collected* saliva samples are accurate enough for most clinical purposes. Theophylline distributes freely into umbilical cord blood, breast milk (not clinically significant for the infant), and cerebrospinal fluid.

Theophylline is metabolized by biotransformation in the liver via a cytochrome P450–dependent microsomal mixed-function oxidase. Metabolism occurs via both first-order (linear) and nonlinear capacity-dependent processes. Some patients show disproportionate dose-dependent changes in theophylline serum concentration, particularly at the higher doses, owing to the nonlinear elimination. About 10–15% of theophylline is excreted unchanged in urine (50% in prematures). There is substantial intersubject variation in the rate of theophylline body clearance. Intrasubject variations in clearance also occur.

TABLE 143–1 Factors That Affect Theophylline Clearance

Factor	Decreased Clearance: Increased Levels	Increased Clearance: Decreased Levels
Disease	Liver disease (cirrhosis, acute hepatitis)	Hyperthyroidism
	Congestive heart failure	Cystic fibrosis
	Acute pulmonary edema	
	Febrile viral respiratory illness	
	Renal failure	
Drugs	Troleandomycin	Carbamazepine
	Erythromycin	Phenytoin
	Clarithromycin	Rifampin
	Fluoroquinolones	Phenobarbital
	Cimetidine	Terbutaline
	Ranitidine (less than cimetidine)	Isoproterenol (intravenous)
	Oral contraceptives	Sulfinpyrazone
	Ketoconazole	
	Mexiletine	
	Pentoxifylline	
	Allopurinol	
	Ticlopidine	
	Thiabendazole	
	Propranolol	
	Influenza vaccine	
Habits	High carbohydrate, low protein	Smoking (tobacco or marijuana)
Diet	Dietary xanthines	High protein, low carbohydrate
		Charcoal-broiled meats

As with other drugs eliminated by hepatic metabolism, many environmental and disease factors alter the rate of elimination (Table 143–1). Most of the factors listed tend to decrease clearance, with increased theophylline concentration and risk of adverse effect. The clinical relevance of the factors varies: cigarette smoking, hepatic or heart disease, some drugs (macrolide antibiotics, cimetidine, allopurinol, carbamazepine, phenytoin, rifampin) have substantial effects, whereas others are probably of less clinical relevance (phenobarbital, ranitidine, protein-carbohydrate dietary content, ingestion of charcoal-broiled meats). Average theophylline clearance also varies with age, and dosage is based on this fact (Table 143–2).

Pharmacodynamics. The logarithmic relationship between the theophylline bronchodilator effect and serum concentration in the 5–20 μg/mL range is well documented. The serum concentration that provides optimal bronchodilator effect probably varies from patient to patient. The physician should use the patient's response rather than the theophylline blood level as a guide to increases in dosage, but dosage should not exceed the average doses for the age group without determination of peak serum theophylline concentrations to ensure safety. Some patients receive good bronchodilator effect with serum concentrations less than 10 μg/mL; in such cases, there is no need to increase the theophylline dose. Regular administration of SR theophylline to maintain trough serum concentrations of 8 to 15 μg/mL can afford symptomatic control of mild to moderate asthma comparable to that achievable with inhaled beclomethasone dipropionate, 84 μg four times each day.

Toxicity. Theophylline toxicity is a major clinical problem. Signs and symptoms of acute theophylline intoxication vary from mild nausea, insomnia, irritability, tremors, and headache to severe seizures and death. Gastrointestinal symptoms (nausea, vomiting, hematemesis, cramping) are usually the earliest to appear and generally precede the more serious central nervous system (seizures, coma) manifestations of toxicity. Uncommonly, seizures may appear as the first sign of theophylline intoxication. Disturbances in cardiac rate, most often tachycardia, rhythm disturbances (atrial and ventricular premature contractions or tachycardia), and hypotension are commonly observed with serious toxicity. Additional problems include hypokalemia, hyperglycemia, ataxia, and hallucinations. Signs and symptoms of theophylline intoxication are, by and large, serum concentration–dependent, but concentrations associated with symptoms of serious toxicity vary widely. In adults with seizures, the mean serum concentration has been reported to be approximately 50 μg/mL with a range of 20–70 μg/mL. Several infants with theophylline-induced seizures have been reported to have very high serum theophylline concentrations (180 μg/mL in one case) with no apparent permanent sequelae. Healthy adolescents who ingest theophylline in suicide attempts may tolerate very high theophylline serum concentrations (>100 μg/mL) with no permanent sequelae if treated appropriately. Conversely, children who survive serious theophylline intoxication also may be left with severe brain damage that resembles the sequelae of anoxic encephalopathy.

Treatment of theophylline intoxication should begin with measures designed to induce emesis (e.g., immediate administration of ipecac, if the patient is not already vomiting) or gavage, followed by a slurry of 30 g of activated charcoal to adsorb the theophylline remaining in the gastrointestinal tract. Activated charcoal can also remove serum theophylline that has already been absorbed from the gastrointestinal tract. It may be best to delay administration of charcoal until ipecac has induced emesis because the charcoal also adsorbs ipecac. After ingestion of SR theophylline, repeated administration of charcoal at 2–3 hr intervals is advisable. The addition of a nonabsorbed saline cathartic is effective for decreasing intestinal transit time when SR products have been ingested. Peritoneal dialysis can remove theophylline from intoxicated patients, but hemoperfusion using a specially prepared charcoal column is the method of choice. The indications for charcoal hemoperfusion are not completely defined; they depend both on the serum concentration and on clinical considerations. Diazepam is effective therapy for seizures, propranolol is help-

TABLE 143–2 Usual Theophylline Dosage Requirements After the Neonatal Period

Age (yr)	Total Daily Dose (mg/kg/24 Hr)
<1	5 + 0.2 × age in weeks
1–16	16
>16	12–13

Initial dosage should be one-half to two-thirds the usual final dosage for age. Later changes in dosage should be determined by clinical response and guided by serum theophylline determinations to achieve serum concentrations of 5–15 μg/mL at steady state (after at least 48 hr at given dosage).

ful for treating hypotension or supraventricular or ventricular arrhythmias (lidocaine is also effective for ventricular tachycardia), and ranitidine may be helpful in controlling gastric acid–induced emesis.

Chronic theophylline use may produce or exacerbate subtle behavioral changes, such as hyperactivity and sleep disturbances. These effects are dose-dependent. Theophylline has no adverse effect on cognitive function.

ANTIHISTAMINES. These drugs compete with histamine for receptors in various tissues. There are at least three histamine receptors: H_1, H_2, and H_3. Initially, only H_1-receptor blockers were used in treatment of allergic disorders. A combination of H_1 and H_2 antagonists, however, may be beneficial in some patients with chronic urticaria and in treatment of anaphylactoid reactions such as those caused by intravenous injections of contrast media for urography. Cimetidine and probably ranitidine (H_2 antagonists) inhibit delayed-type hypersensitivity skin responses, suggesting that H_2-receptor blocking agents may modulate cell-mediated immune injury. The H_1-type antihistamines, as a group, are nitrogenous bases with aliphatic side chains that resemble histamine. The side chains are attached to cyclic or heterocyclic rings of various configurations. The antihistamines may be classified as follows:

Type I—ethylenediamines (tripelennamine [Pyribenzamine], methapyrilene [Histadyl])
Type II—ethanolamines (diphenhydramine [Benadryl], carbinoxamine [Clistin, Rondec])
Type III—alkylamines (chlorpheniramine [Chlor-Trimeton, Teldrin, Novahistine, Demazin], brompheniramine [Dimetane, Bromfed], triprolidine [Actidil, Actifed])
Type IV—piperazines (cyclizine [Manezine], meclizine [Bonine])
Type V—piperidines (cyproheptadine [Periactin], azatadine [Trinalin])
Type VI—phenothiazines (promethazine [Phenergan])

Hydroxyzine (Atarax, Vistaril), which has potent antihistaminic activity, and some second-generation H_1 antihistamines do not fit well into any of these types. Second-generation antihistamines such as terfenadine, astemizole, loratadine, acrivastine, azelastine, fexofenadine (an active metabolite of terfenadine), and cetirizine (an active metabolite of hydroxyzine) are effective in suppressing the signs and symptoms of allergic rhinitis, do not cross the blood-brain barrier (because they are lipophobic), and have fewer sedative effects than other antihistamines. This is an important distinction; first-generation antihistamines can cause impairment of function even in patients who perceive no sedation or impairment from the drug. *The antihistamines may be found alone or in combination with decongestants.* The chemical classification of antihistamines does not usually have functional significance and, except for cyproheptadine, which also has antiserotonin activity, drugs from each class have equal antihistaminic activity.

In general, the H_1 antagonists are rapidly absorbed after oral administration, with onset of action within 30 min, peak plasma concentration within 1 hr, and complete absorption within 4 hr. Antihistamines are eliminated by biotransformation in the liver; little nonmetabolized drug is found in urine. Some antihistamines (diphenhydramine and chlorcyclizine) stimulate liver microsomal drug-metabolizing enzymes in animals and may accelerate their own metabolism and that of other drugs. There have been relatively few pharmacokinetic studies of the antihistamines; most of the prescribing patterns are empirically based on clinical experience. Diphenhydramine has a relatively short serum half-life of 3–4 hr, yet the drug is effective in suppressing the wheal and flare response to allergy skin testing for more than 24 hr. Thus, with this antihistamine there appears to be little correlation between serum concentration and therapeutic effect in the tissue. A study of chlorpheniramine in children showed a mean serum half-life of 13.7 hr (range, 6–34 hr). Significant suppression of clinical symptoms of allergic rhinitis was observed for as long as 30 hr after injection of a single dose, at which time chlorpheniramine was not detectable in the serum. Data indicate that chlorpheniramine, brompheniramine, and hydroxyzine may not need to be given three or four times a day but that twice or even once a day may suffice. In addition to histamine antagonism, the antihistamines have pharmacologic effects on exocrine secretions, the central nervous system, and the cardiovascular system. Some have anticholinergic-like side effects (Benadryl), whereas others are sedatives (hydroxyzine); both groups have the potential to produce drowsiness.

Because antihistamines act as competitive antagonists, they are more effective in preventing than in reversing the action of histamine. To be most effective, they must be administered at doses and intervals that keep tissue histamine receptor sites saturated. Histamine is released explosively at the site of an IgE-mediated reaction; accordingly, antihistamines are less potent in antagonizing the effects of endogenous than of exogenous histamine. Their relative inefficacy in patients with asthma is related not only to this and to the fact that mediators of bronchoconstriction other than histamine are involved in allergic reactions in the lung but also to limitation by sedation to ineffective doses. Second-generation antihistamines may afford protection against bronchoconstriction induced by a variety of stimuli, including allergens, exercise, and histamine. Many antihistamines possess anticholinergic activity, which is valuable in allergic rhinitis for controlling rhinorrhea. Anticholinergic activity may account for some of the response of asthma to some first-generation antihistamines. In children, antihistamines usually have neither favorable nor deleterious effects on the course of asthma.

There is little reason to choose one antihistamine over another, except for avoidance of adverse effects, including sedation and impairment of function, which are of great importance for students as well as drivers. Excessive doses of either first-generation or two second-generation antihistamines can have adverse cardiac effects. Very large doses of terfenadine (no longer available in the United States) or astemizole have elicited cardiac arrest secondary to prolongation of the QT interval and ventricular tachycardia (torsades de pointes) in rare patients. This has occurred in a few patients who denied ingesting an excessive dosage of the astemizole. There has been no evidence of any similar cardiac arrhythmia with loratadine acrivastine, azelastine, fexofenadine, or cetirizine. Patients with prolonged serum elimination of antihistamines may be at increased risk for adverse effects. These patients include those with impaired hepatic function or patients receiving concurrent treatment with an inhibitor of cytochrome P450 enzymes, including erythromycin and other macrolide antibiotics, ketoconazole, itraconazole, or the antidepressants nefazodone and fluvoxamine.

In general, antihistamines are extraordinarily safe, and most are sold without prescription. They can have other adverse effects, especially in high dosages. Combinations of antihistamines with other central nervous system depressants (e.g., alcohol) should be avoided. In high doses or in certain sensitive patients, the anticholinergic properties of antihistamines cause undesirable adverse reactions. These include excitation, nervousness, tachycardia, palpitations, dryness of the mouth, urinary retention, and constipation. Seizures are common in antihistamine poisoning. Skin eruptions, blood dyscrasias, fever, and neuropathy are rarely observed.

CROMOLYN SODIUM (DISODIUM CROMOGLYCATE). Cromolyn sodium is the disodium salt of 1,3,-*bis* (2-carboxychromon-5-yloxy)-2-hydroxypropane. It is soluble in water but insoluble in lipids; only 1% is absorbed from the gastrointestinal tract. The drug is administered as a powder (Intal) with a special turboinhaler, the Spinhaler, or as a 1% (20 mg/2 mL) solution for nebulization, or by metered-dose inhaler (800 μg/actuation). It is used principally in asthma but has some value in allergic rhinitis, for which it is available without prescription for delivery as a nasal spray. It has been used with varying results in patients with aphthous ulcers, food allergy, systemic mastocytosis, ulcerative colitis, and chronic proctitis. The drug has no bronchodilator properties; therefore, it is not effective for treatment of acute asthma but is given prophylactically, in a 20-mg dose two to four times each day by Spinhaler or nebulization or 1.6 mg two to four times each day by metered-dose inhaler. It prevents both antibody-mediated and non–antibody-mediated mast cell degranulation and mediator release. This effect may be due to the ability of cromolyn to block antigen-stimulated calcium transport across the mast cell membrane. Cromolyn inhibition of histamine release may also occur by regulation of phosphorylation of a mast cell protein. The drug also has weak phosphodiesterase inhibitor activity. Cromolyn appears to reduce airway hyper-reactivity by a mechanism that is not yet understood, and it can prevent late-phase asthmatic responses when administered before allergen challenge. It inhibits bronchoconstriction produced by nonimmunologic stimuli such as frigid air, exercise, and sulfur dioxide. Some of these stimuli do not cause release of mast cell–derived mediators; accordingly, cromolyn may directly affect neural control of the airway by inhibiting reflex bronchoconstriction through inhibition of the transmission of neural impulses by myelinated afferent nerve fibers.

Cromolyn is of greatest value in allergic or extrinsic asthma, but patients with nonallergic or intrinsic asthma who use it may also improve. Patients with mild degrees of asthma respond more favorably than those with severe disease. About 70% of asthmatic patients receive some benefit from inhalation of the drug. The incidence of toxic reactions to cromolyn is extremely low; dry throat and transient bronchoconstriction have been the most frequently reported side effects. The latter is most likely due to inhalation of the dry powder into irritable airways and is not an intrinsic effect of the drug itself. Rare reports have associated urticaria, angioedema, and pulmonary eosinophilia with the use of cromolyn. There are no known contraindications to its use except that during acute asthma in some patients, the powder may rarely act as an airway irritant.

NEDOCROMIL SODIUM. This is a pyranoquinoline dicarboxylic acid, chemically remote from cromolyn, which has antiallergic and anti-inflammatory activity. Like cromolyn, it inhibits release of mediators from human lung mast cells and suppresses activation of eosinophils, neutrophils, and macrophages. It inhibits both early- and late-phase asthmatic and rhinitic responses and associated increases in airway hyperresponsiveness as well as seasonal increases in nonspecific bronchial responsiveness. It can inhibit bronchoconstrictive effects of exercise; hyperventilation with cold air; inhalation of ultrasonically nebulized distilled water, sulfur dioxide, or adenosine. It can reduce airway hyperresponsiveness in asthmatic patients. Nedocromil, 4 mg four times a day, has a prophylactic effect equivalent to that of inhaled beclomethasone dipropionate at a total daily dose of 400 μg but is less effective than beclomethasone at a total daily dose of 800 μg in asthmatic adults. There are few studies of nedocromil in children; inhalation of 4 mg has been reported to have a protective effect against exercise-induced asthma comparable to that of cromolyn, 10 mg, by metered-dose inhaler in asthmatic children. Such treatment (4 mg four times a day) elicits improvement within 3–4 wk. Some adults have complained of unpleasant taste. Less frequent adverse effects have included coughing, sore throat, rhinitis, headache, and nausea; these occasional side effects have been of minor significance.

IPRATROPIUM BROMIDE. This is an anticholinergic agent that inhibits vagally mediated reflexes by antagonizing the action of acetylcholine at muscarinic receptors. It is a quarternary amine, poorly absorbed from the nasal, airway, and gastrointestinal mucosa and does not cross the blood-brain barrier readily. Inhalation of ipratropium bromide aerosol can enhance bronchodilation elicited by maximal doses of inhaled albuterol, especially in patients with severe airway obstruction due to acute asthma. Treatment of children at least 5 yr of age with nebulized ipratropium bromide, three doses of 250 μg each at 20-min intervals combined with nebulized albuterol is safe and effective. Administration as a nasal spray (0.03% or 0.06%) is effective in reducing rhinorrhea due to perennial nonallergic rhinitis or the common cold; there may be improvement in nasal congestion, sneezing, and postnasal drip in patients with perennial rhinitis. There are few associated side effects. Nasal dryness and epistaxis are the most frequent side effects of the nasal spray, occuring in less than 10% of patients; coughing has occurred in less than 6% of patients after inhalation of the aerosol.

LEUKOTRIENE INHIBITORS AND ANTAGONISTS. These agents improve pulmonary function and reduce symptoms of asthma. They afford protection against bronchoconstriction induced by exercise, cold air, platelet-activating factor, and allergens. Cysteinyl leukotriene antagonists inhibit late-phase asthmatic responses to inhaled allergen and the subsequent increase in bronchial responsiveness. They may have additive effects in patients treated with corticosteroids and may substitutes for low doses of inhaled corticosteroids in patients whose asthma requires continual treatment.

The leukotriene antagonist *zafirlukast* can inhibit exercise-induced bronchoconstriction 2 hr after oral administration but has less protective effect at 4 hr and still less at 8 hr. *Montelukast* can inhibit exercise-induced bronchoconstriction as long as 24 hr after oral administration.

Zileuton, a 5-lipoxygenase synthesis inhibitor, can prevent not only bronchoconstriction but also the nasal and gastrointestinal symptoms and angioedema that can follow aspirin challenge in aspirin-sensitive patients.

Zafirlukast and zileuton are labeled for use in patients at least 12 yr of age. Zafirlukast should be administered twice each day, at least 1 hr before or at least 2 hr after meals because food interferes with its absorption. Zileuton usually is administered at least four times each day initially. Montelukast requires administration only once each day. Erythromycin, terfenadine, and theophylline may decrease bioavailability of zafirlukast. Zileuton can decrease clearance of terfenadine, warfarin, and theophylline; when initiating treatment with zileuton, it is prudent to decrease theophylline dosage by half and monitor plasma theophylline concentrations. Elevations of hepatic enzymes in occasional patients treated with zileuton necessitate periodic monitoring of serum alanine aminotransferase levels and observation for signs or symptoms of hepatitis in patients treated with zileuton. *Churg-Strauss syndrome*, an allergic granulomatous vasculitis affecting small and medium-sized arteries with a predilection for the lungs, has been found in rare patients treated with zafirlukast or montelukast when dosages of oral corticosteroids are tapered. No causal relationship with zafirlukast or montelukast has been established. Churg-Strauss syndrome can present with fever, myalgia, headache, respiratory distress, and weight loss.

LODOXAMIDE TROMETHAMINE. This is a mast cell stabilizer that is more effective than topical cromolyn sodium in alleviating signs and symptoms of allergic ocular disease. It is used in children older than 2 yr for vernal keratoconjunctivitis, vernal conjunctivitis, and vernal keratitis. Occasional adverse effects have included transient burning or stinging after instillation.

OLOPATADINE HYDROCHLORIDE. This is both a mast cell stabilizer and an H_1-receptor antagonist effective in relieving signs and symptoms of allergic conjunctivitis after topical instillation. It is labeled for use in children at least 3 yr of age. Headaches have occurred in 7% of patients treated; burning and stinging have occurred in fewer than 5%.

CORTICOSTEROIDS. Corticosteroids are the most potent drugs available for treatment of allergic disorders. Following administration of prednisone, peak plasma concentration is attained at 1–2 hr. The systemic availability of the drug is more than 80% of the oral dose. Regardless of the route of administration, there is interconversion of prednisone and prednisolone (the active form), with prednisolone concentrations 4–10 times those of prednisone. There is little effect of liver disease or renal insufficiency on the conversion of prednisone to prednisolone or on prednisolone disposition. The volume of distribution, metabolic clearance, and renal clearance of prednisone increase with increasing doses owing to the partially saturable binding of prednisolone to transcortin in plasma, which provides more unbound drug at higher plasma concentrations of this steroid.

Some effects of prednisolone are evident within 2 hr after oral or intravenous administration (fall in peripheral eosinophils and lymphocytes); others may be delayed 6–8 hr or longer (e.g., hyperglycemia and improvement in pulmonary function in asthmatics). The delayed responses reflect the indirect mechanism of action of glucocorticoids. It is newly synthesized enzymes that mediate some of the effects of glucocorticoids. The *biologic half-life of the steroid* is determined by the turnover time of the newly synthesized enzymes, not by steroid plasma concentrations. Plasma half-lives of commonly used steroids vary from 1.5–5 hr, whereas biologic half-lives vary from 8–54 hr. Clinically significant drug interactions occur with phenobarbital and phenytoin, both of which increase steroid clearance.

The anti-inflammatory actions of glucocorticoids result from (1) alteration in leukocyte number and activity (redistribution, suppression of migration to sites of inflammation, decreased response to mitogens, decreased cytotoxicity, and suppression of delayed hypersensitivity responses in the skin), (2) suppression of mediator release (decreased histamine synthesis and release, decreased synthesis of prostaglandins and other products of arachidonic acid metabolism), (3) enhanced response to agents that increase cyclic adenosine monophosphate (prostaglandin E_2 and histamine via the H_2 receptor), and (4) enhanced response to β-adrenergic agonists (increased synthesis of β-adrenergic receptors, increased availability of epinephrine as a result of decreased extraneuronal uptake of catecholamines). The anti-inflammatory effects of glucocorticoids may be due to inhibition of synthesis of cytokines, including interleukin (IL)-1β, tumor necrosis factor-α, granulocyte-macrophage colony stimulating factor, IL-2, IL-3, IL-4, IL-5, and IL-6, and inhibition of synthesis of the chemokines IL-8, RANTES, and macrophage inflammatory protein-1α.

Topical steroids have direct local effects that include decreased inflammation, edema, mucus production, vascular permeability, and mucosal IgE levels. There is also less local accumulation of neutrophils, eosinophils, basophils, and mast cells and an attenuation of airway hyperresponsiveness. Topical steroids may reduce early- and late-phase reactions, whereas systemic steroids predominantly inhibit late-phase response to antigen. Possible complications of inhaled steroids include oropharyngeal candidiasis, dysphonia, disseminated varicella and, at high doses, suppression of the hypothalamic-pituitary-adrenal axis. Total daily dosage of not more than 400 μg budesonide or 200 μg fluticasone does not suppress linear growth in the majority of asthmatic children; larger doses may affect growth, but uncontrolled asthma can also impair growth. Beclomethasone may be more likely than other inhaled or intranasal steroids to reduce growth velocity slightly. Growth impairment from inhaled steroids at total daily dosage as high as 800 μg is less than that from oral prednisone, 2.5 mg daily. Suppressive effects of steroids on growth depend on dosage and duration of treatment; attainment of normal height is possible after discontinuation of steroids, but prolonged administration of large doses of systemic steroids can cause permanent short stature.

The few available clinical comparisons of inhaled corticosteroids suggest equivalent activity of beclomethasone dipropionate, triamcinolone acetonide, flunisolide, and budesonide delivered by metered-dose inhaler. Turbuhaler doubles delivery of budesonide to the airway as compared with metered-dose inhaler. Effects of fluticasone propionate have been comparable to twice the dose of beclomethasone dipropionate or budesonide by metered-dose inhaler (Table 143–3). Spacers or chambers, which are recommended for corticosteroid metered-dose inhalers to minimize pharyngeal deposition, enhance delivery to the airways.

The short-term use of *systemic corticosteroids* in self-limited allergic conditions such as contact dermatitis due to poison ivy or occasional episodes of severe asthma is not associated with significant adverse effects. Long-term use, in contrast, especially if daily administration is required, may have substantial undesirable side effects. In children, the most common adverse effect is suppression of linear growth. Posterior subcapsular cataracts develop occasionally in children receiving long-term steroid therapy. Other untoward effects of steroids include osteoporosis (vertebral collapse), hypertension, diabetes mellitus, cushingoid habitus, infections (particularly disseminated varicella or *Pneumocystis carinii*) pancreatitis, gastritis, and myopathy (see also Chapter 728).

Before any decision is made to initiate long-term, systemic corticosteroid therapy, all other modalities of management should be tried. Nevertheless, a small proportion of asthmatic children have severe and continuing symptoms that interfere with normal school attendance, play activities, and sports participation. The judicious use of glucocorticoids can produce substantial improvement in such children with little adverse effect, especially if they are administered as prednisone, prednisolone, or methylprednisolone, in single doses on alternate mornings.

TABLE 143–3 Estimated Comparative Daily Dosages for Inhaled Corticosteroids

Drug	Dose/Puff (μg)	Dosage for Children (μg)			Dosage for Adults (μg)		
		Low	*Medium*	*High*	*Low*	*Medium*	*High*
Beclomethasone dipropionate	42, 84						
Flunisolide	250	<550	550–800	>800	<1100	1100–2000	>2000
Triamcinolone acetonide*	100						
Budesonide Turbuhaler	200	200	200–400	>400	200–400	400–600	>600
Fluticasone propionate:							
Metered-Dose Inhaler	44, 110, 220						
Dry Powder Inhaler	50, 100, 250	<250	250–500	>500	<550	550–1000	>1000

**The Expert Panel concluded beclomethasone dipropionate was equivalent to twice the dose of triamcinolone acetonide, for which they estimated the low dosage for children at 400–1000 μg, medium dosage at 1000–2000 μg, and high dosage at more than 2000 μg.*

Modified from National Heart, Lung, and Blood Institute: Washington, DC, Expert Panel Report 2: Guidelines for the Diagnosis and Management of Asthma. NIH Pub. No. 97–4051, 1997.

A few considerations in the systemic use of corticosteroids bear emphasis.

1. When given in equivalent anti-inflammatory doses, available drugs do not differ qualitatively in anti-inflammatory effects. Adverse effects are related to dose, dosing interval, and duration of treatment. Prednisone or prednisolone is the preferred drug for oral administration and methylprednisolone for intravenous use. Other steroids with longer durations of biologic activity have greater propensities for certain adverse effects, are not suitable for alternate-day therapy, and are more expensive.

2. When corticosteroid therapy is initiated, a sufficient amount should be given daily in three to four divided doses to bring the disease under control. An attempt should then be made to adjust the dose and the dosing interval to suppress activity of the disease without adverse effects. Whenever possible, alternate-day regimens using prednisone or prednisolone should be tried. In the alternate-day regimen, the drug is given usually as a single dose every 48 hr between 6:00 and 8:00 A.M.. If daily steroid medication is required, a single dose usually has been given, again between 6:00 and 8:00 A.M.; this regimen mimics endogenous cortisol secretion and may cause less suppression of the hypothalamic-pituitary-adrenal axis and fewer other adverse side effects than the same daily dose of drug given in divided doses. Limited data in adults indicate administration of oral prednisone as a single dose at 3:00 P.M. may afford better control of asthma, especially nocturnal asthma, than administration in the morning or evening; the safety of such a regimen remains to be established. Administration of the total daily dose of inhaled triamcinolone acetonide at 3:00–5:30 P.M. may be as effective in adults as administration in four divided doses during the day and more effective than administration of a single dose in the morning without any increased adverse systemic effect. When exacerbations of asthma occur during low-dose oral maintenance therapy, high-dose suppressive therapy is indicated for a few days, with prompt return to low-dose alternate-day treatment as soon as the acute process is under control.

3. Short-term steroid therapy (<7 days) for exacerbations of asthma or poison ivy suppresses the pituitary-adrenal axis only briefly and can be stopped abruptly without tapering the dose. Patients receiving steroids for longer periods require gradual reduction of the dose to avoid precipitating an acute adrenal crisis.

ADDITIONAL PHARMACOLOGIC AGENTS. *Ketotifen,* a benzocycloheptathiophene, is an antihistamine with mast cell–stabilizing properties and a leukotriene antagonist. This drug is an anti-anaphylactic agent, inhibits IgE-dependent mediator release, and attenuates platelet-activating factor–induced bronchoconstriction. Ketotifen is a potentially useful drug, but limited experience with it has been recorded in allergic children.

Methotrexate, an immunosuppressant antagonist of folic acid, has anti-inflammatory effects when given in low doses and has been demonstrated to reduce the required doses of steroids among patients with severe chronic asthma. Methotrexate has also been effective in reducing the dose of steroids in patients with severe psoriasis and rheumatoid arthritis. The long-term risks of methotrexate use in children with severe allergic diseases have not been determined. Methotrexate remains an experimental therapy for patients with severe steroid-dependent asthma.

Monoclonal anti-IgE antibodies are undergoing clinical trials in patients with allergen-induced asthma and hold promise as a future therapy.

Barnes PJ: Molecular mechanisms of steroid action in asthma. J Allergy Clin Immunol 97:159, 1996.

Bollinger ME, Wood RA, Chen P, et al: Measurement of cat allergen levels in the home by use of an amplified ELISA. J Allergy Clin Immunol 101:124, 1998.

Boulet L, Chapman K, Cote J, et al: Inhibitory effects of anti-IgE antibody E25 on allergen-induced early asthmatic response. Am J Respir Crit Care Med 155:1835, 1997.

Drazen JM: Pharmacology of leukotriene receptor antagonists and 5-lipoxygenase inhibitors in the management of asthma. Pharmacother 17:22S, 1997.

Lemanske RF Jr, Busse WW: Asthma. JAMA 278:1855, 1997.

McCubbin MM, Milavetz G, Grandgeorge S, et al: A bioassay for topical and systemic effect of three inhaled corticosteroids. Clin Pharmacol Ther 57:455, 1995.

Pincus DJ, Humeston TR, Martin RJ: Further studies on the chronotherapy of asthma with inhaled steroids: The effect of dosage timing on drug efficacy. J Allergy Clin Immunol 100:771, 1997.

Schuh S, Johnson DW, Callahan S, et al: Efficacy of frequent nebulized ipratropium bromide added to frequent high-dose albuterol therapy in severe childhood asthma. J Pediatr 126:639, 1995.

Shapiro G, Bronsky EA, La Force CF, et al: Dose-related efficacy of budesonide administered via dry powder inhaler in the treatment of children with moderate to severe persistent asthma. J Pediatr 132:976, 1998.

Wechsler ME, Garpestad E, Flier SR, et al: Pulmonary infiltrates, eosinophilia, and cardiomyopathy following corticosteroid withdrawal in patients with asthma receiving zafirlukast. JAMA 279:455, 1998.

Yanni JM, Miller ST, Gamache DA, et al: Comparative effects of topical ocular anti-allergy drugs on human conjunctival mast cells. Ann Allergy Asthma Immunol 79:541, 1997.

143.2 Immunotherapy

IMMUNOLOGIC CHANGES. In the early weeks following the institution of regular injections of ragweed pollen extract, IgE antibody against ragweed pollen antigen increases; as treatment continues, however, the titer of anti–ragweed IgE antibody decreases. In untreated patients with ragweed hay fever, a rise and fall of anti–ragweed IgE occurs during the year; the rise occurs with the seasonal exposure to ragweed. Injection therapy blunts this anamnestic rise. With continuing treatment, ragweed antibodies of the IgG class ("blocking" or "antigen binding") appear in the serum; the ultimate titer achieved is related to the quantity of ragweed extract injected but does not necessarily correlate with clinical changes, if any occur.

Immunotherapy also can inhibit histamine release from leukocytes (basophils) on challenge in vitro with ragweed antigen E. Leukocytes from treated individuals require exposure to increased amounts of antigen E in order to release the same amount of histamine as they did prior to therapy. Leukocyte preparations from some treated patients behave as if they have been completely desensitized and do not release histamine on challenge with ragweed antigen E at any concentration. The basis for this change in cell sensitivity is unknown; it does not appear to be related to titers of either anti–ragweed IgE or IgG. There may be some intrinsic change in receptors for IgE or in the biochemical pathways that cause histamine release. Changes in ratios of helper to suppressor T cells in control of B cells, with an increase in antigen-specific suppressor T cells, have been reported in experimental animals undergoing immunotherapy and to a lesser extent in humans. Immunotherapy decreases production of IL-2 and reduces the number of IL-2 receptors. Immunotherapy inhibits the late-phase asthmatic response to allergenic challenge and decreases bronchial hyperresponsiveness.

STUDIES OF EFFICACY. Critical review of placebo-controlled, double-blind studies of treatment of ragweed hay fever by ragweed extract injections indicates that most patients improve with immunotherapy. Data supporting the efficacy of grass and tree pollen, house dust mite, and *Alternaria* immunotherapy in rhinitis induced by these allergens are fewer, but the results appear similar to those with ragweed. Controlled, randomized, double-blind studies of treatment of asthmatic patients with extracts of ragweed, mountain cedar, grass pollen, house dust mites, *Cladosporium,* and cat allergen have shown beneficial effects in most participants. A meta-analysis of 20 randomized, placebo-controlled, double-blind trials of immunotherapy for asthma disclosed significant improvement in symptoms and pulmonary function with decreased use of medications and reduced bronchial hyperresponsiveness. Nonetheless, other studies are not as conclusive. Partly because of the multiple factors that can trigger asthma (cold, exercise, smoke, cholinergic agents), immunotherapy does not cause complete remission of symptoms. Immunotherapy with Hymenoptera venom in patients having anaphylactic sensitivity to such stinging insect venom protects against anaphylaxis on subsequent sting.

The cost of immunotherapy, its inconvenience, the possibility of making the disease worse, the risk of inducing anaphylaxis, and other factors must be considered. There is no conclusive evidence for efficacy of injection therapy with allergens other than those just noted with the possible exceptions of birch, dog, and cockroach. Specifically, the injection of other epidermoids, most molds, bacterial vaccines, occupational allergens, synthetic antigens, whole-insect extracts, or food extracts has not been shown to influence favorably the course of rhinitis, anaphylaxis, or asthma.

INDICATIONS, MATERIALS, AND PROCEDURE. Immunotherapy is indicated in patients suffering from allergic rhinitis, IgE-mediated asthma, or allergy to stinging insects. Atopic dermatitis and food allergy are not improved by immunotherapy. A patient is a candidate for a trial of immunotherapy when good correlation exists between symptoms and exposure to an inhalant allergen that cannot be adequately avoided, when the patient has evidence of IgE-mediated allergy by either in vivo (skin testing) or in vitro testing, and when disabling symptoms are not easily controlled with medication. There should also be a reasonable likelihood of good compliance with the regimen because treatment requires injections of allergenic extracts at regular intervals for several years.

Aqueous extracts are used most commonly. Extracts usually contain many different antigens in addition to the specific allergen. In ragweed pollen, the allergen, antigen E, represents 8.5% of the protein extract. Pelt or skin proteins constitute the predominant allergens for patients sensitive to a cat or dog, whereas proteins in house dust mite feces are responsible for most dust hypersensitivity. The cat pelt protein, Fel d1, is the most important cat allergen. Alum-precipitated pollen extracts and alum-precipitated pyridine-extracted extracts (Allpyral) do not appear to offer any substantial advantages over aqueous extract therapy. Furthermore, the immunogenicity of one Allpyral extract (ragweed) has been questioned. Allergenic extracts are considered drugs by the U.S. Food and Drug Administration, but standards of potency exist for only a few. Some extracts sold in the United States for diagnosis and therapy have been totally lacking in allergenic activity when tested by radioallergosorbent test inhibition. Some of the antigens in allergenic extracts (e.g., ragweed antigen E) are quite labile. Methods of extraction, antigen concentration, and storage temperature are all critical factors in determining the activity and shelf life of an allergenic extract. Pollen extracts are being modified in attempts to reduce their allergenicity without reducing their immunogenicity. Allergens polymerized with glutaraldehyde retain their immunogenicity but are less allergenic. Thus, the initial dose of extract may be substantially increased, the maintenance dose can be reached within 2 mo compared with 5–6 mo with conventional therapy, and there is a greatly reduced incidence of local and systemic reactions. Such modified extracts have not yet been approved in the United States.

In practice, immunotherapy with aqueous extracts involves the repeated injection of increasing amounts of extract until the patient reaches an "optimal" maintenance dose. The dose considered optimal is often arbitrary; clinical trials involving ragweed have reported better results with "high-dose" than with "low-dose" treatment. High-dose therapy is possible only when limited numbers of allergens are included in the extract. No more than 10, and preferably fewer than 6 allergens should be included in a single injection. Children tolerate the same doses as adults.

The injections are given one to three times each week until the patient reaches the maintenance dose, usually after 5–6 mo. In the "rush" method of immunotherapy, the initial injection period is compressed into a few days with apparently satisfactory results. The interval between injections is then extended to 2, 3, and then 4 wk. If more than 1 wk has elapsed since the last dose, the dose is not increased. If more than 6 wk have elapsed between injections, the subsequent dose is reduced to avoid the possibility of a systemic reaction. There is little reason to continue weekly injections for prolonged periods after reaching maintenance dosage. During the course of the initial injections, the patient is observed carefully for evidence of excessive local reactions. Large local reactions may sometimes predict systemic reactions, but this is uncertain. If an extensive local reaction or a systemic reaction occurs, the subsequent dose is reduced and then cautiously increased according to the patient's tolerance. Failure to see a local reaction at any time suggests either that the patient is not allergic to the constituents of the extract or that the extract is inactive. Beneficial results often do not become evident until after 6 mo of therapy. Improvement may continue for several years.

Perennial treatment, in which injections are given throughout the year, is preferred to preseasonal treatment, in which the treatment regimen is renewed each year, beginning several months before the pollen season. During the pollen season, the maintenance dose of extract is unchanged except for the patient in whom systemic reactions develop presumably because of combined exposure to seasonal and injected allergen. For such patients, the dose may need to be reduced.

The optimal duration of treatment is not known and probably differs from patient to patient. Many allergists believe that if the patient is significantly improved after 3 yr of therapy, it is reasonable to discontinue the injections and observe for recurrence of symptoms. Some children have received "allergy shots" for many years with no evidence that they have been beneficial. Immunotherapy should not be continued if there is no substantial improvement within 2 yr in the condition for which the patient is being treated. Since skin reactivity changes little during the early years of immunotherapy, it is unnecessary to retest the child yearly.

PRECAUTIONS AND ADVERSE REACTIONS. Allergenic extracts should *always* be administered in a physician's office where treatment of a systemic reaction or anaphylactic shock is readily available. The patient should always remain under observation for at least 20 min after each injection because life-threatening reactions are most likely to occur within this time. Occasionally children will have delayed symptoms; for example, an exacerbation of asthma may occur in the evening of the day on which an injection of extract was given. Rarely, because of distance from a physician's office, it may be necessary to administer allergenic extracts in another setting. Under such circumstances, however, the nonphysician who administers an injection must be prepared to treat a systemic reaction.

Immunotherapy should not be administered during uncontrolled asthma because of diminished pulmonary reserve in the event of a systemic reaction to the allergenic extract. Allergenic extracts are best replaced at intervals of little more than 6 mo because of loss of potency. Dilute extracts lose potency rapidly. Extracts should be kept refrigerated at approximately 4°C. Dilution with 0.03% human serum albumin minimizes loss of potency. Because of anticipated potency loss, the initial dose of newly prepared allergenic extract should be reduced by at least 50% to minimize the risk of a systemic reaction. Except for the possibility of constitutional reactions, no short- or long-term adverse effects of administration of allergenic extracts to children are known.

Abramson MJ, Puy RM, Weiner JM: Is allergen immunotherapy effective in asthma? A meta-analysis of randomized controlled trials. Am J Respir Crit Care Med 151:969, 1995.
Adkinson N, Eggleston P, Eney D, et al: A controlled trial of immunotherapy for asthma in allergic children. N Engl J Med 336:324, 1997.
Frew A: Injection immunotherapy. Br Med J 307:919, 1993.
Iliopoulis O, Proud D, Adkinson NF Jr, et al: Effects of immunotherapy on the early, late, and rechallenge nasal reaction to provocation with allergen: Changes in inflammatory mediators and cells. J Allergy Clin Immunol 87:855, 1991.

CHAPTER 144
Allergic Rhinitis

Seasonal allergic rhinitis, seasonal pollinosis, and hay fever all describe a symptom complex that follows sensitization to wind-borne pollens of trees, grasses, and weeds. Estimates indicate that 5–9% of children in unselected samples meet diagnostic criteria. Prevalence increases with age; seasonal allergic rhinitis and perennial rhinitis together exceed 20% among adolescents. Ragweed hay fever is rarely observed before 4–5 yr of age.

In *perennial allergic rhinitis* the patient has symptoms year-round. The causative agents, when they can be identified, are generally allergens to which the patient is exposed more or less continually, although exposure may vary during the year. Indoor inhalant allergens are implicated most often. These include components of house dust, feathers, allergens or danders of household pets, and mold spores. In an occasional patient, foods cause symptoms of allergic rhinitis. Some patients may be able to ingest certain foods with impunity except during a pollen season, when ingestion causes an aggravation of nasal symptoms. The prognosis is not good. Follow-up of children with allergic rhinitis 5–10 yr later disclosed that only 10–20% were free of symptoms; asthma or wheezing develops in 10–19% within 8–11 yr.

PATHOPHYSIOLOGY. Inhaled pollens, mold spores, and animal or mite antigens are deposited on the nasal mucosa. Water-soluble antigens diffuse into the epithelium and, in genetically predisposed atopic individuals, initiate the production of local IgE. IgE-stimulated release of mast cell mediators, synthesis of new mast cell mediators, and subsequent recruitment of neutrophils, eosinophils, basophils, and lymphocytes are responsible for the early- and late-phase reactions to inhalant allergens. These reactions result in mucus, edema, inflammation, pruritus, and vasodilation. Delayed inflammation may contribute to nasal hyperresponsiveness to specific allergens, a priming effect, and to nonspecific stimuli such as irritants and strong odors.

DIAGNOSIS AND CLINICAL MANIFESTATIONS. The symptoms of allergic rhinitis include sneezing, which is frequently paroxysmal; rhinorrhea, which is often watery and profuse; nasal obstruction; and itching of the nose, palate, pharynx, and ears. Itching, redness, and tearing of the eyes may also occur, causing severe discomfort.

The typical patient with allergic rhinitis presents with bilateral nasal obstruction resulting from boggy edema of the mucous membranes. Frequently, redundant mucosa is piled up on the floor of the nose. The mucous membranes are bluish and rather pale, and there is a clear mucoid nasal discharge. The child often has mannerisms caused by itching of the nose or attempts to improve the airway. The child wrinkles the nose (rabbit nose) and may rub it in characteristic ways (allergic salute). Rubbing in an upward direction may lead to a horizontal crease at the junction of the bulbous tip of the nose with the more rigid bridge. Dark circles under the eyes have been attributed to venous stasis resulting from interference with blood flow caused by edematous nasal mucous membranes. Mouth breathing is common. Fever is unusual except when sinusitis or otitis media complicates allergic rhinitis.

The diagnosis of allergic rhinitis is substantiated by the finding of a predominance of eosinophils in a smear made of the nasal secretions. There is often a personal or family history of eczema or asthma.

DIFFERENTIAL DIAGNOSIS. *Eosinophilic nonallergic rhinitis* occurs mostly in adults. Symptoms are perennial; the mucous membranes are pale, and there may be associated nasal polyps or sinus disease. Eosinophils are found in the nasal smear, but serum IgE levels are normal and allergy skin test results are generally negative. *Primary nasal mastocytosis,* with onset most often in adulthood, presents with perennial nasal blockage and rhinorrhea. Mast cells are found in the nasal smear, and allergy skin test results are negative. *Neutrophilic (infectious) rhinitis* occurs during the early years of childhood when allergic rhinitis is uncommon; there are complaints of chronic rhinorrhea and nasal blockage, mostly during cold weather. Nasal secretions are commonly mucopurulent, and the nasal smear shows neutrophils, bacteria, and debris. A posterior pharyngeal discharge is often present. Radiographic studies of the maxillary sinuses or computed tomographic scans may show evidence of sinusitis. The condition appears to result from recurrent viral respiratory illnesses complicated by bacterial infections, but the possibility of underlying disease such as humoral antibody deficiency, ciliary dyskinesia, or cystic fibrosis should be considered. *Vasomotor rhinitis* designates a poorly understood disorder presumably resulting from an imbalance of autonomic nervous system control of mucosal vasculature and mucous glands, in which symptoms suggest allergic rhinitis, but an allergic cause cannot be identified. Nasal obstruction is the predominant symptom, with minimal itching, sneezing, and rhinorrhea. The obstruction is aggravated by environmental changes in temperature or humidity and by exposure to irritants such as tobacco smoke. The patients do not have eosinophils in their nasal secretions.

Other causes of nasal obstruction include *unilateral choanal atresia* in infants who have a unilateral nasal discharge, *deviated septum, hypertrophy of the adenoids, encephalocele,* and *nasal polyposis.* Nasal polyposis occurs in as many as 20% of children with cystic fibrosis. Fewer than 0.5% of patients in a typical allergy practice have nasal polyps resulting from allergic rhinitis. Nasal polyposis occurs in *ciliary dyskinesia* immotile cilia syndrome (Chapter 417), and in *immunologic deficiencies.* The syndrome of nasal polyps, asthma, and aspirin intolerance is known as *triad asthma.* A foul-smelling, unilateral purulent, or blood-tinged purulent nasal discharge in a child suggests a *foreign body.* A persistent bloody discharge always suggests *malignancy;* nasal obstruction with epistaxis in a male in late childhood or early adolescence suggests *benign nasopharyngeal fibroma* also known as *angiofibroma.* Nasal obstruction occurs in *hypothyroidism.* Adolescents may suffer from *rhinitis of pregnancy.* A profuse, clear nasal discharge should suggest *cerebrospinal fluid rhinorrhea,* which can be confirmed by measuring the level of glucose in the fluid. Excessive use of vasoconstrictor nose drops or sprays can lead to *rhinitis medicamentosa,* in which nasal obstruction can be severe. Chronic cocaine abuse may produce rhinitis with or without secondary infection or nasal septum perforation. Additional, rarer causes of rhinitis-like symptoms include syphilis, diphtheria, Wegener's granulomatosis, sarcoidosis, and various malignancies.

Swelling of the mucous membranes of the sinuses frequently occurs with allergic rhinitis in childhood and may be seen in roentgenograms of the involved sinuses, occasionally with fluid levels. The sinuses appear abnormal so often on roentgenography, not only in children with allergic rhinitis but also in those with viral upper respiratory tract infections and in entirely asymptomatic children, that such examination must be carefully interpreted. Sinus infection may complicate allergic rhinitis; the symptoms generally are nocturnal coughing, fetid breath, and persistent mucopurulent nasal and pharyngeal discharge. Headache and facial pain and swelling are prominent symptoms of sinusitis in older children.

TREATMENT. Treatment of either seasonal or perennial allergic rhinitis includes avoidance of exposure to suspected allergens and irritants, immunotherapy for those who cannot avoid inhalant allergens, and drug therapy.

Avoidance. It is difficult or impractical to avoid exposure to seasonal pollens, but much can be done to eliminate exposure to indoor inhalant factors such as house dust, danders, and molds. Control of house dust, with special attention to the child's bedroom, often ameliorates symptoms in the dust-allergic child. Elimination of exposure to danders and feathers is mandatory for a child with perennial allergic rhinitis when these factors contribute to the symptoms. For the child sensitive to indoor molds, avoidance of damp basements and measures to discourage mold growth in the house frequently are beneficial. These measures include dehumidifiers, air conditioners with efficient filters, and air-cleaning devices, either the electronic precipitator type or one containing a high-efficiency particulate air filter. A 1:750 solution of zephiran chloride is effective in controlling mold growth; a 1:10 dilution of household bleach (sodium hypochlorite) also can be helpful. In areas that can be closed off, such as damp cellars, volatilization of paraformaldehyde from several open jars is also frequently effective in inhibiting growth of mold. For infants with persistent rhinorrhea and nasal obstruction, dietary elimination of milk, egg, or wheat is rarely helpful unless allergy skin testing or in vitro testing has confirmed food allergy.

Immunotherapy is discussed in Chapter 143.2.

Drug Therapy. Appropriate drugs usually relieve symptoms of allergic rhinitis. *Antihistamines* are useful, especially in the treatment of seasonal allergic rhinitis (Chapter 143.1). It may be necessary to increase the dosage beyond that routinely recommended until relief of symptoms or side effects occur. Nasal itching, sneezing, and rhinorrhea are usually well controlled by antihistamine therapy, whereas nasal obstruction is relieved to a lesser degree. The major adverse side effect of antihistamine therapy is somnolence, which usually lessens with continued use. Nonsedating antihistamines (acrivastine, astemizole, fexofenadine, loratadine) should be used if possible because of evidence that first-generation antihistamines often cause impairment of function even in patients unaware of somnolence and can interfere with learning.

If nasal obstruction is particularly troublesome, a decongestant such as pseudoephedrine or phenylpropanolamine may be administered alone or in combination with an antihistamine. Insomnia and irritability are the most frequent side effects; phenylpropanolamine has been implicated as a cause of acute hypertension, headache, toxic encephalopathy, intracranial hemorrhage, and convulsions, as well as acute psychosis with visual hallucinations. Dosage of pseudoephedrine usually should not exceed 15 mg every 6 hr for children 2 to 5 yr of age, 30 mg for children 6 to 12 yr of age, and 60 mg every 6 hr for children older than 12 yr of age.

Nose drops or sprays containing sympathomimetic drugs should be avoided except for short-term use; continued use may lead to progressively severe nasal obstruction due to rebound vasodilation. Treatment of this latter complication requires complete cessation of use of medicated nose drops and the substitution of nose drops of physiologic saline solution.

Cromolyn nasal solution (4%) is useful both in seasonal and in perennial allergic rhinitis. In children with hay fever, use of the nasal spray is best begun before the pollen season. The dose varies from one to two sprays in each nostril three to six times per day. As with the powder, cromolyn nasal solution is used prophylactically (Chapter 143.1).

By far the most effective treatment of allergic rhinitis is topical use of *corticosteroids*. Beclomethasone, budesonide, flunisolide, fluticasone, or mometasone should be used in children whose nasal symptoms are resistant to antihistamine-decongestant therapy or as an alternative. The initial dosage is usually one to two sprays in each nostril two to three times per day (budesonide, two sprays to each nostril twice each day; fluticasone or mometasone, two sprays to each nostril daily). After 3–4 days, as symptoms improve, the dose and frequency of use are reduced until a minimal effective dosage, one to two sprays once or twice each day, is reached and continued as maintenance therapy. Complications of topical nasal steroids include local burning, irritation, and epistaxis. There is little systemic absorption, and nasal or pharyngeal candidiasis and mucosal atrophy are not problems. Regular use of intranasal beclomethasone can cause a slight suppression of growth velocity; fluticasone and monetasone may not have such an effect. Occasionally, temporary use of corticosteroid eye drops is necessary in a child with hay fever and particularly severe eye symptoms, but this is best prescribed by an ophthalmologist who can observe the patient for any possible adverse effects. Treatment with olopatadine hydrochloride (Patanol) eyedrops twice each day or 0.1% lodoxamide tromethamine (Alomide) eye drops four times each day is safer and is often effective in preventing symptoms of allergic conjunctivitis (Chapter 143.1). Treatment of allergic conjunctivitis with 0.05% levocabastine hydrochloride eye drops four times each day is also effective, but this H_1 antihistamine is not labeled for use in children younger than 12 yr.

Leukotriene antagonists, labeled only for treatment of asthma, also can help control symptoms of allergic rhinitis and conjunctivitis.

For children who suffer from persistent neutrophilic (infectious) rhinitis with or without sinusitis, a 2-wk course of a broad-spectrum antibiotic (amoxicillin) frequently is effective. Nasal irrigation with a warm saline solution using a bulb syringe or with an adaptation of the Water Pik device (1 tsp of salt to a full reservoir of warm water) is helpful symptomatically in patients with nonallergic chronic rhinitis.

Dykewicz MS, Fineman S, Skoner DP, et al: Diagnosis and management of rhinitis: Complete guidelines of the Joint Task Force on practice parameters in allergy, asthma and immunology. Ann Allergy Asthma Immunol 81:478, 1998.

Fahy GT, Easty DL, Collum LM, et al: Randomised double-masked trial of lodoxamide and sodium cromoglycate in allergic eye disease: A multicentre study. Eur J Ophthalmol 2:144, 1992.

Linna O, Kokkonen J, Lukin M: A 10-year prognosis for childhood allergic rhinitis. Acta Paediatr 81:100, 1992.

Malmstrom K, Meltzer E, Prenner B, et al: Effects of montelukast (a leukotriene receptor antagonist), loratadine, montelukast + loratadine, and placebo in seasonal allergic rhinitis and conjunctivitis. J Allergy Clin Immunol 101:S97, 1998.

Milgrom H, Bender B: Adverse effects of medications for rhinitis. Ann Allergy Asthma Immunol 78:439, 1997.

Naclerio R, Solomon W: Rhinitis and inhalant allergens. JAMA 278:1842, 1997.

Simons FE: Allergic rhinitis: Recent advances. Pediatr Clin North Am 35:1053, 1988.

CHAPTER 145
Asthma

Asthma is a leading cause of chronic illness in childhood. It is responsible for a significant proportion of school days lost because of chronic illness. Asthma is the most frequent admitting diagnosis in children's hospitals and results nationally in 5–7 lost school days/yr/child. As many as 10–15% of boys and 7–10% of girls may have asthma at some time during childhood. Before puberty, approximately twice as many boys as girls are affected; thereafter, the sex incidence is equal. Asthma can lead to severe psychosocial disturbances in the family. With proper treatment, however, satisfactory control of symptoms is usually possible. There is no universally accepted definition of asthma; it may be regarded as a diffuse, obstructive lung disease with (1) hyperreactivity of the airways to a variety of stimuli and (2) a high degree of reversibility of the obstructive process, which may occur either spontaneously or as a result of treatment. Also known as *reactive airway disease,* the asthma complex probably includes wheezy bronchitis, viral-associated wheezing, and atopic-related asthma. In addition to bronchoconstriction, inflammation is an important pathophysiologic factor. Mast cells, eosinophils, activated T lymphocytes, macrophages, and neutrophils have key roles in the chronic inflammation of asthma.

Both large (>2 mm) and small (<2 mm) airways may be involved to varying degrees. Irritability or hyperreactivity of the airways, although not limited to asthmatic patients, appears to be an intrinsic part of the disease and is present to some degree in almost all asthmatic individuals. This hyperresponsiveness manifests itself as bronchoconstriction following exercise; on natural exposures to strong odors or irritant fumes such as sulfur dioxide, tobacco smoke, or cold air; and on intentional exposures in the laboratory to inhalations of histamine or parasympathomimetic agents such as methacholine (Mecholyl). This heightened airway irritability is a sensitive objective indicator of asthma and is present to some degree when patients are asymptomatic, free of abnormal physical findings, and capable of normal findings on spirometry. Airway hyperreactivity relates to the overall severity of the disease. It varies from patient to patient but generally is relatively stable over time in the same patient except for temporary fluctuations; increased reactivity occurs during viral respiratory infections, following exposure to air pollutants and allergens or to occupational chemicals in sensitized individuals, and following administration of β-receptor antagonists. An acute decrease in airway irritability follows administration of β-receptor agonists, theophylline, and anticholinergics, and decreased irritability follows chronic administration of cromolyn, nedocromil, or systemic or inhaled corticosteroids.

Data on the inheritance of asthma are most compatible with polygenic or multifactorial determinants. A child with one affected parent has about a 25% risk of having asthma; the risk increases to about 50% if both parents are asthmatic. However, asthma is not universally present among monozygotic twins. Lability of bronchoconstriction with exercise is concordant in identical twins but not in dizygotic twins. Bronchial lability in response to exercise testing also has been demonstrated in healthy relatives of asthmatic children. A genetic predisposition combined with environmental factors may explain most cases of childhood asthma.

EPIDEMIOLOGY. Asthma may have its onset at any age; 30% of patients are symptomatic by 1 yr of age, whereas 80–90% of asthmatic children have their first symptoms before 4–5 yr of age. The course and severity of asthma are difficult to predict. The majority of affected children have only occasional attacks of slight to moderate severity, which are managed with relative ease. A minority experience severe, intractable asthma, usually perennial rather than seasonal; it is incapacitating and interferes with school attendance, play activity, and day-to-day functioning. The relationship of age of onset to prognosis is uncertain; most severely affected children have an onset of wheezing during the first yr of life and a family history of asthma and other allergic diseases (particularly atopic dermatitis). These children may have growth retardation unrelated to corticosteroid administration (although ultimate height attainment usually is normal), chest deformity secondary to chronic hyperinflation, and persistent abnormalities on pulmonary function testing.

The prognosis for young asthmatic children is generally good. Ultimate remission depends partly on growth in the cross-sectional diameter of the airways. Longitudinal studies indicate that about 50% of all asthmatic children are virtually free of symptoms within 10–20 yr, but recurrences are common in adulthood. In children who have mild asthma with onset between 2 yr and puberty, the remission rate is about 50%, and only 5% experience severe disease. In contrast, resolution is rare in children with severe asthma characterized by chronic steroid-dependent disease with frequent hospitalizations; about 95% become asthmatic adults. Whether the hyperirritability of the airways ever disappears is unknown; abnormal responsiveness to methacholine inhalation in formerly asthmatic patients has been found as long as 20 yr after symptoms have abated.

Both prevalence and mortality from asthma have increased during the last three decades. The 1988 Health Interview Survey indicated a prevalence of asthma of nearly 5% in the United States among children 10 to 17 yr of age, but a 1993 survey of a group of Detroit school children in grades 3 to 5, who were nearly all black, disclosed that 17% had physician-diagnosed asthma; an additional 14% had significant decreases in FEV_1 after exercise challenge or at least three episodes of symptoms suggestive of asthma within the previous 12 mo. Increases in prevalence have been reported from England, Wales, Israel, New Zealand (from 26% in 1975 to 34% in 1989 among adolescents), and Australia (from 19% in 1964 to 46% in 1990 among 7-yr-old children in Melbourne). The causes of the increased prevalence are unknown, but some of the factors associated with both onset of asthma and increased mortality have been identified. Risk factors for the occurrence of asthma include poverty, black race, maternal age less than 20 yr at the time of birth, birthweight less than 2,500 g, maternal smoking (more than one-half pack per day), small home size (<eight rooms), large family size (≥six members), and intense allergenic exposure in infancy (more than 10 μg of house dust mite allergen *Der p* I per gram of dust collected from homes). Additional risk factors may include frequent respiratory infections in early childhood, overweight in black and hispanic inner-city children, and less than optimal parenting. Sensitization to inhalant allergens can occur in infancy, but it becomes increasingly frequent beyond 2 yr of age and is demonstrable in most children beyond 4 yr of age who require emergency room visits for wheezing. Risk factors for death from asthma include underestimation of severity of asthma, delay in implementation of appropriate treatment, underuse of bronchodilators and corticosteroids, black race, noncompliance with recommendations for management, psychosocial dysfunction and stress that may interfere with compliance or perception of increasing airway obstruction, sedation, and excessive allergenic exposure. Recent emergency treatment or recent admission to a hospital for asthma increases the risk of fatal asthma. Patients subject to sudden, severe airway obstruction and those with chronic, steroid-dependent asthma are at especially high risk for fatal asthma.

PATHOPHYSIOLOGY. Manifestations of the airway obstruction in asthma are due to bronchoconstriction, hypersecretion of mucus, mucosal edema, cellular infiltration, and desquamation of epithelial and inflammatory cells. Various allergic and nonspecific stimuli, in the presence of hyperreactive airways, initiate the bronchoconstriction and inflammatory response. These stimuli include inhaled allergens (dust mites, pollens, molds, cockroach, cat or dog allergens), vegetable proteins, viral infection, cigarette smoke, air pollutants, odors, drugs (nonsteroidal anti-inflammatory agents, β-receptor antagonists, metabisulfite), cold air, and exercise.

The pathology of severe asthma includes bronchoconstriction, bronchial smooth muscle hypertrophy, mucous gland hypertrophy, mucosal edema, infiltration of inflammatory cells (eosinophils, neutrophils, basophils, macrophages), and desquamation. Pathognomonic findings include Charcot-Leyden crystals (lysophospholipase from eosinophil membranes), Curschmann spirals (bronchial mucous casts), and Creola bodies (desquamated epithelial cells).

Newly synthesized and stored mediators are released from local mucosal mast cells following nonspecific stimulation or the binding of allergens to specific mast cell–associated IgE. Mediators such as histamine, leukotrienes C_4, D_4, and E_4, and platelet-activating factor initiate bronchoconstriction, mucosal edema, and the immune responses (see Chapter 141). The early immune response results in bronchoconstriction, is treatable with β_2-receptor agonists, and may be prevented by mast cell-stabilizing agents (cromolyn or nedocromil). The late-phase reaction occurs 6–8 hr later, produces a continued state of airway hyperresponsiveness with eosinophilic and neutrophilic infiltration, can be treated and prevented by steroids, and can be prevented by cromolyn or nedocromil.

Obstruction is most severe during expiration because the intrathoracic airways normally become smaller during expiration. Although the airway obstruction is diffuse, it is not entirely uniform throughout the lungs. Segmental or subsegmental atelectasis may occur, aggravating mismatching of ventilation and perfusion (Fig. 145–1). Hyperinflation causes decreased compliance, with consequent increased work of breathing. Increased transpulmonary pressures, necessary for expiration through obstructed airways, may cause further narrowing or complete premature closure of some airways during expiration, thus increasing the risk of pneumothorax. Increased intrathoracic pressure may interfere with venous return and reduce cardiac output, which may be manifested as a pulsus paradoxus.

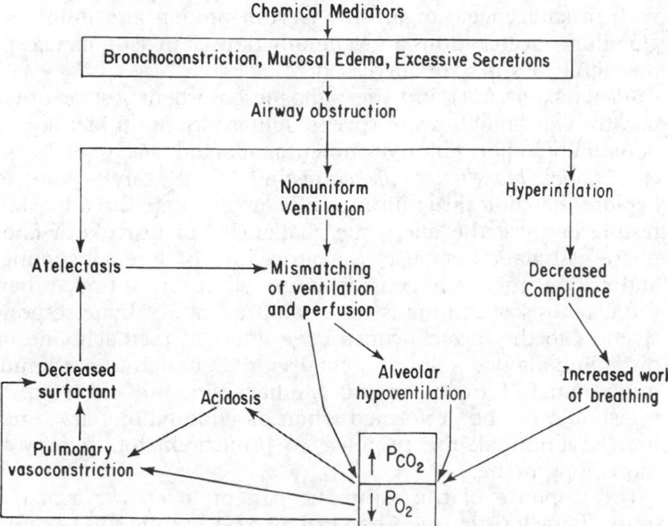

Figure 145–1 The pathophysiology of asthma. (Po_2 = partial pressure of oxygen; Pco_2 = partial pressure of carbon dioxide.) (Modified from Siegel SC: Bronchial Asthma. *In:* Kelley VC [ed]: Practice of Pediatrics. Chapter 74. Vol 2. Hagerstown, MD, Harper & Row, 1987.)

Mismatching of ventilation with perfusion, alveolar hypoventilation, and increased work of breathing cause changes in blood gases (see Fig. 145–1). Hyperventilation of some regions of the lung compensates initially for the higher carbon dioxide tension in blood that perfuses poorly ventilated regions. However, it cannot compensate for hypoxemia while breathing room air because of the patient's inability to increase the partial pressure of oxygen and oxyhemoglobulin saturation. Further progression of airway obstruction causes more alveolar hypoventilation, and hypercapnia may occur suddenly. Hypoxia interferes with conversion of lactic acid to carbon dioxide and water, causing metabolic acidosis. Hypercapnia increases carbonic acid, which dissociates into hydrogen ions and bicarbonate ions, causing respiratory acidosis.

Hypoxia and acidosis can cause pulmonary vasoconstriction, but cor pulmonale resulting from sustained pulmonary hypertension is not a common complication of asthma. Hypoxia and vasoconstriction may damage type II alveolar cells, diminishing production of surfactant, which normally stabilizes alveoli. Thus, this process may aggravate the tendency toward atelectasis.

ETIOLOGY. Asthma is a complex disorder involving autonomic, immunologic, infectious, endocrine, and psychologic factors in varying degrees in different individuals. The control of the diameter of the airways may be considered a balance of neural and humoral forces. Neural bronchoconstrictor activity is mediated through the cholinergic portion of the autonomic nervous system. Vagal sensory endings in airway epithelium, termed *cough* or *irritant receptors,* depending on their location, initiate the afferent limb of a reflex arc, which at the efferent end stimulates bronchial smooth muscle contraction. Vasoactive intestinal peptide neurotransmission initiates bronchial smooth muscle relaxation. Vasoactive intestinal peptide may be a dominant neuropeptide involved in maintaining airway patency. Humoral factors favoring bronchodilation include the endogenous catecholamines that act on β-adrenergic receptors to produce relaxation in bronchial smooth muscle. When local humoral substances such as histamine and leukotrienes are released through immunologically mediated reactions, they produce bronchoconstriction, either by direct action on smooth muscle or by stimulation of the vagal sensory receptors. Locally produced adenosine, which binds to a specific receptor, may contribute to bronchoconstriction. Methylxanthines are competitive antagonists of adenosine.

Asthma may be due to abnormal β-adrenergic receptor–adenylate cyclase function, with decreased adrenergic responsiveness. Reports of decreased numbers of β-adrenergic receptors on leukocytes or genetic polymorphisms of the β-receptor of asthmatic patients may provide a structural basis for hyporesponsiveness to β-agonists. Alternatively, increased cholinergic activity in the airway has been proposed as a defect in asthma, perhaps due to some intrinsic or acquired abnormality in irritant receptors, which seem in asthmatic patients to have lower than normal thresholds for response to stimulation. Neither theory reconciles all the data. In individual patients, a number of factors generally contribute in varying degrees to the activity of the asthmatic process.

Immunologic Factors. In some patients with so-called *extrinsic* or *allergic asthma,* exacerbations follow exposure to environmental factors such as dust, pollens, and danders. Often, but not always, such patients have increased concentrations of both total IgE and specific IgE against the allergen implicated. In other patients with clinically similar asthma, there is no evidence of IgE involvement; skin test results are negative and IgE concentrations low. This form of asthma, which is seen most often in the first 2 yr of life and in older adults (late-onset asthma), has been called *intrinsic.* The distinction between intrinsic and extrinsic asthma may be artificial because the basic immune mediator–induced mucosal injury is similar in both groups. Extrinsic asthma may be associated with more easily identified stimuli of mediator release than intrinsic asthma. Patients of all ages with asthma usually have elevated serum IgE levels, suggesting an allergic-extrinsic component in most patients. Although increased IgE levels may be due to atopy, chronic nonspecific stimulation of the mast cell allergen-induced late-phase immune reactions creates a prolonged nonspecific airway hyperreactivity, which can produce bronchospasm in the absence of identifiable extrinsic factors.

Viral agents are the most important infectious triggers of asthma. Early in life, respiratory syncytial virus (RSV) and parainfluenza virus are most often involved; in older children rhinoviruses have also been implicated. Influenza virus infection assumes importance with increasing age. Viral agents may act to initiate asthma through stimulation of afferent vagal receptors of the cholinergic system in the airways. An IgE response to RSV can occur in infants and children with RSV-associated wheezing but not in those whose RSV respiratory disease is without associated wheezing. Wheezing with RSV infection may unmask a predisposition to asthma.

Endocrine Factors. Asthma may worsen in relation to pregnancy and menses, especially premenstrually, or may have its onset in women at menopause. It improves in some children at puberty. Little else is known about the role of endocrine factors in the etiology or pathogenesis of asthma. Thyrotoxicosis increases the severity of asthma; the mechanism is unknown.

Psychologic Factors. Emotional factors can trigger symptoms in many asthmatic children and adults, but "deviant" emotional or behavioral characteristics are not more common among asthmatic children than among children with other chronic disabling illnesses. Conversely, the effects of severe chronic illness such as asthma on children's views of themselves, their parents' views of them, or their lives in general can be devastating. Emotional or behavioral disturbances are related more closely to poor control of asthma than to the severity of the attack itself; accordingly, skillful medical intervention can have an important impact.

CLINICAL MANIFESTATIONS. The onset of an asthma exacerbation may be acute or insidious. Acute episodes are most often caused by exposure to irritants such as cold air and noxious fumes (smoke, wet paint) or exposure to allergens or simple chemicals, for example, aspirin or sulfites. When airway obstruction develops rapidly in a few minutes, it is most likely due to smooth muscle spasm in large airways. Exacerbations precipitated by viral respiratory infections are slower in onset, with gradual increases in frequency and severity of cough and wheezing over a few days. Because airway patency decreases at night, many children have acute asthma at this time. The signs and symptoms of asthma include cough, which sounds tight and is nonproductive early in the course of an attack; wheezing, tachypnea, and dyspnea with prolonged expiration and use of accessory muscles of respiration; cyanosis; hyperinflation of the chest; and tachycardia and pulsus paradoxus, which may be present to varying degrees depending on the stage and severity of the attack. Cough may be present without wheezing, or wheezing may be present without cough; tachypnea also may be present without wheezing. Manifestations will vary depending on the severity of the exacerbation (Table 145–1).

When the patient is in extreme respiratory distress, the cardinal sign of asthma—wheezing—may be strikingly absent; in such patients, only after bronchodilator treatment gives partial relief of the airway obstruction can enough movement of air occur to evoke wheezing. Shortness of breath may be so severe that the child has difficulty walking or even talking. The patient with severe obstruction may assume a hunched-over, tripod-like sitting position that makes it easier to breathe. Expiration is typically more difficult because of premature expiratory closure of the airway, but many children complain of inspiratory difficulty as well. Abdominal pain is common, particularly in younger children, and is presumably due to the strenuous use of abdominal muscles and the diaphragm. The liver and spleen may be palpable because of hyperinflation of the lungs. Vomiting is common and may be followed by temporary relief of symptoms.

During severe airway obstruction, respiratory effort may be great, and the child may sweat profusely; a low-grade fever may develop simply from the enormous work of breathing; fatigue may become severe. Between exacerbations, the child may be entirely free of symptoms and have no evidence of pulmonary disease on physical examination. A barrel chest deformity is a sign of the chronic, unremitting airway obstruction of severe asthma. Harrison sulci, an anterolateral depression of the thorax at the insertion of the diaphragm, may be present in children with recurrent severe retractions. Clubbing of the fingers is rarely observed in uncomplicated asthma, even in severe asthma. Clubbing suggests other causes of chronic obstructive lung disease such as cystic fibrosis.

DIAGNOSIS. Recurrent episodes of coughing and wheezing, especially if aggravated or triggered by exercise, viral infection, or inhaled allergens, are highly suggestive of asthma. However, asthma can also cause persistent coughing in children with no history of wheezing because flow rates are insufficient to generate wheezing, airway obstruction is relatively mild, or caretakers are unable to recognize wheezing. Symptoms may have been ascribed erroneously to "allergic cough," "allergic bronchitis," "wheezy bronchitis," or "chronic bronchitis." Pulmonary function testing before and after administration of methacholine or a bronchodilator or before and after exercise may help establish the diagnosis of asthma. Examination during an episode of severe symptoms may also be helpful if improvement occurs following bronchodilator therapy. Furthermore, when treated by measures that are specific for asthma, affected children show remarkable improvement, strongly suggesting that the cough is a sign of asthma.

Laboratory Evaluation. *Eosinophilia* of the blood and sputum occurs with asthma. Blood eosinophilia of more than 250–400 cells/mm^3 is usual. Asthmatic sputum is grossly tenacious, rubbery, and whitish. An eosin-methylene blue stain usually discloses numerous eosinophils and the granules from disrupted cells. Few diseases in children other than asthma are likely to cause eosinophilia in sputum. Sputum cultures are generally not helpful in asthmatic children because bacterial superinfection is rare and cultures are frequently contaminated with oropharyngeal organisms. Serum protein and immunoglobulin concentrations are generally normal in asthma, except that IgE levels may be increased.

Allergy skin testing and the radioallergosorbent test or other in vitro determinations of specific IgE are useful in identifying potentially important environmental allergens (Chapter 142).

Inhalation bronchial challenge testing is only rarely done to explore the clinical significance of allergens implicated by skin testing because the allergenic challenge can provoke a late-phase asthmatic response, the procedure is time-consuming, and only a single allergen can be tested at one sitting. When the diagnosis of asthma is uncertain, testing for hyperresponsiveness to the bronchoconstrictive effect of methacholine or histamine may be helpful in children old enough to cooperate in pulmonary function testing. Methacholine provocative testing should not be performed when baseline pulmonary function is abnormal; the response to bronchodilator therapy is more appropriate.

The response of the asthmatic patient to *exercise testing* is quite characteristic (see Chapter 430.5). Running for 1–2 min often causes bronchodilation in patients with asthma, but prolonged strenuous exercise causes bronchoconstriction in virtually all asthmatic subjects when breathing dry, relatively cold air. Demonstration of this abnormal response to exercise is

TABLE 145–1 Classification of Severity of Acute Asthma Exacerbations

	Mild	Moderate	Severe	Respiratory Arrest Imminent
Symptoms				
Breathlessness	While walking	While talking (infant—softer, shorter cry; difficulty feeding)	While at rest (infant—stops feeding)	
	Can lie down	Prefers sitting	Sits upright	
Talks in	Sentences	Phrases	Words	
Alertness	May be agitated	Usually agitated	Usually agitated	Drowsy or confused
Signs				
Respiratory rate	Increased	Increased Guide to rates of breathing in awake children: **Age** — **Normal Rate** <2 month — <60/minute 2–12 months — <50/minute 1–5 years — <40/minute 6–8 years — <30/minute	Often >30/min	
Use of accessory muscles; suprasternal retractions	Usually not	Commonly	Usually	Paradoxical thoracoabdominal movement
Wheeze	Moderate, often only end expiratory	Loud; throughout exhalation	Usually loud; throughout inhalation and exhalation	Absence of wheeze
Pulse/minute	<100	100–120 Guide to normal pulse rates in children: **Age** — **Normal Rate** 2–12 months — <160/minute 1–2 years — <120/minute 2–8 years — <110/minute	>120	Bradycardia
Pulsus paradoxus	Absent <10 mg Hg	May be present 10–25 mm Hg	Often present >25 mm Hg (adult) 20–40 mm Hg (child)	Absence suggests respiratory muscle fatigue
Functional Assessment				
PEF % predicted or % personal best	80%	Approx. 50–80%	<50% predicted or personal best or response lasts <2 hr	
Pa_{O_2} (on air)	Normal (test not usually necessary)	>60 mm Hg (test not usually necessary)	<60 mm Hg: possible cyanosis	
and/or				
P_{CO_2}	<42 mm Hg (test not usually necessary)	<42 mm Hg (test not usually necessary)	≥42 mm Hg: possible respiratory failure	
Sa_{O_2} % (on air) at sea level	>95% (test not usually necessary)	91–95%	<91%	

Hypercapnia (hypoventilation) develops more readily in young children than in adults and adolescents.

NOTE:
- The presence of several parameters, but not necessarily all, indicates the general classification of the exacerbation.
- Many of these parameters have not been systematically studied, so they serve only as general guides.

From National Asthma Education and Prevention Program, National Heart, Lung, and Blood Institute, Expert Panel Report 2: Guidelines for the Diagnosis and Management of Asthma. NIH Publication No. 97–4051, July 1997.

diagnostically helpful and helps to convince patients and parents of the importance of preventive treatment. Treadmill running at 3–4 miles/hr up a 15% grade while breathing through the mouth for at least 6 min elicits airway obstruction in most patients with asthma, especially if the exercise has caused an increase in pulse rate to at least 180 beats/min. Measurement of pulmonary function immediately before exercise, immediately after exercise, and 5 and 10 min later usually discloses decreases in peak expiratory flow rate (PEFR) or forced expiratory volume in 1 sec (FEV_1) of at least 15% without premedication. If exercise causes no airway obstruction, repeat testing on other days when relative humidity is low usually elicits a positive response in patients with asthma. Exercise testing should be deferred whenever significant airway obstruction is already present. If possible, bronchodilators and cromolyn should be withheld for at least 8 hr before testing; slow-release theophylline and most leukotriene antagonists should not be administered 12–24 hr prior to testing; 36 hr for montelukast.

Every child suspected of having asthma does not require *roentgenograms of the chest*, but these are often appropriate to exclude other possible diagnoses or complications, such as atelectasis or pneumonia. Lung markings are commonly increased in asthma. Hyperinflation occurs during acute asthma and may become chronic when airway obstruction is persistent. Atelectasis may occur in as many as 6% of children during acute exacerbations and is especially likely to involve the right middle lobe, where it may persist for months. Repeated chest roentgenograms during exacerbations usually are not indicated in the absence of fever, unless there is suspicion of a pneumothorax, or there is tachypnea greater than 60 beats/min, tachycardia of more than 160 beats/min, localized rales or wheezing, or decreased breath sounds.

Pulmonary function testing (see Chapters 375 and 377) is valuable in the evaluation of children in whom asthma is suspected. In those known to have asthma, such tests are useful in assessing the degree of airway obstruction and the disturbance in gas exchange, in measuring response of the airways to inhaled allergens and chemicals or exercise (bronchial provocation testing), in assessing the response to therapeutic agents, and in evaluating the long-term course of the disease. Assessments of pulmonary function in asthma are most valuable when made before and after administration of an aerosol bronchodilator, a procedure that indicates the degree of reversibility of the airway obstruction at the time of the testing

(Chapters 142 and 375). An increase of at least 10% in PEFR or FEV_1 after aerosol therapy is strongly suggestive of asthma. Failure to respond does not exclude asthma and may be due to status asthmaticus or to nearly maximal pulmonary function.

In mild cases of asthma in remission, no abnormalities may be detected. In others, a variety of abnormalities may be found (see Table 145–1). Total lung capacity, functional residual capacity, and residual volume are increased. Vital capacity is usually decreased. Dynamic tests of air flow, forced vital capacity, FEV_1, PEFR, and maximal expiratory flow between 25 and 75% of the vital capacity ($FEF_{25-75\%}$) may also show reduced values, which return toward normal after administration of aerosolized bronchodilators. With the availability of small, relatively inexpensive instruments that measure peak expiratory flow rate (Mini-Wright Peak Flow Meter, Health Scan Assess Plus peak flow meter, Astech Peak-Flow Meter), it is feasible to monitor expiratory flow rate at home two to three times each day. This provides objective measurements of the degree of airway obstruction between office visits. A fall in peak expiratory flow predicts the onset of an exacerbation and encourages early intervention with additional drug therapy. Results can be compared with normal populations (Fig. 145–2), but it is best to establish the normal peak for each patient by determining the best of three efforts in the early afternoon daily for 2 wk when asymptomatic or after a bronchodilator inhalation when symptoms are mild. The PEFR is usually lowest on awakening in the morning and highest in the early afternoon in asthmatic patients. Measurement at these times before treatment can establish diurnal variability; increases in variability of more than 30% indicate increased bronchial responsiveness and worsening asthma with increased susceptibility to airway obstruction.

Determination of arterial blood gases and pH is important in evaluating the patient with asthma during an exacerbation requiring hospitalization. During remission, Po_2, Pco_2, and pH may be normal. In symptomatic periods, low Po_2 is regularly found and may persist days to weeks after an acute episode is over. Determination of oxygen saturation by pulse oximetry is helpful in determining the severity of an acute exacerbation. Pco_2 is generally low during the early stages of acute asthma. As the obstruction worsens, Pco_2 rises; this is an ominous sign. Blood pH remains normal (or sometimes slightly alkalotic owing to hyperventilation) until the buffering capacity of the blood is exhausted, and then acidosis develops. As airway obstruction and hypoxia become more severe, a mixed respiratory and metabolic acidosis develops owing to hypercarbia and lactic acidosis, respectively.

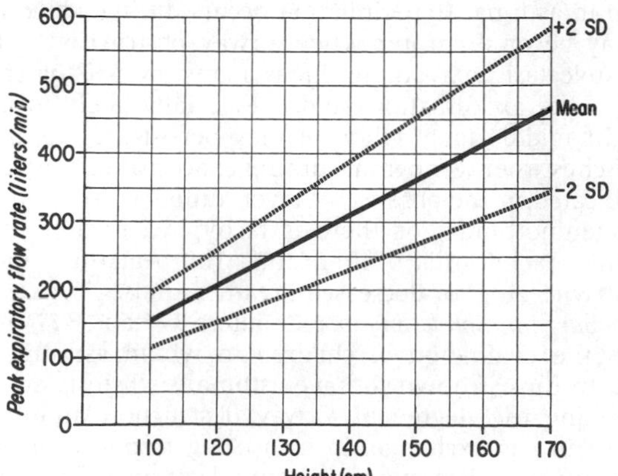

Figure 145–2 Mean peak expiratory flow rate (Wright Peak Flow Meter, adult model) as a function of height in normal boys and girls. From data collected by Polgar G and Promadhat V: Pulmonary Function Testing in Children: Techniques and Standards. Philadelphia, WB Saunders, 1971. (From Sly RM: Pediatric Allergy. New Hyde Park, NY, Medical Examination Publishing Company, 1985.)

DIFFERENTIAL DIAGNOSIS. Most children who have recurrent episodes of coughing and wheezing have asthma. Other causes of airway obstruction include congenital malformations (of the respiratory, cardiovascular, or gastrointestinal systems), foreign bodies in the airway or esophagus, infectious bronchiolitis, cystic fibrosis, immunologic deficiency diseases, hypersensitivity pneumonitis, allergic bronchopulmonary aspergillosis, and a variety of rarer conditions that compromise the airway, including endobronchial tuberculosis, fungal diseases, and bronchial adenoma (Table 145–2). Rarely in the United States, tropical eosinophilia and other parasitic infections may involve the lung and mimic asthma.

ASTHMA IN EARLY LIFE. Wheezing in the infant merits special mention because it is common and presents substantial diagnostic and therapeutic problems. A significant number of children subsequently shown to have asthma have had symptoms of obstructive airway disease early in life (30% younger than 1 yr and 50–55% younger than 2 yr).

A number of anatomic and physiologic peculiarities of early life predispose to obstructive airway disease: (1) a decreased amount of smooth muscle in the peripheral airways compared with adults may result in less support; (2) mucous gland hyperplasia in the major bronchi compared with adults favors increased intraluminal mucus production; (3) disproportionately narrow peripheral airways up to 5 yr of age result in decreased conductance relative to adults and render the infant and young child vulnerable to disease affecting the small airways; (4) decreased static elastic recoil of the young lung prediposes to early airway closure during tidal breathing and results in mismatching of ventilation and perfusion and hypoxemia; (5) highly compliant rib cage and mechanically disadvantageous angle of insertion of diaphragm to rib cage (horizontal vs. oblique in the adult) increase diaphragmatic work of breathing; (6) decreased number of fatigue-resistant skeletal muscle fibers in the diaphragm leave the diaphragm poorly equipped to maintain high work output; and (7) deficient collateral ventilation with the pores of Kohn and the Lambert canals deficient in number and size. The infant and young child are therefore predisposed to the development of atelectasis distal to obstructed airways. The combination of these factors with the normal susceptibility of infants and children to viral respiratory infections renders this age group particularly vulnerable to lower respiratory tract obstructive disease.

The clinical, roentgenographic, and blood gas findings in asthma and bronchiolitis are similar. It is helpful to remember that the incidence of bronchiolitis caused by RSV peaks during the first 6 mo of life, principally during the cold weather months, and that second and third attacks are uncommon. The onset of symptoms is rather typical. Previously well infants or young children develop what may seem to be a cold with rhinorrhea, rapidly followed by irritability, cough, tachypnea, and wheezing. The symptoms may progress rapidly and often require hospitalization.

During infancy, respiratory tract infections with viruses or *Chlamydia* may cause symptoms of airway obstruction that can be confused with asthma. Bacterial infections of the lower airway are rare, and the concept that allergic reactions to bacteria cause asthma is unproved. A child with recurrent episodes of coughing and wheezing associated with bacterial infections should be investigated for cystic fibrosis or immunologic deficiency. Chronic aspiration caused by swallowing dysfunction (usually in developmentally delayed children) or gastroesophageal reflux also may cause recurrent cough and wheezing in early life. Symptoms of respiratory distress often occur with or shortly after feeding, and a chest roentgenogram is commonly abnormal. Rarer causes of obstructive airway disease in early life include obliterative bronchiolitis (usually a sequela of a severe viral insult, most often adenovirus) and bronchopulmonary dysplasia (see Table 145–2).

The role of food allergy as a major cause of obstructive

TABLE 145–2 Differential Diagnosis of Childhood Asthma

Disease	Comment
Infections	
Bronchiolitis (RSV)	Atopic individuals may have predisposition to wheeze with RSV
Pneumonia	Acute febrile illness
Croup	Barking cough, stridor, more than wheezing
Tuberculosis, histoplasmosis	Lymphadenopathy compresses bronchi with wheezing
Bronchiectasis	Congenital, acquired, 1st- or 2nd-degree infections
Bronchiolitis obliterans	Postinfections process (influenza, adenovirus, measles)
Bronchitis	Probably asthma
Sinusitis	Cough usually worse at night; may trigger asthma
Anatomic, Congenital	
Cystic fibrosis	Persistent symptoms, clubbing, *Staphylococcus aureus, Pseudomonas aeruginosa, P. cepacia*
Vascular rings	Associated esophageal abnormalities
Ciliary dyskinesia	Chronic, recurrent infections, situs inversus
B lymphocyte immune defect	Recurrent sinopulmonary infection
Congestive heart failure	Murmur, large left-to-right shunt
Laryngotracheomalacia	Stridor, noisy respirations from birth
Tumor, lymphoma	Bronchial obstruction
H-type tracheoesophageal fistula	Rare, difficult to diagnose, recurrent aspiration pneumonia from birth
Repaired tracheoesophageal fistula	Patients have increased risk of reflux and wheezing, possibly asthma
Gastroesophageal reflux	May also exacerbate true asthma
Vasculitis, Hypersensitivity	
Allergic bronchopulmonary aspergillosis	Marked eosinophilia, high serum IgE levels; sputum positive for aspergillosis
Allergic alveolitis, hypersensitivity pneumonitis	Reaction to foreign antigen (fungi, bird protein, plants); occupational
Churg-Strauss syndrome	Allergic angitis and granulomatosis, eosinophilia
Periarteritis nodosa	Multisystem (kidney, lung, nerves), eosinophilia
Other	
Foreign body aspiration	Sudden cough, gagging, *localized* wheezing and diminished breath sounds
Pulmonary thromboembolism	Acute chest pain, hypoxia
Psychogenic cough	Absent during sleep
Sarcoidosis	Lymphadenopathy-induced bronchial obstruction
Bronchopulmonary dysplasia	History of prematurity, may predispose to asthma
Vocal cord dysfunction	Recurrent, severe shortness of breath and wheezing; flow-volume loop shows inspiratory obstruction; may mimic or complicate asthma; visualization of vocal cords necessary for diagnosis; oxygen saturation and spirometry normal during exacerbations.

RSV = respiratory syncytial virus; IgE = immunoglobulin E.

airway symptoms during early life is controversial. Positive skin test results for IgE-mediated sensitivity to foods are unusual in asthmatic infants, but when present, they indicate the need for temporary elimination of the suspected food, usually milk, wheat, or egg from the diet of the asthmatic patient. After elimination from the diet for 3 wk, challenge with the implicated food may be appropriate to confirm the clinical relevance of the positive skin test result. Challenge may be necessary two or three times after temporary dietary elimination to ensure clinical relevance. Challenge is contraindicated in patients with a history of anaphylaxis after ingestion of the food. Confirmed food allergy indicates a need for dietary elimination for at least 6 mo (see Chapters 143 and 153).

For an infant who has had several episodes of obstructive airway disease, a history of asthma, hay fever, or atopic dermatitis in mother, father, or siblings is an important predictor of subsequent obstructive airway problems. Eczema is also frequently associated with the subsequent appearance of asthma. Eosinophilia greater than 400 cells/mm³ (and especially greater than 700 cells/mm³) and high serum IgE concentrations predict continuing respiratory tract problems.

TREATMENT. Asthma therapy includes basic concepts of avoiding allergens, improving bronchodilation, and reducing mediator-induced inflammation. Systemic or topical inhaled medications are used, depending on the severity of the episode. The principles of avoidance of allergens outlined under treatment of allergic rhinitis also serve the child with asthma. The hyperreactivity of the asthmatic airway as an additional factor is dealt with by minimizing exposure to nonspecific irritants such as tobacco smoke, smoke from wood-burning stoves, and fumes from kerosene heaters and to strong odors such as wet paint and disinfectants, and by avoiding ice-cold drinks and rapid changes in temperature and humidity. Maintenance of humidified air is important in dry, cold climates in the winter, but relative humidity should not exceed 50% because house dust mites thrive at higher humidity. If the clinical history suggests IgE-mediated sensitivity to inhalant allergens that cannot be avoided or can be only partially avoided, immunotherapy should be considered; its indications and evidence for its efficacy in asthma are discussed in Chapter 143.

Treatment of acute asthma based on severity and location (home, emergency department, in hospital) is summarized in Figures 145–3 and 145–4.

Pharmacologic therapy is the mainstay of treatment of asthma. Oxygen administered by mask or nasal prongs at 2–3 L/min is indicated in most children during acute asthma. Not only is the Po_2 reduced during an acute episode but also drugs used in therapy (β-adrenergic agonists or intravenous aminophylline) may cause a transient fall in Po_2 secondary to worsening of ventilation-perfusion mismatching, which occurs because these agents cause pulmonary vasodilation and increased cardiac output. Injection of epinephrine was the treatment of choice for acute asthma for many years, but bronchodilator aerosols are now preferable.

When epinephrine is used, a dose of 0.01 mL/kg of the 1:1,000 (1.0 mg/mL) concentration of the aqueous preparation may be given. It may be necessary to repeat the same dose once or twice at intervals of 20 min to obtain optimal relief. In infants and small children, a dose of 0.05 mL is often effective. The unpleasant side effects of epinephrine (pallor, tremor, anxiety, palpitations, and headache) can frequently be minimized if doses of no more than 0.3 mL are given at any age. Terbutaline, a more selective β_2-agonist (see Chapter 143), is available in an injectable form and is an alternative to epinephrine. The usual dose of 0.01 mL/kg of the 1:1,000 (1 mg/mL) concentration does not cause peripheral vasoconstric-

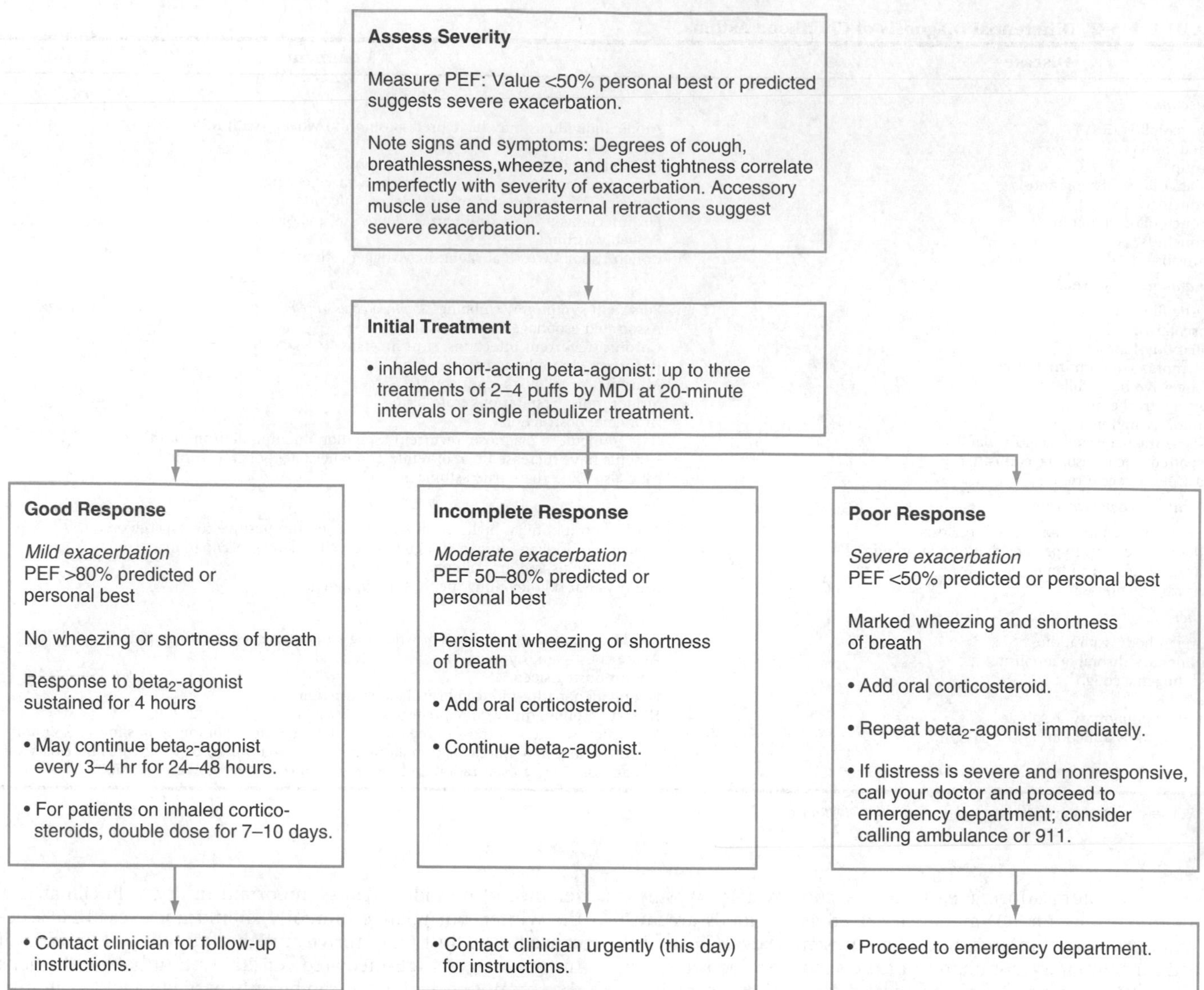

Figure 145–3 Home management of acute asthma. PEF, peak expiratory flow rate; MDI, metered dose inhaler. (Modified from National Asthma Education and Prevention Program, National Heart, Lung, and Blood Institute, Expert Panel Report 2: Guidelines for the Diagnosis and Management of Asthma. NIH Publication No. 97-4051, July 1997.)

tion and has a longer duration of activity, up to 4 hr. The maximal dose of terbutaline by subcutaneous injection is 0.25 mL; this dose may be repeated once, if necessary, after 20 min.

Inhalation of bronchodilator aerosols is rapidly effective in relieving the signs and symptoms of asthma. Aerosols have the advantage that substantially less drug is given than would be required by the subcutaneous route; and the unpleasant side effects of injected drugs such as epinephrine are avoided. Furthermore, despite airway obstruction, which may limit aerosol delivery to peripheral airways, aerosol therapy is probably more effective than epinephrine in reversing bronchoconstriction. Albuterol (Proventil, Ventolin) solution is safe and effective at a dose of 0.15 mg/kg (maximum 5 mg) followed by 0.05–0.15 mg/kg at intervals of 20–30 min until response is adequate. Albuterol is available as a 0.5% solution (5 mg/mL) to be diluted with 2–3 mL normal saline and as a prediluted 2.5-mg unit dose, 0.083% (0.83 mg/mL). Nebulization with oxygen at 6 L/min prevents hypoxemia that might be related to the treatment. Edetate disodium and benzalkonium chloride, found in some solutions of albuterol and metaproterenol for nebulization, can cause bronchoconstriction in occasional asthmatic patients; Ventolin Nebules and levalbuterol contain neither.

Delivery of inhaled albuterol by metered-dose inhaler, 3 to 10 puffs per dose, with a spacer such as Aerochamber, can be as effective as delivery by nebulizer, although nebulization is more effective for patients unable to coordinate inhalation sufficiently with actuation of the inhaler. Treatment with doses of 6 to 10 puffs has been evaluated only with delivery of all the drug into the spacer before inhalation, although more medication reaches the patient with inhalation from the spacer immediately after delivery of each puff, a method found effective for the dose of three puffs.

If response to the β_2-agonist is not adequate, treatment with both a β_2-agonist and nebulized ipratropium bromide, 250–500 μg, may be more effective. Both can be administered safely at intervals of 20 min for three doses and subsequently at intervals of 2 to 4 hr if necessary for children 6 yr of age or older.

Theophylline does not provide additional benefit for patients receiving optimal treatment with an inhaled β_2-agonist but should be considered for patients who have been receiving maintenance treatment with theophylline and for those unable to tolerate maximal treatment with inhaled β_2-agonists. If indicated, aminophylline may be given intravenously in a dose of 5 mg/kg for 5–15 min at a rate no greater than 25 mg/min. This dose (which will increase the serum theophylline

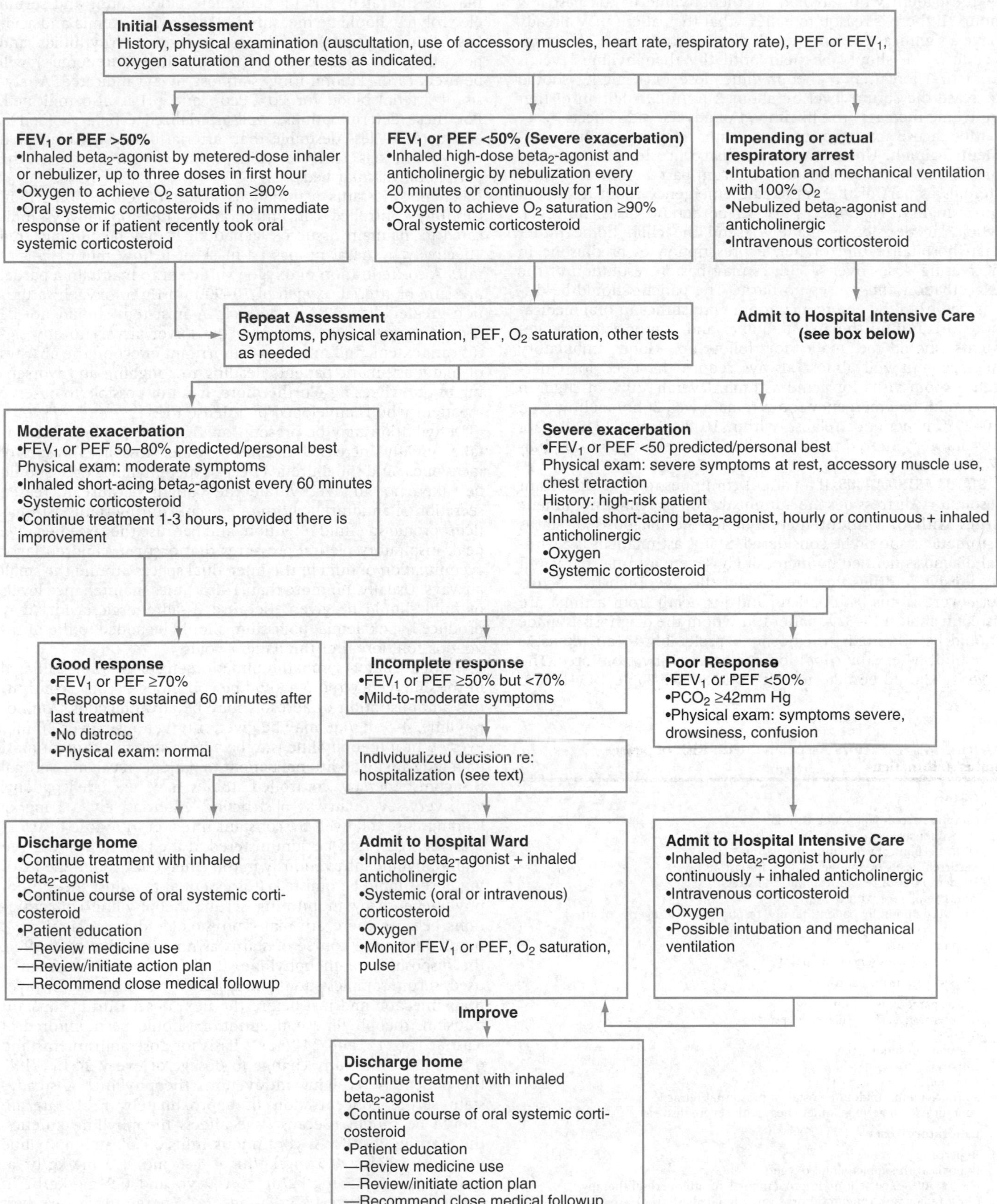

Figure 145–4 Emergency department and hospital-based care of acute asthma. (From National Asthma Education and Prevention Program, National Heart, Lung, and Blood Institute, Expert Panel Report 2: Guidelines for the Diagnosis and Management of Asthma. NIH Publication No. 97-4051, July 1997.)

concentration by no more than 10 μg/mL at the peak) is safe in the patient who has had no theophylline in the past few hours. If there is reason to believe that the patient may already have a significant serum theophylline concentration, the intravenous dose should be held until the theophylline level is known. Thereafter, a theophylline dose of 1 mg/kg should increase the serum level by about 2 μg/mL. Addition of theophylline increases the likelihood of adverse side effects.

Most acute exacerbations of asthma respond to this treatment regimen. Unless the patient is corticosteroid-dependent or has had corticosteroids in the recent past, administration of steroids as part of the immediate emergency room treatment program may be unnecessary. In borderline cases, however, when the decision is made to send the child home rather than hospitalize him or her, a prescription of prednisone in decreasing doses over 5–7 days may hasten resolution of the exacerbation and causes no harm. The patient should be discharged from the emergency room with sufficient oral medication to continue therapy at home, and appropriate arrangements should be made for follow-up. Good ambulatory management will almost always reduce the need for emergency room visits for acute asthma. Overall, 70% of children treated in the emergency room remain well at home; however, 10–20% experience relapse within 10 days, and 15–20% are hospitalized. Steroid therapy reduces the relapse and hospitalization rates.

STATUS ASTHMATICUS. If a patient continues to have significant respiratory distress despite administration of sympathomimetic drugs with or without theophylline, the diagnosis of status asthmaticus should be considered. Status asthmaticus is a clinical diagnosis defined by increasingly severe asthma that is not responsive to drugs that are usually effective. High-risk factors for severe status asthmaticus and for death from asthma are listed in Table 145–3. A patient in whom the diagnosis is made should be admitted to a hospital, preferably to an intensive care unit, where the condition can be carefully monitored. The severity should be determined initially (see Table 145–1) and monitored at regular intervals. An indwelling arterial catheter may be indicated. Baseline complete blood count and serum electrolytes should be measured. Because hypoxemia and acid-base disturbances may predispose to cardiac arrhythmias, and potentially cardiotoxic drugs (theophylline, adrenergics) will be used, cardiac monitoring is almost always indicated. Analysis of arterial blood for Po_2, Pco_2, and pH is also indicated. For these determinations, well-arterialized capillary blood is adequate but less desirable than arterial blood, particularly if the patient has received epinephrine, which constricts the peripheral vascular bed.

TABLE 145–3 Factors Associated with Risk of Severe Status Asthmaticus

History
Chronic steroid-dependent asthma
Prior intensive care admission
Prior mechanical ventilation for asthma
Recurrent visits to emergency unit in past 48 hr
Sudden onset of severe respiratory distress
Poor compliance with therapy
Poor recognition by patient, family, or physician, of severity of attack
Family dysfunction, crisis
Respiratory arrest
Hypoxic seizures, encephalopathy
Physical Examination
Pulsus paradoxus >20 mm Hg
Hypotension, tachycardia, tachypnea
Cyanosis
1–2 word dyspnea
Lethargy
Agitation
Sternocleidomastoid, intercostal, suprasternal retractions
Poor air exchange (e.g., quiet chest with severe distress)
Laboratory Tests
Hypercarbia
Hypoxia with supplemental oxygen
FEV_1 <30% expected; no improvement 1 hr after aerosol therapy
Chest radiograph (pneumothorax, pneumomediastinum)
Therapy
Overreliance on aerosol, inhalter therapy
Delayed use of systemic corticosteroids
Sedation
Delayed admission to hospital or intensive care unit

FEV_1 = forced expiratory volume in 1 sec.

Patients in status asthmaticus are hypoxemic. Oxygen in carefully controlled concentrations is therefore always indicated to maintain tissue oxygenation. It may be administered effectively by nasal prongs or mask at a flow rate of 2–3 L/min. A concentration of oxygen sufficient to maintain a partial pressure of arterial oxygen of 70–90 mm Hg or oxygen saturation greater than 92% is optimal. A mist tent should not be used; the water does not reach the lower airway to any significant extent, and mists have an irritant effect on the airways of many asthmatic patients, leading to coughing and worsening of the wheezing. Furthermore, it is not possible to observe a patient who is enveloped in a dense fog.

Dehydration may be present, owing to inadequate fluid intake, greatly increased insensible water loss as a result of tachypnea, and the diuretic effect of theophylline. Care should be taken not to overhydrate the patient because increased secretion of antidiuretic hormone occurs during status asthmaticus, promoting fluid retention, and because the large negative peak-inspiratory pleural pressures that occur in children favor accumulation of fluid in the interstitial spaces around the small airways. Usually, no more than 1–1.5 times maintenance levels of fluid should be given. Because β_2-adrenergic agents may produce hypokalemia, potassium should be added to the intravenous solution after the patient voids.

Bronchodilator sympathomimetic aerosol therapy initiated in the emergency room should be continued because continuous administration of aerosols may be advantageous. Aminophylline, 4–5 mg/kg, may be given intravenously over 20 min every 6 hr if theophylline is to be administered; although most data indicate no additional benefit to patients receiving optimal β_2-agonist therapy, controlled studies have excluded patients with very severe airway obstruction. Alternatively, a 5 mg/kg loading dose followed by constant infusion in a dose of 0.75–1.25 mg/kg/hr may be administered. If the patient has received aminophylline intravenously in the emergency room, the loading dose should be omitted. It is essential to adjust the aminophylline dose by monitoring serum theophylline concentrations because there are many physiologic derangements that occur during the course of status asthmaticus that may affect the disposition of theophylline. If the every 6-hr regimen is used, serum samples should be obtained 1 hr after the intravenous injection and just before the next dose. During constant infusion, theophylline concentration should be monitored at least at 1, 6, 12, and 24 hr as a basis for dose adjustments and 6 and 12 hr after any change in dosage or every 24 hr while the patient is receiving intravenous theophylline. A steady-state serum concentration of approximately 12–15 μg/mL should be sought. Because age affects theophylline kinetics, the starting dose for a continuous infusion of aminophylline varies as follows: 0.5 mg/kg/hr at 1–6 mo, 1.0 mg/kg/hr at 6–11 mo, 1.2–1.5 mg/kg/hr at 1–9 yr, and 0.9 mg/kg/hr in children older than 10 yr of age. Adrenergic drugs are best administered by aerosol as previously described. Administration of β-agonists by inhalation at intervals of 20 min or continually is safer than administration by intravenous infusion and is probably equally effective. Nonetheless, some authorities recommend terbutaline by subcutaneous (0.01 mg/kg; 0.3 mg maximum) or intravenous (10 μg/kg bolus; 0.4–0.6

μg/kg/min continuous infusion increasing by 0.2 μg/kg/min to 3–6 μg/kg/min) administration for severe status asthmaticus.

Treatment with nebulized ipratropium bromide given in combination with a nebulized β-agonist can be more effective than treatment with either alone, although the peak bronchodilation from ipratropium may be reached more slowly than that of the β-agonist. Nebulization of ipratropium bromide at doses of 250–500 μg at intervals of 20 min for three doses followed by administration at intervals of 2–4 hr is safe and effective for children at least 6 yr of age.

Corticosteroids, such as methylprednisolone (Solu-Medrol), 1 mg/kg every 6 hr should be administered for the first 48 hr followed by 1–2 mg/kg/24 hr (maximum 60 mg/24 hr for a child, 60–80 mg for an adult) in two divided doses until the PEFR is 70% of the personal best or predicted. Because it has less effect on mineral metabolism when given in high doses and a lower cost for an equivalent anti-inflammatory dose, methylprednisolone is preferable to hydrocortisone. Corticosteroids can sometimes reverse tolerance to β-agonists within 1 hr, but maximal effects of steroids are usually delayed for 6 hr. Steroids improve oxygenation, decrease airway obstruction, and shorten the time needed for recovery.

Treatment is guided by serial measurement of blood gases and pH every few hours, or more often if indicated. If gas and pH analysis both indicate that respiratory failure is impending, an anesthesiologist should be alerted, and facilities and equipment should be available for tracheal intubation and respiratory support.

Mechanical ventilation should be anticipated; elective tracheal intubation with diazepam (Valium), vecuronium, and atropine premedication is safer than emergency intubation. Respiratory care should include patient paralysis on a volume-cycled ventilator with short inspiratory and long expiratory times, a 10- to 15-mL/kg tidal volume, 8–15 breaths/min, and peak pressures of less than 60 cm H_2O. The goals are to improve oxygenation, maintain P_{CO_2} between 40 and 60 mm Hg, and avoid barotrauma. Positive end-expiratory pressure is added in the recovery phase to prevent atelectasis. Mild or moderate hypercapnia with treatment of associated respiratory acidosis with intravenous sodium bicarbonate is preferable to minimize lung injury from high ventilatory pressures. Sedation during mechanical ventilation may be accomplished with diazepam, midazolam (Versed), or ketamine (which at doses of 1–2.5 mg/kg/hr is a sedative-analgesic-anesthetic with bronchodilator activity). Halothane anesthesia produces prompt bronchodilation but is difficult to administer in an intensive care unit. It should be reserved for the most severe cases of status asthmaticus.

Breathing heliox, an 80:20 blend of helium to oxygen, to reduce airway resistance may reduce pulsus paradoxus in severe asthma, with improvement of PEFR, and may avert the need for intubation and mechanical ventilation. Intravenous administration of magnesium sulfate has not been found effective in most studies, although it may be helpful in rare patients; infusion of 25 mg/kg, maximum 2 g, over 20 min has elicited improvement in pulmonary function in some children at least 6 yr of age with moderate to severe acute asthma.

Sedation of nonventilated patients with status asthmaticus is hazardous. Tranquilizers, morphine, and other opiates are also contraindicated because of their depressant effects on the respiratory center. The best sedative for the patient is the presence of a competent, compassionate physician and nurse at the bedside and decreased airway obstruction with relief of hypoxia and hypercarbia. Chest roentgenograms should be obtained in all severe cases and repeated as indicated to detect complications such as mediastinal emphysema or pneumothorax. Routine administration of antibiotics has not been shown to alter the course of status asthmaticus in children or to reduce the incidence of infectious complications.

DAILY MANAGEMENT OF THE ASTHMATIC CHILD. On the basis of the history, physical examination, laboratory data, pulmonary function testing, and need for medication, patients may be classified as having mild intermittent, mild persistent, moderate persistent, or severe persistent asthma (Table 145–4). Classification is convenient for describing a stepwise approach to therapy (see Chapter 143 and Figs. 145–3 and 145–4).

Mild Intermittent Asthma. Children with mild intermittent asthma have exacerbations of varying frequency, up to twice each week, with decreases in PEFR of not more than 20%; they respond to bronchodilator treatment within 24–48 hr. Gener-

TABLE 145–4 Classification of Asthma Severity

Clinical Features Before Treatment*	Symptoms†	Nighttime Symptoms	Lung Function
Step 4			
Severe Persistent	Continual symptoms Limited physical activity Frequent exacerbations	Frequent	■ FEV_1 or PEFR ≤60% predicted ■ PEFR variability >30%
Step 3			
Moderate Persistent	Daily symptoms Daily use of inhaled short-acting β_2-Agonist Exacerbations affect activity Exacerbations ≥2 times a week; may last days	>1 time a week	■ FEV_1 or PEFR >60%–<80% predicted ■ PEFR variability >30%
Step 2			
Mild Persistent	Symptoms >2 times a week but <1 time a day Exacerbations may affect activity	>2 times a month	■ FEV_1 or PEFR ≥80% predicted ■ PEFR variability 20–30%
Step 1			
Mild Intermittent	Symptoms ≤2 times a week Asymptomatic and normal PEFR between exacerbations Exacerbations brief (from a few hours to a few days); intensity may vary	≤2 times a month	■ FEV_1 or PEFR ≥80% predicted ■ PEFR variability <20%

**The presence of one of the features of severity is sufficient to place a patient in that category. An individual should be assigned to the most severe grade in which any feature occurs. The characteristics noted in this figure are general and may overlap because asthma is highly variable. Furthermore, an individual's classification may change over time.*

†Patients at any level of severity can have mild, moderate, or severe exacerbations. Some patients with intermittent asthma experience severe and life-threatening exacerbations separated by long periods of normal lung function and no symptoms.

PEFR = peak expiratory flow rate.

Modified from National Asthma Education and Prevention Program, National Heart, Lung, and Blood Institute, Expert Panel Report 2: Guidelines for the Diagnosis and Management of Asthma. Washington, DC, NIH Publication No. 97-4051, July, 1997.

ally, medication is not required between exacerbations for mild asthma with symptoms less than every 2 wk, when the child is essentially free of symptoms of airway obstruction. Children with mild asthma have good school attendance, good exercise tolerance, and little or no interruption of sleep by asthma. They have no hyperinflation of the chest; their chest roentgenograms are essentially normal. Pulmonary function testing may show mild, reversible airway obstruction, with little or no increase in lung volume (Table 145–4).

Whatever the severity or frequency of the asthma, a partnership with the patient and parents should be established. They should learn about asthma and its causes and prevention. They should know the purposes and side effects of medications and how to use inhalers and holding chambers or spacers. Written daily management plans can be helpful; written action plans based on symptoms and PEFRs to guide treatment of acute asthma can be lifesaving. Action plans should include telephone numbers of physicians and emergency departments, sources of rapid transportation to emergency care, and others who can provide emergency assistance (Fig. 145–5).

General guidelines to the stepwise approach to management appear in Figures 145–6 and 145–7.

Mild Persistent Asthma. Symptoms more than twice each week but less often than daily indicate mild persistent asthma. Nocturnal symptoms may occur more than twice each month. The PEFR or FEV_1 is at least 80% predicted. Daily variations in PEFR may be as great as 30% (see Table 145–4). These patients usually require daily anti-inflammatory therapy, usually cromolyn or nedocromil, although inhaled corticosteroids may be more effective. Sustained release theophylline is a less expensive alternative. A leukotriene antagonist (montelukast, zafirlukast) is another oral alternative, depending on the age of the patient (see Figs. 145–6 and 145–7).

Moderate Persistent Asthma. Children with moderate persistent asthma have symptoms more frequently than those with mild disease and often have cough and mild wheezing between more severe exacerbations. School attendance may be impaired, exercise tolerance will be diminished because of coughing and wheezing, and the child may lose sleep at night, particularly during exacerbations. Such children will generally require continuous treatment with cromolyn, nedocromil, or an inhaled corticosteroid to achieve satisfactory control of symptoms. Hyperinflation may be evident clinically and roentgenographically. The FEV_1 or PEFR may be between 60 and 80% of predicted normal, and the daily PEFR variability may exceed 30%.

Severe Persistent Asthma. Children with severe persistent asthma have virtually daily wheezing and more frequent and more severe exacerbations; they require recurrent hospitalization, which is rarely required for mild or moderate asthma. Severely affected children may miss significant amounts of school, have their sleep interrupted often by asthma, and have poor exercise tolerance. They may have increased anteroposterior diameter of the chest as a result of chronic hyperinflation, evident on roentgenograms. Anti-inflammatory medication will be required continuously, and regimens should include regularly inhaled corticosteroids and may include systemic corticosteroids. Pulmonary function testing will show more severe airway obstruction than in mild or moderate asthma with FEV_1 or PEFR less than 60% of predicted normal and less reversibility in response to inhaled bronchodilator.

Guide to Management of Asthma for ____________________

____

Regular medicines: ____________________

____

____

____

____

Before exercise: ____________________

For mild coughing, wheezing, shortness of breath, tightness of chest,

Peak expiratory flow rate (PEFR) reduced by 10 to 30%:

Get away from possible cause (smoke, dust, animal, pollen).

Inhale bronchodilator (____________________) every 4 hours.

For more severe symptoms,

PFR reduced by 30 to 50%:

Inhale bronchodilator (____________________) every 20 minutes for 1 hour if necessary.

If unimproved, continue bronchodilator (____________________) every 2 hours, double your dose of inhaled corticosteroid (____________________), contact physician, and start oral prednisone (____________________).

For very severe symptoms, struggling to breathe, blue or gray lips or fingernails, difficulty walking or talking, chest and neck sucked in with each breath,

PFR reduced by 50% or more:

Inhale bronchodilator (____________________) every 20 minutes and go immediately to physician or emergency room.

Telephone Numbers: Dr. XXX (____________________)

Dr. YYY (____________________)

Emergency Room (____________________)

Emergency Transportation (____________________)

Figure 145–5 Personalized crisis plan for management of asthma. Indications for intervention can be individualized based upon the patient's usual PEFR variability.

TREATMENT OF ACUTE ASTHMA. Figures 145–3 and 145–4 summarize treatment of acute asthma. Children with mild asthma should receive bronchodilator medication only when symptomatic, and most exacerbations may be satisfactorily treated with adrenergic agents, preferably by aerosol (albuterol, levalbuterol, metaproterenol, terbutaline, pirbuterol, or bitolterol) or, rarely, by injection (aqueous epinephrine, terbutaline). Levalbuterol, the first single-isomeric β-adrenergic agonist, has less effect than albuterol on heart rate and serum potassium. Use of a chamber such as an AeroChamber or InspirEase enhances delivery of drug to the lower airways when a metered-dose inhaler is used by younger children who are unable to coordinate actuation of the inhaler with inhalation. Such chambers permit effective administration of β-agonists from metered-dose inhalers to children as young as 3 yr of age. Slow inhalation also increases delivery to the lungs because a rapid inhalation causes impaction of drug particles in the pharynx. Breath holding for up to 10 sec after inhalation of the drug also favors deposition in the lungs. When moderate or severe airway obstruction is present, nebulization with an air compressor such as the Proneb with PARI-LC jet or the DeVilbiss No. 561 Pulmo-Aide is often more effective than use of a metered-dose inhaler with a chamber. The apparent advantage of nebulization over metered-dose inhaler is largely due to the different doses administered. Nebulization with such a compressor permits effective delivery of aerosols even to infants. The Aerochamber with Mask may permit delivery of medication from metered-dose inhalers to young children and infants. β-Agonist liquids for oral administration are also available for treatment of infants and young children. Theophylline may be added to an oral regimen when indicated. Drug therapy usually can be discontinued after a few days.

EXERCISE-INDUCED ASTHMA. Exercise-induced asthma is most effectively prevented by inhalation of a β_2-agonist immediately

Preferred treatments are in bold print.

	Long-Term Control	Quick Relief	Education
STEP 4 Severe Persistent	Daily medication: • **Anti-inflammatory: inhaled corticosteroid (high dose)** AND • Long-acting bronchodilator: either **long-acting inhaled beta$_2$-agonist**, sustained-release theophylline, or long-acting beta$_2$-agonist tablets AND • Corticosteroid tablets or syrup long term (make repeat attempts to reduce systemic steroids and maintain control with high dose inhaled steroids)	• Short-acting bronchodilator: **inhaled beta$_2$-agonists** as needed for symptoms. • Intensity of treatment will depend on severity of exacerbation; see Figs. 145-3 and 145-4. • Use of short-acting inhaled beta$_2$-agonists on a daily basis, or increasing use, indicates the need for additional long-term-control therapy.	Steps 2 and 3 actions plus: • Refer to individual education/counseling
STEP 3 Moderate Persistent	Daily medication: • Either **Anti-inflammatory: inhaled corticosteroid (medium dose)** OR Inhaled corticosteroid (low-medium dose) and add a long-acting bronchodilator, especially for nighttime symptoms; either **long-acting inhaled beta$_2$-agonist,** sustained-release thephylline, or long-acting beta$_2$-agonist tablets. • If needed Anti-inflammatory: **inhaled corticosteroids (medium-high dose)** AND **Long-acting bronchodilator,** especially for nighttime symptoms; either **long-acting inhaled beta$_2$-agonist,** sustained release theophylline, or long-acting beta$_2$-agonist tablets.	• Short-acting bronchodilator: **inhaled beta$_2$-agonists** as needed for symptoms. • Intensity of treatment will depend on severity of exacerbation; see Figs. 145-3 and 145-4. • Use of short-acting inhaled beta$_2$-agonists on a daily basis, or increasing use, indicates the need for additional long-term-control therapy.	Step 1 actions plus: • Teach self-monitoring • Refer to group education if available • Review and update self-management plan
STEP 2 Mild Persistent	One daily medication: • Anti-inflammatory: either **inhaled corticosteroid** (low doses) or **cromolyn or nedocromil** (children usually begin with a trial of cromolyn or nedocromil). • Sustained-release theophylline to serum concentration of 5–15 μg/mL is an alternative, but not preferred, therapy. Zafirlukast or zileuton may also be considered for patients ≥12 years of age, montelukast for patients ≥6 yr of age, although their position in therapy is not fully established.	• Short-acting bronchodilator: **inhaled beta$_2$-agonists** as needed for symptoms. • Intensity of treatment will depend on severity of exacerbation: see Figs. 145-3 and 145-4. • Use of short-acting inhaled beta$_2$-agonists on a daily basis, or increasing use, indicates the need for additional long-term-control therapy.	Step 1 actions plus: • Teach self-monitoring • Refer to group education if available • Review and update self-management plan

Figure 145–6 *See legend on following page*

STEP 1 Mild Intermittent	• No daily medication needed.	• Short-acting bronchodilator: **inhaled beta$_2$-agonists** as needed for symptoms. • Intensity of treatment will depend on severity of exacerbation; see Figs. 145–3 and 145–4. • Use of short-acting inhaled beta$_2$-agonists more than 2 times a week may indicate the need to initiate long-term-control therapy.	• Teach basic facts about asthma • Teach inhaler/spacer/holding chamber technique • Discuss roles of medications • Develop self-managment plan • Develop action plan for when and how to take rescue actions, especially for patients with a history of severe exacerbations • Discuss appropriate environmental control measures to avoid exposure to known allergens and irritants

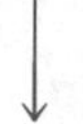

Step down
Review treatment every 1 to 6 months; a gradual stepwise reduction in treatment may be possible.

Step up
If control is not maintained, consider step up. First, review patient medication technique, adherence, and environmental control (avoidance of allergens or other factors that contribute to asthma severity).

Note:

- **The stepwise approach presents general guidelines to assist clinical decision making; it is not intended to be a specific prescription. Asthma is highly variable; clinicians should tailor specific medication plans to the needs and circumstances of individual patients.**
- Gain control as quickly as possible; then decrease treatment to the least medication necessary to maintain control. Gaining control may be accomplished by either starting treatment at the step most appropriate to the initial severity of the condition or starting at a higher level of therapy (e.g., a course of systemic corticosteroids or higher dose of inhaled corticosteroids).
- A rescue course of systemic corticosteroids may be needed at any time and at any step.
- Some patients with intermittent asthma experience severe and life-threatening exacerbations separated by long periods of normal lung function and no symptoms. This may be especially common with exacerbations provoked by respiratory infections. A short course of systemic corticosteroids is recommended.
- At each step, patients should control their enviroment to avoid or control factors that make their asthma worse (e.g., allergens, irritants); this requires specific diagnosis and education.
- Referral to an asthma specialist for consultation or comanagement is *recommended* if there are difficulties achieving or maintaining control of asthma or if the patient requires step 4 care. Referral may be *considered* if the patient requires step 3 care.

Figure 145–6 Stepwise approach to the management of asthma in adults and children more than 5 yr of age. (Modified from National Asthma Education and Prevention Program, National Heart, Lung, and Blood Institute, Expert Panel Report 2: Guidelines for the Diagnosis and Management of Asthma. NIH Publication No. 97-4051, July 1997.)

before exercise. Use of a muffler or cold weather mask to warm and humidify air before inhalation also is effective. Inhaled albuterol usually affords protection for 4 hr; inhaled salmeterol (not labeled for patients younger than 12 yr by the U.S. Food and Drug Administration [FDA]), for 12 hr. Duration and extent of protection by salmeterol may become less after patients have received it continuously for 1 wk even if used only once each day. Salmeterol should be administered at least 30 min before exercise. Inhalation of cromolyn or nedocromil shortly before exercise is also effective in preventing exercise-induced asthma but is usually most effective only for the first hour. Oral leukotriene antagonists also inhibit exercise-induced asthma, for example, montelukast for up to 24 hr with no loss of protective effect after daily treatment for as long as 12 wk. Theophylline also is effective but would require either an unusually large dose or continual administration to maintain adequate serum concentrations. When treatment with a single drug is inadequate, a combination of two or three is more effective.

THEOPHYLLINE. For children with persistent asthma, theophylline can be a less expensive alternative to cromolyn, nedocromil, low-dose inhaled corticosteroid, or a long-acting inhaled β-agonist. It can be especially helpful for control of nocturnal asthma. Sustained-release theophylline twice each day can be nearly as effective as inhaled beclomethasone dipropionate, 84 μg 4 times/day for control of mild to moderate asthma. Addition of sustained-release theophylline to low-dose inhaled corticosteroid can be as effective and less expensive than treatment with high-dose inhaled corticosteroid (see Table 143–3 for inhaled corticosteroid dosage classification). Dose and dosing regimen should be individualized. Some experienced allergists reserve monitoring of serum theophylline concentrations for those patients who fail to show a favorable bronchodilator response or who have symptoms of toxicity (gastrointestinal or central nervous system) with average dosages. When sustained-release formulations of theophylline such as Slo-bid Gyrocaps or Theo-Dur tablets are used, the peak plasma concentration (assuming that a constant fraction of drug is absorbed, which may not be the case) occurs 4–8 hr after the dose, at which time a blood sample for monitoring should be obtained. Peak concentration may not occur until 12 hr after a bedtime dose of an sustained-release preparation because of delayed nocturnal absorption. Blood sampling should be delayed until after a day or so of therapy with sustained-release drugs to ensure that a steady state has been achieved. Some children can be treated successfully on an every 12-hr schedule, but others metabolize theophylline particularly rapidly and experience marked fluctuations in serum concentration. These peaks and troughs of concentration are minimized by dividing the 24-hr dose into equal 8-hr doses.

Younger children (aged 1–9 yr) generally eliminate theophylline more rapidly than do older children and adolescents and hence require a higher daily dose on a milligram/kilogram basis. Nonetheless, it is safest to begin with a dose of 10 mg/kg/24 hr in most children. If this dose is well tolerated, one may increase by 25% increments at 3- to 4-day intervals to average doses for age as necessary to control symptoms (see Table 143–2). If adequate control of symptoms is not achieved

	Long-term control	Quick Relief
STEP 4 Severe Persistent	• Daily anti-inflammatory medicine —High-dose inhaled corticosteroid with spacer/holding chamber and face mask —If needed, add systemic corticosteroids 2 mg/kg/day and reduce to lowest daily or alternate-day dose that stabilizes symptoms	• Bronchodilator as needed for symptoms (see step 1) up to 3 times a day
STEP 3 Moderate Persistent	• Daily anti-inflammatory medication. Either: —Medium-dose inhaled corticosteroid with spacer/holding chamber and face mask OR, once control is established: —Medium-dose inhaled corticosteroid and nedocromil OR —Medium-dose inhaled corticosteroid and long-acting bronchodilator (theophylline)	• Bronchodilator as needed for symptoms (see step 1) up to 3 times a day
STEP 2 Mild Persistent	• Daily anti-inflammatory medication. Either: —Cromolyn (nebulizer is preferred; or MDI) or nedoromil (MDI only) —Infants and young children usually begin with a trial of cromolyn or nedocromil OR —Low-dose inhaled corticosteroid with spacer/holding chamber and face mask	• Bronchodilator as needed for symptoms (see step 1)
STEP 1 Mild Intermittent	• No daily medication needed.	• Bronchodilator as needed for symptoms $\leq$2 times a week. Intensity of treatment will depend upon severity of exacerbation. Either: —Inhaled short-acting beta$_2$-agonist by nebulizer or face mask and spacer/holding chamber OR —Oral beta$_2$-agonist for symptoms • With viral respiratory infection —Bronchodilator q 4–6 hours up to 24 hours (longer with physician consult) but, in general, repeat no more than once every 6 weeks —Consider systemic corticosteroid if • Current exacerbation is severe OR • Patient has history of previous severe exacerbations

↓ **Step down**
Review treatment every 1 to 6 months. If control is sustained for at least 3 months, a gradual stepwise reduction in treatment may be possible.

↑ **Step up**
If control is not achieved, consider step up. But first: review patient medication technique, adherence and environmental control (avoidance of allergens or other precipitant factors).

Note:

- **The stepwise approach presents guidelines to assist clinical decision making. Asthma is highly variable; clinicians should tailor specific medication plans to the needs and circumstances of individual patients.**
- Gain control as quickly as possible; then decrease treatment to the least medication necessary to maintain control. Gaining control may be accomplished by either starting treatment at the step most appropriate to the initial severity of their condition or by starting at a higher level of therapy (e.g., a course of systemic corticosteroids or higher dose of inhaled corticosteroids).
- A rescue course of systemic corticosteroid (prednisolone) may be needed at any time and step.
- In general, use of short-acting beta$_2$-agonist on a daily basis indicates the need for additional long-term-control therapy.
- It is important to remember that there are very few studies on asthma therapy for infants.
- Consultation with an asthma specialist is *recommended* for patients with moderate or severe persistent asthma in this age group. Consultation should be *considered* for all patients with mild persistent asthma.

Figure 145–7 Stepwise approach to the management of asthma in infants and children less than 6 yr of age. (Modified from National Asthma Education and Prevention Program, National Heart, Lung, and Blood Institute, Expert Panel Report 2: Guidelines for the Diagnosis and Management of Asthma. NIH Publication No. 97-4051, July 1997.)

at the maximal doses or if adverse effects become evident, adjustment in the dosing regimen must be guided by determination of the serum theophylline concentration.

Rapidly absorbed liquids and uncoated tablets, although suitable for children with mild asthma who require a few days of therapy for an exacerbation, have no place in the therapeutic regimen of children who require round-the-clock theophylline therapy because wide fluctuations in serum theophylline concentrations are observed when rapidly absorbed products are used. Which of the sustained-release products to use depends on the dosage form (tablet vs capsule) and the amount of drug needed. Capsule formulations that can be opened are virtually tasteless, should not be chewed, may be mixed with *moist* food, and are particularly suitable for young children. Crushing a sustained-release tablet destroys its constant-release properties. Exacerbations of asthma in patients receiving round-the-clock theophylline medication should be treated with adrenergic drugs, as described earlier (see Fig. 145–3 and 145–4).

CROMOLYN AND NEDOCROMIL. Cromolyn powder inhaled four times a day from a Spinhaler or cromolyn aerosol delivered by a metered-dose inhaler or nedocromil (not FDA-labeled for patients younger than 12 yr) is useful in children with persistent asthma (see Chapter 143.1). A solution of cromolyn is available for home nebulization regimens for young children subject to recurrent attacks of asthma. Cromolyn and albuterol or metaproterenol solutions may be mixed together in the nebulizer for ease of administration if concurrent administration of a bronchodilator is necessary. Most data show little if any benefit of continuing treatment with cromolyn in patients who require inhaled corticosteroids, but continued treatment with nedocromil may reduce dosage requirements of inhaled corticosteroids.

CORTICOSTEROIDS. In certain children with moderate asthma, significant flare-ups occur from time to time that may require the use of corticosteroids for a few days. Early use of steroids in the child who is known to become severely ill may reduce the need for hospitalization. Early intervention with bronchodilator drugs (with or without steroids, depending on the clinical setting) is important in the management of all asthmatic children, regardless of the severity of their conditions. Steroids should be given in adequate doses (1–2 mg/kg/24 hr of prednisone or prednisolone in two to three doses) and should be discontinued as quickly as possible, for example, within 5–7 days; a long "weaning" period following acute asthma is unnecessary. In patients who only rarely require steroid administration, return of normal hypothalamic-pituitary-adrenal function is hastened by the *prompt* discontinuation of the drug when the acute episode is over. Inhaled topical steroid preparations are also effective for children with severe persistent asthma.

In a minority of children who have severe asthma despite the management guidelines outlined here, unacceptable degrees of coughing and wheezing persist, severely limiting the child's play activities and school attendance. In such children, the judicious administration of oral corticosteroids on an alternate-day basis and as an inhaled aerosol frequently results in significant amelioration of symptoms and allows the child to lead a normal life without suffering the adverse effects of corticosteroids. If alternate-day therapy is indicated because of either chronic disability or the severity or frequency of attacks of status asthmaticus, the patient is given 5–7 days of intensive daily therapy and then switched to an alternate-day regimen with a short-acting steroid (prednisone, prednisolone, or methylprednisolone). A 12-yr-old child might be given 60 mg, 40 mg, 30 mg, 20 mg, and 10 mg of prednisone/24 hr over a 5-day period for an exacerbation of asthma, to be followed by alternate-day therapy at a dose of 20 mg/24 hr given as a single dose at 7.00–8.00 A.M. every 48 hr or 3:00–5:30 P.M. if adherence to administration in late afternoon is possible. If the patient responds well to this regimen, the prednisone may be reduced by 5 mg per dose at 10- to 14-day intervals until the lowest dose compatible with acceptable control of symptoms is reached, usually 5–10 mg on alternate days. Concurrent therapy with long-acting adrenergic drugs, theophylline, or nedocromil should be continued because this reduces the dose of steroid required. Low-dose alternate-day therapy is associated with minimal adverse effects and thus may be justified in a disease that can be life: threatening. Use of steroid therapy should *not*, however, substitute for or delay comprehensive management of the disease.

Inhalational corticosteroids, such as beclomethasone dipropionate (Vanceril, Beclovent), budesonide (Pulmicort), flunisolide (AeroBid), fluticasone propionate (Flovent), and triamcinolone (Azmacort), are indicated for children with moderate or severe persistent asthma. They also are appropriate for children with mild persistent asthma, especially if uncontrolled with cromolyn, nedocromil, sustained-release theophylline, or a leukotriene antagonist (Accolate or Singulair) (see Figs. 145–6 and 145–7). Table 143–3 indicates relative clinical potency of inhaled corticosteroids. Beclomethasone, which is effective in microgram doses, is rapidly inactivated in the liver into metabolites devoid of glucocorticoid activity. Accordingly, systemic effects in children given less than 14 μg/kg/24 hr (usual dose is two inhalations or 84 μg four times a day) are minimal. Intrapulmonary metabolism to the active monopropionate may account for slight suppression of growth velocity as compared with equivalent dosages of budesonide. Oropharyngeal candidiasis rarely occurs. Its frequency and that of other adverse effects are diminished by rinsing the mouth and expectorating after inhaling the aerosol and inhaling the aerosol through a chamber or spacer. Effective use of inhaled steroid requires a degree of compliance by the patient not often found in children younger than 6–7 yr. Studies of adults who have received beclomethasone for up to 7 yr have shown no evidence of epithelial atrophy or thinning of underlying connective tissue, and there have been no long-term adverse effects of the drug on the pharynx and airways.

Continual treatment with an inhaled corticosteroid, nedocromil, or cromolyn is appropriate for any child with symptoms of asthma occurring as frequently as weekly except for exercise-induced asthma preventable by pretreatment with a β-agonist, cromolyn, nedocromil, theophylline, or a leukotriene antagonist, although the Expert Panel guidelines recommend continual treatment only when symptoms recur at least twice each week (see Table 145–4 and Figs. 145–6 and 145–7).

Home monitoring of peak expiratory flow rate two to three times a day facilitates early detection of airway obstruction in patients with severe asthma and in patients with infrequent symptoms that may progress to severe airway obstruction. Graphing the results of monitoring will establish the child's diurnal variation and permit the physician to suggest treatment guidelines that anticipate decreases in peak expiratory flow rate. Daily changes in flow rate may also indicate a need for changes in continual treatment regimens. Whatever the degree of severity of the asthma, a personalized, written crisis plan is helpful (see Fig. 145–5). This can remind patients and parents about what to do in an emergency.

EMOTIONS. Emotional tensions surrounding asthma are best handled by unhurried discussion with the parents of the child's difficulty, by avoidance of overdramatization of the child's illness, and by careful examinations with the parents of those areas in which parent and child seem to be in conflict. The use of tranquilizers or sedatives as a substitute for more direct attempts to solve emotional problems should be avoided. As the asthma is brought under control, the emotional climate is often improved.

FACTORS THAT AFFECT SEVERITY. Various factors may exacerbate asthma or make the disease difficult to treat: gastroesophageal reflux, allergic bronchopulmonary aspergillosis, nonsteroidal anti-inflammatory agents, pregnancy, and sinusitis. Chronic sinusitis may be due to noninfectious immune-mediated inflammation or to bacterial infection. Treatment of sinusitis with antibiotics, intranasal steroids, and oral or topical (3–5 days) decongestants for 3 wk may improve bronchoconstriction as well as sinusitis.

EDUCATION. Asthma education programs, for example, ACT (*A*sthma *C*are *T*raining) and You Can Control Asthma (available from Asthma and Allergy Foundation of America, 1125 15th St., NW, Suite 502, Washington, DC 20005) or Open Airways at School (American Lung Association), are being used in comprehensive asthma management. Their goal is to increase knowledge of asthma and its treatment on the part of both the child and parent, to improve communication within the family and with the physician and nurse, to improve compliance with the treatment plan, and to decrease the need for use of emergency room or hospital.

PREVENTION OF DEATHS FROM ASTHMA. Death from childhood asthma is rare, but asthma mortality rates have been increasing. In the United States asthma mortality rates increased from 1.2/100,000 general population in 1979 to 2.1/100,000 in 1994 and 1995. Numbers of deaths from asthma in children less than 15 yr of age increased from 54 in 1977 to 164 in 1995 (Fig. 145–8). Among children 10–14 yr old the asthma mortality rate increased from 0.1/100,000 in 1979 to 0.5/100,000 in 1987, the greatest proportional increase for any age group. Rates have been three to nine times as high in black children as in whites. Increases have also occurred in many other countries.

Reasons for these increases in mortality are unknown. Possible causes include increased prevalence of asthma; increased indoor air pollution as a result of tighter construction of homes with emphasis on energy conservation; excessive exposure to allergen; psychosocial dysfunction that may interfere with perception of airway obstruction and with compliance with recommended management; delays in implementation of appropriate treatment for acute asthma; lack of access or utilization of medical care, including preventive care; overreliance on bronchodilator inhalers leading to delayed treatment with steroids or other therapy until patients are in extremis; unavailability of epinephrine for patients unable to use inhalers effectively; inappropriate use of the metered-dose inhaler; and failure to provide continuity of care or education about what to do for an unusually severe episode of asthma. Introduction of β-agonist inhalers that release no propellant after exhaustion of the supply of medication should help patients recognize the need for replacing the inhaler.

Most but not all deaths from asthma are preventable with appropriate care. It is possible to identify many of those at greatest risk for death from their histories, for example, respiratory failure with hypercapnia, loss of consciousness caused by asthma, or psychosocial dysfunction in the patient or family. These patients require especially close monitoring and psychotherapy when indicated. Each should carry a written emergency protocol indicating current medications and recommended emergency treatment as guidance for emergency personnel who may be unfamiliar with the patient. They should also have a written crisis plan indicating what they should do in an emergency. This should include which medications to use, which doses to use at what intervals, how to reach their physicians, and where to get further assistance. A Medic-Alert emblem can be helpful if such a patient is found unconscious or unable to indicate the nature of the illness. Such patients should be provided with injectable epinephrine in a convenient preparation (e.g., EpiPen or EpiPen Jr.) for use in an emergency when inhalation therapy is ineffective or inappropriate, but use of the EpiPen should not delay transport to an emergency facility.

REFERRAL FOR CONSULTATION. National Guidelines for the Diagnosis and Management of Asthma include recommendations for referral to an asthma specialist for consultation or management (Table 145–5). Such specialists usually are allergists or pulmonologists, but nasal complications may necessitate referral to an otolaryngologist, and psychiatric or psychosocial dysfunction may require referral to a mental health professional.

TABLE 145–5 Possible Indications for Referral to an Asthma Specialist

Severe, acute asthma that has caused loss of consciousness, hypoxia, respiratory failure, convulsions, or near death
Poorly controlled asthma as indicated by admission to a hospital, frequent need for emergency care, need for oral corticosteroids, absence from school or work, disruption of sleep, interference with quality of life
Severe, persistent asthma requiring step 4 care (consider for patients who require step 3 care)
Patient less than 3 years old who requires step 3 or 4 care* (consider for patient less than 3 years old who requires step 2 care)
Requirement for continuous oral corticosteroids or high-dose inhaled corticosteroids or more than two short courses of oral corticosteroids within 1 year
Need for additional diagnostic testing such as allergy skin testing, rhinoscopy, provocative challenge, complete pulmonary function testing, bronchoscopy
Consideration for immunotherapy
Need for additional education regarding asthma, complications of asthma and treatment of asthma, problems with adherence to management recommendations, or allergen avoidance
Uncertainty of diagnosis
Complications of asthma, including sinusitis, nasal polyposis, aspergillosis, severe rhinitis, vocal cord dysfunction, gastroesophageal reflux

Modified from National Asthma Education and Prevention Program, National Heart, Lung, and Blood Institute, Expert Panel Report 2: Guidelines for the Diagnosis and Management of Asthma. Washington, DC, NIH Publication No. 97-4051, July, 1997.

**See Table 145–4 for definition of steps.*

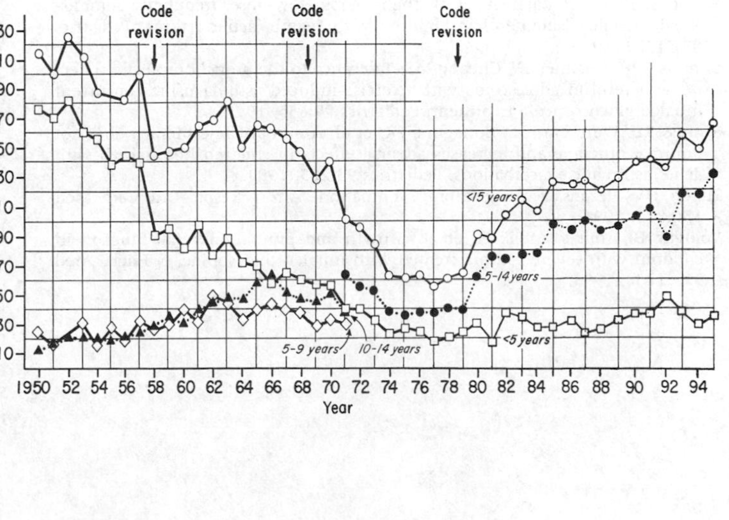

Figure 145–8 Deaths from asthma in children less than 15 years of age by age group. (Modified from Sly RM: Textbook of Pediatric Allergy. New Hyde Park, NY, Medical Examination Publishing Company, 1985.)

Adinoff A, Cummings N: Sinusitis and its relationship to asthma. Pediatr Ann 18:785, 1989.
Allen DB, Brensky EA, LaForce CF, et al: Growth in asthmatic children treated with fluticasone propionate. J Pediatr 132:472, 1998.
Carter E, Cruz M, Chesrown S, et al: Efficacy of intravenously administered theophylline in children hospitalized with severe asthma. J Pediatr 122:470, 1993.
Chou KJ, Cunningham SJ, Crain EF: Metered-dose inhalers with spacers vs nebulizers for pediatric asthma. Arch Pediatr Adolesc Med 149:201, 1995.
Ciarallo L, Sauer AH, Shannon MW: Intravenous magnesium therapy for moderate to severe pediatric asthma: Results of a randomized, placebo-controlled trial. J Pediatr 129:809, 1996.
Connett GJ, Warde C, Wooler E, et al: Prednisolone and salbutamol in the hospital treatment of acute asthma. Arch Dis Child 70:170, 1994.
Duff AL, Pomeranz ES, Gelber LE, et al: Risk factors for acute wheezing in infants and children: Viruses, passive smoke, and IgE antibodies to inhalant allergens. Pediatrics 92:535, 1993.
Evans DJ, Taylor DA, Zetterstrom O, et al: A comparison of low-dose inhaled budesonide plus theophylline and high-dose inhaled budesonide for moderate asthma. N Engl J Med 337:1412, 1997.
Gershel J, Goldman H, Stein R, et al: The usefulness of chest radiographs in first asthma attacks. N Engl J Med 309:336, 1983.
Goren AI, Hellmann S: Changing prevalence of asthma among schoolchildren in Israel. Eur Respir J 10:2279, 1997.
Joseph CLM, Foxman B, Leickly FE, et al: Prevalence of possible undiagnosed asthma and associated morbidity among urban schoolchildren. J Pediatr 129:735, 1996.
Kerem E, Levison H, Schuh S, et al: Efficacy of albuterol administered by nebulizer versus spacer device in children with acute asthma. J Pediatr 123:313, 1993.
Knorr B, Matz J, Bernstein JA, et al: Montelukast for chronic asthma in 6- to 14-year-old children. JAMA 279:1181, 1998.
Landwehr LP, Wood RP II, Blager FB, et al: Vocal cord dysfunction mimicking exercise-induced bronchospasm in adolescents. Pediatrics 98:971, 1996.
Larsen GL: Asthma in children. N Engl J Med 326:1540, 1992.
Leff JA, Bronsky EA, Kemp J, et al: Montelukast (MK-0476) inhibits exercise-induced bronchoconstriction (EIB) over 12-weeks without causing tolerance. Am J Respir Crit Care Med 155:A977, 1997.
Manthous CA, Hall JB, Melmed A, et al: Heliox improves pulsus paradoxus and peak expiratory flow in nonintubated patients with severe asthma. Am J Respir Crit Care Med 151:310, 1995.
Martinez FD, Wright AL, Taussig LM, et al: Asthma and wheezing in the first six years of life. N Engl J Med 332:133, 1995.
McFadden ER, Gilbert IA: Exercise-induced asthma. N Engl J Med 330:1362, 1994.
National Asthma Education Program, National Heart, Lung, and Blood Institute, Expert Panel Report: Guidelines for the Diagnosis and Management of Asthma (NIH pub no 97-4051). Bethesda, MD, U.S. Department of Health and Human Services, 1997.
Nelson HS, Bensch G, Pleskow WW, et al: Improved bronchodilation with levalbuterol compared with racemic albuterol in patients with asthma. J Allergy Clin Immunol 102:943, 1998.
Provisional Committee on Quality Improvement: Practice parameters: The office management of acute exacerbations of asthma in children. Pediatrics 93:119, 1994.
Reed CE, Offord KP, Nelson HS, et al: Aerosol beclomethasone dipropionate spray compared with theophylline as primary treatment for chronic mild-to-moderate asthma. J Allergy Clin Immunol 101:14, 1998.
Rock M, De LaRocha S, L'Hommedieu S, et al: Use of ketamine in asthmatic children to treat respiratory failure refractory to conventional therapy. Crit Care Med 14:514, 1986.
Scarfone RJ, Fuchs SM, Nager AL, et al: Controlled trial of oral prednisone in the emergency department treatment of children with acute asthma. Pediatrics 92:513, 1993.
Schuh S, Johnson DW, Callahan S, et al: Efficacy of frequent nebulized ipratropium bromide added to frequent high-dose albuterol therapy in severe childhood asthma. J Pediatr 126:639, 1995.
Schuh S, Parkin P, Rajan A, et al: High- versus low-dose, frequently administered, nebulized albuterol in children with severe, acute asthma. Pediatrics 83:513, 1989.
Simons FER, Gerstner TV, Cheang MS: Tolerance to the bronchoprotective effect of salmeterol in adolescents with exercise-induced asthma using concurrent inhaled glucocorticoid treatment. Pediatrics 99:655, 1997.
Strauss RE, Wertheim DL, Bonagura VR, et al: Aminophylline therapy does not improve outcome and increases adverse effects in children hospitalized with acute asthmatic exacerbations. Pediatrics 93:205, 1994.
Tuxen DV: Permissive hypercapnic ventilation. Am J Respir Crit Care Med 150:870, 1994.
Volovitz B, Amir J, Malik H, et al: Growth and pituitary-adrenal function in children with severe asthma treated with inhaled budesonide. N Engl J Med 329:1703, 1993.

CHAPTER 146

Atopic Dermatitis

(Infantile or Atopic Eczema)

Atopic dermatitis is an inflammatory skin disorder characterized by erythema, edema, intense pruritus, exudation, crusting, and scaling. In the acute stages, intraepidermal vesiculation (spongiosis) is present. There appears to be a genetically determined predilection. Infants with atopic dermatitis tend to experience allergic rhinitis and asthma subsequently (see also Chapter 663).

About 80% of patients with atopic dermatitis have serum IgE concentrations increased 5- to 10-fold above normal. There is conflicting evidence as to whether the level of IgE is related to either the severity or the extent of the dermatitis. The concentration of IgE does, however, fluctuate with the stage of the disease. The level returns to normal when the disease has been quiescent for several years. It is not established that atopic dermatitis is primarily an IgE-mediated allergic disorder; it is difficult to demonstrate consistently a role for allergens, whether foods or inhalants, in the pathogenesis of eczema. Children with atopic dermatitis and food hypersensitivity have high rates of spontaneous basophil histamine release. This phenomenon returns to normal following a food elimination diet and is mediated by a monocyte cytokine (histamine-releasing factor), which interacts with a specific subtype of IgE bound to basophils. Typical lesions of atopic dermatitis may occur in individuals with X-linked agammaglobulinemia, who have virtually no IgE.

Increased concentrations of IgE in atopic dermatitis may be related to a deficiency of IgE isotype-specific "suppressor" T-cell function. Impairment of cell-mediated immunity in some patients with atopic dermatitis is indicated by (1) absence of the reactions of delayed hypersensitivity on intradermal skin testing with certain antigens; (2) inability to be sensitized with potent contact sensitizers (e.g., poison ivy, dinitrochlorobenzene); (3) diminished proliferative response of lymphocytes to mitogens such as phytohemagglutinin; and (4) variable phagocytic and chemotactic defects of monocytes and neutrophils.

Potential primary immune abnormalities include an increased frequency of allergen-specific Th2 cells that secrete various interleukins (IL-4, IL-5, IL-13) and reduced numbers of Th1 cells. Th2-type cytokines may initiate the acute inflammatory response. Allergen-reactive T cells, which express the cutaneous lymphocyte-associated antogen may migrate to the skin and initiate disease.

The hyperreactive skin of atopic dermatitis differs from normal skin in its response to a variety of physical and pharmacologic stimuli. For example, within 1 min a light mechanical stroke results in a white line with a surrounding blanched area. This phenomenon ("white dermographism") is not seen in normal skin, which becomes red. Involved skin has abnormal rates of cooling and warming in response to temperature changes, particularly in flexural areas. Paradoxical responses occur to injections of various pharmacologic agents, such as histamine, acetylcholine (blanching rather than erythema), and nicotinic acid ester. Adrenergic responses are decreased in lymphocytes and granulocytes in atopic dermatitis, suggesting that autonomic imbalance may be a basis for the abnormalities in the skin. The abnormal reactivity of the skin has a counterpart in the airway hyperreactivity of asthma; in both disorders, such hyperreactivity seems to be intrinsic to the disease, which may, in part, be due to the late-phase immune response (see

Chapter 141). In addition to its genetic and atopic features, eczema is also characterized by cutaneous dysregulation of the autonomic nervous system, a reduced threshold for secondary skin infections (*Staphylococcus aureus* molluscum), skin hyperirritability, and exacerbation by stress.

CLINICAL MANIFESTATIONS. Atopic dermatitis affects 2–10% of children and typically occurs in three stages with fairly distinctive features. The disease most often begins in infancy, usually during the first 2–3 mo of life. The onset is sometimes delayed until the 2nd or 3rd yr; 60% of patients are affected by 1 yr of age and 90% by 5 yr of age. The earliest lesions are erythematous, weepy patches on the cheeks, with subsequent extension to the remainder of the face, neck, wrists, hands, abdomen, and extensor aspects of the extremities. Involvement of flexural areas characteristically appears later but may occur as popliteal and antecubital dermatitis in early life (Fig. 146–1).

Pruritus is marked; the affected infant makes incessant efforts to scratch by rubbing the face on bedclothes and against the sides of the crib. This trauma to the skin rapidly leads to weeping and crusting; secondary infection is common and may be extensive.

The onset of dermatitis frequently coincides with the introduction of certain foods into the infant's diet, especially cow milk, wheat, soy, peanuts, fish, or eggs. Cutaneous symptoms develop after food challenges in 50–90% of infants and children who have dermatitis and high IgE serum concentrations. Overall, about 20–30% of patients with eczema have food hypersensitivity to one or more of the six common allergens. There is unequivocal evidence of reaginic sensitivity in certain infants who have urticaria, colic, and a diffuse erythematous flush following ingestion of the offending food. The erythematous flush appears to be accompanied by intense itching, which results in scratching and then in the appearance of the skin lesions characteristic of eczema. The major role of scratching in the production of skin lesions has been demonstrated when one extremity has been encased in surgical dressings and the other left uncovered; the lesions of atopic dermatitis occur only in the uncovered extremity.

Atopic dermatitis shows a tendency to remission at 3–5 yr of age. In most cases, the disease becomes less prominent by the age of 5 yr; in some, a mild to moderate eczema may persist in the antecubital and popliteal fossae, on the wrists, behind the ears, and on the face and neck. During childhood, antecubital and popliteal involvement becomes common; extensor surfaces of the extremities may still be actively affected. With increasing age, there is a tendency toward drying and thickening of the skin in the involved areas, especially in the antecubital and popliteal fossae, and on the neck, forehead, eyelids, wrists, and the dorsa of the hands and feet. The face takes on a whitish hue as increased capillary permeability and dilatation result in edema and blanching of surrounding tissues, sometimes called the "mask of atopic dermatitis." Hyperpigmentation of the skin, scaling, and lichenification (a particular kind of popular thickening of the skin, with accentuation of the normal surface lines) become prominent. Prognosis is poorest in children with severe dermatitis, family histories of atopic dermatitis, associated asthma or allergic rhinitis, onset before 1 yr of age, and in females. There is a marked tendency toward lasting remission in the 4th and 5th decades of life.

DIAGNOSIS. When pruritus is intense and the lesions characteristic, the diagnosis of atopic dermatitis may be easy. A family history of asthma, hay fever, or atopic dermatitis; the finding of elevated serum IgE concentrations and of reaginic antibodies to a variety of foods and inhalants; the presence of eosinophilia; and the demonstration of white dermographism support the diagnosis. Some patients have accentuated lines or grooves below the margin of the lower eyelids (atopic pleat, Dennie's line, or Morgan's fold) and an increased number of creases of the skin of the palm. The skin has an abnormal tendency to lichenify in response to chronic irritation or rubbing. Generalized dryness of the skin, even in uninvolved areas, and sparsity of the hair of the lateral portion of the eyebrows, thought to be secondary to chronic rubbing, are also characteristic. Specific diagnosis criteria are provided in Tables 146–1 and 146–2.

DIFFERENTIAL DIAGNOSIS. The eczematoid skin reaction characterized by erythema, edema, exudation, crusting, and scaling is not specific for atopic dermatitis. In infants and children, the differential diagnosis includes seborrheic dermatitis, scabies, primary irritant dermatitis, allergic contact dermatitis, infectious eczematoid dermatitis, ichthyosis, phenylketonuria, acrodermatitis enteropathica, histiocytosis X, and two primary immunologic deficiency disorders: the Wiskott-Aldrich syndrome and X-linked agammaglobulinemia. Eczematous lesions may also be noted in ataxia-telangiectasia, Job's syndrome, hyper-IgE syndrome, and biotinidase deficiency.

Seborrheic dermatitis typically begins on the scalp, often as "cradle cap," and involves the ear and contiguous skin, the sides of the nose, and eyebrows and eyelids with greasy, brownish scales. These are usually distinguished easily from

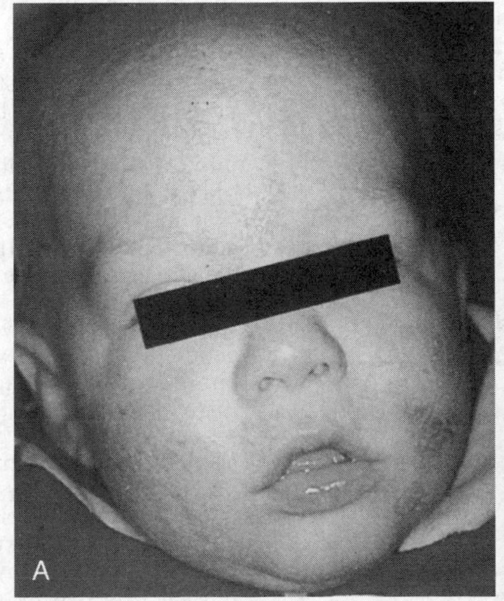

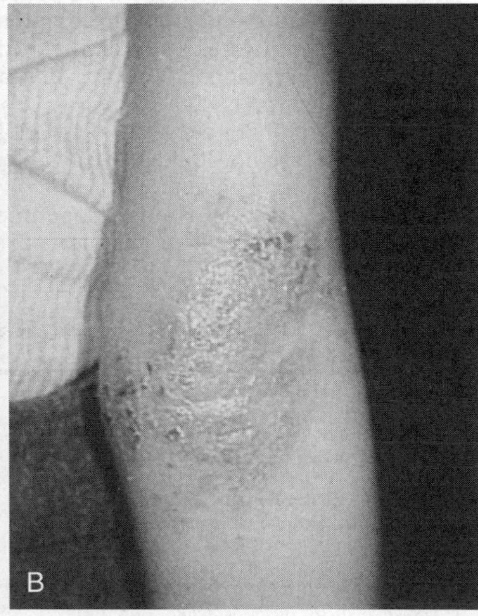

Figure 146–1 (A–B) Infantile atopic dermatitis begins typically as a pruritic, erythematous, papulovesicular eruption over the cheeks but may also involve the wrists and extensor aspects of the extremities or may become generalized, usually sparing the diaper area. By 2 yr of age, involvement of antecubital and popliteal spaces, neck, wrists, and ankles is common with scaling, excoriations, lichenification, and hyperpigmentation. Crusting indicates superimposed infection. (From The Dermatologic Dozen, 1980. Used with permission of Westwood Pharmaceuticals, Inc.) See also color section.

TABLE 146–1 Diagnostic Features of Atopic Dermatitis

Must have three or more major features:
Pruritus
Typical morphologic appearance and distribution
  Flexural lichenification or linearity in adults
  Facial and extensor involvement in infants and children
Chronic or chronically relapsing course
Personal or family history of atopy (asthma, allergic rhinitis, or atopic dermatitis)

Must also have three or more minor features:
Xerosis
Ichthyosis, palmar hyperlinearity, keratosis pilaris
Immediate (type I) skin test reactivity
Elevated serum IgE
Early age of onset
Tendency toward cutaneous infections (especially *Staphylococcus aureus* and herpes simplex)/impaired cell-mediated immunity
Tendency toward nonspecific hand or foot dermatitis
Nipple eczema
Cheilitis
Recurrent conjunctivitis
Dennie-Morgan infraorbital fold
Keratoconus
Anterior subcapsular cataracts
Orbital darkening
Facial pallor, facial erythema
Pityriasis alba
Itch when sweating
Intolerance to wool and lipid solvents
Perifollicular accentuation
Food hypersensitivity
Course influenced by environmental, emotional factors
White dermographism, delayed blach

From Sampson HA: Atopic dermatitis. Ann Allergy 69:469, 1992.

the erythematous, weeping, crusted lesions of infantile atopic dermatitis, but sometimes during the first few months of life it is difficult to distinguish clearly between seborrhea and atopic dermatitis, particularly when the face is primarily involved. Seborrhea in infancy has a shorter course than that of atopic eczema and responds much more rapidly to treatment. The difficulty in differentiating the two conditions is indicated by the use of the term *seborrheic eczema* by some dermatologists. In infancy, scabies may be confused with atopic dermatitis. The location of the lesions helps to differentiate the two. Atopic dermatitis most often begins on the cheeks and does not involve the palms and soles, whereas scabies commonly starts with large papules on the upper back and vesicles on the palms and soles. The mite of scabies or its ova can be seen in scrapings from the vesicles.

Primary irritant dermatitis is a nonallergic reaction caused by various irritants and is most common in infancy in the perioral (from fruit juices) and diaper areas. The location and rapid response of lesions to therapy indicate the correct diagnosis.

The lesions of allergic contact dermatitis (poison ivy is the prototype) are usually limited to sites of exposure to the offending allergen and do not typically involve the flexural areas. Occasionally, contact dermatitis is superimposed on atopic dermatitis after sensitization to chemicals in topical agents such as neomycin, the parabens (used as preservatives in many ointments), or iodochlorohydroxyquin (Vioform).

TABLE 146–2 Criteria Modified for Diagnosis of Atopic Dermatitis in Infants

Must have three major features:
Family history of atopic disease
Typical facial or extensor eczematous or lichenified dermatitis
Evidence of pruritus

Must also have three minor features:
Xerosis, ichthyosis, hyperlinear palms
Postauricular fissures
Chronic scaling of scalp

From Sampson HA: Atopic dermatitis. Ann Allergy 69:469, 1992.

Infectious eczematoid dermatitis may follow discharge of purulent material from a draining ear or other site of infection. The typical location of the lesions and rapid response to therapy support the diagnosis.

In ichthyosis vulgaris, dryness of the skin may lead to confusion with atopic dermatitis, but the scales of ichthyosis are usually larger than those of atopic dermatitis, and the pruritus of ichthyosis, if any, is generally mild. The two disorders may be associated. Infants and children with untreated phenylketonuria acquire an eczematous dermatitis often confused with atopic eczema. The rash of phenylketonuria is responsive to a diet low in phenylalanine.

Histiocytosis X (Letterer-Siwe disease—Langerham cell histiocytosis) and acrodermatitis enteropathica are serious systemic diseases occurring early in life. Failure to thrive is prominent. Hemorrhagic manifestations are common in the eczematous eruption of histiocytosis X. In acrodermatitis, the skin around the oral, nasal, genitourinary, and rectal orifices is typically involved.

Patients with Wiskott-Aldrich syndrome and X-linked agammaglobulinemia may have an eczema that is indistinguishable from atopic dermatitis.

COMPLICATIONS. During early infancy and childhood, secondary infection of the lesions of atopic dermatitis with bacterial, fungal, or viral agents is common. Staphylococci and β-hemolytic streptococci are the bacterial agents most often recovered from infected lesions. Herpes simplex (Kaposi's varicelliform eruption) is also of particular concern. Infants and children with eczema should not be exposed to adults with herpes simplex infection ("cold sores"). Infections with common wart and molluscum contagiosum viruses may also occur. Keratoconus is occasionally seen in children with atopic dermatitis, perhaps owing to chronic rubbing of the eyelids. Cataracts occur in 5–10% of adults with severe atopic dermatitis but are rarely seen during childhood.

TREATMENT. Effective treatment of atopic dermatitis requires control of the environmental precipitants of the itch-scratch-itch cycle that perpetuates the disease, beginning with avoidance of ingestant, injectant, contactant, and atmospheric factors that can trigger itching or scratching. Extremes of temperature and humidity should be avoided. A warm climate of moderate humidity is optimal for most patients. Sweating leads to itching and aggravation of the disease. Exposure to sunlight and salt water is of benefit to many patients.

Garments should be made of a smooth-textured cotton; wool should be avoided. Infants should not be allowed to crawl on wool carpeting.

For the dry skin of atopic dermatitis, use of soaps and detergents that defat the skin should be avoided as much as possible. Bathing should be kept to a minimum. The purpose of bath oil or other creams applied to the skin is to seal water into the skin; bath oil is added to the tub after the patient has soaked for 20 min, thus sealing the moisture in the hydrated skin instead of excluding it as would occur if the oil were added before the patient enters the bath. The same principle applies to application of creams and lotions; they should be applied to the damp skin following a bath. Soaking in tepid water for 30 min two or three times each day followed by gentle drying of the skin and application within 3 min of an ointment base (Aquaphor) or a cream base (Acid Mantle) to maintain hydration of the skin is often helpful. Should bathing appear to make the condition worse, a nondrying, cleansing agent such as Cetaphil, a commercially available nonlipid lotion, can be used.

If a food aggravates itching, it should be excluded from the diet. Skin testing by the prick method is useful in excluding IgE-mediated food hypersensitivity. Positive skin test results must be assessed by properly controlled food challenges (see

TABLE 146–3 Potency of Selected Topical Corticosteroids

Potency	Corticosteroid	Brand
Superpotent	Betamethasone dipropionate	Diprolene ointment, 0.05%
	Clobetasol propionate	Temovate ointment, 0.05%
Very highly potent	Betamethasone dipropionate	Diprosone ointment, 0.05%
	Halcinonide	Halog ointment, 0.1%
	Fluocinonide	Lidex cream, 0.05%
Highly potent	Triamcinolone acetonide	Aristocort cream (HP), 0.5%
	Betamethasone dipropionate	Diprosone cream, 0.05%
	Betamethasone valerate	Valisone ointment, 0.1%
Somewhat less highly potent	Hydrocortisone valerate	Westcort ointment, 0.2%
	Triamcinolone acetonide	Aristocort ointment, 0.1%
	Flurandrenolide	Cordran ointment, 0.05%
Mild potency	Betamethasone valerate	Valisone cream, 0.1%
Milder potency	Mometasone furoate	Elocon cream and ointment, 0.1%
	Alclometasone dipropionate	Aclovate cream and ointment, 0.05%
Low potency	Fluocinolone acetonide	Synalar solution, 0.01%
	Desonide	Tridesilon cream, 0.05%
Lowest potency	Hydrocortisone	Hytone cream and ointment, 1.0%, 2.5%

Chapter 153). Arbitrary exclusion of numerous foods from the diets of infants with atopic dermatitis without clear evidence that they are involved in the disease is irrational and can lead to malnutrition. Double-blind food elimination and provocative testing may identify the offending food (see Chapter 153). Subsequent elimination of the identified food from the diet will decrease symptoms (peanut, soy, egg, milk). Some children "outgrow" these food-induced symptoms, although allergy to peanut may be lifelong. Thus, reintroducing the offending foods may be possible within 2–4 yr. Food allergen sensitization can be reduced by breast-feeding and by delaying the introduction of solid foods until after 6 mo of age. Breast-feeding mothers should avoid ingesting high-risk foods because some food allergens appear in human milk and can potentially sensitize an atopic infant.

House dust mite specific lymphocyte stimulation is greatly elevated in infants with atopic dermatitis, and IL-5 production by their mite-stimulated peripheral blood monocytes is increased. Avoidance of mite allergens can improve control of atopic dermatitis. Such precautions (see Chapter 143) may be appropriate whether or not specific sensitization to mites is demonstrable. Other aeroallergens also can aggravate atopic dermatitis beyond infancy.

Local therapy is the mainstay of management of atopic dermatitis. During acute flare-ups of the disease, wet dressings (e.g., Burow's solution, 1:20) have an antipruritic and anti-inflammatory effect. Topical corticosteroid lotions or creams may be applied between changes of wet dressings. The continuous application of wet dressings also has the advantage of immobilizing and protecting the affected parts and preventing scratching. Unless scratching can be controlled, it is almost impossible to manage the disease successfully, especially during infancy and early childhood. Fingernails must be kept cut as short as possible; restraints for the elbows to keep the hands from the face are sometimes necessary to control scratching at night. Itching is difficult to control with drugs. Drugs with both sedative and antihistamine activity, such as diphenhydramine (Benadryl), hydroxyzine (Atarax, Vistaril), or promethazine (Phenergan), are of value, but a nonsedating (Claritin) or low sedating (Zyrtec) antihistamine can also be effective without adverse effects on behavior, learning, or quality of sleep. In some patients, aspirin has a marked antipruritic effect.

When infection is present (acute weeping or crusting), antibiotics should be given systemically. Erythromycin or cephalexin is a prudent choice because of frequent resistance to penicillin of the infecting *S. aureus.* Antibiotics in topical medications not only are of little therapeutic value but also can lead to sensitization to the agents applied, particularly in the case of neomycin. Mupirocin (Bactroban) is an exception and is often helpful for localized infections. The possibility of superimposed contact sensitization must be considered when there is sudden exacerbation of atopic dermatitis to which a topical medicament has been applied. Parabens, mercurial compounds, and lanolin can all cause contact sensitization.

After the acute phase has subsided, topical application of corticosteroid creams and ointments is of great value in managing the disease. Topical triamcinolone acetonide ointment, 0.1%, is often useful but is best limited to 1–3 wk at a time; after improvement, substitute an even less potent corticosteroid if possible (Table 146–3). It is safest to prescribe the least potent corticosteroid that affords adequate control. Their cost may be a serious problem. Cost can be reduced by purchasing relatively concentrated preparations in bulk, which the pharmacist can dilute to half strength with Aquaphor or a moisturizer (Eucerin), rather than purchasing equivalent material in 15- or 30-g amounts. Small amounts of steroid rubbed in well at frequent intervals give better results than large amounts applied only infrequently. Percutaneous absorption of corticosteroid occurs but is not generally clinically significant. Long-term topical use of steroids leads to an increase in growth of hair in some patients and to atrophy of the skin. The more potent topical steroids should not be applied to the face, genitals, or intertriginous areas, or to large areas for prolonged periods. Application of 0.5% or 1% hydrocortisone to the face is safe.

Systemic administration of corticosteroids for treatment of atopic dermatitis should be avoided except briefly in the most severely affected patients while awaiting response to other therapies.

Topical treatment with corticosteroids has largely superseded the use of coal tar preparations. Tars stain clothes and skin and compliance of the patient in their use is often poor. Application at night and removal by washing the next morning improves acceptability to patients. Tar preparations should not be applied to acutely inflamed skin. Tars are considerably less expensive for long-term topical use than corticosteroids. Coal tar is photosensitizing, and occasionally its use results in a sterile, pustular folliculitis.

Short-term treatment with oral corticosteroids affords rapid but temporary relief, with rapid recurrence with discontinuation. Accordingly, topical therapy should be intensified as the oral steroid is tapered. Immunotherapy usually has not been helpful, often aggravating the dermatitis.

Cyclosporine is beneficial for severe atopic dermatitis unresponsive to topical corticosteroids but has been limited by side effects, including nausea, hypertrichosis, hypertension, paresthesias, and hepatic and renal toxicity. Tacrolimus, an immunosuppressive ointment, is effective and safe; limited data suggest azathioprine may be beneficial.

Indications for consultation with an allergist or dermatologist are listed in Table 146–4.

TABLE 146–4 Indications for Consultation with a Specialist

Severe or persistent atopic dermatitis (20% general skin involvement or 10% skin involvement affecting eyelids, hands, intertriginous areas and not responsive to first-line therapy)
Erythroderma or extensive exfoliation
Requires more than one course of systemic corticosteroids
Requires admission to hospital for atopic dermatitis
Identification of allergens and triggers
Intensive education
Associated asthma or rhinitis
Impaired quality of life (lost school days, sleep disturbance, poorly controlled pruritus)
Infection
Ocular complications
Psychosocial complications
Uncertainty of diagnosis

Modified from Leung DYM, Hanifin JM, Charlesworth EN, et al: Disease management of atopic dermatitis: A practice parameter. Ann Allergy Asthma Immunol 79:197, 1997.

PROGNOSIS. With adequate control of factors known to trigger itching, appropriate local treatment, and understanding support for the parents of a child for whom no immediate cure is expected, reasonable control of atopic dermatitis is usually possible. Improvement usually occurs within 5 yr.

Bos JD, Kapsenberg ML, Sillevis Smitt JH: Pathogenesis of atopic eczema. Lancet 343:1338, 1994.

Burks A, James J, Hiegel A, et al: Atopic dermatitis and food hypersensitivity reactions. J Pediatr 132:132, 1998.

Hoeger PH, Lenz W, Boutonnier A, et al: Staphylococcal skin colonization in children with atopic dermatitis: Prevalence, persistence, and transmission of toxigenic and nontoxigenic strains. J Infect Dis 165:1064, 1992.

Kimura M, Tsuruta S, Yoshida T: Correlation of house dust mite–specific lymphocyte proliferation with IL-5 production, eosinophilia, and the severity of symptoms in infants with atopic dermatitis. J Allergy Clin Immunol 101:84, 1998.

Lear JT, English JSC, Jones P, et al: Retrospective review of the use of azathioprine in severe atopic dermatitis. J Am Acad Dermatol 35:642, 1996.

Leung DYM, Hanifin JM, Charlesworth EN, et al: Disease management of atopic dermatitis: A practice parameter. Ann Allergy Asthma Immunol 79:197, 1997.

Przybilla B, Eberlein-Konig B, Rueff F: Practical management of atopic eczema. Lancet 343:1342, 1994.

Sampson HA: Atopic dermatitis. Ann Allergy 69:469, 1992.

CHAPTER 147

Urticaria-Angioedema

(Hives)

CLINICAL MANIFESTATIONS. Urticaria, or hives, is a common skin disorder characterized by usually well-circumscribed but sometimes coalescent, localized or generalized, erythematous, raised skin lesions (wheals or welts) of various sizes. The lesions may be intensely pruritic or itch little, if at all. The individual hive usually resolves within 48 hr, but new ones may continue to appear singly or in crops. When urticaria persists for longer than 6 wk, the condition is arbitrarily deemed chronic. Urticaria has been attributed to edema of the upper corium as a result of dilatation and increased permeability of the capillaries.

In angioedema (angioneurotic edema), the deeper layers of skin or submucosa and subcutaneous or other tissues are involved; the upper respiratory tract and the gastrointestinal tract are common target organs. The distinction between urticaria and angioedema is frequently not clear; the lesions appear to differ only in the depth of tissue involvement.

INCIDENCE. As many as 20% of individuals experience hives at some time during life. Urticaria is somewhat more frequent in females than in males.

PATHOGENESIS. The principal noncytotoxic mechanism for urticaria and angioedema is interaction of antigen with mast cell– or basophil-bound IgE antibodies. The release of histamine from these cells causes vasodilation and increased vascular permeability and stimulates an axon reflex, which produces a typical wheal and flare reaction. Leukotrienes may contribute to the edema of the IgE-mediated reaction. A second mediator pathway for urticaria involves the complement system. Two complement component split products, C3a and C5a, act as anaphylatoxins (see Chapter 133) and trigger histamine release from mast cells and basophils by direct action on the cell surfaces, independent of antibodies. C3a and C5a can be generated through both the classic and alternative complement pathways. A third mediator pathway involves the plasma kinin-forming system of the coagulation scheme. Bradykinin is at least as potent as histamine in increasing vascular permeability. Both non-IgE immunologic reactions and nonimmunologic events can cause urticaria and angioedema when they activate the complement and kinin-forming systems. Autoimmune chronic urticaria, a subgroup of chronic urticaria, is due to IgG autoantibodies directed against the α subunit of the IgE receptor of mast cells and basophils.

ETIOLOGY. A clinical classification of urticaria is given in Table 147–1.

DIFFERENTIAL DIAGNOSIS. With a few exceptions, no laboratory tests establish or exclude the diagnosis of urticaria and angioedema. Allergy skin testing is generally not helpful except when specific drug (penicillin) or food allergies are identified. Dermographism is frequent in patients with urticaria, is associated with increased cutaneous responsiveness to histamine, and can complicate allergy skin testing. In the absence of any clue suggesting an ingestant cause, elimination diets generally are not useful. The diagnosis is clinical and requires that the physician be aware of the various forms of urticaria. A careful history usually identifies the type. Except when there are obvious associations with IgE-mediated reactions, naming the "cause" of urticaria may be difficult. Drugs and foods are the most common causes of urticaria. The cause of chronic urticaria is identified in only 10% of cases; some patients demonstrate autoantibodies to the IgE receptor.

Some forms of urticaria need special mention. Papular urticaria usually occurs in small children, generally on the extremities and other exposed parts at the sites of insect bites. Cholinergic urticaria appears as wheals 1–2 mm in diameter surrounded by large areas of erythema (flares) and frequently involves the skin of the neck. It is caused by exercise, hot showers, and occasionally by anxiety. Affected individuals have increased sensitivity to cholinergic mediators, which can be demonstrated when an intradermal injection of 0.01 mg of methacholine (Mecholyl) in 0.1 ml of saline causes a localized hive surrounded by smaller, satellite lesions. Urticaria is probably more often due to viral infection than is commonly recognized. It is particularly associated with hepatitis, especially during the prodromal stages, and with infectious mononucleosis. Viral infections can also produce erythema multiforme, often confused with urticaria, in which typical iris or target lesions occur and mucosal involvement is common. In some patients, typical hives change spontaneously into lesions of erythema multiforme, which can be a sign of drug allergy (see Chapter 150).

Urticaria pigmentosa typically occurs during the first few years of childhood and has a distinctive presentation. Systemic mastocytosis is a serious form of urticaria pigmentosa in which mast cells infiltrate skeleton, liver, spleen, and lymph nodes. In adults, and rarely in children, urticaria may be associated with malignancy or collagen-vascular disorders.

Cold urticaria is the most common form caused by physical factors. Urticarial lesions, which may be pruritic or painful or burning, appear on exposure to cold and are confined to the exposed parts of the body. The lesions develop not only on

TABLE 147–1 Types of Urticaria (Angioedema)

Caused by ingestants (IgE mechanism in some cases)
- Foods, particularly fish, shellfish, nuts, eggs, and peanuts; food additives (tartrazine, azo dyes, benzoates)
- *Anisakis simplex*, a parasite of seafoods
- Drugs (penicillin, aspirin, sulfonamides, codeine, angiotensin-converting enzyme inhibitors)

Caused by contactants (IgE mechanism in some cases)
- Plant substances (e.g., stinging nettle)
- Animal, insect (tarantula hairs, Portuguese man-of-war, cat scratch, moth scales)
- Drugs applied to the skin
- Animal saliva

Caused by injectants (IgE mechanism in some cases)
- Drugs (particularly penicillin), transfused blood, therapeutic antisera, insect stings and bites (papular urticaria), allergenic extracts

Caused by inhalants (IgE mechanism)
- Pollens, danders, and ? molds

Caused by infectious agents (mechanism unknown)
- Parasites
- Viruses (e.g., hepatitis, infectious mononucleosis)
- Bacteria (*Streptococcus*, mycoplasma)
- ? Fungi

Caused by physical factors (mechanism mostly unknown)
- Dermographism
- Cold urticaria
- Delayed pressure urticaria
- Solar urticaria
- Aquagenic urticaria
- Local heat urticaria
- Exercise induced
- Vibratory angioedema

Episodic angioedema with eosinophilia (? a distinct entity)

Cholinergic urticaria (a distinct entity)

Associated with systemic diseases (mechanism mostly unknown)
- Collagen-vascular (systemic lupus erythematosus, cryoglobulinuria, Sjögren's syndrome)
- Cutaneous vasculitis
- Serum sickness–like disease
- Malignancy (leukemia-lymphoma)
- Hyperthyroidism
- Urticaria pigmentosa (systemic mastocytosis)

Associated with genetic disorders (various mechanisms)
- Familial cold urticaria
- Hereditary angioedema
- Amyloidosis with deafness and urticaria
- C3b inactivator deficiency

Chronic urticaria and angioedema (mechanism unknown)

Psychogenic urticaria (existence as an entity uncertain)

exposure to cold weather but also with local application of cold. The cooling of skin associated with evaporation on emerging from water can produce urticaria. Swimming in cold water is hazardous; death may occur in patients so exposed. There are two forms: a primary acquired form and a familial form. Cold urticaria can occur in adults with systemic diseases such as cryofibrinogenemia, cryoglobulinemia, cold-agglutinin disease, and secondary syphilis. In some cases of primary acquired urticaria, the phenomenon has been passively transferred using purified IgE and IgM fractions of serum from affected patients. After appropriate cold challenge, there are also increased concentrations of histamine, eosinophil and neutrophil chemotactic factors, and platelet-activating factor in venous blood draining the challenge site. Primary acquired cold urticaria appears and disappears spontaneously; in some cases, its onset occurs with a viral illness.

Hereditary angioedema, a potentially life-threatening form of angioedema is the most important familial form of angioedema (see Chapter 134.3).

A syndrome of episodic angioedema—urticaria and fever with associated eosinophilia—has been described in both adults and children. In contrast to other hypereosinophilic syndromes, this entity has a benign course.

Exercise-induced anaphylaxis presents with varying combinations of pruritus, urticaria, angioedema, wheezing, laryngeal obstruction, or hypotension after exercise. Cholinergic urticaria is differentiated by positive results on heat challenge tests and the rare occurrence of anaphylactic shock. The combination of ingestion of various food allergens (shrimp, celery, wheat) and postprandial exercise results in cutaneous mast cell degranulation; food or exercise alone may not produce this reaction.

Skin biopsy for diagnosis of possible *urticarial vasculitis* is recommended for urticarial lesions that persist at the same location for more than 24 hr or those with pigmented or purpuric components. Additional features suggestive of urticarial vasculitis include painful lesions, poor response to antihistamines, a high erythrocyte sedimentation rate, and features of systemic inflammation (fever).

TREATMENT. In most instances, urticaria is a self-limited illness requiring little treatment other than antihistamines. Hydroxyzine (Atarax), 0.5 mg/kg, is one of the most effective antihistamines for control of urticaria, but diphenhydramine (Benadryl), 1.25 mg/kg, and other antihistamines are also effective at the expense of sedation. Loratadine or cetirizine also can be effective and are preferable because of reduced frequency of impairment of function and learning.

Epinephrine 1:1,000, 0.01 mL/kg, maximum of 0.3 mL, usually affords rapid relief of acute, severe urticaria. Hydroxyzine (0.5 mg/kg every 4–6 hr) has been the drug of choice for cholinergic and chronic urticaria, but a nonsedating antihistamine such as loratadine is preferable. The combined use of H_1- and H_2-type antihistamines is sometimes helpful to control chronic urticaria; doxepin, an antagonist of both H_1 and H_2 receptors, can be helpful. H_2 antihistamines alone may exacerbate urticaria. Cyproheptadine (Periactin) (2–4 mg every 8–12 hr) is especially useful as a prophylactic agent for cold urticaria, but a nonsedating antihistamine is preferable. Cyproheptadine can cause appetite stimulation and weight gain in some patients. Sunscreens are the only effective treatment for solar urticaria. Corticosteroids have varying effects on chronic urticaria; the doses required to control the urticaria are often so large that they cause serious side effects. Treatment with small doses of cyclosporine has been effective in a few adults with chronic urticaria, but use of large doses has been limited by nephrotoxicity. Chronic urticaria does not often respond favorably to dietary manipulation. Treatment of autoimmune chronic urticaria includes intravenous immunoglobulin or plasmapheresis, or both. Unfortunately, chronic urticaria may persist for years. For treatment of hereditary angioedema, see Chapter 134.3.

Bellanti JA, Kadlec JV, Escobar-Gutiérrez A: Cytokines and the immune response. Pediatr Clin North Am 41:597, 1994.

Charlesworth EN: Urticaria and angioedema: A clinical spectrum. Ann Allergy Asthma Immunol 76:484, 1996.

Galli SJ: Seminars in medicine of the Beth Israel Hospital, Boston. N Engl J Med 328:257, 1993.

Greaves M, Sabroe R: Allergy and the skin I-Urticaria. Br Med J 316:1147, 1998.

Henz BM, Jeep S, Ziegert FS, et al: Dermal and bronchial hyperreactivity in urticarial dermographism and urticaria factitia. Allergy 51:171, 1996.

Hide M, Francis DM, Grattan CEH, et al: Autoantibodies against the high-affinity IgE receptor as a cause of histamine release in chronic urticaria. N Engl J Med 328:1599, 1993.

Leung DYM: Mechanisms of the human allergic response: Clinical implications. Pediatr Clin North Am 41:727, 1994.

Leung DYM, Diaz LA, DeLeo V, Soter NA: Allergic and immunologic skin disorders. JAMA 278:1914, 1997.

Moreno-Ancillo A, Caballero MT, Cabanas R, et al: Allergic reactions to *Anisakis simplex* parasitizing seafood. Ann Allergy Asthma Immunol 79:246, 1997.

Orfan NA, Kolski GB: Physical urticarias. Ann Allergy 71:205, 1993.

Toubi E, Blant A, Kessel A, et al: Low-dose cyclosporin A in the treatment of severe chronic idiopathic urticaria. Allergy 52:312, 1997.

Chapter 148
Anaphylaxis

DEFINITION. Anaphylaxis is an acute, potentially life-threatening reaction caused by rapid release of mediators from mast cells and basophils that follows the interaction of allergen with specific, cell-bound IgE.

ETIOLOGY. Virtually any foreign substance is capable of eliciting anaphylaxis under appropriate circumstances (Table 148–1). Most anaphylactic reactions are due to drug, food, or Hymenoptera venom allergy. Following IgE production in response to antigen stimulus, re-exposure to the offending antigen may result in a systemic reaction. Exercise can provoke anaphylaxis in occasional patients; in some, it occurs only after antecedent ingestion of a specific food or possibly alcohol or aspirin. Intensive evaluation has failed to identify a cause of recurrent anaphylaxis in occasional patients with idiopathic anaphylaxis, most of whom have had concomitant allergy or asthma not obviously related to the recurrent anaphylaxis.

Anaphylaxis from latex is a significant problem among patients chronically exposed to this compound (repeated operations or urinary catheterization, e.g., in spina bifida). Intraoperative anaphylaxis may be due to anesthetics, muscle-relaxing agents, other drugs, or blood products, but latex is one of the most frequent causes. Patients with latex hypersensitivity may have had cutaneous reactions to adhesive tape and cutaneous or systemic reactions to balloons and latex in toys or clothing. There can be cross-reactivity with banana, avocado, chestnut, kiwi and, less frequently, hazelnut, peanut, celery, papaya, melons, potato, fig, passion fruit, pineapple, cherry, peaches, plums, tomato, and grapes.

PATHOGENESIS. When IgE-mediated anaphylactic sensitivity to an antigen has developed, subsequent administration of even minute amounts of the antigen may result in an explosive antigen-antibody reaction with massive release of chemical mediators such as histamine. The action of the mediators on various tissue receptors throughout the body produces the symptoms. Histamine plays a central role in the pathogenesis of human anaphylaxis, but other vasoactive substances (arachidonic acid metabolites, kinins, platelet-activating factor) may also have roles. Decreased levels of factor V and factor VIII have been reported, suggesting consumption of coagulation factors as a result of intravascular coagulation. Several patients studied during severe episodes of systemic anaphylaxis have had low levels of high molecular weight kininogen, C3, and C4. When an immunologic mechanism cannot be identified (anaphylactoid reactions, see Table 148–1), it is presumed that mediator release occurs as a direct effect of the causative agent on basophils and mast cells or perhaps by activation of the alternative complement pathway, with generation of anaphylatoxins (see prior discussion).

TABLE 148–1 Etiology of Anaphylaxis

Drugs (penicillin, cephalosporins, chemotherapy, muscle relaxants)
Foods (seafood, nuts, legumes, egg, celery, milk food containing mold)
Insect Stings (Hymenoptera: kissing bug, deerfly, fire ants)
Biological Agents (L-asparaginase, allergen extracts, blood products, insulin, immunoglobulins)
Food Additives (metabisulfite, monosodium glutamate, aspartame, carmine dye)
Latex
Exercise-Induced
Pseudoallergic* (iodinated radiocontrast media, opiates, D-tubocurarine, thiamine, aspirin, captopril)
Idiopathic

**Pseudoallergic or anaphylactoid is not necessarily IgE mediated. Substances can produce direct mast cell degranulation.*

CLINICAL MANIFESTATIONS. Anaphylactic reactions are characteristically explosive, particularly when the antigen is injected. Surviving patients describe a "feeling of impending doom." The more rapidly symptoms appear after administration of the foreign material, the more serious is the reaction. Often the first symptom noted is a tingling sensation around the mouth or face, followed by a feeling of warmth, difficulty in swallowing, and tightness in the throat or chest. There may be apprehension, weakness, and diaphoresis followed by generalized pruritus. The patient becomes flushed; urticaria and angioedema then appear, along with varying degrees of hoarseness, inspiratory stridor, dysphagia, nasal congestion, itching of the eyes, sneezing, and wheezing. Abdominal cramps, diarrhea, and contractions of the uterus and other organs of smooth muscle may also occur. The patient may lose consciousness and, on examination, be hypotensive, with feeble heart sounds, bradycardia, and sometimes an arrhythmia. Cardiorespiratory arrest and death may ensue. In fatal cases, death has most often resulted from acute upper airway obstruction, although profound circulatory collapse may occur without upper airway obstruction.

Most anaphylactic reactions begin within 30 min of exposure to the allergen, especially if by injection. Signs and symptoms usually resolve within a few hours in surviving patients. Some patients experience biphasic reactions with recurrence of signs and symptoms 1–8 hr after initial resolution in response to therapy; this may be due to a limited duration of action of initially administered pharmacologic agents. In a third group of patients, signs and symptoms of anaphylaxis may continue for many hours or days despite aggressive treatment. Protracted anaphylaxis is more likely to follow oral administration than injection of the offending agent. Biphasic or protracted anaphylaxis is more likely when initial manifestations have occurred more than 30 min after exposure.

Food-dependent, exercise-induced anaphylaxis occurs during exercise within 2 hr of ingestion of the food to which the patient has specific IgE (shellfish, wheat, vegetables, fruit) or following the ingestion of any food. Exercise typically is tolerated 3 hr or more after ingestion; the food has no adverse effect without subsequent exercise. Exercise-induced anaphylaxis may also occur after ingestion of aspirin or other nonsteroidal anti-inflammatory drugs.

DIAGNOSIS. Diagnosis depends on recognition of the typical manifestations but sometimes may be uncertain, especially when the victim is found dead. Vasovagal reactions may be confused with anaphylaxis. They are characterized by nausea, pallor, diaphoresis, bradycardia, hypotension, weakness, and occasionally syncope but lack pruritus, urticaria, angioedema, tachycardia, and bronchospasm. Bradycardia can rarely occur with anaphylaxis.

When there has been loss of consciousness and there are no cutaneous manifestations of anaphylaxis, the differential diagnosis also includes pulmonary embolism; cardiac arrhythmia; cerebrovascular hemorrhage, embolism, or thrombosis; convulsive disorder; foreign body aspiration; and acute poisoning. Systemic mastocytosis can cause symptoms of anaphylaxis occasionally, usually with a history of flushing and maculopapular lesions that urticate with stroking. Hereditary angioneurotic edema can cause laryngeal edema, but associated angioedema is nonpruritic and usually develops gradually over a period of hours. Sudden vascular collapse can occur after exposure to cold in patients with cold urticaria and may be associated with urticaria or airway obstruction; it usually follows swimming in cold water.

Determination of plasma or serum tryptase concentrations can be helpful in the diagnosis of anaphylaxis. Concentrations of 10 ng/ml or more indicate mast cell activation. Increased concentrations may not occur during the first 30 min but tend to peak at 1–2 hr and then decline with a half-time of 2 hr. Plasma histamine (H) concentrations, in contrast, peak within 5 to 10 min after a bee sting challenge and return to baseline within 30 min. Therefore, determination of plasma or serum tryptase concentration is usually more helpful in the diagnosis of anaphylaxis. Other causes of increased tryptase concentrations include asthma (e.g., provoked by a nonsteroidal anti-inflammatory drug) and systemic mastocytosis.

Patients with systemic mastocytosis have elevated plasma histamine concentrations when they are asymptomatic. Patients with hereditary angioneurotic edema have absent or dysfunctional C1 inhibitor, and plasma C4 concentrations are usually low both during and between exacerbations.

In vitro detection of specific IgE is safer than allergy skin testing, but allergy skin testing is more sensitive and with appropriate precautions is safe for allergy to penicillin and Hymenoptera venom. In vitro testing is not available for all allergens.

TREATMENT. Effective treatment depends on prompt diagnosis and rapid implementation of appropriate therapy. The treatment of choice is aqueous epinephrine, 1:1,000, 0.01 mL/kg (maximum 0.3 mL for a child or 0.5 mL for an adult) by intramuscular injection, which can result in higher plasma concentrations and more rapid attainment of effective concentrations than can subcutaneous administration. If necessary, this dose may be repeated at 15-min intervals. If the reaction is to injection of an allergen extract or to a Hymenoptera sting on an extremity, one half of this dose of epinephrine may be diluted in 2 mL normal saline and infiltrated subcutaneously at the site of the injection or sting to slow absorption. A tourniquet above the site can also slow systemic distribution of the allergen. The tourniquet can be loosened after improvement or briefly at intervals of 3 min.

A persistent, serious reaction can be treated cautiously with careful cardiac monitoring of the intravenous infusion of epinephrine at an initial infusion rate of 0.1 μg/kg/min in a child (or 2 μg/min in an adult) to sustain a systolic blood pressure of 80 mm Hg

Supplemental oxygen (100%, 4–6 L/min) is indicated. Extension of the neck and use of an oropharyngeal airway may be helpful for upper airway obstruction. Endotracheal intubation may be necessary; if this cannot be accomplished, cricothyrotomy is indicated for laryngeal obstruction. Nebulized albuterol and intravenous aminophylline are effective for treatment of lower airway obstruction as in the treatment of asthma.

If hypotension is unresponsive to administration of epinephrine by subcutaneous injection, rapid intravenous administration of isotonic saline is indicated (up to 100 mL/min to a limit of 3 L for an adult). A supine position with the feet elevated is helpful. Extreme or persistent hypotension may require treatment with norepinephrine by intravenous infusion or dopamine.

An H_1 antagonist such as diphenhydramine, 1 mg/kg, by intramuscular injection or intravenous infusion may be helpful for hypotension as well as urticaria. Combined use of an H_1 antagonist and an H_2 antagonist such as cimetidine, 4 mg/kg (maximum 300 mg), infused intravenously over at least 5 min, may be more helpful than diphenhydramine alone.

Systemic adrenal corticosteroids are appropriate after treatment of the initial manifestations of anaphylaxis, although it is uncertain whether they are helpful in preventing biphasic reactions.

If the only manifestations of anaphylaxis have been urticaria or angioedema and the patient will not be far from medical care, observation is not necessary long after resolution of the cutaneous signs and symptoms; it is prudent for such patients to receive epinephrine initially because of possible progression of involvement to other systems. It is safest to continue observation of patients who have had hypotension or airway obstruction for at least 12 hr because of possible recurrence of the initial life-threatening manifestations.

PREVENTION. Serious anaphylactoid reactions to intravenous radiocontrast media are less common in children than in adults but occur occasionally. A prophylactic regimen for patients known to be at risk by virtue of previous reactions consists of prednisone, 50 mg orally every 6 hr for three doses, ending 1 hr before the procedure, and diphenhydramine, 50 mg, given by intramuscular injection 1 hr before the procedure. This regimen prevents adverse reactions of any degree in more than 90% of high-risk adult patients.

The incidence of drug-induced anaphylaxis would drop substantially if drugs were given only when indicated and only by the oral route unless some compelling reason for injection exists. Not only is anaphylactic sensitivity more easily induced by injection of drugs than by oral administration but also in the sensitized patient anaphylaxis occurs more commonly following parenteral than oral administration. The incidence of anaphylaxis following Hymenoptera stings can be reduced significantly by the appropriate use of venom immunotherapy (see Chapters 143 and 151).

Patients with histories of systemic anaphylaxis after eating egg may rarely be at special risk for anaphylaxis after administration of vaccines that contain egg protein, including influenza vaccine and yellow fever vaccine. The Committee on Infectious Diseases of the American Academy of Pediatrics has recommended administration of such vaccines to patients with such histories only after prick and intradermal testing with the vaccine has not elicited a positive reaction or administration with desensitization if a skin test with the vaccine has produced positive results. Measles, mumps, and measles-mumps-rubella (MMR) vaccines previously were included among vaccines with such precautions, but anaphylaxis can follow administration of these vaccines whether or not there is a history of allergy to egg, and the vast majority of egg allergic children can tolerate MMR vaccine without any significant adverse reaction. Such reactions may be due to allergy to gelatin, suggesting a need for caution in patients who have reacted adversely to gum drops or Jell-O. It is prudent to perform skin tests on egg-allergic children with influenza vaccine or yellow fever vaccine to evaluate the safety of administration of the vaccine, but skin testing with MMR vaccine is not necessary. Administration of any of these vaccines in all children should be supervised carefully with preparations for treatment of anaphylaxis if it should occur.

Only powder-free, low-allergen latex gloves should be use in health care facilities to reduce the risk to patients and health care personnel. Patients with latex allergy should be cautioned about sources of exposure and potential cross-reacting foods and are advised to acquire a supply of latex-free examination gloves to carry with them to health facilities that may not be appropriately equipped.

All patients who have had anaphylaxis should always be equipped with injectable epinephrine for use in an emergency and advised that its purpose is to enable them to reach an emergency facility. They should wear Medic-Alert emblems to identify their risks of anaphylaxis.

Patients who have had food-dependent, exercise-induced anaphylaxis should defer strenuous exercise for at least 6 hr after eating a meal and for 12 hr after consuming a previously implicated specific food.

American College of Allergy, Asthma and Immunology and American Academy of Allergy, Asthma and Immunology: AAAI and ACAAI Joint Statement concerning the use of powdered and non-powdered natural rubber latex gloves. Ann Allergy Asthma Immunol 79:487, 1997.

Baldwin JL, Chou AH, Solomon WR: Popsicle-induced anaphylaxis due to carmine dye allergy. Ann Allergy Asthma Immunol 79:415, 1997.

Ditto AM, Krasnick J, Greenberger PA, et al: Pediatric idiopatic anaphylaxis: Experience with 22 patients. J Allergy Clin Immunol 100:320, 1997.

Kelly KJ, Pearson ML, Kurup VP, et al: A cluster of anaphylactic reactions in children with spina bifida during general anesthesia: Epidemiologic features, risk factors, and latex hypersensitivity. J Allergy Clin Immunol 94:53, 1994.

Landwehr LP, Boguniewicz M: Current perspectives on latex allergy. J Pediatr 128:305, 1996.

Novembre E, Cianferoni A, Bernardini R, et al: Anaphylaxis in children. Clinical and allergologic features. Pediatrics 101:1, 1998.

Romano A, Di Fonso M, Giuffreda F, et al: Diagnostic work-up for food-dependent, exercise-induced anaphylaxis. Allergy 50:817, 1995.

Simons FER, Roberts JR, Gu X, Simons KJ: Epinephrine absorption in children with a history of anaphylaxis. J Allergy Clin Immunol 101:33, 1998.

Tiles S, Schocket A, Milgrom H: Exercise-induced anaphylaxis related to specific foods. J Pediatr 127:587, 1995.

CHAPTER 149

Serum Sickness

Serum sickness is a hypersensitivity vasculitis that follows the administration of foreign antigenic material.

ETIOLOGY. The disorder was first described as a consequence of antitoxin therapy for diseases such as diphtheria and tetanus. The illness was shown to be due to an adverse reaction to the serum proteins of the animal in which the antitoxin was prepared. Therapeutic antisera of animal origin, especially equine, are still occasionally used, but today the major cause of the serum sickness syndrome is drug allergy, particularly that caused by penicillin. Instances have also followed the use of other therapeutic agents, including human gamma globulin and even Hymenoptera stings. Preparations of immunoglobulin of human origin are available for treatment of diphtheria and tetanus (and prophylaxis of rabies) in humans, but antitoxins for treatment of crotalid envenomation and clostridial intoxication (botulism, gas gangrene) are still prepared in the horse.

PATHOGENESIS. Serum sickness is the classic example of a type III hypersensitivity, "immune complex" disease in the experimental animal. The symptoms of serum sickness occur coincidentally with the appearance of antibody formed against the injected antigen, at a time when the latter is still present in the circulation. Antigen-antibody complexes formed under conditions of moderate antigen excess lodge in small vessels and in filtering organs throughout the body (deposition being aided in the rabbit by the actions of IgE antibody, basophils, and platelet-activating factor and by the release of vasoactive amines that increase the permeability of blood vessels); these complexes activate the complement sequence. Complement components bound at the site of immune complex deposition promote accumulation of neutrophils through at least two general processes: adherence of neutrophils to the site of bound complement and chemotactic activity of the C567 complex and C3a and C5a fragments. Tissue injury results from the liberation of toxic molecules from the neutrophils. Healing of the lesions occurs following elimination of the complexes from the circulation.

Serum sickness demonstrates how the differing biologic activities of the several species of antibodies formed against a complex antigen may be responsible for diverse parts of the clinical picture; the urticaria of serum sickness is thought to be due to IgE antibody molecules reacting with horse serum proteins, whereas the joint symptoms are thought to occur as a result of deposition of antigen-antibody complexes of the IgG and IgM classes. It is suspected that histamine release from basophils and mast cells, mediated by IgE antibodies, facilitates the deposition of immune complexes through increases in vascular permeability.

CLINICAL MANIFESTATIONS. Typically, the symptoms of serum sickness begin 7–12 days following injection of the foreign material but may appear as late as 3 wk afterward. If there has been earlier exposure or previous allergic reaction to the same foreign antigen, symptoms may appear in accelerated fashion, within 1–3 days following injection, or as anaphylaxis. Fever and malaise are almost always present, as are cutaneous eruptions. Urticaria, usually generalized, is a common finding. Faint erythema with a serpiginous border at the margins of palmar or plantar skin of the hands, fingers, feet, and toes may precede the generalized cutaneous eruption. This characteristic cutaneous lesion may become purpuric with time. Edema, particularly around the face and neck, facial flushing, myalgia, lymphadenopathy, arthralgia, or arthritis involving multiple joints (ankle, knee, wrist, fingers, toes), and gastrointestinal complaints (cramping, diarrhea, nausea) also occur. Intense pruritus accompanying the urticaria is the most distressing symptoms in many patients. The site of injection of the foreign material generally becomes red and swollen, commonly 1–3 days before systemic symptoms appear. The disease generally runs a self-limited course, and the patient recovers in 7–10 days. Carditis and glomerulonephritis occur rarely; the most serious complications of serum sickness are Guillain-Barré syndrome and peripheral neuritis, especially involving the brachial plexus (C5–6).

LABORATORY MANIFESTATIONS. The blood leukocyte and eosinophil counts are variable; marked thrombocytopenia is often found. Mild proteinuria, hemoglobinuria, and microscopic hematuria may be seen. Plasma cells have been found in blood. The erythrocyte sedimentation rate is often increased. A sheep cell agglutinin titer of the Forssman type is usually elevated. Serum complement levels (C3 and C4) are variably depressed and may fall to low concentrations around the 10th day. C3a anaphylatoxin may be increased. In serum sickness caused by horse serum proteins, antibodies of the IgG, IgA, IgM, and IgE classes may be found directed against various horse serum proteins. Direct immunofluorescence studies of skin lesions often reveal immune deposits of IgM, IgA, IgE, or C3.

TREATMENT. Patients generally respond well to aspirin and antihistamines. When the symptoms are especially severe, corticosteroids have been used with great efficacy. High doses are given and rapidly reduced as the patient improves. Plasmapheresis can be helpful for severe serum sickness not responsive to these measures.

PREVENTION. The use of horse serum or other animal serum in therapy should be limited to cases for which no alternative is available. When only equine antitoxin is available, skin tests should be employed prior to administration of serum, beginning with a puncture test using a 1:10 dilution. If the reaction is negative, one may then begin intradermal testing with 0.02 mL of a 1:10,000 dilution. If there is no reaction, a subsequent skin test should be performed with a 1:1,000 dilution. If a negative result again is obtained, a final intradermal test with a 1:100 dilution of horse serum is performed. A negative reaction to the strongest solution indicates that anaphylactic sensitivity to horse serum is unlikely; skin tests do not predict the likelihood of development of serum sickness.

Occasionally, patients who have evidence of anaphylactic sensitivity to horse serum by virtue of either a previous reaction or a positive immediate wheal and flare skin test require treatment with horse serum. In such a case, the antitoxin can be successfully administered by a process of rapid desensitization. Some allergists medicate the patient with epinephrine and antihistamines before beginning the desensitization procedure. Others prefer not to mask possible evidence of a reaction at an early stage when it still might be of a minor degree and serve as a warning to proceed more slowly with the desensitization. The desensitization process is begun with 0.1-mL amounts of antitoxin, diluted to 1:100,000–1:10,000, depending on an estimate of the degree of the patient's sensitivity, and injected intravenously at 20-min intervals. If the patient tolerates the previous injection without adverse reactions, the amount administered may be doubled every 20 min. Generally, the entire amount of antitoxin can be administered safely over a 4- to 6-hr period. The desensitization, unfortunately, is transient, and the patient often regains the previous anaphylactic sensitivity within a few months. Administration of methylprednisolone in doses of 1–1.5 mg/kg/24 hr has not prevented the development of serum sickness.

Bielory L, Gascon P, Lawley T, et al: Human serum sickness: A prospective analysis of 35 patients treated with equine antithymocyte globulin for bone marrow failure. Medicine 67:40, 1988.
Kunnamo I, Kallio P, Pelkonen P, et al: Serum sickness–like disease is a common cause of acute arthritis in children. Acta Pediatr Scand 75:964, 1986.
Ledford DK: Immunologic aspects of vasculitis and cardiovascular disease. JAMA 278:1962, 1997.
Reisman RE, Livingston A: Late-onset allergic reactions, including serum sickness, after insect stings. J Allergy Clin Immunol 84:331, 1989.

CHAPTER 150
Adverse Reactions to Drugs

(See Chapter 727)

DEFINITION. An adverse reaction to a drug may be defined as any unwanted consequence of administration of the agent during or following a course of therapy. Adverse reactions fall into two broad categories: those dependent on pharmacologic mechanisms and those dependent on immunologic mechanisms (Table 150–1). The majority of adverse drug reactions are pharmacologic; only 6% have an allergic basis. In a study of hospitalized children who had adverse drug reactions, no more than 15% were thought to be of an allergic nature.

Certain generalities apply to adverse drug reactions: (1) Virtually any organ system may be involved. (2) After the neonatal period, children are affected less often than are adults. (3) The incidence of reactions increases almost exponentially with the number of drugs given concurrently. (4) Certain diseases predispose to adverse drug reactions, especially those in which multiple drug therapy is common (cardiovascular, infectious, and psychiatric illnesses). Diseases that affect organs responsible for absorption (gastrointestinal tract), metabolism (liver), or excretion of drugs (kidney) also increase the likelihood of adverse reactions. (5) The pharmacokinetic properties of a drug (e.g., the extent of protein binding) also affect the incidence of adverse reactions.

CLASSIFICATION. Adverse drug reactions can be classified in terms of their underlying mechanisms. Toxicity may result from a high concentration of drug in the body caused by excessive intake—accidental or intentional—or from abnormalities in absorption, metabolism, or excretion of the drug. Various diseases, genetic factors, or drug interactions may permit accumulation of a drug. Some patients, for unknown reasons, have excessive pharmacologic responses (intolerance) to average drug doses. The signs and symptoms are generally intensifications of the expected pharmacologic effects of the agent.

Side effects are undesirable but essentially unavoidable effects of drugs and largely reflect the fact that a given drug rarely affects only one tissue. When theophylline is given as a bronchodilator agent in asthma, for example, central nervous system stimulation is considered a side effect, although this latter effect of theophylline warrants its use in neonatal apnea. Secondary effects of drugs are those not related to their primary pharmacologic actions. An example is disturbance of the bacterial flora of the intestine as a consequence of antibiotic therapy. In drug idiosyncrasy, the signs and symptoms of the reaction are unrelated to the known pharmacologic properties of the agent, sometimes because of metabolic abnormalities. An example is the hemolytic anemia that follows ingestion of primaquine in patients with glucose-6-phosphate dehydrogenase deficiency (see Chapter 469.3).

Drug interactions are discussed in Chapter 727; see also Table 728–1.

Allergic drug reactions occur on the basis of recognized models of immune injury. These include (1) IgE-mediated reactions; (2) cytotoxic reactions resulting from hapten binding to cell membranes and subsequent reaction with antihapten antibodies; (3) immune complex reactions in which drug-antibody immune complexes with affinity for cell membranes activate the complement system, resulting in cell membrane damage; (4) reactions caused by autoantibody formation; and (5) reactions caused by cell-mediated mechanisms. Most drugs are simple chemicals with molecular weights of less than 1,000d and are rarely immunogenic. Substances with low molecular weights may act as haptens and become immunogenic after covalent chemical binding with tissue proteins to form drug-protein conjugates. Hapten–protein complex formation is necessary for the macrophage–T cell–B cell interaction that leads to formation of hapten-specific humoral antibodies and cellular immunity. In general, only drugs (or their degradative or metabolic products) with sufficient chemical reactivity to bind irreversibly with proteins are capable of inducing hypersensitivity reactions. The major impediment to both study and diagnosis of drug allergy is that the chemically reactive substance is often not the native drug itself but a metabolic or degradative product. Because little is known about the metabolic fate of many drugs in common use, it is often impossible to identify the chemically reactive intermediates necessary for investigative or diagnostic use.

The complexities of understanding allergic reactions to drugs are illustrated by considering the penicillin model. Benzyl penicillin (penicillin G) has produced a wide variety of allergic reactions, including systemic responses such as anaphylaxis, serum sickness, and vasculitis; hematologic disorders, including hemolytic anemia, thrombocytopenia, and granulocytopenia; a broad spectrum of cutaneous eruptions; pulmonary disease; and renal disease (see Table 150–1). Under physiologic conditions, both in vivo and in vitro, a number of highly protein-reactive compounds are formed from penicillin. These metabolic products become immunogenic following conjugation with tissue proteins, as described earlier. The penicilloyl group, formed by the combination of benzyl penicillenic acid with amino groups of proteins, is the antigenic determinant formed in largest amounts. Ninety-five per cent of all benzyl penicillin that conjugates with tissue proteins in vivo forms benzylpenicilloyl haptenic groups (BPO), and thus benzyl penicillin has been designated the "major" haptenic determinant of penicillin hypersensitivity. A large percentage of individuals who have been treated with penicillin possess antibodies to the BPO determinant, but most do not experience symptoms of penicillin allergy. BPO-specific IgE antibodies can be detected through a BPO-polylysine skin test reagent in which BPO haptenic groups are attached to a "backbone" of lysine. BPO polylysine is available as a skin test reagent and for coupling to cyanogen bromide-activated disks in the radioallergosorbent test (RAST).

Unfortunately, the most feared consequence of penicillin allergy, anaphylaxis, usually is not due to IgE sensitization to the major BPO haptenic group but to less well defined, so-called minor haptenic determinants. These include penicilloate, penilloate, and penicillenate and its oxidation products. Although only 5% or less of the benzyl penicillin that reacts with proteins forms minor haptenic determinants, they have major clinical significance; unfortunately, antigens with minor

TABLE 150–1 Adverse Drug Reactions

Reaction	Example	Comment
Drug Allergy		
Type I IgE–mediated hypersensitivity	Penicillin, insulin, cephalosporins	Urticaria, wheezing, anaphylaxis
Type II cytotoxic antibodies	Penicillin—hemolytic anemia Quinidine—thrombocytopenia	Drug-hapten interaction
Type III immune complex	Penicillin, sulfonamides, cephalosporins (especially cefaclor)	Serum sickness
Type IV cell-mediated	Neosporin contact dermatitis, topical antihistamines	T lymphocyte–dependent
Possibly Allergic–Immune		
Drug-induced systemic lupus erythematosus	Hydralazine, phenytoin, penicillamine, INH	Immune complex; low incidence of cerebral, renal disease; positive antihistone antibodies
Anticonvulsant hypersensitivity	Phenytoin, phenobarbital, carbamazepine-induced rash, hepatitis, lymphadenopathy, pneumonitis, fever	Hereditary abnormal drug metabolism produces toxic metabolites that damage target cells such as lymphocytes
Sulfonamide hypersensitivity	Rash, fever, lymphadenopathy	Same as above
Drug fever	Antibiotic, phenytoin	± Eosinophilia, recurrence with rechallenge
Mucocutaneous reactions	Stevens-Johnson syndrome (sulfonamides) Toxic epidermal necrolysis (penicillin, sulfonamides, phenytoin) Fixed drug eruption (penicillin) Erythema nodosum (oral contraceptive agents) Photoallergic reactions (sulfonamides) Trimethoprim-sulfamethoxazole–induced rash, neutropenia in AIDS	Presumed allergy but mechanisms undetermined
Pulmonary hypersensitivity	Asthma (aspirin) Pulmonary infiltrates with eosinophilia (sulfonamides)	Alters prostaglandin production Unknown, possible lymphocyte sensitization
Hepatic hypersensitivity	Cholestasis (phenothiazine, sulfonamides) Hepatocellular (INH, hydralazine)	Unknown
Renal hypersensitivity	Interstitial nephritis (penicillins)	High IgE, eosinophiluria
Pseudoallergic		
Anaphylactoid	Radiocontrast, D-tubocurarine, opiates	Direct mast cell degranulation
Ampicillin rash	With or without EBV infection	Unknown cause; onset 7th day without EBV infection
β-Blocking agents	Asthma	Bronchoconstriction
Nonallergic		
Drug overdose	Acetaminophen	Toxic metabolite
Drug-drug interaction	Erythromycin-theophylline	Toxic theophylline levels as erythromycin inhibits cytochrome P450 metabolism
Drug side effect	Sedation—antihistamines Impaired excretion	Predictable Renal-hepatic insufficiency
Secondary effects	Antibiotics—perianal candidiasis	Predictable
Drug idiosyncrasy	Phenytoin Glucose-6-phosphate dehydrogenase deficiency and hemolysis (sulfonamides) Malignant hyperthermia (halothane)	May be genetically determined (see above) Genetically determined enzyme deficiency Genetic abnormality in muscle contraction
Drug teratogenicity	Thalidomide	Maturational-differential effects in fetus
Coincidental	Development of viral rash while receiving therapy with antibiotics	Common in children
Psychogenic	Nausea, abdominal pain despite placebo, or drug unlikely to produce symptoms Placebo effect	

INH = isoniazid; AIDS = acquired immunodeficiency syndrome; EBV = Epstein-Barr virus.

determinant specificity are not readily available for testing either in vivo or in vitro.

Allergy to benzyl penicillin is further complicated by the development of related semisynthetic penicillins and cephalosporins that share a degree of immunologic cross-reactivity. Among the penicillins, the specificity of the antibody formed by the patient (e.g., whether directed toward the 6-aminopenicillin acid core common to all penicillins or directed toward a unique determinant on a distinctive side chain) determines the degree of cross-allergenicity. Thus, some patients allergic to benzyl penicillin can tolerate the semisynthetic penicillins and vice versa. Although substantially different structurally, penicillin and cephalosporins share the highly protein-reactive β-lactam ring structure. As many as 5.6% of patients with a history of reactions to penicillin and positive skin test results to penicillin who receive a cephalosporin may have allergic reactions, including anaphylaxis, compared with 1.7% of those with negative skin test results to penicillin. Early reports of reactions to first-generation cephalosporins may overestimate the risk because of contamination with small amounts of penicillin. Postmarketing data from pharmaceutical companies indicate overall adverse reaction rates to cephalosporins of 1 to 10%, with rates of anaphylaxis less than 0.02% and little or no increase in rates for patients with a history of allergy to penicillin.

Adverse reactions to ampicillin occur in 10% of patients who receive the drug and merit special consideration. The typical ampicillin rash is not urticarial and appears in 90% of patients with infectious mononucleosis and also in patients with hyperuricemia. That the rash causes no other ill effects and typically disappears with continuing therapy casts doubt on its immunologic nature; the pathogenesis of ampicillin rash remains an enigma. However, allergy to ampicillin manifested by an urticarial eruption may occur in 1% of children treated with the drug.

RISK FACTORS. As many as 25% of children with at least one parent with allergy to an antimicrobial drug may be at risk for the development of allergy to antibiotics compared with less than 2% when neither parent has drug allergy. Atopic patients are not at increased risk for drug allergy but may be at risk for more severe reactions if they do acquire drug allergy. Patients with a history of allergy to an antibiotic may have as much as a ninefold increased risk of allergy developing to an unrelated antibiotic.

More than half of patients with acquired immunodeficiency syndrome experience adverse reactions to trimethoprim-sulfamethoxazole, and more than half of patients infected with human immunodeficiency virus and CD4+ cell counts of less than 200/μL may experience cutaneous eruptions during treatment with amoxicillin-clavulanate. The susceptibility of such patients to adverse reactions to drugs may be due to impairment of T-cell regulation of IgE production.

Other risk factors include the dose of the drug, route of administration, and duration and frequency of administration. Penicillin-induced hemolytic anemia follows administration of large doses. Topical administration of a drug is more likely to elicit sensitization than is parenteral administration; oral administration is least likely to sensitize. Prolonged, continual treatment is less likely to cause sensitization than frequent, intermittent therapy.

CLINICAL MANIFESTATIONS. Cutaneous eruptions are the most common manifestation of adverse drug reactions in children. Urticarial, exanthematous, and eczematoid eruptions predominate, but almost any morphologic condition can occur: exfoliative dermatitis (penicillin, sulfonamides, phenothiazines, anticonvulsants), bullous dermatoses (including epidermal necrolysis), erythema multiforme, Stevens-Johnson syndrome (sulfonamides, penicillin, barbiturates, anticonvulsants, phenytoin in particular), petechial eruptions, Lyell's syndrome (penicillin, barbiturates, anticonvulsants, isoniazid), acneiform eruptions (iodides in postpubertal patients), lichenoid eruptions, photodermatitis (demethylchlortetracycline and phenothiazines), and fixed drug eruptions.

Renal or pulmonary disease following drug therapy rarely occurs during childhood. There have been occasional reports of interstitial nephritis associated with phenytoin with in vitro evidence of a cellular immune reaction. In a child being treated with nitrofurantoin, fever, cough, and pulmonary infiltration strongly suggest an adverse drug reaction.

When a child who has received prolonged antimicrobial therapy has persistent fever without other cause, drug fever should be considered. Drug fever is often suspected but rarely proved and does not generally occur as the sole manifestation of an adverse drug reaction. There is often a concomitant rash; there may be eosinophilia, leukocytosis, and an increased erythrocyte sedimentation rate. The diagnosis is easily made when the drug is discontinued and defervescence occurs within 24–48 hr.

Immunologically mediated, drug-induced reactions involving the liver are extremely rare in children, unlike the case in adults. The same is true for drug-induced disorders of granulocytes and platelets; the overwhelming majority of these are toxic.

DIAGNOSIS. Diagnosis of an allergic drug reaction depends on a careful history. Urticaria or angioedema following use of a drug is more relevant than nondescript rashes, because urticaria is often due to IgE-mediated reactions. Even under the best of circumstances, however, a definitive diagnosis of an allergic drug reaction is frequently difficult to establish.

Penicillin is the only drug for which allergy skin testing is of well-established reliability in identifying anaphylactic hypersensitivity. Skin testing with benzylpenicilloyl-polylysine (BPL; PrePen) and penicillin G identifies the overwhelming majority of children who are at risk for anaphylactic reactions following penicillin administration. The BPL is tested in a concentration of 6.0×10^{-5} M (as supplied by the manufacturer), first by prick or puncture test and, if negative, by intradermal test according to the manufacturer's instructions. Benzyl penicillin (penicillin G) supplied as potassium penicillin G for injection, USP 1,000,000 U/vial is freshly diluted with saline to a concentration of 10,000 U/mL. It is prudent to begin testing with a further 100-fold dilution of penicillin G if there is a history of a life-threatening, systemic reaction to penicillin within the previous year. Penicillin G is first tested by prick or puncture and then by intradermal technique up to a final concentration of 10,000 U/mL. If the skin test results (interpreted in much the same way as skin tests with pollen or other allergenic extracts; see Chapter 143.2) are negative, anaphylaxis is highly unlikely and, if there is a compelling reason to do so, treatment may be initiated with a small test dose, usually one tenth of the usual dose, given either intravenously or orally. It is, however, impossible to exclude anaphylactic sensitivity due to other haptenic determinants formed in vivo from penicillin for which no skin test reagents are available. Furthermore, penicillin skin tests are predictive only of anaphylaxis and not of serum sickness or other reactions associated with use of the drug. Skin testing with cephalosporins and other β-lactam antibiotics has not been standardized, although some authorities have recommended prick and intradermal testing with concentrations no stronger than 3 mg/mL.

Patch testing to determine delayed hypersensitivity to a drug is helpful; it should be carried out by someone familiar with the technique to avoid both false-positive and false-negative reactions resulting from improper procedure.

In vitro testing for detection of BPO-specific IgE antibodies is as specific as skin testing but less sensitive. RAST for the other haptenic determinants of penicillin allergy is not available. As is the case with other allergens, the properly performed skin test is preferred to RAST because of speed, sensitivity, and cost. Search for serum antibodies to formed elements of the blood in patients with what appear to be drug-induced blood disorders is rarely productive. Assays of cellular immunity have been used in the investigation of drug allergy. Their validity in this context has not been established.

TREATMENT. Therapy depends on the mechanism of drug reaction and the clinical manifestations. Discontinuation of the drug is usually indicated. Under certain conditions, especially in infants and small children who experience rashes while receiving antibiotics, the circumstances may support a decision to continue administration of the drug until the cause of the rash becomes clear. If, for example, an infant or small child with a febrile illness experiences an exanthematous and non-urticarial rash on first exposure to penicillin, ampicillin, or another antibiotic, the rash is more likely that of a viral illness than a cutaneous manifestation of allergy to the drug. Rather than labeling the child allergic to the drug on tenuous grounds and compromising its future use, it may be reasonable to continue therapy for a further period while the course of the rash is observed. If the history suggests that an adverse reaction has a pharmacologic basis, the drug may be introduced at a later date, at a lower dosage, or at a longer interval between doses while the serum concentration of the drug is measured, if possible. Ampicillin presents a special problem. There is little to suggest an allergic basis to the most common rash. If there are special circumstances that dictate the need for the drug, therapy may be continued with the expectation that the rash will disappear and no other problems will develop.

Conversely, if an allergic cause is likely, the drug should not be reintroduced into the patient, and an alternative drug should be sought. Usually, there are many possible alternative drugs available for treatment of patients with allergy to penicillin and cephalosporins. Imipenem often has allergenic cross-reactivity with penicillin but aztreonam does not. Patients allergic to ampicillin but not to penicillin may be allergic to cephalexin; those allergic to amoxicillin but not to penicillin may be allergic to cephadroxil, although most tolerate cephadroxil. Other cephalosporins have unique side chains and probably are unlikely to have allergenic cross-reactivity. Most patients with allergy to semisynthetic penicillins are allergic to penicillin, but in some, allergy is due to the unique side chain, and they may tolerate penicillin. Allergy to phenoxymethylpenicillin (penicillin V) can rarely occur without allergy to penicillin G. Erythromycin, azithromycin, clarithromycin, sulfonamides, a tetracycline, clindamycin, vancomycin, or chloramphenicol may be a suitable alternative for patients with allergy to penicillins and multiple cephalosporins.

When treatment with penicillin is mandatory despite documented allergy to the drug, desensitization may be possible. Fatal anaphylaxis has occurred during parenteral desensitization with penicillin. Oral desensitization is probably safer (Table 150–2). No fatal or life-threatening reactions have been reported in association with oral desensitization to penicillin, but pruritus and cutaneous eruptions have occurred commonly, and serum sickness has occurred rarely. A history of toxic epidermal necrolysis, Stevens-Johnson syndrome, or erythema multiforme is a contraindication to desensitization or challenge with the drug; occurrence of any of these during desensitization indicates a need for immediate discontinuation. Treatment of systemic anaphylaxis is discussed in Chapter 148.

Cutaneous eruptions are the most common manifestation of drug allergy in children. The eruptions are generally self-limited and disappear when the drugs are discontinued. Treatment is therefore symptomatic. Antihistamines are most useful for urticarial rashes. Diphenhydramine (Benadryl) and hydroxyzine (Atarax, Vistaril) have both antihistaminic and sedative properties, which may be useful; loratadine or cetirizine is appropriate when sedation is not desirable. Epinephrine 1:1,000 in doses of 0.1–0.3 mL provides short-term relief. For a more sustained effect, a suspension of epinephrine (Sus-Phrine) in doses of 0.1–0.2 mL may be given subcutaneously every 6 hr. Corticosteroids are reserved for severe cases not relieved by the foregoing measures. The dose and dosage interval are determined by the severity of the reaction.

TABLE 150–2 Oral Desensitization to Penicillin and Other β-Lactam Antibiotics in Patients with Specific Anaphylactic Hypersensitivity to the Drug*

Step	Drug Concentration (mg/mL)	Volume (mL)	Dose Administered (mg)
1	0.5	0.1	0.05
2	0.5	0.2	0.10
3	0.5	0.4	0.20
4	0.5	0.8	0.40
5	0.5	1.6	0.80
6	0.5	3.2	1.60
7	0.5	6.4	3.20
8	5.0	1.2	6.00
9	5.0	2.4	12.00
10	5.0	4.8	24.00
11	50.0	1.0	50.00
12	50.0	2.0	100.00
13	50.0	4.0	200.00
14	50.0	8.0	400.00

**Dilute successive doses in 30 mL of water and administer by mouth at intervals of 15 min. Observe the patient for 30 min after completion of desensitization and then administer 1 g of the same drug by intravenous infusion.*

PREVENTION. To minimize adverse drug reactions, physicians should use drugs only when indicated, be wary of new drugs, and know the relationships between drugs. Anaphylaxis to penicillin can follow nontherapeutic exposure, including sexual intercourse with a partner receiving penicillin and handling penicillin formulations. Concurrent use of two or more drugs should be avoided unless definitely indicated. Oral administration is less sensitizing than parenteral administration and is preferred whenever possible. Topical application should be avoided when possible because of increased risk of sensitization by this route. Drug interactions should be anticipated, and patients should be warned against self-medication.

Anne S, Reisman RE: Risk of administering cephalosporin antibiotics to patients with histories of penicillin allergy. Ann Allergy Asthma Immunol 74:167, 1995.

Blanca M, Carmona MJ, Moreno F, et al: Selective immediate allergic response to penicillin V. Allergy 51:960, 1996.

Blanca M, Garcia J, Vega JM, et al: Anaphylaxis to penicillins after non-therapeutic exposure: An immunological investigation. Clin Exp Allergy 26:335, 1996.

deShazo RD, Kemp SF: Allergic reactions to drugs and biologic agents. JAMA 278:1895, 1997.

Marcos Bravo C, Luna Ortiz I, Gonzalez Vazquez R: Hypersensitivity to cefuroxime with good tolerance to other betalactams. Allergy 50:359, 1995.

Matthews KP: Clinical spectrum of allergic and pseudoallergic drug reactions. J Allergy Clin Immunol 74:558, 1984.

Sastre J, Quijano L-D, Novalbos A, et al: Clinical cross-reactivity between amoxicillin and cephadroxil in patients allergic to amoxicillin and with good tolerance of penicillin. Allergy 51:383, 1996.

Stark BJ, Earl HS, Gross GN, et al: Acute and chronic desensitization of penicillin-allergic patients using oral penicillin. J Allergy Clin Immunol 79:523, 1987.

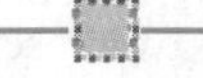

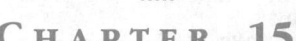

CHAPTER 151
Insect Allergy

(See also Chapter 724)

Allergic reactions to insects can cause (1) symptoms of respiratory allergy as a result of inhalation of particulate matter of insect origin, (2) local cutaneous reactions to insect bites, and (3) anaphylactic reactions to stinging insects.

ETIOLOGY. Sensitization to antigenic material found in the debris and disintegrated bodies of dead insects can cause conjunctivitis, rhinitis, or asthma. Inhalation of scales from the wings of insects such as the mayfly, caddis fly, and moths is a particularly common cause of respiratory symptoms in the U.S. Great Lakes area, where large numbers of these insects appear each summer. Local cutaneous reactions commonly follow bites by mosquitoes, flies, and various insects. Anaphylactic reactions of both immediate (IgE-mediated) and delayed (T lymphocyte) hypersensitivity resulting from insect allergy are almost entirely caused by Hymenoptera, including the apids (honeybee, bumblebee), the vespids (wasp, hornet, yellow jacket) and, rarely, the ant family. About 0.4–0.8% of individuals give histories of systemic reactions to stinging insects, which cause approximately 40 deaths each year in the United States.

PATHOGENESIS. Inhalant allergy to insects is in many cases due to IgE-mediated sensitivity to antigenic materials found in the insects' bodies. The antigenic components responsible for respiratory symptoms have not been thoroughly studied, but the allergenic material appears usually to reside in the cuticle or integument of the insect's body.

In the case of biting insects, the local reaction is frequently a wheal and flare lesion; it appears to be due to vasoactive or irritant materials deposited in the skin while the insect is feeding. There is no evidence for IgE involvement in the local reaction. The mechanism of late or persisting cutaneous reactions is unknown.

Stinging insect venoms contain at least nine components that may contribute to adverse reactions. They include vasoactive materials such as histamine, acetylcholine, and kinins; a number of enzymes (phospholipase A and B, hyaluronidase); apamine; melitin; and formic acid. Phospholipase A, hyaluronidase, melitin, and probably acid phosphatase are the four major allergens of honeybee venom. Phospholipase, hyaluronidase, and antigen 5 are the three major allergens of vespid venoms. Some antigens in Hymenoptera venom and whole body extracts are common to the Hymenoptera order; others are family-specific. There is substantial cross-reactivity among vespid venoms. The majority of patients who experience systemic reactions following Hymenoptera stings have IgE-mediated sensitivity to antigenic material in the venom. There are, however, patients with convincing histories of sting anaphylaxis in whom both skin test and radioallergosorbent test (RAST) results to venoms are negative. Children may have a systemic reaction with the first sting.

CLINICAL MANIFESTATIONS. The clinical findings in inhalant allergy caused by insects are similar to those seen with the usual inhalant allergens such as pollens. Rhinitis, conjunctivitis, and asthma have all been described.

The cutaneous reactions to biting insects are most often urticarial but may be papular, vesicular, and erythematous, particularly as the lesion progresses. Lesions that resemble typical delayed hypersensitivity reactions also occur.

Clinical reactions to stinging venomous insects range in severity from minimal pain and local erythema to life-threatening anaphylactic episodes. The usual reaction is swelling of less than 4–5 cm, lasting less than 24 hr. Large local reactions have more swelling and are of longer duration than the usual reaction. Systemic non–life-threatening reactions include multiple cutaneous lesions distal to the site of envenomation (e.g., generalized urticaria, angioedema, pruritus). Life-threatening, immediate systemic reactions are similar to anaphylaxis (laryngeal edema, bronchospasm, hypotension, urticaria). Children with large local or mild systemic reactions rarely experience subsequent severe anaphylaxis. A toxic nonallergic reaction of fever, malaise, emesis, and nausea often follows multiple stings and is rarely fatal. Serum sickness, nephrotic syndrome, vasculitis, neuritis, or encephalopathy may be seen as late sequelae of the reaction to stinging insects.

DIAGNOSIS. The diagnosis is usually easily made from the history and, in the case of biting insects, by examination of skin lesions. Papular urticaria, which is common in children, is almost always the result of insect bites, especially of mosquitoes, fleas, and bedbugs.

Venoms of five Hymenoptera (honeybee, yellow jacket, yellow hornet, white-faced hornet, and wasp) are available for skin testing and treatment. The skin tests should be performed in accordance with the manufacturer's recommendations. There is a consensus that appropriately performed skin testing with potent materials is useful in identifying children at risk for systemic anaphylaxis, but venom skin test–negative subjects have been reported to experience anaphylaxis when stung. Moreover, as many as 40% of skin test–positive, nonimmunized subjects may *not* experience anaphylaxis on sting challenge. In vitro testing with RAST has not substantially improved the ability to predict anaphylaxis when compared with skin testing. With venom RAST, there is a 20% incidence of both false-positive and false-negative results. Skin testing is indicated for children with systemic reactions. Skin testing is deferred for at least 4 wk after a systemic reaction to minimize false-negative responses, although testing may be accurate within 1 wk after the sting.

TREATMENT. Immunotherapy is occasionally undertaken when it can be established that inhalant allergy is due to a specific insect such as the mayfly or caddis fly. Beneficial results from such treatment have not been thoroughly documented, and avoidance of the insect is the preferred management.

For cutaneous reactions caused by biting insects, treatment with topical medicaments to relieve itching and local discomfort and occasionally the systemic use of an antihistamine are appropriate. Mosquito extract immunotherapy is not of established effectiveness.

In case of an anaphylactic reaction following a Hymenoptera sting, the acute treatment is essentially the same as that for anaphylaxis. Epinephrine 1:1,000 in a dose of 0.01 mL/kg, maximum 0.3 mL, by intramuscular injection is effective for relief of laryngeal edema, bronchoconstriction, and peripheral vascular collapse. Blood volume expanders must be given for persistent hypotension. An antihistamine (e.g., diphenhydramine, 25–50 mg) may be given, although its efficacy has not been established. Corticosteroids are of little use in treatment of the acute systemic reaction but may be useful for treatment of sequelae. See Chapter 148 for further details of treatment of anaphylaxis.

Children (or their parents) who have had previous severe or anaphylactic reactions to Hymenoptera stings should be equipped with an EpiPen or EpiPen Jr, which facilitates rapid delivery of an injection of epinephrine, or with a kit that includes epinephrine for injection and an antihistamine tablet for emergency use. Patients at risk for anaphylaxis from an insect sting should also wear an identification bracelet (Medic-Alert) indicating their allergy.

Children and youth at risk from insect stings should avoid using perfumes or cosmetics and wearing bright or pastel-colored clothing when outdoors. They should always wear gloves when gardening and long pants or slacks and shoes when walking in the grass or through fields. Typical insect repellents are of little use against Hymenoptera.

Venom immunotherapy has an uncertain status because the natural history of venom reactivity is not adequately understood. IgE-mediated reactivity as measured by skin test or RAST may decline spontaneously in untreated patients. During the first months of venom therapy, venom-specific IgE antibodies increase by as much as three times, but usually fall to pretreatment levels over 1–2 yr of therapy. Whether the patient's clinical sensitivity is increased during the early course of immunotherapy is unknown. Venom-specific IgG antibody, which correlates with protection against anaphylaxis in most patients, peaks at 2–4 mo following initiation of immunotherapy and declines according to the half-life of the immunoglobulin; therefore, monthly injections of aqueous extracts are indicated. IgE antibodies may remain detectable for many years in the serum of treated patients. Those who experience severe systemic reactions (airway involvement or hypotension) and have a positive skin test result should receive immunotherapy. Immunotherapy is not considered indicated for children in whom stings have caused only urticarial or local reactions, although their risk for mild anaphylaxis after a subsequent sting may be as high as 9.2% compared with only 1.2% in similar patients treated with immunotherapy. However, therapy is indicated in adolescents and adults if skin test results are positive to venom and there is a history of a non–life-threatening or life-threatening systemic reaction. Immunotherapy is not indicated in patients with a history of sting anaphylaxis and negative skin test and RAST results; one would not know which venom to use. The incidence of side effects during the course of treatment is significant (50% of treated adults experience large local reactions and about 7%, systemic reactions). The incidence of both local and systemic reactions is much lower in children. A major problem is the high cost (related to the difficulty in obtaining vespid and polistes venom) of venom immunotherapy. It is uncertain how long immunotherapy with Hymenoptera venom should continue, but nearly all adults who have received 5 yr of therapy tolerate challenge stings without systemic reactions for several years after completion of treatment.

In children with hypersensitivity to fire ant venom, systemic anaphylaxis may follow the sting of fire ants, *Solenopsis richteri* or *S. invicta,* which are members of the order Hymenoptera. Fire ants are found throughout the southeastern United States. Fire ant venom is more sensitive than whole body extract for identification of allergic patients, but only whole body extract is commercially available for diagnosis by allergy skin testing and for treatment by immunotherapy. Immunotherapy has been successful, but there is considerable variation in the venom content of the commercially available whole body extracts.

Goldberg A, Confino-Cohen R: Timing of venom skin tests and IgE determinations after insect sting anaphylaxis. J Allergy Clin Immunol 100:182, 1997.

Golden DBK, Kwiterovich KA, Kagey-Sobotka A, et al: Discontinuing venom immunotherapy: Outcome after five years. J Allergy Clin Immunol 97:579, 1996.

Graft DF: Venom immunotherapy: Indications, selection of venoms, techniques, and efficacy. *In:* Levine MI, Lockey RF (eds): Monograph on Insect Allergy, 3d ed. Milwaukee, American Academy of Allergy and Immunology, 1995, p 73.

Stafford CT: Hypersensitivity to fire ant venom. Ann Allergy Asthma Immunol 77:87, 1996.

CHAPTER 152
Ocular Allergies

Allergic reactions involving the eye occur much less commonly in children than in adults. The eye may be involved as part of a generalized allergic reaction in atopic dermatitis, urticaria, or angioedema, for example, or the eye alone may be affected. Allergic reactions in the eye are known to occur on the basis of IgE-mediated allergy, as conjunctivitis in a child with ragweed hay fever, for example, or on the basis of a cell-mediated (delayed hypersensitivity) immune reaction, as in contact dermatitis of the eyelids.

EYELIDS. Eyelids are particularly prone to swelling because of their loose areolar connective tissue. Swelling may result from contact dermatitis to a variety of environmental substances. The lids are particularly involved because of the frequency with which offending contact sensitizers are carried to the eyelids with the hands. Occasionally, contact dermatitis appears as a result of sensitization to medication applied to the eyes. Cosmetics and topical ophthalmic medications are common sensitizing agents. Sulfonamides, neomycin, scopolamine, atropine, pilocarpine, contact lens solution, and topical anesthetics cause contact sensitization. The lids become inflamed and indurated, and a scaly, eczematoid reaction is evident. The conjunctiva becomes red, and a follicular conjunctivitis may develop.

Blepharitis. This is an inflammatory eczematous reaction of the eyelid margins that may be caused by infection or allergy, or both. A chronic staphylococcal infection has been implicated as the major cause of chronic eczema of the eyelid margins. The lid margins, particularly of the lower lids, are affected with an itchy, scaly, erythematous eruption with exudate at the base of the lashes. This gives the appearance of "granulated eyelids." The eyelids may be crusted together in the morning. The diagnosis is confirmed by slit-lamp examination.

ALLERGIC CONJUNCTIVITIS. This frequently accompanies allergic rhinitis in patients with hay fever, especially when caused by pollens. In affected children, both eyes itch, the conjunctivae are reddened and edematous, and there may be profuse tearing. Rubbing of the eyes aggravates the condition. There is no photophobia or other signs of corneal involvement. Occasionally, edema of the conjunctiva is so severe that the conjunctiva prolapses over the lower lid in a gelatinous-appearing mass (chemosis) that causes great concern to parents. The secretions are frequently watery but, if persistent, may appear purulent. Even discharges that appear purulent, however, contain predominantly eosinophils, which permits differentiation from infectious conjunctivitis, in which the discharge contains mostly polymorphonuclear leukocytes and bacteria.

Atopic Keratoconjunctivitis. This condition occurs in patients with atopic dermatitis who have extreme ocular itching, red eyes, swollen and thickened eyelids and, when the cornea is involved, photophobia. Onset is not before late adolescence. Symptoms are perennial. Keratoconus, a central corneal ectasia, is thought to be due to repeated eye rubbing; cataracts can occur.

Vernal Conjunctivitis. This inflammation is more common in children, with a 3:1 male to female predominance, than in adults (80% of patients are less than 14 yr old at onset). It appears most often in warm climates and during the spring and summer. The disease affects both eyes and occurs in palpebral and limbal forms. In the palpebral form, which is most common, the tarsal plate of the upper lid presents a characteristic "cobblestone" appearance as a result of hyperplasia and thickening of the conjunctiva. The hyperplasia may cause pseudoptosis. A thick, ropy, whitish discharge may be present over the hypertrophied, giant papillae giving the "cobblestone" appearance. In the limbal form, the junction of the cornea and sclera is involved, with thickening and opacity of the tissue in the area. Whitish Trantas dots, present on the corneoscleral limbus, which represent accumulations of eosinophils, are pathognomonic of the disease. Progression of the limbal form may scar the cornea and lead to blindness in the most severe cases. Symptoms of vernal conjunctivitis include lacrimation, extreme itching, burning, and a particularly distressing photophobia. The seasonal occurrence, the finding of eosinophils, and the frequent coexistence with other atopic diseases such as asthma, hay fever, and eczema suggest that IgE-mediated sensitivity is responsible for the condition, but detailed study of patients with the condition usually fails to identify any cause, and immunotherapy is of little if any value. The symptoms and signs of vernal conjunctivitis are mimicked in a syndrome induced by the wearing of hard or soft contact lenses: giant papillary conjunctivitis.

Red Eye Syndrome. Other causes of red eyes include infection, self-limited conditions or those that are rapidly responsive to a topical antibiotic; iritis, associated with photophobia, poorly reactive pupils, blurred vision, and often pain; keratitis, with photophobia, pain, and extreme lacrimation; giant papillary conjunctivitis due to soft contact lenses; overuse of vasoconstrictor drops; and the dry eye syndrome, which may be associated with a dry mouth and a collagen vascular disorder (Sjögren's syndrome). Application of strips of filter paper over the eyelid margins to measure the amount of wetting by tears within 5 min is diagnostic of dry eyes when the result is less than 5 mm. Artificial tears are effective for treatment of dry eyes. (See also Chapters 626 and 633.)

TREATMENT. Contact dermatitis of the lids is best managed by identification of suspected sensitizers and their elimination. A short course of topical corticosteroids is of value in managing the acute reaction.

Blepharitis is best treated by good lid hygiene, using cotton-tripped applicators and half-strength baby shampoo mixed with water to remove scales and exudate, followed by the use of antistaphylococcal ointments. If an excessive reaction to the treatment results, steroids are applied topically for a few days. Since the disease tends to recur, regular lid care is indicated, often for a lifetime.

Allergic conjunctivitis in the patient with hay fever generally responds well to topical application of sympathomimetics (naphazoline or phenylephrine) in the form of eye drops; 0.05% levocabastine hydrochloride eye drops (Livostin, not labeled for use by the U.S. Food and Drug Administration [FDA] in patients younger than 12 yr); 0.1% lodoxamide tromethamine eye drops (Alomide, not FDA labeled for use in patients younger than 2 yr); or, in more severe cases, to eye drops or ointments containing corticosteroids. Lodoxamide is FDA labeled only for treatment of vernal conjunctivitis. Olopatadine (Patanol, labeled for use in children older than 2 yr) has both antihistaminic and antiallergic properties, inhibiting release of mediators from conjunctival mast cells, and is effective for administration twice each day. Topical nedocromil and lodoxamide may be more effective than cromolyn; topical levocabastine is more effective than both cromolyn and nedocromil. Except for use of a topical steroid, olopatadine may prove to be most effective. As noted further on, steroids should be used in the eyes with caution. Immunotherapy for allergic conjunctivitis in the absence of allergic rhinitis usually gives poor results.

Atopic keratoconjunctivitis requires the use of topical steroids, particularly if the cornea is involved. Referral to an ophthalmologist is indicated.

Vernal conjunctivitis may be treated with topical vasoconstrictors, antihistamines, cold compresses, and 0.1% lodoxamide tromethamine eye drops or, if necessary, with sparing use of corticosteroid eye drops or ointments. Fluorometholone or medrysone, a topically active, poorly absorbed corticosteroid, in a dose of 1–2 drops four times a day, is particularly indicated in allergic conjunctivitis when there is involvement of only the superficial layers of the eye. The drug is less likely to cause increased intraocular pressure than are the more readily absorbed preparations such as dexamethasone or methylprednisolone. Whenever topical steroids are used in the eye for more than a few days, intraocular pressure should be monitored. In addition, prolonged topical steroid administration may predispose the patient to cataracts and opportunistic infections.

Abelson MB, George MA, Garofalo C: Differential diagnosis of ocular allergic disorders. Ann Allergy 70:95, 1993.

Casey R, Abelson MB: Atopic keratoconjunctivitis. Int Ophthalmol Clin 37(2):111, 1997.

Hammann C, Kammerer R, Gerber M, Spertini F: Comparison of effects of topical levocabastine and nedocromil sodium on the early response in a conjunctival provocation test with allergen. J Allergy Clin Immunol 98:1045, 1996.

Michelson PE: Red eye unresponsive to treatment. West J Med 166:145, 1997.

CHAPTER 153
Adverse Reactions to Foods

The incidence of adverse reactions to foods is not known and unquestionably varies in different parts of the world. The average U.S. diet contains many food antigens, chemical food additives, antibiotics, and other substances; accordingly, a significant frequency of adverse reactions to foods should not be surprising. Food reactions caused by allergic mechanisms are estimated to occur in 0.3–0.7% of individuals, but the prevalence of food allergy in infancy may be as high as 8%. Allergy to many foods may resolve within 1 or 2 yr, but allergy to peanuts may be lifelong. Most adverse reactions to food do not have an immunologic basis. In these cases the use of immunologic methods of diagnosis (skin testing or provocative testing [injection or oral administration of food antigen]) is inappropriate.

TABLE 153–1 Differential Diagnosis of Adverse Reactions to Foods

Condition	Example
Food allergy	Anaphylaxis, urticaria-angioedema, eosinophilic colitis, eczema; nuts, eggs, seafood, milk, celery, soy
Immune-mediated	Celiac disease
Food additives	Dyes (tartrazine), flavoring (MSG), preservatives (metabisulfite)
Food poisoning (toxins)	Botulism, *Bacillus cereus, Clostridium perfringens Staphylococcus aureus,* Scombroid, Ciguatera, paralytic shellfish
Infections	*Salmonella, Shigella, Escherichia coli, Yersinia, Campylobacter, Giardia, rotavirus,* Norwalk agents, AIDS
Contaminants	Heavy metals, antibiotics (penicillin)
Pharmacologic agents	Caffeine, tyramine, alcohol, histamine
Gastrointestinal disorders	Gastroesophageal reflux, pyloric stenosis, tracheoesophageal fistula, malrotation, peptic ulceration, inflammatory bowel disease
Enzyme deficiencies	Galactosemia, urea cycle defects, phenylketonuria
Malabsorption syndromes	Lactase deficiency, cystic fibrosis, cholestasis
Psychologic	School phobia
Functional	Irritable bowel syndrome, chronic nonspecific diarrhea of infancy

MSG = monosodium glutamate; AIDS = acquired immunodeficiency syndrome.

ETIOLOGY. Possible mechanisms for adverse reactions to foods include not only allergy but also enzyme deficiencies and nonimmunologic reactions to tyramine, nitrites, and monosodium glutamate (Table 153–1). There is little doubt that intact macromolecules may pass through the epithelium of the gastrointestinal tract and gain access to the systemic circulation, particularly during the first few months of life. Secretory IgA limits the intestinal absorption of intact macromolecules. Children with IgA deficiency have higher levels of antibodies to cow milk proteins and of immune complexes containing milk antigens than do normal controls. IgE-mediated reactions are characteristically rapid in onset and may present as angioedema of the lips, mouth, uvula, or glottis; as generalized urticaria; as asthma; or occasionally as shock. In such cases, the patient usually recognizes that the symptoms have followed ingestion of a certain food. Persons with such IgE-mediated food allergy are at constant risk of exposure to the offending food hidden in a food mixture. For example, a nut-sensitive individual may have a serious reaction to ingestion of a cookie made with almond extract.

Individuals with IgE-mediated food reactions consistently show positive skin test results to the suspected food. In fact, skin testing itself, particularly if performed by the intracutaneous technique, can precipitate the clinical reaction in individuals with anaphylactic allergy to a food. Foods that have the highest potential to cause IgE-mediated sensitivity are fish, shellfish, peanuts (a legume), various nuts and seeds, eggs, cow milk, soy, wheat, and corn.

More difficult to diagnose are reactions that begin a few hr to 24 hr after ingestion of the offending food. Such reactions have been attributed without much convincing evidence to allergy to a digestive product of the food such as a protease or polypeptide. The roles of antigen-antibody complexes and cell-mediated immunity (delayed hypersensitivity) in the pathogenesis of these late-occurring reactions are unknown.

A variety of reactions have been reported to follow ingestion of cow milk by infants and children. In some cases, an IgE mechanism has been established. In others, however, even with antibodies to milk proteins (particularly α-lactalbumin,

TABLE 153–2 Dietary Sources of Cow Milk

Batter-fried foods	Margarine
Biscuits	Meatloaf*
Bread	Muesli
Butter	Muffins
Cakes	Packaged soups
Candy	Pancakes
Cereals	Pies
Cheese	Puddings
Chocolate	Rolls
Cookies	Rusks
Cream sauces	Sausages
Cream soups	Sherbet
Custard	Soup mixes
Fish fried in batter	Soups, canned
Frankfurters*	Soy cheese
Gravies	Sweets
Ice cream	Vegetarian cheese
Imitation sour cream	Waffles
Instant mashed potatoes	Yogurt
Luncheon meats*	

May contain butter, margarine, or skim milk as a binder.
Modified from Steinman HA: "Hidden" allergies in foods. J Allergy Clin Immunol 98:241, 1996.

β-lactoglobulin, and casein) present in sufficient quantities to be demonstrable by gel diffusion methods, no immunologic mechanism has been established. During the first yr of life, vomiting and watery, blood-streaked, mucoid diarrhea may follow cow milk ingestion. Cow milk allergy can contribute to gastroesophageal reflux, especially when associated with diarrhea or atopic dermatitis. An enteropathy with loss of both protein and blood has been found in other young infants fed large volumes of whole pasteurized milk (but not heat-processed formula). In older infants, ingestion of cow milk has been associated with occult fecal blood loss, recurrent roentgenographic pulmonary infiltrates, and multiple precipitating antibodies to cow milk proteins (see Chapter 338). Some cases of pulmonary hemosiderosis are said to be responsive to withdrawal of milk from the diet.

Adverse reactions to milk caused by disaccharidase deficiencies are discussed in Chapter 340.11. For food-dependent, exercise-induced anaphylaxis see Chapter 148.

A number of enteropathies with varying combinations of malabsorption, steatorrhea, hypoalbuminemia, and fecal blood loss have been reported as a result of cow milk or wheat intolerance. Despite close associations between symptoms or signs and the feeding of these foods, a precise mechanism of immunologic injury has not been identified. It is not known whether wheat-sensitive individuals who have adverse symptoms from the gluten fraction of wheat are reacting to α-gliadin as a toxin or as an antigen in an immune-complex type of injury.

During the first 3 yr of life, rashes and diarrhea following ingestion of fruits and juices are common. There is no evidence of an immunologic mechanism.

Sulfites can cause modest bronchoconstriction in some asthmatic patients and severe, life-threatening airway obstruction in a few, probably in part because of increased airway hyperresponsiveness. Sulfites rarely can cause anaphylactic reactions. In the United States, a ban on the use of sulfiting agents on raw fruit and vegetables has greatly reduced this hazard.

Other nonimmunologic adverse reactions to foods, principally in adults, include headaches after ingestion of wine and cheese (tyramine), cured meat or "hot dog" headache (sodium nitrite), or the Chinese restaurant syndrome (monosodium glutamate). Affected individuals apparently have idiosyncratic, but not allergic, reactions to these simple chemicals. In other cases, nonimmunologic adverse reactions may be due to food additives, including the dyes used in foods and drugs. A report of the National Advisory Committee on Hyperkinesis and Food Additives concluded that there was no direct causal connection between artificial food colors and flavors and hyperactivity in children.

DIAGNOSIS. An etiologic diagnosis in a child suspected of an adverse food reaction requires careful objective study. Elimination from the diet for a period of 7–10 days of a food causing difficulty should generally result in improvement in the patient's symptoms. Reintroduction of the food, initially in small quantities and then in increasing amounts, should result in the return of symptoms in a reasonable period, within 7 days at most. If symptoms are produced, the food is eliminated from the diet for several months. Reintroduction of the food (except in cases of anaphylactic sensitivity) should be attempted at regular intervals.

The critical testing of foods by the elimination and provocation method is difficult if either patient or parent anticipates an unfavorable reaction because of the emotional bias incident to the ingestion of the suspected food. Food challenges are best performed in a blind manner, the food being given in a disguised form, for example in opaque capsules or mixed with another food. When symptoms have been continual, dietary elimination of the offending food should cause prompt improvement. Conversely, when symptoms such as headache have been intermittent, results of elimination and provocation testing are frequently equivocal.

Skin testing with properly prepared food antigens reveals the presence of any IgE antibody to the test antigen. A negative prick skin test result with properly prepared potent food extracts has a predictive accuracy of at least 95%. Conversely, a positive skin test result does not necessarily indicate that the particular food causes symptoms. Positive test results, especially if they do not correlate with the history, should be confirmed by food challenge. When prick testing with a commercial extract has produced negative results despite a strongly positive history, prick-by-prick testing with the fresh food may elicit a positive reaction. In anaphylactic food allergy, skin tests almost invariably produce a positive reaction to the offending food, but in this instance the history alone usually establishes the diagnosis, and skin testing is superfluous and may be dangerous. Occasionally, a positive result on a skin test to a food not previously suspected of causing symptoms is clinically corroborated when the history is re-examined in light of the positive test result. All too often, undue attention paid to clinically irrelevant skin reactions to food extracts has led to very restricted diets with no attempt made to confirm the clinical importance of suspected foods through elimination and provocative testing. Overdiagnosis of food allergy has sometimes caused malnutrition in infants and children as well as anxiety and depression in mothers who have found it impossible to adhere to severely restrictive diets.

TABLE 153–3 Labeling That May Indicate Presence of Milk Protein

Artificial butter flavor	Lactose
Butter	Milk
Butter fat	Milk derivative
Buttermilk solids	Milk protein
Caramel color	Milk solids
Caramel flavoring	Natural flavoring
Casein	Nondairy substitutes
Caseinate	Pasteurized milk
Cheese	Rennet casein
Cream	Skim milk powder
Curds	Solids
"De-lactosed" whey	Sour cream
Demineralized whey	Sour cream solids
Dried milk	Sour milk solids
Dry milk solids	Whey
Fully creamed milk powder	Whey powder
High-protein flavor	Whey protein concentrate
Lactalbumin	Yogurt
Lactalbumin phosphate	

Modified from Steinman HA: "Hidden" allergies in foods. J Allergy Clin Immunol 98:241, 1996.

TABLE 153–4 Dietary Sources of Egg

Baked goods	Mayonnaise
Baking mixes	Meatballs
Batters	Meatloaf
Bearnaise sauce	Meringues
Bologna	Muffins
Bouillon (in restaurants)	Noodles (egg)
Breakfast cereals	Nougats
Cake flours	Omelettes
Candy	Pancakes
Cookies	Pie crust
Creamy fillings	Pretzels
Custard	Puddings
Doughnuts	Root beer
Egg noodles	Salad dressing
Eggnog	Sausages
French toast	Sherbet
Fritters	Souffles
Hollandaise sauce	Soups
Ice cream	Spaghetti
Lemon curd	Tartar sauce
Macaroni	Truffles
Macaroons	Turkish Delight
Malted cocoa drinks (Ovaltine, Ovomalt)	Waffles
Marshmallows	Wines (if cleared with egg white)

Modified from Steinman HA: "Hidden" allergies in foods. J Allergy Clin Immunol 98:241, 1996.

Radioallergosorbent test (RAST) assay has been used to detect IgE antibodies to foods. The correlation among clinical history, puncture skin test, and RAST is excellent for codfish, egg white, nuts, peanuts, and peas. Positive RAST and skin test results to cereals correlate poorly with the results of cereal challenge. RAST for soybeans and white beans is unreliable, apparently because of nonspecific binding of IgE to the RAST disk. RAST does not appear to offer any substantial advantage over skin testing with potent food extracts.

In the provocative-neutralizing method of diagnosis of food allergy, dilutions of food extracts are injected intracutaneously in an attempt to reproduce the patient's symptoms, which are then said to be relieved by successive intracutaneous injections of other dilutions of the same extract. The techniques vary among users of the method. For example, some users both "provoke" and "neutralize" by sublingual administration of the antigen solutions. The validity of all these methods has not been established, and their use in diagnosis and therapy is unwarranted and experimental at best.

TREATMENT. The treatment of an adverse food reaction is directed at the clinical manifestations, which may be anaphylaxis, urticaria, diarrhea, vomiting, rhinitis, asthma, or atopic dermatitis. Offending foods should be removed from the diet. This may be difficult because of multiple dietary sources of milk and egg (Tables 153–2 to 153–5). Sorbet may be contaminated with cow milk allergens because of processing with equipment used previously for ice cream. Some restaurants thicken chile with peanut butter. Shelled nuts may be contaminated with peanut allergen because of packaging with the same equipment. Although refined peanut oil lacks peanut allergen, it may be contaminated with peanut allergen, so it is prudent for the allergic patient to avoid any peanut oil.

TABLE 153–5 Labeling That May Indicate the Presence of Egg Protein

Albumin	Globulin	Ovamucoid
Binder	Lecithin	Ovovitellin
Coagulant	Livetin	Powdered egg
Egg white	Lysozyme	Vitellin
Egg yolk or yellow	Ovalbumin	Whole egg
Emulsifier	Ovamucin	

From Steinman HA: "Hidden" allergies in foods. J Allergy Clin Immunol 98:241, 1996.

Introduction of the 2S albumin gene of Brazil nuts into soybeans to improve nutritional value also transferred allergenicity, indicating some transgenic foods can be hazardous for allergic patients. If elimination diets are prescribed, care must be taken to ensure that they are nutritionally adequate and do not impair growth. Infants with enteropathy or enterocolitis due to cow milk often are also sensitive to soy protein, so substitution of a soy formula is not prudent; however, most infants with IgE-mediated allergy to cow milk tolerate soy formula well. Because allergy to soy can occur, some children require substitution of a protein hydrolysate (Alimentum, Nutramigen). Occasional infants with extreme allergy to cow milk are unable to tolerate protein hydrolysates, but amino acid–derived infant formulas (Neocate) are satisfactory substitutes for them. For reasons that are unclear, some children who are highly reactive to foods become "tolerant" as they grow older; this is especially likely to occur among infants and young children. Foods most likely to become tolerated with the passage of time are cow milk, eggs, and soy. Hypersensitivity to peanuts, nuts, and fish persists for long periods. Cautious periodic attempts to reintroduce offending foods are appropriate, perhaps at yearly intervals.

Immunotherapy by injection or sublingual or oral administration of extracts of offending foods is not efficacious.

Further information helpful for patients and parents is available from the Food Allergy Network, 703-691-3179.

American Academy of Pediatrics Committee on Nutrition: Soy protein–based formulas: Recommendations for use in infant feeding. Pediatrics 101:148, 1998.

Bernstein IL, Storms WW: Practice parameters for allergy diagnostic testing. Ann Allergy Asthma Immunol 75:553, 1995.

Bock SA: Prospective appraisal of complaints of adverse reaction to foods in children during the first 3 years of life. Pediatrics 79:683, 1987.

Hill DJ, Cameron DJS, Francis DEM, et al: Challenge confirmation of late-onset reactions to extensively hydrolyzed formulas in infants with multiple food protein intolerance. J Allergy Clin Immunol 96:386, 1995.

Hourihane J'OB, Bedwani SJ, Dean TP, et al: Randomised, double blind, crossover challenge study of allergenicity of peanut oils in subjects allergic to peanuts. Br Med J 314:1084, 1997.

Iacono G, Carroccio A, Cavataio F, et al: Gastroesophageal reflux and cow's milk allergy in infants: A prospective study. J Allergy Clin Immunol 97:822, 1996.

Isolauri E, Siitas Y, Solo MK, et al: Elimination diet of cow's milk allergy: Risk for impaired growth in children. J Pediatr 132:1004, 1998.

Nordlee JA, Taylor SL, Townsend JA, et al: Identification of a Brazil nut allergen in transgenic soybeans. N Engl J Med 334:688, 1996.

Sicherer SH, Burks AW, Simpson HA: Clinical features of acute allergic reactions to peanut and tree nuts in children. Pediatrics 102:1998; www. Pediatrics. org/cgi/content/full.

Steinman HA: "Hidden" allergens in foods. J Allergy Clin Immunol 98:241, 1996.

PART XV

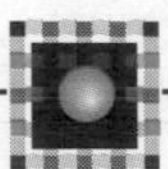

Rheumatic Diseases of Childhood (Connective Tissue Diseases, Collagen-Vascular Diseases)

CHAPTER 154

Evaluation of the Patient with Suspected Rheumatic Disease

Michael L. Miller

Rheumatic diseases result from abnormally regulated immune responses, leading to inflammation of target organs. Because many different organs may be affected, rheumatic diseases must be considered in a wide range of presenting complaints. Often, nonrheumatic diseases that can cause the same symptoms need to be excluded during evaluation.

Early diagnosis may not always be possible, because diagnostic manifestations can take time to develop. Specific diagnostic criteria for rheumatic diseases may not be met for months or, rarely, years. During that time some elements of the clinical evaluation may need to be repeated. Occasionally, a diagnosis will need to be reconsidered. For example, a child meeting diagnostic criteria for juvenile rheumatoid arthritis (JRA) may, after several years, develop anemia, diarrhea, and small bowel biopsy findings consistent with inflammatory bowel disease. Some patients with JRA, particularly those presenting with high titers of antinuclear antibodies (ANAs), may develop lupus years after initial presentation. A child with polyarticular arthritis who later develops weakness disproportionate to synovitis may be found to have an inflammatory myositis, such as juvenile dermatomyositis.

ETIOLOGIES AND PATHOPHYSIOLOGY OF RHEUMATIC DISEASES. Rheumatic diseases are characterized by autoimmune activity that exaggerates the immune response. Normally, the immune system reacts to viruses, bacteria, and other non-self molecules but does not mount a reaction to molecules found in the host's own tissues. This self-tolerance is lost in rheumatic diseases. Two possible reasons for self-reactivity (not mutually exclusive) are (1) similarity between foreign and self molecules as recognized by immune cells (particularly T lymphocytes), and (2) viral infections exaggerating immune responses that are otherwise suppressed. The relative contribution of these mechanisms to the pathogenesis of rheumatic diseases is still being investigated. Genetic factors may increase individual risk for developing rheumatic disease.

A series of abnormal cellular and molecular events is found in many rheumatic diseases. T lymphocytes bearing T-cell receptors recognize viruses and other foreign antigens bound to surfaces of other cells. After the T-cell receptor binds to antigenic molecules resting in the groove of the HLA molecule, molecular signals are released that activate other cells, such as macrophages. Macrophages produce inflammatory cytokines, including tumor necrosis factor-α (TNF-α), interleukin-1 (IL-1), and IL-6. These cytokines can cause tissue damage through direct effects and by attracting additional inflammatory cells to the affected site. Further damage is mediated as B lymphocytes are activated by helper T cells to produce excessive antibody, including autoantibodies that bind to self-antigens. The resulting complement fixation can lead to tissue destruction in some rheumatic diseases. Normal cells in target organs can be destroyed through cytolysis that is mediated by complement, by direct or indirect effects of TNF-α, or by effects of natural killer or cytolytic T lymphocytes.

In children with rheumatic diseases, products of the immune system may affect function of other organs. For example, IL-6 and other cytokines can bind to neuronal receptors in the central nervous system, causing fever. IL-6 can also interfere with osteoblastic activity, resulting in osteopenia, reflected by decreased serum osteocalcin levels. Molecules produced outside the immune system may, in turn, have an effect on immune responses. During a normal immune response, cytokines appear to induce neuroendocrine pathways to produce cortisol, which suppresses cellular and humoral activity. It is possible that defects in these pathways amplify autoimmune responses. The increased incidence of some rheumatic diseases in females may be explained by the ability of female sex hormones to augment cellular immune responses.

CLINICAL MANIFESTATIONS. The history can help distinguish rheumatic conditions from other diseases. For example, parents of children with school phobias are often dubious about the prospect of returning their children to school. In contrast, parents of children with rheumatic diseases, more upset with the school absences themselves, usually are anxious to see their children return to school.

Some symptoms and signs, although not specific, may suggest rheumatic diseases (Table 154–1). Morning stiffness may be reported by children with JRA, as well as postinfectious arthritis. Facial rashes in children with joint complaints or weakness raise the possibility of lupus or dermatomyositis. Raynaud phenomenon can be a presenting complaint of children with scleroderma and overlapping rheumatic syndromes. A history of trauma is sometimes seen in children with JRA. However, if arthritis is monoarticular, near the site of trauma, nonrheumatic disease (e.g., a torn meniscus, osteochondritis) should be considered. A history of travel, family enteric illness, or exposure to sick pets may be found in children with reactive arthritis following an enteric infection. Tick exposure raises the possibility of Lyme arthritis in a child with joint symptoms. Weakness can be found in muscular dystrophies, postviral illnesses, and inflammatory myopathies, of which juvenile dermatomyositis is the most common. Fevers are commonly seen in children with rheumatic diseases; spiking fevers returning to baseline are seen in systemic JRA. However, fever is not specific for rheumatic diseases, and evaluation for infections or malignancies may be necessary. Gait problems are found in

TABLE 154–1 Symptoms Suggestive of Rheumatic Diseases

Symptom	Rheumatic Diseases	Some Possible Nonrheumatic Diseases Causing Similar Symptoms
Fevers	Systemic juvenile rheumatoid arthritis	Malignancies, infections, inflammatory bowel disease
Arthralgia	Juvenile rheumatoid arthritis, systemic lupus erythematosus, juvenile dermatomyositis, scleroderma	Hypothyroidism, trauma, reactive arthritis, infections
Weakness	Juvenile dermatomyositis	Muscular dystrophies
Malar rash	Systemic lupus erythematosus	Photosensitive dermatitis
Chest pain	Juvenile rheumatoid arthritis, systemic lupus erythematosus (with associated pericarditis or costochondritis)	Costochondritis (isolated), rib fracture, spondylolysis, spondylolisthesis
Back pain	Juvenile rheumatoid arthritis, spondyloarthropathy	Vertebral microfracture, diskitis, intraspinal tumor

children with orthopedic problems, such as Legg-Calvé-Perthes disease, as well as JRA. The inability to walk raises the need for immediate attention to exclude conditions such as osteomyelitis or malignancy.

The *physical examination* helps identify the organs involved, supporting a final diagnosis. Because rheumatic diseases may take time to evolve, repeated examinations are often important in detecting new manifestations. The general appearance may suggest certain diagnoses. A depressed or anxious affect may suggest psychiatric disease. Lack of normal movement on the examination table may be a result of muscle weakness, arthritis, central nervous system disease, or skeletal abnormality. Decreased weight may reflect malnutrition from inflammatory bowel disease. Tachycardia is seen in the child with fevers of any cause or with carditis or pericarditis. Nailfold capillaroscopy can detect vasculopathy, reflecting vessel injury in dermatomyositis, scleroderma, and other rheumatic diseases (see Fig. 160–3).

Apparently isolated findings may be clues to target organ involvement in rheumatic diseases. For example, a pericardial friction rub with the inability to lie supine can be seen in pericarditis from lupus or systemic JRA. Persisting oral mucosal lesions are found in lupus; other mucous membrane involvement, such as swollen tongue or lips, raises the possibility of nonrheumatic diseases, including Kawasaki disease, Stevens-Johnson syndrome, and scarlet fever. The eye can be a target in lupus, in which episcleritis may be seen, and JRA, in which posterior synechiae are a later complication of uveitis. Although persisting joint complaints suggest JRA, other rheumatic diseases, including systemic lupus erythematosus (SLE) and dermatomyositis, can also present with arthritis. All children with joint symptoms should be asked about muscle weakness, as muscle involvement is seen in dermatomyositis and mixed connective tissue disease.

The joint examination can detect arthritis (infectious, rheumatic, or secondary to trauma), which is reflected by either swelling of the joint or the combination of pain and limited motion. Pain in a joint with full range of motion can be seen in trauma, psychogenic arthralgia, or early rheumatic disease that cannot yet be diagnosed. The neurologic examination can identify focal deficits resulting from intracranial or intraspinal lesions as well as muscle weakness, seen in many diseases including postviral syndromes, inflammatory myositis and other rheumatic diseases, and muscular dystrophies.

Erythema nodosum, a rash characterized by pretibial tender erythematous nodules found in the deep dermis and subcutaneous tissue (Fig. 154–1), is a hypersensitivity reaction resulting from certain infections, inflammatory diseases, or drugs. The finding of erythema nodosum should lead to consideration of possible underlying causes. Common infectious triggers include streptococcal pharyngitis, tuberculosis, *Yersinia,* histoplasmosis, and coccidioidomycosis. Erythema nodosum is sometimes the first manifestation of inflammatory bowel disease, sarcoidosis, or spondyloarthropathy. The rash may develop after exposure to sulfonamides, phenytoin, or oral contraceptive agents. Lesions may evolve from erythematous to bluish. They may sometimes be flat and in severe cases may be found along the entire length of the legs or even involve the arms. New crops of nodules may develop over several weeks and are sometimes accompanied by fever. Although erythema nodosum is itself a self-limited condition that responds to treatment of the underlying etiology, it must be distinguished from cellulitis, insect bites, thrombophlebitis, and fungal skin infections. When necessary to alleviate pain, supportive treatment includes bed rest, elevation of the legs, and analgesic medication.

LABORATORY FINDINGS. Certain laboratory studies screen for possible rheumatic disease and may contribute to a diagnosis. The erythrocyte sedimentation rate (ESR) is useful to screen for infectious and rheumatic diseases. A normal value does not exclude rheumatic diseases. Although transient infections can increase the ESR, elevations persisting for more than several weeks require explanation, and extensive evaluation may be

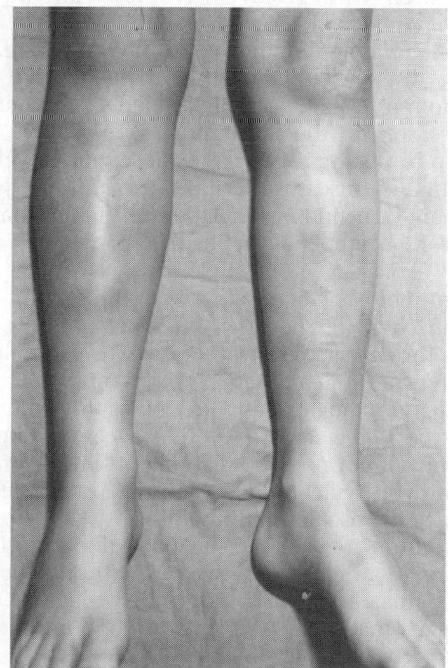

Figure 154–1 Erythematous nodules and plaques are present over both shins. The skin overlying the lesions is red, smooth, and shiny. The nodules are usually tender. Erythema nodosum is considered a hypersensitivity reaction and can be associated with a variety of diseases, including sarcoidosis, group A β-hemolytic streptococcal infection, tuberculosis, coccidioidomycosis, and ulcerative colitis. (Reprinted from the Clinical Slide Collection on the Rheumatic Diseases; Copyright 1991, 1995, 1997. Used by permission of the American College of Rheumatology.)

TABLE 154–2 Specific Antinuclear Antibodies and Associated Diseases

Antigen	Disease
Histone	Drug-induced lupus
Ribonucleoprotein	Mixed connective tissue disease
Pm-Scl	Sclerodermatomyositis
Scl	Scleroderma
Sm	Systemic lupus erythematosus
Ro/SSA	Sjögren's syndrome, congenital heart block, annular erythema
La/SSB	Sjögren's syndrome

The ANA test is a screening test; it does not determine which of various known and unknown nuclear antigens the antinuclear antibody is specific for. Nonspecific elevated ANAs may be detected in healthy children (usually at low titer) and in those with various rheumatic and nonrheumatic diseases. The above specific ANAs are typically found with the corresponding diseases; however, they may sometimes be found in patients without manifestations suggestive of (or diagnostic for) these conditions.

necessary. Usually the symptoms, physical findings, or other laboratory abnormalities will guide the focus of the evaluation.

ANAs are specific for nuclear constituents, some of which have been characterized (Table 154–2). A positive ANA antibody titer (a titer of ≥1:80) is a nonspecific reflection of increased lymphocyte activity. Positive ANA tests are found in children with rheumatic diseases and other diseases such as idiopathic thrombocytopenic purpura, Crohn disease, chronic autoimmune hepatitis, Graves disease, and, rarely, leukemia or lymphoma. Children with positive ANA tests who have nonrheumatic diseases may sometimes develop overlapping rheumatic syndromes, such as lupus. In such cases, other laboratory findings typically appear (e.g., antibodies to DNA in lupus patients). Some drugs, such as anticonvulsant medications (e.g., phenytoin, ethosuximide) and antiarrhythmic agents (e.g., procainamide) can cause positive ANA tests usually without rheumatic disease. Occasionally, lupus will develop in such patients. Malaria and some parasitic infections can also cause positive ANA tests.

Some children with positive ANA tests but no persisting symptoms have normal physical examinations and lack other remarkable laboratory findings. Such children rarely develop a rheumatic disease. Other children with positive ANA tests have been found to have arthralgia related to hyperextensible joints; the reason for the association is unknown. These children need to be distinguished from those who develop JRA or other rheumatic disease. Periodic evaluation will detect changes in physical findings or laboratory abnormalities (e.g., anemia, thrombocytopenia, nephritis) that suggest this possibility.

Other immunologic laboratory tests, although not diagnostic, are useful in characterizing the extent of immune activation and in monitoring response to therapy. For example, levels of total hemolytic complement (CH_{50}), C3, and C4 may be decreased in active lupus or vasculitis syndromes. Immune activation may be reflected by elevated levels of immune complexes, serum immunoglobulins, neopterin (a macrophage product), and von Willebrand factor antigen (a molecule found on the surface of vascular endothelium).

Other laboratory tests may raise consideration of nonrheumatic diagnoses. A decrease in two of the three blood cell lines (e.g., leukopenia, anemia, or thrombocytopenia) in a child with limb pain may be seen in acute lymphocytic leukemia. Lactate dehydrogenase levels may be elevated in rheumatic diseases as a result of cell turnover; marked elevations raise the possibility of malignancy. Thyroid function studies can exclude hypothyroidism, which may cause musculoskeletal symptoms. Decreased albumin and serum protein may be seen in nephrosis or inflammatory bowel disease.

Imaging studies also contribute to evaluation. Bone scans can detect subclinical bone infections or malignancies. MRI studies with gadolinium for joint evaluation and T2-weighted fat suppression for muscle evaluation can reveal tissue abnormalities seen in such diseases as JRA, dermatomyositis, and sarcoidosis. Findings from MRI studies may also suggest nonrheumatic diseases.

Azouz EM, Babyn PS, Mascia AT, et al: MRI of the abnormal pediatric hand and wrist with plain film correlation. J Comput Assist Tomogr 22:252, 1998.
Citera G, Espada G, Maldonado Cocco JA: Sequential development of 2 connective tissue diseases in juvenile patients. J Rheumatol 20:2149, 1993.
Deane PM, Liard G, Siegel DM, et al: The outcome of children referred to a pediatric rheumatology clinic with a positive antinuclear antibody test but without an autoimmune disease. Pediatrics 95:892, 1995.
Malleson PN, Sailer M, Mackinnon MJ: Usefulness of antinuclear antibody testing to screen for rheumatic diseases. Arch Dis Child 77:299, 1997.
ter Meulen DC, Majd M: Bone scintigraphy in the evaluation of children with obscure skeletal pain. Pediatrics 79:587, 1987.
Murray K, Thompson SD, Glass DN: Pathogenesis of juvenile chronic arthritis: Genetic and environmental factors. Arch Dis Child 77:530, 1997.
Passo MH, Fitzgerald JF, Brandt KD: Arthritis associated with inflammatory bowel disease in children. Relationship of joint disease to activity and severity of bowel lesion. Dig Dis Sci 31:492, 1986.
Reed A, Haugen M, Pachman LM, et al: Abnormalities in serum osteocalcin values in children with chronic rheumatic diseases. J Pediatr 116:574, 1990.
Spencer-Green G, Schlesinger M, Bove KE, et al: Nailfold capillary abnormalities in childhood rheumatic diseases. J Pediatr 102:341, 1983.
Wallendal M, Stork L, Hollister JR: The discriminating value of serum lactate dehydrogenase levels in children with malignant neoplasms presenting as joint pain. Arch Pediatr Adolesc Med 150:70, 1996.
Zimmerman SA, Ware RE: Clinical significance of the antinuclear antibody test in selected children with idiopathic thrombocytopenic purpura. J Pediatr Hematol Oncol 19:297, 1997.

CHAPTER 155
Treatment of Rheumatic Diseases

Daniel J. Lovell, Michael L. Miller, and James T. Cassidy

Treatment of children with rheumatic diseases is complex and challenging. The efforts of a team of health care professionals need to be melded into a coordinated system of care that is individualized to meet the needs of each patient and that is sensitive to the capabilities and psychosocial resources of each family. In addition, the rheumatic diseases are not static targets. In each child, disease manifestations vary in severity over time, and treatment needs to be adjusted accordingly. The therapeutic program must provide active treatments for currently symptomatic problems, such as arthritis, and must also include appropriate screening methods for often clinically silent problems such as uveitis in patients with juvenile rheumatoid arthritis (JRA) and early nephritis in patients with systemic lupus erythematosus (SLE). Nor should the treatment regimen focus only on the child with the rheumatic disease. When rheumatic disease afflicts a child, all family members are affected. Indeed, studies have indicated that siblings of a child with a rheumatic disease are often more adversely affected psychosocially than the patient. Furthermore, family dynamics significantly affect treatment outcome. Several studies have shown that the emotional status of the parents at the time of diagnosis of rheumatic disease in their child is one of the strongest predictors of treatment outcomes 5–10 yr later. Fortunately, despite this complex and ever changing therapeutic milieu, current treatment approaches administered by a multidisciplinary team experienced in the care of children with rheumatic diseases (Table 155–1) usually result in acceptable treatment outcomes.

The childhood rheumatic diseases are neither benign nor short lived in the majority of patients. Optimal treatment for these children requires the coordinated efforts of various health care professionals experienced in this specialized area.

TABLE 155–1 Multidisciplinary Team for Care of Children with Rheumatic Diseases

Core Team	Consultant Team
Parents and child	Orthopedic surgeon
Pediatric rheumatologist	Psychologist/psychiatrist
Pediatrician or family physician	Dentist
Nurse	School nurse
Social worker	
Physical therapist	
Occupational therapist	
Dietitian	
Ophthalmologist	

The treatment program includes physical and psychosocial interventions, as well as drugs, and requires tailoring to the needs and severity of each particular child's illness that may vary over time. Current therapies are not curative, as evidenced by the chronicity of these diseases.

PEDIATRIC RHEUMATOLOGY TEAMS AND PRIMARY CARE PHYSICIANS. The goals for treatment are to maximize the daily functional activities of an affected child, relieve discomfort, prevent or reduce organ damage, and avoid or minimize drug toxicity. Although drug therapy is important, nondrug therapy has a large role in the treatment of rheumatic diseases. The role of the physician responsible for treating a child with a rheumatic disease includes, in addition to prescribing and monitoring medications, coordinating the efforts of the other team members and educating the child and family about the treatments and nature and expected course of the disease. A key predictor of long-term outcome is early referral to a rheumatology team experienced in the care of children with rheumatic diseases. For example, significant differences in outcome in patients with JRA even 10 yr after disease onset were evident in those patients referred to a pediatric rheumatology center within 6 mo after disease onset, compared with referral more than 6 mo after disease onset.

The pediatric rheumatology team offers coordinated services needed by children and families. By working closely with the team, the primary care physician helps to monitor compliance with treatment plans and to evaluate symptoms of intercurrent illnesses, to exclude disease exacerbation or concomitant infections. Communicating with subspecialists and teams at tertiary care centers allows intervention when poor compliance occurs and symptoms flare.

Each member of the pediatric rheumatology team contributes to the child's care (Table 155–2). The pediatric rheumatologist establishes the diagnosis, assesses response to treatment, and monitors for change in disease manifestations. With assistance from other team members, the pediatric rheumatologist also monitors a child's health status, including such areas as pain, emotional and behavioral responses to disease, change in roles at home and school, and family response to the child's illness. Nurses provide education about specific chronic illnesses. Occupational and physical therapists assess limitations in joint movement and physical function and provide plans for long-term exercise programs. Physical and occupational therapists prescribe and monitor exercise and splinting programs that families perform at home with the child to improve or maintain joint motion in children with arthritis, as well as in patients with myositis to avoid muscle contractures and improve muscle strength. Splints are used to lessen mechanical stress on joints that is associated with routine daily tasks. Splints may also improve muscle or joint contractures and avoid joint deformities. Ophthalmologists need to examine children with JRA on a regular basis (every 3–12 mo, depending on the type of JRA) to screen for uveitis and to assess for ocular toxicity from certain medications (every 6–12 mo) such as hydroxychloroquine or corticosteroids. Social workers are invaluable aids to families by helping them to confront the significant social and emotional stresses imposed by the illness, to deal with the financial maze of insurance coverage and national and state programs, and to identify community resources needed to provide support. Children with rheumatic diseases are often undernourished because of disease- or medication-related anorexia or overnourished as a result of corticosteroid therapy. Early and ongoing involvement of a nutritionist can significantly improve the health of these patients.

MEDICATIONS. Medications used for treatment of childhood onset rheumatic diseases (Table 155–2) have various mechanisms of action (for some, the mechanism in unknown), but all share the ability to suppress inflammation. Key to satisfactory short- and long-term outcomes in these children is early induction of a significant and sustained suppression of this inflammation.

Nonsteroidal Anti-Inflammatory Drugs (NSAIDs). A large number of NSAIDs are approved by the Food and Drug Administration (FDA) for use in adults with rheumatoid arthritis, but a much smaller number of NSAIDs are FDA-approved for use in children with JRA. The NSAIDs can be prescribed to decrease inflammation in arthritis, pleuritis, pericarditis, uveitis, and some forms of vasculitis. Lower doses, typically those approved for over-the-counter use, or intermittent dosing can result in analgesia but rarely true anti-inflammatory effect. To reduce inflammation requires regular administration of larger doses for longer periods than for analgesia alone. For example, the mean time to achieve an anti-inflammatory effect in the arthritis associated with JRA was 30 days of consistent administration. The NSAIDs work primarily by inhibiting the enzyme cyclooxygenase (COX), which is a critical step in the production of prostaglandins. Prostaglandins are a family of substances that have many physiologic effects including promoting inflammation. Two types of COX receptors have been demonstrated, and several NSAIDs that are in development selectively inhibit those receptors responsible for promoting inflammation (selective COX-2 inhibitors). These selective COX-2 inhibitors may prove to result in greater anti-inflammatory effects with fewer side effects.

The most frequent toxicities with NSAIDs in children are nausea, decreased appetite, and abdominal pain. Gastritis or gastric or duodenal ulceration occurs in children less frequently than in adults. In addition, each of the following side

TABLE 155–2 Cornerstones of Treatment of Children with Rheumatic Diseases

Accurate diagnosis and education of family	Pediatric rheumatologist Pediatrician Nurse Social Worker
Medications	Nonsteroidal anti-inflammatory drugs (NSAIDs) Methotrexate Hydroxychloroquine Sulfasalazine Intravenous immunoglobulin (IVIG) Cyclophosphamide Cyclosporine Corticosteroids (oral, intravenous, pulse, ophthalmic, intra-articular)
Physical medicine and rehabilitation	Physical therapy Occupational therapy Splints/reconstructive surgery
Physical and psychosocial growth and development	Nutrition School integration Peer group relationships Individual and/or family counseling
Coordination of care	Incorporation of patient/family as critical and active members of team Pediatrician Involvement of school and community resources Nurse, social worker, pediatric rheumatologist

effects occurs in 5% or less of children on chronic NSAID therapy: central nervous system (CNS) symptoms (e.g., mood change, sleepiness, irritability, headache, tinnitus), anemia, elevated liver enzymes, proteinuria, and hematuria. Several specific adverse reactions may also occur. Ibuprofen has induced aseptic meningitis in patients with SLE. When used by children, naproxen is far more likely than other NSAIDs to cause a unique skin reaction called *pseudoporphyria* that is characterized by small hypopigmented flat scars occurring in areas of even minor skin trauma (skin fragility), such as fingernail scratches, or after small spontaneous blister lesions. Naproxen-induced pseudoporphyria is more likely to occur in fair-skinned individuals and in sun-exposed areas. The observation of any pseudoporphyria lesions should prompt immediate discontinuation of naproxen, because the scars can persist for several years. NSAIDs should be used very cautiously in patients with dermatomyositis or systemic vasculitis owing to the increased frequency of gastrointestinal (GI) ulceration in these conditions.

The response to NSAIDs varies greatly among individual patients, but overall, approximately 50–60% of children with JRA experience significant improvement in their arthritis with a particular NSAID. Patients often must try several different NSAIDs before finding the NSAID that demonstrates clinical benefit. NSAIDs with longer half-lives or sustained-release formulations have been developed to allow for once- or twice-daily dosing. For patients with JRA or milder cases of SLE, NSAIDs are often a cornerstone of the drug treatment approach. For approximately 30–50% of patients with JRA, NSAIDs are the only drug therapy required to control the arthritis.

Methotrexate. Methotrexate has been used and studied in almost all rheumatic diseases and in many nonrheumatic diseases (e.g., asthma, inflammatory bowel disease, cystic fibrosis, uveitis, and diabetes). It has a central role in the treatment of JRA and is used in approximately 60% of patients with polyarticular JRA. Methotrexate given orally in a dose of 10 mg/m^2 body surface area (BSA) once weekly has been shown to be significantly better than placebo in a randomized, placebo-controlled trial (63% of methotrexate and 36% of placebo patients responded, $p < .001$). In a smaller uncontrolled study, in patients with JRA that failed to respond to the 10 mg/m^2 BSA/wk dose, methotrexate given in higher doses of 23–29 mg/m^2 BSA/wk administered intramuscularly resulted in prolonged clinical improvement in 70% of the patients. Patients who demonstrate clinical improvement in articular inflammation with methotrexate also have improvement in radiologic evaluation of joint damage, growth rate, and functional ability in daily tasks.

Methotrexate is a commonly used drug in treatment of juvenile dermatomyositis that has shown no or inadequate response to corticosteroids. About 70% of patients with dermatomyositis treated with methotrexate show improvement in the myositis. Methotrexate has also been successfully used in patients with SLE to treat arthritis, pleuritis, and, in some cases, nephritis. The dosage used to treat children with SLE is 10–20 mg/m^2 BSA/wk.

Methotrexate is well tolerated by children. Studies of adults have indicated that the mechanism of action in arthritis is *not* primarily suppression of either folic acid metabolism or bone marrow activity. Methotrexate, an analog of folic acid, inhibits dihydrofolate reductase, which is important in purine synthesis, resulting in suppression of inflammation. Because of the lower dose and alternative mechanism(s) of action, toxicity from methotrexate use in rheumatic diseases is much milder and qualitatively different from that observed when methotrexate is used to treat neoplastic diseases. In eight published studies that included 288 patients with JRA on methotrexate therapy, 13% of patients reported GI toxicity, <1% rash, <1% alopecia, 3% stomatitis, 1–2% headache, 15% elevated liver enzymes, 0% hematuria, <1% leukopenia, and <1% interstitial pneumonitis.

Hepatotoxicity observed in adults with rheumatoid arthritis treated long term with methotrexate has raised concern about similar problems occurring in children. In 46 liver biopsies performed in patients with JRA undergoing long-term methotrexate treatment, 95% of specimens were normal, 5% showed mild fibrosis, but none demonstrated even moderate liver damage. Lymphoproliferative disorders have been reported in adults with a rheumatic disease treated with methotrexate, usually after Epstein-Barr virus infection. However, given the large number of adults on methotrexate, the relative risk of lymphoproliferative disease remains low, at approximately 1.0–1.5%. Thus, methotrexate has become one of the cornerstone medications in pediatric rheumatology owing to its potential to induce significant improvement in chronic inflammation and to maintain that improvement for long periods because of low toxicity and high patient acceptance.

Corticosteroids. Corticosteroids are given by various routes for rheumatic diseases, including ocular, oral, intravenous, and intra-articular administration. Ocular steroids are prescribed under the supervision of an ophthalmologist either as drops or injections into the soft tissue surrounding the globe (subtenon injection) for the uveitis associated with JRA. Chronic ocular steroid use can lead to cataract formation and glaucoma. However, current ophthalmic practice has significantly decreased the frequency of blindness as a complication of JRA-associated uveitis.

Oral corticosteroids are a cornerstone of treatment for moderate to severe SLE, dermatomyositis, and most forms of vasculitis. However, long-term oral corticosteroid use always leads to side effects. Corticosteroid therapy in these chronic diseases must be carefully supervised; a responsible plan requires steroid tapering to acceptable doses for long-term use or the introduction of other anti-inflammatory medications to serve as corticosteroid-sparing agents. Intravenous corticosteroids have been used as alternatives to oral corticosteroids to treat the more severe, acute systemic connective tissue diseases such as SLE, dermatomyositis, and vasculitis. The intravenous approach allows for much higher doses of corticosteroid therapy to be given to obtain an immediate, profound anti-inflammatory effect. Methylprednisolone, 10–30 mg/kg/dose up to a maximum of 1 g, has been the drug of choice. Although generally associated with fewer side effects than oral corticosteroids, intravenous corticosteroids are not without significant and occasionally life-threatening toxicities, and they can result in cardiac arrhythmias, acute hypertension, hypotension, and shock.

Intra-articular corticosteroids are prescribed with increasing frequency for children with JRA in whom one or several joints have not responded to standard parenteral drug therapy or as the initial therapy in patients with arthritis involving only one or two joints. Almost all patients have significant improvement in both symptoms and physical findings within 2–3 days; this persists in 60% for at least 6 mo and in 45% for at least 12 mo. Intra-articular corticosteroids may result in subcutaneous atrophy and hypopigmentation of the skin in the area surrounding the injection site, as well as subcutaneous calcifications along the needle tract. It is rare that either of these complications is clinically significant.

Other Drugs. Various other medications are used in the treatment of the rheumatic diseases in selected children. *Hydroxychloroquine sulfate* is an antimalarial drug that has an important role in the treatment of SLE and possibly dermatomyositis. It is used infrequently to treat JRA because a prospective trial in patients with JRA failed to show increased efficacy of hydroxychloroquine compared with placebo. However, blinded withdrawal of hydroxychloroquine in patients with SLE resulted in a significantly higher frequency of disease worsening compared with placebo. It is especially helpful in the treatment of the cutaneous aspects of SLE and dermatomyositis. The dose is 3–6 mg/kg/24 hr; a 3–6-mo trial is necessary to assess therapeutic response. Potential side effects include bone marrow suppression, CNS stimulation, gastric irritation, myasthenia-like weakness, and skin rash. The most significant potential side effect is retinitis, which occurs very rarely but may result in blindness or loss of central vision. Complete ophthalmologic examinations at baseline and every 4–6 mo are mandatory if hydroxychloroquine is used. Fortunately, the frequency of retinal toxicity is rare (approximately 1/5,000).

Sulfasalazine has been used for many years in the treatment of inflammatory bowel disease. In a randomized, double-blinded, placebo-controlled study of children with JRA, sulfasalazine 50 mg/kg/24 hr (maximum 2,000 mg/24 hr) demonstrated significantly greater improvements in joint inflammation, global assessments, and laboratory test results when compared with placebo. However, more than 30% of the sulfasalazine-treated patients withdrew from the study because of adverse side effects, primarily GI irritation and skin rashes. Although none of the side effects in this trial was serious, sulfasalazine has been associated with severe systemic hypersensitivity reactions, especially development of the Stevens-Johnson syndrome. These reactions are much more common in patients with active systemic JRA treated with sulfasalazine. The proper role for sulfasalazine in the treatment scheme is still evolving; in most centers, it is used in polyarticular and pauciarticular JRA and juvenile spondyloarthropathy.

Intravenous immunoglobulin (IVIG) is efficacious in various clinical conditions. IVIG has been shown to significantly improve the short- and long-term natural history of Kawasaki disease. Open studies have supported benefit for SLE-associated thrombocytopenia, systemic JRA, polyarticular JRA, and dermatomyositis. A placebo-controlled crossover study demonstrated significant short-term benefit of IVIG in adults with active myositis. However, the effect was short-lived after cessation of the therapy. Doses of IVIG generally used in these investigations have been large (1–2 g/kg/dose, usually given monthly) and must be given on a regular basis to maintain benefit. In addition to being very expensive and periodically in short supply, IVIG has been associated with severe systemic allergic reactions, transmission of hepatitis C, and postinfusion aseptic meningitis. IVIG seems to hold promise as a treatment for dermatomyositis, although no controlled trials have involved children.

Cyclophosphamide has been evaluated in controlled trials in both SLE and Wegener granulomatosis. Pulse intravenous cyclophosphamide (500–1,000/m^2 BSA/dose) given monthly for 6 mo, then every 3 mo for 12 mo, has been shown to significantly reduce the frequency of renal failure in patients with SLE with diffuse proliferative glomerulonephritis. Open trials suggest efficacy in severe CNS-lupus. Oral cyclophosphamide (2 mg/kg/24 hr) is effective in the treatment of severe Wegener granulomatosis. Cyclophosphamide, an alkylating agent, requires metabolic conversion in the liver to become active. Metabolites alkylate the guanine in DNA that may lead to the observed immunosuppression by the inhibition of the S2 phase of mitosis. Decreases in the numbers of T and B lymphocytes result in decreased humoral and, to various extents, cellular immune responses. Cyclophosphamide is a potent cytotoxic drug associated with significant short- and long-term side effects. It has been used for severe rheumatic illnesses that have not responded to various less toxic treatments. Potential short-term adverse events include alopecia, nausea, vomiting, anorexia, oral and GI ulcerations, cystitis, and bone marrow suppression. Long-term complications include increased risks for cancer (especially leukemias, lymphomas, and bladder cancer) and for sterility.

Cyclosporine has been introduced into the treatment of dermatomyositis and active systemic JRA based on uncontrolled clinical studies. Several drugs commonly used in the past are very seldom used currently. For example, salicylates, gold salts, azathioprine, and D-penicillamine are seldom used in the treatment of JRA at this time.

FUTURE TREATMENTS. Rheumatologists have commonly combined several drugs in the treatment of rheumatic diseases to achieve better disease control, often to permit use of less corticosteroids. However, only in the last few years have prospective studies been performed to test the efficacy of combination drug therapy. In adults with rheumatoid arthritis, the combination of methotrexate, hydroxychloroquine, and sulfasalazine has been shown to be well tolerated. The combination of the three drugs was more efficacious than any of the drugs taken singly or any combination of two of the three drugs. In an open study of children with severe systemic JRA, a combination of intravenous methylprednisolone, intravenous cyclophosphamide, and oral methotrexate demonstrated excellent short-term safety and clinical effect. It is hoped that in the near future, the development of standardized, sensitive outcome measures and large international consortiums of pediatric rheumatologists will allow various combination therapies to be critically evaluated in clinical trials in children with JRA and other rheumatic diseases.

A wide variety of biologic agents that have recently been studied in adults and many more that are in development are thought to affect individual cell populations or molecular species involved in the inflammatory process. Monoclonal antibodies destroy certain T-cell subpopulations, bind particular cytokines or cytokine receptors, or bind anti–double-stranded DNA autoantibodies. These monoclonal antibodies are being widely tested in adults with rheumatic diseases, primarily rheumatoid arthritis and SLE. For example, subcutaneous injection of a synthesized monoclonal antibody to tumor necrosis factor-α, which is often present in high levels in inflamed joints, improves symptoms in adults with rheumatoid arthritis. This medication shows promise for finding a similar role in the treatment of some children with severe polyarticular JRA refractory to conventional therapy. The potential for these therapies in children with rheumatic diseases is great but largely untested at this time.

Boumpas DT, Austin HA, Fessler BJ, et al: Systemic lupus erythematosus: Renal, neuropsychiatric, cardiovascular, pulmonary and hematologic disease. Ann Intern Med 122:940, 1995.

Cassidy JT, Petty RE: Basic concepts of drug therapy. *In*: Cassidy JT, Petty RE (eds): Textbook of Pediatric Rheumatology, 3rd ed. Philadelphia, WB Saunders, 1995, pp 65–107.

Frank RG, Hagglund KJ, Schopp LH: Disease and family contributors to adaptation in juvenile rheumatoid arthritis and juvenile diabetes. Arthritis Care Res 11:166, 1998.

Giannini EH, Brewer EF, Kuzmina N, et al: Methotrexate in resistant juvenile rheumatoid arthritis. N Engl J Med 320:1043, 1992.

Giannini EH, Cawkwell GD: Drug treatment in children with juvenile rheumatoid arthritis past, present, and future. Pediatr Clin North Am 42:1099, 1995.

Lehman TJA: A practical guide to systemic lupus erythematosus. Pediatr Clin North Am 42:1223, 1995.

Lovell DJ: Juvenile rheumatoid arthritis and juvenile spondyloarthropathy. *In*: Klippel JH (ed): Primer on the Rheumatic Diseases, 11th ed. Atlanta, Arthritis Foundation, 1997, pp 393–398.

van Rossum MA, Fiselier TJ, Franssen MJ, et al: Sulfasalazine in the treatment of juvenile chronic arthritis: A randomized, double-blind, placebo-controlled, multicenter study. Arthritis Rheum 41:808, 1998.

Wallace CA: The use of methotrexate in childhood rheumatic diseases. Arthritis Rheum 41:381, 1998.

White PH, Shear ES: Transition/job readiness for adolescents with juvenile arthritis and other chronic illness. J Rheumatol 19:28, 1992.

CHAPTER 156
Juvenile Rheumatoid Arthritis

Michael L. Miller and James T. Cassidy

Juvenile rheumatoid arthritis (JRA) is one of the most common rheumatic diseases of children and a major cause of chronic disability. It is characterized by an idiopathic synovitis of the peripheral joints, associated with soft tissue swelling and effusion. In the classification criteria of the American College of Rheumatology, JRA is regarded not as a single disease but a category of diseases with three principal types of onset: (1) oligoarthritis (pauciarticular disease); (2) polyarthritis; and (3) systemic-onset disease (Table 156–1). Nine distinct course subtypes have also been identified. The European League Against Rheumatism (EULAR) has also published classification criteria for a similar constellation of diseases, identified as juvenile chronic arthritis. The International League Against Rheumatism (ILAR) is in the process of developing new criteria for the classification of seven specific types of onset of peripheral arthritis in children.

ETIOLOGY. The etiology of the diseases classified under JRA is unknown. At least two events are considered necessary: immunogenetic susceptibility and an external, presumably environmental, trigger. Specific HLA subtypes have been identified as rendering the child at risk, and these may confer varying degrees of susceptibility, or indeed protection, depending upon the age of the child. Possible triggers for JRA include certain viruses (e.g., parvovirus B19, rubella, Epstein-Barr virus); host hyperreactivity to specific self-antigens (type II collagen); and enhanced T-cell reactivity to bacterial or mycobacterial heat shock proteins.

EPIDEMIOLOGY. Although difficult to determine with precision, the incidence of JRA is approximately 13.9/100,000 children (15 yr of age or less)/yr, with a prevalence of approximately 113/100,000 children. A report from Australia, however, provided a much higher estimate of prevalence based on examination of school children by a pediatric rheumatologist. This study suggested a need for increased identification and referral of children with arthritis to pediatric rheumatology treatment centers. Different racial and ethnic groups appear to have varying frequencies of the subtypes of JRA. One study reported that black American children with JRA were older at presentation and less likely to have antinuclear antibody (ANA) seropositivity or uveitis.

TABLE 156–1 Criteria for the Classification of Juvenile Rheumatoid Arthritis

Age at onset <16 yr
Arthritis (swelling or effusion, or presence of two or more of the following signs: limitation of range of motion, tenderness or pain on motion, and increased heat) in one or more joints
Duration of disease 6 wk or longer
Onset type defined by type of disease in first 6 mo:
Polyarthritis: 5 or more inflamed joints
Oligoarthritis: <5 inflamed joints
Systemic: arthritis with characteristic fever
Exclusion of other forms of juvenile arthritis

Modified from Cassidy JT, Levison JE, Bass JC, et al: A study of classification criteria for a diagnosis of juvenile rheumatoid arthritis. Arthritis Rheum 29;174, 1986.

PATHOGENESIS. The synovitis of JRA is characterized by villous hypertrophy and hyperplasia with hyperemia and edema of the subsynovial tissues. Vascular endothelial hyperplasia is prominent and characterized by infiltration of mononuclear and plasma cells (Fig. 156–1). Pannus formation occurs in advanced or uncontrolled disease and results in progressive erosion of articular cartilage and contiguous bone (Fig. 156–2).

Although the etiology is unknown, studies suggest excessive immune reactivity of several types of cells in predisposed children, suspected but not proved to be in reaction to exposure to certain viruses. The onset may be triggered by a preceding infection. Although trauma may be cited by the parents as a trigger, it is more likely the result than cause of arthritis. Studies of T-cell receptor expression confirm recruitment of T cells specific for antigens (unknown) present in joint synovium. Specific populations of T cells appear to change over time, sometimes with clonal expansion of cells that may be protective (e.g., those reactive toward certain heat shock pro-

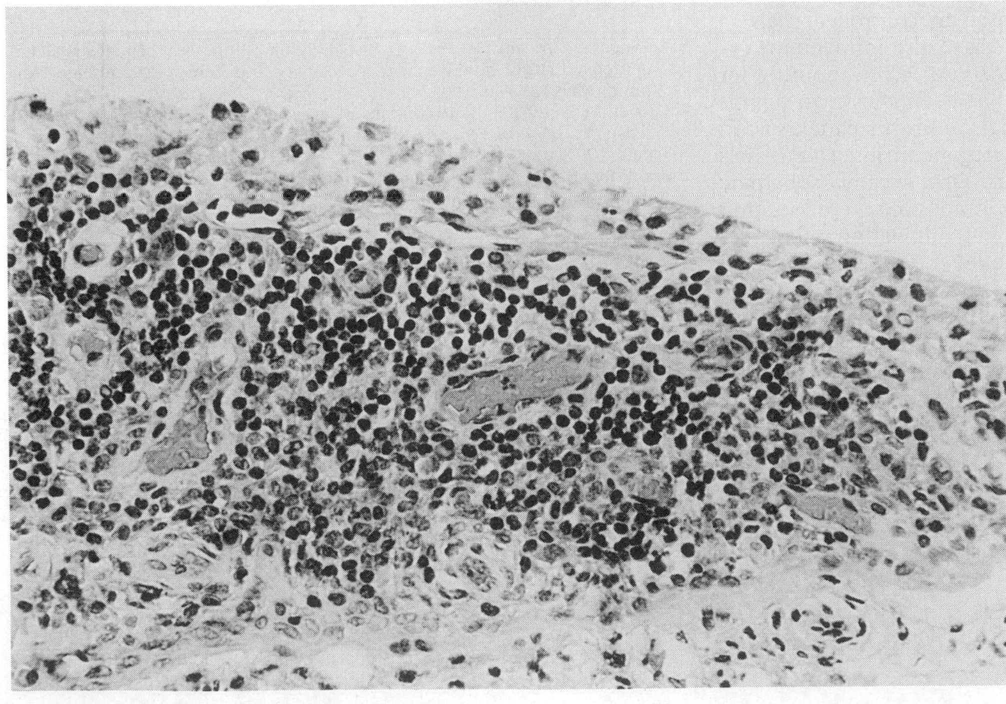

Figure 156–1 Synovial biopsy from a 10-yr-old child with pauciarticular juvenile rheumatoid arthritis. There is a dense infiltration of lymphocytes and plasma cells in the synovium.

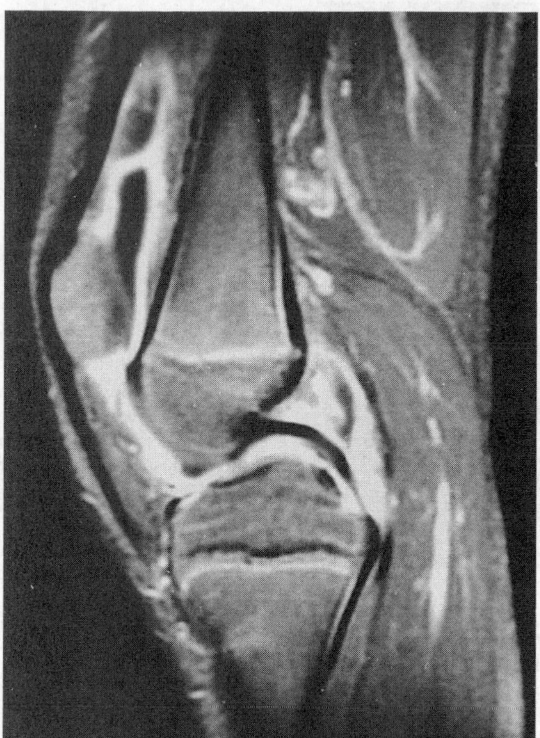

Figure 156–2 MRI scan with gadolinium of a 10-yr-old child with juvenile rheumatoid arthritis (same patient as in Fig. 156–1). The dense white signal in the synovium near the distal femur, proximal tibia, and patella reflects inflammation. MRI is useful to exclude ligamentous injury, chondromalacia of the patella, or tumor.

teins) and associated with improved responsiveness to medical treatment.

The recruitment of these T cells is made possible by certain HLA types found with increased frequency in affected children. HLA-DR4 (particularly the DRB1*0401 allele) is associated with polyarticular disease; pauciarticular JRA has been associated with HLA alleles at the DR8 (particularly DRB1*0801) and DR5 (particularly DRB1*1104) loci.

T-cell activation results in a cascade of events leading to tissue damage in joints and other affected tissues, including B-cell activation, complement consumption, and, in particular, release of interleukin-6 (IL-6), tumor necrosis factor-α (TNFα), and other pro-inflammatory cytokines, possibly under the control of specific genetic alleles.

CLINICAL MANIFESTATIONS. Initial symptoms often include morning stiffness and gelling, ease of fatigue particularly after school in the early afternoon, joint pain later in the day, and joint swelling. The involved joint is often warm, lacks full range of motion, and is occasionally painful on motion but usually not erythematous.

Oligoarthritis (pauciarticular disease) predominantly affects the joints of the lower extremities, such as the knees and ankles (see Fig. 156–2; Fig. 156–3). Involvement of upper extremity large joints, while seen, is not characteristic of this type of onset. Involvement of the hip is almost never a presenting sign of JRA. However, hip disease may occur later, particularly in polyarticular JRA, and is often the first sign of a deteriorating functional course (Fig. 156–4).

Polyarthritis (polyarticular disease) is generally characterized by involvement of both large and small joints (Figs. 156–5 and 156–6). As many as 20 to 40 separate joints are often affected, although inflammation of only five or more joints is required as a criterion for classification of this type of onset or course. Polyarticular disease often resembles the usual presentation of adult rheumatoid arthritis. Rheumatoid nodules found on extensor surfaces of elbows and over the Achilles tendon are associated with a more severe course. Micrognathia reflects chronic temporomandibular joint involvement. Cervical spine involvement of the apophyseal joints (Fig. 156–7) occurs frequently, with risk of atlantoaxial subluxation.

Systemic-onset disease is characterized by a quotidian fever with daily temperature spikes to at least 39°C for a minimum of 2 wk. Each febrile episode is often accompanied by a characteristic faint erythematous macular rash; lesions may be linear or circular, from 2 to 5 mm in size, distributed most commonly over the trunk and proximal extremities (Fig. 156–8). In addition to arthritis, patients with systemic-onset disease often have prominent visceral involvement including hepatosplenomegaly, lymphadenopathy, and serositis, such as a pericardial effusion.

DIAGNOSIS. The diagnosis of JRA is greatly aided by the American College of Rheumatology classification criteria and its subclassification of courses of disease (see Table 156–1) and by the meticulous exclusion of other articular diseases. There is no one pathognomonic finding for these diseases in children. However, the classic intermittent fever in association with the typical rash and objective arthritis is highly suggestive of systemic-onset JRA. Diagnosis is based upon a history compatible with inflammatory joint disease and a physical examination that confirms the presence of objective arthritis, as defined by the classification criteria. Laboratory abnormalities characteristic of inflammation (elevated erythrocyte sedimentation rate [ESR] and C-reactive protein [CRP]), the presence of leukocytosis, thrombocytosis, and the anemia of chronic disease support the diagnosis in the absence of results that would suggest a different disease.

Differential Diagnosis. Arthritis can be the presenting manifestation for any of the rheumatic diseases of childhood, including systemic lupus erythematosus (Chapter 159), juvenile dermatomyositis (Chapter 160), and the vasculitis syndromes (Chapter 167). Diagnosis of these diseases will depend upon specifically associated manifestations. In scleroderma, swelling along the digits early in the disease is not confined to the joints;

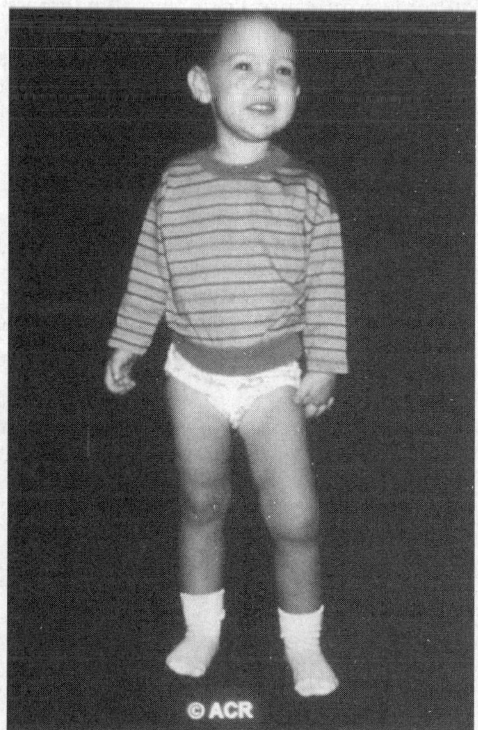

Figure 156–3 Pauciarticular juvenile rheumatoid arthritis with involvement of the left knee and hands. (Reprinted from the Clinical Slide Collection on the Rheumatic Diseases; Copyright 1991, 1995, 1997. Used by permission of the American College of Rheumatology.)

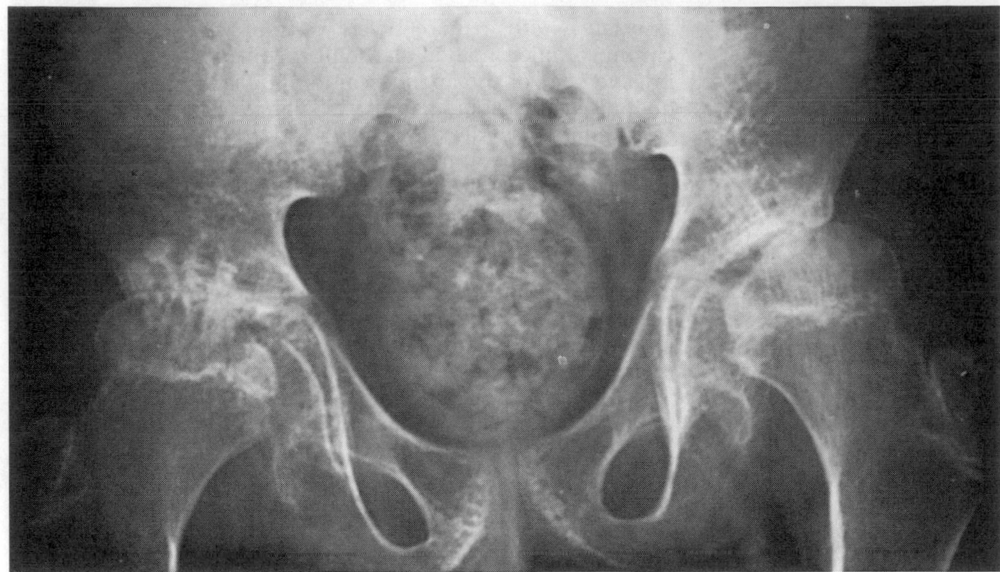

Figure 156–4 Severe hip disease in a 13-yr-old boy with active, systemic-onset juvenile rheumatoid arthritis. X-ray shows destruction of the femoral head and acetabula, joint space narrowing, and subluxation of left hip. The patient had received corticosteroids systemically for 9 yr.

subsequent loss of motion occurs without articular swelling. Rheumatic fever is characterized by exquisite joint tenderness, high spiking fevers, and a polyarthritis that is usually migratory but may also be additive. Joint pain and swelling can be produced by trauma or infection; correlation with history, laboratory, and radiologic findings will help exclude these possibilities. Autoimmune hepatitis can be associated with arthritis. Lyme disease (Chapter 219) should be considered in children living in or visiting endemic areas who present with oligoarticular arthritis. Although a history of tick exposure, preceding flulike illness, and subsequent rash should be sought, these are not always found.

Physical findings may suggest other diagnoses. Fluid in the knee joint resulting in a ballotable patella can be found in JRA but also raises the possibility of infection when a single joint is involved. Chondromalacia of the patella or related femoropatellar syndromes can cause knee pain. Tenderness over insertion of ligaments and tendons raises the possibility of a spondyloarthropathy. Pauciarticular arthritis occurring in an unusual distribution (e.g., small joints of the hand and ankle) can be seen in psoriatic arthritis. However, until psoriasis develops (which may occur years after arthritis presents), that diagnosis can only be suspected.

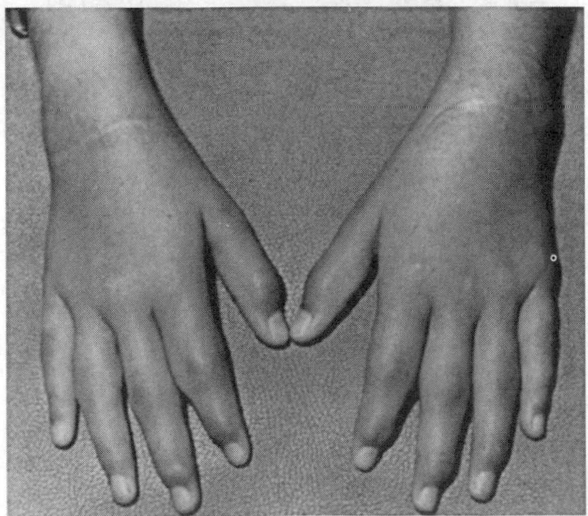

Figure 156–5 Hands and wrists of a girl with rheumatoid factor-negative polyarticular juvenile rheumatoid arthritis. Notice the symmetric involvement of the metacarpophalangeal joints, proximal interphalangeal joints, and distal interphalangeal joints. Both wrists are affected.

Some children will have persistent arthralgia despite repeated normal physical examination. Although these children usually do not have JRA, a diagnosis of JRA may sometimes be confirmed as long as 2 yr after initial presentation. Until persisting joint swelling develops, other diagnoses will need to be considered. Episodes of joint pain and swelling, usually lasting no longer than 1 wk, with complete resolution between episodes, can be seen in juvenile episodic arthritis, often attributed to hypermobility syndrome. Inflammatory bowel disease may present with pauciarticular arthritis, usually affecting joints in the lower extremities. The presence of diarrhea in a child with arthritis can also follow an enteric infection (Chapter 158). A fear of returning to school suggests school phobia.

Less commonly, other diseases can produce joint symptoms and abnormal joint examination. Children with leukemia may have joint pain resulting from metaphyseal expansion of malignant bone marrow, sometimes months before expression of peripheral blood lymphoblasts. Examination of such a child usually reveals a deeper pain to palpation of the bone; bone marrow aspiration will yield the diagnosis. Some diseases, such as cystic fibrosis, diabetes mellitus, and glycogen storage diseases, have associated arthropathies. Swelling that extends beyond the joint can be seen in lymphedema (which may rarely coexist with JRA) and in Henoch-Schönlein purpura. A peripheral arthritis indistinguishable from types of JRA occurs in the presence of humoral immunodeficiency, such as common variable immunodeficiency and selective IgA deficiency.

Laboratory Findings. Hematologic abnormalities often reflect the degree of systemic or articular inflammation, with elevated white blood cell and platelet counts and decreased hemoglobin concentration and mean corpuscular volume. The ESR usually mirrors these findings, along with elevation of CRP, serum globulins, and serum immunoglobulins. However, it is not unusual for the ESR to be normal in some children with JRA, probably when most activated lymphocytes responsible for disease have left the bloodstream and entered the synovium.

ANAs are present in at least 40 to 85% of all children with pauciarticular or polyarticular JRA but are unusual in children with systemic-onset disease. ANAs, usually with homogeneous or speckled pattern, are associated with increased risk for the development of chronic uveitis. The precise specificities for various ANA patterns have not been determined. A positive rheumatoid factor (RF) is often associated with onset of the disease in an older child with polyarticular involvement (approximately 8%) and portends a poor prognosis, the development of rheumatoid nodules, and eventual functional disability. Both ANA and RF can occur in association with transient

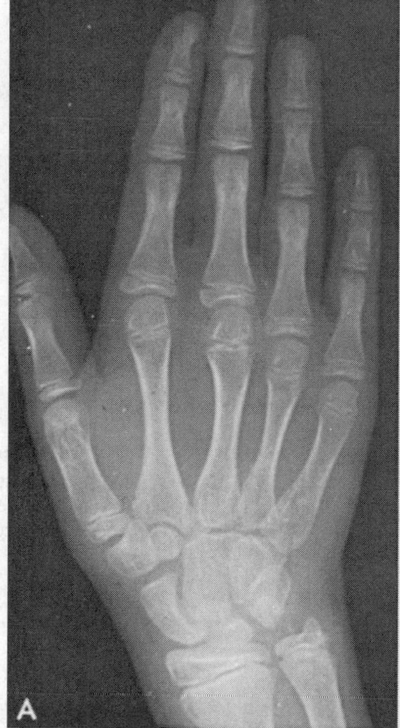

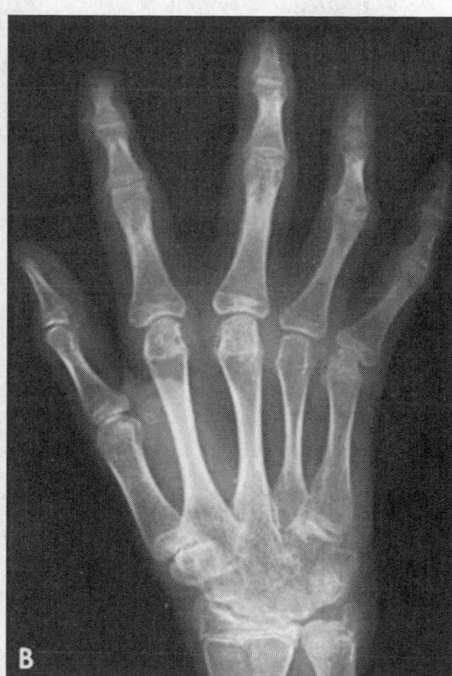

Figure 156–6 Progression of joint destruction in a girl with rheumatoid factor-positive juvenile rheumatoid arthritis despite doses of corticosteroids sufficient to suppress symptoms in the interval between *A* and *B*. *A*, Roentgenogram of the hand at onset. *B*, Roentgenogram 4 yr later, showing a loss of articular cartilage and destruction changes in the distal and proximal interphalangeal and metacarpophalangeal joints and destruction and fusion of wrist bones.

events during childhood, such as viral infections (particularly Epstein-Barr virus); therefore, seropositivity must be defined at a specific titer within a laboratory in relation to accepted positive and negative controls and on the basis of consecutive positive tests over a defined period.

Bone mineral metabolism is often abnormal in children with JRA, relatively independent of onset type or course subtype, and predominantly affects appendicular cortical bone, with less effect upon the normal age-related development of trabecular bone. Increased levels of cytokines such as IL-6 may decrease bone formation (reflected by decreased serum levels of osteocalcin and bone-specific alkaline phosphatase) to a greater extent than bone resorption (which may also be decreased, as reflected by decreased levels of tartrate-resistant acid phosphatase). Corresponding abnormalities of skeletal growth become most prominent during the pubertal growth spurt and in postpubertal children (Tanner stages IV–V).

Early radiographic changes include soft tissue swelling, osteoporosis, and periostitis about the affected joints (Fig. 156–9). Regional epiphyseal closure may be accelerated and the local bone growth increased or decreased. Continued disease may lead to subchondral erosions and narrowing of cartilage space, with varying degrees of bony destruction and fusion. Characteristic late radiographic changes of JRA are seen in the hands and cervical spine, most frequently in the neural arch joints at C2–C3 (see Fig. 156–7). MRI studies may be helpful to evaluate both joint and soft tissues (see Fig. 156–2).

PROGNOSIS. Although the course of JRA in an individual child is unpredictable, some general statements can be made concerning onset type and outcome (Table 156–2). Studies from the United States indicate that, despite current management, approximately 45% of JRA patients have active disease

Figure 156–7 Radiograph of the cervical spine of a patient with active juvenile rheumatoid arthritis, showing fusion of the neural arch between joints C2-C3, narrowing and erosion of the remaining neural arch joints, obliteration of the apophyseal space, and loss of the normal lordosis.

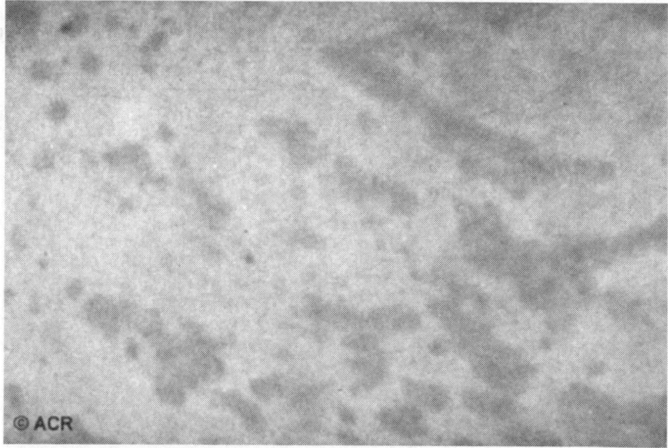

Figure 156–8 The rash of systemic-onset juvenile rheumatoid arthritis. The rash is salmon colored, macular, and nonpruritic. Individual lesions are transient and occur in crops over the trunk and extremities. (Reprinted from the Clinical Slide Collection on the Rheumatic Diseases; Copyright 1991, 1995, 1997. Used by permission of the American College of Rheumatology.)

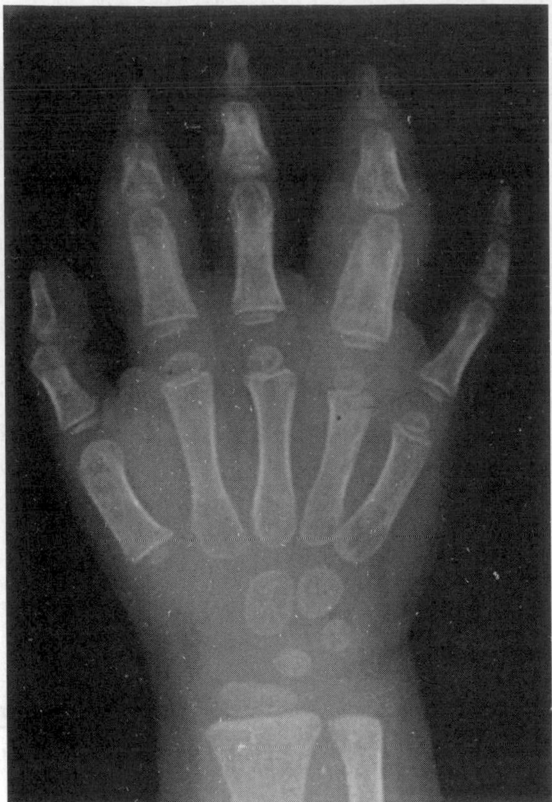

Figure 156–9 Early (6-mo duration) radiographic changes of juvenile rheumatoid arthritis, soft tissue swelling, and periosteal new bone formation appear adjacent to the 2nd and 4th proximal interphalangeal joints.

persisting into early adulthood, often with severe limitations of physical function.

The child with oligoarticular disease, particularly a girl with early onset of arthritis at <6 yr of age, is at risk to develop chronic uveitis. There is usually no association in the course of the arthritis and the chronic uveitis (Fig. 156–10). Uveitis in children with pauciarticular disease can result in posterior synechiae; untreated or refractory disease can result in blindness, which has decreased with more frequent monitoring by slit-lamp examination to exclude asymptomatic uveitis. Many of these children do well, however, with early remission.

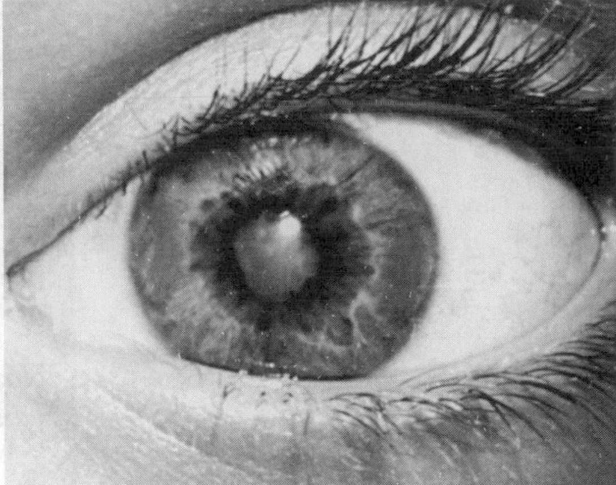

Figure 156–10 Chronic iridocyclitis of juvenile rheumatoid arthritis. Extensive posterior synechiae have resulted in a small, irregular pupil. There is a well-developed cataract and early band keratopathy at the medial and lateral margins of the cornea.

The child with polyarticular disease often has a more prolonged course. Functional risk has been associated with older age of onset, the presence of rheumatoid factor seropositivity or rheumatoid nodules, or the early development of specific articular disease, such as that affecting the cervical spine or hips.

The child with systemic onset is often the most difficult to manage in terms of both articular and systemic manifestations. However, systemic manifestations are usually present only during the first few years after onset. The prognosis after that time is dependent on the number of joints involved and severity of the arthritis.

Anemia, common in active disease or disease of prolonged duration, is usually unresponsive to administration of oral or parenteral iron. Anemia may be exacerbated by gastrointestinal bleeding associated with the use of nonsteroidal anti-inflammatory drugs (NSAIDs). Specific complications may occur in subsets of the disease, such as the development of systemic lupus erythematosus (SLE) during the course of children with polyarticular JRA. Anemia associated with decreases in other blood cell lines raises the possibility of malignancy. Rarely, anemia is a result of hemolytic anemia. Anemia associated with thrombocytopenia or leukopenia in a child with fevers, lymphadenopathy, and hepatosplenomegaly suggests macro-

TABLE 156–2 Prognosis of Juvenile Rheumatoid Arthritis by Type of Onset

Onset Type	Course Subtype	Profile	Outcome
Polyarthritis	RF-seropositive	Female Older age Hand/wrist Erosions Nodules Unremitting	Poor
	ANA-seropositive	Female Young age	Good
	Seronegative	—	Variable
Oligoarthritis	ANA-seropositive	Female Young age Chronic uveitis	Excellent (except eyes)
	RF-seropositive	Polyarthritis Erosions Unremitting	Poor
	HLA-B27–positive	Male Older age	Good
	Seronegative	—	Good
Systemic disease	Oligoarthritis	—	Good
	Polyarthritis	Erosions	Poor

From Cassidy JT, Petty RE: Juvenile rheumatoid arthritis. In *Textbook of Pediatric Rheumatology, 3rd ed. Philadelphia, WB Saunders, 1995.*

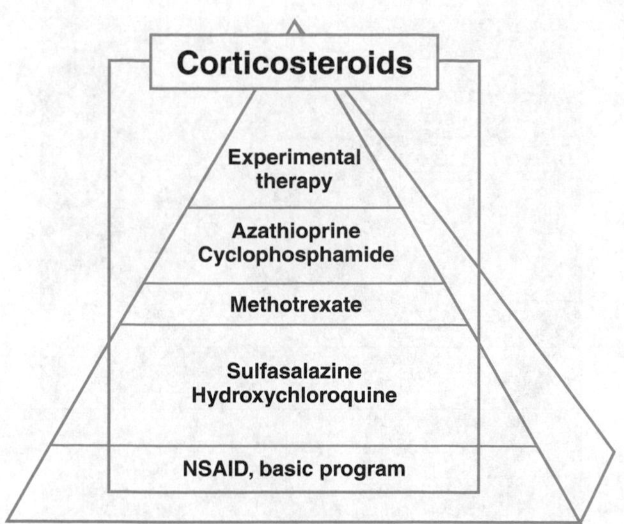

Figure 156–11 The "therapeutic pyramid" of juvenile rheumatoid arthritis. (Adapted from Cassidy JT, Petty RE: Juvenile rheumatoid arthritis. *In:* Textbook of Pediatric Rheumatology, 3rd ed. Philadelphia, WB Saunders, 1995.)

phage activation syndrome, a rare complication of systemic JRA. Diagnosis is confirmed by liver or bone marrow biopsy. Treatment with cyclosporine has been effective in many patients. The development of manifestations of other rheumatic diseases suggests that the diagnosis has changed to an overlapping syndrome or a specific disease, such as SLE or dermatomyositis.

Orthopedic complications include leg length discrepancy, which can be treated with a shoe lift on the shorter side; popliteal cysts, which require no treatment if small; and flexion contractures, particularly of the knees, hips, and wrists. Contractures require medical control of arthritis, appropriate splinting, and a physical therapy program to allow stretching of affected tendons.

Psychosocial adaptation may be affected by JRA. Studies from Scandinavia and the United States indicate that, compared with controls, many of these children have problems with lifetime adjustments and obtaining employment. Disability, not directly associated with arthritis, may continue into young adulthood in as many as 20% of patients, together with continuing chronic pain syndromes in a similar frequency. Psychologic complications, including problems with school attendance and socialization, may respond to counseling by mental health professionals.

TREATMENT. The long-term treatment of children with JRA is initiated and subsequently modified according to disease subtype, severity of the disease, specific manifestations of the illness, and response to therapy. The objectives of treatment are to establish the child in a pattern of adaptation that is as normal as possible and to accomplish this goal with minimal risk of side effects.

A pyramid of therapeutic approach should be considered; combination therapy should begin with the least toxic medications, usually NSAIDs, and proceeding through hydroxychloroquine, methotrexate, or possibly immunosuppressive or experimental drugs (Fig. 156–11). Medications that place the child's present and future health most at risk, such as azathioprine, and cyclophosphamide, are reserved for the very few children who do not respond to less aggressive therapy. Newer modes of treatment may prove to be more specific for synovial inflammatory disease and potentially less toxic than current medications, e.g., the experimental use of soluble TNF-α receptor antagonists.

Corticosteroids are used for management of overwhelming systemic illness, in lower doses for "bridge therapy" for the child who has not yet responded, to the addition of a drug such as methotrexate, and for ophthalmic and intra-articular use. Corticosteroids are very powerful anti-inflammatory drugs, perhaps the most efficacious in current use but impose upon the child the risk of severe toxicity, including Cushing syndrome, growth retardation, and osteopenia.

Methotrexate is considered the safest, most efficacious, and least toxic of the currently available second-line agents. It may be given either orally or subcutaneously once weekly. Intramuscular gold therapy has been generally supplanted by methotrexate. Sulfasalazine may have potential when added to the treatment in selected patients.

Nonmedical aspects of treatment include routine slit-lamp ophthalmic examination of all patients with JRA to exclude asymptomatic uveitis, dietary evaluation and counseling to assure appropriate calcium intake, and physical and occupational therapy.

Aasland A, Flato B, Vandvik IH: Psychosocial outcome in juvenile chronic arthritis: A nine-year follow-up. Clin Exp Rheumatol 15:561, 1997.

Cassidy JT, Levinson JE, Bass JC, et al: A study of classification criteria for a diagnosis of juvenile rheumatoid arthritis. Arthritis Rheum 29:274, 1986.

De Benedetti F, Ravelli A, Martini A: Cytokines in juvenile rheumatoid arthritis. Curr Opin Rheumatol 9:428, 1997.

Denardo BA, Tucker LB, Miller LC, et al: Demography of a regional pediatric rheumatology patient population. J Rheumatol 21:1553, 1994.

Feldman BM, Birdi N, Boone JE, et al: Seasonal onset of systemic-onset juvenile rheumatoid arthritis. J Pediatr 129:513, 1996.

Fernandez-Vina M, Fink CW, Stastny P: HLA associations in juvenile arthritis. Clin Exp Rheumatol 12:205, 1994.

Gare BA: Epidemiology of rheumatic disease in children. Curr Opin Rheumatol 8:449, 1996.

Giannini EH, Brewer EJ Jr, Kuzmina N, et al: Methotrexate in resistant juvenile rheumatoid arthritis. Results of the U.S.A.–U.S.S.R. double-blind, placebo-controlled trial. N Engl J Med 326:1043, 1992.

Grom AA, Murray KJ, Luyrink L, et al: Patterns of expression of tumor necrosis factor alpha, tumor necrosis factor beta, and their receptors in synovia of patients with juvenile rheumatoid arthritis and juvenile spondyloarthropathy. Arthritis Rheum 39:1703, 1996.

Manners PJ, Diepeveen DA: Prevalence of juvenile chronic arthritis in a population of 12-year-old children in urban Australia. Pediatrics 98:84, 1996.

Mouy R, Stephan JL, Pillet P, et al: Efficacy of cyclosporin A in the treatment of macrophage activation syndrome in juvenile arthritis: Report of five cases. J Pediatr 129:750, 1996.

Pepmueller PH, Cassidy JT, Allen SH, et al: Bone mineralization and bone mineral metabolism in children with juvenile rheumatoid arthritis. Arthritis Rheum 39:746, 1996.

Peterson LS, Mason T, Nelson AM, et al: Juvenile rheumatoid arthritis in Rochester, Minnesota 1960–1993. Is the epidemiology changing? Arthritis Rheum 39:1385, 1996.

Peterson LS, Mason T, Nelson AM, et al: Psychosocial outcomes and health status of adults who have had juvenile rheumatoid arthritis: A controlled, population-based study. Arthritis Rheum 40:2235, 1997.

Prakken AB, van Eden W, Rijkers GT, et al: Autoreactivity to human heat-shock protein 60 predicts disease remission in oligoarticular juvenile rheumatoid arthritis. Arthritis Rheum 39:1826, 1996.

Ragsdale CG, Petty RE, Cassidy JT, et al: The clinical progression of apparent juvenile rheumatoid arthritis to systemic lupus erythematosus. J Rheumatol 7:50, 1980.

Schwartz MM, Simpson P, Kerr KL, et al: Juvenile rheumatoid arthritis in African Americans. J Rheumatol 24:1826, 1997.

Sullivan DB, Cassidy JT, Petty RE: Pathogenic implications of age of onset in juvenile rheumatoid arthritis. Arthritis Rheum 18:251, 1975.

Thompson SD, Murray KJ, Grom AA, et al: Comparative sequence analysis of the human T cell receptor beta chain in juvenile rheumatoid arthritis and juvenile spondyloarthropathies: Evidence for antigenic selection of T cells in the synovium. Arthritis Rheum 41:482, 1998.

Walco GA, Varni JW, Ilowite NT: Cognitive-behavioral pain management in children with juvenile rheumatoid arthritis. Pediatrics 89:1075, 1992.

Zhang H, Phang D, Laxer RM, et al: Evolution of the T cell receptor beta repertoire from synovial fluid T cells of patients with juvenile onset rheumatoid arthritis. J Rheumatol 24:1396, 1997.

CHAPTER 157
Ankylosing Spondylitis and Other Spondyloarthropathies

Michael L. Miller and Ross E. Petty

The diseases collectively referred to as spondyloarthropathies include ankylosing spondylitis, the psoriatic arthritides, arthritis accompanying inflammatory bowel diseases, and chronic reactive arthritis following enteric or genitourinary (GU) tract infections. They are characterized by inflammation of joints of the axial skeleton as well as the limbs, by the presence of enthesitis (inflammation at the sites of attachments of ligaments, tendons, fascias, and capsules to bone), and by the absence of rheumatoid factor.

EPIDEMIOLOGY. Estimates of the prevalence of juvenile ankylosing spondylitis (JAS) range from 11–86/100,000 children and of psoriatic arthritis from 10–15/100,000 children. JAS occurs most frequently in older boys, adolescents, and young adults. The histocompatibility antigen HLA-B27 is strongly associated with JAS (>90%), and is also found in increased frequency in persons having spondyloarthropathies with inflammation of the axial skeleton. As a consequence, these disorders are frequently familial.

Psoriatic arthritis is particularly common in young girls. The arthropathies of inflammatory bowel diseases, reactive arthritis, and Reiter syndrome are much less common in childhood; they can affect children of any age and are somewhat more common in boys.

PATHOGENESIS. The histologic appearance of the synovium in spondyloarthropathies is indistinguishable from that of other idiopathic chronic arthritides. Tenosynovitis may be present, and periostitis may occur. Enthesitis is characterized by chronic inflammation and, in advanced disease, usually found in adults, by calcification of ligaments and fusion of joints.

Chronic reactive arthritis may follow enteric infection with *Salmonella enteritidis, Salmonella oranienburg, Salmonella typhimurium, Shigella flexneri, Yersinia enterocolitica,* or *Campylobacter jejuni,* or GU tract infection with *Chlamydia trachomatis.* The cause of the other spondyloarthropathies is unknown. It is postulated that similarity between self-antigens and bacterial antigens (molecular mimicry) permits the development of an autoimmune process in genetically predisposed individuals.

CLINICAL MANIFESTATIONS

Juvenile Ankylosing Spondylitis. Early JAS is most frequently characterized by oligoarthritis and enthesitis. Joints of the legs are more frequently affected than those of the arms, and abnormalities of the axial skeleton including sacroiliac joints are usually absent until later in the disease course. Loss of spinal flexibility may eventually be noted (Fig. 157–1). Hip joint arthritis at onset is particularly suggestive of early JAS. Enthesitis, presenting as localized tenderness at characteristic locations around the foot and knee, is particularly common and has led to the description of a syndrome of seronegativity (absence of rheumatoid factor), enthesitis, and arthritis (SEA syndrome), which is probably the most common initial presentation of JAS. The disease course is often characterized by long periods of apparent disease remission. Systemic symptoms such as low-grade fever and weight loss raise questions about the possibility of occult inflammatory bowel disease.

Psoriatic Arthritis. The most common pattern of psoriatic arthritis is oligoarthritis affecting large and small joints in an asymmetric pattern. Patients with psoriatic arthritis occasionally have symmetric distal interphalangeal joint disease or sacroiliitis that is associated with HLA-B27. The presence of nail pitting (Fig. 157–2), dactylitis, onycholysis, or a family history of psoriasis supports the diagnosis of psoriatic arthritis in a child with oligoarthritis or polyarthritis.

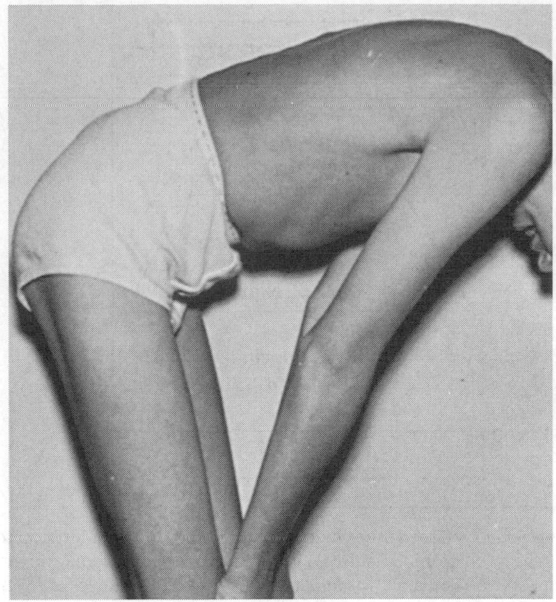

Figure 157–1 Loss of lumbodorsal spine mobility in a boy with ankylosing spondylitis: The lower spine remains straight when the patient bends forward.

Arthritis with Inflammatory Bowel Disease. Two patterns of arthritis complicate Crohn disease and ulcerative colitis. A polyarthritis affecting large and small joints, which reflects the activity of the intestinal inflammation, is most common and is not truly a spondylarthritis because it does not affect joints of the spine and is not associated with HLA-B27. Less commonly, arthritis of the sacroiliac joints and other peripheral joints (in a pattern similar to that in ankylosing spondylitis) occurs, accompanied in most instances by HLA-B27. Its severity is independent of the activity of the gastrointestinal (GI) inflammation.

Reactive Arthritis. Reactive arthritis, which includes Reiter syndrome (arthritis, urethritis, and conjunctivitis), is usually preceded by GI or GU infection. The arthritis is usually oligoarticular and may be quite severe, with considerable swelling, pain, and even erythema. Joints of the lower limbs are most commonly affected. Unlike the more common clinical forms of

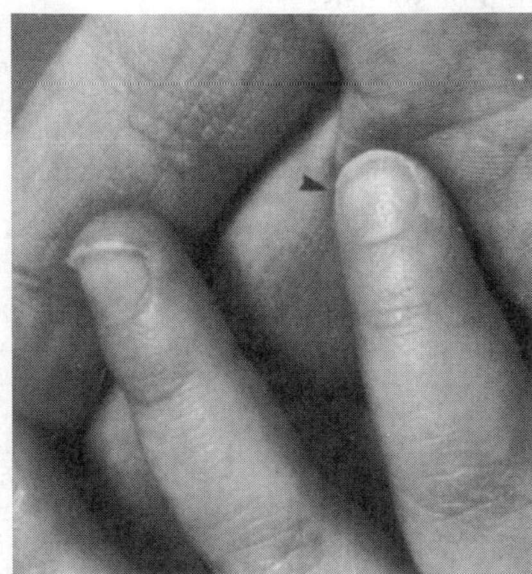

Figure 157–2 Nail pitting *(arrow)* and "sausage digit" (dactylitis) of the left index finger of a girl with juvenile psoriatic arthritis. (From Petty RE, Malleson P: Spondyloarthropathies of childhood. Pediatr Clin North Am 33;1079, 1986.)

self-limited reactive arthritis (Chapter 158), the arthritis may become chronic, with a duration of arthritis that ranges from several weeks to years. Enthesitis may be prominent.

DIAGNOSIS. The diagnosis of a spondyloarthropathy is suggested by the onset in an older child, particularly a boy, of oligoarthritis that predominantly affects the hips, knees, ankles or feet, and particularly the intertarsal joints, especially if accompanied by enthesitis. A diagnosis of ankylosing spondylitis is confirmed if there is radiographic evidence of sacroiliitis. Because radiographic changes seldom occur at onset, it may be difficult to differentiate a spondylarthritis from oligoarticular juvenile rheumatoid arthritis (JRA) early during the disease course. The presence of synovitis in the upper extremities tends to be more common in patients with JRA than with spondyloarthropathies. The presence of erythema nodosum, pyoderma gangrenosum, significant fever, weight loss, or anorexia suggests inflammatory bowel disease. The acute onset of arthritis, a recent history of diarrhea, and symptoms of urethritis or conjunctivitis may suggest reactive arthritis. Psoriasis, nail changes (see Fig. 157–2), or a family history of psoriasis suggests the diagnosis of psoriatic arthritis in a child (often a young girl) with oligoarthritis or polyarthritis. Early differentiation among the spondyloarthropathies by laboratory or radiographic means is difficult. Sacroiliac joint change or enthesitis may be seen on technetium-99 bone scan, but results of this examination are often difficult to interpret in children and adolescents.

Back pain may occur in children with early ankylosing spondylitis but could also be caused by septic arthritis of the sacroiliac joint, osteomyelitis of the pelvis or spine, osteoid osteoma of the posterior elements of the spine, or malignancies such as osteogenic sarcoma, Ewing sarcoma, or leukemia. In addition, mechanical causes such as spondylolysis, spondylolisthesis, and Scheuermann disease should be considered. Back pain secondary to fibromyalgia usually affects the soft tissues of the upper back in a symmetric pattern, as well as other well-localized tender points.

Hip joint arthritis is characterized by pain over the inguinal ligament and loss of internal rotation of the hip joint. Legg-Calvé-Perthes disease, slipped capital femoral epiphysis, and chondrolysis may have a similar presentation.

LABORATORY FINDINGS. Laboratory evidence of systemic inflammation is often present at the onset of disease, with elevated erythrocyte sedimentation rate and mild increase in white blood cell count and platelet count. Rheumatoid factor is absent in all children with spondyloarthropathies. Antinuclear antibodies are absent except in children with psoriatic arthritis, in whom antinuclear autoantibodies occur in as many as 50%. HLA-B27 is present in more than 90% of children with JAS but is probably not increased significantly in those with other types of spondylarthritis unless sacroiliitis or acute anterior uveitis is present.

Radiographic changes include periarticular osteoporosis, loss of sharp cortical margins in areas of enthesitis (which may eventually show erosions or bony spurs), sclerosis and indistinct margins of the sacroiliac joints (Fig. 157–3), and, rarely, squaring of the corners of the vertebral bodies. The characteristic "bamboo" spine caused by calcification of ligaments so characteristic of advanced ankylosing spondylitis in adults is very rare in childhood.

COMPLICATIONS. Acute iridocyclitis occurs in as many as 25% of patients with JAS. Chronic iridocyclitis similar to that in JRA occurs in approximately 15% of children with psoriatic arthritis. Aortic valve insufficiency is a rare but important complication of ankylosing spondylitis. Atlantoaxial subluxation has also been reported.

TREATMENT. The aims of therapy are to minimize pain, control inflammation, and preserve function. These are accomplished by a combination of anti-inflammatory medications, physical therapy, and psychosocial support. Nonsteroidal anti-inflammatory drugs may be sufficient. It may be necessary to add sulfasalazine (up to 50 mg/kg/24 hr, no more than 3 g/24 hr in adolescents). Intra-articular triamcinolone hexacetonide is useful for controlling localized joint inflammation. Exercises to maintain range of motion in the back, thorax, and affected joints should be instituted early in the disease course. Custom-fitted insoles are particularly useful in management of painful entheses around the feet.

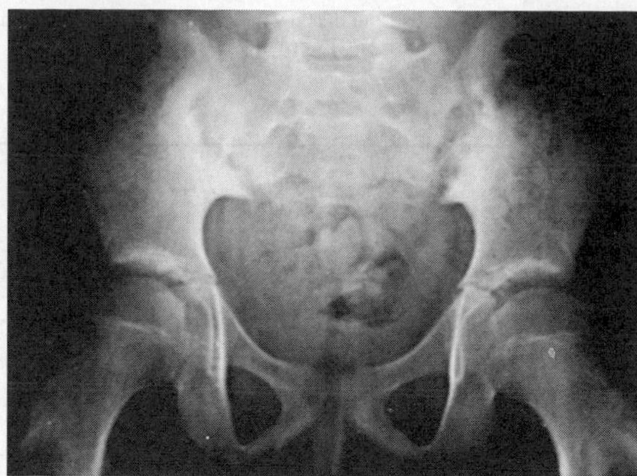

Figure 157–3 Well-developed sacroiliitis in a boy with ankylosing spondylitis; both sacroiliac joints show extensive sclerosis, erosion of joint margins, and apparent widening of the joint space.

PROGNOSIS. There is little reliable information about long-term outcome of the spondyloarthropathies in childhood. These are chronic diseases with highly variable clinical courses. JAS is often characterized by long periods of active disease followed by long periods of inactivity. Most studies have shown that over many years, the disease progresses to involve joints of the spine and sacroiliac joints and may cause fusion and significant disability. Psoriatic arthritis tends to be a chronic unremitting disease. Reactive arthritis may be very brief (several weeks or months) but may become chronic and progress to ankylosing spondylitis. In children with inflammatory bowel disease, the peripheral arthritis is usually controlled when the GI inflammation is controlled; if the arthritis is associated with HLA-B27, the course tends to be more chronic.

Burgos-Vargas R, Vazquez-Mellado J: The early clinical recognition of juvenile-onset ankylosing spondylitis and its differentiation from juvenile rheumatoid arthritis. Arthritis Rheum 38:835, 1995.

Cabral DA, Oen KG, Petty RE: SEA syndrome revisited: A long-term followup of children with a syndrome of seronegative enthesopathy and arthropathy. J Rheumatol 19:1282, 1992.

Flato B, Aasland A, Vinje O, et al: Outcome and predictive factors in juvenile rheumatoid arthritis and juvenile spondyloarthropathy. J Rheumatol 25:366, 1998.

Foster HE, Cairns RA, Burnell RH, et al: Atlantoaxial subluxation in children with seronegative enthesopathy and arthropathy syndrome: 2 case reports and a review of the literature. J Rheumatol 22:548, 1995.

Jacobs JC, Berdon WE, Johnston AD: HLA-B27-associated spondyloarthritis and enthesopathy in childhood: Clinical, pathologic, and radiographic observations in 58 patients. J Pediatr 100:521, 1982.

Mielants H, Veys EM, Cuvelier C, et al: Gut inflammation in children with late onset pauciarticular juvenile chronic arthritis and evolution to adult spondyloarthropathy—a prospective study. J Rheumatol 20:1567, 1993.

Peh WC, Ho WY, Luk KD: Applications of bone scintigraphy in ankylosing spondylitis. Clin Imaging 21:54, 1997.

Roberton DM, Cabral DA, Malleson PN, et al: Juvenile psoriatic arthritis: Follow-up and evaluation of diagnostic criteria. J Rheumatol 23:166, 1996.

Rosenberg AM, Petty RE: A syndrome of seronegative enthesopathy and arthropathy in children. Arthritis Rheum 25:1041, 1982.

Schaller J, Bitnum S, Wedgwood RJ: Ankylosing spondylitis with childhood onset. J Pediatr 74:505, 1969.

Sheerin KA, Giannini EH, Brewer EJ Jr, et al: HLA-B27-associated arthropathy in childhood: Long-term clinical and diagnostic outcome. Arthritis Rheum 31:1165, 1988.

Shore A, Ansell BM: Juvenile psoriatic arthritis—an analysis of 60 cases. J Pediatr 100:529, 1982.

Southwood TR, Petty RE, Malleson PN, et al: Psoriatic arthritis in children. Arthritis Rheum 32:1007, 1989.

Stamato T, Laxer RM, de Freitas C, et al: Prevalence of cardiac manifestations of juvenile ankylosing spondylitis. Am J Cardiol 75:744, 1995.

CHAPTER 158
Postinfectious Arthritis and Related Conditions

Michael L. Miller and James T. Cassidy

Infections have been associated with arthritis during their course and as a postinfectious reaction observed several weeks or months afterward. Although certain infectious organisms have been suspected but not proved to trigger juvenile rheumatoid arthritis (JRA), other agents that have been identified are often associated with a transient arthritis that does not satisfy the classification criteria for JRA. *Reactive arthritis* follows an infection outside the joint, particularly the gastrointestinal (GI) or genitourinary (GU) tract. The course of reactive arthritis is variable and may progress to chronic spondyloarthropathy (Chapter 157). *Postinfectious arthritis* follows infections that are usually viral in origin and of shorter duration than reactive arthritis.

PATHOGENESIS. Reactive arthritis may follow enteric infection with *Salmonella enteritidis, S. oranienburg, S. typhimurium, Shigella flexneri, Yersinia enterocolitica,* or *Campylobacter jejuni,* or GU tract infection with *Chlamydia trachomatis.* Reactive arthritis most likely represents an autoimmune response involving T lymphocytes that are cross-reactive to antigens in joints. A study of synovial fluid from patients with reactive arthritis suggested that T cells may be more engaged in promoting inflammation than in eliminating bacteria through cytotoxic mechanisms. However, the origin of these abnormal cells may be from outside the joint. Studies of joint fluid from patients with reactive arthritis, using polymerase chain reaction (PCR) amplification, have failed to demonstrate bacterial DNA.

Several viruses (rubella, varicella-zoster, herpes simplex, and cytomegalovirus) have been isolated from the joint space. Antigens from other viruses (hepatitis B, adenovirus 7) have been identified in immune complexes from joint tissue. Postinfectious arthritis following viral infections appears to involve the deposition in joints of immune complexes containing viral antigens.

Certain HLA types may predispose to development of reactive arthritis, possibly by triggering autoreactive T lymphocytes. Adolescents and adults with reactive arthritis following enteric infections have shown persistent gut inflammation even after resolution of GI manifestations, particularly in HLA-B27–positive individuals. Uveitis complicating reactive arthritis to *Yersinia* enteritis has also been associated with HLA-B27. Some children with reactive arthritis (often HLA-B27 positive) eventually develop spondyloarthropathy, further suggesting that HLA antigens have a role in pathogenesis.

CLINICAL MANIFESTATIONS. Bacterial enteritis caused by *Shigella, Salmonella, Yersinia,* and *Campylobacter* can be followed within days to several weeks by the development of arthritis and sometimes enthesitis in a syndrome similar to spondyloarthropathy and overlapping with it (Chapter 157). Although the erythrocyte sedimentation rate may be elevated, fever and leukocytosis are often absent. Urethritis and conjunctivitis (Reiter syndrome) will also develop occasionally. Postinfectious arthritis following less apparent illness, such as viral upper respiratory tract infections, may precede arthralgia and arthritis by 1–2 mo. Symptoms of arthralgia and joint swelling are transient, usually lasting less than 6 wk.

Certain viruses associated with arthritis (Table 158–1) may result in particular patterns of joint involvement. Rubella and hepatitis B virus typically affect the small joints, and mumps and varicella often involve large joints, in particular the knees. The hepatitis B arthritis-dermatitis syndrome is characterized by rash and arthritis resembling serum sickness. Rubella-associated arthropathy follows natural rubella infection and, infrequently, rubella immunization. It typically occurs in young women, with increased incidence with advancing age, and is uncommon in preadolescent children and in males. Arthralgias of the knees and hands usually begin within 7 days of onset of the rash or 10–28 days after immunization. Parvovirus B19, responsible for erythema infectiosum (fifth disease), can cause arthralgia, symmetric joint swelling, and morning stiffness in adults, particularly women, and less frequently in children. Arthritis is rare after Epstein-Barr virus infection but occurs occasionally during cytomegalovirus infection and may occur during varicella infections. Varicella may also be complicated by septic arthritis, usually due to group A *Streptococcus.*

Arthritis has been reported in children with severe truncal acne, usually in male adolescents. Patients often have fever and superficial infection of skin lesions. Recurrent episodes may be associated with myopathy and may last for as long as several months. Infective endocarditis can be associated with arthralgia, arthritis, or signs suggestive of vasculitis, such as Osler nodes, Janeway lesions, and Roth spots. Arthritis has also occurred in children with *Mycoplasma pneumoniae* infections.

Poststreptococcal arthritis may follow infection with either group A or group G *Streptococcus.* Because valvular lesions have been documented by echocardiography after the acute illness in some of these children, some clinicians consider this to be an incomplete form of acute rheumatic fever (Chapter 184.1). Certain HLA-DRB1 types may predispose children to develop either poststreptococcal arthritis or classic rheumatic fever. Poststreptococcal arthritis is pauciarticular, may affect the small and large joints, and persists for months, compared with the typical course of migratory polyarthritis of rheumatic fever. The symptoms are usually mild and tend to resolve completely.

Transient synovitis (toxic synovitis) typically affects the hip, often after a respiratory infection. Boys from 3–10 yr of age are most commonly affected and have complaints of pain in the hip, thigh, or knee. The erythrocyte sedimentation rate and white blood cell count are usually normal. Radiologic or ultrasound examination may reveal widening of the joint space of the hip. Aspiration of the hip may be necessary to exclude septic arthritis. The cause of this relatively common syndrome is not known, but it is presumed to be a viral or postinfectious arthritis.

DIAGNOSIS. The diagnosis of reactive postinfectious arthritis is made by exclusion after arthritis has resolved. Arthritis affecting a single joint may result from septic arthritis; osteomyelitis

TABLE 158–1 Viruses Associated with Arthritis

Togaviruses	Adenoviruses
Rubivirus	Adenovirus 7
Rubella	Herpesviruses
Alphaviruses	Epstein-Barr
Ross River	Cytomegalovirus
Chikungunya	Varicella-zoster
O'nyong-nyong	Herpes simplex
Mayaro	Paramyxoviruses
Sindbis	Mumps
Ockelbo	Enteroviruses
Pogosta	Echovirus
Parvovirus	Coxsackievirus B
B19	Orthopoxviruses
Hepadnavirus	Variola virus (smallpox)
Hepatitis B	Vaccinia virus

Adapted from Cassidy JT, Petty RE: Arthritis related to infection. In: *Textbook of Pediatric Rheumatology. Philadelphia, WB Saunders, 1995, p 503.*

may cause joint pain but more often is associated with pain over the site of infection. Arthritis associated with GI symptoms or elevated liver function test results may be caused by infectious or autoimmune hepatitis. Arthritis or spondyloarthritis may occur in some children with inflammatory bowel disease, either Crohn disease or chronic ulcerative colitis (Chapter 337). When two or more blood cell lines show a progressive decrease in a child with arthritis, parvovirus infection, macrophage activation syndrome, and leukemia need to be considered. Persisting arthritis suggests the possibility of rheumatic disease, including JRA, spondyloarthropathy, and systemic lupus erythematosus.

COMPLICATIONS. Postinfectious arthritis following viral infections usually resolves without complications unless it is part of a severe viral infection affecting other organs (e.g., in children with encephalomyelitis). Reactive arthritis, especially after bacterial enteric infection or GU tract infection with *C. trachomatis*, has the potential for evolving to a chronic arthritis and spondyloarthropathy (Chapter 157). Children with reactive arthritis following enteric infections occasionally develop inflammatory bowel disease months to years after onset. Both uveitis and carditis have been reported in some children with reactive arthritis.

TREATMENT. No specific treatment is necessary for postinfectious arthritis, except that directed at relief of pain and the functional limitations of arthritis. If swelling or arthralgia recurs, further evaluation may be necessary to preclude active infection or evolving rheumatic disease, such as spondyloarthropathy, JRA, or systemic lupus erythematosus.

Ahmed S, Ayoub EM, Scornik JC, et al: Poststreptococcal reactive arthritis: Clinical characteristics and association with HLA-DR alleles. Arthritis Rheum 41:1096, 1998.

Birdi N, Allen U, D'Astous J: Poststreptococcal reactive arthritis mimicking acute septic arthritis: A hospital-based study. J Pediatr Orthoped 15:661, 1995.

Carroll WL, Balistreri WF, Brilli R, et al: Spectrum of *Salmonella*-associated arthritis. Pediatrics 68:717, 1981.

Chantler JK, Tingle AJ, Petty RE: Persistent rubella virus infection associated with chronic arthritis in children. N Engl J Med 313:1117, 1985.

Cron RQ, Sherry DD: Reiter's syndrome associated with cryptosporidial gastroenteritis. J Rheumatol 22:1962, 1995.

De Cunto CL, Giannini EH, Fink CW, et al: Prognosis of children with poststreptococcal reactive arthritis. Pediatr Infect Dis J 7:683, 1988.

Huppertz HI, Sandhage K: Reactive arthritis due to *Salmonella enteritidis* complicated by carditis. Acta Paediatr 83:1230, 1994.

Mertz AK, Ugrinovic S, Lauster R, et al: Characterization of the synovial T cell response to various recombinant Yersinia antigens in *Yersinia enterocolitica*–triggered reactive arthritis. Heat-shock protein 60 drives a major immune response. Arthritis Rheum 41:315, 1998.

Moon RY, Greene MG, Rehe GT, et al: Poststreptococcal reactive arthritis in children: A potential predecessor of rheumatic heart disease. J Rheumatol 22:529, 1995.

Petty RE, Tingle AJ: Arthritis and viral infection. J Pediatr 113:948, 1988.

Poggio TV, Orlando N, Galanternik L, et al: Microbiology of acute arthropathies among children in Argentina: *Mycoplasma pneumoniae* and *hominis* and *Ureaplasma urealyticum*. Pediatr Infect Dis J 17:304, 1998.

Schaad UB: Reactive arthritis associated with *Campylobacter enteritis*. Pediatr Infect Dis 1:328, 1982.

Tingle AJ, Allen M, Petty RE, et al: Rubella-associated arthritis. I. Comparative study of joint manifestations associated with natural rubella infection and RA 27/3 rubella immunization. Ann Rheum Dis 45:110, 1986.

Yin Z, Braun J, Neure L, et al: Crucial role of interleukin-10/interleukin-12 balance in the regulation of the type 2 T helper cytokine response in reactive arthritis. Arthritis Rheum 40:1788, 1997.

CHAPTER 159

Systemic Lupus Erythematosus

Marisa S. Klein-Gitelman and Michael L. Miller

Systemic lupus erythematosus (SLE, or lupus), a rheumatic disease of unknown cause, is characterized by autoantibodies directed against self-antigens and resulting inflammatory damage to target organs including the kidneys, blood cells, and the central nervous system (CNS). The natural history of SLE is unpredictable; patients may present with many years of symptoms or with acute, life-threatening disease. Untreated SLE may be followed by spontaneous remission, years of smoldering disease, or rapid death. Because of its possible manifestations, SLE must be considered in the differential diagnosis of many problems, ranging from fevers of unknown origin to arthralgia, anemia, and nephritis. Early diagnosis and treatment tailored to the particular problems of an individual patient can greatly improve the prognosis for what used to be a fatal disease.

ETIOLOGY. The cause and disease mechanisms of SLE remain unknown. Research suggests that many factors, including genetics, hormones, and the environment, contribute to immune dysregulation in lupus. The hallmark is autoantibody production against many self-antigens, particularly DNA, as well as other nuclear antigens, ribosomes, platelets, coagulation factors, immunoglobulin, erythrocytes, and leukocytes. Elevated levels of autoantibodies, particularly anti-DNA antibodies, are associated with circulating and tissue-bound immune complexes. These result in complement fixation and recruitment of inflammatory cells, leading to tissue injury.

Polyclonal activation of B lymphocytes results in elevated immunoglobulin levels, which may be one cause of elevated autoantibody levels. The mechanism for polyclonal activation is not yet understood. Possible causes include nonspecific response to an antigenic stimulus such as a viral agent or loss of tolerance to self-antigens by loss of suppressor T-lymphocyte function. Investigations have focused on the normal phenomenon of programmed cell death or apoptosis. Apoptosis is regulated by several proteins including *fas* and *bcl*-2. Dysregulation of apoptosis in SLE may lead to the presence of self-reactive lymphocytes that normally undergo apoptosis before birth.

Other mechanisms may have a role in amplifying the effects of SLE. Defects in macrophage phagocytosis and handling of immune complexes have been described. The effects of sex hormones may be responsible for the predominance of females with SLE; one study found higher follicle-stimulating hormone and luteinizing hormone levels and lower free androgen levels in postpubertal boys and girls with SLE. SLE has been associated with complement abnormalities including C1q, C2, and C4 deficiency, a high incidence of C4 null genes, and abnormal complement receptors. Exposure to the ultraviolet rays in sunlight can exacerbate SLE manifestations, perhaps through damage to nuclear material, resulting in release of DNA, which complexes with circulating anti-DNA antibodies.

Genetic associations in SLE are suggested by the frequent findings of antinuclear antibodies (ANA), hypergammaglobulinemia, and SLE or other autoimmune diseases in family members of patients with SLE. Some HLA types (e.g., B8, DR2, and DR3) may occur with increased frequency among patients with SLE, depending on the racial and ethnic backgrounds of patients studied. Lupus-like disease also occurs after exposure to certain drugs, notably anticonvulsants, sulfonamides, and antiarrhythmic agents. Their similar structure to histone proteins may be one cause, because antihistone antibodies are found in many patients with drug-induced lupus.

EPIDEMIOLOGY. The incidence of SLE is not known but varies by location and ethnicity. Prevalence rates of 4–250/100,000 have been found, with decreased prevalence in white compared with Native American, Asian, Latin, and black American patients. Although onset before age 8 years is unusual, SLE has been diagnosed during the first year of life. Female predominance varies from 4:1 or less before puberty to 8:1 afterward.

PATHOLOGY. Fibrinoid deposits are found in blood vessel walls of affected organs, whose parenchyma may contain hematoxylin bodies, most likely representing degenerated cell nuclei.

TABLE 159–1 Presenting Manifestations of Systemic Lupus Erythematosus

Target Organ	Manifestations
Constitutional	Fatigue, anorexia, weight loss, prolonged fever, lymphadenopathy
Musculoskeletal	Arthralgias, arthritis
Skin	Malar rash, discoid lesions, livedo reticularis
Renal	Glomerulonephritis, nephrotic syndrome, hypertension, renal failure
Cardiovascular	Pericarditis (cardiac tamponade)
Neurologic	Seizures, psychosis, stroke, cerebral venous thrombosis, pseudotumor cerebri, aseptic meningitis, chorea, global cognitive deficits, mood disorders, transverse myelitis, peripheral neuritis
Pulmonary	Pleuritic pain, pulmonary hemorrhage
Hematologic	Coombs-positive hemolytic anemia, anemia of chronic disease, thrombocytopenia, leukopenia

Rheumatoid nodules and granulomas are also sometimes found in affected tissues. Also see Chapter 521.

CLINICAL MANIFESTATIONS. Patients can present with various manifestations (Table 159–1). Children most frequently present with fever, fatigue, arthralgia or arthritis, and rash. Symptoms may be intermittent or persistent. A detailed history and physical and laboratory examination can lead to early diagnosis and treatment.

Cutaneous manifestations are frequently present. The characteristic malar or butterfly rash includes the nasal bridge and varies from an erythematous blush to thickened epidermis to scaly patches (Fig. 159–1). Rashes may be photosensitive and extend to all sun-exposed areas. Mucous membrane changes from vasculitic erythema to ulcers occur particularly on palatal and nasal mucosa (Fig. 159–2). Discoid lesions are unusual in childhood. Other cutaneous manifestations include vasculitic-appearing erythematous macular eruptions (particularly on fingers, palms, and soles), purpura, livedo reticularis (Fig. 159–3) and Raynaud phenomenon. Less common findings include subacute psoriasiform or annular skin lesions, bullous lesions, and alopecia.

Musculoskeletal findings include arthralgia, arthritis, tendinitis, and myositis. Deforming arthritis is unusual; hand arthritis can lead to ligament damage and severely lax joints. Avascular necrosis of bone is common and is presumed secondary to vasculopathy or corticosteroid treatment.

Serositis can affect pleural, pericardial, and peritoneal surfaces. Hepatosplenomegaly and adenopathy are often found. Other gastrointestinal manifestations, most often resulting from vasculitis, include pain, diarrhea, infarction and melena, inflammatory bowel disease, and hepatitis. Cardiac involvement may affect all tissues and include valvular thickening and

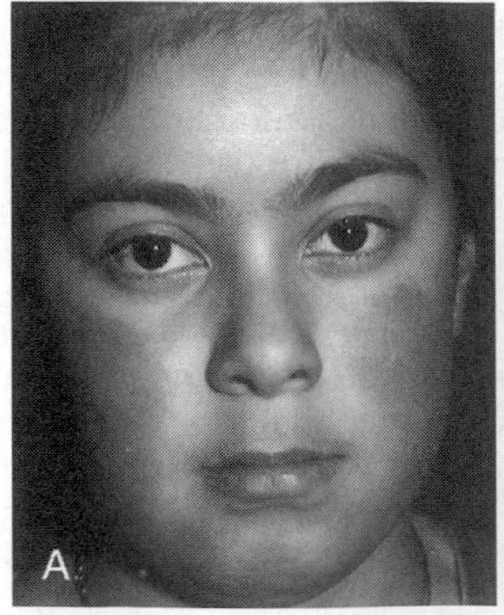

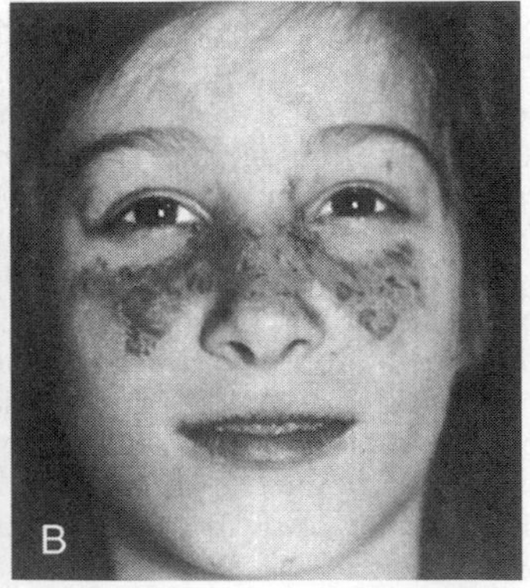

Figure 159–1 The butterfly rash of systemic lupus erythematosus. The rash can vary from an erythematous blush *(A)* to thickened epidermis to scaly patches *(B)*. See also color section.

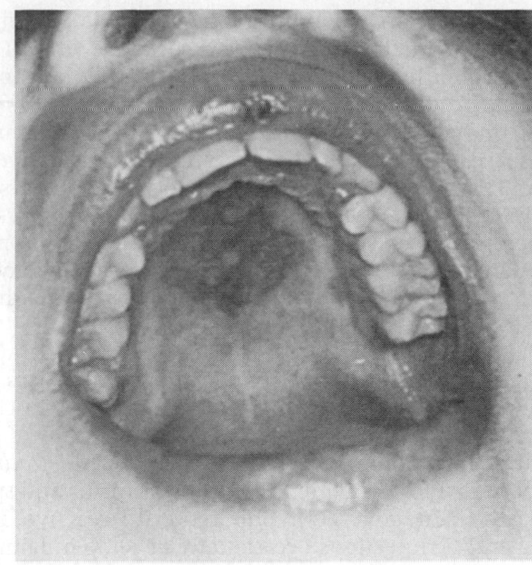

Figure 159–2 Erythematous lesion involving the hard palate in a patient with systemic lupus erythematosus. (From Moschella S, Hurley H (eds): Dermatology, 3rd ed. Philadelphia, WB Saunders, 1992.)

verrucous endocarditis (Libman-Sacks disease), cardiomegaly, myocarditis, conduction abnormalities, and heart failure (caused by coronary artery vasculitis and thrombosis). Pulmonary manifestations include acute pulmonary hemorrhage, pulmonary infiltrates (sometimes with superimposed infection), and chronic fibrosis.

Neurologic manifestations can include the CNS and peripheral nervous system (see Table 159–1). It is likely that many patients with SLE experience memory loss or other cognitive dysfunction during their disease course. The occurrence of arterial or venous thrombosis (Fig. 159–4), suggestive of antiphospholipid antibody syndrome, can occur in any organ and can be associated with recurrent fetal loss, livedo reticularis, thrombocytopenia, and Raynaud phenomenon.

Renal disease is manifested by hypertension, peripheral edema, retinal vascular changes, and clinical manifestations in association with electrolyte abnormalities, nephrosis, or acute renal failure (see Chapter 521).

LABORATORY FINDINGS. ANA is often present in children with active SLE and is an excellent screening tool; however, ANA can be found without any disease or can be associated with rheumatic and other conditions (Table 159–2). Levels of anti–

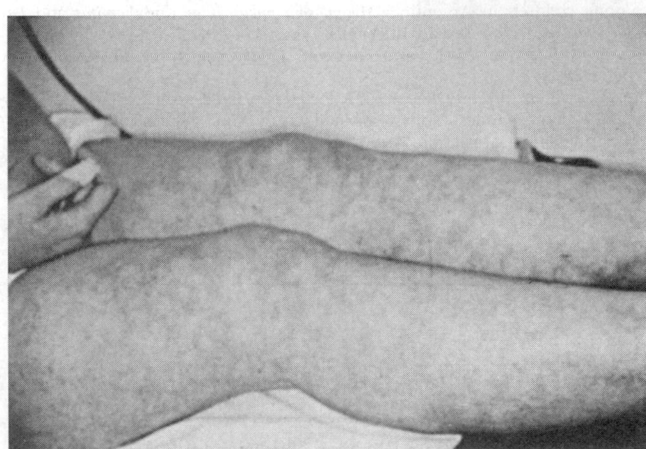

Figure 159–3 Livedo reticularis. Lacelike bluish, purplish, or erythematous discoloration of the skin indicating vascular instability. (From Moschella S, Hurley H (eds): Dermatology, 3rd ed. Philadelphia, WB Saunders, 1992.)

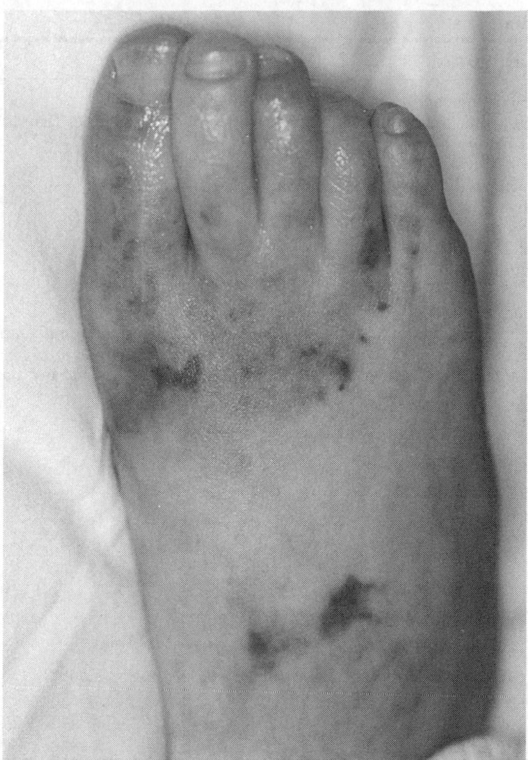

Figure 159–4 A 12-yr-old girl with systemic lupus erythematosus and antiphospholipid antibodies with painful cutaneous vasculitis of the right foot. Arterial thrombosis documented by angiography resulted in cyanosis of the large toe. Symptoms resolved with treatment with heparin and corticosteroids.

double-stranded DNA, more specific for lupus, reflect the degree of disease activity. Serum levels of total hemolytic complement (CH_{50}), C3, and C4 are decreased in active disease and provide a second measure of disease activity. Anti-Smith antibody, found only in patients with SLE, does not measure disease activity. When present, anti-SSA and anti-SSB antibodies are often associated with Sjögren's syndrome. Many autoantibodies can be found (Table 159–3). Hypergammaglobulinemia is also frequent.

DIAGNOSIS. The diagnosis is confirmed by the combination of clinical and laboratory manifestations revealing multisystem disease. Criteria for the diagnosis of SLE require the presence of 4 of 11 criteria serially or simultaneously (Table 159–4). A positive ANA test result is not required for diagnosis; however, its absence is rare. Hypocomplementemia is not diagnostic; extremely low levels or absence of total hemolytic complement suggests the possibility of complement component deficiency. Renal biopsy is used to confirm diagnosis of lupus nephritis and to determine treatment.

TREATMENT. The treatment regimen depends on the affected target organs and disease severity. Patients are treated to support clinical well-being, using serologic markers of disease activity as guidelines, and to normalize serum complement levels. Nonsteroidal anti-inflammatory agents, used to treat arthralgia and arthritis, are used with caution because patients with SLE are more susceptible to hepatotoxicity. The antimalarial agent hydroxychloroquine may be used to treat mild manifestations, including skin lesions, fatigue, arthritis, and arthralgia.

TABLE 159–2 Conditions Associated with Antinuclear Antibodies (ANAs)

Systemic lupus erythematosus	Scleroderma
Drug-induced lupus	Infectious mononucleosis
Juvenile arthritis	Chronic active hepatitis
Juvenile dermatomyositis	Hyperextensibility
Vasculitis syndromes	

TABLE 159–3 Autoantibodies Found in Systemic Lupus Erythematosus

Antibody	Manifestation
Coombs antibodies	Hemolytic anemia
Antiphospholipid antibodies	Antiphospholipid antibody syndrome
Lupus anticoagulant	Coagulopathy
Antithyroid antibodies	Hypothyroidism
Antiribosomal P antibody	Lupus cerebritis

Patients with thrombosis and antiphospholipid antibodies should receive anticoagulant medication at least until SLE is in remission. Low molecular weight heparin is the anticoagulant of choice; however, warfarin can also be used.

Corticosteroids have been demonstrated to control symptoms and autoantibody production in SLE. Treatment with corticosteroids has improved kidney disease and the rate of survival. Corticosteroids, however, can make diagnosis of tuberculosis difficult; all patients should have PPD and control skin tests, when possible, before corticosteroids are initiated. The optimal dose and route of administration of corticosteroids are controversial. Patients with systemic disease are often started on 1–2 mg/kg/24 hr of oral prednisone in divided doses. When complement levels rise to within the normal range, the dose is carefully tapered over 2–3 yr to the lowest effective dose. One method is to use alternate-day high-dose corticosteroids to prevent the adverse effects of daily corticosteroid administration. Severely ill patients may require pulse intravenous corticosteroid therapy (30 mg/kg/dose, not greater than 1 g, given over 60 min once per day, for 3 days). Pulse therapy in combination with low-dose daily corticosteroids has been used as an alternative regimen in some centers. Adverse effects of corticosteroids include hypertension, gastritis, cataracts, osteopenia, and cushingoid body habitus.

Patients with severe disease may require cytotoxic therapy Pulse intravenous cyclophosphamide has maintained renal function and prevented progression in patients with lupus nephritis, particularly diffuse proliferative glomerulonephritis. Cyclophosphamide has been used to treat vasculitis, pulmonary hemorrhage, and CNS disease refractory to corticosteroids. Azathioprine has been used to prevent renal disease progression. Little is known about the long-term sequelae of cytotoxic medications, particularly in children. Adverse effects include secondary infections, gonadal dysfunction, and possibly increased risk of malignancies later in life. Prepubertal children, compared with those who have entered puberty, may be at less risk for subsequent gonadal dysfunction from cytotoxic agents.

Other interventions are being proposed for the treatment of SLE. The role of methotrexate, cyclosporine, and mycophenolate mofetil remains undetermined. Hormonal therapy and autologous and cord stem cell marrow transplantation for patients with severe, persistent disease are undergoing clinical trials in adult patients with SLE. Biologic agents that target cytokine production are also being developed and studied.

The extent of renal involvement may be out of proportion to findings on urinalysis, and renal biopsy for staging can help determine whether an immunosuppressive agent such as cyclophosphamide needs to be added to a corticosteroid regimen (see Chapter 521). Biopsy findings according to the World Health Organization classification correlate with morbidity and mortality. Class I is defined as the absence of abnormalities on light microscopy, immunofluorescence studies, and electron microscopy. Class IIA shows minimal immunoglobulin and complement deposition in mesangium on immunofluores-

TABLE 159–4 1982 Revised Criteria for Diagnosis of Systemic Lupus Erythematosus

Criterion*	Definition
Malar rash	Fixed erythema, flat or raised, over the malar eminences, tending to spare the nasolabial folds
Discoid rash	Erythematous raised patches with adherent keratotic scaling and follicular plugging; atrophic scarring may occur in older lesions
Photosensitivity	Rash as a result of unusual reaction to sunlight (elicited by patient history or physician observation)
Oral ulcers	Oral or nasopharyngeal ulceration, usually painless, observed by a physician
Arthritis	Nonerosive arthritis involving two or more peripheral joints, characterized by tenderness, swelling, or effusion
Serositis	Pleuritis—convincing history of pleuritic pain or rub heard by a physician or evidence of pleural effusion or Pericarditis—documented by ECG or rub or evidence of pericardial effusion
Renal disorder	Persistent proteinuria > 0.5 g/day or > 3-plus (+ + +) if quantitation not performed or Cellular casts—may be red blood cell, hemoglobin, granular, tubular, or mixed
Neurologic disorder	Seizures—in the absence of offending drugs or known metabolic derangements (e.g., uremia, ketoacidosis, or electrolyte imbalance) or Psychosis—in the absence of offending drugs or known metabolic derangements (e.g., uremia, ketoacidosis, or electrolyte imbalance)
Hematologic disorder	Hemolytic anemia—with reticulocytosis or Leukopenia—< 4,000/mm^3 total on two or more occasions or Lymphopenia—< 1,500/mm^3 on two or more occasions or Thrombocytopenia—< 100,000/mm^3
Immunologic disorder	Positive LE cell preparation or Anti-DNA antibody to native DNA in abnormal titer or Anti-Sm—presence of antibody to Sm nuclear antigen or False-positive serologic test result for syphilis known to be positive for at least 6 mo and confirmed by *Treponema pallidum* immobilization or fluorescent treponemal antibody absorption test
Antinuclear antibody	An abnormal titer of antinuclear antibody by immunofluorescence or an equivalent assay at any time and in the absence of drugs known to be associated with "drug-induced lupus syndrome"

**The proposed classification is based on 11 criteria. For the purpose of identifying patients in clinical studies, a person shall be said to have systemic lupus erythematosus if any 4 or more of the 11 criteria are present, serially or simultaneously, during any interval of observation.*

From Tan EM, Cohen AS, Fries JF, et al: The 1982 revised criteria for the classification of systemic lupus erythematosus. Arthritis Rheum 25:1271, 1982.

cence and is associated with good prognosis for renal function. Class IIB (mesangial glomerulonephritis) shows increased lymphocytic infiltration of the mesangium and has a variable prognosis; it occasionally progresses to more extensive renal involvement. Class III (focal and segmental proliferative glomerulonephritis) is characterized by focal, segmental proliferation of cells near capillaries, with necrosis and lymphocytic infiltration, and is often associated with chronic renal disease. Class IV (diffuse proliferative glomerulonephritis) shows a majority of each glomerulus affected by cellular infiltration, mesangial cellular proliferation, and crescent formation corresponding to scarring and has been correlated with increased risk for developing end-stage renal disease in adulthood; intravenous pulse cyclophosphamide can decrease this risk. Class V disease (membranous glomerulonephritis) shows thickened capillary walls on light microscopy and subepithelial deposits on electron microscopy along the basement membrane. These changes have been associated with proteinuria, which can occur with the other types of lupus nephritis, and variable chronic renal disease, often poorly responsive to treatment.

The most important management tool in the treatment of SLE is meticulous and frequent re-evaluation of patients. This includes clinical and laboratory evaluation, especially for renal and serologic flare of disease. Prompt recognition and treatment of disease flare is essential to patient outcome. Lupus is a lifelong illness, and patients must be monitored indefinitely.

PROGNOSIS. Childhood SLE was initially viewed as a uniformly fatal disease. With progress in diagnosis and treatment, the 5-yr survival rate is 90%. However, a significant proportion of patients die later of the disease. Major causes of death in patients with SLE currently include infection, nephritis, CNS disease, pulmonary hemorrhage, and myocardial infarction; the latter complication may be a result of chronic corticosteroid administration.

159.1 Neonatal Lupus

Lupus in newborns results from maternal transfer of IgG autoantibodies (usually anti-Ro) between the 12th and 16th wk of gestation. Manifestations include congenital heart block, cutaneous lesions, liver disease, thrombocytopenia, neutropenia, and pulmonary and neurologic disease. Treatment is supportive. Most manifestations resolve; however, congenital heart block is permanent and often requires cardiac pacing, either after birth or, when detected and severe, antenatally. Even infants of mothers with lupus who are asymptomatic may have slightly prolonged PR intervals. Cardiomyopathy is a rare serious sequela, sometimes requiring heart transplantation.

Neonatal lupus is distinguished from infantile multisystem inflammatory disease, a rare syndrome characterized by fever, rash, arthropathy, chronic meningitis, seizures, uveitis, and lymphadenopathy. This syndrome is difficult to treat and usually requires long-term immunosuppression.

Arisaka O, Obinata K, Sasaki H, et al: Chorea as an initial manifestation of systemic lupus erythematosus. A case report of a 10-year-old girl. Clin Pediatr 23:298, 1984.

De Cunto CL, Liberatore DI, San Roman JL, et al: Infantile-onset multisystem inflammatory disease: A differential diagnosis of systemic juvenile rheumatoid arthritis. J Pediatr 130:551, 1997.

Dungan DD, Jay MS: Stroke in an early adolescent with systemic lupus erythematosus and coexistent antiphospholipid antibodies. Pediatrics 90:96, 1992.

Eberhard BA, Laxer RM, Eddy AA, et al: Presence of thyroid abnormalities in children with systemic lupus erythematosus. J Pediatr 119:277, 1991.

Gazarian M, Feldman BM, Benson LN, et al: Assessment of myocardial perfusion and function in childhood systemic lupus erythematosus. J Pediatr 132:109, 1998.

Lane AT, Watson RM: Neonatal lupus. Am J Dis Child 138:663, 1984.

Lehman TJ, Sherry DD, Wagner-Weiner L, et al: Intermittent intravenous cyclophosphamide therapy for lupus nephritis. J Pediatr 114:1055, 1989.

Lehman TJ, McCurdy DK, Bernstein BH, et al: Systemic lupus erythematosus in the first decade of life. Pediatrics 83:235, 1989.
Lehman TJ, Hanson V, Singsen BH, et al: The role of antibodies directed against double-stranded DNA in the manifestations of systemic lupus erythematosus in childhood. J Pediatr 96:657, 1980.
Miller RW, Salcedo JR, Fink RJ, et al: Pulmonary hemorrhage in pediatric patients with systemic lupus erythematosus. J Pediatr 108:576, 1986.
Reed BR, Lee LA, Harmon C, et al: Autoantibodies to SS-A/Ro in infants with congenital heart block. J Pediatr 103:889, 1983.
Seaman DE, Londino AV Jr, Kwoh CK, et al: Antiphospholipid antibodies in pediatric systemic lupus erythematosus. Pediatrics 96:1040, 1995.
Uziel Y, Laxer RM, Blaser S, et al: Cerebral vein thrombosis in childhood systemic lupus erythematosus. J Pediatr 126:722, 1995.

CHAPTER 160

Juvenile Dermatomyositis

Lauren M. Pachman

Juvenile dermatomyositis (JDM), the most common of the pediatric inflammatory myopathies, is a systemic vasculopathy with characteristic cutaneous findings and focal areas of myositis resulting in progressive proximal muscle weakness that is responsive to immunosuppressive therapy.

ETIOLOGY. The disease onset may be triggered by an infectious process in a genetically susceptible host. The putative agent appears to cause episodic disease; new cases of JDM may occur in clusters. Enterovirus (coxsackievirus B) has been implicated in new-onset JDM, both in the United Kingdom by RNA detection and in the United States by rise in complement-fixing and neutralizing antibody titers. JDM has followed documented infection with group A β-hemolytic streptococci. Case-control serologic studies of other potential infectious triggers such as *Toxoplasma gondii*, herpes simplex virus, or hepatitis B virus have not substantiated an association with JDM. A national epidemiology study is ongoing (Telephone contact: 773-880-3333).

EPIDEMIOLOGY. Exposure to sun may be a cofactor; the rash often occurs in the summer months in the United States. The pediatric age distribution is bimodal (5–9 and 10–14 yr of age), with three to four cases per million children per year for polymyositis/dermatomyositis (PM/DM), as well as a separate peak in adulthood. The average age of onset is 6 yr; those with disease onset before age 7 yr may have a milder course. In the United States, the female:male ratio is 2:1, with a white predominance, although children of black or Asian origin may be at increased risk. Genetic variation appears to predispose to varied disease susceptibility and expression. Numerous cases of myositis in a kindred are very rare, and familial autoimmune disease is not increased in JDM (as opposed to juvenile rheumatoid arthritis).

PATHOGENESIS. Disease chronicity appears to be associated with a gene related to HLA antigen DQA1*0501, which is found in more than 80% of JDM children in the United States. Endothelial cell activation by the putative antigen and/or immune complexes is accompanied by deposition of immunoglobulin and terminal complement components with release of von Willebrand factor antigen from the damaged endothelium. Occlusion of capillaries with subsequent capillary dropout, local infarction of tissue, perifascicular atrophy, and a mononuclear cellular infiltrate confirm the histologic diagnosis of JDM. The perivascular mononuclear infiltrate is primarily composed of CD19+ B cells, occasionally occurring in clusters. New-onset, untreated JDM has four times as many CD56+ natural killer (NK) cells in the muscle as in matched peripheral blood, suggesting a role for NK cells. Other T-cell subsets are also represented in diseased muscle; the number of monocytes/macrophages (CD14+) correlates with serum levels of neopterin, a macrophage-derived T-cell factor. Extensive fibrosis and microscopic collections of calcium precipitate are components of chronic inflammation. With healing, both new blood vessels and muscle fibers regenerate. In affected skin, the epidermis is thinned, and the dermis demonstrates edema and vascular inflammation.

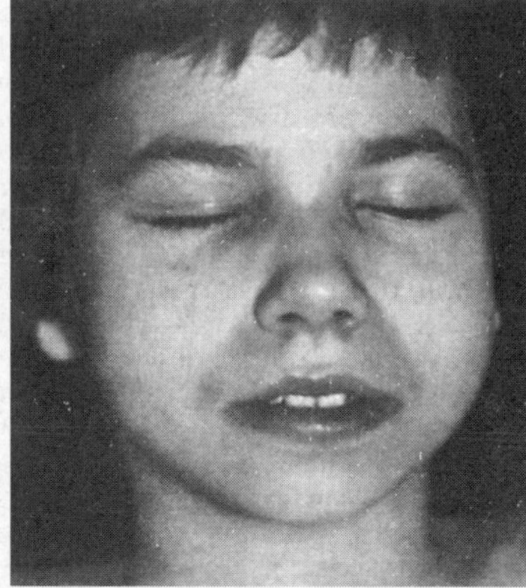

Figure 160–1 The facial rash of juvenile dermatomyositis. There is erythema over the bridge of the nose and malar areas, with violaceous (heliotropic) discoloration of the upper eyelids. See also color section.

CLINICAL MANIFESTATIONS. Disease onset is often insidious; constitutional symptoms of fatigue, low-grade fever, weight loss, and irritability are common. The characteristic rash usually appears first, particularly over sun-exposed areas, followed by proximal muscle weakness after a median of 2 mo. Periorbital violaceous (heliotropic) erythema (heliotrope eyelids) may cross the nasal bridge (Fig. 160–1). Periorbital and facial edema may be associated. The rash may involve the upper torso, the extensor surfaces of the arms and legs, the medial malleoli of the ankles, and the buttocks. Facial edema and eyelid telangiectasia occur in 50–90% of cases. Partial baldness is a consequence of chronic scalp inflammation. The skin over the metacarpal and proximal interphalangeal joints may be hypertrophic and pale red (Gottron papules) during active disease, with a papular, alligator skin–like appearance (Fig. 160–2), which evolves into atrophic colorless bands. Children with the amyopathic form of JDM (rash only) initially often develop

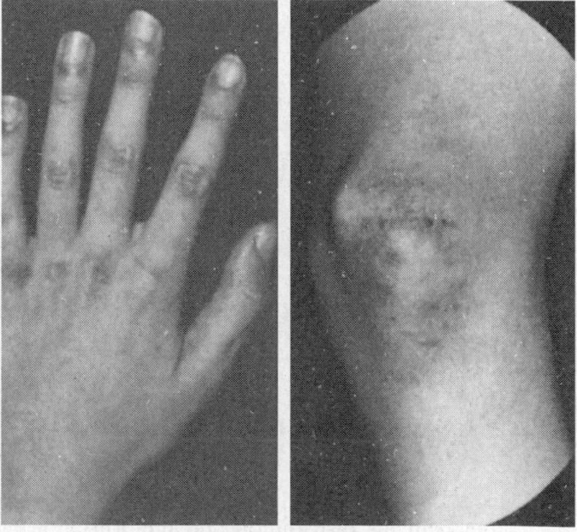

Figure 160–2 The rash of juvenile dermatomyositis. The skin over the metacarpal and proximal interphalangeal joints may be hypertrophic and pale red (Gottron papules). See also color section.

myositis and subsequent calcinosis later in their disease course. Diffuse vasculopathy (e.g., nail bed telangiectasia, infarction of oral epithelium and skinfolds, or digital ulceration) is clearly associated with more severe disease; healing is manifested by hyperpigmentation or vitiligo.

The onset of proximal muscle weakness is insidious and difficult to recognize. It is often detected by difficulty in climbing stairs, combing hair, or standing from a sitting position or rising unassisted from the floor without "climbing up the body" (Gowers sign). Neck flexor weakness (inability to raise the head from the bed) or abdominal muscle weakness (inability to perform a sit-up) identifies inflamed muscles that are often tender on compression. Derangement of upper airway function can be detected by hoarseness, a nasal quality to the speech, or difficulty in handling secretions. Dysphagia is a severe prognostic sign and should prompt immediate aggressive therapeutic intervention. Complaints of constipation reflect impaired gastrointestinal (GI) smooth muscle function, and abdominal pain or diarrhea may indicate occult GI bleeding, which can progress and be life threatening. Cardiac involvement with conduction abnormality is frequent at diagnosis; dilated cardiomyopathy has been reported. Lymphadenopathy is not uncommon.

Children with antibody to the polymyositis/scleroderma (Pm/Scl) antigen often have bambooing of the digits with loss of cutaneous elasticity, similar to scleroderma. "Mechanic's hands," with thickened skin, cuticle overgrowth, and range losses, are indicators of a subset of refractory inflammatory myopathy more common in adults, who have severe lung involvement and characteristic circulating antibody (Jo-1) to tRNA synthetase.

Less frequent findings include hepatosplenomegaly, retinitis, iritis, central nervous system (CNS) involvement with seizures and depression, and evidence of renal impairment. Association with malignancy at disease onset is frequent in adults with dermatomyositis, but not in children.

DIAGNOSIS. The characteristic rash facilitates early diagnosis but should be differentiated from other connective tissue diseases such as systemic lupus erythematosus, scleroderma, or mixed connective tissue disease by both the specific antibody tests and clinical findings associated with each of these disorders. Careful examination of the nailfold capillaries usually documents periungual avascularity with capillary dropout and vessel dilatation with characteristic terminal bush formation (Fig. 160–3).

If the initial symptom is weakness, other causes of myopathy should be considered, including acute polymyositis associated with influenza B infection, the muscular dystrophies (including Duchenne and Becker muscular dystrophies), myasthenia gravis, Guillain-Barré syndrome, and endocrine or metabolic disorders. Infections associated with muscular symptoms, such as poliomyelitis, trichinosis, or toxoplasmosis, also should be considered. Blunt trauma and crush injuries may lead to transient rhabdomyolysis with myoglobinuria. Other events associated with myositis in children include vaccinations, drugs, growth hormone, and bone marrow transplantation, in which graft versus host myositis occurs as a component of immune activation (Chapter 137).

LABORATORY FINDINGS. Elevated serum levels of muscle-derived enzymes—creatine kinase (CK), aldolase, serum glutamic-oxaloacetic transaminase (SGOT), and lactic acid dehydrogenase (LDH)—reflect the leaky muscle membranes. Antinuclear antibody (ANA) with a speckled pattern (unknown specificity) is present in more than 60% of children and, initially, may be of high titer. Tests for antibodies to SSA, SSB, Sm, RNP, and DNA are negative. Other myositis-specific antibodies, which rarely occur in children, identify those with a protracted disease course; antibodies to Pm/Scl are most frequent. The erythrocyte sedimentation rate may be elevated or normal, with a Coombs-negative anemia; the rheumatoid factor is negative.

Indicators of immunologic activation in JDM include increased peripheral blood CD19+ B cells (despite being lymphopenic); von Willebrand factor antigen (vWf:Ag), which is released by damaged endothelial cells; and neopterin, which is released by activated macrophages.

MRI using T2 weighted images and fat suppression (Fig. 160–4) can localize the active site of disease for diagnostic muscle biopsy and electromyogram, both of which are nondiagnostic in 20% of instances if not directed by MRI. Extensive rash and abnormal MRI findings are not uncommon despite normal serum levels of muscle-derived enzymes. Muscle biopsy often demonstrates evidence of disease activity and chronicity that is not suspected from serum enzyme levels alone.

A rehabilitation cookie swallow documents significant palatorespiratory dysfunction and an unprotected airway. Pulmonary function testing of the diffusion capacity of the lung for

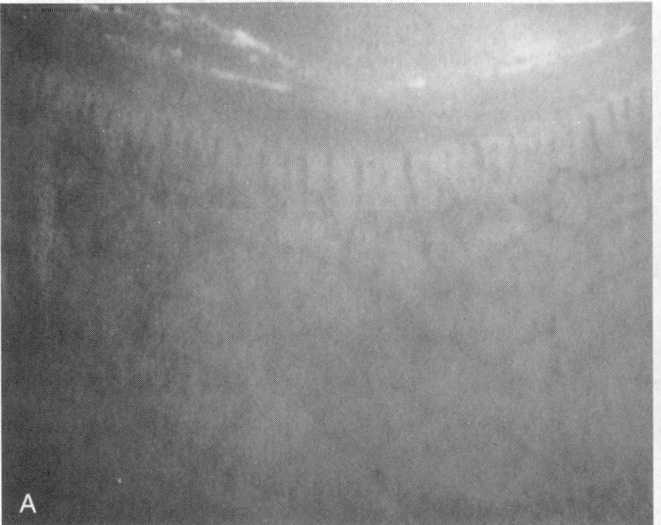

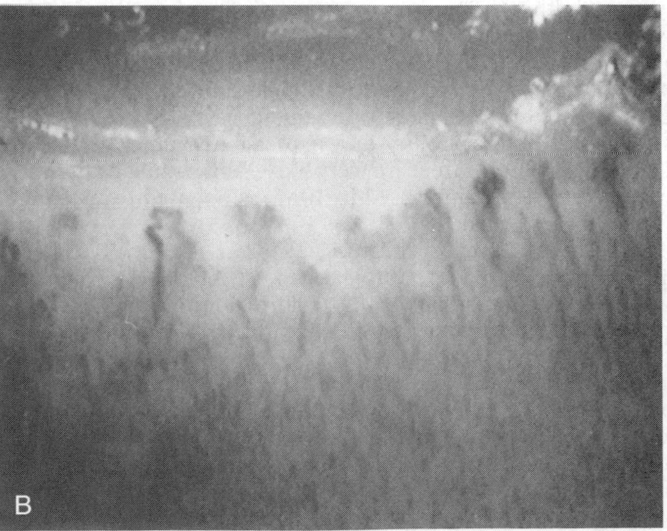

Figure 160–3 Nailfold capillary pattern in rheumatic diseases. *A*, Normal nailfold capillary pattern in a healthy child, with a homogeneous distribution and uniform appearance of capillary loops. *B*, The nailfold capillary pattern in a child with juvenile dermatomyositis that shows dropout of capillary end-loops resulting in a wide band of avascularity. Dilated, tortuous capillaries are also seen, some with terminal bush formation that is found in patients with juvenile dermatomyositis, with scleroderma, and with Raynaud phenomenon that may progress to scleroderma.

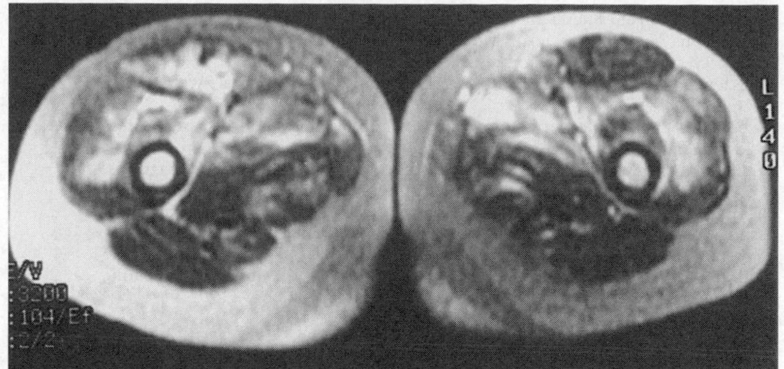

Figure 160–4 An MRI scan, with T2 weighted image with fat suppression, of the proximal muscle of the lower extremities of a child with juvenile dermatomyositis with normal muscle enzymes. There is focal inflammatory myopathy. The white areas reflect the inflammatory response in involved muscle; those areas that are darker are more normal. Identification of the involved areas by MRI aids in directing the location of the muscle biopsy or electromyogram (EMG).

carbon monoxide (DLCO) (for children >6 yr detects decreased respiratory muscle strength as well as alveolar fibrosis associated with other connective tissue diseases. Active disease is frequently associated with decreased bone density with abnormal findings on densitometry and low osteocalcin and vitamin D levels. Calcinosis is detected best by plain radiographs.

COMPLICATIONS. Aspiration pneumonia is a frequent major complication associated with unrecognized impairment in swallowing fluids. Progressive bowel infarction can lead to perforation and death. Depression and mood swings are part of the disease spectrum of CNS involvement and may be accentuated by steroid administration.

Calcinosis is present in 3–20% of patients at diagnosis and is associated with increased morbidity and mortality. It is probably a consequence of disease chronicity, fostered by either delay in initiation of therapy or insufficient suppression of inflammation. The calcium deposits form in muscle, subcutaneous tissue, and fascia; they may drain a white cheesy material and resolve or serve as a nidus for infection (most frequently staphylococcal), which can progress to septicemia and death. Calcinosis decreases with aggressive therapy.

Partial lipodystrophy develops in more than 10% of cases of chronic JDM and is characterized by loss of subcutaneous fat on the extremities, giving a hypermuscular appearance; acanthosis nigricans; weakened abdominal muscles resulting in a potbelly appearance; and abnormal glucose and lipid metabolism. Sterility may result if disease onset is before puberty.

TREATMENT. All children with JDM should use a sunscreen (*p*-aminobenzoic acid free) that provides maximal protection (ultraviolet A and B). Vitamin D, at the dose appropriate for weight, with a diet sufficient in calcium, repairs osteopenia and decreases the frequency of bone fracture.

The aid of an experienced pediatric rheumatologist is essential in assessing the need for therapeutic intervention. Children with only cutaneous findings and a negative family history of color blindness may take hydroxychloroquine (maximum dose of 2 mg/kg/24 hr), with a low daily dose or oral corticosteroids (prednisone, 0.5 mg/kg/24 hr) if needed. These children should be monitored for the development of muscle involvement by repeat determination of serum muscle enzymes and MRI.

With mild muscle damage, oral corticosteroids (prednisone, 1–2 mg/kg/24 hr) may suffice, with rapid normalization of the serum levels of muscle-derived enzymes. More intensive therapy may be necessary if the more resistant indicators of inflammation (CD19+ B cells, neopterin, vWf:Ag) remain elevated. With severe disease at onset, prompt institution of high-dose intermittent intravenous methylprednisolone therapy may be lifesaving. Inhibitors of gastric acid secretion are usually also administered to minimize gastric bleeding. Pulse intravenous corticosteroid therapy (30 mg/kg/24 hr of methylprednisolone, not greater than 1 g daily, for 3 days) usually is initially given; thereafter, the frequency of methylprednisolone administration ranges from three times per week to once each week until indicators of inflammation normalize. Low-dose oral prednisone (0.5 mg/kg/24 hr) is given on non–intravenous methylprednisolone days. Methotrexate can be added (15–20 mg/M^2) if laboratory values fail to normalize as rapidly as expected but should be given in conjunction with folic acid (1 mg/24 hr). Cyclophosphamide (500 mg/M^2), given with mesna for bladder protection) is considered for children unresponsive to intravenous methylprednisolone and methotrexate. The associated immunosuppression may result in decreased levels of IgG (<300 mg%) and replacement immune globulin (0.4 g/kg/mo) may be required to help prevent infections. High-dose intravenous immune globulin may initially diminish cutaneous symptoms, but it is not clear that the disease course is altered. Cyclosporine has been successful in some resistant cases.

Children with dysphagia require a soft diet, or nasogastric feedings if necessary, until treatment restores a functional, protected airway. In rare cases, a respirator and tracheostomy or even extracorporeal membrane oxygenation are required. Absorption of calories and medication may be impaired by extensive GI vasculitis, requiring parenteral hyperalimentation and intravenous administration of drugs. Renal damage secondary to massive creatinine excretion can be averted by appropriate intravenous hydration.

Physical and occupational therapy provide passive stretching early in the disease course and, once active inflammation has resolved, direct reconditioning of muscles to regain strength and range of motion. Bed rest is not indicated; weight bearing improves bone density. Social work services may help facilitate adjustment to the frustration of physical impairment in a previously active child.

PROGNOSIS. Before the advent of corticosteroids, one third of affected children died and another third were disabled. The mortality rate is currently about 3%. Although the disease is classified as "chronic," little is known about the persistence of vascular inflammation. The period of active symptoms has decreased from about 3.5 yr to less than 1.5 yr with more aggressive immunosuppressive therapy. Unlike many adults with inflammatory myopathies, children with JDM appear able to repair their vasculature and muscle damage, but follow-up biopsy studies await analysis. The impact of partial lipodystrophy on adult morbidity is not known. Overall, with newer tests to monitor inflammation and disease activity and guide more aggressive therapy, the prognosis for this illness has markedly improved.

Bohan A, Peter JB: Polymyositis and dermatomyositis (parts 1 and 2). N Engl J Med 292:344, 403, 1975.

DeBenedetti F, DeAmici M, Aramini L, et al: Correlations of serum neopterin concentrations with disease activity in juvenile dermatomyositis. Arch Dis Child 69:232, 1993.

Eisenstein DM, O'Gorman MR, Pachman LM: Correlations between change in disease activity and changes in peripheral blood lymphocyte subsets in patients with juvenile dermatomyositis. J Rheumatol 24:1830, 1997.

Feldman BM, Reichlin M, Laxer RM, et al: Clinical significance of specific autoantibodies in juvenile dermatomyositis. J Rheumatol 23:1794, 1996.

Martini AA, Ravelli S, Albani S, et al: Recurrent juvenile dermatomyositis and cutaneous necrotizing arteritis with molecular mimicry between streptococcal type 5M protein and human skeletal myosin. J Pediatr 121:739, 1992.
Mejlszenkier JD, Safran SE, Healy JJ: The myositis of influenza. Arch Neurol 29:441, 1973.
Pachman LM: Juvenile dermatomyositis: Pathophysiology and disease expression. Pediatr Clin North Am 23:619, 1995.
Pachman LM, Hayford JR, Chung A, et al: Juvenile dermatomyositis at diagnosis: Clinical characteristics of 79 children. J Rheumatol 25:1198, 1998.
Pachman LM, Hayford JR, Hochberg MC, et al: New-onset juvenile dermatomyositis: Comparisons with a healthy cohort and children with juvenile rheumatoid arthritis. Arthritis Rheum 40:1526, 1997.
Rider LG, Miller FW: Classification and treatment of the juvenile idiopathic inflammatory myopathies. Rheum Dis Clin North Am 23:619, 1997.

CHAPTER 161
Scleroderma

Michael L. Miller

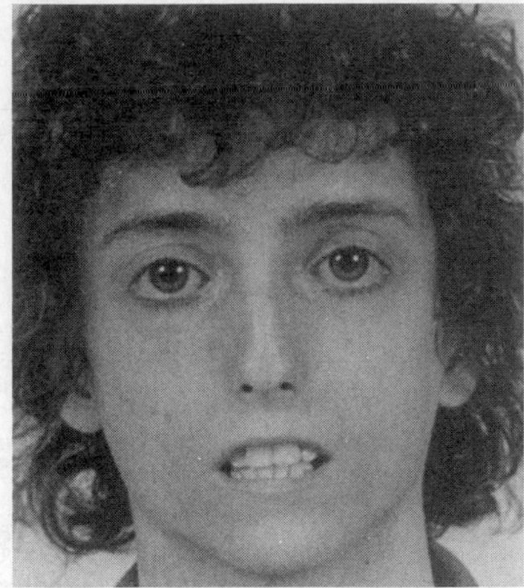

Figure 161–1 Facial changes in a 16-yr-old boy with scleroderma. There is a small mouth with puckering of the lips, pinched nose, and hyperpigmentation of the neck. (From Uziel Y, Miller ML, Laxer RM: Scleroderma in children. Pediatr Clin North Am 42:1177, 1995.)

Scleroderma, a chronic disease of unknown cause, is characterized by fibrosis affecting the dermis and arteries of the lungs, kidneys, and gastrointestinal (GI) tract. Antinuclear antibodies (ANA) specific for topoisomerase 1 (SCL70) and the centromere are found in many patients; this observation suggests that autoimmune processes have a role in pathogenesis. Scleroderma is classified according to the pattern of skin and internal organ involvement (Table 161–1).

EPIDEMIOLOGY. Scleroderma is a rare disease. The peak age at onset for systemic sclerosis is 30–50 yr, with a female:male ratio of 3:1. Children represent fewer than 10% of all cases. The cause is unknown but involves injury to vascular endothelium. Rare cases have been reported after exposure to polyvinyl chloride, bleomycin, and pentazocine. Reports of scleroderma in adult women after breast implants may reflect nonrelated conditions, because medical devices (e.g., ventriculoperitoneal shunts) containing silicone have been implanted for many years without reports of similar complications. In children, localized scleroderma is more common than systemic sclerosis.

PATHOGENESIS. Scleroderma is associated with destruction of vascular endothelium and an increase in the basal lamina. During the initial stages of disease, lymphocytes, macrophages, mast cells, plasma cells, and eosinophils infiltrate the dermis. Fibroblast proliferation increases collagen synthesis, resulting in fibrosis of the dermis, subcutaneous fat, and sometimes muscle.

Studies suggest that a yet unidentified agent injures vascular endothelial cells, resulting in increased expression of adhesion molecules on their surfaces. These molecules entrap platelets and inflammatory cells, resulting in vascular changes of the type associated with such manifestations as Raynaud phenomenon, renovascular hypertension, and pulmonary hypertension. Recruitment of lymphocytes to areas of vascular damage may be the event that leads to specific autoantibody production in many patients. After these events, macrophages and other inflammatory cells appear to leave blood vessels and migrate into tissues affected in scleroderma. These cells secrete interleukin 1 (IL-1), causing platelets to release platelet-derived growth factor (PDGF). These and other molecules induce fibroblasts to reproduce and synthesize excessive amounts of collagen, resulting in fibrosis.

TABLE 161–1 Classification of Scleroderma

Systemic Sclerosis
Diffuse: systemic widespread skin fibrosis, including proximal limbs, trunk, and face; early internal organ involvement
Limited (CREST): systemic distal skin involvement, often face, with late, if any, internal organ involvement
Overlap: Sclerodermal skin changes with features of other connective tissue disorders
Localized Scleroderma
Morphea
Generalized morphea
Linear scleroderma
On face, forehead, or scalp *(coup de sabre)*
On extremity
Eosinophilic Fasciitis
Secondary Forms
Drug induced
Chemically induced
Pseudoscleroderma

From Uziel Y, Miller ML, Laxer RM: Scleroderma in children. Pediatr Clin North Am 42:1171, 1995.

CLINICAL MANIFESTATIONS. Raynaud phenomenon, resulting from digital arterial spasm, is often the earliest manifestation and may precede extensive skin and internal organ involvement by months or years. Induced by exposure to cold, Raynaud phenomenon affects the fingers, toes, and occasionally the ears and the tip of the nose. It has three stages: pallor, cyanosis, and finally erythema. Two of three stages are considered sufficient for identifying this manifestation. Episodes can vary in duration from minutes to hours.

Systemic Sclerosis. Systemic sclerosis also often presents with a preliminary edematous phase that can last several months before chronic fibrosis develops. These early changes include puffiness around the fingers, on the dorsum of the hands, and sometimes on the face. An eventual decrease in edema is associated with tightening of the skin. Skin changes tend to spread proximally from the hands. Loss of subcutaneous tissue in the face can result in a small oral stoma with decreased distance between the upper and lower teeth when the mouth is opened wide (Fig. 161–1). Skin ulceration over pressure points, such as the elbows, may be associated with subcutaneous calcifications. Later, atrophic skin can become shiny and waxy in appearance. Loss of tissue at the fingertips may be associated with ulceration if Raynaud phenomenon is severe (Fig. 161–2). The distal phalanges may exhibit resorption of the distal tufts (acro-osteolysis). The fingers take on a tapered appearance associated with tightened skin (sclerodactyly) and eventual development of secondary and often severe flexion

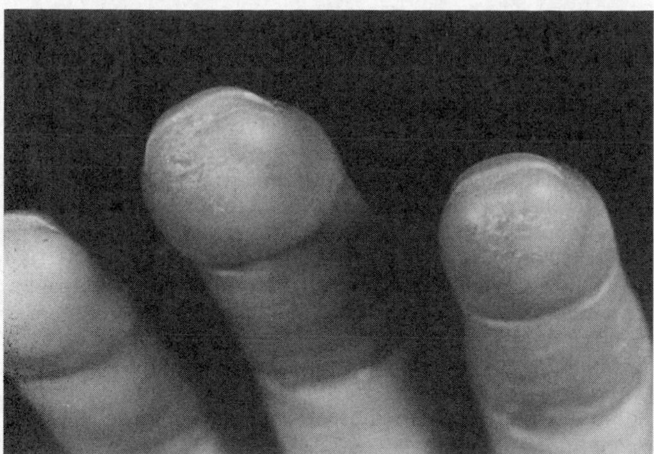

Figure 161–2 Tiny digital pitting scars and loss of pulp space resulting from digital ischemia in a 15-yr-old boy with scleroderma. (From Uziel Y, Miller ML, Laxer RM: Scleroderma in children. Pediatr Clin North Am 42:1178, 1995.)

contractures and limitation of motion (Fig. 161–3). As lesions spread proximally, flexion contractures in the elbows, hips, and knees may be associated with secondary muscle weakness and atrophy. Other chronic changes include epidermal thinning, hair loss, and decreased sweating. Hyperpigmented postinflammatory changes surrounded by atrophic depigmentation may give a salt-and-pepper appearance to some skin lesions. Over a period of years, remodeling of lesions sometimes results in focal improvement in skin thickening at the same time fibrosis extends elsewhere.

Pulmonary disease includes arterial and interstitial involvement and can vary from minimal disease to a progressive course that eventually results in decreased exercise tolerance, dyspnea at rest, and right-sided heart failure. Chest roentgenograms may appear normal early in the course. Evidence of early involvement may be found only by performing pulmonary function tests, including evaluation of oxygen diffusion by diffusion of carbon monoxide capacity (DLCO). High-resolution CT may also detect changes associated with interstitial disease before they become apparent on chest roentgenograms.

Scleroderma can also affect other organs. Renal arterial disease can cause chronic or severe episodic hypertension. Esophageal dilatation caused by fibrosis can cause dysphagia. Dilated

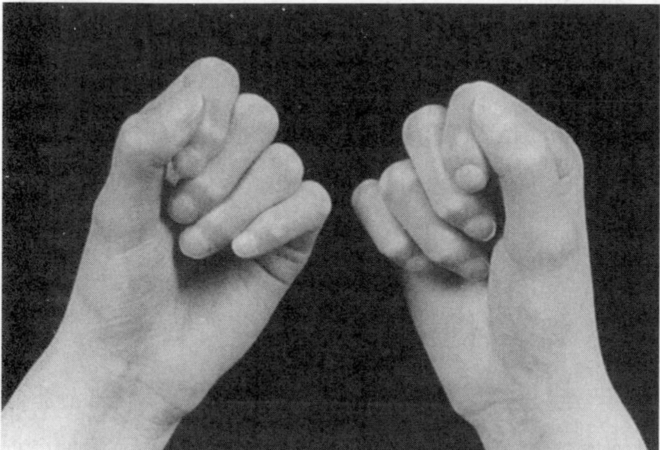

Figure 161–3 Inability to make a full fist due to skin and soft tissue tightening in a 10-yr-old girl with scleroderma. (From Uziel Y, Miller ML, Laxer RM: Scleroderma in children. Pediatr Clin North Am 42:1176, 1995.)

intestinal loops can result in malabsorption and failure to thrive. Cardiac fibrosis has been associated with arrhythmias, ventricular hypertrophy, and decreased cardiac function.

Scleroderma can present with less extensive involvement. In limited systemic scleroderma, children have less prominent fibrosis that is limited to the distal extremities, face, and neck. Telangiectasias may appear on the fingertips, face, chest wall, and inner surface of lips. The CREST syndrome refers to the manifestations of calcinosis, Raynaud phenomenon, esophageal involvement, sclerosis of the skin, and telangiectasias. Severe pulmonary hypertension develops in some patients with CREST syndrome.

Morphea and Linear Scleroderma. In localized scleroderma, the involvement is restricted to the skin; progression to systemic sclerosis is rare. In children with *morphea*, a form of localized scleroderma, lesions are typically discrete and may occur anywhere on the body but particularly on the face. Early inflammation is followed by indurated, depigmented, atrophic lesions. Children with *linear scleroderma* have lesions affecting the length of extremities; these lesions vary in size from several centimeters to the entire length of the extremity. Fibrosis in the dermis can sometimes extend to muscle, resulting in some instances in total loss of muscle tissue between the dermis and bone. Resulting leg-length discrepancies, joint flexion contractures (Fig. 161–4), or cosmetic deformities of the face, forehead, or scalp with scarring alopecia (*coup de sabre*) may require surgical intervention.

DIAGNOSIS. Scleroderma should be suspected in children who develop Raynaud phenomenon or skin changes suggestive of sclerodactyly. If Raynaud phenomenon is present for years before classic disease expression, antinuclear autoantibodies (particularly anti-SCL70) are typically found. Subclinical pulmonary fibrosis, suspected if decreased DLCO is found on pul-

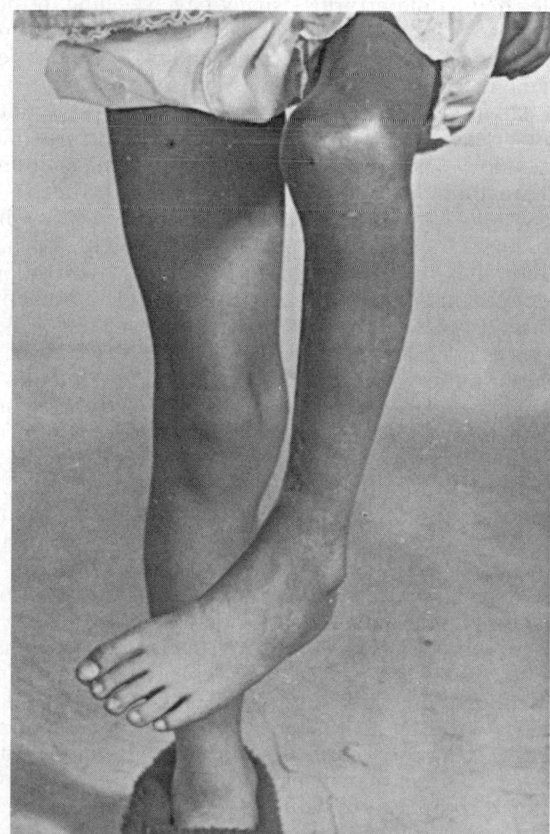

Figure 161–4 Extensive morphea involving the entire left leg causing shortening and flexion contractures. The skin has a shiny appearance with patches of hyperpigmentation and vitiligo.

TABLE 161–2 Diagnostic Criteria of Scleroderma*

Major Criterion

Proximal scleroderma: typical sclerodermatous skin changes (tightness, thickening, and nonpitting induration, excluding localized forms of scleroderma) involving areas proximal to the metacarpophalangeal or metatarsophalangeal joints

Minor Criteria

Sclerodactyly: sclerodermatous skin changes limited to digits
Digital pitting scars resulting from digital ischemia
Bibasilar pulmonary fibrosis not attributable to primary lung disease

**The diagnosis of scleroderma requires the presence of the major criterion or two of the three minor criteria.*

From Subcommittee for scleroderma criteria of the American Rheumatism Association Diagnostic and Therapeutic Criteria Committee: Preliminary criteria for the classification of systemic sclerosis (scleroderma). Arthritis Rheum 23:581, 1980.

monary function testing, may be confirmed by high-resolution CT. Nail fold capillaroscopy of patients with Raynaud phenomenon before progression of disease may reveal a loss of capillaries or abnormal capillary dilatation resulting from vasculopathy (see Fig. 160–3).

According to diagnostic criteria used in adults, the diagnosis of scleroderma requires the presence of the single major criterion (sclerodermatous skin changes proximal to the metacarpophalangeal or metatarsophalangeal joints) or two of the three minor criteria (Table 161–2). The evaluation in these patients should include pulmonary function tests, contrast studies of the upper GI tract to evaluate esophageal motility, and echocardiography to preclude pulmonary arterial hypertension.

Differential Diagnosis. Several conditions present with findings similar to those of scleroderma. Diffuse finger swelling extending to the dorsum of the hands can be seen in Henoch-Schönlein purpura and with allergic reactions. Patients with juvenile rheumatoid arthritis usually have swelling in the fingers that is restricted to the joints. Flexion contractures in these patients are a result of chronic tendinitis without dermal involvement; therefore, the skin is not tight, compared with that of patients with scleroderma. Manifestations of graft versus host disease after bone marrow transplantation (Chapter 137) include erythema affecting the face and distal extremities, sclerodermatous skin changes, hepatitis, and diarrhea.

In *Raynaud disease,* Raynaud phenomenon occurs without the subsequent development of skin or internal organ changes of scleroderma. Such patients usually do not have anti-SCL70 or other autoantibodies, and their Raynaud phenomenon does not worsen over time. Weakness, sometimes related to flexion contractures, in patients with skin changes suggestive of early scleroderma raises the possibility of juvenile dermatomyositis or overlap syndromes in which elements of several rheumatic diseases (e.g., systemic lupus erythematosus, dermatomyositis, arthritis, and scleroderma) may be present.

Patients with eosinophilic fasciitis develop changes similar to those in localized scleroderma. However, laboratory evaluation shows a striking eosinophilia, elevated erythrocyte sedimentation rate, and occasionally hypergammaglobulinemia. Full-thickness skin biopsy, which extends to and includes muscle fascia, shows a predominately eosinophilic inflammatory infiltration in the dermis and fascial tissues that confirms the diagnosis. Progression to systemic sclerosis is rare. Corticosteroid treatment often ameliorates or prevents progression of lesions. However, some patients develop severe contracting fibrosis involving the entire length of the extremities. Limited experience suggests that it may be possible in some cases to prevent this complication with the use of methotrexate.

Pseudoscleroderma comprises unrelated diseases characterized by patchy or diffuse cutaneous fibrosis without the other manifestations of scleroderma. Patients with phenylketonuria can develop such lesions as well as eczematous changes. Scleredema of Buschke is a transient disease of sudden onset often following a febrile illness (especially streptococcal infections) in which patchy sclerodermatous lesions occur on the neck and shoulders, often extending to the face, trunk, and down the arms. These findings usually resolve spontaneously within several months.

LABORATORY FINDINGS. Inflammation early in systemic disease may be reflected by anemia and sometimes eosinophilia. Immunoglobulin levels may be nonspecifically elevated. ANA are often present, with a speckled or nucleolar pattern. If present, anti-SCL70 (specific for topoisomerase 1) and anticentromere autoantibodies are strongly suggestive of a diagnosis of scleroderma. Autoantibodies usually found in systemic lupus erythematosus (anti-DNA) or mixed connective tissue disease (antiribonucleoprotein) suggest the presence of an overlap syndrome. In the early phase of the disease, levels of von Willebrand factor antigen, a marker for vascular endothelial damage, may be elevated. In localized scleroderma, laboratory abnormalities are usually restricted to positive ANA (with anti-SCL70 and anticentromere antibodies much less common than in systemic sclerosis) and, on occasion, eosinophilia.

COMPLICATIONS. Raynaud phenomenon can become severe enough to lead to early gangrenous changes with the threat of autoamputation of the digits. Arterial disease can also cause esophageal rupture, renovascular hypertensive crises, and pulmonary arterial hypertension with cor pulmonale. Chronic pulmonary insufficiency can result from pulmonary parenchymal disease and pulmonary arterial hypertension. Renal disease and chronic pulmonary arterial hypertension can lead to death. GI involvement can result in malabsorption and failure to thrive.

TREATMENT. Although there is no specific treatment, immunosuppressive agents, including methotrexate and corticosteroids, in the early stages of the disease may be helpful in curbing inflammation. However, corticosteroids later in the course of the disease do not appear to be effective and may exacerbate hypertension. Additional treatment includes physical and occupational therapy to improve flexion contractures and maintain muscle strength.

If Raynaud phenomenon persists despite local measures (e.g., keeping hands warm during cold exposure with Mylar or sheepskin gloves), calcium channel blockers (e.g., nifedipine, amlodipine besylate) or angiotensin-converting enzyme inhibitors (e.g., captopril, enalapril), and topical vasodilators (e.g., nitroglycerin paste) may be successful in preventing or ameliorating fingertip ulcerations. Vascular compromise threatening to lead to gangrene and autoamputation of the distal digits may be responsive to central administration of prostaglandin E_1 (alprostadil).

PROGNOSIS. The course of scleroderma is variable, and findings at presentation are not predictive. Some patients stabilize after several years and have no new skin or visceral involvement. Others show unrelenting progression of disease, with death, either in childhood or later in life, resulting from end-stage pulmonary, cardiac, or renal vascular disease.

Britt WJ, Duray PH, Dahl MV, et al: Diffuse fasciitis with eosinophilia: A steroid-responsive variant of scleroderma. J Pediatr 97:432, 1980.
Garty BZ, Athreya BH, Wilmott R, et al: Pulmonary functions in children with progressive systemic sclerosis. Pediatrics 88:1161, 1991.
Gerbracht DD, Steen VD, Ziegler GL, et al: Evolution of primary Raynaud's phenomenon (Raynaud's disease) to connective tissue disease. Arthritis Rheum 28:87, 1985.
Flick JA, Boyle JT, Tuchman DN, et al: Esophageal motor abnormalities in children and adolescents with scleroderma and mixed connective tissue disease. Pediatrics 82:107, 1988.
Itzkowitch D, Alexander M, Famaey JP, et al: Overlapping connective tissue diseases in children. Clin Rheumatol 2:375, 1983.
Seely JM, Jones LT, Wallace C, et al: Systemic sclerosis: Using high-resolution CT to detect lung disease in children. AJR Am J Roentgenol 170:691, 1998.
Shanks MJ, Blane CE, Adler DD, et al: Radiographic findings of scleroderma in childhood. AJR Am J Roentgenol 141:657, 1983.

Sheiner NM, Small P: Isolated Raynaud phenomenon—a benign disorder. Ann Allergy 58:114, 1987.

Subcommittee for scleroderma criteria of the American Rheumatism Association Diagnostic and Therapeutic Criteria Committee: Preliminary criteria for the classification of systemic sclerosis (scleroderma). Arthritis Rheum 23:581, 1980.

CHAPTER 162
Behçet's Disease

Abraham Gedalia

Behçet's disease, a multisystem disorder originally described as recurrent oral and genital ulceration with relapsing iritis or uveitis, is often characterized by cutaneous, arthritic, neurologic, vascular, and gastrointestinal manifestations. Fever, orchitis, myositis, pericarditis, nephritis, splenomegaly, and amyloidosis are rare associated manifestations. The disease is commonly reported in the Mediterranean basin and Asia and is relatively rare in Europe and the United States. The condition is uncommon in children, who account for only an estimated 5% of all cases.

The *cause* of Behçet's disease is unknown, although an association with HLA-B5 and B51 is clear. A few cases of transient neonatal Behçet's disease in offspring of mothers with the disorder have been described, suggesting that an antibody-mediated immune process also may have a role in the pathogenesis. The basic pathologic lesion is vasculitis of small- and medium-sized arteries with cellular infiltrations leading to fibrinoid necrosis and narrowing and obliteration of the vessel lumens. Necrotizing and granulomatous inflammation of a large vessel such as the aorta or pulmonary artery also may occur.

The *clinical course* is highly variable, with recurrent exacerbations and disease-free intervals of uncertain duration. Painful oral ulcers, usually 2–10 mm in diameter with surrounding erythema, develop in all patients, persist for days to weeks, and then heal without scarring. These necrotic ulcers may occur singly or in crops over the oronasal cavity and upper airway. Genital ulcers occur in most patients and follow a parallel course but may heal with scars. Skin manifestations occur in most patients and include erythema nodosum, pseudofolliculitis, papulopustular lesions, and acneiform nodules. Cutaneous pathergy occurs as an erythematous sterile pustule after 24–48 hr at a needle-prick skin site. Ocular manifestations, including anterior or posterior uveitis and retinal vasculitis, occur less frequently in children than in adults but are more severe in the pediatric population and may progress to blindness. Arthritis is common and is usually acute, recurrent, asymmetric, and polyarticular, involving the large joints. Central nervous system abnormalities such as meningoencephalitis, cranial nerve palsies, and psychosis usually occur later in the course of the disease and indicate a poor prognosis.

Laboratory findings are not diagnostic, although HLA-B5/B51 may support the diagnosis.

Treatment is based on anecdotal reports. Systemic corticosteroids, colchicine, chlorambucil, azathioprine, and cyclosporine have been effective in some patients. Of these agents, colchicine is the most promising, showing higher efficacy in children than in adults, especially for oral ulcers, skin rash, joint symptoms, and occasionally eye disease.

Lang BA, Laxer RM, Thorner P, et al: Pediatric onset of Behçet's syndrome with myositis: Case report and literature review illustrating unusual features. Arthritis Rheum 33:418, 1990.

International Study Group for Behçet's Disease: Criteria for diagnosis of Behçet's disease. Lancet 335:1078, 1990.

Kone-Paut I, Yurdakul S, Bahabri SA, et al: Clinical features of Behçet's disease in children: An international collaborative study of 86 cases. J Pediatr 132:721, 1998.

Krause I, Uziel Y, Guedj D, et al: Colchicine treatment in Behçet's disease: Diverse efficacy in adults and children. Arthritis Rheum 40:S67, 1997.

CHAPTER 163
Sjögren's Syndrome

Abraham Gedalia

Sjögren's syndrome is a chronic inflammatory autoimmune disease characterized by progressive lymphocytic and plasma cell infiltration of the salivary and lacrimal glands leading to dry eyes (keratoconjunctivitis sicca, xerophthalmia), dry mouth (xerostomia), and associated connective tissue disease features. Sjögren's syndrome typically occurs in women (female:male ratio of 9:1) between 35–45 yr of age. It is uncommon in the pediatric age group, although more than 50 cases in children have been reported.

Clinical manifestations are related to exocrine disease of the epithelial surfaces of the eyes, mouth, nose, larynx and trachea, vagina, and skin, leading to the common symptoms of photophobia, burning and itching eyes, and blurred vision; painless unilateral or bilateral enlargement of the parotid glands; decreased sense of taste; dental caries; dysphagia; fissured tongue; and angular cheilitis. Additional manifestations may include a decreased sense of smell and epistaxis; hoarseness; chronic otitis media; and internal organ exocrine disease involving the lungs, hepatobiliary system, pancreas, gastrointestinal tract, and kidneys.

Nonexocrine disease manifestations of Sjögren's syndrome may be related to inflammatory vascular disease (in skin, muscle and joints, serosae, peripheral and central nervous system), noninflammatory vascular disease (Raynaud phenomenon), mediator-induced disease (hematologic cytopenias, fatigue, fever), and autoimmune endocrinopathy (thyroiditis). Because monoclonal B-lymphocyte disease originates chiefly from lymphocytic foci within salivary glands or from parenchymal internal organs, lymphoproliferative forms of Sjögren's syndrome occur in adults with potential lymphoid malignancy. Parotitis at onset is much more frequent in children than in adults with Sjögren's syndrome. However, positive antinuclear antibodies and articular manifestations are significantly more frequent in adults.

Sjögren's syndrome can occur as a secondary form in the context of rheumatoid arthritis or systemic lupus erythematosus. It precedes the associated autoimmune disease by years in half of the cases.

The *diagnosis* is based on clinical features supported by biopsy of the lip or glands demonstrating foci of lymphocytic infiltration, elevated IgG serum levels, cryoglobulinemia, positive rheumatoid factor, and the presence of antibodies to La/SSB and Ro/SSA. Maternal Sjögren's syndrome can be an antecedent to the neonatal lupus syndrome. European criteria for the diagnosis of Sjögren's syndrome in adult patients have been developed, but whether these criteria can be applied to children remains to be determined.

The *differential diagnosis* of Sjögren's syndrome in children includes chronic recurrent parotitis, infectious parotitis, and tumors. In these conditions, sicca complex, rash, arthralgia, and antinuclear antibodies are usually absent.

Treatment is symptomatic, with use of artificial tears, oral lozenges, and fluids to limit the damaging effects of decreased secretions. Corticosteroids with or without immunosuppressive agents may be indicated for severe functional disorders and life-threatening complications.

Anaya J-M, Ogawa N, Talal N: Sjögren syndrome in childhood. J Rheumatol 22:1152, 1995.

Manthrope R, Asmussen K, Oxholm P: Primary Sjögren syndrome: Diagnostic criteria, clinical features, and disease activity. J Rheumatol 24(Suppl 50):8, 1997.

Vitali C, Bombardieri S, Moutsopoulos HM, et al: Preliminary criteria for the classification of Sjögren syndrome. Results of a prospective concerted action supported by the European community. Arthritis Rheum 36:340, 1993.

CHAPTER 164

Familial Mediterranean Fever

Abraham Gedalia

Familial Mediterranean fever (FMF) is an inherited disorder characterized by brief acute self-limited episodes of fever and polyserositis recurring at irregular intervals, as well as development of amyloidosis (Chapter 165), which if untreated leads to end-stage renal failure. FMF appears to be transmitted as an autosomal recessive disease and essentially occurs among ethnic groups of Mediterranean origin, mainly Sephardic Jews, Armenians, Arabs, and individuals of Turkish descent. In these populations, the carrier frequency is estimated to be as high as one in five persons. Greeks, Hispanics, and Italians are less commonly affected. FMF is rare among Ashkenazi Jews, Germans, and Anglo-Saxons; other ethnic groups report only sporadic cases.

The *gene* responsible for FMF was first mapped to a small interval on the short arm of chromosome 16 between the gene responsible for adult-onset polycystic kidney disease and the gene linked to Rubinstein-Taybi syndrome. The FMF gene, designated *MEFV,* was then identified and cloned, and five disease-related mutations were discovered. Haplotype and mutational analyses showed ancestral relationships among carrier chromosomes that have been separated for centuries. *MEFV* is a new member of the RoRet gene family; it is approximately 10 kb with 10 exons that express a 3.7-kb transcript encoding a 781 amino acid protein known as *pyrin* that is expressed in neutrophils. Two of the five sequence variations occur most commonly: the methionine-694-valine mutation, which is associated with a higher disease severity index and also a higher incidence of amyloidosis; and the valine-726-alanine mutation, which is associated with milder disease and a lower incidence of amyloidosis. This suggests that phenotypic differences may be related to different mutations. Cloning and identification of the FMF gene now make it possible to establish a diagnosis of FMF, especially in areas where the disease is rare and less familiar to physicians.

The onset of *clinical manifestations* occurs before age 5 yr in 63–68% of cases and before age 20 yr in 90% of cases. The onset may be as early as 6 mo of age. The typical acute episode includes fever and one or more symptoms of peritonitis manifested by abdominal pain (90%), arthritis or arthralgia (85%), and pleuritis manifested by chest pain (20%). Other serosal tissues such as the pericardium and tunica vaginalis testis are rarely affected. Erysipelas-like skin rash, myalgia, splenomegaly, scrotal involvement in boys, neurologic involvement, Henoch-Schönlein purpura, and hypothyroidism are other less common clinical manifestations. In about one third to one half of untreated patients with FMF, amyloidosis of AA type develops and is manifested by proteinuria that progresses to nephrotic syndrome and renal failure over a period of months to several years. Death results from infection, thromboembolism, or uremia. Amyloidosis is common among Sephardic Jews and Turks and less common in Armenians. However, Armenians living in Armenia are reported to have a significantly higher incidence of amyloidosis than do their counterparts in North America, suggesting that environmental factors may also have a role.

The exact *pathogenesis* of the acute episodes of FMF is still not known, although some immunologic abnormalities have been reported. Of special interest is the finding of a C5a inhibitor (inactivating enzyme) deficiency in peritoneal and synovial fluids of patients with FMF. C5a is a fragment of complement, an anaphylatoxin, and a potent chemotactic agent. Normally, small amounts of C5a may be released into serosal cavities and are subsequently neutralized by the inactivating enzyme before they precipitate overt inflammation. One hypothesis is that a deficiency of C5a inhibitor, which is a consequence of pyrin dysfunction in patients with FMF, allows further accumulation of C5a, leading to the acute attack. Better understanding of pyrin function will shed light on its interactions with other proteins involved in the regulation of the inflammatory response.

Attacks of FMF can be *prevented* by prophylactic colchicine therapy at a dose of 0.02–0.03 mg/kg/24 hr (maximum of 2 mg/24 hr) in one or two divided doses. Colchicine therapy not only reduces the frequency of acute attacks but also greatly decreases the probability of development of amyloidosis and may lead to partial regression of existing amyloidosis. Colchicine therapy for FMF during pregnancy has not been reported to harm either the mother or her fetus.

Babior BM, Matzner Y: The familial Mediterranean fever gene—cloned at last. N Engl J Med 337:1548, 1997.

Eisenberg S, Aksentijevich I, Deng Z, et al: Diagnosis of familial Mediterranean fever by a molecular genetics method. Ann Intern Med 129:539, 1998.

Gedalia A, Adar A, Gorodischer R: Familial Mediterranean fever in children. J Rheumatol 19(Suppl 35):1, 1992.

The French FMF Consortium: A candidate gene for familial Mediterranean fever. Nature Genet 17:25, 1997.

The International FMF Consortium: Ancient missense mutations in a new member of the RoRet gene family are likely to cause familial Mediterranean fever. Cell 90:797, 1997.

CHAPTER 165

Amyloidosis

Abraham Gedalia

Amyloidosis comprises a group of diseases characterized by extracellular deposition of insoluble fibrous amyloid proteins in various body tissues. The deposits are composed of seemingly homogeneous eosinophilic material that stains with Congo red dye and in polarized light demonstrates the pathognomonic apple-green birefringence of amyloid. Amyloid material is composed of microscopic fibrils that are biochemically heterogeneous, with at least 15 different types of protein compositions. However, all amyloid deposits contain an identical nonfibrillar component, serum amyloid P. Amyloid fibril deposition may have no apparent consequences, or it may ultimately interfere with organ function. Various disease states result from deposition of different types of amyloid material, and different patterns of tissue deposition result in various patterns of organ dysfunction. Regardless of the cause of amyloidosis, the clinical diagnosis is usually not made until the disease is far advanced.

Classifications of the amyloid proteins and the various amyloid diseases are complex. The systemic amyloidoses are multisystem diseases that correspond to clinical patterns of primary, secondary, familial, and dialysis-related amyloidosis. The localized or organ-limited amyloidoses are associated with aging and diabetes and occur in isolated organs such as endocrine glands, without evidence of systemic involvement. The most common types of amyloidosis are those related to primary idiopathic amyloidosis and multiple myeloma, with deposition of amyloid composed of pieces of monoclonal light chain of immunoglobulin (AL type). Secondary or reactive amyloidosis occurs in individuals with familial Mediterranean fever (FMF) and chronic inflammatory diseases related to another protein, amyloid A protein (AA type). Finally, a group of amyloid conditions, including those associated with aging (e.g., Alzheimer disease), and several rare familial types of amyloidosis are associated with other amyloid protein precursors.

Primary amyloidosis is extremely rare in children. Only secondary amyloidosis affects children in appreciable numbers, and it occurs in some individuals with FMF and after chronic inflammatory diseases, including juvenile rheumatoid arthritis (JRA), rheumatoid arthritis, ankylosing spondylitis, inflammatory bowel disease, chronic infections such as tuberculosis, and cystic fibrosis. Amyloid A protein isolated from amyloid found in these diseases is an N-terminus fragment of serum amyloid A. Because serum amyloid A protein acts as an acute-phase reactant, increased amounts of this material resulting from chronic inflammation may provide an explanation for the occurrence of this form of secondary amyloidosis. Other inflammatory diseases such as lupus erythematosus or dermatomyositis, which are associated with shorter periods of inflammation, are not associated with secondary amyloidosis. Similar to FMF, secondary amyloidosis affects as many as 10% of children with JRA in some European countries but is rarely seen as a complication of seemingly similar disease in children in the United States and Canada. Explanations for this difference are unknown, although environmental factors may have a role. Secondary amyloidosis usually begins some years after the onset of inflammatory disease and is manifested by hepatosplenomegaly, proteinuria, and progression to nephrotic syndrome and eventual renal failure.

The diagnosis of amyloidosis is established by demonstration of amyloid in affected tissues. Renal biopsies are considered hazardous in the presence of amyloidosis because of potential bleeding. The spleen is often affected but is not a suitable site for biopsy. More accessible biopsy sites include the rectal mucosa and gingival tissue. A method of scintigraphy using serum amyloid P component has been described as a useful diagnostic tool and as a tool for monitoring the status of amyloidosis. Patients with JRA and secondary amyloidosis usually show elevated acute-phase reactants and high levels of immunoglobulins.

Unlike amyloidosis associated with FMF, amyloidosis associated with JRA does not respond to colchicine therapy but instead to chlorambucil, which reverses renal findings and prolongs life. Chlorambucil is associated with chromosome breakage and an unknown risk of subsequent malignancy. There is little experience with other cytotoxic agents and with the therapy for secondary amyloidosis associated with other conditions.

Benson MD: Amyloidosis. *In*: Koopman WJ (ed): Arthritis and Allied Conditions. Baltimore, Williams & Wilkins, 1997, pp 1661–1687.

David J, Vouyiouka O, Ansell BM, et al: Amyloidosis in juvenile chronic arthritis: A morbidity and mortality study. Clin Exp Rheumatol 11:85, 1993.

Hawkins PN, Richardson S, Vigushin DM, et al: Serum amyloid P component scintigraphy and turnover studies for diagnosis and quantitative monitoring of AA amyloidosis in juvenile rheumatoid arthritis. Arthritis Rheum 36:842, 1993.

Saatci U, Bakkaloglu A, Ozen S, et al: Familial Mediterranean fever and amyloidosis in children. Acta Paediatr 81:705, 1993.

Woo P: Amyloidosis in children. Baillieres Clin Rheumatol 8:691, 1994.

Chapter 166
Kawasaki Disease

Anne H. Rowley and Stanford T. Shulman

Kawasaki disease (formerly known as mucocutaneous lymph node syndrome or infantile polyarteritis nodosa) is an acute febrile vasculitis of childhood first described by Dr. Tomisaku Kawasaki in Japan in 1967. The disorder occurs worldwide, with Asians at highest risk. Approximately 20% of untreated patients develop coronary artery abnormalities including aneurysms, with the potential for the development of coronary thrombosis, stenosis, myocardial infarction, and sudden death. Kawasaki disease has replaced acute rheumatic fever as the leading cause of acquired heart disease in children in the United States and Japan.

ETIOLOGY. The cause of the illness remains unknown, but clinical and epidemiologic features strongly support an infectious origin. These features include the age group affected, the occurrence of periodic epidemics with a wavelike geographic spread of illness during the epidemic, the self-limited nature of the illness, and the clinical features of fever, rash, enanthem, conjunctival injection, and cervical adenopathy. One hypothesis is that a ubiquitous agent causes Kawasaki disease and that symptomatic illness occurs only in genetically predisposed hosts. The infrequent occurrence of the illness in infants younger than 4 mo may be due to passive maternal antibody, and the virtual absence of cases in adults due to widespread immunity.

EPIDEMIOLOGY. It is estimated that at least 3,000 cases are diagnosed annually in the United States. The incidence of Kawasaki disease in Asian children is substantially higher than in other racial groups, but the illness occurs worldwide in all ethnic groups. In Japan, more than 150,000 cases have been reported since the 1960s. Kawasaki disease is not a new illness; autopsy reports of infantile periarteritis nodosa before the 1960s appear in retrospect to have represented fatal Kawasaki disease. The disorder bears marked similarities to measles infection and may have been particularly difficult to identify before the development of measles vaccine. The illness occurs predominantly in young children; 80% of patients are younger than 5 yr, and only occasionally are teenagers and adults affected.

PATHOGENESIS. Kawasaki disease causes a severe vasculitis of all blood vessels but predominantly affecting the medium-sized arteries, with predilection for the coronary arteries. Pathologic examination of fatal cases in the acute or subacute stages reveals edema of endothelial and smooth muscle cells with intense inflammatory infiltration of the vascular wall, initially by polymorphonuclear cells but rapidly changing to mononuclear cells, lymphocytes (which are largely T cells), and plasma cells. IgA plasma cells are prominent in the inflammatory infiltrate. In the most severely affected vessels, inflammation involves all three layers of the vascular wall, with destruction of the internal elastic lamina. The vessel loses its structural integrity and weakens, resulting in dilatation or aneurysm formation. Thrombi may form in the lumen and obstruct blood flow. In the healing phase, the lesion becomes progressively fibrotic, with marked intimal proliferation, which may result in stenotic occlusion of the vessel over time.

In the subacute phase of illness, elevated levels of all the serum immunoglobulins are present, suggesting that a vigorous antibody response occurs. It is unclear whether the etiologic agent, the host immune response, or both are the major factors leading to coronary disease.

CLINICAL MANIFESTATIONS. Fever is generally high spiking (to 104°F or higher), remittent, and unresponsive to antibiotics. The duration of fever is generally 1–2 wk without treatment but may persist for 3–4 wk. Prolonged fever has been shown to be a risk factor for the development of coronary artery disease. The other characteristic features of the illness are bilateral bulbar conjunctival injection, usually without exudate; erythema of the oral and pharyngeal mucosa with "strawberry" tongue and dry, cracked lips; erythema and swelling of the hands and feet; rash of various forms (maculopapular, erythema multiforme, or scarlatiniform) with accentuation in the groin area; and nonsuppurative cervical lymphadenopathy, usually unilateral, with a node size of 1.5 cm or greater in diameter. One to 3 wk after the onset of illness, periungual desquamation of the fingers and toes begins and may progress to involve the entire hand and foot. Perineal desquamation is common.

Other features include extreme irritability, especially in infants, aseptic meningitis, diarrhea, mild hepatitis, hydrops of the gallbladder, urethritis and meatitis with sterile pyuria, otitis media, and arthritis. Arthritis is more common in girls and may occur early in the illness with fever and other acute manifestations or may develop during the 2nd–3rd week, generally affecting hands, knees, ankles, or hips.

Cardiac involvement is the most important manifestation of Kawasaki disease. Myocarditis manifested by tachycardia and decreased ventricular function occurs in at least 50% of patients. Pericarditis with a small pericardial effusion is common during the acute illness. Coronary artery aneurysms generally develop during the 2nd–3rd wk of illness and can be detected by two-dimensional echocardiography. Valvular regurgitation and systemic artery aneurysms may occur but are uncommon. Giant coronary artery aneurysms (≥8 mm internal diameter) pose the greatest risk for rupture, thrombosis or stenosis, and myocardial infarction.

Kawasaki disease is generally divided into three clinical phases. The acute febrile phase, which usually lasts for 1–2 wk, is characterized by fever and the other acute signs of illness. The subacute phase begins when fever and other acute signs have abated, but irritability, anorexia, and conjunctival injection may persist. The subacute phase is associated with desquamation, thrombocytosis, the development of coronary aneurysms, and the highest risk of sudden death. This phase generally lasts until about the 4th wk. The convalescent stage begins when all clinical signs of illness have disappeared and continues until the erythrocyte sedimentation rate (ESR) returns to normal, at approximately 6–8 wk after the onset of illness.

DIAGNOSIS. The diagnosis of Kawasaki disease is based on demonstration of characteristic clinical signs (Table 166–1). The diagnostic criteria require the presence of fever for at least 5 days and at least four of five of the other characteristic clinical features of illness. Atypical or incomplete cases in which a patient has fever with fewer than four other features of the illness and then develops coronary artery disease have been described worldwide. Atypical cases are most frequent in infants, who unfortunately have the highest likelihood of developing coronary artery disease.

Recognition depends on a high index of suspicion and knowledge of the characteristic clinical features of the illness. Unfortunately, if the diagnosis is not made and treatment instituted, a patient may suffer sudden death secondary to myocardial infarction or coronary aneurysm rupture or may develop serious asymptomatic coronary disease that is not diagnosed until symptoms develop in young adulthood.

DIFFERENTIAL DIAGNOSIS. The differential diagnosis of Kawasaki disease includes scarlet fever, toxic shock syndrome, measles, drug hypersensitivity reactions including Stevens-Johnson syndrome, juvenile rheumatoid arthritis, and, more rarely, Rocky Mountain spotted fever and leptospirosis. Some features of uncomplicated measles that help to distinguish it from Kawasaki disease include the presence of exudative conjunctivitis, Koplik spots, rash that begins on the face behind the ears, and a low white blood cell count and ESR. Some features of drug reactions, such as the presence of periorbital edema, oral lesions, and a low ESR, may help to distinguish these reactions from Kawasaki disease. Toxic shock syndrome may be distinguished by the presence of hypotension, renal involvement, elevated creatine phosphokinase level, and a focus of staphylococcal infection, which are features of this illness but not of Kawasaki disease. A common clinical problem is the differentiation of scarlet fever from Kawasaki disease in a child who is a group A streptococcal carrier. Because patients with scarlet fever have a rapid clinical response to penicillin therapy, treatment with this therapy for 24–48 hr with clinical reassessment at that time generally clarifies the diagnosis. The presence of lymphadenopathy, hepatosplenomegaly, and evanescent, salmon-colored rash suggests a diagnosis of juvenile rheumatoid arthritis. Accurate diagnosis of atypical cases remains a significant challenge for clinicians. Unusual cases should be referred to a center with experience in the diagnosis of Kawasaki disease.

LABORATORY FINDINGS. No specific diagnostic test for the illness exists, but certain laboratory findings are characteristic. The white blood cell count is normal to elevated, with a predominance of neutrophils and immature forms. An elevated ESR, C-reactive protein, and other acute phase reactants are almost universally present in the acute phase of illness and may persist for 4–6 wk. Normocytic anemia is common. The platelet count is generally normal in the 1st wk of illness and rapidly rises by the 2nd–3rd wk of illness and may exceed 1,000,000/mm^3. Antinuclear antibody and rheumatoid factor are not detectable. Sterile pyuria, mild elevations of the hepatic transaminases, and cerebrospinal fluid pleocytosis may be present.

Two-dimensional echocardiography is the most useful test to monitor the potential development of coronary artery abnormalities and should be performed by a pediatric cardiologist. The test should be performed at diagnosis and again after 2–3 wk of illness. If results of both of these are normal, a repeat study is performed 6–8 wk after onset of illness. If coronary abnormalities are not detected by echocardiography by 6–8 wk after onset of illness, when the ESR has normalized, additional follow-up studies are optional. Some centers routinely perform echocardiography again 1 yr after onset of illness. However, Kawasaki disease is an acute vasculitis; there is no convincing evidence of long-term cardiovascular sequelae in children who do not develop coronary abnormalities within 2 mo after the onset of illness.

For patients who develop coronary artery abnormalities, more frequent echocardiographic studies and potentially angiography may be indicated. Treatment of such patients should be determined in consultation with a pediatric cardiologist.

TREATMENT. Patients with acute Kawasaki disease should be treated with intravenous immune globulin (IVIG) and high-

TABLE 166–1 Diagnostic Criteria for Kawasaki Disease

Fever lasting for at least 5 days*
Presence of at least four of the following five signs:

1. Bilateral bulbar conjunctival injection, generally nonpurulent
2. Changes in the mucosa of the oropharynx, including injected pharynx, injected and/or dry fissured lips, strawberry tongue
3. Changes of the peripheral extremities, such as edema and/or erythema of the hands or feet in the acute phase; or periungual desquamation in the subacute phase
4. Rash, primarily truncal; polymorphous but nonvesicular
5. Cervical adenopathy, ≥1.5 cm, usually unilateral lymphadenopathy

Illness not explained by other known disease process

**Experienced physicians may make the diagnosis of Kawasaki disease (and institute treatment) before the 5th day of fever in patients with classic features of the illness.*

TABLE 166–2 Treatment of Kawasaki Disease

Acute Stage

Intravenous immune globulin 2 g/kg over 10–12 hr *with* aspirin 80–100 mg/kg/24 hr divided every 6 hr orally until 14th illness day

Convalescent Stage

Aspirin 3–5 mg/kg once daily orally until 6–8 wk after illness onset

Long-Term Therapy for Those with Coronary Abnormalities

Aspirin 3–5 mg/kg once daily, orally
± dipyridamole 4–6 mg/kg/24 hr divided in two or three doses orally (some experts add warfarin for those patients at particularly high risk of thrombosis)

Acute Coronary Thrombosis

Prompt fibrinolytic therapy with tissue plasminogen activator, streptokinase, or urokinase under supervision of a pediatric cardiologist

dose aspirin as soon as possible after diagnosis (Table 166–2). The mechanism of action of IVIG in Kawasaki disease is unknown, but treatment results in rapid defervescence and resolution of clinical signs of illness in most patients. IVIG reduces the prevalence of coronary disease from 20–25% in children treated with aspirin alone to 2–4% in those treated with IVIG and aspirin within the 1st 10 days of illness. In addition, consideration should be given to treatment of patients diagnosed after the 10th illness day if fever has persisted, because the anti-inflammatory effect may be helpful, although the effect of such therapy on the risk of developing coronary aneurysms is unknown. Aspirin is decreased from anti-inflammatory to antithrombotic doses (3–5 mg/kg/24 hr as a single dose) on the 14th illness day or when a patient has been afebrile for at least 3–4 days. Aspirin is continued for its antithrombotic effect until 6–8 wk after onset, when the ESR has normalized, in patients who have not developed abnormalities detected by echocardiography.

Occasional patients do not respond to an initial IVIG infusion or have only a partial response. Strong consideration should be given to re-treatment of these patients with an additional infusion of IVIG, although the efficacy of such treatment remains unproven. The use of corticosteroids in Kawasaki disease remains controversial and is not generally recommended at this time. Patients treated with IVIG should have measles-mumps-rubella and varicella vaccines delayed for 11 mo because the presence of specific antiviral antibody in IVIG may interfere with the immune response to parenteral live-virus vaccines.

Patients with a small solitary aneurysm should continue aspirin indefinitely. Patients with larger or numerous aneurysms may require the addition of dipyridamole or warfarin therapy; such decisions should be made in consultation with a pediatric cardiologist. Acute thrombosis may occasionally occur in an aneurysmal coronary artery. Thrombolytic therapy may be lifesaving in this circumstance. Long-term follow-up of patients with aneurysms should include echocardiography, stress testing, and potentially angiography.

Patients receiving long-term aspirin therapy are candidates for influenza vaccine to reduce the risk of Reye syndrome. The risk of Reye syndrome in children who take salicylates and who receive varicella vaccine is believed to be much lower than with wild-type varicella. Physicians must weigh the relative risk of vaccine in children on long-term aspirin therapy against the risk of natural varicella infection.

COMPLICATIONS AND PROGNOSIS. Recovery is complete and without apparent long-term effects for patients who do not develop coronary disease. Recurrent illness occurs in only 1–3% of cases. The prognosis for patients with coronary abnormalities depends on the severity of coronary disease. In Japan, fatality rates are now less than 0.1%. Overall, 50% of coronary artery aneurysms resolve echocardiographically by 1–2 yr after the illness. However, intravascular ultrasonography has demonstrated that resolved aneurysms are associated with marked intimal thickening and abnormal functional behavior of the vessel. Giant aneurysms are unlikely to resolve and most often lead to thrombosis or stenosis. Coronary artery bypass grafting may be required if myocardial perfusion is significantly impaired, and it is best accomplished with the use of arterial grafts, which grow with the child and are more likely to remain patent than venous grafts. Heart transplantation has been required in rare cases in which revascularization is not feasible because of distal coronary stenosis or aneurysms or severe myocardial dysfunction. Whether the presence of coronary artery abnormalities resulting from Kawasaki disease predisposes to the development of atherosclerotic heart disease in young adulthood is unknown.

Dajani AS, Taubert KA, Gerber MA, et al: Diagnosis and therapy of Kawasaki disease in children. Circulation 87:1776, 1993.
Dajani AS, Taubert KA, Takahashi M, et al: Guidelines for long-term management of patients with Kawasaki disease. Circulation 89:916, 1994.
Kato H, Sugimura T, Akagi T, et al: Long-term consequences of Kawasaki disease. Circulation 94:1379, 1996.
Melish ME: Kawasaki syndrome. Pediatr Rev 17:153, 1996.
Naoe S, Shibuya K, Takahashi K, et al: Pathologic observations concerning the cardiovascular lesions in Kawasaki disease. Cardiol Young 1:212, 1991.
Newburger JW, Takahashi M, Beiser AS, et al: A single intravenous infusion of gamma globulin as compared with four infusions in the treatment of acute Kawasaki syndrome. N Engl J Med 324:1633, 1991.
Rosenfeld EA, Corydon KE, Shulman ST: Kawasaki disease in infants less than one year of age. J Pediatr 126:524, 1995.
Rowley AH, Eckerley CA, Jack H-M, et al: IgA plasma cells in vascular tissue of patients with Kawasaki syndrome. J Immunol 159:5946, 1997.
Rowley AH, Shulman ST: Kawasaki syndrome. Clin Microbiol Rev 11:405, 1998.

CHAPTER 167
Vasculitis Syndromes

Michael L. Miller and Lauren M. Pachman

Vasculitis in childhood is a result of a spectrum of causes ranging from idiopathic conditions with primary vessel inflammation to syndromes following exposure to known antigens (e.g., infectious agents, drugs causing hypersensitivity reactions). Vasculitis is also a component of many autoimmune diseases. The extent of vessel damage can range from moderate, as in most children with Henoch-Schönlein purpura (HSP), to severe, as in children with polyarteritis nodosa. Most classifications of the vasculitic syndromes are based on the size and location of the blood vessels that are primarily involved, as well as the type of inflammatory infiltrate. The affected target vessels range in size from large afferent vessels, in Takayasu arteritis, to capillary and arteriolar occlusion, characteristic of juvenile dermatomyositis. The inflammatory infiltrate can include various amounts of polymorphonuclear, mononuclear, and eosinophilic cells.

Immune complexes have a key role in the pathophysiology of many vasculitic syndromes. Immune complexes activate complement, releasing chemotactic fragments (C3a, C5a) that attract inflammatory cells. It is speculated in many vasculitic syndromes that immune complexes, after binding to endothelial cells, increase synthesis of adhesion molecules on the cell surfaces. These adhesion molecules bind to other adhesion molecules on circulating polymorphonuclear leukocytes attracted to the vicinity by chemotactic molecules. Subsequent lysosomal release of digestive enzymes from these leukocytes in many vasculitic syndromes destroys the cellular matrix of the blood vessels and surrounding tissues. In the process of

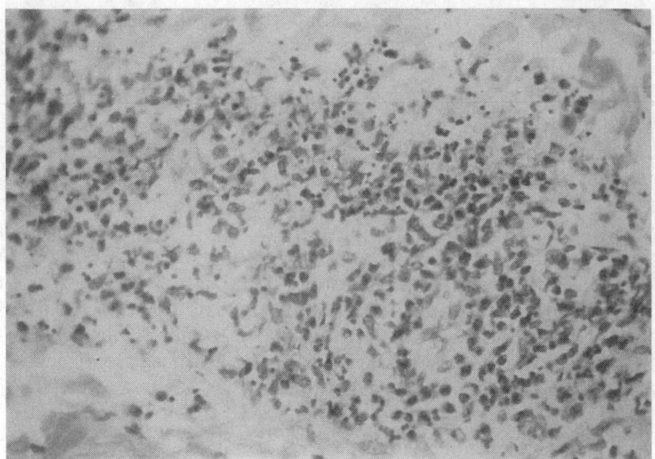

Figure 167–1 Histopathology of a skin biopsy from a patient with Henoch-Schönlein purpura showing leukocytoclastic vasculitis with nuclear degeneration ("nuclear dust").

degranulation, the polymorphonuclear leukocytes may disintegrate to the "nuclear dust" typical of leukocytoclastic angiitis (Fig. 167–1).

The signs and symptoms of the vasculitic syndromes are nonspecific and tend to overlap, but certain clinical features are useful in distinguishing the type of vasculature that is primarily affected. Palpable purpura suggests small vessel vasculitis located deep in the papillary dermis, whereas a circumscribed tender nodule is more likely a result of involvement of medium-sized vessels.

167.1 Henoch-Schönlein Purpura

HSP, also known as anaphylactoid purpura, is a vasculitis of small vessels. It is the most common cause of nonthrombocytopenic purpura in children.

EPIDEMIOLOGY. The cause of HSP is unknown, but HSP typically follows an upper respiratory tract infection. The incidence and prevalence of HSP are probably underestimated because cases are not reported to public health agencies. However, of 31,333 new patients seen at 54 pediatric rheumatology centers in the United States, 1,120 had some form of vasculitis and 558 were classified as HSP. Although HSP accounted for 1% of hospital admissions in the past, changes in medical practice have reduced the frequency of admissions; 0.06% of admissions (62/9,083 in 1997) were for HSP at one large Midwestern pediatric center. This illness is more frequent in children than adults, with most cases occurring between 2–8 yr of age, most frequently in the winter months. Males are affected twice as frequently as females. The overall incidence is estimated to be 9/100,000 population.

PATHOGENESIS. The specific pathogenesis of HSP is not known. The cytokines tumor necrosis factor-α (TNF-α) and interleukin 6 (IL-6) have been implicated in active disease. In one study, almost half of the patients had elevated antistreptolysin O (ASO) antibodies, implicating group A β-hemolytic streptococci. This illness is considered by histopathology to be an IgA-mediated vasculitis of small vessels. Immunofluorescence techniques show deposition of IgA and C3 in the small vessels of the skin and the renal glomeruli, but the role of complement activation is controversial.

CLINICAL MANIFESTATIONS. The disease onset may be acute, with the appearance of several manifestations simultaneously, or insidious, with sequential occurrence of symptoms over a period of weeks or months. Low-grade fever and fatigue occur in more than half of affected children. The typical rash and the clinical symptoms of HSP are a consequence of the usual location of the acute small vessel damage primarily in the skin, gastrointestinal (GI) tract, and kidneys.

The hallmark of the disease is the rash, beginning as pinkish maculopapules that initially blanch on pressure and progress to petechiae or purpura, characterized clinically as palpable purpura that evolve from red to purple to rusty brown before they eventually fade (Fig. 167–2). The lesions tend to occur in crops, last from 3–10 days, and may appear at intervals that vary from a few days to as long as 3–4 mo. In fewer than 10% of children, recurrence of the rash may not end until as late as a year, and rarely several years, after the initial episode. Damage to cutaneous vessels also results in local angioedema, which may precede the palpable purpura. Edema occurs primarily in dependent areas—for example, below the waist, over the buttocks (or on the back and posterior scalp in the infant), or in areas of greater tissue distensibility, such as the eyelids, lips, scrotum, or the dorsum of the hands and feet.

Arthritis, present in more than two thirds of children with HSP, is usually localized to the knees and ankles and appears to be a concomitant of edema. The effusions are serous, not hemorrhagic, in nature and resolve after a few days without residual deformity or articular damage. They may recur during a subsequent active phase of the disease.

Edema and damage to the vasculature of the GI tract may also lead to intermittent abdominal pain that is often colicky in nature. More than half of patients have occult heme-positive stools, diarrhea (with or without blood), or hematemesis. The recognition of peritoneal exudate, enlarged mesenteric lymph nodes, segmental edema, and hemorrhage into the bowel may prevent unnecessary laparotomy for acute abdominal pain. Intussusception may occur; it may be suggested by an empty right lower abdominal quadrant on physical examination or by currant jelly stools, which may be followed by complete obstruction or infarction with bowel perforation.

Several other organ systems may be involved during the acute phase of disease. Renal involvement occurs in 25–50% of children, and hepatosplenomegaly and lymphadenopathy may be found during active disease. A rare but potentially serious outcome of central nervous system (CNS) involvement is the development of seizures, paresis, or coma. Other rare complications include rheumatoid-like nodules, cardiac and eye involvement, mononeuropathies, pancreatitis, and pulmonary or intramuscular hemorrhage.

DIAGNOSIS. The pattern of crops of palpable lesions of similar hue in dependent areas of the body is characteristic. Diagnostic uncertainty arises when the symptom complex of edema, rash, arthritis with abdominal complaints, and renal findings occurs for a prolonged period. HSP can occur with other forms of

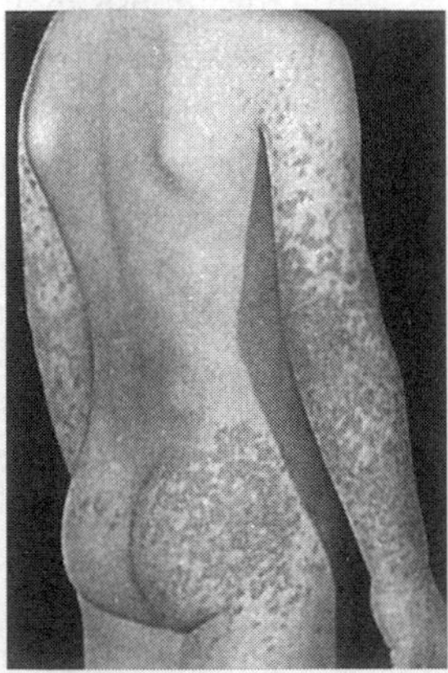

Figure 167–2 Henoch-Schönlein purpura. (From Korting GW: Hautkrankheiten bei Kindern und Jugendlichen, 3rd ed. Stuttgart, FK Schattauer Verlag, 1982.) See also color section.

vasculitis or autoimmune disease such as familial Mediterranean fever or inflammatory bowel disease. In polyarteritis nodosa, the cutaneous manifestations are different, and peripheral neurologic and cardiac manifestations are more common. Palpable purpura can occur in meningococcemia, if there are pre-existing coagulation abnormalities (such as factor V Leiden, protein S, or protein C deficiency). The presentation of unremitting fever, a maculopapular rash that does not reappear in crops but is prominent on the lower extremities, and peripheral arthritis suggests Kawasaki disease. HSP must be distinguished from systemic-onset juvenile rheumatoid arthritis. The salmon-pink rash is evanescent and maculopapular, and swelling does not extend beyond the joint.

LABORATORY FINDINGS. Routine laboratory tests are neither specific nor diagnostic. Affected children often have a moderate thrombocytosis and leukocytosis. The erythrocyte sedimentation rate (ESR) may be elevated. Anemia may result from chronic or acute GI blood loss. Immune complexes are often present, and 50% of active sera contain elevated concentrations of IgA as well as IgM but are usually negative for antinuclear antibodies (ANA), antibodies to nuclear cytoplasmic antigens (ANCA), and rheumatoid factor (even in the presence of rheumatoid nodules). Anticardiolipin or antiphospholipid antibodies may be present and contribute to the intravascular coagulopathy. Intussusception is usually ileo-ileal in location; barium enema may be used for both identification and nonsurgical reduction. Renal involvement is manifested by red blood cells, white blood cells, casts, or albumin in the urine.

Definitive diagnosis of vasculitis, confirmed by biopsy of an involved cutaneous site, shows leukoclastic angiitis. Renal biopsy may show IgA mesangial deposition and occasionally IgM, C3, and fibrin.

TREATMENT. Symptomatic treatment, including adequate hydration, bland diet, and pain control with acetaminophen, is provided for self-limited complaints of arthritis, edema, fever, and malaise. Avoidance of competitive activities and of maintaining the lower extremities in persistent dependence may decrease local edema. If edema involves the scrotum, elevation of the scrotum and local cooling, as tolerated, may decrease discomfort.

Intestinal complications (e.g., hemorrhage, obstruction, and intussusception) may be life threatening and managed with corticosteroids and, when necessary, barium enema reduction or surgical reduction or resection of the intussusception. Therapy with oral or intravenous corticosteroids (1–2 mg/kg/24 hr) is often associated with dramatic improvement of both GI and CNS complications.

Management of renal involvement is the same as for other forms of acute glomerulonephritis (Chapter 519). If anticardiolipin or antiphospholipid antibodies are identified and thrombotic events have occurred, aspirin (81 mg; "baby" aspirin) given once may decrease the risk associated with a hypercoagulable state. Rheumatoid nodules may respond to alternate-day colchicine (0.6 mg/24 hr).

COMPLICATIONS. The major complications of HSP are renal involvement with development of the nephrotic syndrome or bowel perforation. An infrequent complication of scrotal edema is testicular torsion, which may be suggested by pain and must be treated promptly.

PROGNOSIS. The overall prognosis is excellent for this relatively common, self-limited vasculitic disease. Chronic renal disease may result in morbidity in a few children: A population-based study indicated that fewer than 1% of patients with HSP develop persistent renal disease and fewer than 0.1% develop serious renal disease. Rarely, death may occur during the acute phase of the disease as a result of bowel infarction, CNS involvement, or renal disease.

167.2 Takayasu Arteritis

Takayasu arteritis (TA), or pulseless disease, is a chronic vasculitis of large vessels.

EPIDEMIOLOGY. TA is infrequently reported in children in the United States but is more common in Asian and Indian populations. Children of all ethnic backgrounds have been affected. After HSP and Kawasaki disease, TA may be the third most common form of childhood vasculitis in the world. There is a 2.5:1 female:male ratio. About one third of cases have onset before age 20 yr, and symptoms usually appear after age 10 yr, although children as young as 8 mo have been affected. The interval from initial presentation to diagnosis in children has been reported to be as long as 19 mo, almost four times the interval reported for adults.

PATHOGENESIS. TA is a chronic inflammatory and obliterative disease of large vessels, with preference for the aorta and its major branches. Renal lesions include mesangial proliferative, membranoproliferative, and crescentic glomerulonephritis as well as amyloidosis.

Although the antigen responsible for inciting TA has yet to be defined, exposure to tuberculosis has been reported to be associated with the disease in some studies in Asia. Identification of critical amino acid residues of the HLA-B molecule at position 63(Glu) and 67(Ser) suggests a specific antigen-binding site in some cases. Association with specific HLA markers has not been verified in non-Asian populations. Immune complex formation and complement activation have been frequently identified, but it is uncertain why only large vessels are affected.

CLINICAL MANIFESTATIONS. Early disease manifestations (prepulseless phase) include night sweats, anorexia, weight loss, fatigue, myalgia, and arthritis, often followed by unexplained hypertension. During the pulseless phase, systemic symptoms are twice as frequent in children compared with adults; splenomegaly may be found. Dermatologic features include erythema nodosum, a malar rash, and erythema induratum. Cardiac involvement includes dilated cardiomyopathy, myocarditis, and pericarditis. Other associated conditions include interstitial lung disease, pneumonic consolidation, ulcerative colitis, rheumatoid arthritis, and polymyositis.

During the pulseless phase, a characteristic bruit, often over the carotid or subclavian arteries, may be present on auscultation. Children may have diminished or absent radial pulses; limb claudication appears less frequently than in adults. If these symptoms occur in the 1st yr of life, arterial damage may be accompanied by papular rash, uveitis, symmetric polyarthritis, and granulomatous lesions typical of sarcoid, a condition termed *juvenile systemic granulomatosis* by some investigators.

DIAGNOSIS. Prompt diagnosis with institution of therapy is essential and may prevent progression of vascular lesions. The presence of intermittent unexplained systemic symptoms of variable duration in conjunction with an elevated ESR should prompt periodic auscultation of large arteries and blood pressure measurements in all four limbs.

This illness must be differentiated from acute rheumatic fever or juvenile arthritis. Because aortitis and aortic regurgitation may develop in TA, other disorders with these findings must also be considered, including Behçet's disease, Cogan syndrome, relapsing polychondritis, ankylosing spondylitis, seropositive rheumatoid arthritis, or Reiter syndrome. Juvenile temporal arteritis is rare, may be associated with a normal ESR, and is not associated with systemic symptoms.

LABORATORY FINDINGS. The ESR is significantly elevated (typically ≥60 [Westergren]), and a microcytic hypochromic anemia with a leukocytosis is usual. A polyclonal hypergammaglobulinemia is present in one third of cases. Complement activation results in elevated levels of C3a and C5a, which may be used as a guide to adjusting therapy.

The diagnosis can be confirmed by angiography, which often outlines a massively dilated aortic arch, with aneurysmal dilatation and stenosis of various large vessels—carotids, subclavian, abdominal aorta, or rarely in children, lesions of the

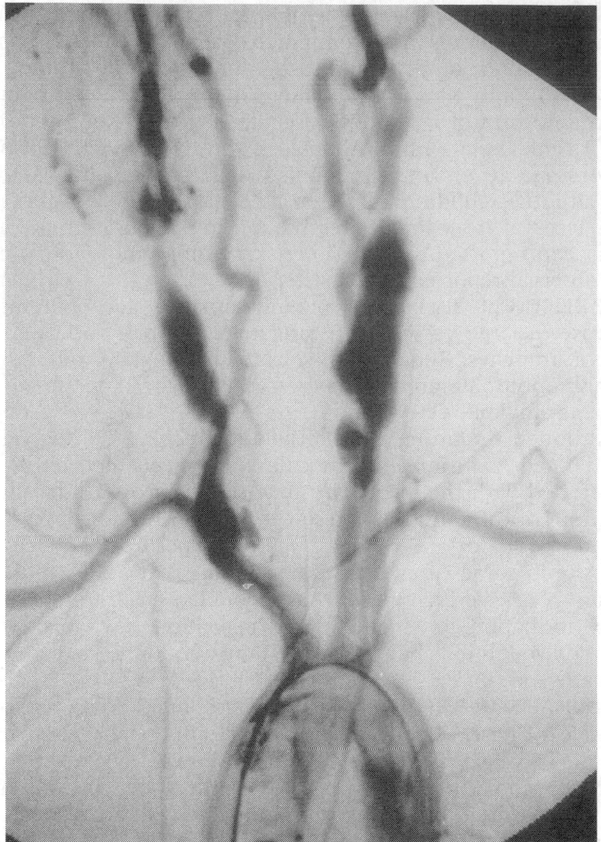

Figure 167–3 Angiogram of a child with Takayasu arteritis showing massive bilateral carotid dilatation, stenosis, and poststenotic dilatation.

coronary artery (Fig. 167–3). Magnetic resonance angiography may be helpful as a noninvasive test for subsequent monitoring of affected vessels.

TREATMENT. Early identification and surgical excision of the predominant lesions are essential, in conjunction with institution of appropriate immunosuppressive therapy. Prednisone (orally or intravenously) is administered in conjunction with other agents. Methotrexate has been useful in some situations, but cyclophosphamide (orally or intravenously) may often be needed to control the intense inflammatory response. More than 50% of cases achieve remission after the 1st course of therapy, but about one fourth of cases never achieve remission. The 5-yr mortality has been reported to be as high as 35%. Supportive care includes management of hypertension and psychologic support. There is no basis for genetic counseling.

COMPLICATIONS. The most dreaded complication of this often fatal illness is an aneurysmal rupture. Therefore, the dilated area is often excised and replaced with an ileal vascular graft. Prevention of chronic hypertension and decreased perfusion can sometimes be accomplished by excision of a stenotic area with graft replacement or by insertion of an intraluminal stent to forestall the redevelopment of stenosis.

PROGNOSIS. In the past, the mortality rate has been quite high. The outlook for these children remains guarded. The best outcome appears to be associated with early diagnosis and institution of medical and surgical therapy.

167.3 *Polyarteritis Nodosa*

Polyarteritis nodosa (PAN) is a necrotizing vasculitis affecting small- and medium-sized arteries. Aneurysms and nodules may form at irregular intervals throughout affected arteries.

EPIDEMIOLOGY. PAN occurs rarely during childhood. Boys and girls appear to be equally affected, with a peak at 10 yr of age. The cause is unknown, although the occurrence of PAN after upper respiratory tract infections, streptococcal infection, and chronic hepatitis B infection suggests that PAN represents a postinfectious autoimmune response to these agents in susceptible individuals. Other infections, including infectious mononucleosis, tuberculosis, cytomegalovirus, and parvovirus, have also been associated with PAN.

PATHOLOGY. Biopsy reveals a necrotizing vasculitis with lymphocytic infiltration affecting all layers of small and medium-sized muscular arteries (Fig. 167–4). Involvement is usually segmental, including bifurcations of vessels. Different stages of inflammation are found, ranging from mild inflammation to extensive fibrinoid necrosis associated with thrombosis and infarction. Aneurysm formation is common. Vascular occlusion may also occur as a result of postinflammatory fibrosis. Renal arterial involvement is found in the majority of patients; glomerular involvement is variable.

CLINICAL MANIFESTATIONS. The clinical presentation is variable but generally reflects the location of vessels that have become inflamed. Children may present with fever of unknown origin before other findings develop. Weight loss and severe abdominal pain suggest mesenteric arterial inflammation and possible thrombosis. Renovascular arteritis can result in hypertension, hematuria, or proteinuria. Vasculitis affecting the skin may be manifested by purpura, edema, and linear erythema with palpable, painful nodules along the course of affected arteries. In cutaneous PAN, the findings are limited to the skin. Arteritis affecting the nervous system may result in cerebrovascular accidents, transient ischemic attacks, psychosis, and ischemic peripheral neuropathy (e.g., with peripheral paresthesias or weakness). Cardiac involvement characterized by myocarditis may result in myocardial ischemia and heart failure; pericarditis and arrhythmias have also been reported. Less common findings include testicular pain (simulating testicular torsion), bone pain, and retinal arteritis, which may cause blindness. Arthralgia, arthritis, or myalgias may be encountered.

DIAGNOSIS. Diagnosis of PAN requires demonstration of findings characteristic of vasculitis on biopsy or angiography. Biopsy of suggestive cutaneous lesions may reveal vasculitis (see Fig. 167–4). Renal biopsy in patients with renal manifestations may show characteristic necrotizing arteritis. Electromyography in children with peripheral neuropathy may identify af-

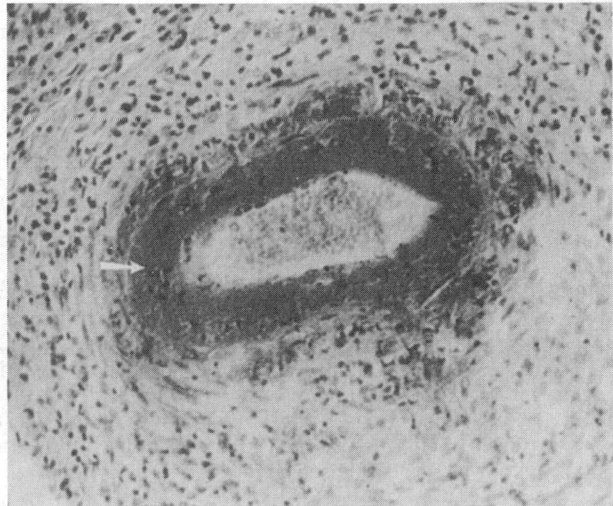

Figure 167–4 Biopsy of a medium-sized muscular artery that exhibits marked fibrinoid necrosis of the vessel wall *(arrow)*. (From Cassidy JT, Petty RE: Juvenile rheumatoid arthritis. *In*: Textbook of Pediatric Rheumatology, 3rd ed. Philadelphia, WB Saunders, 1995.)

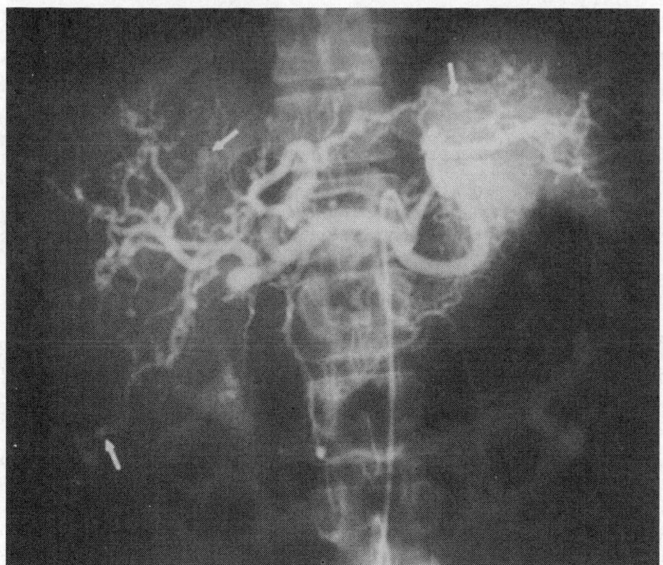

Figure 167–5 Celiac angiography of an 18-yr-old boy showing aneurysms in multiple vessels. (From Cassidy JT, Petty RE: Juvenile rheumatoid arthritis. *In*: Textbook of Pediatric Rheumatology, 3rd ed. Philadelphia, WB Saunders, 1995.)

fected sites; sural nerve biopsy may show an associated diagnostic vasculitis.

Angiography demonstrates areas of aneurysmal dilatation, at branch points of arteries, or segmental stenosis (Fig. 167–5). The renal and mesenteric arteries are often involved.

Evidence for previous or active infection should be sought in children with suspected PAN.

Differential Diagnosis. Early skin lesions may resemble those of HSP; the finding of nodular lesions and systemic findings distinguish PAN. Pulmonary lesions suggest Wegener granulomatosis (WG) or Goodpasture syndrome. Eosinophilia is noted in Churg-Strauss syndrome and eosinophilic fasciitis. Other rheumatic diseases, including systemic lupus erythematosus, dermatomyositis, and scleroderma, have characteristic target organ involvement distinct from PAN. Prolonged fever and weight loss can also characterize inflammatory bowel disease or malignancies.

LABORATORY FINDINGS. An elevated ESR is often the earliest finding. Anemia and leukocytosis are usually present eventually. Hypergammaglobulinemia reflects polyclonal B-cell activation. Abnormal urine sediment, proteinuria, and hematuria indicate renal disease. Markers of vasculitis may be useful in monitoring response to therapy. Von Willebrand factor antigen, a molecule found in vascular subendothelium, is released in increased amounts from inflamed vessels. Neopterin is released from macrophages that are activated in some patients with vasculitis. Levels of immune complexes, measured by the Raji cell and C1q assay, may also be elevated. Elevated hepatic enzymes suggest hepatitis B infection, which is more common in adults than in children.

TREATMENT. Oral and intravenous corticosteroids have been used, sometimes in combination with oral or intravenous cyclophosphamide. Iloprost, a prostacyclin analog, may be used for endarteritis that results in vascular compromise in the extremities.

COMPLICATIONS. Cutaneous nodules may ulcerate, posing a risk of infection. Hypertension may develop from renal arterial involvement. Cardiac involvement may lead to decreased cardiac function or coronary arterial disease. Hepatic aneurysmal rupture is a rare complication.

PROGNOSIS. The course of PAN varies from mild disease with few complications to a severe overwhelming multiorgan disease leading to death. However, aggressive immunosuppressive therapy has resulted in clinical remission.

167.4 Wegener Granulomatosis

WG is a vasculitis affecting the upper and lower respiratory tract and kidneys, characterized by necrotizing granulomas.

EPIDEMIOLOGY. The heterogeneity of clinical presentations suggests that a specific agent is unlikely. Although most cases occur in adults, children can develop WG, which predominates in Caucasians. The cause is unknown; however, proteinase 3 (PR3), normally restricted to neutrophil alpha granules, has been found on the surface of neutrophils of patients with WG. Those ANCA that bind to PR3 are specific for WG, suggesting an etiologic role for abnormal PR3 expression. Interaction of PR3 with the PiZ variant of α_1-antitrypsin has in some studies been found to increase the risk of developing WG.

PATHOLOGY. Necrotizing granulomas are found in affected organs, including the nasal and sinus mucosa, skin, and lower respiratory tract. In the lungs, infiltrates, alveolar hemorrhage, and vasculitis may also be found. Renal involvement can vary from focal proliferative glomerulonephritis to necrotic crescentic glomerulonephritis.

CLINICAL MANIFESTATIONS. Children initially often complain of nonspecific constitutional symptoms of fever, malaise, weight loss, myalgia, and arthralgia. Many affected children have seasonal allergies. Later symptoms include cough, congestion, and nasal discharge from chronic sinusitis (often with mucosal ulceration and bone destruction from necrotizing granulomas), and hemoptysis and dyspnea from pulmonary lesions (Fig. 167–6). Ophthalmic involvement includes conjunctival and corneal lesions, uveitis, and an invasive orbital pseudotumor. Cranial and peripheral neuropathies due to intracranial granulomas and peripheral granulomatous lesions have been reported. Hematuria and proteinuria due to glomerulonephritis

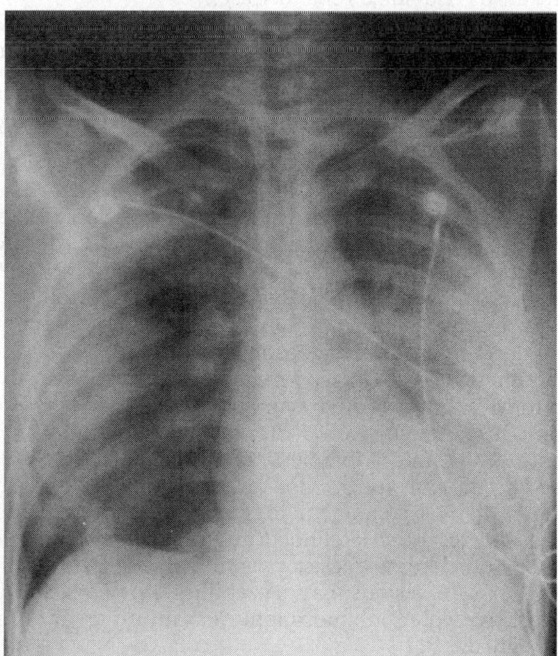

Figure 167–6 Chest radiograph of a 14-yr-old girl with Wegener granulomatosis showing widespread infiltrates suggestive of pulmonary hemorrhage. There were considerable day-to-day variability and eventual total resolution of these abnormalities after treatment with prednisone and cyclophosphamide. (From Cassidy JT, Petty RE: Juvenile rheumatoid arthritis. *In*: Textbook of Pediatric Rheumatology, 3rd ed. Philadelphia, WB Saunders, 1995.)

is often a later manifestation. Cutaneous lesions may include palpable purpuric nodules and ulcers.

DIAGNOSIS. The diagnosis of WG should be suspected in children who have severe sinusitis and who develop radiographic pulmonary findings suggestive of granulomas or renal findings consistent with nephritis. High-resolution CT imaging of the chest may reveal interstitial densities consistent with vasculitis or pulmonary hemorrhage. The diagnosis is confirmed by the presence of anti-PR3 ANCA and the finding of necrotizing granulomatous angiitis on pulmonary, sinus, or renal biopsy.

Differential Diagnosis. Granulomatous lesions can be found in sarcoidosis, in which antibodies to ANCA are absent. Other granulomatous diseases (e.g., tuberculosis) also lack antibodies to ANCA. *Churg-Strauss syndrome* is a vasculitis that can cause chronic sinus lesions; a history of asthma, circulating eosinophilia, and an eosinophilic cutaneous vasculitis distinguish this syndrome from WG.

The lesions in Churg-Strauss syndrome are not usually associated with destructive upper airway disease. Other vasculitic syndromes lack the characteristic granulomas on biopsy of affected organs.

LABORATORY FINDINGS. Elevated ESR, leukocytosis, thrombocytosis, and anemia may be found. Antibodies to ANCA directed toward PR3 are specific for WG. These antibodies, usually of IgG class, are found on immunofluorescence to be distributed in a diffuse granular staining throughout the cytoplasm (c-ANCA); staining for myeloperoxidase by ANCA in a perinuclear pattern (p-ANCA) is not specific for WG.

TREATMENT. Oral and intravenous corticosteroids and cyclophosphamide have been effective in many patients. Methotrexate has also been used.

COMPLICATIONS. Enlarging granulomas may disrupt local anatomy: Intrasinus lesions can invade the orbit; lesions in the ear can result in unilateral deafness. Respiratory complications include pulmonary hemorrhage and upper airway obstruction due to subglottic stenosis. Infectious complications include sinusitis (either as superinfections of granulomatous lesions or after obstruction) and pneumonia. Chronic glomerulonephritis may result in end-stage renal disease.

PROGNOSIS. The course is variable. Mortality has been reduced with the introduction of cyclophosphamide and other immunosuppressive agents.

167.5 Other Vasculitic Syndromes

Leukocytoclastic vasculitis is a term used to refer to a spectrum of vasculitic syndromes, including HSP, as well as to specific biopsy findings. It is characterized by cutaneous vessel inflammation affecting both small arteries and postcapillary venules. Purpura and occasionally urticaria are found, particularly on the extremities. The diagnostic term *leukocytoclastic vasculitis* is sometimes used for cases similar to HSP but with atypical distribution and associated symptoms. *Hypersensitivity angiitis* is cutaneous vasculitis following exposure to drugs, such as sulfonamides. Clinical manifestations include fever, myalgia, and arthralgia but rarely visceral involvement. Subsequent development of systemic findings indicating more extensive vasculitis suggests the likelihood of another diagnosis such as PAN. For both leukocytoclastic vasculitis and hypersensitivity angiitis, biopsy of lesions may reveal fibrinoid necrosis of blood vessels, perivascular polymorphonuclear infiltrate, and nuclear debris or dust.

Athreya B: Vasculitis in children. Pediatr Clin North Am 42:1239, 1995.
Connolly B, Manson D, Eberhard A, et al: CT appearance of pulmonary vasculitis in children. Am J Roentgenol 167:901, 1996.

Henoch-Schönlein Purpura

Amoroso A, Berrino M, Canale L, et al: Immunogenetics of Henoch-Schoenlein disease. Eur J Immunogenet 24:323, 1997.
Besbas N, Saatci U, Ruacan S, et al: The role of cytokines in Henoch-Schönlein purpura. Scand J Rheumatol 26:56, 1997.
Smith GC, Davidson JE, Hughes DA, et al: Complement activation in Henoch-Schönlein purpura. Pediatr Nephrol 11:477, 1997.

Takayasu Arteritis

Hoffman GS: Takayasu arteritis: Lessons from the American National Institutes of Health experience. Int J Cardiol 54:S99, 1996.
Kerr GS, Hallahan CW, Giordano J, et al: Takayasu arteritis. Ann Intern Med 120:919, 1994.
Martini A: Behçet's disease and Takayasu disease in children. Curr Opin Rheumatol 7:449, 1995.
Sharma BK, Jain S, Sagar S: Systemic manifestations of Takayasu arteritis: The expanding spectrum. Int J Cardiol 54:S149, 1996.

Polyarteritis Nodosa

Sheth AP, Olson JC, Esterly NB: Cutaneous polyarteritis nodosa of childhood. J Am Acad Dermatol 31:561, 1994.
David J, Ansell BM, Woo P: Polyarteritis nodosa associated with streptococcus. Arch Dis Child 69:685, 1993.
Ozen S, Besbas N, Saatci U, et al: Diagnostic criteria for polyarteritis nodosa in childhood. J Pediatr 120:206, 1992.

Wegener Granulomatosis

Gottlieb BS, Miller LC, Ilowite NT: Methotrexate treatment of Wegener granulomatosis in children. J Pediatr 129:604, 1996.
Rottem M, Fauci AS, Hallahan CW, et al: Wegener granulomatosis in children and adolescents: Clinical presentation and outcome. J Pediatr 122:26, 1993.
Valentini RP, Smoyer WE, Sedman AB, et al: Outcome of antineutrophil cytoplasmic autoantibodies-positive glomerulonephritis and vasculitis in children: A single-center experience. J Pediatr 132:325, 1998.
Wadsworth DT, Siegel MJ, Day DL: Wegener's granulomatosis in children: Chest radiographic manifestations. Am J Roentgenol 163:901, 1994.

CHAPTER 168
Musculoskeletal Pain Syndromes

Michael L. Miller

Children with poorly localized pain involving the extremities and with normal findings on physical examination and unremarkable laboratory findings can be considered to have a musculoskeletal pain syndrome (MSPS). Fibromyalgia is considered a subset of MSPS. Clinical manifestations of MSPS overlap other conditions including reflex sympathetic dystrophy, erythromelalgia, and chronic fatigue syndrome (Chapter 717). Clinical management of these conditions is remarkably similar.

CLINICAL MANIFESTATIONS. The history is often related almost entirely by a parent who notes the child to have pain at rest. The pain can vary from regional (affecting a single extremity) to generalized. Patients often complain of pain refractory to nonsteroidal anti-inflammatory drugs and analgesic agents. Physical therapy programs may have been tried without success.

Other symptoms associated with pain syndromes include fatigue, sleep problems, and poor school attendance. In contrast to many children with pain due to rheumatic diseases, children with MSPS tend to be depressed at the thought of returning to school rather than staying home from school. Excellent academic performance often precedes prolonged school absences; it is possible that symptoms result when a child is unable to maintain continuing academic demands. Parents may have a history of organic or functional pain, sometimes in the same anatomic region that is symptomatic in the child.

Results of the physical examination are unremarkable, with normal strength and no joint swelling or limitation of motion. However, exquisite tenderness to light touch is often elicited over various parts of the extremities and may not be reproducible on repeat examination. Cold, clammy, cyanotic distal extremities occasionally suggest autonomic dysfunction, such as in reflex sympathetic dystrophy. These findings may improve after a child has exercised.

Fibromyalgia is distinguished by localized areas of tenderness to palpation. These trigger points are not always reproducible. One study found many children with fibromyalgia to have hypermobile joints.

There are no specific *laboratory findings*. Anemia and hypothyroidism should be ruled out. Imaging studies, particularly plain radiographs, may be necessary to rule out fractures or other pathology; MRI studies may be necessary to preclude ligamentous injury. The need for additional tests is individualized, depending on specific symptoms and physical findings.

DIAGNOSIS. The diagnosis of musculoskeletal pain syndromes is one of exclusion. When careful, repeated physical examination and laboratory testing do not reveal a cause, a diagnosis of MSPS can be made. A history of pain associated with sleep problems and tenderness over trigger points on examination suggests fibromyalgia.

Differential Diagnosis. Because psychiatric disorders can overlap and present with symptoms of MSPS, psychiatric evaluation should be considered for children with these syndromes. Prolonged school absence suggests school phobia (Chapter 22). When fatigue is more prominent than pain, chronic fatigue syndrome may be considered (Chapter 717). Physical and sexual abuse may also be manifested by pain syndromes; adolescent girls may have accompanying dizziness. In Munchausen syndrome by proxy (Chapter 35.3), reports of pain are emphasized with the intent of obtaining unnecessary (often interventional) evaluation.

Repeated physical examinations may reveal eventual development of manifestations suggestive of other diseases. Imaging studies, including plain radiographs, MRI, and technetium-99m bone scan, may identify focal pathology resulting from infection, malignancy, or trauma. Weakness may result from thyroid disease, inflammatory myositis, muscular dystrophies, or neurologic disease. Chest pain may be a manifestation of costochondritis, pericarditis, coronary arterial abnormality, or aortic stenosis. Proximal leg pain, often occurring at night, may occur in osteoid osteoma. Back pain may indicate local pathology including spondylolisthesis, diskitis, and vertebral microfractures. When children with poorly localized pain develop tender entheses, ankylosing spondyloarthropathy should be considered (Chapter 157).

TREATMENT. Successful outcome requires that any underlying psychiatric disorder be identified and treated. Therapy should be directed toward emotional support for the patient and family, relief of symptoms, and minimizing unnecessary and misleading diagnostic and therapeutic tests. This may include a combination of restoration of a normal sleep pattern, rehabilitation strategies including exercise for fatigue, and optimism. Children have been found to improve if the physician and other health care providers can overcome parental resistance to a vigorous physical therapy program for stretching and joint protection. Increasing physical activity at home to improve level of physical fitness can also help. Some centers use bedtime doses of antidepressants for MSPS. However, if their use is required for more than several weeks, psychiatric evaluation may be necessary to rule out depression. For children with persisting symptoms, a rehabilitation program by a physiatrist or referral to a pain clinic may be indicated.

COMPLICATIONS. Untreated musculoskeletal pain syndromes can result in impaired physical fitness, decreased socialization leading to isolation, prolonged school absences, and lost opportunities for college or vocational training. When families avoid psychologic evaluation or recommendations, children are at risk for developing or exacerbating depression.

168.1 Reflex Sympathetic Dystrophy

Reflex sympathetic (or neurovascular) dystrophy (RSD), a condition of unknown cause, is characterized by diffuse limb pain with color and temperature changes thought to result from autonomic nervous system dysfunction. RSD is often a response to physical or emotional distress. A history of physical activities (e.g., ballet dancing) causing repeated impact on extremities or severe or prolonged emotional trauma (e.g., divorce of the parents, death of a sibling) may be elicited. Children complain of pain worsened by touch or movement, often with dysesthesia and a sensation of temperature changes and swelling. They tend to maintain the hand or foot in a rigid, unusual position, refusing to allow passive motion. Prolonged disuse of the extremity can cause osteopenia; imaging studies (e.g., Doppler flow studies, technetium-99m bone scan) may show either increased or decreased blood flow. Assurance, physical therapy, and, when indicated, counseling can result in resolution of symptoms and physical findings. Relaxation techniques provided by a psychologist may also be useful. When these measures are unsuccessful, sympathetic blocks may be considered.

168.2 Erythromelalgia

Children with erythromelalgia experience episodes of intense pain, erythema, and heat in the distal portion of their legs (rarely, the hands). Mild heat exposure may trigger symptoms that can last for hours and occasionally for days. Although most cases are sporadic, an autosomal dominant hereditary form has been reported. Erythromelalgia can also be associated with peripheral neuropathy, frostbite, hypertension, and rheumatic disease. Treatment includes avoidance of heat exposure and application of cold during attacks. Propranolol, carbamazepine, or sodium nitroprusside may be effective for some affected children.

Finley WH, Lindsey JR Jr, Fine JD, et al: Autosomal dominant erythromelalgia. Am J Med Genet 42:310, 1992.

Gedalia A, Press J, Klein M, et al: Joint hypermobility and fibromyalgia in school children. Ann Rheum Dis 52:494, 1993.

Mikkelsson M, Sourander A, Piha J, et al: Psychiatric symptoms in preadolescents with musculoskeletal pain and fibromyalgia. Pediatrics 100:220, 1997.

Reid GJ, Lang BA, McGrath PJ: Primary juvenile fibromyalgia: Psychological adjustment, family functioning, coping, and functional disability. Arthritis Rheum 40:752, 1997.

Schanberg LE, Keefe FJ, Lefebvre JC, et al: Pain coping strategies in children with juvenile primary fibromyalgia syndrome: Correlation with pain, physical function, and psychological distress. Arthritis Care Res 9:89, 1996.

Sherry DD: Musculoskeletal pain in children. Curr Opin Rheumatol 9:465, 1997.

Siegel DM, Janeway D, Baum J: Fibromyalgia syndrome in children and adolescents: Clinical features at presentation and status at follow-up. Pediatrics 101:377, 1998.

Stanton RP, Malcolm JR, Wesdock KA, et al: Reflex sympathetic dystrophy in children: An orthopedic perspective. Orthopedics 16:773, 1993.

Wilder RT, Berde CB, Wolohan M, et al: Reflex sympathetic dystrophy in children. Clinical characteristics and follow-up of seventy patients. J Bone Joint Surg Am 74:910, 1992.

Yunus MB, Masi AT: Juvenile primary fibromyalgia syndrome. A clinical study of thirty-three patients and matched normal controls. Arthritis Rheum 28:138, 1985.

CHAPTER 169

Miscellaneous Conditions Associated with Arthritis

Michael L. Miller

Inflammation of joints or connective tissue may be a manifestation of nonrheumatic conditions. These conditions need to be considered in children with joint complaints whose history, clinical findings, or clinical course are not consistent with rheumatic diseases.

RELAPSING POLYCHONDRITIS. Relapsing polychondritis is characterized by episodic necrotizing inflammation of cartilage in the outer ear, trachea, and nose. Patients may also develop polyarticular arthritis, ocular inflammation, and hearing loss resulting from inflammation near the auditory and vestibular nerves. Children may initially relate only episodes of intense erythema over the outer ears. Later, inflammation may be so severe that it causes loss of cartilage from the outer ear, nose, or trachea. Diagnostic criteria established for adults are useful guidelines for evaluating children who develop suggestive symptoms (Table 169–1). The differential diagnosis includes Cogan syndrome (characterized by auditory nerve inflammation and keratitis but not chondritis) and Wegener granulomatosis (Chapter 164.7). The clinical course is variable; although some patients respond to corticosteroids, others experience a relentless, progressive course, culminating in death due to airway obstruction.

MUCHA-HABERMANN DISEASE. Mucha-Habermann disease, or *pityriasis lichenoides et varioliformis acuta* (PLEVA), is characterized by recurrent arthritis associated with episodes of vesicular cutaneous lesions, fever, and elevated erythrocyte sedimentation rate. The diagnosis is confirmed by biopsy of skin lesions, which reveals a lymphocytic vasculitis affecting capillaries and venules in the upper dermis.

SWEET SYNDROME. Sweet syndrome, or acute febrile neutrophilic dermatosis, occurs most often in young women and is rare in children. It is characterized by recurrent fever and raised, tender erythematous plaques over the face, extremities, and trunk. Some children also have arthritis. The syndrome may be idiopathic or secondary to malignancy, Behçet's disease (Chapter 162), or chronic recurrent multifocal osteomyelitis (Chapter 178). Skin biopsy reveals neutrophilic perivascular infiltrates. The condition is usually responsive to treatment with corticosteroids.

HYPERTROPHIC OSTEOARTHROPATHY (HOA). Some children with clubbing develop soft tissue swelling over the hands, particularly the distal digits, with arthritis in the distal interphalangeal joints and tender periosteal new bone formation along tubular long bones and bones in the hand. This complication, HOA, can be found in some children with chronic pulmonary disease (e.g., cystic fibrosis), congenital heart disease, gastrointestinal diseases (e.g., malabsorption syndromes, biliary atresia, and inflammatory bowel disease), and malignancies (e.g., nasopharyngeal sarcoma, osteosarcoma, and Hodgkin disease). Although the cause is unknown, some studies suggest that in diseases underlying HOA, platelet fragments escape the pulmonary circulation and interact with peripheral endothelial cells and other tissues. The resulting release of fibroblast and related growth factors causes the clinical manifestations. The symptoms of HOA may improve if the underlying condition can be successfully treated. Evaluation of children presenting with HOA should include a chest radiograph to eliminate pulmonary disease or intrathoracic mass.

PLANT THORN SYNOVITIS. Puncture wounds due to plant thorns or similar foreign objects that penetrate the synovium can cause acute synovitis that may progress to chronic arthritis. The episode of initial trauma often is forgotten. The diagnosis should be considered in children with chronic monoarticular arthritis unresponsive to anti-inflammatory medication. Diagnosis may require MRI or arthroscopy. Histology often reveals a granulomatous synovitis. Treatment is removal of the foreign body, which may be accomplished by irrigation of the joint during arthroscopy. Chronic synovitis may require synovectomy.

DIABETES MELLITUS. Diabetic cheiroarthropathy is a complication of juvenile-onset diabetes mellitus, which occurs most often in late childhood or adolescence. The soft tissues of the hands and fingers undergo progressive thickening and tightening, leading to contractures of the small joints in the hand but without the tapering and loss of digital pulp over the fingertips characteristic of sclerodactyly seen in patients with scleroderma (Chapter 161). Occupational therapy can improve loss of motion in affected joints. Diabetic cheiroarthropathy needs to be distinguished from polyarticular juvenile rheumatoid arthritis, which can coexist with unrelated chronic conditions and in which joint swelling typically precedes flexion contractures.

CYSTIC FIBROSIS ARTHROPATHY. In addition to hypertrophic osteoarthropathy, some patients with cystic fibrosis experience either episodic or persistent arthritis. The cause is unknown but may reflect synovitis resulting from deposition of immune complexes formed in response to recurrent pulmonary infections. It is also possible that persistent arthritis is a result of expression of coexisting, unrelated juvenile rheumatoid arthritis.

ACUTE PANCREATITIS AND ARTHRITIS. Periostitis, nodular skin lesions, and synovial fat necrosis may develop as a result of lipases released during pancreatitis. Affected children may have fever, arthritis, and bone pain for several weeks after blunt abdominal trauma (including child abuse) or other causes of pancreatitis. Elevated serum lipase and amylase levels, periosteal new bone formation, and abnormal findings on bone scintigraphy (revealing fat-induced infarcts) may be found. Drainage of pancreatic pseudocysts may alleviate symptoms of arthritis in some patients.

IMMUNODEFICIENCY. Some children with B- and T-lymphocyte immunodeficiencies develop rheumatic diseases. There are several potential mechanisms. Defective mucosal immunity in children with B-cell diseases (e.g., IgA deficiency, X-linked hypogammaglobulinemia, and common variable immunodeficiency) may permit entry from the gut into the circulation of viruses that are either cross-reactive with self antigens or capable of causing infective synovitis. T-cell defects may result in the loss of T-lymphocyte control over autoreactive T lymphocytes. Arthritis, both episodic and chronic, has been described in children with various types of hypogammaglobulinemia, IgA deficiency, and DiGeorge syndrome. IgA deficiency has also been associated with other rheumatic diseases, including lupus, dermatomyositis, scleroderma, and spondyloarthropathy. Patients with Wiskott-Aldrich syndrome have been reported to develop arthritis, vasculitis, and other rheumatic manifestations. The differential diagnosis of arthritis in children with immunodeficiencies includes septic arthritis and osteomyelitis.

TABLE 169–1 Diagnostic Criteria for Relapsing Polychondritis

At least three of the following:
Bilateral auricular chondritis
Nonerosive seronegative inflammatory polyarthritis
Nasal chondritis
Ocular inflammation
Respiratory tract chondritis
Audiovestibular chondritis

From McAdam LP, O'Hanlan MA, Bluestone R, et al: Relapsing polychondritis: Prospective study of 23 patients and a review of the literature. Medicine 55:193, 1976.

Akman IO, Ostrov BE, Neudorf S: Autoimmune manifestations of the Wiskott-Aldrich syndrome. Semin Arthritis Rheum 27:218, 1998.

Ansell BM: Hypertrophic osteoarthropathy in the paediatric age. Clin Exp Rheumatol 10(Suppl 7):15, 1992.

Conley ME, Park CL, Douglas SD: Childhood common variable immunodeficiency with autoimmune disease. J Pediatr 108:915, 1986.

Diren HB, Kutluk MT, Karabent A, et al: Primary hypertrophic osteoarthropathy. Pediatr Radiol 16:231, 1986.

Luberti AA, Rabinowitz LG, Ververeli KO: Severe febrile Mucha-Habermann's disease in children: Case report and review of the literature. Pediatr Dermatol 8:51, 1991.

Maillot F, Goupille P, Valat JP: Plant thorn synovitis diagnosed by magnetic resonance imaging. Scand J Rheumatol 23:154, 1994.

McAdam LP, O'Hanlan MA, Bluestone R, et al: Relapsing polychondritis: Prospective study of 23 patients and a review of the literature. Medicine 55:193, 1976.

Marhaug G, Hvidsten D: Arthritis complicating acute pancreatitis—a rare but important condition to be distinguished from juvenile rheumatoid arthritis. Scand J Rheumatol 17:397, 1988.

Oddone M, Toma P, Taccone A, et al: Relapsing polychondritis in childhood: A rare observation studied by CT and MRI. Pediatr Radiol 22:537, 1992.

Staalman CR, Umans U: Hypertrophic osteoarthropathy in childhood malignancy. Med Pediatr Oncol 21:676, 1993.

Sullivan KE, McDonald-McGinn DM, Driscoll DA, et al: Juvenile rheumatoid arthritis–like polyarthritis in chromosome 22q11.2 deletion syndrome (DiGeorge anomalad/velocardiofacial syndrome/conotruncal anomaly face syndrome). Arthritis Rheum 40:430, 1997.

Wulffraat NM, de Graeff-Meeder ER, Rijkers GT, et al: Prevalence of circulating immune complexes in patients with cystic fibrosis and arthritis. J Pediatr 125:374, 1994.

PART XVI

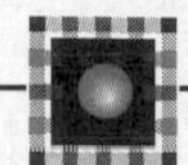

Infectious Diseases

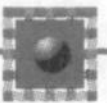

SECTION 1

General Considerations

CHAPTER 170
Fever

Keith R. Powell

Body temperature is regulated by thermosensitive neurons located in the preoptic or anterior hypothalamus. These neurons respond to changes in blood temperature as well as to direct neural connections with cold and warm receptors located in skin and muscle. Thermoregulatory responses include redirecting blood to or from cutaneous vascular beds, increased or decreased sweating, extracellular fluid volume regulation (via arginine vasopressin), and behavioral responses, such as seeking a warmer or cooler environmental temperature. Normal body temperature also varies in a regular pattern each day. This circadian temperature rhythm, or diurnal variation, results in lower body temperatures in the early morning and temperatures approximately 1°C higher in the late afternoon or early evening.

Fever is a controlled increase in body temperature over the normal values for an individual. Fever is regulated in the same manner as normal temperature is maintained in a cool environment, the difference being that the body's thermostat has been reset at a higher temperature. Regardless of whether fever is associated with infection, connective tissue disease, or malignancy, the thermostat is reset in response to endogenous pyrogens including the cytokines interleukin (IL)-1β and IL-6, tumor necrosis factor-α (TNF-α), and interferon (IFN)-β and IFN-γ. Stimulated leukocytes and other cells produce lipids that also serve as endogenous pyrogens. The best-studied lipid mediator is prostaglandin E_2. Most endogenous pyrogen molecules are too large to cross the blood-brain barrier in an efficient manner. However, circumventricular organs in close proximity to the hypothalamus lack a blood-brain barrier and allow for neuronal contact with circulating factors through fenestrated capillaries.

Microbes, microbial toxins, or other products of microbes are the most common "exogenous pyrogens," which are substances that come from outside of the body, stimulate macrophages and other cells to produce endogenous pyrogens, and result in fever. Some substances produced within the body are not pyrogens but are capable of stimulating endogenous pyrogens. Such substances include antigen-antibody complexes in the presence of complement, complement components, lymphocyte products, bile acids, and androgenic steroid metabolites. Endotoxin is one of the few substances that can directly affect thermoregulation in the hypothalamus as well as stimulate endogenous pyrogen release. Fever may be caused by infection, vaccines, biologic agents (granulocyte-macrophage colony-stimulating factor, interferons, interleukins), tissue injury (infarction pulmonary emboli, trauma, intramuscular injections, burns), malignancy (leukemia, lymphoma, hepatoma, metastatic disease), drugs (drug fever, cocaine, amphotericin B), immunologic-rheumatologic disorders (systemic lupus erythematosus, rheumatoid arthritis), inflammatory diseases (inflammatory bowel disease), granulomatous diseases (sarcoidosis), endocrine disorders (thyrotoxicosis, pheochromocytoma), metabolic disorders (gout, uremia, Fabry disease, type 1 hyperlipidemia), genetic disorders (familial Mediterranean fever), and unknown or poorly understood entities. Factitious (self-induced) fever may be due to intentional manipulation of the thermometer or injection of pyrogenic material. The pathogenesis of fever is summarized in Figure 170–1.

Increasing body temperature in response to microbial pathogens is a response observed in reptiles, fish, birds, and mammals. When fish are given an exogenous pyrogen, they swim to warmer water to raise their body temperature. In a similar fashion, lizards given exotoxin lie in the sun until they have raised their body temperature to the febrile range. In humans, increased temperatures are associated with decreased microbial reproduction and an increased inflammatory response. Thus, most evidence suggests that fever is an adaptive response and should be treated only in selected circumstances. Heat production associated with fever increases oxygen consumption, carbon dioxide production, and cardiac output. Thus, fever may exacerbate cardiac insufficiency in patients with heart disease or chronic anemia (e.g., sickle cell disease), pulmonary insufficiency in those with chronic lung disease, and metabolic instability in children with diabetes mellitus or inborn errors of metabolism. Furthermore, children between the ages of 6 mo and 5 yr are at increased risk of benign febrile seizures, whereas those with idiopathic epilepsy may have an increased frequency of seizures associated with a febrile illness (Chapter 602).

CLINICAL MANIFESTATIONS. Although fever patterns per se are not often helpful in determining a specific diagnosis, observing the clinical characteristics of fever can provide useful information. In general, a single isolated fever spike is not associated with an infectious disease. Such a spike can be attributed to the infusion of blood products, some drugs, some procedures, or manipulation of a catheter on a colonized or infected body surface. Similarly, temperatures in excess of 41°C are seldom associated with an infectious cause. Causes of very high temperatures (>41°C) include central fevers (resulting from central nervous system dysfunction that involves the hypothalamus), malignant hyperthermia, malignant neuroleptic syndrome, drug fever, or heatstroke. Temperatures that are

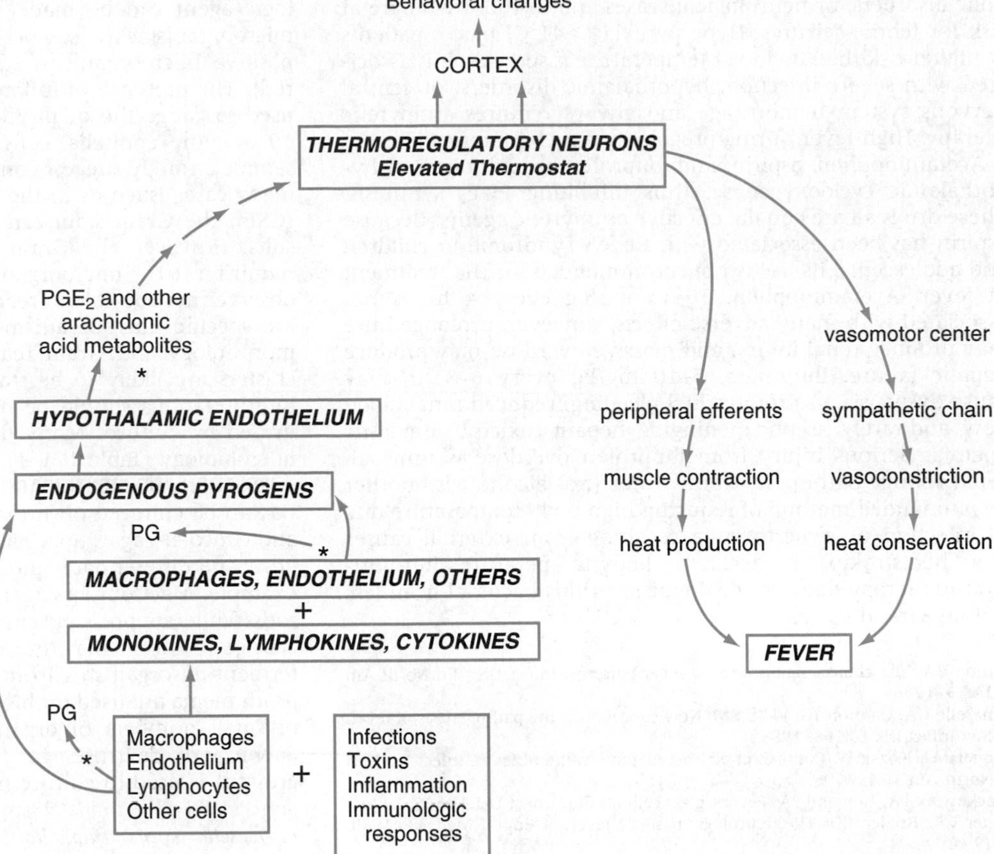

Figure 170–1 The pathogenesis of fever. Various infectious toxins and other mediators induce the production of endogenous pyrogens by host inflammatory cells. Endogenous pyrogens include the cytokines interleukin (IL)-1β and IL-6, tumor necrosis factor-α (TNF-α), and interferon (IFN)-β and IFN-γ. Endogenous pyrogenic cytokines directly stimulate the hypothalamus to produce prostaglandin (PG) E_2 (PGE_2), which then resets the temperature regulatory set point. Neuronal transmission from the hypothalamus leads to conservation and generation of heat, thus raising core body temperature. (From Dinarello CA, Cannon JG, Wolff SM: New concepts on the pathogenesis of fever. Rev Infect Dis 10:183, 1988.)

lower than normal (<36°C) can be associated with overwhelming sepsis but are more commonly related to cold exposure, hypothyroidism, or overuse of antipyretics.

An exaggerated circadian rhythm that includes a period of normal temperatures on most days is termed *intermittent fever;* extremely wide fluctuations may be termed *septic* or *hectic fever.* A sustained fever is persistent and does not vary by more than 0.5°C/day. A remittent fever varies by more than 0.5°C during the course of a day but does not return to normal. Relapsing fevers are separated by intervals of normal temperature; tertian fevers occur on the 1st and 3rd days (*Plasmodium vivax*), and quartan fevers occur on the first and fourth days (*Plasmodium malariae*). Diseases characterized by relapsing fevers are distinguished from infectious diseases with a tendency to relapse (Table 170–1). A biphasic fever indicates a single illness with two distinct periods of fever over 1 or more weeks (camelback fever pattern); poliomyelitis is the classic example. A biphasic course is also characteristic of leptospirosis, dengue fever, yellow fever, Colorado tick fever, spirillary rat-bite fever (*Spirillum minus*), and the African hemorrhagic fevers (Marburg, Ebola, and Lassa fever).

The relationship between a patient's pulse rate and temperature can be informative. Relative tachycardia, when the pulse rate is elevated out of proportion to the temperature, is usually due to noninfectious diseases or infectious diseases in which a toxin is responsible for the clinical manifestations. Relative bradycardia (temperature-pulse dissociation), when the pulse rate remains low in the presence of fever, suggests drug fever, typhoid fever, brucellosis, or leptospirosis. Bradycardia in the presence of fever also may be a result of a conduction defect resulting from cardiac involvement with acute rheumatic fever, Lyme disease, viral myocarditis, or infective endocarditis.

Most infections result in some type of injury that induces an inflammatory response and subsequently results in the release of endogenous pyrogens. Administration of antimicrobial agents can result in a very rapid elimination of bacteria. However, if tissue injury has been extensive, the inflammatory response and fever can continue for days after all microbes have been eradicated.

TREATMENT. Fever with temperatures less than 39°C in healthy children generally do not require treatment. As temperatures become higher, patients tend to become more uncomfortable and administration of antipyretics often makes patients feel better. Other than providing symptomatic relief, antipyretic therapy does not change the course of infectious diseases in normal children. Antipyretic therapy is beneficial in high-risk patients who have chronic cardiopulmonary diseases, meta-

TABLE 170–1 Fevers Prone to Relapse

Infectious Causes	
Relapsing fever (*Borrelia recurrentis*)	Colorado tick fever
Trench fever (*Rochalimaea quintana*)	Leptospirosis
Q Fever	Brucellosis
Typhoid fever	Bartonellosis (Oroyo fever)
Syphilis	Acute rheumatic fever
Tuberculosis	Rat-bite fever (*Spirillum minus*)
Histoplasmosis	Visceral leishmaniasis
Coccidioidomycosis	Lyme disease
Blastomycosis	Malaria
Pseudomonas pseudomallei (melioidosis)	Babesiosis
Lymphocytic choriomeningitis (LCM virus)	Noninfluenzal respiratory viruses
Dengue fever	Epstein-Barr virus
Yellow fever	Cytomegalovirus
Chronic meningococcemia	
Noninfectious Causes	
Behçet's disease	Familial Mediterranean fever
Crohn disease	Fever, adenitis, pharyngitis, aphthous ulcer syndrome
Weber-Christian disease (panniculitis)	Systemic lupus erythematosus
Leukoclastic angiitis	Hyper IgD syndrome
Sweet syndrome	

From Cunha BA: The clinical significance of fever patterns. Infect Dis Clin North Am 10:36, 1996.

bolic disorders, or neurologic diseases and in those who are at risk for febrile seizures. Hyperpyrexia (>41°C) places patients at higher risk than do lower temperature responses. It is associated with severe infection, hypothalamic disorders, or central nervous system hemorrhage and always requires antipyretic therapy. High fever during pregnancy may be teratogenic.

Acetaminophen, aspirin, and ibuprofen are inhibitors of hypothalamic cyclooxygenase, thus inhibiting PGE_2 synthesis. These drugs all are equally effective antipyretic agents. Because aspirin has been associated with Reye's syndrome in children and adolescents, its use is not recommended for the treatment of fever. Acetaminophen, 10–15 mg/kg every 4 hr, is not associated with many adverse effects; however, prolonged use may produce renal injury, and massive overdose may produce hepatic failure. Ibuprofen, 5–10 mg/kg every 6–8 hr, may cause dyspepsia, gastrointestinal bleeding, reduced renal blood flow, and rarely, aseptic meningitis, hepatic toxicity, or aplastic anemia. Serious injury from ibuprofen overdose is unusual. Tepid sponge bathing in warm water (not alcohol) is another recommended method of reducing high body temperature due to infection or hyperthermia resulting from external causes (e.g., heatstroke). The decline of body temperature after antipyretic therapy does not distinguish serious bacterial from less serious viral diseases.

Cunha BA: The clinical significance of fever patterns. Infect Dis Clin North Am 10:33, 1996.
Dinarello CA, Cannon JG, Wolff SM: New concepts on the pathogenesis of fever. Rev Infect Dis 10:168, 1988.
Kluger MJ, Kozak W, Conn C, et al: The adaptive value of fever. Infect Dis Clin North Am 10:1, 1996.
Mackowiak PA, Bouland JA: Fever's glass ceiling. Clin Infect Dis 22:525, 1996.
Saper CB, Breder CD: The neurologic basis of fever. N Engl J Med 330:1880, 1994.

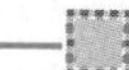

CHAPTER 171
Diagnostic Microbiology

Anita K. M. Zaidi and Donald A. Goldmann

Laboratory diagnosis of infectious diseases is based on one or more of the following: (1) direct examination of specimens by microscopic or antigenic techniques, (2) isolation of microorganisms in culture, (3) serologic testing for development of antibodies (serodiagnosis), and (4) molecular genetic detection. Clinicians must select the appropriate tests and specimens and, when possible, suggest the suspected etiologic agents to the microbiologist, because this facilitates selection of the most cost-effective diagnostic approach. Additional roles of the microbiology laboratory include testing for antimicrobial susceptibility and assisting the hospital epidemiologist in detecting and clarifying the epidemiology of nosocomial infections.

LABORATORY DIAGNOSIS OF BACTERIAL AND FUNGAL INFECTIONS

Diagnosis of bacterial and fungal infections relies mainly on direct demonstration of the microorganisms by microscopic examination or antigen detection and on growth of microorganisms on nutrient culture media. Molecular diagnostic methods for direct detection of certain pathogens are being developed.

MICROSCOPY. The Gram stain remains an extremely useful diagnostic technique because it is a rapid, inexpensive method for demonstrating the presence of bacteria and fungi, as well as inflammatory cells. A preliminary assessment of the etiologic agent can be made by noting the morphology of the microorganisms (e.g., cocci vs rods) and their color (gram-positive microorganisms stain blue, and gram-negative stain red). The presence of inflammatory and epithelial cells can be used to gauge the quality of certain specimens. For example, 10 or more epithelial cells per low-power field in a sputum sample strongly suggest contamination from oral secretions. In many cases, such as in the examination of cerebrospinal fluid (CSF), the Gram stain can provide very rapid and useful results. However, the Gram stain is an insensitive technique, requiring 10^{4-5} microorganisms/mL for detection. A trained observer may be able to reach a tentative conclusion that there are specific microorganisms in the specimen based on their morphology and Gram reaction (e.g., gram-positive cocci in clusters are likely to be staphylococci), but such preliminary interpretations should be made cautiously and must be confirmed by culture. Many different stains are used in clinical microbiology (Table 171–1).

ISOLATION AND IDENTIFICATION. Most medically important bacteria can be cultured on nutrient-rich media such as blood agar and chocolate agar. Specialized agar may be used selectively to grow and differentiate among organisms of different types. For example, MacConkey's agar supports growth of gram-negative rods while suppressing gram-positive organisms, and a color change in the media from clear to pink distinguishes lactose-fermenting organisms from other gram-negative rods. Liquid broth media are used for blood cultures and to enhance growth of small numbers of organisms in other clinical specimens. Sabouraud's dextrose agar (with antibiotics to inhibit bacterial growth) is used to culture most fungi. However, many pathogens such as *Bartonella* spp, *Bordetella pertussis*, *Brucella* spp, *Francisella* spp, *Legionella* spp, mycobacteria, certain fungal

TABLE 171–1 Stains Used for Microscopic Examination

Stain	Clinical Use
Gram stain	Stains bacteria, fungi, leukocytes, and epithelial cells.
Potassium hydroxide (KOH)	A 10% KOH solution dissolves cellular and organic debris and facilitates detection of fungal elements.
Calcofluor white stain	Nonspecific fluorochrome that binds to cellulose and chitin in fungal cell walls. Can be combined with 10% KOH to dissolve cellular material.
Ziehl-Neelson and Kinyoun stains	Acid-fast stains using basic carbol fuchsin, followed by acid-alcohol decolorization and methylene blue counterstaining. Acid-fast organisms (e.g., *Mycobacterium*, *Cryptosporidium*, and *Cyclospora*) resist decolorization and stain pink. A weaker decolorizing agent is used for partially acid-fast organisms (e.g., *Nocardia*).
Acridine orange stain	Fluorescent dye that intercalates into DNA. At acid pH, bacteria and fungi stain orange and background cellular material green.
Auramine-rhodamine stain	Acid-fast stain using fluorochromes that bind to mycolic acid in mycobacterial cell walls and resist acid-alcohol decolorization. Acid-fast organisms stain orange-yellow against a black background.
India ink stain	Detects *Cryptococcus neoformans*, which is an encapsulated yeast, by excluding ink particles from the polysaccharide capsule. (Direct testing for cryptococcal antigen in specimens is much more sensitive than India ink preparations.)
Methenamine silver stain	Stains fungal elements, *Pneumocystis carinii* cysts in tissues. Primarily performed in surgical pathology laboratories.
Lugol iodine stain	Added to wet preparations of fecal specimens for ova and parasites to enhance contrast of the internal structures (nuclei, glycogen vacuoles).
Wright and Giemsa stains	Primarily for detecting blood parasites (*Plasmodium*, *Babesia*, and *Leishmania* spp) and fungi in tissues (yeasts, *Histoplasma*).
Trichrome stain	Stains stool specimens for identification of protozoa.
Direct fluorescent-antibody stain	Used for direct detection of various organisms in clinical specimens by using specific fluorescein-labeled antibodies (e.g., *Bordetella pertussis*, *Legionella* spp, *Chlamydia trachomatis*, *Pneumocystis carinii*, many viruses).

pathogens such as *Malassezia furfur, Mycoplasma* spp, and *Chlamydia* spp require specialized growth media or incubation conditions. Consultation with the laboratory is advised when these pathogens are suspected.

After isolation in culture, microbial identity can be confirmed by a series of biochemical tests, by the ability of the organism to grow in the presence of certain substances that inhibit growth of other microorganisms (e.g., selective antibiotics, salt, bile), or by antigen detection. Molecular probes can also be used.

Blood Culture. Several different blood culture systems are available; most use 50–100-mL bottles containing broth that enhances the growth of bacteria and fungi (mainly yeast). Bottles with smaller volumes are also available specifically for pediatric use. Media containing resins are often used to adsorb antibiotics that may be present in a patient's blood and to improve microbial detection. Many laboratories now use automated systems that greatly reduce the time to microbial detection.

Proper skin disinfection before blood collection is essential. Povidone-iodine may be used, but this agent must be allowed to dry completely for maximum activity. Alcohol is rapidly bactericidal and is a suitable alternative agent. Iodine is effective but must be wiped off with alcohol to avoid skin reactions. The practice of obtaining blood for culture from intravascular catheters without accompanying peripheral venous blood cultures should be discouraged because it is difficult to determine the significance of coagulase-negative staphylococci and other skin flora isolated from blood obtained from "through-the-line" cultures. For patients with suspected bacteremia and fungemia, two or three separate blood cultures are preferred. More than three blood cultures rarely are indicated, even in endocarditis. Whenever possible, at least 2 mL of blood should be obtained for culture before administration of antibiotics. Obtaining a larger volume of blood is necessary to maximize yield from blood cultures, because 10–20% of pediatric patients may have low-grade bloodstream infections. For most patients, the most effective approach is to culture the entire volume of blood in a single aerobic bottle because anaerobic bacteremia is rare in children. Blood should also be cultured anaerobically for patients at increased risk for anaerobic sepsis, such as children who are immunocompromised or who have head and neck or abdominal infections. Detection of mycobacteria in severely immunocompromised patients can be enhanced by culturing blood in special systems, such as the modified Middlebrook blood culture system (Myco/F, Becton-Dickinson, Sparks, MD). Detection of fungi can be aided by lysis-centrifugation techniques, such as the Isolator 1.5 system (Wampole, Cranbury, NJ).

CSF Culture. CSF should be transported quickly to the laboratory, where it is centrifuged to concentrate organisms for microscopic examination. Rapid antigen tests for bacterial pathogens are not routinely necessary but are useful if a patient has been receiving antibiotic therapy. CSF is routinely plated on blood and chocolate agar, which support the growth of common pathogens causing meningitis. If tuberculosis is suspected, cultures for mycobacteria should be specifically requested.

Urine Culture. Urine for culture and colony count can be obtained by collecting clean-voided midstream specimens, by catheterization, or by suprapubic aspiration. Urine samples collected by placing bags on the perineum are unacceptable for culture because of frequent contamination, which renders the results uninterpretable. Rapid transport of urine to the laboratory is imperative because gram-negative enteric pathogens have generation times of 20–30 min, and any delay in transport or plating renders colony counts unreliable. Refrigeration can be used when delay is unavoidable. Culture systems using media-coated "paddles" permit prompt inoculation of the specimen, but confluent growth may be difficult to detect; moreover, accurate antibiotic susceptibility testing requires the presence of individual discrete colonies. Urine obtained by suprapubic puncture should normally be sterile. Urine collected by catheterization is likely to reflect infection if there are 10^3 or more organisms/mL. Clean-voided urine is considered abnormal if $\geq 10^5$ or more organisms/mL are present and possibly abnormal if 10^4–10^5 organisms/mL are present. However, lower counts are sometimes found in urinary tract infections in adolescent girls and young women, especially those with bacterial urethritis, or in patients with fungal infections. A Gram stain of unspun urine with at least one bacterium per oil immersion field correlates well with the presence of 10^5 or more bacterial colonies/mL in urine.

Genital Culture. Specimens from the genital tract include urethral, cervical, and anorectal swabs. *Neisseria gonorrhoeae* organisms are fragile, and rapid inoculation at the bedside onto Thayer-Martin medium (warmed to room temperature) or one of its modifications is crucial. Ordinarily, specimens should be obtained from genital, anorectal, and pharyngeal sources to achieve maximum yield. Specimens for *Chlamydia trachomatis* culture are obtained by cotton-tipped, aluminum-shafted urethral swabs. Endocervical specimens, using swabs with aluminum or plastic shafts, should be collected by rubbing the swab vigorously against the endocervical wall to obtain as much cellular material as possible. *C. trachomatis* is cultured by inoculation into cell culture systems, followed by immunofluorescent staining with monoclonal antibody against the organism. However, nonculture methods, such as enzyme immunoassay (EIA) tests, direct immunofluorescent staining by monoclonal antibodies, and DNA amplification methods are now widely used and tend to be more cost effective than culture.

Throat and Respiratory Cultures. Obtaining a throat swab for culture is the most reliable method of diagnosing group A streptococcal pharyngitis and tonsillitis. Vigorous swabbing of the tonsillar area and posterior pharynx is necessary for maximum detection. Even then, a single swab detects only approximately 90% of infections. The pharynx contains many normal flora; thus, most laboratories screen cultures only for the presence of group A β-hemolytic streptococci. Some laboratories do not use selective procedures, however, and may report the presence of meningococci, usually nontypable, nonpathogenic strains, but occasionally typable meningococci and other potential pathogens. Most patients harboring such bacteria are carriers, and the culture report serves only to create needless alarm. The laboratory should be alerted if diphtheria, pertussis, gonococcal pharyngitis, or infection with *Arcanobacterium haemolyticum* is clinically suspected. Cultures for *B. pertussis* are obtained by aspiration or a Dacron or flexible wire calcium alginate swab (Calgiswab) of the nasopharynx and inoculation onto special charcoal-blood (Regan-Lowe) or Bordet-Gengou media.

The cause of lower respiratory tract disease in children is not easy to confirm microbiologically because of difficulty in obtaining adequate sputum specimens and lack of correlation between upper respiratory tract flora and organisms causing lower respiratory tract disease. Gram-stained smears of specimens with large numbers of epithelial cells or with few neutrophils are unsuitable for culture. Patients with cystic fibrosis can usually provide adequate expectorated sputum, and special media should be used to detect important cystic fibrosis pathogens, such as *Burkholderia cepacia*.

Endotracheal aspirates from intubated patients may be useful if the Gram stain shows abundant neutrophils and bacteria, although pathogens recovered from such specimens may still reflect only contamination from the endotracheal tube or upper airway. Quantitative cultures of bronchoalveolar lavage fluid or bronchial brush specimens may be valuable for distinguishing upper respiratory tract contamination from lower tract disease in special circumstances.

The diagnosis of pulmonary tuberculosis in young children is best made by culture of early morning gastric aspirates, obtained on 3 successive days, rather than by sputum cultures.

Acid-fast stains of gastric aspirates from children are rarely positive. Cultures for *Mycobacterium tuberculosis* should be processed only in laboratories equipped with appropriate biologic safety cabinets and containment facilities.

Stool Culture. Most laboratories in North America routinely culture stool for the presence of *Salmonella, Shigella,* and *Campylobacter* by inoculation onto selective agar (to decrease the growth of normal fecal flora) and differential agar (to help distinguish pathogenic enteric flora from normal enteric flora). Freshly passed stool is preferred, but rectal swabs may be acceptable. Cultures for *Escherichia coli* O157:H7, *Vibrio cholerae, Yersinia enterocolitica, Aeromonas,* and *Plesiomonas* should be specifically requested when these organisms are suspected. Isolation of enterotoxigenic *E. coli,* the commonest cause of traveler's diarrhea, and other pathogenic types of *E. coli* except for *E. coli* O157:H7, is not routinely attempted. Bacterial stool cultures in the United States rarely yield useful results in patients who have been hospitalized for more than 3 days. Cultures for *Clostridium difficile,* the most common bacterial cause of nosocomial diarrhea, have largely been replaced by tests that detect toxin production, such as cell culture assays for cytotoxicity, or EIAs.

Culture of Other Fluids and Tissues. Abscesses, wounds, pleural fluid, peritoneal fluid, joint fluid, and other purulent fluids are cultured onto routine solid agar and broth media. Whenever possible, fluid rather than swabs from infected sites should be sent to the laboratory because culture of a larger volume of fluid may detect organisms present in low concentration. Anaerobic organisms are involved in many abdominal and wound abscesses. These specimens should be collected and transported rapidly under anaerobic conditions, preferably in anaerobic transport tubes.

ANTIMICROBIAL SUSCEPTIBILITY TESTING. Antimicrobial susceptibility tests are generally performed on all organisms of clinical significance except for a few that have predictable antimicrobial susceptibility patterns (e.g., group A streptococci are currently universally susceptible to penicillin). The most common technique is the agar disk diffusion method (Bauer-Kirby method), in which a standardized inoculum of the organism is seeded onto an agar plate. Antibiotic-impregnated filter paper disks are then placed on the agar surface. After 18–24 hr of incubation, the zone of inhibition of bacterial growth around each disk is measured and compared with nationally determined standards for susceptibility or resistance.

The other widely used technique for susceptibility testing is dilution testing. A standard concentration of a microorganism is inoculated into serially diluted concentrations of antibiotic, and the minimum inhibitory concentration (MIC) in μg/mL, the lowest concentration of antibiotic required to inhibit growth of the microorganism, is determined. Dilution testing also permits determination of the minimum bactericidal concentration (MBC), the lowest concentration of antibiotic required to kill the organism. The MBC is sometimes determined to exclude the possibility of bacterial tolerance (MBC $>$ 4 times the MIC). Automated methods that use microtiter wells with premade dilutions of antibiotics are now used commonly. However, MICs from automated systems should be interpreted with caution for certain pathogen-antibiotic combinations (e.g., pneumococci resistant to penicillin, enterococci with low-level resistance to vancomycin). Screening agar plate tests, such as oxacillin disk susceptibility to detect penicillin-resistant pneumococci, followed by confirmatory tests, are recommended. The E-test is a new method of measuring MICs of individual antibiotics on an agar plate. It uses a paper strip impregnated with a known continuous concentration gradient of antibiotic that diffuses across the agar surface, inhibiting microbial growth in an elliptic zone. The MIC is read off the printed strip at the point at which the zone intersects the strip. Major advantages of the E-test are reliable interpretation, reproducibility, and applicability to organisms that require special media or growth conditions, including anaerobic bacteria. However, the cost precludes its use as the principal testing system in clinical laboratories.

OFFICE BACTERIOLOGY. Many office practices perform rapid antigen testing for detection of group A streptococcal pharyngitis. Susceptibility depends on the type of kit used and on the concentration of streptococci present in the sample. As many as 30% of test results may be false-negative; therefore, all negative results should be confirmed by culture.

Other microbiologic tests may be performed in the office setting, provided the site is certified as meeting appropriate quality assurance standards specified by the Clinical Laboratory Improvement Amendments (CLIA) Act of 1988. These include procedures listed under the category of "physician-performed microscopy" (e.g., wet mounts, potassium hydroxide [KOH] preparations, pinworm examinations, fecal leukocyte examinations, and urine sediment analysis). Office laboratories licensed for this category are limited to performing these tests but avoid having to undergo inspections and proficiency testing, although they are still subject to CLIA certification requirements specific to these tests. Gram staining, culture inoculation, and isolation of bacteria are considered moderately to highly complex tests under CLIA specifications. Any office laboratory performing Gram stains or cultures must comply with the same requirements and inspections for quality assurance, proficiency testing, and personnel requirements as fully licensed microbiology laboratories.

LABORATORY DIAGNOSIS OF VIRAL INFECTIONS

Specimens for viral diagnosis are selected on the basis of knowledge of the site that is most likely to yield the suspected pathogen. Specimens should be collected early in the course of infection when viral shedding is maximal. Fluids and respiratory secretions should be collected in sterile containers and delivered to the laboratory promptly. Swabs should be rubbed vigorously against mucosal or skin surfaces to obtain as much cellular material as possible, and sent in viral transport media that contain antibiotics to inhibit bacterial growth. Rectal swabs should not be heavily covered with feces because the antibiotics present in viral transport media may be insufficient to kill a large inoculum of bacteria. All specimens should be transported on ice. Freezing specimens can result in a significant decrease in culture sensitivity. Consultation with the laboratory is advised for any unusual specimens or suspected pathogens.

Laboratory diagnosis of viral infections may be by electron microscopy, antigen detection, virus isolation in culture, serologic testing, or detection of virus genomes by molecular biology techniques. Serologic and molecular tests are the mainstay of diagnosis of viruses such as HIV and Epstein-Barr virus (EBV).

RAPID ANTIGEN TESTS. Immunofluorescent-antibody (IFA) techniques or other methods such as EIA that use antibodies to detect viral antigens directly in clinical specimens permit rapid identification of viruses. For example, smears of cellular material from respiratory secretions stained by immunologic reagents can identify the antigens of respiratory syncytial virus (RSV), adenovirus, influenza virus, and parainfluenza virus within 2–3 hr after the specimen is received. In comparison with isolation in cell culture, IFA is approximately 95% sensitive and 98% specific for the diagnosis of RSV and parainfluenza virus type 3 in reference laboratories; the sensitivity of IFA for influenza viruses and adenoviruses is considerably lower. Sensitive IFA staining techniques are also commercially available for identification of varicella-zoster virus (VZV) and herpes simplex virus (HSV). These specific methods have supplanted the Tzanck smear for multinucleated giant cells characteristic of VZV or HSV infections. A method for detecting cytomegalovirus (CMV) antigen in blood of high-risk patients also has been developed. IFA is not useful for detecting virus in specimens that do not contain an adequate number of infected cells. When possible, an accompanying specimen for virus isolation usually is advisable.

In addition to providing rapid diagnosis, antigen detection EIA tests are commonly used for the diagnosis of viruses that are difficult or impossible to culture, such as rotavirus, Norwalk virus, and hepatitis B virus.

ISOLATION AND IDENTIFICATION. Viruses require living cells for propagation; the cells used most often are human or animal-derived tissue culture monolayers, such as human embryonic lung fibroblasts or monkey kidney cells. In vivo methods for isolation are sometimes necessary (e.g., suckling mice inoculation for culture of arboviruses and rabies virus). Because viruses require various cell culture systems for isolation, it is important for clinicians to provide relevant clinical information to the laboratory to facilitate selection of appropriate cell lines.

Viral growth in susceptible cell cultures can be detected in several ways. Many viruses produce a characteristic cytopathic effect (CPE) visible by light microscopy under low magnification. For example, RSV and HSV produce multinucleated giant cells and syncytia formation. Other viruses (e.g., influenza and mumps) can be detected by hemadsorption because hemagglutinins on infected cell membranes permit adherence of erythrocytes to infected cells. The most reliable confirmatory method for viral detection in cell culture involves fluorescein- or enzyme-labeled monoclonal antibody staining of infected cell monolayers.

LABORATORY DIAGNOSIS OF PARASITIC INFECTIONS

Most parasites are detected by microscopic examination of clinical specimens. For example, *Plasmodium* and *Babesia* spp can be detected in stained blood smears, *Leishmania* spp in bone marrow smears, helminth eggs and *Entamoeba histolytica* and *Giardia lamblia* cysts and trophozoites in fecal smears (Table 172–1). Serologic tests are important in documenting exposure to certain parasites that are difficult to demonstrate in clinical specimens, such as *Trichinella* and *Toxoplasma* spp. Serologic testing also has a role in the diagnosis of intestinal strongyloidiasis, given the insensitivity of stool examinations.

Fecal specimens should not be contaminated with water or urine because water may contain free-living organisms that can be confused with human parasites, and urine may destroy motile organisms. Mineral oil, barium, and bismuth interfere with the detection of parasites, and specimen collection should be delayed for 7–10 days after ingestion of these substances. Because *Giardia* and many worm eggs are shed intermittently into feces, a minimum number of three specimens is required for an adequate examination. It is recommended that the three specimens be collected on separate days, preferably on alternate days. Because many protozoan parasites are easily destroyed, collection kits with stool preservatives should be used if delay between time of specimen collection and transport to the laboratory is anticipated.

Ova and parasite examination of fecal specimens includes a wet mount (to detect motile organisms if fresh stool is received), concentration (to improve yield), and permanent staining, such as trichrome, for microscopic examination. These techniques may miss parasites such as *Cryptosporidium, Cyclospora,* and microsporidia (*Enterocytozoon bieneusi* and *Septata intestinalis*). *Cryptosporidium* and *Cyclospora* are detected by modified acid-fast stain and microsporidia by a modification of the trichrome stain. The laboratory should be alerted if these parasites are suspected. Detection of certain parasites, especially *Giardia* and *Cryptosporidium,* can be simplified by using sensitive EIA antigen detection tests.

SEROLOGIC DIAGNOSIS

Serologic tests are primarily used in the diagnosis of infectious agents that are difficult to culture in vitro or detect by direct examination, such as *Bartonella, Legionella, Borrelia, Treponema pallidum, Mycoplasma, Rickettsia, Ehrlichia,* some viruses (HIV, EBV, hepatitis A and B viruses), and parasites (*Toxoplasma, Trichinella*).

Antibody tests may be specific for immunoglobulin G (IgG) or M (IgM) or may measure antibody response regardless of immunoglobulin class. The IgM response occurs earlier in the illness, generally peaking at 7–10 days after infection, and usually disappears within a few weeks but for some infections (e.g., hepatitis A) may persist for months. The IgG response peaks at 4–6 wk and in most cases persists for life. Because the IgM response is transient, the presence of IgM antibody in most cases correlates with recent infection; therefore, a single positive serum specimen is considered diagnostic. Methods for IgM antibody detection are difficult to standardize, however, and false-positive results frequently occur with some tests. The presence of IgG antibody may indicate new seroconversion or past exposure to the pathogen. To confirm a new infection using IgG testing, it is essential to demonstrate either seroconversion or a rising IgG titer. A fourfold increase in a convalescent titer obtained 2–3 wk after the acute titer is considered diagnostic in most situations. However, for some infections (e.g., *Bartonella, Legionella,* and rickettsiae) a single positive IgG titer is sufficient for diagnosis.

MOLECULAR DIAGNOSTIC TECHNIQUES (also see Chapter 76)

Molecular diagnostic techniques are most useful for detecting and identifying pathogens for which culture and serologic tests are difficult, slow, or not available. Two of the widely used techniques in clinical microbiology are DNA probes for direct detection and nucleic acid amplification using polymerase chain reaction (PCR).

DNA probes detect or identify organisms by hybridization of the probe to complementary sequences in DNA or ribosomal RNA. Detection of pathogen nucleic acid directly in clinical specimens requires the presence of relatively large numbers of organisms in the specimen. With the exception of commercially available probes for direct detection of *Chlamydia* and gonococci, the principal use of DNA probe technology remains rapid identification of organisms that already have been isolated in culture but require additional time-consuming or complex confirmation procedures. For example, probes for mycobacterial species can rapidly distinguish *M. tuberculosis* from *M. avium-intracellulare* growing in broth cultures.

The high sensitivity and specificity of PCR amplification make this the method of choice for direct detection of microbial nucleic acid from clinical specimens. The PCR method is based on the ability of thermostable DNA or RNA polymerase to copy targeted gene sequences using complementary nucleotides as primers to amplify a conserved region of the genome. The reaction takes place in a thermal cycler, and theoretically, each cycle of the reaction doubles the amount of target nucleic acid, resulting in more than a million-fold amplification in 30 cycles of PCR. The number of pathogens that can be detected by PCR is increasing rapidly. PCR tests are available using commercial reagents for HIV, hepatitis C virus, *M. tuberculosis,* and *C. trachomatis.* Additionally, experimental PCR protocols for detection of *Bartonella, B. pertussis, Legionella, M. pneumoniae, Chlamydia pneumoniae,* HSV, and CMV are available in some reference laboratories.

Specimens for PCR should be sent in separate sterile containers and rapidly transported. PCR methods are technically complex and labor intensive. False-positive reactions are a major problem because the extreme sensitivity of the assay can lead to amplification of target nucleic acid from extraneous sources or from crossover contamination from other positive specimens. Clinically relevant diagnostic PCR testing should be performed only in reference laboratories using adequate quality control measures.

Maxson S, Lewno MJ, Schutze GE: Clinical usefulness of cerebrospinal fluid bacterial antigen studies. J Pediatr 125:235, 1994.
Murray PR, Baron EJ, Pfaller MA, et al (eds): Manual of Clinical Microbiology, 6th ed. Washington, DC, American Society for Microbiology, 1995.
Paisley PW, Lauer BA: Pediatric blood cultures. Clin Lab Med 14:17, 1994.
Perkins MD, Mirrett S, Reller LB: Rapid bacterial antigen detection is not clinically useful. J Clin Microbiol 33:1486, 1995.
Persing DH: In vitro nucleic acid amplification techniques. *In:* Persing DH, Smith T, Tenover FC, White T (eds): Diagnostic Molecular Microbiology. Principles and Applications. Washington, DC, American Society for Microbiology, 1993, pp 51–87.
Ray CG, Minnich LL: Efficiency of immunofluorescence for rapid detection of common respiratory viruses. J Clin Microbiol 25:355, 1987.
Rogers WO, Waites KB, Friedberg RC: Microbiology testing and the pediatrician's office. Pediatr Infect Dis J 16:339, 1997.
Stamm WE: Quantitative urine cultures revisited. Eur J Clin Microbiol 3:279, 1984.
Tenover FC, Unger ER: Nucleic acid probes for detection and identification of infectious agents. *In:* Persing DH, Smith T, Tenover FC, White T (eds): Diagnostic Molecular Microbiology. Principles and Applications. Washington, DC, American Society for Microbiology, 1993, pp 3–25.
Zaidi AKM, Knaut AL, Mirrett S, et al. Value of routine anaerobic blood cultures for pediatric patients. J Pediatr 127:263, 1995.

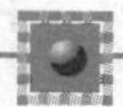

SECTION 2

Clinical Syndromes

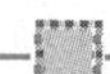

CHAPTER 172
Fever Without a Focus

Keith R. Powell

FEVER AS A MANIFESTATION OF INFECTIOUS DISEASE. Fever is a common manifestation of various infectious diseases with a wide range of severity. Benign febrile diseases in normal hosts include common viral infections (e.g., rhinitis, pharyngitis, pneumonia) and bacterial diseases (e.g., otitis media, pharyngitis, impetigo) that usually respond well to appropriate antimicrobial or supportive therapy and are not life threatening. Several bacterial infections, if untreated, may have significant morbidity or mortality; such diseases include sepsis, meningitis, pneumonia, osteoarticular infections, and pyelonephritis. Many febrile episodes are associated with self-limited infections, which in a normal host have minimal signs of toxicity and require a careful history and physical examination but few if any laboratory tests. However, there are well-defined high-risk groups that, on the basis of age, associated diseases, or immunodeficiency status, require a more extensive evaluation and, in certain situations, prompt antimicrobial therapy before a pathogen is identified (Table 172–1).

FEVER WITHOUT A FOCUS. Fever without localizing signs or symptoms is a common diagnostic dilemma for pediatricians caring for infants younger than 36 mo. Fever is usually of acute onset and is present for less than 1 wk. Infants younger than 1 mo may acquire community pathogens but may also suffer late-onset bacterial diseases or perinatally acquired herpes simplex virus infection (Table 172–1). Infants younger than 3 mo (60 days) demonstrate a limited array of signs with infection, often making it difficult for the clinician to distinguish between serious bacterial infections and self-limited viral illnesses.

Infants Younger Than 3 Mo. Fever in an infant younger than 3 mo should always suggest the possibility of serious bacterial disease. An infectious agent, usually viral, is identified in 70% of these infants, and the remainder are presumed to have had self-limited nonspecific viral infections. Serious bacterial infections are present in 10–15% of infants who were born at term and were previously healthy who have rectal temperatures of 38°C or greater. These infections include sepsis, meningitis, urinary tract infections, gastroenteritis, osteomyelitis, and septic arthritis. Bacteremia is present in 5% of febrile infants younger than 3 mo; organisms responsible for bacteremia include group B streptococci and *Listeria monocytogenes* (late-onset neonatal sepsis and meningitis) and community-acquired pathogens including *Salmonella* spp (gastroenteritis); *Escherichia coli* (urinary tract infection); *Neisseria meningitidis, Streptococcus pneumoniae,* and *Haemophilus influenzae* type b (sepsis and meningitis); and *Staphylococcus aureus* (osteoarticular infection). Pyelonephritis is more common in uncircumcised infant boys, neonates and infants with urinary tract anomalies, and young girls. Other potential bacterial diseases in this age group include otitis media, pneumonia, omphalitis, mastitis, and other skin and soft tissue infections.

Viral pathogens can be identified in 40–60% of febrile infants younger than 3 mo. In contrast to bacterial infections, which have no seasonal pattern, viral diseases have a distinct pattern:

TABLE 172–1 Febrile Patients at Increased Risk for Serious Bacterial Infections

Condition	Comment
Immunocompetent Patients	
Neonates (<28 days)	Sepsis and meningitis caused by group B streptococci, *Escherichia coli, Listeria monocytogenes,* herpes simplex virus
Infants <3 mo	Serious bacterial disease (10–15%); bacteremia in 5% of febrile infants
Infants and children 3–36 mo	Occult bacteremia in 4%; increased risk with temperature >39°C and white blood cell count >15,000/μL
Hyperpyrexia (>41°C)	Meningitis, bacteremia, pneumonia, heatstroke, hemorrhagic shock–encephalopathy syndrome
Fever with petechiae	Bacteremia and meningitis caused by *Neisseria meningitidis, Haemophilus influenzae* type b, *Streptococcus pneumoniae*
Immunocompromised Patients	
Sickle cell anemia	Pneumococcal sepsis, meningitis
Asplenia	Encapsulated bacteria
Complement/properdin deficiency	Meningococcal sepsis
Agammaglobulinemia	Bacteremia, sinopulmonary infection
AIDS	*S. pneumoniae, H. influenzae* type b, *Salmonella*
Congenital heart disease	Increased risk of endocarditis
Central venous line	*Staphylococcus aureus,* coagulase-negative staphylococci, *Candida*
Malignancy	Gram negative enteric bacteria, *S. aureus,* coagulase-negative staphylococci, *Candida*

respiratory syncytial and influenza A virus infections are more common during the winter, whereas enterovirus infections usually occur in the summer and fall.

The approach to febrile patients younger than 3 mo should include a careful history and physical examination. Infants who appear generally well; who have been previously healthy; who have no evidence of skin, soft tissue, bone, joint, or ear infection; and who have a total white blood cell (WBC) count from 5,000–15,000 cells/μL, an absolute band count of less than 1,500 cells/μL, and normal urinalysis results are unlikely to have a serious bacterial infection. The negative predictive value of these criteria for any serious bacterial infection is greater than 98%, and greater than 99% for bacteremia, with 95% confidence.

Ill-appearing (toxic) febrile infants younger than 3 mo require prompt hospitalization; cultures of blood, urine, and cerebrospinal fluid (CSF); and immediate parenteral antimicrobial therapy. Ceftriaxone (50 mg/kg given once daily with normal CSF or 80 mg/kg once daily with CSF pleocytosis) or cefotaxime (50 mg/kg/dose administered q 6 hr) and ampicillin (50 mg/kg/dose given q 6 hr) (for *L. monocytogenes* and enterococci) are effective antimicrobial agents for the initial therapy of ill-appearing patients without focal signs. This regimen is effective against bacterial pathogens producing sepsis, urinary tract infection, and gastroenteritis. However, if meningitis caused by *S. pneumoniae* resistant to penicillin is a possibility, vancomycin (15 mg/kg/dose administered q 6 hr) should be given in addition to the ampicillin and ceftriaxone until the results of culture and susceptibility tests are known.

Occult Bacteremia in Children Age 3 mo–3 yr. Approximately 30% of febrile children 3 mo–3 yr of age have no localizing signs of infection. Occult bacteremia (bacteremia without an obvious focus of infection) due to *S. pneumoniae, H. influenzae* type b, *N. meningitidis,* and *Salmonella* spp occurs in approximately 4% of relatively well-appearing children between 3 and 36 mo of age with fever (rectal temperature ≥38.0°C). *S. pneumoniae* accounts for 85% of cases of occult bacteremia, with *H. influenzae* type b, *N. meningitidis,* and *Salmonella* spp accounting for the remaining positive cultures. The incidence of *H. influenzae* type b infections of all types has decreased dramatically in regions where the conjugate *H. influenzae* type b vaccine is administered to infants. Common bacterial infections among children between 3 and 36 mo who do have localizing signs include otitis media, upper respiratory tract infection, pneumonia, gastroenteritis, urinary tract infection, osteomyelitis, and meningitis. In this age group, bacteremia is present in 11% of febrile children with pneumonia and 1.5% of febrile children with otitis media or pharyngitis.

Risk factors indicating increased probability of occult bacteremia include temperature exceeding 39°C, total WBC count greater than 15,000/μL, or an elevated absolute neutrophil count, band count, erythrocyte sedimentation rate, or C-reactive protein. The incidence of bacteremia among infants between 3 and 36 mo increases as the temperature and WBC count increase, to 13.0% if the temperature is higher than 39.0°C and the WBC count exceeds 15,000/μL. However, no combination of laboratory tests or clinical assessment is completely accurate in predicting the presence of occult bacteremia. Socioeconomic status, race, sex, and age (within the range of 3–36 mo) do not affect the risk for occult bacteremia. The increased incidence of bacteremia among febrile 3- to 36-mo-old children may be due in part to a maturational immune deficiency in the production of opsonic IgG antibodies to the polysaccharide antigens present on these encapsulated bacteria.

Without therapy, occult bacteremia may resolve spontaneously without sequelae, may persist, or may lead to localized infections, such as meningitis, pneumonia, cellulitis, or septic arthritis. The pattern of sequelae may be related to both host factors and the offending organism. In some children, the occult bacteremic illness may represent the early signs of serious localized infection rather than a transient disease state. Bacteremia due to *H. influenzae* type b is of a higher grade, as determined by quantitative blood culture techniques, and is associated with a higher risk of localized serious infection than is bacteremia due to *S. pneumoniae*. Hospitalized children with *H. influenzae* type b bacteremia often develop focal infections, such as meningitis, epiglottitis, cellulitis, or osteoarticular infection, whereas fewer than 5% of these bacteremias can be considered transient or occult. In contrast, among all patients with pneumococcal bacteremia (occult, symptomatic, or focal), the incidence of transient bacteremia with spontaneous resolution is 30–40%. Occult pneumococcal bacteremia, in a well-appearing child, has a higher rate of spontaneous resolution. Two studies of bacteremic children 3–36 mo of age conducted since 1987 showed that only 1/215 children with occult pneumococcal bacteremia went on to develop meningitis. All children in the two studies were treated with oral amoxicillin or amoxicillin/potassium clavulanate or with intramuscular ceftriaxone.

Treatment of toxic-appearing febrile children from 3–36 mo of age who do not have focal signs of infection includes hospitalization; cultures of blood, urine, and CSF; and prompt institution of antimicrobial therapy. Meningitis in patients with occult bacteremia that develops after a lumbar puncture does not represent inoculation of bacteria by the puncture but is coincidental and represents meningeal infection that was developing before the lumbar puncture.

Practice guidelines published in 1993 recommended that infants 3–36 months of age who have a temperature less than 39°C and who do not appear toxic can be observed as outpatients without performing diagnostic tests or administering antimicrobial agents. For non–toxic-appearing infants with a rectal temperature of 39°C or greater, two options are suggested: (1) Obtain a blood culture and give empirical antimicrobial therapy (ceftriaxone, 50 mg/kg once daily, not to exceed 1 g) ; or (2) obtain a complete blood cell count, and if the WBC count is 15,000 or more cells/μL, obtain a blood culture and give empirical antimicrobial therapy. A third option, not offered in these guidelines, is to observe selected infants as outpatients without empirical antimicrobial therapy after blood for culture has been obtained. The family should be instructed to return to the office or clinic within 24 hr if the fever persists or immediately if the child's condition deteriorates.

If pneumococci are found in the first blood culture, the child should return to the physician as soon as the culture results have been reported. If the child appears well and is afebrile and the physical findings are normal, a second blood culture should be obtained, and the child may return home without treatment. If the child appears ill and continues to have fever with no identifiable focus of infection, or if *H. influenzae* or *N. meningitidis* is present in the initial blood culture, the child should have a repeat blood culture, be evaluated for meningitis including lumbar puncture, and receive treatment in the hospital with appropriate antimicrobial agents. If the child develops a localized infection, therapy is directed toward the specific pathogen and the particular site.

FEVER WITH PETECHIAE. Independent of age, fever with petechiae with or without localizing signs indicates high risk for life-threatening bacterial infections such as bacteremia, sepsis, and meningitis. From 8–20% of patients with fever and petechiae have a serious bacterial infection, and 7–10% have meningococcal sepsis or meningitis. *H. influenzae* type b disease can also present with fever and petechiae. Management includes prompt hospitalization, culture of blood and CSF, and administration of appropriate parenteral antimicrobial agents. See Chapters 191 and 193 for treatment.

FEVER IN PATIENTS WITH SICKLE CELL ANEMIA. Infection is the most common cause of death among children with sickle cell anemia (Chapter 468.1). The incidence of infection is greatest among infants younger than 5 yr. The increased risk of infection in these children is due in part to functional asplenia and a defect in the properdin (alternate complement) pathway. Fever without a focus is a common presenting sign of sepsis or meningitis due to pneumococcus in patients with sickle cell anemia. *H. influenzae* type b (meningitis), *Salmonella* (osteomyelitis), and *E. coli* (pyelonephritis) are additional pathogens that may present initially as fever without localizing signs.

The treatment of patients with sickle cell hemoglobinopathies requires culture of blood and, if indicated, CSF, stool, and bone, and administration of antimicrobial agents. Children who appear seriously ill, have a temperature greater than 40°C or WBC counts less than 5,000/μL or greater than 30,000/μL, or who have pulmonary infiltrates or complications of sickle cell disease or severe pain should be hospitalized. Other febrile infants with sickle cell disease can be given intramuscular ceftriaxone and cared for as outpatients after specimens have been obtained for culture. These children should be seen again in 24 hr or earlier if their condition deteriorates.

Prevention of pneumococcal sepsis is possible by instituting long-term penicillin therapy continued until adolescence (oral penicillin V potassium, 250 mg twice daily or long-acting intramuscular, penicillin G benzathine, 600,000 units every 3–4 wk). Pneumococcal and *H. influenzae* vaccines may provide additional protection, but these vaccines should not be used in place of long-term antimicrobial therapy.

HYPERPYREXIA. Hyperpyrexia (temperature >41°C) is uncommon and is not associated with higher rates of serious bacterial infections than temperatures of 39.1–40.0°C or 40.1–41.0°C. Infants and children with hyperpyrexia should be carefully evaluated, but evaluation and management need not differ from that of other children with lesser degrees of fever in excess of 39.0°C.

FEVER OF UNKNOWN ORIGIN. Many physicians use the term *fever of unknown origin* (FUO) to describe the condition of any febrile child admitted to the hospital with neither an apparent site of infection nor a noninfectious diagnosis. In most of these children, the development of additional clinical manifestations over a relatively short period makes the infectious nature of the illness apparent. Therefore, the term is better reserved for children with a fever documented by a health care provider and for which the cause could not be identified after 3 wk of evaluation as an outpatient or after a 1-wk evaluation in hospital.

The principal causes of FUO in children, using more restrictive criteria, are infections and connective tissue (autoimmune or rheumatologic) diseases (Table 172–2). Neoplastic disorders should also be seriously considered, although most children with malignancies do not have fever alone. The possibility of drug fever should be considered if a patient is receiving any drug. Drug fever is not usually associated with other symptoms, and temperature remains elevated at a relatively constant level. Withdrawal of the drug is associated with resolution of the fever, generally within 72 hr, although certain drugs, such as iodides, are excreted for a prolonged period and fever may persist for as long as 1 mo after drug withdrawal.

Most fevers of unknown or unrecognized origin result from atypical presentations of common diseases. In some cases, the presentation of FUO is typical of the disease (juvenile rheumatoid arthritis [JRA]), but a definitive diagnosis can be established only after prolonged observation because initially there are no associated findings on physical examination and all laboratory results are negative or normal.

In the United States, the systemic infectious diseases most commonly implicated in children with FUO (by the more rigorous definition) are salmonellosis, tuberculosis, rickettsial diseases, syphilis, Lyme disease, cat-scratch disease, atypical prolonged presentations of common viral diseases, infectious mononucleosis, cytomegalovirus (CMV) infection, hepatitis, coccidioidomycosis, histoplasmosis, malaria, and toxoplasmosis. Less common infectious causes of FUO include tularemia, brucellosis, leptospirosis, and rat-bite fever. AIDS alone is not usually responsible for FUO, although febrile illnesses frequently occur in patients with AIDS as a result of opportunistic infections.

JRA and systemic lupus erythematosus are the connective tissue diseases associated most frequently with FUO. Inflammatory bowel disease, rheumatic fever, and Kawasaki disease are also commonly reported as causes of FUO. If factitious fever (inoculation of pyogenic material or manipulation of the thermometer by the patient or parent) is suspected, the presence and pattern of fever should be documented in the hospital. Prolonged and continuous observation of patients is imperative. FUO lasting more than 6 mo is uncommon in children and should suggest granulomatosis or autoimmune disease. Repetitive interval evaluation, including history, physical examination, and roentgenographic studies, may be required.

DIAGNOSTIC CLUES IN A CHILD WITH FEVER OF UNKNOWN ORIGIN

History. The *age* of the patient is helpful in evaluating FUO. Children younger than 6 yr often have a respiratory or genitourinary tract infection, localized infection (abscess, osteomyelitis), JRA, or, rarely, leukemia. Adolescent patients are more likely to have tuberculosis, inflammatory bowel disease, autoimmune processes, and lymphoma, in addition to the causes of FUO found in younger children.

A history of *exposure to wild or domestic animals* should be solicited. Zoonotic infections in the United States are increasing in frequency, frequently acquired from pets that are not overtly ill. Immunization of dogs against specific disorders such as leptospirosis may prevent canine disease but does not always prevent the animal from carrying and shedding leptospires, which may be transmitted to household contacts. A history of ingestion of rabbit or squirrel meat may provide a clue to the diagnosis of oropharyngeal, glandular, or typhoidal tularemia. A history of tick bite or travel to tick- or parasite-infested areas should be obtained.

Any history of *pica* should be elicited. Ingestion of dirt is a particularly important clue to infection with *Toxocara* (visceral larva migrans) or *Toxoplasma gondii* (toxoplasmosis).

A history of unusual dietary habits or travel as early as the birth of the child should be sought. Malaria, histoplasmosis, and coccidioidomycosis may re-emerge years after visiting or living in an endemic area. It is important to ask about prophylactic immunizations and precautions taken by the individual against ingestion of contaminated water or food during foreign travel. Rocks, dirt, and artifacts from geographically distant regions that have been collected and brought into the home as souvenirs may serve as vectors of disease.

A *medication history* should be pursued rigorously. This should include over-the-counter preparations and topical agents, including eye drops (atropine-induced fever).

The *genetic background* of a patient also is important. Descendants of the Ulster Scots may have FUO because they are afflicted with nephrogenic diabetes insipidus. Familial dysautonomia (Riley-Day syndrome), a disorder in which hyperthermia is recurrent, is more frequent among Jews than other population groups. Ancestry from the Mediterranean should suggest the possibility of familial Mediterranean fever.

Physical Examination. Sweating in a febrile child should be noted. The continuing absence of sweat in the presence of an elevated or changing body temperature suggests dehydration due to vomiting, diarrhea, or central or nephrogenic diabetes insipidus. It also should suggest anhidrotic ectodermal dysplasia, familial dysautonomia, or exposure to atropine.

A careful ophthalmic examination is important. Red, weeping eyes may be a sign of connective tissue disease, particularly polyarteritis nodosa. Palpebral conjunctivitis in a febrile patient may be a clue to measles, coxsackievirus infection, tuberculosis, infectious mononucleosis, lymphogranuloma venereum,

TABLE 172–2 Causes of Fever of Unknown Origin in Children

Infections

Bacteria

Caused by Specific Organism

Actinomycosis
Bartonellosis (cat-scratch disease)
Brucellosis
Campylobacter
Listeriosis
Meningococcemia (chronic)
Mycoplasma
Salmonellosis
Streptobacillus moniliformis (rat-bite fever)
Tuberculosis
Tularemia
Yersiniosis

Localized Infections

Abscesses: abdominal, brain, dental, hepatic, pelvic, perinephric, rectal, subphrenic
Cholangitis
Endocarditis
Mastoiditis
Osteomyelitis
Pneumonia
Pyelonephritis
Sinusitis

Spirochetes

Relapsing fever (*Borrelia recurrentis*)
Leptospirosis
Lyme disease (*Borrelia burgdorferi*)
Spirillum minus
Syphilis

Viruses

Cytomegalovirus
Hepatitis
HIV
Infectious mononucleosis (Epstein-Barr virus)

Chlamydia

Lymphogranuloma venereum
Psittacosis

Rickettsia

Ehrlichia canis
Q fever
Rocky Mountain spotted fever
Tick-borne typhus

Fungal Diseases

Blastomycosis (extrapulmonary)
Coccidioidomycosis (disseminated)
Histoplasmosis (disseminated)

Parasitic Diseases

Amebiasis
Babesiosis
Giardiasis
Malaria
Toxoplasmosis
Trichinosis
Trypanosomiasis
Visceral larva migrans

Rheumatologic Diseases

Behçet's disease
Juvenile dermatomyositis
Juvenile rheumatoid arthritis
Rheumatic fever
Systemic lupus erythematosus

Hypersensitivity Diseases

Drug fever
Hypersensitivity pneumonitis
Pancreatitis
Serum sickness
Weber-Christian disease

Neoplasms

Atrial myxoma
Cholesterol granuloma
Hodgkin disease
Inflammatory pseudotumor
Leukemia
Lymphoma
Neuroblastoma
Wilms tumor

Granulomatous Diseases

Crohn disease
Granulomatous hepatitis
Sarcoidosis

Familial-Hereditary Diseases

Anhidrotic ectodermal dysplasia
Fabry disease
Familial dysautonomia
Familial Mediterranean fever
Hypertriglyceridemia
Ichthyosis
Sickle cell crisis

Miscellaneous

Chronic active hepatitis
Diabetes insipidus (non-nephrogenic and nephrogenic)
Factitious fever
Hypothalamic-central fever
Infantile cortical hyperostosis
Inflammatory bowel disease
Kawasaki disease
Kikuchi-Fujimoto disease
Pancreatitis
Periodic fever
Poisoning
Pulmonary embolism
Thrombophlebitis
Thyrotoxicosis

Recurrent or Relapsing Fever

See Table 170–1

Undiagnosed Fever

Persistent
Recurrent
Resolved

cat-scratch disease, or Newcastle disease virus infection. In contrast, bulbar conjunctivitis in a child with FUO suggests Kawasaki syndrome or leptospirosis. Petechial conjunctival hemorrhages suggest endocarditis. Uveitis suggests sarcoidosis, JRA, systemic lupus erythematosus, Kawasaki syndrome, Behçet's disease, and vasculitis. Chorioretinitis suggests CMV, toxoplasmosis, and syphilis. Proptosis suggests orbital tumor, thyrotoxicosis, metastasis (neuroblastoma), orbital infection, Wegener granulomatosis, or pseudotumor.

The ophthalmoscope should also be used to examine for nail fold capillary abnormalities that are associated with connective tissue diseases such as juvenile dermatomyositis and systemic scleroderma (see Fig. 160–3). Immersion oil or lubricating jelly is placed on the skin adjacent to the nail bed, and the capillary pattern is observed with the ophthalmoscope set on +40.

FUO is sometimes due to hypothalamic dysfunction. A clue to this disorder is failure of pupillary constriction due to absence of the sphincter constrictor muscle of the eye. This muscle develops embryologically when hypothalamic structure and function also are undergoing differentiation.

Fever resulting from familial dysautonomia may be suggested by lack of tears or an absent corneal reflex or by a smooth tongue with absence of fungiform papillae. Tenderness to tapping over the sinuses and teeth should be sought, and the sinuses should be transilluminated. Recurrent oral candidiasis may be a clue to various disorders of the immune system.

Fever blisters are common findings in patients with pneumococcal, streptococcal, malarial, and rickettsial infection. They also are common in children with meningococcal meningitis (which usually does not present as FUO) but rarely are seen in children with meningococcemia. Fever blisters also are rarely seen with *Salmonella* or staphylococcal infections.

Hyperemia of the pharynx, with or without exudate, may suggest infectious mononucleosis, CMV infection, toxoplasmosis, salmonellosis, tularemia, Kawasaki syndrome, or leptospirosis.

The muscles and bones should be palpated carefully. Point tenderness over a bone may suggest occult osteomyelitis or bone marrow invasion from neoplastic disease. Tenderness over the trapezius muscle may be a clue to subdiaphragmatic abscess. Generalized muscle tenderness suggests dermatomyositis, trichinosis, polyarteritis, Kawaski syndrome, or mycoplasmal or arboviral infection.

Rectal examination may reveal perirectal lymphadenopathy or tenderness, which suggests a deep pelvic abscess, iliac adenitis, or pelvic osteomyelitis. A guaiac test should be obtained; occult blood loss may suggest granulomatous colitis or ulcerative colitis as the cause of FUO.

Repetitive chills and temperature spikes are common in children with septicemia (regardless of cause), particularly when associated with renal disease, liver or biliary disease, endocarditis, malaria, brucellosis, rat-bite fever, or loculated collection of pus. The general activity of the patient and the presence or absence of rashes should be noted. Hyperactive deep tendon reflexes may suggest thyrotoxicosis as the cause of FUO.

Laboratory Findings. Ordering a large number of diagnostic tests in every child with FUO according to a predetermined list may waste time and money. Alternatively, prolonged hospitalization for sequential tests may be more costly. The tempo of diagnostic evaluation should be adjusted to the tempo of the illness; haste may be imperative in a critically ill patient, but if the illness is more chronic, the evaluation can proceed more slowly and deliberately and, usually, in an ambulatory setting.

A complete blood cell count with a differential cell count and a urinalysis should be part of the initial laboratory evaluation. An absolute neutrophil count less than 5,000/μL is evidence against indolent bacterial infection other than typhoid fever. Conversely, patients with polymorphonuclear leukocytes greater than 10,000/μL or nonsegmented polymorphonuclear leukocytes greater than 500/μL have a high likelihood of having a severe bacterial infection. Direct examination of the blood smear with Giemsa or Wright stain may reveal malaria, trypanosomiasis, babesiosis, or relapsing fever.

An *erythrocyte sedimentation rate* (ESR) exceeding 30 mm/hr indicates inflammation and the need for further evaluation for infectious, autoimmune, or malignant diseases. An ESR greater than 100 mm/hr suggests tuberculosis, Kawasaki syndrome, malignancy, or autoimmune disease. A low ESR does not eliminate the possibility of infection or JRA.

Blood cultures should be obtained aerobically. Anaerobic blood cultures have an extremely low yield and should be obtained only if there are specific reasons to suspect an anaerobic infection. Repeated blood cultures may be required to diagnose endocarditis, osteomyelitis, or deep-seated abscesses producing bacteremia. Polymicrobial bacteremia suggests factitious self-induced infection or gastrointestinal (GI) pathology. The isolation of leptospires, *Francisella*, or *Yersinia* may require selective media or specific conditions not routinely used. *Urine culture* should be obtained routinely.

Tuberculin *skin testing* should be performed with intradermal placement of 5 units of purified protein derivative (PPD) that has been kept appropriately refrigerated.

Roentgenographic examination of the chest, sinuses, mastoids, or GI tract may be indicated by specific historical or physical findings. Roentgenographic evaluation of the GI tract for inflammatory bowel disease may be helpful in evaluating selected children with FUO and no other localizing signs or symptoms.

Examination of the *bone marrow* may reveal leukemia; metastatic neoplasm; mycobacterial, fungal, or parasitic diseases; and histiocytosis, hemophagocytosis, or storage diseases. If a bone marrow aspirate is performed, cultures for bacteria, *Mycobacterium*, and fungi should be obtained.

Serologic tests may aid in the diagnosis of infectious mononucleosis, CMV disease, toxoplasmosis, salmonellosis, tularemia, brucellosis, leptospirosis, cat-scratch disease, Lyme disease, rickettsial disease, and, on some occasions, JRA. As serologic tests for more diseases become available through commercial laboratories, it is important to ascertain the sensitivity and specificity of each test before relying on these results to make a diagnosis. Serologic tests for Lyme disease outside of reference laboratories have been generally unreliable.

Radionuclide scans may be helpful in detecting osteomyelitis and abdominal abscesses. Gallium citrate (^{67}Ga) localizes in inflammatory tissues (leukocytes) associated with tumors or abscesses. ^{99m}Tc phosphate is useful for detecting osteomyelitis before plain roentgenograms demonstrate bone lesions. Granulocytes tagged with indium (^{111}In) or iodinated IgG may be useful in detecting localized pyogenic processes. *Echocardiograms* may demonstrate the presence of vegetation on the leaflets of heart valves, suggesting infective endocarditis. *Ultrasonography* may identify intra-abdominal abscesses of the liver, subphrenic space, pelvis, or spleen.

Total body CT or MRI permits detection of neoplasms and collections of purulent material without the use of surgical exploration or radioisotopes. CT and MRI are helpful in identifying lesions of the head, neck, chest, retroperitoneal spaces, liver, spleen, intra-abdominal and intrathoracic lymph nodes, kidneys, pelvis, and mediastinum. CT or ultrasound-guided aspiration or biopsy of suspicious lesions has reduced the need for exploratory laparotomy or thoracotomy. Diagnostic imaging can be very helpful in confirming or evaluating a suspected diagnosis but rarely leads to an unsuspected cause.

Biopsy is occasionally helpful in establishing a diagnosis of FUO. Bronchoscopy, laparoscopy, mediastinoscopy, and GI endoscopy may provide direct visualization and biopsy material when organ-specific manifestations are present.

Treatment. Fever and infection in children are not synonymous; antimicrobial agents should not be used as antipyretics, and empirical trials of medication should generally be avoided. An exception may be the use of antituberculous treatment in critically ill children with possible disseminated tuberculosis. Empirical trials of other antimicrobial agents may be dangerous and can obscure the diagnosis of endocarditis, meningitis, parameningeal infection, or osteomyelitis. Hospitalization may be required for laboratory or roentgenographic studies that are unavailable or impractical in an ambulatory setting, for more careful observation, or for temporary relief of parental anxiety. After a complete evaluation, antipyretics may be indicated to control fever and for symptomatic relief (Chapter 170).

Prognosis. Children with FUO have a better prognosis than do adults. The outcome in a child is dependent on the primary disease process, which is usually an atypical presentation of a common childhood illness. In many cases, no diagnosis can be established and fever abates spontaneously. In as many as 25% of cases in which fever persists, the cause of the fever remains unclear, even after thorough evaluation.

Baker RC, Sequin JH, Leslie N, et al: Fever and petechiae in children. Pediatrics 84:1051, 1989.

Baraff LJ, Bass JW, Fleisher GR, et al: Practice guidelines for the management of infants and children 0–36 months of age with fever without a source. Pediatrics 92:1, 1993; Ann Emerg Med 22:1198, 1993.

Bass JW, Steele RW, Wittler RR, et al: Antimicrobial treatment of occult bacteremia: A multicenter cooperative study. Pediatr Infect Dis J 12:466, 1993.

Dagan R, Hall CB, Powell KR, et al: Epidemiology and laboratory diagnosis of infection with viral and bacterial pathogens in infants hospitalized for suspected sepsis. J Pediatr 115:351, 1989

Fleisher GR, Rosenberg N, Vinci R, et al: Intramuscular versus oral antibiotic therapy for the prevention of meningitis and other bacterial sequelae in young febrile children at risk for occult bacteremia. J Pediatr 124:504, 1994.

Jaskiewicz JA, McCarthy CA, Richardson AC, et al: Febrile infants at low risk for serious bacterial infection—an appraisal of the Rochester criteria and implications for management. Pediatrics 94:390, 1994.

Knockaert DC, Vanneste LJ, Bobbaers HJ: Recurrent or episodic fever of unknown origin. Review of 45 cases and survey of the literature. Medicine 72:184, 1993.

Kramer MS, Shapiro ED: Management of the young febrile child: A commentary on recent pediatric guidelines (pp 128–134); Baroff LJ, Schriger DL, Bass JW, et al: Commentary on pediatric guidelines (pp 134–135); Bauchner H, Pelton SI: Managment of the young febrile child: A continuing controversy (pp 137–138). Pediatrics 100:128, 1997.

Lohr JA, Hendley JO: Prolonged fever of unknown origin. A record of experiences with 54 childhood patients. Clin Pediatr 16:768, 1977.

McClung HJ: Prolonged fever of unknown origin in children. Am J Dis Child 124:544, 1972.

Miller ML, Szer I, Yogev R, et al: Fever of unknown origin. Pediatr Clin North Am 42:999, 1995.

Norris AH, Krasinskas AM, Salhany KE, et al: Kikuchi-Fujimoto disease: A benign cause of fever and lymphadenopathy. Am J Med 171:401, 1996.

Pizzo PA, Lovejoy FH Jr, Smith DH: Prolonged fever in children: Review of 100 cases. Pediatrics 55:468, 1975.

Powell KR: Evaluation and management of febrile infants younger than 60 days of age. Pediatr Infect Dis J 9:153, 1990.

Steele RW, Jones SM, Lowe BA, et al: Usefulness of scanning procedures for diagnosis of fever of unknown origin in children. J Pediatr 119:526, 1991.

Wilimas JA, Flynn PM, Harris S, et al: A randomized study of outpatient treatment with ceftriaxone for selected febrile children with sickle cell disease. N Engl J Med 329:472, 1993.

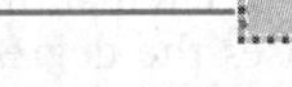

CHAPTER 173
Sepsis and Shock

Keith R. Powell

The recovery of bacteria in a blood culture, *bacteremia,* may be a transient phenomenon not associated with disease or may be the serious extension of an invasive bacterial infection originating elsewhere. Local infections, such as meningitis, osteomyelitis, endocarditis, epiglottitis, and facial cellulitis, usually follow or are concomitant with bacteremia. *Transient bacteremia* may follow instrumentation of the respiratory, gastrointestinal, or genitourinary tracts. Bacteremia may be asymptomatic or associated with few symptoms. When bacteria are not effectively cleared by host defense mechanisms, a systemic inflammatory response is set into motion and can progress independently of the original infection. *Sepsis* is the systemic response to infection with bacteria, viruses, fungi, protozoa, or rickettsiae. Sepsis is one of the causes of the *systemic inflammatory response syndrome (SIRS),* which has noninfectious causes as well. If not recognized and treated early, sepsis can progress to severe sepsis, septic shock (sepsis with hypotension), *multiple organ dysfunction syndrome (MODS),* and death (Fig. 173–1). However, the varied clinical manifestations of sepsis may result in a broad differential diagnosis that includes many noninfectious etiologies (Table 173–1).

EPIDEMIOLOGY. Sepsis may develop as a complication of localized community-acquired infections (Table 173–1) or may follow colonization and local mucosal invasion by virulent pathogens (*Neisseria meningitidis, Streptococcus pneumoniae, Haemophilus influenzae* type b, *Salmonella* spp). Children age 3 mo–3 yr are at risk for occult bacteremia, which occasionally progresses to sepsis (Chapter 172).

Immunocompromised patients (see Table 172–1) are at increased risk for serious nosocomial sepsis. Hospitalized patients develop sepsis caused by *Streptococcus aureus* or coagulase-negative staphylococci associated with intravenous catheters (Chapter 180) or surgical wounds, whereas serious gram-negative (*Escherichia coli, Pseudomonas, Acinetobacter, Klebsiella-Enterobacter, Serratia*) sepsis or fungemia is characteristic of immunocompromised neutropenic patients or acutely ill patients receiving intensive care. Polymicrobial sepsis also occurs in high-risk patients and is associated with central venous catheterization, gastrointestinal disease, neutropenia, and malignancy. Unusual pathogens should be considered in severely immunocompromised patients and in patients who have traveled to or been exposed to products from distant lands. When unusual or uncommon pathogens are identified, an expert in infectious diseases should be consulted.

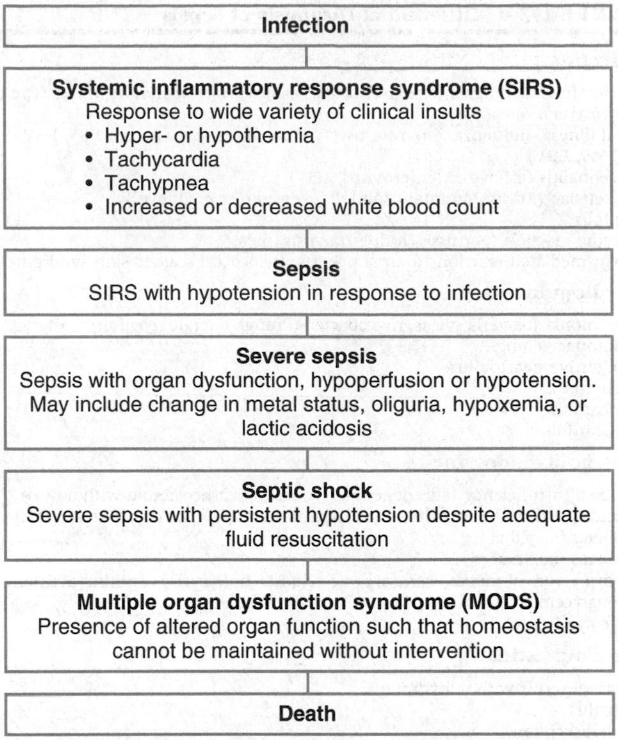

Pseudobacteremia may be associated with contaminated solutions such as heparin flush solutions, intravenous infusates, albumin, cryoprecipitate, and contaminated infusion equipment. Unusual water-associated organisms such as *Burkholderia cepacia, Pseudomonas aeruginosa,* or *Serratia* are often found.

Infection

Systemic inflammatory response syndrome (SIRS)
Response to wide variety of clinical insults
- Hyper- or hypothermia
- Tachycardia
- Tachypnea
- Increased or decreased white blood count

Sepsis
SIRS with hypotension in response to infection

Severe sepsis
Sepsis with organ dysfunction, hypoperfusion or hypotension. May include change in metal status, oliguria, hypoxemia, or lactic acidosis

Septic shock
Severe sepsis with persistent hypotension despite adequate fluid resuscitation

Multiple organ dysfunction syndrome (MODS)
Presence of altered organ function such that homeostasis cannot be maintained without intervention

Death

Figure 173–1 Progression from infection to sepsis (systemic inflammatory response syndrome [SIRS]) and its complications. WBC, white blood cell; MODS, multiorgan dysfunction syndrome. (Modified from Sáez-Llorens X, McCracken GH Jr: Sepsis syndrome and septic shock in pediatrics: Current concepts of terminology, pathophysiology, and management. J Pediatr 123: 498, 1993.)

PATHOGENESIS. SIRS related to sepsis (Fig. 173–1) results from tissue damage following the host response to bacterial products such as endotoxin from gram-negative bacteria and the lipoteichoic acid-peptidoglycan complex from gram-positive bacteria. The cardiopulmonary manifestations of gram-negative (e.g., *H. influenzae, N. meningitidis, E. coli, Pseudomonas*) sepsis can be mimicked by injection of endotoxin or tumor necrosis factor (TNF). Inhibition of TNF action by monoclonal anti-TNF antibody greatly attenuates the manifestations of septic shock in experimental models. When bacterial cell wall components are released into the bloodstream, cytokines are activated, and these in turn can lead to further physiologic derangements (Fig. 173–2). Endogenous mediators of sepsis continue to be identified and currently include TNF-α; interleukin (IL-1, -2, -4, -6, and -8); platelet-activating factor (PAF); interferon-γ; eicosanoids (leukotrienes B_4, C_4, D_4, E_4; thromboxane A2; prostaglandins E_2, I_2); granulocyte-macrophage colony-stimu-

TABLE 173–1 Differential Diagnosis of Sepsis

Infection

Bacteremia/meningitis (*Streptococcus pneumoniae, Haemophilus influenzae* type b, *Neisseria meningitidis*)
Viral illness (influenza, enteroviruses, hemorrhagic fever group, HSV, RSV, CMV, EBV)
Encephalitis (arbovirus, enterovirus, HSV)
Rickettsiae (Rocky Mountain spotted fever, *Ehrlichia,* Q fever)
Syphilis
Vaccine reaction (pertussis, influenza virus, measles)
Toxin-mediated reaction (toxic shock, staphylococcal scalded skin syndrome)

Cardiopulmonary

Pneumonia (bacteria, virus, mycobacteria, fungi, allergic reaction)
Pulmonary emboli
Congestive heart failure
Arrhythmia
Pericarditis
Myocarditis

Metabolic-Endocrine

Adrenal insufficiency (adrenogenital syndrome, corticosteroid withdrawal)
Electrolyte disturbances (hypo- or hypernatremia; hypo- or hypercalcemia)
Diabetes insipidus
Diabetes mellitus
Inborn errors of metabolism (organic acidosis, urea cycle, carnitine deficiency)
Hypoglycemia
Reye syndrome

Gastrointestinal

Gastroenteritis with dehydration
Volvulus
Intussusception
Appendicitis
Peritonitis (spontaneous, associated with perforation or peritoneal dialysis)
Hepatitis
Hemorrhage

Hematologic

Anemia (sickle cell, blood loss, nutritional)
Methemoglobinemia
Splenic sequestration crisis
Leukemia or lymphoma

Neurologic

Intoxication (drugs, carbon monoxide, intentional or accidental overdose)
Intracranial hemorrhage
Infant botulism
Trauma (child abuse, accidental)
Guillain-Barré syndrome
Myasthenia gravis

Other

Anaphylaxis (food, drug, insect sting)
Hemolytic-uremic syndrome
Kawasaki syndrome
Erythema multiforme
Hemorrhagic shock–encephalopathy syndrome

HSV = herpes simplex virus; RSV = respiratory syncytial virus; CMV = cytomegalovirus; EBV = Epstein-Barr virus.

lating factor (GM-CSF); endothelium-derived relaxing factor; endothelin-1; complement fragments C3a and C5a; toxic oxygen radicals and proteolytic enzymes from polymorphonuclear neutrophils; adhesion molecules; platelets; transforming growth factor-β; vascular permeability factor; macrophage-derived procoagulant and inflammatory cytokine; bradykinin; thrombin; coagulation factors; fibrin; plasminogen activator inhibitors; myocardial depressant substance; β-endorphin; and heat shock proteins.

Alone or in combination, bacterial products and proinflammatory cytokines trigger physiologic responses to inhibit microbial invaders. These responses include (1) activation of the complement system; (2) activation of Hageman factor (factor XII), which then initiates the coagulation cascade; (3) adrenocorticotrophic hormone and β-endorphin release; (4) stimulation of polymorphonuclear neutrophils; and (5) stimulation of the kallikrein-kinin system (Fig. 173–2). TNF and other inflammatory mediators increase vascular permeability, producing diffuse capillary leakage, reduced vascular tone, and an imbalance between perfusion and the increased metabolic requirements of tissues. Inflammatory mediator activity or over-responsiveness contributes to the pathogenesis of sepsis.

Current hypotheses on the pathophysiology of sepsis suggest that the proinflammatory molecules that initiate SIRS trigger the release of anti-inflammatory molecules to limit the inflammatory response. The anti-inflammatory response is referred to as the compensatory anti-inflammatory response syndrome. Anti-inflammatory molecules include IL-4, IL-10, IL-11, IL-13, TNF-α receptors, transforming growth factor-β, and IL-1 receptor antagonists. If the response is not purely proinflammatory or anti-inflammatory, it is termed a mixed antagonists responses syndrome (Fig. 173–3).

Shock is defined as a disruption in circulatory function leading to poor perfusion and inadequate delivery of oxygen nutrients to tissues. Shock is not diagnosed by a decrease in blood pressure (BP) because compensatory mechanisms maintain BP by altering vascular tone even as cardiac output decreases. Low BP may be an ominous sign that compensatory mechanisms have failed.

In the early phases of sepsis there is a decrease in systemic vascular resistance and a decline in preload, which results in tachycardia, increased cardiac output, and widened pulse pressure due to low diastolic pressures. Cytokine-induced endothelial damage leads to loss of circulating fluids into tissues (third-space losses) and increases the degree of relative hypovolemia. Clinically, patients are warm and have bounding pulses with brisk capillary refill. In later phases of septic shock, patients have cool extremities with poor peripheral pulses and decreased BP reflecting myocardial depression and decreased cardiac output. As tissue oxygen consumption exceeds oxygen delivery, the resultant tissue hypoxia leads to lactic acidosis.

Pulmonary function is often severely impaired, and the development of adult respiratory distress syndrome (ARDS), or "shock lung," is associated with a poor prognosis. Acute renal failure, hepatic failure, central nervous system dysfunction, and disseminated intravascular coagulation can occur alone or in combination in MODS. Also see Chapters 64.2 and 65.

CLINICAL MANIFESTATIONS. The primary signs and symptoms of sepsis and its complications include fever, shaking chills, hyperventilation, tachycardia, hypothermia, cutaneous lesions (e.g., petechiae, ecchymoses, ecthyma gangrenosum, diffuse erythema), and changes in mental status such as confusion, agitation, anxiety, excitation, lethargy, obtundation, or coma. Secondary manifestations include hypotension, cyanosis, symmetric peripheral gangrene (purpura fulminans), oliguria or anuria, jaundice (direct hyperbilirubinemia), and signs of heart failure. There may be evidence of focal infection such as meningitis, pneumonia, arthritis, cellulitis, or pyelonephritis or of an immunocompromised status such as malignancy, T- or B-lymphocyte defects, or prior splenectomy.

LABORATORY FINDINGS. The laboratory manifestations of sepsis include positive blood cultures; Gram, Wright, methylene blue, or acridine orange stain of the buffy coat or petechial lesions demonstrating microorganisms; metabolic acidosis; thrombocytopenia; prolonged prothrombin and partial thromboplastin times; reduced serum fibrinogen levels; anemia; decreased Pa_{O_2} and Pa_{CO_2}; and alterations in the morphology and number of neutrophils. Elevated neutrophil count and band count (increased immature white blood cells or "shift to the left") suggest bacterial infection, and neutropenia is an ominous sign of fulminant septic shock. Vacuolation of neutrophils, toxic granulations, and Döhle bodies are also suggestive of bacterial sepsis. Examination of the cerebrospinal fluid (CSF) may reveal neutrophils and bacteria. In early stages of meningitis, it may occasionally demonstrate only bacteria before the devel-

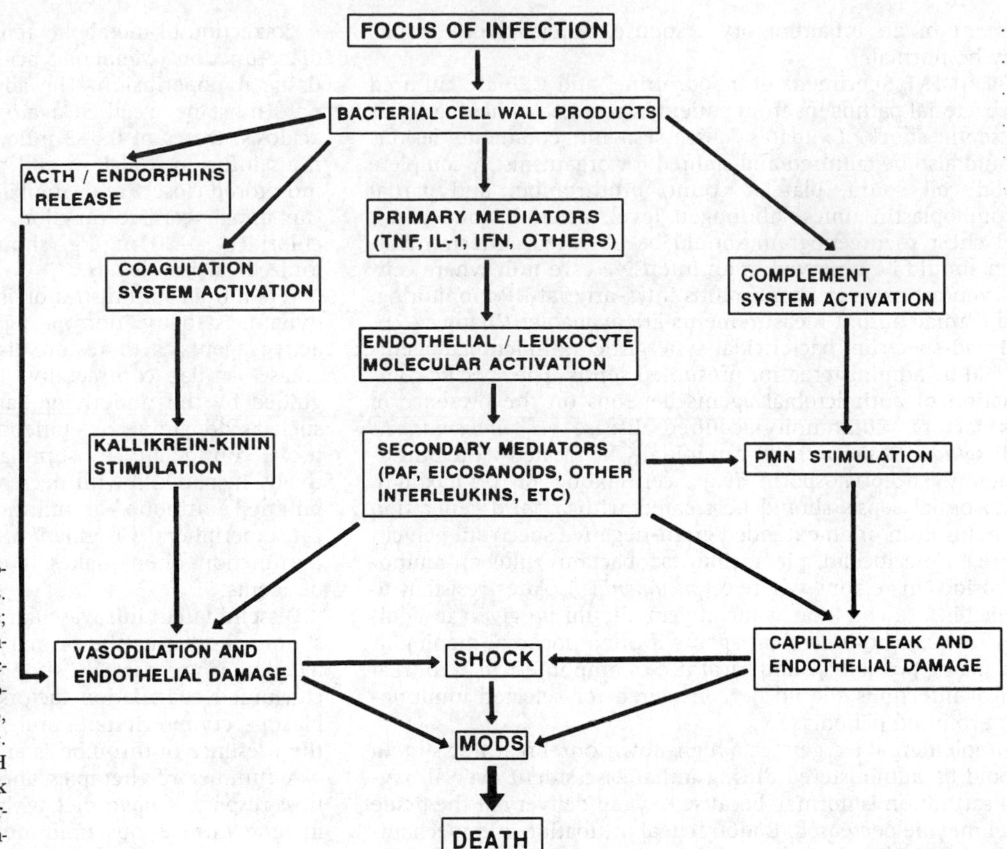

Figure 173–2 Hypothetical pathophysiology of the septic process. ACTH, adrenocorticotropic hormone; TNF, tumor necrosis factor; IL-1, interleukin-1; PAF, platelet activating factor; PMN, polymorphonuclear lymphocytes; IFN, interferon gamma; MODS, multiorgan dysfunction syndrome. (From Sáez-Llorens X, McCracken GH Jr: Sepsis syndrome and septic shock in pediatrics: Current concepts of terminology, pathophysiology, and management. J Pediatr 123:499, 1993.)

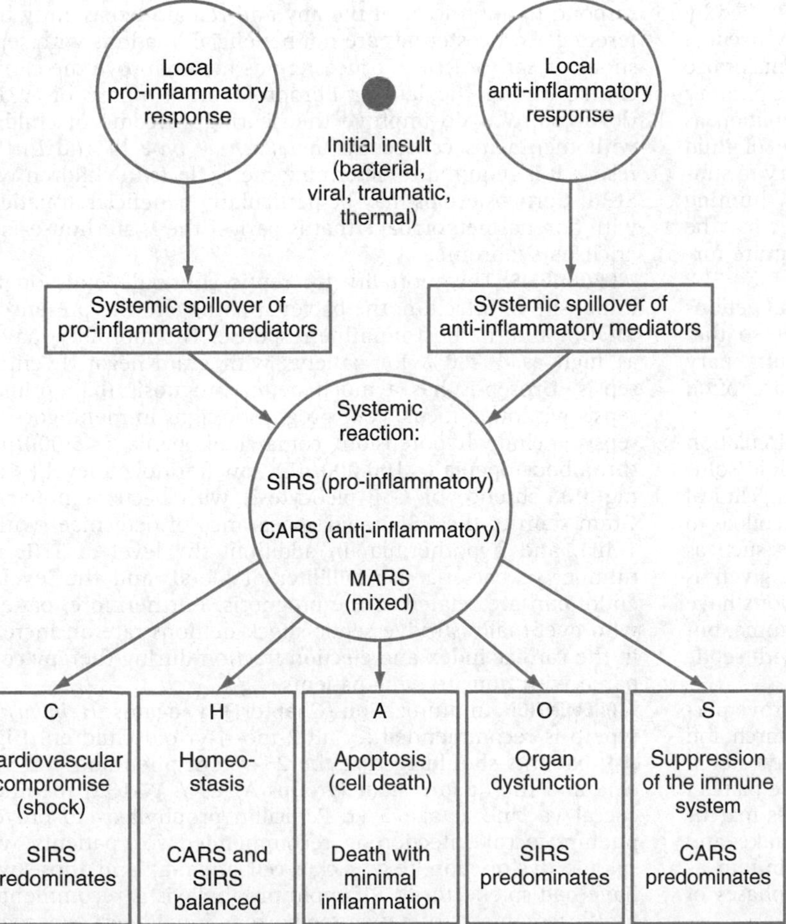

Figure 173–3 The hypothetical relationships between pro-inflammatory responses of the systemic inflammatory response syndrome (SIRS), compensatory anti-inflammatory syndrome (CARS), mixed anti-inflammatory syndrome (MARS), and the ensuing "CHAOS" are illustrated. (From Bone RC, Grodzin CJ, Balk RA: Sepsis: A new hypothesis for pathogenesis of the disease process. Chest 112:240, 1997.)

opment of an inflammatory response. Alternatively, results may be normal.

TREATMENT. Specimens of blood, urine, and CSF are cultured for bacterial pathogens from patients suspected of having sepsis or septic shock. Exudates, abscesses, and cutaneous lesions should also be cultured and stained for organisms. A complete blood cell count, platelet count, prothrombin and partial thromboplastin times, fibrinogen level, arterial blood gases, and chest roentgenogram should be obtained. Affected children should be observed in an intensive care unit where central venous pressure, continuous intra-arterial BP monitoring, and cardiac output measurements are available (Chapter 62).

Broad-spectrum bactericidal synergistic antimicrobial agents should be administered for presumed sepsis. The specific combination of antimicrobial agents depends on the presence of risk factors. Community-acquired disease (*H. influenzae, N. meningitidis, S. pneumoniae*) can initially be treated with a third-generation cephalosporin (e.g., ceftriaxone or cefotaxime). Nosocomial sepsis should be treated with a third-generation cephalosporin or an extended gram-negative spectrum penicillin (e.g., mezlocillin, piperacillin-tazobactam), plus an aminoglycoside. In regions where *S. pneumoniae* isolates resistant to penicillin are common, vancomycin should be given in addition to other antimicrobial agents if pneumococcal meningitis is a strong possibility. Empirical use of amphotericin B to treat fungal infections should be considered for selected immunocompromised patients.

Supplemental oxygen via a high-flow nonrebreathing system should be administered during initial assessment even if oxygen saturation is normal, because oxygen delivery at the tissue level may be decreased. Endotracheal intubation and mechanical ventilation may be necessary despite normal carbon dioxide levels and acceptable oxygenation because of the increased work of breathing and the increased oxygen consumption by respiratory muscles. When possible, the airway in patients with a deteriorating clinical condition should be controlled by elective intubation rather than waiting until urgently needed. Initially, 100% oxygen should be administered to maximize oxygen content and oxygen delivery. Positive end-expiratory pressure (PEEP) may be required to improve oxygenation as increased vascular permeability leads to the escape of fluid into the pulmonary interstitium. Hypoxemia refractory to supplemental oxygen suggests severe intrapulmonary shunting and the diagnosis of ARDS. Diffuse alveolar infiltrates may be seen on roentgenogram. Patients with ARDS may require further increases in PEEP. The cardiovascular effects of PEEP should be monitored by measuring pulmonary central venous pressures and pulmonary capillary wedge pressures so that fluids can be given without causing deterioration in pulmonary oxygen capacity. Sedation and muscle relaxation are often needed.

Once the airway and breathing are stabilized, the circulation should be addressed. Although only 25% of crystalloid solutions will remain in the intravascular compartment, clinical studies do not provide evidence of the superiority of colloid to crystalloid for volume expansion. Isotonic solutions such as normal saline and lactated Ringer solution should be given as rapid infusions of 20 mL/kg. Hypertonic saline solutions have been beneficial in patients suffering from burns or trauma, but there is limited experience in resuscitating patients with septic shock using hypertonic saline.

When crystalloid infusions are not sufficient to improve perfusion, 5% albumin should be given. Hydroxyethyl starch and dextran are not widely used in children. Hydroxyethyl starch can inhibit platelet aggregation, and dextran can cause platelet dysfunction, renal failure, and interfere with the cross matching of blood. With increased fluid losses, decreased intake, and increased microvascular permeability, volumes of albumin as large as 120 mL/kg may be required in the initial phases of resuscitation (Chapter 64.2).

Correction of metabolic abnormalities can also improve cardiac function. Metabolic acidosis often occurs secondary to tissue hypoperfusion. The adverse effects of sodium bicarbonate must be weighed against the benefits of correcting the acidosis. Doses of 0.5–2 mEq/kg are given slowly by intravenous infusion. Calcium and potassium levels should then be monitored closely and supplemented as needed. Hypocalcemia can impair cardiac function. Calcium given as 10% calcium chloride, 10–20 mg/kg, should be given to restore normal ionized calcium levels.

When fluid administration is unsuccessful in restoring hemodynamic stability, inotropic agents are added. The goal of vasoactive agents is to restore tissue perfusion pressure and increase cardiac contractility. The choice of agent should be guided by the underlying cardiovascular parameters. Agents such as dopamine or epinephrine increase afterload and improve contractility by stimulating α and β receptors, respectively. In patients with decreased peripheral perfusion, dobutamine, amrinone, or milrinone may increase inotropy and cause peripheral vasodilation. The complex etiology of cardiac dysfunction often makes it necessary to use a combination of agents.

Disseminated intravascular coagulation (DIC), if present, should resolve as the primary infectious disease is treated. If bleeding is present, DIC should be treated with replacement of consumed coagulation factors by transfusion of fresh frozen plasma, cryoprecipitate, and platelets. Heparin is indicated in the presence of thrombosis and peripheral gangrene.

A number of therapies aimed at modifying overexuberant host responses have met with limited success. Such therapies include intravenous immunoglobulin, monoclonal antiendotoxin antibodies, polyclonal antiendotoxin anticore antibodies, anti–TNF-α, IL-1 receptor antagonist, and granulocyte transfusions. Granulocyte transfusions are reserved for patients who have neutropenia before the septic episode and who do not respond to antimicrobial therapy and remain persistently bacteremic. Corticosteroids are not beneficial in adults with septic shock or early ARDS. Corticosteroids may improve the clinical course during the late or fibroproliferative phase of ARDS. Corticosteroids do improve the hearing outcome of children with meningitis caused by *H. influenzae* type b, and further research is required to determine their effects in children with SIRS. Corticosteroids may be particularly beneficial in patients with adrenal hemorrhage that is part of the Waterhouse-Friderichsen syndrome.

PROGNOSIS. The mortality for septic shock depends on the initial site of infection, the bacterial pathogen, the presence of MODS, and the host immune response. The mortality may be as high as 40–60% for patients with gram-negative enteric sepsis. Urosepsis has a much better prognosis than primary sepsis without a focus. Poor prognostic signs in meningococcal sepsis include hypotension, coma, leukopenia ($<5,000/\mu L$), thrombocytopenia ($<100,000/\mu L$), low fibrinogen level (<150 mg/dL), absence of CSF pleocytosis with bacteria noted on Gram stain of the CSF, rapid appearance of petechiae (within 1 hr), and hypothermia. In addition, the level of TNF, the number of bacteria per milliliter of blood, and the level of endotoxin are related to the prognosis. Furthermore, patients who eventually survive septic shock demonstrate an increase in the cardiac index and ejection fraction during therapy compared with nonsurviving patients.

PREVENTION. Immunization (Chapter 301) against *H. influenzae* type b is recommended for all 2-mo–4-yr-old children. High-risk patients should receive the 23-valent pneumococcal vaccine and the quadrivalent (groups A, C, Y, W-135) meningococcal vaccine at age 2 yr. Penicillin prophylaxis to prevent pneumococcal infection is recommended for patients with splenic dysfunction (e.g., sickle cell anemia) and those who have had splenectomy. Rifampin prophylaxis is recommended for close contacts of patients who may have been exposed to invasive *H. influenzae* or meningococcal disease (Chapters 191 and 193). Prevention of infection and sepsis in immunocompromised patients is discussed in Chapter 179.

Bone RC: Gram-positive organisms and sepsis. Arch Intern Med 154:26, 1994.
Bone RC, Grodzin LI, Balk RA: Sepsis: A new hypothesis for pathogenesis of the disease process. Chest 112:235, 1997.
Casey LC, Balk RA, Bone RC: Plasma cytokine and endotoxin levels correlate with survival in patients with sepsis syndrome. Ann Intern Med 119:771, 1993.
Davies MG, Hagen PO: Systemic inflammatory response syndrome. Br J Surg 84:920, 1997.
Dinarello CA, Wolf SM: The role of interleukin-1 in disease. N Engl J Med 328:106, 1993.
Dorinsky PM (ed): The sepsis syndrome. Clin Chest Med 17:175, 1996.
Kornelisse RF, Hazelzet JA, Hop WCJ, et al: Meningococcal septic shock in children: Clinical and laboratory features, outcome, and development of a prognostic score. Clin Infect Dis 25:640, 1997.
Sáez-Llorens X, McCracken GH Jr: Sepsis syndrome and septic shock in pediatrics: Current concepts of terminology, pathophysiology, and management. J Pediatr 123:497, 1993.

Chapter 174
Central Nervous System Infections

Charles G. Prober

Acute infection of the central nervous system (CNS) is the most common cause of fever associated with signs and symptoms of CNS disease in children. Infection may be caused by virtually any microbe, the specific pathogen being influenced by the age and immune status of the host and the epidemiology of the pathogen. In general, viral infections of the CNS are much more common than bacterial infections, which in turn are more common than fungal and parasitic infections. Infections caused by rickettsiae (e.g., Rocky Mountain spotted fever and *Ehrlichia*) are relatively uncommon but assume important roles under certain epidemiologic circumstances. *Mycoplasma* spp also can cause infections of the CNS, although their precise contribution often is difficult to determine.

Regardless of etiology, most patients with acute CNS infection have similar clinical syndromes. Common symptoms include headache, nausea, vomiting, anorexia, restlessness, and irritability. Unfortunately, most of these symptoms are quite nonspecific. Common signs of CNS infection, in addition to fever, include photophobia, neck pain and rigidity, obtundation, stupor, coma, seizures, and focal neurologic deficits. The severity and constellation of signs are determined by the specific pathogen, the host, and the anatomic distribution of the infection. The anatomic distribution of infection may be diffuse or focal. Meningitis and encephalitis are examples of diffuse infection. Meningitis implies primary involvement of the meninges, whereas encephalitis indicates brain parenchymal involvement. Because these anatomic boundaries are often not distinct, many patients have evidence of both meningeal and parenchymal involvement and should be considered to have meningoencephalitis. Brain abscess is the best example of a focal infection of the CNS. The neurologic expression of this infection is determined by the site and extent of the abscess(es).

The diagnosis of diffuse CNS infections depends on careful examination of cerebrospinal fluid (CSF) obtained by lumbar puncture (LP). Table 174–1 provides an overview of the expected CSF abnormalities with various CNS disorders.

174.1 Acute Bacterial Meningitis Beyond the Neonatal Period

Bacterial meningitis is one of the most potentially serious infections in infants and older children. This infection is associated with a high rate of acute complications and risk of chronic morbidity. The pattern of bacterial meningitis and its treatment during the neonatal period (0–28 days) are generally distinct from those in older infants and children (Chapters 105 and 106). Nonetheless, the clinical patterns of meningitis in the neonatal and postneonatal periods may overlap, especially in 1- to 2-mo-old patients, in whom group B *Streptococcus, Streptococcus pneumoniae* (pneumococcus), *Neisseria meningitidis* (meningococcus), and *Haemophilus influenzae* type b all may cause meningitis.

The incidence of bacterial meningitis is sufficiently high that it should be included in the differential diagnosis of altered mental status such as lethargy or irritability, or evidence of other neurologic dysfunction, in febrile infants.

ETIOLOGY. During the first 2 mo of life, the bacteria that cause meningitis in normal infants reflect the maternal flora or the environment of the infant (i.e., group B *Streptococcus*, gram-negative enteric bacilli, and *Listeria monocytogenes*). In addition, meningitis in this age group may occasionally be due to *H. influenzae* (both type b and nontypable strains) and the other pathogens usually found in older patients.

Bacterial meningitis in children 2 mo–12 yr of age is usually due to *S. pneumoniae, N. meningitidis,* or *H. influenzae* type b. Before the widespread use of *H. influenzae* type b vaccines, approximately 70% of cases of bacterial meningitis among children younger than 5 yr were due to *H. influenzae* type b. Subsequent to the implementation of universal immunization against these bacteria, beginning at about 2 mo of age, the incidence of *H. influenzae* type b meningitis dropped precipitously. The median age of bacterial meningitis in the United States increased from age 15 mo in 1986 to 25 yr in 1995; meningitis now is usually due to *S. pneumoniae* or *N. meningitidis*.

Alterations of host defense due to anatomic defects or immune deficits increase the risk of meningitis from less common pathogens such as *Pseudomonas aeruginosa, Staphylococcus aureus,* coagulase-negative staphylococci, *Salmonella* spp, and *L. monocytogenes.*

EPIDEMIOLOGY. A major risk factor for meningitis is the lack of immunity to specific pathogens associated with young age. Additional risks include recent colonization with pathogenic bacteria, close contact (e.g., household, daycare centers, schools, military barracks) with individuals having invasive disease, crowding, poverty, black race, male sex, and possibly absence of breast-feeding for infants 2–5 mo of age. The mode of transmission is probably person to person contact through respiratory tract secretions or droplets. The risk of meningitis is increased among infants and young children with occult bacteremia (Chapter 172); the odds ratio is greater for meningococcus (85 times) and *H. influenzae* type b (12 times) relative to that for pneumococcus. Specific host defense defects due to altered immunoglobulin production in response to encapsulated pathogens may be responsible for the increased risk of bacterial meningitis in Native Americans and Eskimos, whereas defects of the complement system (C5–C8) have been associated with recurrent meningococcal infection, and defects of the properdin system have been associated with a significant risk of lethal meningococcal disease. Splenic dysfunction (sickle cell anemia) or asplenia (due to trauma, congenital defect, staging of Hodgkin disease) is associated with an increased risk of pneumococcal, *H. influenzae* type b (to some extent), and, rarely, meningococcal sepsis and meningitis. T-lymphocyte defects (congenital or acquired by chemotherapy, AIDS, or malignancy) are associated with an increased risk of

L. monocytogenes infections of the CNS. Congenital or acquired CSF leak across a mucocutaneous barrier, such as cranial or midline facial defects (cribriform plate) and middle ear (stapedial foot plate) or inner ear fistulas (oval window, internal auditory canal, cochlear aqueduct), or CSF leakage through a rupture of the meninges due to a basal skull fracture into the cribriform plate or paranasal sinus, is associated with an increased risk of pneumococcal meningitis. Lumbosacral dermal sinus and meningomyelocele are associated with staphylococcal and gram-negative enteric bacterial meningitis. Penetrating cranial trauma and CSF shunt infections increase the risk of meningitis due to staphylococci (especially coagulase-negative species) and other cutaneous bacteria.

Streptococcus pneumoniae. The risk of sepsis and meningitis due to pneumococcus depends, at least in part, on the infecting serotype. Throat or nasopharyngeal carriage of *S. pneumoniae* is acquired from family contacts after birth, is transient (2–4 mo), is often associated with homotype antibody production, and, if recent (<1 mo), is a risk factor for serious infection. The incidence of pneumococcal meningitis is 1–3/100,000 persons; infection may occur throughout life. The midwinter months are the peak season. The risk of meningitis is 5- to 36-fold greater among blacks than whites, especially among blacks with sickle cell anemia, who have a more than 300-fold increased incidence compared with white children. Approximately 4% of children with sickle cell anemia develop pneumococcal meningitis before the age of 5 yr if they are not given prophylactic antibiotics. Additional risk factors for contracting pneumococcal meningitis include otitis media, sinusitis, pneumonia, CSF otorrhea or rhinorrhea, splenectomy, HIV infection, and chronic graft versus host disease following bone marrow transplantation.

Neisseria meningitidis. Meningococcal meningitis may be sporadic or may occur in epidemics. In the absence of an epidemic, most infections are due to group B. Epidemics usually are caused by groups A and C. Cases occur throughout the year but may be more common in the winter and spring. Nasopharyngeal carriage of *N. meningitidis* occurs in 1–15% of adults. Colonization may last weeks to months; recent colonization places nonimmune younger children at greatest risk for meningitis. The incidence of simultaneous disease occurring in association with an index case in the family is 1%, a rate that is 1,000-fold the risk in the general population. The risk of secondary cases occurring in contacts at daycare centers is about 1/1,000. Most infections of children are acquired from a contact in a daycare facility, a colonized adult family member, or an ill patient with meningococcal disease.

***Haemophilus influenzae* type b.** Before universal *H. influenzae* type b vaccination in the United States, invasive infections occurred primarily in infants 2 mo–2 yr of age; peak incidence was at 6–9 mo of age, and 50% of cases occurred in the 1st yr of life. The risk to children was markedly increased among family or daycare center contacts of patients with *H. influenzae* type b disease. Unvaccinated individuals and those with blunted immunologic responses to vaccine (e.g., children with HIV infection) remain at risk for *H. influenzae* type b meningitis.

PATHOLOGY. A meningeal exudate of varying thickness may be distributed around the cerebral veins, venous sinuses, convexity of the brain, and cerebellum and in the sulci, sylvian fissures, basal cisterns, and spinal cord. Ventriculitis with bacteria and inflammatory cells in ventricular fluid may be present, as may subdural effusions and, rarely, empyema. Perivascular inflammatory infiltrates may also be present, and the ependymal membrane may be disrupted. Vascular and parenchymal cerebral changes characterized by polymorphonuclear infiltrates extending to the subintimal region of the small arteries and veins, vasculitis, thrombosis of small cortical veins, occlusion of major venous sinuses, necrotizing arteritis producing subarachnoid hemorrhage, and, rarely, cerebral cortical necrosis in the absence of identifiable thrombosis have been described at autopsy. Cerebral infarction is a frequent sequela of vascular occlusion from inflammation, vasospasm, and thrombosis. Infarct size ranges from microscopic to involvement of an entire hemisphere.

Inflammation of spinal nerves and roots produces meningeal signs, and inflammation of the cranial nerves produces cranial neuropathies of optic, oculomotor, facial, and auditory nerves. Increased intracranial pressure (ICP) also produces oculomotor nerve palsy due to the presence of temporal lobe compression of the nerve during tentorial herniation. Abducens nerve palsy may be a nonlocalizing sign of raised ICP.

Increased ICP is due to cell death (cytotoxic cerebral edema), cytokine-induced increased capillary vascular permeability (vasogenic cerebral edema), and, possibly, increased hydrostatic pressure (interstitial cerebral edema) after obstructed reabsorption of CSF in the arachnoid villus or obstruction of the flow of fluid from the ventricles. ICP often exceeds 300 mm H_2O; cerebral perfusion may be further compromised if the cerebral perfusion pressure (mean arterial pressure minus ICP) is less than 50 cm H_2O owing to reduced cerebral blood flow. Syndrome of inappropriate antidiuretic hormone secretion (SIADH) may produce excessive water retention, increasing the risk of raised ICP. Hypotonicity of brain extracellular spaces may cause cytotoxic edema after cell swelling and lysis. Tentorial, falx, or cerebellar herniation does not usually occur because the increased ICP is transmitted to the entire subarachnoid space and there is little structural displacement. Furthermore, if the fontanels are still patent, increased ICP is readily dissipated.

Hydrocephalus is an uncommon acute complication of meningitis occurring after the neonatal period. It most often takes the form of a communicating hydrocephalus due to adhesive thickening of the arachnoid villi around the cisterns at the base of the brain. Thus, there is interference with the normal resorption of CSF. Less often, obstructive hydrocephalus develops after fibrosis and gliosis of the aqueduct of Sylvius or the foramina of Magendie and Luschka.

Raised CSF protein levels are due in part to increased vascular permeability of the blood-brain barrier and the loss of albumin-rich fluid from the capillaries and veins traversing the subdural space. Continued transudation may result in subdural effusions, usually found in the later phase of acute bacterial meningitis. Hypoglycorrhachia (reduced CSF glucose levels) is due to decreased glucose transport by the cerebral tissue.

Damage to the cerebral cortex may be due to the focal or diffuse effects of vascular occlusion (infarction, necrosis, lactic acidosis), hypoxia, bacterial invasion (cerebritis), toxic encephalopathy (bacterial toxins), raised ICP, ventriculitis, and transudation (subdural effusions). These pathologic factors result in the clinical manifestations of impaired consciousness, seizures, hydrocephalus, cranial nerve deficits, motor and sensory deficits, and later psychomotor retardation.

PATHOGENESIS. Bacterial meningitis most commonly results from hematogenous dissemination of microorganisms from a distant site of infection; bacteremia usually precedes meningitis or occurs concomitantly. Bacterial colonization of the nasopharynx with a potentially pathogenic microorganism is the usual source of the bacteremia. There may be prolonged carriage of the colonizing organisms without disease or, more likely, rapid invasion after recent colonization. Prior or concurrent viral upper respiratory tract infection may enhance the pathogenicity of bacteria producing meningitis.

N. meningitidis and *H. influenzae* type b attach to mucosal epithelial cell receptors by pili. After attachment to epithelial cells, bacteria breach the mucosa and enter the circulation. *N. meningitidis* may be transported across the mucosal surface within a phagocytic vacuole after ingestion by the epithelial cell. Bacterial survival in the bloodstream is enhanced by large bacterial capsules that interfere with opsonic phagocytosis and are associated with increased virulence. Host-related developmental defects in bacterial opsonic phagocytosis also contribute to the bacteremia. In young, nonimmune hosts, the defect may be due to an absence of preformed IgM or IgG anticapsular antibodies, whereas in immunodeficient patients, various deficiencies of components of the complement or properdin system may interfere with effective opsonic phagocytosis. Direct activation of the antibody-independent properdin system is one mechanism that counteracts the effects of antibody deficiency and the antiphagocytic properties of the bacterial capsule. Splenic dysfunction also may reduce opsonic phagocytosis by the reticuloendothelial system.

Bacteria gain entry to the CSF through the choroid plexus of the lateral ventricles and the meninges and then circulate to the extracerebral CSF and subarachnoid space. Bacteria rapidly multiply because the CSF concentrations of complement and antibody are inadequate to contain bacterial proliferation. Chemotactic factors then incite a local inflammatory response characterized by polymorphonuclear cell infiltration. The presence of bacterial cell wall lipopolysaccharide (endotoxin) of gram-negative bacteria (*H. influenzae* type b, *N. meningitidis*) and of pneumococcal cell wall components (teichoic acid, peptidoglycan) stimulates a marked inflammatory response, with local production of tumor necrosis factor, interleukin-1, prostaglandin E, and other cytokine inflammatory mediators. The subsequent inflammatory response, directly related to the presence of these inflammatory mediators, is characterized by neutrophilic infiltration, increased vascular permeability, alterations of the blood-brain barrier, and vascular thrombosis. Excessive cytokine-induced inflammation continues after the CSF has been sterilized and is thought to be partly responsible for the chronic inflammatory sequelae of pyogenic meningitis.

Meningitis may rarely follow bacterial invasion from a contiguous focus of infection such as paranasal sinusitis, otitis media, mastoiditis, orbital cellulitis, or cranial or vertebral osteomyelitis or may occur after introduction of bacteria via penetrating cranial trauma, dermal sinus tracts, or meningomyeloceles. Meningitis may occur during endocarditis, pneumonia, or thrombophlebitis. It also may be associated with severe burns, indwelling catheters, or contaminated infusion equipment.

CLINICAL MANIFESTATIONS. The onset of acute meningitis has two predominant patterns. The more dramatic and, fortunately, less common presentation is sudden onset with rapidly progressive manifestations of shock, purpura, disseminated intravascular coagulation (DIC) and reduced levels of consciousness frequently resulting in death within 24 hr. More often, meningitis is preceded by several days of upper respiratory tract or gastrointestinal symptoms, followed by nonspecific signs of CNS infection such as increasing lethargy and irritability.

The signs and symptoms of meningitis are related to the nonspecific findings associated with a systemic infection and to manifestations of meningeal irritation. Nonspecific findings include fever (present in 90–95%), anorexia and poor feeding, symptoms of upper respiratory tract infection, myalgias, arthralgias, tachycardia, hypotension, and various cutaneous signs, such as petechiae, purpura, or an erythematous macular rash. Meningeal irritation is manifested as nuchal rigidity, back pain, Kernig sign (flexion of the hip 90 degrees with subsequent pain with extension of the leg), and Brudzinski sign (involuntary flexion of the knees and hips after passive flexion of the neck while supine). In some children, particularly in those younger than 12–18 mo, Kernig and Brudzinski signs may not be evident with meningitis. Increased ICP is suggested by headache, emesis, bulging fontanel or diastasis (widening) of the sutures, oculomotor or abducens nerve paralysis, hypertension with bradycardia, apnea or hyperventilation, decorticate or decerebrate posturing, stupor, coma, or signs of herniation. Papilledema is uncommon in uncomplicated meningitis and should suggest a more chronic process, such as the presence of an intracranial abscess, subdural empyema, or occlusion of a dural venous sinus. Focal neurologic signs usually are due to vascular occlusion. Cranial neuropathies of the ocular, oculomotor, abducens, facial, and auditory nerves also may be due to focal inflammation. Overall, about 10–20% of children with bacterial meningitis have focal neurologic signs. This frequency increases to more than 30% with pneumococcal meningitis, because this organism tends to stimulate the most vigorous inflammatory response.

Seizures (focal or generalized) due to cerebritis, infarction, or electrolyte disturbances occur in 20–30% of patients with meningitis. Seizures that occur on presentation or within the first 4 days of onset are usually of no prognostic significance. Seizures that persist after the 4th day of illness and those that are difficult to treat are associated with a poor prognosis.

Alterations of mental status and a reduced level of consciousness are common among patients with meningitis and may be due to increased ICP, cerebritis, or hypotension; manifestations include irritability, lethargy, stupor, obtundation, and coma. Comatose patients have a poor prognosis. Additional manifestations of meningitis include photophobia and tache cérébrale, which is elicited by stroking the skin with a blunt object and observing a raised red streak within 30–60 sec.

DIAGNOSIS. The diagnosis of acute pyogenic meningitis is confirmed by analysis of the CSF, which reveals microorganisms on Gram stain and culture, a neutrophilic pleocytosis, elevated protein, and reduced glucose concentrations (Table 174–1). LP should be performed when bacterial meningitis is suspected. Contraindications for an immediate LP include (1) evidence of increased ICP (other than a bulging fontanel), such as 3rd or 6th cranial nerve palsy with a depressed level of consciousness, or hypertension and bradycardia with respiratory abnormalities; (2) severe cardiopulmonary compromise requiring prompt resuscitative measures for shock or in patients in whom positioning for the LP would further compromise cardiopulmonary function; and (3) infection of the skin overlying the site of the LP. Thrombocytopenia is a relative contraindication for immediate LP. If an LP is delayed, immediate empirical therapy should be initiated. CT scanning for evidence of a brain abscess or increased ICP also should not delay therapy. LP may be performed after increased ICP has been treated or a brain abscess has been excluded.

A number of bacterial antigen detection systems have been developed, the most popular and widely used being based on latex particle agglutination. In the presence of bacterial meningitis, antigen is most consistently detected in the CSF. Antigenuria also is quite common. Serum is not a useful specimen for antigen detection because false-positive reactions are common. Tests for antigen are best reserved for patients who were receiving antibiotics when their cultures were obtained, because antigen may remain detectable for several days after the initiation of antibiotics, whereas cultures may be negative. Recent immunization with the *H. influenzae* type b polysaccharide vaccine may produce a false-positive result of the antigen test in serum and urine but not in CSF.

Blood cultures should be performed in all patients with suspected meningitis. Blood cultures may reveal the responsible bacteria in 80–90% of cases of childhood meningitis.

Lumbar Puncture. LP is usually performed with a patient in the flexed lateral decubitus position; the styletted needle is passed into the L3–L4 or L4–L5 intervertebral space. After entry into the subarachnoid space, the patient's position is changed to a more extended one to measure the opening CSF pressure, although an accurate reading may not be able to be determined in a crying child. When the pressure is high, only a small volume of CSF should be removed to avoid a precipitous decline in ICP.

The CSF leukocyte count in bacterial meningitis is usually elevated to greater than 1,000/mm^3 and reveals a neutrophilic predominance (75–95%). Turbid CSF is present when the CSF leukocyte count exceeds 200–400/mm³. Normal healthy neonates may have as many as 30 leukocytes/mm³, and older children without viral or bacterial meningitis may have 5 leukocytes/mm³ in the CSF; in both age groups there is a predominance of lymphocytes or monocytes.

A CSF leukocyte count less than 250/mm³ may be present in as many as 20% of patients with acute bacterial meningitis; pleocytosis may be absent in patients with severe overwhelming sepsis and meningitis and is a poor prognostic sign. Pleocytosis with a lymphocyte predominance may be present during the early stage of acute bacterial meningitis; conversely, neutrophilic pleocytosis may be present in patients during the early stages of acute viral meningitis. The shift to lymphocytic-monocytic predominance in viral meningitis invariably occurs within 12–24 hr of the initial LP. The Gram stain is positive in most (70–90%) patients with bacterial meningitis.

Traumatic LP complicates the diagnosis of meningitis. Repeat LP at another interspace may produce less hemorrhagic fluid, but this fluid usually also contains red blood cells. Interpretation of CSF leukocytes and protein concentration are affected by LPs that are traumatic, although the gram stain, culture, and glucose level may not be influenced. Although methods for correcting for the presence of red blood cells have been proposed, it is prudent to rely on the bacteriologic results rather than to attempt to interpret the CSF leukocyte and protein results of a traumatic LP.

Differential Diagnosis. In addition to *S. pneumoniae, N. meningitidis,* and *H. influenzae* type b, many other microorganisms can cause generalized infection of the CNS with similar clinical manifestations. These organisms include less typical bacteria, such as *Mycobacterium tuberculosis, Nocardia, Treponema pallidum* (syphilis), and *Borrelia burgdorferi* (Lyme disease); fungi, such as those endemic to specific geographic areas (*Coccidioides, Histoplasma,* and *Blastomyces*) and those responsible for infections in compromised hosts (*Candida, Cryptococcus,* and *Aspergillus*); parasites, such as *Toxoplasma gondii* and those that cause cysticercosis, resulting from infection with the larval stages (*Cysticercus cellulosae*) of the pork tapeworm *Taenia solium*; and, most frequently, viruses. Focal infections of the CNS including brain abscess and parameningeal abscess (subdural empyema, cranial and spinal epidural abscess) also may be confused with meningitis. Noninfectious illnesses also can cause generalized inflammation of the CNS. These disorders are uncommon relative to infections and include malignancy, collagen vascular syndromes, and exposure to toxins.

Determining the specific cause is facilitated by careful examination of the CSF with specific stains (Kinyoun carbol fuchsin for mycobacteria, India ink for fungi), cytology, antigen detection (bacteria, *Cryptococcus*), serology (syphilis), and viral culture (enterovirus). Other potentially valuable diagnostic tests include CT or MRI of the brain, blood cultures, serologic tests, and possibly brain biopsy. Acute viral meningoencephalitis is the most likely infection to be confused with bacterial meningitis. Although, in general, children with viral meningoencephalitis appear less ill than those with bacterial meningitis, both types of infection have a spectrum of severity. Some children with bacterial meningitis may have relatively mild signs and symptoms, whereas some with viral meningoencephalitis may be critically ill. The classic CSF profiles associated with bacterial versus viral infection tend to be distinct (Table 174–1), but as with clinical manifestations, specific test results may have considerable overlap.

Another diagnostic conundrum in the evaluation of children with suspected bacterial meningitis is the analysis of CSF obtained from children already receiving antibiotic therapy. This is an important issue, because 25–50% of children being evaluated for bacterial meningitis are receiving oral antibiotics when their CSF is obtained. Such partial treatment of a patient with acute bacterial meningitis usually does not substantially alter the typical bacterial CSF profile. Although the frequency of positive CSF Gram stain results and ability to grow the bacteria may be reduced, the concentration of CSF glucose and protein and the neutrophil profile are not substantially altered by pretreatment.

TREATMENT. The therapeutic approach to patients with presumed bacterial meningitis depends on the nature of the initial manifestations of the illness. A child with rapidly progressing disease of less than 24 hr duration, in the absence of increased ICP, should receive antibiotics immediately after an LP is performed. If there are signs of increased ICP or focal neurologic findings, antibiotics should be given without performing an LP and before obtaining a CT scan. Increased ICP should be treated simultaneously. Immediate treatment of associated multiple organ system failure, such as shock and adult respiratory distress syndrome, is also indicated.

Patients who have a more protracted subacute course and become ill over a 1- to 7-day period should also be evaluated for signs of increased ICP and focal neurologic deficits. Unilateral headache, papilledema, and other signs of increased ICP suggest a focal lesion such as a brain or epidural abscess, or subdural empyema. Under these circumstances, antibiotic therapy should be initiated before LP and CT scanning. If no signs of increased ICP are evident, an LP should be performed.

Initial Antibiotic Therapy. The initial (empiric) choice of therapy for meningitis in immunocompetent infants and children should be based on the antibiotic susceptibilities of *S. pneumoniae, N. meningitidis,* and *H. influenzae* type b. Selected antibiotic(s) should achieve bactericidal levels in the CSF. Although there are substantial geographic differences in the frequency of resistance of *S. pneumoniae* to antibiotics, rates are increasing throughout the world. In the United States, 25–50% of strains of *S. pneumoniae* are currently resistant to penicillin; relative resistance (MIC, 0.1–1.0 μg/mL) is more common than high-level resistance (MIC > 2.0 μg/mL). Resistance to cefotaxime and ceftriaxone also is evident in 5–10% of isolates. Most strains of *N. meningitidis* are sensitive to penicillin and cephalosporins, although rare resistant isolates have been reported. Approximately 30–40% of isolates of *H. influenzae* type b produce β-lactamases and therefore are resistant to ampicillin. These β-lactamase–producing strains remain sensitive to the extended-spectrum cephalosporins.

The increasing frequency of *S. pneumoniae* resistance to β-lactam drugs has necessitated a change in empirical therapy in most regions of the United States. Currently, either of the third-generation cephalosporins, cefotaxime (200 mg/kg/24 hr, given every 6 hr) or ceftriaxone (100 mg/kg/24 hr administered once per day or 50 mg/kg/dose, given every 12 hr), combined with vancomycin (60 mg/kg/24 hr, given every 6 hr) is recommended. Patients allergic to β-lactam antibiotics should be treated with chloramphenicol, 100 mg/kg/24 hr, given every 6 hr.

If *L. monocytogenes* infection is suspected, as in infants 1–2 mo old or patients with a T-lymphocyte deficiency, ampicillin (200 mg/kg/24 hr, given every 6 hr) should be given with ceftriaxone or cefotaxime because all cephalosporins are inactive against *L. monocytogenes.* Intravenous trimethoprim-sulfamethoxazole is an alternate treatment for *L. monocytogenes.*

If a patient is immunocompromised and gram-negative bacterial meningitis is suspected, initial therapy might include ceftazidime and an aminoglycoside.

Duration of Antibiotic Therapy. Therapy for uncomplicated penicillin-sensitive *S. pneumoniae* meningitis should be completed with a third-generation cephalosporin or intravenous penicillin (300,000 U/kg/24 hr, given every 4–6 hr) for 10–14 days. If the isolate is resistant to penicillin and the third-generation cephalosporin, therapy should be completed with vancomycin. Intravenous penicillin (300,000 U/kg/24 hr) for 5–7 days is the treatment of choice for uncomplicated *N. meningitidis* meningitis. Uncomplicated *H. influenzae* type b meningitis should be treated for a total of 7–10 days. Ampicillin should be used to complete the course of therapy if the isolate is found to be sensitive.

Patients who receive intravenous or oral antibiotics before LP and who do not have an identifiable pathogen (on Gram stain, culture, or antigen detection) but do have evidence of an acute bacterial infection on the basis of their CSF profile should continue to receive therapy with ceftriaxone or cefotaxime for 7–10 days. If focal signs are present or the child does not respond to treatment, a parameningeal focus may be present and a CT or MRI scan should be performed.

A routine repeat LP is not indicated in patients with uncomplicated meningitis due to antibiotic-sensitive *S. pneumoniae, N. meningitidis*, or *H. influenzae* type b. Repeat examination of CSF is indicated in some neonates, in patients with gram-negative bacillary meningitis, or in infection caused by a β-lactam–resistant *S. pneumoniae*. Improvement in the CSF profile is indicated by an increase in CSF glucose concentration and the appearance of lymphocyte-monocyte cells. The CSF should be sterile within 24–48 hr of initiation of appropriate antibiotic therapy.

Meningitis due to *E. coli* or *P. aeruginosa* requires therapy with a third-generation cephalosporin active against the isolate in vitro. Most isolates of *E. coli* are sensitive to cefotaxime or ceftriaxone, whereas most isolates of *P. aeruginosa* are sensitive to ceftazidime. Gram-negative bacillary meningitis should be treated for 3 wk or for at least 2 wk after CSF sterilization, which may occur after 2–10 days of treatment.

Side effects of antibiotic therapy of meningitis include phlebitis, drug fever, rash, emesis, oral candidiasis, and diarrhea. Ceftriaxone may cause reversible gallbladder pseudolithiasis, detectable by abdominal ultrasonography. This is usually asymptomatic but may produce emesis and right upper quadrant pain.

Corticosteroids. Rapid killing of bacteria in the CSF effectively sterilizes the meningeal infection but releases toxic cell products after cell lysis (cell wall endotoxin) that precipitates the cytokine-mediated inflammatory response. The resultant edema formation and neutrophilic infiltration may produce additional neurologic injury with worsening of CNS signs and symptoms. Therefore, agents that limit production of inflammatory mediators may be of benefit to patients with bacterial meningitis.

Data support the use of intravenous dexamethasone, 0.15 mg/kg/dose given every 6 hr for 2 days, in the treatment of children older than 6 wk with acute bacterial meningitis, especially for *H. influenzae* type b. A regimen of 0.4 mg/kg/dose given every 12 hr for 2 days is also appropriate. Corticosteroid recipients have less fever, lower CSF protein and lactate levels, and a reduction in permanent auditory nerve damage, as manifested by sensorineural hearing loss, than do placebo recipients. Most experience with dexamethasone treatment has been with *H. influenzae* type b infection, and extrapolation to other bacterial pathogens should be done with caution, balancing potential benefits against risks. Corticosteroids appear to have maximum benefit if given just before antibiotics and should be administered with 1–2 hr of antibiotics. Complications of the 2-day regimen are uncommon but may include gastrointestinal bleeding, hypertension, hyperglycemia, leukocytosis, and rebound fever after the last dose. No evidence shows that dexamethasone for longer than 2 days offers additional benefit, and it appears to be associated with an increased incidence of gastrointestinal bleeding.

Supportive Care. Repeated medical and neurologic assessments of patients with bacterial meningitis are essential to identify early signs of cardiovascular, CNS, and metabolic complications. Pulse rate, blood pressure, and respiratory rate should be monitored frequently. Neurologic assessment, including pupillary reflexes, level of consciousness, motor strength, cranial nerve signs, and evaluation for seizures, should be made frequently during the first 72 hr, when the risk of neurologic complications is greatest. Thereafter, neurologic assessment should be performed once a day. Important laboratory studies include an assessment of blood urea nitrogen; serum sodium, chloride, potassium, and bicarbonate levels; urine output and specific gravity; complete blood and platelet counts; and coagulation factors (fibrinogen, prothrombin, and partial thromboplastin times) in the presence of petechiae, purpura, or abnormal bleeding.

Patients should initially receive nothing by mouth. If a patient is judged to be normovolemic, with normal blood pressure, intravenous fluid administration should be restricted to one half to two thirds of maintenance, or 800–1,000 mL/m²/24 hr, until it can be established that increased ICP or SIADH is not present. Fluid administration may be returned to normal (1,500–1,700 mL/m²/24 hr) when serum sodium levels are normal. Fluid restriction is not appropriate in the presence of systemic hypotension because reduced blood pressure may result in a cerebral perfusion pressure of less than 50 cm H_2O, with subsequent CNS ischemia. Therefore, shock must be treated aggressively to prevent brain and other organ dysfunction (acute tubular necrosis, adult respiratory distress syndrome). Patients with shock, a markedly raised ICP, coma, and refractory seizures require intensive monitoring with central arterial and venous access and frequent vital signs, necessitating admission to a pediatric intensive care unit. Patients with septic shock require fluid resuscitation and therapy with vasoactive agents such as dopamine, epinephrine, and sodium nitroprusside (Chapter 173). The goal of such therapy in patients with meningitis is to avoid excessive increases in ICP without compromising blood flow and oxygen delivery to vital organs (brain, heart, lung, kidney).

Neurologic complications include increased ICP with subsequent herniation, seizures, and an enlarging head circumference due to a subdural effusion or hydrocephalus. Signs of increased ICP (other than a bulging fontanel or isolated coma) should be treated emergently with endotracheal intubation and hyperventilation (to maintain the P_{CO_2} at approximately 25 mm Hg). In addition, intravenous furosemide (Lasix, 1 mg/kg) and mannitol (0.5–1 g/kg) osmotherapy may reduce ICP (Chapter 64.7). Furosemide may reduce brain swelling by venodilation and diuresis without increasing intracranial blood volume, whereas mannitol produces an osmolar gradient between the brain and plasma, thus shifting fluid from the CNS to the plasma with subsequent excretion during an osmotic diuresis.

Seizures are common during the course of bacterial meningitis. Immediate therapy for seizures includes intravenous diazepam (0.1–0.2 mg/kg/dose) or lorazepam (0.05 mg/kg/dose), paying careful attention to the risk of respiratory suppression. Serum glucose, calcium, and sodium levels should be monitored to determine if hypoglycemia, hypocalcemia, or hyponatremia is precipitating seizures. After immediate management of seizures, patients should receive phenytoin (15–20 mg/kg loading dose, 5 mg/kg/24 hr maintenance) to reduce the likelihood of recurrence. Phenytoin is preferred to phenobarbital because it produces less CNS depression and permits assessment of a patient's level of consciousness. Serum phenytoin levels should be monitored to maintain them in the therapeutic range (10–20 μg/mL).

COMPLICATIONS. During the treatment of meningitis, complications due to CNS or systemic effects of infection are common. Neurologic complications include seizures, increased ICP, cranial nerve palsies, stroke, cerebral or cerebellar herniation, transverse myelitis, ataxia, thrombosis of dural venous sinuses, and subdural effusions.

Collections of fluid in the subdural space develop in 10–30% of patients with meningitis and are asymptomatic in 85–90% of patients. Subdural effusions are especially common in infants. Symptomatic subdural effusions may result in a bulging fontanel, diastasis of sutures, enlarging head circumference, emesis, seizures, fever, and abnormal results of cranial transillumination. However, many of these manifestations are also present in patients with meningitis without subdural effusion. CT or MRI scanning confirms the presence of a subdural effusion. In the presence of increased ICP or a depressed level of consciousness, symptomatic subdural effusion should be treated by aspiration through the open fontanel. Fever alone is not an indication for aspiration.

SIADH occurs in the majority of patients with meningitis, resulting in hyponatremia and reduced serum osmolality in 30–50%. This may exacerbate cerebral edema or independently produce hyponatremic seizures. Later in the course of therapy, central diabetes insipidus may develop as a result of hypothalamic or pituitary dysfunction.

Fever associated with bacterial meningitis usually resolves within 5–7 days of the onset of therapy. Prolonged fever (>10 days) is noted in about 10% of patients. Prolonged fever usually is due to intercurrent viral infection, nosocomial or secondary bacterial infection, thrombophlebitis, or drug reaction. Pericarditis or arthritis may occur in patients being treated for meningitis. Involvement of these sites may result either from bacterial dissemination or from immune complex deposition. In general, infectious pericarditis or arthritis occurs earlier in the course of treatment than does immune-mediated disease. Secondary fever refers to the recrudescence of elevated temperature after an afebrile interval. Nosocomial infections are especially important to consider in the evaluation of these patients.

Thrombocytosis, eosinophilia, and anemia may develop during therapy for meningitis. Anemia may be due to hemolysis or bone marrow suppression. DIC is most often associated with the rapidly progressive pattern of presentation and is noted most commonly in patients with shock and purpura (purpura fulminans). The combination of endotoxemia and severe hypotension initiates the coagulation cascade; the coexistence of ongoing thrombosis may produce symmetric peripheral gangrene.

PROGNOSIS. Appropriate recognition, prompt antibiotic therapy, and supportive care have reduced the mortality of bacterial meningitis after the neonatal period to 1–8%. The highest mortality rates are observed with pneumococcal meningitis. Severe neurodevelopmental sequelae may occur in 10–20% of patients recovering from bacterial meningitis, and as many as 50% have some, albeit subtle, neurobehavioral morbidity. The prognosis is poorest among infants younger than 6 mo and in those with more than 10^6 colony-forming units of bacteria/mL in their CSF. Those with seizures occurring more than 4 days into therapy or with coma or focal neurologic signs on presentation also tend to have more long-term sequelae. There does not appear to be a correlation between duration of symptoms before diagnosis of meningitis and outcome.

The most common neurologic sequelae include hearing loss, mental retardation, seizures, delay in acquisition of language, visual impairment, and behavioral problems. Sensorineural hearing loss is the most common sequela of bacterial meningitis. It is due to labyrinthitis following cochlear infection and occurs in as many as 30% of patients with pneumococcal meningitis, 10% with meningococcal, and 5–20% of those with *H. influenzae* type b meningitis. Hearing loss may also be due to direct inflammation of the auditory nerve. Adjunctive therapy with dexamethasone appears to reduce the incidence of severe hearing loss, at least for meningitis caused by *H. influenzae* type b. Regardless of the bacterial agent, type of antibiotic therapy, or use of dexamethasone, all patients with bacterial meningitis should undergo careful audiologic assessment before or soon after discharge from the hospital. Frequent reassessment on an outpatient basis is indicated for all patients who have a hearing deficit.

Repeated episodes of meningitis are rare but have three distinct patterns. Recrudescence is the reappearance of infection during therapy with appropriate antibiotics. CSF culture reveals the growth of bacteria that have developed antibiotic resistance. Relapse occurs between 3 days and 3 wk after therapy and represents persistent bacterial infection in the CNS (subdural empyema, ventriculitis, cerebral abscess) or other site (mastoid, cranial osteomyelitis, orbital infection). Relapse is often associated with an inadequate choice, dose, or duration of antibiotic therapy. Recurrence is a new episode of meningitis due to reinfection with the same bacterial species or another pyogenic pathogen. Recurrent meningitis suggests the presence of an acquired or congenital anatomic communication between the CSF and a mucocutaneous site. Defects in immune host defense also predispose to recurrent meningitis.

PREVENTION. Vaccination and antibiotic prophylaxis of susceptible at-risk contacts represent the two available means of reducing the likelihood of bacterial meningitis. The availability and application of each of these approaches are different for each of the three major causes of bacterial meningitis in children.

Neisseria meningitidis. Chemoprophylaxis is recommended for all close contacts of patients with meningococcal meningitis regardless of age or immunization status. Close contacts should be treated with rifampin 10 mg/kg/dose every 12 hr (maximum dose of 600 mg) for 2 days as soon as possible after identification of a case of suspected meningococcal meningitis or sepsis. Close contacts include household, daycare center, and nursery school contacts and health care workers who have direct exposure to oral secretions (e.g., mouth-to-mouth resuscitation, suctioning, intubation). Exposed contacts should be treated immediately on suspicion of infection in the index patient; bacteriologic confirmation of infection should not be awaited. In addition, all contacts should be educated about the early signs of meningococcal disease and the need to seek prompt medical attention if these signs develop.

Meningococcal quadrivalent vaccine against serogroups A, C, Y, and W135 is recommended for high-risk children older than 2 yr. High-risk patients include those with anatomic or functional asplenia or deficiencies of terminal complement proteins. The vaccine may also be used as an adjunct with chemoprophylaxis for exposed contacts and during epidemics of meningococcal disease. Unfortunately, most cases of endemic meningococcal meningitis are due to group B, for which there currently is no effective vaccine.

***Haemophilus influenzae* type b.** Rifampin prophylaxis should be given to all household contacts, including adults, if any close family member younger than 48 mo has not been fully immunized or if an immunocompromised child resides in the household. A household contact is one who lives in the residence of the index case or who has spent a minimum of 4 hr with the index case for at least 5 of 7 days preceding the patient's hospitalization. Family members should receive rifampin prophylaxis immediately after the diagnosis is suspected in the index case because more than 50% of secondary family cases occur in the 1st wk after the index patient has been hospitalized.

The risk of secondary cases of *H. influenzae* type b infection in daycare center contacts is less than that for household contacts and probably greater than that for the general population. The risk is exceedingly low for daycare center children who are not classroom contacts and those older than 2 yr. The efficacy of chemoprophylaxis in daycare centers is uncertain, and there are difficulties in ensuring that all at-risk daycare center attendees receive the drug. Chemoprophylaxis for children and adults in daycare centers that resemble households (e.g., >25 hr/wk of close contact) should be provided to all adults and children if two or more cases of *H. influenzae* type b infection occur within 60 days and some of the children are younger than 2 yr and not fully immunized.

The dose of rifampin is 20 mg/kg/24 hr (maximum dose of

600 mg) given once each day for 4 days. Rifampin discolors the urine and sweat red-orange, stains contact lenses, and reduces the serum concentrations of some drugs, including oral contraceptives. Rifampin is contraindicated during pregnancy. In addition to receiving prophylaxis, daycare center workers and parents should be educated about the signs of serious *H. influenzae* infection and the importance of seeking prompt medical attention for fever or other potential manifestations of *H. influenzae* disease.

H. influenzae type b nasopharyngeal colonization may not be eradicated in the index case despite 10 days of appropriate parenteral antibiotic therapy. Therefore, before discharge from the hospital, patients should receive rifampin (20 mg/kg/dose every day for 4 days) to prevent introduction or reintroduction of the organism into the household or daycare center.

The most exciting advance in the prevention of childhood bacterial meningitis is the development and licensure of vaccines against *H. influenzae* type b. Four conjugate vaccines are licensed in the United States. Although each vaccine elicits different profiles of antibody response in infants immunized at 2–6 mo of age, all three result in protective levels of antibody with efficacy rates ranging from 70–100%. Efficacy is not as consistent in Native American populations, a group recognized as having an extremely high incidence of disease. As a result, all children should be immunized with *H. influenzae* type b conjugate vaccine beginning at 2 mo of age.

Streptococcus pneumoniae. No chemoprophylaxis or vaccination is required for normal hosts who may be contacts of patients with pneumococcal meningitis, because secondary cases rarely have occurred. High-risk patients age 2 yr or older should receive the 23-valent pneumococcal vaccine, and patients with sickle cell anemia should also receive chemoprophylaxis with daily oral penicillin, amoxicillin, or trimethoprim-sulfamethoxazole (Chapter 468.1).

174.2 *Viral Meningoencephalitis*

Viral meningoencephalitis is an acute inflammatory process involving the meninges and, to a variable degree, brain tissue. These infections are relatively common and may be caused by a number of different agents. The CSF is characterized by pleocytosis and the absence of microorganisms on Gram stain and routine bacterial culture. In most instances, the infections are self-limited; in some cases, however, substantial morbidity and mortality may be observed.

ETIOLOGY. Although the specific etiologic agent is not identified in most cases, clinical and research experience indicate that viruses are usually the responsible pathogens, accounting for the seasonal pattern of disease. Enteroviruses cause more than 80% of all cases. Other frequent causes of infection include arboviruses and herpesviruses. Mumps is a common pathogen in regions where mumps vaccine is not widely used.

Enteroviruses are small RNA-containing viruses; almost 70 specific serotypes have been identified. The severity of disease ranges from mild, self-limited illness with primarily meningeal involvement to severe encephalitis with death or significant sequelae. Epidemics, some devastating, have occurred among newborns.

Arboviruses are zoonoses in which humans, not being essential in the viral life cycle, are infected accidentally by an arthropod vector. Most commonly, mosquitoes or ticks acquire arboviruses by biting infected birds or small mammals, which often have prolonged viremia without illness. The insect vectors transmit the virus to other vertebrates, including humans and horses. Encephalitis in horses ("blind staggers") may be the first indication of an incipient epidemic. Although rural exposure is most common, urban and suburban outbreaks are also frequent. The most common arboviruses responsible for CNS infection in the United States are St. Louis and California encephalitis viruses (Chapter 258).

Herpes simplex virus type 1 (HSV-1) is an important cause of severe, sporadic encephalitis in children and adults. Brain involvement usually is focal; progression to coma and death occurs in 70% of cases without antiviral therapy. Severe encephalitis with diffuse brain involvement is caused by herpes simplex virus type 2 (HSV-2) in neonates who usually contract the virus from their mothers at delivery. A mild transient form of meningoencephalitis may accompany genital herpes infection in sexually active adolescents; most of these infections are caused by HSV-2. Varicella-zoster virus (VZV) may cause CNS infection in close temporal relationship with chickenpox. The most common manifestation of CNS involvement is cerebellar ataxia, and the most severe is an acute encephalitis. After primary infection, VZV becomes latent in spinal and cranial nerve roots and ganglia, expressing itself later as herpes zoster, often with accompanying mild meningoencephalitis. Cytomegalovirus (CMV) infection of the CNS may be part of congenital infection or disseminated disease in immunocompromised hosts, but it does not cause meningoencephalitis in normal infants and children. Epstein-Barr virus (EBV) has been associated with myriad CNS syndromes (Chapter 247).

Mumps meningoencephalitis is mild, but deafness due to damage of the 8th cranial nerve is not uncommon. Meningoencephalitis is caused occasionally by respiratory viruses, rubeola, rubella, or rabies.

EPIDEMIOLOGY. The epidemiologic pattern of viral meningoencephalitis reflects the prevalence of the enteroviruses, the primary etiology. Infection with enteroviruses is spread directly from person to person, with a usual incubation period of 4–6 days. Most cases in temperate climates occur in the summer and fall. Epidemiologic considerations in aseptic meningitis due to agents other than enteroviruses also include season, geography, climatic conditions, animal exposures, and factors related to the specific pathogen.

PATHOGENESIS. The sequence of events varies with the infecting agent and host. In general, viruses enter the lymphatic system, either through ingestion of enteroviruses; by inoculation of mucous membranes by measles, rubella, VZV, or HSV; or by hematogenous spread from a mosquito or other insect bite. There, multiplication begins, and seeding of the bloodstream leads to infection of several organs. At this stage (the extraneural phase), a systemic febrile illness is present, but if further viral multiplication takes place in the seeded organs, a secondary propagation of large amounts of virus may occur. Invasion of the CNS is followed by clinical evidence of neurologic disease. HSV-1 probably reaches the brain by direct spread along neuronal axons.

Neurologic damage is caused by direct invasion and destruction of neural tissues by actively multiplying viruses or by a host reaction to viral antigens. Most neuronal destruction is probably due directly to viral invasion, whereas the host's vigorous tissue response induces demyelination and vascular and perivascular destruction.

Tissue sections of the brain generally are characterized by meningeal congestion and mononuclear infiltration, perivascular cuffs of lymphocytes and plasma cells, some perivascular tissue necrosis with myelin breakdown, and neuronal disruption in various stages, including ultimately neuronophagia and endothelial proliferation or necrosis. A marked degree of demyelination with preservation of neurons and their axons is considered predominantly to represent "postinfectious" or "allergic" encephalitis. The cerebral cortex, especially the temporal lobe, is often severely affected by HSV; the arboviruses tend to affect the entire brain; rabies has a predilection for the basal structures. Involvement of the spinal cord, nerve roots, and peripheral nerves is variable.

CLINICAL MANIFESTATIONS. The progression and ultimate severity of the clinical course are very much determined by the relative degree of meningeal and parenchymal involvement, which in turn is determined, at least in part, by the specific infectious agents. However, the clinical manifestations have as wide range of severity, even with the same etiologic agent. Some children may appear to be mildly affected initially, only to lapse into coma and die suddenly. In others, the illness may be ushered in by high fever, violent convulsions interspersed with bizarre movements, and hallucinations alternating with brief periods of clarity, but then complete recovery.

The onset of illness is generally acute, although CNS signs and symptoms often are preceded by a nonspecific acute febrile illness of a few days duration. The presenting manifestations in older children are headache and hyperesthesia, and in infants, irritability and lethargy. Headache is most often frontal or generalized; adolescents frequently note retrobulbar pain. Fever, nausea and vomiting, photophobia, and pain in the neck, back, and legs are common. As body temperature rises, there may be mental dullness, eventuating in stupor in combination with bizarre movements and convulsions. Focal neurologic signs may be stationary, progressive, or fluctuating. Loss of bowel and bladder control and unprovoked emotional bursts may occur.

Exanthems often precede or accompany the CNS signs, especially with echoviruses, coxsackieviruses, VZV, measles, and rubella. Examination often reveals nuchal rigidity without significant localizing neurologic changes, at least at the onset.

Specific forms or complicating manifestations of CNS viral infection include Guillain-Barré syndrome, acute transverse myelitis, acute hemiplegia, and acute cerebellar ataxia.

DIAGNOSIS. The diagnosis of viral encephalitis is usually made on the clinical presentation of nonspecific prodrome followed by progressive CNS symptoms. The diagnosis is supported by examination of the CSF, which usually shows a mild mononuclear predominance (Table 174–1). Other tests of potential value in the evaluation of patients with suspected viral meningoencephalitis include an electroencephalogram (EEG) and neuroimaging studies. The EEG typically shows diffuse slow-wave activity, usually without focal changes. Neuroimaging studies (CT or MRI) may show swelling of the brain parenchyma. Focal seizures or focal findings on EEG or CT or MRI, especially involving the temporal lobes, suggest HSV encephalitis.

Differential Diagnosis. A number of clinical conditions that cause CNS inflammation mimic viral meningoencephalitis. The most important group of alternate infectious agents to consider is bacteria. Most children with bacterial infections of the CNS have a more acute onset and appear more critically ill, but this is not always the case. Bacterial meningitis caused by *S. pneumoniae, N. meningitidis,* and *H. influenzae* type b may be insidious in onset. CNS infection caused by other bacteria, such as tuberculosis, *T. pallidum* (syphilis), *Borrelia burgdorferi* (Lyme disease), and *Bartonella henselae,* the bacillus associated with cat-scratch disease, also may have very indolent courses. Analysis of CSF and appropriate serologic tests is necessary to differentiate these various pathogens. Parameningeal bacterial infections, such as brain abscess or subdural or epidural empyema, may have features similar to viral CNS infections. CNS imaging procedures are critical for the diagnosis of these processes.

Nonbacterial infectious agents also need to be considered in the differential diagnosis of CNS infections. These agents include fungi, rickettsiae, *Mycoplasma,* protozoa, and other parasites. Consideration of these agents usually arises as a result of accompanying symptoms, geographic locality of infection, or host immune factors.

Various noninfectious disorders also may be associated with CNS inflammation and have manifestations overlapping with those associated with viral meningoencephalitis. Some of these disorders include malignancy, collagen vascular diseases, intracranial hemorrhage, and exposure to certain drugs or toxins. Attention to history and other organ involvement usually allows early elimination of these diagnostic possibilities. Recent exposure to possibly infected persons, animals, mosquitoes, or ticks and any recent travel should be noted. Inquiry should also be made about recent injections of biologic substances and about the possibilities of exposure to heavy metals, pesticides, or noxious substances.

LABORATORY FINDINGS. The CSF contains from a few to several thousand cells per cubic millimeter. Early in the disease, the cells are often polymorphonuclear; later, mononuclear cells predominate. This change in cellular type is often demonstrated in CSF samples obtained as little as 8–12 hr apart. The protein concentration in CSF tends to be normal or slightly elevated, but concentrations may be very high if brain destruction is extensive, as illustrated by HSV encephalitis. The glucose level is usually normal, although with certain viruses, for example, mumps, a substantial depression of CSF glucose concentrations is often observed.

The CSF should be cultured for viruses, bacteria, fungi, and mycobacteria; in some instances, special examinations are indicated for protozoa, *Mycoplasma,* and other pathogens. The success of isolating viruses from the CSF of children with viral meningoencephalitis is determined by the time in the clinical course that the specimen is obtained, the specific etiologic agent, whether the infection is a meningitic as opposed to a localized encephalitic process, and the skill of the diagnostic laboratory. Isolating a virus is more likely early in the illness, and the enteroviruses tend to be the easiest to isolate, although recovery of these agents from the CSF rarely exceeds 70%. To increase the likelihood of identifying the putative viral pathogen, specimens for culture also should be obtained from nasopharyngeal swabs, feces, and urine. Although isolating a virus from one or more of these sites does not prove causality, it is highly suggestive.

A serum specimen should be obtained early in the course of illness and, if viral cultures are not diagnostic, again 2–3 wk later for serologic studies. Serologic methods are not practical for diagnosing CNS infections caused by the enteroviruses because there are too many serotypes. However, this approach may be useful to confirm that a case is caused by a known circulating viral type. Serologic tests also may be of value in determining the etiology of nonenteroviral CNS infection. Newer diagnostic techniques for suspected viral meningoencephalitis that use polymerase chain reaction to detect viral DNA or RNA in CSF are promising.

TREATMENT. Until a bacterial cause is excluded by culture of blood and CSF, parenteral antibiotic therapy should be administered. With the exception of the use of acyclovir for HSV encephalitis, treatment of viral meningoencephalitis is nonspecific. Treatment of mild disease may require only symptomatic relief. Headache and hyperesthesia are treated with rest, non–aspirin-containing analgesics, and a reduction in room light, noise, and visitors. Acetaminophen is recommended for fever. Codeine, morphine, and the phenothiazine derivatives may be necessary for pain and vomiting, but if possible, their use in children should be minimized because they may induce misleading signs and symptoms. Intravenous fluids are occasionally necessary because of poor oral intake. More severe disease may require hospitalization and intensive care.

It is important to anticipate and be prepared for convulsions, cerebral edema, hyperpyrexia, inadequate respiratory exchange, disturbed fluid and electrolyte balance, aspiration and asphyxia, and cardiac or respiratory arrest of central origin. Therefore, all patients with severe encephalitis should be monitored closely. In patients with evidence of increased ICP, placement of a pressure transducer in the epidural space may be indicated for monitoring ICP. The risks of cardiac and respiratory failure or arrest are high with severe disease. All fluids, electrolytes, and medications are initially given parenterally. In prolonged states of coma, parenteral alimentation is indicated.

TABLE 174–1 Cerebrospinal Fluid Findings in Central Nervous System Disorders

Condition	Pressure (mm H_2O)	Leukocytes (mm³)	Protein (mg/dL)	Glucose (mg/dL)	Comments
Normal	50–80	<5, ≥75% lymphocytes	20–45	>50 (or 75% serum glucose)	
Common Forms of Meningitis					
Acute bacterial meningitis	Usually elevated (100–300)	100–10,000 or more; usually 300–2,000; PMNs predominate	Usually 100–500	Decreased, usually <40 (or <66% serum glucose)	Organisms usually seen on Gram stain and recovered by culture. Latex agglutination of CSF usually positive
Partially treated bacterial meningitis	Normal or elevated	5–10,000; PMNs usual but mononuclear cells may predominate if pretreated for extended period of time	Usually 100–500	Normal or decreased	Organisms may be seen on Gram stain. Latex agglutination CSF may be positive. Pretreatment may render CSF sterile
Viral meningitis or meningoencephalitis	Normal or slightly elevated (80–150)	Rarely >1,000 cells. Eastern equine encephalitis and lymphocytic choriomeningitis (LCM) may have cell counts of several thousand. PMNs early but mononuclear cells predominate through most of the course	Usually 50–200	Generally normal; may be decreased to <40 in some viral diseases, particularly mumps (15–20% of cases)	HSV encephalitis is suggested by focal seizures or by focal findings on CT or MRI scans or EEG. Enteroviruses and HSV infrequently recovered from CSF. HSV and enteroviruses may be detected by PCR of CSF
Uncommon Forms of Meningitis					
Tuberculous meningitis	Usually elevated	10–500; PMNs early, but lymphocytes predominate through most of the course	100–3,000; may be higher in presence of block	<50 in most cases; decreases with time if treatment is not provided	Acid-fast organisms almost never seen on smear. Organisms may be recovered in culture of large volumes of CSF. *Mycobacterium tuberculosis* may be detected by PCR of CSF
Fungal meningitis	Usually elevated	5–500; PMNs early but mononuclear cells predominate through most of the course. Cryptococcal meningitis may have no cellular inflammatory response	25–500	<50; decreases with time if treatment is not provided	Budding yeast may be seen. Organisms may be recovered in culture. Cryptococcal antigen (CSF and serum) may be positive in cryptococcal infection
Syphilis (acute) and leptospirosis	Usually elevated	50–500; lymphocytes predominate	50–200	Usually normal	Positive CSF serology. Spirochetes not demonstrable by usual techniques of smear or culture; darkfield examination may be positive
Amebic (*Naegleria*) meningoencephalitis	Elevated	1,000–10,000 or more; PMNs predominate	50–500	Normal or slightly decreased	Mobile amebae may be seen by hanging-drop examination of CSF at room temperature
Brain and Parameningeal Abscesses					
Brain abscess	Usually elevated (100–300)	5–200; CSF rarely acellular; lymphocytes predominate; if abscess ruptures into ventricle, PMNs predominate and cell count may reach >100,000	75–500	Normal unless abscess ruptures into ventricular system	No organisms on smear or culture unless abscess ruptures into ventricular system
Subdural empyema	Usually elevated (100–300)	100–5,000; PMNs predominate	100–500	Normal	No organisms on smear or culture of CSF unless meningitis also present; organisms found on tap of subdural fluid
Cerebral epidural abscess	Normal to slightly elevated	10–500; lymphocytes predominate	50–200	Normal	No organisms on smear or culture of CSF
Spinal epidural abscess	Usually low, with spinal block	10–100; lymphocytes predominate	50–400	Normal	No organisms on smear or culture of CSF
Chemical (drugs, dermoid cysts, myelography dye)	Usually elevated	100–1,000 or more; PMNs predominate	50–100	Normal or slightly decreased	Epithelial cells may be seen within CSF by use of polarized light in some children with dermoids
Noninfectious Causes					
Sarcoidosis	Normal or elevated slightly	0–100; mononuclear	40–100	Normal	No specific findings
Systemic lupus erythematosus with CNS involvement	Slightly elevated	0–500; PMNs usually predominate; lymphocytes may be present	100	Normal or slightly decreased	No organisms on smear or culture. LE preparation may be positive. Positive neuronal and ribosomal P protein antibodies in CSF
Tumor, leukemia	Slightly elevated to very high	0–100 or more; mononuclear or blast cells	50–1,000	Normal to decreased (20–40)	Cytology may be positive

PMN = polymorphonuclear neutrophils; CSF = cerebrospinal fluid; EEG = electroencephalogram; HSV = herpes simplex virus; PCR = polymerase chain reaction.

SIADH is quite common in acute CNS disorders; thus, constant evaluation is required for its early detection (Chapter 569.1). Normal blood levels of glucose, magnesium, and calcium must be maintained to minimize the threat of convulsions. If cerebral edema or seizures become evident, vigorous treatment should be instituted.

PROGNOSIS. Supportive and rehabilitative efforts are very important after patients recover. Motor incoordination, convulsive disorders, total or partial deafness, and behavioral disturbances may appear only after an interval of time. Visual disturbances due to chorioretinopathy and perceptual amblyopia may also have a delayed appearance. Special facilities and, at times, institutional placement may become necessary. Some sequelae of infection may be very subtle. Therefore, neurodevelopmental and audiologic evaluations should be part of the routine follow-up of children who have recovered from viral meningoencephalitis.

Most children completely recover from viral infections of the CNS, although the prognosis depends on the severity of the clinical illness, the specific cause, and the age of the child. If the clinical illness is severe and substantial parenchymal involvement is evident, the prognosis is poor, with potential deficits being intellectual, motor, psychiatric, epileptic, visual, or auditory in nature. Severe sequelae also should be anticipated in those with infection caused by HSV. Although some literature suggests that infants who contract viral meningoencephalitis have a poorer long-term outcome than older children, other data refute this observation. Although about 10% of children younger than 2 yr with enteroviral CNS infections suffer an acute complication such as seizures, increased ICP, or coma, almost all have favorable long-term neurologic outcomes.

PREVENTION. Widespread use of effective attenuated viral vaccines for polio, measles, mumps, rubella, and varicella has almost eliminated CNS complications from these diseases in the United States. The availability of domestic animal vaccine programs against rabies has reduced the frequency of rabies encephalitis. Control of encephalitis due to arboviruses has been less successful because specific vaccines for the arboviral diseases that occur in North America are not available. However, control of insect vectors by suitable spraying methods and eradication of insect breeding sites reduce the incidence of these infections.

174.3 Eosinophilic Meningitis

Eosinophilic meningitis is defined as 10 or more eosinophils/mm^3 of CSF. The most common cause worldwide of eosinophilic pleocytosis is CNS infection with helminthic parasites. However, in countries such as the United States, where helminthic infestation is uncommon, the differential diagnosis of CSF eosinophilic pleocytosis is broad.

ETIOLOGY. Although any tissue-migrating helminth may cause eosinophilic meningitis, the most common cause is human infection with the rat lungworm *Angiostrongylus cantonensis* (Chapter 289). Other parasites that can cause eosinophilic meningitis include *Gnathostoma spinigerum* (dog and cat roundworm) (Chapter 293), *Baylisascaris procyonis* (raccoon roundworm), *Ascaris lumbricoides* (human roundworm), *Trichinella spiralis, Toxocara canis, Toxoplasma gondii, Paragonimus westermani, Echinococcus granulosus, Schistosoma japonicum, Onchocerca volvulus,* and *T. solium.* Eosinophilic meningitis also may occur as an unusual manifestation of more common viral, bacterial, or fungal infections of the CNS. Noninfectious causes of eosinophilic meningitis include multiple sclerosis, malignancy, hypereosinophilic syndrome, or a reaction to medications or a ventriculoperitoneal shunt.

EPIDEMIOLOGY. *A. cantonensis* is found in Southeast Asia, the South Pacific, Japan, Taiwan, Egypt, Ivory Coast, and Cuba. Infection is acquired by eating raw or undercooked freshwater snails, slugs, prawns, or crabs containing infectious third-stage larvae. *Gnathostoma* infections are found in Japan, China, India, Bangladesh, and Southeast Asia. Gnathostomiasis is acquired by eating undercooked or raw fish, frog, bird, or snake meat.

CLINICAL MANIFESTATIONS. When eosinophilic meningitis results from helminthic infestation, patients become ill 1–3 wk after exposure, as the parasites migrate from the gastrointestinal tract to the CNS. Common concomitant findings include fever, peripheral eosinophilia, vomiting, abdominal pain, creeping skin eruptions, or pleurisy. Neurologic symptoms may include headache, meningismus, ataxia, cranial nerve palsies, and paresthesias. Paraparesis or incontinence can result from radiculitis or myelitis.

DIAGNOSIS. The presumptive diagnosis of helminth-induced eosinophilic meningitis is made by travel and exposure history in the presence of typical clinical and laboratory findings.

TREATMENT. Treatment is supportive, because infection is self-limited and anthelmintic drugs do not appear to influence the outcome of infection. Analgesics should be given for headache and radiculitis, and CSF removal or shunting should be performed to relieve hydrocephalus, if present.

PROGNOSIS. The prognosis is good; 70% of patients improve sufficiently to leave the hospital in 1–2 wk. Mortality associated with eosinophilic meningitis is less than 1%.

Acute Bacterial Meningitis

Baraff LJ, Lee SI, Schriger DL: Outcomes of bacterial meningitis in children: A meta-analysis. Pediatr Infect Dis J 12:389, 1993.

Blazer S, Berant M, Alon U: Bacterial meningitis: Effect of antibiotic treatment on cerebrospinal fluid. J Clin Pathol 80:386, 1983.

Dodge PR, Davis H, Feigin RD, et al: Prospective evaluation of hearing impairment as a sequela of acute bacterial meningitis. N Engl J Med 311:869, 1984.

Feigin RD, McCracken GH, Klein JO: Diagnosis and management of meningitis. Pediatr Infect Dis J 11:785, 1992.

Fijen C, Hanneman AJ, Kuiper E, et al: Complement deficiencies in patients over ten years old with meningococcal disease due to uncommon serogroups. Lancet 2:585, 1989.

Grimwood K, Anderson VA, Bond L, et al: Adverse outcomes of bacterial meningitis in school-age survivors. Pediatrics 95:646, 1995.

Kilpi T, Anttila M, Kallio MJT, et al: Severity of childhood bacterial meningitis and duration of illness before diagnosis. Lancet 338:406, 1991.

Kilpi T, Anttila M, Kallio MJT, et al: Length of prediagnostic history related to the course and sequelae of childhood bacterial meningitis. Pediatr Infect Dis J 12:184, 1993.

McIntyre PB, Berkey CS, King SM, et al: Dexamethasone as adjunctive therapy in bacterial meningitis. A meta-analysis of randomized clinical trials since 1988. JAMA 278:925, 1997.

Pomeroy SL, Holmes SJ, Dodge PR, et al: Seizures and other neurologic sequelae of bacterial meningitis in children. N Engl J Med 323:1651, 1990.

Quagliarello V, Sheld WM: Treatment of bacterial meningitis. N Engl J Med 336:708, 1997.

Radetsky M: Duration of symptoms and outcome in bacterial meningitis: An analysis of causation and the implications of a delay in diagnosis. Pediatr Infect Dis J 11:694, 1992.

Rodriguez WJ, Khan WN, Cocchetto D, et al: Treatment of *Pseudomonas* meningitis with ceftazidime with or without concurrent therapy. Pediatr Infect Dis J 9:83, 1990.

Saez-Llorens X, Ramilo O, Mustafa M, et al: Molecular pathophysiology of bacterial meningitis: Current concepts and therapeutic implications. J Pediatr 116:671, 1990.

Schuchat A, Robinson K, Wenger JD, et al: Bacterial meningitis in the United States in 1995. N Engl J Med 337:970, 1997.

Spanos A, Harrell FE, Durack DT: Differential diagnosis of acute meningitis: An analysis of the predictive value of initial observations. JAMA 262:2700, 1989.

Syrogiannopoulos GA, Nelson JD, McCracken GH: Subdural collections of fluid in acute bacterial meningitis: A review of 136 cases. Pediatr Infect Dis 5:343, 1986.

Talan DA, Guterman JJ, Overturf GD, et al: Analysis of emergency department management of suspected bacterial meningitis. Ann Emerg Med 18:856, 1989.

Viral Meningoencephalitis

Rautonen J, Koskiniemi M, Vaheri A: Prognostic factors in childhood encephalitis. Pediatr Infect Dis J 10:441, 1991.

Rorabaugh ML, Berlin LE, Heldrich F, et al: Aseptic meningitis in infants younger than 2 years of age: Acute illness and neurologic complications. Pediatrics 92:206, 1993.

Strikas RA, Anderson LJ, Parker RA: Temporal and geographic patterns of iso-

lates of nonpolio enterovirus in the United States, 1970–1983. J Infect Dis 153:346, 1986.
Whitley RJ: Viral encephalitis. N Engl J Med 323:242, 1990.
Wilfert CM, Lehrman SN, Katz SL: Enteroviruses and meningitis. Pediatr Infect Dis 2:333, 1983.

Eosinophilic Meningitis

Hsu W, Chen J, Chien C, et al: Eosinophilic meningitis caused by *Angiostrongylus cantonensis*. Pediatr Infect Dis J 9:443, 1990.
Vejjajiva A: Eosinophilic meningitis. *In:* Warren KS, Mahmoud AAF (eds): Tropical and Geographical Medicine, 2nd ed. New York, McGraw-Hill, 1990, p 455.
Weller PF: Eosinophilic meningitis. Am J Med 95:250, 1993.

CHAPTER 175
Pneumonia

Charles G. Prober

Pneumonia is an inflammation of the parenchyma of the lungs. Most cases of pneumonia are caused by microorganisms, but a number of noninfectious causes sometimes need to be considered. These noninfectious causes include but are not limited to aspiration of food or gastric acid, foreign bodies, hydrocarbons, and lipoid substances; hypersensitivity reactions; and drug- or radiation-induced pneumonitis. Infections in neonates and other compromised hosts (Chapter 179) are distinct from infections occurring in otherwise normal infants and children. The most common microbiologic causes of pneumonia in normal children include respiratory viruses, *Mycoplasma pneumoniae*, and selected bacteria. Less common causes of infectious pneumonia include nonrespiratory viruses (e.g., varicella-zoster virus), enteric gram-negative bacteria, mycobacteria, *Chlamydia*, rickettsiae, *Pneumocystis carinii*, and fungi.

Pneumonia has been classified on an anatomic basis as a lobar or lobular, alveolar, or interstitial process, but classification of infectious pneumonia on the basis of presumed or proven etiology is diagnostically and therapeutically more relevant.

Respiratory viruses are the most common cause of pneumonia during the first several years of life. *M. pneumoniae* assumes a predominant role in the etiology of pneumonia in school-aged and older children. Although bacteria are numerically less important as causes of pneumonia, they tend to be responsible for more severe infections than those caused by the nonbacterial agents. The most common bacterial causes of pneumonia in normal children are *S. pneumoniae*, *Streptococcus pyogenes* (group A *Streptococcus*), and *Staphylococcus aureus*. *Haemophilus influenzae* type b also has been responsible for bacterial pneumonia in young children in the past but has become much less common with the routine use of effective vaccines.

VIRAL PNEUMONIA

ETIOLOGY. The most common viruses causing pneumonia include respiratory syncytial virus (RSV), parainfluenza, influenza, and adenoviruses. RSV is the most common cause of viral pneumonia, especially during infancy. In general, lower respiratory tract viral infections are much more common during the winter months. The type and severity of the illness are influenced by several factors including age, season of the year, immune status of the host, and environmental factors such as crowding. Unlike bronchiolitis, for which the peak attack rate is within the 1st yr, the peak attack rate for viral pneumonia is between the ages of 2 and 3 yr and decreases slowly thereafter.

CLINICAL MANIFESTATIONS. Most viral pneumonias are preceded by several days of upper respiratory tract symptoms, typically rhinitis and cough. Other family members are frequently ill with similar symptoms. Although fever usually is present, temperatures are generally lower than in bacterial pneumonia. Tachypnea accompanied by intercostal, subcostal, and suprasternal retractions, nasal flaring, and use of accessory muscles is common. Severe infection may be accompanied by cyanosis and respiratory fatigue, especially in infants. Chest auscultation may reveal widespread rales and wheezing, but it often is difficult to localize the source of these adventitious sounds in very young children with hyper-resonant chests. Viral pneumonia cannot be definitely differentiated from mycoplasmal disease on clinical grounds and may, on occasion, be difficult to distinguish from bacterial pneumonia. Furthermore, evidence of viral upper respiratory tract infection is present in many patients who have confirmed bacterial pneumonia.

DIAGNOSIS. The chest roentgenogram is characterized by diffuse infiltrates (Fig. 175–1). In some patients, transient lobar infiltrates may also be present or even dominate the picture. Hyperinflation is common. There may be substantial between-observer differences in the interpretation of chest radiograms. Therefore, clinical correlation of radiographic findings is always necessary. The peripheral white blood cell count of children with viral pneumonia tends to be normal or only slightly elevated ($<$20,000/mm^3), with a predominance of lymphocytes. Acute phase reactants (e.g., erythrocyte sedimentation rate [ESR] or C-reactive protein [CRP]) usually are normal or only slightly elevated. However, there is substantial overlap of test results between children with viral and bacterial pneumonia, underscoring the importance of clinical judgment.

Definitive diagnosis requires isolation of a virus from a specimen obtained from the respiratory tract. Growth of a respiratory virus in tissue culture usually requires 5–10 days. However, an immediate diagnosis can be established by rapid diagnostic tests that use labeled virus-specific antibodies to detect viral antigens in respiratory secretions. Reliable reagents for the rapid detection of RSV, parainfluenza, influenza, and adenoviruses are available. Finally, serologic techniques can be used to diagnose a recent respiratory viral infection. Acute and convalescent serum samples are collected, and a rise in antibodies to a specific viral agent is sought. This diagnostic

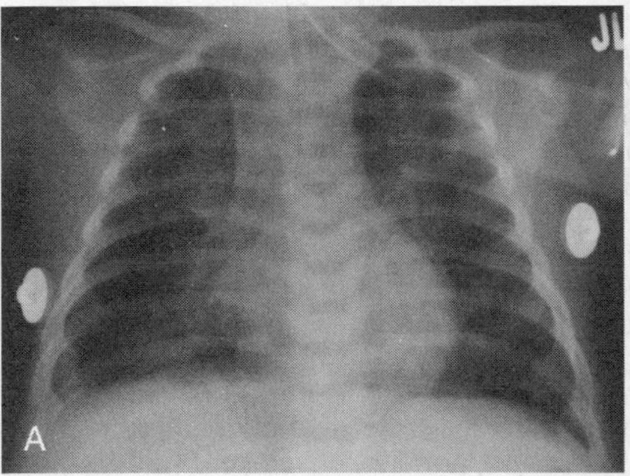

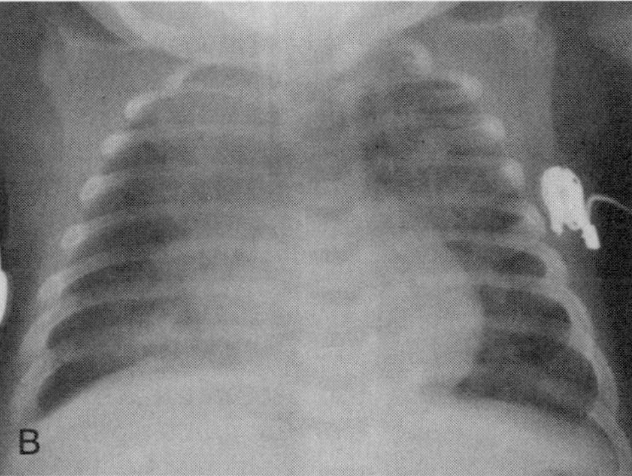

Figure 175–1 *A*, Roentgenographic findings characteristic of RSV pneumonia in a 6-mo-old infant with rapid respirations and fever. An anteroposterior (AP) radiograph of the chest shows hyperexpansion of the lungs with bilateral fine air space disease and streaks of density, indicating the presence of both pneumonia and atelectasis. An endotracheal tube is in place. *B*, One day later the AP radiograph of the chest shows increased bilateral pneumonia.

technique is laborious, slow, and not generally clinically useful, because the infection usually resolves by the time it is confirmed serologically. Nevertheless, serology may be valuable as an epidemiologic tool to define the incidence and prevalence of the various respiratory viral pathogens.

TREATMENT. Many patients are given antibiotic agents initially if bacterial pneumonia is suspected. Failure to respond to antibiotic treatment is additional evidence of a viral cause. Usually, only minimal supportive measures are required, although some patients need hospitalization for intravenous fluids, oxygen, or even assisted ventilation.

The only specific agents available for the treatment of respiratory viral infections are oral amantadine (or rimantadine) and aerosolized ribavirin. Amantadine and rimantadine are active against influenza A isolates. They have demonstrable efficacy in preventing influenza A infections in exposed, susceptible individuals and in the treatment of patients infected with influenza A virus. Treatment appears to be beneficial only if started within 48 hr of the onset of the infection. Ribavirin is active in vitro against RSV and appears to be beneficial for selected infants hospitalized with lower respiratory tract infection caused by RSV. It is, however, an expensive agent that needs to be administered by aerosolization. Limited clinical circumstances under which ribavirin therapy should be considered have been suggested by the Committee on Infectious Diseases of the American Academy of Pediatrics to include children with serious RSV disease and congenital heart disease, bronchopulmonary dysplasia or other chronic lung disease, or underlying immunosuppressive disease or therapy. The role of ribavirin for hospitalized RSV-infected infants is a subject of debate.

PROGNOSIS. Most children with viral pneumonia recover uneventfully and have no sequelae, although the course may be prolonged, especially in infants. Nonetheless, life-threatening lower respiratory tract infections caused by RSV do occur, especially among infants younger than 6 wk and those with underlying cardiorespiratory conditions or immunosuppression. In addition, adenovirus, especially types 1, 3, 4, 7, and 21, can cause fatal acute fulminant pneumonia or chronic lung disease associated with bronchiolitis obliterans.

MYCOPLASMAL PNEUMONIA. See Chapter 220.

BACTERIAL PNEUMONIA

Bacterial pneumonia during childhood is not a common infection, in the absence of an underlying chronic illness, such as cystic fibrosis or immunologic deficiency.

The most common event disturbing the defense mechanisms of the lungs is a viral infection that alters the properties of normal secretions, inhibits phagocytosis, modifies the bacterial flora, and may temporarily disrupt the normal epithelial layer of the respiratory passages. A viral respiratory disease often precedes the development of bacterial pneumonia by a few days.

An underlying disorder should be considered if a child experiences recurrent bacterial pneumonia. Defects to consider include abnormalities of antibody production (e.g., agammaglobulinemia) or polymorphonuclear leukocytes, cystic fibrosis, congenital bronchiectasis, ciliary dyskinesia, tracheoesophageal fistula, increased pulmonary blood flow, or deficient gag reflex. Trauma, anesthesia, and aspiration are factors that promote pulmonary infection.

PNEUMOCOCCAL PNEUMONIA. Although the incidence of pneumococcal pneumonia has declined during the past several decades, *S. pneumoniae* is still the most common cause of bacterial infection of the lungs.

Pathogenesis. Pneumococcal organisms are probably aspirated into the periphery of the lung from the upper airway or nasopharynx. Initially, a reactive edema that occurs supports proliferation of the organisms and aids in their spread into adjacent portions of the lung. One or more lobes or parts of lobes are usually involved, leaving the remaining bronchopulmonary system uninvolved. However, this pattern of lobar pneumonia is often not present in infants, who may have a more patchy and diffuse disease that follows a bronchial distribution and is characterized by many areas of consolidation around the smaller airways. Permanent injury is rare.

Clinical Manifestations. The classic history of sudden onset with a shaking chill followed by a high fever, cough, and chest pain described in adults with pneumococcal pneumonia may be noted in older children, but it is rarely observed in infants and young children, in whom the clinical pattern is considerably more variable.

INFANTS. A mild upper respiratory tract infection characterized by stuffy nose, fretfulness, and diminished appetite usually precedes the onset of pneumococcal pneumonia in infants. This mild prodrome of several days duration ends with abrupt onset of fever, restlessness, apprehension, and respiratory distress. Patients appear ill, with moderate to severe air hunger and often cyanosis. The respiratory distress is manifested by grunting; nasal flaring; retractions of the supraclavicular, intercostal, and subcostal areas; tachypnea; and tachycardia.

Physical examination of the chest is often unrevealing. Dullness to percussion overlying an area of consolidation associated with bronchial breath sounds and rales may be found. Abdominal distention may be prominent because of gastric dilation from swallowed air or ileus. The liver may seem enlarged because of downward displacement of the right diaphragm or superimposed congestive heart failure. Nuchal rigidity without meningeal infection may also be prominent, especially with involvement of the right upper lobe. Physical findings in the lungs usually change little during the course of illness, although more rales may become audible during resolution.

CHILDREN AND ADOLESCENTS. The signs and symptoms are similar to those in adults. A brief, mild upper respiratory tract infection is often followed by onset of a shaking chill and then by high fever. This is accompanied by drowsiness with intermittent periods of restlessness; rapid respirations; a dry, hacking, unproductive cough; anxiety; and occasionally delirium. Circumoral cyanosis may be observed. Many children are noted to be splinting on the affected side to minimize pleuritic pain and improve ventilation; they may lie on their side with their knees drawn up to their chest. Abnormal chest findings include retractions, nasal flaring, dullness to percussion, diminished tactile and vocal fremitus, bronchial breath sounds, and rales. As resolution occurs, moist rales are heard, and the cough loosens and becomes productive of large amounts of blood-tinged mucus.

The development of a pleural effusion or empyema may cause a visible lag in respiration on the affected side, with exaggerated excursion on the opposite side. Dullness to percussion is usually found over the area of the effusion, with diminished fremitus and breath sounds. Tubular breathing is often noted immediately above the fluid level and on the unaffected side.

Diagnosis. Pneumococcal pneumonia cannot be differentiated from other bacterial and viral pneumonias without appropriate microbiologic studies. Conditions possibly confused with pneumonia are bronchiolitis, allergic bronchitis, congestive heart failure, acute exacerbations of bronchiectasis, aspiration of a foreign body, sequestered lobe, atelectasis, and pulmonary abscess.

An older child with right lower lobe pneumonia may have diaphragmatic irritation with pain referred to the right lower quadrant of the abdomen. Because ileus may accompany pneumonia, right lower quadrant pain and absent bowel sounds may be misinterpreted as acute appendicitis.

LABORATORY FINDINGS. The white blood cell count is usually elevated to 15,000–40,000 cells/mm^3, with a preponderance of polymorphonuclear cells. The hemoglobin value is usually normal or only slightly diminished. Arterial blood samples usually show hypoxemia without hypercapnia.

Pneumococci can be isolated from the nasopharyngeal secretions in most patients. This finding cannot be considered proof of a causative relation because 10–15% of the population may be colonized with *S. pneumoniae.* However, isolation of the bacteria from blood or pleural fluid is diagnostic of infection. Bacteremia is present in 10–30% of patients with pneumococcal pneumonia.

Roentgenographic Findings. The roentgenographic changes (Fig. 175–2) do not always correspond to the clinical observations. Consolidation may be demonstrated by roentgenography before it can be detected by physical examination. Lobar consolidation is not as common in infants and young children as in older children. Pleural reaction with the presence of fluid is common. Radiographic resolution of the infiltrate may not be complete until several weeks after a child is clinically well. Therefore, unless there is evidence of clinical deterioration, it is not prudent to perform many radiographs early in the illness.

Treatment. The drug of choice is penicillin G (100,000 units/kg/24 hr). A third-generation cephalosporin (cefotaxime, 150 mg/kg/24 hr, or ceftriaxone, 75 mg/kg/24 hr) should be used if the isolate of *S. pneumoniae* is resistant to penicillin (MIC > 2.0 μg/mL) but sensitive to the cephalosporin. Vancomycin (40 mg/kg/24 hr) should be used if the isolate is resistant to both penicillin and third-generation cephalosporins. The majority of older children with pneumococcal pneumonia can be treated at home; the decision to hospitalize depends on the severity of the illness. Pneumonia in young infants is best treated in the hospital, because fluids and antibiotics may have to be administered intravenously. Furthermore, the course of illness in young infants is more variable and complications are more common. Patients with pneumonia associated with pleural effusion or empyema also should be hospitalized. Oxygen administered promptly to patients with respiratory distress greatly reduces the need for sedatives and analgesics; it should be given before patients become cyanotic.

Complications. With the use of antibiotic therapy, complications of bacterial pneumonia have become unusual. Although concomitant pneumococcal infection in other locations may be present before the onset of the symptoms of pneumonia, metastatic infection after the initiation of antibiotic treatment is infrequent. Empyema may occur as a result of extension of infection to the pleural surfaces. It is more common in infants than in older children.

Prognosis. In the preantibiotic era, the mortality rate in infants and small children ranged from 20–50% and in older children from 3–5%. Furthermore, the incidence of chronic empyema with altered pulmonary function was relatively high. With appropriate antibiotic therapy instituted early in the course of the illness, the mortality rate during infancy and childhood is now less than 1%, and long-term morbidity is low.

GROUP A STREPTOCOCCAL PNEUMONIA. Group A streptococci most commonly cause disease limited to the upper respiratory tract (pharyngitis), but the organisms may spread to other areas of the body including the lower respiratory tract. Streptococcal pneumonia and tracheobronchitis are uncommon, but certain viral infections, particularly those causing exanthems and epidemic influenza, predispose to these diseases, which are encountered most frequently in children 3–5 yr of age.

Pathogenesis. Streptococcal infections of the lower respiratory tract result in tracheitis, bronchitis, or interstitial pneumonia. Lobar pneumonia is uncommon. Lesions consist of necrosis of the tracheobronchial mucosa with the formation of ragged ulcers and large amounts of exudate, edema, and localized hemorrhage. The process may extend to the interalveolar septa and involve lymphatic vessels. Pleural involvement is relatively common; the effusion is often large and serous, occasionally serosanguineous, or thinly purulent, with less fibrin than the exudate of pneumococcal pneumonia.

Clinical Manifestations. The signs and symptoms of streptococcal pneumonia are similar to those of pneumococcal pneumonia. The onset may be sudden, characterized by high fever, chills, signs of respiratory distress, and, at times, extreme prostration. However, it may occasionally be more insidious, and a child may appear only mildly ill, with cough and low-grade fever.

Diagnosis. The clinical course and roentgenographic findings of streptococcal pneumonia are similar to those of staphylococcal pneumonia. Pleural effusions and pneumatoceles may occur in both conditions. The roentgenographic changes of uncomplicated streptococcal pneumonia may be indistinguishable from other interstitial pneumonitides, including those caused by *M. pneumoniae.*

Laboratory Findings. Leukocytosis occurs as in pneumococcal pneumonia. A rise in serum antistreptolysin (ASO) titer is supportive diagnostic evidence. The disease may be suspected if large amounts of group A β-hemolytic streptococci are isolated from a throat swab, nasopharyngeal secretions, bronchial washings, or sputum, but definitive diagnosis rests on recovery of the organism from pleural fluid, blood, or lung aspirate. Bacteremia occurs in about 10% of patients.

Roentgenographic Findings. Chest roentgenograms usually show diffuse bronchopneumonia, often with a large pleural effusion. Final roentgenographic resolution may not be complete for more than 10 wk.

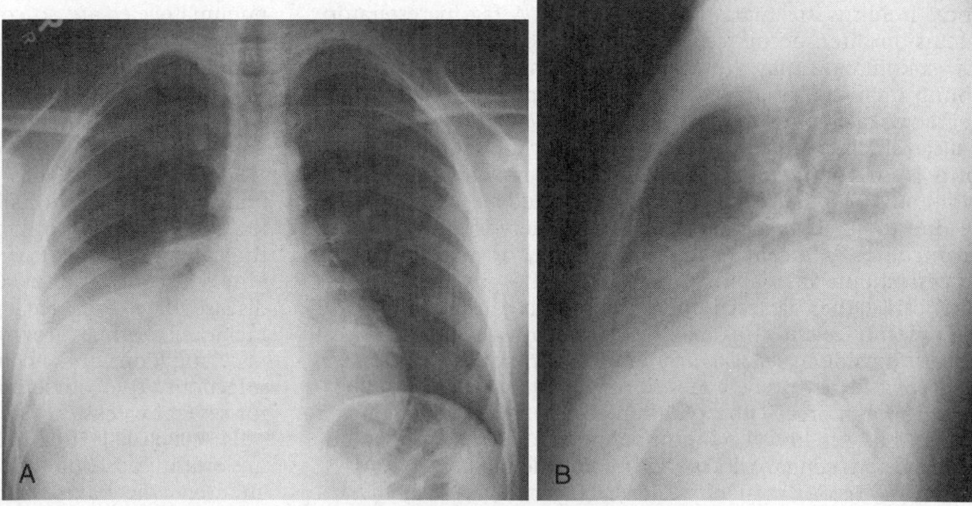

Figure 175–2 Roentgenographic findings characteristic of pneumococcal pneumonia in a 14-yr-old male with cough and fever. Posteroanterior *(A)* and lateral *(B)* chest radiographs reveal consolidation in the right lower lobe, strongly suggesting bacterial pneumonia.

Treatment. The drug of choice is penicillin G (100,000 units/kg/24 hr). Parenteral penicillin is used initially, and a 2–3-wk course may be completed orally after clinical improvement has begun in the hospital. If empyema develops, thoracentesis should be performed for diagnostic purposes and for removal of fluid. On occasion, repeated thoracentesis or closed drainage with indwelling chest tubes may be required if the fluid reaccumulates.

Complications. Bacterial complications and long-term morbidity are common in untreated patients but rare after antibiotic treatment is begun. Empyema occurs in 20% of children, and septic foci occasionally develop in other areas, such as the bones or joints; otherwise, extension of the disease is uncommon.

STAPHYLOCOCCAL PNEUMONIA. Pneumonia caused by *S. aureus* is a serious and rapidly progressive infection. It occurs less frequently than viral or pneumococcal pneumonia.

Epidemiology. Most cases occur between October and May. As with other bacterial pneumonias, staphylococcal pneumonia is frequently preceded by a viral upper respiratory tract infection. Although it may occur at any age, 30% of all patients are younger than 3 mo and 70% are younger than 1 yr. Boys are affected more commonly than girls.

Pathogenesis. Staphylococci cause confluent bronchopneumonia that is often unilateral or more prominent on one side than the other and is characterized by the presence of extensive areas of hemorrhagic necrosis and irregular areas of cavitation. The pleural surface is usually covered by a thick layer of fibrinopurulent exudate. Numerous abscesses occur, containing clusters of staphylococci, leukocytes, erythrocytes, and necrotic debris. Rupture of a small subpleural abscess may result in pyopneumothorax, which in turn may erode into a bronchus, producing a bronchopleural fistula.

Clinical Manifestations. Infants younger than 1 yr are most commonly affected and typically have a history of an upper respiratory tract infection for several days to 1 wk. An infant's condition changes abruptly, with the onset of high fever, cough, and evidence of respiratory distress. Signs and symptoms include tachypnea, grunting respirations, sternal and subcostal retractions, nasal flaring, cyanosis, and anxiety. If left undisturbed, infants are lethargic but on arousal are irritable and appear toxic. They may develop severe dyspnea and a shocklike state. Some infants have associated gastrointestinal disturbances, characterized by vomiting, anorexia, diarrhea, and abdominal distention secondary to a paralytic ileus. A rapid progression of symptoms is characteristic.

Physical findings depend on the stage of pneumonia. Early in the course of illness, diminished breath sounds, scattered rales, and rhonchi are commonly heard over the affected lung. With the development of effusion, empyema, or pyopneumothorax, dullness on percussion is noted, and breath sounds and vocal fremitus are markedly diminished. A lag in respiratory excursion often occurs on the affected side. Results of physical examination may, however, be misleading, particularly in young infants, with meager findings disproportionate to the degree of tachypnea.

Diagnosis. Recognizing early staphylococcal pneumonia in infants is often difficult. Abrupt onset and rapid progression of symptoms of pneumonia in infants should be considered to be due to staphylococci until proved otherwise. A history of furunculosis, a recent hospital admission, or maternal breast abscess should also alert physicians to the possibility of this diagnosis. Other bacterial pneumonias that cause empyema or pneumatoceles and thus may be confused with staphylococcal disease include *S. pneumoniae,* group A *Streptococcus, Klebsiella, H. influenzae* (both type b and nontypable), and primary tuberculous pneumonia with cavitation. Aspiration of a radiolucent foreign body followed by pulmonary abscesses may occasionally lead to a similar clinical and radiologic picture.

Laboratory Findings. Leukocytosis usually occurs, with the increase primarily among the polymorphonuclear cells. Mild to moderate anemia is common.

Material for diagnostic cultures should be obtained by tracheal aspiration or pleural tap; Gram stain frequently reveals gram-positive cocci in clusters. The finding of staphylococci in the nasopharynx is of no diagnostic value, but results of blood cultures may be positive. Pleural fluid typically reveals an exudate with polymorphonuclear cell counts of 300–100,000/mm^3, protein above 2.5 g/dL, and a low glucose concentration.

Roentgenographic Findings. Most patients with staphylococcal pneumonia have roentgenographic evidence of nonspecific bronchopneumonia early in the illness. The infiltrate may soon become patchy and limited in extent or may be dense and homogeneous and involve an entire lobe or hemithorax. The right lung alone is involved in about 65% of cases; bilateral involvement occurs in fewer than 20% of patients. A pleural effusion or empyema is noted during the course in most patients; pyopneumothorax occurs in approximately 25%. Pneumatoceles of various sizes are common.

Although no roentgenographic change can be considered diagnostic, rapid progression from bronchopneumonia to effusion or pyopneumothorax with or without pneumatoceles is highly suggestive of staphylococcal pneumonia. Chest films should be obtained at frequent intervals if the diagnosis is suspected. Clinical improvement usually precedes roentgenographic clearing by weeks, and pneumatoceles may persist for months.

Treatment. Therapy consists of appropriate antibiotics and drainage of collections of pus. Infants should be given oxygen and placed in a semireclining position to relieve cyanosis and anxiety. During the acute phase, intravenous hydration and nutrition are indicated. Assisted ventilation may occasionally be needed.

A semisynthetic, penicillinase-resistant penicillin should be administered intravenously immediately after cultures are obtained (e.g., nafcillin, 200 mg/kg/24 hr).

Although patients with staphylococcal pneumonia may occasionally recover completely without chest tube drainage, it is recommended, even if only a small effusion or empyema is present, in order to reduce the chance of bronchopleural fistula and the need for repeated pleural taps. Generally, pus reaccumulates so rapidly and becomes so viscous or loculated that closed drainage with a chest tube of the largest possible caliber is required. The appearance of pyopneumothorax is another indication for immediate insertion of a catheter into the pleural space. It is often necessary to use several chest tubes when loculation occurs. Once an infant begins to improve and the lung has re-expanded, the tubes can be removed, even if they are still draining small amounts of pus. Decortication procedures are rarely needed.

Complications. Because empyema, pyopneumothorax, and pneumatoceles are so common with staphylococcal pneumonia, they are considered part of the natural course of the illness and not complications. Septic lesions outside the respiratory tract occur rarely, except in young infants, in whom staphylococcal pericarditis, meningitis, osteomyelitis, and numerous metastatic abscesses in soft tissue may occur.

Prognosis. Survival has improved substantially with current management, but mortality still ranges from 10–30% and varies with the length of illness before hospitalization, the age of the patient, the adequacy of therapy, and the presence of other illness or complications. Children who do not have underlying disease have an excellent prognosis for complete recovery, including normal growth and development, normal pulmonary function, and no increased susceptibility to pulmonary infections. The course may be prolonged, with hospitalization for several weeks.

HAEMOPHILUS INFLUENZAE PNEUMONIA. *H. influenzae* type b is an important cause of serious bacterial infection in infants and children who have not received *H. influenzae* type b vaccine.

Pneumonia is second in frequency to meningitis in children with invasive *H. influenzae* disease; most cases occur during winter and spring.

Clinical Manifestations. *H. influenzae* pneumonia is usually lobar in distribution, but there is no characteristic chest roentgenogram. Segmental infiltrates, single or multiple lobe involvement, pleural effusion, and pneumatoceles occur. Pathologically, involved areas show a polymorphonuclear or lymphocytic inflammatory reaction with extensive destruction of the epithelium of smaller airways, interstitial inflammation, and marked, often hemorrhagic edema.

Although the clinical manifestations may be difficult to distinguish from those of pneumococcal pneumonia, *H. influenzae* pneumonia is more often insidious in onset, and the course is usually prolonged over several weeks. Many patients are already receiving treatment for otitis media at the time of diagnosis. Cough is almost always present but may not be productive, and patients are febrile and often tachypneic, with nasal flaring and retractions. Localized dullness to percussion and rales and bronchial breath sounds may be noted; pleural fluid is often present on roentgenogram in young infants.

Diagnosis. The diagnosis is established by isolating the organism from the blood, pleural fluid, or lung aspirate. Moderate leukocytosis is usually found. In the absence of a positive culture, a positive urine latex agglutination test result supports the diagnosis of this infection.

Treatment. Treatment consists of the same symptomatic and supportive measures used in pneumococcal and staphylococcal pneumonias. When *H. influenzae* is suspected as the causative agent, ceftriaxone (75 mg/kg/24 hr) or cefotaxime (150 mg/kg/24 hr) should be included in the initial antibiotic therapy until it is known whether the organism produces penicillinase; if the strain is sensitive, ampicillin (100 mg/kg/24 hr) may be administered. Effusion and pyarthrosis may require drainage. Needle thoracentesis is often adequate for effusion drainage, but the procedure may occasionally have to be repeated. Closed chest drainage may be required if purulent pleural fluid is present, but open drainage is infrequently needed. If the initial response to antibiotics is good, oral treatment can be instituted to complete a 10- to 14-day course. Roentgenographic demonstration of complete resolution may be delayed for several weeks.

Complications. Complications are frequent, particularly in young infants, and include bacteremia, pericarditis, cellulitis, empyema, meningitis, and suppurative arthritis.

American Academy of Pediatrics, Committee on Infectious Diseases: Reassessment of the indications for ribavirin therapy in respiratory syncytial virus infections. Pediatrics 97:137, 1996.

Davies HD, Wang EEL, Manson D, et al: Reliability of the chest radiograph in the diagnosis of lower respiratory infections in young children. Pediatr Infect Dis J 15:600, 1996.

Isaacs D: Problems in determining the etiology of community-acquired childhood pneumonia. Pediatr Infect Dis J 8:143, 1989.

Knight GJ, Carmen PG: Primary staphylococcal pneumonia in childhood: A review of 69 cases. J Paediatr Child Health 28:447, 1992.

Nohynek H, Valkeila E, Leinonen M, et al: Erythrocyte sedimentation rate, white blood cell count and serum C-reactive protein in assessing etiologic diagnosis of acute lower respiratory infections in children. Pediatr Infect Dis J 14:484, 1995.

Peter G: The child with pneumonia: Diagnostic and therapeutic considerations. Pediatr Infect Dis J 7:453, 1988.

Ray CG, Holberg CJ, Minnich LL, et al: Acute lower respiratory illnesses during the first three years of life: Potential roles for various etiologic agents. Pediatr Infect Dis J 12:10, 1993.

Schutze GE, Jacobs RF: Management of community-acquired bacterial pneumonia in hospitalized children. Pediatr Infect Dis J 11:160, 1992.

Turner RB, Lande AE, Chase P, et al: Pneumonia in pediatric outpatients: Cause and clinical manifestations. J Pediatr 111:194, 1987.

CHAPTER 176
Gastroenteritis

Larry K. Pickering and John D. Snyder

Infections of the gastrointestinal (GI) tract are caused by a wide variety of enteropathogens, including bacteria, viruses, and parasites (Table 176–1). Clinical manifestations depend on the organism and host and include asymptomatic infection, watery diarrhea, bloody diarrhea, chronic diarrhea, and extraintestinal manifestations of infection. A presumptive etiologic diagnosis can be made from epidemiologic clues, clinical manifestations, physical examination, and knowledge of the pathophysiologic mechanism of enteropathogens. The two basic types of acute infectious diarrhea are inflammatory and noninflammatory. Enteropathogens elicit noninflammatory diarrhea through enterotoxin production by some bacteria, destruction of villus (surface) cells by viruses, adherence by parasites, and adherence and/or translocation by bacteria. Inflammatory diarrhea is usually caused by bacteria that invade the intestine directly or produce cytotoxins. Some enteropathogens possess more than one of these virulence properties.

Laboratory studies to identify diarrheal pathogens are often not required because most episodes are self-limited. All patients with diarrhea require fluid and electrolyte therapy, a few need other nonspecific support, and some may benefit from antimicrobial therapy.

EPIDEMIOLOGY. Diarrheal diseases are one of the leading causes of morbidity and mortality in children worldwide, causing 1 billion episodes of illness and 3–5 million deaths annually. In the United States, 20–35 million episodes of diarrhea occur each year among the 16.5 million children younger than 5 yr, resulting in 2.1–3.7 million physician visits, 220,000 hospitalizations, 924,000 hospital days, and 300–400 deaths. The major mechanisms of transmission for diarrheal pathogens are person to person through the fecal-oral route or by ingestion of contaminated food or water. Enteropathogens that are infectious in a small inoculum (*Shigella*, enteric viruses, *Giardia lamblia*, *Cryptosporidium parvum*, *Entamoeba histolytica*, and *Escherichia coli* 0157:H7) may be transmitted by person-to-person contact. Factors that increase susceptibility to infection with enteropathogens include young age, immune deficiency, measles, malnutrition, travel to an endemic area, lack of breastfeeding, exposure to unsanitary conditions, ingestion of contaminated food or water, level of maternal education, and child-care center attendance.

ETIOLOGY. The relative importance and epidemiologic charac-

TABLE 176–1 Causative Agents of Gastroenteritis

Bacteria	Viruses	Parasites
Aeromonas spp	Astrovirus	*Blastocystis hominis*
*Bacillus cereus**	Caliciviruses	*Cryptosporidium parvum*
Campylobacter jejuni	Enteric adenovirus	*Cyclospora cayetanensis*
*Clostridium perfringens**	Rotavirus	*Entamoeba histolytica*
Clostridium difficile	Cytomegalovirus and herpes simplex virus†	*Enterocytozoon bieneusi*
Escherichia coli		*Giardi lamblia*
Plesiomonas shigelloides		*Isospora belli*
Salmonella spp		Microsporidia (*Enterocytozoon bieneusi* and *Enterocytozoon intestinalis*)
Shigella spp		
*Staphylococcus aureus**		
Vibrio cholerae		
Vibrio parahaemolyticus		
Yersinia enterocolitica		*Strongyloides stercoralis*

**Generally associated only with food-borne outbreaks.*
†Generally associated only with immunocompromised hosts.

teristics of diarrheal pathogens vary by geographic location. Children in developing countries become infected with a diverse group of bacterial and parasitic pathogens, whereas all children in developed as well as developing countries acquire rotavirus and, in many cases, the other viral enteropathogens and *G. lamblia* during their first 5 yr of life. Acute diarrhea or diarrhea of short duration may be associated with any of the bacteria, viruses, or parasites listed in Table 176–1. Chronic or persistent diarrhea lasting 14 days or longer may be due to (1) an infectious agent, including *G. lamblia, Cryptosporidium,* and enteroaggregative or enteropathogenic *E. coli;* (2) any enteropathogen that infects an immunocompromised host; or (3) residual symptoms due to damage to the intestine by an enteropathogen following an acute infection. There are also many noninfectious causes of diarrhea in children (Table 176–2).

Bacterial Enteropathogens. Bacterial enteropathogens may cause either inflammatory or noninflammatory diarrhea, and specific enteropathogens may be associated with either clinical manifestation. Generally, inflammatory diarrhea is associated with *Aeromonas* spp, *Campylobacter jejuni, Clostridium difficile,* enteroinvasive *E. coli,* enterohemorrhagic *E. coli, Plesiomonas shigelloides, Salmonella* spp, *Shigella* spp, *Vibrio parahaemolyticus,* and *Yersinia enterocolitica.* Noninflammatory diarrhea may be caused by enteropathogenic *E. coli,* enterotoxigenic *E. coli, Vibrio cholerae,* and several of the pathogens associated with inflammatory diarrhea. Antimicrobial therapy is administered to selected patients with diarrhea to shorten the clinical course, to decrease excretion of the causative organism, or to prevent complications. Indications for specific antimicrobial therapy of patients infected with bacterial enteropathogens are shown in Table 176–3. Discussion of *Helicobacter pylori,* which infects gastric mucosa and is associated with ulcer disease, can be found in Chapter 336.

Parasitic Enteropathogens. *G. lamblia* is the most common parasitic cause of diarrhea in the United States; other pathogens include *C. parvum, Cyclospora cayetanensis, E. histolytica, Strongyloides stercoralis, Isospora belli, Enterocytozoon bieneusi,* and *Enterocytozoon intestinalis.* The latter three agents have been found most often in persons with AIDS. The role of *Dientamoeba fragilis* and *Blastocystis hominis* as causes of diarrhea has not been fully defined. Patients with diarrhea normally do not need to have their stools examined for ova and parasites unless they have a history of recent travel to an endemic area, stool cultures are negative for other enteropathogens, and diarrhea persists for more than 1 wk; or unless they are part of an outbreak of diarrhea; or unless they are immunocompromised. Examination of more than one stool specimen may be necessary to establish a diagnosis. Certain medications, antidiarrheal compounds, and barium may interfere with identification of parasitic enteropathogens. Treatment of these organisms depends on the clinical condition and availability of effective therapy (Table 176–4).

TABLE 176–2 Noninfectious Causes of Diarrhea

Feeding Difficulty

Anatomic Defects
- Malrotation
- Intestinal duplications
- Hirschsprung disease
- Fecal impaction
- Short bowel syndrome
- Microvillus atrophy
- Strictures

Malabsorption
- Disaccharidase deficiencies
  - Glucose-galactose monosaccharide malabsorption
- Pancreatic insufficiency
  - Cystic fibrosis
  - Shwachman syndrome
- Reduced intraluminal bile salts
  - Cholestasis
- Hereditary fructose intolerance
- Abetalipoproteinemia
- Celiac disease

Endocrinopathies
- Thyrotoxicosis
- Addison disease
- Adrenogenital syndrome

Food Poisoning
- Heavy metals
- Scombroid
- Ciguatera
- Mushrooms

Neoplasms
- Neuroblastomas
- Ganglioneuromas
- Pheochromocytomas
- Carcinoid
- Zollinger-Ellison syndrome
- Vasoactive intestinal peptide syndrome

Miscellaneous
- Milk allergy
- Crohn disease (regional enteritis)
- Familial dysautonomia
- Immune deficiency disease
- Protein-losing enteropathy
- Ulcerative colitis
- Acrodermatitis enteropathica
- Hartnup disease
- Laxative abuse
- Motility disorders

TABLE 176–3 Antimicrobial Therapy for Bacterial Enteropathogens in Children

Organism	Antimicrobial Agent	Indication for Antimicrobial Therapy
Aeromonas	TMP/SMX	Dysentery-like illness, prolonged diarrhea
Campylobacter	Erythromycin*	Early in the course of illness
Clostridium difficile	Metronidazole or vancomycin	Moderate to severe disease
Escherichia coli		
Enterotoxigenic	TMP/SMX*	Severe or prolonged illness
Enteropathogenic	TMP/SMX	Nursery epidemics, life-threatening illness
Enteroinvasive	TMP/SMX*	All cases if organism susceptible
Salmonella	Ampicillin or chloramphenicol or TMP/SMX or cefotaxime*	Infants <3 mo, immunodeficient patients, typhoid fever (*Salmonella typhi*), bacteremia, dissemination with localized suppuration
Shigella	TMP/SMX; cefixime or ceftriaxone for resistant strains*	All cases if organism susceptible
Vibrio cholerae	Tetracycline or doxycycline	All cases

**Quinolones (ciprofloxacin or ofloxacin) are recommended for persons ≥18 yr of age. TMP-SMX = trimethoprim and sulfamethoxazole.*

Viral Enteropathogens. The four causes of viral gastroenteritis include rotavirus, enteric adenovirus, astrovirus, and calicivirus. Cytomegalovirus and herpes simplex virus have been associated with diarrhea and other GI tract signs and symptoms, generally in immunocompromised hosts.

GENERAL APPROACH TO CHILDREN WITH ACUTE DIARRHEA. Enteric infections cause signs of GI tract involvement as well as systemic manifestations and complications. GI tract involvement may include diarrhea, cramps, and emesis. Systemic manifestations may include fever, malaise, and seizures. Extraintestinal infections related to bacterial enteric pathogens include local spread, causing vulvovaginitis, urinary tract infection, and keratoconjunctivitis. Remote spread can result in endocarditis, osteomyelitis, meningitis, pneumonia, hepatitis, peritonitis, chorioamnionitis, soft tissue infection, and septic thrombophlebitis. Immune-mediated extraintestinal manifestations of enteric pathogens usually occur after diarrhea has resolved (Table 176–5).

The main objectives in the approach to a child with acute

TABLE 176–4 Antimicrobial Therapy for Enteric Parasites in Children

Organism	Antimicrobial Agent
Giardia lamblia	Metronidazole or furazolidone or paromomycin
Entamoeba histolytica	Metronidazole followed by iodoquinol
Blastocystis hominis	Metronidazole or iodoquinol
Cryptosporidium parvum	None*
Cyclospora cayetanensis	Trimethoprim/sulfamethoxazole (TMP/SMX)
Isospora belli	TMP/SMX
Enterocytozoon bieneusi	Albendazole
Enterocytozoon intestinalis	Albendazole
Strongyloides stercoralis	Thiabendazole

**Paromomycin or azithromycin may be indicated in immunocompromised hosts.*

TABLE 176–5 Immune-Mediated Extraintestinal Manifestations of Enteric Pathogens

Manifestation	Related Enteric Pathogen(s)
Reactive arthritis	*Salmonella, Shigella, Yersinia, Campylobacter, Cryptosporidium, Clostridium difficile*
Guillain-Barré syndrome	*Campylobacter*
Glomerulonephritis	*Shigella, Campylobacter, Yersinia*
IgA nephropathy	*Campylobacter*
Erythema nodosum	*Yersinia, Campylobacter, Salmonella*
Hemolytic anemia	*Campylobacter, Yersinia*

diarrhea are to (1) assess the degree of dehydration and provide fluid and electrolyte replacement, (2) prevent spread of the enteropathogen, and (3) in select episodes determine the etiologic agent and provide specific therapy if indicated. Information about oral intake, frequency and volume of stool output, general appearance and activity of the child, and frequency of urination must be obtained. Information should be obtained about child-care center attendance, recent travel to a diarrhea endemic area, use of antimicrobial agents, exposure to contacts with similar symptoms, and intake of seafood, unwashed vegetables, unpasteurized milk, contaminated water, or uncooked meats. The duration and severity of diarrhea, stool consistency, presence of mucus and blood, and other associated symptomatology, such as fever, vomiting, and seizures, should be determined. Fever is suggestive of an inflammatory process and also occurs as a result of dehydration. Nausea and emesis are nonspecific symptoms, but vomiting suggests organisms that infect the upper intestine, such as viruses, enterotoxin-producing bacteria, *Giardia,* and *Cryptosporidium.* Fever is common in patients with inflammatory diarrhea, abdominal pain is more severe, and tenesmus may occur in the lower abdomen and rectum, indicating involvement of the large intestine. Emesis is common in noninflammatory diarrhea; fever usually is absent or low grade; pain is crampy, periumbilical, and not severe; and diarrhea is watery, indicating upper intestinal tract involvement. Because immunocompromised patients require special consideration, information about an underlying immunodeficiency or chronic disease is important. Chronic diarrhea is defined as diarrhea lasting more than 14 days.

Examination of Stool. Stool specimens should be examined for mucus, blood, and leukocytes, the presence of which indicates colitis. Fecal leukocytes are produced in response to bacteria that invade the colonic mucosa diffusely. A positive fecal leukocyte examination indicates the presence of an invasive or cytotoxin-producing organism such as *Shigella, Salmonella, C. jejuni,* invasive *E. coli, C. difficile, Y. enterocolitica, V. parahaemolyticus,* and possibly an *Aeromonas* species or *P. shigelloides.* Not all patients with colitis have positive results on leukocyte examination. Patients infected with enterohemorrhagic *E. coli* and *E. histolytica* generally have minimal to no fecal leukocytes.

Stool cultures should be obtained as early in the course of the disease as possible from patients in whom the diagnosis of hemolytic uremic syndrome (HUS) is suspected, in patients with bloody diarrhea, if stools contain fecal leukocytes, during outbreaks of diarrhea, and in persons who have diarrhea and are immunosuppressed. Fecal specimens that cannot immediately be plated for culture can be transported to the laboratory in a non–nutrient-holding medium such as Cary-Blair to prevent drying or overgrowth of specific organisms.

Because certain bacterial agents, such as *Y. enterocolitica, V. cholerae, V. parahaemolyticus, Aeromonas* spp, *C. difficile,* and *Campylobacter* spp., require modified laboratory procedures for identification, laboratory personnel should be notified when one of these organisms is the suspected etiologic agent. Serotype and toxin assays are available for further characterization of *E. coli.* Detection of *C. difficile* toxins is valuable in the diagnosis of antimicrobial-associated colitis. Proctosigmoidoscopy may be helpful in establishing a diagnosis in patients in whom symptoms of colitis are severe or the cause of an inflammatory enteritis syndrome remains obscure after initial laboratory evaluation.

Management of Fluids and Electrolytes and Refeeding. Also see Chapters 54 and 55.1. Management of dehydration remains the cornerstone of therapy of diarrhea. Children, especially infants, are more susceptible than adults to dehydration because of the greater basal fluid and electrolyte requirements per kilogram and because they are dependent on others to meet these demands. Patients with diarrhea and possible dehydration should be evaluated to assess the degree of dehydration as evident from clinical signs and symptoms, ongoing losses, and daily requirements.

Oral hydration usually is the treatment of choice for all but the most severely dehydrated patients whose caretakers cannot administer fluids. Rapid rehydration with replacement of ongoing losses during the first 4–6 hr should be carried out using an appropriate oral rehydration solution. Once a patient is rehydrated, an orally administered maintenance solution should be used (see Table 54–1). Home remedies including decarbonated soda beverages, fruit juices, Jell-O, Kool-Aid, and tea are not suitable for use because they contain inappropriately high osmolalities due to excessive carbohydrate concentrations, which may exacerbate diarrhea; low sodium concentrations, which may cause hyponatremia; and inappropriate carbohydrate to sodium ratios. Once rehydration is complete, food should be reintroduced while the oral electrolyte solution is continued to replace ongoing losses from stools and for maintenance. Breast-feeding of infants should be resumed as soon as possible. Older children should be refed as soon as they can tolerate feeding. Foods with complex carbohydrates (rice, wheat, potatoes, bread, and cereals), lean meats, yogurt, fruits, and vegetables are better tolerated. Fatty foods or foods high in simple sugars (including juices and carbonated sodas) should be avoided.

Antidiarrheal Compounds. These agents are classified by their mechanism of action, which includes alteration of intestinal motility, adsorption of fluid or toxins, alteration of intestinal microflora, and alteration of fluid and electrolyte secretion. Antidiarrheal compounds are generally not recommended for use in children with diarrhea because of their minimal benefit and potential for side effects.

PREVENTION. Patients who are hospitalized should be placed under contact precautions, including handwashing before and after patient contact, gowns when soiling is likely, and gloves when touching infected material. Patients and their families should be educated about the mode of acquisition of enteropathogens and methods to decrease transmission. Patients who attend child-care centers should be excluded from the center or cared for in a separate area until diarrhea has subsided. Cases of diarrhea caused by *E. histolytica,* episodes secondary to *E. coli* 0157:H7, *Giardia, Campylobacter, Salmonella, Shigella, V. cholerae,* and *V. parahaemolytica* should be reported to the local health department.

Vaccines are available to prevent or modify infection by rotavirus, which is recommended for all infants, and *Salmonella typhi,* which is recommended for international travelers to endemic areas of developing countries. Cholera vaccine induces incomplete, unreliable protection of short duration and is not recommended.

ACUTE FOOD-BORNE AND WATER-BORNE DISEASE. Food-borne and water-borne disease is a major cause of morbidity and mortality in all developed countries, including the United States. Changes in food production, flaws in inspection systems, rapid international distribution of food, alterations in dietary habits, and lack of recognition of methods of prevention magnify these problems. Food-borne illness in the United States is estimated to cause 6–81 million cases of gastroenteritis yearly,

TABLE 176–6 Characteristics of Food-Borne Illness by Symptoms and Incubation Period

Symptoms	Incubation Period (hr)	Cause
Nausea and vomiting	<1–6	*Staphylococcus aureus, Bacillus cereus*, heavy metals
Paresthesia	0–6	Fish and shellfish, monosodium glutamate, niacin
Neurologic, gastroenteritis	0–2	Mushroom (early onset)
Watery diarrhea, abdominal cramps	8–16	*B. cereus, C. perfringens*
	16–48	Caliciviruses, enterotoxigenic *E. coli, Vibrio cholerae* 01 and non-01, *Cryptosporidium, Cyclospora*
Diarrhea, fever, abdominal cramps	16–72	*Salmonella, Shigella, Clostridium jejuni, Yersinia enterocolitica*, enteroinvasive *E. coli, Vibrio parahaemolyticus*
Bloody diarrhea, abdominal cramps	72–120	Enterohemorrhagic *E. coli*
Neurologic, hepatorenal	6–24	Mushroom (late onset)
Paralysis, nausea, vomiting	18–48	*Clostridium botulinum*

to cause 500–7,000 annual deaths, and to cost $8–23 billion yearly in medical costs and lost productivity.

The diagnosis of a food-borne or water-borne illness should be considered when two or more persons who have ingested common food or water develop a similar acute illness that usually is characterized by nausea, emesis, diarrhea, or neurologic symptoms. Pathogenesis and severity of bacterial disease depend on whether organisms have preformed toxins (*Staphylococcus aureus, Bacillus cereus*), produce toxins, or are invasive and whether they replicate in food. The severity of disease due to viral, parasitic, and chemical causes depends on the amount inoculated into the food or water. The epidemiology of outbreaks often suggests specific etiologic agents. Determination of the incubation period and the specific clinical syndrome often leads to the correct diagnosis. Confirmation is established by specific laboratory testing of food, stool, or emesis. As a general rule, when outbreaks are grouped by incubation period of illness, those less than 1 hr are associated with chemical poisoning, toxins from fish or shellfish, or preformed toxins of *S. aureus* or *B. cereus*. Enterotoxin-producing bacteria, invasive bacteria, calicivirus, and some forms of mushroom poisoning have longer incubation periods.

Clinical Syndromes. Several clinical syndromes follow ingestion of contaminated food or water, including nausea and vomiting within 6 hr; paresthesia within 6 hr; neurologic and GI tract symptoms within 2 hr; abdominal cramps and watery diarrhea within 16–48 hr; fever, abdominal cramps and diarrhea within 8–72 hr; abdominal cramps and bloody diarrhea without fever within 72–120 hr; neurologic signs and symptoms within 6–24 hr; and nausea, vomiting, and paralysis within 18–48 hr (Table 176–6).

Short incubation periods with vomiting as the major sign are associated with toxins that produce direct gastric irritation, such as heavy metals, or with preformed toxins of *B. cereus* or *S. aureus*; *B. cereus* also produces an enterotoxin. Paresthesias after a brief incubation period are suggestive of scombroid (histamine fish poisoning), paralytic or neurotoxic shellfish poisoning, Chinese restaurant syndrome (monosodium glutamate poisoning), niacin poisoning, or ciguatera fish poisoning. The early-onset syndrome associated with ingestion of toxic mushrooms ranges from gastroenteritis to neurologic symptoms that include parasympathetic hyperactivity, confusion, visual disturbances, and hallucinations to hepatic or hepatorenal failure, which occurs after a 6–24-hr incubation period.

Watery diarrhea and abdominal cramps after an 8–16-hr incubation period are associated with enterotoxin-producing *Clostridium perfringens* and *B. cereus*. Abdominal cramps and watery diarrhea following a 16–48-hr incubation period can be associated with calicivirus, several enterotoxin-producing bacteria, *Cryptosporidium* and *Cyclospora*. *Salmonella, Shigella, C. jejuni, Y. enterocolitica*, enteroinvasive *E. coli* and *V. parahaemolyticus* are associated with diarrhea that may contain fecal leukocytes, abdominal cramps, and fever, although these organisms can cause watery diarrhea without fever. Bloody diarrhea and abdominal cramps following a 72–120-hr incubation period are associated with enterohemorrhagic *E. coli*, such as *E. coli* 0157:H7. Hemolytic-uremic syndrome (Chapter 198) is a sequela of infection with enterohemorrhagic *E. coli*. The combination of GI tract symptoms followed by blurred vision, dry mouth, dysarthria, diplopia, or descending paralysis should suggest *Clostridium botulinum* as the cause.

Therapy of most persons with food-borne disease is supportive, because the majority of these illnesses are self-limited. The exceptions are botulism, paralytic shellfish poisoning, and long-acting mushroom poisoning, all of which may be fatal in previously healthy persons. If a food-borne or water-borne outbreak is suspected, public health officials should be notified.

American Academy of Pediatrics, Subcommittee on Acute Gastroenteritis: Practice parameter: The management of acute gastroenteritis in young children. Pediatrics 97:424, 1996.

Brown KH, Peerson JM, Fontaine O: Use of nonhuman milks in the dietary management of young children with acute diarrhea: A meta-analysis of clinical trials. Pediatrics 93:17, 1994.

Centers for Disease Control and Prevention: Surveillance for waterborne disease outbreaks—United States, 1995–1996. MMWR 47(SS-5):1, 1998.

Cicirello HG, Glass RI: Current concepts of the epidemiology of diarrheal diseases. Semin Pediatr Infect Dis 5:163, 1994.

Goodgame RW: Understanding intestinal spore-forming protozoa: Cryptosporidia, microsporidia, isospora and cyclospora. Ann Intern Med 124:429, 1996.

Guerrant RL: Lessons from diarrheal diseases: Demography to molecular pharmacology. J Infect Dis 169:1206, 1994.

International Study Group on reduced-osmolarity ORS solutions: Multicentre evaluation of reduced-osmolarity oral rehydration salts solution. Lancet 345:282, 1995.

Nataro JP, Kaper JB: Diarrheagenic *Escherichia coli*. Clin Microbiol Rev 11:142, 1998.

Pavia AT: Approach to acute foodborne and waterborne disease. Semin Pediatr Infect Dis 5:222, 1994.

Pickering LK: Emerging antibiotic resistance in enteric bacterial pathogens. Semin Pediatr Infect Dis 7:272, 1996.

Pickering LK, Morrow AL: Factors in human milk that protect against diarrheal disease. Infection 21:355, 1993.

Sears CL, Kaper JB: Enteric bacterial toxins: Mechanisms of action and linkage to intestinal secretion. Microbiol Rev 60:167, 1996.

Snyder J: The continuing evolution of oral therapy for diarrhea. Semin Pediatr Infect Dis 5:231, 1994.

CHAPTER 177
Viral Hepatitis

John D. Snyder and Larry K. Pickering

Viral hepatitis continues to be a major health problem in developing and developed countries. Advances in the field of molecular biology have aided identification and understanding of the pathogenesis of the six viruses that are now known to cause hepatitis as their primary disease manifestation. These hepatotropic viruses are designated hepatitis A, B, C, D, E and G (Table 177–1). Many other viruses can cause hepatitis as part of their clinical spectrum, including herpes simplex virus (HSV), cytomegalovirus (CMV), Epstein-Barr virus, varicella, HIV, rubella, adenoviruses, enteroviruses, parvovirus B19, and arboviruses. However the hepatic involvement with these viruses is usually only one component of a multisystem disease.

The six hepatotropic viruses are a heterogeneous group of viruses that cause similar acute clinical illness, except for the

TABLE 177–1 Viral Hepatitis Nomenclature

Hepatotropic Viruses	Antigens	Identified Antibodies
Hepatitis A virus (HAV)	HAV	anti-HAV*
		IgM anti-HAV
Hepatitis B virus (HBV)	HBsAg*	anti-HBsAg*
		IgM anti-HBsAg*
	HBcAg	anti-HBcAg*
	HBeAg*	anti-HBeAg*
Hepatitis C virus (HCV)		anti-HCV*
Hepatitis D virus (HDV)	HDAg	anti-HDV*
Hepatitis E virus (HEV)		anti-HEV
		IgM anti-HEV
Hepatitis G virus (HGV)		anti-HGV

**Assays are commercially available.*

most recently discovered virus, HGV, which appears to cause no or mild disease. HBV is a DNA virus, while HAV, HCV, HDV, HEV, and HGV are RNA viruses representing four different families (Table 177–2). HAV and HEV are not known to cause chronic illness, whereas HB-DV, HB, C, and D viruses can cause important morbidity and mortality through chronic infections. HGV can cause chronic infections but with little morbidity or mortality yet reported. In the United States, HAV appears to cause most cases of hepatitis in children. HBV probably accounts for about one third of the cases in children, whereas HCV is found in approximately 20%. HDV occurs in only a small percentage of children who must also have HBV infection. HEV has not been reported in children who have lived and traveled only in the United States. Because HGV is newly recognized, its role is not yet completely known, but the virus appears to account for a small percentage of the cases of non–HA-EV (or non-HAV-HEV).

DIFFERENTIAL DIAGNOSIS. The probable causes of hepatitis vary somewhat by age. Physiologic jaundice, hemolytic disease, and sepsis in neonates usually are distinguished easily from hepatitis. In the newborn period, infection remains an important cause of hyperbilirubinemia but metabolic and anatomic causes (biliary atresia and choledochal cysts) also must be considered. The introduction of pigmented vegetables into an infant's diet may result in carotenemia, which may be mistaken for jaundice.

In later infancy and childhood, hemolytic-uremic syndrome may be initially mistaken for hepatitis (see Chapter 526). Reye and Reye-like syndromes present in a similar fashion to acute fulminating hepatitis (Chapter 360). Jaundice also may occur with malaria, leptospirosis, and brucellosis and with severe infection in older children, particularly in children with malignancy or immunodeficiency. Gallstones may obstruct biliary drainage and cause jaundice in adolescents as well as in children with chronic hemolytic processes. Hepatitis may be the initial presentation of Wilson's disease, cystic fibrosis, and Jamaican vomiting sickness. The liver may be involved in collagen diseases including systemic lupus erythematosus.

Medications, including acetaminophen overdose, valproic acid, and various hepatotoxins, can be associated with a hepatitis-like picture. Drugs well tolerated in healthy children may cause problems in children with certain illnesses.

HEPATITIS A

ETIOLOGY. HAV is a 27-nm-diameter, RNA-containing virus that is a member of the Picornavirus family. It originally was isolated from stools of infected patients. Laboratory strains of HAV have been propagated in tissue culture. Acute infection is diagnosed by detecting immunoglobulin M (IgM) antibodies (anti-HAV) by radioimmunoassay or, rarely, by identifying viral particles in stool.

EPIDEMIOLOGY. HAV infections occur throughout the world but are found most commonly in developing countries, where the prevalence rate approaches 100% in children by age 5 yr. In the United States, approximately 30–40% of the adult population has evidence for previous HAV infection, with the rates of infection being similar in the first, second, and third decades of life. Hepatitis A causes only acute hepatitis and accounts for approximately 50% of clinically apparent acute viral hepatitis in the United States. The illness is much more likely to be symptomatic in adults than in children. Most infections in children younger than 5 yr are asymptomatic or have mild, nonspecific manifestations. Transmission of HAV is almost always by person-to-person contact. Spread is predominantly by the fecal-oral route; percutaneous transmission is a rare occurrence, and maternal-neonatal transmission is not recognized as an epidemiologic entity. HAV infection during pregnancy or at the time of delivery does not appear to result in increased complications of pregnancy or increased clinical disease in the newborn. The infectivity of human saliva, urine, and semen is unknown. In the United States, increased risk of infection is found in contacts of infected persons, child-care centers, household contacts of children in child-care, and homosexual populations and is associated with contact with contaminated food or water and travel to endemic areas. However, no known source is found in about half of the cases. Common source food-borne and water-borne outbreaks have occurred, including several due to contaminated shellfish. Fecal excretion of the virus occurs late in the incubation period, reaches its peak just before the onset of symptoms, and is minimal in the week after the onset of jaundice (Fig. 177–1). The mean incubation period for HAV is about 4 wk, with a range of 15–50 days.

PATHOGENESIS. The acute response of the liver to HAV is similar to that of the hepatotropic viruses (HBV-HEV). The entire liver is involved with necrosis, most markedly in the centrilobular areas, and increased cellularity, which is predominant in the portal areas. The lobular architecture remains intact, although balloon degeneration and necrosis of single or groups of parenchymal cells occur initially. Fatty change is rare. A diffuse mononuclear cell inflammatory reaction causes expansion in the portal tracts; bile duct proliferation is common, but bile duct damage is not often found. Diffuse Kupffer cell hyperplasia is present in the sinusoids, along with infiltration of polymorphonuclear leukocytes and eosinophils. Neonates respond to hepatic injury by forming giant cells. In fulminant

TABLE 177–2 Features of the Six Hepatotropic Viruses

	HAV	HBV	HCV	HDV	HEV	HGV
Nucleic acid	RNA	DNA	RNA	RNA	RNA	RNA
Incubation (mean)	30 days	100–120 days	7–9 wk	2–4 mo	40 days	Unknown
Transmission						
Percutaneous	Rare	Common	Common	Common	No	Common
Fecal-oral	Common	No	No	No	Common	No
Sexual	Rare	Common	Rare	Rare	Rare	Rare
Transplacental	No	Common	Rare	No	Probably no	Rare
Chronic infection	No	Yes	Yes	Yes	No	Yes
Fulminant disease	Rare	Yes	Rare	Yes	Rare	Probably no

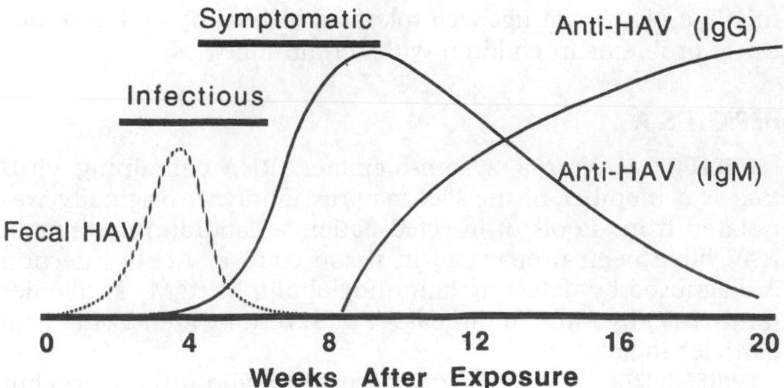

Figure 177–1 Pattern of response to hepatitis A virus (HAV) infection. (IgM = immunoglobulin M; IgG = immunoglobulin G.)

hepatitis, total destruction of the parenchyma occurs, leaving only connective tissue septa. By 3 mo after the onset of acute hepatitis due to HAV, the liver usually is normal morphologically.

Other organ systems can be affected during HAV infection. Regional lymph nodes and the spleen may be enlarged. The bone marrow may be moderately hypoplastic, and aplastic anemia has been reported. Small intestine tissue may show changes in villous structure, and ulceration of the gastrointestinal tract can occur, especially in fatal cases. Acute pancreatitis and myocarditis have been reported rarely, and nephritis, arthritis, vasculitis, and cryoglobulinemia may result from circulating immune complexes.

Injury in acute hepatitis caused by hepatotropic viruses is evidenced in three main ways. The first is a reflection of cytopathic injury to the hepatocytes, which release alanine aminotransferase (ALT, formerly serum glutamic-pyruvic transaminase) and aspartate aminotransferase (AST, formerly serum glutamic-oxaloacetic transaminase) into the bloodstream. ALT is more specific to the liver than AST, which also can be elevated after injury to erythrocytes, skeletal muscle, or myocardial cells. The height of elevation does not correlate with the extent of hepatocellular necrosis and has little prognostic value. In some cases, a falling aminotransferase level may predict a poor outcome if the decline occurs in conjunction with a rising bilirubin level and prolonged prothrombin time (PT). This combination of findings indicates that massive hepatic injury has occurred, resulting in few functioning hepatocytes. Another enzyme, lactic dehydrogenase (LDH), is even less specific to liver than AST and usually is not helpful in evaluating liver injury. The second mechanism of injury in viral hepatitis results from cholestatic jaundice, in which both direct and indirect bilirubin levels are elevated. Jaundice results from obstruction of biliary flow and damage to hepatocytes. Elevations of serum alkaline phosphatase (ALP), 5′-nucleotidase, γ-glutamyl transpeptidase (GGT), and urobilinogen all can reflect injury to the biliary system. Abnormal protein synthesis is reflected by increased PT. Because of the short half-life of these proteins, the PT is a sensitive indicator of damage to the liver. Serum albumin is another liver-manufactured serum protein, but its longer half-life limits its role in monitoring acute liver injury. Cholestasis results in a decreased intestinal bile acid pool and decreased absorption of fat-soluble vitamins. The third mechanism of hepatic injury by HAV is related to changes that occur in carbohydrate, ammonia, and drug metabolism. Although circulating immune complexes commonly occur in HAV infection, no direct evidence shows that they induce hepatic necrosis or viral clearance.

CLINICAL MANIFESTATIONS. The onset of HAV infection usually is abrupt and is accompanied by systemic complaints of fever, malaise, nausea, emesis, anorexia, and abdominal discomfort. This prodrome may be mild and often goes unnoticed in infants and preschool-aged children. Diarrhea often occurs in children, but constipation is more common in adults. Jaundice may be so subtle in young children that it can be detected only by laboratory tests. When jaundice and dark urine occur, they usually develop after the systemic symptoms. In contrast to infections in children, most HAV infections in adults are symptomatic and can be severe. Symptoms of HAV infection include right upper quadrant pain, dark-colored urine, and jaundice. The duration of symptoms usually is less than 1 mo, and appetite, exercise tolerance, and a feeling of well-being gradually return. Almost all patients with HAV infection recover completely, but a relapsing course can occur for several months. Fulminant hepatitis leading to death is rare. HAV is not associated with chronic liver disease, persistent viremia, or an intestinal carrier state.

DIAGNOSIS. The diagnosis of HAV infection should be considered when a history of jaundice exists in family contacts, friends, schoolmates, or child-care playmates or personnel or if the child or family have traveled to an area endemic for HAV. The diagnosis is made by serologic criteria; liver biopsies rarely are performed. Anti-HAV is detected at the onset of symptoms of acute hepatitis A and persists for life (see Fig. 177–1). The acute infection is diagnosed by the presence of IgM anti-HAV, which is present at the onset of illness and usually disappears within 4 mo but may persist for 6 mo or longer. Thereafter, IgG anti-HAV is detectable. IgM antibody is seldom detected after immunization. The virus is excreted in stools from 2 wk before to 1 wk after the onset of illness. Rises are almost universally found in ALT, AST, bilirubin, ALP, 5′-nucleotidase, and GGT and do not help to differentiate the etiology. The PT should always be measured in a child with hepatitis to help assess the extent of liver injury; prolongation is a serious sign mandating hospitalization.

COMPLICATIONS. Children almost universally recover from HAV infections. Rarely, fulminant hepatitis (see Chapter 363) can occur, in which a progressive rise in serum bilirubin is accompanied by an initial rise in aminotransferases followed by a fall to normal or low values despite disease progression. Hepatic synthetic function decreases, and the PT becomes prolonged and is often accompanied by bleeding. The serum albumin level falls, causing edema and ascites. The ammonia level usually rises, and the sensorium becomes altered, progressing from drowsiness to stupor and then deep coma. End-stage disease and death can occur in less than 1 wk or can develop more insidiously.

PREVENTION. Persons infected with HAV are contagious for about 7 days after the onset of jaundice and should be excluded from school, child care, or work during this period. Careful handwashing is necessary, particularly after changing diapers and before preparing or serving food. In hospital settings, contact as well as standard precautions, including strict handwashing, are recommended for diapered or incontinent patients for 1 wk after onset of symptoms.

Vaccine. The availability of two inactivated, highly immunogenic and safe HAV vaccines marks a major advance in the prevention of HAV infection. Both vaccines are approved for persons age 2 yr or older. They are administered intramuscularly in a two-dose schedule, with the second dose given 6–12 mo after the first dose. Seroconversion rates in children exceed 90% after an initial dose and approach 100% after the second dose. The immune response in immunocompromised persons may be suboptimal. HAV vaccine may be administered simultaneously with other vaccines at separate sites. Recommended use of HAV vaccine in the United States is primarily for susceptible persons traveling to or working in countries where HAV is endemic. For persons age 2 yr or older, vaccine is preferable to immunoglobulin (IG) for pre-exposure prophylaxis (Table 177–3). Other candidates for HAV immunization include (1) children age 2 or older in defined and circumscribed communities with endemic rates or periodic outbreaks of HAV infection (i.e., Native Americans or Alaskan Natives); (2) patients with

TABLE 177–3 Hepatitis A Virus Prophylaxis

Age	Exposure	Dose
Pre-Exposure Prophylaxis (Travelers to Endemic Regions)		
< 2 yr	Expected < 3 mo	IG 0.02 mL/kg
	Expected 3–5 mo	IG 0.06 mL/kg
	Expected long term	IG 0.06 mL/kg at departure and every 5 mo thereafter
≥ 2 yr	Expected < 3 mo	HAV vaccine* OR IG 0.02 mL/kg
	Expected 3–5 mo	HAV vaccine* OR IG 0.06 mL/kg
	Expected long term	HAV vaccine*
Postexposure Prophylaxis		
	Future exposure likely	
≥ 2 yr	≤ 2 wk since exposure	IG 0.02 mL/kg and HAV vaccine
	> 2 wk since exposure	HAV vaccine*
	Future exposure unlikely	
All ages	≤ 2 wk since exposure	IG 0.02 mL/kg and HAV vaccine should be considered (if ≥ 2 years)
	> 2 wk since exposure	No prophylaxis

**Two inactivated vaccines are approved for use in persons ≥ 2 yr of age.*
IG = Immunoglobulin.

chronic liver disease; (3) homosexual or bisexual men; (4) users of injection and illicit drugs; (5) individuals at occupational risk of exposure.

Immunoglobulin. Indications for intramuscular administration of IG include pre-exposure and postexposure prophylaxis (Table 177–3). Intravenous IG (IVIG) is likely to be effective against HAV infection, but appropriate dose, efficacy, and duration of protection have not been defined. IG is recommended for pre-exposure prophylaxis for all susceptible travelers to countries where HAV is endemic. For individuals age 2 yr and older, HAV immunization is preferred if the interval before departure is more than 1 mo after dose one. IG as prophylaxis in postexposure situations is used in (1) household and sexual contacts of HAV cases; (2) newborn infants of HAV-infected mothers; (3) child-care center staff, employees, children and their household contacts during an outbreak; and (4) outbreaks in institutions and hospitals. The use of IG more than 2 wk after exposure is not indicated.

IG is not recommended routinely for sporadic nonhousehold exposure (e.g., protection of hospital personnel or schoolmates). Mass immunization of school children has been used when epidemics have been school centered. Available data are not sufficient to recommend HAV vaccine alone for postexposure prophylaxis.

HEPATITIS B

ETIOLOGY. HBV is a 42-nm-diameter member of the Hepadnaviridae family, a noncytopathogenic, hepatotropic group of DNA viruses. HBV has a circular, partially double-stranded DNA genome composed of approximately 3,200 nucleotides. Four genes have been identified, the S (surface), C (core), X, and P (polymer) genes. The surface of the virus includes two particles designated hepatitis B surface antigen (HBsAg): a 22-nm-diameter spherical particle and a 22-nm-wide tubular particle with a variable length of up to 200 nm. The inner portion of the virion contains hepatitis B core antigen (HBcAg), the nucleocapsid that encodes the viral DNA, and a nonstructural antigen called hepatitis B e antigen (HBeAg), a nonparticulate soluble antigen derived from HBcAg by proteolytic self-cleavage. HBeAg serves as a marker of active viral replication. Replication of HBV occurs predominantly in the liver but also occurs in the lymphocytes, spleen, kidney, and pancreas.

EPIDEMIOLOGY. Worldwide, the areas of highest prevalence of HBV infection are sub-Saharan Africa, China, parts of the Middle East, the Amazon basin, and the Pacific Islands. In the United States, the Eskimo population in Alaska has the highest prevalence rate. An estimated 300,000 new cases of HBV infection occur in the United States each year, with the 20–39-yr-old age group at greatest risk. The number of new cases in children reported each year is thought to be low but is difficult to estimate because the majority of infections in children are asymptomatic. The risk of chronic infection is related inversely to age; although fewer than 10% of infections occur in children, these infections account for 20–30% of all chronic cases.

The most important risk factor for acquisition of HBV in children is perinatal exposure to an HBsAg-positive mother. The risk of transmission is greatest if the mother also is HBeAg positive; 70–90% of their infants become chronically infected if untreated. During the neonatal period, hepatitis B antigen is present in blood of 2.5% of infants born to affected mothers, indicating that intrauterine infection occurred. In most cases, antigenemia appears later, suggesting that transmission occurred at the time of delivery; virus contained in amniotic fluid or in maternal feces or blood may be the source. Although most infants born to infected mothers become antigenemic from 2–5 mo of age, some infants of HBsAg-positive mothers are not affected until later ages. Of the 22,000 infants born each year to HBsAg-positive mothers in the United States, more than 98% receive immunoprophylaxis and are protected from infection.

HBsAg has been demonstrated inconsistently in human milk of infected mothers. Breast-feeding of unimmunized infants by infected mothers does not appear to confer a greater risk of hepatitis on offspring than does formula feeding, despite the possibility that cracked nipples may result in ingestion of contaminated maternal blood by a nursing infant.

Other important risk factors for HBV infection in children and adolescents include intravenous acquisition by drugs or blood products, sexual contact, institutional care, and contact with carriers. No risk factors are identified in about 40% of cases.

The risk of developing chronic HBV infection, defined as being positive for HBsAg for 6 mo or more or being negative for IgM anti-HBc and positive for HBsAg, is related inversely to age; the older the age of acquisition, the lower the risk of chronic disease. Chronic infection is associated with chronic liver disease and primary hepatocellular carcinoma, which is the most important cause of cancer-related death in Asia.

HBV is present in high concentrations in blood, serum, and serous exudates and in moderate concentrations in saliva, vaginal fluid, and semen. For these reasons, efficient transmission occurs through blood exposure and sexual contact. The incubation period ranges from 45–160 days, with a mean of about 120 days.

PATHOGENESIS. The acute response of the liver to HBV is the same as for all the hepatotropic viruses. Persistence of histologic changes in patients with hepatitis B, C, or D indicates development of chronic liver disease (Chapter 361).

HBV, unlike the other hepatotropic viruses, is a noncytopathogenic virus that causes injury by immune-mediated processes. The severity of hepatocyte injury reflects the degree of the immune response, with the most complete immune response being associated with the greatest likelihood of viral clearance and the most severe injury to hepatocytes. The first step in the process of acute hepatitis is infection of hepatocytes by HBV, resulting in viral antigens on the cell surface. The most important of these viral antigens may be the nucleocapsid antigens, HBcAg and HBeAg. These antigens, in combination with class I major histocompatibility (MHC) proteins, make the cell a target for cytotoxic T-cell lysis.

The mechanism for development of chronic hepatitis is less well understood. To permit hepatocytes to continue to be infected, the core protein or MHC class I protein may not be recognized, the cytotoxic lymphocytes may not be activated, or some other yet unknown mechanism may interfere with destruction of hepatocytes. For cell-to-cell infection to continue, some virus-containing hepatocytes must remain alive.

Immune-mediated mechanisms also are involved in the extrahepatic conditions that can be associated with HBV infections. Circulating immune complexes containing HBsAg can occur in patients who develop associated polyarteritis nodosa, membranous or membranoproliferative glomerulonephritis, polymyalgia rheumatica, leukocytoclastic vasculitis, and Guillain-Barré syndrome.

Mutations of HBV are more common than for the usual DNA viruses, and a series of mutant strains have been recognized. The most important mutation, which does not affect replication, is one that results in failure to express HBeAg and has been associated with development of severe hepatitis and perhaps more severe exacerbations of chronic HBV infection. Other core-related mutations yielding similar results have been noted.

CLINICAL MANIFESTATIONS. Many cases of HBV infection are asymptomatic, as evidenced by the high carriage rate of serum markers in persons who have no history of acute hepatitis. The usual acute symptomatic episode is similar to HAV and HCV infections but may be more severe and is more likely to include involvement of skin and joints. The first clinical evidence of HBV infection is elevation of ALT level, which begins to rise just before development of lethargy, anorexia, and malaise, which occur about 6–7 wk after exposure. The illness may be preceded in a few children by a serum sickness–like prodrome marked by arthralgia or skin lesions, including urticarial, purpuric, macular, or maculopapular rashes. Papular acrodermatitis, the Gianotti-Crosti syndrome, also may occur. Other extrahepatic conditions associated with HBV infections in children can include polyarteritis, glomerulonephritis, and aplastic anemia. Jaundice, which may be present in about 25% of infected individuals, usually begins about 8 wk after exposure and lasts for about 4 wk. In the usual course of resolving HBV infection, symptoms are present for 6–8 wk. The percentage of children in whom clinical evidence of hepatitis develops is higher for HBV than for HAV, and the rate of fulminant hepatitis also is greater. Chronic hepatitis also occurs, and the chronic active form can result in cirrhosis and hepatocellular carcinoma, which occurs almost exclusively in patients with cirrhosis, typically 25–30 yr after HBV infection.

On physical examination, symptomatic infection results in skin and mucous membranes that are icteric, especially the sclera and the mucosa under the tongue. The liver usually is enlarged and tender to palpation. When the liver is not palpable below the costal margin, tenderness can be demonstrated by gently striking the rib cage over the liver with a closed fist. Splenomegaly and lymphadenopathy are common.

DIAGNOSIS. The serologic pattern for HBV is more complex than for HAV and differs depending on whether the disease is acute, subclinical, or chronic (Fig. 177–2). Table 177–1 summarizes the several antigens and antibodies that can be used to confirm the diagnosis of acute HBV infection. Routine screening for HBV infection requires assay of at least two serologic markers. HBsAg is the first serologic marker of infection to appear and is found in almost all infected persons; its rise closely coincides with the onset of symptoms. HBeAg is often present during the acute phase and indicates a highly infectious state. Because HBsAg levels fall before the end of symptoms, IgM antibody to HBcAg (IgM anti-HBcAg) also is required because it rises early after infection and persists for many months before being replaced by IgG anti-HBcAg, which persists for years. IgM anti-HBcAg usually is not present in perinatal HBV infections. Anti-HBcAg is the most valuable single serologic marker of acute HBV infection because it is present almost as early as HBsAg and continues to be present later in the course of the disease when HBsAg has disappeared. Only anti-HBsAg is present in persons immunized with hepatitis B vaccine, whereas anti-HBsAg and anti-HBcAg are detected in persons with resolved infection.

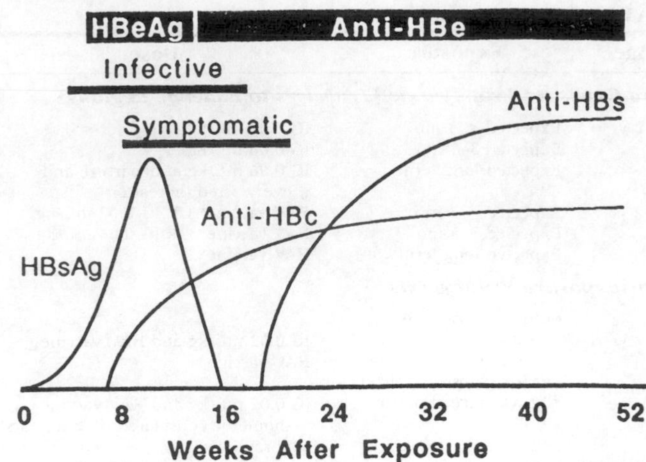

Figure 177–2 Pattern of response to hepatitis B virus infection. (HBeAg = hepatitis B e antigen: HBsAg = hepatitis B surface antigen HBc = hepatitis B core antigen.)

TREATMENT. No available medical therapy is successful in the majority of persons infected with HBV. Interferon-α-2b (IFN-α2b) is approved for treatment of chronic hepatitis B in patients age 18 yr or older with compensated liver disease and HBV replication. IFN-α2b also has been used in children, with long-term eradication rates similar to the 25% rate reported in adults. Recombinant interferons have immunomodulatory and antiviral effects. Persons most likely to respond have low serum HBV DNA titers, HBeAg, active inflammation, and recently acquired disease. Remissions generally are sustained without further treatment. Liver transplantation also has been used to treat patients with end-stage HBV infection.

COMPLICATIONS. Acute fulminant hepatitis with coagulopathy, encephalopathy, and cerebral edema occurs more frequently with HBV than with the other hepatotropic viruses, and the risk of fulminant hepatitis is further increased when there is co-infection or superinfection with HDV. Mortality due to fulminant hepatitis is greater than 30%. Liver transplantation is the only effective intervention; supportive care aimed at sustaining patients while providing the time needed for regeneration of hepatic cells is the only other option.

HBV infections also can result in chronic hepatitis, which can lead to cirrhosis and primary hepatocellular carcinoma (Chapter 510.2). Membranous glomerulonephritis with deposition of complement and HBeAg in glomerular capillaries is a rare complication of HBV infection. Immunization to decrease the carrier rate in the population has resulted in a marked decline in the incidence of hepatocellular carcinoma in children in Taiwan.

PREVENTION. Hepatitis B vaccine and hepatitis B immunoglobulin (HBIG) are available for prevention of HBV infection. Two recombinant DNA vaccines are available in the United States, and both are highly immunogenic in children. Universal immunization of all infants with hepatitis B vaccine is recommended in both pre-exposure and postexposure situations and provides long-term protection. In addition, all children who have not previously received the vaccine should be immunized by or before 11–12 yr of age, and catch-up programs should be implemented for unimmunized adolescents and high-risk adults. HBIG is indicated only for specific postexposure circumstances and provides temporary protection.

Infants born to HBsAg-positive women should receive vaccine at birth, 1–2 mo, and 6 mo of age (Table 177–4). The first dose should be accompanied by administration of 0.5 mL of HBIG as soon after delivery as possible, because the effective-

TABLE 177–4 Indications and Dosing Schedule for Hepatitis B Vaccine and Hepatitis B Immune Globulin

Groups	Vaccine			HBIG	
	Recombivax HB (μg)	*Engerix-B* (μg)	*Schedule*	*Dose* (mL)	*Schedule*
Neonates					
Infants of HBsAg-positive women	5	10	Birth, 1, 6 mo	0.5	Within 12 hr of birth
Infants of HBsAg-negative women	5	10	Birth, 1–2, 6–18 mo	None	
Children and adolescents (11–19 yr)	5	10	0, 1, and 6 mo	None	
Contact with acute HBV					
Intimate					
0–19 yr old	5	10	Exposure, 1 and 6 mo	0.06/kg	At exposure
>19 yr old	10	20	Exposure, 1 and 6 mo	0.06/kg	At exposure
Household	None	None	None	None	
Casual	None	None	None	None	
Contact with chronic HBV					
Intimate and household					
0–19 yr old	5	10	Exposure, 1 and 6 mo	None	
>19 yr old	10	20	Exposure, 1 and 6 mo	None	
Casual	None	None		None	
Immunosuppressed or hemodialysis patients	40	40	Exposure, 1 and 6 mo	None	

ness decreases rapidly with increased time after birth. Postvaccination testing for HBsAg and anti-HBs should be at 9–15 mo. If positive for anti-HBs, the child is immune to HBV. If positive for HBsAg only, the parent should be counseled and the child evaluated by a pediatric hepatologist. If negative for both HBsAg and anti-HBs, a second complete hepatitis B vaccine series should be administered, followed by testing for anti-HBs to determine if subsequent doses are needed.

Infants born to HBsAg-negative women should receive the vaccine at 0–2 mo, 1–4 mo, and at 6–18 mo of age. Routine postvaccination testing of immunized infants born to HBsAg-negative women or with anti-HBs is not recommended. The three-dose series can be completed regardless of the intervals between doses.

Recommendations for postexposure prophylaxis for prevention of hepatitis B infection depend on the conditions under which the person is exposed to HBV (Table 177–4).

HEPATITIS C

ETIOLOGY. HCV is now recognized as the cause of almost all parenterally acquired cases of what was previously known as non-A, non-B hepatitis. The virus has not been isolated but was cloned in 1988 using recombinant DNA technology. HCV is a single-stranded RNA virus, classified as a separate genus within the Flaviviridae family, with marked genetic heterogeneity. It has six major genotypes and numerous subtypes and quasi-species, which may permit it to escape host immune surveillance. Genetic variation may partially explain the differences in clinical course.

EPIDEMIOLOGY. The most important risk factor for HCV transmission in the United States is intravenous or intranasal drug use with exposure to blood or blood products from HCV-infected persons. Other risk factors include sexual contacts with an infected person, multiple sexual partners, imprisonment, and occupational exposure. Approximately 10% of new infections are unexplained. Perinatal transmission has been described but is uncommon except when the mother is HIV infected or has a high titer of HCV RNA. Since the introduction of routine blood tests for HCV in 1985–1990, the risk of HCV infection from a blood transfusion is now less than 0.01% per unit transfused. It is estimated that about 4 million people in the United States are infected with HCV. Approximately 85% of infected individuals remain persistently infected, even in the absence of biochemical evidence of liver disease. The incubation period is 7–9 wk (range of 2–24 wk).

PATHOGENESIS. The pattern of acute hepatic injury is similar to that of the other hepatotropic viruses. In chronic cases, lymphoid aggregates or follicles in portal tracts are found, either alone or as part of a general inflammatory infiltration of the tracts. HCV appears to cause injury primarily by cytopathic mechanisms, but immune-mediated injury also may occur. The cytopathic component appears to be mild, because the acute illness is typically the least severe of all hepatotropic virus infections except HGV.

CLINICAL MANIFESTATIONS. The clinical pattern of the acute infection is similar to that of the other hepatitis viruses. Acute disease tends to be mild and insidious in onset in adults and children. Fulminant liver failure rarely occurs. HCV is the most likely hepatotropic virus to cause chronic infection; about 85% of cases become chronic, with a fluctuating pattern of elevated hepatic transaminases. After approximately 20–30 yr, about 25% ultimately progress to cirrhosis, liver failure, and occasionally primary hepatocellular carcinoma. Hepatocellular carcinoma associated with HCV, which is less effective than HBV in causing primary hepatocellular carcinoma, almost always occurs in the presence of cirrhosis and probably results from chronic inflammation and necrosis rather than an oncogenic effect of the virus.

Chronic HCV infection may be associated with small vessel vasculitis and is a common cause of essential mixed cryoglobulinemia. Other extrahepatic manifestations include cutaneous vasculitis, peripheral neuropathy, cerebritis, membranoproliferative glomerulonephritis, and nephrotic syndrome.

DIAGNOSIS. The clinically available assays for detection of HCV infection are based on detection of antibodies to HCV antigens or testing directly for the virus RNA; diagnostic tests are not available for HCV viral protein. The antibody assays are mainly used for detection of chronic HCV infection, because antibodies remain negative for as long as 1–3 mo after clinical onset of illness. The current second-generation assays detect three of the five known antigenic epitopes. These second-generation assays have improved sensitivity over the first-generation tests but still have a 5–10% false-negative rate. Anti-HCV antibody is not a protective antibody, does not confer immunity, and is usually present simultaneously with the virus.

Assays for viral RNA using reverse-transcriptase polymerase chain reaction (RT-PCR) permit detection of small amounts of HCV RNA in serum and tissue samples within days of infection, but they are costly. PCR detection is especially useful in patients with recent or perinatal infection, hypogammaglobulinemia, or immunosuppression. Methods for determining HCV genotype are available, but the clinical utility of typing is limited.

The presence of HCV-associated liver disease is indicated by an elevated serum ALT level and confirmed by histologic examination of liver biopsy. Chronic HCV infection in patients with anti-HCV is defined by persistently elevated levels of ALT in the presence of hepatic fibrosis and by the presence of HCV RNA in the blood. Currently there is no means to identify patients who will have progressive disease; a liver biopsy is the only means to assess the presence and extent of hepatic fibrosis. Most patients with chronic HCV hepatitis have 10^{5-7} genome copies/mL of HCV RNA in their serum.

The following individuals have HCV risk factors and should be screened: persons who have used any illegal drugs (even if only once); recipients of clotting factors made before 1987 (when inactivation procedures were introduced), patients undergoing hemodialysis; persons with persistently abnormal (even slightly) ALT levels; persons who have been notified that they received blood from an HCV-positive donor; and recipients of any blood transfusion, blood component, or organ transplant before 1992. Persons with clinical hepatitis not due to hepatitis A or hepatitis B should be tested for anti-HCV. Routine screening of all pregnant women is not recommended. Children born to HCV-infected women should be tested for anti-HCV after 12 mo of age; RT-PCR testing is not generally available. Neither national nor international adoptees are at increased risk, although adoptees should be tested if the mother was known to be at high risk.

TREATMENT. Treatment of HCV infection is provided to prevent progression to future complications. IFN-α2b is approved for treatment of chronic HCV in patients who are age 18 yr or older and who have compensated liver disease and a history of blood or blood product exposure or are anti-HCV positive. This treatment has also been used in children with a long-term response rate similar to the 25% rate reported in adults. Factors associated with improved response include mild liver histopathologic abnormalities, low serum HCV RNA levels, and infection with a genotype other than genotype 1, which is the predominant type in the United States. Response to treatment as measured by lowered serum ALT level occurs in about 50% of patients by the end of 6 mos of therapy, but only 10–15% of patients are "sustained responders," defined as having normal ALT levels and negative RT-PCR results 6 mo after therapy. "Relapsers" initially show a response, but virus is again detectable 6 mo after therapy is discontinued. "Nonresponders" never lose detectable virus. Combination therapy with IFN-α2b and ribavirin results in higher frequency of sustained response and in histologic improvement.

COMPLICATIONS. The risk of fulminant hepatitis is low with HCV, but the risk of chronic hepatitis is the highest of the hepatotropic viruses. Risk factors for progression to hepatic fibrosis include older age, male sex, and even moderate alcohol ingestion (two 1-oz drinks per day). Infected adults should refrain from using alcohol to prevent additional hepatic injury. Persons infected with HCV should be immunized with hepatitis A and hepatitis B vaccines to minimize further hepatic injury. The usual chronic course is a mild one even when cirrhosis develops; long-term follow-up indicates that the overall mortality of persons with transfusion-acquired HCV is no different from that of noninfected controls.

PREVENTION. No vaccine is available to prevent HCV. Immunoglobulin has not proved to be of benefit. Immunoglobulin produced in the United States does not contain antibodies to HCV because blood and plasma donors are screened for anti-HCV and excluded from the donor pool.

To minimize transmission, persons with HCV should use condoms, not share toothbrushes or razors, and not donate blood or organs.

HEPATITIS D

ETIOLOGY. HDV, the smallest known animal virus, is considered defective because it cannot produce infection without a concurrent HBV infection. The 36-nm-diameter virus is incapable of making its own coat protein; its outer coat is composed of excess HBsAg from HBV. The inner core of the virus is single-stranded circular RNA that expresses the HDV antigen.

EPIDEMIOLOGY. HDV cannot produce infection without HBV as a helper virus. HDV can cause an infection at the same time as the initial HBV infection (co-infection), or HDV can infect a person who is already infected with HBV (superinfection). Transmission usually occurs by intrafamilial or intimate contact in areas of high prevalence, which are primarily developing countries. In areas of low prevalence, such as the United States, the percutaneous route is far more common. HDV infections are uncommon in children in the United States but must be considered when fulminant hepatitis occurs. In the United States, HDV infection is found most frequently in parenteral drug abusers, patients with hemophilia, and persons emigrating from areas that include southern Italy, parts of eastern Europe, South America, Africa, and the Middle East. HDV is uncommon in the Far East where HBV infection is common. The incubation period for HDV superinfection is about 2–8 wk; with co-infection, the incubation period is similar to that of HBV infection.

PATHOGENESIS. Liver pathology in HDV hepatitis has no distinguishing features except that damage is usually more severe. In contrast to HBV, HDV causes injury directly by cytopathic mechanisms. Many of the most severe cases of HBV infection appear to be a result of co-infection of HBV and HDV. HDV superinfection of a person who has chronic HBV infection is more common in developed countries.

CLINICAL MANIFESTATIONS. The symptoms of hepatitis D infection are similar to but usually more severe than those of the other hepatotropic viruses. The clinical outcome for HDV infection depends on the mechanism of infection. In co-infection, acute hepatitis, which is much more severe than for HBV alone, is common but the risk of developing chronic hepatitis is low. In superinfection, acute illness is rare and chronic hepatitis is common. However, the risk of fulminant hepatitis is highest in superinfection. Hepatitis D should be considered in any child who experiences acute hepatic failure.

DIAGNOSIS. HDV has not been isolated, and no circulating antigen has been identified. The diagnosis is made by detecting IgM antibody to HDV; the antibodies to HDV develop about 2–4 wk after co-infection and about 10 wk after a superinfection. A test for anti-HDV antibody is commercially available. PCR assays for viral RNA are available only as a research tool.

COMPLICATIONS. HDV must be considered in all cases of fulminant hepatitis.

PREVENTION. There is no vaccine for hepatitis D. However, because HDV replication cannot occur without hepatitis B co-infection, immunization against HBV also prevents HDV infection. Hepatitis B vaccines and HBIG are used for the same indications as for hepatitis B alone (see Table 177–3).

HEPATITIS E

ETIOLOGY. HEV has not been isolated but has been cloned using molecular techniques. This RNA virus has a nonenveloped sphere shape with spikes and is similar in structure to the caliciviruses.

EPIDEMIOLOGY. Hepatitis E is the epidemic form of what was formally called non-A, non-B hepatitis. Transmission is associated with shedding of 27–34-nm particles in the stool. The highest prevalence of HEV infection has been reported in the Indian subcontinent, the Middle East, Southeast Asia, and Mexico, especially in areas with poor sanitation. In the United States, the only reported cases have been in persons who have visited or emigrated from endemic areas. The mean incubation period is about 40 days (range of 15–60 days).

PATHOGENESIS. HEV appears to act as a cytopathic virus. The pathologic findings are similar to those of the other hepatitis viruses.

CLINICAL MANIFESTATIONS. The clinical illness associated with

HEV infection is similar to HAV, the other enterically transmitted virus, but is often more severe. Both viruses produce only acute disease; chronic illness does not occur. In addition to often causing a more severe episode than HAV, HEV affects older patients with a peak age between 15 and 34 yr. Another important clinical difference is that HEV has a high case fatality rate in pregnant women.

DIAGNOSIS. Recombinant DNA technology has resulted in development of antibodies to HEV particles, and IgM and IgG assays are available to distinguish between acute and resolved infections. IgM antibody to viral antigen becomes positive after about 1 wk of illness. Viral RNA can be detected in stool and serum by PCR.

COMPLICATIONS. HEV is associated with a high prevalence of death in pregnant women.

PREVENTION. No vaccines are available, and no evidence shows that immunoglobulin is effective in preventing HEV infections. However, immunoglobulin pooled from patients in endemic areas may prove to be effective.

HEPATITIS F

In 1994, French researchers reported the isolation of an enteric agent responsible for sporadic cases of non-A–E hepatitis and named the virus hepatitis F (HFV), for hepatitis French virus. However, their findings have not been confirmed by others and the term HFV is currently unclaimed.

HEPATITIS G

ETIOLOGY. Hepatitis G virus (HGV), which includes HGV and GBV-C virus, is the most recently discovered of the hepatitis viruses and was identified by RT-PCR of the plasma of a patient with chronic hepatitis. HGV is a single-stranded RNA virus that is included in the Flaviviridae family and shares a 27% homology with HCV. The virus has not yet been isolated, but PCR testing indicates that it has a worldwide distribution and can cause chronic infection and viremia.

EPIDEMIOLOGY. HGV has been reported in adults and children from all population groups and is found in about 1.5% of blood donors in the United States. Infection has been reported in 10–20% of adults with chronic hepatitis B and hepatitis C, indicating that co-infection is a common occurrence. The primary route of spread is thought to be through transfusions, but HGV also can be transmitted by organ transplantation. Other important risk factors for infection include injection drug use, hemodialysis, and homosexual and bisexual relationships, indicating that sexual transmission also occurs. Vertical transmission also may occur.

PATHOGENESIS. Most infected persons have evidence of persistent viremia, but histologic evidence of HGV infection is rare and ALT values usually are normal. To date, little evidence shows that infections with HGV cause symptomatic disease. The detection of HGV in lymphocytes suggests that the virus may behave biologically like Epstein-Barr virus or CMV. No cases of chronic hepatitis have developed in patients infected with HGV alone.

CLINICAL MANIFESTATIONS. HGV accounts for only a small proportion of cases of non-A–E hepatitis. Most HGV infections are not associated with hepatic inflammation, and co-infection does not seem to worsen the course of concurrent HBV or HCV infection. Because the virus is distributed so widely and is associated with only mild or no disease, it is not yet clear whether HGV is a pathogen.

DIAGNOSIS. The only diagnostic tests for HGV infection are PCR assays used to detect HGV RNA. Development of serologic tests will greatly improve our understanding of this virus.

COMPLICATIONS. No conclusive evidence shows that HGV causes fulminant or chronic disease.

PREVENTION. There is currently no method to prevent infection with HGV.

177.1 Hepatitis in Neonates

Various infectious agents have been implicated in hepatic inflammation in neonates, including bacterial and viral pathogens. Hepatitis in neonates due to specific causes usually is distinguished from the term "neonatal hepatitis," which has been used to designate hepatic inflammation of unknown cause (Chapter 356.1).

ETIOLOGY. The six hepatotropic viruses that cause hepatitis as their primary disease manifestation rarely cause clinical hepatitis in neonates. Transplacental and perinatal transmission of HAV, HDV, and HEV is rare. The greatest risk of perinatal transmission of any hepatotropic virus occurs with HBV, but almost all neonates infected with HBV are asymptomatic. Perinatal transmission rarely is associated with HCV, but the risk is increased in neonates of HIV-infected mothers or mothers with high titers of HCV; symptomatic infection is rare. HGV infection has been reported in neonates, but clinical illness has not been associated with infection.

Most cases of neonatal hepatitis are a result of systemic disease. Sepsis caused by systemic and extrahepatic bacterial and viral infections must always be considered when hepatitis is present in a newborn infant. Gram-negative bacterial infections are especially important causes of sepsis in newborn infants and require immediate, appropriate therapy. The pathogenesis of hepatic involvement is not understood completely, but the cholestatic effects of bacterial endotoxins appear to have an important role. Sepsis caused by gram-positive organisms and viruses can also be associated with hepatitis. In most infants, bilirubin elevation, predominantly conjugated, is of much greater magnitude than that of the aminotransferases or ALP.

Many other viruses, including enteroviruses, CMV, HSV, and HIV, must be considered in the etiology of neonatal hepatitis. Hepatitis associated with these viruses occurs as part of a systemic illness. Nonviral infectious causes of hepatitis in neonates include congenital syphilis and congenital toxoplasmosis.

CLINICAL MANIFESTATIONS. Hepatitis in neonates may be characterized by jaundice, vomiting, poor feeding, and elevated hepatic enzyme levels. When infection is caused by an organism other than one of the six hepatotropic viruses, evidence of diffuse illness usually is present and may involve the skin, central nervous, cardiorespiratory, and musculoskeletal systems. A spectrum of illness, ranging from mild to fulminant disease, can occur with any of the infecting agents listed. Fulminant hepatitis is characterized by rapid progression to very high hepatic enzyme levels, decreased production of coagulation proteins, elevated serum ammonia level, shock, coma, or death. The levels of the serum bilirubin and aminotransferase levels are poor predictors of outcome. Because of the short half-life of the coagulation proteins, the PT is the best prognostic indicator.

HBV, the most common hepatotropic virus that infects neonates, usually results in an asymptomatic infection. The most common sequence of events is for an infant to have no clinical evidence of disease and to become chronically infected and positive for HBsAg. These children often have normal or only mildly abnormal hepatic enzyme values. Liver biopsy findings may be normal initially, but chronic infection can lead to cirrhosis usually in the 3rd to 4th decades of life, greatly increasing the risk of developing primary hepatocellular carcinoma.

The differential diagnosis of hepatitis in neonates must include infectious causes, many of which are treatable, and noninfectious causes including anatomic (intrahepatic and extrahepatic biliary atresia and choledochal cyst), metabolic (cystic fibrosis, disorders of bile acid metabolism, galactosemia, tyrosinosis, and α_1-antitrypsin deficiency), and toxic (drugs, hyperalimentation) disorders.

TREATMENT. In addition to effective antimicrobial therapy for bacteria-associated hepatitis, acyclovir is effective against HSV and varicella virus, and ganciclovir and foscarnet can be used to treat CMV infections.

PREVENTION. Women should be tested for HBsAg during routine prenatal care, and infants born to women who are HBsAg positive should receive hepatitis B vaccine and HBIG (see Table 177–4) within 12 hr of birth. Additional doses of vaccine are administered at ages 1 and 6 mo. Hepatitis B vaccine should be administered to all other infants, beginning in the first 2 mo of life. After administration of the first dose to HBsAg-negative mothers, the second dose should be administered 1 mo after the first dose but not before age 6 mo. Routine postvaccination testing of infants to determine the presence of anti-HBs is not recommended. However, testing is advised 1–2 mo after the third vaccine dose for infants born to HBsAg-positive mothers.

Alter MJ, Gallagher M, Morris TT, et al: Acute non-A–E hepatitis in the United States and the role of hepatitis G virus infection. N Engl J Med 336:741, 1997.
Alter MJ, Mast EE: The epidemiology of viral hepatitis in the United States. Gastroenterol Clin North Am 23:437, 1994.
American Academy of Pediatrics, Committee on Infectious Diseases: Prevention of hepatitis A infections: Guidelines for use of hepatitis A vaccine and immune globulin. Pediatrics 98:1207, 1996.
American Academy of Pediatrics, Committee on Infectious Diseases: Hepatitis C virus infection. Pediatrics 101:481, 1998.
Centers for Disease Control and Prevention: Recommendations for prevention and control of hepatitis C virus (HCV) infection and HCV-related chronic disease. MMWR 47(RR-19):1, 1998.
Fishman LN, Jonas MM, Lavine JE: Update on viral hepatitis in children. Pediatr Clin North Am 43:57, 1996.
Hall AJ: Hepatitis in travellers: Epidemiology and prevention. Br Med Bull 49:382, 1993.
Hoofnagle JH, DiBisceglie AM: The treatment of chronic viral hepatitis. N Engl J Med 336:347, 1997.
Lee WM: Hepatitis B virus infection. N Engl J Med 337:1733, 1997.
McHutchison JG, Gordon SC, Schiff ER, et al: Interferon alfa-2b alone or in combination with ribavirin as initial treatment for chronic hepatitis C. N Engl J Med 339:1485, 1998.
Ohto H, Terazawa S, Saski N, et al: Transmission of hepatitis C virus from mothers to infants. N Engl J Med 330:774, 1994.
Polish LB, Gallagher M, Fields HA, et al: Delta hepatitis: Molecular biology and clinical and epidemiological features. Clin Microbiol Rev 6:211, 1993.
Rizetto M, Durazzo M: Hepatitis delta virus infections: Epidemiological and clinical heterogeneity. J Hepatol 13:S116, 1991.
Sjogren MH: Serologic diagnosis of viral hepatitis. Med Clin North Am 80:929, 1996.
Zwiener RJ, Fielman BA, Cochran C, et al: Interferon-α-2b treatment of chronic hepatitis C in children with hemophilia. Pediatr Infect Dis J 15:906, 1996.

CHAPTER 178
Osteomyelitis and Suppurative Arthritis

John D. Nelson

Suppurative infections of bones and joints in children are not common, but they are important because of their potential to cause permanent disability. The risk is greatest if the physis (the growth plate of bone) or the synovium is damaged. As with most infectious diseases, the frequency of skeletal infection is greater in infants and toddlers than in older children. Recognition of osteomyelitis or arthritis in young patients before extensive infection has occurred is often difficult, yet early institution of appropriate medical and surgical therapy is probably necessary to minimize permanent damage.

ETIOLOGY. Bacteria are the usual pathogens in acute skeletal infections. Fungal infections usually occur as part of multisystem disseminated disease, and *Candida* arthritis or osteomyelitis sometimes complicates bloodstream infection in neonates with indwelling vascular catheters. Infection with atypical *Mycobacteria* can occur after penetrating injuries. Primary viral infections of bones or joints are exceedingly rare, but arthralgia or arthritis accompanies many viral syndromes, suggesting immune-mediated symptoms.

A microbial cause is defined in about two thirds of cases of suppurative arthritis and three fourths of cases of osteomyelitis. The yield of bacterial growth for synovial fluid and bone aspirates is disappointingly small. Some negative cultures are explained by prior antibiotic therapy and some by the inhibitory effect of pus on microorganisms. It is likely that some cases treated as bacterial arthritis are actually reactive arthritis (Chapter 158) rather than primary infection.

In osteomyelitis, *Staphylococcus aureus* is the most common infecting organism in all age groups, including newborns. Group B *Streptococcus* and gram-negative enteric bacilli are also prominent pathogens in neonates. Group A *Streptococcus* is next in frequency but constitutes fewer than 10% of all cases. After 6 yr of age, most cases of osteomyelitis are caused by gram-positive cocci or *Pseudomonas aeruginosa*. The *Pseudomonas* cases are related almost exclusively to puncture wounds of the foot.

The microbial spectrum is diverse in suppurative arthritis, but staphylococcal infection is most common. Before widespread vaccination of infants for *Haemophilus influenzae* type b infection, that organism accounted for more than half of all cases of bacterial arthritis in infants. Invasive group A *Streptococcus* disease and *Streptococcus pneumoniae* (pneumococcus) infection occur in 10–20% of cases.

EPIDEMIOLOGY. Infection of bones and joints can follow penetrating injuries or various medical and surgical maneuvers such as arthroscopy, prosthetic joint surgery, intra-articular steroid injection, and various orthopedic surgeries on bones, but these are uncommon. Various factors of impaired host defenses also increase the risk of skeletal infection. However, the majority of infections in otherwise healthy children are of hematogenous origin. Trauma is a common preceding event in cases of osteomyelitis, occurring in about one third of patients.

PATHOGENESIS. Supporting the role of trauma in pathogenesis are animal models of experimental osteomyelitis that are based on inflicting trauma to a bone of an animal that is bacteremic. The unique anatomy of the ends of long bones explains the predilection for localization of blood-borne bacteria. In the metaphysis are tiny vascular loops in which blood flow is sluggish and oxygen tension is low. Rupture of some of these vessels as a result of trauma provides a favorable environment for the multiplication of bacteria.

In newborn and young infants, blood vessels connect the metaphysis and epiphysis, so it is common for pus from the metaphysis to enter the joint space. In the latter part of the 1st yr of life, the physis forms, obliterating these transphyseal blood vessels. Bone is not distensible, and because pus under pressure is prevented from decompressing into the joint in these children, purulent material moves laterally through cortical vascular channels and accumulates under the loosely attached periosteum. After growth ceases, transphyseal blood vessels are re-established.

Preceding trauma is less common in suppurative arthritis, and the pathogenesis of hematogenous arthritis is poorly understood. The synovium is rich in blood vessels, and it may be that insignificant, unremembered trauma has a role in pathogenesis. In addition, synovial membrane receptors for bacteria may play a part in localization because certain bacterial genera have a predilection for causing arthritis. Once bacteria reach the synovium, a series of events occurs. The synovium contains no basement membrane. Bacteria are deposited in the subsynovial capillary vessel network, with migration of bacteria and blood products into the joint space. If the host's immune system contains the infection, the arthritis does not progress and the process is aborted; however, if bacterial multiplication remains unchecked, the inflammatory cascade is triggered, resulting in joint damage and possible sequelae. This inflammation results from the outpouring of white blood cells into the synovial fluid, with release of proteolytic enzymes and toxic products produced by polymorphonuclear cells, synovial lining cells, and bacteria themselves. Chondrocytes also have a role in the destruction of articular cartilage. In experimental arthritis, ultrastructural analysis of chondrocytes has shown an increase in the lysosomal electron-dense bodies, suggestive of the production of proteolytic enzymes. Chondrocytes, which contain acid and neutral proteases, may be stimulated to release these enzymes by either bacterial lipopolysaccharides or interleukin-1. In turn, interleukin-1 may lead to increasing amounts of prostaglandin E and collagenase from the synoviocyte and chondrocyte. Articular cartilage degradation occurs because of depletion of collagen and proteoglycan (glycosaminoglycan). Pus in the joint increases intracapsular pressure, with resulting decrease in blood flow to the epiphysis, which can lead to irreversible ischemic damage when the pressure is not relieved promptly.

Both conditions are most common in young children. This is particularly true of arthritis, in which half of all cases occur in the first 2 yr of life and three fourths of all cases occur by 5 yr of age. The figures for osteomyelitis in these two age groups are about one third and one half, respectively. In all reported series, skeletal infections are consistently more common in boys than in girls, usually by a factor of 2:1. It may be that the lifestyle of boys predisposes to traumatic events. There appears to be no particular predilection for arthritis or osteomyelitis based on race. In most reported series, the racial distribution of cases reflects that of the local population.

CLINICAL MANIFESTATIONS. The earliest signs and symptoms of skeletal infection are often subtle. This is particularly true of neonates, who characteristically do not appear ill and in half of cases do not have fever. Infants may have only pseudoparalysis of an extremity or apparent pain on movement of the affected extremity. Most older infants and children have fever and localizing signs.

Redness and swelling of the skin and soft tissue overlying the site of infection tend to be seen earlier in arthritis than in osteomyelitis. The bulging, infected synovium is relatively near the surface, whereas the metaphysis is located deeper under the soft tissues. The exception to this is septic arthritis of the hip, in which external signs are usually absent because of the deep location of the hip joint. Local swelling and redness with osteomyelitis mean that the infection has spread out of the metaphysis into the subperiosteal space and denote a secondary soft tissue inflammatory response.

Nonspecific systemic signs of infection such as nausea, vomiting, diarrhea, and headache are not prominent features of skeletal infections, even though many of the patients are bacteremic. If those signs are present, a disseminated infectious syndrome with multiple foci of disease should be suspected; this is most likely to occur with *S. aureus* infection.

Long bones are principally involved in osteomyelitis (Table 178–1). The femur and tibia are equally affected and together constitute almost half of all cases. The bones of the upper extremities account for one fourth of all cases. Flat bones are less commonly affected. Joints of the lower extremity constitute three quarters of all cases of arthritis (Table 178–2). The elbow, wrist, and shoulder joints are involved in about 25% of cases, and small joints are uncommonly infected. In bone or joint infection, a single locus is usually involved. Several bones or joints are infected in fewer than 10% of cases. Exceptions are gonococcal infections, which typically affect many joints, and osteomyelitis in neonates, in whom two or more bones are involved in almost half of the cases.

TABLE 178–1 Distribution of Affected Bones in Acute Hematogenous Osteomyelitis

Bone	No.	Per Cent
Tibia	107	24.3
Femur	105	23.8
Humerus	58	13.2
Fibula	26	5.9
Radius	17	3.9
Ulna	10	2.3
Vertebra	9	2.0
Foot bones	33	7.5
Pelvic bones	30	6.8
Hand bones	27	6.1
Chest bones	13	2.9
Head bones	6	1.4

Based on the author's series of 372 patients with 441 infected bones.

DIAGNOSIS. The diagnosis is most directly confirmed by needle aspiration of infected material for examination and culture when the history and physical findings indicate a strong likelihood of suppurative bone or joint disease.

Analysis of aspirated synovial fluid for cells, protein, and glucose in cases of bacterial arthritis has limited usefulness because noninfectious inflammatory diseases, such as rheumatic fever and rheumatoid arthritis, can cause exuberant reaction of cells and protein and decrease of glucose. Most joint spaces are easy to enter, but the hip can pose technical problems. Sonographic guidance can facilitate aspiration. If no fluid is obtained, a small amount of air or contrast material is injected and a roentgenogram is obtained to make sure that the needle tip is in the joint cavity. In cases of osteomyelitis, a steel needle is needed to penetrate the cortex into the metaphysis. If pus is encountered in the subperiosteal space, there is no need to go further. Aspiration of joint or bone pus not only serves to confirm the diagnosis of infection but provides the best specimen for bacteriologic culture.

Routine tests of inflammation such as white blood cell count, erythrocyte sedimentation rate (ESR), and C-reactive protein value are nonspecific and not helpful in distinguishing between skeletal infection and other inflammatory processes. Furthermore, the leukocyte count and ESR may be normal during the first few days of infection. Normal test results do not preclude the diagnosis of skeletal infection.

Roentgenographic Findings. Radiologic studies are often helpful in evaluating suspected osteomyelitis and arthritis, but normal results of standard roentgenograms do not preclude those diagnoses. In osteomyelitis, destructive changes in bone do not appear radiographically for at least 10 days; however, effacement of normal deep soft tissue planes around bone is indicative of an inflammatory process.

TABLE 178–2 Distribution of Affected Joints in Acute Suppurative Arthritis

Joint	No.	Per Cent
Knee	309	39.6
Hip	173	22.2
Elbow	109	14.0
Ankle	104	13.3
Shoulder	37	4.7
Wrist	34	4.4
Sacroiliac	5	0.6
Interphalangeal	4	0.5
Metatarsal	3	0.4
Acromioclavicular	1	0.1
Sternoclavicular	1	0.1
Metacarpal	1	0.1

Based on the author's series of 725 patients with 781 infected joints.

The findings on routine roentgenograms in suppurative arthritis are a result of swelling of the capsule. Joint space widening and soft tissue swelling may be found. In the case of hip involvement, roentgenograms should be obtained in the frog-leg position, as well as with the legs extended at the knees and slightly internally rotated. Other findings that help in the radiologic diagnosis of hip joint infection are the obturator sign, in which the margins of the muscle are displaced medially into the pelvis as the obturator internus passes over the capsule; displacement or obliteration of the gluteal fat lines, displacement of the femoral head laterally and upward; and elevation of the femoral portion of the Shenton line and widening of the arc.

Sonography is most useful in evaluating suppurative arthritis of the hip and may be used to guide closed arthrocentesis to obtain joint fluid.

Radionuclide imaging is not necessary in most cases, but it can be very useful when in doubt about the diagnosis or localization of infection (Fig. 178–1). Technetium-99m diphosphonate bone scans accurately identify the joint involved in 90% of patients and differentiate joint from bone involvement. Results of radionuclide bone scans are positive in approximately three fourths of cases of osteomyelitis during the 1st wk of illness but by the 2nd wk are positive in 95% or more of cases. Advanced cases may show decreased instead of the usual increased uptake of the isotope because of infarction and poor blood flow. Both gallium-67 and indium-111 scans may be useful if the technetium scan is nondiagnostic. MRI is very sensitive, detecting signs of osteomyelitis reflected in the bone marrow and soft tissues (Fig. 178–1).

Differential Diagnosis. A great many noninfectious disorders affect the musculoskeletal system. It is common for children with acute leukemia to have bone or joint pain as an initial manifestation of disease. Bone involvement in neuroblastoma is often mistaken as osteomyelitis. Primary bone tumors are not associated with fever or other systemic signs of illness and do not cause diagnostic confusion.

The differential diagnosis of suppurative arthritis depends on the age of the patient and the joint involved. In the hip joint, considerations are transient synovitis (toxic synovitis), Legg-Calvé-Perthes disease, slipped capital femoral epiphysis, psoas abscess (from communication between the psoas sheath and the hip joint, although in some cases the infected hip joint may decompress into the iliopsoas muscle), proximal femoral or vertebral osteomyelitis, and diskitis. In the knee, the differential diagnosis includes distal femoral or proximal tibial osteomyelitis or referred pain from the hip. Other conditions that should be considered in any child with an inflamed joint are cellulitis, pyomyositis, other infectious arthritis (e.g., viral, mycoplasmal, mycobacterial, fungal, Lyme disease), sickle cell disease, hemophilia, trauma, collagen vascular diseases, and Henoch-Schönlein purpura. When patients present with involvement of several joints, conditions such as rheumatic fever, serum sickness, Henoch-Schönlein purpura, and collagen vascular disease also must be considered. Most cases of collagen vascular disease are preceded by a history of a chronic or intermittent process with involvement of other organs and failure to respond to antibiotic therapy.

Reactive arthritis following gastrointestinal infections, streptococcal pharyngitis, or viral hepatitis can be extraordinarily difficult to distinguish from acute suppurative arthritis. The interval between the inciting infection and arthritis is usually

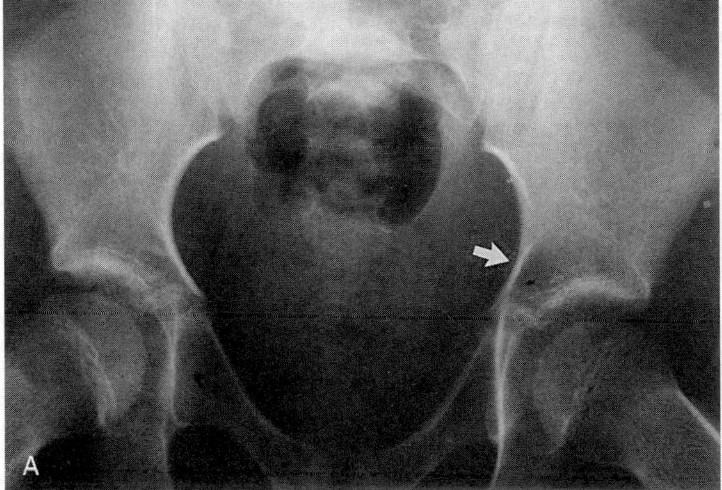

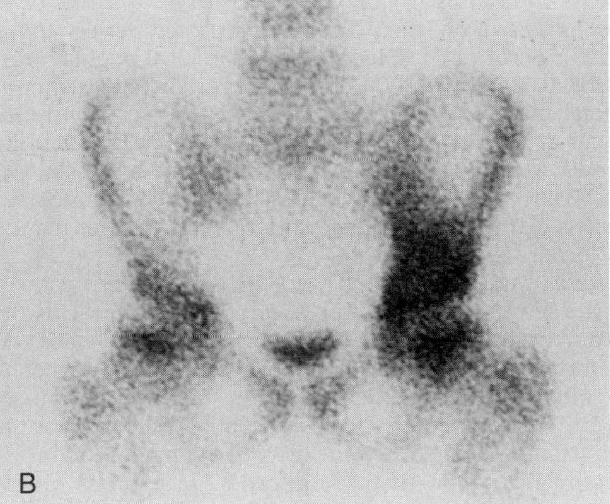

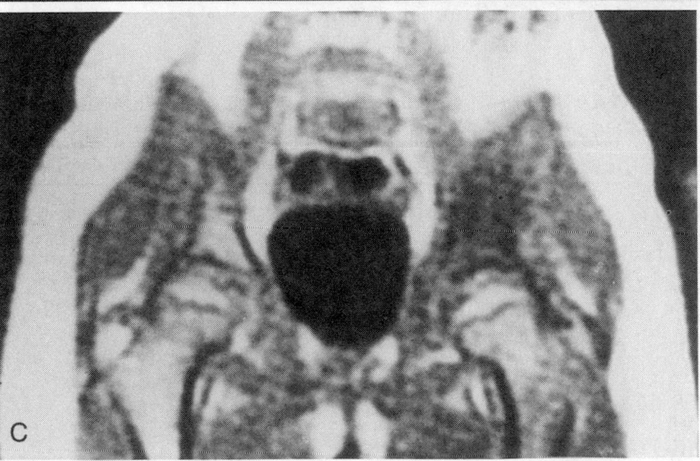

Figure 178–1 Pelvic osteomyelitis of the left iliac bone in a 12-yr-old girl with pain in the left hip region of 1–2 wk duration. *A*, Frontal radiograph of the pelvis shows mild demineralization of the acetabular portion of the iliac bone adjacent to the triradiate cartilage. There is very subtle periosteal reaction *(arrow)* along the margin of the sciatic notch. *B*, Technetium-99m bone scan shows increased uptake in the left iliac bone and mild increased uptake in the femoral head. *C*, Coronal MRI shows decreased signal from the marrow of the left iliac bone compared with the bright signal from the normal fatty marrow on the right. The femoral head is normal, and there is no joint effusion. Needle aspiration of the iliac bone yielded *Staphylococcus aureus*; the patient responded well to antimicrobial therapy. (From Markowitz RI: Diagnostic imaging. *In*: Jenson HB, Baltimore RS [eds]: Pediatric Infectious Diseases: Principles and Practice. Norwalk, CT, Appleton & Lange, 1995.)

2 wk or longer; thus, the association is overlooked by the patient and physician and the synovial fluid analysis mimics that of bacterial infection.

Children with hemophilia are at increased risk because hemarthrosis predisposes to joint infection, most commonly with pneumococci. Patients with sickle cell disease often have episodes of aseptic bone infarction that have the clinical appearance of infection.

Suppurative bursitis is very rare in children and is usually in the prepatellar bursa. It can easily be misdiagnosed as arthritis. Similarly, acute or subacute epiphyseal osteomyelitis often elicits a sterile effusion in the knee joint and is misdiagnosed as arthritis.

Chronic recurrent multifocal osteomyelitis is an inflammatory syndrome of unknown cause afflicting older children and young adults. In addition to long bones, bones rarely infected in bacterial osteomyelitis, such as the clavicle and spine, are commonly involved in this syndrome. It remits and relapses for many months or years. Patients with this syndrome commonly have chronic inflammatory skin conditions such as psoriasis, pustulosis palmaris et plantaris, and Sweet syndrome.

TREATMENT. Optimal treatment of skeletal infections requires collaborative efforts of a pediatrician, orthopedic surgeon, and physiatrist.

Antibiotic Therapy. The initial empirical antibiotic therapy is based on knowledge of likely bacterial pathogens at various ages, the results of the Gram stain of aspirated material, and special considerations. In newborns, an antistaphylococcal penicillin, such as oxacillin (150–200 mg/kg/24 hr in 3–4 divided doses), and a broad-spectrum cephalosporin, such as cefotaxime (100–150 mg/kg/24 hr in 3–4 divided doses), provide coverage for the anticipated *S. aureus*, group B *Streptococcus*, and gram-negative bacilli. An aminoglycoside could be used in place of the cephalosporin, but aminoglycoside antibiotics have somewhat reduced antibacterial activity in sites with decreased oxygen tension and pH, conditions that are present in tissue infections. If the neonate is a small premature baby or has a central vascular catheter, one must consider the possibility of nosocomial bacteria or fungi.

In infants and children up to about 4–5 yr of age, the principal pathogens of infection are *S. aureus*, streptococci, and *H. influenzae* type b in children who have not received the *H. influenzae* vaccine. Several antibiotics are useful for these types of infection. Most experience has been with cefuroxime (100–150 mg/kg/24 hr in 3 divided doses) or a third-generation cephalosporin (cefotaxime [150 mg/kg/24 hr in 3 divided doses] or ceftriaxone [50 mg/kg/24 hr given once daily]). Beyond 5 yr of age and in the absence of special circumstances, virtually all cases of osteomyelitis are caused by gram-positive cocci, so an antistaphylococcal antibiotic such as nafcillin (150 mg/kg/24 hr in 4 divided doses) or cephalothin (100–150 mg/kg/24 hr in 4 divided doses) can be used; however, in children who have arthritis and who are older than 5 yr, the etiologic bacteria are more varied and broader-spectrum drugs (cefuroxime or a third-generation cephalosporin) are generally given unless gram-positive cocci are seen in the stain of synovial fluid.

Special situations dictate deviations from the usual empirical antibiotic selection. In patients with sickle cell anemia with osteomyelitis, gram-negative enteric bacteria are common pathogens, so a broad-spectrum cephalosporin such as cefotaxime or ceftriaxone should be used in addition to an antistaphylococcal drug. Clindamycin (30–40 mg/kg/24 hr in 3–4 divided doses) is a useful alternative drug for patients allergic to β-lactam drugs. In addition to good antistaphylococcal activity, clindamycin has broad activity against anaerobes; thus, it is useful for the treatment of infections secondary to penetrating injuries or compound fractures. Vancomycin (40 mg/kg/24 hr in 4 divided doses) is used in place of a β-lactam antibiotic whenever the clinical situation raises the possibility of methicillin-resistant staphylococcal infection.

For immunocompromised patients, combination therapy is usually initiated. Several combinations of two or three drugs such as vancomycin with ceftazidime or ticarcillin-clavulanate with an aminoglycoside are used.

When the pathogen is identified, appropriate adjustments in antibiotics are made, if necessary. If a pathogen is not identified and a patient's condition is improving, therapy is continued with the antibiotic selected initially. Under these circumstances, consideration should be given to the possibility of a noninfectious inflammatory condition. Similarly, if a pathogen is not identified and a patient's condition is not improving, reaspiration or biopsy and the possibility of a noninfectious condition should be considered.

When pus is drained and appropriate antibiotic therapy is given, the improvement in signs and symptoms is rapid. Failure to improve or worsening by 72 hr requires review of the appropriateness of the antibiotic therapy, the need for surgical intervention, or the correctness of the diagnosis. Acute-phase reactants have been evaluated as monitors. The serum C-reactive protein typically normalizes within 7 days after start of treatment, whereas the ESR typically rises for 5–7 days, falls slowly during the next few days, and drops sharply after 10–14 days. Failure of either of these nonspecific reactants to follow the usual course should raise concerns about the adequacy of therapy.

In the past, prolonged courses of antibiotic therapy were recommended, but a trend now is toward shorter courses. For infections caused by group A *Streptococcus*, pneumococcus, or *H. influenzae* type b, antibiotics are given for a minimum of 10–14 days, provided that (1) the patient shows prompt resolution of signs and symptoms (5–7 days) and (2) the ESR has normalized. For *S. aureus* or gram-negative bacillary infections, the minimum duration of antibiotics is 21 days, with the same provisos. For gonococcal *(Neisseria gonorrhoeae)* tenosynovitis, the Centers for Disease Control and Prevention guidelines for treatment of sexually transmitted diseases recommend 7 days of therapy. Seven postoperative days of treatment is adequate for *Pseudomonas* osteochondritis or arthritis when thorough curettage of infected tissue has been performed. Immunocompromised patients generally require prolonged courses of therapy, as do patients with fungal or tuberculous disease.

It has become commonplace in pediatric medicine to change antibiotics from the parenteral route to oral administration when a patient's condition has stabilized, which is generally after 1 wk of parenteral therapy. For the oral antibiotic regimen with β-lactam drugs for staphylococcal or streptococcal infection, a dose two to three times that used for mild infections is prescribed. The adequacy of the dose is assessed by testing serum for peak bactericidal activity 45–60 min after a dose of suspension or 1½–2 hr after a capsule or tablet. A serum bactericidal titer of 1:8 or greater is considered desirable. Alternatively, serum antibiotic concentration is measured. Peak concentrations of β-lactam antibiotics greater than 20 μg/mL are desired. The oral regimen decreases the risk of nosocomial infections related to prolonged intravenous therapy, is more comfortable for patients, and permits treatment outside the hospital if therapeutic compliance can be ensured.

Surgical Therapy. Surgical measures for skeletal infections have not been subjected to randomized prospective study comparing two or more surgical procedures.

Hip joint infection is considered a surgical emergency because of the vulnerability of the blood supply to the head of the femur. After a penetrating injury and when a foreign body is likely to be involved, surgical intervention is also indicated. In other situations, the need for surgery is individualized.

For joints other than the hip, daily percutaneous needle aspirations of synovial fluid are required. Generally, one or two subsequent aspirations suffice. If fluid is still accumulating after 4–5 days, arthrotomy is needed. At the time of surgery, the joint is flushed with sterile saline solution. Antibiotics are not instilled, because they are irritating to synovial tissue and adequate amounts of antibiotic are achieved in joint fluid with systemic administration. When frank pus is obtained from subperiosteal or metaphyseal aspiration, the patient usually needs a surgical drainage procedure.

Treatment of chronic osteomyelitis consists of surgical removal of sinus tracts and sequestrum, if present. Antibiotic therapy is continued for several months until clinical and radiographic findings suggest that healing has occurred.

Physical Therapy. The major role of physical medicine is a preventive one. If a child is allowed to lie in bed with an extremity in flexion, limitation of extension may develop within a few days. The affected extremity should be kept in extension with sandbags, splints, or, if necessary, casts. Casts are also indicated when there is a potential for pathologic fracture. After 2–3 days, when pain is easing, passive range of motion exercises are started and continued until the child resumes normal activity. In neglected cases with flexion contractures, prolonged physical therapy is required.

PROGNOSIS. Recurrence of disease and development of chronic infection after treatment occur in fewer than 10% of patients.

Because children are in a dynamic state of growth, sequelae of skeletal infections may not become apparent for months or years; therefore, long-term follow-up is necessary with close attention to range of motion of joints and bone length. Infection of the hip joint carries the worst prognosis for anatomic and functional impairment, which develop in one quarter to one half of patients. If the physis was affected, bone growth is retarded and orthopedic corrective procedures may be needed. Limitation of motion after joint infection occurs in approximately one fifth of patients.

Although firm data about the impact of delayed treatment on outcome are not available, it appears that initiation of medical and surgical therapy within a week of onset of symptoms provides a better prognosis than delayed treatment.

Bradley JS, Kaplan SL, Tan TQ, et al: Pediatric pneumococcal bone and joint infections. Pediatrics 102:1376, 1998.
Burnett MW, Bass JW, Cook BA: Etiology of osteomyelitis complicating sickle cell disease. Pediatrics 101:296, 1998.
Dubey L, Krasinski K, Hernanz-Schulman M: Osteomyelitis secondary to trauma or infected contiguous soft tissue. Pediatr Infect Dis J 7:26, 1988.
Jacobs RF, McCarthy RE, Elser JM: *Pseudomonas* osteochondritis complicating puncture wounds of the foot in children. J Infect Dis 160:657, 1989.
Jaramillo D, Treves ST, Kasser JR: Osteomyelitis and septic arthritis in children: Appropriate use of imaging to guide treatment. Am J Roentgenol 165:399, 1995.
Kai T, Ishii E, Matsuzaki A, et al: Clinical and prognostic implications of bone lesions in childhood leukemia at diagnosis. Leuk Lymphoma 23:119, 1996.
Karwowska A, Davies HD, Jadavji T: Epidemiology and outcome of osteomyelitis in the era of sequential intravenous-oral therapy. Pediatr Infect Dis J 17:1021, 1998.
Knudsen CJM, Hoffman EB: Neonatal osteomyelitis. J Bone Joint Surg 72:846, 1990.
Lew DP, Waldvogel FA: Osteomyelitis. N Engl J Med 336:999, 1997.
Nelson JD: Skeletal infections in children. Adv Pediatr Infect Dis 6:59, 1991.
Nelson JD: Toward simple but safe management of osteomyelitis. Pediatrics 99:883, 1997.
Pappo AS, Buchanan GR, Johnson A: Septic arthritis in children with hemophilia. Am J Dis Child 143:1226, 1989.
Peltola H, Unkila-Kallio L, Kallio MJ: Simplified treatment of acute staphylococcal osteomyelitis of childhood. Pediatrics 99:846, 1997.
Syrogiannopoulos GA, Nelson JD: Duration of antimicrobial therapy for acute suppurative osteoarticular infections. Lancet 9:37, 1988.
Trujillo M, Nelson JD: Suppurative and reactive arthritis in children. Semin Pediatr Infect Dis 8:242, 1997.
Unkila-Kallio L, Kallio MJ, Eskola J, et al: Serum C-reactive protein, erythrocyte sedimentation rate, and white blood cell count in acute hematogenous osteomyelitis of children. Pediatrics 93:59, 1994.
Wong M, Isaacs D, Howman-Giles R, et al: Clinical and diagnostic features of osteomyelitis in the first three months of life. Pediatr Infect Dis J 14:1047, 1995.

CHAPTER 179
Infections in Immunocompromised Hosts

Walter Hughes and Philip A. Pizzo

A compromised host is one who, at the time of microbial exposure, has a pre-existing condition that reduces one or more mechanisms for normal defense against infection. The compromise may be due to a defect or dysfunction of the immune system per se or to other factors that heighten susceptibility to infection. Although such a categorization allows a conceptual basis for evaluation, compromised patients with infection often do not fit completely into one group or the other. More than one defect in the body's defense mechanisms may be affected. For example, patients with a specific T-lymphocyte defect caused by HIV may also have neutropenia caused by drugs used for antiviral therapy or by breech of the integrity of the skin and mucous membranes from indwelling central lines or intravenous drug abuse; or by secondary malignancy, malnutrition, and increased exposure to infections such as tuberculosis and sexually transmitted diseases, including hepatitis. However, knowledge of the primary defect of a compromised host is useful in predicting the types of infections that might occur and in establishing strategies for evaluating and managing infectious episodes. Children with one type of immune deficiency disorder may be prone to specific infections, even though the defect is not limited solely to these pathogens. An immunocompromised host is also at risk for all of the infections that occur in otherwise healthy children.

CAUSES OF IMMUNOCOMPROMISE AND INFECTION. The major causes of increased risk for infection in immunocompromised hosts are listed in Table 179–1, and the most common causative organisms are listed in Table 179–2.

Whether or not a child becomes infected on exposure to a microbial organism depends on a critical balance between the child's immunocompetence and the number and virulence of the organism (infection = virulence × number of organisms/

TABLE 179–1 Major Causes of Increased Risk for Infection in Immunocompromised Hosts

Primary	Secondary
Antibody deficiency (B-cell defects)	Human immunodeficiency virus
X-linked agammaglobulinemia	Malignancies
IgG subclass deficiencies	Transplantation
Common variable immunodeficiency	■ Bone marrow
Selective IgA deficiency	■ Solid organ
Cell-mediated deficiency (T-cell defects)	Burns
DiGeorge syndrome	Sickle cell disease
Hyper-IgM	Cystic fibrosis
CD8 lymphopenia	Diabetes mellitus
Cytokine deficiencies	Drugs: immunosuppressive
Defective T-cell receptor	Asplenia
T-cell activation defects	Implanted foreign body
Combined B- and T-cell defects	Malnutrition
■ Severe combined immunodeficiency	
■ Wiskott-Aldrich syndrome	
■ Ataxia telangiectasia	
■ Hyper-IgE syndrome	
■ Omenn syndrome	
Phagocyte defects	
■ Chronic granulomatous disease	
■ Congenital neutropenias	
■ Leukocyte adhesion disorder	
■ Other	
Complement deficiencies	

TABLE 179–2 Most Common Causes of Infections in Immunocompromised Children

Bacteria	Viruses
Escherichia coli	Varicella-zoster virus
Pseudomonas aeruginosa	Cytomegalovirus
Klebsiella spp	Herpes simplex virus
Enterobacter spp	Epstein-Barr virus
Haemophilus influenzae	Human herpesvirus 6
Staphylococcus aureus	Respiratory and enteric viruses
Staphylococcus, coagulase-negative	**Protozoa**
Streptococcus pneumoniae	
Bacillus spp	*Pneumocystis carinii*
Corynebacterium spp	*Toxoplasma gondii*
Viridans streptococcus group	*Cryptosporidium parvum*
Listeria monocytogenes	
Enterococcus faecalis	
Mycobacterium spp	
Nocardia spp	
Fungi	
Candida albicans	
Candida, not *albicans*	
Aspergillus spp	
Cryptococcus neoformans	
Zygomycetes	

host resistance). The greater frequency of infections due to low-virulence organisms in compromised hosts is probably because of the constant exposure to the large nonvirulent, commensal flora of the environment (opportunistic organisms) in contrast to a much more sparse distribution of virulent organisms required to infect otherwise normal hosts.

UNIQUE CLINICAL MANIFESTATIONS. The clinical features of infections in a compromised child as well as in an otherwise normal child depend primarily on the host responses to the invading microbe. The causative organisms are limited by their tissue or cellular tropism and virulence in eliciting specific clinical manifestations of disease. The basic clinical responses of a normal host are fever and the acute inflammatory reaction. The acute inflammatory reaction stems from granulocytic infiltrations, hyperemia, and capillary leakage, evidenced as cellulitis if involving the skin, pneumonitis in the lungs, and meningitis in the central nervous system. Defects in the normal host response may be reflected in clinical manifestations. For example, extensive bacterial infection may occur in the lungs of severely neutropenic patients without an infiltrate discernible by chest radiography; the swelling and erythema of cellulitis may not be evident, and anemic and neutropenic patients may have acute otitis media without erythema and congestion of the tympanic membrane. Diagnostic evaluation may be complicated when the defect is in the humoral immune function, such as agammaglobulinemia, because serologic tests for antibody responses are of the little value. With an impaired cell-mediated immune response, antigenic skin tests are often nonreactive.

Several general axioms about clinical features of infection in immunocompromised hosts can be formulated. Any organism is a potential pathogen in an immunosuppressed host. A microbiologist in a laboratory cannot always determine whether or not a microbial isolate is the cause of disease. Physicians must always assess an individual case to delineate a relationship between clinical findings and microbiologic laboratory results, or the lack of them.

Fever is a sensitive and specific sign of an infectious disease, even in an immunocompromised host. Almost all infections of significance are associated with a febrile response. Immunosuppressive drugs, such as corticosteroids and anticancer drugs, do not necessarily mask febrile responses during infections. Thus, fever in an immunocompromised host must be considered of infectious cause until proved otherwise. Aside from fever, characteristic signs and symptoms of infection may be absent in a compromised host.

Microbes of low virulence and even components of the normal flora of the skin and mucous membranes may cause severe, life-threatening infections. Some organisms may directly evoke signs and symptoms due to specific tropism or toxin production, such as pneumonitis from *Pneumocystis carinii,* diarrhea from *Cryptosporidium parvum* or *Clostridium difficile,* and thrush from *Candida albicans.*

Extreme granulocytopenia with absolute neutrophil counts of ≤500 cells/mm^3 is predictive of impending infection. With counts between 500 and 1,000 cells/mm^3, the risk of infection is still increased above that of normal individuals but is less than with lower counts. Generally, with counts ≤500 cells/mm^3, the risk for serious infection is directly proportional to the duration of the neutropenia. Infections in neutropenic patients are usually caused by bacteria or fungi.

A CD4$^+$ T-lymphocyte count of <500 cells/mm^3 (<15%) in children 1–5 yr of age, and <200 cells/mm^3 (<15%) in older children and adolescents indicates high risk for *P. carinii* pneumonitis in HIV-infected patients. The reliability of CD4$^+$ counts in predicting *P. carinii* pneumonitis is low in infants, particularly infants <6 mo of age.

Multiple infections, either concomitant or sequential, are especially common in patients with prolonged immunocompromise.

Known and suspected bacterial infections should be treated promptly with antibacterial antibiotics given intravenously in maximum tolerated doses. Often drugs must be given empirically before a diagnosis has been established.

A number of the drugs required for the treatment of infections in immunocompromised hosts can have toxic side effects.

Primary Immune Deficiencies

INFECTIONS WITH PRIMARY ANTIBODY IMMUNODEFICIENCY (B-CELL DEFECTS). Patients with X-linked agammaglobulinemia and common variable immunodeficiency are unable to generate adequate immunoglobulins. They are especially susceptible to encapsulated pyogenic bacterial infection with *Staphylococcus aureus, Haemophilus influenzae,* and *Streptococcus pneumoniae* as well as infection with other bacteria (Table 179–2). To a lesser extent, progressive viral and protozoan infections may affect these patients. Infections of the upper and lower respiratory tracts are the most frequent types encountered. Chronic and recurrent pulmonary infections lead to bronchiectasis. Arthritis and pneumonitis may also be caused by *Mycoplasma* spp. *Salmonella* and *Campylobacter* species cause enteritis. Chronic rotavirus and *Giardia lamblia* are common. Pyoderma, sepsis, pneumonia, meningitis, and otitis media are often due to pyogenic bacteria. A chronic enteroviral meningoencephalitis, often with hepatitis, may lead to progressive neurologic symptoms. Also, patients may develop paralytic polio from exposure to oral polio vaccine.

Patients with selective IgA deficiency lack secretory IgA at the mucosal barrier. Most patients have no increased susceptibility to infection, but some may have recurrent bacterial infections of mild to moderate severity.

Patients with hyper-IgM syndrome have decreased levels of IgG, IgA, and IgE and often neutropenia. In addition to the bacterial sinopulmonary infections that are characteristic of agammaglobulinemia, *P. carinii* pneumonitis and *Cryptosporidium* infection also pose an increased risk to these children.

The IgG subclass deficiencies are not clearly understood but are associated with mild to severe cases of sinopulmonary diseases, meningitis, bacteremia, osteomyelitis, and pyoderma. In IgG subclass 2 deficiency, poor antibody responses follow infections with polysaccharide-encapsulated bacteria, such as *H. influenzae* and pneumococcus, as well as immunization with the polysaccharide bacterial vaccines.

INFECTIONS WITH PRIMARY DEFECTS IN CELL-MEDIATED IMMUNITY. Patients with congenital T-lymphocyte or combined T- and B-lymphocyte immunodeficiency states develop infection soon after birth because T-lymphocyte function is greatly reduced and protection by passive transfer of maternal IgG is transient. Early infectious complications include chronic mucocutaneous candidiasis, chronic rhinitis and otitis media, recurrent pneumonia, and diarrhea. Because of the marked heterogeneity of the immunodeficiency state in DiGeorge syndrome, some children may have minor infections, whereas others who survive after early severe infections may have less frequent or less serious infections as the immune defect spontaneously improves. A few patients with DiGeorge anomaly may have chronic infections in the form of pneumonia, diarrhea, cutaneous candidiasis, and serious infections with herpesviruses and *P. carinii*.

The most commonly acquired disorder resulting from a predominantly T-lymphocyte defect is AIDS. Antibody production is also deficient in patients with AIDS owing to a defect of helper T-lymphocyte function. Therefore, patients with AIDS are at increased risk for infections with microorganisms that typically infect patients with both T- and B-cell deficiencies (see Chapter 268).

A presumed primary immunodeficiency identified as chronic mucocutaneous candidiasis is uncommon. It is rarely associated with systemic candidiasis. Impaired cell-mediated responses also predispose to other infections, including histoplasmosis.

INFECTIONS WITH PRIMARY COMBINED B- AND T-CELL DEFECTS. Patients with severe combined immunodeficiency syndrome (SCID), Wiskott-Aldrich syndrome, and ataxia-telangiectasia suffer from high frequencies of infections (Table 179–2). Patients with SCID have acute and chronic infections with all classes of microbes. Bacterial infections are less likely in early infancy than later because of maternally acquired IgG. Surface and systemic candidiasis, cytomegalovirus (CMV) infection, bacterial infections, and *P. carinii* pneumonitis may be life threatening. Fatal Epstein-Barr virus (EBV)–associated lymphocyte proliferative disease has been encountered in patients with SCID either before or after bone marrow transplants. Even live-attenuated vaccines for polio and measles may cause serious disease. The Wiskott-Aldrich syndrome has a pattern of infectious diseases similar to the other combined cell-mediated and humoral immunodeficiencies. Late-onset sinopulmonary infections from streptococcus, enterococcus, *H. influenzae*, and respiratory viruses are found in ataxia-telangiectasia.

INFECTIONS WITH PRIMARY LYMPHOCYTE-PHAGOCYTE DEFECTS. Infants with the leukocyte adhesion deficiency have delayed separation of the umbilical cord, cellulitis, gingivitis, and necrotic skin lesions. *S. aureus* and *Pseudomonas aeruginosa* often cause severe recurrent bacterial infections of the skin and mucous surfaces and gastrointestinal tract.

INFECTIONS WITH COMPLEMENT DEFICIENCY. Deficiencies of complement components are associated with familial susceptibility to rheumatologic disorders and increased risk for recurrent pneumococcemia, meningococcemia, and gonococcemia. Fulminant infections due to *Neisseria meningitidis* or *S. pneumoniae* are also noted in patients with defects of the alternate pathway (Chapter 134.1).

INFECTIONS WITH PRIMARY PHAGOCYTE-NEUTROPHIL DEFECTS. Infants and children with quantitative or qualitative defects in neutrophils and phagocytes (Table 179–1) have increased susceptibility to *S. aureus* and other gram-positive bacteria, *P. aeruginosa*, enteric gram-negative bacilli, and opportunistic fungi, especially *C. albicans* and *Aspergillus* spp, but can acquire other infections to otherwise low-virulence organisms. The skin and mucous membranes are frequently the sites of bacterial infections and candidiasis. Systemic bacterial infection with sepsis, pneumonia, and meningitis may also occur. Chronic and recurrent pyogenic lymphadenitis, hepatic abscesses, gingivitis, pneumonia, and osteomyelitis are characteristic of patients with impaired neutrophil microbicidal activity.

The risks of infection increase as the neutrophil count decreases below 1,000/mm^3. Neutropenia may be congenital or acquired. The neutropenia associated with common febrile viral illnesses is usually benign. Neutropenia may be isolated, or it may be a sign of more significant bone marrow deficiency (aplastic anemia, leukemia).

Patients with chronic granulomatous disease (CGD) have persistent and recurrent suppurative infections of soft tissues, liver, or perirectal abscesses. In addition, these patients are susceptible to pneumonia, osteomyelitis, lymphadenitis, and involvement of any organ of the body. The infections are often caused by catalase-positive bacteria and fungi. *Aspergillus* spp infections occur with frequency.

In Chédiak-Higashi syndrome, recurrent infection of the respiratory tract and skin are the most common sites of involvement. *S. aureus* is the most frequent cause of these infections. Prophylactic antibiotics have had little if any success, in contrast to the benefits observed in patients with CGD.

Leukocyte adhesion deficiency is associated with severe gingivitis, periodontitis, and skin and mucosal lesions of *ecthyma gangrenosum* and *pyoderma gangrenosum*. Despite marked granulocytosis, abscesses with pus do not form.

The clinical manifestations of infection include fever, chills, sore throat, and localizing signs and symptoms, such as local erythema, tenderness, pain, swelling, and limitation of motion. Neutropenia may attenuate or eliminate the local manifestations of infection and can mute the more typical manifestations of cellulitis, pharyngitis, catheter tract infection, meningitis and perirectal abscess. Patients with severe neutropenia (<500 neutrophils), in the absence of other host defense defects, are at a high risk of fulminant bacterial sepsis, which may be associated only with fever or which may also be accompanied by fever, chills, disorientation, lethargy, warm-pink or cold-cyanotic extremities, and hypotension.

Treatment. The treatment of infection in patients with congenital or acquired neutropenia depends on the microorganisms responsible for the infection, the duration and severity of the neutropenia, the possibility of bone marrow recovery, and any other associated impairment(s) of host defense. Empirical therapy for bacterial sepsis is necessary for febrile patients with high-risk granulocyte disorders, such as leukocyte adhesion defects, CGD, and congenital neutropenia. The antibiotic regimens described later in this chapter for empirical treatment of febrile neutropenic patients with cancer can usually be applied to other neutrophil disorders and to absolute neutrophil counts of less than 500 cells/μL. In addition to antibiotics, corticosteroids may help to resolve granulomas in patients with CGD. Granulocyte transfusions should be reserved for patients with documented bacterial or fungal infections unresponsive to conventional therapy with intravenous antibacterial drugs and other forms of supportive therapy. Although granulocyte transfusions may be beneficial in some cases, they are expensive and include the risk of transmission of CMV, allosensitization to HLA antigens, graft versus host disease (GVHD) in immunosuppressed patients, pulmonary infiltrates and hypoxia if given in conjunction with amphotericin B, and transfusion reactions (especially in patients with X-linked CGD who lack the X-$_k$Kell-related antigen).

The role of recombinant colony-stimulating factors (G-CSF; GM-CSF) has not been well delineated. However, small studies show G-CSF to induce beneficial responses in children with cyclic neutropenia, chronic idiopathic neutropenia, and neutropenia with aplastic anemia.

Prevention. Prevention of infection in patients with neutrophil functional defects may occasionally be accomplished with the use of prophylactic antibiotics. Intracellular penetration of the broad-spectrum antibiotic combination trimethoprim-sulfamethoxazole improves phagocytic killing in patients with CGD. Recombinant human interferon-γ in a dose of 50 μg/M^2 SC three times per week plus oral trimethoprim-sulfamethoxazole has been reported to significantly reduce the infection rate in CGD.

INFECTIONS WITH DEFECTIVE OPSONIZATION. Splenectomy, congenital asplenia, and splenic dysfunction due to sickle cell disease are associated with an increased risk for serious bacterial infections. *S. pneumoniae, H. influenzae,* and *Salmonella* spp are common causative organisms of sepsis, pneumonia, meningitis, and osteomyelitis. Impaired phagocytic function and defective complement-mediated opsonization are some of the underlying defects. The efficacy of penicillin prophylaxis has been demonstrated for sickle cell disease and is recommended for patients at 3 mo of age and continued for at least the first 5 yr of age. In addition to routine immunizations, the 23-valent pneumococcal vaccine should be given at 2 yr of age, with the expectation that only modest protective efficacy will be attained. Influenza virus vaccine is also recommended each autumn for children 6 mo of age and older.

Acquired Immune Deficiencies

INFECTIONS WITH ORGAN AND TISSUE TRANSPLANTATIONS. Transplantation of bone marrow, liver, kidney, lungs, and heart has achieved acceptance as a therapeutic modality for selected diseases and at medical centers with special competence. GVHD disease and infectious complications pose the major barriers to successful outcome. Although the organisms causing infections in transplant recipients are the same as those responsible for infections in other immunocompromised hosts, the relative frequencies of occurrence, magnitude of disease, and response to therapy may vary (Table 179–2). The extent of donor-recipient match, the organ or tissue to be transplanted, and the intensity of immunosuppressive preparatory regimens influence infectious complications.

Autologous Bone Marrow Transplantation. Autologous bone marrow transplantation involves using a patient's own bone marrow to re-establish hematopoietic cell function after intensive chemotherapy or irradiation. The risk for infection is relatively small, but infection may occur in 5–10% of patients during the period required for hematologic recovery. These infections most often affect the lungs and may be due to the organisms described for allogeneic transplants. Prophylactic precautions used for allogeneic transplantation should also be used with autologous transplant recipients until the functional marrow has been re-established.

Allogeneic Bone Marrow Transplantation. *Allogeneic* transplantation involves transplantation of bone marrow from one person to another. If the donor and recipient are identical twins, the transplantation is *syngeneic.* Infection and GVHD are the major serious complications of allogeneic transplantation. Infection limits the extent of immunosuppression possible for control of graft rejection; infection is less likely in the absence of GVHD infection.

Preparative immunosuppressive management for allogeneic transplantation usually combines either one or two chemotherapy drugs with total body irradiation or the use of cytotoxic drugs without irradiation. During the pretransplantation period, the type and extent of infections depend in part on the primary underlying disease, the harboring of subclinical or unresolved infection when preparative immunosuppression is started, and the intensity of the preparative regimen. Bacterial infections are common, especially during the period of neutropenia that occurs after the preparative regimen is administered. Cellulitis, mucositis, pneumonia, urinary tract infection, and sepsis may occur (Table 179–3), although fatal infections during this time are uncommon. Antibiotic therapy is essential and should be administered empirically at the earliest sign of infection because gram-negative bacilli and gram-positive cocci cause most of these infections.

During the month after transplantation, granulocytopenia, as well as compromise of all immune responses, is profound and is a major determinant in the type and extent of infections. Damage to mucous membranes resulting in mucositis and a breach of the skin barrier by indwelling catheters provide portals of entry for gram-positive cocci, gram-negative bacilli, and opportunistic fungi. Respiratory syncytial virus (RSV) may cause upper and lower respiratory tract infection. RSV pneumonitis has serious consequences during the early post-transplantation period.

TABLE 179–3 Infections with Bone Marrow Transplantation

Stage	Compromised Defense Mechanism	Most Common Infections
Pretransplant days 0–14	Skin and mucous membranes integrity Neutropenia	Mucositis, cellulitis Sepsis, pneumonia UTI
Post-transplant before engraftment days 0–30	Skin and mucous membranes integrity Neutropenia Change in microbial flora Acute GVHD	Oral thrush, herpes simplex virus Bacterial sepsis; coagulase-negative staphylococci, *S. aureus,* streptococci, *Corynebacterium* spp; Gram-negative bacilli Fungal infections: *Candida* spp, *Aspergillus* spp Pneumonia: bacterial, fungal, RSV, parainfluenza Sinusitis: bacterial, fungal
Post-transplant, postengraftment days 30–100	Impaired cell-mediated immunity Hypogammaglobulinemia Impaired neutrophil and phagocytic function Acute GVHD	CMV infection: pneumonitis, hepatitis, gastroenteritis, esophagitis, retinitis Diffuse interstitial pneumonia: RSV, parainfluenza, adenovirus EBV infection Cystitis: adenovirus, BK papovavirus Systemic candidiasis, aspergillosis *Pneumocystis carinii* pneumonia Toxoplasmosis Viral hepatitis
Post-transplant, postengraftment days 100–365	Impaired cell-mediated immunity Impaired humoral immunity Reticuloendothelial tissue abnormalities Chronic GVHD	Varicella (chickenpox) Herpes zoster CMV disease Viral hepatitis *P. carinii* pneumonia Toxoplasmosis Common bacterial infection: *Streptococcus pneumoniae, Haemophilus influenzae* (type b and non-typable)

GVHD = graft versus host disease; UTI = urinary tract infection; CMV = cytomegalovirus; RSV = respiratory syncytial virus; EBV = Epstein-Barr virus.

Infections occurring between about 30 and 100 days after transplantation are usually not due to granulocytopenia but to other derangements in the immune system (Table 179–3); graft rejection or GVHD adds to the risk of infection. CMV may cause disease in 50–60% of patients if no prophylaxis is used.

Interstitial pneumonia is common in patients with leukemia, occurs about the 60th day after transplantation, and may be due to CMV, *P. carinii*, or RSV; in 30% of patients it is idiopathic. Idiopathic interstitial pneumonia may be due to GVHD or prior conditioning irradiation or chemotherapy and has a significant mortality.

The pattern of infection changes after about the 100th posttransplant day, when chronic graft versus host–associated antibody deficiency predisposes the recipient to pneumococcal sepsis or meningitis, and sinopulmonary infections. In addition, varicella-zoster virus reactivation occurs with increased frequency in this later period. Additional infections include hemorrhagic cystitis due to reactivation of papovavirus BK, rotavirus enteritis, pseudomembranous colitis due to *C. difficile*, and possibly human herpesvirus virus-6 infection.

TREATMENT. The treatment of infection after bone marrow transplantation depends on the amount of time elapsed since transplantation and the presence of neutropenia or of acute or chronic GVHD. The approach to febrile neutropenic transplant recipients is similar to that of febrile neutropenic patients with malignancy and includes prompt institution of empirical bactericidal broad-spectrum antibiotics, which are usually continued until the neutrophil count exceeds 500 cells/mm^3.

Acyclovir is effective therapy for herpes simplex and varicella-zoster virus infections, which are usually reactivations of latent virus. Ganciclovir and CMV hyperimmune globulin have improved the survival of patients with serious primary CMV pneumonitis. Foscarnet and cidofovir are alternatives for patients who do not respond to ganciclovir therapy.

PREVENTION. Prevention of early bacterial infection has been attempted by administering intravenous immunoglobulin and fluorinated quinolones and by preventing acute GVHD. Because of the emergence of drug-resistant bacteria related to antibiotic use, efforts should be focused on minimizing unnecessary use of antibiotics, especially vancomycin. Prevention of CMV infection has been attempted by avoiding administration of blood products from CMV-positive donors to CMV-negative recipients and minimizing the incidence of GVHD. Prophylactic use of ganciclovir for recipients who are seropositive or who are seronegative and receive marrow from a seropositive donor is warranted during the period of high risk for CMV infection. Also, acyclovir may be used during the early recovery phase to prevent activation of herpes simplex infections. When the neutrophil count recovers to 500 cells/mm^3 or greater, trimethoprim-sulfamethoxazole prophylaxis for *P. carinii* pneumonia should be started. Fluconazole has been shown to be effective in preventing infections due to *Candida* spp and may be indicated when there is an unusually high risk for systemic candidiasis. Reimmunization with routine childhood vaccines after successful transplantation is recommended on the basis of serologic tests for specific antibodies.

Infections in Liver Transplant Recipients. More than half of pediatric liver transplant recipients will have one or more infections from bacteria, fungi, protozoa, and viruses after the transplantation. The highest risk for infection is during the 1st mo after transplantation, when an average of 2.5 episodes of infection occur per patient. During the 2nd and 3rd mo, the rates decrease to about 0.35 and 0.17 episodes per patient, respectively. In addition to immunocompromise due to suppressive drugs, liver transplant recipients have the additional risk of having undergone a surgical procedure that enhances access of the microbial flora of the gastrointestinal tract to the biliary tract and liver.

Common early infections include gram-negative enteric bacterial pneumonia, soft tissue and wound infections, intra-abdominal abscesses due to enterococci and anaerobic and gram-negative enteric bacteria, peritonitis, disseminated candidiasis, and cholangitis. The latter characteristically presents with Charcot's triad of fever, abdominal pain, and jaundice; it should be distinguished from liver graft rejection by microscopic examination of a liver biopsy, Gram stain, and culture. Hepatic abscesses are often due to biliary or vascular obstruction, whereas cholangitis may be related to biliary stricture or the use of endoscopic retrograde cholangiopancreatography. Ischemic injury to the bile ducts due to hepatic artery occlusion or bile duct anatomic breakdown may produce bile leakage and gram-negative bacillary or candidal peritonitis, which are detected by culture of the abdominal drains.

CMV infections occur in 30–60% of children who receive liver transplants. Most of these are found in the first 3 mo after transplantation. As many as 15% of children who are transplant recipients will have CMV hepatitis. Pneumonitis and gastroenteritis may also be caused by this virus. Studies show human herpesvirus-6 to be a cause of fever in liver transplant recipients.

Reactivation of EBV may produce a mononucleosis-like syndrome, or it may progress to a late-onset lymphoproliferative syndrome that may improve by reducing the dose of immunosuppressive therapy.

Evaluation of the febrile liver transplant recipient for infection includes cultures of blood and abdominal drains, chest roentgenogram, abdominal ultrasonography and CT imaging, and Doppler assessment of hepatic artery blood flow. Percutaneous liver biopsy is needed to diagnose cholangitis and to preclude the possibility of rejection. Antibiotic prophylaxis should be used before biopsy and cholangiogram and continued 24–48 hr but no longer.

TREATMENT. Treatment is directed at the specific infectious complication present and may include broad-spectrum antibiotics and aspiration or drainage of abscesses.

PREVENTION. Prevention of infection has been attempted by using prophylactic antimicrobial agents, avoiding neutropenia due to azathioprine, and maintaining good surgical technique. Perioperative antibiotics, such as cefotaxime, or cefotaxime plus ampicillin, are used in most centers but should not be continued more than 2 days. Trimethoprim-sulfamethoxazole, ganciclovir, and acyclovir are used in some centers but not all.

Infections in Renal Transplant Recipients. Encountered by other severely immunocompromised patients, infection is the major cause of death in children with renal transplants. Urinary tract infection is the most common infection, with the highest incidence (10%) during the 1st mo after transplantation. During this time, *P. aeruginosa* is the most common cause, but after the 1st mo, *Escherichia coli* is more frequent.

The risk of CMV infection has been reduced by prophylactic use of antiviral drugs, administration of CMV antibody–negative blood products, and selection of seronegative organ donors. In one series of 70 children, the overall incidence of infection was only 10%, and no cases were fatal. The most common clinical pattern is a syndrome occurring 1–4 mo after transplantation, with fever, malaise, myalgia, arthralgia, and leukopenia. Hepatitis and pneumonitis may occur, as well as infrequent involvement of other organs. Infections with other herpesviruses (herpes simplex, varicella-zoster, EBV), *P. carinii, Aspergillus* spp, *Candida* spp, and viral hepatitis pose additional hazards of low frequency.

TREATMENT. Treatment of infection is directed at the specific manifestation (e.g., pneumonia or urinary tract infection) and the responsible microbiologic agent. Urine, blood, and sputum should be cultured before antibiotic therapy. Biopsy of the transplanted kidney may be needed to differentiate infection from rejection.

PREVENTION. Prevention of infection is similar to that used for other transplant recipients. Perioperative antibiotics may be used and continued for 2–5 days. Prophylactic trimethoprim-sulfamethoxazole may reduce the incidence of pyelonephritis as well as *P. carinii* pneumonitis. Careful evaluation of the urinary tract for abnormalities, such as urethral, ureteral, and vesicoureteral strictures; ureteral reflux; lymphocele; and neurogenic bladder, may identify the cause of recurrent urinary tract infections. Primary CMV infection can be prevented by avoiding the use of CMV-positive blood products as well as transplantation from a CMV-positive donor to a CMV-negative recipient. Prophylactic ganciclovir may be used in high-risk patients.

Infections in Heart Transplant Recipients. Heart transplant recipients are at risk for the same infections as patients with other organ transplants. In addition, mediastinitis caused by *S. aureus*, coagulase-negative staphylococci, or gram-negative bacilli may result from an infected surgical wound. Fever, sternal tenderness, erythema, and purulent drainage with bone destruction suggest the diagnosis of mediastinitis. Treatment is directed at the specific pathogen, and the precautions and prophylaxis used in other organ transplantations are indicated.

INFECTIONS IN PATIENTS WITH CANCER. Children with malignancy may be severely compromised from immunodeficiency caused by the cancer, the therapy, or both. Increased risk for infection is also associated with damage to the skin and mucous membranes, indwelling catheters, malnutrition, prolonged antibiotic use, and hospitalization.

Because the immunodeficiency is related primarily to anticancer therapy, the risk of infection is related to the type, intensity, and duration of chemotherapy. More than one dysfunction of the immune system is usually involved. For example, corticosteroid drugs and radiation cause destruction of both T and B lymphocytes; methotrexate and other folate antagonists inhibit DNA synthesis; alkylating agents such as cyclophosphamide block DNA replication; and 6-mercaptopurine interferes with purine synthesis. All of these agents inhibit the inflammatory response to invading microbes. The organisms causing infections in patients with cancer are listed in Table 179–2.

The significance of the neutrophil count in predicting the risk and response to infections was clearly elucidated in the 1960s. This parameter serves as the basis for management of infections in children with malignancies. While CD+ T-lymphocyte counts are dependable predictors of certain infections in patients with AIDS, no studies to date have used this measure in patients with cancer. Infections in children with cancer are categorized as those occurring in neutropenia and non-neutropenic patients, keeping in mind that exceptions occur with each category.

Infections in Non-neutropenic Patients with Cancer. Organisms that may cause infection in non-neutropenic patients with cancer include the viral infections listed in Table 179–2, *P. carinii, Toxoplasma gondii*, and certain fungal infections such as histoplasmosis, cryptococcosis, and coccidioidomycosis. These patients are also at risk for infections encountered in an otherwise normal host, such as pneumococcal pneumonia, otitis media, streptococcal pharyngitis, and urinary tract infection. Infections with coagulase-negative staphylococci, *P. aeruginosa, Serratia marcescens, Candida* spp, and *Aspergillus* spp are rare.

Although the need to start specific antimicrobial therapy is urgent, the empirical antibiotic therapy used for neutropenic patients is usually not initiated until after an attempt to establish an etiologic diagnosis has been made.

Infections in Neutropenic Patients with Cancer. When the granulocyte (neutrophil) count is 500 cells/mm^3 or less, the patient is at heightened risk for a serious infection, usually of bacterial etiology. The risk is less at counts of 500–1,000 cell/mm^3 but is greater than for normal children. As the count remains below 500 cells/mm^3, the risk for infection increases proportionately. Because of the granulocytopenia and the poor inflammatory response, fever is often the only manifestation of infection.

Because the cause of infection in febrile granulocytopenic patients cannot be predicted from physical signs and symptoms, initial antibiotic treatment requires broad-spectrum antibiotics. Gram-positive cocci have emerged as the most frequent cause of febrile episodes in recent years, but gram-negative bacilli continue to have a significant role in these serious infections (Table 179–2). Coagulase-negative staphylococci, *S. aureus*, and α-hemolytic streptococci are the most frequent organisms cultured from the blood of febrile children with neutropenia. In some cases of α-hemolytic streptococcal bacteremia, an acute septic shock syndrome may occur, resembling the adult respiratory distress syndrome (ARDS); this manifestation is most common in children receiving cytarabine or quinolone drugs. *P. aeruginosa, E. coli*, and *Klebsiella pneumoniae* are the most common gram-negative bacillary infections. Antibiotic therapy is usually effective in controlling bacterial infections, but the need for prolonged antibiotic therapy predisposes patients to opportunistic fungal infections, especially from species of *Candida* and *Aspergillus*.

Gram-negative bacillary sepsis is typically more severe than that due to *Staphylococcus epidermidis. E. coli*, or *Pseudomonas* infection results in septic shock in 30–50% of episodes. Oropharyngeal infection is manifested as ulcerating stomatitis, gingivitis, and periodontal lesions. Mucositis may be drug induced or due to anaerobic bacteria, herpes simplex, *Candida* spp, or a mixed infection. Esophagitis may be due to these same microorganisms or to CMV and may be associated with mucositis or may occur independently. Cutaneous lesions may occur as perirectal cellulitis at sites of central venous catheter insertion, venipuncture, lumbar puncture, bone marrow biopsy, or abrasions or as infection of sweat glands and paronychia. Cutaneous signs of disseminated infection include ecthyma gangrenosum (*P. aeruginosa* and other microorganisms), nodules (*Candida* spp, mucormycosis), gangrenous cellulitis (*Aspergillus*, mucormycosis), and thrombotic arterial occlusion with distal ischemia due to *Aspergillus* spp.

Pneumonia in granulocytopenic patients with cancer may be subtle and manifested as local rales, tachypnea, chest pain, or ARDS. Pulmonary infiltrates may be absent or faint, only to appear more obvious when the neutrophil count increases above 500 cells/mm^3. Pneumonia is usually due to gram-negative enteric bacteria but may also be due to fungi. *Aspergillus* may produce a characteristic wedge-shaped infiltrate typical of arterial invasion and subsequent thrombotic pulmonary infraction. Pulmonary cavitation is suggestive of aspergillosis, mucormycosis, and, rarely, infection with gram-negative enteric bacteria. Pulmonary infiltrates in neutropenic patients with cancer may also represent noninfectious disorders, such as hemorrhage, malignancy, emboli, edema, reactions to granulocyte transfusions, and radiation- or chemotherapy-induced pneumonitis.

Additional infectious complications include sinusitis with possible intracranial extension due to aspergillosis, mucormycosis, or mixed bacteria; hepatic and splenic candidiasis in the absence of candidemia; candidal endophthalmitis; and severe diarrhea due to *C. difficile*.

Blood samples for cultures should be drawn from a peripheral vein and from each lumen of the central venous catheter. Cultures or biopsies should be made of local cutaneous lesions, and a chest roentgenogram should be examined for infiltrates, infarction, or cavitation. In higher risk patients (i.e., neutrophil count $<500/mm^3$ for >10 days), nasal secretions and sputum should be cultured for the presence of *Aspergillus*. Sinus roentgenograms or CT may reveal asymptomatic sinusitis. Esophageal endoscopy may be indicated to identify the cause of odynophagia. If pseudohyphae are demonstrated from esophageal lesions, a presumptive diagnosis of disseminated candidiasis is suggested. Serum C-reactive protein levels of greater than 40 mg/L suggest bacterial infection.

Meningitis is unusual in granulocytopenic febrile patients

with cancer. Lumbar puncture should be obtained in the presence of significant signs of central venous system infection, realizing that neutrophils may be absent even when bacteria are present.

In certain situations, fiberoptic bronchoscopy, bronchoalveolar lavage, transbronchial biopsy, or open lung biopsy may be required to identify the microorganism responsible for pneumonia.

TREATMENT. Treatment of infections in febrile granulocytopenic patients with cancer requires prompt initiation of empirical broad-spectrum bactericidal antibiotics to decrease the risks of septic shock, ARDS, hypotension, renal and other organ dysfunction, and death.

Many effective antibiotics and antibiotic combinations are available. In 1997, the Infectious Diseases Society of America published *Guidelines for the Use of Antimicrobial Agents in Neutropenic Patients with Unexplained Fever.* These guidelines apply to children and adults and provide detailed suggestions for management (Fig. 179–1). Any of three initial regimens is acceptable, and the overall outcome is expected to be similar; however, one may be more appropriate for certain patients and in certain institutions than are the others. These are (1) a single-drug therapy (monotherapy); (2) two-drug therapy without vancomycin (duotherapy), and (3) vancomycin plus one or two other drugs. The most important difference in these regimens is the use of vancomycin. Because of the emerging development of organisms that are susceptible only to vancomycin, efforts are made to reduce the unnecessary use of this drug and to reserve it for only indicated use. The selection of drugs for initial therapy must include consideration about whether or not the patient has indications for the use of vancomycin. Patients who have severe mucositis; who have received quinolone drugs for prophylaxis; who are known to be colonized with methicillin-resistant *S. aureus* or penicillin-cephalosporin-resistant pneumococci; who have obvious catheter-related infection; and who are critically ill with hypotension are at high risk for infection by bacteria susceptible only to vancomycin. Patients who qualify should receive vancomycin plus ceftazidime. If vancomycin is not indicated, a single drug such as ceftazidime, imipenem, or meropenem may be used. Alternatively, a combination of an aminoglycoside (gentamicin, tobramycin, and amikacin) plus an antipseudomonal β-lactam drug (ticarcillin, piperacillin) may be used. A disadvantage of the aminoglycoside is infrequent side effects of nephrotoxicity, ototoxicity, and hypokalemia. If the causative organism is identified, the treatment should be modified for optimal susceptibility while continuing broad-spectrum antimicrobial coverage. After 3 days of the initial regimen, a patient is reassessed. If a patient has become afebrile and no cause is identified, consideration is given to changing the antibiotics to be administered by the oral route and allowing the patient to be discharged to complete the 1-wk course of antibiotics. Patients who lacked signs of sepsis (e.g., chills, hypotension) at admission, who have a neutrophil count of 100 cells/mm^3 or greater, and who have no discernible infectious process (pneumonia, cellulitis) are at low risk for recurrence and can be treated after day 2 or 3 as outpatients on an antibiotic such as cefixime. If these risk factors exist in an afebrile patient, then initial intravenous antibiotic regimen should be continued in the hospital. Vancomycin may be discontinued if no organism requiring its use is cultured by day 2 or 3. For patients who persist to have fever during the first 3 days of treatment, the same antibiotics may be continued if the clinical condition has not worsened. The mean time for defervescence is 5 days. If the course is worsening, antibiotics can be changed, especially with the addition of vancomycin if not included in the initial regimen. If fever persists for 5–7 days or more, the addition of amphotericin B is usually indicated because of the risk for systemic fungal infection. Fluconazole may be an acceptable alternative to amphotericin B for some patients at hospitals where drug-resistant *Candida* and *Aspergillus* species are uncommon.

The duration of antibiotic therapy depends on the pattern of fever and neutrophil counts. If a patient becomes afebrile by day 3 and the neutrophil count is less than 500/mm^3 by day 7, antibiotics should be continued for patients in the high-risk category. If a patient is at low risk, the drugs can be discontinued when the patient has been afebrile for 5–7 days.

For patients who have persistent fever after day 3, the drugs may be discontinued 4–5 days after the neutrophil count has increased to 500/mm^3 or greater in the absence of complications. However, for those with persistent fever and neutropenia less than 500/mm^3, antibiotics should be continued for 2 wk and then stopped, with re-evaluation of the patient.

PREVENTION. Prevention of infection in neutropenic patients with cancer is difficult. Methods include reverse isolation and a total protective environment, but these are cumbersome and of limited efficacy. Prophylactic oral nonabsorbable antibiotics, such as colistin, nystatin, and polymyxin; and oral absorbable antibiotics, such as trimethoprim-sulfamethoxazole, the quino-

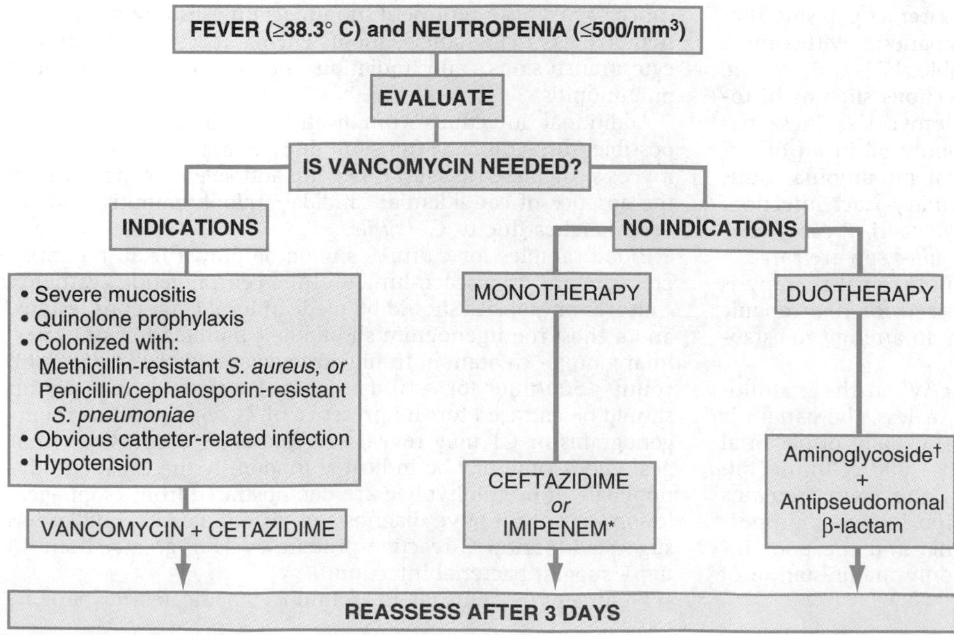

Figure 179–1 Guide to the initial management of the febrile neutropenic patient. *Recent studies suggest that cefepime or meropenem may be as effective as ceftazidime or imipenem as monotherapy. †Aminoglycoside antibiotics should be avoided if patient is also receiving nephrotoxic, ototoxic, or neuromuscular blocking agents; has renal or severe electrolyte dysfunction; or is suspected of having meningitis (poor blood-brain perfusion). (Adapted from Hughes WT, Armstrong D, Bodey GP, et al: Guidelines for the use of antimicrobial agents in neutropenic patients with unexplained fever. Clin Infect Dis 25:551, 1997.)

TABLE 179–4 Defects in Anatomic Barriers That May Contribute to Infection

Skin

Traumatic break (trauma, surgery, burns)
Blockage of sweat excretion
Change in fatty acid components of sebaceous glands
Change in normal microbial flora

Mucous Membranes

Decrease in tears; lysozyme, normal desquamation; mucus production; acidity of stomach, vagina, and skin; flow of urine; ciliary escalation of respiratory tract; coughing and sneezing; salivation; bile salts; and peristaltic activity
Change in the normal microbial flora

Obstruction to Normal Organ Excretion/Secretion

Urinary tract obstruction
Biliary tract obstruction

Impaired Febrile Response

Foreign Body

Intravascular access device

lones, and fluconazole may reduce the risk of infection in severely granulocytopenic (<100 cells/mm^3) patients receiving cancer chemotherapy or bone marrow transplantation. However, because of the lack of effect on the overall mortality rate and the emergence of drug-resistant organisms, no sound consensus is established for prophylaxis except for the use of trimethoprim-sulfamethoxazole in the prevention of *P. carinii* pneumonia.

Indications for recombinant human G-CSF and GM-CSF are not adequately defined. Their use in febrile neutropenic patients appears to reduce the period of granulocytopenia, the incidence of infection, and the number of days for hospitalization and antibiotic therapy, but overall survival from infection has not been affected.

BREECH IN SKIN AND MUCOUS MEMBRANE BARRIERS TO INFECTION. To establish infection, microbial pathogens must first penetrate the important protective covering of the skin, conjunctivas, and mucous membranes. Commensal organisms colonize these surfaces without invasion. The barrier may be overcome by organisms of very high virulence or by a defect in this host barrier (Table 179–4). In addition to being a physical obstacle that few pathogens can penetrate, the skin contains bacteriostatic and bactericidal fatty acids secreted by the sebaceous glands. Mucous membrane secretions contain various enzymes (lactoperoxidase, lysozyme, lactoferrin) and secretory IgA, and specific areas have unfavorable acidic environments (stomach, urine, vagina) that reduce bacterial activity. Furthermore, a normal bacterial flora of mucosal surfaces may prevent local colonization by pathogenic microorganisms. This *colonization resistance* is due to local bacterial production of antimicrobial compounds (bacteriocins), alteration of the redox potential, and competition for nutrients. Additional local defense mechanisms include mucociliary clearance, the cough reflex, unobstructed flow of secretions, and the activity of tissue phagocytic cells and antimicrobial proteins and peptides of the innate immune system. Interference or disruption of any of these local defense mechanisms may predispose to infection. Broad-spectrum antibiotics may alter the normal flora and reduce colonization resistance; therapy intended to increase gastric pH may increase gastric colonization with pathogenic bacteria; obstruction to the flow of urine or lung secretions may cause pyelonephritis or pneumonia, respectively; and surgical incision, burns, or trauma may alter the physical barrier.

Medical devices such as intravenous access devices, cerebrospinal fluid shunts, urethral catheters, peritoneal dialysis catheters, and orthopedic prostheses pose special considerations that predispose to infections (Chapter 180).

Burns. Infections in children with burns (Chapter 70) are related to interruption of the skin and mucous membrane barriers, to the presence of necrotic tissue, which serves as a culture medium, to pulmonary injury, to long-term administration of antibiotics, and to prolonged intravenous or urinary catheterization. Septicemia with *P. aeruginosa, S. aureus,* and coagulase-negative staphylococci is frequent. Burn injury has been associated with abnormal immune response to infection, including neutrophil dysfunction, abnormal antibody responses to specific antigens, and delayed rejection of homografts. The risk of infection is directly related to the extent of the burn, the neutrophil chemotactic defect, and an associated hypogammaglobulinemia. The burn site may aid in selection of antibiotics if evidence of infection occurs, such as fever, cellulitis, or necrosis. Fever may be due to a metabolic response to injury or to infection. Broad-spectrum antibiotic coverage is recommended if infection is suspected. Sepsis is a major cause of death with extensive burns, and *P. aeruginosa* is the most common cause. Occlusive dressings with silver sulfadiazine may be used prophylactically against infection.

Surgery. The surgical incision is an obvious breech in the skin

TABLE 179–5 Immunizations for Immunocompromised Infants and Children

Vaccine	Routine	HIV/AIDS	Severe Immunosuppression*	Asplenia	Renal Failure	Diabetes
			Routine Infant Immunizations			
DTaP/DTP(DT/T/Td)	Recommended	Recommended	Recommended	Recommended	Recommended	Recommended
OPV	Recommended	Contraindicated	Contraindicated	Recommended	Recommended	Recommended
IPV	Recommended	Recommended	Recommended	Use as indicated	Use as indicated	Use as indicated
MMR/MR/M/R	Recommended	Recommended/ considered	Contraindicated	Recommended	Recommended	Recommended
Hib	Recommended	Recommended	Recommended	Recommended	Recommended	Recommended
Hepatitis B	Recommended	Recommended	Recommended	Recommended	Recommended	Recommended
Varicella	Recommended	Contraindicated/ considered§	Contraindicated	Contraindicated	Use if indicated	Use if indicated
Rotavirus	Recommended	Contraindicated	Contraindicated	Contraindicated	Use if indicated	Use if indicated
			Other Childhood Immunizations			
Pneumococcus†	Use if indicated	Recommended	Recommended	Recommended	Recommended	Recommended
Influenza‡	Use if indicated	Recommended	Recommended	Recommended	Recommended	Recommended

**Severe immunosuppression can result from congenital immunodeficiency, HIV infection, leukemia, lymphoma, aplastic anemia, generalized malignancy, alkylating agents, antimetabolites, radiation, or large amounts of corticosteroids.*

†Recommended for persons ≥2 yr of age.

‡Not recommended for infants <6 mo of age.

§Varicella vaccine should be considered for asymptomatic or mildly symptomatic HIV-infected children in CDC class N1 or A1 with age-specific CD4$^+$ T-lymphocyte percentages of ≥25%. Eligible children should receive two doses of varicella vaccine with a 3-mo-interval between doses.

Adapted from Centers for Disease Control and Prevention: Recommendations of the Advisory Committee on Immunization Practices (ACIP): Use of vaccines and immune globulins in persons with altered immunity. MMWR 42(RR-4):15, 1993.

or mucous membrane barrier and introduces an increase in risk for infection, usually bacterial. The risk is proportionate to the number and virulence of microbes entering the wound, the site, and the length of time the incision is open (Chapter 302).

CHRONIC DISEASES. Many chronic diseases and debilitating circumstances render patients at increased risk for infection. These include diseases such as sickle cell anemia, cystic fibrosis, diabetes mellitus, malnutrition, nephrotic syndrome, uremia, cirrhosis, and AIDS.

Immunization in Immunocompromised Infants and Children

Because many immunocompromised children survive into adult life and some may eventually be restored to immunocompetence, immunization with live-attenuated and killed vaccines in general use deserves consideration. Key factors are adverse effects that might result from use of live-attenuated vaccines, such as the oral poliovirus vaccine, and the inability of the host to muster an adequate immune response (Table 179–5). Suboptimal responses may occur in some patients; thus, the guidelines may not apply to certain individual patients.

American Academy of Pediatrics: Immunization in special circumstances. *In*: Peter G (ed): 1997 Redbook: Report of the Committee on Infectious Diseases, 24th ed. Elk Grove Village, IL, American Academy of Pediatrics, 1997, pp 50–58.

Armitage JO: Bone marrow transplantation. N Engl J Med 330:827, 1994.

Bowen RA: Respiratory virus infections after marrow transplant: The Fred Hutchinson Cancer Research Center Experience. Am J Med 102:31, 1997.

Chang FY, Singh N, Gayowski T, et al: Fever in liver transplant recipients: Changing spectrum of etiologic agents. Clin Infect Dis 26:59, 1998.

Chanock SJ, Pizzo PA: Infectious complications of patients undergoing therapy for acute leukemia: Current status and future prospects. Semin Oncol 24:132, 1997.

Dell'Orto M, Rovelli A, Barzaghi A, et al: Febrile complications in the first 100 days after bone marrow transplantation in children: A single center's experience. Pediatr Hematol Oncol 14:335, 1997.

Ezekowitz RAB, Dinauer MC, Jaffe HS, et al: Partial correction of the phagocyte defect in patients with X-linked chronic granulomatous disease by subcutaneous interferon gamma. N Engl J Med 319:146, 1988.

Freifeld AG, Pizzo PA: The outpatient management of febrile neutropenia in cancer patients. Oncol 10:599, 1996.

Hughes WT, Armstrong D, Bodey GP, et al: Guidelines for the use of antimicrobial agents in neutropenic patients with unexplained fever. Clin Infect Dis 25:551, 1997.

Lautenschlager I, Höckerstedt K, Linnavuori K, et al: Human herpesvirus-6 infection after liver transplantation. Clin Infect Dis 26:702, 1998.

Lucas VS, Beighton D, Roberts GJ, et al: Changes in the oral streptococcal flora of children undergoing allogenic bone marrow transplantation. J Infect Dis 35:135, 1997.

Patrick CC: Infections in Immunocompromised Infants and Children. New York, Churchill Livingstone, 1992.

Pizzo PA: Management of fever in patients with cancer and treatment-induced neutropenia. N Engl J Med 328:1323, 1993.

Riikonen P, Saarinen UM, Mäkipernaa A, et al: Recombinant human granulocyte-macrophage colony-stimulating factor in the treatment of febrile neutropenia: A double blind placebo-controlled study in children. Pediatr Infect Dis J 13:197, 1994.

Rowe JM, Ciobanu N, Ascesao J, et al: Recommended guidelines for the management of autologous and allogenic bone marrow transplantation: A report from the Eastern Cooperative Oncology Group. Ann Intern Med 120:143, 1994.

Sable CA, Donowitz GR: Infections in bone marrow transplant recipients. Clin Infect Dis 18:272, 1994.

Sanders JE. Bone marrow transplantation in pediatric oncology. *In*: Pizzo PA, Poplack DG: Principles and Practice of Pediatric Oncology, 3rd ed. Philadelphia, Lippincott-Raven, 1997.

So SKS, Simmons RL: Infections following kidney transplantation in children. *In*: Patrick CC (ed): Infection in Immunosuppressed Infants and Children. New York, Churchill Livingstone, 1992, pp 215–230.

Wong W-Y, Overturf GD, Powars DR: Infections caused by *Streptococcus pneumoniae* in children with sickle cell disease: Epidemiology, immunologic mechanisms, prophylaxis, and vaccination. Clin Infect Dis 14:1124, 1992.

CHAPTER 180
Infection Associated with Medical Devices

Patricia M. Flynn and Fred F. Barrett

Despite the therapeutic successes and convenience of the many synthetic devices used in pediatric patients, infectious complications are problematic. The pathogenesis of device-related infection is not completely defined, but many factors are important, including the susceptibility of the host, the composition of the device, the ability of microorganisms to adhere to the device itself or to the biofilm that quickly forms on it, and environmental factors that include the insertion technique and maintenance of the device.

INTRAVASCULAR DEVICES. Intravascular access devices range from short stainless steel needles to multilumen implantable synthetic plastic catheters that are expected to remain in use for years. Despite the variability in the catheter material, all induce local changes in the surrounding tissues, commonly called a *foreign body reaction*. In this microenvironment, host phagocytes, complement, and proteins interact with the catheter material to establish a milieu that can support adherence and proliferation of microorganisms.

Infectious complications of intravascular devices include localized infections (exit site and tunnel tract infection and suppurative phlebitis) and systemic infections (catheter-related bacteremia and fungemia). The pathogenesis is related to local contamination and subsequent colonization of the catheter rather than primary bacteremia seeding the intravascular device. Infection due to the microbial skin flora at the insertion site may extend along the external surface of the catheter. This route of infection is most common in intravascular catheters in place for less than 30 days. Organisms may also gain access to the intraluminal portion of the catheter through improper handling of the catheter hub or contaminated infusate. This route of infection is thought to be more prevalent in catheters in place longer than 30 days. Gram-positive cocci predominate in both categories; more than half are coagulase-negative staphylococci. Gram-negative enteric bacteria are isolated in approximately 20–30% of episodes, and fungi account for 5–10%.

The *clinical manifestations* of local infection include erythema, tenderness, and purulent discharge at the exit site or along the subcutaneous tunnel tract of the catheter. Catheter-related sepsis may also present as fever without an identifiable focus.

The *diagnosis* of localized infection is made clinically. A Gram stain and culture of exit site drainage should be performed and may help elucidate the cause. The diagnosis of catheter-related sepsis is confirmed by performing simultaneous quantitative blood cultures via the catheter and a peripheral vein. Greater than four times the numbers of organisms isolated from blood obtained via the catheter as compared with that obtained via a peripheral vein is evidence of catheter-related bacteremia or fungemia. Catheter-related sepsis can also be diagnosed by isolation of the same organism from the blood and the catheter tip. This method, however, requires catheter removal and is not optimal for patients with long-term devices.

Short-term peripheral catheters are most commonly used in pediatric patients, and infectious complications occur infrequently. The rate of peripheral catheter-related bacteremia is less than 0.15%. Age less than 1 yr, duration of use greater than 144 hr, and select infusates are associated with increased risk of catheter-related infection.

Central venous catheters (CVCs) are widely used in both

adults and pediatric patients and are responsible for the majority of catheter-related infections. They are commonly used in critically ill patients, including neonates, who often have many risk factors for the development of nosocomial infection. Patients who are in an intensive care unit and who have a CVC in place have a fivefold greater risk of developing a nosocomial bloodstream infection than those without a CVC. Maintenance of these catheters remains controversial. Although prevalence of infection increases with prolonged duration of catheter use, routine replacement of a CVC results in significant morbidity. Current guidelines suggest placement with full barrier precautions without a policy for routine replacement either via a new site or exchange of the catheter over a guide wire.

The use of peripherally inserted central catheters (PICCs) has increased in pediatric patients. This catheter is inserted into a peripheral vein with the distal end in a central vein. Published information about these devices in children is scanty, but adult studies demonstrate a life span of approximately 3 mo and infection rates significantly lower than for CVCs, 1.9 episodes/1,000 catheter-days.

When prolonged intravenous access is required, a cuffed silicone rubber (Silastic) catheter may be inserted into the right atrium through the subclavian, cephalic, or jugular vein. The extravascular segment of the catheter passes through a subcutaneous tunnel before exiting the skin, usually on the superior aspect of the chest (Broviac or Hickman catheters). Totally implanted venous access systems (Mediport, Port-A-Cath, Infuse-A-Port) consist of a reservoir placed in a subcutaneous pocket with a self-sealing silicone septum that permits repeated percutaneous needle insertion and administration of drugs at the distal end. The use of these central venous devices has improved the quality of life of high-risk patients but has also increased the risk of various infections.

The incidence of local (exit site, tunnel, pocket) infection is 0.2–2.8/1,000 catheter-days. The incidence of Broviac or Hickman catheter sepsis is 0.5–6.8/1,000 catheter days, whereas that for implantable systems is 0.3–1.8/1,000 catheter-days. The risk of catheter infection is increased among premature infants, young children, and those receiving total parenteral nutrition.

If either localized or systemic catheter-related infection is diagnosed in a peripheral catheter or CVC, the device should be removed. Antibiotics should be administered in cases of systemic infection, with the exception of uncomplicated coagulase-negative staphylococcal bacteremia in normal hosts.

In patients with long-term vascular access devices in place (Hickman, Broviac, implanted ports), antibiotic treatment is successful in most systemic bacterial infections without removal of the device. Antibiotic therapy should be directed to the isolated pathogen and given for a total of 10–14 days. Until identification and susceptibility testing are available, empirical therapy with a third-generation cephalosporin or aminoglycoside plus vancomycin is indicated. If medical therapy without immediate removal is attempted, daily blood cultures should be obtained to monitor the progress of therapy. If blood cultures remain positive after a patient has received 72 hr of optimal therapy or if a patient deteriorates clinically, the device should be removed. Most experts advocate removal of the device and therapy with systemic antifungals in cases of catheter-related fungemia. Exit-site infections usually respond to local care or systemic antibiotics, but tunnel tract infections require removal of the catheter in approximately two thirds of patients.

Prevention of Infection. Prevention of long-term vascular access device-related infection includes placement using meticulous surgical aseptic technique in an operating room–like environment, use of antibacterial ointment, avoidance of occlusive or semipermeable dressings, avoidance of bathing or swimming, and careful catheter care. The use of central venous catheters impregnated with antibiotics may be a future means to prevent catheter-related infection.

CEREBROSPINAL FLUID SHUNTS. Cerebrospinal fluid (CSF) shunting is required for the treatment of many children with hydrocephalus. The usual procedure uses a silicone rubber device with a proximal portion inserted into the ventricle, a unidirectional valve, and a distant segment that diverts the CSF from the ventricles to either the peritoneal cavity (VP shunt) or right atrium (VA shunt). The incidence of shunt infection ranges from 1–20%, with an average of 10%. The highest rates are reported in young infants. Most infections are a result of intraoperative contamination of the surgical wound by skin flora. Accordingly, coagulase-negative staphylococci are isolated in more than half of the cases. *Staphylococcus aureus* is isolated in approximately 20% and gram-negative bacilli in 15%.

Four distinct clinical syndromes have been described: colonization of the shunt, infection associated with wound infection, distal infection with peritonitis, and infection associated with meningitis.

The most common type of infection is colonization of the shunt. Symptoms associated with colonized VP shunts are usually those of shunt malfunction and include lethargy, headache, vomiting, and a full fontanel. Low-grade fever is common. Symptoms usually occur within months of the surgical procedure. Colonization of a VA shunt results in more severe systemic symptoms and often without symptoms of shunt malfunction. Septic pulmonary emboli, pulmonary hypertension, and endocarditis are reported complications of VA shunt colonization. Chronic VA shunt colonization may cause hypocomplementemic glomerulonephritis due to antigen-antibody complex deposition in the glomeruli, commonly called *shunt nephritis*; clinical findings include hypertension, microscopic hematuria, elevated blood urea nitrogen (BUN) and serum creatinine levels, and anemia. In shunt colonization, CSF obtained from either lumbar or ventricular puncture is often sterile, and the infecting organism is isolated only from the shunt reservoir. Because of this, it is unusual to see signs of ventriculitis, and CSF findings are only minimally abnormal. Blood culture results are usually nondiagnostic in cases of VP colonization but positive in VA shunt colonization.

Wound infection presents with obvious infection or dehiscence along the shunt tract and most often occurs within days to weeks of the surgical procedure. *S. aureus* is the most common isolate. In addition to physical findings, fever is common, and signs of shunt malfunction eventually ensue in most cases.

Distal infection with peritonitis presents with abdominal symptoms, usually without evidence of shunt malfunction. The pathogenesis is likely related to perforation of bowel at the time of VP shunt placement or translocation of bacteria across the bowel wall. Thus, gram-negative isolates predominate and mixed infection is common. The infecting organisms are often isolated from only the distal portion of the shunt.

The usual meningeal pathogens, *Streptococcus pneumoniae, Neisseria meningitidis*, and *Haemophilus influenzae* can also cause bacterial meningitis in patients with shunts in place. Clinical presentation is similar to that for acute bacterial meningitis.

Treatment of shunt colonization and distal infection with peritonitis includes the use of antibiotics against the specific organisms isolated and, in most situations, removal of the shunt. Intrashunt antibiotics are indicated because of the poor penetration of most antibiotics into the CNS across uninflamed meninges. If the isolate is susceptible, a parenteral antistaphylococcal penicillin plus intrashunt vancomycin is the treatment of choice. If the organism is resistant to the penicillins, systemic and intrashunt vancomycin is recommended. In cases of gram-negative infections, a combination of a third-generation cephalosporin and intrashunt aminoglycoside is optimal. When using intrashunt antibiotics, monitoring of levels is necessary to avoid toxicity. The best treatment success occurs with initial systemic and intrashunt antibiotics in combination with exteriorization of the distal end of the shunt. After CSF from the reservoir has remained sterile for 48 hr, shunt replacement on the opposite side can be performed. Partial shunt revision with antibiotic therapy or antibiotic therapy alone has been successful in some series, but the relapse rate is higher. When wound infection is diagnosed, the shunt most always needs to be removed. To allow for continued ventricular drainage, a temporary catheter is often placed, with replacement of a new shunt on the opposite side after the wound infection has healed. Only treatment with systemic antibiotics is necessary for cases of bacterial meningitis in patients with a shunt in place; the shunt does not need to be removed.

Prevention of Infection. Prevention of shunt infection includes meticulous cutaneous preparation and surgical technique. Systemic and intraventricular antibiotics and soaking the shunt tubing in antibiotics have been used to reduce the incidence of infection, with varying success. A meta-analysis of 12 clinical trials involving 1,359 randomized patients showed that perioperative use of an antimicrobial agent in CSF shunt placement reduced the risk for infection, although only 1 of the 12 studies individually revealed an effect and various antimicrobial regimens were used.

URETHRAL CATHETERS. Urinary catheters are a frequent cause of nosocomial infection, about 14 infections per 1,000 admissions. Like other devices, microorganisms adhere to the catheter surface and establish a biofilm that allows proliferation. The physical presence of the catheter reduces the normal host defenses by preventing complete emptying of the bladder, thus providing a medium for growth, distending the urethra, and blocking periurethral glands. Almost all patients catheterized for more than 30 days develop bacteriuria. The urinary tract is considered infected if specimens of urine obtained directly from an indwelling catheter yield a level of 100 or greater colony-forming units. Gram-negative bacilli and enterococci from the gastrointestinal tract are the predominant organisms isolated in catheter-related urinary tract infection; coagulase-negative staphylococci are implicated in about 15%. Symptomatic infection should be treated with antibiotics and catheter removal. Asymptomatic infections can usually be managed with catheter removal alone.

Prevention of Infection. All urinary catheters introduce risk for infection, and their casual use should be avoided. When they are in place, their duration of use should be minimized. Technologic advances have led to development of silver- or antibiotic-impregnated urinary catheters that are associated with lower rates of infection. Prophylactic antibiotics do not reduce the infection rates for long-term indwelling urethral catheters.

PERITONEAL DIALYSIS CATHETERS. During the 1st yr of peritoneal dialysis for end-stage renal disease, 65% of children will have one or more episodes of peritonitis. Bacterial entry comes from luminal or periluminal contamination of the catheter or by translocation across the intestinal wall. Hematogenous infection is a rare event. Infections can be localized at the exit site, associated with peritonitis, or both. Organisms responsible for peritonitis include *Staphylococcus epidermidis* (30–40%), *S. aureus* (10–20%), streptococci (10–15%), *Escherichia coli* (5–10%), *Pseudomonas* spp (5–10%), other gram-negative bacteria (5–15%), enterococci (3–6%), and fungi (2–10%). *S. aureus* is more common in localized exit or tunnel tract infections (42%). Most infectious episodes are due to a patient's own flora, and carriers of *S. aureus* have been shown to have increased rates of infection as compared with noncarriers.

The *clinical manifestations* of peritonitis may be subtle and include low-grade fever, mild abdominal pain, and tenderness. Cloudy peritoneal dialysis fluid may be the first or predominant sign. In peritonitis, the cell count of the fluid is usually greater than 100 cells/μL. When peritonitis is suspected, the effluent dialysate should be submitted for cell count, Gram stain (up to 40% are positive if peritonitis is present) and culture.

Patients with cloudy fluid and clinical symptoms should receive empirical therapy, preferably guided by results of a Gram stain. If no organisms are visualized, vancomycin and either an aminoglycoside or third-generation cephalosporin with antipseudomonal activity should be given via the intraperitoneal route. Patients without cloudy fluid and with minimal symptoms may have therapy withheld pending culture results. Once a cause is defined, changes in the therapeutic regimen may be needed. Oral rifampin may be added for *S. aureus* infections. Fungal peritonitis should be treated with a combination of oral flucytosine and intraperitoneal fluconazole. Duration of therapy is a minimum of 14 days, with longer treatment of 21–28 days for episodes of *S. aureus, Pseudomonas* spp, and fungi. Patients who have a repeat episode of peritonitis within 4 wk of previous therapy are diagnosed with "apparently relapsing" peritonitis. If the patient responds to therapy, a course of up to 6 wk should be administered. In all cases, if the infection fails to clear on appropriate therapy or if a patient's condition is deteriorating, the catheter should be removed. Exit-site and tunnel infections may occur independently of peritonitis or may precede it. Appropriate antibiotics should be administered on the basis of Gram stain and culture findings. Some experts recommend that the catheter be removed if *Pseudomonas* spp or fungal organisms are isolated.

ORTHOPEDIC PROSTHESES. Orthopedic prostheses are uncommonly used in children. However, their use is increasing in limb salvage procedures for osteosarcoma. Infection most often follows introduction of microorganisms at surgery or via hematogenous spread. The former results in early infection (within 12 wk), which accounts for about 40% of all infections. The latter route is more common in late infections. As with other foreign devices, the most common isolates are staphylococci, and they are equally divided between coagulase-negative staphylococci and *S. aureus*. Clinical manifestations can include obvious wound infection, pain at the site of the prosthesis, and fever. Late infection may present only with pain. Radiographic abnormalities may be apparent on plain films and radionucleotide imaging but may be initially difficult to distinguish from postoperative changes. Treatment with antibiotics alone without prosthesis removal is not often effective. The use of systemic antibiotic prophylaxis, antibiotic-containing bone cement, and operating rooms fitted with laminar flow all have been proposed as beneficial in reducing infection. To date, clinical studies are conflicting.

Barrett FF: Cerebrospinal fluid shunt infection. *In*: Schlossberg D (ed): Current Therapy of Infectious Disease. St. Louis, CV Mosby, 1996, pp 245–249.

Keane WF, Everett ED, Golper TA, et al: Peritoneal dialysis-related peritonitis treatment recommendations; 1993 update. Perit Dial Int 13:14, 1993.

Patrick CC (ed): Infections in Immunocompromised Children. New York, Churchill Livingstone, 1992.

Seifert H, Jansen B, Farr BM (eds): Catheter-Related Infections. New York, Marcel Dekker, 1997.

CHAPTER 181
Animal and Human Bites

Charles M. Ginsburg

Mammalian bite injuries account for 0.5–1% of visits to hospital emergency rooms and free-standing emergency centers in the United States. The number of individuals who sustain a bite injury and who seek medical attention in medical offices and primary care clinics is unknown but has been estimated to be at least comparable to the number who seek care in emergency facilities.

EPIDEMIOLOGY. Between 1979 and 1996, 304 fatalities due to dog bites were reported in the United States; 70% of these occurred in children who were younger than 11 yr. The breed of dog involved in the attacks on children varied; however, rottweilers, pit bulls, and German shepherds accounted for greater than 50% of all fatal bite-related injuries.

The majority of dog-related attacks occur in children 6–11 yr old. Boys are attacked more often than girls (1.5:1). Approximately two thirds of attacks occur around the home; 75% of the biting animals are known by the child, and almost half of the attacks are said to be unprovoked. In comparison, the 450,000 reported cat bites per year occur primarily in girls and are inflicted by known household animals. Limited data define the incidence and demographics of human bite injuries. Preschool and early school-aged children appear to be the age group at greatest risk to sustain an injury from a bite by a human. Data suggest that human bites are the leading cause of injury in child-care centers in the United States. Rat bites are not reportable conditions; therefore, a paucity of information is available on the epidemiology of the injuries and the incidence of infection after rat-inflicted bites or scratches.

CLINICAL MANIFESTATIONS. Dog bite–related injuries can be divided almost equally into three categories: abrasions, puncture wounds, and lacerations with or without an associated avulsion of tissue. The most common type of injury from cat and rat bites is a puncture wound. Human bite injuries are of two types, an occlusion injury that is incurred when the upper and lower teeth come together on a body part and, in older children and young adults, a clenched-fist injury that occurs when the fist, usually of the dominant hand, comes in contact with the tooth of another individual.

EVALUATION. Treatment of a bite victim should begin with a thorough history and physical examination. Careful attention should be paid to the circumstances surrounding the bite (type of animal, domestic or sylvatic, provoked or unprovoked, and location of the attack), a history of drug allergies, and the immunization status of the child and animal. During physical examination, meticulous attention should be paid to the type, size, and depth of the injury; the presence of foreign material in the wound; the status of underlying structures; and, in instances where the bite is on an extremity, the range of motion of the affected area. A diagram of the injury(s) should be recorded in a patient's medical record. A roentgenogram of the affected part should be obtained if it is likely that a bone or joint could have been penetrated or fractured or if retained foreign material present is possible. The possibility of a fracture or penetrating injury of the skull should be considered in individuals, particularly infants, who have sustained dog bite injuries of the face and head.

COMPLICATIONS. Infection is the most common complication of bite injuries, regardless of the species of biting animal. Whether to obtain material for culture from a wound depends on the species of the biting animal, the length of time that has transpired since the injury, the depth of the wound, the presence of foreign material contaminating the wound, and whether there is evidence of infection. Although potentially pathogenic bacteria have been isolated from as many as 80% of dog bite wounds that are brought to medical attention within 8 hr after a bite, the infection rate for wounds receiving medical attention in less than 8 hr is small (2.5–20%). Thus, unless they are deep and extensive, dog bite wounds that are less than 8 hr old do not need to be cultured unless contamination or early signs of infection are evident. By contrast, the infection rate in cat bite wounds that receive early medical attention is at least 50%. Therefore, it is prudent to obtain material for culture from all but the most trivial cat-inflicted wounds and from all other animal bite wounds, regardless of species of the biting animal, that are not brought to medical attention within 8 hr.

All human bite wounds, regardless of the mechanism of injury, should be regarded as at high risk for infection; culture is required. Because of the high incidence of anaerobic infection after bite wounds, it is important to obtain material for anaerobic as well as aerobic cultures.

Cat-scratch disease, caused by *Bartonella henselae*, can be transmitted at the time of cat scratches or bites but infrequently presents with wound infections. *Afipia felis* may account for approximately 10% of cases of cat-scratch disease. *B. henselae* typically causes regional lymphadenopathy with a prolonged febrile course, sometimes complicated by distant infection including osteomyelitis or hepatosplenic abscesses (Chapter 207.2).

The rate of infection after rat-bite injuries is not known. The oral flora of the majority of rats is similar to that of other mammals, although *Streptobacillus moniliformis* and *Spirillum minus*, the causative organisms of the two forms of rat-bite fever, are present in the oropharynx of approximately 50% and 25% of rats, respectively.

TREATMENT. After the appropriate material has been obtained or the wound swabbed for bacterial culture, the wound should be anesthetized, cleaned, and vigorously irrigated with copious amounts of normal saline. Irrigation with antibiotic-containing solutions provides no advantage over irrigation with saline alone and has the potential to cause local irritation of the tissues. Puncture wounds should be thoroughly cleaned and gently irrigated with a catheter or blunt-tipped needle; however, high-pressure irrigation should not be used. Avulsed or devitalized tissue should be debrided, and any fluctuant areas incised and drained.

All but the most trivial bite wounds of the hand should be immobilized in a position of function for 3–5 days, and patients with bite wounds of an extremity should be instructed to keep the affected extremity elevated for 24–36 hr or until the edema has resolved. All bite-wound victims should be re-evaluated within 24–36 hr after the injury.

Wound Closure. There is much controversy and few data to determine whether bite wounds should undergo primary closure or delayed primary closure (after 3–5 days) or should be allowed to heal by secondary intention. Factors to be considered are the type, size, and depth of the wound; the anatomic location; the presence of established infection; the time interval since the injury; and the potential for cosmetic disfigurement. Surgical consultation should be obtained for all deep or extensive wounds, those involving the bones and joints, and infected wounds that require open drainage. Although the general agreement is that infected wounds and those that are beyond 24 hr since the time of injury should not be sutured, there is disagreement and varying clinical experience in terms of the efficacy and safety of closing wounds that are within 8 hr from the time of injury with no evidence of infection.

All hand wounds should be considered to be at high risk for infection, particularly if disruption of the tendons or penetration of the bones has occurred; therefore, delayed primary closure is recommended for all but the most trivial bite wounds of the hands. In contrast to hand wounds, facial lacerations are at less risk for secondary infection because of the more abundant blood supply to this region. Many plastic surgeons advocate primary closure of facial bite wounds that have been brought to medical attention within 5 hr and have been thoroughly irrigated and debrided.

Antibiotic Therapy. Few studies unequivocally demonstrate a clear-cut efficacy of antimicrobials for prophylaxis of bite injuries that do not show signs of infection. However, a consensus is that antibiotics should be administered after all human bites and after all but the most trivial of dog, cat, and rat-bite injuries, regardless of whether there is evidence of infection.

The bacteriology of bite-wound infections is primarily a reflection of the oral flora of the biting animal and, to a lesser extent, a reflection of the skin flora of the victim. Because each of the multitude of aerobic and anaerobic bacterial species that colonize the oral cavity of a biting animal has the potential to invade local tissue, multiply, and cause tissue destruction, the majority of bite-wound infections are polymicrobial. Cultures of infected dog- and cat-bite wounds have a median of five bacterial isolates (range, 0–16). Despite the high degree of correlation between the bacterial flora of the oral cavity of humans, dogs, and cats, important differences exist between the biting species, as reflected in the wound infections that occur. The predominant bacterial species isolated from infected dog bite wounds are *Staphylococcus aureus* (20–30%), *Pasteurella canis* (20–30%), *Pasteurella multocida* (10–20%), *Staphylococcus intermedius* (25%), and *Capnocytophagia canimorsus*. Approximately 30–50% of dog-bite wound infections include mixed anaerobes including anaerobic streptococci and *Bacteroides, Fusobacterium,* and *Prevotella* species. Similar species are isolated from infected cat-bite wounds; however, *P. multocida* has a larger role and is the predominant species in at least 50% of cat-bite wound infections. *S. moniliformis* and *S. minus* are found principally in rats. The predominant species in human bite wounds are *Eikenella corrodens, S. aureus*, α-hemolytic streptococci, nontypable strains of *Haemophilus influenzae*, and β-lactamase–producing aerobes (≈50%). Clenched-fist injuries are particularly prone to infection by *E. corrodens* (25%) and anaerobic bacteria (50%).

The choice between an oral and parenteral antimicrobial agent should be based on the severity of the wound, the presence and degree of overt infection, signs of systemic toxicity, and the immune status of the patient. Amoxicillin-clavulanate (40 mg/kg/24 hr amoxicillin) is an excellent choice for empirical oral prophylaxis or therapy of human and animal bite wounds because of its activity against the majority of strains of bacteria that have been isolated from infected bite injuries. Similarly, ticarcillin-clavulanate (200–300 mg/kg/24 hr) or ampicillin-sulbactam (100–200 mg/kg/24 hr) is preferred for patients who require empirical parenteral therapy. Procaine penicillin remains the drug of choice for prophylaxis and treatment of rat-inflicted injuries. First-generation cephalosporins have limited activity against *P. multocida* and *E. corrodens* and therefore should not be used for prophylaxis or empirical initial therapy of bite-wound infections. No regimen is recognized to be effective for prophylaxis of cat-scratch disease *(B. henselae)*.

The therapeutic alternatives for penicillin-allergic patients are limited because the traditional alternative agents are generally inactive against one or more of the many pathogens that cause bite-wound infections. Although erythromycin (40 mg/kg/24 hr) is commonly recommended as an alternative agent for penicillin-allergic patients who have suffered dog and cat bites, it has spotty activity against strains of *P. multocida* and *S. moniliformis* and is not effective against *E. corrodens*. Similarly, clindamycin and the combination trimethoprim-sulfamethoxazole have limited activity against strains of *P. multocida* and anaerobic bacteria, respectively. Tetracycline (25–50 mg/kg/24 hr) is the drug of choice for penicillin-allergic patients who have sustained rat-bite injuries.

Tetanus. Although the occurrence of tetanus after human or animal bite injuries is extremely rare (Chapter 209), it is important to obtain a careful immunization history and to provide tetanus toxoid to all patients who are incompletely immunized or to adults who have not had tetanus immunization for more than 10 yr.

Rabies. The need for postexposure rabies vaccine in victims of dog and cat bites depends on whether or not the biting animal is known to have been vaccinated against rabies and, most importantly, on the local experience with rabid animals in the community (Chapter 265). The local health department should be consulted for advice in all instances when the vaccination status of the biting animal is unknown and in instances when rabies is known to be endemic in the region.

Hepatitis B. Postexposure prophylaxis for hepatitis B should be considered in the rare instance when an individual has sustained a human bite from an individual who is at high risk for hepatitis B (Chapter 177).

PREVENTION. It is not possible to prevent all mammalian bite injuries; however, it is possible to reduce the risk of injury with anticipatory guidance. Parents should be routinely counseled during prenatal visits and routine health maintenance examinations about the risks of having potentially biting pets in the household, and they should be cautioned against harboring exotic animals for pets. Additionally, parents should be made aware of the proclivity of certain breeds of dogs (rottweilers, pit bulls, and German shepherds) to inflict serious injuries, especially to newborns brought into the family. All young children should be closely supervised when in the presence of animals and, from a very early age, taught to respect animals and to be aware of their potential to inflict injury. Reduction of human bite injuries, particularly in child-care centers and schools, can be achieved by close surveillance of the children and by having adequate ratios of supervisory personnel to children.

181.1 Rat-Bite Fever

Rat-bite fever is a generic term that has been applied to at least two distinct clinical syndromes of fever, cutaneous findings, and systemic symptoms, each caused by a different microbial agent.

Streptobacillus moniliformis. The most common form of rat-bite fever in the United States is caused by *S. moniliformis*, a gram-negative bacillus that is present in the nasopharyngeal flora of approximately 50% of rats. Infection with *S. moniliformis* most commonly occurs after the bite of a rat but has also been reported in individuals who have been scratched by rats, in those who have handled dead rats, and in individuals who have ingested milk contaminated with *S. moniliformis* (Haverhill fever).

The incubation period for the streptobacillary form of rat-bite fever is variable, ranging from 3–10 days. The illness is characterized by an abrupt onset of fever, severe throbbing headache, intense myalgia, chills, and vomiting. In virtually all instances, the cutaneous inoculation site has healed by the

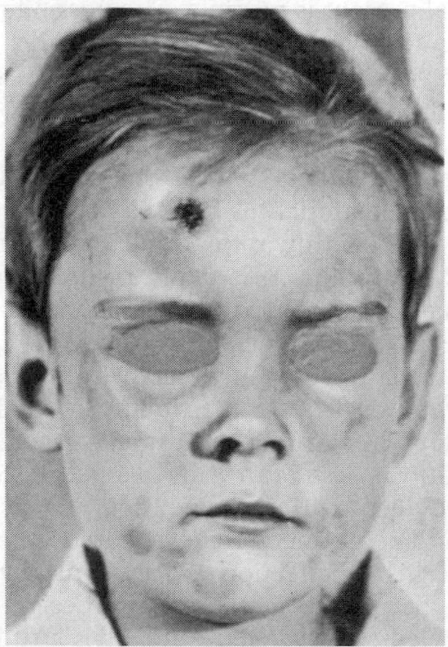

Figure 181–1 Sodoku. A chancre-like indurated ulcer at the site of a rat bite on the forehead. There is also a macular eruption on the face.

time the systemic systems first appear. Shortly after the onset of the fever, a polymorphic rash occurs in up to 75% of patients. In the majority of patients, the rash consists of blotchy red maculopapular lesions that often have a petechial component; the distribution of the rash is variable but is usually most dense on the extremities. Approximately half of patients have arthritis that is first manifested toward the end of the 1st wk of disease; early on, the arthritis may be migratory. If untreated, the fever, rash, and arthritis last from 14–21 days; the fever and arthritis often have a biphasic pattern.

Myriad complications have been reported in patients with rat-bite fever, the most common being pneumonia, arthritis, brain and soft tissue abscesses, and, less commonly, myocarditis or endocarditis.

The diagnosis of the streptobacillary form of rat-bite fever is difficult because the disease is uncommon and it is often confused with Rocky Mountain spotted fever or, less commonly, meningococcemia. A definitive diagnosis is made when the organism is recovered from blood or joint fluid.

Spirillum minus. The less common form of rat-bite fever, sodoku, is caused by *S. minus*, a small spiral aerobic gram-negative organism. The incubation period of sodoku is longer, from 14–21 days, than that of the streptobacillary form of disease, and myalgia and arthritis are less common manifestations.

The hallmark of spirillary rat-bite fever is an indurated, often suppurative, nonhealing ulcerative lesion at the bite site (Fig. 181–1). Lymphadenopathy and lymphadenitis are invariably present in the regional nodes that drain the inoculation site, and many patients may develop a generalized macular rash that is most prominent when fever is present. In untreated patients, sodoku has a relapsing course; after 5–7 days of chills and fever, symptoms abate but recur 7–10 days later. Numerous cycles may ensue if the disease is not recognized and treated. The diagnosis of sodoku is made on clinical grounds because there are no diagnostic serologic tests and *S. minus* has not been cultured on artificial media. Rarely, the organism may be identified in Gram-stained smears from pus from the infected inoculation site.

Penicillin is the drug of choice for both forms of rat-bite fever. Tetracycline or streptomycin is an effective alternative for penicillin-allergic patients.

Centers for Disease Control and Prevention: Dog-bite–related fatalities—United States 1995–1996. MMWR 216:463, 1997.

Dire DJ: Cat bite wounds: Risk factors for infection. Ann Emerg Med 20:973, 1991.

Goldstein EC, Citron DM, Richwald GA: Lack of in-vitro efficacy of oral forms of certain cephalosporins, erythromycin and oxacillin against *Pasteurella multocida*. Antimicrob Agents Chemother 32:213, 1988.

Goldstein EJC: Bite wounds and infection. Clin Infect Dis 14:663, 1992.

Grossman AI, Adams JP, Kunec J: Prophylactic antibiotics in simple hand lacerations. J Emerg Med 245:1055, 1981.

Raffin BJ, Freemark M: Streptobacillary rat-bite fever: A pediatric problem. Pediatrics 64:214, 1979.

Sacks JJ, Lockwood R, Hornreich J, Saitin RW: Fatal dog attacks, 1989–1994. Pediatrics 97:891, 1996.

Strauman-Raymond K, Lie L, Kempf-Berkseth J: Creating a safe environment in daycare. J School Health 63:250, 1993.

Talan DA, Citron D, Abrahamian FM, et al: Bacteriologic analysis of infected dog and cat bites. N Engl J Med 340:85, 1999.

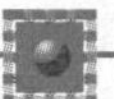

SECTION 3

Gram-Positive Bacterial Infections

CHAPTER 182

Staphylococcal Infections

James K. Todd

Staphylococci are hardy, aerobic, non–spore-forming, ubiquitous bacteria that are present in air, fomites, and dust or as normal flora of humans and animals. They are resistant to heat and drying and may be recovered from nonphysiologic environments weeks to months after inoculation. These organisms are gram positive and grow in clusters, aerobically or as facultative anaerobes. Strains are classified as *Staphylococcus aureus* if they are coagulase positive or as coagulase-negative staphylococci (e.g., *S. epidermidis, S. saprophyticus, S. haemolyticus*). Generally, *S. aureus* produces a yellow pigment and β-hemolysis on blood agar and *S. epidermidis* produces a white pigment with variable hemolysis results, although species confirmation requires further testing. *S. aureus* has many virulence factors that mediate various serious diseases, whereas coagulase-negative staphylococci tend to be less pathogenic unless a foreign body (e.g., intravascular catheter) is present.

182.1 Staphylococcus aureus

S. aureus is the most common cause of pyogenic infection of the skin; it also may cause furuncles, carbuncles, osteomyelitis, septic arthritis, wound infection, abscesses, pneumonia, empyema, endocarditis, pericarditis, meningitis, and toxin-mediated diseases, including food poisoning, scalded skin syndrome, and toxic shock syndrome (TSS).

ETIOLOGY. Disease may be a result of tissue invasion or may reflect injury due to various toxins and enzymes elaborated by different strains of these organisms (Fig. 182–1). Strains of *S. aureus* can be identified by the virulence factors they produce and classified by means of bacteriophage group typing (groups I–IV, miscellaneous). Strains typing in certain phage groups often have similar pathogenic potential (e.g., phage group I is associated with TSS, phage group II with scalded skin syndrome).

Adhesion of *S. aureus* to mucosal cells is mediated by teichoic acid in the cell wall, and exposure to the submucosa or subcutaneous sites increases adhesion to fibrinogen, fibronectin, collagen, and other proteins. Strains of *S. aureus* produce many virulence factors (Table 182–1). These factors have one or more of four different roles: protect the organism from host defenses, localize infection, cause local tissue damage, and act as toxins affecting noninfected tissue sites.

Most strains of *S. aureus* possess factors that protect the organism from host defenses. Many staphylococci produce a loose polysaccharide capsule, or slime layer, which may interfere with opsonophagocytosis. Clumping factor interacts with fibrinogen to cause large clumps of organism to form, interfering with effective phagocytosis. Production of clumping factor or coagulase differentiates *S. aureus* from *S. epidermidis* and other coagulase-negative staphylococci. Coagulase causes plasma to clot by interacting with fibrinogen; this may have

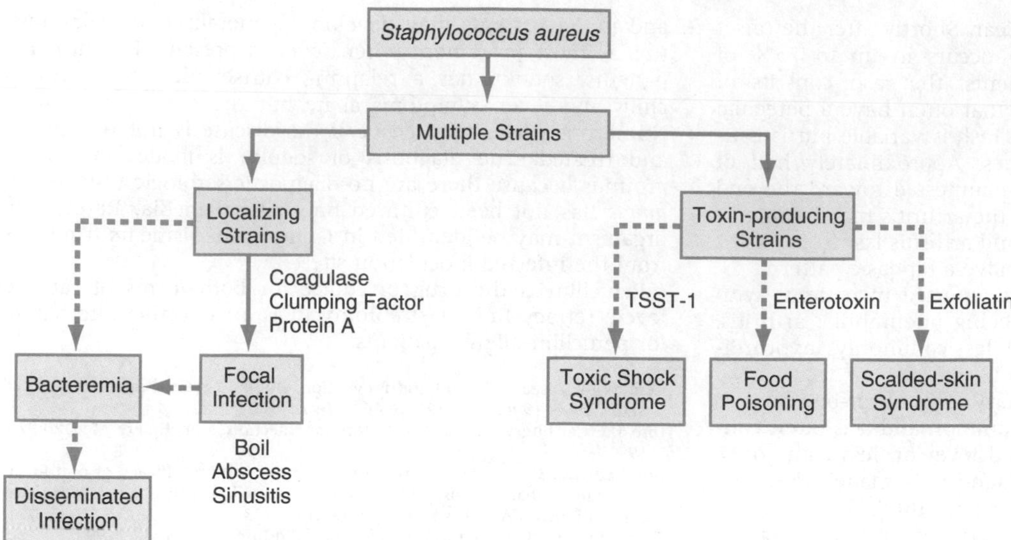

Figure 182–1 Relationship of virulence factors to diseases associated with *Staphylococcus aureus.*

an important role in localization of infection (i.e., abscess formation). Protein A, which is present in most strains of *S. aureus* but not in *S. epidermidis,* reacts specifically with IgG1, IgG2, and IgG4. It is located on the outermost coat of the bacterium and can absorb serum immunoglobulin, preventing antibacterial antibodies from acting as opsonins and thus inhibiting phagocytosis. Other enzymes elaborated by staphylococci include catalase (inactivates hydrogen peroxide, promoting intracellular survival), penicillinase or β-lactamase (inactivates penicillin at the molecular level), and lipase (associated with skin infection). Leukocidin, which is produced by most strains of *S. aureus,* combines with the phospholipid of the phagocytic cell membrane, producing increased permeability, leakage of protein, and eventual death of the neutrophil and macrophage.

Many strains of *S. aureus* produce substances that cause local tissue destruction. A number of immunologically distinct hemolysins have been identified. α-Toxin acts on cell membranes and causes tissue necrosis, injures human leukocytes, and produces aggregation of platelets and spasm of smooth muscle. A β-hemolysin degrades sphingomyelin, causing hemolysis of red blood cells, and a δ-hemolysin disrupts membranes by a detergent-like action.

Many strains of *S. aureus* release exotoxins. Exfoliatins A and B are two serologically distinct proteins that produce localized (e.g., bullous impetigo) or generalized (e.g., scalded skin syndrome, scarlatiniform eruption) dermatologic complications (Chapter 663). Exfoliative toxin produces skin separation by splitting the desmosome and altering the intracellular matrix in the stratum granulosum.

One or more staphylococcal enterotoxins (types A, B, C_1, C_2, D, E) are elaborated by most strains of *S. aureus.* Ingestion of preformed enterotoxin A or B is associated with vomiting and diarrhea and, in some cases, with the development of profound hypotension. Virtually all individuals by the age of 10 yr have antibodies to at least one enterotoxin.

Toxic shock syndrome toxin-1 (TSST-1) is associated with TSS related to menstruation and focal staphylococcal infection. Enterotoxin A and enterotoxin B also may be associated with nonmenstrual TSS. TSST-1 induces production of interleukin 1 and tumor necrosis factor, resulting in hypotension, fever, and multisystem involvement.

EPIDEMIOLOGY. Most neonates are colonized within the first week of life, and 20–30% of normal individuals carry at least one strain of *S. aureus* in the anterior nares.

The organisms may be transmitted from the nose to the

TABLE 182–1 Virulence Factors Produced by *Staphylococcus aureus* and Their Role in Disease

Factor	Location	Action	Pathophysiology
Cell Wall Components			
Peptidoglycan	Cell wall		Aggressin, shock
Teichoic acids	Cell wall		Adhesion to epithelium
Slime (coagulase-negative)	Cell wall	Extracellular matrix	Cements and protects
Capsule	Cell wall	Extracellular matrix	Protect from phagocytosis
Protein A	Cell wall	Binds IgG	Protect from phagocytosis
Clumping factor	Cell wall	Binds fibrin	Large clumps, blocks phagocytosis
Fibronectin-binding	Cell wall	Attaches to fibronectin	Attachment to cell
PBP2a	Cell wall	Alters penicillin binding	Methicillin resistance
Enzymes			
Catalase	Soluble	Catalyzes H_2O_2	Inhibits PMN killing
Coagulase	Soluble	Clots plasma	Forms abscess wall
Leukocidin	Soluble	Destroys PMNs	Protects from phagocytosis
Hemolysins	Soluble	Cytotoxic	Tissue damage
Lipase	Soluble	Lipolysis	Skin infection
β-Lactamase	Soluble	Penase	Penicillin G resistance
Toxins			
Enterotoxin A-E	Soluble	Vagal stimulator	Food poisoning (TSS)
Exfoliatin A-B	Soluble	Granular layer cleavage	Scalded skin syndrome
TSST-1	Soluble	TNF, IL-1 stimulator	TSS

TSST-1 = toxic shock syndrome-1; PMN = polymorphonuclear neutrophil; H_2O_2 = hydrogen peroxide; TNF = tumor necrosis factor; IL-1 = interleukin 1.

skin, where persistent colonization seems to be more transient. Repeated recovery of *S. aureus* from the skin suggests repeated transfer rather than persistent skin colonization. Persistent umbilical and perianal carriage has been described.

Transmission of *S. aureus* generally occurs by direct contact or by spread of heavy particles over a distance of 6 ft or less. Spread by fomites is rare. Heavily colonized individual carriers are particularly effective disseminators. Autoinfection is common, and minor infections (e.g., styes, pustules, and paronychia) may be the source of disseminated infection. Handwashing between contacts with patients decreases the spread of staphylococci from patient to patient. Older children and adults are more resistant than neonates to colonization.

Infection may follow colonization. Antibiotic therapy with a drug to which *S. aureus* is resistant favors colonization and the development of infection. Other factors that increase the likelihood of infection include wounds, skin disease, ventriculoperitoneal shunts, intravenous or intrathecal catheterization, corticosteroid treatment, starvation, acidosis, and azotemia. Viral infections of the respiratory tract also may predispose to secondary bacterial infection with staphylococci.

PATHOGENESIS. The development of staphylococcal disease is related to resistance of the host to infection and to virulence of the organism (see Fig. 182–1). The intact skin and mucous membranes serve as barriers to invasion by staphylococci. Defects in the mucocutaneous barriers produced by trauma, surgery, foreign surfaces (e.g., sutures, shunts, intravascular catheters), and burns increase the risk of infection.

Infants may acquire type-specific humoral immunity to staphylococci transplacentally. Older children and adults develop antibodies to staphylococci as a result of intermittent minor infections of the skin and soft tissues; the antistaphylococcal titer of serum generally increases after overt staphylococcal disease. The presence of antibody, however, does not always protect the individual from staphylococcal disease. There is some indication that disseminated *S. aureus* disease in previously healthy children may occur after a viral infection that suppresses neutrophil or respiratory epithelial cell function.

Individuals with congenital or acquired defects in the complement system required for chemotaxis, defective chemotaxis (Job, Chédiak-Higashi, and Wiskott-Aldrich syndromes), defective phagocytosis, and defective humoral immunity (antibodies required for opsonization), as well as those with an impaired intracellular bactericidal capacity, are at increased risk of infection with staphylococci. Patients with *chronic granulomatous disease,* in which phagocytosis proceeds normally but killing of ingested catalase-positive bacteria is severely impaired, are particularly susceptible to staphylococcal disease. Impaired mobilization of polymorphonuclear leukocytes has been documented in children with diabetic ketoacidosis and in healthy individuals after ingesting alcohol. Patients with HIV infection have neutrophils that are defective in their ability to kill *S. aureus* in vitro.

CLINICAL MANIFESTATIONS. The signs and symptoms vary with the location of the infection, which, although most commonly located on the skin, may involve any tissue. Disease states of various degrees of severity are generally a result of local suppuration, systemic dissemination with metastatic infection, or systemic effects of toxin production. Although the nasopharynx and skin of many persons may be colonized with *S. aureus,* disease due to this organism is relatively uncommon. Lesions, especially those of the skin, are considerably more prevalent among persons living in low socioeconomic circumstances and particularly among those in tropical climates.

Newborn. Staphylococcal neonatal infections are discussed in Chapters 105 and 106; pneumonia in Chapter 175, otitis media in Chapter 646, conjunctivitis in Chapter 633, and osteomyelitis and septic arthritis in Chapter 178.

Skin. Pyogenic skin infections may be primary or secondary to wounds or may be a superinfection of other noninfectious skin disease (eczema) or of impetigo contagiosa.

Impetigo contagiosa, ecthyma, bullous impetigo, folliculitis, hydradenitis, furuncles, carbuncles, staphylococcal scalded skin syndrome (i.e., Ritter's disease), and a syndrome resembling the rash of scarlet fever are described in Chapter 184. Folliculitis (i.e., pyoderma of the hair follicle) may extend to a deep-seated furuncle or carbuncle if more than one hair follicle is involved. *Recurrent furunculosis* is a disorder of unknown cause and is associated with repeated episodes of pyoderma over months to years. Patients should be evaluated for immune defects associated with recurrent infection, especially those involving neutrophil dysfunction. Nosocomial skin lesions are discussed in Chapter 302.

Respiratory Tract. Infections of the upper respiratory tract due to *S. aureus* are rare, considering the frequency with which this area is colonized. Otitis media (see Chapter 646) and sinusitis (see Chapter 381.2) due to *S. aureus* may rarely occur. Staphylococcal sinusitis is relatively common in children with cystic fibrosis or defects in white blood cell (WBC) function. Suppurative parotitis is a rare infection, but *S. aureus* is a common cause. Staphylococcal tonsillopharyngitis is rare in otherwise normal children. Bacterial tracheitis that complicates viral croup may be caused by *S. aureus* but also by other organisms. Patients typically have high fever, leukocytosis, and evidence of severe upper airway obstruction. Direct laryngoscopy or bronchoscopy shows a normal epiglottis with subglottic narrowing and thick, purulent secretions within the trachea. Treatment requires antibiotics and careful airway management.

Pneumonia (see Chapter 175) due to *S. aureus* may be primary (hematogenous) or secondary after a viral infection such as influenza. Hematogenous pneumonia may be secondary to septic emboli, right-sided endocarditis, or the presence of intravascular devices. Inhalation pneumonia is caused by alterations of mucociliary clearance, leukocyte dysfunction, or bacterial adherence initiated by a viral infection. More common are high fever, abdominal pain, tachypnea, dyspnea, and localized or diffuse bronchopneumonia or lobar disease. Staphylococci cause a necrotizing pneumonitis; empyema, pneumatoceles, pyopneumothorax, and bronchopleural fistulas develop frequently. Staphylococcal pneumonia occasionally produces a diffuse interstitial disease characterized by extreme dyspnea, tachypnea, and cyanosis. Cough may be nonproductive. *S. aureus* is an important pathogen of pneumonia in patients with cystic fibrosis (Chapter 363).

Sepsis. Staphylococcal bacteremia and sepsis (Chapter 173) may be associated with any localized infection. The onset may be acute and marked by nausea, vomiting, myalgia, fever, and chills. Organisms may localize subsequently at any site but are found especially in the lungs, heart, joints, bones, kidneys, and brain. If appropriate antibiotic therapy is provided, blood cultures may remain positive for 24–48 hr. Fever begins to decrease at a median time of 22 hr (range, 8–90 hr), and body temperature returns to normal at a median time of 58 hr (range, 12–180 hr) in patients with *S. aureus* septicemia. Differentiating sepsis from endocarditis may be difficult. Echocardiographic evidence of vegetations, intravenous drug abuse, the presence of immune complexes and antistaphylococcal antibodies, and the absence of a primary focus of infection suggest endocarditis.

In some instances, especially in young adolescent males, disseminated staphylococcal disease occurs, characterized by fever, persistent bacteremia despite antibiotics, and focal involvement of two or more separate tissue sites (e.g., skin, bone, joint, kidney, lung, liver, heart).

Muscle. Localized staphylococcal abscesses in muscle associated with elevation of muscle enzymes but without septicemia have been called *tropical pyomyositis.* Although this disorder has been reported most frequently from tropical areas, it also has occurred in the United States in otherwise healthy children. Multiple abscesses occur in 30–40% of cases. Prodromal symptoms may include coryza, pharyngitis, diarrhea, or prior trauma at the site of the abscess. Surgical drainage and appropriate antibiotic therapy are essential.

Bones and Joints. *S. aureus* is the most common cause of osteomyelitis and suppurative arthritis in children (Chapter 178).

Central Nervous System. Meningitis (Chapter 174.1) due to *S. aureus* is not common; it is associated with cranial trauma and neurosurgical procedures (e.g., craniotomy, cerebrospinal fluid [CSF] shunt placement) and less frequently with endocarditis, parameningeal foci (e.g., epidural or brain abscess), diabetes mellitus, or malignancy. The CSF profile in *S. aureus* meningitis is indistinguishable from that in other bacterial causes of meningitis.

Heart. Acute bacterial endocarditis (Chapter 443) may follow staphylococcal bacteremia. *S. aureus* is a common cause of acute virulent endocarditis on native valves. Perforation of heart valves, myocardial abscesses, heart failure, conduction disturbances, acute hemopericardium, purulent pericarditis, and sudden death may ensue.

Kidney. *S. aureus* is a common cause of renal and perinephric abscess (Chapter 546). Urinary tract infection due to *S. aureus* is unusual.

Toxic Shock Syndrome. *S. aureus* is the principal cause of TSS (Chapter 182.2).

Intestinal Tract. Staphylococcal enterocolitis follows overgrowth of normal bowel flora by staphylococci. Although uncommon, this can follow use of broad-spectrum oral antibiotic therapy. Diarrhea is associated with blood and mucus.

Peritonitis associated with *S. aureus* in patients receiving long-term ambulatory peritoneal dialysis usually involves the catheter tunnel. Removal of the catheter is required to achieve a bacteriologic cure.

Food poisoning (Chapter 176) may be caused by ingestion of preformed enterotoxins preformed by staphylococci contaminating foods. Approximately 2–7 hr after ingestion of the toxin, sudden, severe vomiting begins. Watery diarrhea may develop, but fever is absent or low. Symptoms rarely persist longer than 12–24 hr. Rarely, shock and death may occur.

DIAGNOSIS. The diagnosis of staphylococcal infection depends on isolation of the organisms from nonpermissive sites such as skin lesions, abscess cavities, blood, or other sites of infection. Isolation from the nose or skin does not necessarily imply causation because these are normally colonized sites. The organisms can be grown readily in liquid and on solid media. After isolation, identification is made on the basis of Gram stain and coagulase, clumping factor, and protein A reactivity. Patterns of susceptibility to antibiotics should be assessed in serious cases.

Diagnosis of staphylococcal food poisoning generally is made on the basis of epidemiologic and clinical findings. Food suspected of contamination should be examined by Gram stain, cultured, and tested for enterotoxin. Enterotoxin testing can be carried out by the Centers for Disease Control and Prevention.

Differential Diagnosis. Skin lesions due to *S. aureus* and those due to group A β-hemolytic streptococci may be indistinguishable. Staphylococcal pneumonia can be suspected on the basis of chest roentgenograms that may reveal pneumatoceles, pyopneumothorax, or lung abscess. These changes suggesting a necrotizing pneumonitis are not pathognomonic for staphylococcal infection and may be noted in patients with pneumonia due to other bacteria, including *Klebsiella* and many anaerobes. Fluctuant skin and soft tissue lesions also can be caused by many organisms, including *Mycobacterium tuberculosis*, atypical mycobacteria, *Bartonella henselae* (cat-scratch disease), *Francisella tularensis*, and various fungi.

TREATMENT. Antibiotic therapy alone is rarely effective in individuals with undrained abscesses or with infected foreign bodies. Loculated collections of purulent material should be relieved by incision and drainage. Foreign bodies should be removed, if possible. Therapy always should be initiated with a penicillinase-resistant antibiotic because more than 90% of all staphylococci isolated, regardless of source, are resistant to penicillin.

For serious infections, parenteral treatment is indicated, at least at the outset, until symptoms are controlled. Serious staphylococcal infections, with or without abscesses, tend to persist and recur, necessitating prolonged therapy.

The antibiotic used as well as the dose, route, and duration of treatment depends on the site of infection, the response of the patient to treatment, and the sensitivity of the organisms recovered from blood or from local sites of infection. In a patient with staphylococcal pneumonia, intravenous treatment is recommended until the patient has been afebrile for 72 hr and other signs of infection have disappeared. Oral therapy is continued for a total of 3 wk, longer in selected cases. Treatment of staphylococcal osteomyelitis (see Chapter 178), meningitis (see Chapter 174.1), and endocarditis (see Chapter 443) are discussed in their respective chapters.

In all of these infections, oral treatment may be provided to complete the course of treatment when parenteral therapy has been discontinued; dicloxacillin is penicillinase resistant, absorbed well orally, and quite effective. This drug is administered in a dose of 50–100 mg/kg/24 hr in four divided oral doses. Amoxicillin combined with the β-lactamase inhibitor clavulanic acid also is effective at a dose based on the amoxicillin component of 40–80 mg/kg/24 hr in three divided doses. First-generation cephalosporins and trimethoprim-sulfamethoxazole administered orally may also be effective. The duration of oral therapy also depends on a patient's response as determined by the clinical, roentgenographic, and laboratory findings and by culture results.

Skin and soft tissue infection and minor upper respiratory tract infection may be managed by oral therapy alone or by an initial brief course of antibiotics provided parenterally, followed by oral medication. In patients with very mild, localized skin infection, repeated cleansing with a mild antiseptic and use of topical antibiotics (e.g., mupirocin) may be effective.

Individuals sensitive to penicillin and its derivatives must be treated with other antibiotics or desensitized to the penicillin derivative to be used. About 5% of penicillin-sensitive children are also sensitive to cephalosporins. Clindamycin has proved effective for the treatment of skin, soft tissue, bone, and joint infections due to *S. aureus* if the organism is susceptible. Clindamycin may be provided in three to four divided doses parenterally or orally (total daily dose, 30–40 mg/kg/24 hr). Clindamycin should *not* be used to treat endocarditis, brain abscess, or meningitis due to *S. aureus*. Vancomycin can be used to treat penicillin-sensitive individuals with serious *S. aureus* infections, but serum levels of this antibiotic should be monitored when it is used. Peak serum concentrations should be 25–40 μg/mL. It can be administered in a dose of 10–15 mg/kg/dose given every 6 hr intravenously. Vancomycin or teicoplanin (a vancomycin derivative) should be used to treat bacteremic staphylococcal infections when the organism is resistant to semisynthetic penicillin derivatives—so-called methicillin-resistant *S. aureus* (MRSA). Despite in vitro susceptibility of *S. aureus* to ciprofloxacin and other quinolone antibiotics, these agents should not be used in serious staphylococcal infections, because their use has not consistently been associated with high cure rates.

Serious staphylococcal infections (e.g., endocarditis, central nervous system infections, disseminated staphylococcal septicemia) can be treated by intravenous methicillin or nafcillin and, in penicillin-allergic children, by vancomycin, trimethoprim-sulfamethoxazole, or imipenem. Rifampin or gentamicin may be added for synergy.

Methicillin-Resistant *Staphylococcus aureus*. MRSA has become a major nosocomial pathogen. Patients at risk for MRSA infection are the seriously ill (e.g., those with burns, surgical wounds, chronic venous access, lengthy hospitalizations, contact with other MRSA-infected patients, and premature infants). Most MRSA strains belong to phage group II; however, outbreaks with nontypable and phage group I strains have been reported.

The resistance to semisynthetic penicillins is thought to be related to a novel penicillin-binding protein that is relatively insensitive to antibiotics containing a β-lactam ring. MRSA strains appear to be as virulent as their methicillin-sensitive counterparts. Vancomycin and its derivative, teicoplanin, are highly effective in the treatment of these infections. Vancomycin is the drug of choice if MRSA is considered a possible cause of infection or if MRSA has been isolated. MRSA is also resistant to cephalosporins and imipenem but often remains sensitive to trimethoprim-sulfamethoxazole and ciprofloxacin.

When MRSA is recovered, strict isolation of affected patients has been shown to be the most effective method for preventing nosocomial spread of infection. Thereafter, control measures should be directed toward identification of new isolates and strict isolation of newly colonized or infected patients. It also may be necessary to identify colonized hospital personnel and eradicate carriage in affected individuals.

Strains of *S. aureus* resistant to vancomycin with limited other treatment options have been reported, emphasizing the need for restricting the prescription of unnecessary antibiotics and the importance of isolation of the causative organism and susceptibility testing in serious infections.

PROGNOSIS. Untreated staphylococcal septicemia is associated with a mortality rate of 80% or greater. Mortality rates have been reduced significantly by appropriate antibiotic treatment. Staphylococcal pneumonia can be fatal at any age but is more likely to be associated with high morbidity and mortality in young infants or in patients whose therapy has been delayed.

A total WBC count below 5,000/mm^3 or a polymorphonuclear leukocyte response of less than 50% is a grave prognostic sign. Prognosis also may be influenced by numerous host factors, including nutrition, immunologic competence, and the presence or absence of other debilitating diseases. In most cases with abscess formation, surgical drainage will be necessary.

PREVENTION. Staphylococcal infection is transmitted primarily by direct contact. *Strict attention to handwashing techniques* is the most effective measure for preventing the spread of staphylococci from one individual to another (Chapter 302). Use of a detergent containing an iodophor, chlorhexidine, or hexachlorophene is recommended. In hospitals or other institutional settings, all persons with acute staphylococcal infections should be isolated until they have been treated adequately. There should be constant surveillance for nosocomial staphylococcal infections within hospitals.

Patients with recurrent staphylococcal furunculosis may be treated with hexachlorophene washes and dicloxacillin or clindamycin and nasal mupirocin to prevent recurrences.

Food poisoning (Chapter 176) may be prevented by excluding individuals with staphylococcal infections of the skin from the preparation and handling of food. Prepared foods should be eaten immediately or refrigerated appropriately to prevent multiplication of staphylococci with which the food may have been contaminated.

182.2 Toxic Shock Syndrome

TSS is an acute multisystemic disease characterized by high fever, hypotension, vomiting, diarrhea, myalgias, nonfocal neurologic abnormalities, conjunctival hyperemia, strawberry tongue, and an erythematous rash with subsequent desquamation on the hands and feet.

ETIOLOGY AND EPIDEMIOLOGY. Many cases occur in menstruating women who are 15–25 yr of age and who use tampons or other vaginal devices (e.g., diaphragm, contraceptive sponge) in the presence of vaginal colonization or infection with toxin-producing strains of *S. aureus*. TSS, however, also occurs in children, nonmenstruating women, and men. Nonmenstrual TSS has been associated with wound infection, nasal packing, sinusitis, tracheitis, pneumonia, empyema, abscesses, burns, osteomyelitis, and primary bacteremia. Without antimicrobial therapy, menstrual TSS has a high recurrence rate (30%), with secondary cases being milder and occurring within 3 mo of the original episode; the overall mortality rate is 3%.

PATHOGENESIS. A majority of *S. aureus* strains isolated from confirmed cases are phage group I and produce a number of extracellular toxins. The primary toxin associated with TSS is TSST-1. TSST-1 causes massive loss of fluid from the intravascular space directly or after production of interleukin 1 and tumor necrosis factor. However, TSST-1–negative strains have been isolated from patients with TSS, suggesting that other toxins (primarily the enterotoxins) have a role in TSS (especially nonmenstrual). Epidemiologic and in vitro studies suggest that these toxins are selectively produced in a clinical environment consisting of a neutral pH, a high P_{CO_2}, and an "aerobic" P_{O_2}, which are the conditions found in the vagina with tampon use during menstruation. This may explain why 90% of adults have antibody to TSST-1 without a history of clinical TSS—that is, they became colonized with a toxin-producing organism at a site (e.g., anterior nares) where low-grade or inactive toxin exposure resulted in an immune response without disease. The risk factors for symptomatic disease require a nonimmune host colonized with a toxin-producing organism, which is exposed to focal growth conditions (e.g., menstruation plus tampon use or abscess), which induce toxin production.

CLINICAL MANIFESTATIONS. The diagnosis of TSS is based on clinical manifestations (Table 182–2). The onset is abrupt, with high fever, vomiting, and diarrhea, and is accompanied by sore throat, headache, and myalgias. A diffuse erythematous macular rash (sunburn-like or scarlatiniform) appears within 24 hr and may be associated with hyperemia of pharyngeal, conjunctival, and vaginal mucous membranes. A strawberry tongue is common. Symptoms often include alterations in the level of consciousness, oliguria, and hypotension, which in severe cases may progress to shock and disseminated intravascular coagulation. Complications including adult respiratory distress syndrome, myocardial failure, and renal failure are commensurate with the degree of shock. Recovery occurs within 7–10 days and is associated with desquamation, particularly of palms and soles; hair and nail loss have also been observed after 1–2 mo.

DIAGNOSIS. There is no specific laboratory test; appropriate

TABLE 182–2 Diagnostic Criteria of Staphylococcal Toxic Shock Syndrome

Criteria
Major Criteria (All Required)
Acute fever >38.8°C
Hypotension (orthostatic or shock)
Rash (erythroderma with late desquamation)
Minor Criteria (Any 3)
Mucous membrane inflammation
Vomiting, diarrhea
Liver abnormalities
Renal abnormalities
Muscle abnormalities
Central nervous system abnormalities
Low platelets
Exclusionary Criteria
Absence of another explanation
Negative blood cultures (except for *S. aureus*)

selective tests reveal involvement of multiple organ systems including the hepatic, renal, muscular, gastrointestinal, cardiopulmonary, and central nervous systems. Bacterial cultures of the associated focus (e.g., vagina, abscess) before administration of antibiotics usually yield *S. aureus*, although this is not a required element of the definition.

Differential Diagnosis. Group A *Streptococcus* can cause a similar TSS-like illness, termed *streptococcal TSS* (Chapter 184), which is often associated with streptococcal bacteremia or a focal streptococcal infection such as cellulitis or pneumonia.

Kawasaki disease closely resembles TSS clinically but is usually not as severe or rapidly progressive. Both are associated with fever unresponsive to antibiotics, hyperemia of mucous membranes, and an erythematous rash with subsequent desquamation. Many of the clinical features of TSS, however, are absent or rare in Kawasaki disease, including diffuse myalgia, vomiting, abdominal pain, diarrhea, azotemia, hypotension, adult respiratory distress syndrome (see Chapter 166), and shock. Kawasaki disease typically occurs in children younger than 5 yr—some cases of "adult Kawasaki disease" may be TSS. Scarlet fever, Rocky Mountain spotted fever, leptospirosis, toxic epidermal necrolysis, sepsis, and measles must also be considered in the differential diagnosis.

TREATMENT. Parenteral administration of a β-lactamase–resistant antistaphylococcal antibiotic (e.g., nafcillin or a first-generation cephalosporin) is recommended after appropriate cultures have been obtained. The addition of clindamycin in severe or unresponsive cases may terminate toxin production. Drainage of the vagina, by removal of any retained tampons in menstrual TSS, and of infected or colonized sites in nonmenstrual TSS is indicated. Antistaphylococcal therapy may also reduce the risk of recurrence in menstrual TSS.

Fluid replacement should be aggressive to prevent or treat hypotension, renal failure, and cardiovascular collapse. Inotropic agents may be needed to treat shock; corticosteroids and intravenous immune globulin are reserved for severe cases.

PREVENTION. The low risk of acquiring TSS (6.2 cases/100,000 menstruating women) can be reduced by not using tampons or by using them intermittently during each menstrual period. If a fever, rash, or dizziness develops during menstruation, any tampon should be removed immediately and medical attention sought.

182.3 Coagulase-Negative Staphylococci

S. epidermidis is one of many recognized species of coagulase-negative staphylococci (CONS) affecting or colonizing humans. Originally thought to be avirulent commensal bacteria, CONS, particularly *S. epidermidis*, is now known to produce nosocomial infections in patients with indwelling foreign devices (intravenous catheters—sepsis; hemodialysis shunts and grafts—sepsis; CSF shunts—meningitis; peritoneal dialysis catheters—peritonitis; pacemaker wires and electrodes—pocket infection; prosthetic cardiac valves—endocarditis; urinary catheters—pyelonephritis; prosthetic joints—arthritis), surgical trauma (sternal osteomyelitis, endophthalmitis), immunocompromised states (malignancy, granulocytopenia, neonates), and, rarely, community-acquired disease in patients with no underlying disease (urinary tract infection, osteomyelitis). *S. haemolyticus*, another CONS species, is an important cause of invasive infection and may develop resistance to vancomycin and teicoplanin.

EPIDEMIOLOGY. CONS consist of normal inhabitants of the human skin, throat, mouth, vagina, and urethra. *S. epidermidis* is the most common and persistent species, representing 65–90% of staphylococci present on the skin and mucous membranes. Colonization, sometimes with strains acquired from hospital staff, precedes infection; alternatively, direct inoculation during surgery may initiate infection through CSF shunts or prosthetic valves. For epidemiologic purposes, CONS can be identified on the basis of phage typing, antibiotic sensitivities, slime layer production, and molecular DNA methods (chromosomal and phage DNA hybridization–restriction enzyme analysis).

PATHOGENESIS. *S. epidermidis* produces an exopolysaccharide protective biofilm (slime) that surrounds the organism and may enhance adhesion to foreign surfaces, resist phagocytosis, and impair penetration of antibiotics.

CLINICAL MANIFESTATIONS. The low virulence of CONS usually requires the presence of another factor, such as immune compromise or a foreign body, for development of clinical disease.

Bacteremia. CONS, specifically *S. epidermidis*, are the most common cause of nosocomial bacteremia. In neonates, *S. epidermidis* bacteremia, with or without a central venous catheter, may be manifested as apnea, bradycardia, temperature instability, abdominal distention, hematochezia, meningitis in the absence of CSF pleocytosis, cutaneous abscesses, and persistence of positive blood cultures for as long as 2 wk despite adequate antimicrobial therapy. *S. epidermidis* bacteremia in patients with bone marrow transplantation and malignancy (e.g., leukemia, lymphoma) is associated with neutropenia, central venous access (Hickman's or Broviac's catheter), and gastrointestinal colonization. In most circumstances, *S. epidermidis* bacteremia is indolent and is not usually associated with overwhelming septic shock.

Endocarditis. Infection of native heart valves or the right atrial wall secondary to an infected thrombosis at the end of a central line may produce endocarditis. *S. epidermidis* and other CONS may also produce native valve subacute indolent endocarditis in previously normal patients without a central venous catheter. *S. epidermidis* is a common cause of prosthetic valve endocarditis, presumably due to inoculation at the time of surgery. Infection of the valve sewing ring, with abscess formation and dissection, produces valve dysfunction, dehiscence, arrhythmias, or valve obstruction. See Chapter 443 for clinical manifestations.

Central Venous Catheter Infection. Central venous catheters become infected through the exit site and subcutaneous tunnel, which provide a direct path to the bloodstream. *S. epidermidis* is the most common CONS, owing in part to its high rate of cutaneous colonization. Line sepsis is manifested as fever, leukocytosis, tenderness and erythema at the exit site or along the subcutaneous tunnel, and catheter thrombosis.

Cerebrospinal Fluid Shunts. *S. epidermidis*, introduced at the time of surgery, is the most common pathogen associated with CSF shunt meningitis. Most (70–80%) infections occur within 2 mo of the operation and are manifested by signs of meningeal irritation, fever, increased intracranial pressure (headache), and peritonitis due to the intra-abdominal position of the distal end of the shunt tubing.

Urinary Tract Infection. *S. epidermidis* causes asymptomatic urinary tract infection in hospitalized patients with urinary catheters and after urinary tract surgery or transplantation. *S. saprophyticus* is a common cause of symptomatic urinary tract infection in previously healthy, sexually active teenage girls after urethral colonization. Manifestations are similar to those characteristic of urinary tract infection due to *Escherichia coli* (Chapter 546).

S. epidermidis is the most common pathogen producing peritonitis in patients on continuous ambulatory peritoneal dialysis. Manifestations of infection include abdominal pain, fever, more than 100 neutrophils/mm^3, and a positive culture or Gram stain.

DIAGNOSIS. Because *S. epidermidis* is a common skin inhabitant and may contaminate poorly collected blood cultures, differentiating bacteremia from contamination may be difficult. Similarly, it may be difficult to differentiate bacteremia due to line sepsis from sepsis not associated with central venous line colonization. Bacteremia should be suspected when blood cultures grow rapidly (within 24 hr), when two or more blood cultures are positive with the same CONS, when the peripheral venous blood culture has a quantitative colony count comparable to that drawn from a central venous catheter, and when clinical and laboratory signs and symptoms compatible with CONS sepsis are present and subsequently resolve with appropriate therapy. No blood culture that is positive for *S. epidermidis* in a neonate or patient with intravascular catheter should be considered contaminated without careful assessment of the foregoing criteria and examination of the patient.

TREATMENT. Most *S. epidermidis* is resistant to methicillin. Vancomycin is the drug of choice for methicillin-resistant *S. epidermidis*. The new quinolones and teicoplanin have some activity against CONS, and the addition of rifampin or gentamicin to vancomycin may increase antimicrobial efficacy. In many cases of CONS infection associated with foreign bodies, the catheter, valve, or shunt must be removed to ensure a cure. Prosthetic heart valves and CSF shunts usually have to be removed to treat the infection adequately.

Antibiotic therapy given through an infected central venous catheter (through each lumen) may effectively cure *S. epidermidis* line sepsis. If the catheter or reservoir is no longer needed, it should be removed. Unfortunately, this is not always possible owing to the therapeutic requirements of the underlying disease (nutrition for short bowel syndrome, chemotherapy for malignancy). A trial of intravenous vancomycin is indicated to preserve the use of the central line.

Peritonitis due to *S. epidermidis* in patients on continuous ambulatory peritoneal dialysis is another infection that may be treated with intravenous or intraperitoneal antibiotics without removing the dialysis catheter. If the organism is resistant to methicillin, vancomycin adjusted for renal function is appropriate therapy.

PROGNOSIS. Most episodes of CONS bacteremia respond successfully to antibiotics and removal of any foreign body that is present. Poor prognosis is associated with malignancy, neutropenia, and infected prosthetic or native heart valves. CONS increases morbidity, the duration of hospitalization, and mortality rates among patients with underlying complicated illnesses.

Staphylococcus aureus

Bille J: Medical treatment of staphylococcal infective endocarditis. Eur Heart J 16(Suppl B):80, 1995.
Centers for Disease Control and Prevention: Interim guidelines for prevention and control of staphylococcal infection associated with reduced susceptibility to vancomycin. MMWR 46:626, 1997.
Centers for Disease Control and Prevention: Update: *Staphylococcus aureus* with reduced susceptibility to vancomycin—United States, 1997. MMWR 46:813, 1998.
Herold BC, Immergluck LC, Maranan MC, et al: Community-acquired methicillin-resistant *Staphylococcus aureus* in children with no identified predisposing risk. JAMA 279:593, 1998.
Hodes DS, Barzilai A: Invasive and toxin mediated *Staphylococcus aureus* diseases in children. Adv Pediatr Infect Dis 5:35, 1990.
Lowy FD: *Staphylococcus aureus* infections. N Engl J Med 339:520, 1998.
Saiman L, Jakob K, Holmes KW, et al: Molecular epidemiology of staphylococcal scalded skin syndrome in premature infants. Pediatr Infect Dis J 17:329, 1998.
Todd JK: Staphylococcal scalded skin syndrome. *In:* Kaplan SL (ed): Current Therapy in Pediatric Infectious Disease. St. Louis, Mosby–Year Book, 1993.
Vaquero F: Gram-positive resistance: Challenge for the development of new antibiotics. J Antimicrob Chemother 39(Suppl A):1, 1997.

Toxic Shock Syndrome

Bohach GA, Fast DJ, Nelson RD, et al: Staphylococcal and streptococcal pyogenic toxins involved in toxic shock syndrome and related illnesses. Crit Rev Microbiol 17:251, 1990.
Ferguson MA, Todd JK: Toxic shock syndrome associated with *Staphylococcus aureus* sinusitis in children. J Infect Dis 161:953, 1990.
Stevens DL: Streptococcal toxic shock syndrome: Spectrum of disease, pathogenesis, and new concepts in treatment. Emerg Infect Dis 1:69, 1995.
Todd JK: Therapy of toxic shock syndrome. Drugs 39:856, 1990.
Todd JK, Todd BH, Franco-Buff A, et al: Influence of focal infection conditions on the pathogenesis of toxic shock syndrome. J Infect Dis 155:673, 1987.

Coagulase-Negative Staphylococci

Matrai-Kovalskis Y, Greenberg D, Shinwell ES, et al: Positive blood cultures for coagulase-negative staphylococci in neonates: Does highly selective vancomycin usage affect outcome? Infection 26:85, 1998.
Meskin I: Staphylococcus epidermidis. Pediatr Rev 19:105, 1998.
Patrick CC: Coagulase-negative staphylococci: Pathogens with increasing clinical significance. J Pediatr 116:497, 1990.
Patrick CC, Kaplan SL, Baker CJ, et al: Persistent bacteremia due to coagulase-negative staphylococci in low birth weight neonates. Pediatrics 84:977, 1989.
Younger JJ, Christensen GD, Bartley DL, et al: Coagulase-negative staphylococci isolated from cerebrospinal fluid shunts: Importance of slime production, species identification, and shunt removal to clinical outcome. J Infect Dis 156:548, 1987.

CHAPTER 183
Streptococcus pneumoniae (*Pneumococcus*)

James K. Todd

The pneumococcus (*Streptococcus pneumoniae*), a normal inhabitant of the upper respiratory tract, can cause local respiratory tract disease (otitis, sinusitis) and can also be an invasive pathogen (pneumonia, bacteremia, meningitis). *S. pneumoniae* is the most common cause of community-acquired bacterial pneumonia and otitis media and, with the widespread use of conjugated *Haemophilus influenzae* type b vaccines, has become the second most common cause of bacterial meningitis in children. *S. pneumoniae* is the most common cause of meningitis in adults. The significance of this agent is accentuated by the emergence of penicillin-resistant and multidrug-resistant strains in many communities.

ETIOLOGY. *S. pneumoniae* is a gram-positive, lancet-shaped, encapsulated diplococcus. In body fluids and culture media, the organisms also may be found as individual cocci or as chains. Serotypes (90) are identified by their type-specific capsular polysaccharides. Antisera to some pneumococcal capsular polysaccharides cross react with other pneumococcal types or with other bacterial species (e.g., *Escherichia coli*, group B streptococci, and *H. influenzae* type b). Only smooth, encapsulated strains cause serious disease in humans. Virulence is related in part to the size of the capsule, but pneumococcal types with capsules of identical size may vary widely in virulence. Fully encapsulated strains (e.g., type 3) are extraordinarily virulent. Capsular material impedes phagocytosis.

On solid media, pneumococci form unpigmented, umbilicated colonies surrounded by a zone of incomplete (α) hemolysis. Pneumococcal capsules can be seen and the organisms typed by exposing them to type-specific antisera that combine with their respective capsular polysaccharides, rendering the capsules refractile (i.e., quellung reaction). In humans, antibodies to the capsular polysaccharide are protective by promoting opsonization and phagocytosis.

C substance is a cell wall antigen that is related to species rather than to specific pneumococcal serotypes. It is a teichoic acid–containing phosphocholine and galactosamine-6-phosphate. C substance precipitates with an acute β-globulin, the C-reactive protein, which may activate complement and stimulate phagocytosis.

EPIDEMIOLOGY. Many healthy individuals carry *S. pneumoniae* in their upper respiratory tracts. As many as 91% of children between 6 mo and 4.5 yr of age carry *S. pneumoniae* at some time. Serotypes 4, 6B, 9V, 14, 18C, 19F, and 23F constitute the majority of invasive isolates in children. Of these, types 6B, 9V, 14, 19A, and 19F, are often found to be resistant to penicillin. Frequently, the same serotype is carried continuously for extended periods (45 days–6 mo). Carriage of a particular serotype does not consistently induce local or systemic immunity sufficient to prevent later reacquisition of the same serotype. Multiple serotypes may coexist in the same nasopharynx. Pneumococcal isolation rates peak during the first 2 yr of life and decline gradually thereafter; carriage rates are highest in institutional settings and in the winter and lowest in the summer.

S. pneumoniae is the most frequent bacterial cause of bacteremia, pneumonia, and otitis media and the second most common cause of meningitis in infants and children. The decreased ability to produce antibody to polysaccharide capsule antigens in children less than 2 yr of age and the high frequency of colonization may explain, in part, the increased susceptibility to pneumococcal infection and the decreased vaccine effectiveness in this age group. Males are more commonly affected than females, and native Americans and blacks more than whites; the unusual susceptibility of black children is not entirely explained by the increased risk associated with sickle cell disease.

Pneumococcal disease generally occurs sporadically. *S. pneumoniae* is spread from person to person by respiratory droplet transmission. Its frequency and severity are increased in patients with sickle cell disease, asplenia, splenosis, deficiencies in humoral (B cell) immunity, acquired immunodeficiency syndrome, malignancy (e.g., leukemia, lymphoma), and complement deficiencies.

PATHOGENESIS. Pneumococci must invade to produce disease. Nonspecific host defense mechanisms, including the presence of other bacteria in the nasopharynx, usually limit the multiplication of pneumococci. Aspiration of secretions containing pneumococci is hindered by the epiglottic reflex and by the cilia of the respiratory epithelium, which continuously move infected mucus upward toward the pharynx. Similarly, the normal flow of fluid from the middle ear down the internal auditory tube and from the sinus to the nasopharynx prevents infection with nasopharyngeal flora, including pneumococci. Interference with these normal clearance mechanisms by allergy, viral infection, or irritants (e.g. smoke) may allow colonization and ultimate infection with these organisms in what otherwise would normally be sterile sites.

Whether disease develops when pneumococci reach the alveoli depends on the outcome of the interaction of the bacteria with the alveolar macrophages. Pneumococci are highly resistant to phagocytosis by alveolar macrophages.

Pneumococcal disease frequently follows a viral respiratory tract infection that may produce mucosal damage, diminish the epithelial ciliary activity, and depress the function of alveolar macrophages. Phagocytosis may be impeded by respiratory secretions and the alveolar exudate. In the tissues, pneumococci multiply and spread through the lymphatics or bloodstream (bacteremia) or by direct extension from a local site of infection.

The severity of disease is related to the virulence and number of organisms causing bacteremia and to the integrity of specific host defenses. Generally, a poor prognosis correlates with very large numbers of pneumococci or significant concentrations of capsular polysaccharide in the circulation; despite effective antibiotic therapy, patients with heavy antigenemia may have severe and protracted illness.

Deficiency of the terminal components of complement (C–C9) has been associated classically with recurrent pyogenic infection, which includes those caused by *S. pneumoniae.* C2 deficiency also appears to be associated with *S. pneumoniae* infection. The propensity for pneumococcal disease in asplenic persons is presumed to relate to deficient opsonization of pneumococci as well as to absence of the filtering function of the spleen on circulating bacteria. Pneumococcal disease is more prevalent in patients with sickle cell disease and other hemoglobinopathies. This risk is greatest in infants younger than 2 yr when antibody production is attenuated. Patients with sickle cell anemia have a deficit in the antibody-independent properdin (alternate) pathway of complement activation. Properdin deficiency and deficient antibody production result in defects in antibody-independent and antibody-dependent opsonophagocytosis of pneumococci. With advancing age, patients with sickle cell anemia produce anticapsular antibody, augmenting antibody-dependent opsonophagocytosis and reducing but not eliminating the risk of severe pneumococcal disease.

The efficacy of phagocytosis also is diminished in patients with B- and T-cell immunodeficiency syndrome because of a lack of opsonic anticapsular antibody and a failure to produce lysis and agglutination of bacteria. These observations suggest that opsonization of pneumococci depends on the classic and the properdin (or alternative) complement pathways and that recovery from pneumococcal disease depends on the development of anticapsular antibodies that act as opsonins, enhancing phagocytosis and ultimately killing the pneumococci.

In the lungs and other body tissues, the spread of infection is enhanced by the antiphagocytic properties of the pneumococcal capsule. The surface fluid of the respiratory tract contains only small amounts of IgG and is deficient in complement. Both are necessary for opsonization of encapsulated microorganisms. After inflammation has been established in the lungs, there is an influx of IgG, complement, and polymorphonuclear neutrophils. Phagocytosis of bacteria by neutrophils may occur, but even normal human serum may not be able to opsonize pneumococci to prepare them for phagocytosis by alveolar macrophages. Macrophages eventually replace the leukocytes in the exudate, and the lesion resolves. The sequence of events evolves over 7–10 days but may be modified by appropriate antibiotic therapy or by administration of *type*-specific serum.

CLINICAL MANIFESTATIONS. The signs and symptoms are related to the site of infection. Common infections include pneumonia (Chapter 175), otitis media (Chapter 646), sinusitis and pharyngitis, abscesses of the upper airway (Chapter 381), laryngotracheobronchitis (Chapter 385), peritonitis, and bacteremia, especially in young children with fever without localizing signs (Chapter 172). Local spread of infection may occur, causing empyema, pericarditis, mastoiditis, epidural abscess, or, rarely, meningitis. Colonizing pneumococci may spread through the eustachian tube, producing otitis media, and aspiration of infected pharyngeal secretions may produce pneumonia. Bacteremia may be followed by meningitis (Chapter 174.1), septic arthritis and osteomyelitis (Chapter 178), endocarditis (Chapter 443), and brain abscess (Chapter 610).

Hemolytic-uremic syndrome (Chapter 526) and disseminated intravascular coagulation also occur as rare manifestations of pneumococcal disease.

DIAGNOSIS. The diagnosis is established by recovery of pneumococci from the site of infection or the blood. However, pneumococci found in the nose or throat of patients with otitis media, pneumonia, septicemia, or meningitis may not be related causally to their disease.

Blood cultures should be obtained for all children with pneumonia, meningitis, arthritis, osteomyelitis, peritonitis, pericarditis, or gangrenous skin lesions. It may also be advisable to obtain blood cultures in children who are 1–24 mo of age and who have fever but no localized signs of infection if they are not consolable, are toxic, or have leukocytosis (Chapter 172).

Pneumococci can be identified in body fluids as gram-positive, lancet-shaped diplococci. Early in the course of pneumococcal meningitis, many bacteria may be seen in a relatively acellular cerebrospinal fluid. The latex particle agglutination test may be helpful in establishing a diagnosis rapidly; however, it is not necessary if organisms are seen on the Gram stain. The latex test for pneumococcus is not as sensitive for other organisms and is usually not helpful in patients with localized disease (e.g., pneumonia, otitis media).

Leukocytosis generally is pronounced, with total white blood cell counts often greater than 15,000/mm³, a common occurrence; however, severe cases (including meningitis) may have a low white count with a shift to the left.

TREATMENT. Penicillin has historically been the treatment of choice for pneumococcal infection. The incidences of relative and complete penicillin resistance and multidrug resistance (e.g., penicillin, tetracycline, chloramphenicol, rifampin, erythromycin, sulfonamides, clindamycin) have increased during the past decade. Intermediate resistance varies but may be as high as 40% in some areas of North America. Multiply resistant strains have been identified in South Africa, Spain, Great Britain, Australia, and the United States. Resistance to antibiotics is most often noted in the pneumococcal serotypes 6, 9, 14, 19 and 23—the serotypes that most often cause disease in children.

Problems in treatment may be encountered by organisms that are intermediately resistant to penicillin (minimum inhibitory concentration [MIC] 0.1–1.0 mg/L), organisms that are highly resistant to penicillin (MIC ≥ 2.0 mg/L), and organisms that are resistant to several antibiotics. Because of varying patterns of resistance, all isolates from patients with severe infections should be tested for susceptibility to antibiotics. The use of an E-test or MIC is the preferred method for measuring penicillin susceptibility because it identifies intermediately resistant strains more specifically. Many penicillin-resistant strains are also resistant to the cephalosporins. Vancomycin resistance has not been reported.

Empirical treatment of pneumococcal disease should be based on knowledge of susceptibility patterns in specific communities. Penicillin G is the drug of choice for penicillin-susceptible strains. Oral penicillin V (50–100 mg/kg/24 hr every 6–8 hr) for minor infections, intravenous penicillin G (200,000–250,000 U/kg/24 hr every 4–6 hr) for bacteremia or pneumonia, and intravenous penicillin G (300,000 U/kg/24 hr every 4–6 hr) for meningitis are recommended. For serious infections (e.g., meningitis) with strains that are intermediately resistant to penicillin and for all infections with highly penicillin-resistant strains, vancomycin (60 mg/kg/24 hr, every 6 hr) is the treatment of choice. Rifampin (20 mg/kg/24 hr every 12 hours) may be added in severe or unresponsive cases. Resistance to the third-generation cephalosporins, such as cefotaxime and ceftriaxone, is common in penicillin-resistant strains, and treatment failures have been reported. In areas with an increasing incidence of penicillin-resistant pneumococci, vancomycin should be given as initial treatment for any suspected pneumococcal meningitis and other severe disease.

For susceptible strains and patients without noninvasive infection, clindamycin, erythromycin, cephalosporins, trimethoprim-sulfamethoxazole, and chloramphenicol may provide effective alternative therapy for individuals who are allergic to penicillin.

PROGNOSIS. The prognosis depends on the integrity of host defenses, the virulence of the infecting organism, the age of the host, the site and extent of the infection, and the adequacy of treatment.

PREVENTION. Polyvalent pneumococcal vaccines have proved to be immunologic and associated with few untoward reactions in older children and adults. However, responsiveness to pneumococcal polysaccharide is unpredictable in children younger than 2 yr. A licensed 23-valent pneumococcal vaccine contains purified polysaccharide from 23 pneumococcal serotypes responsible for more than 95% of cases of bacteremia and meningitis and for 85% of cases of otitis media in children. The clinical efficacy of the vaccine is controversial; several large studies have yielded conflicting results. In children, the mean postimmunization antibody titers after vaccine administration are, on the average, lower than those in healthy adults. In addition, antigens 6A, 14, 19F, and 23F are poorly immunogenic in children younger than 6 yr. Pneumococcal serotype 6A is one of the strains most likely to produce disease in children.

Immunization is recommended for children who are older than 2 yr and who have sickle cell anemia, functional or anatomic asplenia, nephrotic syndrome, splenectomy after staging laparotomy for Hodgkin's disease, cerebrospinal fluid leaks, HIV infection, and chronic cardiovascular, pulmonary, or liver disease. Vaccine is not recommended for prevention of recurrent otitis media or sinusitis. The need for revaccination is uncertain. A single revaccination 3 yr after the first dose may be considered for children 10 yr of age or younger at the time of revaccination and 5 yr or more after the first dose for children 10 yr of age or older at the time of revaccination.

Immunization does not prevent pneumococcal disease related to serotypes not found in the vaccine and does not invariably prevent infection from a pneumococcal strain that is serotypically identical to one of the vaccine strains. Many reports of serious and even fatal infections in vaccinated children have been described.

New, protein-conjugate pneumococcal polysaccharide vaccines are being evaluated; these appear to offer a higher degree of immunization in children 2 yr old or younger. Once licensed, these may result in a decrease in severe pneumococcal disease similar to the success with *H. influenzae* type b vaccines.

Penicillin prophylaxis is still warranted in children at risk of pneumococcal sepsis. Penicillin V potassium (125 mg bid for children <5 yr and 250 mg bid for children ≥5 yr) substantially decreases the incidence of pneumococcal sepsis in children with sickle cell anemia. In addition, once-monthly intramuscular benzathine penicillin may be efficacious in preventing overwhelming sepsis. Erythromycin may be used in children with penicillin allergy. Prophylaxis is usually continued for at least 2 yr after splenectomy, or up to 6 yr of age, and may be continued into adulthood for high-risk patients. If oral prophylaxis is used, strict compliance must be encouraged. Given the rapid emergence of penicillin-resistant pneumococci, especially in children receiving long-term low-dose therapy, prophylaxis cannot be relied on to prevent disease. High-risk children with fever should be promptly evaluated and treated regardless of vaccination or penicillin prophylaxis.

Alario AJ, Nelson EW, Shapiro ED: Blood cultures in the management of febrile outpatients later found to have bacteremia. J Pediatr 115:195, 1989.

Guillemot C, Carbon C, Balkau B, et al: Low dosage and long treatment duration of β-lactam: Risk factors for carriage of penicillin-resistant *Streptococcus pneumoniae.* JAMA 279:365, 1998.

Jacobs MR, Dagan R, Appelbaum PC, et al: Prevalence of antimicrobial-resistant pathogens in middle ear fluid: Multinational study of 917 children with acute otitis media. Antimicrob Agents Chemother 42:589, 1998.

Kaplan SL, Mason EO Jr, Barson WJ, et al: Three-year multicenter surveillance of systemic pneumococcal infections in children. Pediatrics 102:538, 1998.

Lovgren M, Spika JS, Talbot JA, et al: Invasive *Streptococcus pneumoniae* infections: Serotype distribution and antimicrobial resistance in Canada, 1992–1995. Can Med Assoc J 158:327, 1998.

Pastor P, Medley F, Murphy TV, et al: Invasive pneumococcal disease in Dallas County, Texas: Results from population-based surveillance in 1995. Clin Infect Dis 26:590, 1998.

Rennels MB, Edwards KM, Keyserling HL, et al: Safety and immunogenicity of heptavalent pneumococcal vaccine conjugated to CRM197 in United States infants. Pediatrics 101:604, 1998.

Tan TQ, Mason EO Jr, Kaplan SL: Penicillin-resistant systemic pneumococcal infection in children: A retrospective case-control study. Pediatrics 92:761, 1993.

Wong WY, Overturf GD, Powars DR: Infection caused by *Streptococcus pneumoniae* in children with sickle cell disease: Epidemiology, immunologic mechanisms, prophylaxis, and vaccination. Clin Infect Dis 14:1124, 1992.

Yagupsky P, Porat N, Fraser D, et al: Acquisition, carriage, and transmission of pneumococci with decreased antibiotic susceptibility in young children attending a day care facility in southern Israel. J Infect Dis 177:1003, 1998.

CHAPTER 184
Group A Streptococcus

James K. Todd

Streptococci are among the most common causes of bacterial infection in infancy and childhood. Group A *Streptococcus,* the most common bacterial cause of acute pharyngitis, also produces diverse other infections as well as nonsuppurative sequelae such as rheumatic fever (Chapter 184.1) and glomerulonephritis (Chapter 519.1). Infection during the first 3 mo of life with group B β-hemolytic streptococci is common and may present as bacteremia, meningitis, osteomyelitis, or septic arthritis (Chapter 185).

ETIOLOGY. Streptococci are gram-positive cocci that grow in pairs or variable-length chains, classified on the basis of their ability to hemolyze red blood cells: those with hemolysins producing complete hemolysis β-*hemolytic*), those producing partial (green) hemolysis (α-*hemolytic*), and those producing no hemolysis (γ-*hemolytic*).

Because hemolysis alone does not define pathogenicity, Lancefield further separated the streptococci on the basis of differences in carbohydrate components (C-carbohydrate) within the cell wall; streptococcal groups A through H and K through V have been identified so far (Chapter 181). In group A streptococci, the cell wall is composed of three distinct layers. The outer portion contains several antigenic proteins; the most important is M protein (Table 184–1). Group A β-hemolytic streptococci can be divided into more than 80 immunologically distinct types based on differences in the M protein. M antigen appears to be the major virulence factor, having a role in attachment to epithelial cells and resistance to phagocytosis. Lipoteichoic acid, another cell wall constituent, is another virulence factor that promotes colonization by binding to fibronectin on the surface of epithelial cells. The hyaluronic acid capsule resists phagocytosis, further facilitating virulence. Acquired immunity is directed at the M protein.

Streptococci elaborate toxins, enzymes, and hemolysins. More than 20 extracellular antigens released by group A hemolytic streptococci growing in human tissues have been identified. The extracellular products of greatest clinical significance are pyrogenic (formerly erythrogenic) exotoxins (A, B, and C), streptolysin O, streptolysin S, streptokinases, deoxyribonuclease (DNase), hyaluronidase, and proteinase. Pyogenic exotoxins are responsible for the rash of scarlet fever and for shock in toxic shock–like illness. Generally, the elaboration of pyogenic exotoxins depends on bacteriophage infection (lysogeny) of the streptococcus. Streptolysin S is largely cell bound and damages the membranes of neutrophils and platelets. Streptolysin O is produced by most group A and some group G streptococci. It lyses red blood cells and is toxic to neutrophils, platelets, and mammalian heart muscle. Elaboration of streptolysins S and O produces the clear zone of hemolysis permitting classification of the organisms as β-hemolytic strains. Extracellular digestive enzymes facilitate rapid spreading of streptococci through tissue planes: Streptokinase lyses fibrin, DNase B helps liquefy pus, and hyaluronidase breaks down ground substance. The proteinase, in particular, is associated with tissue destruction of severe invasive streptococcal disease (Fig. 184–1). Antibodies to streptolysin O (ASO), DNase B, hyaluronidase, and streptokinase are useful in the serodiagnosis of group A streptococcal disease. M-type specific antibodies are detectable 4–8 wk after infection; antibiotic therapy ablates this response.

EPIDEMIOLOGY. The incidence of suppurative and nonsuppurative sequelae from group A streptococci increased in the late 1980s and 1990s. The reason for this resurgence of serious streptococcal disease is unknown but is suspected to be related to an increased prevalence of streptococcal strains that produce more of the aforementioned virulence factors. Group A streptococci are normal inhabitants of the oropharynx; colonization rates in children vary from 15–20%. The incidence of disease depends on the age of the child, the season of the year, the climate and geographic location, and the degree of contact with infected individuals.

Generally, incidence is lowest among infants, who may be protected by transplacental acquisition of type-specific antibodies and a lack of pharyngeal receptors for streptococcal binding. Streptococcal infection of the skin is most common in children younger than 6 yr; streptococcal pharyngitis is most common between 5 and 15 yr of age. Streptococcal disease, including scarlet fever, is uncommon in children younger than 3 yr, but in families with known streptococcal infection, it may present as nonspecific upper respiratory tract infection, pharyngitis, and otitis media, with or without impetigo. Severe, invasive group A streptococcal infection can occur at any age. The incidence of streptococcal pharyngitis is higher in temperate climates; incidence and severity appear to increase in cold weather, typically during the school year. Impetigo is more prevalent in tropical climates and in warmer weather in temperate climates.

Group A β-hemolytic streptococci are spread from person to person. Infection may be spread by droplets; pharyngeal carriers are effective disseminators. Infection also may be spread by contact with skin lesions or transmitted by food, milk, and water.

Acquisition of streptococci generally is associated with crowding in the home, school, military installation, or other institution. Disruption of the cutaneous epithelium predisposes to streptococcal pyoderma or impetigo. Concomitant varicella creates many breaks in the integument; these serve as a portal of entry and may decrease the host response to subsequent streptococcal infection. Acquisition from an infected individual is most common during the acute illness (3–5 days) and decreases during the colonization stage. Colonization (pharyngeal) may precede or follow (2–6 wk) overt infection. Immu-

TABLE 184–1 Virulence Factors Associated with Group A Streptococcal Infections

Factor	Location	Action	Pathophysiology
Hyaluronic acid	Capsule	Mucoid strains	Resists phagocytosis
M protein	Cell wall	Attachment	Colonization Resists phagocytosis
Lipoteichoic acids/proteins	Cell wall	Attachment	Colonization
DNase B	Soluble	DNase	Spreading factor
Streptokinase	Soluble	Fibrinolysin	Spreading factor
Hyaluronidase	Soluble	Cleaves ground substance	Spreading factor
Proteinase	Soluble	Protein cleavage	Necrotizing factor
Pyrogenic exotoxin A–C (erythrogenic toxins)	Soluble	TNF, IL-1 stimulator	Scarlet fever toxin Toxic shock syndrome

DNase = deoxyribonuclease; TNF = tumor necrosis factor; IL-1 = interleukin 1.

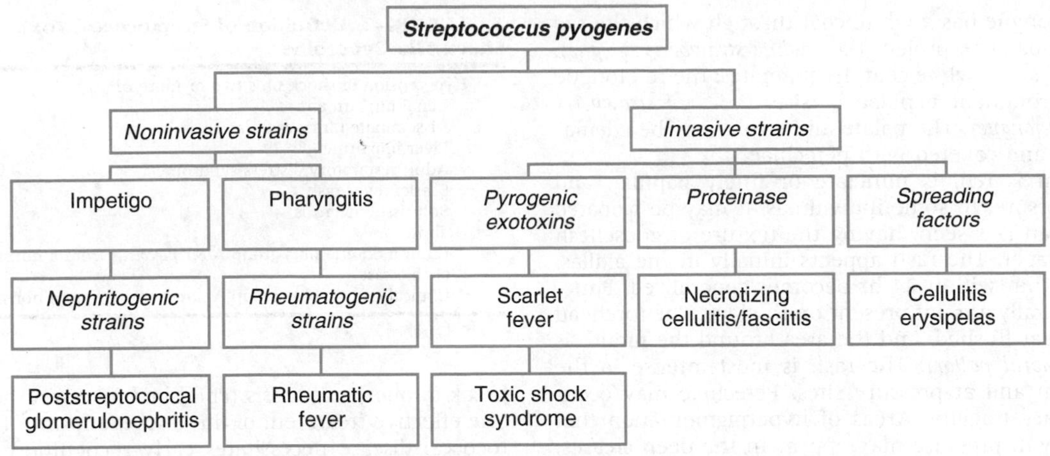

Figure 184–1 Relationship of virulence factors with diseases associated with different group A streptococcal strains.

nity, which is type specific, may be induced either by carriage of the organism or by overt infection. The risk of streptococcal disease diminishes during adult life as immunity develops to the more prevalent serotypes.

PATHOGENESIS. After inhalation or ingestion, streptococci attach themselves to respiratory epithelial cells by their surface fibrils and cell wall lipoteichoic acid. Fibrils contain antiphagocytic epitopes of type-specific M proteins, which with capsular hyaluronic acid resist phagocytosis. Extracellular digestive enzymes facilitate the spread of infection by interfering with local thrombosis (streptolysins) and pus formation (DNase) and enhancing connective tissue digestion (hyaluronidase, proteinase). Suppurative complications follow local inflammation (peritonsillar abscess, retropharyngeal abscess), direct extension (otitis media, sinusitis), lymphangitic spread (lymphadenitis), or bacteremia (sepsis, osteomyelitis, pneumonia).

Scarlet fever–producing streptococci lead to clinical manifestations that are similar to those produced by nonpyrogenic exotoxin-containing strains with the addition of a scarlatiniform rash. Serologically distinct pyrogenic exotoxins (A–C) produce the rash in nonimmune hosts. Rash production is dependent in part on a host hypersensitivity reaction and is decreased by host synthesis of specific antitoxins. These toxins also exhibit pyrogenicity and cytotoxicity, enhance the effects of endotoxin, and have been associated with toxic shock–like illness. Streptococcal pyrogenic exotoxin A has partial amino acid homology with staphylococcal enterotoxin B, which is associated with staphylococcal toxic shock syndrome (TSS).

CLINICAL MANIFESTATIONS. The most common infections caused by group A β-hemolytic streptococci involve the respiratory tract, skin, soft tissues, and blood.

Respiratory Tract Infection (Including Pharyngitis). See Chapter 381.

Pneumonia. See Chapter 175.

Skin Infections. The most common form of skin infection due to group A β-hemolytic streptococci is superficial pyoderma (impetigo) (Chapter 671). Colonization of unbroken skin precedes pyoderma by about 10 days. Skin lesions such as impetigo, ecthyma, and cellulitis develop after intradermal inoculation by insect bites, scabies, or minor trauma. Skin colonization or pyoderma may predispose patients to later pharyngeal colonization with the same strain.

Deeper soft tissue infections may occur. Erysipelas is an acute, well-demarcated infection of the skin with lymphangitis involving the face (associated with pharyngitis) and extremities (wounds). The skin is erythematous and indurated; the advancing margins of the lesions have raised, firm borders. The skin lesion usually is associated with fever, vomiting, and irritability.

Streptococcal cellulitis is a painful, erythematous, indurated infection of the skin and subcutaneous tissues that commonly follows some injury to the skin. Certain streptococcal strains (i.e., those producing proteinase) may cause a more severe necrotizing fasciitis or myositis that results in a rapidly spreading tissue-destructive process that causes necrosis of involved soft tissues including skin, fat, fascia, and muscle. Lymphangitis and regional lymphadenitis are common.

In some cases, streptococci break through the lymphatic barrier, and subcutaneous abscesses, bacteremia, and metastatic foci of infection are observed. Bacteremia and death have been associated with streptococcal cellulitis, and progression may be so rapid that there is no response to treatment with penicillin.

Vaginitis. β-Hemolytic streptococci are a common cause of vaginitis in prepubertal girls (Chapter 557). Patients usually have a serous discharge and marked erythema and irritation of the vulvar area, accompanied by discomfort in walking and in urination.

Perianal Disease. Perianal streptococcal cellulitis produces local itching, pain, blood-streaked stools, erythema, and proctitis.

Bacteremia and Sepsis. Bacteremia may follow a localized cutaneous (wounds, cellulitis, varicella lesions, hemangioma, abscess) or respiratory (pharyngitis, otitis media, sinusitis, pneumonia) infection in previously healthy or immunocompromised (malnutrition, malignancy) patients. It has also occurred in children with no obvious focus of infection (Chapter 172). Sepsis may be rapidly progressive, leading to a toxic shock–like illness with hypotension, fever, leukocytosis, disseminated intravascular coagulation, and peripheral gangrene. Metastatic foci may result in meningitis, brain abscess, osteomyelitis, septic arthritis, pneumonia, and peritonitis. Rarely, endocarditis may complicate group A streptococcal bacteremia. The prognosis is poorest for patients with an underlying disease such as malignancy.

Scarlet Fever. This disease is a result of infection by streptococci that elaborate one of three pyrogenic (erythrogenic) exotoxins. The incubation period ranges from 1–7 days, with an average of 3 days. The onset is acute and is characterized by fever, vomiting, headache, toxicity, pharyngitis, and chills. Abdominal pain may be present; when this is associated with vomiting before the appearance of the rash, an abdominal surgical condition may be suggested. Within 12–48 hr, the typical rash appears.

Generally, temperature increases abruptly, may peak at 39.6–40°C (103–104°F) on the 2nd day, and gradually returns to normal within 5–7 days in untreated patients; it is usually normal within 12–24 hr after initiation of penicillin therapy. The tonsils are hyperemic and edematous and may be covered with a gray-white exudate. The pharynx is inflamed and covered by a membrane in severe cases. The tongue may be edematous and reddened. During the early days of illness, the dorsum of the tongue has a white coat through which the red and edematous papillae project (i.e., *white strawberry tongue*). After several days, the white coat desquamates; the red tongue studded with prominent papillae persists (i.e., *red strawberry tongue, raspberry tongue*). The palate and uvula may be edematous, reddened, and covered with petechiae.

The exanthem is red, is punctate or finely papular, and blanches on pressure. In some individuals, it may be palpated more readily than it is seen, having the texture of gooseflesh or coarse sandpaper. The rash appears initially in the axillas, groin, and neck but within 24 hr becomes generalized. Punctate lesions generally are not present on the face. The forehead and cheeks appear flushed, and the area around the mouth is pale (i.e., *circumoral pallor*). The rash is most intense in the axillas and groin and at pressure sites. Petechiae may occur owing to capillary fragility. Areas of hyperpigmentation that do not blanch with pressure may appear in the deep creases, particularly in the antecubital fossae (i.e., *Pastia's lines*). In severe disease, small vesicular lesions *(miliary sudamina)* may appear over the abdomen, hands, and feet.

Desquamation begins on the face in fine flakes toward the end of the 1st wk and proceeds over the trunk and finally to the hands and feet. The duration and extent of desquamation vary with the intensity of the rash; it may continue for as long as 6 wk.

Scarlet fever may follow infection of wounds (i.e., surgical scarlet fever), burns, or streptococcal skin infection. Clinical manifestations including the strawberry tongue are similar to those just described, but the tonsils and posterior pharynx generally are not involved. A similar picture may be observed with certain strains of staphylococci that produce an exfoliative toxin, although a strawberry tongue is usually absent.

Scarlet fever must be differentiated from other exanthematous diseases, including measles (characterized by its prodrome of conjunctivitis, photophobia, dry cough, and Koplik spots), rubella (disease is mild, postauricular lymphadenopathy usually is present, and throat culture is negative), and other viral exanthems. Patients with infectious mononucleosis have pharyngitis, rash, lymphadenopathy, and splenomegaly as well as atypical lymphocytes. The exanthems produced by several enteroviruses can be confused with scarlet fever, but differentiation can be established by the course of the disease, the associated symptoms, and the results of culture. Roseola usually occurs in younger children and is characterized by the cessation of fever with the onset of rash and the transient nature of the exanthem. Kawasaki disease, drug eruption, and TSS must also be considered.

Scarlet fever may be differentiated from Kawasaki's disease by an older age at onset, absence of conjunctival involvement, and recovery of group A streptococci. *Arcanobacterium haemolyticum* (formerly *Corynebacterium haemolyticum*) also produces tonsillitis, pharyngitis (without a strawberry tongue), and a scarlatiniform rash in adolescents and young adults. Severe sunburn can also be confused with scarlet fever.

Streptococcal Toxic Shock–Like Syndrome. Streptococcal toxic shock–like syndrome is associated with streptococcal strains that produce the pyrogenic exotoxins and is characterized by hypotension accompanied by multiorgan-system dysfunction (Table 184–2). It is often difficult to distinguish from staphylococcal TSS until results of cultures are obtained. A focus of group A streptococcal infection is usually present (e.g., bacteremia, pneumonia, cellulitis). Pharyngitis is commonly absent, and results of throat cultures may be negative despite isolation of the organism from other sites.

TABLE 184–2 Definition of Streptococcal Toxic Shock–Like Syndrome

Hypotension of shock plus two or more of
- Renal impairment
- Disseminated intravascular coagulation
- Liver impairment
- Adult respiratory distress syndrome
- Scarlet fever rash
- Soft tissue necrosis

Definite case
- Clinical criteria plus group A *Streptococcus* from a normally sterile site

Probable case
- Clinical criteria plus group A *Streptococcus* from a nonsterile site

Severe Invasive Streptococcal Disease. A group of the more severe group A streptococcal diseases including puerperal sepsis, severe scarlet fever, necrotizing fasciitis, TSS, and septicemia have increased worldwide, probably because of the increased prevalence of more toxigenic streptococcal strains. These strains may be similar to those that caused a worldwide outbreak of puerperal sepsis (child-bed fever) in the 18th century. The effective treatment of these severe forms of group A streptococcal disease necessitates early recognition and aggressive therapy.

DIAGNOSIS. Colonization of the throat with group A streptococci may occur in 10–20% of normal school-aged children. These carriers are not actively infected and are not at risk of developing rheumatic fever. Although 30% of children with sore throat have a positive throat culture result for group A streptococci, only half of these have a positive antibody response indicative of active infection rather than colonization. Streptococcal pharyngitis is suggested by age greater than 5 yr, high fever, exudates, tender anterior cervical lymphadenopathy, scarlatiniform rash, and a history of exposure. However, many children with active infection may have milder symptoms. Clinical judgment does not predict which children may have streptococcal infection and which must undergo throat culture or antigen detection.

Throat culture is the most useful laboratory aid in reaching a diagnosis in patients with acute tonsillitis or pharyngitis. Vigorous swabbing of the tonsils and posterior pharynx is essential to get an adequate sample for testing. Selective media culture often gives a higher yield than sheep blood agar plates. β-Hemolytic colonies can be confirmed as streptococci by the absence of bubbling in the presence of 3% hydrogen peroxide (a negative catalase test) and confirmed as group A streptococci by inhibition by a bacitracin disk or latex agglutination. Because hemolytic streptococci are common inhabitants of the pharynx in well children, isolation of group A *Streptococcus* from the pharynx of a child with pharyngeal infection does not necessarily indicate that the disease is caused by this organism. When streptococci are isolated from children who have moderate or severe exudative pharyngitis and who have petechiae on the palate and cervical adenitis, the diagnosis is more secure. Current rapid antigen detection tests are not sufficiently sensitive to be used without a backup culture; however, a positive result is usually reliable. *Treatment is, however, recommended for all children with pharyngitis and a positive result of throat culture or rapid antigen test for group A streptococci, even though in some cases the streptococci represent colonization.*

The white blood cell count may or may not be elevated in patients with streptococcal disease. Because leukocytosis may occur in many bacterial and viral diseases, this finding is nonspecific. Similarly, elevations in the erythrocyte sedimentation rate (ESR) and C-reactive protein (CPR) do not help to establish a specific diagnosis.

The immunologic response of the host after exposure to streptococcal antigen can be assessed by measuring ASO and anti-DNase B (ADB) titers. An increase in ASO titer to greater than 166 Todd units occurs in more than 80% of untreated children with streptococcal pharyngitis within the first 3–6 wk after infection. This response may be modified or abolished by early and effective antibiotic therapy. ASO titers may be very high in patients with rheumatic fever; in contrast, they are weakly positive or not elevated at all in patients with streptococcal pyoderma; responses in patients with glomerulonephritis are variable. Group A β-hemolytic streptococci also may be recovered from the pharynx of asymptomatic individuals who develop an antibody response to this organism, indicating that subclinical infection has occured.

Individuals with impetigo may react more strongly to stimulation by other streptococcal extracellular products. Anti-DNase B provides the best serologic test for streptococcal pyoderma; levels begin to rise 6–8 wk after infection. Many patients with streptococcal pharyngitis also develop elevated titers to this enzyme. Patients with pyoderma and pharyngitis also may develop antibody responses to hyaluronidase, but antihyaluronidase (AH) titers are elevated with less regularity than are ASO titers. When it is important to document a recent streptococcal infection, titers to multiple streptococcal products should be considered (e.g., ASO and ADB).

Differential Diagnosis. Acute pharyngitis that is indistinguishable clinically from that caused by group A β-hemolytic streptococci may be caused by many viruses, including adenovirus and Epstein-Barr virus (infectious mononucleosis). A viral cause may be suggested by failure to isolate streptococci and can be identified specifically by viral culture and serologic studies. Infectious mononucleosis may be suggested by the clinical manifestations, the presence of atypical lymphocytes in the peripheral blood, and a rise in heterophil and Epstein-Barr viral antibody titers. Acute pharyngitis similar to that caused by β-hemolytic streptococci may rarely occur in patients with diphtheria, tularemia, and mycoplasmal infections. These diseases can be differentiated by appropriate cultures and serologic tests.

Streptococcal pyoderma must be differentiated from staphylococcal skin disease. These bacterial species often coexist. The lesions produced are clinically indistinguishable; distinction is made only by culture.

Streptococcal septicemia, meningitis, septic arthritis, and pneumonia present signs and symptoms similar to those produced by other bacterial organisms. The offending pathogen can be established only by culture.

COMPLICATIONS. Complications generally reflect extension of streptococcal infection from the nasopharynx. This may result in sinusitis, otitis media, mastoiditis, cervical adenitis, retropharyngeal or parapharyngeal abscess, or bronchopneumonia. Hematogenous dissemination of streptococci may cause meningitis, osteomyelitis, or septic arthritis. Nonsuppurative late complications include rheumatic fever and glomerulonephritis.

TREATMENT. The goals of therapy are to decrease symptoms and prevent septic, suppurative, and nonsuppurative complications. Penicillin is the drug of choice for the treatment of streptococcal infections. All strains of group A β-hemolytic streptococci isolated to date have been sensitive to concentrations of penicillin (and many cephalosporins) achievable in vivo. Variable levels of resistance have been reported to erythromycin, depending on the frequency of that antibiotic's use, and rarely to clindamycin. Failure to respond to penicillin treatment owing to slowly growing organisms at the site of deep group A streptococcal infections (e.g., necrotizing fasciitis) has been called the "eagle effect."

Blood and tissue levels of penicillin sufficient to kill streptococci should be maintained for at least 10 days. Children with streptococcal pharyngitis should be treated with penicillin (250–500 mg/dose bid–tid) for 10 days. Penicillin G or penicillin V may be used; the latter is preferable because satisfactory blood levels are achieved even when the stomach is not empty. A single intramuscular injection of a long-acting benzathine penicillin G (600,000 U for children <60 lb and 1,200,000 U for children >60 lb) may be more effective for treatment or prevention of relapse and is indicated for all noncompliant patients or those having nausea, vomiting, or diarrhea.

Erythromycin (40 mg/kg/24 hr), clindamycin (30 mg/kg/24 hr), or the first-generation cephalosporins may be used for treating streptococcal pharyngitis in patients who are allergic to penicillin. Generally, relapse rates are lower with regimens other than penicillin. Tetracyclines and sulfonamides should not be used for treatment, although sulfonamides may be used for prophylaxis of rheumatic fever. Successful treatment with shorter courses (5 days) of azithromycin or cefpodoxime has been reported.

Treatment failure, defined as persistence of streptococci after a complete course of penicillin, occurs in 5–20% of children and is more common with oral than with intramuscular therapy. It may be due to poor compliance, reinfection, the presence of β-lactamase–producing oral flora, tolerant streptococci, or the presence of a carrier state. Persistent carriage of streptococci predisposes a small number of patients to symptomatic relapse. Repeating the throat culture after a course of penicillin therapy is indicated only in high-risk situations, such as in patients with a history of previous rheumatic fever or apparent frequent streptococcal infections. If the throat culture result is again positive for group A streptococci, some clinicians recommend a second course of treatment. Persistence after a second course of antibiotics probably indicates a carrier state, which poses a low risk for development of rheumatic fever and does not require further therapy.

Patients with severe scarlet fever, streptococcal bacteremia, pneumonia, meningitis, deep soft tissue infections, erysipelas, streptococcal toxic shock–like syndrome, or complications of streptococcal pharyngitis should be treated parenterally with penicillin, preferably intravenously. The dose and duration of therapy must be tailored to the nature of the disease process, with daily doses as high as 400,000 U/kg/24 hr required in the most severe infections. One study suggests that deep or necrotizing infections may require the addition of a second antibiotic (e.g., clindamycin) to ensure complete bacterial killing. TSS may require additional therapies (Chapter 182.2) that may include aggressive fluid management, intravenous immunoglobulin, or steroids.

PREVENTION. Administration of penicillin prevents most cases of streptococcal disease if the drug is provided before the onset of symptoms. Except for rheumatic fever (Chapter 179.1), indications for prophylaxis are not clear. Oral penicillin G or V (400,000 U/dose) may be provided four times each day for 10 days. Alternatively, 600,000 U of benzathine penicillin in combination with 600,000 U of aqueous procaine penicillin may be given as a single intramuscular injection. This approach should be used for institutional epidemics. Children exposed to an individual case at school may be observed carefully.

Treatment of carriers of group A β-hemolytic streptococci is controversial. It has been suggested that treatment of the carrier precludes the development of type-specific immunity, thereby leaving the individual susceptible to reinfection later in life. It is probably unnecessary to re-treat asymptomatic convalescent patients with persistently positive throat cultures for group A streptococci, because they are generally carriers who do not have persistent or recurrent streptococcal infections. Children thought to have recurrent streptococcal infections may be carriers who have frequent viral respiratory infections masquerading as streptococcal infections. Parental anxiety may be high after several such episodes. Treatment with a nonpenicillin antibiotic (e.g., cephalosporin, erythromycin, clindamycin) may be useful in eradicating the carrier state but should be reserved for the rare problem case.

No group A streptococcal vaccines are available for clinical use.

PROGNOSIS. The prognosis for adequately treated streptococcal infections is excellent; most suppurative complications are prevented or readily treated. When therapy is provided promptly, nonsuppurative complications are prevented and complete recovery is the rule. In rare instances, particularly in neonates or in children whose response to infection is compromised, fulminant pneumonia, septicemia, and death may occur despite usually adequate therapy.

184.1 Rheumatic Fever

In the early 1960s, rheumatic fever and its major complication, valvular heart disease, were major problems worldwide. During the decades of the late 1960s and 1970s, this disease almost disappeared in the United States and Western Europe, although it continues unabated in developing countries. However, the recent resurgence of acute rheumatic fever noted in the United States in the middle and late 1980s has once again emphasized the threat of this nonsuppurative sequela of group A streptococcal pharyngitis. The resurgence of rheumatic fever in the United States has also re-emphasized the need for better understanding of its pathogenesis so that appropriate public health and other preventive measures can be more effective.

ETIOLOGY. Group A β-hemolytic *Streptococcus* is the inciting agent leading to the development of acute rheumatic fever, although the exact pathogenetic mechanisms remain unexplained. Not all of the serotypes of group A streptococci can cause rheumatic fever. When some strains (e.g., M type 4) were present in a very susceptible rheumatic population, no recurrences of rheumatic fever ensued. In contrast, other serotypes prevalent in the same population caused recurrence attack rates of 20–50% of those with pharyngitis. The concept of "rheumatogenicity" is further supported by studies suggesting that those serotypes of group A streptococci that were frequently associated with skin infection, usually the higher serotypes, were frequently isolated from the upper respiratory tract but seldom caused recurrences of rheumatic fever in individuals with a previous history of rheumatic fever. Further, certain serotypes of group A streptococci (e.g., M types 1, 3, 5, 6, 18, 24) are more frequently isolated from patients with acute rheumatic fever than are other serotypes. However, because the serotype is unknown at the time of clinical diagnosis of streptococcal pharyngitis, clinicians must assume that all group A streptococci have the capacity to cause rheumatic fever, and all episodes of streptococcal pharyngitis should be treated accordingly.

EPIDEMIOLOGY. The epidemiology of acute rheumatic fever is essentially the epidemiology of group A streptococcal pharyngitis. Rheumatic fever is most frequently observed in the age group most susceptible to group A streptococcal infections, children from 5–15 yr of age. However, susceptibility to rheumatic fever is also evident in older age groups, as is noted by the outbreaks of acute rheumatic fever that have occurred in specific closed populations such as military recruits. Increased numbers of cases also occur in socially and economically disadvantaged groups. This has been attributed to crowding, which is more frequent in this segment of the population. Furthermore, the increased incidence of group A streptococcal pharyngitis in the fall, winter, and early spring is associated with an increased number of cases of acute rheumatic fever during these same periods of the year.

Group A streptococcal impetigo does not result in acute rheumatic fever, but infection of the upper respiratory tract or the skin may lead to another nonsuppurative complication of streptococcal infection, acute poststreptococcal glomerulonephritis. The reasons for this are not fully understood. Hypotheses relating to differences in rheumatogenic potential of "skin strains" and "throat strains," as well as observed differences in the immunologic response to group A streptococcal impetigo compared with streptococcal upper respiratory tract infection, have been proposed to explain the contrast.

The major epidemiologic risk factor for development of acute rheumatic fever is group A streptococcal pharyngitis. The attack rate of acute rheumatic fever after group A upper respiratory tract infection depends on the number of individuals with untreated or inadequately treated infection, the strain of infecting organism, and certain host factors. Many children who harbor group A *Streptococcus* are carriers of group A streptococci in their upper respiratory tract. Group A streptococcal carriers are at much reduced risk for development of acute rheumatic fever and for spread of the organism to close family or school contacts.

Of particular epidemiologic interest is the resurgence of acute rheumatic fever that occurred in the United States in the middle and late 1980s. Although the annual incidence of acute rheumatic fever in many communities in the United States was less than 1/100,000 in the years through the early 1980s, beginning in the mid-1980s, outbreaks of acute rheumatic fever occurred in numerous areas across the United States. The initial and largest outbreak was reported from Utah, but subsequent reports from eastern states, including Ohio and Pennsylvania, indicated that this resurgence was multifocal. One survey of pediatric cardiologists in large referral medical centers in the United States suggested that an increase in numbers of cases of acute rheumatic fever between 1985 and 1989 occurred in approximately 25 states. At least two outbreaks of acute rheumatic fever also occurred in military recruit populations in the United States between 1985 and 1988.

The reasons for this resurgence of acute rheumatic fever in the United States remain unknown. Although rheumatic fever has been associated with socially and economically disadvantaged populations, the 1980s' resurgence has been associated with middle-class, often suburban and rural, families. In addition, serotypes of group A streptococci that have been isolated only rarely during the previous 2 or 3 decades have emerged and spread. These serotypes began to be isolated in greater numbers when rheumatic fever cases were being reported. An increased number of isolates from patients with rheumatic fever or simultaneously from their household contacts and siblings were shown to be M types 1, 3, 5, 6, and 18. These types have historically been associated with rheumatic fever. Very mucoid strains, especially strains of M type 18 group A streptococci, have appeared in a number of communities before the appearance of rheumatic fever. Mucoid strains have historically been associated with virulence.

PATHOGENESIS. Despite remarkable increases in our knowledge of the biology of the group A streptococci and of the human host and despite important observations about the epidemiologic association between group A streptococci and the human host, the pathogenetic mechanism responsible for the development of acute rheumatic fever remains unknown. Two basic theories are postulated to explain the development of this sequel to group A streptococcal pharyngitis: a toxic effect produced by an extracellular toxin of group A streptococci on target organs such as myocardium, valves, synovium, and brain; and an abnormal immune response by the human host. The search for the correct hypothesis has been severely hampered by the fact that there is no adequate animal model.

The most popular hypotheses are those that postulate an abnormal immune response by the human host to some still undefined component of group A streptococci. The resulting antibodies might then cause the immunologic damage leading to clinical manifestations. The latent period, usually 1–3 wk between the onset of the actual group A streptococcal infection and the onset of symptoms of acute rheumatic fever, lends support to an immunologic mechanism of tissue damage. Although the specific antigen or antigens responsible for inciting such an immune response have still to be identified, several possibilities exist. Group A *Streptococcus* is a complex microorganism producing a large number of somatic and extracellular antigens that evoke brisk immune responses. This theory is further supported by the observation that different humans appear to respond quantitatively differently to streptococcal antigens. For example, in vitro studies with human lymphocytes show that individuals can be divided into high and low responders to streptococcal blastogen A, an extracellular product of the organism. This finding is compatible with the clinical and epidemiologic observations that not all people appear to be susceptible to developing rheumatic fever.

The possibility of an abnormal immune response is also based on cross reactivity between group A streptococci M protein and human tissue. The M protein is the virulence factor that is responsible for the organism's ability to resist phagocytosis. In addition, after infections with group A streptococci, type-specific immunity is conferred against the specific M protein type. The group A streptococcal M protein shares certain amino acid sequences with some human tissues, and this has been proposed as a possible source of cross reactivity between the organism and its human host, leading to the abnormal immune response. One of the two classes of M protein correlates with serotypes of group A streptococci that are frequently isolated from patients with acute rheumatic fever.

In patients with Sydenham chorea, common antibodies to antigens are found in the group A streptococcal cell membrane and the caudate nucleus of the brain. This observation further supports the concept of an abnormal autoimmune mechanism for the central nervous system manifestations of rheumatic fever and Sydenham chorea.

An understanding of the pathogenesis of rheumatic fever must encompass the differences in human susceptibility to the development of acute rheumatic fever, including an unusual incidence of rheumatic fever and rheumatic heart disease among members of certain family groups. In regard to this genetic influence, a specific alloantigen is present on the surface of non–T lymphocytes in 70–90% of rheumatic individuals, but fewer than 30% of "control" nonrheumatic individuals have the marker. The marker is more common in families in which there is an index case of rheumatic fever than in nonaffected members of "control" families.

Although humans may have genetic differences in rheumatic susceptibility, the exact mechanism remains unknown. It is unlikely that the recent outbreaks of acute rheumatic fever in the United States are caused by an increasingly susceptible population based only on genetics. It is most likely that the pathogenetic mechanism for the development of rheumatic fever after upper respiratory tract infection with group A β-hemolytic streptococci involves a combination of specific characteristics of the organism and some yet incompletely defined genetic predisposition in the human host.

CLINICAL MANIFESTATIONS. No single specific clinical manifestation or specific laboratory test unequivocally establishes the diagnosis of rheumatic fever.

Carditis. This important finding in acute rheumatic fever is a pancarditis that involves the pericardium, epicardium, myocardium, and endocardium (Chapter 444). Carditis is the only residual of acute rheumatic fever that results in chronic changes. Common manifestations include evidence of valvular insufficiency, most frequently affecting the mitral valve, but the mitral and the aortic valve may be affected. Isolated involvement of the aortic valve is rare. Tricuspid valve or pulmonary valve involvement is unusual. Valvular insufficiency is present in the acute state of the disease. Later, in the chronic stage, scarring of the valve with either typical "fish-mouth" abnormality or even calcified valve tissue may lead to stenosis. A combination of insufficiency and stenosis is often found. Carditis occurs in 40–80% of patients with rheumatic fever. In the recent outbreaks in the United States, more than 80% of patients in one of the large series had evidence of carditis.

Other manifestations of carditis include pericarditis, pericardial effusion, and arrhythmias (usually first-degree heart block, but third-degree or complete heart block may occur). The carditis of rheumatic fever may be mild or very severe, leading to intractable heart failure; rarely, surgical intervention, even in the acute stage of the disease, may be necessary if medical management cannot control the heart failure. These patients usually have myocardial involvement and significant valvular insufficiency.

Polyarthritis. This is the most confusing of the major criteria and probably leads to more diagnostic errors than any of the other manifestations. The arthritis of acute rheumatic fever is exquisitely tender. It is not uncommon for children with this form of arthritis to refuse to allow even bed sheets or clothing to cover an affected joint. The joints are red, warm, and swollen. The arthritis is migratory and affects several different joints: the elbows, knees, ankles, and wrists. It rarely occurs in the fingers, toes, or spine. It need *not* be symmetric. Effusions may be present. If the joint is aspirated, a leukocytosis is usually found; polymorphonuclear leukocytes are the cells found most frequently. However, there are no specific laboratory findings in the synovial fluid.

The arthritis does *not* result in chronic joint disease. After anti-inflammatory therapy is begun, the arthritis may disappear in 12–24 hr. Untreated, it may persist for a week or more. In many patients with early arthritis of rheumatic fever, because of treatment with anti-inflammatory drugs, the classic migratory polyarthritis does not develop, confusing the diagnosis.

Chorea. Sydenham chorea, a unique part of the rheumatic fever syndrome, occurs much later than other manifestations. These choreoathetoid movements may begin very subtly. The latent period following streptococcal pharyngitis may be as long as several months, and the movements are often very difficult to detect at the onset. However, careful questioning of parents and teachers usually reveals evidence of increased clumsiness. One of the best signs of this in school-aged children is a marked deterioration in their handwriting. Emotional lability is a frequent finding. Sydenham chorea may affect all four extremities or may be unilateral. Although at one time it could be seen in as many as one half of patients with acute rheumatic fever, more recent evidence suggests that it occurs, at least in the United States, in 10% or fewer cases. Sydenham chorea frequently is the only symptom of rheumatic fever. It usually disappears within weeks to months. It may return, but this has become a rare occurrence.

Erythema Marginatum. This unique rash seen in patients with rheumatic fever is another of the major manifestations that can be very difficult to diagnose. It occurs very infrequently, and therefore few clinicians have had extensive experience in recognizing it. Although early in the disease it may be manifested as nonspecific pink macules that are usually seen over the trunk, later in its fully developed form, blanching occurs in the middle of the lesions, sometimes with fusing of the borders, resulting in a serpiginous-looking lesion. This rash can be made worse with application of heat, but characteristically it is evanescent. The rash does not itch. It often occurs in patients with chronic carditis. The rash of erythema marginatum can be mistaken for the rash seen with Lyme disease.

Subcutaneous Nodules. These lesions occur infrequently and are most commonly observed in patients with severe carditis. These pea-sized nodules are firm and nontender, and there is no inflammation. They are characteristically seen on the extensor surfaces of the joints, such as the knees and elbows, and over the spine.

Minor Manifestations. The minor manifestations are much less specific but may be necessary to confirm a diagnosis of rheumatic fever. They include the clinical findings of fever and arthralgia. Arthralgia is present if a patient feels discomfort in a joint in the absence of objective findings (e.g., pain, redness, warmth) on physical examination. Fever, usually a temperature no higher than 101–102°F, may be present. High temperature of 103–104°F requires careful re-evaluation and consideration of other diagnoses.

DIAGNOSIS. A number of selective clinical findings, the Jones criteria, are used to determine the diagnosis of acute rheumatic fever. Although the Jones criteria have been changed several times since their original publication, they have remained basically stable and are the accepted method by which the diagnosis of this disease is confirmed (Table 184–3).

The five major criteria are considered to be the most specific findings of acute rheumatic fever. Sydenham chorea frequently is the only symptom of rheumatic fever, and for this reason, this symptom alone is adequate to satisfy the Jones criteria. Included in the minor criteria are symptoms and results of several laboratory tests. Arthralgia cannot be counted as a minor manifestation if arthritis is used as a major manifestation. Levels of acute-phase reactants, such as the ESR or CRP, may be elevated. Results of these tests may remain elevated for prolonged periods (months) and are used by some clinicians as a guideline for modifying doses of anti-inflammatory drugs (see later). A prolonged PR interval on the ECG is also included among the minor criteria. This also is a nonspecific finding and should be used only after careful consideration. An echocardiogram is useful in evaluating patients suspected of having rheumatic fever or rheumatic heart disease.

Evidence of Group A Streptococcal Infection. This is one of the most important aspects of the Jones criteria. There must be evidence of a preceding group A streptococcal infection documented by a positive throat culture, a history of scarlet fever, or elevated streptococcal antibodies such as ASO, ADB, or AH. A diagnosis of rheumatic fever should *not* be seriously considered in patients without evidence of a recent group A streptococcal infection (see later exceptions for chorea and indolent carditis). Approximately 80% of individuals with rheumatic fever have an elevated ASO titer, but if the titers of two additional streptococcal antibodies are also elevated or rising, an elevation of at least one antibody is found in more than 95% of patients with rheumatic fever.

In three situations, acute rheumatic fever may be diagnosed even in the absence of two major criteria or one major and two minor criteria, as required by the revised Jones criteria (Table 184–3). Rheumatic fever should be strongly considered if chorea or indolent carditis is present with no other likely cause. In addition, a recurrence of rheumatic fever should be considered in patients with prior rheumatic fever or rheumatic heart disease and with evidence of a recent streptococcal infection with one major or two minor criteria.

Laboratory Findings. No single specific laboratory test can confirm the diagnosis of acute rheumatic fever. Laboratory evidence of a previous streptococcal infection is confirmed by a search for the organism itself (i.e., culture) or evidence of an immune response to a group A streptococcal antigen. The throat culture remains the gold standard for confirmation of the presence of group A streptococci, although rapid antigen detection tests are available. All patients suspected of having acute rheumatic fever should have at least one throat culture performed before beginning antibiotic therapy. Rapid antigen detection tests may be used if it is recognized that these tests have reduced sensitivity. For small numbers of group A streptococci, the test may be falsely negative. On the other hand, because the specificity of most of these tests is quite accurate, a positive result of a rapid antigen detection test provides evidence of group A streptococci. If a rapid antigen detection test result is negative, a throat culture should be obtained in patients in whom rheumatic fever is suspected.

Streptococcal antibody tests are another method of documenting the presence of a previous group A streptococcal infection. The most commonly used test is the ASO test. Other tests that may be used are the ADB test and the AH test. A commercially available agglutination screening test is less satisfactory because of its technical difficulties. An elevated streptococcal antibody titer is clear evidence of a previous group A streptococcal infection, but a more reliable way of demonstrating the earlier infection is by showing a rise in titer between acute and convalescent sera. The ASO test result reaches its peak 3–6 wk after infection, whereas the ADB test result reaches its peak slightly later (6–8 wk). Acute and convalescent sera, if available, should be tested simultaneously. There is some variation with the age of the patient, the interval since the streptococcal infection, and the population.

Acute-phase reactants such as the ESR or CRP are usually elevated at the onset of acute rheumatic fever. However, these tests are nonspecific. Determination of rheumatoid factor, tests for the presence of antinuclear antibody, and determination of the complement level are rarely helpful in making a diagnosis of acute rheumatic fever. Nonspecific elevations of serum gamma globulin may occasionally be encountered.

An electrocardiogram (ECG) may indicate a first-degree heart block (prolonged PR interval), and on rare occasions, second- or third-degree block may also be present. In first attacks, ECG findings are otherwise usually unremarkable. In patients with chronic rheumatic heart disease, ECG manifestations of resulting cardiac disease, such as left atrial enlargement, may be evident.

No specific findings are revealed by the common chest roentgenogram, but cardiomegaly is common, especially in individuals with significant carditis.

Some individuals with subclinical evidence of valvular disease may show valvular regurgitation on two-dimensional Doppler echocardiography. This observation may explain why many patients without evidence of carditis at the time of the acute attack present in the 4th or 5th decade of life with evidence of mitral valve disease.

Differential Diagnosis. The differential diagnosis is extensive because so many of the clinical and laboratory findings associated with rheumatic fever are not specific and no single laboratory test can confirm the diagnosis. Juvenile rheumatoid arthritis or other connective tissue diseases often need to be considered. Infective endocarditis is frequently confused with rheumatic fever, especially in patients with recurrences of rheumatic fever. Patients with a previous history of rheumatic fever or rheumatic valvular heart disease should be carefully evaluated for infective endocarditis before a diagnosis of recurrent rheumatic fever is made. This may be difficult because such patients may be taking an antibiotic for secondary rheumatic fever prophylaxis in a dose high enough to prevent blood cultures from becoming positive. The typical rash of Lyme disease may be confused with erythema marginatum.

COMPLICATIONS. The major complication of acute rheumatic

TABLE 184–3 The Jones Criteria for Diagnosis of an Initial Attack of Rheumatic Fever

Major Criteria*	Minor Criteria
Carditis	Fever
Polyarthritis, migratory	Arthralgia
Erythema marginatum	Elevated acute-phase reactants (erythrocyte sedimentation rate, C-reactive protein)
Chorea	Prolonged PR interval on an electrocardiogram
Subcutaneous nodules	
Plus	
Evidence of a preceding group A streptococcal infection (culture, rapid antigen, antibody rise/elevation)	

**Two major criteria or one major and two minor criteria plus evidence of a preceding streptococcal infection indicate a high probability of rheumatic fever. In the three special categories listed below, the diagnosis of rheumatic fever is acceptable without two major or one major and two minor criteria. However, only for 1 and 2 can the requirement for evidence of a preceding streptococcal infection be ignored.*

1. *Chorea,* if other causes have been precluded.
2. *Insidious or late-onset carditis* with no other explanation.
3. *Rheumatic recurrence: In patients with documented rheumatic heart disease or prior rheumatic fever, the presence of one major criterion or of fever, arthralgia, or elevated acute-phase reactants suggests a presumptive diagnosis of recurrence. Evidence of previous streptococcal infection is needed here.*

From Special Writing Group of the Committee on Rheumatic Fever, Endocarditis, and Kawasaki Disease of the Council on Cardiovascular Disease in the Young of the American Heart Association: Guidelines for the diagnosis of rheumatic fever. JAMA 268:2069, 1992.

fever is the development of rheumatic valvular heart disease. None of the other manifestations results in a chronic disease. The mitral valve is most frequently involved, but the aortic and tricuspid valves also may be affected. The tricuspid valve usually becomes involved only in patients who have significant mitral or aortic disease resulting in pulmonary hypertension.

TREATMENT. Management of acute rheumatic fever can be divided into three approaches: treatment of the group A streptococcal infection that led to the disease, use of anti-inflammatory agents to control the clinical manifestations of the disease, and other supportive therapy, including management of congestive heart failure, if that has occurred.

All patients presenting with acute rheumatic fever should be treated for a group A streptococcal infection at the time the diagnosis is made, whether or not the organism is initially isolated from the patient. The organism can be difficult to recover from a patient at onset because of the latent period, especially in patients with chorea. Ten full days of an appropriate oral agent or a single intramuscular injection of 1,200,000 units of benzathine penicillin G is recommended. Treatment for group A β-hemolytic streptococcal infections is discussed in more detail in Chapter 184. Because some patients receiving intramuscular benzathine penicillin G may experience nonspecific rises in the ESR, some clinicians elect to treat patients initially with oral penicillin, especially if they are monitoring the ESR as a measure of the effectiveness of anti-inflammatory therapy given for other rheumatic manifestations. Sulfadiazine is not an appropriate agent for treatment of acute streptococcal pharyngitis.

Therapy is given acutely for three systemic manifestations of acute rheumatic fever. These are arthritis, carditis, and Sydenham chorea. Salicylates provide prompt and dramatic relief for patients with the arthritis of acute rheumatic fever. The exquisitely tender migratory polyarthritis can be relieved in 12–24 hr by the use of salicylates. Early administration of salicylates to patients suspected of having rheumatic fever before the diagnosis is established with certainty may obscure the diagnosis by interrupting the development of migratory arthritis. Therefore, salicylates or other anti-inflammatory agents should be withheld until the clinical course of the disease has adequately defined itself. For patients with very painful arthritis, comfort can be provided by the use of small doses of codeine or similar drugs, because they do not interfere with the progression of the disease and its subsequent diagnosis. Corticosteroids are seldom indicated for the treatment of arthritis or rheumatic fever. No studies document the efficacy of other nonsteroidal anti-inflammatory agents in the treatment of rheumatic fever.

For patients with mild carditis without evidence of congestive heart failure, salicylates alone are indicated. However, in patients with congestive heart failure or other significant manifestations of carditis, corticosteroids are required. No definitive evidence shows that the use of salicylates or corticosteroids is beneficial in preventing the subsequent development of rheumatic heart disease. This is in contrast to the clinical impression that corticosteroids may have a beneficial effect in patients with moderate to severe carditis. It is appropriate to restrict the use of corticosteroids to patients who have moderate or severe carditis, especially those with evidence of heart failure.

Administration of corticosteroids should be limited both in amount and in duration to reduce their untoward side effects. For most children, a total dose of 2.5 mg/kg/24 hr of prednisone divided into two doses is appropriate. A short course of corticosteroids over 2–3 wk is usually sufficient, depending on a patient's response clinically and on laboratory tests (e.g., ESR, CRP). Even with short courses of steroids in these doses, side effects may occur, including some cushingoid changes and hypertension. Alternate-day steroids may reduce the side effects, but controlled studies have not been carried out. The dose should be tapered rather than abruptly stopped.

Salicylates should be given in a dose that results in blood levels of 20–25 mg/dL. Usually 90–120 mg/kg/24 hr in four divided doses is adequate to reach this level in children. However, serum salicylate levels should be carefully monitored to reduce the possibility of toxicity. Liver function should also be monitored. In patients who are receiving corticosteroids for therapy of carditis, it is advisable to add salicylates to the corticosteroids, especially when the doses are being tapered, to prevent the possibility of rheumatic rebound. The salicylates should be given during the last week of corticosteroid therapy and continued for approximately 3–4 wk after the steroids have been discontinued. The duration of salicylate therapy depends on a patient's response and clinical course.

Congestive heart failure should be treated by conventional techniques (Chapter 448). Diuretics are indicated in patients with severe congestive heart failure. Cardiac glycosides such as digitalis also may be used, although usually in relatively small doses. Long periods of bed rest are not necessary for most patients. In the past, bed rest was used primarily for patients with arthritis or carditis. Arthritis usually responds quickly to therapy and is not a significant factor after 24 hr of salicylate therapy. Strict bed rest is not needed. Bed rest is indicated for the therapy of patients with carditis and congestive heart failure, but prolonged bed rest is usually unnecessary. It is, however, preferable to keep patients at bed rest until the ESR approaches normal and congestive heart failure has been controlled. Corticosteroids, bed rest, and cardiac medications occasionally are not effective in treating with carditis of rheumatic fever. In these rare cases, cardiovascular surgery with replacement of the valve or valvuloplasty may be required.

The treatment of Sydenham chorea has been controversial. Phenobarbital or other sedatives were originally used; then chlorpromazine became popular. Diazepam, a benzodiazepine derivative, is prescribed for patients with mild chorea. In patients with severe chorea, haloperidol has been used successfully. These children must be closely observed, because severe toxic reactions to this drug have been reported.

There is no specific therapy for erythema marginatum or the subcutaneous nodules of acute rheumatic fever.

PREVENTION. Prevention and treatment of group A streptococcal infection can prevent rheumatic fever. The two forms of prevention for acute rheumatic fever are primary prophylaxis and secondary prophylaxis.

Primary prophylaxis refers to antibiotic treatment of the streptococcal upper respiratory tract infection to prevent an initial attack of rheumatic fever. Appropriate diagnosis and adequate antibiotic therapy with eradication of group A streptococci from the upper respiratory tract reduce the risk of developing rheumatic fever to near zero. Antibiotic therapy initiated up to approximately 1 wk after onset of the streptococcal sore throat can prevent rheumatic fever. See Chapter 184 for treatment of group A streptococcal infections. However, antibiotic therapy must be adequate. Ten full days of oral therapy is essential if the oral method is used.

Secondary prophylaxis (Table 184–4) refers to the prevention of colonization or infection of the upper respiratory tract with group A β-hemolytic streptococci in individuals who have already had a previous attack of acute rheumatic fever. Patients who receive antibiotics continuously and who do not have group A streptococcal infections do not have recurrences of rheumatic fever. The recommended methods of secondary prevention include regular monthly (every 3–4 wk) injections of intramuscular benzathine penicillin G, daily administration of oral penicillin, daily administration of oral sulfadiazine, or daily oral administration of erythromycin (for individuals who cannot take any of the previously recommended antibiotics). Although sulfadiazine or other sulfa drugs should *never* be

TABLE 184–4 Secondary Prevention of Rheumatic Fever

Route of Administration	Antibiotic	Dose	Frequency
Intramuscular	Benzathine penicillin G	1,200,000 units	Every 3–4 wk
Oral	Penicillin V	250 mg	Twice daily
	Sulfadiazine	500–1000 mg	Daily
	Erythromycin	250 mg	Twice daily
Do not use tetracycline antibiotics			

used for the treatment of group A streptococcal infections (because a high percentage of organisms are resistant to these antimicrobial agents), sulfadiazine *is* effective in preventing colonization of the upper respiratory tract and is an acceptable form of oral secondary prophylaxis. Regular injections of intramuscular benzathine penicillin G are preferable to oral secondary prophylaxis because of better compliance. Individuals at high risk for rheumatic recurrence should be given 1,200,000 units IM every 3 wk. Penicillin levels during the 4th wk after injection may be lower than the minimal inhibitory concentration for group A β-hemolytic streptococci. However, in most instances in the United States, 4-wk intervals for injections are sufficient because the risk of recurrence of rheumatic fever is small.

The necessary duration of secondary prophylaxis in individuals with a documented history of rheumatic fever or with rheumatic heart disease is controversial. Recurrences of acute rheumatic fever are less frequent 5 yr or more after the most recent attack, and, for this reason, some clinicians think that patients may not need secondary prophylaxis more than 5 yr after the most recent attack or when they reach their 21st birthday, whichever comes last. Others recommend that for patients who have significant rheumatic heart disease or who have a significant risk of contracting group A streptococcal upper respiratory tract infection (e.g., medical professionals, school teachers, those living in crowded conditions), the duration of secondary prophylaxis should be longer. Some recommend that treatment be continued for at least 10 yr in patients with residual rheumatic valvular heart disease and at least until the age of 40 yr (others recommend lifelong prophylaxis). Recommendations for each patient must be individualized, depending on a patient's condition and the living and working environment.

No streptococcal vaccine is available. Physicians and public health authorities must still depend on the accurate and timely diagnosis and therapy of group A streptococcal upper respiratory tract infections and avoidance of recurrent infections in known rheumatic patients to prevent the crippling effects of rheumatic fever and rheumatic heart disease.

Group A Streptococcus

American Academy of Pediatrics, Committee on Infectious Diseases: Severe invasive group A streptococcal infections: A subject review. Pediatrics 101:136, 1998.

Hodge CW, Schwartz B, Talkington DF, et al: The changing epidemiology of invasive group A streptococcal infections and the emergence of streptococcal toxic shock-like syndrome. JAMA 269:384, 1993.

Kokx NP, Comstock JA, Facklam RR: Streptococcal perianal disease in children. Pediatrics 80:659, 1987.

Miller RA, Brancato F, Holmes KK: *Corynebacterium hemolyticum* as a cause of pharyngitis and scarlatiniform rash in young adults. Ann Intern Med 105:867, 1986.

Pichichero ME, Disney FA, Talpey WB, et al: Adverse and beneficial effects of immediate treatment for Group A beta-hemolytic streptococcal pharyngitis with penicillin. Pediatr Infect Dis J 6:635, 1987.

Pichichero ME, Margolis PA: A comparison of cephalosporins and penicillins in the treatment of Group A beta-hemolytic streptococcal pharyngitis: A meta-analysis supporting the concept of microbial copathogenicity. Pediatr Infect Dis J 10:275, 1991.

Radetsky M, Solomon JA, Todd JK: Identification of streptococcal pharyngitis in the office laboratory: Reassessment of new technology. Pediatr Infect Dis J 6:556, 1987.

Stevens DL: Streptococcal toxic shock syndrome: Spectrum of disease, pathogenesis, and new concepts in treatment. Emerg Infect Dis 1:69, 1995.

Todd JK: The sore throat: Pharyngitis and epiglottitis. Infect Dis Clin North Am 2:149, 1988.

Wheeler MC, Roe MH, Kaplan EL, et al: Clinical, epidemiological, and microbiological correlates of an outbreak of group A streptococcal septicemia in children. JAMA 266:533, 1991.

The Working Group: Defining the group A streptococcal toxic shock syndrome. JAMA 269:390, 1993.

Rheumatic Fever

Berrios X, del Campo E, Guzman B, Bisno AL: Discontinuing rheumatic fever prophylaxis in selected adolescents and young adults: A prospective study. Ann Intern Med 118:401, 1993.

Dajani AS, Ayoub E, Bierman FZ, et al: Guidelines for the diagnosis of rheumatic fever: Jones Criteria, update 1993. Circulation 87:302, 1993.

Dajani A, Taubert K, Ferrieri P, et al: Treatment of acute streptococcal pharyngitis and prevention of rheumatic fever: A statement for health professionals. Pediatrics 96:758, 1995.

Denny FW Jr, Wannamaker LW, Brink WR, et al: Prevention of rheumatic fever: Treatment of the preceding streptococcal infection. JAMA 143:151, 1950.

Dudding BA, Ayoub EM: Persistence of streptococcal group A antibody in patients with rheumatic valvular disease. J Exp Med 128:1081, 1968.

Kaplan EL: The rapid identification of group A beta-hemolytic streptococci in the upper respiratory tract. Pediatr Clin North Am 35:535, 1988.

Kaplan EL, Berrios X, Speth J, et al: Pharmacokinetics of benzathine penicillin G: Serum levels during the 28 days after intramuscular injection of 1,200,000 units. J Pediatr 115:146, 1989.

Kaplan EL, Johnson DR, Cleary PP: Group A streptococcal serotypes isolated from patients and sibling contacts during the resurgence of rheumatic fever in the United States in the mid-1980s. J Infect Dis 159:101, 1989.

Kavey RW, Kaplan EL: Resurgence of acute rheumatic fever. Pediatrics 84:585, 1989.

Secord E, Emre U, Shah BR, Tunnessen WW Jr: Picture of the month: Erythema marginatum in acute rheumatic fever. Am J Dis Child 146:637, 1992.

Special Writing Group of the Committee on Rheumatic Fever, Endocarditis, and Kawasaki Disease of the Council on Cardiovascular Disease in the Young of the American Heart Association: Guidelines for the diagnosis of rheumatic fever. JAMA 268:2069, 1992.

Swedo SE, Leonard HL, Schapiro MB, et al: Sydenham's chorea: Physical and psychological symptoms of St. Vitus dance. Pediatrics 91:706, 1993.

Veasy LG, Tani LY, Hill HR: Persistence of acute rheumatic fever in the intermountain area of the United States. J Pediatr 124:9, 1994.

CHAPTER 185
Group B Streptococcus

Samuel P. Gotoff

Group B *Streptococcus* (GBS) is a major cause of severe systemic and focal infections in newborns.

ETIOLOGY. *Streptococcus agalactiae* is the species of streptococci belonging to Lancefield group B. It is a facultative, encapsulated gram-positive diplococcus that produces a narrow zone of β-hemolysis on blood agar. Occasional strains are nonhemolytic. Most strains are resistant to bacitracin and show a positive CAMP test result. Strains of GBS are classified serologically by capsular polysaccharide and protein antigens and include types Ia, Ib, Ia/c, II, III, IV, V, VI, VII, and VIII. Early-onset disease may be due to any serotype, whereas late-onset disease is due to type III in 90% of cases. GBS produces extracellular substances, which include hemolysin, CAMP factor, hippuricase, nucleases, protease, neuraminidase, and lipoteichoic acid. The only factor associated with increased virulence is the quantity of type-specific capsular polysaccharide that inhibits opsonophagocytic killing in vitro.

EPIDEMIOLOGY. The organism is a common inhabitant of the maternal genital and gastrointestinal tracts and colonizes approximately 20% (range 4–40%) of pregnant women. Pregnant women who are colonized are usually asymptomatic but may have urinary tract infections, chorioamnionitis, or endometritis. Colonization at birth is noted in 40–70% of infants born to colonized mothers. Infants born of women who are heavily colonized are more likely to become colonized. Colonization rates are increased in women younger than 20 yr, in blacks, and in lower socioeconomic groups. Maternal colonization may be chronic, transient, or intermittent. Nearly 50% of sexual partners of genitally colonized women have positive cultures for GBS, which is evidence for sexual transmission. Women colonized in the 2nd trimester may have negative findings at delivery (30%), and women with negative results in the 2nd trimester may be colonized at delivery (8%). Concordance of prenatal cultures and cultures at delivery is related to the interval between prenatal culture and delivery. Cultures after 35 wk of gestation have a negative predictive value of 97% and a positive predictive value of 89% for colonization at delivery.

The incidence of neonatal GBS disease varies from 0.2–3.7/1,000 live births. With increased use of maternal chemoprophylaxis, these rates are diminishing. From 0.5–2% of newborn infants born to colonized mothers become infected. Early-onset GBS disease occurs within the 1st wk of life, usually before 72 hr. Late-onset GBS disease accounts for about 20% of cases, with cases appearing up to 6 mo of age. Cases after 1 mo of age occur primarily in premature infants and those with immunodeficiencies. Many infants (50%) with early-onset GBS are symptomatic at birth, indicating infection was established in utero. Before implementation of maternal chemoprophylaxis, the highest attack rate of early-onset GBS disease occurred among very low birthweight infants; the incidence was more than 8/1,000 in infants weighing less than 1,500 g and less than 1/1,000 in infants weighing more than 2,500 g. In the 1990s, full-term infants usually accounted for more than 50% of cases, probably as a result of the increasing use of chemoprophylaxis in women with premature labor. The rate of neonatal infection is also influenced by prolonged rupture of the amniotic membranes, prolonged labor, and most importantly by maternal chorioamnionitis (fever, tender uterus, leukocytosis). The presence of maternal urinary tract infection indicates either gastrointestinal or vaginal colonization or both. A previous delivery with GBS disease increases the likelihood of colonization and has tremendous psychologic implications for a subsequent pregnancy. Late-onset GBS disease is due to acquisition from maternal and nonmaternal sites (nursery personnel, community) and is not associated with obstetric risk factors.

The rate of early-onset GBS disease is also related to the degree of colonization at birth. Heavily colonized infants are 12 times as likely to have early-onset disease as lightly colonized infants. Case fatality rates for early- and late-onset disease have fallen below 15%.

GBS is a major cause of chorioamnionitis and puerperal infection. GBS also causes infections in nonpregnant adults, particularly those with chronic medical problems and advanced age.

PATHOGENESIS. Early-onset GBS infection is acquired through vertical transmission. Ascending infection usually occurs through ruptured amniotic membranes, but occasionally there is no history of rupture. GBS infection or colonization may also occur during passage through a colonized birth canal. Identical serotypes are found in mother and newborn. The rate of vertical transmission is approximately 50% and varies with the inoculum size. However, lightly colonized women may deliver infected infants. There is a direct correlation between duration of membrane rupture and incidence of early-onset GBS infection. Neonates may also acquire GBS after horizontal transmission in the nursery or from adults other than their mothers. Infant-to-infant and adult-to-infant spread has produced colonization, late-onset GBS disease, and, rarely, epidemics of GBS in nurseries.

Early-onset GBS disease is associated with immature host defense mechanisms, particularly among low birthweight infants, and exposure to a heavily colonized maternal genital tract (ascending vertical transmission through ruptured amniotic membranes). GBS may cause local inflammation of intact membranes, leading to subsequent weakness and rupture of amniotic fluid membranes, thus initiating premature labor. The attack rate of early-onset GBS disease is 1.1/1,000, with membrane rupture occurring at less than 18 hr and 7.6/1,000 with rupture occurring at 18 hr or more after delivery. Fetal infection may also develop through intact membranes. Amniotic fluid contains low levels of type-specific GBS antibodies, complement, phagocytic cells, and other nonspecific defense components and is a favorable culture medium for GBS. On occasion, fetal aspiration of infected amniotic fluid may initiate fetal and subsequent neonatal pneumonia, bacteremia, and septic shock.

Opsonophagocytic defects present in neonatal phagocytes are further compromised in infants with GBS infection as a result of a deficiency of maternally derived type-specific antibody. Serum levels of greater than 1–2 μg/mL of IgG antibody to type-specific capsular polysaccharides of GBS are associated with effective opsonophagocytosis and killing of GBS and protection in animal models of infection. Only 10–20% of adult women have antibody levels of this magnitude. In premature infants, transplacental passage of antibody is impaired. At 28 and 32 wk of gestation, levels of type-specific anticapsular GBS antibodies are 33% and 50% of maternal levels, respectively. Although newborns with early-onset GBS infection are deficient in type-specific antibody, other colonized infants with similar levels remain well. Thus, other factors mediating virulence and host defense mechanisms affect pathogenesis.

Early-onset GBS disease is usually characterized by pneumonia with bacteremia and complicated by pulmonary hypertension. The latter may be attenuated by inhibition of thromboxane synthesis, suggesting a role for the activity of the pulmonary cyclooxygenase pathway in the pathogenesis of GBS-associated pulmonary hypertension. The development of pulmonary hypertension in full-term babies is apparently related to the adult respiratory distress syndrome (ARDS).

Intrauterine death may occur at any time during gestation. In intrauterine and early-onset infections, pulmonary inflammation is characterized by interstitial or alveolar neutrophil exudates, vascular congestion, edema, and various degrees of pulmonary hemorrhage. Premature and full-term infants who die of early-onset sepsis frequently have hyaline membranes. This may be a result of surfactant deficiency in premature infants and ARDS in full-term and perhaps premature infants owing to sepsis.

The inflammatory response in early-onset disease is variable, in part because of the duration of illness and an infant's diminished ability to mount an inflammatory response. In early-onset meningitis, infants may have little evidence of inflammation. Bacteria are prominent, and thrombosis, hemorrhage, and perivascular inflammation are noted. Periventricular leukomalacia may be found in infants with central nervous system infection and those who survive GBS septic shock.

The pathophysiology of late-onset GBS may be related to an initial colonization, alterations of the mucosal barrier by a prior viral respiratory tract infection, elaboration of large amounts of GBS type III capsular polysaccharide, and possibly reduced amounts of maternal antibody. The pathophysiology of late-onset GBS osteomyelitis is atypical and may be related to an early-onset asymptomatic bacteremia, inoculation into a traumatized bone, and subsequent late onset of a single site of osteomyelitis. Affected infants usually have few systemic symptoms. The presence of type-specific IgG antibody to GBS type III suggests that the infant produced antibodies and restricted the infection to a metaphyseal location. Acquisition of type-specific IgM antibodies may explain the age-specific incidence of GBS disease.

Although late-onset sepsis may be rapid, with pathologic features similar to early-onset disease, the inflammatory response is usually similar to that in older infants who die of pyogenic infections. A substantial inflammatory response occurs, and abscess formation is common.

CLINICAL MANIFESTATIONS. The spectrum of early-onset infections ranges from asymptomatic bacteremia to septic shock (Chapter 106). Early-onset disease may present at birth, and most infants become ill within 6 hr of age. In utero infection may result in fetal asphyxia, coma, or shock. Respiratory symptoms are prominent and include cyanosis, apnea, tachypnea, grunting, flaring, retractions, and roentgenographic findings consisting of a reticulogranular pattern (50%), patchy pneumonic infiltrates (30%), and, less commonly, pleural effusions, pulmonary edema, cardiomegaly, and increased pulmonary vascular markings. Persistent fetal circulation or ARDS may develop. Bacteremia or sepsis without localization is noted in 30–40% of infants. Apnea or hypotension may be the initial presentation of sepsis.

Meningitis occurs in about 10% of infants with early-onset infection. Patients with meningeal involvement may have seizures, lethargy, coma, and a bulging fontanel, but meningitis may be present without signs of meningeal involvement.

Late-onset GBS infection is manifested as bacteremia without a focus (55%), meningitis (35%), osteoarthritis, and soft tissue infection and is predominantly caused by the type III serotype. Additional manifestations of late-onset GBS are noted in Table 106–3. The presenting signs of late-onset GBS meningitis are usually fever and lethargy. Bulging fontanel and nuchal rigidity are more common in late-onset than early-onset meningitis.

DIAGNOSIS. The differential diagnosis of early-onset GBS infection includes hyaline membrane disease; amniotic fluid aspiration syndrome; sepsis from other vertically transmitted ascending infections (*Escherichia coli,* herpes simplex virus), and those metabolic (hypoglycemia, hyperammonemia), anatomic (congenital heart disease, diaphragmatic hernia), or other conditions that produce manifestations of sepsis. The probability of infection increases with the presence of risk factors and colonization in the mother if untreated during labor. Diagnosis of GBS infection is confirmed by culture.

Laboratory Findings. The diagnosis is established by isolation and identification of the organism from normally sterile sites. CSF should be examined in all patients suspected of having meningitis or sepsis. Early in the course of early-onset meningitis, the culture may be positive in the absence of pleocytosis. The demonstration of gram-positive organisms in pairs or chains in buffy coat or other normally sterile fluids is evidence of infection, which is most commonly due to GBS. Gram-positive cocci in gastric or tracheal aspirates indicate colonization. Isolation of GBS from skin or mucous membranes also indicates colonization and not invasive infection.

Antigen detection of GBS is possible with latex particle agglutination, but the test is less sensitive than culture and is most useful if the mother or infant has had prior antibiotic therapy, and in sepsis without bacteremia. Urine samples may need to be pretreated to remove cross-reacting ABO antigens. Urine samples collected by bag frequently yield false-positive results in healthy but colonized neonates owing to contamination by GBS organisms, which colonize the perineum or rectum. Thus, a urine latex test must be performed on a catheterized or aspirated urine specimen. The test should not be performed on asymptomatic newborn infants; the amount of antigen in urine needed for a positive test result is associated with signs of infection. Rapid antigen detection tests have been used for screening women at the time of delivery. One study showed that only 40% of colonized women would be detected.

Nonspecific laboratory tests may include an increased band count, increased ratio of immature to total white blood cells (>0.20), neutropenia, thrombocytopenia, leukocytosis, elevated serum C-reactive protein level, and pneumonia or osteomyelitis on roentgenogram.

TREATMENT. GBS is uniformly sensitive to penicillin G, which is the treatment of choice of confirmed GBS infection. Empirical antimicrobial therapy is initiated with a penicillin (usually ampicillin) and an aminoglycoside until GBS has been identified by culture. In vitro, a combination of penicillin and gentamicin provides synergistic bactericidal activity against GBS despite resistance of GBS to aminoglycosides. Some authorities recommend continuation of ampicillin plus gentamicin for several days until a good clinical response occurs or the CSF becomes sterile.

GBS demonstrates a minimal inhibitory concentration (MIC) (0.01–0.4 mg/mL) for penicillin G that is 4- to 10-fold greater than that of group A streptococci. An inoculum effect (higher GBS colonies per milliliter require more penicillin) may have clinical implications because CSF may contain as many as 10^7–10^8 colony-forming units per milliliter. Rarely (4–6%), GBS demonstrates tolerance (minimal bactericidal concentration >16–32 times the MIC), which may correlate with delayed killing and recurrent infection. The significance of in vitro tolerance among GBS remains speculative.

GBS is also susceptible to vancomycin, semi-synthetic penicillins, cefotaxime, ceftriaxone, and imipenem. These agents are not superior to penicillin or ampicillin and should not be used to treat documented GBS infection. Penicillin should be used in high doses for the treatment of GBS meningitis (i.e., 300,000 units/kg/24 hr of penicillin G or 300 mg/kg/24 hr of ampicillin). These higher than usual doses are recommended because of a relatively higher MIC, high CSF inoculum, reports of relapse of GBS meningitis in patients treated with 200,000 units/kg/24 hr of penicillin G, and the relative safety of penicillins in neonates. CSF should be obtained within 48 hr of therapy of documented meningitis to determine whether persistent infection is present (>90% are sterile within 36 hr), owing to a high inoculum effect or tolerant GBS. If GBS continue to grow from the CSF, some authorities continue giving a combination of penicillin (or ampicillin) and gentamicin (for synergism) for the duration of treatment (2–3 wk). Failure to document sterile CSF within 48 hr of therapy may also signify subdural empyema, brain abscess, ventriculitis, suppurative dural sinus thrombosis, or an insufficient dose of a bactericidal antibiotic.

Treatment of bacteremia with a soft tissue focus or pneumonia may be discontinued after 10 days. Arthritis may be treated in 2–3 wk and osteomyelitis and endocarditis in 3–4 wk.

Recurrent infection is uncommon. It is more likely due to persistent mucosal colonization rather than a sequestered focus, particularly if the interval to recrudescence is longer than 3–4 days. Re-treatment with a full course of a penicillin and aminoglycoside may be followed by rifampin, 10 mg/kg/24 hr for 5–7 days, in an attempt to eradicate colonization. The sequence is important because antagonism between penicillin and rifampin against GBS has been demonstrated in vitro. Because mother's milk may be a source of recurrent late-onset GBS infection, cultures should be obtained and rifampin may be considered for the mother as well as the infant.

Supportive care of infants with GBS infection is important (Chapter 106), including the treatment of hypoxia and shock, disseminated intravascular coagulation, seizures, increased intracranial pressure, and inappropriate secretion of antidiuretic hormone. Extracorporeal membrane oxygenation may be an effective adjunctive therapy for full-term or large preterm hypoxic infants who are unresponsive to conventional mechanical ventilation.

Adjunctive therapy with currently available intravenous immunoglobulin (IVIG) has not demonstrated marked efficacy, likely because of low levels of protective antibody, although a meta-analysis of studies of IVIG for neonatal sepsis did show a benefit in improved mortality. Hyperimmune IVIG or human monoclonal antibodies would overcome this limitation. Although granulocyte transfusion may be beneficial in neutropenic infants with neutrophil storage pool depletion, there are associated risks (viral infection, pulmonary sequestration, graft versus host disease) and logistical problems. A study of the use of granulocyte colony-stimulating factor (G-CSF) in infants with neutropenia and clinical signs of early-onset sepsis did not show a difference in circulating neutrophils, the neutrophil storage pool, or clinical outcome. It is important to remember that antibody, complement, and phagocytes are required for optimal killing.

COMPLICATIONS. The mortality rate for neonatal GBS disease ranges from 5–15%; the mortality rate is highest in very low birthweight infants and in those with septic shock or a delay in instituting antimicrobial therapy. Because of increased awareness, earlier diagnosis and treatment, and the increased use of intrapartum chemoprophylaxis by obstetricians, the incidence and mortality rates from GBS early-onset disease appear to have declined. The mortality rate from GBS-associated persistent fetal circulation has dramatically decreased owing to the use of extracorporeal membrane oxygenation. Neurologic sequelae after meningitis are severe in 20–30% of cases and include mental retardation, quadriplegia, repeated uncontrollable seizures, hypothalamic dysfunction, cortical blindness, hydrocephalus, bilateral deafness, and hemiplegia. Additional neurodevelopmental sequelae are noted in 15–25% of patients and include mild mental retardation, mild cortical atrophy, a stable seizure disorder, delay in receptive and expressive speech and language development, and other learning disabilities.

Sequelae of focal infections (arthritis, osteomyelitis) are usually localized and are not as significant as those associated with sepsis and meningitis.

PROGNOSIS. Mortality due to GBS disease is currently close to 10%. The principal predictor of mortality and morbidity is septic shock. Periventricular leukomalacia may develop in the absence of meningitis, and survivors have significant developmental delay. Major neurologic sequelae, consisting of cortical blindness, spasticity, and global mental retardation, occur in 12–30% of infants who survive meningitis. Less severe complications include motor deficits, deafness, and mild mental retardation. With the exclusion of these children, survivors of GBS meningitis are comparable to siblings relative to intellectual performance.

PREVENTION. Selective intrapartum chemoprophylaxis (SIC) has been repeatedly demonstrated to decrease the incidence of GBS early-onset disease but not late-onset disease. Intravenous penicillin G [(5 million units initially and then 2.5 million units every 4 hr until delivery)] or ampicillin (2 g initially and then 1 g every 4 hr until delivery) is given immediately to selected women at the onset of labor or when prolongation of membrane rupture is anticipated. Clindamycin (900 mg IV every 8 hr) is recommended for penicillin-allergic mothers. SIC reduces colonization and provides bactericidal levels of penicillin in neonates in the immediate peripartum period. A single dose of penicillin may not prevent colonization of newborns if there is insufficient time (<4 hr) to achieve bactericidal levels in amniotic fluid before delivery. If intrauterine infection of the infant has already occurred, SIC represents initial therapy. Therefore, a few infants will have symptomatic or asymptomatic partially treated early-onset infection.

SIC should be implemented in communities and hospitals where GBS perinatal disease is prevalent. The selection of women for SIC remains controversial, and several strategies have been recommended. In all cases, maternal chorioamnionitis is an indication for treatment of the mother with broad-spectrum antibiotics. In 1996, the Centers for Disease Control and Prevention, the American Academy of Pediatrics, and the American College of Obstetricians and Gynecologists approved consensus recommendations offering a choice between two strategies: (1) SIC based on risk factors, followed by anogenital cultures for group GBS at 35–37 wk of gestation for women without risk factors, or (2) SIC based solely on risk factors (Fig. 185–1). These strategies are not equivalent. Depending on the proportion of prenatally colonized women without risk factors who are identified and who agree to intrapartum penicillin, the first CDC strategy has a predicted efficacy of 60 to 90%. If all colonized women accept chemoprophylaxis, approximately 30% (1.2 million/yr) of all parturients will receive a penicillin and be at risk (estimated to be 0.01%) for fatal anaphylaxis. In contrast, the risk-based approach leads to unnecessary penicillin exposure for four noncolonized women for each colonized woman with a risk factor and has a predicted efficacy of 60%.

All infants whose mothers received SIC should be observed for 48 hr for signs of infection. Individual circumstances may indicate the need for a full or limited evaluation and empirical therapy (Fig. 185–2). Symptomatic newborn infants require diagnostic evaluations and antimicrobial therapy. If the mother of a symptomatic infant was treated with an antibiotic for longer than 24 hr, the possibility of an antibiotic-resistant infection should be considered. If evidence supports a neonatal infection, treatment should be continued for 5–7 days. If an infant remains well, laboratory test results are normal, and cultures are negative, it is possible to discontinue antibiotics and discharge the baby. If the mother had chorioamnionitis and her infant is asymptomatic, the infant's blood culture should be negative because an antibiotic-resistant infection is unlikely. If the mother did not have chorioamnionitis but received SIC for risk factors or a positive culture, then intrauterine infection of the infant is very unlikely and SIC should be sufficient (Fig. 185–2).

An alternative algorithm for mothers and infants to the CDC algorithms employs a combined approach. Women with chorioamnionitis, labor <35 wk, and positive or unknown culture status with risk factors are selected for antimicrobial intervention, *and* asymptomatic newborns of women with positive or unknown culture status receive 50,000 units of penicillin G intramuscularly prophylactically at birth regardless of risk factors or maternal chemoprophylaxis (Fig. 185–3). The predicted efficacy of this combined strategy is 90%, but fewer women would receive penicillin, lowering the risk of reactions.

Other approaches to prevention of GBS infection are much less attractive. Attempts to eradicate GBS colonization during pregnancy have been ineffective. Neonatal prophylaxis alone does not prevent infections acquired in utero. Rapid antigen detection of vaginal GBS at the time of labor is less sensitive than culture and does not allow enough time for SIC.

In theory, early- and late-onset GBS disease might be prevented by immunoprophylaxis. Because colonized mothers, and thus infants with GBS infection, often lack type-specific IgG antibody, it has been proposed that active immunization of the mother or possibly passive IgG administration to the newborn infant might prevent GBS disease. Sera containing type-specific antibody facilitate opsonophagocytosis against the individual GBS type in the presence of complement and neutrophils. Passive immune therapy would require development of hyperimmune type-specific GBS sera because the currently available commercial preparations of standard IVIG have variable and potentially inadequate levels of GBS IgG antibody. Type-specific active immunization is possible using purified capsular polysaccharides from type Ia, II, or III strains. Pregnant women without demonstrable antibodies to GBS respond to injection of type III-specific polysaccharide conjugate

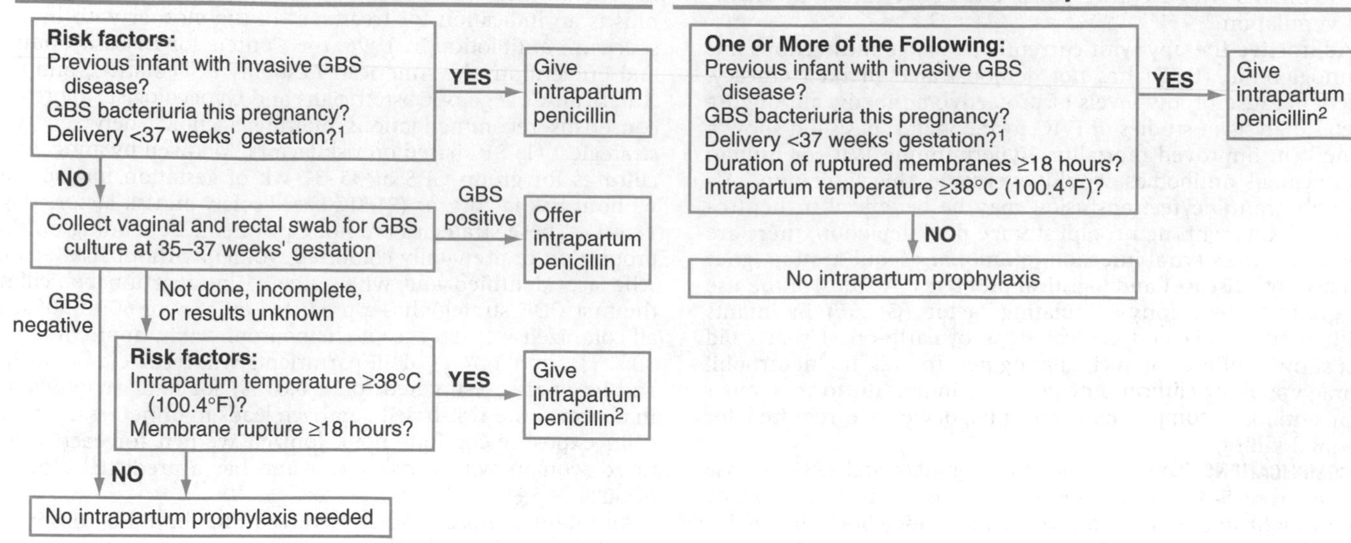

Risk Factor and Culture-Based Screening
Risk factors:
Previous infant with invasive GBS disease?
GBS bacteriuria this pregnancy?
Delivery <37 weeks' gestation?1
YES
Give intrapartum penicillin
NO
Collect vaginal and rectal swab for GBS culture at 35–37 weeks' gestation
GBS positive
Offer intrapartum penicillin
GBS negative
Not done, incomplete, or results unknown
Risk factors:
Intrapartum temperature ≥38°C (100.4°F)?
Membrane rupture ≥18 hours?
YES
Give intrapartum penicillin2
NO
No intrapartum prophylaxis needed
Risk Factors Only
One or More of the Following:
Previous infant with invasive GBS disease?
GBS bacteriuria this pregnancy?
Delivery <37 weeks' gestation?1
Duration of ruptured membranes ≥18 hours?
Intrapartum temperature ≥38°C (100.4°F)?
YES
Give intrapartum penicillin2
NO
No intrapartum prophylaxis

[1]If membranes rupture at <37 wks' gestation, and the mother has not begun labor, collect GBS culture and either (a) administer antibotics until cultures are completed and the results are negative, or (b) begin antibotics only when cultures become positive. No prophylaxis is needed if culture obtained at 35–37 wks' gestation was negative.

[2]Broad-spectrum antibotics may be considered at the discretion of the physician based on clinical indications.

Figure 185–1 The Centers for Disease Control and Prevention algorithms for prevention of group B *Streptococcus* (GBS) infections using risk factors and culture-based screening *(left)* or risk factors only *(right)*. (Adapted from Centers for Disease Control and Prevention: Prevention of perinatal group B streptococcal disease: A public health perspective. MMWR 45[RR-7]:16, 19, 1996.)

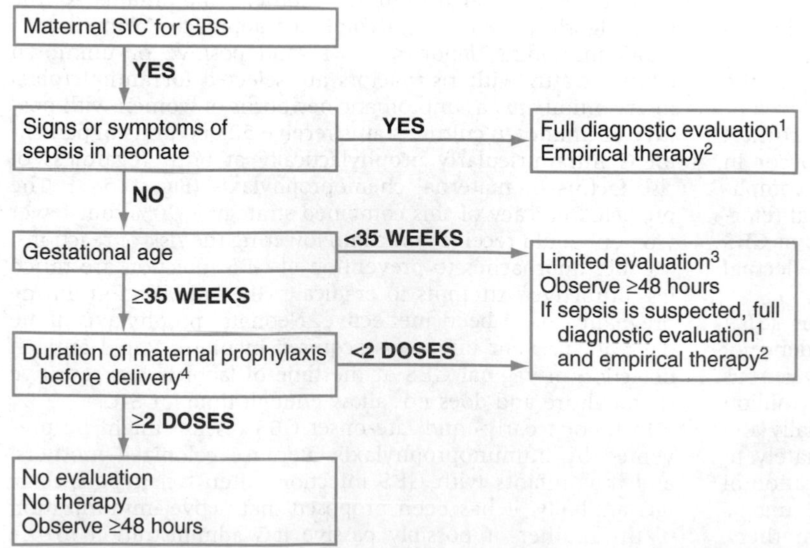

Maternal SIC for GBS
YES
Signs or symptoms of sepsis in neonate
YES
Full diagnostic evaluation1
Empirical therapy2
NO
Gestational age
<35 WEEKS
Limited evaluation3
Observe ≥48 hours
If sepsis is suspected, full diagnostic evaluation1 and empirical therapy2
≥35 WEEKS
Duration of maternal prophylaxis before delivery4
<2 DOSES
≥2 DOSES
No evaluation
No therapy
Observe ≥48 hours

[1]Includes CBC and differential, blood culture, and chest radiograph if respiratory symptoms are present. A lumbar puncture is performed at the discretion of the physician.
[2]Duration of therapy will vary depending on results of blood culture and CSF findings (if obtained), as well as on the clinical course of the infant. If laboratory results and clinical course are unremarkable, duration may be as short as 48–72 hours.
[3]CBC and differential, blood cultures.
[4]Duration of penicillin or ampicillin chemoprophylaxis. Duration relates to number of doses administered; one dose is given every 4 hr.

Figure 185–2 Management of the neonate whose mother received group B *Streptococcus* (GBS) intrapartum prophylaxis according to the Centers for Disease Control and Prevention prevention algorithms (see Fig. 185–1). SIC = selective intrapartum chemoprophylaxis. CBC = complete blood count; CSF, cerebrospinal fluid. (Adapted from Centers for Disease Control and Prevention: Prevention of perinatal group B streptococcal disease: A public health perspective. MMWR 45[RR-7]:20, 1996 [published erratum appears in MMWR 45:679, 1996].)

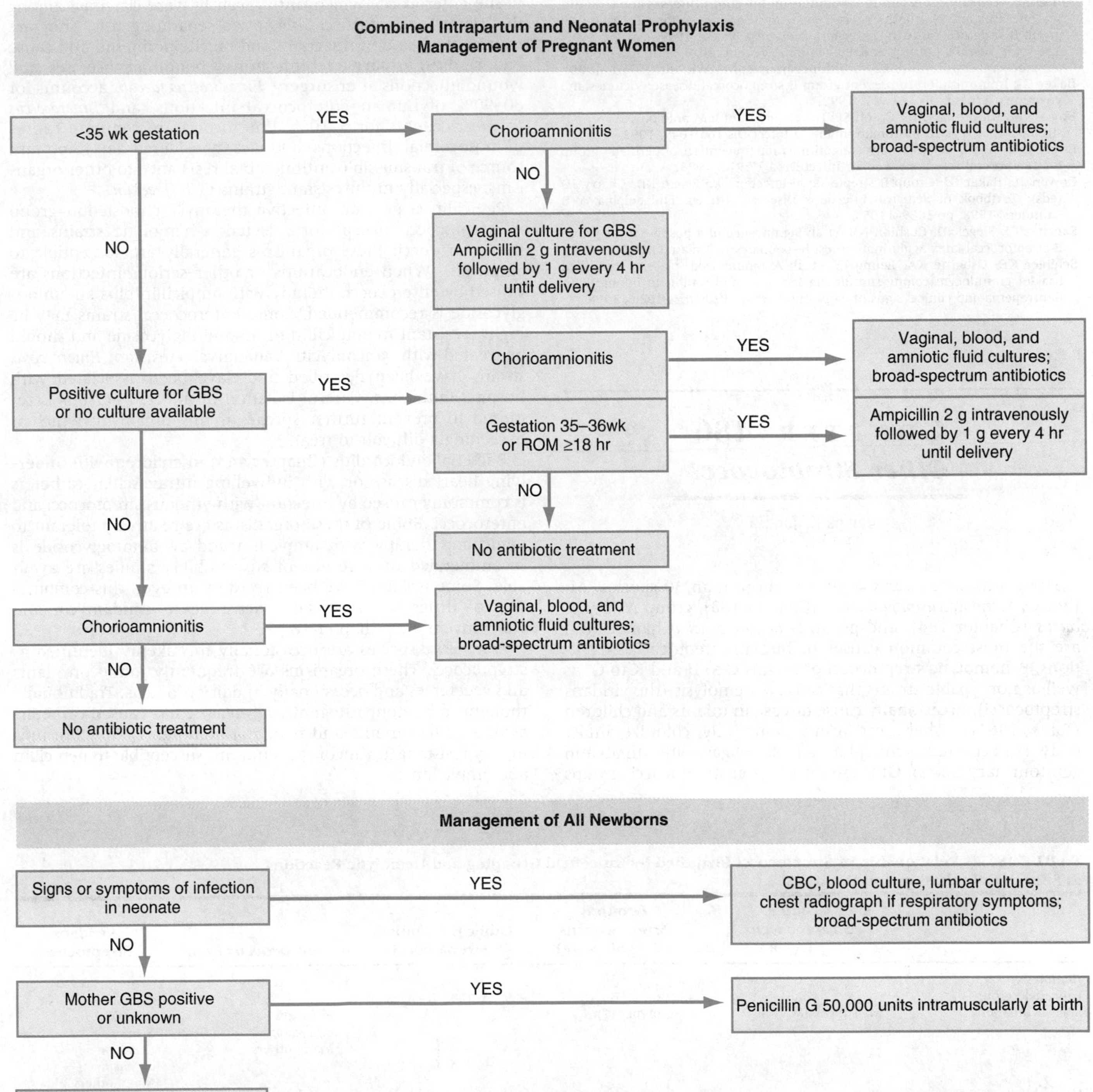

Figure 185–3 An alternative algorithm for prevention of group B *Streptococcus* (GBS) infections, combining intrapartum and neonatal prophylaxis. Infants born to women with probable or confirmed chorioamnionitis should be evaluated with a complete blood count (CBC) and blood culture and treated with broad-spectrum antibiotics. Infants of mothers with possible chorioamnionitis should be considered for neonatal chemoprophylaxis without diagnostic evaluation. (Adapted from Boyer KM, Gotoff SP: Alternative algorithms for prevention of perinatal group B streptococcal infections. Pediatr Infect Dis J 17:973, 1998.)

vaccines with a significant rise in antibody, which is transferred to cord sera and persists for 1–2 mo in the infant. Clinical trials are in progress.

American Academy of Pediatrics, Committee on Infectious Diseases and Committee on Fetus and Newborn: Revised guidelines for prevention of early-onset group B streptococcal (GBS) infection. Pediatrics 99:489, 1997.

Centers for Disease Control and Prevention: Prevention of perinatal group B streptococcal disease: A public health perspective. MMWR 45(RR-7):1, 1996.

Baker CJ: Immunization to prevent group B streptococcal disease: Victories and vexations. J Infect Dis 161:917, 1990.

Boyer KM, Klegerman ME, Gotoff SP: Development of IgM antibody to group B streptococcus type III in human infants. J Infect Dis 165:1049, 1992.

Boyer KM, Gotoff SP: Alternative algorithms for prevention of perinatal group B streptococcal infections. Pediatr Infect Dis J 17:973, 1998.

Rowen JL, Baker CJ: Group B streptococcal infection. *In*: Feigin RD, Cherry JD (eds): Textbook of Pediatric Infectious Diseases, 4th ed. Philadelphia, WB Saunders, 1998, pp 1089–1105.

Sanchez PJ, Siegel JD, Cushion NB, et al: Significance of a positive urine group B streptococcal latex agglutination test in neonates. J Pediatr 116:601, 1990.

Schibler KR, Osborne KA, Leung LY, et al: A randomized, placebo-controlled trial of granulocyte colony-stimulating factor administration to infants with neutropenia and clinical signs of early-onset sepsis. Pediatrics 102:6, 1998.

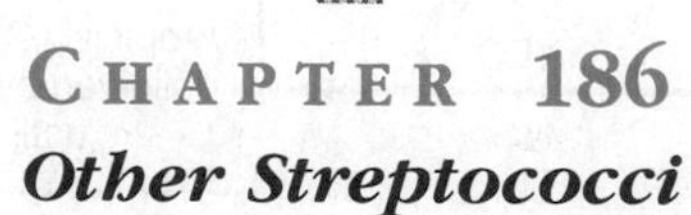

CHAPTER 186
Other Streptococci

James K. Todd

The genus *Streptococcus* comprises more than 30 species. Although *Streptococcus pneumoniae* (Chapter 183), group A *Streptococcus* (Chapter 184), and group B *Streptococcus* (Chapter 185) are the most common causes of human streptococcal infections, β-hemolytic streptococci of groups C to H and K to O, as well as nontypable strains that cause α-hemolysis (the viridans streptococci), occasionally cause disease in infants and children (Table 186–1). These organisms commonly colonize intact body surfaces (e.g., the pharynx, skin, gastrointestinal and genitourinary tracts). Of these uncommon streptococci, groups D and G most frequently cause human disease. They act as opportunists, causing infections such as endocarditis on damaged heart valves, cellulitis after human bites, or surgical wound infections.

The enterococci, which until recently were classified among the group D streptococci, are now a separate genus. They are commonly found in the colon and on the perineum and cause endocarditis, urinary tract infections, abdominal abscesses, and wound infections after surgery. *Enterococcus faecalis* accounts for 80–90% of human enterococcal infections, and *Enterococcus faecium* accounts for 5–10%. Enterococci are common causes of nosocomial infections and are considered an important source of transmissible antimicrobial resistance to other organisms, especially multiresistant strains of *E. faecium*.

Penicillin G provides effective therapy for most non–group A streptococci, except for selected α-hemolytic strains and the enterococci; these organisms generally are susceptible to ampicillin. When endocarditis or other serious infections are caused by enterococci, therapy with ampicillin plus an aminoglycoside is recommended. Some enterococcal strains may be highly resistant to ampicillin or an aminoglycoside and should be treated with vancomycin. Vancomycin-resistant *Enterococcus* strains have been described and have been associated with hospital outbreaks. Careful isolation of infected persons is required to prevent further spread of this organism, which is exceedingly difficult to treat.

Bacterial endocarditis (Chapter 443) in children with underlying heart disease or with indwelling intravascular catheters is commonly caused by infection with viridans streptococci and enterococci. Some of these organisms are relatively tolerant to penicillin; therapy with ampicillin and an aminoglycoside is recommended until results of susceptibility studies are available. Some isolates have been resistant to even this combination of drugs but have been sensitive to clindamycin and vancomycin. See Chapter 182.1.

Leuconostoc species are occasionally mistakenly identified as streptococci. These organisms are frequently found on plants and vegetables and occasionally in dairy products. Traditionally thought to be nonpathogenic, *Leuconostoc* has caused catheter-associated bacteremia and neonatal meningitis. They are uniformly resistant to vancomycin but are susceptible to penicillin and ampicillin.

TABLE 186–1 Relationship of Streptococci Identified by Lancefield Grouping and Hemolytic Reactions to Sites of Colonization and Disease

	Group A *Streptococcus* (*S. pyogenes*)	Group B *Streptococcus* (*S. agalactiae*)	Other β-Hemolytic Streptococci	*Enterococcus* spp.	Viridans Streptococci
Hemolysis	β	β	β	α, β, γ	α
Lancefield group	A	B	C–H, K–V		
Species or strains	M, T types (80)	Serotypes (7)		*E. faecalis* *E. faecium* Many others	*S. bovis* *S. mitis* *S. mutans* *S. sanguis* Many others
Normal flora	Pharynx, skin, anus	Gastrointestinal and genitourinary tracts	Pharynx, skin, gastrointestinal and genitourinary tracts	Gastrointestinal and genitourinary tracts	Pharynx, nose, skin, genitourinary tract
Common human diseases	Pharyngitis, tonsillitis, erysipelas, impetigo, septicemia, wound infections, necrotizing fasciitis, cellulitis, meningitis, pneumonia, scarlet fever, toxic shock–like syndrome, rheumatic fever, acute glomerulonephritis	Puerperal sepsis, chorioamnionitis, endocarditis, neonatal sepsis, meningitis, osteomyelitis, pneumonia	Wound infections, puerperal sepsis, cellulitis, sinusitis, endocarditis, brain abscess, sepsis, nosocomial infections, opportunistic infections	Endocarditis, urinary tract infections, biliary tract infections, peritonitis, wound infections	Endocarditis, human bite infections

α = partial hemolysis; β = complete hemolysis; γ = no hemolysis (nonhemolytic).

Centers for Disease Control and Prevention: Recommendations for preventing the spread of vancomycin resistance. Recommendations of the Hospital Infection Control Practices Advisory Committee (HICPAC). MMWR 44(RR-12):1, 1995.

Nourse C, Murphy H, Byrne C, et al: Control of a nosocomial outbreak of vancomycin resistant *Enterococcus faecium* in a paediatric oncology unit: Risk factors for colonisation. Eur J Pediatr 157:20, 1998.

Pfaller MA, Jones RN, Marshall SA, et al: Nosocomial streptococcal blood stream infections in the SCOPE Program: Species occurrence and antimicrobial resistance. The SCOPE Hospital Study Group. Diagn Microbiol Infect Dis 29:259, 1997.

Shay DK, Goldmann DA, Jarvis JW, et al: Reducing the spread of antimicrobial-resistant microorganisms: Control of vancomycin-resistant enterococci. Pediatr Clin North Am 42:703, 1995.

Tuohy M, Washington JA: Antimicrobial susceptibility of viridans group streptococci. Diagn Microbiol Infect Dis 29:277, 1997.

Wilson WR, Karchmer AW, Dajani AS, et al: Antibiotic treatment of adults with infective endocarditis due to streptococci, enterococci, staphylococci, and HACEK microorganisms. American Heart Association. JAMA 274:1706, 1995.

CHAPTER 187

Diphtheria (Corynebacterium diphtheriae)

Sarah S. Long

Diphtheria is an acute toxicoinfection caused by *Corynebacterium diphtheriae*. Diphtheria was the first infectious disease to be conquered on the basis of principles of microbiology and public health. Although diphtheria was reduced from a major cause of childhood death in the West in the early 20th century to a medical rarity, modern reminders of the fragility of such success underscore the need to apply those same principles assiduously in an era of vaccine dependence and a single global community.

ETIOLOGY. *Corynebacterium* species are aerobic, nonencapsulated, non–spore-forming, mostly nonmotile, pleomorphic, gram-positive bacilli. Not fastidious in growth requirements, their isolation is enhanced by selective media (i.e., cystine-tellurite blood agar) that inhibit growth of competing organisms and, when reduced by *C. dipththeriae*, renders colonies gray-black. Three biotypes (i.e., *mitis, gravis,* and *intermedius*), each capable of causing diphtheria, are differentiated by colonial morphology, hemolysis, and fermentation reactions. A lysogenic bacteriophage carrying the gene that encodes for production of exotoxin confers diphtheria-producing potential to strains of *C. diphtheriae*, but it provides no essential protein to the bacterium. Investigation of outbreaks of diphtheria in England and the United States using a molecular technique suggested that indigenous nontoxigenic *C. diphtheriae* had been rendered toxigenic and disease producing after importation of toxigenic *C. diphtheriae*. Diphtheritic toxin can be demonstrated in vitro by the agar immunoprecipitin technique (Elek test), by polymerase chain reaction, or by the in vivo toxin neutralization test in guinea pigs (lethality test). Toxigenic strains are indistinguishable by colony type, microscopy, or biochemical tests.

EPIDEMIOLOGY. Unlike other diphtheroids (coryneform bacteria), which are ubiquitous in nature, *C. diphtheriae* is an exclusive inhabitant of human mucous membranes and skin. Spread is primarily by airborne respiratory droplets, direct contact with respiratory secretions of symptomatic individuals, or exudate from infected skin lesions. Asymptomatic respiratory tract carriers are important in transmission. Where diphtheria is endemic, 3–5% of healthy individuals may harbor toxigenic organisms, but carriage is exceedingly rare if diphtheria is rare. Skin infection and skin carriage are silent reservoirs of diphtheria. Viability in dust and on fomites for up to 6 mo has less epidemiologic significance. Transmission through contaminated milk and an infected food handler has been proved or suspected.

In the 1920s, more than 125,000 cases and 10,000 deaths due to diphtheria were reported annually in the United States, with highest fatality rates among very young and elderly patients. From 1921–1924, diphtheria was the leading cause of death among Canadian children 2–14 yr of age. The incidence began to fall, and with the widespread use of diphtheria toxoid in the United States after World War II, it declined steadily, with dramatic reductions in the latter 1970s. Since then, there have been zero to five cases per year and no epidemics of respiratory tract diphtheria. Similar decreases have occurred in Europe. Although disease incidence has fallen worldwide, diphtheria remains endemic in many developing countries. The sustained low incidence of diphtheria and high level of childhood vaccination have led authorities to set a goal to eliminate diphtheria among persons 25 yr of age or younger in the United States by the year 2000.

When diphtheria was endemic, it primarily affected children younger than 15 yr, but epidemiology has shifted to adults who lack natural exposure to toxigenic *C. diphtheriae* in the vaccine era and have low rates of booster vaccinations. In the 27 sporadic cases of respiratory tract diphtheria reported in the United States in the 1980s, 70% occurred in persons older than 25 yr. The largest outbreak of diphtheria in the developed world since the 1960s occurred from 1990–1995 throughout the states of the former Soviet Union, where more than 47,000 cases and 1,700 deaths occurred in 1994 alone. This outbreak was due to lack of immunization, use of suboptimal antigen dose, and social factors (including population movements). Most affected individuals were older than 14 yr. Smaller epidemiologically similar outbreaks followed in Denmark and Sweden. Since 1994, public health authorities in the Russian federation have initiated aggressive efforts to vaccinate adults, and in 1995 the number of reported cases decreased.

Most proven cases of respiratory tract diphtheria in the United States in the past decade have been associated with importation of toxigenic *C. diphtheriae*, the organism believed to have become rare or to have disappeared from the United States. Enhanced surveillance surrounding the rare indigenous cases, however, shows that *C. diphtheriae* can continue to circulate in areas with previously endemic diphtheria. Protection from serious disease depends on immunization.

The estimated minimum protective level of diphtheria antitoxin is 0.01 IU/mL. It has been considered advisable that an antitoxin level of at least 0.1 IU/mL should be achieved after primary immunization to secure long-term protection. In serosurveys, in the United States and other developed countries with almost universal immunization during childhood, such as Sweden, Italy, and Denmark, significant percentages of adults and especially the elderly lack protective antitoxin levels. Booster doses of diphtheria-containing vaccine are recommended every 10 yr for adults in the United States.

Cutaneous diphtheria, a curiosity when diphtheria was common, accounted for more than 50% of *C. diphtheriae* isolates reported in the United States by 1975 and featured prominently in the changing epidemiology of diphtheria in the 1990s. An indolent local infection with infrequent toxic complications, cutaneous infection, compared with mucosal infection, is associated with more prolonged bacterial shedding, increased contamination of the environment, and increased transmission to the pharynx and skin of close contacts. Outbreaks are associated with homelessness, crowding, poverty, alcoholism, poor hygiene, contaminated fomites, underlying dermatosis, and introduction of new strains from exogenous sources. No longer a tropical or subtropical disease, 1,100 *C. diphtheriae* infections were documented in a neighborhood in Seattle, Washington, from 1971–1982; 86% were cutaneous, and 40% involved toxigenic strains. Cutaneous diphtheria is the important reservoir for toxigenic *C. diphtheriae* in the United States and a frequent mode of importation of source cases for subsequent sporadic respiratory tract diphtheria. In an attempt to focus attention on respiratory tract diphtheria, which is much more likely to cause acute obstructive complications and toxic manifestations, skin isolates of *C. diphtheriae* were removed from annual diphtheria statistics reported by the Centers for Disease Control and Prevention (CDC) after 1979.

PATHOGENESIS. Toxigenic and nontoxigenic *C. diphtheriae* organisms cause skin and mucosal infection and some cases of distant infection after bacteremia. The organism usually remains in the superficial layers of skin lesions or respiratory tract mucosa, inducing local inflammatory reaction. The major virulence of the organism lies in its ability to produce the potent 62-kd polypeptide exotoxin, which inhibits protein synthesis and causes local tissue necrosis. Within the first few days of respiratory tract infection, a dense necrotic coagulum of organisms, epithelial cells, fibrin, leukocytes, and erythrocytes forms, advances, and becomes a gray-brown adherent pseudomembrane. Removal is difficult and reveals a bleeding edematous submucosa. Paralysis of the palate and hypopharynx is an early local effect of the toxin. Toxin absorption can lead to necrosis of kidney tubules, thrombocytopenia, cardiomyopathy, and demyelination of nerves. Because the latter two complications can occur 2–10 wk after mucocutaneous infection, the pathophysiologic mechanism in some cases may be immunologically mediated.

CLINICAL MANIFESTATIONS. The manifestations of *C. diphtheriae* infection are influenced by the anatomic site of infection, the immune status of the host, and the production and systemic distribution of toxin.

Respiratory Tract Diphtheria. In the classic description of 1,400 cases of diphtheria in California in 1954, the primary focus of infection was the tonsils or pharynx in 94%, with the nose and larynx the next two most common sites. After an average incubation period of 2–4 days, local signs and symptoms of inflammation develop. Temperature is rarely higher than 39°C. Infection of the anterior nares (more common in infants) causes serosanguineous, purulent, erosive rhinitis with membrane formation. Shallow ulceration of the external nares and upper lip is characteristic. In tonsillar and pharyngeal diphtheria, sore throat is a universal early symptom, but only half of patients have fever, and fewer have dysphagia, hoarseness, malaise, or headache. Mild pharyngeal injection is followed by unilateral or bilateral tonsillar membrane formation, which extends variably to affect the uvula, soft palate, posterior oropharynx, hypopharynx, and glottic areas. Underlying soft tissue edema and enlarged lymph nodes can cause a bull-neck appearance. The degree of local extension correlates directly with profound prostration, bull-neck appearance, and fatality due to airway compromise or toxin-mediated complications.

The leather-like adherent membrane, extension beyond the faucial area, relative lack of fever, and dysphagia help differentiate diphtheria from exudative pharyngitis due to *Streptococcus pyogenes* and Epstein-Barr virus. Vincent's angina, infective phlebitis and thrombosis of the jugular veins, and mucositis in patients undergoing cancer chemotherapy are usually differentiated by the clinical setting. Infection of the larynx, trachea, and bronchi can be primary or a secondary extension from the pharyngeal infection. Hoarseness, stridor, dyspnea, and croupy cough are clues. Differentiation from bacterial epiglottitis, severe viral laryngotracheobronchitis, and staphylococcal or streptococcal tracheitis hinges partially on the relative paucity of other signs and symptoms in patients with diphtheria and primarily on visualization of the adherent pseudomembrane at the time of laryngoscopy and intubation.

Patients with laryngeal diphtheria are highly prone to suffocation because of edema of soft tissues and the obstructing dense cast of respiratory epithelium and necrotic coagulum. Establishment of an artificial airway and resection of the pseudomembrane are lifesaving, but further obstructive complications are common, and systemic toxic complications are inevitable.

Cutaneous Diphtheria. Classic cutaneous diphtheria is an indolent, nonprogressive infection characterized by a superficial, ecthymic, nonhealing ulcer with a gray-brown membrane. Diphtheritic skin infections cannot always be differentiated from streptococcal or staphylococcal impetigo, and they frequently coexist. In most cases, underlying dermatoses, lacerations, burns, bites, or impetigo have become secondarily contaminated. Extremities are more often affected than the trunk or head. Pain, tenderness, erythema, and exudate are typical. Local hyperesthesia or hypesthesia is unusual. Respiratory tract colonization or symptomatic infection and toxic complications occur in the minority of patients with cutaneous diphtheria. Among infected Seattle adults, 3% with cutaneous infections and 21% with symptomatic nasopharyngeal infection, with or without skin involvement, had toxic myocarditis, neuropathy, or obstructive respiratory tract complications. All had received at least 20,000 U of equine antitoxin at the time of hospitalization.

Infection at Other Sites. *C. diphtheriae* occasionally causes mucocutaneous infections at other sites, such as the ear (otitis externa), eye (purulent and ulcerative conjunctivitis), and genital tract (purulent and ulcerative vulvovaginitis). The clinical setting, ulceration, membrane formation, and submucosal bleeding help differentiate diphtheria from other bacterial and viral causes. Rare cases of septicemia are described and are universally fatal. Sporadic cases of endocarditis occur, and clusters among intravenous drug users have been reported in several countries; skin was the probable portal of entry, and almost all strains were nontoxigenic. Sporadic cases of pyogenic arthritis, mainly due to nontoxigenic strains, are reported in adults and children. Diphtheroids isolated from sterile body sites should not be dismissed as contaminants without careful consideration of the clinical setting.

Toxic Cardiomyopathy. Toxic cardiomyopathy occurs in approximately 10–25% of patients with diphtheria and is responsible for 50–60% of deaths. Subtle signs of myocarditis can be detected in most patients, especially the elderly, but the risk for significant complications correlates directly with the extent and severity of exudative local oropharyngeal disease and delay in administration of antitoxin. The first evidence of cardiac toxicity characteristically occurs in the 2nd–3rd wk of illness as pharyngeal disease improves but can appear acutely as early as the 1st wk, when a fatal outcome is likely, or insidiously as late as the 6th wk of illness. Tachycardia out of proportion to fever is common and may be evidence of cardiac toxicity or autonomic nervous system dysfunction. A prolonged PR interval and changes in the ST-T wave on an electrocardiographic tracing are relatively frequent findings, and dilated and hypertrophic cardiomyopathy detected by echocardiogram have been described. Single or progressive cardiac dysrhythmias can occur, such as first-, second-, and third-degree heart block; atrioventricular dissociation; and ventricular tachycardia. Clinical congestive heart failure may have an insidious or acute onset. Elevation of the serum aspartate aminotransferase concentration closely parallels the severity of myonecrosis. Severe dysrhythmia portends death. Histologic postmortem findings may show little or diffuse myonecrosis with acute inflammatory response. Survivors of more severe dysrhythmias can have permanent conduction defects; for others, recovery from toxic myocardiopathy is usually complete.

Toxic Neuropathy. Neurologic complications parallel the extent of primary infection and are multiphasic in onset. Acutely or 2–3 wk after onset of oropharyngeal inflammation, hypesthesia and local paralysis of the soft palate occur commonly. Weakness of the posterior pharyngeal, laryngeal, and facial nerves may follow, causing a nasal quality in the voice, difficulty in swallowing, and risk of death due to aspiration. Cranial neuropathies characteristically occur in the 5th wk and lead to oculomotor and ciliary paralysis, which are manifested as strabismus, blurred vision, or difficulty with accommodation. Symmetric polyneuropathy has its onset 10 days–3 mo after oropharyngeal infection and causes principally motor deficits with diminished deep tendon reflexes. Proximal muscle weakness of the extremities progressing distally and, more commonly, distal weakness progressing proximally are described. Clinical and cerebrospinal fluid findings in the latter are indistinguishable from those of polyneuropathy of Guillain-Barré syndrome. Paralysis of the diaphragm can ensue. Complete recovery is likely. Rarely, 2–3 wk after onset of illness, dysfunction of the vasomotor centers can cause hypotension or cardiac failure.

DIAGNOSIS. Specimens for culture should be obtained from the nose and throat and any other mucocutaneous lesion. A portion of membrane should be removed and submitted with underlying exudate. The laboratory must be notified to use selective medium. *C. diphtheriae* survives drying. In remote areas, a swab specimen can be placed in a silica gel pack and sent to a reference laboratory. Evaluation of a direct smear using Gram stain or specific fluorescent antibody is unreliable. Culture isolates of coryneform organisms should be identified to the species level, and toxigenicity and antimicrobial susceptibility tests should be performed for *C. diphtheriae* isolates.

TREATMENT. Specific antitoxin is the mainstay of therapy and should be administered on the basis of clinical diagnosis, because it neutralizes only free toxin. Efficacy diminishes with elapsing time after the onset of mucocutaneous symptoms. Diphtheria antitoxin is no longer commercially available in the United States but may be obtained for treatment of suspected cases of diphtheria through the CDC (24-hr telephone [404] 639–2889). Antitoxin is administered once at empirical dose based on the degree of toxicity, site and size of the membrane, and duration of illness. Antitoxin is probably of no value for local manifestations of cutaneous diphtheria, but its use is prudent because toxic sequelae can occur. Commercially available immunoglobulin preparations for intravenous use contain low titers of antibodies to diphtheria toxin; their use for therapy of diphtheria is not proved or approved. Antitoxin is not recommended for asymptomatic carriers.

Antimicrobial therapy is indicated to halt toxin production, treat localized infection, and prevent transmission of the organism to contacts. *C. diphtheriae* is usually susceptible to various agents in vitro, including penicillins, erythromycin, clindamycin, rifampin, and tetracycline. Resistance to erythromycin is common in closed populations if the drug has been used broadly. Only penicillin or erythromycin is recommended; erythromycin is marginally superior to penicillin for eradication of nasopharyngeal carriage. Appropriate therapy is erythromycin given orally or parenterally (40–50 mg/kg/24 hr; maximum, 2 g/24 hr), aqueous crystalline penicillin G given intramuscularly or intravenously (100,000–150,000 U/kg/24 hr divided in four doses), or procaine penicillin (25,000–50,000 U/kg/24 hr divided in two doses) given intramuscularly. Antibiotic therapy is not a substitute for antitoxin therapy. Therapy is given for 14 days. Some patients with cutaneous diphtheria have been treated for 7–10 days. Elimination of the organism should be documented by at least two successive cultures from the nose and throat (or skin) taken 24 hr apart after completion of therapy. Treatment with erythromycin is repeated if the culture result is positive.

Patients with pharyngeal diphtheria are placed in respiratory isolation, and patients with cutaneous diphtheria are placed in contact isolation until the cultures taken after cessation of therapy are negative. Cutaneous wounds are cleaned thoroughly with soap and water. Bed rest is essential during the acute phase of disease, usually for at least 2 wk until the risk of symptomatic cardiac damage has passed, with a return to physical activity guided by the degree of toxicity and cardiac involvement.

COMPLICATIONS. Respiratory tract obstruction by pseudomembranes may require bronchoscopy or intubation and mechanical ventilation to maintain a patent airway. Recovery from the myocarditis and neuritis is often slow but usually complete. Corticosteroids do not diminish these complications and are not recommended.

PROGNOSIS. The prognosis for patients with diphtheria depends on the virulence of the organism (subspecies *gravis* has the highest fatality), age, immunization status, site of infection, and speed of administration of the antitoxin. Mechanical obstruction from laryngeal diphtheria or bull-neck diphtheria and the complications of myocarditis account for most diphtheria-related deaths. The case-fatality rate of almost 10% for respiratory tract diphtheria has not changed in 50 yr; the rate was 18% in the Swedish outbreak. At recovery, administration of diphtheria toxoid is indicated to complete the primary series or booster doses of immunization, because not all patients develop antibodies after infection.

PREVENTION. Local public health officials should be notified promptly when a diagnosis of diphtheria is suspected or proved. Investigation is aimed at preventing secondary cases in exposed individuals and at determining the source and carriers to halt spread to unexposed individuals. Reported rates of carriage in household contacts of case patients have been 0–25%. The risk of developing diphtheria after household exposure to a case is approximately 2%, and the risk is 0.3% after similar exposure to a carrier.

Asymptomatic Case Contacts. All household contacts and those who have had intimate respiratory or habitual physical contact with a patient are closely monitored for illness through the 7-day incubation period. Cultures of the nose, throat, and any cutaneous lesions are performed. Antimicrobial prophylaxis is given, regardless of immunization status, using oral erythromycin (40–50 mg/kg/24 hr for 7–10 days; maximum, 2 g/24 hr) or, if intolerant of erythromycin or if complete compliance is not ensured, using intramuscular benzathine penicillin (600,000 U for those <30 kg or 1,200,000 U for those ≥30 kg). The efficacy of antimicrobial prophylaxis is presumed but not proved. Diphtheria toxoid vaccine, in age-appropriate form, is given to immunized individuals who have not received a booster dose within 5 yr. Some experts suggest that the longevity of protective antibody is variable enough that a booster should be given to close contacts if 1 yr has elapsed since immunization. Children who have not received their fourth dose should be vaccinated. Those who have received fewer than three doses of diphtheria toxoid or with uncertain immunization status are immunized with age-appropriate preparation on a primary schedule.

Asymptomatic Carriers. When an asymptomatic carrier is identified, antimicrobial prophylaxis is given for 7–10 days and an age-appropriate preparation of diphtheria toxoid is administered immediately if a booster has not been given within 1 yr. Individuals are placed in respiratory isolation (respiratory tract colonization) or contact isolation (cutaneous colonization only) until at least two subsequent cultures taken 24 hr apart after cessation of therapy are negative. Repeat cultures are performed 2 wk or more after completion of therapy for cases and carriers, and if positive, an additional 10-day course of oral erythromycin should be given and follow-up cultures performed. Neither antimicrobial agent eradicates carriage in 100% of individuals. In one report, 21% of carriers had failure of eradication after a single course of therapy. Antitoxin is not recommended for asymptomatic close contacts or carriers, even if inadequately immunized. Transmission of diphtheria in modern hospitals is rare. Only those with an unusual contact with respiratory or oral secretions should be managed as contacts. Investigation of the casual contacts of patients and carriers or persons in the community without known exposure has yielded extremely low carriage rates and is not routinely recommended.

Vaccine. Universal immunization with diphtheria toxoid throughout life to provide constant protective antitoxin levels and to reduce indigenous *C. diphtheriae* is the only effective control measure. Although immunization does not preclude subsequent respiratory or cutaneous carriage of toxigenic *C. diphtheriae*, it decreases local tissue spread, prevents toxic complications, diminishes transmission of the organism, and provides herd immunity when at least 70–80% of a population is immunized. Serum antitoxin concentration of 0.01 IU/mL is conventionally accepted as the minimum protective level, and 0.1 IU/mL provides the certain protective level.

Diphtheria toxoid is prepared by formaldehyde treatment of toxin, standardized for potency, and adsorbed to aluminum salts, which enhance immunogenicity. Two preparations of diphtheria toxoids are formulated according to the limit of flocculation (Lf) content, a measure of the quantity of toxoid. The pediatric preparation (i.e., DTaP, DT, DTP) contains 6.7–12.5 Lf units of diphtheria toxoid per 0.5-mL dose; the adult preparation (i.e., Td) contains no more than 2 Lf units of toxoid per 0.5-mL dose. The higher-potency (i.e., D) formulation of toxoid is used for primary series and booster doses for children through 6 yr of age because of superior immunogenicity and minimal reactogenicity. For individuals 7 yr of age and older, Td is recommended for the primary series and booster doses, because the lower concentration of diphtheria toxoid is adequately immunogenic and because increasing the content of diphtheria toxoid heightens reactogenicity with increasing age.

For children from 6 wk to the seventh birthday, five 0.5-mL doses of diphtheria-containing (D) vaccine are given in a primary series, including three doses at approximately 2, 4, and 6 mo of age, with a fourth dose, an integral part of the primary series, at 6–12 mo after the third dose. A booster dose is given at 4–6 yr (unless the fourth primary dose was administered after the fourth birthday). For persons 7 yr of age or older, three 0.5-mL doses of diphtheria-containing (D) vaccine are given in a primary series of two doses 4–8 wk apart and a third dose 6–12 mo after the second dose. The only contraindication to tetanus and diphtheria toxoid is a history of neurologic or severe hypersensitivity reaction after a previous dose. For children in whom pertussis immunization is contraindicated, DT or Td is used. Those begun with DTaP, DTP, or DT at before 1 yr of age should have a total of five 0.5-mL doses of diphtheria-containing (D) vaccines by 6 yr. For those beginning at or after 1 yr of age, the primary series is three 0.5-mL doses of diphtheria-containing (D) vaccine, with a booster given at 4–6 yr, unless the third dose was given after the fourth birthday.

Further reduction in the number of cases of diphtheria in industrialized countries will require universal booster immunization throughout life. Booster doses of 0.5 mL of Td should be given every 10 yr starting at 11–12 yr of age. Vaccination with diphtheria toxoid should be used whenever tetanus toxoid is indicated to ensure continuing diphtheria immunity.

There is no known association of DT or Td with increased risk of convulsions. Local side effects alone do not preclude continued use. Persons who experience Arthus-type hypersensitivity reactions or a temperature of 103°F (39.4°C) after a dose of Td (rare in childhood) usually have high serum tetanus antitoxin levels and should not be given Td more frequently than every 10 yr, even if a significant tetanus-prone injury is sustained. DT preparations and Td can be given concurrently with other vaccines. *Haemophilus influenzae* conjugate vaccines containing diphtheria toxoid (PRP-D) or the variant of diphtheria toxin, CRM_{197} protein (HbOC), are not substitutes for diphtheria toxoid immunization and do not affect reactogenicity.

Bisgard KM, Handy IRB, Popovic T, et al: Respiratory diphtheria in the United States, 1980 through 1995. Am J Public Health 88:787, 1998.

Centers for Disease Control and Prevention: Diphtheria, tetanus, and pertussis: Recommendations for vaccine use and other preventive measures. Recommendations of the Immunization Practices Advisory Committee (ACIP). MMWR 40(RR-10):1, 1991.

Centers for Disease Control and Prevention: Update: Diphtheria epidemic—New independent states of the former Soviet Union, January 1995–March 1996. MMWR 45:693, 1996.

Centers for Disease Control and Prevention: Availability of diphtheria antitoxin through an investigational new drug protocol. MMWR 46:380, 1997.

Committee on Infectious Diseases, American Academy of Pediatrics: Diphtheria. *In*: Peter G (ed): (Red Book) Report of the Committee on Infectious Diseases, 24th ed. Elk Grove Village, IL, American Academy of Pediatrics, 1997.

Expanded Program on Immunization, World Health Organization: Outbreak of diphtheria, update. Wkly Epidemiol Rec 68:134, 1993.

Farizo KM, Strebel PM, Chen RT, et al: Fatal respiratory disease due to *Corynebacterium diphtheriae*: Case report and review of guidelines for management, investigation, and control. Clin Infect Dis 16:59, 1993.

Gupta RK, Griffin P Jr, Xu J, et al: Diphtheria antitoxin levels in US blood and plasma donors. J Infect Dis 173:1493, 1996.

Harnisch JP, Tronca E, Nolan CM, et al: Diphtheria among alcoholic urban adults: A decade of experience in Seattle. Ann Intern Med 111:71, 1989.

Popovic T, Wharton M, Wenger JD, et al: Are we ready for diphtheria? A report from the Diphtheria Diagnostic Workshop, Atlanta, 11 and 12 July, 1994. J Infect Dis 171:765, 1995.

Thisyakorn U, Wongvanich J, Kumpeng V: Failure of corticosteroid therapy to prevent diphtheritic myocarditis or neuritis. Pediatr Infect Dis 3:126, 1984.

Chapter 188
Listeria monocytogenes

Robert S. Baltimore

Listeriosis in humans is caused principally by *Listeria monocytogenes*, one of seven species of the genus *Listeria* that are widely distributed in the environment and throughout the food chain. Infection occurs most commonly at the extremes of age. In the pediatric population, perinatal infections predominate and usually occur secondary to maternal infection or colonization. Outside the newborn period, disease is most commonly encountered in immunosuppressed children and adults and in the elderly. In the United States, food-borne outbreaks are caused by improperly processed dairy products and contaminated vegetables, and they principally affect the same individuals at risk for sporadic disease.

ETIOLOGY. Members of the genus *Listeria* are facultatively anaerobic, non–spore-forming, motile, gram-positive bacilli. The seven *Listeria* species are divided into two genomically distinct groups based on DNA-DNA hybridization studies. One group contains the species *L. murrayi* and *L. grayi*, considered nonpathogenic. The second group contains five species: the nonhemolytic species *L. innocua* and *L. welshimeri* and the hemolytic species *L. monocytogenes, L. seeligeri*, and *L. ivanovii*. *L. ivanovii* is pathogenic primarily in animals, and the vast majority of both human and animal disease is due to *L. monocytogenes*.

Subtyping of *L. monocytogenes* isolates for epidemiologic purposes has been attempted using heat-stable somatic O and heat-labile flagellar H antigens, phage typing, ribotyping, and multilocus enzyme electrophoresis. Electrophoretic typing demonstrates the clonal structure of populations of *L. monocytogenes*, as well as the sharing of populations between human and animal sources.

Selected biochemical tests together with the demonstration of "tumbling" motility, "umbrella"-type formation below the surface in semisolid medium, hemolysis, and a typical cyclic adenosine monophosphate (cAMP) test are usually sufficient to establish a presumptive identification of *L. monocytogenes* from among the gram-positive bacilli.

EPIDEMIOLOGY. *L. monocytogenes* is widespread in nature, has been isolated throughout the environment, and is associated with epizootic disease and asymptomatic carriage in more than 42 species of wild and domestic animals and 22 avian species. Epizootic disease in large animals such as sheep and cattle is associated with abortion and "circling disease," a form of basilar meningitis. *L. monocytogenes* is isolated from sewage, silage, and soil, where it survives for more than 295 days. The rate of disease in the United States is approximately 0.7 cases per 100,000 population but varies between states. Epidemic human listeriosis has been associated with food-borne transmission in several large outbreaks, especially associated with aged soft cheeses; improperly pasteurized milk and milk products; contaminated raw and ready-to-eat beef, pork, poultry, and packaged meats; and vegetables grown on farms where the ground is contaminated with the feces of colonized animals. The ability of *L. monocytogenes* to grow at temperatures as low as 4°C increases the risk of transmission from aged soft cheeses and stored contaminated food. Small clusters of nosocomial person-to-person transmission have occurred in hospital nurseries and obstetric suites. Sporadic endemic listeriosis is less well characterized. Likely routes include food-borne infection, zoonotic spread, and person-to-person transmission. Zoonotic transmission with cutaneous infections occurs in veterinarians and farmers who handle sick animals.

Reported cases of listeriosis are clustered at the extremes of age, and some studies have shown higher rates in males and a seasonal predominance in the late summer and fall in the Northern Hemisphere. Outside the newborn period and during pregnancy, disease is usually reported in patients with underlying immunosuppression, with a 100–300 times increased risk in HIV-infected persons and in the elderly (Table 188–1).

The incubation period is defined only for common-source food-borne disease and is 21–30 days. Asymptomatic carriage and fecal excretion are reported in 1% of normal people and 5% of abattoir workers, but duration of excretion, when studied, is short (<1 mo).

PATHOGENESIS. *L. monocytogenes* produces multisystem disease, particularly pyogenic meningitis. Granulomatous reactions and microabscess formation have been reported in many organs, including the liver, lungs, adrenals, kidneys, central nervous system (CNS), and, notably, the placenta. Animal models demonstrate translocation, the transfer of intraluminal organisms across intact intestinal mucosa; whether or not this occurs in humans is not known.

Studies of intracellular and intercellular spread of *L. monocytogenes* have revealed a complex pathogenesis. Four pathogenic steps are described: internalization, escape from the phagocytic vacuole, nucleation of actin filaments, and cell-to-cell spread. Genes involved in each step are known, and isogenic mutants have been shown to have reduced virulence. Listeriolysin, a hemolysin and the best-characterized virulence factor, probably mediates lysis of vacuoles and is responsible for the zone of hemolysis when grown on blood-containing solid media. In cell-to-cell spread, locomotion proceeds via cytochalasin-sensitive polymerization of actin filaments, which extrude the bacteria in pseudopods, which are phagocytosed by adjacent cells, necessitating escape from a double-membrane vacuole. This mechanism protects intracellular bacteria from the humoral arm of immunity and is responsible for the well-known requirement of T-cell–mediated activation of monocytes by lymphokines for clearance of infection and establishment of immunity. The role of opsonizing antibody in protecting against infection is unclear.

TABLE 188–1 Types of *Listeria monocytogenes* Infections

- Listeriosis in pregnancy
- Neonatal listeriosis
  - Early onset
  - Late onset
- Food-borne outbreaks
- Listeriosis in normal children and adults (rare)
- Listeriosis in immunocompromised persons
  - Lymphohematogenous malignancies
  - Collagen vascular diseases
  - Diabetes mellitus
  - HIV infection
  - Transplant recipients
- Listeriosis in the elderly

TABLE 188–2 Characteristic Features of Early- and Late-Onset Neonatal Listeriosis

Early Onset (<5 days)	Late Onset (≥5 days)
Premature delivery	Term delivery
Low birthweight	Normal birthweight
Neonatal sepsis	Neonatal meningitis
Mean age at onset 1.5 days	Mean age at onset 14.2 days
Mortality rate >30%	Mortality rate <10%
Obstetric complications	Uncomplicated pregnancy
Maternal *Listeria* isolates	Nosocomial outbreaks

CLINICAL MANIFESTATIONS. The clinical presentation of listeriosis is highly dependent on the age of the patient and the circumstances of the infection.

Listeriosis in Pregnancy. Early gestational listeriosis is not well understood. *L. monocytogenes* has been grown from placental and fetal cultures of pregnancies ending in spontaneous abortion. The usual presentation in the 2nd and 3rd trimesters is a flulike illness that may result in bacteremia seeding the uterine contents. Rarely is maternal listeriosis severe, but meningitis in pregnancy has been reported. Recognition and treatment at this stage has been associated with normal pregnancy outcomes, but the fetus may not be infected even if listeriosis in the mother is not treated. In other instances, placental listeriosis develops with infection of the fetus and onset of premature labor and delivery and may be associated with stillbirth. Delivery of an infected premature fetus is associated with 50–90% infant mortality. Disseminated disease is apparent at birth, often with a diffuse pustular rash. Infection in the mother usually resolves without specific therapy after delivery, but postpartum fever and infected lochia may occur.

Neonatal Listeriosis. Two clinical presentations are recognized for neonatal listeriosis: an early-onset (<5 days, usually within 1–2 days) predominantly septicemic form and a late-onset (>5 days, mean 14 days) predominantly meningitic form. The principal characteristics of the two presentations (Table 188–2) resemble the clinical syndromes described for group B *Streptococcus* (Chapter 185).

Early-onset disease occurs from milder transplacental or ascending infections from the female genital tract. There is a strong association with prematurity, obstetric complications, recovery of *L. monocytogenes* from the maternal genital tract, and sepsis without CNS localization. The mortality rate is approximately 30%.

The epidemiology of late-onset disease is poorly understood. Onset is usually after 5 days but before 30 days of age. Affected infants frequently are term, and the mothers are asymptomatic and culture negative. The presenting syndrome is usually that of purulent meningitis, which, if adequately treated, has a mortality rate of less than 20%.

Postneonatal Infections. Listeriosis beyond the newborn period may rarely occur in otherwise healthy children but is most often encountered in association with underlying malignancies or immunosuppression. The clinical presentation is usually meningitis, less commonly sepsis, and rarely other CNS involvement such as cerebritis, meningoencephalitis, brain abscess, spinal cord abscess, or a focus outside the CNS such as septic arthritis, osteomyelitis, or liver abscess. It is not known if the frequent gastrointestinal signs and symptoms result from enteric infection, because the mode of acquisition is unknown.

DIAGNOSIS. Listeriosis should be included in the differential diagnosis of infections in pregnancy, neonatal sepsis and meningitis, and of sepsis or meningitis in older children with underlying malignancies or receiving immunosuppressive therapy. The diagnosis is established by culture of *L. monocytogenes* from blood and cerebrospinal fluid (CSF). Cultures from the maternal cervix, vagina, or lochia and, if possible, placenta, should be obtained when intrauterine infections lead to premature delivery or in early-onset neonatal sepsis. It is helpful to alert the laboratory to suspected cases so that *Listeria* isolates are not discarded as contaminating diphtheroids. Cold-enrichment procedures are rarely used for clinical specimens but improve isolation rates from heavily contaminated sources, such as feces, food, or environmental samples.

Histologic examination of the placenta is useful. Polymerase chain reaction assays detect *L. monocytogenes*, but commercial assays are not available. Serodiagnostic tests have not proved useful.

Differential Diagnosis. Listeriosis is indistinguishable clinically from sepsis and pyogenic meningitis due to other organisms. The presence of increased peripheral blood monocytes should alert one to the possibility of listeriosis. Monocytosis or lymphocytosis may be modest or striking. Beyond the neonatal period *L. monocytogenes* CNS infection is associated with fever, headache, seizures, and signs of meningeal irritation. The brain stem characteristically may be affected. The white blood cell concentration may vary from normal to slightly elevated, and the CSF laboratory findings are variable. Polymorphonuclear leukocytes or mononuclear cells may predominate, with shifts from polymorphonuclear to mononuclear cells in sequential lumbar punctures. A low CSF glucose level that mirrors the severity of disease is usually found. The CSF protein is moderately elevated. *L. monocytogenes* is isolated from the blood in 40–75% of cases of meningitis due to the organism. Deep focal infections, such as endocarditis, osteomyelitis, and liver abscess, due to *L. monocytogenes*, are also indistinguishable clinically from the more common organisms associated with these sites. Cutaneous infections should be suspected in patients with a history of contact with animals, especially products of conception.

TREATMENT. The emergence of multiple antibiotic resistance makes routine susceptibility testing of isolates mandatory. Ampicillin alone (100–200 mg/kg/24 hr, divided in four doses; 200–400 mg/kg/24 hr if meningitis is present) or in combination with an aminoglycoside (5–7.5 mg/kg/24 hr, divided in three doses) is the therapy of choice. Special attention to dosing is required for neonates, who need longer dosing intervals due to the longer half-lives of the antibiotics. Combination therapy is recommended for severe infections. Isolates usually demonstrate tolerance (the minimum bactericidal concentration is ≥32 times the minimum inhibitory concentration) to ampicillin as well as penicillin, erythromycin, and tetracycline. Addition of gentamicin lowers the minimum bactericidal concentration. *L. monocytogenes* is not susceptible to the cephalosporins, including third-generation cephalosporins. If these agents are used for empirical therapy for sepsis in a newborn, it is essential to add ampicillin for possible *L. monocytogenes* infection. Vancomycin, or vancomycin and an aminoglycoside, is an alternative, as are trimethoprim-sulfamethoxazole and erythromycin. The duration of therapy is usually 2 wk and may be longer (3 wk) in immunosuppressed patients or those with meningitis.

PROGNOSIS. Early gestational listeriosis may be associated with abortion or stillbirth, although maternal infection with sparing of the fetus has been reported. No convincing evidence shows that *L. monocytogenes* is associated with repeated abortions in humans. The mortality rate exceeds 50% for premature infants infected in utero and is 30% for early-onset neonatal sepsis, 15% for late-onset neonatal meningitis, and less than 10% in older children with prompt institution of appropriate antimicrobial therapy. Mental retardation, hydrocephalus, and other CNS sequelae are reported in survivors of *Listeria* meningitis.

PREVENTION. Consumption of unpasteurized or improperly processed dairy products, especially aged soft cheeses, uncooked and precooked meat products that have been stored at 4°C for extended periods, and unwashed vegetables should be avoided. This is particularly important during pregnancy and for immunosuppressed patients. Infected domestic animals should be avoided when possible. Careful handwashing is essential to prevent nosocomial spread within obstetric and neonatal units.

Appleman MD, Cherubin CE, Heseltine PNR, et al: Susceptibility testing of *Listeria monocytogenes*: A reassessment of bactericidal activity as a predictor for clinical outcome. Diagn Microbiol Infect Dis 14:311, 1991.

Linnan MJ, Mascola L, Lou XD, et al: Epidemic listeriosis associated with Mexican-style cheese. N Engl J Med 319:823, 1988.

Lorber B: Listeriosis. Clin Infect Dis 24:1, 1997.

McLauchlin J: Human listeriosis in Britain, 1987–85, a summary of 722 cases: I. Listeriosis during pregnancy and in the newborn. II. Listeriosis in non-pregnant individuals, a changing pattern of infection and seasonal incidence. Epidemiol Infect 104:181, 191, 1990.

Michelet C, Avril JL, Cartier F, et al: Inhibition of intracellular growth of *Listeria monocytogenes* by antibiotics. Antimicrob Agents Chemother 38:438, 1994.

Portnoy DA, Chakraborty T, Goebel W, et al: Molecular determinants of *Listeria monocytogenes* pathogenesis. Infect Immun 60:1263, 1992.

Schuchat A, Swaminathan B, Broome CV: Epidemiology of human listeriosis. Clin Microbiol Rev 4:169, 1991.

Skogberg K, Syrjanen J, Jahkola M, et al: Clinical presentation and outcome of listeriosis in patients with and without immunosuppressive therapy. Clin Infect Dis 14:815, 1992.

Southwick FS, Purich DL: Intracellular pathogenesis of listeriosis. N Engl J Med 334:770, 1996.

Topalovski M, Yang SS, Boonpasat Y: Listeriosis of the placenta: Clinicopathologic study of seven cases. Am J Obstet Gynecol 169:616, 1993.

CHAPTER 189
Actinomycosis

Richard F. Jacobs and Gordon E. Schutze

Actinomyces species are slow-growing, gram-positive bacteria that are part of the normal oral flora in humans. Their filamentous structure gives them a fungus-like appearance, and infections that are caused by these bacteria are termed *actinomycosis.* The disease actinomycosis is a chronic, granulomatous, suppurative disease characterized by peripheral spread with extension to contiguous tissue in the formation of numerous draining sinus tracts. These infections usually involve the cervicofacial, thoracic, abdominal, or pelvic regions.

ETIOLOGY. *Actinomyces israelii* is the predominant organism causing actinomycoses in humans. Other implicated species, in order of importance, include *Propionibacterium propionicus* (originally described as *A. propionicus), A. odontolyticus, A. meyeri, A. naeslundii, A. viscosus, A. gerencseriae, A. georgiae, A. pyogenes,* and *A. graevenitzii.*

Actinomyces are non–spore-forming gram-positive, facultative, or strict anaerobes with a variable morphology. The irregular morphology ranges from diphtheroid to mycelial. The organisms are found in clinical specimens, such as sputum, purulent exudates, and tissues obtained surgically or at necropsy. Staining of crushed tissue specimens rinsed with sterile saline or purulent exudate stained by Gram or acid-fast procedures can reveal organisms within the classic sulfur granules. Cultures on brain-heart infusion agar incubated at 37°C anaerobically (95% nitrogen and 5% carbon dioxide) and a separate set incubated aerobically reveal organisms within the lines of streak at 24–48 hr. *A. israelii* colonies appear as loose masses of delicate branching filaments with a characteristic spider-like growth. Colonies of *A. naeslundii, A. viscosus,* and *A. propionicus* may have similar growth characteristics. Owing to the similarity in growth characteristics from colony morphology, various biochemical tests are performed to identify the specific organism.

EPIDEMIOLOGY. Actinomycosis occurs worldwide without relation to age, sex, race, season, or occupation. In a review of 85 cases of actinomycosis, 27% were in persons younger than 20 yr, with 7% of the patients younger than 10 yr. The youngest patient in this description was 28 days old. Although actinomycosis is usually not an opportunistic infection, disease has been described in patients receiving steroids and those with leukemia, renal failure, congenital immunodeficiency diseases, HIV infection, and AIDS. Antecedent disease and surgery predisposed 81 of 181 subjects to infection. The source of human infection is almost always endogenous flora.

Actinomycosis, even in closed infections, is usually part of a polymicrobial infection involving mixed bacteria. In a large study of more than 650 cases, Holm was unable to identify a single infection in which *Actinomyces* occurred in pure culture; *Actinomyces* was identified with other bacteria, most notably *Actinobacillus actinomycetemcomitans* and *Haemophilus aphrophilus,* as well as other local flora.

PATHOGENESIS. The organism infects the host after introduction into the tissue by trauma or aspiration into the lung. It spreads locally and, rarely, hematogenously. Actinomycosis is a chronic, suppurative, scarring inflammatory process. Sites of infection show dense cellular infiltrates and suppuration that form many interconnecting abscesses and sinus tracts. This may be followed by cicatricial healing from which the organism then spreads by burrowing along fascial planes. This causes deep communicating scarred sinus tracts. Characteristic sulfur granules have an adherent mass of polymorphonuclear neutrophils that are attached to the radially arranged eosinophilic clubs of the granule. A fuzzy outer coat of hairlike fimbrias has been considered to contribute to failure of endodontic therapy due to *A. israelii.*

The three important sites of *Actinomyces* infection in order of frequency are cervicofacial, abdominal, and thoracic. Many less common infections occur, involving every organ in the body. Actinomycosis must be differentiated from several other chronic inflammatory diseases, including tuberculosis, mycotic infections, *Yersinia enterocolitica* "pseudoappendicitis," appendicitis, amebiasis, hepatic abscess, osteomyelitis, nocardiosis, and other chronic bacterial infections. In addition to introduction at wound sites, another route is through use of intrauterine devices (IUD), which permit the development of pelvic and gastrointestinal (GI) actinomycosis. Pulmonary actinomycosis occurs after inhalation or aspiration of organisms, introduction of a colonized foreign body, or spread from an existing cervicofacial or abdominal actinomycotic infection. These masslike lesions may present as a tumor requiring invasive approaches for differentiation.

CLINICAL MANIFESTATIONS. The three major forms of actinomycosis—cervicofacial, abdominal and pelvic, and pulmonary infections—arise by different routes but may predispose to other forms of the disease. The diagnosis of actinomycosis in children should raise suspicion of an underlying immunodeficiency disease state, especially chronic granulomatous disease.

Cervicofacial Actinomycosis. In cervicofacial actinomycosis, the organisms enter the tissue through trauma to the mucous membranes of the mouth or pharynx by way of caries or through tonsillar tissue. Clinical characteristics are pain, trismus, firm swelling, and fistula with drainage containing the characteristic sulfur granules. Cervicofacial actinomycosis is usually painless, slow growing, with a hard mass that can produce cutaneous fistulas, a condition commonly known as *lumpy jaw* (Fig. 189–1). Less frequently, cervicofacial actinomycosis can present as an acute, tender, fluctuant mass suggestive of an acute pyogenic infection. Bone is not involved early in the disease, but a periostitis, mandibular osteomyelitis, or perimandibular abscess may later develop. Infection may spread via sinus tracts to the cranial bones, which may give rise to meningitis. The ability of the organisms in this disease to burrow through tissue planes and even bone is a key differentiating point between actinomycosis and nocardiosis. The cervicofacial type of actinomycosis has the best prognosis, and the disease is usually cured with surgical debridement and excision as an adjunct to proper antibiotic therapy.

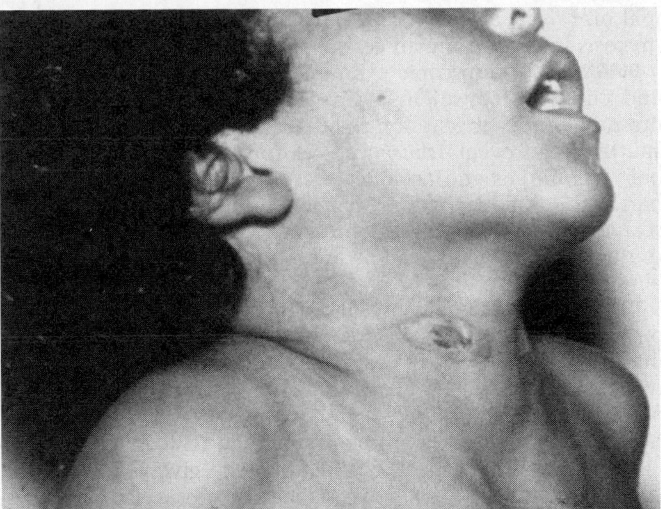

Figure 189–1 A 2-yr-old HIV-infected male with cervicofacial actinomycosis and a chronic draining fistula.

Abdominal and Pelvic Actinomycosis. This disease usually develops as a result of an acute perforative GI disease or after trauma to the abdomen. Of all the forms of actinomycosis, a delayed diagnosis is typical for abdominal or pelvic disease. GI disease occurs as appendicitis in 25% of cases but can be manifested as various ulcerative diseases. Infection classically appears after appendectomy as a hard, irregular mass in the ileocecal area that softens and then drains to the outside via a fistula. Hepatic involvement has been described in approximately 15% of abdominal actinomycosis cases as solitary or multiple liver abscesses or in a miliary pattern. The clinical course is indolent, with chills, fever, night sweats, and weight loss, and is similar to the presentation of tuberculous peritonitis. Extension from this focus is usually by direct continuity or, rarely, hematogenously to involve any tissue or organ, including muscle, spleen, kidneys, fallopian tubes, ovaries, uterus, testes, bladder, or rectum.

Pulmonary Actinomycosis. Neither the clinical nor radiographic presentation of pulmonary actinomycosis is specific. Principal symptoms include fever, productive cough, chest pain, and weight loss. Infection frequently dissects along tissue planes and may extend through the chest wall or diaphragm, producing numerous sinuses. These characteristic sinus tracts contain small abscesses and purulent drainage. Other complications include bony destruction of adjacent ribs, sternum, and vertebral bodies. Pyogenic mediastinitis has been attributed to *A. odontolyticus* in lung transplant recipients. Multiple lobe involvement is occasionally found in the lung. Associated conditions, such as dental caries, aspiration, inhalation injury, introduction of a colonized foreign body, or pre-existing cervicofacial or abdominal disease, should heighten the index of suspicion. Accurate diagnosis can be more difficult with the propensity of *Actinomyces* to infect pre-existing pulmonary cavities. A specific diagnosis can be made by examining purulent sinus tract drainage for sulfur granules and by appropriate cultures. The presence of *Actinomyces* in sputum or bronchoscopy specimens is hampered because these organisms are normal oral flora. The differential diagnosis of pulmonary actinomycosis includes lung abscess and tuberculosis.

DIAGNOSIS. Microscopic examination with appropriate stains and culture of purulent drainage from fistulas, abscesses, or draining sinus tracts, along with bronchoalveolar lavage and sputum, can reveal *Actinomyces*. Appropriate anaerobic and aerobic techniques and an index of suspicion for *Actinomyces* enhance the yield on microbiologic cultures. An abdominal CT scan can be helpful in the presence of a contrast-enhancing multicystic lesion that can be approached by CT-guided needle biopsy and culture.

TREATMENT. The mainstay of treatment for actinomycosis is prolonged antibiotic therapy and an appropriate surgical approach to sinus tracts and abscesses. Prompt use of antibiotics results in a high rate of cure. Actinomycosis is treated with penicillin (250,000 U/kg/24 hr intravenously divided every 4 hr). Other appropriate antibiotics include tetracycline, clindamycin, chloramphenicol, and imipenem, given parenterally. Although controversy still exists about the dosage and duration of therapy, appropriate therapy usually includes parenteral antibiotics for 2–6 wk followed by oral antibiotics for 3–12 mo. The oral antibiotic of choice is penicillin (100 mg/kg/24 hr divided every 6 hr). Although most *A. israelii* strains are sensitive to penicillin with minimum inhibitory concentrations in the 0.03–0.5 mg/mL range, some resistant strains have been identified. Antibiotic susceptibility testing should be performed on all patients with significant disease or with an underlying immunocompromised disease state. Hepatic abscesses or other deep tissue infections need to be treated for 6–12 mo. Large abscesses usually require surgical excision. Removal of chronically infected tonsils and treatment of pyorrhea or caries may eliminate possible sources of infection. Generally, the prognosis is excellent with adequate therapy and early diagnosis.

Bassiri AG, Girgis RE, Theodore J: *Actinomyces odontolyticus* thoracopulmonary infections: Two cases in lung and heart-lung transplant recipients and a review of the literature. Chest 109:1109, 1996.

Bates M, Cruikshank G: Thoracic actinomycosis. Thorax 12:99, 1952.

Brown JR: Human actinomycosis: A study of 181 subjects. Hum Pathol 4:319, 1973.

Cintron JR, Del Pino A, Duarte B, Wood D: Abdominal actinomycosis. Dis Colon Rectum 39:105, 1996.

Feder HM Jr: Actinomycosis manifesting as an acute painless lump of the jaw. Pediatrics 85:858, 1990.

Holm G: Studies on the etiology of human actinomycosis: I. The other microbes of actinomycosis and their importance. Acta Pathol Microbiol Scand 27:736, 1950.

Ramos CP, Falsen E, Alvarez N, et al: *Actinomyces graevenitzii* sp. Nov., isolated from human clinical specimens. Int J Syst Bacteriol 47:885, 1997.

Reddy I, Ferguson DA Jr, Sarubbi FA: Endocarditis due to *Actinomyces pyogenes*. Clin Infect Dis 25:1476, 1997.

Schaal KP, Lee HJ: Actinomycete infections in humans—a review. Gene 115:201, 1992.

Weisse WC, Smith I: A study of 57 cases of actinomycosis over a 36-year period. Arch Intern Med 135:1562, 1975.

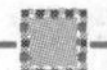

CHAPTER 190
Nocardia

Richard F. Jacobs and Gordon E. Schutze

Nocardiosis is an acute, subacute, or chronic suppurative infection with a tendency for remissions and exacerbations. Nocardiosis is uncommon in children, presenting primarily as lung disease in immunocompromised hosts. Hematogenous dissemination to other body sites, most notably brain and skin, may also occur. *Nocardia* is a member of the order Actinomycetales, which includes gram-positive filamentous bacteria such as *Actinomyces, Streptomyces,* and mycobacteria. Soil and decaying vegetable matter are their natural habitat. Infection in humans occurs by the respiratory route or by direct skin inoculation.

ETIOLOGY. Numerous taxonomic studies have established the heterogeneity of the species *Nocardia asteroides* and has led to the description of *N. asteroides* complex. Current methods of recognition of *N. asteroides* in the clinical laboratory include microscopic and colonial morphology and inability to hydrolyze casein, tyrosine, xanthine, and hypoxanthine, with resistance to lysozyme. Unfortunately, the species *N. asteroides, N. farcinica, N. otidis-caviarum, N. nova,* and *N. transvalensis* share similar features and have contributed to the apparent heterogeneity of *N. asteroides*. New identification and rapid diagnostic schemes use molecular typing and identification of preformed enzymes.

In 1988, a susceptibility study of 78 clinical isolates of the *N. asteroides* complex from the United States found that 95% of strains exhibited one of five antibiotic resistance patterns. The first pattern studied (type 5) was found in approximately 20% of isolates, including essentially all isolates in the *N. asteroides* complex that were resistant to cefotaxime, ceftriaxone, and cefamandole. Subsequent studies established these isolates as *N. farcinica*. The second group (type 3) comprises approximately 20% of the strains and was characterized by susceptibility to ampicillin and erythromycin. Isolates with this susceptibility pattern were determined to be *N. nova*. The remaining groups had susceptibility patterns that included resistance to broad-spectrum cephalosporins, susceptibility to ampicillin and carbenicillin, but intermediate susceptibility to imipenem; the most common group, occurring in 35% of isolates, was resistant to ampicillin but susceptible to the broad-spectrum cephalosporins and imipenem. The most active parenteral agents were amikacin (95%), imipenem (88%), ceftriaxone (82%), and cefotaxime (82%). The most active oral agents were the sulfonamides (100%), minocycline (100%), and ampicillin (40%).

Systemic nocardiosis is caused most frequently by the bacteria in the *N. asteroides* complex. *N. brasiliensis* is the principal cause of localized, chronic mycetoma but has been described in the United States and worldwide as a form of pulmonary and systemic disease, especially in immunocompromised patients. *Actinomadura madurae* (Madura foot), *N. farcinica, N. nova,* and *N. transvalensis* are also causes of human disease. *N. asteroides* complex includes the most common agents of systemic nocardiosis in the United States, whereas *N. brasiliensis* is found more commonly in Central America, South America, and Asia. These agents are similar morphologically and can be distinguished only by biochemical and serologic procedures.

EPIDEMIOLOGY. Nocardiosis was once thought to be a rare cause of human disease but is now being recognized more frequently. It has been diagnosed in individuals ranging from 4 wk–82 yr of age. Almost all of the patients have one or more severe underlying diseases, usually accompanied by compromised cellular immunity due to steroids, primary immunodeficiency (chronic granulomatous disease), organ transplantation, cytotoxic chemotherapy, or HIV infection and AIDS. Although nocardiosis is not considered an AIDS-defining infection, HIV-infected patients are at increased risk. *Nocardia* infections in bone marrow transplant recipients have been associated with a high rate of invasive fungal infection and a lack of protection by trimethoprim-sulfamethoxazole prophylaxis.

Soil is the natural habitat of *Nocardia*, and it has been isolated throughout the world. The organism is inhaled in aerosolized dust and causes pulmonary infection with widespread dissemination in susceptible hosts. Although communicability from human to human has not been proved to be common, a description of human-to-human transmission of *N. farcinica* resulting in sternal wound infections in patients undergoing open heart surgery has raised concern about *Nocardia* as a nosocomial pathogen.

PATHOGENESIS. *N. asteroides* complex and *N. brasiliensis* organisms are obligate aerobes and grow on ordinary culture media. These organisms are sensitive to various antibiotics; thus, media containing these specific drugs do not support growth. Many isolates of *Nocardia* are thermophilic and can grow at temperatures up to 50°C; however, best growth is achieved at 37°C. At 25°C, the organisms grow very slowly. Colonies appear within 1–2 wk on brain-heart infusion agar and Lowenstein-Jensen media, usually as waxy, folded, or heaped colonies at the edges. With further incubation, these colonies develop aerial hyphae that tend to give them a white, chalky appearance. Classifications of species of *Nocardia* are based on physiologic reactions with various substrates and antibiotic susceptibility testing. An isolated 55-kd protein that has apparent specificity for *N. asteroides* complex is used in an enzyme immunoassay. In biopsy specimens or clinical body fluids using the modified Kinyoun's acid-fast staining technique, *Nocardia* demonstrates fragmented bacilli with stain concentrated in a beaded fashion along portions of the branching filaments.

The primary infection of *Nocardia* is pulmonary, and the disease becomes systemic by hematogenous spread. Direct inoculation from soil into traumatized skin (Madura foot) is also a frequent cause of *Nocardia* infection. In patients with impaired cellular immunity, direct spread from lungs or hematogenous spread to brain, skin, and other organs can occur.

CLINICAL MANIFESTATIONS. Nocardiosis is a pulmonary disease in 75% of all cases. Almost all cases occur in immunocompromised patients or patients with underlying pulmonary disease, especially alveolar proteinosis. Demonstration of tissue invasion is important for identifying active infection because the organism can occasionally exist as a respiratory saprophyte. Clinical manifestations include pneumonia and necrotizing pneumonia with single or numerous abscesses. Diagnosis is established in one third of cases by sputum analysis and culture in adults. Bronchoalveolar lavage or lung biopsy may be required to establish the diagnosis in the remaining two thirds of adults and in children. The mortality with nocardiosis generally exceeds 50% but may be lower when the diagnosis is made early in infection.

Metastatic lesions may occur anywhere in the body, but the brain is the most common secondary site, affected in 15–40% of cases. Brain lesions may be numerous or single. Brain abscess is the most common presentation, with meningitis the second most common, as manifested by pleocytosis (lymphocytes or neutrophils), elevated cerebrospinal fluid protein, and hypoglycorrhachia. Persistent neutrophilic meningitis with sterile cultures is classic for central nervous system (CNS) *Nocardia* infection. The onset of CNS infection may be gradual or sudden and includes manifestations varying from headache to coma. Cranial CT is recommended in all immunocompromised patients with pulmonary nocardiosis, even when asymptomatic, because of the frequency of CNS involvement, and should be considered in all patients with pulmonary nocardiosis.

The skin is the third most commonly involved organ. Renal nocardiosis is the fourth most common site, presenting with dysuria, hematuria, or pyuria. Lesions may extend from the cortex into the medulla. Gastrointestinal involvement may also be associated, with nausea, vomiting, diarrhea, abdominal distention, and melena. Infection may metastasize to skin, pericardium, myocardium, spleen, liver, or adrenal glands; bone involvement is rare. Almost all of the involved organs have several abscesses, but in contrast to actinomycosis, granules are rarely found. Keratitis due to *N. farcinica* has been associated with the use of semipermeable rigid contact lenses.

DIAGNOSIS. Laboratory diagnosis of nocardiosis requires direct examination of clinical material for characteristic gram-positive, acid-fast organisms and isolation by culture methods. Smears of clinical material are Gram stained or stained by the modified Kinyoun's acid-fast technique. *N. asteroides* complex and *N. brasiliensis* appear as delicately branched gram-positive structures that tend to fragment and may have a coccoid to bacillary shape. In properly stained and decolorized acid-fast smears, the organisms may appear as fragmented bacilli with the stain concentrated in a beaded fashion along the portions of the filaments. Antibody titers to the 55-kd *Nocardia* protein of 1:256 or greater appear sensitive and specific for diagnosis and have also been used to monitor response to medical treatment.

TREATMENT. Sulfonamides are the treatment of choice in human nocardiosis. Trisulfapyrimidines or sulfasoxazole (120–150 mg/kg/24 hr divided every 6 hr) therapy for 3–6 mo is standard. For severe infections, amikacin (15–30 mg/kg/24 hr divided every 8 hr) as a single agent or in combination with a β-lactam antibiotic (cefotaxime, ceftriaxone, or imipenem) can be used. In addition, and for specific *N. asteroides* complex isolates with in vitro susceptibility testing, alternative drug combinations may include erythromycin and newer macrolides (azithromycin and clarithromycin), carbapenems, streptomycin, minocycline, quinolones, or third-generation cephalosporins. Clinical trials have shown ampicillin or amoxicillin-clavulanate to be effective in *N. brasiliensis* infections. Antibiotic resistance has become an important issue in many *Nocardia* infections, with resistance to cotrimoxazole, streptomycin, and ampicillin reported. Antibiotic susceptibility testing may need to be performed in selected patients. Relapses of *Nocardia* have been demonstrated in patients who were treated for less than 3 mo. Patients with AIDS probably should be treated indefinitely. Surgical drainage of abscesses is important. Despite adequate therapy, the overall mortality is approximately 50%, which may be secondary to a delay in diagnosis or to the debilitated state of patients with severely compromised host defenses.

Angeles AM, Sugar AM: Rapid diagnosis of nocardiosis with an enzyme immunoassay. J Infect Dis 155:292, 1987.

Baghdadlian H, Sorger S, Knowles K, et al: *Nocardia transvalensis* pneumonia in a child. Pediatr Infect Dis J 8:470, 1989.

Biehle JR, Cavalieri SJ, Felland T, et al: Novel method for rapid identification of *Nocardia* species by detection of preformed enzymes. J Clin Microbiol 34:103, 1996.

Burucoa C, Breton I, Ramassamy A, et al: Western blot monitoring of disseminated *Nocardia nova* infection treated with clarithromycin, imipenem, and surgical drainage. Eur J Clin Microbiol Infect Dis 15:943, 1996.

Law BJ, Marks MI: Pediatric nocardiosis. Pediatrics 70:560, 1982.

McNeil MM, Brown JM, Georghiou PR, et al: Infections due to *Nocardia transvalensis*: Clinical spectrum and antimicrobial therapy. Clin Infect Dis 15:453, 1992.

Pinkhas J, Oliver I, deVries A, et al: Pulmonary nocardiosis complicating malignant lymphomas successfully treated with chemotherapy. Chest 63:367, 1973.

Steingrube VA, Brown BA, Gibson JL, et al: DNA amplification and restriction endonuclease analysis for differentiation of 12 species and taxa of *Nocardia*, including recognition of four new taxa within the *Nocardia asteroides* complex. J Clin Microbiol 33:3096, 1995.

Van Burik JA, Hackman RC, Nadeem SQ, et al: Nocardiosis after bone marrow transplantation: A retrospective study. Clin Infect Dis 24:1154, 1997.

Wallace RJ, Brown BA, Tsukamura M, et al: Clinical and laboratory features of *Nocardia nova*. J Clin Microbiol 29:2407, 1991.

Wallace RJ, Septimus EJ, Williams TW, et al: Use of trimethoprim-sulfamethoxazole for treatment of infections due to *Nocardia*. Rev Infect Dis 4:315, 1982.

Wallace RJ, Steele LC, Sumter G, et al: Antimicrobial susceptibility patterns of *Nocardia asteroides*. Antimicrob Agents Chemother 32:1776, 1988.

Wallace RJ, Tsukamura M, Brown BA, et al: Cefotaxime-resistant *Nocardia asteroides* strains are isolates of the controversial species *Nocardia farcinica*. J Clin Microbiol 28:2726, 1990.

Young LS, Armstrong D, Blevins A, et al: *Nocardia asteroides* infection complicating neoplastic disease. Am J Med 50:356, 1971.

SECTION 4

Gram-Negative Bacterial Infections

CHAPTER 191

Neisseria meningitidis *(Meningococcus)*

Michele Estabrook

Meningococcal disease, first described by Vieusseaux in 1805 as epidemic cerebrospinal fever, remains a significant health problem, particularly in the developing world. Although nasopharyngeal colonization rarely leads to disseminated disease, the fulminant, rapidly fatal course of meningococcemia is not soon forgotten.

ETIOLOGY. *Neisseria meningitidis* is a gram-negative diplococcus that is often described as biscuit shaped. It is a common commensal organism of the human nasopharynx and has not been isolated from animal or environmental sources. The meningococcus is fastidious, and growth is facilitated in a moist environment at 35–37°C in an atmosphere of 5–10% carbon dioxide. It grows well on several enriched media, including supplemented chocolate agar. Mueller-Hinton agar, blood agar base, and trypticase soy agar. On solid media, colonies are transparent, nonpigmented, and nonhemolytic. *N. meningitidis* is identified by its ability to ferment glucose and maltose to acid and its inability to ferment sucrose or lactose. Indole and hydrogen sulfide are not formed. The cell wall contains cytochrome oxidase, which results in a positive oxidase test result.

The meningococci have been divided into serogroups based on antigenic differences in their capsular polysaccharides. Although 13 serogroups are currently recognized, groups A, B, C, W135, and Y account for most meningococcal disease. The other serogroups often colonize the nasopharynx but rarely disseminate. Lipooligosaccharides (e.g., endotoxin) and proteins found in the outer membrane complex are also used to serotype meningococcal strains.

EPIDEMIOLOGY. Meningococcal dissemination occurs as endemic disease punctuated by outbreaks of cases that are often clustered geographically. True epidemics have become rare in developed countries but remain a significant problem in much of the developing world. Endemic disease appears to be caused by a heterogeneous group of meningococcal serotypes, and epidemics are caused by a single serotype. Analysis with multilocus enzyme genetic methods has confirmed that a meningococcal epidemic is caused by strains derived from a single clonotype.

The Centers for Disease Control (CDC) reported the results of a laboratory-based surveillance for meningococcal disease in a large United States population for the years 1989–1991. The average annual rate of invasive disease was 1.1/100,000 population, with an estimated 2,600 cases of meningococcal disease annually in the United States. The highest attack rates were during the winter and early spring months. Males accounted for 55% of the total cases, and 29% of the cases occurred in children younger than 1 yr, with the peak incidence of disease being 26/100,000 infants younger than 4 mo. Forty-six per cent of the cases occurred in children 2 yr of age or younger, and an additional 25% of the cases occurred in persons 30 yr of age or older. Serogroup B and serogroup C meningococci accounted for nearly equal proportions of disease (46% and 45%, respectively), but 69% of group C disease occurred in persons older than 2 yr. Fifty-eight per cent of the patients were reported to have meningitis. *N. meningitidis* was isolated from blood in 66% of cases, cerebrospinal fluid (CSF) in 51%, and joint fluid in 1%.

Subsequent data indicate that the proportion of cases caused by serogroup Y is increasing. The United States has also experienced an increased incidence of outbreaks of serogroup C disease. Eight outbreaks occurred during 1992–1993, and most of these outbreaks had attack rates exceeding 10 cases per 100,000 population.

Meningococcal disease, particularly group A, remains a major health problem in much of the developing world. Many areas, such as China and Africa, have an endemic rate of disease of 10–25/100,000 persons and major periodic epidemics (100–500/100,000). Epidemic disease typically involves individuals who are older than those with endemic disease.

PATHOGENESIS. *N. meningitidis* is thought to be acquired by a respiratory route. Colonization of the nasopharynx with meningococci usually leads to asymptomatic carriage, and only rarely does dissemination occur. Colonization can persist for weeks to months. Carriage rates vary from 2–30% in a normal population during nonepidemic periods but are higher among children in daycare centers and in conditions of crowding. The carriage rate can approach 100% in a closed population during an epidemic.

Meningococcal nasopharyngeal colonization is facilitated by the secretion of proteases that cleave the proline-rich hinge region of secretory IgA and render it nonfunctional. Meningococci and gonococci produce this enzyme, but nonpathogenic *Neisseria* organisms do not. Meningococci then adhere selectively to nonciliated epithelial cells. Pili appear to be of major importance in the attachment of meningococci to the human nasopharynx. The bacteria enter nonciliated epithelial cells by endocytosis and are carried across the cell in membrane-bound vacuoles.

Meningococci disseminate from the upper respiratory tract through the bloodstream. Serum antibody leading to complement-mediated bacterial lysis has been shown to block this dissemination, and a deficiency of antimeningococcal antibody is associated with the development of meningococcemia. Bactericidal antibody is directed against the capsular polysaccharide, subcapsular protein, and lipooligosaccharide antigens. Newborn infants have protective antibody that is primarily IgG of maternal origin. As this antibody wanes, infants 3–24 mo of age experience the highest incidence of meningococcal disease. By adulthood, most individuals have developed natural immunity against *N. meningitidis* from nasopharyngeal colonization with *N. meningitidis* and colonization of the gastrointestinal tract with enteric bacteria that express cross-reactive antigens. Infants have a high carriage rate of an unencapsulated, nonpathogenic neisserial strain, *N. lactamica*, that leads to the development of bactericidal antibody against the meningococcus.

The importance of the complement system in host defense against *N. meningitidis* is underscored by the fact that individuals with primary or acquired complement deficiency have an increased risk of developing meningococcal disease, and 50–

60% of individuals with properdin, factor D, or terminal-component deficiencies develop bacterial infections that are caused almost solely by *N. meningitidis*. Recurrent infection is common with terminal component deficiencies but is uncommon with properdin deficiency. Acquired complement deficiency also carries an increased risk and can be seen with systemic diseases that deplete serum complement. Examples are systemic lupus erythematosus, nephrotic syndrome, multiple myeloma, and hepatic failure.

The group B capsule is a homopolymer of sialic acid, which is known to inhibit alternative complement pathway activation. Antibody that activates the classic pathway can overcome this inhibition. The lack of specific antibody coupled with inhibition of the alternative pathway may explain the prevalence of serogroup B meningococcal disease in young children.

PATHOLOGY. Disseminated meningococcal disease is associated with an acute inflammatory response. Hemorrhage and necrosis may be seen in any organ system and appear to be mediated by intravascular coagulation with deposition of fibrin in small vessels. The major organ systems involved in fatal cases of meningococcemia are the heart, central nervous system, skin, mucous and serous membranes, and adrenals. Myocarditis is found in more than 50% of patients who die of meningococcal disease. Cutaneous hemorrhages, ranging from petechiae to purpura, occur in most fatal infections and are associated with acute vasculitis with fibrin deposition in arterioles and capillaries. Diffuse adrenal hemorrhage may occur in patients with fulminant meningococcemia (i.e., Waterhouse-Friderichsen syndrome). Meningitis is characterized by acute inflammatory cells in the leptomeninges and perivascular spaces. Focal cerebral involvement is uncommon.

The interaction of endotoxin released by *N. meningitidis* and the complement system probably is key in the pathogenesis of the clinical manifestations of meningococcal disease. Complement activation correlates with the concentration of meningococcal lipooligosaccharide in the plasma. The concentration of circulating endotoxin is directly correlated with activation of the fibrinolytic system, development of disseminated intravascular coagulopathy (DIC), multiple organ system failure, septic shock, and death. The level of endotoxemia correlates with the concentration of circulating cytokines, which are released from endotoxin-stimulated monocytes and macrophages. The concentrations of tumor necrosis factor-α and interleukins have been directly associated with fatal meningococcal disease.

CLINICAL MANIFESTATIONS. The spectrum of meningococcal disease can vary widely, from fever and occult bacteremia to sepsis, shock, and death. Recognized patterns of disease are bacteremia without sepsis, meningococcemic sepsis without meningitis, meningitis with or without meningococcemia, meningoencephalitis, and infection of specific organs.

A well-recognized entity is occult bacteremia in a febrile child (Chapter 172). Upper respiratory or gastrointestinal symptoms or a maculopapular rash can be evident. The child often is sent home on no antibiotics or oral antibiotics for a minor infection. Spontaneous recovery without antibiotics has been reported, but some children have developed meningitis.

Acute meningococcemia initially can mimic a virus-like illness with pharyngitis, fever, myalgias, weakness, and headache. With widespread hematogenous dissemination, the disease rapidly progresses to septic shock characterized by hypotension, DIC, acidosis, adrenal hemorrhage, renal failure, myocardial failure, and coma. Meningitis may or may not develop. Concomitant pneumonia, myocarditis, purulent pericarditis, and septic arthritis have been described. More often, meningococcal disease is manifested as acute meningitis that responds to appropriate antibiotics and supportive therapy. Seizures and focal neurologic signs occur less frequently than in patients with meningitis caused by pneumococcus or *Haemophilus influenzae* type b. Rarely, meningoencephalitis can occur with diffuse brain involvement.

A review of 100 children with invasive meningococcal disease revealed that 71% presented with fever, 4% with hypothermia, and 42% with shock. Skin lesions occurred in 71% of the cases with petechiae and/or purpura and in 49% with both. Purpura fulminans developed in 16%. Other rashes described were maculopapular, pustular, and bullous lesions. Additional presenting symptoms and signs were irritability in 21%, lethargy in 30%, and emesis in 34%. Diarrhea, cough, rhinorrhea, seizure, and arthritis occurred much less frequently (6–10%). Leukopenia and low platelet counts affected 21% and 14%, respectively, and the white blood cell counts ranged from 900–46,000/mm^3. *N. meningitidis* was isolated in blood culture from 48% of the children, and meningitis was diagnosed in 55%. Six children had meningococci isolated from CSF in the absence of CSF pleocytosis, hypoglycorrhachia, or organisms detected by Gram stain. Five of eight children who presented with arthritis had *N. meningitidis* isolated from joint aspiration fluid. Eight per cent of the children had radiographic evidence of pneumonia on presentation.

Uncommon manifestations of meningococcal disease include endocarditis, purulent pericarditis, pneumonia, septic arthritis, endophthalmitis, mesenteric lymphodenitis, and osteomyelitis. Primary purulent conjunctivitis can lead to invasive disease. Sinusitis, otitis media, and periorbital cellulitis also can be caused by the meningococcus. Primary meningococcal pneumonia is associated with pleural effusions or empyema in 15% of cases. *N. meningitidis* is a rare isolate of the genitourinary tract in asymptomatic or symptomatic individuals and has been the causal organism in urethritis, cervicitis, vaginitis, and proctitis.

Chronic meningococcemia is a rare manifestation of meningococcal disease that can occur in children and adults. It is characterized by fever, nontoxic appearance, arthralgias, headache, and rash. The rash resembles that of disseminated gonococcal infection. Symptoms are intermittent, with the rash often appearing with fever. The mean duration of illness is 6–8 wk. Blood cultures may initially be sterile. Without specific therapy, complications such as meningitis can result.

DIAGNOSIS. Definitive diagnosis of meningococcal disease is made by isolation of the organism from a usually sterile body fluid such as blood, CSF, or synovial fluid. Isolation of meningococci from the nasopharynx is not diagnostic for disseminated disease. Blood and CSF are the usual sources of organism isolation. The blood culture yields *N. meningitidis* in about half of the cases of disseminated disease, and culture or Gram stain usually reveals the organism in those with meningitis. Culture or Gram stain of petechial or papular lesions has been variably successful in identifying meningococci. Bacteria can occasionally be seen on Gram stain of the buffy coat layer of a spun blood sample.

In meningitis, the morphologic and clinical characteristics of CSF are those of acute bacterial meningitis (Chapter 174.1). CSF cultures can be positive in patients with meningococcemia but without clinical evidence of meningitis or CSF pleocytosis. CSF cultures may be negative if the patient has received previous antibiotic treatment.

Particle agglutination using latex beads, which has replaced counterimmunoelectrophoresis, can detect meningococcal capsular polysaccharide in CSF, serum, joint fluid, or urine. This is especially useful when results are positive in the setting of partially treated infections with negative cultures. The available latex agglutination tests do not detect group B meningococcus, the most common cause of endemic meningococcal infections, and therefore have limited usefulness. Latex agglutination is not a substitute for proper Gram stain and culture techniques.

Other laboratory findings may include elevated sedimentation rate and C-reactive protein, leukocytopenia or leukocytosis, thrombocytopenia, proteinuria, and hematuria. Patients with DIC coagulation have decreased serum concentrations of prothrombin and fibrinogen.

Differential Diagnosis. This includes acute bacterial or viral meningitis, *Mycoplasma* infection, leptospirosis, syphilis, acute hemorrhagic encephalitis, encephalopathies, serum sickness, collagen vascular diseases, Henoch-Schönlein purpura, hemolytic-uremic syndrome, and ingestion of various poisons. The petechial or purpuric rash of meningococcemia is similar to that in any patient with a disease characterized by generalized vasculitis. These diseases include septicemia due to many gram-negative organisms; overwhelming septicemia with gram-positive organisms; bacterial endocarditis; Rocky Mountain spotted fever; epidemic typhus; *Ehrlichia canis* infection; infections with echoviruses, particularly types 6, 9, and 16; coxsackievirus infections, predominantly of types A2, A4, A9, and A16; rubella; rubeola and atypical rubeola; Henoch-Schönlein purpura; Kawasaki's disease; idiopathic thrombocytopenia; and erythema multiforme or erythema nodosum due to drugs or infectious or noninfectious disease processes. The morbilliform rash occasionally observed may be confused with any macular or maculopapular viral exanthem.

TREATMENT. Aqueous penicillin G is the drug of choice and should be given in doses of 250,000–300,000 U/kg/24 hr, administered intravenously in six divided doses. Cefotaxime (200 mg/kg/24 hr) and ceftriaxone (100 mg/kg/24 hr) are acceptable alternatives. Chloramphenicol sodium succinate (75–100 mg/kg/24 hr IV in four divided doses) provides effective treatment for patients who are allergic to β-lactam antibiotics. Therapy is continued for 5–7 days.

Isolates of *N. meningitidis* have been reported from Spain, South Africa, and Canada as being relatively resistant to penicillin, defined as having a minimal inhibitory concentration of penicillin of 0.1–1.0 μ/mL. Moderate resistance is caused, at least in part, by altered penicillin-binding protein 2. High-level resistance due to β-lactamase production has been reported from South Africa. The CDC estimated that about 4% of meningococcal disease in 1991 in the United States was caused by *N. meningitidis* strains that were relatively resistant to penicillin. None of the strains isolated produced β-lactamase. The clinical significance of moderate penicillin resistance is unknown. The CDC decided that routine susceptibility testing of clinical meningococcal isolates is probably not indicated in the United States at this time, but continued surveillance is necessary.

Patients with acute meningococcal infections should be monitored carefully. Supportive care and other therapy are discussed in Chapter 64).

COMPLICATIONS. Acute complications are related to the inflammatory changes, vasculitis, DIC, and hypotension of invasive meningococcal disease. These can include adrenal hemorrhage, arthritis, myocarditis, pneumonia, lung abscess, peritonitis, and renal infarcts. The vasculitis can lead to skin loss with secondary infection, tissue necrosis, and gangrene. Skin sloughing can necessitate the use of skin grafts. Bone involvement can lead to growth disturbance and late skeletal deformities secondary to epiphyseal avascular necrosis and epiphyseal-metaphyseal defects. Limb amputation has been reported for patients with purpura fulminans.

Meningitis rarely is complicated by subdural effusion or empyema or by brain abscess. Deafness is the most frequent neurologic sequela, but the reported incidence varies from 0–38%. Other rare sequelae include ataxia, seizures, blindness, cranial nerve palsies, hemiparesis or quadriparesis, and obstructive hydrocephalus.

The late complications of meningococcal disease are thought to be immune complex mediated and become apparent 4–9 days after the onset of illness. The usual manifestations are arthritis and cutaneous vasculitis. The arthritis is usually monarticular or oligoarticular. Effusions are usually sterile and respond to nonsteroidal anti-inflammatory agents. Permanent joint deformity is uncommon. Because most patients with meningococcal meningitis are afebrile by the 7th hospital day, the persistence or recrudescence of fever after 5 days of antibiotics warrants an evaluation for immune complex–mediated complications.

PROGNOSIS. Despite the use of appropriate antibiotics, the mortality rate for disseminated meningococcal disease remains at 8–13% in the United States. Poor prognostic factors include hypothermia, hypotension, purpura fulminans, seizures or shock on presentation, leukopenia, thrombocytopenia, and high circulating levels of endotoxin and tumor necrosis factor. The presence of petechiae for less than 12 hr before admission, hyperpyrexia, and the absence of meningitis reflect rapid progression and poorer prognosis.

Screening for complement deficiency after resolution of the acute infection is recommended for individuals with meningococcal disease. In one series of 20 patients with a first episode of meningococcal meningitis, meningococcemia, or meningococcal pericarditis, three had a deficiency of a terminal-pathway component and three had deficiencies of multiple complement components associated with underlying systemic diseases.

PREVENTION. Close contacts of patients with meningococcal disease are at increased risk of infection and should be carefully monitored and brought to medical attention if fever develops. Prophylaxis is indicated as soon as possible for household, daycare, and nursery school contacts. Prophylaxis is also recommended for persons who have had contact with patients' oral secretions. Prophylaxis is not routinely recommended for medical personnel except those with intimate exposure, such as with mouth-to-mouth resuscitation, intubation, or suctioning before antibiotic therapy was begun. Rifampin is given (10 mg/kg; maximum dose, 600 mg) orally every 12 hr for 2 days (total of four doses). The dose is reduced to 5 mg/kg for infants younger than 1 mo. Other effective antimicrobial agents are ciprofloxacin (500 mg orally as a single dose for adults) and ceftriaxone as a single intramuscular dose (125 mg for children < 15 yr and 250 mg for adults). Penicillin does not eradicate nasopharyngeal carriage, and patients treated with penicillin should receive chemoprophylactic antibiotics before hospital discharge.

Vaccine. A quadrivalent vaccine composed of capsular polysaccharide of meningococcal groups A, C, Y, and W135 is licensed in the United States. The vaccine is immunogenic in adults but is unreliable in children younger than 2 yr. The group B polysaccharide is poorly immunogenic in children and adults, and no vaccine is available against this serogroup. Routine immunization of the United States population is not recommended at this time, but the vaccine is routinely given to all American military recruits.

Immunization is useful to control outbreaks of meningococcal disease of the serogroups represented in the quadrivalent vaccine. It is also recommended for travelers to countries with a high incidence of meningococcal disease. Immunization of close contacts of individuals with A, C, Y, or W135 disease should be considered, because it has been useful in the prevention of secondary cases. Individuals with anatomic or functional asplenia and those with complement component deficiencies should be immunized.

Polysaccharide-protein conjugate vaccines are being developed for the prevention of meningococcal disease, and subcapsular proteins and detoxified lipooligosaccharides are being investigated as possible vaccines.

American Academy of Pediatrics, Committee on Infectious Diseases: Meningococcal disease prevention and control strategies for practice-based physicians. Pediatrics 97:404, 1996.

Barquet N, Domingo P, Caylà JA, et al: Prognostic factors in meningococcal disease: Development of a bedside predictive model and scoring system. JAMA 278:491, 1997.

Centers for Disease Control: Laboratory-based surveillance for meningococcal disease in selected areas—United States, 1989–1991. MMWR 42:21, 1993.

Centers for Disease Control and Prevention: Control and prevention of meningococcal disease. Recommendations of the Advisory Committee on Immunization Practices (ACIP). MMWR 46(RR-5):1, 1997.

Centers for Disease Control and Prevention: Control and prevention of serogroup C meningococcal disease: Evaluation and management of suspected outbreaks: Recommendations of the Advisory Committee on Immunization Practices (ACIP). MMWR 46(RR-5):13, 1997.

DeVoe IW: The meningoccus and mechanisms of pathogenicity. Microbiol Rev 46:162, 1982.

Edwards MS, Baker CJ: Complications and sequelae of meningococcal infections in children. J Pediatr 99:540, 1981.

Ellison RT, Kohler PF, Gurd JG, et al: Prevalence of congenital or acquired complement deficiency in patients with sporadic meningococcal disease. N Engl J Med 308:913, 1983.

Gedde-Dahl TW, Bjark P, Hoiby EA, et al: Severity of meningococcal disease: Assessment by factors and scores and implications for patient management. Rev Infect Dis 12:973, 1990.

Jackson LA, Schuchat A, Reeves MW, et al: Serogroup C meningococcal outbreaks in the United States, an emerging threat. JAMA 273:383, 1995.

Kornelisse RF, Hazelzet JA, Hop WCJ, et al: Meningococcal septic shock in children: Clinical and laboratory features, outcome, and development of a prognostic score. Clin Infect Dis 25:640, 1997.

Leggiadro RJ: Prevalence of complement deficiencies in children with systemic meningococcal infections. Pediatr Infect Dis J 6:75, 1987.

Oppenheim BA: Antibiotic resistance in *Neisseria meningitidis*. Clin Infect Dis 24(Suppl 1):598, 1997.

Wong VK, Hitchcock W, Mason WH: Meningococcal infections in children: A review of 100 cases. Pediatr Infect Dis 8:224, 1989.

CHAPTER 192

Neisseria gonorrhoeae (*Gonococcus*)

Michele Estabrook

Neisseria gonorrhoeae produces various forms of gonorrhea, an infection of the genitourinary tract mucous membranes and rarely of the mucosa of the rectum, oropharynx, and conjunctiva. Gonorrhea transmitted by sexual contact or perinatally is the most frequently reported communicable disease in the United States and affects children of all ages. This high prevalence and the development of antibiotic-resistant strains have produced significant morbidity in adolescents.

ETIOLOGY. *N. gonorrhoeae* is a nonmotile, aerobic, non–spore-forming, gram-negative intracellular diplococcus with flattened adjacent surfaces. Optimal growth occurs at 35–37°C and at pH 7.2–7.6 in an atmosphere of 3–5% carbon dioxide. The specimen should be inoculated immediately on to fresh, moist modified Thayer-Martin or specialized transport media because gonococci do not tolerate drying. Presumptive identification may be based on colony appearance, Gram stain, and production of cytochrome oxidase. Gonococci are differentiated from other *Neisseria* species by the fermentation of glucose but not maltose, sucrose, or lactose. Gram-negative diplococci are seen in infected material, often within polymorphonuclear leukocytes.

The cell surface of the gonococcus is similar to that of other gram-negative bacteria and contains pili, outer membrane proteins, and lipooligosaccharides (endotoxin), which contribute to cell adherence, tissue invasion, and resistance to host defenses. *N. gonorrhoeae* may be subdivided on the basis of the presence of pili, serologic typing, colony appearance, and nutritional requirements. The two systems primarily used to characterize gonococcal strains are auxotyping (i.e., nutritional requirements) and serotyping. The most widely used serotyping system is based on antigenic differences in protein I found in the outer membrane. Protein I can be antigenically classified into two groups: IA and IB. Monoclonal antibodies are used to further subdivide strains as serovars (e.g., IA-1, IB-12).

EPIDEMIOLOGY. *N. gonorrhoeae* infection occurs only in humans. The organism is shed in the exudate and secretions of infected mucosal surfaces and is transmitted through intimate contact, such as sexual contact or parturition and, rarely, by contact with fomites. Gonococcal infections in the newborn period generally are acquired during delivery. Gonococcal infections in children after the newborn period and before puberty are acquired rarely through household exposure to infected caretakers. In such cases, the possibility of sexual abuse should be seriously considered.

It is estimated that 600,000 new cases of gonococcal infections occur annually in the United States. Reported cases have declined from 323/100,000 population in 1987 to 123/100,000 population in 1996. The highest incidence of gonococcal infection is reported for adolescent males and females 15–19 yr of age. Risk factors include nonwhite race, homosexuality, increased number of sexual partners, prostitution, presence of other sexually transmitted diseases (STDs), unmarried status, poverty, and failure to use condoms. Peak incidence occurs in July–September, and the nadir is January–April. Techniques of auxotyping and serotyping can be used together to analyze the spread of individual strains of *N. gonorrhoeae* within a community.

Maintenance and subsequent spread of gonococcal infections in a community require a hyperendemic, high-risk core group such as prostitutes or adolescents with multiple sexual partners. Proper education, contact identification, and local treatment clinics may limit transmission.

Gonococcal infection of neonates usually results from peripartum exposure to infected exudate from the cervix of the mother. An acute infection begins 2–5 days after birth. The incidence of neonatal infection depends on the prevalence of gonococcal infection among pregnant women, prenatal screening for gonorrhea, and neonatal ophthalmic prophylaxis. The prevalence of gonorrhea is less than 1% in most U.S. prenatal populations but may be higher in some areas.

PATHOGENESIS AND PATHOLOGY. Mucosal invasion by gonococci results in a local inflammatory response that produces a purulent exudate consisting of polymorphonuclear leukocytes, serum, and desquamated epithelium. The gonococcal lipooligosaccharide (endotoxin) exhibits direct cytotoxicity, causing ciliostatis and sloughing of ciliated epithelial cells. Once the gonococcus traverses the mucosal barrier, the lipooligosaccharide binds bactericidal IgM antibody and serum complement, causing an acute inflammatory response in the subepithelial space. Tumor necrosis factor and other cytokines are thought to mediate the cytotoxicity of gonococcal infections.

The purulent discharge produced by urogenital gonococcal infection may block the ducts of paraurethral (Skene) or vaginal (Bartholin) glands, causing cysts or abscesses. In untreated patients, the inflammatory exudate is replaced by fibroblasts, and fibrous tissue may lead to stricture of the urethra. Gonococci may ascend the urogenital tract, causing acute endometritis, salpingitis, and peritonitis (collectively termed acute pelvic inflammatory disease [PID]) in postpubertal females and urethritis or epididymitis in postpubertal males. Perihepatitis (Fitz-Hugh–Curtis syndrome) follows dissemination through the peritoneum from the fallopian tubes to the liver capsule. Gonococci that invade the lymphatics and blood vessels may lead to inguinal lymphadenopathy; to perineal, perianal, ischiorectal, and periprostatic abscesses; and to disseminated gonococcal infection (DGI).

A number of gonococcal virulence and host immune factors are involved in the penetration of the mucosal barrier and subsequent manifestations of local and systemic infection. Selective pressure from different mucosal environments probably leads to changes in the outer membrane of the organism, including expression of variants of pili, opacity or Opa proteins (formerly protein II), and lipooligosaccharides. These changes may enhance gonococcal attachment, invasion of human cells, replication, and evasion of the host's immune response.

For infection to occur, the gonococcus must first attach to

host cells. A gonococcal IgA protease inactivates IgA1 by cleaving the molecule in the hinge region and may be an important factor in colonization or invasion of host mucosal surfaces. Gonococci adhere to the microvilli of nonciliated epithelial cells by hairlike protein structures (pili) that extend from the cell wall. Pili are thought to protect the gonococcus from phagocytosis and complement-mediated killing. Pili undergo high-frequency antigenic variation that may aid in the organism's escape from the host immune response and may provide specific ligands for different cell receptors. Opacity proteins, most of which confer an opaque appearance to colonies, are also thought to function as ligands to facilitate binding to human cells. Gonococci that express certain Opa proteins adhere and are phagocytosed by human neutrophils in the absence of serum.

Other phenotypic changes that occur in response to environmental stresses allow gonococci to establish infection. Examples include iron-repressible proteins for binding transferrin or lactoferrin, anaerobically expressed proteins, and synthesis of proteins that is mediated by contact with epithelial cells. Gonococci may grow in vivo under anaerobic conditions or in an environment with relative lack of iron.

Approximately 24 hr after attachment, the epithelial cell surface invaginates and surrounds the gonococcus in a phagocytic vacuole. This phenomenon is thought to be mediated by the gonococcal outer membrane protein I inserting into the host cell and causing alterations in membrane permeability. Subsequently, phagocytic vacuoles begin releasing gonococci into the subepithelial space by means of exocytosis. Viable organisms may then cause local disease (i.e., salpingitis) or disseminate through the bloodstream or lymphatics.

Serum IgG and IgM directed against gonococcal proteins and lipooligosaccharides lead to complement-mediated bacterial lysis. Stable serum resistance to this bactericidal antibody probably results from the particular type of porin protein expressed in gonococci, and these strains are often the cause of disseminated disease. Other strains are sensitive when grown in vitro but are not killed in vivo because of blocking antibodies directed against protein III or sialylation of lipooligosaccharide that probably interferes with complement fixation. Gonococcal adaptation also appears to be important in the evasion of killing by neutrophils. Examples include sialylation of lipooligosaccharides, increases in catalase production, and changes in the expression of surface proteins.

N. gonorrhoeae isolates from patients with DGI share common features that distinguish them from other gonococci. Most gonococci that produce DGI form transparent colonies (Opa −). Most contain outer membrane protein IA. They are resistant to the bactericidal activity of normal human serum. Genital infections with these organisms fail to elicit an inflammatory response and are asymptomatic. Human IgG antibodies ("blocking antibodies") that do bind to DGI gonococci may interfere with bactericidal antibody- and complement-mediated lysis. DGI isolates have unique nutritional requirements (58% belong to the Arg−Hyx−Ura−auxotype) and greater sensitivity to penicillin. These strains have occurred infrequently in the United States in the past decade.

Host factors may influence the incidence and manifestations of gonococcal infection. Prepubertal girls are susceptible to vulvovaginitis and, rarely, experience salpingitis. *N. gonorrhoeae* infects noncornified epithelium, and the thin noncornified vaginal epithelium and alkaline pH of the vaginal mucin predispose this age group to infection of the lower genital tract. Estrogen-induced cornification of the vaginal epithelium in neonates and mature females resists infection. Postpubertal females are more susceptible to salpingitis, especially during menses, when diminished bactericidal activity of the cervical mucus and the reflux of blood from the uterine cavity into the fallopian tubes facilitate passage of gonococci into the upper reproductive tract.

Populations at risk for DGI include asymptomatic carriers; neonates; menstruating, pregnant, and postpartum women; homosexuals; and immunocompromised hosts. The asymptomatic carrier state implies failure of the host immune system to recognize the gonococcus as a pathogen, the capacity of the gonococcus to avoid being killed, or both. Pharyngeal colonization has been proposed as a risk factor for DGI. The high rate of asymptomatic infection in pharyngeal gonorrhea may account for this phenomenon. Women are at greater risk for developing DGI during menstruation and pregnancy and postpartum, presumably because of the maximal endocervical shedding and decreased peroxidase bactericidal activity of the cervical mucus during these periods. A lack of neonatal bactericidal IgM antibody is thought to account for a neonate's increased susceptibility to DGI. Persons with terminal complement component deficiencies (C5–C9) are at considerable risk of developing recurrent episodes of DGI.

CLINICAL MANIFESTATIONS. Gonorrhea is manifested by a spectrum of clinical presentations from asymptomatic carriage, to the characteristic localized urogenital infections, to disseminated systemic infection.

Asymptomatic Gonorrhea. The incidence of this form of gonorrhea in children has not been ascertained. Gonococci have been isolated from the oropharynx of young children who have been abused sexually by male contacts; oropharyngeal symptoms are usually absent. Most genital tract infections produce symptoms in children. However, as many as 80% of sexually mature females with urogenital gonorrhea infections are asymptomatic; asymptomatic rectal carriage of *N. gonorrhoeae* has been documented in 40–60% of females with urogenital infection. At least 20% of rectal infections are asymptomatic, and 78% of pharyngeal gonococcal infections are asymptomatic in homosexual men. Individuals with asymptomatic gonorrhea are an important reservoir of infection and may develop disseminated disease.

Uncomplicated Gonorrhea. Genital gonorrhea has an incubation period of 2–5 days in men and 5–10 days in women. Primary infection develops in the urethra of males, the vulva and vagina of prepubertal females, and the cervix of postpubertal females. Neonatal ophthalmitis occurs in both sexes.

Urethritis is usually characterized by a purulent discharge and by burning on urination without urgency or frequency. Untreated urethritis in males resolves spontaneously in several weeks or may be complicated by epididymitis, penile edema, lymphangitis, prostatitis, or seminal vesiculitis. Gram-negative intracellular diplococci are found in the discharge.

In prepubertal females, vulvovaginitis usually is characterized by a purulent vaginal discharge with a swollen, erythematous, tender, and excoriated vulva. Dysuria may occur. In postpubertal females, symptomatic gonococcal cervicitis and urethritis are characterized by purulent discharge, suprapubic pain, dysuria, intermenstrual bleeding, and dyspareunia. The cervix may be inflamed and tender. In urogenital gonorrhea limited to the lower genital tract, pain is not enhanced by moving the cervix, and the adnexa are not tender to palpation. Purulent material may be expressed from the urethra or ducts of the Bartholin's gland. Rectal gonorrhea, although often asymptomatic, may cause proctitis with symptoms of anal discharge, pruritus, bleeding, pain, tenesmus, and constipation. Asymptomatic rectal gonorrhea may not be due to anal intercourse but may represent colonization from vaginal infection.

Gonococcal ophthalmitis may be unilateral or bilateral. It may occur in any age group after inoculation of the eye with infected secretions. Ophthalmia neonatorum due to *N. gonorrhoeae* usually appears from 1–4 days after birth (Chapter 633). Ocular infection in older patients results from inoculation or autoinoculation from a genital site. The infection begins with mild inflammation and a serosanguineous discharge. Within 24 hr, the discharge becomes thick and purulent, and tense edema of the eyelids with marked chemosis occurs. If the disease is not treated promptly, corneal ulceration, rupture, and blindness may follow.

Disseminated Gonococcal Infection. Hematogenous dissemination occurs in 1–3% of all gonococcal infections, more frequently after asymptomatic primary infections than symptomatic infections. Women account for the majority of cases, with symptoms beginning 7–30 days after infection and within 7 days of menstruation. The most common manifestations are asymmetric arthralgia, petechial or pustular acral skin lesions, tenosynovitis, suppurative arthritis, and, rarely, carditis, meningitis, and osteomyelitis. The most common initial symptoms are acute onset of polyarthralgia with fever. Only 25% of patients complain of skin lesions. Most deny genitourinary symptoms; however, primary mucosal infection is documented by genitourinary cultures. Approximately 80–90% of cervical cultures are positive in women with DGI. In males, urethral cultures are positive in 50–60%, pharyngeal cultures are positive in 10–20%, and rectal cultures are positive in 15% of cases.

DGI has been classified into two clinical syndromes that have some overlapping features. The first and more common is the tenosynovitis-dermatitis syndrome, which is characterized by fever, chills, skin lesions, and polyarthralgias predominantly involving the wrists, hands, and fingers. Blood culture results are positive in approximately 30–40% of cases, and synovial fluid cultures are almost uniformly negative. The second syndrome is the suppurative arthritis syndrome, in which systemic symptoms and signs are less prominent and a monarticular arthritis, often involving the knee, is more common. A polyarthral phase may precede the monarticular infection. In cases of monarticular involvement, synovial fluid culture results are positive in approximately 45–55%, whereas blood culture results are usually negative. DGI in neonates usually occurs as a polyarticular septic arthritis.

Dermatologic lesions usually begin as painful, discrete, 1- to 20-mm pink or red macules that progress to maculopapular, vesicular, bullous, pustular, or petechial lesions. The typical necrotic pustule on an erythematous base is distributed unevenly over the extremities, including the palmar and plantar surfaces, usually sparing the face and scalp. The lesions number between 5 and 40; 20–30% may contain gonococci. Although immune complexes may be present in DGI, complement levels are normal, and the role of the immune complexes in pathogenesis is uncertain.

Acute endocarditis is an uncommon (1–2%) but often fatal manifestation of DGI that usually leads to rapid destruction of the aortic valve. Acute pericarditis is a rarely described entity in patients with disseminated gonorrhea. Meningitis with *N. gonorrhoeae* has been documented. Signs and symptoms are similar to those of any acute bacterial meningitis.

DIAGNOSIS. It is not possible to distinguish gonococcal from nongonococcal urethritis on the basis of symptoms and signs alone. Gonococcal urethritis and vulvovaginitis must be distinguished from other infections that produce a purulent discharge, including β-hemolytic streptococci, *C. trachomatis, Mycoplasma hominis, Trichomonas vaginalis,* and *Candida albicans.* Rarely, infection with human herpesvirus type 2 may produce symptoms similar to those of gonorrhea.

In males with symptomatic urethritis, a presumptive diagnosis of gonorrhea can be made by identification of gram-negative intracellular diplococci (within leukocytes) in the urethral discharge. A similar finding in females is not sufficient because *Mima polymorpha* and *Moraxella,* which are normal vaginal flora, have a similar appearance. The sensitivity of the Gram stain for diagnosing gonococcal cervicitis and asymptomatic infections is also low. The presence of commensal *Neisseria* species in the oropharynx prevents the use of the Gram stain for diagnosis of pharyngeal gonorrhea. Nonpathogenic *Neisseria* are not intracellular.

Diagnosis of gonococcal disease depends on isolation of *N. gonorrhoeae.* Male urethral specimens are obtained by placing a small swab 2–3 cm into the urethra. Material for cervical cultures is obtained after wiping the exocervix and placing a swab in the cervical os and rotating it gently for several seconds. For optimal culture results, specimens should be obtained with noncotton swabs, inoculated directly onto culture plates, and incubated immediately. Samples from the urethra should be cultured for heterosexual men, and samples from the endocervix and rectum should be cultured for all females, regardless of the absence of a history of anal intercourse. Symptomatic sites plus the pharynx should be cultured in patients with orogenital exposure. Specimens from sites (e.g., cervix, rectum, pharynx) that normally are colonized by other organisms should be inoculated on a selective culture medium, such as modified Thayer-Martin medium (fortified with vancomycin, colistin, nyastatin, and trimethoprim to inhibit growth of indigenous flora). Specimens from sites that are normally sterile or minimally contaminated (i.e., synovial fluid, blood, cerebrospinal fluid [CSF]) should be inoculated on a nonselective chocolate agar medium. If DGI is suspected, blood, pharynx, rectum, urethra, cervix, and synovial fluid (if involved) should be cultured. Cultured specimens should be incubated promptly at 35–37°C in 3–5% carbon dioxide. When specimens must be transported to a central laboratory for culture plating, a reduced, nonnutrient holding medium (i.e., Amies modified Stuart medium) preserves specimens with minimal loss of viability for up to 6 hr. When transport may delay culture plating by more than 6 hr, it is preferable to inoculate the sample directly onto a culture medium and transport it at an ambient temperature in a candle jar. The Transgrow and JEMBEC systems of modified Thayer-Martin medium are alternative transport systems.

When microbiology laboratory facilities are not readily available or when patients may be unavailable for follow-up, rapid diagnostic techniques may prove efficacious. Care must be taken in selecting and interpreting results because many rapid tests are less specific than cultures. Nonculture tests include enzyme immunoassay (EIA; polyclonal antigonococcal antibodies for detection of gonococcal antigen), ELISA (monoclonal antibodies), DNA probes, and nucleic acid amplification tests (polymerase chain reaction or ligase chain reaction). These tests appear to be less reliable than culture in low-risk asymptomatic patients, for nongenital specimens, and for specimens obtained from children. Nucleic acid amplification tests and DNA probes may prove to be comparable to culture in sensitivity and specificity. Nonculture tests cannot replace bacteriologic cultures for definitive diagnosis of *N. gonorrhoeae* or for animicrobial susceptibility testing and may be more expensive. They may serve as useful adjuvant diagnostic tools in high-prevalence, transient populations (i.e., in adolescent STD clinics), in which a rapid and accurate presumptive diagnosis is required for prompt institution of therapy.

Gonococcal arthritis must be distinguished from other forms of septic arthritis as well as from rheumatic fever, rheumatoid arthritis, inflammatory bowel disease, and arthritis secondary to rubella or rubella immunization. Gonococcal conjunctivitis in the newborn period must be differentiated from chemical conjunctivitis caused by silver nitrate drops as well as from conjunctivitis caused by *C. trachomatis, Staphylococcus aureus,* group A or B streptococcus, *Pseudomonas aeruginosa,* or human herpesvirus type 2.

TREATMENT. General principles in the treatment of gonorrhea include the need to consider therapy for coexisting STDs (syphilis, *Chlamydia* infection, HIV) and infection due to resistant *N. gonorrhoeae.* The incidence of *Chlamydia* co-infection is 15–25% among males and 35–50% among females. It is recommended that *Chlamydia* infection be treated simultaneously with gonorrhea (Chapter 223.2). Sexual partners exposed in the preceding 30 days should be examined, cultures should be taken, and presumptive treatment started.

Because of the increased prevalence of resistance of *N. gonor-*

rhoeae to penicillin, a third-generation cephalosporin, specifically ceftriaxone, is recommended as initial therapy for all ages. Routine culture and antimicrobial susceptibility testing should be used as guides to therapy. A single intramuscular injection of ceftiaxone (125 mg) for children and adults is the treatment of choice for uncomplicated urethritis, vulvovaginitis, proctitis, or pharyngitis. Alternative regimens shown to be effective for adults and children weighing 45 kg or more are cefixime (400 mg), ciprofloxacin (500 mg), or ofloxacin (400 mg) PO in a single dose. Spectinomycin (40 mg/kg, maximum dose 2 g) in a single intramuscular dose is another alternative but is expensive and is not recommended for pharyngeal infections. Ceftriaxone may also be effective against incubating syphilis but is ineffective against *Chlamydia* infections. In sexually active individuals infected with *N. gonorrhoeae*, simultaneous infection with *C. trachomatis* is common, accounts for most postgonococcal urethritis, and contributes to fallopian tube scarring and infertility. The addition of doxycycline (100 mg PO bid for 7 days) or azithromycin 1 g PO in a single dose is recommended. Children younger than 9 yr and pregnant women should not be given tetracycline drugs, and erythromycin is recommended for them.

Several options exist for treating uncomplicated gonorrhea in penicillin-allergic individuals. A single intramuscular dose of spectinomycin may be given (40 mg/kg for children, 2 g for adults). It is relatively ineffective for pharyngeal gonorrhea, is ineffective against incubating syphilis or *Chlamydia* infections, but is effective against penicillinase-producing *N. gonorrhoeae*. Spectinomycin must be followed by a course of doxycycline. Alternatively, ceftriaxone may be used because the incidence of cross reactivity to cephalosporins is low. Additional therapy for penicillin-allergic patients includes ciprofloxacin (500 mg PO in a single dose). During pregnancy, erythromycin should be added to spectinomycin or ceftriaxone. Tetracyclines should not be used as single-drug therapy for gonorrhea.

Ceftriaxone is recommended as the treatment of choice for DGI. Hospitalization is recommended. A 7-day course of parenteral ceftriaxone (50 mg/kg/24 hr; maximum 1 g/24 hr) given intravenously or intramuscularly is recommended. Alternatives for adults and older adolescents include intravenous cefotaxime 1 g every 8 hr or ceftizoxime 1 g every 8 hr, for 7 days. Ciprofloxacin, ofloxacin, and spectinomycin are alternatives for patients with β-lactam allergy. For adults, parenteral therapy may be discontinued 24–48 hr after improvement occurs and a 7-day course completed with an appropriate oral antibiotic such as cefixime (400 mg), ciprofloxacin (500 mg), or ofloxacin (400 mg) orally twice a day. Endocarditis or meningitis should be treated with 50 mg/kg of ceftriaxone (maximum dose, 2 g) twice daily for children and 1–2 g every 12 hr for adults. Endocarditis is treated for at least 4 wk, and meningitis is treated for 10–14 days. Concurrent therapy for treatment of genital *Chlamydia* infection is important.

Neonates with gonococcal ophthalmitis must be hospitalized and evaluated for DGI. Nondisseminated infections including ophthalmia neonatorum should be treated with ceftriaxone (25–50 mg/kg IV or IM, not to exceed 125 mg) given once. A single dose of cefotaxime (100 mg/kg) is an acceptable alternative. Concomitant saline irrigation of the eyes is recommended. Infants with arthritis or septicemia should be treated for 7 days. Infants with meningitis should receive 10–14 days of therapy.

PID requires hospitalization for evaluation and initiation of treatment. PID encompasses a spectrum of infectious diseases of the upper genital tract due to *N. gonorrhoeae, C. trachomatis*, and endogenous flora (streptococci, anaerobes, gram-negative bacilli). Therapy must cover a broad spectrum and must be given to adolescents as inpatients. A commonly recommended therapeutic regimen is 2 g of cefoxitin IV every 6 hr or 2 g of cefotetan IV every 12 hr, plus 100 mg of doxycyline PO or IV every 12 hr. Therapy is continued for at least 48 hr after a patient shows improvement. Thereafter, oral doxycycline is continued for a total of 10–14 days. An alternative recommended regimen is clindamycin (900 mg IV every 8 hr) plus a loading dose of gentamicin (2 mg/kg IV), followed by maintenance gentamicin (1.5 mg/kg every 8 hr). Therapy is then continued for 48 hr after a patient improves and is followed by oral doxycycline for 10–14 days. If an intrauterine device is present, it must be removed and an alternative form of birth control used. Sexual partners should be examined and treated for uncomplicated gonorrhea. Follow-up culture (test of cure) of cephalosporin-doxycycline therapy of gonococcal STD is not recommended owing to the low treatment failure rate. A follow-up examination and culture are recommended in 1–2 mo to evaluate the possibility of reinfection or, rarely, treatment failure.

COMPLICATIONS. Complications of gonorrhea result from the spread of gonococci from a local site of invasion. The interval between primary infection and development of a complication is usually days to weeks. In postpubertal females, endometritis may occur, especially during menses. This may progress to salpingitis and peritonitis (PID). Manifestations of PID include signs of lower genital tract infection (e.g., vaginal discharge, suprapubic pain, cervical tenderness) and upper genital tract infection (e.g., fever, leukocytosis, elevated erythrocyte sedimentation rate, and adnexal tenderness or mass). The differential diagnosis includes gynecologic (ovarian cyst, ovarian tumor, ectopic pregnancy) and intra-abdominal (appendicitis, urinary tract infection, inflammatory bowel disease) pathology.

Once inside the peritoneum, gonococci may seed the liver capsule, causing a perihepatitis. The resultant right upper quadrant pain, with or without signs of salpingitis, is known as the Fitz-Hugh–Curtis syndrome. Perihepatitis may also be caused by *Chlamydia trachomatis*. Progression to PID occurs in about 20% of cases of gonococcal cervicitis. *N. gonorrhoeae* is isolated in approximately 40% of cases of PID in the United States. Untreated cases may lead to hydrosalpinx, pyosalpinx, tubo-ovarian abscess, and eventual sterility. Even with adequate treatment of PID, the risk of sterility caused by bilateral tubal occlusion approaches 20% after one episode of salpingitis and exceeds 60% with three or more episodes. The risk of ectopic pregnancy is increased approximately sevenfold after one or more episodes of salpingitis. Additional sequelae of PID include chronic pain, dyspareunia, and increased risk of recurrent PID.

Urogenital gonococcal infection acquired during the 1st trimester of pregnancy carries a high risk of septic abortion. After 16 wk, infection causes chorioamnionitis, a major cause of premature rupture of the membranes and premature delivery.

Because these patients are at high risk for other STDs, all patients with gonorrhea should have a serologic test for syphilis and be evaluated and treated for recurrent *C. trachomatis* infection at the time of diagnosis. HIV testing is also indicated. The Venereal Disease Research Laboratory test should be repeated 3 mo later.

PROGNOSIS. Prompt diagnosis and correct therapy ensure complete recovery from uncomplicated gonococcal disease. Complications and permanent sequelae may be associated with delayed treatment, recurrent infection, metastatic sites of infection (meninges, aortic valve), and delayed or topical therapy of gonococcal ophthalmia.

PREVENTION. Efforts to develop a gonococcal pilus vaccine have been unsuccessful thus far. The high degree of inter- and intrastrain antigenic variability of pili poses a formidable deterrent to the development of a single effective pilus vaccine. Other gonococcal surface structures such as the porin protein, stress proteins, and lipooligosaccharides may prove more promising as vaccine candidates. In the absence of a vaccine, prevention of gonorrhea can be achieved through education, use of barrier contraceptives (especially condoms and spermicides), intensive epidemiologic and bacteriologic surveillance (screening sexual contacts), and early identification and treatment of infected contacts.

Gonococcal ophthalmia neonatorum can be prevented by instilling 2 drops of a 1% solution of silver nitrate into each conjunctival sac shortly after birth (see Chapter 633). Erythromycin (0.5%) or tetracycline (1%) ophthalmic ointment may also be used. Infants born to mothers with active gonorrhea are at high risk for developing gonococcal ophthalmitis and should be given a single 125-mg intramuscular injection of ceftriaxone for prophylaxis; for low birthweight infants, the dose is 25–50 mg/kg. A single dose of cefotaxime (100 mg/kg IV or IM) is an alternative.

Cates W, Wasserheit JN: Gonorrhea, chlamydia, and pelvic inflammatory disease. Curr Opin Infect Dis 3:10, 1990.
Centers for Disease Control and Prevention: 1998 guidelines for treatment of sexually transmitted diseases. MMWR 47(RR-1):1, 1998.
Cohen MS, Sparling PF: Mucosal infection with *Neisseria gonorrhoeae*, bacterial adaptation and mucosal defenses. J Clin Invest 89:1699, 1992.
Fox KK, Knapp JS, Holmes KK, et al: Antimicrobial resistance in *Neisseria gonorrhoeae* in the United States, 1988–1994: The emergence of decreased susceptibility to the fluoroquinolones. J Infect Dis 175:1396, 1997.
Hook EW, Holmes KK: Gonococcal infections. Ann Intern Med 102:229, 1985.
Lind I: Antimicrobial resistance in *Neisseria gonorrhoeae*. Clin Infect Dis 24(Suppl 1):593, 1997.
Moran JS, Levine WC: Drugs of choice for the treatment of uncomplicated gonococcal infections. Clin Infect Dis 20(Suppl 1):547, 1995.
O'Brien JP, Goldenberg DL, Rice PA: Disseminated gonococcal infection: A prospective analysis of 49 patients and a review of pathophysiology and immune mechanisms. Medicine (Baltimore) 62:395, 1983.
Whitington WL, et al: Incorrect identification of *Neisseria gonorrhoeae* from infants and children. Pediatr Infect Dis J 7:34, 1988.

CHAPTER 193

Haemophilus influenzae

Robert S. Daum

Approximately 100 yr after the recognition of *Haemophilus influenzae* as the cause of several important syndromes in childhood, an effective vaccine to prevent these illnesses was introduced in the United States, resulting in a dramatic decrease in the prevalence of infections due to this organism. However, mortality and morbidity from *H. influenzae* type b infection remain a problem worldwide, primarily in unimmunized populations.

ETIOLOGY. *H. influenzae* is a fastidious, gram-negative, pleomorphic coccobacillus that requires factors X (hematin) and V (phosphopyridine nucleotide) for growth. These factors are present within erythrocytes, and the demonstration of their requirement for growth is the basis for speciating *H. influenzae* in the laboratory.

Some *H. influenzae* isolates are surrounded by a polysaccharide capsule. Such isolates can be serotyped into six antigenically and biochemically distinct types, designated a–f. The most virulent isolates belong to serotype b.

EPIDEMIOLOGY. Before the advent of effective conjugate vaccine use in 1988, *H. influenzae* was a major cause of certain invasive diseases in children. Serotype b organisms accounted for more than 95% of these cases. There was a striking age distribution of cases; more than 90% occurred in children younger than 5 yr, and the majority occurred in children younger than 2 yr. The annual attack rate of invasive disease was estimated to be 64–129 cases/100,000 children less than 5 yr of age/yr. Invasive disease caused by other capsular serotypes was much less frequent; the incidence of invasive disease was estimated at 0.7 cases/100,000 children less than 5 yr of age/yr. Nonencapsulated (nontypable) *H. influenzae* organisms cause invasive disease in neonates, immunocompromised children, and children in certain developing countries. Nontypable isolates are common etiologic agents in otitis media, sinusitis, and in chronic bronchitis in adults.

Humans are the only natural hosts for *H. influenzae*. This species is a constituent of the normal respiratory flora in 60–90% of healthy children. Most isolates are nontypable. Colonization by serotype b organisms is infrequent. Before the advent of conjugate vaccine immunization, *H. influenzae* type b could be isolated from the pharynx of 2–5% of healthy preschool and school-aged children; lower rates occurred among infants younger than 1 yr and adults. Such asymptomatic colonization with *H. influenzae* type b probably occurs at lower rates in immunized populations, although, importantly, the bacterium continues to circulate.

From 1989–1997, the incidence of invasive *H. influenzae* type b disease among children younger than 5 yr declined 99%, from 34 to 0.4 cases/100,000 children/yr. Because a similar decline in invasive *H. influenzae* disease due to other serotypes or due to nontypable organisms has not occurred, the proportion of cases due to serotype b organisms has also declined and accounted for only 32–41% of reported cases in 1996–1997.

The few cases of serotype b invasive disease that occurred in 1996–1997 occurred in both unvaccinated and fully vaccinated children; 48% occurred in infants younger than 6 mo, too young to have received a three-dose primary series. Among those cases age-eligible to have received such a series, 36% had received at least a three-dose primary series, about half of these had also received a booster dose.

Certain groups and individuals have been identified to have an increased incidence of invasive disease, including Alaskan Eskimos, Apaches, Navajos, and blacks. In these populations, the proportion of cases of invasive disease in children younger than 12 mo has been relatively high. Persons known to be at an increased risk for invasive disease have also included those with sickle cell disease, asplenia, congenital and acquired immunodeficiencies, and malignancies. Nonvaccinated infants younger than 12 mo who had previously documented invasive infection are at increased risk for recurrence.

Socioeconomic risk factors for invasive *H. influenzae* type b disease include child care outside the home, the presence of siblings of elementary school age or younger, short duration of breast-feeding, and parental smoking. Previous hospitalization for invasive *H. influenzae* type b disease and a history of otitis media are associated with an increased risk for invasive disease. Much less is known about the epidemiology of *H. influenzae* infections other than serotype b.

The mode of transmission is most commonly by direct contact or inhalation of respiratory tract droplets containing *H. influenzae*. The incubation period for invasive disease is variable, and the exact period of communicability is unknown. Most children with invasive *H. influenzae* type b disease are colonized in the nasopharynx before initiation of antimicrobial therapy; 25–40% may remain colonized during the first 24 hr of therapy.

Among age-susceptible household contacts who have been exposed to a case of invasive *H. influenzae* type b disease, the risk of secondary cases of invasive disease in the first 30 days is estimated at 0.26%. The attack rate for secondary *H. influenzae* type b cases in household contacts has been highest in susceptible children younger than 24 mo (3.2%) and rare (<0.1%) in contacts older than 47 mo. Whether such an increase in risk occurs in individuals exposed to patients with invasive disease caused by nonserotype b organisms is not known.

PATHOGENESIS. The precise mechanisms that facilitate successful colonization of the respiratory epithelium have not been identified. In an organ culture of human nasopharyngeal tissue, type b and non-b strains of *H. influenzae* organisms attach to nonciliated columnar epithelial cells and subsequently can be seen within those cells and in the intercellular spaces.

The events that result in entry into the intravascular compartment by serotype b organisms are unclear. Once there, however, type b strains resist intravascular clearance mechanisms more readily than do strains of other serotypes and nonencapsulated organisms. Whether it is the type b PRP capsule itself that confers the potential for invasive disease or another closely linked virulence factor is not certain. An undeciphered clue may lie in the predilection of genes encoding for PRP to be present in an unusual tandem arrangement on the genome of 98% of clinical isolates.

Once established, the magnitude of *H. influenzae* type b bacteremia and its duration are independent variables that determine the likelihood of dissemination of bacteria into sites such as the meninges or joints. The bacterial and host mechanisms that determine the magnitude of bacteremia are poorly understood.

Noninvasive *H. influenzae* infections such as otitis media, sinusitis, and bronchitis, usually caused by nontypable strains, probably gain access to sites such as the middle ear and sinus cavities by direct extension from the pharynx. The factors facilitating spread from the pharynx include eustachian tube dysfunction and antecedent viral infections of the upper respiratory tract.

Antibiotic Resistance. Isolates that produced β-lactamase were identified for the first time in 1974, and their incidence increased in the subsequent decade. The most recent multicenter collaborative surveillance study conducted in the United States in 1994–1995 showed that 36.5% of *H. influenzae* isolates produced a β-lactamase and were resistant to ampicillin. About 4% of β-lactamase–negative isolates are ampicillin resistant but do not produce β-lactamase. The mechanism of resistance in this instance is the production of a penicillin-binding protein with decreased affinity for β-lactam compounds.

Chloramphenicol is effective against most isolates of *H. influenzae* regardless of β-lactamase production. The disadvantages of chloramphenicol include the need for complex monitoring strategies and the rare occurrence of idiosyncratic aplastic anemia. Isolates of *H. influenzae* type b have been identified as resistant to chloramphenicol; resistance is usually mediated by the action of chloramphenicol acetyltransferase (CAT), although a few isolates do not produce this enzyme. Chloramphenicol-resistant isolates have remained relatively rare (about 0.2% of isolates) in the United States and throughout the world, although they have been reported to be more common in a few locales such as Barcelona and Taiwan. Isolates resistant to both chloramphenicol and ampicillin have been identified rarely. In the United States, fewer than 1% of isolates were resistant to both compounds. Resistance to trimethoprim-sulfamethoxazole (TMP-SMX) occurred in 9% of clinical isolates.

Until recently, amoxacillin-clavulanate was considered uniformly active against *H. influenzae* clinical isolates. However, about 3% of β-lactamase–positive isolates are resistant to amoxacillin-clavulanate. Furthermore, amoxacillin-clavulanate offers no apparent synergy against ampicillin-resistant isolates that do not elaborate β-lactamase. Among the newer macrolides, 99% and 78% of *H. influenzae* isolates were susceptible to azithromycin and clarithromycin, respectively, whereas the activity of erythromycin against *H. influenzae* clinical isolates has been considered to be poor. Resistance to quinolones, first recognized in 1993, is believed to be infrequent. Resistance to extended-spectrum cephalosporins, which are commonly used in therapy, has not been documented.

Immunity. The most important element of host defense is antibody directed against the type b capsular polysaccharide, PRP. In the prevaccination era anti-PRP antibody was acquired in an age-related fashion; its mechanism of action is to facilitate clearance of *H. influenzae* type b from blood. This is related in part to its opsonic activity; other antibodies directed against antigens such as outer membrane proteins or lipopolysaccharides may also have a role in opsonization. Both the classic and alternative complement pathways are important in the opsonization of *H. influenzae* type b. The macrophages of the reticuloendothelial system aid in intravascular clearance of *H. influenzae* type b by affecting intracellular killing after opsonization.

Before the introduction of vaccination and among recipients of unconjugated PRP vaccines, protection from *H. influenzae* type b infection was presumed to correlate with the concentration of circulating anti-PRP antibody at the time of exposure. A serum antibody concentration of 0.15–1.0 μg/mL was considered protective against invasive infection; the higher concentration in vaccinees may predict maintenance of a level of more than 0.15 μg/mL over time. Most infants lack an anti-PRP antibody concentration of this magnitude and are susceptible to disease on encounter with *H. influenzae* type b. This lack of antibody in young infants may reflect a maturational delay in the immunologic response to thymus-independent type 2 (TI-2) antigens such as unconjugated PRP, and it was thought to explain the high incidence of serotype b infections in young infants in the prevaccination era.

Unlike the PRP unconjugated vaccine, the conjugate vaccines—with the exception of PRP-OMP, which also has thymus-independent type 1 (TI-1) properties—act as thymus-dependent (TD) antigens (Table 193–1). They elicit serum antibody responses in young infants, although repeat doses may be required, and prime memory antibody responses on subsequent encounters with PRP. The concentration of circulating anti-PRP antibody in a child primed by a conjugate vaccine may not correlate precisely with protection, because a memory response may occur rapidly on exposure to PRP and provide protection.

Less is known about immunity to nontypable *H. influenzae*. Evidence suggests that antibodies directed against one or more outer membrane proteins (OMP) are bactericidal and protect against experimental challenge. For example, P6, a major OMP, is present in all strains of *H. influenzae* and is highly conserved among encapsulated and nontypable strains. In infant rats, antibody to P6 is bactericidal for encapsulated and nontypable *H. influenzae* and is protective against *H. influenzae* type b disease. Another OMP, P2, has substantial interstrain heterogeneity. Antibody elicited to the nonconserved regions of P2 had complement-dependent bactericidal activity to the homologous strain. Monoclonal antibodies directed against a group of surface-exposed high molecular weight OMPs have provided protection in experimental infection in animals.

DIAGNOSIS. Presumptive identification of *H. influenzae* is made by direct examination of the collected specimen after Gram staining. Because of its small size, pleomorphism, poor uptake of stain by some isolates, and the tendency for fluids, particularly when proteinaceous, to have a red background, *H. influenzae* is sometimes difficult to visualize; staining with methylene blue may be helpful. With this technique, *H. influenzae* appears as a blue-black coccobacillus against a light blue-gray background. Because identification of microorganisms on smear by either technique requires at least 10^5 bacteria/mL, failure to visualize them does not preclude their presence.

Culture of *H. influenzae* requires prompt transport and processing of specimens, because the organism is fastidious. Specimens should not be exposed to drying or temperature extremes. Primary isolation of *H. influenzae* can be accomplished on chocolate agar, *Haemophilus* isolation agar, or on blood agar plates using the *Staphylococcus* streak technique.

Serotyping of *H. influenzae* is accomplished by slide agglutination with type-specific antisera. Accurate serotyping is essential to monitor progress toward elimination of serotype b invasive disease. Timely reporting of cases to public health authorities should be ensured.

TABLE 193–1 ***Haemophilus influenzae* type b Conjugate Vaccines**

Abbreviation	Trade Name	Manufacturer	Protein Carrier
HbOC*	HibTITER	Lederle	CRM_{197} (a nontoxic naturally occurring mutant of diphtheria toxin)
PRP-OMP†	PedvaxHIB	Merck	OMP (an outer membrane protein complex of *Neisseria meningitidis*)
PRP-T‡	ActHIB	Pasteur-Mérieux Connaught	Tetanus toxoid
	OmniHIB	SmithKline Beecham	
PRP-D§	ProHIBiT	Connaught	Diphtheria toxoid

**HbOC is also available as a combination vaccine with whole-cell pertussis DTP (Tetramune), which can be used for all doses in children.*
†PRP-OMP is also available as a combination vaccine with hepatitis B vaccine (Comvax). This should not be used for hepatitis B immunization at birth.
‡PRP-T can be reconstituted with Connaught whole cell DTP immediately before administration in a single syringe, which can be used for all doses in children. PRP-T can also be reconstituted with Connaught DTaP vaccine (Tripedia), a combination marketed as TriHIBit, which is acceptable only for the booster (4th) dose in infants ≥15 mo of age.
§PRP-D is recommended only for children ≥12 mo of age. HbOC, PRP-OMP, and PRP-T are recommended for infants beginning at 2 mo of age.

Detection of PRP in cerebrospinal fluid (CSF), serum, urine, or other relevant body fluids using latex particle agglutination (LA) and enzyme immunoassay is useful in the diagnosis of serotype b infections. LA is perhaps the most sensitive, versatile, and accessible method for direct detection of PRP. Detection of type b PRP capsular antigen is most helpful for diagnosing *H. influenzae* type b infections in patients who received prior antimicrobial therapy when culture results may not be revealing. Recent immunization against *H. influenzae* type b is often associated with antigenuria of variable duration (usually <7 days) and occasionally antigenemia of very short duration (<3 days); this may confound the diagnostic use of PRP detecting techniques for a short time after immunization.

CLINICAL MANIFESTATIONS AND TREATMENT. The clinical manifestations and treatment of all invasive *H. influenzae* disease are similar regardless of serotype. The initial antibiotic therapy of invasive infections possibly due to *H. influenzae* type b should be a parenterally administered antimicrobial agent effective in sterilizing all foci of infection and effective against ampicillin-resistant strains. Extended-spectrum cephalosporins, such as cefotaxime or ceftriaxone, have been used as the initial antimicrobial agent when *H. influenzae* type b is considered a likely pathogen, and they have achieved popularity because of their relative lack of serious adverse effects and ease of administration. Alternatively, chloramphenicol can be used with ampicillin. After the antimicrobial susceptibility of the isolate has been determined, an appropriate agent can be selected to complete the therapy. Ampicillin remains the drug of choice for the therapy of infections caused by susceptible isolates. If the isolate is resistant to ampicillin, extended-spectrum cephalosporins such as cefotaxime or ceftriaxone are useful; the latter can be administered once daily in selected circumstances for outpatient therapy. Chloramphenicol also has extensive clinical experience.

Oral antimicrobial agents are sometimes used to complete a course of therapy initiated by the parenteral route. If the organism is susceptible to ampicillin, amoxicillin is the drug of choice. An oral third-generation cephalosporin (e.g., cefixime, cefpodoxime) or amoxicillin-clavulanate may be used when the isolate is resistant to ampicillin. Chloramphenicol is another option that continues to enjoy popularity in some countries because of its low cost.

Meningitis (see Chapter 174.1). Before the development of *H. influenzae* type b conjugate vaccines, *H. influenzae* type b was the leading cause of bacterial meningitis in children in the United States. Clinically, meningitis due to *H. influenzae* type b cannot be differentiated from that due to *Neisseria meningitidis* or *Streptococcus pneumoniae* and may be complicated by other foci of infection, such as the lungs, joints, bones, or pericardium.

Antimicrobial therapy should be administered parenterally for 7–14 days for uncomplicated cases. Cefotaxime, ceftriaxone, ampicillin, and chloramphenicol all are thought to cross the blood-brain barrier during acute inflammation in concentrations adequate to render them effective for *H. influenzae* meningitis. Chloramphenicol has been administered orally to complete a therapeutic regimen for meningitis.

The prognosis of *H. influenzae* type b meningitis depends on the age at presentation, the duration of illness before appropriate antimicrobial therapy, the CSF capsular polysaccharide concentration, and the rapidity with which it is cleared from CSF, blood, and urine. Low intelligence quotients correlate with clinically manifested inappropriate secretion of antidiuretic hormone and evidence of focal neurologic deficits at presentation. About 6% of patients with *H. influenzae* type b meningitis are left with some hearing impairment, probably because of inflammation of the cochlea and the labyrinth. Dexamethasone (0.6 mg/kg/24 hr divided every 6 hr for 2 days), particularly when given shortly before or concurrent with the initiation of antimicrobial therapy, decreases the incidence of hearing loss associated with *H. influenzae* type b meningitis. Major neurologic sequelae of *H. influenzae* type b meningitis include behavior problems, language disorders, delayed development of language, impaired vision, mental retardation, motor abnormalities, ataxia, seizures, and hydrocephalus.

Cellulitis. Children with *H. influenzae* cellulitis often have an antecedent upper respiratory tract infection. They usually have no prior history of trauma, and the infection is thought to represent seeding of the organism to the involved soft tissues during bacteremia. The head and neck, particularly the cheek and preseptal region, are the most common sites of involvement. The involved region generally has indistinct margins and is tender and indurated. Buccal cellulitis is classically erythematous with a violaceous hue, although this sign may be absent. *H. influenzae* may often be recovered directly from an aspirate with or without prior injection of 0.1 mL of a nonbacteriostatic sterile solution into the area of involvement. The blood culture may reveal the causative organism. Other foci of infection may be present concomitantly, particularly in a patient is younger than 18 mo or one who is febrile. A diagnostic lumbar puncture should be considered at the time of diagnosis for these children.

Parenteral antimicrobial therapy is indicated until patients become afebrile. Prolonged fever may be a sign of distant foci (e.g., meningitis, arthritis). After patients become afebrile and the signs of inflammation decrease, an appropriate orally administered antimicrobial agent may be substituted. A 7–10-day course is customary.

Preseptal Cellulitis. Infection involving the superficial tissue layers anterior to the orbital septum is termed preseptal cellulitis, which may be caused by *H. influenzae*. Uncomplicated preseptal cellulitis does not imply a risk for visual impairment or direct central nervous system extension. However, concurrent bacteremia may be associated with the development of meningitis. *H. influenzae* preseptal cellulitis is characterized by fever, edema, tenderness, warmth of the lid, and, occasionally, purple discoloration. Evidence of interruption of the integument is usually absent. Conjunctival drainage may be associated. *S. pneumoniae, Staphylococcus aureus,* and group A β-hemolytic streptococci cause clinically indistinguishable preseptal cellulitis. The latter two pathogens are more likely when fever is absent and with an interruption of the integument (e.g., an insect bite).

Those with preseptal cellulitis in whom *H. influenzae* or *S. pneumoniae* are etiologic considerations (i.e., young age, high fever, intact integument) should have blood submitted for culture, and a diagnostic lumbar puncture should be considered.

Parenteral antibiotics are indicated for preseptal cellulitis. Because *S. aureus, S. pneumoniae,* and group A β-hemolytic streptococci are other causes, empirical therapy should include agents active against these pathogens. Patients with preseptal cellulitis without concurrent meningitis should receive parenteral therapy for about 5 days until fever and erythema have abated. In uncomplicated cases, antimicrobial therapy should be given for a total of 10 days.

Orbital Cellulitis. Infections of the orbit are infrequent and usually complicate acute ethmoid and sphenoid sinusitis. Orbital cellulitis may present with lid edema but is distinguished by the presence of proptosis, chemosis, impaired vision, limitation of the extraocular movements, decreased mobility of the globe, or pain on movement of the globe. The distinction between preseptal and orbital cellulitis may be difficult. The extent of the infection is best delineated by CT.

Orbital infections are treated with parenteral therapy for at least 14 days. Underlying sinusitis may require surgical drainage. Abscesses in the orbit usually require prompt surgical drainage and more prolonged antimicrobial therapy. If no abscess is found at the initial evaluation, the need for surgical exploration to drain a subperiosteal or orbital abscess should be reconsidered if the response to therapy is not prompt.

Supraglottitis or Acute Epiglottitis (see Chapter 385). Epiglottitis is a cellulitis of the tissues comprising the laryngeal inlet that include the epiglottis, aryepiglottic folds, and arytenoid cartilage. It has become exceedingly rare. Direct invasion of the involved tissues by *H. influenzae* type b is probably the initiating pathophysiologic event. This dramatic, potentially lethal condition usually occurs in children 2–7 yr old. Because of the risk of sudden, unpredictable airway obstruction, supraglottitis is a medical emergency. Pneumonia is detected by chest radiograph in about 25% of cases. Other foci of infection, such as meningitis, are rare. Antimicrobial therapy directed against *H. influenzae* type b should be administered parenterally but only after the airway is secured, and therapy should be continued until patients are able to take fluids by mouth. The duration of antimicrobial therapy typically is 7 days.

Pneumonia (see Chapter 175). The true incidence of *H. influenzae* type b pneumonia in children is unknown because invasive procedures are required to obtain cultures and are seldom performed. The signs and symptoms of pneumonia due to *H. influenzae* cannot be differentiated from those of pneumonia caused by many other microorganisms. Other foci of infection may be present concomitantly. Antigen detection tests performed on blood or urine may aid in diagnosis if serotype b organisms are the cause.

Children suspected of having *H. influenzae* type b pneumonia who are younger than 12 mo should receive parenteral antimicrobial therapy initially because of their increased risk for bacteremia and its complications. Older children who do not appear severely ill may be managed with an orally administered antimicrobial. Therapy is continued for 7–10 days of combined parenteral-oral therapy.

Uncomplicated pleural effusion associated with *H. influenzae* pneumonia requires no special intervention. However, if empyema develops, insertion of a chest tube and a more prolonged course of antimicrobial therapy may be necessary.

Suppurative Arthritis (see Chapter 178). Large joints, such as the knee, hip, ankle, and elbow, are affected most commonly. Other foci of infection may be present concomitantly. Although single joint involvement is the rule, multiple joint involvement occurs in about 6% of cases. The signs and symptoms of septic arthritis due to *H. influenzae* are indistinguishable from those of arthritis caused by other bacteria.

Uncomplicated septic arthritis should be treated with an appropriate antimicrobial administered parenterally for at least 5–7 days. If the clinical response is satisfactory (i.e., defervescence, decreased signs of inflammation, and a decrease in the C-reactive protein or the erythrocyte sedimentation rate) the remainder of the course of antimicrobial treatment may be given orally. Ensuring compliance is an important consideration in the selection of candidates for oral therapy. Therapy is typically given for 3 wk for uncomplicated septic arthritis, but it may be continued beyond 3 wk until the erythrocyte sedimentation rate is normal.

Pericarditis (see Chapter 446). *H. influenzae* is a rare cause of bacterial pericarditis. Affected children often have had an antecedent upper respiratory tract infection. Fever, respiratory distress, and tachycardia are consistent findings. Other foci of infection may be present concomitantly.

The diagnosis may be established by recovery of the organism from blood or pericardial fluid. Gram stain or detection of PRP in pericardial fluid, blood, or urine (when serotype b organisms are the cause) may aid the diagnosis. Antimicrobials should be provided parenterally in a regimen similar to that used for meningitis (see Chapter 174.1). Pericardiectomy is useful for draining the purulent material effectively and preventing tamponade and constrictive pericarditis.

Bacteremia Without an Associated Focus (see Chapter 172). Bacteremia due to *H. influenzae* type b may be associated with fever without any apparent focus of infection. In this situation, risk factors for "occult" bacteremia include the magnitude of fever (≥ 39°C) and the presence of leukocytosis (≥ 15,000 cells/μL). It is estimated that 26.6% of children with occult *H. influenzae* type b bacteremia develop meningitis if left untreated. In the vaccine era, this *H. influenzae* type b infection has become exceedingly rare. When it does occur, however, the child should be re-evaluated for a focus of infection and a second blood culture obtained. The child should be hospitalized and given parenteral antimicrobial therapy after a diagnostic lumbar puncture and chest radiograph are obtained. If no focus is identified, oral antimicrobial therapy may be substituted after 2–5 days to complete a 7–10-day course.

If no source is found at the time of re-evaluation and a child is afebrile and appears well, a follow-up blood culture should also be obtained. In this instance, further diagnostic evaluation (e.g., lumbar puncture) may not be necessary. However, many experts believe that oral antimicrobial therapy may not be adequate because of the risk of serious focal infection. Therefore, a daily dose of ceftriaxone (50 mg/kg) may be given. Children should be closely monitored until it is apparent that the fever has not recurred, the second blood culture is known to be sterile, and no focus of infection has developed.

Miscellaneous Infections. Urinary tract infection, epididymo-orchitis, cervical adenitis, acute glossitis, infected thyroglossal duct cysts, uvulitis endocarditis, endophthalmitis, primary peritonitis, osteomyelitis and periappendiceal abscess are rarely caused by *H. influenzae*.

Invasive Disease in Neonates. In neonates with invasive *H. influenzae* infection, nontypable isolates are more common than serotype b isolates, although both are rare. When illness occurs in the first 24 hr of life, especially in association with maternal chorioamnionitis or prolonged rupture of membranes, transmission of the organism to the infant is likely to have occurred through the maternal genital tract, which may be (<1%) colonized with nontypable *H. influenzae*. Transmission to neonates by colonized mothers may occur at a rate of up to 50%. Manifestations of neonatal invasive infection include bacteremia with sepsis, pneumonia, respiratory distress syndrome with shock, conjunctivitis, scalp abscess or cellulitis, or meningitis. Less commonly, mastoiditis, septic arthritis, or a congenital vesicular eruption may occur.

Otitis Media (see Chapter 646). Acute otitis media is one of the most common infectious diseases of childhood. It is thought to result from the spread of bacteria from the nasopharynx through the eustachian tube into the middle-ear cavity. Usually because of a preceding viral upper respiratory tract infection, the mucosa in the area becomes hyperemic and swollen, resulting in obstruction and an opportunity for bacterial multiplication in the middle ear.

The most common bacterial pathogens are *S. pneumoniae, H. influenzae,* and *Moraxella catarrhalis*. Most *H. influenzae* isolates are nontypable. Amoxicillin (80–90 mg/kg/24 hr) is a suitable first-line oral antimicrobial agent; the combined probability of the causative isolate being resistant to amoxicillin and of invasive potential is sufficiently low to continue to justify this approach. Alternatively, a single dose of ceftriaxone may constitute adequate therapy.

In the case of treatment failure or if a β-lactamase–producing isolate is obtained by tympanocentesis or from drainage fluid, amoxicillin-clavulanate, erythromycin-sulfisoxazole, and cefaclor are among the available alternatives. The latter combination may be useful as first-line agents for patients allergic to β-lactam compounds.

Conjunctivitis (see Chapter 633). Acute infection of the conjunctiva is the most common eye infection in childhood. In neonates, *H. influenzae* is an infrequent cause. However, it is an important pathogen in older children, as are *S. pneumoniae* and *S. aureus*. Most *H. influenzae* isolates associated with conjunctivitis are nontypable, although serotype b isolates and other microorganisms are occasionally found. Empirical treatment of conjunctivitis beyond the neonatal period usually consists of topical antimicrobial therapy with sulfacetamide and erythromycin.

Sinusitis (see Chapter 381). *H. influenzae* is an important cause of acute sinusitis in children, second in frequency only to *S. pneumoniae*. Chronic sinusitis lasting longer than 1 yr or severe sinusitis requiring hospitalization is often caused by *S. aureus* or anaerobes such as *Peptococcus, Peptostreptococcus,* or *Bacteroides* species. Nontypable *H. influenzae* and viridans group *streptococci* are also frequently recovered.

For uncomplicated sinusitis, amoxicillin is acceptable initial therapy. However, if clinical improvement does not occur, a broader-spectrum regimen may be appropriate, such as amoxicillin-clavulanate; hospitalization with parenteral therapy is occasionally required. For uncomplicated sinusitis, a 10-day course is sufficient.

PREVENTION OF SEROTYPE B INFECTIONS

Chemoprophylaxis. Unvaccinated close contacts younger than 48 mo of patients with invasive *H. influenzae* type b infections are at increased risk of invasive infection when exposed to an index case. The risk of secondary disease is inversely related to age (for children >3 mo of age). About half of the cases of secondary disease among susceptible household contacts occur in the 1st wk after hospitalization of the index patient. Because many children are now protected against *H. influenzae* type b by prior immunization, the need for chemoprophylaxis has greatly decreased.

The goal of chemoprophylaxis is to prevent a susceptible child from acquiring *H. influenzae* type b from contacts by eliminating colonization in the close contacts. Rifampin prophylaxis is indicated for all members of the close contact group, including the index patient, if one or more children younger than 48 mo are not fully immunized, defined as having received at least one dose of a *H. influenzae* type b conjugate vaccine at 15 mo of age or older, two doses at 12–14 mo of age, two or more doses at 12 mo of age or older, or three doses while younger than 12 mo of age and one dose at 12 mo of age. An exception is made when the household contact group includes a fully vaccinated immunocompromised child, because the vaccination may have been ineffective. The household contact group is defined as individuals residing with the index patient or a nonresident who has spent 4 hr or more with the index patient for at least 5 of the 7 days preceding the day of hospitalization of the index patient.

Parents of children hospitalized for invasive *H. influenzae* type b disease should be told that there is an increased risk for secondary infection due to this organism in other young children in the same household if they are partially immunized. The parents should be alerted to any signs or symptoms that might be related to such an infection and should be instructed to seek prompt medical attention when such signs do appear. Although parents of children exposed to a single case of invasive *H. influenzae* type b disease in a child-care center or nursery school should be similarly warned, there is disagreement about the use of rifampin for these children. Because the data on the risk of secondary *H. influenzae* type b infection among children who attend group daycare are conflicting, some experts believe that the risk is too low to justify chemoprophylaxis. It is difficult to institute a uniform policy that would include all the many different caretakers and physicians involved.

A few guidelines for chemoprophylaxis are useful in evaluating a childcare setting for possible rifampin administration. In childcare settings resembling households, such as those with children younger than 2 yr in which contact is at least 25 hr/wk, rifampin prophylaxis may be of benefit. When two or more cases of invasive disease have occurred within 60 days among attendees, regardless of the size of the care facility, administering rifampin to all attendees and supervisory personnel is recommended. If all childcare contacts are older than 2 yr, chemoprophylaxis need not be given.

For chemoprophylaxis, children should be given rifampin orally (0–1 mo of age, 10 mg/kg/dose; >1 mo, 20 mg/kg/dose, not to exceed 600 mg/dose), once each a day for 4 consecutive days. The adult dose is 600 mg once daily. It is not recommended for pregnant women, because the effects on a fetus are not established. Because rifampin induces enzymes that metabolize oral contraceptives, other methods of contraception should be implemented during the period of rifampin administration. Rifampin turns body fluids (e.g., urine, saliva, tears) reddish orange and may permanently stain soft contact lenses.

Vaccine (see Chapter 301). The first-generation unconjugated PRP vaccine has been replaced by four licensed *H. influenzae* type b conjugate vaccines that differ in the carrier protein used, the saccharide molecular size, and the method of conjugating the saccharide to the protein (see Table 193–1). Combination vaccines consisting of a *H. influenzae* type b conjugate vaccine and one or more other vaccines recommended for routine administration in childhood are under development. Currently available combinations are PRP-OMP combined with hepatitis B vaccine (Comvax) and HbOC combined with DTP (whole-cell pertussis vaccine) (Tetramune). Attempts to combine DTaP (acellular pertussis vaccine) with a *H. influenzae* type b conjugate vaccine have resulted in decreased anti-PRP antibody, and to date, no such combination vaccine has been licensed.

Barbour ML: Conjugate vaccines and the carriage of *Haemophilus influenzae* type b. Emerg Infect Dis 3:176, 1996.

Bisgard KM, Kao A, Leake J, et al: *Haemophilus influenzae* invasive disease in the United States, 1994–1995: Near disappearance of a vaccine-preventable childhood disease. Emerg Infect Dis 4:229, 1998.

Centers for Disease Control and Prevention: Progress toward eliminating *Haemophilus influenzae* type b disease among infants and children—United States, 1987–1997. MMWR 47:993, 1998.

Daum RS, Granoff DM: Lessons from the evaluation of the immunogenicity. *In*: Ellis RW, Granoff DM (eds): Development and Clinical Uses of Haemophilus b Conjugate Vaccines. New York, Marcel Dekker, 1994, pp 291–312.

McIntyre PB, Berkey CS, King SM, et al: Dexamethoasone as adjunctive therapy in bacterial meningitis. A meta-analysis of randomized clinical trials since 1988. JAMA 278:925, 1997.

Murphy TV, White KE, Pastor P, et al: Declining incidence of *Haemophilus influenzae* type b diseases since introduction of vaccination. JAMA 269:246, 1993.

Schuchat A, Robinson K, Wenger JD et al: Bacterial meningitis in the United States in 1995. N Engl J Med 337:970–976, 1997.

CHAPTER 194

Chancroid (Haemophilus ducreyi)

Parvin Azimi

Chancroid is a sexually transmitted disease characterized by painful genital ulceration and inguinal lymphadenopathy that is caused by *Haemophilus ducreyi*, a fastidious gram-negative bacillus. Chancroid is prevalent in many countries and endemic in some areas of the United States; it is a risk factor for transmission of HIV. No cases have been reported in children.

Infection begins with a small inflammatory papule on the preputial orifice or frenulum in men and on the labia, fourchette, or perineal region in women. The lesion becomes pustular, eroded, and ulcerative within 2–3 days. Painful, tender inguinal lymphadenopathy occurs in more than 50% of cases. Unlike lymphogranuloma venereum (Chapter 223.4), the ulcer of chancroid is concurrent with lymphadenopathy.

Diagnosis is usually established by the clinical presentation in the absence of both *Treponema pallidum* and herpes simplex virus infections. Culture requires special media and is 80% or less sensitive. Polymerase chain reaction may become the best means for diagnosis.

Most *H. ducreyi* organisms are resistant to penicillin and ampicillin because of plasmid-mediated β-lactamase production. Spread of plasmid-mediated resistance among *H. ducreyi* has resulted in lack of efficacy of previously useful drugs such as sulfonamides and tetracyclines as well. The recommended treatment of chancroid is azithromycin (1 g as a single dose orally) or ceftriaxone (250 mg as a single dose intramuscularly). Alternative regimens include ciprofloxacin (500 mg PO bid for 3 days, for persons ≥18 yr of age) or erythromycin (500 mg PO qid for 7 days). Fluctuant nodes may require drainage. Symptoms usually resolve within 3–7 days. Relapses can usually be treated successfully with the original treatment regimen. Patients with HIV infection may require longer duration of treatment.

Patients with chancroid should be evaluated for other sexually transmitted diseases; an estimated 10% of patients have concomitant syphilis or genital herpes. Sexual contacts of patients with chancroid should be evaluated and treated.

Mertz KJ, Weiss JB, Webb RM, et al: An investigation of genital ulcers in Jackson, Mississippi, with use of a multiplex polymerase chain reaction assay: High prevalence of chancroid and human immunodeficiency virus infection. J Infect Dis 178:1060, 1998.

Trees DL, Morse SA: Chancroid and *Haemophilus ducreyi*: An update. Clin Microbiol Rev 8:357, 1995.

CHAPTER 195

Pertussis (Bordetella pertussis *and* B. parapertussis)

Sarah S. Long

Pertussis is an acute respiratory tract infection that was well described in the 1500s. Current worldwide prevalence is diminished only by active immunization. Sydenham first used the term *pertussis* (intense cough) in 1670; it is preferable to "whooping cough," because most infected individuals do not whoop.

ETIOLOGY. *Bordetella pertussis* is the sole cause of epidemic pertussis and the usual cause of sporadic pertussis. *B. parapertussis* is an occasional cause of pertussis, accounting for fewer than 5% of isolates of *Bordetella* species in the United States. *B. parapertussis* contributes significantly to total cases of pertussis in other areas such as Scandinavia, the Czech Republic, Slovakia, and the Russian federation. *B. pertussis* and *B. parapertussis* are exclusive pathogens of humans (and some primates). *B. bronchiseptica* is a common animal pathogen; occasional case reports in humans involve any body site and typically occur in immunocompromised patients or young children with unusual exposure to animals. Protracted coughing can be caused by *Mycoplasma*, parainfluenza or influenza viruses, enteroviruses, respiratory syncytial virus, or adenoviruses. None is an important cause of pertussis.

EPIDEMIOLOGY. Sixty million cases of pertussis a year occur worldwide, with more than half a million deaths. During the prevaccine era of 1922–1948, pertussis was the leading cause of death due to communicable disease among children under 14 yr of age in the United States. Widespread use of pertussis vaccine led to a greater than 99% decline in cases. The high incidence of disease in developing and developed countries, such as Italy and certain regions of Germany, where vaccine coverage is low, or Nova Scotia, where a less potent vaccine may have been used, and the dramatic resurgence of disease when immunization was halted attest to the pivotal role of vaccination. In the United States, lax implementation of policy is partially responsible for the rise in annual pertussis incidence to 1.2 cases/100,000 population from 1980 through 1989 and epidemic pertussis in many states in 1989–1990, 1993, and 1996. The more than 7,500 cases reported to the Centers for Disease Control and Prevention in 1996 are the highest incidence since 1967.

Pertussis is endemic, with superimposed epidemic cycles every 3–4 yr after accumulation of a sizable susceptible cohort. The majority of cases occur from July through October. Pertussis is extremely contagious, with attack rates as high as 100% in susceptible individuals exposed to aerosol droplets at close range. *B. pertussis* does not survive for prolonged periods in the environment. Chronic carriage by humans is not documented. After intense exposure as in households, the rate of subclinical infection is as high as 80% in fully immunized and naturally immune individuals. When carefully sought, a symptomatic source case can be found for most patients.

Neither natural disease nor vaccination provides complete or lifelong immunity against reinfection or disease. Protection against typical disease begins to wane 3–5 yr after vaccination and is unmeasurable after 12 yr. Subclinical reinfection undoubtedly contributes significantly to immunity against disease ascribed to both vaccine and prior infection. Adults in the United States have inadequate antibody to *B. pertussis*. Despite history of disease or complete immunization, outbreaks of pertussis have occurred in the elderly, in nursing homes, in residential facilities with limited exposures, in highly immunized suburbia, and in adolescents and adults with lapsing time since immunization. Coughing adolescents and adults (usually not recognized as having pertussis) currently are the major reservoir for *B. pertussis* and are the usual sources for "index cases" in infants and children.

In the prevaccine era and in countries such as Germany, Sweden, and Italy with limited immunization, the peak incidence of pertussis is in children 1–5 yr of age; infants younger than 1 yr account for fewer than 15% of cases. In contrast, in the United States in recent years, approximately one-half of cases have occurred in infants younger than 1 yr of age, and one quarter in adolescents and adults. Possible explanations for increases in disease incidence and ages affected include decreased vaccine efficacy, waning immunity, increased awareness and diagnosis, and enhanced surveillance. Without natural reinfection with *B. pertussis* or repeated booster vaccinations, adolescents and adults are susceptible to clinical disease if exposed, and mothers provide little if any passive protection to young infants. The latter observation provides correction to an old tenet that there was little transplacental protection against pertussis.

PATHOGENESIS. *Bordetella* organisms are tiny gram-negative coccobacilli that grow aerobically on starch blood agar or completely synthetic media with nicotinamide growth factor, amino acids for energy, and charcoal or cyclodextrin resin to absorb noxious substances. *Bordetella* species share a high degree of DNA homology among virulence genes, and whether sufficient diversity exists to warrant classification as distinct species is controversial. Only *B. pertussis* expresses pertussis toxin (PT), the major virulence protein. Serotyping is dependent on heat-labile K agglutinogens. Of 14 agglutinogens, 6 are specific to *B. pertussis.* Serotypes vary geographically and over time.

B. pertussis produces an array of biologically active substances, many of which are postulated to have a role in disease and immunity. After aerosol acquisition, filamentous hemagglutinin (FHA), some agglutinogens (especially fimbriae [Fim] types 2 and 3), and a 69-kd nonfimbrial surface protein called pertactin (Pn) are important for attachment to ciliated respiratory epithelial cells. Tracheal cytotoxin, adenylate cyclase, and PT appear to inhibit clearance of organisms. Tracheal cytotoxin, dermonecrotic factor, and adenylate cyclase are postulated to be predominantly responsible for the local epithelial damage that produces respiratory symptoms and facilitates absorption of PT. PT has numerous proven biologic activities (e.g., histamine sensitivity, insulin secretion, leukocyte dysfunction), some of which may account for systemic manifestations of disease. PT causes lymphocytosis immediately in experimental animals by rerouting lymphocytes to remain in the circulating blood pool. PT appears to have a central but not a singular role in pathogenesis.

CLINICAL MANIFESTATIONS. Pertussis is a lengthy disease, divided into catarrhal, paroxysmal, and convalescent stages, each lasting 2 wk. Classically, after an incubation period ranging from 3–12 days, nondistinctive catarrhal symptoms of congestion and rhinorrhea occur, variably accompanied by low-grade fever, sneezing, lacrimation, and conjunctival suffusion. As symptoms wane, coughing begins first as a dry, intermittent, irritative hack and evolves into the inexorable paroxysms that are the hallmark of pertussis. After the most insignificant startle from a draught, light, sound, sucking, or stretching, a well-appearing young infant begins to choke, gasp, and flail extremities, eyes watering and bulging, face reddened. Cough (expiratory grunt) may not be prominent at this stage. Whoop (forceful inspiratory gasp) infrequently occurs in infants under 3 mo who are exhausted or lack muscular strength to create sudden negative intrathoracic pressure. A well-appearing, playful toddler with similarly insignificant provocation suddenly expresses an anxious aura and may clutch a parent or comforting adult before beginning a machine-gun burst of uninterrupted coughs, chin and chest held forward, tongue protruding maximally, eyes bulging and watering, face purple, until at the seeming last moment of consciousness, coughing ceases and a loud whoop follows as inspired air traverses the still partially closed airway. The episode may end with expulsion of a thick plug of inspissated tracheal secretions, denuded cilia, and necrotic epithelium. Adults describe a sudden feeling of strangulation followed by uninterrupted coughs, feeling of suffocation, bursting headache, diminished awareness, and then a gasping breath, usually without a whoop. Post-tussive emesis is common in pertussis at all ages and is a major clue to the diagnosis in adolescents and adults. Post-tussive exhaustion is universal. The number and severity of paroxysms progress over days to a week (more rapidly in young infants) and remain at that plateau for days to weeks (longer in young infants). At the peak of the paroxysmal stage, patients may have more than one episode hourly. As paroxysmal stage fades into convalescence, the number, severity, and duration of episodes diminish. Paradoxically in infants, with growth and increased strength, cough and whoops may become louder and more classic in convalescence.

Immunized children have foreshortening of all stages of pertussis. Adults have no distinct stages. In infants younger than 3 mo, the catarrhal phase is usually a few days or not recognized at all when apnea, choking, or gasping cough herald the onset of disease; convalescence includes intermittent paroxysmal coughing throughout the 1st yr of life, including "recurrences" with subsequent respiratory illnesses; these are not due to recurrent infection or reactivation of *B. pertussis.*

Findings on physical examination generally are uninformative. Signs of lower respiratory tract disease are not expected. Conjunctival hemorrhages and petechiae on the upper body are common.

DIAGNOSIS. Pertussis should be suspected in any individual who has pure or predominant complaint of cough, especially if the following are absent: fever, malaise or myalgia, exanthem or enanthem, sore throat, hoarseness, tachypnea, wheezes, and rales. For sporadic cases, a clinical case definition of cough of 14 or more days' duration with at least one associated symptom of paroxysms, whoop, or post-tussive vomiting has sensitivity of 81% and specificity of 58% for culture confirmation. Approximately 20% of university students who were studied on many continents, who had no known contact with pertussis, and who had coughing illness for more than 7 days had pertussis. Apnea or cyanosis (before appreciation of cough) is a clue in infants younger than 3 mo. *B. pertussis* is an occasional cause of sudden infant death.

Adenoviral infections are usually distinguishable by associated features, such as fever, sore throat, and conjunctivitis. *Mycoplasma* causes protracted episodic coughing, but patients usually have a history of fever, headache, and systemic symptoms at the onset of disease as well as frequent finding of rales on auscultation of the chest. Although pertussis is often included in the laboratory evaluation of young infants with "afebrile pneumonia," *B. pertussis* is associated uncommonly with staccato cough (breath with every cough), purulent conjunctivitis, tachypnea, rales or wheezes that typify infection due to *Chlamydia trachomatis*, or predominant lower respiratory tract signs that typify infection due to respiratory syncytial virus. Unless an infant with pertussis has secondary pneumonia (and is then ill appearing), the examination findings between paroxysms are entirely normal, including respiratory rate.

Leukocytosis (15,000–100,000 cells/mm^3) due to absolute lymphocytosis is a characteristic in late catarrhal and paroxysmal stages. Lymphocytes are of T- and B-cell origin and are normal small cells, rather than the large atypical lymphocytes seen with viral infections. Adults and partially immune children have less impressive lymphocytosis. Absolute increase in neutrophils suggests a different diagnosis or secondary bacterial infection. Eosinophilia is not common in pertussis, even in young infants. A severe course and death are correlated with extreme leukocytosis (median peak white cell count fatal vs nonfatal cases, 94 vs 18 $\times$ 10^9 cells/L) and thrombocytosis (median peak platelet count fatal vs nonfatal cases, 782 vs 556 $\times$ 10^9/L). Mild hyperinsulinemia and reduced glycemic response to epinephrine have been demonstrated; hypoglycemia is reported only occasionally. The chest radiograph appearance is mildly abnormal in the majority of hospitalized infants, showing perihilar infiltrate or edema (sometimes with a butterfly appearance) and variable atelectasis. Parenchymal consolidation suggests secondary bacterial infection. Pneumothorax, pneumomediastinum, and air in soft tissues can be seen occasionally.

All current methods for confirmation of infection due to *B. pertussis* have limitations in sensitivity, specificity, or practical-ity. Isolation of *B. pertussis* in culture remains the gold standard and is a more sensitive and specific method of diagnosis than direct fluorescent antibody (DFA) testing of nasopharyngeal secretions if careful attention is paid to specimen collection, transport, and isolation technique. Culture results are positive during the catarrhal stage and escalating paroxysmal stage but are less likely to be positive in partially immune individuals and in those who have received amoxicillin or erythromycin. The specimen is obtained by deep nasopharyngeal aspiration or by use of a flexible swab (Dacron or calcium alginate preferred) held in the posterior nasopharynx for 15–30 sec. (or until coughing). A 1.0% casamino acid liquid is acceptable for holding a specimen up to 2 hr; Stainer-Scholte broth or Regan-Lowe semisolid transport medium is used for longer periods, up to 4 days. Regan-Lowe charcoal agar with 10% horse blood and 5–40 μg/mL cephalexin or Stainer-Scholte media with cyclodextrin resins are the preferred isolation media. Cultures are incubated at 35–37°F in humid environment (with or without 5% carbon dioxide) and examined daily for 7 days for slow-growing, tiny glistening colonies. DFA testing of potential isolates using specific antibody for *B. pertussis* and *B. parapertussis* maximizes recovery. Direct testing of nasopharyngeal secretions by DFA is a rapid test, especially helpful in patients who have received antibiotics, but is reliable only in laboratories with continuous experience. Experience with the polymerase chain reaction to test nasopharyngeal specimens is increasing. Serologic tests for detection of various antibodies to components of the organism in acute and convalescent samples are the most sensitive tests and are useful epidemiologically. They are not generally available, are not helpful during acute illness, and are difficult to interpret in immunized individuals.

TREATMENT. Goals of therapy are to limit the number of paroxysms, to observe the severity of the cough to provide assistance when necessary, and to maximize nutrition, rest, and recovery without sequelae (Table 195–1). Infants younger than 3 mo are admitted to hospital almost without exception, at between 3 and 6 mo unless witnessed paroxysms are not severe, and at any age if significant complications occur. Prematurely born young infants and children with underlying cardiac, pulmonary, muscular, or neurologic disorders have a high risk for severe disease.

The specific, limited goals of hospitalization are to (1) assess progression of disease and likelihood of life-threatening events at peak of disease, (2) prevent or treat complications, and (3) educate parents in the natural history of the disease and in care that will be given at home. Heart rate, respiratory rate, and pulse oximetry are monitored continuously with alarm settings so that paroxysms can be witnessed by health care personnel. Detailed cough records and documentation of feeding, vomiting, and weight change provide data to assess severity. Typical paroxysms that are not life threatening have the following features: duration less than 45 sec; red but not blue color change; tachycardia, bradycardia (not <60 beats/min in infants), or oxygen desaturation that spontaneously resolves at the end of the paroxysm; whooping or strength for self-rescue at the end of the paroxysm; self-expectorated mucus plug; and post-tussive exhaustion but not unresponsiveness. Assessing the need to provide oxygen, stimulation, or suctioning requires skilled personnel who can document an infant's ability for self-rescue but who will intervene rapidly and expertly when necessary. Infants whose paroxysms repeatedly lead to life-threatening events despite passive delivery of oxygen or whose fatigue leads to hypercarbia require intubation, paralysis, and ventilation. Subsequent management is complex, with frequent need to suction the airway and intervene when bradycardia or secondary pulmonary processes occur. Mist by tent, specifically avoided by some experts, can be useful in some infants with thick, tenacious secretions and excessively irritable airways. The benefit of a quiet, dimly lighted, undisturbed, comforting environment cannot be overestimated or forfeited in a desire to monitor and intervene. Feeding children with pertussis is challenging. The risk of precipitating cough by nipple feeding does not warrant nasogastric, nasojejunal, or parenteral alimentation in most infants. The composition or thickness of formula does not affect the quality of secretions, cough, or retention. Large-volume feedings are avoided.

TABLE 195–1 Caveats in Assessment and Care of Infants with Pertussis

Infants with potentially fatal pertussis may appear completely well between episodes.

In making the decision between hospital and home care, a paroxysm must be witnessed.

Only careful compilation and analysis of cough record permits assessment of severity and progression of illness.

Suctioning of nose, oropharynx, or trachea always precipitates coughing, occasionally causes bronchospasm or apnea, and should not be performed on a "preventive" schedule.

If a patient is alert and has retained strength after a coughing episode, feeding is best taken and retained during this brief refractory period for coughing.

At hospitalization, family support begins with empathy for the child's and family's experience to date, transfer of the burden of responsibility for the child's life to the health care team, and delineation of assessments and treatments to be performed.

Family education, recruitment as part of the team, and continued support after discharge are essential.

Hospital discharge is appropriate if over a 48 hr period disease severity is unchanged or diminished, no intervention is required during paroxysms, nutrition is adequate, no complication has occurred, and parents are adequately prepared for care at home.

Within 48–72 hr, the direction and severity of disease are usually obvious by analysis of recorded information. Many infants have marked improvement upon hospitalization and antibiotic therapy, especially if they are early in the course of disease or have been removed from aggravating environmental smoke, excessive stimulation, or a dry or polluting heat source. Apnea and seizures occur in the incremental phase of illness and in those with complicated disease. Portable oxygen, monitoring, or suction apparatus should not be needed at home.

Antimicrobial Agents. An antimicrobial agent is always given when pertussis is suspected or confirmed for potential clinical benefit and to limit the spread of infection. Erythromycin, 40–50 mg/kg/24 hr PO in four divided doses (maximum 2 g/24 hr) for 14 days is standard treatment. Limited studies of erythromycin salts dosed twice or three times a day for 14 days, erythromycin estolate (40 mg/kg/24 hr; maximum 1 g/24 hr) for 7 days, clarithromycin (10 mg/kg/24 hr) divided into two doses for 7 days; and azithromycin (10 mg/kg/24 hr) once a day for 5 days have compared favorably with standard treatment for elimination of organisms. Ampicillin, rifampin, and trimethoprim-sulfamethoxazole are modestly active, but first- and second-generation cephalosporins are not. In clinical studies, erythromycins are superior to amoxicillin for eradication of *B. pertussis* and are the only agents with proven efficacy.

Salbutamol. A handful of small clinical trials and reports suggest a modest reduction of symptoms from the β_2-adrenergic stimulant salbutamol (albuterol). No rigorous clinical trial has demonstrated a beneficial effect; one small study showed no effect. Fussing associated with aerosol treatment triggers paroxysms.

Corticosteroids. No randomized, blinded clinical trial of sufficient size has been performed to evaluate the usefulness of corticosteroids in the management of pertussis. Studies of animals have shown a salutary effect on disease manifestations that do not have a corollary in respiratory infection in humans. Their clinical use is not warranted.

Pertussis Immune Globulin. Hyperimmune serum, derived from adults convalescing from pertussis, was widely prescribed and regarded as beneficial in the 1930s and 1940s; later studies and the only placebo-controlled trial demonstrated little or no value. In a double-blind study in Sweden using large intramuscular doses of hyperimmune serum (raised by immunization of adults), whooping (but not cough or vomiting) was significantly reduced in patients treated in the 1st wk of disease compared with patients given placebo. A multicenter placebo-controlled treatment trial of a hyperimmune pertussis immune globulin, intravenous, is under way in Canada and the United States. Standard intravenous immunoglobulin is not recommended for treatment of pertussis.

Isolation. Patients are placed in respiratory isolation for at least 5 days after initiation of erythromycin therapy.

Care of Household and Other Close Contacts. Erythromycin, 40–50 mg/kg/24 hr PO in four divided doses (maximum 2 g/24 hr) for 14 days should be given promptly to all household contacts and other close contacts, such as those in daycare, regardless of age, history of immunization, or symptoms. Visitation and movement of coughing family members in the hospital must be assiduously controlled until erythromycin has been taken for 5 days. Close contacts younger than 7 yr who are underimmunized should be given a pertussis-containing vaccine, with further doses to complete recommended series. Children younger than 7 yr who received a third dose 6 mo or more before exposure or a fourth dose 3 yr or more before exposure should receive a booster dose. If infection with *B. pertussis* is proved, the individual usually is exempted from routine pertussis immunization. Some experts recommend immunization after pertussis in infants, whose response to infection may be suboptimal. Antimicrobial prophylaxis is not routinely recommended for exposed health care workers. Coughing health care workers, with or without known exposure to pertussis, should be promptly tested for pertussis. For major hospital outbreaks, multifaceted control procedures have included targeted erythromycin treatment of coughing individuals and subsequent mass erythromycin prophylaxis.

COMPLICATIONS. Rates of complications are difficult to establish because severe outcomes are preferentially reported, but infants younger than 6 mo have excessive mortality and morbidity. Those younger than 2 mo have the highest reported rates of pertussis-associated hospitalization (82%), pneumonia (25%), seizures (4%), encephalopathy (1%), and death (1%). Among 23 fatal cases in the United States in 1992–1993, approximately 80% were less than 6 mo of age. Preterm birth and young maternal age were significantly associated with pertussis, and pneumonia complicated more than 95% cases.

The principal complications of pertussis are apnea, secondary infections (such as otitis media and pneumonia), and physical sequelae of forceful coughing. The need for intensive care and artificial ventilation is usually limited to infants younger than 3 mo. Apnea, cyanosis, and secondary bacterial pneumonia are events precipitating intubation and ventilation. Bacterial pneumonia or adult respiratory distress syndrome is the usual cause of death at any age; pulmonary hemorrhage has occurred in neonates. Fever, tachypnea or respiratory distress between paroxysms, and absolute neutrophilia are clues to pneumonia. Expected pathogens include *Staphylococcus aureus, S. pneumoniae,* and bacteria of mouth flora. Bronchiectasis has been reported rarely after pertussis. Abnormal pulmonary function may persist for 12 mo after uncomplicated pertussis in children younger than 2 yr.

Increased intrathoracic and intra-abdominal pressure during coughing can result in conjunctival and scleral hemorrhages, petechiae on the upper body, epistaxis, hemorrhage in the central nervous system (CNS) and retina, pneumothorax and subcutaneous emphysema, and umbilical and inguinal hernias. Laceration of the lingual frenulum is not uncommon. Rectal prolapse, once reported as a frequent complication of pertussis, was probably due to pertussis in malnourished children or missed diagnosis of cystic fibrosis. It is distinctly unusual and should elicit evaluation for underlying condition. Especially in infants in developing countries, dehydration and malnutrition following post-tussive vomiting can have a severe impact. Tetany has been associated with profound post-tussive alkalosis.

CNS abnormalities occur at a relatively high frequency and are almost always a result of hypoxemia or hemorrhage associated with coughing or apnea in young infants. Apnea or bradycardia or both may result from apparent laryngospasm or vagal stimulation just before a coughing episode, from obstruction during an episode, or from hypoxemia following an episode. Lack of associated signs in some young infants with apnea raises the possibility of a primary effect of PT on the CNS. Seizures are usually a result of hypoxemia, but hyponatremia from excessive secretion of antidiuretic hormone during pneumonia can occur. Although hypoglycemia, a direct effect of PT, and secondary infection due to neurotropic virus have been postulated mechanisms for neurologic symptoms, no animal data support such theories, and the only neuropathology documented in humans is parenchymal hemorrhage and ischemic necrosis.

PREVENTION (see Chapter 301). Universal immunization of children with pertussis vaccine, beginning in infancy, is central to the control of pertussis. Despite enormous effort, the critical mechanism(s) of immunity following disease or vaccination, a serologic correlate of protection, and the cause of vaccine-associated adverse events are not known. The only current standards for vaccine usefulness are clinical efficacy and safety. Current goals of immunization are protection of the individual from a significant coughing illness and control of endemic and epidemic disease.

Whole-Cell Vaccine. Diphtheria and tetanus toxoids combined with whole-cell pertussis (DTP) vaccine currently are licensed for use in the United States and are recommended by the World Health Organization for use throughout most of the world. Vaccines of this type are prepared from suspension of inactivated *B. pertussis* bacterial cells, the potency and safety of which are assayed to contain 4–12 protective units and not more than 16 opacity units per 0.5 mL dose, respectively. Based on controlled efficacy trials conducted in the 1940s and on subsequent observational efficacy data, a primary series comprising four doses of whole-cell DTP vaccine has been considered 70–90% effective in preventing serious pertussis disease.

Whole-cell pertussis vaccines commonly are associated with local adverse events (e.g., erythema, swelling and pain at the injection site), fever, and other mild systemic events (e.g., fretfulness, drowsiness, and anorexia). More serious systemic events (e.g., seizures and hypotonic hyporesponsive episodes) occur in approximately 1/1,750 doses administered. Acute encephalopathy occurs even more rarely (0–10.5 cases in 1 million doses administered). Experts disagree on whether whole-cell pertussis vaccine causes lasting brain damage but agree that if the vaccine causes such damage, it does so rarely. Concerns about safety of DTP vaccine prompted the development of purified (acellular) pertussis vaccines.

Acellular Vaccine. Multiple diphtheria and tetanus toxoids combined with acellular pertussis (DTaP) vaccines currently are licensed in the United States and are preferred over DTP because of fewer adverse reactions. Acellular pertussis vaccines contain inactivated PT and may contain one or more other bacterial components (FHA, Pn, Fim 2 and 3). PT is detoxified either chemically or using molecular genetic techniques. Lacking serologic criteria for protection, licensure has been based on clinical efficacy trials conducted in Europe and Africa since 1991 to evaluate 8 DTaP vaccines administered to infants. The vaccines, produced by different manufacturers, contained various types, numbers, and quantities of antigens. (All contained inactivated PT.) Because of differences in study design, case definition, and laboratory confirmation of pertussis cases, comparison among studies is difficult. Within certain studies, efficacy of DTaP vs DTP vaccines can be compared directly. The efficacy of acellular pertussis vaccines in preventing moderate to severe pertussis diseases was within the range expected, more than most whole-cell DTP vaccines, and is superior to one currently licensed DTP vaccine. Mild local and systemic adverse events as well as more serious events (including high fever, persistent crying of 3 hr or longer duration, hypotonic hyporesponsive episodes, and seizures) occurred significantly less frequently among infants who received DTaP compared with DTP vaccine. The number of subjects included in these studies (although exceeding 70,000) was insufficient to estimate a risk for rare potential events such as encephalopathy or anaphylactic shock.

Although efficacy trials have not demonstrated a direct correlation between antibody response and protection against pertussis disease, antibody studies are useful to compare immune responses elicited by a single product under different conditions or in different studies. Limited data support simultaneous administration of DTaP with other vaccines used in standard schedules for children. Combination vaccines that include DTaP in place of DTP can affect immunogenicity of products. Combination vaccine(s) should be used only in the dosing series and age group for which each is licensed. When feasible, until further data are available, the same brand of DTaP vaccine is recommended for all doses of the vaccination series.

The same special considerations, precautions, contraindications, and reporting requirements for serious adverse events that exist for DTP vaccination apply to DTaP as well. Acellular pertussis vaccines are now licensed for use only among children through 6 yr of age.

American Academy of Pediatrics: Pertussis. *In*: Peter G (ed): 1997 Red Book: Report of the Committee on Infectious Diseases, 24th ed. Elk Grove Village, IL, American Academy of Pediatrics, 1997, pp 394–407.

American Academy of Pediatrics, Committee on Infectious Diseases: Acellular pertussis vaccine: Recommendations for use as the initial series in infants and children. Pediatrics 99:282, 1997.

Centers for Disease Control and Prevention: Recommendations of the Advisory Committee on Immunization Practices (ACIP): Pertussis vaccination: Use of acellular pertussis vaccines among infants and young children. MMWR 46:RR–7, 1997.

Christie CDC, Marx ML, Marchant CD, et al: The 1993 epidemic of pertussis in Cincinnati: Resurgence of disease in a highly immunized population of children. N Engl J Med 331:16, 1994.

Edwards KM, Decker MD, Graham BS, et al: Adult immunization with acellular pertussis vaccine. JAMA 269:53, 1993.

Farizo KM, Cochi SL, Zell ER, et al: Epidemiologic features of pertussis in the United States, 1980–1989. Clin Infect Dis 14:708, 1992.

Gale JL, Thapa PB, Wassilak SGF, et al: Risk of serious acute neurological illness after immunization with diphtheria-tetanus-pertussis vaccine: A population-based case-control study. JAMA 271:37, 1994.

He Q, Viljanen MK, Arvilommi H, et al: Whooping cough caused by *Bordetella pertussis* and *Bordetella parapertussis* in an immunized population. JAMA 280:635, 1998.

Howson CP, Fineberg HV: Adverse events following pertussis and rubella vaccines: Summary of a report of the Institute of Medicine. JAMA 267:392, 1992.

Long SS, Welkon CJ, Clark JL: Widespread silent transmission of pertussis in families: Antibody correlates of infection and symptomatology. J Infect Dis 161:480, 1990.

Mink CAM, Sirota NM, Nugent S: Outbreak of pertussis in a fully immunized adolescent and adult population. Arch Pediatr Adolesc Med 148:153, 1994.

Sutter RW, Cochi SL: Pertussis hospitalizations and mortality in the United States, 1985–1988: Evaluation of the completeness of national reporting. JAMA 267:386, 1992.

Wortis N, Strebel PM, Wharton M, et al: Pertussis deaths: Report of 23 cases in the United States, 1992 and 1993. Pediatrics 97:607, 1996.

CHAPTER 196
Salmonella

Thomas G. Cleary

Salmonella infections occur worldwide. Acute gastroenteritis, the most frequent presentation, is usually self-limited, although bacteremia and focal extraintestinal infections may develop, especially in immunocompromised patients. The latter group has become more important and complex because of the increasing number of children who are compromised by AIDS, organ transplant, or chemotherapy. Enteric fever, a severe systemic disease typically caused by *Salmonella typhi*, is found mainly in developing countries, but it is encountered worldwide because of international travel.

Salmonella is a genus that belongs to the family Enterobacteriaceae and contains three species: *S. typhi*, *S. choleraesuis*, and *S. enteritidis*. The former two species have one serotype each, but *S. enteritidis* contains more than 1,800 distinct serotypes. For convenience, serotypes are sometimes artificially identified as if they were *Salmonella* species (e.g., *S. typhimurium*).

Salmonellae are motile, nonsporulating, nonencapsulated, gram-negative rods. Most strains ferment glucose, mannose, and mannitol to produce acid and gas, but they do not ferment lactose or sucrose. *S. typhi* does not produce gas. *Salmonella* organisms grow aerobically and are capable of facultative anaerobic growth. They are resistant to many physical agents but can be killed by heating to 130°F (54.4°C) for 1 hr or 140°F (60°C) for 15 min. They remain viable at ambient or reduced temperatures for days and may survive for weeks in sewage, dried foodstuffs, pharmaceutical agents, and fecal material. Like other members of the Enterobacteriaceae, *Salmonella* possesses somatic O antigens and flagellar H antigens. The O antigens are the heat-stable lipopolysaccharide components of cell wall; the H antigens are heat-labile proteins that can be present in phase 1 or 2. The Kauffmann-White scheme commonly used to classify salmonellae serotypes is based on O and H antigens. Serotyping is important clinically because certain serotypes tend to be associated with specific clinical syndromes and because detection of an unusual serotype is sometimes useful in recognizing a common-source outbreak. A virulence capsular polysaccharide (Vi), present on *S. typhi*, is also found on strains of *S. dublin* and *S. paratyphi* C (*S. hirschfeldii*).

These classification schemes are based on biochemical and antigenic relationships. Molecular technology has enabled classification at the gene level. DNA analysis has proved that all *Salmonella* organisms are closely related genetically as a single species with six subgroups; most isolates causing human or animal disease belong to subgroup 1.

196.1 Nontyphoidal Salmonellosis

EPIDEMIOLOGY. About 50,000 cases of culture-proven salmonellosis, approximately 98% of which are caused by nontyphoidal salmonellae, are reported annually in the United States. Because culturing and reporting are incomplete, the actual number of cases has been estimated as 1–5 million/yr. These figures are higher than those of the 1970s and may be related to modern practices of mass food production, which increase the potential for epidemic salmonellosis. About half of the reported cases occur in persons younger than 20 yr, and one third occur in children 4 yr of age or younger; the highest isolation rate is for infants younger than 1 yr. Nontyphoidal *Salmonella* infections have a worldwide distribution, with an incidence related to water potability, sewage disposal, and food preparation practices.

Salmonella infections occur with highest frequency in the warm months, July through November in the United States. Although most reported cases of nontyphoidal salmonellosis occur sporadically, food-borne outbreaks are common. Each year, about 500 food-borne *Salmonella* outbreaks are reported, representing more than 50% of all gastroenteritis outbreaks with a documented bacterial cause. Some of the *Salmonella* outbreaks are widespread—interstate or even international—and affect thousands of individuals. Refinement of outbreak tracing has improved with the development of molecular epidemiology techniques, such as plasmid analysis and endonucleases digestion of chromosomal genes for recognition of small differences in chromosomal structure. These can "fingerprint" a particular clone and are especially useful in tracing outbreaks caused by common serotypes. The *Salmonella* serotypes most often encountered in the United States include *S. typhimurium, S. enteritidis, S. heidelberg,* and *S. newport.*

Animals constitute the principal source of human nontyphoidal *Salmonella* disease. Infected animals are often asymptomatic. *Salmonella* has been isolated from many animals, including poultry (i.e., chickens, turkeys, ducks), sheep, cows, pigs, pets, and birds. Specific serotypes are associated with particular animal hosts. For example, children with *S. marina* typically have exposure to pet iguanas. Animal-to-animal transmission may occur. Animal feeds containing fish meal or bone meal contaminated with *Salmonella* spp are an important source of infection for animals. Moreover, subtherapeutic concentrations of antibiotics are often added to animal feed. Such practices promote the emergence of antibiotic-resistant bacteria, including *Salmonella,* in the gut flora of the animals. During slaughtering, these gut organisms may contaminate the meat, which is subsequently consumed by humans. Data suggest that animal antibiotic exposure may be responsible for antibiotic-resistant *Salmonella* infections in humans.

Poultry and poultry products (mainly eggs) caused about half of the common-source outbreaks. Foods containing raw or undercooked eggs (e.g., Caesar salad, egg-dipped bread, and homemade eggnog) are of special importance. *Salmonella* infections in chickens increase the risk for contamination of eggs. Salmonellae can contaminate the shell surface, penetrate the egg, or be transmitted from an ovarian infection directly to the egg yolk. *Salmonella* serotypes have been isolated in as many as 50% of poultry, 16% of pork, 5% of beef, and 40% of frozen egg products purchased in retain stores. Meats, especially beef and pork, caused about 13% of the outbreaks, and raw or powdered milk and dairy products were the source of about 5% of the outbreaks. Food product–related outbreaks are often caused by contaminated equipment in processing plants or infected food handlers. Pets, especially turtles, caused about 3% of the outbreaks.

The estimated number of bacteria that must be ingested to cause symptomatic disease in healthy adults is 10^6–10^8 *Salmonella* organisms. In infants and in persons with certain underlying conditions, the inoculum size that can produce disease is smaller. Because of the relatively high inoculum size of *Salmonella* infection, ingestion of contaminated food, in which the organisms can multiply, is a major source of human infection. Because of the high infecting dose, person-to-person transmission by direct fecal-oral spread is unusual but can occur, especially in young children who are not yet toilet trained and do not maintain proper hygiene. Perinatal transmission during vaginal delivery has been reported.

Nosocomial infections have been related to contaminated medical instruments (particularly endoscopes) and diagnostic or pharmacologic preparations, particularly those of animal origin (e.g., pancreatic extracts, pituitary extracts, bile salts, pepsin, gelatin, vitamins, carmine dye). Food-borne nosocomial transmission is also possible. Hospitalized patients are at increased risk of severe and complicated *Salmonella* infections. Intravenous transmission by platelet transfusion has been reported.

After infection, nontyphoidal salmonellae are excreted in feces for a median of 5 wk. In young children and in individuals with symptomatic infections, the excretion period is longer. Prolonged carriage of *Salmonella* organisms is rare in healthy children but has been reported in those with underlying immune deficiency. During the period of *Salmonella* excretion, the individual may infect others, directly by the fecal-oral route or indirectly by contaminating foods.

PATHOGENESIS. Enterocolitis is the typical disorder caused by nontyphoidal *Salmonella* infection. Findings include diffuse mucosal inflammation and edema, sometimes with erosions and microabscesses. Although *Salmonella* organisms are capable of penetrating the intestinal mucosa, neither destruction of epithelial cells nor production of ulcers is usually found. Intestinal inflammation, with polymorphonuclear leukocytes and macrophages, usually involves the lamina propria. Underlying intestinal lymphoid tissue and mesenteric lymph nodes enlarge and may develop small areas of necrosis. Such lymphoid hypertrophy may cause interference with the blood supply to the gut mucosa. Hyperplasia of the reticuloendothelial system is also noted within the liver and spleen. If bacteremia develops, it may lead to localized infection and suppuration in almost any organ.

The development of disease after infection with *Salmonella* depends on the number of infecting organisms, on their virulence traits, and on several host defense factors. Ingested *Salmonella* organisms reach the stomach, where acid is the first protective barrier. The acidity inhibits multiplication of the salmonellae, and when gastric pH reaches 2.0, most organisms are rapidly killed. Achlorhydria, buffering medications, rapid gastric emptying after gastrectomy or gastroenterostomy, and a large inoculum enable viable organisms to reach the small intestine. Neonates and young infants have hypochlorhydria and rapid gastric emptying, which contribute to their increased vulnerability to symptomatic salmonellosis. Because the transit time through the stomach is faster for drinks than for foods, a lower inoculum may cause disease in water-borne infection.

In the small and large intestines, salmonellae have to compete with normal bacterial flora to multiply and cause disease; prior antibiotic therapy disrupts this competitive relationship. Decreased intestinal motility due to anatomic causes or medications increases the contact time of the ingested salmonellae with the mucosa and the likelihood of symptomatic disease. After multiplication within the lumen, the organisms penetrate the mucosa, typically at the distal part of the ileum and the proximal part of the colon, with subsequent localization in the Peyer's patches. The penetration process includes specific attachment to the luminal surface of epithelial cells, internalization into the cell by receptor-mediated endocytosis, cytoplasmic translocation of the infected endosome to the basal epithelial membrane, and release of the salmonellae in the lamina propria. Penetration usually occurs without destroying epithelial cells, and ulcers are not produced.

Heat-labile cholera-like enterotoxin is produced by many *Salmonella* isolates. This toxin and the prostaglandins that are produced locally increase cyclic adenosine monophosphate levels within intestinal crypts, causing a net efflux of electrolytes and water into the intestinal lumen.

Genes code for adherence to epithelial cells, invasion of epithelial cells, a cholera toxin–like enterotoxin, spread beyond the Peyer's patches to mesenteric lymph nodes, intracellular growth in the liver and spleen, survival in macrophages, serum resistance, and complement resistance. The genes causing invasion of intestinal cells are closely related to the *Shigella* invasion genes. However, *Shigella* spp lack the genes for spread beyond the intestine and survival in the bloodstream. These genetic differences explain the higher frequency of bacteremia in *Salmonella* infection. Some virulence traits are shared by all salmonellae, but others are serotype restricted. These virulence traits have been defined in tissue culture and murine models; it is likely that clinical features of human *Salmonella* infection will eventually be related to specific DNA sequences.

With most diarrhea-associated nontyphoidal salmonelloses, the infection does not extend beyond the lamina propria and the local lymphatics. *S. dublin* and *S. choleraesuis* rapidly invade the bloodstream with little or no intestinal involvement. Specific virulence genes are related to the ability to cause bacteremia. These genes are found significantly more often in strains of *S. typhimurium* isolated from the blood than the feces of humans. Bacteremia, however, is possible with any *Salmonella* strain, especially in individuals with reduced host defenses. An impaired reticuloendothelial or cellular immune response is important. Children with chronic granulomatous disease, other white cell disorders, and AIDS are at increased risk. Children with sickle cell disease are prone to *Salmonella* septicemia and osteomyelitis. The numerous infarcted areas in the gastrointestinal tract, bones, and reticuloendothelial system may initially permit organisms greater access to the circulation from the intestine and then furnish an optimal environment for localization. The decreased phagocytic and opsonizing capacity of patients with sickle cell disease also contributes to the high infection rate.

Chronic infection is associated with cholelithiasis, *Schistosoma mansoni* hepatosplenic involvement, and urinary tract *Schistosoma hematobium* infection. Localized infections are more common in areas with impaired local defenses (e.g., effusions, tumors, hematomas).

CLINICAL MANIFESTATIONS. Several distinct clinical syndromes can develop in children infected with nontyphoidal *Salmonella*, depending on host factors and the specific serotype involved.

Acute Gastroenteritis. (Also see Chapter 176.) This is the most common clinical presentation. After an incubation period of 6–72 hr (mean, 24 hr), there is an abrupt onset of nausea, vomiting, and crampy abdominal pain primarily in the periumbilical area and right lower quadrant, followed by mild to severe watery diarrhea and sometimes by diarrhea containing blood and mucus. Moderate fever (temperature of 101–102°F [38.5–39°C]) affects about 70% of patients. Some children develop severe disease with high fever, headache, drowsiness, confusion, meningismus, seizures, and abdominal distention. Abdominal examination reveals some tenderness. The stool typically contains a moderate number of polymorphonuclear leukocytes and occult blood. Mild leukocytosis may be detected. Symptoms subside within 2–7 days in healthy children; fatalities are rare.

In certain high-risk groups, the course of *Salmonella* gastroenteritis may be more complicated. Neonates, young infants, and children with primary or secondary immune deficiency may have symptoms persisting for several weeks. In patients with AIDS, the infection may become widespread and overwhelming, causing multisystem involvement, septic shock, and death. In patients with inflammatory bowel disease, especially active ulcerative colitis, *Salmonella* gastroenteritis may cause invasion of the bowel with rapid development of toxic megacolon, systemic toxicity, and death. Patients with schistosomiasis have increased susceptibility to salmonellosis and exhibit persistence of infection unless the schistosomiasis is also treated. *Salmonella* organisms are able to multiply within the schistosomes, where they are protected from antibiotics.

Bacteremia. Transient bacteremia during nontyphoidal *Salmonella* gastroenteritis is thought to occur in 1–5% of patients. The precise incidence is unclear, because blood cultures often are not obtained from patients with *Salmonella* gastroenteritis, especially those who are not hospitalized, and because most data are from retrospective studies. *Salmonella* bacteremia is associated with fever, chills, and often with a toxic appearance. Bacteremia has been documented, however, in afebrile, well-appearing children, especially neonates. Prolonged or intermittent bacteremia is associated with low-grade fever, anorexia, weight loss, diaphoresis, and myalgias. Children with certain underlying conditions and *Salmonella* gastroenteritis are at increased risk of bacteremia (Table 196–1), which may lead to extraintestinal infection. Children who have no underlying disease may be at increased risk of bacteremia if they have been treated with antibiotics in the month before acquisition of *Salmonella* infection. Bacteremic disease after antibiotic treatment is more likely to be due to a resistant *Salmonella* spp. In patients with AIDS, recurrent septicemia appears despite antibiotic therapy, often with a negative stool culture for *Salmonella* and sometimes with no identifiable focus of infection. Prolonged or recurrent bacteremia also occurs in patients with schistosomiasis. Hemolytic anemias, malaria, and bartonellosis are associated with an increased risk of bacteremia, presumably because of reticuloendothelial system dysfunction. In pregnancy, *Salmonella* septicemia and fetal loss have been reported. *S. typhimurium* is the most common serotype causing *Salmonella* bacteremia in the United States.

TABLE 196–1 Conditions That Increase the Risk of *Salmonella* Bacteremia During *Salmonella* Gastroenteritis

Neonates and young infants (≤3 mo)
AIDS, chronic granulomatous disease, and other immune deficiencies
Malignancies, especially leukemia and lymphoma
Immunosuppressive and corticosteroid therapy
Hemolytic anemia, including sickle cell disease, malaria, and bartonellosis
Collagen vascular disease
Inflammatory bowel disease
Gastrectomy or gastroenterostomy
Achlorhydria or antacid medication use
Impaired intestinal motility
Schistosomiasis
Malnutrition

Extraintestinal Focal Infections. After salmonellae have entered the bloodstream, they have a unique capability to metastasize and cause a focal suppurative infection of almost any organ. Sites of pre-existing abnormalities are often involved. Extraintestinal infections are most common in the first 3 mo of life, in those with sickle cell disease, and in those who have had prior gastrointestinal surgery. The most common focal infections involve the skeletal system, meninges, and intravascular sites. *Salmonella* is a common cause of osteomyelitis in children with sickle cell disease. *Salmonella* osteomyelitis and suppurative arthritis also occur in sites of previous trauma or skeletal prosthesis. Reactive arthritis may follow *Salmonella* gastroenteritis, usually in children with the HLA-B27 antigen. Meningitis appears mainly in infants. Patients may present with little or no fever and minimal symptoms, but rapid deterioration, a high mortality rate, and neurologic sequelae occur despite appropriate antibiotic therapy. *Salmonella* meningitis occurs also in patients with AIDS, for whom the mortality rate is more than 50%, and relapse and brain abscesses can occur. Persistent bacteremia suggests endocarditis, arteritis, or an infected aneurysm.

DIAGNOSIS. Definitive diagnosis of the various clinical syndromes is still based on culturing and subsequent identification of *Salmonella* organisms. In children with gastroenteritis, cultures of stools have higher yields than rectal swabs. In patients with sites of local suppuration, aspirated specimens should be Gram stained and cultured. *Salmonella* organisms grow well on nonselective or enriched media, such as blood agar, chocolate agar, or nutrient broth. Normally sterile body fluids (e.g., cerebrospinal fluid, joint fluid, urine) can be cultured on any of these. For specimens normally containing mixed bacterial flora (e.g., stools), selective media, such as MacConkey, XLD, bismuth sulfite (BBL), or *Salmonella-Shigella* (SS) agar, which inhibit the growth of normal flora, should be used.

Several methods are being developed to answer the need for rapid diagnosis. Two tests, based on latex agglutination and fluorescence, are commercially available for the rapid diagnosis of *Salmonella* colonies growing in stool culture enrichment broth or culture plates. Clinical experience is limited. Alternatively, chromosomal fragments that are unique to the genus *Salmonella* have been used as DNA probes to detect *Salmonella* species. Serologic assay for detecting antibodies against *S. typhi-*

murium and *S. enteritidis* has been reported, but clinical usefulness is still unclear.

Differential Diagnosis. *Salmonella* gastroenteritis should be differentiated from other bacterial, viral, and parasitic causes of diarrhea. The presentation of inflammatory diarrhea with moderate fever should be particularly differentiated from *Shigella,* enteroinvasive *Escherichia coli, Yersinia enterocolitica,* and *Clostridium difficile* infections. Rotavirus infections in infants can mimic *Salmonella* enterocolitis. Etiologic diagnosis on the basis of the clinical picture is seldom possible. Epidemiologic data may be helpful. If abdominal pain and tenderness are severe, appendicitis, perforated viscus, and ulcerative colitis merit consideration in the differential diagnosis.

TREATMENT. Appropriate therapy depends on the specific clinical presentation of *Salmonella* infection. Assessment of the hydration status, correction of dehydration and electrolyte disturbances, and supportive care (Chapters 54 and 55) are the most important aspects of managing *Salmonella* gastroenteritis in children. Antimotility agents prolong intestinal transit time and are thought to increase the risk of invasion; they should not be used when salmonellosis is suspected. In patients with gastroenteritis, antimicrobial agents do not shorten the clinical course, nor do they eliminate fecal excretion of *Salmonella.* By suppressing normal intestinal flora, antimicrobial agents may prolong the excretion of *Salmonella* and increase the risk of creating the chronic carrier state. Antibiotics therefore are not indicated routinely in treating *Salmonella* gastroenteritis. They should be used in young infants (≤3 mo of age) and other children who are at increased risk of a disseminated disease (Table 196–1) and in those with a severe or protracted course.

Children with bacteremia or extraintestinal focal *Salmonella* infections should receive antimicrobial therapy. Ampicillin (200 mg/kg/24 hr in four divided doses) is efficacious and used to be the drug of choice; trimethoprim-sulfamethoxazole (TMP-SMX; 10–50 mg/kg/24 hr in two divided doses) and chloramphenicol (75 mg/kg/24 hr in four divided doses) are also effective. Because of the increasing worldwide antibiotic resistance of *Salmonella* strains, it is necessary to perform susceptibility tests on all human isolates. About 20% of *Salmonella* isolates in the United States are resistant to ampicillin. Multiresistance to ampicillin, TMP-SMX, and chloramphenicol has been reported. The third-generation cephalosporins cefotaxime (150–200 mg/kg/24 hr in three to four divided doses) or ceftriaxone (100 mg/kg/24 hr in one or two doses) are effective if the isolate is susceptible. Quinolones are also effective, but they are not approved for use in children because of the potential damage to growing cartilage. In children with severe disease, initial treatment with a third-generation cephalosporin is recommended until antibiotic susceptibility is known. Thereafter, antibiotics should be changed on the basis of susceptibility data and clinical syndrome.

The duration of antimicrobial therapy is 10–14 days for children with bacteremia, 4–6 wk for acute osteomyelitis, and 4 wk for meningitis. For children with a focal suppurative process, surgical drainage is necessary in addition to antibiotic treatment. Surgical intervention is often necessary in intravascular *Salmonella* infections and in cases of chronic osteomyelitis.

PROGNOSIS. Complete recovery is the rule in healthy children who develop *Salmonella* gastroenteritis. Young infants and immunocompromised patients often have systemic involvement, a prolonged course, and extraintestinal foci. The prognosis is poor for children with *Salmonella* meningitis or endocarditis.

Chronic Carrier State. After clinical recovery from *Salmonella* gastroenteritis, asymptomatic fecal excretion of salmonellae occurs for several months, particularly in younger children or those treated with antibiotics. A chronic carrier state is defined as asymptomatic excretion of *Salmonella* organisms for more than 1 yr. A prolonged carrier state after nontyphoidal salmonellosis is rare (<1%); it is more common in patients with biliary tract disease (e.g., cholelithiasis). The only significance of asymptomatic fecal excretion of nontyphoidal *Salmonella* is the potential transmission of the infection to other individuals.

PREVENTION. Chlorinated water, proper sanitary systems, and adequate food hygiene practices are necessary to prevent nontyphoidal salmonellosis in humans. Handwashing is of paramount importance in controlling person-to-person transmission by means of food. In hospitalized patients, enteric precautions should be used for the duration of illness. Individuals with symptomatic or asymptomatic excretion of *Salmonella* strains should be excluded from activities that involve food preparation or child care until repeated stool cultures are negative. Breast-feeding has been shown to reduce infection.

Control of the transmission of *Salmonella* infections to humans requires control of the infection in the animal reservoir, judicious use of antibiotics in dairy and livestock farming, prevention of contamination of foodstuffs prepared from animals, and use of appropriate standards in food processing in commercial and private kitchens. Whenever cooking practices prevent food from reaching a temperature greater than 150°F (65.5°C) for more than 12 min, *Salmonella* may remain viable. Because large outbreaks are often related to mass food production, it should be recognized that contamination of just one piece of machinery used in food processing may cause an outbreak; meticulous cleaning of equipment is essential. No vaccine against nontyphoidal *Salmonella* infections is available. Infections should be reported to public health authorities so that outbreaks can be recognized and investigated.

196.2 Enteric Fever

Enteric fever is a systemic syndrome produced by certain *Salmonella* organisms. It encompasses typhoid fever, caused by *S. typhi,* and paratyphoid fever, caused by *S. paratyphi* A, *S. schottmuelleri* (formerly *S. paratyphi* B), *S. hirschfeldii* (formerly *S. paratyphi* C), and occasionally other *Salmonella* serotypes. Typhoid fever, the most frequent enteric fever, tends to be more severe than the other forms.

EPIDEMIOLOGY. The incidence, mode of transmission, and consequences of enteric fever differ significantly in developed and developing countries. The incidence has decreased markedly in developed countries. In the United States, about 400 cases of typhoid fever are reported each year, giving an annual incidence of less than 0.2/100,000, which is similar to that in Western Europe and Japan. In Southern Europe, the annual incidence is 4.3–14.5/100,000. In developing countries, *S. typhi* is often the most common *Salmonella* isolate, with an incidence that can reach 500/100,000 (0.5%) and a high mortality rate. The World Health Organization has estimated that 12.5 million cases occur annually worldwide (excluding China).

Because humans are the only natural reservoir of *S. typhi,* direct or indirect contact with an infected person (sick or chronic carrier) is necessary for infection. Ingestion of foods or water contaminated with human feces is the most common mode of transmission. Water-borne outbreaks due to poor sanitation and direct fecal-oral spread due to poor personal hygiene are encountered, mainly in developing countries. Oysters and other shellfish cultivated in water contaminated by sewage are also a source of widespread infection. In the United States, about 65% of the cases result from international travel. Travel to Asia (especially to India) and Central or South America (especially Mexico) is usually implicated. Domestically acquired enteric fever is most frequent in the southern and western United States and is usually caused by consumption of foods contaminated by individuals who are chronic carriers. Congenital transmission of enteric fever can occur by transplacental infection from a bacteremic mother to her fetus. Intrapartum transmission is also possible, occurring by a fecal-oral route from a carrier mother.

PATHOGENESIS. In younger children, the morphologic changes of *S. typhi* infection are less prominent than in older children and adults. Hyperplasia of Peyer's patches with necrosis and sloughing of overlying epithelium, producing ulcers that may bleed, is typical. The mucosa and lymphatic tissue of the intestinal tract are severely inflamed and necrotic. Ulceration that heals without scarring is common. Strictures and intestinal obstruction virtually never occur after typhoid fever. The inflammatory lesion may occasionally penetrate the muscularis and serosa of the intestine and produce perforation. The mesenteric lymph nodes, liver, and spleen are hyperemic and generally reveal areas of focal necrosis. Hyperplasia of reticuloendothelial tissue with proliferation of mononuclear cells is the predominant finding. A mononuclear response may be seen in the bone marrow in association with areas of focal necrosis. Inflammation of the gallbladder is focal, inconstant, and modest in proportion to the extent of local bacterial multiplication. Bronchitis is common. Inflammation also may be observed in the form of localized abscesses, pneumonia, septic arthritis, osteomyelitis, pyelonephritis, endophthalmitis, and meningitis.

Bloodstream invasion is necessary to produce the enteric fever syndrome. The inoculum size required to cause disease in volunteers is 10^5–10^9 *S. typhi* organisms. These estimates may be higher than in naturally acquired infection because the volunteers ingested the organisms in milk; stomach acidity is an important determinant of susceptibility to salmonella. After attachment to the microvilli of the ileal brush borders, the bacteria ivade intestinal epithelium, apparently through the Peyer's patches. Organisms are transported to intestinal lymph nodes, where multiplication takes place within the mononuclear cells. Monocytes, unable to destroy the bacilli early in the disease process, carry these organisms into the mesenteric lymph nodes. Organisms then reach the bloodstream through the thoracic duct, causing a transient bacteremia. Circulating organisms reach the reticuloendothelial cells in the liver, spleen, and bone marrow and may seed other organs. After proliferation in the reticuloendothelial system, bacteremia recurs. The gallbladder is particularly susceptible to being infected. Local multiplication in the walls of the gallbladder produces large numbers of salmonellae, which reach the intestine through the bile.

Several virulence factors seem to be important. Invasion of Peyer's patches is encoded by genes closely related to the invasion genes of *Shigella* spp and enteroinvasive *E. coli*. However, *S. typhi* possesses a number of additional genes not found in *Shigella* that are responsible for the features of typhoid fever. The surface Vi capsular antigen found in *S. typhi* interferes with phagocytosis by preventing the binding of C3 to the surface of the bacterium. The ability of organisms to survive within macrophages after phagocytosis is an important virulence trait encoded by the *phoP* regulon; it may be related to metabolic effects on host cells. Circulating endotoxin, a lipopolysaccharide component of the bacterial cell wall, is thought to cause the prolonged fever and toxic symptoms of enteric fever, although its levels in symptomatic patients are low. Alternatively, endotoxin-induced cytokine production by human macrophages may cause the systemic symptoms. The occasional occurrence of diarrhea may be explained by presence of a toxin related to cholera toxin and *E. coli* heat-labile enterotoxin.

Cell-mediated immunity is important in protecting the human host against typhoid fever. Decreased numbers of T lymphocytes are found in patients who are critically ill with typhoid fever. Carriers show impaired cellular reactivity to *S. typhi* antigens in the leukocyte migration inhibition test. In carriers, a large number of virulent bacilli pass into the intestine daily and are excreted in the stool, without entering the epithelium of the host.

CLINICAL MANIFESTATIONS. The incubation period is usually 7–14 days, but it may range from 3–30 days, depending mainly on the size of the ingested inoculum. The clinical manifestations of enteric fever depend on age.

School-Age Children and Adolescents. The onset of symptoms is insidious. Initial symptoms of fever, malaise, anorexia, myalgia, headache, and abdominal pain develop over 2–3 days. Although diarrhea having a pea soup consistency may be present during the early course of the disease, constipation later becomes a more prominent symptom. Nausea and vomiting if occurring in the 2nd or 3rd wk suggest a complication. Cough and epistaxis may ensue. Severe lethargy may develop in some children. Temperature, which rises in a stepwise fashion, becomes an unremitting and high fever within 1 wk, often reaching 40°C (104°F).

During the 2nd wk of illness, high fever is sustained, and fatigue, anorexia, cough, and abdominal symptoms increase in severity. Patients appear acutely ill, disoriented, and lethargic. Delirium and stupor may be observed. Physical findings include a relative bradycardia, which is disproportionate to the high fever. Hepatomegaly, splenomegaly, and distended abdomen with diffuse tenderness are very common. In about 50% of patients with enteric fever, a macular or maculopapular rash (i.e., rose spots) appears on about the 7th–10th day. Lesions are usually discrete, erythematous, and 1–5 mm in diameter; the lesions are slightly raised, and blanch on pressure. They appear in crops of 10–15 lesions on the lower chest and abdomen and last 2–3 days. They leave a slight brownish discoloration of the skin on healing. Cultures of the lesions have a 60% yield for *Salmonella* organisms. Rhonchi and scattered rales may be heard on auscultation of the chest. If no complications occur, the symptoms and physical findings gradually resolve within 2–4 wk, but malaise and lethargy may persist for an additional 1–2 mo. Patients may be emaciated by the end of the illness. Enteric fever caused by nontyphoidal *Salmonella* is usually milder, with a shorter duration of fever and a lower rate of complications.

Infants and Young Children (<5 yr). Enteric fever is relatively rare in this age group in endemic areas. In the United States, those 0–5 yr of age are over-represented. Although clinical sepsis can occur, the disease is surprisingly mild at presentation, making the diagnosis difficult. Mild fever and malaise, misinterpreted as a viral syndrome, occur in infants with culture-proven typhoid fever. Diarrhea is more common in young children with typhoid fever than in adults, leading to a diagnosis of acute gastroenteritis. Other children may present with signs and symptoms of lower respiratory tract infection.

Neonates. In addition to its ability to cause abortion and premature delivery, enteric fever during late pregnancy may be transmitted vertically. The neonatal disease usually begins within 3 days of delivery. Vomiting, diarrhea, and abdominal distention are common. Temperature is variable but may be as high as 40.5°C (104.9°F). Seizures may occur. Hepatomegaly, jaundice, anorexia, and weight loss can be marked.

DIAGNOSIS. Culturing the *Salmonella* strain involved is usually the basis for confirming the diagnosis. Results of blood cultures are positive in 40–60% of the patients seen early in the course of the disease, and stool and urine cultures become positive after the first week. The stool culture result is also occasionally positive during the incubation period. Because of the intermittent and low-level bacteremia, repeated blood cultures should be obtained in suspect cases. Cultures of bone marrow often yield positive results during later stages of the disease, when blood cultures may be sterile; although seldom obtained, cultures of mesenteric lymph nodes, liver, and spleen may also have positive results at this point. A culture of bone marrow is the single most sensitive method of diagnosis (positive in 85–90%) and is less influenced by prior antimicrobial therapy. Results of stool and sometimes urine cultures are positive in chronic carriers. In suspected cases with negative results of stool cultures, a culture of aspirated duodenal fluid or of a duodenal string capsule may be helpful in confirming infection. However, the duodenal string culture test cannot be performed on those too young or too ill to cooperate.

Because identification of *S. typhi* from culture usually takes several days, several methods for earlier diagnosis are being developed. Direct detection of *S. typhi*–specific antigens in the serum or *S. typhi* Vi antigen in the urine has been attempted by immunologic methods, often using monoclonal antibodies. Polymerase chain reaction has been used to amplify specific genes of *S. typhi* in the blood of patients, enabling diagnosis within a few hours. This method is specific and more sensitive than blood cultures, given the low level of bacteremia in enteric fever. Serology is of little help in establishing the diagnosis, but it may be useful in epidemiologic studies. The classic Widal's test measures antibodies against O and H antigens of *S. typhi*. Because many false-positive and false-negative results occur, diagnosis of typhoid fever by Widal's test alone is prone to error. Experience is still limited with new serologic assays.

Laboratory Findings. A normochromic, normocytic anemia often develops after several weeks of illness and is related to intestinal blood loss or bone marrow suppression. Blood leukocyte counts are frequently low in relation to the fever and toxicity, but there is a wide range in counts; leukopenia, usually not below 2,500 cells/mm^3, is often found after the 1st or 2nd wk of illness. When pyogenic abscesses develop, leukocytosis may reach 20,000–25,000/mm^3. Thrombocytopenia may be striking and persist for as long as 1 wk. Liver function test results are often disturbed. Proteinuria is common. Fecal leukocytes and fecal blood are very common.

Differential Diagnosis. During the initial stage of enteric fever, the clinical diagnosis may mistakenly be gastroenteritis, viral syndrome, bronchitis, or bronchopneumonia. Subsequently, the differential diagnosis includes sepsis with other bacterial pathogens; infections caused by intracellular microorganisms, such as tuberculosis, brucellosis, tularemia, leptospirosis, and rickettsial diseases; viral infections, such as infectious mononucleosis and anicteric hepatitis; and malignancies, such as leukemia and lymphoma.

TREATMENT. Antimicrobial therapy is essential in treating enteric fever. Because of increasing antibiotic resistance, however, choosing the appropriate empirical therapy is problematic and controversial. Although antibiotic resistance of *S. typhi* isolates in the United States is relatively low (3–4%), most infections are acquired abroad, where resistance occurs. Increasing rates of plasmid-mediated antibiotic resistance of *S. typhi* have been reported from Southeast Asia, Mexico, and certain countries in the Middle East. Reports from India describe multiresistance to chloramphenicol, ampicillin, and TMP-SMX in 49–83% of *S. typhi* isolates. Resistant strains are usually susceptible to third-generation cephalosporins. Fluoroquinolones are efficacious but are not approved for children. Most antibiotic regimens are associated with a 5–20% recurrence risk. Chloramphenicol (50 mg/kg/24 hr PO or 75 mg/kg/24 hr IV in four equal doses), ampicillin (200 mg/kg/24 hr IV in four to six doses), amoxicillin (100 mg/kg/24 hr PO in three doses), and trimethoprim-sulfamethoxazole (10 mg of TMP and 50 mg of SMX/kg/24 hr PO in two doses) have demonstrated good clinical efficacy. Although chloramphenicol therapy is associated with a more rapid defervescence and sterilization of blood, the rate of relapse is somewhat higher, and this agent can cause potentially serious adverse effects. Most children become afebrile within 7 days; treatment of uncomplicated cases should be continued for at least 14 days, or 5–7 days after defervescence. Data suggest that very short courses of therapy may be adequate with oral cefixime (20 mg/kg/24 hr in two divided doses for 8 days), ceftriaxone (50 mg/kg/24 hr IM for 5 days) or oral ofloxacin (15 mg/kg/24 hr for 2 days). Chloramphenicol remains the gold standard. However, despite its low cost, ease of administration, and efficacy, these new treatment options may eventually supplant chloramphenicol as more data are published.

In adults, ciprofloxacin at a dose of 500 mg bid for 7–10 days is effective and associated with a low relapse rate. In children with suspected resistant strains, we recommend empirical therapy with ceftriaxone (or cefotaxime) until antibiotic susceptibility patterns are available.

In addition to antibiotic therapy, a short course of dexamethasone, using 3 mg/kg for the initial dose, followed by 1 mg/kg every 6 hr for 48 hr, improves the survival rate of patients with shock, obtundation, stupor, or coma. This does not increase the incidence of complications if antibiotic therapy is adequate. Supportive treatment and maintenance of appropriate fluid and electrolyte balance are essential. When intestinal hemorrhage is severe, blood transfusion is needed. Surgical intervention with broad-spectrum antibiotics is recommended for intestinal perforation. Platelet transfusions have been suggested for the treatment of thrombocytopenia that is sufficiently severe to cause intestinal hemorrhage in patients for whom surgery is contemplated.

Although attempts to eradicate chronic carriage of *S. typhi* are recommended for public health considerations, eradication is difficult despite in vitro susceptibility to the antibiotic used. A course of 4–6 wk of high-dose ampicillin (or amoxicillin) plus probenecid or TMP-SMX results in an approximately 80% cure rate of carriers if no biliary tract disease is present. Ciprofloxacin has been used successfully in adults. In the presence of cholelithiasis or cholecystitis, antibiotics alone are unlikely to be successful; cholecystectomy within 14 days of antibiotic treatment is recommended.

COMPLICATIONS. Severe intestinal hemorrhage and intestinal perforation occur in 1–10% and 0.5–3% of the patients, respectively. These and most other complications usually occur after the 1st wk of the disease. Hemorrhage, which usually precedes perforation, is manifested by a drop in temperature and blood pressure and an increase in the pulse rate. Perforations, which are usually pinpoint size but may be as large as several centimeters, typically occur in the distal ileum and are accompanied by a marked increase in abdominal pain, tenderness, vomiting, and signs of peritonitis. Sepsis with various enteric aerobic gram-negative bacilli and anaerobes may develop. Although disturbed liver function test results are found for many patients with enteric fever, overt hepatitis and cholecystitis are considered complications. An increase in serum amylase levels may sometimes accompany clinically obvious pancreatitis.

Pneumonia often caused by superinfection with organisms other than *Salmonella* is more common in children than in adults. In children, pneumonia or bronchitis is common (approximately 10%). Toxic myocarditis with fatty infiltration and necrosis of the myocardium may be manifested by arrhythmias, sinoatrial block, ST-T changes on the electrocardiogram, or cardiogenic shock. Thrombosis and phlebitis occur rarely. Neurologic complications include increased intracranial pressure, cerebral thrombosis, acute cerebellar ataxia, chorea, aphasia, deafness, psychosis, and transverse myelitis. Peripheral and optic neuritis have been reported. Permanent sequelae are rare. Other reported complications include fatal bone marrow necrosis, pyelonephritis, nephrotic syndrome, meningitis, endocarditis, parotitis, orchitis, and suppurative lymphadenitis. Although osteomyelitis and septic arthritis can occur in a normal host, they are more common in children with hemoglobinopathies.

PROGNOSIS. The prognosis for a patient with enteric fever depends on prompt therapy, the age of the patient, previous state of health, the causative *Salmonella* serotype, and the appearance of complications. In developed countries, with appropriate antimicrobial therapy, the mortality rate is less than 1%. In developing countries, the mortality rate is higher than 10%, usually because of delays in diagnosis, hospitalization, and treatment. Infants 1 yr of age or younger and children with underlying debilitating disorders are at higher risk. The appearance of complications, such as gastrointestinal perforation or severe hemorrhage, meningitis, endocarditis, and pneumonia, is associated with high morbidity and mortality rates.

Relapse after the initial clinical response occurs in 4–8% of the patients who are not treated with antibiotics. In patients who have received appropriate antimicrobial therapy, the clinical manifestations of relapse become apparent about 2 wk after stopping antibiotics and resemble the acute illness. The relapse, however, is usually milder and of shorter duration. Numerous relapses may occur. Individuals who excrete *S. typhi* 3 mo or longer after infection are usually excretors at 1 yr and defined as chronic carriers. The risk of becoming a carrier is low in children and increases with age; of all patients with typhoid fever, 1–5% become chronic carriers. The incidence of biliary tract diseases is higher in chronic carriers than in the general population. Although chronic urinary carriage may also occur, it is rare and found mainly in individuals with schistosomiasis.

PREVENTION. In endemic areas, improved sanitation and clean running water are essential to control enteric fever. To minimize person-to-person transmission and food contamination, personal hygiene measures, handwashing, and attention to food preparation practices are necessary. Efforts to eradicate *S. typhi* from carriers are recommended, because humans are the only reservoir of *S. typhi*. When such efforts are unsuccessful, carriers should be prevented from working in food- or water-processing activities, in kitchens, and in occupations related to patient care. These individuals should be made aware of the potential contagiousness of their condition and of the importance of handwashing and attentive personal hygiene.

Vaccine. Three vaccines against *S. typhi* are commercially available. A parenteral heat-phenol inactivated vaccine confers limited protection (51–76% efficacy) and is associated with adverse effects, including fever, local reactions, and headache in at least 25% of recipients. It is approved for children 6 mo of age or older. Two doses (0.25 mL for persons 6 mo–10 yr; 0.5 mL for persons ≥10 yr of age) are administered subcutaneously 4 wk or more apart. Booster doses are necessary every 3 yr. A second vaccine is an oral, live-attenuated preparation of the Ty21a strain of *S. typhi*. Several large studies have shown good efficacy (67–82%). Four enteric-coated capsules are given on alternate days, and the entire series is repeated every 5 yr. Significant adverse effects are rare. The oral vaccine is not recommended for children 6 yr of age or younger because of limited experience. Infants and toddlers do not develop immune responses with this preparation. It should not be used in persons with immunodeficiency syndromes. A third vaccine against typhoid fever is made from the Vi capsular polysaccharide and can be used in persons 2 yr of age or older. It is given as a single intramuscular dose, with a booster every 2 yr.

Typhoid vaccination is recommended to travelers to endemic areas, especially Latin America, Southeast Asia, and Africa. Such travelers need to be cautioned that the vaccine is not a substitute for personal hygiene and careful selection of foods and drinks, because none of the vaccines has efficacy approaching 100%. Vaccination is also recommended to individuals with intimate exposure to a documented carrier and for control of outbreaks.

Nontyphoidal Salmonellosis

Cohen JI, Bartlett JA, Corey GP: Extra-intestinal manifestations of *Salmonella* infections. Medicine (Baltimore) 66:349, 1987.

Goldberg MB, Rubin RH: The spectrum of *Salmonella* infection. Infect Dis Clin North Am 2:571, 1988.

Hedberg CW, David MJ, White KE, et al: Role of egg consumption in sporadic *Salmonella enteritis* and *Salmonella typhimurium* infection in Minnesota. J Infect Dis 167:107, 1993.

Isomaki O, Vuento R, Granfors K: Serologic diagnosis of *Salmonella* infections by enzyme immunoassay. Lancet 1:1411, 1989.

Lee LA, Puhr ND, Maloney EK, et al: Increase in antimicrobial-resistant *Salmonella* infections in the United States, 1989–1990. J Infect Dis 170:128, 1994.

Schutze GE, Schutze SE, Kirby RS: Extra-Intestinal salmonellosis in a children's hospital. Pediatr Infect Dis J 16:482, 1997.

Sperber SJ, Schleupner CJ: Salmonellosis during infection with human immunodeficiency virus. Rev Infect Dis 9:925, 1987.

St. Geme JW, Hodes HL, Marcy SM, et al: Consensus: Management of *Salmonella* infection in the first year of life. Pediatr Infect Dis J 7:615, 1988.

Enteric Fever

Bhutta ZA, Khan IA, Molla AM: Therapy of multiply resistant typhoid fever with oral cefixime vs intravenous ceftriaxone. Pediatr Infect Dis J 13:990, 1994.

Butler T, Islam A, Kabir I, et al: Patterns of morbidity and mortality in typhoid fever dependent on age and gender. A review of 552 patients hospitalized with diarrhea. Rev Infect Dis 13:85, 1991.

Centers for Disease Control and Prevention: Typhoid immunization: Recommendations of the Immunization Practices Advisory Committee (ACIP). MMWR 43(RR-14):1, 1994.

Girgis NI, Sultan Y, Hammad O, et al: Comparison of the efficacy, safety and cost of cefixime, ceftriaxone and aztreonam in the treatment of multidrug-resistant *Salmonella typhi* septicemia in children. Pediatr Infect Dis J 14:603, 1995.

Mahle WT, Levine MM: *Salmonella typhi* infection in children younger than five years of age. Pediatr Infect Dis J 12:627, 1993.

Mermin JH, Townes JM, Gerber M, et al: Typhoid Fever in the United States, 1985–1994. Changing risks of international travel and increasing antimicrobial resistance. Arch Intern Med 158:633, 1998.

Misra S, Diaz PS, Rowley AH: Characteristics of typhoid fever in children and adolescents in a major metropolitan area in the United States. Clin Infect Dis 24:998, 1997.

Mosley JG, Chaudhuri AK: Surgery and *Salmonella*: Complications require prompt diagnosis and treatment. Br Med J 300:552, 1990.

Soe GB, Overturf GD: Treatment of typhoid fever and other systemic salmonelloses with cefotaxime, ceftriaxone, cefoperazone and other newer cephalosporins. Rev Infect Dis 9:719, 1987.

Song JH, Cho H, Park MY, et al: Detection of *Salmonella typhi* in the blood of patients with typhoid fever by polymerase chain reaction. J Clin Microbiol 31:1439, 1993.

Thisyakorn U, Mansuwan P, Taylor DN: Typhoid and paratyphoid fever in 192 hospitalized children in Thailand. Am J Dis Child 141:862, 1987.

CHAPTER 197
Shigella

Henry F. Gomez and Thomas G. Cleary

Although dysenteric syndromes have long been recognized as a scourge of humans, it is only in the past century that the bacteriology of the most common form of epidemic dysentery has been appreciated. Four species of *Shigella* are responsible for illness: *S. dysenteriae* (serogroup A), *S. flexneri* (serogroup B), *S. boydii* (serogroup C), and *S. sonnei* (serogroup D). There are 13 serotypes in group A, 6 serotypes and 13 subserotypes in group B, 18 serotypes in group C, and 1 serotype in group D.

EPIDEMIOLOGY. Infection with shigellae occurs most often during the warm months in temperate climates and during the rainy season in tropical climates. The sexes are affected equally. Although infection can occur at any age, it is most common in the 2nd and 3rd yr of life. Infection in the first 6 mo is rare for reasons that are not clear. Breast milk, which in endemic areas contains antibodies to both virulence plasmid-coded antigens and lipopolysaccharides, may partially explain the age-related incidence. Asymptomatic infection of children and adults occurs commonly in endemic areas.

In industrialized societies, *S. sonnei* is the most common cause of bacillary dysentery, with *S. flexneri* second in frequency; in preindustrial societies, *S. flexneri* is most common, with *S. sonnei* second in frequency. *S. dysenteriae* serotype 1 tends to occur in massive epidemics, although it is also endemic in Asia.

Contaminated food (often a salad or other item requiring extensive handling of the ingredients) and water are important vectors. However, person-to-person transmission is probably the major mechanism of infection in most areas of the world.

Spread within families, custodial institutions, and child-care centers demonstrates the ability of low numbers of organisms to cause disease on a person-to-person basis.

PATHOGENESIS. The basic virulence trait shared by all shigellae is the ability to invade colonic epithelial cells. This characteristic is encoded on a large (120–140 MD) plasmid that is responsible for synthesis of a group of polypeptides involved in cell invasion and killing. Shigellae that lose the virulence plasmid no longer act as pathogens. *Escherichia coli* that harbor this plasmid [enteroinvasive *E. coli*] behave like shigellae. In addition to the major plasmid-encoded virulence traits, chromosomally encoded factors are also required for full virulence; some of these chromosomal traits are important for all shigellae (e.g., lipopolysaccharide synthesis), whereas others are important only in some serotypes (e.g., shigatoxin synthesis by *S. dysenteriae* serotype 1 and ShET-1 by *S. flexneri* 2a). Shigatoxin, a potent protein synthesis–inhibiting exotoxin, is produced in significant amounts only by *S. dysenteriae* serotype 1 and certain *E. coli* (shigatoxin-producing *E. coli [STEC]*). The watery diarrhea phase of shigellosis may be caused by unique enterotoxins: shigella enterotoxin 1 (ShET-1), encoded on the bacterial chromosome of *S. flexneri* 2a, and *sen*, an enterotoxin produced by nearly all shigellae and enteroinvasive *E. coli*.

Shigellae require very low inocula to cause illness. Ingestion of as few as 10 *S. dysenteriae* serotype 1 organisms can cause dysentery in some susceptible individuals. This is in contrast to organisms such as *Vibrio cholerae*, which require ingestion of 10^8–10^{10} organisms to cause illness. The inoculum effect explains the ease of person-to-person transmission of shigellae in contrast to *V. cholerae*.

The pathologic changes of shigellosis take place primarily in the colon, the target organ for shigellae. The changes are most intense in the distal colon, although pancolitis may occur. Grossly, localized or diffuse mucosal edema, ulcerations, friable mucosa, bleeding, and exudate may be seen. Microscopically, ulcerations, pseudomembranes, epithelial cell death, infiltration extending from the mucosa to the muscularis mucosae by polymorphonuclear and mononuclear cells, and submucosal edema occur.

Immune Responses. Secretory IgA and serum antibodies develop within days to weeks after infection with *Shigella*. Although both antilipopolysaccharide and antivirulence plasmid polypeptide antibodies have been described, identification of the major determinant of protection against subsequent infection remains unclear. Evidence shows that protection is serotype specific, but there is also the suggestion that a degree of cross-protection against all shigellae follows infection with a given serotype. Cell-mediated immunity may also have a role in protection.

CLINICAL MANIFESTATIONS. Bacillary dysentery is clinically similar regardless of whether the disease is caused by an enteroinvasive *E. coli* (Chapter 198) or any of the four species of *Shigella*; however, there are some clinical differences, particularly relating to the severity and risk of complications with *S. dysenteriae* serotype 1 infection.

Ingestion of shigellae is followed by an incubation period of 12 hr to several days before symptoms ensue. Severe abdominal pain, high fever, emesis, anorexia, generalized toxicity, urgency, and painful defecation characteristically occur. Physical examination at this point may show abdominal distention and tenderness, hyperactive bowel sounds, and a tender rectum on digital examination.

The diarrhea may be watery and of large volume initially, evolving into frequent small-volume, bloody mucoid stools; however, some children never progress to the stage of bloody diarrhea, whereas in others the first stools are bloody. Significant dehydration related to the fluid and electrolyte losses in both feces and emesis can occur. Untreated diarrhea may last 1–2 wk; only about 10% of patients have diarrhea persisting for more than 10 days. Chronic diarrhea is uncommon except in malnourished infants or those with AIDS.

Neurologic findings are among the most common extraintestinal manifestations of bacillary dysentery, occurring in as many as 40% of hospitalized infected children. Enteroinvasive *E. coli* can cause similar neurologic toxicity. Convulsions, headache, lethargy, confusion, nuchal rigidity, or hallucinations may be present before or after the onset of diarrhea. The cause of these neurologic findings is not understood. In the past, these symptoms were attributed to the neurotoxicity of shigatoxin, but it is now clear that that explanation is wrong. Seizures sometimes occur when little fever is present, suggesting that simple febrile convulsions do not explain their appearance. Hypocalcemia or hyponatremia may be associated with seizures in a small number of patients. Although symptoms often suggest central nervous system infection, and cerebrospinal fluid pleocytosis with minimally elevated protein levels can occur, meningitis due to shigellae is rare.

The most common complication of shigellosis is dehydration, with its attendant risks of renal failure and death. Inappropriate secretion of antidiuretic hormone with profound hyponatremia may complicate dysentery, particularly when *S. dysenteriae* is the etiologic agent. Hypoglycemia and protein-loosing enteropathy are common.

Other major complications, particularly in very young, malnourished children, include sepsis and disseminated intravascular coagulation. Given that these organisms penetrate the intestinal mucosal barrier, these events are surprisingly uncommon. Shigellae and sometimes other gram-negative enterics are recovered from blood cultures in 1–5% of patients in whom blood cultures are taken; because patients selected for blood cultures represent a biased sample, the risk in unselected cases of shigellosis is presumably lower. Bacteremia is more common with *S. dysenteriae* serotype 1 than with other shigellae. The mortality rate is high when sepsis occurs.

In those who have *S. dysenteriae* serotype 1 infection, hemolysis, anemia, and hemolytic-uremic syndrome are common complications. This syndrome is caused by shigatoxin-mediated endothelial injury; *E. coli* that produce shigatoxin (e.g., *E. coli* 0157:H7, *E. coli* 0111:NM, *E. coli* 026:H11, and others) also cause hemolytic-uremic syndrome (Chapter 526).

Rectal prolapse, toxic megacolon or pseudomembranous colitis (usually associated with *S. dysenteriae*), cholestatic hepatitis, conjunctivitis, iritis, corneal ulcers, pneumonia, arthritis (usually 2–5 wk after enteritis), Reiter's syndrome, cystitis, myocarditis, and vaginitis (typically with a blood-tinged discharge associated with *S. flexneri*) are uncommon events. The rare syndrome of extreme toxicity, convulsions, extreme hyperpyrexia, and headache followed by brain edema and a rapidly fatal outcome without sepsis or significant dehydration (Ekiri's syndrome or "lethal toxic encephalopathy") is not well understood. Death is a rare outcome in well-nourished older children; malnutrition, illness in the 1st yr of life, hypothermia, severe dehydration, thrombocytopenia, hyponatremia, renal failure, and bacteremia are common in children who die during bacillary dysentery.

DIAGNOSIS. Although clinical features suggest shigellosis, they are insufficiently specific to allow confident diagnosis. Infection by *Campylobacter jejuni, Salmonella* spp, enteroinvasive *E. coli*, shigatoxin-producing *E. coli* such as *E. coli* 0157:H7, *Yersinia enterocolitica, Clostridium difficile*, and *Entamoeba histolytica* as well as inflammatory bowel disease may cause confusion. Presumptive data supporting a diagnosis of bacillary dysentery include the finding of fecal leukocytes (confirming the presence of colitis), fecal blood, and demonstration in peripheral blood of leukocytosis with a dramatic left shift (often with more bands than segmented neutrophils). The total peripheral white blood cell count is usually 5,000–15,000 cells/mm³, although leukopenia and leukemoid reactions occur.

Culture of both stool and rectal swab specimens optimizes

the chance of diagnosing *Shigella* infection. Culture media should include MacConkey's agar as well as selective media such as xylose-lysine deoxycholate (XLD) and SS agar. Transport media should be used if specimens cannot be cultured promptly. Appropriate media should be used to exclude *Campylobacter* and other agents. Culture is the gold standard for diagnosis, but it is not absolute. Unfortunately, the laboratory is often not able to confirm the clinical suspicion of shigellosis even when the pathogen is present. Stool cultures of adult volunteers with dysentery after ingestion of shigellae failed to detect the organism in nearly 20% of subjects. Studies of food-borne outbreaks in closed populations suggest that a single culture leads to diagnosis in about half of symptomatic patients with shigellosis. Although additional tools to improve diagnosis (e.g., gene probes) are being developed, the diagnostic inadequacy of cultures makes it incumbent on the clinician to use judgment in the management of clinical syndromes consistent with shigellosis. In children who appear to be toxic, blood cultures should be obtained; this is particularly important in very young or malnourished infants because of their increased risk of bacteremia.

TREATMENT. As with gastroenteritis of other causes, the first concern about a child with suspected shigellosis should be for fluid and electrolyte correction and maintenance (Chapters 54 and 55.6). Drugs that retard intestinal motility (e.g., diphenoxylate hydrochloride with atropine [Lomotil] or loperamide [Imodium]) should not be used because of the risk of prolonging the illness.

The next concern is a decision about the use of antibiotics. Although some authorities recommend withholding antibacterial therapy because of the self-limited nature of the infection, the cost of drugs, and the risk of emergence of resistant organisms, there is a persuasive logic in favor of empirical treatment of all children in whom shigellosis is strongly suspected. Even if not fatal, the untreated illness may cause a child to be quite ill for 2 wk or more; chronic or recurrent diarrhea may ensue. A risk is that malnutrition will develop or worsen during prolonged illness, particularly in children in developing countries. The risk of continued excretion and subsequent infection of family contacts further argues against the strategy of withholding antibiotics.

There are major geographic variations in antibiotic susceptibility of shigellae. In the United States, shigellae are so frequently resistant to ampicillin that it is not effective for empirical therapy. However, oral ampicillin (100 mg/kg/24 hr divided into four doses) may be used if the strain is known to be susceptible. Amoxicillin, because of better gastrointestinal absorption, is less effective than ampicillin in therapy of ampicillin-sensitive strains. Many regions of the United States now harbor strains that are also resistant to trimethoprim-sulfamethoxazole (TMP-SMX), and it also is a poor choice for empirical therapy. Cefixime (8 mg/kg/24 hr PO in two divided doses for 5 days) or another oral third-generation cephalosporin, or ceftriaxone (50 mg/kg/24 hr as a single daily dose given parenterally for 2–5 days) can be used for empirical therapy. Nalidixic acid (55 mg/kg/24 hr in four divided doses for 5 days) is also an acceptable alternate drug. Quinolones such as ciprofloxacin, norfloxacin, or ofloxacin, which have been recommended for use in persons 18 yr of age or older, is not routinely used for children because of the putative risk of arthropathy; use of these agents is reserved for seriously ill children with bacillary dysentery whose organism is suspected or known to be resistant to other agents. Treatment regimens are for a 5-day course. Oral first- and second-generation cephalosporins are inadequate as alternative drugs.

Treatment of patients suspected on clinical grounds of having *Shigella* infection should be initiated when patients are first examined. Stool culture is obtained to preclude other pathogens and to assist in antibiotic changes should a child fail to respond to empirical therapy. A child who has typical dysentery and who responds to initial empirical antibiotic treatment should be continued on that drug for a full 5-day course even if the stool culture is negative. The logic of this recommendation is based on the difficulty of culturing *Shigella* from stools. Furthermore in those patients in parts of the world where enteroinvasive *E. coli* is common, they cause dysentery indistinguishable from that due to shigellae and cannot be diagnosed in routine clinical microbiology laboratories. In a child who fails to respond to therapy of a dysenteric syndrome in the presence of initially negative stool culture results, cultures should be retaken and the child re-evaluated for other possible diagnoses.

PREVENTION. Two simple measures decrease the risk of shigellosis in children. The first is to encourage prolonged breast-feeding in regions in which shigellosis is common. Breast-feeding decreases the risk of symptomatic shigellosis and lessens its severity in infants who acquire infection despite breast-feeding. The second measure is to educate families and child-care center personnel in handwashing techniques, especially after defecation and before food preparation and consumption. Other public health measures, including water and sewage treatment, are expensive and are unlikely to be universally available in the near future in developing countries.

Ashkenazi S, Amir J, Waisman Y, et al: A randomized, double-blind study comparing cefixime and trimethoprim sulfamethoxazole in the treatment of childhood shigellosis. J Pediatr 123:817, 1993.

Bennish ML: Potentially lethal complications of shigellosis. Rev Infect Dis 13:319, 1991.

Nelson JD, Kusmiesz H, Shelton S: Oral or intravenous trimethoprim-sulfamethoxazole therapy for shigellosis. Rev Infect Dis 4:546, 1982.

Salam MA, Bennish ML: Therapy for shigellosis: I. Randomized, double-blind trial of nalidixic acid in childhood shigellosis. J Pediatr 113:901, 1988.

Varsano I, Eidlitz-Marcus T, Nussinovitch M, et al: Comparative efficacy of ceftriaxone and ampicillin for treatment of severe shigellosis in children. J Pediatr 118:627, 1991.

CHAPTER 198
Escherichia coli

Jane T. Atkins and Thomas G. Cleary

Escherichia coli organisms are ubiquitous in the environment. They are a major component of the normal intestinal flora but are relatively uncommon on other body sites. They are important causes of enteric infections, urinary tract infections (Chapter 546), and bacteremia and sepsis in immunocompromised patients (Chapter 179) and in patients with intravascular devices (Chapter 180).

E. coli species are members of the Enterobacteriaceae family. They are oxidase-positive, facultatively anaerobic, gram-negative bacilli. Fermentation of lactose is variable.

ETIOLOGY. Five classes of *E. coli* are recognized as agents associated with pediatric gastroenteritis (Chapter 176). Because *E. coli* organisms are normal fecal flora, demonstration of virulence characteristics is the usual way by which the diarrheogenic *E. coli* can be defined. The mechanism by which *E. coli* produces diarrhea typically involves adherence of organisms to a glycoprotein or glycolipid receptor, followed by production of some noxious substance that injures gut cells or disturbs their function. The genes for virulence properties and for antibiotic resistance are often carried on transferable plasmids or bacteriophages.

Enterotoxigenic *E. coli*. Enterotoxigenic *E. coli* (ETEC) strains produce a heat-labile enterotoxin (LT) and/or a heat-stable enterotoxin (ST). LT, a large molecule consisting of five receptor-binding subunits and one enzymatically active subunit, is structurally, functionally, and immunologically related to cholera toxin produced by *Vibrio cholerae*. ST is a small molecule (18–19 amino acids) not related to LT or cholera toxin, although it is related to an enterotoxin produced by some strains of *Yersinia enterocolitica*. These toxins do not injure or kill cells; rather, they disturb cyclic nucleotide-regulated fluid and electrolyte absorption. ST stimulates guanylate cyclase, resulting in increased cyclic guanosine monophosphate, but LT (like cholera toxin) stimulates adenylate cyclase, resulting in increased cyclic adenosine monophosphate. The ETEC strains typically also possess fimbria or colonization factor antigens (CFAs) that allow them to adhere tightly to intestinal epithelium, thereby efficiently colonizing and delivering toxin to the epithelium. Several CFAs have been recognized as important in effecting the adherence of ETEC to gut mucosal cells. These CFAs are called CFA I, CFA II, CFA III, CFA IV, CS7, CS17, 2230, 8786, PCF 09, PCF 0166, PCF 0148, and PCF 0159. A second plasmid-encoded pilus termed "longus" is very common among ETEC from widely separated geographic regions. Longus is more common in ETEC producing only ST. After colonization of intestinal epithelium, the ETEC release ST or LT. The genes for both colonization factors and enterotoxins are typically encoded on the same plasmid. Of the more than 170 *E. coli* serogroups, only a relatively small number typically are ETEC; these serogroups (06, 08, 015, 020, 025, 027, 063, 078, 080, 085, 0115, 0128ac [but not subgroups 0128ab or 0128ad], 0139, 0148, 0153, 0159, and 0167) are generally different from those found in the other diarrhea-associated *E. coli*.

Enteroinvasive *E. coli*. The enteroinvasive *E. coli* (EIEC) strains behave like shigellae in their capacity to invade gut epithelium and produce a dysentery-like illness. This *Shigella*-like behavior occurs because these *E. coli* possess a large virulence plasmid closely related to the plasmid that endows *Shigella* with its invasiveness (Chapter 197). Invasion of epithelium causes cell death and a brisk inflammatory response that is clinically recognizable as colitis. The bacterial product that kills intestinal cells is not known. EIEC encompass a small number of serogroups (028ac, 029, 0124, 0136, 0143, 0144, 0152, 0164, 0167, and some untypable strains). These serogroups have lipopolysaccharide (LPS) antigens related to *Shigella* LPS, and, like shigellae, the organisms are nonmotile (they lack H or flagellar antigens) and are usually non–lactose fermenters.

Enteropathogenic *E. coli*. The enteropathogenic *E. coli* (EPEC) belong to serogroups (O antigen or LPS antigen) that have been associated with outbreaks of infantile gastroenteritis but do not produce conventional enterotoxins or invade epithelial cells. However, confusion has arisen because organisms within these serogroups also frequently have been isolated from well individuals. The EPEC adhere to the intestinal mucosa in a distinctive way. This pattern of adherence, seen on transmission electron microscopy, has been called "close attaching and effacing" adherence or "pedestal-forming" adherence. The lesion consists of loss of microvilli with adherence of bacteria to the epithelial cells, which form a cup or pedestal in which the bacteria can be seen. Chronic inflammation with flattened villi may also be seen on small bowel biopsy of affected children. EPEC cause localized adherence based on HEp-2 cell assays. EPEC with localized adherence attach loosely to the microvilli of the epithelial cell through ropelike structures called *bundle-forming pili*, which are encoded on a plasmid (EAF plasmid), followed by attachment to the epithelial cell through intimin, the product of the *eae* gene (*E. coli* attaching-effacing). Attachment results in increased intracellular calcium concentration and dense polymerization of actin at the site of attachment. How these cytoskeletal changes cause diarrhea is not clear, although decreased fluid absorption due to loss of microvilli may explain the clinical features. EPEC, which are diffusely adherent in the HEp-2 cell assay system, produce an adhesin involved in diffuse adherence (AIDA-I), which has homology to a *S. flexneri* protein associated with intercellular spread (VirG). Some serogroups are associated with localized adherence and are EAF probe positive (055, 086, 0111, 0119, 0125, 0126, 0127, 0128ab, and 0142), whereas others are nonadherent or diffusely adherent to HEp-2 cells and are usually EAF probe negative (018, 044, 0112, and 0114). There is more evidence that EPEC with localized adherence are true enteropathogens than there is for those with diffuse adherence.

Shigatoxin-Producing *E. coli*. The shigatoxin-producing *E. coli* (STEC) produce one or more toxins that kill mammalian cells. They have also been called enterocytotoxic *E. coli*, *Shiga*-like toxin-producing *E. coli* (SLT-EC), enterohemorrhagic *E. coli* (EHEC), and verotoxin-producing *E. coli* (VTEC). Two major toxins are produced by STEC. One (Stx_1) is essentially identical to shigatoxin, the protein synthesis-inhibiting exotoxin of *Shigella dysenteriae* serotype 1. The second (Stx_2) is more distantly related to shigatoxin, with only 55% amino acid homology. The first toxin has also been called SLT-I or VT-1, and the second SLT-II or VT-2. Numerous variants of Stx_2 probably exist. Some STEC produce only Stx_1 and others only Stx_2, but most STEC produce both toxins. These toxins kill cells by cleaving an adenine residue from ribosomal RNA at the site where elongation factor 1–dependent attachment of aminoacyl tRNA occurs; the result is protein synthesis inhibition and cell death. STEC adhere to intestinal cells and produce attaching-effacing lesions that resemble, on electron microscopy, those seen with EPEC, although they are more restricted in their distribution (being found primarily in the colon) compared with EPEC (which infest the entire intestine). The protein product of the *eae* gene of STEC is closely related but not identical to intimin, the product of the *eae* gene of EPEC, and to invasin, produced by *Yersinia pseudotuberculosis*. The most common serotypes are *E. coli* O157:H7, *E. coli* 0111:NM, and *E. coli* 026:H11, although a number of other STEC serotypes have also been described. Some *E. coli* 026:H11 and *E. coli* 0111:NM strains produce shigatoxin, but others do not. STEC are associated with the hemolytic-uremic syndrome (Chapter 526).

Enteroaggregative *E. coli*. The enteroaggregative *E. coli* (EAggEC) have the ability to adhere to HEp-2 cells in tissue culture. They are also referred to as autoagglutinating and enteroadherent-aggregative *E. coli*. It is likely that this group will be further subdivided, and some of these organisms will be shown to be nonpathogens. EAggEC attach to HEp-2 cells and colonic epithelial cells by plasmid-encoded enteroaggregative adherence fimbriae (AAF/I). These organisms do not possess the *eae* genes or produce attaching-effacing lesions. A heat-stable toxin, EAST 1, related to the heat-stable toxin of ETEC, is encoded on a plasmid. This toxin, originally found only in EAggEC, is now known to be common among *E. coli*. A second toxin is a 120-kd heat-labile protein related to the pore-forming cytolytic toxin family, which contains the *Bordetella pertussis* adenylate cyclase hemolysin. This heat-labile toxin increases intracellular levels of calcium. The role of these toxins in EAggEC pathogenesis is unknown. Virulence is incompletely understood in this group. Some EAggEC belong to serogroups formerly considered to be EPEC.

EPIDEMIOLOGY. In the developing world, the various diarrheogenic serogroups of *E. coli* cause frequent infections in the first few years of life. They occur with increased frequency during the warm months in temperate climates and during rainy season months in tropical climates. Most *E. coli* strains (except STEC and perhaps some EPEC) require a large inoculum of organisms to induce disease; person-to-person spread is atypical, but food-borne or water-borne illness is common. Infection is most likely when food-handling or sewage-disposal practices are suboptimal. Although infection occurs in children in the United States, it is more common in those who live in or have recently visited the developing world. STEC and EPEC organisms are transmitted person to person as well as by food and water, suggesting that ingestion of a lower number of these organisms is sufficient to cause disease. Poorly cooked hamburger is a common cause of food-borne outbreaks of STEC, although other foods including apple cider, lettuce, salami, and unpasteurized dairy products have also been incriminated.

PATHOGENESIS. ETEC cause few or no structural alterations in the gut mucosa. EIEC cause colonic lesions like those of bacillary dysentery; ulcerations, hemorrhage, and infiltration of polymorphonuclear leukocytes with mucosal and submucosal edema are typical. EPEC are associated with blunting of villi, inflammatory changes and sloughing of superficial mucosal cells on light microscopy, and attaching and effacing changes on transmission electron microscopy; these lesions are found from the duodenum through the colon. STEC affect the colon most severely. These organisms cause edema, fibrin deposits, hemorrhage in the submucosa, mucosal ulceration, neutrophil infiltration, and microvascular thrombi. Pseudomembranous colitis may be seen. Some of these effects may result from a synergistic action of shigatoxin and LPS.

CLINICAL MANIFESTATIONS. The clinical features of *E. coli*-associated diarrhea vary in relation to the different mechanisms of disease production.

ETEC are a major cause of dehydrating infantile diarrhea in the developing world. The typical signs and symptoms include explosive watery diarrhea, abdominal pain, nausea, vomiting, and little or no fever. Resolution usually occurs in a matter of days. These infections have an untoward effect on infant nutritional status.

EIEC cause an illness that is indistinguishable from classic bacillary dysentery. Fever, systemic toxicity, crampy abdominal pain, tenesmus, and urgency with watery or bloody diarrhea are characteristic.

EPEC usually are isolated from infants and children who are in the first 2 yr of life and who have a nonbloody diarrhea with mucus; fever may occur. Unlike ETEC, EIEC, or STEC, these organisms often cause a prolonged diarrheal disease, particularly in the 1st yr of life.

STEC may cause a nondescript diarrheal illness or an illness characterized by abdominal pain with diarrhea that is initially watery but within a few days becomes blood-streaked or grossly bloody (hemorrhagic colitis). Although this pattern resembles that of shigellosis or EIEC disease, it differs in that fever is an uncommon manifestation. The major risk with STEC is that approximately 5–8% of symptomatic infections are complicated by development of hemolytic-uremic syndrome.

EAggEC cause significant fluid loss with dehydration, but vomiting and grossly bloody stools are relatively infrequent. These organisms, like the EPEC, are often associated with prolonged diarrhea. Severe colicky pain lasting 2–4 wk is common.

DIAGNOSIS. The clinical features of illness are seldom distinctive enough to allow confident diagnosis, and routine laboratory studies are of very limited value. Diagnosis currently depends heavily on laboratory studies that are not readily available to practitioners. Routine stool cultures from which *E. coli* organisms are isolated are interpreted as showing "normal flora". Biochemical criteria (e.g., fermentation patterns) are of minimal value. STEC serotype O157:H7 is suggested by failure of a suspect colony to ferment sorbitol on MacConkey's sorbitol medium; latex agglutination confirms that the organism contains O157 LPS. The other STEC can be detected in routine hospital laboratories using commercially available enzyme immunoassays or toxin-specific latex agglutination that detect shigatoxins. Culture of duodenal fluid may be helpful in the diagnosis of EPEC because of their tendency to colonize the small intestine. This study is generally indicated only in children with chronic diarrhea.

Other laboratory data are at best nonspecific indicators of etiology. Fecal leukocyte examination of the stool is usually positive with the EIEC but negative with all other diarrheogenic *E. coli*. Blood counts, especially with EIEC and STEC, often show an elevated leukocyte count with a left shift. Electrolyte changes are nonspecific, reflecting only fluid loss.

The traditional methods of identification of these organisms require animal or tissue culture models that are unacceptably cumbersome and expensive for routine use by hospital laboratories. Some of these organisms, especially the EPEC, could theoretically be defined serologically. However, the frequency of cross reactions, the unavailability of suitable reagents, and the infrequency with which the serogroup alone is adequate to define a pathogen make these methods unsuitable. DNA probes for genes encoding the various virulence traits hold the greatest promise for the future; they have been developed for ETEC, EIEC, EPEC, EAggEC, and STEC but are currently available only as a research tool.

Suspected organisms should be forwarded to reference or research laboratories for definitive evaluation. Such efforts are seldom necessary, but they may be critical for correct diagnosis when a child has severe or life-threatening complications or for the occasional outbreak investigation.

TREATMENT. The cornerstone of proper management is related to fluid and electrolyte therapy. In general, this therapy should include oral replacement and maintenance with rehydrating solutions such as those specified by the World Health Organization. Early refeeding (within 8–12 hr of initiation of rehydration) with breast milk or dilute formula should be encouraged. Prolonged withholding of feeding frequently leads to chronic diarrhea and malnutrition.

Specific antimicrobial therapy of diarrheogenic *E. coli* is problematic because of the difficulty of making an accurate diagnosis of these pathogens and the unpredictability of antibiotic susceptibilities. ETEC respond to antimicrobial agents such as trimethoprim-sulfamethoxazole (TMP-SMX) when the *E. coli* strains are susceptible. However, other than for a child recently returning from travel in the developing world, empirical treatment of severe watery diarrhea with antibiotics is seldom appropriate. Although treatment of EPEC infection with TMP-SMX (5–10 mg/kg/24 hr of the trimethoprim component in four divided doses) intravenously or orally for 5 days is effective in speeding resolution, the lack of a rapid diagnostic test makes treatment decisions difficult. EIEC infections are usually treated before the availability of culture results because the clinician typically suspects shigellosis and begins empirical therapy. If the organisms are susceptible, TMP-SMX is an appropriate choice. The STEC represent a particularly difficult therapeutic dilemma. The data suggest that antibiotic treatment, particularly with sulfa-containing regimens, may increase the risk of hemolytic-uremic syndrome (Chapter 526); however, the lack of large prospective controlled trials makes these observations questionable. It is too early to assess the usefulness of antibiotics in the treatment of EAggEC.

Antibiotic resistance is often encoded on the same plasmids that carry virulence properties and continues to make rational decisions about antibiotic therapy difficult. Because emergence of resistance to widely used regimens is typical, new antimicrobial agents must continue to be evaluated.

Prophylactic antibiotic therapy, although effective in adult travelers, has not been studied in children and is not recommended. Public health measures, including sewage disposal and food-handling practices, have made pathogens that require large inoculums to produce illness relatively uncommon in industrialized countries. Food-borne outbreaks of STEC are a problem for which no adequate solution has been found. During the occasional hospital outbreak of EPEC disease, attention to enteric isolation precautions and cohorting may be critical.

COMPLICATIONS. The major complications of diarrheal illness are related to dehydration and electrolyte loss. Some complications are related to specific pathogens. EPEC and EAggEC are likely to cause persistent diarrhea. Infection with STEC is frequently associated with the hemolytic-uremic syndrome (Chapter 526).

PREVENTION. In the developing world, prevention of disease caused by diarrheogenic *E. coli* is probably best done by maintaining prolonged breast-feeding, paying careful attention to personal hygiene, and following proper food- and water-handling procedures. Children traveling to these places can be best protected by paying careful attention to diet, particularly by consuming only processed water, bottled beverages, breads, fruit juices, fruits that can be peeled, or foods that are served steaming hot.

Gomez HF, Cleary TG: *Escherichia coli* as a cause of diarrhea in children. Semin Pediatr Infect Dis 5:175, 1994.

Levine MM: *Escherichia coli* that cause diarrhea: Enterotoxigenic, enteropathogenic, enteroinvasive, enterohemorrhagic, and enteroadherent. J Infect Dis 155:377, 1987.

Parry SM, Salmon RL, Willshaw GA, et al: Risk factors for and prevention of sporadic infections with vero cytotoxin (shiga toxin) producing *Escherichia coli* O157. Lancet 351:1019, 1998.

Robins-Browne R: Traditional enteropathogenic *Escherichia coli* of infantile diarrhea. Rev Infect Dis 9:28, 1987.

Slutsker L, Ries AA, Greene KD, et al: *Escherichia coli* O157:H7 diarrhea in the United States: Clinical and epidemiologic features. Ann Intern Med 126:505, 1997.

Willshaw GA, Scotland SM, Smith HR, et al: Properties of Vero cytotoxin-producing *Escherichia coli* of human origin of O serogroups other than O157. J Infect Dis 166:797, 1992.

CHAPTER 199
Cholera (Vibrio cholerae)

Henry F. Gomez and Thomas G. Cleary

The 1990s heralded dramatic changes in the understanding of cholera. The major developments are the spread of epidemic cholera to the Western Hemisphere, the emergence in India of a new and unique strain of *Vibrio cholerae*, and the discovery of new virulence genes in *V. cholerae*. Cholera is acute watery diarrhea caused by a group of toxins produced by *V. cholerae* serotype O1 or serotype O139 (Bengal). The clinical spectrum includes asymptomatic infection, mild watery diarrhea, and severe watery diarrhea with vomiting that rapidly leads to hypovolemic shock, metabolic acidosis, and death.

ETIOLOGY. *V. cholerae* are gram-negative, non–spore-forming, motile, slightly curved rods (1.5–3.0 × 0.5 μm), each with a polar flagellum. They grow in alkaline media with bile salts. The two biogroups (i.e., biotypes) of *V. cholerae* O1 are classified as classic and El Tor based on hemolysin, hemagglutination, susceptibility to polymyxin B, and susceptibility to bacteriophages. They are also subdivided into serogroups (i.e., serovars) based on the somatic or O antigen. *V. cholerae* O1 has two major O antigenic types (Ogawa and Inaba) and unstable intermediate type (Hikojima). The new epidemic strain, *V. cholerae* O139 (Bengal), does not agglutinate with O1-O138 antisera but is closely related to the El Tor biotype. Since this strain has arisen, it has become clear that *V. cholerae* has continuous reassortment of genes. Non-O1 *V. cholerae* (nonagglutinating *V. cholerae*, or NAG) has long been present in the Gulf States of the United States, but unlike the new O139 strain, the NAG *V. cholerae* is not associated with epidemic cholera.

EPIDEMIOLOGY. *V. cholerae* organisms survive in warm salty water with nutrients and oxygen. They have been found in roots of plants, undercooked shellfish (e.g., shrimp, crabs), and raw bivalves (e.g., clams, oysters, mussels). Direct person-to-person transmission is rare because the inoculum required to cause disease is high. Volunteer studies found that 70–80% of those who ingest 10^6 *V. cholerae* O1 El Tor or *V. cholerae* O139 develop illness. Lower inoculums cause illness less often. In endemic areas, *V. cholerae* O1 primarily affects children 2–15 yr of age whereas *V. cholerae* O139 primarily affects adults. Breast milk may have a role in protecting children from severe cholera during the first 2 yr of life.

In January 1991, epidemic cholera appeared in the Western Hemisphere for the first time in this century. It began on the north coast of Peru and rapidly spread through much of South and Central America. As of 1993, a total of 948,429 cases were reported. Although the number of cases subsequently decreased, epidemic disease re-emerged in 1998. This epidemic has been characterized by rapid spread, high attack rates (300–900 cases/100,000 inhabitants), and low mortality rates. The low case-fatality rate (0.8%) reflects the success of current therapy rather than decreased virulence of the epidemic strain. Mortality rates have been high where medical care has been unavailable. Children and adults have been affected. Several outbreaks of cholera have occurred in the United States as a result of this epidemic.

In 1992, *V. cholerae* strains of a new serotype, *V. cholerae* O139, were isolated during an outbreak in Madras, India. This outbreak represented the first time that epidemic cholera was due to an organism that was not serotype O1. By early 1993, 107,297 cases with 1,473 deaths were reported. Since its emergence in India, this new pathogen has caused epidemics in Bangladesh and Thailand as well as sporadic imported cases in other countries including the United States. Illness due to this pathogen is indistinguishable from typical cholera in its clinical features and potential for epidemic spread. Data suggest that this new strain is hardier than O1 and may therefore pose a greater risk of transmission. The outbreaks are characterized by high frequency of secondary infection, a high ratio of symptomatic to asymptomatic infection, and high attack rates in adults. However, in the 2 yr after emergence of this new strain, O1 El Tor again became the predominant cause of cholera in India.

PATHOGENESIS. Vibrios are very acid sensitive; the stomach is a formidable barrier in preventing these organisms from reaching the small bowel. Vibrios must colonize the small bowel to establish infection and cause disease. They attach to small bowel mucosa and proliferate, to 10^7–10^8 organisms/mL of intestinal fluid. The mucous layer contains factors that are chemotactic for vibrios. The vibrios produce proteolytic enzymes, including mucinase. Motility has also been postulated as an important virulence trait. Colonization of the duodenum and jejunum, followed by enterotoxin-mediated fluid secretion, is responsible for the clinical features. The mucosa is not destroyed during this process, although edema fills the interstitial spaces, and the capillaries and lymphatics in the tips of villi become dilated. A few inflammatory cells are present in the lamina propria. The fluid lost is isotonic with plasma and has high concentrations of bicarbonate and potassium. Although there is some impairment of jejunal disaccharidases, including lactase, glucose absorption is usually preserved.

The fluid losses in cholera result from production of enterotoxins encoded on the bacterial chromosome in a virulence cassette. The most important of these toxins is cholera toxin, a large periplasmic protein whose structural genes (*ctxA* and *ctxB*) encode an enzymatically active A subunit and cell-binding B subunit. Differences in the number of copies of choleratoxin structural genes are strain related. The receptor for subunit B is the ganglioside GM_1. The A1 portion of A subunit is an adenosine diphosphate–ribosyltransferase that activates the α-subunit of the stimulatory G protein to bind and activate adenylate cyclase, resulting in prolonged elevation of cyclic adenosine monophosphate (cAMP) levels. The high cAMP level causes a decrease in active absorption of sodium and chloride by villous cells and an increase in active secretion of chloride by crypt cells.

The role of a second toxin produced by *V. cholerae* is evident from vaccine studies in which genetically engineered strains with a deletion of cholera toxin A subunit still cause diarrhea. This factor alters the intercellular tight junctions by decreasing the strand complexity of the zonula occludens, resulting in fewer strand intersections. The function of intestinal zonula occludens is to restrict or prevent diffusion of water-soluble molecules through the intercellular space back into the lumen. When this function is altered by the zonula occludens toxin *(zot),* the mucosa becomes more permeable, and water and electrolytes leak into the lumen because of hydrostatic pressure and cause diarrhea. This toxin affects only the small intestine.

A third potential enterotoxin (accessory cholera enterotoxin *[ace]*) gene shows striking similarity to eukaryotic ion-transporting adenosine triphosphatases, including the product of the cystic fibrosis transmembrane conductance gene *(CFTR).* The *ctx, zot,* and *ace* genes, along with the pilin genes, flanked by a transposable element called *RS1,* represent a "virulence cassette" of *V. cholerae.* The severity of fluid and electrolyte losses in cholera compared with losses due to other enteropathogens that produce enterotoxins closely related to cholera toxin (e.g., enterotoxigenic *Escherichia coli, Campylobacter, Salmonella*) may be a result of these other toxins in the *V. cholerae* virulence cassette.

The non-O1, non-O139 *V. cholerae* (NAG) produce an enterotoxin unrelated to cholera toxin. This toxin is heat stable and is related to a heat-stable enterotoxin produced by *Yersinia enterocolitica.*

CLINICAL MANIFESTATIONS. Watery diarrhea and vomiting develop after an incubation period of 6 hr–5 days (average, 2–3 days). Low-grade fever occurs in some children. In severe cases, patients have profuse, painless, watery diarrhea having a rice-water consistency with a fishy odor, sometimes with flecks of mucus but no blood. The fluid and electrolyte losses lead to thirst and tachycardia, followed by tachypnea, irritability, a sunken anterior fontanel, and poor skin turgor, and progress to circulatory collapse, stupor, and renal failure if untreated. Diarrhea may be so massive that vascular collapse occurs less than 24 hr after onset. Fluid losses may continue for as long as 1 wk.

DIAGNOSIS. In endemic areas, any child with severe watery diarrhea should be considered to have a possible case of cholera pending laboratory investigations. In the United States, the diagnosis should be suspected in any child with severe watery diarrhea and a history of recent travel to an endemic area.

Two selective media are used for culturing *V. cholerae*: thiosulfate-citrate-bile-sucrose (TCBS) and tellurite-taurocholate-gelatin agar (TTGA). On TCBS, *V. cholerae* organisms stand out as large smooth yellow colonies against the bluish-green background of the medium. On TTGA, the colonies are small and opaque, with a zone of cloudiness around them. Colonies of O139 strains grown in TTGA are described as grayish opaque colonies with dark centers. Biotyping of *V. cholerae* into classic or El Tor can be obtained on the basis of direct hemagglutination with chicken or sheep red blood cells (i.e., El Tor strains agglutinate), sensitivity to polymyxin B (i.e., classic strains are sensitive), or susceptibility to cholera-phage group IV (i.e., classic strains are susceptible). Various enzyme-linked immunosorbent assays for toxin detection and DNA methods (e.g., probes, polymerase chain reaction) are being evaluated as tools for rapid diagnosis. Serologic assays can be used for retrospective detection of vibriocidal, agglutinating, or toxin-neutralizing antibodies 7–14 days after the onset of illness.

TREATMENT. The mainstay of treatment for cholera is fluid and electrolyte replacement (Chapter 55.1). Per liter, the World Health Organization Oral Rehydration Solution (WHO-ORS) contains 90 mmol of Na^+, 20 mmol of K^+, 80 mmol of Cl^-, 111 mmol of glucose, and 30 mmol of bicarbonate (citrate can be substituted for bicarbonate). Although rice-based ORS may be superior to WHO-ORS, it presents more logistical problems because it requires boiling rice flour (50 g/L boiled for 7 min) before adding the salts and because it should be discarded and prepared fresh every 8 hr. Oral rehydration given ad libitum is the treatment of choice, unless the child is obtunded, has an ileus, or is in shock; in these cases, intravenous saline or lactated Ringer's solution rather than oral rehydration is appropriate. Vomiting is not a contraindication to oral rehydration. Although all patients with cholera should be carefully monitored, attention to intake and output is especially important in infants who can take orally only those fluids that are offered. Food should be restarted as soon as deficits are replaced to minimize the nutritional impact of the illness; refeeding does not affect purging rates or the duration of diarrhea. The success of oral rehydration was well demonstrated when epidemic cholera arrived in Peru in 1991; the mortality rate was less than 1% despite the fact that this massive outbreak was totally unanticipated.

Antibiotics represent therapy of secondary importance, although they are useful in shortening the duration of illness due to either 01 or 0139 strains. Antibiotic resistance is common. Asian strains are often resistant to trimethoprim-sulfamethoxazole (TMP-SMX). Doxycycline is preferable to tetracycline for Asian strains because 01 strains (but not 0139 strains) are often resistant. South American isolates tend to be more susceptible to numerous antibiotics. Some African isolates (from Uganda) have been reported to be resistant to TMP-SMX, tetracycline, chloramphenicol, ampicillin, and streptomycin. The antimicrobial regimens used are TMP-SMX (10 mg/kg/24 hr of trimethoprim and 50 mg/kg/24 hr of sulfamethoxazole as two divided doses for 3 days) or, in older children, tetracycline (50 mg/kg/24 hr divided in four doses for 2–3 days) or doxycycline (6 mg/kg, 300 mg maximum) as a single dose. Adults are better treated with a quinolone such as ciprofloxacin.

COMPLICATIONS. Lethargy, seizures, altered consciousness, fever, hypoglycemia, hyperglycemia, and death occur more frequently in children than adults. Inadequate fluid and electrolyte replacement may lead to acute tubular necrosis. In severely ill children with potassium depletion and acidosis, hypokalemic arrhythmia can cause sudden death. Children with low potassium levels can develop paralytic ileus and abdominal distention that may make oral rehydration impossible. In as many as 10% of small children, prolonged drowsiness, coma, or seizures occur. When the seizures are associated with hypoglycemia, they are often followed by coma and death; 14.3% of children with cholera complicated by hypoglycemia died, compared with 0.7% of children without hypoglycemia. Hyperglycemia can be caused by secretion of epinephrine, norepinephrine, cortisol, glucagon, and C peptide in response to the stress of hypovolemia. Pulmonary edema occurs in some children, probably because of fluid overload during rehydration. Transient tetany may occur during correction of electrolyte imbalances. In children treated with excessive sugar and salt, hypernatremia can be observed. Despite its high sodium content, WHO-ORS is not associated with hypernatremia if used properly; it can be used to treat children with hypernatremic dehydration.

PREVENTION. The most practical method of preventing life-threatening cholera in infants is prolonged breast-feeding. Safe food and water and proper handling of sewage are the long-term solutions to the problem. Cost, ignorance, and politics have kept these basic needs from being met, and for the immediate future, development of an improved vaccine is a high priority.

Vaccine. The currently available vaccine uses killed organisms administered parenterally as a two-dose primary series followed by boosters every 6 mo. This vaccine has about 50% efficacy by 3–6 mo after vaccination. Because of its low efficacy and high frequency of reactions (i.e., pain, erythema, local induration, fever, headaches), this vaccine should be used only in very high-risk hosts (e.g., those with achlorhydria) with a very high probability of exposure. It is not recommended for children younger than 6 mo.

No country or territory currently requires cholera vaccination as a condition for entry. Local authorities, however, may continue to require documentation of cholera vaccination; in such cases, a single dose of vaccine is sufficient to satisfy local requirements. Travelers to cholera-infected areas should take appropriate food precautions (Chapter 304). Persons who follow the usual tourist itinerary and who use standard accommodations in countries reporting cholera are at virtually no risk of infection.

Vibriocidal antibodies (directed primarily to lipopolysaccharide), rather than anti-cholera toxin antibodies, appear to be of primary importance in protection from severe disease. This fact, coupled with the experience with *V. cholerae* O139 (Bengal), in which adults in cholera-endemic areas have developed severe cholera, suggests that current vaccines are unlikely to be effective against this new epidemic strain.

Bhattacharya SK, Bhattacharya MK, Balakrish-Nair G, et al: Clinical profile of acute diarrhoea cases infected with the new epidemic strain of *Vibrio cholerae* O139: Designation of the disease as cholera. J Infect 27:11, 1993.

Calia KE, Murtagh M, Ferraro MJ, et al: Comparison of *Vibrio cholerae* O139 with *V. cholerae* O1 classical and El Tor biotypes. Infect Immun 62:1504, 1994.

Fasano A, Baudry B, Pumplin DW, et al: *Vibrio cholerae* produces a second enterotoxin, which affects intestinal tight junctions. Proc Natl Acad Sci U S A 88:5242, 1991.

Swerdlow DL, Ries AA: Cholera in the Americas. JAMA 267:1495, 1992.

Trucksis M, Galen JE, Michalski J, et al: Accessory cholera enterotoxin (Ace), the third toxin of a *Vibrio cholerae* virulence cassette. Proc Natl Acad Sci U S A 90:5267, 1993.

World Health Organization: WHO Guidelines for Cholera Control. Geneva, World Health Organization, 1993.

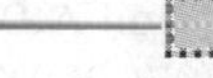

CHAPTER 200
Campylobacter

Gloria P. Heresi, James R. Murphy, and Thomas G. Cleary

The genus *Campylobacter* (meaning a curved rod) includes 18 species. Those known or considered pathogenic for humans include *C. jejuni, C. fetus, C. coli, C. hyointestinalis, C. lari, C. upsaliensis, C. concisus, C. sputorum, C. rectus, C. mucosalis, C. jejuni* subspecies *doylei, C. curvus, C. gracilis,* and *C. cryaerophila.* Additional *Campylobacter* spp have been isolated from clinical specimens, but their roles as pathogens have not been proved. More than 90 serotypes of *C. jejuni* have been identified. The organisms previously classified as *C. pylori, C. fennelliae,* and *C. cinaedi* are now classified as *Helicobacter pylori* (Chapter 336), *H. fennelliae,* and *H. cinaedi,* respectively.

ETIOLOGY. *Campylobacter* organisms are thin, curved, gram-negative non–spore-forming rods that usually have tapered ends; they can be short and S shaped or long, multispiraled, and filamentous. In older cultures, coccal forms may be seen. The organisms are motile, with a flagellum at one or both poles and form small (0.5–1 mm), slightly raised, smooth colonies on solid media. Visible growth in blood culture is often not apparent until 5–14 days after inoculation. Most *Campylobacter* organisms are microaerophilic. They neither oxidize nor ferment carbohydrates. Selective culture media developed to enhance isolation of *C. jejuni* may not support the growth of other *Campylobacter* species and may even inhibit it.

Clinical presentations associated with *Campylobacter* differ, in part, by species (Table 200–1). Intestinal disease is usually associated with *C. jejuni* and *C. coli,* and extraintestinal and systemic infections are usually associated with *C. fetus.* However, *C. jejuni* septicemia is increasingly recognized; this at times occurs without signs. Less frequently, enteritis is recognized in association with isolation of *C. lari, C. fetus,* and other species.

EPIDEMIOLOGY. Human campylobacterioses most commonly result from ingestion of contaminated food or water, from direct acquisition from other environmental sources (i.e., a pet), or from person-to-person transmission.

Campylobacter organisms are global in distribution and are ubiquitous in the environment. Although chickens are the classic source of *Campylobacter,* essentially all animal sources of food for humans have been shown to harbor or can harbor *Campylobacter*; oysters and mussels have recently been shown to harbor organisms. Additionally, many animals kept as human pets can carry *Campylobacter.* Puppies with diarrhea have been associated with human illness. Beetles and flies that frequent chicken farms may harbor *C. jejuni.* Direct or indirect exposure to this plethora of environmental sources is thought to be the primary route by which humans get infection.

Direct transmission of *Campylobacter* between humans is possible. The classic enteric *C. jejuni* and *C. coli* may spread person to person perinatally and where diapered toddlers are present. Individuals infected with *C. jejuni* usually shed the organism for weeks but may shed for months. The minimum human infectious dose for *C. jejuni* is as low as a few hundred colony-forming units in some volunteers; however, very large inoculums fail to make some individuals sick. The infectious dose for other species is unknown.

PATHOGENESIS. Widely disparate pathology results from infections with *Campylobacter.* Evidence from the well-studied species *C. jejuni* suggests that most infections (colonizations) do not cause symptoms. The frequency of asymptomatic infections with other *Campylobacter* species is less well known.

When pathology follows *Campylobacter* colonization, the pathology generally reflects the site at which the bacteria localize, whether or not septicemia occurs and whether immunoreactive complications are triggered. Species of *Campylobacter* differ markedly in preferred sites of colonization and in propensity to cause bacteremia.

The spectrum of *C. jejuni* infection includes fever, watery diarrhea, invasive enteritis, and systemic infection. Acute watery diarrhea may occur without grossly visible pathology. Acute inflammation of the colon and rectum is the hallmark of *C. jejuni* invasive enteritis, although hemorrhagic jejunitis and ileitis may occur. In those patients who have undergone proctoscopy, a normal mucosa is found in approximately 50%; in the rest, mucosal edema, congestion, friability, and granularity are seen. The spectrum of histologic change ranges from edema with acute and chronic inflammatory cells without vascular congestion to moderate inflammation, cryptitis, and crypt abscess formation. Acute appendicitis, mesenteric lymphadenitis, and ileocolitis have been reported in patients who have had appendectomies during *C. jejuni* infection. The pathology associated with less-studied *C. coli* appears similar to that with *C. jejuni.*

C. fetus shows a predilection for systemic infection. The organism preferentially associates with endovascular surfaces in adults and the central nervous system in neonates. At sites of colonization, inflammation, microabscesses, necrosis, and disruption of blood flow are pathologic hallmarks. *C. fetus* has affinity for pregnant hosts and may infect an infant hematogenously or by ascending infection during amnionitis and premature rupture of membranes. In either case, the consequences for a fetus may be severe.

TABLE 200–1 *Campylobacter* **Species Associated with Human Disease**

Species	Clinical Illnesses in Humans	Common Sources
C. jejuni	Gastroenteritis, bacteremia	Poultry, raw milk, cats, dogs, cattle, swine, monkeys, water
C. coli	Gastroenteritis, bacteremia	Poultry, raw milk, cats, dogs, cattle, swine, monkeys, oysters, water
C. fetus	Bacteremia, meningitis, endocarditis, mycotic aneurysm, diarrhea, relapsing fevers, abortions	Sheep, cattle, birds
C. hyointestinalis	Diarrhea, bacteremia, proctitis	Swine, cattle, deer, raw milk, oysters
C. lari	Diarrhea, colitis, appendicitis, bacteremia, urinary tract infection	Seagulls, water, poultry, cattle, oysters, mussels
C. upsaliensis	Diarrhea, bacteremia, abscesses, enteritis, colitis, hemolytic-uremic syndrome, abortion	Cats, other domestic pets
C. concisus	Diarrhea, gastritis, enteritis, periodontitis	
C. sputorum	Diarrhea, bedsores, abscesses, periodontitis	Swine
C. rectus	Periodontitis	
C. mucosalis	Enteritis	Swine
C. jejuni subspecies *doylei*	Diarrhea, gastritis, bacteremia	
C. curvus	Gingivitis	
C. gracilis	Abscesses (head and neck, abdominal, empyema)	
C. cryaerophila	Diarrhea	Swine

C. upsaliensis, C. lari, C. hyointestinalis, and *C. jejuni* subspecies *doylei* cause diarrhea and bacteremia and may cause abscesses, colitis, and appendicitis similar to that caused by *C. jejuni. C. sputorum* is known primarily as a cause of abscesses of the lungs, perianal region, groin, and axilla. *C. rectus, C. curvus,* and *C. concisus* have been associated with periodontitis, osteomyelitis, and diarrhea, but definitive proof that these organisms are pathogens for immunologically intact humans is lacking.

C. jejuni and possibly other *Campylobacter* spp can trigger damaging host responses. *Campylobacter*-associated Guillain-Barré syndrome is characterized by wallerian-like neural degeneration. Similar pathology has been induced in a chicken model by feeding *Campylobacter* isolated from patients with Guillain-Barré.

Some studies suggest that in vitro invasion of cultured cells corresponds to isolates from patients with colitis, but others have failed to show relationships between in vitro invasion and clinical disease.

A cholera-like enterotoxin that has been described can be detected with ganglioside GM_1-based enzyme-linked immunosorbent assay (ELISA) causes fluid accumulation in intestinal loop assays and fluid secretion into intestines in an animal model.

Campylobacter exhibits various cytotoxic activities (including cytolethal distending toxin, shiga-like toxin, and hemolysin). Because the inflammatory pathology in some *Campylobacter* infections is consistent with cytotoxins, a role for these in human disease is postulated. As with the enterotoxin, direct evidence of a role for cytotoxins in human disease is not available.

C. fetus possesses a high molecular weight S-layer protein that endows this species with high-level resistance to serum-mediated killing and phagocytosis and is thus thought to be responsible for its propensity to bacteremia. *C. jejuni* and *C. coli* isolates are mostly sensitive to serum-mediated killing, but variants of greater resistance exist, and it has been suggested that these serum-killing–resistant variants may be more capable of systemic dissemination.

A strong association between Guillain-Barré syndrome and preceding infection with some serotypes of *C. jejuni* is noted. The core oligosaccharides of the lipopolysaccharide (LPS) of the neuropathic serotypes contain tetrasaccharides or pertasaccharides identical with those of several gangliosides including GM_1, GD_{1a}, and GQ_{1b}. Molecular mimicry between nerve tissue and this group of infectious agents may be the triggering factor in *Campylobacter*-associated Guillain-Barré syndrome and Miller-Fisher syndrome, a variant of Guillain-Barré syndrome characterized by ataxia, areflexia, and ophthalmoplegia.

CLINICAL MANIFESTATIONS. Several clinical presentations of *Campylobacter* infections are possible, depending on the species involved and host factors, such as age, immunocompetence, and underlying conditions.

Acute Gastroenteritis. Diarrhea is usually caused by *C. jejuni* (90–95%) or *C. coli* and rarely by *C. lari, C. hyointestinalis,* and *C. upsaliensis.* The incubation period is 1–7 days. Patients may have loose, watery stools or bloody and mucus-containing stools (dysentery). Blood appears in the stools 2–4 days after the onset of symptoms. Fever, vomiting, malaise, and myalgia are common. Fever may be the only initial manifestation, but 60–90% of older children also complain of abdominal pain. The abdominal pain is periumbilical; cramping may precede other symptoms or persist after the stools return to normal. Abdominal pain may mimic appendicitis or intussusception.

Mild infection lasts only 1–2 days and resembles viral gastroenteritis. Most patients recover in less than 1 wk, although 20–30% remain ill for 2 wk and 5–10% longer. Persistent or recurrent *Campylobacter* gastroenteritis and emergence of erythromycin resistance during therapy have been reported both in normal hosts and in patients with hypogammaglobulinemia (congenital or acquired) and AIDS. Persistent infection may mimic chronic inflammatory bowel disease. Fecal shedding of the organisms in untreated patients usually lasts for 2–3 wk. The range may be from a few days to several months. Young children tend to shed the organisms for longer periods.

Bacteremia. Bacteremia occurs in malnourished children, in patients with chronic illnesses, in those with immunodeficiency, and at the extremes of age. *C. fetus* may cause bacteremia in adults with or without identifiable focal infection. Most have underlying conditions such as malignancy or diabetes mellitus. Bacteremia, when symptomatic, is associated with fever, headache, and malaise. Relapsing or intermittent fever is associated with night sweats, chills, and weight loss when the illness is prolonged. Lethargy and confusion can occur, but focal neurologic signs are unusual without cerebrovascular disease or meningitis. Abdominal pain is frequent; diarrhea, jaundice, and hepatomegaly are less common. A cough may occur, but pulmonary parenchymal involvement is unusual. Results of the physical examination are unimpressive except for the ill appearance of the patient. Moderate leukocytosis may be found. Both transient asymptomatic bacteremia and rapidly fatal septicemia have been described. A prolonged bacteremia of 8–13 wk has been described, with spontaneous remissions and relapses, especially in immunocompromised hosts. Occasional reports describe bacteremia with *C. upsaliensis.*

Focal Extraintestinal Infections. Focal infections caused by *C. jejuni* occur mainly in neonates or immunocompromised patients. These include meningitis, pancreatitis, cholecystitis, ileocecitis with right lower quadrant pain mimicking appendicitis, urinary tract infection, arthritis, and peritonitis. *C. fetus* shows a predilection for vascular endothelium, causing endocarditis, pericarditis, thrombophlebitis, and mycotic aneurysms; focal infections include meningitis, septic arthritis, osteomyelitis, urinary tract infections, lung abscess, and cholangitis. *C. hyointestinalis* has been associated with proctitis, *C. upsaliensis* with breast abscesses, and *C. rectus* with periodontitis.

Perinatal Infections. Severe perinatal infections, although uncommon, are usually caused by *C. fetus* and, rarely, by *C. jejuni.* Maternal *C. fetus* and *C. jejuni* infections, which may be asymptomatic, may result in abortion, stillbirth, premature delivery, or neonatal infection with sepsis and meningitis. Newborn infection with *C. jejuni* is associated with diarrhea that may be bloody; *C. fetus* rarely causes diarrhea.

DIAGNOSIS. The clinical presentation of *Campylobacter* enteritis is similar to that of enteritis caused by other bacterial enteropathogens. Differential diagnosis should include *Shigella, Salmonella,* invasive *Escherichia coli, E. coli* O157:H7, *Yersinia enterocolitica, Aeromonas, Vibrio parahaemolyticus,* and amebiasis. Fecal leukocytes are found in as many as 75% of cases and fecal blood in 50%.

The diagnosis of *Campylobacter* is usually confirmed by identification of the organism in culture. Selective media, such as Skirrow's or Butzler's, and microaerophilic conditions (5–10% oxygen) are commonly used. Some *C. jejuni* grow best at 42°C. Filtration methods are available and can preferentially enrich for *Campylobacter* by selecting for their smaller size. These methods allow for subsequent culture of the enriched sample on antibiotic free media. This enhances rates of isolation of those *Campylobacter* inhibited by the antibiotics included in standard selective media.

For rapid diagnosis of *Campylobacter* enteritis, direct carbolfuchsin stain of fecal smear, indirect fluorescence antibody test, darkfield microscopy, or latex agglutination can be used, but the sensitivity of these methods is generally low. Species-specific DNA probes and specific gene amplification by polymerase chain reaction have been described, although clinical experience is limited. Serologic diagnoses may be made with enzyme-linked immunoassays to measure the antibody (IgG, IgM, IgA) levels to *C. jejuni.*

TREATMENT. Fluid replacement, correction of electrolyte imbalance, and supportive care are the mainstays of treatment of children with *Campylobacter* gastroenteritis. Antimotility agents may cause prolonged or fatal disease and should not be used.

The need for antibiotic therapy in patients with uncomplicated gastroenteritis is controversial. Some data suggest a shortened duration of symptoms and intestinal shedding if erythromycin ethylsuccinate suspension is initiated early in the disease in patients with the dysenteric form of *Campylobacter* enteritis.

Most *Campylobacter* are susceptible to macrolides, quinolones, aminoglycosides, chloramphenicol, tetracycline, and clindamycin and resistant to cephalosporins, rifampin, penicillin, trimethoprim, and vancomycin. Quinolone resistance developing after initiation of therapy has been reported. The new macrolides clarithromycin and azithromycin show good in vitro activity, but clinical evaluation is limited. Antibiotics are recommended for patients with the dysenteric form of the disease, high fever, or a severe course and for children who are immunosuppressed or have underlying diseases.

Extraintestinal infection caused by *Campylobacter* requires parenteral antibiotic therapy with an aminoglycoside. In patients with *C. fetus* bacteremia, prolonged therapy is advised. *C. fetus* isolates resistant to erythromycin have been reported.

COMPLICATIONS. Severe, prolonged *C. jejuni* infection can occur in patients with immunodeficiencies including hypogammaglobulinemia and malnutrition. In patients with AIDS, an increased frequency and severity of *C. jejuni* infection have been reported; severity correlates inversely with CD4 count.

Reactive Arthritis. Reactive arthritis may accompany *Campylobacter* enteritis in adolescents and adults, especially those who are positive for HLA-B27. It appears 5–40 days after the onset of diarrhea, involves mainly large joints, and resolves in 1–21 wk without any sequelae. The arthritis typically is migratory, but the child is afebrile. Synovial fluid is always sterile. Reiter's syndrome (i.e., reactive arthritis with conjunctivitis, urethritis, and rash) and erythema nodosum are less common. IgA nephropathy and immune complex glomerulonephritis with *C. jejuni* antigens in the kidneys have been reported. Other complications are hemolytic anemia and rectal bleeding.

Guillain-Barré Syndrome. Guillain-Barré syndrome has been reported 1–12 wk after culture-proven *C. jejuni* gastroenteritis. Stool cultures obtained from patients with Guillain-Barré syndrome at the onset of neurologic symptoms have yielded *C. jejuni* in more than 25% of the cases. Serologic studies suggest that 20–45% of patients with Guillain-Barré syndrome have evidence of recent *C. jejuni* infection. The management of Guillain-Barré syndrome includes supportive care, plasma exchange, and intravenous immunoglobulin (Chapter 623).

PROGNOSIS. Although *Campylobacter* gastroenteritis is usually self-limited, immunosuppressed children, including those with AIDS, may experience a protracted or a severe course. Septicemia in newborns and immunocompromised hosts has a poor prognosis, with an estimated mortality rate of 30–40%.

PREVENTION. Most human campylobacterioses are acquired indirectly or directly from infected animals. Interventions to minimize transmission include preparing food under conditions that kill *Campylobacter* and that prevent recontamination after cooking (not using the same surfaces, utensils, or containers for both uncooked and cooked food), ensuring that water sources are not contaminated and that water is kept in clean containers, and taking steps to prevent direct transmission from infected persons or infected domestic pets. Breast-feeding appears to decrease symptomatic *Campylobacter* disease but does not reduce colonization.

Several approaches at immunization are being studied, including the use of live-attenuated organisms, subunit vaccines, and killed whole-cell vaccines. A candidate whole-cell vaccine in combination with an oral adjuvant is currently in clinical trials.

Allos BM: Association between *Campylobacter* infection and Guillain-Barré syndrome. J Infect Dis 176:S125, 1997.

Allos BM, Blaser MJ: *Campylobacter jejuni* and the expanding spectrum of related infections. Clin Infect Dis 20:1092, 1995.

Ketley JM: Pathogenesis of enteric infection by *Campylobacter.* Microbiology 143:5, 1997.

Mishu B, Blaser MJ: Role of infection due to *Campylobacter jejuni* in the initiation of Guillain-Barré syndrome. Infect Dis 17:104, 1993.

Reina J, Borrell N, Serra A: Emergence of resistance to erythromycin and fluoroquinolones in thermotolerant *Campylobacter* strains isolated from feces, 1987–1991. Eur J Clin Microbiol Infect Dis 11:1163, 1992.

Ruiz-Palacios GM, Calva JJ, Pickering LK, et al: Protection of breast-fed infants against *Campylobacter* diarrhea by antibodies in human milk. J Pediatr 116:707, 1990.

Yuki N, Taki T, Inagaki F, et al: A bacterium lipopolysaccharide that elicits Guillain-Barré syndrome has a GM_1 ganglioside-like structure. J Exp Med 178:1771, 1993.

CHAPTER 201
Yersinia

Thomas G. Cleary

Yersinia infections are enzootic in many animal species, including birds, rodents, and wild and domestic mammals. The genus *Yersinia* has many named species, but only three species are known to be regularly transmitted to humans: *Yersinia enterocolitica, Y. pseudotuberculosis,* and *Y. pestis.* Infections due to *Y. enterocolitica* far outnumber infections due to *Y. pseudotuberculosis* and *Y. pestis.* Domestic animals, especially swine, and household pets, such as cats and dogs, are major reservoirs for *Y. enterocolitica* and *Y. pseudotuberculosis. Y. pestis* is endemic in wild rodents in the western United States and in many other areas of the world. Humans are accidental hosts for *Y. enterocolitica* and *Y. pseudotuberculosis* and are usually infected by handling contaminated animal tissues or ingesting contaminated meat, water, or milk. *Y. pestis* is transmitted to humans from infected rodents by flea bites.

The genus *Yersinia* was transferred from the family Pasteurellaceae to the family Enterobacteriaceae on the basis of DNA hybridization studies and the presence of the enterobacterial common antigen. They resemble "atypical" coliforms morphologically and biochemically.

201.1 Yersinia enterocolitica

ETIOLOGY. *Y. enterocolitica* organisms are oxidase-negative, non-lactose-fermenting, gram-negative bacilli that are motile at 22°C but not at 37°C. Strains resembling *Y. enterocolitica* are isolated from extraintestinal infections and stool from asymptomatic patients or patients with mild gastroenteritis. These strains are considered to be nonenteropathogenic in that they lack the genes required for invasion and have now been assigned to a new species.

EPIDEMIOLOGY. Animals, food, and water are the major reservoirs for *Y. enterocolitica.* Many animal species harbor *Yersinia,* but swine, cattle, goats, dogs, and cats are more commonly involved. *Y. enterocolitica* has been isolated or detected by the polymerase chain reaction in commercial meat products, especially chitterlings and other pork products. Infections occur primarily in children and young adults, with most occurring in children younger than 7 yr. Infecting serogroups show variable geographic distributions, with O:3, O:5, 27, O:8, and O:9 strains predominant. Disease is more common in the colder months and in males than females. Common-source outbreaks due to contaminated food or water are reported, with incubation periods ranging from 1–11 days. Institutional and hospital spread, including neonatal transmission from a symptomatic mother and transfusion-related disease from red blood cell–containing products, are reported. Extraintestinal infections due to *Y. enterocolitica* are rare.

PATHOGENESIS. *Y. enterocolitica* pathogenesis is multifactorial, involving chromosomal and plasmid genes. All strains pathogenic for humans carry a related virulence plasmid that encodes several calcium- and thermally regulated virulence factors. The essential mechanisms involved in pathogenesis appear to be adherence, toxin production, and invasion. Pathologic changes include a superficial ulcerative ileocolitis with mesenteric lymphadenitis, lymphoid hyperplasia, and abscesses of Peyer's patches. The appendix usually is normal or minimally inflamed.

Several features of the organism are important for transfusion-acquired disease. First, pathogenic strains require iron and survive best in red blood cell–containing products. The role of iron is supported by reports of septicemia in patients with hemochromatosis, thalassemia, and sickle cell anemia and after accidental overdose of oral iron in previously healthy children. The organism can use iron bound to deferoxamine; thus, sepsis may also occur during chelation therapy of iron overload. Second, the risk of transfusion-associated disease increases with blood stored for more than 2 wk. *Y. enterocolitica* grows better than other common bacteria at 4°C, and release of organisms from the phagocytic cell fraction in aging units allows the organism to proliferate under normal storage conditions. This cold-enhanced growth is useful for isolating the organism from mixed sources, such as stool, but increases the bacterial load in stored meat products and blood products.

CLINICAL MANIFESTATIONS. Disease is usually manifested in younger children as an acute enteritis. The most common presenting signs and symptoms are fever (40–50%), occasionally to 40°C, abdominal pain (20–80%) that is usually colicky and sometimes localized to the right lower quadrant, and diarrhea (80–95%). Stools may be mucoid and bloody or, less commonly, watery, usually with fecal leukocytes. Illness may be as short as 2 days or may persist for 3–4 wk. It is usually self-limited in older children, but bacteremia develops in 20–30% of infants 3 mo of age or younger. Fever occurs in 40–50% of cases, abdominal pain in 20–80%, and diarrhea in 80–95%. Older children may present with mesenteric lymphadenitis with fever, right lower quadrant pain, and abdominal tenderness, which may mimic appendicitis (pseudoappendicitis). Asymptomatic infections are frequently detected in family contacts.

DIAGNOSIS. The history may suggest enterocolitis due to *Y. enterocolitica* based on contact with animals or ingestion of uncooked meat products, especially pork. Direct examination of diarrheal stool for fecal leukocytes is helpful in establishing that an invasive pathogen is present. Culture is the most useful diagnostic test. Because many laboratories do not routinely culture for *Yersinia,* it is important to notify the laboratory of suspected cases. *Yersinia*-selective agar (cefsulodin-irgasan-novobiocin [CIN agar]) is inoculated with stool and incubated at reduced temperatures of 25°C or 32°C. Some laboratories use cold enrichment methods and subculture material held at 4°C for as long as 3–4 wk. Isolations from nonstool sources and sterile body fluids may be made on routine media. Speciation from nonenteric sources is important. Pathogenic stool strains of *Y. enterocolitica* can be differentiated from nonpathogenic strains using Congo red–magnesium oxalate agar, the pyrazinamidase test, salicin fermentation, and esculin hydrolysis.

Serotyping of isolates and serodiagnosis in culture-negative cases is of value for epidemiologic purposes only.

Differential Diagnosis. Enterocolitis due to *Y. enterocolitica* is similar in clinical presentation to invasive diarrheal disease due to other enteric pathogens, such as *Shigella, Salmonella* spp, *Campylobacter* spp, *C. difficile,* or enteroinvasive *Escherichia coli* or inflammatory bowel disease. The pseudoappendicitis syndrome can also be caused by *Y. pseudotuberculosis.*

TREATMENT. Uncomplicated enterocolitis due to *Y. enterocolitica* is a self-limited disease, and the benefit of antimicrobial therapy has not been established. Patients with culture-proven septicemia at any age and patients 3 mo of age or younger who have a high rate of septicemia should be treated. In one retrospective study, aminoglycosides in combination with third-generation cephalosporins, quinolones, or other agents, such as rifampin and trimethoprim-sulfamethoxazole, were effective, whereas other β-lactams, such as amoxicillin with or without clavulanate, benzylpenicillin, erythromycin, and clindamycin were associated with treatment failures.

COMPLICATIONS. Complications are uncommon in children. The most frequent complication, reactive arthritis, usually occurs in older children, affecting one to four joints of the extremities. Intact organisms are not detected in synovial specimens known to contain bacterial antigen. This observation suggests that only stable degradation products or immune complexes trapped from the circulation are associated with *Yersinia*-triggered reactive arthritis. Resolution usually occurs in a few weeks. Erythema nodosum, erythema multiforme, hemolytic anemia, thrombocytopenia, and bacteremic spread to other sites with meningitis, hepatic abscess, and pneumonia all have been reported.

PREVENTION. Infection is preventable by careful attention to the preparation of meat, especially the slaughter of swine, and by avoiding ingestion of uncooked meat, precooked pork products held at 4°C, potable water of questionable purity, and unpasteurized milk or milk products made from unpasteurized milk. Vaccines are not available.

201.2 Yersinia pseudotuberculosis

Infection due to *Y. pseudotuberculosis* is most often found as a pseudoappendicitis syndrome without diarrhea. It also causes a Kawasaki's syndrome–like illness and occasionally septicemia.

ETIOLOGY. *Y. pseudotuberculosis* is differentiated biochemically from *Y. enterocolitica* on the basis of ornithine decarboxylase activity, fermentation of sucrose, sorbitol, cellobiose, and other tests, although some overlap between species may be noted. Antisera to somatic O antigens and sensitivity to *Yersinia* phages may also be used to differentiate the two species. Subspecies-specific DNA sequences that allow direct probe- and primer-specific differentiation of *Y. pestis, Y. pseudotuberculosis,* and *Y. enterocolitica* have been described. *Y. pseudotuberculosis* is more closely related to *Y. pestis* than to *Y. enterocolitica.*

EPIDEMIOLOGY. Less is known of the epidemiology of *Y. pseudotuberculosis* infections than for *Y. enterocolitica* or *Y. pestis.* The seasonal incidence in humans parallels that in wild and domestic animals. Transmission from cats and cat-contaminated substances is established. Consumption of contaminated water is sometimes the source of infection.

PATHOGENESIS. The pathology is similar to that described for *Y. enterocolitica,* with ileal and colonic mucosal ulceration and mesenteric lymphadenitis. Necrotizing epithelioid granulomas are seen in the mesenteric nodes. The appendix is frequently grossly and microscopically normal. Mesenteric nodes are frequently the only source of positive culture results. *Y. pseudotuberculosis* antigens bind directly to HLA class II molecules and function as superantigens, which may partly explain the clinical illness resembling Kawasaki's syndrome caused by this organism.

CLINICAL MANIFESTATIONS. Children usually present with fever and abdominal pain that is diffuse or localized to the right lower quadrant. Tenderness is frequently elicited over the McBurney's point, and appendicitis is strongly suspected on a clinical basis. At surgery, the terminal ileum is thickened and shiny with enlarged mesenteric lymph nodes, which may appear necrotic. The appendix is normal or only mildly inflamed.

Enterocolitis is uncommon. Fever, strawberry tongue, pharyngeal erythema, a scarletiniform rash, cracked red swollen lips, conjunctivitis, sterile pyuria, periungual desquamation, and thrombocytosis may mimic Kawasaki's syndrome. Coronary aneurysms have been described in *Y. pseudotuberculosis* infection. Septicemia may occur in iron overload states just as with *Y. enterocolitica.* Renal involvement is distinctive; azotemia, pyuria, and glucosuria occur, sometimes with oliguria. Renal biopsy specimens show tubulointerstitial nephritis. Recovery occurs within 1 mo.

DIAGNOSIS. Mesenteric lymphadenitis should be suspected in children with unexplained fever and abdominal pain. A characteristic picture of enlarged mesenteric lymph nodes, thickening of the terminal ileum, and no image of the appendix may appear on ultrasonography. *Y. pseudotuberculosis* is rarely isolated. It is almost never isolated from stools, and the best source is an involved mesenteric node. Culture conditions are the same as for *Y. enterocolitica.*

Tubulointerstitial nephritis can be suspected when ultrasound examination of the kidneys shows them to be enlarged and to have cortical hyperechogenicity.

Differential Diagnosis. Appendicitis is the most common diagnostic consideration. Inflammatory bowel disease and other intra-abdominal infections are also considered. Kawasaki syndrome, staphylococcal or streptococcal disease, leptospirosis, Stevens-Johnson syndrome, and collagen vascular diseases including acute-onset juvenile rheumatoid arthritis can mimic the syndrome with prolonged fever and rash.

TREATMENT. Uncomplicated mesenteric lymphadenitis due to *Y. pseudotuberculosis* is a self-limited disease, and antimicrobial therapy is not required. Culture-confirmed bacteremia should be treated with an aminoglycoside, ampicillin, chloramphenicol, or a third-generation cephalosporin.

PREVENTION. Specific preventive measures other than avoiding exposure to potentially infected animals and careful food-handling practices are not apparent. Vaccines for prevention of *Y. pseudotuberculosis* have not been developed.

201.3 Yersinia pestis

ETIOLOGY. *Y. pestis* was first described by Yersin in 1894. Based on DNA hybridization analysis, *Y. pestis* and *Y. pseudotuberculosis* are subspecies of the same species. *Y. pestis* shares with *Y. pseudotuberculosis* characteristic bipolar (safety pin) staining but is differentiated from *Y. pseudotuberculosis* by biochemical reactions, serology, and susceptibility to selected *Yersinia* phage.

EPIDEMIOLOGY. The first pandemic of plague (Black Death) was described in 541 A.D. Subsequent pandemics through the Middle Ages devastated portions of Europe, with losses of 30–50% of the population.

Sylvatic plague occurs as a stable enzootic infection or as epizootic disease with a high mortality rate for the host, usually rodent, population. Hibernating animals are able to maintain the infection over winter, and transmission from animal to animal is achieved by way of a rodent-flea cycle. Different species of fleas show variable efficiencies of transmission, based on their relative preference for other hosts and whether or not they regurgitate infected material when they feed. Humans are at greatest risk when infected rats die, forcing rat fleas to seek alternate hosts.

Y. pestis was introduced into the western United States in the 1800s from infected rats carried by ships returning from Asia. In the United States, plague has slowly migrated eastward and is now endemic as far east as western Nebraska, western North Dakota, and eastern Texas. However, human disease in these areas is rare. About 90% of cases are reported from Arizona, California, Colorado, and New Mexico. Outside the United States, plague is found in Asia, Africa, the Americas, and southeastern Europe near the Caspian Sea. Plague is typically transmitted to humans by the bite of fleas that have fed on infected animals, or less often by direct contact with infected domestic or wild animals, or by direct inhalation of infected droplets from patients or animals with the pneumonic form of the disease. Domestic cats that roam freely have become an important source of human plague because they are more likely to cause pneumonic plague than other sources of infection. These cats typically have signs of infection (oral lesions, swollen tongue, lymphadenopathy, or pneumonia).

PATHOGENESIS. *Y. pestis* ingested by fleas proliferate in the intestine and are regurgitated into the dermal lymphatics of the host when fleas next feed. Organisms are initially trapped in the regional lymph nodes, which become enlarged and tender (i.e., buboes). In severe bubonic plague, organisms gain access to the efferent lymphatics and disseminate, causing septicemia, meningitis, and secondary pneumonia. Organisms are readily demonstrated in buboes and on direct smear of peripheral blood in septicemia.

Primary pneumonic plague occurs when infected material is inhaled. The organism is highly transmissible from person to person and from domestic cat to person in this form. Droplets containing large numbers of organisms are expelled and may cause fulminant fatal infections when inhaled.

Y. pestis carries three virulence plasmids, two of which are shared by *Y. enterocolitica* and *Y. pseudotuberculosis* and that promote intracellular survival and suppression of cytokine synthesis. One plasmid unique to *Y. pestis* enhances dissemination and resistance to phagocytosis. The adhesin and invasin genes found in the enteropathogenic species are cryptic in *Y. pestis*.

CLINICAL MANIFESTATIONS. Infection with *Y. pestis* can be subclinical (positive serology without disease), bubonic, septicemic, pneumonic, or rarely meningitic. The incubation period of bubonic plague is 2–8 days, and that of pneumonic plague is 1–3 days. Most cases in children are bubonic plague. Sudden onset of fever, chills, headache, weakness, prostration, and extraordinarily painful lymphadenopathy (buboes) are common. Femoral, inguinal, axillary, and cervical nodes may be involved, depending on the site of inoculation. Tender hepatosplenomegaly and shock may be found on examination. Skin lesions are uncommon, although pustules, papules, eschars, or vesicles at the inoculation site may occur. Disseminated intravascular coagulation may cause the purpuric lesions that were the basis for the term Black Death. Meningitis may present after starting therapy for bubonic plague, particularly when streptomycin is used as a sole agent, and occurs in association with axillary and cervical buboes or septicemia without apparent lymphadenopathy. Undifferentiated septicemia is reported more often in adults. Secondary pneumonia occurs in as many as 25% of patients with bubonic or septicemic plague. Primary pneumonic plague acquired by inhalation of infected droplets from person-to-person or animal-to-human transmission is rare. Pulmonary signs and symptoms may not be apparent until just before death. Gastrointestinal symptoms and signs, including abdominal pain, nausea, vomiting, and bloody diarrhea, occur in more than 50% of patients with plague. Cutaneous manifestations have included nonspecific petechial or purpuric and vesicular or pustular rashes.

DIAGNOSIS. The diagnosis of sporadic plague depends on a high index of suspicion. Outside of endemic areas, a history of travel to an endemic area, especially including camping, or contact with ground squirrels and the presence of flea bites are very important clues to the clinical diagnosis. Case-fatality rates are higher in patients outside of endemic areas, probably because of missed or delayed diagnosis. Sputum, blood, purulent exudates, and lymph node aspirates should be examined directly with Gram and Giemsa or Wayson's stains for bipolar staining organisms and should be cultured for *Y. pestis*. During septicemia, the load of organisms may be so high that bacteria can be seen on smears of peripheral blood. Bubo aspirates are best obtained by injecting sterile nonbacteriostatic saline and immediately withdrawing it for Gram and Wayson's stain and culture. Commercial identification systems may not identify *Y. pestis*. Suspected isolates of *Y. pestis* should be forwarded to a public health laboratory for confirmation. Serologic tests are not clinically useful in diagnosing the acute disease but may help to establish a retrospective diagnosis in patients inadvertently treated with appropriate antibiotics.

Differential Diagnosis. Mild and subacute forms of bubonic plague may be confused with other disorders causing localized lymphadenitis and lymphadenopathy. However, the unusual tenderness coupled with a patient's toxicity should raise the index of suspicion in endemic areas. Septicemic plague may be indistinguishable from other forms of overwhelming bacterial sepsis.

TREATMENT. The treatment of choice for bubonic plague has been intramuscular streptomycin (30 mg/kg/24 hr divided every 12 hr) for 10 days. However, intramuscular streptomycin is inappropriate for septicemia because absorption from muscles may be erratic when perfusion is poor. The poor central nervous system penetration of streptomycin makes this an inappropriate drug for meningitis. Therefore, septicemia and meningitis are usually treated with intravenous chloramphenicol (60–100 mg/kg/24 hr divided every 6 hr). Resistance to these agents and relapses are rare. Mild disease may be treated with oral chloramphenicol or tetracycline in children older than 10 yr. Prophylaxis or expectant treatment should be given to close contacts of patients with pneumonic plague. Recommended regimens include a 7-day course of tetracycline, doxycycline, or trimethoprim-sulfamethoxazole. Contacts of cases of uncomplicated bubonic plague do not require prophylaxis.

PROGNOSIS. Acute bubonic plague progresses to delirium, shock, and death within 3–5 days if untreated. The overall mortality rate for untreated bubonic plague is 60–90%. The progression of pneumonic plague is rapid and almost always fatal within 24–48 hr if untreated. Septicemic plague not associated with a bubo also has a high mortality rate because plague is not suspected and empirical therapy therefore is often inadequate.

When bubonic plague is treated early, the mortality rate is less than 10%. The prognosis in primary pneumonic plague remains poor if specific treatment is not provided within 18 hr of onset.

PREVENTION. Primary prevention requires avoidance of exposure to infected animals and their fleas. In endemic areas, the public should be educated to avoid rodent burrows, to refrain from handling sick or dead rodents, to deflea household pets, and to reduce the domestic rat habitat. The prevalence and distribution of plague can be determined in wild rodent populations by surveillance for disease or by using the polymerase chain reaction to detect *Y. pestis* in fleas.

Patients with plague should be quarantined until treated and kept under strict respiratory isolation if they have pulmonary symptoms. Infected material should be handled with extreme caution, and the laboratory should be notified of suspected cases.

A killed whole-cell vaccine is available for laboratory and field personnel working directly with the organism, persons engaged in aerosol experiments, and persons engaged in field operations where enzootic plague is known and preventing exposure to rodents and fleas is not possible. Routine immunization of children in endemic areas is not recommended.

Yersinia enterocolitica

Adamkiewicz TV, Berkovitch M, Krishnan C, et al: Infection due to *Yersinia enterocolitica* in a series of patients with β-thalassemia: Incidence and predisposing factors. Clin Infect Dis 27:1362, 1998.

Gayraud M, Scavizzi MR, Mollaret HH, et al: Antibiotic treatment of *Yersinia enterocolitica* septicemia: A retrospective review of 43 cases. Clin Infect Dis 17:405, 1993.

Gong J, Hogman CF, Hambraeus A, et al: Transfusion-transmitted *Yersinia enterocolitica* infection. Vox Sang 65:42, 1993.

Kane DR, Reuman PD: *Yersinia enterocolitica* causing pneumonia and empyema in a child and a review of the literature. Pediatr Infect Dis J 11:591, 1992.

Krogstad P, Mendelman PM, Miller VL, et al: Clinical and microbiologic characteristics of cutaneous infection with *Yersinia enterocolitica*. J Infect Dis 165:740, 1992.

Naqvi SH, Swierkosz EM, Gerard J, et al: Presentation of *Yersinia enterocolitica* enteritis in children. Pediatr Infect Dis J 12:386, 1993.

Nikkari S, Merilahti-Palo R, Saario R, et al: *Yersinia*-triggered reactive arthritis. Arthritis Rheum 35:682, 1992.

Yersinia pseudotuberculosis

Sato K, Ouchi K, Taki M: *Yersinia pseudotuberculosis* infection in children, resembling Izumi fever and Kawasaki syndrome. Pediatr Infect Dis J 2:123, 1983.

Tertti R, Vuento R, Mikkola P, et al: Clinical manifestations of *Yersinia pseudotuberculosis* infection in children. Eur J Clin Microbiol Infect Dis 8:587, 1989.

Uchiyama T, Miyoshi-Akiyama T, Kato H, et al: Superantigenic properties of a novel mitogenic substance produced by *Yersinia pseudotuberculosis* isolated from patients manifesting acute and systemic symptoms. J Immunol 151:4407, 1993.

Weber J, Finlayson NB, Mark JBD: Mesenteric lymphadenitis and terminal ileitis due to *Yersinia pseudotuberculosis*. N Engl J Med 283:172, 1970.

Yersinia pestis

Butler T: The black death past and present: I. Plague in the 1980s. Trans R Soc Trop Med Hyg 83:458, 1989.

Centers for Disease Control and Prevention: Prevention of plague. Recommendations of the Advisory Committee on Immunization Practices (ACIP). MMWR 45(RR-14):1, 1996.

Galimand M, Guiyoule A, Gerbaud G, et al: Multidrug resistance in *Yersinia pestis* mediated by a transferable plasmid. N Engl J Med 337:677, 1997.

CHAPTER 202
Aeromonas *and* Plesiomonas

Jane T. Atkins and Thomas G. Cleary

Similar to *Vibrio*, *Aeromonas* and *Plesiomonas* are indigenous to salt and estuarine waters and are more prevalent in the summer when the water is warm. Both organisms are associated with diarrheal disease but occasionally cause invasive infections.

202.1 Aeromonas

Aeromonas species infect a wide variety of warm- and cold-blooded animals. In humans, infection with *Aeromonas* spp is associated with three distinct syndromes: (1) gastroenteritis, (2) skin and soft tissue infections, and (3) septicemia. *Aeromonas* strains are divided into two major groups: the nonmotile psychrophilic organisms that infect cold-blooded animals and the motile mesophilic organisms that infect humans and other warm-blooded animals. The species most often associated with human infection are *A. hydrophila*, *A. veronii* biotype *sobria*, and *A. caviae*.

Aeromonas species are members of the Vibrionaceae family. They are oxidase-positive, facultatively anaerobic, gram-negative bacilli. Fermentation of lactose is variable.

EPIDEMIOLOGY. *Aeromonas* spp are ubiquitous. They are isolated from numerous environmental aquatic sources including well water, sewage, fresh water, and salt water. They are often cultivated from aquatic sources during warm-weather months, correlating with the peak incidence of human disease during these months. *Aeromonas* spp have been isolated from red meat, poultry, fish, vegetables, and unpasteurized milk. Most human illness is associated with drinking contaminated fresh water or with swimming or bathing in it. Pretreatment with ampicillin is often associated with symptomatic infection. Asymptomatic infection with *Aeromonas* spp occurs in humans and is more common in inhabitants of tropical regions.

PATHOGENESIS. Clinical and epidemiologic data demonstrate that many *Aeromonas* spp are enteric pathogens. However, adult volunteers fed 10^4–10^{10} colony-forming units of *Aeromonas* did not develop diarrhea or become colonized. *Aeromonas* spp possess various potential virulence factors including α- and β-hemolysin, adherence fimbriae, enterotoxin, protease, and chitinase. The β-hemolysin has been shown to be cytotoxic to various cell lines. Enterotoxin causes fluid accumulation in rabbit ileal loops, increases intracellular cyclic adenosine monophosphate cAMP in rabbit intestinal epithelium, and cross reacts immunologically with cholera toxin. The protease cleaves peptide bonds and may have a role in extraintestinal manifestation of *Aeromonas* infections. A few strains produce shigatoxin. It is not clear which of the potential virulence traits defines strains that cause illness.

CLINICAL MANIFESTATIONS. The spectrum of illness includes gastroenteritis, focal invasive infections, and septicemia in susceptible hosts.

Gastroenteritis. The most common clinical manifestation of infection with *Aeromonas* spp is gastroenteritis (Chapter 176). It occurs primarily in children younger than 3 yr. Some studies suggest that it is the third or fourth most common cause of childhood bacterial diarrhea. *Aeromonas* spp have been isolated from 2–10% of patients with diarrhea and 1–5% of asymptomatic controls in various studies. The diarrheal illness is often watery and self-limited, although a dysentery-like syndrome with blood and mucus in the stool has also been described. Fever is common in children. Gastroenteritis caused by *A. hydrophila* and *A. sobria* tends to be acute and self-limited, whereas a third of the patients with *A. caviae* gastroenteritis have chronic or intermittent diarrhea that may last weeks. Complications of *Aeromonas* gastroenteritis include intussusception, failure to thrive, hemolytic-uremic syndrome, and bacteremia.

Skin and Soft Tissue Infection. *A. hydrophila* is the predominant species associated with skin and soft tissue infections, with peak incidence during the summer months. Predisposing factors include local trauma and exposure to contaminated fresh water. *Aeromonas* soft tissue infections have been reported to result from alligator bites, water-sport injuries, and the use of medicinal leech therapy. The spectrum of skin and soft tissue infections is broad, ranging from a localized skin nodule to life-threatening necrotizing fasciitis and myonecrosis. *Aeromonas* cellulitis is indistinguishable from that due to other bacterial pathogens that cause cellulitis but should be suspected in wounds in contact with a water source, especially during the summer. Mixed infections with other organisms occur in more than 80% of trauma-associated cases.

Septicemia. *Aeromonas* spp septicemia is associated with a high mortality rate (reported range 27–73%). *Aeromonas* septicemia usually occurs in patients with underlying conditions such as hepatobiliary disease or malignancy but may occur in an immunocompetent host. *Aeromonas* may be the only organism isolated or may be part of a polymicrobial bacteremic syndrome. *A. hydrophila* and *A. sobria* are the most common species causing septicemia.

Other Infections. Less common infections associated with *Aeromonas* spp include endocarditis, meningitis, osteomyelitis, septic arthritis, endophthalmitis, urinary tract infection, peritonitis, and pneumonia. *Aeromonas* can be associated with aspiration pneumonia after a near-drowning event.

DIAGNOSIS. Isolation of the organisms from the stool or a normally sterile body site is paramount for the diagnosis of infection with *Aeromonas* spp. The organisms are readily isolated from sterile sites but usually require enriched or selective media to adequately detect them in the stool. The organisms are easily cultivated on media routinely used in clinical laboratories such as blood agar and MacConkey's agar. Most strains produce β-hemolysis on blood agar. Lactose-fermenting strains of *Aeromonas* may be overlooked in stool specimens if the clinical laboratory does not routinely perform oxidase tests on lactose fermenters isolated on MacConkey's or does not routinely use selective media for the isolation of *Aeromonas* spp. Isolation of *Aeromonas* spp from the stool is best achieved by using selective or enriched media such as ampicillin-blood agar, cefsulodin-irgasan-novobiocin agar, or MacConkey's agar supplemented with Tween 80 and ampicillin.

TREATMENT *Aeromonas* gastroenteritis is usually self-limited, and antimicrobial therapy may not be indicated. No controlled trials have been carried out; however, data from uncontrolled trials suggest that antimicrobial therapy shortens the course of the illness. Antimicrobial therapy is reasonable to consider in patients with protracted diarrhea, a dysentery-like illness, or underlying conditions such as hepatobiliary disease or immunocompromise. Most isolates are resistant to ampicillin. Septicemia should be treated with an aminoglycoside or a third-generation cephalosporin. Other options include aztreonam, imipenem, chloramphenicol and trimethoprim-sulfamethoxazole (TMP-SMX).

202.2 Plesiomonas shigelloides

Plesiomonas shigelloides causes acute gastroenteritis and rarely extraintestinal infections.

P. shigelloides is an oxidase-positive, facultatively anaerobic, motile, gram-negative bacillus. *P. shigelloides* is currently classified as a member of the Vibrionaceae family. This is based on phenotypic characteristics, such as oxidase production, polar flagella, and fermentation properties. However, analysis of the sequence of 5S rRNA, 16S rRNA, and 16S rDNA suggests that *P. shigelloides* is closely related to Enterobacteriaceae.

EPIDEMIOLOGY. *P. shigelloides* inhabits the gut of various warm- and cold-blooded animals including cats, dogs, pigs, cows, vultures, fish, shellfish, snakes, and newts. *P. shigelloides* has been isolated from fresh water, estuaries, and salt water. Infections in humans are associated with consumption of contaminated food (especially oysters or shellfish) or water or with contact with colonized animals. *P. shigelloides* gastroenteritis is more common in tropical and subtropical regions of Africa, Asia, and Australia than in the United States or Europe.

PATHOGENESIS. Strong epidemiologic evidence shows that *P. shigelloides* is an enteropathogen. However, diarrhea failed to develop in human volunteers fed *P. shigelloides*. Both in vitro and in vivo studies of pathogenicity suggest a low virulence potential.

CLINICAL MANIFESTATIONS. *Plesiomonas* gastroenteritis is usually secretory but occasionally is dysenteric, with blood and mucus. Symptoms include fever, headache, abdominal cramping, vomiting, and diarrhea. The illness usually resolves in 1–2 wk, but reports describe diarrhea lasting 4 wk or longer.

Extraintestinal infections are rare and usually occur in patients with underlying conditions such as immunodeficiency, malignancy, sickle cell disease, or cirrhosis. Extraintestinal disease includes septicemia, meningitis, osteomyelitis, septic arthritis, reactive arthritis, cellulitis, endophthalmitis, pseudoappendicitis, pseudomembranous colitis, proctitis, and cholecystitis. Early-onset neonatal sepsis and meningitis is rare; it has a very high mortality rate (88%).

DIAGNOSIS. Isolation of the organism from stool or sterile body fluids is essential for diagnosis. *P. shigelloides* grows well on traditional enteric media such as MacConkey's SS media, Hektoen agar, and deoxycholate citrate agar. It may be underrecognized by clinical laboratories that do not routinely perform an oxidase test. Fecal leukocytes are often present in the stool.

TREATMENT. Gastroenteritis due to *P. shigelloides* is usually self-limited. Antimicrobial therapy is reserved for those patients with prolonged or bloody diarrhea. Data from uncontrolled trials suggest that antimicrobial therapy decreases the duration of symptoms. *P. shigelloides* is susceptible to TMP-SMX and quinolones (not approved for use in the United States in children <17 yr of age).

Antibiotics are essential for therapy of extraintestinal disease. Empirical therapy with a third-generation cephalosporin is reasonable, because most isolates are susceptible in vitro. Definitive therapy should be guided by the susceptibility of the individual isolate.

Aeromonas

Gold WL, Salit IE: *Aeromonas hydrophila* infections of skin and soft tissue: Report of 11 cases and review. Clin Infect Dis 16:69, 1993.

Holmberg SD, Schell WL, Fanning GR: *Aeromonas* intestinal infections in the United States. Ann Intern Med 105:683, 1988.

Janda JM, Abbott SL: Evolving concepts regarding the genus *Aeromonas*: An expanding panorama of species, disease presentations, and unanswered questions. Clin Infect Dis 27:332, 1998.

Janda JM, Guthertz LS, Kokka RP, et al: *Aeromonas* species in septicemia: Laboratory characteristics and clinical observations. Clin Infect Dis 19:77, 1994.

Ko WC, Chuang YC: *Aeromonas* bacteremia: Review of 59 episodes. Clin Infect Dis 20:1298, 1995.

San Joaquin VVH, Pickett DA: *Aeromonas*-associated gastroenteritis in children. Pediatr Infect Dis J 7:53, 1988.

Plesiomonas shigelloides

Brenden RA, Miller MA, Janda JM: Clinical disease spectrum and pathogenic factors associated with *Plesiomonas shigelloides* infections in humans. Rev Infect Dis 10:303, 1988.

Sack DA, Hoque AT, Huq A, et al: Is protection against shigellosis induced by natural infection with *Plesiomonas shigelloides*? Lancet 343:1413, 1994.

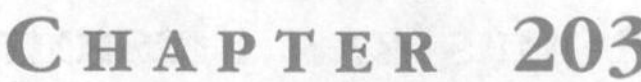

CHAPTER 203
Pseudomonas, Burkholderia, *and* Stenotrophomonas

Robert S. Baltimore

Pseudomonas and *Burkholderia* species live abundantly in soil and water and on plants and are widespread throughout nature. Most human infections due to these species are opportunistic and occur among low birthweight infants and in older infants and children with impaired host defenses, such as those with traumatic wounds, cystic fibrosis, malignancies, extensive burns, malnutrition (especially in impoverished populations), and primary immunodeficiencies as well as those receiving immunosuppressive therapy. *Pseudomonas aeruginosa* is an important cause of nosocomial infections.

A number of species formerly considered under the genus *Pseudomonas* were reclassified on the basis of rRNA homology. Species formerly classified as *P. cepacia, P. mallei,* and *P. pseodomallei* are now *Burkholderia cepacia, B. mallei,* and *B. pseudomallei. P. maltophilia* is now *Stenotrophomonas maltophilia.*

A large number of *Pseudomonas, Burkholderia,* and related organisms have been identified, but only a few are pathogenic for humans; of these, *P. aeruginosa* is by far the most common. Other species occasionally recognized as human pathogens include *B. cepacia, S. maltophilia, P. fluorescens, B. putrefaciens, B. pseudomallei,* and *B. mallei.*

203.1 Pseudomonas aeruginosa

P. aeruginosa is a gram-negative rod and is a strict aerobe. It can multiply in most moist environments that contain minimal amounts of organic compounds because it can use any source of carbon. Strains from clinical specimens may produce β-hemolysis on blood agar; more than 90% of strains produce a bluish-green phenazine pigment (blue pus) as well as fluorescein, which is yellow-green and fluoresces. These pigments diffuse into and color the medium surrounding the colonies. Strains of *Pseudomonas* can be differentiated for epidemiologic purposes by serologic, phage, and pyocin typing and by genome restriction fragment length polymorphisms using pulsed-field gel electrophoresis.

EPIDEMIOLOGY. *P. aeruginosa* and other pseudomonads frequently enter the hospital environment on the clothes, skin, or shoes of patients or hospital personnel, with plants or vegetables brought into the hospital, and in the gastrointestinal (GI) tracts of patients. Colonization of any moist or liquid substance may ensue; for example, the organisms may be found growing in distilled water, hospital kitchens and laundries, some antiseptic solutions, and equipment used for respiratory therapy. Colonization of patients' skin, throat, stool, and nasal mucosa is low at admission to the hospital but increases to as high as 50–70% with prolonged hospitalization and the use of broad-spectrum antibiotics, chemotherapy, mechanical ventilation, and urinary catheters. Patients' intestinal microbial flora may be altered by the use of broad-spectrum antibiotics, with reduced resistance to colonization permitting *P. aeruginosa* in the environment to populate the GI tract. Intestinal mucosal breakdown associated with medications, especially cytotoxic agents, and nosocomial enteritis may provide a pathway by which *P. aeruginosa* spreads to the lymphatics or bloodstream.

PATHOGENESIS. The requirement of oxygen for growth may account for the lack of invasiveness of *Pseudomonas* after it has colonized or even infected the skin. Invasiveness of *P. aeruginosa* is mediated by a host of virulence factors. It produces endotoxin that is weak compared with that of other gram-negative bacilli. It also produces numerous exotoxins, including exotoxin A, which causes local necrosis and facilitates systemic bacterial invasion, and exoenzyme S, which acts as both an adhesin and a cellular toxin. *Pseudomonas* produces disease in three stages. Bacterial colonization and attachment are facilitated by pili or fimbriae and by opportunistic adhesion to epithelium damaged by prior injury or infection. A mucopolysaccharide may inhibit phagocytosis, whereas extracellular proteins, proteases, elastases, and cytotoxin (formerly leukocidin) digest cell membranes, and antibodies produce capillary vascular permeability and inhibit leukocyte function. Dissemination and bloodstream invasion follow extension of local tissue damage and are facilitated by the antiphagocytic properties of endotoxin, the mucoid exopolysaccharide, and protease cleavage of IgG. The host responds to infection by producing antibodies to *Pseudomonas* exotoxin (exotoxin A) and lipopolysaccharide. Compromised host defense mechanisms (owing to trauma, neutropenia, mucositis, immunosuppression, impaired mucociliary transport) explain the predominant role of this organism in producing opportunistic infections.

CLINICAL MANIFESTATIONS. Most clinical patterns (Table 203–1) are related to opportunistic infections (see Chapter 179) or are associated with shunts and indwelling catheters (see Chapter 180 and Table 203–1). *P. aeruginosa* may be introduced into a minor wound of a healthy person as a secondary invader, and cellulitis and a localized abscess that exudes green or blue pus may follow. The characteristic skin lesions of *Pseudomonas,* ecthyma gangrenosum, whether caused by direct inoculation or secondary to septicemia, begin as pink macules and progress to hemorrhagic nodules and eventually to ulcers with ecchymotic and gangrenous centers with eschar formation, surrounded by an intense red areola.

TABLE 203–1 *Pseudomonas aeruginosa* **Infections**

Infection	Common Clinical Characteristics
Endocarditis	Native right-sided (tricuspid) valve disease in intravenous drug addicts
Pneumonia	Compromised local (lung) or systemic host defense mechanisms. Nosocomial (respiratory), bacteremic (malignancy), or abnormal mucociliary clearance (cystic fibrosis) may be pathogenetic. Cystic fibrosis is associated with mucoid *P. aeruginosa* organisms producing capsular slime and *B. cepacia*
Central nervous system infection	Meningitis, brain abscess; contiguous spread (mastoiditis, dermal sinus tracts, sinusitis); bacteremia or direct inoculation (trauma, surgery)
External otitis	Swimmer's ear; humid warm climates, swimming pool contamination
Malignant otitis externa	Invasive, indolent, febrile toxic, destructive necrotizing lesion in young infants, immunosuppressed neutropenic patients, or diabetic patients; associated seventh nerve palsy and mastoiditis
Chronic mastoiditis	Ear drainage, swelling, erythema; perforated tympanic membrane
Keratitis	Corneal ulceration; contact lens keratitis
Endophthalmitis	Penetrating trauma, surgery, penetrating corneal ulceration; fulminant progression
Osteomyelitis/septic arthritis	Puncture wounds of foot and osteochondritis; intravenous drug abuse; fibrocartilaginous joints, sternum, vertebrae, pelvis; open fracture osteomyelitis; indolent; pyelonephritis and vertebral osteomyelitis
Urinary tract infection	Iatrogenic, nosocomial; recurrent urinary tract infections in children, instrumented patients, and those with obstruction or stones
Gastrointestinal tract infection	Immunocompromise, neutropenia, typhlitis, rectal abscess, ulceration, rarely diarrhea; peritonitis in peritoneal dialysis
Ecthyma gangrenosum	Metastatic dissemination; hemorrhage, necrosis, erythema, eschar, discrete lesions with bacterial invasion of blood vessels; also subcutaneous nodules, cellulitis, pustules, deep abscesses
Primary and secondary skin infections	Local infection; burns, trauma, decubitus ulcers, toe web infection, green nail (paronychia); whirlpool dermatitis: diffuse, pruritic, folliculitis, vesiculopustular or maculopapular, erythematous lesions

Outbreaks of dermatitis and urinary tract infections caused by *P. aeruginosa* have been reported in healthy persons after use of community swimming pools, recreational whirlpools, or family-owned hot tubs. Skin lesions of folliculitis develop several hours to 2 days after contact with these water sources. Skin lesions may be erythematous, macular, papular, or pustular. Illness may vary from a few scattered lesions to extensive truncal involvement. In some children, malaise, fever, vomiting, sore throat, conjunctivitis, rhinitis, and swollen breasts may be associated with dermal lesions.

Pseudomonads other than *P. aeruginosa* rarely cause disease in healthy children, but pneumonia and abscesses due to *B. cepacia,* otitis media due to *P. putrefaciens* or *P. stutzeri,* abscesses due to *P. fluorescens,* and cellulitis and septicemia and osteomyelitis due to *S. maltophilia* have been reported. Septicemia and endocarditis due to *S. maltophilia* have also been associated with intravenous abuse of drugs.

Burns and Wound Infection. The surfaces of burns or wounds are frequently populated by *Pseudomonas* and other gram-negative organisms; this initial colonization with a low number of adherent organisms is a necessary prerequisite to invasive disease. Administration of antibiotics may diminish the susceptible microbiologic flora, permitting strains of *Pseudomonas* to flourish. Multiplication of organisms in devitalized tissues or associated with prolonged use of intravenous or urinary catheters increases the risk of septicemia with *P. aeruginosa,* a major problem in burned patients (see Chapter 70).

Cystic Fibrosis. *P aeruginosa* is common in children with cystic fibrosis; prevalence increases with increasing age and severity of pulmonary disease. Mucoid strains of *P. aeruginosa* predominate in patients with cystic fibrosis but are rarely encountered in other conditions. The infection begins insidiously or even asymptomatically, and the progression has a highly variable pace. In children with cystic fibrosis, antibody does not eradicate the organism and antibiotics are only partially effective, thus, infection becomes chronic (see Chapter 416).

Immunocompromised Persons. Children with leukemia or other debilitating malignancies, particularly those who are receiving immunosuppressive therapy and who are neutropenic, are extremely susceptible to septicemia due to invasion of the bloodstream by *Pseudomonas* with which the patient is already colonized, usually in the respiratory or GI tract. Signs of sepsis are often accompanied by a generalized vasculitis, and hemorrhagic necrotic lesions may be found in all organs, including the skin, where they appear as purple nodules or ecchymotic areas that become gangrenous (ecthyma gangrenosum). Hemorrhagic or gangrenous perirectal cellulitis or abscesses may occur, associated with ileus and profound hypotension.

Nosocomial Pneumonia. Although not a significant cause of community-acquired pneumonia in children, *P. aeruginosa* is an important cause of nosocomial pneumonia, especially ventilator-associated pneumonia. *P. aeruginosa* has historically been found to contaminate ventilators, tubing, and humidifiers, but this is uncommon today with appropriate disinfection and routine changing of equipment. Nevertheless, colonization of the upper respiratory tract and the GI tract may be followed by aspiration of *P. aeruginosa*-contaminated secretions, resulting in severe pneumonia. One of the most challenging situations is distinguishing between colonization and pneumonia in intubated patients. This can often only be resolved by using invasive culture techniques such as bronchoscopy with bronchial brushing.

Infants. *P. aeruginosa* is an occasional cause of nosocomial bacteremia in newborns and accounts for 2–5% of positive blood culture results in neonatal intensive care units. A frequent focus preceding bacteremia is conjunctivitis. Older infants may occasionally present with community-acquired sepsis due to *P. aeruginosa*, but this is uncommon. In the few reports describing this sepsis, preceding conditions included ecthyma-like skin lesions, virus-associated transient neutropenia, and prolonged contact with contaminated bath water.

DIAGNOSIS. *P. aeruginosa* infection is rarely clinically distinctive. Diagnosis depends on recovery of the organism from the blood, cerebrospinal fluid, urine, or needle aspirate of the lung or from purulent material obtained by aspiration of subcutaneous abscesses or areas of cellulitis. An exception is ecthyma gangrenosum, which is characteristic of *Pseudomonas* infection of the skin. Rarely, similar skin lesions may follow septicemia due to *Aeromonas hydrophila*, other gram-negative bacilli, and *Aspergillus*.

TREATMENT. Systemic infections with *Pseudomonas* should be treated promptly with an antibiotic to which the organism is susceptible *in vitro*. Response to treatment may be limited, and prolonged treatment may be necessary for systemic infection in compromised hosts.

Septicemia and other aggressive infections should be treated with either one or two bactericidal agents. Little evidence shows that more than one agent is needed for individuals with normal immunity or when treating urinary tract infections, but dual therapy is often used for a synergistic effect in immunocompromised patients or when the susceptibility of the organism is in doubt. Appropriate single agents include ceftazidime, cefoperazone, ticarcillin-clavulanate, and piperacillin-tazobactam. Gentamicin or another aminoglycoside may be used concomitantly for synergistic effect. Carbenicillin, ticarcillin, and mezlocillin alone are not recommended because strains of the organism rapidly become resistant to these agents.

Ceftazidime has proved to be extremely effective in patients with cystic fibrosis (150–200 mg/kg/24 hr in three or four divided doses). Azlocillin, mezlocillin, or piperacillin (300–450 mg/kg/24 hr IV in three or four divided doses) also have proved to be effective therapy for susceptible strains of *P. aeruginosa* when combined with an aminoglycoside. Additional effective antibiotics include imipenem, aztreonam, and ciprofloxacin, but these are not approved for infants and young children at this time.

Meningitis is best treated with ceftazidine in combination with gentamicin, given intravenously. Concomitant intraventricular or intrathecal treatment with gentamicin (1–2 mg once daily, independent of body weight, until the cerebrospinal fluid is sterile) may be required when intravenous therapy fails but is not recommended for routine use.

PROGNOSIS. The prognosis is dependent in large part on the nature of the underlying disease. In severely immunocompromised patients, the prognosis for patients with *P. aeruginosa* sepsis is poor unless susceptibility factors such as neutropenia or hypogammaglobulinemia can be reversed. The outcome is improved by combined antimicrobial therapy, a urinary tract portal of entry, absence of neutropenia or recovery from neutropenia, and drainage of local sites of infection. *Pseudomonas* is recovered from the lungs of most children who die of cystic fibrosis and may be responsible for the slow deterioration of these patients; *B. cepacia*, which is frequently resistant to standard antimicrobial agents, has been associated with a more rapid decline in pulmonary function and lower survival. The prognosis for normal development is poor in the few infants who survive *Pseudomonas* meningitis.

PREVENTION. Prevention of infections due to *P. aeruginosa* is not a concern for healthy individuals outside of the hospital but is dependent on limiting contamination of the health care environment and preventing transmission to patients. Effective hospital infection control programs are necessary to identify and eradicate sources of the organism as quickly as possible. *Pseudomonas* may grow in distilled water, some disinfectants, parenteral alimentation solutions, and medications. In newborn nurseries, infection generally has been transmitted to the infants by the hands of personnel, from washbasin surfaces, from catheters, and from solutions used to rinse suction catheters.

Strict attention to handwashing, particularly with an iodophor-containing solution, before and between contacts with neonates may prevent or interdict epidemic disease. Meticulous care and sterile procedures in suctioning of endotracheal tubes, insertion and care of indwelling catheters, preparation of intravenous solutions especially those for total parenteral alimentation, and regular replacement of intravenous administration tubing greatly reduce the hazard of extrinsic contamination by *Pseudomonas* and other gram-negative organisms.

Prevention of follicular dermatitis caused by *Pseudomonas* contamination of whirlpools or hot tubs is possible by maintaining pool water at a pH of 7.2–7.8 and free chlorine concentration at 70.5 mg/L.

Infections in burned patients may be minimized by protective isolation, debridement of devitalized tissue, and topical application of sulfadiazine or 10% mafenide acetate cream. Administration of intravenous immunoglobulin may be used. Approaches under investigation to prevent infection include development of *Pseudomonas* vaccine and development of hyperimmune globulin.

Pseudomonas infection of dermal sinuses communicating with the cerebrospinal space can be prevented by early identification and surgical repair. *Pseudomonas* infection of the urinary tract may be minimized or prevented by early identification and corrective surgery of obstructive lesions.

203.2 Burkholderia

B. cepacia. *B. cepacia* is a filamentous gram-negative rod. It may be difficult to isolate from respiratory specimens in the laboratory, requiring an enriched, selective media (OFPBL) and as long as 3 days of incubation.

B. cepacia is a classic opportunist that rarely infects normal tissue but can be a pathogen for individuals with pre-existing damage to respiratory epithelium, especially persons with cystic fibrosis. Although it is found throughout the environment, human-to-human spread among patients with cystic fibrosis occurs either directly by inhalation of aerosols or indirectly from contaminated equipment or surfaces. This has led to cohorting of patients with cystic fibrosis in clinics, hospital wards, and social gatherings on the basis of *B. cepacia* colonization. *B. cepacia* in persons with cystic fibrosis is associated with an acute respiratory syndrome of fever, leukocytosis, and progressive respiratory failure. This is in contradistinction to *P. aeruginosa* in cystic fibrosis, which is insidious and rarely communicable.

Treatment in hospitals should include standard precautions and avoidance of placing colonized and uncolonized patients in the same room. Persons who have cystic fibrosis and who visit or provide care and are not infected or colonized with *B. cepacia* may elect to wear a mask when within 3 ft of a colonized patient. The use of antibiotics is guided by susceptibility studies of a patient's isolates because the susceptibility pattern of this species is quite variable. Ureidopenicillins (piperacillin, mezlocillin), aminoglycosides, ceftazidime, ciprofloxacin, and cotrimoxazole frequently show good activity. Resistance to aminoglycosides is the rule and presence of inducible beta-lactamase in many strains is probably the cause of clinical failures reported with ureidopenicillins and ceftazidime. Treatment with two or three agents may be necessary to control the infection and avoid the development of resistance.

***B. mallei* (Glanders).** Glanders is a severe infectious disease of horses and other domestic and farm animals due to *B. mallei*, a nonmotile gram-negative bacillus that is occasionally transmitted to humans. It may be acquired by inoculation into the skin or inhalation of aerosols. Laboratory workers may acquire it from clinical specimens. The disease is relatively common in Asia, Africa, and the Middle East. The clinical manifestations include septicemia, acute or chronic pneumonitis, and hemorrhagic necrotic lesions of the skin, nasal mucous membranes, and lymph nodes. Glanders is treated with sulfadiazine, tetracycline, or chloramphenicol and streptomycin over a period of many months.

***B. pseudomallei* (Melioidosis).** This important disease of Southeast Asia and northern Australia occurs in the United States mainly in persons returning from endemic areas. The causative agent is *B. pseudomallei*, an inhabitant of soil and water in the tropics. It is ubiquitous in endemic areas; infection follows inhalation of dust or direct contamination of abrasions or wounds. Human-to-human transmission has only rarely been reported. Serologic surveys demonstrate that asymptomatic infection occurs in endemic areas. The disease may remain latent and appear when host resistance is reduced, sometimes years after the initial exposure.

Melioidosis may present as a single primary skin lesion (vesicle, bulla, or urticaria). Pulmonary infection may be subacute and mimic tuberculosis or it may present as an acute necrotizing pneumonia. Occasionally, septicemia occurs and numerous abscesses are noted in various organs of the body. Myocarditis, pericarditis, endocarditis, intestinal abscess, cholecystitis, acute gastroenteritis, urinary tract infections, septic arthritis, paraspinal abscess, osteomyelitis, and generalized lymphadenopathy all have been observed. Melioidosis may also present as an encephalitic illness with fever and seizures.

Diagnosis is based on visualization of characteristic small gram-negative rods in exudates or growth on laboratory media such as eosin methylene blue (EMB) or MacConkey's agar. Serologic tests are available, and diagnosis can be established by a fourfold or greater rise in antibody titer in an individual with an appropriate syndrome.

B. pseudomallei is susceptible to many antimicrobial agents, including third-generation cephalosporins, aminoglycosides, tetracycline, cotrimoxazole, sulfisoxazole, chloramphenicol, and amoxicillin-clavulanate. Therapy should be guided by antimicrobial susceptibility tests. Two or three agents such as ceftazidime or chloramphenicol plus either cotrimoxazole, sulfisoxazole, or an aminoglycoside are usually chosen for severe or septicemic disease. For severe disease, prolonged treatment of 2–6 mo is recommended to prevent relapses. Appropriate antibiotic therapy generally results in recovery.

203.3 Stenotrophomonas

S. maltophilia (formerly *Xanthomonas maltophilia* or *Pseudomonas maltophilia)* is a short to medium-sized straight gram-negative bacillus. It is ubiquitous in nature and can be found in the hospital environment. Strains isolated in the laboratory may be contaminants, may be a commensal from the colonized surface of a patient, or may represent an invasive pathogen. The species is an opportunist; serious infections usually afflict those requiring intensive care, typically patients with ventilator-associated pneumonia or catheter-associated infections. Common types of infection include pneumonia, urinary tract infection, endocarditis, and osteomyelitis. Strains vary as to antibiotic susceptibility. Treatment should be based on the results of susceptibility testing. Trimethoprim-sulfamethoxazole, minocycline, doxycycline, ticarcillin-clavulanate, and chloramphenicol frequently show good activity. Aminoglycosides, cephalosporins, and carbapenems are usually inactive. Among the quinolone antibiotics, ciprofloxacin often has good activity and has been used clinically, and the newer agents sparfloxacin and levofloxacin usually show good activity in vitro.

Baltimore RS, Christie CDC, Smith GJW: Immunohistopathologic localization of *Pseudomonas aeruginosa* in lungs from patients with cystic fibrosis: Implications for the pathogenesis of progressive lung deterioration. Am Rev Respir Dis 140:1650, 1989.

Chaowagul W, White NJ, Dance DAB, et al: Melioidosis: A major cause of community-acquired septicemia in northeastern Thailand. J Infect Dis 159:890, 1989.

Chusid MJ, Hillmann SM: Community-acquired *Pseudomonas* sepsis in previously healthy infants. Pediatr Infect Dis J 6:681, 1987.

Feder HM Jr, Grant-Kels JM, Tilton RG: *Pseudomonas* whirlpool dermatitis. Clin Pediatr 22:638, 1983.

Hilf M, Yu VL, Sharp JS, et al: Antibiotic therapy for *Pseudomonas aeruginosa* bacteremia: Outcome correlations in a prospective study of 200 patients. Am J Med 87:540, 1989.

Isles A, Maclusky I, Corey M, et al: *Pseudomonas cepacia* infection in cystic fibrosis: An emerging problem. J Pediatr 104:206, 1984.

Kerem E, Corey M, Gold R, et al: Pulmonary function and clinical course in patients with cystic fibrosis after pulmonary colonization with *Pseudomonas aeruginosa*. J Pediatr 116:714, 1990.

Kusne S, Eibling DE, Yu VL, et al: Gangrenous cellulitis associated with gram-negative bacilli in pancytopenic patients: Dilemma with respect to effective therapy. Am J Med 85:490, 1988.

McManus AT, Mason AD, McManus WF, et al: Twenty-five year review of *Pseudomonas aeruginosa* bacteremia in a burn center. Eur J Clin Microbiol 4:219, 1985.

Reed MD, Stern RC, O'Brien CA, et al: Randomized double blind evaluation of ceftazidime dose ranging in hospitalized patients with cystic fibrosis. Antimicrob Agents Chemother 31:698, 1987.

Rodriguez WJ, Khan WN, Cocchetto DM, et al: Treatment of *Pseudomonas* meningitis with or without concurrent therapy. Pediatr Infect Dis J 9:83, 1990.

Salmen T, Dwyer DM, Vorse H, et al: Whirlpool associated *Pseudomonas aeruginosa* urinary tract infections. JAMA 15:2025, 1983.

CHAPTER 204
Tularemia (Francisella tularensis)

Gordon E. Schutze and Richard F. Jacobs

Tularemia is a zoonotic infection caused by the gram-negative bacterium *Francisella tularensis*. Tularemia is primarily a disease of wild animals; human disease is incidental and usually results from contact with blood-sucking insects or wild animals. The illness caused by *F. tularensis* is manifested by different clinical syndromes, the most common of which consists of an ulcerative lesion at the site of inoculation with regional lymphadenopathy or lymphadenitis.

ETIOLOGY. *F. tularensis*, the causative agent of tularemia, is a small, nonmotile, pleomorphic, gram-negative coccobacillus. The two main biovars are *F. tularensis* biovar tularensis (Jellison's type A) and *F. tularensis* biovar *palearctica* (Jellison's type B). Type A produces more serious disease in humans and is most commonly found in North America; type B may be found in North America, Europe, and Asia and produces a less virulent disease. Type A is associated with ticks and lagomorphs (rabbits, hares); type B can be associated with mosquitoes, rodents, and water and marine animals.

EPIDEMIOLOGY. Of all the zoonotic diseases, tularemia is unusual because of the different modes of transmission of disease. A large number of animals serve as a reservoir for this organism, which can penetrate both intact skin and mucous membranes. Transmission can occur through the bite of infected ticks or other biting insects, by contact with infected animals or their carcasses, by consumption of contaminated foods or water, or through inhalation, as might occur in a laboratory setting. This organism is not, however, transmitted from person to person. In the United States, rabbits and ticks are the principal reservoirs. Most disease due to rabbit exposure occurs in the winter, and disease due to tick exposure occurs in the warmer months (April–September). *Amblyomma americanum* (Lone Star tick), *Dermacentor variabilis* (dog tick), and *Dermacentor andersoni* (wood tick) are the most common tick vectors. These ticks usually feed on infected small rodents and later feed on humans. Taking that blood meal through a fecally contaminated field transmits the infection.

PATHOGENESIS. The most common portal of entry for human infection is through the skin or mucous membrane. This may occur through the bite of an infected insect or via inapparent abrasions. Inhalation or ingestion of *F. tularensis* can also result in infection. More than 10^8 organisms are usually required to produce infection if they are ingested, but as few as 10 organisms may cause disease if they are inhaled or injected into the skin. Within 48–72 h after injection into the skin, an erythematous, tender, or pruritic papule may appear at the portal of entry. This papule may enlarge and form an ulcer with a black base, followed by regional lymphadenopathy. Once *F. tularensis* reaches the lymph nodes, the organism may multiply and form granulomas. Bacteremia may also be present, and although any organ of the body may be involved, the reticuloendothelial system is the most commonly affected.

Conjunctival inoculation may result in infection of the eye with preauricular lymphadenopathy (Parinaud's oculoglandular syndrome). Inhalation, aerosolization, or hematogenous spread of the organisms can result in pneumonia. Chest roentgenograms of such patients may reveal patchy infiltrates rather than areas of consolidation. Pleural effusions may also be present and may contain blood. In pulmonary infections, mediastinal adenopathy may be present; in oropharyngeal disease, patients may develop cervical lymphadenopathy. *Typhoidal tularemia* may be used to describe severe bacteremic disease, irrespective of the mode of transmission or portal of entry.

Infection with tularemia stimulates the host to produce antibodies. This antibody response, however, has only a minor role in fighting this infection. The body is dependent on cell-mediated immunity to contain and eradicate this infection. Infection is usually followed by specific protection; thus, chronic infection or reinfection is unlikely.

CLINICAL MANIFESTATIONS. Although it may vary, the average incubation period from infection until clinical symptoms appear is 3 days (range, 1–21 days). A sudden onset of fever with other associated symptoms is quite common (Table 204–1). Physical examination may include lymphadenopathy, hepatosplenomegaly, or skin lesions. Various skin lesions have been described, including erythema multiforme and erythema nodosum. Approximately 20% of patients may develop a generalized maculopapular rash that occasionally becomes pustular. These clinical manifestations of tularemia have been divided into various syndromes (Table 204–2).

Ulceroglandular and glandular disease are the two most common forms of tularemia diagnosed in children. The most common glands involved are usually the cervical or posterior auricular nodes owing to a tick bite on the head or neck. If an ulcer is present, it is erythematous and painful and may last from 1–3 wk. The ulcer is located at the portal of entry. After the ulcer develops, regional lymphadenopathy ensues. These nodes may vary in size from 0.5–10 cm and may appear singly or in clusters. These affected nodes may become fluctuant and drain spontaneously, but most usually resolve with treatment. Late suppuration of the involved nodes has been described in 25–30% of patients despite effective therapy. Examination of this material from such lymph nodes usually reveals sterile necrotic material.

TABLE 204–1 Common Clinical Manifestations of Tularemia in Children

Sign or Symptom	% With Sign/Symptom
Lymphadenopathy	96
Fever (>38.3°C)	87
Ulcer/eschar/papule	45
Pharyngitis	43
Myalgias/arthralgias	39
Nausea/vomiting	35
Hepatosplenomegaly	35

TABLE 204–2 Clinical Syndromes of Tularemia in Children

Clinical Syndrome	% With Syndrome
Ulceroglandular	45
Glandular	25
Pneumonia	14
Oropharyngeal	4
Oculoglandular	2
Typhoidal	2
Other*	6

Includes meningitis, pericarditis, hepatitis, peritonitis, endocarditis, osteomyelitis.

Pneumonia due to *F. tularensis* usually presents as variable parenchymal infiltrates that are unresponsive to β-lactam antimicrobial agents. Inhalation-related infection has been described in laboratory workers who are working with the organism; it results in a relatively high mortality rate. Aerosols from farming activities involving rodent contamination (e.g., haying, threshing) or carcass destruction with lawnmowers have been reported to cause pneumonia as well. Patchy parenchymal infiltrates can also be demonstrated in other forms of tularemia. Patchy segmental infiltrates, hilar adenopathy, and pleural effusions are the most common abnormalities demonstrated on chest roentgenograms. Patients may also complain of a nonproductive cough, dyspnea, or pleuritic chest pain.

Oropharyngeal tularemia results from consumption of poorly cooked meats or contaminated water. This syndrome is characterized by acute pharyngitis, with or without tonsillitis, and cervical adenitis. Infected tonsils may become large and develop a yellowish-white membrane that may resemble the membranes associated with diphtheria. Gastrointestinal disease may also occur and usually presents with mild, unexplained diarrhea but may progress to rapidly fulminant and fatal disease.

Oculoglandular tularemia is uncommon, but when it does occur, the portal of entry is the conjunctiva. Contact with contaminated fingers or debris from crushed insects is the most common way of applying the organisms to the conjunctiva. The conjunctiva is painful and inflamed, with yellowish nodules and pinpoint ulcerations. This purulent conjunctivitis with regional lymphadenopathy (ipsilateral preauricular or submandiular nodes) is referred to as Parinaud's oculoglandular syndrome.

Typhoidal tularemia is usually associated with a large inoculum of organisms and usually presents with fever, headaches, and signs or symptoms of endotoxemia. Patients typically are critically ill, and symptoms mimic those with other forms of sepsis. Clinicians practicing in tularemia-endemic regions must always consider this diagnosis in critically ill children.

DIAGNOSIS. The history and physical examination of the patient may suggest the diagnosis of tularemia, especially if the patient lives in or has visited an endemic region. A history of animal or tick exposure may be especially helpful. Hematologic data are nondiagnostic, and results of routine cultures and smears are usually not helpful and are positive only about 10% of the time. Tularemia can be grown in the microbiology laboratory on cysteine–glucose–blood agar, but care should be taken to alert the personnel in the laboratory if this is attempted so they can take the proper precautions to protect themselves from acquiring infection.

The diagnosis of tularemia is most commonly established through the use of a standard and highly reliable serum agglutination test. In the standard tube agglutination test, a single titer of 1:160 or greater in a patient with a compatible history and physical findings can establish the diagnosis. A fourfold increase in titer from paired serum samples collected 2–3 wk apart is also diagnostic. False-negative serologic responses can be obtained early in the infection, and as many as 30% of individuals require longer than 3 wk before testing positive. Once infected, patients may have a positive agglutination test result (1:20–1:80) that may persist for a life time.

Other testing techniques available include a microagglutination test, an enzyme-linked immunosorbent assay, an analysis of urine for tularemia antigen, and polymerase chain reaction. These techniques may become more popular in the future but at this time have a limited role in establishing the diagnosis of tularemia.

Differential Diagnosis. When diagnosing a case of ulceroglandular or glandular tularemia, the following entities should be considered: cat-scratch disease *(Bartonella henselae)*; infectious mononucleosis; Kawasaki's syndrome; lymphadenopathy due to *Staphylococcus aureus*, group A *Streptococcus, Mycobacterium tuberculosis, Toxoplasma gondii*, and the nontuberculous mycobacteria, along with *Sporothrix schenckii*; plague; anthrax; melioidosis; and rat-bite fever.

Oculoglandular disease may also be demonstrated with other infectious agents, such as *Treponema pallidum, Coccidioides immitis*, herpes simplex virus, adenovirus, and the bacterial agents responsible for purulent conjunctivitis. Oropharyngeal tularemia must be differentiated from the same diseases that cause ulceroglandular/glandular disease and from cytomegalovirus, herpes simplex, adenovirus, and other viral or bacterial etiologies. Pneumonic tularemia must be differentiated from the other non–β-lactam-responsive organisms such as *Mycoplasma, Chlamydia*, mycobacteria, fungi, and rickettsia. Typhoidal tularemia must be differentiated from other forms of sepsis as well as from enteric fever (typhoid and paratyphoid fever) and brucellosis.

TREATMENT. All strains of *F. tularensis* are susceptible to gentamicin and streptomycin. Gentamicin (5 m/kg/24 hr bid or tid) has become the drug of choice for the treatment of tularemia in children. This has come about because of the limited availability of streptomycin (30–40 mg/kg/24 hr bid) and the fewer side effects of gentamicin. Therapy is typically continued for 7–10 days, but in mild cases, a 5- to 7-day course may be effective. Chloramphenicol and tetracyclines have been used in the past, but the high relapse rate has limited their use in children. Early data suggested that *F. tularensis* would be susceptible to the third-generation cephalosporins (e.g., cefotaxime, ceftriaxone), but clinical case reports demonstrate a nearly universal failure rate with these agents. Patients typically have defervescence within 24–48 hr after starting therapy, and relapses are uncommon if gentamicin or streptomycin is used. Patients who have not started on appropriate therapy early may respond more slowly to antimicrobial therapy. Late suppuration of involved lymph nodes may occur despite adequate therapy but usually contains sterile material.

PROGNOSIS. Poor outcomes are associated with a delay in recognition and treatment but with rapid recognition and treatment, fatalities are exceedingly rare. The mortality rate for severe untreated disease (e.g., pneumonia, typhoidal disease) can be as high as 30% in these situations, but in general, the overall mortality rate is less than 1%.

PREVENTION. Prevention of tularemia is based on avoiding exposure. Children living in tick-endemic regions should be taught to avoid tick-infested areas, and families should have a tick control plan for their immediate environment and for their pets. Protective clothing should be worn when entering a tick-infested area, but more importantly, children should undergo frequent tick checks during and after their time in these areas. Skin repellents such as *N-N*-diethyl-M-toluamide (DEET) can be used but have been described to cause systemic reactions if used incorrectly on small infants. Avoiding taking young infants into tick-endemic regions is the most prudent approach. If DEET-containing compounds are used, they should be used sparingly on the exposed skin, avoiding the hands and face. The repellent should be washed off completely after leaving the high-risk region. Clothing repellents that use permethrin have been demonstrated to be an effective addition to the use of protective clothing. If ticks are found on the child, forceps should be used to pull the tick straight out. The skin should be cleansed before and after this procedure.

Children should also be taught to avoid sick and dead animals. Dogs and cats are most likely to bring these animals to a child's attention. Children should be encouraged to wear gloves while cleaning wild game. A vaccine is available for adults with high-risk vocations (e.g., veterinarians), but there are no recommendations for use in children. Prophylactic antimicrobial agents are not effective in preventing tularemia and should not be used after exposure.

Cross JT, Jacobs RF: Tularemia: Treatment failures with outpatient use of ceftriaxone. Clin Infect Dis 17:976, 1993.

Cross JT, Schutze GE, Jacobs RF: Treatment of tularemia with gentamicin in pediatric patients. Pediatr Infect Dis J 14:151, 1995.

Enderlin G, Morales L, Jacobs RF, et al: Streptomycin and alternative agents for the treatment of tularemia: Review of the literature. Clin Infect Dis 19:42, 1994.

Jacobs RF, Condrey YM, Yamauchi T: Tularemia in adults and children: A changing presentation. Pediatrics 76:818, 1985.

Jacobs RF, Narain JP: Tularemia in children. Pediatr Infect Dis J 2:487, 1983.

Risi GF, Pombo DJ: Relapse of tularemia after aminoglycoside therapy: Case report and discussion of therapeutic options. Clin Infect Dis 20:174, 1995.

Sotiropoulos SV: Tularemia. Semin Pediatr Infect Dis 5:102, 1994.

Uhari M, Syrjala H, Salminen A: Tularemia in children caused by *Francisella tularensis* biovar *palaeartica*. Pediatr Infect Dis J 9:80, 1990.

CHAPTER 205
Brucella

Gordon E. Schutze and Richard F. Jacobs

Human brucellosis, caused by organisms of the genus *Brucella*, continues to be a major public health problem worldwide. Humans are accidental hosts and acquire this zoonotic disease from direct contact with an infected animal or consumption of products of an infected animal. Although brucellosis is widely recognized as an occupational risk among adults working with livestock, much of the brucellosis in children is food-borne and is associated with consumption of unpasteurized milk products.

ETIOLOGY. Human brucellosis is caused by one of four biovars of the genus *Brucella*. *Brucella abortus* (cattle), *B. melitensis* (goat/sheep), *B. suis* (swine), and *B. canis* (dog) are the most common organisms responsible for human disease. These organisms are small, aerobic, non–spore-forming, nonmotile, gram-negative coccobacillary bacteria that are fastidious in their growth but can be grown on various laboratory media including blood and chocolate agars. When brucellosis is suspected, however, the clinical laboratory should be alerted so the cultures can be maintained for 21 days or longer to ensure growth if the organism is present.

EPIDEMIOLOGY. Brucellosis exists worldwide but is especially prevalent in the Mediterranean basin, Arabian gulf, the Indian subcontinent, and parts of Mexico and Central and South America. In industrialized countries, recreational or occupational exposure to infected animals is a major risk factor for the development of disease. Among children, however, geographic locations that are endemic for *B. melitensis* remain areas of increased risk for the development of infection. In such locations, unpasteurized milk from goats or camels may be used to feed children, thus leading to the development of brucellosis. Consequently, a history of travel to endemic regions or consumption of exotic food or unpasteurized dairy or dairy products may be an important clue to the diagnosis of human brucellosis.

PATHOGENESIS. Routes of infection for these organisms include inoculation through cuts or abrasions in the skin, inoculation of the conjunctival sac of the eye, inhalation of infectious aerosols, or ingestion of contaminated meat or dairy products. The risk of infection depends on the nutritional and immune status of the host, the route of inoculum, and the species of *Brucella*. For reasons that remain unclear, *B. melitensis* and *B. suis* tend to be more virulent than *B. abortus* or *B. canis*.

The major virulence factor for *Brucella* appears to be its cell wall lipopolysaccharide. Strains containing smooth lipopolysaccharide have been demonstrated to have greater virulence and are more resistant to killing by polymorphonuclear leukocytes. These organisms are facultative intracellular pathogens that can survive and replicate within the mononuclear phagocytic cells (monocytes, macrophages) of the reticuloendothelial system. Even though *Brucella* are chemotactic for leukocytes entry into the body, the leukocytes are less efficient in killing these organisms than other bacteria despite the assistance of serum factors such as complement.

Organisms that are not phagocytosed by the leukocytes are ingested by the macrophages and become localized within the reticuloendothelial system. Specifically, they reside within the liver, spleen, lymph nodes, and bone marrow and result in granuloma formation. Antibodies are produced against the lipopolysaccharide and other cell wall antigens. This provides a means of diagnosis and probably has a role in long-term immunity. The major factor in recovery from infection appears to be development of a cell-mediated response resulting in macrophage activation and enhanced intracellular killing. Specifically, sensitized T lymphocytes release cytokines (e.g., interferon-γ and tumor necrosis factor-α), which activate the macrophages and enhance their intracellular killing capacity.

CLINICAL MANIFESTATIONS. Brucellosis is a systemic illness that can be very difficult to diagnose in children without a history of animal or food exposure. Symptoms can be acute or insidious in nature and are usually nonspecific, beginning 2–4 wk after inoculation. Although the clinical manifestations do vary, the classic triad of fever, arthralgia/arthritis, and hepatosplenomegaly can be demonstrated in most patients. Other associated symptoms include abdominal pain, headache, diarrhea, rash, night sweats, weakness/fatigue, vomiting, cough, and pharyngitis. A common constellation of symptoms in children is refusal to eat, lassitude, refusal to bear weight, and failure to thrive. Besides hepatosplenomegaly, the physical findings on examination are usually few, with the exception of arthritis. The fever pattern can vary widely, and virtually any organ or tissue can be involved.

If abnormalities are demonstrated on physical examination, the bones and joint frequently are involved, with the sacroiliac joint as well as the hips, knees, and ankles being the most common. Although headache, mental inattention, and depression may be demonstrated in patients with brucellosis, invasion of the nervous system occurs in only about 1% of cases. Congenital infections with these organisms have also been described. These have been attributed to both transplacental and breast milk transmission, and the signs and symptoms associated with this infection are very vague and nonpathognomonic.

DIAGNOSIS. Routine laboratory examinations of the blood are not helpful, with the exception of the white blood cell count, which may be low or normal. A history of exposure to animals or ingestion of unpasteurized dairy products may be more helpful. A definitive diagnosis is established by recovering the organisms in the blood, bone marrow, or other tissues. Although automated culture systems and the use of the lysis-centrifugation method have shortened the isolation time from weeks to days, it is prudent to alert the clinical microbiology laboratory that brucellosis is suspected. Isolation of the organism still may require as long as 4 wk from a blood culture sample. Caution is also advised when using automated bacterial identification systems, because isolates have been misidentified as other gram-negative organisms (e.g., *Haemophilus influenzae* type b).

In the absence of positive culture results, various serologic tests have been applied to the diagnosis of brucellosis. The serum agglutination test (SAT) is the most widely used and detects antibodies against *B. abortus, B. melitensis*, and *B. suis*. This method does not detect antibodies against *B. canis* because this organism lacks the smooth lipopolysaccharide. No single titer is ever diagnostic, but most patients with acute infections have titers of 1:160 or greater. Low titers may be found early in the course of the illness, requiring the use of acute and convalescent sera testing to confirm the diagnosis. Because patients with active infection have both an IgM and an IgG response and the SAT measures the total quantity of agglutinating antibodies, the total quantity of IgG is measured by treatment of the serum with 2-mercaptoethanol. This fractionation is important in determining the significance of the antibody titer because low levels of IgM can remain in the serum for weeks to months after the infection has been treated. It is important to remember that all titers must be interpreted in light of a patient's history and physical examination. False-positive results due to cross-reacting antibodies to other gram-negative organisms such as *Yersinia enterocolitica, Francisella tularensis*, and *Vibrio cholerae* can occur. In addition, the prozone effect can give false-negative results in the presence of high titers of antibody. To avoid this issue, serum that is being tested should be diluted to 1:320 or higher.

Among newer tests, the enzyme immunoassay appears to be the most sensitive method for detecting *Brucella* antibodies. Polymerase chain reaction assays are also becoming available but at this time are mostly limited to research facilities.

Differential Diagnosis. Brucellosis may be confused with other infections such as tularemia, cat-scratch disease, typhoid fever, and fungal infections due to histoplasmosis, blastomycosis, or coccidioidomycosis. Infections due to *Mycobacterium tuberculosis*, atypical mycobacteria, rickettsiae, and *Yersinia* can present in a similar fashion to brucellosis.

TREATMENT. Many antimicrobial agents are active in vitro against the *Brucella* species, but the clinical effectiveness does not always correlate with these results. Doxycycline is the most useful antimicrobial agent and, when combined with an aminoglycoside, is associated with the fewest relapses (Table 205–1). Treatment failures with β-lactam antimicrobial agents, including the third-generation cephalosporins, may be due to the intracellular nature of the organism. Agents that provide intracellular killing are required for eradication of this infection. Likewise, it is apparent that prolonged treatment is the key to preventing disease relapse. Relapse is confirmed by isolation of *Brucella* within weeks to months after therapy has ended and is usually not associated with antimicrobial resistance.

The onset of initial antimicrobial therapy may precipitate a Jarisch-Herxheimer–like reaction presumably due to a large antigen load. It is rarely severe enough to require corticosteroid therapy.

PROGNOSIS. Before the use of antimicrobial agents, the course of brucellosis was often prolonged and may have led to death.

TABLE 205–1 Recommended Treatment of Brucellosis

<8 Years of Age

TMP-SMX 10 mg/kg/24 hr of trimethoprim (maximum daily dose, 480 mg/24 hr) and 50 mg/kg/24 hr of sulfamethoxazole (maximum daily dose: 2.4 g/24 hr) PO for 45 days
plus
Rifampin 15–20 mg/kg/24 hr PO for 45 days

>8 Years of Age

Doxycycline 200 mg/24 hr PO for 6 wk
plus
Streptomycin 1 g/24 hr IM for 1–2 wk
or gentamicin 3–5 mg/kg/24 hr IM or IV for 1–2 wk

Alternative:
Doxycycline 200 mg/24 hr PO for 6 wk
plus
Rifampin 600–900 mg/24 hr PO for 6 wk

Meningitis, Osteomyelitis, or Endocarditis

Doxycycline 200 mg/24 hr PO for 4–6 mo
plus
Streptomycin 1 g/24 hr IM for 4–6 mo or gentamicin
plus/minus
Rifampin 15–20 mg/kg/24 hr (<8 yr) or 600–900 mg/24 hr (>8 yr) PO for 4–6 mo

Since the institution of specific therapy, most deaths are due to specific organ system involvement (e.g., endocarditis) in complicated cases. The prognosis after specific therapy is excellent if patients are compliant with the prolonged therapy.

PREVENTION. Prevention of brucellosis is dependent on effective eradication of the organism from cattle, goats, and swine herds as well as from other animals. Pasteurization of milk and dairy products for human consumption remains an important aspect of prevention. No vaccine currently exists for use in children; therefore, education of the public continues to have a prominent role in prevention of this disease.

Al-Eissa YA, Al-Mofada SM: Congenital brucellosis. Pediatr Infect Dis J 11:667, 1992.

Al-Eissa YA, Kambal A, Al-Nasser MN, et al: Childhood brucellosis: A study of 102 cases. Pediatr Infect Dis J 9:74, 1990.

Chheda S, Lopez SM, Sanderson EP: Congenital brucellosis in a premature infant. Pediatr Infect Dis J 16:81, 1997.

Chomel BB, DeBess EE, Mangiamele DM, et al: Changing trends in the epidemiology of human brucellosis in California from 1973 to 1992: A shift toward foodborne transmission. J Infect Dis 170:1216, 1994.

Gottesman G, Vanunu D, Maayan MC, et al: Childhood brucellosis in Israel. Pediatr Infect Dis J 15:610, 1996.

Khuri-Bulos NA, Daoud AH, Azab SM: Treatment of childhood brucellosis: Results of a prospective trial on 113 children. Pediatr Infect Dis J 12:377, 1993.

Lubani MM, Dudin KI, Araj GF, et al: Neurobrucellosis in children. Pediatr Infect Dis J 8:79, 1989.

Lubani MM, Dudin KI, Sharda DC, et al: A multicenter therapeutic study of 1100 children with brucellosis. Pediatr Infect Dis J 8:75, 1989.

Young EJ: Serologic diagnosis of human brucellosis: Analysis of 214 cases by agglutination tests and review of the literature. Rev Infect Dis 13:359, 1991.

Young EJ: An overview of human brucellosis. Clin Infect Dis 21:283, 1995.

CHAPTER 206
Legionella

Lucy Tompkins

Legionellosis comprises Legionnaires' disease (pneumonia), other invasive extrapulmonary infections, and an acute flulike illness known as Pontiac fever. In contrast to the syndromes associated with invasive disease, Pontiac fever is a self-limiting illness that develops after aerosol exposure and may represent a toxic or hypersensitivity response to *Legionella*.

ETIOLOGY. Legionellaceae are aerobic, non–spore-forming unencapsulated gram-negative bacilli that stain poorly with Gram stain when performed on smears from clinical specimens. Microorganisms in tissue can be better visualized with the Gimenez or silver stains (Dieterle or Warthin-Starry). Stained smears of *Legionella pneumophila* taken from colonial growth resemble *Pseudomonas*. Unlike other *Legionella* species, *L. micdadei* stains acid fast. Although more than 30 species of the genus have now been identified, the majority (90%) of clinical infections are caused by *L. pneumophila*, and most of the remainder are caused by *L. micdadei, L. bozemanii, L. dumoffii*, and *L. longbeachae*.

The organisms are fastidious and require L-cysteine, ferric ion, and α-keto acids for growth. Colonies develop within 3–5 days on buffered charcoal yeast extract agar (BCYE), which may contain selected antibiotics to inhibit overgrowth by other microorganisms; *Legionella* rarely grows on routine laboratory media.

EPIDEMIOLOGY. Fresh water (lakes, streams, thermally polluted waters, potable water) is the environmental reservoir of *Legionella* in nature, and invasive pneumonia (Legionnaires' disease) is related to exposure to potable water or to aerosols containing the bacteria. Growth of *Legionella* occurs more readily in hot water, and exposure to warm water sources is an important risk factor for disease. *Legionella* organisms are facultative intracellular parasites and grow inside protozoans present in biofilms consisting of organic and inorganic material found in plumbing and water storage tanks and various other bacterial species. Sporadic cases of community-acquired Legionnaires' disease can be attributed to potable water in the local environment of the patient. Risk factors for acquisition of sporadic community-acquired pneumonia include nonmunicipal water supply, residential plumbing repairs, and lower water heater temperatures which facilitate growth of bacteria or lead to release of a bolus of biofilm containing *Legionella* into potable water. The mode of transmission may be via inhalation of aerosols or by aspiration. Outbreaks of Legionnaires' disease have been associated with protozoans in the implicated water source; replication within these eukaryotic cells presumably amplifies and maintains *Legionella* within the potable water distribution system. Outbreaks of community-acquired pneumonia and some nosocomial outbreaks have been linked to common sources, including evaporative condensers cooling towers whirlpool baths, humidifiers, nebulizers, and showers.

Hospital-acquired infections are most often linked to potable water. Exposure may occur through two general mechanisms: (1) aspiration of ingested microorganisms, including those in gastric feedings, that are mixed with contaminated tap water; and (2) aerosols from showers and sinks. Extrapulmonary legionellosis may occur through topical application of contaminated tap water into surgical or traumatic wounds. In contrast to Legionnaires' disease, Pontiac fever outbreaks have occurred through exposure to aerosols from whirlpool baths, ultrasonic humidifiers, and ventilation systems.

The incidence of community-acquired Legionnaires' disease caused by *L. pneumophila* occurring sporadically in adults is estimated at 7–20 cases/100,000/yr and demonstrates geographic differences. *Legionella* infections have no seasonal pattern. In one large community-based study of adults, *Legionella* was associated with 3% of pneumonia cases. Taken together, *Mycoplasma pneumoniae, Chlamydia pneumoniae*, and *Legionella pneumophila* accounted for 10–38% of all community acquired pneumonia. Therefore, empiric therapy includes macrolides or quinolones. Approximately 0.5–5.0% of those exposed to a common source become clinically ill, whereas the attack rate in Pontiac fever outbreaks is very high (85–100%).

As estimated by seroconversion to *L. peumophila* among children hospitalized with pneumonia, the Legionnaires' disease rate was found to be quite low. Community-acquired pneumonia occurs most often in children over 4 yr of age. Most nosocomial infections have been reported as case reports; therefore, the true incidence of disease in children is unknown. Nosocomial infection rates in adults are difficult to determine since many hospital laboratories do not attempt to isolate *Legionella* by culture. Hospital-acquired legionellosis in children is associated with clinical risk factors and with environmental exposure. Acquisition of antibodies to *L. pneumophila* in healthy children occurs progressively over time, although this presumably reflects subclinical infection or mild respiratory disease or antibodies that cross react with other bacterial species.

PATHOGENESIS. *Legionella* organisms are facultative intracellular parasites of eukaryotic cells. In humans, the target cell is the alveolar macrophage, although other cell types may also be invaded. Although *Legionella* can be grown on artificial media, the intracellular environment provides the definitive site of growth. Growth in macrophages occurs to the point of cell death, followed by reinfection of new cells, until these cells are activated and can subsequently kill intracellular microorganisms. Acute, severe infection of the lung provokes an acute inflammatory response and necrosis; early on, more bacteria are found in extracellular spaces. Subsequently, macrophage activation and other immune responses produce intense infiltration of tissue by macrophages that contain intracellular bacteria. Corticosteriod therapy poses a high risk of infection by interfering with T cell and macrophage function. Legionnaires' disease rarely occurs in healthy immunocompetent patients with no evidence of respiratory tract disease or dysfunction.

Although certain bacterial factors have been postulated to have a role in virulence, the contribution of each of these to overall pathogenesis is unclear. As in other diseases caused by facultative intracellular microorganisms, the outcome is critically dependent on the specific and nonspecific immune responses of the host, in particular, macrophage and T-cell responses.

CLINICAL MANIFESTATIONS. Legionnaires' disease was originally believed to cause a clinical syndrome called atypical pneumonia and was associated with extrapulmonary signs and symptoms, including diarrhea, hyponatremia, hypophosphatemia, abnormal results of liver function tests, confusion, and renal dysfunction. Although a subset of patients may exhibit "classic" manifestations, *Legionella* infection typically causes pneumonia that is indistinguishable from disease produced by other infectious agents. Fever, cough, and chest pain are common presenting symptoms; the cough may be productive of purulent sputum or may be nonproductive. Although the classic chest radiographic appearance showed rapidly progressive alveolar filling infiltrates, in usual cases of pneumonia the chest radiographic appearance is widely variable, appearing as tumor-like shadows, evidence of nodular infiltrates, unilateral or bilateral infiltrates, or cavitation, although cavitation is rarely seen in nonimmunocompromised patients. This picture overlaps substantially with disease caused by *Streptococcus pneumoniae*. Although pleural effusion is less commonly associated with Legionnaires' disease, its frequency varies so widely that neither the presence or absence of effusion is helpful in differential diagnosis. If present, pleural fluid should be obtained for culture.

A few clinical features may help to differentiate *Legionella* pneumonia from other causes. *Legionella* pueumonia produces an acute-onset febrile illness, the radiograph shows alveolar filling infiltrates, and there is no clinical response to broad-spectrum β-lactam (penicillins and cephalosporins) or aminoglycoside antibiotics.

Concomitant infection with other pathogens occurs in 5–10% of cases of Legionnaires' disease; therefore, culture of another potential pulmonary pathogen does not preclude the diagnosis of legionellosis.

Reports of nosocomial *Legionella* pneumonia in children demonstrate that rapid onset, temperature greater than 38.5°C, cough, pleuritic chest pain, and dyspnea are present in most. Abdominal pain, headache, and diarrhea are also common. Chest radiographs reveal lobar consolidations or diffuse bilateral infiltrates, and pleural effusions are noted. Symptoms do not respond to treatment with β-lactam antibiotics or aminoglycosides.

Risk factors for infection in adults include chronic diseases of the lung (smoking, bronchitis, others), older age, other chronic diseases, including diabetes and renal failure, immunosuppression associated with organ transplantation, and episodes of aspiration. The number of reported cases of community-acquired Legionnaires' disease in children is small. Among these, immunocompromised status and exposure to contaminated potable water are the major risk factors. Infection in a few children with chronic pulmonary disease without immune deficiency has also been reported. Apparently, infection in children lacking any risk factors is very uncommon. The modes of transmission of community-acquired disease in children include exposure to mists, water coolers, and other aerosol-generating apparatuses. Nosocomial *Legionella* infection occurs more frequently than community-acquired disease in children, and the modes of acquisition include microaspiration, frequently associated with nasogastric tubes, and aerosol inhalation. Bronchopulmonary *Legionella* infections occur in patients with cystic fibrosis and have been associated with aerosol therapy or mist tents. Legionnaires' disease is also reported in pediatric patients with asthma and tracheal stenosis. Chronic steroid therapy for asthma is a reported risk factor for *Legionella* sp. infections in children.

Pontiac fever in adults and children is characterized by high fever, myalgia, headache, and extreme debilitation, lasting for a few days. Cough, breathlessness, diarrhea, confusion, and chest pain may occur, but there is no evidence for invasive infection. The disease is self-limited without sequelae. Virtually all exposed individuals seroconvert to *Legionella* antigens. A very large outbreak in Scotland that affected 35 children was attributed to *L. micdadei*, which was isolated from a whirlpool spa. The onset of illness was 1–7 days (median, 3 days), and all exposed children developed significant titers of specific antibodies to *L. micdadei*. The pathogenesis of Pontiac fever is not known. In the absence of evidence of true infection, the most likely hypothesis is that this syndrome is caused by a toxic or hypersensitivity reaction to microbial, or protozoan, antigens.

LABORATORY FINDINGS. Culture of *Legionella* from sputum, other respiratory tract specimens, blood, or tissue is the gold standard against which indirect methods of detection should be compared. Specimens obtained from the respiratory tract that are contaminated with oral flora must be treated and processed to reduce contaminants and plated onto selective media. Because these are costly and time-consuming methods, many laboratories do not process specimens for culture. The microorganisms can be identified presumptively by direct immunofluorescence antibody screening, although the sensitivity of the test is generally low in most laboratories, in part because of the lack of antisera directed against other *Legionella* serogroups and species. This method failed to detect the infection in several well-documented pediatric cases. Retrospective diagnosis can be made serologically using the indirect immunofluorescence assay to detect specific antibody production. Seroconversion may not occur for several weeks after onset of infection, and the available serologic assays do not detect all strains of *L. pneumophila* or all species. The urinary antigen assay that detects *L. pneumophila* serogroup I has an 80% sensitivity and 99% specificity. Thus, the assay is a useful method in the prompt diagnosis of Legionnaires' disease caused by this serogroup which accounts for the majority of symptomatic infections. In view of the low sensitivity of direct detection and the slow growth of the microorganism in culture, the diagnosis of legionellosis should be pursued actively when there is suggestive clinical evidence, including the lack of response to "usual" antibiotics, even when results of other laboratory studies are negative.

TREATMENT. Erythromycin (40 mg/kg/24 hr parenterally and orally), with or without rifampin (15 mg/kg/24 hr), has been empirically established as effective therapy. The macrolides (azithromycin [10 mg/kg on day 1, then 5 mg/kg daily for 4 days] and clarithromycin [15 mg/kg/24 hr orally]) and the quinolones (ciprofloxacin, levofloxacin, trovafloxacin, and sparfloxacin) have excellent activity in vitro, although quinolones are not approved for children < 18 yr of age. In serious infections or in high-risk patients, parenteral therapy is recommended initially; a switch to oral therapy can be made when a patient has had a clinical response. Acute hearing loss, which is reversible, is associated with high dose parenteral erythromycin therapy. The duration of therapy for Legionnaires' disease is 2–3 wk. Treatment of extrapulmonary infections, including prosthetic valve endocarditis and sternal wound infections, may require prolonged therapy. Alternative antibiotics include doxycycline (2–4 mg/kg/24 hr) and trimethoprim-sulfamethoxazole (TMP-SMZ; 15 mg TMP/kg/24 hr). β-lactams and aminoglycosides and other antibiotics that do not penetrate mammalian cells are not clinically effective. Relapse (recrudescence) may occur after cessation of erythromycin therapy.

PROGNOSIS. The mortality rate of community-acquired Legionnaires' disease in adults who are hospitalized is approximately 15%. The prognosis depends on underlying host factors and possibly on the duration of the illness before appropriate therapy is begun. Despite appropriate antibiotic therapy, patients may succumb to respiratory complications, such as acute respiratory distress syndrome, associated with artificial ventilation and intubation.

Anderson RD, Lauer BA, Fraser DW, et al: Infections with *Legionella pneumophila* in children. J Infect Dis 143:386, 1981.
Brady MT: Nosocomial Legionnaires' disease in a children's hospital. J Pediatr 115:46, 1989.
Edelstein PH: Legionnaires' disease. Clin Infect Dis 16:741, 1993.
Famiglietti RF, Bakerman PR, Sanbolle MA, et al: Cavitary legionellosis in two immunocompetent infants. Pediatrics 99:899, 1997.
Goldberg DJ, Collier PW, Fallon RJ, et al: Lochgoilhead fever: Outbreak of nonpneumonic legionellosis due to *Legionella micdadei*. Lancet 1:316, 1989.
Holmberg RE Jr, Pavia AT: Nosocomial *Legionella* pneumonia in the neonate. Pediatrics 92:450, 1993.
Lowry PW, Tompkins LS: Nosocomial legionellosis: A review of pulmonary and extrapulmonary syndromes. Am J Infect Control 21:21, 1993.
Marston BJ, Plouffe JF, File TM, et al: Incidence of community-acquired pneumonia requiring hospitalization. Arch Intern Med 157:1709, 1997.
Stout JE, Yu V: Legionellosis. N Engl J Med 337:682, 1997.
Straus WL, Plouffe JF, File TM, et al: Risk factors for domestic acquisition of Legionnaires disease. Arch Intern Med 156:1685, 1996.

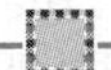

CHAPTER 207
Bartonella

Barbara W. Stechenberg

The spectrum of disease resulting from human infection with *Bartonella* species has expanded rapidly in the past 2 decades, including the association of bacillary angiomatosis with AIDS and cat-scratch disease (CSD) with the fastidious gram-negative rod initially identified as *Rochalimaea henselae*. However, like *Bartonella bacilliformis*, which has been identified for many years, *Rochalimaea* species grow on the surface of eukaryotic host cells and on blood agar. On the basis of these findings, 16S ribosomal RNA gene sequencing, and other molecular genetic homologies, the Rochalimaea genus was transferred to the genus *Bartonella*, as part of the alpha subdivision of proteobacteria. Five *Bartonella* species have been found to be pathogenic for humans: *B. bacilliformis, B. henselae, B. quintana, B. elizabethae,* and most recently *B. clarridgeiae*. Seven other *Bartonella* species have been found in animals, particularly rodents and moles (Table 207–1).

Members of the genus *Bartonella* are gram-negative, oxidase-negative, fastidious aerobic rods that ferment no carbohydrates. Only one species, *B. bacilliformis*, is motile by means of polar flagella. Optimal growth is obtained on fresh media containing 5% or more sheep or horse blood in the presence of 5% carbondioxide. The use of lysis-centrifugation for specimens from blood on chocolate agar for extended periods (2–6 wk) enhances recovery.

207.1 Bartonellosis (Bartonella bacilliformis)

The first human *Bartonella* infection described was bartonellosis, a geographically distinct disease caused by *B. bacilliformis*, which causes two predominant forms of illness: Oroya fever, a severe, febrile hemolytic anemia; and verruca peruana (verruga peruana), an eruption of hemangioma-like lesions. The organism also causes asymptomatic infection. Bartonellosis is also called Carrión's disease in honor of the Peruvian medical student who inoculated himself with blood from a verruca and 21 days later developed Oroya fever. He died 39 days after inoculation, thus proving the unitary etiology of the two clinical illnesses.

ETIOLOGY. *B. bacilliformis* is a small, motile gram-negative organism with a brush of 10 or more unipolar flagella, which appear to be important components for invasiveness. An obligate aerobe, it grows best or 28°C in semisolid nutrient agar containing rabbit serum and hemoglobin.

EPIDEMIOLOGY. Bartonellosis is a zoonosis found only in mountain valleys of the Andes Mountains in Peru, Ecuador, Colombia, Chile, and Bolivia at altitudes and environmental conditions favorable for the vector, which is the sandfly, *Phlebotomus noguchi*.

PATHOGENESIS. After the bite, *Bartonella* organisms enter the endothelial cells of blood vessels, where they proliferate. Found throughout the reticuloendothelial system, they then re-enter the bloodstream and parasitize the erythrocytes. They bind on the cells, deform the membranes, and then enter intracellular vacuoles. The resultant hemolytic anemia may involve as many as 90% of the erythrocytes. Patients who survive this acute phase may or may not develop the cutaneous manifestations, which are nodular hemangiomatous le-

TABLE 207–1 Bartonella Causing Human Disease

Disease	Organism	Vector	Primary Risk Factor
Bartonellosis	*B. bacilliformis*	Sandfly (*Phlebotomus noguchi*)	Living in endemic area (Andes Mountains)
Cat-scratch disease	*B. henselae* *B. clarridgeiae* (1 case)	Cat	Cat scratch or bite
Trench fever	*B. quintana*	Human body louse	Body louse infestation during outbreak
Bacteremia, endocarditis	*B. henselae* *B. quintana* *B. elizabethae*	Cat for *B. henselae*	Severely immunocompromised
Bacillary angiomatosis	*B. henselae* *B. quintana*	Cat for *B. henselae*	Severely immunocompromised
Peliosis hepatis	*B. henselae* *B. quintana*	Cat for *B. henselae*	Severely immunocompromised

sions or verrucae ranging in size from a few millimeters to several centimeters.

CLINICAL MANIFESTATIONS. The incubation period is 2–14 wk. Patients may be totally asymptomatic or may have nonspecific symptoms such as headache and malaise without anemia. Patients with Oroya fever are febrile, rapid development of anemia. Clouding of the sensorium and delirium are common symptoms and may progress to overt psychosis. Physical examination demonstrates signs of severe anemia, icterus, and pallor, which may be associated with generalized lymphadenopathy.

In the pre-eruptive stage, patients may complain of arthralgias, myalgias, and paresthesias. Inflammatory reactions such as phlebitis, pleuritis, erythema nodosum, and encephalitis may develop. The appearance of verrucae is pathognomonic of the eruptive phase. They vary greatly in size and number.

DIAGNOSIS. The diagnosis is made on clinical grounds in conjunction with a blood smear demonstrating organisms, or by blood culture. The anemia is macrocytic and hypochromic, with reticulocyte counts as high as 50%. *B. bacilliformis* may be seen on Giemsa's stain as red-violet rods in the erythrocytes. In the recovery phase, these organisms change to a mere coccoid form and disappear from the blood. In the absence of anemia, the diagnosis depends on blood cultures. In the eruptive phase, the typical verruca confirms the diagnosis. Antibody testing has been used to document infection.

TREATMENT. *B. bacilliformis* is sensitive to many antibiotics, including penicillin, tetracycline, and chloramphenicol. Treatment is very effective in rapidly lowering fever and eradicating the organism from the blood. Chloramphenicol (50–75 mg/kg/24 hr) is considered the drug of choice, because it also is useful in the treatment of intercurrent infections such as *Salmonella*. Blood transfusions and supportive care are critical in patients with severe anemia. Treatment for verruca peruana is not necessary unless large lesions are disfiguring or interfere with function; then, surgical excision may be needed. Oral tetracycline may aid in healing of lesions.

PREVENTION. Prevention depends on avoidance of the vector, particularly at night, by the use of protective clothing and insect repellents (Chapter 297).

207.2 Cat-Scratch Disease (Bartonella henselae)

The most common presentation of *Bartonella* infection is CSD, a subacute, regional lymphadenitis caused by *B. henselae*. It is the most common cause of chronic lymphadenitis, lasting for more than 3 wk.

ETIOLOGY. In 1983, small pleomorphic gram-negative bacilli were first visualized by Warthin-Starry stain in affected lymph nodes from patients with CSD. A putative causative organism, *Afipia felis*, was cultured and initially presumed to be the agent of CSD, but most patients with CSD did not develop an immune response to this organism. *A. felis* has not been cultured from lymph node tissue of a patient with CSD. In 1992, *B. henselae* was cultured from the blood of a healthy cat and was used in serologic studies that indicated *B. henselae* as the cause of CSD. Development of serologic tests that showed prevalence of antibodies in 84–100% of cases of CSD, culturing of *B. henselae* from CSD nodes, and detection of *B. henselae* by polymerase chain reaction in the majority of lymph node samples and pus from patients with CSD confirmed the organism as the cause of CSD. Occasional cases of CSD may be caused by other organisms; one report described a veterinarian with CSD caused by *B. clarridgeiae*.

EPIDEMIOLOGY. CSD is very common, with more than 24,000 estimated cases per year in the United States. It is transmitted by cutaneous inoculation. Most (87–99%) patients have had contact with cats, many of which are kittens younger than 6 mo. More than 50% have a definite history of a cat scratch or bite. Cats have a high-level *Bartonella* bacteremia for months without any clinical symptoms; kittens are more frequently bacteremic than adult cats. The precise mechanism of cat-to-human transmission remains unclear. Transmission between cats is arthropod borne by the cat flea, *Ctenocephalides felis*. In temperate zones, the majority of cases occur between September and March. This may be related to the seasonal breeding of domestic cats or to close proximity to family pets in the fall and winter. In tropical zones, there is no seasonal prevalence. Distribution is worldwide and infection occurs in all races.

Cat scratches appear to be more common among children, and boys are affected more often than girls. CSD is a sporadic illness; only one family member usually is affected, even though many siblings play with the same kitten. However, clusters do occur with family cases within weeks of one another. Anecdotal reports have implicated other sources such as dog scratches, wood splinters, fishhooks, cactus spines, and porcupine quills.

PATHOGENESIS. The pathologic findings in the primary inoculation papule and affected lymph nodes are similar. Both show a central avascular necrotic area with surrounding lymphocytes, giant cells, and histiocytes. Three stages of involvement occur in affected nodes, although they may coexist in the same node. First is generalized enlargement with thickening of the cortex and germinal center hypertrophy. Lymphocytes predominate. Epithelioid granulomas with Langhans' giant cells are scattered throughout the node. In the middle stage, granulomas become denser, fuse, and become infiltrated with polymorphonuclear leukocytes. Central necrosis of these granulomas begins in this stage, progressing to the last stage with formation of large pus-filled sinuses. This purulent material may rupture into surrounding tissue. Similar granulomas have been found in the liver and osteolytic lesions of bone when those organs are involved.

CLINICAL MANIFESTATIONS. After an incubation period of 7–12 days (range 3–30 days), one or more 3–5 mm red papules develop at the site of cutaneous inoculation, often reflecting a linear cat scratch. Because of their small size, these lesions are often overlooked but with careful search are found in at least two thirds of patients. Lymphadenopathy generally is evident within a period of 1–4 wk. Chronic regional lymphadenitis is the hallmark, affecting the first or second set of nodes draining the entry site. Affected lymph nodes in order of frequency include the axillary, cervical, submandibular, preauricular, epitrochlear, femoral, and inguinal nodes. Involvement of more than one group occurs in 10–20% of patients, although at a given site, half the cases involve several nodes.

Nodes involved are usually tender and have overlying erythema but without cellulitis. They usually range between 1–5 cm in size, although they can become much larger. Between 10–40% eventually suppurate. The duration of enlargement is usually 1–2 mo, with persistence up to 1 yr in rare cases. Fever, usually a temperature of 38–39°C, occurs in about 30% of patients. Other nonspecific symptoms including malaise, anorexia, fatigue, and headache affect less than one third of patients. Transient rashes may occur in about 5% of patients. These consist mainly of truncal maculopapular rashes; erythema nodosum, erythema multiforme and erythema annulare are also reported.

The most common atypical presentation, noted in 2–17% of patients, is Parinaud's occuloglandular syndrome, which is unilateral conjunctivitis followed by preauricular lymphadenopathy. Direct eye inoculation as a result of rubbing with the hands after cat contact is the presumed mode of spread. A conjunctival granuloma may be found at the inoculation site. The involved eye is usually not painful and has little or no discharge, but it may be quite red and swollen. Submandibular or cervical lymphadenopathy may also occur. CSD is usually a self-limited infection with spontaneous resolution within a few weeks to months.

More severe, disseminated illness occurs in a small percentage of patients. These patients present with high fever often persisting for several weeks. Although systemic symptoms are usually more pronounced than with isolated lymphadenitis, they often seem mild relative to fever, the exception being abdominal pain and weight loss, both of which can be dramatic. Hepatosplenomegaly may occur, although hepatic dysfunction is rare. Granulomatous changes may be seen in the liver and spleen. Another common site of dissemination is bone, with the development of granulomatous osteolytic lesions. These are usually associated with localized pain, without erythema, tenderness, or swelling.

DIAGNOSIS. In most cases, the diagnosis can be strongly suspected on clinical grounds with the history of exposure to a cat. Several serologic assays have been developed. The Centers for Disease Control and Prevention has developed an indirect immunofluorescent assay (IFA) that has shown good correlation with disease. Other IFA and enzyme-linked immunoassay (EIA) tests are commercially available, although little comparative data are available. Most patients have elevated antibody titers at presentation. There is cross reactivity among Bartonella species, particularly *B. henselae* and *B. quintana*.

If tissue specimens are obtained, bacilli may be visualized with Warthin-Starry and Brown-Hopp's tissue Gram stains. *Bartonella* DNA can be identified by polymerase chain reaction, but this test is not available in most hospitals. Culturing of the organism is not practical for clinical diagnosis.

Use of a skin test antigen prepared by heat-treating purulent aspirate from a CSD node is strongly discouraged because of lack of standardization and potential transmission of infectious agents.

Differential Diagnosis. The differential diagnosis of CSD includes virtually all causes of lymphadenopathy (Chapter 496). The more common entities include pyogenic lymphadenitis primarily from staphylococcal or streptococcal infections, atypical mycobacterial infections, and malignancy. less common entities include tularemia, brucellosis, or sporotrichosis. Epstein-Barr virus, cytomegalovirus, or *Toxoplasma gondii* infections usually cause more generalized lymphadenopathy.

LABORATORY FINDINGS. Routine laboratory tests are not helpful. The erythrocyte sedimentation rate is often elevated. The white blood cell count may be normal or mildly elevated. Hepatic transaminases may be elevated in systemic disease. Ultrasonography or CT may reveal many granulomatous nodules in the liver and spleen, appearing as hypodense round irregular lesions.

TREATMENT. Treatment of CSD with antibiotics is not clearly beneficial. For the majority of patients, treatment includes conservative symptomatic care and observation. Studies show a significant discordance between in vitro activity of antibiotics and clinical effectiveness. For many patients, diagnosis is considered in the context of failure to respond to β-lactam antibiotic treatment of presumed staphylococcal lymphadenitis. A small prospective study of azithromycin (500 mg on day 1, then 250 mg on days 2–5; for smaller children, 10 mg/kg/24 hr on day 1 and 5 mg/kg/24 hr day 2–5) showed a decrease in initial lymph node volume in 50% of patients during the first 30 days, but after 30 days there was no difference in lymph node volume. No other clinical benefit was found. It is clear that for the majority of patients, the disease is self-limited, with resolution occurring over weeks to months, and that treatment affords minimal, if any, clinical benefit.

Suppurative lymph nodes that become tense and extremely painful should be drained by needle aspiration, which may need to be repeated. Incision and drainage of nonsuppurative nodes should be avoided because chronic draining sinuses may result. Surgical excision of the node rarely is necessary.

COMPLICATIONS. Encephalopathy can occur in as many as 5% of patients. Typically occurring 1–3 wk after the onset of lymphadenitis is the sudden onset of neurologic symptoms, which often include seizures, combative or bizarre behavior, and altered level of consciousness. Imaging studies are generally normal. The cerebrospinal fluid is normal or shows minimal pleocytosis or protein elevation. Recovery occurs without sequelae in nearly all patients but takes place slowly over many months.

Other neurologic manifestations include myelitis, radiculitis, compression neuropathy, and cerebellar ataxia. One patient with encephalopathy with persistent cognitive impairment and memory loss has been reported.

Stellate macular retinopathy has been associated with several infections, including CSD. Children and young adults present with unilateral or rarely bilateral loss of vision with central scotoma, optic disc swelling, and macular star formation from exudates radiating out from the macula. The findings resolve completely, with recovery of vision, usually within 2–3 mo.

Hematologic manifestations include hemolytic anemia, thrombocytopenic purpura, nonthrombocytopenic purpura, and eosinophilia. Leukocytoclastic vasculitis similar to Henoch-Schönlein purpura has been reported in association with CSD in one child. A systemic presentation of CSD with pleurisy, arthralgia or arthritis, mediastinal masses, enlarged nodes at the head of the pancreas, and atypical pneumonia has also been reported.

PROGNOSIS. The prognosis for CSD in a normal host is generally excellent, with resolution of clinical findings over several months. Recovery occasionally is slower and may take as long as a year.

PREVENTION. Person-to-person spread of *Bartonella* infections is not known. Isolation is not necessary. Prevention would require elimination of cats from our households, which is not practical or necessarily desirable. Awareness of the risk of cat (and particularly kitten) scratches should be emphasized to parents.

207.3 Trench Fever (Bartonella quintana)

The causative agent of trench fever was first designated as *Rickettsia quintana*, then assigned to the genus *Rochalimaea*, and has been reassigned as *B. quintana*.

EPIDEMIOLOGY. Trench fever was first recognized as a distinct clinical entity during World War I, when more than a million troops in the trenches were infected. The disease became quiescent until World War II, when it again was epidemic. It is extremely rare in the United States.

Humans are the only known reservoir. No other animal is naturally infected, nor are the usual laboratory animals susceptible. The human body louse, *Pediculus humanus* var. *corporis*, is the vector, capable of transmission to a new host 5–6 days after feeding on an infected person. Lice excrete the organism for life; transovarian passage does not occur. Humans may have prolonged asymptomatic bacteremia for years.

CLINICAL MANIFESTATIONS. The incubation period averages about 22 days (range, 4–35 days). The clinical presentation is highly variable. Symptoms can be very mild and brief. About half of infected persons have a single febrile illness with abrupt onset lasting 3–6 days. In others, prolonged, sustained fever may occur. More commonly, patients have periodic febrile illness with three to eight episodes lasting 4–5 days each, sometimes occurring over a period of a year or more. This form is reminiscent of malaria or relapsing fever *(Borrelia recurrentis)*. Afebrile bacteremia can occur.

Clinical findings usually include fever (usually 38.5–40°C), malaise, chills, sweats, anorexia, and severe headache. Common findings include marked conjunctival injection, tachycardia, myalgias, arthralgias, and severe pain in the neck, back, and legs. Crops of erythematous macules or papules may occur or the trunk in as many as 80% of patients. Splenomegaly and mild liver enlargement may be noted.

DIAGNOSIS. In nonepidemic situations, it is impossible to establish a diagnosis of trench fever on clinical grounds because the findings are not distinctive. A history of body louse infection or having been in an area of epidemic disease should heighten suspicions. *B. quintana* can be cultured from the blood with modification to include culture on epithelial cells. *Serologic* tests for *B. quintana* are available, but there is cross reaction with *B. henselae*.

TREATMENT. There are no controlled trials of treatment; however, patients with trench fever have responded dramatically to tetracycline and chloramphenicol with rapid defervescence.

207.4 Bacillary Angiomatosis and Bacillary Peliosis Hepatis (Bartonella henselae *and* Bartonella quintana)

Both *B. henselae* and *B. quintana* cause two vascular proliferative diseases, bacillary angiomatosis and bacillary peliosis, in severely immunocompromised persons, primarily adult patients with AIDS or cancer and organ transplant recipients. Subcutaneous and lytic bone lesions are strongly associated with *B. quintana*, whereas peliosis hepatis is associated exclusively with *B. henselae*.

Bacillary Angiomatosis. Lesions of cutaneous bacillary angiomatosis (BA), also known as epithelioid angiomatosis, are the most easily identified and recognized form of *Bartonella* infection in immunocompromised hosts. They are found primarily in patients with AIDS with very low CD4+ counts. The clinical appearance can be quite diverse. The vasoproliferative lesions of BA may be cutaneous or subcutaneous and resemble the vascular lesions (verruca peruana) of *B. bacilliformis* in immunocompetent persons. They are erythematous papules on an erythematous base with a collarette of scale. They may enlarge to form large pedunculated lesions. Ulceration may occur, as can profuse bleeding after trauma.

BA may be clinically indistinguishable form Kaposi's sarcoma. Other considerations in the differential diagnosis are pyogenic granuloma and verruca peruana *(B. bacilliformis)*. Deep soft tissue masses caused by BA may mimic a malignancy.

Osseous BA lesions commonly involve the long bones. These lytic lesions are very painful and highly vascular. Occasionally found is an erythematous plaque over the lesion. The high degree of vascularity, which produces a very positive result on a technetium-99m methylene diphosphonate bone scan, resembles a malignant lesion.

Lesions can be found in virtually any organ, producing similar vascular proliferative lesions. They may appear raised, nodular, or ulcerative when seen on endoscopy or bronchoscopy. They may be associated with enlarged lymph nodes with or without an obvious local cutaneous lesion. Lesions in one brain parenchyma have been described.

Bacillary Peliosis. Bacillary peliosis affects the reticuloendothelial system, primarily the liver (peliosis hepatis) and less frequently the spleen and lymph nodes. It is a vasoproliferative disorder characterized by random proliferation of venous lakes surrounded by fibromyxoid stroma harboring numerous bacillary organisms. Clinical findings include fever and abdominal pain in association with abnormal results of liver function tests, particularly a markedly increased alkaline phosphatase level. Cutaneous BA or splenomegaly may be associated, with or without thrombocytopenia or pancytopenia. The vascular proliferative lesions in the liver and spleen appear on CT scan as hypodense lesions scattered throughout the parenchyma. The differential diagnosis includes hepatic Kaposi's sarcoma, lymphoma, and disseminated infection with *Pneumocystis carinii* or *Mycobacterium avium* complex.

Bacteremia and Endocarditis. *B. henselae*, *B. quintana*, and *B. elizabethae* all have been reported to cause bacteremia or endocarditis. They are associated with symptoms of prolonged fevers, night sweats, and profound weight loss. A cluster of cases in Seattle in 1993 occurred in a homeless population with chronic alcoholism. These patients with high fever or hypothermia were thought to represent "urban trench fever," but no body louse infestation was associated. Some cases of culture-negative endocarditis may represent *Bartonella* endocarditis. One report described central nervous system involvement with *B. quintana* in two children.

DIAGNOSIS. Diagnosis of bacillary angiomatosis is made initially by biopsy. The characteristic small vessel proliferation with mixed inflammatory response and the staining of bacilli by Warthin-Starry silver staining distinguish it from Kaposi's sarcoma or pyogenic granuloma. Travel history can usually preclude verruca peruana.

Culture is impractical for CSD but is the diagnostic procedure for suspected bacteremia or endocarditis. The use of lysis-centrifugation technique or fresh chocolate or heart infusion agar with 5% rabbit blood with prolonged incubation may increase the yield of culture.

TREATMENT. *Bartonella* infections in immunocompromised hosts caused by both *B. henselae* and *B. quintana* have been treated successfully with antimicrobial agents. Rigorous studies have not been published; thus, therapy is guided by clinical experience. BA responds rapidly to erythromycin or to macrolides, azithromycin or clarithromycin, which are the drugs of choice. An alternative choice is doxycycline or tetracycline. Severely ill patients with peliosis hepatis, endocarditis, or osteomyelitis may be treated initially with intravenous erythromycin or doxycycline with the addition of rifampin or gentamicin. A Jarisch-Herxheimer reaction may occur. Relapses may follow; prolonged treatment for several months may be necessary.

PREVENTION. Immunocompromised persons should consider the potential risks of cat ownership because of the risks of *Bartonella* infections, as well as toxoplasmosis and enteric infections. Those who elect to obtain a cat should try to adopt or purchase a cat older than 1 yr and in good health.

Adal KA, Cockerell CJ, Petri WA: Cat scratch disease, bacillary angiomatosis and other infections due to *Rochalimaea*. N Engl J Med 330:1509, 1994.

Anderson BE, Newman NA: *Bartonella* spp. as emerging human pathogens. Clin Microbiol Rev 10:203, 1997.

Baoto E, Payne M, Slater LN, et al: Culture-negative endocarditis caused by *Bartonella henselae*. J Pediatr 132:1051, 1998.

Bass JW, Freitas BC, Freitas AD, et al: Prospective randomized double blind placebo-controlled evaluation of azithromycin for treatment of cat-scratch disease. Pediatr Infect Dis J 17;447, 1998.

Bass JW, Vincent JM, Person DA: The expanding spectrum of *Bartonella* infections: I Bartonellosis and trench fever. Pediatr Infect Dis J 16:2, 1997.

Bass JW, Vincent JM, Person DA: The expanding spectrum of *Bartonella* infections: II cat scratch disease. Pediatr Infect Dis J 16:163, 1997.

Carithers HA: Cat scratch disease an overview based on a study of 1,200 patients. Am J Dis Child 139:1124, 1985.

Carithers HA, Margileth Am: Cat scratch disease: Acute encephalopathy and other neurologic manifestations. Am J Dis Child 145:98, 1991.

Dunn MW, Berkowitz FE, Miller JJ, et al: Hepatosplenic cat-scratch disease and abdominal pain. Pediatr Infect Dis J 16:269, 1997.

Gray GC, Johnson AA, Thornton SA, et al: An epidemic of Oroyo fever in the Peruvian Andes. Am J Trop Hyg 42:215, 1990.

Jacobs R, Schutze G: *Bartonella henselae* as a cause of prolonged fever and fever of unknown origin in children. Clin Infect Dis 26:80, 1998.

Koehler JE, Sanchez MA, Garrido CS, et al: Molecular epidemiology of *Bartonella* infections in patients with bacillary angiomatosis-peliosis. N Engl J Med 337:1876, 1997.

Ricketts WE: Clinical manifestations of Carrion's disease. Arch Intern Med 84:751, 1949.

Szelc-Kelly CM, Goral S, Perez-Perez GI, et al: Serologic responses to *Bartonella* and *Afipia* antigens in patients with cat scratch disease. Pediatrics 96;1137, 1995.

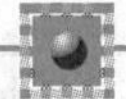

SECTION 5

Anaerobic Bacterial Infections

CHAPTER 208

*Botulism**

Robert Schechter and Stephen S. Arnon

Botulism is the acute, flaccid paralytic illness caused by the neurotoxin produced by *Clostridium botulinum* or, rarely, an equivalent neurotoxin produced by unique strains of *C. butyricum* and *C. baratii*. Three forms of human botulism are known: infant botulism (the most common in the United States), food-borne (classic) botulism, and wound botulism.

ETIOLOGY. *Clostridium botulinum* is a gram-positive, spore-forming obligate anaerobe whose natural habitat worldwide is soil, dust, and marine sediments. It is found in a wide variety of fresh and cooked agricultural products. Spores of some *C. botulinum* strains survive boiling for several hours, which enables the organism to survive human efforts at food preservation. In contrast, botulinum toxin is heat labile and easily destroyed by heating at 80°C or higher for 10 min. Little is known about the ecology of neurotoxigenic strains of *C. butyricum* and *C. baratii*.

Botulinum toxin is the most poisonous substance known, the parenteral human lethal dose being estimated at 10^{-7} mg/kg. The toxin blocks neuromuscular transmission and causes death through airway and respiratory muscle paralysis. Seven antigenic toxin types, assigned the letters A–G, are distinguished by the inability of protective (neutralizing) antibody against one toxin type to protect against a different type. The seven toxin types serve as convenient clinical and epidemiologic markers. Neurotoxigenic *C. butyricum* strains produce a type E toxin, whereas neurotoxigenic *C. baratii* strains produce a type F toxin. Toxin types A, B, E, and F are well-established causes of human botulism, whereas types C and D cause illness in other animals. Type G has not been established as a cause of either human or animal disease.

Botulinum toxin is a simple di-chain protein consisting of a 100 kd heavy chain that contains the neuronal attachment sites and a 50 kd light chain that is taken into the cell after binding. The phenomenal potency of botulinum toxin is explained by the fact that its seven light chains are Zn^{2+}-endopeptidases, whose substrates are one or two of three protein components of the docking complex by which synaptic vesicles fuse with the terminal cell membrane and release acetylcholine into the synaptic cleft.

EPIDEMIOLOGY. *Infant botulism* has been reported from all inhabited continents except Africa. Notably, the infant is the only family member ill. The most striking epidemiologic feature of infant botulism is its age distribution, in which in 95% of cases the infants are between 3 wk and 6 mo of age, with a broad peak between 2–4 mo of age. This pattern is matched only by one other condition, the sudden infant death syndrome. However, cases in infants as young as 3 days or as old as 382 days at onset have been reported. The male:female ratio of cases is essentially 1:1, and cases have occurred in all major racial and ethnic groups.

Infant botulism is an uncommon and often unrecognized illness. In the United States 75–100 cases are diagnosed annually; 1,448 cases were reported from 1976 to 1996. Almost half of U.S. cases were reported from California. Consistent with the known asymmetry of the soil distribution of toxin types of *C. botulinum*, most cases west of the Mississippi River have been caused by type A strains, whereas most cases east of it have been caused by type B strains. One case each in the states of New Mexico and Washington resulted from *C. baratii* and type F toxin, whereas cases in Italy resulted from *C. butyricum* and type E toxin. Identified risk factors for the illness include the ingestion of honey and a slow intestinal transit time (less than one stool per day). Breast-feeding appears to provide protection against fulminant, sudden death from infant botulism. Under rare circumstances of altered intestinal anatomy, physiology, and microflora, older children and adults may contract infant-type botulism.

Food-borne botulism results from the ingestion of a food in which *C. botulinum* has multiplied and produced its toxin. Recent outbreaks in North America associated with restaurants in which foods such as baked potatoes, sautéed onions, and chopped garlic were implicated have revised the traditional view of food-borne botulism as resulting mainly from home-canned foods. Other U.S. outbreaks have occurred from commercial foods sealed in plastic pouches that relied solely on refrigeration to prevent outgrowth of *C. botulinum* spores. Non-canned foods responsible for recent food-borne botulism episodes include peyote tea, the hazelnut flavoring added to yogurt, sweet cream cheese, sautéed onions in "patty melt" sandwiches, potato salad, and fresh and dried fish. A recent trend toward a single case per outbreak or of cases presenting separately in different cities or hospitals has meant that the physician cannot rely on the temporal and geographic clustering of illness (often in a family) to suggest the diagnosis.

Most preserved foods have been implicated in food-borne botulism, but the usual offenders in the United States are the "low-acid" (pH 6.0 and above) home-canned foods such as jalapẽno peppers, asparagus, olives, and beans. The potential for foodborne botulism exists throughout the world, but outbreaks occur most commonly in the temperate zones rather than the tropics, where preservation of fruits, vegetables, and other foods is less common.

In the past 10 yr, approximately 250 cases of food-borne botulism from about 150 outbreaks have occurred in the United States. Most of the continental U.S. outbreaks resulted from either proteolytic type A or type B strains, which produce a strongly putrefactive odor in the food that some people find necessary to verify by tasting. In contrast, in Alaska and Canada most food-borne outbreaks have resulted from nonproteolytic type E strains in Native American foods, such as fermented salmon eggs and seal flippers, that do not exhibit signs of spoilage. A further hazard of type E strains is their ability to grow at temperatures as low as 5°C, the temperature of household refrigerators.

Wound botulism is an exceptionally rare disease, with fewer than 200 cases reported worldwide, but it is important to pediatrics because adolescents and children are disproportionately affected. Many cases have occurred in young, physically active males at greatest risk of traumatic injury, but wound botulism also occurs with crush injuries in which no break in

*All material in this chapter is in the public domain, with the exception of any borrowed figures or tables.

the skin is evident. In the last 10 yr wound botulism from injection has become increasingly common in adult drug (heroin) abusers in the western United States, not always with evident abscess formation.

PATHOGENESIS. All three forms of botulism produce disease through a final common pathway: botulinum toxin is carried by the bloodstream to peripheral cholinergic synapses, where it binds irreversibly, blocking acetylcholine release and causing impaired neuromuscular and autonomic transmission. *Infant botulism* is an infectious disease that results from ingesting the spores of any of the three botulinum toxin–producing clostridial strains, with subsequent spore germination, multiplication, and production of botulinum toxin in the large intestine. *Food-borne botulism* is an intoxication that results when preformed botulinum toxin contained in an improperly preserved or cooked food is swallowed. *Wound botulism* results from spore germination and colonization of traumatized tissue by *C. botulinum*; it is the analog of tetanus.

Because botulinum toxin is not a cytotoxin, it causes no overt macroscopic or microscopic pathology. However, secondary pathologic changes (e.g., pneumonia, petechiae on intrathoracic organs) may be found at autopsy. No diagnostic technique is available to identify botulinum toxin bound at the neuromuscular junction. The healing process in botulism consists of sprouting of new terminal unmyelinated motor neurons. Movement resumes when these new twigs locate noncontracting muscle fibers and reinnervate them by inducing formation of a new motor end-plate. In experimental animals this process takes about 4 wk.

CLINICAL MANIFESTATIONS. Botulinum toxin is distributed hematogenously. Because relative blood flow and density of innervation are greatest in the bulbar musculature, all three forms of botulism manifest neurologically as a symmetric, descending flaccid paralysis of the cranial nerve musculature. *It is not possible to have botulism without having multiple bulbar palsies*, yet in infants such symptoms as poor feeding, weak suck, feeble cry, drooling, and even obstructive apnea are often not recognized as bulbar in origin. Patients with evolving illness may already have generalized weakness and hypotonia in addition to bulbar palsies when first seen.

In older children with food-borne or wound botulism, the onset of neurologic symptoms follows a characteristic pattern of diplopia, blurred vision, ptosis, dry mouth, dysphagia, dysphonia, and dysarthria, with deceased gag and corneal reflexes. Importantly, because the toxin acts only on motor nerves, paresthesias are not seen in botulism, except when a patient hyperventilates from anxiety. The sensorium remains clear, but this may be difficult to ascertain because of the slurred speech.

Food-borne botulism begins with gastrointestinal symptoms of nausea, vomiting, or diarrhea in about one third of cases. These symptoms are thought to result from metabolic byproducts of growth of *C. botulinum* or from the presence of other toxic contaminants in the food, because gastrointestinal distress is not seen in wound botulism. Constipation is common in food-borne botulism once flaccid paralysis becomes evident. Illness usually begins 18–36 hr after ingestion of the contaminated food but can range from as little as 2 hr to as long as 8 days. The incubation period in wound botulism is 4–14 days. Fever may be present in wound botulism but is absent in food-borne botulism unless a secondary infection (e.g., pneumonia) is present. All three forms of botulism display a wide spectrum in their clinical severity, from the very mild with minimal ptosis, flattened facial expression, minor dysphagia, and dysphonia to the fulminant, with rapid onset of extensive paralysis, respiratory distress, and frank apnea. *Fatigability with repetitive muscle activity is the clinical hallmark of botulism.*

Infant botulism differs in apparent initial symptoms of illness only because the infant cannot verbalize them. Usually, the first indication of illness is a decreased frequency or even abscence of defecation, although this sign is frequently overlooked. Parents typically notice inability to feed, lethargy, listlessness, weak cry, and diminished spontaneous movement. Dysphagia may be evident as secretions drooling from the mouth. Gag, suck, and corneal reflexes diminish as the paralysis advances. Oculomotor palsies may be evident only with sustained observation. Paradoxically, the pupillary light reflex may be unaffected until the child is severely paralyzed, or it may be initially sluggish. Loss of head control is typically a prominent sign. Respiratory arrest may occur suddenly from airway occlusion by unswallowed secretions or from obstructive flaccid pharyngeal musculature. Occasionally, the diagnosis of infant botulism is suggested by a respiratory arrest that occurs after the infant is curled into position for lumbar puncture.

In mild cases or in the early stages of illness, the physical signs of infant botulism may be subtle and easily missed. Eliciting cranial nerve palsies and fatigability of muscular function requires careful examination. Ptosis may not be seen unless the head of the child is kept erect. The presence of decreased anal sphincter tone may suggest a generalized neuromuscular disease.

DIAGNOSIS. The classic picture of botulism is the acute onset of a flaccid descending paralysis with clear sensorium, no fever, and no paresthesias. The rarity of foodborne and wound botulism makes them easily confused with other diseases (Table 208–1). Routine laboratory studies, including those of the cerebrospinal fluid (CSF), are normal in botulism unless dehydration or starvation ketosis are present. Electromyography (EMG) may demonstrate a defect in neuromuscular transmission, and the distinctive EMG finding in food-borne and wound botulism is facilitation (potentiation) of the evoked muscle action potential at high-frequency (50 Hz) stimulation. In infant botulism a characteristic pattern, known by the acronym BSAP (*b*rief, *s*mall, *a*bundant motor-unit action *p*otentials), is present only in clinically weak muscles. Nerve conduction velocity and sensory nerve function are normal in botulism.

Food-borne and wound botulism are often difficult to distinguish from myasthenia gravis and Guillain-Barré syndrome (GBS). The edrophonium (Tensilon) test helps with the former, and a lumbar puncture helps with the latter. In GBS, CSF protein concentration usually has become elevated and nerve conduction velocity has slowed by 4–6 wk after onset. Paresthesias are common in GBS. Possible organophosphate intoxication should be pursued aggressively because a specific antidote (PAM) is available and because the patient may be part of a commonly exposed group, some of whom have yet to develop illness.

Infant botulism requires a high index of suspicion for early diagnosis (Table 208–2). Even today, >20 yr after its recognition, "rule-out sepsis" is the most common admission diagnosis. If a previously healthy infant, usually 2–4 mo of age, develops weakness with difficulty in sucking, swallowing, crying, or breathing, infant botulism should be considered a likely diagnosis. A careful cranial nerve examination is then quite helpful.

The diagnosis of botulism is unequivocally established by

TABLE 208–1 Differential Diagnoses of Food-borne and Wound Botulism

Acute gastroenteritis	Aminoglycoside-associated paralysis
Myasthenia gravis	Tick paralysis
Guillain-Barré syndrome	Hypocalcemia
Organophosphate poisoning	Hypermagnesemia
Meningitis	Carbon monoxide poisoning
Encephalitis	Hyperemesis gravidarum
Psychiatric illness	Laryngeal trauma
Cerebrovascular accident	Diabetic complications
Poliomyelitis	Inflammatory myopathy
Hypothyroidism	Overexertion

TABLE 208–2 Differential Diagnosis of Infant Botulism

Admission Diagnosis	Common Subsequent Diagnoses
Suspected sepsis	Guillain-Barré syndrome
Pneumonia	Myasthenia gravis
Dehydration	Disorders of amino acid metabolism
Viral syndrome	Hypothyroidism
Hypotonia of unknown etiology	Drug ingestion
Constipation	Brain stem encephalitis
Failure to thrive	Heavy metal poisoning (Pb, Mg, As)
Werdnig-Hoffmann disease	Poliomyelitis
	Viral polyneuritis
	Hirschsprung's disease
	Metabolic encephalopathy
	Medium chain acetyl-CoA dehydrogenase (MCAD) deficiency

demonstrating the presence of botulinum toxin in serum or of *C. botulinum* toxin or organisms in wound material or feces. *C. botulinum* is not part of the normal resident intestinal flora of humans, and its presence in the setting of acute flaccid paralysis is diagnostic. State health departments (first call) and the Centers for Disease Contol and Prevention (second call; phone: 404-639-2206 workdays and 404-639-2888 at other times) can arrange for specimen testing, epidemiologic investigation, and provision of equine antitoxin. *Suspected botulism represents a medical and public health emergency that is immediately reportable in virtually all U.S. health jurisdictions.* An epidemiologic diagnosis of food-borne botulism can be made when *C. botulinum* organisms and toxin are found in food eaten by patients.

TREATMENT. Management of botulism rests on three principles: (1) fatigability with repetitive muscle activity is the clinical hallmark of the disease; (2) complications are best avoided by anticipating them; and (3) meticulous supportive care is a necessity. The first principle applies mainly to feeding and breathing. Correct positioning is imperative to protect the airway and improve respiratory mechanics. The patient is placed face up on a *rigid-bottomed crib* (or bed), the head of which is tilted at 30 degrees. A small cloth roll is placed under the cervical vertebrae to tilt the head back so that secretions drain to the posterior pharynx and away from the airway. In this tilted position the abdominal viscera pull the diaphragm down, thereby improving respiratory mechanics. The patient's head and torso should not be elevated by bending the middle of the bed; if this is done, the hypotonic thorax will slump into the abdomen and breathing will be compromised.

About one half of patients will require endotracheal intubation, which is best done prophylactically. The indications include diminished gag and cough reflexes and progressive airway obstruction by secretions. With meticulous management technique (especially proper tube diameter), monitoring, and positioning, patients have tolerated months of intubation without subglottic stenosis or need for tracheostomy.

Feeding should be done by a nasogastric or nasojejunal tube until sufficient oropharyngeal strength and coordination enables feeding by breast or bottle. Expressed breast milk is the most desirable food, in part because of its immunologic components (sIgA, lactoferrin, leukocytes). Tube feeding also assists in the restoration of peristalsis, a nonspecific but probably essential part of eliminating *C. botulinum* from the intestinal flora. Intravenous feeding (hyperalimentation) is discouraged because of the potential for infection and the advantages to tube feeding.

Antibiotic therapy is not part of the treatment of uncomplicated infant or foodborne botulism because the toxin is primarily an intracellular molecule that is released into the intestinal lumen with vegetative bacterial cell death and lysis. Antibiotics are reserved for the treatment of secondary infections, and in the absence of antibody therapy a nonclostridiocidal antibiotic such as trimethoprim/sulfamethoxazole is preferred. Aminoglycoside antibiotics should be avoided because they may potentiate the blocking action of botulinum toxin at the neuromuscular junction. However, wound botulism requires aggressive treatment with antibiotics and antitoxin in a manner analogous to tetanus (see Chapter 209). The currently licensed botulinum antitoxin used in foodborne and wound botulism is a horse serum–derived product that has side effects of serum sickness, anaphylaxis, and potential lifelong sensitization to equine proteins; its use in children requires careful consideration.

Specific treatment for infant botulism is now available. In California a recently completed 5-year, randomized, double-blind, placebo-controlled treatment trial demonstrated the apparent safety and efficacy of human-derived botulinum antitoxin, formally known as botulism immune globulin (BIG). Use of BIG reduced mean hospital stay from approximately 5.5 weeks to approximately 2.5 weeks and reduced mean hospitalization cost by approximately $70,000. Treatment with BIG should be started as early in the illness as possible. In the United States, BIG may be obtained from the California Department of Health Services (24-hour telephone: 510-540-2646) under a U.S. Food and Drug Administration–approved investigational new drug (IND) protocol.

Because sensation remains intact, providing auditory, tactile, and visual stimuli is beneficial. Maintaining strong central respiratory drive is essential, so sedatives or central nervous system depressants (e.g., metoclopramide [Reglan]) are contraindicated. Full hydration and stool softeners may mitigate the protracted constipation. Cathartics are not recommended. Patients with foodborne and infant botulism excrete *C. botulinum* toxin and organisms in their feces, often for weeks, and care should be taken in handling their excreta. When bladder palsy occurs, gentle suprapubic pressure with the patient in the sitting position with the head supported may help attain complete voiding and reduce the risk of urinary tract infection.

COMPLICATIONS. Avoidance of complications is best accomplished by noting past experience (Table 208–3). Even so, some critically ill, paralyzed patients who must spend weeks or months on ventilators in intensive care units will inevitably develop complications. All of the complications listed in Table 208–3 were nosocomially acquired; some of them were iatrogenic. Infant botulism does not have a relapsing course, and suspected "relapses" usually reflect premature hospital discharge, an undiscovered underlying complication, such as pneumonia, or perhaps additional toxemia.

PROGNOSIS. In the absence of complications, particularly those related to hypoxia, the prognosis in infant botulism is for full and complete recovery. Hospital stay in infant botulism averages approximately 1 mo but differs significantly by toxin type, with type B cases being hospitalized a mean of 3.7 wk and type A cases 5.6 wk. When the regenerating nerve endings have induced formation of a new motor end-plate, neuromuscular transmission is restored. In the United States, the case-fatality ratio for hospitalized infant botulism is <1%. The case-fatality ratio in foodborne and wound botulism varies by age, with younger patients having the best prognosis. Some adults with botulism have reported chronic weakness and fatigue as sequelae. After recovery, infant botulism patients appear to

TABLE 208–3 Complications of Infant Botulism

Adult respiratory distress syndrome	Recurrent atelectasis
Aspiration	Seizures secondary to hyponatremia
Fracture of the femur	Sepsis
Inappropriate antidiuretic hormone secretion	Tension pneumothorax
Misplaced or plugged endotracheal tube	Transfusion reaction
Clostridium difficile enterocolitis	Urinary tract infection
Otitis media	Subglottic stenosis
Pneumonia	Tracheal granuloma
	Tracheitis

have an increased incidence of strabismus that requires timely screening and treatment.

PREVENTION. Food-borne botulism is best prevented by adhering to safe methods of home canning (pressure cooker and acidification), by avoiding suspicious foods, and by heating all homecanned foods to 80°C for at least 5 min. Wound botulism is best prevented by thorough cleansing and surgical debridement of contaminated traumatic injuries with provision of appropriate antibiotics and by not using illicit drugs.

Most infant botulism patients probably inhale and then swallow airborne clostridial spores; these cases are unpreventable. The one identified, avoidable source of botulinum spores for infants in *honey*. Honey is an unsafe food for any child younger than 1 yr old. Corn syrups were once thought to be a possible source of botulinum spores, but recent evidence indicates otherwise. Breast-feeding appears to slow the onset of infant botulism and to diminish the risk of sudden death in infants in whom the disease develops.

Arnon SS: Infant botulism: Anticipating the second decade. J Infect Dis 154:201, 1986.

Arnon SS, Damus K, Chin J: Infant botulism: Epidemiology and relation to sudden infant death syndrome. Epidemiol Rev 3:45, 1981.

Arnon SS, Damus K, Thompson B, et al: Protective role of human milk against sudden death from infant botulism. J Pediatr 100:568, 1982.

Arnon SS, Werner SB, Faber HK, Farr WH: Infant botulism in 1931: Discovery of a misclassified case. Am J Dis Child 133:580, 1979.

Aureli P, Fenicia L, Pasolini B, et al: Two cases of type E infant botulism in Italy caused by neurotoxigenic *Clostridium butyricum*. J Infect Dis 54:207, 1986.

Hurst DL, Marsh WW: Early severe infantile botulism. J Pediatr 122:909, 1993.

Long SS: Epidemiologic study of infant botulism in Pennsylvania: Report of the infant botulism study group. J Pediatr 75:928, 1985.

Long SS, Gajeweski JL, Brown LW, Gilligan PH: Clinical, laboratory, and environmental features of infant botulism in southeastern Pennsylvania. Pediatrics 75:935, 1985.

Montecucco C, Schiavo G: Tetanus and botulism neurotoxins: A new group of zinc proteases. Trends Biochem Sci 18:324, 1993.

Paisley JW, Lauer BA, Arnon SS: A second case of infant botulism type F caused by *Clostridium baratii*. Pediatr Infect Dis J 14:912, 1995.

Passaro DJ, Werner SB, McGee J, et al: Wound botulism associated with black tar heroin among injecting drug users. JAMA 279:859, 1998.

Schreiner MS, Field E, Ruddy R: Infant botulism: A review of 12 years' experience at the Children's Hospital of Philadelphia. Pediatrics 87:159, 1991.

Shapiro RL, Hatheway C, Swerdlow DL: Botulism in the United States: A clinical and epidemiological review. Ann Intern Med 129:221, 1998.

Smith LDS, Sugiyama H: Botulism: The Organism, its Toxins, the Disease, 2nd ed. Springfield, IL, Charles C. Thomas, 1988.

Thilo EH, Townsend SF, Deacon J: Infant botulism at 1 week of age: Report of two cases. Pediatrics 92:151, 1993.

Weber JT, Goodpasture HC, Alexander H, et al: Wound botulism in a patient with a tooth abscess: Case report and review. Clin Infect Dis 16:635, 1993.

Woodruff BA, Griffin PM, McCroskey LM, et al: Clinical and laboratory comparisons of botulism from toxin types A, B, and E in the United States, 1975–88. J Infect Dis 166:1281, 1992.

CHAPTER 209
Tetanus*

Stephen S. Arnon

Tetanus (lockjaw) is an acute, spastic paralytic illness caused by tetanus toxin (tetanospasmin), the neurotoxin produced by *Clostridium tetani*.

ETIOLOGY. *C. tetani* is a motile, gram-positive, spore-forming obligate anaerobe whose natural habitat worldwide is soil, dust, and the alimentary tracts of various animals. It forms spores terminally, thus producing a drumstick or tennis racket appearance microscopically. Tetanus spores can survive boiling but not autoclaving, whereas the vegetative cells are killed by antibiotics, heat, and standard disinfectants. Unlike many clostridia, *C. tetani* is not a tissue-invasive organism; instead it causes illness through the effects of a single toxin, tetanospasmin, more commonly referred to as tetanus toxin. Tetanus toxin is the second most poisonous substance known, being surpassed in potency only by botulinum toxin; the human lethal dose of tetanus toxin is estimated to be 10^{-6} mg/kg.

EPIDEMIOLOGY. Tetanus occurs worldwide and is endemic in 90 developing countries, but its incidence varies considerably. The most common form, neonatal (umbilical) tetanus, kills approximately 500,000 infants each year because the mother was not immunized; about 80% of these deaths occur in just 12 tropical Asian and African countries. In addition, an estimated 15,000–30,000 unimmunized women worldwide die each year from maternal tetanus that results from postpartum, postabortal, or postsurgical wound infection with *C. tetani*. Approximately 50 cases of tetanus are reported each year in the United States, mostly in persons age 60 yr or older, but toddler-aged and neonatal cases also occur. One fifth of children in the United States aged 10–16 yr lack a protective antibody level.

Most non-neonatal cases of tetanus are associated with a traumatic injury, often a penetrating wound inflicted by a dirty object, such as a nail, splinter, fragment of glass or unsterile injection, but a rare case may have no history of trauma. Tetanus occurring after illicit drug injection is becoming more common, whereas uncommon settings include animal bites, abscesses (including dental abscesses), ear piercing, chronic skin ulceration, burns, compound fractures, frostbite, gangrene, intestinal surgery, ritual scarification, and female circumcision. The disease also occurs after the use of contaminated suture material or after intramuscular injection of medicines, most notably quinine for chloroquine-resistant falciparum malaria.

PATHOGENESIS. Tetanus occurs after introduced spores germinate, multiply, and produce tetanus toxin in the low oxidation-reduction potential (E_h) of an infected injury site. A plasmid carries the toxin gene; the toxin is released with vegetative bacterial cell death and subsequent lysis. Tetanus toxins (and the botulinum toxins) are 150 kd simple proteins consisting of a heavy (100 kd) and a light (50 kd) chain joined by a single disulfide bond. Tetanus toxin binds at the neuromuscular junction and is then endocytosed by the motor nerve, after which it undergoes retrograde axonal transport to the cytoplasm of the alpha-motoneuron. In the sciatic nerve the transport rate was found to be 3.4 mm/hr. The toxin exits the motoneuron in the spinal cord and next enters adjacent, spinal inhibitory interneurons, where it prevents neurotransmitter release. Tetanus toxin thus blocks the normal inhibition of antagonistic muscles that is the basis of voluntary coordinated movement; in consequence, affected muscles sustain maximal contraction. The autonomic nervous system is also rendered unstable in tetanus.

The phenomenal potency of tetanus toxin is enzymatic in nature. The light chain of tetanus toxin (and of several of the botulinum toxins) is a Zn^{2+}-containing endoprotease whose substrate is synaptobrevin, a constituent protein of the docking complex that enables the synaptic vesicle to fuse with the terminal cell membrane. The heavy chain of the toxin contains its binding domain.

C. tetani is not an invasive organism and its toxin-producing vegetative cells remain where introduced into the wound, which may or may not display local inflammatory changes and a mixed infectious flora.

CLINICAL MANIFESTATIONS. Tetanus may be either localized or generalized, the latter being more common. The incubation period typically is 2–14 days, but it may be as long as months after the injury. In *generalized tetanus*, trismus (masseter muscle spasm, or "lockjaw") is the presenting symptom in about half

*All material in this chapter is in the public domain, with the exception of any borrowed figures or tables.

the cases. Headache, restlessness, and irritability are early symptoms, often followed by stiffness, difficulty chewing, dysphagia, and neck muscle spasm. The so-called sardonic smile of tetanus (risus sardonicus) results from intractable spasm of facial and buccal muscles. When the paralysis extends to abdominal, lumbar, hip, and thigh muscles, the patient may assume an arched posture, opisthotonos, in which only the back of the head and the heels touch ground. Opisthotonos is an equilibrium position that results from unrelenting total contraction of opposing muscles, all of which display the typical "boardlike" rigidity of tetanus. Laryngeal and respiratory muscle spasm can lead to airway obstruction and asphyxiation. Because tetanus toxin does not affect sensory nerves or cortical function, the patient unfortunately remains conscious, in extreme pain, and in fearful anticipation of the next tetanic seizure. These seizures are characterized by sudden, severe tonic contractions of the muscles, with fist clenching, flexion, and adduction of the arms and hyperextension of the legs. Without treatment, the seizures range from a few seconds to a few minutes in length with intervening respite periods, but as the illness progresses the spasms become sustained and exhausting. The smallest disturbance by sight, sound, or touch may trigger a tetanic spasm. Dysuria and urinary retention result from bladder sphincter spasm; forced defecation may occur. Fever, occasionally with a temperature as high as 40°C, is common because of the substantial metabolic energy consumed by spastic muscles. Notable autonomic effects include tachycardia, arrhythmias, labile hypertension, diaphoresis, and cutaneous vasoconstriction. The tetanic paralysis usually becomes more severe in the 1st wk after onset, stabilizes in the 2nd wk, and ameliorates gradually over the ensuing 1–4 wk.

Neonatal tetanus (tetanus neonatorum), the infantile form of generalized tetanus, typically manifests within 3–12 days of birth as progressive difficulty in feeding (i.e., sucking and swallowing), with associated hunger and crying. Paralysis or diminished movement, stiffness to the touch, and spasms, with or without opisthotonos, characterize the disease. The umbilical stump may hold remnants of dirt, dung, clotted blood or serum, or it may appear relatively benign.

Localized tetanus results in painful spasms of the muscles adjacent to the wound site and may precede generalized tetanus. *Cephalic tetanus* is a rare form of localized tetanus involving the bulbar musculature that occurs with wounds or foreign bodies in the head, nostrils, or face. It also occurs in association with chronic otitis media. Cephalic tetanus is characterized by retracted eyelids, deviated gaze, trismus, risus sardonicus, and spastic paralysis of tongue and pharyngeal musculature.

DIAGNOSIS. The picture of tetanus is one of the most dramatic in medicine, and the diagnosis may be made clinically. The typical setting is an unimmunized patient (and/or mother) who was injured or born within the preceding 2 wk and who presents with trismus, other rigid muscles, and a clear sensorium.

Regular laboratory studies are usually normal. A peripheral leukocytosis may result from a secondary bacterial infection of the wound or may be stress induced from the sustained tetanic spasms. The cerebrospinal fluid (CSF) is normal, although the intense muscle contractions may raise its pressure. Neither the electroencephalogram nor the electromyogram show a characteristic pattern. *C. tetani* is not always visible on Gram stain of wound material, and it is isolated in only about one third of cases.

Fully developed, generalized tetanus cannot be mistaken for any other disease. However, trismus may result from parapharyngeal, retropharyngeal, or dental abscesses, or rarely, from acute encephalitis involving the brain stem. Either rabies or tetanus may follow an animal bite, and rabies may present as trismus with seizures. However, rabies may be distinguished from tetanus by its hydrophobia, marked dysphagia, predominantly clonic seizures, and CSF pleocytosis. Although strychnine poisoning may result in tonic muscle spasms and generalized seizure activity, it seldom produces trismus, and unlike tetanus general relaxation usually occurs between spasms. Hypocalcemia may produce *tetany,* characterized by laryngeal and carpopedal spasms, but trismus will be absent. Occasionally, epileptic seizures, narcotic withdrawal, or other drug reactions may suggest tetanus.

TREATMENT. Management of tetanus requires eradication of *C. tetani* and the wound environment conducive to its anaerobic multiplication, neutralization of all accessible tetanus toxin, control of seizures and respiration, palliation and provision of meticulous supportive care, and, finally, prevention of recurrences.

Surgical wound excision and debridement is often needed to remove the foreign body or devitalized tissue that created anaerobic growth conditions. Surgery should be done promptly, after the administration of human tetanus immune globulin (TIG) and antibiotics. Excision of the umbilical stump in neonatal tetanus is no longer recommended.

Once tetanus toxin has begun its axonal ascent to the spinal cord it cannot be neutralized by TIG. Accordingly, TIG is given as soon as possible to neutralize toxin that diffuses from the wound into the circulation before the toxin can bind at distant muscle groups. An optimal dose of TIG has not been determined. A single intramuscular injection of 500 U of TIG is sufficient to neutralize systemic tetanus toxin, but doses as high as 3,000–6,000 U are also recommended. Infiltration of TIG into the wound is now considered unnecessary. If TIG is unavailable, use of human intravenous immune globulin (IVIG), which contains 4–90 U/mL of TIG, or of equine- or bovine-derived tetanus antitoxin (TAT), may be necessary. However, the optimal dosage of IVIG is not known, and it is not approved for this usage. The usual dose of TAT is 50,000–100,000 U, with half given intramuscularly and half intravenously, but as little as 10,000 U may be sufficient. Approximately 15% of patients given the usual dose of TAT will experience serum sickness. When using TAT, it is essential to check for possible sensitivity to horse serum and desensitization may be needed. The human-derived immune globulins are much preferred because of their longer half-life (30 days) and the virtual absence of allergic and serum sickness side effects. Intrathecal TIG, given to neutralize tetanus toxin in the spinal cord, is not effective.

Penicillin G remains the antibiotic of choice because of its effective clostridiocidal action and its diffusability, an important consideration because blood flow to injured tissue may be compromised. The dose is 100,000 U/kg/24 hr divided and administered in 4–6 hr intervals for 10–14 days. Metronidazole, 500 mg of 8 hr, appears to be equally effective. Erythromycin and tetracycline (in patients ≥8 yr old) are alternatives for penicillin-allergic patients.

All patients with generalized tetanus need muscle relaxants. Diazepam proivides both relaxation and seizure control; the initial dose of 0.1–0.2 /kg every 3–6 hr given intravenously is then titrated to control the tetanic spasms, after which it is sustained for 2–6 wk before its tapered withdrawal. Magnesium sulfate, other benzodiazepines (e.g., midazolam), chlorpromazine, dantrolene, and baclofen are also used. Intrathecal baclofen produces such complete muscle relaxation that apnea often ensues; like most other agents listed, baclofen should be used only in an intensive care unit setting. The best survival rates in generalized tetanus are achieved with neuromuscular blocking agents such as vecuronium and pancuronium, which produce a general flaccid paralysis that is then managed by mechanical ventilation. Autonomic instability is regulated with standard α- and β- (or both) blocking agents; morphine has also proved useful.

Meticulous supportive care in a quiet, dark, secluded setting is most desirable. Because tetanic spasms may be triggered by minor stimuli, the patient should be sedated and protected from all unnecessary sounds, sights, and touch; and all therapeutic and other manipulations must be carefully scheduled and coordinated. Endotracheal intubation may not be required, but it should be done to prevent aspiration of secretions before laryngospasm develops. A tracheotomy kit should be immediately at hand for unintubated patients. However, endotracheal intubation and suctioning easily provoke reflex tetanic seizures and spasms, and early tracheostomy deserves consideration in severe cases not managed by pharmacologically induced flaccid paralysis. Cardiorespiratory monitoring, frequent suctioning, and maintenance of the substantial fluid, electrolyte, and caloric needs are fundamental. Careful nursing attention to mouth, skin, bladder, and bowel function is needed to avoid ulceration, infection, and obstipation. Prophylactic subcutaneous heparin use is sensible.

COMPLICATIONS. The seizures and the severe, sustained rigid paralysis of tetanus predispose the patient to many complications. Aspiration of secretions and pneumonia may have begun before the first medical attention is received. Maintaining airway patency often mandates endotracheal intubation and mechanical ventilation with their attendant hazards, including pneumothorax and mediastinal emphysema. The seizures may result in lacerations of the mouth or tongue, in intramuscular hematomas or rhabdomyolysis with myoglobinuria and renal failure, or in long bone or spinal fractures. Venous thrombosis, pulmonary embolism, gastric ulceration with or without hemorrhage, paralytic ileus, and decubitus ulceration are constant hazards. Excessive use of muscle relaxants, an integral part of care, may produce iatrogenic apnea. Cardiac arrhythmias, including asystole, unstable blood pressure, and labile temperature regulation reflect disordered autonomic nervous system control that may be aggravated by inattention to maintenance of intravascular volume needs.

PROGNOSIS. Recovery in tetanus occurs through regeneration of synapses within the spinal cord and thereby the restoration of muscle relaxation. However, because an episode of tetanus does not result in the production of toxin-neutralizing antibodies, active immunization with tetanus toxoid at discharge with provision for completion of the primary series is mandatory.

The most important factor influencing outcome is the quality of supportive care. Mortality is highest in the very young and the very old. A favorable prognosis is associated with a long incubation period, with the absence of fever, and with localized disease. An unfavorable prognosis is associated with a week or less between the injury and the onset of trismus and with 3 days or less between trismus and the onset of generalized tetanic spasms. Sequelae of hypoxic brain injury, especially in infants, include cerebral palsy, diminished mental abilities, and behavioral difficulties. Most fatalities occur within the 1st wk of illness. Reported case fatality rates for generalized tetanus range between 5% and 35% and for neonatal tetanus extend from <10% with intensive care treatment to >75% without it. Cephalic tetanus has an especially poor prognosis because of breathing and feeding difficulties.

PREVENTION. Tetanus is an entirely preventable disease; a serum antibody titer of ≥0.01 U/mL is considered protective. Active immunization should begin in early infancy with combined diphtheria toxoid–tetanus toxoid–pertussis (DTaP is preferred over DTP) vaccine at 2, 4, and 6 mo of age, with a booster at 4–6 yr of age and at 10 yr intervals thereafter throughout adult life with tetanus-diphtheria (Td) toxoids. Immunization of women with tetanus toxoid prevents neonatal tetanus, and the World Health Organization is currently engaged in a global elimination of neonatal tetanus campaign through maternal immunization with at least two doses of tetanus toxoid. For unimmunized persons 7 yr old or older, the primary immunization series consists of three doses of Td toxoid given intramuscularly, the second 4–6 wk after the first and the third 6–12 mo after the second.

Wound Management. Tetanus prevention measures after trauma consist of inducing active immunity to tetanus toxin and of passively providing antitoxic antibody (Table 209–1). Tetanus prophylaxis is an essential part of all wound management, but specific measures depend on the nature of the injury and the immunization status of the patient. Tetanus toxoid should always be given after a dog or other animal bite, even though *C. tetani* is infrequently found in canine mouth flora. All nonminor wounds require human TIG except those in a fully immunized patient. In any other circumstances (e.g., patients with an unknown or incomplete immunization history; or crush, puncture, or projectile wounds; wounds contaminated with saliva, soil, or feces; avulsion injuries; compound fractures; or frostbite), 250 U of TIG should be given intramuscularly, and increased to 500 U for highly tetanus-prone wounds (i.e., undebridable, with substantial bacterial contamination, or >24 hr old). If TIG is unavailable, then use of human IGIV may be considered. If neither of these products is available, then 3,000–5,000 U of equine- or bovine-derived tetanus antitoxin (TAT) may be given intramuscularly after testing for hypersensitivity; even at this dose, serum sickness may occur.

The wound should have immediate, thorough surgical cleansing and debridement to remove foreign bodies and any necrotic tissue in which anaerobic conditions might develop. Tetanus toxoid should be given to stimulate active immunity and may be administered concurrently with TIG (or TAT) if given in separate syringes at separate sites. A tetanus toxoid booster (preferably Td) is given to all persons with *any* wound if their tetanus immunization status is unknown or incomplete. A booster is given to injured persons who have completed their primary immunization series if (1) the wound is clean and minor but ≥10 yr have passed since the last booster, or (2) the wound is more serious and ≥5 yr have passed since the last booster. With delayed wound care, active immunization should be started at once. Although fluid tetanus toxoid produces a more rapid immune response than the adsorbed or precipitated toxoids, the adsorbed toxoid results in a more durable titer.

TABLE 209–1 Tetanus Prophylaxis in Wound Management

	Clean, Minor Wounds		Other Wounds*	
Prior Tetanus Doses	**Td†**	**TIG‡**	**Td†**	**TIG‡**
Uncertain, or <3	Yes	No	Yes	Yes
Three or more	No§	No	No‖	No

Adapted from Centers for Disease Control. Diphtheria, tetanus, and pertussis: Recommendations for vaccine use and other preventive measures. Recommendations of the Immunization Practices Advisory Committee (ACIP). MMWR 41 (RR-10):21, 1991.

**Such as, but not limited to: wounds contaminated with dirt, feces, and saliva; puncture wounds; avulsions; wounds resulting from missiles, crushing, burns, and frostbite; and wounds extending into muscle.*

†For children <7 yr, DTaP or DTP is preferred to tetanus toxoid alone if < 3 doses of DTaP/DTP have been previously given; if pertussis vaccine is contraindicated, DT is given. For persons ≥ 7 yr, Td is preferred to tetanus toxoid alone.

‡TIG = tetanus immune globulin. TIG should be administered for tetanus-prone wounds in HIV-1–infected patients regardless of the history of tetanus immunizations.

§Yes, if ≥ 10 yr since the last dose.

‖Yes, if ≥ 5 yr since the last dose. (More frequent boosters are not needed and can accentuate adverse events.)

Abrutyn E, Berlin JA: Intrathecal therapy in tetanus: A meta-analysis. JAMA 226:2262, 1991.

Centers for Disease Control: Diphtheria, tetanus, and pertussis: Recommendations for vaccine use and other preventive measures. Recommendations of the Immunization Practices Advisory Committee (ACIP). MMWR 41(RR-10):1, 1991.

Centers for Disease Control and Prevention: Tetanus surveillance—United States, 1991–1994. MMWR 45(SS-2):15, 1997.

Ernst ME, Klepser ME, Fouts M, Marangos MN: Tetanus: Pathophysiology and management. Ann Pharmacother 31:1507, 1997.

Expanded Program on Immunization: Progress toward the global elimination of neonatal tetanus, 1989–1993. MMWR 43:885–887, 893–894, 1994.

Fauveau V, Mamdani M, Steinglass R, et al: Maternal tetanus: magnitude, epidemiology and potential control measures. Int J Gynecol Obstet 40:3, 1993.
Gergen PJ, McQuillan GM, Kiely M, et al: A population-based serologic survey of immunity to tetanus in the United States. N Engl J Med 332:761, 1995.
Lee DC, Lederman HM: Anti-tetanus antibodies in intravenous gamma globulin: An alternative to tetanus immune globulin. J Infect Dis 166:642, 1992.
Montecucco C, Schiavo G: Tetanus and botulism neurotoxins: a new group of zinc proteases. Trends Biochem Sci 18:324, 1993.
Muguti GI, Dixon MS: Tetanus following human bite. Br J Plastic Surg 45:614, 1992.
Sesardic D, Wong MY, Gaines Das RE, et al: The first international standard for antitetanus globulin, human; pharmaceutical evaluation and international collaborative study. Biologicals 21:67, 1993.
Thayaparan B, Nicoll A: Prevention and control of tetanus in childhood. Curr Opin Pediatr 10:4, 1998.
Wesley AG, Pather M: Tetanus in children: An 11-year review. Ann Trop Pediatr 7:32, 1987.
Wright DK, Lalloo UG, Nayiger S, et al: Autonomic nervous system dysfunction in severe tetanus: current perspectives. Crit Care Med 17:371, 1989.
Yen LM, Dao LM, Day NPJ, et al: Role of quinine in the high mortality of intramuscular injection tetanus. Lancet 344:786, 1994.

CHAPTER 210
Pseudomembranous Colitis (Clostridium difficile)

Margaret C. Fisher

Clostridium difficile–associated diarrhea, also known as pseudomembranous colitis or antibiotic-associated diarrhea, is a major cause of nosocomial diarrhea. It appears that *Staphylococcus aureus* or *Clostridium perfringens* can also rarely cause antibiotic-associated diarrhea.

ETIOLOGY. *C. difficile* is a spore-forming gram-positive anaerobic bacillus that is ubiquitous in the environment in the soil. The organism produces two toxins: toxin A (enterotoxin) acts on the intestinal mucosa to produce diarrhea; toxin B (cytotoxin) increases vascular permeability in low doses and is lethal to experimental animals in high doses. With rare exceptions, strains either produce both toxins or neither toxin.

EPIDEMIOLOGY. *C. difficile*–associated diarrhea rarely, if ever, occurs in the absence of recent or current antimicrobial therapy. Virtually all known antibiotics (vancomycin being an exception) have been implicated. Pseudomembranous colitis is more commonly seen in patients receiving penicillin, cephalosporins, or clindamycin, usually after oral therapy but occasionally after parenteral therapy.

Newborns are often colonized with *C. difficile* during the first 2 weeks of life. Colonization is found in approximately half of healthy infants during the first year of life. Many of these strains produce toxin. The carriage rate decreases to the adult carriage rate of 1–3% by 2 yr of age. This toxin-mediated disease is unique in children in that *C. difficile* and its toxin rarely cause illness in neonates and young children. The basis for this is unknown. Asymptomatic carriers are not at increased risk for disease unless given antibiotics.

PATHOGENESIS. The two toxins are markers for disease, in the appropriate clinical setting, but it is not known if they are responsible, alone or acting together, for disease in humans.

Normal gut flora appears to be protective. The administration of antibiotics that impair growth of normal flora but not *C. difficile* is the most common risk factor, but any process that disrupts the normal bowel flora (e.g., chemotherapy) or bowel motility (e.g., bowel stasis, bowel surgery) predisposes to *C. difficile*–associated diarrhea.

CLINICAL MANIFESTATIONS. Clinical symptoms vary widely. Patients more commonly have a mild self-limited diarrhea without pseudomembranes, or explosive watery diarrhea with occult blood, or the classic picture of pseudomembranous colitis with blood and mucus accompanied by fever, cramps, abdominal pain, nausea, and vomiting. Disease occurs during and as long as weeks after antibiotic therapy.

DIAGNOSIS. The diagnosis is confirmed by detecting *C. difficile* or its toxin in the stool of a patient with significant diarrhea or colitis in the setting of prior or current antimicrobial use.

It has been recommended in adult patients that the diagnosis of *C. difficile*–associated diarrhea be considered in any patient with diarrhea (three or more watery or unformed stools in 24 hr) or abdominal pain who has received antibiotics within 2 mo or whose diarrhea began >72 hr after hospitalization.

Identification of toxin in a single stool specimen is the laboratory test usually used for diagnosis. Inoculation of stool filtrates into cell culture to detect cytotoxicity is considered the reference method; however, this is a labor-intensive method that requires 2 days. Many clinical laboratories use enzyme immunoassay tests that detect toxin A only, or toxin A plus B. Culture of the stool for *C. difficile* is time consuming and does not differentiate toxin-producing from non–toxin-producing strains. The interpretation of positive *C. difficile* culture or toxin in stool from children <1 yr old requires clinical correlation.

Sigmoidoscopy or colonoscopy will demonstrate the pseudomembranous nodules and plaques characteristic of toxin-related colitis, but this is not necessary unless required for evaluation for other colonic diseases.

Fecal leukocytes are present in approximately half of cases. The stool may have occult of frank blood.

TREATMENT. The first and essential step in treatment is the discontinuation of the current antibiotics, if at all possible. In most instances this course combined with appropriate fluid and electrolyte replacement is sufficient. If symptoms persist, antibiotics cannot be discontinued, or the illness is severe, then oral metronidazole (20–50 mg/kg/24 hr, divided every 6–8 hr) or vancomycin (25–50 mg/kg/24 hr divided every 6 hr) should be given for a 7–10 day course. Oral metronidazole is the preferred therapy for most children; it is less expensive, has an excellent response rate, and minimizes the emergence of vancomycin-resistant enterococci, which is especially important in hospitalized or institutionalized patients.

PROGNOSIS. The initial response rate is >95%, but 5–30% of patients will have clinical relapse, usually within 1–2 wk of treatment. These patients should be re evaluated and usually respond to the original treatment. A small proportion of patients develop multiple recurrences, with short-lived responses to repeated treatment. Treatment strategies for these patients include oral cholestyramine, oral bacitracin, oral immune globulin, reconstitution of bowel flora with oral lactobacilli, baker's yeast, or instillation of fecal flora by tube feeding or enemas. None of these methods works for all cases.

PREVENTION. *C. difficile* is often acquired nosocomially or in childcare settings. The spores of the organism are resistant to drying and to some disinfectants and frequently contaminate bathrooms and diaper changing areas of hospital rooms or childcare areas. Prevention of *C. difficile*–associated diarrhea requires meticulous hand washing, appropriate environmental cleaning, and appropriate use of antimicrobial agents.

Cerquetti M, Biol D, Luzzi I, et al: Role of *Clostridium difficile* in childhood diarrhea. Pediatr Infect Dis J 14:598, 1995.
Fekety R: Guidelines for the diagnosis and management of *Clostridium difficile*–associated diarrhea and colitis. Am J Gastroenterol 92:739, 1997.
Hirschhorn LR, Trnka Y, Onderdonk A, et al: Epidemiology of community-acquired *Clostridium difficile*–associated diarrhea. J Infect Dis 169:127, 1994.
Johnson S, Gerding DN: *Clostridium difficile*–associated diarrhea. Clin Infect Dis 26:1027, 1998.
Manabe YC, Vinetz JM, Moore RD, et al: *Clostridium difficile* colitis: An efficient clinical approach to diagnosis. Ann Intern Med 123:835, 1995.
Wenisch C, Parschalk B, Hasenhundl M, et al: Comparison of vancomycin, teicoplanin, metronidazole, and fusidic acid for the treatment of *Clostridium difficile*–associated diarrhea. Clin Infect Dis 22:813, 1996.

CHAPTER 211
Other Anaerobic Infections

Margaret C. Fisher

Anaerobic bacteria are the most numerous organisms colonizing humans. Anaerobes are present in soil and are normal inhabitants of all living animals, but infections caused by anaerobes are relatively uncommon. Anaerobes are relatively or entirely intolerant of exposure to oxygen. The ability to survive in the presence of oxygen varies greatly, with the majority of organisms being facultative anaerobes, that is, able to survive in the presence of oxygen but growing better when oxygen tension is reduced. Some anaerobes are obligate anaerobes and will not survive any exposure to oxygen.

Infections with anaerobes occur most commonly adjacent to mucosal surfaces and as mixed infections with aerobes. Optimal conditions for proliferation of anaerobes are circumstances with reduced oxygen tension. Traumatized areas, devascularized areas, and areas of crush injury are all ideal sites for anaerobic infections. Often aerobic flora and anaerobic flora are initially inoculated but local extension and bacteremia are most often due to the more virulent aerobes. Abscess formation is usually due to mixed aerobes and anaerobes. Examples of such infections include appendicitis, appendiceal abscess, perirectal abscess, peritonsillar abscess, lung abscess, and dental abscess. Septic thrombophlebitis is a common consequence of infections such as appendicitis, chronic sinusitis or otitis media, and Lemierre's syndrome.

Anaerobic infection is due to endogenous flora rather than acquisition of a virulent pathogen. Combinations of altered physical barriers to infection, compromised tissue viability, alterations in endogenous flora, defects in host immunity, and anaerobic bacterial virulence factors contribute to infection with these inhabitants of mucous membranes. Virulence factors include capsules, toxins, and production of enzymes and fatty acids.

CLINICAL MANIFESTATIONS. Anaerobic infections occur in a variety of sites throughout the body (Table 211–1). Anaerobes exist synergistically with aerobes; infections with anaerobes are almost always polymicrobial and include aerobes.

Central Nervous System. Meningitis is rare, but it has occurred in neonates and as a complication of *Fusobacterium* infections of the ear and neck. Brain abscess and subdural empyema are usually polymicrobial, with anaerobes commonly involved. Brain abscess occurs most commonly after contiguous spread of infection from sinuses, middle ear, or lung.

Upper Respiratory Tract. The respiratory tract is colonized by both aerobes and anaerobes. Anaerobic bacteria are involved in chronic sinusitis, chronic otitis media, peritonsillar infections, periodontal infections, necrotizing pneumonia, and lung abscess. Anaerobic periodontal disease is most common in patients with poor dental hygiene and in those who are receiving drugs that result in hypertrophy of the gums. Vincent's angina or trench mouth is an acute, fulminating, necrotizing infection of the gums and floor of the mouth. The disease is characterized by pain, foul breath, and pseudomembrane formation. Ludwig's angina is a life-threatening cellulitis of the sublingual and submandibular spaces; disease spreads rapidly in the neck, and airway obstruction can occur. Retropharyngeal abscesses involve mixed normal flora, which includes anaerobes.

Lemierre's syndrome, or postanginal sepsis, is a suppurative infection of the lateral pharyngeal space and septic thrombophlebitis of the jugular vein leading to septic embolization to the lungs and central nervous system. Clinical signs include neck swelling and pain, trismus, dysphagia, and severe toxicity. *Fusobacterium necrophorum* is the most commonly involved organism; polymicrobial infection is common.

Lower Respiratory Tract. Lung abscess and anaerobic pneumonia are most common in children with swallowing dysfunction and in those with an increased incidence of aspiration or an increased volume of aspiration. All children and adults aspirate during sleep or during periods of unconsciousness. In most cases, the lung cilia and phagocytes clear particulate matter and microbes. If the aspiration is of high volume or high frequency, the ability of lung clearance mechanisms are overcome and infection ensues.

Intra-abdominal. The digestive tract is colonized throughout by anaerobes. The density of organisms is highest in the colon, where anaerobes outnumber aerobes by 1,000 to 1. Rupture of the gut leads to spillage of gut flora into the peritoneum, resulting in peritonitis that involves both aerobes and anaerobes. Bacteremia due to aerobes occurs early. As the infection is walled off in the peritoneum, an abscess is often formed that usually contains both aerobes and anaerobes. Liver abscesses are rare in children; the predisposing illnesses are usually appendicitis, inflammatory bowel disease, or biliary tract disease. In children with malignancies who are receiving chemotherapy, the gut mucosa is often damaged, leading to translocation of bacteria and focal invasion of bowel flora. Typhlitis, or necrotizing colitis, is a mixed infection of the gut wall usually beginning in the colon; abdominal pain, diarrhea, fever, and abdominal distention are common features. Empirical therapy for fever and neutropenia is usually not optimal against the anaerobes involved in typhlitis.

Genital Tract. Genital tract infections in women often involve anaerobes. Pelvic inflammatory disease and tubo-ovarian abscesses are frequently due to mixed aerobes and anaerobes. Vaginitis can be caused by overgrowth of anaerobic flora. Anaerobes frequently contribute to chorioamnionitis and may result in anaerobic bacteremia in the neonate. Although most of these bacteremias are transient, anaerobes occasionally cause invasive disease in the newborn.

Skin and Soft Tissue. Anaerobic skin infections occur in the setting of bites or skin and tissue ulceration due to pressure necrosis or lack of adequate blood supply. Animal bites and human bites inoculate animal oral flora and human skin flora into the subcutaneous tissues that may include anaerobes, but the more virulent aerobic infections are responsible for most clinical infections (see Chapter 181). The extent of the infection depends on the depth of the bite and the associated crush injury to the tissues.

Clostridial myonecrosis, or gas gangrene, is a rapidly progressive infection associated with *Clostridium perfringens*. Necrotizing fasciitis is a polymicrobial infection with acute onset and rapid progression, with significant morbidity and mortality. Group A streptococcus and *Staphylococcus aureus* are occasionally the sole pathogens. Synergistic gangrene is caused by synergistic infection between *S. aureus* or gram-negative bacilli and anaerobic streptococci. All of these are uncommon infections in healthy children. Early recognition with aggressive surgical debridement and antimicrobial therapy is necessary to limit morbidity and mortality.

Other Sites. Occasionally the bone adjacent to anaerobic infection becomes infected by direct extension from contiguous infections or by direct inoculation associated with trauma. Anaerobic infections of the kidneys (renal and perirenal abscesses) and heart (pericarditis) are rare.

DIAGNOSIS. The diagnosis of anaerobic infection requires a high index of suspicion and the collection of appropriate and adequate specimens for culture (Table 211–2). Cultures should be obtained in a manner that protects the specimen from contamination with mucosal bacteria and from exposure to ambient oxygen. Swab cultures of mucosal surfaces or of nasal secretions, respiratory specimens, and stool should not be sent

TABLE 211–1 Infections Associated with Anaerobic Bacteria

Site and Infection	Major Risk Factors	Anaerobic Bacteria*
Central Nervous System		
Cerebral abscess Subdural empyema Epidural abscess	Direct extension from contiguous sinusitis, otitis media, mastoiditis	(Polymicrobial) *B. fragilis*† *Fusobacterium* *Peptostreptococcus* *Veillonella*
Upper Respiratory Tract		
Dental abscess Ludwig angina (cellulitis of sublingual-submandibular space) Necrotizing gingivitis (Vincent stomatitis) Chronic otitis-mastoiditis-sinusitis Peritonsillar abscess Retropharyngeal abscess	Poor periodontal hygiene Drugs that cause gum hypertrophy	*Peptostreptococcus* *Fusobacterium* *P. melaninogenica*
Lower Respiratory Tract		
Aspiration pneumonia Necrotizing pneumonitis Lung abscess Pulmonary empyema	Periodontal disease Bronchial obstruction Altered gag or consciousness	(Polymicrobial) *P. melaninogenica* *B. intermedius* *Fusobacterium* *Peptostreptococcus, Eubacterium* *B. fragilis, Veillonella*
Intra-abdominal		
Abscess Secondary peritonitis	Appendicitis Penetrating trauma (especially of the colon)	(Polymicrobial) *B. fragilis* Other *Bacteroides* species *Clostridium* species *Peptostreptococcus* *Eubacterium* *Fusobacterium*
Female Genital Tract		
Bartholin abscess Tubo-ovarian abscess Endometritis Pelvic cellulitis or thrombophlebitis Salpingitis Chorioamnionitis Septic abortion	Vaginosis Intrauterine device	*B. fragilis* *B. bivius* Peptostreptococcus *Clostridium* species *Mobiluncus* Actinomycosis
Skin and Soft Tissue		
Cellulitis Perirectal cellulitis Myonecrosis (gas gangrene) Necrotizing fasciitis Synergistic gangrene	Decubitus ulcers Abdominal wounds Pilonidal sinus Trauma Human and animal bites Immunosuppressed or neutropenic patients	(Varies with site and contamination with mouth or enteric flora) *Clostridium perfringens (myonecrosis)* *Bacteroides* *Fusobacterium* *Clostridium tertium* *C. septicum* Anaerobic streptococci
Bacteremia	Secondary to intra-abdominal infection, abscess, myonecrosis, or necrotizing fasciitis	*B. fragilis* *Clostridium* Anaerobic streptococci

**Infections may also be due to or involve aerobic bacteria as the sole or part of a mixed infection: brain abscess may contain microaerophilic streptococci; intra-abdominal infections may contain gram-negative enteric organisms and enterococci; and salpingitis may contain* Neisseria gonorrhoeae, *and* Chylamydia trachomatis.

†Bacteroides fragilis *is usually isolated from infections below the diaphragm except for brain abscesses.*

for anaerobic culture because these sites normally harbor anaerobes. Aspirates of infected sites, abscess material, and biopsy specimens are ideal. The specimen should be protected from oxygen and transported to the laboratory immediately. A transport medium is used to increase the recovery of obligate anaerobes. Gram stains are useful; anaerobic infections are usually polymicrobial. Susceptibility testing of anaerobes is not always performed because it is labor intensive and time consuming, although several methods are available. A rapid and easy screening test is available to detect β-lactamase production.

TREATMENT. Treatment of anaerobic infections requires adequate drainage and appropriate antimicrobial therapy. Antibiotic therapy varies depending on the suspected or proven anaerobe involved. Some oral anaerobic flora are susceptible to penicillins, whereas some produce β-lactamase. The drugs that are active against these organisms include metronidazole, penicillins combined with β-lactamase inhibitors (ticarcillin-clavulanic acid, ampicillin-sulbactam, and piperacillin-tazobactam), carbapenems (imipenem and meropenem), clindamycin, cefoxitin, and chloramphenicol. Penicillin and vancomycin are active against the gram-positive anaerobes.

Aerobes are usually present with the anaerobes in soft tissue infections, necessitating broad-spectrum antibiotic combinations for empirical therapy.

For soft tissue infections, providing perfusion to the area is key to success; at times a muscle flap or skin flap procedure will be needed to ensure that nutrients and antimicrobial agents are brought to the affected area. Drainage of infected areas is often necessary for cure. Bacteria may survive in abscesses due to high bacterial inoculum, lack of bactericidal activity, and local conditions that facilitate bacterial proliferation. Aspiration is sometimes effective for small collections whereas incision and drainage may be required for larger abscesses. Broad debridement and resection of all devitalized tissue is needed to control fasciitis and myonecrosis.

TABLE 211–2 Clues to Presumptive Diagnosis of Anaerobic Infections*

Infection that is contiguous to or in proximity with a mucosal surface colonized with anaerobic bacteria (oropharynx, intestinal-genitourinary tract)
Foul-smelling, putrid odor (present in 50% of anaerobic infections)
Severe tissue necrosis, abscesses, gangrene, or fasciitis
Gas formation in tissues (crepitus or on radiograph)
Failure to recover organisms using conventional aerobic microbiologic methods
Failure of organisms to grow after pretreatment with antibiotics effective against anaerobics
Failure of organisms to respond to antibiotics with poor efficacy against anaerobic bacteria (e.g., aminoglycosides)
Toxin-mediated syndromes (botulism, tetanus, gas gangrene, *Clostridium perfringens* food poisoning, *C. difficile* pseudomembranous colitis)
Typical infections associated with anaerobic bacteria (see Table 211–1)
Sterile pus
Septic thrombophlebitis
Septicemic syndrome with jaundice or intravascular hemolysis
Mixed polymorphic organisms on Gram stain
Typical Gram stain appearance:
Bacteroides species—small, delicate, pleomorphic, pale, gram-negative bacilli
Fusobacterium nucleatum—thin gram-negative bacilli with fusiform shape, pointed ends
F. necrophorum—pleomorphism gram-negative bacilli with rounded ends
Peptostreptococcus—gram-positive cocci similar to aerobic cocci
C. perfringens—large, short, fat (boxcar-shaped) gram-positive bacilli

**Suspicion of anaerobic infection is critical before specimens are cultured to ensure optimal microbiologic techniques and prompt, appropriate therapy.*

COMMON ANAEROBIC PATHOGENS

CLOSTRIDIUM PERFRINGENS. Strains of *Clostridium* cause disease by infection, production of toxins, or both. More than 60 species have been identified, but only a few cause diseases in humans. The most commonly recovered organisms are *Clostridium difficile* (see Chapter 210) and *C. perfringens*; other species encountered in human-disease include *C. botulinum* (see Chapter 208), *C. tetani* (see Chapter 209), *C. butyricum, C. septicum, C. sordellii, C. tertium,* and *C. histolyticus*.

Clostridium perfringens produces a variety of toxins and virulence factors. Strains of *C. perfringens* are designated A through E. Alpha toxin is a phospholipase that hydrolyzes sphingomyelin and lecithin and is produced by all strains. This toxin causes hemolysis, platelet lysis, increased capillary permeability, and hepatotoxicity. Beta toxin, produced by strains B and C, causes hemorrhagic necrosis of the small bowel. Epsilon toxin, produced by B and D strains, injures vascular endothelial cells leading to increased vascular permeability, edema, and organ dysfunction. Iota toxin, produced by E strains, causes dermal edema. An enterotoxin is produced by type A and some type C and D strains. Hemolysins and a variety of enzymes are produced by many *C. perfringens* strains.

Myonecrosis. *C. perfringens* is the major cause of myonecrosis, or gas gangrene, a rapidly progressive infection of soft tissue. In compromised hosts, especially patients receiving cancer chemotherapy, *C. septicum* is a cause of rapidly fatal gas gangrene. A clue to the diagnosis is pain out of proportion to the clinical appearance of the wound. Infection progresses rapidly with edema, swelling, myonecrosis, and sometimes crepitation of the soft tissue. Hypotension, mental confusion, shock, and renal failure are common. A characteristic sweet odor is present in the serosanguineous discharge. Gram stain of the exudate reveals gram-positive rods and a few white blood cells. Early and complete debridement with excision of necrotic tissue is key to controlling the infection. High-dose penicillin (250,000 units/kg/24 hr IV, divided every 4–6 hr) or clindamycin (25–40 mg/kg/24 hr IV, divided every 6–8 hr) should be started immediately. The role of hyperbaric oxygen remains unclear but has been beneficial in several studies. The prognosis is poor even with early, aggressive therapy.

Food Poisoning. *C. perfringens* type A produces an enterotoxin that causes food poisoning. The intoxication results in the acute onset of watery diarrhea and crampy abdominal pain. The usual foods containing toxin are improperly prepared meats and gravies. A specific diagnosis is rarely made in children with food poisoning. Therapy consists of rehydration and electrolyte replacement if necessary. The illness resolves spontaneously within 24 hr of onset. Prevention requires the maintenance of hot food at a temperature of ≥74°C. See also Chapter 723.

Gastroenteritis. A severe gastroenteritis, termed *pig-bel* or *enteritis necroticans,* is caused by type C strains of *C. perfringens* that produce beta toxin. The disease occurs in Papua, New Guinea, and is related to particular dietary habits and malnutrition.

BACTEROIDES AND PREVOTELLA. *Bacteroides fragilis* is one of the more virulent of the anaerobes. It is an anaerobic pathogen that is most frequently recovered from blood cultures and cultures of tissue or pus. The most common infection in children is infection associated with appendicitis. The organism is part of normal colonic flora but is not common in the mouth or respiratory tract. *B. fragilis* is usually found as part of a polymicrobial appendiceal and other intra-abdominal abscesses and is also involved in genital tract infections such as pelvic inflammatory disease and tubo-ovarian abscess. *Prevotella* species are normal oral flora; infection involves gums, teeth, and tonsils. Both organisms are sometimes involved in anaerobic pneumonia and lung abscess.

Strains of *B. fragilis* and *P. melaninogenica* produce β-lactamase and thus are resistant to penicillin. Antibiotics of choice include clindamycin, chloramphenicol, ticarcillin/clavulanic acid, piperacillin/tazobactam, cefoxitin, imipenem, meropenem, and metronidazole. Many strains have become resistant to piperacillin and clindamycin. Chloramphenicol is rarely used because of toxicity and failure of therapy for intra-abdominal infection. Most infections involving these organisms are polymicrobial, and therefore therapy should include antimicrobial agents active against the probable aerobic pathogens as well. Drainage of abscesses and debridement of necrotic tissue are often required for control of these infections.

FUSOBACTERIUM. *Fusobacterium* species inhabit the intestine and respiratory and female genital tracts. These organisms are more virulent than most of the normal anaerobic flora and have been reported to cause bacteremia and a variety of rapidly progressive infections. Lemierre's syndrome, bone and joint infection, and abdominal and genital tract infections are most common. Some strains produce β-lactamase and are thus resistant to penicillins.

VEILLONELLA. *Veillonella* species are normal flora of the mouth, upper respiratory tract, intestine, and vagina. These anaerobes rarely cause infection; strains are recovered as part of the polymicrobial flora causing abscess, chronic sinusitis, empyema, peritonitis, and wound infection. *Veillonella* species are susceptible to penicillins, cephalosporins, clindamycin, metronidazole, and carbapenems.

ANAEROBIC COCCI. *Peptostreptococcus* species are normal flora of the skin, respiratory tract, and gut. These organisms are often present in brain abscesses, chronic sinusitis, chronic otitis, and lung abscesses. Such infections are often polymicrobial, and therapy is aimed at the accompanying aerobes as well as the anaerobes. Most of the gram-positive cocci are susceptible to penicillin, cephalosporins, carbapenems, and vancomycin.

Brook I: *Veillonella* infections in children. J Clin Microbiol 34:1283, 1996.

Brook I, Frazier EH: Clinical and microbiological features of necrotizing fasciitis. J Clin Microbiol 33:2382, 1995.

Chow AW: Life-threatening infections of the head and neck. Clin Infect Dis 14:991, 1992.

Citron DM, Goldstein EJC, Kenner MA, et al: Activity of ampicillin/sulbactam, ticarcillin/clavulanate, clarithromycin, and eleven other antimicrobial agents against anaerobic bacteria isolated from infections in children. Clin Infect Dis 20 (Suppl 2):S356, 1995.

Finegold SM, George WI (eds): Anaerobic Infections in Humans. New York, Academic Press, 1989.

Goldstein EJC, Citron DM, Goldman RJ: National hospital survey of anaerobic culture and susceptibility testing methods: Results and recommendations for improvement. J Clin Microbiol 30:1529, 1992.

Rathore MH, Barton LL, Dunkle LM: The spectrum of fusobacterial infections in children. Pediatr Infect Dis J 9:505, 1990.
Sloas MM, Flynn PM, Kaste SC, Patrick CC: Typhlitis in children with cancer: A 30-year experience. Clin Infect Dis 17:484, 1993.
Tibbles PM, Edelsberg JS: Hyperbaric-oxygen therapy. N Engl J Med 334:1642, 1996.
Wexler HM: Susceptibility testing of anaerobic bacteria: The state of the art. Clin Infect Dis 16:S328, 1993.

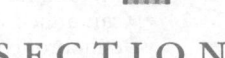

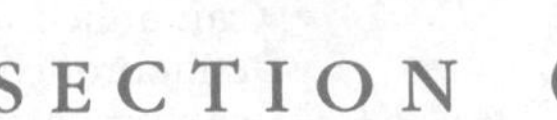

SECTION 6

Mycobacterial Infections

CHAPTER 212
Tuberculosis

Jeffrey R. Starke and Flor Munoz

After decades of decline in the incidence of tuberculosis, the number of tuberculosis cases has increased dramatically over the past decade. Almost 1.3 million cases and 450,000 deaths occur among children each year. The incidence of childhood tuberculosis increased by 35% in the United States from 1987 to 1996 as a consequence of poverty, immigration from high prevalence countries, the epidemic of HIV infection, and limitations in health care services to high-risk populations.

ETIOLOGY. The agents of tuberculosis, *Mycobacterium tuberculosis, Mycobacterium bovis,* and *Mycobacterium africanum,* are members of the order Actinomycetales and the family Mycobacteriaceae. The tubercle bacilli are non–spore forming, nonmotile, pleomorphic, weakly gram-positive curved rods 2–4 μm long. They may appear beaded or clumped in stained clinical specimens or culture media. They are obligate aerobes that grow in synthetic media containing glycerol as the carbon source and ammonium salts as the nitrogen source. These mycobacteria grow best at 37–41°C, produce niacin, and lack pigmentation. A lipid-rich cell wall accounts for resistance to the bactericidal actions of antibody and complement. A hallmark of all mycobacteria is acid-fastness—the capacity to form stable mycolate complexes with arylmethane dyes such as crystal violet, carbolfuchsin, auramine, and rhodamine. Once stained, they resist decoloration with ethanol and hydrochloric or other acids.

Mycobacteria grow slowly, their generation time being 12–24 hr. Isolation from clinical specimens on solid synthetic media usually takes 3–6 wk, and drug-susceptibility testing requires an additional 4 wk. However, growth can be detected in 1–3 wk in selective liquid medium using radiolabeled nutrients (the BACTEC radiometric system), and drug susceptibilities can be determined in an additional 3–5 days. The presence of *M. tuberculosis* in clinical specimens can be detected within hours using nucleic acid amplification (NAA) that employs a DNA probe that is complementary to mycobacterial DNA or RNA. Data from children are limited, but the sensitivity of some NAA techniques is similar to that for culture.

EPIDEMIOLOGY. Infection and Disease. Tuberculosis *infection* occurs after the inhalation of infective droplet nuclei containing *M. tuberculosis.* A reactive tuberculin skin test and the absence of clinical and radiographic manifestations are the hallmark of this stage. Tuberculosis *disease* occurs when signs and symptoms or radiographic changes become apparent. The word "tuberculosis" refers to disease. The World Health Organization estimates that one third of the world's population—2 billion people—are infected with *M. tuberculosis.* Infection rates are highest in Southeast Asia, China, India, Africa, and Latin America. Ten to 20 million people living in the United States harbor the tubercle bacillus. If left untreated, 5–10% of these individuals will develop tuberculosis disease in the future.

Tuberculosis case rates fell during the first half of the century long before the advent of antituberculosis drugs as a result of improved living conditions. The incidence began to rise in the United States in 1985 (Fig. 212–1). Most people in developed countries remain at low risk for tuberculosis except for certain fairly well-defined groups (Table 212–1). Cities with populations of greater than 250,000 account for 18% of the U.S. population but more than 45% of tuberculosis cases. At every age, tuberculosis case rates are strikingly higher in foreign born and nonwhite individuals. Genetics may play a small role, but environmental factors such as socioeconomic status, overcrowding, poor nutrition, and inadequate health care undoubtedly play the major role in the incidence.

Among adults, two thirds of cases occur in males, but there is a slight predominance of tuberculosis among females in childhood. Tuberculosis rates are highest among the elderly in white populations in the United States; these individuals acquired the infection decades ago. In contrast, among nonwhite populations tuberculosis is most common in young adults and children <5 yr of age. The age range of 5–14 yr is often called the "favored age" because in all human populations this group has the lowest rate of tuberculosis disease.

In the United States, most children are infected with *M. tuberculosis* in their home by someone close to them, but outbreaks of childhood tuberculosis also occur in elementary

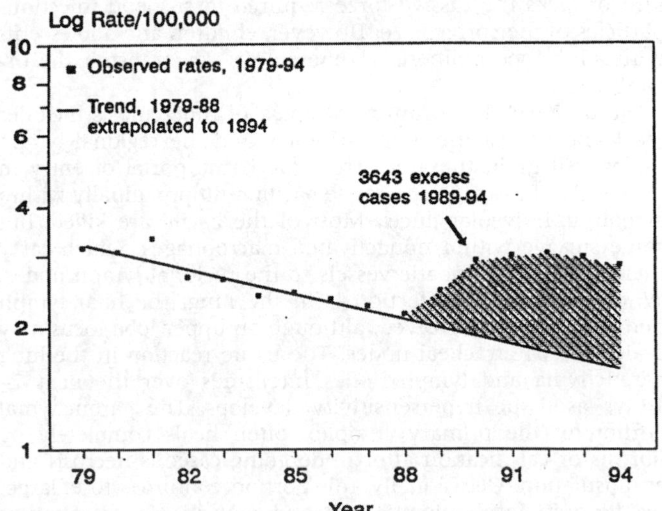

Figure 212–1 Observed rates of childhood tuberculosis in the United States, 1979–1994. Compared with the number of cases expected from previous trends, 3,643 excess cases were reported from 1988 to 1994. (Data from the Centers for Disease Control and Prevention, 1996.)

TABLE 212–1 Groups at High Risk for Tuberculosis Infection and Disease in Developed Countries

Tuberculosis Infection
Foreign-born persons from high-incidence countries
Poor and indigent persons, especially in large cities
Present and former residents of correctional institutions
Homeless persons
Injecting drug users
Health care workers caring for high-risk patients
Children exposed to high-risk adults
Tuberculosis Disease Once Infected
Coinfection with the human immunodeficiency virus
Other immunocompromising diseases, esp. malignancy
Immunosuppressive medical treatments
Infants and children ≤3 yr of age

and high schools, nursery schools, daycare centers, homes, churches, school buses, and sports teams. HIV-infected adults with tuberculosis can transmit *M. tuberculosis* to children, some of whom develop tuberculosis disease, and children with HIV infection probably are at increased risk of developing tuberculosis after infection.

The incidence of drug-resistant tuberculosis has increased dramatically throughout the world. In the United States, about 11% of *M. tuberculosis* isolates are resistant to at least one drug, whereas 2% are resistant to both isoniazid and rifampin. However, in some countries drug resistance rates range from 20–50%. The major reasons for the development of drug resistance are poor patient adherence to treatment and provision of inadequate drug regimens by the physician or national tuberculosis program.

Transmission. Transmission of *M. tuberculosis* is person to person, usually by airborne mucus droplet nuclei. Transmission rarely occurs by direct contact with an infected discharge or a contaminated fomite. The chance of transmission increases when the patient has an acid-fast smear of sputum, an extensive upper lobe infiltrate or cavity, copious production of thin sputum, and severe and forceful cough. Environmental factors, especially poor air circulation, enhance transmission. Most adults no longer transmit the organism within several days to 2 wk after beginning adequate chemotherapy, but some patients remain infectious for many weeks. Young children with tuberculosis rarely, if ever, infect other children or adults. Tubercle bacilli are sparse in the endobronchial secretions of children with pulmonary tuberculosis, and cough is often absent or lacks the tussive force required to suspend infectious particles of the correct size. However, children and adolescents with adult-type pulmonary tuberculosis can transmit the organism.

PATHOGENESIS. The primary complex of tuberculosis includes local infection at the portal of entry and the regional lymph nodes that drain the area. The lung is the portal of entry in over 98% of cases. The tubercle bacilli multiply initially within alveoli and alveolar ducts. Most of the bacilli are killed, but some survive within nonactivated macrophages, which carry them through lymphatic vessels to the regional lymph nodes. When the primary infection is in the lung, the hilar lymph nodes usually are involved, although an upper lobe focus may drain into paratracheal nodes. The tissue reaction in the lung parenchyma and lymph nodes intensifies over the next 2–12 wk as tissue hypersensitivity develops. The parenchymal portion of the primary complex often heals completely by fibrosis or calcification after undergoing caseous necrosis and encapsulation. Occasionally, this portion continues to enlarge, resulting in focal pneumonitis and pleuritis. If caseation is intense, the center of the lesion liquefies and empties into the associated bronchus, leaving a residual cavity.

The foci of infection in the regional lymph nodes develop some fibrosis and encapsulation, but healing is usually less complete than in the parenchymal lesion. Viable *M. tuberculosis* can persist for decades within these foci. In most cases of initial tuberculosis infection the lymph nodes remain normal in size. However, hilar and paratracheal nodes that enlarge significantly as part of the host inflammatory reaction may encroach on a regional bronchus or bronchiole. Partial obstruction of the bronchus caused by external compression may cause hyperinflation in the distal lung segment. Inflamed caseous nodes can attach to the bronchial wall and erode through it, causing endobronchial tuberculosis or a fistula tract. The caseum causes complete obstruction of the bronchus. The resulting lesion, a combination of pneumonitis and atelectasis, has been called a collapse-consolidation or segmental lesion (Fig. 212–2).

During the development of the primary complex, tubercle bacilli are carried to most tissues of the body through the blood and lymphatic vessels. Disseminated tuberculosis occurs if the number of circulating bacilli is large and the host response is inadequate. More often the number of bacilli is small, leading to clinically inapparent metastatic foci in many organs. These remote foci usually become encapsulated, but they may be the origin of both extrapulmonary tuberculosis and reactivation tuberculosis in some individuals.

The time between initial infection and clinically apparent disease is quite variable. Disseminated or meningeal tuberculosis are early manifestations, often occurring within 2–6 mo of the infection. Clinically significant lymph node or endobronchial tuberculosis usually appears within 3–9 mo. Lesions of the bones and joints take several years to develop, whereas renal lesions may become evident decades after infection. Pulmonary tuberculosis that occurs more than a year after the primary infection is usually caused by endogenous regrowth of bacilli persisting in partially encapsulated lesions. This reactivation tuberculosis is rare in children but is common among adolescents and young adults. The most common form is an infiltrate or cavity in the apex of the upper lobes, where oxygen tension and blood flow are great. Dissemination during reactivation tuberculosis is rare in immunocompetent hosts but is common in adults with AIDS. Only 5–10% of immunocompetent adults who become infected with *M. tuberculosis* ever develop clinical disease. However, approximately 40% of

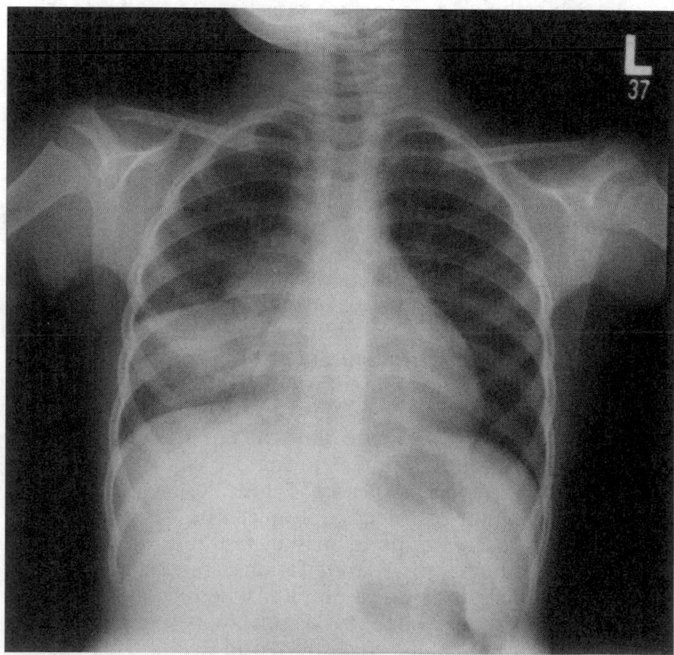

Figure 212–2 Right-sided hilar adenopathy and collapse-consolidation lesions of primary tuberculosis in a 4-yr-old child.

infants with untreated infection develop disease within 1–2 yr. The risk declines throughout childhood. Twenty-five to 35 percent of children with tuberculosis develop extrapulmonary manifestations compared with about 10% of immunocompetent adults.

Pregnancy and the Newborn. Congenital tuberculosis is rare because the most common result of female genital tract tuberculosis is infertility. Congenital transmission occurs most commonly from a lesion in the placenta through the umbilical vein. Primary infection in the mother just before or during pregnancy is more likely to cause congenital infection than is reactivation of a previous infection. The tubercle bacilli first reach the fetal liver, where a primary focus with periportal lymph node involvement may occur. Organisms pass through the liver into the main fetal circulation and infect many organs. The bacilli in the lung usually remain dormant until after birth, when oxygenation and pulmonary circulation increase significantly.

Congenital tuberculosis may also be caused by aspiration or ingestion of infected amniotic fluid. However, the most common route of infection for the neonate is postnatal airborne transmission from an adult with infectious pulmonary tuberculosis.

Immunity. Conditions that adversely affect cell-mediated immunity predispose to progression from tuberculosis infection to disease. Tuberculosis is associated with a vast antibody response, but these antibodies appear to play little role in host defense. In the first several weeks after infection, tubercle bacilli undergo a short period of uninhibited growth in both free alveolar spaces and within inactivated alveolar macrophages. Sulfatides in the mycobacterial cell wall inhibit fusion of the macrophage phagosome and lysosomes, allowing the organisms to escape destruction by intracellular enzymes. Cell-mediated immunity develops 4–8 wk after infection, at about the same time that tissue hypersensitivity begins. A small population of lymphocytes that recognize mycobacterial antigens after macrophage processing proliferate and secrete lymphokines and other mediators that attract other lymphocytes and macrophages to the area. Certain lymphokines activate macrophages, causing them to develop high concentrations of lytic enzymes that enhance their mycobactericidal capacity. A discrete subset of regulator helper and suppressor lymphocytes modulates the immune response. Development of specific cellular immunity prevents progression of the initial infection in most individuals.

The pathologic events in the initial tuberculosis infection seem to depend on the balance among the mycobacterial antigen load; cell-mediated immunity, which enhances intracellular killing; and tissue hypersensitivity, which promotes extracellular killing. When the antigen load is small and the degree of tissue sensitivity is high, granuloma formation results from the organization of lymphocytes, macrophages, and fibroblasts. When both antigen load and the degree of sensitivity are high, granuloma formation is less organized. Tissue necrosis is incomplete, resulting in formation of caseous material. When the degree of tissue sensitivity is low, as is often the case in infants or immunocompromised individuals, the reaction is diffuse and the infection is not well contained, leading to dissemination and local tissue destruction. Tissue necrosis factor and other cytokines released by specific lymphocytes promote cellular destruction and tissue damage in susceptible individuals.

Tuberculin Skin Tests. The development of delayed-type hypersensitivity (DTH) in most individuals infected with the tubercle bacillus makes the tuberculin skin test a useful diagnostic tool. Multipuncture tests (MPTs) are not as accurate as the Mantoux test because the exact dose of tuberculin antigen introduced into the skin cannot be controlled. The MPTs should no longer be used in pediatric practice.

The Mantoux tuberculin skin test is the intradermal injection of 0.1 mL containing 5 tuberculin units (TU) of purified protein derivative (PPD) stabilized with Tween 80. The amount of induration in response to the test should be measured by a trained person 48–72 hr after administration. Occasional patients will have the onset of induration more than 72 hr after placement of the test; this is a positive result. Tuberculin sensitivity develops 3 wk to 3 mo—most often in 4–8 wk—after inhalation of organisms. Host-related factors, including very young age, malnutrition, immunosuppression by disease or drugs, viral infections (measles, mumps, varicella, influenza), live-virus vaccines, and overwhelming tuberculosis, can depress the skin test reaction in a child infected with *M. tuberculosis*. Corticosteroid therapy may decrease the reaction to tuberculin, but the effect is variable. Tuberculin skin testing done at the time of initiating corticosteroid therapy is usually reliable. Approximately 10% of immunocompetent children with tuberculosis disease—up to 50% of those with meningitis or disseminated disease—do not react initially to PPD; most become reactive after several months of antituberculosis therapy. Nonreactivity may be specific to tuberculin or more global to a variety of antigens, so positive "control" skin tests with a negative tuberculin test never rule out tuberculosis. The most common reasons for a false-negative skin test are poor technique or misreading the results.

False-positive reactions to tuberculin can be caused by cross-sensitization to antigens of nontuberculous mycobacteria (NTM), which generally are more prevalent in the environment as one approaches the equator. These cross reactions are usually transient over months to years and produce less than 10–12 mm of induration. Previous vaccination with bacille Calmette-Guèrin (BCG) also can cause a reaction to a tuberculin skin test. Approximately one half of infants who receive a BCG vaccine never develop a reactive tuberculin skin test, and the reactivity usually wanes in 2–3 yr in those with initially positive skin tests. Older children and adults who receive a BCG vaccine are more likely to develop tuberculin reactivity, but most lose the reactivity by 5–10 yr after vaccination. When skin test reactivity is present, it usually causes less than 10 mm of induration, although larger reactions occur in some individuals. In general, a tuberculin skin reaction ≥10 mm in a BCG-vaccinated child or adult indicates infection with *M. tuberculosis*, which necessitates further diagnostic evaluation and treatment. Prior vaccination with BCG is never a contraindication to tuberculin testing.

The appropriate size of induration indicating a positive Mantoux tuberculin skin test varies with related epidemiologic and risk factors. In children with no risk factors for tuberculosis, skin test reactions are usually false-positive results. For this reason, the American Academy of Pediatrics (AAP) and Centers for Disease Control and Prevention (CDC) discourage routine testing of children with no specific risk factors. Possible exposure to an adult with or at high risk for infectious pulmonary tuberculosis is the most crucial factor for determining risk for children. To minimize false results, reaction size limits for determining a positive result vary with the individual's risk of infection. For adults and children at the highest risk of having infection progress to disease—those with recent contact with infectious persons, clinical illnesses consistent with tuberculosis, or HIV infection or other immunosuppression—a reactive area ≥5 mm is classified as a positive result, indicating infection with *M. tuberculosis*. For other high-risk groups (see Table 212–1), a reactive area ≥10 mm is considered positive. For low-risk persons, especially these residing in communities where the prevalence of tuberculosis is low, the cutoff point for a positive reaction may be ≥15 mm. Classifying children with this scheme depends on the willingness and ability of the clinician and family to develop a thorough exposure history for the child and the adults who care for the child. To interpret the tuberculin skin test correctly, the clinician must clearly understand the epidemiology of tuberculosis in the community and the correct indication for tuberculin testing of the individual.

CLINICAL MANIFESTATIONS AND DIAGNOSIS

Primary Pulmonary Disease. The primary pulmonary complex includes the parenchymal focus and the regional lymph nodes. About 70% of lung foci are subpleural, and localized pleurisy is common. The initial parenchymal inflammation usually is not visible on chest radiograph, but a localized, nonspecific infiltrate may be seen before the development of tissue hypersensitivity. All lobar segments of the lung are at equal risk of initial infection. Two or more primary foci are present in 25% of cases. The hallmark of primary tuberculosis in the lung is the relatively large size of the regional lymphadenitis compared with the relatively small size of the initial lung focus. In most cases, the parenchymal infiltrate and adenitis resolve early. As DTH develops, the hilar lymph nodes continue to enlarge in some children, especially infants, compressing the regional bronchus and causing obstruction. The common sequence is hilar adenopathy, focal hyperinflation, and then atelectasis. The resulting radiographic shadows have been called collapse-consolidation or segmental tuberculosis (see Fig. 212–2). These radiographic findings are similar to those seen with foreign body aspiration but are different from typical cases of bacterial pneumonia in children.

Rarely, inflamed caseous nodes attach to the endobronchial wall and erode through it, causing endobronchial tuberculosis or a fistula tract. The caseum causes complete obstruction of the bronchus, resulting in extensive infiltrate and collapse.

Most cases of tuberculous bronchial obstruction in children resolve fully with appropriate treatment. Occasionally, there is residual calcification of the primary focus or regional lymph nodes. The appearance of calcification implies that the lesion has been present for at least 6–12 mo. Healing of the segment is rarely complicated by scarring or contraction associated with cylindrical bronchiectasis.

Children may have lobar pneumonia without impressive hilar adenopathy. If the primary infection is progressively destructive, liquefaction of the lung parenchyma can lead to formation of a thin-walled primary tuberculosis cavity. Rarely, bullous tuberculous lesions can occur in the lungs and lead to pneumothorax if they rupture. Enlargement of the subcarinal lymph nodes can cause compression of the esophagus and, rarely, a bronchoesophageal fistula.

The symptoms and physical signs of primary pulmonary tuberculosis in children are surprisingly meager considering the degree of radiographic changes often seen. More than 50% of infants and children with radiographically moderate to severe pulmonary tuberculosis have no physical findings and are discovered only by contact tracing. Infants are more likely to experience signs and symptoms. Nonproductive cough and mild dyspnea are the most common symptoms. Systemic complaints such as fever, night sweats, anorexia, and decreased activity occur less often. Some infants have difficulty gaining weight or develop a true failure-to-thrive syndrome that often does not improve significantly until several months of effective treatment have been taken. Pulmonary signs are even less common. Some infants and young children with bronchial obstruction have localized wheezing or decreased breath sounds that may be accompanied by tachypnea or, rarely, respiratory distress. These pulmonary symptoms and signs are occasionally alleviated by antibiotics, suggesting bacterial superinfection.

The most specific confirmation of pulmonary tuberculosis is isolation of *M. tuberculosis*. The best culture specimen is usually the early morning gastric acid obtained before the child has arisen and peristalsis has emptied the stomach of the pooled secretions that have been swallowed overnight. Unfortunately, even under optimal conditions, three consecutive morning gastric aspirates yield the organisms in less than 50% of cases. The culture yield from bronchoscopy is even lower, but this procedure may demonstrate the presence of endobronchial disease or a fistula. Negative cultures never exclude the diagnosis of tuberculosis in a child. For most children, the presence of a positive tuberculin skin test, an abnormal chest radiograph consistent with tuberculosis, and history of exposure to an adult with infectious tuberculosis is adequate proof that the disease is present. The drug susceptibility test results from the adult source case's isolate can be used to determine the best therapeutic regimen for the child. Cultures should be obtained from the child whenever the source case is unknown or the source case has possible drug-resistant tuberculosis.

Progressive Primary Pulmonary Disease. A rare but serious complication of tuberculosis in a child occurs when the primary focus enlarges steadily and develops a large caseous center. Liquefaction may cause formation of a primary cavity associated with large numbers of tubercle bacilli. The enlarging focus may slough necrotic debris into the adjacent bronchus, leading to further intrapulmonary dissemination. Significant signs or symptoms are frequent in locally progressive disease in children. High fever, severe cough with sputum production, weight loss, and night sweats are common. Physical signs include diminished breath sounds, rales, and dullness or egophony over the cavity. The prognosis for full but usually slow recovery is excellent with appropriate therapy.

Reactivation Tuberculosis. Pulmonary tuberculosis in adults usually represents endogenous reactivation of a site of tuberculosis infection established previously in the body. This form of tuberculosis is rare in childhood but may occur in adolescence. Children with a healed tuberculosis infection acquired before age 2 yr rarely develop chronic reactivation pulmonary disease, which is more common in those who acquire the initial infection after 7 yr of age. The most frequent pulmonary sites are the original parenchymal focus, lymph nodes, or the apical seedings (Simon foci) established during the hematogenous phase of the early infection. This form of disease usually remains localized to the lungs because the established immune response prevents further extrapulmonary spread. The most common radiographic presentation of this type of tuberculosis is extensive infiltrates or thick-walled cavities in the upper lobes.

Older children and adolescents with reactivation tuberculosis are more likely to experience fever, anorexia, malaise, weight loss, night sweats, productive cough, hemoptysis, and chest pain than children with primary pulmonary tuberculosis. However, physical examination findings usually are minor or absent, even when cavities or large infiltrates are present. Most signs and symptoms improve within several weeks of starting effective treatment, although the cough may last for several months. This form of tuberculosis may be highly contagious if there is significant sputum production and cough. The prognosis for full recovery is excellent when patients are given appropriate therapy.

Pleural Effusion. Tuberculous pleural effusions, which can be local or general, originate in the discharge of bacilli into the pleural space from a subpleural pulmonary focus or caseated lymph node. Asymptomatic local pleural effusion is so frequent in primary tuberculosis that it is basically a component of the primary complex. Larger and clinically significant effusions occur months to years after the primary infection. Tuberculous pleural effusion is infrequent in children <6 yr of age and rare in those <2 yr of age. Effusions are usually unilateral but can be bilateral. They are virtually never associated with a segmental pulmonary lesion and are rare in disseminated tuberculosis. Often the radiographic abnormality is more extensive than would be suggested by physical findings or symptoms (Fig. 212–3).

Clinical onset of tuberculous pleurisy is often sudden, characterized by low to high fever, shortness of breath, chest pain on deep inspiration, and diminished breath sounds. The fever and other symptoms may last for several weeks after the start

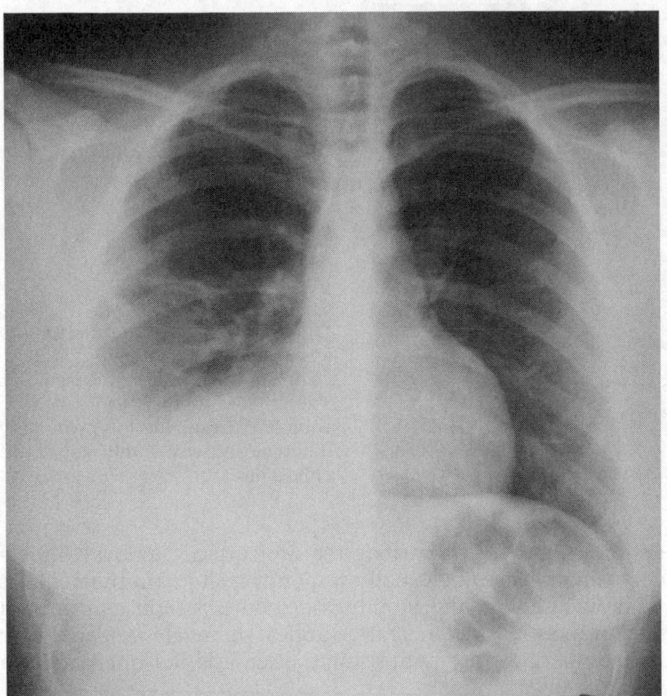

Figure 212–3 Pleural tuberculosis in a 16-yr-old girl.

of antituberculosis chemotherapy. The tuberculin skin test is positive in only 70–80% of cases. The prognosis is excellent, but radiographic resolution often takes months. Scoliosis is a rare complication from a long-standing effusion.

Examination of pleural fluid and the pleural membrane is important to establish the diagnosis of tuberculous pleurisy. The pleural fluid is usually yellow and only occasionally tinged with blood. The specific gravity is usually 1.012–1.025, the protein level is usually 2–4 g/dL, and the glucose concentration may be low, although it is usually in the low-normal range (20–40 mg/dL). Typically there are several hundred to several thousand white blood cells per cubic millimeter with an early predominance of polymorphonuclear cells followed by a high percentage of lymphocytes. Acid-fast smears of the pleural fluid are almost never positive. Cultures of the fluid are positive in only <30% of cases. Biopsy of the pleural membrane is more likely to yield a positive acid-fast stain or culture, and granuloma formation usually can be demonstrated.

Pericardial Disease. The most common form of cardiac tuberculosis is pericarditis. It is rare, occurring in 0.5–4% of tuberculosis cases in children. Pericarditis usually arises from direct invasion or lymphatic drainage from subcarinal lymph nodes. The presenting symptoms are usually nonspecific, including low-grade fever, malaise, and weight loss. Chest pain is unusual in children. A pericardial friction rub or distant heart sounds with pulsus paradoxus may be present. The pericardial fluid is typically serofibrinous or hemorrhagic. Acid-fast smear of the fluid rarely reveals the organism, but cultures are positive in 30–70% of cases. The culture yield from pericardial biopsy may be higher, and the presence of granulomas often suggests the diagnosis. Partial or complete pericardiectomy may be required when constrictive pericarditis develops.

Lymphohematogenous (Disseminated) Disease. Tubercle bacilli are disseminated to distant sites, including liver, spleen, skin, and lung apices, in all cases of tuberculosis infection. The clinical picture produced by lymphohematogenous dissemination depends on the quantity of organisms released from the primary focus and the adequacy of the host immune response. Lymphohematogenous spread is usually asymptomatic. Rare patients experience protracted hematogenous tuberculosis caused by the intermittent release of tubercle bacilli as a caseous focus erodes through the wall of a blood vessel in the lung. Although the clinical picture may be acute, more often it is indolent and prolonged, with spiking fever accompanying the release of organisms into the bloodstream. Multiple organ involvement is common, leading to hepatomegaly, splenomegaly, lymphadenitis in superficial or deep nodes, and papulonecrotic tuberculids appearing on the skin. Bones and joints or kidneys also may become involved. Meningitis occurs only late in the course of the disease. Early pulmonary involvement is surprisingly mild, but diffuse involvement becomes apparent with prolonged infection.

The most clinically significant form of disseminated tuberculosis is miliary disease, which occurs when massive numbers of tubercle bacilli are released into the bloodstream, causing disease in two or more organs. Miliary tuberculosis usually complicates the primary infection, occurring within 2–6 mo of the initial infection. Although this form of disease is most common in infants and young children, it is also found in adolescents and older adults, resulting from the breakdown of a previously healed primary pulmonary lesion. The clinical manifestations of miliary tuberculosis are protean, depending on the load of organisms that disseminate and where they lodge. Lesions are often larger and more numerous in the lungs, spleen, liver, and bone marrow than other tissues. Because this form of tuberculosis is most common in infants and malnourished or immunosuppressed patients, the host's immune incompetency probably also plays a role in pathogenesis.

The onset of miliary tuberculosis is sometimes explosive, and the patient may become gravely ill in several days. More often, the onset is insidious with early systemic signs, including anorexia, weight loss, and low-grade fever. At this time abnormal physical signs are usually absent. Generalized lymphadenopathy and hepatosplenomegaly develop within several weeks in about 50% of cases. The fever may then become higher and more sustained, although the chest radiograph usually is normal and respiratory symptoms are minor or absent. Within several more weeks, the lungs may become filled with tubercles and dyspnea, cough, rales, or wheezing occur. The lesions of miliary tuberculosis are usually smaller than 2–3 mm in diameter when first visible on chest radiograph (Fig. 212–4). The smaller lesions coalesce to form larger lesions and sometimes extensive infiltrates. As the pulmonary disease progresses, an alveolar-airblock syndrome may result in frank respiratory distress, hypoxia, and pneumothorax, or pneumomediastinum. Signs or symptoms of meningitis or peritonitis are found in 20–40% of patients with advanced disease. Chronic or recurrent headache in a patient with miliary tuberculosis usually indicates the presence of meningitis, whereas the onset of abdominal pain or tenderness is a sign of tuberculous peritonitis. Cutaneous lesions include papulonecrotic tuberculids, nodules, or purpura. Choroid tubercles occur in 13–87% of patients and are highly specific for the diagnosis of miliary tuberculosis. Unfortunately, the tuberculin skin test is nonreactive in up to 40% of patients with disseminated tuberculosis.

Diagnosis of disseminated tuberculosis can be difficult, and a high index of suspicion by the clinician is required. Often the patient presents with fever of unknown origin. Early sputum or gastric aspirate cultures have a low sensitivity. Biopsy of the liver or bone marrow with appropriate bacteriologic and histologic examinations more often yields an early diagnosis. The most important clue is usually history of recent exposure to an adult with infectious tuberculosis.

The resolution of miliary tuberculosis is slow, even with proper therapy. Fever usually declines within 2–3 wk of starting chemotherapy, but the chest radiographic abnormalities may not resolve for many months. Occasionally, corticosteroids hasten symptomatic relief, especially when airblock, peritoni-

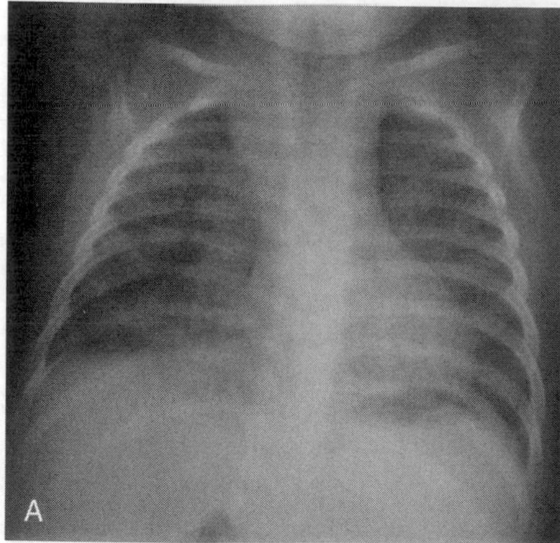

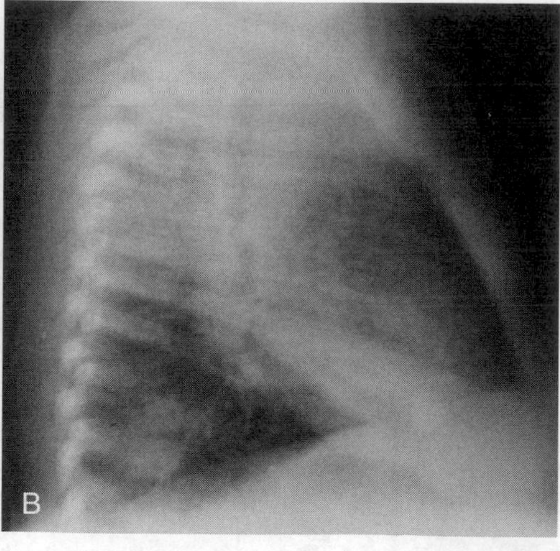

Figure 212–4 Posteroanterior *(A)* and lateral *(B)* chest radiographs of an infant with miliary tuberculosis. The child's mother had failed to complete treatment for pulmonary tuberculosis twice within 3 yr of this child's birth.

tis, or meningitis is present. The prognosis is excellent if the diagnosis is made early and adequate chemotherapy is given.

Upper Respiratory Tract Disease. Tuberculosis of the upper respiratory tract is rare in developed countries but is still observed in developing countries. Children with laryngeal tuberculosis have a croupy cough, sore throat, hoarseness, and dysphagia. Most children with laryngeal tuberculosis have extensive upper lobe pulmonary disease, but occasional patients have primary laryngeal disease with a normal chest radiograph. Tuberculosis of the middle ear results from aspiration of infected pulmonary secretions into the middle ear or from hematogenous dissemination in older children. The most common signs and symptoms are painless unilateral otorrhea, tinnitus, decreased hearing, facial paralysis, and a perforated tympanic membrane. Enlargement of lymph nodes in the preauricular or anterior cervical chains may accompany this infection. Diagnosis is difficult because stains and cultures of ear fluid are frequently negative and histology of the affected tissue often shows a nonspecific acute and chronic inflammation without granuloma formation.

Lymph Node Disease. Tuberculosis of the superficial lymph nodes, often referred to as scrofula, is the most common form of extrapulmonary tuberculosis in children. Historically, scrofula was usually caused by drinking unpasteurized cow's milk laden with *M. bovis*. Most current cases occur within 6–9 mo of initial infection by *M. tuberculosis*, although some cases appear years later. The tonsillar, anterior cervical, submandibular, and supraclavicular nodes become involved secondary to extension of a primary lesion of the upper lung fields or abdomen. Infected nodes in the inguinal, epitrochlear, or axillary regions result from regional lymphadenitis associated with tuberculosis of the skin or skeletal system. The nodes usually enlarge gradually in the early stages of lymph node disease. They are firm but not hard, discrete, and nontender. The nodes often feel fixed to underlying or overlying tissue. Disease is most often unilateral, but bilateral involvement may occur because of the crossover drainage patterns of lymphatic vessels in the chest and lower neck. As infection progresses, multiple nodes are infected, resulting in a mass of matted nodes. Systemic signs and symptoms other than a low-grade fever are usually absent. The tuberculin skin test is usually reactive. The chest radiograph is normal in 70% of cases. The onset of illness is occasionally more acute, with rapid enlargement of lymph nodes, high fever, tenderness, and fluctuance. The initial presentation is rarely a fluctuant mass with overlying cellulitis or skin discoloration.

Lymph node tuberculosis may resolve if left untreated but more often progresses to caseation and necrosis. The capsule of the node breaks down, resulting in the spread of infection to adjacent nodes. Rupture of the node usually results in a draining sinus tract that may require surgical removal. Tuberculous lymphadenitis usually responds well to antituberculosis therapy, although the lymph nodes do not return to normal size for months or even years. Surgical removal is not adequate therapy because the lymph node disease is but one part of a systemic infection.

A definitive diagnosis of tuberculous adenitis usually requires histologic or bacteriologic confirmation, which is best accomplished by excisional biopsy of the involved node. Culture of lymph node tissue yields the organism in only about 50% of cases. Many other conditions can be confused with tuberculous adenitis, including infection due to nontuberculous mycobacteria (NTM), cat-scratch disease, tularemia, brucellosis, toxoplasmosis, tumor, branchial cleft cyst, cystic hygroma, and pyogenic infection. The most frequent problem is distinguishing infection due to *M. tuberculosis* from lymphadenitis due to NTM in geographic areas where NTM are common. Both conditions are usually associated with a normal chest radiograph and a reactive tuberculin skin test. An important clue to the diagnosis of tuberculous adenitis is an epidemiologic link to an adult with infectious tuberculosis. In areas where both diseases are common, the only way to distinguish them may be culture of the involved tissue.

Central Nervous System Disease. Tuberculosis of the central nervous system is the most serious complication in children and is fatal without effective treatment. Tuberculous meningitis usually arises from the formation of a metastatic caseous lesion in the cerebral cortex or meninges that develops during the lymphohematogenous dissemination of the primary infection. This initial lesion increases in size and discharges small numbers of tubercle bacilli into the subarachnoid space. The resulting gelatinous exudate infiltrates the corticomeningeal blood vessels, producing inflammation, obstruction, and subsequent infarction of cerebral cortex. The brain stem is often the site of greatest involvement, which accounts for the frequently associated dysfunction of cranial nerves III, VI, and VII. The exudate also interferes with the normal flow of cerebrospinal fluid (CSF) in and out of the ventricular system at the level of the basilar cisterns, leading to a communicating hydrocephalus. The combination of vasculitis, infarction, cerebral edema, and hydrocephalus results in the severe damage that can occur gradually or rapidly. Profound abnormalities in electrolyte metabolism, due to salt wasting or the syndrome of inappropriate antidiuretic hormone secretion, also contribute to the pathophysiology of tuberculous meningitis.

Tuberculous meningitis complicates about 0.3% of untreated tuberculosis infections in children. It is most common in children between 6 mo and 4 yr of age. Occasionally, tuberculous meningitis occurs many years after the infection, when rupture of one or more of the subependymal tubercles discharges tubercle bacilli into the subarachnoid space. The clinical progression of tuberculous meningitis may be rapid or gradual. Rapid progression tends to occur more often in infants and young children, who may experience symptoms for only several days before the onset of acute hydrocephalus, seizures, and cerebral edema. More commonly, the signs and symptoms progress slowly over several weeks and can be divided into three stages. The *1st stage,* which typically lasts 1–2 wk, is characterized by nonspecific symptoms, such as fever, headache, irritability, drowsiness, and malaise. Focal neurologic signs are absent, but infants may experience a stagnation or loss of developmental milestones. The *2nd stage* usually begins more abruptly. The most common features are lethargy, nuchal rigidity, seizures, positive Kernig or Brudzinski signs, hypertonia, vomiting, cranial nerve palsies, and other focal neurologic signs. The accelerating clinical illness usually correlates with the development of hydrocephalus, increased intracranial pressure, and vasculitis. Some children have no evidence of meningeal irritation but may have signs of encephalitis, such as disorientation, movement disorders, or speech impairment. The *3rd stage* is marked by coma, hemiplegia or paraplegia, hypertension, decerebrate posturing, deterioration of vital signs, and, eventually, death. The prognosis of tuberculous meningitis correlates most closely with the clinical stage of illness at the time treatment is initiated. The majority of patients in stage 1 have an excellent outcome, whereas most patients in stage 3 who survive have permanent disabilities, including blindness, deafness, paraplegia, diabetes insipidus, or mental retardation. The prognosis for young infants is generally worse than for older children. It is imperative that antituberculosis treatment be considered for any child who develops basilar meningitis and hydrocephalus, cranial nerve palsy, or stroke with no other apparent etiology. Often the key to the correct diagnosis is identifying an adult in contact with the child who has infectious tuberculosis. Because of the short incubation period of tuberculous meningitis, the ill adult has not yet been diagnosed in many cases.

The diagnosis of tuberculous meningitis can be difficult early in its course requiring a high degree of suspicion on the part of the clinician. The tuberculin skin test is nonreactive in up to 50% of cases and 20–50% of children have a normal chest radiograph. The most important laboratory test for the diagnosis of tuberculous meningitis is examination and culture of the lumbar CSF. The CSF leukocyte count usually ranges from 10–500 cells/mm^3. Polymorphonuclear leukocytes may be present initially, but lymphocytes predominate in the majority of cases. The CSF glucose is typically <40 mg/dL but rarely <20 mg/dL. The protein level is elevated and may be markedly high (400–5,000 mg/dL) secondary to hydrocephalus and spinal block. Although the lumbar CSF is grossly abnormal, ventricular CSF may have normal chemistries and cell counts because this fluid is obtained from a site proximal to the inflammation and obstruction. The success of the microscopic examination of acid-fast stained CSF and mycobacterial culture is related directly to the volume of the CSF sample. Examinations or culture of small amounts of CSF are unlikely to demonstrate *M. tuberculosis*. When 5–10 mL of lumbar CSF can be obtained, the acid-fast stain of the CSF sediment is positive in up to 30% of cases and the culture is positive in 50–70% of cases. Cultures of other fluids, such as gastric aspirates or urine, may help confirm the diagnosis. Radiographic studies may aid in the diagnosis of tuberculous meningitis. Computed tomography (CT) or magnetic resonance imaging (MRI) of the brain of patients with tuberculous meningitis may be normal during early stages of the disease. As disease progresses, basilar enhancement and communicating hydrocephalus with signs of cerebral edema or early focal ischemia are the most common findings. Some small children with tuberculous meningitis may have one or several clinically silent tuberculomas, occurring most often in the cerebral cortex or thalamic regions.

Another manifestation of central nervous system tuberculosis is the *tuberculoma,* which usually presents clinically as a brain tumor. Tuberculomas account for up to 40% of brain tumors in some areas of the world, but they are rare in North America. In adults tuberculomas are most often supratentorial, but in children they are often infratentorial, located at the base of the brain near the cerebellum. Lesions are most often singular but may be multiple. The most common symptoms are headache, fever, and convulsions. The tuberculin skin test is usually reactive, but the chest radiograph is usually normal. Surgical excision is often necessary to distinguish tuberculoma from other causes of brain tumor. However, surgical removal is not necessary because most tuberculomas resolve with medical management. Corticosteroids are usually administered during the first few weeks of treatment or in the immediate postoperative period to decrease cerebral edema. On CT or MRI of the brain, tuberculomas usually appear as discrete lesions with a significant amount of surrounding edema. Contrast medium enhancement is often impressive and may result in a ringlike lesion. Since the advent of CT, the paradoxical development of tuberculomas in patients with tuberculous meningitis who are receiving ultimately effective chemotherapy has been recognized. The cause and nature of these tuberculomas are poorly understood, but they do not represent failure of drug treatment. This phenomenon should be considered whenever a child with tuberculous meningitis deteriorates or develops focal neurologic findings while on treatment. Corticosteroids may help alleviate the occasionally severe clinical signs and symptoms that occur. These lesions may persist for months or even years.

Cutaneous Disease. See Chapter 671.

Bone and Joint Disease. Bone and joint infection complicating tuberculosis is most likely to involve the vertebrae. The classic manifestation of tuberculous spondylitis is progression to Pott's disease, in which destruction of the vertebral bodies leads to gibbus deformity and kyphosis (Chapter 685.4). Skeletal tuberculosis is a late complication of tuberculosis and has become a rare entity since antituberculosis therapy became available.

Abdominal and Gastrointestinal Disease. Tuberculosis of the oral cavity or pharynx is quite unusual. The most common lesion is a painless ulcer on the mucosa, palate, or tonsil with enlargement of the regional lymph nodes. Tuberculosis of the esophagus is rare in children but may be associated with a tracheoesophageal fistula in infants. These forms of tuberculosis are usually associated with extensive pulmonary disease and swallowing of infectious respiratory secretions. However, they can occur in the absence of pulmonary disease, presumably by spread from mediastinal or peritoneal lymph nodes.

Tuberculous peritonitis, which occurs most often in young men, is uncommon in adolescents and rare in children. Generalized peritonitis may arise from subclinical or miliary hematogenous dissemination. Localized peritonitis is caused by direct extension from an abdominal lymph node, intestinal focus, or genitourinary tuberculosis. Pain and tenderness are mild initially. Rarely, the lymph nodes, omentum, and peritoneum become matted and can be palpated as a "doughy" irregular nontender mass. Ascites and low-grade fever commonly accompany this complication. The tuberculin skin test is usually reactive. The diagnosis can be confirmed by paracentesis with appropriate stains and cultures, but this procedure must be performed carefully to avoid entering a bowel that is intertwined with the matted omentum.

Tuberculous enteritis is caused by hematogenous dissemination or by swallowing tubercle bacilli discharged from the patient's own lungs. The jejunum and ileum near Peyer's patches and the appendix are the most common sites of involvement. The typical findings are shallow ulcers that cause pain, diarrhea or constipation, and weight loss with low-grade fever. Mesenteric adenitis usually complicates the infection.

The enlarged nodes may cause intestinal obstruction or erode through the omentum to cause generalized peritonitis. The clinical presentation of tuberculous enteritis is nonspecific, mimicking other infections and conditions that cause diarrhea. The disease should be suspected in any child with chronic gastrointestinal complaints and a reactive tuberculin skin test. Biopsy, acid-fast stain, and culture of the lesions are usually necessary to confirm the diagnosis.

Genitourinary Disease. Renal tuberculosis is rare in children because the incubation period is several years or longer. Tubercle bacilli usually reach the kidney during lymphohematogenous dissemination. The organisms often can be recovered from the urine in cases of miliary tuberculosis and in some patients with pulmonary tuberculosis in the absence of renal parenchymal disease. In true renal tuberculosis, small caseous foci develop in the renal parenchyma and release *M. tuberculosis* into the tubules. A large mass develops near the renal cortex that discharges bacteria through a fistula into the renal pelvis. Infection then spreads locally to the ureters, prostate, or epididymis. Renal tuberculosis is often clinically silent in its early stages, marked only by sterile pyuria and microscopic hematuria. Dysuria, flank or abdominal pain, and gross hematuria develop as the disease progresses. Superinfection by other bacteria, which often causes more acute symptoms, occurs frequently but may also delay recognition of the underlying tuberculosis. Hydronephrosis or ureteral strictures may complicate the disease. Urine cultures for *M. tuberculosis* are positive in 80–90% of cases, and acid-fast stains of large volumes of urine sediment are positive in 50–70% of cases. The tuberculin skin test is nonreactive in up to 20% of patients. An intravenous pyelogram often reveals mass lesions, dilatation of the proximal ureters, multiple small filling defects, and hydronephrosis if ureteral stricture is present. Disease is most often unilateral.

Tuberculosis of the genital tract is uncommon in both males and females before puberty. This condition usually originates from lymphohematogenous spread, although it can be caused by direct spread from the intestinal tract or bone. Adolescent girls may develop genital tract tuberculosis during the primary infection. The fallopian tubes are most often involved (90–100% of cases) followed by the endometrium (50%), ovaries (25%), and cervix (5%). The most common symptoms are lower abdominal pain and dysmenorrhea or amenorrhea. Systemic manifestations are usually absent and the chest radiograph is normal in the majority of cases. The tuberculin skin test is usually reactive. Genital tuberculosis in adolescent males causes epididymitis or orchitis. The condition usually manifests as a unilateral nodular painless swelling of the scrotum. Involvement of the glans penis is extremely rare. Genital abnormalities and a positive tuberculin skin test in an adolescent male or female should suggest the diagnosis of genital tract tuberculosis.

Disease in HIV-Infected Children. Most cases of tuberculosis in HIV-infected children have been described in developing countries. Establishing the diagnosis of tuberculosis in an HIV-infected child may be difficult because skin test reactivity is often absent, culture confirmation is difficult, and the clinical features of tuberculosis are similar to many other HIV-related infections and conditions. Tuberculosis in HIV-infected children is often more severe, progressive, and likely to occur in extrapulmonary sites. Radiographic findings are similar to those in children with normal immune systems, but lobar disease and lung cavitation are more common. Nonspecific respiratory symptoms, fever, and weight loss are the most common complaints. Rates of drug-resistant tuberculosis are higher in HIV-infected adults and, probably, are also higher in HIV-infected children. The mortality rate of HIV-infected children with tuberculosis is high, especially as the CD4 lymphocyte numbers fall. In adults, tuberculosis appears to accelerate the immune suppression caused by HIV.

Perinatal Disease. Symptoms of congenital tuberculosis may be present at birth but more commonly begin by the 2nd or 3rd wk of life. The most common signs and symptoms are respiratory distress, fever, hepatic or splenic enlargement, poor feeding, lethargy or irritability, lymphadenopathy, abdominal distention, failure to thrive, ear drainage, and skin lesions. The clinical manifestations vary in relation to the site and size of the caseous lesions. Many infants have an abnormal chest radiograph, most often a miliary pattern. Some infants with no pulmonary findings early in the course of the disease later develop profound radiographic and clinical abnormalities. Hilar and mediastinal lymphadenopathy and lung infiltrates are common. Generalized lymphadenopathy and meningitis occur in 30–50% of patients.

The clinical presentation of tuberculosis in newborns is similar to that caused by bacterial sepsis and other congenital infections, such as syphilis, toxoplasmosis, and cytomegalovirus. The diagnosis should be suspected in an infant with signs and symptoms of bacterial or congenital infection whose response to antibiotic and supportive therapy is poor and evaluation for other infections is unrevealing. The most important clue for rapid diagnosis of congenital tuberculosis is a maternal or family history of tuberculosis. Frequently, the mother's disease is discovered only after the neonate's diagnosis is suspected. The infant's tuberculin skin test is negative initially but may become positive in 1–3 mo. A positive acid-fast stain of an early morning gastric aspirate from a newborn usually indicates tuberculosis. Direct acid-fast stains on middle-ear discharge, bone marrow, tracheal aspirate, or biopsy tissue (especially liver) can be useful. The CSF should be examined and cultured, although the yield for isolating *M. tuberculosis* is low. The mortality rate of congenital tuberculosis remains very high because of delayed diagnosis; many children will have a complete recovery if the diagnosis is made promptly and adequate chemotherapy is started.

TREATMENT. Tubercle bacilli can be killed only during replication. Individual organisms that are naturally resistant to each antimycobacterial drug are present within large populations of *M. tuberculosis*. All known genes that encode for drug resistance within *M. tuberculosis* are located on a chromosome; transfer between organisms does not occur. The estimated frequency of these naturally drug-resistant organisms is about 10^{-6} but varies among drugs: with streptomycin (STM) it is 10^{-5}; with isoniazid (INH), 10^{-6}; and with rifampin (RIF), 10^{-8}. A cavity containing 10^9 tubercle bacilli has thousands of drug-resistant organisms, whereas a closed caseous lesion with its much smaller population contains few, if any, naturally resistant organisms. Fortunately, the natural occurrence of resistance to one drug is independent of resistance to any other drug. The chance that an organism is naturally resistant to both INH and RIF is on the order of 10^{-14}. Because populations of this size do not occur in patients, organisms naturally resistant to two drugs are essentially nonexistent.

The major biologic determinant of the success of antituberculosis chemotherapy is the size of the bacillary population within the host. For patients with large bacterial populations, such as adults with cavities or extensive infiltrates, many naturally drug-resistant organisms are present and at least two antituberculosis drugs must be used to effect a cure. Conversely for patients with infection (reactive skin test) but no disease, the bacterial population is small, drug-resistant organisms are rare or nonexistent, and a single drug can be used. Children with pulmonary tuberculosis and most patients with extrapulmonary tuberculosis have medium-sized populations in which significant numbers of naturally drug-resistant organisms may or may not be present. In general, these patients are treated with at least two drugs. The phenomena of drug resistance mutation and microbial population size explain why poor patient adherence to treatment or an inadequate treatment regimen can lead to the development of drug-resistant tuberculosis. If a patient with extensive pulmonary tuberculosis is given a single medication, the subpopulation of bacilli susceptible to that drug will be eliminated but the subpopulation of bacilli resistant to the drug have the opportunity to multiply and become the predominant strain. The patient will temporarily improve but will suffer a relapse from tuberculosis completely resistant to that drug. With treatment using two drugs to which the *M. tuberculosis* isolate is susceptible, drug X eliminates the subpopulation of bacilli resistant to drug Y and drug Y eliminates the subpopulation of bacilli resistant to drug X. If all the organisms have initial resistance to a certain medication (called primary resistance) and the patient is treated with that plus one other medication, only one effective medication is being used and the patient will eventually relapse with tuberculosis that is resistant to both drugs.

The various antituberculosis drugs (Table 212–2) differ in their primary site of activity and their actions. INH and RIF are highly bactericidal for *M. tuberculosis*. STM and several other aminoglycoside antibiotics are also bactericidal for extracellular tubercle bacilli, but their penetration into macrophages is poor. Pyrazinamide (PZA) cannot be shown to be bactericidal in the laboratory but clearly contributes to the killing of *M. tuberculosis* within the patient. Other antituberculosis drugs, such as ethambutol (EMB) at low doses (15 mg/kg/24 hr), ethionamide (ETH), and cycloserine, are bacteriostatic for *M. tuberculosis* and their primary purpose in the therapeutic regimen is to prevent emergence of resistance to other drugs. EMB at 25 mg/kg/24 hr has some bactericidal activity, which may be important in treating cases of drug-resistant tuberculosis. INH, RIF, and EMB are also effective in preventing emergence of resistance to other drugs, but pyrazinamide has almost no similar activity.

Isoniazid. INH is inexpensive, diffuses into all tissues and body fluids, and has a very low rate of adverse reactions. It can be administered either orally or intramuscularly. At the usual daily dose of 10 mg/kg, serum concentrations greatly exceed the minimum inhibitory concentration for *M. tuberculosis*. Peak concentrations in blood, sputum, and CSF are reached within a few hours and persist for at least 6–8 hr. INH is metabolized by acetylation in the liver. Rapid acetylation is more frequent among African-Americans and Asians than among whites. There is no correlation between acetylation rate and either efficacy or adverse reactions in children.

INH has two principal toxic effects, both of which are rare in children. Peripheral neuritis results from competitive inhibition of pyridoxine utilization. Pyridoxine levels are decreased in children taking INH, but clinical manifestations are rare and pyridoxine administration is not generally recommended. However, teenagers with inadequate diets, children from groups with low levels of milk and meat intake, and breastfeeding infants require supplemental pyridoxine. The most common physical manifestation of peripheral neuritis is numbness and tingling in the hands or feet. CNS toxicity from INH is rare, occurring usually when there is a significant overdose. The major toxic effect of INH is hepatotoxicity, which is also rare in children but increases with age. Three to 10 percent of children taking INH experience transient elevated serum transaminase levels. Clinically significant hepatotoxicity is very rare, being more likely to occur in adolescents or children with severe forms of tuberculosis. For most children, routine biochemical monitoring is not necessary, and toxicity can be monitored using clinical signs and symptoms. Allergic manifestations or hypersensitivity reactions caused by INH are very rare. INH can increase phenytoin levels and lead to toxicity by blocking its metabolism. Occasionally, INH interacts with theophylline, requiring modification of the dosage. Rare side effects of INH include pellagra, hemolytic anemia in patients with glucose-6-phosphate dehydrogenase deficiency, and a lupus-like reaction with rash and arthritis.

Rifampin. RIF is well absorbed from the gastrointestinal tract during fasting, with peak serum levels achieved within 2 hr. Oral and intravenous forms of RIF are now readily available. Like INH, rifampin is distributed widely in tissues and body fluids, including the CSF. Whereas excretion is mainly through the biliary tract, effective levels are reached in the kidneys and urine. Side effects are more common than with INH and include orange discoloration of urine and tears (with permanent staining of contact lenses), gastrointestinal disturbances, and hepatotoxicity, usually manifested as asymptomatic elevations in serum transaminase levels. When RIF is administered with INH, there is an increased risk of hepatotoxicity, which can be minimized by lowering the daily dose of INH to 10 mg/kg/24 hr. RIF has been associated with thrombocytopenia. It can render oral contraceptives ineffective and interacts with several drugs, including quinidine, cyclosporine, sodium warfarin, and corticosteroids. RIF is generally available in 150 mg and 300 mg capsules that, unfortunately, are inconvenient for many weight ranges of children. A suspension can be made using a variety of carriers but should not be taken with food because of malabsorption. A preparation called Rifamate contains both INH (150 mg) and RIF (300 mg); this preparation helps to ensure that the patient gets both INH and RIF or neither drug so that selective drug resistance is not created.

Pyrazinamide. In adults, a once-daily dose of PZA, 30 mg/kg/24 hr, produces serum levels of 20 μg/mL and little liver toxicity. The optimal dose in children is unknown, but this same dose causes high CSF levels, is well tolerated by children, and correlates with clinical success in treatment trials of tuberculosis in children. Extensive experience with PZA in children has verified its safety. Approximately 10% of adults treated with PZA develop arthralgias, arthritis, or gout due to hyperuricemia. Although uric acid levels are slightly elevated in children taking PZA, clinical manifestations of the hyperuricemia are extremely rare. Hypersensitivity reactions are rare in chil-

TABLE 212–2 Most Commonly Used Antituberculosis Drugs

Drug	Daily Dose (mg/kg/24 hr)	Twice-Weekly Dose (mg/kg/dose)	Maximum Dose
Isoniazid*	10–15	20–30	Daily: 300 mg; twice weekly: 900 mg
Rifampin*	10–20	10–20	600 mg
Pyrazinamide*	20–40	40–60	2 g
Streptomycin (IM)	20–40	20–40	1 g
Ethambutol	15–25	25–50	2.5 g
Ethionamide	15–20 (1–3 divided doses)	—	1 g
Cycloserine	10–20 (1–2 divided doses)	—	1 g
Kanamycin or capreomycin (IM)	15–30	15–30	1 g
Amikacin (IV)	15–30	15–30	1 g

IM = intramuscular; IV = intravenous.

**Isoniazid (150 mg) and rifampin (300 mg) are combined in one preparation called Rifamate. Isoniazid, rifampin, and pyrazinamide are combined in one preparation called Rifater.*

dren. The only dosage form of PZA is a rather large 500 mg tablet, which produces some dosing problems for children, especially infants. These pills can be crushed and given with food in the same manner as INH, but formal pharmacokinetic studies using this method have not been reported.

Streptomycin. STM is used less frequently than in the past for the treatment of childhood tuberculosis but is important for the treatment of drug-resistant disease. It may be given intramuscularly or intravenously. STM penetrates inflamed meninges fairly well but does not cross uninflamed meninges. Its major current use is when initial INH resistance is suspected or when the child has a life-threatening form of tuberculosis. The major toxicity of STM is to the vestibular and auditory portions of the 8th cranial nerve. Renal toxicity is much less frequent. STM is contraindicated in pregnant women because up to 30% of their infants will suffer severe hearing loss.

Ethambutol. EMB has received little attention in children because of its potential toxicity to the eye. At a dose of 15 mg/kg/24 hr it is primarily bacteriostatic, and its historic purpose has been to prevent emergence of resistance to other drugs. However, at 25 mg/kg/24 hr EMB has some bactericidal activity, which may be important in the treatment of drug-resistant disease. It is well tolerated by both adults and children when given orally as a once- or twice-a-day dose. The major potential toxicity is optic neuritis and red-green color blindness. There have been no reports of optic toxicity in children, but the drug has not been widely used because of the inability to routinely test visual fields and acuity in young children. EMB is not recommended for general use in young children for whom vision cannot be adequately examined but should be considered for children with suspected drug-resistant tuberculosis when other agents are not available or cannot be used.

Ethionamide. ETH is a bacteriostatic drug whose major purpose is treatment of drug-resistant tuberculosis. ETH penetrates into CSF very well and may be particularly useful in cases of tuberculous meningitis. It is generally well tolerated by children but often must be given in two or three divided daily doses because of gastrointestinal disturbance. ETH is chemically similar to INH and can cause significant hepatitis.

Other Drugs. These drugs are used less commonly for tuberculosis because they are significantly less effective or more toxic. Several aminoglycosides, especially kanamycin and amikacin, have significant antituberculosis activity and are used in cases of streptomycin-resistant tuberculosis. A closely related drug, capreomycin, is used more commonly in adults. These drugs can be given either intramuscularly or intravenously, are bactericidal, and usually do not demonstrate cross resistance with STM. Cycloserine is an effective antituberculosis drug in adults but has been used infrequently in children because of its major side effects of impairment with thought processes and tendency to cause depression and other psychiatric abnormalities. The drug is usually given in one or two divided doses, and most experts recommend monitoring serum levels during administration. Pyridoxine supplementation should be given when cycloserine is used. Ciprofloxacin and ofloxacin are fluoroquinolones with significant antituberculosis activity that are used commonly for drug-resistant tuberculosis in adults. These drugs are generally contraindicated in children because they cause destruction of growing cartilage in some animal models. However, they have been used effectively in some cases of multi–drug-resistant tuberculosis in children when few other effective agents were available.

Treatment Regimens for Disease. The basic principles of management of tuberculosis in children and adolescents are the same as those in adults. Several drugs are used to effect a relatively rapid cure and prevent the emergence of secondary drug resistance during therapy. Over the past 20 yr, a number of trials of antituberculosis therapy for children with drug-susceptible tuberculosis have demonstrated that a 9-mo regimen of INH and RIF is highly successful. Medication should be given daily initially but may be administered twice weekly during the final months of treatment. The major drawbacks of this two-drug, 9-mo regimen are the necessary length of treatment, the need for good adherence by the patient, and the relative lack of protection against possible initial drug resistance. Several clinical trials have shown that a 6-mo duration of INH and RIF, supplemented during the first 2 mo of treatment with PZA, yields a success rate approaching 100% with an incidence of clinically significant adverse reactions of less than 2%. Based on the reported studies, the AAP and CDC have endorsed a regimen of 6 mo of INH and RIF supplemented during the first 2 mo by PZA as standard therapy of intrathoracic tuberculosis in children. Most experts recommend that all drug administration be directly observed, meaning that a health care worker is physically present when the medications are administered to the patients. When directly observed therapy is used, intermittent (twice-weekly) administration of drugs after an initial period as short as 2 wk of daily therapy is as effective in children as daily therapy for the entire course. In locales where the community rate of INH resistance is greater than 5–10%, or when the adult source case is at increased risk for drug-resistant tuberculosis, most experts recommend adding a 4th drug—usually STM, EMB, or ETH—to the initial regimen. The reason to add the 4th drug is that PZA is not effective in preventing the emergence of RIF resistance during therapy when INH resistance already exists.

Controlled clinical trials for treating various forms of extrapulmonary tuberculosis are virtually nonexistent. Extrapulmonary tuberculosis is usually caused by small numbers of mycobacteria. In general, the treatment for most forms of extrapulmonary tuberculosis in children is the same as for pulmonary tuberculosis. Exceptions are bone and joint, disseminated, and CNS tuberculosis for which there are inadequate data to recommend 6-mo therapy. These cases usually are treated for 9–12 mo. Surgical debridement in bone and joint disease and ventriculoperitoneal shunting in CNS disease are frequently necessary.

The optimal treatment of tuberculosis in HIV-infected children has not been established. Adults with tuberculosis who are HIV seropositive can be treated successfully with standard regimens that include INH, RIF, and PZA. The total duration of therapy should be 6–9 mo or 6 mo after culture of sputum becomes sterile, whichever is longer. Data for children are limited to isolated case reports and small series. It may be difficult to determine whether a pulmonary infiltrate in an HIV-infected child who has a positive tuberculin reaction or history of exposure to an adult with infectious tuberculosis is being caused by *M. tuberculosis*. The radiographic appearance of other pulmonary complications of HIV infection in children, such as lymphoid interstitial pneumonitis and bacterial pneumonia, may be similar to that of tuberculosis. Treatment is often empirical based on epidemiologic and radiographic information. Therapy should be considered when tuberculosis cannot be excluded. Most experts believe that HIV-seropositive children with drug-susceptible tuberculosis should receive at least INH, RIF, and PZA for 2 mo followed by INH and RIF to complete a total treatment duration of 6–12 mo. It is recommended that all children with tuberculosis be evaluated for HIV infection because the presence of HIV may necessitate a longer duration of treatment. Children with HIV infection appear to have more frequent adverse reactions to antituberculosis drugs and must be monitored closely during therapy.

Drug-Resistant Tuberculosis. The incidence of drug-resistant tuberculosis is increasing in many areas of the world, including North America. There are two major types of drug resistance. Primary resistance occurs when an individual is infected with *M. tuberculosis* that is already resistant to a particular drug. Secondary resistance occurs when drug-resistant organisms emerge as the dominant population during treatment. The major causes of secondary drug resistance are poor adherence with the medication by the patient or inadequate treatment regimens prescribed by the physician. Nonadherence with one drug is more likely to lead to secondary resistance than failure to take all drugs. Secondary resistance is rare in children because of the small size of their mycobacterial population. Therefore, most drug resistance in children is primary, and patterns of drug resistance among children tend to mirror those found among adults in the same population. The main predictors of drug-resistant tuberculosis among adults are history of previous antituberculosis treatment, co-infection with HIV, and exposure to another adult with infectious drug-resistant tuberculosis.

Treatment of drug-resistant tuberculosis is successful only when at least two bactericidal drugs are given to which the infecting strain of *M. tuberculosis* is susceptible. When a child has possible drug-resistant tuberculosis, at least three and usually four or five drugs should be administered initially until the susceptibility pattern is determined and a more specific regimen can be designed. The specific treatment plan must be individualized for each patient according to the results of susceptibility testing on the isolates from the child or the adult source case. Treatment of 9 mo duration with RIF, PZA, and EMB is usually adequate for INH-resistant tuberculosis in children. When resistance to INH and RIF is present, the total duration of therapy often must be extended to 12–18 mo. The prognosis of single or multi–drug-resistant tuberculosis in children is usually good if the drug resistance is identified early in the treatment, appropriate drugs are administered under directly observed therapy, adverse reactions from the drugs do not occur, and the child and family are in a supportive environment. The treatment of drug-resistant tuberculosis in children always should be undertaken by a clinician with specific expertise in the treatment of tuberculosis.

Corticosteroids. These are useful in the treatment of some children with tuberculosis disease. They are most beneficial when the host inflammatory reaction contributes significantly to tissue damage or impairment of organ function. There is convincing evidence that corticosteroids decrease mortality rates and long-term neurologic sequelae in some patients with tuberculous meningitis by reducing vasculitis, inflammation, and, ultimately, intracranial pressure. Lowering the intracranial pressure limits tissue damage and favors circulation of antituberculosis drugs through the brain and meninges. Short courses of corticosteroids also may be effective for children with endobronchial tuberculosis that causes respiratory distress, localized emphysema, or segmental pulmonary lesions. Several randomized clinical trials have shown that corticosteroids can help relieve symptoms and constriction associated with acute tuberculous pericardial effusion. Corticosteroids may cause dramatic improvement in symptoms in some patients with tuberculous pleural effusion and shift of the mediastinum. However, the long-term course of disease is probably unaffected. Some children with severe miliary tuberculosis have dramatic improvement with corticosteroid therapy if the inflammatory reaction is so severe that alveolocapillary block is present. There is no convincing evidence that one corticosteroid preparation is better than another. The most commonly prescribed regimen is prednisone, 1–2 mg/kg/24 hr in one to two divided doses for 4–6 wk with gradual tapering.

Supportive Care. Children receiving treatment should be followed carefully to promote adherence with therapy, to monitor for toxic reactions to medications, and to ensure that the tuberculosis is being adequately treated. Adequate nutrition is important. Patients should be seen at monthly intervals and should be given just enough medication to last until the next visit. Anticipatory guidance with regard to the administration of medications to children is crucial. The physician should foresee difficulties that the family might have in introducing several new medications in inconvenient dosage forms to a young child. The clinician must report all cases of suspected tuberculosis in a child to the local health department to be sure that the child and family receive appropriate care and evaluation.

Nonadherence to treatment is the major problem in tuberculosis therapy. The patient and family must know what is expected of them through verbal and written instructions in their primary language. At least 30–50% of patients taking long-term treatment are significantly nonadherent with medications, and clinicians are usually not able to determine in advance which patients will be nonadherent. If the clinician suspects any chance of nonadherence with daily self-administered medications, directly observed therapy should be instituted with the help of the local health department.

Treatment of Tuberculosis Infection Without Disease. The treatment of children with asymptomatic tuberculosis infection (reactive tuberculin skin test, normal chest radiograph, normal physical examination) to prevent the development of tuberculosis disease is an established practice. The effectiveness of INH therapy in children has approached 100% and has lasted for at least 30 yr. INH therapy should be given to any child with a positive tuberculin skin test but no clinical or radiographic evidence of disease. The currently recommended regimen is 9 mo of daily INH therapy. INH can be given twice weekly under direct observation if adherence with daily treatment is likely to be poor. INH therapy also should be started for children <6 yr of age with a negative tuberculin skin test who have had recent exposure to an adult with infectious tuberculosis, including infants born to mothers who have tuberculosis. These children may already be infected with *M. tuberculosis* but have not yet developed delayed hypersensitivity. Significant tuberculosis disease may develop simultaneously with skin test reactivity in small children and infants, and the illness may develop before the positive skin test is recognized. In exposed children, tuberculin skin testing is repeated 3 mo after contact with the adult source case has been interrupted. If the repeat tuberculin skin test is negative, INH can be discontinued; if the second skin test is reactive (≥5 mm), the child has tuberculosis infection and a full course of INH therapy can be administered. Children with HIV infection or other causes of immune suppression should receive 12 months of treatment.

The optimal treatment for asymptomatic tuberculosis infection caused by drug-resistant strains of *M. tuberculosis* has not been established. For infections with strains that are INH resistant only, most experts recommend a 6–9 mo course of RIF. No data from controlled clinical trials support this practice, however. Similarly, no data are available concerning treatment of tuberculosis infection caused by organisms that are resistant to both INH and RIF. Some experts have recommended a combination of a fluoroquinolone and PZA for 6–9 mo. An alternative regimen is high-dose EMB and PZA for a similar period of time. For infection with isolates that are resistant to many drugs, the clinician usually administers two drugs to which the organism is susceptible. The efficacy and safety of these regimens in children are not established, and an expert in pediatric tuberculosis should be consulted for treatment of multi–drug-resistant tuberculosis infection in children.

PREVENTION. The highest priority of any tuberculosis control program should be case finding and treatment, which interrupts transmission of infection between close contacts. The children and adults in close contact with an adult suspected of having infectious pulmonary tuberculosis should be tuberculin skin tested and examined as soon as possible. On average, 30–50% of household contacts to infectious cases will be tuberculin skin test positive, and 1% of contacts already have overt disease. This scheme relies on effective and adequate public health response and resources. Children, particularly young infants, should receive high priority during contact investigations because their risk of infection is high and they are more likely to rapidly develop severe forms of tuberculosis.

Mass testing of large groups of children for tuberculosis

infection is an inefficient process. When large groups of children at low risk for tuberculosis are tested, the vast majority of skin test reactions are actually false-positive reactions due to biologic variability or cross sensitization with NTM. However, testing of high-risk groups of adults or children should be encouraged because most of these individuals with positive tuberculin skin tests have tuberculosis infection. Testing should take place only if effective mechanisms are in place to ensure adequate evaluation and treatment of the individuals who test positive.

Bacille Calmette-Guérin Vaccination. The only available vaccine against tuberculosis is the bacille Calmette-Guérin (BCG), named for the two French investigators responsible for its development. The original vaccine organism was a strain of *M. bovis* attenuated by subculture every 3 wk for 13 yr. This strain was distributed to dozens of laboratories that continued to subculture the organism on different media under various conditions. The result has been production of many BCG vaccines that differ widely in morphology, growth characteristics, sensitizing potency, and animal virulence. The route of administration and dosing schedule for the BCG vaccines are important variables for efficacy. The preferred route of administration is intradermal injection with a syringe and needle because it is the only method that permits accurate measurement of an individual dose. However, the intradermal route is expensive and needles and syringes are reused in developing countries, creating a danger of HIV and hepatitis virus transmission. A unit-dose multipuncture technique is the only technique available in the United States and many other parts of the world.

The BCG vaccines are extremely safe in immunocompetent hosts. Local ulceration and regional suppurative adenitis occur in 0.1–1% of vaccine recipients. Local lesions do not suggest underlying host immune defects and do not affect the level of protection afforded by the vaccine. They usually resolve spontaneously, but chemotherapy is needed occasionally. Surgical excision of a suppurative draining node is rarely necessary and should be avoided if possible. Osteitis is a rare complication of BCG vaccination that appears to be related to certain strains of the vaccine that are no longer in wide use. Systemic complaints such as fever, convulsions, loss of appetite, and irritability are extraordinarily rare after BCG vaccination. Profoundly immunocompromised patients may develop disseminated BCG infection after vaccination. Children with HIV infection appear to have rates of local adverse reactions to BCG vaccines that are comparable to rates in immunocompetent children. However, the incidence in these children of disseminated infection months to years after vaccination is currently unknown.

Recommended vaccine schedules vary widely among countries. The official recommendation of the World Health Organization is a single dose administered during infancy, including in areas where HIV infection is prevalent. In some countries repeat vaccination is universal. In others it is based on either tuberculin skin testing or the absence of a typical scar. The optimal age for administration and dosing schedule are unknown because adequate comparative trials have not been performed.

Although dozens of BOG trials have been reported in various human populations, the most useful data have come from several controlled trials. The results of these studies have been disparate. Some demonstrated a great deal of protection from BCG vaccines, but others showed no efficacy at all. A recent meta-analysis of published BCG vaccination trials suggested that BCG is 50% effective in preventing pulmonary tuberculosis in adults and children. The protective effect for disseminated and meningeal tuberculosis appears to be slightly higher, with BCG preventing 50–80% of cases. A variety of explanations for the varied responses to BCG vaccines have been proposed, including methodologic and statistical variations within the trials, interaction with NTM that either enhances or decreases the protection afforded by BCG, different potencies among the various BCG vaccines, and genetic factors for BCG response within the study populations. BCG vaccination administered during infancy has little effect on the ultimate incidence of tuberculosis in adults, suggesting that the effect of the vaccine is time limited.

In summary, BCG vaccination has worked well in some situations but poorly in others. Clearly, BCG vaccination has had little effect on the ultimate control of tuberculosis throughout the world because more than 5 billion doses have been administered but tuberculosis remains epidemic in most regions. BCG vaccination does not substantially influence the chain of transmission because those cases of contagious pulmonary tuberculosis in adults that can be prevented by BCG vaccination constitute a rather small fraction of the sources of infection in a population. The best use of BCG vaccination appears to be prevention of life-threatening forms of tuberculosis in infants and young children.

BCG vaccination has never been adopted as part of the strategy for the control of tuberculosis in the United States. Widespread use of the vaccine would render subsequent tuberculin skin testing less useful. However, BCG vaccination may contribute to tuberculosis control in selected population groups. BCG is recommended for tuberculin skin test–negative infants and children who (1) are at high risk of intimate and prolonged exposure to persistently untreated or ineffectively treated adults with infectious pulmonary tuberculosis and cannot be removed from the source of infection or placed on long-term preventive therapy or (2) are continuously exposed to persons with tuberculosis who have bacilli that are resistant to INH and RIF. Any child receiving BCG vaccination should have a documented negative tuberculin skin test before receiving the vaccine. After receiving the vaccine, the child should be separated from the possible sources of infection until it can be demonstrated that the child has had a vaccine response (demonstrated by tuberculin reactivity, which usually develops within 1–3 mo). Occasionally, a second BCG vaccination must be given to children who fail to develop skin test reactivity after the first dose.

Perinatal Tuberculosis. The most effective way of preventing tuberculosis infection and disease in the neonate or young infant is through appropriate testing and treatment of the mother and other family members. High-risk pregnant women should be tested with a tuberculin skin test, and those with a positive test should receive a chest radiograph with appropriate abdominal shielding. If the mother has a negative chest radiograph and is clinically well, no separation of the infant and mother is needed after delivery. The child needs no special evaluation or treatment if he or she remains asymptomatic. Other household members should receive tuberculin skin testing and further evaluation as indicated.

If the mother has suspected tuberculosis at the time of delivery, the newborn should be separated from the mother until the chest radiograph is taken. If the mother's chest radiograph is abnormal, separation should be maintained until the mother has been evaluated thoroughly, including examination of the sputum. If the mother's chest radiograph is abnormal but the history, physical examination, sputum examination, and evaluation of the radiograph show no evidence of current active tuberculosis, it is reasonable to assume that the infant is at low risk for infection. The mother should receive appropriate treatment, and she and her infant should receive careful follow-up care. In addition, all household members should be evaluated for tuberculosis.

If the mother's chest radiograph or acid-fast sputum smear shows evidence of current tuberculosis disease, additional steps are necessary to protect the infant. INH therapy for newborns has been so effective that separation of the mother and infant is no longer considered mandatory. Separation should occur only if the mother is ill enough to require hospitalization, she has been or is expected to become nonadherent with her treatment, or there is strong suspicion that she has drug-resistant tuberculosis. INH treatment for the infant should be continued until the mother has been shown to be sputum culture negative for at least 3 mo. At that time, a Mantoux tuberculin skin test should be placed on the child. If positive, INH is continued for a total duration of 9–12 mo; if negative, INH can be discontinued. Because INH resistance is increasing in the United States, it is not always clear that INH therapy will be effective for the neonate. If INH resistance is suspected or the mother's adherence to medication is in question, separation of the infant from the mother should be considered. The duration of separation must be at least as long as is necessary to render the mother noninfectious. An expert in tuberculosis should be consulted if the young infant has potential exposure to the mother or another adult with tuberculous disease caused by an INH-resistant strain of *M. tuberculosis*.

Although INH is not thought to be teratogenic, the treatment of pregnant women with asymptomatic tuberculosis infection is often deferred until after delivery. However, symptomatic pregnant women or those with radiographic evidence of tuberculous disease should be appropriately evaluated. Because pulmonary tuberculosis is harmful to both the mother and the fetus, and it represents a great danger to the infant after delivery, tuberculosis in pregnant women always should be treated. The most common regimen for drug-susceptible tuberculosis is INH, RIF, and EMB. The aminoglycosides and ETH should be avoided because of their teratogenic effect. The safety of PZA in pregnancy has not been established.

American Academy of Pediatrics, Committee on Infectious Diseases: Chemotherapy for tuberculosis in infants and children. Pediatrics 89:161, 1992.

American Academy of Pediatrics, Committee on Infectious Diseases: Screening for tuberculosis in infants and children. Pediatrics 93:131, 1994.

American Thoracic Society: Diagnostic standards and classification of tuberculosis. Am Rev Respir Dis 142:725, 1990.

American Thoracic Society: Treatment of tuberculosis and tuberculous infection in adults and children. Am J Respir Crit Care Med 149:1359, 1994.

Brudney K, Dobkin J: Resurgent tuberculosis in New York City. Human immunodeficiency virus, homelessness, and the decline of tuberculosis control programs. Am Rev Respir Dis 144:745, 1991.

Centers for Disease Control and Prevention: Initial therapy for tuberculosis in the era of multidrug resistance: Recommendations of the Advisory Council for the Elimination of Tuberculosis. MMWR 42:1, 1993.

Centers for Disease Control and Prevention: Anergy skin testing and preventive therapy for HIV-infected persons: Revised recommendations. MMWR 46 (RR-15):1, 1997.

Centers for Disease Control and Prevention: Screening for tuberculosis and tuberculosis infection in high-risk populations: Recommendations of the Advisory Committee for the Elimination of Tuberculosis. MMWR 44 (RR-11):19, 1995.

Colditz GA, Brewer TF, Berkey CS, et al: Efficacy of BCG vaccine in the prevention of tuberculosis: Meta-analysis of the published literature. JAMA 271:698, 1994.

Hsu KHK: Thirty years after isoniazid: Its impact on tuberculosis in children and adolescents. JAMA 251:1283, 1984.

Hussey G, Chisholm T, Kibel M: Miliary tuberculosis in children: A review of 94 cases. Pediatr Infect Dis J 10:832, 1991.

Mukadi Yu, Wiktor SZ, Nulibaly H, et al: The impact of HIV infection on the development, clinical presentation and outcome of tuberculosis among children in Abidjon, Cote d'Ivoire. AIDS 11:1151, 1997.

O'Brien R, Long M, Cross F, et al: Hepatotoxicity from isoniazid and rifampin among children treated for tuberculosis. Pediatrics 72:491, 1983.

Pineda PR, Leung A, Muller NL, et al: Intrathoracic paediatric tuberculosis: A report of 202 cases. Tubercle Lung Dis 74:261, 1993.

Starke JR, Correa AG: Management of mycobacterial infection and disease in children. Pediatr Infect Dis J 14:455, 1995.

Starke JR, Jacobs RF, Jereb J: Resurgence of tuberculosis in children. J Pediatr 120:839, 1992.

Steiner P, Rao M: Drug-resistant tuberculosis in children. Semin Pediatr Infect Dis 4:275, 1993.

Ussery XT, Valway SE, McKenna M, et al: Epidemiology of tuberculosis among children in the United States, 1985 to 1994. Pediatr Infect Dis J 15:697, 1996.

Vallejo JG, Starke JR: Tuberculosis and pregnancy. Clin Chest Med 13:693, 1992.

Vallejo JG, Ong LT, Starke JR: Clinical features, diagnosis and treatment of tuberculosis in infants. Pediatrics 94:1, 1994.

Waecker NJ, Conner JD: Tuberculous meningitis in 30 children. Pediatr Infect Dis J 9:539, 1990.

CHAPTER 213

Leprosy

(Hansen Disease)

Dwight A. Powell

Leprosy is a chronic disease resulting from infection with *Mycobacterium leprae* and the ensuing host response. The organs most prominently affected are the skin and the peripheral nervous system, but upper respiratory, testicular, and ocular involvement are also relatively common. Humans were long believed to be the sole host of *M. leprae*, but naturally acquired infection has been documented in armadillos in the southeastern United States and experimental infection has been established in primates, nude mice, and armadillos.

Chronic skin lesions, madarosis, sensory neuropathy resulting in the loss of digits or limbs, and paresis secondary to motor nerve dysfunction are among the sequelae of leprosy. The highly visible nature of these debilities led to the historical stigmatization of the "leper." The psychologic and sociologic sequelae of this stigma can be as debilitating as the disease itself and may result in delays in seeking medical attention. To combat this prejudice, the term *leprosy patient* has replaced the word *leper* and *Hansen disease* has become an accepted designation.

ETIOLOGY. *M. leprae* is an acid-fast bacillus of the family Mycobacteriaceae. The exceedingly slow multiplication of *M. leprae* observed in animal models may partially explain the long incubation period seen in human disease; a period of 3–5 yr is believed to be typical. The rare occurrence of leprosy in infants as young as 3 mo of age suggests that in utero transmission may occur or that very short incubation periods may be possible in certain situations. Possible modes of transmission include contact with desquamated infected epidermis, ingestion of infected breast milk, and bites of mosquitoes or other vectors. At present, however, transmission by means of infected nasal secretions appears to be the basis for most infections. Extensive involvement of the nasopharynx manifested as chronic rhinitis is common in lepromatous disease.

EPIDEMIOLOGY. After the introduction of multidrug therapy (MDT) by the World Health Organization (WHO) in 1982, there has been a steady decline in the prevalence of leprosy. On a global scale, the estimated prevalence has reduced 75–80% from 10–12 million cases in 1985 to 2.4 million cases in 1994. This decrease may be due in part to the shorter duration of disease after MDT and may not reflect a significant decrease in the annual incidence of new cases. In 1992, 690,000 new cases were detected, a number no different than previous years. However, in some long-standing, well-organized control programs in which there has been a prolonged high level of MDT, there has been a significant decline in case-detection rates. More than 95% of the world's leprosy patients reside in 16 major endemic countries in Africa, India, Southeast Asia, and Central and South America. Human-to-human transmission accounts for an overwhelming majority of cases; a high percentage of them occur in family members or in close contacts of known patients. Approximately 200 cases are reported annually in the United States, of which 90% are in immigrants. The remaining 10% develop in localized foci along the Gulf coast, in Hawaii, and in the Micronesian territories.

Leprosy occurs at all ages, but infections in infants are extremely rare; incidence rates peak during childhood and early adulthood in endemic areas. HIV infection may alter the risk of leprosy in areas of high prevalence for both pathogens.

PATHOGENESIS. Damage is mediated through many pathways,

some of which are release of humoral mediators of inflammation by activated lymphocytes and macrophages, nerve compression by enlarging granulomas, and deposition of immune complexes. Multiple mechanisms may operate simultaneously or sequentially.

The site of entry of *M. leprae* into the human host is unknown. Direct invasion through skin injury has been thought to be the most likely route of infection, but several reports have suggested the respiratory tract may be more important than previously thought. Growth and multiplication of *M. leprae* are maximal at 34–35°C. Nothing is known of the host immune responses in the initial period after infection, but skin testing (Mitsuda reaction, see later) and serologic studies suggest that up to 80–90% of those infected develop immunity without ever manifesting clinical disease. Most of the remaining patients, after a highly variable incubation period averaging 3–5 yr, develop typical skin lesions of *indeterminate leprosy.* Studies in endemic areas using the polymerase chain reaction show widespread presence of the organism in nasal secretions from asymptomatic individuals.

Fully developed clinical leprosy is classified into five categories that can be aligned on a spectrum representing the range of intensity and efficacy of the cellular limb of the host immune response.

One end of the spectrum is *tuberculoid leprosy,* in which there is a vigorous and specific cell-mediated immune response. In tissue biopsies there are tightly organized granulomas composed of epithelioid cells and lymphocytes but bacilli are scant or absent. Macrophages, when present, do not contain intracellular organisms. Caseation is rare. Heavy cellular infiltration is found in the dermis with destruction of cutaneous nerve fibers.

At the other end of the spectrum is *lepromatous leprosy,* in which there is total and specific anergy to *M. leprae* both by skin testing and by in vitro assays of cell-mediated immunity. Large amounts of circulating and tissue-based antibody to mycobacterial antigens are present, but they afford no protective immunity. Bacilli are found in enormous numbers in the skin, nasal mucosa, and peripheral nerves. There is continual bacillemia as well as bacillary invasion of all major organs except the central nervous system. Tissue granulomas are poorly formed and are composed chiefly of loose aggregates of foamy histiocytes. Macrophages teeming with undigested bacilli (globi) are common. There is extensive, symmetric involvement of peripheral nerves, although the cutaneous nerve endings are usually spared.

An *M. leprae*–specific suppressor T-cell population is found in the circulation of patients with lepromatous leprosy, and increased numbers of suppressor T cells are found in their skin granulomas. T cells from lepromatous patients also produce less interleukin 2 and less gamma interferon after stimulation with *M. leprae* antigens than do T cells from tuberculoid patients or normal controls. These findings may relate to the underlying cellular defect that permits development of clinical leprosy in the susceptible individual.

Borderline or *dimorphous leprosy* is subdivided into three subclasses that lie between the tuberculoid and lepromatous poles on the clinical spectrum.

CLINICAL MANIFESTATIONS

Indeterminate Leprosy (I). This is the earliest clinically detectable form of leprosy. Although it is observed in only 10–20% of infected individuals, it is a stage through which most patients with advanced leprosy have passed. Usually there is a single hypopigmented macule, 2–4 cm in diameter, with a poorly defined border but having no erythema or induration. Anesthesia is minimal or absent, particularly if the lesion is on the face. Tissue samples may contain granulomas, but bacilli are rarely demonstrable. The histopathology is not distinctive; the diagnosis is usually made by exclusion of other skin disorders in contacts (especially children) of leprosy patients. In 50–75% of patients with indeterminate leprosy, the lesions heal spontaneously; in the remainder, they progress to one of the classic forms.

Tuberculoid Leprosy (TT). There is usually a single, large (often over 10 cm in diameter) lesion with a well-demarcated, elevated erythematous rim. The interior of the lesion is flat, atrophic, hypopigmented, and anesthetic. Rarely, there may be as many as four lesions. The closest superficial nerve is often impressively thickened. The ulnar, posterior tibial, and great auricular nerves are most commonly affected. Periodic examination of all leprosy patients and their contacts should include palpation of these nerves. Without therapy, the skin lesion tends to enlarge slowly, but documented instances of spontaneous resolution exist. The coloration of the rim slowly fades with therapy, and the induration resolves, resulting in a flat lesion with central hypopigmentation and a ring of postinflammatory hyperpigmentation. Loss of hair follicles, sweat glands, cutaneous nerve receptors, and sensation in the central portion of the lesion is irreversible. Marked improvement should be apparent within 1–2 mo after initiating therapy, but complete resolution may take up to 8–12 mo. There is an entity of "pure neural" tuberculoid leprosy, which presents as a mononeuropathy with prominent nerve thickening but no cutaneous lesions. Histopathology is mandatory to establish this diagnosis. Nerve trunk size varies widely, and overdiagnosis of "enlarged" nerves is common among inexperienced observers. Nodular or fusiform nerve thickening has greater diagnostic value than a palpable nerve that is smooth and symmetric.

Borderline Leprosy. The clinical and histologic criteria for the three subdivisions of borderline leprosy are less well defined than are those of the two polar categories. In contrast to the tuberculoid and lepromatous patterns, those in the borderline divisions are unstable. For example, host or bacterial factors can result in downgrading the clinical condition toward the lepromatous pattern or upgrading it toward the tuberculoid pattern. Therapy is the most common cause of upgrading reactions; downgrading can be seen in conditions that compromise host immunity, for example, pregnancy. Clinical characteristics of the three generally accepted borderline subclasses are as follows.

In the *borderline tuberculoid* (BT) pattern the lesions are greater in number but smaller in size than in tuberculoid leprosy. There may be small satellite lesions around older lesions, and the margins of the borderline tuberculoid lesions are less distinct. There is usually thickening of two or more superficial nerves.

In the *borderline* (BB) pattern the lesions are more numerous and more heterogeneous in appearance. They may become confluent, and plaques may be present. The borders are poorly defined, and the erythematous rim fades into the surrounding skin. There may be anesthesia, but hypesthesia is more common. Mild to moderate nerve thickening is common, but severe muscle wasting and neuropathy are unusual.

In the *borderline lepromatous* (BL) pattern, there are a large number of asymmetrically distributed lesions that are heterogeneous in appearance. Macules, papules, plaques, and nodules may all coexist. Individual lesions are small unless confluent. Anesthesia is mild and superficial nerve trunks are spared. The initial response to therapy is often dramatic; nodules and plaques flatten within 2–3 mo. With continued therapy the lesions become macular and almost invisible.

Lepromatous Leprosy (LL). The lesions are innumerable, often confluent, and symmetric. Initially there may be only vague macules or even uniform, diffuse skin infiltrations without discernible lesions. As the disease progresses, the lesions become increasingly papular and nodular, so that with the diffuse thickening and infiltration of the skin, the characteristic leonine facies accompanied by loss of the eyebrows and distortion of the earlobes becomes apparent. Anesthesia of the lesions either does not occur or is mild, but a symmetric peripheral sensory neuropathy may develop. Testicular infiltration leading to azoospermia, infertility, and gynecomastia is common in adults but not in children. Bacilli are demonstrable in most internal organs other than the central nervous system, but tissue damage or interference with function is infrequent. Glomerulonephritis, when it occurs, is believed to be secondary to immune complex deposition rather than to infection per se. The initial response to therapy may be encouraging but is often followed by a long (2–5 yr) period of very slow improvement. In true lepromatous leprosy, the specific anergy to the leprosy bacillus persists despite therapy, thus making the patient theoretically susceptible to relapse if even a single viable bacillus remains at the end of therapy.

Reactional States. Acute clinical exacerbations are common in leprosy and are believed to reflect abrupt changes in the host-parasite immunologic balance. Although these reactional states do occur in the absence of therapy, they are especially common during the initial years of treatment. Up to 50% of patients receiving effective chemotherapy can develop reactions, and, unless adequately treated, they will result in crippling deformities. Two major variants are recognized.

Type 1 (reversal) reactions are observed predominantly in borderline leprosy. Acute tenderness and swelling at the site of existing cutaneous and neural lesions and the development of new lesions are the major manifestations. Existing or new skin lesions often ulcerate to leave hideous scars. Fever and systemic toxicity are uncommon, but the acute neuritis that can present either as a severe painful episode or be insidious and painless can lead to irreversible nerve injury (anesthesia, facial paralysis, claw hand, footdrop) if not treated immediately. Reversal reactions constitute perhaps the only medical emergency related to leprosy per se. Patients should be instructed to contact their physicians immediately if signs of a reaction appear. A sudden increase in effective cell-mediated immunity in response to *(M. leprae)* antigens after rapid killing of bacilli is the initiating event.

Type 2 (erythema nodosum leprosum) reactions occur in the majority of patients with polar lepromatous leprosy and in 25–40% of borderline lepromatous cases. Tender dermal nodules, clinically resembling erythema nodosum, are the hallmark of this syndrome. High fever, migrating polyarthralgia, orchitis, iridocyclitis, and, rarely, nephritis may occur. Circulating and tissue-based immune complexes are frequently present and may explain the resemblance to other immune complex disorders, but the underlying mechanism appears to involve the activation of a helper T-cell subset. There is a strong tendency to recurrence, and there is a risk of amyloidosis and renal failure if treatment is inadequate.

DIAGNOSIS. The critical factor in the diagnosis of leprosy is its inclusion in the differential diagnosis of a skin disorder in anyone who has resided in an endemic leprosy region. Anesthetic skin lesions with or without thickened peripheral nerves are virtually pathognomonic of leprosy. A full-thickness skin biopsy from an active lesion (stained with both a standard histologic stain and an acid-fast stain such as Fite-Faraco) is the optimal procedure for confirmation of the diagnosis and accurate disease classification. Acid-fast bacilli are rarely found in patients with indeterminate or tuberculoid disease, so diagnosis in these cases is based on the clinical picture and the presence of typical dermal granulomas. For purposes of assigning patients to the appropriate WHO MDT regimen, slit skin smears are assessed to determine whether patients have paucibacillary or multibacillary infections. Other routine clinical, microbiologic, and radiologic tests have little or no role in the diagnosis of leprosy, although they may be useful in the exclusion of other diagnoses. Various assays for serum antibodies directed against unique antigens of *M. leprae* have been developed, but current tests lack sufficient sensitivity and specificity for active disease to be useful for clinical diagnostic purposes.

Lepromin is a suspension of killed *M. leprae* obtained from infected human or armadillo tissue. After intradermal inoculation, early (48 hr, Fernandez reaction) as well as late (3–4 wk, Mitsuda reaction) reactions may be seen. The Mitsuda reaction, a granulomatous response to the antigen, is more consistent. Patients with tuberculoid leprosy have strongly positive (5 mm) responses, whereas patients with lepromatous leprosy do not respond. The test is not useful in the diagnosis of leprosy, because the majority of the population in both endemic and nonendemic leprosy areas will be Mitsuda positive. Lepromin is not available in the United States.

Many diseases endemic in developing countries can mimic the appearance of leprosy; these include secondary syphilis, cutaneous leishmaniasis, yaws, and cutaneous fungal infections. None of these entities involve paresthesia/anesthesia localized to the skin lesions or cause thickening of peripheral nerves. The presence of nerve thickening with skin lesions also differentiates leprosy from primary neurologic disease. Indeterminate leprosy may present as minimal anesthesia, no nerve thickening, and equivocal histopathology suggesting a superficial fungal infection, particularly tinea versicolor. The diagnosis of indeterminate leprosy should be considered one of exclusion and will rarely be made in anyone other than a close contact of a known patient.

TREATMENT. Physicians considering the diagnosis or treatment of leprosy are strongly encouraged to obtain consultation and assistance in patient management from the Gillis W. Long Hansen's Disease Center (Carville, Louisiana) or its regional centers.

Only three antimycobacterial agents have proven to be consistently effective in the treatment of leprosy. Since the early 1940s, *dapsone* (diaminodiphenylsulfone) has remained the cornerstone of therapy because of its low cost, minimal toxicity, and wide availability. Unfortunately, secondary resistance tends to develop when it is used as the sole agent. More worrisome is the increasing incidence of primary resistance, which has been reported in up to 30% of newly diagnosed patients in Malaysia and Ethiopia. Dermatitis, hepatitis, and methemoglobinemia are the most common side effects; granulocytopenia is rare but potentially fatal. Dose-related hemolytic anemia, which can be severe, is seen in patients with glucose-6-phosphate dehydrogenase deficiency, methemoglobin reductase deficiency, or hemoglobin M. Pregnancy studies have not shown an increased risk of fetal abnormalities.

Rifampin is the most rapidly mycobactericidal drug for *M. leprae*, achieving excellent levels inside cells, where most leprosy bacilli reside. Resistance has been reported infrequently. The widespread use of rifampin has been limited by cost more than by toxicity. Hepatitis is the most common side effect that necessitates discontinuance.

Clofazimine, a phenazine dye with both antimycobacterial and anti-inflammatory activity, is particularly useful in cases of dapsone resistance or when recurrent reactional states have developed. The pharmacokinetics are poorly understood, but the half-life is several days. The drug is avidly taken up by epithelial cells, a feature that may be important for its activity but also results in cutaneous hyperpigmentation, ichthyosis, xerosis, and enteritis. The intense reddish-brown discoloration of the skin is cosmetically a deterrent to use and often results in discontinuation or poor compliance.

The increasing incidence of drug-resistant *M. leprae* has led to an intensified search for alternative therapeutic agents. Minocycline, certain 2nd-generation quinolones, and some new macrolide derivatives such as clarithromycin have shown promise in experimental models or preliminary human trials.

Delineation of the optimal therapeutic regimens for leprosy has been hampered by deficient patient compliance, the long durations of therapy required, and inadequacies in the long-term follow-up for late relapses. All patients with leprosy should receive multidrug therapy to reduce the emergence of resistance and eradicate persistent *M. leprae* that are the usual cause for relapse. Data collected by the WHO from several countries on cohorts of patients completing the recommended MDT regimens between 1981 and 1993 have presented very favorable results. Of a total of 20,141 multibacillary patients and 51,553 paucibacillary patients followed over 9 years, cumulative relapse rates were 0.74% and 1.09%, respectively. In comparison, among multibacillary patients treated with dapsone monotherapy, the expected relapse rate would be 10–20%. Thus, in 1993, the WHO study group on chemotherapy of leprosy restated support for the WHO MDT regimen. For adults with multibacillary leprosy (all BL and lepromatous patients), therapy is recommended for 24 mo to include rifampin, 600 mg once a mo, supervised; dapsone, 100 mg daily, self-administered; and clofazimine, 300 mg monthly, supervised, and 50 mg daily, self-administered. For adults with paucibacillary leprosy (all indeterminate, TT, and most BT patients), therapy is recommended for 6 mo with rifampin 600 mg once a mo, supervised, and dapsone 100 mg daily, self-administered. Patients who experience relapse are re-treated with the same regimens except those multibacillary patients with proven rifampin-resistant *M. leprae*. Such patients are treated daily for 6 mo with clofazimine, 50 mg, and two of the following: ofloxacin, 400 mg, minocycline, 100 mg, or clarithromycin, 500 mg. This is followed by an additional 18-mo period of therapy of daily clofazimine, 50 mg, with minocycline, 100 mg, or ofloxacin, 400 mg. Appropriate daily pediatric doses of the three main antileprosy medications are dapsone, 1 mg/ kg/24 hr; rifampin, 10 mg/kg/24 hr; and clofazimine, 1 mg/kg/24 hr. Patients treated in the United States often receive regimens that vary from WHO recommendations, and expert consultation is advised.

Therapy for reactional states can become very complicated and generally requires expert consultation. Erythema nodosum leprosum usually responds to corticosteroid therapy (1 mg/kg/24 hr of prednisone) but often relapses when the drug is discontinued. Clinical remission of acute and suppression of chronic erythema nodosum can be achieved with thalidomide. *Thalidomide is absolutely contraindicated in women of child-bearing age*; otherwise it is much safer than corticosteroids for chronic use. The major side effect is fatigue. Pediatric dosages have not been established. Clofazimine is also useful in managing chronic erythema nodosum. Reversal reactions are optimally treated with corticosteroids. Alternate-day regimens may be effective in patients with frequent relapses.

PROGNOSIS. The prognosis for arresting progression of tissue and nerve damage is good, but recovery of lost sensory and motor function is variable and generally incomplete; hyperpigmentation, hypopigmentation, and loss of skin organs persist. Intercurrent reactional states, poor compliance, and emergence of drug resistance can all lead to clinical exacerbations or relapses necessitating close follow-up of patients. Much of the chronic debility results from repeated trauma to anesthetic digits and limbs. Careful counseling of patients and consultation with physical and occupational therapy services is essential for an optimal outcome.

PREVENTION. Two approaches are advocated for interrupting leprosy transmission in endemic areas. The first is directed at the risk of infection among household contacts of leprosy patients, especially those with multibacillary disease. It is based on regular periodic examination of contacts and early treatment at the first evidence of leprosy. Through a vigorous program of case detection and administration of MDT, the WHO has established a goal of eliminating leprosy by the year 2000. It is estimated that 2.4 million cases of leprosy must be treated between 1996–2000 to accomplish that goal.

One historical practice that has fortunately been abandoned is the forcing of leprosy patients into leprosariums. Mouse footpad inoculation studies have demonstrated that viability of *M. leprae* in skin biopsies falls sharply within 3 wk of initiating therapy with dapsone and rifampin. This rapid drop in infectivity combined with the high probability that family members have had prolonged exposure to the patient before the diagnosis makes physical isolation of leprosy patients unnecessary.

Brubaker ML, Meyers WM, Bourland J: Leprosy in children one year of age and under. Int J Lepr 53:517, 1985.

Chemotherapy of leprosy. Report of a WHO study group. WHO Tech Rep Ser 847:1, 1994.

Dayal R: Early detection of leprosy in children. J Trop Pediatr 37:310, 1991.

Ladhani, Shamez: Leprosy disabilities: The impact of multidrug therapy. Int J Dermatol 36:561, 1997.

Leprosy elimination campaigns reaching every patient in every village. WHO Weekly Epidemiol Record 28:205, 1997.

Neill MA, Hightower AL, Broome CV: Leprosy in the United States, 1971–1981. J Infect Dis 152:1064, 1985.

Orege PA, Fine PE, Lucas SB, et al: A case control study on human immunodeficiency virus-1 (HIV-1) infection as a risk factor for tuberculosis and leprosy in western Kenya. Tuber Lung Dis 74:377, 1993.

Ridley DS, Jopling WH: Classification of leprosy according to immunity: A five-group system. Int J Lepr 34:255, 1966.

Sehgal VN, Srivastava G: Leprosy in children. Int J Dermatol 26:557, 1987.

van Beers SM, Izumi S, Madjid B, et al: An epidemiological study of leprosy infection by serology and polymerase chain reaction. Int J Lepr Other Mycobact Dis 62:1, 1994.

CHAPTER 214
Atypical Mycobacteria

Dwight A. Powell

Nontuberculous, nonleprous *Mycobacterium* species (NTM), which are also referred to as atypical mycobacteria, mycobacteria other than tuberculosis (MOTT), or potentially pathogenic environmental mycobacteria are members of the family of Mycobacteriaceae. They differ from *M. tuberculosis* in their nutritional requirements, ability to produce pigments, enzymatic activity, and susceptibility patterns to antituberculous drugs. In contrast to *M. tuberculosis*, NTM are generally acquired from contact with the environment rather than by person-to-person spread.

ETIOLOGY. Thirteen strains of NTM are associated with human infections. Phenotypically, they are divided into four groups described by Runyon in 1959 (Table 214–1) based on their colony growth and morphology on solid media. Groups I, II, and III are slow growing (>7 days to detect growth); group IV is rapid growing (<7 days to detect growth). Photochromogens form pigment after exposure to light, scotochromogens form pigment in the dark, and nonchromogens fail to produce pig-

TABLE 214–1 Nontuberculous Mycobacteria Associated with Human Disease

Runyon Group	Mycobacteria
III. Photochromogens	*M. kansasii* *M. marinum* *M. simiae*
III. Scotochromogens	*M. scrofulaceum* *M. xenopi* *M. szulgai*
III. Nonchromogens	*M. avium* *M. intracellulare* *M. malmoense* *M. haemophilum* *M. ulcerans*
IV. Rapid growers	*M. chelonei* *M. fortuitum*

ment. Species and serovars of NTM are now defined by biochemical reactions, antibody specificity, radiolabeled DNA probes, DNA restriction fragment length polymorphism, or ribosomal-RNA sequencing. Biochemically and immunologically related species that are difficult for clinical laboratories to differentiate are referred to as "complexes," for example, the *M. fortuitum* complex *(M. fortuitum* and *M. chelonae)* and the *M. avium* complex *(M. avium* and *M. intracellulare)*.

EPIDEMIOLOGY. NTM are distributed worldwide and are ubiquitous in the environment, existing as saprophytes in soil and water; as pathogens in swine, birds, and cattle; and as part of the normal human pharyngeal flora. Some NTM have well-defined ecologic niches that help explain transmission patterns. The natural reservoir for *M. marinum* is fish and other cold-blooded animals, so infections follow injury in an aquatic environment. *M. fortuitum* and *M. chelonae* are ubiquitous in the hospital environment and have caused clusters of nosocomial surgical wound and venous catheter-related infections. *M. ulcerans* is recovered only from soils and waters of rain forests and is associated with chronic skin infections in the tropics. *M. avium* complex is found in abundance in the waters, soils, and aerosols of the acid, brown-water swamps of the southeastern United States. In rural countries in this region, asymptomatic infections with *M. avium* complex approach 70% by adulthood.

With the exception of cervical lymphadenitis, illness related to NTM infections is relatively uncommon in children. Infection with NTM, particularly *M. avium* complex, is one of the most common terminal infections in patients with AIDS.

PATHOGENESIS. The histologic appearances of lesions produced by *M. tuberculosis* and NTM are often indistinguishable. Mycolic acids and other lipids in the cell wall of mycobacteria give them their hallmark trait of acid-fastness with the Ziehl-Neelsen or Kinyoun stains. They may also be identified with the fluorochrome stain auramine-rhodamine. The sensitivity of these stains for detecting NTM in tissue samples is less than with the tubercle bacilli. As with *M. tuberculosis*, the classic pathologic lesion consists of caseating granulomas. However, NTM infections are more likely to result in granulomas that are noncaseating, ill-defined (nonpalisading), and irregular or serpiginous. Granulomas may be absent, with only chronic inflammatory changes observed. In patients with AIDS and disseminated NTM infection, the inflammatory reaction is usually scant and tissues are filled with large numbers of histiocytes packed with acid-fast bacilli.

CLINICAL MANIFESTATIONS. Lymphadenitis of the superior anterior cervical or submandibular nodes is the most frequent manifestation of NTM infection in children. Preauricular, posterior cervical, axillary, and inguinal nodes are involved occasionally. This infection is most common in children 1–5 yr of age because of their tendency to put objects contaminated with soil, dust, or standing water into their mouths. Affected children usually lack constitutional symptoms and present with a unilateral subacute and slowly enlarging lymph node or group of closely approximated nodes >1.5 cm that are firm, painless, freely movable, and not erythematous (Fig. 214–1). The involved nodes occasionally resolve without treatment, but most undergo rapid suppuration after several weeks. The center of the node becomes fluctuant, and the overlying skin becomes erythematous and thin. Eventually, the nodes rupture and form cutaneous sinus tracts that drain for months or years, resembling the classic scrofula of tuberculosis (Fig. 214–2). In the United States, *M. avium* complex accounts for approximately 80% of NTM lymphadenitis in children. *M. scrofulaceum* and *M. kansasii* account for most other cases, particularly in the southwestern United States. Rarely, *M. xenopi, M. malmoense, M. haemophilum*, and *M. szulgai* are described.

Cutaneous disease due to NTM is rare in children. Infection usually follows percutaneous inoculation with fresh or salt water contaminated by *M. marinum*. Within several weeks of exposure, a solitary nodule develops at the site of minor abrasions on the elbows, knees, or feet ("swimming pool granuloma") and on the hands and fingers of fish fanciers ("fish tank granuloma"). The lesions are usually nontender and enlarge over 3–5 wk to ulcerated granuloma or warty lesions, as seen in cutaneous tuberculosis. The lesions sometimes resemble sporotrichosis; satellite lesions near the site of entry extend along the skin following the superficial lymphatics. Lymphadenopathy is usually absent. Although most infections remain localized to skin, penetrating *M. marinum* infections may result in tenosynovitis, bursitis, osteomyelitis, or arthritis.

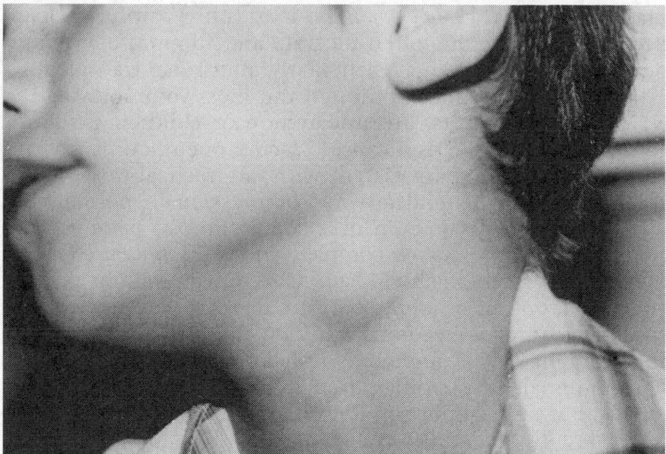

Figure 214–1 An enlarging cervical lymph node with atypical mycobacterial infection, which is firm, painless, freely movable, and not erythematous.

M. ulcerans also causes cutaneous infection in children living in tropical countries (Africa, Australia, Asia, and South America). Infection follows percutaneous inoculation and presents as a painless erythematous nodule, most frequently on a leg, which undergoes central necrosis and ulceration. The lesion, often called a Buruli ulcer after the region in Uganda where most cases are reported, has a characteristic undermined edge, gradually expands, and may result in extensive soft tissue destruction with secondary bacterial infection. The lesion may heal slowly over 6–9 mo or may continue to spread, leading to deformities and contractures.

Skin and soft tissue infections due to *M. fortuitum* and *M. chelonae* are rare in children and usually follow percutaneous inoculation due to puncture wounds and minor abrasions. Clinical disease usually arises after a 4–6 wk incubation period and presents as a localized cellulitis, painful nodules, or a

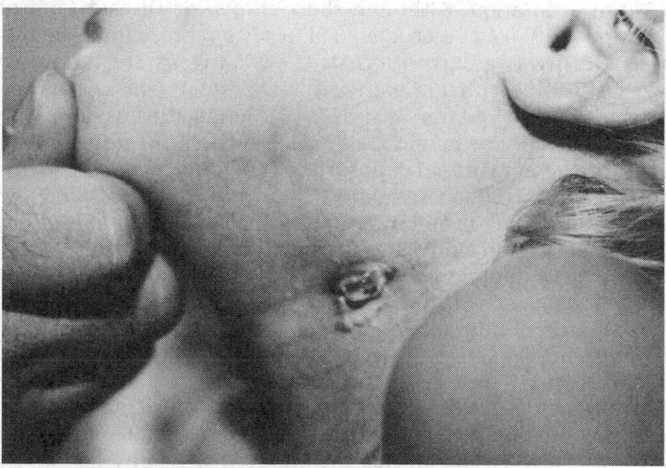

Figure 214–2 A ruptured cervical lymph node with atypical mycobacterial infection, which resembles the classic scrofula of tuberculosis.

draining abscess. *M. haemophilum* may cause painful subcutaneous nodules, which often ulcerate and suppurate in immunocompromised patients, particularly after renal transplant.

Pulmonary infections, although the most common cause of NTM illness in adults, are uncommon in children. *M. avium* complex is described as a cause of acute pneumonitis, chronic cough, or wheezing associated with paratracheal or peribronchial lymphadenitis and airway compression in normal children. Chronic infections in older cystic fibrosis patients have been caused by *M. avium* complex and *M. fortuitum* complex. *M. kansasii, M. xenopi,* and *M. szulgai* are uncommon in children and usually occur in adults with underlying chronic lung disease. The onset is insidious and consists of low-grade fever, cough, night sweats, and general malaise. Thin-walled cavities with minimal surrounding parenchymal infiltrates are characteristic, but radiographic findings may resemble those of tuberculosis.

In unusual circumstances, NTM cause bone and joint infections that are indistinguishable from those produced by *M. tuberculosis* or bacterial agents. Such infections usually result from operative incision or accidental puncture wounds. *M. fortuitum* infections from puncture wounds of the foot resemble infections caused by *Pseudomonas aeruginosa* and *Staphylococcus aureus.*

Disseminated disease, usually associated with *M. avium* complex infections, occurs occasionally in children without any apparent immunodeficiency. Some of these patients have defective interferon gamma production. The majority of disseminated NTM infections occur in patients with AIDS, usually late in the illness when CD4 cell counts are <100 cells/mm^3. Colonization of the respiratory or gastrointestinal tract probably precedes disseminated *M. avium* complex infections, but screening studies of respiratory secretions or stool samples are not useful to predict dissemination. Continuous high-grade bacteremia is usual, and multiple organs are infected, including most commonly lymph nodes, liver, spleen, bone marrow, and gastrointestinal tract; thyroid, pancreas, adrenal gland, kidney, muscle, and brain may be involved. The most common signs and symptoms of disseminated *M. avium* complex infections are fever, night sweats, chills, anorexia, marked weight loss, wasting, weakness, generalized lymphadenopathy, and hepatosplenomegaly. Jaundice, elevated alkaline phosphatase level, anemia, and neutropenia may occur. In children with AIDS, the mean survival time after isolation of *M. avium* complex from a body source is 5–9 mo.

DIAGNOSIS. The differential diagnosis of NTM lymphadenitis includes tuberculosis, cat-scratch disease, mononucleosis, toxoplasmosis, brucellosis, tularemia, and malignancies, especially lymphomas. An intermediate strength tuberculin skin test (5 tuberculin units) is usually weakly positive with 3–15 mm induration. Although the Centers for Disease Control and Prevention have produced skin tests representing the different Runyon groups of NTM, these antigens are no longer available. Differentiation between NTM and *M. tuberculosis* may be difficult, but children with NTM lymphadenitis usually have unilateral anterior cervical node involvement, a normal lung roentgenogram, and no exposure to tuberculosis; children with tuberculous lymphadenitis most often have bilateral posterior cervical node involvement, an abnormal lung roentgenogram, and exposure to adult tuberculosis. Definitive diagnosis requires excision of involved nodes and recovery of the responsible pathogen.

Diagnosis of cutaneous infections depends on isolating the responsible microorganisms from an excised lesion because acid-fast stains are rarely positive. The diagnosis of pulmonary NTM infection in children is also difficult because many species of NTM, including *M. avium* complex, can be isolated from oral and gastric secretions of healthy children. Definitive diagnosis requires invasive procedures such as bronchoscopy and pulmonary or endobronchial biopsy.

Blood cultures are 90–95% sensitive in AIDS patients with disseminated infection. *M. avium* complex may be detected within 7 days of inoculation in nearly all patients with the BACTEC radiometric blood culture system. Commercially available DNA probes differentiate NTM from *M. tuberculosis.* Identification of histiocytes containing numerous acid-fast bacilli from bone marrow and other biopsy tissues provides a rapid presumptive diagnosis of disseminated mycobacterial infection.

TREATMENT. Therapy for NTM infections involves medical, surgical, or combined treatment. Isolation of the infecting strain with susceptibility testing is ideal because susceptibility patterns vary. *M. kansasii, M. marinum, M. xenopi, M. ulcerans,* and *M. malmoense* are usually susceptible to some standard antituberculous drugs. *M. fortuitum, M. chelonae, M. scrofulaceum,* and *M. avium* complex are often resistant to standard antituberculous drugs but have variable susceptibility to newer antibiotics such as quinolones and macrolides. Multiple drug therapy is essential to avoid development of resistance.

The preferred treatment of NTM lymphadenitis is complete surgical excision. Nodes should be removed while still firm and encapsulated. Excision is more difficult if extensive caseation with extension to surrounding tissue has occurred, and complications of facial nerve damage or recurrent infection are more likely. Incomplete surgical excision is not advised because chronic drainage may develop. Antituberculous medications are not necessary with complete excision, but if there is concern for *M. tuberculosis* infection, therapy with isoniazid, rifampin, and pyrazinamide should be given until cultures confirm the cause. If chronic drainage develops, a 6 mo regimen of daily clarithromycin, 15 mg/kg/24 hr, plus rifabutin, 5 mg/kg/24 hr, may be curative.

Cutaneous NTM lesions usually heal spontaneously after incision and drainage without other therapy. *M. marinum* is susceptible to rifampin, amikacin, ethambutol, sulfonamides, trimethoprim/sulfamethoxazole, and tetracyclines. Therapy with one or a combination of these drugs should be given for 3–4 mo. Corticosteroid injections should not be used. Superficial infections with *M. fortuitum* or *M. chelonae* usually resolve after surgical incision and open drainage, but deep-seated or catheter-related infections require removal of infected central lines and therapy with parenteral amikacin and cefoxitin or clarithromycin. Pulmonary infections should be treated initially with isoniazid, rifampin, and pyrazinamide pending culture identification and susceptibility testing. Chemotherapy for disseminated disease due to *M. avium* complex does not cure the infection, but various multiple drug combinations of clarithromycin, azithromycin, clofazimine, rifabutin, rifampin, ciprofloxacin, and ethambutol may limit progression. Interferon gamma may be beneficial in selected patients.

In adults with AIDS, daily prophylaxis with azithromycin with or without rifabutin reduces infection with *M. avium* complex by over 50%. Although pediatric studies are lacking, the U.S. Public Health Service recommends either azithromycin (20 mg/kg/wk) or clarithromycin (7.5 mg/kg twice daily) for HIV-infected children with the following indications: for children $\geq$6 yr, CD4$^+$ count $<50/\mu L$; aged 2–6 yr, CD4$^+$ count $<75/\mu L$; aged 1–2 yr, CD4$^+$ count $<500/\mu L$; aged <1 yr, CD4$^+$ count <750 μL.

Centers for Disease Control and Prevention: 1997 USPHSHS/IDSA guidelines for the prevention of opportunistic infections in persons infected with human immunodeficiency virus. MMWR 46(RR-12):1, 1997.

Berger C, Pfyffer GE, Nadal D: Treatment of nontuberculous mycobacterial lymphadenitis with clarithromycin plus rifabutin. J Pediatr 128:383, 1996.

Brady RC, Sheth A, Mayer T, et al: Facial sporotrichoid infection with *Mycobacterium marimum.* J Pediatr 130:324, 1997.

Correa AG, Starke JG: Nontuberculous mycobacterial disease in children. Semin Respir Infect 11:262, 1996.

Fergie JE, Milligan TW, Henderson BM, Stafford WW: Intrathoracic *Mycobacterium avium* complex infection in immunocompetent children: Case report and review. Clin Infect Dis 24:250, 1997.

Frucht DM, Holland SM: Defective monocyte costimulation for IFN-gamma production in familial disseminated *Mycobacterium avium* complex infection: Abnormal IL-12 regulation. J Immunol 157:411, 1996.
Havlir DV, Dube MP, Sattler FR, et al: Prophylaxis against disseminated *Mycobacterium avium* complex with weekly azithromycin, daily rifabutin, or both. N Engl J Med 335:392, 1996.
Holland SM, Eisenstein EM, Kuhus DB, et al: Treatment of refractory disseminated nontuberculous mycobacterial infection with interferon gamma: A preliminary report. N Engl J Med 330:1348, 1994.
Horsburgh CR Jr: *Mycobacterium avium* complex in the acquired immunodeficiency syndrome. N Engl J Med 324:1332, 1991.
Kilby JM, Gilligan PH, Yankaskas JR, et al: Nontuberculous mycobacteria in adult patients with cystic fibrosis. Chest 102:70, 1992.
Levin RH, Bolinger AM: Treatment of non-tuberculous mycobacterial infections in pediatric patients. Clin Pharm 7:545, 1988.
Lewis LL, Butler KM, Husson RN, et al: Defining the population of human immunodeficiency virus–infected children at risk for *Mycobacterium avium-intracellulare* infection. J Pediatr 121:677, 1992.
Margileth AM, Chandra R, Altman P: Chronic lymphadenopathy due to mycobacterial infection. Am J Dis Child 138:917, 1984.
Peloquin CA: Controversies in the management of *Mycobacterium avium* complex infection in AIDS patients. Ann Pharmacother 27:928, 1993.
Raad II, Vartivarian S, Khan A, et al: Catheter-related infections caused by the *Mycobacterium fortuitum* complex: 15 cases and review. Rev Infect Dis 13:1120, 1991.
Wallace RJ Jr, Tanner D, Brennan PJ, et al: Clinical trial of clarithromycin for cutaneous (disseminated) infection due to *Mycobacterium chelonae*. Ann Intern Med 119:482, 1993.
Wolinsky E: Mycobacterial diseases other than tuberculosis. Clin Infect Dis 15:1, 1992.

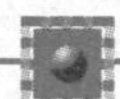

SECTION 7

Spirochetal Infections

CHAPTER 215

Syphilis (Treponema pallidum)

Parvin Azimi

ETIOLOGY. Syphilis is a systemic communicable infection caused by *Treponema pallidum*, a long, slender, tightly coiled, motile spirochete with finely tapered ends belonging to the family Spirochaetaceae. The pathogenic members of this genus include *T. pallidum* (venereal syphilis), *T. pertenue* (yaws), *T. pallidum* subsp. *endemicum* (endemic syphilis), and *T. carateum* (pinta). Because these microorganisms stain poorly, detection in clinical specimens requires darkfield microscopy or direct immunofluorescent staining techniques. *T. pallidum* cannot be cultured in vitro but has been propagated by intratesticular inoculation in rabbits. Transmission occurs by sexual contact or transplacentally. Other modes of transmission include transfusion of contaminated blood or by direct contact with infected tissues.

EPIDEMIOLOGY. Two forms of syphilis are encountered in children. *Acquired* syphilis is transmitted almost exclusively by sexual contact. After an epidemic resurgence of primary and secondary syphilis in the 1980s in the United States that peaked in 1989, the annual rate has declined and in 1997 was the lowest since reporting for syphilis began in 1941. Despite these declines, syphilis remains endemic in parts of the south, where it is many times more common (6.6 per 100,000 population) than in the midwest (2.0), northeast (1.1), and west (1.0). The rates for primary and secondary syphilis remain substantially higher for blacks (22.0 per 100,000 population) than for nonwhite Hispanics (1.6) and for non-Hispanic whites (0.5).

Congenital syphilis results from transplacental transmission of spirochetes. Pregnant women with primary and secondary syphilis and spirochetemia are more likely to transmit infection to the fetus than are women with latent infection. Transmission can occur at any stage of pregnancy. The incidence of congenital infection in the offspring of untreated infected women remains highest during the first 4 yr after acquisition of primary infection, secondary, and early latent disease. The risk factors most commonly associated with congenital syphilis are lack of prenatal care and cocaine drug abuse, which is associated with prostitution, unprotected sex, and trading of sex for drugs, in addition to inadequate prenatal care of pregnant addicts.

CLINICAL MANIFESTATIONS. *Primary syphilis* is characterized by syphilitic chancre and regional lymphadenitis. A painless papule appears at the site of inoculation 2–6 wk after *T. pallidum* has been introduced. The papule soon develops into a clean, painless ulcer with raised borders called a chancre. The chancre, usually on the genitals, contains viable *T. pallidum* and is highly contagious. Extragenital chancres can also be seen, depending on the site of primary inoculation. Adjacent lymph nodes are generally enlarged. The chancre heals spontaneously within 4–6 wk, leaving a thin scar. Untreated patients develop manifestations of *secondary syphilis* 2–10 wk after the chancre heals. Manifestations of secondary syphilis are related to spirochetemia and include a nonpruritic maculopapular rash, which can cover the entire body involving palms and soles; pustular lesions may also develop. Condylomata lata (gray-white to erythematous wartlike plaques) can occur in moist areas around the anus and vagina, and white plaques called mucous patches may be found in mucous membranes.

A flulike illness with low-grade fever, headache, malaise, anorexia, weight loss, sore throat, myalgias, and arthralgias, and generalized lymphadenopathy is often present. Renal, hepatic, and ophthalmologic manifestations may be present, as well as meningitis. Meningitis occurs in 30% of patients with secondary syphilis, manifested by cerebrospinal fluid (CSF) pleocytosis and elevated protein, but the patient may not show neurologic symptoms. Secondary infection becomes *latent* within 1–2 mo after the onset of the rash. Relapses with secondary manifestations can be seen during the 1st year of latency. This period is referred to as the early latent period. No relapses occur after the 1st year; what follows is late syphilis, which may be either asymptomatic *(late latent)* or symptomatic *(tertiary)*. At this stage, patients may begin showing the manifestations of tertiary disease, which include neurologic, cardiovascular, and gummatous lesions. The latter are granulomas of the skin and musculoskeletal system resulting from the host's delayed hypersensitivity reaction.

Congenital Infection. Syphilis during pregnancy has a transmission rate approaching 100%. Fetal or perinatal death occurs in 40% of affected infants. Among survivors, manifestations have traditionally been divided into early and late stages. The former appear during the first 2 yr of life, whereas the latter appear gradually during the first 2 decades. Early manifestations result from transplacental spirochetemia and are analogous to the secondary stage of acquired syphilis. Approximately two thirds of infants are asymptomatic at the time of birth and are identified only by routine prenatal screening; if they are untreated, symptoms develop within weeks or months.

The early manifestations of congenital infection are varied and involve multiple organ systems. Hepatosplenomegaly, jaundice, and elevated liver enzymes are common. Histologically, liver involvement includes bile stasis, fibrosis, and extramedullary hematopoiesis. Lymphadenopathy tends to be diffuse and resolve spontaneously; shotty nodes may persist. Coomb-negative hemolytic anemia is characteristic. Thrombocytopenia is often associated with platelet trapping in an enlarged spleen. Characteristic osteochondritis and periostitis (Fig. 215–1) and mucocutaneous rash (Fig. 215–2), presenting with erythematous maculopapular or bullous lesions, followed by desquamation involving hands and feet, are common. Mucous patches, rhinitis (snuffles), and condylomatous lesions are highly characteristic features of mucous membrane involvement in congenital syphilis. Bone involvement occurs frequently. Roentgenographic abnormalities include multiple sites of osteochondritis at the wrists, elbows, ankles, and knees; and periostitis of the long bones, and rarely the skull. The osteochondritis is painful and often results in irritability and refusal to move the involved extremity (pseudoparalysis of Parrot). Central nervous system (CNS) abnormalities, failure to thrive, chorioretinitis, nephritis, and nephrotic syndrome may also be seen. Clinical manifestations of renal involvement include hypertension, hematuria, proteinuria, hypoproteinemia, hypercholesterolemia, and hypocomplementemia. They appear to be related to glomerular deposition of circulating immune complexes. Less common clinical manifestations of early congenital syphilis include gastroenteritis, peritonitis, pancreatitis, pneumonia, eye involvement (glaucoma and chorioretinitis), nonimmune hydrops, and testicular masses.

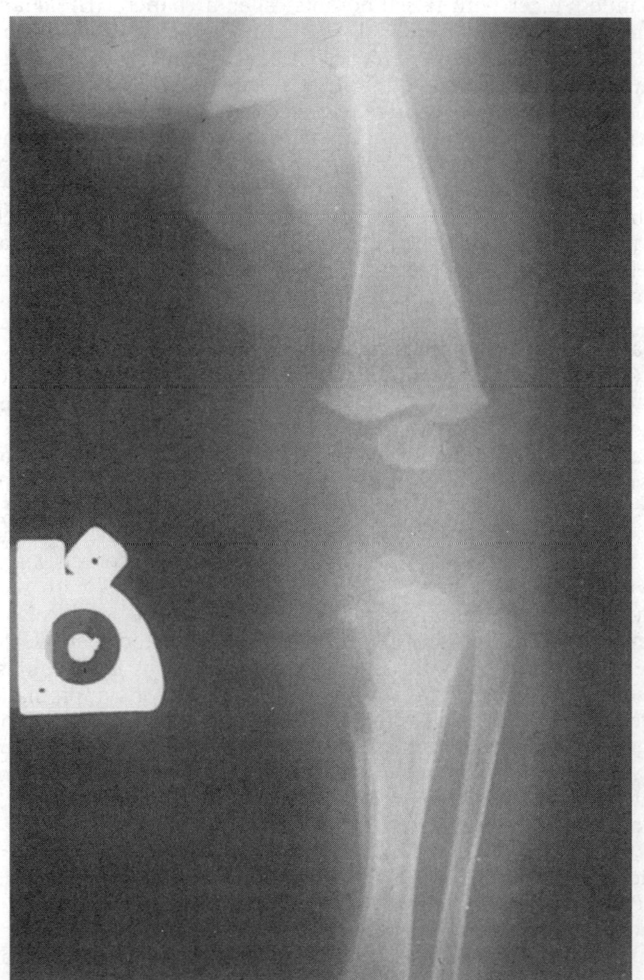

Figure 215–1 Osteochondritis and periostitis in a newborn with congenital syphilis.

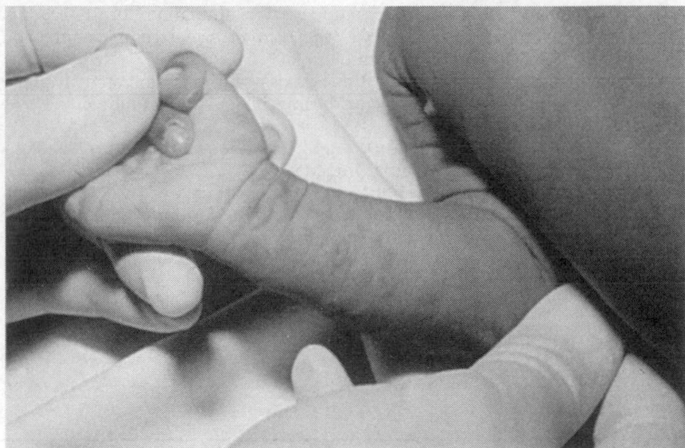

Figure 215–2 The mucocutaneous rash of congenital syphilis. See also color section.

The late manifestations result primarily from chronic inflammation of bone, teeth, and the CNS. Skeletal changes due to persistent or recurrent periostitis and associated thickening of bone include frontal bossing, a bony prominence of the forehead ("olympian brow"); unilateral or bilateral thickening of the sternoclavicular portion of the clavicle (Higoumenakis sign); an anterior bowing of the midportion of the tibia (saber shins); and scaphoid scapula, a convexity along its medial border. Dental abnormalities are common and include (1) Hutchinson teeth (Fig. 215–3), which are the peg or barrel-shaped upper central incisors that erupt during the 6th yr of life; (2) abnormal enamel, which results in a notch along the biting surface; and (3) mulberry molars, abnormal 1st lower (6 yr) molars, characterized by a small biting surface and an excessive number of cusps. Defects in enamel formation lead to repeated caries and eventual tooth destruction.

A saddle nose (Fig. 215–4), a depression of the nasal root, is a result of syphilitic rhinitis that destroys the adjacent bone and cartilage. A perforated nasal septum is an associated abnormality. Rhagades are linear scars that extend in a spokelike pattern from previous mucocutaneous fissures of the mouth, anus and genitalia. Juvenile paresis, an uncommon latent meningovascular infection, typically presents during adolescence with behavioral changes, focal seizures, or loss of intellectual function. Juvenile tabes with spinal cord involvement and cardiovascular involvement with aortitis are extremely rarc.

Other late manifestations of congenital syphilis may repre-

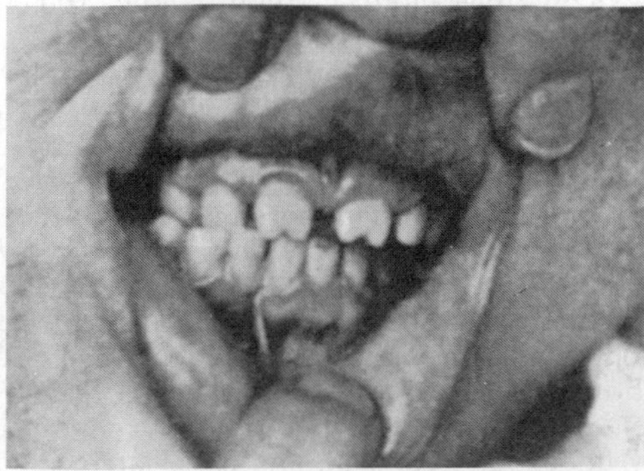

Figure 215–3 Hutchinson teeth as a late manifestation of congenital syphilis.

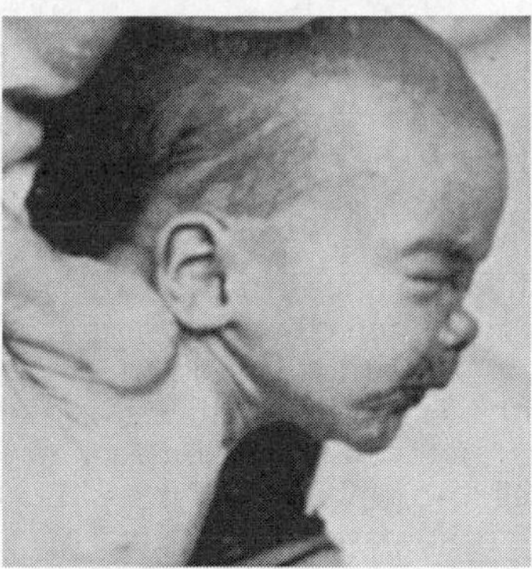

Figure 215–4 Saddle nose in a newborn with congenital syphilis.

sent a hypersensitivity phenomenon. These include unilateral or bilateral interstitial keratitis with symptoms such as intense photophobia and lacrimation, followed within weeks or months by corneal opacification and complete blindness. Less common ocular manifestations include choroiditis, retinitis, vascular occlusion, and optic atrophy. Eighth nerve deafness may be unilateral or bilateral, appears at any age, presents initially as vertigo and high-tone hearing loss, and progresses to permanent deafness. The Clutton joint represents a unilateral or bilateral synovitis involving the lower extremities (usually the knee), which presents as painless joint swelling with sterile synovial fluid; spontaneous remission usually occurs after a period of several weeks. Soft tissue gummas (identical to those of acquired disease) and paroxysmal cold hemoglobinuria are rare hypersensitivity phenomena.

DIAGNOSIS. Diagnosis of primary syphilis is made with certainty when *T. pallidum* is demonstrated by darkfield microscopy or direct immunofluorescence on specimens from skin lesions, placenta, or umbilicus. However, serologic tests for syphilis are the principal means for diagnosis.

Nontreponemal tests, such as the Venereal Disease Research Laboratory (VDRL) and rapid plasma reagin (RPR) tests, detect antibodies against a cardiolipin-cholesterol-lecithin complex, not specific for syphilis. The quantitative results of these nontreponemal tests tend to correlate with disease activity and therefore are very helpful in screening. Titers rise when disease is active (including treatment failure or reinfection) and fall when treatment is adequate. Serum usually becomes nonreactive in the nontreponemal tests within 1 yr of adequate therapy for primary syphilis and within 2 yr of treatment for secondary disease. In congenital infection, these tests become nonreactive within a few months after adequate treatment. Certain conditions such as autoimmune diseases may give false-positive VDRL results in the serum (but not in the CSF), although false-positive results are less common since the introduction of purified cardiolipin-lecithin-cholesterol antigen. Pregnancy itself does not give a false-positive VDRL result; all positve maternal serologic tests for syphilis, regardless of the titer, necessitate thorough investigation.

Treponemal tests, which measure antibody specific for *T. pallidum*, include the *T. pallidum* immobilization test (TPI), the fluorescent treponemal antibody absorption test (FTA-ABS), and the microhemagglutination assay for antibodies to *T. pallidum* (MHA-TP). Treponemal tests are used as confirmatory testing of positive results from the nontreponemal antibody tests. The MHA-TP has few false-positive test results (<1% of healthy persons) and is the treponemal test used by most clinical laboratories. Treponemal antibody titers become positive soon after initial infection and usually remain positive for life, even with adequate therapy. These antibody titers do not correlate with disease activity and are not quantified. They are useful for diagnosis of a first episode of syphilis and for distinguishing false-positive results of nontreponemal antibody tests but are of limited usefulness in the evaluation of response to therapy and possible reinfections.

There is limited cross-reactivity of treponemal antibody tests with the causative organisms of Lyme disease *(Borrelia burgdorferi)*, yaws (*T. pallidum* subsp. *pertenue*), endemic syphilis (*T. pallidum* subsp. *endemicum*), and pinta *(T. carateum)*. Only venereal syphilis *(T. pallidum)* and Lyme disease are found in the United States. The nontreponemal tests (VDRL, RPR) are uniformly nonreactive in Lyme disease.

Tests for IgM antibodies have been developed, including FTA-ABS 19S-IgM, IgM capture enzyme-linked immunosorbent assay (ELISA), and Western immunoblotting assays, but these have been relatively insensitive and are not generally available. Tests for *T. pallidum* using polymerase chain reaction (PCR) amplification are also being developed.

The interpretation of nontreponemal and treponemal serologic tests in the newborn may be confounded by maternal IgG antibodies that are transferred to the fetus. Passively acquired antibody is suggested by neonatal titer at least fourfold (i.e., a two-tube dilution) less than the maternal titer. This can be verified by gradual decline in antibody in the infant, usually becoming undetectable by 3–6 mo of age.

The diagnosis of neurosyphilis in acquired disease is made by demonstrating pleocytosis and increased protein in the CSF, and a positive CSF VDRL along with neurologic symptoms. The CSF VDRL is very specific but relatively insensitive (22–69%) for neurosyphilis.

Darkfield microscopy of scrapings from primary lesions or congenital or secondary lesions can reveal *T. pallidum*, often before serology becomes positive, but this technique is usually not available in clinical practice. Similarly, rabbit infectivity testing, used for measuring the sensitivity of investigational tests such as PCR and Western immunoblotting, is not widely available. Placental examination by gross and microscopic techniques can be useful in the diagnosis of congenital syphilis. The disproportionately large placentas are characterized histologically by focal proliferative villitis, endovascular and perivascular arteritis, and focal or diffuse immaturity of placental villi.

Congenital Syphilis. The asymptomatic infant considered at risk for congenital syphilis because the maternal nontreponemal and treponmal serology is positive should be evaluated: if maternal treatment was inadequate, unknown, or undocumented; ≤30 days before delivery; if the mother was treated with erythromycin or other nonpenicillin regimen; or if the maternal nontreponemal titers did not decrease sufficiently to demonstrate a cure (fourfold or greater). If the maternal treatment was adequate and ≥1 mo before delivery and the infant's positive nontreponemal test represents passively acquired antibody, the infant does not need treatment at delivery, but follow-up serology should be obtained. If the maternal evaluation is unable to be completed, these infants must be assumed to be infected and treated.

The diagnosis of neurosyphilis in the newborn with syphilitic infection is difficult owing to the poor sensitivity of the CSF VDRL in this age group and the lack of CSF abnormalities. In general, a positive CSF VDRL in a newborn warrants treatment for neurosyphilis, even though it might reflect passive transfer of antibodies from serum to CSF. More importantly, it is now accepted that all infants with a presumptive diagnosis of congenital syphilis should be treated with regimens effective for neurosyphilis because this cannot be reliably excluded.

The Centers for Disease Control and Prevention (CDC) recommends that infants be treated if (1) they were born to mothers who had untreated syphilis at delivery; (2) there is evidence of maternal relapse or reinfection; (3) there is physical evidence of active disease; (4) there is radiologic evidence of syphilis; (5) there is a reactive CSF VDRL or, for infants born to seropositive mothers, an abnormal CSF white blood cell count or protein, regardless of CSF serology; or (6) a serum quantitative nontreponemal serologic titer in the infant is at least fourfold greater than the mother's titer.

TREATMENT. *T. pallidum* is extremely sensitive to penicillin, and there is no evidence of increasing penicillin resistance. A concentration 0.018 μg/mL (0.03 U/mL) of penicillin is needed to ensure killing of spirochetes in serum and CSF. Table 215–1 presents the recommended therapeutic regimens for syphilis. Although nonpenicillin regimens are available to the penicillin-allergic patient, desensitization followed by penicillin therapy is the most reliable strategy. An acute systemic febrile reaction, the *Jarisch-Herxheimer reaction,* with exacerbation of lesions, occurs in 15–20% of all patients with acquired or congenital syphilis who are treated with penicillin. It is not an indication for discontinuation of penicillin therapy.

Acquired Syphilis. Primary, secondary, and early latent disease are treated with a single intramuscular dose of benzathine penicillin G (50,000 units/kg; maximum 2.4 million units). Nonpregnant penicillin-allergic patients without neurosyphilis may be treated with either doxycycline (100 mg orally two times a day for 2 wk) or tetracycline (500 mg orally four times a day for 2 wk).

Patients who are also infected with HIV are at increased risk for neurologic complications and have higher rates of treatment failures. The CDC guidelines recommend the same treatment of primary and secondary syphilis as for non–HIV-infected persons, but some experts recommend three weekly doses of benzathine penicillin G. HIV-infected patients with late latent syphilis or latent syphilis of unknown duration should have a CSF evaluation for neurosyphilis before treatment.

Incubating syphilis may be effectively treated with the currently recommended penicillin regimens for gonorrhea, and all patients treated for gonorrhea should have serologic testing for syphilis at the time of treatment and at follow up 6–8 weeks later. Therapy with ampicillin, amoxicillin, or ceftriaxone is probably also effective. Spectinomycin therapy will not cure incubating syphilis. Because of the high risk of acquiring infection, "prophylactic treatment" should be given to sexual contacts of persons with infectious syphilis within the preceding 3 mo, regardless of serology. Three additional elements of syphilis therapy are obligatory: (1) Follow-up serology should be performed on treated individuals to establish adequacy of therapy; (2) sexual contacts should be identified and treated; and (3) testing for other sexually transmitted diseases (STDs), including HIV, should be performed on all patients.

Syphilis in Pregnancy. When clinical or serologic findings suggest active infection or when the diagnosis of active syphilis cannot be excluded with certainty, treatment is indicated. Patients should be treated with the penicillin regimen appropriate for the woman's stage of syphilis. Women who have been adequately treated in the past do not require additional therapy unless quantitative serology suggests evidence of reinfection (fourfold rise in titer). Doxycycline and tetracycline should not be administered during pregnancy, and erythromycin does not effectively treat fetal infection.

Congenital Syphilis. Adequate maternal therapy should eliminate the risk of congenital syphilis. All infants born to mothers with syphilis should be followed until nontreponemal serology is negative. The infant should be treated if there is an uncertainty about the adequacy of the mother's treatment.

Current recommendations for treatment of congenital syphilis include regimens of IV aqueous penicillin G (100,000–150,000 U/kg/24 hr) and IM procaine penicillin (50,000 U/kg/24 hr) given for 10–14 days. Higher concentrations of penicillin are achieved in the CSF of infants treated with IV aqueous penicillin G than in those treated with IM procaine penicillin. Both penicillin regimens are still recognized as adequate therapy for congenital syphilis. Treated infants should be followed serologically to confirm decreasing nontreponemal antibody titers.

PREVENTION. Testing is indicated at any time for persons with suspicious lesions, a history of recent sexual exposure to a person with syphilis, or diagnosis of another sexually transmitted infection, including HIV infection.

Congenital Syphilis. Routine prenatal screening for syphilis remains the most important factor in the identification of infants at risk for development of congenital syphilis and is legally required at the beginning of prenatal care in all states. In pregnant women without optimal prenatal care, serologic screening for syphilis should be performed at the time pregnancy is diagnosed. Any woman who is delivered of a stillborn infant ≥20 wk of gestation should be tested for syphilis. In communities and populations with a high prevalence of syphilis, or for patients at high risk, testing should be performed at least two additional times, at the beginning of the third trimester (28 wk) and at delivery. Some states mandate repeat testing at delivery for all women. Women at high risk for syphilis should possibly be screened more frequently, either monthly or pragmatically because of inconsistent prenatal care, at every medical encounter because they may have repeat infections during pregnancy or reinfection late in pregnancy.

No newborn should leave the hospital without the maternal serologic status having been determined at least once during pregnancy. In states conducting newborn screening for syphilis, both the mother's and infant's serologic results should be known before discharge. Testing of the mother's serum is preferred to testing cord blood or the infant's serum because the titers are frequently lower in the infant and may be nonreactive if the mother was infected late in pregnancy.

TABLE 215–1 Treatment of Syphilis

Stage	Treatment and Dosage	Alternatives
Primary, secondary, or early latent (<1 yr)	Penicillin G benzathine, 2.4 million U IM, in one dose	Tetracycline (500 mg PO qid for 2 wk) or doxycycline (100 mg PO bid for 2 wk) or erythromycin (500 mg PO qid for 2 wk)
Late latent (>1 yr), latent of unknown duration, or tertiary (gumma or cardiovascular syphilis)	Penicillin G benzathine, 2.4 million U IM, weekly for 3 doses	Tetracycline (500 mg PO qid for 4 wk) or doxycycline (100 mg PO bid for 4 wk)
Neurosyphilis	Aqueous crystalline penicillin G (12–24 million U/24 hr IV given as 2.4 million U every 4 hr) for 10–14 days	Penicillin G procaine (2.4 million U/day IM) *plus* probenicid (500 mg PO qid). Both for 10–14 days
Congenital syphilis	Aqueous crystalline penicillin G (100,000–150,000 U/kg/24 hr, given as 50,000 U/kg IV every 12 hr for the first 7 days and every 8 hr thereafter) for 10–14 days or Procaine penicillin G (50,000 U/kg IM daily in a single dose) for 10–14 days	

Azimi PH, Janner D, Berne P, et al: Concentrations of procaine and aqueous penicillin in the cerebrospinal fluid of infants treated for congenital syphilis. J Pediatr 124:649, 1994.

Beck-Sague C, Alexander ER: Failure of benzathine penicillin G treatment in early congenital syphilis. Pediatr Infect Dis J 6:1061, 1987.

Centers for Disease Control: 1998 Guidelines for treatment of sexually transmitted diseases. MMWR 47(RR-1):1, 1998.

Centers for Disease Control: Syphilis and congenital syphilis—United States, 1985–1988. MMWR 37:486, 1989.

Centers for Disease Control and Prevention: Primary and secondary syphilis—United States, 1997. MMWR 47:493, 1998.
Larsen SA, Steiner BM, Rudolph AH: Laboratory diagnosis and interpretation of tests for syphilis. Clin Microbiol Rev 8:1, 1995.
Moyer VA, Schneider V, Yetman R, et al: Contribution of long-bone radiographs to the management of congenital syphilis in the newborn infant. Arch Pediatr Adolesc Med 152:353, 1998.
Musher DM: Syphilis, neurosyphilis, penicillin, and AIDS. J Infect Dis 163:1201, 1991.
Sison CG, Ostrea Jr EM, Reyes MP, et al: The resurgence of congenital syphilis: A cocaine-related problem. J Pediatr 130:289, 1997.
Zenker PN, Berman SM: Congenital syphilis: Trends and recommendations for evaluation and management. Pediatr Infect Dis J 1:105, 1991.

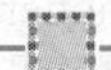

CHAPTER 216
Nonvenereal Treponemal Infections

Parvin Azimi

Several variants of endemic syphilis are recognized by their geographic distribution. These diseases, which include yaws, bejel, and pinta, are caused by spirochetes belonging to the genus *Treponema* that are morphologically and immunologically identical to *T. pallidum* and extremely sensitive to penicillin. They cause diseases that are differentiated primarily on the basis of clinical findings. Yaws is the most common of the nonvenereal spirochetal diseases.

216.1 Yaws

(*Treponema pertenue*)

Yaws is a chronic relapsing infection involving the skin and bony structures caused by the spirochete *T. pertenue*, which cannot be differentiated microscopically or serologically from *T. pallidum*. It is found in the warm, humid tropical regions of Africa, Asia, South America, and Oceania, and almost all cases occur in children. A high percentage of the population is infected in endemic areas.

T. pertenue cannot penetrate intact skin and is transmitted by direct contact from an infected lesion through a skin abrasion or laceration. Transmission is facilitated by overcrowding and poor personal hygiene. The initial papular lesion (the "mother yaw") occurs 2–8 wk after inoculation. The papule develops into a raised raspberry-like papilloma, which is often associated with regional lymphadenopathy. Secondary lesions erupt before or after the ulceration and healing of the mother yaw. With the healing of the mother yaw, there is hypopigmented scar formation. Secondary papillomas may appear anywhere and can be associated with lymphadenopathy, anorexia, and malaise. Ulcerated lesions are covered by exudates containing treponemes. Secondary lesions heal without scarring, but relapses are common within 5 yr after the primary lesion.

The lesions and exacerbations are often associated with bone pain and underlying periostitis or osteomyelitis, especially in the fingers, nose, and tibia. After the initial period of clinical activity, the patient enters a 5–10 yr period of latency. This is followed by the appearance of tertiary lesions at puberty, which are often solitary and destructive. These present as painful papillomas on the hands and feet, gummatous skin ulcerations, or osteitis. Bony destruction and deformity are common, as are juxta-articular nodules, depigmentation, and painful hyperkeratosis ("dry crab yaws") of the palms and soles.

Diagnosis depends on the clinical manifestations of the disease in an endemic area. Darkfield examination of cutaneous lesions and serologic tests for syphilis, both treponemal and nontreponemal, are confirmatory.

Treatment of patients and all contacts consists of a single intramuscular dose of benzathine penicillin (1.2 million U), which cures the lesions of active yaws, renders them noninfectious, and prevents relapse. Eradication of yaws from endemic foci may be accomplished by treating the entire population with penicillin. Patients allergic to penicillin may be treated with erythromycin or tetracycline.

216.2 Endemic Syphilis

(*Treponema pallidum* subsp. *endemicum*)

Endemic syphilis, or bejel, affects children living in the Saharan regions of Africa and the Middle East. Infection with *Treponema pallidum* subsp. *endemicum* follows penetration of the spirochete through traumatized skin or mucous membranes. In experimental infections, a primary papule forms at the inoculation site after an incubation period of 3 wk; in human infections a primary lesion is almost never visualized.

The *clinical manifestations* of the secondary stage of bejel are confined to the skin and mucous membranes and consist of highly infectious mucous patches on the oral mucosa and condyloma-like lesions on the moist areas of the body, especially the axilla and anus. These mucocutaneous lesions resolve spontaneously over a period of several months, but recurrences are common. The secondary stage is followed by a variable latency period before the onset of late or tertiary bejel. The late complications, identical to those of yaws, include gumma formation in skin, subcutaneous tissue, and bone, resulting in painful destructive ulcerations, swelling, and deformity.

Diagnosis is suspected on epidemiologic and clinical grounds and is confirmed either by darkfield examination of the skin and mucous membrane lesions or by serologic testing (positive Venereal Disease Research Laboratory, *T. pallidum* immobilization test, and fluorescent treponemal antibody absorption tests). Differentiation from venereal syphilis is extremely difficult in an endemic area. Bejel can be suspected by the absence of a primary chancre and lack of involvement of the central nervous system and cardiovascular system during the late stage.

Treatment of early injection consists of a single intramuscular dose of benzathine penicillin (1.2 million U); late infection is treated with three injections, each of the same dose at intervals of 7 days. Patients allergic to penicillin may be treated with erythromycin or tetracycline.

216.3 Pinta

(*Treponema carateum*)

Pinta is a chronic, nonvenereally transmitted injection caused by *Treponema carateum*, a spirochete morphologically and serologically indistinguishable from other human treponemes. The disease is endemic in Mexico, Central America, South America, and parts of the West Indies. Infection follows direct inoculation of the treponeme through abraded skin. After a variable incubation period of days, a primary lesion appears at the inoculation site as a small asymptomatic erythematous papule resembling localized psoriasis or eczema. The regional lymph nodes are often enlarged, and spirochetes can be visualized on darkfield examination of skin scrapings or of the involved lymph nodes. After a period of enlargement, the primary lesion disappears. Secondary lesions follow within 6–8 mo; they consist of small macules and papules on the face, scalp, and other exposed portions of the body. These pigmented lesions are scaly and nonpruritic and may coalesce to form large plaquelike elevations resembling psoriasis. In the late stage, atrophic and depigmented lesions develop on the hands, wrists, ankles, feet, face, and scalp. Hyperkeratosis of palms and soles is uncommon. *Diagnosis* is confirmed by darkfield examination of early lesions and a positive serologic test for syphilis. *Treatment* consists of a single intramuscular dose of benzathine penicillin (1.2 million U). Tetracycline and erythromycin are alternatives for patients allergic to penicillin.

CHAPTER 217
Leptospira

Parvin Azimi

ETIOLOGY. Leptospirosis is a generalized infection of humans and animals caused by spirochetes of the genus *Leptospira*. The pathogenic leptospires belong to a single species, *Leprospira interrogans*, which contains approximately 200 distinct serovars. A single serovar may produce a variety of distinct syndromes, and a single clinical manifestation (e.g., aseptic meningitis) may be caused by multiple serotypes. The organisms are aerobic bacteria, 6–20 μm long and 0.1 μm wide with terminal hooks. They can be visualized by darkfield examination and by silver impregnation staining. A special medium is required for their growth, and it may take weeks for cultures to become positive.

EPIDEMIOLOGY. Leptospirosis is a zoonosis of worldwide distribution. Leptospires infect many species of wild and domestic animals and have been isolated from birds, fish, and reptiles. The rat is the principal source of human infection. Other important animal reservoirs include dogs, cats, livestock, and wild animals. Animal infection varies from inapparent to fatal. Once infected, animals excrete spirochetes in urine for an extended period of time. Leptospire survival outside the animal host is dependent on the moisture content, temperature, and pH of the soil or water into which they are shed. The majority of human cases worldwide result from occupational exposure to rat-contaminated water or soil. Occupational groups with a high incidence of leptospirosis include agricultural workers, persons who live or work in rat-infested environments, individuals involved in animal husbandry or veterinary medicine, and laboratory workers. In the United States, the major animal reservoir is the dog, and contact with spirochetes is often associated with recreational activities that result in contact with contaminated soil or water during the summer months.

PATHOGENESIS. Leptospires enter humans through moist and preferably abraded skin or through mucous membranes. After penetration of the skin or mucous membranes, leptospires circulate in the bloodstream and spread to all organs of the body. The primary lesion caused by leptospires is damage to the endothelial lining of small blood vessels with resultant ischemic damage to the liver, kidneys, meninges, and muscles. After an incubation period of 7–12 days, an initial *septicemic phase* begins in which leptospires can be isolated from the blood, cerebrospinal fluid (CSF) and other tissues. Initial symptoms, which last 2–7 days, may be followed by a brief period of well-being and a second symptomatic or *immune phase*. The immune phase is associated with the appearance of circulating antibody, the disappearance of organisms from the blood and CSF, and the appearance of additional signs and symptoms. Despite the presence of circulating antibody, leptospires may persist in the kidney, urine, and aqueous humor. The immune or leptospiruric phase may last for several weeks.

CLINICAL MANIFESTATIONS. Most cases of human leptospirosis are subclinical, with inapparent infection particularly common in high-risk occupational groups such as farmers and their families. Symptomatic infection may present as an acute febrile illness with nonspecific signs and symptoms (70%), as meningitis (20%), or as hepatorenal dysfunction (10%). The onset is typically sudden, and the illness tends to follow a biphasic course (Fig. 217–1).

Anicteric Leptospirosis. The onset of the initial or septicemic phase is abrupt, with fever, shaking chills, severe headache, malaise, nausea, vomiting, and severe, often debilitating muscular pain. Circulatory collapse is uncommon, but some patients have bradycardia and hypotension. Typically, the child is lethargic, with mild to moderate dehydration. Additional physical findings include extreme muscle tenderness, which is most prominent in the lower extremities, the lumbosacral spine, and the abdomen. Conjunctival suffusion with photophobia and orbital pain (in the absence of chemosis and purulent exudate), generalized lymphadenopathy, and hepatosplenomegaly may also be present. Cutaneous lesions are common (10%), usually consisting of a truncal erythematous maculopapular rash, but they may be urticarial, petechial, purpuric, or desquamating. Less common manifestations include pharyngitis, pneumonitis, arthritis, carditis, cholecystitis, and orchitis. The second or immune phase may follow a brief asymptomatic interlude and is characterized by recurrence of fever. Aseptic meningitis is the hallmark of this phase. Despite abnormal CSF profiles in 80% of infected children, only 50% have meningeal manifestations. CSF abnormalities include a modest elevation in pressure, a mononuclear pleocytosis rarely exceeding 500 cells/mm^3 (polymorphonuclear leukocytes predominate initially), normal or slightly elevated protein levels, and normal glucose values. Encephalitis, cranial and peripheral neuropathies, papilledema, and paralysis are uncommon. Symptoms referable to the central nervous system resolve spontaneously within a week or so. Uveitis may occur during this phase; it can be unilateral or bilateral and is usually self-limited, rarely resulting in permanent visual impairment.

Icteric Leptospirosis (Weil's Syndrome). This severe form of leptospirosis occurs in <10% of affected children. The initial manifestations are similar to those described for anicteric leptospirosis. The immune phase, however, is distinctive, being characterized by clinical and laboratory evidence of hepatic and renal dysfunction. In fulminating cases, hemorrhagic phenomena and cardiovascular collapse also occur. Hepatic abnormalities include right upper quadrant pain, hepatomegaly, direct and indirect hyperbilirubinemia, and modest elevation of levels of serum liver enzymes. Renal manifestations are common, may dominate the clinical picture, and are the principal cause of death in fatal cases; all patients have abnormal findings on urinalysis (hematuria, proteinuria, and casts), and azotemia is common, often associated with oliguria or anuria. Congestive heart failure is uncommon; however, abnormal electrocardiograms are present in 90% of affected children. Hemorrhagic manifestations are rare but when present may include epistaxis, hemoptysis, and gastrointestinal and adrenal hemorrhage. Thrombocytopenia and hypoprothrombinemia also occur.

DIAGNOSIS. Leptospirosis should be considered in the differential diagnosis of any acute febrile illness when there is a history of direct contact with animals or with soil or water contaminated with animal urine, and especially when the onset is abrupt with chills, fever, severe myalgias, conjunctival suffusion, headache, nausea, and vomiting. Isolation of the infecting organism from clinical specimens or a fourfold rise in antibody titer in the presence of clinical symptoms compatible with leptospirosis establishes the diagnosis. A presumptive diagnosis is made in symptomatic children with stable titers of 1:100 or greater in two or more specimens and in asymptomatic children with evidence of exposure and a seroconversion (i.e., a fourfold rise in antibody titer in specimens obtained 2 or more

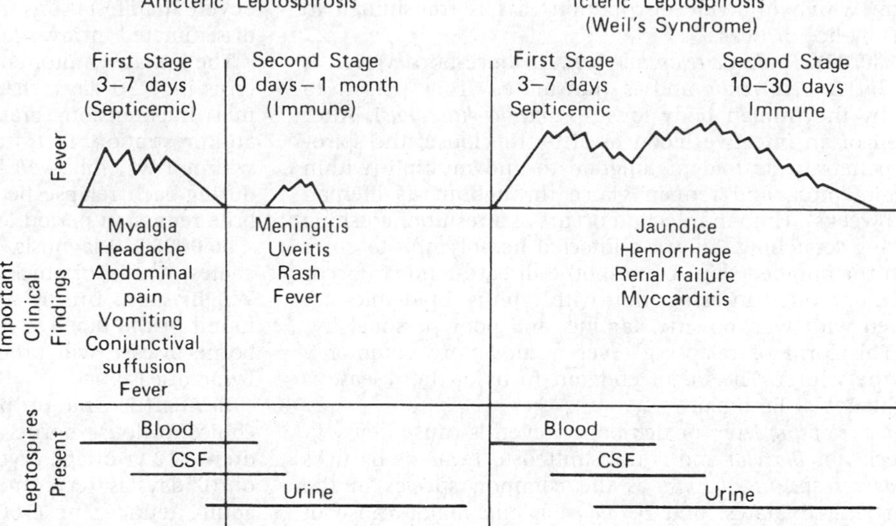

Figure 217–1 Stages of anicteric and icteric leptospirosis. Correlation between clinical findings and presence of leptospires in body fluids. (Reprinted with permission from Feigin RD, Anderson DC: CRC Crit Rev Clin Lab Sci 5:413, 1975. Copyright CRC Press, Inc., Boca Raton, FL.)

wk apart). Several serologic tests are available for the detection of antibodies. These include microscopic agglutination tests in research laboratories using live organisms. Macroscopic agglutination tests that utilize killed antigens are widely available. This test is useful in screening for recent or recurrent infection. Enzyme-linked immunosorbent assay (ELISA) and dot-ELISA procedures have been developed for identification of serovars.

Silver impregnation and fluorescent antibody techniques permit identification of leptospires in infected tissue or body fluids. Spirochetes may also be demonstrated by phase-contrast or darkfield microscopy, however, the skill required and the high frequency of artifacts found with these tests limit their use. Unlike other pathogenic spirochetes, leptospires are easily cultured on commercially available media.

Media containing rabbit serum or bovine serum albumin and long-chain fatty acids are suitable. Repeated blood cultures in the 1st wk of infection with very small inocula of blood are recommended. A small inoculum (i.e., one drop in 5 mL of medium) is used to minimize growth inhibitory factors. They can be recovered from the blood or CSF during the first 10 days of illness and from urine after the 2nd wk. The number of leptospires in clinical specimens is small and their growth rate is slow; leptospires may be seen in several days, although cultures may not become positive for 2–4 mo. Prolonged incubation is thus required.

The diagnosis is most often established by serologic testing. A microscopic slide-agglutination test utilizing killed antigen is the most useful screening test. A microscopic slide-agglutination test with a live or formalin-treated antigen may be used to determine antibody titer and tentatively identify the infecting serotype. Agglutinins usually appear by the 12th day of illness and reach a maximum titer by the 3rd wk. Low titers may persist for years. Approximately 10% of infected persons do not have detectable agglutinins, presumably because available antisera do not identify all *Leptospira* serotypes. The indirect hemagglutination test or the highly specific and sensitive ELISA and dot-ELISA tests have replaced the conventional slide agglutination tests.

TREATMENT. Despite the in vitro sensitivity of *Leptospira* to penicillin and tetracycline and the efficacy of these agents in treating experimental infection, their effectiveness in human leptospirosis remains controversial. It does appear that initiation of treatment before the 7th day will probably shorten the clinical course and decrease the severity of the infection. On this basis, treatment with penicillin or tetracycline (in children >8 yr of age) should be instituted as soon as the diagnosis is suspected. Parenteral penicillin G, 6–8 million U/m²/24 hr in six divided doses for 7 days is recommended. In patients allergic to penicillin, tetracycyline (10–20 mg/kg/24 hr) should be administered orally or intravenously in four divided doses for 7 days.

PREVENTION. Prevention of human leptospirosis is possible by instituting rodent control measures and avoiding contaminated water and soil. Immunization of livestock and family pets has been recommended as a means of eliminating animal reservoirs, but these programs have met with limited success. A formalin-killed polyvalent human vaccine has been used in "at risk" occupation groups in Europe and Asia; however, there have been no clinical trials to determine its efficacy. Leptospirosis has been prevented in American servicemen stationed in the tropics by administering doxycycline, 200 mg orally once a week, as prophylaxis. This schedule may be similarly effective for the traveler entering a highly endemic area for a limited period of time.

Farr RW: Leptospirosis. Clin Infect Dis 21:1–8, 1995.
Heath CW Jr, Alexander AD, Galton MM: Leptospirosis in the United States: Analysis of 483 cases in man, 1949–1961. N Engl J Med 273:857, 1965.
Jackson LA, Kaufmann AF, Adams WG, et al: Outbreak of leptospirosis associated with swimming. Pediatr Infect Dis J 12:48, 1993.
Takafnji ET, Kirkpatrick JW, Miller RN, et al: An efficacy trial of doxycycline chemoprophylaxis against leptospirosis. N Engl J Med 310:497, 1984.
Vinetz JM, Glass GE, Flexner CE, et al: Sporadic urban leptospirosis. Ann Intern Med 125:794, 1996.
Watt G, Alquiza LM, Padre LP, et al: The rapid diagnosis of leptospirosis: A prospective comparison of the dot enzyme-linked immunosorbent assay and the genus-specific microscopic agglutination test at different stages of illness. J Infect Dis 157:4, 1993.
Wong ML, Kaplan S, Dunkle LM, et al: Leptospirosis: A childhood disease. J Pediatr 90:532, 1977.

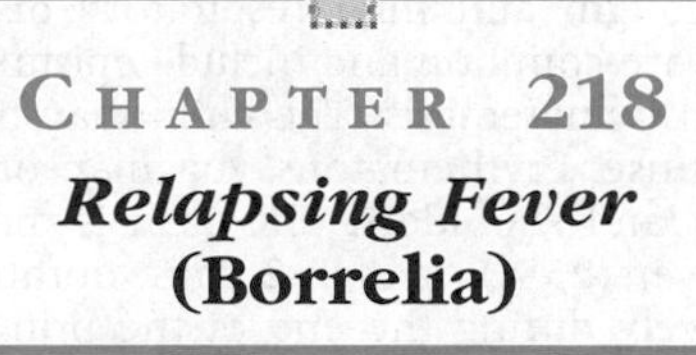

CHAPTER 218
Relapsing Fever (Borrelia)

Parvin Azimi

ETIOLOGY. Relapsing fever is an uncommon arthropod-borne infection characterized by recurrent episodes of fever. It is caused by spirochetes of the genus *Borrelia*, a fastidious microorganism with worldwide distribution that is transmitted to humans by lice or ticks.

EPIDEMIOLOGY. *Epidemic relapsing fever,* or louse-borne fever, is caused by *B. recurrentis* and is transmitted from person to person by the human body louse *(Pediculus humanus).* After ingestion of an infective blood meal by the louse, the spirochetes penetrate its midgut, migrate to and multiply within the hemolymph, and remain viable throughout its lifespan (several weeks). Human infection occurs as a result of crushing lice during scratching, allowing infected hemolymph to enter through the abraded skin. Louse-borne disease tends to occur in epidemics, often in association with typhus. Epidemics are associated with war, poverty, famine, and poor personal hygiene. This form of relapsing fever occurs more commonly during the winter. The major endemic focus of the disease is the highlands of Ethiopia.

Endemic relapsing fever, or tick-borne fever, is caused by several species of *Borrelia* and is transmitted to humans by ticks (*Ornithodoros* sp.). *B. hermsii* is the common species in the western United States, and *B. dugesi* is the major cause of disease in Mexico and Central America. After ingestion of an infective blood meal, spirochetes invade all tissues of their arthropod hosts, including the salivary glands and reproductive tract. The latter permits transovarian passage of infected spirochetes, perpetuating arthropod infection in successive generations. Human infection occurs when saliva, coxal fluid, or excrement is released by the tick during feeding, thereby permitting spirochetes to penetrate the skin and mucous membranes. *Ornithodoros* is distributed worldwide (including the western United States), prefers warm, humid environments and high altitudes, and is found in rodent burrows, caves, and other nesting sites; rodents are the principal reservoirs. Infected ticks gain access to human dwellings on the rodent host. Human contact is often unnoticed because these ticks are nocturnal feeders, have a painless bite, and detach immediately after a short blood meal.

PATHOGENESIS. The cyclic nature of relapsing fever is explained by the ability of *Borrelia* organisms to continually undergo antigenic (phase) variation. Multiple variants evolve simultaneously during the first relapse, with one type becoming predominant. Spirochetes isolated during the primary febrile episode differ antigenetically from those recovered during a subsequent relapse. During febrile episodes, spirochetes enter the bloodstream, induce the development of specific IgM and IgG antibody, and undergo agglutination, immobilization, lysis, and phagocytosis. During remission, *Borrelia* spirochetes may remain in the bloodstream, but spirochetemia is insufficient to produce symptoms. The number of relapses in untreated patients depends on the number of antigenic variants of the infecting strain.

CLINICAL MANIFESTATIONS. Louse-borne disease has a longer incubation period, longer periods of pyrexia, fewer relapses, and longer remission periods than tick-borne disease. Each illness is associated with sudden onset of high fever, headache, photophobia, nausea, vomiting, myalgia, and arthralgia. Additional symptoms may appear later and include abdominal pain, a productive cough, and mild respiratory distress. Bleeding manifestations are common and include epistaxis, hemoptysis, hematuria, and hematemesis. The child may be lethargic and often has a diffuse, erythematous, macular, or petechial rash over the trunk and shoulders. This rash is more common in louse-borne fever (25%), is of 1–2 days' duration, and occurs almost exclusively during the end of the primary febrile episode. There may also be lymphadenopathy, pneumonia, and splenomegaly. Hepatic tenderness associated with hepatomegaly is a common sign. Jaundice may occur in half of affected children. Central nervous system manifestations may be the principal feature of late relapses in tick-borne disease; they include lethargy, stupor, meningismus, convulsions, peripheral neuritis, focal neurologic deficits, and cranial nerve paralysis. Severe manifestations include myocarditis, hepatic failure, and disseminated intravascular coagulopathy.

The initial symptomatic period characteristically ends with a crisis in 4–10 days, marked by abrupt diaphoresis, hypothermia, hypotension, bradycardia, profound muscle weakness, and prostration. In untreated patients, the first relapse occurs within 1 wk, followed by up to five relapses with symptoms during each relapse becoming milder and shorter as the afebrile remission period lengthens.

DIAGNOSIS. Diagnosis depends on demonstration of spirochetes in thin or thick blood smears stained with Giemsa or Wright stain. During afebrile remissions, spirochetes are not found in the blood. Serologic tests are being evaluated. Tick-borne disease will produce a false-positive serologic test for Lyme disease.

TREATMENT. Oral or parenteral tetracycline is the drug of choice for louse-borne and tick-borne relapsing fever. In children <12 yr of age erythromycin (50 mg/kg/24 hr) for a total of 10 days is recommended. For older children and young adults, tetracycline (500 mg every 6 hr) for 10 days has been effective. Single-dose treatment with erythromycin or tetracycline (a single 500-mg oral dose) is efficacious in adults, but experience in children is limited.

Resolution of each febrile episode either by natural crisis or as a result of antimicrobial treatment is usually accompanied within 2 hr by the Jarisch-Herxheimer reaction, which is associated with clearing of the spirochetemia. Attempts to control this reaction by prior treatment with corticosteroids or antipyretics have met with limited success.

PROGNOSIS. With adequate therapy the mortality rate for relapsing fever is <5%. A majority of patients recover from their illness with or without treatment after the appearance of antiborrelial antibodies, which agglutinate, kill, or opsonize the spirochete.

PREVENTION. No vaccine is available. Disease control requires avoidance or elimination of the arthropod vectors. In epidemics of louse-borne disease, dissemination can be prevented by good personal hygiene and delousing of persons, dwellings, and clothing with commercially available insecticides.

Butler T: Relapsing fever: New lessons about antibiotic action. Ann Intern Med 102:397, 1985.
Butler T, Jones PK, Wallace CK: *Borrelia recurrentis* infection. Single dose antibiotic regimens and management of Jarisch-Herxheimer reaction. J Infect Dis 137:573, 1978.
Perine PL, Teklu B: Antibiotic treatment of louse-borne relapsing fever in Ethiopia: A report of 377 cases. Am J Trop Med Hyg 32:1096, 1983.
Stoennerita DT, Larcen C: Antigenic variation in *Borrelia hermsii.* J Exp Med 156:1297, 1982.

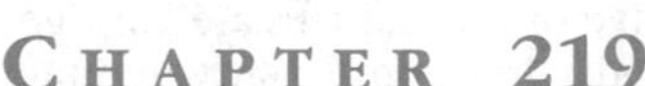

CHAPTER 219
Lyme Disease (Borrelia burgdorferi)

Eugene D. Shapiro

Lyme disease is the most common vector-borne disease in the United States. Although Lyme disease is a public health concern, extensive publicity as well as a very high frequency of misdiagnoses have resulted in a degree of anxiety about Lyme disease that is out of proportion to the actual morbidity that it causes.

ETIOLOGY. Lyme disease is caused by the spirochete *Borrelia burgdorferi.* The organism is a fastidious, microaerophilic bacterium that replicates very slowly and requires special media for in vitro growth. *B. burgdorferi* is a cylindrically shaped organism, the cell membrane of which is covered by flagella and a loosely associated outer membrane. The three major outer-surface proteins—OspA, OspB, and OspC (which are highly charged basic proteins of molecular weights of about 31, 34, and 23 kd, respectively)—as well as the 41 kd flagellar protein, are important targets for the immune response. Differences in the molecular structure of *B. burgdorferi* strains, especially between isolates from Europe and the United States, are well documented. Clinical manifestations of Lyme borreliosis in Europe and in the United States, such as the greater frequency of radiculoneuritis in Europe, may be attributable to these differences.

EPIDEMIOLOGY. Lyme disease has been reported from 49 states and from more than 50 countries. In the United States, most of the cases of Lyme disease occur in southern New England, the eastern parts of the Middle Atlantic states, and the upper Midwest. There is a smaller endemic focus of Lyme disease along the Pacific coast. In Europe, most cases occur in the Scandinavian countries and in central Europe, especially Germany, Austria, and Switzerland. Estimates of the incidence of Lyme disease are complicated by passive systems for reporting of Lyme disease and the high frequency of misdiagnosis of this illness. In endemic areas, the reported annual incidence ranges from 20–100 cases/100,000 population, although this figure may be as high as 1,000 cases/100,000 population in hyperendemic areas such as Lyme, Connecticut. The reported incidence is highest among children 5–10 yr of age, which is almost twice as high as the incidence among older children and adults.

Transmission. Lyme disease is a zoonosis caused by the transmission of *B. burgdorferi* to humans through the bite of an infected tick of the *Ixodes* species. In the eastern and midwestern United States the vector is *Ixodes scapularis* (formerly known as *Ixodes dammini*), the black-legged tick that is commonly known as the deer tick, which is responsible for most cases of Lyme disease in the United States. The vector on the Pacific Coast is *Ixodes pacificus*, the western black-legged tick. *Ixodes* has a 2 yr, three-stage life cycle. The larvae hatch in the early summer and are usually uninfected with *B. burgdorferi*. The tick may become infected at any stage of its life cycle by feeding on a host, usually a small mammal such as the white-footed mouse *(Peromyscus leucopus)*, which is a natural reservoir for *B. burgdorferi*. The larvae overwinter and emerge the following spring in the nymphal stage, which is the stage of the tick that is most likely to transmit the infection. The nymphs molt to adults in the fall. The females lay their eggs the following spring before they die, and the 2 yr life cycle begins again.

Several factors are associated with increased risk of transmission of *B. burgdorferi* from ticks to humans. The proportion of infected ticks varies by geographic area and for each stage of the tick's life cycle. In endemic areas in the northeastern and midwestern United States, 15–20% of nymphal ticks and 35–40% of the adult ticks are infected with *B. burgdorferi*. There are small foci in which the rate of infection of adult deer ticks is 60–80% or even higher. By contrast, *Ixodes pacificus* often feeds on lizards, which are not a competent reservoir for *B. burgdorferi*. Only 1–3% of these ticks, even in the nymphal and adult stages, are infected with *B. burgdorferi*. The risk of transmission of *B. burgdorferi* from infected *Ixodes* ticks is related to the duration of feeding. It takes hours for the mouthparts of ticks to implant fully in the host and much longer (days) for the tick to become fully engorged. Experiments in animals have shown that nymphal ticks must feed for ≥36–48 hr, and infected adults must feed for ≥48–72 hr before the risk of transmission of *B. burgdorferi* becomes substantial. Most individuals who are bitten by a tick will recognize and remove the tick before the transmission of *B. burgdorferi* can occur. Persons with increased occupational, recreational, or residential exposure to tick-infested woods or fields (the preferred habitat of ticks) in endemic areas are at increased risk of developing Lyme disease. Other risk factors, such as age, race, or gender, have not been studied adequately.

PATHOGENESIS. The skin is the initial target of infection by *B. burgdorferi*. Inflammation induced by *B. burgdorferi* leads to the development of the characteristic rash, erythema migrans. Early disseminated Lyme disease is caused by the spread of spirochetes, through the bloodstream, to tissues throughout the body. The spirochete adheres to the surfaces of a wide variety of different types of cells, which may be responsible for the involvement of many organs. Because the organism may persist in tissues for prolonged periods of time, symptoms may appear very late after initial infection.

The symptoms of early disseminated as well as of late Lyme disease are due to inflammation mediated by interleukin 1 and other lymphokines in response to the presence of the organism. It is likely that relatively few organisms actually invade the host, but cytokines serve to amplify the inflammatory response and lead to much of the tissue damage. The refractory symptoms of late Lyme disease may have an immunogenetic basis. Patients with the HLA-DR2, DR3, and DR4 allotypes may be genetically predisposed to develop chronic recurrent Lyme arthritis. These class II histocompatibility molecules located on macrophages and B cells are involved in the presentation of antigens to T-helper cells that initiate the immune response. In genetically susceptible individuals, *B. burgdorferi* may initiate an autoimmune response that causes persistent inflammation and clinical symptoms long after the bacteria have been killed.

Histologically, Lyme disease is characterized by inflammatory lesions that contain both T and B lymphocytes, macrophages, plasma cells, and some mast cells. The erythema migrans rash consists of a moderately dense infiltrate of lymphocytes, plasma cells, and occasional macrophages, located around the small blood vessels of the upper dermis. Lyme myocarditis is a transmyocarditis with a widespread interstitial lymphocytic and plasma cell infiltrate. Similar infiltrates have been seen in the meninges and cerebral cortex. There are few reports of the histology of synovial tissue during the acute stages of Lyme arthritis. At this stage of the illness the synovial fluid often has a marked predominance of polymorphonuclear cells, suggesting that the synovial tissue also will have a polymorphonu clear inflammatory infiltrate. By contrast, chronic, recurrent arthritis is characterized by a chronic hypertrophic synovitis. This nonspecific abnormality, also found in other disorders such as rheumatoid arthritis, is marked by hyperplasia of the synovial cells with varying degrees of lymphocytic infiltrates that sometimes form abortive germinal centers and follicles. Plasma cells are present at the periphery of the lymphoid aggregates. In advanced disease, neovascularization (a nonspecific response to chronic inflammation) may occur.

CLINICAL MANIFESTATIONS. The clinical manifestations of Lyme disease are divided into early and late stages. Early Lyme disease is further classified as early localized or early disseminated disease. Untreated patients may progressively develop clinical symptoms of each stage of the disease, or they may present with early disseminated or with late disease without apparently having had any symptoms of the earlier stages of Lyme disease.

Early Localized Disease. The first clinical manifestation of Lyme disease is the typical annular rash, named erythema migrans. Although it usually occurs 7–14 days after the bite, the onset of the rash has been reported from 3–32 days later. The initial lesion occurs at the site of the bite. The rash may be uniformly erythematous, or it may appear as a target lesion with central clearing or central vesicular or necrotic areas. Occasionally the rash may be itchy or painful. The lesion can occur anywhere on the body, although the most common locations are the axilla, the periumbilical area, the thigh, and the groin. Erythema migrans may be associated with systemic features including fever, myalgia, headache, or malaise. Without treatment, the rash gradually expands (hence the name *migrans*) to an average diameter of 15 cm and remains present for at least 1–2 wk.

Early Disseminated Disease. In the United States a substantial proportion of patients with acute *B. burgdorferi* infection develop secondary erythema migrans lesions, a common manifestation of early disseminated Lyme disease caused by hematogenous spread of the organisms to multiple skin sites. The secondary lesions, which may develop several days or even weeks after the first lesion, usually are smaller than the primary lesion and are often accompanied by fever, myalgia, headache, and malaise; conjunctivitis and lymphadenopathy also may develop. Occasionally, when the erythema migrans rash resolves, new evanescent lesions, which usually are small (1–3 cm), erythematous annular lesions that do not expand, continue to appear for several weeks. Other manifestations may include aseptic meningitis, with signs of meningeal irritation such as nuchal rigidity; uveitis; focal neurologic findings, especially cranioneuropathies; and, rarely, carditis, with varying degrees of heart block. Paralysis of the facial (7th) cranial nerve is relatively common in children and may be the initial or the only manifestation of Lyme disease. The paralysis usually lasts 2–8 wk and resolves completely in most cases. There is no evidence that the clinical course of the facial palsy is affected by antimicrobial treatment.

Late Disease. Arthritis, beginning months after the initial infection, is the usual manifestation of late Lyme disease. Arthritis typically involves the large joints, especially the knee, which is affected in >90% of cases, but any joint may be affected. The joint is swollen and tender but patients do not experience the exquisite pain that is typical of bacterial arthritis. Although it may last for several weeks, the joint swelling usually resolves within 1–2 wk before recurring, often in other joints. If the disease is not treated, the episodes of arthritis often increase in duration, sometimes lasting for months; but in most cases the disease eventually resolves, even in patients who are untreated and who have had many recurrences of arthritis.

Late manifestations of Lyme disease involving the central nervous system (CNS) (sometimes termed *tertiary neuroborreliosis*) are rarely reported in children. In adults, chronic demyelinating encephalitis, polyneuritis, and impairment of memory have been attributed to Lyme disease.

Congenital Lyme Disease. Although *B. burgdorferi* has been identified from several abortuses and from a few live-born children with congenital anomalies, the placentas and the abortuses in which the spirochete was identified usually did not show histologic evidence of inflammation. No consistent pattern of fetal damage has been identified to suggest a clinical syndrome of congenital infection. Furthermore, studies conducted in endemic areas have indicated that there is no difference in the prevalence of congenital malformations among the offspring of women with serum antibodies against *B. burgdorferi* and the offspring of those without such antibodies. If congenital Lyme disease does exist, it must be extremely rare.

DIAGNOSIS. The clinical manifestations of Lyme disease, other than erythema migrans, are not specific. The monoarticular or pauciarticular arthritis may mimic either an acute septic joint or other causes of arthritis in children, such as juvenile rheumatoid arthritis or rheumatic fever. Clinically, 7th nerve palsy due to Lyme disease is indistinguishable from idiopathic Bell palsy, and Lyme meningitis may mimic enteroviral meningitis. The diagnosis of erythema migrans may be difficult because the rash initially may be confused with nummular eczema, tinea, granuloma annulare, an insect bite, or cellulitis. However, the relatively rapid expansion of erythema migrans helps to distinguish it from these other conditions.

Although attempts have been made to develop antigen-based diagnostic tests, including the polymerase chain reaction, all of these tests are experimental. None of the tests for *B. burgdorferi* antigens that have been adequately evaluated are sufficiently sensitive and specific to be clinically useful. Consequently, the confirmation of Lyme disease usually is based on the demonstration of antibodies to *B. burgdorferi* in the patient's serum.

Serology. Specific IgM antibodies appear first usually at 3–4 wk, peak at 6–8 wk, and subsequently decline, although a prolonged elevation of IgM antibodies sometimes occurs despite effective antimicrobial treatment. Consequently, the results of tests for specific IgM antibodies should not be used as an indicator of either active or recent infection. Specific IgG antibodies usually appear at 6–8 wk, peak after 4–6 mo, and may remain elevated indefinitely. The antibody response to *B. burgdorferi* may be abrogated in patients with early Lyme disease who are treated promptly with an effective antimicrobial agent, but in most patients IgG antibodies remain detectable for many years after treatment and clinical resolution of the illness.

Because the immunofluorescent antibody test requires subjective interpretation and is time consuming to perform, it has been replaced by enzyme-linked immunosorbent assays (ELISA) for the detection of antibodies against *B. burgdorferi*. The ELISA method sometimes produces false-positive results because of cross-reactive antibodies to other spirochetal infections (e.g., syphilis, leptospirosis, or relapsing fever), to certain viral infections (e.g., varicella), against spirochetes that comprise part of the normal oral flora, and with certain autoimmune diseases (e.g., systemic lupus erythematosus).

Western immunoblotting is also used as a diagnostic test for Lyme disease, although there is still some debate about its interpretation. For example, many people who do not have Lyme disease have antibodies against the 41 kd protein (the flagellar protein) of *B. burgdorferi*. The immunoblot is most useful to validate a positive or equivocal ELISA in a patient with a low likelihood of having Lyme disease. Official recommendations for serologic tests for Lyme disease are to perform a quantitative test (such as ELISA) and a confirmatory Western immunoblot test if the ELISA result is either positive or equivocal.

The currently available serologic tests, especially widely used commercial kits, are poor and have an estimated mean sensitivity of 26–57% and mean specificity of 12–60%. Use of these commercial diagnostic serologic tests will result in a high rate of misdiagnosis.

In contrast, the serologic tests for Lyme disease performed by reference laboratories are relatively accurate. Even with these tests, the predictive value still depends primarily on the probability that the patient has Lyme disease based on the clinical and epidemiologic history and the physical examination (the "pretest probability"). With few exceptions, the pretest probability that a patient has Lyme disease will be very low in areas in which Lyme disease is rare. Even in areas with a high prevalence of Lyme disease, patients with nonspecific signs and symptoms, such as fatigue, headache, and arthralgia, are not likely to have Lyme disease; most positive serologic tests in such patients are false-positive results.

Serologic tests for Lyme disease, using reference laboratories, should be obtained for patients from populations with a relatively high prevalence of Lyme disease who have specific clinical findings that are suggestive of Lyme disease so that the predictive value of a positive test is high.

Even though a symptomatic patient has antibodies to *B. burgdorferi*, Lyme disease may not be the cause of the patient's symptoms. The test may be falsely positive, or the patient may have been infected previously. Once serum antibodies to *B. burgdorferi* develop, they may persist for many years despite adequate treatment and clinical cure of the disease. Because many people who become infected with *B. burgdorferi* are asymptomatic, the background rate of seropositivity among patients who have never had clinically apparent Lyme disease is substantial in endemic areas.

Culture. The isolation of *B. burgdorferi* from a symptomatic patient is considered diagnostic of Lyme disease. Although *B. burgdorferi* has been isolated from blood, skin, cerebrospinal fluid (CSF), myocardium, and the synovium of patients with Lyme disease, the medium in which *B. burgdorferi* is cultured is expensive, it can take as long as 4 wk for the bacteria to grow in culture, and the frequency of isolation of *B. burgdorferi* from patients with active Lyme disease is low. It usually is necessary for patients to undergo an invasive procedure, such as a skin biopsy or a lumbar puncture, to obtain appropriate tissue or fluid for culture. *B. burgdorferi* has been identified with silver stains (Warthin-Starry or modified Dieterle) and with immunohistochemical stains (using monoclonal or polyclonal antibodies) in skin, synovial, and myocardial biopsy specimens. However, *B. burgdorferi* can be confused with normal tissue structures or it can be missed because it usually is present in low concentrations.

Laboratory Findings. Routine laboratory tests rarely are helpful in diagnosing Lyme disease because the associated laboratory abnormalities usually are nonspecific. The peripheral white blood cell count may be either normal or elevated. The erythrocyte sedimentation rate usually is elevated. The white blood cell concentration in joint fluid may range from 25,000–125,000/mL, often with a preponderance of polymorphonuclear cells. When the central nervous system is involved, there usually is a mild pleocytosis with a lymphocytic predominance. The CSF protein level may be elevated, but the glucose concentration usually is normal.

TREATMENT. No clinical trials of treatment for Lyme disease have been conducted in children. Recommendations for the treatment of children (Table 219–1) are extrapolated from studies of adults. Children <8 yr of age should not be treated with doxycycline because it may cause permanent discoloration of their teeth. Patients who are treated with doxycycline should be alerted to the risk of developing dermatitis in sun-exposed areas while taking the medication. Cefuroxime is also licensed for the treatment of Lyme disease and is an alternative for persons who cannot take doxycycline and who are allergic to penicillin. Preliminary results with azithromycin have been disappointing. There is little need to use newer agents because the results of treatment with either amoxicillin or doxycycline have been good.

Some patients may develop a Jarisch-Herxheimer reaction soon after treatment is initiated. The manifestations of this reaction are increased temperature, sweats, and myalgia. These symptoms resolve spontaneously, although administration of nonsteroidal anti-inflammatory drugs often is beneficial. Nonsteroidal anti-inflammatory agents also may be useful in treating symptoms of early Lyme disease and of Lyme arthritis.

Fatigue, arthralgia, and myalgia, which may accompany or follow more specific symptoms and signs of Lyme disease but almost never are the sole presenting manifestations of Lyme disease, sometimes persist after treatment but generally resolve over a period of weeks to months. There is little evidence that these symptoms are related to persistence of the organism. There is no evidence that either repeated or prolonged courses of antimicrobial agents hasten the resolution of such symptoms. Because antibodies against *B. burgdorferi* persist after successful treatment, there is no reason to obtain follow-up serologic tests.

PROGNOSIS. There is a widespread misconception that Lyme disease is difficult to treat successfully and that chronic symptoms and clinical recurrences are common. In fact, the most common reason for apparent treatment failure is misdiagnosis in patients who do not have Lyme disease. The impression that Lyme disease requires prolonged treatment, including intravenous antimicrobial therapy, and that treatment is often unsuccessful can be attributed to the treatment of patients whose symptoms were not due to Lyme disease.

The prognosis for children treated for Lyme disease is excellent. Children treated for erythema migrans do not progress to late Lyme disease. The long-term prognosis for patients who are treated beginning in the late phase of Lyme disease also is excellent. Although recurrences of arthritis do occur rarely, especially among patients with the DR2, DR3, or DR4 HLA allotypes, most children who are treated for Lyme arthritis are permanently cured. Although there are rare reports of adults who have developed late neuroborreliosis after being treated for Lyme disease, no similar cases have been reported in children.

PREVENTION. Children in endemic areas are often bitten by deer ticks, but the overall risk of acquiring Lyme disease is low (1–2%), even in these areas. Even if the patient is bitten by a nymphal-stage deer tick infected with *B. burgdorferi*, the risk of acquiring Lyme disease is only 8–10%. If infection develops treatment of the infection is highly effective. The effectiveness of antimicrobial prophylaxis for persons bitten by a deer tick is not known, and it is not recommended. The routine testing of ticks that have been removed from humans for infection with *B. burgdorferi* is not recommended because the predictive value of a positive test for infection in the human host is unknown.

The most reasonable approach to preventing Lyme disease is to wear appropriate protective clothing when entering tick-infested areas and to check for and remove ticks after spending time in such areas. Insect repellents may provide temporary protection, but they may be absorbed from the skin and, if used frequently or in large doses, they may produce significant toxicity, especially in children.

Vaccine. Lyme vaccines composed of recombinant OspA protein are effective and safe, although local adverse effects such as pain and swelling at the site of the injection are common. The first of these vaccines has been licensed for persons ≥15 yr of age living in endemic areas of the Northeast (Massachusetts to Maryland), the upper Midwest (Minnesota and Wisconsin), or the West Coast (California and Oregon) who engage in

TABLE 219–1 Antimicrobial Treatment of Lyme Borreliosis

Early Disease

Erythema Migrans and Disseminated Early Disease Without Focal Findings

Doxycycline, 100 mg twice daily for 14–21 days (do not use in children <8 yr)

or

Amoxicillin, 50 mg/kg/24 hr in 3 divided doses (maximum 500 mg/dose) for 14–21 days

Alternative agents for those who cannot take either amoxicillin or doxycycline are either erythromycin, 30–50 mg/kg/24 hr in 4 divided doses (maximum: 250 mg/dose) for 14–21 days, or cefuroxime, 30 mg/kg/24 hr in 2 divided doses (maximum: 500 mg/dose) for 14–21 days

Palsy of the Cranial Nerves (Including 7th Nerve Palsy)

Treat as for erythema migrans for 21–30 days. Do not use corticosteroids.

Carditis

Treat as for late neurologic disease.

Meningitis

Treat as for late neurologic disease.

Late Disease

Neurologic Disease*

Ceftriaxone, 50–80 mg/kg/24 hr in a single dose (maximum: 2 g) intravenously or intramuscularly for 14–21 days, or penicillin G, 200,000–400,000 U/kg/24 hr (maximum: 20 million units/24 hr) divided every 4 hr intravenously for 14–21 days.

Arthritis

Initial treatment is the same as for erythema migrans except treatment is continued for 30 days. If symptoms fail to resolve after 2 mo or there is a recurrence, then give either a second course or orally administered antimicrobial agents for 30 days or treat as for late neurologic disease.

**For isolated palsy of the facial nerve or of other cranial nerves, see Palsy of the Cranial Nerves.*

outdoor recreation or have a high risk occupation that requires spending much time in rural or wooded areas. Three doses (0, 1, and 12 mo) provided 76% protection against Lyme disease. Protective efficacy after 2 doses was only 50%. Use in children requires completion of safety and efficacy trials. Many experts have reservations about the advisability of routine use of a vaccine for a disease that is relatively rare and that is usually easily treated.

American College of Physicians: Guidelines for Laboratory Evaluation in the Diagnosis of Lyme Disease. Ann Intern Med 127:1106, 1997.

American College of Rheumatology and the Council of the Infectious Diseases Society of America: Appropriateness of parenteral antibiotic treatment for patients with presumed Lyme disease. Ann Intern Med 119:518, 1993.

Centers for Disease Control and Prevention: Lyme Disease—United States, 1996. MMWR 46:531, 1997.

Dattwyler RJ, Luft BJ, Kunkel MJ, et al: Ceftriaxone compared with doxycycline for the treatment of acute disseminated Lyme disease. N Engl J Med 337:289, 1997.

Eckman MH, Steere AC, Kalish RA, et al: Cost effectiveness of oral as compared with intravenous antibiotic therapy for patients with early Lyme disease or Lyme arthritis. N Engl J Med 337:357, 1997.

Eppes SC, Nelson DK, Lewis LL, Klein JD: Characterization of Lyme meningitis and comparison with viral meningitis in children. Pediatrics 103:957, 1999.

Gerber MA, Shapiro ED: Diagnosis of Lyme disease in children. J Pediatr 121:157, 1992.

Gerber MA, Shapiro ED, Burke GS, et al: Lyme disease in children in Southeastern Connecticut. N Engl J Med 335:1270, 1996.

Gerber MA, Zemel LS, Shapiro ED: Lyme arthritis in children: Clinical epidemiology and long-term outcomes. Pediatrics 102:905, 1998.

Massarotti EM, Luger SW, Rahn DW, et al: Treatment of early Lyme disease. Am J Med 92:396, 1992.

Reid MC, Schoen RT, Evans J, et al: The consequences of overdiagnosis and overtreatment of Lyme disease: An observational study. Ann Intern Med 128:354, 1998.

Seltzer EG, Shapiro ED: Misdiagnosis of Lyme disease: When not to order serologic tests. Pediatr Infect Dis J 15:762, 1996.

Shapiro ED, Gerber MA, Holabird N, et al: A controlled trial of antimicrobial prophylaxis for Lyme disease after deer-tick bites. N Engl J Med 327:1769, 1992.

Tugwell P, Dennis DT, Steere AC, et al: Laboratory evaluation in the diagnosis of Lyme disease. Ann Intern Med 127:1109,1997.

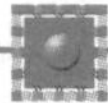

SECTION 8

Mycoplasmal Infections

CHAPTER 220
Mycoplasma pneumoniae

Dwight A. Powell

Among the five *Mycoplasma* species isolated from the human respiratory tract, *Mycoplasma pneumoniae* is the only known human pathogen. It is a major cause of respiratory infections in school-aged children and young adults.

ETIOLOGY. *M. pneumoniae*, originally thought to be a virus and called the Eaton agent, was found to be a *Mycoplasma* in the early 1960s. Mycoplasmas are the smallest self-replicating biologic system and are dependent on attachment to host cells for obtaining essential precursors such as nucleotides, fatty acids, sterols, and amino acids. They contain double-stranded DNA with genome sizes ranging from 577–1380 kb. Growth of *M. pneumoniae* in commercially available culture systems is fastidious and generally too slow to be of practical clinical use.

EPIDEMIOLOGY. *M. pneumoniae* infections occur worldwide. In contrast to the acute, short-lived epidemics of some respiratory agents, *M. pneumoniae* infection is endemic in larger communities, with epidemic outbreaks occurring every 4–7 yr. In smaller communities, infections are sporadic with long-lasting and smoldering outbreaks occurring at irregular intervals. Infections occur throughout the year.

The occurrence of mycoplasmal illness is related, in part, to the age and immune status of the patient. Overt illness is unusual before 3–4 yr of age; younger children appear to have frequent mild or subclinical infections, and reinfections appear to be common. The peak incidence of illness occurs in school-aged children: *M. pneumoniae* accounts for 33% and 70% of all pneumonias in children aged 5–9 yr and 9–15 yr, respectively. Recurrent infections occur infrequently but are well documented to occur in adults at intervals of 4–7 yr.

M. pneumoniae infections are not highly communicable, as evidenced by the slow rate at which susceptible family contacts become infected; such periods may extend for weeks or months. Infection occurs through the respiratory route by large droplet spread, and the incubation period is thought to be 1–3 wk. Explosive epidemics have been reported among military recruits and summer camps for children.

PATHOGENESIS. Cells of the ciliated respiratory epithelium are the target cells of *M. pneumoniae* infection. The organism is an elongated snakelike structure with an attachment tip characterized by an electron-dense core and a trilaminar outer membrane. Attachment to the ciliary membrane is mediated by a complex network of interactive adhesion and adherence—accessory proteins localized to this specialized attachment tip. These proteins cooperate structurally and functionally to mobilize and concentrate adhesions at the tip and permit mycoplasmal colonization of mucous membranes. Avirulent phenotypes that arise through spontaneous mutations at high frequency cannot synthesize specific cytoadherence-related proteins or are unable to stabilize them at the tip organelle.

Virulent organisms attach to ciliated respiratory epithelial cell surfaces through sialated glycoprotein receptors and burrow down between cells, resulting in ciliastasis and eventual sloughing of the cells. Although the mechanisms of cytopathology have not been determined, intracellular organisms have not been found, and *M. pneumoniae* rarely invade beyond the basement membrane.

A variety of serologic responses occur after *M. pneumoniae* infection. Nonspecific cold hemagglutinins reacting to the I antigen of red blood cell glycoproteins are usually the first antibodies detected. Appearing with titers of at least 1:32 in approximately 50% of patients, cold hemagglutinins develop late in the 1st or 2nd wk of illness and increase fourfold or more by the 3rd wk. They disappear in about 6 wk. The presence of elevated titers of cold hemagglutinins and the height of the titer correlate with the severity of the illness. Specific immunologic reactions to *M. pneumoniae* can be measured by a variety of techniques and persist for long periods of time.

Although the presence of circulating antibodies in humans can be correlated with protection against *M. pneumoniae* infections, studies in the hamster have shown that circulating antibody alone, in the absence of other forms of immunity, is incompletely protective. In hamsters, most of the peribronchial mononuclear cells are laden with antibody. However, ablation of the T-cell system with antithymocyte serum completely prevents the development of pneumonia. Thus, the disease produced by *M. pneumoniae* is very complex; the immunologic response of the host may be responsible for the disease itself as well as for protection against it, depending on the qualitative and quantitative balance of humoral and cellular immunity. Patients with immunodeficiency states such as hypogammaglobulinemia and sickle cell anemia may have more severe mycoplasmal pneumonia than do normal hosts. *M. pneumoniae* is the most common infectious cause of acute chest syndrome in sickle cell patients but is not prevalent in patients with AIDS.

CLINICAL MANIFESTATIONS. Bronchopneumonia is the most commonly recognized clinical syndrome occurring after *M. pneumoniae* infections. Although the onset of illness may be abrupt, it is usually characterized by gradual onset of headache, malaise, fever, rhinorrhea, and sore throat, with progression of lower respiratory symptoms, including hoarseness and cough. Coryza is unusual in *M. pneumoniae* pneumonia and usually suggests a viral etiology. Although the clinical course in untreated individuals is variable, coughing usually worsens during the first 2 wk of illness, and then all symptoms gradually resolve within 3–4 wk. The cough is initially nonproductive, but older children and adolescents may produce a frothy white sputum. The severity of symptoms is usually greater than the condition suggested by the physical signs, which appear later in the disease. Crackles or rales, which are often fine and crackling and resemble those heard in asthma and bronchiolitis, are the most prominent sign. With progression of the disease, the fever intensifies, the cough becomes more troublesome, and the patient may become dyspneic.

Roentgenographic findings are not specific. Pneumonia is usually described as interstitial or bronchopneumonic; involvement is most common in the lower lobes, with unilateral centrally dense infiltrates described in 75% of cases. Lobar pneumonia is seen infrequently. Hilar lymphadenopathy may be described in up to 33% of patients. Significant amounts of pleural fluid are unusual, but patients with large effusions due to *M. pneumoniae* have been described as having more severe and prolonged illness compared with those without pleural involvement. The white blood cell and differential counts are usually normal, whereas the sedimentation rate is usually elevated.

Additional respiratory illnesses caused infrequently by *M. pneumoniae* include undifferentiated upper respiratory tract infections, pharyngitis, sinusitis, croup, bronchitis, and bronchiolitis. *M. pneumoniae* is a common inducer of wheezing in asthmatic children. Otitis media and bullous myringitis have been described but are rarely seen without associated lower respiratory tract infection.

DIAGNOSIS. No specific clinical, epidemiologic, or laboratory observations permit a definite diagnosis of mycoplasmal infection early in the clinical course. Certain observations, however, are suggestive and can be helpful to the astute physician. For example, pneumonia in school-aged children and young adults, especially if cough is a prominent finding, is always suggestive of *M. pneumoniae* disease. Cultures of the throat or sputum on special media may demonstrate *M. pneumoniae*, but growth is rarely detected earlier than 1 wk. Serum cold hemagglutinins in a titer of 1:64 or greater or a positive IgM *M. pneumoniae* antibody support the diagnosis. A rise or fall in convalescent-phase complement-fixing serum antibody to *M. pneumoniae* obtained after 10 days to 3 wk is diagnostic. Rapid diagnostic tests to detect the presence of *M. pneumoniae* antigens or DNA are not commercially available, but several promising approaches such as polymerase chain reaction and hybridization to radioactive as nonradioactive DNA probes are emerging. When *M. pneumoniae* is confirmed in the community in a few patients, the probability of the existence of other mycoplasmal illnesses is greatly increased.

TREATMENT. In general, *M. pneumoniae* illness is mild, and hospitalization is infrequently required. *M. pneumoniae* is exceptionally sensitive to erythromycin, clarithromycin, azithromycin, and the tetracyclines in vitro; because of the absence of a cell wall, the organism is resistant to the penicillins and cephalosporins. Erythromycin, clarithromycin, azithromycin, and the tetracyclines are effective in shortening the course of mycoplasmal illnesses. Two multicenter studies of pediatric community-acquired pneumonia demonstrated equal efficacy between erythromycin and clarithromycin or azithromycin. These newer macrolides were better tolerated and more effective at eradiction of *M. pneumoniae* from the respiratory tract. Clarithromycin (15 mg/kg/24 hr given in two divided doses for 10 days) or azithromycin (10 mg/kg on day 1, and 5 mg/kg/24 hr on days 2–5) eradicated *M. pneumoniae* in 100% of patients studied.

COMPLICATIONS. Complications are unusual, as is bacterial superinfection. Despite the rare isolation of *M. pneumoniae* from nonrespiratory sites such as joints, pleural fluid, and CSF, nonrespiratory illness is generally believed to involve autoimmune mechanisms rather than direct organism invasion. Patients with respiratory infections may occasionally manifest illness involving the skin, central nervous system, blood, heart, gastrointestinal tract, and joints. Skin lesions include a variety of exanthems, most notably maculopapular rashes, erythema multiforme, and the Stevens-Johnson syndrome. Stevens-Johnson syndrome associated with *M. pneumoniae* usually develops 3–21 days after initial respiratory symptoms, lasts less than 14 days, and is rarely associated with severe complications. Central nervous system complications include meningoencephalitis, transverse myelitis, aseptic meningitis, cerebellar ataxia, Bell's palsy, deafness, brain stem syndrome, and Guillain-Barré syndrome. Neurologic complications occur 3–23 days (mean 10 days) after respiratory illness but may not be preceded by respiratory illness in 20% of cases. Encephalitis most commonly manifests as seizures (50%), impaired consciousness (75%), and meningeal signs (85%). The CSF is usually normal, and diagnosis is usually based on a rise in serum antibody titer. Brain imaging studies include diffuse edema or multifocal white matter inflammatory lesions on magnetic resonance imaging consistent with postinfectious demyelinating encephalomyelitis. Common hematologic complications include mild degrees of hemolysis with positive Coombs test and minor reticulocytosis 2–3 wk after the onset of illness. Severe hemolysis, associated with high titers of cold hemagglutinins (≥1:512), is rare, as are thrombocytopenia and coagulation defects. Mild hepatitis, pancreatitis, and protein-losing hypertrophic gastropathy are reported gastrointestinal complications. Myocarditis, pericarditis, and a rheumatic fever–like syndrome are uncommon manifestations, but arrhythmias, ST- and T-wave changes, and cardiac dilation with heart failure may accompany *M. pneumoniae* infection in adults more commonly than children. Transient monoarticular arthritis was described in 1% of patients in one large series.

PROGNOSIS. Virtually all patients have complete recovery without complications. Fatal infections are very rare.

Abele-Horn M, Franck W, Busch U, et al: Transverse myelitis associated with *Mycoplasma pneumoniae* infection. Clin Infect Dis 26:909, 1998.

Baseman JB, Tully JG: Mycoplasmas: Sophisticated, reemerging and burdened by their notoriety. Emerg Infect Dis 3:21, 1997.

Denny FW, Clyde WA Jr, Glezen WP: *Mycoplasma pneumoniae* disease: Clinical spectrum, pathophysiology, epidemiology, and control. J Infect Dis 123:74, 1971.

Fernald GW, Collier AM, Clyde WA Jr: Respiratory infections due to *Mycoplasma pneumoniae* in infants and children. Pediatrics 55:327, 1975.

Koskiniemi M: CNS manifestations associated with *Mycoplasma pneumoniae* infections: Summary of cases at the University of Helsinki and review. Clin Infect Dis 17(Suppl 1):S52, 1993.

Levy M, Shear NH: *Mycoplasma pneumoniae* infections and Stevens-Johnson syndrome. Clin Pediatr 30:42, 1991.

Luby JP: Pneumonia caused by *Mycoplasma pneumoniae* infection. Clin Chest Med 12:237, 1991.
Murray BJ: Nonrespiratory complications of *M. pneumoniae* infection. Am Fam Physician 37:127, 1988.
Poncz M, Kane E, Gill FM: Acute chest syndrome in sickle cell disease: Etiology and clinical correlates. J Pediatr 107:861, 1985.
Roiman CM, Rao CP, Lederman HW, et al: Increased susceptibility to *Mycoplasma* infection in patients with hypogammaglobulinemia. Am J Med 80:590, 1986.
Taylor-Robinson D: Infections due to species of *Mycoplasma and Ureaplasma*: An update. Clin Infect Dis 23:671, 1996.

CHAPTER 221
Genital Mycoplasmas (Mycoplasma hominis *and* Ureaplasma urealyticum)

Dwight A. Powell

Two *Mycoplasma* species, *Mycoplasma hominis* and *Ureaplasma urealyticum*, are human urogenital pathogens. They are often associated with sexually transmitted diseases such as nongonococcal urethritis or puerperal infections such as endometritis. Both organisms commonly colonize the female genital tract and are capable of causing chorioamnionitis, colonization of neonates, and perinatal infections. *M. genitalium* has been implicated as a possible cause of nongonococcal urethritis. Two other genital *Mycoplasma* species, *M. fermentans* and *M. penetrans*, have recently been identified in respiratory or genitourinary secretions with greater frequency in patients infected with HIV than in those without HIV. This has led to speculation, as yet unproved, that these mycoplasmas may play a role as cofactors in progression of HIV infection.

ETIOLOGY. *M. hominis* and *U. urealyticum* require sterols for growth and can grow in cell-free media. They produce characteristic colonies on agar (*U. urealyticum*: 16–60 μm; *M. hominis*: 200–300 μm, with "fried egg" appearance). Lacking a cell wall and not producing folic acid, they are resistant to β-lactams, sulfonamides, and trimethoprim. All seven serovars of *M. hominis* are susceptible to clindamycin, moderately susceptible to chloramphenicol, and resistant to erythromycin and rifampin. Aminoglycosides have limited activity, and increasing numbers of tetracycline-resistant strains are being reported. There are 14 serovars of *U. urealyticum*, and most are susceptible to erythromycin, clarithromycin, and the newer quinolones but resistant to lincomycin or clindamycin. Susceptibility to aminoglycosides and tetracyclines is variable.

EPIDEMIOLOGY. *M. hominis* and *U. urealyticum* colonize the genital and urinary tracts of postpubertal females and males. Female colonization is maximal in the vagina and less frequently in the endocervix, urethra, or endometrium. Male colonization occurs primarily in the urethra. Colonization rates are directly related to sexual activity, with colonization occurring in <10% of prepubertal children and sexually inactive adults. Rates are highest in those with multiple sexual partners. Colonization of pregnant females varies from 40–90%, and vertical transmission rates of 25–60% are observed in neonates born to colonized women. Contamination by colonized amniotic fluid or during vaginal delivery is the route of neonatal acquisition. Neonatal colonization can occur in the presence of intact amniotic fluid membranes and with delivery by cesarean section. Colonization rates are highest in infants weighing <1,500 g, in the presence of clinical chorioamnionitis and in mothers of lower socioeconomic status. Organisms are recovered from the newborn's throat, vagina, rectum, or, occasionally, eye for as long as 3 mo after birth.

PATHOGENESIS. Genital mycoplasmas can produce chronic inflammation of the genitourinary tract and amniotic fluid membranes. Ureaplasmas may infect the amniotic sac early in gestation without rupturing the fetal membranes, resulting in a clinically silent, chronic chorioamnionitis characterized by an intense inflammatory response. Attachment to fetal human tracheal epithelium has been shown to cause ciliary disarray, clumping, and loss of epithelial cells. *U. urealyticum* expresses a specific human immunoglobulin A_1 protease that cleaves immunoglobulin A_1 to intact Fab and Fc fragments. Immunity appears to require serotype-specific antibody. Thus, a lack of maternal antibody may account for a higher risk of disease in premature newborns.

CLINICAL MANIFESTATIONS. In older children and adolescents, genital mycoplasmas are commonly associated with other sexually transmitted diseases and uncommonly associated with focal infections outside the genital tract. Patients with systemic lupus erythematosus or hypogammaglobulinemia have developed severe persistent osteomyelitis, arthritis, cellulitis, and chronic respiratory infections. Postsurgical wound, blood, or urine infections have occurred in solid organ transplant patients. *U. urealyticum* is a confirmed pathogen of nongonococcal urethritis; approximately 30% of cases in males are caused by this organism either alone or together with *Chlamydia trachomatis*. Disease is most common in young adults but is also prevalent in sexually active adolescents. The average incubation period is 2–3 wk, with symptoms typically consisting of scanty, mucoid-white urethral discharge, dysuria, or penile discomfort. The discharge is often evident only in the morning or after the urethra is stripped. Rare complications of nongonococcal urethritis are epididymitis, proctitis, and Reiter's syndrome. Females rarely have urethritis; and despite the high vaginal colonization rates, vaginitis or cervicitis is uncommon. *M. hominis* is an occasional contributing cause of pelvic inflammatory disease, and both genital mycoplasmas are associated with endometritis and postpartum sepsis.

Neonates. Genital mycoplasmas are associated with a variety of fetal and neonatal infections, other sexually transmitted diseases, and chronic infections in immunocompromised patients. *U. urealyticum* may cause clinically inapparent chorioamnionitis resulting in an eightfold increase in fetal death or premature delivery. *U. urealyticum* can be recovered from up to 50% of infants <34 wk gestational age from tracheal, blood, cerebrospinal fluid (CSF), or lung biopsy specimens. The role of these organisms causing severe respiratory insufficiency, the need for assisted ventilation, the development of bronchopulmonary dysplasia, or death remains controversial. At least 14 controlled studies have investigated this question. Early studies demonstrated infants weighing <1000 g who had ureaplasmas isolated from tracheal aspirates within the first 24 hr of life were twice as likely to die or develop chronic lung disease compared with uninfected infants of similar birth weight or those weighing >1000 g. More recent studies controlling for gestational age and other factors have shown no correlation between the respiratory isolation of *U. urealyticum* and development of bronchopulmonary dysplasia, duration of ventilatory support, oxygen dependency, or length of hospitalization. Thus, although it is clear that a high percentage of premature infants are colonized with *U. urealyticum*, the pathogenicity of ureaplasmas in premature infants awaits further study.

M. hominis and *U. urealyticum* have been isolated from the CSF of premature and full-term infants in some cases. Simultaneous isolation of other pathogens is unusual, and most infants have no overt signs of central nervous system infection. CSF pleocytosis is not a consistent observation, and spontaneous clearance of mycoplasmas has been documented without specific therapy. *U. urealyticum* meningitis has been associated with intraventricular hemorrhage and hydrocephalus; meningitis due to *M. hominis* may be benign. The day of onset of meningitis varies from 1–196 days of life; organisms may persist in the CSF without therapy for days to weeks. *M. hominis* or *U. urealyticum* has been described to cause neonatal conjunctivitis, lymphadenitis, pharyngitis, pneumonitis, osteomyelitis, and scalp abscesses.

DIAGNOSIS. Diagnosis of a genital tract infection may be difficult because of high colonization rates in the vagina and urethra. Nongonococcal urethritis is confirmed by Gram stain of urethral discharge showing at least three polymorphonuclear leukocytes/oil-immersion field and the absence of gram-negative diplococci. A urethral swab or exudate should be cultured for *C. trachomatis* and *U. urealyticum*.

Neonates. *U. urealyticum* and *M. hominis* have been isolated from urine, blood, CSF, tracheal aspirates, pleural fluid, abscesses, and lung tissue. Premature neonates clinically ill with pneumonitis, focal abscesses, or central nervous system disease, particularly progressive hydrocephalus with or without pleocytosis, for whom bacterial cultures are negative or in whom there is no improvement with standard antibiotic therapy warrant cultures for genital mycoplasmas. Isolation requires special media, and clinical specimens must be cultured immediately or frozen at −80°C to avoid loss of organisms. When inoculated into broth containing arginine *(M. hominis)* or urea *(U. urealyticum)*, growth is indicated by an alkaline pH. Identification of *U. urealyticum* on agar requires 1–2 days of growth and visualization with the dissecting microscope, whereas *M. hominis* is apparent to the eye but may require 1 wk to grow. Surface cultures of the upper respiratory tract are probably meaningless owing to high colonization rates. Cultures of the lower respiratory tract through endotracheal aspirate or biopsy are essential.

TREATMENT. Nongonococcal urethritis in adolescents and adults is treated with azithromycin (1 g orally in a single dose) or doxycycline (100 mg orally twice a day for 7 days). Sexual partners should be treated to avoid recurrent disease.

Neonates. Therapy for neonatal genital *Mycoplasma* infections is indicated in infections associated with a pure growth of the organism and evidence that the disease manifestations are compatible with an infectious process rather than merely colonization with *Mycoplasma*. The role of therapy in diminishing chronic lung disease in very low birthweight infants awaits results of ongoing studies. Treatment is based on predictable antimicrobial sensitivities because susceptibility testing is not readily available. For symptomatic central nervous system infections, doxycycline is recommended. Because the long-term consequences of asymptomatic central nervous system *Mycoplasma* infection, especially in the absence of pleocytosis, are uknown and because mycoplasmas may spontaneously be cleared from the CSF, therapy should involve minimal risks. If erythromycin is used in patients concurrently receiving theophylline, serum theophylline levels should be monitored carefully, because this antibiotic inhibits theophylline metabolism.

Baseman JB, Tully JG: Mycoplasmas: Sophisticated, reemerging and burdened by their notoriety. Emerg Infect Dis 3:21, 1997.

Cassel GH, Waites KB, Watson HL, et al: *Ureaplasma urealyticum* intrauterine infection: Role in prematurity and disease in newborns. Clin Microbiol Rev 6:69, 1993.

DaSilva O, Gregson D, Hammerberg O: Role of *Ureaplasma urealyticum* and *Chlamydia trachomatis* in development of bronchopulmonary dysplasia in very low birth weight infants. Pediatr Infect Dis J 16:364, 1997.

Taylor-Robinson D: Infections due to species of *Mycoplasma* and *Ureaplasma*: An update. Clin Infect Dis 23:671, 1996.

Van Waarde WM, Brus F, Okken A, Kimpen JL: *Ureaplasma urealyticum* colonization, prematurity and bronchopulmonary dysplasia. Eur Respir J 10:886, 1997.

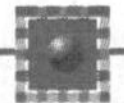

SECTION 9

Chlamydial Infections

CHAPTER 222
Chlamydia pneumoniae

Margaret R. Hammerschlag

Chlamydia pneumoniae is increasingly recognized as a common cause of lower respiratory tract diseases, including pneumonia in children and bronchitis and pneumonia in adults.

ETIOLOGY. Chlamydiae are obligate intracellular bacteria that are distinguished by a unique developmental cycle. Members of the genus possess DNA and RNA, contain their own ribosomes, and have a cell wall (but no detectable peptidoglycan or muramic acid); however, they do have penicillin-binding proteins. Chlamydiae lack the ability to generate adenosine triphosphate and can be considered an energy parasite. All members of the genus share a group lipopolysaccharide (LPS) antigen and a unique developmental cycle that involves an infectious, metabolically inactive extracellular form, the elementary body (EB), and a noninfectious, metabolically active form, the reticulate body (RB). The EBs, which are 200–400 μm in diameter, attach to the surface of the host cell by electrostatic binding or through specific receptor proteins and gain cell entry by endocytosis. The EB remains within a membrane-lined phagosome and inhibits phagosomal-lysosomal fusion during its entire life cycle. Approximately 9–12 hr after ingestion, the EBs differentiate into RBs, which then undergo binary fission, forming the typical intracytoplasmic inclusions of the genus. After approximately 36 hr, the RBs differentiate back into EBs. The total life cycle takes 48–72 hr; release occurs by cytolysis or by a process of exocytosis or extrusion of the whole inclusion, leaving the host cell intact. This process varies from species to species and provides a biologic basis for the ability of *Chlamydia* to cause prolonged, often subclinical infection.

The first isolates of *C. pneumoniae* were obtained during studies of trachoma in the 1960s. Subsequent serologic studies demonstrated that the organism caused an outbreak of mild pneumonia among school children in Finland in 1978. In 1986, the organism was isolated from the respiratory tract of college students with acute respiratory disease. DNA hybridization studies show <5% relatedness between *C. pneumoniae, C. trachomatis*, and *C. psittaci*.

EPIDEMIOLOGY. *C. pneumoniae* appears to be a primary human respiratory pathogen. No zoonotic reservoir has been identified. A recent multicenter study of community-acquired pneumonia in children 3–12 yr of age found evidence of *C. pneumoniae* infection based on culture results in 14% and of *Mycoplasma pneumoniae* in 22%. The prevalence of *C. pneumoniae* infection in children ≤6 yr of age was 15%; in those >6 yr of age it was 18%. Almost 20% of the children with *C. pneumoniae* infection were co-infected with *M. pneumoniae*. The seroprevalence of *C. pneumoniae* reaches 30–45% by adolescence, suggesting that clinically inapparent infection is common.

Transmission probably occurs from person to person through respiratory droplets. Spread of the infection occurs among members in the same household. *C. pneumoniae* may be responsible for 10–20% of community-acquired "atypical" pneumonia, including acute chest syndrome in children with sickle-cell disease, 10% of those with bronchitis, and 5–10% of those with pharyngitis. *C. pneumoniae* appears to affect individuals of all ages.

CLINICAL MANIFESTATIONS. Infections caused by *C. pneumoniae* cannot be readily differentiated from those caused by other respiratory pathogens, especially *M. pneumoniae*. The pneumonia usually presents as a classic atypical (or nonbacterial) pneumonia characterized by mild to moderate constitutional symptoms, including fever, malaise, headache, cough, and frequently pharyngitis.

C. pneumoniae may serve as an infectious trigger for asthma and can cause pulmonary exacerbations in patients with cystic fibrosis. *C. pneumoniae* has also been isolated from middle-ear aspirates of children with acute otitis media but was usually associated with bacteria. Asymptomatic respiratory infection has been documented in 2–5% of adults and children and may persist for 1 yr or longer.

DIAGNOSIS. It is not possible to differentiate *C. pneumoniae* from other causes of atypical pneumonia on the basis of clinical findings. Auscultation reveals the presence of rales and often wheezing. The chest radiograph often appears worse than the patient's clinical status would indicate and may show mild, diffuse involvement or lobar infiltrates with small pleural effusions. The complete blood count is usually unremarkable.

Specific diagnosis of *C. pneumoniae* infection is based on isolation of the organism in tissue culture and on serology. *C. pneumoniae* grows best in cycloheximide-treated HEp-2 and HL cells. The optimum site for culture is the posterior nasopharynx; the specimen is collected with wire-shafted swabs in the same manner as that used for *C. trachomatis*. The organism can be isolated from sputum, throat cultures, bronchoalveolar lavage fluid, and pleural fluid, but few laboratories perform such cultures because of technical difficulties and safety concerns.

Direct detection of EBs in clinical specimens using fluorescent antibody stains is sometimes possible but is not very sensitive or specific. Chlamydial antigen is detected in some clinical specimens by enzyme immunoassay (EIA), which is not very sensitive. All currently available EIA tests can detect *C. pneumoniae* as well as *C. trachomatis* because they use polyclonal genus-specific monoclonal antibodies. Initial reports of the use of polymerase chain reaction (PCR) appear to be promising, but there are still no commercially available kits.

Serologic diagnosis can be accomplished using the microimmunofluorescence (MIF) or the complement fixation (CF) tests. The CF test is genus specific and is also used for diagnosis of lymphogranuloma venereum and psittacosis. Most individuals with oculogenital *C. trachomatis* infection do not have detectable CF antibody. Its sensitivity in hospitalized patients with *C. pneumoniae* infection is variable. Criteria have been suggested for serologic diagnosis of *C. pneumoniae* infection using the MIF test. By these criteria, acute infection is defined by a fourfold or greater increase in IgG titer, a single IgM titer of ≥1:16, or a single IgG titer of ≥1:512. Past or pre-existing infection is defined by an IgG titer of ≥1:16 and <1:512. These criteria are based mainly on data in adults; there is concern about the inconsistent correlation of these data with the culture results. Studies of *C. pneumoniae* infection in children with pneumonia and asthma show that more than 50% of children with culture-documented infection have no detectable MIF antibody.

TREATMENT. The optimum dose and duration of antimicrobial therapy for *C. pneumoniae* infections remain uncertain. Most treatment studies have used serology only for diagnosis, and thus its microbiologic efficacy cannot be assessed. Prolonged therapy (≥2 wk) may be desirable because recrudescent symptoms and persistent positive cultures have been described following 2 wk of erythromycin and 30 days of tetracycline or doxycycline.

Tetracyclines, erythromycin, the newer macrolides (azithromycin and clarithromycin), and quinolones show in vitro activity. Like *C. psittaci*, *C. pneumoniae* is highly resistant to sulfonamides. The results of recent treatment studies have shown that erythromycin (40 mg/kg/24 hr divided into two doses orally for 10 days), clarithromycin (15 mg/kg/24 hr divided in two doses orally for 10 days), and azithromycin (10 mg/kg/24 on day 1, 5 mg/kg/24 hr on days 2–5) are effective for eradication of *C. pneumoniae* from the nasopharynx of children with pneumonia in approximately 80% of cases.

Block S, Hedrick J, Hammerschlag MR, et al: *Mycoplasma pneumoniae* and *Chlamydia pneumoniae* in pediatric community-acquired pneumonia: Comparative efficacy and safety of clarithromycin vs. erythromycin ethylsuccinate. Pediatr Infect Dis J 14:471, 1995.

File TM, Bartlett JG, Cassell GH, et al: The importance of *Chlamydia pneumoniae* as a pathogen: the 1996 consensus conference on *Chlamydia pneumoniae* infections. Infect Dis Clin Prac 6(2 Suppl):S28, 1997.

Gaydos CA, Roblin PM, Hammerschlag MR, et al: Diagnostic utility of PCR-enzyme immunoassay, culture and serology for the detection of *Chlamydia pneumoniae* in symptomatic and asymptomatic patients. J Clin Microbiol 32:903, 1994.

Grayston JT, Campbell LA, Kuo CC, et al: A new respiratory pathogen: *Chlamydia pneumoniae* strain TWAR. J Infect Dis 161:618, 1990.

Hammerschlag MR: Diagnosis of chlamydial infection in the pediatric population. Immunol Invest 26:151, 1997.

Kutlin A, Roblin PM, Hammerschlag MR: Antibody response to *Chlamydia pneumoniae* infection in children with respiratory illness. J Infect Dis 177:720, 1998.

Miller ST, Hammerschlag MR, Chirgwin K, et al: Role of *Chlamydia pneumoniae* in acute chest syndrome of sickle cell disease. J Pediatr 118:30, 1991.

Norman E, Gnarpe J, Bnarpe H, et al: *Chlamydia pneumoniae* in children attending day-care centers in Gävle, Sweden. Pediatr Infect Dis J 17:474, 1998.

Roblin PM, Hammerschlag MR: Microbiologic efficacy of azithromycin and susceptibilities to azithromycin of isolates of Chlamydia pneumoniae from adults and children with community-acquired pneumonia. Antimicrob Agents Chemother 42:194, 1998.

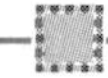

CHAPTER 223
Chlamydia trachomatis

Margaret R. Hammerschlag

The organism *Chlamydia trachomatis* is subdivided into two biovars: lymphogranuloma venereum (LGV) and trachoma (the agent of human oculogenital diseases other than LGV). Although the strains of both biovars have almost complete DNA homology, they differ in growth characteristics and virulence in tissue culture and animals. In developed countries, *C. trachomatis* is the most prevalent sexually transmitted disease, causing urethritis in men, cervicitis and salpingitis in women, and conjunctivitis and pneumonia in infants.

223.1 Trachoma

Trachoma is the most important preventable cause of blindness in the world. It is caused primarily by the A, B, Ba, and C serotypes of *C. trachomatis*. It is endemic in the Middle East and Southeast Asia and among Navajo Indians in the southwestern United States. In areas that are endemic for trachoma such as Egypt, genital chlamydial infection is caused by the serotypes responsible for oculogenital disease: D, E, F, G, H, I, J, and K. The disease is spread from eye to eye. Flies are a frequent vector.

Trachoma starts as a follicular conjunctivitis, usually in early childhood. The follicles heal, leading to conjunctival scarring, which may result in the eyelid turning inward so that the lashes abrade the cornea (entropion). Corneal ulceration secondary to the constant trauma leads to scarring and blindness. Bacterial superinfection may also contribute to scarring. Blindness occurs years after the active disease.

Trachoma can be diagnosed clinically. The World Health Organization suggests that at least two of the following four criteria must be present for a diagnosis of trachoma: (1) lymphoid follicles on the upper tarsal conjunctivae; (2) typical conjunctival scarring; (3) vascular pannus; and (4) limbal follicles. The diagnosis is confirmed by culture or staining methods performed during the active stage of disease. Serologic tests are not helpful clinically because of the long duration of the disease and its high seroprevalence in endemic populations.

Poverty and lack of sanitation are important factors in the spread of trachoma. As socioeconomic conditions improve, the incidence of the disease decreases substantially. Endemic trachoma has been controlled in most instances by administering topical tetracyclines (or, rarely, erythromycin ointment) daily for periods of 6–10 wk or intermittently over a 6-mo period. Although oral doxycycline is effective, it is contraindicated in children <8 yr of age. Oral erythromycin requires frequent dosing, which is impractical in the control of endemic trachoma. A recent study reported that one to six doses of oral azithromycin was equivalent to 30 days of treatment with topical oxytetracycline/polymyxin ointment. However, although topical and systemic treatment temporarily suppresses conjunctival inflammation and chlamydial eye infection, trachoma and chlamydial infection rapidly reappear in a large proportion of those treated.

223.2 Genital Tract Infections

EPIDEMIOLOGY. The trachoma biovar of *C. trachomatis* causes a spectrum of disease in sexually active adolescents and adults. Asymptomatic infections are common, especially in women. *C. trachomatis* is a major cause of epididymitis and is the cause of 23–55% of all cases of nongonococcal urethritis, although the proportion of chlamydial nongonococcal urethritis has been gradually declining. As many as 50% of men with gonorrhea may be co-infected with *C. trachomatis*. The prevalence of chlamydial cervicitis among sexually active women is 2–35%. Rates of infection among adolescent girls exceed 20% in many urban populations but are as high as 15% in suburban populations as well (Chapter 119).

Children who have been sexually abused may acquire anogenital *C. trachomatis* infection. These infections usually are asymptomatic. Because perinatally acquired rectal and vaginal infections may persist for ≥3 yr, the presence of *C. trachomatis* in the vagina or rectum of a prepubertal child is not absolute evidence of sexual abuse. Cultures rather than nonculture methods should be used for diagnosis of specimens from these sites when a prepubertal child is being evaluated to minimize false-positive results.

CLINICAL MANIFESTATIONS. *C. trachomatis* can cause urethritis (acute urethral syndrome), epididymitis, cervicitis, salpingitis, proctitis, and pelvic inflammatory disease. The symptoms of chlamydial genital tract infections are less acute than those of gonorrhea, consisting of a discharge that is usually mucoid rather than purulent. Asymptomatic urethral infection is frequent in sexually active men. Autoinoculation from the genitals to the eyes can lead to inclusion conjunctivitis.

DIAGNOSIS. Definitive diagnosis of genital chlamydial infection is accomplished by isolation of the organism in tissue culture and confirmed by microscopic identification of the characteristic inclusions using fluorescent antibody staining in culture specimens obtained from the urethra in men and the endocervix in women. *C. trachomatis* can be grown in cycloheximide-treated HeLa, McCoy, and HEp-2 cells. *Chlamydia* culture has been further defined by the Centers for Disease Control as isolation of the organism in tissue culture and confirmation of the characteristic inclusions by fluorescent antibody staining. Care should be taken to obtain cells, not discharge.

Alternatively, a nonculture method can be used. The four nonculture methods currently available are the direct fluorescent antibody (DFA) test, in which chlamydial elementary bodies (EBs) are identified directly on a specimen smear stained with a conjugated antichlamydial monoclonal antibody; the enzyme immunoassay (EIA); DNA probe; and nucleic acid amplification (NAA) tests. NAA now include a polymerase chain reaction (PCR) assay, ligase chain reaction (LCR), and a transcription-mediated amplification (TMA) assay. The DFA, EIA, and DNA probes perform best in screening high-prevalence (>7%) populations. All of these assays perform equivalently with sensitivities ranging from 70% to over 90% and specificities of over 95% compared to culture. The NAA tests are probably the most sensitive and specific nonculture tests available; data suggest that the sensitivity of NAA tests exceeds that of culture by 10%. The amplification assays are currently approved for use with cervical specimens from women, urethral specimens from men, and first-voided urine specimens from women and men. The use of urine may greatly facilitate screening in certain populations, especially adolescents.

The etiology of most cases of nonchlamydial nongonococcal urethritis is unknown; *Ureaplasma urealyticum* and possibly *Mycoplasma genitalium* are implicated in up to one-third of cases (see Chapter 221). Proctocolitis may develop in individuals who have a rectal infection with an LGV strain (see Chapter 223.4).

TREATMENT. Recommended treatment regimens for uncomplicated *C. trachomatis* genital infection in men and nonpregnant women are azithromycin (1 g orally in a single dose) or doxycycline (100 mg orally twice a day for 7 days). Neither of these regimens can be used in pregnant women. Alternative regimens are erythromycin base (500 mg orally four times daily for 7 days), erythromycin ethylsuccinate (800 mg orally four times daily for 7 days), and ofloxacin (300 mg orally twice a day for 7 days). The high erythromycin dosages may not be tolerated. Doxycycline and ofloxacin are contraindicated in pregnant women; quinolones are contraindicated in persons <18 yr of age. For pregnant women, the recommended treatment regimen is erythromycin base (500 mg orally four times daily for 7 days) or amoxicillin (500 mg orally three times daily for 7 days). Alternative regimens are erythromycin base (250 mg orally four times daily for 14 days), erythromycin ethylsuccinate (800 mg orally four times daily for 7 days or 400 mg orally four times daily for 14 days) and azithromycin (1 g orally in a single dose). Amoxicillin at this dosage is as effective as any of the erythromycin regimens and is much better tolerated. However, experience with all these regimens is still limited.

Empirical treatment without microbiologic diagnosis is recommended only for patients at high risk for infection who are unlikely to return for follow-up evaluation, which includes adolescents with multiple sexual partners. These patients should be treated empirically for both gonorrhea (see Chapter 192) and *C. trachomatis*.

Sex partners of patients with nongonococcal urethritis should be treated if they have had sexual contact with the patient during the 60 days preceding the onset of symptoms. The most recent sexual partner should be treated even if the last sexual contact was >60 days from onset of symptoms.

COMPLICATIONS. Complications of genital chlamydial infections in women include perihepatitis (Fitz-Hugh-Curtis syndrome) and salpingitis. The latter may cause significant morbidity, leading to infertility and ectopic pregnancy. Adolescent girls may be at higher risk for developing complications, especially salpingitis, than older women. Salpingitis in adolescent girls is also more likely to lead to tubal scarring, subsequent obstruction with secondary infertility, and increased risk of ectopic pregnancy.

223.3 Conjunctivitis and Pneumonia in Newborns

EPIDEMIOLOGY. Chlamydial genital infection is reported in 5–30% of pregnant women. Newborns may acquire *C. trachomatis* at parturition from a mother with chlamydial infection. The risk of vertical transmission is about 50%. The infant may become infected at one or more sites, including the conjunctivae, nasopharynx, rectum, and vagina. Transmission is rare following cesarean section with intact membranes.

CLINICAL MANIFESTATIONS. Approximately 70% of infected infants are infected in the nasopharynx. Clinically, the infant may develop conjunctivitis or pneumonia.

Inclusion Conjunctivitis. *C. trachomatis* is the most frequent identifiable infectious cause of neonatal conjunctivitis, the major clinical manifestation of neonatal chlamydial infection. Approximately 30–50% of infants born to mothers with chlamydial infection develop clinical conjunctivitis. Symptoms usually develop 5–14 days after delivery, or earlier if premature rupture of membranes has occurred. At least 50% of infants with chlamydial conjunctivitis also have nasopharyngeal infection. The presentation is extremely variable and ranges from mild conjunctival injection with scant mucoid discharge to severe conjunctivitis with copious purulent discharge, chemosis, and pseudomembrane formation. The conjunctiva may be very friable and may bleed when stroked with a swab. Chlamydial conjunctivitis must be differentiated from gonococcal ophthalmia, which is sight-threatening.

Pneumonia. Pneumonia due to *C. trachomatis* develops in 10–20% of infants born to women with chlamydial infection. Only about 25% of infants with nasopharyngeal chlamydial infection develop pneumonia. *C. trachomatis* pneumonia of infancy has a very characteristic presentation. Onset usually appears between 1 and 3 mo of age and is often insidious, with persistent cough, tachypnea, and absence of fever. Auscultation reveals rales; wheezing is uncommon. The absence of fever and wheezing helps to distinguish *C. trachomatis* pneumonia from respiratory syncytial virus (RSV) pneumonia. A distinctive laboratory finding is the presence of peripheral eosinophilia (>400 cells/mm^3). The most consistent finding on chest radiograph is hyperinflation accompanied by minimal interstitial or alveolar infiltrates.

Infections at Other Sites. Infants born to *Chlamydia*-positive mothers may develop an infection in the rectum or vagina. Although infection in these sites appears to be totally asymptomatic, it may cause confusion if it is identified at a later date. Perinatally acquired rectal, vaginal, and nasopharyngeal infections may persist for ≥3 yr. *C. pneumoniae* can also be confused with *C. trachomatis* infection in nasopharyngeal cultures if a genus-specific monoclonal antibody is used to confirm the culture.

DIAGNOSIS. Definitive diagnosis is achieved by isolation of *C. trachomatis* in cultures of specimens obtained from the conjunctiva or nasopharynx. Several nonculture methods, using DFA and EIA, are approved for diagnosis of chlamydial conjunctivitis. These tests have sensitivities of ≥90% and specificities of ≥95% for conjunctival specimens compared with culture. Their accuracy for nasopharyngeal specimens is not as good. DNA probe and PCR assays are not approved for tests of any sites in children, including the conjunctiva. Nonculture methods should never be used to test rectal or vaginal specimens obtained from children. Because all available EIA tests use genus-specific antibodies, these tests also detect *C. pneumoniae* if used for tests of respiratory specimens.

TREATMENT. The recommended treatment regimen for *C. trachomatis* conjunctivitis or pneumonia in infants is erythromycin (50 mg/kg/24 hr in two or four divided doses orally for 14 days). The rationale for using oral therapy for conjunctivitis is that 50% or more of these infants have nasopharyngeal infection or disease at other sites. Studies have demonstrated that topical therapy with sulfonamide drops and erythromycin ointment is not effective. The failure rate with oral erythromycin remains 10–20%, and some infants require a second course of treatment. Mothers (and their sexual contacts) of infants with *C. trachomatis* infections should be empirically treated for genital infection.

PREVENTION. The best method of preventing neonatal chlamydial infection is prenatal screening and treatment of pregnant women, as is done for gonococcal infection. Treatment of *C. trachomatis* infection requires 1–2 wk of erythromycin, which causes problems related to compliance and tolerance.

Neonatal gonococcal prophylaxis with topical erythromycin or tetracycline ointment (but not silver nitrate) may also prevent neonatal *C. trachomatis* conjunctivitis, but clinical studies have not confirmed this. Neither agent prevents nasopharyngeal colonization with *C. trachomatis* or chlamydial pneumonia.

223.4 Lymphogranuloma Venereum (LGV)

LGV is a systemic sexually transmitted disease caused by the L_1, L_2, and L_3 serotypes of the LGV biovar of *C. trachomatis*. Unlike strains of the trachoma biovar, LGV strains have a predilection for lymphoid tissue. About 20 cases of LGV have been reported in children, and fewer than 1,000 cases are reported in adults in the United States each year.

CLINICAL MANIFESTATIONS. The first stage of LGV is characterized by the appearance of the primary lesion, a painless, usually transient papule on the genitals. The second stage is characterized by usually unilaterally femoral or inguinal lymphadenitis with enlarging, painful buboes. The nodes may break down and drain, especially in males. In females, the vulvar lymph drains to the retroperitoneal nodes. Fever, myalgia, and headache are common. In the tertiary stage, a genitoanorectal syndrome occurs, with rectovaginal fistulas, rectal strictures, and urethral destruction.

DIAGNOSIS. LGV is diagnosed by culture of *C. trachomatis* from a specimen aspirated from a bubo or by serologic testing. Most patients with LGV have complement-fixing antibody titers of >1:16. Chancroid and herpes simplex virus can be distinguished clinically from LGV by the concurrent presence of painful genital ulcers. Syphilis can be differentiated by serologic tests. However, co-infections can occur.

TREATMENT. Doxycycline (100 mg orally twice daily for 21 days) is the recommended treatment. The alternative regimen is erythromycin base (500 mg four times a day for 21 days). Clinical data are lacking for use of azithromycin. Sex partners of patients with LGV should be treated if they have had sexual contact with the patient during the 30 days preceding the onset of symptoms.

Alexander ER, Harrison HR: Role of *Chlamydia trachomatis* in perinatal infection. Rev Infect Dis 5:713, 1983.

Bell TA, Stamm WE, Wang SP, et al: Chronic *Chlamydia trachomatis* infections in infants. JAMA 267:400, 1992.
Black CM: Current methods for laboratory diagnosis of *Chlamydia trachomatis* infections. Clin Microbiol Rev 10:160, 1997.
Centers for Disease Control and Prevention: 1998 Guidelines for treatment of sexually transmitted diseases. MMWR 47 (RR-1):1, 1998.
Dawson CR, Schachter J, Sallam S, et al: A comparison of oral azithromycin with topical oxytetracycline/polymyxin for the treatment of trachoma in children. J Infect Dis 24:363, 1997.
Eagar RM, Beach RK, Davidson AJ, et al: Epidemiologic and clinical factors of *Chlamydia trachomatis* in black, Hispanic and white female adolescents. West J Med 143:37, 1985.
Hammerschlag MR, Golden NH, Oh MK, et al: Single dose azithromycin for the treatment of genital chlamydial infections in adolescents. J Pediatr 122:961, 1993.
Schachter J, Grossman M, Sweet RL, et al: Prospective study of perinatal transmission of *Chlamydia trachomatis*. JAMA 255:3374, 1986.

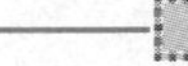

CHAPTER 224
Psittacosis (Chlamydia psittaci)

Margaret R. Hammerschlag

C. psittaci is primarily an animal pathogen. *C. psittaci*, the cause of psittacosis (also known as parrot fever and ornithosis), causes human disease infrequently.

ETIOLOGY. *C. psittaci* is a diverse species that infects approximately 100 avian species (avian chlamydiosis) and many mammalian species as well. The life cycle of *C. psittaci* is the same as that for *C. pneumoniae* (Chapter 222). There is only a 10% DNA homology between *C. psittaci* and *C. trachomatis*. *C. psittaci* can be differentiated from *C. trachomatis* by a lack of glycogen in the inclusions, inclusion morphology, and resistance to sulfonamides. Analysis of strains of *C. psittaci* indicates that there are at least five biovars. The avian biovar contains at least four serovars. Two of these serovars, psittacine and turkey, are of major importance in the avian population of the United States.

EPIDEMIOLOGY. There were 831 reported cases of psittacosis in the United States from 1987 to 1996; 70% of the cases resulted from exposure to caged pet birds, usually psittacine birds such as parrots, macaws, cockatiels, and parakeets. Among caged nonpsittacine birds, chlamydiosis occurs most frequently in pigeons, doves, and mynah birds. Persons at highest risk of acquiring psittacosis include bird fanciers and owners of pet birds (43% of cases) and pet shop employees (10% of cases).

Several major outbreaks of psittacosis have occurred in turkey processing plants. Workers exposed to turkey viscera are at the highest risk of infection. Inhalation of aerosols from feces, fecal dust, and secretions of animals infected with *C. psittaci* is the primary route of infection. Source birds are either asymptomatic or have anorexia, ruffled feathers, lethargy, and watery green droppings.

Psittacosis is uncommon in children. Children may be less likely to have close contact with infected birds.

CLINICAL MANIFESTATIONS. The mean incubation period is 15 days after exposure, with a range of 5–21 days. Onset of disease is usually abrupt with complaints of fever, cough, headache, and malaise. The fever is high and often is associated with rigors and sweats. The headache can be so severe that meningitis is considered. The cough is usually nonproductive. Rales may be heard on auscultation. Chest radiographs are usually abnormal with variable infiltrates, and pleural effusions may be present. The white blood cell count is usually not elevated, but there may be a mild leukocytosis. Abnormal results of liver function tests, including elevations in aspartate aminotransferase, alkaline phosphatase, and bilirubin, are common.

DIAGNOSIS. The diagnosis of psittacosis can be difficult because of the varying clinical presentations. A history of exposure to birds is very important, but as many as 20% of patients with psittacosis have no known contact. Pneumonia due to *C. pneumoniae* should be suspected if there is evidence of person-to-person spread, which is unusual with psittacosis. Other infections that cause pneumonia with high fever, unusually severe headache, and myalgia include *Mycoplasma pneumoniae*, tularemia, Q fever, tuberculosis, fungal infections, legionnaires' disease, and, most commonly, bacterial and viral respiratory infections. The diagnosis of psittacosis in humans is based on clinical presentation, epidemiology, and serology. Culture of *C. psittaci* is not avilable outside of research laboratories.

A *confirmed* case of psittacosis is a compatible clinical illness and laboratory confirmation by (1) *C. psittaci* cultured from respiratory secretions; (2) fourfold or greater increase in antibody titer to ≥1:32, determined by complement fixation or microimmunofluorescence, in paired acute and convalescent serum samples collected ≥2 wk apart; or (3) IgM antibody titer of ≥1:16 detected by microimmunofluorescence. A *probable* case is compatible clinical illness that is (1) epidemiologically linked to a confirmed case of psittacosis, or (2) a single antibody titer of ≥1:32 after onset of symptoms. The CF antibody test is a genus-specific test, and titers of ≥1:32 can result from infection caused by *C. pneumoniae* and *C. trachomatis*. Early treatment of psittacosis with tetracycline may abrogate the antibody response.

The organism can be isolated from sputum or pleural fluid, but few laboratories perform cultures because of technical difficulty and safety concerns.

TREATMENT. Recommended treatment regimens for psittacosis are doxycycline (100 mg twice a day orally) or tetracycline (500 mg every 6 hr orally) for at least 10–14 days after the fever abates. The initial treatment of severely ill patients should be with doxycycline hyclate (2.2 mg/kg/dose intravenously at 12-hr intervals; maximum: 100 mg/dose). Erythromycin (2 g/24 hr orally for 7–10 days) is an alternative drug useful for persons for whom tetracyclines are contraindicated (children <8 yr of age and pregnant women) but may be less effective. Remission is usually evident within 48–72 hours. Relapses can occur.

Centers for Disease Control and Prevention: Compendium of measures to control *Chlamydia psittaci* among humans (psittacosis) and pet birds (avian chlamydiosis), 1998. MMWR 47(RR-10):1, 1998.
Yung AP, Grayson ML: Psittacosis: A review of 135 cases. Med J Austral 148:228, 1988.

SECTION 10

Rickettsial Infections

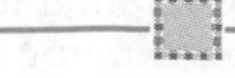

CHAPTER 225

Spotted Fever Group Rickettsioses

J. Stephen Dumler

Many members of the spotted fever group of rickettsiae are pathogenic for humans (Table 225–1). These include the tick-borne agents *Rickettsia rickettsii* (Rocky Mountain spotted fever), *R. conorii* (boutonneuse fever), *R. siberica* (North Asian tick typhus), *R. japonica* (Oriental spotted fever), *R. australis* (Queensland tick typhus), *R. honei* (Flinders Island spotted fever), the unnamed Israeli spotted fever rickettsia, *R. africae* (African tick bite fever), and possibly others. *R. akari* (rickettsialpox) is transmitted by the bite of a mite. Infections with the uncommon members of the spotted fever group rickettsiae present with signs similar to boutonneuse fever (fever, maculopapular rash, and eschar at the initial site of tick attachment). Israeli spotted fever is generally associated with a more severe course, and fatalities in children can occur.

225.1 Rocky Mountain Spotted Fever (*Rickettsia rickettsii*)

Rocky Mountain spotted fever (RMSF) is the most frequently diagnosed rickettsial disease in the United States. While infrequently diagnosed, this potentially rapidly fatal infection is often considered in the differential diagnosis of patients with fever, headache, and rash in the summer months, especially after tick exposure.

ETIOLOGY. The disease is caused by systemic endothelial cell infection by the obligate intracellular bacteria *Rickettsia rickettsii*. Proliferation of the rickettsiae within endothelial cell cytoplasm leads to vasculitis and microvascular leakage, tissue hypoperfusion, and end-organ damage.

EPIDEMIOLOGY. The term *Rocky Mountain* spotted fever is a misnomer because the disease occurs in almost every state of the continental United States, southwestern Canada, Mexico,

TABLE 225–1 Rickettsial Diseases of Humans: Summary of Pertinent Features

Group and Disease	Causative Agent	Arthropod Vector-Transmission	Hosts	Confirmatory Tests*	Geographic Distribution
Spotted Fever					
Rocky Mountain spotted fever	*Rickettsia rickettsii*	Tick bite	Dogs, rodents	IFA, DFA, IH	Western hemisphere
Boutonneuse fever (Mediterranean spotted fever)	*Rickettsia conorii*	Tick bite	Dogs, rodents	IFA, DFA, IH	Africa, Mediterranean region, India, Middle East
Rickettsialpox	*Rickettsia akari*	Mite bite	Mice	IFA	North America, Russia, Ukraine, Adriatic region, Korea, South Africa
Scrub Typhus					
Scrub typhus	*Orientia tsutsugamushi*	Chigger bite	Rodents?	IFA	Southern Asia, Japan, Indonesia, Australia, Korea, Asiatic Russia, India, China
Typhus					
Murine typhus	*Rickettsia typhi/ Rickettsia felis*	Rat flea or cat flea feces	Rats, opossums	IFA, DFA	Worldwide
Epidemic typhus	*Rickettsia prowazekii*	Louse feces	Humans	IFA	Africa, South America, Central America, Mexico, Asia
Brill-Zinsser disease (recrudescent typhus)	*Rickettsia prowazekii*	Reactivation of latent infection	Humans	IFA	Potentially worldwide; United States, Canada, Eastern Europe
Flying squirrel (sylvatic) typhus	*Rickettsia prowazekii*	Louse or flea of flying squirrel	Flying squirrels	IFA	Eastern United States
Ehrlichioses					
Human monocytic ehrlichiosis	*Ehrlichia chaffeensis*	Tick bite	Deer, dogs?	IFA, PCR	United States, Europe, Africa
Human granulocytic ehrlichiosis	*Ehrlichia phagocytophila* group	Tick bite	Rodents	IFA, PCR	United States, Europe
Sennetsu ehrlichiosis	*Ehrlichia sennetsu*	Unknown	Unknown	IFA	Japan, Malaysia
Q fever	*Coxiella burnetii*	Aerosols, ticks?	Cattle, sheep, goats, cats, rabbits	IFA	Worldwide

IFA = indirect fluorescent antibody assay; DFA = direct fluorescent antibody; IH = immunohistology; PCR = polymerase chain reaction.

**DFA or IH test can be used to detect* Rickettsia *in tissue samples. PCR may be performed to detect* Ehrlichia *nucleic acids in acute phase blood using specific oligonucleotide primers. The preferred confirmatory serologic test is IFA. Cultivation may be attempted by specialized health laboratories.*

Central America, and South America. In 1996, the highest numbers of cases were seen in North Carolina, Georgia, Virginia, Tennessee, Oklahoma, and Maryland; however, the changing ecology of tick vectors and climate changes may influence the geographic prevalence over time. The incidence of RMSF varies in a cyclical pattern over decades, the last peak occurring approximately in 1981 and the last nadir in 1996. Since then, the incidence has been rising, which suggests that another peak will occur within the next decade. Although the disease was first recognized as a distinct clinical entity in the Bitterroot region of Montana and areas of Idaho, only a small percentage of all documented cases are currently reported from the Rocky Mountain region. Habitat associations with disease are predicted by those favored by tick vectors including wooded areas or coastal grassland and salt marshes. Foci of infection have also been well documented in rural and some urban settings such as the South Bronx. Most cases in the United States occur during seasons with peak tick activity and potential human exposure, especially April through October. The incidence is highest in children 5–9 yr of age.

Transmission. Ticks are the natural hosts, reservoirs, and vectors of *R. rickettsii*. Ticks maintain the infection naturally by transovarial transmission (passage of the organism from infected ticks to their progeny) and to a lesser extent by acquisition of rickettsiae when a blood meal is taken from transiently rickettsemic animal hosts such as small mammals or dogs. Many species of ticks are capable of sustaining and transmitting the infectious agent to mammalian hosts, including humans, by regurgitation of infected saliva during feeding. The principal tick hosts of *R. rickettsii* are *Dermacentor variabilis* (the dog tick) in the eastern United States and Canada, *D. andersoni* (the wood tick) in the western United States and Canada, *Rhipicephalus sanguineus* (the brown dog tick) in Mexico, and *Amblyomma cajennense* in Central and South America.

Dogs may also serve as reservoir hosts for *R. rickettsii* and are important vehicles for bringing potentially infected ticks into the environment shared by humans. Serologic studies of patients with RMSF indicate that a high percentage may have contracted the illness from ticks carried by the family dog. Infection is largely transmitted via the bite of an infected tick; however, transmission can occur by inoculation of tick fluids or feces into open wounds or conjunctivae from the fingers and hands. Fatalities have occurred in laboratory workers exposed to infectious aerosols.

PATHOGENESIS. Following inoculation into the dermis, the rickettsiae attach to the vascular endothelium via protein ligands and initiate a focal host cell membrane injury due to rickettsial phospholipase activity. The membrane damage induces phagocytosis for repair, and the phagocytosed rickettsia then gains free access to the cytosol by continued phospholipase-mediated vacuolar membrane lysis. Members of the spotted fever serologic group actively initiate intracellular actin polymerization to achieve directional movement, and rickettsiae can thus easily invade neighboring cells while inducing minimal initial host cell damage. The rickettsiae proliferate and damage the host cell by peroxidative membrane alterations or by continued phospholipase activity.

The presence of the infectious agent initiates the inflammatory cascade including release of cytokines such as tumor necrosis factor-α (TNF-α), interleukin-1β, and interferon gamma (IFN-γ), partly by paracrine excretion from adjacent mononuclear phagocytes and lymphocytes and partly by autocrine secretion from infected endothelial cells. Infection of endothelial cells by *R. rickettsii* induces surface E–selectin expression and procoagulant activity. Cytokine release and vascular selectin expression results in infiltration of the damaged endothelial cells by lymphocytes, macrophages, and occasionally neutrophils. Local inflammatory and immune responses have been suspected as contributors to vascular injury in the rickettsioses; however, the benefits of effective inflammation and immunity outweigh any potential damage mediated by host responses directed toward elimination of local infection. Blockade of TNF-α and IFN-γ action in animal models diminishes survival and increases the morbidity of spotted fever group infections, probably by abrogating upregulation of nitric oxide synthase and arginine-dependent intracellular killing events. The *Rickettsia*-mediated endothelial injury that leads to upregulated expression of procoagulant molecules on the surfaces of infected endothelial cells to promote platelet adhesion, leukocyte emigration, and coagulation factor consumption may result in a clinical syndrome similar to disseminated intravascular coagulation.

Initially, a perivascular infiltrate of lymphoid and histiocytic cells and edema without significant endothelial damage is present, coinciding with the development of macules and maculopapules. Thereafter, the characteristic pathologic finding is that of a lymphohistiocytic or leukocytoclastic vasculitis of small venules and capillaries that results in the formation of petechial skin lesions, vascular leakage, organ hypoperfusion, and ischemic injury. Rickettsiae are localized within inflamed vessels that may be eccentrically involved, leading to nonocclusive thrombi. Rarely, small and large vessels become completely obliterated by thrombosis leading to tissue infarction or hemorrhagic necrosis. Significant sequelae result from vascular leakage in the lungs with noncardiogenic pulmonary edema and from meningoencephalitis leading to cerebral edema.

CLINICAL MANIFESTATIONS. The incubation period in children varies from 2–14 days, with a median of 7 days. The illness is initially nonspecific with headache, fever, anorexia, myalgias, and restlessness. Gastrointestinal symptoms such as nausea, vomiting, diarrhea, or abdominal pain occur frequently (39–63%) early in the disease. Often considered the hallmark of rickettsial infection, skin rash is detected usually after the third day of illness, and the typical clinical triad of headache, fever, and rash is documented in only 3% of all patients at presentation. Approximately 10% of patients have no rash or atypical cutaneous manifestations. The site of the tick bite is usually inapparent. Discrete, pale, rose-red blanching macules or maculopapules appear initially, characteristically on the extremities including the ankles, wrists, or lower legs (Fig. 225–1*A*). The rash then spreads rapidly to involve the entire body, including the soles and palms. After several days, the rash becomes more petechial or hemorrhagic, with sometimes a palpable purpura (Fig. 225–1*B*). Fever and headache persist and are accompanied by severe myalgia and malaise. Splenomegaly and hepatomegaly are present in approximately 33% of patients. In severe disease, the petechiae may enlarge into ecchymoses, which may become necrotic. Severe vascular obstruction secondary to the rickettsial vasculitis and thrombosis is very infrequent but may result in gangrene of the digits, ear lobes, scrotum, nose, or an entire limb. Central nervous system infection often produces changes in the sensorium, and delirium or coma may supervene. In addition, patients may manifest ataxia, meningismus, or auditory deficits. Other severe manifestations include facial edema, myocarditis, acute renal failure, vascular collapse, and pneumonitis with noncardiogenic pulmonary edema.

In patients with glucose-6-phosphate dehydrogenase (G6PD) deficiency, a rapid and fulminant infection may develop, leading to death in less than 5 days; the clinical course in these patients is characterized by profound coagulopathy and extensive visceral thrombosis with kidney, liver, or respiratory failure. Clinical features associated with a fatal outcome include hepatomegaly, jaundice, stupor, acute renal failure, respiratory distress, and a disseminated intravascular coagulation-like syndrome.

DIAGNOSIS. Severe or fatal rickettsial infections are associated with delays in diagnosis and treatment. No single laboratory test completely establishes an early diagnosis. Thus, treatment

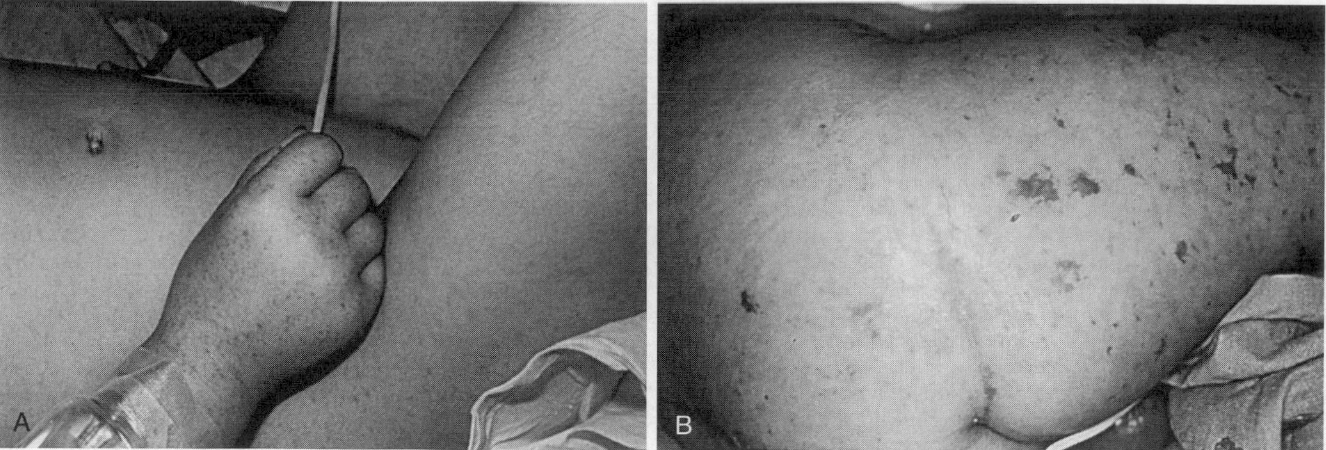

Figure 225–1 Patient with Rocky Mountain spotted fever. *A*, Rash early in the illness that is prominent on the extremities. *B*, Later in the course of Rocky Mountain spotted fever the rash may become hemorrhagic or purpuric. (Courtesy of Debra Karp Skopicki, M.D.) See also color section.

should not be withheld pending laboratory results for a patient with clinically suspected illness.

The diagnosis of RMSF should be considered in patients presenting during the spring through fall with an acute febrile illness accompanied by headache and myalgia, particularly if they were exposed to ticks in known endemic regions, were in forested or tick-infested rural areas, or had contact with a dog. A history of tick exposure and the appearance of a rash, especially on the palms or soles, together with laboratory findings of a low serum sodium concentration, normal or low leukocyte count with a marked left shift, and a relatively low or falling platelet count, are clues that are sometimes helpful in distinguishing RMSF from some other acute infections. In patients with no rash or in dark-skinned individuals in whom a rash may be difficult to appreciate, the diagnosis may be exceptionally elusive and delayed. On occasion, rickettsial vascular infection predominates in a single organ or system, erroneously suggesting a localized process such as appendicitis or cholecystitis. A thorough evaluation usually reveals evidence of a systemic process and can avoid unnecessary and potentially detrimental surgical intervention.

If a rash is present, a vasculotropic rickettsial infection can be diagnosed as early as day 3 of illness by immunohistologic demonstration of specific rickettsial antigen in the endothelium in skin biopsies of petechial lesions. The procedure may be performed by immunofluorescence or immunoperoxidase and is very specific. Unfortunately, the sensitivity of this method is probably not greater than 70%, and it can be adversely influenced by prior antimicrobial therapy, biopsy of skin lesions that are suboptimal, or examination of insufficient tissue because the infection may be very focal. Moreover, because approximately 10–15% of patients with RMSF either do not have a rash or have an atypical rash, selection of an appropriate biopsy site may be difficult. Unfortunately, evaluation of blood for *R. rickettsii* nucleic acids by polymerase chain reaction (PCR) demonstrates little sensitivity beyond that of immunohistology, probably because the level of rickettsemia is generally very low (<6 rickettsia/mL).

Because treatment must be initiated on the clinical diagnosis alone, confirmation is most often accomplished by serology in convalescence. Diagnostic serologic criteria include a fourfold rise in antibody titer (usually indirect fluorescent antibody [IFA] assay) in acute and convalescent sera (2–4 wk apart) or a single elevated IFA titer of ≥1:64 in convalescent serum. A case is considered probable if a single titer of ≥1:128 is found. Weil-Felix antibody testing should not be performed because it lacks both sensitivity and specificity.

Differential Diagnosis. Other rickettsial infections are easily confused with RMSF, especially human monocytic ehrlichiosis, human granulocytic ehrlichiosis, and murine typhus. Although murine typhus may be treated similarly, chloramphenicol therapy for ehrlichiosis is controversial, and thus an accurate and thorough clinical evaluation is mandatory to differentiate the two entities if this therapy is to be used. Rocky Mountain spotted fever can mimic many diseases; among the most important of these are meningococcemia, measles, and enteroviral exanthems. Negative blood cultures may aid in reaching a correct diagnosis; however, *R. rickettsii* may elicit a lymphocytic meningitis, suggesting a viral etiology and further confounding the diagnosis. Other diseases sometimes included in the differential diagnosis are typhoid fever, secondary syphilis, Lyme borreliosis, leptospirosis, scarlet fever, toxic shock syndrome, rheumatic fever, rubella, Kawasaki disease, idiopathic thrombocytopenic purpura, thrombotic thrombocytopenic purpura, Henoch-Schönlein purpura, hemolytic uremic syndrome, aseptic meningitis, acute gastrointestinal illness, acute abdomen, hepatitis, infectious mononucleosis, dengue fever, and drug reactions.

Laboratory Findings. An abnormally low platelet count, normal to slightly low leukocyte count, and low serum sodium concentration are present in about half of these patients and may be early clues to the diagnosis. Most other clinical laboratory findings are nonspecific and vary depending on the degree of specific organ involvement. RMSF may cause meningoencephalitis that presents with a cerebrospinal fluid pleocytosis enriched for mononuclear cells.

TREATMENT. The time-proven effective therapies for RMSF are tetracycline and chloramphenicol. Both agents have drawbacks for pediatric therapy in that tetracycline and doxycycline may be associated with tooth discoloration, while chloramphenicol is rarely associated with aplastic anemia. Recent controversial evaluations of mortality in patients with RMSF reveal that mortality is significantly increased when choramphenicol alone is used compared with tetracycline, even when other factors such as severity are considered. Tetracyclines can be used safely in children <8 yr of age, since tooth discoloration is dose-dependent, and it is unlikely that children <8 yr of age will require multiple courses. Doxycycline is recommended for children because the risk of dental staining with it is less than with other tetracyclines.

Greater morbidity and excess mortality are associated with the use of sulfonamides, and consequently their use should be discouraged. Other antibiotics including penicillins, cephalosporins, and aminoglycosides are not effective. The use of alternative antimicrobial agents such as quinolones and the newer macrolides (azithromycin and clarithromycin) for RMSF has not been evaluated.

Recommended treatment regimens for RMSF are: doxycycline orally or intravenously (two loading doses of 2.2 mg/kg/dose at 12-hr intervals followed by 2.2 mg/kg/24 hr divided in two doses every 12 hr; maximum: 300 mg/dose); tetracycline orally (25–50 mg/kg/24 hr divided in four doses; maximum: 2 g/24 hr) or chloramphenicol (50–100 mg/kg/24 hr divided in four doses; maximum: 3 g/24 hr). Therapy should be continued for a minimum of 5 days and until the patient has been afebrile for at least 2–4 days to avoid relapse, especially in patients who were treated early. Patients treated with one of these regimens usually become afebrile within 48 hr, and thus the entire period of therapy lasts less than 10 days.

COMPLICATIONS. Complications of infection include noncardiogenic pulmonary edema from pulmonary microvascular leakage, cerebral edema from meningoencephalitis, multiorgan damage (hepatitis, pancreatitis, cholecystitis, epidermal necrosis, and gangrene) partly mediated by rickettsial vasculitis or the accumulated effects of hypoperfusion and ischemia (acute renal failure). Long-term neurologic sequelae are more likely to occur in patients who have been hospitalized for ≥2 weeks and include paraparesis, hearing loss, peripheral neuropathy, bladder and bowel incontinence, cerebellar, vestibular, and motor dysfunction, and language disorders.

PROGNOSIS. Delays in diagnosis and therapy are significant factors associated with death or severe illness. Before the advent of effective antimicrobial therapy for RMSF the case fatality rate was 10–40%. More recent statistics show that this rate has stabilized fluctuating between 2% and 7%. Fatalities occur despite the availability of effective therapeutic agents, indicating the need for vigilant clinical suspicion and a low threshold for early and aggressive therapy in clinically suspected cases. Even with administration of tetracycline or chloramphenicol, delays in therapy may allow sufficient vascular or end-organ damage to prevent complete recovery or ensure an inevitable fatal outcome. Early therapy in uncomplicated cases ordinarily leads to rapid defervescence within 1–3 days and recovery within 7–10 days.

PREVENTION. No vaccines are available. Prevention of RMSF is best accomplished by eliminating tick infestations of dogs, avoiding wooded or grassy areas where ticks reside, using insect repellents, wearing protective clothing, and carefully inspecting children who have been playing in the woods or fields.

Prompt and complete removal of attached ticks will help reduce the risk of transmission because complete exchange of infected tick saliva occurs during the later phases of the blood meal. Contrary to popular belief, the application of petroleum jelly, 70% isopropyl alcohol, fingernail polish, or a hot match are not effective in removing ticks from persons or animals. A tick can be safely removed by grasping the mouth parts of the tick at the site of cutaneous contact with a pair of forceps and applying a gentle and steady retraction force to remove the entire tick and mouth parts. The site of attachment should then be disinfected. Ticks should not be squeezed, crushed, or disrupted because their fluids may be infectious. Disposal may be accomplished by soaking the tick in alcohol or flushing it down the toilet, after which one should wash the hands. Prophylactic antimicrobial therapy should not be administered because tetracyclines and chloramphenicol are only rickettsiostatic; such therapy simply delays the onset of illness and confuses the clinical picture by prolonging the incubation period.

225.2 Boutonneuse Fever (*Rickettsia conorii*)

ETIOLOGY. The causative agent of boutonneuse fever, *R. conorii*, is distributed over a large geographic region including India, Pakistan, Russia, Ukraine, Georgia, Israel, Ethiopia, Kenya, South Africa, Morocco, and southern Europe. The disease it causes is known by various geographically recognized names including boutonneuse fever, Mediterranean spotted fever, Kenya tick typhus, and Indian tick typhus. Similar illnesses are distributed globally but are caused by distinct yet related species such as *R. siberica* in Russia, China, Mongolia, and Pakistan, *R. australis* or *R. honei* in Australia, *R. japonica* in Japan, and *R. africae* in South Africa (see Table 225–1). These species are closely related to *R. rickettsii* by analysis of antigens and DNA sequences.

EPIDEMIOLOGY. Boutonneuse fever has demonstrated a steadily increasing incidence since 1980 in southern Europe and has achieved seroprevalence rates of 11–26% in some areas. The peak incidence is seen during July and August in the Mediterranean basin, but in other regions it occurs during warm seasons when ticks are active. Many cases of imported infection have been documented in travelers to endemic regions, especially those who go on safari in regions with high grass and bush land.

Transmission. Transmission occurs after the bite of the brown dog tick, *Rhipicephalus sanguineus*, or other tick species including *Dermacentor, Haemaphysalis, Amblyomma, Hyalomma*, and *Ixodes*. A strong correlation exists among the incidence of boutonneuse fever, infected ticks, and evidence of infection in both dogs and humans, implicating the household dog as a potential vehicle for transmission.

CLINICAL MANIFESTATIONS. Patients with boutonneuse fever typically experience fever, headache, myalgias, and a maculopapular rash, which appears 3–5 days after onset of symptoms. In about 70% of patients, an eschar *(tache noire)* at the initial site of tick attachment and regional lymphadenopathy are present. Although it was previously considered benign and self-limited, this infection may cause severe disease in up to 6% of infected individuals. It is characterized by findings similar to those seen in Rocky Mountain spotted fever, including purpuric skin lesions, neurologic signs, respiratory distress, acute renal failure, severe thrombocytopenia, and death in 1.4–5.6% of cases. As in Rocky Mountain spotted fever, a particularly malignant form occurs in patients with G6PD deficiency and in individuals with other underlying conditions such as alcoholic liver disease or diabetes mellitus.

DIAGNOSIS. Laboratory diagnosis of boutonneuse fever and the other spotted fever group rickettsioses is the same as that for Rocky Mountain spotted fever and may be accomplished by immunohistologic demonstration of rickettsiae on skin biopsy, immunocytologic demonstration of *R. conorii* (and potentially other spotted fever group rickettsiae) in circulating endothelial cells, in vitro cultivation by means of centrifugation-assisted shell vial tissue culture, or the demonstration of serum antibodies to spotted fever group rickettsiae in convalescent patients. Reagents useful for the diagnosis of Rocky Mountain spotted fever in the United States or boutonneuse fever in Europe, Africa, and Asia can be used effectively for the diagnosis of infections by most members of the spotted fever group of rickettsiae.

TREATMENT. Boutonneuse fever is effectively treated with tetracycline, doxycycline, chloramphenicol, ciprofloxacin, ofloxacin, pefloxacin, or levofloxacin.

225.3 Rickettsialpox (*Rickettsia akari*)

Rickettsialpox is caused by *R. akari*, which is transmitted by the mouse mite, *Allodermanyssus sanguineus*. Although the mouse host for this mite is widely distributed in cities in the United States, Europe, and Asia, the disease is relatively mild and is infrequently diagnosed.

Rickettsialpox is generally mild and is best known because

of its association with a varicelliform rash. In fact, this rash is a modified form of an antecedent typical macular or maculopapular rash like those seen in other vasculotropic rickettsioses. At presentation, most patients have fever, headache, and chills. There may be a papular or ulcerative lesion at the initial site of inoculation in up to 90% of cases that may be associated with regional lymphadenopathy. In some patients, the maculopapular rash, which is distributed over the trunk, head, and extremities, may become vesicular. The infection resolves spontaneously even without therapy. Complications and fatalities are rare.

Abramson JS, Givner LB: Rocky Mountain spotted fever. Semin Pediatr Infect Dis 5:131, 1994.

Kass EM, Szaniawski WK, Levy H, et al: Rickettsialpox in a New York City Hospital, 1980 to 1989. N Engl J Med 331:1612–1617, 1994.

Dalton MJ, Clarke MJ, Holman RC, et al: National surveillance for Rocky Mountain spotted fever, 1981–1992: Epidemiologic summary and evaluation of risk factors for fatal outcome. Am J Trop Med Hyg 52:405, 1995.

Dumler JS, Walker DH: Diagnostic tests for Rocky Mountain spotted fever and other rickettsial diseases. Dermatol Clin 12:25, 1994.

Hackstadt T: The biology of rickettsiae. Infect Agents Dis 5:127–43, 1996.

Helmick CG, Bernard KW, D'Angelo LJ: Rocky Mountain spotted fever: Clinical, laboratory, and epidemiological features of 262 cases. J Infect Dis 150:480, 1984.

Kirkland KB, Wilkinson WE, Sexton DJ: Therapeutic delay and mortality in cases of Rocky Mountain spotted fever. Clin Infect Dis 20:1118, 1995.

Raoult D, Drancourt M: Antimicrobial therapy of rickettsial diseases. Antimicrob Agents Chemother 35:2457, 1991.

Walker DH: Rocky Mountain spotted fever: A seasonal alert. Clin Infect Dis 20:1111, 1995.

CHAPTER 226
Scrub Typhus (Orientia tsutsugamushi)

J. Stephen Dumler

ETIOLOGY. *Orientia tsutsugamushi* (formerly *Rickettsia tsutsugamushi*) is the causative agent of scrub typhus, or Tsutsugamushi fever, and is distinct from other spotted fever and typhus group rickettsiae. *O. tsutsugamushi* lacks both lipopolysaccharide and peptidoglycan in its cell wall. However, like other vasculotropic *Rickettsia* spp., *O. tsutsugamushi* infects endothelium and elicits vasculitis, the predominant clinicopathologic feature of the disease.

EPIDEMIOLOGY. Scrub typhus occurs mostly in the Far East, including areas delimited by a triangle connecting Korea, Pakistan, and northern Australia. Aside from infections in these tropical and subtropical regions, the disease occurs in Japan, the Primorye of far eastern Russia, Tadzhikistan, Nepal, and nontropical China including Tibet. Imported cases in the United States have been reported.

Transmission. *O. tsutsugamushi* is transmitted via the bite of a trombiculid mite (*Leptotrombidium* spp.), which serves as both vector and reservoir. Because transovarial transmission occurs efficiently and transmission of the organism to mites from infected animals is poor, the rodent hosts of these mites are not likely to be involved in natural maintenance of the agent. Although multiple serotypes are known, most share antigenic cross reactivity.

CLINICAL MANIFESTATIONS. Scrub typhus may be mild or severe. After an incubation period of 6–21 days, the rickettsiae proliferate at the site of the chigger (mite) bite to form a necrotic eschar with an erythematous rim in <50% of cases. The onset of illness usually becomes manifest by fever, headache, and sometimes myalgia, cough, and gastrointestinal symptoms. Regional or generalized lymphadenopathy is common. A maculopapular rash is present in <50% of patients and involves the trunk and extremities and infrequently the hands or face. Complications include severe meningoencephalitis and interstitial pneumonitis. The case fatality rate in untreated patients may be as high as 7%.

DIAGNOSIS. The diagnosis is usually confirmed by indirect fluorescent antibody assay or immunoperoxidase serologic tests using various serotypes of *O. tsutsugamushi* as antigen.

TREATMENT. Therapy includes doxycycline and chloramphenicol in the same regimens suggested for Rocky Mountain spotted fever or murine typhus (see Chapters 225.1 and 227.1), after which prompt defervescence (within 24–48 hr) occurs; however, some reports suggest that more virulent or potentially doxycycline-resistant strains may have emerged. In vitro data suggest that azithromycin should be a highly effective therapy for scrub typhus.

PREVENTION. Prevention is based on avoidance of the chiggers that transmit *O. tsutsugamushi*. Protective clothing is the next most useful mode of prevention.

Pai H, Sohn S, Seong Y, et al: Central nervous system involvement in patients with scrub typhus. Clin Infect Dis 26:247, 1998.

Silpapojakul K, Chupuppakam S, Yuthasompob S, et al: Scrub and murine typhus in children with obscure fever in the tropics. Pediatr Infect Dis J 10:200, 1991.

Tamura A, Ohashi N, Urakami H, Miyamura S: Classification of *Rickettsia tsutsugamushi* in a new genus, *Orientia* gen. nov., as *Orientia tsutsugamushi* comb. nov. Int J Syst Bacteriol 45:589, 1995.

Wang CL, Yang KD, Cheng SN, Chu ML: Neonatal scrub typhus: A case report. Pediatrics 89:965, 1992.

CHAPTER 227
Typhus Group Rickettsioses

J. Stephen Dumler

227.1 *Murine Typhus* (Rickettsia typhi)

ETIOLOGY. Murine typhus is caused by *Rickettsia typhi*, a typhus group rickettsia that is transmitted from infected fleas to rats or opossums and back to fleas. Transovarial transmission in fleas is inefficient, and thus transmission depends on distribution by the flea to uninfected mammals, which become transiently rickettsemic and in turn transmit the organism to uninfected fleas.

A novel agent within the genus *Rickettsia* has been identified as a cause of murine typhus in south Texas. This new rickettsia, *R. felis*, is genetically related to both *R. typhi* and *R. rickettsii* and is capable of highly efficient transovarial transmission in cat fleas; it may be found in cat fleas obtained from areas endemic for murine typhus in the United States.

EPIDEMIOLOGY. Murine typhus has a worldwide distribution and occurs especially in warm coastal ports where it is maintained in a cycle involving rat fleas *(Xenopsylla cheopis)* and rats *(Rattus species)*. Peak incidence occurs when rat populations are highest during spring, summer, and fall. In the United States, the disease is most prevalent in south Texas and southern California, although sporadic cases have been reported in most other states as well. In the coastal areas of south Texas, the disease is seen predominantly from March through June and is associated with opossums, cats, and cat fleas *(Ctenocephalides felis)*.

Transmission. Human acquisition of murine typhus occurs when rickettsiae-infected flea feces contaminate flea-bite wounds.

PATHOGENESIS. *R. typhi* is a vasculotropic rickettsial species that causes disease in much the same way as does *R. rickettsii* of Rocky Mountain spotted fever (Chapter 225.1). *R. typhi* organisms in flea feces deposited on the skin as part of the flea feeding reflex are inoculated into the pruritic flea bite wound. After an interval during which local proliferation occurs, the rickettsiae spread systemically to infect the endothelium in many tissues. As with spotted fever group rickettsiae, typhus group rickettsiae infect endothelial cells but polymerize actin poorly for intracellular mobility and probably cause cellular injury by simple mechanical lysis owing to the accumulation of large numbers of rickettsiae within the endothelial cell cytoplasm. Intracellular infection leads to endothelial cell damage and recruitment of inflammatory cells and vasculitis. The inflammatory cell infiltrates bring in a number of effector cells, including macrophages that produce proinflammatory cytokines, and CD4+ and CD8+ lymphocytes which may produce immune cytokines such as interferon-γ or participate in cell-mediated cytotoxic responses. Intracellular rickettsial proliferation of typhus group rickettsiae is inhibited by cytokine-mediated, nitric oxide-dependent and -independent mechanisms.

Pathologic findings include the presence of systemic vasculitis in response to the presence of rickettsiae within endothelial cells. This is manifest as interstitial pneumonitis, interstitial nephritis, myocarditis, meningitis, and mild hepatitis with periportal lymphohistiocytic infiltrates. As vasculitis and inflammatory damage accumulate, multi-organ damage may ensue.

CLINICAL MANIFESTATIONS. Murine typhus is a moderately severe infection that is similar to other vasculotropic rickettsioses. The infection in children generally appears to be mild. The incubation period may vary between 1 and 2 wk. The initial presentation is often nonspecific, with fever as the predominant finding. Fewer than half of pediatric patients experience other typically important clues for rickettsiosis including rash (48%), myalgias (29%), vomiting (29%), cough (24%), headache (19%), and diarrhea or abdominal pain (10%). Although neurologic involvement may be a frequent finding in adults with murine typhus, confusion, stupor, coma, seizures, meningismus, and ataxia are seen in <5% of infected children. A petechial rash is infrequent, and the usual appearance is that of macules or maculopapules distributed on the trunk and extremities. The rash may involve both the soles and palms on rare occasions.

DIAGNOSIS. As for other vasculotropic rickettsioses, delays in diagnosis and therapy are associated with increased morbidity and mortality; thus, diagnosis must be based on clinical suspicion. Confirmation of the diagnosis is usually accomplished in convalescence by indirect fluorescent antibody assay serology. Research tools now being evaluated include polymerase chain reaction amplification of rickettsial nucleic acids in acute phase blood, rickettsial culture by the centrifugation-assisted shell vial assay, and immunohistology on skin biopsy.

Occasionally, patients present with findings suggestive of pharyngitis, bronchitis, hepatitis, gastroenteritis, or sepsis; thus, the differential diagnosis may be extensive.

Laboratory Findings. Although they are nonspecific, laboratory findings that may be helpful include mild leukopenia (36%) with a moderate left shift, mild to marked thrombocytopenia (50%), hyponatremia (20%), hypoalbuminemia (57%), and elevated serum concentrations of hepatic transaminases such as aspartate aminotransferase (88%) and alanine aminotransferase (83%). Elevations in serum urea nitrogen are usually due to prerenal mechanisms.

TREATMENT. Therapy for murine typhus includes the use of tetracyclines or chloramphenicol and is similar to that recommended for Rocky Mountain spotted fever. No controlled trials of other antimicrobial agents have been performed; however, ciprofloxacin has been used effectively to treat murine typhus, and in vitro experiments suggest that minimal inhibitory concentrations of azithromycin and clarithromycin for *R. typhi* should be easily achieved.

Recommended treatment regimens for murine typhus include doxycycline orally or intravenously (2.2 mg/kg/24 hr divided in two doses; maximum: 300 mg/dose), tetracycline orally (25–50 mg/kg/24 hr divided in four doses; maximum: 2 g/24 hr, and chloramphenicol (50–100 mg/kg/24 hr divided in four doses; maximum 3 g/24 hr). Therapy should be continued for a minimum of 5 days or until the patient has been afebrile for at least 2–4 days to avoid relapse, especially in patients treated early.

COMPLICATIONS. Complications of murine typhus in pediatric patients are infrequent; however, relapse, stupor, facial edema, dehydration, and cerebrospinal fluid pleocytosis have been reported.

PREVENTION. Control of murine typhus has been dependent on elimination of the rat and rat flea reservoir, and this remains an important component of control. However, with the recognition of cat fleas as potentially significant reservoirs and vectors, the presence of these flea vectors and their mammalian hosts in suburban and urban areas where close human exposures occur will probably pose increasingly important control problems.

227.2 Epidemic Typhus (Rickettsia prowazekii)

ETIOLOGY. Humans have long been considered the principal or only reservoir of *R. prowazekii*, the causative agent of epidemic or louse-borne typhus, also known as recrudescent typhus or sylvatic flying squirrel typhus, and its recrudescent form, Brill-Zinsser disease, also known as Brill's disease or recrudescent typhus.

EPIDEMIOLOGY. The infection is characteristically seen in winter or spring or during times of poor hygienic practices associated with crowding, war, famine, and civil strife. The cause of sporadic cases of a mild, typhus-like illness has been confirmed as *R. prowazekii*; such cases are associated with exposure to flying squirrels harboring infected lice or fleas. The *R. prowazekii* organisms isolated from these squirrels appear to be genetically different from isolates obtained during typical outbreaks.

Most cases of epidemic typhus from 1981–1997 have been sporadic, but outbreaks have been identified in Africa (Ethiopia, Nigeria, Burundi), Mexico, Central America, South America, eastern Europe, Afghanistan, northern India, and China, although reporting of this illness is almost certainly woefully underestimated.

Transmission. Human body lice (*Pediculus humanus* subsp. *corporis*) or head lice (*P. capitis*) become infected by feeding on rickettsemic persons. The ingested rickettsiae infect the midgut epithelial cells of the lice and are passed into the feces, which are introduced in turn into a susceptible human host through abrasions or perforations in the skin, through the conjunctivae, or rarely through inhalation of dried infected louse excreta present in clothing, bedding, or furniture.

CLINICAL MANIFESTATIONS. Epidemic typhus fever may be a mild or severe disease in children. The incubation period is usually <14 days. The clinical manifestations include fever, severe headache, abdominal tenderness, and rash in most patients, as well as chills (82%), myalgias (70%), arthralgias (70%), anorexia (48%), nonproductive cough (38%), dizziness (35%), photophobia (33%), nausea (32%), abdominal pain (30%), tinnitus (23%), constipation (23%) meningismus (17%), visual disturbances (15%), vomiting (10%), and diarrhea (7%). The rash is initially pink or erythematous and blanches. In one third of patients, red, nonblanching macules and petechiae appear predominantly on the trunk. Infections identified during the preantibiotic era typically produced a variety of central nervous system findings including delirium (48%), coma (6%), and seizures (1%). Estimates of case fatality rates range between 3.8% and 20% in outbreaks.

Brill-Zinsser disease is an unusual form of typhus that becomes recrudescent months to years after the primary infection. When rickettsemic, these infected individuals may transmit the agent to lice.

TREATMENT. Recommended treatment regimens for epidemic or sylvatic typhus are identical to those used for murine typhus: doxycycline orally or intravenously (2.2 mg/kg/24 hr divided in two doses; maximum: 300 mg/dose), tetracycline orally (25–50 mg/kg/24 hr divided in four doses; maximum: 2 g/24 hr), or chloramphenicol (50–100 mg/kg/24 hr divided in four doses; maximum 3 g/24 hr). Therapy should be continued for a minimum of 5 days and until the patient has been afebrile for at least 2–4 days to avoid relapse, especially in patients treated early.

PREVENTION. Immediate destruction of vectors with an insecticide is important in the control of an epidemic. Dust containing excreta from infected lice is capable of transmitting typhus, and care must be taken to prevent its inhalation.

Dumler JS: Murine typhus. Semin Pediatr Infect Dis 5:137, 1994.

Dumler JS, Taylor JP, Walker DH: Clinical and laboratory features of murine typhus in south Texas, 1980–1987. JAMA 266:1365, 1991.

Perine PL, Chandler BP, Krause DK, et al: A clinico-epidemiological study of epidemic typhus in Africa. Clin Infect Dis 14:1149, 1992.

Schriefer ME, Sacci JB Jr, Dumler JS, et al: Identification of a novel rickettsial infection in a patient diagnosed with murine typhus. J Clin Microbiol 32:949, 1994.

Silpapojakul K, Chupuppakam S, Yuthasompob S, et al: Scrub and murine typhus in children with obscure fever in the tropics. Pediatr Infect Dis J 10:200, 1991.

CHAPTER 228
Ehrlichioses

J. Stephen Dumler

ETIOLOGY. First recognized as infectious agents of dogs and ruminants, members of the genus *Ehrlichia* were largely ignored as important human pathogens until 1987, when the first case of an *Ehrlichia canis*-like infection was detected in humans. This initial infection was diagnosed when clusters of bacteria confined within cytoplasmic vacuoles of circulating leukocytes (morulae), particularly mononuclear leukocytes, were detected in the peripheral blood of a severely ill patient suffering from suspected Rocky Mountain spotted fever. In 1990, a new rickettsial species, *E. chaffeensis,* was cultivated and identified as the predominant agent of human ehrlichiosis. Seroepidemiologic investigation has shown that in some geographic areas *E. chaffeensis* infections occur more frequently than Rocky Mountain spotted fever, and the infection is strongly associated with tick bites.

In 1994, another species of the genus was implicated as an agent of human disease in the United States. This new human infection was recognized by the observation of ehrlichial morulae that were present only in circulating neutrophils. Serologic investigation in these cases revealed the lack of *E. chaffeensis* antibodies, and most of these patients had serologic reactions to *E. phagocytophila* and *E. equi,* which were previously known only as pathogens of ruminant and horse granulocytes, respectively. Accumulating data suggest that this new agent of humans, *E. phagocytophila,* and *E. equi* represent variants of a single species called the *E. phagocytophila* group.

To differentiate between *E. chaffeensis,* which infects predominantly monocytic cells, and infections caused by the human granulocyte ehrlichial pathogen, the names human monocytic ehrlichiosis (HME) and human granulocytic ehrlichiosis (HGE) have been applied.

Ehrlichiae are small, pleomorphic, obligate intracellular bacteria that possess gram-negative-type cell walls. Ehrlichiae induce the endosome to enter a receptor recycling pathway that avoids phagosome-lysosome fusion and allows the growth of a cytoplasmic aggregate of bacteria called a morula. *Ehrlichia* species have no detectable lipopolysaccharide but apparently do contain peptidoglycan in their cell walls. Genetic analysis of the 16S ribosomal RNA and heat shock protein genes, and protein immunoblot investigations indicate that the genus contains at least three separate groups, each denoted by a prototype, *E. canis, E. sennetsu,* and *E. phagocytophila.* These bacteria are pathogens of hematopoietic cells in mammals, and characteristically each species has a specific host cell affinity: *E. chaffeensis* and *E. sennetsu* infect mononuclear phagocytes, and the human granulocytic *Ehrlichia, E. equi,* and *E. phagocytophila* infect neutrophils. Differences in these host cell affinities may in part explain the clinical findings of rare cells with *E. chaffeensis* in circulating leukocytes, whereas infections in patients with the granulocytic *Ehrlichia* are associated with morulae in up to 40% of circulating neutrophils.

EPIDEMIOLOGY. Infections with *E. chaffeensis* have been detected in many southeastern and south central states in a distribution that parallels that of Rocky Mountain spotted fever. However, infections have also been documented in patients from more northern states, including Washington, New York, and Connecticut. Additional suspected cases with appropriate serologic findings have been reported in Europe, Africa, and the Far East. Infections with the HGE agent have been recognized mostly in the northeast and upper midwestern United States, but cases or serologic evidence of such infections exist in residents of California, the mid-Atlantic, south Atlantic, and south central United States and broadly across Europe, implying that the agent is very widely distributed.

Although the median age of patients infected with monocytic ehrlichiosis is 42 yr, many pediatric patients have been identified. Definite infections of children with the granulocytic *Ehrlichia* also have been identified, but the median patient age is between 44 and 59 yr. As expected, both infections are highly associated with tick exposure and tick bites, and infections are identified predominantly during May through September, with a second peak of HGE in late October through December.

Transmission. The predominant tick species that harbors *E. chaffeensis* is *Amblyomma americanum,* the Lone Star tick. Additional vectors such as *Dermacentor variabilis,* the American dog tick, have not been proved but may explain the presence of disease outside the known range of *A. americanum.* The tick vectors of HGE are *Ixodes* species, including *I. scapularis* (black-legged or deer tick) in the eastern United States, *I. pacificus* (western black-legged tick) in the western United States, and *I. ricinus* (sheep tick) in Europe. *Ehrlichia* species are maintained in nature predominantly by horizontal tick to mammal to tick transmission because the organisms do not invade the female tick ovary and do not appear in larvae from infected females. The major reservoir host for *E. chaffeensis* is the white-tailed deer *(Odocoileus virginianus),* which is found abundantly in many parts of the United States. The major reservoir for the *E. phagocytophila* group in the eastern United States appears to be the white-footed mouse, *Peromyscus leucopus,* but white-tailed deer or domestic ruminants may also play a role. This suggests that efficient transmission requires persistent infection of mammalian hosts, a situation long recognized in dogs infected with *E. canis,* goats with *E. phagocytophila,* and other hosts of various ehrlichial species. However, while *E. chaffeensis* and *E. phagocytophila* group may cause persistent infections in animals, these appear to be very infrequent in humans.

PATHOGENESIS. Although patients with human monocytic and granulocytic ehrlichiosis often present with an illness that appears similar to the vasculotropic rickettsioses, the pathogenesis is clearly different because endothelial cell infection and vasculitis are rare in the ehrlichioses. The exact pathogenetic mechanisms are poorly understood, but the end result appears to be a diffuse proliferation of mononuclear phagocytes leading to granuloma formation (HME) or histiocytic infiltrates and activation of the mononuclear phagocyte system with consumption of platelets and leukocytes (HME and HGE). This activation results in moderate to profound leukopenia and thrombocytopenia in the presence of a hypercellular reactive bone marrow, and fatalities are often associated with severe hemorrhage or secondary opportunistic infections. Hepatic or other organ-specific injury occurs by an unknown mechanism that is apparently unrelated to direct infection. An unexplained observation in severe HME and HGE is the occurrence of diffuse alveolar damage that results in the clinical picture of adult respiratory distress syndrome (ARDS), which also appears not to be closely related to direct ehrlichial infection. Lymphohistiocytic meningitis with a mononuclear cell cerebrospinal fluid pleocytosis may be present in HME.

Pathologic findings include diffuse but mild perivascular lymphohistiocytic infiltrates, infrequent hepatocyte apoptoses, Kupffer cell hyperplasia, mild lobular hepatitis, increases in mononuclear phagocyte infiltrates in the spleen, lymph nodes, and bone marrow in which occasional erythrophagocytic cells are present, granulomas of the liver and bone marrow in patients with *E. chaffeensis* infections, and hyperplasia of one or more bone marrow hematopoietic lineages.

CLINICAL MANIFESTATIONS. HME and HGE are distinct clinical entities caused by infection with different *Ehrlichia* species that result in similar illnesses. Many well-defined cases of pediatric infection of variable severity, including a fatality, have been reported. The incubation period after the last preceding tick bite or tick exposure ranges from 2 days to 3 wk, and no tick bite is documented in nearly one fourth of all patients. The disease usually presents with nonspecific findings including fever and headache. The majority of patients also describe myalgias, anorexia, and nausea or vomiting. Unlike adult patients, nearly two thirds of children with HME present with a rash. The rash is usually described as macular or maculopapular, although petechial lesions may occur. Photophobia and conjunctivitis also may occur, and pharyngitis and lymphadenopathy are seen in a minority of patients.

Hepatomegaly and splenomegaly are frequent physical findings. Meningoencephalitis with a mononuclear cell-predominant cerebrospinal fluid pleocytosis is infrequently encountered but can be a severe complication. The presence of arthritis or arthralgias may suggest Lyme borreliosis or meningococcemia, but this presentation appears to be infrequent. Edema of the face, hands, and feet may contribute to diagnostic uncertainty.

The illness ordinarily lasts 4–12 days, and in most published cases hospitalization was required. Well-documented seroconversions in the absence of overt clinical manifestations strongly suggest the occurrence of mild or subclinical infections. Clinically evident infections of children with granulocytic *Ehrlichia* are infrequent; however, the clinical presentation of this illness in adults is very similar to that of adult *E. chaffeensis* infection.

DIAGNOSIS. As for Rocky Mountain spotted fever, a delay in diagnosis or treatment of ehrlichiosis may contribute to increased morbidity or mortality; thus, an early clinical diagnosis is important. Since both HME and HGE have been associated with a fatal outcome, therapy should not be withheld while awaiting confirmatory laboratory test results.

The first patient and several subsequent pediatric patients with *E. chaffeensis* infection were identified presumptively on the basis of typical *Ehrlichia* morulae in peripheral blood leukocytes (Fig. 228–1*A*). This finding has been too infrequent to be considered a useful diagnostic tool. In contrast, granulocytic ehrlichiosis presents with a small but significant percentage (1–40%) of circulating neutrophils (Fig. 228–1*B*) containing typical *Ehrlichia* morulae in 20–60% of patients. The distinction between the two infections relies on polymerase chain reaction (PCR) amplification of species-specific DNA sequences or on the demonstration of specific *E. chaffeensis* or *E. phagocytophila* group antigen serology.

The current diagnostic criteria for *E. chaffeensis* infection include a seroconversion with a titer of ≥1:64, or a single serum titer (usually convalescent serum) of ≥1:128, in the context of a clinically compatible illness. Similarly, granulocytic ehrlichiosis may be confirmed by a seroconversion or single high

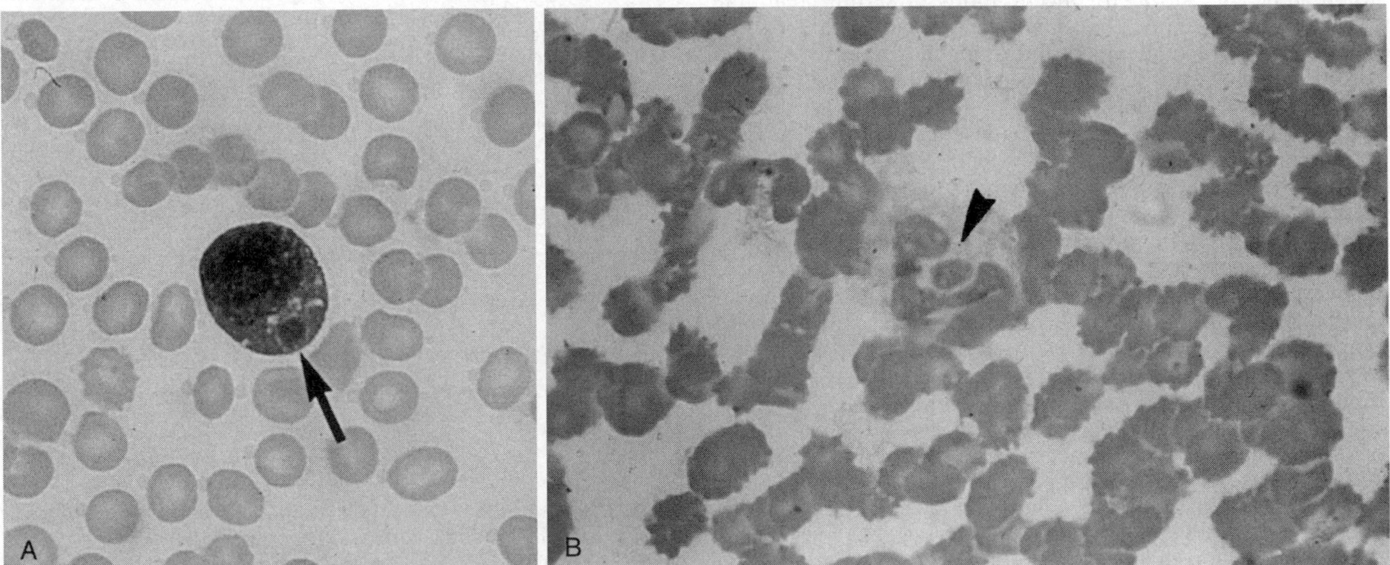

Figure 228–1 *Ehrlichia* morulae in a peripheral blood leukocyte. *A,* A morula *(arrow)* containing *Ehrlichia chaffeensis* in a monocyte. *B,* A morula *(arrowhead)* containing *Ehrlichia phagocytophila* group in a neutrophil. (Wright stains, original magnifications ×1,200). *Ehrlichia chaffeensis* and the human granulocytic ehrlichia have similar morphologies but are serologically and genetically distinct. See also color section.

titer of *E. phagocytophila* group antibodies; some laboratories refer to the causative agent as the HGE agent or *E. equi*. Patients with granulocytic ehrlichiosis experience serologic reactions to *E. chaffeensis* in up to 15% of cases, and thus serodiagnosis of monocytic or granulocytic ehrlichiosis depends on testing with both *E. chaffeensis* and *E. phagocytophila* group antigens. During the acute phase of illness when antibodies may not be detected, PCR amplification of specific *E. chaffeensis* or *E. phagocytophila* group DNA sequences is sensitive in 86% of cases. Immunocytologic and immunohistologic methods have been successfully applied in patients in whom morulae were suspected in peripheral blood or cerebrospinal fluid.

Ehrlichia have been cultivated in tissue culture. Culture for *E. chaffeensis* may take up to 1 month, while culture for the HGE agent is usually more rapid.

Differential Diagnosis. Because of the nonspecific presentation, ehrlichiosis may be mimicked by other arthropod-borne infections such as Rocky Mountain spotted fever, tularemia, babesiosis, Lyme disease, murine typhus, relapsing fever, and Colorado tick fever. When rash and a disseminated intravascular coagulation (DIC)–like clinical picture predominate, meningococcemia, bacterial sepsis, and toxic shock syndrome may be suspected. Other potential diagnoses considered include otitis media, streptococcal pharyngitis, infectious mononucleosis, Kawasaki disease, endocarditis, viral syndromes, hepatitis, leptospirosis, Q fever, collagen-vascular diseases, and leukemia. Meningoencephalitis may suggest enterovirus or herpes simplex virus infections, bacterial meningitis, or Rocky Mountain spotted fever, while severe respiratory disease may be confused with bacterial, viral, or fungal pneumonitis.

Laboratory Findings. Characteristically, most children with monocytic ehrlichiosis present with leukopenia (72%), lymphopenia (78%), or thrombocytopenia (80%). Leukocytosis may also occur. Despite the presence of pancytopenia, examination usually reveals a cellular or reactive bone marrow in adults. Interestingly, granulomas and granulomatous inflammation are identified in nearly 75% of bone marrow specimens examined from patients with proven cases of *E. chaffeensis* infection, but this finding is not present in patients with HGE. Mild to severe hepatic injury is documented by the frequent (83%) finding of elevated serum aspartate aminotransferase levels. Hyponatremia is present in a minority of cases. Although not yet documented in children, severely affected adults may experience varying degrees of renal failure accompanied by elevated concentrations of serum creatinine and urea nitrogen. A clinical picture similar to that of DIC with prolonged activated partial thromboplastin time and prothrombin time and hypofibrinogenemia has been demonstrated in several patients.

TREATMENT. Both HME and HGE are effectively treated with tetracyclines, and the majority of patients usually improve rapidly (within 48 hr). A comprehensive retrospective evaluation of all patients with HME showed a significantly shorter interval of fever and hospitalization among patients treated with tetracycline or chloramphenicol. However, spontaneous recovery without antimicrobial therapy as well as treatment failures with chloramphenicol in patients who responded to tetracyclines are well recognized. Moreover, in vitro tests document that both *E. chaffeensis* and the HGE agent have minimal inhibitory concentrations above safely achieved chloramphenicol blood levels. Because of these findings, a short course of doxycycline or tetracycline is the recommended regimen. Tetracyclines can be used safely in children <8 yr of age since tooth discoloration is dose-dependent, and the need for multiple courses is unlikely in children <8 yr of age. Doxycycline is recommended for children because the risk of dental staining is less than with other tetracyclines.

The recommended treatment regimen for patients with severe or complicated HME and HGE infections is doxycycline orally or intravenously (two loading doses of 2.2 mg/kg/dose at 12-hr intervals followed by 2.2 mg/kg/24 hr divided in two doses every 12 hr; maximum: 300 mg/dose). The loading doses may be omitted in patients with less severe disease. An alternative regimen is tetracycline orally (25–50 mg/kg/24 hr divided in four doses; maximum: 2 g/24 hr). Therapy should be continued for a minimum of 5 days and until the patient has been afebrile for at least 2–4 days.

Other broad-spectrum antibiotics including penicillins, cephalosporins, aminoglycosides, and macrolides are not effective. The HGE agent is not susceptible to azithromycin, but in vitro studies suggest a potential role for rifamycin in HME and HGE. The new quinolone trovafloxacin has a very low minimal inhibitory concentration for the HGE agent in vitro.

COMPLICATIONS. Fatal monocytic ehrlichiosis has been reported in only one pediatric patient to date. In this patient ehrlichiosis was initially dominated by pulmonary involvement with respiratory failure that was complicated by subsequent nosocomial bacterial pneumonia. The pattern of severe pulmonary involvement culminating in diffuse alveolar damage and ARDS and secondary nosocomial or opportunistic infections is now well documented with HME and HGE in adults. Other severe complications include a toxic shock–like illness, meningoencephalitis with long-term neurologic sequelae, myocarditis, rhabdomyolysis, and brachial plexopathy. Patients with underlying immune compromise (HIV infection, high-dose corticosteroid therapy, cancer chemotherapy, or organ transplantation) are at high risk for fulminant infection.

PREVENTION. Because both HME and HGE are tick-borne diseases, any activity that allows exposure to the appropriate tick vectors must be considered risky. Avoidance of tick-infested areas, the use of appropriate light-colored clothing and tick repellents sprayed on clothing, careful inspection for ticks after exposure, and prompt removal of any attached ticks diminish the risk of acquisition of either HME or HGE. During the approximately 48 hr interval after attachment when the tick is still flat, transmission of the infectious agents can be interrupted by simply removing the tick. After 48 hr, or if the tick is engorged, the risk of development of infection is increased. The role of prophylactic therapy for HME and HGE after tick bites has not been investigated.

Bakken JS, Krueth J, Wilson-Nordskog C, et al: Clinical and laboratory characteristics of human granulocytic ehrlichiosis. *JAMA* 275:199, 1996.

Edwards ME: Ehrlichiosis in children. Semin Pediatr Infect Dis 5:143, 1994.

Everett ED, Evans KA, Henry RB, et al: Human ehrlichiosis in adults after tick exposure: Diagnosis using polymerase chain reaction. Ann Intern Med 120:730, 1994.

Fishbein DB, Dawson JE, Robinson LE: Human ehrlichiosis in the United States, 1985 to 1990. Ann Intern Med 120:736, 1994.

Horowitz HW, Kilchevsky E, Haber S, et al: Perinatal transmission of the agent of human granulocytic ehrlichiosis. N Engl J Med 339:375, 1998.

Schutze GE, Jacobs RF: Human monocytic ehrlichiosis in children. Pediatrics 100(1)E10, 1997.

CHAPTER 229

Q Fever (Coxiella burnetii)

J. Stephen Dumler

Q fever (for "query" fever) is a febrile disease, often with no rash, that presents in acute and chronic forms.

ETIOLOGY. The causative organism of Q fever, *Coxiella burnetii*, is genetically distinct from members of the genera *Rickettsia* and *Ehrlichia* and is more closely related to *Legionella pneumophila* and the arthropod symbiont *Francisella* (formerly *Wolbachia*) *persica*. *C. burnetii* is highly infectious for humans and animals; even a single organism can cause infection. The organism, unlike *Rickettsia*, is highly resistant to chemical and physical treatments.

C. burnetii resides intracellularly within phagolysosomes. Unlike *Ehrlichia*, *C. burnetii* tolerates and actively proliferates within the acidified phagolysosome to form aggregates that often contain in excess of 100 bacteria. *C. burnetii* organisms undergo a lipopolysaccharide "phase variation" similar to that described for smooth and rough strains of Enterobacteriaceae.

EPIDEMIOLOGY. The disease is reported worldwide. The relative risk of disease is correlated with increasing age, so that infected children are identified infrequently.

Serologic surveys in the United States and elsewhere indicate that many more cases of Q fever occur each year than are recognized. This is not surprising because acute Q fever is nonspecific, specialized laboratory diagnostic tests are required, and it is not currently a notifiable disease in many states. *C. burnetii* may be the cause of 0.5–3% of serologically investigated acute respiratory illnesses or hepatitides in some areas of the United States. In Japan, *C. burnetii* is implicated as a cause of atypical pneumonia in 40% of pediatric patients. Immune compromise secondary to cancer therapies, acquired immunodeficiency syndrome (AIDS), organ transplantation, hemodialysis, alcoholic liver disease, chronic granulomatous disease, or underlying cardiac valve or vascular damage or prostheses is identified as an underlying factor in more than 20% of patients with acute or chronic Q fever.

Transmission. In contrast to other rickettsial infections, humans acquire *C. burnetii* predominantly after inhalation of infectious aerosols; arthropod vectors are rarely implicated in transmission. Domestic livestock (cattle, sheep, and goats), parturient cats, wild animals such as rabbits, and rarely ticks serve as reservoirs. The usual mode of transmission is via aerosols from dust, straw, cloth contaminated with organisms from birth tissues, or processing of animal products (in abattoirs, hides, wool), or by ingestion of contaminated raw dairy products (fresh cheese or unpasteurized milk). In Nova Scotia and Maine, exposure to newborn animals (chiefly kittens) has been associated with small outbreaks of Q fever in family settings. In Europe and Australia, exposure to domestic ruminants is the major risk; however, many urban dwellers in France, who presumably lack significant exposure to farm animals, acquire Q fever. Human placental infection is sometimes associated with intrauterine growth retardation or death and may result from primary or reactivation of maternal infection. Obstetric health care workers are at risk for acquiring infection because of the quantity of *C. burnetii* released from infected products of conception.

PATHOGENESIS. After inhalation of infectious aerosols, pulmonary infection elicits a mild interstitial lymphocytic pneumonitis with a dense macrophage-rich intra-alveolar exudate that is heavily infected with *C. burnetii*. The infection may elicit granulomas in liver, bone marrow, and other organs, all signs of an acute and usually self-limited infection. Chronic Q fever endocarditis is characterized by macrophage and lymphocyte-rich infiltrates in necrotic fibrinous valvular vegetations and by the absence of granulomas.

As with many other obligate intracellular pathogens, recovery from acute infection may result in nonsterile immunity. It is likely that development of debilitating chronic Q fever results after recovery from a mild or inapparent episode of acute Q fever during which the agent is not cleared. The persistence of *C. burnetii* in tissue macrophages at sites of pre-existing tissue damage causes a low-grade smoldering inflammation, which eventually leads to irreversible cardiac valve damage or persistent vascular injury.

CLINICAL MANIFESTATIONS. Two forms of Q fever occur. The most frequent is acute Q fever, a self-limited form that is usually associated with an influenza-like illness, interstitial pneumonitis, or granulomatous hepatitis. Chronic Q fever results from low-level, persistent infection and smoldering inflammation, usually of the heart valves; it is diagnosed clinically as culture-negative endocarditis and often results in death.

Acute Q fever. Acute Q fever develops about 3 wk (range, 14–39 days) after exposure to the causative agent. The severity of illness in children ranges from subclinical infection to a febrile systemic illness characterized by severe frontal headache, arthralgia, and myalgia, often accompanied by respiratory symptoms. Fewer than half of patients have cough or pneumonia. Most pediatric patients present with fever of unknown origin. In adults, the pneumonia usually resembles primary atypical or viral pneumonitis or legionnaires' disease with a nonproductive cough. Other prominent clinical findings that may lead to diagnostic confusion include fatigue, vomiting, abdominal pain, and meningismus. Hepatomegaly and splenomegaly may be detected in some patients.

In a review of 170 adult French patients with acute Q fever, 81.8% had fever, 62% had elevated serum hepatic transaminase levels, 46% had respiratory involvement, 18% had cutaneous findings, and 11% had neurologic findings that required lumbar puncture for evaluation. Nearly 20% of these patients were afebrile and presented with one or more hepatic, pulmonic, cutaneous, or neurologic findings. Other series of patients indicate that pulmonary involvement is the most frequent manifestation.

Laboratory findings in acute Q fever are usually normal but may reveal leukopenia with a left shift (>5%) in 50% of patients and thrombocytopenia, which is infrequent. Most children have elevated serum hepatic aminotransferase levels that spontaneously return to normal after 20–30 days. The pulmonary consolidations on radiographs become round and resolve slowly.

In children, acute Q fever is usually a self-limited illness that lasts 2–3 wk. However, severe infections including acute encephalopathy with impairment of consciousness and an abnormal pattern on electroencephalogram and computed tomographic scans of the brain have been reported.

Chronic Q fever. The risk of development of chronic Q fever is strongly correlated with advancing age; thus, children are infrequently diagnosed with chronic Q fever. Chronic Q fever endocarditis has not been diagnosed in a child. Chronic Q fever tends to be resistent to therapy and often (23–65%) results in death. Endocarditis, which usually develops on damaged or prosthetic valves, may occur months to years after acute Q fever or in the absence of any history of acute Q fever. Less frequently, chronic Q fever may present as an infection of vascular prostheses and aneurysms, osteomyelitis, myocarditis, undifferentiated fever, pneumonia, and hepatitis or as an isolated purpuric rash. The clinical presentation in children is similar to that in adults. In Q fever endocarditis, fever may be absent in up to 15% of cases, and more than 75% of all identified patients have congestive heart failure. Other frequently observed features include marked clubbing of the fingers, hepatomegaly, and splenomegaly.

Frequent laboratory abnormalities in patients with chronic Q fever include erythrocyte sedimentation rate >20 mm/hr (80% of cases), hypergammaglobulinemia (54%), and hyperfibrinogenemia (67%). The presence of rheumatoid factor in >50% of cases and circulating immune complexes in nearly 90%, plus the frequent findings of antiplatelet antibodies, anti-smooth muscle antibodies, antimitochondrial antibodies, circulating anticoagulants, and positive direct Coombs' test results may suggest an autoimmune process. A variety of other clinical syndromes have been associated with Q fever, including meningoencephalitis, inflammatory pseudotumor of the lung, glomerulonephritis, immune complex vasculitis, hemolytic anemia, and autoimmune disorders.

DIAGNOSIS. Although it is infrequently diagnosed, Q fever should be considered in children with fever of unknown origin or culture-negative endocarditis who live in rural areas or who are in close contact with domestic livestock, cats, or their products.

Q fever is most easily diagnosed serologically. The diagnosis of Q fever can be confirmed serologically in acute and convalescent sera (2–4 wk apart), which show a fourfold increase in indirect fluorescent antibody titers to phase I and phase II antigens or a fourfold increase in complement fixation antibody titers. The inability of the complement fixation test to discriminate between recent and remote infection diminishes its usefulness when acute phase sera are not available. Elevated or rising titers of phase II antibody alone are characteristic of acute Q fever, and the appearance and persistence of elevated titers of phase I and phase II antibody are indicative of chronic Q fever. Elevated titers of phase I immunoglobulin (Ig) A antibody are reported to be diagnostic for Q fever endocarditis; however, one evaluation showed that a phase II IgG titer of $\geq$1:200 is indicative of *C. burnetii* infection and that a phase I IgG titer of $<$1:800 is inconsistent with chronic Q fever.

C. burnetii has been cultivated in tissue culture cells, which may become positive within 48 hr, but isolation and antimicrobial susceptibility testing of *C. burnetii* should be attempted only in specialized biohazard facilities.

Differential Diagnosis. The differential diagnosis depends on the clinical presentation. For respiratory disease, *Mycoplasma* pneumonia, legionellosis, psittacosis, and Epstein-Barr virus infection should be considered. For granulomatous hepatitis, mycobacterial infections, salmonellosis, visceral leishmaniasis, toxoplasmosis, Hodgkin's disease, ehrlichiosis, brucellosis, or autoimmune disorders including sarcoidosis should be considered. Culture-negative endocarditis also suggests infection with *Brucella* species or *Bartonella* species, or nonbacterial endocarditis.

TREATMENT. Most pediatric patients with Q fever experience a self-limited illness that is identified only on retrospective serologic evaluation. However, to prevent potential complications, patients with acute Q fever should be treated within 3 days of onset of symptoms with tetracycline (25–50 mg/kg/24 hr divided in four doses) or doxycycline (2.2 mg/kg/24 hr divided in two doses). Later therapy has little effect on the course of the acute infection. Because early laboratory confirmation is not currently available, empirical therapy is warranted in clinically suspected cases. The quinolones ofloxacin and pefloxacin have proved effective, and success with a combination of pefloxacin and rifampin has also been achieved with prolonged (16–21 days) therapy. The efficacy of erythromycin is controversial. Most β-lactams are ineffective; however, individual reports document success with a wide variety of agents including chloramphenicol, trimethoprim-sulfamethoxazole, and ceftriaxone. In anecdotal cases of hepatitis associated with "autoimmune" laboratory findings, prednisone was reported to provide additional clinical benefit.

For chronic Q fever, especially endocarditis, prolonged therapy is mandatory. This usually requires prolonged use of the rickettsiostatic drugs tetracycline or doxycycline in combination with rickettsicidal drugs such as rifampin, ofloxacin, or pefloxacin. The use of lysosomotropic alkalinizing agents such as chloroquine may aid in maintaining the activity of pH-sensitive antimicrobial agents in the phagolysosomal environment of *C. burnetii*. For patients with heart failure, valve replacement may be warranted and should be accompanied by an effective antibiotic regimen to avoid reinfection of the prosthetic valves. Therapy should be monitored by periodic serologic evaluation; phase I titers of less than 200 for IgG and an absent IgA titer indicate cure. Even with such evaluation, cure of chronic Q fever in less than 2 yr is unlikely, and thus therapy should be continued for at least 3 yr.

PREVENTION. Recognition of the disease in livestock should alert communities to the risk of human infection. Milk from infected herds must be pasteurized at temperatures sufficient to destroy *C. burnetii*. In contrast to *Rickettsia*, *C. burnetii* is resistant to significant environmental conditions but may be inactivated with a solution of 1% Lysol, 1% formaldehyde, or 5% hydrogen peroxide. Special isolation measures are not required because person-to-person transmission is rare except during exposure to infected products of conception.

Ruiz-Contreras J, Montero RG, Amador JTR, et al: Q fever in children. Am J Dis Child 146:300, 1993.

Richardus JH, Dumas AM, Huisman J, et al: Q fever in infancy: A review of 18 cases. Pediatr Infect Dis 4:369, 1985.

Sawyer LA, Fishbein DB, McDade JE: Q fever: Current concepts. Rev Infect Dis 9:935, 1987.

Tissot-DuPont H, Raoult D, Brouqui P, et al: Epidemiologic features and clinical presentation of acute Q fever in hospitalized patients: 323 French cases. Am J Med 93:427, 1992.

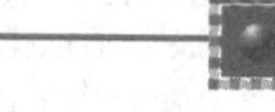

SECTION 11

Mycotic Infections

CHAPTER 230
Candida

Martin Weisse and Stephen C. Aronoff

Candidiasis is caused by several species of the genus *Candida*. The former genus name was *Monilia*, and the term moniliasis is still used occasionally to describe skin or mucous membrane infection. *Candida* exists in three morphologic forms: oval to round blastospores or yeast cells (3–6 mm in diameter); double-walled chlamydospores (7–17 mm in diameter) usually at the terminal end of a pseudohyphae; and pseudomycelium, which is a mass of pseudohyphae and represents the tissue phase of *Candida*. Pseudohyphae are filamentous processes that elongate from the yeast cell. Candida grows aerobically on routine laboratory media but may require several days for incubation.

C. albicans accounts for most human infections, but *C. parapsilosis, C. tropicalis, C. krusei, C. lusitaniae, C. glabrata* (formerly *Torulopsis glabrata*) and several other species have been reported as pathogens with increasing frequency. Because *C. albicans* is the most frequently isolated pathogen, a rapid germ tube test should be performed before further identification tests are ordered. *C. albicans* is the only species that forms a germ tube when suspended in rabbit or human serum and incubated for 1–2 hr. The other clinically important species can be identified within 48 hr on the basis of biochemical test results.

Treatment of invasive *Candida* infections has become complicated with the emergence of these non-*albicans* strains. Amphotericin is inactive against approximately 20% of strains of *C. lusitaniae*. Fluconazole may be useful for selected *Candida* infections but is inactive against all strains of *C. krusei* and approximately 20% of strains of *C. glabrata*. These species are usually susceptible to ketoconazole and itraconazole, but cross resistance to other azoles does occur. Susceptibility testing of these clinical isolates is recommended.

230.1 *Neonatal Infections*

Candida species are a common cause of oral mucous membrane infections (thrush) and perineal skin infections (diaper dermatitis) in newborn infants. With the improved survival of very low birthweight infants, disseminated *Candida* infections have become more frequent in special care nurseries; the incidence can be as high as 5% in very low birthweight infants.

EPIDEMIOLOGY. *C. albicans* is commonly isolated from the gastrointestinal and vaginal flora of adults. Pregnancy increases the rate of vaginal colonization from <20% to >30%. In approximately 10% of term infants the gastrointestinal and respiratory tracts are colonized in the first 5 days of life; the colonization rate in infants weighing <1,500 g approaches 30%. Skin colonization is common after 2 wk of age.

Systemic candidiasis is predominantly an infection of very low birthweight infants, in whom the attack rate is estimated to be 2–5%. Risk factors in neonates of any gestational age include abdominal surgery, prolonged ventilatory support, prolonged intravenous catheterization, use of intravenous alimentation, and especially broad-spectrum antibiotic administration.

PATHOGENESIS. Overgrowth of *Candida* on mucocutaneous surfaces and colonization of intravenous catheter tips favor entry and penetration; clinical infection is related to inoculum size. The inability of the newborn infant to localize, control, and eradicate *Candida* infections appears to be related to the relative impairment of specific and nonspecific host defense mechanisms. Hematogenous spread leads to vasculitis and miliary nodules in many organs. The lungs, kidneys, gastrointestinal tract, heart, eyes, and meninges are commonly involved.

CLINICAL MANIFESTATIONS. Neonates may develop thrush and candidal diaper dermatitis (see Section 230.2, Infections in the Normal Host).

The manifestations of systemic infection vary in acuteness and severity. Fungemia may be asymptomatic or may be associated with sepsis and shock. *Candida* causes significant disseminated disease in 2–5% of premature infants weighing <1,500 g. Risk factors associated with candidal sepsis include prolonged antibiotic therapy, prolonged use of intravascular catheters, intravenous hyperalimentation, and poor nutrition. The presentation of disseminated candidiasis mimics that of bacterial sepsis, with respiratory distress, apnea, bradycardia, temperature instability, glucose intolerance, and abdominal signs or symptoms.

Cutaneous evidence of *Candida* infection may be seen in as many as half of these patients and manifests as a diffuse erythroderma or vesiculopustules from which the organism can be cultured. Renal involvement is found in >50% of patients and may be subclinical with persistent candiduria or may become manifest with a flank mass, hypertension, renal failure, renal abscesses, papillary necrosis, or fungal balls in the collecting system resulting in obstruction and hydronephrosis. Ultrasonography is most useful in evaluating patients with urinary tract involvement. Ultrasonography or computed tomography may also be helpful in identifying foci in the liver and spleen.

Central nervous system involvement occurs in as many as one third of cases and may involve the meninges, ventricles, or cerebral cortex with abscess formation. Clinical manifestations of central nervous system disease may be inapparent, mandating evaluation of the cerebrospinal fluid in all patients with disseminated candidiasis regardless of central nervous system signs or symptoms. Because endophthalmitis is seen in 20–50% of cases, retinal examinations should be performed in neonates with systemic candidiasis; repeat examinations are necessary to monitor resolution of the retinal lesions. Endophthalmitis begins as chorioretinitis and may extend to the vitreous. Cotton ball exudates are typical of *Candida* retinal pathologic conditions. Osteoarthritis is a complication in 20% of cases.

Vascular disease ranges from vasculitis of the aorta or vena cava to endocarditis. Infected thrombi in vessels and the right atrium are not uncommon. Candidal endocarditis is an infrequent complication but should be considered in patients with central venous catheters that extend into the atrium as well as in those with persistent candidemia. Pneumonia occurs in as many as 70% of patients with disseminated candidemia on the basis of autopsy studies, although some patients do not have radiographic evidence of pneumonia on initial evaluation. Cultures from the endotracheal tube are not predictive of pulmonary involvement.

Congenital Candidiasis. Congenital candidiasis, which is rare, occurs in otherwise normal neonates and presents at birth as widespread skin involvement, especially in the intertriginous areas. The pathogenesis of congenital candidiasis is ascending infection from a mother with heavy colonization or vulvar infection with *Candida*. The newborn rash is maculopapular; *Candida* may be recovered from some vesicles and pustules. There is usually little or no mucous membrane involvement. Topical antifungal therapy is usually all that is necessary unless the neonate shows evidence of systemic infection. Preterm infants more frequently have systemic disease characterized by pneumonia, leukocytosis, and shock, which are associated with a high mortality rate.

DIAGNOSIS. Isolation of fungi from cultures of normally sterile body fluids is the basis for diagnosis of invasive candidiasis. Buffy coat smears of blood may show yeast, allowing a preliminary diagnosis. Skin scrapings of generalized rashes in very low birthweight infants with suspected systemic candidiasis should be examined microscopically for yeast. Because cultures of blood and cerebrospinal fluid are often intermittently positive, multiple samples should be obtained. Cerebrospinal fluid cultures are positive in one third of infants with systemic infection. Cultures should be taken from peripheral veins to differentiate true positive cultures from contaminated catheters. Urine specimens for culture must also be obtained by catheterization or suprapubic tap to differentiate perineal colonization. Transient candidemia and disseminated candidiasis may be associated with a contaminated intravascular catheter, which must be removed.

Ultrasonography is useful for localization of *Candida* infection in the cardiovascular, renal, and central nervous systems. Radiographs of the chest may reveal pneumonia.

TREATMENT. Amphotericin B (0.5–1.0 mg/kg/24 hr intravenously) is the drug of choice for systemic candidiasis and is active against both yeast and mycelial forms. The duration of therapy varies widely according to the extent of infection, clinical response, and drug toxicity. The total recommended dose is 20–30 mg/kg. Nephrotoxicity is common in the newborn infant and generally presents with oliguria, azotemia, and hyperkalemia. Liposomal amphotericin B (5 mg/kg/24 hr) is associated with less renal toxicity and is indicated in neonates with significant renal compromise or in whom desoxycholate amphotericin causes creatinine levels to double. In addition to amphotericin, flucytosine (100–150 mg/kg/24 hr divided every 6 hr orally) is recommended for the treatment of central nervous system and parenchymal kidney infections. Patients must be observed for bone marrow, gastrointestinal, and hepatic toxicities.

Fluconazole may be useful for selected *Candida* infections but is inactive against all strains of *C. krusei* and approximately 20% of strains of *C. glabrata*. These are usually susceptible to ketoconazole and itraconazole, but cross resistance to other azoles does occur. The susceptibility of these clinical isolates should be tested if treatment with azoles is contemplated.

Vascular catheters associated with transient fungemia or disseminated infection should be removed, and the patient should then be treated with amphotericin B for 2–3 wk. Infected intracardiac and intravascular thrombi usually must be resected, but resolution without surgery has been described.

230.2 Infections in Immunocompetent Children and Adolescents

ORAL CANDIDIASIS. Oral thrush, or oral pseudomembranous candidiasis, is a superficial mucous membrane infection that affects approximately 2–5% of normal newborns. Infants acquire *Candida* from their mothers at delivery and remain colonized. Thrush may develop as early as 7–10 days of age. The use of antibiotics, especially in the first year of life, may lead to recurrent or persistent thrush. The plaques of thrush invade the mucosa superficially and may be found on the lips, buccal mucosa, tongue, and palate. Removal of plaques from these surfaces may cause mild punctate areas of bleeding, which helps to confirm the diagnosis. Thrush may be asymptomatic or may cause pain, fussiness, and decreased feeding. It is uncommon after 12 mo of age but may occur in children treated with oral antibiotics. Persistent or recurrent thrush with no obvious predisposing reason, such as recent antibiotic treatment, warrants investigation of an underlying condition such as diabetes mellitus or immunodeficiency, especially vertically transmitted human immunodeficiency virus (HIV) infection.

Treatment of mild cases may not be necessary. When treatment is warranted, the most commonly prescribed antifungal agent is nystatin. Many other treatments are also effective including (in decreasing order of efficacy) miconazole gel, amphotericin B suspension, gentian violet, and nystatin suspension. Clotrimazole troches may also be effective, although clinical studies of such treatment are lacking. Miconazole gel is currently unavailable in the United States.

DIAPER DERMATITIS. Diaper dermatitis is the most common infection caused by *Candida*. Primary infection generally occurs in the intertriginous areas of the perineum and presents as a confluent papular erythema with red satellite papules. *Candida* diaper dermatitis often complicates oral antibiotic treatment of otitis media as well as other noninfectious diaper dermatitides. Many physicians presumptively treat any diaper rash that has been present for >3 days for *Candida*.

Treatment is usually performed with nystatin cream, powder, or ointment, clotrimazole 1% cream, miconazole 2% ointment, or amphotericin cream or ointment. If significant inflammation is present, the addition of hydrocortisone 1% may be useful for the first day or two. Combination drugs with topical corticosteroids, such as clotrimazole/triamcinolone, should be used cautiously or not at all in infants because the relatively potent topical corticosteroid may lead to unwanted local side effects. Frequent diaper changes and periods without diapers are important adjuncts to treatments.

Periungual Infections. Paronychia and onychomycosis may be due to *Candida*, although this agent is much less common than *Trichophyton* or *Epidermophyton* as a cause of periungual infection. Candidal onychomycosis differs from tinea infections by its propensity to affect the fingernails and not the toenails and by the associated paronychia. Candidal infections often respond to treatment that consists of keeping the hands dry and using a topical antifungal agent. A short course of systemic therapy with an oral azole antifungal drug may be necessary.

VULVOVAGINITIS. Vulvovaginitis is a common candidal infection of pubertal and postpubertal females that affects as many as 75% of females at one time or another (see Chapter 557). Predisposing factors include pregnancy, oral contraceptive use, poor hygiene, and use of oral antibiotics. Prepubertal girls with candidal vulvovaginitis usually have a predisposing factor such as diabetes mellitus or prolonged antibiotic treatment. Clinical manifestations may include pain or itching, dysuria, vulvar or vaginal erythema, an opaque white or cheesy exudate, and thrushlike mucosal plaques.

Candidal vulvovaginitis can be effectively treated with either vaginal creams or troches of nystatin, clotrimazole, or miconazole. Oral therapy with single-dose fluconazole has been found to be as effective as clotrimazole in women and may be useful in adolescent girls.

230.3 Infections in Immunocompromised Children and Adolescents

ETIOLOGY. Most cases of candidemia in immunocompromised patients are due to *C. albicans* (70–90%). Other species commonly involved include *C. tropicalis* (5–15%), *C. parapsilosis* (3–13%), *C. glabrata* (0–4%), *C. lusitaniae*, *C. krusei*, and *C. guilliermondii* (all <2%).

CLINCAL MANIFESTATIONS. *Candida* infections in immunocompromised patients vary from superficial mucocutaneous infections to life-threatening sepsis and shock.

HIV-Infected Children. Oral thrush and diaper dermatitis are the most common candidal infections in HIV-infected children, occurring in as many as 50–85% of patients. Infants with symptomatic HIV infection are more than twice as likely to have thrush, which is often much more extensive in these infants than in normal children. Besides oral candidiasis, three other clinical variants of candidal infection may be observed in HIV-infected children: *atrophic candidiasis*, which presents as a fiery erythema of the mucosa or loss of papilla of the tongue; *chronic hyperplastic candidiasis*, which presents with oral symmetric white plaques that cannot be rubbed away; and *angular cheilitis*, in which there is erythema and fissuring of the angles of the mouth. Topical therapy may be effective, but systemic treatment with fluconazole or itraconazole is usually necessary. Symptoms of dysphagia or poor oral intake may indicate that the infection has progressed to candidal esophagitis, necessitating systemic therapy with either itraconazole or fluconazole.

Candidal dermatitis and onychomycosis are also more common in HIV-infected children. These infections are generally more severe than they are in immunocompetent children and require more aggressive or prolonged topical, and sometimes oral, therapy.

Cancer and Transplant Patients. Fungal infections, especially *Candida* and *Aspergillus* infections, are a significant problem in oncology patients with chemotherapy-associated neutropenia (see Chapter 179). Although the greatest risk for these patients is from bacterial pathogens, the risk of candidemia increases dramatically after 5–7 days of neutropenia and fever. If fever persists for ≥5–7 days, amphotericin B is usually indicated because of the risk of systemic fungal infection. Fluconazole may be an acceptable alternative to amphotericin B for some patients in hospitals where drug-resistant *Candida* and *Aspergillus* species are uncommon.

Patients undergoing bone marrow transplantation have a much higher risk of fungal infection because of the dramatically increased duration of neutropenia. Prophylactic use of fluconazole has been shown to decrease the incidence of candidemia in bone marrow transplant patients but not in leukemia patients undergoing chemotherapy. An increased incidence of infection with *C. krusei*, which is resistant to fluconazole, has been noted. The use of granulocyte colony-stimulating factor affects the duration of neutropenia after chemotherapy and is associated with decreased risk for candidemia. When *Candida* infection occurs, the lung, spleen, kidney, and liver are involved in >50% of cases.

Patients undergoing solid organ transplantation are also at increased risk for superficial and invasive candidal infections. Studies in liver transplant patients demonstrate the utility of antifungal prophylaxis with either amphotericin B or fluconazole.

Catheter-Associated Infections. Central venous catheter infections occur most often in oncology patients but may affect any patient with a central catheter (see Chapter 180). Neutropenia, use of broad-spectrum antibiotics, and hyperalimentation are associated with increased risk of candidal central catheter infection. Recovery of *Candida* from the central catheter alone poses the same risk of disseminated infection as culture of the organism from both the central catheter and peripheral blood. Treatment requires removal of the catheter as well as a 2–3 wk course of amphotericin B (1 mg/kg/24 hr, to a total dose of 20 mg/kg).

DIAGNOSIS. Diagnosis may be presumptive in neutropenic patients with prolonged fever because positive blood cultures are seen only in a minority of patients who are later found to have disseminated infection. *Candida* grows readily on routine blood culture media; 90% or more of positive cultures are identified by 72 hr, and 97% or more are identified by 7 days. *Candida* recovered from urine or tracheal secretions may represent colonization or infection. It is important to remember that when *Candida* infects one organ system it is very likely that other organs are involved as well.

TREATMENT. Amphotericin B remains the treatment of choice for systemic candidal infections, alone or with the addition of flucytosine or fluconazole, which is especially useful for central nervous system infections and parenchymal kidney infections. In one study in adults, fluconazole was as effective as amphotericin B for disseminated candidal infections and had fewer adverse effects. Fluconazole may be useful for selected candidal infections but is not effective against *C. krusei* and many strains of *C. glabrata*. Amphotericin is inactive against approximately 20% of strains of *C. lusitaniae*; susceptibility testing should be performed for all strains. Liposomal amphotericin B (5 mg/kg/24 hr) may be useful in patients with compromised renal function if the creatinine level doubles while on amphotericin B or who otherwise cannot tolerate desoxycholate amphotericin B.

230.4 Chronic Mucocutaneous Candidiasis

Chronic mucocutaneous candidiasis is a heterogeneous group of immune disorders, all of which involve a primary defect of T-lymphocyte responsiveness to candidal antigen. Endocrinopathies (hypoparathyroidism, Addison's disease) and autoimmune disorders are associated with this disorder in some patients. Symptoms may begin in the first few months of life or as late as the second decade of life. The disorder is characterized by chronic and severe skin and mucous membrane infections with *Candida*. Systemic candidiasis is rarely a complication; occasionally other dermatophytes cause chronic infection as well. Topical antifungal therapy may provide limited improvement early in the course of the disease, but repeated courses of ketoconazole or fluconazole, or occasionally amphotericin B, are usually necessary. The infection usually responds temporarily to treatment but is not eradicated and recurs.

Baley JE: Neonatal candidiasis: The current challenge. Clin Perinatol 18:263, 1991.
Como KA, Dismukes WE: Oral azole drugs as systemic antifungal therapy. N Engl J Med 330:263, 1994.
Darouiche RO: Oropharyngeal and esophageal candidiasis in immunocompromised patients: Treatment issues. Clin Infect Dis 26:259, 1998.
Edwards JE, Filler SG: Current strategies for treating invasive candidiasis: Emphasis on infections in nonneutropenic patients. Clin Infect Dis 14(Suppl):S106, 1992.
Eppes SC, Troutman JL, Gutman LT: Outcome of treatment of candidemia in children whose central catheters were removed or retained. Pediatr Infect Dis J 8:99, 1989.
Hoppe JE: Treatment of oropharyngeal candidiasis and candidal diaper dermatitis in neonates and infants: Review and reappraisal. Pediatr Infect Dis J 16:885, 1997.
Hughes WT: Systemic candidiasis: A study of 109 fatal cases. Pediatr Infect Dis J 1:11, 1982.
Prose NS: Mucocutaneous disease in pediatric human immunodeficiency virus infection. Pediatr Clin North Am 38:977, 1991.
van den Anker JN, van Popele NML, Sauer PJJ: Antifungal agents in neonatal systemic candidiasis. Antimicrob Agents Chemother 39:1391, 1995.
Wong-Beringer A, Jacobs RA, Guglielmo BJ: Lipid formulations of amphotericin B: Clinical efficacy and toxicities. Clin Infect Dis 27:603, 1998.

CHAPTER 231
Cryptococcus neoformans

Stephen C. Aronoff

ETIOLOGY. Cryptococcosis is an invasive fungal disease caused by a monomorphic, encapsulated yeast. *Cryptococcus neoformans* var. *neoformans* is the most common etiologic agent worldwide and is the predominant pathogenic fungal infection among individuals infected with human immunodeficiency virus (HIV).

EPIDEMIOLOGY. *C. neoformans* var. *neoformans* predominates in temperate climates and is found in soil contaminated with avian droppings, on fruits and vegetables, and may be carried by cockroaches. *C. neoformans* var. *gatti* is found mostly in the tropics under flowering river red gum trees *(Eucalyptus camaldulensis)*. This species causes endemic disease in the tropics in non-HIV-infected individuals. *C. albidus* and *C. laurentii* are rare human pathogens.

Cryptococcosis is an unusual disease in immunocompetent persons and is rare in children. Pigeon breeders and laboratory personnel who work with *Cryptococcus* are at greatest risk. Seroprevalence studies of cryptococcal exposure show no evidence of exposure in young infants, but exposure occurs in <5% in children >5 yr of age and in 60% of adults. Cryptococcosis is also rare (<1%) among HIV-infected children but occurs in 5–10% of HIV-infected adults; higher rates of infection have been reported from less developed countries. Pediatric cases of cryptococcosis are evenly divided among immunocompetent and immunocompromised individuals.

PATHOGENESIS. In most cases *C. neoformans* is acquired by inhalation of fungal spores. Local inoculation rarely leads to cutaneous or ophthalmic infection. In most immunocompetent individuals, infection is limited to the lung. When the immune system fails to contain the infection, dissemination follows with potential involvement of the brain, meninges, skin, eyes, and skeletal system.

Pulmonary cryptococcosis produces granulomas that are often subpleural in location and contain yeast forms. Cystic cryptococcomas occur in the central nervous system (CNS) in 20% of non-HIV-infected patients with disseminated disease and may be found in the absence of overt meningitis. Granulomas and microabscesses containing yeast occur in patients with cutaneous and bony infection.

CLINICAL MANIFESTATIONS. Pneumonia. Pneumonia is the most common form of cryptococcosis. Asymptomatic pulmonary infections occur frequently, especially among pigeon breeders, bird fanciers, and laboratory workers. Asymptomatic carriage may occur in patients with underlying chronic lung disease. Progressive pulmonary disease is symptomatic and often precedes disseminated infection in the immunocompromised host. Fever, cough, pleuritic chest pain, and constitutional symptoms occur. Chest radiographs may demonstrate a poorly localized bronchopneumonia, nodular changes, or lobar consolidations; cavities and pleural effusions are rare.

Disseminated Infection. Disseminated infection follows primary pulmonary disease and is seen most often in immunocompromised individuals. HIV infection is the most common predisposing factor for disseminated cryptococcosis; other major predisposing conditions include acute lymphoblastic leukemia, allogeneic bone marrow transplantation, primary immunodeficiencies affecting both T- and B-cell lineages, immunosuppression for rheumatic disorders, and celiac disease.

Meningitis. Subacute or chronic meningitis is the most common clinical manifestation of disseminated cryptococcal infection. The clinical presentation is variable and prognostic. Good outcomes are associated with headache as the initial symptom; normal mental status; absence of a predisposing condition; normal cerebrospinal fluid (CSF) opening pressure; normal CSF glucose; CSF white cell count of <20 cells/μL; negative India ink stain; absence of extraneural infection by culture; and cryptococcal antigen titers in CSF and serum of <1:32. Overt symptoms of meningitis and HIV infection are predictors of a poor outcome. HIV-infected patients typically present with unexplained fevers, headache, and malaise; cryptococcal antigen titers in these individuals are often >1:1,024. Computed tomography of the brain identifies cryptococcomas in as many as 30% of patients with disseminated infection and no clinical signs of CNS involvement. The mortality rate for cryptococcal meningitis is 15–30%, with most deaths occurring within several weeks of diagnosis. The fatality rates are higher in HIV-infected individuals, who have relapse rates of >50%. Relapse is unusual in adequately treated, non-HIV-infected patients. Postinfectious sequelae are common and include hydrocephalus, changes in visual acuity, deafness, cranial nerve palsies, seizures, and ataxia.

Sepsis Syndrome. Sepsis syndrome is a rare manifestation of cryptococcosis and occurs almost exclusively in HIV-infected patients. Fever is followed by respiratory distress and multiorgan system disease. This syndrome is often fatal.

Cutaneous Infection. Cutaneous disease may accompany disseminated cryptococcosis or local infection. Early lesions are erythematous, may be single or multiple, and are variably indurated and tender. Lesions often become ulcerated with central necrosis and raised borders. Cutaneous cryptococcosis in HIV-infected patients may resemble molluscum contagiosum.

Skeletal Infection. Skeletal infection occurs in approximately 5% of individuals with disseminated infection but rarely in HIV-infected patients. The onset of symptoms is insidious and chronic. Bony involvement is typified by soft tissue swelling and tenderness, and arthritis is characterized by effusion, erythema, and pain on motion. Skeletal disease is unifocal in approximately 75% of cases. The vertebrae are the most common sites of infection followed by the tibia, ileum, rib, femur, and humerus. Concomitant bone and joint disease results from contiguous spread.

Ocular Infection. Chorioretinitis is rare, occurs primarily in adults, and is usually a manifestation of disseminated disease, although direct inoculation of the eye has been described. Eye infection is characterized by the acute loss of visual acuity, eye pain, visual floaters, and photophobia. On examination, choroiditis with or without retinitis is usually noted. Retinal and vitreal masses and anterior uveitis are seen less commonly. Because eye disease is often a manifestation of disseminated infection, the mortality rate is >20%. Only 15% of survivors recover full vision.

Lymph Nodes. Lymphonodular disease has been reported in two children, one of whom had an underlying immunodeficiency. Lymphonodular cryptococcosis is characterized by disseminated lymphadenopathy including thoracic and abdominal nodes, subcutaneous lesions, liver granulomas, and concomitant pulmonary disease.

DIAGNOSIS. Recovery of the fungus by culture or demonstration of the fungus in histologic sections of infected tissue is diagnostically definitive. A latex agglutination test, which detects cryptococcal antigen in serum and CSF, is the most useful diagnostic test. India ink preparations of CSF are useful prognostically but are less sensitive than culture and antigen detection. Skin test antigens are poorly characterized, and the sensitivity and specificity of this test are unknown.

TREATMENT. The immunocompetent host with asymptomatic or mild disease limited to the lungs may be closely observed without therapy or, alternatively, treated with oral fluconazole (200–400 mg/24 hr) for 3–6 mo. Immunocompetent hosts with progressive pulmonary disease or non-HIV-infected immunosuppressed patients with disease limited to the lungs can be treated with amphotericin B (15 mg/kg to a maximum of 1.5 g total dose) alone or in combination with flucytosine.

Combination therapy using amphotericin B and flucytosine is recommended for the treatment of CNS and other manifestations of disseminated infection in non-HIV-infected individuals. The total dosage of amphotericin B should exceed 15 mg/kg. Flucytosine (50–150 mg/kg/24 hr) is administered concurrently, and the dosage should be adjusted to maintain serum concentrations between 50 and 150 μg/mL. Effectiveness of therapy is monitored by serial cryptococcal antigen testing; serum or CSF values of ≥1:8 are predictive of relapse. Ventriculoperitoneal shunts may be required for patients with hydrocephalus, and aggressive medical management of increased intracranial pressure may also be required.

Because of the high rate of relapse, CNS or disseminated cryptococcal infections in HIV-infected patients require induction and maintenance therapy. Several induction therapies have been described, but data from comparative trials are still forthcoming. Amphotericin B with or without flucytosine in doses similar to those used for non-HIV-infected individuals is the best studied regimen for initial therapy. High rates of adverse events with flucytosine may preclude its use in HIV-infected patients. Lifelong maintenance therapy with fluconazole is currently recommended for HIV-infected patients.

Cutaneous infections are usually treated medically, although surgical biopsy may be required for diagnosis. Skeletal infections generally require surgical debridement in addition to systemic antifungal therapy. Chorioretinitis also requires systemic antifungal therapy with amphotericin B and either fluconazole or flucytosine, both of which achieve high drug concentrations in the vitreous.

Dismukes WE: Management of cryptococcosis. Clin Infect Dis 17(Suppl 2):S507, 1993.

Dromer F, Mathoulin S, Dupont B, et al: Epidemiology of cryptococcosis in France: A 9-year survey (1985–1993). Clin Infect Dis 23:82, 1996.

Gonzalez CE, Shetty D, Lewis LL, et al: *Cryptococcus* in human immunodeficiency virus-infected children. Pediatr Infect Dis J 15:796, 1996.

Leggiadro RJ, Barrett FF, Hughes WT: Extrapulmonary cryptococcosis in immunocompromised infants and children. Pediatr Infect Dis J 11:43, 1992.

Leggiadro RJ, Kline MW, Hughes WT: Extrapulmonary cryptococcosis in children with acquired immunodeficiency syndrome. Pediatr Infect Dis J 10:658, 1991.

Moncino MD, Gutman LT: Severe systemic cryptococcal disease in a child: Review of prognostic indicators predicting treatment failure and an approach to maintenance therapy with oral fluconazole. Pediatr Infect Dis J 9:363, 1990.

Speed BR, Kaldor J: Rarity of cryptococcal infection in children. Pediatr Infect Dis J 16:536, 1997.

CHAPTER 232
Malassezia furfur

Martin E. Weisse

Malassezia furfur is the cause of the fungal dermatosis tinea versicolor (see Chapter 672). It has emerged as an infrequent cause of fungemia in patients with indwelling catheters.

M. furfur is a commensal lipophilic yeast with a predilection for the sebum-rich areas of skin. Because the yeast forms may be either oval or round, they were earlier designated *Pityrosporum ovale* and *P. orbiculare*. Transformation of the yeast to hyphal forms facilitates invasive disease. The clusters of thick-walled blastopores together with the hyphae produce the characteristic "spaghetti and meatballs" appearance.

Catheter-related *Malassezia* fungemia occurs almost exclusively in patients receiving intravenous lipids. Infection is most common in premature infants, although older patients with malignancy or immune compromise may also be infected. Symptoms of catheter-associated fungemia are indistinguishable from other causes of catheter-associated infections (see Chapter 180) but should be suspected in patients, especially neonates, receiving intravenous lipid infusions. *Malassezia* does not grow readily on standard fungal media, and successful culture requires overlaying the agar with olive oil. Recovery of *Malassezia* from blood culture is optimized by supplementing the media with olive oil or palmitic acid.

Fungemia due to *M. furfur* can be successfully treated in most cases by immediately discontinuing the lipid infusion and removing the infected catheter. For persistent or invasive infections, amphotericin B and imidazoles are effective.

Powell DA, Aungst J, Snedden S, et al: Broviac catheter-related *Malassezia furfur* sepsis in five infants receiving intravenous fat emulsions. J Pediatr 105:987, 1984.

Powell DA, Hayes J, Durrell DE, et al: *Malassezia furfur* skin colonization of infants hospitalized in intensive care units. J Pediatr 111:217, 1987.

Richet HM, McNeil MM, Edwards MC, Jarvis WR: Cluster of *Malassezia furfur* pulmonary infections in infants in a neonatal intensive-care unit. J Clin Microbiol 27:1197, 1989.

CHAPTER 233
Aspergillus

Stephen C. Aronoff

Aspergillosis refers to a group of diseases caused by monomorphic, mycelial fungi of the genus *Aspergillus*. Most diseases in children are caused by *A. fumigatus*; less frequently, *A. flavus* and *A. niger* are the causative agents. *A. nidulans* and *A. terreus* have also been reported in pediatric infections. Aspergilli are distributed worldwide, and spores (conidia) are readily isolated from soil and decaying plants. Outbreaks of invasive disease among immunosuppressed children may occur after they have been exposed to aerosolized conidia at construction sites near hospitals and clinics. Infection is usually acquired from inhalation of airborne spores, which colonize the upper and lower respiratory tracts. Immunocompromised persons are at risk for hematogenous dissemination. Cutaneous infection is also common and may follow wound contamination, intradermal inoculation, or hematogenous dissemination. Ingestion and aspiration may also produce disease. *Aspergillus*-associated diseases may be immunoglobulin (Ig) E mediated (hypersensitivity syndromes), saprophytic (noninvasive), or invasive.

233.1 Hypersensitivity Syndromes

ASTHMA. Atopic asthma (see Chapter 145) may be precipitated by inhalation of *Aspergillus* spores, which triggers an IgE-mediated response and bronchospasm. The clinical symptoms are nonspecific and include the acute onset of wheezing in the absence of pulmonary infiltrates or fever.

EXTRINSIC ALVEOLAR ALVEOLITIS. Extrinsic alveolar alveolitis is a hypersensitivity pneumonitis that occurs in nonatopic individuals after repeated exposures to organic dust. *Aspergillus* is one of many organic substances that produce this syndrome ("malt worker's" or "farmer's" lung). The pathogenesis is unknown but is similar to the alveolitis caused by other immunogens and may represent an immune complex disease. The clinical manifestations typically follow exposure by 4–6 hr and include fever, cough, and dyspnea. Physical examination often reveals rhonchi without wheezes. Eosinophilia is absent from blood and sputum, and chest radiograph often shows diffuse interstitial infiltrates. Chronic exposure gradually leads to irreversible pulmonary fibrosis.

ALLERGIC BRONCHOPULMONARY ASPERGILLOSIS. Allergic bronchopulmonary aspergillosis complicates chronic pulmonary disease in approximately 10% of children with asthma or cystic fibrosis. Chronic mucosal colonization with *A. fumigatus* produces an exaggerated IgG and IgE response, which results in recurrent bronchospasm and proximal cylindrical bronchiectasis. The diagnosis should be considered in patients with asthma or cystic fibrosis who have recurrent bronchospasm and transient pulmonary infiltrates. Expectoration of mucous spirals containing mycelia is a hallmark of this illness; peripheral eosinophilia is common. The diagnosis of allergic bronchopulmonary aspergillosis requires fulfillment of the following criteria: (1) reversible paroxysmal bronchiolar obstruction (asthma); (2) immediate cutaneous reactivity to *A. fumigatus* antigens or specific serum IgE to *A. fumigatus* (radioallergosorbent [RAST] test); (3) elevated total serum IgE; (4) peripheral blood eosinophilia; (5) precipitating serum antibodies against *A. fumigatus*; and (6) proximal bronchiectasis.

TREATMENT. Treatment of the hypersensitivity pulmonary syndromes focuses on anti-inflammatory agents, notably corticosteroids, and bronchodilator therapy. Growing experience with itraconazole in older adolescents and young adults with allergic bronchopulmonary dysplasia has demonstrated the potential benefit of this drug when used in combination with corticosteroid therapy.

233.2 Saprophytic (Noninvasive) Syndromes

OTOMYCOSIS. Otomycosis is a chronic condition that is found predominantly in tropical and subtropical regions and is rare in infants and children. Most infections are due to *A. niger* or, less commonly, *A. fumigatus*; coinfection with *Staphylococcus aureus* or *Pseudomonas* species occurs in one third of cases. Most cases are unilateral, and patients present with ear pain, itching of the auditory canal, and a sense of fullness. Otorrhea, decreased hearing, and tinnitus are less common. Examination of the auditory canal typically shows conidial "forests" or mycelial mats. Topical antifungal agents such as nystatin, tolnaftate, dilute acetic acid, and topical corticosteroids are therapeutic. Oral itraconazole has also been effective, but experience with it is limited.

SINUSITIS. *Aspergillus* noninvasive sinonasal disease may present in three forms. Chronic or indolent sinusitis is confined to one sinus and presents as a chronic infection that is unresponsive to antibacterial therapy. Sinus radiograms are nonspecific, showing mucosal thickening without bony changes. Endoscopic surgery is curative in most cases. Sinus aspergilloma, which is rare in children, presents with long-standing nasal symptoms. Sinus radiographs demonstrate a solitary mass in the ethmoid or maxillary sinus. Bony destruction is variable. Surgical removal of the mass, often endoscopically, is the treatment of choice. Allergic fungal sinusitis involves multiple sinuses and occurs in immunocompetent individuals who usually have a history of multiple preceding sinus surgeries and nasal polyposis. *Aspergillus* species and less often *Curvularia lunata* are the usual etiologic agents. Histology of nasal secretions in these patients reveals thick mucin, eosinophils, and few fungal hyphae. Sinus imaging typically shows involvement of multiple sinuses with hypodense areas, occasional calcifications, and occasional bony erosions. Criteria for the diagnosis of allergic fungal sinusitis are immunologic and are identical to those listed for allergic bronchopulmonary aspergillosis, which may complicate allergic fungal sinusitis. Treatment includes surgical drainage and debridement as well as corticosteroid therapy.

ASPERGILLOMA. Pulmonary aspergillomas develop in poorly drained bronchi or pre-existing pulmonary cavities and may complicate pulmonary tuberculosis, histoplasmosis, blastomycosis, or sarcoidosis; rarely, aspergillomas complicate invasive *Aspergillus* pulmonary disease. Colonization and fungal proliferation occur in the cavity, but no vascular invasion occurs; an amorphous mycelial mass (mycetoma, fungus ball) results. Affected children are often asymptomatic, although cough and hemoptysis may be reported. Chest radiographs characteristically demonstrate the air shadow of a pulmonary cavity outlining a rounded mass; these findings may be confirmed by computed tomography of the chest. Management is controversial and may range from watchful waiting for asymptomatic and otherwise healthy children to surgical resection in patients with symptoms.

233.3 Invasive Disease

Invasive *Aspergillus* infection is characterized by hyphal infiltration of vascular structures, thrombosis, and focal necrosis. Invasive disease occurs most commonly in immunocompromised patients, particularly neutropenic children with leukemia, children with human immunodeficiency virus (HIV) infection, bone marrow transplant recipients, and, less commonly, solid organ recipients. Primary invasive disease may occur at any site in which airborne conidia may colonize and germinate, such as the respiratory tract or skin. In the severely neutropenic child, dissemination follows direct extension from the primary site and hematogenous seeding of distant sites. Sinonasal disease, pulmonary disease, and cutaneous disease are the most common primary infections in children. Otitis media is rare. Although systemic amphotericin B (either desoxycholate or the liposomal formulations) remains the recommended treatment for most established *Aspergillus* infections, the outcome appears to hinge on resolution of the underlying immunocompromised state. Itraconazole, a triazole antifungal agent, has appreciable in vitro activity against *Aspergillus* species, but experience with this agent for the treatment of aspergillosis in children is limited. Aerosolized amphotericin B is currently under investigation for prophylaxis in cancer patients during periods of profound neutropenia.

OTITIS EXTERNA. Otitis externa associated with *Aspergillus* infection is rare, occurs in immunosuppressed individuals, and is associated with hearing loss and spread to the petrous portion of the temporal bone and the pinna. Therapy includes amphotericin B and surgical debridement; experience with itraconazole is limited.

SINUSITIS. Nasosinusitis occurs almost exclusively in patients with profound neutropenia associated with chemotherapy for cancer and is rare in children. Fever, cough, epistaxis, headache, and sinus pain are the most common clinical signs. Examination typically shows nasal crusting with rhinorrhea, sinus tenderness, nasal or oral ulceration, and duskiness or necrosis of the nasal septum or inferior turbinates. Multiple sinus involvement with opacification or air-fluid levels can be demonstrated radiographically or by computed tomography. Scrapings of the nasal or sinus mucosa demonstrate large numbers of hyphae, and fungal cultures typically yield *A. fumigatus*, *A. flavus*, or, less often, *Rhizopus* or *Candida* species.

Treatment is not standardized but often includes surgical drainage, intravenous and intranasal amphotericin B, and removal of devascularized necrotic tissue. Extensive surgical procedures are often hampered by underlying thrombocytopenia and extensive and at times life-threatening hemorrhage. Sporadic treatment successes and failures have been reported with itraconazole; however, comparative data with amphotericin B are not available. Invasive sinusitis has a poor prognosis for children with leukemia in relapse; better outcomes occur with resolution of the granulocytopenia or remission of the underlying disease.

PNEUMONIA AND DISSEMINATED INFECTION. Invasive pulmonary aspergillosis is the most common form of *Aspergillus* infection and usually occurs in immunocompromised patients. The onset is often insidious. In both immunocompetent and immunocompromised patients, symptomatic infection presents acutely with fever, cough, dyspnea, and abnormal chest findings; pleuritic chest pain is an infrequent complaint. Chest radiographs often show nodular infiltrates. Coexisting sinusitis is a common finding in neutropenic children. In children with chronic granulomatous disease, direct extension from the lungs to the chest wall has been reported.

The diagnosis is confirmed by histologic demonstration of hyphal invasion of blood vessels and recovery of the fungus by culture of the biopsy specimen. Recovery of a pure culture of *Aspergillus* species from two sputum samples from immunocompromised patients with nodular, cavitary, or wedge-shaped lesions on chest radiographs is highly suggestive of invasive disease.

Treatment with high-dose amphotericin B (1 mg/kg/24 hr) for 4–6 wk, or until the neutropenia resolves or the underlying disease goes into remission, is recommended. Experience with itraconazole is limited.

SKIN. Cutaneous aspergillosis is a common manifestation of invasive aspergillosis in immunocompromised children. Lesions are typically seen at sites of local trauma such as intravenous sites. Cutaneous disease may result either from direct inoculation of the skin or, more frequently, from hematogenous dissemination. The lesions appear initially as tender erythematous plaques that progress to necrotic eschars or hemorrhagic bullae (ecthyma gangrenosum). In the majority of children with profound neutropenia, cutaneous aspergillosis is a sentinel marker of disseminated disease and indicates a poor outcome. Treatment with high-dose amphotericin B (1 mg/kg/24 hr) is recommended for 4–6 wk, or until the neutropenia resolves or the underlying disease goes into remission. Local debridement and topical amphotericin have also been used. Experience with itraconazole is limited.

EYE. Fungal endophthalmitis is an important diagnostic finding in immunosuppressed children with disseminated *Aspergillus* infection. Although most patients have no ocular symptoms, pain, photophobia, and diminished visual acuity may occur. Examination of the retina shows focal retinitis, an overlying vitreitis, and retinal hemorrhage. Treatment of the underlying immunosuppressive illness, systemic antifungal therapy, vitrectomy, and intraocular amphotericin B are recommended. Amphotericin B and itraconazole achieve poor intraocular concentrations.

Orbital cellulitis rarely complicates invasive sinusitis and follows destruction of the orbital walls and fungal extension into the retro-orbital space. Diplopia, periorbital edema, proptosis, and pain on lateral gaze may occur. Treatment requires a combination of surgical debridement, systemic antifungal therapy, and resolution of the underlying immunocompromised state.

Fungal keratitis and episcleritis are rare problems and follow direct inoculation of spores into the eye. In the absence of significant disseminated disease, topical and intrascleral amphotericin B therapy is recommended.

CENTRAL NERVOUS SYSTEM. Cerebral aspergillosis is a rare and almost uniformly fatal complication of disseminated disease. In most cases, infection involves single or multiple foci within the cerebral hemispheres or cerebellum. Focal neurologic deficits begin acutely, most often hemiparesis, anterior cranial nerve palsies, or seizures. Progression to herniation is rapid. Meningeal signs are rare, and at autopsy arachnoiditis is limited to the area adjacent to the cerebral focus. Cerebrospinal fluid shows a mild mononuclear pleocytosis, elevated CSF protein, and variable degrees of hypoglycorrhachia. Imaging studies demonstrate focal central nervous system lesions with edema and variable enhancement. The diagnosis can be established by the acute appearance of neurologic symptoms in a patient with proven or suspected invasive aspergillosis or occasionally by cerebrospinal fluid or brain biopsy culture. High-dose amphotericin B combined with flucytosine has been effective in a paucity of cases.

Epidural abscess is a rare complication of vertebral osteomyelitis caused by *Aspergillus* species. In two children with epidural abscess, vertebral osteomyelitis and cord compression, surgical decompression, and high-dose amphotericin B were curative.

BONE. Aspergillosis of the bone is an extremely rare disease and follows direct extension of infection from a surgical or traumatic wound or hematogenous seeding. Involvement of the vertebrae is most common. Osteomyelitis of the rib is rare, occurs in children with chronic granulomatous disease, and represents extension from a pulmonary focus. Surgical drainage is often required. Although comparative studies are not available, initial therapy with amphotericin B plus flucytosine followed by itraconazole is a promising approach.

HEART. Endocarditis is a rare form of aspergillosis and can follow contamination at the time of surgery or implantation of a contaminated graft, or, uncommonly, it may be a manifestation of disseminated aspergillosis. High-dose amphotericin B therapy coupled with surgical removal of infected grafts or prostheses is recommended.

Denning DW, Stevens DA: Antifungal and surgical treatment of invasive aspergillosis: Review of 2121 published cases. Rev Infect Dis 12:1147, 1990.

Horvath JA, Dummer S: The use of respiratory tract cultures in the diagnosis of invasive pulmonary aspergillosis. Am J Med 100:171, 1996.

Neijens HJ, Frenkel J, et al: Invasive *Aspergillus* infection in chronic granulomatous disease: Treatment with itraconazole. J Pediatr 115:1016, 1989.

Walmsley S, Devi S, King S, et al: Invasive *Aspergillus* infections in a pediatric hospital: A ten-year review. Pediatr Infect Dis J 12:673, 1993.

Wong-Beringer A, Jacobs RA, Guglielmo BJ: Lipid formulations of amphotericin B: Clinical efficacy and toxicities. Clin Infect Dis 27:603, 1998.

CHAPTER 234

Histoplasmosis (Histoplasma capsulatum)

Stephen C. Aronoff

ETIOLOGY. Histoplasmosis is caused by *Histoplasma capsulatum*, a dimorphic fungus found in nature in the mycelial (saprophytic) form and in human tissue in the parasitic form as yeast.

EPIDEMIOLOGY. The saprophytic form is found in soil throughout the midwestern United States, primarily along the Ohio and Mississippi rivers; sporadic cases of human and animal histoplasmosis have been reported from 31 of the 48 contiguous states. In parts of Kentucky and Tennessee, almost 90% of the population >20 yr of age have positive skin tests to histoplasmin.

H. capsulatum thrives in soil rich in nitrates such as areas that are heavily contaminated with bird droppings or decayed wood. Fungal spores are often carried on the wings of birds. Focal outbreaks of histoplasmosis have been reported after aerosolization of microconidia resulting from construction in areas previously occupied by starling roosts or chicken coops or by chopping decayed wood. Unlike birds, bats are actively infected with *Histoplasma*. Focal outbreaks of histoplasmosis have also been reported after intense exposure to bat guano in caves and along bridges frequented by bats.

PATHOGENESIS. Inhalation of microconidia is the initial stage of human infection. The conidia reach the alveoli, germinate, and proliferate as yeast. The initial infection is a bronchopneumonia. As the initial pulmonary lesion ages, giant cells form, and these are followed by formation of granuloma and central necrosis. At the time of spore germination, yeast cells gain access to the reticuloendothelial system via the pulmonary lymphatic system and hilar lymph nodes. Dissemination with splenic involvement typically follows the primary pulmonary infection. In normal hosts, an immune response follows in approximately 2 wk. The initial pulmonary lesion resolves within 2–4 mo but may undergo calcification resembling the Ghon complex of tuberculosis; alternatively, "buckshot" calcifications involving the lung and spleen may be seen. Unlike tuberculosis, reinfection with *H. capsulatum* occurs and may lead to exaggerated host responses in some cases.

CLINICAL MANIFESTATIONS. There are three forms of human histoplasmosis: acute pulmonary infection, chronic pulmonary histoplasmosis, and progressive disseminated histoplasmosis. *Acute pulmonary histoplasmosis* follows initial or recurrent respiratory exposure to microconidia. The majority of patients are asymptomatic. Symptomatic disease occurs more often in young children; in older individuals symptoms follow exposure to large inocula in closed spaces (e.g., chicken coops or caves) or prolonged exposure (e.g., camping on contaminated soil, chopping decayed wood). The prodrome is not specific and usually consists of flulike symptoms: headache, fever, chest pain, and cough. Hepatosplenomegaly occurs more often in infants and young children. Symptomatic infections may be associated with significant respiratory distress and hypoxia and may require intubation, ventilation, and steroid therapy. Acute pulmonary disease may also present with a prolonged illness (10 days to 3 wk) consisting of weight loss, dyspnea, high fever, asthenia, and fatigue. Ten per cent of patients with acute pulmonary infection present with a sarcoid-like disease that includes arthritis or arthralgia, erythema nodosum, keratoconjunctivitis, or iridocyclitis and pericarditis. Most children with acute pulmonary disease have normal chest radiographs. Individuals with symptomatic disease typically have a patchy bronchopneumonia; hilar adenopathy is variably present. In young children, the pneumonia may coalesce. Focal or buckshot calcifications are convalescent findings in patients with acute pulmonary infection.

Exaggerated host responses to fungal antigens within the lung parenchyma or hilar lymph nodes produce thoracic complications of acute pulmonary histoplasmosis. Histoplasmomas are of parenchymal origin and are usually asymptomatic. These fibroma-like lesions are often concentrically calcified and single. Rarely, these lesions may produce broncholithiasis associated with "stone spitting," wheezing, and hemoptysis. In endemic regions, these lesions may mimic parenchymal tumors and are occasionally diagnosed at lung biopsy. *Mediastinal granulomas* form when reactive hilar lymph nodes coalesce and mat together. Although these lesions are usually asymptomatic, huge granulomas may compress the mediastinal structures, producing symptoms of esophageal, bronchial, or vena caval obstruction. Local extension and necrosis may produce pericarditis or pleural effusions. *Mediastinal fibrosis* is a rare complication of mediastinal granulomas and represents an uncontrolled fibrotic reaction arising from the hilar nodes. Structures within the mediastinum become encased within a fibrotic mass, producing obstructive symptomatology. Superior vena cava syndrome, pulmonary venous obstruction with a mitral stenosis-like syndrome, and pulmonary artery obstruction with congestive heart failure have been described. Dysphagia accompanies esophageal entrapment, and a syndrome of cough, wheeze, hemoptysis, and dyspnea accompanies bronchial obstruction.

Chronic pulmonary histoplasmosis is an opportunistic infection in adult patients with centrilobular emphysema. This entity is rare in children.

Progressive disseminated histoplasmosis is a disease that affects infants and immunosuppressed individuals. Disseminated disease of infancy occurs almost exclusively in infants younger than 1 yr and follows primary pulmonary infection. Fever is the most common finding and may last for weeks to months before the condition is diagnosed. The majority of patients have hepatosplenomegaly, anemia, and thrombocytopenia. Pneumonia and pancytopenia are variably present. Although radiographs of the chest are normal in more than half of these children, the yeast can frequently be identified on bone marrow examination.

Children who are immunosuppressed (e.g., oncology patients, organ transplant recipients, those with human immunodeficiency virus [HIV] infection) are at increased risk for disseminated histoplasmosis. In non-HIV-infected individuals, disseminated disease presents with unexplained fevers, weight loss, lymphadenopathy, and interstitial pulmonary disease. Extrapulmonary infection is a characteristic of disseminated disease and may include destructive bony lesions, oropharyngeal ulcers, Addison's disease, meningitis, cutaneous infection, and endocarditis. Elevated liver function test results and high serum concentrations of angiotensin-converting enzyme may be observed.

Disseminated histoplasmosis in an HIV-infected individual is an acquired immunodeficiency syndrome (AIDS)-defining illness. Disseminated disease is often preceded or followed by another opportunistic infection in this patient population. Fever and weight loss occur in most individuals. In the majority of patients pulmonary disease develops; hepatosplenomegaly, lymphadenopathy, skin rashes, and meningoencephalitis are variably present. A sepsis-like syndrome has been identified in a small number of HIV-infected patients with disseminated histoplasmosis and is characterized by the rapid onset of shock, multiorgan failure, and coagulopathy.

DIAGNOSIS. Recovery of *H. capsulatum* by culture differs with the form of infection. In normal hosts with symptomatic or asymptomatic acute pulmonary histoplasmosis, sputum cultures are rarely obtained and are variably positive; cultures of bronchoalveolar lavage fluid appear to have a slightly higher yield than sputa. Blood cultures are sterile in patients with acute pulmonary histoplasmosis, and cultures from any source are typically sterile in individuals with the sarcoid form of the disease. Yeast forms may be demonstrated histologically in tissue from patients with complicated forms of acute pulmonary disease (mediastinal granuloma, mediastinal fibrosis, and histoplasmoma). Sputum cultures are positive in 60% of adults with chronic pulmonary histoplasmosis. The yeast can be recovered from blood or bone marrow in >90% of patients with progressive disseminated histoplasmosis.

Detection of fungal antigen by radioimmunoassay is the best diagnostic study in patients in whom progressive disseminated histoplasmosis is suspected. In HIV-infected patients as well as others at risk for disseminated disease, histoplasma-associated antigen can be demonstrated in the urine or blood in more than 90% of cases. False-positive results may occur in individuals with blastomycosis, coccidioidomycosis, and paracoccidioidomycosis. Sequential measurement of antigen in patients with disseminated disease is useful for monitoring response to therapy. Serum and urine from individuals with acute or chronic pulmonary infections are variably antigen positive.

Seroconversion continues to be useful for the diagnosis of acute pulmonary histoplasmosis, its complications, and chronic pulmonary disease. Serum antibody to yeast and mycelium-associated antigens is classically measured by complement fixation. Although titers >1:8 are found in more than 80% of patients with histoplasmosis, titers of ≥1:32 are most significant for the diagnosis of recent infection. Complement fixation antibody titers are often not significant early in the infection and do not become positive until 4–6 wk after exposure. Complement fixation titers may be falsely positive in patients with other systemic mycoses and may be falsely negative in immunocompromised patients. Antibody detection by immunodiffusion is less sensitive than complement fixation and is used to confirm questionably positive complement fixation titers. Skin testing is useful only for epidemiologic studies because cutaneous reactivity is lifelong, and intradermal injection may elicit an immune response in otherwise seronegative individuals.

TREATMENT. Antifungal therapy is not warranted for persons with asymptomatic or mildly symptomatic acute pulmonary histoplasmosis. Mediastinal complications of acute pulmonary infection often require surgical therapy. Sarcoid-like disease with or without pericarditis may be treated with nonsteroidal anti-inflammatory agents.

Amphotericin B continues to be the cornerstone of therapy for patients with progressive disseminated histoplasmosis. In immunocompromised adults and infants with disseminated disease, 35–40 mg/kg total dose is required to minimize relapses. Both ketoconazole and itraconazole have been used successfully to treat progressive disseminated disease in immunocompromised adults. Oral itraconazole alone was shown to be effective for the treatment of disseminated disease in seven children treated in an uncontrolled fashion. No comparative data with amphotericin B are available. Serial measurement of fungal antigen in urine or serum is recommended to ensure adequate treatment.

Relapses in HIV-infected individuals with progressive disseminated histoplasmosis are common. Currently, induction therapy with amphotericin B (10–15 mg/kg total dose; total dose >500 mg in adults) is recommended. Lifelong suppressive therapy may be accomplished with daily itraconazole (200 mg/24 hr in adults). Ketoconazole is not effective in HIV-infected individuals. For severely immunocompromised, HIV-infected children living in endemic regions, itraconazole (2–5 mg/kg every 12–24 hr) may be used prophylactically. Care must be taken to avoid interactions between antifungal azoles and protease inhibitors.

Goodwin RA, Loyd JE, Des Prez R: Histoplasmosis in normal hosts. Medicine 60:231, 1981.

Leggiadro RJ, Barrett FF, Hughes WT: Disseminated histoplasmosis of infancy. Pediatr Infect Dis J 7:799, 1988.
Tobon AM, Franco L, Espinal D, et al: Disseminated histoplasmosis in children: The role of itraconazole therapy. Pediatr Infect Dis J 15:1002, 1996.
Wheat J, Hafner R, Wulfsohn M, et al: Prevention of relapse of histoplasmosis with itraconazole in patients with the acquired immunodeficiency syndrome: The NIAID Clinical Trials and Mycoses Study Group Collaborators. Ann Intern Med 118:610, 1993.
Wheat LJ: Histoplasmosis in Indianapolis. Clin Infect Dis 14(Suppl 1):S91, 1992.
USPHS/IDSA Working Group: 1997 USPHS/IDSA Guidelines for the Prevention of Opportunistic Infections in Persons Infected with HIV: Disease-Specific Recommendations. Clin Infect Dis 25(Suppl 3):S313, 1997.

CHAPTER 235
Blastomycosis (Blastomyces dermatitidis)

Stephen C. Aronoff

ETIOLOGY. Blastomycosis is an uncommon fungal disease caused by *Blastomyces dermatitidis,* a dimorphic fungus that is found in nature in the mycelial (saprophytic) form and in human tissue in the parasitic form as yeast.

EPIDEMIOLOGY. Blastomycosis in children is unusual, but children <15 yr of age constitute 2–10% of reported cases. Sporadic infection in endemic regions accounts for the majority of cases of human and canine blastomycosis. The fungus is found throughout the midwestern and southeastern portions of the United States, particularly along the Ohio and Mississippi River valleys, north central Wisconsin, North Carolina, Minnesota, and Illinois. Blastomycosis is rarely reported outside of North America, primarily from Africa. Although difficult to isolate from soil, *B. dermatitidis* has been recovered from earth enriched with rotted wood, bird droppings, or animal droppings. Soil surrounding bodies of water within the endemic region is particularly rich in fungi. Epidemics are unusual but have been described after excavation of contaminated soil in endemic regions. Individuals who spend large amounts of time in wooded areas within endemic regions, such as hunters or forestry workers, are at highest risk for infection.

PATHOGENESIS. The pathogenesis of blastomycosis is similar to that of histoplasmosis. Inhalation of spores results in alveolar inoculation and germination to yeast forms. Although pulmonary macrophages eliminate the majority of spores before infection occurs, those that survive produce pneumonitis and may disseminate hematogenously. The immune response to infection consists of neutrophil and macrophage migration into infected tissue. The resulting "pyogranulomatous" response with associated necrosis and fibrosis is characteristic of blastomycosis.

CLINICAL MANIFESTATIONS. Human blastomycosis presents as a pulmonary or extrapulmonary infection. Three forms of pulmonary infection have been described. *Asymptomatic infection* is rarely identified because of the lack of an inexpensive, reliable screening test. Subclinical infections have been identified serologically during investigations of epidemics; individuals may exhibit nonspecific symptoms such as weight loss, unexplained fever, and malaise. Chest radiographs often demonstrate an alveolar process that may resemble a parenchymal mass. *Acute pneumonia* is the most common form of human blastomycosis. These patients present with an acute onset of fever, chills, and productive cough; hemoptysis is variably identified. Pleural effusions occur in approximately 25–50% of cases, and erythema nodosum may occur during resolution. Alveolar or reticulonodular patterns without hilar lymphadenopathy are often seen on chest radiographs. Diffuse pulmonary disease associated with adult respiratory distress syndrome (ARDS) has been described in a few immunocompetent adults with acute pneumonia. *Chronic pneumonia* is characterized by several months of weight loss, cough, night sweats, and fever. The cough becomes productive and may be associated with chest pain; cavitary disease is an uncommon complication of this form of infection.

Extrapulmonary or disseminated disease occurs in immunocompetent individuals and is usually preceded by pulmonary symptoms. Laryngeal blastomycosis is relatively common, usually following primary infection of the upper airway, and presents as a laryngeal mass. Cutaneous disease follows hematogenous or direct inoculation of the subcutaneous tissue and appears as either verrucous or ulcerative lesions. Osteomyelitis occurs in one quarter of patients with extrapulmonary infections and usually involves flat bones such as the skull, vertebrae, and ribs. Central nervous system infection occurs in 10% of patients with extrapulmonary infections and is typified by intracranial abscesses or, rarely, meningitis. Prostatitis and orchitis in males are unusual; endometrial disease is sexually transmitted. Fungal abscesses may form anywhere, including the heart and its surrounding structures, the orbit, and the sinuses.

DIAGNOSIS. Because colonization with *B. dermatitidis* does not occur, recovery of the fungus from sputum, bronchoalveolar lavage fluid, pleural fluid, or other sterile sites is diagnostic. Similarly, histologic demonstration of the characteristic yeast is diagnostic. Serologic diagnosis using complement fixation or immunodiffusion is insensitive and is complicated by the high rate of cross reactivity with anti-*Histoplasma* antibody. Enzyme-linked immunosorbent assay (ELISA) is the most specific serologic test and is positive in >75% of cases. Skin testing is unreliable because reactivity wanes over time at an unpredictable rate.

TREATMENT. Uncomplicated acute pneumonia may resolve spontaneously. Itraconazole (200–400 mg/24 hr) or fluconazole (400–800 mg/24 hr) for ≥6 mo is curative in the majority of adults with mild to moderate acute lung disease, osteomyelitis, or laryngeal or cutaneous infection. Itraconazole (5–7 mg/kg/24 hr) has been used successfully to treat a small number of children with non-life-threatening infections. Amphotericin B remains the drug of choice for life-threatening and central nervous system infections in children. Amphotericin B alone (35 mg/kg total dose) or short courses of amphotericin B (5–10 mg/kg total dose) followed by itraconazole for 6 mo may be used to treat extrapulmonary disease. Neither fluconazole nor itraconazole is beneficial in treating central nervous system blastomycosis. Acute pneumonia associated with ARDS and extrapulmonary disease is treated with moderate doses of amphotericin B (>1.5 g total dose) or induction courses of amphotericin B (500 mg total dose) followed by 5–6 mo of itraconazole therapy. Immunocompromised persons, especially patients with AIDS, may require chronic suppressive therapy.

Dismukes WE, Bradsher RW, Cloud GC, et al: Itraconazole therapy for blastomycosis and histoplasmosis. Am J Med 93:489, 1992.
Istorico LJ, Sanders M, Jacobs RF, et al: Otitis media due to blastomycosis: Report of two cases. Clin Infect Dis 14:355, 1992.
Meyer KC, McManus EJ, Maki DG: Overwhelming pulmonary blastomycosis associated with the adult respiratory distress syndrome. N Engl J Med 329:1231, 1993.
Pappas PG, Bradsher RW, Kauffman CA, et al: Treatment of blastomycosis with higher doses of fluconazole. Clin Infect Dis 25:200, 1997.
Schutze GE, Hickerson SL, Fortin EM, et al: Blastomycosis in children. Clin Infect Dis 22:496, 1996.

CHAPTER 236
Coccidioidomycosis (Coccidioides immitis)

Demosthenes Pappagianis

ETIOLOGY. Coccidioidomycosis (San Joaquin fever, Valley fever, desert rheumatism, coccidioidal granuloma) is an infection caused by the fungus *Coccidioides immitis*, which is found in the soil of the New World. *C. immitis* is a dimorphic fungus that is found as a mold or filamentous form in nature, but in tissue it transforms into a large, thick-walled spherule containing endospores. Although *C. immitis* is a dimorphic fungus, the parasitic form is not a yeast as with other dimorphic fungi.

EPIDEMIOLOGY. Within the arid endemic areas of California's San Joaquin Valley, in scattered regions in northern and southern California, in central and southern Arizona, and even in southwestern Texas, many long-time residents have been infected, along with cattle, sheep, dogs, horses, llamas, and wild rodents. Recovery from infection confers permanent immunity except in persons with acquired (natural or iatrogenic) immunodeficiency. Population shifts bring susceptible individuals into endemic areas.

PATHOGENESIS. The minute arthroconidia of the *C. immitis* mycelial saprophytic phase that are airborne in dust are inhaled or, rarely, enter the host through injured skin. In the infected host they round up into spherules, which develop endospores. Liberation of the latter leads to formation of new spherules, which spread within a host but not to a new host. Viable *C. immitis* does occur in pulmonary cavities, often in the mycelial as well as spherule form, but no cases of person-to-person infection have been discovered. However, the arthroconidia that occur in nature and on the surface of cultures are highly infectious. Although isolation of the patient is unnecessary, precautions should be taken with dressings and casts over open lesions to preclude the development of infective arthroconidia, which occurs in 4–5 days on surface cultures.

CLINICAL MANIFESTATIONS. Human infection takes three forms (Fig. 236–1): (1) a benign, self-limited, primary infection (60% of infected persons show no clinical manifestations); (2) residual pulmonary lesions; and (3) a rare, disseminating, sometimes fatal disease. The disease tends to be milder in children; however, in children requiring medical attention, dissemination to the bones and meninges is fairly common and approaches the incidence of these complications in adults. Laryngeal coccidioidomycosis, although not frequent, has been detected at a proportionately higher rate in children. Maternal-fetal and maternal-neonatal infection has been reported.

Primary Coccidioidomycosis. The incubation period varies from 1–4 wk, with an average of 10–16 days. Symptoms are flulike; the onset may be insidious or abrupt with malaise, chills, and fever. Chest pain is frequent and may vary from a mere sense of constriction to excruciating pain. Night sweats and anorexia are common. On occasion, there is a persistent dry cough, and the throat may be painful. There also may be headache or backache.

A generalized, fine, macular erythema or urticarial eruption may appear within the first day or so. It may be evanescent and present only in the groin. Rarely, a vesicular, varicella-like rash has been noted. Most frequently, tibial erythema nodosum occurs with or without erythema multiforme. These lesions develop when sensitivity to coccidioidin is maximal, 3–21 days after onset of symptoms. These rashes characteristic of the acute infection do not contain the organism and may result from hypersensitivity to coccidioidal antigen. Skin lesions may occur, however, in persons who are otherwise asymptomatic. Other allergic manifestations, arthritis, and phlyctenular conjunctivitis may occur concomitantly.

Chest examination rarely discloses abnormal findings, even though roentgenography reveals extensive consolidation. Dullness, a friction rub, or fine rales may be detected infrequently. Pleural effusions occasionally occur and may be massive enough to compromise respiratory status; they may develop without preceding respiratory symptoms.

Residual Pulmonary Coccidioidomycosis. Infrequently, a cavity may develop in an area of pulmonary consolidation during the primary infection and then regress. More often, however, after a variably prolonged period a persistent cavity may form. There are often no symptoms, and the diagnosis is made roentgenographically. Occasionally there is mild to moderate hemoptysis, which may recur and be alarming. Rarely, fatal hemorrhage occurs. Dissemination of the fungus from cavities to other areas is rare. Pulmonary residual "granulomas" sometimes persist. They are not harmful but do pose problems of differentiation from tuberculosis or neoplasms. Infrequently, a chronic progressive fibrocavitary pulmonary disease is seen.

Disseminated or Progressive Coccidioidomycosis (Coccidioidal Granuloma). Certain persons are unable to localize coccidioidal infection. Dissemination, which is rare and occurs mainly in males, especially Filipinos, other Asians, and blacks, usually follows the initial illness within 6 mo, often without any interlude. This is analogous to the course of progressive primary tuberculosis. Persons with blood group B may be particularly disposed to dissemination. Certain immunosuppressed states enhance dissemination or bring about relapse of apparently arrested coccidioidomycosis. Dissemination is enhanced if coccidioidal infection is acquired during pregnancy. Skin lesions and cold abscesses, both subcutaneous and osseous, occur. Meningitis is the most serious of the disseminated lesions and is clinically similar to tuberculous meningitis. In whites it is not unusual for meningitis to be the only extrapulmonary lesion. Miliary dissemination and peritonitis may be distinguishable from tuberculosis only by demonstration of the causative agent, though coccidioidal peritonitis may present as a very mild disease. The mortality rate of untreated meningitis is practically 100% but varies with other forms of disseminated coccidioidomycosis.

DIAGNOSIS. Diagnosis of the disseminated infection may be established by biopsy or at autopsy. Sputum is generally so scanty in patients with the primary infection that bronchoalveolar lavage or gastric aspirates may be advisable, especially in children. The diagnosis is confirmed if histologic examination demonstrates the characteristic double-contoured spherules with endospores and without budding. Demonstration of the fungus by culture and confirmation by DNA probe, exoantigen test, or animal inoculation are also diagnostic. Only specially qualified laboratories should undertake culture because of safety concerns.

The erythrocyte sedimentation rate is elevated in patients with primary or disseminated infection and is helpful in evaluating clinical status. Eosinophilia is common and is proportion-

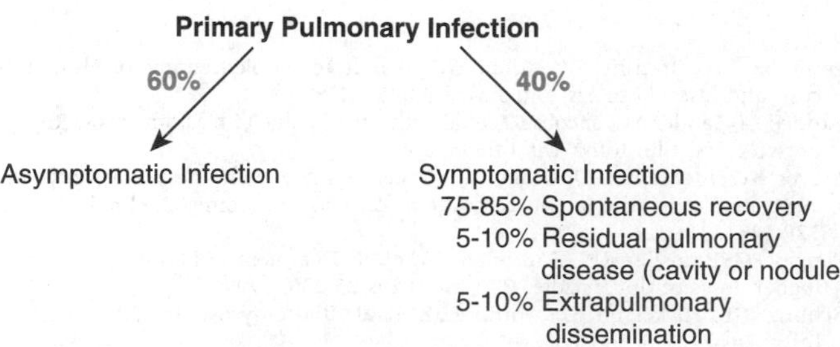

Figure 236–1 Natural history of coccidioidomycoses.

ately higher in patients with more severe infections. Serum alkaline phosphatase may be elevated in acute coccidioidomycosis even in the absence of obvious systemic dissemination. The cerebrospinal fluid findings in patients with *C. immitis* meningitis are similar to those characteristic of tuberculous meningitis (see Chapter 212).

Concomitant coccidioidomycosis and other infections (e.g., tuberculosis) can be confounding.

Skin Test. Tests with coccidioidin or spherulin are specific except for occasional cross reactions with histoplasmosis and blastomycosis. A positive reaction does not distinguish between a recent and an old infection unless it has been preceded within a reasonably short time by a negative test result. However, *a negative skin test does not exclude coccidioidal infection.* Coccidioidin or the equivalent dose of spherulin is administered intradermally as 0.1 mL of a 1:1,000, 1:100, or even 1:10 dilution. The reaction generally reaches its peak at 36 hr and should be read at 24 hr and 48 hr. An area of induration >5 mm in diameter is positive. Patients with suspected coccidioidal erythema nodosum are likely to be hypersensitive and should receive the 1:1,000 dilution. Patients with disseminated infections are much less sensitive; even a 1:10 dilution may not elicit a reaction. Dermal sensitivity to coccidioidin is less durable than sensitivity to tuberculin. There is no danger of disseminating or activating a coccidioidal infection by producing a strong coccidioidin reaction, although there may be a systemic reaction as well as a local one. Coccidioidin does not evoke antibodies in the human; therefore, the skin test may precede serologic tests and will provide information useful in their interpretation. However, a negative skin test should not preclude serologic tests. A positive skin test in a healthy individual indicates resistance to reinfection with *C. immitis*.

Serology. Antibodies to *C. immitis* are generally not demonstrable in persons with asymptomatic acute infections. Serum precipitins (immunoglobulin [Ig] M) and complement fixation (IgG) antibodies are detectable in early coccidioidomycosis and may persist in those with disseminated coccidioidomycosis. In general, more severe infections are associated with higher complement fixation titers. Rarely, serologic tests may be negative in patients with active coccidioidomycosis, especially if they are immunosuppressed.

Antibodies detectable by complement fixation do not pass the blood-brain barrier (although immunodiffusion may reveal their presence) but are found in cord blood at the same titer as in the mother's blood. Passively transferred antibody disappears from the infant within 6 mo. Coccidioidal precipitin (IgM) has been detected in some neonates of mothers with coccidioidomycosis when there has been no manifestation of disease in the infants.

C. immitis antibodies in cerebrospinal fluid are measured by complement fixation. Cerebrospinal fluid antibodies occur in 95% of patients with coccidioidal meningitis, are usually diagnostic, and are occasionally present in patients with epidural coccidioidal lesions. Complement-fixing antibody is more frequently detected in cisternal and lumbar fluid but may be deceptively absent from the ventricular fluid.

Roentgenography. During the primary infection roentgenograms of the chest may not reveal pulmonary changes. Hilar lymphadenopathy is frequent, and there may be single or multiple, sharply circumscribed or soft, feathery, small pulmonary densities or larger consolidated areas. Acute respiratory insufficiency may result. Pulmonary cavities, which occur less frequently in children than in adults, tend to be thin-walled when present. Pleural effusions vary in extent. Osseous lesions, which are usually multiple and have a predilection for cancellous bone, often are widespread and are generally indistinguishable from those of tuberculosis.

TREATMENT. Because most primary coccidioidal infections resolve spontaneously over a variable time period, they have historically been treated conservatively; the patient's activity and symptomatic measures are restricted until the erythrocyte sedimentation rate returns to normal, clinical and roentgenographic improvement is noted, serum precipitins (IgM) become undetectable, and the serum complement fixation (IgG) titer decreases. With the advent of the relatively benign oral azoles, physicians have often initiated therapy as soon as coccidioidomycosis is suspected or confirmed. This has been done despite any evidence that such treatment for primary coccidioidomycosis hastens recovery or decreases the risk of pulmonary dissemination or development of pulmonary residua (e.g., cavity or solitary nodule).

Antifungal chemotherapy is indicated for those at high risk of severe coccidioidomycosis (though there is no assurance that this will prevent dissemination) and those who have recognized pulmonary dissemination. Currently available chemotherapeutic agents are amphotericin B, as a desoxycholate suspension or in a liposomal or lipid complex form; fluconazole, oral or intravenous; and ketoconazole or itraconazole, both in oral forms. Indications for the choice of medications are not clearly defined. However, in the patient with rapidly progressing coccidioidomycosis, amphotericin B (0.1–1.0 mg/kg/24 hr) should be administered. Once the full dose has been achieved, it can be given every other day or two to three times a week to minimize renal toxicity.

Amphotericin B does not cross the blood-brain barrier in therapeutic amounts for *C. immitis*, but it may mask the presence of meningitis. Intrathecal (cisternal or lumbar) or intraventricular administration of amphotericin B had been the mainstay of treatment of coccidioidal meningitis. Orally administered fluconazole readily penetrates from the blood into the cerebrospinal fluid, whereas itraconazole does not. Both fluconazole and itraconazole have proved useful in the treatment of coccidioidal meningitis, although the duration of the treatment and of arrest of the meningitis has not yet been defined. The sole indication for parenteral miconazole is intrathecal or intraventricular administration for treatment of *C. immitis* meningitis.

Ketoconazole (3–15 mg/kg/24 hr), fluconazole (3–12 mg/kg/24 hr), or itraconazole (3–6 mg/kg/24 hr) administered orally has been useful in treating disseminated coccidioidomycosis outside the central nervous system that is neither extensive nor progressing rapidly. The higher doses may be required for the treatment of meningitis. Although the azoles have increasingly been used to treat children as well as adults with coccidioidomycosis, there is limited information about their effects in younger patients. While ketoconazole can cause hepatic dysfunction and inhibit testosterone synthesis in adults, these effects have not been adequately evaluated in children. Fluconazole is primarily excreted by the kidneys, and itraconazole is metabolized in the liver; these drugs do not significantly affect testosterone or adrenocorticoid synthesis. On the basis of limited experience, coccidioidomycosis in pregnant women should be treated with amphotericin B, which has no apparent adverse effect on the fetus. Until more data are available, azoles should not be given to pregnant patients. The duration of therapy needed with the azoles has not been clearly defined and must be determined individually. Relapses have occurred in some patients after favorable clinical responses have been seen following therapy for >1 yr.

Surgery. Chronic pulmonary coccidioidal disease, cavitary or fibrocavitary, has not been consistently improved by the azoles or by amphotericin B. Pulmonary cavities frequently close spontaneously and are often best left alone, but when a cavity persists or is located peripherally, or when there is recurrent bleeding or rupture of the cavity through the pleura, excision should be considered. Coccidioidal cavities that have a fluid level or are accompanied by fever or hemoptysis should initially be treated with antibacterial antibiotics. Infrequently, bronchopleural fistulas or recurrent cavitation may occur as surgical complications; rarely, dissemination may result. When thoracic surgery is required, perioperative intravenous therapy with amphotericin B may be desirable.

Other surgical procedures include drainage of cold abscesses, removal of infected synovial membranes, and curettage or excision of osseous lesions. Local as well as systemic administration of amphotericin B can be used to treat coccidioidal osseous and articular disease.

PREVENTION. Avoidance of exposure to the arthroconidia, although often impractical, is the only means of preventing infection. An available whole killed cell vaccine did not prevent coccidioidomycosis in humans.

Ampel NM, Wieden MA, Galgiani JN: Coccidioidomycosis: A clinical update. Rev Infect Dis 11:897, 1989.

Bickel KD, Press BH, Hovey LM: Successful treatment of coccidioidomycosis osteomyelitis in an infant. Ann Plast Surg 30:462, 1993.

Boyle JO, Coulthard SW, Mandel RM: Laryngeal involvement in disseminated coccidioidomycosis. Arch Otolaryngol 117:433, 1991.

Dewsnups DH, Galgiani JN, Graybill SR, et al: Is it ever safe to stop azole therapy for *Coccidioides immitis* meningitis? Ann Intern Med 124:305, 1996.

Galgiani JN: Coccidioidomycosis. West J Med 159:153, 1993.

Harrison HR, Galgiani JN, Reynolds AF Jr, et al: Amphotericin B and imidazole therapy for coccidioidal meningitis in children. Pediatr Infect Dis 2:216, 1983.

Kafka JA, Catanzaro A: Disseminated coccidioidomycosis in children. J Pediatr 98:355, 1981.

Labadie EL, Hamilton RH: Survival improvement in coccidioidal meningitis by high-dose intrathecal amphotericin B. Arch Intern Med 146:2013, 1986.

Pappagianis D: Coccidioidomycosis. *In*: Balows A, et al (eds): Laboratory Diagnosis of Infectious Diseases. New York, Springer-Verlag, 1988.

Pappagianis D, Zimmer BL: Serology of coccidioidomycosis. Clin Microbiol Rev 3:247, 1990.

Peterson CM, Schuppert K, Kelly PC, et al: Coccidioidomycosis and pregnancy. Obstet Gynecol Surg 48:149, 1993.

Shafai T: Neonatal coccidioidomycosis in premature twins. Am J Dis Child 132:634, 1978.

Tucker RM, Williams PL, Arathoon EG, et al: Treatment of mycoses with itraconazole. Ann NY Acad Sci 544:451, 1988.

CHAPTER 237
Paracoccidioides brasiliensis

Stephen C. Aronoff

ETIOLOGY. Paracoccidioidomycosis (South American blastomycosis, Brazilian blastomycosis, Lutz-Splendore-Almeida blastomycosis) is an uncommon fungal infection in Central and South America caused by *Paracoccidioides brasiliensis*, a dimorphic fungus found in nature in the mycelial (saprophytic) form and in human tissue in the parasitic form as a yeast.

EPIDEMIOLOGY. *P. brasiliensis* is ecologically unique to Central and South America. Endemic outbreaks occur mainly in the tropical rainforests of Brazil with scattered cases in Argentina, Colombia, and Venezuela. No known animal vectors have been described. Infection typically follows inhalation of conidia; there is no evidence of person-to-person transmission.

CLINICAL MANIFESTATIONS. There are two clinical forms of disease. The acute form is rare, occurs almost exclusively in children and persons with immunodeficiency, and targets the mononuclear phagocytic system. Pulmonary symptoms are typically absent, although chest radiographs often show patchy, confluent, or nodular densities. Patients typically present acutely with fever, lymphadenopathy, hepatosplenomegaly, and gastrointestinal complaints as a result of intra-abdominal lymphadenopathy. Multiple areas of osteomyelitis, arthritis, and pericardial effusions can also occur. This form of the disease has a 25% mortality rate.

Adults develop a more chronic, less explosive illness that presents initially with flulike symptoms, fever, and weight loss. Pulmonary infection is the most common complaint and is seen primarily in adult agrarians. Dyspnea, cough, chest pain, and hemoptysis are among the typical presenting symptoms. Findings on physical examination are scant, although chest radiographs may show infiltrates that are out of proportion to the clinical findings. Mucositis involving the mouth and its structures as well as the nose may become manifest with localized pain, change in voice, or dysphagia. Lesions may extend beyond the oral cavity onto the skin. Generalized lymphadenopathy, hepatosplenomegaly, and Addison's disease may also be seen.

DIAGNOSIS. Demonstration of the fungus by potassium hydroxide wet mount preparation of sputum, exudate, or pus establishes the diagnosis in most patients. Gomori stain of biopsy material is also diagnostic. The fungus can also be recovered on Sabouraud-dextrose or yeast extract agar. Antibodies to *P. brasiliensis* can be demonstrated in the sera of most patients. Serial antibody titers and lymphocyte proliferative responses to fungal antigens are useful in monitoring the response to therapy. Skin testing with paracoccidioidin is not reliable, since one third of patients with active disease have test results that are nonreactive.

TREATMENT. Amphotericin B (total dose 3–6 g) followed by maintenance sulfonamide administration for a total of 18 mo is the traditional approach to therapy in adults; the outcome with 18 mo of ketoconazole therapy is comparable. Fluconazole (200–400 mg/24 hr for 6–18 mo) and itraconazole (50 mg/24 hr for 12 mo) are potentially useful alternatives, although comparative trials have not been performed.

Benard G, Orii NM, Marques HHS, et al: Severe acute paracoccidioidomycosis in children. Pediatr Infect Dis J 13:510, 1994.

Borelli D: A clinical trial of itraconazole in the treatment of deep mycoses and leishmaniasis. Rev Infect Dis 9 (suppl 1): S57, 1987.

Brummer E, Castenada E, Restrepo A: Paracoccidioidomycosis: An update. Clin Microbiol Rev 6:89, 1993.

Diaz M, Negroni R, Montero-Gei F, et al: A pan-American study of fluconazole therapy for deep mycoses in the immunocompetent host. Clin Infect Dis 14 (Suppl 1):S68, 1992.

Marques SA, Dillon NL, Franco MF, et al: Paracoccidioidomycosis: A comparative study of the evolutionary serologic, clinical and radiologic results for patients treated with ketoconazole or amphotericin B plus sulfonamides. Mycopathologia 89:19, 1985.

CHAPTER 238
Sporotrichosis (Sporothrix schenckii)

Stephen C. Aronoff

ETIOLOGY. Sporotrichosis is an uncommon chronic fungal infection caused by *Sporothrix schenckii*, a dimorphic fungus that is found in nature in the mycelial (saprophytic) form and in human tissue in the parasitic form as yeast.

EPIDEMIOLOGY. The fungus is ubiquitous, although it predominates in the Missouri and Mississippi river valleys and exists in its saprophytic form in living and rotting plant matter. Cutaneous sporotrichosis follows intradermal inoculation with spores after fomite contact (sphagnum moss, barberry, rosebushes, and some grasses) or animal contact (cats, dogs, rodents, insects, or fish). Sporotrichosis is often an occupational disease among farmers, gardeners, veterinarians, and pet owners. Human-to-human spread has not been reported. Disseminated infection is unusual but can occur in immunocompromised patients following ingestion or inhalation of spores.

PATHOGENESIS. Sporotrichosis is characterized histologically by noncaseating granulomas and microabscess formation. Oval or cigar-shaped forms are rarely seen in biopsy specimens because of the small number and size of the organisms and the lack of specific staining techniques.

CLINICAL MANIFESTATIONS. Cutaneous sporotrichosis is the most common form of disease in infants and children. Lymphocutaneous sporotrichosis accounts for >75% of reported cases and occurs after traumatic subcutaneous inoculation. After a variable and often prolonged incubation period (1–12 wk), an isolated, painless erythematous papule develops at the inoculation site, usually on an extremity. The initial lesion enlarges and ulcerates. Although the infection may remain limited to the inoculation site (fixed cutaneous sporotrichosis), satellite lesions follow lymphangitic spread and appear as multiple, tender, subcutaneous nodules tracking the lymphatic channels that drain the lesion. These secondary nodules are subcutaneous granulomas that adhere to the overlying skin and subsequently ulcerate. Sporotrichosis does not heal spontaneously, and these ulcerative lesions may persist for years if they are untreated. Systemic signs and symptoms are uncommon.

Extracutaneous sporotrichosis is rare in children; pulmonary sporotrichosis, meningitis, osteomyelitis, arthritis, and disseminated disease have been reported in immunocompromised adults.

DIAGNOSIS. Cutaneous and lymphocutaneous sporotrichosis must be differentiated from other causes of nodular lymphangitis: *Mycobacterium marinum* and other atypical mycobacteria, *Nocardia, Leishmania brasilieiensis,* tularemia, other systemic mycoses including coccidioidomycosis, melioidosis, and cutaneous anthrax. Definitive diagnosis requires isolation of the fungus from the site of infection. In cases of disseminated disease, demonstration of serum antibody against *S. schenckii*-related antigens is diagnostically useful.

TREATMENT. Although comparative trials and extensive experience in children are not available, itraconazole appears to be the treatment of choice for infections outside the central nervous system. Dosages of 100–200 mg/24 hr for up to 2 years may be required for complete resolution. Alternatively, younger children with cutaneous disease only may be treated with a saturated solution of potassium iodide (SSKI) given orally once daily begining at 5–10 drops three times per day. The dose is gradually advanced to 25 40 drops three times per day for children, or 40–50 drops three times per day for adolescents and adults. Therapy is continued until the cutaneous lesions have resolved, which usually takes 6–12 wk. Amphotericin B, usually in combination with flucytosine, is used for central nervous system infections.

Cabezas C, Bustamante B, et al: Treatment of cutaneous sporotrichosis with one daily dose of potassium iodide. Pediatr Infect Dis 15:352, 1996.

Kostman JR, DiNubile MJ: Nodular lymphangitis: A distinctive but often unrecognized syndrome. Ann Intern Med 118:883, 1993.

Kauffman CA: Old and new therapies for sporotrichosis. Clin Infect Dis 21:981, 1995.

Restrepo A, Robledo J, Gomez I, et al: Itraconazole therapy in lymphangitic and cutaneous sporotrichosis. Arch Dermatol 122:413, 1986.

Sharkey-Mathis PK, Kauffman CA, Graybill JR, et al: Treatment of sporotrichosis with itraconazole: NIAID mycoses study. Am J Med 95:279, 1993.

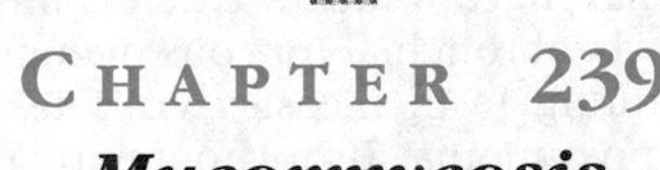

CHAPTER 239
Mucormycosis

Stephen C. Aronoff

ETIOLOGY. Mucormycosis (zygomycosis) refers to a group of opportunistic mycotic infections characterized by vascular invasion, thrombosis, and necrosis associated with dimorphic fungi of the class Zygomycetes and the order Mucorales. Members of the genera *Rhizopus, Absidia, Cunninghamella,* and *Mucor* are ubiquitous and are found in soil, in decayed plant or animal matter, and on moldy cheese, fruit, or bread. Colonies of Mucorales grow on laboratory media as fluffy white, gray, or brown molds.

EPIDEMIOLOGY. Exposure to fungal spores is common, but infections in children are rare. They occasionally cause disease in normal children after insect bites or penetrating injuries, especially on farms. Invasive disease is unusual and occurs almost exclusively in immunocompromised children including those with diabetes, persistent acidosis, or leukemia, those receiving corticosteroids, organ transplant recipients, and those with human immunodeficiency virus (HIV) infection. Person-to-person spread does not occur.

PATHOGENESIS. Rhinocerebral and pulmonary infections occur after spores are inhaled from the environment. Inhalation is followed by germination and local invasion of the nasal mucosa or lung, or both. In severely immunosuppressed individuals or those with poorly controlled diabetes, the fungus disseminates hematogenously. Cutaneous infection follows inoculation or contact with contaminated materials.

CLINICAL MANIFESTATIONS. Rhinocerebral mucormycosis occurs primarily in individuals with leukemia, diabetes mellitus, or Fanconi's anemia. Headache, retro-orbital pain, fever, and nasal discharge are the initial complaints in infected patients. Eye examination demonstrates periorbital edema, proptosis, ptosis, and ophthalmoplegia. The nasal discharge is often dark and bloody; examination of the nasal mucosa reveals black, necrotic areas. Extension beyond the nasal cavity is common. Destructive paranasal sinusitis with intracranial extension can be demonstrated by CT or MRI scanning. Brain abscesses can occur in patients with rhinocerebral infection that extends directly from the nasal cavity and sinuses, usually to the frontal or frontotemporal lobes, or in those with disseminated disease, which may involve the occipital lobe or brain stem. Gastrointestinal mucormycosis may occur as a complication of disseminated disease or as an isolated intestinal infection in diabetics, immunosuppressed or malnourished children, or preterm infants. Abdominal distention, pneumoperitoneum, or obstruction are often seen in children with perforated ulcers caused by *Mucor.*

Pulmonary mucormycosis is characterized by fever, tachypnea, and productive cough; pleuritic chest pain and hemoptysis occur variably. Signs of consolidation are found on physical examination. Lobar pneumonia or bilateral infiltrates may be seen on chest radiographs; pleural effusions are not rare.

Cutaneous mucormycosis can complicate burns or surgical wounds. An outbreak among preterm infants followed the use of contaminated wooden tongue depressors to immobilize the extremities. Infection presents as an erythematous papule that ulcerates, leaving a black necrotic center.

DIAGNOSIS. Identification of the fungus histologically or recovery of the fungus by culture is required for diagnosis. In lung biopsy specimens and other tissue samples, Mucorales appear as thick-walled, nonseptate, right angle-branched hyphae when stained with silver. At gastrointestinal endoscopy, the lesions appear as black ulcers with deep erythematous margins. Vascular invasion is a hallmark of the disease. These fungi may also be identified in secretions by suspending the clinical material in a solution of 20% potassium hydrochloride before microscopic examination is performed. The fungi may be grown on standard laboratory media from sputum, bronchoalveolar lavage fluid, skin lesions, or biopsy material.

TREATMENT. The optimal therapy for mucormycosis in children has not been established. Rhinocerebral mucormycosis and brain abscesses caused by Mucorales have high fatality rates.

Correction of the underlying disease, if possible, is a major therapeutic requirement. Extensive surgical debridement and high-dose amphotericin B therapy (1–1.5 mg/kg/24 hr to a total dose of 70 mg/kg) have been associated with successful outcomes. Hyperbaric oxygen has been used as an adjunctive therapy. Pulmonary mucormycosis has been treated successfully in adults with intermediate doses of amphotericin B (30 mg/kg total dose). Cutaneous mucormycosis requires local debridement and intermediate dosages of amphotericin B (0.5–1 mg/kg/24 hr to a total dose of 30 mg/kg).

Cohen-Abbo A, Bozeman PM, Patrick CC: *Cunninghamella* infections: Review and report of two cases of *Cunninghamella* in immunocompromised children. Clin Infect Dis 17:173, 1993.

Kline MW: Mucormycosis in children: Review of the literature and report of cases. Pediatr Infect Dis J 4:672, 1985.

Mitchell SJ, Gray J, Morgan MEI, et al: Nosocomial infection with *Rhizopus microsporus* in preterm infants: Association with wooden tongue depressors. Lancet 348:441, 1996.

Mooney JE, Wanger A: Mucormycosis of the gastrointestinal tract in children: Report of a case and review of the literature. Pediatr Infect Dis J 12:872, 1993.

Shah PD, Peters KR, Reuman PD: Recovery from rhinocerebral mucormycosis with carotid artery occlusion: A pediatric case and review of the literature. Pediatr Infect Dis 16:68, 1997.

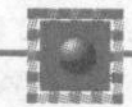

SECTION 12

Viral Infections

CHAPTER 240

Measles

Yvonne Maldonado

Measles (rubeola) is an important childhood disease that was historically widespread but is now very infrequent. It is an acute viral infection characterized by a final stage with a maculopapular rash erupting successively over the neck and face, body, arms, and legs and accompanied by a high fever.

ETIOLOGY. Measles virus, the cause of measles, is an RNA virus of the genus *Morbillivirus* in the family Paramyxoviridae. Only one serotype is known. During the prodromal period and for a short time after the rash appears, it is found in nasopharyngeal secretions, blood, and urine. It can remain active for at least 34 hr at room temperature.

EPIDEMIOLOGY. Measles is endemic throughout the world. In the past, epidemics tended to occur irregularly, appearing in the spring in large cities at 2–4 yr intervals as new groups of susceptible children were exposed. It is rarely subclinical. Prior to the use of measles vaccine, the age of peak incidence was 5–10 yr. Individuals born before 1957 are considered to be immune from natural infection.

In the United States, during the 1980s the incidence of measles rose, probably due to inadequate vaccination as well as vaccine failure. The reported numbers of measles cases dropped by >99.7% from 894, 134 cases in 1941 by >99.7% to an all-time low of 138 cases in 1997, probably as a result of intensified efforts to ensure appropriate vaccination. Measles now occurs most often in unimmunized preschool-aged children, as occasional epidemics in high schools and colleges, and as imported cases. Because measles is still a common disease in many countries, infective persons entering this country may infect United States residents, and Americans traveling abroad risk exposure there. More than half of the recent cases seen in the United States are imported or due to exposure to imported cases.

The Pan American Health Organization has established the goal of eliminating measles from the Western hemisphere by the year 2000. The many similarities among the biologic features of measles and smallpox suggest the possibility that measles might be eradicated. These features are (1) a distinctive rash as a sentinel marker, (2) no animal reservoir, (3) no vector, (4) seasonal occurrence with disease-free periods, (5) no transmissible latent virus, (6) one serotype, and (7) an effective vaccine. A prevalence of more than 90% immunization of infants has been shown to produce disease-free zones.

Transmission. Measles is very contagious; approximately 90% of susceptible family contacts acquire the disease. Maximal dissemination of virus occurs by droplet spray during the prodromal period (catarrhal stage). Transmission to susceptible contacts often occurs prior to diagnosis of the original case.

Infants acquire immunity transplacentally from mothers who have had measles or measles immunization. This immunity is usually complete for the first 4–6 mo of life and disappears at a variable rate. Although maternal antibody levels are generally undetectable in the infant by the usual tests performed after 9 mo of age, some protection persists, which may interfere with immunization administered to infants prior to 12 mo of age. Most women of childbearing age in the United States now have measles immunity by means of immunization rather than disease. Some studies now suggest that infants of mothers with measles vaccine-induced immunity lose passive antibody at a younger age than infants of mothers who had measles infection. Infants of mothers who are susceptible to measles have no measles immunity and may contract the disease with the mother before or after delivery.

PATHOGENESIS. The essential lesion of measles is found in the skin; in the mucous membranes of the nasopharynx, bronchi, and intestinal tract; and in the conjunctivae. Serous exudate and proliferation of mononuclear cells and a few polymorphonuclear cells occur around the capillaries. Hyperplasia of lymphoid tissue usually occurs, particularly in the appendix, where multinucleated giant cells of up to 100 μm in diameter (Warthin-Finkeldey reticuloendothelial giant cells) may be found. In the skin, the reaction is particularly notable about the sebaceous glands and hair follicles. Koplik spots consist of serous exudate and proliferation of endothelial cells similar to those in the skin lesions. A general inflammatory reaction of the buccal and pharyngeal mucosa extends into the lymphoid tissue and the tracheobronchial mucous membrane. Interstitial pneumonitis resulting from measles virus takes the form of Hecht giant cell pneumonia. Bronchopneumonia may be due to secondary bacterial infection. In fatal cases of encephalomyelitis, perivascular demyelinization occurs in areas of the brain and spinal cord. In subacute sclerosing panencephalitis (SSPE), there may be degeneration of the cortex and white matter with intranuclear and intracytoplasmic inclusion bodies (see Chapter 240.1).

CLINICAL MANIFESTATIONS. Measles has three clinical stages: an incubation stage, a prodromal stage with an enanthem (Koplik spots) and mild symptoms, and a final stage with a maculopapular rash accompanied by high fever. The incubation period lasts approximately 10–12 days to the first prodromal symptoms and another 2–4 days to the appearance of the rash; rarely, it may be as short as 6–10 days. The temperature may increase slightly 9–10 days from the date of infection and then subside for 24 hr or so. The patient may transmit the virus by the 9th–10th day after exposure and occasionally as early as the 7th day, before the illness can be diagnosed.

The prodromal phase usually lasts 3–5 days and is characterized by a low-grade to moderate fever, a dry cough, coryza, and conjunctivitis. These symptoms nearly always precede the appearance of Koplik spots, the pathognomonic sign of measles, by 2–3 days. An enanthem or red mottling is usually present on the hard and soft palates. Koplik spots are grayish white dots, usually as small as grains of sand, that have slight, reddish areolae; occasionally they are hemorrhagic. They tend to occur opposite the lower molars but may spread irregularly over the rest of the buccal mucosa. Rarely they are found within the midportion of the lower lip, on the palate, and on the lacrimal caruncle. They appear and disappear rapidly, usually within 12–18 hr. As they fade a red, spotty discoloration of the mucosa may remain. The conjunctival inflammation and photophobia may suggest measles before Koplik spots appear. In particular, a transverse line of conjunctival inflammation, sharply demarcated along the eyelid margin, may be of diagnostic assistance in the prodromal stage. As the entire conjunctiva becomes involved, the line disappears.

Occasionally, the prodromal phase may be severe, being ushered in by a sudden high fever, sometimes with convulsions and even pneumonia. Usually the coryza, fever, and cough are increasingly severe up to the time the rash has covered the body.

The temperature rises abruptly as the rash appears and often reaches 40°C (104°F) or higher. In uncomplicated cases, as the rash appears on the legs and feet the symptoms subside rapidly within about 2 days usually with an abrupt drop in temperature to normal. Patients up to this point may appear desperately ill, but within 24 hr after the temperature drops, they appear essentially well.

The rash usually starts as faint macules on the upper lateral parts of the neck, behind the ears, along the hairline, and on the posterior parts of the cheek. The individual lesions become increasingly maculopapular as the rash spreads rapidly over the entire face, neck, upper arms, and upper part of the chest within approximately the first 24 hr (Fig. 240–1). During the succeeding 24 hr it spreads over the back, abdomen, entire arm, and thighs. As it finally reaches the feet on the 2nd–3rd day, it begins to fade on the face. The rash fades downward in the same sequence in which it appeared. The severity of the disease is directly related to the extent and confluence of the rash. In mild measles the rash tends not to be confluent, and in very mild cases there are few, if any, lesions on the legs. In severe cases the rash is confluent, the skin is completely covered, including the palms and soles, and the face is swollen and disfigured.

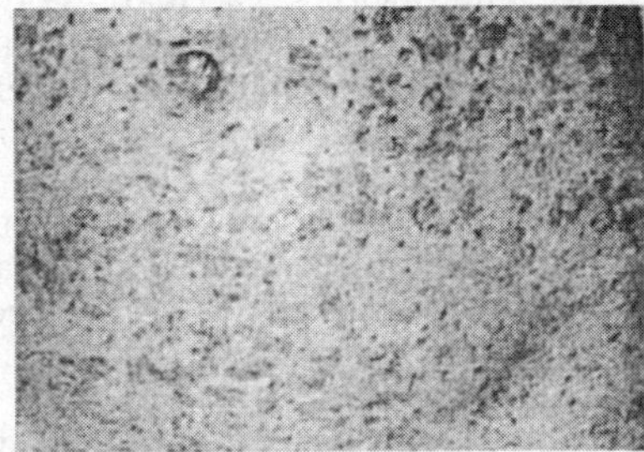

Figure 240–1 Maculopapular rash of measles. (From Korting GW: Hautkrankheiten bei Kindern und Jugendlichen, 3rd ed. Stuttgart, FK Schattauer Verlag, 1982.) See also color section.

The rash is often slightly hemorrhagic; in severe cases with a confluent rash, petechiae may be present in large numbers, and there may be extensive ecchymoses. Itching is generally slight. As the rash fades, branny desquamation and brownish discoloration occur and then disappear within 7–10 days.

The appearance of the rash may vary markedly. Infrequently a slight urticarial, faint macular, or scarlatiniform rash may appear during the early prodromal stage, disappearing in advance of the typical rash. Complete absence of rash is rare except in patients to whom immune globulin products have been administered during the incubation period, in some patients with HIV infection, and occasionally in infants <9 mo who have appreciable levels of maternal antibody. In the hemorrhagic type of measles (black measles), bleeding may occur from the mouth, nose, or bowel. In mild cases the rash may be less macular and more nearly pinpoint, somewhat resembling that of scarlet fever or rubella.

Lymph nodes at the angle of the jaw and in the posterior cervical region are usually enlarged, and slight splenomegaly may be noted. Mesenteric lymphadenopathy may cause abdominal pain. Characteristic pathologic changes of measles in the mucosa of the appendix may cause obliteration of the lumen and symptoms of appendicitis. Changes of this type tend to subside as the Koplik spots disappear. Otitis media, bronchopneumonia, and gastrointestinal symptoms such as diarrhea and vomiting are more common in infants and small children (especially if they are malnourished) than in older children.

Atypical Measles. Atypical measles occurs in recipients of killed measles virus vaccine, which was used from 1963 to 1967, who later come in contact with wild-type measles virus. Measles prodromal symptoms, except for fever, occur infrequently. Atypical measles is distinguished by severe headache, severe abdominal pain, often with vomiting, myalgias, respiratory symptoms, pneumonia with pleural effusion, and an exanthem that is very different from the typical measles rash. The atypical measles rash first appears on the palms, wrists, soles, and ankles, and progresses in a centripetal direction. The lesions are initially maculopapular but become vesicular and later may become purpuric or hemorrhagic. Koplik spots rarely appear in patients with atypical measles.

DIAGNOSIS. The diagnosis is usually apparent from the characteristic clinical picture; laboratory confirmation is rarely needed. During the prodromal stage multinucleated giant cells can be demonstrated in smears of the nasal mucosa. Antibodies become detectable when the rash appears; testing of acute and convalescent sera shows the diagnostic seroconversion or fourfold increase in titer. Measles virus can be isolated by tissue culture in human embryonic or rhesus monkey kidney cells. Cytopathic changes, visible in 5–10 days, consist of multinucleated giant cells with intranuclear inclusions.

The white blood cell count tends to be low with a relative lymphocytosis. Cerebrospinal fluid in patients with measles encephalitis usually shows an increase in protein and a small increase in lymphocytes. The glucose level is normal.

The diagnosis of measles is frequently delayed in adults because practitioners providing health care for adults are not used to encountering the disease and rarely include it in the differential diagnosis. The clinical picture is similar to that seen in children. Liver involvement, with abdominal pain, mild to moderate elevation of aspartate aminotransferase (AST) levels, and occasionally jaundice, is common in adults.

Differential Diagnosis. The rash of rubeola must be differentiated from that of rubella; roseola infantum (human herpesvirus 6); infections resulting from echovirus, coxsackievirus, and adenovirus; infectious mononucleosis; toxoplasmosis; meningococcemia; scarlet fever; rickettsial diseases; Kawasaki disease; serum sickness; and drug rashes.

Koplik spots are pathognomonic for measles. The rashes of rubella and of enteroviral and adenoviral infections tend to be less striking than that of measles, as do the degree of fever and severity of illness. The rash of roseola infantum appears as the fever disappears, whereas in measles they appear concomitantly. Although cough is present in many rickettsial infections, the rash usually spares the face, which is characteristically involved in measles. The absence of administration of a drug in the history usually serves to exclude serum sickness or drug rashes. Meningococcemia may be accompanied by a rash that is somewhat similar to that of measles, but cough and conjunctivitis are usually absent. In acute meningococcemia the rash is characteristically petechial and purpuric. The diffuse, finely papular rash of scarlet fever has a "goose flesh" texture on an erythematous base and is relatively easy to differentiate from the maculopapular rash of measles.

TREATMENT. There is no specific antiviral therapy; treatment is entirely supportive. Antipyretics (acetaminophen or ibuprofen) for fever, bed rest, and maintenance of an adequate fluid intake are indicated. Humidification of the room may be necessary for those with laryngitis or an excessively irritating cough, and it is best to keep the room comfortably warm rather than cool. Patients with photophobia should be protected from exposure to strong light. The complications of otitis media and pneumonia require appropriate antimicrobial therapy.

Complications such as encephalitis, subacute sclerosing panencephalitis, giant cell pneumonia, and disseminated intravascular coagulation must be assessed individually. Good supportive care is essential. Immune globulin and corticosteroids are of limited value. Currently available antiviral compounds are not effective.

Vitamin A. Hyporetinemia is present in over 90% of cases of measles in Africa and in approximately 22–72% of children with measles in the United States; there is an apparent inverse correlation between retinol concentration and measles severity. Treatment with oral vitamin A reduces morbidity and mortality in children with severe measles in the developing world. Although data to determine the need for vitamin A supplementation for children with measles in the United States are incomplete, the American Academy of Pediatrics recommends consideration of vitamin A supplementation for children 6 mo to 2 yr of age who are hospitalized for measles and its complications and for children >6 mo of age with measles and: immunodeficiency; ophthalmologic evidence of vitamin A deficiency (e.g., night blindness, Bitot's spots. or evidence of xerophthalmia); impaired intestinal absorption (e.g., biliary obstruction, short-bowel syndrome, cystic fibrosis); moderate to severe malnutrition; or recent immigration from areas where high mortality rates from measles have been observed. The recommended regimen is a single dose of 100,000 IU orally for children 6 mo to 1 yr, and 200,000 IU for children ≥1 yr of age. Children with ophthalmologic evidence of vitamin A deficiency should be given additional doses the next day and 4 wk later.

COMPLICATIONS. The chief complications of measles are otitis media, pneumonia, and encephalitis. Noma of the cheeks may occur in rare instances. Gangrene elsewhere appears to be secondary to purpura fulminans or disseminated intravascular coagulation following measles. Interstitial pneumonia may be caused by the measles virus (giant cell pneumonia). Measles pneumonia in HIV-infected patients is often fatal and is not always accompanied by rash. Bacterial superinfection and bronchopneumonia is more frequent, however, usually with pneumococcus, group A *Streptococcus*, *Staphylococcus aureus*, and *Haemophilus influenzae* type b. Laryngitis, tracheitis, and bronchitis are common and may be due to the virus alone.

Measles may exacerbate underlying *Mycobacterium tuberculosis* infection. There may also be a temporary loss of hypersensitivity reaction to tuberculin skin testing.

Myocarditis is an infrequent serious complication, although transient electrocardiographic changes may be relatively common.

Neurologic complications are more common in measles than in any of the other exanthematous diseases. The incidence of encephalomyelitis is estimated to be 1–2/1,000 cases of measles. There is no correlation between the severity of the rash illness and that of the neurologic involvement, or between the severity of the initial encephalitic process and the prognosis. Infrequently, encephalitic involvement is manifest in the pre-eruptive period, but more often its onset occurs 2–5 days after the appearance of the rash. The cause of measles encephalitis remains controversial. It has been suggested that direct viral invasion may be operative for encephalitis early in the course of the disease, although measles virus has rarely been isolated from brain tissue. Encephalitis that occurs later is predominantly demyelinating and may reflect an immunologic reaction. In this demyelinating type the symptoms and course do not differ from those of other parainfectious encephalitides. Fatal encephalitis has occurred in children receiving immunosuppressive treatment. Other central nervous system complications, including Guillain-Barré syndrome, hemiplegia, cerebral thrombophlebitis, and retrobulbar neuritis, occur rarely.

PROGNOSIS. Case fatality rates in the United States have decreased in recent years to low levels for all age groups, largely because of improved socioeconomic conditions but also because of effective antibacterial therapy for the treatment of secondary bacterial infections. Despite the decline in measles cases and fatalities in the United States, the case fatality rate is still 1–2/1,000 cases. Deaths are primarily due to pneumonia or secondary bacterial infections. In developing countries measles frequently occurs in infants; possibly because of concomitant malnutrition, the disease is very severe in these locations and has a high mortality.

When measles is introduced into a highly susceptible population, the results may be disastrous. Such an occurrence in the Faroe Islands in 1846 resulted in the deaths of about one fourth, nearly 2,000, of the total population. At Ungava Bay, Canada, where 99% of 900 persons contracted measles, the mortality rate was 7%.

PREVENTION. Isolation precautions, especially in hospitals and other institutions, should be maintained from the 7th day after exposure until 5 days after the rash has appeared.

Vaccine. The initial measles immunization, usually as measles-mumps-rubella (MMR) vaccine, is recommended at 12–15 mo of age but may be given for measles postexposure and outbreak prophylaxis as early as 6 mo of age. A second immunization, also as MMR, is recommended routinely at 4–6 yr of age but may be administered at any time during childhood provided at least 4 wk have elapsed since the first dose. Children who have not previously received the second dose should be immunized by 11–12 yr of age. Adolescents entering college or the work force should have received a second measles immunization.

The response to live measles vaccine may be abrogated if immune globulin has been recently administered (see Chapter 301). Anergy to tuberculin skin testing may develop and can persist for >1 mo after measles vaccination. Children with active tuberculous infection should be receiving antituberculosis treatment when measles vaccine is administered. A tuberculin test prior to or concurrent with active immunization against measles is desirable.

Measles vaccine is not recommended for pregnant women, children with primary immunodeficiency, untreated tuberculosis, cancer, or organ transplantation, those receiving long-term immunosuppressive therapy, or severely immunocompromised HIV-infected children.

Postexposure Prophylaxis. Passive immunization with immune globulin is effective for prevention and attenuation of measles within 6 days of exposure. Susceptible household and hospital contacts who are <12 mo of age or who are pregnant should receive immune globulin (0.25 mL/kg; maximum: 15 mL) intramuscularly as soon as possible after exposure, but within 5 days. Immunocompromised persons should receive immune globulin (0.5 mL/kg; maximum: 15 mL) intramuscularly regardless of immunization status. Infants ≤6 mo of age born to nonimmune mothers should receive immune globulin; infants ≤6 mo of age born to immune mothers are considered protected by maternal antibody. Susceptible children 6–12 mo of age should also be vaccinated; this vaccination does not count as one of the 2 required measles vaccinations. Susceptible children ≥12 mo of age should receive vaccine alone within 72 hr. Pregnant women and immunocompromised persons should receive immune globulin but not vaccine.

240.1 Subacute Sclerosing Panencephalitis

ETIOLOGY. Subacute sclerosing panencephalitis (Dawson's encephalitis) is a chronic encephalitis caused by persistent measles virus infection of the central nervous system. Dawson was the first to describe it clearly and to postulate a viral cause. Subsequently, measles virus was isolated from the brains of patients with subacute sclerosing panencephalitis (SSPE).

EPIDEMIOLOGY. SSPE is a rare disease that occurs worldwide. The disease has been diagnosed in patients aged 6 mo to older than 30 yr of age, but it affects primarily children and young adolescents. In more than 85% of cases, onset occurs from 5–15 yr of age. Infection with measles before the age of 18 mo seems to increase the risk of SSPE substantially. The risk among boys is more than twice that among girls, and it is higher among rural children than city children, children with two or more siblings, and children of lower socioeconomic status. SSPE was once especially common in the southeastern United States, the Ohio River valley, and some New England states. Recently, cases have been more common in the western United States and in New York City, especially among Hispanic immigrant children. Exposure to birds and other animals has been reported with abnormal frequency in the histories of patients with SSPE; the reason is not clear.

The annual incidence of SSPE in the United States fell markedly from 0.61 cases per 1 million persons younger than 20 yr in 1960 to 0.06 cases per 1 million in 1980. Since 1982 only five or fewer new cases in the entire country have been registered with the U.S. National SSPE Registry each year. The decrease roughly parallels the progressive decline in the annual number of measles cases diagnosed since the introduction of live attenuated measles vaccine in the United States in 1963. The risk of SSPE has been estimated at 8.5 SSPE cases per 1 million cases of measles for a 6-yr period, during which the estimated risk after measles vaccination was only 0.7 cases per 1 million doses of vaccine. The overwhelming advantage of measles vaccination in preventing SSPE is clear.

In a recent case control study, the lack of vaccination was a highly significant risk factor for SSPE, and in a survey in England and Wales the relative risk of SSPE after measles infection was 29 times that of the risk of SSPE after measles vaccination. In cases occurring in vaccinated children, it has not been determined whether SSPE resulted from persistent infection with the attenuated measles virus of the vaccine, from undiagnosed wild-type measles infection preceding vaccination, or from vaccine failure and subsequent undiagnosed measles. SSPE continues to occur in areas of the world where measles remains unchecked and may be anticipated to increase wherever compliance with vaccination protocols diminishes.

Children with SSPE generally have a history of typical measles with full recovery several years before the onset of neurologic disease. Measles may have been either mild or severe. Some patients with SSPE have had measles pneumonia, but none have had a history of typical measles encephalitis. The mean interval between measles and onset of SSPE was formerly about 7 yr, but recently it has increased to 12 yr. In vaccinated patients without a history of measles, the mean interval between vaccination and onset of SSPE was 5 yr before 1980 and 7.7 yr between 1980 and 1986.

PATHOGENESIS. The histopathology of SSPE consists of inflammation, necrosis, and repair. Brain biopsy performed in the early stages of SSPE shows mild inflammation of the meninges and a panencephalitis involving cortical and subcortical gray matter as well as white matter, with cuffs of plasma cells and lymphocytes around blood vessels (Fig. 240–2) and increased numbers of glia throughout. Neuronal loss may not be marked until later in the course of the illness, when loss of myelin secondary to neuronal degeneration may be apparent. Intranuclear inclusion bodies surrounded by clear halos (Cowdry type A) may be seen within the nuclei of neurons, astrocytes, and oligodendrocytes. On electron microscopy, the inclusions are seen to contain tubular structures typical of the nucleocapsids of paramyxoviruses. Measles viral antigens can be demonstrated by labeled antibody techniques within the inclusions as well as in cells without inclusions. Lesions may be unevenly distributed throughout the brain, and biopsy is not always diagnostic.

The same findings of inclusion-body panencephalitis are generally present at autopsy; however, late in the disease it may be difficult to find typical areas of inflammation, and the main histopathologic changes are necrosis and gliosis. The disease is believed to begin in the cortical gray matter, progressing then to the subcortical white and gray matter (myoclonus probably results from extrapyramidal involvement) and finally to the lower structures. Although persistent infection of lymphoid tissues with measles virus has been reported, these show no pathologic changes.

It has been proposed that viral mutation may render the measles virus more likely to establish persistent CNS infection, and multiple mutations have been found in isolates from patients with SSPE. However, no consistent genomic abnormalities have been identified in those isolates, and clusters of SSPE cases suggestive of strains of special virulence have been described only rarely. It has also been theorized that patients with SSPE have subtle predisposing immune deficiency; the markedly increased risk of SSPE after measles in infancy suggests that either immunologic immaturity or persistence of maternal antibodies to measles virus is involved in the later occurrence of the disease.

Complete measles virus particles are not found in the brains

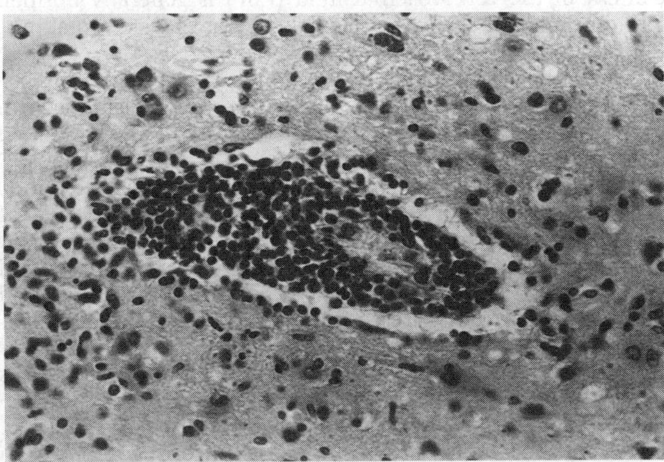

Figure 240–2 A cuff of inflammatory cells surrounds a blood vessel in the cerebral cortex of a child with subacute sclerosing panencephalitis. (Courtesy of Janice Stevens, MD, National Institute of Mental Health, and Peggy Swoveland, MD, University of Maryland School of Medicine.)

of patients with SSPE, and the matrix (M) protein required for the final assembly and budding of virus from the host cells is missing not only from the brain tissue of patients but also from cells cultured from their brains; however, the full complement of genetic material needed to code for all proteins, including the M protein, is present and functional. Several studies have suggested that M proteins are encoded but that because of a variety of mutations they cannot bind to nucleocapsid, resulting in accumulation of incomplete measles virus that cannot be cleared either by antibodies or by cell-mediated immunity.

CLINICAL MANIFESTATIONS. The clinical picture of SSPE tends to be quite stereotypical; almost 70% of cases have an acute, subacute, or chronic progressive course; fewer than 10% have remissions. The onset is usually insidious and is marked by subtle changes in behavior and deterioration of schoolwork; this is followed by more overtly bizarre behavior and finally by frank dementia.

There is no fever, photophobia, or other findings of acute encephalitis except for occasional complaints of headache. Diffuse neurologic disease becomes progressively more severe. The appearance of massive, repetitive myoclonic jerks, generally symmetric, involving especially the axial musculature and occurring at 5–10 sec intervals, marks the onset of the second clinical stage of SSPE. The myoclonic jerks appear to be abnormal movements rather than epileptic seizures, but true convulsions can also occur at any stage of the illness. In addition to myoclonic jerks, which tend to disappear as the disease progresses, a variety of other abnormal movements and dystonias have been observed. Cerebellar ataxia may occur. Retinopathy and optic atrophy may appear, sometimes even before the behavioral changes. Dementia progresses to stupor and coma, sometimes with autonomic insufficiency. Patients may be rigid or spastic with decorticate postures, or they may be flaccid.

The speed of progression is highly variable, but in at least 60% of patients the course is inexorable and relatively rapid. The total duration of illness may be as short as a few months, but most patients survive for 1–3 yr after diagnosis, with a mean of about 18 mo. Occasional patients show some spontaneous improvement and live for more than 10 yr. In recent years, the few patients diagnosed with SSPE in the United States have tended to have a relatively long survival, perhaps because of improvements in chronic care.

DIAGNOSIS. Blood tests are normal except for elevated titers of antibodies to measles virus; antibodies are of the immunoglobulin (Ig) G and IgM classes and are directed against all the component proteins of measles virus except the M protein. Cell content of the cerebrospinal fluid (CSF) is generally normal, although stained sediments may show plasma cells. Total protein content of the CSF is normal or only slightly elevated; however, the gamma globulin fraction is greatly elevated (usually comprising at least 20% of total protein), resulting in a paretic type of colloidal gold curve. When the CSF is examined by electrophoresis or isoelectric focusing, oligoclonal bands of Ig are often observed. IgG and IgM antibodies to measles virus, not normally found in unconcentrated CSF, make up most of the Ig, and these can often be detected in dilutions of 1:8 or more. The complement fixation test has been especially useful for demonstrating antibodies in CSF, but hemagglutination inhibition, immunofluorescence, and other serologic tests, including enzyme-labeled immunosorbent assays (ELISA), are also satisfactory. The normal ratio of titer in serum to CSF is reduced (<200) for measles antibodies, whereas serum-CSF ratios are normal for other viral antibodies and for albumin, indicating that the increased amounts of measles antibodies in the CSF of patients with SSPE result from synthesis within the nervous system and that the blood-brain barrier is normal.

Early in the course of disease, the electroencephalogram (EEG) may be normal or show only moderate nonspecific slowing. In the myoclonic stage, most patients with SSPE have "suppression-burst episodes" in which high-amplitude slow and sharp waves recur at intervals of 3–5 sec on a slow background; however, this pattern is not unique to SSPE. Later in the illness, the EEG becomes increasingly disorganized and shows high-amplitude, random dysrhythmic slowing; in terminal disease, the amplitude may fall.

CT or MRI scans of patients with SSPE may show variable cortical atrophy and ventricular enlargement, and there may be focal or multifocal low-density lesions in the white matter. However, these studies may be normal, especially early in the disease.

Brain biopsy is no longer needed to diagnose SSPE. When performed, it often shows the typical histopathologic findings described earlier. Examination of frozen sections by immunofluorescence techniques may demonstrate the presence of measles viral antigens. Persistence of measles virus infection in cultures may be demonstrated by labeled antibody techniques before the complete virus appears. Many specimens fail to yield complete virus. Modifications of the polymerase chain reaction can detect various regions of the measles virus RNA in frozen and even paraffin-embedded brain tissue specimens of patients with SSPE. Nucleic acid hybridization techniques have also been used to demonstrate the measles viral genome.

Differential Diagnosis. It is most important to rule out potentially treatable illnesses such as bacterial infections and tumors. The diverse cerebral storage diseases and nonstorage poliodystrophies, leukodystrophies, and demyelinating diseases of childhood can also produce progressive dementia with seizures and paralysis resembling SSPE. Early in the course of illness, SSPE must be distinguished from atypical acute viral encephalitides. Other slow viral infections, such as Creutzfeldt-Jakob disease (CJD) and progressive rubella panencephalitis, must be considered in appropriate age groups. The presence of a typical EEG pattern suggests SSPE, as do unusually high levels of measles antibodies in serum. The diagnosis is practically confirmed if measles antibodies are detected in CSF.

The persistent measles infection seen in SSPE does not result in complete virus particles. Patients with SSPE, therefore, pose no hazard of infection to others, and no special precautions need ordinarily be taken. Blood precautions might be justified under special circumstances.

TREATMENT. Administration of inosiplex (100 mg/kg/24 hr) may prolong survival and may produce some clinical improvement in the degree of disability. Other treatments have been ineffective. The use of anticonvulsants, maintenance of nutritional status, prompt treatment of secondary bacterial infections, physical therapy, and other supportive care may also prolong survival and improve the quality of life for the patient and family. Information on current therapeutic trials can be obtained from the U.S. National SSPE Registry (Dr. Paul R. Dyken, Institute for Research in Childhood Neurodegenerative Diseases, Mobile, Alabama; Telephone 334-478-6424).

COMPLICATIONS. Patients with SSPE have the usual secondary complications associated with incapacitating neurologic diseases, such as recurrent pneumonias and decubitus ulcers.

PROGNOSIS. Few patients live for >3 yr after the diagnosis of SSPE, and those who do survive longer are usually disabled.

PREVENTION. Measles vaccination is the most important measure to prevent SSPE.

American Academy of Pediatrics, Committee on Infectious Diseases: Age of routine administration of the second dose of measles-mumps-rubella vaccine. Pediatrics 101:129, 1998.

American Academy of Pediatrics, Committee on Infectious Diseases: Vitamin A treatment of measles. Pediatrics 91:1014, 1993.

Aicardi J: Acute measles encephalitis in children with immunosuppression. Pediatrics 59:232, 1977.

Brem J: Koplik spots for the record: An illustrated historical note. Clin Pediatr 11:161, 1972.

Centers for Disease Control and Prevention: Advances in global measles control

and elimination. Summary of the 1997 international meeting. MMWR 47 (RR-11):1, 1998.
Gustafson TL, Brunell PA, Lievens, AW, et al: Measles outbreak in a "fully immunized" secondary school population. N Engl J Med 316:771, 1987.
Hussey G, Klein N: A randomized trial of vitamin A in children with severe measles. N Engl J Med 323:160, 1990.
Jabbour JT, Duenas DA, Sever JL, et al: Epidemiology of subacute sclerosing panencephalitis (SSPE). A report of the SSPE registry. JAMA 220:959, 1972.
Markowitz LE, Preblud SR, Orenstein WA, et al: Patterns of transmission in measles outbreaks in the United States, 1985–1986. N Engl J Med 320:75, 1989.
Mathias RG, Meeklson WC, Arcand TA, et al: The role of secondary vaccine failures in measles outbreaks. Am J Public Health 79:474, 1989.
McLaughlin M, Thomas P, Onorato I, et al: Live virus vaccines in human immunodeficiency virus-infected children: A retrospective study. Pediatrics 82:229, 1988.
Modlin JF: Epidemiologic studies of measles, measles vaccine, SSPE. Pediatrics 59:505, 1977.
Payne FE, Baublis JV, Itabashi HH: Isolation of measles virus from cell cultures of brain from a patient with subacute sclerosing panencephalitis. N Engl J Med 281:11, 1969.
Quiambao BP, Gatchalian SR, Halonen P, et al: Coinfection is common in measles-associated pneumonia. Pediatr Infect Dis J 17:89, 1998.
Vitek CR, Redd SC, Redd SB, et al: Trends in importation of measles to the United States, 1986–1994. JAMA 277:1952, 1997.

CHAPTER 241
Rubella

Yvonne Maldonado

Rubella (German or three-day measles) is an important childhood disease that was historically widespread but is now very infrequent. It is an acute viral infection ordinarily characterized by mild constitutional symptoms, a rash similar to that of mild rubeola or scarlet fever, and enlargement and tenderness of the postoccipital, retroauricular, and posterior cervical lymph nodes. Rubella in early pregnancy may cause the congenital rubella syndrome, a serious multisystem disease with a wide spectrum of clinical expression and sequelae.

ETIOLOGY. Rubella virus, the cause of rubella, is an RNA virus of the genus *Rubivirus* in the family Togaviridae.

EPIDEMIOLOGY. Humans are the only natural host of rubella virus, which is spread either by oral droplet or transplacentally to the fetus causing congenital infection. It is distributed worldwide and affects both sexes equally. Before introduction of the rubella vaccine in 1969, pandemics of rubella occurred every 6–9 yr, with most cases occurring in the spring. In 1964–1965, an epidemic in the United States caused more than 12 million cases of rubella and an additional 20,000 infants with congenital rubella syndrome. The peak incidence of rubella was in children 5–14 yr of age. Now most cases occur in susceptible teenagers and young adults. Outbreaks have been reported among college students and in unvaccinated populations, such as Amish communities. In closed populations, such as institutions and military barracks, almost 100% of susceptible individuals may become infected. In family settings the spread of the virus is less; 50–60% of susceptible family members acquire the disease.

Indigenous rubella and congenital rubella syndrome have been targeted for elimination in the United States by the year 2000. From a peak of 57,686 cases in 1969 through 1989, the numbers of annual reported cases have decreased, with a slight resurgence during 1990–1991, by 99.7% to 128–192 cases of rubella and 4–11 cases of congenital rubella syndrome annually from 1992 to 1997.

During clinical illness the virus is present in nasopharyngeal secretions, blood, feces, and urine. Virus has been recovered from the nasopharynx 7 days before exanthem and 7–8 days after its disappearance. Patients with subclinical disease are also infectious.

PATHOGENESIS. The pathogenesis of rubella is not well understood. Virus can be found from both infected and uninfected areas of skin, suggesting that immune processes may be important.

The risk for congenital defects and disease is greatest with primary maternal infection during the first trimester. Congenital defects occur in about 90% of infants whose mothers acquire maternal infection before the 11th week of pregnancy, diminishing to about 10–20% by the end of the first trimester, with an overall risk for the trimester being about 70%. Maternal infection after the 16th week of pregnancy, poses a low risk for congenital defects, although infection of the fetus may occur.

CLINICAL MANIFESTATIONS. The incubation period is 14–21 days. The prodromal phase of mild catarrhal symptoms is shorter than that of measles and may be so mild that it goes unnoticed. Approximately two thirds of infections are subclinical.

The most characteristic sign is retroauricular, posterior cervical, and postoccipital lymphadenopathy. No other disease causes the tender enlargement of these nodes to the extent that rubella does. An enanthem appears in 20% of patients just before the onset of the skin rash. It consists of discrete rose spots on the soft palate (Forchheimer spots) that may coalesce into a red blush and extend over the fauces.

Lymphadenopathy is evident at least 24 hr before the rash appears and may remain for 1 wk or more. The exanthem is more variable than that of rubeola. It begins on the face (Fig. 241–1) and spreads quickly. Its evolution is so rapid that the rash may be fading on the face by the time it appears on the trunk. Discrete maculopapules are present in large numbers; there are also large areas of flushing that spread rapidly over the entire body, usually within 24 hr. The rash may be confluent, particularly on the face. During the second day the rash may assume a pinpoint appearance, especially over the trunk, resembling that of scarlet fever. Mild itching may occur. The eruption usually clears by the third day. Desquamation is minimal. Rubella without a rash has been described.

The pharyngeal mucosa and the conjunctivae are slightly inflamed. In contrast to rubeola, there is no photophobia. Fever is low grade or absent during the rash and persists for 1, 2, or occasionally 3 days. Anorexia, headache, and malaise are not common.

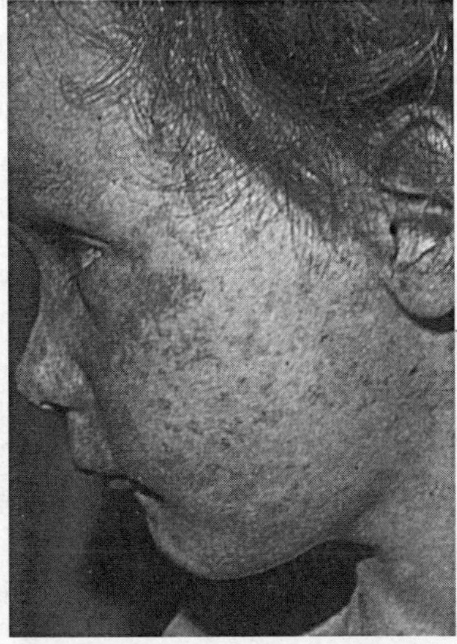

Figure 241–1 Rash of rubella (German measles). (From Korting GW: Hautkrankheiten bei Kindern und Jugendlichen, 3rd ed. Stuttgart, Germany, FK Schattauer Verlag, 1982.) See also color section.

Especially in older girls and women, polyarthritis may occur with arthralgia, swelling, tenderness, and effusion but usually without any residuum. Any joint may be involved, but the small joints of the hands are affected most frequently. The duration is usually several days to 2 wk; rarely it persists for months. Paresthesia also has been reported.

Congenital rubella affects virtually all organ systems. The most common manifestation is intrauterine growth retardation. Other common findings are: cataracts, bilateral or unilateral, which are frequently associated with microphthalmia; myocarditis and structural cardiac defects (e.g., patent ductus arteriosus or pulmonary artery stenosis); "blueberry muffin" skin lesions, similar to those in congenital cytomegalovirus infection; hearing loss from sensorineural deafness; and meningoencephalitis. Persistent infection leads to pneumonia, hepatitis, bone lucencies, thrombocytopenic purpura, and anemia. Later sequelae include motor and mental retardation.

DIAGNOSIS. The diagnosis of rubella may be apparent from the clinical symptoms and physical examination, but it is usually confirmed by serology or virus culture.

The spleen is often slightly enlarged. The white blood cell count is normal or slightly reduced; thrombocytopenia is rare, with or without purpura.

Hemagglutination-inhibition (HI) antibody has been the reference method of determining immunity to rubella, but newer methods that are easier to perform are now used more commonly. Latex agglutination, enzyme immunoassay, passive hemagglutination, and fluorescent immunoassay appear to be equal or superior to the HI test in sensitivity. Immunoglobulin (Ig) M antibodies are detectable in the first few days of illness and are considered diagnostic. Detection of IgM antibodies, which do not cross the placenta, in the newborn is especially useful for the diagnosis of congenital rubella syndrome. Seroconversion, or a fourfold increase in IgG titer, is diagnostic.

Rubella virus can be cultured from the nasopharynx and blood. It is detected by the ability of rubella-infected African green monkey kidney (AGMK) cells to resist challenge with enterovirus.

Differential Diagnosis. Because similar symptoms and rashes can occur with many other viral infections, rubella is a difficult disease to diagnose clinically except when the patient is seen during an epidemic. A history of having had rubella or rubella vaccine is unreliable; immunity should be determined by antibody testing. Particularly in its more severe forms, rubella may be confused with the mild types of scarlet fever and rubeola. Roseola infantum (exanthem subitum) is distinguished by a higher fever and the appearance of the rash at the end of the febrile episode rather than at the height of the signs and symptoms. Infectious mononucleosis may have a rash but is associated with generalized lymphadenopathy and characteristic atypical lymphocytosis. Enteroviral infections accompanied by a rash can be differentiated in some instances by accompanying respiratory or gastrointestinal manifestations and the absence of retroauricular lymphadenopathy. Drug rashes may be extremly difficult to differentiate from the rash of rubella, but the characteristic enlargement of the lymph nodes strongly supports a diagnosis of rubella.

TREATMENT. There is no specific antiviral therapy; treatment is entirely supportive. Antipyretics (acetaminophen or ibuprofen) are indicated for fever.

COMPLICATIONS. Complications are relatively uncommon in childhood. Encephalitis similar to that seen with measles occurs in about 1/6,000 cases. The severity is highly variable, and there is an overall mortality rate of 20%. Symptoms in survivors usually resolve within 1–3 wk without neurologic sequeale. Thrombocytopenic purpura occurs at an overall rate of 1/3,000 cases.

The most important consequence of rubella in a pregnant woman is congenital rubella syndrome. Progressive rubella panencephalitis is a persistent, slowly progressive rubella infection of the central nervous system (see Chapter 241.1).

Congenital Rubella Syndrome. Congenital rubella affects virtually all organ systems. The most common manifestation is intrauterine growth retardation. Other common findings are: cataracts, bilateral or unilateral, which are frequently associated with microphthalmia; myocarditis and structural cardiac defects (e.g., patent ductus arteriosus or pulmonary artery stenosis); "blueberry muffin" skin lesions, similar to those seen in congenital cytomegalovirus infection; hearing loss from sensorineural deafness; and meningoencephalitis. Persistent infection leads to pneumonia, hepatitis, bone lucencies, thrombocytopenic purpura, and anemia. Later sequelae include motor and mental retardation.

The diagnosis is confirmed by finding rubella-specific IgM antibody in the neonatal serum, or by culturing rubella virus from the infant (nasopharynx, urine, or tissues). Virus can be shed in the urine for 1 yr or longer. Prenatal diagnosis of fetal rubella infection can be made either by isolating the virus from amniotic fluid or by identification of rubella-specific IgM in cord blood.

Infants with the complete spectrum of the congenital rubella syndrome have a grim prognosis, especially when the neurologic symptoms continue to progress throughout infancy. The prognosis is better for infants with fewer stigmata of the syndrome, presumably those who were initially infected later in gestation. Only about 30% of infants with encephalitis appear to escape residual neuromotor deficitis, including an autistic syndrome.

PROGNOSIS. The prognosis of rubella in childhood is excellent. Infection usually confers permanent immunity, although reinfection may occur.

Reinfection. The incidence of reinfection on exposure to wild virus is 3–10% among those with a history of previous rubella and 14–18% among those immunized with the RA 27/3 vaccine. Reinfection may lead only to an IgG booster response, to both an IgM and IgG response, or to clinical rubella. Maternal reinfection during pregnancy has resulted in congenital rubella syndrome. The significance of rubella reinfection is controversial.

PREVENTION. Rubella vaccine is derived from the RA 27/3 strain of rubella virus, which is attenuated by serial passage tissue culture in WI-38 and MRC-5 human diploid cells. The vaccine induces antibody in >99% of seronegative recipients and has protective efficacy in >90%. Vaccine virus may be shed from the nasopharynx in low titers for as long as 18–25 days after vaccination, although there is no evidence of communicability.

The initial rubella immunization, usually as measles-mumps-rubella (MMR), is recommend at 12–15 mo of age. A second immunization, also as MMR, is recommended routinely at 4–6 yr of age but may be administered at any time during childhood provided at least 4 wk have elasped since the first dose. Children who have not previously received the second dose should be immunized by 11–12 yr of age. It is especially important for girls to have immunity to rubella before they reach childbearing age.

Pregnant women should not be given live rubella virus vaccine and should avoid becoming pregnant for 3 mo after they have been vaccinated. Routine serologic testing of postpubertal women before rubella immunization is not necessary. Inadvertent immunization is not ordinarily a reason to interrupt the pregnancy. No cases of congenital rubella syndrome have been reported in >200 women immunized during pregnancy with RA 27/3 vaccine who have been studied. Other contraindications include allergy to a vaccine component (anaphylaxis to neomycin), moderate or severe acute illness with or without fever, immunodeficiency (primary immunodeficiency, cancer and cancer therapy, long-term high-dose corticosteroids, severely immunocompromised, including those with HIV infection), and recent immune globulin administration (see Chapter 301).

Symptoms that may follow rubella immunization include fever (5–15%), rash (5%), lymphadenopathy, and arthralgias and arthritis. Joint involvement, usually seen in the small peripheral joints 10–21 days after vaccination, is uncommon in children but occurs frequently in postpubertal females with both arthralgias (25%) and transient arthritis (10%) being reported. It may last for weeks. Transient peripheral paresthesia and pain in the arms and legs are reported rarely.

All health care workers should be immune to rubella as well as to measles and varicella. Persons born before 1957 can be considered immune to rubella, except women of childbearing age who could become pregnant. Adolescent girls and premenopausal women should either be vaccinated or have documented laboratory evidence of immunity. Maternal antibody is protective for the infant for the first 6 mo of life.

Postexposure Prophylaxis. Nonpregnant susceptible contacts of persons with rubella should be vaccinated. This does not prevent infection but ensures protection for future rubella exposures.

All pregnant women, regardless of immunization history, should make every effort to avoid exposure to rubella. If a pregnant woman whose immune status is unknown is exposed to rubella, an antibody test should be performed immediately. Immune women should be reassured. Susceptible pregnant women exposed to rubella should not receive vaccine because of the potential risk of transmission of vaccine virus to the fetus. Susceptible women should undergo repeat serologic testing 3–4 wk after exposure, and, if they are still seronegative, again 6 wk after exposure. Seroconversion on either specimen indicates infection, and the mother should be counseled about the risk of transmission to the fetus and the resulting anomalies. Routine immune globulin administration for postexposure prophylaxis in pregnancy is not recommended but should be considered if termination of the pregnancy is not an option. For the susceptible pregnant woman exposed to measles for whom termination of pregnancy is a viable option and for whom timing permits documentaion of seroconversion within the period of time when abortion is possible, immune globulin is not recommended, since it may provide an unjustified sense of security, and precludes a positive serologic diagnosis as the basis for termination of pregnancy. However, for the susceptible pregnant woman exposed to rubella for whom abortion is not an option, immunoglobulin should be administered in a dose of 0.55 mL/kg, which reduces the attack rate but does not eliminate the risk of fetal infection. Fetal infection may occur even in the absence of clinical signs in the mother. The use of intravenous immunoglobulin (IVIG) may be an alternative but has not been studied.

241.1 Progressive Rubella Panencephalitis

EPIDEMIOLOGY. Progressive rubella panencephalitis is an exceedingly rare form of chronic encephalitis associated with persistent rubella virus infection of the brain. Since the disease was first recognized in 1974 20 cases have been reported, all involving males 8–21 yr of age at onset. Most had typical stigmata of the congenital rubella syndrome including cataracts, deafness, and mental retardation, but two had apparently had childhood rubella from which they made a full recovery. No new cases have been described in the United States in recent years, presumably because of effective childhood rubella immunization programs.

PATHOGENESIS. Rubella virus has been isolated from brain cell cultures and from blood lymphocytes. The histopathologic changes seen in the brain are similar to those seen in SSPE, with cuffs of lymphocytes and plasma cells around blood vessels, glial nodules in the cortex, some loss of neurons, an increase in astrocytes throughout the gray matter, and an even greater increase in the white matter. However, in progressive rubella panencephalitis, there are no inclusion bodies, and deposits of material that stains with the periodic acid-Schiff reaction are found around vessels in subcortical white matter.

CLINICAL MANIFESTATIONS. At onset, progressive rubella panencephalitis resembles subacute sclerosing panencephalitis (SSPE; see Chapter 240.1), with insidious changes in behavior and deteriorating school performance. Subsequently, frank dementia and other signs of multifocal brain disease occur, including seizures, cerebellar ataxia, and spastic weakness. Myoclonus and other abnormal movements may occur but are not as common as those seen in SSPE. Retinopathy and optic atrophy may occur.

DIAGNOSIS. Early in the course of illness, progressive rubella panencephalitis must be distinguished from atypical acute viral encephalitides. Other slow viral infections, such as Creutzfeldt-Jakob disease (CJD) and SSPE, must be considered in appropriate age groups. The stigmata of congenital rubella syndrome or rubella infection suggests the diagnosis of progressive rubella panencephalitis.

Remarkable laboratory abnormalities include elevated antibody titers to rubella virus, a normal or slightly elevated CSF cell count, and a slightly elevated CSF protein concentration with a marked increase in globulin, which may constitute >50% of the total protein. Oligoclonal electrophoretic bands of globulin consist of antibodies to rubella virus antigens. Antibodies to rubela virus are readily detectable in CSF, often at dilutions of 1:8 or higher. The hemagglutination inhibition, complement fixation, and enzyme immunoassay techniques should be satisfactory for testing the cerebrospinal fluid. Most of the rubella antibodies in the CSF are IgG, although some IgM antibodies have also been detected early in the course of progressive rubella panencephalitis. There is a high CSF: serum ratio of rubella antibody titers compared to ratio of titers to measles and other viruses. Isolation of rubella virus from blood lymphocytes may be attempted, but brain biopsy should not be needed to establish the diagnosis.

The EEG shows a generalized slowing with occasional high voltage activity, but the suppression-burst pattern of SSPE has not been seen in progressive rubella panencephalitis. Encephalograms (computed tomography was not available when published cases were studied) show enlargement of all ventricles, especially the fourth, with prominent atrophy of the cerebellum.

PROGNOSIS. The course of progressive rubella panencephalitis is similar to that seen in SSPE, progressing to coma, spasticity, brain stem involvement, and death in 2–5 yr.

Patients with progressive rubella panencephalitis pose no substantial risk of infection to others. Rubella viruria has not been detected.

PREVENTION. Rubella vaccination is the most important measure to prevent rubella panencephalitis.

Centers for Disease Control and Prevention: Measles, mumps, and rubella—vaccine use and strategies for elimination of measles, rubella, and congenital rubella syndrome and control of mumps. Recommendations of the Advisory Committee on Immunization Practices (ACIP). MMWR 47 (RR-8):1, 1998.

Centers for Disease Control and Prevention: Rubella and congenital rubella syndrome—United States, 1994–1997. MMWR 46:350, 1997.

Chang TW: Rubella reinfection and intrauterine involvement. J Pediatr 84:617, 1974.

Dudgeon JA: Congenital rubella. J Pediatr 87:1078, 1975.

Howson CP, Katz M, Johnston RB, et al: Chronic arthritis after rubella vaccination. Clin Infect Dis 15:307, 1992.

Lee SH, Ewert DP, Frederick PD, et al: Resurgence of congenital rubella syndrome in the 1990s. JAMA 267:2616, 1992.

Miller E, Cradock-Watson JE, Pollock TM: Consequences of confirmed maternal rubella at successive stages of pregnancy. Lancet 2:781, 1982.

Rawls WE, Desmyter J, Melnick JL: Serologic diagnosis and fetal involvement in maternal rubella. JAMA 203:627, 1968.

Rawls WE, Phillips CA, Melnick JL, et al: Persistent virus infection in congenital rubella. Arch Ophthalmol 77:430, 1967.

Tardieu M, Grospierre B, Durandy A, et al: Circulating immune complexes containing rubella antigens in late-onset rubella syndrome. J Pediatr 97:370, 1980.
Townsend JJ: Progressive rubella panencephalitis: Late onset after congenital rubella. N Engl J Med 292:990, 1975.
Weibel RE, Benor DE: Chronic arthropathy and musculoskeletal symptoms associated with rubella vaccines. Arthritis Rheum 39:1529, 1996.

CHAPTER 242
Mumps

Yvonne Maldonado

Mumps is an important childhood disease that was historically widespread but now occurs very infrequently. It is an acute viral infection characterized by painful enlargement of the salivary glands, chiefly the parotids, as the usual presenting sign.

ETIOLOGY. Mumps virus, the cause of mumps, is an RNA virus of the genus *Paramyxovirus* in the family paramyxoviridae, which also includes the parainfluenza viruses. Only one serotype is known.

EPIDEMIOLOGY. Mumps is endemic in most unvaccinated populations; the virus is spread from human reservoir by direct contact, airborne droplets, fomites contaminated by saliva, and possibly by urine. It is distributed worldwide and affects both sexes equally. Before introduction of the vaccine in 1967, the peak incidence of the disease occurred in children 5–9 yr of age; 85% of infections occurred in children <15 yr of age. Now most cases occur in young adults, producing outbreaks in colleges or in the workplace. Outbreaks appear to be primarily related to a lack of immunization, especially in an underimmunized cohort of children born from 1967–1977, rather than to waning to immunity. Epidemics occur at all seasons but are slightly more frequent in late winter and spring.

There has been a dramatic decrease in the incidence of mumps since the introduction of the mumps vaccine in 1968. Except for a small increase in 1987, the incidence of mumps has steadily decreased in the United States. In 1997 there were 683 reported cases of mumps (0.27/100,000 population), a >99% reduction from the 152,209 cases reported in 1968.

Virus has been isolated from saliva as long as 6 days before and up to 9 days after appearance of salivary gland swelling. Transmission does not seem to occur more than 24 hr before the appearance of the swelling or later than 3 days after it has subsided. Virus has been isolated from urine from the 1st–14th day after the onset of salivary gland swelling.

PATHOGENESIS. After entry into the last and initial multiplication in the cells of the respiratory tract, the virus is bloodborne to many tissues, among which the salivary and other glands are the most susceptible.

CLINICAL MANIFESTATIONS. The incubation period ranges from 14–24 days, with a peak at 17–18 days. Approximately 30–40% of infections are subclinical. In children, prodromal manifestations are rare but may be manifest by fever, muscular pain (especially in the neck), headache, and malaise.

Salivary Glands. The onset is usually characterized by pain and swelling in one or both parotid glands. The parotid swells characteristically; it first fills the space between the posterior border of the mandible and the mastoid and then extends in a series of crescents downward and forward, being limited above by the zygoma. Edema of the skin and soft tissues usually extends further and obscures the limit of the glandular swelling, so that the swelling is more readily appreciated by sight than by palpation. Swelling may proceed extremely rapidly, reaching a maximum within a few hours, although it usually peaks in 1–3 days. The swollen tissues push the ear lobe upward and outward, and the angle of the mandible is no longer visible. Swelling slowly subsides within 3–7 days but occasionally lasts longer. One parotid gland usually swells a day or two before the other, but in approximately one quarter of cases the disease remains unilateral. The swollen area is tender and painful, pain being elicited especially by tasting sour liquids such as lemon juice or vinegar. Redness and swelling about the opening of the Stensen duct are common. Edema of the homolateral pharynx and soft palate accompanies the parotid swelling and displaces the tonsil medially; acute edema of the larynx has also been described. Edema over the manubrium and upper chest wall may occur, probably because of lymphatic obstruction. The parotid swelling is usually accompanied by low-grade fever, but this may be absent.

Although the parotid glands alone are affected in the majority of patients, swelling of the submandibular glands occurs frequently and usually accompanies or closely follows that of the parotid glands. In 10–15% of patients only the submandibular gland(s) may be swollen. Little pain is associated with the submandibular infection, but the swelling subsides more slowly than that of the parotids. Redness and swelling at the orifice of the Wharton duct frequently accompany swelling of the gland. Least commonly, the sublingual glands are infected, usually bilaterally; the swelling is evident in the submental region and in the floor of the mouth.

DIAGNOSIS. The diagnosis of mumps parotitis is usually apparent from the clinical symptoms and physical examination. When the clinical manifestations are limited to less common lesions, the diagnosis is less clear but may be suspected during an outbreak.

Routine laboratory tests are nonspecific; usually leukopenia is present with relative lymphocytosis. An elevation in serum amylase levels is common; the rise tends to parallel the parotid swelling and then to return to normal within 2 wk.

The microbiologic diagnosis is by serology or virus culture. Enzyme immunoassay for mumps immunoglobulin (Ig) G and IgM antibodies are most commonly used for diagnosis. IgM antibodies are detectable in the first few days of illness and are considered diagnostic. They may remain elevated for weeks to months. IgG antibodies are directed primarily against the fusion (F) protein; cross reactions with parainfluenza viruses may occur. Seroconversion, or a fourfold increase in IgG titer, is diagnostic.

Mumps virus can be cultured from the saliva, cerebrospinal fluid, blood, urine, brain, and other infected tissues. Primary cultures of human or monkey kidney cells are used for viral isolation. Cytopathic effect is occasionally observed, but hemadsorption is the most sensitive indicator of infection.

The mumps skin test is unreliable for diagnosis of mumps and for determination of susceptibility to infection.

Differential Diagnosis. Other viral causes of parotitis include human immunodeficiency virus (HIV) infection, influenza, parainfluenza viruses 1 and 3, cytomegalovirus, and Coxsackieviruses. Acute suppurative parotitis is a bacterial infection usually caused by *Staphylococcus aureus* in which pus can often be expressed from the duct. A salivary calculus obstructing either a parotid or, more commonly, a submandibular duct causes intermittent swelling. Preauricular or anterior cervical lymphadenitis can be differentiated by the well-defined borders of the lymph node and a location that is completely posterior to the angle of the mandible. Orchitis may also be caused by Coxsackieviruses.

TREATMENT. There is no specific antiviral therapy; treatment is entirely supportive. Antipyretics (acetaminophen or ibuprofen) are indicated for fever. Bed rest should be guided by the patient's needs, but no evidence indicates that it prevents complications. The diet should be adjusted to the patient's ability to chew. Orchitis should be treated with local support and bed rest. Mumps arthritis may respond to a 2-wk course of a nonsteroidal anti-inflammatory agent or corticosteroids. Salicylates do not appear to be effective.

COMPLICATIONS. Viremia early in the infection probably accounts for the widespread complications. There is no firm evidence that maternal infection is damaging to the fetus; a possible relationship to endocardial fibroelastosis has not been firmly established. Mumps in early pregnancy does increase the chance of abortion.

Meningoencephalomyelitis. This is the most frequent complication in childhood. Its true incidence is hard to estimate because subclinical infection of the central nervous system, as evidenced by cerebrospinal fluid pleocytosis, has been reported in >65% of patients with mumps parotitis. Clinical manifestations occur in >10% of patients. The incidence of mumps meningoencephalitis is approximately 250/100,000 cases; 10% of these cases occurred in patients >20 yr of age. The mortality rate is about 2%. Males are affected three to five times as frequently as females.

The pathogenesis of mumps meningoencephalitis may be either a primary infection of neurons or a postinfectious encephalitis with demyelination. In the first type, parotitis frequently appears at the same time or following the onset of encephalitis. In the latter type, encephalitis follows parotitis by an average of 10 days. Parotitis may in some cases be absent. Aqueductal stenosis and hydrocephalus have been associated with mumps infection. Injecting mumps virus into suckling hamsters has produced similar lesions.

Mumps meningoencephalitis is clinically indistinguishable from meningoencephalitis of other origins (see Chapter 174.2). Moderate stiffness of the neck is seen, but the remaining findings on neurologic examination are usually normal. The cerebrospinal fluid may show a lymphocytic pleocytosis of <500 cells/ mm^3, although occasionally the count may exceed 2,000 cells/mm^3.

Orchitis and Epididymitis. These complications rarely occur in prepubescent boys but are common (14–35%) in adolescents and adults. The testis is most often infected with or without epididymitis; epididymitis may also occur alone. Bilateral orchitis occurs in approximately 30% of patients. Rarely, there is a hydrocele. The orchitis usually follows parotitis within 8 days. Orchitis may also occur without evidence of salivary gland infection. The onset is usually abrupt, with a rise in temperature, chills, headache, nausea, and lower abdominal pain; when the right testis is implicated, appendicitis may be suggested as a diagnostic possibility. The affected testis becomes tender and swollen, and the adjacent skin is edematous and red. The average duration of illness is 4 days. Approximately 30–40% of affected testes atrophy, leaving a cosmetic imbalance. Infertility is rare even with bilateral orchitis.

Oophoritis. Pelvic pain and tenderness are noted in about 7% of postpubertal female patients. There is no evidence of impairment of fertility.

Pancreatitis. Mild or subclinical pancreatic involvement is common, but severe pancreatitis is rare. It may be unassociated with salivary gland manifestations and may be misdiagnosed as gastroenteritis. Epigastric pain and tenderness, which are suggestive, may be accompanied by fever, chills, vomiting, and prostration. An elevated serum amylase value is characteristically present in patients with mumps, with or without clinical manifestations of pancreatitis.

Thyroiditis. Although it is uncommon in children, a diffuse, tender swelling of the thyroid may occur about 1 wk after the onset of parotitis; antithyroid antibodies subsequently develop.

Myocarditis. Serious cardiac manifestations are extremely rare, but mild infection of the myocardium may be more common than is recognized. Electrocardiographic tracings revealed changes, mostly depression of the ST segment, in 13% of adults in one series. Such involvement may explain the precordial pain, bradycardia, and fatigue sometimes noted among adolescents and adults with mumps.

Deafness. Unilateral, rarely bilateral, nerve deafness may occur; although the incidence is low (1/15,000 cases), mumps was historically a leading cause of unilateral nerve deafness. The hearing loss may be transient or permanent.

Ocular Complications. Dacryoadenitis may occur with painful swelling, usually bilateral, of the lacrimal glands. Optic neuritis (papillitis) may occur; symptoms vary from loss of vision to mild blurring, and recovery occurs in 10–20 days.

Arthritis. Migratory polyarthralgia and even arthritis are occasionally seen in adults with mumps but are rare in children. The knees, ankles, shoulders, and wrists are most commonly affected. The symptoms last from a few days to 3 mo, with a median duration of 2 wk.

PROGNOSIS. The prognosis of rubella in childhood is excellent. Infection usually confers permanent immunity, although reinfections have been documented.

PREVENTION. Mumps vaccine is derived from the Jeryl Lynn strain of mumps virus, which is attenuated by serial passage in embryonated hens' eggs and chick embryo cell culture. The vaccine induces antibody in 96% of seronegative recipients and has 97% protective efficacy.

The initial mumps immunization, usually as measles-mumps-rubella (MMR) vaccine, is recommended at 12–15 mo of age. A second immunization, also as MMR, is recommended routinely at 4–6 yr of age but may be administered at any time during childhood provided at least 4 wk have elapsed since the first dose. Children who have not previously received the second dose should be immunized by 11–12 yr of age. Women should avoid becoming pregnant for 30 days after monovalent mumps vaccination (3 mo if vaccination was performed with rubella vaccine). Other contraindications to vaccination include allergy to a vaccine component (anaphylaxis to neomycin), moderate or severe acute illnesses with or without fever, immunodeficiency (primary immunodeficiencies, cancer and cancer therapy, long-term high-dose corticosteroid therapy, severely immunocompromised, including those with HIV infection), and recent immune globulin administration (see Chapter 301).

Rarely, parotitis and low-grade fever can develop 10–14 days after vaccination. Vaccinees do not shed virus.

Persons born before 1957 can be considered immune to mumps. Maternal antibody is protective in the infant in the first 6 mo of life.

Bistrian B, Phillips CA, Kaye IS: Fatal mumps meningoencephalitis: Isolation of virus premortem and postmortem. JAMA 222:478, 1972.

Centers for Disease Control and Prevention: Measles, mumps, and rubella—vaccine use and strategies for elimination of measles, rubella, and congenital rubella syndrome and control of mumps. Recommendations of the Advisory Committee on Immunization Practices (ACIP). MMWR 47 (RR-8):1, 1998.

Centers for Disease Control and Prevention: Mumps surveillance—United States, 1988–1993. MMWR 44(SS-3):1, 1995.

Cochi SI, Preblud SR, Orenstein WA: Perspectives in the relative resurgence of mumps in the United States. Am J Dis Child 142:499, 1988.

Gordon SC, Lauter CB: Mumps arthritis: A review of the literature. Rev Infect Dis 6:338, 1984.

Ni J, Bowles NE, Kim YH, et al: Viral infection of the myocardium in endocardial fibroelastosis: Molecular evidence for the role of mumps virus as an etiologic agent. Circulation 95:133, 1997.

Quast U, Hennessen W, Widmark RM: Vaccine-induced mumps-like disease. Develop Biol Standard 43:269, 1979.

Chapter 243
Enteroviruses

Abraham Morag and Pearay L. Ogra

Enteroviruses are a large group of viral agents that inhabit the intestinal tract and are responsible for significant and frequent human illnesses that produce protean clinical manifestations.

ETIOLOGY. Enteroviruses are RNA viruses belonging to the Picornaviridae family. The original enteroviral subgroups—Coxsackieviruses, echoviruses, and polioviruses—were differentiated by their effects in tissue culture and animals (Table 243–1). Coxsackieviruses are named after the town of Coxsackie, New York, where they were first isolated in 1948, as nonpolio enteroviruses causing paralysis in children. Echoviruses (enteric cytopathogenic human orphan viruses) were not recognized initially to cause any disease in animals or humans. The Coxsackieviruses consist of two groups, A and B. Since 1970 new enteroviral types (68–72) have been classified by enteroviral numbers. Hepatitis A virus is classified as enterovirus 72 but is antigenically distinct from all other enteroviruses.

Enteroviruses retain activity for several days at room temperature and can be stored indefinitely at ordinary freezer temperatures (−20°C). They are rapidly inactivated by heat (>56°C), formaldehyde, chlorination, and ultraviolet light. Enteroviruses, except for most members of Coxsackie group A, grow well in many cell cultures and cause cytopathic effects that are different from those caused by herpesvirus, adenoviruses, and reoviruses. Coxsackie A viruses are identified by their pathologic effects in suckling mice.

243.1 Polioviruses

ETIOLOGY. There are three antigenically distinct serotypes of poliovirus (types 1, 2, and 3).

EPIDEMIOLOGY. In 1952 there were more than 57,879 cases of polio in the United States, including 21,269 cases of paralytic polio that resulted in more than 3,000 deaths. The use of poliovirus vaccine has eliminated, since 1979, wild poliovirus in the United States. The last case of wild poliovirus in the Americas occurred in Peru, in 1991. In 1994 the World Health Organization declared that polio had been eradicated from the Western hemisphere.

However, poliomyelitis still occurs in many regions of the developing world. In countries where vaccines are not available and economic conditions are poor, poliomyelitis remains a significant disease of infants and young children, with several thousand cases annually worldwide. A changing epidemiologic pattern is emerging in some underdeveloped countries as economic standards improve. Significant outbreaks occasionally occur in these countries where paralytic poliomyelitis had become rare.

TABLE 243–1 Human Enteroviruses

Polioviruses: Types 1–3
Coxsackieviruses A: Types A1–A24 (A23 has been reclassified as echovirus 9)
Coxsackieviruses B: Types B1–B6
Echoviruses: Types 1–33 (echovirus 10 has been reclassified as reovirus 1; echovirus 28 has been reclassified as rhinovirus 1A)
Enteroviruses: Types 68–72 (hepatitis A virus is classified as enterovirus 72 but is antigenically distinct from all other enteroviruses)

From 1980 to 1994, 133 cases of paralytic poliomyelitis were reported in the United States. Of these, 125 cases were associated with oral poliovirus vaccine, six cases were imported, and two cases were indeterminate. Approximately four to eight cases of vaccine-associated paralytic poliomyelitis (VAPP) occur annually in the United States.

PATHOGENESIS. The neuropathy of poliomyelitis and other paralytic diseases caused by nonpolio enteroviruses is due to direct cellular destruction. Secondary damage may be due to immunologic mechanisms. In poliomyelitis, neuronal lesions occur in the (1) spinal cord (chiefly in the anterior horn cells and to a lesser degree in the intermediate and dorsal horn and dorsal root ganglia); (2) medulla (vestibular nuclei, cranial nerve nuclei, and the reticular formation, which contains the vital centers controlling respiration and circulation); (3) cerebellum (nuclei in the roof and vermis only); (4) midbrain (chiefly the gray matter but also the substantia nigra and occasionally the red nucleus); (5) thalamus and hypothalamus; (6) pallidum; and (7) cerebral cortex (motor cortex). Areas that are spared include (1) the entire cerebral cortex except the motor area; (2) the cerebellum except the vermis and deep midline nuclei; and (3) the white matter of the spinal cord.

Infants acquire immunity transplacentally from their mothers. This immunity is usually complete during the first 4–6 mo of life and disappears at a variable rate. Active immunity, after natural infection, probably lasts for life. Neutralizing antibodies against polioviruses develop within several days after exposure, often before the onset of illness. The early production of immunoglobulin (Ig) G antibodies is a result of replication of the virus in the intestinal tract and deep lymphatic tissues, which occurs before the central nervous system is invaded. Local (mucosal) immunity, conferred mainly by secretory IgA, is an important defense against polioviral infection.

CLINICAL MANIFESTATIONS. Poliovirus infections may follow one of several courses: inapparent infection, which occurs in 90–95% of cases and causes no disease and no sequelae, abortive poliomyelitis, nonparalytic poliomyelitis, or paralytic poliomyelitis.

Abortive Poliomyelitis. Abortive poliomyelitis is a brief febrile illness with one or more symptoms of malaise, anorexia, nausea, vomiting, headache, sore throat, constipation, and diffuse abdominal pain. Coryza, cough, pharyngeal exudate, diarrhea, and localized abdominal tenderness and rigidity are uncommon. The fever seldom exceeds 39.5°C (103°F), and the pharynx appears normal despite the frequent complaint of sore throat.

Nonparalytic Poliomyelitis. The symptoms in this form of poliovirus infection are the same as those enumerated for abortive poliomyelitis except that headache, nausea, and vomiting are more intense, and there is soreness and stiffness of the posterior muscles of the neck, trunk, and limbs. Fleeting paralysis of the bladder is not uncommon, and constipation is frequent. Approximately two thirds of these children have a short symptom-free interlude between the first phase (minor illness) and the second phase (central nervous system disease or major illness). This two-phase course is less common in adults, in whom the evolution of symptoms is more insidious. Nuchal and spinal rigidity are the basis for the diagnosis of nonparalytic poliomyelitis during the second phase.

Physical examination reveals nuchal-spinal signs and changes in superficial and deep reflexes. In cooperative patients the nuchal-spinal signs are first sought by active tests. The child is asked to sit up unassisted. If this causes undue effort and if the knees flex upward and the patient writhes a bit from side to side in sitting up and uses the hands on the bed to assume the tripod supporting position, there is unmistakable spinal rigidity. Still sitting, the patient is asked to flex the chin to the chest and is observed for nuchal rigidity. Alternatively, in the supine position, with the knees held down gently, the patient is asked to sit up and kiss his or her knees.

If the knees draw up sharply or if the maneuver cannot be adequately completed, there is stiffness of the spine as a result of muscle spasm. If the diagnosis is still uncertain, attempts should be made to elicit the Kerning and Brudzinski signs. Gentle forward flexion of the occiput and neck will elicit nuchal rigidity, which may precede spinal rigidity. Head drop may be demonstrated by placing the hands under the patient's shoulders and raising the trunk. Normally the head follows the plane of the trunk, but in poliomyelitis it often falls backward limply. The head-drop sign is not due to true paresis of the neck flexors. In struggling infants it may be difficult to distinguish voluntary resistance from clinically important involuntary nuchal rigidity. One may place the infant's shoulders flush with the edge of the table, support the weight of the occiput in the hand, and then flex the head anteriorly. Nuchal rigidity that persists during this maneuver may be interpreted as involuntary. When not closed, the anterior fontanel may be tense or bulging as in meningitis.

In the early stages the reflexes are normally active and remain so unless paralysis supervenes. Changes in reflexes, either an increase or depression, may precede weakness by 12–24 hr; hence, it is important to detect them, especially in nonparalytic patients managed at home. The superficial reflexes, that is, the cremasteric and abdominal reflexes and the reflexes of the spinal and gluteal muscles, are usually the first to be diminished. The spinal and gluteal reflexes may disappear before the abdominal and cremasteric ones do. Changes in the deep tendon reflexes generally occur 8–24 hr after the superficial reflexes are depressed and indicate impending paresis of the extremities. Tendon reflexes are absent with paralysis. Sensory defects do not occur in poliomyelitis.

Paralytic Poliomyelitis. The manifestations are those enumerated for nonparalytic poliomyelitis plus weakness of one or more muscle groups, either skeletal or cranial. These symptoms may be followed by a symptom-free interlude of several days and then a recurrence of disease culminating in paralysis. Bladder paralysis lasting 1–3 days occurs in approximately 20% of patients, and bowel atony is common, occasionally to the point of paralytic ileus. In some patients muscular paralysis may be the initial presentation.

Flaccid paralysis is the most obvious clinical expression of the neuronal injury. The ensuing muscular atrophy is due to denervation plus the atrophy of disuse. The pain, spasticity, nuchal and spinal rigidity, and hypertonia early in the illness are probably due to lesions of the brain stem, spinal ganglia, and posterior columns. Respiratory and cardiac arrhythmias, blood pressure and vasomotor changes, and the like reflect damage to the vital centers in the medulla.

On physical examination the distribution of paralysis is characteristically spotty. To detect mild muscular weakness, it is often necessary to apply gentle resistance in opposition to the muscle group being tested. In the spinal form there is weakness of some of the muscles of the neck, abdomen, trunk, diaphragm, thorax, or extremities. In the bulbar form there is weakness in the motor distribution of one or more cranial nerves with or without dysfunction of the vital centers controlling respiration and circulation. Components of both the preceding forms occur together in bulbospinal poliomyelitis. In the encephalitic form irritability, disorientation, drowsiness, and coarse tremors not explained by inadequate ventilation are noted; peripheral or cranial nerve paralysis coexists or ensues. Hypoxia and hypercapnia caused by inadequate ventilation due to respiratory insufficiency may produce disorientation without true encephalitis.

A number of components acting together may produce insufficiency of ventilation, resulting in hypoxia and hypercapnia, which may produce profound effects on many other systems. Because respiratory insufficiency may develop rapidly, continued clinical evaluation is essential. Despite weakness of the respiratory muscles, the patient may respond with so much respiratory effort (associated with anxiety and fear) that overventilation may occur at the outset, resulting in respiratory alkalosis. Such effort is fatiguing and soon leads to respiratory failure.

There are certain characteristic patterns of disease. *Pure spinal poliomyelitis* with respiratory insufficiency involves tightness, weakness, or paralysis of the respiratory muscles (chiefly the diaphragm and intercostals) without discernible clinical involvement of the cranial nerves or vital centers that control respiration, circulation, and body temperature. The cervical and thoracic spinal cord segments are chiefly affected. *Pure bulbar poliomyelitis* involves paralysis of the motor cranial nerve nuclei with or without involvement of the vital centers. Involvement of the 9th, 10th, and 12th cranial nerves results in paralysis of the pharynx, tongue, and larynx with consequent airway obstruction. *Bulbospinal poliomyelitis* with respiratory insufficiency affects the respiratory muscles and results in coexisting bulbar paralysis.

The clinical findings associated with involvement of the respiratory muscles include (1) anxious expression; (2) inability to speak without frequent pauses, resulting in short, jerky, "breathless" sentences; (3) increased respiratory rate; (4) movement of the alae nasi and of the accessory muscles of respiration; (5) inability to cough or sniff with full depth; (6) paradoxical abdominal movements caused by diaphragmatic immobility due to spasm or weakness of one or both leaves; (7) relative immobility of the intercostal spaces, which may be segmental, unilateral, or bilateral. When the arms are weak, and especially when deltoid paralysis occurs, there may be impending respiratory paralysis because the phrenic nerve nuclei are in adjacent areas of the spinal cord. Observation of the patient's capacity for thoracic breathing while the abdominal muscles are splinted manually indicates minor degrees of paresis. Light manual splinting of the thoracic cage will help to assess the effectiveness of diaphragmatic movement.

The clinical findings seen with bulbar poliomyelitis with respiratory difficulty (other than paralysis of extraocular, facial, and masticatory muscles) include (1) nasal twang to the voice or cry caused by palatal and pharyngeal weakness (hard-consonant words such as "cookie" or "candy" bring this out best); (2) inability to swallow smoothly, resulting in accumulation of saliva in the pharynx, indicates partial immobility (holding the larynx lightly and asking the patient to swallow will confirm such immobility); (3) accumulated pharyngeal secretions, which may cause irregular respirations because each inspiration must be "planned" to avoid aspirating; the respirations may thus appear interrupted and abnormal even to the point of falsely simulating intercostal or diaphragmatic weakness; (4) absence of effective coughing, shown by constant fatiguing efforts to clear the throat; (5) nasal regurgitation of saliva and fluids as a result of palatal paralysis, with inability to separate the oropharynx from the nasopharynx during swallowing; (6) deviation of the palate, uvula, or tongue; (7) involvement of vital centers in the medulla, which are manifested by irregularities in rate, depth, and rhythm of respiration; by cardiovascular alterations including blood pressure changes (especially increased blood pressure), alternate flushing and mottling of the skin, and cardiac arrhythmias; and by rapid changes in body temperature; (8) paralysis of one or both vocal cords, causing hoarseness, aphonia, and ultimately asphyxia unless this is recognized by laryngoscopy and managed by immediate tracheostomy; and (9) the "rope sign," an acute angulation between the chin and larynx caused by weakness of the hyoid muscles (the hyoid bone is pulled posteriorly, narrowing the hypopharyngeal inlet).

DIAGNOSIS. Poliomyelitis should be considered in any unimmunized or incompletely immunized child with nonspecific febrile illness, aseptic meningitis, or paralytic disease. The combination of fever, headache, neck and back pain, asymmetric flaccid paralysis without sensory loss, and pleocytosis is not regularly seen in any other illness.

The cerebrospinal fluid, while often normal during the minor illness, demonstrates a pleocytosis between 20–300 cells/mm^3 with central nervous system involvement; the cells may be polymorphonuclear early in the disease but shift to mononuclear cells soon afterward. By the second week of the major illness, the total WBC count falls to near-normal values. In contrast, the cerebrospinal fluid protein is normal or only slightly elevated at the outset of central nervous system disease but usually rises to between 50–100 mg/dL by the second week of illness.

Serologic testing demonstrates seroconversion or a fourfold or greater increase in antibody titers. Poliovirus is easily cultured from the stool and nasopharynx and infrequently from the cerebrospinal fluid. Isolates should be submitted to the Centers for Disease Control and Prevention for DNA sequence analysis, which can distinguish wild poliovirus from the strains used in the oral poliovirus vaccine.

Differential Diagnosis. Several other conditions of muscular weakness should be considered. Guillain-Barré syndrome is the most common disease and the most difficult to distinguish from poliomyelitis. Paralysis is characteristically symmetric, and sensory changes and pyramidal tract signs are common in Guillain-Barré syndrome absent in poliomyelitis. Fever, headache, and meningeal signs are less notable, and there are few cells but an elevated protein level in the cerebrospinal fluid. Peripheral neuritis may be due to lead toxicity, cranial nerve herpes zoster, or postdiphtheritic neuropathy. Arthropod-borne viral encephalitis, rabies, and tetanus have been confused with bulbar poliomyelitis. Botulism may closely simulate bulbar poliomyelitis, but nuchal-spinal rigidity and pleocytosis are absent. Demyelinating types of encephalomyelitis are associated with or follow the exanthems and other infections or occur as an untoward sequel of antirabies vaccination. Neoplasms originating in and around the spinal cord rarely have a fairly abrupt onset. Familial periodic paralysis, myasthenia gravis, and acute porphyria are uncommon causes of muscle weakness. Hysteria and malingering are rare in children.

Conditions causing pseudoparalysis do not present with nuchal-spinal rigidity or pleocytosis. These causes include unrecognized trauma, transient (toxic) synovitis, acute osteomyelitis, acute rheumatic fever, scurvy, and congenital syphilis (pseudoparalysis of Parrot).

TREATMENT. The broad principles of management are to allay fear, to minimize ensuing skeletal deformities, to anticipate and meet complications that may occur in addition to the neuromusculoskeletal problems, and to prepare the child and family for the prolonged treatment that may be required and for permanent disability if this seems likely. Patients with the nonparalytic and mildly paralytic forms of poliomyelitis may be treated at home.

Abortive Poliomyelitis. Supportive treatment with analgesics, sedatives, an attractive diet, and bed rest until the child's temperature is normal for several days is usually sufficient. Avoidance of exertion for the ensuing 2 wk is desirable, and there should be a careful neuromusculoskeletal examination 2 mo later to detect any minor involvement.

Nonparalytic Poliomyelitis. Treatment for the nonparalytic form is similar to that for the abortive form; in particular, relief is indicated for the discomfort of muscle tightness and spasm of the neck, trunk, and extremities. Analgesics are more effective when they are combined with the application of hot packs for 15–30 min every 2–4 hr. Hot tub baths are sometimes useful. A firm bed is desirable and can be improvised at home by placing table leaves or a sheet of plywood beneath the mattress. A footboard should be used to keep the feet at a right angle to the legs. Because muscular discomfort and spasm may continue for some weeks, even in the nonparalytic form, hot packs and gentle physical therapy may be necessary. Such patients should also be carefully examined 2 mo after apparent recovery to detect minor residual effects that might cause postural problems in later years.

Paralytic Poliomyelitis. Most patients with the paralytic form require hospitalization. A calm atmosphere is desirable. Suitable body alignment is necessary to avoid excessive skeletal deformity. A neutral position with the feet at a right angle to the legs, knees slightly flexed, and hips and spine straight is achieved by use of boards, sandbags, and, occasionally, light splint shells. Active and passive motions are indicated as soon as the pain has disappeared. Opiates and sedatives are permissible only if no impairment of ventilation is present or impending. Constipation is common, and fecal impaction should be prevented. When bladder paralysis occurs, a parasympathetic stimulant such as bethanechol (5–10 mg orally or 2.5–5.0 mg subcutaneously) may induce voiding in 15–30 min; some patients do not respond, and others respond with nausea, vomiting, and palpitations. Bladder paresis rarely lasts more than a few days. If bethanechol fails, manual compression of the bladder and the psychologic effect of running water should be tried. If catheterization must be performed, care must be taken to prevent urinary tract infections. An appealing diet and a relatively high fluid intake should be started at once unless the patient is vomiting. Additional salt should be provided if the environmental temperature is high or if the application of hot packs induces sweating. Anorexia is common initially. Adequate dietary and fluid intake can be maintained by placement of a central venous catheter. An orthopedist and a physiatrist should see these patients as early in the course of the illness as possible and should assume responsibility for their care before fixed deformities develop.

The management of pure bulbar poliomyelitis consists of maintaining the airway and avoiding all risk of inhalation of saliva, food, or vomitus. Gravity drainage of accumulated secretions is favored by using the head-low (foot of bed elevated 20–25 degrees) prone position with the face to one side. Aspirators with rigid or semirigid tips are preferred for direct oral and pharyngeal aspiration, and soft, flexible catheters may be used for nasopharyngeal aspiration. Fluid and electrolyte equilibrium is best maintained by intravenous infusion because tube or oral feeding in the first few days may incite vomiting. In addition to close observation for respiratory insufficiency, the blood pressure should be taken at least twice daily because hypertensionis not uncommon and occasionally leads to hypertensive encephalopathy. Patients with pure bulbar poliomyelitis may require tracheostomy because of vocal cord paralysis or constriction of the hypopharynx; most patients who recover have little residual impairment, although some exhibit mild dysphagia and occasional vocal fatigue with slurring of speech.

Impaired ventilation must be recognized early; mounting anxiety, restlessness, and fatigue are early indications for preemptive intervention. Tracheostomy is indicated for some patients with pure bulbar poliomyelitis, spinal respiratory muscle paralysis, and bulbospinal paralysis because these patients are generally unable to cough, sometimes for many months. Mechanical respirators are often needed.

COMPLICATIONS. Paralytic poliomyelitis may be associated with numerous complications. Melena severe enough to require transfusion may result from single or multiple superficial intestinal erosions; perforation is rare. Acute gastric dilatation may occur abruptly during the acute or convalescent stage, causing further respiratory embarrassment; immediate gastric aspiration and external application of ice bags are indicated. Mild hypertension of a few days or weeks duration is common in the acute stage, probably related to lesions of the vasoregulatory centers in the medulla and especially to underventilation. In the later stages, because of immobilization, hypertension may occur along with hypercalcemia, nephrocalcinosis, and vascular lesions. Dimness of vision, headache, and a light-headed feeling associated with hypertension should be regarded as premonitory of a frank convulsion. Cardiac irregularities are uncommon, but electrocardiographic abnormalities suggesting myocarditis are not rare. Acute pulmonary edema occurs occasionally, particularly in patients with arterial hypertension. Pulmonary embolism is uncommon despite the immobilization. Skeletal decalcification begins soon after immobilization and results in hypercalciuria, which in turn predisposes the patient to urinary calculi, especially when urinary stasis and infection are present. A high fluid intake is the only effective prophylactic measure. The patient should be mobilized as much and as early as possible.

PROGNOSIS. Mortality in poliomyelitis epidemics in the United States prior to vaccine use was 5–7%. Most deaths occur within the first 2 wk after onset. Mortality and the degree of disability are greater after the age of puberty. In general, the more extensive the paralysis in the first 10 days of illness, the more severe is the ultimate disability. Unexpected improvement may appear soon after defervescence and again about 6 wk after onset, a time that corresponds to functional restoration of temporarily inactive neurons. The degree of functional recovery also depends upon the adequacy and promptness of supportive therapy: proper body positioning, active motion, use of assistive devices, and, of great importance, the psychologic motivation of the patient to return to as full and normal a life as possible.

Postpolio Syndrome. After an interval of 30–40 yr, as many as 30–40% of persons who survived paralytic poliomyelitis in childhood may experience muscle pain and exacerbation of existing weakness, or they may develop new weakness or paralysis. This entity, which is referred to as *postpolio syndrome*, has been reported only in persons who were infected in the era of wild poliovirus circulation. Risk factors for postpolio syndrome include increasing length of time since acute poliovirus infection, presence of permanent residual impairment after recovery from acute illness, and female sex.

PREVENTION. Vaccination is the only effective method of preventing poliomyelitis. Hygienic measures help limit the spread of the infection among young children, but immunization is necessary to control transmission among all age groups. Both the inactivated polio vaccine (IPV), which is currently produced using improved methods compared to the original vaccine and is sometimes referred to as enhanced IPV, and the live, attenuated, orally administered polio vaccine (OPV) have established efficacy in preventing poliovirus infection and paralytic poliomyelitis. Both vaccines induce production of antibodies against the three strains of poliovirus. IPV elicits higher serum immunoglobulin (Ig) G antibody titers, but OPV also induces significantly greater mucosal IgA immunity in the oropharynx and gastrointestinal tract that limits replication of the wild poliovirus at these sites. Transmission of wild poliovirus by fecal spread is limited in OPV recipients. The immunogenicity of IPV is not affected by the presence of maternal antibodies.

IPV has no adverse effects. Live vaccine may undergo reversion to neurovirulence as it multiplies in the human intestinal tract and may cause vaccine-associated paralytic poliomyelitis (VAPP) in vaccinees or in their contacts. This risk is very low, but since 1979 VAPP accounts for all of the four to eight cases of paralytic poliomyelitis that have occurred annually in the United States. The overall risk of VAPP is low (1 case/2.4 million doses) but is higher after the first dose for children (1/750,000 first doses) and for all first-dose recipients (1/1.2 million first doses). Based on doses distributed, the overall risk for recipients is 1 case/6.2 million doses.

Many countries rely on OPV, whereas Sweden, Finland, and Holland use only IPV as the standard vaccine preparation. IPV and OPV are used in a combined regimen in Denmark and Israel.

In the United States, the Centers for Disease Control and the American Academy of Pediatrics in 1999 revised poliomyelitis vaccine recommendations to increase reliance on IPV. The relative benefits of OPV on the United States population have diminished because of the elimination of wild poliovirus in the Western hemisphere and the reduced threat of poliovirus importation into the United States. Thus, the risk of vaccine-associated poliomyelitis caused by OPV is now judged less acceptable. A transition policy has been implemented that will increase the use of IPV and decrease the use of OPV; recommendation of an IPV-only immunization schedule for children is anticipated by 2001.

As of January, 2000, the IPV-only schedule is recommended for routine polio vaccination in the United States. All children should receive four doses of IPV at 2 mo, 4 mo, 6–18 mo, and 4–6 yr of age. OPV should be used only for (1) mass vaccination campaigns to control outbreaks; (2) unvaccinated children who will be traveling within 4 wk to areas where polio is endemic; and (3) children of parents who do not accept the recommended number of vaccine injections; these children may receive OPV only for the third or fourth dose or both. Health care providers should administer OPV only after discussing the risk of VAPP with parents or caregivers. OPV is contraindicated for use in immunocompromised persons as well as in all their household contacts, because of the risk of VAPP; these persons should receive only IPV. OPV remains the vaccine of choice in countries where polio is endemic.

243.2 Nonpolio Enteroviruses

EPIDEMIOLOGY. Humans are the only known reservoir for the human enteroviruses. Viruses related to human enteroviruses have been isolated from dogs and cats, but there is no evidence of spread from animals to humans. These viruses are spread from person to person by fecal-oral and possibly oral-oral (respiratory) routes. The enteroviruses infect the human gastrointestinal tract, but they do not colonize it. Even during the season of greater prevalence, very few strains circulate, probably as a result of interference among the virus types.

Children are immunologically susceptible, and their unhygienic habits facilitate spread. Transmission occurs from child to child (via feces to skin to mouth) and then within family groups. Even when an enterovirus is spreading through a community, it is often confined to households with young children. Rapid and extensive spread occurs in other similar environments such as summer camps and day-care centers. Recovery of enteroviruses is inversely related to age, and prevalence of specific antibodies is directly related to age. The incidence of infections and the prevalence of antibodies do not differ between boys and girls, but significant disease is more common in boys. Enteroviruses are often isolated from sewage and survive for up to 6 mo in wet soil, but person-to-person spread is the primary mode of transmission. Environmental contamination is probably the result rather than the cause of human infection.

Enteroviruses have a worldwide distribution. In tropical and semitropical areas, they are found year round. In temperate climates, they are detected during winter and spring but are more common during summer and fall, with peaks from August to October. Winter outbreaks are rare. Infection and acquisition of postinfection immunity occur with greater frequency and at earlier ages in crowded, economically deprived populations. Under such conditions, the incidence of infection with one or more enterovirus serotypes may exceed 50%; mixed infections are common.

Although there are 68 identified enteroviruses (see Table 243–1), most illness in the United States is due to about a dozen nonpolio enteroviral types. Recently, the most prevalent types have been echoviruses 4, 6, 9, 11, and 30, Coxsackieviruses A9, A16, and B2–B5, and enteroviruses 70 and 71.

PATHOGENESIS. Following the acquisition of virus by the oral or respiratory route, initial viral replication occurs in the pharynx and the lower gastrointestinal tract (Fig. 243–1). Cell surface macromolecules serve as virus receptors in the gastrointestinal tract for several enteroviruses: poliovirus receptor (PVR) and integrin (VLA-2) for echoviruses 1 and 8; decay accelerating factor (DAF, CD55) for echovirus 7 and Coxsackie B viruses. Virus receptors for enteroviruses appear to be expressed on both the apical and the basolateral surfaces of intestinal epithelial cells.

The environmental conditions of the gastrointestinal tract, low pH, the presence of proteolytic enzymes, and bile salts favor the viability and local infection of certain viruses over some others. The detergent-like action of bile salts is especially detrimental to enveloped viruses and explains the fact that intestinal infections are mainly due to nonenveloped viruses (e.g., enteroviruses and rotaviruses). Two or more enteroviruses may invade and replicate at the same time in the gastrointestinal tract, but replication of one type often interferes with the growth of the heterologous type. Interference has been documented between echovirus, Coxsackievirus, and poliovirus, including vaccine strains. Within 1 day the infection extends to the regional lymph nodes. On about the third day minor viremia occurs, involving many secondary sites. Multiplication of virus in these sites coincides with the onset of clinical symptoms. Illness can vary from minor to fatal infections. Major viremia occurs during the period of multiplication of virus in the secondary sites and usually lasts from the 3rd to the 7th day of infection. In many enteroviral infections central nervous system involvement occurs at the same time as other secondary organ involvement, but the occasional delay in appearance of central nervous system symptoms suggests that seeding occurred later in association with the major viremia or by another pathway such as autonomic nerve fibers. Cessation of viremia correlates with the appearance of serum antibody. The viral concentration in secondary sites begins to diminish on about the 7th day. However, infection continues in the lower intestinal tract for prolonged periods (Fig. 243–2).

Enteroviruses have been detected in some cases of myopericarditis. The pathogenesis of enterovirus-associated nephritis, myositis, polyradiculitis, pancreatitis, hepatitis, pneumonitis, and other syndromes is unclear; these disorders may be due to the inflammatory response to viral antigens or to virus-induced tissue damage. Enteroviral RNA sequences have been demonstrated in cardiac tissues from patients with cardiomyopathies, but a causal relationship has not been established. Some peptide sequences that constitute viral epitopes are shared by host tissues, which may provide a mechanism for autoimmune reactions in enteroviral infection.

Certain viral infections, most notably Coxsackievirus B and other enterovirus infections, have been implicated in the pathogenesis of childhood (insulin-dependent) diabetes mellitus. These viruses can induce β cell damage in mice, but their causal role remains undefined. There is no conclusive evidence to support an association of enteroviral infection with chronic fatigue syndrome (see Chapter 717).

Neutralizing antibodies against enteroviruses form within several days after exposure, often before the onset of illness. This early production of IgG antibodies is a result of replication of the virus in the intestinal tract and deep lymphatic tissues, which occurs before the target organs, such as the central nervous system, are invaded. Mucosal immunity, conferred mainly by secretory immunoglobulin IgA, is an important defense against enteroviral infection, mediating protection against intestinal reinfection after recovery from natural infection.

CLINICAL MANIFESTATIONS. Coxsackieviral and echoviral infections are exceedingly common, and their spectrum of disease is protean. Because many of the clinical-virologic associations are based on a limited number of cases and because enteroviruses are frequently carried asymptomatically in the gastrointestinal tract for relatively long periods of time, some of the observed illnesses and coincidentally recovered viruses may represent a causal relationship. However, repeated observations have confirmed many virus-illness associations, even though their occurrence has been sporadic. More than 90% of infections caused by nonpolio enteroviruses are asymptomatic or result in undifferentiated febrile illnesses. Some clinical

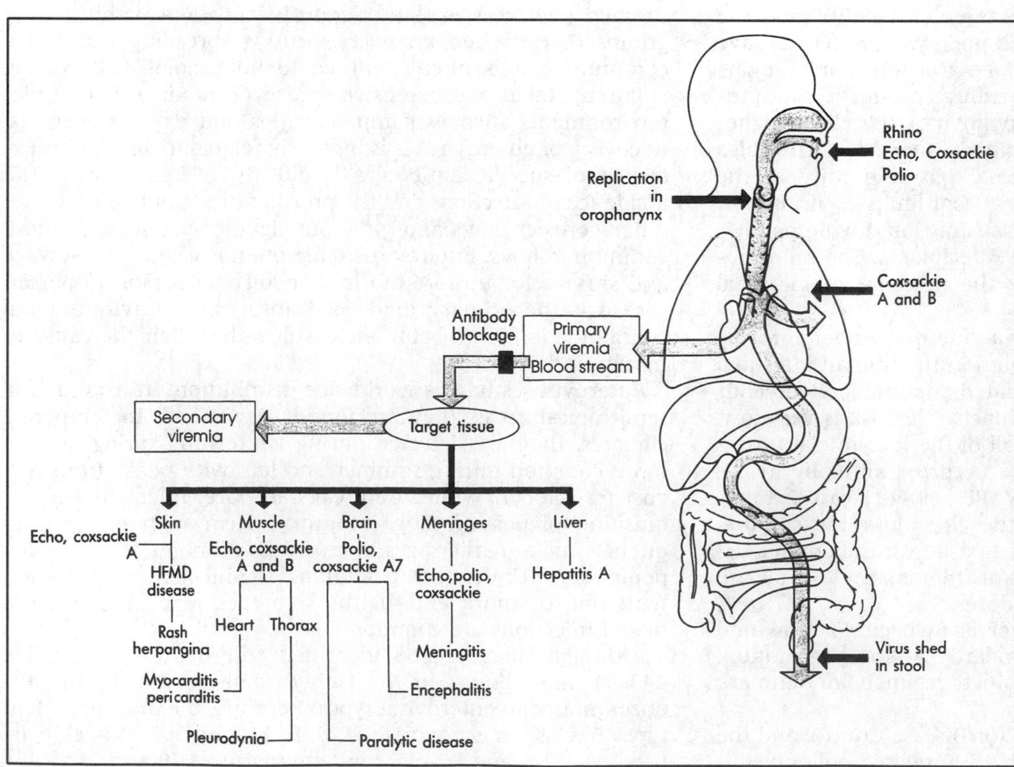

Figure 243–1 The pathogenesis of enteroviral infections. (HFMD = hand, foot, and mouth disease.)

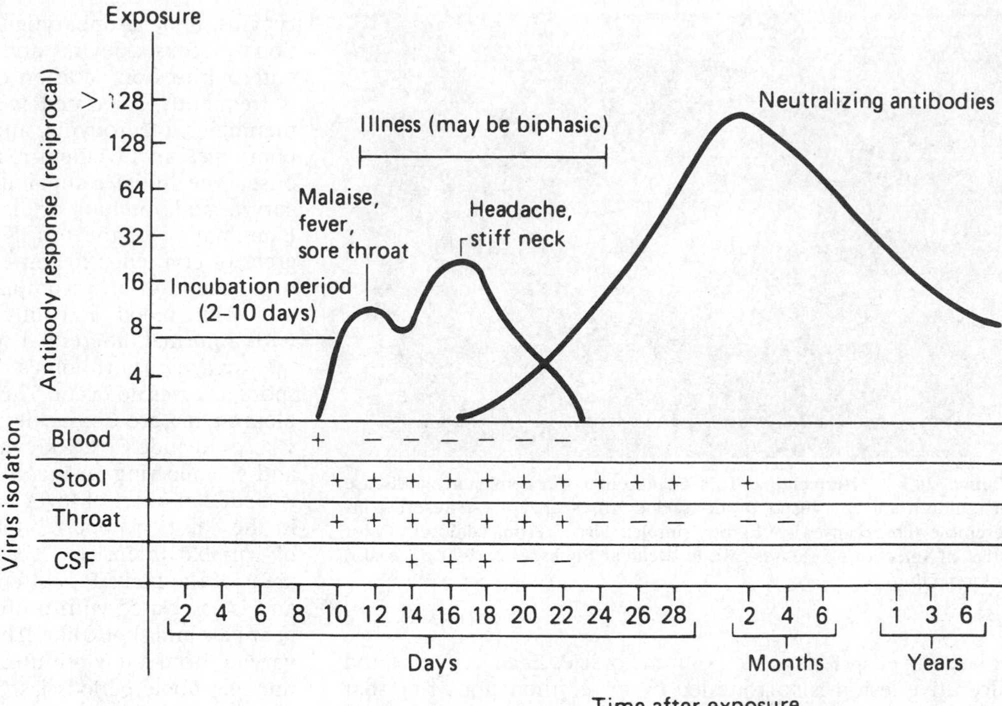

Figure 243–2 Time course of clinical and laboratory manifestations of enteroviral infections. (CSF = cerebrospinal fluid.)

syndromes are highly but not exclusively associated with certain serotypes.

Asymptomatic Infection. Coxsackieviruses and echoviruses are frequently recovered from the stools of healthy children, but there are few data on the rate of asymptomatic infection with nonpolio enteroviruses. The isolation of enteroviruses from the stool cannot be equated with asymptomatic infection because illness, if it occurs, happens shortly after the virus is acquired and is of short duration, whereas viral shedding may continue for 1–3 mo. In general, the more carefully clinical symptomatology is sought, the lower the percentage of truly asymptomatic infections that is found. Clinical expression is also inversely related to age and varies by viral type. Overall, probably <50% of all infections are asymptomatic.

Nonspecific Febrile Illness. Nonspecific febrile illness is the most common manifestation of enteroviral infections. All viral types cause this clinical presentation, but the frequency varies considerably among individual viruses. Onset of illness is usually abrupt and has no prodrome. In young children the initial finding is fever that may be associated with malaise. In older children headache and myalgia are usually also noted. The temperature ranges from 38.5–40°C (101–104°F) and has a mean duration of 3 days. In some instances the fever is biphasic; it occurs for 1 day, is absent for 2–3 days, and then recurs for an additional 2–4 days. Malaise and anorexia are often related to the degree of temperature elevation, as is headache in older patients. The complaint of a sore or scratchy feeling in the throat is common, but significant pharyngeal inflammation is not present. Other nonspecific symptoms that may be present include nausea and vomiting at the onset of illness, mild abdominal discomfort, loose stools, and myalgia. Findings on physical examination are generally nonspecific and include minimal conjunctivitis, injection of the pharynx, and cervical lymphadenopathy. The duration of illness varies from 24 hr to 6 days with an average of 3–4 days. White blood cell count and other routine laboratory tests are normal.

Nonpolio enteroviruses are common causes of a large variety of skin manifestations. In the summer and fall they are the leading cause of nonspecific exanthems. There is a marked variation in the rates at which exanthems occur among the various viral types and also among different age groups of the host. In general, the frequency is inversely related to the age of the infected patient, and several different agents can produce similar skin manifestations. The relative importance of enteroviruses as causative agents of exanthems in children in developed countries is due to immunization programs, which have decreased the classic childhood exanthems such as measles and rubella.

Hand, Foot, and Mouth Disease. Coxsackievirus A16 is the major cause of the hand, foot, and mouth disease, which has a typically enteroviral pattern with a short incubation period (4–6 days) and a summer and fall seasonal pattern. The clinical expression rate of the enanthem-exanthem complex is high, being close to 100% in young children, 38% in school children, and 11% in adults. The intraoral lesions are ulcerative and average about 4–8 mm in size. The tongue and buccal mucosa are most frequently involved. The hands are more commonly involved than the feet. Buttock lesions are also common, but these do not usually progress to vesiculation. The lesions on the hands and feet are usually tender and vesicular and vary in size from 3–7 mm; they are generally more common on the dorsal surfaces but frequently occur on the palms and soles as well. They clear by absorption of the fluid in about 1 wk. Coxsackievirus A16 is frequently associated with subacute, chronic, and recurring skin lesions. Recently, enterovirus 71 has been the etiologic agent in several outbreaks of hand, foot, and mouth disease. Illness with this virus is frequently more severe than that due to Coxsackievirus A16; aseptic meningitis, encephalitis, and paralytic disease are common.

Herpangina. Herpangina is usually characterized by a sudden onset of fever, although the initial temperature can be quite variable, ranging from normal to 41°C (106°F). The temperature tends to be higher in younger patients. Older children frequently complain of headache and backache. Vomiting occurs in about 25% of children <5 yr of age. In the majority of children the oropharyngeal lesions are present on the first examination at the time or shortly after fever is observed (Fig. 243–3). The characteristic lesions are small, 1–2 mm vesicles and ulcers. They are usually discrete and number about five per patient; some patients have only one or two lesions but others have 15 or more. When seen early, the vesicular lesions

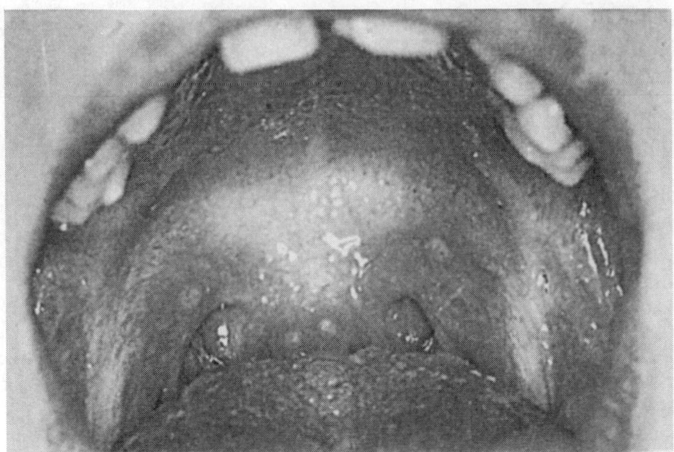

Figure 243–3 Herpangina. This enanthem is predominantly a disease of children and is caused by coxsackieviruses group A. These lesions resemble those caused by herpes simplex virus. (From Edmond's Color Atlas of Infectious Diseases. Wolfe Medical Publishers, 1990.) See also color section.

enlarge over 2–3 days to 3–4 mm in size. Each vesicular and ulcerative lesion is surrounded by an erythematous ring that varies in size up to 10 mm in diameter. The major site of the lesions is the anterior tonsillar pillars. They also occur on the soft palate, uvula, tonsils, pharyngeal wall, and occasionally the posterior buccal surfaces. Aside from these lesions, the remainder of the throat appears either normal or minimally erythematous. Although herpangina is occasionally associated with aseptic meningitis or other more severe enteroviral illnesses, most cases of herpangina are mild and have no complications. The usual duration of signs and symptoms is 3–6 days.

Echovirus type 9 is the most prevalent nonpolio enterovirus and usually causes a nonspecific febrile illness or aseptic meningitis, but an exanthem occurs in about one third of cases; 57% of children <5 yr of age have rash compared to 6% of those >10 yr of age. The rash is most frequently rubelliform, but patechiae frequently occur in addition to or as the sole manifestation. Rash and fever usually appear at about the same time, and frequently the illness closely mimics meningococcemia. The rash usually lasts 3–5 days. The disease may be confused with measles in some patients in whom the lesions of the oral mucosa resemble Koplik spots and patchy rash, but the coryza and conjunctivitis of measles are absent.

Acute Hemorrhagic Conjunctivitis. Enterovirus 70 has been the cause of a majority of epidemics of acute hemorrhagic conjunctivitis. It has a sudden onset that is accompanied by severe eye pain associated with photophobia, blurred vision, lacrimation, erythema and congestion of the eye, and edematous and chemotic lids. There are subconjunctival hemorrhages of varying size and frequently a transient punctate epithelial keratitis, conjunctival follicles, and preauricular lymphadenopathy. Eye discharge is initially serous but becomes mucopurulent with secondary bacterial infection. Systemic symptoms (including fever) are rare. Occasionally, a picture suggestive of pharyngoconjunctival fever occurs. A small number of patients have a polyradiculoneuropathy or paralytic poliomyelitis following enterovirus 70 acute hemorrhagic conjunctivitis. Persons 20–50 yr of age have the highest attack rates, and children are less often involved. Initially, most epidemics occurred in the coastal areas of tropical countries toward the end of hot rainy periods. More recently, outbreaks of disease have occurred in temperate climates, including many areas of the United States. Epidemics are explosive and are spread mainly by the eye-hand-fomite-eye route.

Respiratory Manifestations. Pharyngitis, tonsillitis, tonsillopharyngitis, and nasopharyngitis are common clinical manifestations of coxsackieviral and echoviral infections; probably all enteroviruses on occasion cause mild pharyngitis. Pharyngitis is frequently associated with other clinical findings such as meningitis, pleurodynia, and exanthem. Although evidence of pharyngeal involvement may be present at the time of disease onset, the initial complaint is most often fever. Sore throat, coryza, and vomiting or diarrhea, or both, may also be noted. Examination of the tonsils and pharynx reveals varying degrees of erythema; in some, patches of exudate are seen. The usual duration of uncomplicated pharyngitis is 3–6 days. The total white blood cell count may be normal or slightly elevated with a normal differential count.

Pleurodynia (Bornholm's disease) is an epidemic disease, but sporadic cases do occur. The major etiologic agents in epidemic pleurodynia are Coxsackieviruses B3 and B5; other associated viruses include Coxsackieviruses B1 and B2 and echoviruses 1 and 6. Following an incubation period of about 4 days, there is a sudden onset of fever and pain. The typical pain is located in the chest or upper abdomen, is muscular in origin, and is of variable intensity. Occasionally, the pain occurs in other areas of the body. It is often excruciatingly severe and sudden and is associated with profuse sweating. The patient may appear pale and shock-like. The pain is spasmodic, with durations varying from a few minutes to several hours. Most commonly, the spasmodic periods last about 15–30 min. During spasms, the respirations are usually rapid, shallow, and grunting, suggesting pneumonia of pleural inflammation. Pleural friction rubs may be noted on auscultation, and they may appear and disappear with the coming and going of the pain episodes. Coughing, sneezing, or deep breathing makes the pain worse. In older children and adults the pain is described as stabbing or knife-like. When pain is localized to the abdomen, it is frequently crampy and suggests colic in the younger child. The child may double over and refuse to walk or move. Occasionally, the abdominal pain in association with a pale, sweaty, shock-like appearance suggests acute intestinal obstruction. Splitting and guarding of the abdomen also suggest appendicitis and peritonitis. Tenderness to some degree is present in areas of pain, but frank myositis with muscle swelling is not observed. Fever and pain usually last 1–2 days. Frequently, however, the illness is biphasic; after the initial febrile period the patient is asymptomatic for several days, and then the pain and fever recur. Rarely, patients have several recurrent episodes over a period of a few weeks. In these cases fever is less prominent during the recurrences.

In epidemics both children and adults are afflicted, with the majority of cases occurring in persons <30 yr of age. Most children have other signs of enteroviral infection such as anorexia, nausea, vomiting, headache, and sore throat. The white blood cell count is variable, but polymorphonuclear neutrophils are increased and band forms are frequent. The erythrocyte sedimentation rate may be normal to extremely high. The chest roentgenogram is most often normal.

Complications in pleurodynia are uncommon. Aseptic meningitis has been noted, and adult males have experienced orchitis. Myocarditis and pericarditis may also complicate pleurodynia.

A variety of nonpolio enteroviruses have been associated with sporadic instances of parotitis, croup, bronchitis, bronchiolitis, infectious asthma, and pneumonia as well as outbreaks of lymphonodular pharyngitis, stomatitis, and other lesions in the anterior mouth.

Gastrointestinal Manifestations. Gastrointestinal manifestations are common (7–30%) in patients with enteroviral infections. Vomiting is a common manifestation of infections due to many coxsackieviral and echoviral types, but it is rarely the major complaint of the patient or the parent. Except for the hand, foot, and mouth syndrome (Coxsackievirus A16), in which vomiting is uncommon, this manifestation occurs in about

50% of all cases seen in epidemic enteroviral disease. Vomiting is most common in meningitis and least common in pleurodynia and uncomplicated exanthematous disease.

Diarrhea occurs commonly in coxsackieviral and echoviral infections as one of many manifestations of the systemic illness. It is rarely severe. In most instances loose stools occur for 2–4 days. The stools are rarely watery and never bloody and number less than six to eight per day.

Abdominal pain is also a common complaint in many enteroviral infections. About 10% of patients with hand, foot, and mouth syndrome (Coxsackievirus A16) complain of abdominal pain. Coxsackieviral and echoviral meningitis is associated with abdominal pain in about 25% of cases. The severity of pain in enteroviral infections is quite variable and on occasion may suggest a surgical abdomen. The pain is most often periumbilical; it may be either constant or colicky. The associated fever is most often higher than 38.3°C (101°F).

Nonpolio enteroviruses have been associated with a variety of other gastrointestinal and abdominal complaints. In most situations these findings are just one manifestation of a more typical enteroviral illness.

Neurologic Manifestations. Aseptic meningitis resulting from enteroviruses occurs in epidemics and as isolated cases (see Chapter 174.2). Epidemics have occurred most commonly with Coxsackievirus B5 and echoviruses 4, 6, 9, and 11. In general, illness is more common in children than in adults. Virtually all patients have fever, and many have mild pharyngitis; other respiratory manifestations are also common. Rash is common but varies with the specific viral agents; 30–50% of all patients with echovirus 9 meningitis have exanthem. Frequently, the rash is petechial, thus suggesting meningococcemia. Except for the occurrence of rash, herpangina, pleurodynia, or myocarditis, there is little clinical evidence that helps in identifying the cause in a sporadic case of aseptic meningitis. Generalized muscle stiffness or spasm is usually observed, although the degree varies considerably; Kernig and Brudzinski signs are positive in fewer than half the cases. Deep tendon reflexes are usually normal.

The duration of illness is variable. In the majority of instances the temperature returns to normal within 4–6 days, and disability resulting from neurologic involvement lasts 1–2 wk. Occasionally, a biphasic illness pattern occurs consisting of an initial period with fever, headache, nausea, vomiting, and muscle aches and pains of a few days duration followed by general recovery; then the same symptoms return with more pronounced neurologic involvement.

About 2% of reported cases of encephalitis (see Chapter 174.2) in the United States have an enteroviral cause. This is probably an underestimate of the number of severe cases, which may total >1,000/yr. Echovirus type 9 is the most common cause of enteroviral encephalitis; other commonly associated enteroviral types are echoviruses 3, 4, 6, and 11 and Coxsackieviruses B2, B4, and B5. In general, the prognosis in encephalitis caused by enteroviral infections is good, but fatalities have been associated with disease due to Coxsackieviruses B3 and B6, echoviruses 2, 9, 17, and 25, and enterovirus 71.

Paralysis on the basis of anterior horn cell disease occasionally results from infection with nonpolio enteroviruses. Many coxsackieviruses and echoviruses have been associated with the Guillain-Barré syndrome. Cerebellar ataxia has been noted in association with Coxsackieviruses A4, A7, A9, B3, and B4 and with echoviruses 6, 9, and 16. Peripheral neuritis has been reported with echovirus 9 infection, and Coxsackievirus A9 has been associated with a focal encephalitis and acute hemiplegia.

Pericarditis and Myocarditis. Cardiac manifestations have been noted in association with 27 different nonpolio enteroviruses. The group B Coxsackieviruses have been most frequently implicated, and B5 has been the most common causative agent. Of the echoviruses, echovirus 6 has been most frequently associated with cardiac involvement. Hepatitis, pneumonia, nephritis, meningitis, and orchitis have also been occasional associated findings with Coxsackievirus B. The mortality resulting from acute coxsackieviral and echoviral heart disease is significant. In nonfatal cases recovery is usually complete without residual disability; occasionally, constrictive pericarditis occurs as well as other sequelae.

Orchitis and Epididymitis. Group B Coxsackieviruses are second only to mumps as causative agents of orchitis; B5 is the most commonly associated Coxsackievirus, but B2 and B4 have also been implicated on many occasions. In almost all instances the orchitis is a secondary event, most commonly associated with pleurodynia. The illness is frequently biphasic; fever and pleurodynia or meningitis are followed by apparent recovery and then by orchitis about 2 wk after onset. Many patients also have epididymitis. In epidemics of disease resulting from group B Coxsackieviruses, the occurrence of testicular involvement is quite variable. Generally, orchitis is infrequent, but in one B2 outbreak 17% of the postpubertal males had orchitis, and 7% also had eipdidymitis.

Myositis and Arthritis. Myalgia is a common complaint accompanying many coxsackieviral and echoviral illnesses. However, there is almost no direct (demonstration of virus in muscle) or indirect (muscle enzyme elevations) evidence of muscle involvement in routine enteroviral illnesses. Coxsackievirus A2 has been associated with myositis, and Coxsackievirus A9 and echovirus 18 have been associated with polymyositis. A dermatomyositis-like syndrome has been associated with immune deficiency and enteroviral infection. Arthritis has occurred rarely in enterovirus infection.

Neonatal Infections. Nonpolio enteroviral infections in neonatal infants result in a wide variety of clinical manifestations ranging from asymptomatic infection to sepsis-like illness, fatal encephalitis, and myocarditis. The illness usually begins within the first 2 wk of life after perinatal transmission from the mother, usually by transplacental transmission immediately prior to delivery. Nursery outbreaks also occur. Coxsackieviruses B1–B5 are associated with neonatal myocarditis. The onset of neonatal myocarditis is sudden and associated with acute respiratory illness. Other symptoms are fever, feeding difficulties, respiratory distress, cyanosis, and lethargy. Later signs include cardiomegaly, hepatomegaly, and electrocardiographic changes. Cardiovascular signs are accompanied by various neurologic manifestations in up to a third of cases. The prognosis is poor despite extensive supportive care.

DIAGNOSIS. The clinical differentiation of enteroviral disease from treatable bacterial illnesses is frequently very difficult, although when all circumstances of a particular illness are considered, enteroviral diseases often can be suspected on clinical grounds. The most important factors in clinical diagnosis are season of the year, geographic location, exposure, incubation period, and clinical symptoms. In temperate climates enteroviral prevalence is distinctly seasonal; therefore, disease is usually seen in the summer and fall and is unlikely to occur in the winter; in the tropics enteroviruses are prevalent throughout the year. A mother's nonspecific mild febrile illness at the time of a delivery that occurs in the summer and fall suggests the possibility of neonatal enteroviral infection.

Most viral diagnostic laboratories have facilities for recovering the majority of enteroviruses that cause illness. Tissue culture systems allow the isolation of polioviruses, group B Coxsackieviruses, echoviruses, and Coxsackieviruses A9 and A16. Enteroviral growth in tissue culture takes only a few days in many cases and less than a week in most; identification of type frequently takes much more time. A complete diagnostic isolation spectrum can be obtained using suckling mouse inoculation. Specimens for virus isolation should be obtained from the throat and rectum (feces) and any other clinically involved site. Virus isolation from all sites except the feces can usually be considered causally related to a specific illness.

Virus cultures of cerebrospinal fluid of patients suffering from enterovirus meningitis are often negative. Recently the use of reverse transcriptase polymerase chain reaction (RT-PCR) has been shown to increase sensitivity and accelerate the diagnosis of enterovirus infections. The results by RT-PCR can be obtained in 1–2 days. This method also permits genotyping for epidemiological investigations.

Demonstration of a rise in neutralizing antibody titer to a virus recovered from the feces indicates recent infection and may confirm a causal role for the isolated virus. Serum should be collected and stored frozen as soon as possible after the onset of illness and then again 2–4 wk later. Serologic testing usually requires a viral isolate to determine which enterovirus serologies should be tested.

Differential Diagnosis. The differential diagnosis of enteroviral infections depends on the clinical manifestations. It is most important to distinguish bacterial diseases such as those commonly associated with pharyngitis, pneumonia, pericarditis, meningitis, and septicemia, although other viral illnesses must also be considered.

COMPLICATIONS. Complications of enteroviral infections such as those associated with myocarditis or encephalitis are presented in other sections of this text.

PREVENTION. Vaccines for enteroviruses other than polioviruses are not available. However, passive protection with pooled human immune globulin (0.2 mL/kg intramuscularly) may be useful in preventing disease in virulent nursery outbreaks. Intravenous immune globulin (IVIG) can be expected to contain antibodies against Coxsackievirus types B1–B5, offering protection to infants who lack transplacentally acquired specific antibody and have not yet become infected.

TREATMENT. There is no specific therapy for any enterovirus infection. In severe, catastrophic, and generalized neonatal infections, it is reasonable to administer intravenous immune globulin to the infant, although there are no studies that demonstrate its efficacy.

Corticosteroids should not be given during acute severe enteroviral infections, such as neonatal myocarditis or encephalitis, although some authors believe this therapy has been beneficial in patients with Coxsackievirus myocarditis. The use of corticosteroids has had deleterious effects in experimental coxsackieviral infections of mice and has not shown benefit in human myocarditis. Because the possibility of bacterial sepsis cannot be ruled out in many instances of enteroviral infections, antibiotics should frequently be administered for the most likely potential bacterial pathogens.

PROGNOSIS. The prognosis in nonpolio enteroviral infections in the vast majority of instances is excellent. Morbidity and mortality are related almost entirely to perinatal disseminated disease in neonates and to myocarditis and encephalitis in older children.

Polioviruses

American Academy of Pediatrics, Committee on Infectious Diseases: Poliomyelitis prevention: Revised recommendations for use of inactivated and live oral poliovirus vaccines. Pediatrics 103:171, 1999.

Centers for Disease Control and Prevention: Certification of poliomyelitis eradication—the Americas, 1994. MMWR 43:720, 1994.

Centers for Disease Control and Prevention: Paralytic poliomyelitis—United States, 1980–1994. MMWR 46:79, 1997.

Centers for Disease Control and Prevention: Poliomyelitis prevention in the United States: Introduction of a sequential vaccination schedule of inactivated poliovirus vaccine followed by oral poliovirus vaccine. Recommendations of the Advisory Committee on Immunization Practices (ACIP). MMWR 46(RR-3):1, 1997.

Dalakas MC, Elder G, Hallett M, et al: A long-term follow-up study of patients with post-poliomyelitis neuromuscular symptom. N Engl J Med 314:959,1986.

Faden H, Modlin JF, Thomas ML, et al: Comparative evaluation of immunization with live attenuated and enhanced-potency inactivated trivalent poliovirus vaccines in childhood: Systemic and local immune responses. J Infect Dis 162:1291, 1990.

Strebel PM, Sutter RW, Cochi SL, et al: Epidemiology of poliomyelitis in the United States one decade after the last reported case of indigenous wild virus-associated disease. Clin Infect Dis 14:568, 1992.

Nonpolio Enteroviruses

Abzug MJ, Keyserling HL, Lee ML, et al: Neonatal enterovirus infection: Virology, serology, and effects of intravenous immune globulin. Clin Infect Dis 20:1201, 1995.

Abzug MJ, Levin MF, Rotbart HA: Profile of enterovirus disease in the first two weeks of life. Pediatr Infect Dis J 12:820, 1993.

Ahmed A, Brito F, Goto C, et al: Clinical utility of the polymerase chain reaction for diagnosis of enteroviral meningitis in infancy. J Pediatr 131:393, 1997.

Dagan R, Hall CB, Powell KR, et al: Epidemiology and laboratory diagnosis of infection with viral and bacterial pathogens in infants hospitalized for suspected sepsis. J Pediatr 115:351, 1989.

Hayward JC, Gillespie SM, Kaplan KM, et al: Outbreak of poliomyelitis-like paralysis associated with enterovirus 71. Pediatr Infect Dis J 8:611, 1989.

Kaplan MH, Klein SW, McPhee J, et al: Group B coxsackievirus infections in infants younger than three months of age: A serious childhood illness. Rev Infect Dis 5:1019, 1983.

Modlin JF: Perinatal echovirus infection: Insights from a literature review of 61 cases of serious infection and 16 outbreaks in nurseries. Rev Infect Dis 8:918, 1986.

Ogra PL, Garofalo R: Secretory antibody response to viral vaccines. Prog Med Virol 37:156, 1990.

Rotbart H: Enteroviral infections of the central nervous system. Clin Infect Dis 20:971, 1995.

Strikas RA, Anderson LJ, Parker RA: Temporal and geographic patterns of isolates of nonpolio enterovirus in the United States, 1970–1983. J Infect Dis 153:346, 1986.

Yin-Murphy M: Acute hemorrhagic conjunctivitis. Prog Med Virol 29:23, 1984.

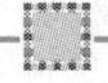

Chapter 244
Parvovirus B19

William C. Koch

ETIOLOGY. Parvovirus B19, which was discovered in 1975, is a member of the genus *Erythrovirus* in the family Parvoviridae. Parvoviruses are small DNA viruses that infect a variety of animal species. Parvoviruses are recognized as important causes of disease in animals, including canine parvovirus and feline panleukopenia virus. Parvovirus B19 is the only strain that is pathogenic in humans. It does not infect other animals, and animal parvoviruses do not infect humans.

B19 is composed of an icosahedral protein capsid without an envelope that contains single-stranded DNA approximately 5.5 kb in length. It is relatively heat- and solvent-resistant. It is antigenically distinct from other mammalian parvoviruses, and there is only one known serotype. Parvoviruses replicate in mitotically active cells. Because of their limited genome, they require host cell factors present in late S phase to replicate. B19 can be propagated only in erythropoietin-stimulated erythropoietic cells derived from human bone marrow, umbilical cord blood, or primary fetal liver culture.

EPIDEMIOLOGY. The frequency of B19 infection in the general pediatric population was not recognized until 1983, when Anderson and colleagues identified B19 as the cause of erythema infectiosum.

Infections with parvovirus B19 are common and worldwide. Clinically apparent infections (rash illness and aplastic crisis) are most prevalent in school-aged children, with 70% of cases occurring between 5 and 15 yr of age. Seasonal peaks occur in the late winter and spring; sporadic infections occur throughout the year. Seroprevalence increases with age; 40–60% of adults have evidence of prior infection.

Transmission of B19 is by the respiratory route, presumably via large droplet spread, from nasopharyngeal viral shedding. The transmission rate in households ranges from 15 to 30% in susceptible contacts; mothers are more commonly infected than fathers. In outbreaks of erythema infectiosum in elementary schools, the secondary attack rates range from 10 to 60%. Nosocomial outbreaks are described, with secondary attack rates of 30% in susceptible health care workers.

Although respiratory spread is the primary mode of transmission, B19 is transmissible in blood and blood products, as shown in hemophiliac children receiving pooled donor clotting factor. Given its resistance to solvents, fomite transmission could be important in child care and other group settings, but this mode of transmission is not documented.

PATHOGENESIS. The primary target of B19 infection is the erythroid cell line, specifically erythroid precursors near the pronormoblast stage. The virus lyses these cells, leading to a progressive depletion and a transient arrest of erythropoiesis. The virus has no apparent effect on the myeloid cell line. The tropism for erythroid cells is related to the erythrocyte P blood group antigen, which serves as a virus receptor. Endothelial cells and myocardial cells also possess this antigen. Thrombocytopenia and neutropenia are often observed, but their pathogenesis is unexplained.

Experimental infection of normal volunteers revealed a biphasic illness. From 7 to 11 days after inoculation, the subjects had viremia and nasopharyngeal viral shedding and experienced fever, malaise, and rhinorrhea. Their reticulocyte counts dropped to <0.1% but resulted only in a mild, clinically insignificant fall in serum hemoglobin. Symptoms resolved and hemoglobin returned to normal with the appearance of specific antibodies. Several subjects experienced a rash associated with arthralgia 17 or 18 days after inoculation. Some manifestations of B19 infection, such as transient aplastic crisis, appear to be a direct result of viral infection, whereas others, including the exanthem and arthritis, appear to be postinfectious phenomena related to the immune response. Skin biopsy results from patients with erythema infectiosum are compatible with an immune process, showing edema in the epidermis and a perivascular mononuclear infiltrate.

Individuals with chronic hemolytic anemia and increased red cell turnover are very susceptible to perturbations in erythropoiesis. Infection with B19 leads to a transient arrest in red cell production and a precipitous fall in serum hemoglobin, often requiring transfusion. The reticulocyte count falls to near zero, reflecting the lysis of infected erythroid precursors. Humoral immunity is crucial in controlling infection. Specific immunoglobulin M (IgM) appears within 1 to 2 days followed by anti-B19 IgG, leading to control of the infection and restoration of reticulocytosis and a rise in serum hemoglobin.

Individuals with impaired humoral immunity are at increased risk for more serious or persistent infection with B19, which usually manifests as chronic red cell aplasia, but neutropenia, thrombocytopenia, and marrow failure are also described. Children on chemotherapy for leukemia, those with congenital immunodeficiency states, and those with AIDS are at risk for chronic B19 infections.

Infections in the fetus and neonate are somewhat analogous to infections in the immunocompromised host. B19 is associated with nonimmune fetal hydrops and stillbirth in women experiencing a primary infection but does not appear to be teratogenic. Like most mammalian parvoviruses, B19 can cross the placenta and cause fetal infection during primary maternal infection. Parvoviral cytopathic effects are seen primarily in erythroblasts of the bone marrow and sites of extramedullary hematopoiesis in the liver and spleen. Fetal infection can presumably occur as early as 6 wk of gestation, when erythroblasts are first found in the fetal liver; after the fourth gestational month hematopoiesis switches to the bone marrow. In some cases, fetal infection leads to a profound fetal anemia and subsequent high-output cardiac failure (Chapter 99). Fetal hydrops ensues, often associated with fetal mortality. There may also be a direct effect of the virus on myocardial tissue that contributes to the cardiac failure. However, most infections during pregnancy result in normal deliveries at term. Some of these asymptomatic infants have been reported to have chronic postnatal infection with B19 that is of unknown significance.

CLINICAL MANIFESTATIONS. Many infections are clinically inapparent. Children characteristically develop erythema infectiosum. Adults, especially women, frequently develop acute arthralgias with or without erythema infectiosum.

Erythema Infectiosum (Fifth Disease). The most common manifestation of parvovirus B19 is erythema infectiosum, also known as fifth disease, which is a benign, self-limited exanthematous illness of childhood. It was the fifth in a classification scheme of childhood exanthems; the others were rubella, measles, scarlet fever, Filatov-Dukes disease (atypical scarlet fever), and roseola infantum.

The incubation period for erythema infectiosum ranges from 4 to 28 days (average, 16–17 days). The prodromal phase is mild and consists of low-grade fever, headache, and symptoms of mild upper respiratory tract infection. The hallmark of erythema infectiosum is the characteristic rash, which occurs in three stages that are not always distinguishable. The initial stage is an erythematous facial flushing, often described as a "slapped-cheek" appearance. The rash spreads rapidly or concurrently to the trunk and proximal extremities as a diffuse macular erythema in the second stage. Central clearing of macular lesions occurs promptly, giving the rash a lacy, reticulated appearance. Palms and soles are spared, and the rash tends to be more prominent on extensor surfaces. Affected children are afebrile and not ill-appearing. Older children and adults often complain of mild pruritus. The rash resolves spontaneously without desquamation but tends to wax and wane over 1–3 wk. It can recur with exposure to sunlight, heat, exercise, and stress. Lymphadenopathy and atypical papular, purpuric, vesicular rashes are also described.

Arthropathy. Arthritis and arthralgia occur as a complication of fifth disease or as the only clinical manifestation of B19 infection. Joint symptoms are much more common in adults and older adolescents. Females are affected more frequently than males. In one outbreak of fifth disease, 60% of adults and 80% of adult women reported joint symptoms. Joint symptoms range from diffuse arthralgias with morning stiffness to frank arthritis. The joints most often affected are the hands, wrists, knees, and ankles, but practically all have been reported. The joint symptoms are self-limited and, in the majority of patients, resolve within 2–4 wk. Some patients have a prolonged course of many months, suggesting rheumatoid arthritis. Transient rheumatoid factor positivity is reported in some of these patients but with no joint destruction.

Transient Aplastic Crisis. The incubation period for transient aplastic crisis is shorter than for erythema infectiosum because it occurs coincident with the viremia. The transient arrest of erythropoiesis and absolute reticulocytopenia induced by B19 infection leads to a sudden fall in serum hemoglobin in individuals with chronic hemolytic conditions. B19-induced aplastic crises occur in patients with all types of chronic hemolysis, including sickle cell disease, thalassemia, hereditary spherocytosis, and pyruvate kinase deficiency. In contrast to children with erythema infectiosum, these patients are ill with fever, malaise, and lethargy and have signs and symptoms of profound anemia, such as pallor, tachycardia, and tachypnea. Rash is rarely present. Children with sickle cell hemoglobinopathies may also have a concurrent vaso-occlusive pain crisis.

Immunocompromised Hosts. Patients with impaired humoral immunity are at risk for chronic infections with parvovirus B19. Chronic anemia is the most common manifestation, sometimes accompanied by neutropenia, thrombocytopenia, or complete marrow suppression. Chronic infections are seen in children with cancer receiving cytotoxic chemotherapy, children with congenital immunodeficiencies, children (and adults) with AIDS, and patients with subtle defects in IgG production who are unable to generate neutralizing antibodies.

Fetus. Primary maternal infection is associated with nonimmune fetal hydrops and intrauterine fetal demise, estimated at <5%. The mechanism of fetal disease appears to be a viral-induced red cell aplasia at a time when the fetal erythroid fraction is rapidly expanding. This can lead to profound anemia, high-output cardiac failure, and hydrops. Viral DNA has been detected in infected abortuses. The second trimester seems to be the most sensitive period, but fetal losses are reported at every stage of gestation. Most infants infected in utero are born normally at term, even some with ultrasonographic evidence of hydrops. Some of these infants may acquire a chronic or persistent postnatal infection with B19, but its significance is unknown. Congenital anemia associated with intrauterine B19 infection has been reported in a few cases, sometimes following intrauterine hydrops. This process may mimic other forms of congenital hypoplastic anemia (i.e., Diamond-Blackfan syndrome). Fetal infection with B19 has not been associated with other birth defects. B19 is only one of many causes of hydrops fetalis (Chapter 99).

DIAGNOSIS. Laboratory tests for the diagnosis of B19 infection are not routinely available. Diagnosis of erythema infectiosum is usually based on clinical presentation of the typical rash and exclusion of other conditions. IgM develops rapidly after infection and persists for up to 6–8 wk. Anti-B19 IgG serves as a marker of past infection or immunity. Determination of anti-B19 IgM is the best marker of recent or acute infection; seroconversion of anti-B19 IgG antibodies in paired sera can also be used to confirm recent infection. Serologic diagnosis is unreliable in patients with immunodeficiencies.

The virus cannot be isolated by culture. Methods to detect viral particles or viral DNA such as polymerase chain reaction or nucleic acid hybridization are necessary to establish the diagnosis. Prenatal diagnosis of B19-induced fetal hydrops can be accomplished by detection of viral DNA in fetal blood by these methods or visualization of viral particles by immune electron microscopy.

Differential Diagnosis. The rash of erythema infectiosum must be differentiated from that of rubella, measles, enteroviral infections, and drug reactions. Rash and arthritis in older children should prompt consideration of juvenile rheumatoid arthritis, systemic lupus erythematosus, and other connective tissue disorders.

TREATMENT. There is no specific antiviral therapy. Commercial lots of intravenous immunoglobulin (IVIG) have been used with some success to treat B19-related episodes of anemia and bone marrow failure in immunocompromised children. Specific antibody may facilitate clearance of the virus; it is not always necessary, however, because cessation of cytotoxic chemotherapy will often suffice. In patients whose immune status is not likely to improve, such as AIDS patients, administration of IVIG may give only a temporary remission, and periodic re-infusions may be required.

B19-infected fetuses with anemia and hydrops can be managed successfully with intrauterine transfusions, but this has significant attendant risks. Once fetal hydrops is diagnosed, regardless of the suspected etiology, the mother should be referred to a fetal therapy center for further evaluation because of the high risk for serious complications (Chapter 99).

COMPLICATIONS. Erythema infectiosum is often accompanied by arthralgias or arthritis in adolescents and adults, which may persist after resolution of the rash. B19 causes thrombocytopenic purpura and, rarely, aseptic meningitis in normal individuals after erythema infectiosum. B19 is also a cause of virus-associated hemophagocytic syndrome, usually in immunocompromised patients.

PREVENTION. Children with erythema infectiosum are not likely to be infectious at presentation because the rash and arthropathy represent immune-mediated, postinfectious phenomenon. Isolation and exclusion from school or childcare are unnecessary and ineffective after diagnosis.

Children with B19-induced red cell aplasia (aplastic crisis) are infectious when they present and demonstrate a more intense viremia. Most of these children require transfusions and supportive care until their hematologic status stabilizes. They should be isolated in the hospital to prevent spread to susceptible patients and staff. Isolation should continue for at least 1 wk and until the patient is afebrile. Pregnant caregivers should not be assigned to these patients. Exclusion of pregnant women from workplaces where children with erythema infectiosum may be present (e.g., schools) is not recommended as a general policy because it is unlikely to reduce their risk. There are no data to support the use of IVIG for postexposure prophylaxis in pregnant caregivers or immunocompromised children. No vaccine is available.

Anand A, Gray ES, Brown T, et al: Human parvovirus infection in pregnancy and hydrops fetalis. N Engl J Med 316:183, 1987.

Anderson MJ, Jones SE, Fisher-Hoch SP, et al: Human parvovirus, the cause of erythema infectiosum (fifth disease)? Lancet 1:1378, 1983.

Chorba T, Coccia R, Holman RC, et al: The role of parvovirus B19 in aplastic crisis and erythema infectiosum (fifth disease). J Infect Dis 154:383, 1986.

Gratacos E, Torres PJ, Vidal J, et al: The incidence of human parvovirus B19 infection during pregnancy and its impact on perinatal outcome. J Infect Dis 171:1360, 1995.

Harger J, Adler SP, Koch WC, et al: Prospective evaluation of 618 pregnant women exposed to parvovirus B19: Risks and symptoms. Obstet Gynecol 91:413, 1998.

Koch WC, Harger JH, Barnstein B, Adler SP: Serologic and virologic evidence for frequent intrauterine transmission of human parvovirus B19 with a primary maternal infection during pregnancy. Pediatr Infect Dis J 17:489, 1998.

Koch WC, Massey G, Russell CE, Adler SP: Manifestations and treatment of human parvovirus B19 infection in immunocompromised patients. J Pediatr 116:355, 1990.

Schowengerdt KO, Ni J, Denfield SW, et al: Association of parvovirus B19 genome in children with myocarditis and cardiac allograft rejection: Diagnosis using the polymerase chain reaction. Circulation 96:3549, 1997.

Török TJ: Parvovirus B19 and human disease. Adv Intern Med 37:431, 1992.

CHAPTER 245
Herpes Simplex Virus

Steve Kohl

Herpes simplex virus (HSV) is common among humans and has a variety of clinical manifestations involving the skin, mucous membranes, eye, central nervous system (CNS), and genital tract. It also causes generalized systemic disease. Disease manifestations are in large part determined by the immune competence of the host. Two strains of the virus are identified: HSV-1 commonly infects skin and mucous membranes above the waist, and HSV-2 commonly infects the genitals and the neonate.

Three types of infection are recognized: primary infection; first infection, nonprimary; and recurrent. Primary infection is the HSV seronegative, susceptible host's first experience with the virus, which in most instances is a subclinical infection; otherwise there are usually local superficial lesions (see later discussion) accompanied by varying degrees of systemic reaction. In newborns, immunocompromised children, and severely malnourished infants, a serious systemic infection, often without superficial lesions, may occur. Circulating antibodies and a cell-mediated response develop in nonfatal cases.

First infection, nonprimary is the infection in a person with immunity to one type of HSV (e.g., type 1) and infection by a second type (e.g., type 2). These infections are usually less severe than primary infection. In pregnant women near delivery, first infection nonprimary disease can lead to severe infection in the newborn owing to the absence of type-specific antibody.

Recurrent herpetic lesions represent reactivation of a latent infection in an immune host with circulating antibodies. Reactivation follows such nonspecific stimuli as changes in the external milleu (e.g., cold, ultraviolet light) or in the internal milieu (e.g., menstruation, fever, or emotional stress). The lesions tend to be localized and, generally, are not associated with systemic reactions. In immunocompromised individuals, especially with T- or natural killer lymphocyte defects, lesions may be progressive without therapy. Viral reactivation may take place in the absence of clinical recurrence, leading to asymptomatic viral shedding.

ETIOLOGY. HSV is a double-stranded DNA-containing enveloped virus. The icosahedral protein core is surrounded by a lipid envelope in which are embedded a number of viral glycoproteins (e.g., glycoproteins B, C, D, E, G, I, J, K) responsible for viral–target cell interaction and infection. These glycoproteins are also key targets for the host humoral and cellular immune response. HSV grows rapidly in human and nonhuman cell lines and produces characteristic cytopathic changes. HSV-1 and HSV-2 are about 50% homologous by nucleic acid analysis and share immunologic cross reactivity but may be differentiated by DNA analysis (endonuclease restriction analysis) and commercially by reactivity with type-specific monoclonal antibodies in a variety of fluorescent and enzyme-linked immunosorbent (ELISA) assays. Several enzymes important for viral DNA synthesis, such as thymidine kinase and DNA polymerase, are useful targets for antiviral agents.

EPIDEMIOLOGY. The virus develops an extremely compatible relationship with its host. In about 85% of instances the infection is subclinical. Even when clinical manifestations are present, the host is only rarely seriously disabled. Occasionally, the primary or recurrent infection may lead to institutional or family outbreaks of stomatitis. This has been reported in orphanages and daycare center settings. HSV may also be transmitted by infection of digits (herpetic whitlow), during contact sports such as rugby or wrestling (herpes gladiatorum), and rarely in the hospital setting. The incubation period is 2–12 days (average, 6 days). The spread of infection appears to be determined by two factors: close body contact and trauma such as teething or a break in the skin.

The higher incidence of HSV antibodies in lower socioeconomic groups correlates with crowded living conditions. The epidemiology differs for the two types of HSV. Detailed serologic studies have been done in low-income groups, in which most infants have transplacental antibody for about the first 6 mo of life. From 1–4 yr, there is a sharp rise in antibodies to HSV-1 and then a much slower rate of acquisition up to 14 yr. At this time, there is a second sharp rise in antibodies, mostly to HSV-2. By adult life, HSV antibodies are seen in by far the majority of persons in the lower socioeconomic groups. HSV-1 antibodies are found in 30% of university students. HSV-2 antibodies are found in up to 60% of the lower socioeconomic status adults. The incidence of type 2 antibody in higher socioeconomic groups is 10–30% and in nuns about 3%. Recent serologic studies have indicated a rise in the prevalence of HSV-2 antibody in the United States to 21.7%. Ten per cent of HSV-2 seropositive individuals will infect their HSV-2 seronegative sexual partners with HSV-2 each year.

Once infected, the majority of individuals continue to carry the virus in a latent state in neuronal ganglia and maintain an almost constant level of circulating antibodies. The initial level of antibodies reached after a primary infection may fall and several subclinical recurrences may occur before a stable antibody level is established. Carriers may distribute the virus without having any manifest lesion. HSV can be isolated from the pharynx of 1–2% of asymptomatic adults.

PATHOGENESIS. The pathologic changes vary with the tissue infected. In general, a specific lesion is characterized by the presence of intranuclear inclusion bodies, which are homogeneous masses lying in the middle of a severely disorganized nucleus in which the basic chromatin has marginated to the nuclear membrane. Around the specific lesion there is always evidence of an acute inflammatory reaction. In the skin and mucous membranes the typical lesion is a unilocular vesicle. In the skin, the vesicle is tense. Ballooned epithelial cells containing intranuclear inclusions can best be seen at the margins of the vesicle. The vesicular fluid contains infected epithelial cells, including multinucleated giant cells and leukocytes. In the corium there is no necrosis, but capillaries are dilated and there is infiltration with mononuclear and polymorphonuclear cells. In the mucous membrane, because of maceration, there is early leakage of the vesicular fluid, resulting in a collapsed vesicle, mainly filled with fibrin. The edematous roof cells form a gray membrane over the ulcerated lesion.

In otherwise healthy persons, the lesions are confined to the skin and mucous membranes; viremia has rarely been described. Bloodstream spread of the virus with resultant widely disseminated disease occurs mainly in the newborn, in severely malnourished children, in persons with skin diseases such as eczema, and in those with defects in cell-mediated immunity. In these patients the virus spreads hematogenously from the portal of entry to susceptible organs. Virus increases within these organs, and secondary viremia occurs with evidence of extensive cell destruction. It is probable, however, that most cases of HSV-1 encephalitis other than in the newborn are caused by neurogenic transmission of the virus to the brain. Healing begins with clearing of the viremia and a decrease in the production of virus within the cells.

CLINICAL MANIFESTATIONS. HSV characteristically produces a vesicular lesion. Only rarely is there a viremic distribution that results in widespread systemic disease or neurogenic transmission that leads to meningoencephalitis. Furthermore, although the occurrence of primary and recurrent lesions is an accepted characteristic of herpetic infection, their distinction clinically is often not possible without knowledge of the presence or absence of homologous type-specific serum antibodies in the patient.

Lesions of the Skin and Mucous Membranes. On the skin the lesion consists of aggregates of thin-walled vesicles on an erythematous base. These rupture, scab, and heal within 7–10 days without leaving a scar except after repeated attacks or secondary bacterial infections; temporary depigmentation may occur in darkly pigmented individuals. The lesions may be preceded by mild irritation or burning at the local site or by severe neuralgic pain in the region. The vesicles may become secondarily infected, introducing impetigo into the differential diagnosis. The lesions tend to recur at the same site, particularly at mucocutaneous junctions, but may occur anywhere.

Primary infection, especially in the immunocompromised patient, may, uncommonly, result in a generalized vesicular eruption in which the lesions are small and may continue to appear over a period of 2–3 wk. If the systemic manifestations are mild, the infection must be differentiated from varicella.

Traumatic lesions of the skin or burns can be infected by HSV. Primary lesions can also occur on apparently unbroken skin, as, for example, on the chin of a drooling infant with herpetic stomatitis, in whom scattered isolated vesicles appear, in contrast to the grouped vesicles of recurrent attacks. When the skin of a limb is infected, vesicles appear in 2–3 days at the site of trauma. There is often centripetal spread along lymph channels, causing enlargement of regional lymph nodes and scattered vesicles on the intervening undamaged skin. This clinical picture may be mistaken for that of *herpes zoster,* especially if accompanied by neuralgic pain, unless the lesions are recognized as not being confined to a dermatome. The lesions heal slowly, often taking 3 wk. Recurrences at the site of local trauma are common and may assume a bullous pattern. Wrestlers and medical personnel are prone to herpetic infections of superficial abrasions (herpes gladiatorum and her-

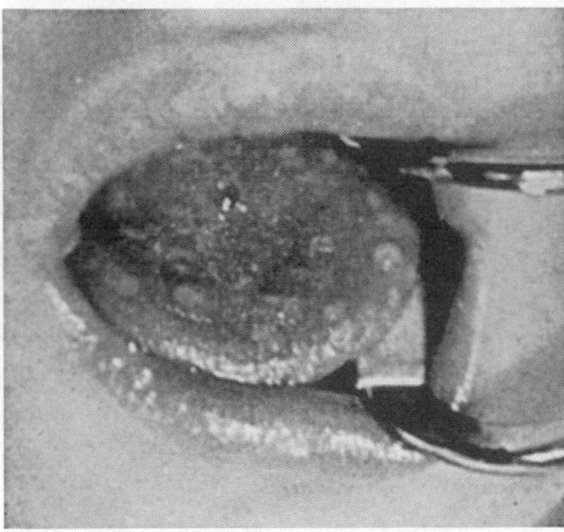

Figure 245–1 Lesions of herpetic stomatitis on the tongue.

petic whitlow). In the latter, infection of minor trauma about the nails leads to extremely painful, deep-seated spreading lesions with vesicles that resolve spontaneously in 2–3 wk. Similar lesions occur on the fingers of thumb suckers who are suffering from herpetic gingivostomatitis. The lesions must be differentiated from bacterial infection and should not be incised.

Acute Herpetic Gingivostomatitis. This primary infection, probably the most common cause of stomatitis in children 1–3 yr of age, can also occur in older children and adults. The symptoms may appear abruptly, with pain in the mouth, salivation, fetor oris, refusal to eat, and fever, often as high as 40–40.6°C (104–105°F). The onset may be insidious, with fever and irritability preceding the oral lesions by 1–2 days. The initial lesion is a vesicle (Fig. 245–1), which is seldom seen because of its early rupture. The residual lesion is 2–10 mm in diameter and is covered with a yellow-gray membrane (Fig. 245–2). When this membrane sloughs, a true ulcer remains. Although the tongue and cheeks are most commonly involved, no part of the oral lining is exempt. Except in edentulous infants, acute gingivitis is characteristic of the disease and may precede the appearance of mucosal vesicles. Submaxillary lymphadenitis is common. The acute phase lasts 4–9 days and is self-limited. Pain tends to disappear 2–4 days before healing of the ulcers is complete. In some instances the tonsillar regions are involved early and appear exudative, and acute tonsillitis of bacterial origin or enterovirus-induced herpangina may be suspected. Negative cultures for group A *Streptococcus* and other bacterial pathogens and failure of the lesion to respond to antibiotic therapy differentiate a bacterial infection. The spread of the vesiculation to the buccal mucosa and anterior portion of the mouth is atypical for herpangina (see Chapter 243.2).

Recurrent Stomatitis and Herpes Labialis. The typical oral recurrence of HSV is one or a few vesicles grouped at the mucocutaneous junction. Lesions are usually accompanied by local pain, tingling, or itching and last 3–7 days. Systemic symptoms are unusual. Less commonly, localized lesions may occur on the palate in association with a febrile illness or on the mucosa adjacent to a lesion on the lip. Recurrent aphthous ulcers, however, are not caused by HSV. In some persons a generalized stomatitis recurs consistently 7–10 days after a recurrent herpetic lesion of the lip or elsewhere and is often accompanied by skin lesions of erythema multiforme. Indeed, recurrent HSV infection is the most common causes of recurrent erythema multiforme.

Eczema Herpeticum (Kaposi Varicelliform Eruption). This, the most serious manifestation of "traumatic herpes," results from a widespread infection of the eczematous skin with HSV. The severity of this complication varies; the lesion may be so mild as to be overlooked, or it may be fatal. In a typical severe primary attack, vesicles develop abruptly in large numbers over the area of eczematous skin. They continue to appear in crops for as long as 7–9 days. Isolated at first, they later become grouped and may occur on adjoining areas of normal skin (Fig. 245–3). Wide denudation of the epidermis may occur. Scabs eventually form, and epithelialization occurs. The systemic reaction varies, but temperatures of 39.4–40.6°C (103–105°F) for 7–10 days are not uncommon. Recurrent attacks develop on chronic atopic skin lesions. Death may result from profound physiologic disturbances from loss of fluid, electrolytes, and protein through the skin; from dissemination of the virus to the brain and other organs; or from secondary bacterial invasion usually with *Staphylococcus* or *Streptococcus.* A differentiation from *eczema vaccinatum* can usually be made by determining with reasonable certainty that the child has not been exposed to vaccinia and by the occurrence of crops of vesicles in herpes. The diagnosis can be accurately established by examination of vesicular fluid with rapid viral diagnostic techniques.

Ocular Infections. *Conjunctivitis* and *keratoconjunctivitis* may occur as manifestations of either a primary or a recurrent infection. The conjunctiva appears congested and swollen, but there

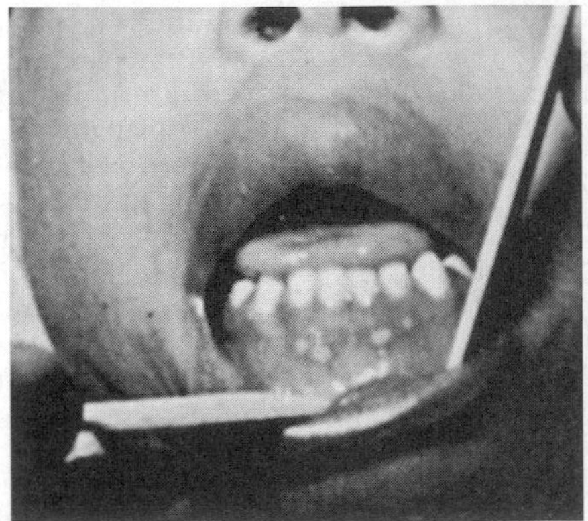

Figure 245–2 Herpetic stomatitis.

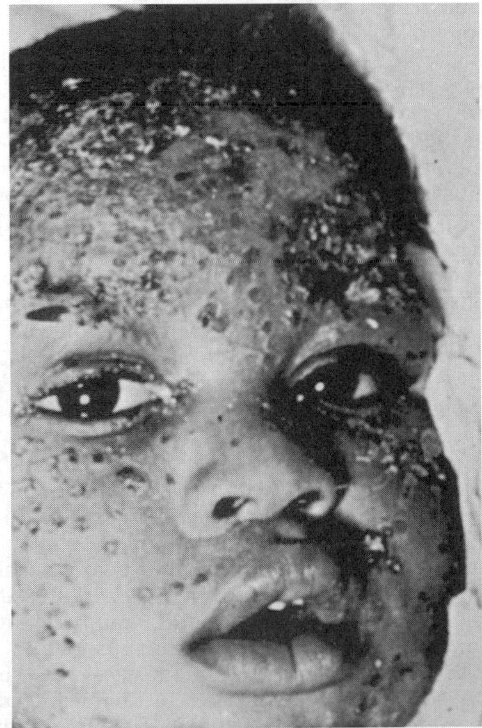

Figure 245–3 Eczema herpeticum (Kaposi varicelliform eruption).

is little, if any, purulent discharge. In primary infection the preauricular node is usually enlarged and tender. Cataracts, uveitis, and chorioretinitis have been described in newborns and in the immunocompromised.

Corneal lesions may be superficial, in the form of a dendritic ulcer, or deep, as a disciform keratitis. Dendritic keratitis is unique to HSV eye involvement. The diagnosis is suggested by the presence of herpetic vesicles on the lids; it is established by the isolation of the virus. Topical corticosteroid use will worsen HSV ocular disease. The highly contagious *epidemic keratoconjunctivitis* (shipyard conjunctivitis) caused by any of several serotypes of adenovirus or enterovirus induced conjunctivitis must be considered in the differential diagnosis. Recurrent herpetic corneal infection may result in scarring of the cornea and vision impairment.

Genital Herpes. Genital infections with herpesvirus occur most commonly in adolescents and young adults, are usually due to HSV-2, and are usually spread by sexual activity. Although hand to genital infection and autoinoculation are possible, genital or rectal herpes in a young child warrants a sensitive and careful appraisal of the possibility of child abuse. Ten to 25 per cent of cases of primary genital herpes are caused by HSV-1. Almost all cases of recurrent genital herpes are due to HSV-2. In primary genital infection, when the patient has no antibody to either type of herpes (approximately 30% of cases), systemic symptoms such as fever, regional adenopathy, and dysuria are more likely to occur. In adult women, the vulva and vagina may be involved with vesicles and ulcers, but the cervix is the primary site of infection. Recurrence is common. Both primary and recurrent disease are frequently subclinical, but virus shed during this time may infect a sex partner or an infant during passage through the birth canal.

In males herpetic vesicles or ulcers are usually seen on the glans penis, prepuce, or shaft of the penis. The scrotum is less frequently involved. Genital HSV is a risk factor for HIV infection.

Central Nervous System Infections. HSV has a predilection to infect the nervous system. Both types 1 and 2 may cause a meningoencephalitis as part of neonatal HSV. In patients with primary genital herpes, usually resulting from HSV 2, an aseptic meningitis syndrome may complicate the course. The cerebrospinal fluid (CSF) reveals a lymphocytic pleocytosis, and the virus may be cultured from it in patients with this self-limited syndrome. HSV-1 is an unusual cause of the aseptic meningitis syndrome, but it is the most common cause of fatal sporadic encephalitis. It has a striking predilection to involve the frontal and parietal areas. Typical signs and symptoms include fever, altered consciousness, headache, personality changes, seizures, dysphasia, and focal neurologic signs. If untreated, the mortality rate is 75%, with severe sequelae in survivors. HSV is the cause of some cases of recurrent aseptic meningitis (Mollaret meningitis), based on demonstration of HSV DNA in the CSF by polymerase chain reaction (PCR).

Immunocompromised Persons. Unusually severe HSV infection may occur in a variety of persons, including the newborn; the severely malnourished; and children with malignancies or other conditions necessitating immunosuppressive therapy, with AIDS, with burns, or with primary immunodeficiency diseases that particularly impair cell-mediated immunity. In children receiving therapy for cancer or organ transplantation, the risk of severe HSV infection coincides with the time of maximum immunosuppression. The most common syndrome is local and chronic oral or genital mucocutaneous disease. The lesions may resemble typical vesicles and ulcers or progress to large necrotic painful erosions or atypical exophytic, wartlike lesions. Mucositis, esophagitis, proctitis, and pneumonitis are less common. The most severe manifestation, usually a result of primary infection in the immunocompromised child, is widespread disseminated disease involving the liver, lungs, adrenal gland, and CNS. These patients have a sepsis-like syndrome with leukopenia, hepatitis, disseminated intravascular coagulopathy, fever, or hypothermia and progression to death. Skin lesions may be localized to mucous membranes, widely disseminated, resembling varicella infection, or absent. This form of HSV infection has a high mortality rate even with therapy.

Perinatal Infections. Most cases of neonatal herpes occur due to infection during delivery, and 75–80% are HSV type 2. At delivery, 0.2–0.4% of women shed HSV in their genital tract, a number that increases to 1–2% if there is a history of genital herpes in the woman. The classification of maternal genital disease greatly determines the attack rate of the newborn delivered vaginally to a woman shedding virus. Maternal primary or first episode genital herpes (no antibody present against the type of virus shed) has an attack rate of 33–50%. Recurrent maternal disease has an attack rate of only 1–3%. Only 15–20% of women delivered of infants with neonatal herpes have a history of infection, and approximately only 25% have some relevant symptoms at delivery.

Rarely (5%), cases are true intrauterine infection, and about 10% of infants acquire their infection post partum, not necessarily from the mother, but usually from another close family member shedding HSV (often type 1), from fever blisters, finger infections, or lesions at other sites.

Infection manifests in the first month of life, with 25% on the first day, and in two thirds by the first week. Of the three major categories, localized skin, eye, and mouth infection and also disseminated infection occur at a mean of 11 days post partum, whereas localized CNS infection occurs later at a mean of 17 days post partum. The hallmark of neonatal HSV infection—the vesicular, ulcerative skin lesions (Fig. 245–4)—are present in only 30–43% of children at presentation; one third will never manifest skin lesions. Symptoms of CNS involvement are found in 48–79% and include lethargy, poor feeding, irritability, poor tone, and seizures. Fever (7–14%) and respiratory distress (5–19%) may be present.

Particular attention should additionally be directed to sites of fetal monitoring for the signs of pustular-vesicular infection unresponsive to antibiotics and to the eyes for signs of herpetic keratoconjunctivitis. Unfortunately whereas a large percentage of neonates begin with localized infection, if not treated 70% will progress to CNS or disseminated disease.

The clinician must consider neonatal HSV infection in any child with suggestive signs born to a parent (mother or father) with a history of genital herpes. Also suspect is the child with antibiotic-unresponsive sepsis especially with thrombocytopenia, elevated results of liver function tests, disseminated intravascular coagulopathy, or early pneumonitis. The neonate

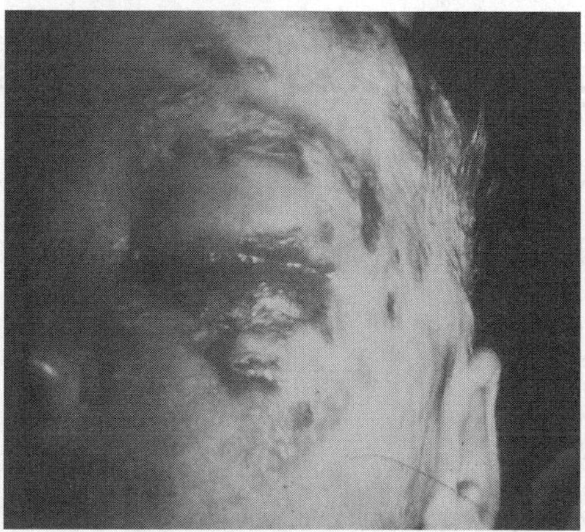

Figure 245–4 Vesicular-pustular lesions on the face of an HSV-infected neonate. (From Kohl S: Neonatal herpes simplex virus infection. Clin Perinatol 24:129, 1997.) See also color section.

with unexplained lymphocytic meningitis and the child with a vesiculoulcerative eruption must be treated for HSV pending diagnostic evaluation.

The infant born with a congenital infection syndrome, especially with skin vesicles or scars, chorioretinitis, microphthalmia, and microcephaly, should be evaluated for both congenital HSV and varicella, as well as other agents of congenital infection.

The risk of mortality due to HSV increases with CNS (15%) or disseminated (57%) disease. It is also increased in infants with coma, disseminated intravascular coagulopathy, prematurity, and pneumonitis. Morbidity among survivors increases with CNS or disseminated diseases, seizures, infection with type 2 virus, and frequent cutaneous recurrences.

The differential diagnosis of a vesicular-ulcerative eruption in the neonate is extensive (Table 245–1). Often an experienced pediatric dermatologist is invaluable help for diagnosis of some of the more arcane syndromes listed.

DIAGNOSIS. The diagnosis is based on any two of the following: (1) a compatible clinical pattern; (2) isolation of the virus; (3) development of specific antibodies; and (4) demonstration of characteristic cells, histologic changes, viral antigen, or HSV DNA in scrapings, CSF, or biopsy material. A rise in CSF HSV antibody occurs in HSV encephalitis, but it is late in the illness and is useful only for retrospective diagnosis. HSV serologic changes (fourfold rise or seroconversion from negative to positive) usually occur after the critical period for diagnosis and therapy. Illnesses resulting from HSV recurrence may not demonstrate a diagnostic serologic rise, and neonates or severely immunocompromised individuals may fail to produce antibody during primary infection. Reliable antibody tests to differentiate serologic response to HSV-1 from HSV-2 are not commercially available. HSV-1 and HSV-2 viral isolates may be typed by a variety of readily available antigen (ELISA, fluorescent antibody) and molecular techniques. HSV isolates that are unrelated epidemiologically are all slightly different at the nucleic acid level, as discerned by DNA endonuclease restriction analysis. Using this technique, it is possible to confirm infection of one individual by another and to demonstrate that apparent nosocomial outbreaks or viral transmission represent a chance collection of unrelated cases, which may be extremely important for counseling and medicolegal reasons.

The use of PCR analysis of CSF and perhaps blood may be critical to diagnose neonatal HSV infection, especially in the absence of skin lesions. Serology is not a useful tool for rapid diagnosis of HSV infection in the neonate, and as in the older child, because of transplacental maternal antibodies; MRI of the brain is often abnormal in neonates with CNS involvement and suggestive of HSV infection.

TABLE 245–1 Differential Diagnosis of Vesicular Eruption in the Neonate

Infectious Etiologies	
Herpes simplex virus	*Aspergillus*
Staphylococcus aureus	Varicella-zoster virus
Pseudomonas	Cytomegalovirus
Haemophilus influenzae	*Listeria monocytogenes*
Treponema pallidum	Group B *Streptococcus*
Candida	
Noninfectious Conditions	
Erythema toxicum	Herpes gestationis
Pustular melanosis	Incontinentia pigmenti
Miliaria	Neonatal lupus
Letterer-Siwe disease	Epidermolysis bullosa
Urticaria pigmentosa	Epidermolytic hyperkeratosis
Bullous mastocytosis	Acropustulosis
Dermatitis herpetiformis	Neonatal bullous dermatitis
Pemphigus vulgaris	Langerhans' cell histiocytosis

Data from Clinical pathology exercise. N Engl J Med 320:1399, 1989; 334:1591, 1996. From Kohl S: Neonatal herpes simplex virus infection. Clin Perinatol 24:129, 1997.

Laboratory Findings. Microscopic examination of scrapings from lesions (Tzanck stain) reveals multinuclear giant cells and intranuclear inclusions approximately 50% of the time. Specific antigen detection methods such as ELISA and immunofluorescent techniques applied to these specimens can be useful in rapidly diagnosing herpes infection and in differentiating the two types of herpes. Virus can be readily isolated from vesicles and from conjunctival swabs in 1–4 days. The CSF is positive for virus in about one third of infected neonates but is rarely positive in older children with encephalitis. PCR permits detection of viral DNA in CSF and, if positive, will make brain biopsy unnecessary. Brain biopsy may be necessary if PCR is negative for definitive diagnosis and exclusion of other treatable entities. At this time, PCR for HSV is available through specialized laboratories only.

Moderate polymorphonuclear leukocytosis occurs in acute herpetic gingivostomatitis, eczema herpeticum, and meningoencephalitis. In meningoencephalitis there are frequently red cells in the CSF and an increase in lymphocytes, usually $<100/mm^3$ but occasionally up to $1,000/mm^3$; the protein level is elevated, and the glucose is usually within the normal range but may be reduced. Electroencephalography (EEG) and magnetic resonance imaging (MRI) may demonstrate a temporal lobe lesion in early encephalitis. Computed tomography (CT) may be normal in early encephalitis but becomes abnormal as the disease progresses. Thrombocytopenia and elevated levels of liver function tests often occur with systemic infection.

TREATMENT. Acyclovir (9-[-2-hydroxyethoxymethyl] guanine, a purine nucleoside analog) is the mainstay of therapy for HSV. Viral thymidine kinase phosphorylates acyclovir, which is then triphosphorylated by cellular enzymes to act as an HSV DNA polymerase inhibitor and DNA chain terminator. Thymidine kinase-negative HSV isolates are resistant to acyclovir.

Two recently licensed oral anti-herpes drugs simplify the therapy for genital herpes. Valacyclovir, a prodrug of acyclovir, and famciclovir, a prodrug of penciclovir, have excellent oral bioavailability (55–80%) and are converted in vivo to acyclovir and penciclovir, respectively. As with acyclovir, penciclovir is phosphorylated by HSV thymidine kinase and then cellular enzymes to the triphosphate active agents. Due to excellent oral adsorption these drugs may be used less frequently than acyclovir. The ease of use is offset by the increased cost compared with generic acyclovir. Ongoing studies using these new agents in immunocompromised patients in whom larger doses reach serum levels obtained with intravenous acyclovir have facilitated oral therapy and prophylaxis of more severe forms of HSV infection.

Acyclovir-resistant HSV is rare in the normal host but occurs in the immunocompromised host treated with long-term or multiple, intermittent courses of acyclovir. When immunocompromised patients have unresponsive or worsening HSV infection despite acyclovir therapy, the virus should be forwarded to reference laboratories for drug susceptibility testing. Pending laboratory results (resistance to acyclovir is associated with inhibitory levels equal to or greater than 2 μg/mL), the drug of choice for acyclovir-resistant HSV is intravenous foscarnet (phosphonoformic acid), 40 mg/kg/dose every 8 hr. This drug has serious side effects (azotemia, electrolyte disturbance, anemia, and granulocytopenia). Cidofovir has been successfully used in a small number of cases of resistant virus. Acyclovir and foscarnet dosages must be modified in patients with renal impairment.

Topical acyclovir therapy for oral or genital herpes may decrease the period of viral shedding but has little effect on symptoms and is not recommended. Topical penciclovir, another nucleoside analog, reduces symptoms of oral recurrent herpes only modestly.

Topical trifluorothymidine, vidarabine, and idoxuridine are all usually effective in treating herpetic keratitis but do not reduce the recurrence rate. Topical corticosteroids may increase ocular involvement, if used alone, and should only be used with antiviral therapy.

The child or adolescent with recurrent oral or genital herpes may have severe psychologic problems and may benefit from anticipatory guidance or formal counseling. Genital disease should be destigmatized and safer sex practices emphasized. Parents of children with most types of HSV infection, such as gingivostomatitis or skin infection, should be reassured that common childhood HSV infections are not related to sexual activity or abuse.

Lesions of the Skin and Mucous Membranes. Oral acyclovir (15 mg/kg five times a day with a maximum dose of 1 g/24 hr for 7 days) started within 72 hr of onset of lesions has significant benefits in children with primary herpetic gingivostomatitis by decreasing drooling, gum swelling, pain, eating and drinking difficulties, and duration of lesions. Therapy for recurrent oral herpes with oral acyclovir has limited effects.

Symptomatic and supportive therapy is of great importance. Oral lavage should be used for mouth care; Ceepryn 1:4,000 or Zephiran 1:1,000 may be useful. Local analgesics, such as viscous lidocaine or benzocaine lozenges, are not advocated because they may cause the child to damage friable and anesthetized parts of the mouth. Food and fluid intake will be facilitated by acquiescing to the child's whims. Ice-cold fluids, ice slush, or semisolids are often accepted when other food is refused. In infants especially, eczema herpeticum and stomatitis may lead to severe dehydration, shock, and hypoproteinemia, requiring intravenous replacement of fluids, electrolytes, and proteins.

Acyclovir has no effect on HSV-associated erythema multiforme. Suppression of the HSV infection by prophylactic therapy as for genital disease prevents the erythema multiforme recurrences.

Oral acyclovir is beneficial for treating primary and recurrent herpes whitlow and rectal herpes.

Genital Herpes. Patients with primary genital infection who are treated with oral acyclovir (200 mg five times daily for 10 days) have significantly less pain, itching, and time to crusting; a shorter duration of viral shedding, and fewer new lesions compared with control patients. Those with recurrent genital infections who are treated similarly with oral acyclovir have a shorter duration of viral shedding and heal faster. Therapy for primary attacks does not prevent recurrences. However, daily prophylactic administration of oral acyclovir can diminish the number of recurrences and may be prescribed if recurrences are frequent or severe.

The recommended treatment regimen for initial genital herpes is valacyclovir (1,000 mg/dose) or famciclovir (500 mg/dose) given twice daily for 10 days; these are equivalent to acyclovir five times a day. For HSV genital recurrence, valacyclovir (500 mg/dose) and famciclovir (125 mg/dose) given twice daily for 5 days are equivalent to acyclovir five times a day. Daily suppressive therapy reduces the frequency of genital herpes recurrences by ≥75% among persons with ≥6 recurrences per year. Recommended regimens for daily suppressive therapy are famciclovir (250 mg) twice a day, valacyclovir (500 mg or 1000 mg) once a day, or acyclovir (400 mg) twice a day. These are doses for adults and older adolescents. Pediatric doses and formulations have not been established.

Genital lesions may be made less painful by using sitz baths. Local drying agents prolong healing and may increase secondary infection. Analgesics should be used systemically as required. Antibiotics are useful only in treating secondary bacterial infections.

Central Nervous System and Systemic Infections. Intravenously administered acyclovir (10 mg/kg/dose given over 1 hr every 8 hr for 14–21 days) is the treatment of choice for herpes encephalitis. The drug is well tolerated. The best results are obtained when treatment is started early. Patients <30 yr of age and those who are only lethargic compared with those who have progressed to coma have a better prognosis. Supportive care to minimize increased intracranial pressure, seizure activity, and respiratory compromise requires an intensive care setting and a team of experts.

Intravenous acyclovir (5–10 mg/kg/dose given over 1 hr every 8 hr [duration depending on clinical response]) is recommended for treatment of HSV infections in the immunocompromised host. The larger doses are used for severe and systemic infections. The lower dose may be used for localized mucocutaneous disease. As the patient responds, therapy may be switched to the oral route. Oral acyclovir, as used in genital disease, may be used to suppress HSV recurrences in seropositive patients during periods of maximum immunosuppression after organ or marrow transplantation or during induction therapy for leukemia, lymphoma, or solid tumors. Immunosuppressed patients with frequently recurring HSV infection, such as those with AIDS or primary immunodeficiencies, benefit from chronic suppressive oral therapy. Valacyclovir should not be used in immunocompromised children due to unusual side effects.

Perinatal Infections. As in other serious forms of HSV infection, intravenous acyclovir (60 mg/kg/24 hr in three divided doses for 14–21 days) is the drug of choice for neonatal HSV infection. For the neonate with HSV infection, intensive care is necessary initially to observe for signs of disseminated or CNS disease necessitating ventilatory control, seizure management, and intensive supportive care. There is preliminary evidence to suggest extending therapy of HSV neonatal encephalitis for longer than 21 days until the HSV CSF PCR becomes negative. Preliminary data suggest that the use of daily oral acyclovir (300 mg/m^2 three times a day) for 6 mo can suppress the common cutaneous recurrences associated with poor outcome, but the effects on central nervous system infection and long-term prognosis are unproved. Recurrence of cutaneous infection soon after cessation of suppressive therapy is frequent. Prolonged treatment has been associated with neutropenia and emergence in at least one instance of acyclovir-resistant virus.

PROGNOSIS. Primary localized infections with HSV in the normal host are self-limited, usually lasting 1–2 wk. Mortality rates are high in newborns who also have systemic infection and in older infants who are severely immunocompromised or malnourished. In patients with meningoencephalitis the prognosis for survival or for recovery without serious permanent residuals is guarded. Outcome is improved with early diagnosis and therapy.

Attacks may frequently recur, but they seldom cause more than temporary inconvenience except in the eye, where they may eventually cause scarring of the cornea and blindness. Recurrent herpes lesions can be a significant problem in immunocompromised patients. Recurrent genital disease may be associated with significant discomfort and psychologic morbidity. The major complication of any form of genital HSV infection in a woman is infection of her newborn.

PREVENTION. Acyclovir administered during periods of high risk in immunocompromised hosts and administered chronically in individuals with frequently recurrent genital or oral disease markedly decreases the rate of recurrence. Acyclovir administered before a known trigger factor, such as intense sunlight, usually prevents recurrences.

HSV spread can be limited by standard methods of infection control. Open lesions on skin, hands, and mucous membranes should be well covered. Wrestlers with possible HSV cutaneous lesions should be excluded from practice and competition until they are healed. Wrestling mats should be cleansed with a bleach solution at least daily. Children with immunodeficiencies or chronic skin diseases that predispose to severe HSV infection should not be cared for by persons with herpetic whitlow or active uncovered fever blisters. Active herpes le-

TABLE 245–2 Management of the Child Born to a Woman with Active Genital HSV Infection

Maternal Primary or First-Episode Infection

Cesarean section within 24 (preferably 4) hours of ruptured membranes
- Culture eyes, nose, mouth, urine, stool at 48 hours.
- Treat with acyclovir if any culture is positive or there are signs of neonatal HSV.*

Unavoidable vaginal delivery
- Culture eyes, nose, mouth, urine, stool, and cerebrospinal fluid.
- Treat with acyclovir.

Recurrent Infection, Active at Delivery

Cesarean section within 24 (preferably 4) hours of ruptured membranes
- Culture eyes, nose, mouth, urine, and stool at 48 hours.
- Treat with acyclovir if any culture is positive or there are signs of HSV infection.*

Unavoidable vaginal delivery
- Culture eyes, nose, mouth, urine, and stool at 48 hours.
- Treat with acyclovir if any culture is positive or there are signs of HSV infection.*

**If infant is to be treated with acyclovir, a cerebrospinal fluid analysis, culture, and polymerase chain reaction for HSV DNA are indicated.*

From Kohl S: Neonatal herpes simplex virus infection. Clin Perinatol 24:129, 1997.

sions that can be covered are not a reason to exclude children from daycare or school activities.

There is active research to develop a vaccine to prevent HSV infection. HSV may be prevented in some animal models by live, attenuated, naked DNA, or subunit viral particle vaccines. Several purified HSV glycoprotein vaccines are antigenic in humans, but to date these vaccines have lacked efficacy in clinical trials.

Obstetric Management of the Woman with Genital HSV Infection. The major aims of obstetric care of the woman with genital HSV infection are to ameliorate the symptoms of infection in the mother and to lessen the risk of neonatal HSV infection in the neonate. A reliable history of genital HSV infections must be determined for all women presenting for prenatal care.

Acyclovir is a pregnancy category C medication (should not be used during pregnancy unless the potential benefit justifies the potential risk to the fetus). In a registry of >600 women exposed to acyclovir during pregnancy, no increased rate of fetal malformations or unusual pattern of malformations has been noted, although this number is too low to detect a low-level or rare teratogenic effect. It is clear that primary HSV infection in the pregnant woman carries an increased risk of life-threatening dissemination, and intravenous acyclovir should be administered if there are any signs of disseminated HSV disease.

Recommendations of both the American Academy of Pediatrics and the American College of Obstetrics and Gynecology are for a cesarean section if primary, first-episode, or recurrent HSV lesions are present at the onset of labor (Table 245–2). This recommendation for recurrent infection is controversial: given the low attack rate of HSV to the neonate in the case of maternal recurrent disease, nearly 1,600 excess cesarean deliveries will be performed for every prevention of poor neonatal outcome, at a cost of $2.5 million per case of neonatal herpes prevented and a possible excess of maternal deaths outnumbering prevented deaths in neonates.

If no lesions can be demonstrated at delivery, the child may be delivered via the vaginal route. For women with a history of recurrent genital herpes who have no obvious lesions at the time of delivery, it is not universally agreed that routine HSV cultures taken at delivery of mother or newborn are useful, although some experts advocate routine cultures. If cultures at delivery are positive for HSV, most experts recommend obtaining cultures from the neonate at 24–48 hr of life (eyes, mouth, urine, stool) and treating with acyclovir if any cultures are positive or if the neonate has any signs of HSV infection in the ensuing 4 wk (see Table 245–2).

In pregnant women with a history of genital herpes, there are preliminary data to demonstrate that suppressive acyclovir therapy administered near delivery reduces viral shedding and the need for cesarean section. This strategy of prophylactic maternal acyclovir needs further confirmation before it can be universally recommended.

Primary and first-episode genital infections are probably associated with some increased risk of spontaneous abortion, and with increased risk of premature delivery of 30–50%. Intrauterine infection is a rare consequence of genital infection.

In the neonate inadvertently born vaginally to a woman with active primary or first-episode HSV infection, positive cultures at 24–48 hr of life (eyes, mouth, urine, stool, and CSF), abnormal CSF findings, or any signs of HSV in the first 4 weeks of life mandate acyclovir therapy (see Table 245–2). Many experts recommend anticipatory use of acyclovir therapy after delivery in this setting because of the high attack rate, although there are no data to demonstrate reduction of neonatal infection, and several case reports had demonstrated failure of early neonatal therapy.

Cesarean section is not completely protective, because 20–30% of infants with neonatal HSV infection are born by abdominal delivery. Thus, all newborns of women with primary or first-episode genital HSV infection also should have cultures taken at 48 hr of life and be followed for signs of infection regardless of the route of delivery.

Most women who are delivered of a neonate with HSV infection are not aware of their own HSV infection and usually have no symptoms at delivery. It also may be difficult to determine clinically if a genital infection at delivery represents a recurrence or a more severe primary or first-episode infection. Determination of serologic status of these women and their partners with type-specific antibody, and a rapid antigen or PCR strategy for genital viral detection, may be useful in the future.

Amir J, Harel L, Smetana Z, Varsano I: Treatment of herpes simplex gingivostomatitis with acyclovir in children: A randomized double-blind placebo-controlled study. BMJ 314:1800, 1997.

Aurelius E, Johansson B, Skoldenberg B, et al: Rapid diagnosis of herpes simplex encephalitis by nested polymerase chain reaction assay of cerebral spinal fluid. Lancet 337:189, 1991.

Benedetti J, Corey L, Ashley R: Recurrence rates in genital herpes after symptomatic first-episode infection. Ann Intern Med 121:847, 1994.

Diaz-Mitoma F, Sibbald RG, Shafran SD, et al: Oral famciclovir for the suppression of recurrent genital herpes: A randomized controlled trial. JAMA 280:887, 1998.

Fleming DT, McQuillan GM, Johnson RE, et al: Herpes simplex virus type 2 in the United States, 1976 to 1994. N Engl J Med 337:1105, 1997.

Frenck RW, Kohl S: Herpes simplex virus in the immunocompromised child. *In* Patrick CC (ed): Infections in Immunocompromised Infants and Children. New York, Churchill Livingstone, 1992, pp 603–624.

Kimberlin DW, Lakeman FD, Arvin AM, et al: Application of the polymerase chain reaction to the diagnosis and management of neonatal herpes simplex virus disease. J Infect Dis 174:1162, 1996.

Kimberlin D, Powell D, Gruber W, et al: Administration of oral acyclovir suppressive therapy after neonatal herpes simplex virus disease limited to the skin, eye and mouth: Results of a phase I/II trial. Pediatr Infect Dis J 15:247, 1996.

Kohl S: Neonatal herpes simplex virus infection. Clin Perinatol 24:129, 1997.

Kohl S: Herpes simplex virus encephalitis in children. Pediatr Clin North Am 35:465, 1988.

Whitley RJ, Arvin A, Prober C, et al: Predictors of morbidity and mortality in neonates with herpes simplex virus infections. N Engl J Med 324:450, 1991.

CHAPTER 246
Varicella-Zoster Virus

Martin G. Myers and Lawrence R. Stanberry

Varicella-zoster virus (VZV) causes primary, latent, and recurrent infections. The primary infection is manifested as varicella (chickenpox) and results in establishment of a lifelong latent infection of sensory ganglion neurons. Reactivation of the latent infection causes herpes zoster (shingles). Although often a mild illness of childhood, chickenpox can cause increased morbidity and mortality in adolescents and immunocompromised persons and predisposes to severe group A *Streptococcus* and *Staphylococcus aureus* infections. Chickenpox and zoster can be treated with antiviral drugs. Infection can be prevented by immunization with a live-attenuated VZV vaccine. Gestational chickenpox can be severe in the mother and can cause a rare but distinct intrauterine syndrome. Chickenpox in the newborn can be severe and life threatening.

ETIOLOGY. VZV is a neurotropic human herpesvirus with similarities to another α-herpesvirus, herpes simplex virus (HSV). These viruses are enveloped with double-stranded DNA genomes that encode more than 70 proteins, including proteins that are targets of cellular and humoral immunity.

EPIDEMIOLOGY. The epidemiology of varicella is different in temperate and tropical countries; in temperate countries such as the United States, in the pre-vaccine era, 90–95% of individuals acquired VZV infection in childhood. In contrast, individuals from tropical countries may not acquire infection until later in life. In the United States, annual varicella epidemics occur in winter and spring. Within households with a case of varicella, transmission of VZV to susceptible individuals occurs at a rate of 80–90%; more casual contact, such as occurs in a school classroom, is associated with attack rates of ≤30%. Patients with varicella are contagious from 24–48 hr before the rash appears and until vesicles are crusted, usually 3–7 days after onset of rash. Susceptible children may also acquire varicella after close, direct contact with adults who have herpes zoster.

Herpes zoster, because it is due to the reactivation of latent VZV, is uncommon in childhood and shows no seasonal variation in incidence. The lifetime risk for herpes zoster for individuals with a history of varicella is 10%, with 75% of cases occurring after 45 yr of age. Despite anecdotal reports, epidemiologic studies demonstrate that exposure to varicella does not cause herpes zoster. Herpes zoster is very rare in healthy children <10 years of age except for those infected in utero or in the first year of life; herpes zoster in these children tends to be mild. However, herpes zoster occurs more frequently, occasionally multiple times, and may be severe in children receiving immunosuppressive therapy for malignancy or other diseases and in those who have HIV infection.

PATHOGENESIS. VZV is transmitted in respiratory secretions and in the fluid of skin lesions either by airborne spread or through direct contact. Primary infection (varicella) results from the respiratory inoculation of virus in a susceptible child. During the early part of the incubation period, which lasts 10–21 days, virus replicates in the respiratory tract followed by a brief subclinical viremia. Widespread cutaneous lesions occur during a second viremic phase. Peripheral blood mononuclear cells carry infectious virus, generating new crops of vesicles for 3–7 days. VZV is also transported back to respiratory mucosal sites during the late incubation period, permitting spread to susceptible contacts before the appearance of rash. Host immune responses limit viral replication and facilitate recovery from infection. In the immunocompromised child, the failure of immune responses, especially the cell-mediated immune response, results in continued viral replication with resultant injury to lungs, liver, brain, and other organs.

VZV establishes latent infection in sensory ganglia cells in all individuals who experience primary infection. Subsequent reactivation of latent virus causes herpes zoster, a vesicular rash that usually is dermatomal in distribution. During herpes zoster, necrotic changes may be produced in the associated ganglia. The skin lesions of varicella and herpes zoster have identical histopathology, and infectious VZV is present in both. Varicella elicits humoral and cell-mediated immunity that is highly protective against symptomatic re-infection. Suppression of cell-mediated immunity to VZV correlates with an increased risk of VZV reactivation as herpes zoster.

CLINICAL MANIFESTATIONS. Varicella is an acute febrile illness, common in children who have not been immunized, which has variable severity and that is usually self-limited. It may be associated with several complications, including congenital infection and perinatal transmission causing life-threatening infection in the fetus. Herpes zoster, uncommon in children, causes localized cutaneous symptoms, but may disseminate in immunocompromised patients.

Varicella. The illness usually begins 14–16 days after exposure, although the incubation period can range from 10–21 days. Subclinical varicella is rare; almost all exposed, susceptible children experience a rash, but illness may be limited to only a few lesions. Prodromal symptoms may be present, particularly in older children. Fever, malaise, anorexia, headache, and occasionally mild abdominal pain may occur 24–48 hr before the rash appears. Temperature elevation is usually moderate, usually from 100–102°F but may be as high as 106°F; fever and other systemic symptoms persist during the first 2–4 days after the onset of the rash.

Varicella lesions often appear first on the scalp, face, or trunk. The initial exanthem consists of intensely pruritic erythematous macules that evolve to form clear, fluid-filled vesicles. Clouding and umbilication of the lesions begin in 24–48 hr. While the initial lesions are crusting, new crops form on the trunk and then the extremities; the simultaneous presence of lesions in various stages of evolution is characteristic of varicella (Fig. 246–1). Ulcerative lesions involving the oropharynx and vagina are also common; many children have vesicular lesions on the eyelids and conjunctivae, but corneal involvement and serious ocular disease is rare. The average number of varicella lesions is about 300, but healthy children may have <10 to >1,500 lesions. In cases resulting from secondary household spread and in older children, more lesions usually occur, and new crops of lesions may continue to develop for a longer period of time. The exanthem may be much more extensive in children with skin disorders, such as eczema or recent sunburn. Hypopigmentation or hyperpigmentation of lesion sites persists for days to weeks in some children, but scarring is unusual unless the lesions were secondarily infected.

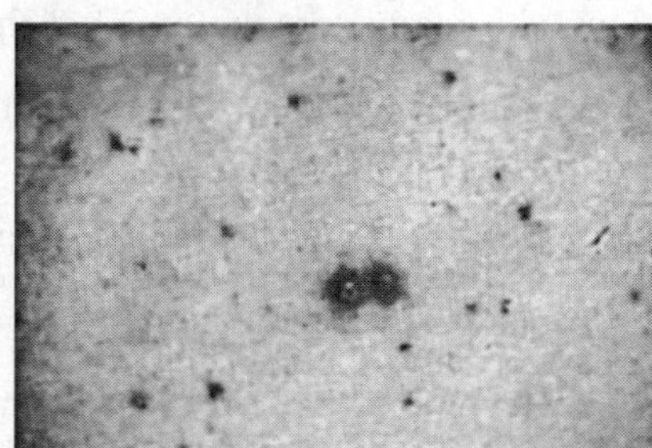

Figure 246–1 Skin lesions of chickenpox. Note the varying stages of development (macules, papules, and vesicles) present at the same time. See also color section. (Courtesy of PF Lucchesi.)

The differential diagnosis of varicella includes vesicular rashes caused by other infectious agents, such as herpes simplex virus, enterovirus, or *Staphylococcus aureus*; drug reactions; contact dermatitis; and insect bites.

Progressive Varicella. Progressive varicella, with visceral organ involvement, coagulopathy, severe hemorrhage, and continued lesion development is a dreaded complication of primary VZV infection. Severe abdominal pain and the appearance of hemorrhagic vesicles in otherwise healthy adolescents and adults, immunocompromised children, pregnant women, and newborns may herald this. The risk of progressive varicella is highest in children with congenital cellular immune deficiency disorders and those with malignancy, particularly if chemotherapy was given during the incubation period and the absolute lymphocyte count is <500 cells/mm³. In one large series, the mortality rate for children who acquired varicella while undergoing treatment for malignancy and who were not treated with antiviral therapy was 7%. In this series all varicella-related deaths occurred within 3 days after the diagnosis of varicella pneumonia. Children who acquire varicella after organ transplantation are also at risk for progressive VZV infection. Children on long-term, low-dose corticosteroid therapy usually have no complications, but progressive varicella does occur in patients receiving high-dose corticosteroids and has been reported in patients receiving inhaled corticosteroids. Unusual clinical findings of varicella, including lesions that develop a unique hyperkeratotic appearance and the continued new lesion formation for weeks or months, have been described in children with HIV infection.

Neonatal Chickenpox. Delivery within 1 wk before or after the onset of maternal varicella frequently results in the newborn developing varicella, which may be severe. The initial infection is intrauterine, although the newborn often develops clinical chickenpox post partum. The risk to the newborn is dependent on the amount of maternal anti-VZV antibody that the fetus acquired transplacentally before birth. If there was ≥1 wk interval between maternal chickenpox and parturition, it is likely that the newborn received sufficient transplacental antibody to VZV to ameliorate neonatal infection. Alternatively, if the interval was <1 wk, the newborn will be unlikely to have protective VZV antibody and neonatal chickenpox may be exceptionally severe.

The recommendations for varicella-zoster immune globulin (VZIG) reflect the differing risks to the exposed infant. Newborns whose mothers develop varicella 5 days before to 2 days after delivery should receive one vial. Although neonatal varicella may occur in about half of these infants despite administration of VZIG, it is usually mild. Every premature infant born to a mother with active chickenpox at delivery (even if present >1 wk) should receive VZIG. Perinatally acquired varicella may be life threatening and should be treated with acyclovir (10 mg/kg per dose given every 8 hr) intravenously.

Many infants with severe manifestations of congenital varicella syndrome have severe neurologic deficiencies. However, some may have only isolated stigmata, amenable to treatment, and develop normally throughout childhood. Infants with neonatal chickenpox who receive prompt antiviral therapy have an excellent prognosis.

Neonatal chickenpox can also follow a post-partum exposure of an infant delivered to a mother who was susceptible to VZV, although the frequency of complications declines rapidly in the weeks after birth. Infants with community-acquired chickenpox who develop signs of pneumonia, hepatitis, or encephalitis, should also receive treatment with intravenous acyclovir (10 mg/kg per dose given every 8 hr).

Congenital Varicella Syndrome. When pregnant women contract chickenpox, about 25% of the fetuses may become infected, although not every infected fetus is clinically affected. However, up to 2% of fetuses whose mothers had varicella between 8–20 wk of pregnancy may demonstrate VZV embryopathy. The period of greatest risk to the fetus (8–20 wk of gestation) correlates with the gestational period when there is major development and innervation of the limb buds and maturation of the eyes. Fetuses infected at 6–12 wk of gestation appear to have maximal interruption with limb development; fetuses infected at 16–20 wk may have eye and brain involvement. In addition, viral damage to the sympathetic fibers in the cervical and lumbosacral cord may lead to divergent effects such as Horner's syndrome and dysfunction of the urethral or anal sphincters.

Most of the stigmata can be attributed to virus-induced injury to the nervous system, although there is no obvious explanation why certain regions of the body are preferentially infected during fetal VZV infection. The virus may select tissues that are in a rapid developmental stage, such as the limb buds. Histologic examination of the brain demonstrates necrotizing cerebral lesions involving the leptomeninges, the cortex, and the adjacent white matter. The characteristic cicatricial scarring may represent the cutaneous residua of VZV infection of the sensory nerves, analogous to herpes zoster.

The stigmata involve mainly the skin, extremities, eyes, and brain (Table 246–1). The characteristic cutaneous lesion has been called a cicatrix, a zigzag scarring, often in a dermatomal distribution. The other hallmark of this syndrome is one or more shortened and malformed extremities (Fig. 246–2). Frequently, the atrophic extremity is covered with a cicatrix. The remainder of the torso may be entirely normal in appearance. Alternatively, there may be neither skin nor limb abnormalities but the infant may show cataracts or even extensive aplasia of the entire brain. Occasionally, calcifications are evident within a microcephalic head (Fig. 246–3).

The diagnosis of VZV fetopathy is based mainly on the history of gestational chickenpox combined with the stigmata seen in the fetus. Virus cannot be cultured from the affected newborn, but viral DNA can be detected in tissue samples by PCR. Some infants have VZV-specific IgM antibody detectable in the cord blood sample, although the IgM titer drops quickly post partum. Chorionic villus sampling and fetal blood collection for the detection of viral DNA, virus, or antibody have been used in an attempt to diagnose fetal infection and embryopathy. The usefulness of these tests for patient management and counseling has not been defined. Because these tests may not distinguish between infection and disease, their utility may primarily be that of reassurance when the test is negative.

Although VZIG is often administered to the susceptible mother exposed to chickenpox, it is uncertain as to whether this modifies infection in the fetus. Similarly, acyclovir treatment may be given to the mother with severe varicella; however, neither its safety nor its efficacy for the fetus is known. The damage caused by fetal VZV infection does not progress post partum, an indication that there is no persistent viral

TABLE 246–1 Stigmata of Varicella-Zoster Virus Fetopathy

Damage to Sensory Nerves
Cicatricial skin lesions
Hypopigmentation
Damage to Optic Stalk and Lens Vesicle
Microphthalmia
Cataracts
Chorioretinitis
Optic atrophy
Damage to Brain/Encephalitis
Microcephaly
Hydrocephaly
Calcifications
Aplasia of brain
Damage to Cervical or Lumbosacral Cord
Hypoplasia of an extremity
Motor and sensory deficits
Absent deep tendon reflexes
Anisocoria
Horner's syndrome
Anal/urinary sphincter dysfunction

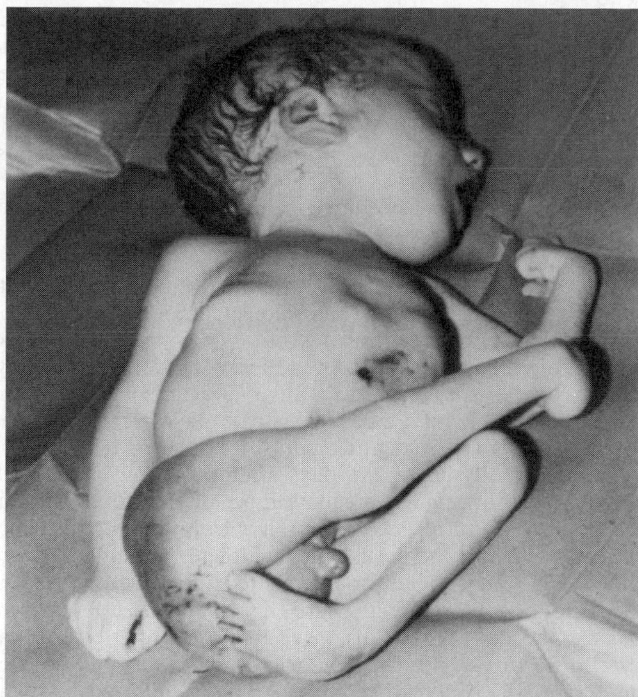

Figure 246–2 Newborn with congenital varicella syndrome. The infant had severe malformations of both lower extremities and cicatricial scarring over his left abdomen.

replication. Thus, antiviral treatment of infants with congenital VZV syndrome is not indicated.

Herpes Zoster. Herpes zoster is manifested as vesicular lesions clustered within one or less commonly two adjacent dermatomes (Fig. 246–4). Unlike zoster in adults, zoster in children is infrequently associated with localized pain, hyperesthesias, pruritus, and low-grade fever. In children, the rash is mild, with new lesions appearing for a few days; symptoms of acute neuritis are minimal; and complete resolution usually occurs within 1–2 wk. In contrast to adults, postherpetic neuralgia is very unusual in children. Approximately 4% of patients suffer a second episode of herpes zoster; ≥3 episodes are rare. Transverse myelitis with transient paralysis is a rare complication of herpes zoster.

Immunocompromised children may have more severe herpes zoster that is similar to that in adults, including post herpetic neuralgia. Immunocompromised patients may also experience disseminated cutaneous disease that mimics varicella, as well as visceral dissemination with pneumonia, hepatitis, encephalitis, and disseminated intravascular coagulopathy. Severely immunocompromised children, particularly those with HIV infection, may have unusual, chronic, or relapsing cutaneous disease, retinitis, or central nervous system disease without rash.

DIAGNOSIS. Laboratory evaluation is not necessary for the diagnosis or management of healthy children with varicella or herpes zoster. Leukopenia is typical during the first 72 hours; it is followed by a relative and absolute lymphocytosis. Results of liver function tests are also usually (75%) mildly elevated. Patients with neurologic complications of varicella or uncomplicated herpes zoster have a mild lymphocytic pleocytosis and a slight to moderate increase in protein in the cerebrospinal fluid; the glucose concentration is usually normal.

Rapid laboratory diagnosis of VZV is often important in high-risk patients and is sometimes important for infection control. VZV can be identified quickly by polymerase chain reaction (PCR) amplification testing or by direct immunohistochemical staining of cells from cutaneous lesions. Although multinucleated giant cells can be detected with nonspecific stains (Tzanck smears), they have poor sensitivity and do not differentiate

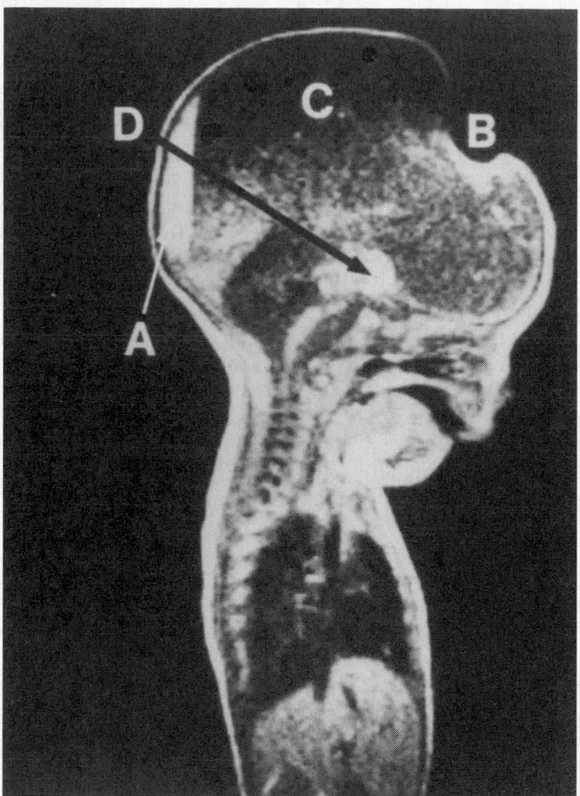

Figure 246–3 Magnetic resonance image of newborn with encephalitis secondary to congenital varicella syndrome. The intrauterine infection occurred about 3 mo ante partum, at which time there was extensive necrosis of the cerebral hemispheres. The image of the newborn head was taken with the patient supine; therefore, there is a fluid/fluid interface in the dependent occiput *(A)*. The hydrocephalus *(C)* and calcifications in the basal ganglia *(D)* are visible; a cranial artifact *(B)* is seen secondary to a scalp vein needle.

VZV and HSV infections. Infectious virus may be recovered using tissue culture methods, but this typically requires 7–10 days. VZV immunoglobulin G (IgG) antibodies can be detected by several methods, but serologic diagnosis is retrospective. However, VZV IgG antibody tests can be valuable to determine the immune status of individuals whose clinical history of varicella is unknown or equivocal. Testing for VZV IgM antibodies is not useful for clinical diagnosis because commercially available methods are unreliable.

TREATMENT. Antiviral treatment modifies the course of both varicella and herpes zoster. Antiviral drug resistance is rare but has occurred in children with HIV infection who have been treated. Foscarnet is the only drug now available for the treatment of acyclovir-resistant VZV infections.

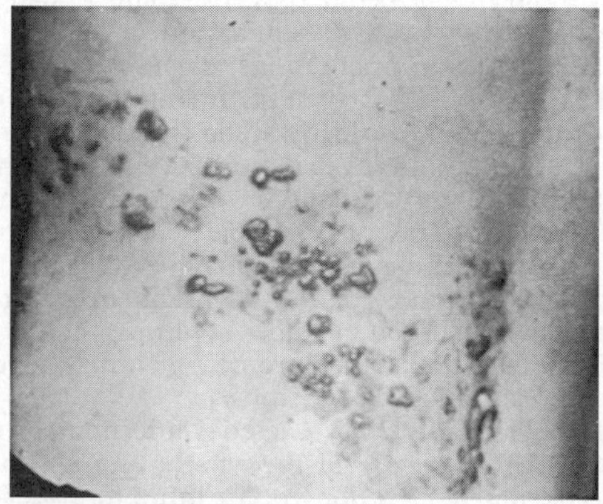

Figure 246–4 Herpes zoster.

Varicella. The only antiviral drug available in liquid formulation and that is licensed for pediatric use is acyclovir. Given the safety profile of acyclovir and its demonstrated efficacy in the treatment of varicella, treatment of all children, adolescents, and adults with varicella is acceptable. However, acyclovir therapy is not recommended routinely by the American Academy of Pediatrics for treatment of uncomplicated varicella in the otherwise healthy child because of the marginal benefit, the cost of the drug, and the low risk of complications. Oral therapy with acyclovir (20 mg/kg/dose; maximum of 800 mg/dose) given as four doses per day for 5 days should be used to treat uncomplicated varicella in nonpregnant individuals ≥13 yr of age and children ≥12 mo of age: with chronic cutaneous or pulmonary disorders; receiving short-term, intermittent, or aerosolized corticosteroids; receiving long-term salicylate therapy; and possibly second cases in household contacts. To be most effective treatment should be initiated as early as possible, preferably ≤48 hr of the onset of the exanthem. There is dubious clinical benefit if initiation of treatment is delayed ≤72 hr after onset of the exanthem. Acyclovir therapy does not interfere with the induction of VZV immunity.

Intravenous therapy is indicated for severe disease and for varicella in immunocompromised patients. Acyclovir has been used to treat varicella in pregnant women; however, its safety for the fetus has not been established. Any patient who has signs of disseminated VZV including pneumonia, severe hepatitis, thrombocytopenia, or encephalitis should receive immediate treatment. Intravenous acyclovir (500 mg/m^2 every 8 hr) therapy initiated ≤72 hr of development of initial symptoms decreases the likelihood of progressive varicella and visceral dissemination in high-risk patients. Treatment is continued for 7 days or until no new lesions have appeared for 48 hr. Delaying antiviral treatment until prolonged new lesion formation is evident is not advisable because visceral dissemination occurs during the same time period.

Herpes Zoster. Antiviral drugs are effective for treatment of herpes zoster. In healthy adults, acyclovir (800 mg five times a day for 5 days), famciclovir (500 mg three times a day for 7 days), and valacyclovir (1,000 mg three times a day for 7 days) reduce the duration of the illness and the risk of developing postherpetic neuralgia; concomitant corticosteroid usage improves the quality of life in the elderly. In otherwise healthy children, however, herpes zoster is a less severe disease and postherpetic neuralgia is rare. Therefore, treatment of uncomplicated herpes zoster in the child with an antiviral agent may not always be necessary, although some experts would treat with oral acyclovir (20 mg/kg/dose; maximum 800 mg/dose) to shorten the duration of the illness. Use of corticosteroids for herpes zoster is not recommended.

In contrast, herpes zoster in immunocompromised children can be severe and disseminated disease may be life threatening. Patients at high risk for disseminated disease should receive acyclovir (500 mg/m^2 or 10 mg/kg every 8 hr) intravenously. Oral acyclovir is an option for immunocompromised patients with uncomplicated herpes zoster and who are considered at low-risk for visceral dissemination.

COMPLICATIONS. The complications of VZV infection occur with varicella, or with reactivation of infection in immunocompromised patients. Mild varicella hepatitis is relatively common but rarely clinically symptomatic. Mild thrombocytopenia occurs in 1–2% of children with varicella and may be associated with transient petechiae. Purpura, hemorrhagic vesicles, hematuria, and gastrointestinal bleeding are rare complications that may have serious consequences. Other rare complications of varicella include nephritis, nephrotic syndrome, hemolytic-uremic syndrome, arthritis, myocarditis, pericarditis, pancreatitis, and orchitis.

Bacterial Infections. Secondary bacterial infections of the skin, usually caused by *Streptococcus pyogenes* (group A β-hemolytic streptococcus or *S. aureus*), may occur in up to 5% of children with varicella. These range from superficial impetigo to cellulitis, lymphadenitis, and subcutaneous abscesses. An early manifestation of secondary bacterial infection is erythema of the base of a new vesicle. Recrudescence of fever 3–4 days after the initial exanthem may also herald a secondary bacterial infection. The more invasive infections such as varicella gangrenosa, bacterial sepsis, pneumonia, arthritis, osteomyelitis, and necrotizing fasciitis account for much of the morbidity and mortality of varicella in otherwise healthy children. Bacterial toxin-mediated diseases (e.g., toxic shock syndrome) also may complicate varicella.

Encephalitis and Cerebellar Ataxia. Encephalitis and acute cerebellar ataxia are well-described neurologic complications of varicella; morbidity from central nervous system complications is highest among patients <5 yr or >20 yr of age. Nuchal rigidity, altered consciousness, and seizures characterize meningoencephalitis. Patients with cerebellar ataxia have a gradual onset of gait disturbance, nystagmus, and slurred speech. Neurologic symptoms usually begin 2–6 days after the onset of the rash but may occur during the incubation period or after resolution of the rash. Clinical recovery is typically rapid, occurring within 24–72 hr, and is usually complete. Although severe hemorrhagic encephalitis, analogous to that caused by HSV, is very rare in children with varicella, the consequences are similar to herpes encephalitis. Reye syndrome of encephalopathy and hepatic dysfunction associated with varicella has become rare since salicylates are no longer routinely used as antipyretics (Chapter 360).

Pneumonia. Varicella pneumonia is very rare in children, but this complication accounts for most of the increased morbidity and mortality in adults and other high-risk populations. Respiratory symptoms, which may include cough, dyspnea, cyanosis, pleuritic chest pain, and hemoptysis, usually begin within 1–6 days after the onset of the rash. Adults are at increased risk for severe pneumonia complicating varicella. The frequency of this complication may be greater in the parturient and may lead to premature termination of pregnancy.

PROGNOSIS. Primary varicella has a mortality rate of <2 per 100,000 cases. Approximately 80–100 deaths, usually from secondary bacterial sepsis or pneumonia, occurred in the United States annually before the introduction of the VZV vaccine. The mortality rate of untreated primary infection in immunocompromised children is 7–14% and may approach 50% in adults.

Neuritis with herpes zoster should be managed with appropriate analgesics. Postherpetic neuralgia can be a severe problem in adults and may persist for months, requiring care by a specialist in pain management.

PREVENTION. VZV transmission is difficult to prevent because the infection is contagious for 24–48 hr before the rash appears. Infection control practices, including caring for infected patients in isolation rooms with filtered air systems, are essential in hospitals that treat immunocompromised children. All health care workers should have documented VZV immunization or immunity. Susceptible health care workers who have had a close exposure to VZV should not care for high-risk patients during the incubation period.

Vaccine. Varicella is a vaccine-preventable disease. Live virus vaccine is recommended for routine administration in children at 12–18 mo of age. Older individuals without a history of VZV infection should also be immunized. Children 12 mo to 12 yr receive a single vaccine dose; adolescents and adults require two vaccine doses, a minimum of 4 wk apart. Live virus vaccine is contraindicated in immunocompromised children. Vaccine is 85–95% effective at preventing disease. Illness may occur in about 6% of vaccinated children subsequently exposed to VZV but is usually very mild ("breakthrough varicella"). The illness usually consists of only a few macules or vesicles and is usually without fever. Vaccine virus establishes latent infection; the risk of developing subsequent herpes zoster is no greater than after natural VZV infection. Ongoing studies of the persistence of immunity after vaccination may ultimately demonstrate a need for children to receive a booster dose of vaccine.

Postexposure Prophylaxis. Varicella-zoster immune globulin (VZIG) postexposure prophylaxis is recommended for immunocompromised children, pregnant women, and newborns exposed to maternal varicella. VZIG is distributed by the American Red Cross Blood Services. The dosage is 1 vial (125 units) for each 10 kg increment (maximum: 625 units) given intramuscularly as soon as possible but within 96 hr after exposure.

Newborns whose mothers develop varicella 5 days before to 2 days after delivery should receive one vial. Adults should be tested for VZV IgG antibodies before VZIG administration because many adults with no clinical history of varicella are immune. VZIG prophylaxis may ameliorate disease but does not eliminate the possibility of progressive disease; patients should be monitored and treated with acyclovir if necessary. Immunocompromised patients who have received high-dose intravenous immune globulin (100–400 mg/kg) for other indications within 2–3 wk before the exposure can be expected to have serum antibodies to VZV.

Close contact between a susceptible high-risk patient and a patient with herpes zoster is also an indication for VZIG prophylaxis. Passive antibody administration or treatment does not reduce the risk of herpes zoster or alter the clinical course of varicella or herpes zoster when given after the onset of symptoms.

Vaccine given to normal children within 3 days exposure may be effective in preventing varicella; although the effectiveness of this strategy requires further study, its use in this fashion should present little or no risk. Oral acyclovir administered late in the incubation period may modify subsequent varicella in the normal child. However, its use in this manner is not recommended until it can be further evaluated.

Arvin AM: Varicella-zoster virus. Clin Microbiol Rev 9:361, 1996.

Brunell PA: Varicella in pregnancy, the fetus and the newborn: Problems in management. J Infect Dis 166(Suppl 1):S42, 1992.

Centers for Disease Control and Prevention: Prevention of varicella. Recommendations of the Advisory Committee on Immunization Practices (ACIP). MMWR 45 (RR-11):1, 1996.

Centers for Disease Control and Prevention: Varicella-related deaths among adults—United States, 1997. MMWR 46:409, 1997.

Choo PT, Donahue JG, Manson JE: The epidemiology of varicella and its complications. J Infect Dis 172:706:1995.

Connelly BL, Stanberry LR, Bernstein DI: Detection of varicella-zoster virus DNA in nasopharyngeal secretions of immune household contacts of varicella. J Infect Dis 168:1253, 1993.

Dunkle LM, Arvin AM, Whitley RJ, et al: A controlled trial of acyclovir for chickenpox in normal children. N Engl J Med 325:1539, 1991.

Enders G, Miller E. Cradock-Watson J, et al: Consequences of varicella and herpes zoster in pregnancy: Prospective study of 1739 cases. Lancet 343: 1548, 1994.

Gershon AA, LaRussa P: Varicella vaccine. Pediatr Infect Dis J 17:248, 1998.

Gershon AA, Mervish N, LaRussa P, et al: Varicella-zoster virus infection in children with underlying human immunodeficiency virus infection. J Infect Dis 176:1496, 1997.

Grose C: Congenital infections caused by varicella zoster virus and herpes simplex virus. Semin Pediatr Neurol 1:43, 1994.

Guess HA, Broughton DD, Melton LJ II, et al: Population-based studies of varicella complications. Pediatrics 78:723, 1987.

Kustermann A, Zoppini C, Tassis B, et al: Prenatal diagnosis of congenital varicella infection. Prenat Diagn 16:71, 1996.

Nader S, Bergen R, Sharp M, et al: Age-related differences in cell-mediated immunity to varicella zoster virus among children and adults immunized with live attenuated varicella vaccine. J Infect Dis 171:13, 1995.

Pastuszak AL, Levy M, Schick B, et al: Outcome after maternal varicella infection in the first 20 weeks of pregnancy. N Engl J Med 330:901, 1994.

Peterson CL, Mascola L, Chao SM, et al: Children hospitalized for varicella: A prevaccine review. J Pediatr 129:529, 1996.

Petursson G, Helgason S, Gudmundsson S, et al: Herpes zoster in children and adolescents. Pediatr Infect Dis J 17:905, 1998.

Whatson BM, Piercy SA, Plotkin SA, Starr SE: Modified chickenpox in children immunized with the Oka/Merck varicella vaccine. Pediatrics 91:17, 1993.

Wood MJ, Johnson RW, McKendrick MW, et al: A randomized trial of acyclovir for 7 days or 21 days with and without prednisolone for treatment of acute herpes zoster. N Engl J Med 330:896, 1994.

Zerboni L, Nader S, Aoki K, Arvin A: Analysis of the persistence of humoral and cellular immunity in children and adults immunized with varicella vaccine. J Infect Dis 177:1701, 1998.

CHAPTER 247
Epstein-Barr Virus

Hal B. Jenson

Infectious mononucleosis is the best-known clinical syndrome caused by Epstein-Barr virus (EBV). It is characterized by systemic somatic complaints consisting primarily of fatigue, malaise, fever, sore throat, and generalized lymphadenopathy. Originally described as *glandular fever,* it derives its name from the mononuclear lymphocytosis with atypical-appearing lymphocytes that accompany the illness. Other infections may cause infectious mononucleosis–like illnesses.

ETIOLOGY. EBV, a member of the γ-herpesviruses, causes more than 90% of infectious mononucleosis cases. Five to 10 per cent of infectious mononucleosis–like illnesses are caused by primary infection with cytomegalovirus, *Toxoplasma gondii,* adenovirus, viral hepatitis, HIV, and possibly rubella virus. In the majority of EBV-negative infectious mononucleosis–like illnesses, the exact cause remains unknown.

EPIDEMIOLOGY. The epidemiology of infectious mononucleosis is related to the epidemiology and age of acquisition of EBV infection. EBV infects >95% of the world's population. It is transmitted in oral secretions by close contact such as kissing or exchange of saliva from child to child, such as occurs between children in out-of-home childcare. Nonintimate contact, environmental sources, or fomites do not contribute to spread of EBV.

EBV is shed in oral secretions for >6 mo after acute infection and then intermittently for life. Twenty to 30 per cent of healthy EBV-infected persons are excreting virus at any particular time. Immunosuppression permits reactivation of latent EBV; 60–90% of EBV-infected immunosuppressed patients shed the virus. EBV is also found in the genital tract of women and may be spread by sexual contact.

Infection with EBV in developing countries and among socioeconomically disadvantaged populations of developed countries usually occurs during infancy and early childhood. In central Africa, almost all children are infected by 3 yr of age. Primary infection with EBV during childhood is usually inapparent or indistinguishable from other childhood infections; the clinical syndrome of infectious mononucleosis is practically unknown in undeveloped regions of the world. Among more affluent populations in industrialized countries, infection during childhood is still most common, but approximately one third of cases occur during adolescence and young adulthood. Primary EBV infection in adolescents and adults is manifest in >50% of cases by the classic triad of fatigue, pharyngitis, and generalized lymphadenopathy, which constitute the major clinical manifestations of infectious mononucleosis. This syndrome may be seen at all ages but is rarely apparent in children <4 yr of age, when most EBV infections are asymptomatic, or in adults >40 yr of age, when most individuals have already been infected by EBV. The true incidence of the syndrome of infectious mononucleosis is unknown but is estimated to occur in 20–70/100,000 persons/yr; in young adults the incidence rises to about 1/1,000 persons/yr. The prevalence of serologic evidence of past EBV infection increases with age; almost all adults in the United States are seropositive.

PATHOGENESIS. After acquisition in the oral cavity, EBV initially infects oral epithelial cells; this may contribute to the symptoms of pharyngitis. After intracellular viral replication and cell lysis with release of new virions, virus spreads to contiguous structures such as the salivary glands with eventual viremia and infection of B lymphocytes in the peripheral blood and the entire lymphoreticular system, including the liver and spleen. The atypical lymphocytes that are characteristic of infectious mononucleosis are $CD8^+$ T lymphocytes, which exhibit both suppressor and cytotoxic functions that develop in response to the infected B lymphocytes.This relative as well as absolute increase in $CD8^+$ lymphocytes results in a transient reversal of the normal 2:1 $CD4^+/CD8^+$ (helper-suppressor) T-lymphocyte ratio. Many of the clinical manifestations of infectious mononucleosis may result, at least in part, from the host immune response, which is effective in reducing the number of EBV-infected B lymphocytes to less than 1 per 10^6 of circulating B lymphocytes.

Epithelial cells of the uterine cervix may become infected by sexual transmission of the virus, although neither local symptoms nor infectious mononucleosis have been described after sexual transmission.

EBV, like the other herpesviruses, establishes lifelong latent infection after the primary illness. The latent virus is carried in oropharyngeal epithelial cells and systemic B lymphocytes as multiple episomes in the nucleus. The viral episomes replicate with cell division and are distributed to both daughter cells. Viral integration into the cell genome is not typical. Only a few viral proteins, including the EBV-determined nuclear antigens (EBNA), are produced during latency. These proteins are important in maintaining the viral episome during the latent state. Progression to viral replication begins with production of EBV early antigens (EA), proceeds to viral DNA replication, followed by production of viral capsid antigen (VCA), and culminates in cell death and release of mature virions. Reactivation with viral replication occurs at a low rate in populations of latently infected cells and is responsible for intermittent viral shedding in oropharyngeal secretions of infected individuals. Reactivation is apparently asymptomatic and not recognized to be accompanied by distinctive clinical symptoms.

Oncogenesis. EBV was the first human virus to be associated with malignancy and, therefore, was the first virus to be identified as a human tumor virus. EBV infection may result in a spectrum of proliferative disorders ranging from self-limited, usually benign disease such as infectious mononucleosis to aggressive, nonmalignant proliferations such as the virus-associated hemophagocytic syndrome to lymphoid and epithelial cell malignancies. Benign EBV-associated proliferations include oral hairy leukoplakia, primarily in adults with AIDS, and lymphoid interstitial pneumonitis, primarily in children with AIDS. Malignant EBV-associated proliferations include nasopharyngeal carcinoma, Burkitt lymphoma, Hodgkin disease, lymphoproliferative disorders, and leiomyosarcoma in immunodeficient states, including AIDS.

Nasopharyngeal carcinoma occurs worldwide but is 10 times more common in persons in southern China, where it is the most common malignant tumor among adult men. It is also common among whites in North Africa and Inuits in North America. All malignant cells of undifferentiated nasopharyngeal carcinoma contain a high copy number of EBV episomes. Persons with undifferentiated and partially differentiated, nonkeratinizing nasopharyngeal carcinomas have elevated EBV antibody titers that are both diagnostic and prognostic. High levels of immunoglobulin (Ig) A antibody to EA and VCA may be detected in asymptomatic individuals and can be used to follow response to tumor therapy (Table 247–1). Cells of well-differentiated, keratinizing nasopharyngeal carcinoma contain a low or zero copy number of EBV genomes and these persons have EBV serologic patterns similar to those of the general population.

Endemic (African) Burkitt lymphoma, often found in the jaw, is the most common childhood cancer in equatorial East African and New Guinea. The median age at onset is 5 yr. These regions are holoendemic for *Plasmodium falciparum* malaria and have a high rate of EBV infection early in life. The constant malarial exposure acts as a B-lymphocyte mitogen that contributes to the polyclonal B-lymphocyte proliferation with EBV infection. It also impairs the T-lymphocyte control of EBV-infected B lymphocytes. Approximately 98% of cases of endemic Burkitt lymphoma contain the EBV genome compared with only 20% of nonendemic (sporadic or American) Burkitt lymphoma cases. Individuals with Burkitt lymphoma have unusually and characteristically high levels of antibody to VCA and EA that correlate with the risk of developing tumor (see Table 247–1).

All cases of Burkitt lymphoma, including those that are EBV negative, are monoclonal and demonstrate chromosomal translocation of the c-*myc* proto-oncogene to the constant region of the immunoglobulin heavy-chain locus, t(8;14), to the kappa constant light-chain locus, t(2;8), or to the lambda constant light-chain locus, t(8;22). This results in the deregulation and constitutive transcription of the c-*myc* gene with overproduction of a normal c-*myc* product that autosuppresses c-*myc* production on the untranslocated chromosome.

The incidence of *Hodgkin disease* peaks in childhood in developing countries and in young adulthood in developed countries. Levels of EBV antibodies are consistently elevated preceding development of Hodgkin disease; only a small minority of patients are seronegative for EBV. Infection with EBV appears to increase the risk of Hodgkin disease by a factor of 2 to 4. EBV is associated with more than one half of cases of mixed-cellularity Hodgkin disease and approximately one fourth of cases of the nodular sclerosing subtype and is rarely associated with lymphocyte-predominant Hodgkin disease. Immunohistochemical studies have localized EBV to the Reed-Sternberg cells and their variants, the pathognomonic malignant cells of Hodgkin disease.

Failure to control EBV infection may result from host immunologic deficits. The prototype is the *X-linked lymphoproliferative syndrome (Duncan's syndrome),* an X chromosome–linked recessive disorder of the immune system associated with severe, persistent, and sometimes fatal EBV infection (Chapter 124.7). Approximately two thirds of these male patients die of disseminated and fulminating lymphoproliferation involving multiple organs at the time of primary EBV infection. Surviving patients acquire hypogammaglobulinemia, B-cell lymphoma, or both. Most patients die within 10 yr.

A number of other congenital and acquired immunodeficiency syndromes are associated with an increased incidence of EBV-associated B-lymphocyte lymphoma, particularly central nervous system lymphoma. The incidence of lymphoproliferative syndromes parallels the degree of immunosuppression. A decline in T-cell function evidently permits EBV to escape from immune surveillance. Congenital immunodeficiencies predisposing to EBV-associated lymphoproliferations include the X-linked lymphoproliferative syndrome, common-variable immunodeficiency, ataxia-telangiectasia, Wiskott-Aldrich syndrome, and Chédiak-Higashi syndrome. Individuals with acquired immunodeficiencies resulting from anticancer chemotherapy, immunosuppression after solid organ or bone marrow transplantation, or HIV infection have a significantly increased risk of EBV-associated lymphoproliferations. The lymphomas may be focal or diffuse, and they are usually histologically polyclonal but may become monoclonal. Their growth is not reversed on cessation of immunosuppression.

EBV has been credibly linked to leiomyosarcomas in HIV-infected patients and transplant patients, primary central nervous system lymphoma, and carcinoma of the salivary glands. Other tumors putatively associated with EBV include some T-lymphocyte lymphomas (including lethal midline), angioimmunoblastic lymphadenopathy-like lymphoma, thymomas and thymic carcinomas derived from thymic epithelial cells, supraglottic laryngeal carcinomas, lymphoepithelial tumors of the respiratory tract and gastrointestinal tract, and gastric adenocarcinoma. The precise contribution of EBV to these various malignancies is not well defined.

TABLE 247–1 Correlation of Clinical Status and Serologic Responses to EBV Infection

	Serologic Response					
	Heterophile Antibodies	*EBV-Specific Antibody*				
Clinical Status	*(Qualitative Test)*	**IgM-VCA**	**IgG-VCA**	**EA-D**	**EA-R**	**EBNA**
Negative reaction	−	<1:8*	<1:10*	<1:10*	<1:10*	<1:2.5*
Susceptible	−	−	−	−	−†	−
Acute primary infection: infectious mononucleosis	+	1:32 to 1:256	1:160 to 1:640	1:40 to 1:160	−†	− to 1:2.5
Recent primary infection: infectious mononucleosis	+/−	− to 1:32	1:320 to 1:1,280	1:40 to 1:160	−†	1:5 to 1:10
Remote infection	−	−	1:40 to 1:160	−‡	− to 1:40	1:10 to 1:40
Reactivation: immunosuppressed or immunocompromised	−	−	1:320 to 1:1,280	−‡	1:80 to 1:320	− to 1:160
Burkitt's lymphoma	−	−	1:320 to 1:1,280	−‡	1:80 to 1:320	1:10 to 1:80
Nasopharyngeal carcinoma	−	−	1:320 to 1:1,280	1:40 to 1:160	−§	1:20 to 1:160

The data were obtained from numerous studies. Individual responses outside the characteristic range may occur.
**Or the lowest test dilution.*
†In young children and adults with asymptomatic seroconversion, the anti–early antigen response may be mainly to the EA-R component.
‡A minority of individuals will have the anti–early antigen response mainly to the EA-D component.
§A minority of individuals will have the anti–early antigen response mainly to the EA-R component.
EBV = Epstein-Barr virus; − = negative; + = positive; IgM = immunoglobulin M; IgG = immunoglobulin G; VCA = viral capsid antigen; EA-D = diffuse staining component of EA; EA-R = cytoplasmic restricted component of early antigen; EBNA = EBV-determined nuclear antigens.
Reprinted with permission from Jenson HB, Ench Y, Sumaya CV: Epstein-Barr virus. In: Rose NR, de Macario EC, Folds JD, et al (eds): Manual of Clinical Laboratory Immunology, 5th ed. Washington, DC, American Society for Microbiology, 1997, p 637.

CLINICAL MANIFESTATIONS. The incubation period of infectious mononucleosis in adolescents is 30–50 days. In children it may be shorter. The majority of cases of primary EBV infection in infants and young children are clinically silent. In older patients, the onset of illness is usually insidious and vague. Patients may complain of malaise, fatigue, fever, headache, sore throat, nausea, abdominal pain, and myalgia. This prodromal period may last 1–2 wk. The complaints of sore throat and fever gradually increase until patients seek medical care. Splenic enlargement may be rapid enough to cause left upper quadrant abdominal discomfort and tenderness, which may be the presenting complaint.

The physical examination is characterized by generalized lymphadenopathy (90% of cases), splenomegaly (50% of cases), and hepatomegaly (10% of cases). Lymphadenopathy occurs most commonly in the anterior and posterior cervical nodes and the submandibular lymph nodes and less commonly in the axillary and inguinal lymph nodes. Epitrochlear lymphadenopathy is particularly suggestive of infectious mononucleosis. Symptomatic hepatitis or jaundice is uncommon. Splenomegaly to 2–3 cm below the costal margin is typical; massive enlargement is uncommon.

The sore throat is often accompanied by moderate to severe pharyngitis with marked tonsillar enlargement, occasionally with exudates (Fig. 247–1). Petechiae at the junction of the hard and soft palate are frequently seen. The pharyngitis resembles that caused by streptococcal infection. Other clinical findings may include rashes and edema of the eyelids. Rashes are usually maculopapular and have been reported in 3–15% of patients. Eighty per cent of patients with infectious mononucleosis will experience a rash if treated with ampicillin or amoxicillin; the basis for this phenomenon is unknown.

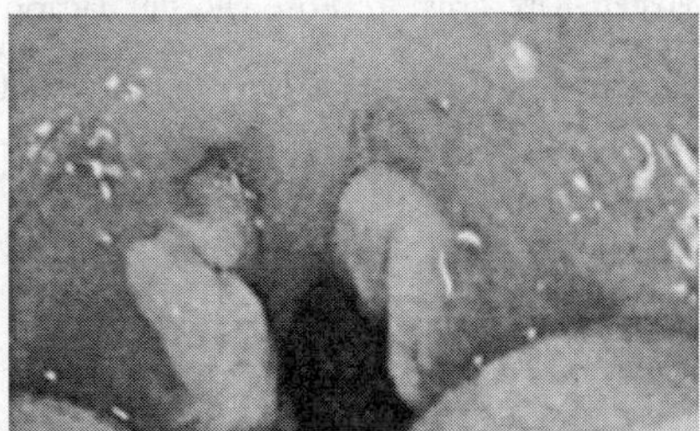

Figure 247–1 Tonsillitis with membrane formation in infectious mononucleosis. See also color section. (Courtesy of Alex J. Steigman, M.D.)

DIAGNOSIS. The diagnosis of infectious mononucleosis implies primary EBV infection. A presumptive diagnosis may be made by the presence of typical clinical symptoms with atypical lymphocytosis in the peripheral blood. The diagnosis is confirmed by serologic testing.

Differential Diagnosis. Infectious mononucleosis–like illnesses may be caused by primary infection with cytomegalovirus, *T. gondii*, adenovirus, viral hepatitis, HIV, or possibly rubella virus. Cytomegalovirus infection is a particularly common cause in adults. Streptococcal pharyngitis may cause sore throat and cervical lymphadenopathy indistinguishable from that of infectious mononucleosis but is not associated with hepatosplenomegaly. Approximately 5% of cases of EBV-associated infectious mononucleosis have positive throat cultures for group A β-hemolytic streptococci; this represents pharyngeal streptococcal carriage. Failure of a patient with streptococcal pharyngitis to improve within 48–72 hr should evoke suspicion of infectious mononucleosis. The most serious problem in the diagnosis of acute illness arises in the occasional patient with extremely high or low white blood cell counts, moderate thrombocytopenia, and even hemolytic anemia. In these patients, bone marrow examination and hematologic consultation are warranted to exclude the possibility of leukemia.

Routine Laboratory Tests. In >90% of cases there is leukocytosis of 10,000–20,000 cells/mm^3, of which at least two thirds are lymphocytes; atypical lymphocytes usually account for 20–40% of the total number. The atypical cells are mature T lymphocytes that have been antigenically activated. Compared with regular lymphocytes microscopically, atypical lymphocytes are larger overall, with larger, eccentrically placed indented and folded nuclei with a lower nuclear-cytoplasm ratio. Although atypical lymphocytosis may be seen with many of the infections usually causing lymphocytosis, the highest degree of atypical lymphocytes is classically seen with EBV infection. Other syndromes associated with atypical lymphocytosis include acquired cytomegalovirus infection (as contrasted to congenital cytomegalovirus infection), toxoplasmosis, viral hepatitis, rubella, roseola, mumps, tuberculosis, typhoid, *Mycoplasma* infection, malaria, as well as some drug reactions. Mild thrombocytopenia to 50,000–200,000 platelets/mm^3 occurs in >50% of patients, but only rarely are values low enough to cause purpura. Mild elevation of hepatic transaminases occurs in approximately 50% of uncomplicated cases but is usually asymptomatic without jaundice.

Heterophile Antibody Test. Heterophile antibodies agglutinate cells from species different from those in the source serum. The transient heterophile antibodies seen in infectious mononucleosis, also known as Paul-Bunnell antibodies, are IgM antibodies detected by the Paul-Bunnell-Davidsohn test for sheep red cell agglutination. The heterophile antibodies of infectious mononucleosis agglutinate sheep or, for greater sensitivity, horse red cells but not guinea pig kidney cells. This adsorption property differentiates this response from the heterophile response found in patients with serum sickness, rheumatic diseases, and some normal individuals. Titers greater than 1:28 or 1:40 (depending on the dilution system used) after absorption with guinea pig cells are considered positive.

The sheep red cell agglutination test is likely to be positive for several months after infectious mononucleosis; the horse red cell agglutination test may be positive for as long as 2 yr. The most widely used method is the qualitative, rapid slide test using horse erythrocytes. It detects heterophile antibody in 90% of cases of EBV-associated infectious mononucleosis in older children and adults but in only up to 50% of cases in children <4 yr because they typically develop a lower titer. Five to 10 per cent of cases of infectious mononucleosis are not caused by EBV and are not uniformly associated with a heterophile antibody response. The false-positive rate is less than 10%, usually resulting from erroneous interpretation. If the heterophile test is negative and an EBV infection is suspected, EBV-specific antibody testing is indicated.

Specific EBV Antibodies. EBV-specific antibody testing is useful to confirm acute EBV infection, especially in heterophile-negative cases, or to confirm past infection and determine susceptibility to future infection. Several distinct EBV antigen systems have been characterized for diagnostic purposes (Fig. 247–2). Table 247–1 summarizes serologic responses that are expected in various situations. The EBNA, EA, and VCA antigen systems are most useful for diagnostic purposes. The acute phase of infectious mononucleosis is characterized by rapid IgM and IgG antibody responses to VCA in all cases and an IgG response to EA in most cases. The IgM response to VCA is transient but can be detected for at least 4 wk and occasionally up to 3 mo. The laboratory must take steps to remove rheumatoid factor, which may cause a false-positive IgM VCA result. The IgG response to VCA usually peaks late in the acute phase, declines slightly over the next several weeks to months, and then persists at a relatively stable level for life.

Anti-EA antibodies are usually detectable for several months but may persist or be detected intermittently at low levels for many years. Antibodies to the diffuse-staining component of EA, EA-D, are found transiently in 80% of patients during the acute phase of infectious mononucleosis and reach high titers in patients with nasopharyngeal carcinoma. Antibodies to the cytoplasmic-restricted component of EA, EA-R, emerge transiently in the convalescence from infectious mononucleosis and often attain high titers in patients with EBV-associated Burkitt lymphoma, which in the terminal stage of the disease may be exceeded by antibodies to EA-D. High levels of antibodies to EA-D or EA-R may be found also in immunocompromised patients with persistent EBV infections and active EBV replication. Anti-EBNA antibodies are the last to develop in infectious mononucleosis and gradually appear 3–4 mo after the onset of illness and remain at low levels for life. Absence of anti-EBNA when other antibodies are present implies recent infection, whereas the presence of anti-EBNA implies infection occurring more than 3–4 mo previously. The wide range of individual antibody responses and the various laboratory methods used can occasionally make interpretation of an antibody profile difficult. The detection of IgM antibody to VCA is the most valuable and specific serologic test for the diagnosis of acute EBV infection and is generally sufficient to confirm the diagnosis.

TREATMENT. There is no specific treatment for infectious mononucleosis. Therapy with high doses of acyclovir, with or without corticosteroids, decreases viral replication and oropharyngeal shedding during the period of administration but does not reduce the severity or duration of symptoms or alter the eventual outcome. Rest and symptomatic therapy are the mainstays of management. Bed rest is necessary only when the patient has debilitating fatigue. As soon as there is definite symptomatic improvement, the patient should be allowed to begin resuming normal activities. Because blunt abdominal trauma may predispose patients to splenic rupture, it is customary and prudent to advise against participation in contact sports and strenuous athletic activities during the first 2–3 wk of illness or while splenomegaly is present.

Short courses of corticosteroids (less than 2 wk) may be helpful for complications of infectious mononucleosis, but this use has not been evaluated critically. Some appropriate indications include incipient airway obstruction, thrombocytopenia with hemorrhaging, autoimmune hemolytic anemia, and seizures and meningitis. A recommended dosage is prednisone, 1 mg/kg/24 hr (maximum 60 mg/24 hr) or equivalent, for 7 days and tapered over another 7 days. There are no controlled data to show efficacy of corticosteroids in any of these conditions. In view of the potential and unknown hazards of immunosuppression for a virus infection with oncogenic

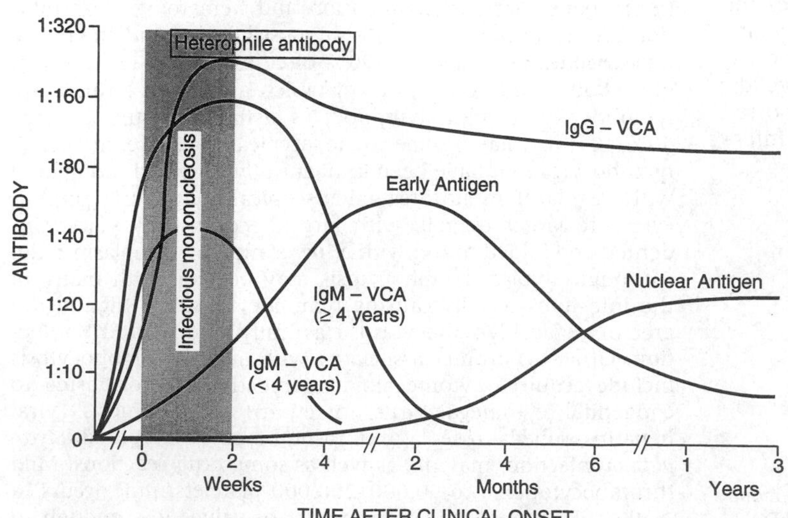

Figure 247–2 Schematic representation of the development of antibodies to various Epstein-Barr virus antigens in patients with infectious mononucleosis. The titers are geometric mean values expressed as reciprocals of the serum dilution. The immunoglobulin M (IgM) response to viral capsid antigen (VCA) is divided because of the significant differences noted according to age of the patient. IgG = immunoglobulin G. (Reprinted with permission from Jenson HB, Ench Y, Sumaya CV: Epstein-Barr virus. *In*: Rose NR, de Macario EC, Folds JD, et al [eds]: Manual of Clinical Laboratory Immunology, 5th ed. Washington, DC, American Society for Microbiology, 1995.)

complications, corticosteroids should not be used in uncomplicated cases of infectious mononucleosis.

COMPLICATIONS. Very few patients with infectious mononucleosis experience complications. The most feared complication is splenic rupture, which occurs most frequently during the 2nd week of the disease. A 0.2% rate has been reported in adults; the rate in children is unknown but is probably much lower. Rupture is commonly related to trauma, which often may be mild. Swelling of the tonsils and oropharyngeal lymphoid tissue may be substantial and cause airway impairment manifest by stridor and interference with breathing. Airway impairment may be treated by administration of corticosteroids; respiratory distress with incipient or actual airway occlusion should be managed by maintaining the airway with intubation in an intensive care setting.

Many uncommon and unusual conditions have been reported to be associated with EBV infectious mononucleosis. Neurologic involvement may be serious with ataxia and seizures. Perceptual distortions of space and size, referred to as the Alice in Wonderland syndrome, may be a presenting symptom. There may be meningitis with nuchal rigidity and mononuclear cells in the cerebrospinal fluid, facial nerve palsy, transverse myelitis, and encephalitis.

Guillain-Barré syndrome or Reye syndrome may follow acute illness. Hemolytic anemia, often with a positive Coombs test and with cold agglutinins specific for red cell antigen i, may occur late in the illness. Aplastic anemia is a rare complication that usually presents 1 mo after the onset of illness. The prognosis for eventual recovery is good, although substantial supportive treatment is necessary during the acute stages. Myocarditis or interstitial pneumonia may occur, both resolving in 3–4 wk. Other rare complications include pancreatitis, parotitis, and orchitis.

PROGNOSIS. The prognosis for complete recovery is excellent if no complications ensue during the acute illness. The major symptoms typically last 2–4 wk, followed by gradual recovery. Second attacks of infectious mononucleosis caused by EBV have not been documented. Fatigue, malaise, and some disability that may wax and wane for several weeks to a few months are common complaints even in otherwise unremarkable cases. Occasional persistence of fatigue for a few years after infectious mononucleosis is well recognized. At present, there is no convincing evidence linking EBV infection or EBV reactivation to chronic fatigue syndrome (see Chapter 717).

Alpert G, Fleisher GR: Complications of infection with Epstein-Barr virus during childhood: A study of children admitted to the hospital. Pediatr Infect Dis 3:304, 1984.

Andiman WA: Epstein-Barr virus-associated syndromes: A critical reexamination. Pediatr Infect Dis 3:198, 1984.

Gaffey MJ, Weiss LM: Association of Epstein-Barr virus with human neoplasia. Pathol Annu 27:55, 1992.

Horwitz CA, Henle W, Henle G, et al: Clinical and laboratory evaluation of cytomegalovirus-induced mononucleosis in previously healthy individuals: Report of 82 cases. Medicine 65:124, 1986.

Jenson H, McIntosh K, Pitt J, et al: Natural history of primary Epstein-Barr virus infection in children of mothers infected with human immunodeficiency virus type 1. J Infect Dis 179:1395, 1999.

Seemayer TA, Gross TG, Egeler RM, et al: X-linked lymphoproliferative disease: Twenty-five years after the discovery. Pediatr Res 38:471, 1995.

Straus SE, Tosato G, Armstrong G, et al: Persisting illness and fatigue in adults with evidence of Epstein-Barr virus infection. Ann Intern Med 102:7, 1985.

Sumaya CV, Ench Y: Epstein-Barr virus infectious mononucleosis in children: I. Clinical and general laboratory findings. Pediatrics 75:1003, 1985.

Sumaya CV, Ench Y: Epstein-Barr virus infectious mononucleosis in children: II. Heterophil antibody and viral-specific responses. Pediatrics 75:1011, 1985.

Tynell E, Aurelius E, Brandell A, et al: Acyclovir and prednisolone treatment of acute infectious mononucleosis: A multicenter, double-blind, placebo-controlled study. J Infect Dis 174:324, 1996.

White PD, Grover SA, Kangro HO, et al: The validity and reliability of the fatigue syndrome that follows glandular fever. Psychol Med 25:917, 1995.

CHAPTER 248
Cytomegalovirus

Sergio Stagno

Human cytomegalovirus (CMV) is a member of the Herpesviridae family with wide distribution. Most CMV infections are inapparent, but the virus can cause a variety of clinical illnesses that range in severity from mild to fatal. CMV is the most common congenital infection, which occasionally causes the syndrome of cytomegalic inclusion disease (hepatosplenomegaly, jaundice, petechia, purpura, and microcephaly). In immunocompetent adults, the infection is occasionally characterized by a mononucleosis-like syndrome. In immunosuppressed individuals, including recipients of transplants and patients with AIDS, CMV pneumonitis, retinitis, and gastrointestinal disease are common and can be fatal.

Primary infection occurs in a seronegative, susceptible host. Recurrent infection represents reactivation of latent infection or reinfection in a seropositive immune host. Disease may result from primary or recurrent CMV infection, but the former is a more common cause of severe disease.

ETIOLOGY. CMV is the largest of the herpesviruses, with a genome of 240 kb and a virus diameter of 200 nm. It contains double-stranded DNA in a 64-nm core enclosed by an icosahedral capsid composed of 162 capsomers. The core is assembled in the nucleus of the host cells. The capsid is surrounded by a poorly defined amorphous tegument, which is itself surrounded by a loosely applied, lipid-containing envelope. The envelope is acquired during the budding process through the nuclear membrane into a cytoplasmic vacuole, which contains the protein components of the envelope. Mature viruses exit the cells by reverse pinocytosis. Serologic tests do not define specific serotypes. In contrast, restriction endonuclease analysis of CMV DNA shows that, although all known human strains are genetically homologous, none are identical unless they were obtained from epidemiologically related cases.

EPIDEMIOLOGY. Seroepidemiologic surveys demonstrate CMV infection in every population examined worldwide. The prevalence of infection, which increases with age, is higher in developing countries and among lower socioeconomic strata of the more developed nations. Transmission sources of CMV include saliva, breast milk, cervical and vaginal secretions, urine, semen, stools, and blood. The spread of CMV requires very close or intimate contact because it is very labile. Transmission occurs by direct person-to-person contact, but indirect transmission is possible via contaminated fomites.

The incidence of congenital infection ranges from 0.2–2.4% of all live births, with the higher rates in populations with a lower standard of living. The fetus may become infected as a consequence of primary and recurrent maternal infection. The risk for fetal infection is greatest with maternal primary CMV infection (40%) and much less likely with recurrent infection (< 1%). In the United States, from 1–4% of pregnant women acquire primary CMV infection, with as many as 8,000 newborns with neurodevelopmental sequelae associated with congenital CMV infection.

Perinatal transmission is common, reaching 10–60% by 6 mo of age. The most important sources of virus are genital tract secretions at delivery and breast milk. Infected infants excrete virus for years in saliva and urine.

After the 1st year of life, the prevalence of infection is dependent on group activities, with child-care centers contributing to the rapid spread of CMV in childhood. Infection rates of 50–80% during childhood are common. For children who are not exposed to other toddlers, the rate of infection increases very slowly throughout the first decade of life. A second peak occurs in adolescence as a result of sexual transmission. Seronegative child-care workers and parents of young children shedding CMV have a 10–20% annual risk of acquiring CMV, which contrasts with 1–3% per year for the general population.

Health care providers are not at increased risk for acquiring CMV infection from patients. Nosocomial infection is a hazard of transfusion of blood and blood products. In a population with a 50% prevalence of CMV infection, the risk has been estimated at 2.7% per unit of whole blood. Leukocyte transfusions pose a much greater risk. Infection is usually asymptomatic, but even in well children and adults there is a risk of disease if the recipient is seronegative and receives multiple units.

Immunocompromised patients and seronegative premature infants have a much higher (10–30%) risk of disease. CMV infection is transmitted in transplanted organs (e.g., kidney, heart, and bone marrow). After transplantation, many patients excrete CMV as a result of infection acquired from the donor organ or from reactivation of latent infection caused by immunosuppression. Seronegative recipients of organs from seropositive donors are at greatest risk for severe disease.

PATHOGENESIS. Cytomegalic cells are strikingly enlarged epithelial or mesenchymal cells with large intranuclear inclusions and smaller intracytoplasmic inclusions, and are pathognomonic for CMV infection. The virus induces focal mononuclear cell infiltrates, which may be present with or without cytomegalic cells. The virus may induce focal necrosis in the brain and liver, which may be extensive and accompanied by granulomatous change with calcifications. The lung, liver, kidney, gastrointestinal tract, and salivary and other exocrine glands are the most commonly affected organs, although the virus has been found in most cell types. The extent of abnormal organ function and the quantity of virus that can be recovered from infected organs are not related to the number of cytomegalic inclusion-bearing cells, which may be few or absent in each organ section examined.

CLINICAL MANIFESTATIONS. The signs and symptoms of CMV infection vary with age, route of transmission, and immunocompetence of the patient. The infection is subclinical in most patients. In young children, primary CMV infection occasionally causes pneumonitis, hepatomegaly, hepatitis, and petechial rashes. In older children, adolescents, and adults, CMV may cause mononucleosis-like syndrome characterized by fatigue, malaise, myalgia, headache, fever, hepatosplenomegaly, abnormal liver function test results, and atypical lymphocytosis. The course of CMV mononucleosis is generally mild, lasting 2–3 wk. An occasional patient may present with persistent fever, overt hepatitis, or morbilliform rash, or a combination. Recurrent infections are asymptomatic in the immunocompetent host.

Immunocompromised Hosts. In immunocompromised individuals, the risk of CMV disease is increased with both primary and recurrent infections (Chapter 179). Illness with a primary infection includes pneumonitis (most common), hepatitis, chorioretinitis, gastrointestinal disease, or fever with leukopenia as isolated entities or as manifestations of generalized disease, which is often fatal. The risk is greatest in bone marrow transplant recipients and in patients with AIDS. Pneumonia, retinitis, and involvement of the central nervous system and gastrointestinal tract are usually severe and progressive. Submucosal ulcerations can occur anywhere in the gastrointestinal tract. Hemorrhage and perforation are known complications, as are pancreatitis and cholecystitis.

Congenital Infection. The condition of symptomatic congenital CMV infection was originally called *cytomegalic inclusion disease*. Only 5% of all congenitally infected infants have severe cytomegalic inclusion disease, another 5% have mild involvement, and 90% are born with subclinical but chronic CMV infection. The most characteristic signs and symptoms include intrauterine growth retardation, prematurity, hepatosplenomegaly and jaundice, thrombocytopenia and purpura, and microcephaly and intracranial calcifications. Other neurologic problems include chorioretinitis, sensorineural hearing loss, and mild increases in cerebrospinal fluid protein. Symptomatic newborns are usually easy to identify. Most symptomatic congenital infections and those resulting in sequelae are caused by primary rather than recurrent infections in pregnant women. Asymptomatic congenital CMV infection is likely a leading cause of sensorineural hearing loss in young children, occurring in approximately 7% of infected infants.

Perinatal Infection. Infections resulting from exposure to CMV in the maternal genital tract at delivery or in breast milk occur despite the presence of maternally derived, passively acquired antibody. Approximately 6–12% of seropositive mothers transmit CMV to their infants by contaminated cervical-vaginal secretions and 50% by breast milk. The majority of infants remain asymptomatic and do not exhibit sequelae. Occasionally, perinatally acquired CMV infection is associated with pneumonitis. Premature and ill full-term infants may have neurologic sequelae and psychomotor retardation. However, the risk of hearing loss, chorioretinitis, and microcephaly does not appear to be increased.

Seronegative premature infants with birth weights of <1,500 g with transfusion-acquired CMV infection have a 40% risk of experiencing hepatosplenomegaly, pneumonitis, gray pallor, jaundice, petechiae, thrombocytopenia, atypical lymphocytosis, and hemolytic anemia.

DIAGNOSIS. Active CMV infection is best demonstrated by virus isolation from urine, saliva, bronchoalveolar washings, breast milk, cervical secretions, buffy coat, and tissues obtained by biopsy. Rapid (24 hr) identification is now routine with the centrifugation-enhanced rapid culture system based on the detection of CMV early antigens using monoclonal antibodies. Several methods are used for rapid detection of CMV antigens, and polymerase chain reaction (PCR) and DNA hybridization techniques are also available for rapid diagnosis. The presence of viral shedding and active infection does not distinguish between primary and recurrent infections. A primary infection is confirmed by seroconversion or the simultaneous detection of immunoglobulin (Ig) M as well as IgG antibodies. Rising IgG antibody titers may be caused by primary and recurrent infection and must be interpreted carefully.

Sensitive and specific serologic tests to measure IgG antibodies are available in diagnostic laboratories. Complement fixation, neutralization, anticomplement immunofluorescence, and indirect immunofluorescence assays are preferable to define increases in antibody titers because they are quantitative. In contrast, radioimmunoassay (RIA) and enzyme-linked immunosorbent assay (ELISA) are less reliable for demonstrating significant changes in titers because most laboratories establish binding ratio (RIA) and absorbance units (ELISA) at a fixed serum dilution to compare the quantities of antibodies present in two sera. A simple increase in antibody titers in initially seropositive patients must be interpreted with caution because these are occasionally seen years after primary infection. IgG antibodies persist for life. IgM antibodies can be demonstrated transiently (4–16 wk) during the acute phase of symptomatic as well as asymptomatic primary infection in adults. RIA, ELISA, and an IgM capture RIA have acceptable specificity and sensitivity to detect primary infections. IgM antibodies are rarely found with these assays (0.2–1%) in patients with recurrent infection.

A recurrent infection is defined by the reappearance of viral excretion in a patient known to have been seropositive in the past. The distinction between reactivation of endogenous virus and reinfection with a different strain of CMV requires restriction enzyme analysis of viral DNA to demonstrate polymorphisms between viral isolates.

In immunocompromised patients, excretion of CMV, increases in IgG titers, and even the presence of IgM antibodies are common, making the distinction between primary and recurrent infections more difficult. Demonstrating viremia by buffy coat culture or detection of CMV DNA implies active disease and worse prognosis regardless of whether the type of infection is primary, recurrent, or uncertain.

Congenital Infection. The definitive method for diagnosis of congenital CMV infection is virus isolation or demonstration of specific DNA sequences by PCR. This must be performed at or shortly after birth. Urine and saliva are the best specimens for culture. Infants with congenital CMV infection may excrete CMV in high titers in the urine for several months. An IgG antibody test is of little diagnostic value because a positive result also reflects maternal antibodies, although a negative result excludes the diagnosis of congenital CMV infection. Demonstration of stable or rising titers in serial specimens during the first year of life does not help because acquired infection in the first few months of life is common. In general, IgM tests lack sensitivity and specificity and are unreliable for diagnosis of congenital CMV infection. Congenital toxoplasmosis and syphilis must also be considered.

CMV infection can be diagnosed in utero by isolation of the virus from the amniotic fluid. A negative culture does not exclude fetal infection because the interval between maternal infection and fetal infection is unknown. Although isolation of CMV by this means documents fetal infection, it does not indicate whether the newborn will have a symptomatic or an asymptomatic infection.

TREATMENT. Ganciclovir combined with immune globulin, either standard intravenous immunoglobulin (IVIG) or hyperimmune CMV IVIG, has been used to treat life-threatening CMV infections in immunocompromised hosts (e.g., bone marrow, heart, and kidney transplant recipients and patients with AIDS). Two published regimens are ganciclovir (7.5 mg/kg/24 hr intravenously divided every 8 hr for 14 days) with CMV IVIG (400 mg/kg on days 1, 2, and 7, and 200 mg/kg on day 14); and ganciclovir (7.5 mg/kg/24 hr intravenously divided every 8 hr for 20 days with IVIG 500 mg/kg every other day for 10 doses).

CMV retinitis and gastrointestinal disease appear to be clinically responsive to therapy but, like viral excretion, often recur on cessation. Toxicity with ganciclovir is frequent and often severe, including neutropenia, thrombocytopenia, liver dysfunction, reduction in spermatogenesis, and gastrointestinal and renal abnormalities. Foscarnet is an alternative antiviral agent, although there is limited information of its use in children.

Congenital Infection. A phase II study with ganciclovir (12 mg/kg 24 hr for a total of 6 wk) showed hearing improvement or stabilization in 5 of 30 infants, suggesting efficacy. A randomized study of symptomatic congenital CMV infection is in progress.

PROGNOSIS. Patients with CMV mononucleosis usually recover fully, although some have a protracted symptomatic illness. Most immunocompromised patients also recover uneventfully, but many experience severe pneumonitis, with a high fatality rate if hypoxemia develops. CMV infection and disease may be terminal events in individuals with increased susceptibility to infections such as patients with AIDS.

Congenital Disease. The prognosis for normal development with symptomatic cytomegalic inclusion disease is poor; more than 90% of these children demonstrate central nervous system and hearing defects in later years. In infants with subclinical infection, the outlook is much better. The primary concern is the subsequent development of sensorineural hearing loss (5–10%), chorioretinitis (3–5%), and other less frequent manifestations such as developmental abnormalities, microcephaly, and neurologic deficits.

PREVENTION. The use of CMV-free blood products, especially for premature newborns, and, whenever possible, the use of organs from CMV-free donors for transplantation represent important measures to prevent CMV infection and disease in patients at high risk.

Pregnant women who are CMV seropositive are at low risk of delivering a symptomatic newborn. If possible, pregnant women should have a CMV serologic test, especially if they care for young children who are potential CMV excreters. Those who are CMV seronegative should be counseled regarding good handwashing and other hygienic measures and avoidance of contact with oral secretions of others.

Passive Immunoprophylaxis. The use of IVIG or CMV IVIG for prophylaxis of infection in solid organ and bone marrow transplant recipients reduces the risk of symptomatic disease but does not prevent infection. The efficacy of prophylaxis is more striking when the hazard of primary CMV infection is greatest, such as in bone marrow transplantation. There is no consensus for a uniform prophylaxis regimen for CMV infection. Recommended regimens include either IVIG (1,000 mg/kg) or CMV IVIG (500 mg/kg) given as a single intravenous dose beginning within 72 hr of transplantation and once weekly thereafter until day 90–120 after transplantation.

Active Immunization. The beneficial role of immunity is substantial, as illustrated by the fact that most severe disease follows primary infection, especially in congenital infection, transfusion-acquired infection, and infection in transplant recipients. Candidates for a CMV vaccine include seronegative women of childbearing age and seronegative transplant recipients. Live, attenuated vaccines such as the Towne strain prototype are immunogenic, but immunity wanes quickly. Vaccine virus does not seem to be transmissible. The vaccine does not protect renal transplant recipients from CMV infection, but appears to reduce the virulence of primary infection. In a study of vaccine efficacy in normal adult women, the Towne strain vaccine did not provide protection against naturally acquired infection. Other types of vaccines, such as subunit and recombinant vaccines, are being evaluated in early clinical trials.

Boppana SB, Fowler KB, Vaid Y, et al: Neuroradiographic findings in the newborn period and long-term outcome in children with symptomatic congenital cytomegalovirus infection. Pediatrics 99:409, 1997.

Emanuel D, Cunningham I, Jules-Elysee K, et al: Cytomegalovirus pneumonia after bone marrow transplantation successfully treated with the combination of ganciclovir and high-dose intravenous immune globulin. Ann Intern Med 109:772, 1988.

Fowler KB, McCollister FP, Dahle AJ, et al: Progressive and fluctuating sensorineural hearing loss in children with asymptomatic congenital cytomegalovirus infection. J Pediatr 130:624, 1997.

Horwitz CA, Henle W, Henle G, et al: Clinical and laboratory evaluation of cytomegalovirus-induced mononucleosis in previously healthy individuals. Report of 82 cases. Medicine (Baltimore) 65:124, 1986.

Istas AS, Demmler GJ, Dobbins JG, et al: Surveillance for congenital cytomegalovirus disease: A report from the National Congenital Cytomegalovirus Disease Registry. Clin Infect Dis 20:665, 1995.

Iversson S-A, Lernmark B, Svanberg L: Ten-year clinical, developmental, and intellectual follow-up of children with congenital cytomegalovirus infection without neurologic symptoms at one year of age. Pediatrics 99:800, 1997.

Levin M: Current approaches to the prevention and treatment of cytomegalovirus disease after bone marrow transplantation: An overview. Semin Hematol 27:1, 1990.

Reed EC, Bowden RA, Dandliker PS, et al: Treatment of cytomegalovirus pneumonia with ganciclovir and intravenous cytomegalovirus immunoglobulin in patients with bone marrow transplants. Ann Intern Med 109:783, 1988.

Rubin RH: Impact of cytomegalovirus infection on organ transplant recipients. Rev Infect Dis 12 (suppl 7): S754, 1990.

Stagno S: Cytomegalovirus. *In:* Remington JS, Klein JO (eds): Infectious Diseases of the Fetus and Newborn Infant, 4th ed. Philadelphia, WB Saunders, 1995, pp 312–353.

Stagno S, Cloud GA: Working parents: The impact of day care and breast feeding on cytomegalovirus infection in offspring. Proc Natl Acad Sci U S A 91:2384, 1994.

CHAPTER 249
Roseola (Human Herpesvirus Types 6 and 7)

Charles T. Leach

Human herpesvirus type 6 (HHV-6) was discovered in 1986, 22 yr after the discovery of the 5th human herpesvirus (Epstein-Barr virus). Six isolates of a new virus were identified in the peripheral blood mononuclear cells (PBMCs) of adult patients with AIDS or lymphoproliferative diseases. In 1990, human herpesvirus 7 (HHV-7) was identified in the peripheral blood mononuclear cells of an HIV-uninfected adult. HHV-6 is the etiologic agent for most cases of roseola infantum (exanthem subitum), and also is associated with other diseases in normal and immunocompromised patients. Disease associations for HHV-7 are fewer; only its role in some cases of roseola is well established. Preliminary evidence links HHV-6 with multiple sclerosis.

ETIOLOGY. Roseola was first established as a distinct illness at the turn of the century. Until recently, no pathogen could be consistently identified as the agent responsible for roseola. However, it now appears that primary infection with HHV-6, and less frequently HHV-7, causes the majority of cases of roseola. In studies of children with roseola from Europe and Asia, HHV-6 was responsible for 45–86% (average 66%) of cases and HHV-7 caused 10–31% (average 23%) of cases. Other viruses (e.g., echovirus 16) probably account for the remainder of cases.

HHV-6 and HHV-7 belong to the β-herpesvirus subfamily of herpesviruses, which also includes human cytomegalovirus (CMV). HHV-6 and HHV-7 share physical and biologic characteristics with other herpesviruses, including a large double-stranded DNA genome (159,000 base pairs and 145,000 base pairs, respectively), the presence of a nucleocapsid, and the establishment of latency after primary infection. HHV-6 is essentially colinear with HHV-7, and both viruses share much homology with CMV. The principal target cells for HHV-6 and HHV-7 infection in vivo are $CD4^+$ T cells; HHV-6 can also infect other cells, including $CD8^+$ (suppressor) T cells, natural killer T cells, δγ T cells, glial cells, epithelial cells, monocytes, megakaryocytes, and endothelial cells. HHV-6 and HHV-7 are typically cultivated in vitro in mitogen-stimulated human mononuclear cells (isolated from cord blood or peripheral blood) and can be identified by the development of large balloon-like cells accompanied by cell lysis. Two distinct types of HHV-6 (types A and B) exist, based on differences in DNA sequence, antigenicity, and laboratory growth requirements. Type B causes more than 99% of HHV-6–associated roseola cases. Type A virus has been found in some immunocompromised patients (particularly adults) but has not yet been linked with any disease.

EPIDEMIOLOGY. Primary HHV-6 infection occurs early in life. More than 90% of newborn infants are HHV-6 seropositive, reflecting transplacental transfer of maternal antibodies. By 4–6 mo of age, the prevalence drops significantly (0–60%). By 12 mo of age, 60–90% of children possess antibodies to HHV-6, and by 3–5 yr, 80–100% of children are seropositive. Peak acquisition of primary HHV-6 infection, from 6–15 mo of age, corresponds with peak acquisition of roseola. However, because the incidence of roseola in the United States is only 30–45%, the majority of HHV-6 infections are not recognizable as roseola. Primary infection with HHV-7 occurs slightly later than HHV-6 infection, with 45–75% of children infected by 2 yr of age and 90% by 7–10 yr of age.

Roseola can develop in children year-round; some series indicate a higher incidence during spring and fall months. Unlike some of the other childhood exanthems, children with roseola rarely report contact with other affected children, and outbreaks are uncommon. Sex, race, and geography do not play an important role in acquisition of roseola. The incubation period averages 10 days (range of 5–15 days).

Most adults excrete HHV-6 and HHV-7 in saliva and may serve as primary sources for virus transmission to children. Women excrete HHV-6 and HHV-7 in the genital tract at low rates (0–19% and 3%, respectively), but sexual transmissibility has not been demonstrated. There is evidence that HHV-6 can be transmitted in utero, although this is a rare occurrence; no congenital HHV-7 infections have been described. Breast milk does not appear to be an important vehicle for transmission of HHV-6.

PATHOGENESIS. Little is known regarding the pathogenesis of infections associated with HHV-6, including roseola. Virus is probably acquired from the saliva of healthy persons and enters the host through the oral, nasal, or conjunctival mucosa. This is supported by the experimental transmission of roseola via the respiratory tract in the 1950s. After HHV-6 replication at an unknown site, a high level of viremia develops in PBMCs. After acute infection, HHV-6 establishes latency in monocytes and macrophages and possibly in the salivary glands, kidneys, lungs, and central nervous system. The basis for the unique pattern of rash after resolution of fever in children with roseola has not been established. There is no information regarding the pathogenesis of HHV-7 infection.

HHV-6 can suppress all cellular lineages within the bone marrow, and active HHV-6 infection is associated with bone marrow suppression in bone marrow transplant patients. Also, in vitro HHV-6 infection suppresses lymphoproliferative responses of PBMCs.

CLINICAL MANIFESTATIONS. Roseola is the prototypical HHV-6 infection, although nonspecific infections are common.

Roseola Infantum (Exanthem Subitum). Roseola is a mild febrile, exanthematous illness occurring almost exclusively during infancy. More than 95% of roseola cases occur in children younger than 3 yr, with a peak at 6–15 mo of age. Transplacental antibodies likely protect most infants until 6 mo of age.

Infants with classic roseola exhibit a unique constellation of findings displayed over a short period of time. Consequently, classic roseola is infrequently confused with other childhood exanthems.

The prodromal period of roseola is usually asymptomatic but may include mild upper respiratory tract signs, among them minimal rhinorrhea, slight pharyngeal inflammation, and mild conjunctival redness. Mild cervical or, less frequently, occipital lymphadenopathy may be noted. Some children may have mild palpebral edema. Physical findings during the prodromal stage have no clear relationship to roseola, and may simply reflect an accompanying respiratory viral infection.

Clinical illness is generally heralded by high temperature, usually ranging from 37.9–40°C (101–106°F), with an average of 39°C (103°F). Some children may become irritable and anorexic during the febrile stage, but most behave normally despite high temperatures. Seizures may occur in 5–10% of children with roseola during this febrile period. Infrequent complaints include rhinorrhea, sore throat, abdominal pain, vomiting, and diarrhea.

Fever persists for 3–5 days, and then typically resolves rather abruptly ("crisis"). Occasionally, the fever may gradually diminish over 24–36 ("lysis"). A rash appears within 12–24 hr of fever resolution. In many cases, the rash develops during defervescence or within a few hours of fever resolution. The rash of roseola is rose colored, as the name implies, and is fairly distinctive. However, it may be confused with exanthems resulting from rubella, measles, or erythema infectiosum. The roseola rash begins as discrete, small (2–5 mm), slightly raised pink lesions on the trunk and usually spreads to the neck, face, and proximal extremities. The rash is not usually pruritic, and no vesicles or pustules develop. Lesions typically remain discrete but occasionally may become almost confluent. After 1–3 days, the rash fades. Some children experience evanescent rashes that resolve within a few hours.

Subtle differences in clinical presentation have been noted between roseola associated with HHV-7 compared with HHV-6. These include a slightly older age, lower mean temperature, and shorter duration of fever in HHV-7–associated cases. However, these differences are insufficient to clinically distinguish HHV-6– from HHV-7–associated roseola. There are reports of children experiencing HHV-6–associated roseola followed later by HHV-7–associated roseola.

Fever in Infants Without Classic Roseola. A significant proportion of nonspecific febrile illnesses in infants is caused by HHV-6. In two large studies examining febrile infants presenting to a hospital emergency room, approximately one third of infants with nonspecific fever or fever with otitis media had primary HHV-6 infection.

Central Nervous System Infections. Like most other herpesviruses, HHV-6 is neurotropic. Primary HHV-6 infection is responsible for one third of febrile seizures in infants. Most of these children (70–80%) do not subsequently experience a rash. One small study also noted febrile seizures occurring frequently in infants with acute HHV-7 infections. HHV-6 is also associated with rare cases of encephalitis and meningoencephalitis, typically during the febrile stage of roseola. Investigators from the Collaborative Antiviral Study Group noted HHV-6 DNA in cerebrospinal fluid from 6% of children and adults with focal encephalitis of unknown cause.

Mononucleosis-Like Illness and Hepatitis. Several heterophile-negative mononucleosis-like infections associated with HHV-6 have been reported in adults. HHV-6 uncommonly causes clinical symptoms of hepatitis, and only one case has been described for HHV-7. One fatal case of hepatitis occurred in a neonate after maternal transmission of HHV-6.

Infections in Immunocompromised Patients. Numerous severe and occasionally fatal HHV-6–associated infections (encephalitis and pneumonitis) have occurred in immunocompromised patients, including patients with AIDS or organ transplants. These have predominately occurred in adults and reflect reactivated HHV-6 infection. Because HHV-6 shares $CD4^+$ cell tropism with HIV, upregulates HIV, and stimulates in vitro replication of HIV, there has been considerable interest in the role of HHV-6 as a cofactor for clinical progression of AIDS. Epidemiologic studies do not support a significant role for HHV-6 as an AIDS cofactor.

Other Diseases Possibly Associated with HHV-6 or HHV-7. Rash illness without fever has been described in a small number of infants with primary HHV-6 infection. Other small studies or case reports have suggested that HHV-6 may be associated with some cases of hemophagocytic syndrome, intussusception, idiopathic thrombocytopenic purpura, recurrent aphthous stomatitis, and disseminated disease. One study suggests a link between HHV-7 and pityriasis rosea, a benign exanthematous illness.

Controversy exists regarding the association of HHV-6 with multiple sclerosis. HHV-6 subtype B has been detected within the plaques of brains from patients with multiple sclerosis; further studies are needed to clarify this putative association.

HHV-6 DNA has been detected in various malignancies, including non-Hodgkin lymphoma, Hodgkin disease, cervical and oral carcinoma, and leukemia. However, no consistent etiologic relationship has been established with any of these cancers. Small studies have suggested a link between HHV-6 and two histiocytic disorders: Langerhans cell histiocytosis and sinus histiocytosis with massive lymphadenopathy (Rosai-Dorfman disease).

DIAGNOSIS. The most important reason for establishing the diagnosis of roseola is to differentiate this generally mild illness from other potentially more serious childhood rash illnesses such as measles. It is also important to identify other, more serious illnesses caused by HHV-6, such as encephalitis and pneumonitis, especially in immunocompromised patients, for timely consideration of antiviral therapy.

The diagnosis of roseola can be established primarily on the basis of age, history, and clinical findings. HHV-6– and HHV-7–associated roseola cases cannot be distinguished on clinical grounds. Specific testing for HHV-6 or HHV-7 infection may be performed using laboratory methods, including serology, virus culture, antigen detection, and polymerase chain reaction (PCR).

A variety of HHV-6 serologic tests are available; no commercial tests are available for HHV-7. An HHV-6 immunoglobulin (Ig) M response typically develops by the 5th–7th day of illness, peaks at 2–3 wk, and resolves within 2 mo. Unfortunately, the accuracy of currently available IgM tests varies widely, and none have been sufficiently evaluated to provide unequivocal evidence of acute HHV-6 infection. Seroconversion of HHV-6 IgG antibodies in serum samples collected 2–3 wk apart is a more reliable means of establishing primary HHV-6 infection. Fourfold increases or decreases in HHV-6 IgG antibodies also suggest active HHV-6 infection (primary or reactivated). Because of the high seroprevalence of HHV-6 in the general population, a single positive HHV-6 IgG test is of no diagnostic significance for diagnosis of acute infection. CMV antibodies can cross-react with HHV-6; therefore, diagnosis of HHV-6 infection by serologic means requires exclusion of CMV infection.

Identification of HHV-6 or HHV-7 in PBMCs by virus culture firmly establishes the presence of active infection in immunocompetent hosts; association with specific disease is more problematic in immunocompromised patients as a result of a low background rate of viremia. Identification of HHV-6 and HHV-7 by culture requires incubation of PBMCs (with or without cocultivation with exogenous PBMCs) for days to several weeks, and is presently available only in research laboratories.

A commercial HHV-6 antigen assay has been described that is comparable in sensitivity to virus culture for detection of active HHV-6 infection.

PCR amplification tests for HHV-6 and HHV-7 are becoming widely available for diagnosis, and may provide more timely information for diagnosis. Active, replicating infection is indicated if viral DNA is detected in noncellular specimens such as serum or cerebrospinal fluid. However, detection at other sites (e.g., PBMCs, saliva, and tissues) does not necessarily indicate active infection, because both viruses exist in latent form in many tissues after primary infection.

Other diagnostic tests for consideration in selected circumstances include in situ hybridization and immunohistochemistry.

Laboratory Findings. Leukocytosis (8,000–9,000 white blood cells [WBCs]/μL) may be found during the first few days of fever in children with roseola, but by the time the exanthem appears, the WBC count falls to 4,000–6,000 with a relative lymphocytosis (70–90%). The cerebrospinal fluid in children with HHV-6–associated febrile seizures typically is normal. The cerebrospinal fluid from rare cases of HHV-6–associated meningoencephalitis and encephalitis is characterized by a mild pleocytosis with predominance of mononuclear cells, normal glucose, and normal to slightly elevated protein.

Differential Diagnosis. Children with roseola typically present at two different stages of the illness: at the time of fever before the rash (pre-eruptive) and after the rash has appeared. During the pre-eruptive stage, many conditions may be confused with roseola. However, the pattern of fever in a generally well child without significant physical findings, rather precipitous defervescence, and a subsequent rash is unique for roseola.

Nonetheless, some patients may not display all these characteristics and may mimic other illnesses.

Roseola is probably most commonly confused with rubella. In contrast to the absence of a distinct prodrome in children with roseola, children with rubella invariably have a mildly symptomatic prodromal period, including prominent occipital and postauricular lymphadenopathy. Lymphadenopathy is an inconsistent finding in roseola; when lymphadenopathy does occur, occipital lymph nodes are more frequently affected than those in the postauricular region. Rubella usually causes only low-grade fever, which is coincident with the exanthem. The rubella rash is typically more extensive than that seen with roseola, and coalescence is more common. A history of exposure is frequently elicited from those in whom rubella develops. Most important, vaccinated persons rarely acquire rubella.

Roseola may be confused with measles. However, the development of an exanthem at the height of the fever, as well as the presence of cough, coryza, conjunctivitis, and Koplik's spots on the buccal mucosa in the early stages of measles should serve to differentiate these two illnesses.

Outbreaks of roseola-like illnesses have been associated with many different viruses, most commonly enteroviruses. In summer and fall months, some cases of roseola-like illnesses may be attributable to enteroviruses.

Scarlet fever may also resemble roseola. Important features of scarlet fever are its rarity in infancy, the simultaneous presence of fever and rash, and the discrete, small, sandpaper-like rash lesions.

Drug hypersensitivity is a common condition resembling roseola. Antibiotics are frequently prescribed to children with roseola during the febrile phase before onset of the rash. A child who acquires a drug rash may do so soon after resolution of the fever, which is the characteristic pattern for children with roseola. However, the usually morbilliform nature, pruritus, and resolution after discontinuation of the implicated drug should distinguish a drug rash.

It may be difficult to distinguish central nervous system disease caused by HHV-6 from other etiologies. Development of a roseola-like illness in association with febrile seizures, meningoencephalitis, or encephalitis makes HHV-6 infection more likely; however, this occurs infrequently.

Hepatitis and heterophile-negative mononucleosis are uncommonly associated with HHV-6, and other causes for these infections should first be sought.

TREATMENT. HHV-6 is inhibited by ganciclovir (but not acyclovir) and foscarnet at levels that are achievable in serum; more limited data have indicated that HHV-7 is inhibited by foscarnet. The clinical efficacy of these drugs, however, has not been evaluated.

The generally benign nature of roseola precludes consideration of antiviral therapy. However, future studies may address the need for specific antiviral therapy in those unusual cases of roseola or other forms of HHV-6 infection in which significant morbidity exists, such as children with neurologic complications of roseola or immunocompromised children with HHV-6 infection.

Children in the febrile, pre-eruptive phase of roseola usually are quite comfortable and require little supportive therapy. Those children who are uncomfortable and irritable, or in whom histories of febrile convulsions exists, may benefit from treatment with acetaminophen or ibuprofen. Adequate fluid balance should be maintained in all affected children. Referral should be considered in those unusual circumstanes in which serious disease develops, such as encephalitis, hepatitis, or pneumonitis.

PROGNOSIS. The prognosis for the great majority of children with roseola is excellent, with no obvious sequelae. Before the discoveries of HHV-6 and HHV-7, rare complications of roseola (hemiparesis, mental retardation) were attributable to brain anoxia during prolonged febrile seizures. However, damage resulting from direct viral invasion of the brain, liver, and other organs has been demonstrated for HHV-6. Deaths directly attributable to HHV-6 have been reported in normal as well as immunocompromised patients in whom encephalitis, hepatitis, pneumonitis, disseminated disease, or hemophagocytosis syndrome developed.

PREVENTION. Very little information is available on which to base guidelines for prevention of HHV-6 or HHV-7 infection. Experimental evidence suggests that roseola may be transmitted via blood or saliva, and both HHV-6 and HHV-7 are shed in the saliva. It is likely that healthy immune carriers with latent viral infections transmit infection to susceptible infants and children. No specific recommendations for prevention can be made until proper studies have been conducted.

Adams O, Krempe C, Kogler G, et al: Congenital infections with human herpesvirus 6. J Infect Dis 178:544, 1998.

Braun DK, Dominguez G, Pellett PE: Human herpesvirus 6. Clin Microbiol Rev 10:521, 1997.

Caserta MT, Hall CB, Schnabel K, et al: Primary human herpesvirus 7 infection: A comparison of human herpesvirus 7 and human herpesvirus 6 infections in children. J Pediatr 133:386, 1998.

Hall CB, Long CE, Schnabel KC, et al: Human herpesvirus-6 infection in children: A prospective study of complications and reactivation. N Engl J Med 331:432, 1994.

Huang LM, Lee CY, Liu MY, et al: Primary infections of human herpesvirus-7 and herpesvirus-6: A comparative, longitudinal study up to 6 years of age. Acta Paediatr 86:604, 1997.

Lanphear BP, Hall CB, Black J, et al: Risk factors for the early acquisition of human herpesvirus 6 and human herpesvirus 7 infections in children. Pediatr Infect Dis J 17:792, 1998.

Leach CT, Brown NA, Sumaya CV: Human herpesvirus-6: Clinical implications of a recently discovered, ubiquitous agent. J Pediatr 121:173, 1992.

Leach CT, Newton ER, McParlin S, et al: Human herpesvirus 6 infection of the female genital tract. J Infect Dis 169:1281, 1994.

McCullers JA, Lakeman FD, Whitley RJ: Human herpesvirus 6 is associated with focal encephalitis. Clin Infect Dis 21:571, 1995.

Pruksananonda P, Hall CB, Insel RA, et al: Primary human herpesvirus 6 infection in young children. N Engl J Med 326:1445, 1992.

Soldan SS, Berti R, Salem N, et al: Association of human herpes virus 6 (HHV6) with multiple sclerosis: Increased IgM response to HHV-6 early antigen and detection of serum HHV-6 DNA. Nat Med 3:1394, 1997.

Suga S, Yoshikawa T, Kajita Y, et al: Prospective study of persistence and excretion of human herpesvirus-6 in patients with exanthem subitum and their parents. Pediatrics 102:900, 1998.

Yamanishi K, Kondo T, Shiraki K, et al: Identification of human herpesvirus-6 as a causal agent for exanthem subitum. Lancet 1:1065, 1988.

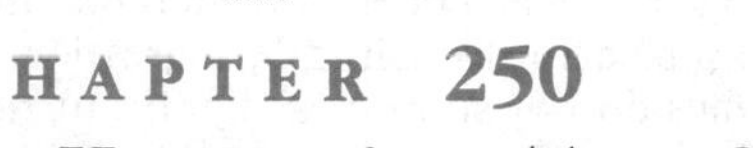

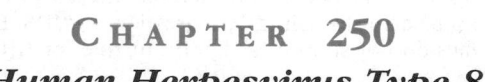

CHAPTER 250
Human Herpesvirus Type 8

Charles T. Leach

The identification of the newest human herpesvirus, human herpesvirus type 8 (HHV-8; also known as Kaposi sarcoma (KS) –associated herpesvirus), in 1994 resulted from a search for an infectious agent responsible for KS in patients with AIDS. Earlier studies suggested that a sexually transmitted infectious virus was responsible for this malignancy. Molecular biologic methods were used to isolate and identify DNA sequences present in malignant (but not normal) tissues from AIDS patients with KS. Comparison of these sequences to other known DNA sequences revealed this new human herpesvirus.

ETIOLOGY. HHV-8 is a member of the γ-herpesviruses, which includes Epstein-Barr virus. HHV-8 is an enveloped DNA virus of approximately 160,000 base pairs, and has a genomic structure typical for other human herpesviruses. Several HHV-8 proteins mimic human cellular genes involved in the regulation of cell growth: viral interferon regulatory factor; homologs to cellular proto-oncogenes, including a D-type cyclin and anti-apoptotic *bcl*-2; interleukin (IL) 6 homologs; and a constitutively active IL-8–like receptor. It is postulated that these proteins contribute to the pathogenesis of HHV-8–associated malignancies.

EPIDEMIOLOGY. HHV-8 infection is rare in healthy children and adults in most developed countries. However, HHV-8 infection is found in 5 to 20% of adults in certain areas of Greece and Italy and in 30 to 60% of adults in Central and East Africa. Approximately one third of HIV-infected homosexual males and more than 80% of HIV-infected homosexual males who acquire KS are infected with the virus. Patients with HIV infection acquired in another manner (e.g., vertically from an HIV-positive mother or through transfusion of blood or blood products) have low rates (0–5%) of HHV-8 infection that are similar to that observed in HIV-uninfected persons and blood donors (0–8%). HHV-8 can be carried in the saliva and reproductive tract of adults. HHV-8 infection has been identified in HIV-infected and HIV-uninfected young children (3–12 yr of age) from Africa with KS, suggesting possible vertical transmission of HHV-8. HHV-8 is potentially transmissible via blood transfusion, but this has not been documented. The virus has been transmitted to kidney transplant recipients via the donor organ.

Manifestations of acute HHV-8 infection are not known, and the incubation period has not been determined. In HIV-infected homosexual males in whom KS develops, HHV-8 infection can be detected up to 6 yr before onset of the malignancy.

CLINICAL MANIFESTATIONS. Three malignancies occurring primarily in adults with AIDS are associated with HHV-8: KS, multicentric Castleman disease, and primary effusion lymphoma. KS is the most common neoplasm associated with AIDS but also occurs in HIV-uninfected persons living in the Mediterranean region (classic KS), in equatorial Africa (endemic KS), and in organ transplant recipients (post-transplant KS). Multicentric Castleman disease is a much rarer, atypical lymphoproliferative skin disorder principally developing in patients with AIDS with concomitant KS. Primary effusion lymphoma is an infrequent form of non-Hodgkin's lymphoma developing predominantly in patients with AIDS that is characterized by a malignant effusion in one or more body cavities, generally in the absence of a primary tumor mass. Although HHV-8 can be identified in malignant tissue from most patients with these disorders, a clear etiologic link has not yet been firmly established. Limited data also suggest that HHV-8 is associated with multiple myeloma, a plasma cell malignancy occurring in elderly persons. It has been suggested that HHV-8 may play an indirect role in these malignancies by providing viral analogues of cellular growth factors.

DIAGNOSIS. HHV-8 infection can be demonstrated in research laboratories by serologic testing using enzyme immunoassay and Western immunoblotting, or detection of HHV-8 DNA sequences by polymerase chain reaction amplification. Commercial tests are not available. The virus is not easily cultivated.

TREATMENT. Several antiviral compounds inhibit HHV-8 in vitro, including ganciclovir, foscarnet, and cidofovir. However, the benefit of antiviral therapy for HHV-8–associated disease has not yet been established.

Chang Y, Cesarman E, Pessin MS, et al: Identification of herpesvirus-like DNA sequences in AIDS-associated Kaposi's sarcoma. Science 266:1865, 1994.
Chang Y, Ziegler J, Wabinga H: Kaposi's sarcoma-associated herpesvirus and Kaposi's sarcoma in Africa. Arch Intern Med 156:202, 1996.
Gao SJ, Alsina M, Deng JH, et al: Antibodies to Kaposi's sarcoma-associated herpesvirus (human herpesvirus 8) in patients with multiple myeloma. J Infect Dis 178:846, 1998.
Goedert JJ, Kedes DH, Ganem D: Antibodies to human herpesvirus 8 in women and infants born in Haiti and the USA. Lancet 349:1368, 1997.
Knowles DM, Cesarman E: The Kaposi's sarcoma-associated herpesvirus (human herpesvirus-8) in Kaposi's sarcoma, malignant lymphoma, and other diseases. Ann Oncol 8 (suppl 2):123, 1997.
Leach CT, Frantz C, Head DR, et al: Human herpesvirus-8 (HHV-8) associated with small noncleaved cell lymphoma in a child with AIDS. Am J Hematol 60:215, 1999.
Regamey N, Tamm M, Wernli M, et al: Transmission of human herpesvirus 8 infection from renal-transplant donors to recipients. N Engl J Med 339:1358, 1998.
Simpson GR, Schulz TF, Whitby D, et al: Prevalence of Kaposi's sarcoma associated herpesvirus infection measured by antibodies to recombinant capsid protein and latent immunofluorescence antigen. Lancet 348:1133, 1996.
Whitby D, Smith NA, Matthews S, et al: Human herpesvirus 8: Seroepidemiology among women and detection in the genital tract of seropositive women. J Infect Dis 179:234, 1999.

CHAPTER 251
Influenza Viruses

Peter Wright

Influenza viral infections cause a broad array of respiratory illnesses that are responsible for significant morbidity and mortality in children.

ETIOLOGY. Influenza viruses are members of the family Orthomyxoviridae. They are large, single-stranded RNA viruses with a segmented genome encased in a lipid-containing envelope. The two major surface proteins that determine the serotype of influenza, hemagglutinin and neuraminidase, project as spikes through the envelope. Influenza viruses are divided into three types: A, B, and C. Influenza types A and B are the primary influenzal pathogens and causes of epidemic disease. Influenza type C is a sporadic cause of predominantly upper respiratory tract disease. Influenza types A and B are further divided into serotypically distinct strains that circulate on a yearly basis through the population.

EPIDEMIOLOGY. Influenza A viruses have a complex epidemiology involving animal hosts that serve as a reservoir for diverse strains with potential for infecting the human population. The segmented nature of the influenza genome allows reassortment to occur between an animal and human virus when coinfection occurs. Thus, potentially any of 15 hemagglutinins (H) and 9 neuraminidases (N) residing in animal reservoirs may be introduced into humans; influenza A viruses behave epidemiologically as though there were many serotypes. Minor changes within a serotype are termed *antigenic drift;* major changes in serotype are termed *antigenic shift.* In addition, migratory avian hosts may be responsible for spread of disease. A recent example occurred in Hong Kong in the winter of 1997 when a small outbreak of avian H5N1 influenza in humans was associated with a high mortality; 6 of 18 patients died. Influenza B has much less capacity for major antigenic change and no identified animal reservoir.

The worldwide epidemiology of influenza viruses demonstrates annual spread from Asia across the Pacific Ocean to North America. When a virus identified by a novel and serologically distinct hemagglutinin or neuraminidase enters the population, there is potential for a pandemic of influenza with excess morbidity and mortality on a global scale in a largely nonimmune population. The most dramatic pandemic in recent history occurred in 1918, when influenza was estimated to have killed more than 20 million people. More common is the almost yearly variation in the antigenic composition of the surface proteins, which confers a selective advantage to a new strain and results in localized epidemics of disease with mortality largely confined to the elderly and to those with underlying cardiopulmonary disease. Each year's strain is novel for infants because they have no pre-existing antibody except for maternally transferred antibody in the very young.

The attack rate and frequency of isolation of influenza is

highest in young children. As many as 30–50% of children have serologic evidence of infection in a typical year. Children undergoing primary exposure to an influenza strain have higher titered and more prolonged shedding of the virus than adults, making them extremely effective transmitters of infection. Influenza is a disease of the colder months of the year in temperate climates; spread appears to occur by small-particle aerosol. Transmission through a community is rapid; the highest incidence of illness occurs within 2–3 wk of introduction. Influenza is marked by increased school absenteeism and the yearly peak in visits to the pediatrician. Influenza has been implicated in hospital spread of infection and may complicate the original illness that required hospitalization.

On a country or global basis, one or two predominant strains spread to create the annual epidemic. At present, influenza type A strains with the H1N1 and H3N2 serotypes and type B strains are co-circulating, and either type may be predominant in any one year, making predictions about the serotype and severity of the upcoming influenza season very difficult. Strain variants are identified by their hemagglutinin and neuraminidase serotypes, by the geographic area from which they were originally isolated, by their isolate number, and by year of isolation. Thus, the influenza vaccine for 1998–1999 was trivalent, having strains identified as A/Sydney/5/97/ (H3N2), A/Beijing/262/95 (H1N1), and B/Harbin/07/94.

PATHOGENESIS. The virus attaches to sialic acid residues on cells via the hemagglutinin and, via endocytosis, makes its way into vacuoles, where, with progressive acidification, there is fusion to the endosomal membrane and release of the viral RNA into the cytoplasm. The RNA is transported to the nucleus and transcribed. Newly synthesized RNA is returned to the cytoplasm and translated into proteins, which are transported to the cell membrane. This is followed by budding of virus through the cell membrane. The packaging mechanisms for the segmented genome are not well understood. A proteolytic cleavage of the hemagglutinin occurs at some point in the assembly and release of the virus, which is essential for successful reinfection and amplification of virus titer. In humans, this replicative cycle is confined to the respiratory epithelium. With primary infection, virus replication continues for 10–14 days. Implicit in successful replication in the respiratory tract is the assumption that key proteolytic enzymes exist at this site. The effective cleavage of hemagglutinin has been demonstrated by respiratory secretions, but the cellular origin of the enzyme remains undefined.

Influenza causes a lytic infection of the respiratory epithelium with loss of ciliary function, decreased mucus production, and desquamation of the epithelial layer. These changes permit secondary bacterial invasion either directly through the epithelium or, in the case of the middle ear space, through obstruction of the normal drainage through the eustachian tube. Influenza types A and B have been reported to cause myocarditis, and influenza type B can cause myositis. Reyes syndrome can result with the use of salicylates for influenza type B infection (Chapter 360).

The exact immune mechanisms involved in termination of primary infection and protection against reinfection are not well understood. The incubation period of influenza can be as short as 48–72 hr. The extremely short incubation period of influenza and its growth on the mucosal surface pose particular problems for invoking a protective immune response. Antigen presentation must be primarily at mucosal sites acting through the bronchial associated lymphoid tract. The major humoral response is directed against the hemagglutinin. High serum antibody levels generated by inactivated vaccine correlate with protection. Mucosally produced immunoglobulin (Ig) A antibodies are presumably directed at the same antigenic sites and are thought to be the most effective and immediate response that can be generated to protect against influenza. Unfortunately, measurable IgA antibodies against influenza persist for a relatively short period, and symptomatic reinfection with influenza can be seen at intervals of 3–4 yr. Although heterotypic immunity can be demonstrated in the mouse through cell-mediated immune mechanisms directed toward common internal proteins, heterotypic immunity has not been shown in humans.

CLINICAL MANIFESTATIONS. Influenza types A and B cause predominantly a respiratory illness. The onset of illness is abrupt and is marked by coryza, conjunctivitis, pharyngitis, and dry cough (Table 251–1). The predominant symptoms may localize anywhere in the respiratory tract, producing an isolated upper respiratory tract illness, croup, bronchiolitis, or pneumonia. More so than any of the other respiratory viruses, influenza is accompanied by systemic signs of high temperature, myalgia, malaise, and headache. Many of these symptoms may be mediated through cytokine production by the respiratory tract epithelium instead of reflecting systemic spread of the virus. The typical duration of the febrile illness is 2–4 days. Cough may persist for longer periods of time, and evidence of small airway dysfunction is often found weeks later. Other family members or close contacts often have a similar illness. Influenza is a less distinct illness in younger children and infants; manifestations may be localized to any region of the respiratory tract. The children may be highly febrile and toxic in appearance, prompting a full diagnostic work-up. In spite of the distinctive features of influenza, the illness is often indistinguishable from that caused by other respiratory viruses such as respiratory syncytial virus, parainfluenza viruses, and adenoviruses.

DIAGNOSIS. The diagnosis of influenza depends on epidemiologic and clinical considerations. In the context of an epidemic, the clinical diagnosis of influenza in a young child with fever, malaise, and respiratory symptoms can be made with some certainty. The laboratory confirmation of influenza can be made in three ways. If seen early in the illness, virus can be isolated from the nasopharynx by inoculation of the specimen into embryonated eggs or a limited number of cell lines that support the growth of influenza. The presence of influenza in the culture is confirmed by hemadsorption, which depends on the capacity of the hemagglutinin to bind red cells. Rapid diagnostic tests for influenza A are available in some centers that use antigen capture in an enzyme-linked immunosorbent assay. The diagnosis can be confirmed serologically with acute and convalescent sera drawn at about the time of illness and tested by hemagglutination inhibition.

Laboratory Findings. The clinical laboratory abnormalities associated with influenza are nonspecific. A relative leukopenia is

TABLE 251–1 Relative Frequency of Symptoms and Signs During Classic Influenza in Older Children and Adolescents

Variable	Occurrence
Symptoms	
Chilly sensation	++++
Cough	+++
Headache	+++
Sore throat	+++
Prostration	++
Nasal stuffiness	++
Diarrhea	++
Dizziness	+
Eye irritation or pain	+
Vomiting	+
Myalgia	+
Signs	
Fever	++++
Pharyngitis	+++
Conjunctivitis (mild)	++
Rhinitis	++
Cervical lymphadenopathy	+
Pulmonary rales, wheezes, or rhonchi	+

++++ = *76–100%;* +++ = *51–75%;* ++ = *26–50%;* + = *1–25%.*

frequently seen. Chest radiographs show evidence of atelectasis or infiltrate in about 10% of children.

TREATMENT. Amantadine and rimantadine can be used in the prophylaxis and treatment of influenza type A outbreaks, in institutions, and in individual cases, including patients with underlying conditions that predispose them to severe or complicated influenza infection (Table 251–2). These antivirals are not effective against influenza B and are not approved for use in children younger than 1 yr. If given within the first 48 hr, they decrease the severity and duration of influenzal symptoms. Confusion and inability to concentrate or sleep are seen in some patients given amantadine. Drug resistance develops fairly quickly during a course of therapy, but it is not widespread among circulating viruses. Both influenza A and B viruses are susceptible to ribavirin in vitro, but ribavirin is not approved for treatment of influenza infections. Drugs under investigation are modeled to fit in the crystallographic structure of the neuraminidase pocket to inhibit neuraminidase activity.

Adequate fluid intake and rest are important components in the management of influenza. Acetaminophen or ibuprofen, but not salicylates because of the risk of Reye syndrome, should be used as antipyretics to control fever. The most difficult question for parents is the appropriate timing of consultation with a health care provider. Bacterial superinfections are common, and antibiotic therapy should be administered. Bacterial superinfections should be suspected with recrudescence of fever, prolonged fever, or deterioration in clinical status. With uncomplicated influenza, children should feel at their worst over the first 48 hr.

COMPLICATIONS. Otitis media and pneumonia are common complications of influenza in young children. Acute otitis media may be seen in up to 25% of cases of culture-documented influenza. Pneumonia accompanying influenza may be a primary viral process. An acute hemorrhagic pneumonia may be seen in the most severe cases, as may have been frequent with the highly virulent strain seen in 1918. The more common cause of pneumonia is probably secondary bacterial infection through the damaged epithelial layer. Unusual clinical manifestations of influenza include acute myositis seen with influenza type B, which follows the acute respiratory illness by 5 7 days and is marked by muscle weakness and pain, particularly in the thigh muscles, and myoglobinuria. Myocarditis also follows influenza, and toxic shock syndrome is associated with influenza type B and staphylococcal colonization. Influenza is particularly severe in children with underlying cardiopulmonary disease, including congenital and acquired valvular disease, cardiomyopathy, bronchopulmonary dysplasia, asthma, cystic fibrosis, and neuromuscular diseases affecting the accessory muscles of breathing. Virus is shed for longer periods of time in children receiving cancer chemotherapy and children with immunodeficiency.

PROGNOSIS. The prognosis for recovery is excellent, although full return to normal levels of activity and freedom from cough usually requires weeks rather than days.

PREVENTION. Influenza vaccine of targeted high-risk populations is the best means of prevention of severe disease from influenza. Chemoprophylaxis is a less desirable alternative, and is only effective against influenza A.

Vaccine. An inactivated influenza vaccine becomes available each summer incorporating changes in formulation that reflect the strains anticipated to circulate in the coming winter. The American Committee on Immunization Practices publishes guidelines for their use each year when the vaccines are formulated and released. Current guidelines include the administration of vaccine intramuscularly to children at least 6 mo of age in chronic care facilities; with chronic disorders of the pulmonary or cardiovascular system, including asthma; with chronic metabolic diseases (including diabetes mellitus), renal dysfunction, hemoglobinopathies, or immunosuppression (including immunosuppression caused by medications); and receiving long-term aspirin therapy who may be at risk for Reye's syndrome after influenza. Vaccination is also recommended for women who will be in the second or third trimester (≥14 wk gestation) of pregnancy during the influenza season (December–March). In addition, vaccine is recommended for individuals who may transmit influenza to persons at high risk, including health care workers and household members.

Because of the decreased potential for causing febrile reactions, only the split-virus vaccine is recommended for children younger than 12 yr. Two doses of vaccine (0.25 mL for 6–36 mo of age; 0.5 mL for 3–8 yr of age) at least 1 mo apart are recommended for primary immunization of children younger than 9 yr. Live, attenuated vaccines that are administered intranasally are in clinical trials and have been demonstrated to have an efficacy comparable to that of inactivated vaccine in adults. Trials in children have shown efficacy of 90%. These vaccines are likely to be licensed soon. Their ease of administration could serve to increase influenza vaccination among children.

Chemoprophylaxis. Amantadine and rimantadine are licensed for prophylaxis of influenza A infections (see Table 251–2). They are recommended for prophylaxis for vaccinated and

TABLE 251–2 Amantadine and Rimantadine Treatment and Prophylaxis of Influenza A

Antiviral Agent	Age (yr) 1–9	10–13	14–64	≥ 65
Amantadine*				
Treatment	5 mg/kg/day (maximum daily dose, 150 mg) orally in 2 divided doses	100 mg orally twice daily‡	100 mg orally twice daily	≤ 100 mg/day
Prophylaxis†	5 mg/kg/day (maximum daily dose, 150 mg) orally in 2 divided doses	100 mg orally twice daily‡		≤ 100 mg/day
Rimantadine*				
Treatment	Not approved	Not approved	100 mg orally twice daily	100 or 200 mg/day§
Prophylaxis†	5 mg/kg/day (maximum daily dose, 150 mg) orally in 2 divided doses	100 mg orally twice daily‡	100 mg orally twice daily	100 or 200 mg/day§

Adapted from Centers for Disease Control and Prevention: Prevention and control of influenza: Recommendations of the Advisory Committee on Immunization Practices (ACIP). MMWR *48(RR-4):18, 1999.*

**The package insert should be consulted for dosage recommendations for administering amantadine to persons with impaired renal function (both drugs) or impaired hepatic function (rimantadine).*

†To be maximally effective as prophylaxis, amantadine or rimantadine must be taken each day for the duration of influenza activity in the community. However, to be most cost effective, prophylaxis should be taken only during the period of peak influenza activity in a community.

‡Children ≥10 yr of age or who weigh <40 kg should be administered amantadine or rimantadine at a dose of 5 mg/kg/day.

§Elderly nursing home residents should be given only 100 mg of rimantadine per day. A reduction in dose to 100 mg/day should be considered for all persons ≥ 65 yr if they experience side effects when taking 200 mg/day.

unvaccinated high-risk patients and their unvaccinated health care providers during influenza A outbreaks in closed settings, unvaccinated persons and health care providers during community influenza A outbreaks, and during the period of peak influenza A activity in immunodeficient persons and those for whom the influenza vaccine is contraindicated.

Belse RB, Mendelman PM, Treanor J, et al: The efficacy of live attenuated, cold-adapted, trivalent, intranasal influenza virus vaccine in children. N Engl J Med 338:1405, 1998.
Centers for Disease Control and Prevention: Control and prevention of influenza: Recommendations of the Advisory Committee on Immunization Practices (ACIP). MMWR Morb Mortal Wkly Rep 48(RR-4):1, 1999.
Glezen PW, Couch RB: Interpandemic influenza in the Houston area (1974-76). N Engl J Med 298:587, 1978.
Glezen WP, Taber LH, Frank AL, et al: Influenza virus infection in infants. Pediatr Infect Dis J 16:1065, 1997.
Hall CB, Dolin R, Gala CL, et al: Children with influenza A infection: Treatment with rimantadine. Pediatrics 80:275, 1987.
Subbarao K, Klimov A, Katz J, et al: Characterization of an avian influenza A (H5N1) virus isolated from a child with a fatal respiratory illness. Science 279:393, 1998.
Webster RG, Bean WJ, Gorman OT, et al: Evolution and ecology of influenza A viruses. Microbiol Rev 56:152, 1992.
Wright PF, Bryant JD, Karzon DT: Comparison of influenza B/Hong Kong virus infections among infants, children and young adults. J Infect Dis 141:430, 1980.
Wright PF, Ross KB, Thompson J, et al: Influenza A infections in young children. N Engl J Med 296:829, 1977.

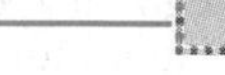

CHAPTER 252
Parainfluenza Viruses

Peter Wright

Viruses in the parainfluenza family are common causes of respiratory illness in infants and young children. They cause a spectrum of upper and lower respiratory tract illnesses, but are particularly associated with laryngotracheitis, bronchitis, and croup.

ETIOLOGY. The parainfluenza viruses are members of the Paramyxoviridae family. There are four viruses in the parainfluenza group that cause illness in humans, designated types 1–4. The viruses have a nonsegmented, single-stranded RNA genome with a lipid-containing envelope derived from budding through the cell membrane. The major antigenic moieties are envelope spike proteins that exhibit hemagglutinating (HN protein) and cell fusion (F protein) properties.

EPIDEMIOLOGY. Parainfluenza viruses are spread from the respiratory tract by aerosolized secretions or direct hand contact with secretions. By 3 yr of age, most children have experienced infection with types 1, 2, and 3. Type 3 is endemic and can cause disease in the infant younger than 6 mo. Serious illness is seen with parainfluenza type 3 in immunocompromised patients. Types 1 and 2 occur in a seasonal pattern in the summer and fall and alternate years in which their serotype is most prevalent. Parainfluenza type 4 is more difficult to grow in tissue culture; thus, its epidemiology is less well defined. However, it does not appear to be a major cause of illness.

PATHOGENESIS. Parainfluenza viruses replicate in the respiratory epithelium without evidence of systemic spread. The propensity to cause illness in the upper large airways is presumably related to enhanced replication in the larynx, trachea, and bronchi compared with other viruses. The destruction of cells in the upper airways can lead to secondary bacterial invasion and resultant bacterial tracheitis. Eustachian tube obstruction can lead to secondary bacterial invasion of the middle-ear space and acute otitis media.

Illness caused by parainfluenza occurs shortly after inoculation with the virus. The mechanisms by which viral injury occurs are not known. Some parainfluenza viruses induce cell-to-cell fusion. During the budding process, cell membrane integrity is lost, and viruses can induce cell death through the process of apoptosis. The severity of illness correlates with the amount of viral shedding. Immune destruction of virally infected cells may also occur, but appears to be less important with mucosal than systemic infection. The level of immunoglobulin A antibody is the best predictor of susceptibility to infection. Reinfection is seen particularly with parainfluenza type 3 as mucosal immunity wanes. The inability of children with serious T-cell defects to clear parainfluenza type 3 suggests a cell-mediated component of immunity.

CLINICAL MANIFESTATIONS. Most parainfluenza virus infections are confined to the upper respiratory tract. Selected signs, symptoms, and clinical diagnoses, based on cultures from young children with respiratory illness are shown in Table 252–1. This relatively mild-appearing illness is belied by a spectrum of rarer but more serious illnesses that result in hospitalization. The parainfluenza viruses account for 50% of hospitalizations for croup and 15% of cases of bronchiolitis and pneumonia. Parainfluenza type 1 causes more cases of croup, whereas parainfluenza type 3 causes a broad spectrum of lower respiratory tract diseases.

Parainfluenza virus infections are not associated with fever. Aside from low-grade fever, systemic complaints are rare. The illness usually lasts 4–5 days; however, virus may be recovered in low titers for 2–3 wk. Rarely, parainfluenza viruses have been implicated in parotitis.

DIAGNOSIS. The diagnosis of parainfluenza virus infection in children is usually based only on clinical and epidemiologic criteria. The virus should be specifically sought in persistent pneumonias in immunosuppressed children. The radiographic

TABLE 252–1 Diagnoses and Signs and Symptoms of Children Younger than 5 Yr of Age with Parainfluenza Infections

Diagnoses	Type 1 (n = 77)	Type 2 (n = 33)	Type 3 (n = 157)	Other (n = 19)
Upper Respiratory	90%	94%	89%	84%
Common cold	31%	42%	32%	42%
Pharyngitis	21%	18%	10%	11%*
Acute otitis media	38%	30%	52%	32%†
Lower Respiratory	17%	15%	15%	21%
Croup (laryngotracheobronchitis)	16%	6%	5%	21%‡
Bronchiolitis	1%	9%	6%	0%
Signs and Symptoms				
Coryza	74%	75%	83%	83%
Conjunctivitis	36%	36%	36%	44%
Cough	73%	67%	81%	77%
Hoarseness	28%	18%	11%	39%§
Rales or rhonchi	6%	15%	15%	11%
Wheezing	9%	12%	4%	5%
Temperature > 38°C	33%	16%	38%	6%‖
Temperature > 39°C	8%	6%	10%	0%
Irritability	47%	30%	54%	72%¶
Anorexia	36%	36%	36%	44%
Vomiting	15%	15%	24%	22%
Diarrhea	21%	15%	14%	22%

From Reed G, Jewett PH, Thompson J, et al: Epidemiology and clinical impact of parainfluenza virus infections in otherwise healthy infants and young children < 5 years old. J Infect Dis 175:808, 1997. Used with permission.

Note that p values are for Fisher's exact test for the null hypothesis that all types are alike.

* $p = .09$
† $p = .03$
‡ $p = .01$
§ $p = .001$
‖ $p = .004$
¶ $p = .02$

"steeple sign" of progressive narrowing of the subglottic region is characteristic of parainfluenza virus respiratory tract infections.

Laboratory Findings. There are no distinctive laboratory findings. The laboratory diagnosis of parainfluenza virus infection can be accomplished by inoculation of nasal secretions into tissue culture, with presumptive diagnosis based on finding a hemadsorbing agent and final serotypic diagnosis based on hemadsorption inhibition. Direct immunofluorescent staining is available in some centers for rapid identification of virus antigen in oropharyngeal sections.

TREATMENT. The possibility of rapid respiratory compromise during severe croup should influence the level of care given (Chapter 385). Careful attention to symptomatic care is important. Parents should be provided a description of the parameters of increasing respiratory distress that should lead to reassessment by a health care provider. Humidification and exposure to cold air are both classically associated with a decrease in mucosal edema and liquefaction of secretions that may help to relieve obstruction; however, their value has never been proved in a controlled trial. Aerosolized racemic epinephrine may temporarily improve aeration, but has the possibility of rebound. Aerosolized or systemic corticosteroids are helpful in the management of croup in the emergency room setting and after hospitalization. The indications for antibiotics are limited to well-documented secondary bacterial infections of the middle ears or lower respiratory tract.

Ribavirin has some antiviral activity against parainfluenza virus, and should be considered in the immunocompromised child with persistent parainfluenza viral pneumonia.

COMPLICATIONS. In children with fever or more severe respiratory compromise, the possibility of a bacterial tracheitis with purulent infection below the epiglottis and vocal cords should be considered. The high frequency of otitis media complicating parainfluenza virus indicates that careful pneumatic otoscopy should be performed in all children with suspected parainfluenza virus infection.

PROGNOSIS. The prognosis for full recovery is excellent in the normal child. No long-term pulmonary residua of parainfluenza virus infection have been described.

PREVENTION. Work is progressing with both live and subunit parainfluenza type 3 vaccines. The live vaccines include a cold-adapted virus of human origin and a bovine parainfluenza virus, which is attenuated because of host range adaptation. The measure of protection afforded by vaccines will be difficult to assess because symptomatic reinfection is seen and the frequency of serious infection in the general population is low. Nonetheless, it is clear that prevention of acute respiratory illness that results from parainfluenza virus is a worthwhile goal.

Denny FW, Murphy TF, Clyde WA Jr, et al: An 11-year study in a pediatric practice. Pediatrics 71:871, 1983.

Hall CB, Geiman JM, Breese BB, et al: Parainfluenza infections in children: Correlation of shedding with clinical manifestations. J Pediatr 91:194, 1993.

Henrickson KJ, Kuhn SM, Savatski LL: Epidemiology and cost of infection with human parainfluenza virus types 1 and 2 in young children. Clin Infect Dis 18:770, 1994.

Knott AM, Long CE, Hall CB: Parainfluenza viral infections in pediatric outpatients: Seasonal patterns and clinical characteristics. Pediatr Infect Dis J 13:269, 1994.

Landau LI, Geelhoed GC: Aerosolized steroids for croup. N Engl J Med 33:322, 1994.

Reed G, Jewett PH, Thompson J, et al: Epidemiology and clinical impact of parainfluenza virus infections in otherwise healthy infants and young children < 5 years old. J Infect Dis 175:807, 1997.

Skolnik NS: Treatment of croup: A critical review. Am J Dis Child 143:1045, 1989.

Smith CB, Purcell RH, Bellanti JA, et al: Protective effect of antibody to parainfluenza type 1 virus. N Engl J Med 275:1145, 1966.

CHAPTER 253
Respiratory Syncytial Virus

Kenneth McIntosh

Respiratory syncytial virus (RSV) is the major cause of bronchiolitis (Chapter 391) and pneumonia in children younger than 1 yr. It is the most important respiratory tract pathogen of early childhood.

ETIOLOGY. RSV is a medium-sized, membrane-bound RNA virus that develops in the cytoplasm of infected cells and matures by budding from the plasma membrane. It belongs to the family Paramyxoviridae, along with parainfluenza, mumps, and measles viruses, but is the sole member of the genus *Pneumovirus*. Although different strains of RSV show some antigenic heterogeneity, this variation is primarily in one of the two surface glycoproteins, and it is not clear that this degree of difference is clinically or epidemiologically significant.

RSV grows in a number of types of tissue culture, in which it produces characteristic syncytial cytopathology. Specimens for culture should be delivered rapidly on wet ice to the laboratory because the virus is heat labile and very susceptible to destruction by freezing and thawing.

EPIDEMIOLOGY. The occurrence of annual outbreaks and the high incidence of infection during the first months of life are unique among human viruses. RSV is distributed worldwide and appears in yearly epidemics. In temperate climates, these epidemics occur each winter and last 4–5 mo. During the remainder of the year, infections are sporadic and uncommon. In the Northern Hemisphere, epidemics usually peak in January, February, or March, but peaks have been recognized as early as December and as late as June. At these times, hospital admissions for bronchiolitis and pneumonia of children younger than 1 yr increase and decrease in proportion to the number of RSV infections in the community. In the tropics, the epidemic pattern is less clear.

Placentally transmitted anti-RSV antibody, when present in high concentration, has some protective effect. This may account for low frequency of severe infections in the first 4–6 wk of life, except in infants born prematurely who receive less than a full complement of maternal immunoglobulin (Ig)G. Nevertheless, serum antibody is not fully protective, and the age at which an infant undergoes first infection depends also on the opportunities for exposure. It is estimated that in an urban setting about half of the susceptible infants undergo primary infection in each epidemic. Thus, infection is almost universal by the 2nd birthday. Reinfection occurs at a rate of 10–20% per epidemic throughout childhood; the frequency is lower in adults. In situations of high exposure such as daycare centers, attack rates are higher: nearly 100% for first infections and 60–80% for second and subsequent infections.

Estimates of the severity of primary infections have emerged from studies of outbreaks in nurseries and institutions. Under these circumstances asymptomatic infection is rare. Most infants experience coryza and pharyngitis, usually with fever and occasionally with otitis media. In 10–40% of patients, the lower respiratory tract is involved to a varying degree. Bronchitis, bronchopneumonia, and bronchiolitis all occur. Calculations based on hospital admissions in the United States and Britain yield a ratio of 1–3 infants hospitalized with bronchiolitis or pneumonia for every 100 primary infections with the virus.

Reinfection may occur as early as a few weeks after recovery, but usually takes place during subsequent annual outbreaks.

The severity of illness during reinfection is usually lower, and appears to be a function of both partial immunity and increased age. Nevertheless, instances of severe RSV bronchiolitis occurring twice in succession have been documented.

Bronchiolitis is the most common clinical diagnosis in infants hospitalized with RSV infections, although the syndrome is often indistinguishable from RSV pneumonia in infants, and, indeed, the two frequently coexist. All RSV diseases of the lower respiratory tract (excluding croup) have their highest incidence from 2–7 mo of age and decrease in frequency thereafter. The syndrome of bronchiolitis becomes uncommon after the 1st birthday; acute infective wheezing attacks after that age are often termed "wheezy bronchitis," "asthmatoid bronchitis," or simply asthma attacks. Viral pneumonia is a persistent problem throughout childhood, although RSV becomes less prominent as the etiologic agent after the 1st year. RSV is responsible for 45–75% of cases of bronchiolitis, 15–25% of childhood pneumonias, and 6–8% of cases of croup.

Bronchiolitis and pneumonia resulting from RSV are more common in boys than in girls by a ratio of about 1.5:1. Racial factors make little difference. Lower respiratory tract involvement occurs more often and earlier in life in lower socioeconomic groups and in crowded living conditions.

The incubation period from exposure to 1st symptoms is about 4 days. The virus is excreted for variable periods, probably depending on severity of illness and immunologic status. Most infants with lower respiratory tract illness shed virus for 5–12 days after hospital admission. Excretion for 3 wk and longer has been documented. Spread of infection occurs when large, infected droplets, either airborne or conveyed on hands, are inoculated in the nose or conjunctiva of a susceptible subject. RSV is probably introduced into most families by schoolchildren undergoing reinfection. Typically, in the space of a few days, older siblings and one or both parents acquire colds, but the infant becomes more severly ill with fever, otitis media, or lower respiratory tract disease.

Nosocomial infection during RSV epidemics is an important concern. Virus is usually spread from child to child on the hands of caregivers. Adults undergoing reinfection have also been implicated in spread of the virus.

PATHOGENESIS. Bronchiolitis is characterized by virus-induced necrosis of the bronchiolar epithelium, hypersecretion of mucus, and round cell infiltration and edema of the surrounding submucosa. These changes result in formation of mucous plugs obstructing bronchioles with consequent hyperinflation or collapse of the distal lung tissue. In interstitial pneumonia, infiltration is more generalized, and epithelial necrosis may extend to both the bronchi and the alveoli. Infants are particularly apt to experience small airway obstruction because of the small size of the normal bronchioles.

Several facts suggest immunologic injury as a factor in the pathogenesis of bronchiolitis caused by RSV: (1) Anti-RSV IgE antibody is found in the secretions of convalescent infants with bronchiolitis; (2) recent studies in infants and in various animal models of RSV infection indicate that a large number of soluble factors (interleukins, leukotrienes, and chemokines) with the potential to stimulate inflammation and tissue damage are liberated during RSV infection; (3) children who received a highly antigenic, inactivated, parenterally administered RSV vaccine experienced, on subsequent exposure to wild-type RSV, more severe and more frequent bronchiolitis than did their age-matched controls; and (4) bronchiolitis merges into asthma in older infants, and RSV is a frequently recognized cause of acute asthma attacks in children 1–5 yr old.

It is not clear how often superimposed bacterial infection plays a pathogenic role in RSV lower respiratory tract disease. The present view is that RSV-induced bronchiolitis in infants is an exclusively viral disease, and that bacteria are of little importance even when the disease is accompanied by atelectasis or interstitial pneumonia.

CLINICAL MANIFESTATIONS. The first signs of infection of the infant with RSV are rhinorrhea and pharyngitis. Cough may appear simultaneously but more often after an interval of 1–3 days, at which time there may also be sneezing and a low-grade fever. Soon after the cough develops, the child begins to wheeze audibly. If the disease is mild, the symptoms may not progress beyond this stage. Auscultation often reveals diffuse rhonchi, fine rales or crackles, and wheezes. Clear rhinorrhea usually persists throughout the illness, with intermittent fever. Roentgenograms of the chest at this stage are frequently normal.

If the illness progresses, cough and wheezing increase and air hunger ensues with increased respiratory rate, intercostal and subcostal retractions, hyperexpansion of the chest, restlessness, and peripheral cyanosis. Signs of severe, life-threatening illness are central cyanosis, tachypnea of more than 70 breaths/min, listlessness, and apneic spells. At this stage, the chest may be greatly hyperexpanded and almost silent to auscultation because of poor air exchange.

Chest roentgenograms of infants hospitalized with RSV bronchiolitis are normal in about 10% of cases; air trapping or hyperexpansion of the chest is evident in about 50%. Peribronchial thickening or interstitial pneumonia is seen in 50–80%. Segmental consolidation occurs in 10–25%. Pleural effusion is rarely, if ever, seen.

In some infants, the course of the illness may be more like that of pneumonia with the prodromal rhinorrhea and cough followed by dyspnea, poor feeding, and listlessness, with a minimum of wheezing and hyperexpansion. Although the clinical diagnosis is pneumonia, wheezing is often present intermittently and the chest roentgenogram may show air trapping.

Fever is an inconstant sign in RSV infection. Rash and conjunctivitis each occur in a few cases. In young infants, particularly those who were born prematurely, periodic breathing and apneic spells have been distressingly frequent signs, even with relatively mild bronchiolitis. It is likely that a small portion of deaths included in the category of sudden infant death syndrome are due to RSV infection.

RSV infections in profoundly immunocompromised hosts may be severe at any age. The mortality associated with RSV pneumonia in the first few weeks after bone marrow or solid organ transplantation is 50% or higher. RSV infection does not seem to be severe in HIV-infected patients.

DIAGNOSIS. Bronchiolitis is a clinical diagnosis. The involvement of RSV in any particular child's disease can be suspected with varying degrees of certainty from the season of the year and the presence of a typical outbreak at the time. Other epidemiologic features that may be helpful are the presence of colds in older household contacts and the age of the child, because, aside from RSV, the only respiratory virus that attacks infants frequently during the first few months of life is parainfluenza virus type 3.

Routine laboratory tests offer little helpful information in most cases of bronchiolitis or pneumonia caused by RSV. The white cell count is normal or elevated, and the differential count may be normal with either a neutrophilic or mononuclear predominance. Bacterial cultures of the throat grow only normal flora. Hypoxemia is frequent, and tends to be more marked than anticipated on the basis of the clinical findings. When it is severe, it is frequently accompanied by hypercapnia and acidosis.

The diagnostic dilemma of greatest import is the question of possible bacterial or chlamydial involvement. When bronchiolitis is clinically mild or when infiltrates are absent by roentgenogram, there is little likelihood of a bacterial component. In infants 1–4 mo of age, interstitial pneumonitis may be caused by *Chlamydia trachomatis* (Chapter 223.3). In *C. tracho-*

matis pneumonia, there may be a history of conjunctivitis, and the illness tends to be of subacute onset. Coughing and rales are prominent; wheezing is not. There may also be eosinophilia. Fever is usually absent.

Consolidation without other signs or with pleural effusion is considered of bacterial origin until proved otherwise. Other signs suggesting bacterial pneumonia are elevation of the neutrophil count, depression of the white cell count in the presence of severe disease, ileus or other abdominal signs, high temperature, and circulatory collapse. In such instances, there is rarely any doubt about the need for antibiotics.

Definitive diagnosis of RSV infection is based on the detection of virus or viral antigens in respiratory secretions. An aspirate of mucus or a nasopharyngeal wash from the child's posterior nasal cavity is the optimal specimen. Nasopharyngeal or throat swabs are less preferred but acceptable. A tracheal aspirate is unnecessary. The specimen should be placed on ice, taken directly to the laboratory, and processed for antigen detection or inoculated onto susceptible cell monolayers.

TREATMENT. In uncomplicated cases of bronchiolitis, treatment is symptomatic. Humidified oxygen is usually indicated for hospitalized infants because most are hypoxic. Many infants are slightly to moderately dehydrated; therefore, fluids should be carefully administered in amounts somewhat greater than maintenance. Often intravenous or tube feeding is helpful when sucking is difficult due to tachypnea. Infants may breathe more easily when propped up at an angle of 10–30 degrees.

A trial of a bronchodilator administered either parenterally or by aerosol may relieve wheezing and improve clinical status, and should be repeated if initial benefit is shown. Studies have indicated that epinephrine is more often useful in bronchiolitis than albuterol. Corticosteroids are not indicated except in older children with an established diagnosis of asthma.

In most instances antibiotics are not useful, and their indiscriminate use in presumed viral bronchiolitis and pneumonia should be discouraged. Interstitial pneumonia in infants 1–4 mo old may be chlamydial; therefore, erythromycin (40 mg/kg/24 hr) or clarithromycin (7.5 mg/kg every 12 hr) may be beneficial. When infants with interstitial pneumonia are older, or when consolidation is found, parenteral antibiotics may be indicated. In the critically ill child, antibiotics may also be indicated.

The antiviral drug ribavirin, delivered by small-particle aerosol and breathed, along with the required concentration of oxygen, for 20 of 24 hr/day for 3–5 days, has a modest beneficial effect on the course of RSV pneumonia. Shortened hospital stay and reduced mortality have not been demonstrated, and long-term effects are still unknown. Its use is, therefore, indicated only in very sick infants or in high-risk infants, such as those with underlying cyanotic congenital heart disease, significant bronchopulmonary dysplasia, or severe immunodeficiency. If indicated, it should be administered early in the course of the infection.

PROGNOSIS. The mortality of hospitalized infants with RSV infection of the lower respiratory tract is about 2%. Almost all deaths occur in young, premature infants or those with underlying disease of the neuromuscular, pulmonary, cardiovascular, or immunologic system.

Many children with asthma have a history of bronchiolitis in infancy. There is recurrent wheezing in 33–50% of children with typical RSV bronchiolitis in infancy. The likelihood of recurrence is increased in the presence of an allergic diathesis (eczema, hay fever, or a family history of asthma). In bronchiolitis, in patients older than 1 yr there is an increasing probability that, although the episode may be virus induced, this is the first of multiple wheezing attacks that will later be called asthma.

PREVENTION. Within the hospital, the most important preventive measures are aimed at blocking nosocomial spread. During RSV season, high-risk infants should be separated from infants with respiratory symptoms. Separate gowns and gloves and careful handwashing should be used for the care of all infants with suspected or established RSV infection.

Passive Immunoprophylaxis. Administration of either palivizumab (15 mg/kg intramuscularly), a monoclonal antibody against RSV, or high-titered RSV intravenous immunoglobulin (RSV-IVIG; 750 mg/kg) is recommended for protecting high-risk children against serious complications from RSV disease. Immunoprophylaxis reduces the frequency and total days of hospitalization for RSV infections in high-risk infants. These agents are administered monthly from the beginning (October–December) to the end (March–May) of the RSV season. Palivizumab is preferred for most children because of ease of intramuscular administration and lack of interference with live virus vaccinations (measles-mumps-rubella and varicella). RSV-IVIG provides some protection against other respiratory pathogens and may be substituted for IVIG during the RSV season for children with immunodeficiency receiving monthly IVIG.

Candidates for immunoprophylaxis include children with lung disease and children who were born very prematurely. Children younger than 2 yr with bronchopulmonary dysplasia requiring supplemental oxygen therapy currently or within the 6 mo before the RSV season should receive prophylaxis for the first two RSV seasons if they have severe lung disease and only the first RSV season for less severe lung disease. Infants without bronchopulmonary dysplasia should receive prophylaxis up to 12 mo of age if they were born at 28 wk of gestation or earlier and up to 6 mo of age if they were born at 29–32 wk of gestation. One dose of immunoprophylaxis may be considered for premature infants to be discharged from the hospital during the RSV season. RSV-IVIG is contraindicated and palivizumab is not recommended for children with cyanotic congenital heart disease. Adverse events with palivizumab are uncommon.

Vaccine. There is not currently a vaccine against RSV. Vaccine development for RSV has proceeded cautiously since the experience in the 1960s with an alum-precipitated formalin-inactivated vaccine. This vaccine was excellent for inducing serum antibodies, but vaccinees had augmented disease after natural infection. Live, attenuated vaccines have produced unacceptable symptoms or reverted to wild-type virus. Current candidate vaccines are either purified subunit vaccines against the fusion (F) protein or attenuated, cold-adapted live vaccines.

American Academy of Pediatrics, Committee on Infectious Diseases: Reassessment of the indications for ribavirin therapy in respiratory syncytial virus infections. Pediatrics 97:137, 1996.

American Academy of Pediatrics, Committee on Infectious Diseases and Committee on Fetus and Newborn: Prevention of respiratory syncytial virus infections: Indications for the use of palivizumab and update on the use of RSV-IGIV. Pediatrics 102:1211, 1998.

Glezen WP, Paredes A, Allison JE, et al: Risk of respiratory syncytial virus infection for infants from low-income families in relationship to age, sex, ethnic group and maternal antibody level. J Pediatr 98:708, 1981.

Hall CB, Douglas RG Jr, Geiman JM, et al: Nosocomial respiratory syncytial virus infections. N Engl J Med 293:1343, 1975.

Henderson FW, Collier AM, Clyde WA Jr, et al: Respiratory-syncytial-virus infections, reinfections and immunity: A prospective, longitudinal study in young children. N Engl J Med 300:530, 1979.

Hertz MI, Englund JA, Snover D, et al: Respiratory syncytial virus-induced acute lung injury in adult patients with bone marrow transplants. Medicine 68:269, 1989.

Holberg CJ, Wright AL, Martinez FD, et al: Risk factors for respiratory syncytial virus-associated lower respiratory illnesses in the first year of life. Am J Epidemiol 133:1135, 1991.

McIntosh K: Bronchiolitis and asthma: Possible common pathogenetic pathways. J Allergy Clin Immunol 57:595, 1976.

PREVENT Study Group: Reduction of respiratory syncytial virus hospitalization among premature infants and infants with bronchopulmonary dysplasia using respiratory virus immune globulin prophylaxis. Pediatrics 99:93, 1997.

Simpson W, Hacking PM, Court SDM, et al: Radiological findings in respiratory syncytial virus infection in children: II. The correlation of radiological categories with clinical and virological findings. Pediatr Radiol 2:155, 1974.

Chapter 254
Adenoviruses

Kenneth McIntosh

Adenoviruses cause 5–8% of acute respiratory disease in infants, plus a wide array of other syndromes, including pharyngoconjunctival fever, follicular conjunctivitis, epidemic keratoconjunctivitis, myocarditis, hemorrhagic cystitis, acute diarrhea, intussusception, and encephalomyelitis. Only a third of the 49 serotypes have been associated with disease. Fatal disease is rare, but is associated with infection by certain serotypes (particularly type 7) and infection in severely immunocompromised hosts.

ETIOLOGY. The Adenoviridae are DNA viruses of intermediate size, which are classified into subgenera A to F. The virion has an icosahedral coat (capsid) made up of 252 subunits (capsomers) of which 240 are "hexons" and 12 are "pentons." The hexons have a cross reacting antigen common to all mammalian adenoviruses. The penton confers type specificity, and antibody to it is protective. It is cytotoxic in tissue culture, and toxic properties have been ascribed to it in vivo as well. Adenoviruses can also be classified by their characteristic DNA "fingerprints" on gels after being digested with restriction endonucleases, and this classification generally conforms to their antigenic types.

All adenovirus types, except types 40 and 41, grow in primary human embryonic kidney cells, and most grow in HEp-2 or HeLa cells, producing a typical destructive cytopathic effect. Types 40 and 41 (and other serotypes as well) grow in 293 cells, a line of human embryonic kidney cells into which certain "early" adenovirus genes have been introduced.

Many adenovirus types, but particularly the common childhood types (1, 2, and 5), are shed for prolonged periods from both the respiratory and gastrointestinal tracts. These types also establish low-level and chronic infection of the tonsils and adenoids.

EPIDEMIOLOGY. Adenoviral infections are distributed worldwide. They occur year-round but are most prevalent in spring or early summer and again in midwinter in temperate climates. Certain types tend to occur in epidemics, notably types 4 and 7 in outbreaks of febrile respiratory disease, types 3, 7, and 21 in severe pneumonia; type 3 in pharyngoconjunctival fever; type 11 in hemorrhagic cystitis; and types 8, 19, and 37 in epidemic keratoconjunctivitis. For unexplained reasons, adenovirus types 3 and 7 cause severe epidemics of pneumonia in the children of northern China and Korea, with mortality rates of 5–15%.

More than 60% of school-age children have antibodies to the common respiratory types. Almost all adults have serum antibody to types 1–7. Infections with types 1 and 2 tend to occur during the 2nd yr of life, and types 3 and 5 occur a little later. Spread occurs by the respiratory and fecal-oral routes, although it is not clear whether spread is by large- or small-particle aerosol. Hospital outbreaks of respiratory disease and keratoconjunctivitis have been described.

PATHOGENESIS. Adenoviruses are among the few "respiratory" viruses that grow well in the epithelium of the small intestine. Although mucosal surfaces are the primary target early in infection and typically the site of the most common pathology, viremia probably occurs frequently, with accompanying fever.

Adenoviral pneumonia produces characteristic microscopic changes, with dense lymphocytic infiltrates, destruction of the bronchial and bronchiolar epithelium, focal necrosis of mucous glands, hyaline membrane formation, and several types of nuclear inclusion bodies.

CLINICAL MANIFESTATIONS. Adenoviruses cause a wide array of clinical syndromes.

Acute Respiratory Disease. This is the most common manifestation of adenovirus infection in children and adults. Acute adenovirus respiratory tract infections in infants and children are not clinically distinctive and are usually caused by types 1, 2, 3, 5, or 6. Primary infections in infants are frequently associated with fever and respiratory symptoms and are complicated by otitis media in more than half of the patients. Adenovirus respiratory infections are associated with a significant incidence of diarrhea.

Pharyngitis due to adenovirus typically has symptoms of coryza, sore throat, and fever. Adenoviruses can be identified in 15–20% of children with isolated pharyngitis, mostly in preschoolers and infants.

Pneumonia is uncommon, but 7–9% of hospitalized children with acute pneumonia have adenovirus infection. Any of the "respiratory" types can cause pneumonia, but severe infections are most likely due to type 3, 7, or 21. Such infections have a mortality as high as 10%, and survivors may have residual airway damage, manifested by bronchiectasis, bronchiolitis obliterans, or, rarely, pulmonary fibrosis. Neonatal adenovirus pneumonia occurs rarely, but may be severe or fatal.

A *pertussis-like syndrome* has been described in association with adenovirus infections. In these cases, adenoviruses frequently accompany *Bordetella pertussis* as coinfecting agents, but occasionally they may also be causative on their own.

Pharyngoconjunctival fever is a clinically distinct syndrome that occurs particularly in association with type 3 adenovirus. Features include a high temperature that lasts 4–5 days, pharyngitis, conjunctivitis, preauricular and cervical lymphadenopathy, and rhinitis. Nonpurulent conjunctivitis occurs in 75% of patients and is manifested by inflammation of both the bulbar and palpebral conjunctivae of one or both eyes; it often persists after the fever and other symptoms have resolved. Headache, malaise, and weakness are common, and there is considerable lethargy after the acute stage.

Conjunctivitis and Keratoconjunctivitis. Adenovirus is one of the most common causes of follicular conjunctivitis and keratoconjunctivitis. The former is a relatively mild illness. The latter, which may occur, in epidemics, is associated with infection by adenovirus types 8, 19, and 37. Keratitis begins as the conjunctivitis wanes, and may cause corneal opacities that last several years.

Myocarditis. In several series of acute myocarditis or idiopathic cardiomyopathy, investigated by the application of polymerase chain reaction (PCR) in the search for microbial agents, adenovirus has been found as commonly as, or more commonly than, nonpolio enteroviruses. It is widely assumed that adenovirus has an important etiologic role in this disease. It has also been associated with heart transplant rejection and with some cases of endocardial fibroelastosis.

Gastrointestinal Infections. Adenoviruses can be found in the stools of 5–9% of children with acute diarrhea. About one half of these are the "enteric" types, 40 or 41. It is also clear that enteric infection with any adenovirus serotype is often asymptomatic, so the causative role in these episodes is frequently uncertain.

The pathogenesis of intussusception is thought by many to include enlarged lymph nodes as an initiating factor. Adenoviruses have been recovered from mesenteric lymph nodes or appendices at surgery and also from surface cultures in a higher percentage of children with intussusception than of controls. Adenoviruses have also been found in the appendices of children with appendicitis.

Hemorrhagic Cystitis. This syndrome has a sudden onset of bacteriologically sterile hematuria, dysuria, frequency, and urgency lasting 1–2 wk. Infection with adenovirus types 11 and 21 has been found in some affected children and young adults.

Reye's Syndrome and Reye's-like Syndromes. Typical Reye's syndrome has followed confirmed adenovirus infection of several serotypes, particularly in very young children. In addition, several cases of a *Reye's-like syndrome* have been reported, all of which are caused by infection with adenovirus type 7. The latter disease, which is frequently fatal, is characterized by severe bronchopneumonia, hepatitis, seizures, and disseminated intravascular coagulation. Circulating adenovirus penton antigen has been found in several patients and has been implicated in the pathogenesis.

Infections in Immunocompromised Hosts. Adenoviruses are important pathogens in immunocompromised hosts with either B- or T-cell deficiencies. In B-cell–deficient (hypogammaglobulinemic) patients, a chronic meningoencephalitis similar to that caused by enteroviruses has been described. In T-cell–deficient patients, regardless of whether this deficiency is congenital, acquired, or iatrogenic, fulminant hepatitis and pneumonia, frequently with a fatal outcome, have been described. There is also a close association between adenovirus infection and both hemorrhagic cystitis and tubulointerstitial nephritis in immunosuppressed children.

DIAGNOSIS. The laboratory diagnosis of adenovirus infection in children may be made by suggestive pathologic changes in biopsy material, detection of virus by culture or PCR, demonstration of a rise in antibody titers, or a combination of virus detection and serologic testing. PCR has proven a very useful method in the detection of adenovirus in biopsy tissues. If virus is found in a "privileged" site, such as blood, urine, or cerebrospinal fluid, or in a biopsy of the lung or liver, the implication of infection with disease and organ damage is strong. Likewise, detection of certain adenovirus types in respiratory secretions (type 7 or 21) probably indicates their etiologic involvement. The presence of untyped virus or the common childhood types (1, 2, and 5) in respiratory secretions or stool does not, however, indicate clinical adenovirus infection because these viruses may be excreted chronically and asymptomatically. In these instances, discovery of a coincident rise in antibody by complement fixation (group specific) or neutralization or hemagglutination inhibition (type specific) is helpful in assigning a specific adenovirus type to disease. Adenovirus infection may also be considered etiologic if a rise in antibody is found between sera drawn in the acute stage and in convalescence from a patient with an appropriate illness. Adenovirus infection often results in a high erythrocyte sedimentation rate and white blood cell count.

TREATMENT. There are at present no recognized antiviral agents that are effective in treating adenovirus infections. Ribavirin can inhibit viral growth of some strains in vitro, but evidence of its clinical efficacy is lacking.

PREVENTION. Vaccines that contain either killed or live virus have been developed to prevent type 4 and 7 infections in military recruits. These vaccines have not, however, been used in children.

Brandt CD, Kim HW, Jeffries BC, et al: Infections in 18,000 infants and children in a controlled study of respiratory tract disease: II. Adenovirus pathogenicity in relation to serologic type and illness syndrome. Am J Epidemiol 90:484, 1970.

Brandt CD, Kim HW, Rodriguez WJ, et al: Adenoviruses and pediatric gastroenteritis. J Infect Dis 151:437, 1985.

Kelsey DS: Adenovirus meningoencephalitis. Pediatrics 61:291, 1978.

Ladisch S, Lovejoy FH, Hierholzer JC, et al: Extrapulmonary manifestations of adenovirus type 7 pneumonia simulating Reye syndrome and the possible role of an adenovirus toxin. Pediatrics 95:348, 1979.

Martin AB, Webber S, Fricker FJ, et al: Acute myocarditis: Rapid diagnosis by PCR in children. Circulation 90:330, 1994.

Michaels MG, Green M, Wald ER, et al: Adenovirus infection in pediatric liver transplant recipients. J Infect Dis 165:170, 1992.

Nelson KE, Gavitt F, Batt MD, et al: The role of adenoviruses in the pertussis syndrome. J Pediatr 86:335, 1975.

Numazaki Y, Kumasaki T, Yano N, et al: Further study on acute hemorrhagic cystitis due to adenovirus type H. N Engl J Med 289:344, 1973.

Ruuskanen O, Meurman O, Sarkkinen H: Adenoviral diseases in children: A study of 105 hospital cases. Pediatrics 76:79, 1985.

Simil S, Ylikorkala O, Wasz-Hockert O: Type 7 adenovirus pneumonia. J Pediatr 79:605, 1971.

Van R, Wun CC, O'Ryan ML, et al: Outbreaks of human enteric adenovirus types 40 and 41 in Houston day care centers. J Pediatr 120:516, 1992.

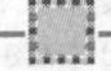

CHAPTER 255

Rhinoviruses

Kenneth McIntosh

Rhinoviruses are collectively the most common cause of the "common cold" in adults. They are also very common in young children, but because of the frequency of other viral respiratory tract infections in this age group, their relative importance is somewhat less than in adults. They are difficult to grow in tissue culture, however, and studies using polymerase chain reaction (PCR) indicate that their frequency and importance in respiratory illnesses are considerably greater than has been thought in the past.

ETIOLOGY. There are 101 serologically distinct rhinoviruses (numbered 1-100, and subtype 1A), members of the Picornaviridae family of small RNA viruses. They are best identified in clinical samples by PCR performed on nasal secretions from infected individuals. Tissue culture is approximately one third as sensitive as PCR. Routine serologic testing for development of antibody is not practical because of the multiplicity of serotypes.

Not all rhinovirus infections are associated with symptoms, even in infants and children. In longitudinal studies, 75% of pediatric rhinovirus infection (detected by culture) is associated with illness, usually rhinitis or pharyngitis. Rhinoviruses have also been associated with serious lower respiratory tract disease, particularly in very young infants and those with underlying illnesses. They are frequent precipitators of asthma in children and of chronic bronchitis in adults.

EPIDEMIOLOGY. Rhinoviruses are distributed worldwide with no predictable pattern of infection by serotype. Multiple types may be present in a community at one time.

In temperate climates the incidence of rhinovirus infection peaks in September and again in April or May, but infections occur year-round. The peak incidence in the tropics occurs during the rainy season.

Rhinoviruses are recovered in highest concentration in nasal secretions, and experimental infection is most easily accomplished by nasal or conjunctival instillation. Virus persists for several hours in secretions on hands or other surfaces. Transmission occurs when infected secretions carried on contaminated fingers are rubbed into the nasal or conjunctival mucosa. Evidence also implicates spread through prolonged contact with aerosols produced by talking, coughing, or sneezing.

PATHOGENESIS. Rhinoviruses, like other picornaviruses, infect cells only after interaction with specific cell receptors. For most rhinovirus types, this is ICAM-1, an intercellular adhesion molecule present on the epithelium covering the adenoids (lymphoepithelium) and on other epithelial cells of the nose after stimulation by various interleukins (interferon-γ, tumor necrosis factor, interleukin 1). Thus, for these types, infection probably begins in the nasopharynx and then, as interleukins are produced, spreads forward to the nasal mucosa. The peak nasal inflammatory response occurs when virus growth is at its greatest, 2–4 days after experimental infection, and is accompanied by the production of multiple proinflammatory mediators. Immune responses include specific nasal immunoglobulin (Ig) A and serum IgG antibody, which may contribute to modifying the illness and limiting viral shedding.

CLINICAL MANIFESTATIONS. The primary clinical response to rhinovirus infection, like that to most respiratory viral infections, is the *common cold* (see Chapter 381.1). There is an incubation period of 2–4 days; then sneezing, nasal obstruction and discharge, and sore throat ensue. Cough and hoarseness occur in 30–40% of cases. Fever is neither as frequent nor as high as in primary infections with respiratory syncytial virus, parainfluenza virus, influenza virus, or adenovirus. Headache and other systemic symptoms are not as common as with influenza virus. Symptoms are worse in the first 2–3 days of illness and last for 1 wk in a majority of patients; they persist for more than 14 days in 35% of young children.

DIAGNOSIS. Because other viral agents can produce the same manifestations, a clinical diagnosis is only presumptive but is usually adequate. Laboratory diagnosis is not practical under ordinary circumstances. Bacterial antigen testing or cultures should be performed to exclude streptococcal nasopharyngitis if this is suspected (Chapter 184).

TREATMENT. Relief of acute symptoms may be provided by acetaminophen or ibuprofen for antipyresis and mild analgesia and by saline or decongestant (in children >6 mo of age) nose drops used for a short time for nasal discharge and obstruction.

Several antiviral drugs have been developed with potent activity against rhinoviruses. Tests in volunteers have shown that, although these reduce the titer of virus in the nose, they do not lessen symptoms or decrease the duration of illness. It seems likely that successful treatment will have to target the host response as well as the virus.

COMPLICATIONS. As with any infection causing edema and inflammation in the nasopharynx, complications include otitis media and sinusitis. In one study rhinoviruses were the most common virus recovered from the middle-ear fluids of infants and children with otitis media. In very young infants bronchiolitis may occur. Rhinoviruses are the most common cause of acute exacerbations of asthma in school-age children.

PREVENTION. The best approach to reducing spread includes careful handwashing and avoidance of manual nose and eye manipulation.

Arola M, Ziegler T, Ruuskanen O, et al: Rhinovirus in acute otitis media. J Pediatr 113:693, 1988.

Dick EC, Jennings LC, Mink KA, et al: Aerosol transmission of rhinovirus colds. J Infect Dis 156:442, 1987.

Johnston SL, Pattemore PK, Sanderson G, et al: Community study of role of viral infections in exacerbations of asthma in 9-11 year old children. BMJ 310:1225, 1995.

Ketler A, Hall CE, Fox JP, et al: The Virus Watch Program: A continuing surveillance of viral infections in metropolitan New York families: VIII. Rhinovirus infections: Observations of virus excretion, intrafamilial spread and clinical response. Am J Epidemiol 90:244, 1969.

McMillan JA, Weiner LB, Higgins AM, et al: Rhinovirus infection associated with serious illness among pediatric patients. Pediatr Infect Dis J 12:321, 1993.

CHAPTER 256

Rotavirus and Other Agents of Viral Gastroenteritis

Dorsey M. Bass

Diarrhea is probably the leading cause of childhood mortality in the world, accounting for 5 million to 10 million deaths per year. In early childhood, the single most important cause of severe dehydrating diarrhea is rotavirus infection. Rotavirus and other gastroenteritis viruses not only are major causes of pediatric mortality but also lead to significant morbidity as a result of malnutrition.

ETIOLOGY. Rotavirus, astrovirus, adenovirus, and caliciviruses, such as the Norwalk agent, are the medically important pathogens of human viral gastroenteritis.

Rotaviruses cause disease in virtually all mammals and birds. The virus is a wheel-like, double-shelled icosahedron containing 11 segments of double-stranded RNA. The diameter of the particles by electron microscopy is approximately 80 nm. Rotaviruses are classified by group (A, B, C, D, E), subgroup (I or II), and serotype. Group A, which has no antigenic relationship to the other groups, includes the common human pathogens as well as a variety of animal viruses. Group B rotavirus is reported as a cause of severe disease in infants and adults in China but not elsewhere. Occasional human outbreaks of group C rotavirus are reported. The other groups are limited to animal strains. Rotavirus strains are species specific and do not cause disease in heterologous hosts. Subgrouping of rotaviruses is determined by the antigenic structure of the inner capsid protein, VP6. Serotyping of rotaviruses, as determined by classic cross-neutralization serology, depends on the outer capsid glycoprotein, VP7. This type of serotype is often referred to as the G type (for glycoprotein). Many investigators have also reported P types for rotavirus (the "P" refers to the structure of the other rotavirus outer capsid protein, VP4). Although both VP4 and VP7 can elicit neutralizing immunoglobulin (Ig) G antibodies, the role of these systemic antibodies compared with mucosal IgA antibodies in protective immunity remains unclear.

Astroviruses are the second most important agent of viral gastroenteritis in young children, with a high incidence in both the developing and the developed worlds. Astroviruses are positive-sense, single-stranded RNA viruses. They are small, approximately 30-nm diameter particles with a characteristic central five- or six-pointed star when viewed by electron microscopy. The capsid consists of three structural proteins. There are eight known human serotypes.

Enteric adenoviruses are another common cause of viral gastroenteritis in infants and children. Although many adenovirus serotypes exist and are found in stool, especially during and after typical upper respiratory tract infections (Chapter 254), only serotypes 40 and 41 cause gastroenteritis. These strains do not cause respiratory symptoms and are very difficult to grow in tissue culture. They are 80-nm diameter, icosahedral viruses with a relatively complex single-stranded DNA genome.

Caliciviruses are small 27- to 35-nm viruses that are the most common cause of gastroenteritis outbreaks in older children and adults. They are positive-sense, single-stranded RNA viruses with a single structural protein. Variant but closely related calici-like viruses have been named for locations of initial outbreaks: Norwalk, Snow Mountain, Montgomery County, Sapporo, and others. Caliciviruses also cause a rotavirus-like illness in young infants. Caliciviruses and astroviruses are sometimes referred to as small, round viruses on the basis of appearance on electron microscopy.

Several other viruses that may cause diarrheal disease in animals have been postulated but not yet well established as human gastroenteritis viruses. These include coronaviruses and pestiviruses. Picobirnaviruses, another group of small 30-nm, double-stranded RNA viruses, have been reported to be found in 10% of patients with HIV-associated diarrhea.

EPIDEMIOLOGY. Worldwide, rotavirus is estimated to cause more than 125 million cases of diarrhea annually in children younger than 5 yr. Eighteen million cases are considered at least moderately severe, with approximately 600,000 deaths per year. Rotavirus causes 3 million cases of diarrhea, 50,000 hospitalizations, and 20–40 deaths annually in the United States.

Rotavirus infection is most common in winter months in temperate climates. In the United States the annual winter peak spreads from west to east (Figure 256–1). Unlike other

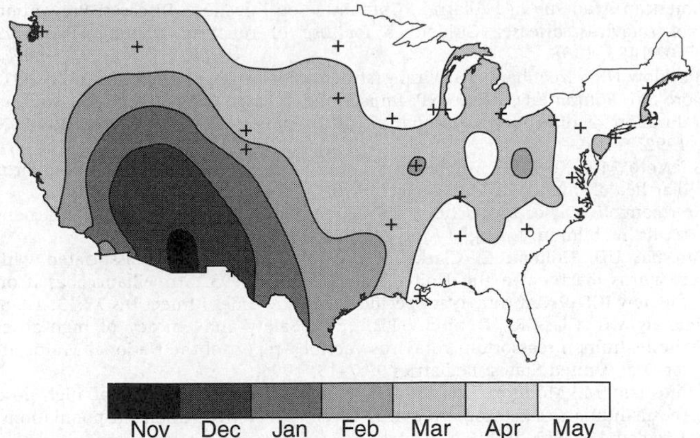

Figure 256–1 Peak rotavirus activity by month in the United States for July 1996 to June 1997. This pattern is typical of the annual rotavirus activity each year. (From Centers for Disease Control and Prevention: Laboratory-based surveillance for rotavirus—United States, July 1996–June 1997. MMWR 46:1093, 1997.)

winter viruses such as influenza, this wave of increased incidence is not due to a single prevalent strain or serotype. Typically, several serotypes predominate in a given community for one or two seasons while nearby locations may harbor unrelated strains. Disease tends to be most severe in patients between 3 and 24 mo of age, although 25% of the cases of severe disease occur after 2 yr of age, with serologic evidence of infection developing in virtually all children by age 4 or 5 yr. Infants younger than 3 mo are relatively protected by transplacental antibody and possibly breast-feeding. Infections in neonates and in adults in close contact with infected children are generally asymptomatic. Some rotavirus strains have stably colonized newborn nurseries for years, infecting virtually all newborns without any overt illness.

Rotavirus and the other gastroenteritis viruses spread efficiently via a fecal-oral route, and outbreaks are common in children's hospitals and child-care centers. The virus is shed in stool at very high concentration before and for days after the clinical illness. Very few infectious virions are needed to cause disease in a susceptible host.

The epidemiology of astroviruses is not as thoroughly studied as rotavirus, but it is a common cause of mild to moderate watery winter diarrhea in children and infants and an uncommon pathogen in adults. Hospital outbreaks are common. Enteric adenovirus gastroenteritis occurs year-round, mostly in children younger than 2 yr. Nosocomial outbreaks occur but are less common than with rotavirus and astrovirus. Calicivirus is best known for causing large, explosive outbreaks among older children and adults, particularly in settings such schools, cruise ships, and hospitals. Often a single food, such as shellfish or water used in food preparation, is identified as a source.

PATHOGENESIS. Viruses that cause human diarrhea selectively infect and destroy villus tip cells in the small intestine. Biopsies of the small intestines show variable degrees of villus blunting and round cell infiltrate in the lamina propria. Pathologic changes may not correlate with the severity of clinical symptoms and usually resolve before the clinical resolution of diarrhea. The gastric mucosa is not affected despite the commonly used term "gastroenteritis," although delayed gastric emptying has been documented during Norwalk virus infection.

In the small intestine, the upper villus enterocytes are differentiated cells, which have both digestive functions, such as hydrolysis of disaccharides, and absorptive functions, such as the transport of water and electrolytes via glucose and amino acid co-transporters. The crypt enterocytes are undifferentiated cells, which lack the brush border hydrolytic enzymes and are net secretors of water and electrolytes. Selective viral infection of intestinal villus tip cells thus leads to (1) an imbalance in the ratio of intestinal fluid absorption to secretion, and (2) malabsorption of complex carbohydrates, particularly lactose. Most evidence supports the first mechanism as the more important factor in the genesis of viral diarrhea.

In the normal host, extraintestinal infection is quite rare, although immunocompromised patients may experience hepatic and renal involvement. The increased vulnerability of infants (compared with older children and adults) to severe morbidity and mortality from gastroenteritis viruses may relate to a number of factors, including decreased intestinal reserve function, lack of specific immunity, and decreased nonspecific host defense mechanisms such as gastric acid and mucus. Viral enteritis greatly enhances intestinal permeability to luminal macromolecules and has been postulated to increase the risk of food allergies.

CLINICAL MANIFESTATIONS (also see Chapter 176). Rotavirus infection typically begins after an incubation period of less than 48 hr, with mild to moderate fever and vomiting followed by the onset of frequent, watery stools. Vomiting and fever typically abate during the second day of illness, but diarrhea often continues for 5–7 days. The stool is without gross blood or white cells. Dehydration may develop and progress rapidly, particularly in infants. Malnourished children and children with underlying intestinal disease such as short-bowel syndrome are particularly likely to acquire severe rotavirus diarrhea. Rarely, immunodeficient children will experience severe and prolonged illness. Although most newborns infected with rotavirus are asymptomatic, some outbreaks of necrotizing enterocolitis have been associated with the appearance of a new rotavirus strain in the affected nurseries.

The clinical course of astrovirus appears to be similar to that of rotavirus, with the notable exception that the disease tends to be milder, with less significant dehydration. Adenovirus enteritis tends to cause diarrhea of longer duration, often 10–14 days. The Norwalk virus has a short (12 hr) incubation period. Vomiting and nausea tend to predominate in illness associated with the Norwalk virus, and the duration is brief, usually 1–3 days of symptoms. The clinical and epidemiologic picture of Norwalk virus often closely resembles so-called food poisoning from preformed toxins such as *Staphylococcus aureus* and *Bacillus cereus*.

DIAGNOSIS. In most cases, a satisfactory diagnosis can be made on the basis of the clinical and epidemiologic features. Enzyme immunoassays, which offer approximately 90% specificity and sensitivity, are available for detection of group A rotavirus and enteric adenovirus in stool samples. More obscure cases can be studied by electron microscopy of stools, RNA electrophoresis, nucleic acid hybridization, and polymerase chain reaction assays. The diagnosis of viral gastroenteritis should always be questioned in patients with persistent high temperature, blood or white cells in the stool, or persistent severe or bilious vomiting (especially in the absence of diarrhea).

Laboratory Findings. Isotonic dehydration with acidosis is the most common finding in children with severe viral enteritis. The stools are free of blood and leukocytes. Although the white blood cell count may be moderately elevated secondary to stress, the marked left shift seen with invasive bacterial enteritis is absent.

Differential Diagnosis. The differential diagnosis includes other infectious causes of enteritis such as bacteria and protozoa. Occasionally, surgical conditions such as appendicitis, bowel obstruction, and intussusception may initially mimic viral gastroenteritis.

TREATMENT. Avoiding and treating dehydration are the main goals in treatment of viral enteritis. A secondary goal is maintenance of the nutritional status of the patient.

There is no role for antiviral drug treatment of viral gastroenteritis. Controlled studies have shown no benefit from antiemetics or antidiarrheal drugs, and there is a significant risk of serious side effects. Antibiotics are similarly of no benefit. Immunoglobulins have been administered orally to both normal and immunodeficient patients with severe rotavirus gastroenteritis, but this treatment is currently considered experimental.

Supportive Treatment. Rehydration can be accomplished in most patients via the oral route. Modern rehydration solutions containing appropriate quantities of sodium and glucose promote optimum absorption of fluid from the intestine (see Table 54–1). There is no evidence that a particular carbohydrate source (e.g., rice) or addition of amino acids improves the efficacy of these solutions for children with viral enteritis. Other clear liquids such as flat soda, fruit juice, and sports drinks are inappropriate for rehydration of young children with significant stool loss. Rehydration via the oral (or nasogastric if needed) route should be done over 6–8 hr and feedings begun immediately thereafter. Rehydration solution should be continued as a supplement to make up for ongoing excessive stool losses. Initial intravenous fluids are required for the infant in shock or the occasional child with intractable vomiting.

After rehydration has been achieved, resumption of a normal diet for age has been shown to result in a more rapid recovery from viral gastroenteritis. Prolonged (>12 hr) administration of exclusive clear liquids or dilute formula is without clinical benefit and actually prolongs the duration of diarrhea. Breast-feeding should be continued even during rehydration. Selected infants may benefit from lactose-free feedings (such as soy formula or lactose-free cow's milk) for several days, although this is not necessary for most children. Hypocaloric diets low in protein and fat such as BRAT (**b**ananas, **r**ice, cereal, **a**pplesauce, and **t**oast) have not been shown to be superior to a regular diet.

PROGNOSIS. Most fatalities occur in infants with poor access to medical care and are attributed to dehydration. Children may be infected with rotavirus several times during their lives but with decreasing severity of subsequent infections. After the initial natural infection, children have limited protection against any subsequent infection (38%) and diarrhea (77%) but have protection against severe diarrhea (87%).

PREVENTION. Good hygiene reduces the transmission of viral gastroenteritis, but even in the most hygienic societies virtually all children become infected as a result of the efficiency of infection of the gastroenteritis viruses, particularly rotavirus. Good handwashing and isolation procedures can help control nosocomial outbreaks. The role of breast-feeding in prevention or amelioration of rotavirus infection may be small given the variable protection observed in a number of studies.

Vaccine. Rotavirus vaccine is a live, attenuated vaccine that contains three reassortant strains and one unaltered rotavirus: Three are single-gene reassortants of the VP7 gene of human origin (types G1, G2, and G4); the fourth strain is rhesus rotavirus (type G3), which is antigenically similar to human G3. Each reassortant contains the gene encoding the G protein of its parent human rotavirus, and the remaining 10 genes are from the parent rhesus rotavirus. Each dose of lyophilized vaccine, containing approximately 1×10^5 plaque-forming units of each of the four strains, is given orally immediately after reconstitution with 2.5 mL of citrate-bicarbonate diluent.

The rotavirus vaccine was licensed in 1998 for oral administration to infants at 2, 4, and 6 mo of age. If given, each dose should be separated by at least 3 wk; at least one dose should be given by 6 mo of age, and the series should be completed no later than 12 mo of age. In 1999, preliminary analysis of ongoing postlicensure surveillance of adverse events identified several cases of intussusception among recipients of rotavirus vaccine, usually occurring during the first wk after immunization and usually after the first dose. Use of the vaccine was suspended in July 1999. Physicians should monitor updated recommendations for use of rotavirus vaccine.

American Academy of Pediatrics, Committee on Infectious Diseases: Prevention of rotavirus disease: Guidelines for use of rotavirus vaccine. Pediatrics 102:1483, 1998.
Blacklow NR, Greenberg HB: Viral gastroenteritis. N Engl J Med 325:252, 1991.
Gore SM, Fontaine O, Pierce NP: Impact of rice based ORS on stool output and duration of diarrhea: Meta-analysis of 13 clinical trials. Br Med J 304:287, 1992.
Guerrero ML, Noel JS, Mitchell DK, et al: A prospective study of astrovirus diarrhea of infancy in Mexico City. Pediatr Infect Dis J 17:723, 1998.
Herrmann JE, Taylor DN, Echeverria P, et al: Astroviruses as a cause of gastroenteritis in children. N Engl J Med 24:1757, 1991.
Parashar UD, Holman C, Clarke MH, et al: Hospitalizations associated with rotavirus diarrhea in the United States, 1993—1995: Surveillance based on the new ICD-9-CM rotavirus-specific diagnostic code. J Infect Dis 77:13, 1998.
Rennels MB, Glass RI, Dennehy PH, et al: Safety and efficacy of high-dose-rhesus-human reassortant rotavirus vaccines–report of the National Multicenter Trial, United States. Pediatrics 97:7–13, 1996.
Santosham M, Moulton LH, Reid R, et al: Efficacy and safety of high-dose rhesus-human reassortant rotavirus vaccine in Native American populations. J Pediatr 131:632, 1997.
Tucker AW, Haddix AC, Bresee JS, et al: Cost-effectiveness analysis of a rotavirus immunization program for the United States. JAMA 279:1371, 1998.

CHAPTER 257
Papillomaviruses

Laura T. Gutman

Human papillomaviruses (HPVs) cause a variety of proliferative cutaneous and mucosal lesions, including common skin warts, benign and malignant genital tract lesions, and life-threatening respiratory papillomas. Most HPV-related infections in children who come to medical attention are external genital warts.

ETIOLOGY. The papillomaviruses are small (55 nm), DNA-containing viruses of the family Papovaviridae that are ubiquitous in nature, infecting most mammalian and many nonmammalian animal species. Strains are almost always species specific. At least 75 different types of HPVs have been identified by sequence homology. The different HPV types typically cause disease in specific anatomic sites; about half of the HPV types have been identified in genital tract specimens.

The inability to propagate these pathogens in tissue culture has prevented the application of traditional virologic culture methods to their study and slowed progress in the field, but newer molecular techniques have spawned a dramatic increase in understanding.

EPIDEMIOLOGY. HPV infections of the skin are very common, and most individuals are probably infected with one or more HPV types at some time. There are no animal reservoirs for HPV, and all transmission is presumably person-to-person or occasionally (probably very rarely) through contaminated fomites. Common warts are frequently seen in children, where they infect the hands, which are areas of frequent minor trauma.

Genital warts (condylomata acuminata) are the most prevalent viral sexually transmitted disease in the United States. They are a very common medical condition of sexually active adolescents, but occur infrequently in preadolescent children. The prevalence rises with increased numbers of sexual partners. Sexual contact is the predominate means of transmission. As with many other genital pathogens, perinatal transmission to newborns also occurs.

In sexually active persons, subclinical infections with HPV are much more common than are clinically apparent lesions. Subclinical infections also occur in exposed children, although probably at rates that are much lower than among adults. In virginal populations, including children who are not sexually abused, rates of both clinical disease and papilloma infection are very low to zero.

Some infants may acquire papillomaviruses during passage through an infected birth canal, leading to recurrent respiratory papillomatosis. Cases have been reported after cesarean section. The maximum incubation period for emergence of clinically apparent lesions (genital warts or laryngeal papillomas) after perinatally acquired infection is unknown, but appears to be at least 6 mo. Genital warts appearing in later childhood often result from sexual abuse, with papillomavirus transmission during the abusive contact. Genital warts may represent a sexually transmitted disease even in some very young children. Their presence is cause to suspect that possibility. A child with genital warts should, therefore, be provided with a complete evaluation for possible abuse, including the presence of other sexually transmitted diseases. See Chapter 35.1 for discussion of sexual abuse and Chapter 556 for the gynecologic examination of a child.

PATHOGENESIS. Epithelial HPV infection causes a failure of the squamous or mucosal keratinocytes to differentiate as they approach the surface layers of the skin. The HPV-infected epithelium shows a proliferation of the spinous layer, causing an increase in the thickness of the epithelium.

Lesions caused by HPV may be broadly grouped into those with little malignant potential and those with greater malignant potential. Certain HPV genotypes (types 6 and 11) cause visible genital warts that are exophytic and very infrequently progress to malignant or premalignant lesions, whereas other genotypes (especially 16 and 18 but also 31, 33, and 35) are strongly associated with cervical dysplasia or malignancy. Lesions may be infected simultaneously with multiple HPV types. Viral infections with the low-risk types have a high rate of spontaneous resolution if there are no apparent lesions, whereas the high-risk types tend to persist. Most children with recognized lesions have exophytic lesions and are infected with the more benign types. There have been only rare reports of HPV-associated genital malignancies occurring in preadolescent children. Nevertheless, there is concern that adolescents appear to be experiencing an increasing incidence of genital HPV diseases with the high-risk genotypes. Prevention of adolescent sexually transmitted diseases, including HPV infections, is a major goal of current public health initiatives.

CLINICAL MANIFESTATIONS. The typical HPV induced lesions of the skin are proliferative, papular, and hyperkeratotic.

Genital Lesions. Genital lesions may be found throughout the perineum around the anus, vagina, and urethra as well as intra-anal and intravaginal. Intra-anal warts occur predominantly in patients who have had receptive anal intercourse, as contrasted with perianal warts that may occur in men and women without a history of anal sex. Lesions caused by genital genotypes can also be found on other mucosal surfaces such as conjunctivae, gingiva, and nasal mucosa. They may be single or multiple and are usually localized to a limited anatomic area. On mucosal epithelium, the lesions are softer. Flat or macular lesions also occur. Infections may also be inapparent to visual inspection. Depending on the size and anatomic location, lesions may be pruritic and painful, cause burning with urination, be friable and bleed, or become superinfected. Children may be very disturbed by the development of genital lesions.

Laryngeal Papillomatosis. The median age of onset of recurrent laryngeal papillomatosis is 3 yr of age. Children present with hoarseness or, in infants, an altered cry and sometimes stridor. Rapid growth of respiratory papillomas can occlude the upper airway, causing respiratory compromise. These lesions may recur within weeks of removal, requiring frequent surgery.

DIAGNOSIS. The diagnosis of external genital warts may be reliably determined by visual inspection of a lesion by an experienced observer. Cytologic evaluation of mucosal lesions may be obtained through examination of exfoliated cells by Papanicolaou (Pap) smear. A biopsy with histologic examination can confirm a clinical diagnosis, but is not required if the lesion is typical and the examiner experienced. A biopsy should be considered if the diagnosis is uncertain, the lesions do not respond to therapy, the lesions worsen during therapy, the patient is immunocompromised, or the warts are pigmented, indurated, fixed, and ulcerated.

There are no serologic tests to assist in the diagnosis of HPV infection. During the past decade, very sensitive tests for the presence of HPV DNA, RNA, and proteins have been developed. These tests are becoming generally available, although they are not required for the diagnosis of external genital warts or related conditions.

Differential Diagnosis. Genital warts can be distinguished from condyloma latum of syphilis by serologic testing for syphilis. Other conditions to consider include molluscum contagiosum, skin tags, melanocytic nevi, psoriasis, and seborrheic dermatitis.

TREATMENT. Most hand warts will resolve spontaneously and usually do not require treatment.

Untreated warts may spontaneously regress, remain unchanged, or increase in size and number. Symptomatic lesions should be removed. Genital warts of children usually remit, but only over an extended period of time. Relatively small lesions may progress to very extensive disease. For this reason, it is recommended that genital lesions be treated by ablative therapy, which involves the destruction of the underlying epidermis. This may be achieved by application of podofilox or trichloracetic acid, cryotherapy, laser vaporization, or surgical excision. No single therapy is superior to other treatments or is ideal for all patients or all lesions.

Some treatments are patient applied, and some are provider administered. Laser vaporization under general anesthesia is often preferred if it is available. Many therapies are painful, and children should not undergo painful genital treatments unless adequate pain control is provided. Parents and patients should not be expected to apply painful therapies themselves. *In adolescents and adults,* recommended patient-applied treatment regimens for external genital warts include topical podofilox and imiquimod. Podofilox 0.5% solution (using a cotton swab) or gel (using a finger) is applied to visible warts in a cycle of applications twice a day for 3 days followed by 4 days of no therapy, repeated for a total of four cycles. Imiquimod 5% cream is applied at bedtime, three times a week for 16 weeks; the treated area should be washed with mild soap and water 6–10 hr after treatment. Neither podofilox or imiquimod are recommended during pregnancy. Provider-administered treatments include cryotherapy with liquid nitrogen or a cryoprobe, podophyllin resin 10–25%, trichloroacetic acid or bichloroacetic acid, or surgical removal. Intralesional, but not systemic, interferon is no more effective than other therapies, and is associated with significant adverse effects.

If exposure as a result of sexual abuse is suspected or known, the clinician should ensure that the child's safety has been achieved and is maintained.

COMPLICATIONS. The presence of these lesions in the genital area may be a cause of profound embarrassment to a child or parent. Complications of therapy are uncommon; chronic pain (vulvodynia) or hypoesthesia may occur at the treatment site. Lesions may heal with hypopigmentation or hyperpigmentation and less commonly with depressed or hypertrophic scars.

Numerous epidemiologic studies of adults, but not children, have demonstrated that papillomavirus infection, especially with types 16 and 18, is a strong risk factor for precancerous lesions and cancer. Respiratory papillomas also may become malignant, especially if they have been treated with radiation.

PROGNOSIS. With all forms of therapy, lesions very commonly recur, and approximately half of children will require a second or third treatment. This appears to be especially true for respiratory papillomatosis. Patients and parents should be warned of this likelihood. Combination therapy does not improve response but may increase complications.

PREVENTION. The only means to prevent infection is to avoid direct contact with lesions.

American Academy of Pediatrics, Committee on Child Abuse and Neglect: Guidelines for the evaluation of sexual abuse of children. Pediatrics 87:254, 1991.

Centers for Disease Control and Prevention: 1998 guidelines for treatment of sexually transmitted diseases. MMWR Morb Mortal Wkly Rep 47(RR-1):1, 1998.

Evander M, Edlund K, Gustafsson A, et al: Human papillomavirus infection is transient in young women: A population-based cohort study. J Infect Dis 171:1026, 1995.

Gutman LT, Herman-Giddens M, Phelps WC: Transmission of genital human papillomavirus disease: Comparison of data from adults and children. Pediatrics 91:31, 1993.

Gutman LT, St. Claire KK, Herman-Giddens ME, et al: Evaluation of intravaginal specimens from sexually abused and unabused girls for human papillomavirus infection. Am J Dis Child 146:694, 1992.

Morrison EAB: Natural history of cervical infection with human papillomaviruses. Clin Infect Dis 18:172, 1994.

Siegfried E, Rasnick-Conley J, Cook S, et al: Human papillomavirus screening in pediatric victims of sexual abuse. Pediatrics 101:43, 1998.

CHAPTER 258

Arboviral Encephalitis in North America

Scott B. Halstead

The *ar*thropod-*bo*rne (*arbo*virus) viral encephalitides are a group of clinically similar severe neurologic infections caused by several different viruses. They are transmitted by mosquitoes during warm weather, and are incurred by outdoor exposure in overlapping regions across most of the United States and much of southern Canada.

ETIOLOGY. The principal causes of the arthropod-borne encephalitides of North America include St. Louis encephalities (SLE), the complex of viruses included in the California (CE) encephalitis group of viruses, and, less frequently, western equine encephalitis (WEE), eastern equine encephalitis (EEE), and Colorado tick fever. The etiologic agents belong to different viral taxa: alphaviruses of the family *Togaviridae* (EEE and WEE), *Flaviviridae* (SLE), the California complex of the *Bunyaviridae* (CE), and *Reoviridae* (Colorado tick fever virus). Alphaviruses are 69-nm enveloped positive-strand RNA viruses that evolved from a common Venezuelan equine encephalitis-like viral ancestor in the Western Hemisphere. Flaviviruses are 40- to 50-nm enveloped positive-strand RNA viruses evolved from a common ancestor, globally distributed, and responsible for many important human viral diseases. The California serogroup, one of 16 Bunyavirus groups, are 75- to 115-nm enveloped viruses possessing a three-segment negative-strand RNA genome. Reoviruses are 60- to 80-nm double-stranded RNA viruses.

EPIDEMIOLOGY. Viral encephalitis cases and outbreaks were only recognized during the 20th century, when human population densities across the United States became relatively high, public health disease reporting systems were maturing, and laboratories were able to discriminate viral from bacterial infections. From the mid-19th century, epizootics of equine encephalitis were observed in the United States. In 1931, WEE was isolated from horse cases in the Central Valley of California. In 1938, the same virus was recovered from the central nervous system from fatal human cases. In the summer of 1932, an epidemic of human encephalitis, first regarded as Von Economo's disease was recognized in Paris, Illinois. The next year, more than 1000 cases were reported from St. Louis County, and several SLE viruses were isolated. In 1933, EEE virus was isolated from a horse epizootic, which occurred in Virginia, Maryland, Delaware, and New Jersey. The same virus was isolated from human cases in 1938. The first CE virus, now called La Crosse virus, was isolated from a fatal case of encephalitis in a 4-yr-old girl in rural Wisconsin. Colorado tick fever was first described as a nosologic entity in 1930.

Eastern Equine Encephalitis. In the United States, EEE is a very low incidence disease, with a median of three cases occurring annually in the Atlantic and Gulf states (Fig. 258–1). Transmission occurs often in focal endemic areas of the coast of Massachusetts, the six southern counties of New Jersey, and northeastern Florida. In North America, the virus is maintained in freshwater swamps in a zoonotic cycle involving *Culiseta melanura* and birds. Various other mosquito species obtain viremic meals from birds and transmit the virus to horses and humans. Virus activity varies markedly from year to year in response to still unknown ecologic factors. Most infections in birds are silent, but infections in pheasants are often fatal, and epizootics in these species are used as sentinels for periods of increased viral activity. Cases have been recognized on Caribbean islands. The case to infection ratio is lowest in children (1:8) and somewhat higher in adults (1:29).

Western Equine Encephalitis. Infections occur principally in the United States and Canada west of the Mississippi River (see Fig. 258–1) mainly in rural areas where water impoundments, irrigated farmland, and naturally flooded land provide breeding sites for *Culex tarsalis.* The virus is transmitted in a cycle involving mosquitoes, birds, and other vertebrate hosts. Humans and horses are susceptible to encephalitis. The case to infection ratio varies by age, having been estimated at 1:58 in children younger than 4 yr, and 1:1,150 in adults. Infections are most severe at the extremes of life; one third of cases occur in children younger than 1 yr. Recurrent human epidemics have been reported from the Yakima Valley in Washington State and the Central Valley of California; the largest outbreak on record—3,400 cases—occurred in Minnesota, North and South Dakota, Nebraska, and Montana and Alberta, Manitoba, and Saskatchewan, Canada. Epizootics in horses precede human epidemics by several weeks. For the past 20 years, possibly as a result of successful mosquito abatement, few cases of WEE have been reported.

St. Louis Encephalitis. Cases are reported from nearly all states; the highest attack rates occur in the Gulf and central states (see Fig. 258–1). Epidemics frequently occur in urban and suburban areas; the largest, in 1975, involved 1,800 persons living in Houston, Chicago, Memphis, and Denver. Cases often cluster in areas where there is ground water or septic systems, which support mosquito breeding. The principal vectors are *Culex pipiens* and *C. quinquefasciatus* in the central Gulf states, *C. nigripalpus* in Florida, and *C. tarsalis* in California. SLE virus is maintained in nature in a bird-mosquito cycle. Viral amplification occurs in bird species abundant in residential areas (e.g., sparrows, blue jays, and doves). Virus is transmitted in the late summer and early fall. The case to infection ratio may be as high as 1:300. Age-specific attack rates are lowest in children and highest in individuals older than 60 yr.

California Encephalitis. La Crosse viral infections are endemic in the United States, occurring annually from July to September principally in the north central and central states (see Fig. 258–1). Infections occur in peridomestic environments as the result of bites from *Aedes triseriatus* mosquitoes, which often breed in tree holes. The virus is maintained vertically in nature by transovarial transmission, and can be spread between mosquitoes by copulation and amplified in mosquito populations by viremic infections in various vertebrate hosts. Amplifying hosts include chipmunks, squirrels, foxes, and woodchucks. A case:infection ratio of 1:22–300 has been surmised. La Crosse

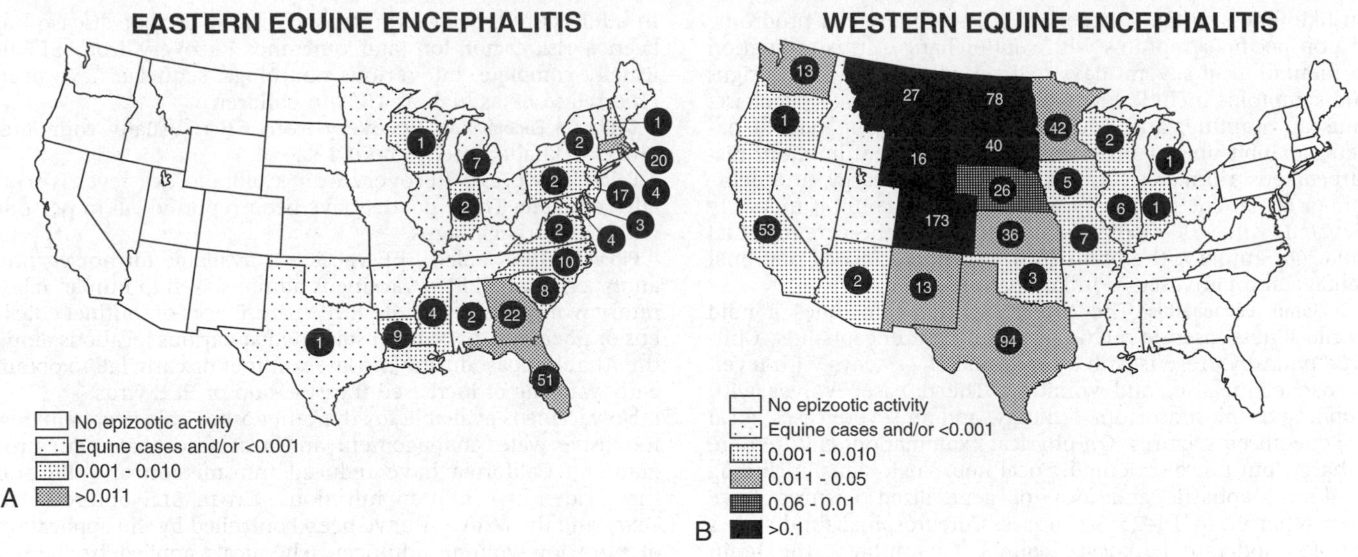

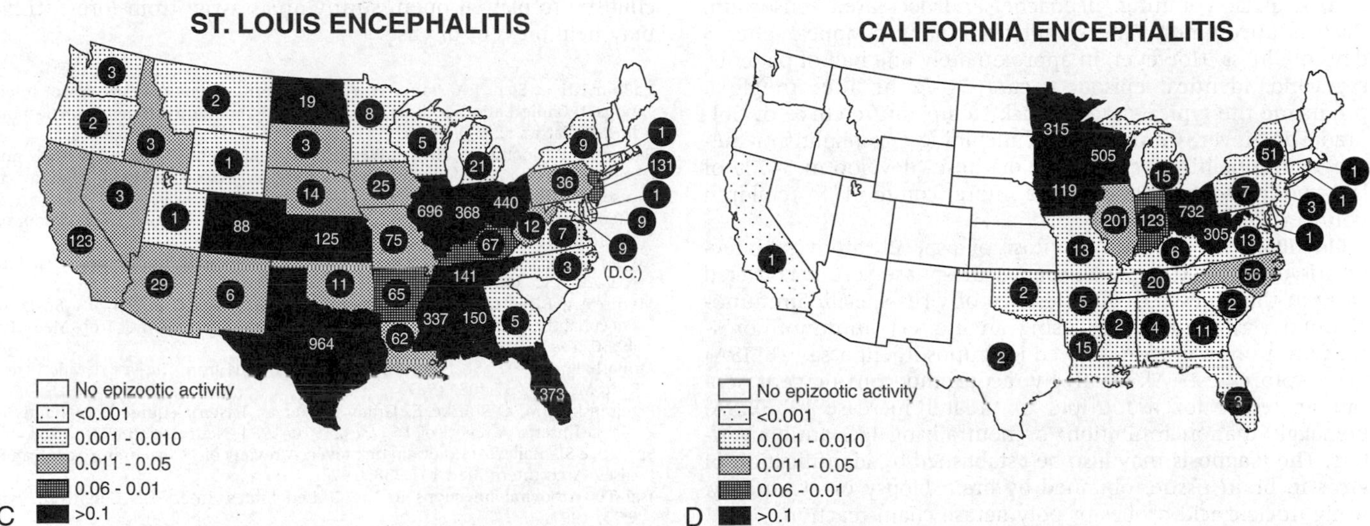

Figure 258–1 The incidence of reported cases of Eastern equine encephalitis (*A*), Western equine encephalitis (*B*), St. Louis encephalitis (*C*), and California encephalitis (*D*) reported to the Centers for Disease Control and Prevention in 1997.

encephalitis is principally a disease of children, who may constitute up to 75% of cases.

Colorado Tick Fever. Colorado tick fever virus is transmitted by the wood tick *Dermacentor andersoni,* which inhabits high-elevation areas of states extending from the central plains to the Pacific coast. The tick is infected with the virus at the larval stage and remains infected for life. Squirrels and chipmunks serve as primary reservoirs. Human infections typically occur in hikers and campers in indigenous areas during the spring and early summer.

CLINICAL MANIFESTATIONS. With the exception of EEE, these arboviruses produce similar symptoms of encephalitis.

Eastern Equine Encephalitis. This is a fulminant encephalitis with a rapid progression to coma and death in one third of cases. In infants and children, abrupt onset of fever, irritability, and headache are followed by lethargy, confusion, seizures, and coma. High temperature, bulging fontanel, stiff neck, and generalized flaccid or spastic paralysis are observed. There may be a brief prodrome of fever, headache, and dizziness. Unlike most other viral encephalitides, the peripheral white blood cell count usually demonstrates a marked leukocytosis, and the cerebrospinal fluid may show marked pleocytosis. Pathologic changes are found in the cortical and gray matter, with viral antigens localized to neurons. There is necrosis of neurons, neutrophilic infiltration, and perivascular cuffing by lymphocytes.

Western Equine Encephalitis. There may be a prodrome with symptoms of an upper respiratory tract infection. The onset is usually sudden with chills, fever, dizziness, drowsiness, increasing headache, malaise, nausea and vomiting, stiff neck, and disorientation. Infants typically present with the sudden cessation of feeding, fussiness, fever, and protracted vomiting. Convulsions and lethargy develop rapidly. On physical examination, patients are somnolent, exhibit meningeal signs, and have generalized motor weakness and reduced deep tendon reflexes. In infants, a bulging fontane, spastic paralysis, and generalized convulsions may be observed. On pathologic examination, disseminated small focal abscesses, small focal hemorrhages, and patchy areas of demyelination are distinctive.

St. Louis Encephalitis. Clinical manifestations vary from a mild flu-like illness to fatal encephalitis. There may be a prodrome of nonspecific symptoms with subtle changes in coordination or mentation of several days to 1 wk in duration. Early signs and symptoms include fever, photophobia, headache, malaise, nausea, vomiting, and neck stiffness. About one half of patients exhibit abrupt onset of weakness, incoordination, disturbed sensorium, restlessness, confusion, lethargy, and delirium or coma. The peripheral white blood cell count is modestly elevated, with 100–200 cells/mm³ found in the cerebrospinal fluid. On autopsy, the brain shows scattered foci of neuronal damage and perivascular inflammation.

California Encephalitis. The clinical spectrum includes a mild febrile illness, aseptic meningitis, and fatal encephalitis. Children typically present with a prodrome of 2–3 days with fever, headache, malaise, and vomiting. The disease evolves with clouding of the sensorium, lethargy, and, in severe cases, focal or generalized seizures. On physical examination, children are lethargic but not disoriented. Focal neurologic signs, including weakness, aphasia, and focal or generalized seizures, have been reported in 16–25% of cases. Cerebrospinal fluid shows low to moderate leukocyte counts. On autopsy, the brain shows focal areas of neuronal degeneration, inflammation, and perivascular cuffing.

Colorado Tick Fever. The illness begins with the abrupt onset of a flu-like illness, including high temperature, malaise, arthralgias and myalgia, vomiting, headache, and decreased sensorium. Rash is uncommon. The symptoms rapidly disappear after 3 days of illness. However, in approximately one half of patients, a second, identical episode recurs 24–72 hr after the first, producing the typical "saddle-back" temperature curve of Colorado tick fever. Complications, including encephalitis or meningoencephalitis or a bleeding diathesis, develop in 3–7% of infected persons and may be more common in children younger than 12 yr.

DIAGNOSIS. The etiologic diagnosis of a specific arboviral infection is established by testing an acute-phase serum collected early in the illness for the presence of virus-specific immunoglobulin (Ig)M antibodies using an indirect immunofluorescence test or an enzyme-linked immunosorbent assay (ELISA) IgM-capture test. Alternatively, acute and convalescent sera can be tested for a fourfold or greater increase in ELISA, hemagglutination inhibition, or neutralizing IgG antibody titers. The diagnosis may also be established by identification of virus in brain tissue, obtained by brain biopsy or at autopsy, using nucleic acid probes or polymerase chain reaction.

The diagnosis of encephalitis may be aided by CT or MRI and by electroencephalography. Focal seizures or focal findings on CT or MRI or electroencephalogram should suggest the possibility of herpes simplex encephalitis, which may be treated with acyclovir (Chapter 245).

TREATMENT. There is no specific treatment for arboviral encephalitides. The treatment of acute arboviral encephalitis is intensive supportive care (Chapter 64.7), including control of seizures (Chapter 602).

PROGNOSIS. With the exception of EEE, the arboviral encephalitides are self-limited and resolve without residua in most, but not all, patients.

Eastern Equine Encephalitis. The prognosis is better in patients with a prolonged prodrome; the occurrence of convulsions conveys a poor prognosis. Patient fatality rates are 33–75% and are highest in the elderly. Residual neurologic defects are common, especially in children.

Western Equine Encephalitis. Patient fatality rates are 3–9%, and are highest in the elderly. Major neurologic sequelae have been reported in up to 13% of cases and may be as high as 30% in infants. Parkinsonian syndrome has been reported as a residual in adult survivors.

St. Louis Encephalitis. The principal risk factor for fatal outcome is advanced age, with patient fatality rates being as high as 80% in early outbreaks. In children, mortality rates are 2–5%. In adults, underlying hypertensive cardiovascular disease has been a risk factor for fatal outcome. Recovery from SLE is usually complete, but serious neurologic sequelae have been reported to be as high as 10% in children.

California Encephalitis. Recovery from CE is usually complete. The case fatality rate is about 1%.

Colorado Tick Fever. Recovery from Colorado tick fever is usually complete. Three deaths have been reported, all in persons with hemorrhagic signs.

PREVENTION. A killed EEE vaccine is available for horses, and an experimental killed vaccine is administered to human laboratory workers who handle EEE virus. Flocks of sentinel chickens or pheasants have been stationed at various locations along the Atlantic coast during the late summer or early fall to obtain early warning of increased transmission of EEE virus.

No vaccine is available for the other arboviral encephalitides. Extensive water management and mosquito abatement programs in California have reduced transmission of WEE and the incidence of human infections. Urban SLE outbreaks in Texas and the Midwest have been controlled by the application of ultra low-volume adulticide chemicals applied from low-flying aircraft.

Because infections in children may occur as the result of summer daytime mosquito biting in residential areas, sealing mosquito breeding sites, using insect repellents, and instructing children to play in open, sunny areas away from forest fringe may help prevent disease.

Balfour HH Jr, Siem RA, Bauer H, et al: California arbovirus (La Crosse) infections. I. Clinical and laboratory findings in 66 children with meningoencephalitis. Pediatrics 52:680, 1973.

Earnest MP, Goolishian HA, Calverley JR, et al: Neurologic, intellectual, and psychologic sequelae following western encephalitis: A follow-up study of 35 cases. Neurology 21:969, 1971.

Griffen DE, Levine B, Ubul S, et al: The effects of alphavirus infection on neurons. Ann Neurol 35:523, 1994.

Komar N, Spielman A: Emergence of eastern encephalitis in Massachusetts. Ann N Y Acad Sci 740:157, 1995.

Marfin AA, Bleed DM, Lofgren JP, et al: Epidemiological aspects of a St. Louis encephalitis epidemic in Jefferson County, Arkansas. Am J Trop Med Hyg 49:30, 1993.

Monath TP, Tsai TF: St. Louis encephalitis: Lessons from the last decade. Am J Trop Med Hyg 37:40S, 1987.

Przelomski MM, O'Rourke E, Grady GE, et al: Eastern equine encephalitis in Massachusetts: A report of 16 cases, 1970–1984. Neurology 38:736, 1988.

Spruance SL, Bailey A: Colorado tick fever: A review of 115 laboratory confirmed cases. Arch Intern Med 131:288, 1973.

Tsai TF: Arboviral infections in the United States. Infect Dis Clin North Am 5:73, 1991.

CHAPTER 259
Arboviral Encephalitis Outside North America

Scott B. Halstead

The principal causes of arboviral encephalitides outside North America are Venezuelan equine encephalitis (VEE) virus, Japanese encephalitis (JE) virus, and tick-borne encephalitis (TBE) virus (Table 259–1).

259.1 Venezuelan Equine Encephalitis

The VEE virus was isolated from an epizootic in Venezuelan horses in 1938. Human cases were first identified in 1943. Hundreds of thousands of equine and human cases have oc-

TABLE 259–1 Vectors and Geographic Distribution of Arboviral Encephalitis Outside North America

Genus	Virus and Disease	Vector	Geographic Distribution
Flavivirus	Japanese encephalitis	*Culex tritaeniorhynchus*	Asia/Japan to Sri Lanka
Flavivirus	Murray Valley encephalitis	*Culex annulirostris*	Eastern Australia
Flavivirus	Rocio	*Psorophora* spp. or *Aedes* spp.	Sao Paulo, Brazil
Flavivirus	Tick-borne encephalitis	*Ixodes ricinus* *I. persulcatus*	Europe Russia
Togavirus	Venezuelan equine encephalitis	*Culex* spp. and others	Northern South America

curred over the past 70 yr. During 1971, epizootics moved through Central America and Mexico to southern Texas. After 2 decades of quiescence, epizootic disease emerged again in Venezuela and Colombia in 1995.

ETIOLOGY. VEE is an alphavirus of the genus *togaviridae*. VEE circulates in nature in six subtypes. Types I and III viruses have multiple antigenic variants. Types IAB and IC have been the cause of epizootics and human epidemics.

EPIDEMIOLOGY. The majority of epizootics resulting from types IAB and IC have occurred in Venezuela and Colombia. The virus resides in ill-defined sylvatic reservoirs in the South American rain forests. Known hosts include rodents and aquatic birds with transmission by *Culex melaconion* species. Vectors for horse-to-horse and horse-to-human transmission include *Aedes taeniorhynchus* and *Psorophora confinnis*. Epizootics move rapidly, up to several miles per day. Human cases are proportional to and follow epizootic occurrences. Viremia levels in human blood are high enough to infect mosquitoes. Because virus can be recovered from human pharyngeal swabs, and household attack rates are often as high as 50%, it is widely believed that person-to-person transmission occurs, although direct evidence is lacking. Types II–VI viruses are restricted to relatively small foci; each has a unique vector-host relationship and rarely result in human infections.

CLINICAL MANIFESTATIONS. The incubation period is 2–5 days followed by the abrupt onset of fever, chills, headache, sore throat, myalgia, malaise, prostration, photophobia, nausea, vomiting, and diarrhea. In 5–10% of cases there is a biphasic illness; the second phase is heralded by seizures, projectile vomiting, ataxia, confusion, agitation, and mild disturbances in consciousness. On physical examination, there is cervical lymphadenopathy and conjunctival suffusion. Cases of meningoencephalitis may demonstrate cranial nerve palsy, motor weakness, paralysis, seizures, and coma. Microscopic examination of tissues reveals inflammatory infiltrates in lymph nodes, spleen, lung, liver, and brain. Lymph nodes show cellular depletion, necrosis of germinal centers, and lymphophagocytosis. The liver shows patchy hepatocellular degeneration, the lungs demonstrate a diffuse interstitial pneumonia with intra-alveolar hemorrhages, and the brain shows patchy cellular infiltrates.

DIAGNOSIS. The etiologic diagnosis of VEE is established by testing an acute-phase serum collected early in the illness for the presence of virus-specific immunoglobulin (Ig)M antibodies or, alternatively, demonstrating a fourfold or greater increase in IgG antibody titers by testing paired acute and convalescent sera. The virus can also be identified by polymerase chain reaction (PCR).

TREATMENT. There is no specific treatment for VEE. The treatment is intensive supportive care (Chapter 64.7), including control of seizures (Chapter 602).

PROGNOSIS. In patients with meningoencephalitis, the fatality rate ranges from 10–25%. Sequelae include nervousness, forgetfulness, recurrent headache, and easy fatigability.

PREVENTION. Several veterinary vaccines are available to protect equines. VEE virus is highly infectious in laboratory settings, and BL-3 containment should be used. An experimental vaccine is available for use in laboratory workers.

259.2 Japanese Encephalitis

Epidemics of encephalitis were reported in Japan from the late 1800s. The JE virus was first isolated by Japanese workers by intracerebral inoculation of monkeys in 1934 and subsequently in mice in 1936. The virus was initially called Japanese B encephalitis to distinguish it from an unusual epidemic of von Economo (type A) encephalitis that occurred in Japan in the 1920s.

ETIOLOGY. JE virus is a positive-sense single-stranded RNA virus and a member of the family *Flaviviridae*.

EPIDEMIOLOGY. JE is a mosquito-borne viral disease of humans as well as horses, swine, and other domestic animals that causes human infections and acute disease in a vast area of Asia, northern Japan, Korea, China, Taiwan, Philippines, and the Indonesian archipelago and from Indo-China through the Indian subcontinent. *Culex tritaeniorhyncus summarosus*, a night-time-biting mosquito that feeds preferentially on large domestic animals and birds but only infrequently on humans, is the principal vector of zoonotic and human JE in northern Asia. A more complex ecology prevails in southern Asia. From Taiwan to India, *Culex tritaeniorhyncus* and members of the closely related *Culex vishnui* group are vectors. Before the introduction of JE vaccine, summer outbreaks of JE occurred regularly in Japan, Korea, China, Okinawa, and Taiwan. Over the past decade, there has been a pattern of steadily enlarging recurrent seasonal outbreaks in Vietnam, Thailand, Nepal, and India, with small outbreaks in the Philippines, Indonesia, and the northern tip of Queensland, Australia. Seasonal rains are accompanied by increases in mosquito populations and increased transmission. Pigs serve as amplifying host.

The annual incidence in endemic areas ranges from 1–10/10,000 population. Children younger than 15 yr are principally affected, with nearly universal exposure by adulthood. The case to infection ratio for JE virus been variously estimated at 1:25–1,000. Higher ratios have been estimated for populations indigenous to enzootic areas. JE occurs in travelers visiting Asia; therefore, a travel history in the diagnosis of encephalitis is critical.

CLINICAL MANIFESTATIONS. After a 4- to 14-day incubation period, patients cases typically progress through four stages: prodromal illness (2–3 days), acute stage (3–4 days), subacute stage (7–10 days), and convalescence (4–7 wk). Onset may be characterized by abrupt onset of fever, headache, respiratory symptoms, anorexia, nausea, abdominal pain, vomiting, and sensory changes, including psychotic episodes. Grand mal seizures are seen in 10–24% of children; parkinsonian-like non-intention tremor and cogwheel rigidity are seen less frequently. Particularly characteristic are rapidly changing central nervous system signs (e.g., hyperreflexia followed by hyporeflexia or plantar responses that change). The sensory status of the patient may vary from confusion, disorientation, delirium, or somnolence, progressing to coma. There is usually a mild pleocytosis (100–1,000 leukocytes/mm^3) in the cerebrospinal fluid, initially polymorphonuclear but in a few days predominantly lymphocytic. Albuminuria is common. Fatal cases usually progress rapidly to coma, and the patient dies within 10 days.

DIAGNOSIS. JE should be suspected in patients reporting exposure to night-biting mosquitoes in endemic areas during the transmission season. The etiologic diagnosis of JE is established by testing an acute-phase serum collected early in the illness for the presence of virus-specific IgM antibodies or, alternatively, demonstrating a fourfold or greater increase in IgG antibody titers by testing paired acute and convalescent sera. The virus can also be identified by PCR.

TREATMENT. There is no specific treatment for JE. The treatment is intensive supportive care (Chapter 64.7), including control of seizures (Chapter 602).

PROGNOSIS. Patient fatality rates are 24–42%, and are highest in children aged 5–9 yr and in persons older than 65 yr. The frequency of sequelae is 5–70% and is directly related to age of the patient and to the severity of disease. Sequelae are most common in patients younger than 10 yr at the onset of disease. The more common sequelae are mental deterioration, severe emotional instability, personality changes, motor abnormalities, and speech disturbances.

PREVENTION. Travelers to endemic country with stays of 1 mo or longer in rural areas of the endemic region during the expected period of seasonal transmission, or those traveling in areas experiencing endemic transmission, should receive JE vaccine. The JE vaccine is given in a three-dose series (0.5 mL for 1–3 yr of age; 1 mL for >3 yr of age) subcutaneously; the first two doses are given 1 wk apart and the third dose 30 days later, with booster doses every 2 yr. Reactions to vaccination, including headache, malaise, myalgia, tenderness, redness, and swelling, occur in about 20% of vaccines. Serious generalized urticaria, facial angioedema, and respiratory distress have been observed in adults. Because vaccine is prepared in mouse brain, surveillance should be maintained for central nervous system disease after JE vaccination. In humans, prior dengue virus infection provides partial protection from clinical JE.

Personal measures should be taken to reduce exposure to mosquito bites, especially for short-term residents in endemic areas. This consists of avoiding evening outdoor exposure, using insect repellents, covering the body with clothing, and using bed nets or house screening.

Commercial pesticides, widely used by rice farmers in Asia, are effective in reducing populations of *C. tritaeniorhyncus*. Fenthion, fenitrothion, and phenthoate are effectively adulticidal and larvicidal. Insecticides may be applied from portable sprayers or from helicopters or light aircraft.

259.3 Tick-Borne Encephalitis

TBE was identified by Russian scientists in 1937 and subsequently shown to be widespread in Europe, where it was identified as the cause of milk-borne encephalitis.

ETIOLOGY. TBE virus is a positive-sense, single-stranded RNA virus and a member of the family *Flaviviridae*.

EPIDEMIOLOGY. Tick-borne encephalitis refers to neurotropic tick-transmitted flaviviral infections occurring across the Eurasian land mass. In the Far East, the disease is called Russian spring-summer encephalitis; the milder, often biphasic form in Europe is simply called tick-borne encephalitis. TBE is found in all countries of Europe except Portugal and the Benelux countries. The incidence is particularly high in Austria, Poland, Hungary, Czech Republic, Slovakia, former Yugoslavia, and Russia. The incidence tends to be very focal. Seroprevalence is as high as 50% in farm and forestry workers. The majority of cases occur in adults, but even young children may be infected while playing in the woods or on picnics or camping trips. The seasonal distribution of cases is midsummer in southern Europe, with a longer season in Scandinavia and the Russian Far East. TBE can be excreted from the milk of goats, sheep, or cows. Before World War II, when milk was consumed unpasteurized, milk-borne cases were common.

Viruses are transmitted principally by hard ticks of the *Ixodes ricinus* in Europe and *Ixodes persulcatus* in the Far East. Viral circulation is maintained by a combination of transmission from ticks to birds, rodents, and larger mammals and transstadial transmission from larval to nymphal and adult stages. In some parts of Europe and Russia, ticks feed actively during the spring and early fall, giving rise to the name spring-summer encephalitis.

CLINICAL MANIFESTATIONS. After an incubation period of 7–14 days, the European form begins as an acute nonspecific febrile illness followed in 5–30% of cases by meningoencephalitis. The Far Eastern variety more often results in encephalitis with higher case fatality and sequelae rates. The first phase of illness is characterized by fever, headache, myalgia, malaise, nausea, and vomiting for 2–7 days. Fever disappears and after 2–8 days may return accompanied by vomiting, photophobia, and signs of meningeal irritation in children and more severe encephalitic signs in adults. This phase rarely lasts more than 1 wk.

DIAGNOSIS. The diagnosis of TBE should be suspected in patients reporting a tick bite in endemic areas during the transmission season. The etiologic diagnosis of TBE is established by testing an acute-phase serum collected early in the illness for the presence of virus-specific IgM antibodies or, alternatively, demonstrating a fourfold or greater increase in IgG antibody titers by testing paired acute and convalescent sera. The virus can also be identified by PCR.

TREATMENT. There is no specific treatment for TBE. The treatment is intensive supportive care (Chapter 64.7), including control of seizures (Chapter 602).

PROGNOSIS. The main risk for fatal outcome is advanced age; the fatality rate in adults is about 1%, but sequelae in children are very rare. Transient unilateral paralysis of an upper extremity is a common finding in adults. Common sequelae include chronic fatigue, headache, sleep disorders, and emotional disturbances.

PREVENTION. Specific Ig has been given to persons with seasonal tick bite exposure, although efficacy of this preventive therapy is not well studied. Effective inactivated vaccines for human use, made from virus grown in tissue culture, are licensed in Russia and Europe. They are administered in a three-dose series, as described for JE vaccine.

Centers for Disease Control: Inactivated Japanese encephalitis virus vaccine. Recommendations of the Advisory Committee on Immunization Practices (ACIP). MMWR Morb Mortal Wkly Rep 42(RR-1):1, 1993.

Innis BL, Nisalak A, Nimmannitya S, et al: An enzyme-linked immunosorbent assay to characterize dengue infections where dengue and Japanese encephalitis co-circulate. Am J Trop med Hyg 40:418, 1989.

Kluger G, Schottler A, Waldvogel K, et al: Tickborne encephalitis despite specific immunoglobulin prophylaxis. Lancet 346:1502, 1995.

McNeil JG, Lednar WM, Stansfield SK, et al: Central European tick-borne encephalitis: Assessment of risk for persons in the Armed Forces and vacationers. J Infect Dis 152:650, 1985.

Paul WS, Moore PS, Karabatsos N, et al: Outbreak of Japanese encephalitis on the island of Saipan, 1990. J Infect Dis 167:1053, 1993.

Poland JD, Cropp CB, Craven RB, et al: Evaluation of the potency and safety of inactivated Japanese encephalitis vaccine in U.S. inhabitants. J Infect Dis 161:878, 1990.

Rico-Hesse R, Weaver SC, Siger de J, et al: Emergence of a new epidemic/epizootic of Venezuelan equine encephalitis virus in South America. Proc Natl Acad Sci U S A 92:5278, 1995.

Tsai TF: Arboviral infections: General considerations for prevention, diagnosis and treatment in travelers. Semin Pediatr Infect Dis 3:62, 1992.

CHAPTER 260

Dengue Fever/Dengue Hemorrhagic Fever

Scott B. Halstead

Dengue fever, a benign syndrome caused by several arthropod-borne viruses, is characterized by biphasic fever, myalgia or arthralgia, rash, leukopenia, and lymphadenopathy. Dengue hemorrhagic fever (Philippine, Thai, or Singapore hemorrhagic fever; hemorrhagic dengue; acute infectious thrombocytopenic purpura) is a severe, often fatal, febrile disease caused by dengue viruses. It is characterized by capillary permeability, abnormalities of hemostasis, and, in severe cases, a protein-losing shock syndrome (dengue shock syndrome). It is currently thought to have an immunopathologic basis.

ETIOLOGY. There are at least four distinct antigenic types of dengue virus, members of the family *Flaviviridae*. In addition, three other *ar*thropod-*bo*rne (*arbo*viruses) cause similar or identical febrile diseases with rash (Table 260–1).

EPIDEMIOLOGY. Dengue viruses are transmitted by mosquitoes of the *Stegomyia* family. *Aedes aegypti*, a daytime biting mosquito, is the principal vector, and all four virus types have been recovered from it. In most tropical areas, *A. aegypti* is highly urbanized, breeding in water stored for drinking or bathing and in rainwater collected in any container. Dengue viruses have also been recovered from *Aedes albopictus*, and outbreaks in the Pacific area have been attributed to several other *Aedes* species. These species breed in water trapped in vegetation. In Southeast Asia and West Africa, dengue may be maintained in a cycle involving canopy-feeding jungle monkeys and *Aedes* species, which feed on monkeys.

Epidemics were common in temperate areas of the Americas, Europe, Australia, and Asia until early in the 20th century. Dengue fever and dengue-like disease are now endemic in tropical Asia, the South Pacific Islands, northern Australia, tropical Africa, the Caribbean, and Central and South America. Dengue fever occurs frequently among travelers to these areas.

Dengue outbreaks in urban areas infested with *A. aegypti* may be explosive; up to 70–80% of the population may be involved. Most disease occurs in older children and adults. Because *A. aegypti* has a limited range, spread of an epidemic occurs mainly through viremic human beings and follows the main lines of transportation. Sentinel cases may infect household mosquitoes; a large number of nearly simultaneous secondary infections give the appearance of a contagious disease. Where dengue is endemic, children and susceptible foreigners may be the only persons to acquire overt disease, adults having become immune.

Dengue-Like Diseases. Dengue-like diseases may also occur in epidemics. Epidemiologic features depend on the vectors and their geographic distribution (see Table 260–1). Chikungunya virus is widespread in the most populous areas of the world.

TABLE 260–1 Vectors and Geographic Distribution of Dengue-Like Diseases

Genus	Virus and Disease	Vector	Geographic Distribution
Togavirus	Chikungunya	*Aedes aegypti* *Aedes africanus*	Africa, India, Southeast Asia
Togavirus	O'nyong-nyong	*Anopheles funestus*	East Africa
Flavivirus	West Nile fever	*Culex molestus* *Culex univittatus*	Africa, Middle East, India

In Asia, *A. aegypti* is the principal vector; in Africa, other *Stegomyia* may be important vectors. In Southeast Asia, dengue and chikungunya outbreaks occur concurrently. Outbreaks of o'nyong-nyong and West Nile fever usually involve villages or small towns, in contrast to the urban outbreaks of dengue and chikungunya.

Dengue Hemorrhagic Fever. Dengue hemorrhagic fever occurs where multiple types of dengue virus are simultaneously or sequentially transmitted. Currently, it is endemic in all of tropical America and Asia, where warm temperatures and the practices of water storage in homes plus outdoor breeding sites result in large, permanent populations of *A. aegypti*. Under these conditions, infections with dengue viruses of all types are common, and second infections with heterologous types are frequent.

Second dengue infections are relatively mild in the majority of instances, ranging from an inapparent infection through an undifferentiated upper respiratory tract or dengue-like disease, but may also progress to dengue hemorrhagic fever. Nonimmune foreigners, adults and children, exposed to dengue virus during outbreaks of hemorrhagic fever have classic dengue fever or even milder disease. The differences in clinical manifestations of dengue infections between natives and foreigners in Southeast Asia are related more to immunologic status than to racial susceptibility. Dengue hemorrhagic fever can occur during primary dengue infections, most frequently in infants whose mothers are immune to dengue.

Dengue 3 virus strains circulating in mainland Southeast Asia since 1983 are associated with a particularly severe clinical syndrome, characterized by encephalopathy, hypoglycemia, markedly elevated liver enzymes, and, occasionally, jaundice.

PATHOGENESIS. The pathogenesis of dengue fever is not clear. Fatalities with chikungunya and West Nile fever infections have been ascribed to viral encephalitis or hemorrhage.

Dengue Hemorrhagic Fever. The pathogenesis is incompletely understood, but epidemiologic studies suggest that it is usually associated with second infections with dengue types 1–4. In the Americas, dengue hemorrhagic fever and dengue shock syndrome have been associated only with dengue 2 strains of recent Southeast Asian origin. The recent occurrence of sizable dengue hemorrhagic fever outbreaks in India and Pakistan also appear to be related to imported dengue strains. There is evidence that non-neutralizing antibodies promote cellular infection and enhance severity of the disease. Dengue viruses demonstrate enhanced growth in cultures of human mononuclear phagocytes prepared from dengue-immune donors or in cultures supplemented with non-neutralizing dengue antibody. Monkeys infected sequentially or receiving small quantities of enhancing antibody have enhanced viremias. Retrospective studies of sera from human mothers whose infants acquired dengue hemorrhagic fever or prospective studies on children acquiring sequential dengue infections have shown that the circulation of infection-enhancing antibodies at the time of infection is the strongest risk factor for development of severe disease. Even low levels of neutralizing antibodies, whether from earlier homotypic infection in mothers or heterotypic infections in children, protect infants or children from dengue hemorrhagic fever. Early in the acute stage of secondary dengue infections, there is rapid activation of the complement system. Shortly before or during shock, blood levels of soluble tumor necrosis factor receptor, interferon-γ, and interleukin 2 are elevated. C1q, C3, C4, C5-C8, and C3 proactivators are depressed, and C3 catabolic rates are elevated. These factors may interact at the endothelial cell to produce increased vascular permeability through the nitric oxide final pathway. The blood clotting and fibrinolytic systems are activated, and levels of factor XII (Hageman factor) are depressed. The mechanism of bleeding in dengue hemorrhagic fever is not known, but a mild degree of disseminated intravascular coagulation, liver damage, and thrombocytopenia may operate synergistically. Capillary damage allows fluid, electrolytes, small proteins, and, in some instances, red cells to leak into extravascular spaces. This internal redistribution of fluid, together with deficits caused by fasting, thirsting, and vomiting, results in hemoconcentration, hypovolemia, increased cardiac work, tissue hypoxia, metabolic acidosis, and hyponatremia.

Usually no pathologic lesions are found to account for death. In rare instances, death may be due to gastrointestinal or intracranial hemorrhages. Minimal to moderate hemorrhages are seen in the upper gastrointestinal tract, and petechial hemorrhages are common in the interventricular septum of the heart, on the pericardium, and on the subserosal surfaces of major viscera. Focal hemorrhages are occasionally seen in the lungs, liver, adrenals, and subarachnoid space. The liver is usually enlarged, often with fatty changes. Yellow, watery, and at times blood-tinged effusions are present in serous cavities in about three fourths of patients.

Microscopically, there is perivascular edema in the soft tissues and widespread diapedesis of red cells. There may be maturational arrest of megakaryocytes in bone marrow, and increased numbers of them are seen in capillaries of the lungs, in renal glomeruli, and in sinusoids of the liver and spleen.

Dengue virus is usually absent in tissues at the time of death; rare isolations have been reported from liver and lymphatic tissues, most often in children younger than 1 yr who have experienced primary infections.

CLINICAL MANIFESTATIONS. The incubation period is 1–7 days. The clinical manifestations are variable and are influenced by the age of the patient. In infants and young children, the disease may be undifferentiated or characterized by fever for 1–5 days, pharyngeal inflammation, rhinitis, and mild cough. A majority of infected older children and adults experience sudden onset of fever, which rapidly rises to 39.4–41.1°C (103–106°F), usually accompanied by frontal or retro-orbital pain, particularly when pressure is applied to the eyes. Occasionally, severe back pain precedes the fever (back-break fever). A *transient*, macular, generalized rash that blanches under pressure may be seen during the first 24–48 hr of fever. The pulse rate may be slow relative to the degree of fever. Myalgia and arthralgia occur soon after the onset and increase in severity. Joint symptoms may be particularly severe in patients with chikungunya or o'nyong-nyong infection. From the 2nd–6th days of fever, nausea and vomiting are apt to occur, and generalized lymphadenopathy, cutaneous hyperesthesia or hyperalgesia, taste aberrations, and pronounced anorexia may develop.

One to 2 days after defervescence, a generalized, morbilliform, maculopapular rash appears, which spares the palms and soles. It disappears in 1–5 days; desquamation may occur. Rarely there is edema of the palms and soles. About the time this second rash appears, the body temperature, which has previously fallen to normal, may become slightly elevated and demonstrate the characteristic biphasic temperature pattern.

Dengue Hemorrhagic Fever. Differentiation between dengue fever and dengue hemorrhagic fever is difficult early in the course of illness. A relatively mild first phase with abrupt onset of fever, malaise, vomiting, headache, anorexia, and cough is followed after 2–5 days by rapid clinical deterioration and collapse. In this second phase, the patient usually has cold, clammy extremities, a warm trunk, flushed face, diaphoresis, restlessness, irritability, and midepigastric pain. Frequently, there are scattered petechiae on the forehead and extremities; spontaneous ecchymoses may appear, and easy bruising and bleeding at sites of venipuncture are common. A macular or maculopapular rash may appear, and there may be circumoral and peripheral cyanosis. Respirations are rapid and often labored. The pulse is weak, rapid, and thready and the heart sounds faint. The liver may enlarge to 4–6 cm below the costal margin and is usually firm and somewhat tender. Approximately 20–30% of cases of dengue hemorrhagic fever are complicated by shock (dengue shock syndrome). Fewer than 10% of patients have gross ecchymosis or gastrointestinal bleeding, usually after a period of uncorrected shock. After a 24- to 36-hr period of crisis, convalescence is fairly rapid in the children who recover. The temperature may return to normal before or during the stage of shock. Bradycardia and ventricular extrasystoles are common during convalescence.

DIAGNOSIS. A clinical diagnosis of dengue fever derives from a high index of suspicion and a knowledge of the geographic distribution and environmental cycles of causal viruses. Because clinical findings vary and there are many possible causative agents, the term "dengue-like disease" should be used until a specific diagnosis is established.

The World Health Organization criteria for dengue hemorrhagic fever are fever, minor or major hemorrhagic manifestations, thrombocytopenia (≤ 100,000/mm^3), and objective evidence of increased capillary permeability (hematocrit increased ≥ 20%), pleural effusion (by chest radiograph), or hypoalbuminemia. Dengue shock syndrome must meet these criteria plus hypotension or narrow pulse pressure (≤ 20 mm Hg).

Virologic diagnosis can be established by serologic tests or by isolation of the virus from blood leukocytes or serum. In both primary and second dengue infections, there is a relatively transient appearance of antidengue immunoglobulin (Ig)M antibodies. These disappear after 6–12 wk, which can be used to time a dengue infection. In second primary dengue infections, most antibody is of the IgG class. Serologic diagnosis depends on a fourfold or greater increase in IgG antibody titer in paired sera by hemagglutination inhibition, complement fixation, enzyme immunoassay, or neutralization test. Carefully standardized immunoglobulin IgM- and IgG-capture enzyme immunoassays are now widely used to identify acute-phase antibodies from patients with primary or secondary dengue infections in single-serum samples. Usually such samples should be collected not earlier than 5 days nor later than 6 wk after onset. It may not be possible to distinguish the infecting virus by serologic methods alone, particularly when there has been prior infection with another member of the same arbovirus group. Virus can be recovered from acute-phase serum after inoculating tissue culture or living mosquitoes. Viral RNA can be detected in blood or tissues by specific complementary DNA probes or amplified first by the polymerase chain reaction.

Differential Diagnosis. The differential diagnosis of dengue fever includes viral respiratory and influenza-like diseases, the early stages of malaria, mild yellow fever, scrub typhus, viral hepatitis, and leptospirosis.

Four arboviral diseases have dengue-like courses but without rash: Colorado tick fever, sandfly fever, Rift Valley fever, and Ross River fever. Colorado tick fever occurs sporadically among campers and hunters in the western United States; sandfly fever in the Mediterranean region, the Middle East, southern Russia, and parts of the Indian subcontinent; and Rift Valley fever in North, East, Central, and South Africa. Ross River fever is endemic in much of eastern Australia with epidemic extension to Fiji. In adults, Ross River fever often produces protracted and crippling arthralgia involving weight-bearing joints.

Because meningococcemia, yellow fever (Chapter 261), other viral hemorrhagic fevers (Chapter 262), many rickettsial diseases, and other severe illnesses caused by a variety of agents may produce a clinical picture similar to dengue hemorrhagic fever, the etiologic diagnosis should be made only when epidemiologic or serologic evidence suggests the possibility of a dengue infection.

Laboratory Findings. In dengue fever, pancytopenia may occur after the 3–4 days of illness. Neutropenia may persist or reappear during the latter stage of the disease and may continue into convalescence; white blood cell counts as low as 2,000/mm^3 have been recorded. Platelets rarely fall below 100,000/mm^3. Venous clotting, bleeding and prothrombin times, and plasma fibrinogen values are within normal ranges. The tourniquet test infrequently is positive. Mild acidosis, hemoconcentration, increased transaminase values, and hypoproteinemia may occur during some primary dengue virus infections. The electrocardiogram may show sinus bradycardia, ectopic ventricular foci, flattened T waves, and prolongation of the P-R interval.

The most common hematologic abnormalities during dengue hemorrhagic fever and dengue shock syndrome are hemoconcentration with an increase of more than 20% in hematocrit, thrombocytopenia, prolonged bleeding time, and moderately decreased prothrombin level that is seldom less than 40% of control. Fibrinogen levels may be subnormal and fibrin split products elevated. Other abnormalities include moderate elevations of the serum transaminase levels, consumption of complement, mild metabolic acidosis with hyponatremia, and occasionally hypochloremia, slight elevation of serum urea nitrogen, and hypoalbuminemia. Roentgenograms of the chest reveal pleural effusions (left > right) in nearly all patients.

TREATMENT. Treatment of uncomplicated dengue fever is supportive. Bed rest is advised during the febrile period. Antipyretics should be used to keep body temperature less than 40°C (104°F). Analgesics or mild sedation may be required to control pain. Aspirin is contraindicated and should not be used because of its effects on hemostasis. Fluid and electrolyte replacement is required for deficits caused by sweating, fasting, thirsting, vomiting, and diarrhea.

Dengue Hemorrhagic Fever. Management of dengue hemorrhagic fever and dengue shock syndrome includes immediate evaluation of vital signs and degrees of hemoconcentration, dehydration, and electrolyte imbalance. Close monitoring is essential for at least 48 hr because shock may occur or recur precipitously early in the disease. Patients who are cyanotic or have labored breathing should be given oxygen. Rapid intravenous replacement of fluids and electrolytes can frequently sustain patients until spontaneous recovery occurs. When elevation of the hematocrit persists after replacement of fluids, plasma or plasma colloid preparations are indicated. Care must be taken to avoid overhydration, which may contribute to cardiac failure. Transfusions of fresh blood or platelets suspended in plasma may be required to control bleeding; they should not be given during hemoconcentration but only after evaluation of hemoglobin or hematocrit values. Salicylates are contraindicated because of their effect on blood clotting.

Paraldehyde or chloral hydrate may be required for children who are markedly agitated. Use of vasopressors has not resulted in a significant reduction of mortality compared with that observed with simple supportive therapy. Disseminated intravascular coagulation may require treatment (Chapter 488). Corticosteroids do not shorten the duration of disease or improve prognosis in children receiving careful supportive therapy.

Hypervolemia during the fluid reabsorptive phase may be life threatening and is heralded by a fall in hematocrit with wide pulse pressure. Diuretics and digitalization may be necessary.

COMPLICATIONS. Primary infections with dengue fever and dengue-like diseases are usually self-limited and benign. Fluid and electrolyte losses, hyperpyrexia, and febrile convulsions are the most frequent complications in infants and young children. Epistaxis, petechiae, and purpuric lesions are uncommon but may occur at any stage. Swallowed blood from epistaxis, vomited or passed by rectum, may be erroneously interpreted as gastrointestinal bleeding. In adults and possibly in children, underlying conditions may lead to clinically significant bleeding. Convulsions may occur during high temperature especially with chikungunya fever. Infrequently, after the febrile stage, prolonged asthenia, mental depression, bradycardia, and ventricular extrasystoles may occur in children.

In endemic areas, dengue hemorrhagic fever should be suspected in children with a febrile illness suggestive of dengue fever who experience hemoconcentration and thrombocytopenia.

PROGNOSIS. The prognosis of dengue fever may be adversely affected by passively acquired antibody or by prior infection with a closely related virus that predisposes to development of dengue hemorrhagic fever.

Dengue Hemorrhagic Fever. Death has occurred in 40–50% of patients with shock, but with adequate intensive care deaths should occur in less than 2% of cases. Survival is directly related to early and intense supportive treatment. Infrequently, there is residual brain damage caused by prolonged shock or occasionally by intracranial hemorrhage.

PREVENTION. Several types of dengue types 1, 2, 3, and 4 vaccines are under development, and a killed vaccine for chikungunya is efficacious but not generally available. Prophylaxis consists of avoiding mosquito bites by use of insecticides, repellents, body covering with clothing, screening of houses, and destruction of *A. aegypti* breeding sites (Chapter 304). If water storage is mandatory, a tight-fitting lid or a thin layer of oil may prevent egg laying or hatching. A larvicide, such as Abate [O,O′-(thiodi-*p*-phenylene) O,O,O,O′-tetramethyl phosphorothioate], available as a 1% sand-granule formation and effective at a concentration of 1 part/million, may be added safely to drinking water. Ultra-low-volume spray equipment effectively dispenses the adulticide malathion from truck or airplane for rapid intervention during an epidemic. Only personal antimosquito measures are effective against mosquitoes in the field, forest, or jungle.

The possibility exists that dengue vaccination may sensitize a recipient so that ensuing dengue infection could result in hemorrhagic fever. Vaccination with yellow fever 17D strain has no effect on the severity of dengue illness, although seroconversion rates to a dengue 2 vaccine were enhanced in yellow fever–immune persons.

Burke DS, Nisalak A, Johnson DE, et al: A prospective study of dengue infections in Bangkok. Am J Trop Med Hyg 38:172, 1988.

Centers for Disease Control and Prevention: Imported Dengue—United States, 1996. MMWR Morb Mortal Wkly Rep 47:544, 1998.

World Health Organization: Dengue Haemorrhagic Fever: Diagnosis, Treatment, Prevention and Control, 2nd ed. Geneva, World Health Organization, 1997.

Kalayanarooj S, Vaughn DW, Nimmannitya S, et al: Early clinical and laboratory indicators of acute dengue illness. J Infect Dis 176:313, 1997.

Halstead SB: Immune enhancement of viral infection. Prog Allergy 31:301, 1982.

Halstead SB: Pathogenesis of dengue: Challenges to molecular biology. Science 239:476, 1988.

Halstead SB: Selective primary health care: Strategies for control of disease in the developing world. XI. Dengue. Rev Infect Dis 6:251, 1984.

Kliks S, Nimmannitya S, Nisalak A, et al: Evidence that maternal dengue antibodies are important in development of dengue hemorrhagic fever in infants. Am J Trop Med Hyg 38:411, 1988.

Kliks S, Nisalak A, Brandt WE, et al: Antibody-dependent enhancement of dengue virus growth in human monocytes as a risk factor for dengue hemorrhagic fever. Am J Trop Med Hyg 40:444, 1989.

Rico-Hesse R, Harrison LM, Salas RA, et al: Origins of dengue type 2 viruses associated with increased pathogenicity in the Americas. Virology 230:244, 1997.

Tassniyom S, Vasanawathana S, Chirawatkul A, et al: Failure of high-dose methylprednisolone in established dengue shock syndrome—A placebo controlled double-blind study. Pediatrics 92:111, 1993.

Thisyakorn U, Nimmannitya S: Nutritional status of children with dengue hemorrhagic fever. Clin Infect Dis 16:295, 1993.

Tsai CJ, Kuo CH, Chen PC, et al: Upper gastrointestinal bleeding in dengue fever. Am J Gastroenterol 86:33, 1991.

CHAPTER 261
Yellow Fever

Scott B. Halstead

Yellow fever is an acute infection characterized in its most severe form by fever, jaundice, proteinuria, and hemorrhage. The virus is mosquito borne and occurs in epidemic or endemic form in South America and Africa. Seasonal epidemics occurred in cities located in temperate areas of Europe and the Americas until 1900; epidemics continue to occur in West, Central, and East Africa.

ETIOLOGY. Yellow fever is the prototype of the *Flavivirus* genus of the family Flaviviridae, which are enveloped single-stranded RNA viruses 35–50 nm in diameter.

Yellow fever circulates zoonotically as three genotypes: type I and IIA in Central and West Africa, respectively and type IIB in South America. The type IIA virus is capable of urban transmission between human beings by *Aedes aegypti*. Sometime in the 1600s, this virus was brought to the American tropics through the African slave trade. Subsequently, yellow fever caused enormous coastal and riverine epidemics until the 20th century, when the virus and its urban and sylvan mosquito cycles were identified and a vaccine and mosquito control developed.

EPIDEMIOLOGY. Human and nonhuman primate hosts acquire the infection by the bite of infected mosquitoes. After an incubation-period of 3–6 days, virus appears in the blood and may serve as a source of infection for other mosquitoes. The virus must replicate in the gut of the mosquito and pass to the salivary gland before the mosquito can transmit the virus. Yellow fever virus is transmitted in an urban cycle—human to *A. aegypti* to human—and a jungle cycle—monkey to jungle mosquitoes to monkey. Classic yellow fever epidemics in the United States, South America, the Caribbean, and parts of Europe were of the urban variety. Present-day African epidemics are primarily urban. Most of the approximately 200 cases reported each year in South America are jungle yellow fever. In colonial times, attack rates in white adults were very high, suggesting that subclinical infections are uncommon in this age group. Yellow fever may be less severe in children, with subclinical infections to clinical case ratios of 2:1 or greater. In areas where outbreaks of urban yellow fever are common, most cases involve children because many adults are immune. Transmission in West Africa is highest during the rainy season, from July to November. The migration of nonimmune laborers into endemic regions is a significant factor in some outbreaks.

In tropical forests, yellow fever virus is maintained in a transmission cycle involving monkeys and tree hole–breeding mosquitoes (*Haemogogus* spp in the Americas, *Aedes africanus* in Africa). In the Americas, most cases involve men who work in forested areas and are exposed to infected mosquitoes. In Africa, the virus is prevalent in moist savanna and savanna transition areas where other tree hole–breeding *Aedes* vectors transmit the virus between monkeys and humans and between humans.

CLINICAL MANIFESTATIONS. In Africa, inapparent, abortive, or clinically mild infections are frequent; some studies suggest that children experience a milder disease than adults do. Abortive infections, characterized by fever and headache, may be unrecognized except during epidemics.

In its classic form, yellow fever begins with sudden onset of fever, headache, myalgia, lumbosacral pain, anorexia, nausea, and vomiting. Physical findings during the early phase of illness, when virus is present in the blood, include prostration, conjunctival injection, flushing of face and neck, reddening of the tongue at the tip and edges, and relative bradycardia. After 2–3 days, there may be a brief period of remission, followed in 6–24 hr by reappearance of fever with vomiting, epigastric pain, jaundice, dehydration, gastrointestinal and other hemorrhages, albuminuria, hypotension, signs of renal failure, delirium, convulsions, and coma. Death may occur between the 7th and 10th days. The fatality rate in severe cases approaches 50%. Some patients who survive the acute phase of illness later succumb to renal failure or myocardial damage. Laboratory abnormalities include leukopenia; prolonged clotting, prothrombin, and partial thromboplastin times; thrombocytopenia; hyperbilirubinemia; elevated serum transaminases; albuminuria; and azotemia. Hypoglycemia may be present in severe cases. Electrocardiogram abnormalities characterized by bradycaria and ST-T changes are described.

PATHOGENESIS. Pathologic changes seen in the liver include (1) coagulative necrosis of hepatocytes in the midzone of the liver lobule, with sparing of cells around the portal areas and central veins; (2) eosinophilic degeneration of hepatocytes (Councilman's bodies); (3) microvacuolar fatty change; and (4) minimal inflammation. The kidneys show acute tubular necrosis. In the heart, myocardial fiber degeneration and fatty infiltration are seen. The brain may show edema and petechial hemorrhages. Direct viral injury to the liver results in impaired ability to carry out its functions of biosynthesis and detoxification. This is the central pathogenic event of yellow fever. Hemorrhage is thought to result from decreased synthesis of vitamin K–dependent clotting factors and, in some cases, disseminated intravascular clotting. Renal dysfunction has been attributed to hemodynamic factors (prerenal failure progressing to acute tubular necrosis). The pathogenesis of shock in patients with yellow fever appears to be similar to that described in dengue shock syndrome and the other viral hemorrhagic fevers.

DIAGNOSIS. Yellow fever should be suspected when fever, headache, vomiting, myalgia, and jaundice appear in residents of endemic areas or in unimmunized visitors who have recently traveled (within 2 wk before onset of symptoms) to endemic areas. Clinically, yellow fever is quite similar to dengue hemorrhagic fever. In contrast to the gradual onset of acute viral hepatitis resulting from types A, B, C, D, or E hepatitis viruses, jaundice in yellow fever appears after 3–5 days of high temperature and is often accompanied by severe prostration. Mild yellow fever is dengue like and cannot be distinguished from a wide variety of other infections. Jaundice and fever may occur in any of several other tropical diseases, including malaria, viral hepatitis, louse-borne relapsing fever, leptospirosis, typhoid fever, rickettsial infections, certain systemic bacterial infections, sickle cell crisis, Rift Valley fever, Crimean-Congo hemorrhagic fever, and other viral hemorrhagic fevers. Outbreaks of yellow fever always include cases with severe gastrointestinal hemorrhage.

Specific diagnosis depends on detection of virus or viral antigen in acute-phase blood samples or antibody assays. The immunoglobulin M enzyme immunoassay is particularly useful. Sera obtained during the first 10 days after onset of symptoms should be kept in an ultra-low-temperature freezer (−70°C) and shipped on dry ice for virus testing. Convalescent-phase samples for antibody tests are managed by conventional means. In handling acute-phase blood specimens, medical personnel must take care to avoid contaminating themselves or others on the evacuation trail (laboratory personnel and others). Postmortem diagnosis is based on virus isolation from liver or blood, identification of Councilman bodies in liver tissue, or detection of antigen or viral genome in liver tissue.

TREATMENT. It is customary to keep yellow fever patients in a mosquito-free area, using mosquito nets if necessary. Patients are viremic during the febrile phase of the illness. Although there is no specific treatment for yellow fever, medical care is directed at maintaining physiologic status: (1) sponging and acetaminophen to reduce high temperature, (2) vigorous fluid replacement of losses resulting from fasting, thirsting, vomiting, or plasma leakage, (3) correcting acid-base imbalance, (4) maintaining nutritional intake to lesson the severity of hypoglycemia, and (5) avoiding drugs that are either metabolized by the liver or toxic to the liver, kidney, or central nervous system.

COMPLICATIONS. Complications of acute yellow fever include severe hemorrhage, liver failure, and acute renal failure. Bleeding should be managed by transfusion of fresh whole blood or fresh plasma with platelet concentrates if necessary. Renal failure may require peritoneal dialysis or hemodialysis.

PREVENTION. Yellow fever 17D is a live, attenuated vaccine with a long record of safety and efficacy. It is administered as a single 0.5-mL subcutaneous injection at least 10 days before arrival in a yellow fever endemic area. All persons traveling to endemic areas should be considered for vaccination, but length of stay, exact locations to be visited, and environmental or occupational exposure may determine the specific risk and individual need for vaccination. Persons traveling from yellow fever–endemic to yellow fever–receptive countries may be required to obtain a yellow fever vaccine (e.g., from South America or Africa to India). Usually countries that require travelers to obtain a yellow fever immunization will not issue a visa without a valid immunization certificate. Vaccination is valid for 10 yr for international travel certification, although immunity lasts at least 40 yr and probably for life.

Yellow fever vaccine should not be administered to persons with symptomatic immunodeficiency diseases and those taking immunosuppressant drugs. Although the vaccine is not known to harm fetuses, its administration during pregnancy is contraindicated. In very young children, there is a small risk of encephalitis and death after yellow fever 17D vaccination. The 17D vaccine should not be administered to infants younger than 4 mo because nearly all neurologic complications occur in this age group. Residence or travel to areas of known or anticipated yellow fever activity (e.g., forested areas in the Amazon basin), which places an individual at high risk, warrants immunization of infants 4–9 mo of age. Immunization of children 9 mo of age and older is routinely recommended before entry into endemic areas. Vaccination should be avoided for persons with a history of egg allergy. Alternatively, a skin test can be performed to determine whether a serious allergy exists that would preclude vaccination.

Centers for Disease Control: Yellow fever vaccine. Recommendations of the Advisory Committee on Immunization Practices (ACIP). MMWR Morb Mortal Wkly Rep 39(RR-6):1, 1990.

Chang GJ, Cropp BC, Kinney RM, et al: Nucleotide sequence variation of the envelope protein gene identifies two distinct types of yellow fever virus. J Virol 69:5773, 1995.

Monath TP: Yellow fever—A medically neglected disease. Rev Infect Dis 9:165, 1987.

Monath TP: Yellow fever and dengue—The interactions of virus, vector and host in the re-emergence of epidemic disease. Sem Virol 5:133, 1994.

Monath TP, Naridi A: Should yellow fever vaccine be included in the expanded program of immunization in Africa—A cost-effectiveness analysis for Nigeria. Am J Trop Med Hyg 48:274, 1993.

Yellow fever—The global situation. Bull WHO 70:667, 1992.

CHAPTER 262
Other Viral Hemorrhagic Fevers

Scott B. Halstead

Viral hemorrhagic fevers are a loosely defined group of clinical syndromes in which hemorrhagic manifestations are either common or especially notable in severe illness (Table 262–1). Both the etiologic agents and clinical features of the syndromes differ, but disseminated intravascular coagulopathy may be a common pathogenetic feature.

ETIOLOGY. Six of the viral hemorrhagic fevers are caused by *ar*thropod-*bo*rne (arboviruses) viruses (see Table 262–1). Four are togaviruses of the family Flaviviridae, including Kyasanur Forest disease, Omsk, dengue (Chapter 260), and yellow fever (Chapter 261) viruses. Three are of the family *Bunyaviridae,* including Congo, Hantaan, and Rift Valley fever viruses. Four are of the family Arenaviridae, including Junin, Machupo, Guanarito, and Lassa viruses. Two are of the family Filoviridae, including Ebola and Marburg viruses. The filoviruses are enveloped, filamentous RNA viruses, which are sometimes branched, unlike any other known virus.

EPIDEMIOLOGY AND CLINICAL MANIFESTATIONS. With some exceptions, the viruses causing viral hemorrhagic fevers are transmitted to humans via a nonhuman entity. The specific ecosystem required for viral survival determines the geographic distribution of disease. Although it is commonly thought that all viral hemorrhagic fevers are arthropod borne, seven may be contracted from environmental contamination caused by animals or animal cells or from infected humans (see Table 262–1). Laboratory and hospital infections have occurred with many of these agents. Lassa fever and Argentine and Bolivian hemorrhagic fevers are reportedly milder in children than in adults.

Crimean-Congo Hemorrhagic Fever. Sporadic human infection in Africa provided the original virus isolation. Natural foci are recognized in Bulgaria, western Crimea, and the Rostov-on-Don and Astrakhan regions; a somewhat similar disease occurs in Kazakhstan and Uzbekistan. Index cases were followed by nosocomial transmission in Pakistan and Afghanistan in 1976, in the Arabian Peninsula in 1983, and in South Africa in 1984. In the Commonwealth of Independent States, the vectors are *Hyalomma marginatum* and *Hyalomma anatolicum,* which, along with hares and birds, may serve as viral reservoirs. Disease occurs from June to September, largely among farmers and dairy workers.

Kyasanur Forest Disease. Human cases occur chiefly in adults in an area of Mysore State, India. The main vectors are two *Ixodidae* ticks, *Haemaphysalis turturis* and *Haemaphysalis spinigera.* Monkeys and forest rodents may be amplifying hosts. Laboratory infections are common.

Omsk Hemorrhagic Fever. The disease occurs throughout south central Russia and northern Romania. Vectors may include *Dermacentor pictus* and *Dermacentor marginatus,* but direct transmission from moles and muskrats to humans seems well established. Human disease occurs in a spring-summer-autumn pattern, paralleling the activity of vectors. This infection occurs most frequently in persons with outdoor occupational exposure. Laboratory infections are common.

Rift Valley Fever. The virus causing Rift Valley fever is responsible for epizootics involving sheep, cattle, buffalo, certain antelopes, and rodents in North, Central, East, and South Africa. The virus is transmitted to domestic animals by *Culex theileri* and several *Aedes* species. Mosquitoes may serve as reservoirs by transovarial transmission. An epizootic in Egypt in 1977–

TABLE 262–1 Viral Hemorrhage Fevers

Mode of Transmission	Disease	Virus
Tick borne	Crimean-Congo HF*	Congo
	Kyasanur Forest disease	Kyasanur Forest disease
	Omsk HF	Omsk
Mosquito borne†	Dengue HF	Dengue (four types)
	Rift Valley fever	Rift Valley fever
	Yellow fever	Yellow fever
Infected animals or materials to humans	Argentine HF	Junin
	Bolivian HF	Machupo
	Lassa fever*	Lassa
	Marburg disease*	Marburg
	Ebola HF*	Ebola
	Hemorrhagic fever with renal syndrome	Hantaan

Patients may be contagious, nosocomial infections are common.
†Chikungunya virus is associated at low frequency with petechiae, petechial hemorrhages, and epistaxis. More severe hemorrhagic manifestations have been reported in some studies.
HF = hemorrhagic fever.

1978 was accompanied by thousands of human infections, principally among veterinarians, farmers, and farm laborers. Smaller outbreaks occurred in Senegal in 1987 and Madagascar in 1990. Humans are most often infected during the slaughter or skinning of sick or dead animals. Laboratory infection is common.

Argentine Hemorrhagic Fever. Prior to introduction of vaccine, hundreds to thousands of cases occurred annually from April through July in the maize-producing area northwest of Buenos Aires that reaches to the eastern margin of the Province of Cordoba. Junin virus has been isolated from the rodents *Mus musculus, Akodon arenicola,* and *Calomys laucha laucha.* It infects migrant laborers who harvest the maize and who inhabit rodent-contaminated shelters.

Bolivian Hemorrhagic Fever. The recognized endemic area consists of the sparsely populated province of Beni in Amazonian Bolivia. Sporadic cases occur in farm families who raise maize, rice, yucca, and beans. In the town of San Joaquin, a disturbance in the domestic rodent ecosystem may have led to an outbreak of household infection caused by *Calomys callosus,* ordinarily a field rodent. Mortality rates are high in young children.

Venezuelan Hemorrhagic Fever. In 1989, an outbreak of hemorrhagic illness occurred in the farming community of Guanarito, Venezuela, 200 miles south of Caracas. Subsequently, in 1990–1991, there were 104 cases reported with 26 deaths. Cotton rats (*Sigmodon alstoni*) and cane rats (*Zygodontomys brevicauda*) have been implicated as likely reservoirs.

Lassa Fever. Lassa virus has an unusual potential for human-to-human spread and has resulted in many small epidemics in Nigeria, Sierra Leone, and Liberia. Medical workers in Africa and the United States have also contracted the disease. Patients with acute Lassa fever have been transported by international aircraft, necessitating extensive surveillance among passengers and crews. The virus is probably maintained in nature in a species of African peridomestic rodent, *Mastomys natalensis.* Rodent-to-rodent transmission and infection of humans probably operate via mechanisms established for other arenaviruses.

Marburg Disease. Until recently, the world experience has been limited to 26 primary and 5 secondary cases in Germany and Yugoslavia in 1967, to small outbreaks in Zimbabwe in 1975, Kenya in 1980 and 1988, South Africa in 1983, and a large outbreak in Congo Republic in 1999. Transmission occurs by direct contact with tissues of the African green monkey, with infected blood, or with human semen. The reservoir and mode of transmission of the virus in nature are unknown.

Ebola Hemorrhagic Fever. Ebola virus was isolated in 1976 from a devastating epidemic involving small villages in northern Zaire and southern Sudan; smaller outbreaks have occurred subsequently. Outbreaks initially have been nosocomial. Attack rates have been highest in the birth to 1–yr and 15– to 50–yr age groups. The virus resembles Marburg virus. Ebola virus has been particularly active recently, with a well-known outbreak in Kikwit, Zaire in 1995, followed by scattered outbreaks in Central and West Africa. The virus has been recovered from chimpanzees, but the vertebrate reservoir and mode of transmission to humans are unknown. Reston virus, related to Ebola, has been recovered from Philippine monkeys and has caused subclinical infections in workers in monkey colonies in the United States.

Hemorrhagic Fever with Renal Syndrome. The endemic area of hemorrhagic fever with renal syndrome (HFRS), also known as epidemic hemorrhagic fever and Korean hemorrhagic fever, includes Japan, Korea, Far Eastern Siberia, north and central China, European and Asian Russia, Scandinavia, Czechoslovakia, Romania, Bulgaria, Yugoslavia, and Greece. Although the incidence and severity of hemorrhagic manifestations and the mortality are lower in Europe than in northeastern Asia, the renal lesion is the same. Disease in Scandinavia, nephropathia epidemica, is caused by a different although antigenically related virus associated with *Clethrionomys glariolus.* Cases occur predominantly in the spring and summer. There appears to be no age factor in susceptibility, but because of occupational hazards, young adult men are most frequently attacked. Rodent plagues and evidence of rodent infestation have accompanied endemic and epidemic occurrences. Hantaan virus has been detected in lung tissue and excreta of *Apodemus agrarius coreae.* Antigenically related agents have been detected in laboratory rats and in urban rat populations around the world, including Prospect Hill virus in the wild rodent *Microtus pennsylvanicus* in North America and Sin Nombre virus, the cause of hantavirus pulmonary syndrome (Chapter 264) in the deer mouse in southern and southwestern United States. Rodent-to-rodent and rodent-to-human transmission presumably occurs via the respiratory route.

CLINICAL MANIFESTATIONS. Dengue hemorrhagic fever (Chapter 260) and yellow fever (Chapter 261) are more frequent causes of similar diseases in children in endemic areas.

Crimean-Congo Hemorrhagic Fever. The incubation period of 3–12 days is followed by a febrile period of 5–12 days and a prolonged convalescence. Illness begins suddenly with fever, severe headache, myalgia, abdominal pain, anorexia, nausea, and vomiting. After 1–2 days, fever may subside until the patient experiences an erythematous facial or truncal flush and injected conjunctivae. A second febrile period of 2–6 days then develops, with a hemorrhagic enanthem on the soft palate and a fine petechial rash on the chest and abdomen. Less frequently, there are large areas of purpura and bleeding from gums, nose, intestine, lungs, or uterus. Hematuria and proteinuria are relatively rare. During the hemorrhagic stage, there is usually tachycardia with diminished heart sounds and occasionally hypotension. The liver is usually enlarged, but there is no icterus. In protracted cases, central nervous system signs may include delirium, somnolence, and progressive clouding of consciousness. Early in the disease leukopenia with relative lymphocytosis, progressively worsening thrombocytopenia, and gradually increasing anemia occur. In convalescence there may be hearing and memory loss. The mortality rate is 2–50%.

Kyasanur Forest Disease and Omsk Hemorrhagic Fever. After an incubation period of 3–8 days, both diseases begin with sudden onset of fever and headache. Kyasanur Forest disease is characterized by severe myalgia, prostration, and bronchiolar involvement; it often presents without hemorrhage but occasionally with severe gastrointestinal bleeding. In Omsk hemorrhagic fever there is moderate epistaxis, hematemesis, and a hemorrhagic enanthem but no profuse hemorrhage; bronchopneumonia is common. In both diseases, severe leukopenia and thrombocytopenia, vascular dilatation, increased vascular permeability, gastrointestinal hemorrhages, and subserosal and interstitial petechial hemorrhages occur. Kyasanur Forest disease may be complicated by acute degeneration of renal tubules and focal liver damage. In many patients, recurrent febrile illness may follow an afebrile period of 7–15 days. This second phase takes the form of a meningoencephalitis.

Rift Valley Fever. Most infections have occurred in adults with disease similar to dengue fever (Chapter 260). Onset is acute, with fever, headache, prostration, myalgia, anorexia, nausea, vomiting, conjunctivitis, and lymphadenopathy. The fever lasts 3–6 days and is often biphasic. Convalescence is often prolonged. In the 1977–1978 outbreak, many patients died after showing signs that included purpura, epistaxis, hematemesis, and melena. At autopsy, there was extensive eosinophilic degeneration of the parenchymal cells of the liver.

Argentine, Venezuelan, and Bolivian Hemorrhagic Fever and Lassa Fever. The incubation period is commonly 7–14 days; the acute illness lasts for 2–4 wk. Clinical illnesses range from undifferentiated fever to the characteristic severe illness. Lassa fever is most often clinically severe in whites. Onset is usually gradual, with increasing fever, headache, diffuse myalgia, and anorexia. During the 1st wk, signs frequently include a sore throat, dysphagia, cough, oropharyngeal ulcers, nausea, vomiting, diarrhea, and pains in chest and abdomen. Pleuritic chest pain may persist for 2–3 wk. In Argentine and Bolivian hemorrhagic fevers, and less frequently in Lassa fever, a petechial enanthem appears on the soft palate 3–5 days after onset and at about the same time on the trunk. The tourniquet test may be positive. The clinical course of Venezuelan hemorrhagic fever has not been well described.

In 35–50% of all patients, these diseases may become severe, with persistent high temperature, increasing toxicity, swelling of face or neck, microscopic hematuria, and frank hemorrhages from the stomach, intestines, nose, gums, and uterus. A syndrome of hypovolemic shock is accompanied by pleural effusion and renal failure. Respiratory distress resulting from airway obstruction, pleural effusion, or congestive heart failure may occur. Ten to 20% of patients experience late neurologic involvement characterized by intention tremor of the tongue and associated speech abnormalities. In severe cases, there may be intention tremors of the extremities, seizures, and delirium. The cerebrospinal fluid is normal. In Lassa fever, nerve deafness occurs in early convalescence in 25% of cases. Prolonged convalescence is accompanied by alopecia and in Argentine and Bolivian hemorrhagic fevers by signs of autonomic nervous system lability, such as postural hypotension, spontaneous flushing or blanching of the skin, and intermittent diaphoresis.

Laboratory studies reveal marked leukopenia, mild to moderate thrombocytopenia, proteinuria, and, in Argentine hemorrhagic fever, moderate abnormalities in blood clotting, decreased fibrinogen, increased fibrinogen split products, and elevated serum transaminases. Pathologically, there is focal, often extensive eosinophilic necrosis of liver parenchyma, focal interstitial pneumonitis, focal necrosis of the distal and collecting tubules, and partial replacement of splenic follicles by amorphous eosinophilic material. Usually bleeding occurs by diapedesis with little inflammatory reaction. The mortality rate is 10–40%.

Marburg Disease and Ebola Hemorrhagic Fever. After an incubation period of 4–7 days, illness begins abruptly with severe frontal headache, malaise, drowsiness, lumbar myalgia, vomiting, nausea, and diarrhea. A maculopapular eruption begins 5–7 days later on the trunk and upper arms. It becomes generalized, often hemorrhagic, and exfoliates during convalescence. The exanthem is accompanied by a dark red enanthem on the hard palate, conjunctivitis, and scrotal or labial edema. Gastrointestinal hemorrhage occurs as the severity of illness increases. Late in the illness, the patient may become tearfully depressed with marked hyperalgesia to tactile stimuli. In fatal cases, patients become hypotensive, restless, and confused and lapse into coma. Convalescent patients may experience alopecia and have paresthesias of the back and trunk. There is a marked leukopenia with necrosis of granulocytes. Disseminated intravascular coagulation and thrombocytopenia are universal and correlate with severity of disease; there are moderate abnormalities in clotting proteins and elevated serum transaminases and amylase. The mortality rate of Marburg disease is 25% and of Ebola hemorrhagic fever, 50–90%.

Hemorrhagic Fever with Renal Syndrome. In most cases, HFRS is characterized by fever, petechiae, mild hemorrhagic phenomena, and mild proteinuria, followed by relatively uneventful recovery. In 20% of recognized cases, the disease may progress through four rather distinct phases. The *febrile phase* is ushered in with fever, malaise, and facial and truncal flushing. It lasts 3–8 days and ends with thrombocytopenia, petechiae, and proteinuria. The *hypotensive phase* of 1–3 days follows defervescence. Loss of fluid from the intravascular compartment may result in marked hemoconcentration. Proteinuria and ecchymoses increase. The *oliguric phase*, usually 3–5 days in duration, is characterized by a low output of protein-rich urine, increasing nitrogen retention, nausea, vomiting, and dehydration. Confusion, extreme restlessness, and hypertension are common. The *diuretic phase*, which may last for days or weeks, usually initiates clinical improvement. The kidneys show little concentrating ability, and rapid loss of fluid may result in severe dehydration and shock. Potassium and sodium depletion may be severe. Fatal cases manifest abundant protein-rich retroperitoneal edema and marked hemorrhagic necrosis of the renal medulla. The mortality rate is 5–10%.

DIAGNOSIS. Diagnosis depends on a high index of suspicion in endemic areas. In nonendemic areas, histories of recent travel, recent laboratory exposure, or exposure to an earlier case should evoke suspicion of a viral hemorrhagic fever.

In all viral hemorrhagic fevers, the viral agent circulates in the blood at least transiently during the early febrile stage. Togaviruses and bunyaviruses can be recovered from acute-phase serum by inoculation into tissue culture or living mosquitoes. Argentine, Bolivian, and Venezuelan hemorrhagic fever viruses can be isolated from acute-phase blood or throat washings by inoculation intracerebrally into guinea pigs, infant hamsters, or infant mice. Lassa virus may be isolated from acute-phase blood or throat washings by inoculation into tissue cultures. For Marburg disease and Ebola hemorrhagic fever, acute-phase throat washings, blood, and urine may be inoculated into tissue culture, guinea pigs, or monkeys. The viruses are readily identified by electron microscopy, with a filamentous structure differentiating them from all other known agents. Specific complement-fixing and immunofluorescent antibodies appear during convalescence. The virus of HFRS is recovered from acute-phase serum or urine by inoculation into tissue culture. A variety of antibody tests using viral subunits are becoming available. Serologic diagnosis depends on demonstrating seroconversion, or a fourfold or greater increase in immunoglobulin G antibody titer in acute and convalescent sera taken 3–4 wk apart. These viruses may also be detected in blood or tissues using DNA probes or by polymerase chain reaction.

Handling blood and other biologic specimens is hazardous and must be performed by specially trained personnel. Blood and autopsy specimens should be placed in tightly sealed metal containers, wrapped in absorbent material inside a sealed plastic bag, and shipped on dry ice to laboratories with biocontainment safety level 4 facilities. Even routine hematologic and biochemical tests should be done with extreme caution.

Differential Diagnosis. Mild cases of hemorrhagic fever may be confused with almost any self-limited systemic bacterial or viral infection. More severe cases may suggest typhoid fever; epidemic, murine, or scrub typhus; leptospirosis; or a rickettsial spotted fever, for which effective chemotherapeutic agents are available. Many of these may be acquired in geographic or ecologic locations endemic for a viral hemorrhagic fever.

TREATMENT. Ribavirin administered intravenously is effective in reducing mortality in Lassa fever and HFRS. Further information and advice about management, control measures, diagnosis, and collection of biohazardous specimens can be obtained from Centers for Disease Control and Prevention, National Center for Infectious Diseases, Special Pathogens Branch, Atlanta, Georgia 30333 (404-639-1115).

The principle involved in all these diseases, especially HFRS, is the reversal of dehydration, hemoconcentration, renal failure, and protein, electrolyte, or blood losses. The contribution of disseminated intravascular coagulopathy to the hemorrhagic manifestations is unknown, and the management of hemorrhage should be individualized. Transfusions of fresh blood and platelets are frequently given. Good results have been reported in a few patients after the administration of clotting factor concentrates. The efficacy of corticosteroids, ε-aminocaproic acid, pressor amines, or α-adrenergic blocking agents has not been established. Sedatives should be selected with regard to the possibility of kidney or liver damage. The successful management of HFRS may require renal dialysis.

PREVENTION. A live, attenuated vaccine (Candid-I) for Argentine hemorrhagic fever is highly efficacious. A form of inactivated mouse brain vaccine is reported to be effective in preventing Omsk hemorrhagic fever. Inactivated Rift Valley fever vaccines are widely used to protect domestic animals and laboratory workers. HFRS inactivated vaccine is licensed in Korea, and killed and live, attenuated vaccines are widely used in China. A vaccinia-vector glycoprotein vaccine provides protection against Lassa fever in monkeys.

Prevention of mosquito-borne and tick-borne infections includes use of repellents, tight-fitting clothing that fully covers the extremities, careful examination of the skin after exposure with removal of any vectors found. Diseases transmitted from a rodent-infected environment can be prevented through methods of rodent control; elimination of refuse and breeding sites is particularly successful in urban or suburban areas.

Crimean-Congo hemorrhagic fever, Lassa fever, Marburg disease, and Ebola hemorrhagic fever may be transmitted in hospital settings. Patients should be isolated until they are virus free or for 3 wk after illness. Patients' urine, sputum, blood, clothing, and bedding should be disinfected. Disposable syringes and needles should be used. Prompt and strict enforcement of barrier nursing may be lifesaving. The mortality rate among medical workers contracting these diseases is 50%.

Centers for Disease Control and Prevention: Update: Management of patients with suspected viral hemorrhagic fever. MMWR Morb Mortal Wkly Rep 44:475, 1995.

Fisher-Hoch SP, Platt GS, Neild GH, et al: Pathophysiology of shock and hemorrhage in a fulminating viral infection (Ebola). J Infect Dis 152:887, 1985.

Huggins JW, Hsiang CM, Cosgriff TM, et al: Prospective, double-blind, concurrent, placebo-controlled trial of intravenous ribavirin therapy of hemorrhagic fever with renal syndrome. J Infect Dis 164:1119, 1991.

McCormick JB, King IJ, Webb PA, et al: A case-control study of the clinical diagnosis and course of Lassa fever. J Infect Dis 155:445, 1987.

McCormick JB, King IJ, Webb PA, et al: Lassa fever: Effective therapy with ribavirin. N Engl J Med 314:20, 1986.

CHAPTER 263

Lymphocytic Choriomeningitis Virus

Hal B. Jenson

ETIOLOGY. Lymphocytic choriomeningitis virus is a member of the family Arenaviridae, which are negative-sense single-stranded RNA viruses. The viruses are round, oval, or pleomorphic, averaging 110–130 nm in diameter, with a range from 50–300 nm.

Rodents are the primary reservoir. The virus establishes persistent infection in utero from maternal viremia that occurs in chronically infected rodents, including the common house mouse, *Mus musculus,* and hamsters. The offspring do not develop an effective immune response and excrete virus continuously throughout life in saliva, nasal secretions, semen, milk, urine, and feces.

EPIDEMIOLOGY. The virus has been found in temperate regions of Europe and the Americas. The epidemiology of rodent infection is highly focal. Human cases are sporadic, and are least common during the summer. Outbreaks have been reported after exposure to infected pet hamsters. A serologic survey of adults attending a sexually transmitted disease clinic in Baltimore found that 4.7% of adults had evidence of past infection.

Transmission from rodents to humans is by aerosol, direct contact with rodents or contaminated food and fluids, and infrequently by rodent bites. There is no evidence of chronic infection in humans or of person-to-person transmission.

PATHOGENESIS. Viral infection of rodents is chronic and appears to lead to chronic glomerulonephritis. After inhalation of virus by humans, there is pulmonary and hilar lymph node viral replication with viremia within 48 hr. The liver, spleen, and lymph nodes are most affected and show lymphoid hyperplasia. The kidneys, heart, skeletal muscle, epididymis, and other organs may show mononuclear infiltration.

CLINICAL MANIFESTATIONS. Infection in humans is inapparent in approximately one third of cases. Symptomatic cases may include a nonspecific flulike illness that is unrecognized as lymphocytic choriomeningitis virus infection, or may be characterized by lymphocytic meningitis or meningoencephalitis of varying severity. The classic course is a biphasic illness with usually 3–5 days of nonspecific illness with fever, malaise, myalgias, nausea and vomiting, sore throat and cough, lymphadenopathy, and occasionally a maculopapular rash. There is defervescence for 2–4 days followed by recurrence of fever and headache. In a small proportion of patients, signs of meningoencephalitis develop, sometimes without the prodromal symptoms. The cerebrospinal fluid pressure is elevated, and shows elevated protein (50–300 mg/dL) with several hundred lymphocytes per microliter. There may be papilledema. Transverse myelitis has also been reported. Extraneural manifestations include arthritis, parotitis, orchitis, rash, and myocarditis.

Leukopenia and thrombocytopenia are typical. There are no associated bleeding diatheses, as occur with other arenaviruses (Junin, Machupo, Guanarito, and Lassa) that are associated with viral hemorrhagic fevers (Chapter 262).

Congenital Infection. Lymphocytic choriomeningitis virus has infrequently caused human congenital infection. Only one half of mothers relate illnesses compatible with lymphocytic choriomeningitis virus during pregnancy, usually with only flulike symptoms but occasionally compatible with aseptic meningitis. Only one quarter of mothers have known exposure to rodents.

The affected offspring typically have chorioretinitis, encephalomalacia, microcephaly, hydrocephalus, punctate intracranial calcifications, and developmental delay. The neonatal presentation is similar to congenital cytomegalovirus and toxoplasmosis, but typically without hepatosplenomegaly, and should be considered if there is a history of maternal rodent exposure. Other ophthalmologic manifestations may include optic atrophy, microphthalmia, vitreitis, leukokoria, and cataracts. Unlike congenital cytomegalovirus infection, hearing loss has not been reported.

The cerebrospinal fluid shows a mild pleocytosis (< 70 white blood cells/μL) and mildly elevated protein (average of 67 mg/dL; range of 9–477 mg/dL). CT and MRI reveal encephalomalacia, ventricular enlargement, and calcifications (by CT) adjacent to the lateral ventricles or in the periventricular white matter.

DIAGNOSIS. The diagnosis is usually suspected by the clinical manifestations after exposure to rodents. Serologic tests using immunofluorescent antibody and enzyme-linked immunosorbent assay methods are available and can confirm the clinical diagnosis. The virus can also be isolated from the blood and cerebrospinal fluid during the first week of illness.

TREATMENT. There is no specific treatment for lymphocytic choriomeningitis virus. Ribavirin is active against lymphocytic choriomeningitis virus and other arenaviruses in vitro. Supportive care includes headache control and intravenous hydration, if necessary.

PROGNOSIS. The illness is usually self-limited without sequelae. Hydrocephalus, probably resulting from arachnoidal and ependymal inflammation, is a characteristic complication of congenital infection, and has also been reported rarely after lymphocytic choriomeningitis virus infection in older children and adults.

PREVENTION. Minimizing direct contact with the rodent hosts, especially excreta, is the best means of prevention. This precaution is especially important for pregnant women and should be emphasized. The prevalence of lymphocytic choriomeningitis virus in laboratory animals and household pets, primarily hamsters, is variable and depends on the breeding and handling conditions. Routine monitoring is not uniformly practiced or mandated.

Barton LL, Budd SC, Morfitt WS: Congenital lymphocytic choriomeningitis virus infection in twins. Pediatr Infect Dis J 12:942, 1993.
Biggar RJ, Woodall JP, Walter PD, et al: Lymphocytic choriomeningitis outbreak associated with pet hamsters: Fifty-seven cases from New York State. JAMA 232:494, 1975.
Childs JE, Glass GE, Ksiazek TG, et al: Human-rodent contact and infection with lymphocytic choriomeningitis and Seoul viruses in an inner city population. Am J Trop Med Hyg 41:117, 1991.
Deibel R, Woodall JP, Decher WJ, Schryver GD: Lymphocytic choriomeningitis virus in man. Serologic evidence of association with pet hamsters. JAMA 232:501, 1975.
Farmer TW, Janeway CA: Infection with the virus of lymphocytic choriomeningitis. Medicine (Baltimore) 21:1, 1942.
Larsen PD, Chartrand SA, Tomashek KM, et al: Hydrocephalus complicating lymphocytic choriomeningitis virus infection. Pediatr Infect Dis J 12:528, 1993.
Wright R, Johnson D, Neumann M, et al: Congenital lymphocytic choriomeningitis virus syndrome: A disease that mimics congenital toxoplasmosis or cytomegalovirus infection. Pediatrics 100(1):E9, 1997.

CHAPTER 264
Hantaviruses

Scott Halstead

In June 1993, a newly recognized hantavirus was identified as the etiologic agent of an outbreak of severe respiratory illness in the southwestern United States. Now called the hantavirus pulmonary syndrome (HPS), more than 200 cases have been identified from 25 states, Canada, and several countries in South America caused by at least five distinct hantaviruses. HPS is characterized by a febrile prodrome followed by the rapid onset of noncardiogenic pulmonary edema and hypotension or shock. More than half of identified patients have died.

ETIOLOGY. Hantaviruses are a genus in the family *Bunyaviridae*, which are lipid-enveloped viruses with a negative-stranded RNA genome composed of three unique segments. Several pathogenic viruses that have been recognized within the genus include Hantaan virus, which causes the most severe form of hemorrhagic fever with renal syndrome (HFRS) seen primarily in mainland Asia; Dobrava virus, which causes the most severe form of HFRS seen primarily in the Balkans; Puumala virus, which causes a milder form of HFRS with a high proportion of subclinical infections and is prevalent in northern Europe; and Seoul virus, which results in moderate HFRS and is transmitted predominantly in Asia by urban rats or worldwide by laboratory rats. Prospect Hill virus, a hantavirus that is widely disseminated in U.S. meadow voles, is not known to cause human disease.

Most cases of HPS have been associated with Sin Nombre virus, isolated originally from deer mice *(Peromyscus maniculatus)* in New Mexico. All HPS agents to date belong to a single genetic group of hantaviruses and are associated with rodents of the family *Muridae*, subfamily *Sigmodontinae*. These rodent species are restricted to the Americas, suggesting that HPS may be a Western Hemisphere disease.

EPIDEMIOLOGY. Persons acquiring HPS generally have a history of recent outdoor exposure or live in an area with large populations of deer mice. Clusters of cases have occurred among individuals who have cleaned houses that were rodent infested. *P. maniculatus* is one of the most common North American mammals and, where found, is frequently the dominant member of the rodent community. About half of cases occur between the months of May and July. Patients are almost exclusively from the 12- to 70-yr age range; 60% of patients are 20–39 yr of age. Rare cases are reported in children younger than 12 yr. Two thirds of patients are males, probably reflecting greater outdoor activities. It is not known whether almost complete absence of disease in young children is a reflection of innate resistance or simply lack of exposure. Evidence of human transmission has been obtained in Argentine outbreaks.

Hantaviruses do not cause apparent illness in their reservoir hosts, which remain asymptomatically infected for life. Infected rodents shed virus in saliva, urine, and feces for many weeks, but the duration of shedding and the period of maximum infectivity are unknown. The presence of infectious virus in saliva, the sensitivity of these animals to parenteral inoculation with hantaviruses, and field observations of infected rodents indicate that biting is important for rodent-to-rodent transmission. Aerosols from infective saliva or excreta of rodents are implicated in the transmission of hantaviruses to humans. Persons visiting animal care areas housing infected rodents have been infected after exposure for as little as 5 min. It is possible that hantaviruses are spread through contaminated food and breaks in skin or mucous membranes; transmission to humans has occurred by rodent bites. Person-to-person transmission is distinctly uncommon but has been documented in Argentina.

PATHOGENESIS. HPS is characterized by sudden and catastrophic pulmonary edema, resulting in anoxia and acute heart failure. The virus is detected in pulmonary capillaries, suggesting that pulmonary edema is the direct consequence of virus-induced capillary damage.

CLINICAL MANIFESTATIONS. The HPS is characterized by a prodrome and a cardiopulmonary phase. The mean duration after the onset of prodromal symptoms to hospitalization is 5.4 days. The mean duration of symptoms to death is 8 days (median of 7 days; range of 2–16 days). The most common prodromal symptoms are fever and myalgia (100%); cough or dyspnea (76%); gastrointestinal symptoms, including vomiting, diarrhea, and midabdominal pain (76%); and headache (71%). The cardiopulmonary phase is heralded by progressive cough and shortness of breath. The most common initial physical findings are tachypnea (100%), tachycardia (94%), and hypotension (50%). Rapidly progressive acute pulmonary edema, anoxemia, and shock develop in most severely ill patients. The clinical course of the illness in patients who die is characterized by pulmonary edema accompanied by severe hypotension, frequently terminating in sinus bradycardia, electromechanical dissociation, ventricular tachycardia, or fibrillation. Hypotension may be progressive even with adequate oxygenation.

DIAGNOSIS. The diagnosis of HPS should be considered in a previously healthy patient presenting with a febrile prodrome and acute respiratory distress. Occurrence of thrombocytopenia with the febrile prodrome and outdoor exposure in the spring and summer months are strongly suggestive of HPS. Specific diagnosis of HPS is made by serologic tests that detect hantavirus immunoglobulin M antibodies. Hantavirus antigen can be detected in tissue by immunohistochemistry and amplification of hantaviral nucleotide sequences detected by reverse transcriptase polymerase chain reaction. The state health department or the Centers for Disease Control and Prevention should be consulted to assist in diagnosis, epidemiologic investigations, and outbreak control.

Laboratory Findings. Laboratory findings include leukocytosis (median of 26,000 cells/μL), an increased hematocrit (resulting from hemoconcentration), thrombocytopenia (median of 64,000/μL), prolonged prothrombin and partial thromboplastin times, elevated serum lactate dehydrogenase concentration, decreased serum protein concentrations, and proteinuria.

Differential Diagnosis. The differential diagnosis includes adult respiratory distress syndrome, pneumonic plague, psittacosis, severe mycoplasmal pneumonia, influenza, leptospirosis, inhalation anthrax, rickettsial infections, pulmonary tularemia, atypical bacterial and viral pneumoniae, legionellosis, meningococcemia, and other sepsis syndromes.

TREATMENT. Management of patients with hantavirus infection requires maintenance of adequate oxygenation and careful monitoring and support of cardiovascular function. The pathophysiology of HPS resembles that of dengue shock syndrome (see Chapter 260). Pressor or inotropic agents should be administered in combination with judicious volume replacement to treat symptomatic hypotension or shock while avoiding exacerbating the pulmonary edema. Intravenous ribavirin, which is lifesaving if given early in the course of HFRS, has been shown to be of no value in HPS.

Further information and advice about management, control measures, diagnosis, and collection of biohazardous specimens can be obtained from Centers for Disease Control and Prevention, National Center for Infectious Diseases, Special Pathogens Branch, Atlanta, Georgia 30333 (404-639-1115).

PROGNOSIS. Patient fatality rates are about 50%. Severe abnormalities in hematocrit, white blood cell count, lactate dehydrogenase, and partial thromboplastin time predict mortality with high specificity and sensitivity.

PREVENTION. Avoiding contact with rodents is the only preventive strategy. Rodent control in and around the home is important. Biosafety level 2 facilities and practices are recommended for laboratory handling of blood, body fluids, and tissues from suspect patients or rodents because the virus may be aerosolized. Barrier nursing is advised.

Armstrong LR, Bryan RT, Sarisky J, et al: Mild hantavirus disease caused by Sin Nombre virus in a four-year-old-child. Pediatr Infect Dis J 12:1108, 1995.

Bryan RT, Doyle TJ, Moolenaar RL, et al: Hantavirus pulmonary syndrome in children. Semin Pediatr Infect Dis 8:1, 1997.

Centers for Disease Control and Prevention: Hantavirus pulmonary syndrome: United States, 1995 and 1996. MMWR Morb Mortal Wkly Rep 45:291, 1996.

Centers for Disease Control and Prevention: Laboratory management of agents associated with hantavirus pulmonary syndrome: Interim biosafety guidelines. MMWR Morb Mortal Wkly Rep 43(RR-7):1, 1994.

Childs JE, Ksiazek TG, Koster FT, et al: Serologic and genetic identification of *Peromyscus maniculatus* as the primary rodent reservoir for a new hantavirus in the southwestern United States. J Infect Dis 169:1271, 1994.

Hughes JM, Peters CJ, Cohen ML, et al: Hantavirus pulmonary syndrome: An emerging infectious disease. Science 262:850, 1994.

Khan AS, Khabbaz RF, Armstrong LR, et al: Hantavirus pulmonary syndrome: The first 100 U.S. cases. J Infect Dis 173:1297, 1996.

CHAPTER 265
Rabies

William G. Adams

Human rabies is a viral infection of the central nervous system usually transmitted by contamination of a wound with saliva from a rabid animal. Rabies transmission can be prevented with postexposure prophylaxis; however, the disease is virtually 100% fatal once symptoms develop.

ETIOLOGY. Rabies virus is a member of the family *Rhabdoviridae*. Rabies and several closely related rabies-like viruses are classified in the genus *Lyssavirus*. Rabies-related viruses are found in Europe and Africa and are relatively rare. The viral particles resemble striated bullets, 70–85 nm in diameter and 130–380 nm in length. They have a lipid-containing envelope with a helical nucleocapsid containing one molecule of the negative-sense single-stranded RNA genome. The envelope contains a glycoprotein that elicits neutralizing antibodies and acts as a protective antigen in animal experiments.

EPIDEMIOLOGY. Rabies infection occurs in warm-blooded animals throughout the world. In the United States, rabies occurs principally in skunks, raccoons, foxes, and bats. Skunks are the principal vectors in the Midwest, Southwest, and California, with distinct northern and southern virus strains. Raccoon rabies is now found throughout the eastern United States. Fox rabies is found in Alaska and the northeastern United States, with a separate strain in the Southwest. Bat rabies is found in practically every state. In Central and South America, dogs are the usual source of exposure. Vampire bats, which bite cattle, are an important part of the cycle of rabies in Latin America. Europe has had an epizootic of fox rabies. In Asia and Africa, the principal problem is the rabid dog.

The production of numerous monoclonal antibodies to rabies virus strains has revealed considerable antigenic variation in both the glycoprotein and nucleocapsid antigens of the virus. The result has been the identification of variant strains (called rabies-related viruses) and antigenic differences among true rabies virus that correlate with host species or geographic location. Strains isolated from cattle rabies in South America resemble bat strains, confirming the transmission of virus from the vampire bat to the cow.

The existence of rabies-free land areas permits health authorities in certain locations to omit postexposure prophylaxis of humans after most dog bites on the grounds that terrestrial rabies has been unknown there for years. The continent of Australia and many islands, including those of the United Kingdom and Hawaii, are free of rabies.

Human rabies is a rare disease in the United States and western Europe, where domestic animals are routinely vaccinated and animal control efforts have been successful. Most human cases in these areas are imported from other countries or follow bat exposure. Regrettably, rabies continues to be a major public health problem in areas where dogs are not controlled. Human rabies occurs routinely in India, Southeast Asia, and Africa. The annual global incidence of human rabies is unknown, but is likely between 40,000 and 100,000 cases. Children are at particularly high risk for rabies exposure and infection because of their shorter stature, fearlessness of animals, and inability to protect themselves.

Transmission. In animals, as in humans, rabies produces encephalitis as the principal symptom followed by spread of virus down nerves away from the brain. It multiplies in many organs, but those most important to transmission are the salivary glands. However, not all rabid animals have virus in the saliva, and even when it is present, the quantity is variable. The incubation period for rabies in infected dogs is variable, from 14–180 days. However, viral shedding in saliva of dogs occurs for only 3–6 days before visible symptoms begin. Rabies transmission to humans from dogs that appeared normal for 10 days or more after a biting incident has not been reported. The variability of virus in saliva explains the low transmissibility; less than half of untreated bites by proven rabid animals will result in rabies.

Transmission of rabies can also occur from nonbite exposures. Scratches by the claws of rabid animals are dangerous because animals lick their claws. Saliva applied to a mucosal surface such as the conjunctiva may be infectious. Furthermore, several cases of human rabies in the United States appear to have been caused by bats without any visible sign of direct contact. Bat excreta contain enough rabies virus to pose a danger of rabies to those who enter infested caves and inhale aerosols created by bats or with insignificant physical contact. Aerosols of rabies virus inadvertently produced in laboratories are dangerous to laboratory workers. Transmission of rabies by corneal transplant from patients with undiagnosed rabies encephalitis to healthy recipients has been recorded with sufficient frequency to warrant exclusion of donors dead from unexplained neurologic disease. Human-to-human transmission is theoretically possible but is poorly documented and occurs rarely, if at all.

PATHOGENESIS. The means by which rabies virus travels from the wound to the brain are only partially understood. Because the virus attaches to and penetrates cells rapidly in vitro, it is unlikely that it remains dormant in the wound for long periods of time. Although the virus ascends along axons from the distal extremities to the spinal cord, the speed of spread (3 mm/hr) is far too rapid to explain the long incubation period of the disease.

After inoculation with contaminated saliva from a bite or scratch, the virus infects and multiplies in striated muscle cells, to which it attaches via several receptors, probably including the nicotinic acetylcholine receptor. It is hypothesized that antibody, interferon, and other host factors act on the virus as it leaves striated muscle; if these factors are insufficiently protective, virus eventually attaches to the nerve. At this stage, the development of rabies may be inevitable. The possibility that the virus must overcome another barrier in passing from the first infected neuron to other neurons is indicated by electron microscopic studies of the brain, which demonstrate contiguous viral passage from cell to cell.

Rabies virus causes neuronal destruction in the brain stem and medulla. The cerebral cortex is usually normal in the absence of prolonged anoxia before death. The hippocampus, thalamus, and basal ganglia often show neuronal destruction and glial infiltrates. The most severe desease is evident in the pons and the floor of the fourth ventricle. The inspiratory muscle spasms that result in the striking symptom of hydrophobia may be due to destruction of brain stem neurons inhibitory to the neurons of the nucleus ambiguus, which control inspiration. Hydrophobia does not occur in other diseases because only rabies combines brain stem encephalitis with an intact cortex and maintenance of consciousness.

The Negri body, long the pathologic hallmark of rabies, is a cytoplasmic inclusion found in neurons; it consists of clumped viral nucleocapsid. The absence of Negri bodies does not exclude rabies; fluorescent antibody stains of brain sections or smears may be positive in their absence.

CLINICAL MANIFESTATIONS. The incubation period of rabies in humans is extremely variable. Exceptionally long incubation periods have been described, including a 7-yr incubation period that was confirmed by strain identification. Conversely, an incubation period of only 9 days has followed severe exposure. Usually, the incubation period is 20–180 days, with the peak at 30–60 days. The incubation period tends to be shorter in children and in individuals in whom rabies develops despite vaccination.

There is usually a prodromal phase of rabies, lasting 2–10 days. Pain, pruritus, or paresthesia at the site of the wound is common. Nonspecific symptoms such as fever, malaise, headache, anorexia, and vomiting are often seen. The patient may also have apprehension, anxiety, agitation, or depression.

The illness then enters an acute neurologic phase, of either the furious or paralytic variety, which lasts 2–21 days. In the former, *hydrophobia* is a pathognomonic sign. Attempts to swallow liquids, including saliva, result in aspiration into the trachea. Hydrophobia appears to be an exaggerated respiratory tract protective reflex, perhaps mediated by neuronal dysfunction in the brain stem. Eventually, a psychological component exacerbates the spasms, and even the sight of water evokes terror. *Aerophobia* may be present and is considered by some also to be pathognomonic of rabies. Aerophobia is elicited by fanning a current of air across the face, which causes violent spasms of the pharyngeal and neck muscles.

The neurologic picture in the typical case may consist of bursts of hyperactivity, disorientation, and bizarre combative behavior, alternating with periods of lucidity. During the lucid periods, the patient may be aware of what is happening and may be able to articulate his or her fears. The facial expression is one of grim hopelessness. Patients may also complain of pharyngeal pain, difficulty in swallowing, and hoarseness. Seizures are common, perhaps on the basis of hypoxia compounded by hyperventilation.

In about 20% of patients, an ascending symmetric paralysis with flaccidity and decreased tendon reflexes dominates the entire acute phase. This course is particularly common after bat bites. In the remainder of patients, paralysis develops toward the end of the acute neurologic phase.

Some rabid patients experience meningism or even opisthotonos. The cerebrospinal fluid may be normal or may reflect meningeal irritation, with varying elevations of cells (predominantly lymphocytes) and protein. The peripheral white blood cell count often shows a polymorphonuclear leukocytosis.

If the patient does not die of cardiorespiratory arrest during the acute stage, coma ensues. With modern intensive care, life may be prolonged, but numerous complications occur during this stage. Most significant is myocarditis, manifested by hypotension and arrhythmias. Rabies virus has been recovered from the heart, which shows inflammation at autopsy. Also prominent is pituitary dysfunction expressed clinically as either diabetes insipidus or inappropriate secretion of antidiuretic hormone.

Humans infected with rabies are infectious for about 1 wk before onset of symptoms and can continue to be infectious for up to 5 wk afterward.

DIAGNOSIS. Rabies should be suspected in patients with a history of an animal bite or proximity to bats, especially involving wounds complicated by paresthesia or dysesthesia surrounding the wound site, central nervous system changes, hydrophobia, or aerophobia.

Laboratory diagnosis is now possible before death. The virus may be demonstrated by fluorescent antibody stain of smears of corneal epithelial cells or sections of skin from the neck at the hairline. These are sensitive tests because virus migrates down the nerves from the brain, and both the cornea and hair follicles are richly innervated. Autopsy examination of the brains of patients with fatal encephalitis should include fluorescent antibody test for rabies.

Serologic diagnosis is also possible if the patient survives beyond the acute period. Neutralizing antibodies develop eventually in both serum and cerebrospinal fluid and rapidly rise to extremely high levels, usually more than 100 IU/mL. Vaccination, even with potent vaccine, is unlikely to raise titers above 20 IU/mL.

Differential Diagnosis. Any disease in which there is encephalitis may occasionally cause mental status changes and confusion, such as the encephalitides caused by arboviruses, enteroviruses, and herpes simplex. Other diagnoses can usually be set aside with signs of brain stem involvement in a patient whose sensorium is basically clear and who has no signs of a space-occupying lesion. Paralytic rabies may be misdiagnosed as Guillain-Barré syndrome, poliomyelitis, or postrabies vaccine encephalomyelitis. Careful neurologic examination and analysis of the cerebrospinal fluid will distinguish these diagnoses.

The spasms of tetanus may represent a diagnostic dilemma, but trismus is not seen in rabies, and hydrophobia is not seen in tetanus. Botulism (wound or ingestion) will cause paralysis, but the absence of sensorineural changes should exclude rabies.

Perhaps the most confusing differential problem is hysteria in an individual who thinks that he or she has rabies. Normal blood gases and the absence of variation in bizarre behavior suggest pseudorabies.

TREATMENT. There is no specific treatment available. Intensive supportive care is often required but is insufficient for recovery. Therapies with antiviral agents, interferon, and high-dose rabies immunoglobulin have only prolonged the clinical course. It is doubtful that any treatment can affect mortality once the virus has already spread to the brain.

PROGNOSIS. Recovery from symptomatic rabies in humans is extremely rare. Several persons in the United States have survived rabies infection, but all appear to have received rabies vaccine before exposure.

PREVENTION. Primary prevention of rabies infection includes avoiding contact with potentially rabid animals and vaccination of all domestic animals. Special efforts should be made to teach children to avoid wild animals, stray animals, and animals with unusual behavior.

Local Wound Care. Regardless of the decision whether to provide immunoprophylaxis, local wound management after exposure to a potentially rabid animal is important. All postexposure treatment begins with immediate thorough cleansing of all wounds with soap and water. Vigorous cleansing has been shown to effectively prevent infection in countries with endemic rabies. Wounds should be irrigated for at least 10 min, preferably with a virucidal agent such as povidone-iodine. Catheters should be used for irrigation of puncture wounds. If the mechanical trauma of the local treatment is painful, local anesthetics (e.g., lidocaine) may be used to infiltrate the area without adding risk.

Evaluation of Exposures. Human exposure to a potentially rabid animal is considered to be present if the person (1) is bitten or scratched (with penetration of skin) by a potentially rabid animal or (2) has contamination of a scratch, abrasion, mucous membranes, or open wound with potentially infectious material such as saliva or central nervous system tissue from a potentially rabid animal. The evaluation of human exposures to potentially rabid animals can be complex and is often compounded by a high degree of anxiety. The decision to give postexposure rabies prophylaxis should be based on several factors (Table 265–1). The local epidemiology of rabies should be considered. The type of animal is important since some animals such as raccoons, skunks, bats, woodchucks, and unvaccinated domestic animals are more likely to be infected with rabies virus in certain areas than other animals, such as vaccinated dogs and cats or small wild animals such as squirrels or rodents. The availability of the responsible animal for testing or quarantine is an important consideration and can determine whether or not postexposure prophylaxis is necessary. The circumstances around the exposure, namely whether the attack was provoked or unprovoked, can be considered, especially in situations involving animals rarely infected with rabies virus such as squirrels or mice.

Postexposure rabies prophylaxis is indicated for all persons with a history of a bat bite, scratch, or mucous membrane exposure unless the bat is available for testing and is negative for evidence of rabies. Postexposure prophylaxis is appropriate after bat exposure even in the absence of known direct contact, when there is a reasonable probability that such contact occurred, such as when a sleeping person awakes to find a bat in the room or when an adult witnesses a bat in the room with a previously unattended child, mentally disabled person, or intoxicated person.

Evaluation of secondary or indirect exposure can be more difficult than the evaluation of the direct exposures outlined previously. Secondary contact is typically considered to occur when a domestic animal has had direct contact with a potentially rabid animal and a human then handles or is licked by the domestic animal. The factors that should be considered include the interval since the pet's exposure, the ambient

TABLE 265–1 Rabies Postexposure Prophylaxis Guide for the United States

Animal	Evaluation and Disposition of Animal	Postexposure Prophylaxis Recommendations
Dogs, cats, ferrets	Healthy and available for 10-day observation	Should not begin prophylaxis unless signs of rabies develop in animal*
	Rabid or suspected rabid	Immediately vaccinate
	Unknown (e.g., escaped)	Consult public health officials
Skunks, racoons, foxes, most other carnivores; bats	Regarded as rabid unless animal proven negative by laboratory tests†	Consider immediate vaccination
Livestock, small rodents, lagomorphs (rabbits and hares), large rodents (woodchucks and beavers), other mammals	Consider individually	Consult public health officials; bites of squirrels, hamsters, guinea pigs, gerbils, chipmunks, rats, mice, other small rodents, rabbits, and hares almost never require antirabies prophylaxis

Modified from Centers for Disease Control: Human rabies prevention—United States, 1999. Recommendations of the Advisory Committee on Immunization Practices (ACIP). MMWR 48(RR-1):7, 1999.

**During the 10-day holding period, begin postexposure prophylaxis with human rabies immune globulin (HRIG) and rabies vaccine (HDCV, PCEC, or RVA) at first sign of rabies in a dog or cat that has bitten someone. If the animal exhibits clinical signs of rabies, it should be euthanized immediately and tested.*

†The animal should be euthanized and tested as soon as possible. Holding for observation is not recommended. Discontinue vaccine if immunofluorescence test results of the animal are negative.

temperature, and whether the domestic animal's contact with the human involved an open wound or mucous membranes.

Postexposure Prophylaxis. If rabies prophylaxis is to be given after exposure, prevention depends on three complementary means of reducing the risk. Local wound care is designed to kill the virus by mechanical and virucidal action. Passive immunization with human rabies immunoglobulin (HRIG) then provides immediate blockage of attachment of virus to the nerve endings. However, passive antibody ultimately disappears and must be replaced by the active immune response induced by vaccine. The vaccine must not only produce a primary antibody response but also overcome the depressive effect of passive antibody on the immune response. When given according to currently recommended protocols, no failure of combined HRIG and approved rabies vaccine has been reported in the United States.

PASSIVE IMMUNIZATION. Passive antibody is available as HRIG; the two available formulations are considered equivalent. The dose for HRIG is 20 IU/kg with as much as possible of the full dose of HRIG thoroughly infiltrated in the area around and into the wound(s). Any remaining volume should be administered intramuscularly at a site distant from vaccine inoculation. In some countries, rabies antibody is in the form of purified equine immune globulin, which is associated with serum sickness reactions in about 1% of recipients. Anaphylaxis is a rare possibility with the equine product, but tests for hypersensitivity should be carried out in the usual manner (consult package insert). The dose for equine immune globulin is 40 IU/kg delivered in the same manner as for HRIG.

Passive immunization should be performed regardless of the interval between rabies exposure and initial treatment. However, if vaccine was started previously, passive immunization should not be given once 8 days have elapsed. Corticosteroids should be avoided if possible in the treatment of reactions because they cause activation of rabies virus in experimental animals.

ACTIVE IMMUNIZATION. Early rabies vaccines were prepared in the central nervous system of animals. Their antigenicity was poor, and multiple injections were required. As a result, postvaccination encephalitis was a frequent problem. Animal nerve tissue vaccines are still in use in many places in the world, in particular, suckling mouse brain vaccine, which gives fewer neurologic reactions than sheep brain vaccines because it contains less myelin.

The major advance in rabies vaccine was the development of cell culture technology, which permitted the production of concentrated vaccines with high antigenic potency and low contamination with cellular proteins. Thus, immunogenicity was improved, allowing reduced numbers of doses, and adverse reactions were reduced. Three cell culture rabies vaccines are available in the United States: human diploid cell vaccine (HDCV), purified chick embryo cell culture vaccine (PCEC), and rabies vaccine, absorbed (RVA), produced in fetal rhesus diploid cells. Outside the United States, vaccines produced in monkey kidney, chick embryo, duck embryo, and other cultured cells are also available.

For previously unvaccinated persons, the schedule for postexposure vaccination is five doses given intramuscularly in the deltoid on days 0, 3, 7, 14, and 28. The dose is not reduced for children, although the anterolateral thigh can be used instead of the deltoid if necessary. Administration of rabies vaccine in the gluteus muscle has been associated with vaccine failure and is to be avoided. Immune responses to the postexposure schedule are regularly seen by the 14th day. However, for effective postexposure prophylaxis to rabies, it is mandatory to provide passive as well as active immunization.

For previously fully vaccinated persons after rabies exposure, two vaccine doses are given at an interval of 3 days. HRIG is not given.

Determination of postvaccination antibody titers is not needed unless the patient is immunosuppressed or is receiving antimalarial therapy, which may suppress the response.

Adverse reaction rates to cell culture vaccines have been low, and neurologic reactions have been rare because no nerve tissue is present in the cell cultures used to grow the virus. Allergic reactions occur in less than 0.1% of cases after primary vaccination with HDCV, and systemic symptoms such as malaise and fever occur in only 5–15%. Administration of boosters is associated with an allergic reaction rate of up to 6%. Individuals at continued risk of rabies exposure should have antibody titers determined every 2 yr, and if inadequate, should be given a booster dose. The RVA and PCEC vaccines may be useful in those who have reactions to HDCV. Although no controlled study has been done, the efficacy of rabies vaccination is evidently high, judging from the known incidence of disease after untreated bites by infected animals (approximately 15%) and the paucity of vaccine failures. When seen, vaccine failure has usually followed incomplete immunizations schedules.

Preexposure Prophylaxis. Persons at high risk, such as veterinarians, laboratory workers, and travelers going to rabies-enzootic areas, should be immunized. For pre-exposure immunization, a three-dose vaccination schedule is followed, consisting of intramuscular doses (1.0 mL) given on days 0, 7, and 28. HDCV vaccine may alternatively be administered by intradermal doses (0.1 mL) over the deltoid.

Baer GM (ed): The Natural History of Rabies, 2nd ed. Boca Raton, CRC Press, 1991.

Centers for Disease Control and Prevention: Compendium of animals rabies control, 1998. National Association of State Public Health Veterinarians, Inc. MMWR Morb Mortal Wkly Rep 44 (RR-9):1, 1998.

Centers for Disease Control and Prevention: Human rabies prevention—United States, 1999. Recommendations of the Advisory Committee on Immunization Practices (ACIP). MMWR Morb Mortal Wkly Rep 48 (RR-1):1, 1999.

Fishbein DB, Robinson LE: Rabies. N Engl J Med 329:1632, 1993.

Houff SA, Burton RC, Wilson RW, et al: Human-to-human transmission of rabies virus by corneal transplant. N Engl J Med 300:603, 1979.

Krebs JW, Smith JS, Rupprecht CE, et al: Rabies surveillance in the United States during 1996. J Am Vet Med Assoc 211:1525, 1997.

Lontai I: The current state of rabies prevention in Europe. Vaccine 15 (suppl):S16, 1997.

Sureau P, Rollin P, Wiktor TJ: Epidemiologic analysis of antigenic variations of street rabies virus: Detection by monoclonal antibodies. Am J Epidemiol 117:605, 1983.

Tsiang H: Pathophysiology of rabies virus infection of the nervous system. Adv Virus Res 42:375, 1993.

Turner GS: A review of the world epidemiology of rabies. Trans R Soc Trop Med Hyg 70:175, 1976.

CHAPTER 266

Polyomaviruses

Hal B. Jenson

The polyomaviruses, that with the papillomaviruses constitute the *Papovaviridae* family, are small, nonenveloped, double-stranded circular DNA viruses. The two polyomaviruses that infect humans, JC virus and BK virus, share 75% genome homology but are antigenically distinct. Both viruses are tropic for renal epithelium; JC virus also infects brain oligodendrocytes and is the etiologic agent of progressive multifocal leukoencephalopathy (PML), a fatal demyelinating disease. Several million persons in the United States were exposed to simian virus 40, an oncogenic polyomavirus of Asian macaques, from contaminated inactivated poliovirus vaccines administered between 1955 and 1963, without recognized sequelae and with no demonstrable increased risk of cancer.

Approximately one half of children in the United States are infected with BK virus by 3–4 yr of age and with JC virus by 10–14 yr of age, and approximately 60–80% of adults are seropositive for one or both viruses. Infection persists throughout life, with the viruses remaining latent in renal epithelium, oligodendrocytes, and peripheral blood lymphocytes. Reactivation and viruria occur with increased frequency with advancing age and are more common in immunocompromised persons. BK and JC viruria, as detected by polymerase chain reaction (PCR), occurs in 2.6% and 13.2%, respectively, of persons younger than 30 yr and in approximately 9% and 50%, respectively, of persons older than 60 yr.

Reactivation of BK virus and JC virus with asymptomatic viruria occurs in 10–50% of bone marrow transplant patients and in 20% of renal transplant patients. The direct cytopathic effect of reactivated BK virus on donor ureter has caused localized ureteral ulceration and ureteral stenosis in a few renal transplant patients. BK virus has also been associated with prolonged hemorrhagic cystitis in bone marrow transplant recipients.

PML is a rare central nervous system demyelinating disease resulting from viral lytic infection of myelin-producing oligodendrocytes and an abortive infection of astrocytes. It occurs almost exclusively in immunocompromised persons. More than one half of cases occur in HIV-infected persons, and PML is found in approximately 5% of autopsied AIDS patients. PML characteristically presents with motor weakness, visual field deficits (typically a homonymous hemianopsia), and speech and cognitive impairment (dementia, confusion, personality change). Less frequent symptoms include ataxia, cranial nerve deficits, and extrapyramidal symptoms. The brain shows multifocal, asymmetric, coalescing focal demyelination of white matter with a characteristic cytologic appearance of hyperchromatic enlarged oligodendroglial nuclei and bizarre astrocytes with enlarged multilobulated nuclei. The lesions on CT scan appear as hypodense, nonenhancing focal lesions without surrounding edema or inflammation. On MRI the lesions are hyperintense on T2 weighted images. The cerebrospinal fluid (CSF) is typically normal, but may show mild elevation of protein and less frequently a mononuclear pleocytosis, usually less than 25 cells/μL. JC virus DNA may be detected by PCR in the CSF. Confirmation of the diagnosis requires brain biopsy for histopathologic examination. Patients rapidly experience severe neurologic deficits, including cortical blindness and quadriparesis, with death ensuing usually within 6 months of initial presentation. There is no specific treatment.

Polyomavirus sequences have been identified in human tumors, including osteosarcomas, mesotheliomas, and brain tumors (ependymomas, glioblastomas, oligodendrogliomas, and others). The etiologic role of these viruses in human oncogenesis remains uncertain.

Bergsagel DJ, Finegold MJ, Butel JS, et al: DNA sequences similar to those of simian virus 40 in ependymomas and choroid plexus tumors of childhood. N Engl J Med 326:988, 1992.

Elsner C, Dorries K: Evidence of human polyomavirus BK and JC infection in normal brain tissue. Virology 191:72, 1992.

Strickler HD, Rosenberg PS, Devesa SS, et al: Contamination of poliovirus vaccines with simian virus 40 (1955–1963) and subsequent cancer rates. JAMA 279:292, 1998.

Sundsfjord A, Flaegstad T, Flø R, et al: BK and JC viruses in human immunodeficiency virus type 1-infected persons: Prevalence, excretion, viremia, and viral regulatory regions. J Infect Dis 1994; 169:485–490.

Tornatore C, Amemiya K, Atwood W, et al: JC virus: Current concepts and controversies in the molecular biology and pathogenesis of progressive multifocal leukoencephalopathy. Rev Med Virol 4:197, 1994.

CHAPTER 267
*Transmissible Spongiform Encephalopathies**

David M. Asher

The transmissible spongiform encephalopathies (TSEs), or slow infections of the human nervous system, consist of at least three diseases of humans (Table 267–1): kuru; Creutzfeldt-Jakob disease (CJD) with its variants—sporadic CJD (sCJD), familial CJD (fCJD), iatrogenic CJD (iCJD), new-variant CJD (vCJD), and the Gerstmann-Sträussler-Scheinker syndrome (GSS); and fatal familial insomnia syndrome (FFI), which was recently added to the list of human TSEs. TSEs also affect animals; the most common and best known TSEs of animals are scrapie in sheep and bovine spongiform encephalopathy ("mad cow disease") (BSE) in cattle. All TSEs have similar clinical manifestations and histopathology, and all are "slow" infections: infections with very long asymptomatic incubation periods of at least a year, typical duration of several months or more, and disease restricted to the nervous system. The most striking neuropathologic change that occurs in each TSE (possibly excepting FFI), to a greater or lesser extent, is spongy degeneration of the cerebral cortical gray matter.

ETIOLOGY. The TSEs are transmissible to susceptible animals by inoculation of tissues from affected subjects. Although the infectious agents replicate in some cell cultures, they do not achieve the high titers of infectivity found in brain tissues or cause recognizable cytopathic effects in cultures. Most studies of TSE agents have utilized in vivo assays, using the appearance of typical neurologic disease in animals as evidence that the agent was present and intact. Inoculation of susceptible recipient animals with small amounts of infectious TSE agent results, months later, in the accumulation in tissues of large amounts of agent with the same physical and biologic properties as the original agent. The TSE agents display a spectrum of extreme resistance to inactivation by a variety of chemical and physical treatments that is unknown among conventional pathogens. This characteristic, as well as their partial sensitivity to protein-disrupting treatments and their habitual association with an abnormal amyloid protein stimulated the hypothesis that the TSE agents are probably subviral in size, composed of protein, and devoid of nucleic acid.

In 1982, S. B. Prusiner suggested the term *prion* as an appropriate name for such agents. The prion hypothesis, in its most recent form, proposes that the molecular mechanism by which

*All material in this chapter is in the public domain, with the exception of any borrowed figures or tables.

TABLE 267–1 Transmissible Spongiform Encephalopathies (TSEs; Prion Diseases) of Humans and Animals

Disease	Naturally Infected Hosts
Creutzfeldt-Jakob disease (CJD)	Humans
Sporadic CJD	
Familial CJD	
Iatrogenic CJD	
New-variant CJD (vCJD)	
Gerstmann-Straussler-Scheinker syndrome	Humans
Fatal familial insomnia syndrome	Humans
Kuru	Humans
Bovine spongiform encephalopathy ("mad cow" disease)	Cattle, zoo ungulates; zoo felines, domestic cats*
Chronic wasting disease	American deer, elk
Scrapie	Sheep, goats
Transmissible mink encephalopathy	Mink

**Some authorities classify the new TSE of house cats and felines in zoos as feline spongiform encephalopathy.*

the pathogen-specific information of TSE agents is propagated involves a self-replicating change in the folding of a host-encoded protein associated with a transition from an α-helix–rich structure in the native protease-sensitive conformation toa β-sheet–rich structure in the protease-resistant conformation associated with infectivity. The existence of a second host-encoded protein—a protein X that participates in the transformation—was also postulated to explain certain otherwise puzzling findings.

The prion hypothesis has been widely accepted and was recognized by the awarding of the Nobel Prize in physiology and medicine to Prusiner in 1997. However, the prion hypothesis has not been universally accepted; it relies on the postulated existence of a genome-like coding mechanism based on differences in protein folding that have not been satisfactorily explained at a molecular level. In addition, it has yet to account for the many biologic strains of TSE agent that have been observed. It fails to explain why pure prion protein uncontaminated with nucleic acid from an uninfected host has not transmitted a typical spongiform encephalopathy associated with a serially self-propagating agent. If the TSE agents ultimately prove to consist of protein and only protein, without any nucleic acid component, then the term prion will indeed be appropriate. If the agents are ultimately found to contain small nucleic acid genomes, then they might better be considered atypical viruses for which the term *virino* has been suggested. Until the actual molecular structure of the infectious TSE pathogens and the presence or absence of a nucleic acid genome are rigorously established, it seems less contentious to continue calling them TSE agents.

The first evidence that abnormal proteins are associated with the TSE was morphologic: Scrapie-associated fibrils (SAFs) were found in extracts of tissues from a variety of patients and animals with spongiform encephalopathies but not in normal tissues. SAFs resemble but are distinguishable from the amyloid fibrils that accumulate in the brains of patients with Alzheimer's disease. A group of antigenically related, protease-resistant proteins, designated PrP^{Sc} (scrapie-type prion protein) or PrP-res, proved to be components of SAF and to be present in the amyloid plaques found in the brains of patients and animals with TSE.

It is not yet clear whether PrP-res constitutes the complete infectious particle of spongiform encephalopathies or a component of those particles, or is simply a pathologic host protein not usually separated from the actual infectious entity by currently used techniques. The demonstration that PrP is encoded by a normal host gene seemed to favor the last possibility. However, several studies have suggested that agent-specific pathogenic information can be transmitted and replicated by different conformations of a protein with the same primary amino acid sequence in the absence of agent-specific nucleic acids. (Properties of two fungal proteins were found to be heritable without encoding in nucleic acid, although those properties have not been transmitted to recipient fungi as infectious elements.) Whatever its relationship to the actual infectious TSE particles, PrP clearly plays a central role in infection, because it must be expressed in animals if they are to acquire a TSE or to sustain replication of the infectious agents.

PrPs are glycoproteins; protease-resistant PrPs (variously designated PrP^{Sc} or PrP-res by different authorities) have the physical properties of amyloid proteins. The PrP proteins of several species of animals are very similar in their amino acid sequences and antigenicity, but are not identical in structure. The primary structure of PrP is encoded by the host, and is not altered by the source of the infectious agent provoking its formation. The function of the protease-sensitive PrP precursor (designated PrP^{c} for normal cellular PrP or PrP-sen for protease-sensitive PrP) in normal cells is unknown; it may play some role in normal synaptic transmission but it is not required for life or for relatively normal cerebral function. As noted, expression of PrP is clearly required both for development of scrapie disease and for replication of the transmissible agent in mice. The degree of homology between amino acid sequences of PrPs in different animal species may correlate with the "species barrier" that affects susceptibility of animals of one species to infection with a TSE agent adapted to grow in another species.

Attempts to find particles consistent with those of viruses or virus-like agents in brain tissues of humans or animals with spongiform encephalopathies have generally been unsuccessful. Peculiar tubulovesicles have been seen in thin sections and unique tiny, round particles demonstrated in negatively stained extracts of infected brain tissue. However, it has never been established that either of those structures is associated with infectivity. Using the new technique of representational-fragment analysis, a number of apparently unique nucleic acid sequences were detected in tissues infected with TSE agents; the relationship of those nucleic acids to the infectious agents also remains unknown.

It has been claimed that two other human diseases—*familial Alzheimer disease* of adults and *Alpers disease* of young children—may be caused by infections with agents similar to those causing the spongiform encephalopathies. The latter is a convulsive disorder associated with hemiatrophy and status spongiosus of the cerebral gray matter. Attempts to confirm these claims have failed.

EPIDEMIOLOGY. Kuru once affected many children 4 yr of age and older, adolescents, and young adults living in one area of Papua New Guinea. Transmission of the infection was interrupted more than 40 years ago, and kuru is now recognized only in older adults. The complete disappearance of kuru among young people suggests that the practice of ritual cannibalism was the most important—probably the only—mechanism by which the infection spread in Papua New Guinea.

CJD, the most common human spongiform encephalopathy, was formerly thought to occur only in older adults; however, iCJD and vCJD have affected adolescents and young adults. GSS and FFI have not been diagnosed in children or adolescents. CJD has been recognized worldwide, at rates of 0.25–2 cases/million population/year (not age adjusted), with foci of considerably higher incidence among Libyan Jews in Israel, in isolated villages of Slovakia, and in other limited areas. Epidemiologic surveys have investigated several hypothetical mechanisms of spread of CJD. Person-to-person spread has been confirmed only for iatrogenic cases. The striking resemblance of CJD to scrapie prompted the suggestion that infected sheep tissues might be a source of spongiform encephalopathy in humans. However, so far, no epidemiologic evidence suggests that exposure to potentially scrapie-contaminated animals, meat, meat products, or experimental preparations of the scrapie agent has transmitted a TSE to people. Unfortunately, the same can no longer be said about BSE. The outbreak of BSE among cattle (apparently infected by eating scrapie-contaminated meat and bone meal), ungulate and feline animals in zoos, and domestic cats in Great Britain raised a fear that some strain of the scrapie agent, having crossed the species barrier from sheep to cattle, had acquired a broadened range of susceptible hosts, posing a potential danger for humans. That seems to be the most plausible explanation for the occurrence of vCJD, first recognized in adolescents in 1995 and now affecting more than 35 people in the United Kingdom and 1 person in France. It has long seemed prudent to avoid exposing children to meat or other products likely to be contaminated with any TSE agent; the BSE agent clearly poses a special danger.

Iatrogenic transmission of CJD has been recognized for more than 20 yr (Table 267–2). Accidental transmissions of CJD have occurred by means of contaminated neurosurgical instruments or operating facilities, cortical electrodes contaminated during epilepsy surgery, injections of human cadaveric pitu-

TABLE 267–2 Iatrogenic Transmission of Creutzfeldt-Jakob Disease by Products of Human Origin

Product	No. Patients	Incubation Mean	Incubation Range
Corneal transplants	2	17 mo	16–18 mo
Dura mater allograft†	48	7.4 yr	1.3–16 yr
Human pituitary extract			
Growth hormone	>95*	12 yr	5–30 yr
Gonadotropin	4	13 yr	12–16 yr

Sixteen cases/≈8000 estimated recipients in United States.
†Cases recently recognized in Japan are not included.

itary growth hormone and gonadotropin, and transplantation of contaminated corneas and allografts of human dura mater. Pharmaceuticals and tissue grafts derived from or contaminated with human neural tissues, particularly when obtained from unselected donors and large pools of donors, pose special risks. Although studies of animals experimentally infected with TSE agents suggest that blood and blood products from humans in whom CJD later develops may pose some theoretical risk of transmitting disease to recipients (and such blood products have been withdrawn as a precaution), no epidemiologic study has identified any subject exposed to such products who was later diagnosed with a TSE.

Spouses and household contacts of patients are at very low risk of acquiring CJD, although two instances of conjugal CJD have been reported. However, medical personnel exposed to brains of patients with CJD may be at increased risk; at least 20 health care workers have been recognized with the disease.

PATHOGENESIS. The probable portal of entry for the kuru agent has been thought to be either through the gastrointestinal tract or lesions in the mouth or integument incidentally exposed to the agent during cannibalism. Subjects with vCJD (such as animals with BSE and related infections) are thought to have been similarly infected with the BSE agent through exposure to some contaminated beef product, possibly through the intestinal tract. The first site of replication of the TSE agents appears to be in tissues of the reticuloendothelial system.

The TSE agents have been detected in low titers in blood of experimentally infected animals, mainly associated with nucleated cells; circulating B lymphocytes were found to carry the scrapie agent in experimentally infected mice. Limited evidence suggests that the scrapie agent also spreads to the central nervous system of mice by ascending peripheral nerves. Several researchers claimed to have detected the CJD agent in human blood, although most attempts have failed.

In human kuru, it seems probable that the only portal of exit of the agent from the body, at least in quantities sufficient to infect others, was through infected tissues exposed during cannibalism. In iatrogenically transmitted CJD, the brain and eye of patients with CJD have been the probable sources of contamination. Kidney, liver, lung, lymph node, spleen, and cerebrospinal fluid (CSF) may also contain the CJD agent. At no time during the course of any TSE have antibodies or cell-mediated immunity to the infectious agents been convincingly demonstrated in either patients or animals. However, interesting findings suggest that mice must be immunologically competent to be infected with the scrapie agent by peripheral routes of inoculation.

Typical changes in TSE include vacuolation and loss of neurons with hypertrophy and proliferation of glial cells, most pronounced in the cerebral cortex in patients with CJD and in the cerebellum in those with kuru. The lesions are usually most severe in or even confined to gray matter, at least early in the disease. Loss of myelin appears to be secondary to degeneration of neurons. There generally is no inflammation, but usually a marked increase in the number and size of astrocytes is noted. Status spongiosus is not a striking autopsy finding in patients with FFI, and neuronal degeneration is largely restricted to thalamic nuclei.

"Amyloid" plaques are found in the brains of all patients with GSS and in at least 70% of those with kuru; they are less common in those with CJD. Amyloid plaques are most commonly found in the cerebellum but occur elsewhere in the brain as well. In brains of patients with CJD, plaques surrounded by halos of vacuoles (described as flower-like or "florid" plaques) have been a consistent finding. TSE plaques react with antiserum prepared against PrP, and, even in the absence of plaques, extracellular PrP can be detected in the brain parenchyma by immunostaining.

CLINICAL MANIFESTATIONS. Kuru is a progressive degenerative disease of the cerebellum and brain stem with less obvious involvement of the cerebral cortex. The first sign of kuru is usually cerebellar ataxia followed by progressive incoordination. Coarse, shivering tremors are characteristic. Variable abnormalities in cranial nerve function appear, frequently with impairment in conjugate gaze and swallowing. Patients die from inanition and pneumonia or from burns from cooking fires, usually 1 yr after onset. Although changes in mentation are common, there is no frank dementia or progression to coma, as in CJD. There are no signs of acute encephalitis such as fever, headaches, and convulsions.

CJD occurs throughout the world. Patients initially have either sensory disturbances or confusion and inappropriate behavior, with progression over weeks or months to frank dementia and ultimately coma. Some patients have cerebellar ataxia early in disease, and most experience myoclonic jerking movements. Mean survival of patients with sCJD has been <1 yr from the earliest signs of illness, although about 10% live for 2 yr. New variant CJD (Table 267–3) differs from the more common sporadic CJD: Patients with vCJD are younger at onset, and more often present with complaints of dysesthesia and more subtle behavioral changes than those seen in sCJD. Severe mental deterioration occurs later in the course of vCJD. Patients with vCJD have survived substantially longer than those with sCJD.

GSS is a familial disease resembling CJD but with more prominent cerebellar ataxia and amyloid plaques; dementia may appear only late in the course, and the average duration of illness is longer than that in typical sCJD. FFI is character-

TABLE 267–3 Clinical and Histopathological Features of Patients with New-Variant Creutzfeldt-Jakob Disease (vCJD) and Typical Sporadic CJD

Clinical Feature	New-Variant CJD (10 Patients)	Sporadic CJD (185 Patients)
Mean age at death (yr)*	29 (19–41)	65
Illness duration (mo)*	12 (8–23)	4
Presenting signs	Abnormal behavior, dysesthesia	Dementia
Later signs	Dementia, ataxia, myoclonus	Ataxia, myoclonus
Periodic complexes on electroencephalogram	None	Most
PRNP codon 129 Met/Met	100%	83%
Histopathologic changes	Vacuolation, neuronal loss, astrocytosis, amyloid plaques (100%)	Vacuolation, neuronal loss, astrocytosis, amyloid plaques (≈15%)
Florid PrP plaques†	100%	None
PrP glycosylation pattern	BSE-like‡	Not BSE-like

Modified from Will RG, Ironside JW, Zeidler M, et al: A new variant of Creutzfeldt-Jakob disease in the UK. Lancet 347:921, 1996.
**Median age and duration for vCJD, averages for typical CJD.*
†Dense plaques, pale periphery, surrounded by vacuolated cells.
‡Characterized by an excess of high-molecular-mass-glycoform PrP-res (Collinge et al., 1996).
BSE = bovine spongiform encephalopathy.

ized by progressively severe insomnia and dysautonomia as well as ataxia, myoclonus, and other signs resembling those of CJD and GSS. Neither GSS nor FFI has been diagnosed in children or adolescents.

DIAGNOSIS. Diagnosis of spongiform encephalopathies is most often determined on clinical grounds after excluding other diseases. The presence of 14-3-3 protein in CSF may aid in distinguishing between CJD and Alzheimer's disease, although this is not a consideration in children. Brain biopsy may be diagnostic of CJD, but it can be recommended only if a potentially treatable disease remains to be excluded or if there is some other compelling reason to make a premortem diagnosis. Definitive diagnosis requires microscopic examination of brain tissue obtained at autopsy. The demonstration of protease-resistant PrP proteins in brain extracts has been useful to confirm histopathologic diagnosis. Transmission of disease to susceptible animals by inoculation of brain suspension must be reserved for cases of special research interest.

Laboratory Findings. Virtually all patients with typical sporadic, iatrogenic, and familial forms of CJD have abnormal electroencephalograms (EEGs) as the disease progresses; the background becomes slow and irregular with diminished amplitude. A variety of paroxysmal discharges may also appear—slow waves, sharp waves, spike and wave complexes—and these may sometimes be unilateral or focal as well as bilaterally synchronous. Paroxysmal discharges may be precipitated by loud noise. Many patients have typical periodic suppression-burst complexes of high-voltage slow activity on EEG at some time during the illness. Patients with the vCJD had only generalized slowing, without periodic bursts of high-voltage discharges on EEG. CT may show cortical atrophy and large ventricles late in the course of CJD.

There may be modest elevation of CSF protein content in patients with TSE. Unusual protein spots were observed in CSF specimens after two-dimensional separation in gels and silver staining; the spots were identified as 14-3-3 proteins, normal proteins abundant in neurons but not ordinarily detected in CSF. However, the finding of 14-3-3 protein in CSF is not specific to CJD; it has also been detected in CSF specimens from some patients with acute viral encephalitides and recent cerebral infarctions. In clinical practice, the usual diagnostic problem is to differentiate between CJD and Alzheimer's disease, and the presence of 14-3-3 proteins in CSF militates against the latter. Finding the 14-3-3 protein in CSF has also been of help in confirming the diagnosis of nvCJD. The 14-3-3 protein, thought to have some function in the stabilization of other proteins, is not related to PrP.

TREATMENT. No treatment is effective. Appropriate supportive care should be provided as for other progressive fatal neurologic diseases. On the basis of experimental studies in animals, several prophylactic postexposure treatment regimens have been suggested, but none has been widely accepted.

Genetic Counseling. TSE sometimes occur in families with a pattern of occurrence consistent with an autosomal dominant mode of inheritance. In patients with a family history of CJD, the clinical and histopathologic findings are the same as those seen in sporadic cases. In the United States, only about 10% of cases are familial. GSS and FFI are always familial. In some affected families, about 50% of siblings and children of a patient with a familial TSE eventually acquire the disease; in other families, the "penetrance" of illness may be less.

The gene coding for PrP is closely linked if not identical to that controlling the incubation periods of scrapie in sheep and both scrapie and CJD in mice. The gene encoding the PrP in humans, currently designated the PRNP gene, is located on the short arm of chromosome 20. It has an open reading frame of 759 nucleotides (253 codons), in which more than 10 different point mutations, as well as a variety of inserted sequences encoding extra tandem-repeated octapeptides, have been linked to the occurrence of spongiform encephalopathy in families.

Although the interpretation of these findings in regard to the prion hypothesis is in dispute, in affected families with an autosomal dominant pattern of CJD or GSS, individuals who are heterozygous for linked mutations in the PRNP gene clearly have a high probability of acquiring spongiform encephalopathy. The significance of mutations in the PRNP genes of individuals from families with no history of spongiform encephalopathy is not known. It seems wise to avoid alarming those who have miscellaneous mutations—several of which appear to represent normal polymorphisms—in the PRNP gene and their families because the implications are not yet clear.

The same nucleotide substitution at codon 178 of the PRNP gene associated with CJD in some families has been found in all patients with FFI; however, it is linked to a different amino acid–encoding sequence at codon 129, a site that is polymorphic in normal individuals. Homozygosity for methionine or for valine at codon 129—especially for methionine—seems to increase susceptibility to iCJD and sCJD, although methionine-valine heterozygotes are also susceptible to both diseases. So far, all patients with vCJD to be genotyped have been PRNP codon-129 methionine homozygous.

PROGNOSIS. The prognosis of spongiform encephalopathies is uniformly poor. About 10% of patients may survive for a 1 yr or more, but their quality of life is poor.

PREVENTION. Standard precautions should be used for handling all human tissues, blood, and body fluids. Materials and surfaces known to be contaminated with tissues or fluids from patients suspected of having CJD must be treated with great care. Whenever possible, contaminated instruments should be discarded by careful packaging and incineration. Contaminated tissues and biologic products probably cannot be completely freed of infectivity without destroying their structural integrity and biologic activity; therefore, the medical and family histories of individual tissue donors should be carefully reviewed to exclude a diagnosis of TSE. Where feasible, histopathologic examination of brain tissues of donors and testing for PrP-res should be performed. Although no method of sterilization can be relied on to remove all infectivity from contaminated surfaces, exposure to moist heat, sodium hydroxide, chlorine bleach, concentrated formic acid, and guanidine salts markedly reduces infectivity.

Aguzzi A, Collinge J, Hill AF, et al: Post-exposure prophylaxis after accidental prion inoculation. Lancet 350:1519, 1997.

Asher DM: Slow viral infections of the human nervous system. *In*: Scheld WM, Whitley RJ, Durack DT (eds): Infections of the Nervous System, 2nd ed. New York, Raven Press, 1997, pp 199–221.

Brown P: The "brave new world" of transmissible spongiform encephalopathy (infectious cerebral amyloidosis). Molec Neurobiol 8:79, 1994.

Brown P, Gibbs CJ Jr, Rodgers-Johnson P, et al: Human spongiform encephalopathy: The NIH series of 300 cases of experimentally transmitted disease. Ann Neurol 35:513, 1994.

Bruce ME, Will RG, Ironside JW, et al: Transmissions to mice indicate that "new variant" CJD is caused by the BSE agent. Nature 389:498, 1997.

Chesebro B: BSE and prions: Uncertainties about the agent. Science 279:42, 1998.

Collee JG, Bradley R: BSE: A decade on. Lancet 349:636, 715, 1997.

Collinge J, Sidle KC, Meads J, et al: Molecular analysis of prion strain variation and the aetiology of "new variant" CJD. Nature 383:685, 1996.

Hsich G, Kenney K, Gibbs CJ, et al: The 14-3-3 brain protein in cerebrospinal fluid as a marker for transmissible spongiform encephalopathies. N Engl J Med 335:924, 1996.

Johnson RT, Gibbs CJ Jr: Creutzfeldt-Jakob disease and related transmissible spongiform encephalopathies. N Engl J Med 339: 1994, 1998.

Mestel R: Putting prions to the test. Science 273:184, 1996.

Occupational Safety and Health Administration, U.S. Department of Labor: Occupational Exposure to Bloodborne Pathogens; Final Rule (29 CFR Part 1910.1030). Federal Register USA 56:64175, 1991.

Prusiner SB: Prion diseases and the BSE crisis. Science 278:245, 1997.

Schonberger LB: New variant Creutzfeldt-Jakob disease and bovine spongiform encephalopathy. Infect Dis Clin North Am 12:111, 1998.

van Duijn CM, Delasnerie-Lauprêtre N, Masullo C, et al: Case-control study of risk factors of Creutzfeldt-Jakob disease in Europe during 1993–95. Lancet 351:1081, 1998.

Will RG, Ironside JW, Zeidler M, et al: A new variant of Creutzfeldt-Jakob disease in the UK. Lancet 347:921, 1996.

CHAPTER 268

Acquired Immunodeficiency Syndrome (Human Immunodeficiency Virus)

Ram Yogev and Ellen Gould Chadwick

Recent advances in research and major improvements in the treatment and management of HIV infection have brought about a substantial decrease in the incidence of new infections and AIDS in children born in the United States and western European countries. Most HIV-infected children are born in developing countries. It is estimated that each year almost 400,000 children are newly infected with HIV, and that by the year 2000 as many as 5–8 million children worldwide will be HIV-infected. In addition, because HIV-infected mothers are likely to die of AIDS, between 10 and 15 million children will be orphaned by the beginning of the next century. HIV infection in children progresses more rapidly than in adults, and some children die within the first 2 yr of life. In general, this rapid progression correlates with higher viral burden and faster depletion of infected $CD4^+$ T lymphocytes in infants and children than in adults. Newer diagnostic tests and the availability of potent drugs to inhibit HIV replication have dramatically increased the ability to prevent and control this devastating disease.

ETIOLOGY. HIV types 1 (HIV-1) and 2 (HIV-2) are members of the *Retroviridae* family and belong to the *Lentivirus* genus, which includes cytopathic viruses causing diverse diseases in several animal species. The HIV genome is single-stranded RNA 9.8 kb in size, with identical regions (long terminal repeats) at both ends of the genome that contain important regulatory genes. The remainder of the genome includes three major coding regions (Fig. 268–1). The GAG region encodes the viral core proteins (p24, p17, p9, and p6), which are derived from the precursor p55. The POL region encodes the viral enzymes reverse transcriptase (p51), protease (p10), and integrase (p32). The ENV region encodes the viral envelope proteins gp120 and gp41, which are derived from the precursor gp160. Other regulatory proteins are involved in transcription (TAT [p14]), viral mRNA expression (REV [p19]), viral enhanced infectivity (NEF [p27]), virus release (VPR [p15]), and proviral DNA synthesis (NIF [p23]).

The major external viral protein of HIV is gp120, a heavily glycosylated protein associated with the transmembrane glycoprotein gp41. The gp41 is very immunogenic and is used to detect HIV antibodies in diagnostic assays. The gp120 is a complex molecule that includes the highly variable V3 loop, which is immunodominant for neutralizing antibodies. The heterogeneity of gp120 is the basis for difficulties in developing an effective HIV vaccine. The gp120 also carries the binding site for the $CD4^+$ molecule, the most common host cell surface receptor that is found primarily on helper T lymphocytes. Secondary receptors for attachment have also been identified, including the fusion-inducing molecule, CXCR-4, which has been shown to act as a co-receptor for HIV attachment to lymphocytes, and CCR-5, a β-chemokine receptor, which facilitates HIV entrance into macrophages. Several chemokine receptors (e.g., CCR-3) can also function as co-receptors.

Other less common mechanisms of attachment of HIV to cells include use of non-neutralizing antiviral antibodies. The Fab portion of these antibodies attaches to the virus surface, and the Fc portion binds to cells that express Fc receptors (e.g., macrophages, fibroblasts), thus facilitating virus entry into the cell. The involvement of complement receptors, with or without the Fc receptor, in presenting HIV to cells has also been suggested as a mechanism of attachment. After viral attachment, gp120 and the $CD4^+$ molecule undergo conformational changes, and gp41 interacts with the fusion receptor on the cell surface. Viral fusion with the cell membrane allows entry of viral RNA into the cell's cytoplasm. Viral DNA copies are then transcribed from the virion RNA by viral reverse transcriptase (RNA-dependent DNA polymerase), producing double-stranded circular DNA. The HIV reverse transcriptase is error prone and lacks error-correcting mechanisms. Many mutations arise, creating wide genetic variation of HIV isolates, even in an individual patient. The circular DNA is transported into the nucleus, where it is integrated into chromosomal DNA and referred to as the provirus. The provirus can remain dormant for extended periods. Depending on the relative expression of the viral regulatory genes (e.g., TAT, REV, NEF), the proviral DNA may encode production of the viral RNA genome, which in turn leads to production of viral proteins necessary for viral assembly.

HIV transcription is followed by translation. A capsid polyprotein is cleaved to produce, among others, the virus-specific protease (p10). This enzyme is critical for HIV assembly. Several HIV antiprotease drugs have been developed targeting the increased sensitivity of the viral protease, which differs from the cellular proteases. The RNA genome is then incorporated into the newly formed viral capsid. As the new virus is formed, it buds through the cell membrane and is released.

HIV-2 is a rare cause of infection in children. It is most prevalent in western and southern Africa. The diagnosis of HIV-2 infection is more difficult because the standard antibody assays are HIV-1 specific, and may give indeterminate results in persons with HIV-2 infection. If HIV-2 is suspected, a test that specifically detects antibody to HIV-2 peptides should be used. Disease progression is slower than with HIV-1, but severe immunodeficiency can occur.

EPIDEMIOLOGY. The World Health Organization (WHO) estimated that more than 30 million persons worldwide were living with HIV infection at the end of 1997, 1.1 million of

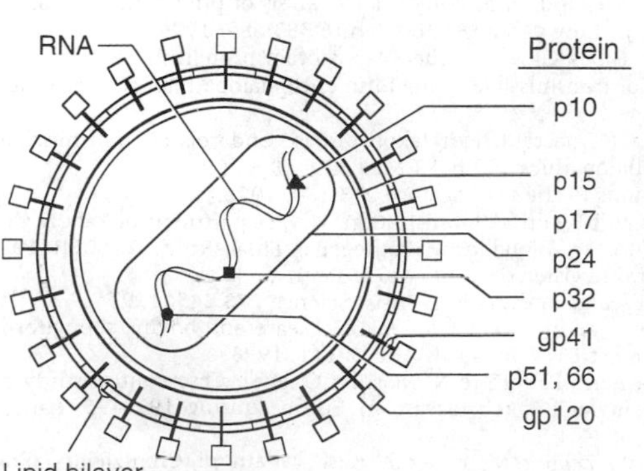

Figure 268–1 Human immunodeficiency virus, its proteins, and their functions.

whom were children younger than 15 yr. In 1997 alone, 5.8 million people acquired HIV and 2.3 million died, including 500,000 children. More than 90% of HIV-infected individuals live in developing nations, where an estimated 350,000 infants are infected through perinatal transmission each year. Sub-Saharan Africa accounts for the fastest growing epidemic, with almost 90% of the world's total population of HIV-infected children. India and Thailand dominate the epidemic in Southeast Asia, with more recent expansion into Vietnam, China, and Cambodia.

Worldwide, 40% of HIV-infected individuals are women, and heterosexual transmission accounts for most HIV spread. In the United States, women account for 23% of reported AIDS cases in 1996. In 1997, the percentage of American women whose exposure category was heterosexual contact (38%) surpassed that of intravenous drug users (32%). However, heterosexual transmission is probably even more common because further investigation of the category "risk not reported or identified" (28%) often leads to reclassification as heterosexual transmission. These are women who have been infected heterosexually by men unrecognized to be infected or to be in a high-risk group. Among mothers giving birth to children with AIDS, heterosexually acquired infection and "risk not reported" are the most common exposure categories, accounting for approximately 80% of the total. The estimated number of children in the United States with AIDS diagnosed each year increased between 1984 and 1992, and then declined by 50% during 1992–1997, despite a relatively stable number of children born to HIV-infected mothers—about 6,000–7,000 children per year—during the latter period. This decline reflects the effectiveness of antiviral prophylaxis in reducing perinatal HIV transmission. Tragically, while the number of HIV-infected infants is decreasing in industrialized nations, the worldwide number of HIV-infected children is increasing dramatically because of lack of funds to provide medications.

In the United States, virtually all HIV infections in children younger than 13 yr are the result of vertical transmission from an HIV-infected mother. A vanishing minority of children was infected through receipt of contaminated blood products or clotting factors (2%), primarily before 1985 when HIV screening of the blood supply was instituted. Children of racial and ethnic minority groups are disproportionally over-represented, particularly non-Hispanic African-Americans and Hispanics. Race and ethnicity are not risk factors for HIV infection per se, but more likely reflect other factors that may be predictive of increased risk for HIV infection, such as lack of educational and economic opportunities and higher rates of injecting drug use. In the United States, the Northeast (44%) and the South (36%) account for most pediatric cases; 85% were diagnosed in metropolitan areas with a population greater than 500,000 persons and 9% in metropolitan areas with populations of 50,000–500,000 persons.

Although adolescents (13–19 yr of age) with AIDS represent only 0.5% of U.S. cases, they constitute one of the fastest growing groups of newly infected persons in the country. Considering the long latency period between the time of infection and the development of clinical symptoms, reliance on AIDS case definition surveillance data severely under-represents the impact of the disease in adolescents. On the basis of a median incubation period of 8–12 yr, it has been estimated that 15–20% of all AIDS cases were acquired between 13 and 19 yr of age. Risk factors for HIV infection vary by gender in adolescents. Whereas 40% of the cumulative number of teenage males with AIDS were infected by contaminated blood or blood products (mostly patients having hemophilia), only 7% of females were infected via this route. As in the adult population, the majority of teenage males with AIDS who acquired HIV through sexual contact had male-to-male transmission. In contrast, more than 50% of adolescent females with AIDS were infected through heterosexual contact and 17% through intravenous drug use compared with 4% and 6%, respectively, in teenage males. As in the pediatric population, adolescent racial and ethnic minority populations are over-represented, especially among females. In addition, a greater proportion of adolescents with AIDS are female (male:female ratio of 1.2:1) than for adults older than 25 yr (male:female ratio of 4.5:1).

Transmission. Transmission of HIV occurs via sexual contact, parenteral exposure to blood, or vertical transmission from mother to child. The primary route of infection in the pediatric population is vertical transmission, accounting for virtually all new cases. Reported rates of transmission of HIV from mother to child have varied; most large studies in the United States and Europe have documented transmission rates in untreated women between 12 and 30%. Reported vertical transmission rates in Africa and Haiti are 25–52%. Perinatal treatment of HIV-infected mothers with antiretroviral drugs has dramatically decreased these rates to less than 8%.

Vertical transmission of HIV can occur before (intrauterine), during (intrapartum), or after (through breast-feeding) delivery. Intrauterine transmission has been suggested by identification of HIV by culture or polymerase chain reaction (PCR) in fetal tissue as early as 10 wk gestation. First-trimester placental tissue from HIV-infected women has been demonstrated to contain HIV by in situ hybridization and immunocytochemistry. It is generally accepted that 30–40% of infected newborns are infected in utero, because this percentage of infants has laboratory evidence of infection (positive viral culture or PCR) within the first week of life. Some studies have found that viral detection soon after birth also correlates with early onset of symptoms and rapid progression to AIDS, consistent with more long-standing infection during gestation.

The highest percentage of HIV-infected children acquire the virus intrapartum, evidenced by the finding that 60–70% of infected infants do not demonstrate detectable virus before 1 wk of age. The mechanism of transmission appears to be exposure to infected blood and cervicovaginal secretions in the birth canal, where HIV is found in high titer during late gestation and at delivery. Furthermore, the international registry of HIV-exposed twins found that first-born twins were three times more likely to be infected, reflecting the longer time that twin A is exposed to maternal secretions in the birth canal.

Several risk factors influence the rate of vertical transmission: preterm delivery (<34 wk gestation), low birth weight, low maternal antenatal $CD4^+$ count (<29%), and intravenous drug use during pregnancy. The single most important variable appears to be more than 4-hr duration of ruptured membranes, which doubles the transmission rate. Cesarean section may confer a protective effect compared with vaginal delivery. A meta-analysis of 15 prospective studies demonstrated that elective cesarean section decreased vertical transmission by 50%. Transmission was reduced by 87% when elective cesarean section was combined with prenatal, intrapartum, and neonatal zidovudine (ZDV) therapy. Importantly, the benefit of cesarean section in these trials was achieved with ZDV monotherapy; the impact of elective cesarean section on transmission in women receiving highly active antiretroviral therapy combination has yet to be determined. Although several studies have shown an overall increased rate of transmission in women with advanced disease (e.g., symptomatic AIDS) or high viral load (>50,000 copies/mL), many transmitting mothers in each series were asymptomatic or had a low viral load.

The least common route of vertical transmission in industrialized nations is breast-feeding; however, this is a very important route of transmission in developing countries. Both cell-associated and cell-free virus have been detected in breast milk from HIV-infected mothers. A meta-analysis of prospective studies found that the increased risk of transmission through breast-feeding in women with HIV infection before pregnancy was 14% compared with a 29% increased risk of transmission in breast-feeding women who acquired HIV postnatally. This suggests that the viremia experienced by the mother during primary HIV infection doubles the risk of transmission by breast-feeding. It, therefore, seems reasonable for women to substitute infant formula for breast milk if they are HIV infected or are at risk for infection from ongoing sexual exposure or intravenous drug use. However, the WHO recommends that in developing countries where other diseases (e.g., diarrhea, pneumonia, and malnutrition) substantially contribute to a high infant mortality rate, the benefit of breast-feeding outweighs the risk of HIV transmission, and HIV-infected women should breast-feed their infants.

Transfusions of contaminated blood or blood products account for 3–6% of all pediatric AIDS cases. The period of highest risk was between 1978 and 1985, before the institution of HIV screening by all blood banks. The prevalence of HIV infection in individuals with hemophilia treated with blood products before 1985 was as high as 70%; HIV screening of blood donors and heat treatment of factor VIII concentrate has virtually eliminated HIV transmission to this group. Blood donor screening has dramatically reduced, but not eliminated, the risk of transfusion-associated HIV infection. The rate of HIV transmission through antibody-screened blood in the United States is estimated to be approximately 1/60,000 transfused units. Unfortunately, in many developing countries screening of blood donors is not uniform, and the risk of transmitting HIV infection via transfusion is substantially higher.

Sexual transmission in the pediatric population is infrequent, but a small number of cases resulting from sexual abuse have been reported. In contrast, sexual contact is a major route of transmission in the adolescent population, being responsible for more than one third of cases.

Although HIV can be isolated rarely from saliva, the titer is very low (< 1 infectious particle/mL), and this has not been implicated as a means of transmission. Studies of hundreds of household contacts of HIV-infected individuals have found that the risk of casual HIV transmission is practically nonexistent. Only a few cases have been reported in which urine and feces have been proposed as possible vehicles of HIV transmission.

PATHOGENESIS. In adults and adolescents, after HIV has entered the circulation, intense viremia ensues, causing flulike symptoms in 50–70% of cases. This primary viremia results in widespread seeding of virus to various organs, including the brain and lymphoid tissues. HIV selectively binds to cells expressing $CD4^+$ molecules on their surface, primarily helper T lymphocytes ($CD4^+$ cells) and cells of the monocyte-macrophage lineage. HIV may also infect other cells bearing $CD4^+$, such as microglia, astrocytes, oligodendroglia, and placental tissue containing villous Hofbauer cells. The $CD4^+$ cells migrate to the lymph nodes, where they become activated and proliferate. This antigen-driven migration and accumulation of $CD4^+$ cells within the lymphoid tissue may contribute to the dramatic decrease in the number of circulating $CD4^+$ cells and the generalized lymphadenopathy characteristic of the *acute retroviral syndrome* in adults and adolescents. With establishment of a cellular and humoral immune response within 2–4 mo, the level of culturable virus from the blood declines substantially, and patients enter a phase characterized by a lack of symptoms and a return of the $CD4^+$ cells to only moderately decreased levels.

Early HIV infection and replication in children have no apparent clinical consequences. Whether tested by virus isolation or by PCR, less than 50% of HIV-infected infants demonstrate evidence of the virus at birth. The virus load increases by 1–4 mo, and almost all HIV-infected infants have detectable HIV in peripheral blood by 4 mo of age.

In adults, the long period of clinical latency, up to 8–12 yr, is not indicative of viral latency. During this seemingly quiescent period, there is a very high turnover of virus and $CD4^+$ cells, more than a billion cells per day, which gradually causes deterioration of the immune system, evidenced particularly by depletion of $CD4^+$ cells. These cells may be destroyed by multiple mechanisms: HIV-mediated single-cell killing, formation of multinucleated giant cells of infected and uninfected $CD4^+$ cells (syncytia formation), virus-specific immune responses, superantigen-mediated activation of T cells (rendering them more susceptible to infection with HIV), and programmed cell death (apoptosis). The viral burden in the lymphoid organs is greater than that in the peripheral blood during the asymptomatic period. As HIV virions and their immune complexes migrate through the lymph nodes, they are trapped in the network of dendritic follicular cells. This trafficking is part of the normal immune response for all antigens to facilitate optimal antigen presentation to competent immune cells; however, because the ability of HIV to replicate in T cells depends on the state of activation of the cells, the immune activation that takes place within the microenvironment of the nodes in HIV disease serves to promote infection of new $CD4^+$ cells as well as subsequent viral replication within the cells. Viral replication in monocytes, which can be infected productively yet resist killing, explains their role as reservoirs of HIV and as effectors of tissue damage in organs such as the brain.

Cell-mediated and humoral responses occur early in the infection. The suppressor T cells ($CD8^+$ cells) play an important role in containing the infection. HIV-specific cytolytic T lymphocytes develop against both the structural (e.g., ENV, POL, GAG) and regulatory (e.g., TAT) viral proteins. In addition, the $CD8^+$ cells release a soluble factor that suppresses viral replication. Neutralizing antibodies appear later during the infection and seem to help in the continued suppression of viral replication during clinical latency. Individual patient differences in the complex immune response directly influence the course of disease.

Several cytokines, including tumor necrosis factor-α (TNF-α), TNF-β, interleukin (IL)-1, IL-3, IL-6, interferon (IFN)-γ, granulocyte-macrophage colony–stimulating factor, and macrophage colony-stimulating factor, play an integral role in upregulating HIV expression from a state of quiescent infection to active viral replication. Other cytokines such as IFN-α, IFN-β, and transforming growth factor D exert a suppressive effect on HIV replication. The local production and interactions among these cytokines, which may not be reflected in plasma cytokine concentrations, influence the concentration of viral particles in the tissues. Even during states of apparent immunologic quiescence, the complex interaction of cytokines sustains a constant level of viral expression, particularly in the lymph nodes.

The progression of disease is related temporally to the gradual disruption of lymph node architecture and degeneration of the follicular dendritic cell network with loss of its ability to trap HIV particles. This frees the virus to recirculate, producing the high levels of viremia seen during the later stages of disease. In addition, biologic properties of HIV also determine the rate of disease progression. Patients with low-replicating, non-syncytium-inducing HIV strains often have the longest symptom-free interval and prolonged survival.

Three distinct patterns of disease have been described in children. From 15–25% of HIV-infected newborns have a rapid disease course, with onset of symptoms and AIDS during the first few months of life and, if untreated, a median survival of 6–9 mo. It has been suggested that, if intrauterine infection coincides with the period of rapid expansion of $CD4^+$ cells in the fetus, this could effectively infect the majority of the immunocompetent cells in the fetus. The normal migration of these cells to the marrow, spleen, and thymus would result in efficient systemic delivery of HIV, unchecked by the immature immune system of the fetus. Thus, widespread infection would be established before the normal ontogenic development of the immune system, causing more severe impairment of immunity. Most children in this group have a positive HIV culture

TABLE 268–1 Pediatric HIV Classification*

Immune Categories	N: No Signs/ Symptoms	A: Mild Signs/ Symptoms	B: Moderate Signs/ Symptoms†	C: Severe Signs/ Symptoms†
1. No evidence of suppression	N1	A1	B1	C1
2. Evidence of moderate suppression	N2	A2	B2	C2
3. Severe suppression	N3	A3	B3	C3

Adapted from Centers for Disease Control and Prevention: 1994 revised classification system for human immunodeficiency virus infection in children less than 13 years of age. MMWR Morb Mortal Wkly Rep 43(RR-12):1, 1994.

**Children whose HIV infection status is not confirmed are classified by using the above grid with a letter E (for perinatally exposed) placed before the appropriate classification code (e.g., EN2).*

†Category C and lymphoid interstitial pneumonitis in category B are reportable to state and local health departments as AIDS.

and/or detectable virus in the plasma in the first 48 hr of life. This evidence of early viral presence suggests that infection occurred in utero. The viral load rapidly increases and peaks by 2–3 mo of age (median of 750,000 copies/mL) and subsequently declines slowly. In contrast to adults, the viral load stays high for at least the first 2 yr of life.

The majority of perinatally infected newborns (60–80%) present with a much slower progression of disease, with a median survival time of 6 yr. Many patients in this group have a negative viral culture or PCR test in the first week of life and are, therefore, considered to be infected intrapartum. The viral load typically increases by 2–3 mo of age (median of 100,000 copies/mL) and slowly declines over a period of 24 mo. The slow decline in viral load is in sharp contrast to the rapid decline after primary infection seen in adults. This observation can be explained only partially by the immaturity of the immune system in newborns and infants.

The third pattern of disease involves the long-term survivors, which occurs in a small percentage (<5%) of perinatally infected children who have minimal or no progression of disease with relatively normal $CD4^+$ counts and very low viral loads for more than 8 yr.

HIV-infected children have similar changes in the immune system as HIV-infected adults. Depletion of $CD4^+$ cells may be less dramatic because infants normally have a relative lymphocytosis. Lymphopenia is relatively rare in perinatally infected children and is usually only found in older children and those with end-stage disease. Although cutaneous anergy is common during HIV infection, it is also frequent in normal children younger than 1 yr; thus, its interpretation is difficult in HIV-infected infants.

B-cell activation occurs in most children early in the infection, as evidenced by hypergammaglobulinemia (> 1.750 g/L) with high levels of anti-HIV antibody. This response may reflect both dysregulation of T-cell suppression of B-cell antibody synthesis and active $CD4^+$ cell enhancement of B-lymphocyte humoral response. Specific antibody production may not occur and if present, may not be protective. Because hypergammaglobulinemia is so common in HIV-infected children, it may serve as a surrogate marker of HIV infection in symptomatic children in whom specific diagnostic tests are not available or too expensive. Hypogammaglobulinemia is very rare (<1%).

Central nervous system involvement is more common in pediatric patients than in adults. Macrophages and microglia play an important role in HIV neuropathogenesis; astrocytes may also be involved. Although the specific mechanisms for encephalopathy in children are not yet clear, the developing brain in young infants, with its delayed myelinization, appears to be more vulnerable to invasion by HIV.

CLINICAL MANIFESTATIONS. The clinical manifestations of HIV infection vary widely among infants, children, and adolescents. In the majority of infants, physical examination at birth is normal. Initial symptoms may be subtle, such as lymphadenopathy and hepatosplenomegaly, or nonspecific, such as failure to thrive, chronic or recurrent diarrhea, interstitial pneumonia, or oral thrush; symptoms may be distinguishable only by their persistence. Whereas systemic and pulmonary findings are common in the United States and Europe, chronic diarrhea, wasting, and severe malnutrition predominate in Africa. Symptoms found more commonly in children than adults with HIV infection include recurrent bacterial infections, chronic parotid swelling, lymphocytic interstitial pneumonitis (LIP), and early onset of progressive neurologic deterioration.

The HIV classification system used to categorize the stage of pediatric disease includes two parameters: clinical status and degree of immunologic impairment (Table 268–1). Among the clinical categories, category A (mild symptoms) includes children with at least two mild symptoms such as lymphadenopathy, parotitis, hepatomegaly, splenomegaly, dermatitis, and recurrent or persistent sinusitis or otitis media. Category B (moderate symptoms) includes, for example, children with any of the following: LIP; oropharyngeal thrush persisting for more than 2 mo; recurrent or chronic diarrhea; persistent fever for more than 1 mo; hepatitis; recurrent herpes simplex virus stomatitis, esophagitis, or pneumonitis; disseminated varicella with visceral involvement; cardiomegaly; or nephropathy. Category C (severe symptoms) includes, for example, children with two serious bacterial infections (e.g., sepsis, meningitis, pneumonia) in a 2-yr period, esophageal or lower respiratory tract candidiasis, cryptococcosis, cryptosporidiosis (>1 mo duration), encephalopathy, malignancies, disseminated mycobacterial infection, *Pneumocystis carinii* pneumonia, cerebral toxoplasmosis (onset after 1 mo of age), and severe weight loss.

The immune classification is based on the absolute $CD4^+$ counts or the percentage of $CD4^+$ cells (Table 268–2). Age adjustment of the absolute $CD4^+$ count is necessary because $CD4^+$ counts are relatively high in normal infants and then decline steadily until 6 yr of age, when they reach adult levels. If there is a discrepancy between the $CD4^+$ count and percentage, the disease is classified into the more severe category. Once a child has met the definition of severe immunosuppression, he or she is henceforth always considered severely immunosuppressed.

Opportunistic infections are generally seen with severe depression of the $CD4^+$ count. In adults, these secondary infections usually represent reactivation of a latent infection acquired early in life. In contrast, young children generally have primary infection with these organisms, and, lacking prior

TABLE 268–2 Centers for Disease Control and Prevention Revised Pediatric HIV Classification: Immunologic Categories Based on $CD4^+$ Counts and Percentage of Total Lymphocytes

	<12 Months		1–5 Years		≥6 Years	
Category	Cells/µL	%	Cells/µL	%	Cells/µL	%
No evidence of immunosuppression	≥1,500	≥25	≥1,000	≥25	≥500	≥25
Evidence of moderate immunosuppression	750–1,499	15–24	500–999	15–24	200–499	15–24
Severe immunosuppression	<750	<15	<500	<15	<200	<15

immunity, often have a more fulminant course. This principle is best illustrated by *P. carinii* pneumonia, the most common opportunistic infection in the pediatric population.

Bacterial Infections. Approximately 20% of AIDS-defining illnesses in children are recurrent bacterial infections caused primarily by encapsulated organisms such as *Streptococcus pneumoniae* and *Salmonella* spp. Other pathogens such as *Staphylococcus, Enterococcus, Pseudomonas aeruginosa, Haemophilus influenzae,* and other gram-negative or gram-positive organisms may also be seen. Most of these infections are the result of HIV-related disturbances in humoral immunity. The most common serious infections are bacteremia, sepsis, and pneumonia, accounting for more than 50% of infections in HIV-infected children. Meningitis, urinary tract infections, deep-seated abscesses, and bone or joint infections occur less frequently. Milder recurrent infections, such as otitis media, sinusitis, and skin and soft tissue infections are very common, and may be chronic with atypical presentations.

Atypical Mycobacterial Infections. Atypical mycobacterial infections, particularly with *Mycobacterium avium* complex (MAC), may cause disseminated disease in HIV-infected children who are severely immunosuppressed. The incidence of MAC infection in HIV-infected children with fewer than 100 $CD4^+$ cells/μL who were not treated with antiretroviral drugs was estimated to be 10%, but MAC infections are rare in children receiving effective antiretroviral therapy. Disseminated MAC infection is characterized by fever, malaise, weight loss, and night sweats; diarrhea, abdominal pain, and rarely intestinal perforation or jaundice (as a result of biliary tract obstruction by lymphadenopathy) may also be present. Diagnosis is by isolation of MAC from blood, bone marrow, or tissue; the isolated presence of MAC in the stool does not confirm a diagnosis of disseminated MAC. Treatment can reduce symptoms and prolong life, but is only capable of suppressing the infection. Therapy should include at least two antimycobacterial drugs, such as clarithromycin (or azithromycin) and ethambutol. A third drug (e.g., rifabutin, rifampin, ciprofloxacin, or amikacin) is generally added to decrease the emergence of drug-resistant isolates. The drug susceptibilities of each isolate should be ascertained and the treatment regimen adjusted accordingly, especially with inadequate clinical response to therapy.

Fungal Infections. Oral candidiasis is the most common fungal infection seen in HIV-infected children. Oral nystatin suspension (100,000 units/mL, 2–5 mL four times a day), is often effective. Clotrimazole troches are an effective alternative. In refractory cases, oral amphotericin suspension should be considered. Oral thrush progresses to involve the esophagus in approximately 20% of children, presenting with symptoms of anorexia, dysphagia, vomiting, and fever. Treatment with oral fluconazole (4–6 mg/kg/24 hr for 14 days) generally results in rapid improvement in symptoms. Disseminated histoplasmosis, coccidioidomycosis, or cryptococcosis are rare in pediatric patients but may occur in endemic areas.

***P. carinii* Pneumonia.** The peak incidence of *P. carinii* pneumonia occurs at 3–6 mo of age, with the highest mortality rate in infants younger than 1 yr. However, newer, more aggressive approaches to treatment have improved the outcome substantially. The classic clinical presentation of *P. carinii* pneumonia includes acute onset of fever, tachypnea, dyspnea, and marked and progressive hypoxemia; however, in some children, more indolent development of hypoxemia may precede other clinical or roentgenographic manifestations. Chest radiography findings most commonly consist of interstitial infiltrates or diffuse alveolar disease, which rapidly progresses. Nodular lesions, streaky or lobar infiltrates, and pleural effusions may occasionally be seen. Diagnosis is by demonstration of *P. carinii* with appropriate silver staining of bronchoalveolar fluid lavage; rarely, an open lung biopsy is necessary.

The first-line therapy of *P. carinii* pneumonia is intravenous trimethoprim (TMP)/sulfamethoxazole (SMZ) (15–20 mg/kg/24 hr of TMP and 75–100 mg/kg/24 hr of SMZ divided every 6 hr) with adjunctive intravenous methylprednisolone (2 mg/kg/24 hr divided every 6 or 12 hr for 5–7 days). After clinical improvment, therapy with oral TMP/SMZ should be continued for a total of 21 days. Historically, up to one third of HIV-infected children have had allergic reactions to TMP/SMZ requiring desensitization, but this is considerably less frequent with the use of adjunctive corticosteroids. Alternative therapy is with intravenous administration of pentamidine (4 mg/kg/24 hr). Other regimens such as TMP plus dapsone, clindamycin plus primaquine, or atovaquone are used as alternatives in adults, but have not been widely used in children.

Other Parasitic Infections. Cryptosporidiosis, microsporidiosis, and rarely isosporiasis or giardiasis are opportunistic infections that cause significant morbidity in HIV-infected patients. Although usually self-limiting diseases in healthy hosts, they cause severe chronic diarrhea, often leading to malnutrition in HIV-infected children with low $CD4^+$ counts. Until recently, there was no effective therapy for cryptosporidiosis, which generally resulted in lifelong infection. Preliminary data on an investigational drug, nitazoxanide, have been promising, with clearance of the infection in some patients. Albendazole was reported to be effective in a few cases of chronic microsporidiosis, and TMP/SMZ seems to be effective for isosporiasis.

Viral Infections. Viral infections, especially with the herpesviruses, pose significant problems for HIV-infected children. Herpes simplex virus causes recurrent gingivostomatitis, which may be complicated by local and distant cutaneous dissemination. Primary varicella-zoster virus infection (chickenpox) may be prolonged and complicated by bacterial infections or visceral dissemination, including pneumonitis. Recurrent, atypical, or chronic episodes of herpes zoster are often debilitating and require prolonged therapy with acyclovir; in rare instances, varicella-zoster virus has developed resistance to acyclovir, requiring the use of foscarnet. Disseminated cytomegalovirus (CMV) infection can occur with fewer than 50 $CD4^+$ cells/μL and may involve single or multiple organs, causing retinitis, pneumonitis, esophagitis, gastritis with pyloric obstruction, hepatitis, colitis, and encephalitis. Ganciclovir (180 mg/kg/24 hr divided every 12 hr) or foscarnet (180 mg/kg/24 hr divided every 8 hr) are the drugs of choice. Measles may occur despite immunization and may present without the typical rash. It often disseminates to the lung or brain with a high mortality rate. Respiratory viruses such as respiratory syncytial virus (RSV) and adenovirus may present with prolonged symptoms and persistent viral shedding.

Central Nervous System. The incidence of central nervous system involvement in perinatally infected children is 40–90%, with a median onset at 19 mo of age. The most common presentation is progressive encephalopathy with loss or plateau of developmental milestones, cognitive deterioration, impaired brain growth resulting in acquired microcephaly, and symmetric motor dysfunction. Encephalopathy may be the initial manifestation of the HIV infection, or it may present much later when severe immune suppression occurs. With progression, marked apathy, spasticity, hyperreflexia, and gait disturbance may occur, as well as loss of language, oral, and fine and gross motor skills. The encephalopathy may progress intermittently, with periods of deterioration followed by transiently stable plateaus. Older children may exhibit behavioral problems and learning disabilities. Associated abnormalities identified by neuroimaging techniques include cerebral atrophy in up to 85% of children with neurologic symptoms, increased ventricular size, basal ganglia calcifications, and, less frequently, leukomalacia.

Focal neurologic signs and seizures are unusual, and may imply a comorbid pathologic process such as a tumor, opportunistic infection, or stroke. Central nervous system lymphoma may present with the new onset of focal neurologic findings, headache, seizures, and mental status changes. Characteristic findings on neuroimaging studies include a hyperdense or isodense mass with variable contrast enhancement or a diffusely infiltrating contrast-enhancing mass. Central nervous system toxoplasmosis is exceedingly rare in young infants, but may occur in HIV-infected adolescents; the overwhelming majority of these cases have serum immunoglobulin (Ig) G anti-*Toxoplasma* as a marker of infection. Other opportunistic infections of the central nervous system are quite rare and include CMV, JC virus (causing progressive multifocal leukoencephalopathy), herpes simplex virus, *Cryptococcus,* and *Coccidioides.* Cerebrovascular disorders (both hemorrhagic and nonhemorrhagic strokes) affect 6–10% of children reported in large clinical series.

Respiratory Tract. Recurrent upper respiratory tract infections such as otitis media and sinusitis are very common. Although the typical pathogens (e.g., *S. pneumoniae, H. influenzae, Moraxella catarrhalis*) are most common, unusual pathogens such as *P. aeruginosa,* yeast, and anaerobes may be present in chronic infections and result in complications such as invasive sinusitis and mastoiditis.

LIP is the most common chronic lower respiratory tract abnormality, occurring in 30–50% of HIV-infected children. LIP is a chronic process with nodular lymphoid hyperplasia in the bronchial and bronchiolar epithelium that often leads to progressive alveolar capillary block developing over months to years. It has a characteristic chronic diffuse reticulonodular pattern on chest radiograph, rarely with hilar lymphadenopathy, which suggests a presumptive diagnosis radiographically, even before the onset of symptoms. Clinically, there is an insidious onset of tachypnea, cough, and mild to moderate hypoxemia with normal auscultatory findings or minimal rales. Progressive disease may be accompanied by digital clubbing and symptomatic hypoxemia, which usually resolves with oral corticosteroid therapy. The cause of LIP has not been proven, although several studies suggest LIP is associated with a primary Epstein-Barr virus infection in the setting of HIV infection.

Most symptomatic HIV-infected children experience at least one episode of pneumonia. *S. pneumoniae* is the most common bacterial pathogen, but gram-negative bacteria may also cause pneumonia; *P. aeruginosa* pneumonia occurs most commonly in severely symptomatic children (C3 category) and is often associated with acute respiratory failure and death. Rarely, bronchiectasis can develop and predispose to recurrent secondary infections. *P. carinii* pneumonia is the most common opportunistic infection, but other pathogens, including CMV, *Aspergillus, Histoplasma,* and *Cryptococcus,* can cause pulmonary disease. Infection with common respiratory viruses, including RSV, influenza, parainfluenza, and adenovirus may occur simultaneously, and have both a protracted clinical course and period of viral shedding from the respiratory tract. Pulmonary and extrapulmonary tuberculosis has been reported with increasing frequency in HIV-infected children, although it is considerably more common in HIV-infected adults.

Cardiovascular System. The incidence of cardiac manifestations has not been assessed accurately, but approximately 20% of HIV-infected children have some degree of cardiac involvement. Children with encephalopathy or other AIDS-defining conditions have the highest rate of cardiac involvement. Hemodynamic abnormalities, dysrhythmias, left ventricular dysfunction, and chronic congestive heart failure are the most frequent findings. Resting sinus tachycardia has been reported in up to 64% and marked sinus arrhythmia in 17% of HIV-infected children. Hemodynamic instability occurs more frequently with advanced HIV disease, especially in patients with severe autonomic neuropathy. Gallop rhythm with tachypnea and hepatosplenomegaly appear to be the best clinical indicators of congestive heart failure in HIV-infected children; anticongestive therapy is generally very effective, especially when initiated early. Electrocardiography and echocardiography are helpful in assessing cardiac function before the onset of clinical symptoms.

Gastrointestinal and Hepatobiliary Tract. Oral manifestations of HIV disease include erythematous or pseudomembranous candidiasis, periodontal disease (e.g., ulcerative gingivitis or periodontitis), salivary gland disease (e.g., swelling, xerostomia), and rarely oral hairy leukoplakia and ulcerations. Lower gastrointestinal tract involvement is common in HIV-infected children and may be caused by bacteria (*Salmonella, Campylobacter,* MAC), protozoa (*Cryptosporidium, Isospora,* microsporidia, and *Giardia*), viruses (CMV, herpes simplex virus, rotavirus), and fungi (*Candida*); MAC and the protozoal infections are most severe and protracted in patients with severe $CD4^+$ cell depletion. Oral or esophageal ulcerations, either viral in origin or idiopathic, are painful and often interfere with eating; lesions that have negative viral cultures may respond to thalidomide (currently investigational) or to short courses of prednisone. AIDS enteropathy, a syndrome of malabsorption with partial villous atrophy not associated with a specific pathogen, has been postulated to be a result of direct HIV infection of the gut. Disaccharide intolerance is common in HIV-infected children with chronic diarrhea.

The most common symptoms of gastrointestinal disease are chronic or recurrent diarrhea with malabsorption, abdominal pain, dysphagia, and failure to thrive. Prompt recognition of weight loss or poor growth velocity in the absence of diarrhea is critical. Linear growth impairment often correlates with the level of HIV viremia. Supplemental enteral feedings should be instituted, either by mouth or with nighttime nasogastric tube feedings in cases associated with more chronic growth problems; placement of a gastrostomy tube for nutritional supplementation may be necessary. The "wasting syndrome," a loss of more than 10% of body weight, is not as common as failure to thrive in pediatric patients. However, the resulting malnutrition is associated with a grave prognosis and generally requires parenteral hyperalimentation.

Chronic liver inflammation, evidenced by fluctuating serum levels of hepatic transaminases with or without cholestasis, is relatively common, often without identification of an etiologic agent. Cryptosporidial cholecystitis is associated with abdominal pain, jaundice, and elevated γ-glutamyl transpeptidase. In some patients, chronic hepatitis caused by CMV, hepatitis B or C, or MAC may lead to portal hypertension and liver failure. Several of the drugs used for patients with AIDS may cause reversible elevation of transaminases, including didanosine (ddI), protease inhibitors, and dapsone.

Pancreatitis with increased pancreatic enzymes with or without abdominal pain, vomiting, and fever may be the result of drug therapy (e.g., pentamidine, ddI, and lamivudine) or rarely, opportunistic infections such as MAC or CMV.

Renal Disease. Nephropathy is an unusual presenting symptom of HIV infection, more commonly occurring in older symptomatic children. A direct effect of HIV on renal epithelial cells has been suggested as the cause, but immune complexes, hyperviscosity of the blood (secondary to hyperglobulinemia), and nephrotoxic drugs are other possible factors. A wide range of histologic abnormalities has been reported, including focal glomerulosclerosis, mesangial hyperplasia, segmental necrotizing glomerulonephritis, and minimal change disease. Focal glomerulosclerosis generally progresses to renal failure within 6–12 mo, but other histologic abnormalities may remain stable without significant renal insufficiency for prolonged periods. Nephrotic syndrome is the most common manifestation of renal disease, with edema, hypoalbuminemia, proteinuria, and azotemia with normal blood pressure. Cases resistant to corticosteroid therapy may benefit from cyclosporine therapy. Polyuria, oliguria, and hematuria have also been observed in some patients.

Skin Manifestations. Many cutaneous manifestations seen in

HIV-infected children are inflammatory or infectious disorders that are not unique to this infection. These disorders tend to be more disseminated and respond less consistently to conventional therapy than in the HIV-uninfected child. Seborrheic dermatitis or eczema that is severe and unresponsive to treatment may be an early nonspecific sign of HIV infection. Recurrent or chronic episodes of herpes simplex virus, herpes zoster, molluscum contagiosum, anogenital warts, and candidal infections are common and may be difficult to control.

Allergic drug eruptions are also common, particularly related to sulfonamides, and generally respond to withdrawal of the drug or to desensitization. Epidermal hyperkeratosis with dry, scaling skin is frequently observed, and sparse hair or hair loss may be seen in the later stages of the disease.

Hematologic Diseases. Anemia occurs in 20–70% of HIV-infected children, more commonly in children with AIDS. The anemia may be due to chronic infection, poor nutrition, autoimmune phenomenon, virus associated hemophagocytic syndrome, parvovirus B19 red cell aplasia, or may be a side effect of drugs (e.g., zidovudine [ZDV]). In children with low erythropoietin levels, subcutaneous recombinant erythropoietin may be successful in treating the anemia.

Leukopenia occurs in almost one third of untreated HIV-infected children, and neutropenia often occurs. In a few cases, antineutrophil antibodies are the cause, and treatment with intravenous immunoglobulin (IVIG) has been successful. Multiple drugs used for treatment or prophylaxis for opportunistic infections such as *P. carinii* pneumonia, MAC, and CMV or antiretroviral drugs (e.g., ZDV) may also cause leukopenia or neutropenia. In many cases, treatment with subcutaneous granulocyte colony-stimulating factor is successful.

Thrombocytopenia occurs in 10–20% of patients. The cause may be immunologic (i.e., circulating immune complexes or antiplatelet antibodies), drug toxicity, or unknown. Treatment with IVIG or anti-D offers temporary improvement in many cases. If ineffective, a 2- to 3-day course of high-dose corticosteroids (30 mg/kg/24 hr) may be an alternative. Antiretroviral therapy may also reverse thrombocytopenia. Deficiency of clotting factors (e.g., factors II, VII, IX) is most often secondary to enteropathy, may occur with advanced disease, and is often correctable with vitamin K.

A novel disease of the thymus has been observed in a few HIV-infected children found to have anterior mediastinal multilocular thymic cysts without clinical symptoms. Histologic examination shows focal cystic changes, follicular hyperplasia, and diffuse plasmocytosis and multinucleated giant cells. Spontaneous thymic involution occurred in some cases.

Malignancy. In contrast to adults, malignant diseases have been reported infrequently in HIV-infected children, representing only 2% of AIDS-defining illnesses. Non-Hodgkin's lymphoma, primary central nervous system lymphoma, and leiomyosarcomas are the most commonly reported neoplasms in children. Epstein-Barr virus is associated with most lymphomas and with all leiomyosarcomas. Kaposi's sarcoma, which frequently occurs in adults and is caused by human herpesvirus type 8 (HHV-8) (Chapter 250), is exceedingly uncommon in HIV-infected children.

DIAGNOSIS. In any child older than 18 mo, demonstration of IgG antibody to HIV by a repeatedly reactive enzyme immunoassay and confirmatory test (e.g., Western immunoblot or immunofluorescence assay) establishes the diagnosis of HIV infection. All infants born to HIV-infected mothers have positive antibody tests at birth because of passive transfer of maternal HIV antibody across the placenta during gestation. Most uninfected infants lose maternal antibody between 6 and 12 mo of age (seroreverters). Because a small proportion of HIV-uninfected infants continue to test positive for HIV antibody for up to 18 mo, positive IgG antibody tests cannot be used for a definitive diagnosis of HIV infection in infants younger than 18 mo. The presence of IgA or IgM anti-HIV in the infant's circulation can indicate HIV infection, because these Ig classes do not cross the placenta. However, detectable quantities of IgA anti-HIV are not generally produced until 3–6 mo of age, limiting the utility of IgA testing; the reported sensitivity is 50–60% at 3 mo and 60–100% at 6 mo. IgM anti-HIV assays have been both insensitive and nonspecific and, therefore, are not valuable for clinical use.

Several viral detection assays are available, including HIV DNA or RNA by PCR, HIV culture, HIV p24 antigen, and immune complex–dissociated p24 antigen (ICD-p24). These are very useful in young infants, allowing a definitive diagnosis in most infected infants by 1–6 mo of age. HIV DNA PCR is the preferred virologic assay in developed countries. Almost 40% of infected newborns have positive tests in the first 2 days of life, with more than 90% testing positive by 2 wk of age.

Plasma HIV RNA assays, which detect viral replication, may prove to be more sensitive than DNA PCR for early diagnosis, but data are limited. HIV culture has similar sensitivity to HIV DNA PCR; however, it is more technically complex and expensive, and results are often not available for 2–4 wk compared with 2–3 days with PCR. The p24 antigen assay is less costly, highly specific, and easy to perform. However, it is not recommended for diagnosis of infection in infants younger than 1 mo because of the high rate of false-positive results. In developing countries, the ICD-p24 test may be considered for older infants; however, a negative result does not exclude infection.

For infants born to HIV-infected mothers, viral diagnostic testing should be performed within the first 2 days of life, at 1–2 mo of age, and at 4–6 mo of age; some also favor testing at age 14 days to maximize early detection of infected infants for initiation of antiretroviral therapy. Infants who have negative virologic assays initially should be retested at these intervals. A single positive virologic assay (detection of HIV by PCR, culture, or p24 antigen) suggests HIV infection and should be confirmed by a repeat test on a second specimen as soon as possible. A diagnosis of HIV infection can be established with two positive virologic tests obtained from different blood samples. Although the perinatal use of prophylactic ZDV to prevent vertical transmission has not affected the predictive value of viral diagnostic testing, the effect of more intensive antiviral combinations in pregnant women on the accuracy of the infant's viral tests is unknown. HIV infection can be reasonably excluded if an infant has had at least two negative virologic tests at 1 mo of age or older, including one performed at 4 mo of age or older. In older infants and children, two or more negative HIV antibody tests performed at least 1 mo apart at 6 mo of age or older in the absence of hypogammaglobulinemia or clinical evidence of HIV disease reasonably excludes HIV infection. The infection can be excluded definitively if the same parameters are met when the infant is 18 mo of age or older.

Complete blood count, differential leukocyte count, and platelet count should be performed at birth for newborns of HIV-infected mothers and, if within normal ranges, repeated monthly for the first 4–6 mo of life. If the child is found to be HIV infected or the HIV status is not clear, these tests should be continued to assess the potential hematologic effect of the disease and its treatment (e.g., prophylactic TMP/SMZ, antiretroviral treatment). $CD4^+$ and $CD8^+$ lymphocyte counts should be performed at 1 and 3 mo of age. If the child is HIV-infected or the HIV status is not clear, the tests should be repeated every 3 mo beginning at 6 mo of age; the frequency should be increased to every 4–6 wk if the $CD4^+$ count or percentage declines rapidly.

TREATMENT. Understanding the compelx relationship between the virus-specific immune responses and the mechanisms used by the virus to survive are crucial for designing therapeutic strategies. Although viral replication can be suppressed by antiretroviral drugs, it will also be important to develop strategies to modulate the immune response.

Antiretroviral Therapy. Decisions about antiretroviral therapy for pediatric HIV-infected patients are based on the magnitude of viral replication (i.e., viral load), $CD4^+$ count and percentage, and clinical condition. As antiretroviral therapies continue to evolve and new drugs and treatment options become available, decisions regarding therapy should be made in consultation with an expert in pediatric HIV infection. Although early treatment trials consisted of single-drug therapy, more recent trials have uniformly confirmed, using virologic, immunologic, and clinical end points, the superiority of multiple-drug combination therapy. Plasma viral load monitoring and measurement of $CD4^+$ cells make it possible to implement rational treatment strategies for viral suppression as well as to assess the efficacy of a particular drug combination.

The following principles form the basis for antiretroviral treatment: (1) Uninterrupted HIV replication causes destruction of the immune system and progression to AIDS; (2) the magnitude of the viral load predicts the rate of disease progression, while the $CD4^+$ count reflects the risk of opportunistic infections and complications; (3) potent combination therapy that suppresses HIV replication to an undetectable level restricts the selection of antiretroviral-resistant mutants; drug-resistant strains are the major factor limiting successful viral suppression and delay of disease progression; (4) the goal of sustainable suppression of HIV replication is best achieved by the simultaneous initiation of combinations of antiretroviral agents to which the patient has not been exposed previously and that are not cross-resistant to drugs with which the patient has been treated previously; and (5) adherence to the complex drug regimens is crucial for a successful outcome.

Rationale for Combination Therapy. Antiretroviral drugs licensed as of 1998 are categorized based on their ability to inhibit the HIV reverse transcriptase or protease enzymes (Table 268–3). The reverse transcriptase inhibitors are further subdivided into nucleoside reverse transcriptase inhibitors (NRTIs) and non-nucleoside reverse transcriptase inhibitors (NNRTIs). Among the NRTIs, thymidine analogs (stavudine [d4T], and ZDV) are found in higher concentrations in "activated" or dividing cells, and nonthymidine analogs (ddI, lamivudine [3TC], and dideoxycytidine [ddC]) have more activity in "resting" cells. Activated cells are thought to produce more than 99% of virions. In contrast, resting cells account for less than 1% of the population, but may serve as a reservoir of HIV; suppression of replication in both populations is thought to be an important component of long-term viral control. NNRTIs (e.g., delavirdine, efavirenz, and nevirapine) act at a different stage of reverse transcription than NRTIs. Protease inhibitors (e.g., ritonavir, nelfinavir, indinavir and saquinavir) are potent agents that are active at a different stage in viral replication, preventing packaging of infectious virions before they leave the infected cell.

Although the principal site of viral replication is lymphoid tissue, sanctuary sites such as the central nervous system may harbor residual virions with the potential of being a source of local or persistent disease. Although data on central nervous system penetration of antiviral agents are presently limited, ZDV, d4T, and 3TC appear to achieve inhibitory concentrations in the brain; indinavir and nevirapine also achieve good levels in the cerebrospinal fluid.

Maximal viral suppression may be feasible by targeting different points in the viral life cycle and stages of cell activation, and delivering drug to all tissue sites. Combinations of three drugs such as a thymidine analog NRTI, a nonthymidine analog NRTI (to suppress replication in both active and resting cells), and a protease inhibitor have been shown in adults and in children to produce prolonged viral suppression. Alternative regimens such as two NRTI with or without an NNRTI have been shown to be beneficial in children. Although not ideal, a less potent combination may be considered when there are concerns about adherence to a complex drug regimen or when the patient or family prefer an alternative regimen. Combination treatment increases the rate of drug toxicities (see Table 268–3), and complex drug-drug interactions exist among many of the antiretroviral drugs. Protease inhibitors are particularly likely to have serious interactions with multiple drug classes, including nonsedating antihistamine, psychotropic, vasoconstrictor, antimycobacterial, cardiovascular, analgesic, and gastrointestinal drugs (e.g., cisapride). Whenever new medications are added to an antiretroviral regimen, especially a protease inhibitor–containing regimen, a pharmacist or AIDS specialist should be consulted to address possible drug interactions.

TABLE 268–3 Antiretroviral Drugs and Adverse Effects

Drug	Adverse Effect: Most Frequent	Adverse Effect: Unusual
Nucleoside Reverse Transcriptase Inhibitors		
Abacavir (ABC)	Gastrointestinal intolerance, headache	Fever, rash, anorexia
Didanosine (ddI)	Gastrointestinal intolerance	Peripheral neuropathy, pancreatitis
Lamivudine (3TC)	Headache, fatigue, gastrointestinal intolerance, rash	Pancreatitis, peripheral neuropathy
Stavudine (d4T)	Headache, gastrointestinal intolerance	Peripheral neuropathy, pancreatitis
Zalcitabine (ddC)	Gastrointestinal intolerance, headache	Peripheral neuropathy, pancreatitis, hepatotoxicity
Zidovudine (ZDV)	Anemia, granulocytopenia	Hepatotoxicity
Nucleotide Reverse Transcriptase Inhibitors		
Adefovir	Gastrointestinal intolerance	Fever, chills
Non-nucleoside Reverse Transcriptase Inhibitors		
Delavirdine (DLV)	Rash (may be severe), gastrointestinal intolerance	Headache
Efavirenz (EFV)		
Nevirapine (NVP)	Rash (may be severe), gastrointestinal intolerance, headache	Hepatotoxicity
Protease Inhibitors*		
Amprenavir†	Gastrointestinal intolerance	Rash, perioral paresthesia
Indinavir†	Gastrointestinal intolerance Hyperbilirubinemia	Nephrolithiasis, taste distortion
Nelfinavir†	Diarrhea	Asthenia, rash, hepatotoxicity
Ritonavir†	Gastrointestinal intolerance, anorexia	Hepatotoxicity, perioral paresthesia
Saquinavir†	Gastrointestinal intolerance, headache, nausea	Hepatotoxicity

**All the protease inhibitors can cause hyperglycemia, increased triglycerides and cholesterol, lipodystrophy, hemolytic anemia, and spontaneous bleeding episodes in patients with hemophilia.*

†Significant drug-drug interactions occur; some may be life-threatening.

Not all adverse effects are listed. See prescribing information in package inserts.

Adherence Issues. Assessment of the likelihood of adherence to treatment is an important factor in deciding whether and when to initiate therapy. Poor adherence to prescribed medication regimens results in subtherapeutic drug concentrations and enhances development of HIV resistance, particularly with protease inhibitors and NNRTI drugs. Antiretroviral therapy has been shown to be most effective in treatment-naive patients, who are less likely to harbor drug-resistant viral strains. Combination antiretroviral regimens require multiple daily doses and are often unpalatable, requiring extreme dedication on the part of the care provider and child; this makes participation of the family in the decision to initiate therapy essential. Intensive education on the relationship of drug adherence to viral suppression, training on drug administration, and frequent follow-up visits are critical for successful antiviral treatment.

Initiation of Therapy. HIV-infected children with symptoms (clinical category A, B, or C) or with evidence of immune dysfunction (immune category 2 or 3) should be treated with antiretroviral therapy regardless of age or viral load. Infants younger than 1 yr are at high risk for disease progression, and immunologic and virologic tests to identify those likely to experience rapidly progressive disease are less predictive than in older children. Therefore, all such infants should be treated with antiretroviral agents as soon as the diagnosis of HIV infection has been confirmed, regardless of clinical or immunologic status or viral load.

Most clinicians advocate treating asymptomatic children older than 1 yr to prevent immunologic deterioration. However, when there are concerns regarding drug adherence, safety, and durability of antiretroviral response, some providers elect to delay treatment in the immunologically normal child older than 1 yr with a low viral load (<20,000 copies/mL), for whom the risk for clinical progression is low. Such children should be monitored regularly for evidence of virologic, immunologic, or clinical progression, at which point therapy should be initiated.

Dosing Issues. Data on antiretroviral drug dosages for neonates are usually limited. Because of the immaturity of the neonatal liver, premature infants and newborns often require an increase in the dosing interval of drugs primarily cleared through hepatic metabolism (glucuronidation).

Adolescents should have antiretroviral dosages prescribed on the basis of Tanner staging of puberty rather than on the basis of age. During early puberty (Tanner stages I, II, and III), pediatric dosing ranges should be used, whereas adolescents in late puberty (Tanner stages IV and V) should follow adult dosing schedules.

Changing Antiretroviral Therapy. Therapy should be changed when the current regimen is judged ineffective, as evidenced by an increase in viral load, a deterioration of the $CD4^+$ count, clinical progression, or development of toxicity or intolerance to drugs. The patient and family should be reassessed for likelihood of adherence when a change is considered. Potential viral cross-resistance suggests that, ideally, all antiretroviral drugs should be changed. However, in many situations (e.g., previous antiretroviral experience, intolerance, toxicity), this is not possible; therefore, at least two antiretroviral drugs should be changed.

Monitoring Antiretroviral Therapy. Virologic and immunologic surveillance (using HIV RNA copy number and $CD4^+$ counts) as well as clinical assessment should be performed regularly in children taking antiretroviral therapy. Initial virologic response usually occurs within 4 wk of initiating antiretroviral therapy, with a maximum response within 12–16 wk. Thus, HIV RNA levels should be measured at 4 wk and 3–4 mo after initiation of therapy. Once an optimal response has occurred, viral load should be measured at least every 3 mo. If the response is unsatisfactory, another viral load should be performed as soon as possible to verify the results before a change in therapy is considered. The $CD4^+$ cells respond more slowly to successful treatment and, therefore, can be monitored less frequently, such as every 3–4 months. Potential toxicity should be monitored closely for the first 8–12 wk. If no clinical or laboratory toxicity is documented, a follow-up visit every 2–3 mo is adequate.

Supportive Care. Even before the new antiretroviral drugs were available, a significant impact on the quality of life and survival of HIV-infected children was achieved with intensive supportive treatment. Because of the frequent changes in supportive care recommendations, physicians providing care to few HIV-exposed or HIV-infected children should periodically consult other physicians with expertise in pediatric HIV infection.

A multidisciplinary team approach is desirable for successful management. Close attention should be given to nutritional status, which is often delicately balanced and may require aggressive pre-emptive intervention (e.g., nasogastric or gastric feedings or parenteral nutrition) to achieve adequate caloric and protein intake. Painful oropharyngeal lesions and dental caries are frequent and may interfere with eating; routine dental evaluations and careful attention to oral hygiene should be encouraged. Development should be evaluated regularly with provision of necessary physical, occupational, and speech therapies. Recognition of pain in the young child may be difficult, and effective pharmacologic and nonpharmacologic protocols for pain management should be instituted, especially during the terminal phase of the disease.

HIV-exposed and infected children can be given most standard pediatric immunizations (Fig. 268–2), although live virus vaccines and live bacterial vaccines (e.g., bacille Calmette-Guérin) are generally contraindicated, especially for severely immunocompromised children (see Table 268–1). Asymptomatic or mildly asymptomatic HIV-infected children in CDC class N1 or A1 should receive their first MMR as soon as possible after reaching their first birthday. Consideration should be given to administering the second dose of MMR vaccine as soon as 1 mo after the first dose, rather than waiting until school entry. Varicella vaccine should be considered for asymptomatic or mildly symptomatic HIV-infected children >1 yr of age in CDC class N1 or A1 with age-specific $CD4^+$ T-lymphocyte percentages of ≥25%. Eligible HIV-infected children should receive two doses of varicella vaccine with a 3-mo interval between doses. Prior immunizations do not always provide protection for HIV-infected children, as evidenced by outbreaks of measles and pertussis in immunized HIV-infected children.

Prophylactic regimens are an integral component for the care of HIV-infected children. All infants between 6 wk and 1 yr of age either born to HIV-infected mothers or proved to be HIV-infected should receive prophylaxis for *P. carinii* regardless of the $CD4^+$ count or percentage (Table 268–4). When the child is older than 12 mo, prophylaxis should be given according to the $CD4^+$ count. The best prophylactic regimen is 150 mg TMP/750 mg SMZ/m^2/24 hr given as two daily doses 3 consecutive days each week. If the patient experiences a rash or mild allergic reaction, desensitization is usually successful to allow daily TMP/SMZ prophylaxis. For severe adverse reactions to TMP/SMZ, alternative prophylaxis regimens include dapsone, atovaquone, or, as a last choice, aerosolized or intravenous pentamidine.

Prophylaxis against *M. avium* complex should be offered to HIV-infected children with advanced immunosuppression (i.e., $CD4^+$ count < 500 cells/μL in children < 1 yr of age; < 75

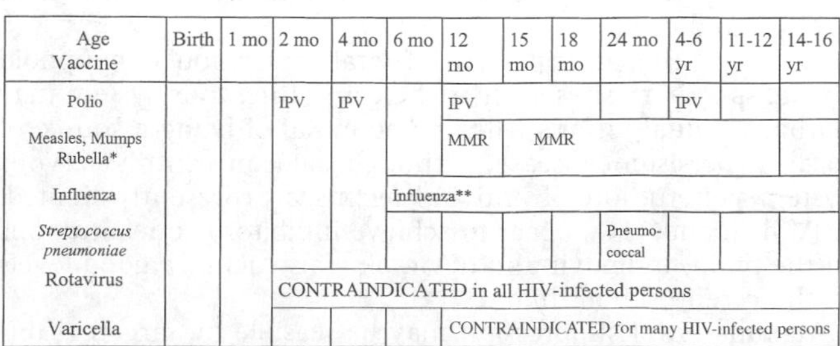

Age / Vaccine	Birth	1 mo	2 mo	4 mo	6 mo	12 mo	15 mo	18 mo	24 mo	4-6 yr	11-12 yr	14-16 yr
Polio			IPV	IPV		IPV				IPV		
Measles, Mumps Rubella*						MMR	MMR					
Influenza					Influenza**							
Streptococcus pneumoniae									Pneumo-coccal			
Rotavirus			CONTRAINDICATED in all HIV-infected persons									
Varicella						CONTRAINDICATED for many HIV-infected persons						

Recommendations for hepatitis B, diphtheria/tetanus/pertussis (DTaP), and *Haemophilus influenzae* type b vaccines are the same as for HIV-infected children (Figure 301–1). Boosters with dT should be every 5 yr during adulthood

* Severely immunocompromised HIV-infected persons (Table 268–2) should not receive measles virus-containing or varicella vaccines.

** Revaccination is required every year

Figure 268–2 Differences in immunization schedule for HIV-infected children.

TABLE 268–4 Recommendations for *Pneumocystis carinii* Pneumonia Prophylaxis and CD4+ Monitoring for HIV-Exposed Infants and HIV-Infected Children, by Age and HIV-Infection Status

Age/HIV Infection Status	*P. carinii* Pneumonia Prophylaxis	CD4+ Monitoring
Birth to 4–6 wk, HIV exposed	No prophylaxis	1 mo
4–6 wk to 4 mo, HIV exposed	Prophylaxis	3 mo
4–12 mo		
HIV-infected or indeterminate	Prophylaxis	6, 9, and 12 mo
HIV infection reasonably excluded*	No prophylaxis	None
1–5 yr, HIV infected	Prophylaxis if $CD4^+$ count is < 500 cells/μL or $CD4^+$ percentage is < 15%†‡	Every 3–4 mo§
6–12 yr, HIV infected	Prophylaxis if $CD4^+$ count is < 200 cells/μL or $CD4^+$ percentage is < 15%‡	Every 3–4 mo§

**HIV infection can be reasonably excluded among children who have had two or more negative HIV diagnostic tests (i.e., HIV culture or polymerase chain reaction), both of which are performed at ≥ 1 mo of age and one of which is performed at ≥ 4 mo of age, or two or more negative HIV antibody tests performed at > 6 mo of age among children who have no clinical evidence of HIV disease.*

†Children 1–2 yr of age who were receiving P. carinii *prophylaxis and had a* $CD4^+$ *count < 750 cells/μL or percentage < 15% at < 12 mo of age should continue prophylaxis.*

‡Prophylaxis should be considered on a case-by-case basis for children who might otherwise be at risk for P. carinii, *such as children with rapidly declining* $CD4^+$ *counts or percentages of children with category C conditions. Children who have had* P. carinii *should receive lifelong* P. carinii *prophylaxis.*

§More frequent monitoring (e.g., monthly) is recommended for children whose $CD4^+$ *counts or percentages are approaching the threshold at which prophylaxis is recommended.*

From Centers for Disease Control and Prevention: 1995 revised guidelines for prophylaxis against Pneumocystis carinii *pneumonia for children infected with or perinatally exposed to human immunodeficiency virus. MMWR Morb Mortal Wkly Rep 44(RR-4):6, 1995.*

cells/μL in children 1 6 yr of age; < 50 cells/μL in children > 6 yr of age). Clarithromycin (15 mg/kg/24 hr divided every 12 hr) is the drug of choice, but azithromycin (20 mg/kg/dose once a week or 5 mg/kg once daily) can be used as an alternative.

IVIG to prevent recurrent serious bacterial infections is recommended for HIV-infected children who (1) have suffered from at least two documented serious bacterial infections within 1 yr, (2) have laboratory-documented inability to make antigen-specific antibodies; or (3) are hypogammaglobulinemic. The dose is 400 mg/kg administered every 4 wk.

All HIV-exposed children should have skin testing for tuberculosis (5 TU of purified protein derivative [PPD]) at 1 yr of age, and be retested every 2 yr. HIV-infected children living in close contact with a person with tuberculosis should be tested annually. To reduce the incidence of other potential infections, parents should be counseled about (1) the importance of good handwashing; (2) avoidance of raw or undercooked food (e.g., *Salmonella*); (3) avoidance of drinking or swimming in lake or river water or being in contact with young farm animals (e.g., *Cryptosporidium*); and (4) the risk of playing with pets (e.g., *Toxoplasma gondii, Salmonella, Bartonella henselae*).

PROGNOSIS. The increased understanding of the pathogenesis of HIV infection in children and the availability of more effective antiretroviral drugs have improved the prognosis considerably. In developed countries where early diagnosis leads to prompt antiretroviral therapy, progression of the disease and mortality during early childhood have markedly diminished. HIV-infected children who are treated live longer with improved quality of life. In general, the best single prognostic indicator is the plasma viral load. Infants with a high viral load (>100,000 copies/mL) with low $CD4^+$ counts tend to have more rapidly progressive disease. Although there is no threshold above which rapid progression can be predicted, it is unusual to see rapid progression in an infant with a viral load of less than 50,000 copies/mL. In addition, a persistently high viral load is associated with greater risk for disease progression and mortality. The $CD4^+$ percentage is another prognostic indicator; the mortality rate is significantly higher in patients with $CD4^+$ percentage less than 15%. The use of both markers—plasma viral load and $CD4^+$ percentage—is recommended for predicting prognosis.

In developing countries where antiretroviral therapy and sophisticated diagnostic tests are scarce, a clinical staging system can be used to predict progression of disease. Children with opportunistic infections (e.g., *P. carinii* pneumonia, MAC), encephalopathy, and wasting syndrome have the worst prognosis; more than 75% die before 3 yr of age. Persistent fever, oral thrush, serious bacterial infections, hepatitis, persistent anemia (< 8.0 g/dL), and thrombocytopenia (< 100,000/μL) also suggest a poor outcome; more than 30% die before 3 yr of age. In contrast, lymphadenopathy, splenomegaly, hepatomegaly, LIP, and parotitis are indicators of better prognosis. The suggested clinical staging is quite similar to the classification recommended in the 1994 revised Centers for Disease Control classification.

PREVENTION. Prevention of sexual transmission involves avoiding the exchange of bodily fluids. Educational efforts about avoidance of risk factors are essential for older school-age children and adolescents and should begin before the onset of sexual activity. In sexually active adolescents, use of condoms should be emphasized to reduce sexually transmitted diseases. Unprotected sex with older partners or with multiple partners and use of illicit drugs is common among HIV-infected adolescents, and these factors increase the risk.

Perinatal Chemoprophylaxis. Interruption of perinatal transmission from mother to child can be achieved by administering ZDV chemoprophylaxis to pregnant women and their offspring. The recommended regimen is ZDV orally to the pregnant woman after the first trimester (100 mg 5 times/day orally), intravenously to the mother in the peripartum period (2 mg/kg loading dose followed by 1 mg/kg/hr), and orally in the newborn (8 mg/kg/24 hr divided every 6 hr) for the first 6 wk of life. This regimen has been documented to decrease the rate of perinatal HIV transmission by more than two thirds, to less than 8% and possibly as low as 3–4%. Toxicity from ZDV therapy in both mothers and infants is minimal. This regimen is effective in asymptomatic women, women not previously taking any antiretroviral therapy, as well as in those with advanced disease, low $CD4^+$ counts, and prior ZDV therapy. Although this regimen is effective, it is logistically complex and expensive. A short-term regimen (300 mg twice daily from 36 wk gestation and 300 mg every 3 hr during delivery) offers a simpler, effective (almost 50% reduction in transmission), and less expensive regimen that can be used in areas where the long-term regimen is difficult to implement.

Oral nevirapine administered once to women in labor and once to the infant during the first 48–72 hr of life capitalizes on the prolonged half-life of this drug and is under investigation. If proved efficacious, this will be a simple and highly cost-effective regimen, providing a feasible intervention in both developed and developing countries.

Combinations of drugs more potent than ZDV are now being used for treatment of HIV infection in nonpregnant women; the role of these agents in prevention of perinatal transmission is under investigation. Decisions regarding use and choice of antiretroviral drugs during pregnancy are complex and require coordination between the HIV specialist and the obstetrician. However, ZDV should be included as a component of all perinatal regimens because it is the only drug that has been demonstrated to prevent perinatal transmission. Intravenous intrapartum ZDV and the 6-wk regimen in the newborn are recommended for HIV-infected women in labor who did not receive antiretroviral therapy during gestation. The 6-wk component is recommended for offspring of HIV-infected mothers who did not receive ZDV during gestation or delivery. ZDV should be instituted in the newborn as soon as possible after delivery, preferably within 12–24 hr, and continued for 6 wk. The ZDV dose for full-term infants is 8 mg/kg/24 hr divided every 6 hr; for preterm infants, the dose is 3 mg/kg/24 hr orally or intravenously divided every 12 hr for the first 2 wk of life and then increased to 6 mg/kg/24 hr divided every 8 hr.

Now that it is clear that perinatal transmission can be reduced dramatically by treating pregnant mothers, a compelling argument exists for prenatal identification of HIV infection in the mother. The benefit of therapy, both for the mother's health and to prevent transmission to the infant, cannot be overemphasized. Eliminating the requirement for extensive HIV counseling and consent for HIV testing for all pregnant women will increase the proportion of pregnant women tested for HIV and will further reduce the number of new infections in many areas of the United States. To meet this goal, universal HIV testing, with patient notification, should become part of the routine prenatal care of all pregnant women.

American Academy of Pediatrics, Committee on Pediatric AIDS: Evaluation and medical treatment of the HIV-exposed infant. Pediatrics 99:909, 1997.

American Academy of Pediatrics, Committee on Pediatric AIDS: Surveillance of pediatric HIV infection. Pediatrics 101:315, 1998.

Centers for Disease Control and Prevention: 1994 revised classification system for human immunodeficiency virus infection in children less than 13 years of age. MMWR Morb Mortal Wkly Rep 43(RR-12):1, 1994.

Centers for Disease Control and Prevention: 1995 revised guidelines for prophylaxis against *Pneumocystis carinii* pneumonia for children infected with or perinatally exposed to human immunodeficiency virus. MMWR Morb Mortal Wkly Rep 44(RR-4):1, 1995.

Centers for Disease Control and Prevention: 1997 USPHS/IDSA guidelines for the prevention of opportunistic infections in persons infected with human immunodeficiency virus. MMWR Morb Mortal Wkly Rep 46(RR-12):1, 1997.

Centers for Disease Control and Prevention: Guidelines for the use of antiretroviral agents in pediatric HIV infection. MMWR Morb Mortal Wkly Rep 47(RR-4):1, 1998.

Centers for Disease Control and Prevention: Human immunodeficiency virus transmission in household settings in United States. MMWR Morb Mortal Wkly Rep 43:347, 1994.

Centers for Disease Control and Prevention: Public Health Service task force recommendations for the use of antiretroviral drugs in pregnant women infected with HIV-1 for maternal health and for reducing perinatal HIV-1 transmission in the United States. MMWR Morb Mortal Wkly Rep 47(RR-2):1, 1998.

Centers for Disease Control and Prevention: Report of the NIH panel to define principles of therapy of HIV infection and guidelines for the use of antiretroviral agents in HIV-infected adults and adolescents. MMWR Morb Mortal Wkly Rep 47(RR-5):1, 1998.

Centers for Disease Control and Prevention: Update: Perinatally acquired HIV-1/AIDS-United States 1997. MMWR Morb Mortal Wkly Rep 46:1086, 1997.

Centers for Disease Control and Prevention: U. S. Public Health Service recommendations for human immunodeficiency virus counseling and voluntary testing for pregnant women. MMWR Morb Mortal Wkly Rep 44(RR-7):1, 1995.

Faye A, Burgard M, Crosnier H, et al: Human immunodeficiency virus type 2 infection in children. J Pediatr 130:994, 1997.

Kahn JO, Walker BD: Acute human immunodeficiency virus type 1 infection. N Engl J Med 339:3, 1998.

Levy JA: HIV and the Pathogenesis of AIDS, 2nd ed. Washington, DC, American Society for Microbiology Press, 1998.

The International Perinatal HIV Group: The mode of delivery and the risk of vertical transmission of human immunodeficiency virus type 1—a meta-analysis of 15 prospective cohort studies. N Engl J Med 340:977, 1999.

CHAPTER 269
Human T-Cell Lymphotropic Viruses Types I and II

Hal B. Jenson

Human T-cell lymphotropic viruses type I (HTLV-I) and type II (HTLV-II), members of the *Oncovirinae* subfamily of the *Retroviridae* family, are single-stranded RNA viruses that encode reverse transcriptase, an RNA-dependent DNA polymerase that transcribes the single-stranded viral RNA into a double-stranded DNA copy. The circular DNA is transported into the nucleus, where it is integrated into chromosomal DNA (provirus), evading the usual mechanisms of immune surveillance and resulting in lifelong infection. HTLV-I and HTVL-II both transform lymphocytes in vitro, and share approximately 65% genome homology. Serologic assays used in early epidemiologic studies were unable to differentiate between the two viruses, but more recent Western immunoblot assays as well as polymerase chain reaction may be used to discriminate infection with these two viruses.

EPIDEMIOLOGY AND CLINICAL MANIFESTATIONS. HTLV-I is the cause of adult T-cell leukemia/lymphoma (ATLL) and a chronic myelopathy that was described separately as HTLV-I–associated myelopathy (HAM) and as tropical spastic paraparesis (TSP) (currently termed HAM/TSP). The geographic epidemiology of ATLL and HAM/TSP are similar. HTLV-I is endemic in southern Japan (where more than 25% of adults are seropositive), Asia, areas of the Caribbean, and in parts of sub-Saharan Africa and Central and South America. There is microclustering with marked variability within small geographic regions. The seroprevalence of HTLV-I and HTLV-II in the United States in the general population is 0.01% for each virus, with higher rates with increasing age. HTLV-I infection correlates greatest with birth from or sexual contact with persons from endemic areas of Japan or the Caribbean, with overall higher prevalence in females and African-American and Hispanic persons. HTLV-II infection correlates with intravenous illicit drug use, with an overall prevalence of approximately 18% in one study of drug users in the United States, often with concomitant HTLV-I or HIV infection.

HTLV-I and II are transmitted as cell-associated virus through sexual contact, contaminated blood products, intravenous illicit drug use, and perinatally, usually via breast milk. Studies in Japan have shown that approximately 25% of children born to infected mothers become infected; more than 90% of HTLV-I–infected children have HTLV-I–infected mothers. Perinatal HTLV-I transmission occurs primarily via breast-feeding from infected mothers, with a threefold increased risk of transmission with breast-feeding for more than 6 mo. Intrauterine and intrapartum transmission probably account for less than 5% of vertical transmission. HTLV-II, like HTLV-I, may also be transmitted via breast-feeding but has a lower breast milk transmission rate, of approximately 14%.

T-Cell Leukemia/Lymphoma. The age distribution of ATLL peaks at approximately 50 yr, underscoring the long latent period of HTLV-I infection. HTLV-I–infected persons remain at risk for ATLL even if they move to an area of low HTLV-I prevalence, with a lifetime risk of ATLL of 2–4%. HTLV-I infects $CD4^+$ lymphocytes with a spectrum of disease from subclinical lymphoproliferation that may spontaneously resolve in approximately half of cases, or progress to chronic leukemia, lymphoma, and culminate in acute ATLL. Chronic, low-grade, HTLV-I–associated lymphoproliferation (pre-ATLL) may persist for years with abnormal lymphocytes with or without peripheral lymphadenopathy before progressing to the acute form. Most cases of ATLL are associated with monoclonal integration of HTLV-I provirus into the cellular genome. ATLL is characterized by hypercalcemia, lytic bone lesions, lymphadenopathy that spares the mediastinum, hepatomegaly, splenomegaly, cutaneous lymphomas, and opportunistic infections. Leukemia may occur with circulating polylobulated malignant lymphocytes possessing mature T-cell markers, called flower cells. Conventional chemotherapy is not curative, and relapses are common, with median survival of 11 mo from diagnosis.

Sequences of the HTLV-I tax gene have been found in lesions of mycosis fungoides, a T-cell lymphoma characterized by proliferation of atypical lymphocytes preferentially in the skin. Patients are usually middle-aged and present with diffuse hypopigmented plaques and patches. Mycosis fungoides may be caused by HTLV-I or a closely related virus.

Myelopathy. HAM/TSP occurs in less than 1% of persons with HTLV-I infection, usually developing during middle age. It is characterized by gradual onset and slowly progressive neurologic degeneration of the corticospinal tracts and, to a lesser extent, the sensory system. Approximately 50% of patients with HAM/TSP have HTLV-I infection; other postulated causes include chronic intoxication of cyanogenic glycosides from the consumption of cassava or from amino acid dietary deficiencies. HAM/TSP is more common in women than in men, and has a relatively short incubation period after HTLV-1 infection: 1–4 yr compared with 40–60 yr for ATLL. Clinical manifestations include permanent evolution of lower extremity spasticity or weakness, lower back pain, and hyperreflexia of the lower extremities with an extensor plantar response. The bladder and intestines may become dysfunctional, and men may become impotent. Some patients may have dysesthesias of the lower extremities with diminished sensation to vibration and pain. Upper extremity function and sensation, cranial nerves, and cognitive function are usually preserved. The cerebrospinal fluid may have a mildly elevated protein and a mild monocytic pleocytosis. Neuroimaging studies are normal or show periventricular lesions in the white matter. Treatment with corticosteroids or danazol, a synthetic androgen, has been reported to benefit some patients.

HTLV-II. HTLV-II was originally identified in patients with hairy cell leukemia, although most patients with hairy cell leukemia are seronegative for HTLV-II infection. HTLV-II has been rarely isolated from patients with leukemias or with myelopathies resembling HAM/TSP, but there is limited evidence of disease specifically associated with HTLV-II infection.

PREVENTION. Routine antibody testing of all blood products using HTLV-I viral lysate began in the United States in 1988, which missed 30–58% of HTLV-II infections, but combination HTLV-I/II antibody testing was implemented in 1997. Formula feeding of infants of HTLV-I–infected mothers is an effective means to control endemic HTLV-I transmission in developed countries.

Centers for Disease Control and Prevention: Recommendations for counseling persons infected with human T-lymphotropic virus, types I and II. MMWR Morb Mortal Wkly Rep 42(RR-9):1, 1993.

Bucher B, Poupard JA, Vernant JC, et al: Tropical neuromyelopathies and retroviruses: A review. Rev Infect Dis 12:890, 1990.

Hollsberg P, Hafler DA: Pathogenesis of diseases induced by human lymphotropic virus type I infection. N Engl J Med 328:1173, 1993.

Kaplan JE, Abrams E, Schaffer N, et al: Low risk of mother-to-child transmission of human lymphotropic virus type II in non-breast-fed infants. J Infect Dis 166:892, 1992.

Van Dyke RB, Heneine W, Perrin ME, et al: Mother-to-child transmission of human T-lymphotropic virus type II. J Pediatr 127:924, 1995.

Zucker-Franklin D, Kosann MK, Pancake BA, et al: Hypopigmented mycosis fungoides associated with human T cell lymphotropic virus type I tax in a pediatric patient. Pediatrics 103:1039, 1999.

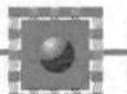

SECTION 13

Protozoan Diseases

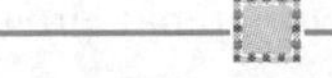

CHAPTER 270

Primary Amebic Meningoencephalitis

Martin Weisse and Stephen Aronoff

Naegleria, Acanthamoeba, and *Balamuthia* spp. are small, free-living amebas that cause human amebic meningoencephalitis. Amebic meningoencephalitis has two distinct clinical presentations. The more common is that of an acute, usually fatal infection of the central nervous system (CNS) caused by *Naegleria* occurring in previously healthy children and young adults. The second form, granulomatous amebic meningoencephalitis, caused by *Acanthamoeba* and *Balamuthia* spp., is a more indolent infection that is more likely to occur in immunocompromised individuals.

ETIOLOGY. *Naegleria* is an ameboflagellate that can exist as cysts, trophozoites, and transient flagellate forms. Temperature and environmental nutrient and ion concentrations are the major factors determining at which stage the ameba is found in the environment. Trophozoites are the only stages that are invasive, although cysts are potentially infective because they can convert to the vegetative form very quickly under the proper environmental stimuli. There are six species of *Naegleria,* of which only *N. fowleri* has been shown to be pathogenic for humans. *Naegleria* meningoencephalitis was first reported in the United States in 1966, and since that time infection has been reported from every continent. Most of the cases have been contracted during the summer months by previously healthy individuals with a history of swimming in or contact with fresh water before their illness. There are usually only one or two cases reported per year in the United States, with a high of eight cases reported in 1980. Most of the reports have come from the southern and southwestern states, with occasional infections occurring in the Midwest and East.

In contrast to *Naegleria* organisms, *Acanthamoeba* has only a cyst and trophozoite form, of which only the trophozoite form is invasive. Of the 13 species of *Acanthamoeba,* 7 are human pathogens. *A. castellani, A. culbertsoni, A. polyphaga,* and *A. rhysodes* have all been recovered from human infections of both the eye and the CNS. *A. astronyxis* and *A. palestinensis* have only been implicated in CNS infections. *A. hatchetti* has only been isolated from the eye. Through 1990, 56 cases of granulomatous amebic encephalitis had been reported worldwide, with 30 in the United States. Nine of these have been in patients with the acquired immunodeficiency syndrome (AIDS), and most of the rest have been associated with other immunomodulating conditions such as diabetes mellitus, alcoholism, or radiation therapy. Cases of *Acanthamoeba* keratitis have usually followed incidents of corneal trauma involving flushing with contaminated water or have occurred in contact lens wearers whose lenses have been contaminated with *Acanthamoeba* spp.

In 1990 an ameba was isolated from the brain of a mandrill baboon that died of meningoencephalitis. On the basis of immunofluorescent staining results, this same organism has been implicated in 35 cases of granulomatous amebic encephalitis that had formerly been without definite diagnosis but attributed to *Acanthamoeba*. This previously undiscovered pathogen has now been named *Balamuthia mandrillaris*. Although the clinical presentation is similar to infection with *Acanthamoeba*, most patients have no known immunocompromising condition.

EPIDEMIOLOGY. The free-living amebas have a worldwide distribution. *Naegleria* has been isolated from a variety of freshwater sources, including ponds and lakes, domestic water supplies, hot springs and spas, thermal discharge of power plants, and groundwater and occasionally from the nasal passages of healthy children. *Acanthamoeba* has been isolated from soil, mushrooms and vegetables, brackish water, and seawater, as well as most of the freshwater sources for *Naegleria*.

PATHOGENESIS. The free-living amebas enter the nasal cavity by inhalation or aspiration of dust or water contaminated with trophozoites or cysts. *Naegleria* gains access to the CNS through the olfactory epithelium and migration via the olfactory nerve to the olfactory bulbs, which are located in the subarachnoid space bathed by the cerebrospinal fluid (CSF). This space is richly vascularized and is the route of spread to other areas of the CNS. In addition to evidence of widespread cerebral edema and hyperemia of the meninges, the olfactory bulbs are necrotic, hemorrhagic, and surrounded by a purulent exudate. Microscopically, the gray matter is the most severely affected, with severe involvement in all cases. Fibrinopurulent exudate may be found throughout the cerebral hemispheres, brain stem, cerebellum, and upper portions of the spinal cord. Pockets of trophozoites may be seen in necrotic neural tissue, usually in the perivascular spaces of arteries and arterioles. No cysts are present in the CNS.

The route of invasion and penetration in cases of granulomatous amebic meningoencephalitis, caused by *Acanthamoeba* and *Balamuthia*, is hematogenous, probably originating from a primary focus in the skin or lungs. Pathologic examination reveals granulomatous encephalitis, with multinucleated giant cells mainly in the posterior fossa structures, basal ganglia, bases of the cerebral hemispheres, and cerebellum. Both trophozoites and cysts may be found in the CNS lesions, primarily located in the perivascular spaces and invading blood vessel walls. The olfactory bulbs and spinal cord are usually spared.

CLINICAL MANIFESTATIONS. The incubation of *Naegleria* infection may be as short as 2 days or as long as 15 days. Symptoms have an acute onset and are rapidly progressive. There is a sudden onset of severe headache, fever, nausea, and vomiting; signs of meningitis; and then encephalitis. Most cases end in death within 1 wk of onset of symptoms.

Granulomatous amebic meningoencephalitis may occur weeks to months after acquiring the organism. The presenting signs and symptoms are often those of single or multiple CNS space-occupying lesions; they include hemiparesis, personality changes, seizures, and drowsiness. Altered mental status is often a prominent symptom. Headache and fever occur only sporadically, but stiff neck is seen in a majority of cases. Palsies of the cranial nerves may be present. Results of neuroimaging studies of the brain usually demonstrate multiple low-density lesions resembling infarcts.

DIAGNOSIS. The CSF in *Naegleria* infection may mimic that of herpes simplex encephalitis early in the disease, and later of acute bacterial meningitis, with a neutrophilic pleocytosis, elevated protein level, and low glucose level. The amebas, which may be motile, may be seen on a wet mount of the CSF but are often mistaken for lymphocytes. A hanging drop examination of CSF and a strong clinical suspicion early in the course of disease affords the best chance for early treatment and cure. *Naegleria* can be grown on agar enriched with gram-negative bacteria, on which they feed.

In granulomatous meningoencephalitis, findings of examination of the CSF resemble those of aseptic meningitis. The isolation and identification of *Acanthamoeba* sp. from the CNS are the best methods of diagnosis. Brain tissue and CSF may be cultured for *Acanthamoeba* using the same agar used for growing *Naegleria* sp., but *Balamuthia* must be grown on mammalian cell cultures. All pediatric cases of *Balamuthia* meningoencephalitis have been diagnosed post mortem. Immunofluorescence staining of brain tissue can differentiate between *Acanthamoeba* and *Balamuthia*.

TREATMENT. *Naegleria* infection is nearly always fatal, and early recognition and early treatment are crucial to successful therapy. There have only been six treatment survivors, five of whom apparently recovered fully. *Naegleria* infections have been successfully treated with regimens of amphotericin B, rifampin, and chloramphenicol; amphotericin B, oral rifampin, and oral ketoconazole; and amphotericin alone. The duration of treatment is uncertain.

Trophozoites and cysts from *Acanthamoeba* keratitis are usually susceptible in vitro to chlorhexidine, polyhexamethyl biguanide (PHMB), propamidine, pentamidine, diminazene, and neomycin, and especially to combinations of these drugs. For treatment of keratitis, oral itraconazole plus topical miconazole, or topical 0.02% PHMB plus 0.1% propamidine, have been successful. PHMB is available as a swimming pool disinfectant.

There is currently no satisfactory treatment for granulomatous amebic meningoencephalitis. Strains of *Acanthamoeba* isolated from fatal cases are usually susceptible in vitro to pentamidine, ketoconazole, flucytosine, and less so to amphotericin B. One patient has been successfully treated with intravenous pentamidine, topical chlorhexidine, and 2% ketoconazole cream, followed by oral itraconazole. Limited success has been demonstrated in *Balamuthia* infection with systemic azole therapy combined with flucytosine. Corticosteroids appear to have a detrimental effect, with rapid progression of disease, and should be avoided.

Brown RL: Successful treatment of primary amebic meningoencephalitis. Arch Intern Med 152:1330, 1992.

Duguid IG, Dart JK, Morlet N, et al: Outcome of acanthamoeba keratitis treated with polyhexamethyl biguanide and propamidine. Ophthalmology 104:1587, 1997.

Ishibashi Y, Matsumoto Y, Kabata T, et al: Oral itraconazole and topical miconazole with debridement for *Acanthamoeba* keratitis. Am J Ophthalmol 109:121, 1990.

Ma P, Visvesvara GS, Martinez AJ, et al: Naegleria and Acanthamoeba infections: Review. Rev Infect Dis 12:490, 1990.

Rowen JL, Doerr CA, Vogel H, et al. *Balamuthia mandrillaris*: A newly recognized agent for amebic meningoencephalitis. Pediatr Infect Dis J 14:705, 1995.

Slater CA, Sickel JZ, Visvesvara GS, et al: Brief report: Successful treatment of disseminated acanthamoeba infection in an immunocompromised patient. N Engl J Med 331:85, 1994.

Visvesvara GS, Schuster FL, Martinez AJ: *Balamuthia mandrillaris*, N.G., n.sp., agent of amebic meningoencephalitis. J Eukaryot Microbiol 40:504, 1993.

Visvesvara GS, Stehr-Green JK: Epidemiology of free-living ameba infections. J Protozool 37:25S, 1990.

Wang A, Kay R, Poon WS, Ng HK: Successful treatment of amoebic meningoencephalitis in a Chinese living in Hong Kong. Clin Neurol Neurosurg 95:249, 1993.

CHAPTER 271
Amebiasis

Sharon B. Weissman and Robert A. Salata

Human infection with *Entamoeba* is prevalent worldwide; endemic foci are particularly common in the tropics, especially in areas with low socioeconomic and sanitary standards. *Entamoeba* parasitizes the lumen of the gastrointestinal tract and causes few or no symptoms or sequelae in most infected subjects. In a small proportion of individuals the organisms invade the intestinal mucosa or may disseminate to other organs, especially the liver.

ETIOLOGY. There are two morphologically identical but genetically distinct species of *Entamoeba* that commonly infect humans. *Entamoeba dispar,* the more prevalent species, is associated only with an asymptomatic carrier state. *Entamoeba histolytica,* the pathogenic species, can become invasive, causing symptomatic disease. Five other species of nonpathogenic *Amoeba* infrequently colonize the human gastrointestinal tract: *E. coli, E. hartmanni, E. gingivalis, E. moshkovskii,* and *E. polecki.*

Infection is established by ingestion of parasite cysts. These cysts, 10–18 μm, contain four nuclei. They are resistant to environmental conditions such as low temperature and the concentrations of chlorine commonly used in water purification; the parasite can be killed by heating to 55°C. Upon ingestion, the cyst, which is resistant to gastric acidity and digestive enzymes, excysts in the small intestine to form eight trophozoites. These are large, actively motile organisms that colonize the lumen of the large intestine and may invade its mucosal lining under conditions that are currently unknown. Infection is not transmitted by trophozoites because of their rapid degeneration outside the body or in the low pH environment of normal gastric contents. Trophozoites have an average diameter of 25 μm, with a single spherical nucleus containing fine peripheral chromatin and a central nucleolus. The endoplasm also contains vacuoles, where, in cases of invasive amebiasis, erythrocytes may be seen.

EPIDEMIOLOGY. The regional prevalence of amebic infections worldwide varies from 5 to 81%, with the highest frequency in the tropics. Humans are the major reservoir. It is estimated that 10%, approximately 480 million people, of the population worldwide is infected with *E. dispar or E. histolytica.* This infection is associated with 50 million cases of symptomatic disease and an annual mortality of 40,000–110,000 deaths; amebiasis is the third leading parasitic cause of death worldwide. *E. dispar* is 10-fold more common than *E. histolytica.* Symptomatic disease occurs in about 10% of individuals with *E. histolytica* infection. Therefore, invasive disease occurs in approximately 1% of persons determined to be infected with *Entamoeba* by light microscopy. Dissemination of the parasites to internal organs such as the liver occurs in an even smaller fraction of infected individuals and is less common in children than in adults.

Although highly endemic in Africa, Latin America, India, and Southeast Asia, amebiasis is not exclusively limited to the tropics. In the United States, amebiasis has been estimated to occur with a prevalence of 1–4% in certain high-risk groups, including chronically institutionalized persons, mentally retarded children, promiscuous homosexual males, emigrants from and travelers to endemic areas, migrant workers, and individuals in lower socioeconomic groups. The majority of children infected with *Entamoeba* fall into these risk groups.

Food or drink contaminated with *Entamoeba* cysts and direct fecal-oral contact are the most common means of infection. Untreated water and human feces used as fertilizer are important sources of infection. Food handlers carrying amebic cysts may, therefore, play a role in spreading the infection. Direct contact with infected feces also may be responsible for person-to-person transmission.

PATHOGENESIS. Trophozoites, which are responsible for tissue invasion and destruction, attach to the colonic mucosa by a galactose-specific lectin receptor. This receptor is also thought to be responsible for resistance to complement-mediated lysis. Once attached to the colonic mucosa, amoebas release a cysteine-rich proteinase that allows for penetration through the epithelial layer. *E. histolytica* trophozoites require direct contact with target cells to cause cell death. Host cells are destroyed by trophozoite release of spore-forming peptides, phospholipases, and hemolysins. Once *E. histolytica* trophozoites invade the intestinal mucosa, they produce tissue destruction (ulcers) with little local inflammatory response because of the cytolytic capacity of the organism. The organisms multiply and spread laterally underneath the intestinal epithelium to produce characteristic flask-shaped ulcers. These lesions are commonly seen in the cecum, transverse colon, and sigmoid colon. Ameba may produce similar lytic lesions if they reach the liver; these lesions are commonly called abscesses although they contain no granulocytes. The disparity between the extent of tissue destruction by ameba and the absence of a local host inflammatory response in the presence of systemic humoral (antibody) and cell-mediated responses remains a major scientific puzzle.

CLINICAL MANIFESTATIONS. Clinical presentations range from asymptomatic cyst passage to amebic colitis, amebic dysentery, ameboma, and extraintestinal disease. To date *E. dispar* has not been associated with symptomatic disease. *E. histolytica* infection is asymptomatic in 90% of persons, but it has the potential to become invasive and thus should be treated. Severe disease is more common in young children, pregnant women, malnourished individuals, and person using corticosteroids.

Extraintestinal disease usually involves only the liver, but rare extraintestinal manifestations include amebic brain abscess, pleuropulmonary disease, and ulcerative skin and genitourinary lesions.

Intestinal Amebiasis. Intestinal amebiasis may occur within 2 wk of infection or be delayed for months. The onset is usually gradual with colicky abdominal pains and frequent bowel movements (six to eight/day). Diarrhea is frequently associated with tenesmus. Stools are blood-stained and contain a fair amount of mucus with few leukocytes. Generalized constitutional symptoms and signs are characteristically absent, with fever documented in only one third of patients. Amebic colitis affects all age groups, but its incidence is strikingly high in children 1–5 yr of age. Severe amebic colitis in infants and young children tends to be rapidly progressive with frequent extraintestinal involvement and high mortality rates, particularly in tropical countries. Occasionally, amebic dysentery is associated with sudden onset of fever, chills, and severe diarrhea, which may result in dehydration and electrolyte disturbances. In a few patients complications such as ameboma, toxic megacolon, extraintestinal extension, or local perforation and peritonitis may occur.

Uncommonly, a chronic form of amebic colitis, which can mimic inflammatory bowel disease with bouts of abdominal pain and bloody diarrhea, often recurring over several years, develops. An ameboma is a nodular focus of proliferative inflammation sometimes developing in chronic amebiasis, usually in the wall of the colon. Chronic amebiasis should be excluded before initiating corticosteroid treatment for inflammatory bowel disease.

Hepatic Amebiasis. Hepatic amebiasis is a very serious manifestation of disseminated infection. Although diffuse liver enlargement has been associated with intestinal amebiasis, liver abscess occurs in < 1% of infected individuals and may appear in patients with no clear history of intestinal disease. In children, fever is the hallmark of amebic liver abscess and is frequently associated with abdominal pain, distention, and enlargement and tenderness of the liver. Changes at the base of the right lung, such as elevation of the diaphragm and atelectasis or effusion, may also occur. Laboratory examination findings are a slight leukocytosis, moderate anemia, high erythrocyte sedimentation rate, and nonspecific elevations of hepatic enzyme (particularly alkaline phosphatase) level. Stool examination for ameba yields negative results in > 50% of patients with documented amebic liver abscess. In most cases, computed tomography (CT), magnetic resonance imaging (MRI), or isotope scans can localize and delineate the size of the abscess cavity. Most patients have a single cavity in the right hepatic lobe, although results of recent studies employing CT have shown an increased rate of multiple abscesses and left lobe involvement. Amebic liver abscess may be associated with rupture into the peritoneum or thorax or through the skin when diagnosis and therapy are delayed.

DIAGNOSIS. Diagnosis is based on detecting the organisms in stool samples, sigmoidoscopically obtained smears, tissue biopsy samples, or, rarely, aspirates of a liver abscess. Examination of three fresh stool samples by experienced laboratory personnel has a sensitivity of 90% for detecting *Entamoeba*. Fresh stool samples should be examined within 30 min of passage and screened for motile trophozoites containing erythrocytes. Whenever amebiasis is suspected, an additional stool sample should be preserved in polyvinyl alcohol for further examination. Endoscopy and biopsies of suspicious areas should be performed when stool sample results are negative and the index of suspicion for amebiasis remains high. Unfortunately, unless phagocytized erythrocytes are seen, microscopy findings do not distinguish between *E. histolytica* and *E. dispar.* Patients with invasive amebic colitis have positive test results for fecal occult blood.

Various serum antiamebic antibody tests are available. Serologic results are positive in 95% of patients with symptomatic disease of > 7 days and in the majority of asymptomatic carriers of pathogenic strains of *Entamoeba*. *E. dispar* does not elicit a humoral response. The most sensitive serologic test, indirect hemagglutination, yields a positive result years after invasive infection. Antigen detection in stool or serum can establish a diagnosis while also distinguishing *E. dispar* from *E. histolytica*. Antigen detection tests are not yet routinely available.

TREATMENT. Two types of drugs are used to treat infection with *E. histolytica*. The luminal amebicides, such as iodoquinol, paromomycin, and diloxanide furoate, are primarily effective in the gut lumen. Metronidazole or other nitroimidazoles, chloroquine, and dehydroemetine are effective in the treatment of invasive amebiasis. All individuals with *E. histolytica* trophozoites or cysts in their stools, whether symptomatic or not, should be treated. Iodoquinol is the first line agent for treating asymptomatic cyst carriers; the recommended regimen is 30–40 mg/kg/24 hr in three divided doses (maximum 650 mg/dose) orally for 20 days. Paromomycin, a nonabsorbable aminoglycoside, is an alternative; the recommended regimen is 25–35 mg/kg/24 hr in three divided doses orally for 7 days. Diloxanide furoate is only available through the Centers for Disease Control and Prevention (CDC). Toxicity is rare, but the drug should not be used in children < 2 yr of age.

Invasive amebiasis of the intestine, liver, or other organs requires the use of metronidazole, a tissue amebicidal drug. The recommended regimen is 30–50 mg/kg/24 hr in three divided doses (maximum: 500–750 mg/dose) orally for 10 days. Two related nitroimidazoles, tinidazole and ornidazole, are available and have been used outside the United States. Adverse effects of metronidazole include nausea, abdominal discomfort, and metallic taste; these are uncommon and disappear after completion of therapy. Metronidazole is also a luminal amebicide but is less effective for this purpose and should be followed by a luminal agent. Metronidazole-resistant *E. histolytica* has not been reported. Nevertheless, for fulminant cases, some experts suggest adding dehydroemetine (available only through the CDC) for the first few days. It is administered either subcutaneously or intramuscularly (never intravenously) in a dose of 1 mg/kg/24 hr. Patients should be hospitalized when this drug is given. If tachycardia, T-wave depression, arrhythmias, or proteinuria develops, the drug should be stopped. Chloroquine, which concentrates in the liver, may be useful in the treatment of amebic hepatic abscess. Aspiration of large lesions or left lobe abscesses may be necessary if rupture is imminent or if the patient shows a poor clinical response 4–6 days after administration of amebicidal drugs.

Stool examination should be repeated every 2 wk until the result is negative after completion of antiamebic therapy to confirm cure.

PROGNOSIS. Most infections evolve to either an asymptomatic carrier state or eradication. Death occurs in about 5% of persons having extraintestinal infection.

PREVENTION. Control of amebiasis can be achieved by exercising proper sanitary measures and avoiding fecal-oral contact. Regular examination of food handlers and thorough investigation of diarrheal episodes may identify the source of infection in some communities. There is no prophylactic drug or vaccine available for amebiasis.

Adams EB, MacLeod IN: Invasive amebiasis. I. Amebic dysentery and its complications. Medicine 56:315, 1997.

Haque R, Neville LM, Hahn O, et al: Rapid diagnosis of *Entamoeba* infection using *Entamoeba* and *Entamoeba histolytica* stool antigen detection kits. J Clin Microbiol 33:2558, 1995.

Li E, Stanley SL: Protozoa, amebiasis. Gastroenterol Clin North Am 25:471, 1996.

Merritt RJ, Coughlin E, Thomas DW, et al: Spectrum of amebiasis in children. Am J Dis Child 136:785, 1982.

Nazir Z, Moazam F: Amebic liver abscess in children. Pediatr Infect Dis J 12:929, 1993.

Ravdin JI: Amebiasis. Clin Infect Dis 20:1453, 1995.

Reed SL: New concepts regarding the pathogenesis of amebiasis. Clin Infect Dis 21(Suppl 2):S182, 1995.

CHAPTER 272
Giardiasis and Balantidiasis

Larry K. Pickering

272.1 Giardia lamblia

Giardia lamblia is a flagellated protozoan that infects the duodenum and small intestine. Infection results in a wide variety of clinical manifestations ranging from asymptomatic colonization to acute or chronic diarrhea and malabsorption. Infection is more prevalent in children than in adults. *Giardia* are endemic in areas of the world with poor levels of sanitation and also are an important cause of morbidity in the developing world, where they are associated with urban child-care centers, residential institutions for the mentally delayed, and waterborne and foodborne outbreaks. *Giardia* is a particularly significant pathogen in people with malnutrition, immunodeficiencies, and cystic fibrosis.

ETIOLOGY. The life cycle of *Giardia* is composed of two stages: trophozoites and cysts. *Giardia* infects humans after ingestion of as few as 10–100 cysts. Ingested cysts, which measure approximately 8–10 μm, each produce two trophozoites in the proximal small intestine. After excystation, trophozoites colonize the lumen of the duodenum and proximal jejunum, where they attach to the brush border of the intestinal epithelial cells and multiply by binary fission. The body of the trophozoite is teardrop shaped, measuring 10–20 μm in length and 5–10 μm in width. It contains two oval nuclei anteriorly, a large ventral disk, a curved median body posteriorly, and four pairs of flagella. As detached trophozoites pass down the intestinal tract, they encyst to form oval cysts that contain four nuclei. Cysts are passed in the stools of infected individuals and may remain viable in water for as long as 2 mo. Their viability is not affected by the usual concentrations of chlorine used to purify water for drinking.

Giardia strains that infect humans are diverse biologically, as shown by differences in antigens, restriction endonuclease patterns, DNA fingerprinting, isoenzyme patterns, and pulsed-field gel electrophoresis. The differences in clinical manifestations and antimicrobial susceptibilities of various strains remain unkown.

EPIDEMIOLOGY. *Giardia* occurs worldwide and is the most common parasite identified in stool specimens in the United States. The age-specific prevalence of giardiasis is high during childhood and begins to decline after adolescence. The asymptomatic carrier rate of *G. lamblia* in the United States is estimated to be 3–7%, and as high as 20% in southern regions and in children < 36 mo of age attending child-care centers. Asymptomatic carriage may persist for several months.

Transmission of *Giardia* is common in certain high-risk groups, including children and employees in child-care centers, consumers of contaminated water, travelers to certain areas of the world, male homosexuals, and persons exposed to certain animals. The major reservoir and vehicle for spread of *Giardia* appears to be water contaminated with *Giardia* cysts, but foodborne transmission is documented with increased frequency. Common to most waterborne outbreaks has been ingestion of surface water treated by faulty or inadequate water purification systems. Drinking untreated mountain stream water presents a major risk to visitors to these areas, as does exposure to contaminated recreational water such as swimming pools. *Giardia* cysts are relatively resistant to chlorination and to ultraviolet light irradiation. Boiling is effective for inactivating cysts.

Person-to-person spread also occurs, particularly in areas of low hygiene standards, frequent fecal-oral contact, and crowding. Individual susceptibility, lack of toilet training, crowding, and fecal contamination of the environment all predispose to transmission of enteropathogens, including *Giardia*, in child-care centers. Child-care centers play an important role in the transmission of urban giardiasis, with secondary attack rates in families as high as 17–30%. Children in child-care centers may pass cysts for several months.

Humoral immunodeficiencies including common variable hypogammaglobulinemia and X-linked agammaglobulinemia predispose humans to chronic symptomatic *Giardia* infection, suggesting the importance of humoral immunity in controlling giardiasis. There is no convincing evidence that patients with acquired immunodeficiency syndrome (AIDS) or selective immunoglobulin A (IgA) deficiency have more severe or prolonged disease. There is a higher incidence of *Giardia* infection in patients with cystic fibrosis, probably due to local factors such as the increased amount of mucus, which may protect the organism against host factors in the duodenum. Human milk contains glycoconjugates and secretory IgA antibodies that may provide protection to nursing infants.

CLINICAL MANIFESTATIONS. The incubation period of *Giardia* infection usually is 1–2 wk but may be longer. A broad spectrum of clinical manifestations occurs, depending on the interaction between *G. lamblia* and the host. Children who are exposed to *G. lamblia* may experience asymptomatic excretion of the organism, acute infectious diarrhea, or chronic diarrhea with persistent gastrointestinal tract signs and symptoms, including failure to thrive. Most infections, in both children and adults, are asymptomatic. There usually is no extraintestinal spread, but occasionally trophozoites may migrate into bile or pancreatic ducts.

Symptomatic infections occur more frequently in children than in adults. Most symptomatic patients usually have a limited period of acute diarrheal disease with or without low-grade fever, nausea, and anorexia; in a small proportion an intermittent or more protracted course characterized by diarrhea, abdominal distention and cramps, bloating, malaise, flatulence, nausea, anorexia, and weight loss develops (Table 272–1). Initially, stools may be profuse and watery and later become greasy and foul-smelling and may float. Stools do not contain blood, mucus, or fecal leukocytes. Varying degrees of malabsorption may occur. Abnormal stool patterns may alternate with periods of constipation and normal bowel movements. Malabsorption of sugars, fats, and fat-soluble vitamins has been well documented and may be responsible for substantial weight loss.

DIAGNOSIS. Giardiasis should be considered in young children in child care or in any person who has had contact with an index case or a history of recent travel to an endemic area who has persistent diarrhea, intermittent diarrhea and constipation, malabsorption, crampy abdominal pain and bloating, or failure to thrive or weight loss.

A definitive diagnosis of giardiasis is established by documentation of trophozoites, cysts, or *Giardia* antigens in stool specimens or duodenal fluid. Several types of specimens from the gastrointestinal tract can be used to diagnose *Giardia* infection. For both trophozoites and cysts of *Giardia* organisms, identification can be made on direct smears of stool or after concentration of stool specimens. Stool specimens should be examined within 1 hr of passage or should be preserved in vials containing polyvinyl alcohol (PVA) or 10% formalin, both of which preserve parasite morphologic characteristics. Trophozoites may be present in unformed stools as a result of rapid bowel transit; they are not stable outside the gastrointestinal tract. Cysts are stable outside the gastrointestinal tract and are the infectious form.

In patients in whom the diagnosis is suspected but in whom examination of stool specimens for *Giardia* yields a negative result, aspiration or biopsy of the duodenum or upper jejunum should be performed. In a fresh specimen, trophozoites usually can be visualized by direct wet mount. An alternate method of directly obtaining duodenal fluid is the commercially available Entero-Test (Hedeco Corp, Mountain View, CA) or duodenal biopsy. The biopsy can be used to make touch preparations and tissue sections for identification of *Giardia* and other enteric pathogens, as well as to visualize changes in histologic features. Biopsy of the small intestine should be considered in patients with characteristic clinical symptoms, negative stool and duodenal fluid specimen findings, and one of the following: abnormal radiographic findings, such as edema and segmentation in the small intestine; abnormal lactose tolerance test result; ab-

TABLE 272–1 Clinical Signs and Symptoms of Giardiasis

Symptom	Frequency (%)
Diarrhea	64–100
Malaise, weakness	72–97
Abdominal distention	42–97
Flatulence	35–97
Abdominal cramps	44–81
Nausea	14–79
Foul-smelling, greasy stools	15–79
Anorexia	41–73
Weight loss	53–73
Vomiting	14–35
Fever	0–28
Constipation	0–27

sent secretory IgA level; hypogammaglobulinemia; or achlorhydria.

Medications, including antibiotics, antacids, antidiarrheals, and enema and laxative preparations, can interfere with identification of the organism by altering their morphologic characteristics or by causing a temporary disappearance of parasites from stool specimens. Patients should not take these compounds for 48–72 hr prior to collection of stool for identification of *Giardia*. Contrast material such as barium also will mask the presence of parasites.

Appropriately conducted direct examination of stool will establish the diagnosis in up to 70% of patients by a single examination, 85% by examination of a second stool specimen, and >90% by examination of three specimens. Comparison of stool examination results with small bowel aspiration results in patients with diarrhea revealed that parasites were detected in 50% of stools of patients in whom a small bowel focus of infection was documented by aspiration. Laboratories can reduce reagent and personnel costs by pooling specimens submitted for detection of *Giardia* prior to evaluation by either microscopy or by enzyme immunoassay (EIA).

Efforts to improve diagnostic testing include the use of polyclonal antisera or monoclonal antibodies against *Giardia* organism–specific antigens in EIA or immunofluorescent assays. Polymerase chain reaction and gene probe–based detection systems specific for *Giardia* have been used in environmental monitoring.

Radiographic contrast studies of the small intestine may show nonspecific findings such as irregular thickening of the mucosal folds. Blood counts usually are normal. Giardiasis is not associated with eosinophilia.

TREATMENT. Children with acute diarrhea in whom *Giardia* organisms are identified should receive therapy. In addition, children who manifest failure to thrive or exhibit malabsorption or gastrointestinal tract symptoms such as chronic diarrhea should be treated.

Asymptomatic excreters generally are not treated except in specific instances such as in outbreak control, for prevention of household transmission by toddlers to pregnant women and patients with hypogammaglobulinemia or cystic fibrosis, and in situations requiring oral antibiotic treatment where *Giardia* may have produced malabsorption of the antibiotic.

There are several drugs available in the United States that are effective in the therapy of patients with giardiasis, including metronidazole, which is the drug of choice, and furazolidone and paromomycin (Table 272–2). Paromomycin, a nonabsorbable aminoglycoside, has been suggested for use in pregnancy but has not been tested thoroughly. Tinidazole is used in other countries as single-dose therapy but is not available in the United States. The cure rate for metronidazole is 92% and for furazolidone is 84%. The only drug available in a liquid preparation for children is furazolidone, which has a cure rate of 92%.

PROGNOSIS. Symptoms recur in some patients, in whom reinfection cannot be documented and in whom an immune deficiency such as an immunoglobulin abnormality is not present, despite use of appropriate therapy. Several studies have demonstrated that variability in antimicrobial susceptibility exists among strains of *Giardia*, and in some instances resistant strains have been demonstrated. Combined therapy may benefit patients in whom infection persists after single-drug therapy, assuming reinfection has not occurred and the medication was taken as prescribed.

TABLE 272–2 Oral Antimicrobial Therapy of Giardiasis

Antimicrobial Agent	Pediatric Dose	Adult Dose
Metronidazole (Flagyl)	15 mg/kg/24 hr in 3 divided doses for 5 days (maximum 750 mg/24 hr)	250 mg 3 times a day for 5 days
Furazolidone (Furoxone)	6 mg/kg/24 hr in 4 divided doses for 10 days (maximum 400 mg/24 hr)	100 mg 4 times a day for 10 days
Paromomycin	Not recommended	30 mg/kg/24 hr in 3 divided doses for 7 days

PREVENTION. Infected persons and persons at risk should practice strict handwashing after any contact with feces. This is especially important for caregivers of diapered infants in child-care centers, where diarrhea is common and *Giardia* organism carriage rates are high.

Methods to purify public water supplies adequately include chlorination, sedimentation, and filtration. The inactivation of *Giardia* cysts by chlorine requires the coordination of multiple variables such as chlorine concentration, water pH, turbidity, temperature, and contact time. These variables cannot be appropriately controlled in all municipalities and are almost impossible to control in swimming pools.

Travelers to endemic areas are advised to avoid uncooked foods that might have been grown, washed, or prepared with water that was potentially contaminated. Purification of drinking water can be achieved by filtration with a pore size ≤1 μm or brisk boiling of water for at least 1 min. Treatment of water with chlorine or iodine is somewhat less effective but may be used as an alternate method when boiling or filtration is not possible.

272.2 Balantidiasis

Balantidium coli is a ciliated protozoan and is the largest protozoan that parasitizes humans. Both trophozoites and cysts may be identified in feces. Disease due to this organism is uncommon in the United States and is generally reported where there is a close association of humans with pigs, which are the natural hosts of the organism. Since the organism infects the large intestine, symptoms are consistent with large bowel disease, similar to those associated with amebiasis, and include nausea, vomiting, lower abdominal pain, and tenesmus. Symptoms associated with chronic infection include abdominal cramps, watery diarrhea with mucus, infrequently bloody diarrhea, and colonic ulcers similar to those associated with *Entamoeba histolytica*. Extraintestinal spread of *B. coli* does not occur.

Diagnosis using direct saline mounts is made by identification of trophozoites (50–100 μm long) or spherical or oval cysts (50–70 μm in diameter) in stool specimens. Trophozoites usually are more numerous than cysts. The recommended treatment regimen is metronidazole (35–50 mg/kg/24 hr divided in three doses; maximum 750 mg/dose) orally for 5 days, or tetracycline (40 mg/kg/24 hr divided in four doses; maximum 500 mg/dose) orally for 10 days in persons ≥8 yr of age; an alternative is iodoquinol (40 mg/kg/24 hr divided in three doses; maximum 650 mg/dose) orally for 20 days. Prevention of contamination of the environment by pig feces is the important means for control.

Adam RD: The biology of Giardia spp. Microbiol Rev 55:706, 1991.
Brodsky RE, Spencer HC Jr, Schultz MG: Giardiasis in American travelers to the Soviet Union. J Infect Dis 130:319, 1974.
Burke JA: Giardiasis in childhood. Am J Dis Child 129:1304, 1975.
Craft JC: Giardia and giardiasis in childhood. Pediatr Infect Dis J 1:196, 1982.
Craft JC, Holt EA, Tan JH: Malabsorption of oral antibiotics in humans and rats with giardiasis. Pediatr Infect Dis J 6:832, 1987.
Davidson RA: Issues in clinical parasitology: The treatment of giardiasis. Am J Gastroenterol 79:256, 1984.
Janoff EN, Craft JC, Pickering LK, et al: Diagnosis of *Giardia lamblia* infection by detection of parasite specific antigens. J Clin Microbiol 27:431, 1989.
Morrow AL, Reves RR, West MS, et al: Protection against infection with *Giardia*

lamblia by breastfeeding in a cohort of Mexican infants. J Pediatr 121:363, 1992.
Murphy TV, Nelson JD: Five vs. ten days therapy with furazolidone for giardiasis. Am J Dis Child 137:267, 1983.
Ortega YR, Adam RD: Giardia: Overview and update. Clin Infect Dis 25:545, 1997.
Pickering LK, Woodward WE, DuPont HL, et al: Occurrence of *Giardia lamblia* in children in day care centers. J Pediatr 104:522, 1984.
Rauch AM, Van R, Bartlett AV, Pickering LK: Longitudinal study of *Giardia lamblia* infection in a day care center population. Pediatr Infect Dis J 9:186, 1990.

CHAPTER 273
Spore-Forming Intestinal Protozoa

Patricia M. Flynn

The spore-forming protozoa—*Cryptosporidium, Isospora, Cyclospora,* and microsporidia—have become increasingly important intestinal pathogens in both immunocompetent and immunocompromised hosts during the past decade. The severity of illness in patients infected with human immunodeficiency virus (HIV) and acquired immunodeficiency syndrome (AIDS), and improved diagnostic capabilities, have helped elucidate the epidemiologic characteristics and clinical manifestations of these organisms. *Cryptosporidium, Isospora,* and *Cyclospora* are coccidian parasites that predominantly infect the epithelial cells lining the digestive tract. Microsporidia are ubiquitous, obligate intracellular protozoa that infect many other organ systems in addition to the gastrointestinal tract and cause a broader spectrum of disease.

273.1 Cryptosporidium

Initially, *Cryptosporidium* was thought to be pathogenic almost exclusively in immunocompromised persons. It is now recognized to be a leading protozoal cause of diarrhea in children worldwide and is a common cause of outbreaks in child-care centers.

ETIOLOGY. Infection with *Cryptosporidium parvum,* the cause of cryptosporidiosis in humans, is initiated by ingestion of infectious oocysts. The oocyst releases four sporozoites that invade enterocytes, primarily in the small intestine. The infection progresses through two stages: the asexual, which allows autoinfection at the luminal surface of the epithelium, and the sexual, which results in production of oocysts that are shed in the stools. The cysts are immediately infectious to other hosts or can reinfect the same host. Ingestion of very few cysts is required to produce infection, even in immunocompetent hosts.

EPIDEMIOLOGY. Cryptosporidiosis is associated with diarrheal illness worldwide and is more prevalent in developing countries and in children <2 yr of age. It has been implicated as an etiologic agent of persistent diarrhea in the developing world and as a cause of significant morbidity and mortality from malnutrition, including permanent effects on growth.

Transmission of *Cryptosporidium* to humans can occur by close association with infected animals, via person-to-person transmission, or from environmentally contaminated water. Although zoonotic transmission, especially from cows, occurs in persons in close association with animals, person-to-person transmission is probably responsible for cryptosporidiosis outbreaks within hospitals and child-care centers, where rates as high as 67% have been reported. Family members of infected child-care center attendees are also infected at approximately 70%. Recommendations to prevent outbreaks in child-care centers include strict handwashing, use of protective clothes or diapers capable of retaining liquid diarrhea, and separation of diapering and food handling areas and responsibilities.

Outbreaks of cryptosporidial infection have been associated with contaminated community water supplies and recreational waters in several states in the United States and in Great Britain. Wastewater, in the form of raw sewage, and runoff from dairies and grazing lands can contaminate both drinking and recreational water sources. It is estimated that *Cryptosporidium* oocysts are present in 65–97% of the surface water in the United States. The organism's small size, 4–6 μm in diameter; resistance to chlorination; and ability to survive for long periods outside a host create problems in public water supplies. A water-borne outbreak in 1993 in Milwaukee, Wisconsin, caused more than 400,000 cases of diarrhea.

CLINICAL MANIFESTATIONS. The incubation period is 2–14 days. Infection with *Cryptosporidium* is associated with profuse, watery, nonbloody diarrhea that can be accompanied by diffuse crampy abdominal pain, nausea, vomiting, and anorexia. Although less common in adults, vomiting occurs in >80% of children with cryptosporidiosis. Nonspecific symptoms such as myalgia, weakness, headache, and anorexia also may occur. Fever occurs in 30–50% of cases. Malabsorption, lactose intolerance, dehydration, weight loss, and malnutrition often occur in severe cases.

In immunocompetent hosts, the disease is usually self-limiting, although diarrhea may persist for several weeks and oocyst shedding may persist many weeks after symptoms resolve. Chronic diarrhea is common in individuals with immunodeficiency, such as congenital hypogammaglobulinemia or HIV infection. Symptoms and oocyst shedding can continue indefinitely and may lead to severe malnutrition, wasting, anorexia, and even death.

Cryptosporidiosis in immunocompromised hosts is often associated with biliary tract disease, characterized by fever, right upper quadrant pain, nausea, vomiting, and diarrhea. It also has been detected in the pancreatic duct of a child with AIDS and has been associated with pancreatitis in an immunocompetent host. Respiratory tract disease, with symptoms of cough, shortness of breath, wheezing, croup, and hoarseness, is very rare.

DIAGNOSIS. Infection is best diagnosed by identifying oocysts in feces or other body fluids or tissues. In stool, they appear as small, spherical bodies, 2–6 μm in size, and stain red when using modified acid-fast staining. Staining for *Cryptosporidium* should be specifically requested so that appropriate concentration and staining techniques can be employed. Because *Cryptosporidium* does not invade below the epithelial layer of the mucosa, fecal leukocytes are not found in stool specimens.

Because oocyst shedding in feces can be intermittent, several fecal specimens (at least three for an immunocompetent host) should be collected for microscopic examination. In addition to the modified acid-fast staining procedure, enzyme immunoassay, indirect immunofluorescence, and polymerase chain reaction testing are available. Serologic diagnosis is not helpful in acute cryptosporidiosis.

In tissue sections, *Cryptosporidium* organisms can be found along the microvillus region of the epithelia that line the gastrointestinal tract. The highest concentration usually is detected in the jejunum. Histologic section results reveal villus atrophy and blunting, epithelial flattening, and inflammation of the lamina propria.

TREATMENT. Since the diarrheal illness due to cryptosporidiosis is self-limited in immunocompetent patients, no specific antimicrobial therapy is required. Treatment should focus on supportive care, consisting of rehydration orally, or, if fluid losses are severe, intravenously.

Immunocompromised patients with severe cryptosporidial enteritis have been treated with a variety of antibiotics, none of which has been consistently effective. Paromomycin, a nonabsorbable aminoglycoside, is recommended for treatment (25–35 mg/kg/24 hr divided in three to four doses) orally; the duration of treatment is uncertain. Combination therapy with paromomycin (1 g twice daily) and azithromycin (600 mg daily) for 4 wk followed by paromomycin monotherapy for 8 wk has also been used in adult patients with AIDS. Treatment with orally administered human serum immunoglobulin or bovine colostrum has been successful in several anecdotal reports.

273.2 Isospora

Like *Cryptosporidium, Isospora belli* has been implicated as a cause of diarrhea in institutional outbreaks and in travelers and has also been linked with contaminated water and food. Unlike *Cryptosporidium* organisms, *Isospora* appears to be more common in tropical and subtropical climates and in developing areas, including South America, Africa, and Southeast Asia. *Isospora* has not been associated with animal contact. It is also an infrequent cause of diarrhea in patients with AIDS in the United States but may infect up to 15% of AIDS patients in Haiti.

The life cycle and pathogenesis of infection with *Isospora* sp. are similar to those of *Cryptosporidium* organisms except that oocysts excreted in the stool are not immediately infectious and must undergo further maturation below 37°C. Histologic appearance of gastrointestinal epithelium reveals blunting and atrophy of the villi, acute and chronic inflammation, and crypt hyperplasia.

The *clinical manifestations* are indistinguishable from cryptosporidiosis although fever may be a more common finding. Eosinophilia, not found with other enteric protozoan infections, may be present. The *diagnosis* is established by detecting the oval, 22–33 μm long by 10–19 μm wide, oocysts by using modified acid-fast staining of the stool. Each oocyst contains two sporocysts with four sporozoites in each. Fecal leukocytes are not detected.

Unlike cryptosporidiosis, isosporiasis responds promptly to *treatment* with oral trimethoprim-sulfamethoxazole (TMP-SMZ) (5 mg TMP, 25 mg SMZ/kg/dose; maximum 160 mg TMP, 800 mg SMZ/dose) orally four times a day for 10 days, then twice a day for 3 wk. In patients with AIDS, relapses are common and often necessitate maintenance therapy. Pyrimethamine, alone or with folinic acid, is effective in patients intolerant of sulfonamide drugs.

273.3 Cyclospora

Cyclospora cayetanensis, previously called cyanobacterium-like body, is a coccidian parasite similar to but larger than *Cryptosporidium parvum.* Cyclosporiasis is endemic in Nepal, Peru, and Haiti but may be found throughout the world. The organism infects both immunocompromised and immunocompetent individuals and is more common in children <18 mo of age. The pathogenesis and pathologic findings of cyclosporiasis are similar to those of isosporiasis. Asymptomatic carriage of the organism has been found, but travelers who harbor the organism almost always have diarrhea. Outbreaks of cyclosporiasis have been linked with contaminated food and water. An outbreak in 1997 in the United States was linked to imported raspberries. Neither person-to-person nor animal-to-person transmission has yet been documented.

The *clinical manifestations* of cyclosporiasis are similar to those of cryptosporidiosis and isosporiasis. Moderate *Cyclospora* illness is characterized by a median of six stools per day with a median duration of 10 days (range, 3–25 days). The diarrhea may not be the presenting complaint and may alternate with constipation. The duration of diarrhea in immunocompetent persons is characteristically longer in cyclosporiasis than in the other intestinal protozoan illnesses. Associated symptoms frequently include fatigue; abdominal bloating or gas; abdominal cramps or pain; nausea; muscle, joint, or body aches; fever; chills; headache; and weight loss. Vomiting may occur. Bloody stools are uncommon. Biliary disease has been reported. After fecal excretion, the oocysts do not sporulate and remain infectious for days to weeks.

Diagnosis is made by identification of oocysts in the stool. Oocysts are wrinkled spheres, measure 8–10 μm in diameter, and resemble large *Cryptosporidium* organisms. Each oocyst contains two sporocysts, each with two sporozoites. The organisms can be seen by using modified acid-fast staining, but stain less consistently than *Cryptosporidium.* They can also be detected with phenosafranin stain and by autofluorescence (strong green or intense blue under ultraviolet [UV] epifluorescence). Fecal leukocytes are not present.

The *treatment* of choice for cyclosporiasis, as for isosporiasis, is trimethoprim-sulfamethoxazole (5 mg TMP, 25 mg SMZ/kg/dose twice a day; maximum 160 mg TMP, 800 mg SMZ/dose) orally for 7 days.

273.4 Microsporidia

Microsporidia are ubiquitous and infect most animal groups, including humans. To date, at least six genera and unclassified organisms of the order *Microsporida* have been linked with human disease in both immunocompetent and immunocompromised hosts. The microsporidian organisms best associated with gastrointestinal disease are *Enterocytozoon bieneusi* and *Septata intestinalis.*

Little is known about the epidemiologic characteristics of these organisms, but they are likely similar to that of the other spore-forming intestinal protozoa. Unlike *Cryptosporidium* and the other protozoa, spores of microsporidia inject their contents into the host cell to establish infection. Intracellular division produces new spores that can spread to nearby cells, disseminate to other host tissues, or be passed into the environment via feces. Spores also have been detected in urine and respiratory epithelium, suggesting that some body fluids may also be infectious. Once in the environment, microsporidial spores remain infectious for up to 4 mo.

Microsporidial intestinal infection has been almost exclusively reported in patients with AIDS, but this finding may be due to the difficulty in diagnosing the infection. Microsporidia-associated diarrhea is intermittent, copious, watery, and nonbloody. Abdominal cramping and weight loss may be present; fever is unusual. Disseminated disease has been reported, and, as in cryptosporidiosis and cyclosporiasis, biliary disease can occur.

Microsporidia stain with hematoxylin-eosin, Giemsa, Gram, periodic acid–Schiff, and acid-fast stains but are often overlooked because of their small size (1–2 μm) and the absence of associated inflammation in surrounding tissues. Electron microscopy remains the reference method of detection, but success with modified trichrome stains and polymerase chain reaction (PCR) is encouraging.

There is no proven therapy for microsporidial intestinal infections. Albendazole (adult dose: 400 mg twice a day for 4 wk) and atovaquone have been reported to decrease symptoms, but controlled clinical trials have not been performed.

Didier ES: Microsporidiosis. Clin Infect Dis 27:1, 1998.

Goodgame RW: Understanding intestinal spore-forming protozoa: *Cryptosporidia, Microsporidia, Isospora* and *Cyclospora.* Ann Intern Med 124:429, 1996.

Herwaldt BL, Ackers ML, and the Cyclospora Working Group: An outbreak of cyclosporiasis associated with imported raspberries. N Engl J Med 336:1548, 1997.

MacKenzie WR, Hoxie NJ, Proctor ME, et al: A massive outbreak in Milwaukee of *Cryptosporidium* infection transmitted through the public water supply. N Engl J Med 331:161, 1994.

Smith NH, Cron S, Valdez LM, et al: Combination drug therapy for cryptosporidiosis in AIDS. J Infect Dis 178:900, 1998.

Wittner M, Tanowitz HB, Weiss LM: Parasitic infections in AIDS patients: Cryptosporidiosis, isosporiasis, microsporidiosis, cyclosporiasis. Infect Dis Clin North Am 7:569, 1993.

CHAPTER 274

Trichomoniasis (Trichomonas vaginalis)

Sharon Weissman and Robert A. Salata

Trichomonas vaginalis is a sexually transmitted protozoan parasite that primarily causes symptomatic vaginitis in women.

EPIDEMIOLOGY. An estimated 3 million American women have trichomoniasis each year; the occurrence in males is unknown. The incidence of trichomoniasis is highest among females with multiple sexual partners and in groups with the highest rates of other sexually transmitted infections. Thus, patients found to harbor *T. vaginalis* should be screened for other sexually transmitted infections. *T. vaginalis* is recovered from > 60% of female partners of infected men and 30–80% of male sexual partners of infected women. Trichomonads can survive for several hours in moist environments, but no case of transmission by indirect exposure has been documented. Vaginal trichomoniasis is rare until menarche. Its presence in a younger child should raise the possibility of sexual abuse.

Trichomoniasis may be transmitted to neonates during passage through an infected birth canal. Neonatal infection is usually self-limited, but rare cases of neonatal vaginitis and respiratory infection have been reported.

PATHOGENESIS. Infected vaginal secretions contain 10^1–10^5 or more protozoa/mL. In fresh preparations, *T. vaginalis* are highly motile and pear shaped and are most easily recognized by their characteristic twitching motility. The organisms reproduce by binary fission and exist only as vegetative cells; cyst forms have not been described. *T. vaginalis* activates the alternative pathway of complement, attracting polymorphonuclear neutrophils, which in turn can kill the protozoon. Monocytes and macrophages have been shown to kill trichomonads in vitro, but their role in natural infection is uncertain. Durable protective immunity does not occur.

CLINICAL MANIFESTATIONS. The incubation period in females is 5–28 days. Symptoms may begin or exacerbate during menses. About 10–50% of women asymptomatically harbor the organism. Signs and symptoms most commonly associated with trichomoniasis include copious malodorous yellow vaginal discharge, vulvovaginal irritation, dysuria, and dyspareunia. On physical examination, a frothy discharge with vaginal erythema and cervical hemorrhages ("strawberry cervix") may be seen. The vaginal discharge has pH > 4.5. Unfortunately, none of these signs and symptoms alone or in combination is specific enough to establish a diagnosis of trichomoniasis confidently. Abdominal discomfort is unusual and should prompt evaluation for pelvic inflammatory disease.

Most males carrying *T. vaginalis* are asymptomatic. The organism can be isolated in 5–15% of men with nongonococcal urethritis; these patients have symptoms that are indistinguishable from those of nongonococcal urethritis of other causes. Symptomatic males usually have dysuria and scant urethral discharge. Trichomonads occasionally cause epididymitis, prostatic involvement, and superficial penile ulceration. Infection in men is often self-limited, spontaneously resolving in 36% of men.

There is growing evidence that trichomoniasis is associated with poor pregnancy outcomes and gynecologic complications. In various studies, trichomoniasis has been shown to be associated with premature rupture of membranes, preterm labor, low birthweight, tubal infertility, and vaginal cuff cellulitis after hysterectomy. There is some evidence to suggest trichomoniasis increases the risk of HIV transmission.

DIAGNOSIS. The accurate diagnosis of trichomoniasis in both sexes is dependent on the demonstration of the protozoan in genital secretions. Trichomonads may be recognized in vaginal secretions by using the wet mount technique, which will identify 60–70% of infected females. Endocervical specimens are unreliable for diagnosis. Wet mount examination of material obtained by platinum loop from the anterior urethra will reveal the organism in 50–90% of infected men. Microscopic examination of urine sediment after prostatic massage is also of high yield in infected men. A negative wet mount finding does not exclude the diagnosis of trichomoniasis. Culture of the organism is the most sensitive (> 95%) method of detection, especially for asymptomatic carriers, but is not routinely available. Serologic testing is plagued by low sensitivity and specificity and has no current role in the evaluation of the individual patient. New diagnostic kits using DNA probes and monoclonal antibodies may prove to be both sensitive and specific tests for detecting trichomonads.

TREATMENT. The treatment of trichomoniasis is a nitroimidazole. In the United States, metronidazole is used; in other countries tinidazole or ornidazole has been used with similar efficacy. Numerous studies have substantiated the efficacy of a metronidazole as a single large dose (2 g) orally in adolescent females; an alternative regimen is metronidazole 250 mg three times a day, or 375 mg two times a day, orally for 7 days. The recommended regimen for infected children is metronidazole 15 mg/kg/24 hr divided in three doses orally for 7 days. Topical metronidazole gel is not efficacious. All sexual partners should be treated simultaneously to prevent reinfection.

There is controversy regarding the safety of metronidazole during the first trimester of pregnancy, although several studies report the safety of this drug in the last two trimesters. It is now recommended to treat trichomoniasis during pregnancy.

The number of putative metronidazole failures appears to be increasing. In some cases metronidazole-resistant *T. vaginalis* has been documented. In most cases, failure is a consequence of reinfection from an untreated sexual partner, or of noncompliance with multidose therapy.

Cotch MF, Pastorek JG, Nugent RP, et al: *Trichomonas vaginalis* associated with low birth weight and preterm delivery. Sex Transm Dis 24:353, 1997.

Heine P, McGregor JA: *Trichomonas vaginalis*: A reemerging pathogen. Clin Obstet Gynecol 36:137, 1993.

CHAPTER 275

Leishmania

Peter C. Melby

The leishmaniases are a diverse group of diseases caused by intracellular protozoan parasites of the genus *Leishmania*, which are transmitted by phlebotomine sandflies. Humans are incidentally infected. Multiple species of *Leishmania* organisms are known to cause human disease involving the skin and mucosal surfaces, and the visceral reticuloendothelial organs.

Cutaneous disease is generally mild but may cause cosmetic disfigurement. Mucosal and visceral leishmaniasis is associated with significant morbidity and mortality rates.

ETIOLOGY. *Leishmania* spp. are members of the Trypanosomatidae family and include two subgenera, *L. (Leishmania)* spp. and *L. (Viannia)* spp. The parasite is dimorphic, existing as a flagellate promastigote in the insect vector and as an aflagellate amastigote that resides and replicates only within mononuclear phagocytes of the vertebrate host. Within the sandfly vector the promastigote undergoes a series of developmental steps from a noninfective procyclic form to an infective metacyclic stage. Fundamental to this transition are changes that take place in the terminal polysaccharides of the surface lipophosphoglycan (LPG), which allow forward migration of the infective parasites from the sandfly midgut to the mouthparts, from which they are inoculated into the host during a blood meal. The metacyclic LPG also plays an important role in the entry and survival of *Leishmania* spp. in the mammalian host by conferring complement resistance and by facilitating entry into the macrophage via the complement receptor 1. Once within the macrophage the promastigote transforms to an amastigote and resides and replicates within a phagolysosome. The parasite is resistant to the acidic, hostile environment of the macrophage and eventually ruptures the cell and goes on to infect other macrophages. Infected macrophages have a diminished capacity to initiate and respond to an inflammatory response, thus providing a safe haven for the intracellular parasite.

EPIDEMIOLOGY. The leishmaniases are estimated to affect 10–50 million people in endemic tropical and subtropical regions on all continents except Australia and Antarctica. The different forms of the disease are distinct in their causes, epidemiologic characteristics, transmission, and geographical distribution. Localized cutaneous leishmaniasis (LCL) is caused by *L. (Leishmania) major* and *L. (L.) tropica* in North Africa, the Middle East, central Asia, and the Indian subcontinent. *L. (L.) aethiopica* is a cause of LCL and diffuse cutaneous leishmaniasis (DCL) in Kenya and Ethiopia. Visceral leishmaniasis (VL) in the Old World is caused by *L. (L.) donovani* in Kenya, Sudan, India, Pakistan, and China, and by *L. (L.) infantum* in the Mediterranean basin, Middle East, and central Asia. *L. infantum* is also a cause of LCL (without visceral disease) in this same geographic distribution. *L. tropica* also has been recognized as an uncommon cause of visceral disease in the Middle East and India. In the New World, *L. (L.) mexicana* causes LCL in a region stretching from southern Texas through Central America. *L. (L.) amazonensis, L. (L.) pifanoi, L. (L.) garnhami, and L. (L.) venezuelensis* are causes of LCL in South America, in the Amazon basin and northward. Members of the *Viannia* subgenus *(L. [V.] braziliensis, L. [V.] panamensis, L. [V.] guyanensis, and L. [V.] peruviana)* are causes of LCL from the northern highlands of Argentina northward to Central America. Members of the *Viannia* subgenus also cause mucosal leishmaniasis (ML) in a similar geographic distribution. VL in the New World is caused by *L. (L.) chagasi,* which is distributed from Mexico (rare) through Central and South America. Like *L. infantum, L. chagasi* can also cause LCL in the absence of visceral disease. The leishmaniases may occur sporadically throughout an endemic region or may occur in epidemic focuses. With only rare exceptions, the *Leishmania* spp. that primarily cause cutaneous disease do not cause visceral disease.

The maintenance of *Leishmania* spp. in most endemic areas is through a zoonotic cycle in which humans are only incidentally infected. In general, the dermatropic strains in both the Old and New Worlds are maintained in rodent reservoirs, and the domestic dog is the usual reservoir for members of the *L. donovani* complex. The transmission between reservoir and sandfly is highly adapted to the specific ecologic characteristics of the endemic region. Human infections occur when their activities bring them in contact with the zoonotic cycle. Anthroponotic transmission, in which humans are the presumed reservoir, occurs with *L. tropica* in some urban areas of the Middle East, and with *L. donovani* in India.

Over the last decade an increased number of cases have been reported from a number of long-standing endemic focuses, and large numbers of cases have been recognized in some new focuses. Severe epidemics with >100,000 deaths from VL have occurred in India and Sudan. The emergence of the leishmaniases in new focuses is the result of (1) movement of a susceptible population into existing endemic areas, usually because of agricultural or industrial development or timber harvesting; (2) increase in vector and/or reservoir populations as a result of agriculture development projects; (3) increase in anthroponotic transmission due to rapid urbanization in some focuses; and (4) increase in sandfly density resulting from a reduction in malaria vector control programs.

PATHOGENESIS. Cellular immune mechanisms determine resistance or susceptibility to *Leishmania* sp. infection. Resistance is mediated by expansion of the T helper 1 (Th1) cell population with interferon-γ production resulting in macrophage activation and parasite killing. Interleukin 12 (IL-12) plays a central role in the development of the protective Th1 response. Susceptibility is associated with expansion of IL-4-producing Th2 cells and the production of IL-10 and transforming growth factor-β, which are potent inhibitors of macrophage activation. Patients with ML exhibit a hyper-responsive cellular immune reaction that may contribute to the prominent tissue destruction seen in this form of the disease. Patients with DCL or active VL demonstrate minimal or absent *Leishmania*-specific cellular immune responses, but these responses resume after successful therapy.

Within endemic areas people who have had a subclinical infection can be identified by a positive delayed-type hypersensitivity response to leishmanial antigens (Montenegro skin test). Subclinical infection occurs considerably more frequently than does active disease, for either cutaneous or visceral disease. Host factors (genetic background, concomitant disease, nutritional status), parasite factors (virulence, size of the inoculum), and possibly vector-specific factors (vector genotype, immunomodulatory salivary constituents) influence the expression as either subclinical infection or active disease. Within endemic areas the prevalence of skin test result positivity increases with age and the incidence of clinical disease decreases with age, indicating that immunity is acquired in the population over time. Individuals with prior active disease or subclinical infection are usually immune to a subsequent clinical infection.

CLINICAL MANIFESTATIONS. The different forms of the disease are distinct in their causes, epidemiologic features, transmission, and geographical distribution.

Localized Cutaneous Leishmaniasis. LCL (oriental sore) can affect individuals of any age, but children are the primary victims in many endemic regions. It typically presents as one or a few papular, nodular, plaquelike, or ulcerative lesions that are usually located on exposed skin, such as the face and extremities. Rarely, cases of >100 lesions have been recorded. The lesions typically begin as a small papule at the site of the sandfly bite, which enlarges to 1–3 cm in diameter and may ulcerate over the course of several weeks to months. The shallow ulcer is usually nontender and surrounded by a sharp, indurated, erythematous margin. There is no drainage unless a bacterial superinfection develops. Lesions caused by *L. major* and *L. mexicana* usually heal spontaneously after 3–6 mo, leaving a depressed scar. Lesions on the ear pinna caused by *L. mexicana,* called *chiclero ulcer* because they were common in chicle harvesters in Mexico and Central America, often follow a chronic, destructive course. In general, lesions caused by *L. (Viannia)* spp. tend to be larger and more chronic. Regional lymphadenopathy and palpable subcutaneous nodules or lymphatic cords (so-called sporotrichoid appearance) are also more common when the patient is infected with organisms of the *Viannia* subgenus. If lesions do not become secondarily infected, there are usually no complications aside from the residual cutaneous scar.

Diffuse Cutaneous Leishmaniasis. DCL is a rare form of leishmaniasis caused by organisms of the *L. mexicana* complex in the New World, and *L. aethiopica* in the Old World. DCL manifests as large nonulcerating macules, papules, nodules, or plaques that often involve large areas of skin and may resemble lepromatous leprosy. The face and extremities are most commonly involved. Dissemination from the initial lesion usually takes place over several years. It is thought that an immunologic defect underlies this severe form of cutaneous leishmaniasis.

Mucosal Leishmaniasis. ML (espundia) is an uncommon but serious manifestation of leishmanial infection resulting from hematogenous metastases to the nasal or oropharyngeal mucosa from a cutaneous infection. ML is usually caused by parasites in the *L. (Viannia)* complex. Approximately half of the patients with mucosal lesions will have had active cutaneous lesions within the preceding 2 yr, but ML may not develop until years after resolution of the primary lesion. ML occurs in <5% of individuals who have, or have had, LCL caused by *L. (V.) braziliensis*. Patients with ML most commonly have nasal mucosal involvement and present with nasal congestion, discharge, and recurrent epistaxis. Oropharyngeal and laryngeal involvement is less common but associated with severe morbidity. Marked soft tissue, cartilage, and even bone destruction occurs late in the course of disease and may lead to visible deformity of the nose or mouth, nasal septal perforation, and tracheal narrowing with airway obstruction.

Visceral Leishmaniasis. VL (kala-azar) typically affects children <5 yr of age in the New World (*L. chagasi*) and Mediterranean region (*L. infantum*), and older children and young adults in Africa and Asia (*L. donovani*). Elegant epidemiologic studies performed in Brazil have defined the clinical evolution of this disease. After inoculation of the organism into the skin by the sandfly, the child may have a completely asymptomatic infection, or an oligosymptomatic illness that either resolves spontaneously or evolves into active kala-azar. Children with asymptomatic infection are transiently seropositive but show no clinical evidence of disease. Children who are oligosymptomatic have mild constitutional symptoms (malaise, intermittent diarrhea, poor activity tolerance) and intermittent fever; most will have a mildly enlarged liver. In most of these children illness will resolve without therapy, but in approximately one fourth of these children it will evolve to active kala-azar within 2–8 mo. Extreme incubation periods of several years have rarely been described. During the first few weeks to months of disease evolution the fever is intermittent, there are loss of energy and weakness, and the spleen begins to enlarge. The classic clinical features of high fever, marked splenomegaly, hepatomegaly, and severe cachexia typically develop approximately 6 mo after the onset of the illness, but a rapid clinical course over 1 mo has been noted in up to 20% of patients in some series. At the terminal stages of kala-azar the hepatosplenomegaly is massive, there is gross wasting, the pancytopenia is profound, and jaundice, edema, and ascites may be present. Anemia may be severe enough to precipitate heart failure. Bleeding episodes, especially epistaxis, are frequent. The late stage of the illness is often complicated by secondary bacterial infections, which frequently are a cause of death. A younger age at the time of infection and underlying malnutrition may be risk factors for the development and more rapid evolution of active VL. Death occurs in >90% of patients without specific antileishmanial treatment.

VL has been increasingly recognized as an opportunistic infection associated with HIV infection. Most cases have occurred in southern Europe and Brazil, but there is potential for many more cases as the endemic regions for HIV and VL converge. Leishmaniasis may also result from reactivation of a long-standing subclinical infection. Frequently there is an atypical clinical presentation of VL in HIV-infected individuals with prominent involvement of the gastrointestinal tract and absence of the typical hepatosplenomegaly.

A small percentage of patients who have previously been treated for VL will have diffuse skin lesions, a condition called *post–kala azar dermal leishmaniasis* (PKDL). These lesions may appear during or shortly after therapy (Africa) or up to several years later (India). The lesions of PKDL are hypopigmented, erythematous, or nodular and commonly involve the face and torso. They may persist for several months or for many years.

DIAGNOSIS. The development of one or several slowly progressive, nontender, nodular, or ulcerative lesions in a patient who had potential exposure in an endemic area should raise suspicion of LCL. Other diseases that should be considered include sporotrichosis, blastomycosis, chromomycosis, lobomycosis, cutaneous tuberculosis, atypical mycobacterial infection, leprosy, ecthyma, syphilis, yaws, and neoplasms. Histopathologic analysis of the LCL lesion shows intense chronic granulomatous inflammation involving the epidermis and dermis. Occasionally neutrophils and even microabscesses can be seen. The lesions of DCL are characterized by dense infiltration with vacuolated macrophages containing abundant amastigotes.

ML is characterized by an intense granulomatous reaction with prominent tissue necrosis, which may include adjacent cartilage or bone. Other infections such as syphilis, tertiary yaws, histoplasmosis, paracoccidioidomycosis, as well as sarcoidosis, Wegener's granulomatosis, midline granuloma, and carcinoma may have clinical features similar to those of ML.

A definitive diagnosis of leishmaniasis is established by the demonstration of amastigotes in tissue specimens or isolation of the organism by culture. Amastigotes can be identified in Giemsa-stained tissue sections, aspirates, or impression smears in about half of the cases of LCL but only rarely in the lesions of ML. Serologic tests for diagnosis of ML or LCL generally have a low sensitivity and specificity and offer little for diagnosis. Culture of a tissue biopsy or aspirate, best performed by using Novy-McNeal-Nicolle (NNN) biphasic blood agar medium, yields a positive finding in only about 65% of cases. A positive culture result allows speciation of the parasite (usually by isoenzyme analysis by a reference laboratory), which may have therapeutic and prognostic significance. Identification of parasites in impression smears, histopathologic sections, or culture medium is more readily accomplished in DCL than in LCL.

VL should be strongly suspected in the patient with prolonged fever, weakness, cachexia, marked splenomegaly, hepatomegaly, cytopenias, and hypergammaglobulinemia who has had potential exposure in an endemic area. The clinical picture may also be consistent with that of malaria, typhoid fever, miliary tuberculosis, schistosomiasis, brucellosis, amebic liver abscess, infectious mononucleosis, lymphoma, and leukemia. In VL there is prominent reticuloendothelial cell hyperplasia in the liver, spleen, bone marrow, and lymph nodes. Amastigotes are abundant in the histiocytes and Kupffer's cells. Late in the course of disease splenic infarcts are common, centrilobular necrosis and fatty infiltration of the liver occur, the normal marrow elements are replaced by parasitized histiocytes, and erythrophagocytosis is present. Results of smears or cultures of material from splenic, bone marrow, or lymph node aspirations are usually diagnostic. In experienced hands, splenic aspiration has a higher diagnostic sensitivity, but it is rarely performed in the United States because of the risk of bleeding complications. Serologic testing by enzyme immunoassay, indirect fluorescence assay, or direct agglutination is very useful in VL because of the very high level of antileishmanial antibodies. An enzyme-linked immunosorbent assay (ELISA) using a recombinant (K39) antigen has a sensitivity and specificity close to 100%. A negative serologic test result in an immunocompetent individual is strong evidence against a diagnosis of VL.

Serodiagnostic tests have positive findings in only about half of the patients who are co-infected with HIV.

Laboratory Findings. Patients with cutaneous or mucosal leishmaniasis generally do not have abnormal laboratory results unless the lesions are secondarily infected with bacteria. Laboratory findings associated with classic kala-azar include anemia (hemoglobin 5–8 mg/dL), thrombocytopenia, leukopenia (2,000–3,000 cells/μL), elevated hepatic transaminase levels, and hyperglobulinemia (>5 g/dL) that is mostly immunoglobulin G (IgG).

TREATMENT. Specific antileishmanial therapy is not routinely indicated for uncomplicated LCL caused by strains that have a high rate of spontaneous resolution and self-healing (*L. major, L. mexicana*). Lesions that are extensive, severely inflamed, located where a scar would result in disability (near a joint) or cosmetic disfigurement (face or ear); that involve the lymphatics; or that do not begin healing within 3–4 mo should be treated. Cutaneous lesions suspected or known to be caused by members of the *Viannia* subgenus (New World) should be treated because of the low rate of spontaneous healing and the potential risk of development of mucosal disease. Similarly, patients with lesions caused by *L. tropica* (Old World), which are typically chronic and nonhealing, should be treated. All patients with VL or ML should receive therapy.

The pentavalent antimony compounds (sodium stibogluconate [Pentostam, Wellcome Foundation, United Kingdom] and meglumine antimoniate [Glucantime, Rhône-Poulenc, France]) have been the mainstay of antileishmanial chemotherapy for more than 40 years. These drugs have similar efficacies, toxicities, and treatment regimens. Currently, for sodium stibogluconate (available in the United States from the Centers for Disease Control and Prevention, Atlanta, GA) the recommended regimen is 20 mg/kg/24 hr intravenously or intramuscularly for 20 days (for LCL and DCL) or 28 days (for ML and VL). Repeated courses of therapy may be necessary in patients with severe cutaneous lesions, ML, or VL. An initial clinical response to therapy usually occurs in the first week of therapy, but complete clinical healing (re-epithelialization and scarring for LCL and ML, and regression of splenomegaly and normalization of cytopenias for VL) is usually not evident for weeks to a few months after completion of therapy. Cure rates with this regimen of 90–100% (LCL), 50–70% (ML), and 80–100% (VL) can be expected. Lower initial cure rates have been noted in patients from regions where clinical resistance to antimony therapy is common, such as India, East Africa, or some parts of Latin America. Relapses are common in patients who do not have an effective antileishmanial cellular immune response, such as those who have DCL or are co-infected with HIV. These patients often require multiple courses of therapy or a chronic suppressive regimen. When clinical relapses occur, they are usually evident within 2 mo after completion of therapy. Adverse effects of antimony therapy are dose- and duration-dependent and commonly include fatigue, arthralgias and myalgias (50%), abdominal discomfort (30%), elevated hepatic transaminase level (30–80%), elevated amylase and lipase levels (almost 100%), mild hematologic changes (slightly decreased white blood cell count, hemoglobin level, and platelet count) (10–30%), and nonspecific T-wave changes on electrocardiograph (30%). Sudden death due to cardiac toxicity is extremely rare and usually associated with use of very high doses of pentavalent antimony.

Several alternative therapies have been used in the treatment of the leishmaniases. Amphotericin B desoxycholate and the newer lipid formulations are very useful in the treatment of antimony-unresponsive VL or ML. Amphotericin B desoxycholate at doses of 0.5–1.0 mg/kg each day or every other day for 14–20 doses achieved a cure rate for VL of close to 100%, but the renal toxicity commonly associated with amphotericin B was evident. The lipid formulations of amphotericin B are especially attractive for treatment of leishmaniasis because the drugs are concentrated in the reticuloendothelial system and are less nephrotoxic. Liposomal amphotericin B (3 mg/kg on days 1–5, and again on day 10) has been shown to be highly effective (90–100% cure rate) for treatment of VL in immunocompetent children, some of whom were refractory to antimony therapy. Treatment of VL with parenteral paromomycin has also shown some success, although it does not appear to be superior to either antimony or amphotericin B. Recombinant human interferon-γ has been successfully used as an adjunct to antimony therapy in treatment of refractory cases of ML and VL. It is not effective alone and has the frequent side effects of fever and flulike symptoms. Pentamidine is an effective alternative treatment for LCL (especially in cases unresponsive to antimony) when given at 2–3 mg/kg every other day for four to seven doses. Treatment of ML and VL with pentamidine requires high doses and a long duration of therapy, making it less attractive than amphotericin B desoxycholate and the lipid formulations. Treatment of LCL with oral drugs has had only modest success. Ketoconazole has been effective in treating adults with LCL caused by *L. major, L. mexicana,* and *L. panamensis,* but not *L. tropica* or *L. braziliensis.* Allopurinol has been used for many years in the treatment of CL, but recent controlled trials indicate that it is probably not effective as monotherapy. It may have a role as adjunct therapy with standard treatment regimens.

PREVENTION. Personal protective measures should include avoidance of exposure to the nocturnal sandflies and when necessary the use of insect repellent and permethrin-impregnated mosquito netting. Where peridomiciliary transmission is present, community-based residual insecticide spraying has had some success in reducing the prevalence of leishmaniasis, but long-term effects are difficult to maintain. Control or elimination of infected reservoir hosts (e.g., seropositive domestic dogs) has had limited success. Where anthroponotic transmission is thought to occur, early recognition and treatment of cases are essential. Vaccination of humans or domestic dogs may have a role in the control of the leishmaniases in the future.

Alvar J, Canavate C, Gutierrez-Solar B, et al: *Leishmania* and human immunodeficiency virus coinfection: The first 10 years. Clin Microbiol Rev 10:198, 1997.

Badaro R, Jones TC, Carvalho EM, et al: New perspectives on a subclinical form of visceral leishmaniasis. J Infect Dis 154:1003, 1986.

Badaro R, Falcoff E, Badaro F, et al: Treatment of visceral leishmaniasis with pentavalent antimony and interferon gamma. N Engl J Med 322:16, 1990

Berman JD: Human leishmaniasis: Clinical, diagnostic, and chemotherapeutic developments in the last 10 years. Clin Infect Dis 24:684, 1997.

di Martino L, Davidson RN, Giacchino R, et al: Treatment of visceral leishmaniasis in children with liposomal amphotericin B. J Pediatr 131:271, 1997.

Dye C, Williams BG: Malnutrition, age, and the risk of parasitic disease: Visceral leishmaniasis revisited. Proc R Soc Lond 254:33, 1993.

Grevelink SA, Lerner EA: Leishmaniasis. J Am Acad Dermatol 34:257, 1996.

Magill AJ, Grogl M, Gasser RA, et al: Visceral infection caused by *Leishmania tropica* in veterans of Operation Desert Storm. N Engl J Med 328:1383, 1993.

McHugh CP, Melby PC, LaFon SG: Leishmaniasis in Texas: Epidemiological and clinical aspects of human cases. Am J Trop Med Hyg 55:547, 1996.

Sundar S, Murray HW: Cure of antimony-unresponsive Indian visceral leishmaniasis with amphotericin B lipid complex. J Infect Dis 173:762, 1996.

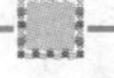

CHAPTER 276

African Trypanosomiasis (Sleeping Sickness; Trypanosoma brucei*)*

Adel A.F. Mahmoud

The trypanosomiases of tropical Africa are a group of diseases of great social and economic importance. Human infections are caused by two subspecies of *Trypanosoma brucei,*

T. b. rhodesiense and *T. b. gambiense,* which are morphologically indistinguishable but differ markedly in their epidemiologic characteristics and the disease syndromes they cause. Infection with *T. b. rhodesiense,* usually results in acute syndromes that have a rapid and, if untreated, fatal course, whereas infection with *T. b. gambiense,* usually has a more chronic course, resulting in the typical syndrome of sleeping sickness.

ETIOLOGY. Human infection is initiated by insect bite; the organisms penetrate intact mucous membranes or skin. The infective metacyclic forms of the trypanosomes are 15 μm long and possess no free flagella. After a period of local multiplication in the skin for 1–3 wk, long and slender forms (12–42 μm) can be seen in the peripheral blood; intermediate and stumpy forms also occur. These are flagellated forms with a well-developed undulating membrane. In the early stages of human infection, the organisms multiply rapidly in the blood and lymph nodes. They appear in waves in the peripheral blood, each wave followed by a febrile crisis. The reappearance of another population of organisms in the blood heralds the formation of a new antigenic variant. Invasion of the central nervous system occurs early in *T. b. rhodesiense* infection but late in the Gambian form.

The insect intermediate vectors are species of the tsetse flies of the genus *Glossina.* Inside the flies, the organisms localize in the posterior part of the midgut, where they multiply for about 10 days, then gradually migrate anteriorly, where they attach to the walls of the salivary ducts and complete the final stages of development into the infective metacyclic forms. The life cycle within the tsetse fly takes 15–35 days.

Direct transmission to humans has also been reported. Transmission is accomplished either mechanically through contact with the contaminated mouthparts of tsetse flies during feeding or congenitally to infants via the placenta of infected mothers.

EPIDEMIOLOGY. Information on the distribution, prevalence, and mortality rate of African trypanosomiasis is unreliable. Human trypanosomiasis in Africa occurs primarily in the region between latitudes 15 degrees north and 15 degrees south, which corresponds roughly to the area where the annual rainfall (500 mm or more) creates optimal climatic conditions for *Glossina* flies. *T. b. rhodesiense* infection is restricted to the eastern third of the endemic area in tropical Africa, stretching from Ethiopia to the northern boundaries of South Africa; *T. b. gambiense* occurs mainly in the western half of the continent's endemic region. African trypanosomiasis affects over 1 million persons.

The insect intermediate vector plays a major role in determining the epidemiologic pattern of trypanosomiasis. Several *Glossina* species transmit the infection in different parts of tropical Africa. *Glossina* captured in endemic foci show a low rate of infection, usually <5%. In the Rhodesian form, which usually has an acute and often fatal course, chances of transmission to tsetse flies are greatly reduced. However, the ability of *T. b. rhodesiense* to multiply enormously in the bloodstream of humans and to infect other species of mammals helps to maintain its life cycle.

T. b. gambiense infection usually have a chronic protracted course with very low levels of parasitemia. Because of low rates of infection in tsetse flies, the Gambian life cycle necessitates close and repeated contact between humans and insects to permit frequent biting. *T. b. gambiense* is found in a variety of animal reservoirs that may play an important role in the endemicity of the Gambian form of infection.

PATHOGENESIS. The initial entry site of the organisms soon develops into a hard, painful, red nodule, a "trypanosomal chancre." Histologically, it contains long, thin trypanosomes multiplying beneath the dermis and is surrounded by a lymphocytic cellular infiltrate. Dissemination into the blood and lymphatic systems follows, with subsequent localization in the central nervous system. The histopathologic findings in the brain are those of meningoencephalitis, with increased cellularity of the pia-arachnoid due to lymphocyte infiltration and perivascular cuffing. In chronic cases the appearance of morular cells (large, strawberry-like cells, supposedly derived from plasma cells) is the most characteristic finding.

CLINICAL MANIFESTATIONS. The clinical presentations vary not only because of the two subspecies of organisms but also because of differences in host response in the indigenous population of endemic areas and in newcomers or visitors. Visitors usually suffer more from the acute symptoms, but in untreated cases death is inevitable for natives and visitors alike. The clinical syndromes of African trypanosomiasis are best described as the trypanosomal chancre, hemolymphatic, and meningoencephalitic stages.

Trypanosomal Chancre. The site of the tsetse fly bite may be the first presenting feature. A nodule or chancre develops in 2–3 days; within 1 wk it becomes a painful, hard, red nodule surrounded by an area of erythema and swelling. These nodules are commonly seen on the lower limbs but sometimes also on the head. They subside spontaneously in about 2 wk, leaving no permanent scar.

Hemolymphatic Stage. The most common presenting features of acute African trypanosomiasis occur at the time of invasion of the bloodstream by the parasites, approximately 2–3 wk after infection. Irregular episodes of fever, each lasting 1–7 days, are the usual early feature, frequently accompanied by headache, sweating, and generalized lymphadenopathy. Attacks may be separated by symptom-free intervals of days or even weeks. Painless, nonmatted lymphadenopathy, most commonly of the posterior cervical and supraclavicular nodes, is one of the most constant signs, particularly in the Gambian form. A common feature of trypanosomiasis in whites is the presence of blotchy, irregular, nonpruritic, erythematous macules, which may appear any time after the first febrile episode, usually within 6–8 wk. The majority of macules have a normal central area, giving the rash a circinate outline. This skin rash is seen mainly on the trunk and is evanescent, fading in one place only to appear at another site. Examination of the blood during this stage may show anemia, leukopenia with relative monocytosis, and elevated levels of immunoglobulin M(IgM).

Meningoencephalitic Stage. Neurologic symptoms and signs are generally nonspecific, including irritability, insomnia, and irrational and inexplicable anxieties with frequent changes in mood and personality. Neurologic symptoms may precede invasion of the central nervous system by the organisms. In untreated *T. b. rhodesiense* infections, invasion of the central nervous system occurs within 3–6 wk and is associated with recurrent bouts of headache, fever, weakness, and signs of acute toxemia. Tachycardia may be evidence of myocarditis. Death occurs in 6–9 mo as a result of secondary infection or cardiac failure.

In the Gambian form, cerebral symptoms can be expected to appear within 2 yr after the onset of acute symptoms. A general increase in drowsiness during the day and insomnia at night reflect the continuous progression of infection, which may be further evidenced by increasing anemia, leukopenia, and wasting of body musculature. Patients with chronic Gambian trypanosomiasis have an increased susceptibility to secondary infections.

The chronic, diffuse meningoencephalitis without localizing symptoms is commonly known as *sleeping sickness.* Drowsiness and an uncontrollable urge to sleep are the major features of this stage of the disease and may become almost continuous in the terminal stages. Associated signs and symptoms, including tremor or rigidity with stiff and ataxic gait, suggest involvement of the basal ganglia. Psychotic changes occur in almost one third of untreated patients.

DIAGNOSIS. Definitive diagnosis can be made during the early stages by examination of a fresh, thick blood smear, which permits visualization of the motile active forms. Dried, Giemsa-stained smears should be examined for the detailed morphologic features of the organisms. If a thick blood or buffy-coat smear yields a negative finding, a simple concentration method may help; 10 mL of heparinized blood is added to 30 mL of 0.87% ammonium chloride, the mixture is centrifuged at 1,000 g for 15 min, and the sediment is examined fresh or by staining dried smears. Aspiration of an enlarged lymph node can also be used to obtain material for parasitologic examination. For every positive result a sample of cerebrospinal fluid should also be examined for the organisms.

TREATMENT. The choice of chemotherapeutic agents depends on the stage of the infection and the causative organisms. The hematogenous forms of both Rhodesian and Gambian trypanosomiasis are susceptible to the action of suramin, which is available as a 10% solution for intravenous administration. A test dose (10 mg for children; 100–200 mg for adults) should first be administered intravenously to detect the rare idiosyncratic reactions of shock and collapse. The dose for subsequent injections is 20 mg/kg (maximum 1 g) intravenously administered on days 1, 3, 7, 14, and 21. Suramin is nephrotoxic; therefore urine should be examined before each administration. The presence of marked proteinuria, blood, or casts is a contraindication to continuation of therapy with suramin.

If central nervous system invasion is present, melarsoprol should be used. Treatment of children is initiated by intravenous administration of 0.36 mg/kg/24 hr and gradual increase in the dose every 1–5 days to 3.6 mg/kg; treatment usually necessitates 10 doses (18–25 mg/kg total dose). Treatment of adults is initiated by 2–3.6 mg/kg for 3 days; after 1 wk, 3.6 mg/kg 24 hr for 3 days, which is repeated after 10–21 days. Mild reactions such as fever and pains in the chest or abdomen may rarely occur immediately or very soon after administration. The most important and serious toxic effects are encephalopathy and, less commonly, exfoliative dermatitis.

PREVENTION. The control of trypanosomiasis in endemic areas of Africa depends on recognition and effective therapy of human infections and on control of the vector. This is complicated by the logistics of applying the available preventive measures particularly in areas of political conflicts and massive population movements.

Pentamidine has been used successfully as a prophylactic drug. A single injection of 3–4 mg/kg will provide protection against Gambian trypanosomiasis for at least 6 mo. Its effect against the Rhodesian form, however, is not certain.

Drugs for parasitic infections. Med Lett Drugs Ther 40:1, 1998.

Hajduk SL, Englund PT, Smith DH: African trypanosomiasis. *In*: Warren KS, Mahmoud AAF (eds): Tropical and Geographical Medicine, 2nd ed. New York, McGraw-Hill, 1990, p 268.

Haller L, Adams H, Merouze F, et al: Clinical and pathological aspects of human African trypanosomiasis *(T. b. gambiense)* with particular reference to reactive arsenical encephalopathy. Am J Trop Med Hyg 35:94, 1986.

Greenwood BM, Whittle HC: The pathogenesis of sleeping sickness. Trans R Soc Trop Med Hyg 74:716, 1980.

WHO: Epidemiology and Control of African Trypanosomiasis. Technical Report Series No. 739, Geneva, WHO, 1986.

CHAPTER 277

American Trypanosomiasis (Chagas' Disease; Trypanosoma cruzi*)*

Robert A. Bonomo and Robert A. Salata

Chagas' disease (American trypanosomiasis) is a zoonosis caused by the parasitic, hemoflagellate protozoan *Trypanosoma cruzi*. Carlos Chagas first described this illness in 1911 in a Brazilian child who had fever, anemia, and lymphadenopathy. Endemic to Central America, Chagas' disease is an emerging problem in North America. Approximately 100,000 immigrants living in the United States from endemic countries may be infected with *T. cruzi*, and several cases have been reported in American cities.

ETIOLOGY. *T. cruzi* has three recognizable morphogenetic phases: amastigotes, trypomastigotes, and epimastigotes. Amastigotes are the intracellular forms found in mammalian tissues; they are spherical and have a short flagellum. Amastigotes form clusters of oval shapes (pseudocysts) within infected tissues. Trypomastigotes are the extracellular nondividing forms; they are spindle shaped, are 20 μm in length, and possess a large kinetoplast. A flagellum arises from the blepharoplast and extends along the outer edge of the undulating membrane until it reaches the anterior end of the body. Trypomastigotes are found in blood and are responsible for transmission of infection to the insect vector and for cell-to-cell spread of infection. Epimastigotes are found in the midgut of the bloodsucking insects *Triatoma, Rhodnius,* and *Panstrongylus* spp. Epimastigotes multiply in the midgut and rectum of arthropods and differentiate into metacyclic trypomastigotes. Metacyclic trypomastigotes, the infectious form for humans, are released onto the skin of a human when the insect defecates close to the site of a bite. Hence, this is an infection caused by contamination, not inoculation. The trypomastigotes enter the skin or damaged mucous membranes and either enter host cells or are phagocytized by macrophages. Once in the host, they multiply intracellularly as amastigotes and are released into the host's circulation when the cell dies. The bloodstream-borne trypomastigotes circulate until they enter another host cell or are taken up by the bite of another insect, completing the life cycle.

EPIDEMIOLOGY. Endemic in South America (particularly Brazil, Argentina, Uruguay, Chile, and Venezuela) and Mexico, Chagas' disease affects over 24 million people, primarily children and young adults. This insect-transmitted illness frequently is asymptomatic and is essentially untreatable, with infection persisting for life. Because of its prevalence, infection by *T. cruzi* is regarded as the most important endemic disease in South America. Over 70,000 individuals die annually as a result of this infection.

The presence of reservoirs and vectors of *T. cruzi* and the socioeconomic and educational levels of the population are the most important risk factors in disease transmission to humans, which occurs via insect vectors. The arthropod vectors for *T. cruzi* are the reduviid insects, variably known as wild bedbugs, assassin bugs, or kissing bugs. Housing conditions are very important in the transmission chain; the incidence and prevalence of infection depend on the adaptation of the triatomids to human dwellings as well as the vector capacity of the species. The animal reservoirs of reduviid bugs are dogs, cats, rats, opossum, guinea pigs, monkeys, bats, and raccoons. In South America, uncontrolled deforestation, increased migration of infected humans from endemic to nonendemic areas, and the presence of domestic reservoir hosts facilitate spread.

Humans can be infected transplacentally, as occurs in 10.5% of infected mothers, causing congenital Chagas' disease. This is associated with premature birth, abortion, and placentitis. Other modes of transmission are via blood transfusion. Seropositivity rates in blood donors from endemic areas are >20%. The risk of transmission through a single blood transfusion from a chagasic donor is 13–23%. Percutaneous injection as a result of laboratory accidents is also a documented mode of transmission. Oral transmission through contaminated food has been reported. Although breast-feeding is a very uncommon mode of transmission, women with acute infections should not nurse until they have been treated.

PATHOGENESIS. Although the pathogenesis of chronic Chagas' disease is unknown, two main mechanisms have been proposed: (1) direct tissue destruction by the parasite and (2) development of an inflammatory reaction resulting from an allergic response to parasitic antigens absorbed by host cells or an autoimmune reaction resulting from shared antigens between host and parasite.

At the site of entry (puncture site) polymorphonuclear neutrophils, lymphocytes, macrophages, and monocytes infiltrate. *T. cruzi* are engulfed by macrophages and are sequestered in membrane-bound vacuoles. Parasite attachment and phagocytosis by macrophages are mediated by protease-sensitive receptors on the surface of the macrophage. Trypanosomes lyse the phagosome membrane, escape into the cytoplasm, and replicate. A local tissue reaction develops (chagoma), and the process extends to a local lymph node. Blood forms appear next and the process disseminates.

T. cruzi strains demonstrate selective parasitism for certain tissues. Most strains are myotropic, invading smooth, skeletal, and heart muscle cells. Attachment is mediated by specific receptors on the trypomastigotes that attach to complementary glycoconjugates on the host cell surface. Attachment to cardiac muscle results in inflammation of the endocardium and myocardium, edema, focal necrosis in the contractile and conducting systems, periganglionitis, and lymphocytic inflammation. The heart becomes enlarged and endocardial thrombosis or aneurysm may result. Right bundle branch block is also commonly seen. Trypanosome parasites also attach to neural cells and reticuloendothelial cells. In individuals with gastrointestinal tract involvement, myenteric plexus destruction leads to organ dilatation (megaesophagus and megacolon).

Immunologic mechanisms for control of parasitism and resistance are not completely understood. Despite strong acquired immunity, there is no parasitologic cure. Antigenic variation that is typical of African trypanosomiasis is not seen with American trypanosomiasis. Antibodies involved with resistance to *T. cruzi* are related to the phase of infection. Immunoglobulin G (IgG) antibodies, probably to several major surface antigens, mediate immunophagocytosis of the parasite by macrophages. Conditions associated with depression of cell-mediated immunity increase the severity of infection with *T. cruzi*. Macrophages probably play a major role in protection against *T. cruzi* infection, especially in the acute phase. Interferon-γ stimulates macrophage killing of amastigotes through oxidative mechanisms.

CLINICAL MANIFESTATIONS. Chagas' disease occurs in acute and chronic forms. Acute Chagas' disease in children is usually asymptomatic or is associated with a mild febrile illness characterized by fever, malaise, facial edema, and lymphadenopathy. Infants often demonstrate local signs of inflammation at the site of parasite entry (chagomas). Approximately 50% of children come to medical attention with Romaña's sign—unilateral, painless eye swelling; conjunctivitis; and preauricular lymphadenitis. Patients complain of fatigue and headache. Fever can persist for 4–5 wk. More severe systemic presentations can occur in children <2 yr of age: lymphadenopathy, hepatosplenomegaly, and meningoencephalitis. A cutaneous morbilliform eruption can accompany the acute syndrome. Anemia, lymphocytosis, hepatitis, and thrombocytopenia have been described.

The heart, central nervous system, peripheral nerve ganglia, and reticuloendothelial system are often heavily parasitized. The heart is the primary target organ. The intense parasitism can result in acute inflammation and in four chamber cardiac dilatation. Diffuse myocarditis and inflammation of the conduction system lead to the development of fibrosis. Histologic examination reveals the characteristic pseudocysts, which are the intracellular aggregates of amastigotes.

Intrauterine infection in pregnant women can cause abortion or premature birth. In children with congenital infection, severe anemia, hepatosplenomegaly, jaundice, and convulsions can mimic congenital cytomegalovirus infection, toxoplasmosis, and erythroblastosis fetalis. *T. cruzi* can be visualized in the cerebrospinal fluid in meningoencephalitis. Children usually undergo spontaneous remission in 8–12 wk and enter an indeterminate phase with lifelong low-grade parasitemia and development of antibodies to many *T. cruzi* cell surface antigens. Mortality rate is 5–10%; deaths are caused by acute myocarditis with resultant heart failure, or meningoencephalitis. Acute Chagas' disease must be differentiated from malaria, schistosomiasis, visceral leishmaniasis, brucellosis, typhoid fever, and infectious mononucleosis.

Chronic Chagas' disease may be asymptomatic or symptomatic. The most common presentation of chronic *T. cruzi* infection is cardiomyopathy, manifested by congestive heart failure, arrhythmia, and thromboembolic events. Electrocardiographically detected abnormalities include partial or complete atrioventricular block and right bundle branch block. Left bundle branch block is unusual. Pathologic examination of infected heart muscle reveals muscle atrophy, myonecrosis, myocytolysis, fibrosis, and lymphocytic infiltration. Myocardial infarction has been reported and may be secondary to left apical aneurysm embolization or necrotizing arteriolitis of the microvasculature. Left ventricular apical aneurysms are pathognomonic of chronic chagasic cardiomypathy.

Autonomic nervous system abnormalities have also been implicated in Chagas' cardiomyopathy. The reduction in acetylcholine and choline acetyltransferase levels in experimental *T. cruzi* infection lends support to this notion.

Autoimmune abnormalities have been reported in Chagas' cardiomyopathy. Depletion of $CD8^+$ cells accelerates infection. *T. cruzi*–infected human peripheral blood mononuclear and endothelial cells synthesize increased levels of interleukin 1B (IL-1B), IL-6, and tumor necrosis factor. These cytokines result in increasing white blood cell recruitment and smooth muscle cell proliferation, which may be responsible for some of the manifestations of the disease. Viral myocarditis, rheumatic heart disease, and endomyocardial fibrosis can mimic chronic chagasic cardiomyopathy.

The gastrointestinal manifestations of chronic Chagas' disease occur in 8–10% of patients and involve a diminution in Auerbach's plexus and Meissner's plexus. There are also preganglionic lesions and a reduction in the number of dorsal motor nuclear cells of the vagus. Characteristically, this involvement presents clinically as megaesophagus and megacolon. Sigmoid dilatation, volvulus, and fecalomas are often found in megacolon. Loss of ganglia in the esophagus results in abnormal dilatation (megaesophagus); the esophagus can reach up to 26 times its normal weight and hold up to 2 L of excess fluid. Megaesophagus presents with dysphagia, odynophagia, and cough. Esophageal body abnormalities occur independently of lower esophageal dysfunction. Megaesophagus can lead to esophagitis and cancer of the esophagus. Aspiration pneumonia and pulmonary tuberculosis are more common in patients with megaesophagus.

Autonomic dysfunction and peripheral neuropathy can occur. Central nervous system involvement in Chagas' disease is uncommon. If granulomatous encephalitis occurs in the acute infection it is usually fatal.

Immunocompromised Persons. *T. cruzi* infections in the immunocompromised child are due to transmission from an asymptomatic donor of blood products or activation of prior infection by immunosuppression. Organ donation to allograft recipients can result in a devastating form of the illness. Cardiac transplantation for Chagas' cardiomyopathy has resulted in reactivation, despite prophylaxis and postoperative treatment with benznidazole. Human immunodeficiency virus (HIV) infection also leads to reactivation; cerebral lesions are more common in these patients and can mimic those of toxoplasmic encephalitis. In immunocompromised patients at risk for reactivation, serologic testing and close monitoring are necessary.

DIAGNOSIS. A careful history with attention to geographic origin and travel is important. Microscopic examination of the peripheral blood smear during the acute phase of illness is diagnostic for Chagas' disease. Motile trypanosomes on a fresh preparation of peripheral blood or Giemsa-stained smear will yield the diagnosis. These are only seen in the peripheral blood in the first 6–12 wk of the illness. Buffy coat smears may improve yield.

Most patients seek medical attention during the chronic phase of the disease, when parasites are not found in the bloodstream and clinical symptoms are not diagnostic. Serologic testing is the best means of diagnosis. Complement fixation is considered the most reliable immunodiagnostic method for establishing the diagnosis. Indirect fluorescent antibody testing is also very accurate and can be used to distinguish acute chagasic infection, with IgM antibodies, from chronic infection, with only IgG antibodies. These tests are available from the Centers for Disease Control and Prevention (CDC). Because false-positive reactions can result from other infections (e.g., malaria, syphilis, and leishmaniasis), it is recommended that a minimum of two independent serologic tests be performed.

Nonimmunologic methods of diagnosis are also available. Mouse inoculation has been used when repeated peripheral smear results are negative. Xenodiagnosis, allowing uninfected reduviid bugs to feed on a patient's blood and examining the intestinal contents of those bugs 30 days after the meal, detects 100% of cases. Detection assays using polymerase chain reaction (PCR) amplification of nuclear and kinetoplast DNA (kDNA) sequences are in development. PCR has a sensitivity of 96–100% and is able to detect a single parasite in 20 mL of blood. Chemiluminescent enzyme-linked immunosorbent assays (ELISAS) are in development and are also reported to be highly sensitive and specific.

TREATMENT. Drug treatment for *T. cruzi* is generally limited to two drugs, nifurtimox and benznidazole. Both are effective against trypomastigotes and amastigotes and have been used to eradicate parasites in the acute stages of infection.

Nifurtimox has been used most extensively, but whether it is effective in the chronic phase of the illness is uncertain. The treatment regimen for children 1–10 yr of age is 15–20 mg/kg/24 hr divided in four doses for 90 days; for children, 11–16 yr of age 12.5–15 mg/kg/24 hr divided in four doses for 90 days; and for children >16 yr of age 8–10 mg/kg/24 hr divided in three to four doses for 90–120 days. Nifurtimox interferes with the parasites' carbohydrate metabolism by disrupting pyruvic acid synthesis. This drug is available from the CDC (404-639-3670 or 404-639-2888). Nifurtimox has been associated with weakness, anorexia, gastrointestinal disturbances, toxic hepatitis, tremors, seizures, and hemolysis in patients with glucose-6-phosphate dehydrogenase (G6PD) deficiency.

Benznidazole is more effective than nifurtimox. The recommended treatment regimen for children <12 yr of age is 10 mg/kg/24 hr divided in two doses for 60 days, and for those ≥12 yr of age 5–7 mg/kg/24 hr for 60 days. In a recent randomized, double-blind, placebo-controlled trial in a rural area of Brazil, a 60 day course of benznidazole was studied in the treatment of early chronic phase *T. cruzi* infection in schoolchildren 7–12 yr of age. The efficacy of benznidazole was 55.8% in producing negative seroconversion. This drug is also associated with significant toxicities, including photosensitivity, peripheral neuritis, and pancytopenia. Of some concern are the reports that detail the development of lymphomas in laboratory animals treated with benznidazole. This finding has not been reported in humans.

Allopurinol, a drug that inhibits hypoxanthine oxidase, has also been used and has been shown to reduce parasitemia. It is ineffective in the acute phase.

Biochemical differences between the metabolism of American trypanosomes and that of mammalian hosts may be exploited for chemotherapy. These trypanosomes are very sensitive to oxidative radicals, and they do not possess catalase or glutathione reductase-glutathione peroxidase, which are key enzymes in scavenging free radicals. All trypanosomes also have an unusual reduced nicotinamide-adenine dinucleotide phosphate–(NADPH)-dependent disulfide reductase. For this reason, drugs that stimulate H_2O_2 generation or prevent its utilization are potential trypanocidal agents.

Treatment of heart failure and arrhythmia, as well as prevention of thromboembolism, requires the use of diuretics, antiarrhythmics, and anticoagulants. Digitalis toxicity occurs frequently in patients with Chagas' cardiomyopathy. Pacemakers may be necessary in cases of severe heart block. A light, balanced diet is recommended for megaesophagus. Surgery or dilation of the lower esophageal sphincter treats megaesophagus; pneumatic dilation is the superior mode of therapy. Nitrates and nifedipine have been used to reduce lower esophageal sphincter pressure in patients with megaesophagus. Treatment of megacolon is surgical and symptomatic.

PREVENTION. Education of residents in endemic areas, use of bed nets, use of insecticides such as dieldrin or lindane, and destruction of adobe houses that harbor reduviid bugs are effective methods to control the bug population. Synthetic pyrethroid insecticides help keep houses free of vectors for 2 yr and have low toxicity for humans. Paints incorporating insecticides have also been used.

Vaccine development has been fruitless. Prophylactic therapy with nifurtimox or benznidazole should be considered only for laboratory accidents.

Since immigrants can carry this disease to nonendemic areas, serologic testing should be performed in blood donors from high-risk populations. Potential seropositive donors can be identified by determining whether they have been or have spent extensive time in an endemic area. Questionnaire-based screening of potentially infected blood donors from areas endemic for infection can reduce the risk of transmission.

Blood transfusions in endemic areas are a significant risk. Gentian violet, an amphophilic cationic agent that acts photodynamically, has been used to kill the parasite in blood. Photoirradiation of blood containing gentian violet and ascorbate generates free radicals and superoxide anions that are trypanocidal. Mepacrine and maprotiline have also been used to eradicate the parasite in blood transfusions.

Potential organ donors from endemic areas should also be screened; seropositivity should be considered a contraindication to organ donation. Although cardiac transplantation has been successful in chagasic patients, further study is warranted.

Almeida IC, Covas DT, Soussumi LM, et al; A highly sensitive and specific chemiluminescent enzyme linked immunoabsorbent assay for the diagnosis of acute *Trypanosoma cruzi* infection. Transfusion 37:850, 1997.

Avila HA, Pereria, Thiemann O: Detection of *Trypanosoma cruzi* in blood samples of chronic chagasic patients by polymerase chain amplification of kinetoplast minicircle DNA: Comparison of serology and xenodiagnosis. J Clin Microbiol 31:2421, 1993.

De Andrade AL, Zicker F, de Olivera RM, et al: Randomized trial of the efficacy of benznidazole in the treatment of early *Trypanosoma cruzi* infection. Lancet 348:1407, 1996

Docompo R, Moreno SN, Cruz FS: Enhancement of the cytotoxicity of crystal violet against *Trypanosoma cruzi* in blood by ascorbate. Mol Biochem Parasitol 27:241, 1998.

Grant IH, Gold JWM, Wittner M, et al: Transfusion associated acute Chagas' disease acquired in the USA. Ann Intern Med 111:849, 1989.

Kirchhoff LV: Trypanosomiasis (Chagas' disease): A tropical disease now in the United States. N Engl J Med 329:639, 1993.

Nickerson P, Orr P, Schroeder ML, et al: Transfusion-associated *Trypanosoma cruzi* in an infection in a non-endemic area. Ann Intern Med 111:851, 1989.

Taenias HB, Kirchhoff LV, Simon D, et al: Chagas' disease. Clin Microbiol Rev 5:400, 1992.

Ramierez LE, Lages-Silva E, Pianett GM, et al: Prevention of transfusion associated Chagas disease by sterilization of infected blood with gentian violet, ascorbic acid and light. Transfusion 35:226, 1995.

Wincker P, Telleria J, Basseno MF, et al: PCR based diagnosis for Chagas disease in Bolivian children living in an active transmission area: Comparison with conventional serological and parasitological diagnosis. Parasitology 114:367, 1997.

CHAPTER 278
Malaria (Plasmodium)

Peter J. Krause

Malaria is an acute and chronic protozoan illness characterized by paroxysms of fever, chills, sweats, fatigue, anemia, and splenomegaly. It has played a major role in human history, having arguably caused more harm to more people than any other infectious disease. Malaria is of overwhelming importance in the developing world today with an estimated 300 million cases and over 1 million deaths each year. Most malarial deaths occur in infants and young children. Although there is no endemic malaria in the United States, approximately 1,000 imported cases are recognized each year. Physicians practicing in nonendemic areas should consider the diagnosis of malaria in any febrile child who has returned from a malaria endemic area within the previous year; delay in diagnosis and treatment can result in severe illness or death.

ETIOLOGY. Malaria is caused by intracellular *Plasmodium* protozoa transmitted to humans by female *Anopheles* mosquitoes. Four species of *Plasmodium* cause malaria in humans: *P. falciparum, P. malariae, P. ovale,* and *P. vivax. Plasmodium* species exist in a variety of forms and have a complex life cycle that enables them to survive in different cellular environments in the human host (asexual phase) and the mosquito vector (sexual phase). A marked amplification of *Plasmodium* organisms from approximately 10^2 to as many as 10^{14} occurs during a two-step process in humans. The first occurs in the cells of the liver (exoerythrocytic phase) and the second in the red cells (erythrocytic phase). The exoerythrocytic phase begins with inoculation of sporozoites into the bloodstream by a female *Anopheles* mosquito. Within minutes, the sporozoites enter the hepatocytes of the liver, where they develop and multiply asexually. The parasite is referred to as a *schizont* at this stage. After 1–2 wk, the hepatocytes rupture and release thousands of merozoites into the circulation. The tissue schizonts of *P. falciparum* and *P. malaria* rupture once and none persists in the liver. There are two types of tissue schizonts for *P. ovale* and *P. vivax.* The primary type ruptures in 6–9 days; a secondary type remains dormant in the liver cell for weeks, months, or as long as 5 years before releasing merozoites, thereby causing *relapses* of infection. The erythrocytic phase of *Plasmodium* sp. asexual development begins when the merozoites from the liver penetrate erythrocytes. Once inside the erythrocyte, the parasite transforms into the ring form, which then enlarges to become a trophozoite. These latter two forms can be identified with Giemsa stain on blood smear, the primary means of confirming the diagnosis of malaria (Fig. 278–1). The trophozoite multiplies asexually to produce many small erythrocytic merozoites. Merozoites are released into the bloodstream when the erythrocyte membrane ruptures, a process associated with fever. Over time, some of the merozoites develop into male and female gametocytes. It is the gametocytes that complete the *Plasmodium* sp. life cycle when they are ingested during a blood meal by the female anopheline mosquito. The male and female gametocytes fuse to form a zygote in the stomach cavity of the mosquito. After a series of further transformations, sporozoites enter the salivary gland of the mosquito and are inoculated into a new host with the next blood meal.

EPIDEMIOLOGY. Malaria is a worldwide problem with transmission occurring in over 100 countries. The principal areas of transmission are Africa, Asia, and South America. *P. falciparum* is the predominant species in Africa, Haiti, and New Guinea.

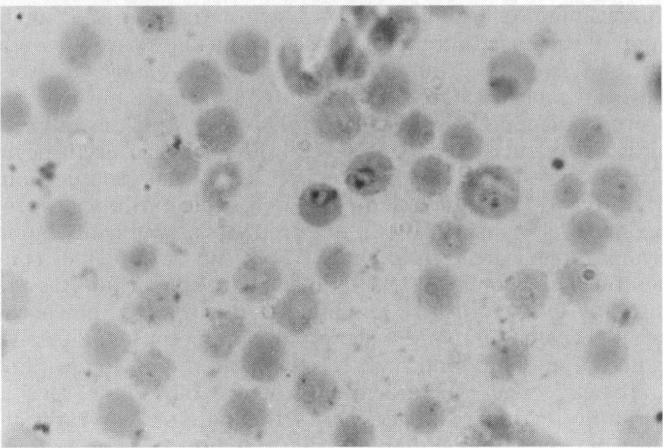

Figure 278–1 Ring forms of *Plasmodium falciparum* within two erythrocytes *(center).*

P. vivax predominates in Bangladesh, Central America, India, Pakistan, and Sri Lanka. *P. vivax* and *P. falciparum* predominate in Southeast Asia, South America, and Oceania. *P. ovale,* the rarest species, is primarily in Africa.

Mosquito transmission of malaria has been eliminated in most of North America (including the United States), Europe, the Caribbean, Australia, Chile, Israel, Japan, Korea, Lebanon, and Taiwan.

Malaria can also be transmitted through blood transfusion and use of contaminated needles, and from a pregnant woman to her fetus. The risk of blood transmission is small and decreasing in the United States but may occur via whole blood, packed red blood cells, platelets, leukocytes, and organ transplantation.

Most cases of malaria in the United States or Europe occur in previously infected visitors from endemic areas, native citizens who travel to endemic areas without taking appropriate chemoprophylactic drugs, and a small number of individuals who have transfusion associated and congenital cases. Since 1986, 11 autochthonous cases have been documented in the United States. It is likely that untreated patients with malaria acquired in an endemic country traveled to the United States and infected local mosquitoes, which subsequently transmitted the disease to others.

PATHOGENESIS. Four important pathologic processes have been identified in patients with malaria: fever, anemia, immunopathologic events, and tissue anoxia resulting from cytoadherence of infected erythrocytes. Fever occurs when erythrocytes rupture and release merozoites into the circulation. Anemia is caused by hemolysis, sequestration of erythrocytes in the spleen and other organs, and suppression of erythrocyte production in the bone marrow. Immunopathologic events that have been documented in patients with malaria include polyclonal activation resulting in both hypergammaglobulinemia and formation of immune complexes, immunosuppression, and release of cytokines such as tumor necrosis factor (TNF) that may be responsible for many of the pathologic features of the disease. Cytoadherence of infected erythrocytes to vascular endothelium occurs in *P. falciparum* malaria. It may lead to obstruction of blood flow and capillary damage with resultant vascular leakage of protein and fluid, and edema and tissue anoxia in the brain, heart, lungs, intestines, and kidneys.

Immunity after *Plasmodium* species infection is incomplete; subsequent severe disease is averted, but complete eradication or prevention of future infection is not achieved. In some cases parasites circulate in small numbers for a long time but are prevented from rapidly multiplying and causing severe illness. Repeated episodes of infection occur because the parasite has developed a number of immunity-evasive strategies such as intracellular replication, rapid antigenic variation, and alteration of the host immune response that includes partial immunosuppression. The human host response to *Plasmodium* species infection includes natural immune mechanisms that prevent infection by other *Plasmodium* species such as those of birds or rodents, as well as several alterations in erythrocyte physiologic processes that prevent or modify malarial infection. Erythrocytes containing hemoglobin S (sickle erythrocytes) resist malarial parasite growth, erythrocytes lacking Duffy blood group antigen are resistant to *P. vivax,* and erythrocytes containing hemoglobin F (fetal hemoglobin) and ovalocytes are resistant to *P. falciparum.* In hyperendemic areas, newborns rarely become ill with malaria, in part because of passive maternal antibody and high levels of fetal hemoglobin. Children between 3 mo and 2–5 yr of age have little specific immunity to malarial species and therefore suffer yearly attacks of debilitating and potentially fatal disease. Severe symptoms of malaria become less common as immunity is acquired. Severe disease may occur during pregnancy or after extended residence outside the endemic region. In general, extracellular *Plasmodium* organisms are targeted by antibody and intracellular organisms are targeted by cellular defenses such as T lymphocytes, macrophages, polymorphonuclear leukocytes, and the spleen.

CLINICAL MANIFESTATIONS. Children and adults are asymptomatic during the initial phase (incubation period) of malarial infection. The usual incubation periods are as follows: *P. falciparum,* 9–14 days; *P. vivax,* 12–17 days; *P. ovale,* 16–18 days; and *P. malariae,* 18–40 days. The incubation period can be as long as 6–12 mo for *P. vivax* and can be prolonged for any *Plasmodium* species in patients with partial immunity or incomplete chemoprophylaxis. A prodrome lasting 2–3 days is noted in some patients before parasites are detected in the blood. Prodromal symptoms include headache, fatigue, anorexia, myalgia, slight fever, and pain in the chest, abdomen, or joints.

The classic presentation of malaria includes febrile paroxysms alternating with periods of fatigue but otherwise relative wellness. This pattern is seldom noted with other infectious diseases. Symptoms associated with febrile paroxysms include high fever, rigors, sweats, and headache, as well as myalgia, back pain, abdominal pain, nausea, vomiting, diarrhea, pallor, and jaundice. Paroxysms coincide with the rupture of schizonts that occurs every 48 hr with *P. vivax* and *P. ovale* and results in daily fever spikes, and occurs every 72 hr with *P. malariae* and results in alternate day or every third day fever spikes. Periodicity is less apparent with *P. falciparum* and mixed infections. Patients with primary infection, such as travelers from nonendemic regions, may also have irregular symptomatic episodes for 2–3 days before regular paroxysms begin. Children with malaria often have special clinical features that differ from those of adults. Symptoms of malaria in children >2 mo of age who are nonimmune vary widely from low grade fever and headache, to fever >104°F with headache, drowsiness, anorexia, nausea, vomiting, diarrhea, pallor, cyanosis, splenomegaly, hepatomegaly, anemia, thrombocytopenia, and a normal or low white blood cell count.

Recrudescence after a primary attack may result from the survival of erythrocyte forms in the bloodstream. Long-term relapse is due to release of merozoites from an exoerythrocytic source in the liver (*P. vivax* and *P. ovale*) or persistence within the erythrocyte (*P. malariae*). A history of typical symptoms in an individual more than a few weeks after return from an endemic area therefore indicates *P. vivax, P. ovale,* or *P. malariae* infection.

P. falciparum malaria is the most severe form and is associated with more intense parasitemia. Fatality rates of up to 25% in nonimmune adults and 30% in nonimmune infants may occur if appropriate therapy is not instituted promptly. *The diagnosis of* P. falciparum *malaria constitutes a medical emergency.* Malaria caused by *P. ovale, P. vivax,* and *P. malariae* usually results in parasitemias of <2%, whereas that of *P. falciparum* can be ≥60% because *P. falciparum* infects immature and mature erythrocytes whereas *P. ovale* and *P. vivax* primarily infect immature erythrocytes, and *P. malariae* infects only mature erythrocytes. *P. falciparum* malaria is the *Plasmodium* malaria most commonly associated with serious complications, although milder or asymptomatic infections occur in those who are partially immune.

P. vivax malaria generally is less severe than *P. falciparum* malaria but may cause death as a result of ruptured spleen or in association with reticulocytosis and high parasitemia after anemia. Relapse of *P. vivax* malaria may occur if antihepatic malarial treatment is not given and is common within 6 mo after an acute attack but may occur as long as 5 yr after initial infection.

P. malariae malaria is the mildest and most chronic of all malarial infections. Recrudescence has been observed 30–50 yr after an acute attack. Although parasitemia is often low, untreated *P. malariae* malaria can cause chronic ill health in addition to acute febrile illness.

P. ovale malaria is the least common type of malaria. It is similar to *P. vivax* malaria and commonly is found in conjunction with *P. falciparum* malaria.

Prenatally or perinatally acquired malaria is a serious problem in tropical areas but is rarely reported in the United States. In endemic areas, congenital malaria is an important cause of spontaneous abortion, miscarriage, stillbirth, premature birth, intrauterine growth retardation, and neonatal death. Congenital malaria usually occurs in a nonimmune mother with *P. vivax* or *P. malariae,* although it can be observed with any of the human malarial species. The first sign or symptom most commonly occurs at 10–30 days of age but may occur at 14 hr to several months of age. Signs and symptoms include fever, restlessness, drowsiness, pallor, jaundice, poor feeding, vomiting, diarrhea, cyanosis, and hepatosplenomegaly. Malaria is often severe during pregnancy and may indirectly have an adverse effect on the fetus or neonate through maternal illness or placental infection even in the absence of transmission from mother to child.

DIAGNOSIS. Any child who has fever or unexplained systemic illness and has traveled or lived in a malarial endemic area within the previous year should be assumed to have life-threatening malaria until proved otherwise. Malaria should be considered regardless of the use of chemoprophylaxis. Important criteria that suggest *P. falciparum* malaria include symptoms occurring <1 mo after return from an endemic area, intense parasitemia (>2%), ring forms with double chromatin dots, and individual erythrocytes infected with more than one parasite.

The diagnosis of malaria is established by identification of organisms on Giemsa-stained smears of peripheral blood. Giemsa stain is superior to Wright's stain or Leishman's stain. Both thick and thin blood smears should be examined. The concentration of erythrocytes on a thick smear is approximately 20–40 times that on a thin smear and is used to scan large numbers of erythrocytes quickly. The thin smear allows for positive identification of the malaria species and determination of the percentage of infected erythrocytes, which is useful in following the response to therapy. Identification of the species is best made by an experienced microscopist and verified against color plates of the various *Plasmodium* species. Although *P. falciparum* is most likely to be identified from blood just after a febrile paroxysm, timing the smears is less important than obtaining them several times a day over a period of 3 successive days. A single negative blood smear finding does not exclude malaria; it may be necessary to repeat the smears as frequently as every 4–6 hr a day in order to establish a diagnosis. Most symptomatic patients with malaria will have detectable parasites on thick blood smears within a 48 hr period. In nonimmune persons, symptoms typically occur 1–2 days before parasites are detectable on blood smear.

A new monoclonal antibody test that is incorporated in a test strip for finger-prick blood samples is as sensitive as a thick smear for detection of *P. falciparum*. Polymerase chain reaction testing is even more sensitive but technically more complex and not generally available.

Differential Diagnosis. The differential diagnosis of malaria is broad and includes viral infections such as influenza and hepatitis, sepsis, pneumonia, meningitis, encephalitis, endocarditis, gastroenteritis, pyelonephritis, babesiosis, brucellosis, leptospirosis, tuberculosis, relapsing fever, typhoid fever, yellow fever, amebic liver abscess, Hodgkin disease, and collagen vascular disease.

TREATMENT. Physicians caring for patients with malaria or traveling to endemic areas need to be aware of current information regarding malaria. Resistance to antimalarial drugs is increasing and has greatly complicated therapy and prophylaxis. The best source for such information is the Centers for Disease Control and Prevention Malaria Hotline, which is available 24 hr a day (888-232-3228).

Any patient with fever without an obvious cause who has left a *P. falciparum* endemic area within the incubation period of 9–14 days and is nonimmune should be considered to constitute a medical emergency. Thick and thin blood smears should immediately be obtained; if the result is positive, the patient should be hospitalized and therapy begun. If blood film results are negative, films should be repeated every few hours, but if the patient is severely ill, antimalarial therapy should be initiated immediately.

Patients with malaria of any type need to be monitored for possible recrudescence, with repeat blood smears at the end of therapy. Recrudescence may occur ≥90 days after therapy with low-grade resistant organisms. For children living in endemic areas, mothers should be encouraged to treat fever with an antimalarial drug. If such children are severely ill, they should be given the same therapy as nonimmune children.

***P. falciparum* Malaria.** Malaria acquired in areas of known or suspected chloroquine resistance should generally be treated with drugs other than chloroquine (Table 278–1). Intravenous quinidine or quinine (quinine is not available in the United States) should be administered when a patient cannot retain oral fluids and medication because of vomiting; has neurologic dysfunction, pulmonary edema, or renal failure; has a peripheral asexual parasitemia that exceeds 5%; or has a peripheral asexual parasitemia of 1–4% with a severe attack. Such patients should be admitted to the intensive care unit for electrocardiogram monitoring to detect arrhythmia, widening QRS complex, or prolonged Q-T interval. Patients should also be monitored for hypotension and other complications. Parenteral therapy should be continued until the parasitemia is <1%, usually within 48 hr, and oral medication can be tolerated. Quinine sulfate is then administered for a total of 3–7 days of combined quinidine/quinine therapy, plus Fansidar (25 mg pyrimethamine and 500 mg sulfadoxine per tablet) in one dose on the last day of therapy. Use of Fansidar is contraindicated in patients with a history of sulfonamide or pyrimethamine intolerance, in infants <2 mo of age, and in pregnant women at term. Patients with less severe disease should be given oral quinine and tetracycline, or alternatively, quinine and Fansidar, or mefloquine alone (Table 278–1). Mefloquine is contraindicated for use in patients with a known hypersensitivity, or with a history of epilepsy or severe psychiatric disorders. Mefloquine may be administered to persons concurrently receiving β blockers if they have no underlying arrhythmia; however, mefloquine is not recommended for persons with cardiac conduction abnormalities. Quinidine or quinine may exacerbate the known side effects of mefloquine; patients who do not respond to mefloquine therapy or mefloquine prophylaxis should be monitored closely if they are treated with quinidine or quinine.

TABLE 278–1 Treatment of Malaria in Children

Drug*	Dosage
***All* Plasmodium *Species Except Chloroquine-Resistant* Plasmodium falciparum**	
Oral drug of choice	
Chloroquine phosphate	10 mg base/kg (maximum: 600 mg base) then 5 mg base/kg (maximum: 300 mg base), 6 hr later, and 5 mg base/kg/24 hr (maximum: 300 mg base) at 24 and 48 hr
Parenteral drug of choice	
Quinidine gluconate	10 mg/kg loading dose (maximum: 600 mg) over 1–2 hr, then 0.02 mg/kg/min continuous infusion until oral therapy can be started
or	
Quinine dihydrochloride (not available in the USA)	20 mg/kg loading dose over 4 hr, then 10 mg/kg over 2–4 hr every 8 hr (maximum: 1,800 mg/24 hr) until oral therapy can be started
P. falciparum *Acquired in Areas of Known Chloroquine Resistance*	
Oral regimen of choice	
Quinine sulfate†	30 mg/kg/24 hr in 3 doses for 3–7 days (maximum: 650 mg/dose)
plus	
Tetracycline‡	20 mg/kg/24 hr divided in 4 doses for 7 days (maximum: 250 mg/dose)
Alternative regimen	
Oral: Quinine sulfate	30 mg/kg in 3 doses for 3 days
Parenteral:	
Quinidine gluconate	Same as for chloroquine-sensitive *P. falciparum*
or	
Quinine dihydrochloride	Same as for chloroquine-sensitive *P. falciparum*
plus	
Pyrimethamine-sulfadoxine (Fansidar)§	<1 yr, single dose of 1/4 tablet 1–3 yr, single dose of 1/2 tablet 4–8 yr, single dose of 1 tablet 9–14 yr, single dose of 2 tablets >14 yr, single dose of 3 tablets
or	
Mefloquine hydrochloride‖	15–25 mg/kg/24 hour) (maximum, 1,250 mg) for 1 day
Prevention of Relapses:* Plasmodium vivax *and* Plasmodium ovale *Only	
Primaquine phosphate**	0.3 mg base/kg/24 hr for 14 days (maximum: 15 mg base [26.3 mg salt])

**Review contraindications and adverse effects before use (see text).*

†For treatment of P. falciparum *infections acquired in Southeast Asia, and possibly in other areas including South America, quinine sulfate should be continued for 7 days.*

‡Physicians must weigh the benefits of tetracycline therapy against the possibility of dental staining in children <8 yr of age.

§Fansidar (25 mg pyrimethamine and 500 mg sulfadoxine per tablet) should not be used for treatment of malaria acquired in Southeast Asia and the Amazon basin because of possible resistance. Carry a single dose for treatment of febrile illness when medical care is not immediately available.

‖Mefloquine is not licensed by the U.S. Food and Drug Administration (FDA) for children who weigh less than 15 kg, but recent Centers for Disease Control and Prevention (CDC) recommendations allow use of the drug to be considered in children without weight restrictions when travel to chloroquine-resistant P. falciparum *areas cannot be avoided. For most patients, 15 mg/kg (maximum: 750 mg) in a single dose is effective therapy, except for those who acquired infection in the areas of the Amazon basin, or the Thailand-Cambodia and Thailand-Myanmar borders. If the 25 mg/kg/24 hr dose is used, 15 mg/kg (maximum: 750 mg) is given followed 8–12 hr later by 10 mg/kg (maximum: 500 mg).*

***Primaquine phosphate can cause hemolytic anemia in patients with glucose-6-phosphate dehydrogenase (G6PD) deficiency. A G6PD screening test should be performed before intiating treatment. Pregnant women should not be administered primaquine.*

Patients with uncomplicated *P. falciparum* malaria acquired in areas without chloroquine resistance should be treated with oral chloroquine (Table 278–1). However, if the parasite count does not drop rapidly (within 24–48 hr) and become negative after 4 days, chloroquine resistance should be assumed and the patient begun on a regimen for chloroquine-resistant malaria. Supportive therapy is very important and includes blood transfusion(s) to maintain the hematocrit >20%, exchange transfusion in life-threatening *P. falciparum* malaria with parasitemia ≥5%, supplemental oxygen and ventilatory support for pulmonary edema or cerebral malaria, careful intravenous rehydration for severe malaria, intravenous glucose for hypoglycemia, anticonvulsants for cerebral malaria with seizures, and dialysis for renal failure. Corticosteroids are no longer recommended for cerebral malaria.

***P. vivax, P. ovale,* or *P. malariae* Malaria.** Non–*Plasmodium falciparum* malaria is treated with chloroquine (Table 278–1) even though a few rare cases of chloroquine-resistant *P. vivax* malaria have been described from Indonesia and New Guinea. Clinical and blood smear responses to therapy should be monitored. If vomiting precludes oral administration, chloroquine can be given by nasogastric tube or, in rare cases and with great care, by intramuscular administration. Sudden death has been attributed to parenteral administration of chloroquine to children. Intravenous quinidine or quinine is given in severe cases. Patients with *P. vivax* or *P. ovale* malaria should be given primaquine once a day for 14 days to prevent relapse. Some strains may require two courses of primaquine. Patients given primaquine must be checked for glucose-6-phosphate dehydrogenase (G6PD) deficiency before initiation of the drug since it can exacerbate hemolytic anemia in such patients.

COMPLICATIONS. Cerebral malaria is a serious complication of *P. falciparum* infection that is especially common in children and nonimmune adults. Cerebral malaria is associated with a fatality rate of 20–40% but rarely causes long-term sequelae if it is treated appropriately. It usually develops after the patient has been ill for several days but may develop precipitously. As with other complications, cerebral malaria is more likely in patients with a parasitemia of >5%. The symptoms always include decreased level of consciousness and range in severity from drowsiness and severe headache to confusion, delirium, hallucinations, or deep coma. Physical findings may be normal or may include fever to 106–108°F, seizures, muscular twitching, rhythmic movement of the head or extremities, contracted or unequal pupils, retinal hemorrhages, hemiplegia, absent or exaggerated deep tendon reflexes, and a positive Babinski's sign. Lumbar puncture reveals increased pressure and cerebrospinal fluid protein level with minimal or no pleocytosis, and normal glucose level. There are no specific electroencephalographic (EEG) findings with cerebral malaria.

Renal failure is a common complication of severe falciparum malaria. It results from deposition of hemoglobin in renal tubules, decreased renal blood flow, and acute tubular necrosis. "Blackwater fever" is a clinical syndrome that consists of severe hemolysis, hemoglobinuria, and renal failure. It is a rare complication that occurs when complement and antibody directed against parasite-laden erythrocytes produce severe hemolytic anemia, hemoglobinuria, oliguria, and jaundice. Renal failure usually requires peritoneal dialysis or hemodialysis.

Pulmonary edema may occur several days after therapy has begun and is commonly associated with excessive intravenous fluid therapy. It can develop rapidly and may be fatal. Care should be taken not to overhydrate patients with *P. falciparum* malaria.

Hypoglycemia is a complication of malaria that is more common in children, pregnant women, and patients receiving quinine therapy. Patients may have decreased level of consciousness that can be confused with cerebral malaria. Hypoglycemia is associated with increased mortality rate and neurologic sequelae.

Thrombocytopenia is a common complication of *P. falciparum* and *P. vivax* malaria. Although significant bleeding is uncommon without disseminated intravascular coagulopathy, platelet counts can diminish to 10,000–20,000/mm^3.

Splenic rupture is a rare complication that may occur with acute infection due to any malaria species. It can occur spontaneously but is usually the result of trauma, including overly vigorous abdominal palpation on physical examination. It causes severe internal hemorrhage and may result in death if splenectomy and blood transfusions are not performed in a timely manner.

Algid malaria is a rare form of *P. falciparum* malaria that occurs with overwhelming infection, hypotension, hypothermia, rapid weak pulse, shallow breathing, pallor, and vascular collapse. Death may occur within a few hours.

PREVENTION. Malaria prevention consists of reducing exposure to infected mosquitoes and using chemoprophylaxis. Travelers to endemic areas should remain in well-screened areas from dusk to dawn, when the risk of transmission is highest. They should sleep under permethrin-treated mosquito netting and spray insecticides indoors at sundown. During the day travelers should wear clothing that covers the arms and legs with trousers tucked into shoes or boots. Mosquito repellent should be applied to thin clothing and exposed areas of the skin with repeated applications every 1–2 hr. A child should not be taken outside from dusk to dawn, but, if that is absolutely necessary, diethyltoluamide (DEET), in a 10–15% solution, should be applied to exposed areas except the eyes, mouth, or hands (hands are often placed in the mouth). The DEET should then be washed off as soon as the child goes back inside. Adverse reactions to DEET include skin rashes, toxic encephalopathy, and seizures. Even with these precautions, a child should be taken to a physician immediately if he or she becomes ill when traveling to a malarious area.

Chemoprophylaxis is necessary for all visitors to and residents of the tropics who have not lived there since infancy (see Table 304–2). Children of non-immune women should have chemoprophylaxis from birth. Chemoprophylaxis should be started 1–2 wk before entering the endemic area (except if doxycycline is used, which can started 1 to 2 days before entrance) and be continued for at least 4 wk after leaving.

Extensive efforts have been made to develop a malaria vaccine, but results to date have been disappointing.

Centers for Disease Control and Prevention: Malaria surveillance—United States, 1994. MMWR 46 (SS-5):1, 1997.

Emanuel B, Aronson N, Shulman S: Malaria in children in Chicago. Pediatrics 92:83, 1993.

Lobel HO, Kozarsky PE: Update on prevention of malaria for travelers. JAMA 278:1767, 1997.

Lynk A, Gold R: Review of 40 children with imported malaria. Pediatr Infect Dis J 8:745, 1989.

McCaslin R, Pikis A, Rodriguez WJ: Pediatric *Plasmodium falciparum* malaria: A ten-year experience from Washington, DC. Pediatr Infect Dis J 13:709, 1994.

Rivera-Matos IR, Atkins JT, Doerr CA, White AC Jr: Pediatric malaria in Houston, Texas. Am J Trop Med Hyg 57:560, 1997.

Stanley J. Malaria. Emerg Med Clin North Am 15:113, 1997.

Zucker JR, Campbell CC: Malaria: Principles of prevention and treatment. Infect Dis Clin North Am 7:547, 1993.

Zucker JR: Changing patterns of autochthonous malaria transmission in the United States: A review of recent outbreaks. Emerg Infect Dis 2:37, 1996.

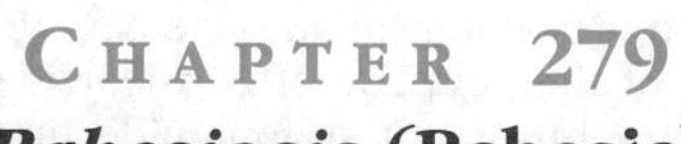

CHAPTER 279
Babesiosis (Babesia)

Peter J. Krause

Babesiosis is an emerging malaria-like disease caused by an intraerythrocytic protozoan that is transmitted by ticks. The clinical manifestations of babesiosis range from subclinical illness to fulminant disease resulting in death.

ETIOLOGY. The causative protozoan was first described in cattle in 1891 by the Hungarian microbiologist Babes. More than 90 species of *Babesia,* which infect a wide variety of wild and domestic animals throughout the world, have been described. At least three *Babesia* species cause disease in humans: *B. microti* (a rodent species), *B. gibsoni* (WA-1, a canine species), and *B. divergens* (*B. bovis*, a cattle species).

EPIDEMIOLOGY. Since the first documented case of human babesial infection was reported in 1957, infection by *B. divergens* has been demonstrated in Europe, and infection by *B. microti* has been documented increasingly in the northeastern and upper midwestern United States. A *Babesia* parasite very closely related to *B. gibsoni* (WA-1) appears to infect humans along the Pacific coast. Human babesiosis cases also have been documented in Taiwan and South Africa.

The primary reservoir for *Babesia microti* is the white-footed mouse (*Peromyscus leucopus*), and the primary vector is the deer tick (*Ixodes dammini*). Deer ticks also transmit *Borrelia burgdorferi*, the etiologic agent of Lyme disease, and may simultaneously transmit both microorganisms. Thus, any area where Lyme disease is found should be considered as a potentially endemic area for babesiosis (Chapter 219). Deer *(Odocoileus virginianus)* serve as the host upon which adult ticks most abundantly feed but are incompetent reservoirs. Rarely, babesiosis is acquired through blood transfusion or transplacentally.

PATHOPHYSIOLOGY. Erythrocyte lysis is responsible for many of the clinical manifestations and complications of the disease, including fever, hemolytic anemia, jaundice, hemoglobinemia, hemoglobinuria, and renal insufficiency. Obstruction of blood vessels by parasitized erythrocytes causes ischemia and necrosis that may result in splenomegaly, hepatomegaly, hepatic dysfunction, and cerebral abnormalities. The spleen has an important role in clearing parasitemia along with antibody, T and B cells, complement, a soluble non-antibody factor, cytokines such as tumor necrosis factor (TNF), macrophages, and polymorphonuclear leukocytes. Immunity is sometimes incomplete since low level parasitemia may exist for as long as 26 mo after symptoms have resolved, and recrudescence may occur. Parasite strain variation also appears to play a role in influencing the course of human infection.

CLINICAL MANIFESTATIONS. Although infection is common in endemic areas, most is asymptomatic or only mild. In some highly endemic areas, moderate to severe disease is frequently observed. In 1994, Nantucket Island reported 21 cases, a total that translates to 280 cases/100,000 population; this proportion categorizes the community burden of disease as "moderately common." The case fatality rate was estimated at 5% in a retrospective study of 136 cases in New York state. Thus, in certain sites, in certain years of high transmission, babesiosis may constitute a significant public health burden.

There is often no recollection of a tick bite because the unengorged *I. dammini* nymph is only about 2 mm in length. In clinically apparent cases, symptoms of babesiosis begin after an incubation period of 1–9 wk from the beginning of tick feeding or 6–9 wk after transfusion. Typical symptoms in moderate to severe infection include intermittent fever to as high as 40°C (104°F) and one or more symptoms of chills, sweats, myalgia, arthralgia, nausea, and vomiting. Less commonly noted are emotional lability, hyperesthesia, headache, sore throat, abdominal pain, conjunctival injection, photophobia, weight loss, and nonproductive cough. The findings on physical examination generally are minimal, often consisting only of fever. Mild splenomegaly, hepatomegaly, or both are noted occasionally but rash seldom is reported.

Risk factors for severe disease include anatomic or functional asplenia, infection with *B. divergens*, age >40 yr, concomitant Lyme disease, or underlying infection with human immunodeficiency virus (HIV). Coinfection with babesiosis and Lyme disease occurs in approximately 10% of Lyme disease cases in parts of southern New England and results in more severe illness than that caused by either disease alone. Moderate to severe babesiosis may occur in children, but infection generally is less severe than in adults.

Four cases of neonatal babesiosis have been described. One infant was severely ill and the others moderately ill with irritability and fever as high as 40°C.

DIAGNOSIS. Diagnosis of *B. microti* infection in human hosts is made by microscopic demonstration of the organism using Giemsa-stained thin blood films. Parasitemias may be exceedingly sparse, especially early in the course of illness. Thick blood smears may be used, but the organisms appear as simple chromatin dots that might be mistaken for stain precipitate or iron inclusion bodies. Subinoculation of a sample of patient's blood into hamsters or gerbils is a specialized test used in reference laboratories. The polymerase chain reaction (PCR) is a sensitive and specific test for detection of *Babesia* DNA that should supplant the hamster inoculation test.

Serologic testing is useful, particularly in diagnosing *B. microti* infection. The indirect immunofluorescence serologic assay (for both immunoglobulin G [IgG] and IgM antibody) is sensitive and specific and may quickly confirm a diagnosis of babesiosis when parasitemia is not detectable.

Laboratory Findings. Abnormal laboratory findings include moderately severe hemolytic anemia, an elevated reticulocyte count, thrombocytopenia, proteinuria, and elevated blood urea nitrogen and creatinine level. The leukocyte count is normal to slightly decreased, with a shift to the left and frequently with lymphopenia. Babesiosis usually lasts for a few weeks to several months, with a prolonged recovery period of up to 18 months in severe cases.

TREATMENT. The recommended treatment of babesiosis in children is a combination of clindamycin (20 mg/kg/24 hr in four divided doses orally; maximum 600 mg/dose) plus quinine (25 mg/kg/24 hr in 3–4 divided doses orally; maximum 650 mg/dose) for 7–10 days. Clindamycin may also be administered intravenously. Adverse reactions, especially tinnitus and abdominal distress, are common. In addition, treatment failures have been reported, particularly in patients with HIV infection. Pentamidine plus trimethoprim-sulfamethoxazole has been used effectively to treat *B. divergens* in humans. Atovaquone plus azithromycin has been used with success to treat *B. microti* in a hamster model. Preliminary studies in humans suggest that this combination may be as efficacious as and safer than clindamycin and quinine.

Exchange blood transfusion can decrease the degree of parasitemia rapidly and remove toxic by-products of *Babesia* infections but should be reserved for patients with severe infections including those with high parasitemia (> 5%), coma, hypotension, congestive heart failure, pulmonary edema, or renal failure. Exchange blood transfusion in addition to clindamycin and quinine is the treatment of choice for all cases of *B. divergens* babesiosis.

PREVENTION. Prevention of babesiosis can be accomplished by avoiding areas where ticks, deer, and mice are known to thrive. Use of clothing that covers the lower part of the body and that is sprayed or impregnated with diethyltoluamide (DEET), dimethyl phthalate, or premethrin (Permanone) is recommended for those who travel and have contact with foliage of endemic areas. Frequent searches for ticks on people and pets should be performed, and the ticks removed by using tweezers to grasp the mouthparts without squeezing the body of the tick.

Prospective blood donors with a history of babesiosis are excluded from giving blood to prevent transfusion-related cases.

Esernio-Jenssen D, Scimeca PG, Benach JL, et al: Transplacental/perinatal babesiosis. J Pediatr 110:570, 1987.

Krause PJ, Telford SR III, Pollack RJ, et al: Babesiosis: An underdiagnosed disease of children. Pediatrics 89:1045, 1992.

Krause PJ, Telford SR III, Spielman A, et al: Concurrent Lyme disease and

babesiosis: Evidence for increased severity and duration of illness. JAMA 275:1657, 1996.
Krause PJ, Spielman A, Telford SR III, et al: Persistent parasitemia after acute babesiosis. N Engl J Med 339:160, 1998.
Scimeca PG, Weinblatt ME, Schonfeld G, et al: Babesiosis in two infants from eastern Long Island, N.Y. Am J Dis Child 140:971, 1986.
White DJ, Talarico J, Chang HG, et al: Human babesiosis in New York state: Review of 139 hospitalized cases and analysis of prognostic factors. Arch Intern Med 158:2149, 1998.

CHAPTER 280
Toxoplasmosis (Toxoplasma gondii)

Rima McLeod and Jack S. Remington

Toxoplasma gondii, an obligate intracellular protozoan, is acquired perorally, transplacentally, or, rarely, parenterally in laboratory accidents; by transfusion; or from a transplanted organ. In the immunologically normal child, the acute acquired infection may be asymptomatic, cause lymphadenopathy, or damage almost any organ. Once acquired, the latent encysted organism persists for the lifetime of the host. In the immunocompromised infant or child, either initial acquisition or recrudescence of latent organisms often causes signs or symptoms related to the central nervous system (CNS). Infection acquired congenitally, if untreated, almost always causes signs or symptoms in the perinatal period or later in life. The most frequent of these signs are due to chorioretinitis and CNS lesions. However, other manifestations, such as intrauterine growth retardation, fever, lymphadenopathy, rash, hearing loss, pneumonitis, hepatitis, and thrombocytopenia, also occur. Congenital toxoplasmosis in infants with human immunodeficiency virus (HIV) infection may be fulminant.

ETIOLOGY. *T. gondii* is a coccidian protozoan. Its tachyzoites are oval or crescent-like, multiply only in living cells, and measure 2–4 × 4–7 μm. Tissue cysts, which are 10–100 μm in diameter, may contain thousands of parasites and remain in tissues, especially the CNS and skeletal and heart muscle, for the life of the host. *Toxoplasma* can multiply in all tissues of mammals and birds, and its disease spectrum is expressed with remarkable similarity in different host species.

Newly infected cats and other Felidae excrete infectious *Toxoplasma* oocysts in their feces. *Toxoplasma* are acquired by susceptible cats by ingestion of infected meat containing encysted brandyzoites or by ingestion of oocysts excreted by other recently infected cats. The parasites then multiply through schizogonic and gametogonic cycles in the distal ileal epithelium of the cat intestine. Oocysts containing two sporocysts are excreted, and under proper conditions of temperature and moisture, each sporocyst matures into four sporozoites. For about 2 wk the cat excretes 10^5–10^7 oocysts/day, which, in a suitable environment, may retain their viability for a year or more. Oocysts sporulate 1–5 days after excretion and are then infectious. Oocysts are killed by drying, boiling, and exposure to some strong chemicals, but not to bleach. Oocysts have been isolated from soil and sand frequented by cats, and outbreaks associated with contaminated water have been reported. Oocysts and tissue cysts are the sources of animal and human infections (Fig. 280–1).

EPIDEMIOLOGY. *Toxoplasma* infection is ubiquitous in animals and is one of the most common latent infections of humans throughout the world. The incidence varies considerably among people and animals in different geographic areas. In many areas of the world, approximately 5.35% of pork, 9–60% of lamb, and 0–9% of beef contain *T. gondii* organisms. Significant antibody titers have been detected in 50–80% of residents of some localities and in < 5% in others. A higher prevalence of infection usually occurs in warmer, more humid climates.

Human infection is usually acquired by the oral route via undercooked or raw meat that contains cysts or by ingestion of oocysts. Freezing meat to −20°C or heating it to 66°C renders the cysts noninfectious. Outbreaks of acute acquired infection have occurred in families who have consumed the same infected food. Except for transplacental infection from mother to fetus and, rarely, by organ transplantation or transfusion, *Toxoplasma* are not transmitted from person to person.

Seronegative transplant recipients who receive an organ (e.g., heart or kidney) from seropositive donors have experienced life-threatening illness requiring therapy. Seropositive recipients may have increased serologic titers without associated disease.

Congenital Toxoplasmosis. Transmission to the fetus usually occurs when the infection is acquired by an immunologically normal mother during gestation. Congenital transmission from immunologically normal women infected prior to pregnancy is extremely rare. Immunocompromised women who are chronically infected have transmitted the infection to their fetuses. The incidence of congenital infection in the United States ranges from 1/1,000 to 1/8,000 live births. The incidence of newly acquired infection in a population of pregnant women depends on the risk of becoming infected in that specific geographic area and the proportion of the population that has not been previously infected.

PATHOGENESIS. *T. gondii* is usually acquired by children and adults from ingesting food that contains cysts or that is contaminated with oocysts usually from acutely infected cats. Oocysts also may be transported to food by flies and cockroaches. When the organism is ingested, bradyzoites are released from cysts or sporozoites from oocysts, and the organisms then enter gastrointestinal cells. They multiply, rupture cells, and infect contiguous cells. They are transported via the lymphatics and disseminated hematogenously throughout the body. Tachyzoites proliferate, producing necrotic focuses surrounded by a cellular reaction. With the development of a normal immune response (humoral and cell-mediated), tachyzoites disappear from tissues. In immunodeficient individuals and some apparently immunologically normal patients, the acute infection progresses and may cause potentially lethal involvement such as pneumonitis, myocarditis, or necrotizing encephalitis.

In acute acquired lymphadenopathic toxoplasmosis, characteristic lymph node changes include reactive follicular hyperplasia with irregular clusters of epithelioid histiocytes that encroach on and blur the margins of germinal centers. Focal distention of sinuses with monocytoid cells also occurs.

Cysts form as early as 7 days after infection and remain for the life span of the host. During latent infection they produce little or no inflammatory response but cause recrudescent disease in immunocompromised patients or chorioretinitis in older children who acquired the infection congenitally.

Congenital Toxoplasmosis. When a mother acquires the infection during gestation, the organism may disseminate hematogenously to the placenta. When this occurs, infection may be transmitted to the fetus transplacentally or during vaginal delivery. Of untreated maternal infections acquired in the first trimester, approximately 17% of fetuses are infected, usually with severe disease. Of untreated maternal infection acquired in the third trimester, approximately 65% of fetuses are infected, usually with disease that is mild or inapparent at birth. These different rates of transmission and outcomes are most likely related to placental blood flow, the virulence and amount of *T. gondii* acquired, and the immunologic ability of the mother to restrict parasitemia.

Examination of the placenta of infected newborns may reveal chronic inflammation and cysts. Tachyzoites can be seen

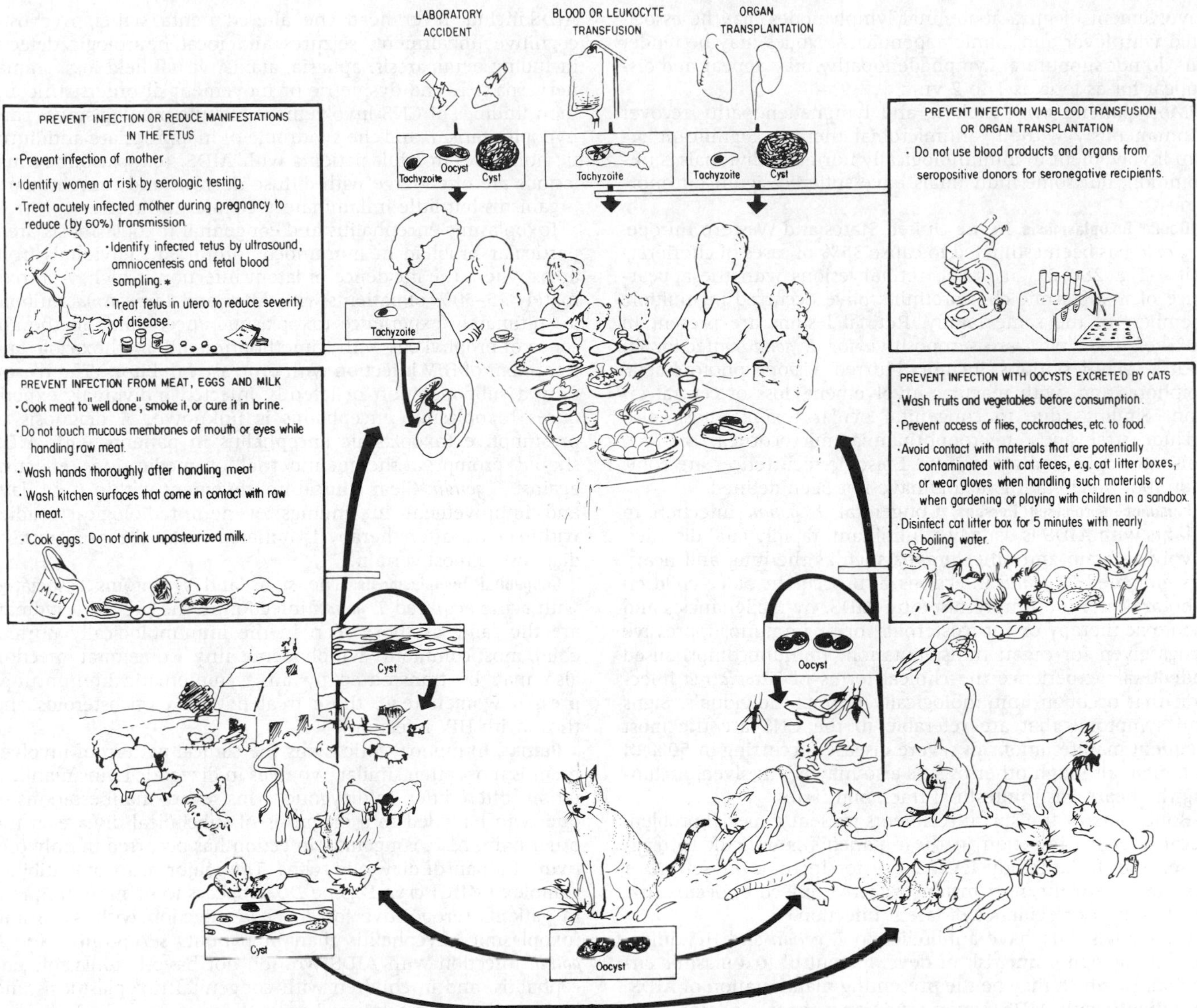

Figure 280–1 Life cycle of *Toxoplasma gondii* and prevention of toxoplasmosis by interruption of transmission to humans.

with Wright or Giemsa stains but are best demonstrated with the immunoperoxidase technique. The tissue cyst stains well with periodic acid–Schiff (PAS) and silver stains as well as with the immunoperoxidase technique. Gross or microscopic areas of necrosis may be present in many tissues, especially the central nervous system, choroid and retina, heart, lungs, skeletal muscle, liver, and spleen. Areas of calcification occur in the brain.

Almost all congenitally infected individuals manifest signs or symptoms of infection, such as chorioretinitis, by adolescence if they are not treated in the newborn period. Some severely involved infants with congenital infection appear to have *Toxoplasma* antigen–specific anergy of their lymphocytes, which may be important in the pathogenesis of their disease. The predilection to predominant involvement of the CNS and eye in congenital infection has not been fully explained.

Immunity. There are profound and prolonged alterations of T-lymphocyte populations during acute acquired *T. gondii* infections, but they have not correlated with outcome. Lymphocytosis, increased $CD8^+$ count, and decreased $CD4^+$:$CD8^+$ ratio are commonly present. Depletion of $CD4^+$ cells in patients with acquired immunodeficiency syndrome (AIDS) may contribute to the severe manifestations of toxoplasmosis seen in these patients.

CLINICAL MANIFESTATIONS. The manifestations of primary infection with *T. gondii* are highly variable and influenced primarily by host immunocompetence. Reactivation of previously asymptomatic congenital toxoplasmosis is usually manifest as ocular toxoplasmosis.

Acquired Toxoplasmosis. Immunologically normal children who acquire the infection postnatally may have no clinically recognizable disease. When clinical manifestations are apparent, they may include almost any combination of fever, stiff neck, myalgia, arthralgia, maculopapular rash that spares the palms and soles, localized or generalized lymphadenopathy, hepatomegaly, hepatitis, reactive lymphocytosis, meningitis, brain abscess, encephalitis, confusion, malaise, pneumonia, polymyositis, pericarditis, pericardial effusion, and myocarditis. Chorioretinitis, usually unilateral, occurs in approximately 1% of cases. Symptoms may be present for a few days only or may persist many months. The most common manifestation is enlargement of one or a few lymph nodes in the cervical region. Cases of *Toxoplasma* lymphadenopathy rarely resemble infectious mononucleosis (due to Epstein-Barr virus or cytomegalovirus), Hodgkin disease, or other lymphadenopathies (Chapter 496). In the pectoral area in older girls and women, the nodes may be confused with breast neoplasms. Mediastinal, mesenteric, and retroperitoneal lymph nodes may be involved.

Involvement of intra-abdominal lymph nodes may be associated with fever and mimic appendicitis. Nodes may be tender but do not suppurate. Lymphadenopathy may appear and disappear for as long as 1 to 2 yr.

Most patients with malaise and lymphadenopathy recover spontaneously without antimicrobial therapy. Significant organ involvement in immunologically normal individuals is uncommon, but some individuals have suffered significant morbidity.

Ocular Toxoplasmosis. In the United States and Western Europe, *T. gondii* has been estimated to cause 35% of cases of chorioretinitis (Fig. 280–2). In Brazil, retinal lesions with the appearance of toxoplasmic chorioretinitis have occurred in multiple members of the same family. Retinal lesions are present in 30% of those who are seropositive for *T. gondii* infection in Brazil. Manifestations include blurred vision, photophobia, epiphora, and, with macular involvement, loss of central vision. Findings due to congenital ocular toxoplasmosis also include strabismus, microophthalmia, microcornea, cataract, anisometropia, and nystagmus. Episodic recurrences are common, but precipitating factors have not been defined.

Immunocompromised Persons. Congenital *T. gondii* infection in infants with AIDS is usually a fulminant, rapidly fatal disorder, involving brain and other organs such as the lung and heart. Disseminated *T. gondii* infections also occur in older children who are immunocompromised by AIDS, by malignancies and cytotoxic therapy or corticosteroids, or by immunosuppressive drugs given for organ transplantation. Immunocompromised individuals experience the clinical forms of *Toxoplasma* infection that occur in immunologically normal individuals. Signs and symptoms that are referable to the CNS are the most frequent manifestations of severe disease (occurring in 50% of patients), although other organs also may be involved, including the heart, gastrointestinal tract, and testes.

Bone marrow transplant recipients present a special problem because active infection in these patients is difficult to diagnose. Specific antibody level may not increase in serum or may be absent. In most instances, active infection occurs in a child with prior evidence of latent infection.

Individuals who have antibodies to *T. gondii* and HIV infection are at significant risk of development of toxoplasmic encephalitis, which may be the presenting manifestation of AIDS. In patients with AIDS, toxoplasmic encephalitis is fatal if not treated. Typical findings of CNS toxoplasmosis in patients with AIDS include fever, headache, altered mental status, psychosis, cognitive impairment, seizures and focal neurologic defects, including hemiparesis, aphasia, ataxia, visual field loss, cranial nerve palsies, and dysmetric or movement disorders. Uncommon findings of CNS involvement include meningismus, panhypopituitarism, and the syndrome of inappropriate antidiuretic hormone. In adult patients with AIDS, toxoplasmic retinal lesions are often large with diffuse necrosis and contain many organisms but little inflammatory cellular infiltrate.

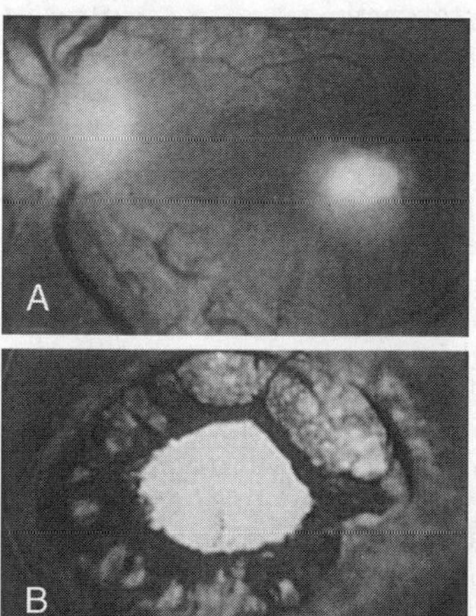

Figure 280–2 Toxoplasmic chorioretinits. *A*, Active acute lesion by indirect ophthalmoscopy. *B*, The healed foci of toxoplasmic chorioretinitis may resemble a colobomatous defect (macular pseudocoloboma). (*B*, adapted from Desmonts G, Remington J: Congenital toxoplasmosis. *In*: Remington JS, Klein JO [eds]: Infectious Diseases of the Fetus and Newborn Infant, 4th ed. Philadelphia, WB Saunders, 1995.) See also color section.

Toxoplasmic encephalitis and congenital toxoplasmosis are a particular problem in immunocompromised individuals from areas where the incidence of latent infection is high. Approximately 25–50% of patients with AIDS and *Toxoplasma* antibodies ultimately experience toxoplasmic encephalitis in the absence of prophylaxis with trimethoprim-sulfamethoxazole and treatment of HIV infection with protease inhibitors. The reason only a subpopulation of latently infected individuals experiences toxoplasmic encephalitis is unknown. A diagnosis of presumptive toxoplasmic encephalitis in patients with AIDS should prompt a therapeutic trial of medications effective against *T. gondii*. Clear clinical improvement within 7–14 days and improvement in findings of neuroradiological studies within 3 wk after therapy is initiated make the presumptive diagnosis almost certain.

Congenital Toxoplasmosis. The signs and symptoms associated with acute acquired *T. gondii* infection in the pregnant woman are the same as those seen in the immunologically normal child, most commonly lymphadenopathy. Congenital infection also may be transmitted by an asymptomatic immunosuppressed woman (e.g., those treated with corticosteroids and those with HIV infection).

GENETICS. In monozygotic twins the clinical pattern of involvement is most often similar, whereas in dizygotic twins manifestations often differ. In dizygotic twins severe manifestations in one twin have led to a diagnosis of subclinical disease in the other twin. Also, congenital infection has occurred in only one twin of a pair of dizygotic twins. The major histocompatibility complex (MHC) class II gene *DQ3* appears to be more frequent in patients seropositive for *T. gondii* infection with AIDS and toxoplasmic encephalitis than in patients seropositive for *T. gondii* infection with AIDS who do not have toxoplasmic encephalitis, and in children with congenital toxoplasmosis and hydrocephalus as compared with those without hydrocephalus.

SPECTRUM AND FREQUENCY OF SIGNS AND SYMPTOMS. Congenital infection may present as a mild or severe neonatal disease, with onset during the 1st month of life, or with sequelae or relapse of a previously undiagnosed infection at any time during infancy or later in life. A wide variety of manifestations of congenital infection occur in the perinatal period. These range from relatively mild signs, such as small size for gestational age, prematurity, peripheral retinal scars, persistent jaundice, mild thrombocytopenia, and cerebrospinal fluid pleocytosis, to the classic triad of signs consisting of chorioretinitis, hydrocephalus, and cerebral calcifications. Infection may result in erythroblastosis, hydrops fetalis, and perinatal death. More than half of congenitally infected infants are considered normal in the perinatal period, but almost all such children will have ocular involvement later in life. Neurologic signs in neonates, which include convulsions, setting-sun sign, and an increase in head circumference due to hydrocephalus, may be associated with substantial cerebral damage. However, such signs also may occur in association with encephalitis without extensive destruction or with relatively mild inflammation adjacent to and obstructing the aqueduct of Sylvius. If such infants are treated promptly, signs and symptoms may resolve, and they may develop normally.

The spectrum and frequency of manifestations that develop in the perinatal period in infants with congenital *Toxoplasma* infection are presented in Table 280–1. Infection in most of these 210 infants was initially suspected because their mothers were identified by a serologic screening program that detected pregnant women with acute acquired *T. gondii* infection. Twenty-one infants (10%) had severe congenital toxoplasmosis with CNS involvement, eye lesions, and general systemic manifestations. Seventy-one (34%) had mild involvement with normal clinical examination results other than retinal scars or isolated intracranial calcifications. One hundred and sixteen (55%) had no detectable manifestations; this may reflect the difficulties associated with funduscopic examination of the peripheral retina in infants and young children. These figures represent an underestimation of the relative frequency of severe congenital infection for the following reasons: The most severe cases, including most of those individuals who died, were not referred; therapeutic abortion was often performed when acute acquired infection of the mother was diagnosed early during pregnancy; in utero spiramycin therapy may have diminished the severity of infection; and only 13 infants had CT brain scans and 23% did not have a cerebrospinal fluid examination. Routine newborn examinations often yield normal findings for congenitally infected infants, but more careful evaluations may reveal significant abnormalities: Specifically, of 28 infants who were detected by a universal state mandated serologic screening program for *T. gondii*–specific immunoglobulin M (IgM), 26 had normal findings of routine newborn examinations and 14 had significant abnormalities detected with more careful evaluation. These abnormalities included retinal scars (7 infants), active chorioretinitis (3 infants), and CNS abnormalities (8 infants).

The clinical spectrum and natural history of untreated congenital toxoplasmosis, which is *clinically apparent* in the first year of life, are presented in Table 280–2. More than 80% of these children had IQ of less than 70, and many had convulsions and severely impaired vision.

SKIN. Cutaneous manifestations in infants with congenital toxoplasmosis include rashes, petechiae, ecchymoses, or large hemorrhages secondary to thrombocytopenia. Rashes may be fine punctate, diffuse maculopapular, lenticular, deep blue-red, sharply defined macular, and diffuse blue papules. Macular rashes involving the entire body, including the palms and soles; exfoliative dermatitis; and cutaneous calcifications have been described. Jaundice due to hepatic involvement with *T. gondii* and/or hemolysis, cyanosis due to interstitial pneumonitis from congenital infection, and edema secondary to myocarditis or nephrotic syndrome may be present. Jaundice and conjugated hyperbilirubinemia may persist for months.

TABLE 280–1 Signs and Symptoms in 210 Infants with Proved Congenital Toxoplasma Infection*

Finding	No. Examined	No. Positive (%)
Prematurity	210	
Birthweight <2,500 g		8 (3.8)
Birthweight 2,500–3,000 g		5 (7.1)
Intrauterine growth retardation		13 (6.2)
Icterus	201	20 (10)
Hepatosplenomegaly	210	9 (4.2)
Thrombocytopenic purpura	210	3 (1.4)
Abnormal blood count (anemia, eosinophilia)	102	9 (4.4)
Microcephaly	210	11 (5.2)
Hydrocephaly	210	8 (3.8)
Hypotonia	210	12 (5.7)
Convulsions	210	8 (3.8)
Psychomotor retardation	210	11 (5.2)
Intracranial calcification x-ray	210	24 (11.4)
Ultrasound	49	5 (10)
Computed tomography	13	11 (84)
Abnormal EEG	191	16 (8.3)
Abnormal CSF	163	56 (34.2)
Microphthalmia	210	6 (2.8)
Strabismus	210	111 (5.2)
Chorioretinitis	210	
Unilateral		34 (16.1)
Bilateral		12 (5.7)

**Infants were identified by prospective study of infants born to women who acquired* Toxoplasma gondii *infection during pregnancy.*

Data are adapted from Couvreur J, et al: Study of homogenous series of 210 cases of congenital toxoplasmosis in infants aged 0 to 11 months detected prospectively. Ann Pediatr 31:815, 1984.

TABLE 280–2 Signs and Symptoms Occurring Prior to Diagnosis or During the Course of Untreated Acute Congenital Toxoplasmosis in 152 Infants (A) and in 101 of These Same Children When They Had Been Followed 4 yr or More (B)

Signs and Symptoms	Frequency of Occurrence in Patients with "Neurologic" Disease*	"Generalized" Disease†
A. Infants	***108 Patients (%)***	***44 Patients (%)***
Chorioretinitis	102 (94)‡	29 (66)
Abnormal CSF	59 (55)	37 (84)
Anemia	55 (51)	34 (77)
Convulsions	54 (50)	8 (18)
Intracranial calcification	54 (50)	2 (4)
Jaundice	31 (29)	35 (80)
Hydrocephalus	30 (28)	0 (0)
Fever	27 (25)	34 (77)
Splenomegaly	23 (21)	40 (90)
Lymphadenopathy	18 (17)	30 (68)
Hepatomegaly	18 (17)	34 (77)
Vomiting	17 (16)	21 (48)
Microcephalus	14 (13)	0 (0)
Diarrhea	7 (6)	11 (25)
Cataracts	5 (5)	0 (0)
Eosinophilia	6 (4)	8 (18)
Abnormal bleeding	3 (3)	8 (18)
Hypothermia	2 (2)	9 (20)
Glaucoma	2 (2)	0 (0)
Optic atrophy	2 (2)	0 (0)
Microphthalmia	2 (2)	0 (0)
Rash	1 (1)	11 (25)
Pneumonitis	0 (0)	18 (41)
B. Children, ≥4 yr of age	***70 Patients (%)***	***31 Patients (%)***
Mental retardation	62 (89)	25 (81)
Convulsions	58 (83)	24 (77)
Spasticity and palsies	53 (76)	18 (58)
Severely impaired vision	48 (69)	13 (42)
Hydrocephalus or microcephalus	31 (44)	2 (6)
Deafness	12 (17)	3 (10)
Normal	6 (9)	5 (16)

Adapted from Eichenwald H: A study of congenital toxoplasmosis. In: Siim JC (ed): Human Toxoplasmosis. Copenhagen, Munksgaard, 1960, pp 41–49. Study performed in 1947. The most severely involved institutionalized patients were not included in the later study of 101 children.

**Patients with otherwise undiagnosed central nervous system disease in the 1st yr of life.*

†Patients with otherwise undiagnosed non-neurologic diseases during the first 2 mo of life.

‡Figure outside parentheses = number; figure inside parentheses = percentage.

SYSTEMIC SIGNS. From 25% to more than 50% of infants with clinically apparent disease at birth are born prematurely. Low Apgar scores also are common. Intrauterine growth retardation and instability of temperature regulation may occur. Other systemic manifestations include lymphadenopathy, hepatosplenomegaly, myocarditis, pneumonitis, nephrotic syndrome, vomiting, diarrhea, and feeding problems. Bands of metaphyseal lucency and irregularity of the line of provisional calcification at the epiphyseal plate may occur without periosteal reaction in the ribs, femurs, and vertebrae. Congenital toxoplasmosis may be confused with isosensitization causing erythroblastosis fetalis; the Coombs test result is usually negative with congenital *T. gondii* infection.

ENDOCRINE ABNORMALITIES. Endocrine abnormalities may occur secondary to hypothalamic or pituitary involvement or end-organ involvement. The following have been reported: myxedema, persistent hypernatremia with vasopressin-sensitive diabetes insipidus without polyuria or polydipsia, sexual precocity, and partial anterior hypopituitarism.

Central Nervous System. Neurologic manifestations of congenital toxoplasmosis vary from massive acute encephalopathy to subtle neurologic syndromes. Toxoplasmosis should be considered as a cause of any undiagnosed neurologic disease in children < 1 yr of age, especially if retinal lesions are present.

Hydrocephalus may be the sole clinical neurologic manifestation of congenital toxoplasmosis and may either be compensated or require shunt placement. Hydrocephalus may present in the perinatal period, progress after the perinatal period, or, less commonly, present later in life. Patterns of seizures are protean and have included focal motor seizures, petit and grand mal seizures, muscular twitching, opisthotonus, and hypsarrhythmia (which may resolve with corticotropin [ACTH] therapy). Spinal or bulbar involvement may be manifested by paralysis of the extremities, difficulty in swallowing, and respiratory distress. Microcephaly usually reflects severe brain damage, but some children with microcephaly due to congenital toxoplasmosis who have been treated appear to function normally in the early years of life. Untreated congenital toxoplasmosis that is symptomatic in the first year of life can cause substantial diminution in cognitive function and developmental delays. Intellectual impairment also occurs in some children with subclinical infection despite treatment with pyrimethamine and sulfonamides for 1 mo. Seizures and focal motor defects may become apparent after the newborn period, even when infection is subclinical at birth.

Cerebrospinal fluid (CSF) abnormalities occur in at least one third of infants with congenital toxoplasmosis. Local production of *T. gondii*–specific antibodies may be demonstrated in CSF fluid of congenitally infected individuals (see later under Diagnosis). CT scan of the brain with contrast enhancement is useful to detect calcifications, determine ventricular size, image active inflammatory lesions and demonstrate porencephalic cystic structures (Fig. 280–3). Calcifications occur throughout the brain, but there appears to be a special propensity for development of such lesions in the caudate nucleus (i.e., especially basal ganglia area), choroid plexus, and subependyma. Ultrasonography may be useful for following ventricular size in congenitally infected babies. Magnetic resonance imaging (MRI), CT with contrast enhancement, and radionucleotide brain scans may be useful for detecting active inflammatory lesions.

Eyes. Almost all untreated congenitally infected individuals will develop chorioretinal lesions by adulthood, and about 50% will have severe visual impairment. *T. gondii* causes a focal necrotizing retinitis in congenitally infected individuals (see Fig. 280–2). Retinal detachment may occur. Any part of the retina may be involved, either unilaterally or bilaterally, including the maculae. The optic nerve may be involved, and toxoplasmic lesions that involve projections of the visual pathways in the brain or the visual cortex also may lead to visual impairment. In association with retinal lesions and vitritis, the anterior uvea may be intensely inflamed, leading to erythema of the external eye. Other ocular findings include cells and protein in the anterior chamber, large keratic precipitates, posterior synechiae, nodules on the iris, and neovascular formation on the surface of the iris, sometimes with an associated increase in intraocular pressure and development of glaucoma. The extraocular musculature may also be involved directly. Other manifestations include strabismus, nystagmus, visual impairment, and micro-ophthalmia. The differential diagnosis of lesions resembling those of ocular toxoplasmosis includes congenital colobomatous defect and other inflammatory lesions due to cytomegalovirus, *Treponema pallidum, Mycobacterium tuberculosis,* or vasculitis. Ocular toxoplasmosis is a recurrent and progressive disease that requires multiple courses of therapy. Couvreur et al. report limited data that suggest that occurrence of lesions in the early years of life may be prevented by instituting antimicrobial treatment (with pyrimethamine and sulfonamides in alternate months with spiramycin) during the first year of life. Bŕzin et al. have noted that treatment of the infected fetus in utero followed by treatment in the first year of life with pyrimethamine, sulfadiazine and leukovorin reduces the incidence and the severity of the retinal disease.

Ears. Sensorineural hearing loss, both mild and severe, may occur. It is not known whether this is a static or progressive disorder. Treatment in the first year of life is associated with diminished occurrence of this sequela.

Concomitant Infections. Congenital toxoplasmosis in infants with HIV infection usually presents as a severe and fulminant illness with substantial CNS involvement but also may be more indolent in its presentation with focal neurologic deficits or systemic manifestations such as pneumonitis.

DIAGNOSIS. Diagnosis of acute *Toxoplasma* infection can be established by isolation of *T. gondii* from blood or body fluids and also by demonstration of tachyzoites in sections or preparations of tissues and body fluids, cysts in the placenta or tissues of a fetus or newborn, and characteristic lymph node histologic features. Serologic tests also are very useful for diagnosis.

Culture. Organisms are isolated by inoculation of body fluids, leukocytes, or tissue specimens into mice or tissue cultures. Body fluids should be processed and inoculated immediately, but *T. gondii* has been isolated from tissues and blood that have been stored at 4°C overnight. Freezing or treatment of specimens with formalin kills *T. gondii.* Six to 10 days after inoculation into mice, or earlier if mice die, peritoneal fluids should be examined for tachyzoites. If they survive for 6 wk and there is antibody in sera of the inoculated mouse, definitive diagnosis is made by visualization of *Toxoplasma* cysts in mouse brain. If cysts are not seen, subinoculations of mouse tissue into other mice are performed.

Microscopic examination of tissue culture inoculated with *T. gondii* shows necrotic, heavily infected cells with numerous extracellular tachyzoites. Isolation of *T. gondii* from blood or body fluids reflects acute infection. Except in the fetus or neonate it is usually not possible to distinguish acute from past infection by isolation of *T. gondii* from tissues such as skeletal muscle, lung, brain, or eye obtained by biopsy or at autopsy.

Diagnosis of acute infection can be made by demonstration of tachyzoites in biopsy tissue sections, bone marrow aspirate, or body fluids such as CSF or amniotic fluid. Immunofluorescent antibody and immunoperoxidase staining techniques may be necessary because it is often difficult to see the tachyzoite with ordinary stains. Tissue cysts are diagnostic of infection but do not differentiate between acute and chronic infection; the presence of many cysts suggests recent acute infection. Cysts in the placenta or tissues of the newborn infant establish the diagnosis of congenital infection. Characteristic histologic features strongly suggest the diagnosis of toxoplasmic lymphadenitis.

Serologic Testing. Multiple serologic tests may be necessary to confirm the diagnosis of congenital or acutely acquired *Toxoplasma* infection. Each laboratory that reports serologic test results must have established values for their tests that diagnose infection in specific clinical settings, provide interpretation of their results, and assure appropriate quality control before therapy is based on serologic test results. Serologic test results used as the basis for therapy should be confirmed in a reference laboratory.

The *Sabin-Feldman dye test* is sensitive and specific. It measures primarily IgG antibodies. Results should be expressed in international units (IU/mL), based on international standard reference sera available from the World Health Organization.

The *IgG indirect fluorescent-antibody (IgG-IFA) test* measures the

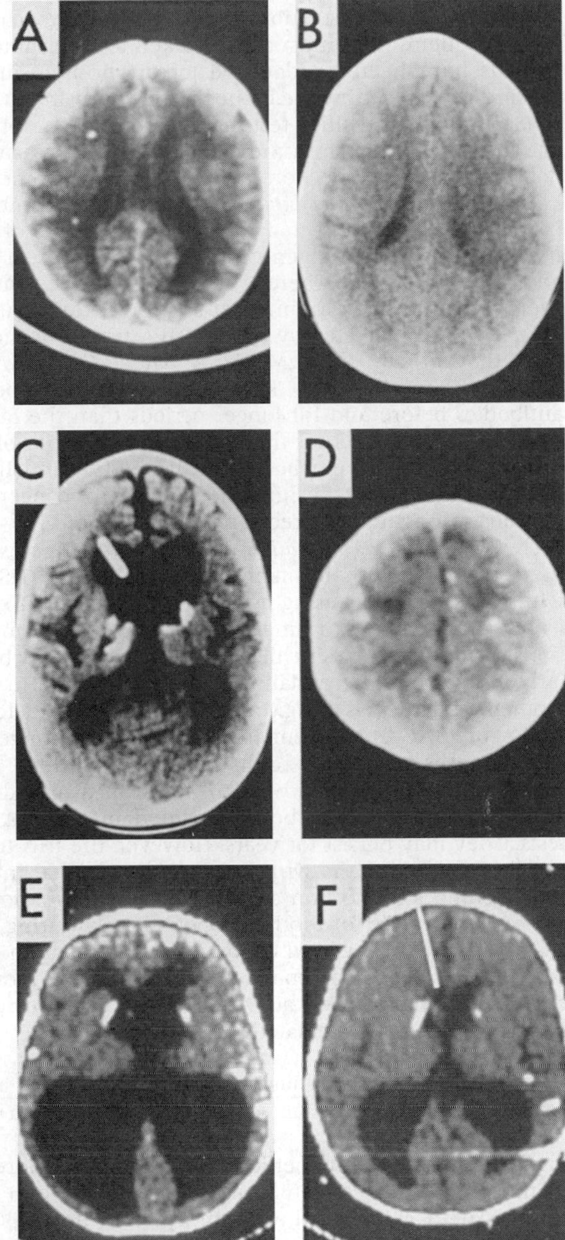

Figure 280–3 Head computed tomography (CT) scans of and historical information in babies with congenital toxoplasmosis. *A*, CT scan at birth that has areas of hypolucency, mildly dilated ventricles, and small calcifications. *B*, CT scan of the same child at 1 yr of age (after antimicrobial therapy for 1 yr. This scan is normal with the exception of two small calcifications. This child's Mental Development Index (MDI) at 1 yr of age was 140 by the Bayley Scale of Infant Development. *C*, CT scan from a 1-yr-old baby who was normal at birth. His meningoencephalitis became symptomatic in the first weeks of life but was not diagnosed correctly and remained untreated during his 1st 3 mo of life. At 3 mo of age, development of hydrocephalus and bilateral macular chorioretinitis led to the diagnosis of congenital toxoplasmosis, and antimicrobial therapy was initiated. This scan shows significant residual atrophy and calcifications. This child has substantial motor dysfunction, development delays, and visual impairment. *D*, CT scan obtained during the 1st mo of life of a microcephalic child. Note the numerous calcifications. This child's intelligence quotient (i.e., using the Stanford-Binet Intelligence Scale for children when she was 3 yr old and the Wechsler Preschool and Primary Scale Intelligence when she was 5 yr old) was 100 and 102, respectively. She received antimicrobial therapy during her 1st yr of life. *E*, CT scan with hydrocephalus owing to aqueductal stenosis (before shunt). *F*, Scan from the same patient as the scan in *E*, after shunt. This child's intelligence quotient (i.e., using the Stanford-Binet Intelligence Scale for children) was approximately 100 when she was 3 and 6 yr old. (Adapted from McAuley J, Boyer K, Patel D, et al: Early and longitudinal evaluations of treated infants and children and untreated historical patients with congenital toxoplasmosis: The Chicago Collaborative Treatment Trial. Clin Infect Dis 18:38, 1994.)

same antibodies as the dye test, and the titers tend to be parallel. These antibodies usually appear 1–2 wk after infection, reach high titers (≥1:1,000) after 6–8 wk, and then decline over months to years. Low titers (1:4 to 1:64) usually persist for life. Antibody titer does not correlate with severity of illness. Approximately half of the commercially available IFA kits for *T. gondii* have been found to be improperly standardized and may yield significant numbers of false-positive and false-negative results.

An *agglutination test* (Bio-Mérieux, Lyon, France) that is available commercially in Europe uses formalin-preserved whole parasites to detect IgM antibodies. This test is accurate, simple to perform, and inexpensive.

The *IgM indirect fluorescent antibody (IgM-IFA) test* is useful for the diagnosis of acute infection with *T. gondii* in the older child because IgM antibodies appear earlier (often by 5 days after infection) and disappear sooner than IgG antibodies. In most instances, antibodies detected by the test rise rapidly (to levels of 1:50 to <1:1,000) and fall to low titers (1:10 or 1:20) or disappear after weeks or months. However, some patients continue to have positive results at low titers for as long as several years. The IgM-IFA test detects *Toxoplasma*-specific IgM in only approximately 25% of congenitally infected infants at birth. IgM antibodies also are often not present in sera of immunodeficient patients with acute toxoplasmosis or in most patients with active toxoplasmosis present only in the eye. The IgM-IFA test may yield false-positive results as a result of rheumatoid factor.

The *double-sandwich enzyme-linked immunosorbent assay (ELISA)* is more sensitive and specific than the IgM-IFA test for detection of *Toxoplasma* IgM antibodies. In the older child, a level of IgM antibodies against *Toxoplasma* in serum of 2.0 or greater (value of one reference laboratory; each laboratory must establish its own values) indicates that *Toxoplasma* infection has most likely been acquired recently. IgM-ELISA detects approximately 75% of infants with congenital infection. IgM-ELISA avoids both the false-positive results due to rheumatoid factor and false-negative results due to high levels of passively transferred maternal IgG antibody in fetal serum, as occurs in the IgM-IFA test. Results obtained with commercial kits must be interpreted with caution since false-positive reactions are not infrequent. Care must also be taken to determine whether the kits have been standardized for diagnosis of infection in specific clinical settings (e.g., in the newborn infant). The *IgA ELISA* is a more sensitive test than the IgM ELISA for detection of congenital infection in the fetus and newborn as well as for detection of acute infection in some pregnant women.

The *immunosorbent agglutination assay (ISAGA)* combines trapping of a patient's IgM to a solid surface and use of formalin-fixed organisms or antigen-coated latex particles. It is read as an agglutination test. There are no false-positive results due to rheumatoid factor or antinuclear antibodies. IgM antibodies to *Toxoplasma* are detected by the IgM-IFA test for a shorter time than they are by the IgM-ELISA. The IgM ISAGA is more sensitive than the IgM ELISA and may detect specific IgM antibodies before and for longer periods than the IgM ELISA. At present, IgM ISAGA is the best test for diagnosis of congenital infection in the newborn. The IgE ELISA and IgE ISAGA are also useful in establishing the diagnosis of congenital toxoplasmosis or acute acquired *T. gondii* infection.

The *differential agglutination test* (HS/SC) compares antibody titers obtained with formalin-fixed tachyzoites (HS antigen) with titers obtained using acetone- or methanol-fixed tachyzoites (AC antigen) to differentiate recent and remote infections in adults and older children. This method may be particularly useful in differentiating remote infection in pregnant women, since levels of IgM and IgA antibodies detectable by ELISA or ISAGA may remain elevated for prolonged periods (e.g., months to years in adults and older children).

The *indirect hemagglutination (IHA) test* measures different *T. gondii* antibodies from those measured in the IFA and dye tests. They may persist for years. However, the IHA test should not be used in infants with suspected congenital infection or in screening for infection acquired during pregnancy because it may be negative for too long a period early during infection.

A relatively higher level of *Toxoplasma* antibody in the aqueous humor or in cerebrospinal fluid demonstrates local production of antibody during active ocular or CNS toxoplasmosis. This comparison is calculated as follows:

$$C = \frac{\text{antibody titer in body fluid}}{\text{antibody titer in serum}} \times \frac{\text{concentration of IgG in serum}}{\text{concentration of IgG in body fluid}}$$

Significant correlation coefficients [C] are 8 or more (eye), 4 or more (CNS for congenital infection), and over 1 (CNS for patients with AIDS). If the serum dye test titer is 300 IU/mL or more, most often it is not possible to demonstrate significant local antibody production using this formula with either the dye test or the IgM-IFA test titer. IgM antibody may be present in CSF.

Toxoplasma antigen has been detected during acute *Toxoplasma* infection but not in sera of uninfected or chronically infected individuals. Antigen was present in the serum, amniotic fluid, and cerebrospinal fluid in the few infants tested with congenital infections.

Comparative *Western immunoblot* tests of sera from a mother and baby may detect congenital infection. Infection is suspected when the mother's serum and her baby's serum contain antibodies that react with different *Toxoplasma* antigens.

Enzyme-linked immunofiltration assay (ELIFA), using micropore membranes, permits simultaneous study of antibody specificity by immunoprecipitation and characterization of antibody isotypes by immunofiltration with enzyme-labeled antibodies. This method may be capable of detecting 85% of cases of congenital infection in the first few days of life. It is still being evaluated.

Polymerase chain reaction (PCR) is used to amplify the DNA of *T. gondii*, which then can be detected by using a DNA probe. Detection of a repetitive *T. gondii* gene, the B1 gene, in amniotic fluid is the procedure of choice for establishing the diagnosis of congenital *Toxoplasma* infection in the fetus. The sensitivity and specificity of this test using amniotic fluid obtained at ≥ 18 weeks gestation are approximately 95%. PCR of vitreous fluid has been used to diagnose ocular toxoplasmosis.

Lymphocyte blastogenesis to *Toxoplasma* antigens has been used to diagnose congenital toxoplasmosis if a question persists concerning the diagnosis and other test results are negative. However, a negative result does not exclude the diagnosis, as many infected infants do not respond to *T. gondii* antigens in the newborn period.

Acquired Toxoplasmosis. Recent infection is diagnosed by seroconversion from a negative to a positive IgG antibody titer (in the absence of transfer of antibody by transfusion); a serial two-tube rise in *Toxoplasma*-specific IgG titer when sera are obtained 3 wk apart and tested in parallel; or the presence of *Toxoplasma*-specific IgM antibody.

Ocular Toxoplasmosis. IgG antibody titers of 1:4 to 1:64 are usual in older children with active toxoplasmic chorioretinitis. When the retinal lesions are characteristic and serologic tests findings are positive, the diagnosis is likely. PCR of vitreous fluid has been used to diagnose ocular toxoplasmosis but is infrequently performed because of the risks associated with obtaining vitreous fluid.

Immunocompromised Persons. IgG antibody titers may be low, and *Toxoplasma*-specific IgM is often absent in immunocompromised individuals with toxoplasmosis. Demonstration of *Toxoplasma* antigens or DNA in serum, blood, and CSF may identify disseminated *Toxoplasma* infection in immunocompromised persons.

Resolution of CNS lesions during a therapeutic trial of pyrimethamine and sulfadiazine has been useful in patients with AIDS. Brain biopsy has been used to establish the diagnosis of toxoplasmic encephalitis when there is no response to this therapeutic trial or to exclude other likely diagnoses.

Congenital Toxoplasmosis. Fetal ultrasound examination, performed every 2 wk during gestation, and PCR analysis of amniotic fluid are used for prenatal diagnosis. *T. gondii* may also be isolated from the placenta.

Serologic tests are the most useful in establishing a diagnosis of congenital toxoplasmosis. Either persistent or rising titers in the dye or IFA test or a positive IgM ELISA or ISAGA result is diagnostic of congenital toxoplasmosis. The half-life of IgM is 3–5 days, so if there is a placental leak, the level of IgM antibodies in the infant's serum falls significantly within 1–2 wk. Passively transferred maternal IgG antibodies may require many months to a year to disappear from the infant's serum, depending on the magnitude of the original titer. Synthesis of *Toxoplasma* antibody is usually demonstrable by the third month of life if the infant is untreated. If the infant is treated, synthesis may be delayed until the ninth month of life, and, infrequently, it may not occur at all. When an infant begins to synthesize antibody, infection may be documented serologically even without demonstration of IgM antibodies by a rise in the ratio of specific serum antibody titer to the total IgG, whereas the ratio will fall if the specific antibody has been passively transferred from the mother.

At birth, when a diagnosis of congenital toxoplasmosis is suspected, the following diagnostic studies should be performed: general, ophthalmologic, and neurologic examinations; head CT scan; attempt to isolate *T. gondii* from the placenta and the infant's white blood cells from umbilical cord blood and buffy coat; measurement of serum *Toxoplasma*-specific IgG, IgM, IgA, and IgE antibodies and the total amount of IgM and IgG in serum; lumbar puncture including analysis of CSF for cells, glucose, protein, *Toxoplasma*-specific IgG and IgM antibodies, and total amount of IgG; and evaluations of CSF for *T. gondii* by PCR and inoculation into mice. The presence of *Toxoplasma*-specific IgM in CSF that is not contaminated with blood, or local antibody production of *Toxoplasma*-

specific IgG antibody demonstrated in CSF establishes the diagnosis of congenital *Toxoplasma* infection.

Many manifestations of congenital toxoplasmosis occur in other perinatal diseases, especially disease caused by cytomegalovirus. Neither cerebral calcification nor chorioretinitis is pathognomonic. Fewer than 50% of children < 5 yr of age with chorioretinitis satisfy the serologic criteria for congenital toxoplasmosis; the causes of most of the other cases are unknown. The clinical picture in the newborn infant may also be compatible with sepsis, aseptic meningitis, syphilis, or hemolytic disease.

TREATMENT. Pyrimethamine plus sulfadiazine or trisulfapyrimidines act synergistically against *Toxoplasma*. Combined therapy is indicated to treat many of the forms of toxoplasmosis. However, use of pyrimethamine is contraindicated during the first trimester of pregnancy. Spiramycin should be used to prevent transmission of infection to the fetus of acutely infected pregnant women and to treat congenital toxoplasmosis. Pyrimethamine inhibits the enzyme dihydrofolate reductase (DHFR), and thus the synthesis of folic acid, and therefore produces a dose-related, reversible, and usually gradual depression of the bone marrow, resulting in thrombocytopenia, leukopenia, and anemia. Neutropenia is the most common side effect in treated infants. All patients treated with pyrimethamine should have platelet and white blood cell counts twice weekly. Seizures may occur with overdosage of pyrimethamine. Folinic acid (calcium leukovorin) should always be administered concomitantly with pyrimethamine to prevent suppression of the bone marrow. Potential toxic effects of sulfonamides (e.g., crystalluria, hematuria, and rash) should be monitored. Hypersensitivity reactions occur, especially in patients with AIDS.

Acquired Toxoplasmosis. Patients with lymphadenopathy do not need specific treatment unless they have severe and persistent symptoms or evidence of damage to vital organs. If such signs and symptoms occur, treatment with pyrimethamine, sulfadiazine, and leukovorin should be initiated. Patients who appear to be immunologically normal but have severe and persistent symptoms or damage to vital organs (e.g., chorioretinitis, myocarditis) need specific therapy until these specific symptoms resolve, followed by therapy for an additional 2 wk. This therapy usually lasts for at least 4–6 wk; the optimal duration of therapy is unknown. A loading dose of pyrimethamine for older children is 2 mg/kg/24 hr (maximum 50 mg), given for the first 2 days of treatment. The maintenance dose is 1 mg/kg/24 hr(maximum: 25 mg/24 hr). Folinic acid is administered orally at a dosage of 5–20 mg three times/wk (or even daily depending on the white blood cell count). Sulfadiazine or trisulfapyrimidine is administered to children >1 yr of age with a loading dose of 75 mg/kg/24 hr followed by 50 mg/kg/24 hr.

Ocular Toxoplasmosis. Patients with ocular toxoplasmosis are usually treated with pyrimethamine, sulfadiazine, and leukovorin for approximately 1 wk after the lesion develops a quiescent appearance (i.e., sharp borders and associated inflammatory cells in the vitreous resolve), which usually occurs in 2–4 wk. Within 7–10 days the borders of the retinal lesions sharpen, and visual acuity usually returns to that noted before development of the acute lesion. Systemic corticosteroids have been administered concomitantly with antimicrobial treatment when lesions involve the macula, optic nerve head, or papillomacular bundle. Photocoagulation has been used to treat active lesions and prevent spread (i.e., most new lesions appear contiguous to old ones). Occasionally vitrectomy and removal of the lens are needed to restore visual acuity.

Immunocompromised Persons. Serologic evidence of acute infection in an immunocompromised patient, regardless of whether signs and symptoms of infection are present or tachyzoites are present in tissue, are indications for therapy similar to that described for immunocompetent children with symptoms of organ injury. It is important to establish the diagnosis as rapidly as possible and institute treatment early. In immunocompromised patients other than those with AIDS, therapy should be continued for at least 4–6 wk beyond complete resolution of all signs and symptoms of active disease. Careful follow-up observation of these patients is imperative because relapse may occur, requiring prompt reinstitution of therapy. Relapse is frequent in patients with AIDS, and suppressive therapy with pyrimethamine and sulfonamides should be continued for life. Therapy usually induces a beneficial response clinically, but it does not eradicate cysts from the CNS and perhaps not from other tissues either. Prophylactic treatment with trimethroprim-sulfamethoxazole for *Pneumocystis carinii* pneumonia appears to reduce the incidence of toxoplasmosis in patients with AIDS.

Treatment of Congenital Toxoplasmosis. All infected newborns should be treated, whether or not they have clinical manifestations of the infection. In infants with congenital infection, treatment may be effective in interrupting acute disease that damages vital organs. Infants should be treated for 1 yr with oral pyrimethamine (1–2 mg/kg/24 hr for 2 days, then 1 mg/kg/24 hr for 2 mo or 6 mo, then 1 mg/kg/24 hr Monday, Wednesday, and Friday), sulfadiazine or triple sulfonamides (100 mg/kg/24 hr loading dose, then 100 mg/kg/24 hr divided in 2 doses) and calcium leukovorin (5–10 mg/kg/24 hr Monday, Wednesday, and Friday). In the U.S. National Collaborative Study, the relative efficacy in reducing sequelae of infection and the safety of treatment, with 2 versus 6 months of the higher dosage of pyrimethamine are being compared. Pyrimethamine, available only in tablet form, may be crushed and administered in a suspension with juice or food. The effectiveness of these regimens has not been proved, but they are considered reasonable empirical recommendations. Information concerning the U.S. National Colloborative Study evaluating these regimens can be obtained from Dr. Rima McLeod by calling (773)-834-4152. Prednisone (1 mg/kg/24 hr orally in divided doses) has been utilized in addition when active chorioretinitis involves the macula or the CSF protein is ≥1,000 mg/dL at birth, but its efficacy also is not established.

Treatment of Pregnant Women with *T. gondii* Infection. The immunologically normal pregnant woman who acquired *T. gondii* before conception does not need treatment to prevent congenital infection of her fetus. Although data are not available to allow for a definitive time interval, if infection occurs in the 6 mo prior to conception, it is reasonable to evaluate the fetus and treat to prevent congenital infection in the fetus in the same manner as described for the acutely infected pregnant patient. Treatment of a pregnant woman who acquires infection at any time during pregnancy reduces the chance of congenital infection in her infant by approximately 60%. The medications used are spiramycin and pyrimethamine in combination with sulfadiazine or triple sulfonamides. Spiramycin is available in the United States through the FDA (telephone 302-443-7580). Because pyrimethamine is potentially teratogenic, spiramycin is administered in the 1st trimester. The dose of spiramycin is 1 g each 8 hr given without food; lower doses are less effective. Toxicity is infrequent. Adverse reactions include paresthesias, rash, nausea, vomiting, and diarrhea. Treatment during the remainder of pregnancy with pyrimethamine and a sulfonamide should be continued at dosages similar to those recommended for therapy of the symptomatic immunocompetent patient with acquired toxoplasmosis. Treatment of the mother of an infected fetus with pyrimethamine and a sulfonamide reduces infection in the placenta and the severity of disease in the newborn.

The approach in France to congenital toxoplasmosis includes systematic serologic screening of all women of childbearing age and again intrapartum. Mothers with acute infection are treated with spiramycin, which decreases the transmission from 60% to 23%. Ultrasound and amniocentesis for PCR after 18 wk gestation are used for fetal diagnosis; they have 97% sensitivity and 100% specificity. Fetal infection is treated with pyrimethamine and sulfadiazine, or by termination of pregnancy. This strategy has excellent outcome with normal development of children. Only 19% have subtle findings of congenital infection, including intracranial calcifications (13%) and chorioretinal scars (6%), although 39% have chorioretinal scars detected at follow-up observation during later childhood.

Chronically infected pregnant women who have been immunocompromised by cytotoxic drugs or corticosteroid therapy have transmitted *T. gondii* to their fetuses. Such women should be treated with spiramycin throughout gestation. The best approach to prevention of congenital toxoplasmosis in the fetus of a pregnant woman with HIV infection and inactive *T. gondii* infection is unknown. If the pregnancy is not terminated, the mother should be treated with spiramycin during the first 17 wk of gestation and then with pyrimethamine and sulfadiazine until term. In a study of adult patients with AIDS, a dose of 75 mg pyrimethamine/24 hr and high dosages of intravenously administered clindamycin (1,200 mg every 6 hr intravenously) appeared equal in efficacy to sulfonamides and pyrimethamine. Other currently experimental agents include the macrolides roxithromycin and azithromycin.

PROGNOSIS. Early institution of specific treatment for congenitally infected infants usually cures the manifestations of toxoplasmosis such as active chorioretinitis, meningitis, encephalitis, hepatitis, splenomegaly, and thrombocytopenia. Hydrocephalus due to aqueductal obstruction may develop or become worse during therapy. Such treatment also may reduce the incidence of some sequelae, such as diminished cognitive or abnormal motor function. Without therapy, chorioretinitis often recurs. Children with extensive involvement at birth may function normally later in life or have mild to severe impairment of vision, hearing, cognitive function, and other neurologic functions. Delays in diagnosis and therapy, perinatal hypoglycemia, hypoxia, hypotension, repeated shunt infections, and severe visual impairment are associated with a poorer prognosis. The prognosis is guarded but is not necessarily poor for infected babies. Treatment with pyrimethamine and sulfadiazine does not eradicate the encysted parasite. No protective vaccine is available.

PREVENTION. Methods of prevention are outlined in Figure 280–1. Counseling women about these methods of preventing transmission of *T. gondii* during pregnancy can substantially reduce acquisition of infection during gestation. Women who do not have specific antibody to *T. gondii* prior to pregnancy should only eat well cooked meat during pregnancy and avoid contact with oocysts excreted by cats. Cats that are kept indoors, maintained on prepared diets, and not fed fresh, uncooked meat should not contact encysted *T. gondii* or shed oocysts. Serologic screening, ultrasound monitoring, and treatment of pregnant women during gestation can also reduce the incidence and manifestations of congenital toxoplasmosis.

Bretagne S. Costa JM, Vidaud M, et al: Detection of *Toxoplasma gondii* by competitive DNA amplification of bronchoalveolar lavage samples. J Infect Dis 168:1585, 1993.

Brooks RG, McCabe RE, Remington JS: Role of serology in the diagnosis of toxoplasic lymphadenopathy. Rev Infect Dis 9:1055, 1987.

Couvreur J, Desmonts G, Tournier G, et al: Study of homogeneous series of 210 cases of congenital toxoplasmosis in infants aged 0 to 11 months detected prospectively. Ann Pediatr 31:815, 1984.

Daffos F, Forestier F, Capella-Pavlovsky M, et al: Prenatal management of 746 pregnancies at risk for congenital toxoplasmosis. N Engl J Med 318:271, 1988.

Dannemann BR, Vaughan WC, Thulliez P, Remington JS: The differential agglutination test for diagnosis of recently acquired infection with *Toxoplasma gondii*. J Clin Microbiol 28:1928, 1990.

Desmonts G, Couvreur J: Natural history of congenital toxoplasmosis. Ann Pediatr 31:799, 1984.

Desmonts G, Forestier F, Thulliez P, et al: Prenatal diagnosis of congenital toxoplasmosis. Lancet 1:500, 1985.

Grover CM, Thulliez P, Remington JS, et al: Rapid prenatal diagnosis of congenital *Toxoplasma* infection by using polymerase chain reaction and amniotic fluid. J Clin Microbiol 28:2297, 1990.

Guerrina NG, Hsu H, Meissner HC, et al: Neonatal seriologic screening and early treatment for congenital *Toxoplasma gondii* infection. N Engl J Med 330:1858, 1994.

Haentjens M, Sacre L, DeMeuter F: Congenital toxoplasmosis after maternal infection before or slightly after conception. Acta Paediatr Scand 75:343, 1986.

Hohlfeld P, Daffos F, Thulliez P, et al: Fetal toxoplasmosis: Outcome of pregnancy and infant follow-up after in utero treatment. J Pediatr 115:765, 1989.

Koppe JG, Loewer-Sieger DH, De Roever-Bonnet H: Results of 20-year follow-up of congenital toxoplasmosis. Lancet 1:254, 1986.

Luft BJ, Remington JS: Toxoplasmic encephalitis in AIDS. Clin infect Dis 15:211, 1992.

McAuley J, Boyer K, Patel D, et al: Early and longitudinal evaluations of treated infants and children and untreated historical patients with congenital toxoplasmosis: The Chicago Collaborative Treatment Trial. Clin Inf Dis 18:38, 1994.

McCabe RE, Brooks RG, Dorfman RF, et al: Clinical spectrum in 107 cases of toxoplasmic lymphadenopathy. Rev Infect Dis 9:754, 1987.

McCabe R, Remington JS: Toxoplasmosis: The time has come. N Engl J Med 318:313, 1988.

McGee T, Wolters C, Stein L, et al: Absence of sensorineural hearing loss in treated infants and children with congenital toxoplasmosis. Otolaryngol Head Neck Surg 106:75, 1992.

Mets MB, Holfels E, Boyer KM, et al: Eye manifestations of congenital toxoplasmosis. Am J Ophthalmol 123:1, 1997.

Montoya JG, Jordan R, Lingamneni S, at al: Toxoplasmic myocarditis and polymyositis in patients with acute acquired toxoplasmosis diagnosed during life. Clin Infect Dis 24:676, 1997.

Montoya JG, Remington JS: Studies on the serodiagnosis of toxoplasmic lyphadenitis. Clin Infect Dis 20:781, 1995.

Mitchell CD, Erlich SS, Mastrucci MT, et al: Congenital toxoplasmosis occurring in infants perinatally infected with human immunodeficiency virus. J Pediatr Infect Dis 9:512, 1990.

Minkoff H, Remington JS, Holman S, et al: Vertical transmission of toxoplasma by human immunodeficiency virus-infected women. Am J Obstet Gynecol 176(3):555, 1997.

Montoya JG, Remington JS: Toxoplasmic chorioretinitis in the setting of acute acquired toxoplasmosis. Clin Infect Dis 23:277, 1996.

Patel DV, Holfels EM, Vogel NP, et al: Resolution of intracerebral calcifications in infants with treated congenital toxoplasmosis. Radiology 199:433, 1996.

Remington JS, McLeod R, Desmonts G: Toxoplasmosis: *In:* Remington J, Klein J (eds): Infectious Diseases of the Fetus and Newborn Infant, 4th ed. Philadelphia, WB Saunders, 1995, pp 140–268.

Roizen N, Swisher C, Boyer K, et al: Developmental and neurologic outcome in congenital toxoplasmosis. Pediatrics 95:11, 1995.

Saxon SA, Knight W, Reynolds DW, et al: Intellectual deficits in children born with subclinical congenital toxoplasmosis: A preliminary report. J Pediatr 8:2792, 1973.

Silveira C, Belfort R Jr, Burnier M Jr, et al: Acquired toxoplasmic infection as the cause of toxoplasmic retinochoroiditis in families. Am J Ophthamol 106:362, 1988.

Wilson CB, Remington JS, Stagno S, et al: Development of adverse sequelae in children born with subclinical congenital *Toxoplasma* infection. Pediatrics 66:767, 1980.

CHAPTER 281
Pneumocystis carinii

Walter T. Hughes

Pneumocystis carinii pneumonia (interstitial plasma cell pneumonitis) in an immunocompromised host is a life-threatening infection. It is believed to result in part from activation of latent organisms acquired in early childhood. Even in the most severe cases, with rare exceptions, the organisms and the disease remain localized to the lungs.

ETIOLOGY. *P. carinii* is a common extracellular parasite found in the lungs of mammals worldwide. The taxonomic placement of this organism has not been established, but it has attributes of fungi and protozoa. Although *P. carinii* DNA has homologic characteristics closer to those of fungi, its morphologic features and susceptibility to drugs are similar to those of protozoa. The natural habitat and mode of transmission to humans are unknown. Experiments in rats have demonstrated animal-to-animal transmission via the airborne route, but animal-to-human transmission is unlikely because of the host-specific nature of *P. carinii*. Person-to-person transmission has been suggested from a few studies but has not been conclusively demonstrated.

EPIDEMIOLOGY. Serologic surveys show most humans become infected with *P. carinii* before 4 yr of age. In the healthy host, these infections are asymptomatic. Pneumonia caused by *P. carinii* occurs almost exclusively in severely immunocompromised hosts including those with congenital or acquired immunodeficiency disorders or malignancies, and in organ transplant recipients.

Without prophylaxis, approximately 40% of infants and children and 70% of adults with the acquired immunodeficiency syndrome (AIDS), 12% of children with leukemia, and 10% of patients with organ transplants experience *P. carinii* pneumonia. Epidemics that occurred among debilitated infants in Europe during and after World War II have been attributed to malnutrition.

PATHOGENESIS. Two forms of *P. carinii* are found in the alveolar space: cysts that are 5–8 nm in diameter and may contain up to eight pleomorphic intracystic sporozoites, and the extracystic trophozoites, which are 2–5 μm delicate cells derived from excysted sporozoites. *P. carinii* attaches to type I alveolar epithelial cells by adhesive proteins such as fibronectin and mannose-dependent ligand. Alveolar macrophages phagocytize and kill opsonized *P. carinii* organisms, releasing tumor necrosis factor. The histopathologic features of *P. carinii* pneumonia are of two types. The first type is infantile interstitial plasma cell pneumonitis, which is seen in epidemic outbreaks in debilitated infants at 3–6 mo of age. Extensive infiltration with thickening of the alveolar septum occurs, and plasma cells are prominent. The second type is a diffuse desquamative alveolar disease found in immunocompromised children and adults. The alveoli contain large numbers of *P. carinii* in a foamy exudate with alveolar macrophages active in the phagocytosis of organisms. The alveolar septum is not infiltrated to the extent it is in the infantile type, and plasma cells are usually absent.

Cell-mediated immunity has the major role in defense against *P. carinii* pneumonia. This is evidenced by the high frequency of *P. carinii* pneumonia in severe combined immunodeficiency disorder, with attack rates >40%, and the infrequency of its occurrence in X-linked agammaglobulinemia. Studies in patients with AIDS show an increase in the occurrence of *P. carinii* pneumonia in the presence of markedly decreased $CD4^+$ T lymphocyte counts. The $CD4^+$ cell count provides a useful indicator for older children and adults of the necessity of prophylaxis for *P. carinii* pneumonia.

CLINICAL MANIFESTATIONS. The epidemic infantile form of *P. carinii* interstitial plasma cell pneumonitis is seen predominantly in infants 3–6 mo of age. The onset of hypoxia and symptoms is subtle with tachypnea but without fever, progressing to intercostal, suprasternal, and infrasternal retractions, nasal flaring, and cyanosis. In the sporadic form of *P. carinii* pneumonia occurring in children and adults with underlying immunodeficiency, the onset of hypoxia and symptoms is usually abrupt with fever, tachypnea, dyspnea, and cough, progressing to nasal flaring and cyanosis. This latter type accounts for the majority of cases, although the severity of clinical expression may vary. Rales are usually not detected on physical examination.

The chest radiograph reveals bilateral diffuse alveolar disease with a granular pattern. The earliest densities are perihilar, and progression proceeds peripherally, sparing the apical areas until last.

DIAGNOSIS. A definitive diagnosis requires the demonstration of *P. carinii* in the lung in the presence of clinical signs and symptoms of the infection. Methods for obtaining appropriate specimens for detecting organisms include bronchoalveolar lavage, tracheal aspirate, transbronchial lung biopsy, bronchial brushings, percutaneous transthoracic needle aspiration, and open lung biopsy. Induced sputum samples are helpful if *P. carinii* is found, but the absence of the organisms in induced sputum does not exclude the infection. The open lung biopsy is the most reliable method, although bronchoalveolar lavage is more practical in most cases. Four stains are in general use: Grocott-Gomori stain and toluidine blue stain for the cyst form, polychrome stains such as Giemsa stain for the trophozoites and sporozoites, and the fluorescein-labeled monoclonal antibody stains for both trophozoites and cysts.

TREATMENT. The recommended therapy is trimethoprim-sulfamethoxazole (TMP-SMZ) (15–20 mg TMP, 75–100 mg SMZ/kg/24 hr divided in four doses) administered intravenously, or orally if there is mild disease and no malabsorption or diarrhea. The duration of treatment is about 3 wk for patients with AIDS, and 2 wk for other patients. Unfortunately, adverse reactions frequently occur with trimethoprim-sulfamethoxazole, including rash and neutropenia, especially in patients with AIDS. For patients who cannot tolerate or fail to respond to trimethoprim-sulfamethoxazole after 5–7 days, pentamidine isethionate (4 mg/kg/24 hr as a single intravenous dose) may be used. Adverse reactions are frequent and include renal and hepatic dysfunction, hyperglycemia or hypoglycemia, rash, and thrombocytopenia. Lamivudine should not be administered concomitantly with pentamidine since both can cause pancreatitis. Atovaquone and trimetrexate glucuronate are alternative treatments that have been used primarily in adults with mild to moderate disease. Pharmacokinetic studies of atovaquone show a dose of 30 mg/kg/24 hr divided in two doses for children ≥2 yr of age is adequate and safe; a dose of 45 mg/kg/24 hr divided in two doses is needed for children <2 yr of age. Other effective therapies include combinations of trimethoprim plus dapsone, and clindamycin plus primaquine.

Studies in adults suggest that administration of corticosteroids in addition to anti–*P. carinii* drugs increases the chances for survival in moderate and severe cases of *P. carinii* pneumonia. The recommended regimen of corticosteroids for adolescents >13 yr of age and adults is oral prednisone, 80 mg/24 hr divided in two doses on days 1–5, 40 mg/24 hr once daily on days 6–10, and 20 mg/24 hr once a day on days 11–21. A regimen for children is oral prednisone, 2 mg/kg/24 hr for the first 7–10 days, followed by a tapering regimen for the next 10–14 days.

COMPLICATIONS. Most complications occur as adverse events associated with the drugs used for treatment. Rarely, *P. carinii* infection affects extrapulmonary sites (e.g., retina, spleen, and bone marrow), but such infections are usually not symptomatic and also respond to treatment. Extrapulmonary focuses are more likely in patients receiving aerosolized pentamidine for prophylaxis, because its effects are limited to the respiratory system.

PROGNOSIS. Without treatment, *P. carinii* pneumonitis is fatal in almost all infected immunocompromised hosts within 3–4 wk of onset. The mortality rate is 10–30% if treatment is initiated early in the course of the pneumonia. Patients remain at risk for *P. carinii* pneumonia as long as they are immunocompromised. Continuous prophylaxis should be initiated or reinstituted at the end of therapy for patients with AIDS.

PREVENTION. Patients at high risk for *P. carinii* pneumonia should be placed on chemoprophylaxis. Prophylaxis of infants born to HIV-infected mothers, and for HIV-infected infants and children, are based on age and $CD4^+$ cell counts (see Table 268–4). Patients with severe combined immunodeficiency syndrome, those with organ transplants, and those receiving intensive immunosuppressive therapy for cancer or other diseases are also candidates for prophylaxis. Trimethoprim-sulfamethoxazole (5 mg TMP, 25 mg SMZ/kg/24 hr orally once daily) is the drug of choice and may be given for 3 consecutive days each week, or, alternatively, each day. Alternatives for prophylaxis include dapsone (2 mg/kg/24 hr orally once daily;

maximum 100 mg/dose), atovaquone (30 mg/kg/24 hr orally once daily), and aerosolized pentamidine (300 mg via Respirgard II nebulizer monthly). The prophylaxis must be continued as long as the patient remains immunocompromised, which may be life-long for patients with AIDS.

Centers for Disease Control and Prevention: 1997 USPHS/IDSA guidelines for the prevention of opportunistic infections in persons infected with human immunodeficiency virus. MMWR 46 (RR-12):1, 1997.
Hughes W, Leoung G, Kramer F, et al: Comparison of atovaquone (566C80) with trimethoprim-sulfamethoxazole to treat *Pneumocystis carinii* pneumonia in patients with AIDS. N Engl J Med 328:1521, 1993.
Hughes WT: Use of dapsone in the prevention and treatment of *Pneumocystis carinii* pneumonia: A review. Clin Infect Dis 27:191, 1998.
Hughes WT, Rivera GK, Schell MJ, et al: Successful intermittent chemoprophylaxis for *Pneumocystis carinii* pneumonia. N Engl J Med 316:1627, 1987.
Kovacs A, Frederick T, Church J, et al: CD_4 T-lymphocyte counts and *Pneumocystis carinii* pneumonia in pediatric HIV infection. JAMA 265:1698, 1991.
Malteqou HC, Petropoulos D, Chorosqy M, et al: Dapsone for *Pneumocystis carinii* prophylaxis in children undergoing bone marrow transplantation. Bone Marrow Transplant 20:879, 1997.
Simmonds RJ, Oxtoby MJ, Caldwell MB, et al: *Pneumocystis carinii* pneumonia among U.S. children with perinatally acquired HIV infection. JAMA 270:470, 1993.

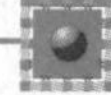

SECTION 14

Helminthic Diseases

CHAPTER 282

Ascariasis (Ascaris lumbricoides)

James W. Kazura

Infection with *Ascaris lumbricoides* is the most prevalent human helminthiasis, causing an estimated 1 billion cases worldwide. Infection is most common in children of preschool or early school age.

ETIOLOGY. The infective stage of *A. lumbricoides* is the mature larva-containing egg. It is broadly oval, has a thick shell with an outer mamillated covering, and measures approximately 40 × 60 μm (Fig. 282–1). Eggs are passed in the feces of infected individuals and mature in 5–10 days under favorable environmental conditions to become infective. Each female has a life span of 1–2 yr and is capable of producing 200,000 eggs/24 hr.

EPIDEMIOLOGY. Ascariasis is ubiquitous; the greatest number of cases occurs in countries having warm climates. Approximately 4 million individuals are infected, mainly children, in North America. Ascariasis is a soil-transmitted infection that depends on dissemination of eggs into environmental conditions that are suitable for their maturation. Promiscuous defecation and use of human manure are the two most important unhygienic practices responsible for the endemicity of ascariasis. The mode of transmission to humans is hand to mouth; the fingers are contaminated by soil contact. Alternatively, food items, particularly those commonly consumed raw, become contaminated by human fertilizers or by flies. Endemicity of *A. lumbricoides* is aided by the extremely high egg output of adult worms and the resistance of eggs to unfavorable environmental conditions. Eggs have been shown to remain infective in soil for months and may survive cool weather (5–10°C) for 2 yr. Transmission of ascariasis may occur throughout the year, with seasonal increases.

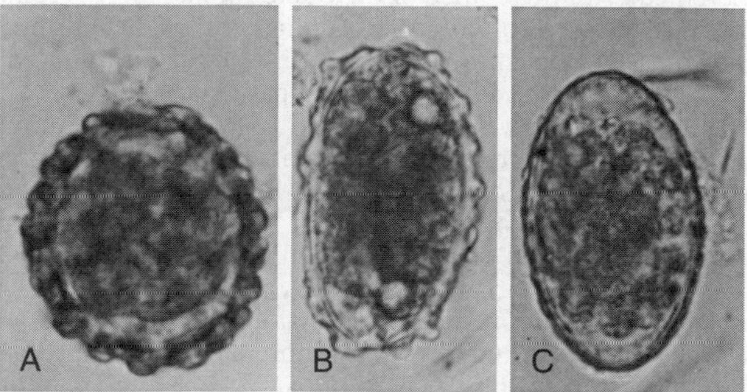

Figure 282–1 Fertilized *(A)* and unfertilized *(B, C)* eggs of *Ascaris lumbricoides* (×400). The egg illustrated in *C* may be mistaken for that of a different nematode or of a trematode.

PATHOGENESIS. After the eggs are ingested by a human host, larvae are released from the eggs and penetrate the intestinal wall before migrating to the lungs via the venous circulation. They then break through the pulmonary tissues into the alveolar spaces, ascend the bronchial tree and trachea, and are reswallowed. On their arrival in the small intestine, the larvae develop into mature adult worms. Males measure 15–25 cm × 3 mm, and females measure 25–35 cm × 4 mm. The pathogenesis of pulmonary ascariasis is not known, although a hypersensitivity phenomenon may be involved. Adult worms may cause gastrointestinal (GI) disease by obstructing the gut or biliary tree and by affecting host nutrition.

CLINICAL MANIFESTATIONS. Although disease occurs in only a small proportion of infected individuals, this is a significant clinical problem because of the high incidence of ascariasis. Morbidity may be manifested during migration of the larvae through the lungs or may be associated with the presence of adult worms in the small intestine. The nutritional status of children with ascariasis may be affected more by their socioeconomic and nutritional background than by the effects of the *Ascaris* infection.

Pulmonary ascariasis may occur after heavy exposure and is also common in individuals who live in areas with seasonal transmission of infection (seasonal pneumonitis). The most characteristic features are cough blood-stained sputum, and eosinophilia. This Löffler's-like syndrome may be associated with transient pulmonary infiltrates. In children, differentiation of this syndrome from visceral larva migrans may be difficult, but abdominal symptoms or signs are very rare in pulmonary ascariasis.

The presence of adult worms in the small intestine is associated with vague complaints such as abdominal pain and distention. Intestinal obstruction, although rare, may be due to a mass of worms in heavily infected children; the peak incidence is in children age 1–6 yr. The onset is usually sudden, with severe colicky abdominal pain and vomiting, which may be bile stained; these symptoms may progress rapidly and follow a course similar to acute intestinal obstruction due to any other cause. Migration of *Ascaris* worms into the biliary tract has also been reported, particularly occurring in China and the

Philippines; the likelihood of this condition increases in heavily infected children. The onset of symptoms is acute, with colicky abdominal pain, nausea, vomiting, and fever. Jaundice is rarely seen.

Steatorrhea and diminished vitamin A absorption may occur in children with ascariasis. A study of Colombian children with moderate infections (30–50 worms) showed that administration of anthelmintic drugs was followed by decreased fat and nitrogen excretion and improved xylose absorption.

DIAGNOSIS. Adult female worms deposit eggs that can be detected by direct fecal smear examination and measured by the Kato's thick smear method. Bisexual infections result in excretion of mature fertile eggs, whereas infertile eggs are found in individuals infected with female worms only (Fig. 282–1 *B* and *C*). Diagnosis of pulmonary ascariasis or GI ascariasis complicated by obstruction is based primarily on clinical symptoms and a high index of suspicion.

TREATMENT. Several chemotherapeutic agents are effective against ascariasis; none, however, is useful during the pulmonary phase of the infection. The recommended treatment of uncomplicated GI ascariasis is albendazole (400 mg PO as a single dose). Alternatives include mebendazole (100 mg bid for 3 days or 500 mg once, for both children and adults) and pyrantel pamoate (11 mg/kg once; maximum, 1 g) orally. Treatment of children with heavy infections should be approached with caution. Piperazine salts (citrate, adipate, or phosphate) cause neuromuscular paralysis of the parasite and relatively rapid expulsion of the worms and are the treatment of choice for ascariasis complicated by intestinal or biliary obstruction. Piperazine is administered orally in a daily dose of 50–75 mg/kg for 2 days. Sporadic hypersensitivity and neurotoxic reactions have been reported with piperazine derivatives. Rarely, surgical treatment may be needed in severe obstructive cases.

PREVENTION. Although ascariasis is the most prevalent worm infection worldwide, little attention has been given to its control, partly because of controversy about its clinical significance and because of its unique epidemiologic features. Attempts at reducing worm loads in humans by mass chemotherapy have shown some promise. Because of the high rate of reinfection, chemotherapy has to be repeated at 3–6-mo intervals. The feasibility and cost of such an undertaking have to be evaluated before it can be widely accepted. Sanitary practices directed at treating human feces before it is used as fertilizer and providing hygienic sewage disposal facilities may be the most effective long-term preventive measures against ascariasis.

Hall A: Intestinal parasitic worms and the growth of children. Trans R Soc Trop Med Hyg 87:241, 1993.
Khuroo MS: Ascariasis. Gastroenterol Clin North Am 25:553, 1996.
Khuroo MS, Zargar SA, Mahajan R: Hepatobiliary and pancreatic ascariasis in India. Lancet 335:1503, 1990.
Louw JH: Abdominal complications of *Ascaris lumbricoides* infestation in children. Br J Surg 53:510, 1966.
Spillman RK: Pulmonary ascariasis in tropical communities. Am J Trop Med Hyg 24:791, 1975.
Watkins WE, Pollitt E: Effect of removing *Ascaris* on the growth of Guatemalan children. Pediatrics 97:871, 1996.

CHAPTER 283
Hookworms (Ancylostoma *and* Necator americanus)

Peter J. Hotez

Hookworm infection is one of the most prevalent infectious diseases of humans, affecting an estimated 1 billion individuals worldwide. Heavily infected children suffer from intestinal blood loss resulting in iron deficiency, which can lead to anemia, as well as protein malnutrition.

Cutaneous larva migrans (creeping eruption) is caused by the larvae of several nematodes, primarily hookworms, which are not usually parasitic for humans.

ETIOLOGY. Two major genera of hookworms infect humans. Hookworms of the genus *Ancylostoma* include the major anthropophilic hookworm *Ancylostoma duodenale,* which causes classical hookworm infection, and the less common zoonotic species *A. ceylanicum, A. caninum,* and *A. braziliense.* Human zoonotic infection with the dog hookworm, *A. caninum,* has been linked to an eosinophilic enteritis syndrome. The larval stage of *A. braziliense,* whose definitive hosts include dogs and cats, is the principal cause of cutaneous larva migrans. *Necator americanus,* the only representative of its genus, is also a major anthropophilic hookworm and causes classic hookworm infection.

The infective larval stages of the anthropophilic hookworms live in a developmentally arrested state in warm, moist, and damp soil. The larvae infect humans either by penetrating through the skin (*N. americanus* and *A. duodenale*) or when they are ingested (*A. duodenale*). Larvae entering the human host by skin penetration undergo extraintestinal migration through the venous circulation and lungs before they are swallowed, whereas orally ingested larvae may either undergo extraintestinal migration or remain in the gastrointestinal tract. Larvae returning to the small intestine undergo two molts to become adult, sexually mature male and female worms ranging in length from 5–13 mm. The buccal capsule of the adult hookworm is armed with teeth (*A. duodenale*) or cutting plates (*N. americanus*) to facilitate attachment to the mucosa and submucosa of the small intestine. Hookworms can remain in the intestine for 1–5 yr, where they mate and produce eggs. Although approximately 2 mo is required for the larval stages of hookworms to undergo extraintestinal migration and develop into mature adults, *A. duodenale* larvae may remain developmentally arrested for many months before resuming development in the intestine. Mature *A. duodenale* female worms produce about 30,000 eggs/24 hr; daily egg production by *N. americanus* is less than 10,000/24 hr. The eggs are thin shelled and ovoid, measuring approximately $40 \times 60\ \mu$. Eggs that are deposited on soil with adequate moisture and shade develop into first-stage larvae and hatch. Over the ensuing several days, under appropriate conditions, the larvae molt twice to the infective stage. Infective larvae are developmentally arrested and nonfeeding. They migrate vertically in the soil until they either infect a new host or exhaust their lipid metabolic reserves and die.

EPIDEMIOLOGY. Because of the requirement for adequate soil moisture, shade, and warmth, hookworm infection is usually confined to rural areas, especially where human feces are used for fertilizer or where sanitation is inadequate. For that reason, hookworm is an infection associated with economic underdevelopment and poverty throughout the tropics and subtropics. High rates of infection are often associated with cultivation of certain agricultural products such as tea in India, mulberry trees in China, coffee in Central and South America, and rubber in Africa. China and India have the highest prevalence of hookworm infection. Wherever hookworm occurs, it is not uncommon to find patients with mixed *N. americanus* and *A. duodenale* infections. *N. americanus* predominates in Central and South America, as well as in South China and southeast Asia, whereas *A. duodenale* predominates in North Africa, in northern India, and in China north of the Yangtze River. The ability of *A. duodenale* to withstand somewhat harsher environmental and climactic conditions may reflect its ability to undergo arrested development in human tissues. *A. ceylanicum* infection occurs in India and Southeast Asia.

Eosinophilic enteritis caused by *A. caninum* was first described in Queensland, Australia, with two reported cases in the United States. Because of its global distribution in dogs, it is anticipated that human *A. caninum* infections will be identified in many locales.

PATHOGENESIS. The major morbidity of human hookworm infection is a direct result of intestinal blood loss. Adult hookworms adhere tenaciously to the mucosa and submucosa of the proximal small intestine by using their teeth (or cutting plates) and a muscular esophagus that creates negative pressure in their buccal capsules. At the attachment site, hookworms downregulate host inflammation by releasing anti-inflammatory polypeptides. Rupture of capillaries in the lamina propria is followed by blood extravasation; some of the blood is directly ingested by the hookworms, which anticoagulate blood through the release of peptides that block factor Xa and VIIa/tissue factor. Each adult *A. duodenale* hookworm causes an estimated 0.2 mL of blood loss per day; blood loss is less for each *N. americanus* hookworm. Individuals with light infections suffer from very little blood loss and, consequently, may have *hookworm infection* but not *hookworm disease*. Hookworm disease results only in individuals with moderate and heavy infections who experience sufficient blood loss to develop iron deficiency and anemia. Hypoalbuminemia and consequent edema and anasarca from the loss of intravascular oncotic pressure can also occur. These features depend heavily on the dietary reserves of the host. Prolonged iron deficiency in childhood may lead to cognitive and intellectual deficits.

CLINICAL MANIFESTATIONS. Anthropophilic hookworm larvae elicit dermatitis sometimes referred to as "ground itch" when they penetrate human skin. The vesiculation and edema of ground itch are exacerbated by repeated infection. Infection with a zoonotic hookworm, especially *A. braziliense*, can result in lateral migration of the larvae to cause the characteristic cutaneous tracts of cutaneous larva migrans (Chapter 283.1). Cough subsequently occurs in *A. duodenale* and *N. americanus* hookworm infection when larvae migrate through the lungs to cause laryngotracheobronchitis, usually about 1 wk after exposure. Pharyngitis also can occur.

Intestinal hookworm infection may occur without specific gastrointestinal complaints, although pain, anorexia, and diarrhea have been attributed to the presence of hookworms. Eosinophilia is often first noticed in the context of asymptomatic infection. The major clinical manifestations are related to intestinal blood loss. Heavily infected children exhibit all of the signs and symptoms of iron deficiency anemia and protein malnutrition. In some cases, children with chronic hookworm disease acquire a yellow-green pallor known as chlorosis.

An infantile form of ancylostomiasis resulting from heavy *A. duodenale* infection has been described. Affected infants experience diarrhea, melena, failure to thrive, and profound anemia. Infantile ancylostomiasis has significant mortality.

Eosinophilic enteritis caused by *A. caninum* is associated with colicky abdominal pain, usually exacerbated by food, which begins in the epigastrium and radiates outward. Extreme cases may mimic acute appendicitis.

DIAGNOSIS. Children with hookworm release eggs that can be detected by direct fecal examination (Fig. 283–1). Quantitative methods are available to determine whether a child has a heavy worm burden that can cause hookworm disease. The eggs of *A. duodenale* and *N. americanus* are morphologically indistinguishable. Species identification typically requires egg hatching and differentiation of third-stage infective larvae; newer methods using polymerase chain reaction methods are under development.

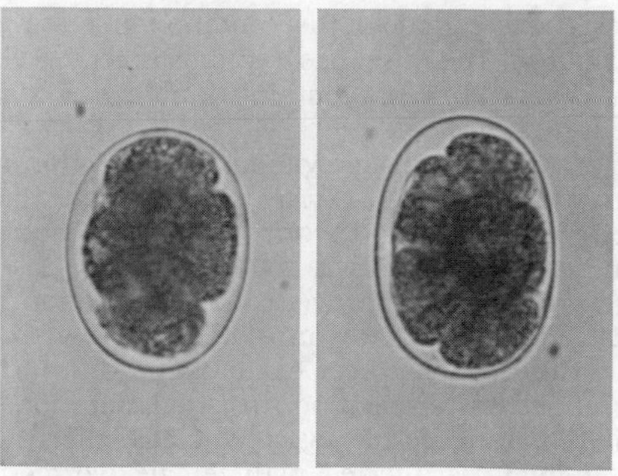

Figure 283–1 Eggs of hookworm *Necator americanus* in early cleavage as seen in freshly passed feces (×400).

In contrast, eggs are generally not present in the feces of patients with eosinophilic enteritis caused by *A. caninum*. Eosinophilic enteritis is often diagnosed by demonstrating ileal and colonic ulcerations by colonoscopy in the presence of significant blood eosinophilia. An adult canine hookworm may occasionally be recovered during colonoscopic biopsy. Patients with this syndrome develop IgG and IgE serologic responses.

TREATMENT. The goals of therapy are removal of the adult hookworms with an anthelmintic drug in addition to nutritional support for children with hookworm-associated iron deficiency and protein malnutrition. The benzimidazole anthelmintics, mebendazole and albendazole, are highly effective at eliminating hookworms from the intestine. A single dose of albendazole (400 mg PO) for children and adults achieves cure rates of up to 95%, although *N. americanus* adult hookworms are sometimes more refractory and require additional doses. Mebendazole (100 mg bid for 3 days, or 500 mg once, for children and adults) is equally effective. Mebendazole is recommended for *A. caninum*–associated eosinophilic enteritis, although recurrences are common. Because the benzimidazoles have been reported to be embryotoxic and teratogenic in laboratory animals, their safety in young children is a potential concern. However, benzimidazole treatment of thousands of children in less-developed countries indicates that these agents are probably safe. Pyrantel pamoate (11 mg/kg once daily for 3 days; maximum, 1 g) is available in liquid form and is an effective alternative to the benzimidazoles. Replacement therapy with an iron salt preparation is often required to correct hookworm iron deficiency.

PREVENTION. Although anthelmintic drugs are effective at eliminating hookworms from the intestine, the high rates of re-infection among children suggest that drug chemotherapy alone is not effective for controlling hookworm in highly endemic areas. Sanitation, health education, avoidance of human feces as fertilizer, and economic development are still critical for reducing endemicity. Work is in progress to genetically engineer hookworm antigens to use as vaccines in humans.

283.1 Cutaneous Larva Migrans

ETIOLOGY. Cutaneous larva migrans is caused by several larval nematodes not usually parasitic for humans. *A. braziliense*, a hookworm of dogs and cats, is the most common cause, but

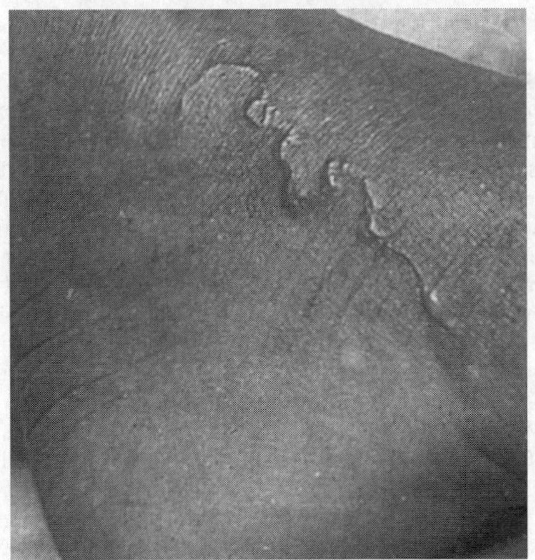

Figure 283–2 Creeping eruption of cutaneous larva migrans. (From Korting GW: Hautkrankheiten bei Kindern und Jugendlichen. Stuttgart, FK Schattauer Verlag, 1969.) See also color section.

other animal hookworms (*A. caninum, Uncinaria stenocephala,* and *Bunostomum phlebotomum*) and human parasites (*N. americanus, A. duodenale,* and *Strongyloides stercoralis*) may also produce the disease.

EPIDEMIOLOGY. Cutaneous larva migrans, which is usually caused by *A. braziliense,* is endemic to the southeastern United States and Puerto Rico.

CLINICAL MANIFESTATIONS. After penetrating the skin, larvae localize at the epidermal-dermal junction and migrate in this plane, moving at a rate of 1–2 cm/24 hr. The response to the parasite is characterized by raised, erythematous, serpiginous tracks, which occasionally form bullas (Fig. 283–2). These lesions may be single or numerous and are usually localized to an extremity, although any area of the body may be affected. As the organism migrates, new areas of involvement may appear every few days. Intense localized pruritus, without any systemic symptoms, may be associated with the lesions.

DIAGNOSIS. Cutaneous larva migrans is diagnosed by clinical examination of the skin. Patients are often able to recall the exact time and location of exposure because the larvae produce intense itching at the site of penetration. Eosinophilia may occur but is uncommon.

TREATMENT. If left untreated, the larvae die, and the syndrome resolves within a few weeks to several months. Topical application of thiabendazole (10% oral suspension qid or oral treatment with ivermectin (150–200 μg once, for children ≥15 kg and adults), albendazole (400 mg once daily for 3 days, for both children and adults), or thiabendazole (50 mg/kg/24 hr divided in two doses for 2–5 days; maximum 3 g/24 hr) hastens resolution and may be used if symptoms warrant treatment. Nausea and vomiting frequently preclude repeated administration of oral thiabendazole.

Davies HD, Sakuls S, Keystone JS: Creeping eruption. A review of clinical presentation and management of 60 cases presenting to a tropical disease unit. Arch Dermatol 129:588, 1993.

Hotez PJ, Ghosh K, Hawdon J, et al: Vaccines for hookworm infection. Pediatr Infect Dis J 16:935, 1997.

Hotez PJ, Pritchard DI: Hookworm infection. Sci Am 272:68, 1995.

Jelinek T, Maiwald H, Nothdurft HD, et al: Cutaneous larva migrans in travelers: Synopsis of histories, symptoms, and treatment of 98 patients. Clin Infect Dis 19:1062, 1994.

CHAPTER 284
Enterobiasis (Pinworm; Enterobius vermicularis*)*

James W. Kazura

Enterobius vermicularis infection occurs worldwide and affects individuals of all ages and socioeconomic levels but is especially common in children. Living in congested districts, institutions, or families with pinworm infections predisposes to enterobiasis. The infection is essentially harmless and causes more social than medical problems in affected children and their families.

ETIOLOGY. Humans are infected by ingesting embryonated eggs, which are usually carried on fingernails, clothing, bedding, or house dust. Eggs hatch in the stomach, and larvae migrate to the cecal region, where they mature into adult worms. *E. vermicularis* organisms are small (1 cm in length) white worms; the gravid females migrate by night to the perianal region to deposit masses of eggs. Pinworm ova are asymmetric, flattened on one side, and measure 30 × 60 μm. After a 6-hr maturation period, a single coiled larva can be seen within each ovum. These larvae may remain viable for 20 days.

Eggs carried under the fingernails are transmitted directly or disseminated in the environment to infect others. Humans are the only natural hosts of *E. vermicularis,* which is an obligate parasite. The prevalence and intensity of infection are low in infants and young children, with the highest prevalence in children 5–14 yr of age; the prevalence decreases in adulthood because of either reduced exposure or acquisition of immunity.

PATHOGENESIS. Perianal irritation during oviposition by female worms, usually at night, induces pruritus.

CLINICAL MANIFESTATIONS. Many local and systemic signs and symptoms have been ascribed to *E. vermicularis* infection; however, a controlled study of infected children 2–12 yr of age failed to document specific syndromes due to *E. vermicularis.* Symptomatic individuals most commonly complain of nocturnal anal pruritus and sleeplessness. The cause and incidence of perianal and perineal irritation are unknown but may be related to the intensity of infection, to the psychologic profile of the infected individual and his or her family, or to an allergic reaction to the parasite. Because tissue invasion does not occur in most cases of enterobiasis, eosinophilia is not observed. Perianal granulomas occur rarely and contain live or dead worms or eggs; surgical excision is not usually required. *E. vermicularis* has been recovered from ectopic sites including the female genital tract and rarely from the appendix, peritoneal cavity, liver, and spleen.

DIAGNOSIS. Definitive diagnosis is established by either finding the parasite eggs or recovering worms. Eggs can be easily detected by pressing adhesive cellophane tape against the perianal region early in the morning and examining it under a microscope. Appropriate collection measures should be used because the eggs are infective. Repeated examination may be necessary, and in certain situations, examination of all family members may be advised. A worm seen in the perianal region should be preserved in 75% ethyl alcohol until microscopic examination can be performed.

TREATMENT. Drug therapy should be administered to all infected and symptomatic individuals. The recommended regimen for enterobiasis is albendazole (400 mg PO for children and adults, with a repeat dose in 2 wk). Alternative treatments include mebendazole (100 mg PO for children and adults with a repeat dose in 2 wk) or pyrantel pamoate (11 mg/kg PO; maximum, 1 g/dose, with a repeat dose in 2 wk).

PREVENTION. Repeated treatments every 3–4 mo may be required in situations in which exposure is constant, such as in children in institutions. Although personal cleanliness is a useful general recommendation, there is no proof that it has a significant role in control of enterobiasis.

Avolio L, Avoltini V, Ceffa F, et al: Perianal granuloma caused by *Enterobius vermicularis*: Report of a new observation and review of the literature. J Pediatr 132:1055, 1998.
Boyer A, Berdknikoff IK: Pinworm infestation in children; the problem and its management. Can Med Assoc J 86:60, 1962.
Weller TH, Sorensen CW: Enterobiasis: Its incidence and symptomatology in a group of 505 children. N Engl J Med 224:131, 1941.

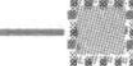

CHAPTER 285
Toxocariasis (Visceral and Ocular Larva Migrans)

James W. Kazura

Visceral larva migrans is a worldwide infection that occurs most frequently in children younger than 10 yr is characterized by fever, hepatomegaly, pulmonary disease, and eosinophilia.

ETIOLOGY. Visceral larva migrans is caused by infection with larvae of the canine ascarid *Toxocara canis* or less commonly the feline ascarid *Toxocara cati.* Infrequent cases include *T. leonina,* from dogs and foxes, and the raccoon ascarid *Baylisascaris procyonis.* These are very common in their definitive hosts. Adult worms of *Toxocara* spp. reside in the gastrointestinal tract of dogs and cats and release large numbers of eggs, which are passed in the feces. Ingestion of eggs by humans is followed by larval penetration of the gastrointestinal tract and migration to the liver, lungs, and occasionally other sites (central nervous system, eyes, kidneys, and heart). *Toxocara* larvae do not develop beyond this stage in human hosts.

EPIDEMIOLOGY. Visceral larva migrans is most common in children 1–4 yr of age, particularly those who engage in pica and have close contact with dogs and cats. Ocular toxocariasis occurs most frequently in older children. Potential sources of infection are widely distributed in the canine and feline population. An estimated 20% of dogs, including almost all puppies, in the United States excrete *T. canis,* and almost all juvenile raccoons excrete *B. procyonis.* Cats and dogs often defecate in areas where children play; in one study, 24% of 800 soil samples taken from public parks in Great Britain were found to contain *Toxocara* eggs.

PATHOGENESIS. *Toxocara* larvae usually elicit a granulomatous response characterized by large numbers of eosinophils, mononuclear cells, and tissue necrosis. These lesions are found in the liver, lungs, and other organs through which the helminth migrates. The inflammatory reaction is much less intense in the eyes, where lesions consist mainly of mononuclear cells and a few eosinophils. Unlike *T. canis* larvae, which do not grow in the aberrant host, the larvae of *B. procyonis* develop considerably in humans and reach sizes as large as 2 mm.

CLINICAL MANIFESTATIONS. Major symptoms depend on the infected organ and commonly include fever (80%), cough with wheezing (60–80%), and seizures (20–30%). Respiratory distress may be severe enough to warrant hospitalization. Abdominal pain has been noted in occasional patients. Physical findings include hepatomegaly (65–87%), rales or rhonchi (40–50%), papular or urticarial skin lesions (20%), and lymph node enlargement (8%). These manifestations subside over a period of several months. Scattered patchy infiltrates are often seen on chest roentgenograms.

Patients with ocular toxocariasis most commonly present with decreased visual acuity (75% of cases) and occasionally with strabismus or periorbital edema. In one study, unilateral blindness was noted in 6 of 17 patients. Most children do not have concurrent signs and symptoms of visceral disease. Funduscopic examination usually reveals solitary granulomatous lesions situated in the retina near the optic disc or macula. These may be mistaken for retinoblastomas and have led to inappropriate enucleation. Peripheral retinal lesions with vitreous bands and involvement of the iris have been documented in a few cases.

Severe eosinophilic meningitis has been reported with *B. procyonis* infection.

DIAGNOSIS. The diagnosis is established on the basis of the clinical manifestations and serologic testing. The only reliable and specific test is an enzyme-linked immunosorbent assay that uses infective eggs of *T. canis* as antigen. This does not reliably measure antibodies against *B. procyonis.* This assay has positive results (serum antibody titer ≥1:32) in 78% of cases of visceral larva migrans and in 45% of individuals with a clinical diagnosis of ocular toxocariasis. An absolute eosinophil count exceeding 500/μL occurs in nearly all patients with the visceral syndrome but is much less common in those with ocular disease. Nonspecific findings include elevations in serum gamma globulins and isohemagglutinins. Although larvae may be found on examination of tissue sections, biopsy of liver or other organs is generally not indicated because clinical and laboratory data provide sufficient information for diagnosis.

TREATMENT. Therapy is not required in the majority of cases, because the signs and symptoms are usually mild and subside over a period of weeks to months. When significant hypoxemia secondary to pulmonary disease occurs, however, administration of anti-inflammatory drugs (prednisone, 5 mg/kg/24 hr until respiratory function improves) is beneficial. When disease is severe or when larvae lodge in critical locations, such as the eye, the use of drugs exhibiting possible larvicidal activity has been advocated. The recommended treatment for ocular larva migrans is diethylcarbamazine (6 mg/kg/24 hr for 7–10 days). Alternative drugs include albendazole (400 mg bid for 3–5 days, for both children and adults) and mebendazole (100–200 mg bid for 5 days, for both children and adults). There is disagreement about the use of anthelmintic drugs, however, because dying larvae theoretically may incite an inflammatory response that produces more tissue damage than encapsulated, dormant parasites.

PREVENTION. Transmission of infection may be prevented by requiring children, particularly those with the habit of pica, to wash their hands after playing with pets and instructing them to avoid areas where dogs and cats defecate. Periodic deworming of dogs, especially puppies younger than 6 mo, also decreases the likelihood of human infection.

Fox AS, Kazacos KR, Gould NS, et al: Fatal eosinophilic meningoencephalitis and visceral larva migrans caused by the raccoon ascarid *Baylisascaris procyonis.* N Engl J Med 312:1619, 1985.
Hotez PJ: Visceral and ocular larva migrans. Semin Neurol 13:175, 1993.
Huntley CC, Costas MC, Lyerly A: Visceral larva migrans syndrome: Clinical characteristics and immunologic studies in 51 patients. Pediatrics 36:623, 1965.
Schantz PM, Glickman LT: Toxocaral visceral larva migrans. N Engl J Med 298:436, 1978.

CHAPTER 286
Strongyloidiasis (Strongyloides stercoralis)

James W. Kazura

Infection with the nematode *Strongyloides stercoralis,* unlike that with other worms, may cause autoinfection with massive parasite invasion of the host (hyperinfection syndrome or disseminated strongyloidiasis) that culminates in death. This complication is more frequent in malnourished or immunosuppressed individuals. *S. stercoralis* infection is widely distributed throughout tropical and temperate regions, although it is less common than infection by other intestinal roundworms.

ETIOLOGY. Infected individuals pass *S. stercoralis* larvae in their stools; these parasites may develop into free-living larvae in the soil or may change into infective filariform larvae, which must penetrate the skin of a host to continue their life cycle. After penetration, they pass through the bloodstream to the lungs and follow a pathway similar to hookworm and *Ascaris* larvae until they reach their final habitat in the upper small intestine. Mature worms (2.2 mm in length) burrow into the intestinal mucosa and begin releasing eggs approximately 4 wk after infection. *S. stercoralis* eggs hatch rapidly, and small larvae (225 × 16 μm) are passed in feces. The larvae must undergo morphologic changes to become infective. These changes usually occur in soil but may also occur as the parasites are being discharged from the body. Larvae are then capable of infecting the same individual by penetrating the intestinal wall or perianal skin. This unique feature of the *Strongyloides* life cycle allows the parasite to survive for many years inside the same host and occasionally to cause overwhelming infection.

EPIDEMIOLOGY. Humans are the primary hosts of *S. stercoralis.* Transmission of infection and its endemicity depend on suitable soil and climatic conditions and poor sanitary habits. Close contact and poor personal hygiene may be important, because the prevalence of infection is much higher in institutions for the mentally retarded. Host factors such as nutrition and immune status may have a crucial role in the development of the hyperinfection syndrome.

PATHOGENESIS. The initial penetration of skin by infective larvae usually produces no apparent pathologic lesions. Repeated skin invasion may, however, result in dermatitis; in cases in which autoinfection is established through the skin, a more extensive skin lesion, *larva currens,* may occur. A Löffler's-like syndrome with eosinophilia may be noted during migration of the larvae through the lungs. Eosinophilia may also occur when adult worms burrow into the intestinal mucosa. Disseminated strongyloidiasis is a complex pathologic entity due to larval invasion and injury of internal organs such as the liver, heart, adrenals, pancreas, kidneys, and central nervous system. It may be accompanied by polymicrobial gram-negative bacteremia.

CLINICAL MANIFESTATIONS. Signs and symptoms of strongyloidiasis occur in only a small proportion of infected individuals or in those with the hyperinfection syndrome. Pulmonary symptoms and skin lesions are usually mild and generally pass unnoticed. Pruritus with a papular erythematous rash may occur. *Larva currens,* a condition due to repeated skin invasion by larvae, is characterized by large erythematous urticarial lesions with rapidly advancing edges. These are usually localized to an area within 30 cm of the anus and have a tendency to recur. Adult worms in the upper small intestine cause the typical symptoms, which include abdominal pain, vomiting, and diarrhea. These symptoms occur with uncertain frequency and may have an abrupt onset with periodic recurrences. Abdominal pain is often epigastric and may be burning, colicky, or dull in nature. Diarrhea with passage of mucus may alternate with periods of constipation. *Chronic strongyloidiasis* may result in a malabsorption-like syndrome with protein-losing enteropathy and weight loss. Blood eosinophilia is usually associated with the intestinal phase of infection and is often the only indication.

Disseminated strongyloidiasis occurs in individuals with predisposing factors such as malnutrition or defects in cell-mediated immunity such as lymphoma, Hodgkin's disease, organ transplantation and AIDS. The onset is usually sudden, with generalized abdominal pain, distention, and fever. It may be accompanied by shock due to gram-negative septicemia. Massive invasion of internal organs by the parasite larvae causes extensive tissue destruction and organ dysfunction. Although leukocytosis may occur in these patients, eosinophilia is often absent.

DIAGNOSIS. Intestinal strongyloidiasis is diagnosed by examining feces or duodenal fluid for the characteristic larvae. Several stool samples should be examined either by direct smear or by a concentration method such as formaldehyde-ether or that of Baermann. Alternatively, duodenal fluid obtained by the enteric string test (Entero-Test) or aspiration may provide samples for definitive diagnosis. In children with hyperinfection syndrome, larvae may be found in sputum, gastric aspirates, or, rarely, in small intestinal biopsy specimens. Strongyloidiasis should also be suspected in immunosuppressed patients who suddenly develop signs and symptoms consistent with disseminated infection. A serologic test for *Strongyloides* antibodies may be more sensitive than parasitologic methods for diagnosing intestinal infection, but the utility of this assay in the hyperinfection syndrome has not been determined.

TREATMENT. Treatment of infected children is directed at eradication of infection; therefore, subsequent stool examination is essential. The recommended treatment is ivermectin (200 μg/kg/24 hr for 1–2 days, for children ≥15 kg and adults). An alternative drug is thiabendazole (50 mg/kg/24 hr divided in 2 doses for 2 days; maximum, 3 g/24 hr PO); this dose is likely to be toxic and may have to be decreased. The use of ivermectin for treatment of disseminated strongyloidiasis has not been established, and thiabendazole may be preferred; it may be necessary to prolong the duration of therapy for up to 2 wk.

PREVENTION. Use of sanitary practices designed to prevent soil and person-to-person transmission are the most effective control measures. Because the infection is uncommon, case detection and treatment are also advisable. Individuals who will be subjected to immunosuppressive therapy should have a screening examination for *S. stercoralis* and, if infected, should be treated with thiabendazole before immunosuppression.

Burke JA: Strongyloidiasis in childhood. Am J Dis Child 132:1130, 1978.
Naguira C, Jimenez G, Guerra JG, et al: Ivermectin for human strongyloidiasis and other intestinal nematodes. Am J Trop Med Hyg 40:304, 1989.
Nucci M, Portugal R, Pulcheri W, et al: Strongyloidiasis in patients with hematologic malignancies. Clin Infect Dis 21:675, 1995.
Smith JD, Goette DK, Odom RB: Larva currens: Cutaneous strongyloidiasis. Arch Dermatol 112:1161, 1976.

Chapter 287
Lymphatic Filariasis (Brugia malayi, Brugia timori, Wuchereria bancrofti)

James W. Kazura

ETIOLOGY. Infection with *Brugia malayi* (Malayan filariasis), *Brugia timori,* or *Wuchereria bancrofti* (bancroftian filariasis) results in similar clinical syndromes of lymphatic filariasis characterized in the early stages by acute lymphangitis and lymphadenitis and later by lymphatic obstruction with hydrocele and elephantiasis.

Filariae are threadlike nematodes. Filarial larvae are introduced into humans in secretions of biting mosquitoes. During a period of several months to a year, this stage of the helminth develops into adult worms that reside in the lymphatics. Sexually mature adult female worms release large numbers of microfilariae that circulate in the bloodstream. The life cycle of the parasite is completed when mosquitoes ingest these organisms in a blood meal.

EPIDEMIOLOGY. More than 120 million people in endemic areas of developing countries, up to 80% of the population, may be infected, although fewer than 10–20% have clinically significant morbidity. Those who live in areas where there is repeated and chronic exposure to larvae-containing mosquitoes, such as in crowded urban areas with poor sanitation, are most at risk for infection. *W. bancrofti* infection is distributed throughout tropical and subtropical Africa, Asia, and South America, whereas infection with *B. malayi* is restricted to the South Pacific and Southeast Asia. *B. timori* infection occurs in Indonesia. Infection of travelers who spend brief periods in endemic areas is rare.

CLINICAL MANIFESTATIONS. The initial infection is characterized by episodes of fever, lymphangitis of an extremity, lymphadenitis, headaches, and myalgias, which last a few days to several weeks. This syndrome is most frequently observed in young persons 10–20 yr of age. Manifestations of chronic disease, such as hydrocele and elephantiasis, occur mostly in adults older than 30 yr and are a direct result of lymphatic fibrosis and obstruction to lymph flow. It is uncommon for children to have clinically significant filariasis. Elephantiasis may involve one or more limbs, the scrotum, the breasts, or the vulva.

Tropical Pulmonary Eosinophilia. The presence of larvae (microfilariae) in the blood is not thought to have any pathologic consequences, except in persons with tropical pulmonary eosinophilia, a syndrome of filarial etiology in which microfilariae can be found in the lungs and lymph nodes. It occurs only in individuals who have lived for at least several months in endemic areas of bancroftian or Malayan filariasis and is most common in Southeast Asia and the South Pacific. Men 20–30 yr of age are most likely to be affected, although this syndrome has been observed in children. Patients present with paroxysmal nonproductive cough, occasional episodes of dyspnea, fever, weight loss, and fatigue. Rales and rhonchi are found on auscultation of the chest; roentgenographic findings may occasionally be normal, but increased bronchovascular markings, discrete opacities in the middle and basal regions of the lung, or diffuse miliary lesions are usually observed. Recurrent untreated episodes may result in interstitial fibrosis and chronic respiratory insufficiency. In children, hepatosplenomegaly and generalized lymphadenopathy are often seen. The diagnosis is suggested by history of exposure, eosinophilia (>2,000/μL), clinical symptoms, increased serum IgE levels (>1,000 IU/mL), and high titers of antimicrofilarial antibodies in the absence of blood-borne helminths. Although microfilariae may be found in sections of lung or lymph node, biopsy is unwarranted in most patients. The clinical response to diethylcarbamazine (5 mg/kg/24 hr for 10 days) is the final criterion for diagnosis; the majority of patients improve with this therapy. If symptoms recur, a second course of the drug should be administered. Patients with chronic symptoms are less likely to show improvement than those who have been ill for a short time.

DIAGNOSIS. Demonstration of microfilariae in the blood is the primary means for confirming diagnosis of lymphatic filariasis. A thick blood smear or 1 mL of blood that is concentrated is obtained at a time of day when the number of parasites in the circulation is expected to be highest (this varies with the geographic strain of filaria and most commonly occurs around midnight) and is examined for the organisms. Infection with *W. bancrofti* in the absence of microfilaremia may also be diagnosed by detection of parasite antigen in the serum.

TREATMENT. The use of antifilarial drugs is controversial. No controlled studies demonstrate that administration of antifilarial chemotherapy, such as diethylcarbamazine, modifies the course of acute lymphangitis. Diethylcarbamazine may be given to asymptomatic microfilaremic persons to lower the intensity of parasitemia, although the effect of the drug on the acute or chronic pathologic manifestations of the infection has not been established. The regimen for children is 1 mg/kg as a single dose on day 1; 3 mg/kg/24 hr divided in three doses on day 2; 3–6 mg/kg/24 hr divided in three doses on day 3; and 6 mg/kg/24 hr divided in three doses on days 4–14. The regimen for adults is 50 mg on day 1; 50 mg tid on day 2; 100 mg tid on day 3; and 6 mg/kg/24 hr divided in three doses on days 4–14. For patients with no microfilaria in the blood, the full dose (6 mg/kg/24 hr) can be given from day one. Repeat doses may be necessary to reduce further the microfilaremia and to kill lymph-dwelling adult parasites. A single dose of ivermectin (20–200 μg/kg, for children ≥15 kg and adults) is as effective as diethylcarbamazine in lowering microfilaremia but does not kill adult worms. Combination ivermectin (200–400 μg/kg, for children ≥15 kg and adults) and albendazole (400 mg), which is also effective in killing adult parasites, has been used and may be more effective than ivermectin alone.

Addiss DG, Beach MJ, Streit TG, et al: Randomised placebo-controlled comparison of ivermectin and albendazole alone and in combination for *Wuchereria bancrofta* microfilaraemia in Haitian children. Lancet 350:480, 1997.

Bockarie MH, Alexander ND, Hyun P, et al: Randomised community-based trial of annual single-dose diethylcarbamazine with or without ivermectin against *Wuchereria bancrofti* infection in human beings and mosquitoes. Lancet 351:162, 1998.

Chapter 288
Infection with Animal Filariae

James W. Kazura

Humans may be infected with three types of animal filariae. *Dirofilaria immitis,* the heartworm of dogs, is found on all continents and is a common parasite of dogs in many parts of the United States. *Dirofilaria tenuis, Brugia beaveri, Brugia lepori,* and other unclassified *Brugia* spp. have also been reported to infect humans. These worms may be introduced into humans by the bite of mosquitoes containing third-stage larvae. The organisms, however, do not undergo normal development in the human host. *D. immitis* organisms are trapped in the lung parenchyma after migrating for several months in the subcutaneous tissues. The pulmonary response consists of granulomas with eosinophils, neutrophils, and tissue necrosis. *D. tenuis* does not leave the subcutaneous tissues, whereas *B. beaveri* eventually localizes to superficial lymph nodes.

Most human infections with *D. immitis* are discovered incidentally when a chest roentgenogram reveals a solitary pulmonary nodule 1–3 cm in diameter. Definitive diagnosis and cure depend on surgical excision and identification of the nematode within the surrounding granulomatous response. *D. tenuis* and *B. beaveri* infections present as painful 1–5-cm rubbery nodules in the skin of the trunk, extremities, and around the orbit. Patients often report having been engaged in activities predisposing to exposure to infected mosquitoes, such as working in swampy areas. Diagnosis and management of these infections is by surgical excision.

Addiss DG, Beach MJ, Streit TG, et al: Randomised placebo-controlled comparison of ivermectin and albendazole alone and in combination for *Wuchereria bancrofti* microfilaraemia in Haitian children. Lancet 350:480, 1997.

Bockanie MH, Alexander ND, Hyun P, et al: Randomised community-based trial of annual single-dose diethylcarbamazine with or without ivermectin against *Wuchereria bancrofti* infection in human beings and mosquitoes. Lancet 351:162, 1998.

Kazura JW: Ivermectin and human lymphatic filariasis. Microb Pathog 14:337, 1993.

Steel C, Guinea A, McCarthy JS, et al: Long-term effect of prenatal exposure to maternal microfilaraemia on immune responsiveness to filarial parasite antigens. Lancet 343:890, 1994.

CHAPTER 289
Angiostrongylus cantonensis

James W. Kazura

The most common infectious cause of eosinophilic meningitis is inadvertent human infection with *Angiostrongylus cantonensis,* the rat lungworm. *Angiostrongylus* is found in Southeast Asia, the South Pacific, Japan, and Taiwan. Infection has also been described in Egypt, Ivory Coast, and Cuba. *Angiostrongylus* is acquired by eating raw or undercooked freshwater snails, slugs, prawns, or crabs containing infectious third-stage larvae.

Patients become ill 1–3 wk after exposure, as the parasites migrate from the gastrointestinal tract to the central nervous system. They may have fever, peripheral eosinophilia, vomiting, abdominal pain, creeping skin eruptions, or pleurisy. Neurologic symptoms include headache, meningismus, ataxia, cranial nerve palsies, and paresthesias. Radiculitis or myelitis may cause paraparesis or incontinence.

The presumptive diagnosis is made by travel and exposure history in the presence of typical clinical and laboratory findings. Eosinophilic pleocytosis (15–90% of a cerebrospinal fluid white blood cell count > 100 cells/μL) is found. The cerebrospinal fluid protein level is elevated, and the glucose level is typically normal. Results of imaging studies are usually negative, although hydrocephalus associated with inflammation may be noted.

Treatment is supportive, because infection is self-limited and anthelmintic drugs do not appear to influence the outcome of infection. Analgesics should be given for headache and radiculitis, and careful removal of cerebrospinal fluid at frequent intervals should be performed to relieve hydrocephalus. Corticosteroids have not shown a consistent beneficial effect. Antiparasitic drugs can exacerbate neurologic symptoms, and most patients recover without drug therapy. Mebendazole (100 mg bid for 5 days for children and adults) has been used.

The prognosis is good, with 70% of patients improving sufficiently to leave the hospital in 1–2 wk. The mortality associated with eosinophilic meningitis is less than 1%.

Koo J, Pien F, Kliks MM: *Angiostrongylus (Parastrongylus)* eosinophilic meningitis. Rev Infect Dis 10:1155, 1988.

CHAPTER 290
Onchocerciasis (Onchocerca volvulus)

James W. Kazura

Infection with *Onchocerca volvulus,* the cause of onchocerciasis or river blindness, is a major cause of blindness in West Africa and Central America. The parasite is introduced into humans by infected blackflies of the genus *Simulium,* which breed in rapidly running water; people who live or work near waterways are thus most likely to be infected. Most individuals are asymptomatic; those with chronic and heavy infections (usually adults >20 yr of age) may suffer from pruritic dermatitis and eye disease (punctate keratitis, corneal pannus formation, chorioretinitis) owing to the presence of microfilariae in subcutaneous and ocular tissues. Firm, nontender subcutaneous nodules containing adult parasites may also be palpable. *O. volvulus* infection is diagnosed by demonstration of parasites in skin snips removed from the buttocks or extremities or by slit-lamp visualization of microfilariae in the cornea or anterior chamber of the eye. Persons with symptomatic skin or eye disease should be treated with ivermectin (150 μg/kg PO as a single dose, for children ≥15 kg and adults). Repeat doses 6–12 mo later should be administered if microfilariae are observed in the skin or eyes. The drug should not be given to persons with disorders of the central nervous system. Annual treatment with ivermectin 150 μg/kg can prevent blindness due to ocular onchocerciasis.

Mabey D, Whitworth JA, Eckstein M, et al: The effects of multiple doses of ivermectin on ocular onchocerciasis. A six-year follow-up. Ophthalmology 103:1001, 1996.

White AT, Newland HS, Taylor HR, et al: Controlled trial and dose finding study of ivermectin for treatment of onchocerciasis. J Infect Dis 156:463, 1987.

CHAPTER 291
Dracunculiasis (Guinea Worm Infection), (Dracunculus medinensis)

James W. Kazura

Dracunculiasis occurs in all areas of the tropics and is especially common in India and West Africa. The parasite *Dracunculus medinensis* infects humans when they swallow larva-containing microscopic crustaceans (copepods) living in communal water sites. Adult worms migrate through the subcutaneous tissues of the lower extremities (or occasionally other sites) and grow to a length of 1 m or more. An ulcer is produced where they penetrate the skin.

The diagnosis is confirmed by identifying larvae contained

in washings from the base of the lesion. Administering mebendazole (25 mg/kg day divided in three doses for 10 days; maximum, 750 mg/dose) diminishes the local inflammatory response and facilitates removal of the helminth. Infection may be prevented by avoiding ingestion of water that humans walk in or use for bathing. Boiling or chlorination kills the organism.

CHAPTER 292
Loiasis (Loa loa)

James W. Kazura

Infection with *Loa loa,* the African eye worm, the cause of loiasis, occurs in the rain forests of West and Central Africa. The parasite is transmitted to humans by infected deerflies of the genus *Chrysops.* Adult worms migrate in the subcutaneous tissues and produce painful transient areas of localized edema known as Calabar swellings, which tend to appear around the joints of the legs and arms. They last for several days to weeks, then subside slowly; they probably represent an immune response. The parasite occasionally may be directly visualized in the conjunctiva, where it produces an intense inflammatory reaction. Microfilariae are present in highest concentrations in the peripheral circulation between 10 A.M. and 2 P.M.; identification in blood samples is diagnostic. Symptomatic individuals should be given gradually increasing doses of diethylcarbamazine as described for lymphatic filariasis (Chapter 284). Therapy should be discontinued and corticosteroids administered if fever, headache, or joint swelling occurs.

Nutman TB, Miller KD, Mulligan M, et al: *Loa loa* infection in temporary residents of enemic regions: Recognition of a hyperresponsive syndrome with characteristic clinical manifestations. J Infect Dis 154:10, 1986.

Rakita RM, White AC Jr, Kielhofner MA: *Loa loa* infection as a cause of migratory angioedema: Report of three cases from the Texas Medical Center. Clin Infect Dis 17:691, 1993.

CHAPTER 293
Gnathostoma spinigerum

James W. Kazura

Human infections with *Gnathostoma spinigerum,* parasites of dogs and cats, are found in Japan, China, India, Bangladesh, and Southeast Asia. Gnathostomiasis is acquired by eating undercooked or raw fish, frog, bird, or snake meat. A few days after ingestion, the larvae migrate through the intestinal wall into the abdominal cavity. Symptoms of epigastric pain, fever, anorexia, and vomiting may persist for weeks and resolve as the characteristic cutaneous manifestations appear, consisting of circumscribed patches of edema, usually on the abdomen, that last a few days and recur at different sites. Eosinophilia is usually identified. Migration of the worms along the nerve tracts, accompanied by severe pain and loss of motor and sensory function, may produce an eosinophilic meningitis. Worms should be surgically removed from accessible loci. Albendazole (400 mg bid for 21 days) has been used.

Ogata K, Nawa Y, Akahane H, et al: Short report: Gnathostomiasis in Mexico. Am J Trop Med Hyg 58:316, 1998.

CHAPTER 294
Trichinosis (Trichinella spiralis)

James W. Kazura

Human infection with *Trichinella spiralis* (trichinosis or trichinellosis) is common worldwide. Infection is transmitted by ingestion of pork or other meat carrying the parasite. Sporadic epidemics have occurred in North America after ingestion of bear meat. Consumption of horse meat in areas of Europe, where this is common, has also been the source of some outbreaks.

ETIOLOGY. Humans are infected by eating flesh contaminated with viable *T. spiralis* larvae. This stage of the parasite excysts in the stomach and matures to form adult worms within the small intestine. Female *T. spiralis* organisms release large numbers of newborn larvae, which penetrate the gut wall and migrate to striated muscles or occasionally to other sites such as the central nervous system and heart. Larvae that enter muscle cells eventually become encysted and may remain viable for years. The life cycle in nature is maintained by hogs or other animals that ingest garbage that contains carcasses of infected rodents.

EPIDEMIOLOGY. *T. spiralis* is found in all areas of the world except Australia and some islands in the South Pacific. Although infection was common in the United States in the past (4% of diaphragms examined post mortem in 1968 contained viable larvae), recent cases have been related to outbreaks resulting from ingestion of undercooked homemade sausage, other pork products, or meat of bears, wild pigs, walruses, and horses. Larvae are destroyed by cooking meat until no trace of pink fluid or flesh remains; this occurs at 55°C or by storage in a freezer at −15°C for 3 wk. Smoked or salted meat may still contain viable parasites.

PATHOGENESIS. Adult worms localize in the upper gastrointestinal tract and induce a mucosal inflammatory reaction characterized by a reduced villus:crypt ratio and the presence of eosinophils, neutrophils, and mononuclear cells. This response peaks within the first week of infection then gradually subsides as adult worms are expelled. In muscle cells, migrating larvae elicit a reaction consisting of large numbers of eosinophils and mononuclear cells. These lesions may eventually calcify.

CLINICAL MANIFESTATIONS. The signs and symptoms appear only in heavily infected individuals. Within the 1st wk, adult worms in the upper gastrointestinal tract produce gastroenteritis and diarrhea associated with abdominal discomfort. Next, during larval invasion of muscle, periorbital or facial edema (80% of cases) and myalgias occur. Pain is associated with muscle activity; it is most common in the masseters, diaphragm, and intercostals. These signs and symptoms are first noted 10–14 days after infection and last for another 2–3 wk. Heart failure and arrhythmias may occur in patients with exceptionally heavy infestation.

DIAGNOSIS. The diagnosis is suggested by findings of periorbital edema, myalgias, fever, and eosinophilia in an individual with a history of eating undercooked meat. A history of similar illness in those sharing the food should be sought. Serologic studies such as the bentonite flocculation test, with a titer of 1:5 or greater, are confirmatory. Biopsy of muscle, usually the deltoid, 3–4 wk after infection may reveal larvae on microscopic examination. Levels of muscle enzymes such as creatine kinase and lactate dehydrogenase are elevated in 50% of patients.

TREATMENT. There is no clinically established therapy for larval invasion of muscles. Mebendazole (200–400 mg tid for 3 days, then 400 mg tid for 10 days) may eliminate adult worms from the gut, but evidence for its efficacy against muscle larvae is not well established. Accordingly, the drug is most clearly indicated for treatment of persons who are known to have been infected in the preceding 1–3 wk. Corticosteroids may be used in critically ill patients, such as those with myocarditis or central nervous system damage, but evidence of their beneficial effect is equivocal.

Bailey TM, Schantz PM: Trends in the incidence and transmission patterns of trichinosis in humans in the United States: Comparison of the periods 1975–1981 and 1982–1986. Rev Infect Dis 12:5, 1990.
MacLean JD, Viallet J, Law C, et al: *Trichinosis* in the Canadian Arctic: Report of five outbreaks and a new clinical syndrome. J Infect Dis 160:513, 1989.
McAuley JB, Michelson MK, Schantz PM: Trichinella infection in travelers. J Infect Dis 164:1013, 1992.
Murrell KD, Bruschi F: Clinical trichinellosis. Prog Clin Parasitol 4:117, 1994.

CHAPTER 295
Trichuriasis (Trichuris trichiura)

James W. Kazura

Trichuris trichiura, or whipworm, causes one of the most common helminthic infections of humans. Approximately half a billion cases occur worldwide. Infection is more common in warm climates, but it does exist in North America.

ETIOLOGY. Infection is due to ingesting parasite eggs (Fig. 295–1), which are passed in the stools of infected individuals and mature in 2–4 wk if moisture and temperature conditions of the soil are optimal. On ingestion by humans, *Trichuris* eggs hatch and larvae penetrate the small intestinal villi, where they remain for 3–10 days before slowly moving down the bowel and maturing into adult worms. The final habitats of *T. trichiura* are the cecum and ascending colon. The body is divided into an anterior whiplike portion (hence the term *whip worm*) and a posterior bulky part and measures approximately 40 mm in length. The worms remain in the gut by anchoring the anterior portion of their body to the intestinal mucosa. Egg deposition by maturing females begins 1–3 mo after infection.

EPIDEMIOLOGY. Trichuriasis is most common in poor rural communities lacking sanitary facilities. Humans are the primary hosts; the highest prevalence and intensity of infection occur in children. Transmission of embryonated eggs occurs by contamination of hands, food, or drink. Eggs may also be carried by flies and other insects.

CLINICAL MANIFESTATIONS. Most infected individuals are asymptomatic; however, vague abdominal complaints, colic, and abdominal distention have been associated with infection. Adult *Trichuris* suck approximately 0.005 mL of blood per worm per day. However, only heavy childhood infections produce mild anemia, bloody diarrhea, or, rarely, rectal prolapse. These cases are referred to as *massive infantile trichuriasis* and are often associated with shigellosis and protozoan infections of the gastrointestinal tract.

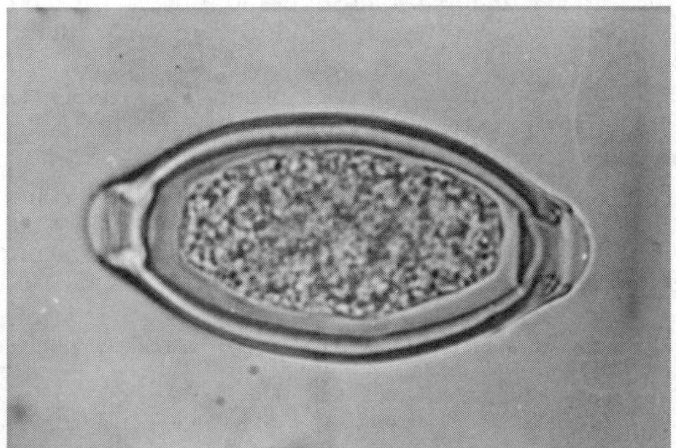

Figure 295–1 Egg of *Trichuris trichiura*, as seen in freshly passed feces (×1,000).

DIAGNOSIS. Examination of stool smears reveals the characteristic eggs of *T. trichiura*.

TREATMENT. An oral course of mebendazole (100 mg bid for 3 days, or 500 mg once, for both children and adults) produces a cure rate of 70–90% and reduces egg output by 90–99%. An alternative is albendazole (400 mg, for both children and adults); therapy with albendazole may have to be extended to 3 days for heavy infection.

Bundy DAP, Cooper ES, Thompson DE, et al: Effect of age and initial infection intensity on the rate of reinfection with *Trichuris trichiura* after treatment. Parasitology 97:469, 1988.
Bundy DAP, Cooper ES: Trichuris and trichuriasis in humans. Adv Parasitol 28:107, 1989.
Cooper ES, Bundy DA, MacDonald TT, Golden MH: Growth suppression in the *Trichuris* dysentery syndrome. Eur J Clin Nutr 44:285, 1990.
MacDonald TT, Choy MY, Spencer J, et al: Histopathology and immunohistochemistry of the caecum in children with the *Trichuris* dysentery syndrome. J Clin Pathol 44:194, 1991.

CHAPTER 296
Schistosomiasis (Schistosoma)

Charles H. King

Schistosoma organisms are the flukes, or trematodes, that parasitize the bloodstream. Five schistosome species infect humans: *Schistosoma haematobium, S. mansoni, S. japonicum, S. intercalatum*, and *S. mekongi*. Schistosomiasis infects >200 million people worldwide, primarily children and young adults. Prevalence is increasing in many areas as population density increases and new irrigation projects provide broader habitats for vector snails.

ETIOLOGY. Humans are infected through contact with water contaminated with cercariae, the free-living infective stage of the parasite. These motile, forked-tail organisms emerge from infected snails and are capable of penetrating intact human skin. In the subcutaneous tissues, cercariae change into the next developmental stage, the schistosomula, and migrate to the lungs and finally the liver. As they reach sexual maturity, adult worms migrate to specific anatomic sites characteristic of each schistosome species: *S. haematobium* adults are found in the perivesical and periureteral venous plexus, *S. mansoni* in the inferior mesenteric, and *S. japonicum* in the superior mesenteric veins. *S. intercalatum* and *S. mekongi* are found in the mesenteric vessels. Adult schistosome worms (1–2 cm in length) are clearly adapted for an intravascular existence. Unlike the other flukes, *Schistosoma* organisms are diecious, and the two sexes are dissimilar in appearance. The female accompanies the male in a groove formed by the lateral edges of its body. On fertilization, female worms begin oviposition in the small venous tributaries. The eggs of the three main schistosome species have characteristic morphologic features: *S. haematobium* has a terminal spine, *S. mansoni* has a lateral spine, and *S. japonicum* has a smaller size with a short, curved spine (Fig. 296–1). Eggs reach the lumen of the urinary tract or intestines and are carried to the outside environment, where they hatch if deposited in fresh water. Motile miracidia

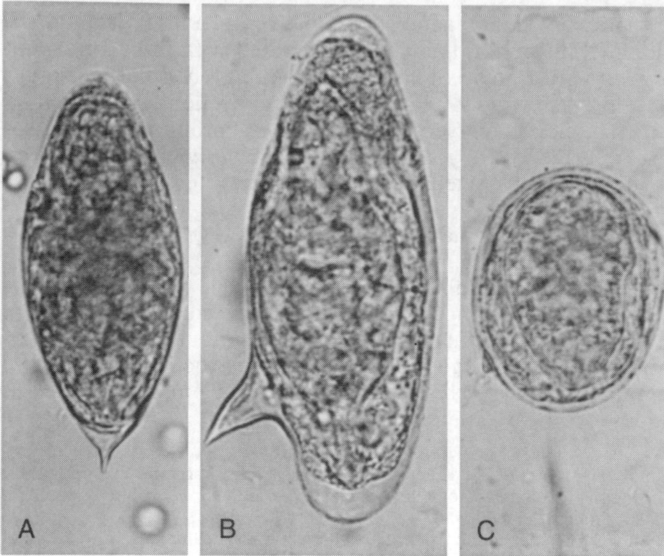

Figure 296–1 Eggs of *Schistosoma haematobium (A)*, *Schistosoma mansoni (B)*, and *Schistosoma japonicum (C)* (×320).

emerge; they infect specific freshwater snail intermediate hosts and divide asexually. In 4–6 wk, the infective cercariae are released in the water.

EPIDEMIOLOGY. Humans are the definitive host for the five clinically important species of schistosomes, although *S. japonicum* may infect some animals such as dogs and cattle. *S. haematobium* is prevalent in Africa and the Middle East; *S. mansoni* in Africa, the Middle East, the Caribbean, and South America; and *S. japonicum* in China, the Philippines, and Indonesia, with some sporadic foci in parts of Southeast Asia. The other two species are less prevalent. *S. intercalatum* is found in West and Central Africa, and *S. mekongi* is found in the Far East.

Transmission depends on disposal of excreta, the presence of specific intermediate snail hosts, and the patterns of water contact and social habits of the population. The distribution of infection in endemic areas shows that prevalence increases with age to a maximum at 10–20 yr of age. Measuring intensity of infection (by quantitative egg count in urine or feces) demonstrates that the heaviest worm loads are found in the younger age groups. Schistosomiasis, therefore, is most prevalent and most severe in children and young adults, who are at maximal risk of suffering from its acute and chronic sequelae.

PATHOGENESIS. The early manifestations of schistosomiasis are immunologically mediated. Acute schistosomiasis (Katayama fever) is a febrile illness that represents an immune complex disease associated with early infection and oviposition.

The major pathology of infection is with chronic schistosomiasis, in which retention of eggs in the host tissues is associated with chronic granulomatous injury. Eggs may be trapped at sites of deposition (urinary bladder, ureters, intestine) or be carried by the bloodstream to other organs, most commonly the liver and less often the lungs and central nervous system. The host response to these eggs involves local as well as systemic manifestations. The cell-mediated immune response leads to granulomas composed of lymphocytes, macrophages, and eosinophils that surround the trapped eggs and add significantly to the degree of tissue destruction. Granuloma formation in the bladder wall and at the ureterovesical junction results in the major disease manifestations of schistosomiasis hematobia: hematuria, dysuria, and obstructive uropathy. Intestinal as well as hepatic granulomas underlie the pathologic sequelae of the other schistosome infections: ulcerations and fibrosis of intestinal wall, hepatosplenomegaly, and portal hypertension due to presinusoidal obstruction of blood flow. Protective immunity against schistosomiasis has been demonstrated in some animal species and may occur in humans.

CLINICAL MANIFESTATIONS. Most infected individuals suffer no apparent ill health; symptoms occur mainly in those who are heavily infected. Cercarial penetration of human skin may result in a papular pruritic rash (schistosomal dermatitis or swimmer's itch). It is more pronounced in previously exposed individuals and is characterized by edema and massive cellular infiltrates in the dermis and epidermis. Acute schistosomiasis (Katayama fever) may occur, particularly in heavily infected individuals 4–8 wk after exposure; this is a serum sickness–like syndrome manifested by the acute onset of fever, chills, sweating, lymphadenopathy, hepatosplenomegaly, and eosinophilia. Acute schistosomiasis most commonly presents in first-time visitors to endemic areas who experience primary infection at an older age.

Symptomatic children with chronic schistosomiasis haematobia usually complain of frequency, dysuria, and hematuria. Urine examination shows erythrocytes, parasite eggs, and occasional leukocytes. In endemic areas, moderate to severe pathologic lesions have been demonstrated in the urinary tract of more than 50% of infected children. The extent of disease correlates with the intensity of infection, but significant morbidity can occur even in lightly infected children. The terminal stages of schistosomiasis haematobia are associated with chronic renal failure, secondary infections, and cancer of the bladder.

Children with chronic schistosomiasis mansoni, japonica, intercalatum, or mekongi may have intestinal symptoms; colicky abdominal pain and bloody diarrhea are the most common. The intestinal phase may, however, pass unnoticed, and the syndrome of hepatosplenomegaly, portal hypertension, ascites, and hematemesis may be the initial presentation. Liver disease is due to granuloma formation and subsequent fibrosis; no appreciable liver cell injury occurs, and hepatic function may be preserved for a long time. Schistosome eggs may escape into the lungs, causing pulmonary hypertension and cor pulmonale. *S. japonicum* worms may migrate to the brain vasculature and produce localized lesions that cause seizures. Transverse myelitis rarely has been reported in children or young adults with chronic *S. haematobium* or *S. mansoni* infection.

DIAGNOSIS. Schistosome eggs are found in the excreta of infected individuals; quantitative methods should be used to provide an indication of the intensity of infection. A volume of 10 mL of urine should be collected around midday, which is the time of maximal egg excretion, and filtered for diagnosis of *S. haematobium* infection. Stool examination by the Kato's thick smear procedure is the method of choice for diagnosis and quantification of other schistosome infections.

TREATMENT. Treatment of children with schistosomiasis should be based on an appreciation of the intensity of infection and the extent of disease. The recommended treatment for schistosomiasis is praziquantel (40 mg/kg/day divided in two doses for 1 day for haematobia, mansoni, and intercalatum; 60 mg/kg/24 hr divided in three doses for 1 day for japonica and mekongi).

PREVENTION. Transmission in endemic areas may be decreased by reducing the parasite load in the population. The availability of oral, single-dose, effective chemotherapeutic agents may help achieve this goal. Other measures, particularly improved sanitation and focal application of molluscicides, may be useful. Control of schistosomiasis is closely linked to economic and social development.

Cheever AW, Yap GS: Immunologic basis of disease and disease regulation in schistosomiasis. Chem Immunol 66:159, 1997.

King CH: Acute and chronic schistosomiasis. Hosp Pract 26:117, 1991.

King CH, Mahmoud AAF: Schistosomiasis. *In*: Guerrant RL, Krogstad DJ, Maguire JH, Walker DH, Weller PF (eds): Tropical Infectious Diseases, Principles, Pathogens and Practice. New York, Churchill Livingstone, 1999.

Pitella JE: Neuroschistosomiasis. Brain Pathol 7:649, 1997.

CHAPTER 297
Flukes (Liver, Lung, and Intestinal)

Charles H. King

The parasitic trematodes, or flukes, are endemic worldwide but are more prevalent in the less developed parts of the world. They include *Schistosoma*, the blood flukes (Chapter 296). Trematodes are characterized by their complex life cycle. Sexual reproduction of adult worms in the definitive host produces eggs that are passed in the stool. Larvae, called miracidia, develop. Asexual multiplication by the larval stages, which requires certain species of molluskan (snails or clams) intermediate hosts, produces cercariae. Some flukes require a second intermediate host such as an insect or fish or must attach to vegetation, producing metacercaria. This "alternation of generations" requires that flukes parasitize more than one host (often three) to complete their life cycle.

FASCIOLIASIS *(FASCIOLA HEPATICA)*. *Fasciola hepatica*, the sheep liver fluke, infects cattle, other ungulates, and occasionally humans. Infection has been reported in many different parts of the world, particularly South America, Europe, Africa, China, Australia, and Cuba. Although *F. hepatica* is enzootic in North America, reported cases are extremely rare. Humans are infected by ingestion of metacercariae attached to vegetation, especially wild watercress. In the duodenum, the parasites excyst and penetrate the intestinal wall, liver capsule, and parenchyma. They wander for a few weeks before entering the bile ducts, where they mature. Adult *F. hepatica* (1 × 2.5 cm) commence oviposition approximately 12 wk after infection; the eggs are large (75 × 140 μm) and operculated. They pass to the intestines with bile and leave the body in the feces (Fig. 297–1). On reaching fresh water, the eggs mature and hatch into miracidia, which infect specific snail intermediate hosts to multiply into many cercariae. These then emerge from infected snails and encyst on aquatic grasses and plants.

Clinical manifestations usually occur either during the liver migratory phase of the parasites or after their arrival at their final habitat in bile canaliculi. Fever, right upper quadrant pain, and hepatosplenomegaly characterize the first phase of illness. Peripheral blood eosinophilia is usually marked. As the worms enter bile ducts, most of the acute symptoms subside. On rare occasions, patients may suffer from obstructive jaundice or biliary cirrhosis. *F. hepatica* infection is diagnosed by identifying the characteristic eggs in fecal smears or duodenal aspirates.

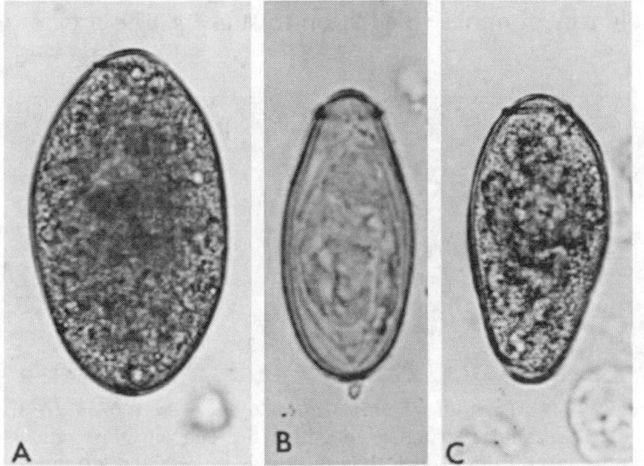

Figure 297–1 Eggs of liver flukes and a lung fluke. *A, Fasciola hepatica* (×400). *B, Clonorchis sinensis* (×1,000). *C, Paragonimus westermani* (×400).

Bithionol (30–50 mg/kg on alternate days for a total of 10–15 doses) is the recommended treatment. In the United States, bithionol is available from the Centers for Disease Control and Prevention, Atlanta, Georgia (telephone: 404-639-3670). The investigational drug, Triclabendazole (Cibas-Geigy) may also be used to treat fascioliasis (see WHO Fact Sheet 191 for availability).

CLONORCHIASIS *(CLONORCHIS SINENSIS)*. Infection of bile passages with *Clonorchis sinensis*, the Chinese or oriental liver fluke, is endemic in China, other parts of East Asia, and Japan. Humans acquire infection by ingestion of raw or inadequately cooked freshwater fish carrying the encysted metacercariae of the parasite under their scales or skin. Metacercariae excyst in the duodenum and pass through the ampulla of Vater to the common bile duct and bile capillaries, where they mature into hermaphroditic adult worms (3 × 15 mm). *C. sinensis* worms deposit small operculated eggs (14 × 30 μm), which are discharged via the bile duct to the intestine and feces (Fig. 297–1). The eggs mature and hatch outside the body, releasing motile miracidia into local freshwater streams, rivers, or ponds. If these are ingested by the appropriate snails, they develop into cercariae, which are in turn released from the snail to encyst under the skin or scales of freshwater fish.

Most individuals with *C. sinensis* infection, particularly those with few organisms, are asymptomatic. In heavily infected individuals, who tend to be older (> 30 yr of age), localized obstruction of a bile duct results from repeated local trauma and inflammation. In these cases, cholangitis and cholangiohepatitis may lead to liver enlargement and jaundice. In Hong Kong, Korea, and other parts of Asia, cholangiocarcinoma is associated with chronic *C. sinensis* infection.

Clonorchiasis is diagnosed by examination of feces or duodenal aspirates for the parasite eggs. The recommended treatment of clonorchiasis is praziquantel (75 mg/kg/24 hr divided in three doses for 1 day). An alternative, used in adults, is albendazole (10 mg/kg for 7 days).

OPISTHORCHIASIS *(OPISTHORCHIS)*. Infections with species of *Opisthorchis* are clinically similar to those by *C. sinensis*. *O. felineus* and *O. viverrini* are liver flukes of cats and dogs that infect humans through ingestion of metacercariae in freshwater fish. Infection with *O. felineus* is endemic in Eastern Europe and Southeast Asia, and *O. viverrini* is found mainly in Thailand. Most individuals are asymptomatic; liver enlargement, relapsing cholangitis, and jaundice may occur in heavily infected individuals. Diagnosis is based on recovering eggs from stools or duodenal aspirates. The recommended treatment of opisthorchiasis is praziquantel (75 mg/kg/24 hr divided in three doses for 1 day).

PARAGONIMIASIS (LUNG FLUKES; PARAGONIMUS). Human infection by the lung fluke *Paragonimus westermani*, and less frequently other species of *Paragonimus*, occurs throughout the Far East, in localized areas of West Africa, and in several parts of Central and South America. The highest incidence of paragonimiasis occurs in older children and adolescents 11–15 yr of age. Although *P. westermani* is found in many carnivores, human cases are relatively rare and seem to be associated with specific dietary habits, such as eating raw freshwater crayfish or crabs. These crustaceans contain the infective metacercariae in their tissues. After ingestion, they excyst in the duodenum, penetrate the intestinal wall, and migrate to their final habitat in the lungs. Adult worms (5 × 10 mm) encapsulate within the lung parenchyma and deposit brown operculated eggs (60 × 100 μm), which pass into the bronchioles and are expectorated by coughing (Fig. 297–1). Ova can be detected in the sputum of infected individuals or in their feces. If eggs reach fresh water, they hatch and undergo asexual multiplication in specific snails. The cercariae encyst in the muscles and viscera of crayfish and freshwater crabs.

Most individuals infected with *P. westermani* harbor low or moderate worm loads and are asymptomatic. Hemoptysis is the principal *clinical manifestation,* occurring in 98% of symptomatic children. Other symptoms include cough and production of rust-colored sputum. There are no characteristic physical findings, but laboratory examination usually demonstrates marked eosinophilia. Chest roentgenogram often reveals small patchy infiltrates or radiolucencies in the middle lung fields; however, the roentgenogram may appear normal in one fifth of infected individuals. In rare circumstances, lung abscess, pleural effusion, or bronchiectasis may develop. Extrapulmonary localization of *P. westermani* in the brain, peritoneum, intestines, or pleura may rarely occur. Cerebral paragonimiasis is encountered primarily in heavily infected individuals living in highly endemic areas of the Far East; the clinical presentation resembles jacksonian epilepsy or cerebral tumors.

Definitive diagnosis of paragonimiasis is established by identification of eggs in fecal or sputum smears. The recommended treatment of paragonimiasis is praziquantel (75 mg/kg divided in three doses for 1 day).

INTESTINAL FLUKES. Several wild and domestic animal intestinal flukes, such as *Fasciolopsis buski, Nanophyetus salmincola,* and *Heterophyes heterophyes,* may accidentally infect humans. *F. buski* is endemic in the Far East. Humans who ingest metacercariae encysted on aquatic plants become infected. These develop into large flukes (1 × 5 cm) that inhabit the duodenum and jejunum. Mature worms produce operculated eggs that pass with feces; the organism completes its life cycle through specific snail intermediate hosts. Individuals with *F. buski* infection are usually asymptomatic; heavily infected subjects complain of abdominal pain and diarrhea and show signs of malabsorption. Diagnosis of fasciolopsiasis and other intestinal fluke infections is established by fecal examination and identification of the eggs. As for other fluke infections, praziquantel (75 mg/kg/24 hr divided in three doses for 1 day) is the drug of choice.

Fischer GW, McGrew GL, Bass JW: Pulmonary paragonimiasis in childhood. JAMA 243:1360, 1980.
King CH: Pulmonary Flukes. *In*: Mahmoud AAF (ed): Parasitic Lung Diseases. New York, Marcel Dekker, 1997, p 157.
Liu LX, Harinasuta KT: Liver and intestinal flukes. Gastroenterol Clin North Am 25:627, 1996.
Price TA, Tuazon CU, Simon GL: Fascioliasis: Case reports and review. Clin Infect Dis 17:426, 1993.

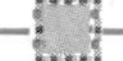

CHAPTER 298
Adult Tapeworm Infections

Ronald Blanton

Infections with cestodes, or tapeworms, are prevalent on every continent except Antarctica. Unlike many parasites that strictly segregate their developmental stages in different host species, some tapeworms can infect humans with the adult worm stage, the invasive intermediate stage, or both. The intermediate stages of some tapeworms are invasive and form cystic structures that result in tissue damage from mass effect or inflammatory reactions, such as echinococcosis (Chapter 300) and cysticercosis (Chapter 299). No signs or symptoms can clearly be attributed to infection with any adult tapeworm except for *Diphyllobothrium latum* infection. Infection with the adult worm can be easily diagnosed by finding eggs or segments of adult worms in the stool, whereas the invasive stage of the parasite cannot be observed in any easily sampled fluid. Infection with an intermediate stage, therefore, must be diagnosed by serologic tests, imaging, or invasive procedures.

TAENIASIS *(Taenia saginata* and *Taenia solium)*

ETIOLOGY. The beef tapeworm (*T. saginata*) and the pork tapeworm (*T. solium*) are large parasites (4–10 m) named for their intermediate hosts that are found only in the adult stage in the human intestine. The body of the adult stage is a connected series of hundreds or thousands of flattened segments, called proglottids, whose most anterior segment, the scolex, anchors the parasite to the bowel wall. New segments arise at the caudal end of the scolex, with sequentially progressive maturation of proglottids farther from the scolex. Both eggs and gravid terminal proglottids, packed with 50,000–100,000 eggs, pass intact in the stool. These two tapeworms differ most significantly in that the intermediate stage of the pork tapeworm (cysticercus) can also infect humans and cause significant morbidity (Chapter 299).

EPIDEMIOLOGY. Both *Taenia* species are distributed worldwide, with the highest risk of infection in Central America, Africa, India, Southeast Asia, and China. The prevalence in adults may not reflect the prevalence in young children, because cultural practices may dictate how well meat is cooked and how much is served to children.

PATHOGENESIS. Uncomplicated infection with the adult beef or pork tapeworm by itself is an infrequent source of symptoms. When children ingest raw or undercooked infected meat, gastric acid and bile release the cystic intermediate stage that attaches to the lumen of the small intestine. The parasite enlarges over 2–3 mo and matures, and gravid segments appear.

CLINICAL MANIFESTATIONS. Adult beef and pork tapeworms cause very little overt morbidity apart from nonspecific abdominal symptoms. The protoscolices of taeniids are visually striking. They are also motile and sometimes produce anal pruritus. They can often be felt as they pass and are thus likely to be noticed and cause a strong emotional reaction in older children and parents when discovered. Taeniids are rare causes of intestinal obstruction, cholangitis, and appendicitis.

DIAGNOSIS. It is important to identify the species of infecting *Taenia* tapeworm. Carriers of adult pork tapeworms are at increased risk of transmitting the pathogenic intermediate stage (cysticercus) to themselves or others, whereas children infected with the beef tapeworm are a risk only to livestock. Because proglottids are generally passed intact, visual examination for gravid proglottids in the stool is the most sensitive test and they may be used to identify species. Eggs, by contrast, are often absent from stool and cannot reliably distinguish between *T. saginata* and *T. solium* (Fig. 298–1). Microscopic examination of a rectal swab specimen or adhesive tape applied near the rectum is more sensitive for detecting eggs. If the parasite is completely expelled, the scolex of each species is diagnostic. The scolex of *T. saginata* has only a set of four anteriorly oriented suckers, whereas *T. solium* is armed with a double row of hooks in addition to suckers. The proglottids of

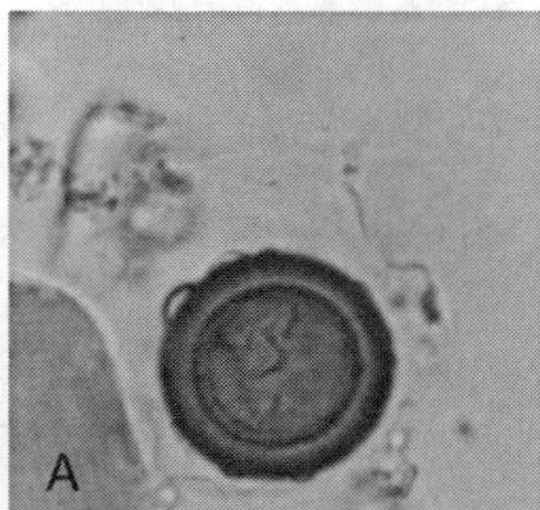

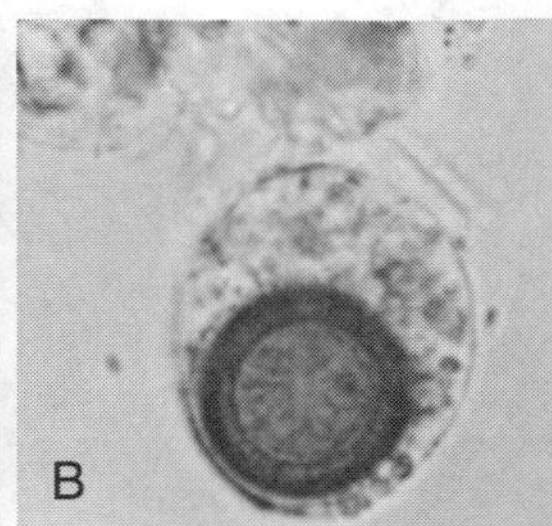

Figure 298–1 Eggs of *Taenia saginata* recovered from fresh feces (×400). The cellular structure in which the egg develops while in the proglottid, more evident in *B* than in *A*, may be retained around the dark prismatic egg membrane that contains the larva. Usually evident in the larva are three pairs of hooklets *(A)*, which may occasionally be seen in motion.

T. saginata have more than 20 uterine branches from a central uterine structure, and those of *T. solium* have 10 or fewer. When in doubt, more proglottids should be obtained or the sample should be referred to a laboratory with parasitologic expertise.

Differential Diagnosis. Anal pruritus may mimic symptoms of pinworm (*Enterobius vermicularis*) infection. *D. latum* or even *Ascaris lumbricoides* might be mistaken for *T. saginata* or *T. solium* in stools.

TREATMENT. Infections with all adult tapeworms respond to praziquantel. The recommended treatment for taeniasis is 5–10 mg/kg PO once Praziquantel tends to cause parasite death and subsequent resorption unless purged. An alternative treatment is niclosamide (1 g PO for children 11–34 lb; 1.5 g PO for 35 lb or greater). The parasite is usually expelled on the day of administration.

PREVENTION. Prolonged freezing or thorough cooking of beef and pork kills the parasite. Appropriate sanitation can interrupt transmission by preventing infection in livestock.

DIPHYLLOBOTHRIASIS (*Diphyllobothrium latum*)

ETIOLOGY. The fish tapeworm, *D. latum,* is the longest human tapeworm (10–20 m) and has an organization similar to that of other adult cestodes. An elongated scolex equipped with slits (bothria) along each side, but no suckers or hooks, is followed by thousands of segments looped in the small bowel. The terminal gravid proglottid detaches periodically but tends to disintegrate before expulsion, thus releasing its eggs into the feces. In contrast to taeniids, the life cycle of *D. latum* requires two intermediate hosts. Eggs hatch in fresh water and release embryos that are swallowed by small crustaceans (copepods). The parasite passes up the food chain as small fish eat the copepods and are in turn eaten by larger fish. In this way, the juvenile parasite becomes concentrated in pike, walleye, perch, salmon, and similar fish. Consumption of raw or undercooked fish leads to human infection with adult worms.

EPIDEMIOLOGY The fish tapeworm is most prevalent in the temperate climates of Europe, North America, and Asia but may be found in cold lakes at high altitude in South America and Africa. In North America, the prevalence is highest in Alaska, Canada, and the northern United States, and the tapeworm is found in fish from those areas brought to market in the continental United States. Persons who prepare raw fish for home or commercial use or who sample fish before cooking are particularly at risk for infection.

PATHOGENESIS. The adult worm efficiently scavenges vitamin B_{12} for its own use in the constant production of large numbers of segments and as many as 1 million eggs per day. The parasite also inhibits vitamin B_{12} uptake by inactivating the B_{12}-intrinsic factor complex. Diphyllobothriasis causes megaloblastic anemia in 2–9% of infections as a result of vitamin B_{12} and folate absorption by the parasite. Children with other causes of vitamin B_{12} or folate deficiency such as chronic infectious diarrhea, celiac disease, or congenital malabsorption are more likely to develop a symptomatic infection.

CLINICAL MANIFESTATIONS. Infection is largely asymptomatic except in those who develop B_{12} or folate deficiency. Megaloblastic anemia with decreased numbers of white blood cells and platelets, glossitis, and signs of spinal cord posterior column degeneration (loss of vibratory sense, proprioception, and coordination) can be evidence of advanced nutritional deficiency due to diphyllobothriasis. The hematologic and neurologic signs may present independently or together.

DIAGNOSIS. Parasitologic examination of the stool is useful because eggs are abundant in the feces and have a morphology distinct from that of all other tapeworms. The eggs are ovoid and have a cap structure at one end, the operculum, that opens to release the embryo (Fig. 298–2). The worm itself has a distinct scolex and proglottid morphology; however, these are not likely to be passed spontaneously.

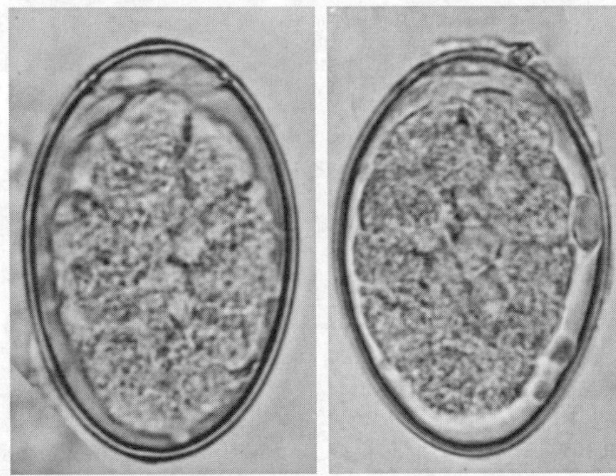

Figure 298–2 Eggs of *Diphyllobothrium latum* as seen in fresh feces (×400). The operculum is usually evident.

Differential Diagnosis. A segment or a whole section of the worm might be confused with *Taenia* or *Ascaris* after it is passed. Pernicious anemia, bone marrow toxins, and dietary restrictions may contribute to or mimic diphyllobothriasis.

TREATMENT. Infections with all adult tapeworms respond to praziquantel. The recommended treatment for diphyllobothriasis is 5–10 mg/kg PO once.

PREVENTION. The intermediate stage is easily eliminated by brief cooking or prolonged freezing. Because humans are the major reservoir for adult worms, health education is one of the most important tools for preventing transmission, together with improved human sanitation.

HYMENOLEPIASIS (*Hymenolepis*)

Infection with *Hymenolepis nana,* the dwarf tapeworm, is very common in developing countries. It is a major cause of eosinophilia, and although it rarely causes overt disease, the presence of *H. nana* eggs in stool may serve as a marker for exposure to poor hygienic conditions. Although the intermediate stage develops in various hosts (rodents, ticks, and fleas), the entire life cycle can be completed in humans. Hyperinfection with thousands of small adult worms in a single child is thus a potential. Less commonly, a similar infection may occur with the species *H. diminuta.* Eggs but not segments may be found in the stool. *H. nana* infection responds to praziquantel (25 mg/kg PO once) or niclosamide (1 g PO for children 11–34 lb, 1.5 g PO for ≥35 lb, for 6 days.

DIPYLIDIASIS (*Dipylidium caninum*)

Dipylidium caninum is a common tapeworm of domestic dogs and cats, yet human infections are relatively rare. Direct transmission between pets and humans does not occur; human infection requires ingestion of the parasite's intermediate host, the dog or cat flea. Infants and small children are particularly susceptible because of their level of hygiene, generally more intimate contact with pets, and activities in areas where fleas can be encountered. Eosinophilia may occur, but no symptoms clearly result from infection. Anal pruritus, vague abdominal pain, and diarrhea have at times been associated with dipylidiasis. Dipylidiasis is effectively treated with a single oral dose of praziquantel (5–10 mg/kg) or niclosamide (1 g for children 11–34 lb; 1.5 g for ≥35 lb). Deworming pets and flea control are the best preventive measures.

Botero D, Tanowitz HB, Weiss LM et al: Taeniasis and cysticercosis. Infect Dis Clin North Am 7:683, 1993.

Chappell CL, Enos JP, Penn HM: *Dipylidium caninum*, an underrecognized infection in infants and children. Pediatr Infect Dis J 9: 745, 1990.

Hamrick HJ, Bowdre JH, Church SM: Rat tapeworm (*Hymenolepsis diminuta*) infection in a child. Pediatr Infect Dis J 9:216, 1990.

CHAPTER 299
Cysticercosis

Ronald Blanton

ETIOLOGY. Cysticercosis is infection with the intermediate stage of *Taenia solium*, the pork tapeworm. The larval form is also called cysticercus, from the previous taxon, *Cysticercus cellulosae*, which was used for this form before the relationship to the adult *T. solium* was recognized. Cysticercosis is the most common parasitic cause of central nervous system (CNS) disease, known as neurocysticercosis. Whereas consumption of infected undercooked pork produces intestinal infection with the adult worm, humans acquire the intermediate form by ingestion of food or water contaminated with the eggs of *T. solium*. The disease may, therefore, develop even in individuals who do not eat pork. Individuals infected with an adult *T. solium* may also infect themselves with eggs by the fecal-oral route. Reverse peristalsis in the small intestine has also been implicated as another means of autoinfection.

In the small intestine, the egg releases an invasive form that crosses the gut wall and spreads hematogenously to many tissues but primarily brain and muscle. Wherever the eggs lodge, they produce small (0.2–0.5 cm) fluid-filled bladders containing a single juvenile-stage parasite (protoscolex).

EPIDEMIOLOGY. The pork tapeworm is distributed worldwide wherever pigs are raised. Intense transmission occurs in Mexico, Central America, India, Indonesia, Korea, and China as well as some areas of Africa. In these areas, 20–50% of cases of epilepsy may be due to cysticercosis. Most cases of cysticercosis in the United States are imported; transmission is uncommon but occurs on occasion.

PATHOGENESIS. The cystic stages of most tapeworms do not provoke a strong immunologic response while they remain alive and intact. Intact viable cysts can be associated with disease when the initial parasite invasion of the brain is massive or when they obstruct the flow of cerebrospinal fluid (CSF). Most cysts remain viable for 5–10 yr and then begin to degenerate, followed by a vigorous host response. The natural history of cysts is for final resolution by complete resorption or calcification.

CLINICAL MANIFESTATIONS. Seizures are the presenting finding in more than 70% of cases, although any cognitive or neurologic abnormality from psychosis to stroke may be a manifestation of cysticercosis. Neurocysticercosis can usually be classified on the basis of its clinical presentation and radiologic appearance as parenchymal, intraventricular, meningeal, spinal, or ocular. Parenchymal disease produces seizures as well as focal neurologic deficits. The seizures are generalized in 80% of cases but frequently begin as simple or complex partial seizures. Rarely, cerebral infarction can result from obstruction of small terminal arteries or vasculitis. With extensive frontal lobe disease, symptoms of intellectual deterioration with dementia or parkinsonism may obfuscate diagnosis until focal signs appear. A fulminant encephalitis-like presentation is also encountered, most frequently in children who have had a massive initial infection.

Intraventricular neurocysticercosis (5–10% of all cases) is associated with hydrocephalus and acute, subacute, or intermittent signs of increased intracranial pressure without localizing signs. The fourth ventricle is the most common site for obstruction and symptoms. Cysts in the laterval ventricles are less likely to cause obstruction. Chronic basilar meningitis is associated with many forms of neurocysticercosis, but some presentations are predominantly meningeal. In this form, in addition to signs of meningeal irritation, increased intracranial pressure results from either edema or inflammation or the presence of a cyst obstructing flow of CSF. Racemose cysticercosis is a form of meningeal cysticercosis in which large, lobulated cysts appear in the basal cisterns. Ocular cysticercosis causes decreased visual acuity due to cysticerci floating in the vitreous, retinal detachment, or iridocyclitis. Spinal neurocysticercosis presents with evidence of spinal cord compression, nerve root pain, transverse myelitis, or meningitis.

Outside of the CNS, cysts can sometimes be palpated under the skin, and very heavy infections in skeletal or heart muscle can result in myositis or carditis.

DIAGNOSIS. Cysticercosis should be suspected in any child with a history of residence in an endemic area or with a care provider from an endemic area, when that person presents with any neurologic, cognitive, or personality disorder. Seizures, hydrocephalus, unilateral visual impairment, or symptoms of encephalitis are particularly suspicious. *Taenia* eggs are observed in feces from only 25% of cases of neurocysticercosis; therefore, imaging studies and serologic tests are necessary to confirm a clinical suspicion.

The most useful diagnostic study is CT. A solitary parenchymal cyst with or without contrast enhancement and numerous calcifications are the most common findings in children (Fig. 299–1). Intraventricular cysts are found in 11–17% of cases of neurocysticercosis. These are difficult to detect because the cyst fluid often has the same density as CSF. Hydrocephalus on CT scan may suggest intraventricular cysts or meningeal inflammation. MRI better detects intraventricular cysts as well as those in the spinal cord by delineating parasite membranes and differences in signal intensity between the fluids and tissues of the cysticercus. The protoscolex may even be visible within the cyst on MRI and provides a pathognomonic sign of cysticercosis. MRI is also more sensitive for detecting evidence of inflammation around a cyst. Plain films may reveal calcifications in muscle or brain consistent with cysticercosis, but these are more often nondiagnostic in children than in adults.

Serologic diagnosis using the enzyme-linked immunotransfer blot (EITB) is available commercially in the United States and through the Centers for Disease Control and Prevention. Serum antibody testing has greater than 90% sensitivity and specificity; thus, a sample of CSF may not be required. Persons with many parenchymal cysts almost always have a positive serum EITB test result. Cases with solitary lesions or old calcified disease may not have detectable antibodies. Cysticercosis is the most important and probably most frequent cause

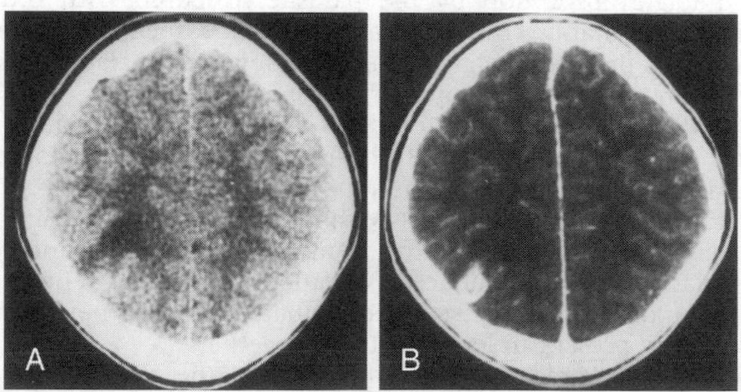

Figure 299–1 Computed tomography (CT) image of a solitary lesion of neurocysticercosis *(A)* with and *(B)* without contrast, showing contrast enhancement. (Courtesy of Dr. Wendy G. Mitchell and Dr. Marvin D. Nelson, Children's Hospital, Los Angeles.)

of eosinophilia in CSF, but this is not a reliable finding and if absent does not preclude the diagnosis.

Differential Diagnosis. Cysticercosis can be confused clinically with encephalitis, stroke, meningitis, and many other conditions. Clinical suspicion is based on travel history or a history of contact with an individual who might carry an adult tapeworm. On imaging studies, cysticerci can be mistaken for calcified tuberculomas, toxoplasmosis, or CNS tumor.

TREATMENT. The specific treatment of neurocysticercosis depends on disease presentation. Some issues concerning when and how to treat are still not resolved. Observation, symptomatic treatment, antiparasitic drugs, and surgery all may have a role. Children with seizures, with no hydrocephalus, and with only calcified, inactive lesions on CT do not require therapy other than antiseizure drugs. If no anticysticercal drugs are administered, however, it is also necessary to determine whether these patients carry adult worms and thus pose a public health risk. Niclosamide used in the treatment of adult worms is not absorbed and does not provoke an inflammatory response to cysticerci. Most seizures associated with inflammation, as demonstrated by CT or MRI, can be controlled using standard antiseizure drugs. If seizures recur or if seizures are associated with inactive lesions, treatment should be extended to 2–3 yr before attempting weaning from anticonvulsants.

Active parenchymal lesions usually resolve spontaneously, and some experts do not treat with anticysticercal drugs. Retrospective studies indicate, however, that anticysticercal chemotherapy is associated with fewer residual seizures on long-term follow-up. Two effective drugs are available, albendazole (15 mg/kg/24 hr divided in two doses for 28 days; maximum, 400 mg/dose), taken with a fatty meal to improve absorption, and praziquantel (50 mg/kg/24 hr divided in three doses for 15 days). Several studies indicate that albendazole produces a somewhat better outcome than praziquantel. A worsening of symptoms can follow the use of either drug as the host responds to the dying parasite with increased inflammation. Corticosteroids given for 2–3 days before and during drug therapy can ameliorate these effects but may decrease praziquantel levels by as much as 50%. An increase of praziquantel to 100 mg/24 hr in three doses or administration of cimetidine, an inhibitor of the cytochrome P450 system, has been advocated when both praziquantel and corticosteroids are used. Albendazole levels, in contrast, increase in the presence of corticosteroids.

Medical therapy may convert quiescent parenchymal lesions to active ones or may worsen ventricular, ocular, or spinal disease. A ventricular shunt must be placed before medical therapy whenever there is evidence of hydrocephalus or ventricular or spinal disease. Surgery should be limited to placement of shunts, removal of large solitary cysts for decompression, removal of mobile cysts causing ventricular obstruction, and some cases that fail to respond to medical therapy. Neuroendoscopy may be used to remove some ventricular cysts. Spillage of cyst contents during surgery is not associated with disseminating the parasite, as it is with echinococcosis. Ocular cysticercosis is essentially a surgical disease. The outcome is not good in any case, and enucleation is frequently required.

PREVENTION. All family members of index cases of cysticercosis, as well as persons handling their food, should be examined for signs of disease or evidence of adult worms. Attention to personal hygiene, proper handwashing by food handlers, and avoidance of fresh fruits and vegetables in areas endemic for *T. solium* help prevent ingestion of eggs. All pork should be cooked thoroughly.

White AC Jr: Neurocysticercosis: A major cause of neurological disease worldwide. Clin Infect Dis 24:101, 1997.

Monteiro L, Nunes B, Mendoça D, et al: Spectrum of epilepsy in neurocysticercosis: A long-term follow-up of 143 patients. Acta Neurol Scand 92:33, 1995.

Dachman WD, Adubofour KO, Bikin DS, et al: Cimetidine-induced rise in praziquantel levels in a patient with neurocysticercosis being treated with anticonvulsants. J Infect Dis 169:689, 1994.

CHAPTER 300
Echinococcosis (Echinococcus granulosus *and* E. multilocularis)

Ronald Blanton

ETIOLOGY. Echinococcosis (hydatid disease or hydatidosis) is the most widespread, serious human cestode infection in the world. It is a zoonosis transmitted from domestic and wild canid animals. Two *Echinococcus* species are responsible for distinct clinical presentations, *E. granulosus* (unilocular or cystic hydatid disease) and the more malignant *E. multilocularis* (alveolar hydatid disease). Dogs, wolves, dingoes, jackals, coyotes, and foxes become infected after eating infected viscera and are the hosts of the small adult worms (2–7 mm). The adult worms, which are composed of two to six proglottids, have a life span of about 5 mo. Eggs from adult worms are passed in stool and contaminate the soil and water, as well as the coats of dogs themselves. In the case of *E. granulosus,* domestic animals such as sheep, goats, cattle, and camels ingest the eggs while grazing. Humans are infected with the intermediate stage of the parasite when they ingest food or water contaminated with eggs or from direct contact with infected dogs. The intermediate forms penetrate the gut and are carried by the vascular or lymphatic systems to the liver, lungs, and less commonly to other tissues. A sylvatic cycle also exists for *E. granulosus* in a wolf/moose cycle in North America, but it is of less importance for transmission to humans. The transmission cycle of *E. multilocularis* is similar to that of *E. granulosus,* except that this species is mainly sylvatic and uses small rodents as its natural intermediate host. The rodents are consumed by foxes, their natural predators, and sometimes by dogs and cats.

EPIDEMIOLOGY. *E. granulosus* thrives in environments as diverse as arctic tundra and the deserts of North Africa. Wherever animals are herded by humans with the help of dogs, there is potential for transmission of this parasite. In urban areas, dogs may be infected by eating entrails remaining after home slaughter of domestic animals. Cysts have been detected in up to 10% of the human population in northern Kenya and Western China. In South America, the disease is prevalent in sheep-herding areas of the Andes, the beef-herding areas of the Brazilian/Argentine Pampas, and Uruguay. Among developed countries, the disease is well known in Italy, Greece, Portugal, Spain, and Australia. In North America, transmission occurs via the sylvatic cycle in Alaska, Canada, and Isle Royale on Lake Superior, as well as in foci of the domestic cycle in sheep-raising areas of the western United States.

Transmission of *E. multilocularis* occurs primarily in temperate climates of Northern Europe, Siberia, Turkey, and China. There is also an extensive area of transmission in Alaska, Canada, and the central United States as far south as Nebraska. Alveolar echinococcosis is, fortunately, uncommon. A separate species (*E. vogeli*) causes polycystic disease similar to alveolar hydatidosis in South America.

PATHOGENESIS. In areas endemic for *E. granulosus,* the parasite is often acquired in childhood, but liver cysts require many years to become large enough to detect or cause symptoms. In children, the lungs appear to be the most common site, although 70% of adults have disease in the right lobe of the liver. Cysts can also be found in bone, the genitourinary system, bowels, subcutaneous tissues, and brain. The host surrounds the primary cyst with a tough, fibrous capsule. Inside this capsule, the parasite produces a thick lamellar layer that supports a thin germinal layer of cells responsible for production of thousands of juvenile-stage parasites (protoscolices) that remain attached to the wall or are free in the cyst fluid. With cystic hydatidosis from *E. granulosus* infection, the established cyst may also produce smaller daughter cysts that remain contained within the primary cysts. The fluid in a healthy cyst is clear and watery. After medical treatment, it may become thick and bile stained.

Reproduction in *E. multilocularis* resembles a malignancy. The secondary reproductive units bud externally and are not confined within a single well-defined structure. Further, the cyst tissues are poorly demarcated from those of the host. This makes these cysts unsuitable for surgical removal. The secondary cysts are also capable of distant metastatic spread. The growing cyst mass eventually replaces a significant portion of the liver and compromises adjacent tissues and structures.

CLINICAL MANIFESTATIONS. The majority of cysts occur in the liver. Many cysts never become symptomatic and regress spontaneously. Those that become symptomatic initially have relatively nonspecific symptoms. Later, increased abdominal girth, hepatomegaly, a palpable mass, vomiting, or abdominal pain ensues. The more serious complications, however, are due to compression of adjacent structures, spillage of cyst contents, and location of cysts in sensitive areas such as the reproductive tract, brain, and bone. Anaphylaxis can occur with cyst rupture or spillage of cyst fluid intraoperatively. Jaundice due to cystic hydatid disease is rare. The second most common site is the lungs, where cysts produce chest pain, coughing, or hemoptysis. Bone cysts may cause pathologic fractures, and in the genitourinary system they can produce hematuria or infertility.

In alveolar hydatid disease, cyst tissue continues to proliferate and may separate and metastasize distantly. The proliferating mass compromises hepatic tissue or the biliary system and causes progressive obstructive jaundice hepatic failure. Symptoms also occur from extrahepatic foci.

DIAGNOSIS. On physical examination, subcutaneous nodules, hepatomegaly, or a palpable abdominal mass may be found. The parasite cannot be recovered from any easily accessible body fluid unless a lung cyst ruptures, after which protoscolices may briefly be seen in sputum. Ultrasonography has proved a very valuable tool in the diagnosis of hydatid disease. Portable machines and generators have made office diagnosis or survey of even isolated populations possible. Benign, simple cysts of the liver are relatively common, but the presence of internal membranes and floating echogenic cyst material (hydatid sand) strongly suggests hydatid disease. Alveolar disease is less cystic in appearance and resembles a diffuse solid tumor. CT findings (Fig. 300–1) are similar to those of ultrasonography and can at times be useful in distinguishing alveolar from cystic hydatid disease in geographic regions where both occur.

Serologic studies can be useful in confirming a diagnosis of echinococcosis, but the false-negative rate may be as high as 50% in cystic hydatid disease of the lungs or when only young, intact liver cysts are present. Most patients with alveolar hydatidosis, however, develop detectable antibody responses. Current tests use crude or partially purified antigens that can cross react in individuals infected with other parasites, such as in cysticercosis or schistosomiasis.

Differential Diagnosis. Cystic hydatid disease can usually be distinguished from benign hepatic cysts on ultrasonography by the presence of either internal structures or hydatid sand. The density of bacterial hepatic abscesses is distinct from the watery cystic fluid characteristic of *E. granulosus* infection, but hydatid cysts may be complicated by secondary bacterial infection. Alveolar echinococcosis is often confused with hepatoma and

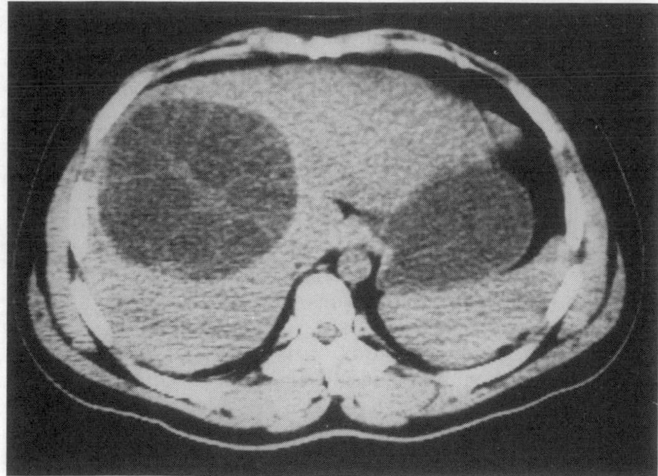

Figure 300–1 Computed tomography (CT) image of an hepatic *Echinococcus granulosus* hydatid cyst. The membranes of multiple internal daughter cysts are visible within the primary cyst structure. (Courtesy of Dr. John R. Haaga, University Hospitals, Cleveland.)

cirrhosis and presents features suggestive of pancreatic carcinoma, metastatic liver disease, and cholangitis.

TREATMENT. Hydatidosis is still primarily a surgical disease. For *E. granulosus* disease, open surgical procedures are rapidly loosing favor to ultrasound- or CT-guided *p*ercutaneous *a*spiration, *i*nstillation of hypertonic saline or another scolicidal agent, and *r*easpiration after 15 min (PAIR). Spillage with PAIR is surprisingly uncommon, but prophylactic albendazole therapy is recommended. At present, PAIR is appropriate for small simple cysts of the liver, but larger more complicated cysts, lung cysts, and renal cysts have been successfully treated. Cysts found to have bile-stained fluid should not be injected with a scolicidal agent because toxicity is increased.

For conventional surgery, the inner cyst wall (laminate and germinal layers) can be easily peeled from the fibrous layer, and only these inner layers need be removed. The cavity is then topically sterilized and either closed or filled with omentum. Considerable care must be taken to avoid spillage of cyst contents, because cyst fluid contains viable protoscolices, each capable of producing secondary cysts wherever it lodges. Another risk is development of anaphylaxis to spilled cyst fluid as a result of surgery, spontaneous rupture, or trauma.

For *E. granulosus* cysts not amenable to PAIR or surgery, albendazole (15 mg/kg/24 hr divided in two doses for 28 days; maximum, 400/dose) is the preferred drug for treatment. A positive response occurs in 40–60% of patients. The course is often repeated for four or more cycles, with 15-day drug-free intervals. Morbid inflammatory response to chemotherapy is not common, as it is in cysticercosis, and corticosteroids thus are not indicated unless patients have anaphylaxis or another allergic response. Ultrasonographic indications of successful therapy are a change in shape from spherical to elliptical or flat, progressive increase in echogenicity, and detachment of membranes from the capsule (water lily sign). Additional CT criteria are reduction in diameter and augmented density of cyst fluid up to that of other tissues.

Alveolar hydatidosis is frequently incurable by any modality, but radical surgery such as partial hepatectomy or lobectomy may cure early limited disease. Medical therapy with albendazole may slow the progression of alveolar hydatidosis, but if at all feasible, removal of the infected tissue is indicated.

PROGNOSIS. Factors predictive of success with chemotherapy are age of the cyst (>2 yr), low internal complexity of the cyst, and small size. The site of the cyst is not important, although cysts in bone respond poorly. For alveolar hydatidosis, if surgical removal is successful, the average mortality is 92% by 10 yr after diagnosis.

PREVENTION. Important measures to interrupt transmission include, above all, thorough handwashing, avoiding contact with dogs in endemic areas, boiling or filtering water when camping, proper disposal of animal carcasses, and proper meat inspection. Strict procedures for proper disposal of refuse from slaughterhouses must be instituted and followed so that dogs or wild carnivores do not have access to entrails. Other useful measures are control or treatment of the feral dog population and regular praziquantel treatment of pets and working dogs in endemic areas.

Filice C, Brunetti E: Use of PAIR in human cystic echinococcosis. Acta Trop 64:95, 1997.
Finlay JC, Speert DP: Sylvatic hydatid disease in children: Case reports and review of endemic *Echinococcus granulosus* infection in Canada and Alaska. Pediatr Infect Dis J 11:322, 1992.
Gottstein B: *Echinococcus multilocularis* infection: Immunology and immunodiagnosis. Adv Parasitol 31:321, 1992.
Kammerer WS, Schantz PM: Echinococcal disease. Infect Dis Clin North Am 7:605, 1993.
Khuroo MS, Wani NA, Javid G, et al: Percutaneous drainage compared with surgery for hepatic hydatid cysts. N Engl J Med 337:881, 1997.
Teggi A, Lastilla MG, De Rosa F: Therapy of human hydatid disease with mebendazole and albendazole. Antimicrob Agents Chemother 37:1679, 1993.

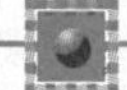

SECTION 15

Preventive Measures

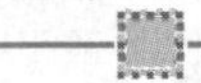

CHAPTER 301

Immunization Practices

Georges Peter

Immunization represents a remarkably successful and very cost-effective means of preventing infectious diseases. As a result of routine childhood immunizations, the occurrence of once common contagious diseases declined markedly in the United States and other countries in the second half of the 20th century. Public health programs based on vaccination have led to global eradication of smallpox, elimination of poliomyelitis from the Americas and possibly from the world in the near future, and greater than 95% reduction in the United States and other countries of invasive *Haemophilus influenzae* type b (Hib) disease. In the United States, immunization has almost eliminated congenital rubella syndrome, tetanus, and diphtheria and has reduced the incidence of rubella and measles to record low rates. Infants and children in this country routinely receive vaccines against 10 diseases: diphtheria, tetanus, pertussis, poliomyelitis, measles, mumps, rubella, Hib infection, hepatitis B, and varicella. Rotavirus vaccine is also recommended, with the realization that universal immunization may require additional time and resources. Hepatitis A vaccine is recommended for some groups of children. More than 50 immunobiologic products are licensed in the United States.

DEFINITIONS AND GENERAL CONCEPTS

Vaccination is administration of any vaccine or toxoid (inactivated toxin) for prevention of disease. Immunization is the process of inducing immunity artificially by either vaccination (active immunization) or administration of antibody (passive immunization). Active immunization involves stimulating the immune system to produce antibodies and cellular immune responses that protect against the infectious agent. Passive immunization consists of providing temporary protection through administration of exogenously produced antibody, such as immune globulin. Passive immunization also occurs naturally through transplacental transmission of antibodies to a fetus, which provides protection against many infectious diseases for the first 3 mo of life.

Immunizing agents include vaccines, toxoids, antitoxins, and immune globulins derived from human or animal donors (Table 301–1). Immune globulins for passive immunization now can be prepared from monoclonally produced antibody. Most of these immunizing agents contain preservatives, stabilizers, antibiotics, adjuvants, and a suspending fluid (Table 301–2).

The current approaches to active immunization are the use of (1) live-attenuated infectious agents and (2) inactivated or detoxified agents, their extracts, or specific recombinant products (e.g., hepatitis B vaccine). For many diseases, such as poliomyelitis and typhoid fever, both approaches have been used. Live-attenuated vaccines are more likely than killed vaccines to induce an immunologic response simulating the response to natural infection. Inactivated or killed vaccines include inactivated whole organisms (e.g., whole-cell pertussis and hepatitis A vaccines), detoxified exotoxins (e.g., tetanus and diphtheria toxoids), purified protein antigens (e.g., acellular pertussis and hepatitis B vaccines), polysaccharide (capsular pneumococcal vaccine), capsular polysaccharide conjugated to a carrier protein (e.g., Hib conjugate vaccines), or components of the organism (e.g., subunit influenza vaccine).

Because the organisms in live vaccines multiply in the recipient until the desired immune response occurs (similar to that which occurs in natural infection), the live-attenuated viral

TABLE 301–1 Immunizing Agents

Agent	Definition
Vaccine	A preparation of proteins, polysaccharides, or nucleic acids of pathogens that are delivered to the immune system as single entities, as part of complex particles, or by live-attenuated agents or vectors, to induce specific responses that inactivate, destroy, or suppress the pathogen
Toxoid	A modified bacterial toxin that has been made nontoxic but retains the capacity to stimulate the formation of antitoxin
Immune globulin	An antibody-containing solution derived from human blood obtained by cold ethanol fractionation of large pools of plasma and used primarily for the maintenance of immunity of immunodeficient persons or for passive immunization; available in intramuscular and intravenous preparations
Antitoxin	An antibody derived from the serum of humans or animals after stimulation with specific antigens; used to provide passive immunity

TABLE 301–2 Constituents of Vaccines

Component	Use and Examples
Preservatives, stabilizers, antibiotics	Constituents can inhibit or prevent bacterial growth or stabilize the antigen. Materials such as mercurials or antibiotics are used. Allergic reactions to any of the additives may occur.
Adjuvants	An aluminum salt is used in some vaccines to enhance the immune response (e.g., toxoids, hepatitis B).
Suspending fluid	Sterile water, saline, or more complex fluids derived from the growing media or biologic system in which the agent is produced (e.g., egg antigens, cell culture ingredients, serum proteins).

vaccines (e.g., measles, rubella, and mumps) are considered likely to confer lifelong protection with a single immunizing dose. In contrast, many inactivated or killed vaccines, which have a lesser antigenic mass, require booster vaccinations to provide protection.

DETERMINANTS OF THE IMMUNE RESPONSE. Responses of individuals to the same vaccine vary because the immune response to specific antigens is genetically determined. The extensive polymorphism of the major histocompatibility complex (MHC) in humans results in recognition by different individuals of different epitopes within a complex protein antigen. To vaccinate a population effectively, a vaccine must contain epitopes that are processed and bound to the product of at least one MHC allele in most, if not all, individuals.

The nature and magnitude of the response to vaccines or toxoids are determined by many factors, including the chemical and physical state of the antigen, the mode of administration, the catabolic rate of the antigen, host factors (e.g., age, nutrition, gender, and pre-existing antibody), and antigen processing as well as the genetic determinants of the host. The age-dependent differences in immune responses are a particularly important consideration in the routine immunization schedule of infants and young children. The presence of high concentrations of maternal antibody in the first few months of life and the relative immaturity of the immune response impair the initial immune response to some vaccines.

The route of administration is another important factor in the immune response. Parenterally administered vaccines may not induce mucosal secretory IgA, whereas vaccines given orally are expected to do so. The immunogenicity of some vaccines is reduced when not given by the proper route; for example, subcutaneous administration of hepatitis B into the fatty tissue of the buttock rather than intramuscularly in the deltoid of adults results in substantially lower seroconversion rates.

IMMUNE RESPONSE TO VACCINE ANTIGENS. Antibodies to vaccine constituents may be of any immunoglobulin class. Important protective antibodies include those that inactivate soluble toxic protein products of bacteria (i.e., antitoxins), facilitate phagocytosis and intracellular digestion of bacteria (i.e., opsonins), interact with components of serum complement to damage the bacterial membrane with resultant bacteriolysis (i.e., lysins), prevent proliferation of infectious virus (i.e., neutralizing antibodies), and interact with components of the bacterial surface to prevent adhesion to mucosal surfaces (i.e., antiadhesins). Antibodies function alone or in conjunction with other components of the immune system by participating directly in the neutralization of a toxin (e.g., diphtheria); by opsonization of virus (e.g., poliovirus); by initiating or combining with complement and promoting phagocytosis (e.g., pneumococcus); by reacting with nonsensitized lymphocytes to stimulate phagocytosis; or by sensitizing macrophages to stimulate phagocytosis.

Many of the structural constituents of microorganisms and exotoxins are antigenic. Most antigens require the interaction of B lymphocytes and T lymphocytes to generate an immune response and thus are termed T (thymus)–dependent antigens. However, some antigens initiate B-cell proliferation and antibody production without the help of T cells and thus are T-independent antigens. In contrast to T-dependent antigens, most T-independent antigens are poor immunogens in children younger than 2 yr. Because many purified polysaccharides are T-independent antigens, vaccines composed of these antigens (e.g., pneumococcal and meningococcal) are often ineffective in infants and young children. However, by conjugation to a protein carrier, a polysaccharide can acquire the antigenic properties of the protein and resulting characteristics of a T-dependent antigen, including immunogenicity in infants. This phenomenon is the basis of the development of Hib conjugate vaccines.

The first step in induction of a T-dependent antibody response is activation of T-helper (CD4+) lymphocytes by presentation of an antigen to mononuclear phagocytes or dendritic cells, a step that may be facilitated by an adjuvant. Antigen presentation triggers the secretion of a cascade of mediators, called cytokines, which stimulate the maturation of naive T-helper cells and communication between leukocytes, using interleukins to regulate the immune response.

In the primary response to a vaccine antigen, a latent period of several days elapses before humoral and cell-mediated immunity can be detected. Serum antibodies initially are detected usually 7–10 days or more after vaccination. The immunoglobulin class of the response evolves and varies with the type of antigen. Early-appearing antibodies are usually IgM; later-appearing antibodies are usually IgG. IgM and IgG antibodies are secreted initially by B lymphocytes in response to thymus-dependent antigens. IgM antibodies are detectable first and fix complement, which facilitates lysis and phagocytosis of microorganisms. The IgM titer diminishes and the IgG titer rises during the 2nd wk or later. IgG responses peak within 2–6 wk. The switch from IgM synthesis to predominately IgG synthesis in B lymphocytes requires T-lymphocyte cooperation. IgG antibodies are produced in high concentrations and are critical to resistance to infections. Their functions include affinity to microorganisms, viral neutralization, precipitation of antigens, and fixation of complement.

Live-virus vaccines given orally (e.g., poliovirus and rotavirus) replicate at mucosal surfaces before host invasion and induce secretory IgA at respiratory, gastrointestinal, and other local sites. IgA antibodies neutralize viruses efficiently, fix complement through the alternative pathway, prevent absorption of organisms to the intestinal wall, and lyse gram-negative bacteria with complement and lysozyme. Most other types of vaccines do not effectively induce secretory IgA antibodies.

Heightened humoral or cell-mediated responses are elicited by a second exposure to the same T-dependent antigen. Secondary responses occur rapidly, usually within 4–5 days, result from immunologic memory mediated by T and B lymphocytes, and are characterized by a marked proliferation of antibody-producing B lymphocytes or effector T lymphocytes. However, T-independent antigens such as polysaccharide vaccines do not evoke these heightened secondary immune responses.

The response to vaccines in clinical practice is assessed by the serum concentration of specific antibody. The presence of circulating antibodies usually correlates with protection, and for some vaccines (e.g., tetanus, diphtheria, and Hib) the specific antibody titers that indicate protection have been established. However, antibody seroconversion and concentrations are only one parameter of the host response. Cellular immunity also is important but is much more difficult to measure and to correlate with protection. Amnestic responses on revaccination, which indicate immunologic memory, suggest that immunity may be persistent. Accordingly, the lack of detectable serum antibody may not mean that the individual is unprotected, particularly with infections that have a long incubation period, such as hepatitis B.

Stimulation of the immune system by vaccination, independent of antibody production, may elicit unanticipated responses, especially hypersensitivity reactions. For example, killed measles vaccine induced incomplete humoral immunity and cell-mediated hypersensitivity, resulting in the development of a syndrome of atypical measles (Chapter 240) in some children after subsequent infection by wild-type virus.

VACCINE RECOMMENDATIONS

Many factors are considered in the development of recommendations and schedules for vaccine administration: the epidemiology of the disease, age-specific morbidity and mortality, vaccine immunogenicity, risks of vaccine-related adverse reactions, cost effectiveness, and the ages of recommended routine health care visits. In general, vaccines for universal administration to children are recommended at the youngest age at which significant risk of disease and its complications exist and at which a protective immunologic response can be expected. Other vaccines are recommended only in special circumstances, such as for children at increased risk for infection during foreign travel (e.g., hepatitis A vaccine), those at increased risk of severe infections (e.g., pneumococcal vaccine for children with sickle cell disease), and those with particular exposure (e.g., rabies vaccine in children bitten by a potentially rabid animal).

In the United States, recommendations for pediatric immunization are formulated by two committees, the Advisory Committee on Immunization Practices (ACIP) of the Centers for Disease Control and Prevention (CDC), and the American Academy of Pediatrics (AAP) Committee on Infectious Diseases. Beginning in 1995, these two committees and the American Academy of Family Physicians (AAFP) have issued an annual national schedule for routinely recommended childhood vaccinations.

VACCINES FOR ROUTINE USE IN CHILDREN AND ADOLESCENTS. The 1999 recommended immunization schedule for infants and children in the United States is given in Figure 301–1. All children should be vaccinated against diphtheria, tetanus, pertussis, poliomyelitis, measles, mumps, rubella, Hib, hepatitis B, and varicella unless contraindicated. Rotavirus vaccine also is recommended by the ACIP and AAP. To complete this schedule by 18 mo of age necessitates a minimum of 11 injections in four visits.

The first dose of hepatitis B is recommended to be given at birth. This is especially important for infants of hepatitis B surface antigen (HBsAg)–positive mothers (Chapter 177).

For poliomyelitis immunization, expanded use of inactivated poliovirus vaccine (IPV) is now recommended in the United States to reduce the risk of vaccine-associated paralytic poliomyelitis associated with oral poliovirus vaccine (OPV). The recommended regimen is IPV only at 2 mo, 4 mo, 6–18 mo, and 4–6 yr of age. OPV may be used for unvaccinated children who will be traveling within 4 wk to areas where polio is endemic and for the third and fourth doses for children whose parents do not accept the number of required vaccine injections. OPV should be used in areas where polio is endemic.

Acellular pertussis vaccine, combined with diphtheria and tetanus toxoids (DTaP), is now the preferred vaccine for pertussis immunization. After the 7th birthday, combined tetanus and diphtheria toxoids in the adult formulation (Td), containing a lesser amount of diphtheria toxoid, are recommended for both primary and booster vaccination. The first booster dose of Td is recommended at 11–12 yr of age and is followed by a booster at 10-yr intervals thereafter.

Both the AAP and ACIP now recommend that the second dose of measles-containing vaccine (given as measles-mumps-rubella [MMR]) should be routinely given before school entry at 4–6 yr of age.

Varicella vaccine is recommended beginning at 12 mo of age and for older children through 12 yr of age if they have not been previously immunized or if they lack a reliable history of chickenpox.

Postlicensure surveillance of rotovirus vaccine identified several cases of intussusception among vaccine recipients. Use of the vaccine was suspended in July 1999. Physicians should monitor updated recommendations for use of rotavirus vaccine.

To enhance the delivery of vaccines to adolescents, a routine visit at 11–12 yr of age has been established for administration of the first Td booster and, if not already immunized, for hepatitis B and varicella vaccination and the second dose of MMR if not previously administered.

Simultaneous Administration of Multiple Vaccines. Most vaccines can be given simultaneously without impairment of effectiveness or safety. Simultaneous administration of vaccines is particularly important for inadequately immunized children in order to ensure timely completion of the recommended schedule. New combination products facilitate administration of multiple vaccines by reducing the number of necessary injections.

Interchangeability of Vaccine Products. Vaccines made by different manufacturers but directed against the same infections are generally considered interchangeable for the primary series and recommended booster doses. The exception is DTaP. Because data are not available on the safety, immunogenicity, and efficacy of different DTaP vaccines given in the primary series, the same product should be used, whenever feasible, for the first three doses of the pertussis vaccination schedule. However, in circumstances in which the type of DTaP product received previously is not known or the previously administered product is not readily available, any licensed product may be used to complete the primary series of three doses.

Lapsed Immunizations. In general, intervals between vaccine doses that exceed those that are recommended do not adversely affect the immunologic response, provided the immunization series is completed. Hence, reinstituting the immunization series or giving additional doses is not indicated under these circumstances.

VACCINES WITH SELECTED INDICATIONS. Vaccines with selected indications for children include influenza, pneumococcal polysaccharide, hepatitis A, meningococcal polysaccharide, rabies, and those given primarily for international travel.

Influenza vaccine should be given annually in the fall to those children 6 mo of age or older who are at increased risk for severe influenza disease or its complications. Major risk factors are asthma and other chronic pulmonary diseases (e.g., cystic fibrosis), congenital heart disease, HIV infection, other immunosuppressive disorders and therapy, sickle cell anemia, and aspirin therapy. Vaccination also should be considered for children with diabetes mellitus, other chronic metabolic disorders, and chronic renal disease and for those traveling to foreign countries where influenza may be occurring.

Pneumococcal vaccine is a 23-valent polysaccharide vaccine with limited but important recommended indications for children with sickle cell disease, asplenia, nephrotic syndrome, renal failure, HIV infection, and organ transplants. Because the vaccine is composed of T-independent antigens, it is not recommended until 2 yr of age. A single revaccination is recommended 3–5 yr later if the child remains at increased risk of severe or frequent infections. For older children who were initially immunized 5 yr or more before, revaccination also is indicated.

A vaccine for Lyme disease, based on recombinant OspA protein, has been licensed in the United States for persons 15 yr of age and older. Protection requires three doses at 0-, 1-, and 12-mo intervals. The vaccine is not approved for use in younger children, although studies are in progress. This vaccine may be considered for use in endemic areas for persons 15 yr of age and older who have frequent or prolonged exposure to ticks.

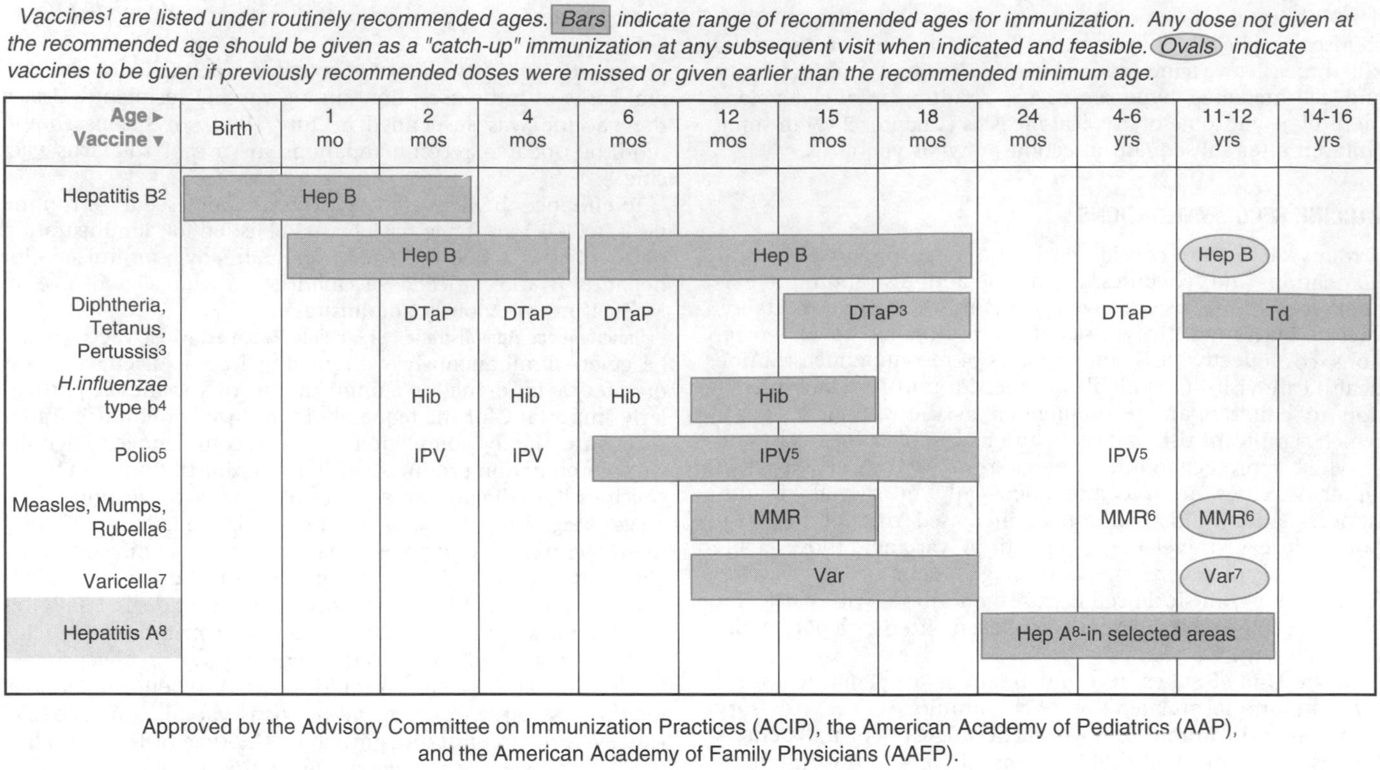

Vaccines[1] are listed under routinely recommended ages. Bars indicate range of recommended ages for immunization. Any dose not given at the recommended age should be given as a "catch-up" immunization at any subsequent visit when indicated and feasible. Ovals indicate vaccines to be given if previously recommended doses were missed or given earlier than the recommended minimum age.

Age ▸ / Vaccine ▾	Birth	1 mo	2 mos	4 mos	6 mos	12 mos	15 mos	18 mos	24 mos	4-6 yrs	11-12 yrs	14-16 yrs
Hepatitis B[2]	Hep B											
			Hep B			Hep B					(Hep B)	
Diphtheria, Tetanus, Pertussis[3]			DTaP	DTaP	DTaP		DTaP[3]			DTaP	Td	
H.influenzae type b[4]			Hib	Hib	Hib	Hib						
Polio[5]			IPV	IPV		IPV[5]				IPV[5]		
Measles, Mumps, Rubella[6]						MMR				MMR[6]	(MMR[6])	
Varicella[7]							Var				(Var[7])	
Hepatitis A[8]										Hep A[8]-in selected areas		

Approved by the Advisory Committee on Immunization Practices (ACIP), the American Academy of Pediatrics (AAP), and the American Academy of Family Physicians (AAFP).

Figure 301–1 Recommended childhood immunization schedule, United States, January-December 2000.

---

[1]This schedule indicates the recommended ages for routine administration of currently licensed childhood vaccines. Any dose not given at the recommended age should be given as a "catch-up" vaccination at any subsequent visit when indicated and feasible. Combination vaccines may be used whenever any components of the combination are indicated and its other components are not contraindicated. Providers should consult the manufacturers' package inserts for detailed recommendations.

[2]*Infants born to HBsAg-negative mothers* should receive the 2nd dose of hepatitis B vaccine at least 1 month after the 1st dose. The 3rd dose should be administered at least 4 months after the 1st dose and at least 2 months after the 2nd dose, but not before 6 months of age for infants.

Infants born to HBsAg-positive mothers should receive hepatitis B vaccine and 0.5 mL hepatitis immune globulin (HBIG) within 12 hours of birth at separate sites. The 2nd dose is recommended at 1–2 months of age and the 3rd dose at 6 months of age.

Infants born to mothers whose HBsAg status is unknown should receive hepatitis B vaccine within 12 hours of birth. Maternal blood should be drawn at the time of delivery to determine the mother's HBsAg status; if the HBsAg test is positive, the infant should receive HBIG as soon as possible (no later than 1 week of age).

All children and adolescents (through 18 years of age) who have not been immunized against hepatitis B may begin the series during any visit. Special efforts should be made to immunize children who were born in or whose parents were born in areas of the world with moderate or high endemicity of HBV infection.

[3]DTaP (diphtheria and tetanus toxoids and acellular pertussis vaccine) is the preferred vaccine for all doses in the immunization series, including completion of the series in children who have received 1 or more doses of whole-cell DTP vaccine. Whole-cell DTP is an acceptable alternative to DTaP. The 4th dose (DTP or DTaP) may be administered as early as 12 months of age, provided 6 months have elapsed since the 3rd dose and if the child is unlikely to return at age 15–18 months. Td (tetanus and diphtheria toxoids) is recommended at 11–12 years of age if at least 5 years have elasped since the last dose of DTP, DTaP, or DT. Subsequent routine Td boosters are recommended every 10 years.

[4]Three *H. influenzae* type b (Hib) conjugate vaccines are licensed for infant use. If PRP-OMP (PedvaxHIB and COMVAX [Merck]) is administered at 2 and 4 months of age, a dose at 6 months is not required. Because clinical studies in infants have demonstrated that using some combination products may induce a lower immune response to the Hib vaccine component, DTaP/Hib combination products should not be used for primary immunization in infants at 2, 4, or 6 months of age, unless FDA approved for these ages.

[5]Two poliovirus-vaccines currently are licensed in the United States: inactivated poliovirus vaccine (IPV) and oral poliovirus vaccine (OPV). The ACIP, AAP and AAFP now recommend that the first two doses of poliovirus vaccine should be IPV. The ACIP continues to recommend a sequential schedule of two doses of IPV administered at ages 2 and 4 months, followed by two doses of OPV at 12–18 months and 4–6 years. Use of IPV for doses also is acceptable and is recommended for immunocompromised persons and their household contacts.

OPV is no longer recommended for the first two doses of the schedule and is acceptable only for special circumstances such as: children of parents who do not accept the recommended number of injections, late initiation of immunization which would require an unacceptable number of injections, and imminent travel to polio-endemic areas. OPV remains the vaccine of choice for mass immunization campaigns to control outbreaks due to wild poliovirus.

[6]Rotavirus (Rv) vaccine is shaded and italicized to indicate: 1) health care providers may require time and resources to incorporate this new vaccine into practice; and 2) the AAFP opinion is that the decision to use rotavirus vaccine should be made by the parent or guardian in consultation with their physician or other health care provider. The first dose of Rv vaccine should not be administered before 6 weeks of age, and the minimum interval between doses is 3 weeks. The Rv vaccine series should not be initiated at 7 months of age or older, and all doses should be completed by the first birthday.

[7]The 2nd dose of measles, mumps, and rubella vaccine (MMR) is recommended routinely at 4–6 years of age but may be administered during any visit, provided at least 4 weeks have elapsed since receipt of the 1st dose and that both doses are administered beginning at or after 12 months of age. Those who have not previously received the second dose should complete the schedule by the 11- to 12-year-old visit.

[8]Varicella vaccine is recommended at any visit on or after the first birthday for susceptible children, i.e, those who lack a reliable history of chickenpox (as judged by a health care provider) and who have not been immunized. Susceptible persons 13 years of age or older should receive 2 doses, given at least 4 weeks apart.

International travel is an indication for vaccines not routinely given to children, in circumstances when the risk of exposure to the diseases is increased in relation to that in their home country. For children living in North America, vaccines include those against hepatitis A, typhoid fever, meningococcal disease, yellow fever, and Japanese encephalitis, depending on the location and circumstances of the travel (Chapter 304). In general, children and adolescents should have received all routinely recommended vaccines for their age before departure. The second dose of measles vaccine (as MMR) should be given to children and adolescents who have received only one dose irrespective of age, provided an interval of 4 wk or more has elapsed since the first dose, because the risk of exposure to cases of measles may be substantial in some countries. Influenza vaccine also should be considered for children traveling to areas where influenza outbreaks are occurring. Some countries may require yellow fever vaccination for entry.

ADVERSE EVENTS AFTER VACCINATION

Modern vaccines, although safe and effective, can be associated with adverse events ranging in severity from mild to life threatening. In addition, because no vaccine can be expected to be completely effective, some persons may develop disease after exposure despite vaccination.

Vaccine components can cause allergic reactions in some recipients. These components include the protective antigens, other components of the microorganisms, animal proteins introduced during vaccine production, antibiotics and other preservatives, or stabilizers such as gelatin. Reactions may be local or systemic, including anaphylaxis and urticaria. Local or systemic reactions result from too frequent administration of some vaccines, such as tetanus toxoids or rabies, and are probably caused by antigen-antibody complexes.

Some adverse events, however, occur coincidentally in temporal association with vaccination and are not caused by the vaccine. Determination of causality of an adverse event in a single child may be difficult. Epidemiologic and related studies are necessary to ascertain the incidence and nature of adverse reactions to vaccines and are important in ensuring a scientific rationale for vaccine use recommendations. The decision to use a vaccine involves assessment of the risk of disease, the benefit of vaccination, and the risk associated with vaccination. Vaccine precautions and contraindications are based on these factors, which may be modified with new information. Thus, continued reassessment of vaccine indications and safety is necessary.

PRECAUTIONS AND CONTRAINDICATIONS

Knowledge of vaccine contraindications and precautions is an important aspect of immunization practice (Table 301–3). A precaution specifies a circumstance in which a vaccine may be indicated if the benefit to an individual is judged to outweigh the risk and consequences of an adverse event. In contrast, a contraindication indicates that the vaccine should not be administered. Applying valid contraindications and precautions helps to minimize the occurrence of adverse reactions and maintain the health of children. Deciding not to vaccinate a child because of an inappropriate contraindication or precaution denies the child the benefit of immunization and is a missed opportunity for vaccination.

Generic contraindications to vaccination include moderate or severe illness, regardless of the presence or absence of fever; an anaphylactic reaction to a previous dose of the same vaccine; and an anaphylactic reaction to a vaccine constituent, such as egg proteins, gelatin, or an antibiotic. Viral vaccines that contain egg proteins, associated with vaccine production using embryonated chicken eggs or chicken embryo fibroblast tissue culture, include measles, mumps, influenza, and yellow fever. Measles and mumps vaccines, however, contain insignificant amounts of egg proteins, and persons with hypersensitivity to eggs are at negligible risk for anaphylactic reactions to these vaccines. As a result, skin testing with measles vaccine is not predictive of a subsequent allergic reaction to vaccination.

Administration of live-virus vaccines (e.g., MMR, OPV, and varicella) is generally contraindicated in immunocompromised persons, including recipients of high-dose corticosteroids. The exception is measles vaccine, which is recommended for HIV-infected persons who are not severely immunosuppressed (Chapter 268).

Because of the theoretical risk to a developing fetus, live-virus vaccines in most cases are not recommended during pregnancy. However, inadvertent vaccination is not necessarily a reason for termination of pregnancy, and some live-virus vaccines (e.g., OPV, influenza, and yellow fever) can be given to pregnant women. Influenza vaccine is specifically recommended for pregnant women who will be in the 2nd or 3rd trimester (≥14 wk gestation) of pregnancy during the influenza season (December through March), because of the increased morbidity of influenza in pregnant women.

In some recipients, vaccines can cause severe reactions that may constitute contraindications or precautions to subsequent administration of the specific vaccine. An example is the contraindication to further doses of DTP or DTaP if encephalopathy occurs within 7 days of administration of a previous dose of either DTP or DTaP. In contrast, a history of a temperature of 40.5°C or greater (≥105°F) within 48 hr of a prior dose is a precaution. In most cases in this circumstance, further doses of DTaP or DTP would not be given. However, if an epidemic of pertussis were occurring in the community, the potential benefit to the child of completing the immunization series may be greater than the risk of recurrence of a severe febrile reaction attributed to pertussis vaccine, the consequences of which are unknown.

VACCINES IN SPECIAL CIRCUMSTANCES

Indications for vaccination also involve considerations of the immunologic status of a child and exposure to infection. As a result, in special circumstances, immunization recommendations may be different from those for most other children.

IMMUNODEFICIENCY. Recommendations for vaccination of immunocompromised persons vary according to the degree and cause of the immunodeficiency, risk of exposure to the disease, and the type of vaccine. Recommendations for immunizations for immunocompromised children are shown in Table 179–5. Recommendations for HIV-infected children are shown in Figure 268–2. Live-bacteria (e.g., oral typhoid) and live-virus vaccines (e.g., MMR, varicella, rotavirus) are contraindicated in most circumstances involving clinically significant immunosuppression. An exception is MMR and varicella vaccination of HIV-infected children who are not severely immunosuppressed (see Chapter 268). Children and adolescents with acute lymphocytic leukemia in remission can receive varicella vaccine under an investigational protocol (Bio-Pharm Clinical Services, 215-283-0770), provided appropriate institutional review board approval and informed consent have been obtained.

OPV is contraindicated in households with immunocompromised persons because of a risk of vaccine-associated paralytic poliomyelitis. For HIV-infected children and other children living in homes with immunocompromised persons, IPV should be given for all doses of the poliomyelitis immunization schedule. Influenza and pneumococcal vaccines are indicated, at the appropriate ages, for household contacts of immunocompromised persons to help prevent spread of infection among these high-risk patients. Although bacillus of Calmette-Guérin (BCG) is contraindicated in HIV-infected children in the United States, the World Health Organization (WHO) rec-

TABLE 301–3 Contraindications to and Precautions in Routine Childhood Vaccinations

True Contraindications and Precautions	Not Contraindications (Vaccines May Be Administered)
General for All Routine Vaccines (DTaP/DTP, OPV, IPV, MMR, Hib, Hepatitis B, Varicella, Rotavirus)	
Contraindications Anaphylactic reaction to a vaccine contraindicates further doses of that vaccine Anaphylactic reaction to a vaccine constituent contraindicates the use of vaccines containing that substance Moderate or severe illnesses with or without a fever	**Not Contraindications** Mild to moderate local reaction (soreness, redness, swelling), after a dose of an injectable antigen Low-grade or moderate fever after a prior vaccine dose Mild acute illness with or without low-grade fever Current antimicrobial therapy Convalescent phase of illness Prematurity (same dose and indications as for normal full-term infants) Recent exposure to an infectious disease History of penicillin or other nonspecific allergies or fact that relatives have such allergies Pregnancy of mother or household contact Unvaccinated household contact
DTaP/DTP	
Contraindications Encephalopathy within 7 days of administration of previous dose of DTaP/DTP **Precautions*** Temperature of ≥40.5°C (105°F) within 48 hr after vaccination with a prior dose of DTaP/DTP and not attributable to another identifiable cause Collapse or shocklike state (hypotonic-hyporesponsive episode) within 48 hr of receiving a prior dose of DTaP/DTP Convulsions within 3 days of receiving a prior dose of DTaP/DTP† Persistent, inconsolable crying lasting ≥3 hr, within 48 hr of receiving a prior dose of DTaP/DTP Guillain-Barré syndrome within 6 wk after a dose‡	**Not Contraindications** Temperature of <40.5°C (105°F) after a previous dose of DTaP/DTP Family history of convulsions† Family history of sudden infant death syndrome Family history of an adverse event after DTaP/DTP administration
OPV	
Contraindications Infection with HIV or a household contact with HIV infection Known immunodeficiency (hematologic and solid tumors; congenital immunodeficiency; long-term immunosuppressive therapy) Immunodeficient household contact **Precaution*** Pregnancy	**Not Contraindications** Breast-feeding Current antimicrobial therapy Mild diarrhea
IPV	
Contraindications Anaphylactic reaction to neomycin, streptomycin, or polymyxin B **Precaution*** Pregnancy	
MMR	
Contraindications Anaphylactic reaction to neomycin or gelatin Pregnancy Known immunodeficiency (hematologic and solid tumors; congenital immunodeficiency; long-term immunosuppressive therapy; HIV infection with evidence of severe immunosuppression) **Precautions*** Recent (within 3–11 mo, depending on product and dose) administration of a blood product or immune globulin preparation Thrombocytopenia* History of thrombocytopenic purpura¶	**Not Contraindications** Tuberculosis or positive PPD test result Simultaneous tuberculin skin testing§ Breast-feeding Pregnancy of mother or household contact of vaccine recipient Immunodeficient family member or household contact HIV infection without evidence of severe immunosuppression Allergic reaction to eggs‖ Nonanaphylactic reactions to neomycin
Hib	
Contraindications None **Precautions** None	
Hepatitis B	
Contraindications Anaphylactic reaction to common baker's yeast **Precautions** None	**Not Contraindications** Pregnancy

TABLE 301–3 Contraindications to and Precautions in Routine Childhood Vaccinations *Continued*

True Contraindications and Precautions	Not Contraindications (Vaccines May Be Administered)
Varicella	
Contraindications	**Not Contraindications**
Anaphylactic reaction to neomycin or gelatin Pregnancy HIV infection with evidence of severe immunosuppression Known immunodeficiency (hematologic and solid tumors; congenital immunodeficiency; long-term immunosuppressive therapy)	Breast-feeding Immunodeficiency in a household contact HIV infection in a household contact Pregnancy of mother or household contact of vaccine recipient
Precautions*	
Recent (within 3–11 mo, depending on product and dose) administration of a blood product or immune globulin preparation Family history of immunodeficiency††	
Rotavirus	
Contraindications	**Not Contraindications**
Hypersensitivity to aminoglycosides, amphotericin B, or monosodium glutamate Moderate or severe febrile illness Known immunodeficiency (hematologic and solid tumors; congenital immunodeficiency; long-term immunosuppressive therapy) Children of HIV-infected mothers, until tests for HIV infection in the infant are negative at ≥2 mo of age by PCR or culture	Breast-feeding Immunodeficiency in a household contact HIV infection in a household contact
Precautions*	
Acute vomiting or diarrhea	

**The events or conditions listed as precautions, although not contraindications, should be carefully reviewed. The benefits and risks of administering a specific vaccine to an individual under the circumstances should be considered. If the risks are believed to outweigh the benefits, the vaccine should be withheld; if the benefits are believed to outweigh the risks (e.g., during an outreak or foreign travel), the vaccine should be administered. Whether and when to administer DTaP/DTP to children with proven or suspected underlying neurologic disorders should be decided on an individual basis. Avoiding administration of certain vaccines to pregnant women is prudent on theoretical grounds. If immediate protection against poliomyelitis is needed, either OPV or IPV is recommended.*

†Acetaminophen administered before DTaP or DTP vaccination and thereafter every 4 hr for 24 hr should be considered for children with a personal or family history of convulsions in siblings or parents.

‡The decision to give additional doses of DTaP or DTP should be based on consideration of the benefit of further vaccination vs the risk of recurrence of Guillain-Barré syndrome. For example, completion of the primary vaccination series in children is justified.

§Measles vaccination may temporarily suppress tuberculin skin test reactivity. MMR vaccine may be administered after or on the same day as Mantoux tuberculin skin testing. If MMR has been given recently, the tuberculin test should be postponed until 4–6 wk after administration of MMR.

‖Recent data suggest that most anaphylactic reactions to measles- and mumps-containing vaccines are not associated with hypersensitivity to egg antigens but to other components of the vaccines, such as gelatin. Because the risk of anaphylactic reactions after administration of measles- or mumps-containing vaccines by persons who are allergic to eggs is extremely low and skin testing with vaccine is not predictive of allergic reactions to these vaccines, skin testing and desensitization are no longer required before administration of MMR vaccine to persons who are allergic to eggs.

¶The decision to vaccinate should be based on consideration of the benefits of immunity to measles, mumps, and rubella vs the risk of recurrence or exacerbation of thrombocytopenia after vaccination, or from natural infections of measles or rubella. In most instances, the benefits of vaccination are much greater than the potential risks and justify giving MMR, particularly in view of the even greater risk of thrombocytopenia after measles or rubella disease. However, if a prior episode of thrombocytopenia occurred in close temporal proximity to vaccination, avoiding a subsequent dose may be prudent.

††Varicella vaccine should not be administered to a member of a household with a family history of immunodeficiency until the immune status of the recipient and other children in the family is documented.

DTaP = diphtheria and tetanus toxoids plus acellular pertussis vaccine; DTP = diphtheria, tetanus, and pertussis vaccine; PPD = purified protein derivative; PCR = polymerase chain reaction; MMR = measles, mumps, and rubella vaccine; OPV = oral poliovirus vaccine; IPV = inactivated poliovirus vaccine; VZIG = varicella-zoster immune globulin.

This information is based on the recommendations of the Advisory Committee on Immunization Practices (ACIP) and of the Committee on Infectious Diseases of the American Academy of Pediatrics (AAP). Some recommendations may vary from those in the manufacturer's product label. For more detailed information, health care providers should consult the published recommendations of the ACIP, AAP, the American Academy of Family Physicians (AAFP), and the manufacturer's product label. These guidelines have been adapted and updated from Centers for Disease Control and Prevention: Update: Vaccine side effects, adverse reactions, contraindications, and precautions. Recommendations of the Advisory Committee on Immunization Practices (ACIP), MMWR 45(RR-12):1, 1996.

ommends giving BCG to asymptomatic HIV-infected children in areas with a high incidence of tuberculosis.

Live-virus vaccines should be administered with caution to children receiving corticosteroids. Children receiving physiologic doses of corticosteroids, or less than 2 mg/kg/24 hr of prednisone or its equivalent or less than 20 mg/24 hr if they weigh more than 10 kg, can be immunized while on treatment. Children receiving greater than or equal to 2 mg/kg/24 hr of daily, alternate-day prednisone or its equivalent, or 20 mg or more daily, if they weigh more than 10 kg, for less than 14 days should have live-virus immunizations deferred until at least discontinuation of corticosteroids; if the duration is 14 days or more, immunization should be deferred until at least 1 mo.

PRETERM INFANTS. The immune response to vaccination is a function of postnatal rather than gestational age. Prematurity does not increase the incidence of vaccine-related adverse events. Hence, preterm infants, including those of very low birthweight, should be vaccinated at the same chronologic age as full-term infants and according to the routine childhood immunization schedule (Fig. 301–1). One exception to this recommendation is hepatitis B vaccination of those born of HBsAg-negative mothers. Initiation of vaccination in this case should be delayed until the infant either weighs 2 kg or is 2 mo of age. Oral rotavirus and OPV, if used instead of IPV, should not be administered to preterm infants until hospital discharge. The dose should not be reduced for any vaccine.

BREAST-FEEDING. Breast-feeding does not adversely affect the immune response of infants and is not a contraindication to any vaccine, including OPV and oral rotavirus vaccine. Most live-virus vaccines, although they replicate in the mother, are not excreted in breast milk. Breast-feeding women also may safely receive vaccines, including receiving OPV and yellow fever vaccines, without interrupting breast-feeding.

POSTEXPOSURE IMMUNOPROPHYLAXIS

For certain infections, active or passive immunization shortly after exposure can prevent or ameliorate disease. For example, postexposure active immunization with rabies vaccine combined with passive immunization with rabies immune globulin (RIG) is highly effective in preventing rabies (Chapter 265). Varicella-zoster immune globulin (VZIG) is indicated after susceptible persons who are immunocompromised are exposed to varicella (Chapter 246). VZIG also is recommended for a newborn infant whose mother had onset of chickenpox within 5 days before to 2 days after delivery (Chapter 246). After a susceptible person is exposed to measles, either measles vaccine given within 72 hr or immune globulin given within 6 days can prevent or modify disease (Chapter 240). Other infections in which passive immunization of a susceptible person is indicated after exposure are tetanus in wound management (Chapter 209) and hepatitis A and hepatitis B (Chapter 177).

PASSIVE IMMUNIZATION. Administration of an immune globulin is indicated in some circumstances for preventing specific infections. The different preparations of globulin include intramuscular immune globulin (IG), intravenous immune globulin (IVIG), and immune globulin preparations termed *hyperimmune globulin* that have high concentrations of specific antibody against a particular pathogen. These products, which were historically prepared from animal sera but today are derived from human sera, include VZIG, RIG, hepatitis B immune globulin (HBIG), cytomegalovirus immune globulin, and respiratory syncytial virus (RSV) immune globulin for intravenous administration (RSV-IGIV).

Monoclonal antibody products may supplant hyperimmune globulin. A monoclonal antibody against RSV, palivizumab, administered intramuscularly at monthly intervals during the RSV season, is recommended for protecting high-risk children against serious complications of RSV disease (Chapter 253).

Prevention of hepatitis A during foreign travel is another indication for passive immunization with IG. For children age 2 yr or older, however, active immunization with hepatitis A vaccine is preferred because the protection is prolonged, if not lifelong, in contrast to the temporary protection afforded by passive immunoprophylaxis.

RECORD KEEPING, PATIENT INFORMATION, AND REPORTING OF ADVERSE EVENTS

Accurate record keeping by physicians is required. Parents should also keep up-to-date immunization records for their children. In the United States, the National Childhood Vaccine Injury Act requires for childhood-mandated vaccines (i.e., those routinely recommended for all children) that health care providers record in a child's medical record the date of administration of the vaccine, manufacturer, lot number, and the name of the health care provider administering the vaccines.

As a general principle, all children and their parents or guardians should be informed about the benefits and risks of vaccines to be administered and the provisions of the National Vaccine Injury Compensation Program. The discussion should be in language understood by the recipient or parent or guardian, and ample opportunity for questions and discussion should be provided. In the United States, a *Vaccine Information Statement* for each childhood-mandated vaccine has been prepared for this purpose by the Department of Health and Human Services; its use is required before each dose of vaccine.

Under the National Childhood Vaccine Injury Act, all temporally associated events severe enough to require a patient to seek medical attention should be reported to the Vaccine Adverse Events Reporting System (VAERS). In addition, specific adverse events in recipients of childhood-mandated vaccines are required to be reported. Additional information can be obtained from the National Vaccine Injury Compensation Program (800-338-2382 and at http://www.hrsa.dhhs.gov/bhpr/vicp/new.htm).

COMPENSATION FOR VACCINE INJURIES. The Vaccine Injury Compensation Program is a no-fault federal program that ensures fairness to persons who have suffered certain vaccine-related injuries and protects federal, state, and local immunization programs, private immunization providers, and vaccine manufacturers. The program is designed to provide prompt and fair compensation to the families of children who have died or have been injured as a result of routinely mandated immunization and to reduce the adverse impact of the tort judicial system on vaccine supply, cost, innovation, and development. This program provides for no-fault compensation for specific adverse effects associated with vaccines (Table 301–4).

DELIVERY OF VACCINES

Success of vaccination in preventing childhood infectious diseases necessitates effective means of vaccine delivery so that children receive recommended immunizations on schedule. In the United States, high rates of immunization in school-aged children have been achieved for the past 2 decades, in part because of state laws requiring immunization for school entry. In contrast to current rates of approximately 95% or higher in school-aged children, immunization rates in infants and young children in the 1980s were significantly lower, with 18–79% having completed vaccinations by the 2nd birthday. Failure to immunize young children was a major factor in the 1989–1991 measles outbreaks in urban areas. Several major barriers to successful infant and childhood immunization were identified in these outbreaks: inadequate access to immunization services, missed opportunities to administer vaccines, inadequate

TABLE 301–4 National Vaccine Injury Compensation Program: Vaccine Injury Table

Vaccine	Adverse Event	Time Period
Tetanus containing	Anaphylaxis	4 hr
	Brachial neuritis	2–28 days
Pertussis containing	Anaphylaxis	4 hr
	Encephalopathy	72 hr
MMR or any component	Anaphylaxis	4 hr
	Encephalopathy	5–15 days
Rubella containing	Chronic arthritis	42 days
Measles containing	Thrombocytopenic purpura	6 mo
	Vaccine-strain measles viral infection in an immunodeficient recipient	
OPV	Paralytic polio from	30 days/6 mo
	vaccine-strain poliovirus infection	30 days/6 mo
IPV	Anaphylaxis	4 hr
Hepatitis B	Anaphylaxis	4 hr
Hib (unconjugated)	Early-onset Hib disease	7 days
Hib (conjugate)	No condition specified	Not applicable†
Varicella	No condition specified	Not applicable†
New vaccines‡	No condition specified	Not applicable†

**Time intervals for immunocompetent/immunodeficient individuals who receive OPV. Contact cases have no time limit.*

†No condition has been identified as requiring inclusion on the Vaccine Injury Table, therefore, compensation for alleged injuries must be pursued on a causation in fact basis.

‡Any new vaccine recommended by the Centers for Disease Control for routine administration to children after publication by the Secretary of Health and Human Services of a notice of coverage.

OPV = oral poliovirus vaccine; IPV = inactivated poliovirus vaccine; Hib = Haemophilus influenzae *type b; MMR = measles, mumps, and rubella vaccine.*

Effective date March 24, 1997. Adapted from Public Health Service, Department of Health and Human Services. National Vaccine Injury Compensation Program: Revisions and additions to the Vaccine Injury Table—II. Federal Register 62:7685, 1997.

TABLE 301–5 Standards for Pediatric Immunization Practices

Standard 1	Immunization servides are **readily available**.
Standard 2	There are **no barriers** or **unnecessary prerequisites** for the receipt of vaccines.
Standard 3	Immunization services are available **free** or for a minimal fee.
Standard 4	Providers use all clinical encounters to **screen** and, when indicated **immunize** children.
Standard 5	Providers **educate** parents or guardians about immunizations in general terms
Standard 6	Providers **question** parents or guardians about **contraindications** and before immunizing a child **inform** them in specific terms about the risks and benefits of the immunization their child is to receive.
Standard 7	Providers follow only true **contraindiations**.
Standard 8	Providers administer **simultaneously** all vaccine doses for which a child is eligible at the time of each visit.
Standard 9	Providers use accurate and complete **recording procedure**.
Standard 10	Providers **co-schedule** immunization appointments in conjunction with appointments for other child health services.
Standard 11	Providers **report adverse events** after immunization promptly, accurately, and completely.
Standard 12	Providers operate a **tracking system**.
Standard 13	Providers adhere to appropriate procedures for **vaccine management**.
Standard 14	Providers conduct semiannual **audits** to assess immunization coverage levels and to **review** immunization records in the patient populations they serve.
Standard 15	Providers maintain up-to-date, easily retrievable **medical protocols** at all locations where vaccines are administered.
Standard 16	Providers operate with **patient-oriented** and **community-based** approaches.
Standard 17	Vaccines are administered by **properly trained** individuals.
Standard 18	Providers receive **ongoing education** and **training** about current immunization recommendations.

resources for public health and preventive programs, and low public awareness and resulting lack of public demand for immunization.

This recognition of low immunization rates prompted a national campaign to achieve the goal of 90% vaccine coverage of children by 2 yr of age. Initiatives have included improved access to vaccines, education of health care providers, and the development of standards for pediatric immunization practices (Table 301–5). These standards serve as guidelines for improving the delivery of vaccines and include evaluation of immunization status of patients at all medical visits, use of valid contraindications, simultaneous administration of all indicated vaccines, and routine audits by providers of the immunization status of their patients. An important principle in these standards is the need to eliminate missed opportunities to vaccinate infants and children.

These and other initiatives have resulted in increasing immunization rates of young children in recent years. According to the National Immunization Survey, coverage rates among children 19–35 mo of age in July 1996 to June 1997 had reached 76% for completion of the schedule of four doses of DTP or DTaP, three of oral poliovirus, three of Hib, and one dose of measles-containing vaccines. All of the national coverage goals for specific vaccines established in the Childhood Immunization Initiative were met, and the composite vaccination rates are the highest ever recorded in the United States for preschool children. This success reflects the collaborative efforts of the public and private sectors in public health.

INTERNATIONAL CONSIDERATIONS

Since the establishment of the Expanded Programme on Immunization (EPI) of the WHO, immunization rates for the basic children's vaccines have risen from 5% to approximately 80% worldwide. At least 2.7 million deaths due to measles, neonatal tetanus, and pertussis and 200,000 cases of paralysis due to poliomyelitis are prevented each year. Despite the successes of the EPI, which include elimination of poliomyelitis from the Americas, some vaccine-preventable diseases, such as measles, pertussis, and neonatal tetanus, remain prevalent in the developing world.

Vaccines against seven diseases are currently recommended by the EPI for routine use in the developing world: BCG, DTP, OPV, measles, and hepatitis B vaccines for children and tetanus toxoid for pregnant women. Hib vaccine is likely to be added in the near future. Yellow fever, Japanese encephalitis, group A meningococcus, mumps, and rubella vaccines are used regionally, depending on the disease epidemiology and resources. Poliomyelitis has been targeted for global eradication by the year 2000.

Because infectious diseases know no geographic or political boundaries, uncontrolled disease anywhere in the world poses a threat to the United States. Vaccines offer the opportunity to control and even eradicate some diseases. Successful eradication means that vaccines are no longer needed. The experience with smallpox demonstrates that the eradication of disease is a remarkably sound economic investment. The total sum spent by the United States for the global smallpox eradication campaign has been recouped in 1968 dollars every 2.5 months since 1971. A similar achievement with poliomyelitis would save the United States more than $300 million each year in vaccine and associated delivery costs.

American Academy of Pediatrics (Peter G [ed]): 1997 Red Book: Report of the Committee on Infectious Diseases, 24th ed. Elk Grove Village, IL: American Academy of Pediatrics, 1997.

Centers for Disease Control and Prevention: Standards for pediatric immunization practices. MMWR 42 (RR-5):1, 1993.

Centers for Disease Control and Prevention: General Recommendations on Immunizations: Recommendations of the Advisory Committee on Immunization Practices (ACIP). MMWR 43 (RR-1):1, 1994.

Centers for Disease Control and Prevention: Update: Vaccine side effects, adverse reactions, contraindications, and precautions. Recommendations of the Advisory Committee on Immunization Practices (ACIP). MMWR 45 (RR-12):1, 1996.

Centers for Disease Control and Prevention: Health Information for International Travel 1996–1997. US Department of Health and Human Services, Public Health Services, 1997.

McDonnell WM, Askari FK: Immunization. JAMA 278:2000, 1997.

Peter G: Childhood immunizations. N Engl J Med 327:1794, 1992.

Plotkin SA, Orenstein WA (eds): Vaccines, 3rd ed. Philadelphia, WB Saunders, 1999.

Watson JC, Peter G: General immunization practices. *In:* Plotkin SA, Orenstein WA (eds): Vaccines, 3rd ed. Philadelphia, WB Saunders, 1999, pp 47–73.

CHAPTER 302
Infection Control and Prophylaxis

Margaret C. Fisher

Infection control is a vital part of pediatric medicine. Controlling infections requires an intact and active public health system, universal immunizations, optimal nutrition, and use of specific methods to prevent transmission of infection from child to child, child to adult, and adult to child. Infection control is the responsibility of every health care provider.

Nosocomial infections are those acquired during hospitalization. An estimated 3–5% of children admitted to hospitals acquire a nosocomial infection; rates are much higher in intensive care units. Infections are also acquired in emergency rooms, physicians' offices, and long-term care settings. Medical devices are increasingly used in the home, and they also require appropriate infection control techniques. Education of home health care providers as well as of families is essential.

Determinants of infection include host factors, prior invasive procedures, use of catheters, use of antibiotics, and exposure to other patients, visitors, or health care providers with contagious diseases. Host factors that increase the risk for infection include anatomic abnormalities (e.g., dermoid sinuses, cleft palate, obstructive uropathy), damage to skin, organ dysfunction, malnutrition, and underlying diseases or co-morbidities. Diseases and therapies that alter immunity are most likely to predispose to infection. Prior procedures may introduce pathogens and damage anatomic host defenses. Intravenous and other catheters bypass host defenses, provide direct access to sterile sites, provide adherence sites for microbes, and may occlude normal ostia such as the eustachian tubes. Antibiotics often alter normal bowel flora and encourage colonization by resistant flora, and they may suppress the bone marrow. Exposure to adults or children with contagious diseases is a clear risk for nosocomial transmission of disease.

Transmission of infectious agents occurs by various routes, but by far the most common and important route is via the hands. Children are constantly placing their own hands in their noses, eyes, and mouths; thus, child-to-child exchange of secretions is common whenever children are together. Bacteria, fungi, viruses, and parasites often travel on hands from one person to another. Medical equipment, toys, and hospital and office furnishings can be contaminated and thus have a role as fomites for transmission of potential pathogens. Thermometers and other equipment that come into contact with mucous membranes are special risks. Some agents are disseminated by airborne transmission, such as varicella virus, measles virus, and Mycobacterium tuberculosis. Food and water can be contaminated and have been involved in hospital outbreaks.

Common causes of nosocomial infections in children are seasonal viruses, staphylococci, and gram-negative bacilli. Fungi and resistant bacteria are frequent causes of infection in immunocompromised children and in those who require intensive care and prolonged hospitalization. Common sites of infection are the respiratory tract, gastrointestinal tract, bloodstream, skin, and urinary tract.

Nosocomial infections cause considerable morbidity and occasional mortality; infections prolong hospital stays and increase health care costs. Surveillance for infection is the first step in identifying nosocomial infections and suggesting methods for prevention. Within hospitals, surveillance is the responsibility of the Infection Control Committee, a multidisciplinary group that collects and reviews surveillance data, establishes policy, and investigates outbreaks. Surveillance within outpatient settings and during home care is often less well established but no less important.

PREVENTION. Prevention of infection is the goal. The most important measure in any infection control program is handwashing. Although much attention is directed at the types of soap used, the important component of handwashing is placement of the hands under water and use of friction with or without soap. Studies show that a 15-sec scrub removes the majority of transient flora but does not alter the permanent flora. Hands should be washed before and after every patient encounter. Studies in childcare settings and schools have determined that handwashing can be taught to children and that the rates of infection are decreased when children as well as care givers regularly wash their hands.

Standard Precautions. Standard precautions, formerly known as universal precautions, are intended to prevent exchange of blood and body fluids (secretions and excretions, excluding sweat) across nonintact skin or mucous membranes and should be used whenever providing care. Infected individuals are often contagious before symptoms of disease develop; further, many infections may be asymptomatic yet the affected person is capable of transmitting the agent. Standard precautions involve the use of barriers—gloves, gowns, masks, goggles, and face shields—as needed to prevent transmission of microbes associated with contact with blood or body fluids.

Isolation. Isolation of patients infected with certain pathogens decreases the risk of nosocomial transmission. The type of isolation depends on the infecting agent and the route of transmission. Contact transmission is the most frequent mode and involves direct contact or contact with a contaminated intermediate object. Droplet transmission is by droplets propelled a short distance through the air and deposited on mucous membranes. Airborne transmission occurs by dissemination of droplet nuclei (≤ 5 μm) of evaporated droplets or dust particles carrying the infectious agent.

Standard precautions are indicated for all patients. In addition, transmission-based precautions are indicated for certain diseases (Table 302–1). Contact precautions include gowns and gloves and single room isolation. Droplet precautions include masks for close contact (<3 ft) and single room isolation. For both contact and droplet precautions, a single room is preferred but is not required for crib-confined patients. Cohorting of children infected with the same pathogen is acceptable. Airborne precautions include masks and single room isolation with negative-pressure ventilation. Transmission-based precautions are continued for as long as a patient is considered to be contagious.

The use of isolation techniques in an outpatient setting has not been studied. Each office must establish policies to ensure that the proper cleaning, disinfection, and sterilization methods are used. Many practices and clinics provide separate waiting areas for sick and well children. Triage of patients is essential to ensure that contagious children or adults are not present in waiting areas. Outbreaks of measles in patients within the waiting area have been reported where airflow allowed the exhaust from the examination room to enter the waiting area. Cleaning the environment is important. Toys and items that are shared between patients should be cleaned between uses; soap and water are sufficient for these items. More complete disinfection or sterilization is required for items that encounter mucous membranes and for all reusable items used for body fluid sampling.

Additional Measures. Other preventive measures include aseptic technique, catheter care, prudent use of antibiotics, isolation of contagious patients, cleaning of the environment, disinfection and sterilization of medical equipment, and establishment of employee health services. Aseptic technique must be used for all invasive procedures; this is especially important during intravenous catheter placement and manipulation. Catheter care also includes limiting the duration and number of catheters as much as possible and removing catheters as soon as they become unnecessary. Prudent use of antibiotics is especially important when these agents are used for prophylaxis.

SURGICAL PROPHYLAXIS. Surgical prophylaxis is appropriate when there is a high risk of postoperative infection or when the consequences of infection are catastrophic. The choice of antibiotic depends on the site and type of surgery (Table 302–2). A useful classification of surgical procedures based on this risk recognizes four categories: clean wounds, clean contaminated wounds, contaminated wounds, and dirty and infected wounds. The following recommendations are standards of the American College of Surgeons, The Surgical Infection Society, and the American Academy of Pediatrics.

Clean wounds are uninfected operative wounds in which no inflammation is noted and the respiratory, alimentary, and genitourinary tracts and the oropharynx are not entered. In addition, the procedure is elective and is performed as primarily closed or drained with closed drainage. Operative incisional wounds following nonpenetrating trauma are included in this category. For clean wounds, prophylactic antimicrobial therapy is not recommended, except in patients at high risk for infection and in circumstances in which the consequences of infection are potentially life threatening (e.g., implantation of a

TABLE 302–1 Selected Diseases and Indications for Transmission-Based Isolation in Addition to Standard Precautions

Clinical Syndrome or Condition	Potential Pathogens	Empirical Precautions
Diarrhea		
Acute diarrhea with a likely infectious cause in an incontinent or diapered patient	*Salmonella, Shigella, Escherichia coli* O157:H7, rotavirus, hepatitis A	Contact
Diarrhea in any patient, especially an adult, with a history of recent antibiotic use	*Clostridum difficile*	Contact
Meningitis	*Neisseria meningitidis, Haemophilus influenzae* type b	Droplet
	Streptococcus pneumoniae	Standard
	Mycobacterium tuberculosis	Standard
Rash or Exanthems		
Petechial/ecchymotic with fever	*N. meningitidis*	Droplet
Vesicular		
Chickenpox	Varicella-zoster virus	Airborne and contact
Zoster (localized in an immunocompetent patient)	Varicella-zoster virus	Standard
Zoster (disseminated or in an immunocompromised patient)	Varicella-zoster virus	Airborne and contact
Maculopapular with coryza and fever	Measles virus	Airborne
Erythema infectiosum	Parvovirus B19	Standard
Parvovirus B19 in an immunocompromised patient	Parvovirus B19	Droplet
Roseola	Human herpesvirus 6	Standard
Rubella	Rubella virus	Droplet
Respiratory Tract Infections		
Cough/fever/upper lobe pulmonary infiltrate in an HIV-negative patient or a patient at low risk for HIV infection	*Mycobacterium tuberculosis*	Airborne
Cough/fever/pulmonary infiltrate in any lung location in an HIV-infected patient or a patient at high risk for HIV infection	*M. tuberculosis*	Airborne
Paroxysmal or severe persistent cough during periods of pertussis activity	*Bordetella pertussis*	Droplet
Bronchiolitis and croup, other lower respiratory tract infections in infants and young children	Respiratory syncytial or parainfluenza virus	Contact
Influenza	Influenza virus	Droplet
Atypical pneumonia	*Mycoplasma pneumoniae*	Droplet
Afebrile pneumonia in young infants	*Chlamydia trachomatis*	Standard
Diphtheria (pharyngeal)	*Corynebacterium diphtheriae*	Droplet
Pneumonic plague	*Yersinia pestis*	Droplet
Pneumococcal pneumonia	*Streptococcus pneumoniae*	Standard
Group A streptococcal pharyngitis, pneumonia, or scarlet fever in infants and young children	Group A *Streptococcus*	Droplet
Skin Diseases		
Skin infections that are highly contagious or that may occur on dry skin (cutaneous diphtheria; herpes simplex virus, neonatal or mucocutaneous; impetigo; major or draining abscesses; cellulitis; decubiti; staphylococcal furunculosis; zoster disseminated or in an immunocompromised host)		Contact
Urinary Tract Infections		Standard
Other Infections		
Infection or colonization with multidrug-resistant organisms	Resistant bacteria	Contact
Invasive *Neisseria meningitidis* disease (meningitis, pneumonia, and sepsis)	*N. meningitidis*	Droplet
Invasive *Haemophilus influenzae* type b disease (meningitis, pneumonia, epiglottitis, and sepsis)	*H. influenzae* type b	Droplet
Viral infections spread by droplet transmission (adenovirus, influenza, mumps, parvovirus B19 in an immunocompromised patient, rubella)		Droplet

Adapted from Garner JS: The Hospital Infection Control Practices Advisory Committee: Guidelines for isolation precautions in hospitals. Infect Control Hosp Epidemiol 17:53, 1996.

prosthetic foreign body such as a prosthetic heart valve; open heart surgery for repair of structural defects; surgery in patients who are immunocompromised as a result of an inherited disease or are receiving corticosteroids or chemotherapy for malignancy; and newborn infants). Systemic antimicrobial agents have been recommended empirically for a clean procedure in patients with infection at another site.

Clean contaminated wounds are operative wounds in which the respiratory, alimentary, or genitourinary tract is entered under controlled conditions and does not have unusual contamination preoperatively. These wounds occur in operations that involve the biliary tract, appendix, vagina, and oropharynx and in which no evidence of infection or major break in technique is encountered, as well as in urgent or emergency surgery in an otherwise clean procedure. In clean but potentially contaminated procedures, the risk of contamination is variable. Recommendations for pediatric patients derived from data on adults suggest that prophylaxis be provided for procedures in patients with obstructive jaundice, certain alimentary tract procedures, and urinary tract surgery or instrumentation in the presence of bacteriuria or obstructive uropathy.

Contaminated wounds include open, fresh, and accidental wounds; major breaks in otherwise sterile operative technique; gross spillage from the gastrointestinal tract; penetrating trauma occurring less than 4 hr earlier; and incisions in which acute nonpurulent inflammation is encountered.

Dirty and infected wounds include penetrating traumatic wounds longer than 4 hr earlier, those with retained devitalized tissue, and those in which clinical infection is apparent or in which the viscera have been perforated. In contaminated and dirty or infected wound procedures, antimicrobial therapy is indicated and may need to be continued for 5–10 days.

TABLE 302–2 Common Surgical Procedures for Which Perioperative Prophylactic Antibiotics are Recommended

Surgical Procedure	Likely Pathogens	Suggested Drug
Clean Wounds		
Cardiac surgery (e.g., open heart surgery) Vascular surgery Neurosurgery Orthopedic surgery (e.g., joint replacement)	Skin flora, enteric gram-negative bacilli	Cefazolin or vancomycin
Clean Contaminated Wounds		
Head and neck surgery entering the oral cavity or pharynx	Skin flora, oral anaerobes, oral streptococci	Cefazolin or clindamycin
Gastrointestinal and genitourinary surgery	Enteric gram-negative bacilli, anaerobes, gram-positive cocci	Cefazolin; if colon involved, consider oral decontamination with neomycin and erythromycin
Contaminated Wounds		
Traumatic wounds (e.g., compound fracture)	Skin flora	Cefazolin
Dirty Wounds		
Appendectomy Colorectal surgery	Enteric gram-negative bacili, anaerobes, gram-positive cocci	Cefoxitin, or clindamycin plus gentamicin

In the truest sense, antimicrobial prophylaxis refers to the use of antibiotics before attachment of contaminating bacteria to the host tissues, as in the clean and potentially contaminated categories. Antibiotics given after the microbial attachment constitute therapy, as in the case of contaminated and dirty wounds.

When used, prophylactic antibiotics should be administered, preferably intravenously, approximately 30 min before the skin incision is made, with the intent of having peak concentrations of the drug at this time. The intent is to maintain adequate plasma and tissue concentration of the drugs until the incision is closed. Repeat doses are necessary only if the surgery lasts longer than 6 hr. Postoperative therapy is usually not necessary; in cases of contaminated surgery, antibiotics are continued as therapy for infection at the site. Drugs administered postoperatively for prophylaxis do not reduce the infection rate. For patients undergoing colonic procedures, additional oral antibiotics may be used and should also be given on the day before surgery.

The selection of antibiotic regimen for prophylaxis is based on the procedure, the expected contaminating organisms, and safety of the drugs. Because of the vast array of antibiotics available now, more than one regimen may be acceptable (Table 302–2). Knowledge of the susceptibilities of the prevalent bacterial causes of nosocomial infections in each hospital is especially important in choosing drugs.

EMPLOYEE HEALTH. Employee health is important because employees are at risk for acquiring infection from patients. This risk is minimized by use of standard precautions and handwashing before and after all patient contacts. Infected employees also pose a risk to patients. Within hospitals, personnel health services or departments of occupational safety and health manage employee health issues. New employees should be screened for the presence of infectious diseases. Their immunization history should be noted and necessary immunizations offered.

All health care workers (medical or nonmedical, paid or volunteer, full time or part time, student or nonstudent, with or without patient care responsibilities) who work in facilities that provide health care to patients (inpatient or outpatient, public or private) should be immune to measles, rubella, and varicella. Facilities that provide care exclusively for elderly patients who are at minimal risk for these diseases are a possible exception. All employees who might be exposed to blood or body fluids should be immunized against hepatitis B. Annual influenza immunizations are recommended for all health care workers who have contact with patients at risk for influenza or its complications. This program lessens staff illness and absenteeism during the influenza season and reduces nosocomial infections. Immunizations should be encouraged and whenever possible should be provided free of charge. Each office and hospital must comply with the rules developed by the Occupational Safety and Health Administration. Further, each office and hospital should have written policies about exclusion of infected staff. Regular educational sessions should be performed to ensure that the staff are aware of infection control methods and that they adhere to infection control policies.

American Academy of Pediatrics, Committee on Infectious Diseases and Committee on Hospital Care: The revised CDC guidelines for isolation precautions in hospitals: Implications for pediatrics. Pediatrics 101:e3, 1998.

Antimicrobial prophylaxis in surgery. Med Lett Drugs Ther 39:97, 1997.

Bennett JV, Brachman PS (eds): Hospital Infections, 3rd ed. Boston, Little, Brown & Co, 1992.

Centers for Disease Control and Prevention: Recommendations of the Advisory Committee on Immunization Practices (ACIP) and the Hospital Infection Control Practices Advisory Committee (HICPAC): Immunization of health-care workers. MMWR 46(RR-18):1, 1997.

Eickhoff TC: Airborne nosocomial infection: A contemporary perspective. Infect Control Hosp Epidemiol 15:663, 1994.

Fisher MC: Nosocomial infections and infection control. In: Jenson HB, Baltimore RS (eds): Pediatric Infectious Diseases. Principles and Practice. Norwalk, CT, Appleton & Lange, 1995.

Garner JS, The Hospital Infection Control Practices Advisory Committee: Guidelines for isolation precautions in hospitals. Infect Control Hosp Epidemiol 17:53, 1996.

Herwaldt LA, Smith SD, Carter CD: Infection control in the outpatient setting. Infect Control Hosp Epidemiol 19:41, 1998.

Lohr JA, Ingram DL, Dudley SM, et al: Hand washing in pediatric ambulatory settings. An inconsistent practice. Am J Dis Child 145:1198, 1991.

Ratula WA: Antisepsis, disinfection, and sterilization in hospitals and related institutions. In: American Society for Microbiology: Manual of Clinical Microbiology. Washington, DC, American Society for Microbiology Press, 1995, pp 227–245.

CHAPTER 303
Child Care and Communicable Diseases

Larry K. Pickering and Danielle J. Laborde

An estimated 13 million children age 5 yr or younger and 60% of school-aged children younger than 13 yr attend some form of child daycare on a regular basis (Chapter 32). Child-care facilities can be classified on the basis of size of enrollment, age of attendees, and health status of the children enrolled. As defined in the United States, child-care facilities consist of child-care centers, child-care homes, and special facilities for ill children or children with special needs. Child-care centers provide care and education for any number of children in a nonresidential setting and are open on a regular basis (i.e., not a drop-in facility). They are licensed and regulated by state governments and care for a mean of 68 children. In contrast, child-care homes may be designated as small (1–6 children) or large (7–12 children), may be full day or part day, may expect regular daily attendance, or may be designed for sporadic use. They generally are not licensed or registered.

Most studies of infectious diseases have been conducted in

child-care centers among infant (6 wk–12 mo of age) and toddler (13–36 mo of age) groups. Almost any organism has the potential to be spread and cause disease in a child-care setting. Epidemiologic studies have established that children in childcare are 2–18 times more likely to acquire certain infectious diseases than children not enrolled in childcare (Table 303–1). In addition, children in childcare are at risk of receiving more courses of antibiotics for longer periods, and acquiring antibiotic-resistant organisms. Transmission of organisms and illness in group care depends on the age and immune status of children involved, the season, hygienic practices, crowding, environmental characteristics of the facilities, and characteristics of particular organisms including infectivity, survivability in the environment, and virulence. Rates of infection, duration of illness, and risk of hospitalization tend to decrease among children in childcare after the first 6 mo of attendance and decline to levels observed among homebound children after 3 yr of age.

EPIDEMIOLOGY. There are several different patterns of occurrence of infectious diseases among children in childcare and their contacts. Respiratory tract infections and diarrhea are the most common diseases associated with childcare. These infections occur in children, child-care staff, and household contacts. Organisms such as enteric pathogens (Chapter 176), which are transmitted by the fecal-oral route, and respiratory tract pathogens can infect both children and adults. Infections due to hepatitis A virus may not be apparent in young children attending childcare but may have a major clinical impact on older children and adult contacts, including child-care staff and household contacts. Other diseases, such as otitis media, varicella, and invasive *Haemophilus influenzae* type b disease, usually affect children rather than adults. Some infections, such as cytomegalovirus (CMV) and parvovirus B19, may have serious consequences for the fetuses of pregnant women or for certain immunosuppressed hosts. Blood-borne pathogens such as hepatitis B virus and HIV (Chapter 268) can infect all ages but have rarely (hepatitis B) or never (HIV) been reported to be transmitted in a child-care setting. Skin infections are acquired through close personal contact and contaminated linens or clothing and more often affect children older than 2 yr.

TABLE 303–1 Infectious Diseases in the Child-Care Setting

Disease	Increased Incidence with Childcare
Respiratory Tract Infections	
Otitis media	Yes
Sinusitis	Probably
Pharyngitis	Probably
Pneumonia	Yes
Gastrointestinal Tract Infections	
Diarrhea (rotavirus, *Giardia lamblia, Shigella, Escherichia coli* O157:H7, and less commonly enteric adenoviruses, *Aeromonas, Campylobacter, Clostridium difficile,* and *Bacillus cereus*)	Yes
Hepatitis A	Yes
Skin Diseases	
Impetigo	Probably
Scabies	Probably
Pediculosis	Probably
Tinea (ringworm)	Probably
Invasive Bacterial Infections	
Haemophilus influenzae type b	Yes
Neisseria meningitidis	Probably
Streptococcus pneumoniae	Yes
Aseptic Meningitis	
Enteroviruses	Probably
Herpesvirus Infections	
Cytomegalovirus	Yes
Varicella-zoster virus	Yes
Herpes simplex virus	Probably
Blood-Borne Infections	
Hepatitis B	Few case reports
HIV	No cases reported
Vaccine-Preventable Diseases	
Measles, mumps, rubella, diphtheria, pertussis, tetanus	Not established
Polio	No
H. influenzae type b	Yes
Varicella	Probably
Rotavirus	Yes

Respiratory Tract Infections. Respiratory tract infections account for the majority of childcare-related illness. Children who are younger than 2 yr and who attend child-care centers have more upper and lower respiratory tract infections than age-matched children not in childcare. The organisms responsible for illness are similar to those that circulate in the community and include respiratory syncytial virus, parainfluenza viruses, adenoviruses, rhinoviruses, coronaviruses, influenza viruses, parvovirus B19, and, infrequently, *Bordetella pertussis* and *Mycobacterium tuberculosis.* The risk of developing otitis media is two to three times greater in children attending childcare than in children receiving home-based care. Otitis media is responsible for most of the antibiotic use in children younger than 3 yr in childcare. These children also are at increased risk for recurrent otitis media, further increasing antibiotic use in this population. Although children in childcare show earlier acquisition of pharyngeal carriage of group A *Streptococcus,* outbreaks of this organism are uncommon.

Gastrointestinal Tract Infections. Acute infectious diarrhea is two to three times more common in children in childcare than in children cared for in their homes. Outbreaks of diarrhea occur frequently in child-care centers and generally are caused by enteric viruses such as rotaviruses, enteric adenoviruses, astroviruses, and caliciviruses or by enteric parasites such as *Giardia lamblia* or *Cryptosporidium.* Low infective doses and high asymptomatic excretion rates characterize the more common enteropathogens, such as rotavirus and *G. lamblia.* Bacterial enteropathogens, such as *Shigella* and *Escherichia coli* O157:H7, and less commonly *Aeromonas, Campylobacter, Clostridium difficile,* and *Bacillus cereus* (from contaminated fried rice) also have caused outbreaks of diarrhea in child-care settings. *Salmonella* is rarely associated with outbreaks of diarrhea in child-care settings. Hepatitis A in children enrolled in childcare has resulted in community-wide outbreaks. Hepatitis A usually is mild or asymptomatic in children and is identified when illness becomes manifested in older children or adults. Enteropathogens and hepatitis A virus are transmitted in child-care facilities by the fecal-oral route and rarely by contaminated food or water. Enteric illness and hepatitis A are more common in centers that care for children who are not toilet trained and where proper hygienic practices are lacking.

Skin Diseases. The most commonly recognized skin infections or infestations in children in childcare are impetigo due to *Staphylococcus aureus* or group A *Streptococcus,* pediculosis, scabies, and tinea capitis and tinea corporis (ringworm). The magnitude of these infections and infestations in children in childcare is not known. Parvovirus B19, which causes erythema infectiosum (fifth disease), is spread through the respiratory route, and outbreaks have occurred in child-care centers. As with CMV, the greatest health hazard is for pregnant women and immunocompromised hosts owing to their respective risks of fetal loss and aplastic crisis.

Invasive Organisms. Primary invasive disease due to *H. influenzae* type b has been shown to be more common in children in childcare; evidence for increased risk of subsequent or secondary disease due to *H. influenzae* type b in a child-care setting is less convincing. Routine immunization against *H. influenzae* type b has greatly reduced the risk of primary invasive infection. There is an indication that the risk of primary disease due to *Neisseria meningitidis* is higher among children in childcare than among children cared for at home. Child-care attendance is associated with nasopharyngeal carriage of penicillin-resistant *Streptococcus pneumoniae* and invasive pneumococcal disease, especially among children with a history of recurrent otitis media and antibiotic use. Secondary spread of *S. pneumoniae* and *N. meningitidis* has been reported, indicating the potential for outbreaks to occur in this setting.

Outbreaks of aseptic meningitis due to echovirus 30 have been reported among children in child-care centers, their parents, and their teachers.

Herpesviruses. Studies of CMV infection in childcare centers have shown that as many as 70% of diapered children shed CMV continuously after acquisition. CMV-infected children often transmit the virus to other children with whom they have contact, as well as to 8–20% of their care providers and mothers per year. Transmission occurs as a result of contact with infected saliva or urine. Varicella frequently has been transmitted in childcare centers, but routine varicella immunization should reduce this risk. The role of childcare facilities in the spread of herpes simplex virus, especially during episodes of gingivostomatitis, requires further clarification.

Blood-Borne Organisms. Concern has arisen about the potential for transmission of two blood-borne organisms in the child-care setting: hepatitis B virus (HBV) and HIV. Hepatitis B transmission among children in childcare has been documented in a few instances, but the potential for transmission of this infection should decline with implementation of universal immunization of infants with HBV vaccine. Issues about HIV in childcare include the potential risk of HIV transmission within the childcare setting and risks to HIV-infected children associated with acquisition of infectious agents. No cases of HIV transmission in out-of-home childcare have been reported. Children with HIV infection enrolled in childcare facilities should be monitored for exposure to infectious diseases, and their health and immune status should be evaluated frequently.

Antibiotic Use and Bacterial Resistance. Antibiotic resistance has become an alarming problem in child-care facilities because the frequency of infection by organisms resistant to frequently used antimicrobial agents has dramatically increased. The estimated annual rate of antibiotic use in children in childcare is from two to four times higher than in age-matched children cared for at home. In addition, the mean duration of antibiotic treatment is four times longer in children in childcare. This frequency of antibiotic use combined with the propensity for person-to-person transmission of pathogens in a crowded environment has resulted in an increased prevalence of antibiotic-resistant bacteria in the respiratory and intestinal tracts, including *S. pneumoniae, H. influenzae, Moraxella catarrhalis, E. coli* 0157:H7, and *Shigella* species.

PREVENTION. Written child-care center policies designed to prevent or control the spread of infectious agents should be available and reviewed regularly. Standards for environmental and personal hygiene should include maintenance of current immunization records for children and staff, appropriate exclusion policies, targeting frequently contaminated areas for environmental cleaning, and appropriate handling of food. Educational strategies for improving adherence to these standards should be implemented.

In the United States, there are 11 diseases for which all children should be immunized unless there are contraindications: diphtheria, pertussis, tetanus, *H. influenzae* type b, measles, mumps, rubella, poliomyelitis, hepatitis B, varicella, and rotavirus. High levels of immunization exist among children in licensed child-care facilities, in part because of laws in almost all states requiring age-appropriate immunizations of children attending licensed childcare programs and in part because of the increased rates of immunization of all children in the United States. The use of vaccines has had a significant beneficial effect on the health of children in child-care settings. Use of *H. influenzae* type b conjugate vaccines has practically eliminated disease due to invasive *H. influenzae* type b organisms. HBV, varicella, and rotavirus vaccines should also benefit children in child-care centers. The role of hepatitis A and influenza vaccines among children and adults in child-care settings requires further evaluation.

Childcare providers should receive all immunizations that are routinely recommended for adults. Local public health authorities should be notified about cases of communicable disease involving children or providers in child-care settings.

STANDARDS. Every state has specific standards for licensing and reviewing child-care centers and family child-care homes. The American Public Health Association and the American Academy of Pediatrics jointly publish comprehensive health and safety performance standards that can be used by pediatricians and other health care professionals to guide decisions about infectious disease and other health matters in childcare facilities (available in print form and at http://nrc.uchsc.edu/).

Alho O-P, Laara E, Oja H: Public health impact of various risk factors for acute otitis media in Northern Finland. Am J Epidemiol 143:1149, 1996.

American Public Health Association and American Academy of Pediatrics: Caring for our children: National health and safety performance standards for out-of-home child care programs. American Public Health Association and American Academy of Pediatrics, Washington, DC, 1992. (Also available at http://nrc.uchsc.edu/).

Belongia EA, Osterholm MT, Soler JT, et al: Transmission of *Escherichia coli* 0157:H7 infection in Minnesota child day-care facilities. JAMA 269:883, 1993.

Cherian T, Steinhoff MC, Harrison LH, et al: A cluster of invasive pneumococcal disease in young children in child care. JAMA 271:695, 1994.

Churchill RB, Pickering LK: Infection control challenges in child care centers. Infect Dis Clin North Am 11:347, 1997.

Engelgau MM, Woernie CH, Schwartz B, et al: Invasive group A streptococcus carriage in a day care centre after a fatal case. Arch Dis Child 71:318, 1994.

Frenck Jr, RW, Glezen WP: Respiratory tract infections in children in day care. Semin Pediatr Infect Dis 1:234, 1990.

Hale FM, Polder JA: The ABCs of safe and healthy child care. Centers for Disease Control and Prevention, Department of Health and Human Services, 1996. (Also available at http://www.cdc.gov/ncidod/hip/abc/abc.htm)

Helfand RF, Khan AS, Pallansch MA, et al: Echovirus 30 infection and aseptic meningitis in parents of children attending a child care center. J Infect Dis 169:1133, 1994.

Holmes SJ, Morrow AL, Pickering LK: Child care practices: Effects of social changes on epidemiology of infectious diseases and antibiotic resistance. Epidemiol Rev 18:10, 1996.

Louhiala PJ, Jaakkola N, Ruotsalainen R, et al: Day-care centers and diarrhea: A public health perspective. J Pediatr 131:476, 1997.

MacDonald JK, Boase J, Stewart LK, et al: Active and passive surveillance for communicable diseases in child care facilities, Seattle-King County, Washington. Am J Public Health 87:1951, 1997.

Osterholm MT: Invasive bacterial diseases and child day care. Semin Pediatr Infect Dis 1:222, 1990.

Pass RF: Day care centers and transmission of cytomegalovirus: New insight into an old problem. Semin Pediatr Infect Dis 1:245, 1990.

Reves RR, Pickering LK: Impact of child day care on infectious diseases in adults. Infect Dis Clin North Am 6:239, 1992.

Reves RR, Jones JA: Antibiotic use and resistance patterns in day care. Semin Pediatr Infect Dis 1:212, 1990.

Shapiro CN, Hadler SC: Significance of hepatitis in children in day care. Semin Pediatr Infect Dis 1:270, 1990.

Simons RJ, Chanock S: Medical issues related to caring for human immunodeficiency virus-infected children in and out of the home. Pediatr Infect Dis J 12:845, 1993.

CHAPTER 304
Health Advice for Children Traveling Internationally

Robert A. Bonomo and Robert A. Salata

The major increase in international travel and the resurgence of malaria and other infectious diseases worldwide bring the issues regarding prevention and management of health problems in travelers into the office of every physician caring for children. Approximately 500 million people will cross international boundaries this year. Many physicians trained in developed countries are unfamiliar with the health hazards and the rapidly changing information and requirements related to international travel. Most children do not become ill until they return home. The risks, needs, and requirements for children who are traveling, particularly those younger than 2 yr, may differ from those of adults.

In the United States, recommendations and vaccine requirements for travel to different countries are provided in the publications by the Centers for Disease Control and Prevention (CDC), including *Health Information for International Travel.* It can be obtained from the Superintendent of Documents, United States Government Printing Office, Washington, DC 20402-9235. Updated information also is available from the CDC at http://www.cdc.gov/travel/index.htm.

GENERAL RECOMMENDATIONS. Parents of traveling children should seek medical consultation well in advance of their departure to obtain a realistic assessment of risks, determine immunization and chemoprophylactic measures, and receive instruction for dealing with disease during travel. Recommendations should be reviewed with a physician at least 4–6 wk before departure to ensure proper scheduling of vaccinations and medications. Traveling with small children, particularly infants, entails special concerns related to incomplete primary immunizations, lack of demonstrated efficacy and safety in infants of many vaccines indicated for travel, and increased morbidity and possible mortality associated with some diseases acquired abroad.

General advice to parents should first include a discussion of eating and drinking habits, because most travel-related health problems result from ingestion of contaminated food or water. Among the bacterial and protozoan infections children can acquire from contaminated water are shigellosis, salmonellosis, *Escherichia coli* infections, cholera, giardiasis, amebiasis, and cryptosporidiosis. Families must be aware that consumption of chlorinated water may not be entirely free of risk (e.g., *Giardia* and amoeba). Boiled water, hot beverages made with boiled water, and canned or bottled carbonated beverages are generally safest. Ice should be avoided, and tap water should not be used when brushing teeth. Boiling water and chemical disinfecting with iodine are the most reliable methods to disinfect water. Disinfection with iodine can be accomplished with use of either tincture of iodine or tetraglycine hydroperiodide tablets, such as Globaline, Portable-Aqua, and others. If water is cloudy, it should first be strained through a clean cloth and treated with twice the usual number of disinfectant tablets. All raw food (e.g., fruits and uncooked vegetables) should be considered contaminated. In particular, children should avoid unpasteurized milk, milk products such as cheese, and uncooked meat or fish. Foods of particular concern include salads, uncooked vegetables, and unpeeled fruit. Fish, especially reef fish, red snapper, and barracuda, are of particular concern because they may possess toxins. Breast-feeding should be encouraged for young children, especially infants younger than 6 mo.

Travel consultation should also include the common problems related to travel, including jet lag, sinus and ear problems, altitude sickness, environmental exposures, the hazards of insects as vectors of many infections (e.g., malaria, yellow fever, dengue, filariasis, trypanosomiasis, and onchocerciasis), and the means to avoid these vectors. Exposure to insect bites can be avoided by restricting high-risk activities, wearing appropriate attire, and using insect repellents containing permethrin and *N,N*-diethyl-M-toluamide (DEET). Insect repellent should be purchased before departure. The higher the concentration of DEET, the longer it lasts as a repellent. Toxic encephalopathy, however, has occurred in children exposed to DEET. Frequent application of products containing high concentrations of DEET (>30% concentration) should be avoided in children.

Injuries and motor vehicle accidents are the major causes of serious disability or loss of life during travel. The use of safety belts for children, preferably sitting in the rear seat, should be emphasized. When possible, child safety-restraint seats should be taken on the trip. Travelers to remote areas should be warned about venomous animals (snake and scorpion bites can be fatal for infants), rabies (predominantly transmitted by domestic dogs and cats), and exposure to rodents (because of plague). Swimming or diving in contaminated water can result in serious injury and can increase the risk of infections including, depending on the locale, leptospirosis, schistosomiasis, and primary amebic meningoencephalitis. Most of the illnesses that develop in traveling children are related to behaviors that can be modified with proper advice and supervision by parents.

Sexually transmitted diseases, including HIV infection and AIDS, are more prevalent in many countries than in the United States. HIV is not transmitted through casual contact, sources of food or water, contact with inanimate objects, mosquitoes, or other insect vectors. The hazards of sexual encounters as well as needle and blood and blood product exposure should be emphasized, especially for adolescents. Blood sources in developing countries can be suspect; systematic screening of blood donations for HIV and other blood-borne infections is not yet feasible in many developing countries. The universal safety of transfusion services abroad cannot be ensured. If resuscitation is needed, colloid and crystalloid plasma expanders can be used as a temporizing measure. Travelers may wish to have their blood typed before departure to determine whether transfusions from family members or travel companions with similar blood types may be possible in dire emergencies. Several agencies can provide emergency medical evacuation to developed countries if the situation dictates.

Children with pre-existing medical problems are traveling more extensively and are in greatest need of consultation before departure. Travel has the greatest impact on children with chronic cardiopulmonary disease, diabetes, allergies, and gastrointestinal problems, especially diarrhea associated with malabsorption or inflammatory bowel disease. Patients with insulin-dependent diabetes or hemophilia should carry an adequate supply of sterile needles, syringes, and disinfectant swabs. Special arrangements should be made for patients with bleeding disorders, those on anticoagulation therapy, and those who require hemodialysis. Biologic products such as clotting factor concentrates or immune globulin should be avoided if manufactured abroad.

Children with medical conditions should take with them a brief medical summary. For children requiring care by specialists, an international directory for that specialty can be consulted. A directory of physicians worldwide who speak English and who have met certain qualifications is available from the International Association for Medical Assistance to Travelers (736 Center St., Lewiston, NY 14092; telephone: [716] 754-4883). If medical care is needed urgently when abroad, sources of information include the American embassy or consulate,

TABLE 304–1 Accelerated Schedule of Routine Childhood Immunizations if Necessary for Travel

Vaccine	Routine Schedule	Accelerated Schedule
Diphtheria, tetanus, pertussis	DTaP: 2, 4, 6, 15–18 mo of age	DTaP: 6 wk of age, with 4 wk between 1st, 2nd, and 3rd doses, and 6 mo between 3rd and 4th doses
	DTaP: 4–6 yr of age (booster)	DTaP: 4 yr of age
	dT every 10 yr	dT every 5 yr if at high risk
Poliomyelitis	IPV/OPV: IPV at 2 and 4 mo, OPV at 12–18 mo and 4–6 yr	OPV: 4 wk of age, with 6 wk between 1st, 2nd, and 3rd doses IPV: 6 wk of age, with 1 mo between 1st and 2nd doses and 6 mo between 2nd and 3rd doses
	No additional boosters unless traveling to an endemic area	A single IPV or OPV lifetime booster for adolescents and adults who have completed primary immunization
Measles, mumps, rubella	MMR: 12–15 mo of age, with second dose at age 4–6 yr	Two doses at ≥12 mo of age, 4 wk apart
	Not routinely recommended for children <12 mo of age	May give first measles as early as age 6 mo, with additional two doses ≥12 mo of age
Haemophilus influenzae type b	2, 4, 6 (if HbOC or PRP-T), and 12–15 mo	HbOC and PRP-T: 6 wk of age, with 1 mo between the 1st and 2nd and the 2nd and 3rd doses; booster at ≥12 mo of age (≥2 mo from the 3rd dose) PRO-OMP: 6 wk of age, with 1 mo between the 1st and 2nd doses; booster at ≥12 mo of age (≥2 mo from the 3rd dose)
Hepatitis B	Birth, 1–2 mo, 6 mo	0, 1, and 4 mo of age
Varicella	12–18 mo of age	12 mo of age (two doses 1 mo apart for persons age ≥13 yr)
Rotavirus	2, 4, 6 mo of age	6 wk of age, with 2nd and 3rd doses each separated by 3 wk

hotel managers, travel agents catering to foreign tourists, and missionary hospitals. Parents should be counseled, however, to take a sufficient supply of prescription medications for their children and to ensure that the bottles are clearly identified. A travel health kit consisting of prescription medications and nonprescription items is often useful. Travelers also need to ascertain whether their health insurance covers medical care abroad.

IMMUNIZATIONS. Immunization is only one component of a comprehensive disease prevention program for traveling children. The routine childhood vaccination schedule can be accelerated to maximize protection for traveling children, especially for unvaccinated and incompletely vaccinated children (Table 304–1; see Chapter 301). Issues related to the minimum age at administration also arise for those immunizations that are considered solely because of specific travel-related needs (e.g., hepatitis A, typhoid, yellow fever, Japanese encephalitis, meningococcus, rabies, and cholera vaccines).

Parents should allow 6 wk before departure for optimal administration of vaccines to their children, because some immunizations require repeated doses for full protection and some immunobiologic agents are incompatible with others. In general, inactivated vaccines can be given simultaneously, although both local and systemic adverse reactions may be cumulative. Live-attenuated viral vaccines should always be administered concurrently, or alternatively, at least 30 days apart to minimize interference. Inactivated and live vaccines can be administered concurrently, with the notable exception of yellow fever and cholera vaccines, which should not be given simultaneously or within 3 wk of each other because the antibody response to both vaccines may be decreased. Measles vaccination should be delayed for 3 mo and varicella for 5 mo, after intramuscular immune globulin, which can interfere with these immunizations. Immune globulin does not interfere with the immune response to oral typhoid, oral poliovirus, or yellow fever vaccines. Immune globulin should not be administered less than 2 wk after measles immunization or less than 3 wk after varicella immunization.

Vaccine products produced in eggs may contain an allergenic substance that causes hypersensitivity responses, including anaphylaxis in persons with known severe egg sensitivity. Screening by history of ability to ingest eggs without adverse effects is a reasonable way to identify those at allergic risk from receiving measles, mumps, influenza, or yellow fever vaccines. Most hypersensitivity reactions to measles and mumps are to gelatin and other components such as preservatives (e.g., thimerosal) and antibiotics (e.g., neomycin).

In general, live-virus vaccines (e.g., oral poliovirus, varicella) and live bacterial vaccines (e.g., bacille Calmette-Guérin [BCG], oral typhoid) are contraindicated in immunocompromised persons (see Table 179–5). An exception is measles and varicella vaccines, which are indicated for all HIV-infected children except those who are severely compromised (Chapter 268). Although children with symptomatic HIV infection should not receive yellow fever vaccine, asymptomatic HIV-infected children may be vaccinated if the risk from yellow fever remains significant. Inactivated vaccines and toxoids are not contraindicated in immunocompromised children. Immunocompromising conditions may, however, reduce immunologic responses to inactivated vaccines and toxoids.

Routine Childhood Vaccinations. All children who travel should be immunized according to routine childhood immunization with all vaccines appropriate for their age (Chapter 301).

DIPHTHERIA, TETANUS, AND PERTUSSIS. Diphtheria is endemic in many developing countries. After the disintegration of the Soviet Union in 1991, diphtheria re-emerged in the new independent states. The highest incidence of diphtheria has been reported from Azerbaijan, Tajikistan, and Latvia. Tetanus is a major cause of worldwide neonatal mortality and is most prevalent in tropical countries. Neonatal tetanus usually occurs in infants born under unhygienic conditions to inadequately vaccinated mothers. Pertussis is common in developing countries and in some developed nations where pertussis immunization is not as widely provided as in the United States.

Protection is attained with four doses of DTaP (or DTP) and a booster at 4–6 yr of age (Chapter 301). The schedule can be accelerated for children traveling internationally (Table 304–1). DT should be used for children who are younger than 7 yr and who have a contraindication to pertussis vaccine. Pertussis vaccination has not been recommended for persons 7 yr of age or older.

POLIOMYELITIS. The risk of poliomyelitis is minimal in most developed nations, and autochthonous polio has been eradicated from the Western hemisphere, but many developing countries are still endemic for poliomyelitis.

The poliovirus vaccination schedule in the United States is with the sequential IPV/OPV regimen, or alternatively with IPV alone or OPV alone, and should be completed for all individuals younger than 18 yr (Chapter 301). Enhanced-potency IPV is indicated for children who are immunocompromised and for close contacts of immunocompromised persons. For very young children, immunization can be started as early as 4–6 wk of age (Table 304–1). A regimen incorporating trivalent OPV is recommended for all infants and children who may travel internationally if there are no contraindications. For unvaccinated adults who are at increased risk of exposure to poliovirus and who cannot complete the recommended IPV regimen (0, 1–2, and 6–12 mo), three doses of IPV should be administered at least 4 wk apart.

Measles, Mumps, and Rubella. Measles is still endemic in many developing countries and in some industrialized nations. Measles vaccine, preferably in combination with mumps and rubella vaccines, should be given to all children at 12–15 mo of age and at 4–6 yr of age, unless there is a contraindication (Chapter 301). The age of the first vaccination should be lowered to 6 mo for children traveling to endemic areas. Infants younger than 6 mo are protected by maternal antibodies. The interval for the second dose for all children can be as soon as 4 wk (Table 304–1). Measles in HIV-infected children can be a devastating illness. Consequently, HIV-infected children who travel abroad should be vaccinated unless severely immunocompromised (see Table 268–2).

Haemophilus Influenzae Type b. Severe *H. influenzae* type b infection is most common in children 6 mo–1 yr of age, but one third of cases of invasive infection are found in children 18 mo of age or older. Before they travel, all unimmunized children younger than 60 mo and all persons with chronic illness at risk for *H. influenzae* type b infections should be vaccinated (Chapter 301).

Hepatitis B. Hepatitis B is highly prevalent in eastern and southeastern Asia, sub-Saharan Africa, and the Pacific Basin. In certain parts of the world, 8–15% of the population may be chronically infected. Situations in which disease transmission can occur include receipt of blood transfusions not screened for hepatitis B surface antigen, exposure to unsterilized needles, or close contact with local children who have open skin lesions. Infants and children traveling to such areas may be at risk if they are exposed directly to blood from the local population. Adolescents may be infected through sexual exposure. Exposure to hepatitis B is more likely for travelers residing for prolonged periods in endemic areas.

Vaccination for hepatitis B is recommended for all children in the United States. The hepatitis B schedule can be accelerated (Table 304–1). Partial protection may be provided by one or two doses.

Varicella. All children who are 12 mo of age or older and who have no history of varicella vaccination or chickenpox should be vaccinated. Infants are generally protected by maternal antibodies. Children younger than 13 yr require only a single dose; children 13 yr of age or older require two doses separated by 4–8 wk.

Rotavirus. Rotavirus vaccine is available and recommended, as resources permit, for all infants in the United States. Infants traveling abroad during the winter-spring rotavirus season are especially appropriate vaccine candidates. The rotavirus vaccine can be given as early as 6 wk of age, and the schedule accelerated with 3 wk between each dose of the three dose regimen (Table 304–1). Vaccination should not be started after 6 mo of age, and all doses should be administered by 12 mo of age.

Special Vaccinations for Travel

Hepatitis A. Hepatitis A is endemic in most of the world, and travelers are at risk even if their travel is restricted to the usual tourist routes. Hepatitis A can occur as a result of ingesting shellfish harvested from sewage-contaminated waters and from unwashed vegetables or fruits. Clinical hepatitis may be asymptomatic in young children; infected children can, however, transmit infection to older children and adults, in whom it is usually symptomatic.

Two inactivated hepatitis A vaccines are currently available. Hepatitis A vaccine in two doses (0.5 mL for 2–17 yr of age; 1 mL for ≥18 yr of age) intramuscularly 6–12 mo apart is recommended for international travelers to countries with intermediate or high hepatitis A endemicity (areas other than the United States, Canada, Australia, New Zealand, Western Europe, and Scandinavia). Protective immunity develops 2–4 wk after receiving the initial vaccine dose.

If immediate protection (before 2 wk) is necessary, intramuscular immune globulin can be given. For short-term protection (1–2 mo), 0.02 mL/kg is given; for long-term protection (3–5 mo), 0.06 mL/kg is given and repeated every 5 mo while exposure to hepatitis A continues. Immune globulin produced in developing countries may not meet the same standards for purity set in developed countries. Immune globulin can be administered with the inactivated vaccine, if necessary, at a separate site and in a separate syringe. Immunization with measles-mumps-rubella vaccine (MMR) should be deferred for 3 mo, and varicella for 5 mo, after immune globulin (0.02 mL/kg or 0.06 mL/kg).

Typhoid. *Salmonella typhi* infection, or typhoid fever, is not uncommon in young children (Chapter 196.2). American international travelers are at risk for contracting typhoid, especially in the Indian subcontinent and western South America. Typhoid vaccination is recommended for persons traveling to endemic areas, especially if exposure to contaminated food and water is likely. Vaccination is also recommended for travelers to areas with *S. typhi* strains that are resistant to antimicrobial agents.

Three typhoid vaccines, including one oral and two parenteral vaccines, are available in the United States. The oral typhoid vaccine is most often used because of its ease of administration but is limited to persons 6 yr of age or older. Parenteral vaccines are used for children younger than 6 yr. The oral vaccine is given as four doses of one enteric-coated capsule on alternate days, with the course repeated as a booster every 5 yr. The oral vaccine is much less immunogenic in children younger than 4 yr and is recommended for persons age 6 yr or older. It is also not recommended for immunocompromised children; the inactivated vaccine should be used for these children. Oral typhoid vaccine should not be given for 24 hr after the most recent dose of antibiotic or mefloquine. The heat-phenol-inactivated vaccine (strain Ty2) has 60–80% efficacy and has been widely used for many years. It is given as two doses (0.25 mL for age 6 mo–10 yr; 0.5 mL for age 10 yr or older) subcutaneously 4 wk apart, with a booster dose every 3 yr. This vaccine can sometimes cause fever (7–24%), headache (10%), and severe local pain (3–35%) at the site of administration. A newer parenteral Vi capsular polysaccharide vaccine (strain Ty2) has fewer adverse effects. It is given as a single dose (0.5 mL IM) for persons age 2 yr or older, with a booster every 2 yr.

Meningococcus. Meningococcal meningitis is a worldwide disease (Chapter 191); epidemic disease has been reported in India, Nepal, Saudi Arabia, and sub-Saharan Africa. Cases in American travelers in such areas are infrequent; however, prolonged contact with the local population could increase the risk of infection, and vaccination is thus a reasonable precaution. Saudi Arabia requires evidence of meningococcal vaccination for travel to parts of that country. Serogroup A is the most common cause of epidemics outside the United States, but serogroup C and, rarely, serogroup B have been associated with epidemics.

One meningococcal vaccine is available in the United States, the quadrivalent polysaccharide A/C/Y/W-135 vaccine. The vaccine is ineffective against serogroup A in infants younger than 3 mo and may be only partially effective in children 3–11 mo of age. Children younger than 2 yr are not protected against serogroup C. The meningococcus vaccine (0.5 mL SC) is recommended for persons age 2 yr or older traveling to or residing in a country with hyperendemic or epidemic meningococcal disease caused by a vaccine serogroup, as well as for children age 3 mo or older traveling to an area with hyperendemic or endemic serogroup A meningococcal disease. Children vaccinated before 4 yr of age should be revaccinated after 2–3 yr if they remain in an endemic area.

INFLUENZA. The risk for exposure to influenza during international travel varies depending on the time of year, destination, and intermingling of persons from different parts of the world where influenza may be circulating. In the tropics, such as the Caribbean, influenza can occur throughout the year. In the temperate regions of the Southern Hemisphere, including Australia and South America, most activity occurs from April through September. In the Northern Hemisphere, including the United States and Canada, influenza generally occurs from November through March. Infection acquired during travel can result in clinical illness during or after travel. Influenza vaccination is recommended for persons at increased risk for complications of influenza, including persons of any age with chronic medical conditions and persons age 65 yr and older (Chapter 301).

RABIES. The risk of rabies is currently the highest in countries where rabies in dogs is uncontrolled, including Colombia, Ecuador, El Salvador, Guatemala, India, Mexico, Nepal, Philippines, Thailand, and Vietnam. Rabies is also endemic in most other countries of Africa, Asia, and Central and South America. Children are at particular risk, because facial bites are more common. Children should be considered for pre-exposure prophylaxis if they will be in endemic areas for longer than 1 mo.

Two inactivated rabies vaccines are available in the United States for pre-exposure vaccination. These vaccines are human diploid cell rabies vaccine (HDCV) and the rabies vaccine absorbed (RVA). The human diploid cell vaccine (HDCV) must be administered by the intradermal route. Pre-exposure prophylaxis is given to individuals at risk either intramuscularly (RVA) as 3 doses (1 mL) on days 0, 7, and 28; or intradermally (HDCV) as 3 doses (0.1 mL) on days 0, 7, and 28. Postexposure prophylaxis, with rabies immune globulin (Chapter 265), is given as five doses (1 mL) on days 0, 3, 7, 14, and 28 if previously unvaccinated, and in two doses (1 mL) on days 0 and 3 if previously vaccinated. Intramuscular administration is the preferred route for pre-exposure travel vaccination and for postexposure. Travelers receiving mefloquine or chloroquine may have limited immune reactions to intradermal rabies vaccines and should be vaccinated intramuscularly.

JAPANESE ENCEPHALITIS. Japanese encephalitis is a mosquito-borne viral disease with a fatality rate of 20%. The disease occurs primarily from June to September in temperate zones and throughout the entire year in tropical zones. Japanese encephalitis is the leading cause of viral encephalitis worldwide and occurs in the People's Republic of China, India, Bangladesh, Nepal, Sri Lanka, Hong Kong, Singapore, Korea, Japan, Taiwan, Philippines, eastern Russia, and Southeast Asia. In endemic areas, the age-specific incidence is highest in young children. The risk for travelers is associated with the extent of exposure to the mosquito vectors. Since 1981, six cases of Japanese encephalitis have been identified among adult expatriate Americans. Fortunately, most cases are asymptomatic, but mortality rates of 50% or significant neurologic sequelae in one third of survivors are associated with symptomatic cases.

The inactivated Japanese encephalitis vaccine, which has an efficacy exceeding 95%, is available in the United States. Anaphylaxis is an infrequent side effect. The vaccine is administered in three doses (0.5 mL for 1–3 yr of age; 1 mL for ≥3 yr of age) subcutaneously on days 0, 7, and 30, to travelers with a high risk of exposure to the mosquito vectors. This includes travelers who will be residing for 1 mo or more in rural endemic areas, especially in areas of rice or pig farming, during transmission season (May to September in temperate climates; variable in subtropical and tropical areas with the rainfall, the rainy season, and the migratory patterns of the avian-amplifying host), and travelers for less than 30 days in areas experiencing endemic transmission.

YELLOW FEVER. Yellow fever (Chapter 261) is a mosquito-borne viral illness resembling other viral hemorrhagic fevers (Chapter 262) but with more prominent hepatic involvement. Yellow fever is present in jungle areas of South America and Africa. In South America, sporadic infection is found in forestry, agricultural, and other workers with occupational exposure. In Africa, the virus is transmitted to young children in the moist savanna zones of West Africa during the rainy season.

Yellow fever vaccine (0.5 mL SC) is a live-attenuated vaccine (17D strain) developed in chick embryos and is extremely safe and effective. However, yellow fever vaccine is associated with an increased risk of encephalitis (1%) and other severe reactions in young infants. Yellow fever vaccine should not be administered to infants younger than 4 mo; infants 4–6 mo of age should be vaccinated only under extreme circumstances; infants 6–9 mo of age should be vaccinated if they cannot avoid traveling to high-risk areas.

Some countries require yellow fever vaccination by law for travelers arriving from endemic areas. Some African countries require evidence of vaccination from all entering travelers. Current recommendations can be obtained by contacting state or local health departments or the Division of Vector-Borne Infectious Diseases of the CDC (telephone: [404] 332-4555). Most countries accept a medical waiver for children who are too young to be vaccinated (<4 mo of age) and for individuals with a contraindication to vaccination, such as immunodeficiency. Children with asymptomatic HIV infection may be vaccinated if exposure to yellow fever virus cannot be avoided.

Long-lived, perhaps lifetime immunity develops; however, international travel certificates require proof of immunization within 10 yr. Cholera vaccine given simultaneously or within 3 wk of yellow fever vaccine reduces but does not prevent an antibody response to yellow fever immunization. Yellow fever vaccine should not be administered to patients with a history of anaphylactic reactions to eggs.

CHOLERA. Cholera is an acute noninflammatory diarrheal illness caused by *Vibrio cholerae* 01 acquired through ingestion of contaminated food or water (Chapter 199). Severe cases can be characterized by watery diarrhea and vomiting, which can progress to dehydration, shock, acidosis, or death. In children younger than 2 yr, cholera is frequently a mild disease. Although its spread has continued since the seventh worldwide pandemic of cholera of 1961, travelers from the United States rarely contract cholera. The reappearance of cholera in South America and Central America poses additional risks to children traveling to these areas.

One cholera vaccine (0.2 mL for 6 mo–4 yr of age; 0.3 mL 5–10 yr of age; 0.5 mL for >10 yr of age; SC or IM, as two doses 1 wk to ≥1 mo apart) is licensed for use in the United States. Although vaccination can reduce the rate of illness by 50%, it provides only short-term protection. Vaccine efficacy is particularly low in children younger than 5 yr. No country or territory currently requires cholera vaccination, although local authorities may continue to require documentation of vaccination; in such cases, a single dose is sufficient to satisfy local requirements. Persons who follow the usual tourist itinerary and who use standard accomodations in countries reporting cholera are at very low risk for infection. The World Health Organization (WHO) and the CDC do not recommend cholera vaccination for international travel. Because cholera vaccination is not recommended for children younger than 6 mo, a medical waiver for these infants should be provided before departure. Breast-feeding should be encouraged in cholera-endemic areas. Several new vaccines, including a killed whole-cell oral vaccine given in two doses and a genetically engineered attenuated strain, are being studied.

LYME DISEASE. A Lyme disease vaccine composed of recombinant OspA protein has been licensed in the United States for persons age 15 yr and older. Protection requires three doses at 0, 1, and 12 mo. The vaccine is not approved for use in children, and no recommendations have been established for international travelers. The dosing regimen, which requires 12 mo to complete, precludes use in most adult travelers.

Plague. The plague vaccine is not currently recommended or required for international travel.

TRAVELER'S DIARRHEA. Traveler's diarrhea, characterized by a twofold or greater increase in the frequency of unformed bowel movements, occurs in as many as 40% of all travelers overseas. Approximately 5 million people per year from developed nations who travel abroad experience this illness. Typical symptoms include nonbloody diarrhea, low-grade fever, nausea, bloating, urgency, and malaise. The disease is usually self-limited and is characterized by 3–5 days of nonbloody diarrhea without significant fever. Careful selection and preparation of food and water can reduce the risk of developing traveler's diarrhea.

Traveler's diarrhea is usually acquired through ingestion of fecally contaminated food and water. Diverse infectious agents (bacteria, viruses, and parasites) have been associated with traveler's diarrhea; enterotoxic *E. coli* is still the most frequent cause. Other bacterial causes include *Shigella, Salmonella, Campylobacter, V. cholerae, Vibrio parahaemolyticus, Aeromonas hydrophilia,* and *Plesiomonas shigelloides.* Protozoan infections such as *Entamoeba histolytica, Giardia lamblia, Cryptosporidium parvum,* and *Isospora* are more common in long-term travelers. Rotavirus has also been associated with traveler's diarrhea. The most important risk factor for traveler's diarrhea is the country of destination. High-risk areas (attack rates of 25–50%) include developing countries of Latin America, Africa, the Middle East, and Asia. Intermediate risk occurs in the Mediterranean, China, and Israel. Low-risk areas include North America, Northern Europe, Australia, and New Zealand.

Few data define the use of antidiarrheal drugs in children. Chemoprophylactic agents for traveler's diarrhea are not recommended for children or adults. Bismuth subsalicylate (Pepto-Bismol) in adults (60 mL or 2 tablets PO qid) appears to be an effective preventive agent, but is not recommended for periods longer than 3 wk or in children, adolescents, or pregnant women. Ingesting such large amounts of bismuth and salicylate is of concern.

Presumptive self-treatment is usually recommended for adults, initiated at the first signs of diarrhea, nausea, bloating, or urgency. For adults and adolescents age 18 yr or older, the recommended regimen is ciprofloxacin (500 mg), norfloxacin (400 mg), or ofloxacin (300 mg) orally twice daily for 3 days. The recommended drug for children age 2 mo or older and an alternative for adults is trimethoprim-sulfamethoxazole (TMP-SMX) (4 mg TMP plus 20 mg SMX/kg/dose; maximum 160 mg TMP plus 800 mg SMX) orally twice daily for 3 days. Antimicrobial therapy for traveler's diarrhea in infants and young children should be administered in consultation with a physician. This is particularly true if the illness is severe, persists for longer than 3 days, or is associated with bloody stools, temperature greater than 102°F, chills, vomiting, or moderate to severe hydration. Resistance to TMP-SMX should be considered. Furazolidone (5 mg/kg/24 hr PO divided in four doses) may be an alternative, given its efficacy against both bacterial pathogens and *G. lamblia.*

Dehydration is the greatest threat presented by a diarrheal illness in a small child. Educating parents about the symptoms and signs of dehydration is necessary. Parents should carry with them prepackaged WHO/UNICEF oral rehydration solution (ORS) packets, which are available at stores or pharmacies in almost all developing countries. Antimotility agents such as diphenoxylate (Lomotil) should be avoided; mortality and morbidity from infection caused by *Salmonella* and *Shigella* are higher with diphenoxylate therapy. Bismuth subsalicylate (5 mL for 3–5 yr of age; 10 mL for 6–8 yr of age; 15 mL for 9–11 yr of age; 30 mL for ≥12 yr of age) as often as every 30 min for eight doses, with no more than eight doses/24 hr, decreases the rate of stooling and shortens the duration of illness. Preexisting gastrointestinal disease such as celiac sprue, ulcerative colitis, Crohn's disease, and immunosuppression due to HIV can place children at great risk, especially for *Salmonella* infection.

MALARIA CHEMOPROPHYLAXIS. Malaria, a mosquito-borne infection, is the leading parasitic cause of death in children worldwide (Chapter 278). Of the four *Plasmodium* species that infect humans, *P. falciparum* causes the greatest morbidity and mortality. Each year, more than 8 million United States citizens visit parts of the world where malaria is endemic (sub-Saharan Africa, Central and South America, India, Southeast Asia, Oceania). Given this major resurgence of malaria, physicians in developed countries are increasingly required to give advice on prevention, diagnosis, and treatment of malaria. The CDC maintains updated information at http://www.cdc.gov/travel/index.htm, as well as a malaria hotline for physicians ([770] 488-7788). Because of continuing changes in the risks of developing malaria in many areas of the world, changing *Plasmodium* resistance patterns, and modifications of recommendations for prophylaxis and treatment, physicians should use these resources for updated information.

Malaria transmission occurs primarily between dusk and dawn. Measures to limit outdoor activities during this time avoid the insect vector and use of appropriate clothing, netting, and insect repellents are extremely important and should be emphasized. Prophylactic chemoprophylaxis has also been shown to be extremely effective but is not a replacement for other protective measures. Chemoprophylaxis should begin 1 wk (1 day if doxycycline is used) before departure, continue during the stay, and for 4 wk after leaving an endemic area. None of the chemoprophylactic drug regimens guarantees complete protection against malaria. Only 28% of the 410 American citizens with *P. falciparum* malaria acquired in Africa between 1980 and 1984 were using a recommended drug for prophylaxis. One survey of 4,042 returning American travelers to Africa and Haiti found that 58% of these individuals did not take recommended prophylactic agents regularly. Travelers are more likely to use prophylactic antimalarial drugs if their physicians provide appropriate recommendations and education before departure. However, in one survey, only 14% of persons who sought medical advice obtained correct information about malaria prevention and prophylaxis.

Resistance of *P. falciparum* to the traditional chemoprophylactic agent, chloroquine, is rapidly increasing worldwide. Because of this growing problem of resistance, other agents are increasingly used. Several factors are important in choosing appropriate chemoprophylactic regimens for malaria. The travel itinerary should be reviewed thoroughly in relation to information about areas of risk within a particular country, especially the risk for acquiring chloroquine-resistant *P. falciparum.* Finally, allergic or other known adverse reactions to antimalarial agents should be considered, as well as the availability of medical care during travel. Malaria chemoprophylaxis for children is problematic because many medications used for adults have not been evaluated in small children or are associated with unacceptable adverse effects. Parents should be discouraged from taking a young child on a trip that will entail evening or nighttime exposure in rural areas of countries with chloroquine- or multidrug-resistant *P. falciparum.*

Chloroquine phosphate is still the mainstay of chemoprophylaxis for travelers to most malaria-endemic areas with chloroquine-sensitive strains of *P. falciparum* (Table 304–2). Chloroquine is available only in tablet form, which tastes bitter. Chloroquine syrup (Nivaquin) is available outside the United States and is well tolerated. *P. falciparum* is fully sensitive to chloroquine only in Haiti, the Dominican Republic, Central America north of the Panama Canal, and the Middle East

TABLE 304–2 Chemoprophylaxis of Malaria in Children

	Drug*	Dosage
Chloroquine-sensitive Areas	Chloroquine phosphate	5 mg/kg base/wk (8.3 mg/kg salt) once per wk (maximum, 300 mg base [500 mg salt])
Chloroquine-resistant Areas	Mefloquine†	<5 kg: 5 mg/kg once per wk 5–9 kg: 1/8 tablet once per wk 10–19 kg: 1/4 tablet once per wk 20–30 kg: 1/2 tablet once per wk 31–45 kg: 3/4 tablet once per wk >45 kg: 1 tablet once per wk
	or	
	Doxycycline‡	2 mg/kg/24 hr (maximum, 100 mg/24 hr) once daily
	Alternatives:	
	Chloroquine phosphate	Same as above
	with or without	
	Proguanil‖	<2 yr of age: 50 mg daily 2–6 yr of age: 100 mg daily 7–10 yr of age: 150 mg daily >10 yr of age: 200 mg daily
	plus	
	Pyrimethamine-sulfadoxine (Fansidar) for presumptive treatment§	<1 yr of age: 1/4 tablet 1–3 yr of age: 1/2 tablet 4–8 yr of age: 1 tablet 9–14 yr of age: 2 tablets >14 yr of age: 3 tablets

**Currently, no drug regimen guarantees protection against malaria. Travelers to countries with risk of malaria should be advised to avoid mosquito bites by using personal protective measures (see text). Prophylaxis is recommended beginning 1 wk (1 day if doxycycline is used) before travel, continuing for the duration of the stay and for 4 wk after last exposure. Review contraindications and adverse effects before use (see text).*

†Mefloquine is not licensed by the US Food and Drug Administration (FDA) for children who weigh <15 kg, but recent recommendations from the Centers for Disease Control and Prevention (CDC) allow use of the drug to be considered in children without weight restrictions when travel to chloroquine-resistant P. falciparum *areas cannot be avoided.*

‡Physicians who prescribe doxycycline as malaria chemoprophylaxis should advise patients to limit their exposure to direct sunlight to minimize the possibility of photosensitivity reaction. Use of doxycycline is contraindicated in pregnant women and usually in children <8 yr of age. Physicians must weigh the benefits of doxycycline therapy against the possibility of dental staining in children <8 yr of age.

§Fansidar tablets contain 25 mg of pyrimethamine and 500 mg of sulfadoxine. Fansidar is contraindicated in patients with a history of pyrimethamine or sulfonamide intolerance, in pregnancy at term, and in infants <2 mo of age, unless circumstances indicate that the potential benefit outweighs the possible risk of hyperbilirubinemia in the infant. Resistance to pyrimethamine-sulfadoxine has been reported from Southeast Asia, the Amazon basin, sub-Saharan Africa, Bangladesh, and Oceania. A single dose of Fansidar can be used for self-treatment of febrile illness if medical care is not available within 24 hours, while promptly seeking medical care.

‖Proguanil (Paludrine), which is not available in the United States but is widely available in Canada and overseas, is recommended primarily for use in sub-Saharan Africa. Failures of prophylaxis with chloroquine and proguanil have been reported commonly, as this combination is only 40–60% effective.

(Egypt). Although the other *Plasmodium* species infecting humans generally remain sensitive to chloroquine, chloroquine resistance among *P. vivax* strains in India and New Guinea has been reported. In areas where *P. falciparum* is developing resistance to chloroquine, sensitive strains coexist. In one study, decreased parasitemia and milder illness were also encountered in individuals who took chloroquine but still developed chloroquine-resistant falciparum malaria.

Mefloquine, a synthetic 4-quinoline related to chloroquine, is highly effective against chloroquine-resistant *P. falciparum*. It is not recommended for children weighing less than 5 kg because of insufficient efficacy and tolerance data.

Doxycycline has been recommended for travelers to areas of multidrug-resistant *P. falciparum* (Thailand, Myranmar, Kampuchea, and the Amazon Basin). Tetracycline is contraindicated in children younger than 8 yr. Patients given doxycycline should limit exposure to direct sunlight to minimize the possibility of photosensitivity.

Proguanil (Paludrine), a dihydrofolate reductase inhibitor, is not available in the United States but is widely available in Canada and overseas. It is recommended by some authorities for prophylaxis against chloroquine-resistant *P. falciparum* in East Africa, especially for children weighing less than 15 kg. Limited data suggest that this drug is not effective in Thailand, the Amazon Basin, Papua New Guinea, and possibly West Africa. Proguanil should only be used in combination with weekly chloroquine phosphate.

Pyrimethamine-sulfadoxine (Fansidar) is no longer recommended for chemoprophylaxis owing to the occasional occurrence of severe adverse effects, including Stevens-Johnson syndrome and even death. Pyrimethamine-sulfadoxine resistance is a problem in sub-Saharan Africa and Southeast Asia. Pyrimethamine-sulfadoxine is still used for presumptive treatment (as a single dose) while travelers seek medical care as quickly as possible.

Primaquine is given to prevent relapses of malaria that occur with *P. vivax* and *P. ovale* infections. Prophylaxis is generally indicated for children who have prolonged exposure in malaria-endemic areas (Table 304–2). Primaquine can cause severe hemolysis in individuals with glucose-6-phosphate dehydrogenase (G6PD) deficiency; patients should be screened for G6PD deficiency before treatment.

Small amounts of antimalarial drugs are secreted into breast milk of lactating women. The amounts of transferred drug are not considered to be either harmful or sufficient to provide adequate prophylaxis against malaria.

Post-travel evaluations are part of travel medicine and continuing care. Testing for tuberculin reactivity, asymptomatic gastrointestinal parasitic infections, hepatitis, and skin lesions should be performed on return to the United States. On leaving a malaria-endemic area after a prolonged visit, travelers may require treatment with primaquine to eliminate the extraerythrocytic forms of *P. vivax* and *P. ovale* to prevent relapses. Malaria should be considered in the evaluation of fever that develops within 1 yr, especially within the first 2 mo, after travel to malarious areas.

Centers for Disease Control: Update: Diphtheria epidemic—new independent states of the former Soviet Union, January 1995–March 1996. MMWR 45:693, 1996.

Centers for Disease Control and Prevention: Health Information for International Travel 1996–1997. Washington, DC, US Department of Health and Human Services, Public Health Services, 1997.

DuPont HL, Ericsson CD: Prevention and treatment of traveler's diarrhea. N Engl J Med 328:1821, 1993.

Fisher PR: Travel with infants and children. Infect Dis Clin North Am 12:355, 1998.

Hill DR, Pearson RD: Health advice for international travel. Ann Intern Med 108:839, 1988.

Jong EC: Immunizations for international travel. Infect Dis Clin North Am 12:249, 1998.

Jong EC, McMullen R: General advice for the international traveler. Infect Dis Clin North Am 6:275, 1992.

Kain KC, Keystone JS: Malaria in travelers: Epidemiology, diseases, and prevention. Infect Dis Clin North Am 12:267, 1998.

Lobel HO, Kozarsky PE: Update on prevention of malaria for travelers. JAMA 278:1767, 1997.

Nahlen BL, Parsonnet J, Preblud SR, et al: International travel and the child younger than two years. II: Recommendations for prevention of travelers' diarrhea and malaria chemoprophylaxis. Pediatr Infect Dis 8:735, 1989.

Preblud SR, Tsai TF, Brink EW, et al: International travel and the child younger than two years. I: Recommendations for immunization. Pediatr Infect Dis 8:416, 1989.

Salata RA, Olds GR: Infectious diseases in travelers and immigrants. *In:* Warren KS, Mahmoud AAF (eds): Tropical and Geographical Medicine, 2nd ed. New York, McGraw-Hill, 1990, pp 228–242.

PART XVII

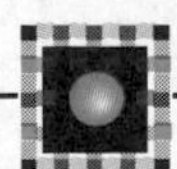

The Digestive System

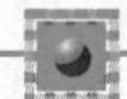

SECTION 1

Clinical Manifestations of Gastrointestinal Disease

Martin Ulshen

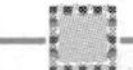

CHAPTER 305

Normal Digestive Tract Phenomena

Gastrointestinal (GI) function varies with maturity; a symptom that might be abnormal at an older age, such as regurgitation, may be normal in an infant. A fetus can swallow amniotic fluid as early as 12 wk gestation, but nutritive sucking in neonates first develops at about 34 wk gestation. The coordinated oral and pharyngeal movements necessary for swallowing solids develop within the 1st mo or two of life in term infants. Before this time, solids are thrust forward by the tongue, and aspiration is a risk from poor coordination of muscle function. By 1 mo of age, infants appear to show preferences for sweet and salty foods. Infants' interest in solids increases at about 4 mo of age. The current recommendation to begin solids at 6 mo of age is based on nutritional concepts rather than maturation of the swallowing process (Chapter 41). Infants swallow air during feeding and must be stimulated to burp to prevent gaseous distention of the stomach.

A number of normal anatomic variations may be noted in the mouth. A short lingual frenulum ("tongue-tie") may be worrisome to parents but only rarely interferes with eating or speech, generally requiring no treatment. Surface furrowing of the tongue (i.e., a geographic or scrotal tongue) is usually a normal finding. A bifid uvula may be normal or associated with a submucous cleft of the soft palate.

Regurgitation, the result of gastroesophageal reflux, occurs commonly in the first 12–18 mo of life. Effortless emesis may dribble out of an infant's mouth but also may be forceful. In an otherwise healthy infant with regurgitation, volumes of emesis are commonly about 15–30 mL but may occasionally be much larger. In contrast to vomiting, the episode of regurgitation from reflux usually surprises both infant and caretaker. Most often, the infant remains happy, although possibly hungry, after an episode of regurgitation. Episodes may occur from less than one to several times per day. If complications develop, gastroesophageal reflux is considered pathologic rather than merely developmental and deserves further evaluation and treatment. These complications include failure to thrive, pulmonary disease (apnea or aspiration pneumonitis), and esophagitis with its sequelae (see Chapters 323 and 324).

Infants and young children may be erratic eaters; this may be a worry to parents. A toddler may eat insatiably after refusing to consume normal amounts of food during previous meals. Infancy and adolescence are periods of rapid growth; high nutrient requirements for growth may be associated with voracious appetites. The reduced appetite of toddlers and preschool children is often a worry to parents who are used to the relatively greater dietary intake during infancy.

The *number, color,* and *consistency of stools* may vary greatly in the same infant and between infants of similar age without apparent explanation. The earliest stools after birth consist of meconium, a dark, viscous, gumlike material. When nursing or formula feedings begin, meconium is replaced by green-brown transition stools, often containing curds, and, after 4–5 days, by yellow-brown milk stools. Stool frequency is extremely variable in normal infants and may vary from none to seven per day. Breast-fed infants may have frequent small, loose stools early (transition stools) and then after 2–3 wk may have very infrequent soft stools. It is possible for a nursing infant not to pass any stool for 1–2 wk and then to have a normal soft bowel movement. The color of stool has little significance except for the presence of blood or absence of bilirubin products. The presence of vegetable matter, such as peas or corn, in the stool of an older infant or toddler ingesting solids is normal and suggests poor chewing and not malabsorption. A pattern of intermittent loose stools, known as "toddler's diarrhea," occurs commonly between 1 and 3 yr of age. These children often drink frequently (especially juices) and snack throughout the day. The stools typically occur during the day and not overnight. The volume of fluid intake is often excessive; eliminating between-meal liquids and snacks often leads to resolution of the pattern of loose stools.

A *protuberant abdomen* is often noted in infants and toddlers, especially after large feedings. This may result from the combination of weak abdominal musculature, relatively large abdominal organs, and lordotic stance. In the 1st yr of life, it is common to palpate the liver up to 2 cm below the right costal margin. The normal liver is soft in consistency and percusses to normal size for age. A Riedel lobe is a thin projection of the right lobe of the liver that may be palpated low in the right lateral abdomen. A soft spleen tip may also be palpable as a normal finding. In thin young children, the vertebral column is easily palpable and an overlying structure may be mistaken for a mass. Commonly, pulsation of the aorta can be appreciated. Normal stool can often be palpated in the left lower quadrant in the descending or sigmoid colon.

Blood loss from GI tract is never normal, but swallowed blood may be misinterpreted as GI bleeding. Maternal blood may be ingested at the time of birth or later by a nursing infant if there is bleeding near the mother's nipple. Nasal or oropharyngeal bleeding is occasionally mistaken for gastrointestinal bleeding. Red dyes in foods or drinks may turn the stool red but do not produce a positive test result for occult blood.

Jaundice is common in neonates, especially among prematures, and usually results from the inability of an immature liver to conjugate bilirubin, leading to an elevated indirect component (Chapter 98.3). Persistent elevation of indirect bilirubin levels in nursing infants may be a result of breast milk jaundice, which is usually a benign entity in full-term infants. Elevated direct bilirubin is never normal and suggests liver disease, although in infants it may be a result of extrahepatic infection (e.g., urinary tract infection). The direct bilirubin fraction should account for no more than 15–20% of the total bilirubin. Indirect hyperbilirubinemia, which occurs commonly in normal newborns, tends to tint the scleras and skin golden yellow, whereas direct hyperbilirubinemia produces a greenish-yellow hue.

CHAPTER 306

Major Symptoms and Signs of Digestive Tract Disorders

Disorders of organs outside of the gastrointestinal (GI) tract can produce symptoms and signs that mimic digestive tract disorders and should be considered in the differential diagnosis (Table 306–1). Understanding the pathogenesis of symptoms is helpful, because specific treatment is not always available and nonspecific management of the symptoms may be necessary.

DISORDERED INGESTION. Disordered ingestion may result from refusal to feed or from swallowing difficulty. Poor weight gain or weight loss suggests a severe process that necessitates further investigation. Dysphagia, or difficulty swallowing, occurs at the level of the mouth, oropharynx, or esophagus and results from a motor disorder (e.g., cerebral palsy or achalasia) or mechanical obstruction (e.g., foreign body, webs, vascular rings, peptic stricture of the esophagus). The dysphagia in motor disorders may be intermittent and may occur with liquids or solids. When solids cause symptoms, they may be washed down with liquids. Ice cold liquids may accentuate symptoms. Liquids pass without difficulty with a mechanical obstruction, but solids that become lodged in the esophagus may require regurgitation. When dysphagia is associated with a delay in passage through the esophagus, a child may be able to point to the level of the chest where the delay occurs; esophageal symptoms may be referred to the suprasternal notch. Therefore, when a child points to the suprasternal notch, the impaction may be found anywhere in the esophagus.

Transfer Dysphagia. A complex sequence of neuromuscular events is involved in the transfer of foods to the upper esophagus. Suckling requires the lips to form a tight seal about the nipple while the tongue is displaced posteriorly. As the glottis closes to guard the airway, the soft palate rises to close the nasopharynx, the cricopharyngeal muscles relax, and food passes to the back of the pharynx. Solids similarly require coordinated actions; for large chunks of solid food, jaw movement and teeth become factors to consider. Salivary secretions, stimulated by the anticipation and act of ingestion, lubricate foods as they pass through the mouth. It is abnormalities of the muscles involved in the ingestion process, their innervation, strength, or coordination that usually cause transfer dysphagia in infants and children. In such cases, an oropharyngeal problem is almost always part of a more generalized neurologic or muscular problem (botulism, diphtheria, cerebral palsy). Painful oral lesions, such as acute viral stomatitis or trauma occasionally interfere with ingestion. If the nasal air passage is seriously obstructed, the need for air causes severe distress when suckling. Although severe structural, dental, and salivary abnormalities would be expected to create difficulties, ingestion proceeds relatively well in most affected children if they are hungry.

TABLE 306–1 Some Nondigestive Tract Causes of Gastrointestinal Symptoms in Children

Anorexia

Systemic disease (e.g., inflammatory, neoplastic)
Cardiorespiratory compromise
Iatrogenic—drug therapy, unpalatable therapeutic diets
Depression
Anorexia nervosa

Vomiting

Inborn errors of metabolism
Medications (erythromycin, chemotherapy)
Increased intracranial pressure
Infection (e.g., urinary tract)
Labyrinthitis
Adrenal insufficiency
Pregnancy
Psychogenic
Abdominal migraine
Toxins

Diarrhea

Infection (e.g., otitis media, urinary)
Uremia
Medications (antibiotics, cisapride)
Tumors (neuroblastoma)

Constipation

Hypothyroidism
Spina bifida
Psychomotor retardation
Dehydration (e.g., diabetes insipidus, renal tubular lesions)
Medications (narcotics)

Abdominal Pain

Pyelonephritis, hydronephrosis, renal colic
Pneumonia
Pelvic inflammatory disease
Porphyria
Angioedema
Endocarditis
Abdominal migraine
Familial Mediterranean fever
Sexual or physical abuse
Systemic lupus erythematosus
School phobia
Sickle cell crisis
Vertebral disk inflammation
Medications (NSAIDs)

Abdominal Distension or Mass

Ascites (e.g., nephrotic syndrome, neoplasm, heart failure)
Discrete mass (e.g., Wilms tumor, hydronephrosis, neuroblastoma, mesenteric cyst, hepatoblastoma)
Pregnancy

Jaundice

Hemolytic disease
Urinary tract infection
Sepsis
Hypothyroidism

Dysphagia. Primary motility disorders causing impaired peristaltic function and dysphagia are rare in children. Motility of the distal esophagus is disordered after repair of tracheoesophageal fistula. Abnormal motility may accompany collagen vascular disorders. Achalasia rarely occurs in children. Esophageal web, tracheobronchial remnant or vascular ring may cause dysphagia in infancy. An esophageal stricture secondary to chronic gastroesophageal reflux and esophagitis occasionally presents with dysphagia as the first manifestation. A Schatzki ring is another mechanical cause of recurrent dysphagia presenting after infancy. An esophageal foreign body or a stricture secondary to a caustic ingestion also causes dysphagia.

Regurgitation. Regurgitation is the effortless movement of stomach contents into the esophagus and mouth. It is not associated with distress, and infants with regurgitation are often hungry immediately after an episode. The lower esophageal sphincter (LES) prevents reflux of gastric contents into the esophagus (Chapter 323). Regurgitation is a result of gastroesophageal reflux through an incompetent or, in infants, immature LES. This is often a developmental process, and regurgitation or "spitting" resolves with maturity. Regurgitation should be differentiated from vomiting, which denotes an active reflex process with a different differential diagnosis (Table 306–2).

Anorexia. Hunger and satiety centers are located in the hypothalamus; it seems likely that afferent nerves from the GI tract to these brain centers are important determinants of the anorexia that characterizes many diseases of the stomach and intestine. For example, satiety is stimulated by distention of the stomach or upper small bowel, the signal being transmitted by sensory afferents, which are especially dense in the upper gut. Chemoreceptors in the intestine, influenced by the assimilation of nutrients, also affect afferent flow to the appetite centers. Impulses reach the hypothalamus from higher centers, possibly influenced by pain or the emotional disturbance of an intestinal disease. Other regulatory factors include hormones, leptin, and plasma glucose, which in turn reflect intestinal function.

VOMITING. Vomiting is a highly coordinated reflex process that may be preceded by increased salivation and begins with involuntary retching. Violent descent of the diaphragm and constriction of the abdominal muscles with relaxation of the gastric cardia actively force gastric contents back up the esophagus. This process is coordinated in the medullary vomiting center, which is influenced directly by afferent innervation and indirectly by the chemoreceptor trigger zone and higher central nervous system (CNS) centers. Many acute or chronic processes can cause vomiting (Table 306–3).

Vomiting caused by obstruction of the GI tract is probably mediated by intestinal visceral afferent nerves stimulating the vomiting center. If obstruction occurs below the second part of the duodenum, vomitus is usually bile stained. With repeated vomiting in the absence of obstruction, however, duodenal contents are refluxed into the stomach and the emesis may become bile stained. Congenital and acquired obstructing lesions are noted in Table 306–3. Nonobstructive lesions of the digestive tract can also cause vomiting; most diseases of the upper bowel, pancreas, liver, or biliary tree are capable of provoking emesis. CNS or metabolic derangements may lead to severe, persistent emesis.

Cyclic vomiting is a syndrome with numerous episodes of vomiting (~ 9 episodes/mo) interspersed with well intervals. The onset is usually between 3–5 yr of age; the episodes last 2–3 days, with four or more emesis episodes per hour. Patients may have a prodrome of nausea, lethargy, and headache or fever. Precipitants include stress and excitement. Idiopathic cyclic vomiting may be a migraine equivalent (abdominal migraine), or it may result from altered intestinal motility or mutations in mitochondrial DNA. The *differential diagnosis* includes GI anomalies (malrotation, duplication cysts, choledochal cysts), CNS disorders (neoplasm, epilepsy, vestibular pathology), nephrolithiasis, cholelithiasis, hydronephrosis, metabolic-endocrine disorders (urea cycle, fatty acid metabolism, Addison disease, porphyria, hereditary angioedema, familial Mediterranean fever), chronic appendicitis, and inflammatory bowel disease. Laboratory evaluation is based on a careful history and physical examination and may include, if indicated, endoscopy, contrast radiography, brain MRI, and

TABLE 306–2 Differential Diagnosis of Emesis During Childhood

Infant	Child	Adolescent
Common		
Gastroenteritis	Gastroenteritis	Gastroenteritis
Gastroesophageal reflux	Systemic infection	Systemic infection
Overfeeding	Toxic ingestion	Toxic ingestion
Anatomic obstruction	Pertussis syndrome	Inflammatory bowel disease
Systemic infection	Medication	Appendicitis
Pertussis syndrome	Reflux	Migraine
		Pregnancy
		Medication
		Ipecac abuse/bulimia
Rare		
Adrenogenital syndrome	Reye syndrome	Reye syndrome
Inborn error of metabolism	Hepatitis	Hepatitis
Brain tumor (increased intracranial pressure)	Peptic ulcer	Peptic ulcer
Subdural hemorrhage	Pancreatitis	Pancreatitis
Food poisoning	Brain tumor	Brain tumor
Rumination	Increased intracranial pressure	Increased intracranial pressure
Renal tubular acidosis	Middle ear disease	Middle ear disease
	Chemotherapy	Chemotherapy
	Achalasia	Cyclic vomiting (migraine)
	Cyclic vomiting (migraine)	Biliary colic
	Esophageal stricture	Renal colic
	Duodenal hematoma	
	Inborn error of metabolism	

TABLE 306–3 Causes of Gastrointestinal Obstruction

Esophagus		
	Congenital:	Esophageal atresia
		Vascular rings
		Schatzki ring
		Tracheobronchial remnant
	Acquired:	Esophageal stricture
		Foreign body
		Achalasia
		Chagas disease
		Collagen vascular disease
Stomach		
	Congenital:	Antral webs
		Pyloric stenosis
	Acquired:	Bezoars/foreign body
		Pyloric stricture (ulcer)
		Chronic granulomatous disease of childhood
		Eosinophilic gastroenteritis
		Crohn disease
		Epidermolysis bullosa
Small Intestine		
	Congenital:	Duodenal atresia
		Annular pancreas
		Malrotation/volvulus
		Malrotation/Ladd bands
		Ileal atresia
		Meconium ileus
		Meckel diverticulum with volvulus or intussusception
		Inguinal hernia
	Acquired:	Postsurgical adhesions
		Crohn disease
		Intussusception
		Distal ileal obstruction syndrome (CF)
		Duodenal hematoma
		Superior mesenteric artery syndrome
Colon		
	Congenital:	Meconium plug
		Hirschsprung disease
		Colonic atresia, stenosis
		Imperforate anus
		Rectal stenosis
		Pseudo-obstruction
		Volvulus
	Acquired:	Ulcerative colitis (toxic megacolon)
		Chagas disease
		Crohn disease
		Fibrosing colonopathy (CF)

CF = cystic fibrosis.

TABLE 306–4 Mechanisms of Diarrhea

Primary Mechanism	Defect	Stool Examination	Examples	Comment
Secretory	Decreased absorption, increased secretion: electrolyte transport	Watery, normal osmolality; osmols = 2 × (Na^+ + K^+)	Cholera, toxigenic *Escherichia coli;* carcinoid, VIP, neuroblastoma, congenital chloride diarrhea, *Clostridium difficile, cryptosporidiosis* (AIDS)	Persists during fasting; bile salt malabsorption also may increase intestinal water secretion; no stool leukocytes
Osmotic	Maldigestion, transport defects, ingestion of unabsorbable solute	Watery, acidic, + reducing substances; increased osmolality; osmosis >2 × (Na^+ + K^+)	Lactase deficiency, glucose-galactose malabsorption, lactulose, laxative abuse	Stops with fasting, increased breath hydrogen with carbohydrate malabsorption, no stool leukocytes
Increased motility	Decreased transit time	Loose to normal-appearing stool, stimulated by gastrocolic reflex	Irritable bowel syndrome, thyrotoxicosis, postvagotomy dumping syndrome	Infection also may contribute to increased motility
Decreased motility	Defect in neuromuscular unit(s) Stasis (bacterial overgrowth)	Loose to normal-appearing stool	Pseudo-obstruction, blind loop	Possible bacterial overgrowth
Decreased surface area (osmotic, motility)	Decreased functional capacity	Watery	Short bowel syndrome, celiac disease, rotavirus enteritis	May require elemental diet plus parenteral alimentation
Mucosal invasion	Inflammation, decreased colonic reabsorption, increased motility	Blood and increased WBCs in stool	*Salmonella, Shigella,* amebiasis, *Yersinia, Campylobacter*	Dysentery = blood, mucus, and WBCs

VIP = vasoactive intestinal peptide; WBC = white blood cell.
Adapted from Behrman RE, Kliegman RM (eds): Nelson Essentials of Pediatrics, 3rd ed. Philadelphia, WB Saunders, 1998.

metabolic studies (lactate, organic acids, ammonia). *Treatment* includes hydration and ondansetron. *Prevention* may be possible with the antimigraine agent amitriptyline or cyproheptadine.

DIARRHEA. Diarrhea is best defined as excessive loss of fluid and electrolyte in the stool. Normally, a young infant has about 5 g/kg of stool output per day; the volume increases to 200 g/24 hr in an adult. The greatest volume of intestinal water is absorbed in the small bowel; the colon concentrates intestinal contents against a high osmotic gradient. The small intestine of an adult may absorb 10–11 L/day of a combination of ingested and secreted fluid, whereas the colon absorbs about 1/2 L. Disorders that interfere with absorption in the small bowel tend to produce voluminous diarrhea, whereas disorders compromising colonic absorption produce lower volume diarrhea. Dysentery (i.e., small volume, frequent bloody stools with mucus, tenemus, and urgency) is the predominant symptom of colitis.

The basis for all diarrhea is disturbed intestinal solute transport; water movement across intestinal membranes is passive and is determined by both active and passive fluxes of solutes, particularly sodium, chloride, and glucose. The pathogenesis

TABLE 306–5 Differential Diagnosis of Diarrhea

	Infant	Child	Adolescent
Acute			
Common	Gastroenteritis Systemic infection Antibiotic associated	Gastroenteritis Food poisoning Systemic infection Antibiotic associated	Gastroenteritis Food poisoning Antibiotic associated
Rare	Primary disaccharidase deficiency Hirschsprung toxic colitis Adrenogenital syndrome	Toxic ingestion	Hyperthyroidism
Chronic			
Common	Postinfectious secondary lactase deficiency Cow's milk/soy protein intolerance Chronic nonspecific diarrhea of infancy Celiac disease Cystic fibrosis AIDS enteropathy	Postinfectious secondary lactase deficiency Irritable bowel syndrome Celiac disease Lactose intolerance Giardiasis Inflammatory bowel disease AIDS enteropathy	Irritable bowel syndrome Inflammatory bowel disease Lactose intolerance Giardiasis Laxative abuse (anorexia nervosa)
Rare	Primary immune defects Familial villous atrophy Secretory tumors Congenital chloridorrhea Acrodermatitis enteropathica Lymphangiectasia Abetalipoproteinemia Eosinophilic gastroenteritis Short bowel syndrome Intractable diarrhea syndrome Autoimmune enteropathy Factitious	Acquired immune defects Secretory tumors Pseudo-obstruction Factitious	Secretory tumor Primary bowel tumor Gay bowel disease

From Behrman RE, Kliegman RM (eds): Nelson Essentials of Pediatrics, 3rd ed. Philadelphia, WB Saunders, 1998.

of most episodes of diarrhea can be explained by secretory, osmotic, or motility abnormalities or a combination of these (Table 306–4).

Secretory diarrhea is often caused by a secretagogue, such as cholera toxin, binding to a receptor on the surface epithelium of the bowel and thereby stimulating intracellular accumulation of cyclic adenosine monophosphate or cyclic guanosine monophosphate. Some intraluminal fatty acids and bile salts cause the colonic mucosa to secrete through this mechanism. Diarrhea not associated with an exogenous secretagogue may also have a secretory component (e.g., congenital microvillus inclusion disease). Secretory diarrhea tends to be watery and of large volume; the osmolality of the stool can be accounted for by the presence of electrolyte. Secretory diarrhea generally persists even when no feedings are given by mouth.

Osmotic diarrhea occurs after ingestion of a poorly absorbed solute. The solute may be one that is normally not well absorbed (e.g., magnesium, phosphate, lactulose, or sorbitol) or one that is not well absorbed because of a disorder of the small bowel (e.g., lactose with lactase deficiency or glucose with rotavirus diarrhea). Malabsorbed carbohydrate is typically fermented in the colon, and short chain fatty acids (SCFAs) are produced. Although SCFAs can be absorbed in the colon and used as an energy source, the net effect is to increase the osmotic solute load. This form of diarrhea is usually of lesser volume than a secretory diarrhea and stops with fasting. The osmolality of the stool is not solely explained by the electrolyte content, because another osmotic component is present [the difference between electrolyte content (sum of [NA^+], [K^+], and associated anions) and stool osmolality is $>$ 50 mOsm] (see Chapter 176). Motility disorders may be associated with rapid or delayed transit and generally are not associated with large volume diarrhea. Slowed motility may be associated with bacterial overgrowth as a cause of diarrhea. The differential diagnosis of common causes of acute and chronic diarrhea are noted in Table 306–5.

CONSTIPATION. Any definition of constipation is relative, dependent on stool consistency, stool frequency, and difficulty in passing the stool. A normal child may have a soft stool only every 2nd or 3rd day without difficulty; this is not constipation. However, a hard stool passed with difficulty every 3rd day should be treated as constipation. Constipation may arise from defects either in filling or emptying the rectum (Table 306–6).

A nursing infant may have very infrequent stools of normal consistency; this is usually a normal pattern. True constipation in the neonatal period is most likely secondary to Hirschsprung disease, intestinal pseudo-obstruction, or hypothyroidism.

Defective rectal filling occurs when colonic peristalsis is ineffective (e.g., in cases of hypothyroidism or opiate use and when bowel obstruction is caused either by a structural anomaly or by Hirschsprung disease). The resultant colonic stasis leads to excessive drying of stool and a failure to initiate reflexes from the rectum that normally trigger evacuation. Emptying the rectum by spontaneous evacuation depends on a defecation reflex initiated by pressure receptors in the rectal muscle. Stool retention, therefore, may also result from lesions involving these rectal muscles, the sacral spinal cord afferent and efferent fibers, or the muscles of the abdomen and pelvic floor. Disorders of anal sphincter relaxation may also contribute to fecal retention.

Constipation tends to be self-perpetuating, whatever its cause. Hard, large stools in the rectum become difficult and even painful to evacuate; thus, more retention occurs and a vicious circle ensues. Distention of the rectum and colon lessens the sensitivity of the defecation reflex and the effectiveness of peristalsis. Eventually, watery content from the proximal colon may percolate around hard retained stool and pass per rectum unperceived by the child. This involuntary *encopresis* may be mistaken for diarrhea. Constipation does not per se have deleterious systemic organic effects. Urinary tract stasis may accompany severe long-standing cases. Constipation may generate anxiety, having a marked emotional impact on the patient and family.

TABLE 306–6 Causes of Constipation

Nonorganic (Functional)—Habit—Retentive

Organic

Intestinal

Hirschsprung disease
Neuronal dysgenesis
Anal-rectal stenosis
Anal stricture
Anterior dislocation of the anus
Cow's milk protein intolerance
Pseudo-obstruction
Collagen vascular diseases
Rectal abscess/fissure
Stricture post-NEC
Volvulus
Milk protein intolerance

Drugs

Lead toxicity
Narcotics
Antidepressants
Psychoactive drugs (chlorpromazine [Thorazine])
Chemotherapeutic agents (vincristine)
Pancreatic enzymes (fibrosing colonopathy)

Metabolic

Dehydration
Cystic fibrosis (meconium ileus equivalent)
Hypothyroidism
Hypokalemia
Hypercalcemia
Renal tubular acidosis

Neuromuscular

Psychomotor retardation
Muscular dystrophy
Spinal cord lesions (tumors or spina bifida)
Infant botulism
Absent abdominal muscle
Chagas disease

Psychiatric

Anorexia nervosa

NEC = necrotizing enterocolitis.
Adapted from Behrman RE, Kliegman RM (eds): Nelson Essentials of Pediatrics, 3rd ed. Philadelphia, WB Saunders, 1998.

ABDOMINAL PAIN. Individual children differ greatly in their perception of and tolerance for abdominal pain. This is one reason the evaluation of chronic abdominal pain is difficult. A child with functional abdominal pain (i.e., no identifiable organic cause) may be as uncomfortable as one with an organic cause. This distinction is an extremely important part of the medical evaluation, guiding how the work-up is approached and the child is treated. The more specific the pain and the more suggestive of a particular diagnosis, the more likely it will have an organic basis. Normal growth and physical examination (including a rectal examination) are reassuring in a child who is suspected of having functional pain.

A specific cause may be difficult to find, but the nature and location of a pain-provoking lesion can usually be determined from the clinical description. Two types of nerve fibers transmit painful stimuli in the abdomen: In skin and muscle, A fibers mediate sharp localized pain, and C fibers from viscera, peritoneum, and muscle transmit poorly localized, dull pain. These afferent fibers have cell bodies in the dorsal root ganglia, and some axons cross the midline and ascend to the medulla, midbrain, and thalamus. Pain is perceived in the cortex of the postcentral gyrus, which can receive impulses arising from both sides of the body.

TABLE 306–7 Recurrent Abdominal Pain in Children

Disorder	Characteristics	Key Evaluations
Nonorganic		
Recurrent abdominal pain syndrome (functional abdominal pain)	Nonspecific pain, often periumbilical	Hx and PE; tests as indicated
Irritable bowel syndrome	Intermittent cramps, diarrhea, and constipation	Hx and PE
Nonulcer dyspepsia	Peptic ulcer-like symptoms without abnormalities on evaluation of the upper GI tract	Hx; esophagogastroduodenoscopy
GI Tract		
Chronic constipation	Hx of stool retention, evidence of constipation on examination	Hx and PE; plain x-ray of abdomen
Lactose intolerance	Symptoms may be associated with lactose ingestion; bloating, gas, cramps, and diarrhea	Trial of lactose-free diet; lactose breath hydrogen test
Parasite infection (especially *Giardia*)	Bloating, gas, cramps, and diarrhea	Stool evaluation for o & p; specific immunoassays for *Giardia*
Excess fructose or sorbitol ingestion	Nonspecific abdominal pain, bloating, gas, and diarrhea	Large intake of apples, fruit juice, or candy/chewing gum sweetened with sorbitol
Crohn disease	See Chapter 337	
Peptic ulcer	Burning or gnawing epigastric pain; worse on awakening or before meals; relieved with antacids	Esophagogastroduodenoscopy or upper GI contrast x-rays
Esophagitis	Epigastric pain with substernal burning	Esophagogastroduodenoscopy
Meckel diverticulum	Periumbilical or lower abdominal pain; may have blood in stool	Meckel scan or enteroclysis
Recurrent intussusception	Paroxysmal severe cramping abdominal pain; blood may be present in stool with episode	Identify intussusception during episode or lead point in intestine between episodes with contrast studies of GI tract
Internal, inguinal, or abdominal wall hernia	Dull abdomen or abdominal wall pain	PE, CT of abdominal wall
Chronic appendicitis or appendiceal mucocele	Recurrent RLQ pain; often incorrectly diagnosed, may be rare cause of abdominal pain	Barium enema, CT
Gallbladder and Pancreas		
Cholelithiasis	RUQ pain, may worsen with meals	Ultrasound of gallbladder
Choledochal cyst	RUQ pain, mass ± elevated bilirubin	Ultrasound or CT of RUQ
Recurrent pancreatitis	Persistent boring pain, may radiate to back, vomiting	Serum amylase and lipase ± serum trypsinogen; ultrasound of pancreas
Genitourinary Tract		
Urinary tract infection	Dull suprapubic pain, flank pain	Urinalysis and urine culture; renal scan
Hydronephrosis	Unilateral abdominal or flank pain	Ultrasound of kidneys
Urolithiasis	Progressive, severe pain: flank to inguinal region to testicle	Urinalysis, ultrasound, IVP, spinal CT
Other genitourinary disorders	Suprapubic or lower abdominal pain; GU symptoms	Ultrasound of kidneys and pelvis; gynecologic evaluation
Miscellaneous Causes		
Abdominal migraine	See text; nausea, family Hx migraine	Hx
Abdominal epilepsy	May have seizure prodrome	EEG (may require more than one study, including sleep-deprived EEG)
Gilbert syndrome	Mild abdominal pain (causal or coincidental?); slightly elevated unconjugated bilirubin	Serum bilirubin
Familial Mediterranean fever	Paroxysmal episodes of fever, severe abdominal pain, and tenderness with other evidence of polyserositis	Hx and PE during an episode, DNA diagnosis
Sickle cell crisis	Anemia	Hematologic evaluation
Lead poisoning	Vague abdominal pain ± constipation	Serum lead level
Henoch-Schönlein purpura	Recurrent, severe crampy abdominal pain, occult blood in stool, characteristic rash, arthritis	Hx, PE, urinalysis
Angioneurotic edema	Swelling of face or airway, crampy pain	Hx, PE, upper GI contrast x-rays serum C1 esterase inhibitor
Acute intermittent porphyria	Severe pain precipitated by drugs, fasting, or infections	Spot urine for porphyrins

o & p = ova and parasites; Hx = history; PE = physical exam; RUQ = right upper quadrant; RLQ = right lower quadrant; IVP = intravenous pyelography; EEG = electroencephalogram; abd = abdominal; GI = gastrointestinal; GU = genitourinary.

Visceral pain tends to be experienced in the dermatome from which the affected organ receives innervation. Painful stimuli originating in the liver, pancreas, biliary tree, stomach, or upper bowel are felt in the epigastrium; pain from the distal small bowel, cecum, appendix, or proximal colon is felt at the umbilicus; and pain from the distal large bowel, urinary tract, or pelvic organs is usually suprapubic. When pain is referred to remote areas supplied by the same neurosegment as the diseased organ, the phenomenon usually means an increased intensity of the provoking stimuli. Parietal pain impulses travel in C fibers of nerves corresponding to dermatomes T6–L1; such pain tends to be more localized and intense than visceral pain.

In the gut, the usual stimulus provoking pain is tension or stretching. Inflammatory lesions may lower the pain threshold, but the mechanisms producing pain of inflammation are not clear. Tissue metabolites released near nerve endings probably account for the pain caused by ischemia. Perception of these painful stimuli can be modulated by input from both cerebral and peripheral sources. Psychologic factors are particularly important. Features of abdominal pain are noted in Tables 306–7 and 306–8.

Gastrointestinal Hemorrhage. Bleeding may occur anywhere along the GI tract, and identification of the site may be challenging (Table 306–9). The small intestine, which is most difficult to

TABLE 306–8 Distinguishing Features of Acute Gastrointestinal Tract Pain in Children

Disease	Onset	Location	Referral	Quality	Comments
Pancreatitis	Acute	Epigastric, left upper quadrant	Back	Constant, sharp, boring	Nausea, emesis, tenderness
Intestinal obstruction	Acute or gradual	Periumbilical—lower abdomen	Back	Alternating cramping (colic) and painless periods	Distention, obstipation, emesis, increased bowel sounds
Appendicitis	Acute	Periumbilical, localized to lower right quadrant; generalized with peritonitis	Back or pelvis if retrocecal	Sharp, steady	Anorexia, nausea, emesis, local tenderness, fever with peritonitis
Intussusception	Acute	Periumbilical—lower abdomen	None	Cramping, with painless periods	Hematochezia, knees in pulled-up position
Urolithiasis	Acute, sudden	Back (unilateral)	Groin	Sharp, intermittent, cramping	Hematuria
Urinary tract infection	Acute, sudden	Back	Bladder	Dull to sharp	Fever, costochondral tenderness, dysuria, urinary frequency

study, is the least likely site of bleeding. The only exception is the painless bleeding of a Meckel diverticulum, which is not difficult to identify. Erosive damage to the mucosa of the GI tract is the most common cause of bleeding, although variceal bleeding secondary to portal hypertension occurs frequently enough to require consideration. Vascular malformations are a rare cause in children; they are difficult to identify.

When bleeding originates in the esophagus, stomach, or duodenum, it may cause *hematemesis.* When exposed to gastric or intestinal juices, blood quickly darkens to resemble coffee grounds; massive bleeding is likely to be red. Red or maroon blood in stools, *hematochezia,* signifies either a distal bleeding site or massive hemorrhage above the distal ileum. Moderate to mild bleeding from sites above the distal ileum tends to cause blackened stools of tarry consistency, *melena,* and major hemorrhages in the duodenum or above can cause melena.

Children can develop iron deficiency anemia from enteric blood loss even when occult blood is not found in stools on random testing. GI hemorrhage, in itself, rarely causes GI symptoms, but brisk duodenal or gastric bleeding may lead to nausea, vomiting, or diarrhea. The breakdown products of intraluminal blood may tip patients into hepatic coma if liver function is already compromised and lead to elevation of serum bilirubin.

ABDOMINAL DISTENTION AND ABDOMINAL MASSES. Enlargement of the abdomen can result from diminished tone of the wall musculature or from increased content—fluid, gas, or solid. Ascites, the accumulation of fluid in the peritoneal cavity, distends the abdomen both in the flanks and anteriorly when it is large in volume. This fluid shifts with movement of the patient and conducts a percussion wave.

Ascitic fluid is usually a transudate with a low-protein concentration resulting from reduced plasma colloid osmotic pressure of hypoalbuminemia, from raised portal venous pressure, or from both. In cases of portal hypertension, the fluid leak probably occurs from lymphatics on the liver surface and from visceral peritoneal capillaries, but ascites does not usually develop until the serum albumin level falls. Sodium excretion in the urine decreases greatly as the ascitic fluid accumulates, and thus additional dietary sodium goes directly to the peritoneal space, taking with it more water. When ascitic fluid contains a high protein concentration, it is usually an exudate caused by an inflammatory or neoplastic lesion.

When fluid distends the gut, either obstruction or imbalance between absorption and secretion should be suspected. The factors causing fluid accumulation in the bowel lumen frequently cause gas to accumulate too. The result may be audible gurgling noises. The source of gas is usually swallowed air, but endogenous flora may increase considerably in malabsorptive states and produce excessive gas when substrate reaches the lower intestine. Gas in the peritoneal cavity (pneumoperitoneum), perhaps signaled by a tympanitic percussion note even over solid organs such as the liver, indicates a perforated viscus.

An abdominal organ may enlarge diffusely or be affected by a discrete mass. In the digestive tract, such discrete masses may occur in the lumen, in the wall, or in the mesentery. In a constipated child, mobile, nontender fecal masses are often

TABLE 306–9 Differential Diagnosis of Gastrointestinal Bleeding in Childhood

Infant	Child	Adolescent
Common		
Bacterial enteritis	Bacterial enteritis	Bacterial enteritis
Milk protein allergy	Anal fissure	Inflammatory bowel disease
Intussusception	Colonic polyps	Peptic ulcer/gastritis
Swallowed maternal blood	Intussusception	Mallory-Weiss syndrome
Anal fissure	Peptic ulcer/gastritis	Colonic polyps
Lymphonodular hyperplasia	Swallowed epistaxis	
	Mallory-Weiss syndrome	
Rare		
Volvulus	Esophageal varices	Hemorroids
Necrotizing enterocolitis	Esophagitis	Esophageal varices
Meckel diverticulum	Meckel diverticulum	Esophagitis
Stress ulcer, stomach	Lymphonodular hyperplasia	Telangiectasia-angiodysplasia
Coagulation disorder (hemorrhagic disease of newborn)	Henoch-Schönlein purpura	Gay bowel disease
	Foreign body	Graft versus host disease
	Hemangioma, arteriovenous malformation	
	Sexual abuse	
	Hemolytic uremic syndrome	
	Inflammatory bowel disease	
	Coagulopathy	

found. The wall of the gut can be affected by anomalies, cysts, or inflammatory disease; gut wall neoplasms are extremely rare in children. The liver may enlarge diffusely in response to many disorders. Discrete liver masses may be islands of regenerating liver tissue in a cirrhotic liver or may be of inflammatory or neoplastic origin.

JAUNDICE (See Chapters 98.3, 98.4, and 356).

Anderson JM, Sugerman KS, Lockhart JR, et al: Effective prophylactic therapy for cyclic vomiting syndrome in children using amitriptyline or cyproheptadine. Pediatrics 100:977, 1997.

Boles RG, Chun N, Senadheera D, et al: Cyclic vomiting syndrome and mitochondrial DNA mutations. Lancet 350:1299, 1997.

Borge A, Nordhagen R, Moe B, et al: Prevalence and persistence of stomach ache and headache among children. Follow-up of a cohort of Norwegian children from 4 to 10 years of age. Acta Paediatr 83:433, 1994.

Castro-Rodriguez J, Salazar-Lindo E, León-Barua R: Differentiation of osmotic and secretory diarrhea by stool carbohydrate and osmolar gap measurements. Arch Dis Child 77:201, 1997.

Cox KC, Ament ME: Upper gastrointestinal bleeding in children and adolescents. Pediatrics 63:408, 1979.

Drossman D: Physical and sexual abuse and gastrointestinal illness: What is the link? Am J Med 97:105, 1994.

Eherer AJ, Fordtran JS: Fecal osmotic gap and pH in experimental diarrhea of various cause. Gastroenterology 103:545, 1992.

Fallon M, O'Neill B: Constipation and diarrhea. Br Med J 315:1293, 1997.

Fitzgerald JF: Cholestatic disorders of infancy. Pediatr Clin North Am 35:357, 1988.

Hamilton JR: The pathogenesis of infectious diarrhea. Mod Concepts Gastroenterol 1:335, 1986.

Hyman PE: Gastroesophageal reflux: One reason why baby won't eat. J Pediatr 125:S103, 1994.

Iacono G, Canataio F, Montalto G, et al: Intolerance of cow's milk and chronic constipation in children. N Engl J Med 339:1100, 1998.

Li BUK, Murray RD, Heitlinger LA, et al: Heterogeneity of diagnoses presenting as cyclic vomiting. Pediatrics 102:583, 1998.

Loening-Baucke V: Chronic constipation in children. Gastroenterology 105:1557, 1993.

Pfau BT, Li BUK, Murray RD, et al: Differentiating cyclic from chronic vomiting patterns in children: Qualitative criteria and diagnostic implications. Pediatrics 97:364, 1996.

Rogers B, Arvedson J, Buck G, et al: Characteristics of dysphagia in children with cerebral palsy. Dysphagia 9:69, 1994.

Vandenplas Y: Reflux esophagitis in infants and children: A report from the working group on gastro-oesophageal reflux disease of the European Society of Paediatric Gastroenterology and Nutrition. J Pediatr Gastroenterol Nutr 18:413, 1994.

Withers GD, Silburn SR, Forbes DA: Precipitants and aetiology of cyclic vomiting syndrome. Acta Paediatr 87:272, 1998.

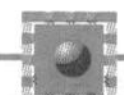

SECTION 2

The Oral Cavity

David Johnsen ■ Norman Tinanoff

The oral cavity is important to the physical and psychologic health of children. Timely diagnosis and treatment require close cooperation between physicians and dentists. School-aged children generally receive periodic dental examinations and treatment; oral problems of infants are frequently recognized first by the physician.

All parents should receive oral health counseling that includes anticipatory guidance, oral hygiene instruction, and diet counseling. Children identified at high risk for dental disease (low socioeconomic setting, inappropriate feeding habits) should be referred for dental care by 1 yr and have periodic dental examinations as frequently at every 3 mo. It is recommended that most children have periodic dental examinations at 6 mo intervals; low risk children can be seen yearly. ■

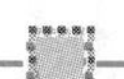

CHAPTER 307

Development and Developmental Anomalies of the Teeth

INITIATION

The primary teeth form in dental crypts that arise from a band of epithelial cells incorporated into each developing jaw. By the 12th wk of fetal life, each of these epithelial bands (the dental laminae) has five areas of rapid growth on each side of the maxilla and the mandible, seen as rounded, bud-like enlargements. Organization of adjacent mesenchyme takes place in each area of epithelial growth, and the two elements together are the beginning of a tooth.

After the formation of these crypts for the 20 primary teeth, another generation of tooth buds forms lingually (toward the tongue), which will develop into the succeeding permanent incisors, cuspids, and premolars that eventually replace the primary teeth. This process takes place from about the 5th gestational month for the central incisors to about the 10th mo of age for the second bicuspids. The permanent first, second, and third molars, on the other hand, arise from extension of the dental laminae backward, beyond the site of the second primary molars. Buds for these teeth develop at approximately 4 mo of gestation, 1 yr of age, and 4 to 5 yr of age, respectively.

Histodifferentiation-Morphodifferentiation. As the epithelial bud proliferates, the deeper surface invaginates, and a mass of mesenchyme becomes partially enclosed. The epithelial cells differentiate into the ameloblasts that form enamel; the mesenchyme forms the vascular, nerve, and lymph structures (dental pulp).

Calcification. After the organic matrix has been laid down, the deposition of the inorganic mineral crystals takes place from several sites of calcification that later coalesce. The characteristics of the inorganic portions of a tooth can be altered by (1) disturbances in formation of the matrix, (2) decreased availability of minerals, or (3) the incorporation of foreign materials. Such disturbances may affect the color, texture, or thickness of the tooth surface. Calcification of primary teeth begins at 3 to 4 mo in utero and concludes postnatally at approximately 12 mo with mineralization of the second primary molars (Table 307–1).

Eruption. At the time of tooth bud formation, each tooth begins a continuous movement outward. The times of eruption of the primary and permanent teeth are listed in Table 307–1.

ANOMALIES ASSOCIATED WITH TOOTH DEVELOPMENT. Both failures and excesses of tooth initiation are observed. *Anodontia,* or absence of teeth, occurs when no tooth buds form (ectodermal dysplasia, or familial missing teeth) or when there is a disturbance of a normal site of initiation (the area of a palatal cleft). The teeth that are most commonly absent include the third molars, the maxillary lateral incisors, and the mandibular second premolars.

TABLE 307–1 Calcification, Crown Completion, Eruption, and Root Completion

	Tooth	First Evidence of Calcification	Crown Completed	Eruption	Root Completed
Primary Dentition					
Maxillary	Central incisor	3–4 mo in utero	4 mo	7 1/2 mo	1 1/2–2 yr
	Lateral incisor	4 1/2 mo in utero	5 mo	8 mo	1 1/2–2 yr
	Canine	5 1/2 mo in utero	9 mo	16–20 mo	2 1/2–3 yr
	First molar	5 mo in utero	6 mo	12–16 mo	2–2 1/2 yr
	Second molar	6 mo in utero	10–12 mo	20–30 mo	3 yr
Mandibular	Central incisor	4 1/2 mo in utero	4 mo	6 1/2 mo	1 1/2–2 yr
	Lateral incisor	4 1/2 mo in utero	4 1/4 mo	7 mo	1 1/2–2 yr
	Canine	5 mo in utero	9 mo	16–20 mo	2 1/2–3 yr
	First molar	5 mo in utero	6 mo	12–16 mo	2–2 1/2 yr
	Second molar	6 mo in utero	10–12 mo	20–30 mo	3 yr
Permanent Dentition					
Maxillary	Central incisor	3–4 mo	4–5 yr	7–8 yr	10 yr
	Lateral incisor	10 mo	4–5 yr	8–9 yr	11 yr
	Canine	4–5 mo	6–7 yr	11–12 yr	13–15 yr
	First premolar	1 1/2–1 3/4 yr	5–6 yr	10–11 yr	12–13 yr
	Second premolar	2–2 1/4 yr	6–7 yr	10–12 yr	12–14 yr
	First molar	At birth	2 1/2–3 yr	6–7 yr	9–10 yr
	Second molar	2 1/2–3 yr	7–8 yr	12–13 yr	14–16 yr
	Third molar	7–9 yr	12–16 yr	17–21 yr	18–25 yr
Mandibular	Central incisor	3–4 mo	4–5 yr	6–7 yr	9 yr
	Lateral incisor	3–4 mo	4–5 yr	7–8 yr	10 yr
	Canine	4–5 mo	6–7 yr	9–10 yr	12–14 yr
	First premolar	1 3/4–2 yr	5–6 yr	10–12 yr	12–13 yr
	Second premolar	2 1/4–2 1/2 yr	6–7 yr	11–12 yr	13–14 yr
	First molar	At birth	2 1/2–3 yr	6–7 yr	9–10 yr
	Second molar	2 1/2–3 yr	7–8 yr	11–13 yr	14–15 yr
	Third molar	8–10 yr	12–16 yr	17–21 yr	8–25 yr

Adapted from Logan WHG, Kronfeld R: Development of the human jaws and surrounding structures from birth to age fifteen years. J Am Dent Assoc 20:379, 1993.

If the dental lamina produces more than the normal number of buds, supernumerary teeth occur, most often in the area between the maxillary central incisors. Because they tend to disrupt the position and eruption of the adjacent normal teeth, their identification by radiographic examination is important. Supernumerary teeth occur with cleidocranial dysostosis (see Chapter 311) and in the area of cleft palates.

Disturbances during differentiation may result in alterations in dental morphology, such as *macrodontia* (large teeth) or *microdontia* (small teeth). The maxillary lateral incisors may assume a slender, tapering shape ("peg-shaped laterals").

Twinning, in which two teeth are joined together, is most often observed in the mandibular incisors of the primary dentition. It may result from gemination, fusion, or concrescence. Gemination is the result of the division of one tooth germ to form a bifid crown on a single root with a common pulp canal; an extra tooth appears to be present in the dental arch. Fusion is the joining of incompletely developed teeth that, owing to pressure or trauma or crowding, continue to develop as one tooth. Fused teeth are sometimes joined through their entire length; in other cases, a single wide crown is supported on two roots. Concrescence is the attachment of the roots of closely approximated adjacent teeth by an excessive deposit of cementum. This type of twinning, unlike the others, is found most often in the maxillary molar region.

Amelogenesis imperfecta, a dominant genetic trait, results in faulty production of the organic matrix. The teeth are covered by only a thin layer of abnormally formed enamel through which the yellow underlying dentin is seen. Usually both primary and permanent teeth are affected. Susceptibility to caries is low, but the enamel is subject to destruction from abrasion. Complete coverage of the crown may be indicated for dentin protection and improved appearance.

Dentinogenesis imperfecta, or hereditary opalescent dentin, is an analogous condition in which the odontoblasts fail to differentiate normally, resulting in poorly calcified dentin. This autosomal dominant disorder may also occur in patients with osteogenesis imperfecta. The junction between the enamel and dentin is altered, the enamel has a tendency to flake away, and the exposed dentin is then susceptible to abrasion. The teeth are opaque and pearly, and the pulp chambers are obliterated by calcification. Both primary and permanent teeth are usually involved. Unless the crowns of these teeth are covered early and completely, the abrasion of chewing often reduces them to the level and contour of the supporting alveolar bone.

Localized disturbances of calcification that correlate with periods of illness, malnutrition, premature birth, or birth trauma are common. An example is *linear hypocalcification or hypoplasia,* expressed as horizontal enamel defects on the permanent central and lateral incisors as well as the canines. Hypocalcification appears as opaque white patches on the tooth; hypoplasia is more severe and manifests as pitting or areas devoid of enamel. Such defects are less common in the primary dentition because intrauterine stress is relatively less frequent compared with illnesses during early infancy. Systemic conditions, such as kidney failure and cystic fibrosis, are associated with enamel defects. Local trauma to the primary incisors also can affect permanent incisor formation.

Mottled enamel is found in people whose early life is spent in areas where the fluoride content of the drinking water is greater than 2.0 parts per million (ppm) and is probably the result of fluoride affecting ameloblastic function. It varies from small inconspicuous white patches to severe, brownish discoloration and hypoplasia; the latter changes are usually seen with fluoride concentrations of greater than 5.0 ppm.

Disturbances due to *mineral deficiency* are rare, but irregular dentin and enlarged pulp chambers have been observed with vitamin D–resistant rickets; hypoplasia has been observed with vitamin D–deficient rickets.

Discolored teeth may result from incorporation of foreign substances into developing enamel. Neonatal *hyperbilirubinemia* may produce blue to black discoloration of the primary teeth, beginning at the neonatal line; the tips of the permanent first molars may also be affected. Porphyria produces a red-brown discoloration. *Tetracyclines* are extensively incorporated into bones and teeth and, if administered during the period of formation of enamel, may result in brown-yellow discoloration and hypoplasia of the enamel. Such teeth fluoresce under ultraviolet light. The period at risk extends from about the 4th mo of gestation to the 7th yr of life. Repeated or prolonged therapy with tetracycline carries the highest risk.

Delayed eruption of all teeth may indicate systemic or nutritional disturbances such as hypopituitarism, hypothyroidism, cleidocranial dysostosis, 21-trisomy, progeria, Albright osteodystrophy, incontinentia pigmenti, rickets, or multiple syndromes. Failure of eruption of single or small groups of teeth may arise from local causes such as malpositioning of teeth, supernumerary teeth, cysts, or retained primary teeth. Premature loss of primary teeth is most commonly caused by premature eruption of teeth. If the entire dentition is advanced for age and sex, precocious puberty or hyperthyroidism should be considered.

Natal teeth are observed in approximately 1 in 2,000 newborn infants; usually there are two in the position of the mandibular central incisors. Natal teeth are present at birth, whereas neonatal teeth erupt in the 1st mo of life. Attachment of natal/neonatal teeth is generally limited to the gingival margin, with little root formation or bony support. They may be a supernumerary or prematurely erupted primary tooth. A radiograph can easily differentiate between the two conditions. Natal teeth are associated with cleft palate, Pierre Robin syndrome, Ellis–van Creveld syndrome, Hallermann-Streiff syndrome, pachyonychia congenita, and other anomalies. A family history of natal teeth or premature eruption is present in 15% to 20% of affected children.

Natal/neonatal teeth may occasionally result in pain and refusal to feed, and at times may produce maternal discomfort because of abrasion or biting of the nipple during nursing. There is a remote danger of detachment, with aspiration of the tooth. Because the tongue lies between the alveolar processes during birth, it may become lacerated, and occasionally the tip is amputated (Riga-Fede disease). Decisions regarding extraction of prematurely erupted primary teeth must be made on an individual basis. Extraction requires careful dissection of the gingival attachment to prevent tearing of the tissue and excessive hemorrhage.

Exfoliation failure occurs when a primary tooth is not shed prior to the eruption of its permanent successor. Occasionally, the primary tooth may need to be extracted if the erupting permanent tooth becomes visible. This occurs most commonly in the mandibular incisor region.

CHAPTER 308
Disorders of the Teeth Associated with Other Conditions

Disorders of the teeth may occur in isolation or in combination with other systemic conditions. Any medical condition that alters the stability of the teeth within the periodontium or alters other tissues such as mucosa (both keratinized and unkeratinized), muscle, or bone can result in changes or lesions seen within the oral environment.

Congenital syphilis affects differentiation of permanent teeth, resulting in screwdriver-shaped incisors, often with central notches in their incisive edges (Hutchinson incisors), and mulberry molars, with lobular occlusal surfaces and narrow, pinched crowns (Chapter 215). Some of the dental problems associated with other medical conditions are noted in Table 308–1.

TABLE 308–1 Dental Problems Associated with Selected Medical Conditions

Medical Condition	Common Associated Dental or Oral Findings
Cleft lip and palate	Missing teeth, extra (supernumerary) teeth, shifting of arch segments, feeding difficulties, speech problems
Kidney failure	Mottled enamel (permanent teeth), facial dysmorphology
Cystic fibrosis	Stained teeth with extensive medication, mottled enamel
Immunosuppression	Oral candidiasis with potential for systemic candidiasis, cyclosporine-induced gingival hyperplasia
Low birthweight with prolonged oral intubation	Palatal groove, narrow arch
Heart defects with BE susceptibility	Bacteremia from dental procedures or trauma
Neutrophil chemotactic deficiency	Juvenile periodontitis (loss of supporting bone around teeth)
Juvenile diabetes (uncontrolled)	Juvenile periodontitis
Neuromotor dysfunction	Oral trauma from falling; malocclusion (open bite); gingivitis from lack of hygiene
Prolonged illness (generalized) during tooth formation	Enamel hypoplasia of crown portions forming during illness
Seizures	Gingival enlargement if phenytoin is used
Maternal viral infections	Syphillis—abnormally shaped teeth
Vitamin D–dependent rickets	Enamel hypoplasia

BE = Bacterial endocarditis.

CHAPTER 309
Malocclusion

The oral cavity is a masticatory instrument. The incisal edges of the anterior teeth are brought into opposition by mandibular closure for the purpose of biting off portions of large food. The cusps of the opposing posterior teeth interdigitate and slide across each other to reduce foodstuffs to a soft, moist bolus. The cheeks and tongue force the food onto the areas of tooth contact.

The masseter and temporal muscles are the main forces of mandibular closure. Acting in conjunction with the internal pterygoid muscles, they allow the mandibular teeth to forcefully contact the maxillary teeth. When teeth meet simultaneously, the force is distributed over a large area of bone-to-tooth attachment. In malocclusion, when only a few teeth touch, the same force is exerted over a smaller area and may contribute to tooth loss in adulthood. Establishing a proper relationship between the mandibular and maxillary teeth is important for physiologic and cosmetic reasons.

Variations in growth patterns are classified into three main types of occlusion determined when the jaws are closed and the mandibular condyles are in the most posterior position within the glenoid fossa (Fig. 309–1). In class I (normal) occlusion, the cusps of the posterior mandibular teeth interdigitate ahead of and inside the corresponding cusps of the opposing maxillary teeth. This relationship provides a normal facial profile. In class II occlusion, the cusps of the posterior mandibular teeth are behind and inside the corresponding cusps of the maxillary teeth. This is the most common occlusal discrepancy, with approximately 45% of the population exhibiting some

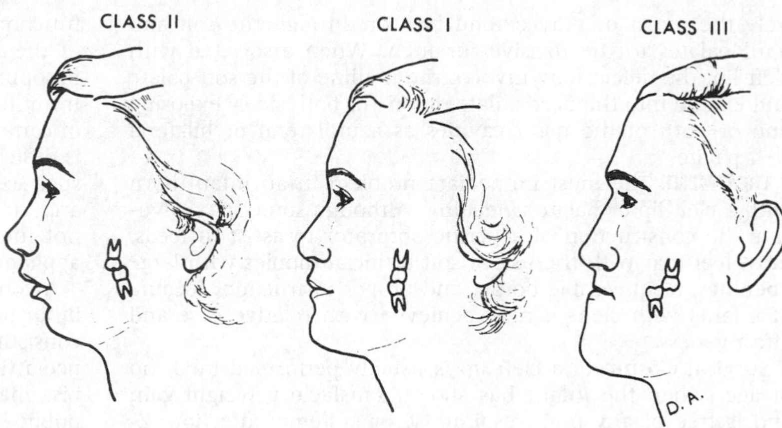

Figure 309–1 Angle classification of occlusion. The typical correspondence between the facial-jaw profile and molar relationship is shown.

degree of this condition. The resultant increased space between upper and lower anterior teeth encourages sucking and tongue-thrust habits. The facial profile often gives the appearance of a "receding chin" (retrognathia). In class III occlusion, the cusps of the posterior mandibular teeth interdigitate a tooth or more ahead of their opposing maxillary counterparts. The anterior teeth appear in cross-bite, with the mandibular incisors protruding beyond the maxillary incisors. The facial profile gives the appearance of a "protruding chin" (prognathia).

CROSS BITE. Normally, the mandibular teeth are in a position just inside the maxillary teeth, so that the outside mandibular cusps or incisal edges meet the central portion of the opposing maxillary teeth. A reversal of this relation is referred to as a *cross-bite.* Cross bites may be anterior, involving the incisors, or posterior, involving the molars.

OPEN AND CLOSED BITES. If the posterior mandibular and maxillary teeth make contact with each other but the anterior teeth are still apart, the condition is called an *open bite.* Open bites may be due to skeletal growth pattern or digit sucking (see below). With prolonged digit sucking, the open bite may not resolve. If mandibular anterior teeth occlude inside the maxillary anterior teeth in an over-closed position, the condition is referred to as a *closed bite.* Treatment of open and closed bites consists of orthodontic correction, generally performed in the pre-teen or teenage years. Some cases require orthognathic surgery to optimally position the jaws in a vertical direction.

DENTAL CROWDING. Overlap of incisors can result when the jaws are too small or the teeth are too large for adequate alignment of the teeth. Growth of the jaws is mostly in the posterior aspects of the mandible and maxilla, and therefore inadequate space for the teeth at 7 or 8 yr of age will not resolve with growth of the jaws. Spacing in the primary dentition is normal and desirable for adequate alignment of successor teeth.

DIGIT SUCKING. Various and conflicting etiologic theories and recommendations for correction have been proposed for digit sucking in children. Prolonged thumb sucking can cause flaring of the maxillary incisor teeth and an open bite. The prevalence of thumb sucking decreases steadily from the age of 2 yr to approximately 10% by the age of 5.

The earlier the habit is discontinued after the eruption of the permanent maxillary incisors (age 7–8), the greater the likelihood that there will be lessening of the incisors flaring and bite opening. Stopping of the habit, however, will not rectify a malocclusion caused by a deviant growth pattern. A variety of treatment protocols have been suggested, including insertion of an appliance with extensions that serves as a reminder when the child attempts to insert the digit. The greatest likelihood of success occurs in cases in which the child desires to stop.

CHAPTER 310
Cleft Lip and Palate

Clefts of the lip and palate are distinct entities closely related embryologically, functionally, and genetically. Cleft of the lip appears because of hypoplasia of the mesenchymal layer, resulting in a failure of the medial nasal and maxillary processes to join. Cleft of the palate appears to represent failure of the palatal shelves to approximate or fuse.

INCIDENCE AND EPIDEMIOLOGY. The incidence of cleft lip with or without cleft palate is about 1 in 750 white births; the incidence of cleft palate alone is about 1 in 2,500 white births. The former is more common in males. Possible etiologies include maternal drug exposure, syndrome-malformation complex, or genetic. Although both may appear to occur sporadically, the inheritance of susceptibility genes allowing the formation of a cleft in certain individuals appears important in the formation of clefts. There are families in which a cleft lip or palate, or both, is inherited in a dominant fashion (van der Woude syndrome), and careful examination of parents is important to distinguish this type from others, since the recurrence risk is 50%. Ethnic factors also affect the incidence of cleft lip and palate. Clefts are highest among Asians and lowest among blacks. The incidence of associated congenital malformations and of impairment in development is increased in children with cleft defects, especially in those with cleft palate alone. These findings are partially explained by an increased incidence of conductive hearing impairment in children with cleft palate, due in part to repeated middle ear infections, and by the frequency of cleft defects among children with chromosomal abnormalities. The risks of recurrence of cleft defects within families are discussed in Chapters 77 and 78.

Animal studies suggest that nongenetic influences may be responsible for clefts in a susceptible host at a critical period of organogenesis. Associated malformations are especially frequent in structures derived from the first branchial arch.

CLINICAL MANIFESTATIONS. Cleft lip may vary from a small notch in the vermilion border to a complete separation extending into the floor of the nose. Clefts may be unilateral (more often on the left side) or bilateral and may involve the alveolar ridge. Deformed, supernumerary, or absent teeth are associated findings. The nasal alar cartilage clefts of the lip are frequently associated with deficiency of the columella and elongation of the vomer, producing a protrusion of the anterior aspect of the cleft premaxillary process.

Isolated cleft palate occurs in the midline and may involve

only the uvula or may extend into or through the soft and hard palates to the incisive foramen. When associated with cleft lip, the defect may involve the midline of the soft palate and extend into the hard palate on one or both sides, exposing one or both of the nasal cavities as a unilateral or bilateral cleft palate.

TREATMENT. The most immediate problem in an infant born with a cleft lip or palate is feeding. Although some may advocate the construction of a plastic obturator to assist in feeds, most feel that with the use of soft artificial nipples with large openings, a squeezable bottle, and proper instruction, feeding of infants with clefts can be achieved with relative ease and effectiveness.

Surgical closure of a cleft lip is usually performed by 3 mo of age, when the infant has shown satisfactory weight gain and is free of any oral, respiratory, or systemic infection. Z-plasty is the most commonly used technique; a staggered suture line minimizes notching of the lip from retraction of scar tissue. The initial repair may be revised at 4 or 5 yr of age. Corrective surgery on the nose may be delayed until adolescence. Nasal surgery can also be performed at the time of the lip repair. Cosmetic results depend on the extent of the original deformity, healing potential of the individual, absence of infection, and the skill of the surgeon.

Because clefts of the palate vary considerably in size, shape, and degree of deformity, the timing of surgical correction should be individualized. Criteria such as width of the cleft, adequacy of the existing palatal segments, morphology of the surrounding areas (such as width of the oropharynx), and neuromuscular function of the soft palate and pharyngeal walls affect the decision. The goals of surgery are the union of the cleft segments, intelligible and pleasant speech, reduction of nasal regurgitation, and avoidance of injury to the growing maxilla.

In an otherwise healthy child, closure of the palate is usually done prior to 1 yr of age to enhance normal speech development. When surgical correction is delayed beyond the 3rd yr, a contoured speech bulb can be attached to the posterior of a maxillary denture so that contraction of the pharyngeal and velopharyngeal muscles can bring tissues into contact with the bulb to accomplish occlusion of the nasopharynx and help the child develop intelligible speech. The cleft usually crosses the alveolar ridge and interferes with the formation of teeth in the maxillary anterior region. The missing elements of the dentition, usually maxillary anterior teeth, must be replaced by prosthetic devices.

PREOPERATIVE AND POSTOPERATIVE MANAGEMENT. Even the suspicion of infection is a contraindication to operation. If the child is in good nutritional condition and in fluid and electrolyte balance, feeding may be permitted to within 6 hr of the operation (see Chapter 73). During the immediate postoperative period, special nursing care is essential. Gentle aspiration of the nasopharynx minimizes the chances of the common complications of atelectasis or pneumonia. The primary considerations in postoperative care are maintenance of a clean suture line and avoidance of tension on the sutures. For these reasons, the infant is fed with a Mead Johnson bottle, and the arms are restrained with elbow cuffs. A fluid or semifluid diet is maintained for 3 wk; feeding is continued with a Mead Johnson bottle or a cup. The patient's hands, toys, and other foreign bodies must be kept away from the surgical site.

COMPLICATIONS. Recurrent otitis media and hearing loss are frequent with cleft palate. Excessive dental decay is common but not inevitable. Displacement of the maxillary arches and malposition of the teeth usually require orthodontic correction.

Speech defects may be present or persist because of inadequate anatomic closure of the palate. Such speech is characterized by the emission of air from the nose and by a hypernasal quality with certain sounds. Both before and sometimes after palatal surgery, the speech defect is due to inadequacies in function of the palatal and pharyngeal muscles. The muscles of the soft palate and the lateral and posterior walls of the nasopharynx constitute a valve that separates the nasopharynx from the oropharynx during swallowing and in the production of certain sounds. If the valve does not function adequately, it is difficult to build up enough pressure in the mouth to make such explosive sounds as p, b, d, t, h, y, or the sibilants s, sh, and ch, and such words as "cats," "boats," and "sisters" are not intelligible. After operation or the insertion of a speech appliance, speech therapy is necessary.

A complete program of habilitation for the child with a cleft lip or palate may require years of special treatment by a team consisting of a pediatrician, plastic surgeon, otolaryngologist, pediatric dentist, prosthodontist, orthodontist, speech therapist, medical social worker, psychologist, child psychiatrist, and public health nurse. The child's physician should be responsible for seeking the coordinated use of specialists and for parental counseling and guidance.

PALATOPHARYNGEAL INCOMPETENCE. The speech disturbance characteristic of the child with a cleft palate can also be produced by other osseous or neuromuscular abnormalities when there is an inability to form an effective seal between oropharynx and nasopharynx during swallowing or phonation. The abnormality may be in the structure of the palate or pharynx or in the muscles attached to these structures. In a child who has the potential for abnormal speech, adenoidectomy may precipitate overt hypernasality. A submucous cleft palate may be the cause of this problem. In such cases, the adenoid mass may have facilitated velopharyngeal closure when the elevated soft palate contacted it. If the neuromuscular function is adequate, compensation in palatopharyngeal movement may take place, and the speech defect may improve, although speech therapy is necessary. In other cases, slow involution of the adenoids may allow for gradual compensation in palatal and pharyngeal muscular function. This may explain why a speech defect does not become apparent in some children who have a submucous cleft palate or similar anomaly predisposing to palatopharyngeal incompetence. Velopharyngeal incompetency (VPI) can also occur in children with an inherent palatal abnormality (velocardiofacial syndrome). VPI should be evaluated by a Craniofacial Disorders Team or a geneticist.

CLINICAL MANIFESTATIONS. Although clinical signs vary, the symptoms of palatopharyngeal incompetence are similar to those of a cleft palate. There may be hypernasal speech (especially noted in the articulation of pressure consonants such as p, b, d, t, h, v, f, and s), conspicuous constricting movement of the nares during speech, inability to whistle, gargle, blow out a candle, or inflate a balloon, loss of liquid through the nose when drinking with the head down, otitis media, and hearing loss. Oral inspection may reveal a cleft palate or a relatively short palate with a large oropharynx; absent, grossly asymmetric, or minimal muscular activity of the soft palate and pharynx during phonation or gagging; or a submucous cleft. The latter is suggested by a bifid uvula, by a translucent membrane in the midline of the soft palate (revealing lack of continuity of muscles), by palpable notching in the posterior border of the hard palate instead of a posterior nasal spinous process, or by forward or V-shaped displacement or grooving on the soft palate during phonation or gagging.

Palatopharyngeal incompetence may also be demonstrated radiographically. The head should be carefully positioned to obtain a true lateral view; one film is obtained with the patient at rest and another during continuous phonation of the vowel "u" as in "boom." The soft palate contacts the posterior pharyngeal wall in normal function, whereas in palatopharyngeal incompetence such contact is absent. Most accurate evaluations of VPI are accomplished by the use of nasoendoscopy.

TREATMENT. In selected cases, the palate may be retropositioned or pharyngoplasty performed using a flap of tissue from the posterior pharyngeal wall. Dental speech appliances have also been used successfully. The type of surgery used is best tailored to the findings on nasoendoscopy.

CHAPTER 311
Syndromes with Oral Manifestations

Many syndromes have distinct or accompanying facial, oral, and dental manifestations (Apert syndrome, Chapter 601; Crouzon disease, Chapter 601; Down syndrome, Chapter 78). The conditions described are examples of some of the common occurring conditions.

Osteogenesis imperfecta is often accompanied by hereditary opalescent dentin, also termed *dentinogenesis imperfecta* (Chapter 307). Depending on the severity of presentation, treatment of the dentition varies from routine preventive and restorative monitoring to covering affected posterior teeth with stainless steel crowns, when the extent of dental involvement is severe. Dentinogenesis can also occur in isolation, but this manifestation cannot be clinically distinguished from the dentinogenesis imperfecta associated with osteogenesis imperfecta.

Another genetic condition, *cleidocranial dysostosis* has orofacial variations such as frontal bossing, mandibular prognathism, and a broad nasal base. Tooth eruption is often delayed. In addition, the primary teeth can be abnormally retained while the permanent teeth remain unerupted. Supernumerary teeth are common, especially in the premolar area. Although the erupted teeth are usually free of hypoplasia, variations in the size and shape of the teeth are common. Restoration of the erupted primary and permanent teeth should be performed when carious lesions are present. It is common to see extensive dental rehabilitation therapy in individuals with this disorder to maintain effective mastication.

Ectodermal dysplasia (Chapter 655) is a heterogeneous group of conditions in which oral manifestations range from little or no involvement (the dentition is completely normal) to cases in which the teeth can be totally or partially absent or malformed. Because alveolar bone does not develop in the absence of teeth, the alveolar processes can be either totally or partially absent, and the resultant overclosure of the mandible causes the lips to protrude. Facial development is otherwise not disturbed. Teeth, when present, can range from normal to small and conical in form. If aplasia of the buccal and labial mucous glands are present, dryness and irritation of the oral mucosa can occur. People with ectodermal dysplasia may need either partial or full dentures, even at a very young age. The vertical height between the jaws is thus restored, improving the position of the lips and facial contours. Masticatory function is restored, and eating habits are therefore improved.

Pierre Robin syndrome consists of micrognathia with a high arched or cleft palate. Posterior displacement of the attachment of the genioglossus muscle to the hypoplastic mandible prevents the normal anchorage of the tongue; in the supine child, under the influence of gravity, the tongue falls back, obstructing the airway. A postalveolar cleft of the hard and soft palates is a common but not constant feature; the palate may be high arched.

The tongue is usually of normal size, but the floor of the mouth is foreshortened. Obstruction of the air passages may occur, particularly on inspiration, and usually requires treatment to prevent suffocation. The infant should be maintained in a prone or partially prone position so that the tongue falls forward to relieve respiratory obstruction. Thirty per cent of the patients require tracheostomy. Sufficient mandibular growth often takes place within a few months to relieve the glossoptosis. The feeding of infants with mandibular hypoplasia requires great care and patience but can usually be accomplished without resorting to gavage. Often the growth of the mandible will achieve an essentially normal profile within 4 to 6 yr. Dental anomalies usually require individualized treatment. Thirty per cent of all children with Pierre Robin syndrome have Sticklers syndrome, an autosomal dominant condition that includes other findings such as early arthritis and ocular problems.

In *mandibulofacial dysostosis* (Treacher Collins syndrome or Franceschetti syndrome), the facial appearance is characterized by palpebral fissures sloping downward, colobomas of the lower eyelids, sunken cheekbones, blind fistulas opening between the angles of the mouth and the ears, deformed pinnae, atypical hair growth extending toward the cheeks, receding chin, and large mouth. Facial clefts, abnormalities of the ears, and deafness are common. The disorder is autosomal dominant, often with incomplete penetrance. The mandible is usually hypoplastic; the ramus may be deficient, and the coronoid and condylar processes are flat or even aplastic. The palatal vault may be either high or cleft. Infrequently, unilateral or bilateral macrostomia, or failure of embryonic fusion of the maxillary and mandibular processes, may occur. Dental malocclusions are frequent. The teeth may be widely separated, hypoplastic, or displaced or have an open bite. Orthodontic and routine dental treatments are indicated.

Hemifacial microsomia is usually characterized by unilateral hypoplasia of the mandible and can be associated with partial paralysis of the facial nerve, macrostomia, blind fistulas between the angles of the mouth and the ears, and deformed external ears. Severe facial asymmetry and malocclusion can develop because of the absence or hypoplasia of the mandibular condyle on the affected side. Congenital condylar deformity tends to increase with age. Early craniofacial surgery may be indicated to minimize the deformity. This disorder can be associated with ocular and vertebral anomalies (oculo-auricula-vertebral spectrum, including Goldenhar syndrome) and therefore radiographs of the vertebrae and ribs should be considered to determine the extent of skeletal involvement.

Facial asymmetries resulting from excessive molding of the cranium or from displacement of the mandible during breech or face presentations are common and are usually self-correcting. Facial asymmetry caused by injury of the growing cartilage or fracture of the condylar head during birth, infancy, or early childhood may be permanent but is frequently of little functional consequences. Traumatic injuries may occur during birth from obstetric forceps placed over the area or may result from blows on the chin during infancy and childhood.

Injuries, acute infections, or arthritis of the growing condylar cartilage may result in partial (fibrous) or complete (bony) *ankylosis of the temporomandibular joint* and failure of that side of the mandible to grow. The normal side, meanwhile, continues to grow and pushes the midline toward the affected side. The midline deviation is exaggerated during mouth opening. Radiographs of the affected side reveal an increased preangular notch or displaced condylar head. Bilateral injuries to the growing cartilage result in failure of the mandible and chin to grow downward and forward, causing the entire mandible to be retruded and smaller than normal.

CHAPTER 312
Dental Caries

ETIOLOGY. The development of dental caries is dependent on inter-relationships between the tooth surface, dietary carbohydrates, and specific oral bacteria. Organic acids produced by bacterial fermentation of dietary carbohydrates reduce the pH of dental plaque adjacent to the tooth to a point at which demineralization occurs. The initial carious lesion appears as an opaque white spot on the enamel; with progressive loss of tooth, mineral cavitation occurs.

A group of microorganisms, mutans type streptococci, are associated with the development of dental caries. These bacteria have the ability to adhere to enamel, produce abundant acid, and survive at low pH. Once the enamel surface cavitates, other oral bacteria (lactobacilli) colonize the tooth, produce acid, and foster further tooth demineralization. Demineralization from acid production is determined more by the frequency of carbohydrate consumption than the actual quantity of carbohydrate eaten. The cariogenic potential of a nursing bottle of a sweetened beverage that is consumed throughout the night or at nap times is much greater than that of the same volume of drink consumed at a single meal. Similarly, sticky candies retained orally for long periods (sucrose in sticky candies) is more cariogenic than the sugar in food products retained for short times.

EPIDEMIOLOGY. Dental caries have generally decreased in developed countries in the past 30 yr but still remain highly prevalent in low-income children and children from developing countries. The decrease is thought to be due to advances in prevention, particularly in the use of fluorides. Still, over half of the children in the United States have dental caries, with most of those having caries primarily in the pits and fissures of the occlusal (biting) surfaces of the molar teeth.

CLINICAL MANIFESTATIONS. The age-related epidemiology is noted in Figure 312–1. Dental caries of the primary dentition usually begin in the pits and fissures. Small lesions may be difficult to diagnose by visual inspection, but larger lesions present as cavitations of the occlusal surface. The second most frequent sites of caries occur on approximal sites (contact surfaces between the teeth), which in many cases can only be detected by intraoral radiographs. Caries lesions of the exposed smooth (buccal and lingual) surfaces are generally found only in children with rampant caries (Fig. 312–2).

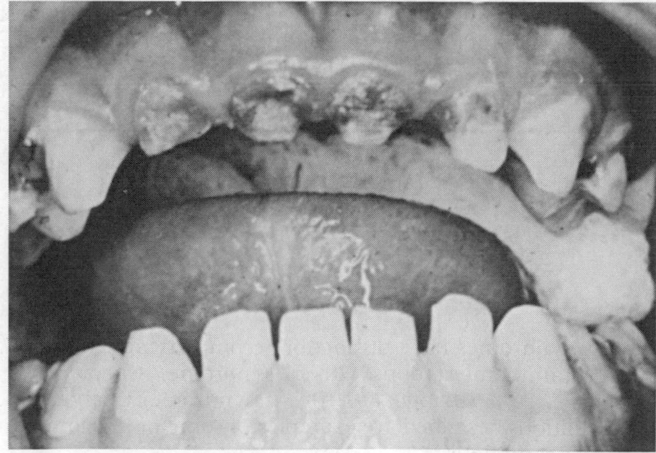

Figure 312–2 Early childhood caries, also called nursing bottle caries or baby bottle tooth decay.

Rampant caries in infants and toddlers, referred to as early childhood caries (ECC), nursing bottle caries, or baby bottle tooth decay, has in the past been ascribed solely to inappropriate bottle-feeding. Although the combination of a child being infected with cariogenic bacteria and the frequent ingestion of sugar, either in the bottle or in solid foods, is critical, other factors such as enamel hypoplasia of primary teeth because of nutritional deficiencies during pregnancy or premature birth may play a role. Reports have also associated "at will" breastfeeding with caries of the maxillary anterior teeth, but the possibility of cariogenic dietary practices other than breastfeeding, in such cases, need further exploration.

Early childhood caries is common, with a reported prevalence of 30% to 50% in children from low socioeconomic backgrounds, and as high as 70% in some Native American groups. ECC is also seen on a regular basis in private pediatric dental offices. It may occur as early as 12 mo of age, long before children visit a dentist. Pediatricians have the responsibility to refer to a dentist those children whom they consider

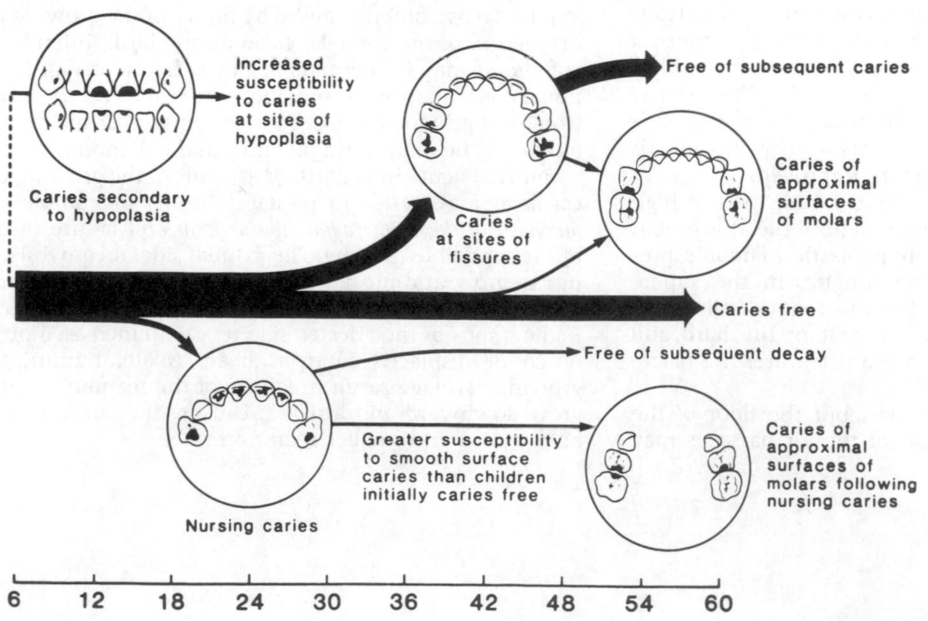

Figure 312–1 Schematic for different kinds of caries and ages when each can start. A significant percentage of children remain caries free. Nursing caries (usually baby bottle tooth decay [BBTD]) begins between 1 and 2 y of age; children with BBTD are at significantly greater risk for future caries than are caries-free children. Pit and fissure caries usually begins after about age 3, with caries of approximating tooth surfaces beginning shortly after. (From Johnsen DC: The role of the pediatrician in identifying and treating dental caries. Pediatr Clin N Am 38:1173, 1991.)

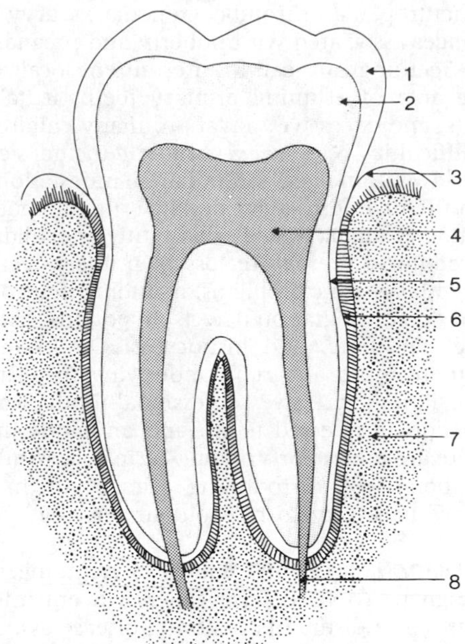

Figure 312–3 Basic dental anatomy: 1 = enamel; 2 = dentin; 3 = gingival margin; 4 = pulp; 5 = cementum; 6 = periodontal ligament; 7 = alveolar bone; 8 = neurovascular bundle.

at risk for ECC (inappropriate feeding habits). Children who develop caries at a young age are known to be at high risk for developing further caries as they get older. Therefore, the appropriate prevention of ECC can result in the elimination of major dental problems in toddlers and less decay in later childhood.

The age at which caries occur is important in dental management. Children under 3 yr of age often require restraint, sedation, or general anesthesia to repair carious teeth. After age 3, children generally can cope with dental restorative care with the use of local anesthesia.

COMPLICATIONS. If left untreated, dental caries usually destroy most of the tooth and invade the dental pulp (Fig. 312–3), leading to an inflammation of the pulp (pulpitis) and significant pain. Pulpitis can progress to necrosis, with bacterial invasion of the alveolar bone (dental abscess; periapical abscess). This process may lead to sepsis and facial space infection (Fig. 312–4). Such periapical infection of a primary tooth may also disrupt normal development of the successor permanent tooth.

TREATMENT. Dental treatment can restore many teeth affected with dental caries, using silver amalgam or plastic restorations and crowns. If caries involve the dental pulp, a partial removal of the pulp (pulpotomy) or complete removal of the pulp (pulpectomy) may be required. If a tooth requires extraction, a space maintainer to prevent migration of teeth may be indicated to prevent impaction or malposition of permanent successor teeth.

Clinical management of the pain and infection associated with untreated dental caries varies with the extent of involvement and the medical status of the patient. Dental infection localized to the dentoalveolar unit can be managed by local measures (extraction, pulpectomy). Oral antibiotics are indicated for dental infections associated with cellulitis or facial swelling. Penicillin is the antibiotic of choice, except in patients with a history of allergy to this agent; clindamycin and erythromycin are suitable alternatives. Oral analgesics, such as acetaminophen with or without codeine, are usually adequate for the pain control. If the infection involves a vital area (submandibular space, which can lead to Ludwig angina; facial triangle, which can lead to cavernous sinus thrombosis; or periorbital space, which can lead to orbital involvement), parenteral antibiotics may be indicated.

PREVENTION

Fluoride. The most effective preventive measure against dental caries is optimizing the fluoride content of communal water supplies to one part per million. In fluoride-deficient water supplies, similar caries prevention benefits are obtained from dietary fluoride supplements (Table 312–1). The fluoride level of a water supply can usually be obtained by calling the local public health department. If the patient uses a private water supply, it is necessary to get the water tested for fluoride levels before prescribing fluoride supplements. To avoid potential overdoses, no fluoride prescription should be written for more than a total of 120 mg of fluoride. Significant overdose of fluoride (greater than 5 mg/kg) needs immediate medical attention. The use of topical fluoride agents, applied professionally or by the patient, are beneficial to children at risk for caries.

Oral Hygiene. Thorough daily brushing and flossing of the teeth

Figure 312–4 *A*, Facial inflammation-infection from the abscess of a maxillary primary molar. *B*, Resolution of the cellulitis in 1 wk with a course of antibiotics and extraction of the tooth.

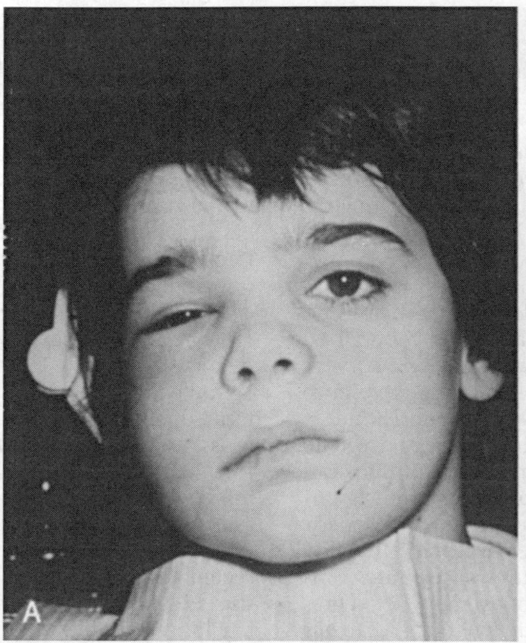

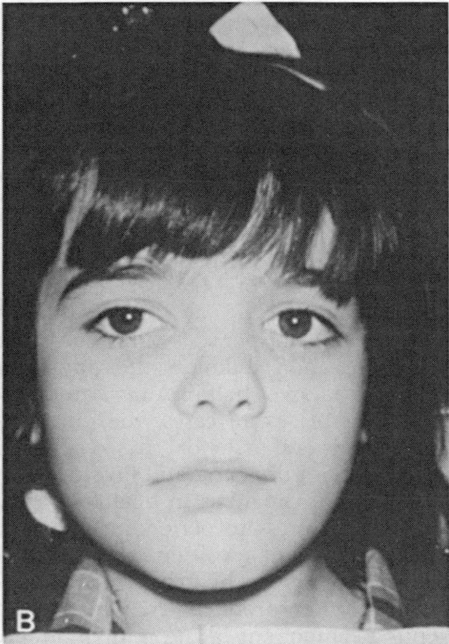

E 312–1 Supplemental Fluoride Dosage Schedule

Age	Fluoride in Home Water (ppm)		
	<0.3	*0.3–0.6*	*>0.6*
6 mo–3 yr	0.25*	0	0
3–6 yr	0.50	0.25	0
6–16 yr	1.00	0.50	0

**Milligrams of fluoride per day.*

may help prevent dental caries and periodontal disease. Studies have shown that most children under 8 yr of age do not have the coordination required for adequate oral hygiene. Accordingly, parents should assume responsibility for the child's oral hygiene, with the degree of parental involvement appropriate to the child's changing abilities.

Diet. Decreasing the frequency of sugar ingestion prevents dental caries. Therefore, using sweetened beverages in the nursing bottle and bedtime bottle should be discouraged, and children at risk for dental caries should reduce between-meal sugar-containing snacks.

Dental Sealants. Plastic dental sealants have been shown to be effective in the prevention of pit and fissure caries. Sealants are most effective when placed soon after the teeth erupt (usually within 1–2 yr) and when used in children with deep grooves and fissures in the molar teeth.

Identification of High-Risk Patients. Intact salivary gland function is the major host defense against dental caries. Impaired salivary function and consequent xerostomia in children are usually due to anticholinergic drugs or head and neck radiation therapy. Additional risk factors for dental caries include low socioeconomic settings, previous history of caries, and presence of high levels of mutans streptococci. Medical conditions associated with high caries risk include gastric reflux, bulimia, rumination, Prader-Willi syndrome, mental retardation, and epidermolysis bullosa. Intensive, preventive therapy must be instituted in such children to prevent rampant dental caries.

CHAPTER 313
Periodontal Diseases

The periodontium includes the gingiva, alveolar bone, cementum, and periodontal ligament (see Fig. 312–3). Several distinct diseases of the periodontium occur during childhood and adolescence. These include gingivitis, teething, prepubertal periodontitis, acute necrotizing ulcerative gingivitis, herpetic gingivostomatitis, cyclosporine- or phenytoin-induced gingival overgrowth, localized juvenile periodontitis, and acute pericoronitis.

GINGIVITIS. Poor oral hygiene results in the accumulation of a dental plaque at the tooth-gingival interface that activates an inflammatory response, expressed as localized or generalized reddening and swelling of the gingiva. Epidemiologic surveys indicate that over half of American school children experience gingivitis. In severe cases, the gingiva spontaneously bleeds and there is oral malodor. *Treatment* is with proper oral hygiene (careful tooth brushing and flossing); complete resolution can be expected. Gingivitis in healthy prepubertal children is unlikely to progress to periodontitis (inflammation of the periodontal ligament resulting in loss of alveolar bone). Inability to resolve gingivitis by oral hygiene measures necessitates considering other problems in which gingivitis may be a presenting component (acute nonlymphocytic leukemia, diabetes mellitus, neutropenia, thrombocytopenia, scurvy, and hormonal changes associated with puberty and pregnancy).

TEETHING. Teething can lead to intermittent localized discomfort in the area of erupting primary teeth, irritability, low-grade fevers, and excessive salivation; many children have no apparent difficulties. *Symptomatic treatment* includes chewing on ice rings and oral analgesics. Similar manifestations can also arise when the first permanent molars erupt at about age 6 yr.

PREPUBERTAL PERIODONTITIS. Periodontitis in children before puberty, leading to premature loss of primary teeth, is often associated with systemic problems, including neutropenia, leukocyte adhesion or migration defects, hypophosphatasia, Papillon-Lefèvre syndrome, and histiocytosis X. In many cases, however, there is no apparent underlying medical problem. *Treatment* includes aggressive professional tooth cleaning, strategic extraction of affected teeth, and antibiotic therapy. Although there are few reports of long-term successful treatment to reverse bone loss surrounding primary teeth, diagnostic work-ups are necessary to rule out underlying systemic disease.

ACUTE NECROTIZING ULCERATIVE GINGIVITIS. Acute necrotizing ulcerative gingivitis (ANUG), also called Vincent infection and trench mouth, is a distinct periodontal disease associated with oral spirochetes and fusobacteria. It is not clear, however, whether bacteria initiate the disease or are secondary invaders. ANUG develops primarily in young adults and adolescents. It rarely develops in healthy children in developed countries. It occurs frequently among children in southern India and certain African countries where affected children usually have protein malnutrition. In such children, the lesion may extend into adjacent tissues, causing necrosis of facial structures (cancrum oris, or noma).

Clinical manifestations of ANUG include (1) necrosis and ulceration of gingiva between the teeth, (2) an adherent grayish pseudomembrane over the affected gingiva, (3) oral malodor, (4) cervical lymphadenopathy, (5) malaise, and (6) fever. The disease is usually localized, with the most common site being the periodontium associated with the mandibular incisor teeth. The condition may be mistaken for acute herpetic gingivostomatitis. Dark-field microscopy of debris obtained from ANUG lesions will demonstrate dense spirochete populations.

Treatment of ANUG is divided into an acute management by antibiotic therapy (penicillin or erythromycin), local debridement, oxygenating agents (direct application of 10% carbamide peroxide in anhydrous glycerol four times a day), and analgesics. Dramatic resolution usually occurs within 48 hr. A second phase of treatment may be necessary if the acute phase of the disease has caused irreversible morphologic damage to the periodontium. Although often regarded otherwise, the disease is not contagious.

HERPETIC GINGIVOSTOMATITIS (See Chapter 245)

Cyclosporine- Or Phenytoin-Induced Gingival Overgrowth. The use of cyclosporine to suppress organ rejection or phenytoin for anticonvulsant therapy and in some cases calcium channel blockers is associated with generalized enlargement of the gingiva. Phenytoin and its metabolites have a direct stimulatory action on gingival fibroblasts, resulting in accelerated synthesis of collagen. Clinical studies indicate that phenytoin induces less gingival hyperplasia in patients who maintain meticulous oral hygiene.

Gingival hyperplasia occurs in 10% to 30% of patients treated with phenytoin. Severe manifestations may include (1) gross enlargement of the gingiva, sometimes covering the teeth; (2) edema and erythema of the gingiva; (3) secondary infection, resulting in abscess formation; (4) migration of teeth; and (5) inhibition of exfoliation of primary teeth and subsequent impaction of permanent teeth. *Treatment* should be directed toward prevention. Ideally, cyclosporine or phenytoin should be discontinued if possible. However, patients undergoing long-term treatment with these drugs should receive frequent dental examinations and oral hygiene care. Severe forms of gingival overgrowth are treated by gingivectomy, but the lesion recurs if drug use is continued.

Localized Juvenile Periodontitis (LJP). Localized juvenile periodontitis is characterized by rapid alveolar bone loss, especially around the permanent incisors and first molars. It is associated with a strain of *Actinobacillus*. In addition, the neutrophils of patients with localized juvenile periodontitis may have chemotactic and phagocytic defects. If left untreated, affected teeth lose their attachment and may exfoliate. *Treatment* varies with the degree of involvement. Patients diagnosed at the onset of the disease are usually managed by local debridement, antibiotic therapy, and meticulous oral hygiene. Patients who have extensive alveolar bone loss at the time of initial diagnosis require extensive periodontal therapy that may include autologous osseous grafting. Prognosis depends on the degree of initial involvement and compliance with therapy.

Acute Pericoronitis. Acute inflammation of the flap of gingiva that partially covers the crown of an incompletely erupted tooth is common in mandibular permanent molars. Accumulation of debris and bacteria between the gingival flap and tooth precipitates the inflammatory response. A variant of this condition is a gingival abscess due to entrapment of bacteria because of orthodontic bands, crowns, and so on. Trismus and severe pain may be associated with the inflammation. Untreated cases may result in facial cellulitis.

Treatment includes local debridement and irrigation, warm saline rinses, and antibiotic therapy. When the acute phase has subsided, extraction of the tooth or resection of the gingival flap prevents recurrence. Early recognition of the partial impaction of mandibular third molars and their subsequent extraction will prevent these areas from having pericoronitis.

CHAPTER 314
Dental Trauma

Traumatic oral injuries may be categorized into three groups: (1) injuries to teeth, (2) injuries to soft tissue (contusions, abrasions, lacerations, punctures, avulsions, burns), and (3) injuries to jaw (mandibular or maxillary fractures or both). This chapter is limited to teeth injuries.

INJURIES TO TEETH. Approximately 10% of children between 18 mo and 18 yr of age will sustain significant tooth trauma. There appear to be three age periods of greatest predilection: (1) toddlers (1–3 yr), usually due to falls or child abuse; (2) school-aged (7–10 yr), usually from bicycle and playground accidents; and (3) adolescents (16–18 yr), often the result of fights, athletic injuries, and automobile accidents. Injuries to teeth are more frequent among children with protruding front teeth. Children with craniofacial abnormalities or neuromuscular deficits are also at increased risk for dental injury. Injuries to teeth may involve the hard dental tissues, the dental pulp (nerve), and injuries to the periodontal structure (surrounding bone and attachment apparatus) (Fig. 314–1; Table 314–1).

Fractures of teeth may be uncomplicated (confined to the hard dental tissues) or complicated (involving the pulp). Exposure of the pulp will result in its bacterial contamination, which can lead to infection and pulp necrosis. Pulp exposure complicates therapy and may lower the likelihood of a favorable outcome.

Trauma to the mouth most often affects the crowns or roots of the maxillary incisor teeth. Uncomplicated crown fractures are treated by covering exposed dentin and by placing an esthetic restoration. Complicated crown fractures usually re-

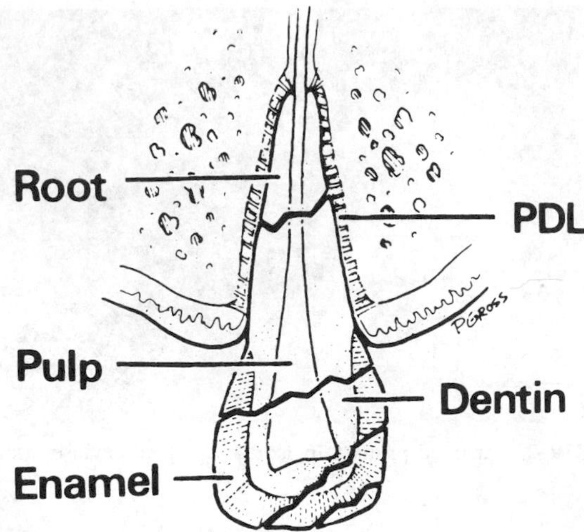

Figure 314–1 Tooth fractures may involve enamel, dentin, or pulp and may occur in the crown or root of a tooth. (From Pinkham JR: Pediatric Dentistry: Infancy Through Adolescence. Philadelphia, WB Saunders, 1988, p 172.)

quire endodontic (root canal) therapy. Crown-root fractures and root fractures usually require extensive dental therapy. Such injuries in the primary dentition may interfere with normal development of the permanent dentition, and therefore, these types of injury of the primary incisor teeth are usually managed by extraction of the fractured segments.

Injuries resulting in fractured teeth should be referred to a dentist as soon as possible. Even when dentition appears intact following oral trauma, the patient should be evaluated promptly by a dentist. Baseline data (radiographs, mobility patterns, responses to specific stimuli, percussion, electricity, hot and cold) enable the dentist to assess the likelihood of future complications.

INJURIES TO PERIODONTAL STRUCTURES. Trauma to teeth with associated injury to periodontal structures usually presents as mobile or displaced teeth. Such injuries are more frequent in the primary than in the permanent dentition. Categories of

TABLE 314–1 Injuries to Crowns of Teeth

Type of Trauma	Description	Treatment and Referral
Enamel infraction (crazing)	Incomplete fracture of enamel without loss of tooth structure.	Initially may not require therapy but should be assessed periodically by dentist.
Enamel fractures	Fracture of only the tooth enamel.	Tooth may be smoothed or treated to replace fragment.
Enamel and dentin fracture	Fracture of enamel and dentinal layer of the tooth. Tooth may be sensitive to cold or air. Pulp may become necrotic, leading to periapical abscess.	Refer as soon as possible. Area should be treated to preserve the integrity of the underlying pulp.
Enamel, dentin fracture involving the pulp	Bacterial contamination may lead to pulpal necrosis and periapical abscess. The tooth may have the appearance of bleeding or may display a small red spot.	Refer immediately. The dental therapy of choice depends on the extent of injury, the condition of the pulp, the development of the tooth, time elapsed from injury, and any other injuries to the supporting structures. Therapy is directed toward minimizing contamination in an effort to improve the prognosis.

From Jossell SD, Abrams RG: Managing common dental problems and emergencies. Pediatr Clin North Am 38:1325, 1991.

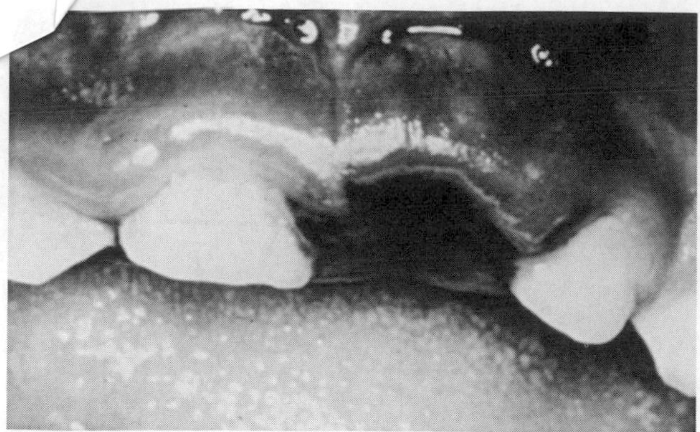

Figure 314–2 Intruded primary incisor that appears evulsed (knocked out).

trauma to the periodontium include (1) concussion, (2) subluxation, (3) intrusive luxation, (4) extrusive luxation, and (5) avulsion.

Concussion. Injuries that produce minor damage to the periodontal ligament are termed concussions. Teeth sustaining such injuries are not mobile or displaced but react markedly to percussion (gentle hitting of the tooth with an instrument). This type of injury usually requires no therapy and resolves without complication. Primary incisors that sustain concussion may change color, indicating pulpal degeneration, and should be evaluated by a dentist.

Subluxation. Subluxated teeth exhibit mild to moderate horizontal mobility, vertical mobility, or both. Hemorrhage is usually evident around the neck of the tooth at the gingival margin. There is no displacement of the tooth. Many subluxated teeth need to be immobilized by acrylic splints to ensure adequate repair of the periodontal ligament. Some of these teeth will develop pulp necrosis. This type of injury should also be referred to a dentist.

Intrusive Luxation. Intruded teeth are pushed up into their socket, sometimes to the point where they are not clinically visible. Intruded primary incisors may give the false appearance of being avulsed (knocked out) (Fig. 314–2). This type of injury is more common in primary teeth. To rule out avulsion, a dental radiograph is indicated (Fig. 314–3). This type of injury should be referred to the dentist as soon as possible.

Extrusive Luxation. This type of injury is characterized by displacement of the tooth from its socket. The tooth is usually displaced to the lingual (tongue) side, with fracture of the wall of the alveolar socket. These teeth need immediate treatment; the longer the delay, the more likely the tooth will be fixed in its displaced position. Therapy is directed at reduction (repositioning the tooth) and fixation (splinting with acrylic). In addition, the pulp of such teeth often becomes necrotic and requires endodontic therapy. Extrusive luxation in the primary dentition is usually managed by extraction because complications of reduction and fixation may result in problems with development of permanent teeth.

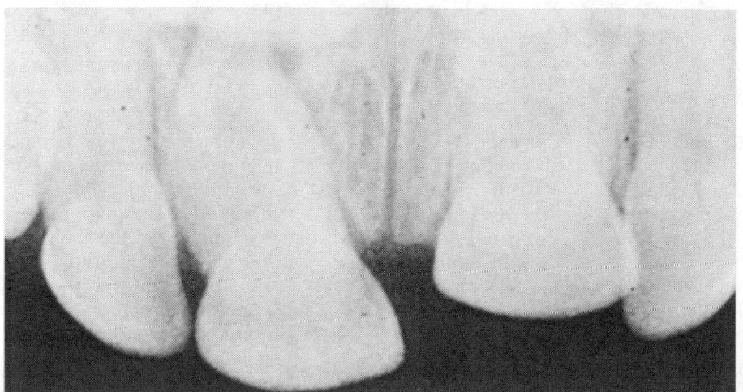

Figure 314–3 Occlusal radiograph documents intrusion of "missing tooth" presented in Figure 314-2.

Avulsion. If avulsed permanent teeth are replanted within 20 min after injury, good success may be achieved; if the delay exceeds 2 hr, however, failure (root resorption, ankylosis) is frequent. The likelihood that normal reattachment will follow replantation of the tooth is related to the viability of the periodontal ligament. Parents confronted with this emergency situation can be instructed to:

1. *Find the tooth.*
2. *Rinse the tooth.* (Do *not* scrub the tooth. Do *not* touch the root. After plugging the sink drain, hold the tooth by the crown and rinse it under running tap water.)
3. *Insert the tooth into the socket.* (Gently place it back into its normal position. Do not be concerned if the tooth extrudes slightly. If the parent or child is too apprehensive for replantation of the tooth, the tooth should be placed in cow's milk. Milk transport medium maintains periodontal ligament viability.)
4. *Go directly to the dentist.* (In transit, the child should hold the tooth in place with a finger. The parent should buckle a seatbelt around the child and drive safely.)

After the tooth is replanted, it must be immobilized (acrylic splint) to facilitate reattachment; endodontic therapy is always required. The initial signs of complications associated with replantation may appear as early as 1 wk post-trauma or as late as several years later. Close dental follow-up is indicated for at least 1 yr.

PREVENTION

To minimize the likelihood of dental injuries:

1. Every child or adolescent who engages in contact sports should wear a mouth guard, which may be constructed by a dentist or purchased at any athletic goods store.
2. Helmets with face guards should be worn by children or adolescents with neuromuscular problems or seizure disorders to protect the head and face during falls.
3. All children or adolescents with protruding incisors should be evaluated by a pediatric dentist or orthodontist.

ADDITIONAL CONSIDERATIONS. Children with dental trauma may also have sustained head and possibly neck trauma; neurologic assessment is warranted. Tetanus prophylaxis should be considered with any injury that disrupts the integrity of the tissues lining the oral cavity. The possibility of child abuse should always be considered.

CHAPTER 315
Common Lesions of the Oral Soft Tissues

OROPHARYNGEAL CANDIDIASIS (Chapter 230.1). Oropharyngeal infection with Candida albicans (thrush, moniliasis) is common in neonates because of contact with the organism in the birth canal. Transmission within the newborn nursery may reach epidemic proportions unless appropriate precautions are instituted. The lesions of oropharyngeal candidiasis (OPC) appear as white plaques covering all or part of the oropharyngeal mucosa. These plaques are removable from the underlying corium, which is characteristically inflamed with pin-point hemorrhages. Discomfort associated with this infection may occasionally interfere with feeding. The diagnosis is confirmed by direct microscopic examination on KOH smears and culture of scrapings from lesions. OPC is usually self-limited in the healthy newborn infant, but treatment with nystatin (1,000,000 units four times a day, applied directly to the lesions) will hasten recovery and reduce the risk of spreading to other infants. Persistent infections should be treated with fluconazole therapy.

Oropharyngeal candidiasis is also a major problem during myelosuppressive therapy. Systemic candidiasis (SC), a major cause of morbidity and mortality during myelosuppressive therapy, develops almost exclusively in patients who have had prior oropharyngeal, esophageal, or intestinal candidiasis. This observation implies that prevention of OPC should reduce the incidence of SC. The use of a multi-agent regimen for OPC prophylaxis in children receiving bone marrow transplants may be effective in preventing OPC, SC, or candidal esophagitis. The multi-agent regimen consists of debriding all mucous membrane surfaces within the oropharyngeal cavity with 0.2% chlorhexidine solution or the use of fluconazole at the beginning of myelosuppressive therapy, or both.

Chronic OPC occurs in children who have certain endocrinopathies and a specific candida immunodeficiency syndrome (associated with cutaneous and nail involvement), the acquired immunodeficiency syndrome (AIDS), or nutritional deficiencies or those who receive broad-spectrum antibiotic therapy that alters the oral flora. In these situations, successful treatment also depends on correction of the underlying problem.

APHTHOUS ULCERS. The aphthous ulcer (Canker sore) is a distinct oral lesion, prone to recurrence (see Chapter 670). The differential diagnosis is noted in Table 315–1.

BOHN NODULES. Bohn nodules are small developmental anomalies located along the buccal and lingual aspects of the mandibular and maxillary ridges and in the hard palate of the neonate. These lesions arise from remnants of mucous gland tissue. Treatment is not necessary, as the nodules disappear within a few weeks.

DENTAL LAMINA CYSTS. Dental lamina cysts are small cystic lesions located along the crest of the mandibular and maxillary ridges of the neonate. These lesions arise from epithelial remnants of the dental lamina. Treatment is not necessary; they will disappear within a few weeks.

MUCOCELE. The mucocele usually appears as a raised bluish vesicle several millimeters in diameter. It occurs most commonly in the lower lip and rarely in the upper lip, palate, buccal mucosa, tongue, or floor of the mouth. It may persist for weeks or months prior to rupture, in which case it usually recurs. This lesion is caused by traumatic laceration of a minor salivary gland duct that permits accumulation of mucus in the soft tissues and subsequent proliferation of granulation tissue to sequester the mucus. Recurrences following surgical excision are largely the result of removing the mucocele without extirpating the minor salivary gland that produced the extravasated mucus.

FORDYCE GRANULES. Almost 80% of adults have multiple, yellow-white granules in clusters or plaque-like areas on the oral mucosa, most commonly on the buccal mucosa or lips. They are aberrant sebaceous glands. The glands are present at birth, but they may hypertrophy and first appear as discrete yellowish papules during the preadolescent period in approximately 50% of children. No treatment is necessary.

CHEILITIS. Dryness of the lips, followed by scaling and cracking and accompanied by a characteristic burning sensation, is common in children. It is usually caused by sensitivity to contact substances (from toys and foods) plus photosensitivity to the sun's rays. It is aggravated by the alternation of wetting with the tongue and drying by the wind, especially in cold weather. Cheilitis often occurs in association with fever. Frequent application of a petroleum jelly facilitates healing and is also preventative.

BLACK HAIRY TONGUE. Black hairy tongue (lingua nigra) is characterized by an elongation of the filiform papillae into hairlike projections. It is generally concentrated in a triangular area in front of the V-shaped line of circumvallate papillae and is associated with accumulation of debris in that region. The patch may vary from brown to black. The condition is usually chronic but will disappear with regular cleansing of the dorsal tongue (see Chapter 670). Hairy tongue may also occur during prolonged antibiotic therapy, especially with oral troches. In addition, oral medications that contain bismuth may produce this benign condition.

GEOGRAPHIC TONGUE. Geographic tongue (migratory glossitis) is a benign and asymptomatic lesion and is characterized by one or more smooth, bright-red patches, often showing a yellow, gray, or white membranous margin on the dorsum of an otherwise normally roughened tongue (see Chapter 670).

FISSURED TONGUE. The fissured tongue (scrotal tongue) is a malformation manifested clinically by numerous small furrows or grooves on the dorsal surface (see Chapter 670).

TABLE 315–1 Differential Diagnosis of Oral Ulceration

Condition	Comment
Common	
Aphthous (canker sore)	Painful
Traumatic	Accidents, chronic cheek biter
Hand, foot, mouth disease	Painful, lesions on tongue, anterior oral cavity, hands and feet
Herpangina	Painful, lesions confined to soft palate and oropharynx
Chemical burns	Alkali, acid, aspirin; painful
Uncommon	
Neutrophil defects	Agranulocytosis, leukemia, cyclic neutropenia; painful
Systemic lupus erythematosus	Recurrent, may be painless
Behçet's syndrome	Resembles aphthous lesions; associated with genital ulcers, uveitis, etc.
Necrotizing ulcerative gingivostomatitis	Vincent stomatitis; painful
Syphilis	Chancre or gumma; painless
Oral Crohn disease	Aphthous-like; painful
Histoplasmosis	Lingual

CHAPTER 316
Diseases of the Salivary Glands and Jaws

With the exception of mumps (Chapter 242), disease of the salivary glands is rare in children. Bilateral enlargement of the submaxillary glands may occur in AIDS, cystic fibrosis, malnutrition, and, transiently, during acute asthmatic attacks. Chronic vomiting may be accompanied by enlargement of the parotid glands. Benign salivary gland hypertrophy has been associated with endocrinopathies: thyroid disease, diabetes, and disorders of the pituitary-adrenal axis.

RECURRENT PAROTITIS. Recurrent idiopathic swelling of the parotid gland may occur in otherwise healthy children. The swelling is usually unilateral, but both glands may be involved simultaneously or alternately; children may have up to 10 or more recurrences. There is little pain; the swelling is limited to the gland and usually lasts 2–3 wk. The incidence appears to be higher in the spring.

[SUP]PURATIVE PAROTITIS. This is usually due to *Staphylococcus [au]reus* and may be primary or a complication of parotitis from another cause. It is usually unilateral and may be accompanied by fever. The gland becomes swollen, tender, and painful. Suppurative parotitis responds to appropriate antibacterial therapy based on culture obtained from the Stensen duct or by surgical drainage, which is infrequently required.

RANULA. Ranula is a cyst associated with a major salivary gland in the sublingual area. A ranula is a large, soft, mucus-containing swelling in the floor of the mouth. It occurs at any age, including infancy. The cyst should be excised, and the severed duct should be exteriorized.

CONGENTIAL LIP PITS. Lip pits are due to fistulous tracts that lead to imbedded mucous glands in the lower lip. They leak saliva, especially with salivary stimulation. Lip pits may be isolated anomalies, or they may be found in patients with cleft lip or palate. Treatment is by surgical excision of the glandular tissue.

XEROSTOMIA. Xerostomia (or dry mouth) may be associated with fever, dehydration, anticholinergic drugs, chronic graft-versus-host disease, Mikulicz disease (leukemia infiltrates), Sjögren's syndrome, or tumoricidal doses of radiation when the salivary glands are within the field. Long-term xerostomia is a high risk factor for dental caries.

SALIVARY GLAND TUMORS. See Chapter 511.1.

CAFFEY DISEASE (Infantile Cortical Hyperostosis). See Chapter 703.

OSTEOMYELITIS (Chapter 178). In the newborn infant, facial osteomyelitis may occur in the area of the premaxillary suture, but during childhood, the mandible is the more common location. The infection is marked by swelling and redness of the oral mucosa or skin and is associated with pain, fever, and lymphadenopathy. Drainage should be established and the exudate cultured so that an appropriate antibiotic may be administered. Large sequestra may require surgical removal.

RETICULOENDOTHELIOSIS (HistiocytosisX) (Chapter 515). Oral lesions may occur in any of the syndromes and may be an early manifestation. Lesions of the jaw may produce pain, swelling, loosening of teeth, and fetid breath. Healing is often delayed after dental extraction.

NEOPLASMS

Benign Tumors. Ossifying fibroma is the most common benign tumor of the jaw. Growth is rapid before puberty, after which it may slow or cease. The lesion is painless, with a unilateral soft tissue swelling being the first sign. Most patients do not require treatment, but if the lesion is extensive, curettage or further surgical correction may be required.

Cysts of the Jaw. These cysts occur with multiple basal cell nevoid syndrome (see Chapter 657).

Malignant Tumors. The malignant primary tumors of the jaws in children include Burkitt lymphoma, osteogenic sarcoma, lymphosarcoma, ameloblastoma, and, more rarely, fibrosarcoma.

CHAPTER 317
Diagnostic Radiology in Dental Assessment

The *panoramic radiograph* provides a single tomographic image of the upper and lower jaw, including all the teeth and supporting structures. The x-ray tube rotates about the patient's head with reciprocal movement of the film or image receptor during the exposure. The panoramic image shows the mandibular bodies, rami and condyles, the maxillary sinuses, and the majority of the facial buttresses. Such images are used to show abnormalities of tooth number, development and eruption pattern, cystic and neoplastic lesions, extensive bone infections, and fractures (Fig. 317–1).

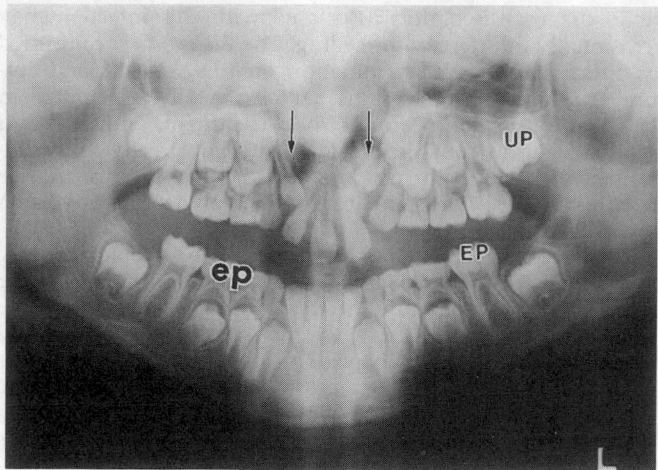

Figure 317–1 A panoramic radiograph of an 8-yr-old patient with a cleft palate showing abnormal numbers and position of teeth in the area of the cleft *(arrows)*. Also shown are erupted primary teeth (ep), erupted permanent teeth (EP), and unerupted permanent teeth (UP).

Cephalometric radiographs are posteroanterior and lateral skull films that are taken using a head positioner (cephalostat) and employ techniques that clearly demonstrate the facial skeleton and soft facial tissues. Similar protocols for positioning children are used throughout the world. From these images, cranial and facial points and planes can be determined and compared to standards derived from thousands of images. A child's facial growth can be assessed serially, because cephalometric radiographs may be taken sequentially. Relationships among the maxilla, mandible, cranial base, and facial skeleton can be determined in a quantitative manner. Additionally, the alignment of the teeth and the relation of the teeth to the supporting bone can be serially measured.

Intraoral dental radiographs are highly detailed, direct exposure films that demonstrate sections of the child's teeth and supporting bone structures. The film or image receptor is placed lingual to the teeth, and the x-ray beam is directed through the teeth and supporting structures. The resulting images are used to detect dental caries, loss of alveolar bone (periodontal disease), abscesses at the roots of the teeth, and trauma to the teeth and alveolar bone and to demonstrate the developmental status and any disorder of the developing permanent teeth within the bone.

Andreasen JO, Andreasen FM: Essentials of Traumatic Injuries to the Teeth. Copenhagen, Munksgaard, 1990.
Berkowitz RJ, Strandjord S, Jones P, et al: Stomatologic complications of bone marrow transplantation in a pediatric population. Pediatr Dent 9:105, 1987.
Committee on Research, Science, and Therapy of the American Academy of Periodontology: Periodontal diseases of children and adolescents. J Periodontol 67:57, 1996.
Dajani AS, Taubert KA, Wilson W, et al: Prevention of bacterial endocarditis. JAMA 277:1794, 1997.
Flaitz CM: Oral pathologic conditions and soft tissue anomalies. *In:* Pinkham JR (ed): Pediatric Dentistry: Infancy Through Adolescence, 2nd ed. Philadelphia, WB Saunders, 1994, p 29.
Greene JC, Louie R, Wycoff SJ: Preventive dentistry. I: Dental caries. JAMA 262:3459, 1989.
Greene JC, Louie R, Wycoff SJ: Preventive dentistry. II: Periodontal diseases, malocclusion, trauma and oral cancer. JAMA 263:421, 1990.
Johnsen D, Nowjack-Raymer R: Baby bottle tooth decay: Issues, assessment, and an opportunity for the nutritionist: J Am Diet Assoc 89:1112, 1989.
Johnsen DC, Tinanoff N: Dental care for the preschool child. Dent Clin North Am, 1995.
Josell SD, Abrams RG: Pediatric oral health. Pediatr Clin North Am 38:1049, 1991.
Kalsbeek H, Verrips GH: Consumption of sweet snacks and caries experience of primary school children. Caries Res 28:447, 1994.
Milerad J, Larson O, Hagberg C, et al: Associated malformations in infants

with cleft lip and palate: A prospective, population-based study. Pediatrics 100:180, 1997.
Nakata M: Genetics in oral-facial growth and disease. Int Dent J 45:227, 1995.
Nelson LP, Shusterman S: Emergency management of oral trauma in children. Curr Opin Pediatr 9:242, 1997.
Serwint JR, Mungo R, Negrete VF, et al: Child-rearing practices and nursing caries. Pediatrics 92:233, 1993.
Tinanoff N: Dental caries: Etiology, pathogenesis, clinical manifestations, and management. *In:* Wei SHY (ed): Pediatric Dentistry: Total Patient Care. Philadelphia, Lea & Febiger, 1988, p 9.

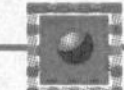

SECTION 3

The Esophagus

John J. Herbst

CHAPTER 318

Development and Function of the Esophagus

The esophagus develops as a pair of folds in the cranial part of the primitive foregut that descends, while a single caudal fold ascends to separate the trachea and esophagus. This is followed by lengthening of the trachea and esophagus. The function of the esophagus is to transport fluids and solids to the stomach and to prevent their regurgitation.

Swallowing has been observed in utero at 20 wk of gestation, and sucking and swallowing seem to be coordinated by 33–34 wk. A full-term newborn infant has short bursts of sucking followed by swallowing. Within a few days (or weeks if premature), an infant is able to swallow and breathe in a coordinated, rhythmic manner during prolonged bursts of sucking.

Swallowing is divided into 3 phases; only the first is under voluntary control. In the first (oral phase), swallowing is initiated by a sudden elevation of the tongue that propels the bolus of food or fluid into the pharynx. In the second phase, superior and anterior displacement of the larynx and positioning of the epiglottis over the trachea protect the laryngeal airway, while the nasopharynx is occluded by the soft palate and uvula. Pharyngeal constrictor muscles help propel food toward the esophagus. In the third phase, the superior esophageal sphincter relaxes and primary peristaltic waves propel food into the stomach. Secondary waves are usually initiated by local distention and serve to empty the esophagus of residual food or gastric contents. Both of these waves empty the esophagus by propulsive efforts. Tertiary waves are nonpropulsive; they are abnormal if present in large numbers and can be associated with chest pains. The lower esophageal sphincter (LES) is a specialized segment of circular musculature in the distal 1–3 cm of the esophagus, where the intraluminal pressure is normally higher than that in the more proximal esophagus or in the stomach. The sphincter prevents gastroesophageal reflux but relaxes during deglutition to allow food to enter the stomach.

The *common clinical manifestations* of esophageal disease are coughing or choking with swallowing, regurgitation or vomiting, dysphagia, complete inability to swallow, pain on swallowing (odynophagia), and hematemesis. Each can be attributed to one or more defects in the complex coordination of the swallowing sequence.

Diagnostic evaluations include conventional barium swallow roentgenographic studies, which may demonstrate masses impinging on the lumen or gastroesophageal reflux. A videoesophagram (oropharyngeal motility study) can evaluate the dynamics of swallowing and reveal abnormalities that are transient. Esophageal manometry permits quantitative measurements of pressures along the esophagus. The pressure in the LES is often decreased in patients with reflux, especially if esophagitis is present. In contrast, pressures are elevated, with poor relaxation, in achalasia (Fig. 318–1). Radionuclide scans evaluate the efficiency of peristalsis in clearing a liquid or solid bolus from the esophagus and test for reflux and aspiration. Prolonged monitoring of distal esophageal pH is a sensitive test for gastric acid reflux. Flexible fiberoptic endoscopy permits biopsy and visualization of the esophagus without general anesthesia; it allows detection and removal of foreign bodies.

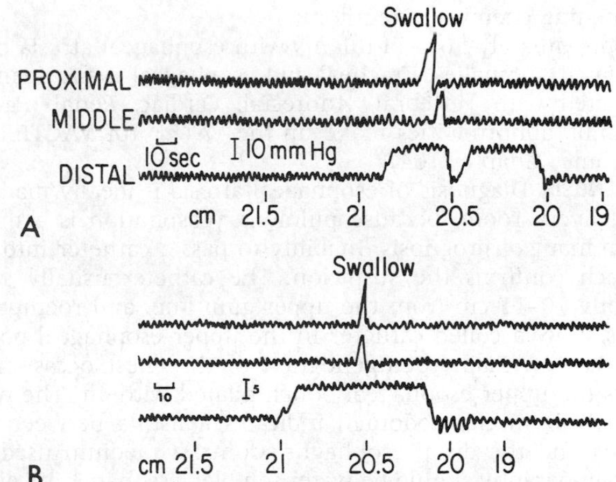

Figure 318–1 *A*, Pressures in the esophagus of a normal infant as recorded with a triple lumen catheter with recording tips 2.5 cm apart. When the distal recording tip was 21.5 cm from the gum line, it was within the lower esophageal sphincter. A swallow initiates a primary peristaltic wave. The pressure wave is detected first in the more proximal catheter and then in the more distal one. A relaxation in the lower esophageal sphincter allows the food to enter the stomach. *B*, Abnormal manometric pattern in a patient demonstrating simultaneous pressure in the two proximal recording tips, characteristic of a tertiary esophageal wave. There is no relaxation of the lower esophageal sphincter. Such a pattern is seen in patients with achalasia.

CHAPTER 319
Atresia and Tracheoesophageal Fistula

Esophageal atresia occurs in 1/3,000–4,500 live births; 30% of affected infants are born prematurely. In more than 85% of cases, a fistula between the trachea and distal esophagus accompanies the atresia (Fig. 319–1*A*). Less commonly, esophageal atresia or tracheoesophageal fistula may occur alone (Fig. 319–1*B, C,*) or in unusual combinations (Fig. 319–1*D,E*). Disorders in the formation and movement of the paired cranial and single caudal folds in the primitive foregut explain the variations in atresia and fistula formation.

CLINICAL MANIFESTATIONS. Atresia of the esophagus should be suspected (1) in cases of maternal polyhydramnios; (2) if a catheter used at birth for resuscitation cannot be inserted into the stomach; (3) if a newborn infant has excessive oral secretions; or (4) if choking, cyanosis, or coughing occurs with an attempt at feeding. Suctioning of excess secretions from the mouth and pharynx frequently results in improvement, but symptoms quickly recur. The diagnosis may not be made until after an infant has aspirated feedings. When a fistula connects the trachea and distal esophagus, air enters the abdomen, which becomes tympanitic; the distention may interfere with breathing. If a fistula connects the proximal esophagus to the trachea, the first attempt at feeding may lead to aspiration. Infants who have atresia but no fistula have scaphoid, airless abdomens. In the rare situation of fistula without atresia (H type) (Fig. 319–1*C*), the usual sign is recurrent coughing with aspiration pneumonia; the diagnosis may be delayed for days or even months. Aspiration of pharyngeal secretions is common among patients with esophageal atresia, but aspiration of gastric contents via a distal fistula causes a more severe, life-threatening chemical pneumonitis.

Approximately 50% of infants with esophageal atresia have associated anomalies. Tracheal and esophageal malformations associated with *V*ertebral, *A*norectal, *C*ardiac, *R*enal, *R*adial, and *L*imb abnormalities make up the VATER (or VACTERAL) syndrome (Chapter 104).

DIAGNOSIS. Diagnosis of esophageal atresia is ideally made in the delivery room, because pulmonary aspiration is a major determinant of prognosis. Inability to pass a catheter into the stomach confirms the suspicion. The catheter usually stops abruptly 10–11 cm from the upper gum line, and roentgenograms show a coiled catheter in the upper esophageal pouch (Fig. 319–2). Plain roentgenogram of the chest occasionally shows the upper esophageal pouch dilated with air. The presence of air in the abdomen indicates a fistula between the trachea and the distal esophagus. Contrast medium used for roentgenography should be water soluble; less than 1 mL given under fluoroscopic control is sufficient to outline the blind upper pouch. The contrast medium should then be withdrawn to prevent overflow into the lungs and development of chemical pneumonitis. A traumatic postintubation pharyngeal pseudodiverticulum may present with drooling and airway obstruction and is identified with contrast radiology. H-type fistulas (Fig. 319–1*C*) may be difficult to demonstrate. A videoesophagram, while filling the esophagus with water-soluble contrast medium, is usually effective. The tracheal orifice of the fistula may be detectable at bronchoscopy. A careful search should be made for associated malformations. Preopera-

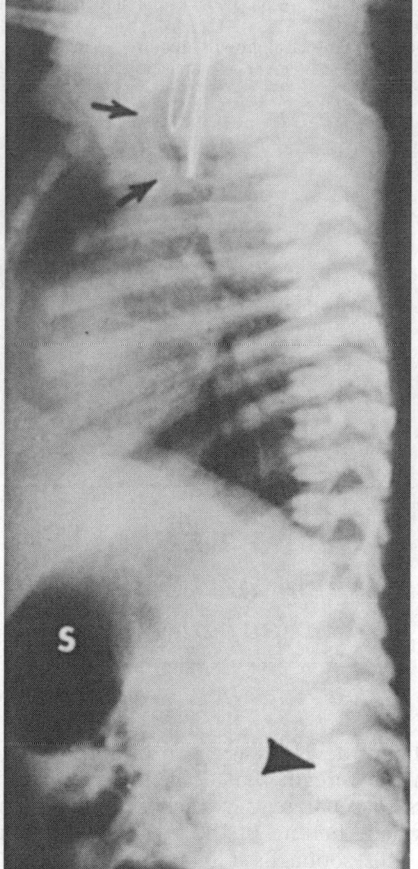

Figure 319–2 Tracheoesophageal fistula. Lateral roentgenogram demonstrating a nasogastric tube coiled *(arrows)* in the proximal segment of an atretic esophagus. The distal fistula is suggested by gaseous dilatation of the stomach (S) and small intestine. The *arrowhead* depicts vertebral fusion, whereas a heart murmur and cardiomegaly suggest the presence of a ventricular septal defect. This patient demonstrated elements of the VATER anomalad. (From Balfe D, Ling D, Siegel M: The esophagus. *In:* Putman CE, Ravin CE (eds): Textbook of Diagnostic Imaging. Philadelphia, WB Saunders, 1988.)

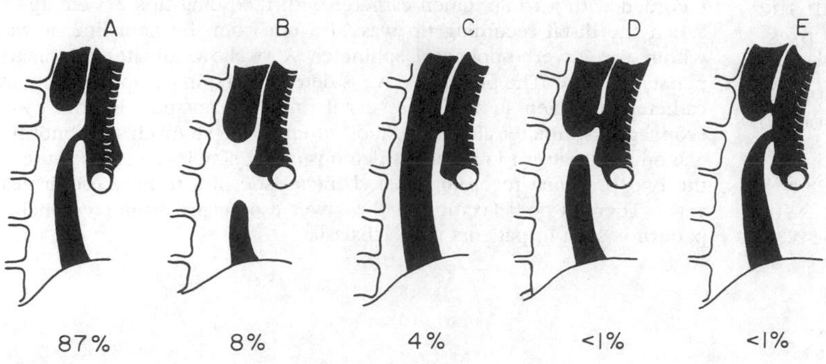

Figure 319–1 Diagrams of the five most commonly encountered forms of esophageal atresia and tracheoesophageal fistula, shown in order of frequency.

tive cardiac ultrasography detects cardiac malformations, which are a significant cause of morbidity.

TREATMENT. Esophageal atresia is a surgical emergency. Preoperatively, patients should be kept prone to decrease any tendency of gastric contents to reach the lungs. The esophageal pouch should be kept empty by constant suction to prevent aspiration of secretions. Careful attention must be given to temperature control, respiratory function, and management of associated anomalies. Occasionally, a patient's condition requires that surgery be performed in stages, the first step usually being ligation of the fistula and insertion of a gastrostomy tube for feeding and the second being anastomosis of the two ends of the esophagus. Eight to 10 days after a primary anastomosis, oral feedings are usually tolerated. Esophagography before feeding determines the status of the anastomosis.

Structural malformations of the trachea are common in patients with esophageal atresia and fistula. Tracheomalacia, recurrent aspiration pneumonia, and reactive airway disease are frequently encountered. Tracheal development is normal if there is no fistula; esophageal stenosis and severe gastroesophageal reflux are more common in these patients. Failure to thrive, slow feeding, coughing, and choking are common sequelae, especially if primary anastomosis cannot be performed in the immediate neonatal period. Stenosis at the anastomotic site is common and may require dilatations.

CHAPTER 320
Other Disorders of the Esophagus

LARYNGOTRACHEOESOPHAGEAL CLEFT. Rarely, the larynx and upper trachea may fail to separate completely from the esophagus for a variable distance. Symptoms of the resultant laryngotracheoesophageal cleft are similar to those of tracheoesophageal fistula; aphonia should suggest the former. Roentgenographic diagnosis using contrast material is difficult; endoscopy is usually required.

EXTERNAL COMPRESSION. The most common masses impinging on the esophagus are enlarged lymph nodes in the subcarinal area, which may be due to tuberculosis, histoplasmosis, other forms of pulmonary suppuration, or lymphoma. Extrinsic pressure may also be caused by vascular anomalies in the mediastinum (Chapter 439.1).

ESOPHAGEAL DUPLICATION CYSTS. These cysts may cause esophageal compression. Their epithelium may be derived from any portion of the intestine, and they do not communicate with the esophagus unless there is ulceration from gastric mucosa in the cyst. Two thirds are on the right side of the esophagus. Rarely, duplication cysts may extend through the diaphragm and communicate with the intestine. Diagnosis is usually made by barium esophagography. Neurenteric cysts are esophageal duplication cysts that contain glial elements; vertebral anomalies usually accompany these cysts.

CONGENITAL STENOSIS AND WEBS. The embryologic development of these rare lesions is probably similar to atresia. Dysphagia is sometimes delayed until solid foods are offered. Fibromuscular stenosis and filamentous webs respond to dilatation but must be distinguished from strictures caused by peptic esophagitis (Chapter 324). If tracheobronchial remnants are found in the stenotic area, resection is indicated.

DYSPHAGIA DUE TO NEUROMUSCULAR DISEASE. Many systemic, neurologic, and muscular disorders may interfere with esophageal motility and give rise to esophageal symptoms. Congenital paralysis of the muscles of deglutition and swallowing as a primary problem or associated with the Möbius syndrome must be considered if no obvious anatomic anomaly is noted. These disorders are listed in Table 320–1 and are discussed elsewhere.

TABLE 320–1 Neuromuscular Disorders That May Cause Dysphagia

Cerebral palsy (more common)
Dermatomyositis
Infections—diphtheria, poliomyelitis, tetanus, botulism
Muscular dystrophy (more common)
Myasthenia gravis
Polyneuritis
Familial dysautonomia (Riley-Day) syndrome
Scleroderma
Specific cranial nerve defects (e.g., Möbius syndrome)
Werdnig-Hoffmann disease

CRICOPHARYNGEAL DYSFUNCTION. Spasm of the cricopharyngeal muscle or achalasia of the superior esophageal sphincter may cause intermittent dysphagia; the increased pressure in the pharynx and upper esophagus may lead to development of a posterior pharyngeal diverticulum. Diagnosis of this idiopathic disorder is made with a videoesophagram or manometric demonstration of failure of the superior esophageal sphincter to relax during deglutition. Symptoms are relieved by myotomy of the cricopharyngeal muscle, analogous to the procedure used in hypertrophic pyloric stenosis (Chapter 329.1).

CRICOPHARYNGEAL INCOORDINATION OF INFANCY. This incoordination is usually evident soon after birth. Sucking is normal, but affected infants tend to choke and aspirate with deglutition; they generally have small jaws that open poorly. Videoradiography shows repetitive to-and-fro movement of the contrast medium in the posterior pharynx. Careful feedings by spoon, gavage, on gastrostomy tube are required until a patient is about 6 mo of age, when symptoms abate. The cause of this disorder is unknown.

BULBAR PALSY (SUPRANUCLEAR OR LOWER MOTOR NEURON). This type of palsy may cause dysphagia. The child sucks liquids poorly and chews and swallows solid food with difficulty. With supranuclear bulbar palsy, the jaw jerk is exaggerated and signs of generalized spastic cerebral palsy usually develop. Lower motor neuron disease with flaccid bulbar palsy and facial diplegia constitutes the Möbius syndrome.

PARALYSIS OF THE SUPERIOR LARYNGEAL NERVE. Paralysis has been reported in ill neonates with dysphagia, diminished esophageal motility, a preference for lying with the head turned to one side, and, in some cases, unilateral facial weakness. The syndrome is thought to be caused when an unusual intrauterine position compresses the nerve between the thyroid cartilage and the hyoid bone. Spontaneous recovery occurs during the 1st yr.

TRANSIENT PHARYNGEAL MUSCLE DYSFUNCTION. This is often associated with palatal dysfunction and may be due to delayed normal development or may be associated with cerebral palsy. Choking during feeding and dribbling of formula are the main symptoms. Paralysis of pharyngeal constrictors and a flaccid soft palate are noted in videoradiographic studies. Gavage on gastrostomy tube feeding can prevent aspiration (the main complication) and may be required for only a few days or for many weeks. Affected infants often have generalized hypotonia; other nervous system dysfunction, especially developmental delays, become evident later.

DIFFUSE ESOPHAGEAL SPASM. This spasm may be a cause of chest pain and dysphagia in adolescents. This primary motility disorder has characteristic esophageal contractions noted on manometry simultaneously with midchest, retrosternal pain after swallowing liquids. Edrophonium (Tensilon) (a cholinergic drug) administration may provoke pain. Treatment is usually not needed, except in severe cases, in which nitrates or calcium channel blocking agents have been successful.

CHAPTER 321
Achalasia

Achalasia is an uncommon motility disorder in which a relative obstruction at the gastroesophageal junction is made worse by a lack of peristaltic waves in the esophagus (see Fig. 318–1*B*). The condition affects primarily adolescents and adults; children younger than 4 yr constitute fewer than 5% of patients. Ganglion cells are frequently decreased in number and are surrounded by inflammatory cells; a heightened response of the esophageal muscles to methacholine has been interpreted as evidence of degeneration hypersensitivity. Only in Chagas disease has the cause been well established.

CLINICAL MANIFESTATIONS AND DIAGNOSIS. Symptoms include difficulty in swallowing, regurgitation of food, cough due to overflow of fluids into the trachea, and failure to gain weight. Pulmonary infections, including bronchiectasis, result from persistent aspiration of esophageal contents. Retention of food in the esophagus may cause esophagitis. Achalasia has been reported in siblings and in association with adrenal insufficiency and alacrima. Air-fluid levels in a dilated esophagus on an upright chest film suggest the diagnosis. Barium swallow reveals abnormal motility with variable but often massive dilatation of the esophagus with tapering (beaking) at the gastric junction. Frequently, there is no air in the stomach (Fig. 321–1). The diagnosis may be confirmed with esophageal manometry, in which the major findings are incomplete or absent relaxation of the lower esophageal sphincter with swallowing, a lack of primary or secondary esophageal propulsive peristaltic waves, and an increased lower esophageal sphincter pressure.

TREATMENT. Nifedipine, a calcium channel blocker, improves esophageal emptying but is recommended only when a brief delay in definitive therapy is indicated. Intrasphincteric injection of botulism toxin also may provide symptomatic relief for as long as 6 mo. Permanent relief of symptoms usually follows surgical division of muscle fibers at the gastroesophageal junction (Heller myotomy). Alternatively, the sphincter may be forcefully dilated with a balloon catheter under fluoroscopic control. Simple bougienage gives only temporary relief and is not recommended. Although surgical or balloon distention of the lower esophageal sphincter permits esophageal emptying, the resulting sphincteric incompetence and the persistence of abnormal esophageal motility may result in esophagitis.

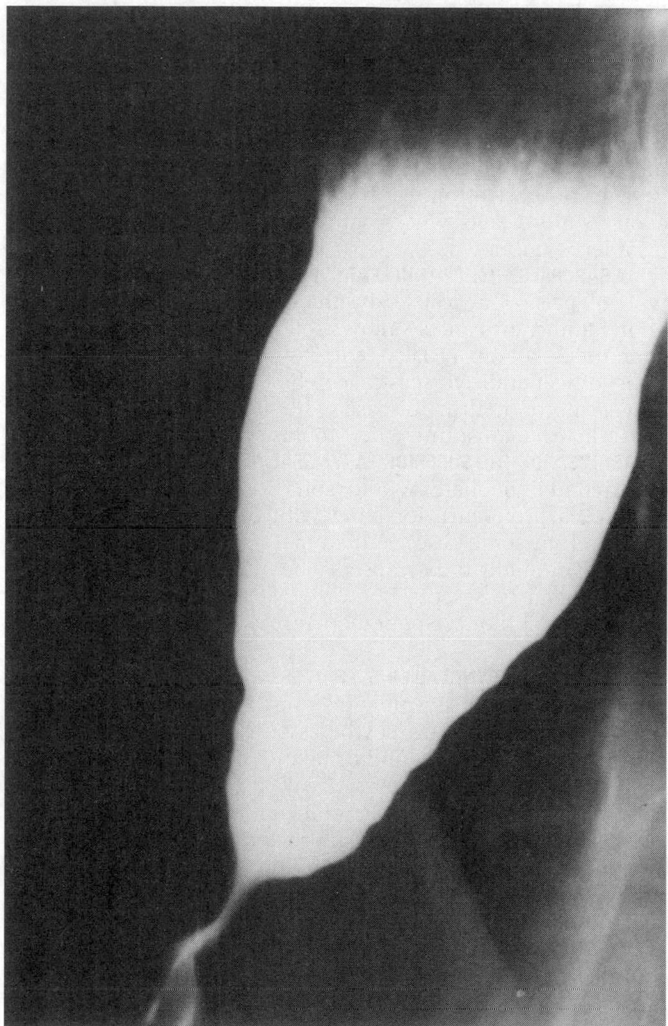

Figure 321–1 Barium esophagogram of a patient with achalasia demonstrating dilated esophagus and narrowing at the lower esophageal sphincter. Note retained secretions layered on top of barium in the esophagus.

CHAPTER 322
Hiatal Hernia

Herniation of the stomach through the esophageal hiatus may occur as a common sliding hernia, in which the gastroesophageal junction slides into the thorax, or it may be paraesophageal, in which a portion of the stomach (usually the fundus) is insinuated inside the gastroesophageal junction in the hiatus (Fig. 322–1). Sliding hernias are frequently associated with gastroesophageal reflux, especially in retarded children. The relationship to hiatal hernias in adults is unclear. Treatment is not directed at the hernia but at the gastroesophageal reflux.

Paraesophageal hernias may be encountered after fundoplication for gastroesophageal reflux, especially if the edges of a dilated esophageal hiatus have not been approximated. Fullness after eating and upper abdominal pain are the usual symptoms. Infarction of the herniated stomach is rare.

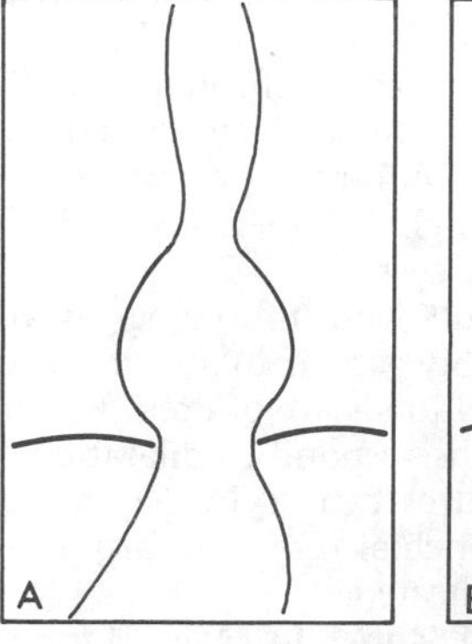

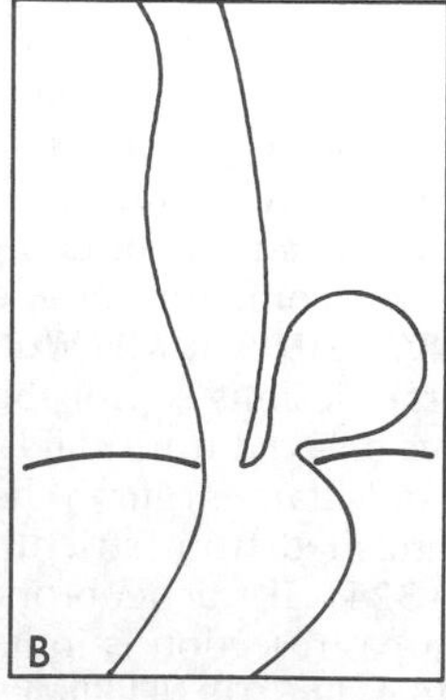

Figure 322–1 Types of esophageal hiatal hernia. *A*, Sliding hiatal hernia, the most common type; *B*, paraesophageal hiatal hernia.

CHAPTER 323
Gastroesophageal Reflux (Chalasia)

When the lower esophageal sphincter (LES) is not competent, passive reflux of gastric contents may cause symptoms. The term *chalasia* describes free reflux across a dilated sphincter. Although many infants have minor degrees of reflux, about 1/300 has significant reflux and associated complications.

ETIOLOGY. Factors contributing to the competence of the LES include abdominal position of the sphincter, angle of insertion of esophagus into the stomach, and sphincter pressure. Frequent spontaneous reductions in sphincter pressure are a major mechanism of reflux, but reflux across a chronically lax sphincter is frequent with esophagitis, whereas reflux with normal pressure may occur with increased abdominal pressure (coughing, crying, defecating). Reflux is common in normal persons after meals. The small reservoir capacity of an infant's esophagus predisposes to vomiting; this is a less common problem in adolescents and adults. Placement of a gastrostomy tube encourages reflux, probably by altering the angle at which the esophagus enters the stomach. Refluxed material is returned to the stomach by secondary peristaltic waves in the esophagus; swallowed saliva neutralizes and washes away the last traces of acid with a primary peristaltic wave.

CLINICAL MANIFESTATIONS. The signs and symptoms relate directly to the exposure of the esophageal epithelium to refluxed gastric contents. In 85% of affected infants, excessive vomiting occurs during the 1st wk of life; an additional 10% have symptoms by 6 wk. Symptoms abate without treatment in 60% by the age of 2 yr as the child assumes a more upright posture and eats solid foods; the remainder continue to have symptoms until at least 4 yr of age. Patients with cerebral palsy, Down syndrome, and other causes of developmental delay have an increased incidence of reflux.

Delayed gastric emptying and occasionally forceful vomiting may occur with pylorospasm. The latter is not typical in most cases of reflux. Aspiration pneumonia occurs in about 30% of patients in infancy; in those in whom symptoms persist until later childhood, chronic cough, wheezing, and recurrent pneumonia are common. There may be rumination (see later). Growth and weight gain are adversely affected in about 60% of patients.

The major manifestation of esophagitis is hemorrhage; the presence of occult blood in the stool is common, hematemesis occurs in some children, but melena is rare. Iron-deficiency anemia is common in patients with severe esophagitis (Chapter 324). Substernal pain is less common, but dysphagia may cause irritability and anorexia in advanced cases. In untreated patients, esophagitis leads to stricture formation in 5% of cases and inanition and pneumonia in another 5%.

Sandifer syndrome, opisthotonos, and other abnormal head posturing, are associated with reflux. The head positioning may be a mechanism to protect the airway or reduce acid-reflux–associated pain. Methylxanthines may exacerbate reflux by lowering sphincter tone.

Reflux may rarely cause laryngospasm, apnea, and bradycardia. The relationship between reflux and acute life-threatening events or sudden infant death syndrome (SIDS) remains controversial and may be coincidental (Chapter 714).

DIAGNOSIS. In mild cases, careful clinical assessment may be sufficient for diagnosis, which is confirmed by assessing the response to therapy. In severe cases, the diagnosis can be confirmed by esophageal pH probe studies and by barium fluoroscopic esophagography. The finding of gastric folds above the diaphragm suggests a hiatal hernia (Fig. 323–1); in children, these folds are detected more readily in a collapsed than in a full esophagus. Gastroesophageal reflux is an episodic event; in symptomatic patients, significant reflux may not be demonstrated initially by roentgenography. It is important to use enough barium to approximate the volume of a normal meal. Special maneuvering of the patient is not necessary. Normal children may have a small amount of reflux that is quickly cleared from the esophagus, but recurrent reflux is abnormal. Strictures are easily demonstrated with barium esophagography. Severe esophagitis may be suspected when a ragged mucosal outline is seen on a roentgenogram, but esophagoscopy with biopsy is a superior diagnostic technique for this disorder. Contrast studies also determine distal obstructive lesions associated with secondary reflux.

Gastric scintiscans may be used to demonstrate aspiration of gastric contents and can demonstrate reflux, but sensitivity for aspiration and specificity for reflux are low. Esophagoscopy evaluates severe reflux and strictures; biopsy is a sensitive test for evidence of reflux. Increased thickness of the germinative layer and increased length of dermal papillas are early changes, but intraepithelial neutrophils, eosinophils, ulcer formation, or presence of columnar epithelium (Barrett esophagitis) are seen with more severe disease. *Barrett esophagitis,* uncommon in children, represents a cellular metaplasia that in rare circum-

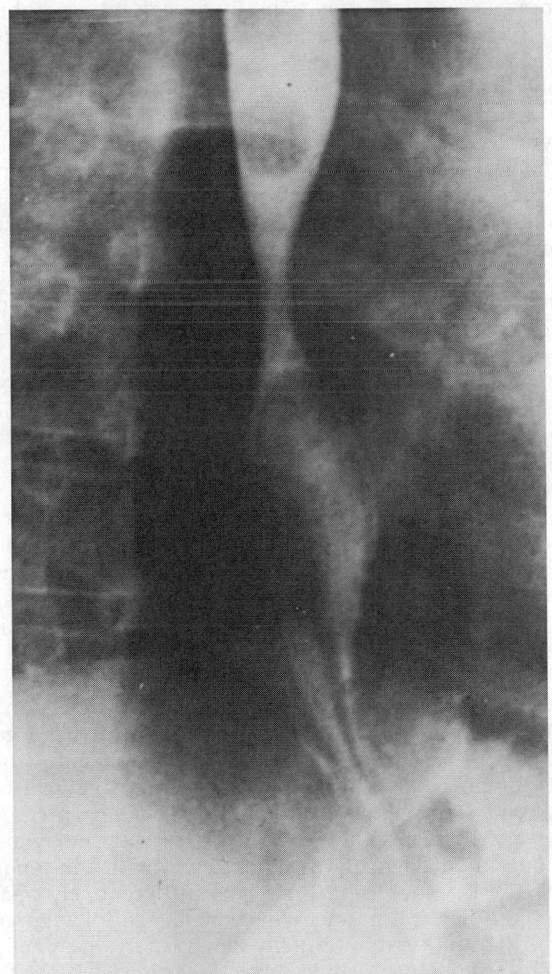

Figure 323–1 Barium esophagogram demonstrating free gastroesophageal reflux. A stricture due to peptic esophagitis is present. Longitudinal gastric folds above the diaphragm indicate the unusual presence of an associated hiatal hernia.

stances leads to adenocarcinoma in children. It is usually found in patients with severe co-morbid conditions including neurologic disease, respiratory conditions, and esophageal atresia. The frequency and duration of reflux can be documented by continuous monitoring of distal esophageal pH. Although a sensitive test, it is not needed for routine diagnosis, and the costs and complexity of obtaining and scoring the data suggest it is best used to investigate patients with atypical symptoms or to determine if unusual events (coughing, choking, stridor, apnea) are temporally related to reflux episodes.

TREATMENT. A long-term cure may be expected in infants. In older children, symptoms are likely to be chronic. Infants with significant symptoms should be kept prone; this exception to the usually recomended supine position is recognized in guidelines from the Academy of Pediatrics. In older infants and children, raising the head of the bed and keeping a child upright are indicated. Thickening an infant's formula with cereal decreases crying and the volume of vomitus. Cisapride (0.2 mg/kg qid) is quite useful and stimulates gastrointestinal motility and decreases mean duration of reflux. Cisapride is a proarrhytmic agent that prolongs the Qtc interval spontaneously or in the presence of drugs that prolong its serum half-life (ketoconazole, erythromycin, astemizole, terfenadine); electrocardiographic monitoring is indicated in at-risk patients. Metoclopramide (0.15 mg/kg qid) also reduces symptoms by stimulating gastric emptying and esophageal motility, but drowsiness, restlessness, and extrapyramidal reaction may occur. If esophagitis is present, antacids, H_2-receptor blockers, or in severe cases the hydrogen pump inhibitors omeprazole or lansoprazole are indicated. The hydrogen pump inhibitors most effectively suppress acid secretion and may be effective in relieving heartburn when H_2 receptors fail, but they are not available in liquid form. Medical therapy is effective in most neurologically normal children.

If symptoms do not improve with a prolonged trial of intensive medical therapy, surgery may be indicated. A shortened trial of medical therapy may be indicated in cases of recurrent aspiration or apnea. Stricture formation due to reflux esophagitis usually requires antireflux therapy in addition to bougienage. The Nissen fundoplication or a variation is used in children. When the procedure is done laprascopically, postoperative recovery is much faster. Reflux is controlled in about 90% of cases. Improvement in respiratory symptoms from reflux depends on the extent to which reflux caused or exacerbated pulmonary problems and if chronic pulmonary disease was initiated by aspiration of refluxed material.

RUMINATION. Repetitive gagging, regurgitation, mouthing, and reswallowing of regurgitated material, often with repetitive head movements and failure to thrive, represent rumination (Chapter 20.1). The cause is unclear. Some cases are associated with mental retardation. Altered interaction with the environment is common, either associated with prolonged lack of stimulation in newborn intensive care units or because of altered relationships with caregivers. There may be an interaction of psychosocial factors and gastroesophageal reflux with esophagitis. Rumination has been noted in association with Sandifer syndrome, the major features of which are gastroesophageal reflux associated with severe esophagitis, iron-deficiency anemia, vomiting, and head tilting. Chewing movements and mouthing of the fingers often precede or accompany the regurgitation. Careful observation may disclose that some infants actively gag themselves with the tongue or fingers. The loss of nutrients may appear deceptively small; an infant often lies continuously in a small pool of regurgitated liquid. A barium swallow usually demonstrates easy reflux or a hiatal hernia and precludes other intestinal lesions such as esophageal stricture, achalasia, or duodenal ulcer. Both behavioral therapy and medical treatment of reflux are indicated. In children not responding to intensive medical therapy, an antireflux surgical procedure stops symptoms.

CHAPTER 324
Esophagitis

Peptic esophagitis due to reflux of gastric acid with pain, blood loss, and occasional stricture formation is the most common form of esophagitis (Chapter 323).

Retroesophageal abscess is rare but may be caused by perforation of the esophagus (Chapter 325), extension of a retropharyngeal abscess, spinal osteomyelitis, pleuritis, suppuration of mediastinal lymph nodes, pericarditis, or pharyngeal diphtheria. The abscess forms behind and around the esophagus, often displacing it to one side, while compressing the more firmly fixed trachea. Symptoms are dyspnea, brassy cough, dysphagia, pain, swelling and redness in the neck, and occasionally, cervical emphysema. An increased retrotracheal space is visible on plain lateral chest films; barium contrast studies are contraindicated if there is cervical perforation. Local extension, exsanguination following erosion into a great vessel, and asphyxia due to tracheal compression are major complications. Appropriate antibiotics and prompt surgical drainage are important. Cervical drainage along the anterior boarder of the sternocleidomastoid is effective to the level of the fourth dorsal vertebra. Antibiotics alone may be adequate in minor instrumental perforations if initiated immediately and if the patient is carefully monitored.

Esophageal candidiasis (moniliasis) is the most common esophageal infection and is not limited to immunocompromised patients. Oral candidiasis is frequently absent. *Torulopsis glabrata*, another fungus, may cause esophageal ulcers in patients with AIDS. Barium esophagography in the most severely affected patients may show mucosal irregularities, but esophagoscopy and biopsy are the most sensitive and accurate diagnostic studies. Ketoconazole 3–6 mg/kg/24 hr as a single daily oral dose is usually effective. In immunocompromised patients and in patients with systemic infection, amphotericin and/or flucytosine may be necessary.

Viral esophagitis is usually caused by herpes simplex virus (HSV), cytomegalovirus (CMV), and occasionally, varicella-zoster. Only HSV is common in the normal host. Severe odynophagia and dysphagia are the main symptoms. More than 90% of patients with AIDS have evidence of CMV dissemination at autopsy, and 10% of liver and kidney transplant recipients develop HSV or CMV esophagitis. Infections are often relatively asymptomatic. Esophagoscopy and biopsy are the best diagnostic tests because superinfection with bacteria and *Candida* is common in immunocompromised hosts. Most immunocompetent hosts require only symptomatic therapy with analgesics and antacids. Acyclovir 750 mg/m^2/24 hr IV in three divided doses is effective for HSV and varicella-zoster. Foscarnet is the drug of choice for immunocompromised patients who have HSV resistant to acyclovir. Ganciclovir 10 mg/kg/24 hr IV bid is effective for CMV.

Bacterial esophagitis may occasionally be due to extension of a pharyngeal diphtheria infection or extension from a tubercular lymph node. In immunocompromised hosts, other bacteria may invade the esophageal mucosa. These lesions do not respond to other therapy for esophagitis and may be a source of sepsis.

CORROSIVE ESOPHAGITIS (see Chapter 722.7). This injury most commonly follows ingestion of household cleaning products. Alkalis (70%), acids (20%), bleaches, detergents, microwave-overheated baby bottles, and button mercuric oxide batteries are common agents. Alkalis produce a severe, deep, liquefaction necrosis that affects all layers of the esophagus. Household liquid alkali agents used as drain-declogging agents contain

8–10% base, industrial strength usually contains 30–35%, and granular agents contain 80% base. Concentrated bases are also used to produce crack cocaine and may be left on the table in poorly labeled containers. Alkalis have no taste; a child may therefore ingest a significant amount.

Acidic agents include toilet bowl cleaners, drain decloggers, and rust and stain removers; they contain various acids (sulfuric, hydrochloric, oxalic, acid sulfates) with a range of concentrations (8–65%). Acids taste bitter, thus limiting the total volume of ingestion. Volatile acids (hydrochloric acid) may produce respiratory symptoms. All acids produce a coagulative necrosis and a thick eschar that usually limits the depth of the esophageal injury to the mucosa and superficial muscularis layers. Alkalis and acids (more likely) can produce severe gastritis.

The peak age of accidental corrosive ingestion is before 5 yr of age. Corrosive solutions stored in innocuous-appearing containers (pop bottles) and in open, unlocked areas are risk factors. If a child has had unobserved access to an open container of such substances, with or without chemical burns of the hands or mouth, the possibility of caustic ingestion should be strongly suggested. Significant ingestion of corrosive substances in adolescents should raise the suspicion of attempted suicide.

Clinical manifestations include salivation, refusal to drink, nausea, vomiting, epigastric pain, oral burns or ulcerations, fever, and leukocytosis that may clear in a few days, as well as, rarely, esophageal perforation. Esophageal strictures may develop over a few weeks and cause dysphagia and weight loss.

Emergency treatment involves oral administration of large quantities of fluid (water or milk) to dilute the corrosive agent. Neutralization, induced emesis, and gastric lavage are contraindicated. Edema of the pharynx, larynx, or airway may require urgent endotracheal intubation or tracheostomy. The child should be hospitalized, receive nothing by mouth, and be given intravenous fluids.

Esophagogastroscopy with a flexible fiberoptic endoscope should be performed in all patients within 48 hr to identify those who do not have burns and who do not need follow-up and to determine the severity of esophageal burns and gastric antral ulceration. Ampicillin may be given for suspected infection; perforation with acute mediastinitis requires broad-spectrum antibiotics and the placement of mediastinal drains. Although prednisone was thought to be effective in reducing the incidence and severity of subsequent stricture formation, a randomized controlled trial did not indicate that prednisone was effective. The risk of stricture formation is related directly to the severity of the injury, as determined by circumferential ulcerations, white plaques, and sloughing of the mucosa. Intraluminal stents may reduce stricture formation in severe esophageal burns.

Early detection and dilatation of developing strictures are an important part of continuing care. Severe strictures that do not respond to dilatation and complete obliteration of the lumen can be treated by colonic interposition. Long-term sequelae, in addition to strictures, include the rare late occurrence of esophageal carcinoma.

Prevention is critical because the morbidity may be great. Corrosive compounds should be kept in their original containers and out of reach of children. Dilute formulations should be used in homes, and industrial strength solutions and solids should be kept at work or locked in a safe, hard-to-reach location.

CHAPTER 325
Esophageal Perforation

Esophageal perforations may be spontaneous or may result from trauma, caustic ingestion, or medical interventions such as endoscopy, esophageal dilitation, erosion of tracheostomy or endotracheal tubes, or difficult tracheal intubation. Many are iatrogenic.

Spontaneous perforation may follow sudden increases in esophageal pressure, which occur with violent retching, in automobile accidents, or even with compression in the birth canal. Ninety-five per cent of perforations occur on the left side of the distal esophagus in children but occur more commonly on the right side in neonates. Common symptoms are vomiting followed by severe substernal pain, cyanosis, and shock. Esophagography shows extraluminal water-soluble contrast material.

Violent retching can tear the esophageal mucosa and submucosa, causing hematemesis (Mallory-Weiss syndrome). Esophagoscopy, if needed, should differentiate this disorder from other more serious forms of upper gastrointestinal bleeding. Blood replacement is usually sufficient because rupture of the esophagus with this condition rarely occurs in children.

CHAPTER 326
Esophageal Varices

Esophageal varices may occur in children as a complication of portal hypertension and may be asymptomatic. The principal signs are recurrent profuse, bright-red hematemesis and tarry stools, with signs of intravascular volume depletion. Children with esophageal varices often have another source for acute gastrointestinal hemorrhage. Roentgenographic studies with barium may outline the varices, but esophagoscopy is more precise in diagnosis. Treatment of portal hypertension and acute gastrointestinal bleeding is discussed in Chapter 366.

CHAPTER 327
Foreign Bodies in the Esophagus

(See Chapter 334)

Children swallow various objects that may lodge in their esophagus, usually below the cricopharyngeal muscle, at the level of the aortic arch or just above the diaphragm. Lodging at any other site should suggest coexistent esophageal disease. Coins are the most commonly ingested object, especially in children younger than 5 yr.

CLINICAL MANIFESTATIONS. Swallowing a foreign body may provoke an attack of coughing, drooling, and choking. Foreign bodies in the esophagus may cause pain, dysphagia (especially with solid foods), and occasionally dyspnea and stridor, due to compression of the trachea or larynx. After an initial symptom-free period, edema and inflammation produce symptoms of esophageal obstruction. Pain, fever, and shock suggest perforation.

DIAGNOSIS. Radiopaque foreign bodies are easily diagnosed. Coins and other flat objects are usually seen on edge on lateral films. Symptomatic patients with esophageal foreign bodies should be examined by endoscopy to remove the object and to examine the esophageal mucosa for injury. Patients, especially infants who swallow radiolucent foreign bodies, should be evaluated with a barium swallow or endoscopy to detect a transiently asymptomatic esophageal foreign body. If the object is identified in the stomach, only careful follow-up for passage in the stool is required.

TREATMENT. The usual treatment is removal of the object under direct vision with esophagoscopy. Roentgenography should be repeated just before the procedure to make sure the foreign body has not passed into the stomach. Sharp objects, such as open safety pins, should be removed emergently, as should disk batteries, because they can cause corrosive injury to the esophagus within 4 hr. Asymptomatic coins in the distal esophagus may be observed for up to 24 hr after ingestion in expectation that they may pass. Another procedure for esophageal coins present for less than 24 hr involves passing a Foley catheter beyond the coin under fluoroscopic control, inflating the balloon, and removing the catheter and coin at the same time. Alternatively, the coin may be pushed into the stomach.

Esophageal Anomalies

Berdon WE, Baker DH: Vascular anomalies and the infant lungs: Rings, slings and other things. Semin Roentgenol 7:39, 1972.

Depaepe A, Dolk H, Lechat M, et al: The epidemiology of tracheoesophageal fistula and oesophageal atresia in Europe. Arch Dis Child 68:743, 1993.

Puntis J, Ritson D, Holden C, et al: Growth and feeding problems after repair of oesophageal atresia. Arch Dis Child 65:84, 1990.

Reyes H, Meller J, Loeff D: Management of esophageal atresia and tracheoesophageal fistula. Clin Perinatol 16:79, 1989.

Hiatal Hernia and Gastroesophageal Reflux

Borgstein E, Heij H, Beugelar J, et al: Risks and benefits of antireflux operations in neurologically impaired children. Eur J Pediatr 153:248, 1994.

Dalla Vecchia LK, Grosfeld JL, West KW, et al: Reoperation after Nissen fundoplication in children with gastroesophageal reflux. Ann Surg 226:315, 1997.

Fonkalsrud E, Ashcraft K, Coran A, et al: Surgical treatment of gastroesophageal reflex in children: a combined hospital study of 7467 patients. Pediatrics 101:419, 1998.

De Giacomo C, Bawa P, Franceschi M, et al: Omeprazole for severe reflux esophagitis in children. J Pediatr Gastroenterol Nutr 24:528, 1997.

Kawahara H, Dent J, Davidson G: Mechanisms of gastroesophageal reflux in Children. Gastroenterology 113:399, 1997.

Laneau S, Evangelista J, Pizzi A, et al: Proarrhythmia—associated with cisapride in children. Pediatrics 101:1053, 1998.

Scott RB, Ferreira C, Smith L, et al: Cisapride in pediatric gastroesophageal reflux. J Pediatr Gastroenterol Nutr 25:499, 1997.

Sulaeman E, Udall J, Brown R, et al: Gastroesophageal reflux and Nissen fundoplication following percutaneous endoscopic gastrostomy in children. J Pediatr Gastroenterol Nutr 26:269, 1998.

Vandenplas Y: Asthma and gastroesophageal reflux. J Pediatr Gastroenterol Nutr 24:89, 1997.

Rumination

Richmond JB, Eddy E, Green M: Rumination: A psychosomatic syndrome of infancy. Pediatrics 22:49, 1958.

Sheagren TG, Mangurten HH, Brea F, et al: Rumination—a new complication of neonatal intensive care. Pediatrics 66:551, 1980.

Achalasia

Azizkham RG, Tapper D, Eraklis A: Achalasia in childhood: A 20-year experience. J Pediatr Surg 15:452, 1980.

Gershman G, Ament ME, Vargas J: Frequency and medical management of esophageal perforation after pneumatic dilatation in achalasia. J Pediatr Gastroenterol Nutr 25:548, 1997.

Khoshoo V, LaGarde DC, Udall JN Jr: Intrasphincteric injection of *botulinum* toxin for treating achalasia in children. J Pediatr Gastroenterol Nutr 24:439, 1997.

Nakayanla DK, Shorter NA, Boyle JT, et al: Pneumatic dilatation and operative treatment of achalasia in children. J Pediatr Surg 22:619, 1987.

Swallowing and Dysphagia

Illingworth RS: Sucking and swallowing difficulties in infancy: Diagnostic problems of dysphagia. Arch Dis Child 44:655, 1969.

Milov D, Cynamon H, Andres J: Chest pain and dysphagia in adolescents caused by diffuse esophageal spasm. J Pediatr Gastroenterol Nutr 9:450, 1989.

Corrosive Esophagitis

Anderson KD, Rouse TM, Randolph JG: A controlled trial of corticosteroids in children with corrosive injury of the esophagus. N Engl J Med 323:637, 1990.

Gorman RL, Kleil-Schwartz W, Oderda GM, et al: Initial symptoms as predictors of esophageal injury in alkaline corrosive ingestions. Am J Emerg Med 10:189, 1992.

Wijburg FA, Heymans HSA, Urbanus NAM: Caustic esophageal lesions in childhood: Prevention of stricture formation. J Pediatr Surg 24:171, 1989.

Foreign Bodies

Campbell JB, Condon VR: Catheter removal of blunt esophageal foreign bodies in children. Pediatr Radiol 19:361, 1989.

Caravati EM, Bennett DL, McElwee NE: Pediatric coin ingestion: A prospective study on the utility of routine roentgenograms. Am J Dis Child 143:549, 1989.

Conners GP, Chamberlain JM, Ochsenschlager DW: Conservative management of pediatric distal esophageal coins. J Emerg Med 14:723, 1996.

Litovitz T, Schmitz BF: Ingestion of cylindrical and button batteries: An analysis of 2382 cases. Pediatrics 89:747, 1992.

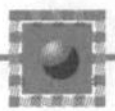

SECTION 4

Stomach and Intestines

CHAPTER 328

Normal Development, Structure, and Function

Martin Ulshen

DEVELOPMENT. The gut matures relatively early in fetal life. In a 4-wk, 3-mm embryo, the primitive foregut and hindgut form a simple tube as the stomach and cecum become distinct. This tube then elongates quickly, protrudes into the umbilical cord, and rotates counterclockwise around the superior mesenteric artery. At 8 wk, the caudal end becomes continuous with the rectum, which has evolved from the cloaca, and at 10 wk the bowel rapidly re-enters the abdomen. Later, the colon achieves its mature conformation. Rotations of the midgut and hindgut are independent events. Most structural anomalies of the stomach and intestine are attributable to a delay or aberration in this complex series of events.

The pyloric musculature of the stomach is seen by the 3rd mo of gestation, and parietal and chief cells appear by 14 wk. Intestinal-type cells found in the gastric mucosa gradually disappear during fetal life. Relatively mature villi are seen along the intestine by 12 wk, and by 20 wk the crypts are deep and enterocytes are columnar with some microvilli. Blood vessels and the nerve supply to the gut are fully developed by 12–13 wk. Intramural ganglia appear first at the proximal end; thus, if their development is interrupted, the effect is seen in the distal regions. Peristalsis has been recognized as early as 8 wk, but motility usually is not fully coordinated until near term. Lymphoid tissue has developed by 20 wk.

Some functions develop relatively early in the fetal gut; others mature in postnatal life. In the stomach, acid secretion is low in the first 5 hr of life and then increases dramatically by 24 hr after birth; acid and pepsin secretion peak during the first 10 days and decrease from 10–30 days after birth. Intrinsic factor secretion rises slowly during the first 2 wk of life, but at term, circulating gastrin levels are inexplicably two- to threefold higher than in adults.

Small intestinal function matures throughout prenatal and postnatal life. Epithelial glucose transport is detectable in the jejunum of a human embryo before 20 wk. In infants, the maximum rate of glucose transport is one quarter that of adults. Disaccharidase activities are measurable in a human fetus at 12 wk; sucrase and maltase achieve maximal activities by the 24th and 32nd wk, respectively; but lactase activity rises later, reaching maximal levels by 36 wk. In many children, particularly of black and Asian races, intestinal lactase activity begins to decline after the first few years of life. Fetal intestine is involved in the daily transport of a large amount of amniotic fluid, and there is significant activity of the Na^+ pump in 10-wk-old human fetal gut. Solute transport is probably adequate but marginal in very young infants. Accordingly, relatively severe functional disturbances in response to small intestinal diseases can be anticipated, whereas older children can be expected to have significant reserve function.

Fat absorption is less efficient in term infants than in older children and even less efficient in premature infants than in those at term. Important determinants of these age-related differences are the relatively slow rates of bile salt synthesis and transport in early life and reduced pancreatic secretion.

The human gut is capable of absorbing antigenically significant quantities of intact protein, particularly during the early weeks of life. Entry of potential protein antigens through the mucosal barrier may have a role in later food- and microbe-induced symptoms.

NORMAL STRUCTURE. The serosal layer of the bowel wall is an extension of the peritoneum that extends distally as far as the rectum. There are two muscle layers: outer longitudinal fibers and inner circular ones; in the colon, the longitudinal fibers form bands, or taeniae. The submucosa is a rich matrix for lymph and vascular plexuses, containing lymphoid cells and macrophages and, in the duodenum, Brunner glands. A complex enteric nervous system is an important factor in regulating not only microvascular flow but epithelial function. The mucosa of the small bowel is well designed to absorb nutrients because its absorptive surface has a very large area owing to a multitude of villi that extend into the lumen, constantly moving in a coordinated fushion. In children, these villi tend to be leaflike rather than finger-shaped projections; thus, the functional surface area of the small intestine probably increases with age. The colonic mucosal surface is flat, with numerous tubular crypts opening into the surface. The lamina propria, a cellular layer just beneath the epithelium that contains cells capable of phagocytosis and immunoglobulin synthesis, provides a connective tissue core for the epithelium and its vascular supply. Lymphoid tissue is concentrated in Peyer patches, which become more numerous in the distal small bowel. There are several types of epithelial cells in the small intestine: The columnar absorptive cell dominates; goblet cells secrete mucus; endocrine cells secrete certain intestinal hormones; Paneth cells secrete granules with antimicrobial action into the crypt lumen; and over areas of lymphoid aggregation, "m" cells have a special capacity to absorb intact, potentially antigenic proteins. The columnar absorptive cell is polarized with a microvillus "brush" border at the luminal surface to which a glycocalyx or "fuzz coat" is tightly adherent. Active cell division of the enterocytes occurs in the crypts, and as cells migrate up the villi, they differentiate. A dramatic shift in gene expression occurs at the crypt-villus junction consistent with differentiation of mature villus enterocytes. The jejunal epithelium is completely renewed in 4–5 days, providing a mechanism for rapid repair after injury; but in very young infants, the process may be slow.

NORMAL FUNCTION. The stomach serves as a reservoir that delivers liquefield, blended, but minimally digested food to the intestine. Initial emulsification of fat and digestion of protein occur here. It also secretes intrinsic factor, essential for the assimilation of vitamin B_{12} in the ileum. The small intestine must process not only ingested nutrients but also a large volume of water and shed epithelial cells. In adults, the quantity of water entering the gut lumen is at least seven times the amount ingested.

Intraluminal digestion depends mainly on the exocrine pancreas. Synthesis and secretion of bicarbonate and digestive enzymes are stimulated by secretin and cholecystokinin, which are released by the upper intestinal mucosa in response to various intraluminal stimuli, among them components of the diet. Digestion is an efficient, fast process, usually completed in the most proximal intestinal segment. Bile salts in the lumen facilitate digestion and are essential for the efficient delivery of products of lipid hydrolysis to the absorptive surface of the epithelium. Emulsification aids digestion, and long-chain monoglycerides and fatty acids usually reach the epithelium in the form of mixed micelles with conjugated bile acids and phospholipid. Sterols such as vitamin D are particularly dependent on these micelles for their absorption; accordingly, diseases such as biliary atresia cause particular difficulties with vitamin D assimilation. Medium-chain triglycerides available in certain specially designed therapeutic diets, on the other hand, do not require micelles, emulsification, or hydrolysis for their absorption.

Carbohydrate, protein, and fat are normally absorbed by the upper half of the small intestine; the distal segments represent a vast reserve of absorptive capacity. Most of the sodium, potassium, chloride, and water is absorbed in the small bowel. Bile salts and vitamin B_{12} are selectively absorbed in the distal ileum, and iron in the duodenum and proximal jejunum.

Disaccharides are hydrolyzed by disaccharidases on the outer surface of the microvillus membranes, and resultant monosaccharides are actively transported across the cell, primarily to portal venous drainage. Dipeptides and larger peptides can be hydrolyzed at the brush border surface but may also enter the cell intact before they contact peptidases. The small bowel has active transport pathways for specific groups of amino acids and for oligopeptides, similar to those in the renal tubule. Monoglycerides and fatty acids enter the epithelium intact; triglycerides are resynthesized, incorporated with phospholipid and lipoprotein into chylomicrons, and released into lymphatics. Medium-chain triglycerides may be taken up intact and released into the portal stream.

The colon extracts additional water and ions from the luminal contents in order to render the stools partially or completely solid. Stools can then be stored in the rectum until distention triggers a defecation reflex that, when assisted by voluntary relaxation of the external sphincter, permits evaluation.

Adibi SA: The oligopeptide transporter (Pept-1) in human intestine: Biology and function. Gastroenterology 113:332, 1997.

Berseth CL: Effect of early feeding on maturation of the preterm infant's small intestine. J Pediatr 120:947, 1992.

Lentze MJ: Molecular and cellular aspects of hydrolysis and absorption. Am J Clin Nutr 61:946S, 1995.

Shi X, Schedl HP, Summers RM, et al: Fructose transport mechanisms in humans. Gastroenterology 113:1171, 1997.
Thompson AB, Wild G: Adaptation of intestinal nutrient transport in health and disease. Part I. Dig Dis Sci 42:453, 1997.
Traber PG: Differentiation of intestinal epithelial cells: Lessons from the study of intestine-specific gene expression. J Lab Clin Med 123:467, 1994.

CHAPTER 329
Pyloric Stenosis and Other Congenital Anomalies of the Stomach

Robert Wyllie

The hallmark of gastric obstruction is nonbilious vomiting. Other symptoms include abdominal pain and nausea. Signs of gastric outlet obstruction include abdominal distention and bleeding from secondary inflammation of the gastric or esophageal mucosa.

The most common cause of nonbilious vomiting is infantile hypertrophic pyloric stenosis. Similar symptoms may be associated with various other gastric malformations including pyloric atresia, antral webs, gastric duplications, and gastric volvulus. The differential diagnosis includes gastroesophageal reflux, peptic ulcer disease, salt-wasting adrenogenital syndrome, bezoars, and various other metabolic and motility abnormalities.

329.1 Hypertrophic Pyloric Stenosis

Hypertrophic pyloric stenosis occurs in approximately 3/1,000 live births in the United States; its frequency may be increasing. It is more common in whites of northern European ancestry, less common in blacks, and rare in Asians. Males (especially first born) are affected approximately four times as often as females. The offspring of a mother and to a lesser extent the father who had pyloric stenosis are at higher risk for pyloric stenosis. Pyloric stenosis develops in approximately 20% of the male and 10% of the female descendants of a mother who had pyloric stenosis. The incidence of pyloric stenosis is increased in infants with type B and O blood groups. Pyloric stenosis is associated with other congenital defects including tracheoesophageal fistula.

ETIOLOGY. The cause of pyloric stenosis is unknown, but many factors have been implicated. Pyloric stenosis is usually not present at birth and is more concordant in monozygotic than dizygotic twins. Abnormal muscle innervation, breast-feeding, and maternal stress in the third trimester all have been implicated. In addition, elevated serum prostaglandins, reduced levels of pyloric nitric oxide synthase, and infant hypergastrinemia have been found. Exogenous administration of prostaglandin E to maintain patency of the ductus arteriosus has been associated with pyloric stenosis, as have eosinophilic gastroenteritis, epidermolysis bullosa, and trisomy 18, and Turner, Smith-Lemli-Opitz, and Cornelia de Lange syndromes.

CLINICAL MANIFESTATIONS. Nonbilious vomiting is the initial symptom of pyloric stenosis. The vomiting may or may not be projectile initially but is usually progressive, occurring immediately after a feeding. Emesis may follow each feeding, or it may be intermittent. The vomiting usually starts after 3 wk of age, but symptoms may develop as early as the 1st wk of life and as late as the 5th mo. After vomiting, the infant is hungry and wants to feed again. As vomiting continues, a progressive loss of fluid, hydrogen ion, and chloride, leads to a hypochloremic metabolic alkalosis. Serum potassium levels are usually maintained, but there may be a total body potassium deficit. Greater awareness of pyloric stenosis has led to earlier identification of patients with fewer instances of chronic malnutrition and severe dehydration.

Jaundice associated with a decreased level of glucuronyl transferase is seen in approximately 5% of affected infants. The jaundice usually resolves promptly after relief of the obstruction.

The *diagnosis* has traditionally been established by palpating the pyloric mass. The mass is firm, movable, approximately 2 cm in length, olive shaped, hard, best palpated from the left side, and located above and to the right of the umbilicus in the midepigastrium beneath the liver edge. In healthy infants, feeding can be an aid to the diagnosis. After feeding, there may be a visible gastric peristaltic wave that progresses across the abdomen (Fig. 329–1). After the infant vomits, the abdominal musculature is more relaxed and the "olive" easier to palpate. Sedation may be used to facilitate examination but is usually unnecessary. The diagnosis can be established clinically approximately 60–80% of the time by an experienced examiner.

Ultrasound examination confirms the diagnosis in the majority of cases, allowing an earlier diagnosis in infants with suspected disease but no pyloric mass on physical examination. Criteria for diagnosis include pyloric muscle thickness greater than 4 mm or an overall pyloric length greater than 14 mm (Fig. 329–2). Ultrasonography has a sensitivity of approximately 90%. When barium studies are performed, they demonstrate an elongated pyloric channel, a bulge of the pyloric muscle into the antrum (shoulder sign), and parallel streaks of barium seen in the narrowed channel, producing a "double tract sign" (Fig. 329–3).

DIFFERENTIAL DIAGNOSIS. The usual case can be diagnosed by the characteristic clinical pattern and the identification of a pyloric mass on physical examination or ultrasonography. Infants who are exceptionally reactive to external stimuli, those fed by inexperienced or anxious caretakers, or those for whom an adequate maternal-infant bonding relationship has not been established may vomit frequently in the early weeks of life. Such infants may come to resemble infants with pyloric stenosis; the vomiting may be persistent and even projectile. Gastric waves are occasionally visible in small, emaciated in-

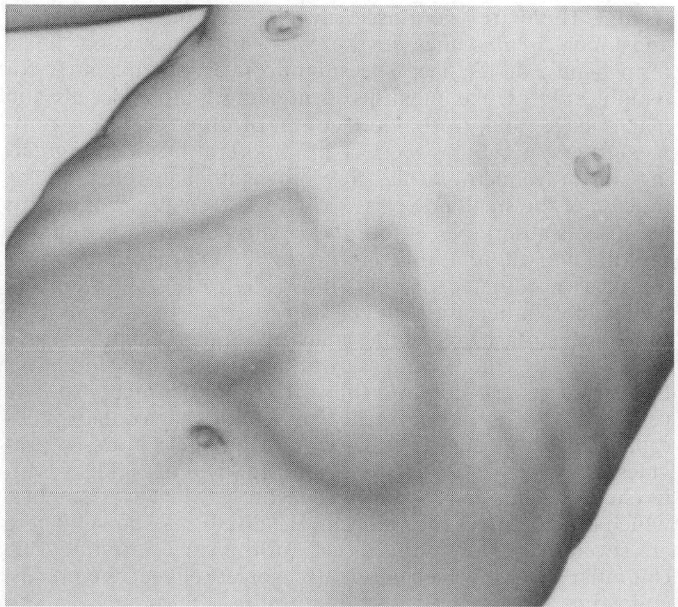

Figure 329–1 Gastric peristaltic wave in an infant with pyloric stenosis.

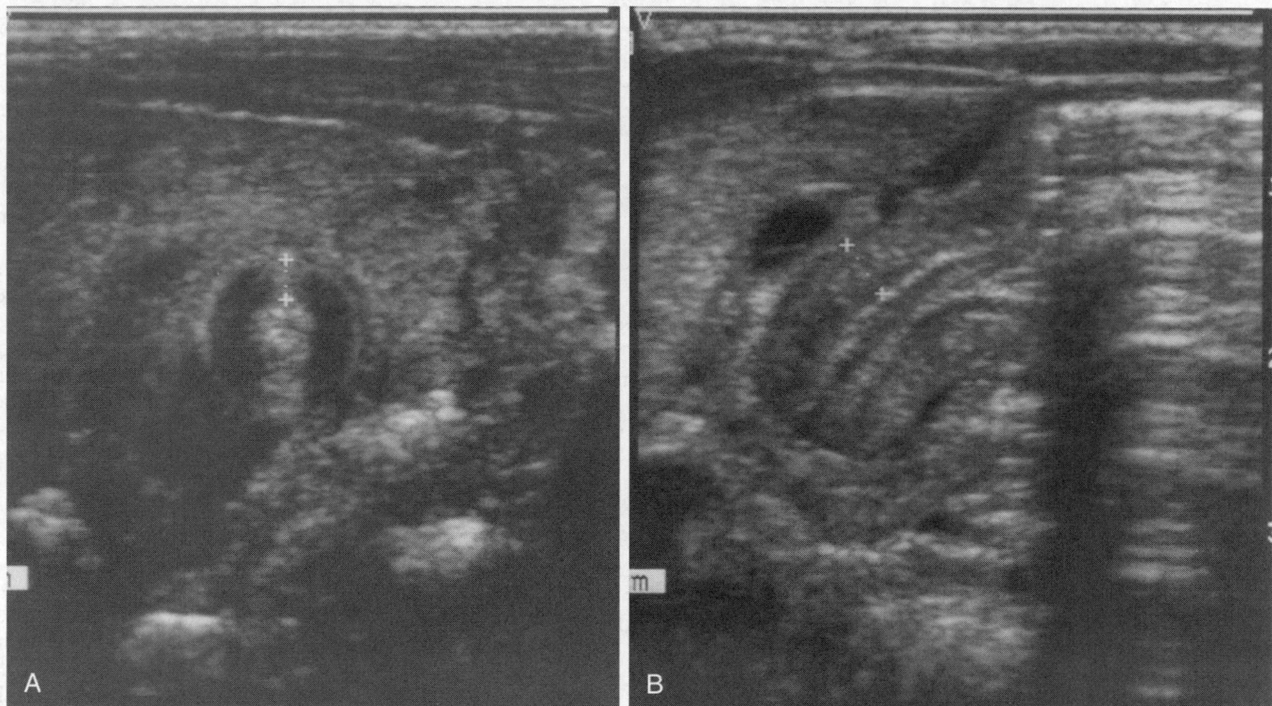

Figure 329–2 *(A)* Transverse sonogram demonstrating a pyloric muscle wall thickness of greater than 4 mm (distance between crosses). *(B)* Horizontal image demonstrating a pyloric channel length greater than 14 mm (wall thickness outlined between crosses) in an infant with pyloric stenosis.

fants who do not have pyloric stenosis. Infrequently, gastroesophageal reflux with or without a hiatal hernia may be confused with pyloric stenosis. Gastroesophageal reflux disease can be differentiated from pyloric stenosis by roentgenographic studies. Adrenal insufficiency may simulate pyloric stenosis, but the absence of a metabolic acidosis and elevated serum potassium and urinary sodium concentrations of adrenal insufficiency aid in differentiation. Inborn errors of metabolism may produce recurrent emesis with alkalosis (urea cycle) or acidosis (organic acidemia) and lethargy, coma, or seizures. Vomiting

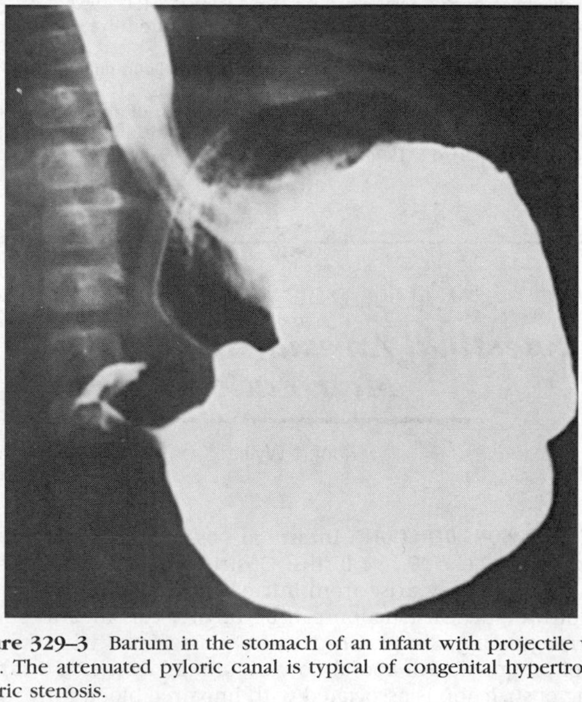

Figure 329–3 Barium in the stomach of an infant with projectile vomiting. The attenuated pyloric canal is typical of congenital hypertrophic pyloric stenosis.

with diarrhea suggests gastroenteritis, but patients with pyloric stenosis occasionally have diarrhea. Very rarely, a pyloric membrane or pyloric duplication may result in projectile vomiting, visible peristalsis, and, in the case of a duplication, a palpable mass. Duodenal stenosis proximal to the ampulla of Vater results in the clinical features of pyloric stenosis but can be differentiated by the presence of a pyloric mass or physical examination or ultrasonography.

TREATMENT. The preoperative treatment is directed toward correcting the fluid, acid-base, and electrolyte losses. Intravenous fluid therapy is begun with 0.45–0.9% saline, in 5–10% dextrose, with the addition of potassium chloride in concentrations of 30–50 mEq/L. Fluid therapy should be continued until the infant is rehydrated and the serum bicarbonate concentration is less than 30 mEq/dL, which implies that the alkalosis has been corrected. Correction of the alkalosis is essential to prevent postoperative apnea, which may be associated with anesthesia. Most infants can be successfully rehydrated within 24 hr. Vomiting usually stops when the stomach is empty, and only an occasional infant requires nasogastric suction.

The surgical procedure of choice is the Ramstedt pyloromyotomy. The procedure is performed through a short transverse incision or laparoscopically. The underlying pyloric mass is split without cutting the mucosa, and the incision closed. Postoperative vomiting may occur in half the infants and is thought to be secondary to edema of the pylorus at the incision site. In most infants, however, feedings can be initiated within 12–24 hr after surgery and advanced to maintenance oral feedings within 36–48 hr of the surgery. Persistent vomiting suggests an incomplete pyloromyotomy, gastritis, gastroesophageal reflux disease, or another cause of the obstruction.

The surgical treatment of pyloric stenosis is curative, with an operative mortality of between 0 and 0.5%. Conservative medical therapy (small frequent feedings, atropine) has been attempted in the past but is associated with slow improvement and a higher mortality. Endoscopic balloon dilation has been successful in infants with persistent vomiting secondary to incomplete pyloromyotomy.

329.2 Congenital Gastric Outlet Obstruction

Gastric outlet obstruction resulting from pyloric atresia and antral webs is uncommon and accounts for less than 1% of all the atresias and diaphragms of the alimentary tract. The cause of the defects is unknown. Pyloric atresia has been associated with epidermolysis bullosa and usually presents in early infancy. The sex distribution is equal.

CLINICAL MANIFESTATIONS. Infants with pyloric atresia present with nonbilious vomiting, feeding difficulties, and abdominal distention during the 1st day of life. Polyhydramnios occurs in the majority of cases, and low birthweight is common. Rupture of the stomach may occur as early as the 1st 12 hr of life. Infants with antral web may present with less dramatic symptoms, depending on the degree of obstruction. Older children with antral webs present with nausea, vomiting, abdominal pain, and weight loss.

DIAGNOSIS. The diagnosis of congenital gastric outlet obstruction is suggested by the finding of a large, dilated stomach on abdominal plain roentgenograms. Upper gastrointestinal contrast series is usually diagnostic and demonstrates a pyloric dimple. An antral web may appear as a thin septum near the pyloric channel. In older children, endoscopy has been helpful in identifying antral webs.

TREATMENT. The treatment of gastric outlet obstruction in neonates starts with the correction of dehydration and hypochloremic alkalosis. Persistent vomiting should be relieved with nasogastric decompression. Surgical or endoscopic repair should be undertaken when a patient is stable.

329.3 Gastric Duplication

Gastric duplications are uncommon cystic or tubular structures that usually occur within the wall of the stomach. Most are smaller than 12 cm in diameter and do not usually communicate with the stomach lumen. Associated anomalies occur in as many as 35% of patients. Duplications have been attributed to a failure of recanalization after the solid stage of intestinal development.

The most common *clinical manifestations* are associated with partial or complete gastric outlet obstruction. In 33% of patients, the cyst may be palpable. Communicating duplications may cause gastric ulceration and be associated with hematemesis or melena.

Gastric duplications are visualized on upper gastrointestinal series as an extrinsic defect usually located along the lesser curve of the stomach. CT or sonography may be helpful in defining a cystic structure. Surgical excision is the treatment for symptomatic gastric duplications.

329.4 Gastric Volvulus

Gastric volvulus presents with a triad of a sudden onset of severe epigastric pain, intractable retching with emesis, and inability to pass a tube into the stomach. The stomach is tethered longitudinally by the gastrohepatic, gastrosplenic, and gastrocolic ligaments. In the transverse axis, it is tethered by the gastrophrenic ligament and the retroperitoneal attachment of the duodenum. A volvulus occurs when one of these attachments is absent or stretched, allowing the stomach to rotate around itself. In most children, other associated defects are present, including intestinal malrotation, diaphragmatic defects, or asplenia. Volvulus may occur along the longitudinal axis, producing organoaxial volvulus, or along the transverse axis, producing mesenteroaxial volvulus.

CLINICAL MANIFESTATIONS. The clinical presentation of gastric volvulus is nonspecific and suggests high intestinal obstruction. Gastric volvulus in infancy is usually associated with nonbilious vomiting. Acute volvulus may advance rapidly to strangulation and perforation. Chronic gastric volvulus is more common in older children, and the children present with a history of emesis, abdominal pain, and early satiety.

The *diagnosis* is suggested in plain abdominal radiographs by the presence of a dilated stomach. Erect abdominal films demonstrate a double fluid level with a characteristic "beak" near the lower esophageal junction in mesenteroaxial volvulus. In organoaxial volvulus, a single air-fluid level is seen without the characteristic beak. *Treatment* of acute gastric volvulus is emergent surgery once a patient is stabilized. In selected cases of chronic volvulus in older patients, endoscopic correction has been successful.

329.5 Hypertrophic Gastropathy

Hypertrophic gastropathy in children is uncommon and, in contrast to that in adults (Menetrier disease), is a transient, benign, self-limited condition, possibly initiated by an infectious agent (cytomegalovirus, herpes simplex virus, *Giardia, Helicobacter pylori*). Clinical manifestations include vomiting, anorexia, upper abdominal pain, diarrhea, edema (hypoproteinemic protein-losing enteropathy), ascites, and rarely hematemesis, if ulceration occurs. Endoscopy with biopsy confirms the diagnosis. The mean age of diagnosis is 5 yr (range 2 days–17 yr); the illness usually lasts 2–4 wk, with complete resolution the rule. The differential diagnosis includes eosinophilic gastroenteritis, gastric lymphoma or carcinoma, Crohn disease, and inflammatory pseudotumor.

Applegate MS, Druschel CM: The epidemiology of infantile hypertrophic pyloric stenosis in New York State, 1983 to 1990. Arch Pediatr Adolesc Med 149:1123, 1995.
Chen EA, Luks FI, Gilchrist BF, et al: Pyloric stenosis in the age of ultrasonography: fading skills, better patients? [See comments.] J Pediatr Surg 31:829, 1996.
Godbole P, Sprigg A, Dickson JA, et al: Ultrasound compared with clinical examination in infantile hypertrophic pyloric stenosis. [See comments.] Arch Dis Child 75:335, 1996.
Hulka F, Harrison MW, Campbell TJ, et al: Complications of pyloromyotomy for infantile hypertrophic pyloric stenosis. Am J Surg 173:450, 1997.
Jacobe S, Lam A, Elliot E: Transient hypertrophic gastropathy. J Pediatr Gastroenterol Nutr 26:211, 1998.
Khoshoo V, Noel RA, LaGarde D, et al: Endoscopic balloon dilatation of failed pyloromyotomy in young infants. J Pediatr Gastroenterol Nutr 23:447, 1996.
Poon TS, Zhang AL, Cartmill T, et al: Changing patterns of diagnosis and treatment of infantile hypertrophic pyloric stenosis: A clinical audit of 303 patients. J Pediatr Surg 31:1611, 1996.

CHAPTER 330
Intestinal Atresia, Stenosis, and Malrotation

Robert Wyllie

GENERAL CONSIDERATIONS. Intestinal obstruction occurs in approximately 1/1,500 live births. Obstruction may be partial or complete and may arise from intrinsic or extrinsic abnormalities of the gut. Obstruction can be further classified as simple or strangulating. Simple obstruction is associated with the failure of progression of aboral flow of luminal contents. Strangulating obstruction is associated with impaired blood flow to the intestine in addition to obstruction of the flow of luminal contents. If strangulating obstruction is not promptly relieved, it may lead to bowel infarction and perforation.

Obstruction is typically associated with an accumulation of ingested food, gas, and intestinal secretions proximal to the point of obstruction, leading to distention of the bowel. As the bowel dilates, intestinal absorption decreases and secretion of fluid and electrolytes increases. The shift in fluid and electrolytes results in isotonic intravascular depletion usually associated with hypokalemia. The gut proximal to the obstruction initially demonstrates an increase in contractile activity, which is followed by a marked decrease with hypoactive bowel sounds. The combination of fluid accumulation and hypomotility is associated with nausea and vomiting.

From an anatomic standpoint, congenital obstructive lesions of the intestines can be viewed as *intrinsic* (e.g., atresia, stenosis, meconium ileus, and aganglionic megacolon) or *extrinsic* (e.g., malrotation, constricting bands, intra-abdominal hernias, and duplications). An attempt should be made to locate the lesion preoperatively in order to guide the surgical approach.

When the obstruction is *complete*, there should be little difficulty in clinical recognition, but when it is *incomplete*, diagnosis may pose considerable difficulty. Polyhydramnios frequently accompanies high intestinal obstruction, as it does esophageal atresia. When polyhydramnios has been noted, the infant's stomach should be aspirated immediately after birth. Aspiration of 15–20 mL or more of gastric fluid, especially if it is bile stained, is suggestive of a high intestinal obstruction.

Meconium stools may be passed initially if the obstruction is in the upper part of the small intestine or if the obstruction developed late in intrauterine life.

When obstruction is *incomplete* (e.g., as with intestinal stenosis, constricting bands, duplications, and incomplete volvulus), signs (vomiting, abdominal distention, obstipation) may appear shortly after birth or may be delayed an indeterminate time. They may approach in severity those of a completely obstructive lesion, or they may be sufficiently mild and infrequent as to be overlooked until either an acute episode or diagnostic studies disclose the lesion. Incomplete obstruction may present as urgent a need for surgical intervention as does complete obstruction.

Atresia refers to complete obstruction of the bowel lumen, and stenosis refers to a partial block of luminal contents. Intestinal atresia is common in the duodenum, jejunum, and ileum and rare in the colon. Intestinal atresia accounts for approximately 33% of all cases of neonatal intestinal obstruction. Atresias affect males and females equally.

Blood flow to the obstructed bowel decreases as the bowel dilates. Blood flow is shifted away from the mucosa, with loss of mucosal integrity. Bacteria proliferate in the stagnant bowel, with a predominance of coliforms and anaerobes. The rapid proliferation of bacteria coupled with the loss of mucosal integrity allows bacterial translocation across the bowel wall, resulting in endotoxemia, bacteremia, and sepsis.

The *clinical presentation* of intestinal obstruction varies with the cause, level of obstruction, and time between the obstructing event and the patient's evaluation. The classic symptoms of obstruction include nausea and vomiting, abdominal distention, and obstipation. Obstruction high in the intestinal tract involving the duodenum or proximal jejunum results in large-volume, frequent, bilious emesis. Pain is intermittent and is usually relieved by vomiting. The pain is localized to the epigastrium or periumbilical area, and there is little abdominal distention. Obstruction in the distal small bowel leads to moderate or marked abdominal distention with emesis that is progressively feculent. Pain is usually diffuse over the entire abdomen.

No laboratory studies are diagnostic of obstruction or differentiate simple obstruction from obstruction associated with bowel infarction. Obstruction high in the gastrointestinal tract is often associated with hypochloremic metabolic alkalosis. Marked leukocytosis with or without thrombocytopenia, metabolic acidosis, and hematochezia suggests bowel infarction. Serum amylase and lipase determinations should be made to rule out pancreatitis.

Bowel obstruction is almost always suggested on the basis of history and physical examination. Imaging is used to confirm the diagnosis and localize the area of obstruction. Plain supine and erect or decubitus roentgenograms are the initial studies.

Valuable information on the location of congenital obstructive lesions in the intestine may often be obtained from flat and upright roentgenograms of the abdomen taken without use of contrast media. With completely obstructing lesions, distention of the bowel is noted above the obstruction, and a series of fluid levels with superimposed gas in the distended loops may be observed in the upright or cross-table lateral position. Pneumoperitoneum may be seen, with free air in the subphrenic regions or over the liver in the left lateral decubitus position. Calcification within the peritoneal cavity usually indicates meconium peritonitis. Rarely, obstruction with intraluminal calcification may be associated with rectourinary fistula, colonic aganglionosis, or intestinal atresia. A characteristic ground-glass appearance in the right lower quadrant with trapped bubbles of air within the obstructing meconium may be seen in patients with meconium ileus. Air is usually demonstrable roentgenographically in the stomach of a normal infant immediately after birth; within 1 hr, air may reach the proximal portion of the small intestine and segments of the colon; air may become visible in the distal parts of the colon as early as the 3rd hr or as late as 18 hr. It is difficult to accurately differentiate small from large bowel obstruction in children younger than 2 yr.

Ultrasonography is helpful in identifying pyloric stenosis and possibly volvulus or intussusception and in differentiating pyloric stenosis from other causes of proximal obstruction. Contrast studies of the bowel are indicated when plain films or ultrasonograms fail to identify the source of obstruction. Water-soluble contrast studies avoid the risk of barium contamination of the peritoneum when there is a significant chance of perforation not detected by the presence of pneumoperitoneum on plain films. Water-soluble contrast enemas are useful in diagnosing malrotation, meconium ileus, meconium plug, and intussusception. In meconium ileus, meconium plug, and intussusception, the enema may be diagnostic and relieve the obstruction. Oral or nasogastric contrast is used to identify obstructing lesions in the proximal bowel (atresia, volvulus, malrotation). Water-soluble agents are used if perforation is suspected.

MANAGEMENT. Infants and children with bowel obstruction suffer from intestinal block and loss of fluid and electrolytes. Those with strangulating vascular obstruction may also suffer intestinal ischemia with sepsis and shock. Initial treatment must be directed at fluid resuscitation and stabilizing the patient. Nasogastric decompression usually provides relief of pain and vomiting. After appropriate cultures, broad-spectrum antibiotics are usually started in neonates with bowel obstruction and those with suspected strangulating infarction. Patients with strangulation must have immediate surgical relief before the bowel infarcts, resulting in gangrene and intestinal perforation. Extensive intestinal necrosis results in short-gut syndrome (Chapter 340.7). Nonoperative conservative management is usually limited to children with suspected adhesions or inflammatory strictures that may resolve with nasogastric decompression or anti-inflammatory medications. If clinical signs of improvement are not evident within 12–24 hr, then operative intervention is usually indicated.

330.1 Duodenal Obstruction

Duodenal atresia is thought to arise from failure to recanalize the lumen after the solid phase of intestinal development during the 4th and 5th wk of gestation. The incidence of duodenal atresia is 1/10,000 births and accounts for approximately 25–40% of all intestinal atresias. Half the patients are born prematurely. Duodenal atresia may take several forms, including an intact membrane obstructing the lumen, a short fibrous cord connecting two blind duodenal pouches, or a gap between the nonconnecting ends of the duodenum. An unusual cause of obstruction is a "windsock" web, which is a distensible flap of tissue associated with anomalies of the biliary tract. The membranous form of atresia is most common, with obstruction occurring distal to the ampulla of Vater in the majority of patients. Duodenal obstruction may also be a result of an extrinsic compression such as an annular pancreas or from Ladd bands in patients with malrotation. Down syndrome occurs in 20–30% of patients with duodenal atresia. Other congenital anomalies that are associated with duodenal atresia include malrotation (20%), esophageal atresia (10–20%), congenital heart disease (10–15%), and anorectal and renal anomalies (5%).

CLINICAL MANIFESTATIONS. The hallmark of duodenal obstruction is bilious vomiting without abdominal distention, which is usually noted on the 1st day of life. Peristaltic waves may be visualized early in the disease process. A history of polyhydramnios is present in half the pregnancies and is caused by a failure of absorption of amniotic fluid in the distal intestine. Jaundice is present in one third of the infants. The diagnosis is suggested by the presence of a "double-bubble sign" on plain abdominal radiographs (Fig. 330–1). The appearance is caused by a distended and gas-filled stomach and proximal duodenum. Contrast studies are usually not necessary and may be associated with aspiration if attempted. Contrast studies may occasionally be needed to preclude malrotation and volvulus because intestinal infarction may occur within 6–12 hr if the volvulus is not relieved. Prenatal diagnosis of duodenal atresia is being made with increasing frequency by fetal ultrasonography.

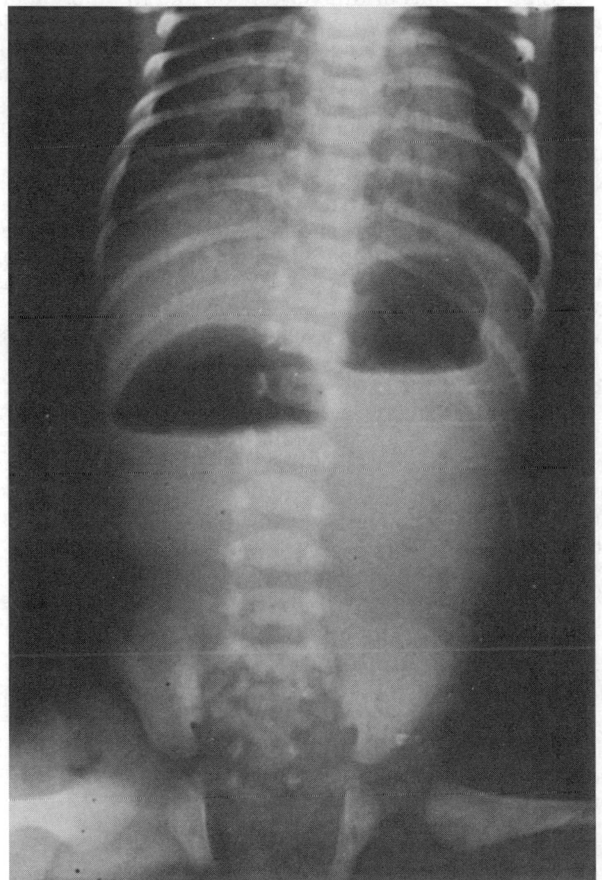

Figure 330–1 Abdominal roentgenogram of a newborn infant held upright. Note the "double bubble" gas shadow above and the absence of gas in the distal bowel in this case of congenital duodenal atresia.

TREATMENT. The initial treatment of infants with duodenal atresia includes naso- or orogastric decompression with intravenous fluid replacement. Echocardiogram and radiology of the chest and spine should be performed to evaluate for associated anomalies. Approximately one third of infants with duodenal atresia have associated life-threatening congenital anomalies. Definitive correction of duodenal atresia is usually postponed to evaluate and treat these life-threatening anomalies.

The usual surgical repair for duodenal atresia is duodenoduodenostomy. The dilated proximal bowel may be tapered in an attempt to improve peristalsis. A gastrostomy tube may be placed to drain the stomach and protect the airway. Intravenous nutritional support or a transanastomotic jejunal tube is needed until infants start to feed orally. The prognosis is primarily dependent on the presence of associated anomalies.

If obstruction is due to Ladd bands with malrotation, an operation is necessary without delay. After division of the abnormal peritoneal folds or bands, the entire large intestine is placed within the left side of the abdomen, after first removing the appendix, with the small bowel on the right—the fetal position of nonrotation. Appendectomy is performed to avoid later misdiagnosis of appendicitis. Malrotation may also coexist with an intrinsic duodenal obstruction, such as a membrane or stenosis; this may be identified by passing a nasogastric balloon-tipped catheter into the jejunum below the site of obstruction, inflating the balloon, and slowly withdrawing the catheter. Annular pancreas is best treated by duodenoduodenostomy without dividing the pancreas, leaving as short a defunctioned loop as possible. Duodenal diaphragmatic obstruction is managed by duodenoplasty. The possibility exists that the common bile duct may open on the diaphragm itself.

330.2 Jejunal and Ileal Atresia and Obstruction

Jejunoileal atresias have been attributed to intrauterine vascular obstructive accidents of the bowel. Four different types of jejunal and ileal atresia are encountered (Fig. 330–2). Type I accounts for 20% of the atresias and is an intraluminal diaphragm that obstructs the lumen while continuity is maintained between the proximal and distal bowel. In type II, a small-diameter solid cord connects the proximal and distal bowel, accounting for about 35% of defects. Type III is divided into two subtypes. Type IIIa accounts for approximately 35% of all atresias and occurs when both ends of the bowel end in blind loops accompanied by a small mesenteric defect. Type IIIb is associated with an extensive mesenteric defect and a loss of the normal blood supply to the distal bowel. The distal ileum coils around the ileocolic artery, from which it derives its entire blood supply, producing an "apple-peel" appearance. This anomaly is associated with prematurity, an unusually short distal ileum, and significant foreshortening of the bowel. Type IV is multiple segments of bowel atresia and accounts for approximately 5% of all bowel atresias. Colon atresia has similarities to jejunoileal atresia but is much less common.

Meconium ileus occurs primarily in newborn infants with cystic fibrosis. Approximately 10% of infants with cystic fibrosis will develop meconium ileus; 80% to 90% of infants presenting with meconium ileus have cystic fibrosis. *In simple meconium ileus,* the last 20–30 cm of ileum is collapsed and filled with pellets of pale-colored stool, above which a dilated loop of varying length appears obstructed by meconium with the consistency of thick syrup or glue. Peristalsis fails to propel

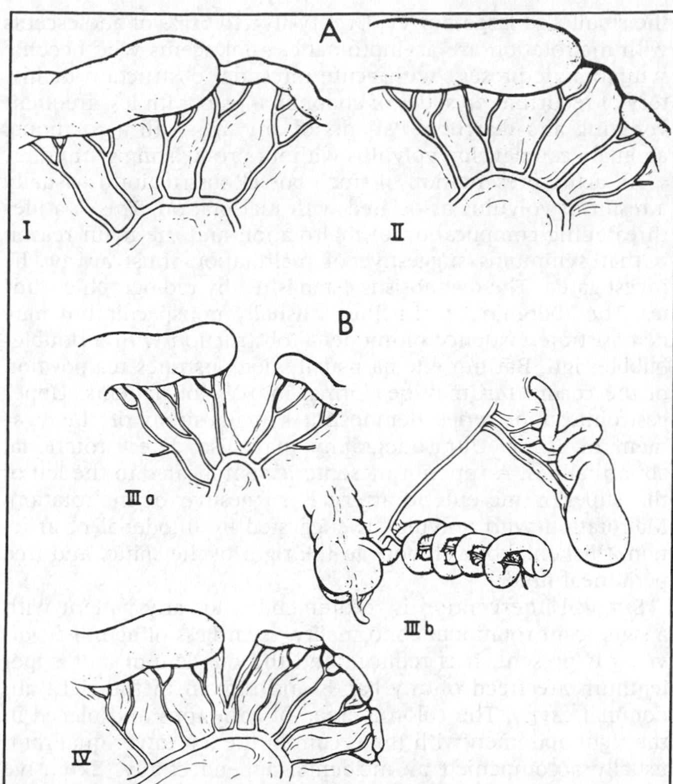

Figure 330–2 *A,* and *B,* Classification of intestinal atresia. Type I: Mucosal obstruction caused by an intraluminal membrane with intact bowel wall and mesentery. Type II: Blind ends are separated by a fibrous cord. Type IIIa: Blind ends are separated by a V-shaped mesenteric defect. Type IIIb: "Apple peel" appearance. Type IV: Multiple atresias. (From Grosfeld J: Jejunoileal atresia and stenosis. *In:* Welch KJ, et al (eds): Pediatric Surgery, 4th ed. Chicago, Year Book Medical Publishers, 1986.)

this very viscid material forward, and it becomes impacted in the ileum. Volvulus, atresia, or perforation of the bowel accompanies *complicated* meconium ileus. Perforation in utero produces meconium peritonitis. Intraperitoneal meconium can cause dense adhesions, leading postnatally to adhesive intestinal obstruction, and may rapidly become calcified.

In 5% of patients with *Hirschsprung disease,* the aganglionic segment involves not only the entire colon but also terminal ileum. This condition causes a dilated small intestine with ganglionated but somewhat hypertrophied walls, a funnel-shaped transitional hypoganglionic zone, and a collapsed distal aganglionic bowel.

CLINICAL MANIFESTATIONS. In contrast to duodenal atresia, extragastrointestinal anomalies are less common in atresias of the remaining intestine. The diagnosis of jejunoileal atresia may be made by prenatal ultrasonograms. Polyhydramnios occurs in 25% of affected patients. Monozygotic twins are at higher risk for atresias than are dizygotic twins or singletons. Premature birth occurs in one third of infants. Most infants become symptomatic during the 1st day of life with abdominal distention and bile-stained emesis or gastric aspirate. Sixty to 75% of the infants fail to pass meconium. Jaundice has been found in one fifth to one third of the patients. Plain radiographs demonstrate many air-fluid levels or peritoneal calcification associated with meconium peritonitis. Contrast studies of the upper and lower bowel delineate the level of obstruction and differentiate atresia from meconium ileus, meconium plug, and Hirschsprung disease.

In meconium ileus, plain films of the abdomen show a typical hazy or ground-glass appearance in the right lower quadrant. Small bubbles of gas trapped in meconium are dispersed within this area. Furthermore, owing to their viscid contents, moderately dilated loops of bowel do not have the air-fluid levels usually seen roentgenographically on the erect projection. If there is meconium peritonitis, patchy calcification may be noted, usually in the flanks. Pneumoperitoneum is most readily seen as free air between the liver and the diaphragm on an upright roentgenogram of the abdomen; if there is a large amount of free air, the entire abdomen may look like a football from distention with air; the ligamentum teres is sometimes clearly visible in the midline.

It is impossible to consistently distinguish small bowel from large bowel by studying plain roentgenograms of the abdomen in newborns and infants. If plain roentgenograms are nonspecific, a water-soluble contrast (Gastrografin, Hypaque) study of the colon may be needed to distinguish small from large intestine obstructions. A small colon, "microcolon," suggests disuse and the presence of obstruction proximal to the ileocecal valve. Water-soluble enemas should be used with caution in the diagnosis and treatment of meconium ileus because their hyperosmolality may result in dehydration, and undue injection pressure may result in perforation.

TREATMENT. Patients with small bowel obstruction should be stable and in adequate fluid and electrolyte balance before operation or roentgenographic attempts at disimpaction unless volvulus is suspected. Infections should be treated with appropriate antibiotics. Prophylactic antibiotics are indicated and should be given intravenously shortly before surgery.

Ileal or jejunal atresia requires resection of the dilated proximal portion of the bowel followed by end-to-end anastomosis. If a simple mucosal diaphragm is present, jejunoplasty or ileoplasty with partial excision of the web is an acceptable alternative to resection. With meconium ileus, an attempt to reduce obstruction with a Gastrografin enema containing polysorbate and a detergent (Tween 80) is usually indicated. The material should be allowed to flow around the pellets of stool in the terminal ileum and into the dilated proximal small bowel containing the obstructing meconium, where it results in an outpouring of fluid from the bowel wall, dilution of the viscid meconium, and diarrhea. The enema may have to be repeated after 8–12 hr. Resection after reduction is not needed if there have been no ischemic complications.

About 50% of patients with simple meconium ileus do not adequately respond to water-soluble enemas and need laparotomy. Operative management is indicated when the obstruction cannot be relieved by repeated attempts at nonoperative management and for infants with complicated meconium ileus. The extent of surgical intervention depends on the degree of pathology. In simple meconium ileus, the plug can be relieved by manipulation or direct enteral irrigation with a *N*-acetylcysteine following an enterotomy. In complicated cases, bowel resection, peritoneal lavage, abdominal drainage, and stoma formation may be necessary. Total parenteral nutrition will be required.

330.3 Malrotation

Malrotation is incomplete rotation of the intestine during fetal development. The gut starts as a straight tube from stomach to rectum. The midbowel (distal duodenum to midtransverse colon) begins to elongate and progressively protrudes into the umbilical cord until it lies totally outside the confines of the abdominal cavity. As the developing bowel rotates in and out of the abdominal cavity, the superior mesenteric artery, which supplies blood to this section of gut, acts as an axis. The duodenum, on re-entering the abdominal cavity, moves to the region of the ligament of Treitz, and the colon that follows is directed to the left upper quadrant. The cecum subsequently rotates counterclockwise within the abdominal cavity and comes to lie in the right lower quadrant. The duodenum becomes fixed to the posterior abdominal wall before the colon is completely rotated. After rotation, the right and left colon and the mesenteric root become fixed to the posterior abdomen. These attachments provide a broad base of support to the mesentery and the superior mesenteric artery, thus preventing twisting of the mesenteric root and kinking of the vascular supply. Abdominal rotation and attachment are completed by 3 mo gestation.

Nonrotation occurs when the bowel fails to rotate after it returns to the abdominal cavity. The first and second portions of the duodenum are in their normal position, but the remainder of the duodenum, jejunum, and ileum occupy the right side of the abdomen while the colon is located on the left. Malrotation and nonrotation are associated with abdominal heterotaxia and the asplenia-polysplenia congenital heart malformation syndrome anomalad (Chapter 438.11).

The most common type of malrotation involves failure of the cecum to move into the right lower quadrant (Fig. 330–3). The usual location of the cecum is in the subhepatic area. Failure of the cecum to rotate properly is associated with failure to form the normal broad-based adherence to the posterior abdominal wall. The mesentery including the superior mesenteric artery is tethered by a narrow stalk, which may twist around itself, producing a midgut volvulus. In addition, bands of tissue (Ladd bands) may extend from the cecum to the right upper quadrant, crossing and possibly obstructing the duodenum.

CLINICAL MANIFESTATIONS. The majority of patients present within the 1st yr of life with symptoms of acute or chronic obstruction. Infants often present within the 1st wk of life with bilious emesis and acute bowel obstruction. Older infants present with episodes of recurrent abdominal pain that may mimic colic. Malrotation in older children may present with recurrent episodes of vomiting, abdominal pain, or both. Patients occasionally present with malabsorption or protein-losing enteropathy associated with bacterial overgrowth. Symptoms are caused by intermittent volvulus or duodenal compression by Ladd bands or other adhesive bands affecting the small and large bowel. Twenty-five to 50% of adolescents with malrotation are asymptomatic. Adolescents who become symptomatic present with acute intestinal obstruction or history of recurrent episodes of abdominal pain with less frequent vomiting and diarrhea. Patients of any age with a rotational anomaly can develop volvulus without pre-existing symptoms.

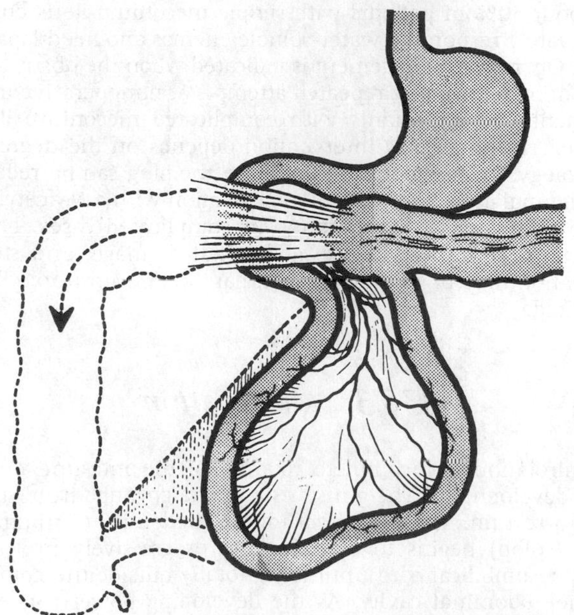

Figure 330–3 The mechanism of intestinal obstruction with incomplete rotation of the midgut (malrotation). The *dotted lines* show the course the cecum should have taken. Failure to rotate has left obstructing bands across the duodenum, and a narrow pedicle for the midgut loop, making it susceptible to volvulus. (From Nixon HH, O'Donnell B: The Essentials of Pediatric Surgery. Philadelphia, JB Lippincott, 1961.)

An acute presentation of small bowel obstruction is usually a result of volvulus associated with malrotation. This is a life-threatening complication of malrotation and the main reason is that symptoms suggestive of malrotation must always be investigated. The diagnosis is established by radiographic studies. The abdominal plain film is usually nonspecific but may demonstrate evidence of duodenal obstruction with a double-bubble sign. Barium enema usually demonstrates malposition of the cecum but may be normal in 10% of patients. Upper gastrointestinal series demonstrates malposition of the ligament of Treitz. Ultrasonography may also detect rotational abnormalities. A superior mesenteric vein located to the left of the superior mesenteric artery is suggestive of malrotation. Malrotation with volvulus is suggested by duodenal obstruction, thickened bowel loops to the right of the spine, and free peritoneal fluid.

Surgical intervention is recommended for any patient with a significant rotational abnormality, regardless of age. If a volvulus is present, it is reduced and the duodenum and upper jejunum are freed of any bands and remain in the right abdominal cavity. The colon is freed of adhesions and placed in the right abdomen with the cecum in the left lower quadrant, usually accompanied by incidental appendectomy. Extensive intestinal ischemia from volvulus produces the short-gut syndrome (Chapter 340.7). Persistent symptoms after repair of malrotation should suggest a pseudo-obstruction–like motility disorder.

Intestinal Atresia

Cragan JD, Martin ML, Waters GD, et al: Increased risk of small intestinal atresia among twins in the United States. Arch Pediatr Adolesc Med 148:733, 1994.

Davenport M: ABC of general surgery in children. Surgically correctable causes of vomiting in infancy. Br Med J 312:236, 1996.

Doolin EJ: Motility abnormality in intestinal atresia. J Pediatr Surg 22:320, 1987.

Duffy LF: Malformation of the gut. Pediatr Rev 13:50, 1992.

Kays DW: Surgical conditions of the neonatal intestinal tract. Clin Perinatol 23:353, 1996.

Kimble RM, Harding J, Kolbe A: Additional congenital anomalies in babies with gut atresia or stenosis: When to investigate, and which investigation. [See comments.] Pediatr Surg Int 12:565, 1997.

Mikaelsson C, Arnbjornsson E, Kullendorff CM: Membranous duodenal stenosis. Acta Paediatr 86:953, 1997.

Smith GHH, Glasson M: Intestinal atresia: Factors affecting survival. Aust N Z J Surg 59:151, 1989.

Malrotation

Devane SP, Coombes R, Smith VV, et al: Persistent gastrointestinal symptoms after correction of malrotation. Arch Dis Child 67:218, 1992.

Ford EG, Senac MO, Srikanth MS, et al: Malrotation of the intestine in children. Ann Surg 215:172, 1992.

Long FR, Kramer SS, Markowitz RI, et al: Radiographic patterns of intestinal malrotation in children. Radiographics 16:547, discussion 556, 1996.

Maxson RT, Franklin PA, Wagner CW: Malrotation in the older child: Surgical management, treatment, and outcome. Am Surg 61:135, 1995.

Rescorla FJ, Shedd FJ, Grosfeld JL, et al: Anomalies of intestinal rotation in childhood: Analysis of 447 cases. Surgery 108:710, 1990.

Seashore JH, Touloukian RJ: Midgut volvulus: An ever-present threat. Arch Pediatr Adolesc Med 148:43, 1994.

Weinberger E, Winters WD, Liddell RM, et al: Sonographic diagnosis of intestinal malrotation in infants: Importance of the relative positions of the superior mesenteric vein and artery. AJR 159:825, 1992.

Meconium Ileus

Kao SC, Franken EA Jr: Nonoperative treatment of simple meconium ileus: A survey of the Society for Pediatric Radiology. Pediatr Radiol 25:97, 1995.

Khoshoo V, Udall JN Jr: Meconium ileus equivalent in children and adults. Am J Gastroenterol 89:153, 1994.

Murshed R, Spitz L, Kiely E, et al: Meconium ileus: A ten-year review of thirty-six patients. Eur J Pediatr Surg 7:275, 1997.

Neal MR, Seibert JJ, Vanderzalm T, et al: Neonatal ultrasonography to distinguish between meconium ileus and ileal atresia. J Ultrasound Med 16:263, quiz 267, 1997.

Ziegler MM: Meconium ileus. Curr Probl Surg 31:731, 1994.

CHAPTER 331

Intestinal Duplications, Meckel Diverticulum, and Other Remnants of the Omphalomesenteric Duct

Robert Wyllie

331.1 Intestinal Duplication

Duplications of the intestinal tract are rare anomalies that consist of well-formed tubular or spherical structures firmly attached to the intestine with a common blood supply. The lining of the duplications resembles that of the gastrointestinal (GI) tract. Duplications are located on the mesenteric border and may communicate with the intestinal lumen. Duplications can be classified into three categories: localized duplications, duplications associated with spinal cord defects and vertebral malformations, and duplications of the colon. Occasionally (10–15%) found are multiple duplications.

Localized duplications may occur in any area of the GI tract but are most common in the ileum and jejunum. They are usually cystic or tubular structures within the wall of the bowel. The cause is unknown, but their development has been attributed to defects in recanalization of the intestinal lumen after the solid stage of embryologic development. Duplication of the intestine occurring in association with vertebral and spinal cord anomalies (hemivertebra, anterior spina bifida, band connection between lesion and cervical or thoracic spine) is thought to arise from splitting of the notochord in the developing embryo. Duplication of the colon is usually associated with anomalies of the urinary tract and genitals. Duplication of the entire colon, rectum, anus, and terminal ileum may occur. The defects are thought to be secondary to caudal twinning with duplication of the hindgut, genital, and lower urinary tracts.

CLINICAL MANIFESTATIONS. Symptoms depend on the size, location, and mucosal lining. Duplications may cause bowel obstruction by compressing the adjacent intestinal lumen, or they may act as the lead point of an intussusception or a site for a volvulus. If they are lined by acid-secreting mucosa, they may cause ulceration, perforation, and hemorrhage of the adjacent bowel. Patients may present with abdominal pain, vomiting, palpable mass, or acute GI hemorrhage. Intestinal duplications in the thorax (neuroenteric cysts) may present with respiratory distress. Duplications of the lower bowel may cause constipation or diarrhea or be associated with recurrent prolapse of the rectum.

The *diagnosis* is suspected on the basis of the history and physical examination. Radiologic studies such as barium studies, ultrasonography, CT, and MRI are helpful but usually nonspecific, demonstrating cystic structures or mass effects. Radioisotope technetium scanning may localize ectopic gastric mucosa. The *treatment* of duplications is surgical resection and management of associated defects.

331.2 Meckel Diverticulum and Other Remnants of the Omphalomesenteric Duct

A Meckel diverticulum is a remnant of the embryonic yolk sac, which may also be referred to as the omphalomesenteric duct or vitelline duct. The omphalomesenteric duct connects the yolk sac to the gut in a developing embryo and provides nutrition until the placenta is established. Between the 5th and 7th wk of gestation, the duct attenuates and separates from the intestine. Just before this involution, the epithelium of the yolk sac develops a lining similar to that of the stomach. Partial or complete failure of involution of the omphalomesenteric duct results in various residual structures. Meckel diverticulum is the most common of these structures and is the most frequent congenital GI anomaly, occurring in 2–3% of all infants. A typical Meckel diverticulum is a 3- to 6-cm outpouching of the ileum along the antimesenteric border approximately 50–75 cm from the ileocecal valve (Fig. 331–1). The distance from the ileocecal valve depends on the age of the patient. Other omphalomesenteric duct remnants occur infrequently, including a persistently patent duct, a solid cord, or a cord with a central cyst or a diverticulum associated with a persistent cord between the diverticulum and the umbilicus.

CLINICAL MANIFESTATIONS. Symptoms of a Meckel diverticulum usually arise within the 1st 2 yr of life, but initial symptoms are common during the 1st decade. The majority of symptomatic Meckel diverticula are lined by an ectopic mucosa, including an acid-secreting mucosa, that causes intermittent painless rectal bleeding by ulceration of the adjacent normal ileal mucosa. Unlike the upper duodenal mucosa, the acid is not neutralized by pancreatic bicarbonate.

The stool is typically described as brick colored or currant jelly colored. Bleeding may cause significant anemia but is usually self-limited because of contraction of the splanchnic vessels as patients become hypovolemic. Bleeding from a Meckel diverticulum can also be less dramatic, with melanotic stools.

Less often, a Meckel diverticulum may be associated with partial or complete bowel obstruction. The most common mechanism of obstruction occurs when the diverticulum acts as the lead point of an intussusception. This presentation is more common in older male children. Other causes of obstruction may result from intraperitoneal bands connecting residual omphalomesenteric duct remnants to the ileum and umbilicus.

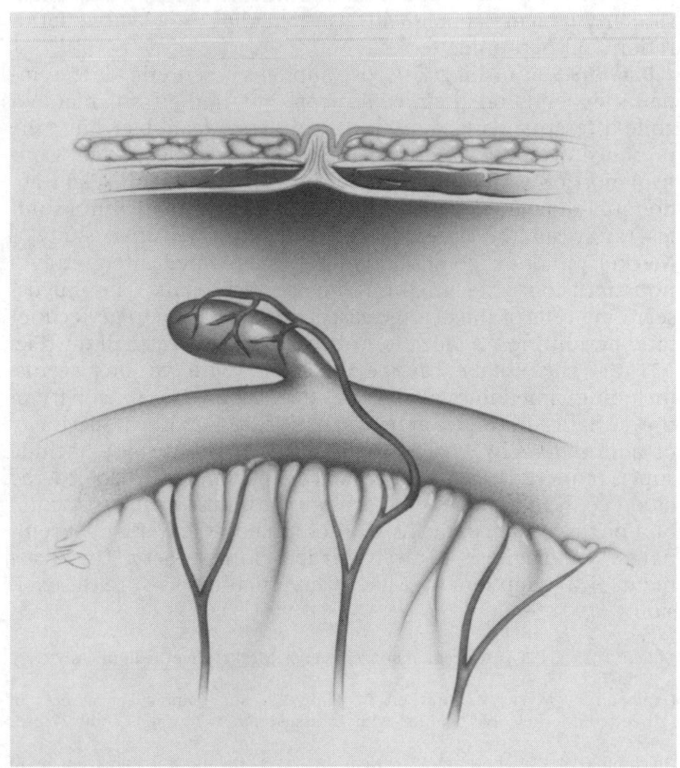

Figure 331–1 Typical Meckel diverticulum located on the antimesenteric border.

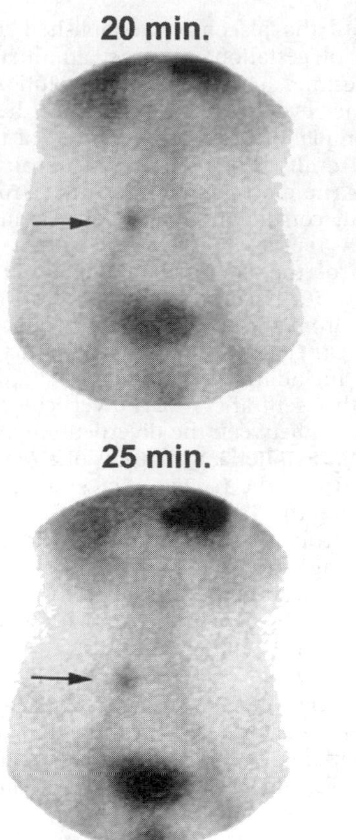

Figure 331–2 Meckel scan demonstrating accumulation of technetium in the stomach superior bladder (inferior) and in the acid-secreting mucosa of a Meckel diverticulum.

These bands cause obstruction by internal herniation or volvulus of the small bowel around the band. A Meckel diverticulum may occasionally become inflamed (diverticulitis) and present similarly to acute appendicitis. Diverticulitis may lead to perforation and peritonitis.

DIAGNOSIS. The diagnosis of omphalomesenteric duct remnants depends on their clinical presentation. If an infant or child presents with significant painless rectal bleeding, the presence of a Meckel diverticulum should be suspected. Confirmation of a Meckel diverticulum can be difficult. Plain abdominal radiographs are of no value, and routine barium studies rarely fill the diverticulum. The most sensitive study is Meckel radionuclide scan, which is performed after intravenous infusion of technetium-99m pertechnetate. The mucus-secreting cells of the ectopic gastric mucosa take up pertechnetate, permitting visualization of the Meckel diverticulum (Fig. 331–2). The uptake can be enhanced with various agents, including cimetidine, glucagon, and gastrin. The sensitivity of the enhanced scan is approximately 85%, with a specificity of approximately 95%. Other methods of detection include superior mesenteric angiography and technetium-labeled red blood cells. In patients who present with intestinal obstruction or a picture of appendicitis with omphalomesenteric duct remnants, the diagnosis is rarely made before surgery. The treatment of a symptomatic Meckel diverticulum is surgical excision.

Cullen JJ, Kelly KA: Current management of Meckel diverticulum. Adv Surg 29:207, 1996.

Daneman A, Myers M, Shuckett B, Alton DJ: Sonographic appearances of inverted Meckel diverticulum with intussusception. Pediatr Radiol 27:295, 1997.

Holcomb GW III, Gheissari A, O'Neill JA Jr, et al: Surgical management of alimentary tract duplications. Ann Surg 209:167, 1989.

Moore TC: Omphalomesenteric duct malformations. Semin Pediatr Surg 5:116, 1996.

Rossi P, Gourtsoyiannis N, Bezzi M, et al: Meckel diverticulum: Imaging diagnosis. [See comments.] AJR Am J Roentgenol 166:567, 1996.

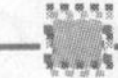

CHAPTER 332
Motility Disorders and Hirschsprung Disease

Robert Wyllie

332.1 Chronic Intestinal Pseudo-Obstruction

Chronic intestinal pseudo-obstruction comprises a group of disorders characterized by signs and symptoms of intestinal obstruction in the absence of an anatomic lesion. Pseudo-obstruction may occur as a primary disease or may be secondary to a large number of conditions that may transiently or permanently alter bowel motility. Pseudo-obstruction represents a wide spectrum of pathologic disorders from abnormal myoelectric activity to abnormalities of the nerves (intestinal neuropathy) or musculature (intestinal myopathy) of the gut. The organs involved may include the entire gastrointestinal (GI) tract or may be limited to certain components such as the stomach or colon. The distinctive pathologic abnormalities are considered together because of their clinical similarities.

Most congenital forms of pseudo-obstruction occur sporadically. A few clusters of autosomal dominant or recessive individuals have been reported as having cases associated with abnormal gut muscle or nerves. Patients with autosomal dominant forms of pseudo-obstruction have variable expressions of the disease. Acquired pseudo-obstruction may follow episodes of acute gastroenteritis presumably resulting in injury to the myenteric plexus.

In congenital pseudo-obstruction, abnormalities of the muscle or nerves can be demonstrated in the majority of cases in which biopsy material is obtained. In muscular disease, the outer longitudinal muscle layer is replaced by fibrous material. In neuronal disease, there may be disorganized or hypo- or hyperganglionosis.

CLINICAL MANIFESTATIONS. More than half the children with congenital pseudo-obstruction experience symptoms within the first few months of life. Two thirds of the infants presenting within the first few days of life are born prematurely, and about 40% have malrotation of the intestine. Seventy-five per cent of the children experience symptoms during the first year of life, and the remainder become symptomatic in the next several years. The most common symptoms are abdominal distention and vomiting, which are present in 75% of affected infants. Constipation, growth failure, and abdominal pain occur in approximately 60% of patients, and diarrhea occurs in 30–40%. The symptoms wax and wane in the majority of the patients; poor nutrition and intercurrent illness tend to exacerbate symptoms.

The diagnosis of pseudo-obstruction is based on the presence of compatible symptoms in the absence of anatomic obstruction. Plain abdominal radiographs demonstrate air-fluid levels in the small intestine. Neonates with evidence of obstruction at birth have a microcolon. Contrast studies demonstrate slow passage of barium, and consideration should be given to using water-soluble agents.

Other studies may provide information on the underlying pathophysiology. Esophageal motility is abnormal in about half the patients. Antroduodenal motility and gastric emptying studies have abnormal results if the upper gut is involved and can be used to distinguish neuropathic and myopathic disease. Colonic motility is abnormal if the colon is involved. Anorectal motility is normal and differentiates pseudo-obstruction from Hirschsprung disease. Intestinal biopsy is not indicated to establish the diagnosis and, if performed, may raise the possibility of future adhesive obstruction with exacerbation of symptoms.

The *differential diagnosis* includes Hirschsprung disease, other causes of mechanical obstruction, psychogenic constipation, neurogenic bladder, and superior mesenteric artery syndrome. Secondary causes of ileus or pseudo-obstruction, such as hypothyroidism, narcotics, scleroderma, Chagas disease, hypokalemia, diabetic neuropathy, amyloidosis, porphyria, angioneurotic edema, and radiation must be excluded.

TREATMENT. Nutritional support is the mainstay of treatment for pseudo-obstruction. Approximately 30–50% require partial or complete parenteral nutrition. Some patients can be treated with intermittent enteral supplementation, whereas others may maintain themselves on selective oral diets. Prokinetic drugs are useful in promoting motility in a small number of children. Cisapride (a 5-hydroxytryptamine receptor antagonist) and erythromycin (a motilin receptor agonist) may enhance gastric emptying and proximal small bowel motility. Isolated gastroparesis may follow episodes of viral gastroenteritis and spontaneously resolves usually within 6–24 mo.

Symptomatic small bowel bacterial overgrowth is usually treated with oral antibiotics. Bacterial overgrowth may be associated with steatorrhea and malabsorption. Antibiotics should be used judiciously, however, because they may lead to the emergence of drug-resistant bacteria. Constipation is treated with enemas, suppositories, or stool softeners. Patients with acid peptic symptoms are treated with acid suppressors (Chapter 336). Surgery, except for gastrostomy or placement of jejunostomy tubes, is generally not helpful. Colectomy in a selective group of children with abnormalities confined to the colon may be curative. Occasional patients with intractable symptoms may need total bowel resection. In the future, bowel transplantation or electromechanical pacing may benefit selected patients, depending on their underlying motility abnormality.

Di Lorenzo C, Flores AF, Buie T, et al: Intestinal motility and jejunal feeding in children with chronic intestinal pseudo-obstruction. Gastroenterology 108:1379, 1995.

Di Lorenzo C, Flores AF, Reddy SN, et al: Colonic manometry in children with chronic intestinal pseudo-obstruction. Gut 34:803, 1993.

Fell JM, Smith VV, Milla PJ: Infantile chronic idiopathic intestinal pseudo-obstruction: The role of small intestinal manometry as a diagnostic tool and prognostic indicator. Gut 39:306, 1996.

Rudolph CD, Hyman PE, Altschuler SM, et al: Diagnosis and treatment of chronic intestinal pseudo-obstruction in children: Report of consensus workshop. [See comments.] J Pediatr Gastroenterol Nutr 24:102, 1997.

Sigurdsson L, Flores A, Putnam PE, et al: Postviral gastroparesis: Presentation, treatment, and outcome. J Pediatr 131:751, 1997.

332.2 Superior Mesenteric Artery Syndrome (Wilkie Syndrome, Cast Syndrome, Arteriomesenteric Duodenal Compression Syndrome)

The existence of the superior mesenteric artery syndrome is debated, with proponents describing an extrinsic compression of the duodenum in children after rapid weight loss and in a supine position. The compression is thought to occur as the mesentery loses its fat and allows the superior mesenteric artery to collapse on the duodenum, compressing it between the superior mesenteric artery anteriorly and the aorta posteriorly. Alternatively, the cause may be that the loss of supporting fat in the second and third portions of the duodenum allows the duodenum to collapse against the spine.

The classic example is an adolescent who starts vomiting after application of a body cast for orthopedic surgery. Other associated factors include anorexia, prolonged bed rest, weight loss, abdominal surgery, and exaggerated lumbar lordosis. The *diagnosis* is established radiologically with the demonstration of a cutoff of the duodenum just to the right of the midline. The duodenal obstruction may be accompanied by proximal duodenal and gastric dilatation.

Treatment of the acute syndrome involves relief of the obstruction and improved nutrition to alter the anatomic relationships of the duodenum with surrounding structures. Positioning patients in a lateral or prone position shifts the duodenum away from potential obstructing structures and may allow resumption of oral intake. Prokinetic agents such as cisapride may be helpful. If repositioning is unsuccessful in relieving symptoms, a nasojejunal tube may be placed past the point of obstruction and feedings begun. Some patients require total parenteral nutrition to replete lost body fat, and occasional patients may need surgical intervention.

332.3 Congenital Aganglionic Megacolon (Hirschsprung Disease)

Hirschsprung disease or congenital aganglionic megacolon is caused by abnormal innervation of the bowel, beginning in the internal anal sphincter and extending proximally to involve a variable length of gut. Hirschsprung disease is the most common cause of lower intestinal obstruction in neonates, with an overall incidence of 1/5,000 live births. Males are affected more often than females (4:1), the disease is uncommon among preterm infants, and there is an increased familial incidence in long segment disease. Hirschsprung disease may be associated with other congenital defects including Down, Laurence Moon Bardet-Biedl, and Waardenburg syndromes and cardiovascular abnormalities.

PATHOLOGY. Hirschsprung disease is result of an absence of ganglion cells in the bowel wall, extending proximally and continuously from the anus for a variable distance. The absence of neural innervation is a consequence of an arrest of neuroblast migration from the proximal to distal bowel. The aganglionic segment is limited to the rectosigmoid in 75% of patients; in 10% the entire colon lacks ganglion cells. Increased nerve endings in the aganglionic bowel result in high concentrations of acetylcholinesterase. Observed histologically is an absence of Meissner and Auerbach plexus and hypertrophied nerve bundles with high concentrations of acetylcholinesterase between the muscular layers and in the submucosa. The disorder, one of the neural crestopathies, has been reproduced in animals by a knockout of the endothelin B receptor.

CLINICAL MANIFESTATIONS. The clinical symptoms of Hirschsprung disease usually begin at birth with the delayed passage of meconium. Ninety-nine per cent of full-term infants pass meconium within 48 hr of birth. Hirschsprung disease should be suspected in any full-term infant (the disease is unusual in preterm infants) with delayed passage of stool. Some infants pass meconium normally but subsequently present with a history of chronic constipation. Failure to thrive, with hypoproteinemia from a protein-losing enteropathy, is a less common presentation now that Hirschsprung disease is usually recognized early in the course of the illness. Breast-fed infants may not suffer as severe a disease as formula-fed infants.

Failure to pass stool leads to dilatation of the proximal bowel and abdominal distention. As the bowel dilates, intraluminal

TABLE 332–1 Distinguishing Features of Hirschsprung Disease and Functional Constipation

Variable	Functional (Acquired)	Hirschsprung Disease
History		
Onset of constipation	After 2 yr of age	At birth
Encopresis	Common	Very rare
Failure to thrive	Uncommon	Possible
Enterocolitis	None	Possible
Forced bowel training	Usual	None
Examination		
Abdominal distention	Rare	Common
Poor weight gain	Rare	Common
Anal tone	Normal	Normal
Rectal examination	Stool in ampulla	Ampulla empty
Malnutrition	None	Possible
Laboratory		
Anorectal manometry	Distention of the rectum causes relaxation of the internal sphincter	No sphincter relaxation or paradoxical increase in pressure
Rectal biopsy	Normal	No ganglion cells Increased acetylcholinesterase staining
Barium enema	Massive amounts of stool, no transition zone	Transition zone, delayed evacuation (>24 hr)

pressure increases, resulting in decreased blood flow and deterioration of the mucosal barrier. Stasis allows proliferation of bacteria, which may lead to enterocolitis (*Clostridium difficile, Staphylococcus aureus,* anaerobes, coliforms) with associated sepsis and signs of bowel obstruction. Early recognition of Hirschsprung disease before the onset of enterocolitis is essential in reducing morbidity and mortality.

Hirschsprung disease in older patients must be distinguished from other causes of abdominal distention and chronic constipation (Table 332–1; Fig. 332–1). The history often reveals increasing difficulty with the passage of stools, starting in the 1st few weeks of life. A large fecal mass is palpable in the left lower abdomen, but on rectal examination the rectum is usually empty of feces. The stools, when passed, may consist of small pellets, may be ribbon-like, or may have a fluid consistency; the large stools and fecal soiling of patients with functional constipation are absent. In infancy, Hirschsprung disease must be differentiated from meconium plug syndrome, meconium ileus, and intestinal atresia.

Rectal examination demonstrates normal anal tone and is usually followed by an explosive discharge of foul-smelling feces and gas. Intermittent attacks of intestinal obstruction from retained feces may be associated with pain and fever.

DIAGNOSIS. Rectal manometry and rectal suction biopsy are the easiest and most reliable indicators of Hirschsprung disease. Anorectal manometry measures the pressure of the internal anal sphincter while a balloon is distended in the rectum. In normal individuals, rectal distention initiates a reflex decline in internal sphincter pressure. In patients with Hirschsprung disease, the pressure fails to drop or there is a paradoxical rise in pressure with rectal distention. The accuracy of this diagnostic test is more than 90%, but it is technically difficult in young infants. A normal response in the course of manometric evaluation precludes a diagnosis of Hirschsprung disease; an equivocal or paradoxical response requires a rectal biopsy.

Rectal suction biopsies should be performed no closer than 2 cm to the dentate line to avoid the normal area of hypoganglionosis at the anal verge. The biopsy material should contain an adequate sample of submucosa to evaluate for the presence of ganglion cells. The biopsy specimen can be stained for acetylcholinesterase, which may facilitate interpretation. Patients with aganglionosis demonstrate a large number of hypertrophied nerve bundles that stain positively for acetylcholinesterase with an absence of ganglion cells.

The roentgenographic diagnosis of Hirschsprung disease is based on the presence of a transition zone between normal dilated proximal colon and a smaller caliber obstructed distal colon caused by the nonrelaxation of the aganglionic bowel. The transition zone is not usually present before 1–2 wk of age and on a radiograph is a funnel-shaped area of intestine between the proximal dilated colon and the constricted distal bowel. Radiologic evaluation should be performed without preparation to prevent transient dilatation of the aganglionic segment. Twenty-four-hour delayed films are helpful (Fig.

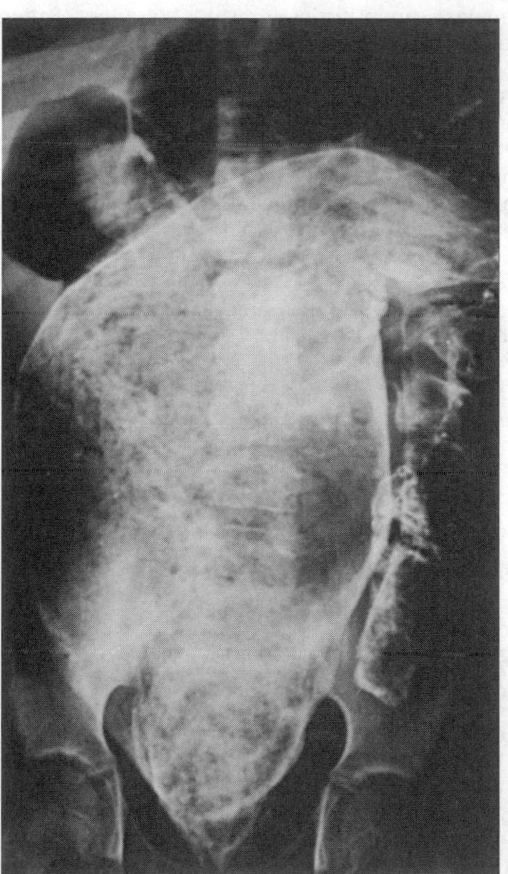

Figure 332–1 Barium enema in a 14-yr-old boy with severe constipation. The enormous dilatation of the rectum and distal colon is typical of acquired functional megacolon.

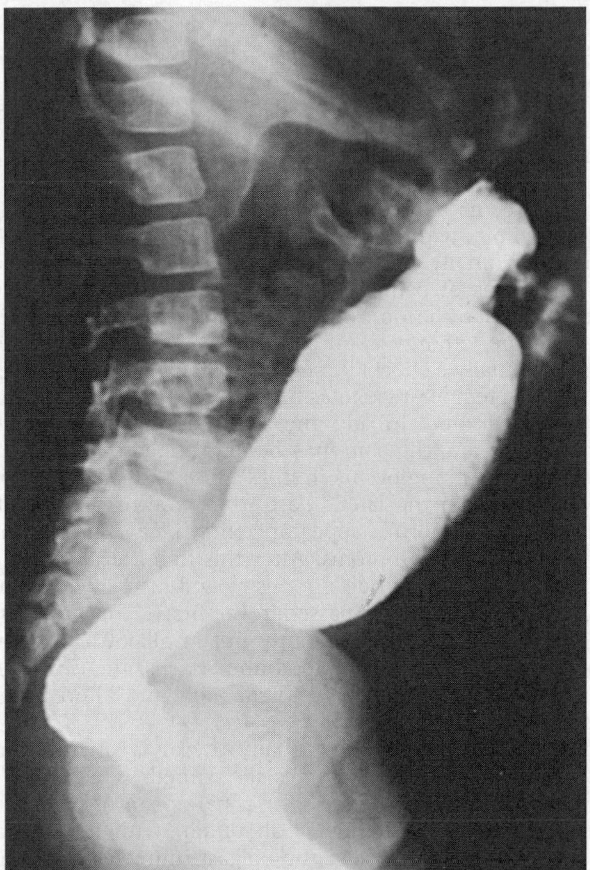

Figure 332–2 Lateral view of a barium enema in a 3-yr-old girl with Hirschsprung disease. The aganglionic distal segment is narrow, with distended normal ganglionic bowel above it.

332–2). If significant barium is still present in the colon, it increases the suspicion of Hirschsprung disease even if a transition zone is not identified. Barium enema examination is useful in determining the extent of aganglionosis before surgery and in evaluating other diseases that present with lower bowel obstruction in a neonate. Full-thickness rectal biopsy may be performed at the time of surgery to confirm the diagnosis and level of involvement.

TREATMENT. Once the diagnosis is established, the definitive treatment is operative intervention. The operative options are to perform a definitive procedure as soon as the diagnosis is established or perform a temporary colostomy and wait until the infant is 6–12 mo old to perform definitive repair. There are three basic surgical options. The first successful surgical procedure, described by Swenson, was to excise the aganglionic segment and anastomose the normal proximal bowel to the rectum 1–2 cm above the dentate line. The operation is technically difficult and led to the development of two other procedures. Duhamel described a procedure to create a neorectum, bringing down normally innervated bowel behind the aganglionic rectum. The neorectum created in this procedure has an anterior aganglionic half with normal sensation and a posterior ganglionic half with normal propulsion. The endorectal pull-through procedure described by Boley involves stripping the mucosa from the aganglionic rectum and bringing normally innervated colon through the residual muscular cuff, thus bypassing the abnormal bowel from within.

In ultrashort segmental Hirschsprung disease, the aganglionic segment is limited to the internal sphincter. The clinical symptoms are similar to those of children with functional constipation. Ganglion cells may be present on rectal suction biopsy, but the rectal motility will be abnormal. Excision of a strip of rectal muscle, including the internal anal sphincter, is diagnostic and therapeutic.

Long-segment Hirschsprung disease involving the entire colon and part of the small bowel represents a difficult problem. Rectal motility studies and rectal suction biopsy demonstrate findings of Hirschsprung disease, but radiologic studies are difficult to interpret because no colonic transition zone can be identified. The extent of aganglionosis can be determined accurately by biopsy at the time of laparotomy.

When the entire colon is aganglionic, often together with a length of terminal ileum, ileal-anal anastomosis is the treatment of choice, preserving part of the aganglionic colon to facilitate water absorption, which helps the stools to become firm.

The prognosis of surgically treated Hirschsprung disease is generally satisfactory; the great majority of patients achieve fecal continence. Postoperative problems include recurrent enterocolitis, stricture, prolapse, perianal abscesses, and fecal soiling.

Catto-Smith AG, Coffey CM, Nolan TM, et al: Fecal incontinence after the surgical treatment of Hirschsprung disease. J Pediatr 127:954, 1995.
Diseth TH, Bjornland K, Novik TS, et al: Bowel function, mental health, and psychosocial function in adolescents with Hirschsprung disease. Arch Dis Child 76:100, 1997.
Fonkalsrud EW: Long-term results after colectomy and ileoanal pull-through procedure in children. Arch Surg 131:881; discussion 885, 1996.
O'Donovan AN, Habra G, Somers S, et al: Diagnosis of Hirschsprung disease. AJR Am J Roentgenol 167:517, 1996.
Skinner MA: Hirschsprung disease. Curr Probl Surg 33:389, 1996.

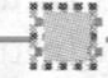

CHAPTER 333
Ileus, Adhesions, Intussusception, and Closed-Loop Obstructions

Robert Wyllie

333.1 Ileus

Ileus is the failure of intestinal peristalsis without evidence of mechanical obstruction. Lack of normal gut motility interferes with aboral movement of intestinal contents and in children is most often associated with abdominal surgery or infection (pneumonia, gastroenteritis, peritonitis). Ileus also accompanies metabolic abnormalities, such as uremia, hypokalemia, or acidosis, and occurs with administration of certain drugs such as vincristine. Ileus may also occur when antimotility drugs such as loperamide are used during episodes of gastroenteritis.

Ileus presents with increasing abdominal distention and initially minimal pain. Pain increases with increasing distention. Bowel sounds are minimal or absent, in contrast to early mechanical obstruction, when they are hyperactive. Plain abdominal radiographs demonstrate many air-fluid levels throughout the abdomen. Serial radiographs usually do not show progressive distention as they do in mechanical obstruction. Contrast radiographs, if performed, demonstrate slow movement of the barium through a patent lumen.

Treatment of ileus involves correction of the underlying abnormality. Nasogastric decompression is used if abdominal distention is associated with pain or to relieve recurrent vomiting. Ileus after abdominal surgical procedures usually results in return of normal intestinal motility within 24–72 hr. Prokinetic agents such as cisapride or erythromycin may stimulate the return of normal bowel motility and be of assistance to children with prolonged ileus.

333.2 Adhesions

Adhesions are fibrous bands of tissue that are a common cause of postoperative small bowel obstruction after abdominal surgery. The risk of forming an adhesion that causes obstructive symptoms in childhood has not been well studied but seems to occur in 2–3% of patients after abdominal surgery. The majority of obstructions are associated with single adhesions and can occur anytime after the 2nd postoperative week.

The *diagnosis* is suspected in patients with abdominal pain and a history of intraperitoneal surgery. Nausea and vomiting quickly follow the development of pain. Bowel sounds initially are hyperactive, and the abdomen is flat. The bowel subsequently dilates, producing abdominal distention in most patients, and bowel sounds disappear. Fever and leukocytosis are suggestive of necrotic bowel and peritonitis. Plain roentgenographs demonstrate obstructive features, and contrast studies may be needed to define the cause of obstruction.

Patients with suspected obstruction should have nasogastric decompression, intravenous fluid resuscitation, and broad-spectrum antibiotics in anticipation of surgery. Nonoperative intervention is contraindicated unless a patient is stable with clear evidence of clinical improvement.

333.3 Intussusception

Intussusception occurs when a portion of the alimentary tract is telescoped into a segment just caudad to it. It is the most common cause of intestinal obstruction between 3 mo and 6 yr of age. Sixty per cent of patients are younger than 1 yr, and 80% of the cases occur before 24 mo; it is rare in neonates. The incidence varies from 1–4/1,000 live births. The male:female ratio is 4:1. A few intussusceptions reduce spontaneously or become autoamputated; if left untreated, most would lead to death.

ETIOLOGY AND EPIDEMIOLOGY. The cause of most intussusceptions is unknown. The seasonal incidence has peaks in spring and autumn. Correlation with adenovirus infections has been noted, and the condition may complicate otitis media, gastroenteritis, or upper respiratory infections. It is postulated that swollen Peyer patches in the ileum may stimulate intestinal peristalsis in an attempt to extrude the mass, thus causing an intussusception. At the peak age of incidence of this condition, an infant's alimentary tract is also being introduced to various new materials. In about 2–10% of patients, recognizable lead points for the intussusception are found, such as inverted appendiceal stump, Meckel diverticulum, an intestinal polyp, duplication, or lymphosarcoma. Uncommonly, the condition complicates Henoch-Schönlein purpura, with an intramural hematoma acting as the apex of the intussusception. Rarely, intussusception is postoperative and then always ileoileal. Intussusception occurs in dehydrated patients with cystic fibrosis. Unusual lesions include metastatic tumors, hemangioma, foreign bodies, parasitic infection, and fecolith; they can occur after cancer chemotherapy. Lead points are more common in very young and older patients. Intrauterine intussusception is associated with the development of intestinal atresia.

PATHOLOGY. Intussusceptions are most often ileocolic and ileoileocolic, less commonly cecocolic, and rarely exclusively ileal. Very rarely, the appendix forms the apex of an intussusception. The upper portion of bowel, the intussusceptum, invaginates into the lower, the intussuscipiens, dragging its mesentery along with it into the enveloping loop. Constriction of the mesentery obstructs venous return; engorgement of the intussusceptum follows, with edema, and bleeding from the mucosa leads to a bloody stool, sometimes containing mucus. The apex of the intussusception may extend into the transverse, descending, or sigmoid colon—even to and through the anus in neglected cases. This presentation must be distinguished from rectal prolapse. Most intussusceptions do not strangulate the bowel within the first 24 hr but may later eventuate in intestinal gangrene and shock.

CLINICAL MANIFESTATIONS. In typical cases there is sudden onset, in a previously well child, of severe paroxysmal colicky pain that recurs at frequent intervals and is accompanied by straining efforts with legs and knees flexed and loud cries. The infant may initially be comfortable and play normally between the paroxysms of pain, but if the intussusception is not reduced, the infant becomes progressively weaker and lethargic. At times, the lethargy is out of proportion to the abdominal signs. Eventually a shocklike state may develop, with an elevation of body temperature to as high as 41°C (106°F). The pulse becomes weak and thready, the respirations become shallow and grunting, and the pain may be manifested only by moaning sounds. Vomiting occurs in most cases and is usually more frequent early. In the later phase, the vomitus becomes bile stained. Stools of normal appearance may be evacuated during the first few hr of symptoms. After this time, fecal excretions are small or more often do not occur, and little or no flatus is passed. Blood generally is passed in the first 12 hr but at times not for 1–2 days and infrequently not at all; 60% of infants pass a stool containing red blood and mucus, the *currant jelly stool.* Some patients have only irritability and alternating or progressive lethargy.

Palpation of the abdomen usually reveals a slightly tender sausage-shaped mass, sometimes ill defined, which may increase in size and firmness during a paroxysm of pain and is most often in the right upper abdomen, with its long axis cephalocaudal. If it is felt in the epigastrium, the long axis is transverse. About 30% of patients do not have a palpable mass. The presence of bloody mucus on the finger as it is withdrawn after rectal examination supports the diagnosis of intussusception. Abdominal distention and tenderness develop as intestinal obstruction becomes more acute. On rare occasions, the advancing intestine prolapses through the anus. This prolapse can be distinguished from prolapse of the rectum by the separation between the protruding intestine and the rectal wall, which does not exist in prolapse of the rectum.

Ileoileal intussusception may have a less typical clinical picture, the symptoms and signs being chiefly those of small intestinal obstruction. *Recurrent intussusception* is noted in 5–8% and is more common after hydrostatic than surgical reduction. *Chronic intussusception,* in which the symptoms exist in milder form at recurrent intervals, is more likely to occur with or after acute enteritis and may arise in older children as well as in infants.

DIAGNOSIS. The clinical history and physical findings are usually sufficiently typical for diagnosis. Plain abdominal roentgenograms may show a density in the area of the intussusception. A barium enema shows a filling defect or cupping in the head of barium where its advance is obstructed by the intussusceptum (Fig. 333–1). A central linear column of barium may be visible in the compressed lumen of the intussusceptum, and a thin rim of barium may be seen trapped around the invaginating intestine in the folds of mucosa within the intussuscipiens (coiled-spring sign), especially after evacuation. Retrogression of the intussusceptum under the pressure of the enema and gaseous distention of the small intestine from obstruction are also useful roentgenographic signs. Ileoileal intussusception is usually not demonstrable by barium enema but is suspected because of gaseous distention of the intestine above the lesion. The use of "air" enemas in the diagnosis and treatment of intussusception is supplanting hydrostatic reduction. Reflux of air into the terminal ileum and the disappearance of the mass at the ileocecal valve document successful reduction. Air reduction is associated with fewer complica-

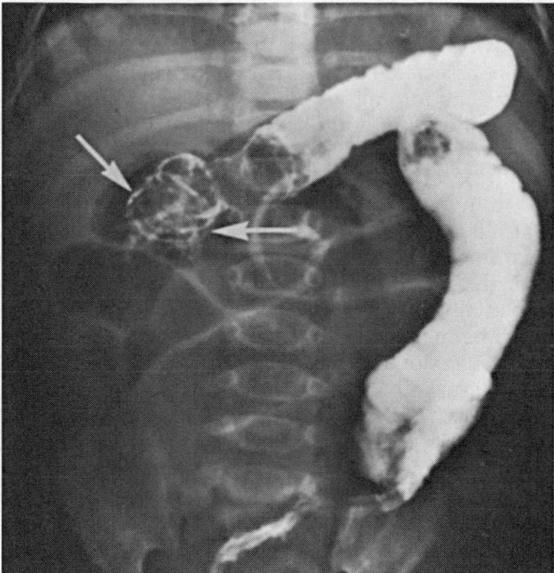

Figure 333–1 Intussusception in an infant. The obstruction is evident in the proximal transverse colon. Contrast material between the intussusceptum and the intussuscipiens is responsible for the coil-spring appearance.

tions and lower radiation exposure than traditional hydrostatic techniques.

Ultrasonography is a sensitive diagnostic tool in the diagnosis of intussusception. It is used in conjunction with hydrostatic or air reduction techniques. The diagnostic findings of intussusception include a tubular mass in longitudinal views and a doughnut or target appearance in transverse images (Fig. 333–2).

DIFFERENTIAL DIAGNOSIS. It may be particularly difficult to diagnose intussusception in a child who already has *gastroenteritis;* a change in the pattern of illness, in the character of pain, or in the nature of vomiting or the onset of rectal bleeding should alert the physician. The bloody stools and abdominal cramps that accompany *enterocolitis* can usually be differentiated from intussusception because the pain is less severe and less regular, there is diarrhea, and the infant is recognizably ill between pains. Bleeding from *Meckel diverticulum* is usually painless. The intestinal hemorrhage of *Henoch-Schönlein purpura* is usually but not invariably accompanied by joint symptoms or purpura elsewhere, and the colicky pain may be similar. Because intussusception may be a complication of this disorder, a barium enema may be required.

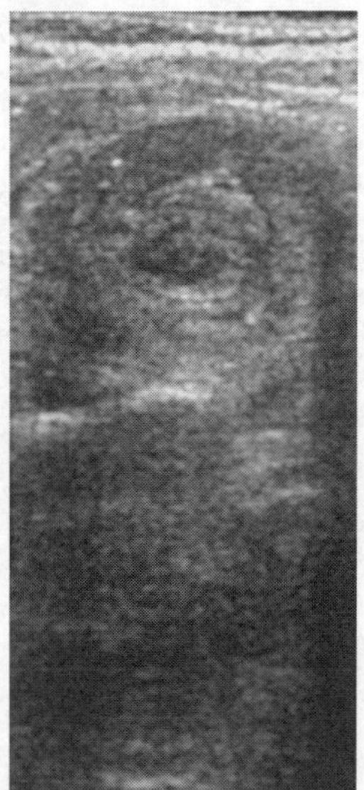

Figure 333–2 Transverse image of an ileocolic intussusception. Note the loops with the loops of bowel.

TREATMENT. Reduction of an acute intussusception is an emergency procedure and performed immediately after diagnosis in preparation for possible surgery. In patients with prolonged intussusception with signs of shock, peritoneal irritation, intestinal perforation, or pneumatosis intestinalis, hydrostatic reduction should not be attempted.

The success rate of hydrostatic reduction under fluoroscopic or ultrasonic guidance is approximately 50% if symptoms are present longer than 48 hr and 75–80% if reduction is done within the first 48 hr. Bowel perforations occur in 0.5–2.5% of attempted barium reductions. The perforation rate with air reduction ranges from 0.1–0.2%.

In an ileoileal intussusception, a barium enema is usually not diagnostic and reduction by the hydrostatic technique may not be possible. Such intussusceptions may develop insidiously as a complication of a laparotomy and require resection. A right-sided transverse paraumbilical or infraumbilical incision gives access to the ascending colon. If manual operative reduction is impossible or the bowel is not viable, resection of the intussusception is necessary, with end-to-end anastomosis.

PROGNOSIS. Untreated intussusception in infants is almost always fatal; the chances of recovery are directly related to the duration of intussusception before reduction. Most infants recover if the intussusception is reduced within the first 24 hr, but the mortality rate rises rapidly after this time, especially after the 2nd day. Spontaneous reduction during preparation for operation is not uncommon.

The recurrence rate after barium enema reduction of intussusceptions is about 10% and after surgical reduction, about 2–5%; none has recurred after surgical resection. It is unlikely that an intussusception caused by a lesion such as lymphosarcoma, polyp, or Meckel diverticulum will be successfully reduced by barium enema. With adequate surgical management, operative reduction carries a very low mortality rate in early cases.

333.4 Closed-Loop Obstructions

Intestinal obstruction may be caused by defects in the mesentery ("internal hernias") through which loops of small bowel may pass and become trapped. Vascular engorgement of the trapped bowel results in intestinal ischemia and gangrene unless promptly relieved. Symptoms include bilious vomiting, abdominal distention, and abdominal pain. Peritoneal signs suggest ischemic bowel. Plain radiographs demonstrate signs of small bowel obstruction or free air if the bowel has perforated. Supportive management includes intravenous fluids, antibiotics, and nasogastric decompression. Prompt surgical relief of the obstruction is indicated if intestinal gangrene is to be prevented. Symptoms can occasionally be transient or recurrent if the herniated bowel slides out of the mesenteric defect, spontaneously relieving the obstruction.

Akgur FM, Tanyel FC, Buyukpamukcu N, Hicsonmez A: Adhesive bowel obstruction in children: The place and predictors of success for conservative treatment. J Pediatr Surg 26:37, 1991.

Carnevale E, Graziani M, Fasanelli S: Post-operative ileo-ileal intussusception: Sonographic approach. Pediatr Radiol 24:161, 1994.

Champoux AN, Del Beccaro MA, Nazar-Stewart V: Recurrent intussusception. Risks and features. Arch Pediatr Adolesc Med 148:474, 1994.

Daneman A, Alton DJ: Intussusception. Issues and controversies related to diagnosis and reduction. Radiol Clin North Am 34:743, 1996.

Eshel G, Barr J, Heiman E, et al: Incidence of recurrent intussusception following barium versus air enema. Acta Paediatr 86:545, 1997.

Harrington L, Connolly B, Hu X, et al: Ultrasonographic and clinical predictors of intussusception. J Pediatr 132:836, 1998.
Lander A, Redkar R, Nicholls G, et al: Cisapride reduces neonatal postoperative ileus: Randomised placebo controlled trial. Arch Dis Child Fetal Neonatal Ed 77:F119, 1997.
Lim HK, Bae SH, Lee KH, et al: Assessment of reducibility of ileocolic intussusception in children: Usefulness of color Doppler sonography. [See comments.] Radiology 191:781, 1994.
Meradji M, Hussain SM, Robben SG, et al: Plain film diagnosis in intussusception. Br J Radiol 67:147, 1994.
Meyer JS, Dangman BC, Buonomo C, et al: Air and liquid contrast agents in the management of intussusception: A controlled, randomized trial. Radiology 188:507, 1993.
Riebel TW, Nasir R, Weber K: US-guided hydrostatic reduction of intussusception in children. Radiology 188:513, 1993.
Stringer MD, Pledger G, Drake DP: Childhood deaths from intussusception in England and Wales, 1984–9. Br Med J 304:737, 1992.

CHAPTER 334
Foreign Bodies and Bezoars

Robert Wyllie

334.1 Foreign Bodies in the Stomach and Intestine

Eighty per cent of all foreign body ingestions occur in children, with a peak incidence between the ages of 6 mo and 3 yr. The exact incidence of foreign bodies ingested is unknown; in the United States, approximately 1,500 people die annually after ingesting a foreign body.

Coins are the most common foreign body ingested by young children. In older children, teenagers, and adults, fish or chicken bones are the most common objects accidentally ingested. The risk of ingestion increases after alcohol consumption or cold liquids because of a decrease in oral sensory acuity. Repeat ingestion may occur in young children and psychiatrically impaired patients. Of the foreign bodies that come to medical attention, 80–90% pass through the gastrointestinal (GI) tract without difficulty. Ten to 20% require endoscopic removal or other conservative management, whereas 1% or less require surgical intervention. Once in the stomach, 95% of all ingested objects pass without difficulty through the remainder of the GI tract. Perforation after foreign body ingestion is estimated to be less than 1% of all objects ingested. Perforation tends to occur in areas of physiologic sphincters (pylorus and ileocecal valve), acute angulation (such as the duodenal sweep), congenital gut malformations (webs, diaphragms, or diverticula), or areas of previous bowel surgery.

Patients with nonfood foreign bodies often describe a history of ingestion. Young children may have a witness to ingestion. Approximately 90% of foreign bodies are opaque. Radiologic examination is routinely performed to determine the type, number, and location of the suspected objects. Contrast radiographs may be necessary to demonstrate some objects such as plastic parts or toys.

Conservative management is indicated in most foreign bodies that have passed through the esophagus and entered the stomach. Most objects pass though the intestine in 4–6 days, although some may take as long as 3–4 wk. While waiting for the object to pass, parents are instructed to continue a regular diet and to observe the stools for the appearance of the ingested object. Cathartics should be avoided. Exceptionally long or sharp objects are usually monitored radiologically. Parents or patients should be instructed to report abdominal pain, vomiting, persistent fever, and hematemesis or melena immediately to their physician. Failure of the object to progress over a 3- to 4-wk period seldom implies an impeding perforation but may be associated with a congenital malformation or acquired bowel abnormality.

In older children and adults, oval objects greater than 5 cm in diameter or 2 cm in thickness tend to lodge in the stomach and should be endoscopically retrieved. Thin objects greater than 10 cm in length fail to negotiate the duodenal sweep and should also be removed. In infants and toddlers, objects longer than 3 cm or larger than 20 mm in diameter usually do not pass through the pylorus and should be removed. Open safety pins should also be endoscopically retrieved, but other sharp objects can be managed conservatively.

Children occasionally place objects in their rectum. Small, blunt objects usually pass spontaneously, but large or sharp objects usually need to be retrieved. Adequate sedation is essential to relax the anal sphincter before attempted endoscopic or speculum removal. If the object is proximal to the rectum, observation for 12–24 hr usually allows the object to descend into the rectum.

Paul RI, Christoffel KK, Binns HJ, et al: Foreign body ingestions in children: Risk of complication varies with site of initial health care contact. Pediatric Practice Research Group. Pediatrics 91:121, 1993.
Shaffer HA Jr, de Lange EE: Gastrointestinal foreign bodies and strictures: Radiologic interventions. Curr Probl Diagn Radiol 23:205, 1994.
Webb WA: Management of foreign bodies of the upper gastrointestinal tract: Update. Gastrointest Endosc 41:39, 1995.

334.2 Bezoars

A bezoar is an accumulation of exogenous matter in the stomach or intestine. Most bezoars have been found in females with underlying personality problems or in neurologically impaired individuals. The peak age of onset of symptoms is the second decade of life. Bezoars are classified on the basis of their composition. Trichobezoars are composed of the patient's own hair, and phytobezoars are composed of a combination of plant and animal material. Lactobezoars were previously found most often in premature infants and may be attributed to the high casein or calcium content of some premature formulas.

Trichobezoars can become large and form casts of the stomach; they may enter into the proximal duodenum. They present with symptoms of gastric outlet or partial intestinal obstruction including vomiting, anorexia, and weight loss. Patients may complain of abdominal pain, distention, and severe halitosis. Physical examination may demonstrate patchy baldness and a firm mass in the left upper quadrant. Patients may occasionally have iron-deficiency anemia, hypoproteinemia, or steatorrhea caused by an associated chronic gastritis. Phytobezoars present in a similar manner.

An abdominal plain film may suggest the presence of a bezoar, which can be confirmed on barium or ultrasound examination. Endoscopy provides a definitive diagnosis and a means of therapeutic disruption and removal of the material. If endoscopy is unsuccessful, surgical intervention may be needed. Lactobezoars usually resolve when feedings are withheld for 24–48 hr.

Byrne WJ: Foreign bodies, bezoars, and caustic ingestion. Gastrointest Endosc Clin North Am 4:99, 1994.

CHAPTER 335
Anorectal Malformations

Alberto Peña

Anorectal malformations refers to a spectrum of defects. Some are complex, difficult to manage, and associated with important anatomic deficiencies and therefore have a poor functional prognosis. Others are minor and easily treated, having an excellent functional prognosis. The main concerns are future bowel control and urinary and sexual function. Anorectal anomalies occur in about 1/4,000 live births and manifest various grades of anal stenosis—agenesis or rectal agenesis—atresia.

EMBRYOLOGY AND PATHOGENESIS. The origin of the anus and the rectum is an embryologic structure called the cloaca. Lateral ingrowths of this structure form the urorectal septum, separating the rectum dorsally from the urinary tract ventrally. Both systems (rectum and urinary tract) become completely separated by the 7th wk of gestation. At this same time, the urogenital portion of the original cloaca already has an external opening, whereas the anal portion is closed by a membrane that opens by the 8th wk of gestation.

Abnormalities in the development of these processes at varying stages provoke a spectrum of anomalies, most of which affect the lower intestinal tract and the genitourinary structures. Persistence of communication between the genitourinary and rectal portions of the cloaca results in fistulas.

PATHOLOGY AND CLASSIFICATION. Figure 335–1 demonstrates a practical, therapeutically oriented classification of these defects.

MALE PATIENTS. Perineal Fistula. Perineal (cutaneous) fistula is the simplest defect in both sexes. Patients have a small orifice located in the perineum, anterior to the center of the external sphincter, close to the scrotum in the male or to the vulva in the female. Male patients frequently have in their perineum a "bucket-handle"–type malformation or a "black ribbon"–type structure that represents a subepithelial fistula filled with meconium. These patients usually have a well-formed sacrum, a prominent midline groove, and a prominent anal dimple. The frequency of associated defects affecting other organs is less than 10%. The diagnosis is established by simple perineal inspection. No further investigations are required, and this defect can be repaired without a protective colostomy.

Rectourethral Fistula. In cases of rectourethral fistula, the rectum communicates with the lower part of the urethra (bulbar urethra) or the upper part of the urethra (prostatic urethra). The sphincteric mechanism usually is satisfactory; a few patients have poor perineal muscles and a flat-looking perineum. The sacrum may have different degrees of hypodevelopment, particularly in cases of rectourethral prostatic fistula. Most of these patients have a well-formed midline perineal groove and an anal dimple. Those with a rectoprostatic fistula have a poorly developed sacrum and frequently a flat perineum. These patients require a protective colostomy during the newborn period. The complete surgical repair is performed later in life. Rectourethral fistula represents the most frequent anorectal defect seen in male patients.

Rectovesical Fistula. In patients having rectovesical fistulas, the rectum communicates with the urinary tract at the level of the bladder neck. The rectal sphincteric mechanism is usually poorly developed. The sacrum is frequently deformed and is often absent. The perineum looks flat. This defect represents 10% of the total number of affected male patients. The prognosis for bowel function is usually poor. A colostomy is mandatory during the newborn period, followed by corrective surgical repair later in life.

Imperforate Anus Without Fistula. This defect has the same characteristics in both sexes. The rectum is completely blind and is usually found approximately 2 cm above the perineal skin. The sacrum and the sphincteric mechanism are usually well developed. The functional prognosis is usually good and is similar to that in those male patients with a rectourethral bulbar fistula. A colostomy is indicated during the newborn period. This defect is frequently associated with Down syndrome. When properly operated on, patients who have this defect and Down syndrome have the same good prognosis for bowel function as chromsomally normal children.

Rectal Atresia. Rectal atresia is a rare defect occurring in only 1% of anorectal anomalies. It has the same characteristics in both sexes. The unique feature of this defect is that affected patients have a normal anal canal and a normal anus. The defect is frequently discovered while a rectal temperature is being taken. An obstruction is present about 2 cm above the skin level. These patients need a protective colostomy. The

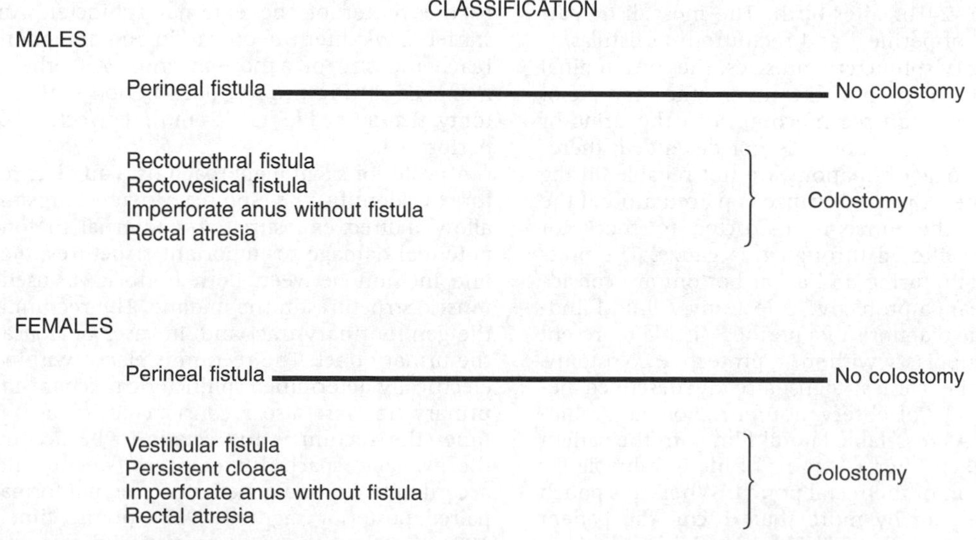

Figure 335–1. Classification of anorectal malformations. (From Kiesewetter WB: *In*: Ravitch MM, et al (eds): Pediatric Surgery, 3rd ed. Chicago, Yearbook, 1979.)

functional prognosis is excellent because they have a normal sphincteric mechanism (and normal sensation), which resides in the anal canal.

FEMALE PATIENTS. Vestibular Fistula. Vestibular fistula is the most frequent defect seen in females. The rectum opens in the vestibule of the female genitalia immediately outside the hymen orifice. Patients are frequently mislabeled as having "rectovaginal fistula." The functional prognosis is excellent. The sacrum is usually normal, and the perineum shows a prominent midline groove and a noticeable anal dimple, all of which indicate that the sphincteric mechanism is intact. A protective colostomy is needed before the corrective surgical procedure, although this colostomy does not need to be performed on an emergency basis because the fistula is frequently competent to decompress the intestinal tract.

Persistent Cloaca. In cases of persistent cloaca, the rectum, vagina, and urinary tract meet and fuse into a single common channel. The perineum shows a single orifice located immediately behind the clitoris. The length of the common channels varies from 1–10 cm; this has important technical and prognostic implications. Patients with short common channels (<3 cm) usually have well-developed sacrums and good sphincters. A common channel longer than 3 cm usually suggests that the patient has a more complex defect and, frequently, has a poor sphincteric mechanism and a poor sacrum. Most patients with cloacas have an abnormally large vagina filled with mucous secretions (hydrocolpos). Different degrees of vaginal and uterine septation also are present. A diverting colostomy is indicated at birth; in addition, patients with a cloaca represent a urologic emergency because approximately 90% have associated urologic defects. Before the colostomy, the urologic diagnosis must be established to decompress the urinary tract, if necessary, at the same time the colostomy is created.

The term *rectovaginal fistula* is not used in this classification because true rectovaginal fistulas are extremely unusual defects. This became obvious after the advent of the posterior sagittal surgical approach, which allowed the surgeon to have a direct view of the anatomy.

DIAGNOSIS AND EARLY MANAGEMENT. The most important decision regarding a newborn with an anorectal malformation is whether the patient needs a diverting-decompression colostomy and emergency urinary diversion for an associated obstructive uropathy.

Male Patients. Good clinical evaluation and a urinalysis provide sufficient information in 80–90% of patients to decide whether a colostomy is needed. If a patient has a perineal or rectourinary fistula, meconium may not be seen at the perineum or in the urine before 16–24 hr after birth. The most distal part of the bowel, in cases of perineal and rectourethral fistulas, is surrounded by voluntary sphincteric muscles; the intraluminal bowel pressure must be high enough to overcome the tone of those muscles before one can see meconium in the urine or in the perineum. At birth, the bowel is not distended; therefore, clinical and radiologic evaluations are not reliable during the first 16–24 hr of life. A piece of gauze is placed around the tip of the penis, and the nurse is instructed to check for particles of meconium filtered through this gauze. The presence of meconium in the urine and a flat bottom are considered indications to create a protective colostomy. Clinical findings consistent with the diagnosis of a perineal fistula represent an indication for an anoplasty without a protective colostomy. Sometimes none of the clinical signs already described becomes evident after 24 hr of observation; a radiologic evaluation is then indicated. A cross-table lateral film with the patient in a prone position taken after 16–24 hr of life is valuable for determining the position of the rectal pouch. When this pouch is separated from the skin by more than 1 cm, the patient needs a colostomy. During the first 24 hrs of life, all these patients need an abdominal ultrasound evaluation to identify an obstructive uropathy.

Female Patients. More than 90% of the time, the diagnosis can be established by a meticulous perineal inspection. These patients must be observed during the first 16–24 hr of life. The presence of a single perineal orifice is pathognomonic of a cloaca. A palpable pelvic mass (hydrocolpos) reinforces the suspicion of a cloaca. The diagnosis of a vestibular fistula can be established by careful separation of the labia to see the vestibule. The rectal orifice is located immediately behind the hymen within the female genitalia and in the vestibule. A perineal fistula is easy to diagnose. The rectal orifice is located somewhere between the female genitalia and the center of the sphincter and is surrounded by skin; the term *anterior anus,* which is sometimes used for this defect, is inadequate because these are abnormal fistula orifices not surrounded by a normal sphincteric mechanism. Fewer than 10% of these patients fail to pass meconium through the genitalia or perineum after 24 hr of observation. Those patients may require a cross-table lateral film. They also need an ultrasound study of the abdomen during the first 24 hr of life, because patients with persistent cloaca have the highest incidence of urologic defects.

ASSOCIATED DEFECTS. About 50% of children with anorectal anomalies have a urologic problem. The more serious and complex the anorectal defect, the more frequently it is associated with a urologic anomaly. Male patients with a rectovesical fistula and patients with a persistent cloaca have a 90% chance of having a urologic defect. On the other hand, patients with a rectoperineal fistula have less than a 10% chance. Urologic evaluation must be established before performing a colostomy. Untreated acidosis and sepsis resulting from an undetected obstructive uropathy are risks.

A good correlation exists between the degree of sacral development and the final functional prognosis. Patients with an absent sacrum have permanent fecal and urinary incontinence. Different degrees of sacral malformations are associated with important functional sequelae. Spinal abnormalities and different degrees of dysraphism are frequently associated with these defects. Tethered cord occurs in approximately 25% of patients with anorectal malformations; severe anorectal defects have a poor prognosis. It is important to establish the diagnosis to aid neurosurgical treatment. The diagnosis of spinal defects can be established during the first 3 mo of life by ultrasound; in older patients, it is necessary to use magnetic resonance imaging. Other associated congenital malformations include esophageal atresia, duodenal atresia, and cardiovascular defects.

TREATMENT. Perineal fistulas are treated by a simple anoplasty without a protective colostomy; the operation is performed during the newborn period. The fistula orifice is moved back to the center of the external sphincter. Anal dilations are started 2 wk after the operation and are gradually increased to reach the size of a normal anus. All other defects are best managed during the newborn period with a protective colostomy. Later in life (1–12 mo), corrective surgical repair is performed.

A posterior sagittal approach uses an electric muscle stimulator to identify the sphincteric mechanism. This approach allows a direct exposure to the internal anatomy, thus avoiding potential damage to important structures and nerves. A midline incision between both buttocks is used to split all the muscle structures in the midline. The rectum is separated from the genitourinary tract and, in cases of cloaca, the vagina and the urinary tract. The rectum is placed within the limits of the electrically determined sphincteric mechanism. The vagina and urinary tract are also reconstructed in cases of cloaca. Sometimes the rectum is too ectatic to be accommodated within the available space; therefore, the rectum has to be tailored accordingly. In male patients, the malformation can be repaired posterior sagittally 90% of the time. The remaining 10% of patients have a rectovesical fistula because the rectum cannot be reached posterior sagittally; a combined posterior sagittal and abdominal approach is needed. In cases of persistent cloaca, the abdomen must be opened in addition to the posterior sagittal approach, in about 30–40% of patients, to mobilize a high rectum or high vagina. Two weeks after corrective surgery, the patients must be subjected to a protocol of anal dilations. These are done twice per day; every week, a larger size dilator is passed to stretch the anus to normal size.

PROGNOSIS. Patients of both sexes with perineal fistula and rectal atresia should have excellent functional results after the repair of their defects; they should be fully continent. Male patients with rectourethral bulbar fistula and patients of both sexes with imperforate anus without a fistula also have good prognosis. About 80% achieve bowel control between 3 and 4 yr of age. A significant number may occasionally suffer from minimal soiling.

Male patients with rectourethral prostatic fistula have about a 60% chance of having bowel control by the age of 3 yr. Male patients with rectovesical fistula have a poor functional prognosis. Only about 20% have voluntary bowel movements by the age of 3 yr.

An extremely abnormal sacrum usually means that the patient will suffer from *fecal incontinence*. An extremely abnormal sacrum is most often associated with rectovesical fistula or rectoprostatic fistula. One rarely finds a good prognostic type of defect, such as perineal or vestibular fistula, associated with a poor sacrum. More than 90% of female patients with rectovestibular fistula have voluntary bowel movements by the age of 3 yr; few have occasional soiling.

Patients with a persistent cloaca with a common channel of less than 3 cm have about an 80% chance of having voluntary bowel movements by the age of 3 yr; most are urine continent. When the common channel is longer than 3 cm, most are fecal incontinent and require intermittent catheterization to empty their bladder. Patients with a persistent cloaca with a common channel longer than 3 cm usually have an extremely abnormal sacrum.

Approximately 25% of all patients have fecal incontinence, and about 70% of those with a cloaca with a long common channel need intermittent catheterization to empty the bladder. When these patients are old enough to be socially active, a medical program for bowel management and urinary control must be implemented. The use of enemas, suppositories, colonic irrigations, specific diets, and sometimes medications to regulate the motility of the colon will allow them to keep clean for 24 hr, thus improving their quality of life. Patients with fecal incontinence who have intractable diarrhea are usually refractory to medical management and require a permanent colostomy.

Most patients subjected to an operation to repair an imperforate anus have varying degrees of constipation. This symptom is more severe in patients with lower and simpler defects. Patients who had inadequate colostomies (loop colostomies that allow the passing of stool from the proximal into the distal limb of the bowel) may subsequently have constipation. These patients need a diet rich in fiber and, sometimes, laxatives to empty the rectum daily. Ineffective medical treatment may exacerbate the problem; the rectosigmoid colon continues to enlarge and becomes inefficient in emptying, making treatment a more difficult task.

Diseth T, Emblem R, Solbraa I, et al: A psychological follow-up of ten adolescents with low anorectal malformation. Acta Paediatr 83:216, 1994.
Levitt MA, Patel M, Rodriguez G, et al: The tethered spinal cord in patients with anorectal malformations. J Pediatr Surg 32:462, 1997.
Peña A: Current management of anorectal anomalies. Surg Clin North Am 72:1393, 1992.
Peña A: The posterior sagittal approach: Implications in adult colorectal surgery. Dis Colon Rectum 37:1, 1994.
Peña A: Anorectal malformations. Semin Pediatric Surgery 4:35, 1995.
Peña A, Guardino K, Tovilla JM, et al: Bowel management for fecal incontinence in patients with anorectal malformations. J Pediatr Surg 33:133, 1998.
Rich MA, Brock WA, Peña A: Spectrum of genitourinary malformations in patients with imperforate anus. Pediatr Surg Int 3:110, 1988.
Torres R, Levitt MA, Tovilla JM, et al: Anorectal malformations and Down's syndrome. J Pediatr Surg 33:194, 1998.
Tsakayannis DE, Shamberger RC: Association of imperforate anus with occult spinal dysraphism. J Pediatr Surg 30:1010, 1995.
Wolf S, Schneble F, Troger J: The conus medullaris: Time of ascendence to normal level. Pediatr Radiol 22:590, 1992.

CHAPTER 336
Ulcer Disease

John J. Herbst

Ulcers and gastritis are classified as primary (peptic) or secondary, caused by factors known to affect the integrity of the gastric or duodenal mucosa. Ulcers and gastritis are closely related. Primary peptic ulcers are usually chronic, duodenal, and related to *Helicobacter pylori* gastritis, whereas secondary ulcers are usually acute and gastric.

PATHOLOGY AND PHYSIOLOGY. An ulcer is a disruption of the intestinal epithelium exposed to acid or pepsin; an erosion is a superficial ulcer. Ulcers are usually 1 cm or less in diameter. A fibrinous coat of leukocytes and red cells covers a zone of fibrinoid necrosis surrounded by an infiltration of acute and chronic inflammatory cells. Gastritis demonstrates inflammation of the gastric mucosa without disruption of the mucosa that may be obvious only by histologic examination. Factors important in the development of gastritis and ulcer disease include mediators of mucosal inflammation such as oxygen free radicals, lymphokines, and monokines. Mucosal defense mechanisms include a surface water–unstirred water layer, intestinal and pancreatobiliary sources of bicarbonate, surface-active hydrophobic phospholipids in the mucosal area, mucosal blood flow, and a rapid rate of cell replacement enhanced by factors such as epidermal growth factor. Prostaglandins help to protect the gastric mucosa from numerous agents including bile, alcohol, and nonsteroidal anti-inflammatory drugs. Prostaglandins directly inhibit parietal cell function and acid secretion, increase bicarbonate and mucous secretion, and maintain mucosal blood flow. Although the presence of acid is vital in the development of ulcers, gastric acidity is often normal or low with gastric ulcers, particularly secondary ulcers. Patients with duodenal ulcers have increased acid secretion; acid secretion does not correlate with ulcer size or duration of symptoms. A family history is noted in 25–50% of children with duodenal ulcers; concordance for duodenal ulcer is 50% for monozygotic twins. This may be partially due to the known clustering of *H. pylori* in families (see later). Other factors that appear to be important include blood type O, cigarette smoking, climatic conditions, dietary habits (consumption of alcohol), and emotional stress. Factors related to acid are more important in duodenal ulcers, and tissue resistance is of greater importance in gastric ulcers.

H. pylori, a spiral gram-negative organism with a smooth surface and multiple unipolar flagella, is an important factor in gastritis and primary peptic ulcer disease. Production of urease is a distinctive characteristic and the basis for several diagnostic tests. Most of the organisms reside in the mucus overlaying the epithelium of the gastric antrum and usually do not invade the mucosa. In adults, the characteristic mucosal reaction is an acute and chronic inflammation of neutrophils and lymphocytes. In children, lymphocytic inflammation, usually associated with lymphonodular hyperplasia, is noted. Characteristics that allow *H. pylori* to exist in the hostile acidic environment of the stomach include urease-mediated ammonia production that neutralizes the acid environment, spiral morphology and flagella that enable peristalsis resistance and penetration of the protective mucous barrier, and adhesion that allows gastric epithelium attachment in a manner similar to the attachment of enteropathic *Escherichia coli* to enterocytes. *H. pylori* strains are genetically diverse. A 40 kb DNA segment, known as the cag pathogenicity island, encodes multiple proteins involved in the ability of cag + strains to induce expression of interleukin-8 in epithelial cells. Other strains differ in the ability to secret a cytotoxin that causes epithelial cell degeneration. Whether the organism causes the ulcer or is important in maintaining the ulcer is unclear; eradication of *H. pylori* is associated with healing and cure of recurrent peptic ulcer disease.

No animal or environmental reservoir exists for *H. pylori*. Overcrowded unsanitary living conditions, sharing of a bed, and lack of running water are major risk factors. Infection rates increase with age; in developing countries, half the children are colonized by 10 yr of age, and more than 80% of adults are colonized. In developed countries such as the United States, colonization in childhood is uncommon, and only 40% of adults are infected. Children of low socioeconomic status have *H. pylori* infection rates similar to those in children in developing countries. The major route of transmission is unknown, but feces, saliva, or vomitus can potentially transmit the organism.

CLINICAL MANIFESTATIONS. Infection with *H. pylori* usually leads to clinically silent gastritis. The gastritis is caused by *H. pylori*, which is not a secondary invader because eradication of the infection results in clearance of the gastritis. A syndrome of abdominal pain, achlorhydria, and neutrophilic gastritis has been observed in adults experimentally infected with *H. pylori* and is rarely seen in clinical practice. Infection is clearly associated with primary ulcer disease in adults and children and also with gastric cancer and gastric mucosa-associated lymphoid tissue lymphoma in adults. *H. pylori* is probably not a cause of dyspepsia or chronic abdominal pain in children.

DIAGNOSIS. Direct culture of mucosal biopsies is a cumbersome standard because it requires an incubation period of up to 7 days. Several rapid tests use the high urease content of the organism by placing biopsy samples on media containing urea and a pH-sensitive indicator to detect ammonia. A positive reaction may be noted within 1 hr, but small amounts of bacteria may not be detected for 24 hr. The test has a sensitivity and specificity in excess of 95% in adults; the test is not quite as sensitive in children, in whom the bacterial load is not as large. Noting spiral organisms on the antral mucosal surface just below the mucous layer may enable the physician to make a presumptive diagnosis. The use of silver, Giemsa, or other special stains can facilitate the search and provide a very sensitive test to diagnosis *H. pylori*. Detection of antibodies to *H. pylori* denotes past infection, but infection is so common that this information is of limited clinical value. The sensitivity of antibody studies is much lower in children than in adults. Immunoglobulin M antibodies may remain elevated for several months after eradication of the organism, making this test of limited usefulness to check for eradication.

Breath tests can detect the presence of the organism. After ingestion of carbon-14 or carbon-13–labeled urea, *H. pylori* metabolizes the urea to produce labeled carbon dioxide, which is detected in the breath. The test is more than 90% sensitive and specific. Tests using carbon-14 suffer from the theoretical disadvantage of use of a minute dose of radioactivity. Tests using the stable carbon-13 isotope avoid this problem. If endoscopy is performed, a rapid test for urease in biopsies or microscopic examination of biopsy samples is most useful. If endoscopy is not performed or if there is a need to test for eradication, the breath tests are most useful.

TREATMENT. Because *H. pylori* colonizes a high proportion of people and is usually asymptomatic, debate exists about which patients need treatment. The eradication of *H. pylori* is strongly recommended if patients have peptic ulcer disease, active or inactive, bleeding or not, on the basis of unequivocal evidence. Effective treatment prevents recurrence of ulcer disease. Eradicating *H. pylori* in patients receiving long-term therapy with proton pump inhibitors for gastroesophageal reflux disease, in patients with low-grade mucosal-associated lymphoma, or after surgical treatment of peptic ulcer disease is advisable based on supportive evidence.

TABLE 336–1 Treatment Regimens for *Helicobacter pylori*

Approved by FDA for Use in Adults
Omeprazole 40 mg qd + clarithromycin tid for 2 wk, then omeprazole 20 mg qd for 2 wk
Ranitidine bismuth citrate 400 mg bid + clarithromycin tid for 2 wk, then ranitidine bismuth citrate 400 mg bid for 2 wk
Pepto-Bismol 525 mg qid + metronidazole 250 mg qid + tetracycline 500 mg qid + H_2-receptor antagonist for 4 wk
Lansoprazole 30 mg + amoxicillin 1 g + clarithromycin 500 mg bid for 2 wk
Acceptable Success in Pediatric Series
Omeprazole + clarithomycin + metronidazole for 2 wk
Metronidazole for 2 wk + 4 wk of bismuth subcitrate
Amoxicillin + bismuth subsalicylate for 6 wk
Amoxicillin + tinidazole for 6 wk

FDA, United States Food and Drug Administration.

Eradication of *H. pylori* usually involves the use of several drugs. Treatment regimens approved for adults by the United States Food and Drug Administration and regimens showing acceptable eradication in pediatric series are noted in Table 336–1. The highest rates of success include the use of omeprazole with two antibiotics (clarithromycin and metronidazole or tinidazole or amoxicillin) with or without bismuth subsalicylate.

336.1 Primary (Peptic) Ulcers

CLINICAL MANIFESTATIONS. The manifestations of peptic ulcer disease include pain, vomiting, acute and chronic gastrointestinal blood loss, and a strong familial incidence. Primary gastritis due to *H. pylori* routinely occurs in conjunction with primary peptic ulcers. Only about 15% of adults with symptoms of dyspepsia thought to be compatible with ulcer disease have ulcers on investigation. The frequency of nonspecific abdominal pain and the rarity of ulcer disease suggest a similar situation in children.

In the 1st mo of life, the two main manifestations are gastrointestinal hemorrhage and perforation. Between the neonatal period and 2 yr of age, recurrent vomiting, slow growth, and gastrointestinal hemorrhage are the major symptoms. In pre–school-aged children, periumbilical postprandial pain is often elicited, whereas vomiting and hemorrhage remain common. After 6 yr of age, the clinical features of ulcer disease are similar to those in adults and commonly include epigastric abdominal pain, acute or chronic gastrointestinal blood loss (hematemesis, hematochezia, or melena) often leading to iron-deficiency anemia, predominantly male gender, and a strong family history of ulcer disease. The pain is often described as dull or aching in character rather than sharp or burning, as in adults. It may last from minutes to hours, and patients have frequent exacerbations and remissions lasting from weeks to months. Nocturnal pain is common. A history of typical ulcer pain with prompt relief after taking antacids is found in fewer than 33% of patients. Rarely, in patients with acute or chronic blood loss, penetration of the ulcer into the abdominal cavity or adjacent organs produces shock, anemia, peritonitis, or pancreatitis. If inflammation and edema are extensive, acute or chronic gastric obstruction may occur.

DIAGNOSIS. Upper gastrointestinal endoscopy is the most useful procedure for investigating children for ulcer disease and gastritis. Although widely available, a barium meal is not sensitive or specific. In one study, a single contrast barium meal identified only one of seven endoscopically demonstrated duodenal ulcers. A barium meal frequently leads to overdiagnosis of peptic ulcer in children. Double contrast studies are more sensitive but increase radiation, and in adult studies, they missed 55% of gastric ulcers and 30% of duodenal ulcers. Nodularity of the antrum is a frequently noted feature of *H. pylori* gastritis in children. Gastritis commonly occurs in mucosa that appears normal at endoscopy, so biopsies should be obtained. Diagnosis of abrasions and superficial ulcers can only be made at endoscopy. Endoscopy can also be used to control bleeding at the time of diagnosis. Plain radiographs allow diagnosis of perforation in acute ulcers. In patients with massively bleeding ulcers whose stomach cannot be lavaged enough to allow endoscopy, angiography can demonstrate the site of bleeding and can permit injection of vasoconstrictors or thrombotic agents to control the bleeding.

The differential diagnosis is extensive and includes esophagitis, giardiasis, pancreatitis, inflammatory bowel disease, cholelithiasis, and recurrent abdominal pain of childhood. Functional, nonspecific pain is common among school-aged children, but it is not associated with weight loss, emesis, blood loss, and preprandial or night pain.

TREATMENT. The goal is to hasten healing of the ulcer, to relieve pain, and to prevent complications. If present, hemorrhagic shock and anemia must be treated as a first priority. Continuous monitoring for signs of continued bleeding and hypovolemia is critical. In cases of recurrent or continuous bleeding in which the stomach can be lavaged sufficiently to allow endoscopy, use of endoscopic cautery (electrocoagulation, heater probe thermal contact) or sclerosis can control bleeding and can decrease the chance of repeated bleeding.

Although antacids, sucralfate, and misoprostol are capable of healing an ulcer, primary ulcers have a high likelihood of recurring unless the associated *H. pylori* gastritis is effectively treated. Acid suppression is used in all the effective treatment regimens, so initiating treatment to eradicate *H. pylori* starts healing of the ulcer and relieves pain while eradicating the organism causing ulcer recurrence.

Surgical treatment is rarely needed but is indicated in patients with perforation, chronic bleeding, loss of more than 30% of the blood volume within 48 hr from hemorrhaging that cannot be controlled, gastric outlet obstruction that does not improve after 72 hr of nasogastric drainage, or chronic intractable pain. Vagotomy and either pyloroplasty or antrectomy are the procedures most often used for chronic ulcer disease. In children with acute hemorrhage or perforation, oversewing the ulcer is usually recommended and is often combined with vagotomy or pyloroplasty.

336.2 Secondary or Stress (Peptic) Ulcer Disease

The underlying causes are not fully understood; multiple factors that interfere with host defense mechanisms are involved. Mucosal blood flow is thought to be important in acute stress ulcers; other factors include mucus production, prostaglandin synthesis, acid production, and cell proliferation.

CLINICAL MANIFESTATIONS. In infants, stress ulcers are usually due to sepsis, respiratory or cardiac insufficiency, trauma, or dehydration. In older children, they are related to trauma or other life-threatening conditions. Stress ulcers and erosions associated with burns are also known as *Curling ulcers.* They are associated with normal gastric secretions and are common in patients with more than 25% body burns. *Cushing ulcers* follow head trauma or surgery and are associated with gastric hypersecretion. Most stress ulcers are asymptomatic, are often multiple, and may be terminal events. They can be associated with severe hemorrhage or perforation. Coagulopathy, hypotension, and need for mechanical respiration are important risk factors for overt clinically important gastrointestinal bleeding. Perforation and, more often, massive hemorrhage are often the initial symptoms.

DRUG-RELATED PEPTIC DISEASE. Nonsteroidal anti-inflammatory drugs, including aspirin, are common causes of gastritis and erosions. These drugs are thought to damage the mucosa by inhibiting prostaglandin synthesis, thereby inhibiting cell proliferation as well as mucosal bicarbonate and mucus secretion.

Alcohol and smoking are known to affect gastroduodenal mucosa adversely. Although results of studies are conflicting, a meta-analysis of available studies indicates a statistical association between corticosteroid use and ulcer disease in children. An inhibitory effect on local production of mucus and prostaglandin is postulated. Other agents that may rarely cause gastritis include iron, calcium salts, potassium chloride, and antibiotics, including chloramphenicol, penicillins, tetracyclines, and cephalosporins.

TREATMENT. Treatment of secondary ulcers is similar to that of primary ulcers. The inciting cause should be removed if possible. Bleeding and, less often, perforation are common presentations and must be addressed immediately. Maintaining gastric pH at more than 3.5 in critically ill patients helps to prevent ulcer formation. Control of gastric acidity is a cornerstone of continuing therapy and should continue for 6 wk if the patient has active disease.

Antacids have been used to neutralize acid once it is secreted. The buffering ability of antacids varies, as do recommendations for their use. The full adult dose of the concentrated liquids is 15 mL per dose. The optimal pediatric dose of antacids is controversial and varies with acid secretion and the buffering capacity of the antacid. Doses of as much as 1 mL/kg/dose have been recommended. Most antacids are mixtures of magnesium and aluminum salts. The magnesium ion causes diarrhea, whereas the aluminum salts may cause constipation. Aluminum hydroxide binds with dietary phosphates and interferes with their absorption. If large doses of aluminum hydroxide are used over a period of time, complications of phosphate depletion and aluminum toxicity including anorexia, osteomalacia, and osteoporosis may occur. Patients with renal disease are especially prone to aluminum toxicity. Calcium antacids can cause increased acid secretion after the buffering effect has stopped.

Histamine (H_2)-receptor blockers that suppress acid secretion are widely used even though they are not approved for children. Cimetidine (20–40 mg/kg/24 hr in four doses) and ranitidine (4–6 mg/kg/24 hr in two doses) are the most frequently used liquid preparations. They are rapidly absorbed and may be taken with meals. They can also be administered intravenously or added to parenteral nutrition solutions.

Hydrogen pump inhibitors, omeprazole and lansoprazole, are the most potent inhibitors of gastric acid secretion and have raised concerns about achlorhydria-related bacterial overgrowth. In adults, healing of ulcers occurs with 4 wk of therapy; hydrogen pump inhibitors are a component of several schemes to eradicate *H. pylori.* The drugs come in capsules containing granules that remain intact in an acid environment. The granules cannot be chewed, although they can be dissolved in sodium bicarbonate for instillation into the small intestine. They are not yet licensed for use in children in the United States.

Sucralfate forms a white pastelike substance in an acid environment that adheres to inflamed mucosa and ulcers. Experience in children is limited. The adult dose is 10 mL of the suspension four times a day on an empty stomach.

Misoprostol, a prostaglandin analog, has been shown in

adults to be effective in preventing and treating ulcers associated with the use of nonsteroidal anti-inflammatory drugs. Its use is limited by gastrointestinal side effects (abdominal pain, diarrhea). Studies in adults indicate that omeprazole is superior in treating erosions and ulcers associated with use of nonsteroidal anti-inflammatory drugs.

336.3 Zollinger-Ellision Syndrome

This rare syndrome can cause multiple recurrent duodenal and jejunal ulcers and is occasionally associated with diarrhea. Gastric secretion is markedly stimulated by serum gastrin and other hormones secreted by an islet cell tumor or hypertrophy. Hypergastrinemia, albeit lower than Zollinger-Ellison syndrome, may be noted in pyloric stenosis, short bowel syndrome, hyperparathyroidism, pheochromocytoma, and multiple endocrine neoplasia. Therapy with H_2 drugs or omeprazole can control gastric acid secretion and can improve symptoms when these slow-growing tumors cannot be entirely removed.

Blaser MJ: *Helicobacter pylori* and gastric diseases. BMJ 316:1507, 1998.
Bode G, Rothenbacher D, Brenner H, et al: *Helicobacter pylori* and abdominal symptoms: A population-based study among preschool children in southern Germany. Pediatrics 101:634, 1998.
Bourke B, Jones N, Sherman P: *Helicobacter pylori* infection and peptic ulcer disease in children. Pediatr Infect Dis J 15:1, 1996.
Buchta RM, Kaplan JM: Zollinger Ellison syndrome in a nine year old child: A case report and review of this entity in childhood. Pediatrics 47:594, 1971.
Cook D, Guyatt G, Marshall J, et al: A comparison of sucralfate and ranitidine for the prevention of upper gastrointestinal bleeding in patients requiring mechanical ventilation. N Engl J Med 338:791, 1998.
Dohil R, Israel DM, Hassall E: Effective 2-wk therapy for *Helicobacter pylori* disease in children. Gastroenterol 92:244, 1997.
Hawkey CJ, Karrasch JA, Szczepanski L, et al: Omeprazole compared with misoprostol for ulcers associated with nonsteroidal anti-inflammatory drugs. N Engl J Med 338:727, 1998.
Judd RH: *Helicobacter pylori*, gastritis, and ulcers in pediatrics. Adv Pediatr 39:283, 1992.
Laine L, Peterson W: Bleeding peptic ulcer. N Engl J Med 331:717, 1994.
Moshkowitz M, Reif S, Brill S, et al: One-week triple therapy with omeprazole, clarithromycin, and nitroimidazole for *Helicobacter pylori* infection in children and adolescents. Pediatrics 102:e14, 1998 URL: http:www.pediatrics.org/cgi/content/full/102/1/e14.
Rauws EAJ, van der Hulst RWM: The management of *H. pylori* infection. BMJ 316:162, 1998.
Rowland M, Lambert I, Gormally S, et al: Carbon 13–labeled urea breath test for the diagnosis of *Helicobacter pylori* infection in children. J Pediatr 131:815, 1997.
Yeomans ND, Tulassay Z, Juhasz L, et al: A comparison of omeprazole with ranitidine for ulcers associated with nonsteriodal anti-inflammatory drugs. N Engl J Med 338:719, 1998.

Chapter 337
Inflammatory Bowel Disease

Martin Ulshen

Inflammatory bowel disease (IBD)—a group of idiopathic, chronic disorders—includes Crohn disease and ulcerative colitis. The etiology is poorly understood, and the natural course is characterized by unpredictable exacerbations and remissions. The most common time of onset of IBD is during adolescence and young adulthood. A bimodal distribution has been shown with an early onset at 15–25 yr of age and a second smaller peak at 50–80 yr of age. Nonetheless, IBD may begin in the 1st yr of life. IBD is more common in urban areas than in rural areas. In developed countries, these disorders are the major causes of chronic intestinal inflammation in children beyond the 1st few yr of life.

Both *genetic and environmental influences* are involved in the pathogenesis of IBD. The incidence among Jews is high but varies geographically. Although incidence rates are low among blacks in Africa, in the United States they are similar to those of whites. The prevalence of Crohn disease in the United States is much lower for Hispanics and Asians than for whites and blacks. The risk of IBD in family members of an affected individual has been reported in the range of 7–22%; a child whose parents both have IBD has a greater than 35% chance of acquiring the disorder. Relatives of an individual with ulcerative colitis have a greater risk of acquiring ulcerative colitis than Crohn disease, whereas relatives of an individual with Crohn disease have a greater risk of acquiring this disorder; the two diseases may occur in the same family. The risk of occurrence of IBD among relatives of individuals with Crohn disease is somewhat greater than for individuals with ulcerative colitis. Within a family, Crohn disease may demonstrate anticipation, developing at an earlier age among the 2nd generation.

The importance of genetic factors in the development of IBD is noted by a higher chance that both twins will be affected if they are monozygotic rather than dizygotic. The concordance rate in twins is higher in Crohn disease than in ulcerative colitis. Genetic disorders that have been associated with IBD include Turner syndrome, the Hermansky-Pudlak syndrome, glycogen storage disease type Ib, and various immunodeficiency disorders. Environmental factors are also important and presumably explain discordance among twins and changes in risk among the same race in different geographic regions; the precise factors remain unknown. Individuals migrating to developed countries often appear to acquire the higher rates of IBD associated with these regions. Cigarette smoking is a risk factor for Crohn disease but paradoxically protects against ulcerative colitis.

Mediators of inflammatory states (cytokines, prostaglandins, reactive oxygen metabolites) may be involved in IBD; therapy is aimed at interfering with these agents. The initiating events that start the inflammatory response remain to be identified.

It is usually possible *to distinguish between ulcerative colitis and Crohn disease* by the clinical presentation and radiologic, endoscopic, and histopathologic findings (Table 337–1). It is not possible to make a definitive diagnosis in as many as 10% of individuals with chronic colitis; this disorder is called *indeterminate colitis.* Occasionally, a child diagnosed with ulcerative colitis on the basis of clinical findings is subsequently diagnosed with Crohn colitis. The treatments of Crohn disease and ulcerative colitis overlap; as refinements in treatment are identified, the distinction between these entities becomes more important.

TABLE 337–1 Comparison of Crohn Disease and Ulcerative Colitis

Feature	Crohn Disease	Ulcerative Colitis
Rectal bleeding	Sometimes	Common
Abdominal mass	Common	Not present
Rectal disease	Occasional	Nearly universal
Ileal involvement	Common	None (backwash ileitis)
Perianal disease	Common	Unusual
Strictures	Common	Unusual
Fistula	Common	Unusual
Discontinuous (skip) lesions	Common	Not present
Transmural involvement	Common	Unusual
Crypt abscesses	Less common	Common
Granulomas	Common	Unusual
Risk for colonic cancer	Slightly increased	Greatly increased
Pyoderma gangrenosum	Less common	Present
Erythema nodosum	Common	Less common
Mouth ulcers	Common	Rare
Cholangitis	Less common	Present
Stroke	Less common	Present

Extraintestinal manifestations occur slightly more commonly with Crohn disease than with ulcerative colitis. Growth retardation may be seen in 15–35% of individuals at diagnosis. Of the extraintestinal manifestations that occur with IBD, joint, skin, eye, mouth, and hepatobiliary involvement tend to be associated with colitis whether ulcerative or Crohn colitis. For some manifestations, activity correlates with activity of the bowel disease, including peripheral arthritis, erythema nodosum, and anemia. Activity of pyoderma gangrenosum correlates less well with activity of the bowel disease, whereas activities of sclerosing cholangitis, ankylosing spondylitis, and sacroiliitis do not correlate with intestinal disease. Arthritis occurs in three patterns: migratory peripheral arthritis involving primarily large joints, ankylosing spondylitis, and sacroiliitis. The peripheral arthritis of IBD tends to be nondestructive. Ankylosing spondylitis begins in the 3rd decade and occurs most commonly in individuals with ulcerative colitis who have the human leukocyte antigen B27 phenotype. Symptoms include low back pain and morning stiffness; back, hips, shoulders, and sacroiliac joints are typically affected. Isolated sacroiliitis is usually asymptomatic but is common when a careful search is performed. Among the skin manifestations, erythema nodosum is most common. Individuals with erythema nodosum or pyoderma gangrenosum have a high likelihood of having arthritis as well. Glomerulonephritis and a hypercoagulable state are other rare manifestations that occur in childhood. Cerebral thromboembolic disease has been described in children with IBD. Uveitis occurs in about 5% of children with IBD and is usually asymptomatic and transient; its occurrence does not correlate with activity of bowel disease.

337.1 *Chronic Ulcerative Colitis*

Ulcerative colitis, an idiopathic chronic inflammatory disorder, is localized to the colon and spares the upper gastrointestinal tract. Disease virtually always begins in the rectum and extends proximally for a variable distance. When it is localized to the rectum, the disease is ulcerative proctitis, whereas disease involving the entire colon is pancolitis. The former disorder is less likely to be associated with systemic manifestations, although it may be less responsive to treatment than more diffuse disease. About 30% of children who present with ulcerative protitis experience proximal spread of the disease. Ulcerative colitis has rarely been noted to present in infancy. Dietary protein intolerance may be easily misdiagnosed as ulcerative colitis in this age group. Dietary protein intolerance (e.g., cow's milk protein) is a transient disorder; symptoms are directly associated with the intake of the offending antigen.

The incidence of ulcerative colitis has remained constant, in contrast to the increase in Crohn disease, but varies with country of origin. Incidence rates are highest in northern European countries and the United States (15/100,000) and lowest in Japan and South Africa (1/100,000). The incidence of ulcerative colitis in Israel varies with the country of origin; those born in Asia or Africa have the lowest risk. The prevalence of ulcerative colitis in northern European countries and the United States varies from 100–200/100,000 population. Men are slightly more likely to acquire ulcerative colitis than are women; the reverse is true for Crohn disease. The incidence of ulcerative proctitis is 20–50% that of ulcerative colitis.

CLINICAL MANIFESTATIONS. Symptoms of mild dysentery (bloody diarrhea with mucus) are the typical presentation of ulcerative colitis. Symptoms such as tenesmus, urgency, crampy abdominal pain (especially with bowel movements), and nocturnal bowel movements suggest a more severe colitis. The onset may be insidious with gradual progression of symptoms but can be fulminant. Fever, severe anemia, hypoalbuminemia, leukocytosis, and stool frequency of more than 6 days all suggest fulminant colitis. Chronicity is an important part of the diagnosis; it is difficult to know whether one is dealing with a subacute, transient colitis or ulcerative colitis when a child has had 3–4 wk of symptoms without an identifiable cause. Symptoms beyond this duration often prove to be secondary to IBD. Occasionally, the presentation of ulcerative colitis may be very mild (mild rectal bleeding without diarrhea due to localized proctitis). Anorexia, weight loss, and growth failure may be present, although systemic manifestations are more typical of Crohn disease.

Extraintestinal manifestations that tend to occur more commonly with ulcerative colitis than with Crohn disease include pyoderma gangrenosum, sclerosing cholangitis, chronic active hepatitis, and ankylosing spondylitis. Any of the extraintestinal disorders described previously for IBD may occur with ulcerative colitis. Iron deficiency may result from chronic blood loss as well as decreased assimilation (due to decreased intake or decreased absorption). Folate deficiency is unusual but may be accentuated in children treated with sulfasalazine, which interferes with folate absorption. Anemia may be the result of chronic disease without an identifiable deficiency. Secondary amenorrhea is common during periods of active disease in older girls.

The clinical course of ulcerative colitis is marked by exacerbations, often without apparent explanation. Typically, the disease may be quieted with medication but eventually it recurs. After initial symptoms, about 5% of children with ulcerative colitis have a prolonged remission (>3 yr). Occasionally, the colitis becomes intractable and may require surgical treatment. The likelihood of eventual colectomy correlates with the severity of disease at onset. It is important to consider the possibility of enteric infection with recurrent symptoms; these infections may mimic a flare-up or actually provoke a recurrence. Nonsteroidal anti-inflammatory drugs may also promote exacerbations.

It is generally believed that the risk of colon cancer begins to increase after 8–10 yr of disease and may then increase by 0.5–1% per yr. The risk is delayed by about 10 yr in individuals with colitis limited to the descending colon. Proctitis alone is associated with virtually no increase in risk over the general population. Childhood onset does not appear to increase the risk further. Because colon cancer is usually preceded by changes of mucosal dysplasia, it is recommended that patients who have had ulcerative colitis more than 10 yr be screened with colonoscopy and biopsy every 1–2 yr. The effectiveness of this approach in preventing colon cancer remains to be established. Two concerns about this plan of management remain unresolved: (1) the original studies may have overestimated the risk of colon cancer and, therefore, the need for surveillance has been overemphasized and (2) screening for dysplasia may not be adequate for the prevention of colon cancer in ulcerative colitis if some cancers are not preceded by dysplasia. Nevertheless, screening and prophylactic colectomy are the only alternatives.

DIFFERENTIAL DIAGNOSIS. The major conditions to exclude are infectious colitis and Crohn colitis. A history of contact with others with gastroenteritis should make one consider an infectious cause. Every child with a new diagnosis of ulcerative colitis should have stool cultured for enteric pathogens, stool evaluation for ova and parasites, and perhaps serologic studies for ameba (Table 337–2). In the setting of antibiotic use, pseudomembranous colitis secondary to *Clostridium difficile* should be considered. The most difficult distinction is from Crohn disease because the colitis of Crohn disease may initially appear identical to that of ulcerative colitis. The appearance of the colitis or development of small bowel disease eventually leads to the correct diagnosis; this may occur years after the initial presentation.

At the onset, the colitis of hemolytic-uremic syndrome may be identical to that of early ulcerative colitis. Ultimately, signs

TABLE 337–2 Infectious Agents Mimicking Inflammatory Bowel Disease

Agent	Manifestations	Diagnosis	Comments
Bacterial			
Campylobacter jejuni	Acute diarrhea, fever, fecal blood, and leukocytes	Culture	Common in adolescents, may relapse
Yersinia enterocolitica	Acute→ chronic diarrhea, right lower quadrant pain, mesenteric adenitis—pseudoappendicitis, fecal blood, and leukocytes Extraintestinal manifestations, mimics Crohn disease	Culture	Common in adolescents as FUO, weight loss, abdominal pain
Clostridium difficile	Postantibiotic onset, watery diarrhea, pseudomembrane on sigmoidoscopy	Cytotoxin assay	May be nosocomial Toxic megacolon possible
Escherichia coli 0157:H7	Colitis, fecal blood, abdominal pain	Culture and typing	Hemolytic-uremic syndrome
Salmonella	Watery→ bloody diarrhea, food borne, fecal leukocytes, cramps	Culture	Usually acute
Shigella	Watery→ bloody diarrhea, fecal leukocytes, fever, pain, cramps	Culture	Dysentery symptoms
Edwardsiella tarda	Bloody diarrhea, cramps	Culture	Ulceration on endoscopy
Aeromonas hydrophila	Cramps, diarrhea, fecal blood	Culture	May be chronic Contaminated drinking water
Plesiomonas	Diarrhea, cramps	Culture	Shellfish source
Tuberculosis	Rarely bovine, now *Mycobacterium tuberculosis* Ileocecal area, fistula formation	Culture, PPD, biopsy	May mimic Crohn disease
Parasites			
Entamoeba histolytica	Acute bloody diarrhea and liver abscess, colic	Trophozoite in stool, colonic mucosal flask ulceration, serologic tests	Travel to endemic area
Giardia lamblia	Foul-smelling, watery diarrhea, cramps, flatulence, weight loss; no colonic involvement	"Owl"-like trophozoite and cysts in stool; rarely duodenal intubation	May be chronic
AIDS-Associated Enteropathy			
Cryptosporidium	Chronic diarrhea, weight loss	Stool microscopy	Mucosal findings not like IBD
Isospora belli	As in *Cryptosporidium*		Tropical location
Cytomegalovirus	Colonic ulceration, pain, bloody diarrhea	Culture, biopsy	

FUO = fever of unknown origin; PPD = purified protein derivative; AIDS = acquired immunodeficiency syndrome; IBD = inflammatory bowel disease.

of microangiopathic hemolysis (the presence of schistocytes on blood smear), thrombocytopenia, and subsequent renal failure should confirm the diagnosis of hemolytic-uremic syndrome. Although Henoch-Schönlein purpura may present with abdominal pain and bloody stools, it is not usually associated with colitis. Behçet's syndrome can be distinguished by its typical features (see Chapters 162 and 337.3). Other considerations are cathartic colitis, radiation proctitis, viral colitis in acquired immunodeficiency syndrome, and ischemic colitis. In infancy, dietary protein intolerance may be confused with ulcerative colitis, although this disorder is a transient problem that resolves on removal of the offending protein. Hirschsprung disease may produce a colitis before or within months after surgical correction; this is unlikely to be confused with ulcerative colitis.

DIAGNOSIS. The diagnosis of ulcerative colitis or ulcerative proctitis requires a typical presentation in the absence of an identifiable specific cause (Table 337–3; also see Table 337–2) and typical endoscopic and radiologic findings (see Table 337–1). The diagnosis is based on the right constellation of history and findings in the context of a chronic disorder. One should be hesitant to make a diagnosis of ulcerative colitis in a child who has experienced symptoms for fewer than 3–4 wk. When the diagnosis is suspected in a child with subacute symptoms, the physician should make a firm diagnosis only when there is evidence of chronicity. Laboratory studies may demonstrate evidence of anemia (either iron deficiency or the anemia of chronic disease) or hypoalbuminemia. Although the sedimentation rate is often elevated, it may be normal even with fulminant colitis. An elevated white count is usually seen only with more severe colitis. Blood antineutrophil cytoplasmic antibodies are present in 65% of the children with ulcerative colitis compared with 20% of those with Crohn disease. This test is not specific enough to make a diagnosis but may be a helpful adjunct. Antibodies persist after colectomy and are also found in healthy relatives of individuals with ulcerative colitis.

Findings of ulcerative colitis can be identified by endoscopic or radiologic examination of the colon, although endoscopy (sigmoidoscopy or colonoscopy) is more sensitive for mild dis-

TABLE 337–3 Chronic Inflammatory Intestinal Disorders

Infection—see Table 337–2
- Bacterial
- Parasite
- AIDS-associated
- Toxin

Immune-Inflammatory
- Congenital immunodeficiency disorders
- Acquired immunodeficiency diseases
- Dietary protein enterocolitis
- Behçet's syndrome
- Lymphoid nodular hyperplasia
- Eosinophilic gastroenteritis
- Graft-versus-host disease

Vascular-Ischemic Disorders
- Systemic vasculitis (SLE, dermatomyositis)
- Henoch-Schönlein purpura
- Hemolytic-uremic syndrome

Other
- Prestenotic colitis
- Diversion colitis
- Radiation colitis
- Neonatal necrotizing enterocolitis
- Typhlitis
- Hirschsprung colitis
- Intestinal lymphoma
- Laxative abuse

AIDS = acquired immunodeficiency syndrome; SLE = systemic lupus erythematosus.

ease and offers the opportunity for simultaneous biopsy. Certain typical features can be seen on either study, including concentric, diffuse colitis starting in the rectum and extending proximally for a variable distance. One should not see skip areas (areas of normal colon between diseased areas); however, the finding of skip areas must be confirmed histologically before it can be used as evidence against a diagnosis of ulcerative colitis. Endoscopic examination should be performed when one suspects this diagnosis. One can use either a flexible sigmoidoscopy to confirm the diagnosis or colonoscopy to evaluate the extent of disease and to rule out evidence of Crohn colitis. A colonoscopy should *not* be performed when fulminant colitis is suspected because of the risk of provoking toxic megacolon or causing a perforation during the procedure. The degree of colitis can be evaluated by the gross appearance of the mucosa. Despite the name, one does not generally see discrete ulcers, which would be more suggestive of Crohn colitis. The endoscopic findings of ulcerative colitis result from microulcers, which give the appearance of a diffuse abnormality. The earliest grossly visible changes are granularity and then loss of the normal vascular pattern. Friability induced on contact with the endoscope may also be seen with mild colitis. More severe changes include erythema, spontaneous friability, and edema of the mucosa with blunting of mucosal folds. With very severe colitis, pseudopolyps may be seen. Perianal disease, with the exception of mild local irritation or anal fissures associated with diarrhea, should make one think of Crohn disease. The biopsy of involved bowel demonstrates evidence of acute and chronic mucosal inflammation. Typical findings are cryptitis, crypt abscesses, separation of crypts by inflammatory cells, foci of acute inflammatory cells, edema, mucus depletion, and branching of crypts. The last finding is a feature not seen in infectious colitis. Granulomas, fissures, or full-thickness involvement of the bowel wall (usually on surgical rather than endoscopic biopsy) suggests Crohn disease. Rectal biopsy can also distinguish chronic IBD from acute self-limiting colitis.

Plain radiographs of the abdomen may demonstrate loss of haustral markings in an air-filled colon or marked dilatation with toxic megacolon. Further radiologic studies are often unnecessary if endoscopy has been performed. A double-contrast barium (air) enema is the best radiographic study to identify ulcerative colitis, although it is not as sensitive as endoscopy for mild colitis. Radiologic findings on barium enema demonstrate diffuse, concentric disease with a finely spiculated border representing the microulceration. The earliest changes are fine granularity followed by more coarse granularity. With severe disease, "collar button" ulcers with submucosal undermining may be seen. Mucosal folds become thickened and may be completely obliterated to give a smooth-appearing surface, sometimes known as a "lead pipe colon." This appearance is sometimes reversible with treatment. The terminal ileum should appear normal, except in children with pancolitis in whom the terminal ileum may be dilatated with a patulous ileocecal valve (known as backwash ileitis). With severe colitis, the colon may become dilated; a diameter of greater than 6 cm, determined radiographically, in an adult suggests toxic megacolon. If it is necessary to examine the colon radiologically in a child with severe colitis (to evaluate the extent of involvement or to try to rule out Crohn disease), it is sometimes helpful to perform an upper gastrointestinal contrast series with small bowel follow-through and then look at delayed films of the colon. This is much safer than performing a barium enema in the situation of potential toxic megacolon.

TREATMENT. A medical cure for ulcerative colitis is not available; treatment is aimed at controlling symptoms and reducing the risk of recurrence. The intensity of treatment varies with the severity of the symptoms. In placebo-controlled studies of therapy, about 20–30% of individuals with ulcerative colitis have spontaneous improvement in symptoms. The first drug to be used with mild colitis is an aminosalicylate. Sulfasalazine has been used extensively over many years, and its effects are well characterized. It is composed of a sulfur moiety linked to the active ingredient 5-aminosalicylate. This linkage prevents the premature absorption of the medication in the upper gastrointestinal tract, allowing it to reach the colon, where the two components are separated by bacterial cleavage. The starting dose of sulfasalazine is 50–75 mg/kg/24 hr (divided into two to four doses). Generally, the dose is not more than 2 to 3 g/24 hr. It is recommended that the dosage gradually increase to full dose over the 1st wk of treatment to avoid gastrointestinal symptoms and to detect sulfa hypersensitivity. Onset of action may be several weeks. Sulfasalazine treats colitis; recurrences may be prevented with its use. It is recommended that the medication be continued even when the disorder is in remission. Hypersensitivity to the sulfa component is the major side effect of sulfasalazine and may occur in up to 10–20% of individuals. Other less allergenic preparations of 5-aminosalicylate have been shown to treat ulcerative colitis and prevent recurrences.

Perhaps 10–20% of individuals who have an allergic reaction to sulfasalazine will have a similar reaction to another 5-aminosalicylate product. On rare occasions, these medications cause exacerbation of colitis. Aminosalicylate may also be given in enema form and is especially useful for proctitis. Hydrocortisone enemas (100 mg) are used to treat proctitis as well. Either form of enema may be administered to older children and is given once a day usually for 2–3 wk. Many children prefer oral medication to enemas.

Children with moderate to severe pancolitis or colitis that is unresponsive to 5-aminosalicylate therapy should be treated with oral corticosteroids, most commonly prednisone. The usual starting dose of prednisone is 1–2 mg/kg/24 hr (60 mg should rarely be exceeded). If symptoms are not severe, this medication may be given in a single morning dose to lessen adrenal suppression. With severe colitis, the daily dose may be divided into three or four doses and may be given intravenously. The goal is to taper to an alternate-day dose within 1–3 mo. Persistent symptoms despite steroid treatment or the inability to taper the dose is an indication for the use of other medications or for surgical management. Prolonged use of daily steroids beyond this period is to be avoided because of the many side effects, including growth retardation, adrenal suppression, cataracts, osteopenia, aseptic necrosis of the head of the femur, glucose intolerance, risk of infection, and cosmetic effects. With medical management, most children are in remission within 3 mo; however, 5–10% continue to have symptoms unresponsive to treatment beyond 6 mo. Colectomy may be necessary in fulminant disease (greater than six to eight stools in 24 hr, passage of stools during the night, fever, elevated white cell count, anemia, hypoalbuminemia, and tender abdomen) that is unresponsive to medical management for 3–4 wk.

No clear benefit of the use of total parenteral nutrition or a continuous enteral elemental diet in the treatment of severe ulcerative colitis has been noted. Nevertheless, parenteral nutrition is often used so that the patient will be ready for surgery if medical management fails. Other agents that have been used in steroid-unresponsive or steroid-dependent colitis include azathioprine, 6-mercaptopurine (6-MP), metronidazole, and cyclosporine. Azathioprine and 6-MP are the slowest to begin to work. Experience with these medications in the treatment of colitis in children is limited. With any medical treatment for ulcerative colitis, one should always weigh the risk of the medication or therapy against the fact that colitis may be successfully treated surgically.

Surgical treatment for intractable or fulminant colitis is total colectomy. The optimal approach is to combine colectomy with an endorectal pull-through. In this procedure, the surgeon retains a segment of distal rectum and strips the mucosa from this region. The distal ileum is pulled down and sutured at the internal anus with a J pouch created from ileum immediately above the rectal cuff. This procedure allows the child to maintain continence. Stool frequency is often increased after the procedure but may be improved with loperamide. The major complication of this operation is "pouchitis," which is a chronic inflammatory reaction in the pouch, leading to bloody diarrhea, abdominal pain, and occasionally low-grade fever. The cause of this complication is unknown, although it is more frequent when the ileal pouch has been constructed for ulcerative colitis than for other indications (familial polyposis coli).

The concept that ulcerative colitis is primarily a psychogenic disorder is untenable. However, emotional stresses may contribute to exacerbations. Difficulty adjusting to a chronic disorder is common, and distorted body image should be considered when evaluating the psychologic profile of a child with this disorder. Psychosocial support is an important part of therapy of this disorder. This may include adequate discussion of the disease manifestations and management between patient and physician, psychologic counseling for the child when necessary, and family support from a social worker or family counselor. Patient support groups have proved helpful for some families. The largest of these is the Crohn and Colitis Foundation of America, which has local chapters throughout the United States. Children with ulcerative colitis should be encouraged to participate fully in age-appropriate activities; however, activity may need to be reduced during periods of decreased stamina.

PROGNOSIS. The course of ulcerative colitis is marked by remissions and exacerbations. Most children with this disorder respond initially to medical management. Many children with mild manifestations continue to respond well to medical management and may stay in remission on a prophylactic 5-aminosalicylate preparation for long periods. However, an occasional child with mild onset experiences intractable symptoms at a later time. The most serious acute complication is toxic megacolon with the risk of perforation. Beyond the 1st decade of disease, the risk of development of colon cancer begins to increase rapidly. However, current thinking is that colon cancer may be prevented with surveillance colonoscopies beginning after 8–10 yr of disease.

Bridger S, Evans N, Parker A, et al: Multiple cerebral venous thromboses in a child with inflammatory bowel disease. J Pediatr Gastroenterol Nutr 25:533, 1997.

Cosgrove M, Al-Atia RF, Jenkins HR: The epidemiology of paediatric inflammatory bowel disease. Arch Dis Child 74:460, 1996.

Dundas SA, Dutton J, Skipworth P: Reliability of rectal biopsy in distinguishing between chronic inflammatory bowel disease and acute self-limiting colitis. Histopathology 31:60, 1997.

Ekbom A, Helmick C, Zack M, et al: Ulcerative colitis and colorectal cancer. N Engl J Med 323:1228, 1990.

Ferry GD, Kirschner BS, Grand RJ, et al: Olsalazine versus sulfasalazine in mild to moderate childhood ulcerative colitis: Results of the Pediatric Gastroenterology Collaborative Research Group Clinical Trial. J Pediatr Gastroenterol Nutr 17:32, 1993.

Galperin C, Gershwin E: Immunopathogenesis of gastrointestinal and hepatobiliary diseases. JAMA 278:1946, 1997.

Hanauer SB, Sninsky CA, Robinson M, et al: An oral preparation of mesalamine as long-term maintenance therapy of ulcerative colitis: A randomized, placebo-controlled trial. Ann Intern Med 124:204, 1996.

Hyams J, Davis P, Lerer T, et al: Clinical outcome of ulcerative proctitis in children. J Pediatr Gastroenterol Nutr 25:149, 1997.

Hyams JS, Davis P, Grancher K, et al: Clinical outcome of ulcerative colitis in children. J Pediatr 129:81, 1996.

Lichtiger S, Present DH, Kornbluth A, et al: Cyclosporine in severe ulcerative colitis refractory to steroid therapy. N Engl J Med 330:1841, 1994.

Pavli P, Cavanaugh J, Grimm M: Inflammatory bowel disease: Germs or genes? Lancet 347:1198, 1996.

Proujansky R, Fawcett PT, Gibney KM, et al: Examination of anti-neutrophil cytoplasmic antibodies in childhood inflammatory bowel disease. J Pediatr Gastroenterol Nutr 17:193, 1993.

Sartor RB: Cytokines in intestinal inflammation: Pathophysiological and clinical considerations. Gastroenterology 106:533, 1994.

Sugita A, Sachar DB, Bodian C, et al: Colorectal cancer in ulcerative colitis: Influence of anatomical extent and age at onset on colitis-cancer interval. Gut 32:167, 1991.

337.2 Crohn Disease (Regional Enteritis, Regional Ileitis, Granulomatous Colitis)

Crohn disease—an idiopathic, chronic inflammatory disorder of the bowel—involves any region of the alimentary tract from the mouth to the anus. Although there are many similarities between ulcerative colitis and Crohn disease, there are also major differences in the clinical course and distribution of the disease in the gastrointestinal tract. The inflammatory process tends to be eccentric and segmental, often with skip areas (normal regions of bowel between inflamed areas). Although inflammation in ulcerative colitis is limited to the mucosa (except in toxic megacolon), gastrointestinal involvement in Crohn disease is transmural. Among children with Crohn disease, the initial presentation most commonly involves ileum and colon (ileocolitis) but may involve the small bowel alone in about 40% (50% of these patients have terminal ileitis alone) or colon alone in about 10% (granulomatous colitis). Crohn disease may rarely present in the 1st yr of life. As with ulcerative colitis, Crohn disease tends to have a bimodal age distribution, with the 1st peak beginning in the late teens. Diagnosis before 20 yr of age is associated with a greater chance of small bowel disease, development of stricture, and eventual need for surgery when compared with diagnosis after 40 yr. Likelihood of Crohn disease in family members is doubled with early diagnosis.

The incidence of Crohn disease has been increasing over the past 10 yr, whereas that of ulcerative colitis has been stable. The proportion of patients with IBD who are being managed for Crohn disease has gradually increased. The reported incidence of Crohn disease is about 3–4/100,000 and the prevalence is 30–100/100,000. The prevalence of Crohn disease in whites and blacks appears to be 3–10 times that of Hispanics and Asians living in the United States.

CLINICAL MANIFESTATIONS. Crohn disease presents in many forms; the manifestations tend to be dictated by the region of bowel involved, the degree of inflammation, and the presence of complications such as stricture or fistula. Children with ileocolitis typically have crampy, abdominal pain and diarrhea, sometimes with blood. Ileitis may present with right lower quadrant abdominal pain alone. Crohn colitis may be associated with bloody diarrhea, tenesmus, and urgency. Systemic signs and symptoms are more common in Crohn disease than in ulcerative colitis. Fever, malaise, and easy fatigability are common. Growth failure with delayed bone maturation and delayed sexual development may precede other symptoms by 1 or 2 yr and are at least twice as likely to occur with Crohn as with ulcerative colitis. Children may present with growth failure as the only manifestation of Crohn disease. Growth retardation is associated with a decrease in lean body mass but preservation of body fat; enteric protein loss and the rate of body protein turnover are increased. Primary or secondary amenorrhea occurs frequently. In contrast to ulcerative colitis, *perianal disease* is common (tags, fistula, abscess). Gastric or duodenal involvement may be associated with recurrent vomiting and epigastric pain. Partial small bowel obstruction, usually secondary to narrowing of the bowel lumen from inflammation or stricture, may cause symptoms of crampy abdominal pain (especially with meals), borborygmus, and intermittent abdominal distention. Stricture should be suspected if the child notes relief of symptoms in association with a sudden sensation of gurgling of intestinal contents through a localized region of the abdomen. Ureteral obstruction secondary to extension of the inflammatory process is a rare complication of Crohn disease.

Enteroenteric or enterocolonic fistulas (between segments of bowel) are often asymptomatic but may contribute to malabsorption if they have high output or result in bacterial overgrowth. Enterovesical fistulas (between bowel and urinary bladder) originate from ileum or sigmoid colon and present with signs of urinary infection, pneumaturia, or fecaluria. Enterovaginal fistulas originate from the rectum, cause feculent vaginal drainage, and are difficult to manage. Enterocutaneous fistulas (between bowel and abdominal skin) often are due to prior surgical anastomoses with leakage. Intra-abdominal abscess may be associated with fever and pain but may have relatively few symptoms. Hepatic or splenic abscess may occur with or without a local fistula. Anorectal abscesses often originate immediately above the anus at the crypts of Morgagni. The patterns of perianal fistulas are complex because of the different tissue planes. Perianal abscess is usually painful, but perianal fistulas tend to produce fewer symptoms than might be anticipated from their appearance. Purulent drainage is commonly associated with perianal fistulas. Psoas abscess secondary to intestinal fistula may present as hip pain, decreased hip extension (psoas sign), and fever.

Extraintestinal manifestations occur more commonly with Crohn disease than with ulcerative colitis; those that are especially associated with Crohn disease include oral aphthous ulcers, peripheral arthritis, erythema nodosum, digital clubbing, episcleritis, renal stones (uric acid, oxalate), and gallstones. Any of the extraintestinal disorders described in the section on IBD may occur with Crohn disease. The peripheral arthritis is nondeforming. In general, the occurrence of extraintestinal manifestations correlates with the presence of colitis. During periods of active disease, secondary amenorrhea is common in older girls.

Extensive involvement of small bowel, especially in association with surgical resection, may lead to short-bowel syndrome, which is rare in children. Complications of terminal ileal dysfunction or resection include bile acid malabsorption with secondary diarrhea and vitamin B_{12} malabsorption. Chronic steatorrhea may lead to oxaluria with secondary renal stones. The risk of cholelithiasis is also increased secondary to bile acid depletion.

A disorder with this diversity of manifestations has a major impact on children's lifestyles. They may repeatedly miss school because of symptoms. The association of pain or diarrhea with eating may limit their interest in participating in many age-appropriate activities. The majority of children with Crohn disease are able to continue with their normal activities, having to limit activity only during periods of increased symptoms.

DIFFERENTIAL DIAGNOSIS. As in patients with ulcerative colitis, the most common diagnoses to be distinguished from Crohn disease are the infectious enteropathies (in the case of Crohn disease: acute terminal ileitis, infectious colitis, enteric parasites, and periappendiceal abscess) (see Tables 337–2 and 337–3). *Yersinia* may cause many of the radiologic and endoscopic findings in the distal small bowel that are seen in Crohn disease. The symptoms of bacterial dysentery are more likely to be mistaken for ulcerative colitis than for Crohn disease. *Giardia* has been noted to produce a Crohnlike presentation including protein-losing enteropathy. Gastrointestinal tuberculosis is rare but can mimic Crohn disease. Foreign body perforation of the bowel (toothpick) may mimic a localized region with Crohn disease. Small bowel lymphoma may mimic Crohn disease but tends to be associated with nodular filling defects of the bowel without ulceration or narrowing of the lumen. In addition, bowel lymphoma is much less common in children than is Crohn disease. Recurrent functional abdominal pain may mimic the pain of small bowel Crohn disease. Lymphoid nodular hyperplasia of the terminal ileum (a normal finding) may be mistaken for Crohn ileitis. Right lower quadrant pain or mass with fever may be the result of periappendiceal abscess. This entity may occasionally be associated with diarrhea as well. Necrotizing jejunitis is a rare condition of transient, acute inflammation of jejunum (or less commonly ileum or colon), which may recur.

Growth failure may be the only manifestation of Crohn disease; other disorders such as growth hormone deficiency or gluten-sensitive enteropathy must be considered. If arthritis precedes the bowel manifestations, an initial diagnosis of juvenile rheumatoid arthritis may be made. Refractory anemia may be the presenting feature and may be mistaken as a primary hematologic disorder. Leukemia may present with abdominal pain in association with an abnormal blood count and initially may be mistaken for Crohn disease. Chronic granulomatous disease of childhood may cause inflammatory changes in the bowel with granulomas seen at biopsy. Antral narrowing in this disorder may be mistaken for a stricture secondary to Crohn disease.

DIAGNOSIS. Crohn disease may present with a variety of symptom combinations. At the onset, symptoms may be subtle (growth retardation or abdominal pain alone); this explains why the diagnosis may not be made until 1 or 2 yr after the start of symptoms. The diagnosis of Crohn disease is dependent on finding typical clinical features of the disorder (history, physical examination, laboratory studies, and endoscopic or radiologic findings), ruling out specific entities that mimic Crohn disease, and demonstrating chronicity. The history may include any combination of abdominal pain (especially right lower quadrant), diarrhea, vomiting, anorexia, weight loss, growth retardation, and extraintestinal manifestations.

Children with Crohn disease often appear chronically ill. They commonly have weight loss and are often malnourished. Linear growth retardation frequently precedes clinical presentation by as much as 1–2 yr; this manifestation may not have been appreciated until the diagnosis is established. Children with Crohn disease often appear pale with decreased energy level and poor appetite; the latter finding sometimes results from an association between meals and abdominal pain or diarrhea. There may be abdominal tenderness that is either diffuse or localized to the right lower quadrant. A tender mass or fullness may be palpable in the right lower quadrant. Perianal disease, when present, may be characteristic. Large anal skin tags (1–3 cm diameter) or perianal fistulas with purulent drainage are suggestive of Crohn disease. Digital clubbing, findings of arthritis, and skin manifestations may be present. A complete blood count commonly demonstrates an anemia, often with a component of iron deficiency. Although the sedimentation rate is often elevated, it may be normal; an elevated platelet count ($>600,000/mm^3$) is seen more commonly. The white cell count may be normal or mildly elevated. The serum albumin level may be low, and stool α_1-antitrypsin may be elevated consistent with a protein-losing enteropathy. Anti-*Saccharomyces cerevisiae* antibodies are identified in 55% of children with Crohn disease but in only 5% of children with ulcerative colitis.

The choice of colonoscopy or a radiologic study depends on the anticipated location of disease. For small bowel involvement, an upper gastrointestinal contrast examination with small bowel follow-through would be the initial study. A variety of findings may be apparent on radiologic studies. Plain films of the abdomen may be normal or may demonstrate findings of partial small bowel obstruction or thumbprinting of the colon wall. An upper gastrointestinal contrast study with small bowel follow-through may show aphthous ulceration and thickened, nodular folds as well as narrowing of the lumen anywhere in the gastrointestinal tract. Linear ulcers may give a cobblestone appearance to the mucosal surface. Bowel loops are often separated as a result of thickening of bowel wall and mesentery. Terminal ileum is most commonly involved and may be evaluated in this fashion or with reflux into the small bowel during a barium enema study. Diseased regions tend to be eccentric, and normal regions may be found between diseased segments (skip areas).

Other manifestations on radiographic studies that suggest more severe Crohn disease are fistulas between bowel (enteroenteric or enterocolonic), sinus tracts, and strictures. Barium enema may demonstrate mucosal changes in the colon similar to those in the small bowel. The cecum and ascending colon tend to be most commonly involved. Strictures, sinus tracts, and fistulas may also be seen in the colon. Ultrasonography and computed tomography (CT) are most useful in identifying intra-abdominal abscess. Thickened bowel wall may be seen on CT. Magnetic resonance imaging can localize areas of active bowel disease, although this study is probably no better for identifying an abscess. MRI is also useful in evaluating Crohn disease during pregnancy because it does not use ionizing radiation.

Colonoscopy with biopsy can be more helpful than radiologic studies in evaluating colon disease and in establishing a diagnosis when it is uncertain. It is often possible to enter the terminal ileum during colonoscopy; this maneuver may be helpful in clarifying an equivocal diagnosis of ileal Crohn disease. Findings on colonoscopy may include patchy, nonspecific inflammatory changes (erythema, friability, loss of vascular pattern), aphthous ulcers, linear ulcers, nodularity, and strictures. Findings on biopsy may be only nonspecific inflammatory changes. When the biopsy findings are less striking than the gross appearance of colitis, one should think of the possibility of Crohn disease in which the abnormalities involve deeper layers of tissue. Noncaseating granulomas, similar to those of sarcoidosis, are the most characteristic histologic findings, although often they are not present. Transmural inflammation is also characteristic but can be identified only in surgical specimens. The presence of colitis or granulomas on blind biopsy of the colon are useful to rule out lymphoma.

TREATMENT. There is no single medical approach to Crohn disease because of the complexity of the disorder and the variety of its manifestations. The aim of treatment is largely to alleviate symptoms; treatment is dictated by the symptoms present. If disease is largely limited to small bowel, oral prednisone, 1–2 mg/kg/24 hr, is often the first treatment (maximum dose of 60 mg). If the activity is severe, the steroid dose may be divided during the day or may be given intravenously. Otherwise, a single morning dose is associated with the least adrenal suppression. The goal is to taper to a single morning alternate-day dose as soon as the disease becomes quiescent. Typically, this occurs by 3–4 wk, although sometimes it may take longer. When an excellent response to the initial prednisone treatment occurs, an immediate change to alternate-day therapy is often well tolerated (changing from prednisone 30 mg every day to 30 mg every other day). Otherwise, it may be necessary to taper more gradually to alternate-day treatment. This approach is well tolerated without apparent side effects. It is sometimes best to continue to treat a child with poorly controlled disease with 1 mg/kg or less every other day. Adolescents may grow better if they continue with alternate-day treatment rather than repeatedly having the medication dose raised and reduced. Side effects of daily steroid treatment tend to occur more rapidly and be more severe when the serum albumin level is reduced. Steroid enemas have been used for distal colon disease. Budesonide is being tried in enema and oral form because of its lower potential for systemic side effects.

Aminosalicylates have been used in the treatment of colon disease and are sometimes more effective than corticosteroids in this region. Sulfasalazine has been used in the same dose as that used for the treatment of ulcerative colitis. A number of other preparations of 5-aminosalicylates that are released in different regions of bowel are available. Aminosalicylate enemas may be used for descending colon disease. The preparation that delivers the highest level of drug to the involved bowel is the best choice in an individual patient. Prophylactic use of 5-aminosalicylates reduces the risk of recurrence. Azathioprine, 1–2 mg/kg/24 hr (or its metabolite 6-MP), may be effective in some individuals who have a poor response to steroids or who are steroid-dependent, although some may not respond to these drugs at all. Metronidazole has also been effective in intractable Crohn disease. Both azathioprine and metronidazole may be helpful in the treatment of perianal fistulas. Ciprofloxacin (in older children) and clarithromycin have been used in this situation. Local care of perianal disease with sitz baths should be performed as well. Application of steroid cream may be helpful for mild perianal disease. Cyclosporine and tacrolimus have been used for intractable disease but should probably be reserved for limited indications. The use of monoclonal antibodies to inhibit inflammatory cytokines (tumor necrosis factor α, infliximab) and the use of inhibitory cytokines (interleukin-10) are under investigation and show promising results. Infliximab is effective in moderate to severe Crohn disease and is effective in closing enterocutaneous fistulas. Diets high in fiber or low in residue or elimination diets have all been tried at one time in the management of Crohn disease, but none is effective. One tries to avoid restricting a child's diet because this often leads to inadequate calorie intake.

The initial onset or a recurrence of Crohn disease may be acute with severe pain, anorexia, fever, abdominal tenderness, and an elevated white cell count. In this situation, it is difficult to rule out an infectious process involving the bowel wall (microperforation). In addition to the use of intravenous steroids, broad-spectrum intravenous antibiotic coverage for bowel flora (gram-negative bacteria and anaerobes) should be started initially and discontinued only if it appears that there is not an infectious process. An ultrasonogram or CT study of the abdomen is often necessary to rule out an intra-abdominal abscess. The development of an enteroenteric or colonic fistula may be identified on CT, although it is best seen on a conventional small bowel contrast study.

Careful use of corticosteroids in Crohn disease does not seem to be associated with growth delays; growth retardation is more commonly related to the presence of the inflammatory process itself. Nevertheless, the injudicious use of daily steroids may lead to many complications, including growth retardation. Supplying adequate calories in the diet usually corrects growth retardation. High-calorie oral supplements, although effective, often are not tolerated because of early satiety or exacerbation of symptoms (abdominal pain, vomiting, or diarrhea). The use of parenteral nutrients in children with Crohn disease was initially shown to promote growth. The continuous administration of nocturnal nasogastric feedings has been effective with a much lower risk of complications. Complex formula may be given at 500–1,000 kcal nightly; treatment with 50–80 kcal/kg/night monthly every 4 mo has been considered equally effective by some.

Nutritional therapy is an effective primary treatment. Total parenteral nutrition is effective not only in nutritional repletion but also in quieting active disease. Controlled trials have compared the use of an elemental diet in active Crohn disease with treatment with corticosteroids or total parenteral nutrition. These studies have suggested that the nutritional approach is both as rapid in onset of response and as effective as the other treatments. An elemental diet has also been compared with complex enteral feedings and was superior in inducing remission. Because these diets are relatively unpalatable, they are administered via a nasogastric or gastrostomy infusion. With severe, acute disease, they may be given continuously as a 24-hr infusion; the treatment may then be cycled to overnight infusion at home. Repletion should be planned for ideal weight to allow for catch-up growth. Most children are hesitant to use nasogastric infusion, but once it is begun most find it is not difficult. The advantages are that it (1) is relatively free of side effects, (2) avoids the problems associated with corticosteroid therapy, and (3) simultaneously addresses the nutritional rehabilitation. Children may participate in normal daytime activities. A major disadvantage of this approach is similar to that of other therapeutic approaches to Crohn disease: early relapse on discontinuing treatment. In addition, perianal and colon disease has not responded well to this treatment. This approach should be reserved for those with severe nutritional depletion, especially with severe growth failure, and for individuals whose disease is unresponsive to conventional treatment. It is possible that remission induced with nutritional therapy may be maintained with delayed-release 5-aminosalicylate or alternate-day steroid therapy.

Surgical therapy should be reserved for very specific indications. Recurrence rate after bowel resection is high (>50% by 5 yr); the risk of requiring additional surgery increases with each operation. Potential complications of surgery include development of fistula or stricture, anastomotic leak, postoperative partial small bowel obstruction secondary to adhesions, and short-bowel syndrome. Nevertheless, there are situations in which surgery is clearly the treatment of choice and include localized disease of small bowel or colon that is unresponsive to medical treatment, bowel perforation, stricture with symptomatic partial small bowel obstruction, and intractable bleeding. Intra-abdominal or liver abscess may sometimes be successfully treated by ultrasonographic or CT-guided catheter drainage and concomitant intravenous antibiotic treatment. Open surgical drainage is necessary if this approach is not successful. Perianal abscess often requires drainage unless it drains spontaneously. In general, perianal fistulas should be managed medically. However, a severely symptomatic perianal fistula may require fistulotomy; this procedure should be considered only if the location allows the sphincter to remain undamaged. Growth retardation was once considered an indication for resection; without other indications, this approach has not been shown to be beneficial, and medical or nutritional therapy, or both, is preferred.

The surgical approach for Crohn disease is to remove as small a region of bowel as possible. There is no evidence that removing bowel up to margins that are free of disease has a better outcome than removing only the most severely involved areas. The latter approach reduces the risk of short-bowel syndrome. One approach to symptomatic small bowel stricture has been to perform a stricturoplasty rather than resection. The surgeon makes a longitudinal incision across the stricture but then closes the incision with sutures in a transverse fashion. This is ideal for short strictures without active disease. The reoperation rate is no higher with this approach than with resection, whereas bowel length is preserved.

Severe perianal disease may be incapacitating and difficult to treat if unresponsive to medical management. Colon diversion may allow the area to be less active, but on reconnection of the colon, disease activity usually recurs. Therefore, surgical treatment of severe perianal disease may require colectomy. Procedures that create a continent ileostomy or endorectal pull-through are generally discouraged in Crohn disease because of the risk of recurrence of the disease in remaining bowel. Generally, with colectomy, a conventional ileostomy is performed.

Psychosocial issues for the child with Crohn disease include a sense of being different, concerns about body image, difficulty in not participating fully in age-appropriate activities, and family conflict brought on by the added stress of this disease. Social support is an important component of the management of Crohn disease. There are active peer support groups for IBD. The largest group is the Crohn and Colitis Foundation of America with local chapters throughout the United States. Parents are often interested in learning about other children with similar problems, but children may be hesitant to participate. Social support and individual psychologic counseling are important in the adjustment to a difficult problem at an age that by itself often has difficult adjustment issues. Marital or family problems may predate the onset of Crohn disease or may be uncovered by the added family stress of this disease. Patients who are socially "connected" fare better. Ongoing education about the disease is an important aspect of management because children generally fare better if they understand and anticipate problems.

PROGNOSIS. Crohn disease is a chronic disorder that is associated with high morbidity but low mortality. Symptoms tend to recur despite treatment and often without apparent explanation. One exception is that symptoms of partial small obstruction may occur after a high-residue meal in the presence of a small bowel stricture. Weight loss and growth failure can usually be improved with treatment and attention to nutritional needs. Up to 15% of individuals with early growth retardation secondary to Crohn disease have a permanent decrease in linear growth. Some of the extraintestinal manifestations may, in themselves, be major causes of morbidity, including sclerosing cholangitis, chronic active hepatitis, pyoderma gangrenosum, and ankylosing spondylitis.

The region of bowel involved may increase with time, although rapid progression typically occurs early and subsequently is slow. Complications of the inflammatory process tend to increase with time and include bowel strictures, fistulas, perianal disease, and intra-abdominal or retroperitoneal abscess. Nearly all individuals with Crohn disease eventually require surgery for one of its many complications; the rate of reoperation is high. The time between the onset of symptoms and the need for surgery appears to be shorter in children than in adults. Surgery is unlikely to be curative and should be avoided except for the specific indications noted previously. Repeated small bowel resection, which may be unavoidable, can lead to malabsorption secondary to short-bowel syndrome. Resection of terminal ileum may result in bile acid malabsorption with diarrhea and vitamin B_{12} malabsorption. Although the risk of colon cancer in individuals with long-standing Crohn colitis may be lower than that associated with ulcerative colitis, it is greater than the risk among the general population.

Despite these complications, most children with Crohn disease lead active, full lives with intermittent flare-up in symptoms.

Bayless TM: Maintenance therapy for Crohn disease. Gastroenterology 110:299, 1996.
Ewe K, Press AG, Singe CC, et al: Azathioprine combined with prednisolone or monotherapy with prednisolone in active Crohn disease. Gastroenterology 105:367, 1993.
Gendre JP, Mary JY, Florent C, et al: Oral mesalamine (Pentasa) as maintenance treatment in Crohn disease: A multicenter placebo-controlled study. Gastroenterology 104:435, 1993.
Kader HA, Raynor SC, Young R, et al: Introduction of 6-mercaptopurine in Crohn disease patients during the perioperative period: A preliminary evaluation of recurrence of disease. J Pediatr Gastroenterol Nutr 25:93, 1997.
Mack DR, Young R, Kaufman SS, et al: Methotrexate in patients with Crohn disease after 6-mercaptopurine. J Pediatr 132:830, 1998.
Mashako MNL, Cezard JP, Navarro J, et al: Crohn disease lesions in the upper gastrointestinal tract: Correlation between clinical, radiological, endoscopic, and histological features in adolescents and children. J Pediatr Gastroenterol Nutr 8:442, 1989.
Motil KJ, Grand RJ, Davis-Kraft L, et al: Growth failure in children with inflammatory bowel disease: A prospective study. Gastroenterology 105:681, 1993.
Oliva L, Wyllie R, Alexander F, et al: The results of strictureplasty in pediatric patients with multifocal Crohn disease. J Pediatr Gastroenterol Nutr 18:306, 1994.
Polito JM, Childs B, Mellits ED, et al: Crohn disease: Influence of age at diagnosis on site and clinical type of disease. Gastroenterology 111:580, 1996.
Polito JM, Rees RC, Childs B, et al: Preliminary evidence for genetic anticipation in Crohn disease. Lancet 347:798, 1996.
Present DH, Rutgeerts P, Targan S, et al: Infliximab for the treatment of fistulas in patients with Crohn's disease. N Engl J Med 340:1398, 1999.
Ruemmele FM, Targan SR, Levy G, et al: Diagnostic accuracy of serological assays in pediatric inflammatory bowel disease. Gastroenterology 115:822, 1998.
Targan SR, Hanauer SB, Van Deventer SJH, et al: A short-term study of chimeric monoclonal antibody cA2 to tumor necrosis factor α for Crohn disease. N Engl J Med 337:1029, 1997.
Taufiq S, Hernanz-Schulman M, Wheeler AV, et al: Recurrent necrotizing jejunitis in a child. J Pediatr 128:246, 1996.
Treem WR, Hyams JS: Cyclosporine therapy in gastrointestinal disease. J Pediatr Gastroenterol Nutr 18:270, 1994.
Walker-Smith JA: Dietary treatment of active Crohn disease: Dietary treatment is best for children. Br Med J 314:1827, 1997.

337.3 Behçet's Syndrome

Behçet's syndrome is a multisystem vasculitis that is rare in children (Chapter 162). Aphthous stomatitis, erythema nodosum, and arthritis are among the most common manifestations. The ulcers are 2–10 mm in diameter and occur anywhere in the mouth or posterior pharynx; intestinal ulceration may mimic Crohn disease. They are covered by white-yellow membranes, have red borders, and are painful. Other signs are genital ulcers, central nervous system involvement, and myositis. Ocular findings (iridocyclitis) are less common in children than in adults. Immunosuppressive drugs have been used with mixed success.

Rakover Y, Adar H, Tal I, et al: Behcet disease: Long-term follow-up of three children and review of the literature. Pediatrics 83:986, 1989.
Stringer DA, Cleghorn GJ, Durie PR, et al: Behcet's syndrome involving the gastrointestinal tract: A diagnostic dilemma in childhood. Pediatr Radiol 16:131, 1986.

CHAPTER 338
Food Allergy (Food Hypersensitivity)

Martin Ulshen

Food allergy is a group of IgE-mediated and non–IgE-mediated disorders in which symptoms result from immunologic responses to specific food antigens. Food allergy occurs in as many as 6% of children during the first 3 yr of life, including the 2–3% of infants and toddlers with cow's milk allergy. Reactions are classified as IgE mediated and non-IgE mediated. IgE-mediated reactions are caused by inflammatory mediators released when food antigen binds to specific IgE antibody on mast cells and basophils. IgE-mediated reactions are associated with rapid development of symptoms. Non–IgE-mediated reactions are cell-mediated and develop over hours to days. Combined IgE-mediated and cell-mediated reactions also occur.

CLINICAL MANIFESTATIONS. Food antigen may provoke respiratory, skin, or gastrointestinal symptoms. Gastrointestinal manifestations can occur anywhere in the alimentary tract and often dominate. Behavioral manifestations have been described but are controversial.

IgE-MEDIATED FOOD HYPERSENSITIVITY

Oral Allergy Syndrome. Contact with the allergen on the oropharynx causes itching or tingling and angioedema of the lips, tongue, palate, and throat. These symptoms may precede other IgE-mediated manifestations of food allergy. Facial erythema from contact with citrus and tomato products is not considered an immune response.

Gastrointestinal Anaphylaxis. Rapid onset of nausea, crampy abdominal pain, vomiting, or diarrhea, or a combination of these conditions occurs after ingestion of an allergen.

Other Nongastrointestinal Manifestations. These include cutaneous urticaria, angioedema and atopic dermatitis (eczema); respiratory, asthma and rhinoconjunctivitis; and systemic anaphylaxis. Life-threatening reactions typically are associated with ingestion of peanuts, nuts, fish, and shellfish.

NON–IgE-MEDIATED FOOD HYPERSENSITIVITY

Allergic Proctocolitis. Infants may present between 1 day and 3 mo of age with spots or streaks of blood and mucus in stool and occasional mild diarrhea. Increased numbers of white blood cells in stool and peripheral eosinophilia may be present. Typically, a patchy, mild colitis is present; nodular lymphoid hyperplasia occurs in about 25% of cases (see Chapter 345). Most often, proctocolitis results from hypersensitivity to cow's milk; soy sensitivity is less common and human milk sensitivity is rare.

Food-Induced Enterocolitis. Protracted vomiting and diarrhea begin between 1 wk and 3 mo of age. Less severe reactions can occur in older children and adults. Stools contain occult blood, neutrophils, and eosinophils. Jejunal biopsy demonstrates flattened villi, edema, and inflammatory cells. Symptoms resolve within 72 hr of removal of the offending food and recur within 1–6 hr of reintroduction. The blood neutrophil count increases by at least 3.5×10^9/L at 4–6 hr after a food challenge. Older infants may develop a poorly characterized syndrome of anemia, hypoproteinemia, and failure to thrive when weaned from nursing or formula to ordinary cow's milk. Eosinophilia is common.

Food-Induced Enteropathy. Malabsorption, protracted diarrhea, vomiting, and failure to thrive caused by food hypersensitivity occur most often during the first mo of life. Small bowel biopsy shows patchy villus atrophy with mononuclear cell inflammatory response. Reaction to food challenge as well as resolution of symptoms on removal of the offending food may take several days to weeks.

Allergic Eosinophilic Gastroenteritis. See Chapter 339.

Allergic (Eosinophilic) Esophagitis. This is an eosinophilic esophagitis that clinically appears to be reflux esophagitis but is unresponsive to conventional treatment and responds to substitution of protein hydrolysate formula for standard formula.

Celiac Disease (Gluten-Sensitive Enteropathy)–Dermatitis Herpetiformis. Both entities occur as an immunologic response to gluten ingestion and the two can occur together. See Chapter 340.8.

Pulmonary Hemosiderosis (Heiner syndrome). A combination of pulmonary infiltrates, gastrointestinal bleeding, iron-deficiency anemia, peripheral eosinophilia, and failure to thrive secondary to food intolerance (often cow's milk protein) resolves on removal of the offending food from the diet.

DIAGNOSIS. Food allergy is suspected when typical symptoms occur with the introduction of specific foods. Other nonallergic mechanisms of food intolerance should be ruled out (compromised digestive or absorptive processes, contamination with microbes or toxins, or pharmacologic activity of foods). Lactose intolerance should be considered when cow's milk allergy is suspected. Elimination diet and subsequent double-blind, placebo-controlled food challenge (DBPCFC) are the gold standard for diagnosis of food allergy. In DBPCFC, suspected foods are administered in capsules in progressively increasing amounts, alternating with placebo, and reactions are evaluated in a blinded fashion. Open food challenges, although commonly performed, are less reliable (except in young infants). Symptoms can be reproduced by DBPCFC in only 40% of children with suspected food allergy. When anaphylaxis has followed ingestion of a food, challenge should not be performed and the child should be evaluated by an allergist.

Skin tests or radioallergosorbent tests evaluate the presence of specific IgE. In a child less than 1 yr of age, a positive skin test result or radioallergosorbent test is likely to be meaningful because IgE is usually not detectable at this age, whereas a negative test result does not rule out allergy. In older children, the reverse is true; a positive test result for specific IgE does not mean that a specific food is the cause of symptoms as children with positive test results are often asymptomatic. However, nearly 100% of children older than 3 yr old with positive DBPCFC results have positive skin test results as well. Total serum IgE is unreliable.

In infancy, hypersensitivity is most often associated with cow's milk or soy protein ingestion. Although nursing may prevent the development of food allergy, manifestations of food allergy, especially proctocolitis, can occur while nursing. Cow's milk in the mother's diet is the most common identifiable cause of food-allergic reactions in nursing infants; reaction to peanut, soy, or egg in the mother's diet occurs less often.

Among infants and children with food allergy, 90% of reactions are to egg, milk, peanuts, soy, and wheat. Seventy-five per cent of children with proven food allergy react only to a single food. Children with allergic eosinophilic gastroenteritis are the exception, often reacting to multiple foods.

TREATMENT AND PROGNOSIS. The only therapy proved effective for food allergy is an elimination diet. Most gastrointestinal manifestations resolve within 3 days, although some may take weeks (food-induced enteropathy). A child at risk for a severe and life-threatening IgE-mediated reaction should have access to injectable epinephrine and an antihistamine.

At least 30% of infants with cow's milk allergy also demonstrate sensitivity to soy protein. Generally, these infants improve with protein hydrolysate formula; less than 5% have persistent symptoms that resolve with the use of protein hydrolysate formulas. Relactation is an alternative when cow's milk allergy presents early. About 50% of infants who experience proctocolitis while nursing improve with removal of cow's milk from the mother's diet. In the others, one must decide whether the symptoms are severe enough (anemia and hypoproteinemia) to warrant a change in the infants diet to a protein hydrolysate formula.

Eight-five per cent of infants with food hypersensitivity to milk proteins no longer have symptoms on food challenge by 3 yr of age. Resolution of symptoms from cow's milk or soy protein hypersensitivity is common by 1 yr of age. When milk is reintroduced, only a teaspoon or less should be offered at first and then increased progressively over a few days if tolerated. Even older children and adults may lose their sensitivity to an offending food when eliminated from the diet for 1 to 2 yr. Symptoms from IgE-mediated allergy to peanut, nuts, fish, or shellfish are the exception and do not resolve.

Bock SA, Sampson HA: Food allergy in infancy. Pediatr Clin North Am 41:1047, 1994

Esteban MM (ed): Adverse reactions to foods in infancy and childhood J Pediatr (Suppl) 121:S1, 1992.

Kelly KJ, Lazenby AJ, Rowe PC, et al: Eosinophilic esophagitis attributed to gastroesophageal reflux: Improvement with an amino acid-based formula. Gastroenterology 109:1503, 1995.

Machida HM, Catto Smith AG, Gall DG, et al: Allergic colitis in infancy: Clinical and pathologic aspects. J Pediatr Gastroenterol Nutr 19:22, 1994.

Odze RD, Wershil BK, Leichtner AM, et al: Allergic colitis in infants. J Pediatr 126:163, 1995.

Sampson HA: Food Allergy. JAMA 278:1888, 1997.

Targan SR, Hanauer SB, Van Deventer SJH, et al: A short-term study of chimeric monoclonal antibody cA2 to tumor necrosis factor α for Crohn's disease. N Engl J Med 337:1029, 1997.

Vanderhoof JA, Murray ND, Kaufman SS, et al: Intolerance to protein hydrolysate infant formulas: An under recognized cause of gastrointestinal symptoms in infants. J Pediatr 131:741, 1997.

CHAPTER 339
Eosinophilic Gastroenteritis

Martin Ulshen

This entity consists of a group of rare and poorly understood disorders that have in common gastric and small intestine infiltration with eosinophils and peripheral eosinophilia. The esophagus and large intestine may also be involved. Tissue eosinophilic infiltration can be seen in mucosa, muscularis, or serosa. Mucosal involvement may produce nausea, vomiting, diarrhea, abdominal pain, gastrointestinal bleeding, protein-losing enteropathy, or malabsorption. Involvement of the muscularis may produce obstruction (especially of the pylorus), whereas serosal activity produces eosinophilic ascites.

This condition clinically overlaps the dietary protein hypersensitivity disorders of the small bowel and colon (see Chapter 338). Allergies to multiple foods are often seen, and serum IgE is commonly elevated. Peripheral eosinophilia is present in more than 50% of individuals with this disorder. The mucosal form is most frequent and is diagnosed by identifying large numbers of eosinophils in biopsies of gastric antrum or small bowel.

The disease usually runs a chronic, debilitating course with sporadic severe exacerbations. Rare patients are helped by elimination diets or the use of cromolyn, but most require systemic administration of corticosteroids. Isolated eosinophilic esophagitis, unresponsive to gastroesophageal reflux therapy, may improve with an elimination diet; in the absence of stomach or small bowel involvement, this may be a separate entity.

Katz AJ, Golman H, Grand RJ: Gastric mucosal biopsy in eosinophilic (allergic) gastroenteritis. Gastroenterology 73:705, 1977.

Kelly KJ, Lazenby AJ, Rowe PC, et al: Eosinophilic esophagitis attributed to gastroesophageal reflux: Improvement with an amino acid–based formula. Gastroenterology 109:1503, 1995.

Whitington PF, Whitington GL: Eosinophilic gastroenteropathy in childhood. J Pediatr Gastroenterol Nutr 7:379, 1988.

CHAPTER 340
Malabsorptive Disorders

Martin Ulshen

Malabsorptive disorders (syndromes) are conditions that cause insufficient assimilation of ingested nutrients as a result either of maldigestion or of malabsorption (Table 340–1). Previously known as celiac syndromes, this term is best avoided because of potential confusion with the specific entity celiac disease (gluten-sensitive enteropathy). Disorders that cause generalized defects in assimilation of nutrients tend to present with similar signs and symptoms: abdominal distention; pale, foul-smelling, bulky stools; muscle wasting; poor weight gain or weight loss; and growth retardation (Fig. 340–1). Stools may appear greasy and may be associated with an oil slick in the toilet; with mild steatorrhea, the stools may appear normal.

Congenital disorders affecting individual intestinal digestive enzymes or transport processes have also been identified. The clinical features of these disorders typically differ from those of the generalized malabsorption syndromes; some present without gastrointestinal symptoms (Table 340–2). The disaccharidase deficiencies are the most common of these entities.

TABLE 340–1 Generalized Malabsorptive States in Childhood

Site	More Common	Less Common
Exocrine pancreas	Cystic fibrosis Chronic protein-calorie malnutrition	Shwachman-Diamond syndrome Chronic pancreatitis
Liver, biliary tree	Biliary atresia	Other cholestatic states (including Alagille syndrome, familial neonatal hepatitis)
Intestine		
Anatomic defects	Massive resection Stagnant loop syndrome	Congenitally short gut
Chronic infection	Giardiasis	Immune deficiency
Others	Celiac disease Dietary protein intolerance (milk, soy)	Tropical sprue Idiopathic diffuse mucosal lesions

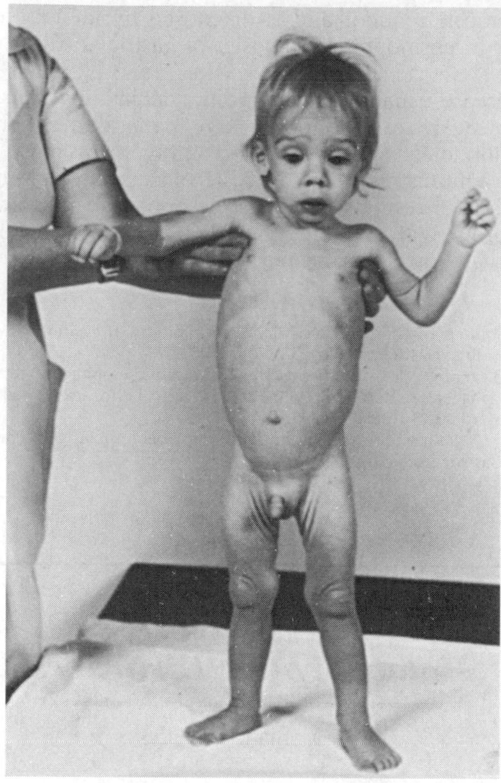

Figure 340–1 An 18-mo-old boy with active celiac disease. Note the loose skin folds, marked proximal muscle wasting, and full abdomen. The child looks ill.

TABLE 340–2 Specific Defects of Digestive-Absorptive Function in Children

Variable	Disease
Intestinal	
Fat	Abetalipoproteinemia
Protein	Enterokinase deficiency Amino acid transport defects (cystinuria, Hartnup disease, methionine malabsorption, blue diaper syndrome)
Carbohydrate	Disaccharidase deficiencies (congenital: sucrase-isomaltase, lactase; developmental: lactase, acquired) Glucose-galactose malabsorption (congenital, acquired) Glucoamylase deficiency (starch malabsorption)
Vitamin	Vitamin B_{12} malabsorption (juvenile pernicious anemia, transcobalamin II deficiency, Imerslund syndrome) Folic acid malabsorption
Ions, trace elements	Chloride-losing diarrhea Congenital sodium diarrhea Acrodermatitis enteropathica (zinc) Menkes syndrome (copper) Vitamin D–dependent rickets Primary hypomagnesemia
Drug-induced	Sulfasalazine (folic acid malabsorption) Cholestyramine (calcium, fat malabsorption) Phenytoin (calcium malabsorption)
Pancreatic	Specific enzyme deficiencies Lipase Trypsinogen

340.1 Evaluation of Children with Suspected Intestinal Malabsorption

CLINICAL MANIFESTATIONS. Although many disorders of malabsorption are inherited, the child without a family history presents the greatest diagnostic challenge. Presentation of congenital disorders may include diarrhea and malabsorption from birth (congenital microvillus inclusion disease, glucose-galactose transport defect, congenital chloride diarrhea). Alternatively, the symptoms may not present until the introduction of a new food (gluten in gluten-sensitive enteropathy, sucrose in congenital sucrase-isomaltase deficiency). A careful history of the time of onset of symptoms and the relation to diet is helpful. Often, well-intended parents may assume that symptoms are associated with events that may, in fact, be coincidental. If a dietary component is important in the cause of the malabsorption, repetition of symptoms should occur on reintroduction of the substance, and improvement should be reproducibly associated with removal of the offending agent. Frequency, looseness, and quantity of stool can be helpful in formulating a differential diagnosis; however, color, other than the pale stool of fat malabsorption, typically does not provide a clue. Failure to thrive can be caused by many systemic or psychosocial disorders, and one must keep this possibility in mind before making a diagnosis of malabsorption. A common example is the child with chronic, nonspecific diarrhea (toddler's diarrhea) who may inadvisedly receive frequent periods of a clear-liquid diet and may lose weight as a result. These children can appear on examination to have a malabsorption syndrome such as gluten-sensitive enteropathy. They typically respond to a return to regular diet with improved weight gain.

The usual growth pattern associated with malabsorption and malnutrition demonstrates an initial decrease in weight followed by a deceleration in height velocity (Fig. 340–2). To make this assessment, it is essential to obtain serial weights and heights. Signs of malnutrition may include lethargy, decreased subcutaneous tissue, muscle wasting, edema, and depigmentation of skin and hair. Initially, many infants with fat malabsorption have a voracious appetite. Other offending foods may produce avoidance behaviors if malabsorption produces gaseous distention (carbohydrates); gluten enteropathy frequently produces anorexia. The examination is typically not helpful in making a specific diagnosis, although occasionally features such as digital clubbing (cystic fibrosis, gluten-sensitive enteropathy), severe growth retardation of Shwachman syndrome, or the facial features of the Johannson-Blizzard syndrome can be helpful. A carotenemic infant or toddler is unlikely to have fat malabsorption.

LABORATORY FINDINGS. The most useful screening test for malabsorption is a microscopic examination of stool for fat. This test can be performed by mixing a small amount of stool with several drops of water or Sudan red stain. Fat droplets separate and can be easily identified, especially with a Sudan stain. The presence of more than six to eight droplets per low-power field is abnormal. Droplets tend to accumulate at the edges of the coverslip. The addition of acetic acid is thought to protonate ionized fatty acids and to increase the number of droplets identified with Sudan stain. In disorders with pancreatic insufficiency (cystic fibrosis or Shwachman syndrome), the fat droplets number in the hundreds to thousands. Some malabsorption syndromes, such as gluten-sensitive enteropathy, may not always be associated with fat in the stool. Serum carotene levels have also been used as a screening test for fat malabsorption, but false-negative and false-positive results are common. The child must be receiving carotene in the diet for the test to be valid.

Steatorrhea is most prominent in disorders associated with pancreatic insufficiency; this finding warrants a sweat chloride test for cystic fibrosis as one of the initial studies. Serum trypsinogen levels have proven to be a good screening test for pancreatic insufficiency. In cystic fibrosis with pancreatic insufficiency, the level is greatly elevated early in life but falls so that by 5–7 yr of age, most patients have subnormal values. The levels in children with cystic fibrosis and pancreatic sufficiency are more variable but tend to be normal or elevated. In

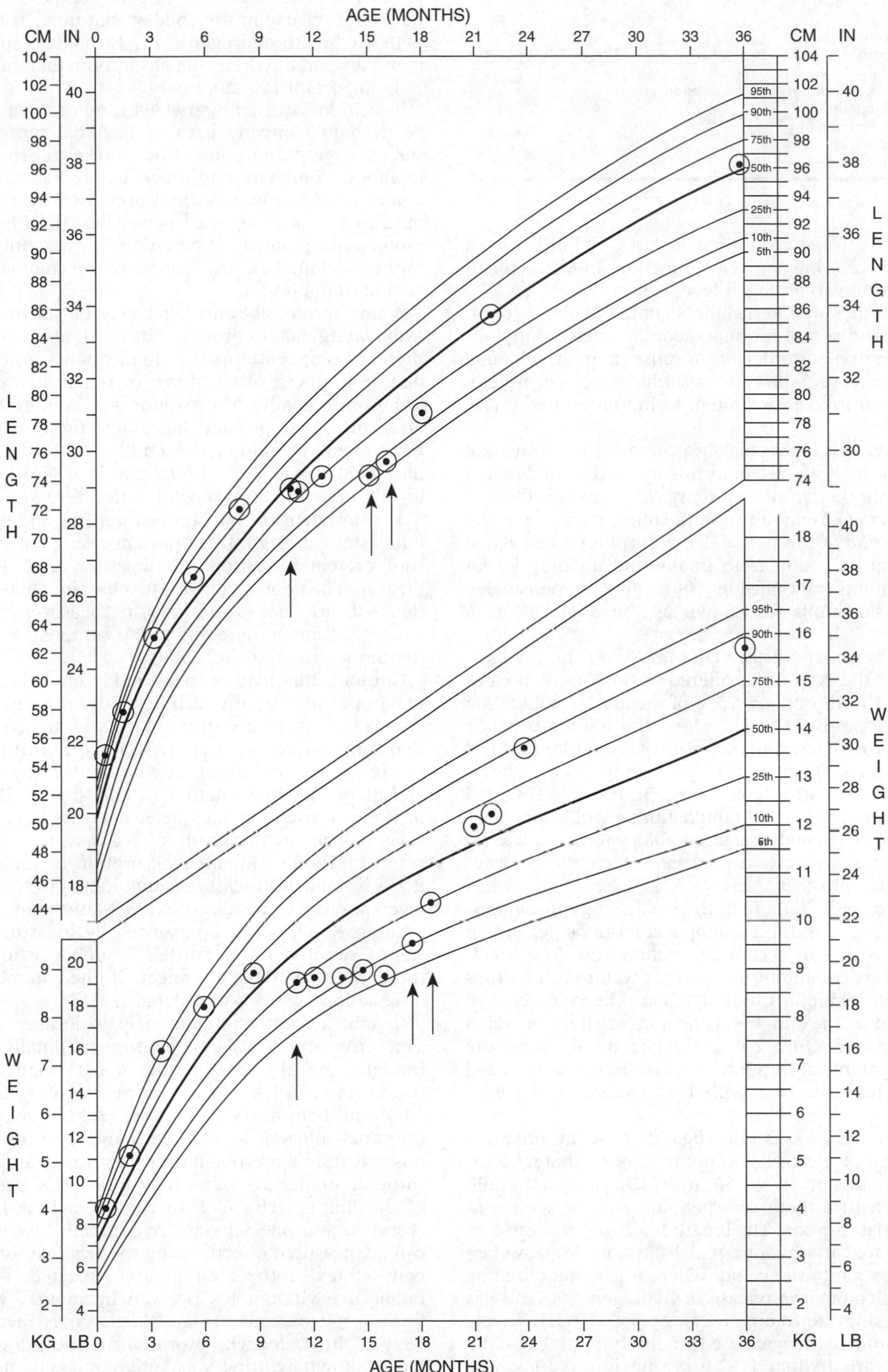

Figure 340–2 Gluten-sensitive enteropathy. Growth curve demonstrates initial normal growth from 0–9 mo, followed by onset of poor appetite with intermittent vomiting and diarrhea after initiation of gluten-containing diet *(single arrow)*. After biopsy-confirmed diagnosis and treatment with gluten-free diet *(double arrow)*, growth improves.

TABLE 340–3 Gastrointestinal Causes of Hypoproteinemia

Inflammatory bowel disease
Gluten-sensitive enteropathy
Cystic fibrosis
Shwachman syndrome
Disorders with secondary small-bowel mucosal damage (e.g., infectious disorders)
Intestinal lymphangiectasia (primary or secondary)
Hypertrophic gastropathy
Eosinophilic gastroenteropathy
Milk protein sensitivity
Trypsinogen or enterokinase deficiency

such children, the trend over time is more helpful than a single value in monitoring pancreatic function. In Shwachman syndrome, the serum trypsinogen level is low.

Other initial studies should include a complete blood count, serum albumin, and serum immunoglobulin levels. Many different gastrointestinal disorders can cause hypoproteinemia as a result of decreased ability to assimilate dietary protein, inadequate protein intake, or protein-losing enteropathy (Table 340–3).

A more sensitive test for fat malabsorption is the 72-hr stool collection for fat analysis. A dietary record during this period is used to calculate the fat intake. Many clinicians use the diet history as an average 3-day intake and collect stools from the beginning to the end of this period. Fat absorption is calculated by subtracting fat excretion from intake and dividing by fat intake; this fraction is multiplied by 100 to give the percentage of intake that is assimilated, known as the *coefficient of fat absorption.*

The ability to assimilate dietary fat varies with the maturity of the infant and the type of fat offered in the diet. A premature infant may absorb only 65–75% of dietary fat, whereas a full-term infant absorbs 90%. Therefore, the finding of fat in the stool on microscopic examination in young infants is not necessarily abnormal. Older children and adults should absorb at least 95% of the fat in a typical diet. Butterfat is absorbed less well than vegetable fat, although human milk fat is absorbed best of all. The mild decreased ability to assimilate fat by infants reflects a decrease in pancreatic secretion or a decrease in duodenal bile acid levels.

Measurement of carbohydrate in the stool using the Clinitest reagent for reducing substances is simple and can be performed at bedside. This is not an accurate screening test. The test is easily performed by combining 10 drops of water with 5 drops of stool and then adding a Clinitest tablet. The color change can be quantified as trace to 4+ using a color sheet provided by the manufacturer. Only 2+ or higher should raise the possibility of sugar malabsorption. Sucrose is not a reducing sugar and requires hydrolysis with hydrochloric acid before analysis.

Stool pH lower than 5.6 is also suggestive of carbohydrate malabsorption. Stool electrolye content (approximately 2 × ([sodium] + [potassium]) + 50 mOsm/L) less than 290 mOsm/L occurs with osmotic diarrhea and may be seen with carbohydrate malabsorption. The breath hydrogen test can also be used to evaluate carbohydrate malabsorption. Malabsorbed carbohydrate passes into the colon, where it is metabolized by bacteria with stoichiometric release of hydrogen gas. This gas is largely absorbed in the colon, enters the portal and systemic venous return, and is then released in the breath. The child ingests a load of carbohydrate (1–2 g/kg, maximum 50 g), and the breath is collected in sealed plastic bags at timed intervals up to 2 hr after ingestion. The hydrogen content of the gas can be easily measured and is reported in parts per million. Malabsorption of any carbohydrate can be evaluated. The child should not be taking antibiotics at the time of the study because these drugs alter the colon flora and suppress hydrogen gas production. If a question exists about the ability of the colonic flora to produce hydrogen gas, the child can ingest the nonabsorbable disaccharide lactulose. A lack of hydrogen production with lactulose implies that the breath hydrogen test is not reliable in the child at that time. The major problem with the breath hydrogen study is that it is so sensitive that it identifies carbohydrate malabsorption that may not be clinically important (asymptomatic).

Protein loss caused by maldigestion or malabsorption cannot be evaluated directly because bacterial protein accounts for such a large proportion of the stool nitrogen. Dietary protein is almost completely absorbed before reaching the terminal ileum. Endogenous intestinal proteins in the small bowel lumen are normally digested as well; less than 1 g of endogenous protein and products of digestion of exogenous protein passes into the colon. As a result, most of the colonic protein content is of bacterial origin.

A low serum albumin level may be the result of difficulty assimilating dietary protein, but it can also occur as a result of protein-losing enteropathy, inadequate protein intake, liver disease (reduced production), or renal disease. With protein-losing enteropathy, the peptide and amino acid products of digestion of the protein that enters the bowel lumen can be reabsorbed. Therefore, the child is not actually in negative nitrogen balance, even though levels of serum proteins including albumin and immunoglobulins are reduced.

Measurement of spot stool α_1-antitrypsin levels is helpful in establishing a diagnosis of protein-losing enteropathy. This serum protein is resistant to digestion and therefore can be measured in stool in contrast to albumin. One- or 2-day collections of stool for α_1-antitrypsin measurement or clearance studies are much more difficult to complete and do not appear to improve the test's reliability.

Nutrients that may be measured in blood include the following: iron, the level of which depends on transferrin concentration as well as on absorption; folic acid, the red cell concentration being a more accurate reflection of nutritional status than the serum concentration; calcium and magnesium; vitamin D and its metabolites; vitamin A; and vitamin B_{12}. If the intake of these nutrients is adequate, decreased concentrations will suggest inadequate absorption. It may take years to deplete stores of vitamin B_{12} after absorption is impaired. Vitamin E levels should be measured simultaneously with serum lipid levels and the value expressed as a ratio to lipid concentration. Vitamin K stores can be assessed by measuring prothrombin (more sensitive) and partial thromboplastin times because these times will be prolonged if the vitamin K–dependent coagulation factors are depleted.

Certain absorptive studies help to localize an intestinal lesion. Iron and D-*xylose,* a pentose minimally metabolized in humans, are absorbed by the upper small bowel. A blood concentration of less than 25 mg/dL of xylose 1 hr after a 14.5 g/m^2 body surface oral dose ($\leq$25 g) suggests a proximal intestinal mucosal lesion, but some false-negative and false-positive results are obtained using this technique. Xylose absorption studies are performed much less frequently because of the limited reliability. In the distal bowel, vitamin B_{12} is absorbed and bile salts are reabsorbed. *Vitamin B_{12} absorption* can be measured directly using the *Schilling test,* in which, after body stores of the vitamin are saturated, a tracer dose of radioactive vitamin B_{12} is given by mouth, with or without intrinsic factor, and urinary excretion is measured over the next 24 hr. Defective absorption in the presence of intrinsic factor, shown by urinary excretion of less than 5% of the dose, occurs when an extensive length of distal ileum is resected or diseased or when bacterial overgrowth occurs within the bowel lumen.

DIAGNOSTIC PROCEDURES. Microbiologic. The only common primary infection causing chronic malabsorption is giardiasis (Chapter 272 and Table 337–2). Techniques to fix and stain specimens have greatly improved the diagnostic value of examining stools for *Giardia* cysts. The trophozoite may be identified in fresh duodenal contents or the duodenal mucosa. Immunoassay techniques are also available to identify *Giardia* antigen in the stool and antibody in the serum. These tests appear sensitive and specific. When enteric clearing of bacteria is impaired, either from stasis of luminal contents or impaired immune function, colony counts from bacterial cultures of proximal intestinal juice may be very high.

Failure to thrive, with chronic diarrhea, may be the first sign of HIV infection (AIDS) (Chapter 268). The cause may be primary infection or parasitic, bacterial, or viral opportunistic enteral pathogens.

Small Bowel Biopsy. Small bowel biopsy identifies diseases of the small bowel mucosa that are associated with histologic findings, including gluten-sensitive enteropathy, abetalipoproteinemia, lymphangiectasia, congenital microvillus inclusion disease, eosinophilic gastroenteritis, infectious disorders, and Whipple disease (rare in children). The biopsy can be safely performed by upper gastrointestinal endoscopy. At the time of biopsy, in addition to mucosa, it is possible to collect aspirates for examination for *Giardia* or bacterial culture. Mucosal samples can be frozen to assay for disaccharidase activities later. Depression of activities of all enzymes tested suggests a secondary deficiency associated with mucosal damage. Reduction of a specific enzyme or group of enzymes is consistent with a specific deficiency (lactase or sucrase-isomaltase deficiency).

Hematologic. A hypochromic, microcytic blood smear indicates iron deficiency; a macrocytic smear suggests deficiency and therefore malabsorption of folic acid or vitamin B_{12}. Acanthocyte transformation of erythrocytes occurs in abetalipoproteinemia. A blood smear may also suggest a lymphocyte defect or neutropenia associated with Shwachman-Diamond syndrome.

Imaging Procedures. Used primarily to identify local lesions in the abdomen, these procedures have limited application to the study of children with malabsorptive disorders. *Plain roentgenograms* and *barium contrast studies* may suggest a site and cause of intestinal stasis. For example, the most common anomaly causing incomplete bowel obstruction is intestinal malrotation, which can be diagnosed with barium contrast studies. Although flocculation of normal barium and dilated bowel with thickened mucosal folds have been attributed to diffuse malabsorptive lesions such as celiac disease, these abnormalities are nonspecific. *Ultrasound* can detect alterations in pancreatic mass, biliary tree abnormalities, and stones. *Retrograde studies* of the *pancreatic* and *biliary tree* using contrast injection via endoscopy are reserved for rare cases requiring careful delineation of the biliary and pancreatic ducts.

340.2 Chronic Malnutrition

Chronic protein-calorie malnutrition can lead to compromise of pancreatic and small bowel function. In developed countries, primary malnutrition is rare and chronic digestive disorders account for many cases of malnutrition in children. Environmental deprivation is also an important cause, as are feeding disorders (improper volume or dilution of formula). Protein-calorie malnutrition appears to contribute to the cycle of protracted diarrhea of infancy perhaps through impairment of the functional capacity of the bowel, impairment of immune function, or the development of small bowel bacterial overgrowth. Worldwide, exocrine pancreatic insufficiency is most often attributable to malnutrition, not to a primary pancreatic disease.

The intestine is remarkably resistant to the effects of protein-calorie malnutrition. Patients with *kwashiorkor* may have a severely flattened small intestinal villi (Chapter 42); these abnormalities are probably attributable to coexisting infections and infestations. In *marasmus,* villus structure is relatively well preserved, although microvillus changes and intracellular electron microscopic abnormalities are observed (Chapter 42). Chronic malnutrition can lead to impaired immune function; bacterial overgrowth of the upper intestine is seen in malnourished subjects (Chapter 42). When oral intake is withheld in experimental animals, intestinal mucosal mass and absorptive function diminish even if nutrient is supplied by the intravenous route. These changes can be reversed by small amounts of oral nutrient. Accordingly, a theoretical advantage exists in delivering nutrients via the gut. Recovery from injury to the gastrointestinal tract (viral gastroenteritis) may be prolonged by chronic malnutrition. Certain nutrients, such as glutamine, soluble fiber, short-chain fatty acids, and short-chain triglycerides, may promote small bowel mucosal growth.

Little is known about the *effect of specific nutritional deficiencies* on the pancreas or intestine; apart from potassium depletion causing ileus and severe dehydration causing constipation, available data suggest a relatively minor clinical effect of a wide range of specific deficiencies. Iron deficiency is associated with enhanced iron uptake at the mucosa and, in a few severe cases, occurrence of mucosal flattening. Deficiencies of vitamin B_{12} and folic acid may cause distortion of enterocyte morphology but no known serious functional abnormalities of the gut. Some hypocalcemic states may be accompanied by steatorrhea and even by ion and water secretion, but this poorly understood relationship is not constant.

Studies from developing countries suggest that vitamin A supplementation reduces childhood mortality. Improved survival during measles and a reduction in relative risk of contracting diarrheal and respiratory diseases have been identified. The explanation for this finding is uncertain, but children with vitamin A deficiency may have T-cell defects (including a low CD4:CD8 ratio), which can be reversed with vitamin supplementation.

340.3 Liver and Biliary Disorders

Cholestatic liver disease and biliary disorders may lead to fat malabsorption by reducing the duodenal bile acid concentration to less than the critical micellar concentration. In addition to steatorrhea, patients with these disorders have a propensity to acquire deficiencies of fat-soluble vitamins (vitamins A, D, E, and K). These deficiencies have no consistent pattern, except vitamin A is least likely to be problematic.

Vitamin E deficiency in patients with chronic cholestasis has been associated with a progressive neurologic syndrome, which includes peripheral neuropathy (presenting as loss of deep tendon reflexes and ophthalmoplegia), cerebellar ataxia, and posterior column dysfunction. Early in the course, findings are partially reversible with treatment; late features may not be reversible. It can be difficult to identify vitamin E deficiency because the elevated blood lipid levels of cholestasis can falsely elevate the serum level of vitamin E. Therefore, it is important to measure the ratio of serum vitamin E to total serum lipids if one suspects this deficiency; the normal level for patients younger than 12 yr is greater than 0.6 and for patients 12 yr and older, greater than 0.8. The neurologic disease can be prevented with the use of an oral water-soluble vitamin E preparation (*d*-α-tocopherol polyethylene glycol-1,000 succinate [TPGS], Liqui-E, Twin Laboratories, Hauppague, NY) at 15–25 IU/kg/24 hr.

Metabolic bone disease can develop secondary to vitamin D deficiency. Simultaneous administration of vitamin D with the water-soluble vitamin E preparation (TPGS) enhances absorption of vitamin D. In young infants, oral vitamin D_3 is given at 1,000 IU/kg/24 hr. After 1 mo, if the serum 25-hydroxyvitamin D level is low, the same dose of oral vitamin D is mixed with TPGS. It has been recommended that 25-hydroxyvitamin D is then monitored every 3 mo, with adjustment of doses as necessary.

Vitamin K deficiency can occur as a result of cholestasis and poor fat absorption. Easy bleeding may be the first sign, or a child may be identified before symptoms develop through routine screening of prothrombin (a more sensitive test) and partial thromboplastin times. It is possible for a patient taking the standard oral preparation to acquire vitamin K–deficient coagulopathy because the currently available oral preparation of vitamin K is not well absorbed.

340.4 Intestinal Infections

Malabsorption is a rare consequence of primary intestinal infection in immunocompetent children. Giardiasis is the most common infectious cause of chronic malabsorption (Chapter 272). Factors that regulate the range of host response to *Giardia* (asymptomatic, acute, or chronic infection) remain to be explained. Symptoms may include diarrhea, vomiting, bloating, and gas. Giardiasis should be suspected if a child with persistent acquired malabsorption has family members who have had transient gastroenteritis symptoms at the onset of the child's illness. Children in day care (especially toddlers) are at special risk for *Giardia,* although they may be asymptomatic and may pass it on to family members. Cryptosporidiosis can also occur in immunocompetent persons, as can coccidiosis. Infectious causes of malabsorption are especially common in immunocompromised persons (Chapters 179, 272, 337, and 340.5).

340.5 Immunodeficiency

Gastrointestinal symptoms are a common manifestation of many immune deficiency states, including AIDS, congenital neutrophil and T- and B-cell immune deficiencies, and conditions of medical immune suppression (cancer and transplantation therapy). Most children with AIDS have diarrhea at some point in their disease. The more common congenital disorders associated with bowel disease include severe combined immunodeficiency, agammaglobulinemia, Wiskott-Aldrich syndrome, common variable immunodeficiency disease, and chronic granulomatous disease. Gastrointestinal symptoms of congenital X-linked hypogammaglobulinemia tend to be milder (chronic rotavirus or enterovirus infection or giardiasis). Malabsorption occurs in about 10% of patients with late-onset common variable hypogammaglobulinemia, a primary disorder that presents later in life. Nodular lymphoid hyperplasia may be noted on small bowel radiographs. T-cell abnormalities can also be associated with malabsorption. Selective immunoglobulin (Ig) A deficiency is common, may not always be associated with gastrointestinal symptoms, but may be associated with an increased incidence of gluten-sensitive enteropathy, nodular lymphoid hyperplasia, inflammatory bowel disease, and giardiasis.

Chronic giardiasis and rotavirus infection have been noted to cause malabsorption in children with immune deficiencies. In addition, in children with AIDS, other organisms, including opportunistic infections, that can interfere with bowel function include *Cryptosporidium parvum,* cytomegalovirus, *Mycobacterium avium-intracellulare, Isospora belli, Enterocytozoon bieneusi, Candida albicans,* astrovirus, calicivirus, adenovirus, and the usual bacterial enteropathogens. Likelihood of infection is related to the CD4 count. *Cryptosporidium* can cause chronic secretory diarrhea and can be carried chronically in the gallbladder. HIV itself appears to be a primary bowel pathogen. Disaccharide intolerance is common in HIV-infected children but does not correlate well with enteric infection. Pancreatic insufficiency with steatorrhea and vitamin B_{12} malabsorption have been described to occur in patients with AIDS. Malnutrition and failure to thrive occur in the majority of untreated children with AIDS; diarrhea is common, although frequently pathogens are not identified. In addition to the range of infectious causes in immunosuppressed children, diarrhea can be a presentation of toxicity to the drug tacrolimus or of immunosuppression-induced lymphoproliferative disease.

Deficiency of neutrophils, congenital cyclic neutropenia, or, more commonly, the neutropenia associated with cancer chemotherapy predisposes children to neutropenic enterocolitis. The colitis can be manifested as mild bloody diarrhea, or it may present with fever, severe right lower quadrant pain, bloody stools, and diarrhea. The latter disorder, known as typhlitis, occurs most often in the lower ileum, cecum, and proximal colon, where vascular compromise, mucosal ulceration, and perforation carry a high mortality. Children with neutropenia are also at risk for fungal infections of the gastrointestinal tract including infections with *Histoplasma, Aspergillus,* and *Mucor.* Enterocolitis may be caused by *Clostridium difficile* in children receiving chemotherapy. In patients with chronic granulomatous disease, phagocytic function is impaired and granulomas may develop throughout the intestine, thus causing diarrhea and malabsorption and mimicking Crohn disease. Inflammation with granulomas, characterized by giant cells and lipid-containing histiocytes, may obstruct the gastric antrum. Children with chronic granulomatous disease are at risk for *Salmonella* infections as well.

340.6 Stagnant Loop Syndrome

(Blind Loop Syndrome: Bacterial Overgrowth Syndrome)

These terms describe a condition associated with stasis of small intestinal contents, particularly in the upper regions. Incomplete bowel obstruction, congenital (malrotation with duodenal bands, stenosis, or a diverticulum) or acquired (postoperative intestinal adhesions, long-standing Crohn disease), impairs intestinal motility or causes loss of the normal intestinal mucosal barrier to microorganisms, allowing enteric bacteria to colonize the upper small bowel. Bacteria deconjugate bile salts, a process that leads to inefficient intraluminal processing of dietary fat and to steatorrhea; they bind vitamin B_{12}, interfering with its absorption; and they may damage the microvillus brush border membrane, diminishing disaccharidase activities.

In addition to symptoms of chronic incomplete bowel obstruction such as distention, pain, and vomiting, the patient may have pale, foul-smelling, bulky stools typical of steatorrhea, megaloblastic anemia from vitamin B_{12} deficiency, or diarrhea from disaccharidase deficiency. Clinical manifestations often do not suggest chronic intestinal obstruction, but laboratory investigations find the aforementioned functional abnormalities as well as bacterial colonization of the upper intestine and deconjugated bile salts in the upper intestinal juice after a fatty meal. Barium contrast roentgenograms may reveal neither the existence nor the cause of obstruction.

Oral administration of antibiotics may be sufficient to control the problem temporarily. At times, cycling of antibiotics may be effective for a longer period of management. Metronidazole has been used for the treatment of bacterial overgrowth. Other alternatives are oral nonabsorbable antibiotics for gram-negative bacteria (gentamicin, colistin) and trimethoprim-sulfamethoxazole. In older teenagers, tetracycline or ciprofloxacin may be used. Operative correction of a partial small bowel obstruction is the ideal approach.

340.7 Short Bowel Syndrome

Short bowel syndrome produces malabsorption and malnutrition after congenital or postnatal loss of at least 50% of the small bowel, with or without loss of a portion of the large intestine. Short bowel results in inadequate absorptive surface and compromised bowel function. The condition may not be permanent because the intestine has the capacity for adaptive growth and increase in functional capacity. Adaptation is a gradual process associated with increase in villus height and small bowel surface, rather than lengthening of the bowel.

The small intestine may be congenitally short in conditions in which bowel is lost in utero (malrotation, gastroschisis, and, in some cases, atresia). Most cases involve some surgical resection of the small intestine. Most occur in the neonatal period (necrotizing enterocolitis), although Crohn disease or trauma can account for later onset.

CLINICAL MANIFESTATIONS. The major clinical manifestations are malabsorption and diarrhea. The ability to assimilate nutrients correlates with the length and location as well as the quality of the residual bowel. Carbohydrate malabsorption and steatorrhea are common features resulting in diarrhea and failure to thrive. Large volumes of fluid and electrolyte are normally secreted into the upper gastrointestinal tract and must be reabsorbed. The capacity to reabsorb fluid and electrolyte is usually inadequate in the short bowel syndrome and results in loss from the gastrointestinal tract with the potential for dehydration, hyponatremia, hypokalemia, and acidosis. The extent of loss is influenced by the presence or absence of the colon in continuity with the small bowel. Trace elements are also poorly absorbed and are lost in excess. D-Lactic acidosis may occur rarely as a result of fermentation of dietary carbohydrate by luminal bacteria in the small bowel caused by bacterial overgrowth. Patients with this manifestation experience confusion, hyperventilation, and acidosis with an anion gap in the absence of elevated serum lactate as measured by standard techniques, which measure L-lactate. Hypersecretion of acid in the stomach occurs as a result of hypergastrinemia for a transient period after small bowel resection. However, this condition does not appear to cause problems in infants and children. These patients often have associated cholestasis resulting from hyperalimentation and other factors. Cholestasis may contribute to ongoing malabsorption of fat and fat-soluble vitamins.

TREATMENT. In the late 1960s, about 50% of infants with short bowel survived. Today, more than 90% survive, even though the infants may have shorter bowel. The use of total parenteral nutrition has dramatically changed the outcome. These infants cannot maintain adequate nutrition by the enteral route alone and initially must have most of their nutrition given intravenously. Very low amounts of enteral nutrients are given at first as a continuous gastric infusion (1–5 mL/hr depending on the size of the infant). Usually an elemental diet is used at regular strength (20 kcal/oz). This approach is important because experimental evidence suggests that exposure to enteral nutrients contributes to adaptive growth of the small bowel. As tolerated, the quantity can be slowly advanced, perhaps by 1–2 mL/hr/24 hr, as the amount of parenteral nutrition is simultaneously decreased. A level is reached at which diarrhea and malabsorption increase, and progression of enteral feedings must be delayed. Bloody diarrhea secondary to patchy, mild colitis may develop during the progression of enteral feedings. The pathogenesis of this "feeding colitis" is unknown, but it is usually benign. Strictures following neonatal necrotizing enterocolitis may also produce bloody stools (see Chapter 98.2).

When possible, an infant may be given a small amount of formula by mouth to maintain an interest in oral feeding. As children age beyond the first year, it is sometimes possible to add a small amount of solids by mouth (cereal, pureed chicken). For infants with an extremely short bowel, it may take several years or more until parenteral nutrition can be stopped. An infant with as little as 15 cm of bowel with an ileocecal valve, or 20 cm without, has the potential to survive and eventually to be weaned from parenteral nutrition.

Certain factors appear to influence the length of time until a child is independent of parenteral nutrition. Infants with less than 40 cm of small bowel take twice as long as infants with 40–80 cm of bowel (average of slightly more than 2 yr vs slightly more than 1 yr). The absence of an ileocecal valve doubles the time to complete adaptation, all other factors being equal. The length of residual ileum is inversely correlated with the time until adaptation. Infants with necrotizing enterocolitis and gastroschisis have more difficulty adapting than children with similar bowel resections for other indications. Identification of small bowel bacterial overgrowth has been associated with prolonged dependence on parenteral nutrition.

Bacterial overgrowth is common in infants with a short bowel and may delay progression of enteral feedings (Chapter 340.6). Metronidazole is used empirically, as are nonabsorbable antibiotics that cover gram-negative organisms. Occasionally, a drug that slows gastrointestinal motility, such as loperamide, can be helpful. However, these drugs often do not appear to alter the course. When the small bowel is in continuity with the colon, bile acid malabsorption can cause colonic fluid secretion. In this situation, cholestyramine, 0.25–1 g every 6–8 hr, may be helpful in reducing the watery diarrhea.

LONG-TERM COMPLICATIONS. Long-term complications include those of parenteral nutrition: central catheter infection, thrombosis, hepatotoxicity, and gallstones. For this reason, a continual effort to advance enteral feedings slowly must be considered. Other long-term complications of short bowel include the potential for late vitamin B_{12} deficiency. Stores of vitamin B_{12} acquired in utero are so great that deficiency may not appear until 1 to 2 yr of age. Therefore, it is important periodically to check vitamin B_{12} levels during and after the 1st years of life. Gallstones were found in 60% of infants receiving chronic parenteral nutrition who had had terminal ileal resection but in none of the children with an intact ileum. Renal stones can occur as a result of hyperoxaluria secondary to steatorrhea with increased oxalate absorption and recurrent dehydration.

FUTURE DIRECTIONS IN MANAGEMENT. Certain nutrients have been considered potential stimulants of adaptive growth in experimental animals, but their role in humans remains to be determined. These include glutamine, soluble fiber, short-chain fatty acids, and short-chain triglycerides. Another area of interest is the role of peptide growth factors in promoting adaptive growth of the bowel. Bowel-lengthening surgical procedures have been performed with mixed results. Small bowel transplantation is used in children who have no hope of ever progressing from parenteral feedings. Small bowel and liver transplantation can be performed and is a particular consideration for the child with severe total parenteral nutrition hepatotoxicity.

340.8 Gluten-Sensitive Enteropathy

(Celiac Disease)

Gluten-sensitive enteropathy is a disorder in which small bowel mucosal damage is the result of a permanent sensitivity to dietary gluten. The disorder does not present until gluten products have been introduced into the diet. Typically, the most common period of presentation is between 6 mo and 2 yr of age. Prevalence varies in different regions (it is more frequent in Europe than in the United States), although the incidence appears to be decreasing. In the United States, the incidence is about 1/10,000 live births.

PATHOGENESIS. Three components interact in the pathogenesis: toxicity of certain cereals, genetic predisposition, and environmental factors. The disorder develops only after long-term dietary exposure to the protein gluten, which is found in wheat, rye, and barley. Oats are not, as previously believed, a cause of this disorder. The activity of gluten resides in the gliadin fraction, which contains certain repetitious amino acid sequences (motifs) that lead to sensitization of lamina propria lymphocytes. A genetic predisposition is suggested because (1) up to 2–5% of first-degree relatives have symptomatic gluten-sensitive enteropathy, (2) as many as 10% of first-degree relatives have asymptomatic damage to small bowel mucosa consistent with this disorder, and (3) the disorder is associated with certain human leukocyte antigen (HLA) types (B8, DR7, DR3, and DQw2). Environmental factors must influence the expression of this genetic predisposition because (1) a 30% rate of discordance in monozygotic twins is reported, (2) a 70% rate of discordance in HLA-identical siblings is noted, (3) the age of onset among siblings is variable, and (4) the onset of symptoms can be precipitated by gastrointestinal surgery, pregnancy, antibiotic use, or a coincidental diarrheal illness.

The immunologic response to gluten results in villus atrophy, crypt hyperplasia, and damage to the surface epithelium in the small bowel. The injury is greatest in the proximal small bowel and extends distally for a variable distance. The latter observation is undoubtedly the explanation for the variable degree of symptoms and findings of malabsorption among persons with gluten-sensitive enteropathy. A decrease in absorptive and digestive capacity results from a decrease in small intestinal surface area and a relative increase in immature epithelial cells. Pancreatic secretion is decreased as a result of lowered serum cholecystokinin and secretin levels.

CLINICAL MANIFESTATIONS. The mode of presentation is variable; most patients present with diarrhea (Table 340–4). Children can have failure to thrive or vomiting as the only manifestation. Perhaps as many as 10% of children referred to endocrinologists for growth retardation without an endocrine or overt gastrointestinal disorder have gluten sensitivity. Anorexia is common and may be the major cause of weight loss or lack of weight gain (see Fig. 340–2). Infants with gluten-sensitive enteropathy are often, but not always, clingy, irritable, unhappy children who are difficult to comfort. In contrast to infants with cystic fibrosis, they are not interested in food, although this is not always the case. Pallor and abdominal distention are common (see Fig. 340–1). Large, bulky stools suggestive of constipation have been described in some children with this condition. Digital clubbing can occur. An increased prevalence of gluten-sensitive enteropathy has been noted in children with selective IgA deficiency, diabetes mellitus, chronic rheumatoid arthritis, and Down syndrome. Lymphocytic gastritis occurs in rare children with gluten-sensitive enteropathy. Pancreatic insufficiency is present in about one third of children with newly diagnosed celiac disease, usually resolving within the first months of treatment. Isolated idiopathic transaminasemia without other hepatic or enteric symptoms may be a manifestation of occult celiac disease.

TABLE 340–4 Active Childhood Celiac Disease: 42 Cases

Symptoms	No. of Patients
Failure to thrive	36
Diarrhea	30
Irritability	30
Vomiting	24
Anorexia	24
Foul stools	21
Abdominal pain	8
Excessive appetite	6
Rectal prolapse	3
Signs	**No. of Patients**
Height <25th percentile	30
Body weight <25th percentile	37
Wasted muscles	40
Abdominal distention	33
Edema	14
Finger clubbing	11

EVALUATION. Screening tests for malabsorption are not particularly helpful because results may be normal in a child with gluten-sensitive enteropathy. Anemia and hypoproteinemia may be present. The first serologic tests, including antigliadin antibodies, were not reliable. However, the sensitivity and specificity of serum IgA-endomysial antibody testing have approached 100% (except in IgA-deficient patients). This antibody recognizes tissue transglutaminase antigen. It is likely that specific assays for antibody against this antigen will replace endomysial antibody tests to diagnose celiac disease. Histologic findings on small bowel biopsy remain the standard for diagnosis, and biopsy should be performed if one has a high suspicion of gluten-sensitive enteropathy or if serum endomysial antibody is found. The strictest approach to diagnosis is to demonstrate that the biopsy returns to normal within 1–2 yr after starting a gluten-free diet and then to rechallenge with a gluten diet and repeat the biopsy. This approach is now in evolution because it is possible to demonstrate antibody conversion while the patient is on a gluten-free diet, and only an initial small bowel biopsy may be necessary.

PATHOLOGY. The diffuse lesion of the upper small intestinal mucosa that characterizes celiac disease is seen on small bowel biopsy. Short, flat villi, deepened crypts, and irregular vacuolated surface epithelium with lymphocytes in the epithelial layer are seen by light microscopy. Similar abnormalities occur in other conditions, but none is likely to be confused with celiac disease. Infections such as rotavirus enteritis, *Giardia lamblia*, or tropical sprue can cause villus flattening and elongated crypts but not the marked abnormalities of enterocytes. Flat mucosa occurs in kwashiorkor but may represent a response to infestation rather than to undernutrition. Tropical sprue, a poorly understood tropical enteropathy, can cause a lesion that is indistinguishable from that of celiac disease. Some cases of cow's milk protein or soy protein intolerance are associated with lesions similar to those of celiac disease in children. In immune deficiency, eosinophilic gastroenteritis, and autoimmune enteropathy, villi can be partially shortened. Infants with familial enteropathy have short villi, but the crypt dimensions are normal.

TREATMENT. Treatment requires a lifelong, strict gluten-free diet. All wheat, rye, and barley products should be eliminated from the diet. Counseling from an experienced dietitian should be provided. Initially, vitamin and iron supplementation is advisable. National celiac support groups provide much specific information about the gluten content of foods and medications. Processed foods must be considered carefully because they commonly contain some gluten. Gluten-free foods are commercially available. When the disorder presents with fulminant diarrhea, initial treatment with oral prednisone can be useful, but it is rarely necessary. Poor weight gain in the first months after diagnosis may improve with pancreatic enzyme treatment.

PROGNOSIS. The clinical response to a gluten-free diet of a child with celiac disease is gratifying. Improvement of mood and appetite is followed by lessening of diarrhea. In most cases, changes occur within 1 wk of starting therapy, but the response may occasionally be delayed. Older patients and extremely ill patients tend to respond slowly, but once in remission, the celiac child should be treated as a well child. Teenagers often become noncompliant. Unfortunately, this is an age when the disorder tends to be symptomatically quiescent, and a teenager may believe that the disorder has resolved. Nevertheless, mucosal damage is present. Subtle manifestations of growth failure or delayed sexual maturation may take place when these patients ingest a gluten-containing diet. Appropriately diagnosed gluten-sensitive enteropathy is a lifelong condition requiring lifelong treatment. The late development of bowel lymphoma in long-standing enteropathy, especially with poor adherence to diet, is possible although controversial. No complications from long-term gluten-free diet treatment are recognized.

340.9 Immunoproliferative Small Intestinal Disease

Immunoproliferative small intestinal disease (Mediterranean lymphoma) occurs most often in 10 to 30 yr olds in the Mediterranean basin, Mideast, the Far East, and Africa. This disorder is an IgA lymphoproliferative disorder that may progress to a B-cell lymphoma. Poverty and frequent episodes of gastroenteritis during infancy are antecedent social and medical problems. In some areas, as socioeconomic conditions have improved, the incidence of this disorder has decreased. Sporadic cases occur in Europe and North and South America, predominantly in immigrants from developing countries, although occasionally in native citizens. A similar disorder has been described in patients with AIDS.

CLINICAL MANIFESTATIONS. Initially, patients have intermittent diarrhea and abdominal pain. Later stages demonstrate persistent chronic diarrhea, malabsorption, protein-losing enteropathy, weight loss, digital clubbing, and growth failure.

DIAGNOSIS. Endoscopic biopsies of multiple duodenal and jejunal mucosal sites aid in the diagnosis. In addition, a serum marker (α heavy-chain paraprotein) of IgA is present in most cases. *Giardia lamblia* may also be present but is not responsible for the lymphoproliferative disorder. Immunosuppressed organ transplant recipients may develop a lymphoproliferative disorder manifesting diarrhea.

TREATMENT. The earliest lesions respond to prolonged (~6 mo) tetracycline or metronidazole therapy. Pre-lymphomatous stages and lymphomas are treated with a combination chemotherapy. Lymphoproliferative disorders in immunosuppressed transplant recipients usually improve with reduction of the immunosuppressive drug dose.

PROGNOSIS. Early therapy of antibiotic responsive lesions produces an excellent outcome. Treatment of the later lymphomatous lesions has resulted in a variable but usually poor outcome.

340.10 Other Malabsorptive Syndromes

PANCREATIC INSUFFICIENCY. Cystic fibrosis is the most common congenital disorder associated with malabsorption. The next most common cause of pancreatic insufficiency in children, although much rarer, is Shwachman syndrome (see Chapters 348, 349, 350).

INTESTINAL LYMPHANGIECTASIA. This group of disorders is characterized by dilatation of intestinal lymphatic vessels and leakage of lymph into the intestinal lumen and, at times, the peritoneal cavity. Because absorbed fat is normally transferred from the intestine via the lymphatic vessels, children with this disorder have steatorrhea with protein-losing enteropathy and may have lymphocyte depletion. Manifestations may include any combination of hypoalbuminemia, hypogammaglobulinemia, edema, lymphocytopenia, fat malabsorption, and chylous ascites. Intestinal lymphangiectasia can be primary or can result from abdominal or thoracic surgical damage to lymphatic vessels, chronic right-sided heart failure, constrictive pericarditis, retroperitoneal tumor, or malrotation with lymphatic obstruction. Primary intestinal lymphangiectasia is the result of a congenital abnormality of lymphatic drainage from the intestine and may be associated with abnormalities in lymphatic drainage from other regions of the body. Turner and Noonan syndromes have been associated with intestinal lymphangiectasia.

The diagnosis is suggested by the typical findings described previously in association with an elevated fecal α_1-antitrypsin level consistent with protein-losing enteropathy. The characteristic radiologic findings of uniform, symmetric thickening of mucosal folds throughout the small intestine are usually, although not always, present on small bowel contrast radiographs. The diagnosis is confirmed by the presence of collections of abnormal dilated lacteals with distortion of villi on peroral small bowel biopsy. The disorder may be seen only in the submucosa, thus requiring surgical biopsy of the intestine.

MICROVILLUS INCLUSION DISEASE (Congenital Microvillus Atrophy). Microvillus inclusion disease is a disorder that presents at birth with intractable, watery diarrhea and severe malabsorption. It appears to be the most common cause of persistent diarrhea that begins in the neonatal period. The disorder seems to be inherited in an autosomal recessive pattern. The findings on small bowel biopsy are the key to the diagnosis and include villus atrophy, crypt hypoplasia, and, on election microscopy, microvillus inclusions in enterocytes. The last finding is also seen in colonocytes. The somatostatin analog octreotide has been used as treatment and may reduce the volume of stool output in some infants. Epidermal growth factor has been used with equivocal results. Infants with this disorder require total parenteral nutrition for survival and may be candidates for bowel transplantation.

AUTOIMMUNE ENTEROPATHY. Autoimmune enteropathy is a poorly characterized syndrome of chronic diarrhea and malabsorption. If symptoms initially develop after the first 6 mo of life, the disorder is likely to be mistaken for gluten-sensitive enteropathy. Typically, the lack of response to a gluten-free diet leads to further evaluation. Histologic findings in the small bowel include partial or complete villous atrophy, crypt hyperplasia, and an increase in chronic inflammatory cells in the lamina propria. Specific serum antienterocyte antibodies may be identified in 50% or more of patients by indirect immunofluorescent staining of normal small bowel mucosa and the kidney. The colon can also be involved. Extraintestinal autoimmune disorders are usual and include arthritis, membranous glomerulonephritis, insulin-dependent diabetes, thrombocytopenia, autoimmune hepatitis, hypothyroidism, and hemolytic anemia. Treatment has included prednisone, azathioprine, cyclophosphamide (Cytoxan), cyclosporine, and tacrolimus.

TUFTING ENTEROPATHY. Tufting enteropathy (intestinal epithelial dysplasia) is a disorder that presents in the first weeks of life with persistent watery diarrhea and appears to account for a small fraction of infants with protracted diarrhea of infancy. Onset of symptoms is not immediately after birth as in microvillus inclusion disease. On small bowel biopsy, the distinctive feature is that 80–90% of the epithelial surface contains focal epithelial "tufts" (teardrop-shaped groups of closely packed enterocytes with apical rounding of the plasma membrane). In other known enteropathies, tufts are seen on 15% or less of the epithelial surface. In this disorder, colonic epithelium shows no abnormality. On electron microscopy of small bowel epithelium, the major finding is shortening of the microvilli. This does not appear to be an autoimmune enteropathy, and no known enteropathogens have been isolated. The intestinal lesion has not responded to removal of dietary antigens, administration of total parenteral nutrition, or use of immunosuppressive therapy. This may be a disorder of cell-cell and cell matrix interactions.

ENDOCRINE DISORDERS. Steatorrhea may occur with a number of endocrine disorders including adrenal insufficiency, hypoparathryroidism, and diabetes mellitus.

TROPICAL SPRUE. This syndrome is characterized by generalized malabsorption associated with a diffuse lesion of the small intestinal mucosa that occurs only in persons who have lived in or visited certain tropical regions. It occurs in some Caribbean countries (not Jamaica), northern South America, Africa, and parts of Asia. Fever and malaise precede the onset of watery diarrhea. In about 1 wk, acute features subside and chronic malabsorption, intermittent diarrhea, and anorexia lead eventually to severe malnutrition. Signs of malnutrition may include night blindness, glossitis, stomatitis, cheilosis, hyperpigmentation, and edema. Muscle wasting is marked, and the abdomen is often distended. Patients have evidence of diffuse malabsorption, including steatorrhea and carbohydrate intolerance. Megaloblastic anemia is the result of folate and vitamin B_{12} deficiencies. Biopsy of the small intestinal mucosa shows villus shortening, increased crypt depth, and an increase in chronic inflammatory cells in the lamina propria. Treatment includes antibiotics (for 3–4 wk) and folate as well as vitamin B_{12} repletion. The response to treatment is usually excellent.

WOLMAN DISEASE. This rare lethal lipid storage disease leads to lipid accumulation in many organs including the small intestine. In addition to vomiting and hepatosplenomegaly, patients may have steatorrhea as the result of lymphatic obstruction (Chapter 83).

340.11 Enzyme Deficiencies

ENTEROKINASE DEFICIENCY

Congenital deficiency of this small intestinal enzyme has been reported in a few children. The disease results in a complete absence of pancreatic proteolytic activity because enterokinase is an essential activator of pancreatic trypsinogens. Affected patients are ill from very early life with severe diarrhea and failure to thrive. Hypoproteinemia is common and may lead to edema. In duodenal fluid, tryptic activity is missing, whereas lipase and amylase are normal; in vitro tryptic activity of the fluid can be restored by the addition of enterokinase. Malabsorption of protein is the major defect, although mild steatorrhea has been reported. Pancreatic enzyme replacements restore normal digestive function; much smaller amounts are needed compared with those required for pancreatic insufficiency.

DISACCHARIDASE DEFICIENCIES

The disaccharidases are located on the brush border membrane surface of the small bowel. Occasionally, congenital deficiencies occur, but abnormal disaccharidase activities in infants and young children have most often been the result of diffuse acquired lesions of the intestinal epithelium, such as those of infection or celiac disease. In older children and adults, late-onset genetic lactase deficiency is the most common condition associated with reduced disaccharidase activity.

The *clinical manifestations* of significant disaccharidase deficiency (disaccharide intolerance) are similar whatever its cause or the enzymes involved. If disaccharide hydrolysis at the brush border is incomplete, the sugar accumulates in the distal intestinal lumen, where organic acids and hydrogen gas are produced by bacteria. The excess intraluminal sugar and organic acids draw water into the lumen, leading to watery osmotic diarrhea with stools that are of low pH (pH < 5.6), contain excess sugar, and tend to excoriate the buttocks. Patients may have bloating and borborygmi, but steatorrhea is rare. In some cases, particularly those beyond infancy, gas production causing crampy abdominal pain is the dominant problem, rather than diarrhea.

If the disaccharide involved is a reducing sugar (lactose), the standard Clinitest examination (Bayer Corp., Elkhart, IN) will be 2+ or greater in most cases. Disaccharidase activities can be assayed in mucosal biopsy specimens. Breath hydrogen excretion after an oral sugar load is a useful noninvasive technique for detecting disaccharide intolerance (see Chapter 340.1).

LACTASE DEFICIENCY. *Congenital* absence of lactase has been reported in few cases. The usual mechanism for primary lactose intolerance relates to the *developmental* pattern of lactase activity. Because lactase activity rises relatively late in fetal life and begins to fall after the age of 3 yr, intolerance to lactose can be anticipated in extremely premature infants and in some older children and adults. Approximately 15% of adult whites, 40% of adult Asians, and 85% of adult blacks in the United States are deficient in intestinal lactase; this is known as "adult-onset hypolactasia" and is an autosomal recessive characteristic. Because lactase activity in the mucosa is at best marginal, this enzyme is particularly likely to be depleted *secondary to diffuse mucosal diseases.*

Clinical manifestations occur in response to ingestion of lactose, the sugar in milk. Explosive watery diarrhea is associated with abdominal distention, borborygmi, flatulence, and an excoriated diaper area. A syndrome of recurrent, vague, crampy abdominal pain has also been attributed to lactose intolerance. School-aged and pre–school-aged children experience episodic mid-abdominal pain. Usually, their general health is unaffected, and they may have no obvious temporal relationship of pain or diarrhea with milk ingestion.

Treatment consists of removal of milk from the diet. In most cases, the elimination need not be total; stopping milk ingestion as a beverage is important. A lactase preparation (LactAid) is available; when added to milk, it allows asymptomatic consumption of modest quantities of milk incubated with the added enzyme. A tablet with lactase activity can also be ingested with meals (LactAid). Live culture yogurt contains bacteria that produce lactase enzyme and is thus tolerated by lactase-deficient individuals.

SUCRASE-ISOMALTASE DEFICIENCY. The only relatively common congenital deficiency of disaccharidase activities, a combined deficiency of sucrase and isomaltase, is inherited as an autosomal recessive trait and occurs in about 0.2% of North Americans. Symptoms usually begin when a sucrose or glucose polymer-containing diet is started. Patients may be intolerant to starch, but because isomaltase acts only on the branch points of the starch molecule, isomaltase deficiency itself is relatively asymptomatic. The symptoms are bloating, watery diarrhea, and failure to thrive. Recurrent abdominal pain has not been attributed to sucrose-isomaltose intolerance. Because sucrose is not a reducing sugar, its presence is not detected in the stool by Clinitest unless the specimen is first hydrolyzed with hydrochloric acid. The morphologic features of the small intestinal mucosa are normal, but enzyme assays show specific deficiencies of sucrase and isomaltase with normal levels of lactase and maltase. Breath testing usually demonstrates increased hydrogen gas after sucrose ingestion. Affected patients improve quickly after dietary sucrose is reduced to minimal amounts.

340.12 Defects of Absorption or Transport

GLUCOSE-GALACTOSE MALABSORPTION. More than 30 different mutations of the sodium/glucose co-transporter (SGLT1) gene have been identified to cause this rare autosomal recessive, congenital disorder of intestinal glucose-galactose absorption. SGLT1 couples glucose and galactose transport to the sodium gradients across intestinal and renal brush borders. Renal tubular epithelium is affected to a lesser degree.

Watery stools follow the ingestion of glucose, breast milk, or conventional formulas because most dietary sugars are polysaccharides or disaccharides with glucose or galactose moieties. The patient may be bloated, and, if diarrhea persists, dehydration and acidosis can be severe, resulting in death. The stools are acidic and contain sugar. Patients with the defect tolerate fructose; their small bowel function and structure are normal in all other aspects. *Treatment* consists of rigorous restriction of glucose and galactose and provision of a fructose-containing formula. Later in life, limited amounts of glucose or sucrose may be tolerated.

Severe diffuse mucosal damage, particularly in a young infant, may also impair the glucose-galactose carrier sufficiently to cause intolerance to these sugars. Usually, if mucosal damage is severe enough to impair glucose transport, other absorptive processes are affected.

ABETALIPOPROTEINEMIA. (Chapter 83.3). This autosomal recessive condition is associated with severe fat malabsorption from birth. Children fail to thrive during the 1st yr of life and their stools are pale, foul smelling, and bulky. The abdomen is distended, and deep tendon reflexes are absent as a result of peripheral neuropathy.

Intellectual development tends to be slow. After 10 yr of age, intestinal symptoms are less severe, ataxia develops, and one sees a loss of position and vibration senses and the onset of intention tremors. These last symptoms reflect involvement of the posterior columns, cerebellum, and basal ganglia. In adolescence, atypical retinitis pigmentosa develops.

Diagnosis rests on finding acanthocytes in the peripheral blood and extremely low plasma levels of cholesterol (<50 mg/dL). Chylomicrons and very-low-density lipoproteins are not detectable, and the low-density lipoprotein (LDL) fraction is virtually absent from the circulation; marked triglyceride accumulation in villus enterocytes occurs in the fasting duodenal mucosa. Usually, steatorrhea occurs in younger patients, but other processes of assimilation are intact. Patients have mutations of the microsomal triglyceride transfer protein (MTP) gene resulting in absence of MTP function in the small bowel. This protein is required for normal assembly and secretion of very-low-density lipoproteins and chylomicrons. The neuropathy is the result of vitamin E deficiency.

Specific *treatment* is not available. Large supplements of the fat-soluble vitamins A, D, E, and K should be given. Vitamin E (100 mg/kg/24 hr) and vitamin A (10,000–25,000 IU/day) may arrest the neurologic degeneration. Limiting long-chain fat intake may alleviate intestinal symptoms; medium-chain triglycerides can be used to supplement the fat intake.

HOMOZYGOUS HYPOBETALIPOPROTEINEMIA. This disorder is transmitted as an autosomal dominant trait; the homozygous form is indistinguishable from abetalipoproteinemia. However, the parents of these patients, as heterozygotes, have reduced plasma LDL and apoprotein-β concentrations, unlike the parents of patients with abetalipoproteinemia, who have normal levels.

CHYLOMICRON RETENTION DISEASE. In this rare recessive disorder, the processes leading up to the release of chylomicrons from enterocytes appear to be defective. These patients have severe intestinal symptoms with steatorrhea and failure to thrive. Acanthocytosis is rare, and neurologic manifestations are less severe than those observed in abetalipoproteinemia. Plasma cholesterol levels are reduced, but moderately so (<75 mg/dL); fasting triglycerides are normal; but the fat-soluble vitamins, particularly A and E, rapidly deplete. Early aggressive therapy with fat-soluble vitamins is indicated, as for abetalipoproteinemia.

AMINO ACID TRANSPORT DEFECTS. In several of the specific congenital disorders of amino acid transport (Chapter 82), defective intestinal amino acid transport occurs. At least three specific small bowel carriers appear to be involved in active transport of amino acids. Amino acid uptake into the intestinal mucosa is defective in *cystinuria,* but these patients have no gastrointestinal symptoms. In *Hartnup disease,* malabsorption of neutral amino acids including tryptophan leads to ataxia, intellectual deterioration, a pellagra-like skin rash, and, at times, diarrhea. *Methionine malabsorption* is associated with episodes of diarrhea in fair-complexioned, retarded children whose urine has a sweet odor and contains excess β-hydroxybutyric acid. In the *blue diaper syndrome,* tryptophan absorption is defective.

VITAMIN B_{12} MALABSORPTION. Several rare congenital defects may affect assimilation of vitamin B_{12}. These conditions are much less common than dietary vitamin B_{12} deficiency or malabsorption secondary to terminal ileal resection or dysfunction. In *juvenile pernicious anemia,* intrinsic factor production in the stomach is defective. Vitamin B_{12} malabsorption results, leading to megaloblastic anemia and growth failure. Gastric structure and function are otherwise normal.

Transcobalamin II deficiency is an inherited defect of a protein necessary for intestinal transport of vitamin B_{12}. The result is severe megaloblastic anemia, diarrhea, and vomiting.

Imerslund syndrome has described patients in whom ileal absorption of vitamin B_{12} is defective. Ileal structure and function are otherwise normal. Megaloblastic anemia develops toward the end of the 1st yr. Proteinuria is commonly associated.

Treatment of these disorders is to administer vitamin B_{12} by injection: 1,000 μg/wk for transcobalamin II deficiency and 100 μg/mo for the others.

CONGENITAL MALABSORPTION OF FOLIC ACID. A few patients have had folic acid deficiency in infancy as the result of a specific defect in folic acid assimilation. In addition to megaloblastic anemia, they have had cerebral degeneration.

CHLORIDE-LOSING DIARRHEA. This rare specific congenital defect of ileal chloride transport is associated with maternal polyhydramnios. The dominant symptom is severe watery diarrhea beginning at birth, the result of accumulation of chloride ion in the intestinal lumen. Watery diarrhea leads to dehydration and a severe electrolyte disturbance characterized by hypokalemia, hypochloremia, and alkalosis, a most unusual pattern for a child with chronic diarrhea. Other aspects of intestinal absorption are normal. Stools contain chloride in excess of the sum of sodium and potassium. No adequate treatment exists. Potassium supplements and some restriction of chloride intake are advisable.

CONGENITAL SODIUM DIARRHEA. A few patients have been described with profuse watery diarrhea from birth. There was maternal polyhydramnios and neonatal abdominal distention; however, unlike chloride diarrhea, this condition was characterized by acidosis and fecal chloride concentration less than sodium concentration. *Treatment* with oral hydration solution was effective in maintaining normal growth. The apparent basis for this rare syndrome is a defect in sodium-hydrogen exchange in the small intestine and colon.

VITAMIN D–DEPENDENT RICKETS. In this autosomal recessive disorder, a specific defect in the metabolism of vitamin D causes malabsorption of calcium (Chapter 712). Intestinal function is otherwise normal.

PRIMARY HYPOMAGNESEMIA. This specific intestinal transport defect in magnesium transport causes severe hypomagnesemia and, secondarily, hypocalcemic tetany in infancy. Other aspects of intestinal function are normal. The findings are reversed by large supplements of magnesium, which must be continued indefinitely.

ACRODERMATITIS ENTEROPATHICA. (see also Chapter 677). This unusual constellation of clinical findings is due to zinc deficiency secondary to zinc malabsorption. Early in life, the patient experiences rashes around mucocutaneous junctions and on the extremities; alopecia, chronic diarrhea, and sometimes steatorrhea may occur. Untreated, the patient fails to thrive. Serum zinc concentration and alkaline phosphatase activity are low. Intestinal mucosal biopsies show Paneth cell inclusions that disappear after treatment. An oral supplement of zinc sulfate, 1–2 mg elemental zinc/kg/24 hr, causes rapid healing of the skin lesions and improvement of diarrhea.

MENKES (KINKY HAIR) SYNDROME. This rare recessively inherited disorder is characterized by growth retardation, abnormal hair, cerebellar degeneration, and early death (Chapter 608.5). Its pathogenesis is unclear, but a widespread defect in cellular copper transport affects the intestine as well as other tissues. Serum copper and ceruloplasmin levels are low, but cellular copper content is increased.

BILE ACID MALABSORPTION. Primary bile acid malabsorption caused by mutations in the ileal sodium-dependent bile acid transporter gene results in diarrhea and steatorrhea from early infancy. These patients have reduced plasma cholesterol levels and severe growth retardation as well.

DRUG-INDUCED ABSORPTIVE DEFECTS. Some drugs have a diffuse impact on the small intestinal epithelium. For example, methotrexate can cause arrest of enterocyte mitoses and can result in a mucosal lesion; large doses of neomycin also affect mucosal structure. *Sulfasalazine* interferes with folic acid absorption. *Cholestyramine* binds bile salts and calcium in the intestinal lumen to cause hypocalcemia and steatorrhea. *Phenytoin* interferes with calcium absorption and can cause rickets.

Malabsorption Syndromes

General Reviews

Ament ME: Malabsorption syndromes in infancy and childhood. J Pediatr 81:685, 1972.

Branski D, Lerner A, Lebenthal E: Chronic diarrhea and malabsorption. Pediatr Clin North Am 43:307, 1996.

Kleinman RE, Klish W, Lebenthal E, et al: Role of juice carbohydrate malabsorption in chronic nonspecific diarrhea in children. J Pediatr 120:825, 1992.

Riby JE, Fujisawa T, Kretchmer N: Fructose absorption. Am J Clin Nutr 58:748S, 1993.

Diagnostic Investigations

Ament ME, Berquist WE, Vargus J, et al: Fiberoptic upper endoscopy in infants and children. Pediatr Clin North Am 35:141, 1988.

Barr RG, Perman JA, Schoeller DA, et al: Breath tests in pediatric gastrointestinal disorders: New diagnostic opportunities. Pediatrics 62:393, 1978.

Ghesh SK, Littlewood JM, Goddard D, et al: Stool microscopy in screening for steatorrhea. J Clin Pathol 30:749, 1977.

Hill RE, Hercz A, Corey MD, et al: Fecal clearance of alpha-1-antitrypsin: A reliable measure of protein loss in children. J Pediatr 99:416, 1981.

Khouri M, Huang G, Shiau Y: Sudan stain of fecal fat: New insight into an old test. Gastroenterology 96:421, 1989.

Murphy MS, Eastham EJ, Nelson R, et al: Non-invasive assessment of intraluminal lipolysis using a $^{13}CO_2$ breath test. Arch Dis Child 65:574, 1990.

Riddlesherger MM: Evaluation of the gastrointestinal tract in the child: CT, MRI, and isotopic studies. Pediatr Clin North Am 35:281, 1988.

Digestive Tract in Chronic Malnutrition

Durie PR, Forstner GG, Gaskin KJ, et al: Elevated serum immunoreactive pancreatic cationic trypsinogen in acute malnutrition: Evidence of pancreatic damage. J Pediatr 106:233, 1985.

Romer H, Cerbach R, Gomez MA, et al: Moderate and severe protein-energy malnutrition in childhood: Effects on jejunal mucosal morphology and disaccharidase activities. J Pediatr Gastroenterol Nutr 2:459, 1983.

Liver and Biliary Disorders

Argao EA, Heubi JE: Fat-soluble vitamin deficiency in infants and children. Curr Opin Pediatr 5:562, 1993.

Hadorn B, Hess J, Troesch V, et al: Role of bile acids in the activation of trypsinogen by enterokinase: Disturbance of trypsinogen activation in patients with intrahepatic biliary atresia. Gastroenterology 66:548, 1974.

Kooh SW, Jones G, Reilly BJ, et al: Pathogenesis of rickets in chronic hepatobiliary disease in children. J Pediatr 94:870, 1979.

Short Small Intestine

Bines J, Francis D, Hill D, et al: Reducing parenteral requirement in children with short bowel syndrome: Impact of an amino acid–based complete infant formula. J Pediatr Gastroenterol Nutr 26:123, 1998.

Caniano DA, Kanoti GA: Newborns with massive intestinal loss: Difficult choices. N Engl J Med 318:703, 1988.

Goulet O: Recent studies on small intestinal transplantation. Curr Opin Gastroenterol 13:500, 1997.

Goulet OJ, Revillon Y, Jan D, et al: Neonatal short bowel syndrome. J Pediatr 119:18, 1991.

Grant D, Wall W, Mimeault R, et al: Successful small-bowel/liver transplantation. Lancet 335:181, 1990.

Kaufman SS, Loseke CA, Lupo JV, et al: Influence of bacterial overgrowth and intestinal inflammation on duration of parenteral nutrition in children with short bowel syndrome. J Pediatr 131:356, 1997.

Leonberg BL, Chuang E, Eicher P, et al: Long-term growth and development in children after home parenteral nutrition. J Pediatr 132:461, 1998.

Taylor SF, Sondheimer JM, Sokol RJ, et al: Noninfectious colitis associated with short gut syndrome in infants. J Pediatr 119:24, 1991.

Stagnant Loop Syndrome

Bayes BJ, Hamilton JR: Blind loop syndrome in children. Acta Dis Child 44:76, 1969.

Gracey M: Intestinal microflora and bacterial overgrowth in early life. J Pediatr Gastroenterol Nutr 1:13, 1982.

Soderlund S: Anomalies of midgut rotation and fixation: Clinical aspects based on sixty-two cases in childhood. Acta Pediatr 51:135, 1966.

Infections Causing Malabsorption

Ament ME: Diagnosis and treatment of giardiasis. J Pediatr 80:663, 1972.

Farthing MJG: The molecular pathogenesis of giardiasis. J Pediatr Gastroenterol Nutr 24:79, 1997.

Liebman WM, Thaler MM, Dehorimier A, et al: Intractable diarrhea of infancy due to intestinal coccidiosis. Gastroenterology 78:579, 1980.

Sood M, Booth I: Is prolonged rotavirus infection a common cause of protracted diarrhoea? Arch Dis Child 80:309, 1999.

Immunodeficiency States and the Intestine

Kotler DP, Francisco A, Clayton F, et al: Small intestinal injury and parasitic diseases in AIDS. Ann Intern Med 113:444, 1990.

Weikel CS, Gaynes BN, Roche JK: Diarrheal disease in the immunocompromised host. *In:* Guerrant R (ed): Ballière's Clinical Tropical Medicine and Communicable Diseases, Vol 3. London, Ballière Tindall, 1988, p 401.

Winter H. Chang TI. Gastrointestinal and nutritional problems in children with immunodeficiency and AIDS. Pediatr Clin North Am 43:573, 1996

Yolken RH, Hart W, Oung I, et al: Gastrointestinal dysfunction and disaccharide intolerance in children infected with human immunodeficiency virus. J Pediatr 118:359, 1991.

Celiac Disease

Carlsson A, Axelsson I, Borulf S, et al: Prevalence of IgA-antigliadin antibodies and IgA-antiendomysium antibodies related to celiac disease in children with Down syndrome. Pediatrics 101:272, 1998.

Carroccio A, Iacono G, Lerro P, et al: Role of pancreatic impairment in growth recovery during gluten-free diet in childhood celiac disease. Gastroenterology 112:1839, 1997.

Chan KN, Phillips AD, Mirakian R, et al: Endomysial antibody screening in children. J Pediatr Gastroenterol Nutr 18:316, 1994.

Dieterich W, Laag E, Schöpper H, et al: Autoantibodies to tissue transglutaminase as predictors of celiac disease. Gastroenterology 115:1317, 1998.

Janatuinen EK, Pikkarainen PH, Kemppainen TA: A comparison of diets with and without oats in adults with celiac disease. N Engl J Med 333:1033, 1995.

Lepore L, Martelossi S, Pennesi M, et al: Prevalence of celiac disease in patients with juvenile chronic arthritis. J Pediatr 129:311, 1996.

Mäki M, Collin P. Coeliac disease. Lancet 349:1755, 1997.

Report to Working Group of European Society of Paediatric Gastroenterology and Nutrition: Revised criteria for diagnosis of coeliac disease. Arch Dis Child 65:909, 1990.

Rossi TM, Albini CH, Kumar V: Incidence of celiac disease identified by the presence of serum endomysial antibodies in children with chronic diarrhea, short stature, or insulin-dependent diabetes mellitus. J Pediatr 123:262, 1993.

Rossi TM, Tjota A: Serologic indicators of celiac disease. J Pediatr Gastroenterol Nutr 26:205, 1998.

Swinson CM, Slavin G, Coles EC, et al: Coeliac disease and malignancy. Lancet 1:111, 1983.

Visakorpi J, Mäki M: Changing clinical features of coeliac disease. Acta Paediatr Suppl 395:10, 1994.

Volta U, De Franceschi L, Lari F, et al: Coeliac disease hidden by cryptogenic hypertransaminasemia. Lancet 352:26, 1998.

Other Syndromes

Bousvaros A, Leichtner AM, Book L, et al: Treatment of pediatric autoimmune enteropathy with tacrolimus (FK506). Gastroenterology 111:237, 1996.

Khojasteh A, Haghighi P: Immunoproliferative small intestinal disease: Portrait of a potentially preventable cancer from the Third World. Am J Med 89:483, 1990.

Mack DR, Forstner GG, Wilschanski M, et al: Shwachman syndrome: Exocrine pancreatic dysfunction and variable phenotypic expression. Gastroenterology 111:1593, 1996.

Patey N, Scoazec JY, Cuenod-Jabri B, et al: Distribution of cell adhesion molecules in infants with intestinal epithelial dysplasia (tufting enteropathy). Gastroenterology 113:833, 1997.

Queloz JM, Capitanio MA, Kirkpatrick JA: Wolman's disease. Radiology 104:357, 1972.

Reifen RM, Cutz E, Griffiths AM, et al: Tufting enteropathy: A newly recognized clinicopathological entity associated with refractory diarrhea in infants. J Pediatr Gastroenterol Nutr 18:379, 1994.

Santiago-Borrero PJ, Maldonado N, Horta E: Tropical sprue in children. J Pediatr 76:470, 1970.

Vardy PA, Lebenthal E, Shwachman H: Intestinal lymphangiectasis: A reappraisal. Pediatrics 55:842, 1975.

Defects of Absorption or Transport

Levy E, Chouraqui JP, Ray CC: Steatorrhea and disorders of chylomicron synthesis and secretion. Pediatr Clin North Am 35:53, 1988.

Muller DPR, Lloyd JK, Bird AC: Long-term management of abetalipoproteinemia. Arch Dis Child 52:209, 1977.

Rader DJ, Brewer B: Abetalipoproteinemia: New insights into lipoprotein assembly and vitamin E metabolism from a rare genetic disease. JAMA 270:865, 1993.

Scott BB, Miller JP, Losowsky MS: Hypobetalipoproteinemia: A variant of the Bassen-Kornzweig syndrome. Gut 20:163, 1979.

Enterokinase Deficiency

Hadorn B, Tarlow M, Lloyd JD, et al: Intestinal enterokinase deficiency. Lancet 1:812, 1969.

Amino Acid Transport Defects

Drummond KN, Michael AF, Ulstrom RA, et al: The blue diaper syndrome: Familial hypercalcemia with nephrocalcinosis and indicanuria. Am J Med 37:928, 1964.
Hooft G, Timmermand J, Snoeck J, et al: Methionine malabsorption syndrome. Ann Pediatr 205:73, 1965.
Milne MD: Hartnup disease. Biochemistry 111:3, 1969.
Morin CL, Thompson MW, Jackson SH, et al: Biochemical and genetic studies in cystinuria: Observations on double heterozygotes of genotype I/II. J Clin Invest 50:1961, 1971.
Whelan DT, Scriver CR: Hyperdibasicaminoaciduria: An inherited disorder of amino acid transport. Pediatr Res 2:525, 1968.

Disaccharidase Deficiencies

Ament ME, Perera DR, Esther L: Sucrase-isomaltase deficiency: A frequently misdiagnosed disease. J Pediatr 83:721, 1973.
Flats G: The genetics of lactose digestion in humans. Adv Hum Genet 16:1, 1987.
Harrison M, Walker-Smith JA: Reinvestigation of lactose intolerant children: Lack of correlation between continuing lactose intolerance and small intestinal morphology, disaccharidase activity and lactose tests. Gut 18:48, 1977.
Newton T, Murphy MS, Booth IW: Glucose polymer as a cause of protracted diarrhea in infants with unsuspected congenital sucrase-isomaltase deficiency. J Pediatr 128:753, 1996.
Ouwendijk J, Moolenaar CE, Peters WJ, et al: Congenital sucrase-isomaltase deficiency: Identification of a glutamine to proline substitution that leads to a transport block of sucrase-isomaltase in a pre-Golgi compartment. J Clin Invest 97:633, 1996.
Treem WR: Congenital sucrase-isomaltase deficiency. J Pediatr Gastroenterol Nutr 21:1, 1995.

Glucose-Galactose Malabsorption

Evans L, Grasset E, Heyman M, et al: Congenital selective malabsorption of glucose and galactose. J Pediatr Gastroenterol Nutr 4:878, 1985.
Fairclough PD, Clark ML, Dawson AM, et al: Absorption of glucose and maltose in congenital glucose-galactose malabsorption. Pediatr Res 12:1112, 1978.
Martin MG, Turk E, Lostao MP: Defects in Na^+/glucose cotransporter (SGLT1) trafficking and function cause glucose-galactose malabsorption. Nat Genet 12:216, 1996.

Vitamin B_{12} Malabsorption

Chanarin I: Disorders of vitamin absorption. Clin Gastroenterol 11:73, 1982.
Hall CA: Congenital disorders of vitamin B_{12} transport and their contribution to concepts. Gastroenterology 65:684, 1973.
Hitzig WH, Dohmann V, Pluss HJ, et al: Hereditary transcobalamin II deficiency: Clinical findings in a new family. J Pediatr 85:622, 1974.
Imerslund O: Idiopathic chronic megaloblastic anaemia in children. Acta Paediatr Suppl 49:119, 1960.
MacKenzie IL, Donaldson RM, Trier JS, et al: Ileal mucosa in familial selective vitamin B_{12} malabsorption. N Engl J Med 286:1021, 1972.

Folate Malabsorption

Poncz M, Colman N, Herbert V, et al: Congenital folate malabsorption. J Pediatr 99:828, 1981.
Urbach J, Abrahamov A, Grossowicz N: Congenital isolated folic acid malabsorption. Arch Dis Child 62:78, 1987.

Chloride-Losing Diarrhea

Bieberdorf FA, Gorden P, Fordtran JS: Pathogenesis of congenital alkalosis with diarrhea: Implications for the physiology of normal ileal electrolyte absorption and secretion. J Clin Invest 51:1958, 1972.
Holmberg C, Perheentupa J, Launiala K, et al: Congenital chloride diarrhea. Arch Dis Child 52:255, 1977.

Congenital Sodium Diarrhea

Booth IW, Murer H, Strange G, et al: Defective jejunal brush border Na^+/H^+ exchange: A cause of congenital secretory diarrhea. Lancet 1:1066, 1985.
Holmberg C, Perheentupa J: Congenital Na^+ diarrhea: A new type of secretory diarrhea. J Pediatr 106:56, 1985.

Vitamin D–Dependent Rickets

Hamilton R, Harrison J, Fraser D, et al: The small intestine in vitamin D dependent rickets. Pediatrics 45:364, 1970.

Primary Hypomagnesemia

Romero R, Meacham LR, Winn KT: Isolated magnesium malabsorption in a 10-year-old boy. Am J Gastroenterol 91:611, 1996.
Stromme JH, Nesbakken R, Normann T, et al: Familial hypomagnesemia. Acta Paediatr Scand 58:433, 1969.

Acrodermatitis Enteropathica

Bohane TD, Cutz E, Hamilton JR, et al: Acrodermatitis enteropathica, zinc and the Paneth cell. Gastroenterology 73:587, 1977.
Moynahan EJ: Acrodermatitis enteropathica: A lethal inherited human zinc-deficiency disorder. Lancet 2:399, 1974.

Menkes Syndrome

Danks DM: Of mice and men, metals and mutations. J Med Genet 23:99, 1986.
Danks DM, Stevens BJ, Campbell PE, et al: Menkes' kinky-hair syndrome. Lancet 1:110, 1972.

Primary Bile Acid Malabsorption

Heubi JE, Balistreri WF, Fondacaro JD, et al: Primary bile acid malabsorption: Defective in vitro ileal active bile acid transport. Gastroenterology 83:804, 1982.
Oelkers P, Kirby LC, Heubi JE, et al: Primary bile acid malabsorption caused by mutations in the ileal sodium-dependent bile acid transporter gene (SLC10A2). J Clin Invest 99:1880, 1997.

Drug-Induced Malabsorption

Franklin JL, Rosenberg HH: Impaired folic acid absorption in inflammatory bowel disease: Effects of salicylazosulfapyridine (Azulfidine). Gastroenterology 64:517, 1973.
Morijiri Y, et al: Factors causing rickets in institutionalized handicapped children on anti-convulsant therapy. Arch Dis Child 56:446, 1981.
Rogers AL, Vloedman DA, Bloom EC, et al: Neomycin-induced steatorrhea. JAMA 197:185, 1966.
Trier JS: Morphologic alterations induced by methotrexate in the mucosa of human proximal intestine. I: Serial observations by light microscopy. Gastroenterology 42:295, 1962.

CHAPTER 341
Chronic Diarrhea
(see also Chapter 340)

Fayez K. Ghishan

Diarrhea in children accounts for approximately 5,000,000 deaths per year in the developing world. In the United States, diarrhea accounts for 10% of all outpatient visits and 14 hospital admissions each year per 1,000 children less than 1 yr of age (see Chapter 176).

DEFINITION. Diarrhea, defined as increased total daily stool output, is usually associated with increased stool water content (see Chapter 306). For infants and children, this would result in stool output greater than 10 g/kg/24 hr or more than the adult limit of 200 g/24 hr. When diarrhea lasts longer than 2 wk, it is considered chronic. Diarrhea results from altered intestinal water and electrolyte transport. The gastrointestinal tract of the infant handles approximately 285 mL/kg/24 hr of fluid (intake plus intestinal secretion) with a stool output of 5–10 g/kg/24 hr. The efficient mechanisms responsible for this absorptive capacity are due to the function of several transport proteins located at the brush border membrane of the small and large intestine. The diffusion of electrolytes across the gastrointestinal tract contributes to the overall absorptive process of the small and large intestine. The stool output in infants and children contains approximately, per liter: 20–25 mEq of sodium, 50–70 mEq of potassium, and 20–25 mEq of chloride. The normal cellular mechanisms responsible for the transport of nutrients and electrolytes across the gastrointestinal tract are noted in Figure 341–1.

FUNCTIONAL ANATOMY OF THE INTESTINAL MUCOSA. The villus, the functional unit of the small intestine, greatly amplifies the absorptive and digestive surface of the intestinal mucosa. The tip of the villus represents the highly differentiated absorptive cells, whereas the crypt epithelia represent undifferentiated secretory cells. The epithelial cells at the villi tip are continually renewed every 4–5 days from the undifferentiated crypt cells.

Normal Transport of Nutrients and Electrolytes Across the Gastrointestinal Tract of an Infant

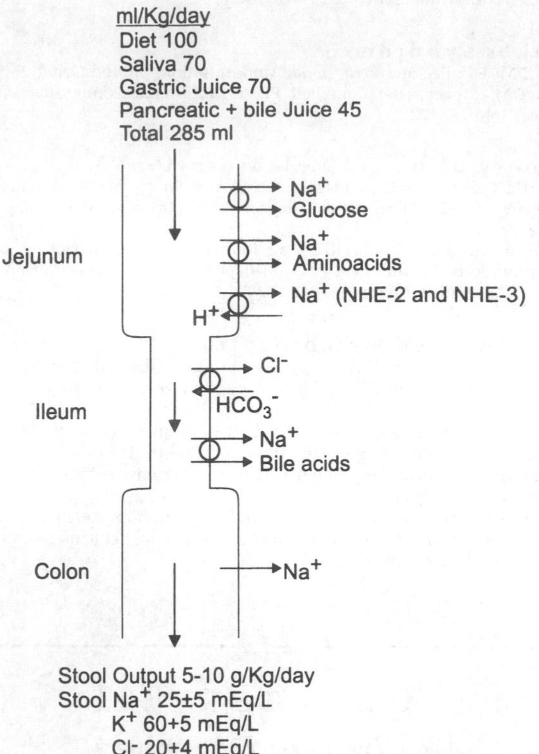

Figure 341–1 The gastrointestinal tract of the infant handles 285 ml/kg/day of dietary and endogenous fluids. The majority of the nutrients and fluids is absorbed via transport protein depicted schematically. NHE-2 and NHE-3 indicate Na^+/H^+ exchanger isoforms 2 and 3. The colon absorbs mainly water and electrolytes via the electroneutral NaCl and the electrogenic Na^+ process.

Digestive enzymes and the transport proteins responsible for the movements of electrolytes across the intestinal mucosa are located at the brush border membrane of the villus cells. The gastrointestinal epithelia are leaky epithelia that adjust the osmotic load presented to the small intestine. Tight junctions, dynamic structures that occur between the epithelial cells, are responsible for movement of water and electrolytes. Transport of electrolytes across the intestinal epithelia occurs through several mechanisms including the glucose-sodium co-transporter. This transport protein requires the presence of a sodium gradient across the brush border membrane that is maintained by the sodium potassium adenosine triphosphatase pump at the basolateral membranes of the enterocyte. The defect in glucose-galactose malabsorption is a missense mutation in the sodium-glucose co-transporter gene (Chapter 340.12).

A second mechanism of electrolyte transport across the intestinal epithelia is the electroneutral sodium chloride–coupled pathway that involves the double exchange mechanism by the sodium-hydrogen exchanger and the chloride-bicarbonate exchanger. Two sodium-hydrogen exchangers (NHE-2 and 3) located at the apical membrane appear to be involved in the transport of sodium. Defects of the genes of sodium-hydrogen and chloride-bicarbonate exchangers are candidates for congenital sodium and chloride diarrhea, respectively. Sodium is absorbed in the colon by the electroneutral sodium chloride–coupled pathway and by an electrogenic mechanism, which is regulated by aldosterone. Intestinal secretion occurs primarily from the crypt cells and is stimulated by an increase in the intracellular level cyclic adenosine monophosphate (cAMP),

A Model for Intestinal Secretion

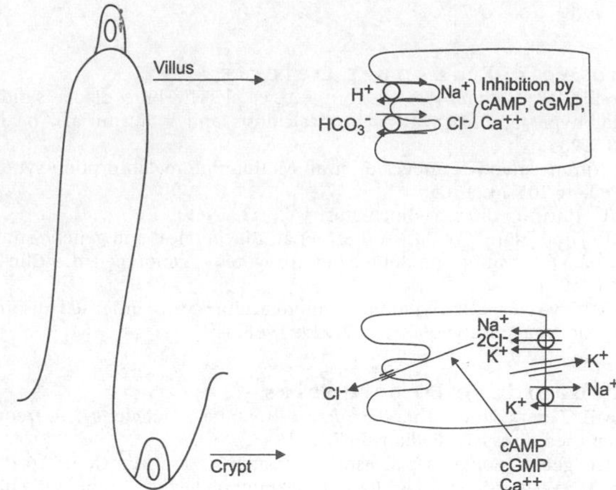

Figure 341–2 Model for intestinal secretion: Enterotoxins increase intracellular mediators (cAMP, cGMP, Ca^{2+}), which open chloride channels in the crypt cells and inhibit the neutral NaCl coupled pathway at the villus cells.

cyclic guanosine monophosphate, (cGMP), and calcium. These mediators inhibit the neutral sodium chloride entry and permit the entry of chloride into the cells through the basolateral membrane via the sodium-potassium-2 chloride transporter (Na^+-K^+-$2Cl^-$). Chloride is then secreted through the opening of chloride channels at the apical membrane of the crypt cells. Sodium and thus water secretion will result in secretory diarrhea. Figure 341–2 depicts a model for intestinal secretion induced by enterotoxins.

PATHOPHYSIOLOGY. The pathophysiologic mechanisms of diarrhea include osmotic diarrhea, secretory diarrhea, mutations in apical membrane transport proteins, a reduction in anatomic surface area, and alteration in intestinal motility (Table 306–4).

Osmotic Diarrhea. Osmotic diarrhea is caused by the presence of nonabsorbable solutes in the gastrointestinal tract (Table 341–1). The classic example of osmotic diarrhea is lactose intolerance due to lactase enzyme deficiency in which lactose is not absorbed in the small intestine and reaches the colon intact (Chapter 340). The colonic bacteria ferment the nonabsorbed lactose to short-chain organic acids generating an osmotic load causing water to be secreted into the lumen. Other examples include ingestion of excessive amounts of carbonated fluids that exceed the transport capacity, especially in toddlers, and ingestion of magnesium hydroxide and sorbitol; both are not absorbed, resulting in an osmotic load. Lactulose, a synthetic therapeutic disaccharide, is not digested in the small intestine and is fermented by the colonic bacteria to form organic acids resulting in osmotic diarrhea. Osmotic diarrhea stops with fasting and has a low pH and is positive for reducing substances. The sum of sodium plus potassium multiplied by

TABLE 341–1 Causes of Osmotic Diarrhea

Causes
Malabsorption of water-soluble nutrients
Glucose-galactose malabsorption
Congenital
Acquired
Disaccharidase deficiencies (lactase and sucrase-isomaltase)
Congenital
Acquired
Excessive intake of carbonated fluids
Excessive intake of nonabsorbable solutes
Sorbitol
Lactulose
Magnesium hydroxide

TABLE 341–2 Differential Diagnosis of Osmotic versus Secretory Diarrhea

	Osmotic Diarrhea	Secretory Diarrhea
Volume of stool	<200 mL/24 hr	>200 mL/24 hr
Response to fasting	Diarrhea stops	Diarrhea continues
Stool Na^+	<70 mEq/L	>70 mEq/L
Reducing substances*	Positive	Negative
Stool pH	<5	>6

**Sucrose is not a reducing agent. Add 5 drops of 0.1 N HCl to a stool sample before adding reducing agent (Clinitest tablet).*

two in the stools will be less than the measured stool osmolarity, a finding suggesting the presence of other osmols in the stool. The main diagnostic points that differentiate osmotic from secretory diarrhea are noted in Table 341–2.

Secretory Diarrhea. The major causes of secretory diarrhea are depicted in Table 341–3. The mechanisms for secretory diarrhea include activation of the intracellular mediators such as cAMP, cGMP, and intracellular calcium, which stimulate active chloride secretion from the crypt cells and inhibit the neutral coupled sodium chloride absorption. These mediators alter the paracellular ion flux because of toxin-mediated injury to the tight junctions. The classic example of secretory diarrhea is that induced by cholera and *Escherichia coli* enterotoxins that bind to a specific enterocyte surface receptor (the monosialoganglioside GM_1); a fragment of the toxin then enters the cell, where it activates adenylate cyclase on the basolateral membrane via interaction with a stimulatory G protein. This increases intracellular cAMP. The enterotoxigenic *E. coli* mediates secretory diarrhea by producing heat-labile toxin (LT) and heat-stable toxin (ST) in the small bowel. The labile toxin is similar in its action to the cholera toxin and binds to the same GM_1 surface receptor. Other causes of secretory diarrhea include vasoactive peptides, which activate G protein–coupled receptors resulting in an increase in intracellular mediators causing secretory diarrhea.

Secretory diarrhea is characterized by high volume; the stools are extremely watery. Stool analysis reveals high sodium and chloride content (>70 mEq/L). Secretory diarrhea continues with fasting.

Mutational Defects in Ion Transport Proteins. Congenital defects of sodium-hydrogen exchange, chloride-bicarbonate exchange, and sodium–bile acid transport proteins result in secretory diarrhea presenting at birth. The defects in chloride-bicarbonate exchange and sodium–bile acid transporters have gene mutations that encode their corresponding transport proteins. The defect in sodium-hydrogen exchange is believed to represent defects in the apical sodium-hydrogen exchanger (NHE-2 or NHE-3). Patients with these defects present with secretory diarrhea and failure to thrive during the neonatal period. The defect in chloride-bicarbonate exchange is well characterized and is more common compared with the defects in sodium-hydrogen exchange and sodium–bile acid transporter (Chapter 340). Patients with chloride diarrhea have hypochloremic metabolic alkalosis with low serum chloride concentration, high stool chloride content coupled with chloride-free urine, low serum potassium, and high serum bicarbonate. Hydramnios is present in the mothers.

Reduction in Anatomic Surface Area. Short bowel syndrome results from resection of the bowel secondary to surgical indications such as necrotizing enterocolitis, midgut volvulus, or intestinal atresia (Chapter 340.7). Celiac disease results in flattening of the proximal intestinal surface area with marked decrease in the digestive and absorptive function of the villus epithelium (Chapter 340.8). Diarrhea is characterized by loss of fluids, electrolytes, macronutrients, and micronutrients.

Alteration in Intestinal Motility. The causes of altered intestinal motility include malnutrition, scleroderma, intestinal pseudo-obstruction syndromes, and diabetes mellitus. Malnutrition, in general, results in hypomotility allowing bacterial overgrowth that leads to deconjugation of bile salts resulting in an increase in the intracellular mediator cAMP leading to, secretory diarrhea.

ETIOLOGY. A simple classification for the etiology of chronic diarrhea is shown in Table 341–4. The two major factors resulting in diarrhea include intraluminal factors and mucosal factors. Intraluminal factors are involved in the digestion process, whereas mucosal factors are involved in the digestion and transport of nutrients across the mucosa. In many situations, both intraluminal and mucosal factors cause diarrhea. The intraluminal factors involve disorders of the pancreas, liver, and the brush border membrane of the enterocytes. In approximately 85% of patients with cystic fibrosis, pancreatic insufficiency results in malabsorption of fats and proteins. Short stature, exocrine pancreatic hypoplasia, normal sweat chloride concentrations, and the variable features of neutro-

TABLE 341–3 Causes of Secretory Diarrhea

Activation of cyclic adenosine monophosphate
- Bacterial toxins: enterotoxins of cholera, *Escherichia coli* (heat-labile), *Shigella, Salmonella, Campylobacter jejuni, Pseudomonas aeruginosa*
- Hormones: vasoactive intestinal peptide, gastrin, secretin
- Anion surfactants: bile acids, ricinoleic acid

Activation of cyclic guanosine monophosphate
- Bacterial toxins: *E. coli* (heat-stable) enterotoxin, *Yersinia enterocolitica* toxin

Calcium-dependent
- Bacterial toxins: *Clostridium difficile* enterotoxin
- Neurotransmitters: acetylcholine, serotonin
- Paracrine agents: bradykinin

TABLE 341–4 Etiology of Chronic Diarrhea

Intraluminal Factors	Mucosal Factors
Pancreatic Disorders	***Altered Integrity***
Cystic fibrosis	Infections: bacterial, viral, fungal
Shwachman-Diamond syndrome	Infestations: parasitic
Johanson-Blizzard syndrome	Cow's and soy protein intolerance
Isolated pancreatic enzyme deficiencies	Inflammatory bowel disease (ulcerative colitis, microscopic colitis, Crohn)
Chronic pancreatitis	
Bile Acid Disorders	***Altered Immune Function***
Chronic cholestasis	Autoimmune enteropathy
Terminal ileum resection	Eosinophilic gastroenteropathy
Bacterial overgrowth	AIDS
Chronic use of bile acid sequestrants	Combined Immunodeficiency
Primary bile acid malabsorption	Immunoglobulin A and G deficiencies
Intestinal Disorders	***Altered Function***
Intraluminal osmolarity	Defects in Cl^-/HCO_3, Na^+/H^+, bile acids, acrodermatitis enteropathica, selective folate deficiency, abetalipoproteinemia
Carbohydrate malabsorption	
Congenital and acquired sucrase, lactase deficiencies	
Congenital and acquired monosaccharide deficiency	
Excessive carbonated fluid intake	
Excessive intake of sorbitol, Mg $(OH)_2$ and lactulose	
	Altered Digestive Function
	Enterokinase deficiency
	Glucoamylase deficiency
	Altered Surface Area
	Celiac disease, postgastroenteritis syndrome
	Microvillus inclusion disease
	Short bowel syndrome
	Altered Secretory Function
	Enterotoxin-producing bacteria
	Tumors secreting vasoactive peptides
	Altered Anatomic Structures
	Hirschsprung disease
	Partial small bowel obstruction
	Malrotation

penia and skeletal changes characterize Shwachman syndrome (Chapter 349). Johannson-Blizzard syndrome is characterized by anal imperforation, agenesis of the nasal cartilage, hair anomalies, mental retardation, deafness, hypothyroidism, and pancreatic insufficiency (Chapter 349). The isolated pancreatic enzyme defects are congenital and result in malabsorption of fat or proteins depending on the defect. These defects include congenital lipase/colipase deficiency and congenital trypsinogen deficiency. Patients with chronic pancreatitis can present with pancreatic insufficiency and insulin-dependent diabetes. Familial pancreatitis, secondary to a mutation in the trypsinogen gene, can result in chronic pancreatitis and pancreatic insufficiency. Disorders of the liver, such as cholestasis, result in a decrease in bile acid pool size with malabsorption of fats. Bile acid loss with fat malabsorption can occur with terminal ileum disease such as Crohn disease or with terminal ileum resection. Primary bile acid malabsorption is a rare disorder secondary to a mutation in the ileal bile acid transporter. Patients present with fat malabsorption and diarrhea. Bacterial overgrowth in the gastrointestinal tract results in deconjugation and dehydroxylation of bile salts resulting in diarrhea. Long-term use of bile acid sequestrants such as cholestyramine can lead to a decrease in bile acid pool size because of the continued loss of bile acids in the stools. Intraluminal osmolarity, resulting from malabsorption of carbohydrates, presents with an osmotic type of diarrhea. The causes of carbohydrate malabsorption include congenital and acquired causes of monosaccharide and disaccharidase deficiencies. Excessive carbonated fluid intake, which exceeds the transport capacity of the small intestine in younger infants, results in nonspecific diarrhea. Excessive intake of nonabsorbable solutes such as sorbitol, magnesium hydroxide, and lactulose results in osmotic diarrhea.

The mucosal factors that lead to chronic diarrhea could be secondary to altered mucosal integrity from infections such as bacterial, viral, parasitic, and fungal agents. Parasitic infestations such as with *Giardia* or cryptosporidia can present with chronic diarrhea. Inflammatory bowel disease such as ulcerative colitis, Crohn disease, and microscopic colitis can lead to the alteration in the mucosal integrity resulting in the decreased absorption of water electrolyte through the gastrointestinal tract. Cow's milk and soy protein intolerance can present with diarrhea secondary to partial villus atrophy or allergic colitis. Altered immune function as seen in patients with agammaglobulinemia, isolated immunoglobulin A deficiency, and combined immunodeficiency disorders can result in diarrhea. Patients with AIDS are more predisposed to bacterial, viral, and fungal infections. Similarly, autoimmune enteropathy and eosinophilic gastroenteropathy are believed to be disorders involving alteration of the mucosal immune function and can result in diarrhea. Altered mucosa transport function, as seen in congenital disorders involving sodium-hydrogen exchange, chloride-bicarbonate exchange, bile acid transport, and glucose galactose transport, results in diarrhea early in the neonatal period. Similarly, defects in the absorption of zinc, such as acrodermatitis enteropathica and folate transport, can result in diarrhea.

Abetalipoproteinemia is characterized by fat malabsorption, neurologic lesions, and ocular abnormalities such as retinitis pigmentosa (Chapter 83.3). The diagnosis is confirmed by the typical hematologic finding of acanthocytosis and the appearance of the small bowel biopsy in which the tip enterocytes are filled with lipid droplets. Altered mucosal digestive function includes congenital enterokinase deficiency that results in loss of activation of trypsinogen to trypsin with protein malabsorption (Chapter 340.11). α-Glucoamylase deficiency is rare and results in loss of hydrolysis of glucose polymers.

Altered mucosal surface area is seen in celiac disease, partial villus atrophy secondary to postgastroenteritis malabsorption syndrome, tropical sprue, microvillus inclusion disease, Whipple disease, and short bowel syndrome. In these disorders, the height and structure of the villi are altered so that the absorptive capacity of the mucosal surface area is markedly decreased. Celiac disease occurs secondary to gluten sensitivity (Chapter 340.8). Postgastroenteritis syndrome is a nutritional disorder that occurs following a prolonged episode of gastroenteritis and decreased energy intake. Microvillus inclusion disease is characterized with diarrhea, failure to thrive, and histologic picture of microvillus inclusions (Chapter 340). The mucosal surface lacks brush border membranes or possesses irregular blunted microvilli. Whipple disease is mainly seen in adults and is secondary to an actinomycete, *Tropheryma whippelii*. Patients present with weight loss, diarrhea, and arthropathy. The diagnosis is established by a small bowel biopsy, and patients respond to prolonged administration of trimethoprim-sulfamethoxazole. Tropical sprue is commonly seen in patients living or returning from trips to developing countries (Chapter 340). Patients present with diarrhea and nutritional deficiencies, especially folate. Alteration in the anatomic structure as seen in Hirschsprung disease, malrotation, and partial small bowel obstruction can result in diarrhea secondary to bacterial overgrowth. Altered mucosal secretory function includes enterotoxin-producing bacteria and tumor-secreting vasoactive peptides.

EVALUATION OF PATIENTS. The evaluation of patients with chronic diarrhea is depicted in Table 341–5. In phase I, the history and physical examination, which include a nutritional assessment, are the initial steps. The clinical history should include the amount and type of fluids ingested per day. If the patient's clinical history suggests excessive carbonated drinks or fruit juices of more than 150 mL/kg/24 hr, with normal growth and height parameters, chronic nonspecific diarrhea needs to be considered. A decrease in the amount of fluid to no more than 90 mL/kg/24 hr will result in resolution of the diarrhea. If the patient is ingesting nonabsorbable nutrients in excessive amounts such as sorbitol, a dietary adjustment needs to be made before extensively investigating the patient.

The stool examination is an integral step in investigating a patient with chronic diarrhea. The most recently evacuated stool, including its liquid content, is useful for diagnostic purposes. Various collection techniques are helpful, including the placement of a urine collection bag over the anus and everting a disposable diaper to collect the stool. Once collected, the stool specimen should be stored in a refrigerator until the examination is performed. Specimens for bacterial culture should be transported immediately to the bacteriology laboratory for inoculation into growth media. The gross examination of the stool should allow the physician to determine whether the patient has diarrhea and whether blood or mucus is pres-

TABLE 341–5 Evaluation of Patients with Chronic Diarrhea

Phase I	Clinical history including specific amounts of fluids ingested per day
	Physical examination including nutritional assessment
	Stool exam (pH, reducing substances, smear for white blood count, fat, ova, and parasites)
	Stool cultures
	Stool for *Clostridium difficile* toxin
	Blood studies (complete blood count, erythrocyte sedimentation rate, electrolytes, blood urea nitrogen, creatinine)
Phase II	Sweat chloride
	72-hr stool collection for fat determination
	Stool electrolytes, osmolality
	Stool for phenolphthalein, magnesium sulfate, phosphate
	Breath H_2 tests
Phase III	Endoscopic studies
	Small bowel biopsy
	Sigmoidoscopy or colonoscopy with biopsies
	Barium studies
Phase IV	Hormonal studies vasoactive intestinal polypeptide, gastrin, secretin, 5-hydroxyindoleacetic assays

ent in the stool, a finding suggesting inflammation of the colon. The color of the stool is rarely helpful unless it is bloody. Occult testing for blood is useful to determine whether the patient has microscopic blood loss. Carbohydrate malabsorption is detected by analysis of the liquid fraction of a fresh specimen. A pH lower than 5 or the presence of moderate reducing substances indicates the presence of reducing carbohydrates (sucrose is not a direct reducing substance). The stools should be sent for electrolytes and osmolality testing if secretory diarrhea is considered (see Table 341–2).

Microscopic examination of the stool helps to determine the presence of white blood cells, which signifies colonic inflammation. The stools could be examined for ova and parasites such as *Giardia*, amoebae, or cryptosporidia. Trichrome stain or acid-fast stain can be of value in identifying *Cryptosporidium* species. Stools should be examined for the presence of *Giardia* antigen. Sudan stain can be used either on a plain stool smear or with the addition of acetic acid and heat to determine the presence of triglycerides and split fats.

In the event that phase I investigation has failed to reveal a cause, a phase II work-up is indicated and includes a sweat chloride test to rule out cystic fibrosis. A 72-hour stool collection for fat determination is the standard to determine whether the patient does have fat malabsorption in the setting of a negative sweat chloride test. Stools could also be checked for phenolphthalein, magnesium, sulfate, and phosphate to determine whether the diarrhea is secondary to the ingestion of laxatives (factitious diarrhea). Breath hydrogen tests can be used to determine a specific carbohydrate malabsorption. A breath hydrogen test for glucose can be used to diagnose bacterial overgrowth.

Phase III investigation includes endoscopic studies for small bowel and colonic biopsies. Barium studies, such an upper gastrointestinal series or a barium enema, can be used to rule out anatomic lesions in the gastrointestinal tract. Finally, if none of these tests is revealing, phase IV evaluation includes hormonal studies and neurohormonal and neurotransmittal studies such as vasoactive intestinal polypeptide, gastrin, secretin, and 5-hydroxyindoleacetic assays.

TREATMENT. Figure 341–3 depicts the general therapeutic approaches to the management of chronic diarrhea. The first principle is to maintain adequate nutritional intake to permit normal growth and development. The height, weight, and nutritional status of the patient must be documented. If nutritional parameters, including weight and height, are normal and the stool examination does not show any fat, the possibility of chronic nonspecific diarrhea needs to be considered. The pathogenesis of this condition includes excessive carbonated fluid intake, nondigestible carbohydrate malabsorption from excessive fruit juice ingestion, and low fat intake.

Chronic nonspecific diarrhea generally presents in well-appearing toddlers between 1 and 3 yr (toddler's diarrhea). The diarrhea is often brown and watery, at times containing undigested food particles. If the child's fluid intake is more than 150 mL/kg/24 hr, fluid intake should be reduced to no more than 90 mL/kg/24 hr. Parents may note that the child is irritable in the first 2 days after the fluid restriction; however, persistence in this approach for several more days results in a decrease in the stool frequency and volume. If the dietary history suggests that the child is ingesting significant amounts of fruit juices, then the offending juices should be decreased. Sorbitol, which is a nonabsorbable sugar, is found in apple, pear, and prune juices and can cause diarrhea in toddlers. Moreover, apple and pear juices contain higher amounts of fructose in excess of glucose concentration, a feature postulated to cause diarrhea in toddlers.

Levels of dietary fat intake may also play a role in chronic diarrhea. If the child's fat intake has been restricted by the parents, then fat intake can be increased to be approximately 40% of the total calories per day.

If the diarrhea is secondary to carbohydrate intolerance, then a trial period of decreased lactose or sucrose may be initiated.

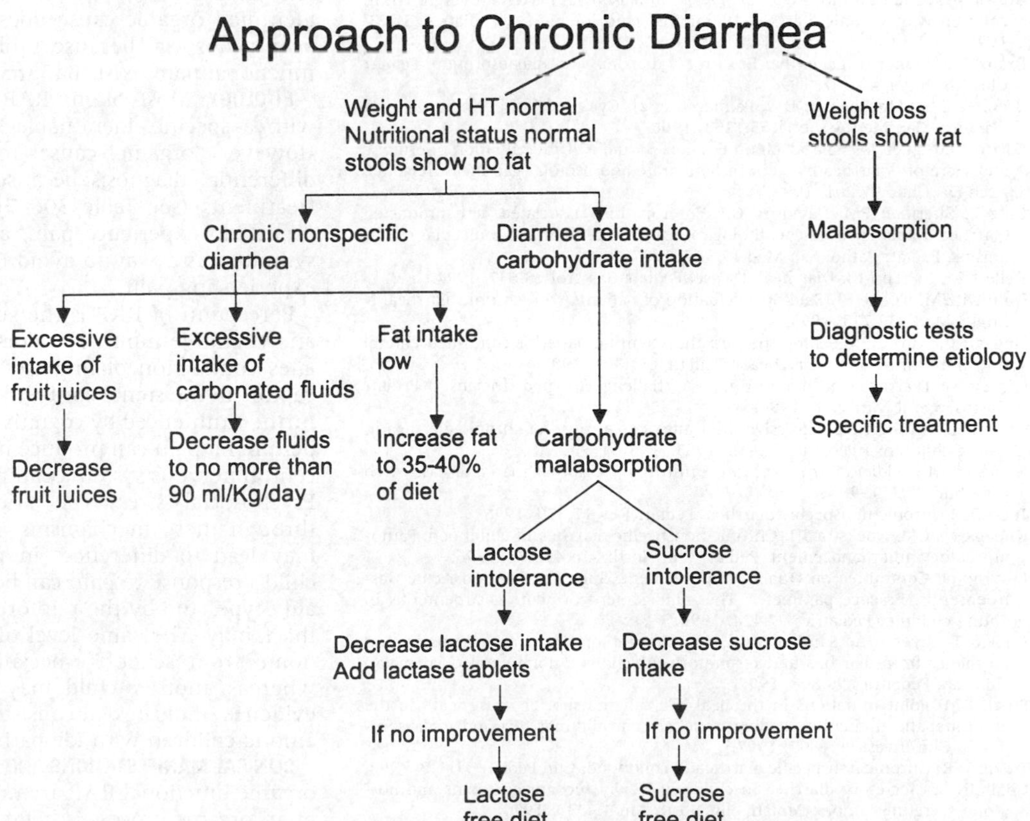

Figure 341–3 General therapeutic approaches to management of chronic diarrhea.

Lactase (LactAid) can be used to aid in the digestion of lactose. If diarrhea persists, a trial of a lactose-free or sucrose-free diet is indicated. Alternatively, breath hydrogen tests can document the presence of lactose or sucrose intolerance. A glucose breath hydrogen test can be used for the diagnosis of bacterial overgrowth.

If the patient presents with weight loss and the stool examination shows fat, the possibility of chronic diarrhea secondary to a malabsorption syndrome needs to be considered. The most common cause of chronic diarrhea associated with the malabsorption is postgastroenteritis malabsorption syndrome. These patients respond well to a predigested formula. In the event that the patient shows intolerance to oral feeding with a predigested formula, such as Pregestimil or Alimentum, nasogastric drip feeding with a elemental formula should be considered for a period of 3–4 wk.

A patient presenting with suspected small intestinal bacterial overgrowth should undergo evaluation for surgical, medical, and nutritional support. Surgical treatment is indicated if the patient has malrotation or partial small bowel obstruction. Antibiotic therapy is usually initiated with metronidazole in combination with ampicillin or trimethoprim-sulfamethoxazole.

Patients presenting with secretory diarrhea, especially during the 1st mo of life, need to be considered for nutritional support, because the most likely cause is a congenital defect in transport proteins. In older children with secretory diarrhea, the cause needs to be identified first, and therapeutic consideration is directed toward the cause of the secretory diarrhea.

Acra S, Ghishan FK: Electrolyte fluxes in the gut and oral rehydration solutions. Pediatr Clin North Am 43:433, 1996.

Barnes GL, Bishop RF: Rotavirus infection and prevention. Curr Opin Pediatr 9:19, 1997.

Bhatnagar S, Bhan MK, Singh KD, et al: Efficacy of milk-based diets in persistent diarrhea: A randomized, controlled trial. Pediatrics 98:1122, 1996.

Bhutta ZA, Hendricks KM: Nutritional management of persistent diarrhea in childhood: A perspective from the developing world. J Pediatr Gastroenterol Nutr 22:17, 1996.

Boissieu D, Chaussain M, Badoual J, et al: Small-bowel bacterial overgrowth in children with chronic diarrhea, abdominal pain, or both. J Pediatr 128:203, 1996.

Branski D, Lerner A, Lebenthal E: Chronic diarrhea and malabsorption. Pediatr Clin North Am 43:307, 1996.

Brennen MK, MacPherson DW, Palmer J, et al: Cyclosporiasis: A new cause of diarrhea. Can Med Assoc J 155:1293, 1996.

Castro-Rodriguez JA, Salazar-Lindo E, Leon-Barua, R: Differentiation of osmotic and secretory diarrhea by stool carbohydrate and osmolar gap measurements. Arch Dis Child 77:201, 1997.

Cutz E, Sherman PM, Davidson GP: Enteropathies associated with protracted diarrhea of infancy: Clinicopathological features, cellular and molecular mechanisms. Pediatr Pathol Lab Med 17:335, 1997.

Dellert SF, Cohen MB: Diarrheal disease. Pediatr Gasterol 23:637, 1994.

Donowitz M, Kokke FT, Saidi R: Evaluation of patients with chronic diarrhea. N Engl J Med 332:725, 1995.

Duggan C, Nurko S: Feeding the gut: the scientific basis for continued enteral nutrition during acute diarrhea. J Pediatr 131:801, 1997.

Gracey M: Diarrhea and malnutrition: A challenge for pediatricians. J Pediatr Gastroenterol Nutr 22:6, 1996.

Green HL, Ghishon FK: Excessive fluid intake as a cause of chronic diarrhea in young children. J Pediatr 102:836, 1983.

Hoekstra JH: Toddler diarrhoea: More a nutritional disorder than a disease. Arch Dis Child 79:2, 1998.

Judd RH: Chronic nonspecific diarrhea. Pediatr Rev 17:379, 1996.

Kneepkens CM, Hoekstra JH: Chronic nonspecific diarrhea of childhood: Pathophysiology and management. Pediatr Clin North Am 43:375, 1996.

Provisional Committee on Quality Improvement, Subcommittee on Acute Gastroenteritis: Practice parameter: The management of acute gastroenteritis in young children. Pediatrics 97:424, 1996.

Ruel MT, Rivera JA, Santizo MC, et al: Impact of zinc supplementation on morbidity from diarrhea and respiratory infections among rural Guatemalan children. Pediatrics 99:808, 1997.

Small DM: Point mutations in the ileal bile salt transporter cause leaks in the enterohepatic circulation leading to severe chronic diarrhea and malabsorption. J Clin Invest 99:1807, 1997.

Treem WR: Chronic nonspecific diarrhea of childhood. Clin Pediatr 31:413, 1992.

Udall JN Jr: Secretory diarrhea in children: Newly recognized toxins and hormone-secreting tumors. Pediatr Clin North Am 43:333, 1996.

Venita J, Edwards V, Halliday W, et al: "Polyphenotypic" tumors in the central nervous system: Problems in nosology and classification. Pediatr Pathol Lab Med 17:369, 1997.

CHAPTER 342
Recurrent Abdominal Pain of Childhood

Martin Ulshen

Recurrent abdominal pain (RAP) is common, occurring in more than 10% of pre–school- and school-aged children. In children younger than 2 yr, the abdominal pain is often associated with an organic cause; however, in older children, only 10% of cases have an organic cause. RAP without an organic cause is often called "functional" abdominal pain. The difficulty for physician, parent, and child is that functional abdominal pain is as uncomfortable and as disruptive to normal activity as organic pain, but it is often more difficult for the physician to evaluate and manage. The family and the child with functional RAP may worry about the inability to identify an organic cause. The tendency is to associate the lack of an obvious organic cause with a more serious prognosis. The possibility that the cause may be emotional rather than physical may be unacceptable to the family. The physician may become frustrated by the difficulty in identifying an obvious cause of the symptoms and by the pressure from the family to "get to the bottom of the problem." The tendency is to perform an excessive evaluation for organic causes when a careful history, social evaluation, and physical examination may suffice. Although it is important to demonstrate that the medical caregivers are considering the symptoms seriously, excessive testing and treatment without closure increase the fear that some serious process is present. The pattern of the pain and the social setting are often typical when abdominal symptoms are functional; extensive investigation is not required. The absence of an identified organic cause does not mean that the cause must be psychosocial because undoubtedly other subtle causes of functional pain exist that are not yet identifiable.

ETIOLOGY. Most often, RAP in childhood is not associated with a specific, identifiable structural or biochemical cause. However, "organic" causes must always be considered in the differential diagnosis because they are amenable to specific treatments (see Table 306–7). Most children with RAP syndrome do experience pain; a child may occasionally use the symptom as a way to avoid certain activities without actually experiencing pain.

Perception of RAP is the summation of sensory, emotional, and cognitive input. The dorsal horn of the spinal cord regulates conduction of impulses from peripheral nociceptive receptors to the spinal cord and brain, and the pain experience is further influenced by cognitive and emotional centers. Chronic peripheral pain can produce increased neural activity in higher central nervous system centers leading to perpetuation of pain. Psychosocial stress can affect pain intensity and quality through these mechanisms. Differences in visceral sensation may lead to differences in perception of pain as well. The child's response to pain can be influenced by stress, by personality type, and by the reinforcement of illness behavior within the family. The same level of discomfort may keep one child home from school, especially if encouraged by caretakers, whereas another child may continue routine activities. No evidence indicates a consistent pattern of psychopathology among children with idiopathic RAP.

CLINICAL MANIFESTATIONS AND DIAGNOSIS. The symptoms of nonorganic functional RAP are nonspecific. This lack of suggestion of an organic process is helpful in making a diagnosis of functional abdominal pain. The symptoms do not have any characteristic temporal pattern. Improvement in symptoms during weekends and school vacations suggests functional pain, but the absence of this pattern does not rule out this diagnosis. Two variants of functional abdominal pain are seen more often in adults but may occur in children. *Irritable bowel syndrome* (IBS) is familial and is characterized by abdominal pain associated with intermittent diarrhea and constipation without an organic basis (see Chapter 341). IBS may occur in as many as 10% of adolescents. IBS is associated with abnormalities of intestinal motility and pain perception. Patients who have symptoms suggestive of peptic disease and seem to respond to antacid treatment but who have no abnormal findings on upper gastrointestinal tract endoscopy are said to have *nonulcer dyspepsia.*

Identification of a relationship between the pain and either meals or bowel movements may be helpful, especially in considering peptic disease, constipation, and IBS. Although the occurrence of nocturnal pain has been considered by some an important indicator of organic cause, children with functional pain may awaken during the night with symptoms. Functional abdominal pain tends to be periumbilical in location and is often difficult for the child to characterize. The child can be distracted from the pain. The child may have good periods with remission of symptoms and then recurrence without any apparent reason. In contrast, in many children, an association with stressful periods may be obvious.

The child appears well between episodes with a normal physical examination and normal growth. The child may appear pale during an episode, but this symptom does not suggest that the cause is more likely to be organic. Children with functional pain may be described as worriers who tend not to share their concerns with others. At school, these are children who are serious about their work and do well or, in contrast, have difficulty. Teachers describe these children as their easiest students because they are compliant and do not complain.

The family may reinforce the symptom by demonstrating excessive concern. This concern may worry the children and may urge physicians to perform more evaluations than would otherwise be considered. The latter approach may further worry the children and parents. Family and child concerns about the possibility of specific organic disorders should always be explored in a nondirective fashion. Often another family member or friend's illness has raised specific concerns.

Children with nonorganic abdominal pain sometimes come from dysfunctional families. Some families focus on a child's abdominal symptoms as an unrecognized way of diverting attention from other stress, such as marital problems. Sexual abuse as a child is a major cause of RAP in adults. This possibility should always be considered, especially in a girl whose abdominal symptoms begin in the preteenage or teenage years. Despite these concerns about psychosocial factors, many children with functional abdominal pain appear to be well adjusted and from well-adapted families.

An initial nondirective interview technique often helps to gain a general sense of the likelihood of organicity. The interviewer should elicit a detailed description of the symptom, including character, temporal pattern, severity on a scale ranging from 1–10, associated symptoms, potential initiating events, limitation of activities, and measures that relieve the pain. Functional abdominal pain is typically not associated with other symptoms, although vomiting or headache is sometimes present as a less striking component. The interviewer should be attuned to possible organic causes and should question more specifically about any of these causes if suggested by the initial history.

The onset of functional RAP may occur at the time of an acute, transient illness, such as gastroenteritis. In this case, the symptoms of the acute illness may serve as a model for ongoing functional symptoms. Family medical history may uncover the possibility of a familial disorder causing abdominal pain but more frequently may uncover models of recurrent abdominal symptoms among close family members. It is common that the relation of the child's symptoms to those of other family members has not occurred to the parents. This process also helps the physician to learn how a family copes with medical illness and about their expectations from the physician. Social history is essential because of the association with family stress and dysfunctional families. Although not always necessary, an assessment by a social worker can be a valuable asset. It is helpful to have an evaluation by a psychologist or psychiatrist when indicated.

During the physical examination, one must keep in mind possible diagnoses raised by the history. A complete examination (including growth parameters) is important because RAP may be a manifestation of many different systemic disorders. Weight loss is not typical of functional pain. Careful assessment of the abdomen for distention, tenderness, organomegaly, or a mass is necessary. A rectal examination should be considered in all children with RAP. Children are unreliable about reporting stool patterns to their parents; the physician may identify a mass of hard stool in the rectum leading to a diagnosis of constipation. Furthermore, a pelvic or abdominal mass may be noted during this examination. Characteristic perianal findings of Crohn disease may be identified at the time of rectal examination. A stool test for occult blood should be done at the time of the rectal examination; otherwise, stool could be collected at home for this evaluation.

Laboratory studies may be unnecessary if the history and physical examination clearly lead to a diagnosis of functional abdominal pain. However, a complete blood count, sedimentation rate, stool test for parasites (especially *Giardia*), and urinalysis are reasonable screening studies. If one suspects inflammatory bowel disease, one must note that as many as 50% of children with this disease may have normal sedimentation rates. The finding of an abnormal sedimentation rate would make one look further for an inflammatory, infectious, or neoplastic disorder. If indicated, an ultrasound examination of the abdomen can give information about kidneys, gallbladder, and pancreas; with lower abdominal pain, a pelvic ultrasonogram may be indicated. An upper gastrointestinal tract x-ray series is indicated if one suspects a disorder of the stomach or small intestine. If peptic disease is suspected, a *Helicobacter pylori* antibody test may be performed first and then esophagogastroduodenoscopy if this test is negative. In the absence of this suspicion, this evaluation is unlikely to identify an abnormality and is usually not necessary.

A wide range of potential organic causes of RAP (see Table 306–7) must be considered before establishing a diagnosis of functional pain. Among the more common causes are chronic constipation, parasitic infection (*Giardia*), and lactase deficiency. Lactose intolerance is so common that the finding may be coincidental; therefore, one must be cautious in attributing chronic abdominal pain to this condition. Pinworms are unlikely to be the cause of abdominal pain. Genitourinary disorders were once considered among the most common causes of RAP, but this diagnosis is less likely. Hydronephrosis can occasionally be the cause of unilateral pain without other symptoms.

Crohn disease typically does not present with pain alone. Nevertheless, if the location and characteristics are suggestive, this diagnosis should be considered. Serum amylase and lipase should be measured during an episode to rule out recurrent pancreatitis. If these results are normal but pancreatitis is still suspected, a serum trypsinogen level is more sensitive. An ultrasonogram may show changes suggestive of pancreatitis and is also helpful to evaluate for gallstones or biliary sludge. Peptic ulcer is an unusual cause of chronic abdominal pain and is diagnosed more frequently than it actually occurs. Persistent pain, perhaps accentuated by meals, should be expected with any of these disorders; intermittent pain lasting less than 30 min. should not be expected. Laparoscopy may have a limited use in the evaluation of carefully selected children with very reproducible, localized, well-characterized chronic abdominal pain when all the standard evaluation methods have not led to a diagnosis. Adhesions (congenital or postoperative), other structure anomalies, or inflammatory lesions may be identified.

Abdominal migraine can cause episodic abdominal pain in children in the absence of headache. The episodes are characteristic and almost always include nausea with or without vomiting. Transient fever or diarrhea is less common but may occur with migraine. The episode can last hours, but it characteristically ends when the child falls asleep and awakens feeling much improved. Episodes may occur several times a week or much less frequently but should not be daily. Patients have a strong family history of migraine headache. No specific tests exist for this disorder; the diagnosis depends on a typical patient and family history. *Abdominal epilepsy* is less common but also can be an unusual cause of RAP. The patient may have a prodrome such as the sense of an unusual aroma at the start of an episode. Abnormalities on electroencephalogram may be identified but may not be seen on a single study; a sleep-deprived electroencephalogram may be required.

The occurrence of chronic *H. pylori* infection is not increased among children with nonspecific RAP. Only peptic ulcer symptoms have been associated with this condition. Therefore, evaluation for *H. pylori* infection and specific treatment should be reserved for children with epigastric pain suggestive of peptic disease (see Chapter 336).

TREATMENT. If functional bowel disease is diagnosed, the most important component of the treatment is reassurance of the children and family members. Specifically, they need to be reassured that no evidence of a serious underlying disorder is present. Cancer is often an unspoken concern. In this context, a careful history and physical examination reassure the parents. Anxiety about the symptom may contribute to focusing on the symptom as well as to reducing the threshold for discomfort. The parents should be instructed to avoid reinforcing the symptom with secondary gain. Furthermore, if children have missed school or have been removed from routine activities because of the pain, it is important that they return to regular activities. Medications are generally unhelpful or, at best, offer transient placebo effect. Gastric acid blockers or visceral muscle relaxants (anticholinergics) may be tried empirically, but they are most often not helpful in the absence of specific indication. Biofeedback and relaxation techniques have been useful in some children with functional pain.

If lactose intolerance is suspected, a trial of a lactose-free diet for 1–2 wk may be both diagnostic and therapeutic. If symptoms improve, the diet should be continued. A fiber supplement often helps the symptoms of irritable bowel. If chronic constipation is identified, it should be treated in the standard fashion (Chapters 20 and 332).

Successful management depends on close follow-up. The family can try new approaches to the child's symptoms without fear that the physician is abandoning them if they know that follow-up by telephone or office visit has been arranged. Often it is during the follow-up visits that one truly comes to know the child and understand the symptoms. It is possible that an organic problem may not have been apparent on the initial visit, but with time, the symptom complex becomes more typical.

These approaches often result in reduction or elimination of the abdominal symptoms. However, children with functional abdominal pain are likely to become adults with functional disorders, although the nature of the symptoms may change.

Apley J: The Child with Abdominal Pain. London, Blackwell Scientific, 1975.
Bode G, Rothenbacher D, Brenner H, et al: *Helicobacter pylori* and abdominal symptoms: A population-based study among preschool children in southern Germany. Pediatrics 101:634, 1998.
Borge A, Nordhagen R, Moe B, et al: Prevalence and persistence of stomachache and headache among children: Follow-up of a cohort of Norwegian children from 4 to 10 years of age. Acta Paediatr 83:433, 1994.
Drossman D: Physical and sexual abuse and gastrointestinal illness: What is the link? Am J Med 97:105, 1994.
Hoffenberg EJ, Rothenberg SS, Bensard D: Outcome after exploratory laparoscopy for unexplained abdominal pain in childhood. Arch Pediatr Adolesc Med 151:993, 1997.
Hyams JS, Hyman PE: Recurrent abdominal pain and the biopsychosocial model of medical practice. J Pediatr 133:473, 1998.
Hyams JS, Burke G, Davis PM, et al: Abdominal pain and irritable bowel syndrome in adolescents: A community-based study. J Pediatr 129:220, 1996.
Maxwell PR, Mendall MA, Kumar D: Irritable bowel syndrome. Lancet 350:1691, 1997.
Murphy MS: Management of recurrent abdominal pain. Arch Dis Child 69:409, 1993.

Chapter 343
Acute Appendicitis

Gary E. Hartman

Acute appendicitis is the most common condition requiring emergency abdominal operation in childhood. Diagnosis is difficult in children, a factor contributing to perforation rates of 30–60%. Fifty per cent of children with perforated appendicitis have been seen by a physician before the diagnosis. The risk of perforation is greatest in 1- to 4-yr-old children (70–75%) and is lowest in the adolescent age group (30–40%), which has the highest age-specific incidence of appendicitis in childhood. The difficulty in distinguishing appendicitis from other common causes of abdominal pain and the increase in morbidity and mortality accompanying perforation keep appendicitis an important concern of clinicians.

EPIDEMIOLOGY. Approximately 80,000 children experience appendicitis in the United States annually, a rate of 4/1,000 children younger than 14 yr. Appendicitis is rare in developing countries, where diets are high in fiber. However, no causal relationship has been established between dietary fiber and appendicitis. The incidence of appendicitis increases with age, peaking in adolescence and rarely occurring in children younger than 1 yr. A familial predilection to appendicitis has been reported. Males predominate, clustering of cases has occurred, and cases occur more often in the autumn and spring.

ETIOLOGY. Experimentally, ligation (obstruction) of the appendix results in a marked increase of intraluminal pressure, which rapidly exceeds systolic blood pressure. Initial venous congestion progresses to thrombosis, necrosis, and perforation. Clinically, obstruction of the lumen is the prime cause of appendicitis. The obstruction is caused by inspissated fecal material (fecalith). The inspissated material may calcify, leading to a radiographically visible appendicolith (15–20%). Obstruction resulting from mucosal edema may be associated with systemic or enteric viral or bacterial *(Yersinia, Salmonella, Shigella)* infections. Abnormal mucus has been suggested as the cause of the increased incidence of appendicitis in children with cystic fibrosis. Carcinoid tumors, foreign bodies, and *Ascaris* have rarely been implicated as causes of appendicitis.

PATHOLOGY. The pathologic changes in appendicitis progress through three predictable phases. Initially, with luminal obstruction, venous congestion progresses to mucosal ischemia, necrosis, and ulceration. Bacterial invasion with inflammatory infiltrate through all layers of the appendiceal wall characterizes the second phase. Organisms can be cultured from the serosal surface before microscopic perforation. Finally, necrosis of the wall results in perforation and contamination of the peritoneum. The perforation usually occurs at the tip of the appendix, distal to the obstructing fecalith.

Subsequent to perforation, the microbiologic fecal contamination may be confined to the pelvis or the right iliac fossa by the omentum and adjacent loops of small bowel, or it may spread throughout the peritoneal cavity. Young children have a poorly developed omentum, and local perforation is not usually confined. Bacterial invasion of the mesenteric veins may result in portal vein sepsis (pylephlebitis) and subsequent liver abscess formation. The inflammatory process associated with perforation may lead to intestinal obstruction or paralytic ileus.

CLINICAL MANIFESTATIONS. The clinical signs and symptoms depend on the pathologic phase of appendicitis at examination. The classic triad consists of pain, vomiting, and fever. In the initial stage of appendiceal obstruction, the pain is periumbilical. Emesis usually follows the onset of pain and is infrequent. Anorexia is more common. Fever is low grade unless perforation with peritonitis has occurred. The sequence of symptoms with pain preceding emesis and fever is important in distinguishing appendicitis from infectious enteritis, which usually begins with vomiting followed by the crampy pain of hyperperistalsis. Diarrhea, if it occurs, is infrequent and consists of small, mucous stools caused by irritation of the sigmoid colon. Similarly, irritation of the bladder may produce urinary symptoms such as frequency and urgency.

As the inflammation progresses to involve the serosa and overlying peritoneum, the pain migrates to the area of peritoneal irritation, usually the right lower quadrant. If the appendix is retrocecal, the pain will be lateral or posterior and may mimic the symptoms associated with septic arthritis of the hip or psoas abscess. With perforation, the pain becomes generalized unless the contamination is well localized to produce a discrete abscess, usually of the right lower quadrant. Palpation of an abdominal or rectal mass indicates abscess formation.

The progression from onset of symptoms to perforation usually occurs over 36–48 hr. If the diagnosis is delayed beyond 36–48 hr, the perforation rate exceeds 65%.

DIAGNOSIS. Physical Examination. History and physical examination should be directed at establishing findings consistent with appendicitis and excluding alternative diagnoses such as viral gastroenteritis, constipation, urinary tract infection, hemolytic-uremic syndrome, Henoch-Schönlein purpura, mesenteric adenitis, and tubo-ovarian disease.

Pertinent aspects of the history favoring a diagnosis of appendicitis include onset of pain before vomiting or diarrhea, loss of appetite, migration of pain from periumbilical to right lower quadrant, and aggravation of pain during the trip to office or hospital. In excluding alternative diagnoses, it is essential to question the history of constipation, urinary tract symptoms, cough and fever suggesting lower lobe pneumonia, profuse diarrhea, headache, myalgias or other constitutional symptoms of viral syndromes, and similar symptoms in other household members. Untreated appendicitis proceeds to perforation within 48–72 hr; therefore, duration of symptoms is important in the interpretation of physical findings and in the determination of a treatment strategy.

Physical examination should begin with inspection of the child's demeanor as well as the appearance of the abdomen. The child with appendicitis frequently moves tentatively and slowly, hunched forward, and often with a slight limp. The child may protect the right lower quadrant with a hand and may be reluctant to climb onto the examining table. Early in appendicitis, the abdomen is flat. Discoloration or bruises should suggest abdominal trauma. Abdominal distention indicates a complication such as perforation or obstruction. Auscultation may reveal normal or hyperactive bowel sounds in early appendicitis to be replaced with hypoactive bowel sounds as it progresses to perforation. Severe gastroenteritis usually produces persistently hyperactive bowel sounds.

Palpation of the abdomen should be gentle after the establishment of rapport and is aided by distraction with conversation or the assistance of a parent. The right lower quadrant (McBurney point) should be palpated last, after the examiner has had an opportunity to judge the response to examination of quadrants that should not be painful. McBurney point is the junction of the lateral and middle thirds of the line joining the right anterior superior ileac spine and the umbilicus. The most important physical finding in appendicitis is persistent direct tenderness to palpation and rigidity of the overlying rectus muscle. If the child is apprehensive or agitated from prior examination, the abdominal muscles may be diffusely tense, making interpretation of this finding impossible.

Testing for rebound tenderness must be done carefully to be meaningful. Deep abdominal palpation with sudden withdrawal of the examining hand causes pain or fear in all children and is not recommended. Gentle finger percussion in all four quadrants is a better test of rebound peritoneal irritation in all age groups but particularly in the frightened child. Testing for rebound tenderness and rectal examination should be the final aspects of the abdominal examination. The value of rectal examination in the diagnosis of appendicitis has been questioned. If the history and abdominal examination are convincing for appendicitis, the rectal examination adds little information. However, if the diagnosis is in doubt, particularly in the very young (younger than 4 yr) or in the female adolescent, rectal examination often yields important information.

After the focused abdominal examination, careful examination of the other body regions, including ears, mucous membranes, lungs, and skin, for signs of other diseases should be noted. Careful attention should be made to identify shock from sepsis, dehydration, or both.

Laboratory Findings. Laboratory evaluation of children with suspected appendicitis usually consists of complete blood count (CBC) and urinalysis. Although many children with appendicitis have leukocytosis or shift in differential, many do not. The primary role of laboratory studies is to exclude alternative diagnoses such as urinary tract infection, hemolytic-uremic syndrome, Henoch-Schönlein purpura, and so on. The proximity of the appendix to the ureter may result in inflammatory cells in the urine. Up to 30 white cells per high-power field and 20 red cells have been reported in suppurative appendicitis. The presence of bacteria or pyuria greater than 30 white cells per high-power field suggests true urinary tract infection. Similarly, the presence of significant proteinuria or cast formation argues against appendicitis. Review of the CBC is directed at identification of microangiopathic anemia, thrombocytosis, or thrombocytopenia, all suggesting diagnoses other than appendicitis.

Imaging Studies. The imaging studies that may be helpful in evaluating children with suspected appendicitis include plain radiographs of the abdomen or chest, ultrasonogram, CT, and rarely barium enema. Findings of appendicitis on abdominal films include calcified appendicolith, small bowel distention or obstruction, and soft tissue mass effect. Severe constipation or lower lobe pneumonia may establish an alternative diagnosis. Graded compression ultrasonography has gained acceptance as a noninvasive study with false-negative and false-positive rates of 8–10% (Fig. 343–1). It is particularly helpful in adolescent girls, whose symptoms may be due to pelvic inflammatory disease, ovarian cysts, or torsion. On rare occasions, when clinical examination and ultrasonography are inconclusive, the diagnosis may be aided by abdominal CT. CT of the abdomen has been used for complicated perforation with multiple intra-abdominal abscesses. Early scanning can improve diagnostic accuracy and can reduce hospitalization in patients with a normal scan. CT will need to be shown superior to ultrasound for it to replace ultrasound as the initial imaging procedure. The value of CT in the diagnosis, localization, and percutaneous drainage of abscesses occurring in the postoperative period is well established. Barium enema findings are those of mass effect on the cecum from the inflammatory process and nonfilling or partial filling of the appendiceal lumen. However,

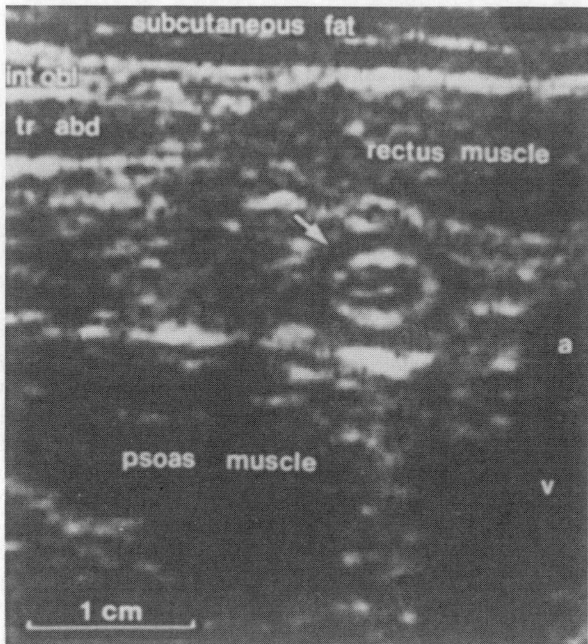

Figure 343–1 A. Graded compression ultrasonogram of acute appendicitis demonstrating edematous enlarged appendix compressed between the abdominal wall and the psoas muscle. (Int obl = internal oblique muscle; tr abd = transverse abdominus muscle; a = right iliac artery; v = right iliac vein.) (From Puylaert JB, Rutgers PH, Laisang RI, et al: A prospective study of ultrasonography in the diagnosis of appendicitis. N Engl J Med 317:666, 1987.)

many healthy children have nonfilling of the appendix, and this finding must be interpreted with caution.

DIFFERENTIAL DIAGNOSIS. Accurate diagnosis of children with abdominal pain is facilitated by a thorough and systematic approach. At the conclusion of the history, physical examination, and initial laboratory studies (CBC, urinalysis), patients fall into three groups: those with definite or highly likely appendicitis, those with a definite alternate diagnosis, and those in whom the diagnosis remains uncertain.

Vomiting preceding the pain, large-volume diarrhea, and high fever suggest gastroenteritis caused by viral or bacterial (*Yersinia, Campylobacter*) agents. Localized right lower quadrant pain in this setting may be mesenteric adenitis. An abnormal hemogram combined with hemorrhagic skin lesions suggests Henoch-Schönlein purpura or hemolytic-uremic syndrome if renal function and urinalysis are abnormal. Weight loss and prolonged symptoms, especially in a teenager, make inflammatory bowel disease a serious consideration. Torsion of an undescended testis is common, and particular note should be made of testicular location. Follicular cysts of the ovary occur in midcycle and may be painful as a result of rupture, rapid enlargement, or hemorrhage. In pelvic inflammatory disease, the pain is usually suprapubic, bilateral, and of longer duration.

Children with cystic fibrosis have a high incidence of appendicitis, but they also have a high incidence of intussusception, constipation, and meconium ileus equivalent. Children with malignancies may experience abdominal pain as a result of their chemotherapy, constipation, typhlitis, or appendicitis. If their malignancy is in remission, the signs and symptoms of appendicitis should be the same as those for healthy children. If the malignancy is not controlled, typhlitis is likely if the child is neutropenic. This entity results from necrotizing enterocolitis involving the terminal ileum and cecum and usually resolves with recovery of the neutrophil count and conservative management.

Those children with an uncertain diagnosis require either further diagnostic studies or observation, depending on the likelihood of appendicitis and the duration of symptoms. Observation may be done at home or in the hospital. If the diagnosis ultimately is appendicitis, the incidence of perforation is significantly higher (60% vs 30%) if observation is carried out at home.

Once the diagnosis of appendicitis is made or highly suspect, the treatment is surgical appendectomy. Meckel diverticulitis may mimic appendicitis and is usually diagnosed at surgery (Chapter 331.2).

TREATMENT. Children with nonperforated appendicitis require minimal preoperative preparation with intravenous fluids and antibiotics. Although the use of antibiotics in uncomplicated, appendicitis is controversial, it has decreased the incidence of postoperative wound infections. Appendectomy should be done within a few hours of establishing the diagnosis and is usually performed through a right lower quadrant incision. Laparoscopic appendectomy has been used in children, although some studies have reported complication rates (intra-abdominal abscess formation) higher than those for open appendectomy. Further evaluation is needed before a definitive comparison of open and laparoscopic appendectomy can be made. In children with an uncertain diagnosis, particularly adolescent females, the laparoscopic approach has the advantage of allowing wider intraperitoneal exploration. Laparoscopy is associated with a shorter recovery period and a lower incidence of wound infection but a longer operative time. Appendectomy for nonperforated appendicitis is associated with a low complication rate, rapid recovery, and short (2–3 days) hospitalization.

If the appendix has perforated, especially with generalized peritonitis, significant fluid resuscitation and broad-spectrum antibiotics may be required a few hours before appendectomy. Nasogastric suction should be used if the patient has significant vomiting or abdominal distention. Antibiotics should cover the commonly encountered organisms (*Bacteroides, Escherichia coli, Klebsiella,* and *Pseudomonas* species). The commonly used intravenous regimens include ampicillin (100 mg/kg/24 hr), gentamicin (5 mg/kg/24 hr), and clindamycin (40 mg/kg/24 hr) or metronidazole (Flagyl) (30 mg/kg/24 hr). Appendectomy is performed with or without drainage of the peritoneal cavity, and antibiotics are continued for 7–10 days. Occasionally, a localized abscess is treated with antibiotics with or without open or percutaneous drainage with appendectomy scheduled as a second, elective procedure in 4–6 wk. If antibiotics are successful, some clinicians question the need for a planned appendectomy. Contrary to nonperforated appendicitis, the postoperative course is characterized by continued fluid requirement, fever, intra-abdominal abscess formation, sepsis, and prolonged (4–5 days) paralytic ileus.

COMPLICATIONS. Complications occur in 25–30% of children with appendicitis, primarily those with perforation. The most effective method of reducing complications of appendicitis is to reduce the incidence of perforation. Mortality from appendicitis is low (0.5–1%). The complications are primarily infectious. Wound infection complicates recovery in 0–2% of children with nonperforated appendicitis and in 10–15% of those with perforated appendicitis. Treatment consists of opening the wound with healing by secondary intention. Further antibiotics are not necessary unless the patient has associated cellulitis or systemic signs of toxicity. Intra-abdominal abscess is rare in simple appendicitis but occurs in 4–6% of children with perforation. Usually, the abscess in the right lower quadrant is solitary and, if needed, can be drained by a CT-guided or ultrasonogram-guided percutaneous approach. Multiple intra-abdominal abscesses are best treated by open laparotomy with drainage. Liver abscess from portal vein sepsis is uncommon but may require multiple drainage procedures.

Intestinal obstruction is a common complication and is usually managed with nasogastric suction if it occurs in the early postoperative period. Infertility caused by adhesions or obstruction of the distal fallopian tube is not associated with simple appendicitis but is three to four times more likely after perforation.

Brender JD, Marcuse EK, Koepsell TD, et al: Childhood appendicitis: Factors associated with perforation. Pediatrics 76:301, 1985.
Chande VT, Kinnane JM: Role of the primary care provider in expediting care of children with acute appendicitis. Arch Pediatr Adolesc Med 150:703, 1996.
Golub R, Siddiqui F, Pohl D: Laparoscopic versus open appendectomy: A meta-analysis. J Am Coll Surg 186:545, 1998.
McCall JL, Sharples K, Jadallah F: Systematic review of randomized controlled trials comparing laparoscopic with open appendicectomy. Br J Surg 84:1045, 1997.
Mollitt DL, Mitchum D, Tepas JJ: Pediatric appendicitis: Efficacy of laboratory and radiologic evaluation. South Med J 81:1477, 1988.
Mueller BA, Daling JR, Moore DE, et al: Appendectomy and the risk of tubal infertility. N Engl J Med 315:1506, 1986.
Rao PM, Rhea JT, Novelline RA, et al: Effect of computed tomography of the appendix on treatment of patients and use of hospital resources. N Engl J Med 338:141, 1998.
Rothrock SG, Skeoch G, Rush JJ, et al: Clinical features of misdiagnosed appendicitis in children. Ann Emerg Med 20:45, 1991.
Rubin SZ, Martin DJ: Ultrasonography in the management of possible appendicitis in childhood. J Pediatr Surg 25:737, 1990.
Ruff M, Friedland I, Hickey S: *Escherichia coli* septicemia in nonperforated appendicitis. Arch Pediatr Adolisc Med 148:853, 1994.
Wagner JM, McKinney WP, Carpenter JL: Does this patient have appendicitis? JAMA 276:1589, 1996.

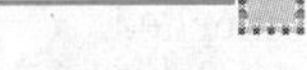

CHAPTER 344

Surgical Conditions of the Anus, Rectum, and Colon

Alberto Peña

In infants and children, close inspection of the anal area is as valuable as a digital rectal examination. *Fissures* can be best identified by having a parent hold the infant's hips in acute flexion so that the examiner can separate the patient's buttocks, using both thumbs, gently stretching the anus and everting the lining to expose the fissure. In all cases of constipation, especially when an obstruction is possible, a digital examination is indicated, after assessing perianal sensation. Properly done, this examination should cause little or no discomfort to the patient. A well-lubricated finger is passed over the anus a few times to accustom the patient to the unusual sensation. Then the pulp of the index or fifth finger is pressed against the anus with increasing flexion of the interphalangeal joints and the finger slips easily into the anal canal.

344.1 Anal Fissure

Anal fissure is a small laceration of the mucocutaneous junction of the anus. It is an acquired lesion secondary to the forceful passage of a hard stool, mainly seen in infancy. Fissures appear to be the consequence and not the cause of constipation.

CLINICAL MANIFESTATIONS. Usually, a history of constipation is elicited. At some point, the patient had a painful bowel movement, which may correspond to the actual event of fissure formation after the passing of hard stool. Then, in addition to the primary cause of constipation, the patient retains stool voluntarily to avoid a painful bowel movement. This exacerbates the constipation, and, eventually, the passing of harder and larger stools creates a vicious cycle. Pain on defecation and bright red blood on the surface of the stool may be observed. The diagnosis is established by inspection of the anal area. For this examination, the infant's hips are held in acute flexion, the patient's buttocks are separated to expand the folds of the perianal skin, and the fissure becomes evident as a minor laceration. Sometimes, peripheral to the laceration, the patient has a little skin appendage that actually represents epithelialized granulomatous tissue, secondary to the chronic inflammation; this is usually known as a "tag."

TREATMENT. The most important element in the treatment of this condition is for the parents to understand the origin of the laceration and the mechanism of the cycle of constipation. The goal of the treatment is to reverse this cycle, which can be achieved only by guaranteeing that the patient has soft stools to avoid overstretching the anus. The healing process may take several days or even several weeks. One single episode of impaction with passing of a hard piece of stool may exacerbate the problem. A stool softener is indicated, but the parents must adjust the dose to the response of the patient. The goal is to avoid both hard stools and diarrhea. Simultaneously, the primary cause of the constipation must be treated when present. No scientific basis supports other types of treatments, including stretching of the anus, "internal" anal sphincterotomy, or excision of the fissure. Chronic anal fissures in older patients have been managed with the local injection of botulinum toxin to treat the associated contraction of the sphincter. The role of this agent in young children is not defined.

344.2 Perianal Abscess and Fistula

Perineal abscess and fistula can be seen in two different groups of pediatric patients with different cause, pathogenesis, and treatment. These include (1) infants with no predisposing conditions and (2) older children with predisposing conditions. The first group is relatively common and includes infants, usually boys younger than 2 yr. This is usually a benign, self-limited condition; the abscess has a communication with one of the crypts of the pectinate line of the anal canal. It is believed that the crypt is the source of contamination; the exact mechanism is unknown. The abscess eventually drains through an orifice in the perianal area. After this drainage, the inflammation subsides, but a fistula remains that communicates with the affected crypt to the perianal external orifice. This condition can be demonstrated during surgical treatment. The fistula becomes chronic but usually disappears spontaneously before 2 yr of age. This fistula is located close to the lumen of the anus, a feature that makes this a very benign condition because the sphincteric mechanism is not affected.

The second group includes patients older than 2 yr with perianal or perirectal abscess and with a predisposing illness, including drug-induced or autoimmune neutropenia, leukemia, AIDS, diabetes mellitus, Crohn disease, prior rectal surgery (Hirschsprung disease, imperforate anus), or sequelae from the use of immunosuppressant drugs. This is considered a much more serious condition; the prognosis is intimately related to that of the predisposing disease. The abscess may be deep and may rapidly expand with severe toxic symptoms, particularly when the predisposing illness is associated with immunosuppression. Bacteriologic examination of abscess material reveals mixed aerobic *(Escherichia coli, Klebsiella pneumoniae, Staphylococcus aureus)* and anaerobic *(Bacteroides species, Clostridium, Veillonella)* flora. Ten to 15% yield pure growth of *E. coli, S. aureus,* or *Bacteroides fragilis.* Neutropenic patients may also have bacteremia that inconsistently has the same organism as the abscess.

CLINICAL MANIFESTATIONS. The infants with no predisposing conditions have mild clinical manifestations, sometimes including low-grade fever, mild rectal pain, and an area of perianal cellulitis. Subsequently, a pustule is formed and the abscess drains through that orifice. This alleviates the symptoms. The inflammation disappears and the pustule heals. However, one or several weeks later, the draining of pus reappears and continues in an intermittent, chronic way. Left alone, this condition usually heals spontaneously before 2 yr of age.

Children with predisposing conditions have a much more serious clinical course. They may or may not have fever depending on their immunologic status. Cellulitis may rapidly expand with warmth, erythema, induration, tenderness, and fluctuation over the ischiorectal fossa, requiring aggressive treatment. Patients may experience severe toxicity and may become septic. In addition, they may show symptoms of the predisposing illness.

TREATMENT. Infants with no predisposing disease usually do not require any treatment because this condition is self-limited. No evidence indicates that antibiotics are useful in these patients. Occasionally, when the patient is extremely uncomfortable, the abscess can be drained under local anesthesia. This alleviates the symptoms of pain and fever but does not eliminate the possibility of a fistula formation. Once a chronic fistula has formed, most clinicians recommend a *fistulotomy* under general anesthesia. The anal canal and lower part of the rectum are exposed with an adequate retractor, and a lacrimal probe is passed through the external orifice of the fistula, coming out through one of the crypts. The tissue between the fistula and the lumen of the anal canal is divided with cautery. The wound is left open to granulate spontaneously. This treatment usually runs a 20% chance of recurrence. Conservative management, (observation) is also accepted because in most cases the fistula disappears spontaneously before 2 yr of age.

Older children with predisposing diseases may require more aggressive treatment and treatment of the predisposing condition. Antibiotics must be administered, including a combination that covers enteric gram-negative organisms, *S. aureus*, and fecal anaerobic flora. Wide excision and drainage are mandatory in cases of sepsis and expanding cellulitis.

Fistulas in older patients are mainly associated with Crohn disease or with a history of pull-through surgery for the treatment of Hirschsprung disease. Those fistulas are difficult to treat. The treatment is the same as that of the predisposing condition.

344.3 Hemorrhoids

Hemorrhoids in children are uncommon and are usually benign. When a hemorrhoid is seen, one must suspect portal hypertension. Infants are sometimes brought for consultation after an incidental finding of a hemorrhoid. These follow a benign course. No reports of thrombosis or other complications of hemorrhoids exist in children; therefore, they should be managed conservatively. Chronic constipation, fecal impaction, or any other kind of irritating local factors must be treated to avoid exacerbation of this condition.

344.4 Rectal Prolapse

Rectal prolapse refers to the exteriorization of the rectal mucosa through the anus. When this extrusion includes all the layers of the rectal wall, it is called *procidentia*. Most cases of rectal tissue protruding through the anus are prolapse and not polyps, intussusception, or other tissue.

Most cases of prolapse are idiopathic. The onset is often between 1 and 5 yr (mean, 3 yr). Predisposing factors include intestinal parasites (particularly in endemic areas), malnutrition, acute diarrhea, ulcerature colitis, pertussis, Ehlers-Danlos syndrome, meningocele (more frequently associated with procidentia owing to the lack of perineal muscle support), cystic fibrosis, and chronic constipation. Patients treated surgically for imperforate anus may have different degrees of rectomucosal prolapse. This is particularly common in patients with poor sphincteric development.

CLINICAL MANIFESTATIONS. Prolapse of the rectum usually occurs during defecation. Afterward, the prolapse is reduced sometimes spontaneously or manually by the patient or parent. In very severe cases, the prolapsed rectum remains chronically exteriorized, becoming congested and edematous, which makes it more difficult to reduce. Rectal prolapse is usually painless or is associated with a mild discomfort. When the rectum remains prolapsed after defecation, it may be traumatized by underwear and may produce bleeding and wetness. Eventually, the exposed rectum becomes ulcerated. The protruding mass varies from bright red to dark red; it may be as long as 10–12 cm. See Chapter 345 for a distinction from a prolapsed polyp.

TREATMENT. The evaluation should include all the necessary tests to rule out the already stated predisposing conditions. *Reduction of protrusion* is aided by pressure with warm compresses. An easy method of reduction is to cover the finger with a piece of toilet paper, introduce it into the lumen of the mass, and gently push it into the patient's rectum. The finger is then immediately withdrawn. The toilet paper adheres to the mucous membrane, permitting release of the finger; the paper, when softened, is later expelled.

General measures should include careful manual reduction of the prolapse after an episode of defecation, attempts to avoid excessive pushing during bowel movements (with patient's feet off the floor), use of laxatives and stool softeners in cases of constipation, avoidance of inflammatory conditions of the rectum, and treatment of intestinal parasitosis when present. If all this fails, surgical treatment may be indicated. None of the existent operations is considered ideal because each has risks and disadvantages. Therefore, medical treatment should always be tried first. Operations include the placement of a subcutaneous, ringlike band in the perianal area to decrease the diameter of the anus. Significant numbers of patients become asymptomatic with this treatment; some may experience megacolon owing to a mechanical anal obstruction. Injection of sclerosing substances in the perirectal area has been reported but has the risk of nerve damage and infection. A posterior incision of the rectum, with anchoring of the rectum to the presacral periosteum, represents a useful alternative in severe cases. In cases of procidentia associated with myelomeningocele, patients may require laparotomy and internal fixation of the rectum to the presacral fascia.

344.5 Pilonidal Sinus and Abscess

A dimple located in the midline intergluteal cleft, at the level of the coccyx, is seen relatively frequently in normal infants. No evidence indicates that this little pilonidal sinus provokes any problems for the patient. Malignant degeneration of pilonidal sinus cyst has been reported only in patients with chronic infections and abscesses. An open dermal sinus is a benign condition and is usually asymptomatic.

Pilonidal abscesses occur in adolescent patients. Why this condition is not seen in younger patients is unknown. The abscess may require incision and drainage during the acute stage, and subsequently, it requires en bloc resection to remove all the epithelial tract that caused the problem.

Ashcraft KW, Garred JL, Holder TM, et al: Rectal prolapse: 17 year experience with the posterior repair and suspension. J Pediatr Surg 15:992, 1990.

Longo WE, Touloukian RJ, Seashore JN: Fistula in ano in infants and children: Implications and management. Pediatrics 87:737, 1991.

Maria G, Cassetta E, Gui D, et al: A comparison of botulinum toxin and saline for the treatment of chronic anal fissure. N Engl J Med 338:217, 1998.
Piazza DJ, Radhakrishnan J: Perianal abscess and fistula-in-ano in children. Dis Colon Rectum 12:1014, 1990.
Pearl RH, Ein SH, Churchill B: Posterior sagittal anorectoplasty for pediatric recurrent rectal prolapse. J Pediatr Surg 24:1100, 1989.
Rakhimov S: Treatment of rectal prolapse in children. Vestn Khir 142:72, 1989.

CHAPTER 345
Tumors of the Digestive Tract

Martin Ulshen

See also Chapter 511.

JUVENILE COLONIC POLYP (Retention Polyp, Inflammatory Polyp). This is the most common childhood bowel tumor, present in 3–4% of people younger than 21 yr. Polyps rarely appear before 1 yr of age. Most present between 2 and 10 yr of age; juvenile polyps are less common beyond 15 yr of age.

Forty per cent or more of these polyps are located proximal to the descending colon. Solitary polyps are common, but two or more juvenile polyps may occur. Most juvenile polyps are erythematous, friable, and pedunculated and range in size from a few millimeters to 3 cm. Histologic examination demonstrates hamartomatous proliferation of glandular and stromal elements, marked vascularity, and infiltration with lymphocytes, eosinophils, and polymorphonuclear and plasma cells. The polyps have characteristic mucus-filled cystic glands and are covered by a fragile, single layer of epithelium. The typical juvenile polyp, with no adenomatous change, has no potential for malignancy. However, juvenile polyps with an adenomatous component have rarely been reported.

Multiple juvenile colonic polyps occur in families as a dominant trait and are associated with congenital anomalies. These polyps are identical to solitary polyps, except for an increased incidence of dysplasia with an increased risk for colonic cancer (see later).

Clinical manifestations include bright red, painless rectal bleeding during or immediately after a bowel movement. Exsanguinating hemorrhage is rare; bleeding often stops spontaneously. Iron-deficiency anemia may be present or, rarely, the initial chief complaint. Lower abdominal pain and cramps are rare and are associated with intussusception or a long pedicle. Prolapse of the polyp appears as a dark, beefy red mass, in distinction to the lighter pink mucosal appearance of rectal prolapse. Spontaneous polyp infarction and self-amputation are common; diarrhea and obstruction are uncommon. The differential diagnosis includes other forms of intestinal polyposis, Meckel diverticulum, fissure in ano, inflammatory bowel disease, intestinal infections, and coagulation disorders.

The *diagnosis* is usually made by colonoscopy. Polyps appear as smooth, pedunculated lesions. Air-contrast barium enema may demonstrate polyps, but even large polyps may not be seen on otherwise adequate barium studies. *Treatment* includes the removal of the polyp at colonoscopy by snare cautery or, rarely, by transabdominal polypectomy. Recurrences occasionally are seen.

FAMILIAL POLYPOSIS SYNDROMES. The familial syndromes associated with intestinal polyposis are important because some of them are premalignant states.

Familial Adenomatous Polyposis Coli. This mendelian dominant, premalignant condition, with reduced penetrance, is characterized by large numbers of adenomatous lesions throughout the colon. It is caused by germ line mutations in the adenomatous polyposis coli (*APC*) gene. The incidence is 1/8,000 persons, with usual onset of polyp development late in the 1st decade of life or during adolescence. By definition, more than 100 (often 1,000) visible adenomas are present when the patient is in the 2nd or 3rd decade. Congenital hypertrophy of retinal pigment epithelial cells is also present from birth in most patients. *APC* gene mutations result in truncated polypeptides. Variability in the clinical features, including extracolonic manifestations, depends on the location of the mutation on the gene. Alterations of the *APC* gene are also responsible for Gardner syndrome and Turcot syndrome (primary brain tumor-medulloblastoma and multiple colorectal polyposis). Some families who do not meet the criteria for familial adenomatous polyposis coli but who have a high frequency of adenomatous polyps and colonic cancer also have a mutation of the *APC* gene.

Initially, the polyps are asymptomatic; many often remain so. When symptomatic, adenomatous polyps cause hematochezia, occasionally cramps, or, rarely, diarrhea. Malignancy arising from preexisting adenomatous polyps may first appear during adolescence, although these lesions usually appear in young adulthood.

The *diagnosis* should be suspected from the family history. In symptomatic patients, the diagnosis is made by direct vision through a colonoscope. The polyps are numerous; biopsies demonstrate the adenomatous nature without the inflammatory and cystic finding of juvenile polyps. *APC* gene mutations are detected in 80% of families with familial polyposis coli, a finding allowing for presymptomatic testing in association with genetic counseling. If a mutation is identified in the index patient, affected family members can be differentiated from unaffected members by gene testing. If the index patient is among the 20% of individuals with this disorder in whom the mutation is not identified, family members should not have the gene test, because a negative result is misleading. For a child with a family history of *APC* and a positive gene test, sigmoidoscopy or colonoscopy is recommended annually after 10 yr of age. A child in a family in which the mutation is not identified should be treated in the same fashion. If the gene test is negative in a family with an identified mutation, it is probably still prudent to screen the patient by endoscopy less frequently, beginning in young adulthood.

For *treatment*, identification of familial polyposis coli requires resection of all colonic mucosa to prevent colorectal cancer. Restoration of bowel continuity is performed by ileorectal pull-through with ileoanal canal anastomosis. Aspirin, sulindac, and complex-resistant starch may slow polyp development; their efficacy is currently unknown.

Gardner Syndrome. This dominantly inherited disorder is characterized by multiple intestinal polyps and tumors of the soft tissue and bone, particularly the mandible. Additional features include dental abnormalities, characteristic bilateral pigmented lesions in the ocular fundus, and extracolonic cancers (hepatoblastoma, central nervous system). Patients with this syndrome have mutations in a specific region on the *APC* gene.

The soft tissue lesions and osteomas may appear during childhood, but intestinal polyps usually do not become apparent until early adult life. These premalignant polyps may develop anywhere along the digestive tract. Accordingly, aggressive surgical treatment of the intestinal lesions is indicated. Children at risk for Gardner syndrome require the same genetic counseling, genetic testing, and colon surveillance as do children having family members with familial polyposis coli. If adenomatous polyps of the colon are identified, colectomy as for familial adenomatous polyposis coli is indicated.

Peutz-Jeghers Syndrome. This rare dominantly inherited syndrome is characterized by mucosal pigmentation of the lips and gums and hamartomas of the stomach and small bowel. Deeply pigmented discrete freckles are seen at birth or appear during infancy on the lips and buccal mucosa and even around the mouth. Evidence of intestinal lesions may come from bleeding but more commonly may arise from crampy pain associated with obstruction or intussusception.

Family studies and genetic counseling may reveal relatives with either partial or complete manifestations of the syndrome. Intestinal lesions should be excised if they are causing significant symptoms; involvement is usually too extensive to remove all the polyps. Fifty per cent of patients have no family member with the disorder, a finding suggesting a high rate of new mutation. Cancer develops in up to 50% of people having Peutz-Jeghers syndrome, most commonly middle-aged adults. Most of these cancers do not occur in the gastrointestinal tract, and typically the hamartomatous polyps do not contain cancer. The Peutz-Jeghers gene encodes a serine/threonine kinase. Peutz-Jeghers is the first cancer-susceptibility syndrome identified as resulting from inactivating mutations of a protein kinase.

HEMANGIOMA OF THE INTESTINE. These rare benign lesions can cause massive, even fatal, hemorrhage. The usual clinical manifestation is painless bleeding beginning in childhood. The blood loss can be subtle and chronic or sudden and massive. Usually, the patient has no additional intestinal symptoms, but if intussusception occurs, obstructive symptoms will occur. About 50% of patients have cutaneous hemangiomas; some have a family history of similar lesions. About half of these lesions are in the colon, where they may be seen by colonoscopy. During a period of bleeding, selective mesenteric arteriography may be useful in locating a lesion.

LEIOMYOMA. This rare benign tumor occurs most commonly in the stomach and jejunum. It remains asymptomatic for long periods, but if it extends into the lumen, it may cause intussusception. Leiomyoma may be confused with leiomyosarcoma, a malignant tumor that occurs rarely in the gastrointestinal tract in children and is associated in some patients with AIDS.

CARCINOMA. Epithelial tumors of the digestive tract are rare in children, and this argues against an aggressive diagnostic approach to many gastrointestinal symptoms in this age group. Several childhood conditions predispose to development of gastrointestinal adenocarcinoma in adult life, for example, familial polyposis, Gardner syndrome, ulcerative colitis, and, to a lesser extent, Crohn disease and disorders associated with chromosomal fragility. The usual site is the colon, but gastric lesions are reported. Symptoms are general ill health, abdominal pain, an abdominal mass, and, less frequently, hemorrhage. The tumors are relatively undifferentiated and highly malignant. Carcinoma of the colon without any predisposing factors is a rare occurrence in children; in some, it is associated with a new mutation of the *APC* gene.

LYMPHOMA. Lymphoma is the most common malignancy of the gastrointestinal tract in children (Chapter 503). About 30% of children with non-Hodgkin lymphoma present with abdominal tumors. Disorders that predispose to lymphoma include AIDS, ataxia-telangiectasia, Wiskott-Aldrich syndrome, agammaglobulinemia, severe combined immunodeficiency syndrome, and long-standing celiac disease. Lymphoma usually occurs in the distal ileum or cecum or appendix and may present with crampy abdominal pain, vomiting, distention, or a palpable abdominal mass. Bowel lymphoma can also present as an acute intussusception. It may be difficult to differentiate symptoms of small bowel lymphoma from Crohn disease.

CARCINOID TUMORS. These tumors of the enterochromaffin cells of the intestine usually occur in the appendix in children and are very low-grade malignancies. They may cause appendicitis or may be found incidentally in the appendix at appendectomy. They do not recur after resection, even when the tumor has extended to the muscularis and lymphatics.

Carcinoid tumors outside the appendix commonly metastasize, and the metastatic lesions give rise to the carcinoid syndrome, which is the result of pharmacologically active secretions produced by the tumor. These produce episodic intestinal hypermotility and diarrhea, vasomotor disturbances, and bronchoconstriction. The most important active agent is serotonin, and the diagnosis is usually made by finding high urinary levels of its metabolite, 5-hydroxyindoleacetic acid. These functioning neoplasms are rare in children.

345.1 Diarrhea from Hormone-Secreting Tumors

Certain hormone-producing tumors cause a marked increase in intestinal secretion leading to severe chronic watery diarrhea (Table 345–1). The secretory diarrhea persists when the patient is placed on nothing by mouth orders. These tumors originate in the APUD cells (*a*mine content, *p*recursor *u*ptake, amino acid *d*ecarboxylation) of the gastroenteropancreatic endocrine system and in adrenal or extra-adrenal neurogenic sites. Neural crest cells are precursors of APUDoma and neurogenic cells.

Diarrhea is massive and results in fluid and electrolyte imbalance and weight loss. Diagnosis is based on the presence

TABLE 345–1 Diarrhea Caused by Hormone-Secreting Tumors

Name	Site	Hormone	Manifestations	Therapy
APUDomas*				
VIPoma	Pancreas	VIP	Watery diarrhea, achlorhydria, hypokalemia	Somatostatin Resection
Somatostatinoma	Pancreas	Somatostatin	Massive diarrhea†	Resection
Gastrinoma	Pancreas	Gastrin	Peptic ulcer, diarrhea	Cimetidine, omeprazole Tumor resection/gastrectomy
Carcinoid	Intestinal argentaffin cells	Serotonin	Diarrhea,† crampy abdominal pain, flushing, wheezing, cardiac valve damage	Somatostatin Resection
Mastocytoma	Cutaneous, intestine, liver, spleen	Histamine, VIP	Pruritus, flushing, apnea, if VIP is positive, diarrhea	H_1- and H_2-blocking agents, cromolyn, steroids Resection if solitary
Medullary carcinoma	Thyroid	Calcitonin, VIP, prostaglandins	Watery diarrhea	Thyroidectomy
Neurogenic				
Ganglioneuroma, ganglioneuroblastoma	Extra-adrenal sites and adrenals	Catecholamines, VIP	Massive watery diarrhea	Resection
Pheochromocytoma	Chromaffin cells; abdominal > other sites	Catecholamines, VIP	Hypertension, tachycardia, sweating, anxiety, watery diarrhea†	Resection

**APUDoma cells are neural crest cell derivatives of the gastroenteropancreatic endocrine system.*
†Reported only in adults.
APUDoma = amine precursor uptake and decarboxylation of amino acids; VIP = vasoactive intestinal polypeptide.

of secretory watery diarrhea, extraintestinal manifestations, measurement of the suspected hormone or its metabolites in serum or urine, and various imaging techniques. If possible, tumor resection is the treatment of choice. Pharmacologic therapy with hormone antagonists may be palliative (see Table 345–1).

NODULAR LYMPHOID HYPERPLASIA. Lymphoid follicles in the lamina propria of the gut normally aggregate in Peyer patches. These areas appear as submucosal nodules, which may be visible on barium contrast roentgenograms and mistaken for an abnormality. Many more Peyer patches are present in the lower than the upper small bowel. In some patients, lymphoid follicles become hyperplastic. The hyperplasia may occur in the colon or may extend to the small bowel. Diffuse small bowel lymphoid hyperplasia may be seen in cases of immunoglobulin deficiency, with and without *Giardia lamblia* infestation. Symptoms are mild. Patients may have rectal bleeding, diarrhea, and abdominal cramps beginning usually by 3 yr of age. In infants with dietary-protein hypersensitivity, lymphoid nodular hyperplasia may occur alone or in association with enterocolitis. Lymphoid nodular hyperplasia also has been noted to occur in inflammatory bowel disease.

The major importance of this entity is the similarity of its manifestations to more serious disorders. Lymphoid nodular hyperplasia usually resolves spontaneously and rarely requires specific treatment. Cyproheptadine or prednisone has been used for extreme bleeding or abdominal pain.

Tumors of the Digestive Tract

Abrahamson J, Shandling B: Intestinal hemangiomata in childhood and a syndrome for diagnosis: A collective review. J Pediatr Surg 8:487, 1973.

Burn J, Chapman P, Eastham E: Familial adenomatous polyposis. Arch Dis Child 71:103, 1994.

Giardiello FM, Brensinger JD, Petersen GM, et al: The use and interpretation of commercial *APC* gene testing for familial adenomatous polyposis. N Engl J Med 336:823, 1997.

Giardiello FM, Offerhaus JA, Krush AJ: Risk of hepatoblastoma in familial adenomatous polyposis. J Pediatr 119:766, 1991.

Giardiello FM, Welsh SB, Hamilton SR, et al: Increased risk of cancer in the Peutz-Jeghers syndrome. N Engl J Med 316:1511, 1987.

Hamilton S, Liu B, Parsons R, et al: The molecular basis of Turcot syndrome. N Engl J Med 332:839, 1995.

Hemminki A, Markie D, Tomlinson I, et al: A serine/threonine kinase gene defective in Peutz-Jeghers syndrome. Nature 391:184, 1998.

Leppert M, Burt R, Hughes JP, et al: Genetic analysis of an inherited predisposition to colon cancer in a family with a variable number of adenomatous polyps. N Engl J Med 322:904, 1990.

Powell SM, Petersen GM, Krush AJ, et al: Molecular diagnosis of familial adenomatous polyposis. N Engl J Med 329:1982, 1993.

Presciuttini S, Varesco L, Sala P, et al: Age of onset in familial adenomatous polyposis: Heterogeneity within families and among *APC* mutations. Ann Hum Genet 58:331, 1994.

Recalde M, Holyoke ED, Elias EG: Carcinoma of the colon, rectum and anal canal in young patients. Surg Gynecol Obstet 139:909, 1974.

Tomlinson IP, Houlston RS: Peutz-Jeghers syndrome. J Med Genet 34:1007, 1997.

Westerman A, Entins MM, de Baar E, et al: Peutz-Jeghers syndrome: 78-year follow-up of the original family. Lancet 353:1211, 1999.

Wu TT, Rezai B, Rashid A, et al: Genetic alterations and epithelial dysplasia in juvenile polyposis syndrome and sporadic juvenile polyps. Am J Pathol 150:939, 1997.

Diarrhea from Hormone-secreting Tumors

Hamilton JR, Radde IC, Johnson G: Diarrhea associated with adrenal ganglioneuroma: New findings related to the pathogenesis of diarrhea. Am J Med 44:473, 1968.

Kaplan SJ, Holbrook CT, McDaniel HE, et al: Vasoactive intestinal peptide secreting tumors of childhood. Am J Dis Child 134:21, 1980.

Mitchell CH, Sinatra FR, Crast FW, et al: Intractable watery diarrhea, ganglioneuroblastoma and vasoactive intestinal peptide. J Pediatr 89:593, 1976.

Rambaud JC, Modigliani R, et al: Pancreatic cholera: studies on tumor secretions and pathophysiology of diarrhea. Gastroenterology 69:110, 1975.

Nodular Lymphoid Dysplasia

Colon AR, DiPalma JS, Leftridge CA: Intestinal lymphonodular hyperplasia of childhood: Patterns of presentation. J Clin Gastroenterol 13:163, 1991.

Hodgson JR, Hoffman HN, Huizenga KA: Roentgenologic features of lymphoid hyperplasia of the small intestine associated with dysgammaglobulinemia. Radiology 88:883, 1967.

Machida HM, Catto Smith AG, Gall DG, et al: Allergic colitis in infancy: Clinical and pathologic aspects. J Pediatr Gastroenterol Nutr 19:22, 1994.

CHAPTER 346
Inguinal Hernias

Stephen J. Shochat

An inguinal hernia is the most common condition requiring operation in the pediatric age group. The incidence of inguinal hernias in children is estimated to be between 10 and 20/1,000 live births. The ratio of boys to girls is 4:1. Approximately 50% will present before 1 yr of age; most are seen in the first 6 mo of life. The most common inguinal hernia in children is an indirect inguinal hernia. Direct hernias are rare, occurring in approximately 1% of all inguinal hernias. Femoral hernias are also rare in the pediatric population. Sixty per cent of inguinal hernias are on the right side, 30% are on the left side, and 10% are bilateral. Premature infants have a higher incidence of inguinal hernia, approaching 30%.

EMBRYOLOGY AND PATHOGENESIS. Most inguinal hernias in infants and children are indirect, resulting from a persistent patency of the processus vaginalis. In the fetus, the gonads begin to develop during the 5th wk of gestation, when the primordial germ cells migrate from the yolk sac to the gonadal ridge. The ligamentous gubernaculum forms and descends on either side of the abdomen at the inferior pole of the gonad and attaches to the internal surface of the labial-scrotal folds. During its course of descent, the gubernaculum passes through the anterior abdominal wall at the site of the future internal inguinal ring and inguinal canal. The processus vaginalis is a diverticular protrusion of the peritoneum that forms just ventral to the gubernaculum and herniates through the abdominal wall with the gubernaculum into the inguinal canal. The testes, which are initially located within the urogenital ridge in the retroperitoneum, descend to the area of the internal ring by approximately 28 wk of gestation. The descent of the testis through the inguinal canal is regulated by androgenic hormones and mechanical factors (increased intra-abdominal pressure). The testes descend into the scrotum by approximately 29 wk of gestation. Each testis descends through the inguinal canal external to the processus vaginalis.

The ovaries also descend into the pelvis from the urogenital ridge, but they do not exit from the abdominal cavity. The cranial portion of the gubernaculum differentiates into the ovarian ligament, and the inferior aspect of the gubernaculum becomes the round ligament, which passes through the internal ring and into the labia majoris. The processus vaginalis in girls extends into the labia majoris through the inguinal canal, also known as the canal of Nuck.

During the last few weeks of gestation or shortly after birth, the layers of the processus vaginalis normally fuse together and obliterate the entrance to the inguinal canal in the vicinity of the internal ring. Failure of obliteration results in a variety of inguinal anomalies (Fig. 346–1). Complete failure of obliteration leads to a complete inguinal hernia. Obliteration distally with patency proximally leads to an indirect inguinal hernia. Obliteration proximally with patency distally leads to an isolated *hydrocele,* also known as a hydrocele of the tunica vaginalis. Obliteration of the processus vaginalis proximally and distally but patency in the midportion of the spermatic cord leads to a hydrocele of the cord. The term *communicating hydrocele* is confusing and should be discarded because this anomaly is synonymous with a complete inguinal hernia (see Fig. 346–1).

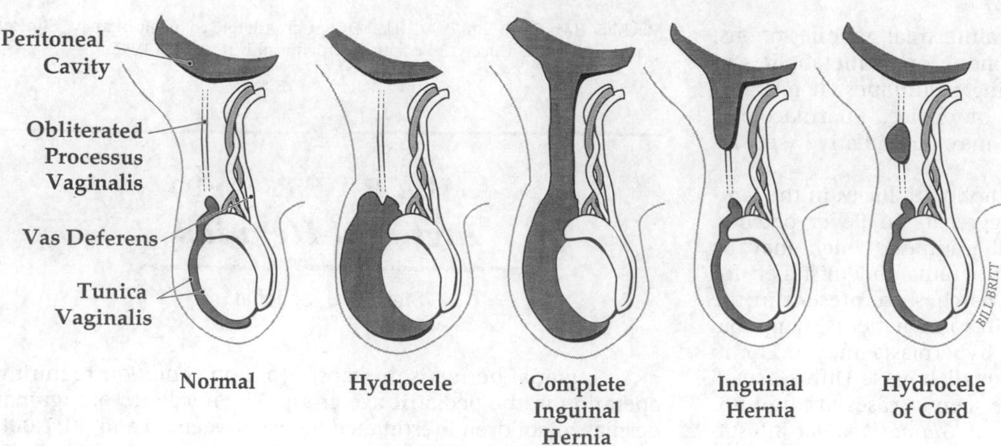

Figure 346–1 Hernias and hydroceles. (Modified from Scherer LR III, Grosfeld JL: Inguinal and umbilical anomalies. Pediatr Clin North Am 40:1122, 1993.)

CLINICAL MANIFESTATIONS. An inguinal hernia usually appears as a bulge in the inguinal region and extends toward or into the scrotum. Occasionally, an infant presents with a swelling of the scrotum without a prior bulge in the inguinal region. The parent is usually the first person to notice this bulge, which may be present only during crying or straining. During sleep or when at rest or relaxed, the hernia reduces spontaneously without a noticeable bulge or enlargement of the scrotum. The history of intermittent groin, labial, or scrotal swelling that spontaneously reduces is classic for an indirect inguinal hernia. Occasionally, an inguinal mass appears suddenly in an infant and is associated with discomfort. The physician must distinguish between a hydrocele of the cord and an incarcerated inguinal hernia, but the hydrocele of the cord is not associated with symptoms of intestinal obstruction such as abdominal distention or vomiting.

Physical examination reveals an inguinal bulge at the level of the internal or external ring or a scrotal swelling that is reducible or fluctuates in size. The classic method of examining an adult for an inguinal hernia by placing the index finger into the inguinal canal is unnecessary in infants and young children and can cause unnecessary discomfort. This is because the internal and external rings are parallel in infants and young children, and a true, well-defined inguinal canal is not present. An inguinal hernia can be identified by having the infant lie supine with extended legs and arms over the head. This usually causes the infant to cry, thereby raising the intra-abdominal pressure, which then demonstrates a bulge over the pubic tubercle (external ring) or a swelling within the scrotum. Older children can be examined while they are standing, a position that also increases the intra-abdominal pressure and demonstrates the hernia. Retractile testes are frequent in young infants and children and can resemble an inguinal hernia with a bulge over the external ring. For this reason, it is important to palpate the testes before palpation of the inguinal bulge. This maneuver allows the differentiation between these two entities and avoids an unnecessary operative procedure.

In difficult diagnostic dilemmas, a rectal examination can be extremely helpful in differentiating acute groin abnormalities. The examiner first examines the internal ring on the uninvolved side and then can sweep the index finger or fifth digit toward the internal ring on the involved side. In cases of an indirect inguinal hernia, an intra-abdominal organ can be palpated extending through the internal ring. This technique is helpful in distinguishing an incarcerated hernia from an acute hydrocele of the cord or other inguinal abnormalities such as inguinal adenitis.

At times, it may be difficult to distinguish a complete inguinal hernia from an isolated hydrocele. These two conditions can usually be differentiated by a careful history. In an infant with a complete inguinal hernia, the scrotal swelling varies during the day, usually being large while the child is crying or straining, and disappears or becomes much smaller during relaxation. The isolated hydrocele does not change in size during the day but may gradually disappear over the 1st yr of life. The hydrocele and the complete inguinal hernia both transilluminate and may be difficult to distinguish from each other because occasionally the complete inguinal hernia cannot be reduced manually as a result of narrowing within a small inguinal canal. In this situation, a classic history is all that is necessary to proceed with operation. In some children with an inguinal hernia, an inguinal bulge or scrotal swelling may not be present at the time of physical examination, and the only finding may be a thickening of the spermatic cord with an associated "silk" sign. The silk sign is elicited by palpating the spermatic cord over the pubic tubercle. The two layers of the peritoneum rubbing together feel like silk. The silk sign in association with a history, of a hernia can be helpful in diagnosing an inguinal hernia. Occasionally, a full bladder occludes the internal inguinal ring so that a hernia cannot be demonstrated. Emptying the bladder may be helpful in this situation.

An increased incidence of indirect inguinal hernias is seen in children with a positive family history of hernias, cystic fibrosis, congenital dislocation of the hip, undescended testes, ambiguous genitalia, hypospadias, epispadias, ascites, and congenital abdominal wall defects. Infants with connective tissue disorders such as Ehlers-Danlos syndrome and mucopolysaccharidosis (Hunter-Hurler syndrome) are at increased risk for inguinal hernia. Female infants with inguinal hernias should be suspected of having testicular feminization because more than 50% of patients with testicular feminization have an inguinal hernia. Conversely, the true incidence of testicular feminization in all female infants with hernias is difficult to determine but is approximately 1%. The diagnosis of testicular feminization can be made at the time of operation either by identifying an abnormal gonad within the hernia sac or by performing a rectal examination to palpate a uterus. In the normal female infant, the uterus is easily palpated as a distinct midline structure beneath the symphysis pubis on rectal examination. Chromosome analysis should be reserved for those infants with definite absence of the uterus. All girls with an inguinal hernia should have a rectal examination and, if needed, a pelvic ultrasound study performed at the time of operation to rule out testicular feminization.

TREATMENT. The treatment of choice is operative repair; an inguinal hernia does not resolve spontaneously. The operation should be carried out electively shortly after diagnosis because of the high risk of later incarceration, especially during the 1st yr of life. Elective inguinal hernia repair can safely be performed in an outpatient setting. Hospitalization should be limited to high-risk patients with cardiac, respiratory, or other medical conditions that would place them at an increased risk after the stress of surgery and anesthesia. Supports and trusses are not indicated and are potentially hazardous. Operation is not indicated for the child with an isolated hydrocele. No indication exists for operating on a hydrocele, except in the infant with a hydrocele of the cord, in which an associated hernia is frequently present. An isolated hydrocele often resolves spontaneously within the 1st yr; if the hydrocele persists beyond this time, the diagnosis is that of a complete inguinal hernia, which should be treated by an inguinal exploration and herniorrhaphy. Hydroceles should not be aspirated.

Controversy exists regarding when to proceed with contralateral groin exploration in infants and children with a unilateral indirect inguinal hernia. The incidence of a patent processus vaginalis is approximately 60% at 2 mo of age and 40% at 2 yr of age. A silent patent processus vaginalis is found in approximately 30% of the general population at autopsy. After unilateral hernia repair in children, a contralateral hernia develops in approximately 30%. If the unilateral repair is on the left side, the chance of developing a subsequent hernia on the right side is 40%, probably because of the late descent of the right testis during fetal life. The risk of developing a contralateral hernia after unilateral repair seems to be higher in younger infants and is as high as 50% in children who underwent unilateral repair within the first year of life. Girls have a higher incidence of a contralateral patent processus vaginalis, approaching 50% in all age groups. The risk of incarceration is high in children younger than 1 yr (approximately 30%), with most occurring in children younger than 6 mo.

On the basis of these data, most pediatric surgeons recommend bilateral inguinal exploration in all boys younger than 1 yr, in patients with conditions associated with an increased risk of an inguinal hernia, and in all girls younger than 2 yr. Boys and girls younger than 2 yr presenting with a left inguinal hernia are at higher risk for the development of a contralateral hernia and should be considered for right-sided surgical exploration. A large series of patients from Japan, followed for several years after unilateral repair in children, revealed an incidence of contralateral hernia of approximately 12%. This series and several smaller series question the wisdom of routine bilateral exploration in children with unilateral hernia. Laparoscopic techniques have been used to visualize the contralateral side, and in experienced hands, this technique has been found to be efficacious, thus avoiding unnecessary contralateral exploration. The decision to perform a bilateral exploration should also depend on the expertise of the surgeon and anesthesiologist and on the general condition of the child.

Antibiotic coverage is an important consideration in infants with congenital heart disease and in children with ventriculoperitoneal shunts before operative repair. Ampicillin and gentamicin are the antibiotics of choice for such children, beginning 2 hr before operation and continued in the immediate postoperative period.

Bilateral absence of the vas deferens at the time of herniorrhaphy is an occasional finding. Although this condition can be an isolated finding, the incidence of cystic fibrosis is higher in children with agenesis of the vas deferens. Children with cystic fibrosis also have an increased incidence of inguinal hernias. A sweat chloride test should be performed in these infants to confirm the diagnosis of cystic fibrosis; DNA testing is also available.

COMPLICATIONS. An *incarcerated hernia* occurs when the contents of the hernia sac cannot be reduced back into the abdominal cavity. The incarcerated organ is usually the intestine, which is associated with signs and symptoms of intestinal obstruction such as vomiting, abdominal distention, constipation, and air-fluid levels on an abdominal radiograph. All infants and young children with unexplained intestinal obstruction should be examined for an unrecognized incarcerated hernia. Although the intestines are the most frequent organs involved in an incarcerated hernia, any intra-abdominal organ can become incarcerated, and in young girls the most common organ is the ovary. Once the blood supply to the organ becomes compromised, a strangulated hernia occurs, a definite indication for emergency operation.

The incidence of incarceration ranges from 9–20%, with the majority seen within the 1st yr of life. The incidence of incarceration is higher in girls and in premature infants of both sexes. Incarcerated hernias present with a tender, firm mass in the inguinal canal or the scrotum. The child is fussy, is intolerant of feedings, and cries inconsolably. The skin over the mass may be edematous and slightly discolored, but it is usually not erythematous or exquisitely tender, as is seen with a strangulated hernia.

The hernia should be promptly reduced, and reduction can be successfully accomplished in approximately 95% of cases. It is unusual for a child with an incarcerated inguinal hernia to require an emergency operation. Reduction of an inguinal hernia is aided by sedation with a short-acting barbiturate or chloral hydrate and placing the patient in the Trendelenburg position. Ice packs are not used and have caused fat necrosis in small infants. Once the child is quiet, a gentle milking of the hernial contents toward the internal or external inguinae rings can be accomplished. After reduction of the hernia, an elective operation should be performed within 24–48 hr once the edema has subsided. Depending on the social situation and the length of time of the incarceration, the infant may have to be admitted to the hospital during this period of observation.

Children with strangulated hernias have systemic signs of vascular compromise such as tachycardia and fever; the groin mass is usually erythematous and exquisitely tender. These children require immediate operative intervention. This condition is a rare occurrence in the pediatric age group. The complication rate, after an emergency operation for an incarcerated or strangulated hernia, is approximately 20 times higher than with an elected procedure.

In young boys with undescended testes and an associated hernia, incarceration is frequently associated with ischemia and infarction of the testis. For this reason, infants with an undescended testis and associated clinical hernia should have an elective orchiopexy and hernia repair at the time of diagnosis. Young girls can have the ovary and fallopian tube incarcerated within the inguinal canal or the labia majora. If the ovary cannot be reduced, early surgical intervention should be considered because of the possibility of infarction of the ovary.

A unique type of hernia that is rare in infants and young children is *Richter hernia*. In Richter hernia, there is an isolated incarceration of the antimesenteric portion of the intestine, and, despite the incarceration and sometimes strangulation, intestinal obstruction is not present. This should be kept in mind when evidence shows incarceration or strangulation without intestinal obstruction. The more common situation is that of strangulated omentum, but both conditions should be considered in the infant with a questionable incarcerated hernia and no signs of intestinal obstruction. The problems can be differentiated by performing a rectal examination to determine whether the patient has evidence of an indirect hernia with contents extending through the internal ring into the inguinal canal.

PREMATURE INFANT. The premature infant has a higher incidence of inguinal hernia and incarceration. Up to 7% of boys born at less than 30 wk of gestation have inguinal hernias compared with only 0.6% of male infants born at later than 36 wk of gestation. In addition, the incidence of hernias in premature infants weighing less than 1,500 g is 20 times greater than in larger infants. Because the incidence of incarceration approaches 30% in this patient population, elective hernia repair should be considered before discharge from the neonatal intensive care nursery.

Postoperative apnea is a life-threatening complication of hernia repair in premature infants. The cause of this apnea is unknown, but it may be due to immaturity of the brain stem ventilatory mechanism. Premature infants with a history of apnea are at extremely high risk for significant respiratory depression after hernia repair. Even premature infants without prior apnea have a significant risk of respiratory arrest and compromise in the postoperative period. The guidelines recommended by pediatric anesthesiologists are that any premature infant younger than 60 wk of postconception age should be hospitalized and requires 24-hr postoperative cardiac and respiratory monitoring after herniorrhaphy. Most of these children require general anesthesia, but local anesthetic methods have been attempted with some success; regional anesthesia may also be effective (see Chapter 73).

PROGNOSIS. The results of inguinal hernia repair in infants and children are excellent. The complication rate after repair of inguinal hernias in children is approximately 2%. The incidence of wound infection approaches 1%, and the recurrence rate is less than 1%. An increased incidence of recurrence is found in children with a history of incarceration or strangulation, in children with connective tissue diseases and chronic respiratory illness, and when intra-abdominal pressure is increased, such as in infants with a ventriculoperitoneal shunt. Injury to the ilioinguinal nerve or the vas deferens is rare. Testicular compromise is seen in 3–5% of boys who present with an incarcerated hernia.

Gallagher TM: Regional anesthesia for surgical treatment of inguinal hernia repair in preterm babies. Arch Dis Child 69:623, 1993.

Holcomb GW: Laparoscopic evaluation for a contralateral inguinal hernia or a nonpalpable testis. Pediatr Ann 22:678, 1993.

Kemmotsu H, Oshima Y, Mouri T, et al: The features of contralateral manifestations after the repair of unilateral inguinal hernia. J Pediatr Surg 33:1099, 1998.

Krieger NR, Shochat SJ, McGowan V, et al: Early hernia repair in the premature infant: Long-term follow-up. J Pediatr Surg 29:978, 1994.

Scherer LR III, Grosfeld JL: Inguinal and umbilical anomalies. Pediatr Clin North Am 40:1121, 1993.

Wulkan ML, Wiener ES, VanBalen N, et al: Laparoscopy through the open ipsilateral sac to evaluate presence of contralateral hernia. J Pediatr Surg 31:1174, 1996.

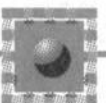

SECTION 5

Exocrine Pancreas

Steven L. Werlin

Excluding cystic fibrosis, disorders of the exocrine pancreas are uncommon in childhood. Pancreatic disease may be based on traumatic, anatomic (annular pancreas, pancreas divisum), metabolic (Reye syndrome, α_1-antitrypsin deficiency), congenital (Shwachman syndrome, enzyme defects), autoimmune (diabetes mellitus), or inflammatory pathology. A comprehensive discussion of cystic fibrosis is found in Chapter 416. ■

CHAPTER 347
Embryology, Anatomy, and Physiology

The human pancreas develops from evaginations of primitive duodenum beginning at about the 5th wk of gestation. Pancreatic agenesis has been associated with a base pair deletion in the *ipf1* HOX gene. The larger dorsal anlage, which develops into the tail, body, and part of the head of the pancreas, grows directly from the duodenum. The smaller ventral anlage develops as one or two buds from the primitive liver and eventually forms the major portion of the head of the pancreas. At about the 17th wk of gestation, the dorsal and ventral anlagen fuse as the buds develop and the gut rotates. The ventral duct forms the proximal portion of the major pancreatic duct of Wirsung, which opens into the ampulla of Vater. The dorsal duct forms the distal portion of the duct of Wirsung and the accessory duct of Santorini, which may empty independently in about 15% of people. Variations in fusion account for pancreatic developmental anomalies.

The pancreas lies transversely in the upper abdomen between the duodenum and the spleen in the retroperitoneum. The head, which rests on the vena cava and renal vein, is adherent to the C-loop of the duodenum and surrounds the distal common bile duct. The tail of the pancreas reaches to the left splenic hilum and passes above the left kidney. The lesser sac separates the tail of the pancreas from the stomach.

By the 13th wk of gestation, exocrine and endocrine cells can be identified. Primitive acini containing immature zymogen granules are found by the 16th wk. Mature zymogen granules containing amylase, trypsinogen, chymotrypsinogen, and lipase are present at the 20th wk. Centroacinar and duct cells, which are responsible for water, electrolyte, and bicarbonate secretion, are also found by the 20th wk. The final three-dimensional structure of the pancreas consists of a complex series of branching ducts surrounded by grapelike clusters of epithelial cells. Cells containing glucagon are present at the 8th wk. Islets of Langerhans appear between the 12th and 16th wks.

347.1 Anatomic Abnormalities

Complete and partial *pancreatic agenesis* are rare conditions. Complete agenesis is associated with severe neonatal diabetes and usually death at an early age. Partial or dorsal pancreatic agenesis is often asymptomatic but may be associated with diabetes, congenital heart disease associated with polysplenia, and recurrent pancreatitis.

An *annular pancreas* results from incomplete rotation of the left (ventral) pancreatic anlage. Patients usually present in infancy with symptoms of complete or partial bowel obstruction. There is frequently a history of maternal polyhydramnios. Some children present with chronic vomiting, pancreatitis, or biliary colic. The treatment of choice is duodenojejunostomy. Division of the pancreatic ring is not attempted, because a duodenal diaphragm or duodenal stenosis frequently accompanies annular pancreas. Annular pancreas may be associated with Down syndrome, intestinal atresia, imperforate anus, pancreatitis, and malrotation.

Ectopic pancreatic rests in the stomach or small intestine occur in approximately 3% of the population. Most cases (70%) are found in the upper intestinal tract. Recognized on barium contrast studies by their typical umbilicated appearance, they are rarely of clinical importance. On endoscopy they are irregular, yellow nodules 2 to 4 mm in diameter. A pancreatic rest may occasionally be the lead point of an intussusception, produce hemorrhage, or cause bowel obstruction.

Pancreas divisum, which occurs in 5 to 15% of the population, is the most common pancreatic developmental anomaly. As the result of failure of the dorsal and ventral pancreatic anlagen to fuse, the tail, body, and part of the head of the pancreas drain through the small accessory duct of Santorini rather than the main duct of Wirsung. It is believed that this anomaly may be associated with recurrent pancreatitis when there is a relative obstruction of the outflow of the ventral pancreas. The treatment of choice of recurrent pancreatitis associated with pancreas divisum is endoscopic insertion of an endoprosthesis. If the episodes stop, surgical sphincterotomy is indicated.

Choledochal cysts are dilatations of the biliary tract and usually cause biliary tract symptoms, such as jaundice, pain, and fever. On occasion, the presentation may be pancreatitis. The diagnosis is usually easily made with ultrasonography, CT scanning, or biliary tract scan. Similarly, a choledochocele, an intraduodenal choledochal cyst, may present with pancreatitis. The diagnosis may be difficult and require endoscopic retrograde cholangiopancreatography.

A number of rare conditions, such as *Ivemark* and *Johanson-Blizzard syndromes,* include pancreatic dysgenesis or dysfunction among their features. Many of these syndromes include renal and hepatic dysgenesis along with the pancreatic anomalies. Absence of islet cells and agenesis of the pancreas produce permanent diabetes mellitus, which begins in the neonatal period (Chapter 599). Pancreatic agenesis is also associated with malabsorption.

Hill ID, Lebenthal E: Congenital abnormalities of the exocrine pancreas. *In:* Go ELW, et al (eds): The Exocrine Pancreas: Biology, Pathology, and Diseases, 2nd ed. New York, Raven Press, 1993, pp 1029–1040.

Lans JI, Geenan JE, Johanson JF, Hogan WJ: Endoscopic therapy in patients with pancreas divisum and acute pancreatitis: A prospective, randomized, controlled clinical trial. Gastrointest Endosc 38:430, 1992.

347.2 Physiology

The acinus is the functional unit of the exocrine pancreas. Acinar cells are arrayed in a semicircle around a lumen. Ducts that drain the acini are lined by centroacinar and ductular cells. This arrangement allows the secretions of the various cell types to mix.

The acinar cell synthesizes, stores, and secretes more than 20 enzymes. These enzymes are stored in zymogen granules, some in inactive forms. The relative concentration of the various enzymes in pancreatic juice is affected and perhaps controlled by the diet, probably by regulating the synthesis of specific messenger RNA. As a general rule, diets high in fat increase the concentration of lipase; a high-protein diet increases pancreatic content of proteases; and a high carbohydrate diet leads to increased content of amylase in the pancreatic juice. *α-Amylase* splits starch into maltose, isomaltose, maltotriose, and dextrins.

Trypsin and *chymotrypsin,* both endopeptidases, and *carboxypeptidase,* an exopeptidase, are secreted by the pancreas as inactive proenzymes. Trypsinogen is activated in the gut lumen by *enterokinase,* a brush border enzyme. Trypsin can then activate trypsinogen, chymotrypsinogen, and procarboxypeptidase into their respective active forms. Enterokinase is thus a key enzyme for exocrine pancreatic function.

Pancreatic *lipase* requires colipase, a coenzyme also found in pancreatic fluid, for activity. Lipase liberates fatty acids from the one and three positions of triglycerides, leaving two monoglycerides.

The stimuli for *exocrine pancreatic secretion* are neural and hormonal. Acetylcholine mediates the cephalic phase; cholecystokinin (CCK) mediates the intestinal phase. CCK is released from the duodenal mucosa by luminal amino acids and fatty acids. Feedback regulation of pancreatic secretion is mediated by pancreatic proteases in the duodenum. Secretion of CCK is inhibited by the digestion of a trypsin-sensitive, CCK-releasing peptide released in the lumen of the small intestine or by a monitor peptide released in pancreatic fluid.

Centroacinar and duct cells secrete water and bicarbonate. Bicarbonate secretion is under feedback control and is regulated by duodenal intraluminal pH. The stimulus for bicarbonate production is *secretin* in concert with CCK. Secretin cells are abundant in the duodenum.

Although normal pancreatic function is required for digestion, maldigestion occurs only after considerable reduction in pancreatic function; lipase and colipase secretion must be decreased by 90 to 98% before fat maldigestion occurs.

Although amylase and lipase are present in the pancreas early in gestation, secretion of both amylase and lipase is low in the infant. Adult levels of these enzymes are not reached in the duodenum until late in the 1st yr of life. Digestion of the starch found in many infant formulas depends on the low levels of salivary amylase that reach the duodenum. This explains the diarrhea that may be seen in infants who are fed formulas high in glucose polymers or starch. Neonatal secretion of trypsinogen and chymotrypsinogen is at about 70% of the level found in the 1-yr-old infant. The low levels of amylase and lipase in duodenal contents of infants may be partially compensated by salivary amylase and lingual lipase. This explains the relative starch and fat intolerance of premature infants.

Lloyd-Still JD, Listernick R, Buentello G: Complex carbohydrate intolerance: Diagnostic pitfalls and approach to management. J Pediatr 112:709, 1988.

Werlin SL: Development of the exocrine pancreas. *In:* Polin RA, Fox WW (eds): Fetal and Neonatal Physiology, 2nd ed. Philadelphia, WB Saunders, 1998, pp 1387–1400.

CHAPTER 348
Pancreatic Function Tests

Pancreatic function can be measured by direct and indirect methods. Direct stimulation of the pancreas with a test (Lundh) meal of corn oil, skimmed milk powder, and dextrose or with secretin plus cholecystokinin can be performed. A triple-lumen tube is used to isolate the pancreatic secretions in the duodenum. Measurement of bicarbonate concentration and enzyme activity (trypsin, chymotrypsin, lipase, amylase) is performed on the aspirated secretions. Normal values for children, excluding infants, are well established. Direct stimulation tests are uncomfortable and are often unnecessary.

A qualitative examination of the stool for *microscopic fat* globules is the most widely practiced screening test for malabsorption (also see Chapter 340). Analysis of random stool specimens by this method may give both false-positive and false-negative results. A 72-hr collection for *quantitative analysis of fat content* is preferable. The collection is usually performed at home, and the parent is asked to keep a careful dietary record, from which fat intake is calculated. A preweighed sealable plastic container is used, which the parent keeps in the freezer. Freezing helps preserve the specimen and reduce the odor. Infants are dressed in disposable diapers with the plastic side facing the skin so that the complete sample can be transferred to the container. Normal fat absorption is greater than 93% of intake.

Pancreatic enzyme activities can be measured in stool or duodenal contents. Stool trypsin has been the most commonly measured but is not as reliable as stool chymotrypsin. Neither test is as reliable as fecal fat analysis. Similarly, a random sample of duodenal fluid can be obtained and analyzed for pancreatic enzyme content. The elevated serum levels of trypsinogen found in neonates with cystic fibrosis form the basis of the newborn screening test in many states. With advancing pancreatic damage, serum trypsinogen levels eventually fall below normal.

Pancreatic function can also be measured by *breath tests.* A labeled triglyceride, most commonly ^{14}C-triolein, is ingested and digested by pancreatic lipase in the duodenum liberating $^{14}CO_2$, which is detected in the expired air. Because of the radioactivity and long half-life of ^{14}C, this test is not appropriate for use in children. Research is now ongoing using triolein-labeled with ^{13}C, a stable, nonradioactive isotope. Although this test is safe for pediatric use, detection of $^{13}CO_2$ requires a mass spectrophotometer, which is generally not available.

Puntis JWL: Assessment of pancreatic function. Arch Dis Child 69:99, 1993.

CHAPTER 349
Disorders of the Exocrine Pancreas

DISORDERS ASSOCIATED WITH PANCREATIC INSUFFICIENCY. Other than cystic fibrosis, conditions that cause pancreatic insufficiency are rare in children. They include Shwachman-Diamond syndrome, isolated enzyme deficiencies, enterokinase deficiency (Chapter 340), chronic pancreatitis, and protein-calorie malnutrition (Chapter 340.2).

Cystic Fibrosis (see Chapter 416). Cystic fibrosis is the most common lethal genetic disease and the most common cause of malabsorption among white American children. By the end of the 1st year of life, 90% of children with cystic fibrosis have pancreatic insufficiency, leading to malnutrition in many cases. Treatment of the associated pancreatic insufficiency leads to improvement in absorption, better growth, and normalized stools. Multiple mutations in the cystic fibrosis gene have been associated with idiopathic chronic pancreatitis.

Shwachman-Diamond Syndrome (see Chapter 131.1). This is an autosomal recessive syndrome (1:20,000 births), consisting of pancreatic insufficiency; neutropenia, which may be intermittent; neutrophil chemotaxis defects; metaphyseal dysostosis; failure to thrive; and short stature. Patients present in infancy with poor growth and greasy, foul-smelling stools that are characteristic of malabsorption. These children can be readily differentiated from those with cystic fibrosis by their normal sweat chloride levels, lack of the cystic fibrosis gene, characteristic metaphyseal lesions, and fatty pancreas on CT examination. Despite adequate pancreatic replacement therapy, poor growth frequently continues. Pancreatic insufficiency is often transient, and steatorrhea may spontaneously improve with age (frequently before 4 yr of age). The neutropenia may be cyclic.

Recurrent pyogenic infections (otitis media, pneumonia, osteomyelitis, dermatitis, sepsis) are common and are a frequent cause of death. Thrombocytopenia is found in 70% of patients and anemia in 50%. Pathologically, the pancreatic acini are replaced by fat with little fibrosis. Islet cells and ducts are normal. The fatty pancreas has a characteristic hypodense appearance on CT and MR scans.

Pearson Syndrome. This is a sporadic mitochondrial DNA mutation affecting oxidative phosphorylation that manifests in infants with severe macrocytic anemia and variable thrombocytopenia. The bone marrow demonstrates vacuoles in erythroid and myeloid precursors as well as ringed sideroblasts. In addition to severe bone marrow failure, pancreatic insufficiency will contribute to growth failure. Other mitochondrial DNA mutations are associated with the development of diabetes mellitus (Kearns-Sayre, chronic progressive external ophthalmoplegia, diabetes with deafness syndromes). Mitochondrial DNA mutations are transmitted through maternal inheritance or are sporadic.

Isolated Enzyme Deficiencies. Isolated deficiencies of trypsinogen, enterokinase, lipase, and colipase have been reported. Although enterokinase is a brush border enzyme, deficiency causes pancreatic insufficiency because pancreatic proteases remain inactive. Deficiencies of trypsinogen or enterokinase manifest with failure to thrive, hypoproteinemia, and edema. Isolated amylase deficiency has not been shown to exist as a primary, permanent enzyme deficiency.

SYNDROMES ASSOCIATED WITH PANCREATIC INSUFFICIENCY. Pancreatic agenesis, the *Johanson-Blizzard syndrome* (pancreatic insufficiency, deafness, low birthweight, microcephaly, midline ectodermal scalp defects, psychomotor retardation, hypothyroidism, dwarfism, absent permanent teeth, and aplasia of the alae nasae), congenital pancreatic hypoplasia, and congenital rubella are rare causes of pancreatic insufficiency. Some children with both syndromic (Alagille) and nonsyndromic paucity of intrahepatic bile ducts may also have pancreatic insufficiency associated with their liver disease. Pancreatic insufficiency has also been reported in duodenal atresia and stenosis and may also be seen in the infant with familial or nonfamilial hyperinsulinemic hypoglycemia (nesidioblastosis) who requires 95% pancreatectomy to control hypoglycemia.

Gaskin KJ, Durie PR, Lee L, et al: Colipase and lipase secretion in childhood-onset pancreatic insufficiency: Delineation of patients with steatorrhea secondary to relative colipase deficiency. Gastroenterology 86:1, 1984.
Mack DR, Forstner GG, Wilchanski M, et al: Shwachman syndrome: Exocrine pancreatic dysfunction and variable phenotypic expression. Gastroenterology 111:1593, 1996.
Rotig A, Cormier V, Blanche S, et al: Pearson's marrow pancreas syndrome. J Clin Invest 86:1601, 1990.
Weizman Z: An update on diseases of the pancreas in children. Curr Opin Pediatr 9:484, 1997.

CHAPTER 350
Treatment of Pancreatic Insufficiency

Treatment of exocrine pancreatic insufficiency by oral enzyme replacement appears simple. However, in practice, although creatorrhea can usually be corrected, steatorrhea is difficult to correct completely. This is due to variability of lipase activity in different commercial preparations, inadequate dosage, incorrect timing of doses, lipase inactivation by gastric acid, and the observation that chymotrypsin in the enzyme preparation digests and thus inactivates lipase. At present, Pancrease, Creon, and Ultrase are the preparations most widely used. These products are enteric-coated preparations that resist gastric acid inactivation.

The dosage of pancreatic replacement for children depends on the amount of food eaten and is established by trial and error. Because these products contain excess protease compared with lipase, the dosage is estimated from the lipase requirement of 1,500 IU/kg/meal. An adequate dose is one that is followed by the return of the stools to normal fat content, size, color, and odor. Enzyme replacement should be given at the beginning of and with the meal. Tablets should be chewed; powder can be mixed with a small quantity of food. Enzyme must also be given with snacks.

When adequate fat absorption is not achieved, gastric acid neutralization with an antacid or an H_2-receptor blocking agent will prevent gastric acid enzyme inactivation and improve delivery of lipase into the intestine. In selected cases, a proton pump inhibitor (omeprazole, lansoprazole) is required. The coating of enteric-coated preparations also protects lipase from acid inactivation.

Untoward effects secondary to pancreatic enzyme replacement therapy include allergic reactions, increased uric acid levels, and kidney stones. *Fibrosing colonopathy,* consisting of colonic fibrosis and strictures, occurs 7–12 mo following high-dose pancreatic supplement therapy (ranging from 6,500 to 58,000 IU lipase/kg/meal).

Smyth RL, Ashby D, O'Hea U, et al: Fibrosing colonopathy in cystic fibrosis: Results of a case control study. Lancet 346:1271, 1995.

CHAPTER 351
Pancreatitis

After cystic fibrosis, acute pancreatitis is probably the most common pancreatic disorder in children. Blunt abdominal injuries, mumps and other viral illnesses, multisystem disease, congenital anomalies, and biliary microlithiasis (sludging) account for most known etiologies; other causes are uncommon (Table 351–1). Many cases are of unknown etiology or are secondary to a systemic disease process. Child abuse is recognized with increased frequency as a cause of traumatic pancreatitis in young children. Disorders newly associated with pancreatitis in children include AIDS, the hemolytic uremic syndrome, organic acidoses, Kawasaki syndrome, refeeding after starvation, pancreas divisum, bone marrow transplantation, brain tumor, and head trauma. Multiple mutated alleles of the cystic fibrosis gene are associated with chronic pancreatitis.

PATHOGENESIS. The precise sequence of events leading to pancreatitis is not well defined. Possibly, following an initial insult such as ductal obstruction, lysosomal hydrolase co-localizes with pancreatic proenzymes within the acinar cell. The pancreatic proenzymes are then activated by cathepsin B, leading to autodigestion, further activation, and release of active proteases. Lecithin is activated by phospholipase A_2 into the toxic lysolecithin. Prophospholipase is unstable and can be activated by minute quantities of trypsin. The healthy pancreas is protected by three factors: (1) the process by which pancreatic proteases are synthesized as inactive proenzymes; (2) the process by which digestive enzymes are segregated into secretory granules at pH 6.2, which minimizes trypsin activity; and (3) the presence of protease inhibitors in both the cytoplasm and the zymogen granules. The histopathologic findings of acute pancreatitis are related to the release of activated proteolytic and lipolytic enzymes. Interstitial edema appears early. Later, as the episode of pancreatitis progresses, localized and confluent necrosis, blood vessel disruption leading to hemorrhage, and an inflammatory response in the peritoneum may develop. The systemic inflammatory response syndrome is noted in most severe cases.

TABLE 351–1 Etiology of Acute Pancreatitis in Children

Drugs and Toxins	Obstructive
Alcohol	Ampullary disease
Acetaminophen overdose	Ascariasis
Azathioprine	Biliary tract malformations
L-Asparaginase	Cholelithiasis and choledocholithiasis (stones or sludge)
Cimetidine	Chlonorchis
Corticosteroids	Duplication cyst
DDC	ERCP complication
DDI	Pancreas divisum
Enalapril	Pancreatic ductal abnormalities
Erythromycin	Postoperative
Estrogen	Sphincter of Oddi dysfunction
Furosemide	Tumor
6-Mercaptopurine	**Systemic Disease**
Mesalamine	Alpha$_1$-antitrypsin deficiency
Methyldopa	Brain tumor
Pentamidine	Collagen vascular diseases
Scorpion bites	Cystic fibrosis
Sulfonamides	Diabetes mellitus
Sulindac	Head trauma
Tetracycline	Hemochromatosis
Thiazides	Hemolytic uremic syndrome
Valproic acid	Hyperlipidemia: types I, IV, V
Vincristine	Hyperparathyroidism
Hereditary Pancreatitis	Kawasaki disease
Infectious	Malnutrition
Ascariasis	Organic acidemia
Coxsackie B virus	Periarteritis nodosa
Epstein-Barr virus	Peptic ulcer
Hepatitis A, B	Renal failure
Influenza A, B	Systemic lupus erythematosus
Leptospirosis	Transplantation: bone marrow, heart, liver, kidney, pancreas
Malaria	Vasculitis
Measles	Venom (spider, scorpion)
Mumps	**Traumatic**
Mycoplasma	Blunt injury
Rubella	Burns
Rubeola	Child abuse
Reye syndrome: varicella, influenza B	Surgical trauma
	Total body cast

CLINICAL MANIFESTATIONS. The patient with acute pancreatitis has abdominal pain, persistent vomiting, and fever. The pain is epigastric and steady, often resulting in the child's assuming an antalgic position with hips and knees flexed, sitting upright, or lying on the side. The child is very uncomfortable and irritable and appears acutely ill. The abdomen may be distended and tender. A mass may be palpable. The pain increases in intensity for 24–48 hr, during which time vomiting may increase and the patient may require hospitalization for dehydration and may need fluid and electrolyte therapy. The prognosis for the acute uncomplicated case is excellent.

Acute hemorrhage pancreatitis, the most severe form of acute pancreatitis, is rare in children. In this life-threatening condition, the patient is acutely ill with severe nausea, vomiting, and abdominal pain. Shock, high fever, jaundice, ascites, hypocalcemia, and pleural effusions may occur. A bluish discoloration may be seen around the umbilicus (Cullen sign) or in the flanks (Grey Turner sign). The pancreas is necrotic and may be transformed into an inflammatory hemorrhagic mass. The mortality rate, which is approximately 50%, is related to the *systemic inflammatory response syndrome* with multiple organ dysfunction: shock, renal failure, acute respiratory distress syndrome, disseminated intravascular coagulation, massive gastrointestinal bleeding, and systemic or intra-abdominal infection. Also see Chapter 64.

DIAGNOSIS. Acute pancreatitis is usually diagnosed by measurement of serum amylase and lipase activities. The serum

TABLE 351–2 Differential Diagnosis of Hyperamylasemia

Pancreatic Pathology
Acute or chronic pancreatitis
Complications of pancreatitis (pseudocyst, ascites, abscess)
Factitious pancreatitis
Salivary Gland Pathology
Parotitis (mumps, *Staphylococcus aureus*, CMV, HIV, EBV)
Sialadenitis (calculus, radiation)
Eating disorders (anorexia nervosa, bulimia)
Intra-Abdominal Pathology
Biliary tract disease (cholelithiasis)
Peptic ulcer perforation
Peritonitis
Intestinal obstruction
Appendicitis
Systemic Diseases
Metabolic acidosis (diabetes mellitus, shock)
Renal insufficiency, transplantation
Burns
Pregnancy
Drugs (morphine)
Head injury
Cardiopulmonary bypass

CMV = cytomegalovirus; HIV = human immunodeficiency virus; EBV = Epstein-Barr virus.

amylase level is typically elevated for up to 4 days. A variety of other conditions may also cause hyperamylasemia without pancreatitis (Table 351–2). Elevation of salivary amylase may mislead the clinician into making the diagnosis of pancreatitis in a child with abdominal pain, but the laboratory can separate amylase isoenzymes into pancreatic and salivary fractions. Initially, serum amylase levels are normal in 10–15% of patients. Serum lipase is more specific than amylase for acute inflammatory pancreatic disease and should be determined when pancreatitis is suspected and the amylase level is normal. The serum lipase typically remains elevated 8–14 days longer than serum amylase. Serum lipase may also be elevated in nonpancreatic diseases.

Other laboratory abnormalities that may be present in acute pancreatitis include hemoconcentration, coagulopathy, leukocytosis, hyperglycemia, glucosuria, hypocalcemia, elevated gamma glutamyl transpeptidase, and hyperbilirubinemia.

Roentgenography of the chest and abdomen may demonstrate nonspecific findings. The chest roentgenogram may demonstrate platelike atelectasis, basilar infiltrates, elevation of the hemidiaphragm, left- (rarely right) sided pleural effusions, pericardial effusion, and pulmonary edema. Abdominal roentgenograms may demonstrate a sentinel loop, dilatation of the transverse colon (cutoff sign), ileus, pancreatic calcification (if recurrent), blurring of the left psoas margin, a pseudocyst, diffuse abdominal haziness (ascites), and peripancreatic extraluminal gas bubbles.

Ultrasound and *CT scanning* have major roles in the diagnosis and follow-up of children with pancreatitis. Findings may include pancreatic enlargement, a hypoechoic, sonolucent edematous pancreas, pancreatic masses, fluid collections, and abscesses (Fig. 351–1); 20% of children with acute pancreatitis initially have normal imaging studies. Endoscopic retrograde cholangiopancreatography (ERCP) is essential in the investigation of recurrent pancreatitis, pancreas divisum, sphincter of Oddi dysfunction, and disease associated with gallbladder pathology. Magnetic resonance cholangiopancreatography (MRCP) and endoscopic ultrasonography are other techniques that visualize the pancreaticobiliary systems.

TREATMENT. The aims of medical management are to relieve pain and restore metabolic homeostasis. Meperidine is the drug of choice for pain relief and should be given in adequate doses. Fluid, electrolyte, and mineral balance should be restored and maintained. Nasogastric suction is useful in patients who are vomiting. The patient should be maintained with nothing by mouth. The routine use of antibiotics is of no benefit during the acute phase unless secondary infection is present. The response to treatment is usually complete over 2–4 days. Refeeding may commence when the serum amylase has normalized and clinical symptoms have resolved.

Although surgical therapy of acute pancreatitis is rarely required, the treatment of severe acute pancreatitis may involve total parenteral nutrition and surgical drainage of necrotic material or abscesses. Other modalities include peritoneal lavage to reduce the risk of secondary infection and the use of trypsin inhibitors. Endoscopic therapy may be of benefit when pancreatitis is caused by anatomic abnormalities, such as strictures or stones.

PROGNOSIS. Children with uncomplicated acute pancreatitis do well and recover over a period of 2–4 days. When pancreatitis is associated with trauma or systemic disease the prognosis is typically related to the associated medical conditions. Measurement of urinary trypsin activation peptide (TAP), the amino terminus peptide split when trypsinogen is activated to trypsin, may be the most sensitive diagnostic test for determining the severity of an episode of acute pancreatitis. TAP measurement is still under study.

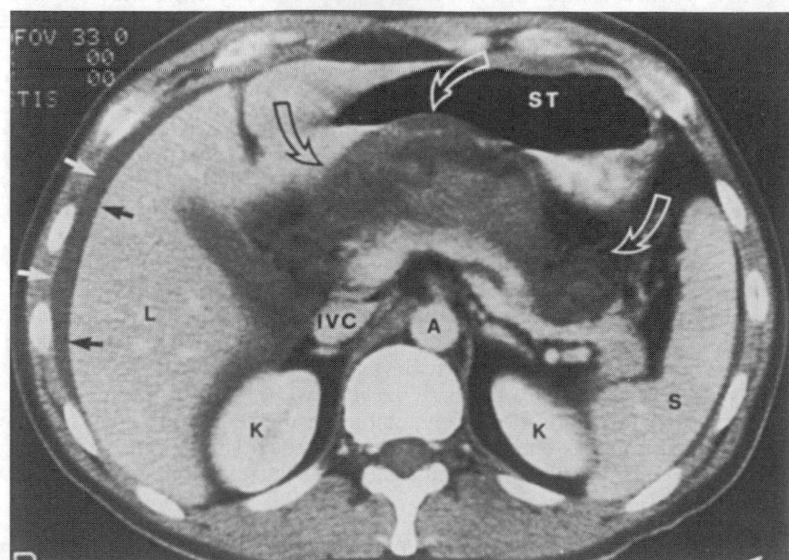

Figure 351–1 Acute pancreatitis. Computed tomography (CT) through the body of the pancreas demonstrates a halo of decreased attenuation around the pancreas that represents a peripancreatic zone of edema and fluid *(curved arrows)*. Note the pancreatic ascites most obvious lateral to the liver *(small arrows)*. If intravenous contrast was administered before the CT scan, the inflamed pancreas would appear more dense (whiter). (L = liver; A = aorta; K = kidney; S = spleen; IVC = inferior vena cava; ST = stomach.) (From Freeny P, Lawson T: The pancreas. *In:* Putman CE, Ravin CE [eds]: Textbook of Diagnostic Imaging. Philadelphia, WB Saunders, 1988.)

Baron T, Morgan D: Acute necrotizing pancreatitis. N Engl J Med 340:1412, 1999.
Blazeby JM, Cooper MJ: Is site of necrosis in acute pancreatitis a predictor of outcome? Lancet 348:1044, 1996.
Greenfield JI, Harmon CM: Acute pancreatitis. Curr Opin Pediatr 9:260, 1997.
Mergener K, Baillie J: Acute pancreatitis. Br Med J 316:44, 1998.
Yeung CY, Lee HC, Huang FY, et al: Pancreatitis in children—experience with 43 cases. Eur J Pediatr 155:458, 1996.

351.1 Chronic Pancreatitis

Chronic, relapsing pancreatitis in children is frequently hereditary or due to congenital anomalies of the pancreatic or biliary ductal system. The former disease is transmitted as an autosomal dominant trait with complete penetrance but variable expressivity. Symptoms frequently begin in the first decade but are usually mild at the onset. Although spontaneous recovery from each attack occurs in 4–7 days, episodes may become progressively severe. Hereditary pancreatitis is diagnosed by the presence of the disease in successive generations of a family. An evaluation during symptom-free intervals may be unrewarding until calcifications, pseudocysts, or pancreatic insufficiency develop. The gene for hereditary pancreatitis has been cloned and mapped to the cationic trypsinogen gene on the long arm of chromosome 7. Cationic trypsinogen has a tendency to autoactivate but has a trypsin-sensitive cleavage site. Loss of this cleavage site in the abnormal protein permits autodigestion of the pancreas.

Other conditions associated with chronic relapsing pancreatitis are hyperlipidemia (types I, IV, and V), hyperparathyroidism, ascariasis, and cystic fibrosis. Most cases of recurrent pancreatitis in childhood are idiopathic; congenital anomalies of the ductal systems, such as pancreas divisum, are probably more common than previously recognized. Mutations of the cystic fibrosis gene have also been associated with chronic idiopathic pancreatitis.

A thorough diagnostic *evaluation* of every child with more than one episode of pancreatitis is indicated. Serum lipid, calcium, and phosphorus levels are determined. Stools are evaluated for *Ascaris*, and a sweat test is performed. Plain abdominal films are evaluated for the presence of pancreatic calcifications. Abdominal ultrasound or CT scanning is performed to detect the presence of a pseudocyst. The biliary tract is evaluated for the presence of stones.

ERCP is a technique that can be used to define the anatomy of the gland and is mandatory whenever surgery is considered. This technique should be performed as part of the evaluation of any child with idiopathic, nonresolving, or recurrent pancreatitis and in patients with a pseudocyst before surgery. In these cases, ERCP may detect a previously undiagnosed anatomic defect that may be amenable to endoscopic or surgical therapy. Endoscopic treatments include sphincterotomy, stone extraction, and insertion of pancreatic or biliary endoprostheses. These treatments allow for successful nonsurgical management of conditions previously requiring surgical intervention. As more experience is gained, MRCP may supplement or replace ERCP.

Brown CB, Werlin SL, Geenen JE, et al: The diagnostic and therapeutic role of endoscopic retrograde cholangiography in children. J Pediatr Gastroenterol Nutr 17:19, 1993.
Durie PR: Pancreatitis and mutations of the cyclic fibrosis gene. N Engl J Med 339:687, 1998.
Mergener K, Baillie J: Chronic pancreatitis. Lancet 350:1379, 1997.
Whitcomb DC, Gorry MC, Preston RA, et al: Hereditary pancreatitis is caused by a mutation in the cationic trypsinogen gene. Nat Genet 14:141, 1996.

CHAPTER 352
Pseudocyst of the Pancreas

Pancreatic pseudocyst formation is an uncommon sequela to acute or chronic pancreatitis. Pseudocysts are sacs delineated by a fibrous wall in the lesser peritoneal sac. They may enlarge or extend in almost any direction, thus producing a wide variety of symptoms (Fig. 352–1).

A pancreatic pseudocyst is suggested when an episode of pancreatitis fails to resolve or when a mass develops after an episode of pancreatitis. Clinical features usually include pain, nausea, and vomiting. The most common signs are a palpable mass in 50% of patients and jaundice in 10%. Other findings include ascites and pleural effusions (usually left-sided).

The most useful diagnostic techniques are ultrasonography, CT scanning, and endoscopic retrograde cholangiopancreatography (ERCP). Because of its ease, availability, and reliability, ultrasonography is the first choice. Sequential ultrasonography studies in adults with pancreatitis suggest that pseudocyst formation is more common than previously thought; most small pseudocysts resolve spontaneously. It is recommended that the patient with acute pancreatitis undergo an ultrasonographic evaluation 2–4 wk after resolution of the acute episode for an evaluation of possible pseudocyst formation.

The treatment for nonresolving, large pseudocysts used to be surgery. Percutaneous and endoscopic drainage of pseudocysts is a safe and effective treatment. A pseudocyst must be allowed to mature for 4–6 wk before surgical drainage is attempted; percutaneous or endoscopic drainage may be attempted earlier. ERCP should precede surgical treatment to help the surgeon plan the approach and define anatomic abnormalities.

Grace PA, Williamson RC: Modern management of pancreatic pseudocysts. Br J Surg 80:573, 1993.
Jaffe RB, Arata IA Jr, Matlak ME: Percutaneous drainage of traumatic pancreatic pseudocysts in children. AJR 152:591, 1989.

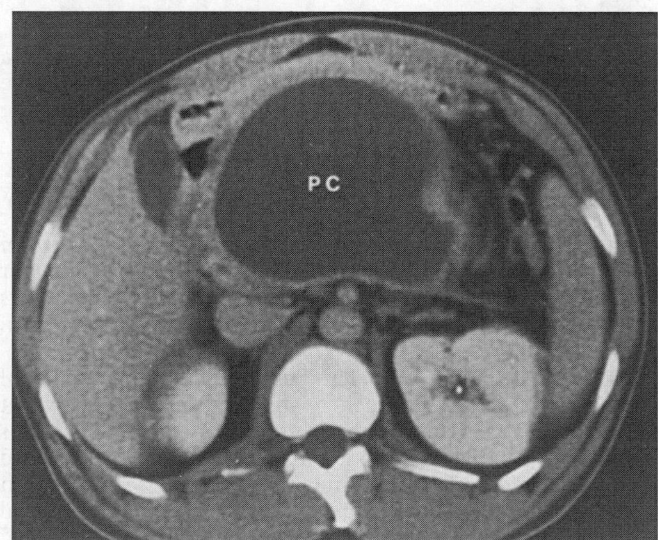

Figure 352–1 Pseudocyst. Follow-up computed tomographic scan 5 mo after the episode of acute pancreatitis demonstrates a large pseudocyst (PC). This large pseudocyst will probably not resolve spontaneously and may need drainage. (From Freeny P, Lawson T: The pancreas. *In:* Putman CE, Ravin CE [eds]: Textbook of Diagnostic Imaging. Philadelphia, WB Saunders, 1988.)

Millar AJW, Rode H, Studen RJ, et al: Management of pancreatic pseudocysts in children. J Pediatr Surg 23:122, 1988.

CHAPTER 353
Pancreatic Tumors

NEOPLASIA. Pancreatic tumors of childhood include α and non-α cell tumors. Non-α cell tumors include gastrinomas and VIPomas. Secretion of gastrin by the gastrinoma produces the Zollinger-Ellison syndrome, with intractable peptic ulcer disease or diarrhea (see Table 345–1). Most gastrinomas arise outside the pancreas. The treatment of choice is surgical removal. If the primary tumor cannot be found or if it has metastasized, cure may not be possible. Treatment with a proton pump inhibitor (omeprazole, lansoprazole), agents that inhibit gastric acid secretion, is then indicated. Gastrectomy is no longer recommended.

The *watery diarrhea–hypokalemia–acidosis syndrome* is usually produced by the secretion of vasoactive intestinal peptide (VIP) by a non-α cell tumor (VIPoma) (see Table 345–1). VIP levels are frequently, but not always, increased in the serum. Treatment is surgical removal of the tumor. When this is not possible, symptoms may be controlled by the use of octreotide acetate (cyclic somatostatin, Sandostatin), a synthetic analog of somatostatin. Pancreatic tumors secreting a variety of hormones, including glucagon, somatostatin, and pancreatic polypeptide, have also been described.

Pancreatoblastomas, pancreatic adenocarcinomas, cystadenomas, and rhabdomyosarcomas are rarely encountered. The *Frantz tumor* is a papillary cystic tumor that is usually found in girls and young women. Presenting symptoms are usually abdominal pain, mass, or jaundice. The treatment of choice is total surgical removal.

Insulinomas and nesidioblastosis or hyperplasia of the β cells produces symptomatic hypoglycemia. Massive subtotal or total pancreatectomy is the treatment of choice when medical treatment fails (Chapter 88). These children may then develop pancreatic insufficiency and diabetes as a complication of treatment.

Maton PN: The management of Zollinger-Ellison syndrome. Aliment Pharmacol Ther 7:467, 1993.

SECTION 6
The Liver and Biliary System

CHAPTER 354
Development and Function

William F. Balistreri

MORPHOGENESIS. The liver and biliary system originate from a cluster of cells that cap a ventral diverticulum in the primitive foregut. The hepatic anlage (pars hepatis) appears during the 4th wk of gestation as a duodenal diverticulum (Fig. 354–1). Within the ventral mesentery proliferation of cells form anastomosing hepatic cords, with the network of primitive liver cells, sinusoids, and septal mesenchyme establishing the basic architectural pattern of liver lobule. The solid *cranial* portion of the hepatic diverticulum eventually forms hepatic glandular tissue and the intrahepatic bile ducts; the *caudal* portion (pars cystica) becomes the gallbladder, cystic duct, and common bile duct.

The hepatic lobules are identifiable at the 6th gestational wk. The liver reaches a peak relative size at the 9th wk at about 10% of the fetal weight. The bile canalicular structures that include microvilli and junctional complexes are specialized loci of the liver cell membrane; these appear very early in gestation, and by 6–7 wk large canaliculi bounded by several hepatocytes are seen. The intrahepatic bile ducts are derived through branching of the hepatic duct; formation is complete by the 3rd mo. The cystic duct and the gallbladder are fully recanalized by the 7th–8th wk.

In the hepatic excretory (biliary) system, intercellular bile canaliculi empty into the smallest bile ductules, which unite to form interlobular bile ducts that follow the terminal branches of the portal vein. At the hilum of the liver, the intrahepatic ducts leave the branches of the portal vein and merge to form the *extrahepatic* biliary system. The ducts of the right and left lobes form the common hepatic duct. The common bile duct is formed from the merger of the common hepatic duct and cystic duct; it extends along the right edge of the lesser omentum, terminating as the intramural papilla of Vater. Union of the biliary tract with the pancreatic ducts forms the ampulla of Vater, which, with the sphincter of Oddi, regulates the flow of bile into the intestine, prevents entry of bile into the pancreatic duct, and inhibits reflux of intestinal contents into the ducts.

The transport and metabolic activities of the liver are facilitated by the structural arrangement of liver cell cords (Fig. 354–1*D*), which are formed by rows of hepatocytes, separated by sinusoids that converge toward the tributaries of the hepatic vein (the central vein) located in the center of the lobule. This establishes the pathways and patterns of flow for substances to and from the liver. Plasma proteins and other plasma components are *secreted* by the liver. Absorbed and circulating nutrients arrive through the portal vein or the hepatic artery and pass through the sinusoids and past the hepatocytes to the systemic circulation at the central vein. Biliary components are transported via the series of enlarging channels from the bile canaliculi through the bile ductule to the common bile duct.

Bile secretion has been noted at the 12th gestational wk. The major components of bile vary with stage of development. Near term, cholesterol and phospholipid content is relatively low; low concentrations of bile acids, the absence of bacterially derived (secondary) bile acids, and the presence of unusual bile acids reflect low rates of bile flow and immature bile acid synthesis.

Fetal hepatic blood flow is derived from the hepatic artery

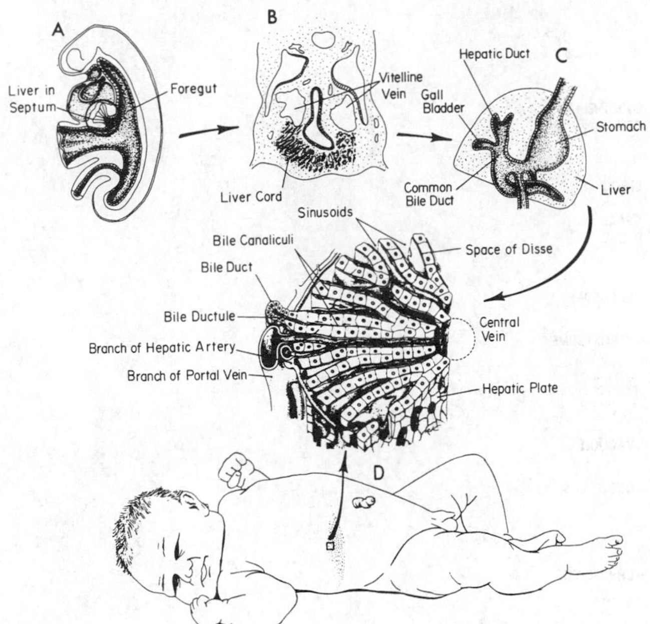

Figure 354–1 Hepatic embryogenesis. *A,* Ventral outgrowth of hepatic diverticulum from foregut endoderm in the 3.5-wk embryo. *B,* Between the two vitelline veins, the enlarging hepatic diverticulum buds off epithelial (liver) cords that become the liver parenchyma, around which the endothelium of capillaries (sinusoids) align (4-wk embryo). *C,* Hemisection of embryo at 7.5 wk demonstrating recanalization of the biliary tract. *D,* Three-dimensional representation of the hepatic lobule as present in the newborn. (From Andres JM, Mathis RK, Walker WA: Liver disease in infants. Parts I and II: Developmental hepatology and mechanisms of liver dysfunction. J Pediatr 90:686 and 964, 1977.)

and from the portal and umbilical veins, which form the portal sinus. The portal venous inflow is directed mainly to the right lobe of the liver; umbilical flow is primarily to the left. The ductus venosus shunts blood from the portal and umbilical veins to the hepatic vein, bypassing the sinusoidal network. The ductus venosus becomes obliterated when oral feedings are initiated. The oxygen saturation is lower in portal than in umbilical venous blood; accordingly, the right hepatic lobe has lower oxygenation and greater hematopoietic activity than the left hepatic lobe. Sinusoidal endothelium is the site of large macrophages, which become the Kupffer (reticuloendothelial) cell network.

The liver constitutes 5% of body weight at birth but only 2% in an adult. Early in gestation (7th wk), hematopoietic cells outnumber functioning hepatocytes in the hepatic anlage. The hepatocytes are smaller (~20 μm) than at maturity (30–35 μm) and contain less glycogen. Near term, the hepatocytes dominate the organ, and cell size and glycogen content increase. Hematopoiesis is virtually absent by the 2nd postnatal month in full-term infants. As the density of hepatocytes increases with gestational age, the relative volume of the sinusoidal network decreases.

ULTRASTRUCTURE. Our understanding of the ultrastructural anatomy of the hepatocyte (Fig. 354–2) has been made possible through electron microscopy and cell fractionation techniques. Various regions of the hepatocyte *plasma membrane* exhibit specialized functions. For example, bidirectional transport occurs at the sinusoidal surface, where materials reaching the liver via the portal system enter and compounds secreted by the liver leave the hepatocyte. Canalicular membranes of adjacent hepatocytes form bile canaliculi, which are bounded by tight junctions preventing transfer of secreted compounds back into the sinusoid. Abundant *mitochondria* are the sites of oxidation and metabolism of heterogeneous classes of substrates, of fatty acid oxidation, of key processes in gluconeogenesis, and of storage and release of energy. The *nucleus* and *nucleolus* are surrounded by a pair of membranes, the outermost of which adjoins the *endoplasmic reticulum.* The latter is a continuous network of rough- and smooth-surfaced tubules and cisternae, which are the site of various processes, including protein and triglyceride synthesis and drug metabolism. The endoplasmic reticulum is the major part of the *microsomal* fraction obtained by ultracentrifugation of liver homogenate. Low fetal activity of microsomal-bound enzymes accounts for a relative inefficiency of xenobiotic (drug) metabolism. The *Golgi apparatus* is active in protein packaging and possibly in bile secretion. Hepatocyte microbodies *(peroxisomes)* are single-membrane-limited cytoplasmic organelles that contain enzymes such as oxidases and catalase and those that have a role in lipid and bile acid metabolism. The *cytoskeleton,* composed of actin filaments, is distributed throughout the cell and concentrated near the plasma membrane. Microfilaments and microtubules may have a role in receptor-mediated endocytosis, in bile secretion, and in maintaining the architecture and motility of the cell. *Lysosomes* contain numerous hydrolases that have a role in intracellular digestion.

FUNCTIONAL DEVELOPMENT. Several of these metabolic processes are immature in a healthy newborn infant, owing in part to the fetal patterns of activity of various enzymatic processes. Many hepatic functions are carried out for a fetus by the maternal liver, which provides nutrients, serves as a route of elimination of metabolic end products, and is a site of biotransformations. Fetal liver metabolism is devoted primarily to the production of proteins for growth requirements. Toward term, primary functions become production and storage of essential nutrients, excretion of bile, and establishment of processes of elimination. Extrauterine adaptation involves de novo enzyme synthesis. Modulation of these processes depends on substrate and hormonal input via the placenta and on dietary and hormonal input in the postnatal period.

354.1 Metabolic Functions of the Liver

CARBOHYDRATE METABOLISM. The liver stores excess carbohydrate as glycogen, a polymer of glucose readily hydrolyzed to glucose during fasting. Immediately after birth, an infant is dependent on hepatic glycogenolysis; thereafter, an infant is capable of both glycogenolysis and gluconeogenesis. Fetal glycogen synthesis begins at about the 9th wk of gestation, with glycogen stores most rapidly accumulated near term, when the liver contains two to three times the amount of glycogen of adult liver. Most of this stored glycogen is used in the immediate postnatal period. Reaccumulation is initiated at about the 2nd wk of postnatal life, and glycogen stores reach adult levels at approximately the 3rd wk in healthy full-term infants. The fluctuations in serum glucose concentration in preterm infants are due in part to the fact that efficient regulation of the synthesis, storage, and degradation of glycogen develops only near the end of full-term gestation. Dietary carbohydrates such as galactose are converted to glucose, but there is a substantial dependence on gluconeogenesis for glucose in early life, especially if glycogen stores are limited. Gluconeogenic activity is present in the fetal liver but increases rapidly after birth.

PROTEIN METABOLISM. During the rapid fetal growth phase, specific decarboxylases that are rate limiting in the biosynthesis of physiologically important polyamines have higher activities than in the mature liver. The rate of synthesis of albumin and secretory proteins in the developing liver parallels the quantitative changes in endoplasmic reticulum. Synthesis of albumin appears at approximately the 7th–8th wk in a human fetus and increases in inverse proportion to that of α-fetoprotein, which is a dominant fetal protein. By the 3rd–4th mo of

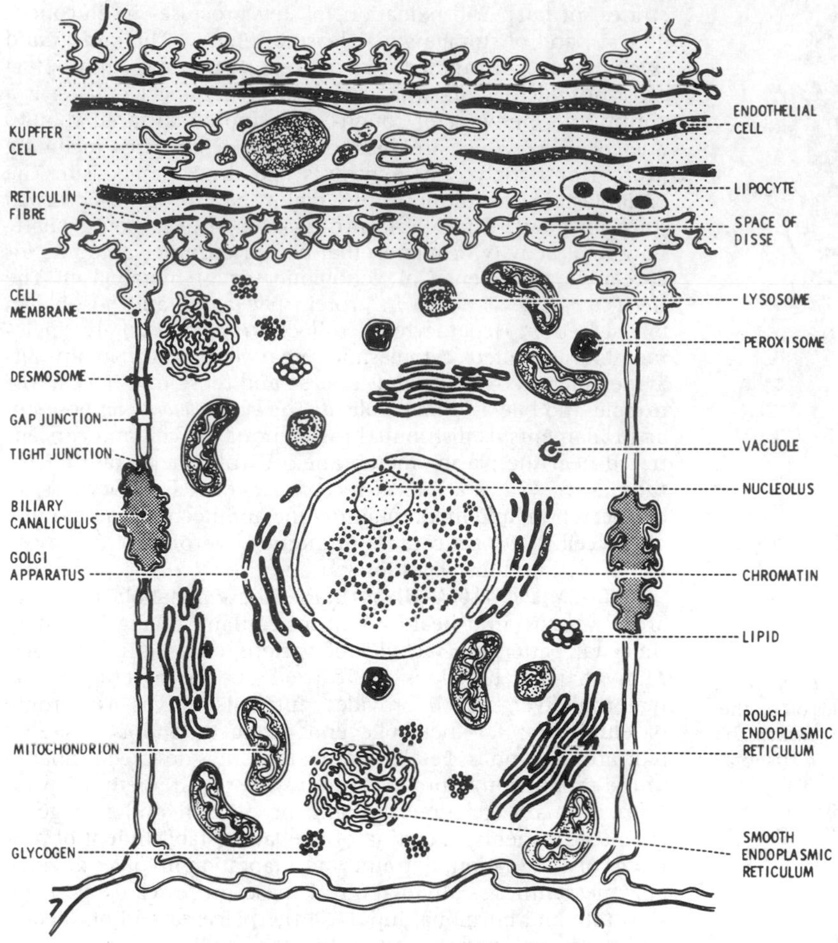

Figure 354–2 Hepatic ultrastructure, conceptualized. Electron microscopic appearance of a normal human liver cell. (From Sherlock S: Hepatic cell structure. *In:* Sherlock S (ed): Diseases of the Liver and Biliary System, Chapter 1. Oxford, Blackwell Scientific, 1981.)

gestation, the fetal liver is able to produce fibrinogen, transferrin, and low-density lipoproteins. From this period on, fetal plasma contains each of the major protein classes, at concentrations considerably below those achieved at maturity.

The *postnatal* patterns of development of various proteins are heterogeneous. Lipoproteins of each class rise abruptly in the 1st wk after birth to reach levels that vary little until puberty. Albumin concentrations are low in a neonate (~2.5 g/dL), reaching adult levels (~3.5 g/dL) after several months. Levels of ceruloplasmin and complement factors increase slowly to adult values during the 1st year. In contrast, transferrin levels at birth are similar to those of an adult, decline for 3–5 mo, and rise thereafter to achieve their final concentrations. Low levels of activity of specific proteins have implications for the nutrition of an infant; for example, a low level of cystathionase activity impairs the trans-sulfuration pathway by which dietary methionine is converted to cystine; accordingly, the latter must be supplied exogenously. Similar dietary requirements may exist for other sulfur-containing amino acids, such as taurine.

LIPID METABOLISM. Fatty acid oxidation provides a major source of energy in early life, complementing glycogenolysis and gluconeogenesis. Newborn infants are relatively intolerant of prolonged fasting, owing in part to a restricted capacity for hepatic ketogenesis. Rapid maturation of the ability of the liver to oxidize fatty acid occurs during the 1st few days of life. Milk provides the major source of calories in early life; this high-fat, low-carbohydrate diet mandates active gluconeogenesis to maintain blood sugar levels. When the glucose supply is limited, ketone body production from endogenous fatty acids may provide energy for hepatic gluconeogenesis and an alternative fuel for brain metabolism. When carbohydrates are in excess, the liver produces triglycerides. Metabolic processes involving lipid and lipoprotein are predominantly hepatic; liver immaturity or disease affects lipid concentrations and lipoproteins.

BIOTRANSFORMATION. Newborn infants have a decreased capacity to metabolize and detoxify certain drugs, owing to underdevelopment of the hepatic microsomal component that is the site of the specific oxidative, reductive, hydrolytic, and conjugation reactions required for these biotransformations (Chapter 727). The major components of the mono-oxygenase system, such as cytochrome P450, the reduced form of nicotinamide-adenine dinucleotide phosphate, and cytochrome-C reductase, are present in low concentrations in fetal microsomal preparations. In full-term infants, hepatic uridine diphosphate (UDP) glucuronyl transferase and enzymes involved in the oxidation of polycyclic aromatic hydrocarbons have very low activities. Age-related differences in pharmacokinetics vary. For example, the half-life of acetaminophen in a newborn is similar to that of an adult, whereas theophylline has a half-life of approximately 100 hr in a premature infant and 5–6 hr in an adult. These physiologic variables taken together with factors such as binding to plasma proteins and renal clearance are important in determining drug dosage and in the production of toxicity. Dramatic examples of the susceptibility of newborn infants to drug toxicity are the responses to chloramphenicol (gray syndrome) or to benzoyl alcohol and its metabolic products, which involve ineffective glucuronide and glycine conjugation, respectively. The low concentrations of antioxidants (vitamin E, superoxide dismutase, and glutathione peroxidase) in the fetal and early newborn liver lead to increased susceptibility to deleterious effects of oxygen toxicity through lipid peroxidation.

Conjugation reactions (which convert drugs or metabolites

TABLE 354–1 Potential Sites for Disturbances in Bile Acid Metabolism

Defective bile acid synthesis may result from:

Specific defects in bile acid synthesis as seen in the following:
- Cerebrotendinous xanthomatosis
- Intrahepatic cholestasis (neonatal hepatitis)
  - Qualitative abnormalities (reductase deficiency, isomerase deficiency)
  - Quantitative abnormalities

Acquired defects in bile acid synthesis (as observed in severe liver disease, such as hepatitis and metabolic liver disease)

Abnormalities of bile acid delivery to the bowel may be seen in:

Celiac sprue (sluggish gallbladder contraction)

Extrahepatic bile duct obstruction caused by the following:
- Biliary atresia
- Stricture
- Stone
- Malignancy

Interruption of the enterohepatic circulation of bile acids may occur with:

An external bile fistula

Ileojejunal exclusion for exogenous obesity or hypercholesterolemia

Cystic fibrosis

Contaminated small bowel syndrome (with bile acid precipitation, increased jejunal absorption, and "short circuiting")

Entrapment of bile acids in intestinal lumen by:
- Cholestyramine
- Trivalent cations (aluminum-containing antacids)
- Fiber

Bile acid malabsorption

Primary bile acid malabsorption (absent or inefficient ileal active transport)
- Intractable diarrhea (infancy)
- Irritable bowel (adults)

Secondary bile acid malabsorption
- Ileal disease or resection
  - Crohn disease
  - Ileal resection
  - Ileal bypass
  - Radiation enteritis
  - Postinfectious enteritis
  - Short-gut syndrome
- Exogenous bile acid administration (e.g., gallstone dissolution)
- Cystic fibrosis

Tertiary bile acid malabsorption
- Postcholecystectomy
- Renal failure
- Drugs

Defective uptake or altered intracellular metabolism

Parenchymal disease (acute hepatitis, cirrhosis)
- Regurgitation from cells
- Portosystemic shunting

Cholestasis

into forms that can be eliminated in bile) also are catalyzed by hepatic microsomal enzymes. For example, newborn infants have decreased activity of UDP-glucuronyl transferase, which converts unconjugated bilirubin to the readily excreted glucuronide conjugate and is the rate-limiting enzyme in the excretion of bilirubin (Chapter 98.3). There is rapid postnatal development of transferase activity, even in prematurely born infants, irrespective of gestational age; this suggests that birth-related rather than age-related factors are of primary importance in the postnatal development of activity of this enzyme. Microsomal activity can be stimulated by administration of phenobarbital or other inducers of cytochrome P450. Alternatively, drugs such as cimetidine may inhibit microsomal P450 activity.

HEPATIC EXCRETORY FUNCTION

Hepatic excretory function and bile flow are closely related to bile acid excretion and recirculation. Bile acids are the major product of degradation of cholesterol. Their incorporation into mixed micelles with cholesterol and phospholipid creates an efficient vehicle for solubilization and intestinal absorption of lipophilic compounds, such as dietary fats and fat-soluble vitamins. Secretion of bile acids is the major determinant of bile flow in the mature animal. Accordingly, the maturity of bile acid metabolic processes affects overall hepatic excretory function, including biliary excretion of endogenous and exogenous compounds.

In humans, two bile acids (cholic and chenodeoxycholic acid—the primary bile acids) are synthesized in the liver. Before excretion, they are conjugated with glycine and taurine. In response to a meal, contraction of the gallbladder delivers bile acids to the intestine to assist in fat digestion and absorption. After mediating fat digestion, the bile acids themselves are reabsorbed from the terminal ileum through specific active transport processes. They return to the liver via portal blood, are taken up by liver cells, and are re-excreted in bile. In an adult, this enterohepatic circulation involves 90–95% of the circulating bile acid pool. Bile acids that escape ileal reabsorption reach the colon, where the bacterial flora, through dehydroxylation and deconjugation, produces the secondary bile acids, deoxycholate and lithocholate. In an adult, the composition of bile reflects the excretion of not only the primary but also the secondary bile acids, which are reabsorbed from the distal intestinal tract.

Neonates have inefficient ileal reabsorption and a low rate of hepatic clearance of bile acids from portal blood. The latter results in elevated serum concentrations of bile acids in healthy newborns, often to levels that would suggest liver disease in older individuals. The size of the bile acid pool in a neonate is about half that of an adult, and the bile acid concentration in the proximal intestinal lumen is similarly decreased to levels that are frequently below the concentration required for micelle formation (2 mM); accordingly, absorption of dietary fats and fat-soluble vitamins is reduced but not sufficiently to produce malabsorption. Transient phases of "physiologic cholestasis" and "physiologic steatorrhea" have a role in the nutrition of low birthweight infants but are of minor importance to healthy full-term newborns.

Beyond the neonatal period, disturbances in bile acid metabolism may be responsible for diverse effects on hepatobiliary and intestinal function (Table 354–1).

Andres JM, Mathis RK, Walker WA: Liver disease in infants: Part I. Developmental hepatology and mechanisms of liver dysfunction. J Pediatr 90:686, 1977.

Andres JM, Mathis RK, Walker WA: Liver disease in infants: Part II. Developmental hepatology and mechanisms of liver dysfunction. J Pediatr 90:964, 1977.

Balistreri WF: Anatomic and biochemical ontogeny of the gastrointestinal tract and liver. *In:* Tsang RC, Nichols BL (eds): Nutrition during Infancy. Philadelphia, Hanley & Belfus, 1987, pp 33–57.

Balistreri WF, Heubi JI, Suchy FJ: Immaturity of the enterohepatic circulation in early life: Factors predisposing to "physiologic" maldigestion and cholestasis. J Pediatr Gastroenterol Nutr 2:346, 1983.

Cox KL, Cheung ATW, Lohse CL, et al: Biliary motility postnatal changes in guinea pigs. Pediatr Res 21:170, 1987.

Desmet VJ: Congenital diseases of intrahepatic bile ducts: Variations on the theme "ductal plate malformation." Hepatology 16:1069, 1992.

Fausto N, Mead JE: Regulation of liver growth: Protooncogenes and transforming growth factors. Lab Invest 60:4, 1989.

Hansen TWR, Mathiesen SBW, Walaas SI: Modulation of the effect of bilirubin on protein phosphorylation by lysine-containing peptides. Pediatr Res 42:615, 1997.

Hutchins GM, Moore GW: Growth and asymmetry of the human liver during the embryonic period. Pediatr Pathol 8:17, 1988.

Provisional Committee for Quality Improvement and Subcommittee on Hyperbilirubinemia. Practice parameter: Management of hyperbilirubinemia in the healthy term newborn. Pediatrics 94:558, 1994.

Rudolph AM: Hepatic and ductus venosus blood flows during fetal life. Hepatology 3:254, 1983.

Shah RD, Gerber MA: Development of intrahepatic bile ducts in humans: Possible role of laminin. Arch Pathol Lab Med 114:597, 1990.

Suchy FJ, Bucuvalas JC, Novak DA: Determinant of bile formation during development: Ontogeny of hepatic bile acid metabolism and transport. Semin Liver Dis 7:77, 1987.

Zaret KS: Molecular genetics of early liver development. Annu Rev Physiol 58:231, 1996.

CHAPTER 355
Manifestations of Liver Disease

William F. Balistreri

PATHOLOGIC MANIFESTATIONS. Alterations in hepatic structure and function can be *acute* or *chronic,* with varying patterns of reaction of the liver to cell injury. The ultimate reaction is cell death, but hepatocytes have a remarkable capacity for regeneration. Collagen is formed during the healing phase of cellular injury, with excessive growth of fibrous tissue being manifested as cirrhosis.

Inflammation or necrosis, or both, of individual hepatocytes can be due to viral infection, drugs or toxins, immunologic disorders, or hypoxia. The evolving process leads to repair, continuing injury with chronic changes, or in rare cases to massive hepatic damage.

Cholestasis is an alternative or concomitant response to injury. It is defined as accumulation in serum of substances normally excreted in bile such as bilirubin, cholesterol, bile acids, and trace elements. A liver biopsy specimen demonstrates accumulation of bile and bile pigment in the parenchyma. In extrahepatic obstruction, bile pigment may be visible in the intralobular bile ducts or throughout the parenchyma as bile lakes or infarcts. Cholestasis may also be seen without evidence of bile duct obstruction, when hepatocyte injury or an alteration in hepatic physiology has led to a reduction in the rate of secretion of solute and water. Likely causes may include alterations in the ultrastructure or cytoskeleton of the hepatocyte, alterations in organelles responsible for bile secretion, alterations in enzymatic activity, or alterations in permeability of the bile canalicular apparatus. The end result is clinically indistinguishable from obstructive cholestasis.

Cirrhosis (defined histologically by the presence of bands of fibrous tissue that link central and portal areas and form parenchymal nodules) is a potential end stage of any acute or chronic liver disease. Cirrhosis may be posthepatitic (after acute or chronic hepatitis) or postnecrotic (after toxic injury), or it may follow chronic biliary obstruction (biliary cirrhosis). Cirrhosis may be **macronodular,** with nodules of various sizes (up to 5 cm) separated by broad septa, or **micronodular,** with nodules of uniform size (<1 cm) separated by fine septa. Mixed forms also occur. The progressive scarring of cirrhosis leads to altered hepatic blood flow, with further impairment of liver cell function. In addition, the restriction of blood flow within the liver leads to portal hypertension.

Primary tumors of the liver are discussed in Chapter 510.

The liver may be **secondarily** involved in neoplastic (metastatic) and non-neoplastic (storage diseases and fat infiltration) and infectious processes. The liver may also be affected by chronic passive congestion or acute hypoxia, with hepatocellular damage.

CLINICAL MANIFESTATIONS

Hepatomegaly. Enlargement of the liver can be due to several mechanisms (Table 355–1). Concepts of normal liver size have been based on age-related clinical indices, such as (1) the degree of extension of the liver edge below the costal margin, (2) the span of dullness to percussion, or (3) the length of the vertical axis of the liver, as estimated from imaging techniques. In children, the normal liver edge can be felt up to 2 cm below the right costal margin. In a newborn infant, extension of the liver edge more than 3.5 cm below the costal margin in the right midclavicular line suggests hepatic enlargement. Measurement of *liver span* is carried out by percussing the upper margin of dullness and by palpating the lower edge in the right midclavicular line; it may be more reliable than an extension of the liver edge alone, and the two measurements may correlate poorly.

TABLE 355–1 Mechanisms of Hepatomegaly

Increase in the Number or Size of the Cells in the Liver

Storage
- *Fat:* malnutrition, obesity, metabolic liver disease (e.g., diseases of fatty acid oxidation and Reye syndrome–like illnesses), lipid infusion (total parenteral nutrition), cystic fibrosis, diabetes mellitus, medication related, pregnancy
- *Specific lipid storage diseases:* Gaucher, Niemann-Pick, Wolman disease
- *Glycogen:* glycogen storage diseases (multiple enzyme defects); total parenteral nutrition; infant of diabetic mother, Beckwith syndrome
- *Miscellaneous:* α_1-antitrypsin deficiency, Wilson disease, hypervitaminosis A, neonatal iron storage

Inflammation

- Hepatocyte enlargement (hepatitis)
  - Viral—acute and chronic
  - Bacterial (sepsis, abscess, cholangitis)
  - Toxic (e.g., drugs)
- Kupffer cell enlargement
- Autoimmune: chronic hepatitis, sarcoidosis, systemic lupus erythematosus, sclerosing cholangitis

Infiltration

- Primary tumors
  - Hepatoblastoma
  - Hepatocellular carcinoma
  - Hemangioma
  - Focal nodular hyperplasia
- Secondary or metastatic tumors
  - Lymphoma
  - Leukemia
  - Histiocytosis
  - Neuroblastoma
  - Wilms tumor

Increased Size of Vascular Space

- Intrahepatic obstruction to hepatic vein outflow
  - Veno-occlusive disease
  - Hepatic vein thrombosis (Budd-Chiari syndrome)
  - Hepatic vein web
- Suprahepatic
  - Congestive heart failure
  - Pericardial disease
  - Tamponade
  - Constrictive pericarditis
  - Hematopoietic: sickle cell anemia, thalassemia

Increased Size of Biliary Space

- Congenital hepatic fibrosis
- Caroli disease
- Extrahepatic obstruction

Idiopathic (? "Benign")

The liver span increases linearly with body weight and age in both sexes. If percussion is used for both the upper and lower borders, the mean liver span is related curvilinearly to age. The span ranges from about 4.5–5 cm at 1 wk of age to approximately 7–8 cm in boys and 6–6.5 cm in girls by 12 yr of age. The expected span of liver dullness in the midclavicular line in both sexes after 12 yr of age can be calculated as follows: in males, span (cm) = 0.032 × weight (pounds) + 0.18 × height (inches) − 7.86; in females, span (cm) = 0.027 × weight (pounds) + 0.22 × height (inches) − 10.75. These formulas are not accurate for newborns or younger children. In some persons, the lower edge of the right lobe of the liver extends downward **(Riedel lobe)** and may be palpable as a broad mass. Downward displacement of the liver by the diaphragm or thoracic organs can create an erroneous impression of hepatomegaly.

Examination of the liver should note the consistency, contour, tenderness, or the presence of any masses or bruits, as well as assessing splenic size.

Ultrasonography can often help in evaluating unexplained hepatomegaly; size and consistency can be assessed. Hyperechogenic hepatic parenchyma can be seen with metabolic disease (glycogen storage disease) or fatty liver (due to malnutrition or hyperalimentation or after corticosteroid therapy).

Ultrasonography can also assess **gallbladder size.** Gallbladder distention may be seen in sick infants who have sepsis. Gallbladder length normally varies from 1.5–5.5 cm (average, 3.0) in infants to 4–8 cm in adolescents; width ranges from 0.5–2.5 cm (mean, 0.8 in neonates) at all ages.

Jaundice. Yellow discoloration of the plasma, skin, and mucous membranes may be the earliest and only sign of hepatic dysfunction; it therefore requires urgent evaluation. Jaundice becomes clinically apparent in children and adults when the serum concentration of bilirubin reaches 2–3 mg/dL. In neonates, higher levels may be found without evident icterus. Icterus may be associated with dark urine or acholic (light-colored) stools.

Bilirubin occurs in plasma in four forms: (1) *unconjugated bilirubin* tightly bound to albumin; (2) *free* or *unbound bilirubin* (the form responsible for kernicterus, because it can cross cell membranes); (3) *conjugated bilirubin* (the only fraction to appear in urine); and (4) δ *fraction* (bilirubin covalently bound to albumin), which appears in serum when hepatic excretion of conjugated bilirubin is impaired in patients with hepatobiliary disease. The δ fraction permits conjugated bilirubin to persist in the circulation and delays resolution of jaundice.

Measurement of serum bilirubin is traditionally via the van den Bergh (diazo) reaction. The terms "direct-reacting" and "indirect-reacting" bilirubin correspond roughly to *conjugated* and *unconjugated* bilirubin, respectively. Routine automated procedures to measure *conjugated* bilirubin significantly overestimate the direct-reacting fraction at relatively low total bilirubin concentrations. Cholestasis can be precluded by measuring serum bile acids, which are elevated in the presence of any form of cholestasis.

Jaundice in an infant or older child may reflect accumulation of either unconjugated or conjugated bilirubin. An increase in unconjugated bilirubin may indicate increased production, hemolysis, reduced hepatic removal, or altered metabolism of bilirubin (Table 355–2). Significant accumulations of conjugated bilirubin (>20% of total) reflect decreased excretion by damaged hepatic parenchymal cells or disease of biliary tract, which may be due to sepsis, endocrine or metabolic disease, inflammation of the liver, or obstruction (Table 355–3). In most patients with diseases that tend to produce **conjugated** hyperbilirubinemia, a portion of the total bilirubin is present in **unconjugated** form, with near-parallel rises in both fractions.

Pruritus. Intense generalized itching may occur in patients with cholestasis (conjugated hyperbilirubinemia), presumably owing to retained components of bile. Symptomatic relief of pruritus follows administration of bile acid–binding agents such as cholestyramine or choleretic agents such as ursodeoxycholic acid. Pruritus is unrelated to the degree of hyperbilirubinemia; deeply jaundiced patients may be asymptomatic, and vice versa.

Spider Angiomas. Vascular spiders (telangiectasias), characterized by central pulsating arterioles from which small, wiry venules radiate, may be seen in patients with chronic liver disease. These are presumably reflective of altered estrogen metabolism in the presence of hepatic dysfunction.

Palmar Erythema. Blotchy erythema, most noticeable over the thenar and hypothenar eminences and on the tips of the fingers, is also noted in patients with chronic liver disease. These may be due to vasodilation and increased blood flow.

Xanthomas. The marked elevation of serum cholesterol (to levels >500 mg/dL) associated with chronic cholestasis may cause the deposition of lipid in the dermis and subcutaneous tissue. Brown nodules may develop first over the extensor surfaces of the extremities; rarely, xanthelasma of the eyelids develops.

Portal Hypertension. The portal vein drains the splanchnic area (abdominal portion of the gastrointestinal tract, pancreas, and

TABLE 355–2 Differential Diagnosis of Unconjugated Hyperbilirubinemia

Increased Production of Unconjugated Bilirubin from Heme

- Hemolytic disease (hereditary or acquired)
  - Isoimmune hemolysis (neonatal; acute or delayed transfusion reaction; autoimmune)
    - Rh incompatibility
    - ABO incompatibility
    - Other blood group incompatibilities
  - Congenital spherocytosis
  - Hereditary elliptocytosis
  - Infantile pyknocytosis
  - Erythrocyte enzyme defects:
    - Glucose-6-phosphate dehydrogenase
    - Pyruvate kinase
    - Hexokinase
  - Hemoglobinopathy
    - Sickle cell anemia
    - Thalassemia
    - Others
  - Sepsis
  - Microangiopathy
    - Hemolytic-uremic syndrome
    - Hemangioma
    - Mechanical trauma (heart valve)
- Ineffective erythropoiesis
- Drugs
- Infection
- Enclosed hematoma
- Polycythemia
  - Diabetic mother
  - Fetal transfusion (recipient)
  - Delayed cord clamping

Decreased Delivery of Unconjugated Bilirubin (in Plasma) to Hepatocyte

- Right-sided congestive heart failure
- Portacaval shunt

Decreased Bilirubin Uptake Across Hepatocyte Membrane

- Presumed enzyme transporter deficiency
- Competitive inhibition
  - Breast milk jaundice
  - Lucey-Driscoll syndrome
  - Drug inhibition (radiocontrast material)
- Miscellaneous
  - Hypothyroidism
  - Hypoxia
  - Acidosis

Decreased Storage of Unconjugated Bilirubin in Cytosol (Decreased Y and Z Proteins)

- Competitive inhibition
- Fever

Decreased Biotransformation (Conjugation)

- Neonatal jaundice (physiologic)
- Inhibition (drugs)
- Hereditary (Crigler-Najjar)
  - Type I (complete enzyme deficiency)
  - Type II (partial deficiency)
- Gilbert disease
- Hepatocellular dysfunction

Enterohepatic Recirculation

- Intestinal obstruction
  - Ileal atresia
  - Hirschsprung disease
  - Cystic fibrosis
  - Pyloric stenosis
- Antibiotic administration

Breast Milk Jaundice

TABLE 355–3 Differential Diagnosis of Neonatal and Infantile Cholestasis

Infectious

- Generalized bacterial sepsis
- Viral hepatitis
  - Hepatitis A, B, C (rare)
  - Cytomegalovirus
  - Rubella virus
  - Herpes virus HSV, HHV_6
  - Varicella virus
  - Coxsackievirus
  - Echovirus
  - Reovirus type 3
  - Parvovirus B19
  - HIV
- Others
  - Toxoplasmosis
  - Syphilis
  - Tuberculosis
  - Listeriosis

Toxic

- Parenteral nutrition related
- Sepsis (e.g., urinary tract) with endotoxemia
- Drug related

Metabolic

- Disorders of **amino acid** metabolism
  - Tyrosinemia
- Disorders of **lipid** metabolism
  - Wolman disease
  - Niemann-Pick disease (type C)
  - Gaucher disease
- Disorders of **carbohydrate** metabolism
  - Galactosemia
  - Fructosemia
  - Glycogenosis IV
- Disorders of **bile acid biosynthesis** (reductase, isomerase deficiency)
- Other metabolic defects
  - α_1-Antitrypsin deficiency
  - Cystic fibrosis
  - Idiopathic hypopituitarism
  - Hypothyroidism
  - Zellweger (cerebrohepatorenal) syndrome
  - Neonatal iron storage disease
  - Indian childhood cirrhosis/infantile copper overload
  - Familial erythrophagocytic lymphohistiocytosis (FELS)
  - Arginase deficiency
  - Mitochrondrial hepatopathies

Genetic/Chromosomal

- Trisomy E
- Down syndrome
- Donahue syndrome (leprechaunism)

Intrahepatic Diseases of Unknown Cause

- Intrahepatic cholestasis—persistent
  - "Idiopathic" neonatal hepatitis
  - Alagillc syndrome (arteriohepatic dysplasia)
  - Intrahepatic biliary hypoplasia or paucity of intrahepatic bile ducts (nonsyndromic)
  - Byler disease (progressive familial intrahepatic cholestasis)
- Intrahepatic cholestasis—recurrent
  - Familial benign recurrent cholestasis associated with lymphedema (Aagenaes)
- Congenital hepatic fibrosis
- Caroli disease (cystic dilatation of intrahepatic ducts)

Extrahepatic Diseases

- Biliary atresia
- Sclerosing cholangitis
- Bile duct stenosis
- Choledochal-pancreaticoductal junction anomaly
- Spontaneous perforation of the bile duct
- Choledochal cyst
- Mass (neoplasia, stone)
- Bile/mucous plug ("inspissated bile")

Miscellaneous

- Histiocytosis X
- Shock and hypoperfusion
- Associated with enteritis
- Associated with intestinal obstruction
- Neonatal lupus erythematosus
- Myeloproliferative disease (21-trisomy)

spleen) into the hepatic sinusoids. Pressure is normally slightly higher (~5–10 mm Hg) in the portal vein than in other venous systems in order to overcome the resistance of the sinusoidal system. Portal hypertension is defined as an increase in portal venous pressure to greater than 20 mm Hg (Chapter 366).

Ascites. Ascites may be associated with urinary tract abnormalities, metabolic diseases (such as lysosomal storage diseases), congenital or acquired heart disease, and hydrops fetalis. Intra-abdominal accumulation of fluid is a common manifestation of end-stage liver disease. In patients with significant hepatic disease, sinusoidal blockade caused by cirrhosis increases hydrostatic pressure and transudation of fluid; this may be worsened by hypoalbuminemia (Chaptesr 366 and 369).

Encephalopathy. Metabolic abnormalities may complicate acute or chronic liver disorders, leading to encephalopathy, with neuropsychiatric disturbances that may include neuromuscular dysfunction, altered mentation, altered consciousness, or coma. With chronic liver disease, hepatic encephalopathy may be recurrent and precipitated by intercurrent illness, drugs, bleeding, or electrolyte and acid-base disturbances.

Hepatic encephalopathy is characterized by profound neural inhibition, which may be due to an interaction between γ-aminobutyric acid (GABA, the primary inhibitory neurotransmitter) and GABA receptors on postsynaptic neurons. With hepatic failure, GABA produced by bacterial flora is not cleared from the blood but crosses the blood-brain barrier and produces inhibition. There may be a simultaneous decrease in excitatory neurotransmission. Other neuroactive or vasoactive compounds, such as glycine or amines, may be synergistic. Alternative theories ascribe a pathogenetic role to ammonia, to synergistic neurotoxins, or to "false neurotransmitters" with plasma amino acid imbalance (Chapter 363).

Endocrine Abnormalities. Endocrine abnormalities are more common in adults with hepatic disease than in children. They reflect alterations in hepatic synthetic, storage, and metabolic functions, including those concerned with hormonal metabolism in the liver. For example, proteins such as those that bind hormones in plasma are synthesized in the liver, and steroid hormones are conjugated in the liver and excreted in the urine; failure of such functions may have clinical consequences. Endocrine abnormalities may also result from malnutrition or specific deficiencies.

Renal Dysfunction. There is a close relationship between hepatic and renal dysfunction. Systemic disease or toxins may affect both organs simultaneously, or parenchymal liver disease may produce secondary impairment of renal function, and vice versa. In hepatobiliary disorders, there may be renal alterations in sodium and water economy, impaired renal concentrating ability, and alterations in potassium metabolism. Ascites in patients with cirrhosis may be related to inappropriate retention of sodium by the kidneys, with expansion of plasma volume, or to sodium retention mediated by diminished effective plasma volume.

Hepatorenal syndrome is defined as renal failure (azotemia and progressive oliguria) in a patient with cirrhosis (often with refractory ascites) and no other demonstrable cause of renal failure. This complication represents a complex sequence of compensation and decompensation in end-stage liver disease. The pathophysiology is poorly defined but seems to involve altered renal blood flow and altered hormone metabolism.

Intense vasoconstriction of the renal cortical vessels is mediated by hemodynamic, humoral, or neurogenic mechanisms. The urinary sodium concentration is low, and the sediment is normal. In management, a trial of volume expansion is warranted to preclude the possibility of prerenal azotemia secondary to volume depletion.

MISCELLANEOUS MANIFESTATIONS OF LIVER DYSFUNCTION. Nonspecific signs of acute and chronic liver disease include (1) anorexia, which often affects patients with anicteric hepatitis and with cirrhosis associated with chronic cholestasis; (2) abdominal pain or distention resulting from ascites, spontaneous peritonitis, or visceromegaly; and (3) bleeding, which may be due to altered synthesis of coagulation factors (biliary obstruction with vitamin K deficiency or excessive hepatic damage) or to portal hypertension. There may be decreased synthesis of specific clotting factors, production of qualitatively abnormal proteins, or alterations in platelet number and function in the presence of hypersplenism. Altered drug metabolism may prolong the biologic half-life of commonly administered medications.

355.1 Evaluation of Patients with Possible Liver Dysfunction

Adequate evaluation of an infant, child, or adolescent with suspected liver disease involves an appropriate and accurate history, a carefully performed physical examination, and skillful interpretation of signs and symptoms. Further evaluation is aided by judicious selection of diagnostic tests, followed by a liver biopsy or the use of imaging modalities. Most of the so-called liver function tests do not measure specific hepatic functions; a rise in serum aminotransferase (transaminase) activity reflects liver cell injury; an increase in immunoglobulin level reflects an immunologic response to injury; or an elevation in serum bilirubin level may reflect any of several disturbances of bilirubin metabolism outlined in Tables 355–2 and 355–3. Any single biochemical assay provides limited information, which must be placed in the context of the entire clinical and historic picture. The most cost efficient approach is for clinicians to become familiar with the rationale, implications, and limitations of a selected group of tests so that specific questions can be answered.

For a patient with suspected liver disease, evaluation addresses the following issues in sequence: (1) Is liver disease present? (2) If so, what is its nature? (3) What is its severity? (4) Is specific treatment available? (5) How can we monitor the response to treatment? and (6) What is the prognosis?

BIOCHEMICAL TESTS. Laboratory tests commonly used to screen for or to confirm a suspicion of liver disease include measurements of serum bilirubin level and of aminotransferase and alkaline phosphatase activities often with determinations of prothrombin time and albumin level. These tests are complementary and provide an estimation of synthetic and excretory functions and may suggest the nature of the disturbance (e.g., inflammation or cholestasis).

Acute liver cell injury (parenchymal disease) in viral hepatitis, drug- or toxin-induced liver disease, shock, hypoxemia, or metabolic disease is best reflected in marked increases in aminotransferase activities. Cholestasis (obstructive disease) involves regurgitation of bile components into serum; accordingly, the serum levels of total and conjugated bilirubin and serum bile acids are elevated. Elevations in serum alkaline phosphatase, 5′ nucleotidase, and γ-glutamyl transpeptidase (GGT) activities are also sensitive indicators of obstructive processes or of inflammation of the biliary tract.

The severity of the liver disease may be reflected in (1) *clinical signs* (occurrence of encephalopathy, variceal hemorrhage, worsening jaundice, apparent shrinkage of liver mass owing to massive necrosis, or onset of ascites) or in (2) *biochemical alterations* (hypoglycemia, hyperammonemia, electrolyte imbalance, continued hyperbilirubinemia, marked hypoalbuminemia, or prolonged prothrombin time unresponsive to parenteral administration of vitamin K).

Measurement of the *conjugated and unconjugated fractions of serum bilirubin* helps to distinguish between elevations caused by hemolysis and those caused by hepatic dysfunction. A predominant elevation in the conjugated fraction provides a relatively sensitive index of hepatocellular disease or hepatic excretory dysfunction. Aminotransferase activities are highly sensitive indices of hepatocellular damage. *Alanine aminotransferase* (ALT, serum glutamate pyruvate transaminase) is liver specific, whereas *aspartate aminotransferase* (AST, serum glutamic-oxaloacetic transaminase) is derived from other organs in addition to the liver. In most cases of hepatic disease there are parallel rises in AST and ALT, but a differential rise or fall can sometimes provide useful information. The most marked rises of aminotransferase activities occur with acute hepatocellular injury, such as acute viral hepatitis, hypoxia or hypoperfusion or toxic injury. After blunt abdominal trauma, elevations in activity of these enzymes may provide an early clue to hepatic injury. In chronic liver disease or in intrahepatic and extrahepatic biliary obstruction, rises in aminotransferase activities may be less marked. In acute hepatitis, the rise in ALT may be greater than that of AST, whereas in alcohol-induced liver injury, in fulminant echovirus infection, and in various metabolic diseases, predominant rises in AST have been reported.

Hepatic synthetic function is reflected in *serum protein* levels and in the *prothrombin time.* Examination of *serum globulin* concentration and of the relative amounts of the globulin fractions may be helpful. Gamma-globulin levels are often high, and increased titers of smooth muscle antibody as well as antimitochondrial antibodies and antinuclear antibodies may be found in patients with autoimmune hepatitis. A resurgence in *α-fetoprotein* levels may suggest hepatoma. Hypoalbuminemia caused by depressed synthesis may complicate severe liver disease and serve as a prognostic factor. Deficiencies of *factor V* and of the *vitamin K–dependent factors* (*II, VII, IX* and *X*) may occur in patients with severe liver disease or fulminant hepatic failure. If the prothrombin time is prolonged as a result of intestinal malabsorption of vitamin K (resulting from cholestasis) or decreased nutritional intake of vitamin K, then parenteral administration of vitamin K should correct the coagulopathy, leading to normalization within 12 hr. Unresponsiveness to vitamin K would suggest hepatic disease. Persistently low levels of factor VII are evidence of a poor prognosis in fulminant liver disease.

Serum levels of *bile acids* are sensitive indicators of hepatobiliary disease, especially in monitoring patients at high risk for liver injury.

Interpretation of results of biochemical tests of hepatic structure and function must be made in the context of age-related changes. The activity of *alkaline phosphatase* varies considerably with age, reflecting predominantly the activity of the isoenzyme that originates in bone. Activity of the liver-specific isoenzyme or of 5′ *nucleotidase* can be measured; the latter has a similar biliary origin and is not found in bone. An isolated increase in alkaline phosphatase does not indicate hepatic or biliary disease if other liver function test results are normal. GTP exhibits high enzyme activity in early life that declines rapidly with age. Cholesterol concentrations increase throughout life. *Cholesterol levels* may be markedly elevated in patients with cholestasis, whether the cause be intrahepatic or extrahepatic. On the other hand, with acute liver disease, such as hepatitis, serum cholesterol levels may be depressed.

Interpretation of *serum ammonia* values must be carried out with caution because of variability in their physiologic determinants and the inherent difficulty in laboratory measurement.

LIVER BIOPSY. The morphologic features of specific hepatic diseases are sufficiently distinctive. Therefore, liver biopsy combined with clinical data can suggest an etiology diagnosis in most cases. Tissue obtained by percutaneous liver biopsy can be used (1) to provide a precise histologic diagnosis (in patients with neonatal cholestasis, chronic active hepatitis, metabolic liver disease, suspected Reye syndrome, intrahepatic cholestasis (paucity of bile ducts), congenital hepatic fibrosis, or undefined portal hypertension); (2) for enzyme analysis to detect inborn errors of metabolism; and (3) for analysis of stored material (e.g., iron, copper, or specific metabolites). Serial assessments of hepatic status by liver biopsies can monitor responses to therapy or detect complications of treatment with potentially hepatotoxic agents, such as aspirin or nonsteroidal anti-inflammatory agents, antimetabolites, or anticonvulsants.

In infants and children, needle biopsy of the liver is easily accomplished through the percutaneous approach. The amount of tissue obtained, even in small infants, is usually sufficient for histologic interpretation and for biochemical analyses (if the latter are deemed necessary). Percutaneous liver biopsy can be performed safely in infants as young as 1 wk. Patients usually require only sedation and *local* anesthesia. Contraindications include prolonged prothrombin time; thrombocytopenia; suspicion of a vascular, cystic, or infectious lesion in the path of the needle; and severe ascites. If administration of fresh frozen plasma or of platelet transfusions fails to correct a prolonged prothrombin time or thrombocytopenia, open surgical (wedge) biopsy may be considered. The risk of development of a complication such as hemorrhage, hematoma, creation of an arteriovenous fistula, pneumothorax, or bile peritonitis is very small.

HEPATIC IMAGING PROCEDURES. Various techniques help define the size, shape, and architecture of the liver and the anatomy of the intrahepatic and extrahepatic biliary trees. Although imaging may not provide a precise histologic and biochemical diagnosis, specific questions can be answered, such as whether hepatomegaly is related to accumulation of fat or glycogen or is due to a tumor or cyst. These studies may direct further evaluation such as percutaneous biopsy and make possible prompt referral of patients with biliary obstruction to a surgeon. Choice of imaging procedure should be part of a carefully formulated diagnostic approach, with avoidance of redundant demonstrations by several techniques.

A *plain roentgenographic study* may suggest hepatomegaly, but a carefully performed physical examination gives a more reliable assessment of liver size. The liver may appear less dense than normal in patients with fatty infiltration or more dense with deposition of heavy metals such as iron. A hepatic or biliary tract mass may displace an air-filled loop of bowel. Calcifications may be evident in the liver (parasitic and neoplastic disease), in the vasculature (with portal vein thrombosis), or in the gallbladder or biliary tree (gallstones). Collections of gas may be seen within the liver (abscess), biliary tract, or portal circulation (necrotizing enterocolitis).

Ultrasonography provides information about the size, composition, and blood flow of the liver. Increased echogenicity is observed with fatty infiltration, and mass lesions as small as 1–2 cm may be shown. Ultrasonography has replaced cholangiography in detecting stones in the gallbladder or biliary tree. Even in neonates, ultrasonography can assess gallbladder size, detect dilatation of the biliary tract, and define a choledochal cyst. In infants with biliary atresia, the gallbladder is usually small or absent and the common duct is not visualized. In patients with portal hypertension, ultrasonography can evaluate patency of the portal vein or demonstrate collateral circulation. Relatively small amounts of ascitic fluid can be detected. The use of Doppler ultrasonography has been helpful in determining vascular patency after orthotopic liver transplantation.

Computed tomography (CT) scanning provides information similar to that obtained by ultrasonography but is less suitable for use in patients younger than 2 yr because of the small size of structures, the paucity of intra-abdominal fat for contrast, and the need for heavy sedation or general anesthesia. *Magnetic resonance imaging (MRI)* is a useful alternative. MR cholangiography can be of value in differentiating biliary tract lesions. CT scan or MRI may be more accurate than ultrasonography in detecting focal lesions such as tumors, cysts, and abscesses. When enhanced by contrast medium, CT scanning may reveal a neoplastic mass density only slightly different from that of a normal liver. When a hepatic tumor is suspected, CT scanning is the best method to define anatomic extent, solid or cystic nature, and vascularity. CT scanning can also reveal subtle differences in density of liver parenchyma, the average liver attenuation coefficient being reduced with fatty infiltration. Increases in density may occur with diffuse iron deposition or with glycogen storage. In differentiating obstructive from nonobstructive cholestasis, CT scanning or MRI identifies the precise level of obstruction more frequently than ultrasonography. Either CT scanning or ultrasonography may be used to guide percutaneously placed fine needles for biopsies, aspiration of specific lesions, or cholangiography.

Radionuclide scanning relies on selective uptake of a radiopharmaceutical agent. Commonly used agents include (1) technetium 99m–labeled sulfur colloid, which undergoes phagocytosis by Kupffer cells; (2) ^{99m}Tc-iminodiacetic acid agents, which are taken up by hepatocytes and excreted into bile; and (3) gallium 67, which is concentrated in inflammatory and neoplastic cells. The anatomic resolution possible with hepatic scintiscans is generally less than that obtained with CT scanning, MRI, or ultrasonography.

The ^{99m}Tc-sulfur colloid scan may detect focal lesions (e.g., tumors, cysts, or abscesses) greater than 2–3 cm in diameter. This modality may help to evaluate patients with possible cirrhosis and with patchy hepatic uptake and a shift of colloid uptake from liver to bone marrow.

The ^{99m}Tc-substituted iminodiacetic acid dyes may differentiate intrahepatic cholestasis from extrahepatic obstruction in neonates. Imaging results are best when scanning is preceded by a 5- to 7-day period of treatment with phenobarbital to stimulate bile flow. After intravenous injection, the isotope is normally detected in the bowel within 1–2 hr. In the presence of extrahepatic obstruction, excretion of the isotope is delayed; accordingly, serial scans should be made for up to 24 hr after injection. Early in the course of biliary atresia, hepatocyte function is usually good; uptake (clearance) occurs rapidly, but excretion into the intestine is absent. In contrast, uptake is poor in parenchymal liver disease, such as neonatal hepatitis, but excretion into the bile and intestine eventually ensues.

In older infants and children who have undergone liver transplantation, scintigraphy may also help to evaluate the gallbladder, bile ducts, and bile flow. In patients with acute cholecystitis, the gallbladder is not visualized but the common duct is opacified.

Cholangiography, direct visualization of the intrahepatic and extrahepatic biliary tree after injection of opaque material, may be required in some patients to evaluate the cause, location, or extent of biliary obstruction. Percutaneous transhepatic cholangiography with a fine needle is the technique of choice in infants and young children. The likelihood of opacifying the biliary tract is excellent in patients in whom CT scanning, MRI, or ultrasonography has shown dilated ducts. Percutaneous transhepatic cholangiography has been used to outline the biliary ductal system.

Endoscopic retrograde cholangiopancreatography (ERCP) is an alternative method of examining the bile ducts in older children. The papilla of Vater is cannulated under direct vision through a fiberoptic endoscope, and contrast material is injected into the biliary and pancreatic ducts to outline the anatomy.

Selective angiography of the celiac, superior mesenteric, or hepatic artery may be used to visualize the hepatic or portal circulation. Both arterial and venous circulatory systems of the liver can be examined. Angiography is frequently required to define the blood supply of tumors before surgery and is useful in the study of patients with known or presumed portal hypertension. The patency of the portal system, the extent of collateral circulation, and the caliber of vessels under consideration for a shunting procedure can be evaluated. MRI can provide similar information.

Alvarez F: Long-term treatment of bleeding caused by portal hypertension in children. J Pediatr 131:798, 1997.
Alvarez F, Bernard O, Brunelle F, et al: Portal obstruction in children. I: Clinical investigation and hemorrhage risk: Portal obstruction in children. J Pediatr 103:696, 1983.
Alvarez F, Bernard O, Brunelle F, et al: Portal obstruction in children. II: Results of surgical portosystemic shunts. J Pediatr 103:703, 1983.
Balistreri WF: Bile acid therapy in pediatric hepatobiliary disease: The role of ursodeoxycholic acid. J Pediatr Gastroenterol Nutr 24:573, 1997.
Balistreri WF, Rej R: Liver function. *In:* Burtis C, Ashwood E (eds): Tietz Textbook of Clinical Chemistry, 2nd ed. Philadelphia, WB Saunders, 1993, pp 1449–1512.
Fonkalsrud EW: Shunt operations for portal hypertension in children. J Pediatr 103:741, 1983.
Laker MF: Liver function tests. Br Med J 301:250, 1990.
Maggiore G, Bernard O, Reily CA, et al: Normal serum β-glutamyl-transpeptidase activity identifies groups of infants with idiopathic cholestasis with poor prognosis. J Pediatr 111:251, 1987.
Newman TB, Easterling J, Goldman ES, et al: Laboratory evaluation of jaundice in newborns. Am J Dis Child 144:364, 1990.
Reiff MI, Osborn LM: Clinical estimation of liver size in newborn infants. Pediatrics 71:46, 1983.
Rosenthal P: Assessing liver function and hyperbilirubinemia in the newborn. Clin Chem 43:228, 1997.
Rosenthal P, Henton D, Felber S, et al: Distribution of serum bilirubin conjugates in pediatric hepatobiliary disease. J Pediatr 110:201, 1987.
Ryckman FC, Alonso MH: Liver transplantation (cadaveric). *In:* Balistreri WF, Ohi R, Todani T, Tsuchida Y (eds): Hepatobiliary, Pancreatic and Splenic Disease in Children: Medical and Surgical Management. New York, Elsevier Science, 1997, pp 391–432.
Schuval S, Bonagura V: Simultaneous percusion auscultation technique for determination of liver span. Arch Pediatr Adolesc Med 148:873, 1994.
Sokol RJ: Medical management of infant or child with chronic liver disease. Semin Liver Dis 7:155, 1987.
Trauner M, Meier PJ, Boyer JL: Molecular pathogenesis of cholestasis. N Engl J Med 339:1217, 1998.

CHAPTER 356
Cholestasis

William F. Balistreri

356.1 Neonatal Cholestasis

Neonatal cholestasis is defined as prolonged elevation of serum levels of conjugated bilirubin beyond the first 14 days of life. Cholestasis in a newborn may be due to infectious, genetic, metabolic, or undefined abnormalities giving rise either to mechanical obstruction of bile flow or to functional impairment of hepatic excretory function and bile secretion (see Table 355–3). An example of the former is stricture or obstruction of the common bile duct; biliary atresia is the prototypic obstructive abnormality. Functional impairment of bile secretion may result from damage to liver cells or to the biliary secretory apparatus. Neonatal cholestasis may be divided into extrahepatic and intrahepatic disease (Fig. 356–1). The clinical features of any form of cholestasis are similar. In an affected neonate, the diagnosis of certain entities, such as galactosemia, sepsis, and hypothyroidism, is relatively simple. In most cases, however, the cause of cholestasis is more obscure. Differentiation among *extrahepatic biliary atresia,* idiopathic *neonatal hepatitis,* and *intrahepatic cholestasis* is often particularly difficult.

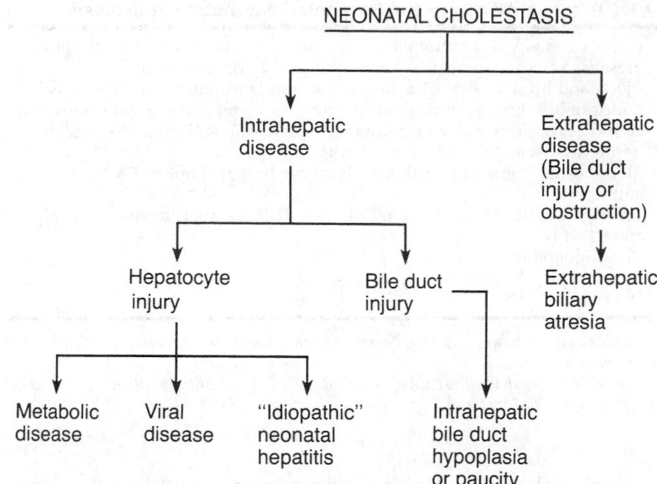

Figure 356–1 Neonatal cholestasis. Conceptual approach to the group of diseases presenting as cholestasis in the neonate. There are areas of overlap—patients with extrahepatic biliary atresia may have some degree of intrahepatic injury. Patients with "idiopathic" neonatal hepatitis may in the future be determined to have a primary metabolic or viral disease.

Mechanisms. The two most likely pathogenetic mechanisms are virus-induced liver injury or metabolic liver disease. There are paradigms for each of these potential mechanisms. For example, metabolic liver disease caused by inborn errors of bile acid metabolism is associated with accumulation of toxic primitive bile acids and the failure to produce normal choleretic and trophic bile acids. The clinical and histologic manifestations are nonspecific and are similar to those in other forms of neonatal hepatobiliary injury. It is also possible that autoimmune mechanisms may be responsible for some of the enigmatic forms of neonatal liver injury. Overall, the mechanisms are not well documented. Some of the histologic manifestations of hepatic injury in early life are not common in older individuals. For example, giant cell transformation of hepatocytes occurs frequently in infants with cholestasis and may occur in any form of neonatal liver injury. It is more frequent and more severe, however, in intrahepatic forms of cholestasis (neonatal hepatitis or intrahepatic bile duct paucity). The clinical and histologic findings thought to exist in patients with neonatal hepatitis and in those with extrahepatic biliary atresia have suggested that these diseases are manifestations of a single basic process, with an undefined initiating insult causing inflammation of the liver cells or of the cells within the biliary tract. If bile duct epithelium is the predominant site of disease, cholangitis may result and lead to progressive sclerosis and narrowing of the biliary tree, the ultimate state being complete obliteration *(extrahepatic biliary atresia).* On the other hand, injury to liver cells may present the clinical and histologic picture of *neonatal hepatitis.* This concept does not account for all phenomena but offers an explanation for well-documented cases of unexpected postnatal evolution of these disease processes; for example, infants initially regarded as having neonatal hepatitis, with a patent biliary system shown on cholangiography, have been later found to have extrahepatic biliary atresia.

TABLE 356–1 Work-up for Suspected Neonatal Cholestasis

1. History and physical examination: size and consistency of liver and spleen; presence of other anomalies (cardiac, renal, skin); stool color
2. Blood and urine analysis: fractionated serum bilirubin; serum bile acids; prothrombin time; α_1-antitrypsin phenotype; metabolic screen-urine/serum amino acids, urine reducing substances; thyroxine and thyroid-stimulating hormone; sweat chloride, serum ferritin
3. Blood, urine, spinal fluid cultures (bacteria, herpes simplex, CMV, enteroviruses)
4. Serologic studies for evidence of infection (HBsAg, specific viral serology,* and VDRL)
5. Ultrasonography
6. Hepatobiliary scintigraphy
7. Liver biopsy

Serology for hepatitis A, B, C, E, herpes simplex, CMV, rubella, HIV, measles, human herpes virus 6, 7.

CMV = cytomegalovirus; HBsAg = hepatitis B surface antigen; VDRL = Venereal Disease Research Laboratories.

Functional abnormalities in the generation of bile flow may also have a role in neonatal cholestasis. Bile flow is directly dependent on effective hepatic bile acid excretion. During the phase of relatively inefficient liver cell transport and metabolism of bile acids in early life, minor degrees of hepatic injury may further decrease bile flow and lead to production of abnormal toxic bile acids. Elective impairment of a single step in the series of events involved in hepatic excretion may produce the full expression of a cholestatic syndrome. A small number of cholestatic syndromes have a familial pattern. For example, Byler disease (progressive familial intrahepatic cholestasis [PFIC]) and benign recurrent cholestasis are presumably related to impaired membrane transport of bile acids. Specific defects in bile acid synthesis have been found in infants with intrahepatic cholestasis and in infants with Zellweger syndrome. Severe forms of familial cholestasis have been associated with neonatal hemochromatosis and an aberration in the contractile proteins that compose the cytoskeleton of he hepatocyte. Sepsis is known to cause cholestasis, presumably mediated by an endotoxin produced by *Escherichia coli*.

Evaluation (Table 356–1.) The clinical features of infants with neonatal cholestasis provide very few clues about etiology. Affected infants have icterus, dark urine, light or acholic stools, and hepatomegaly, all reflecting decreased bile flow resulting from either liver cell injury or bile duct obstruction. Hepatic synthetic dysfunction may lead to hypoprothrombinemia and a bleeding disorder; administration of vitamin K should be considered in the initial treatment of cholestatic infants in order to prevent hemorrhage.

Most infants with neonatal cholestasis come to medical attention in the 1st mo of life. Prompt differentiation of conjugated from unconjugated hyperbilirubinemia is imperative because the findings of cholestasis are more ominous. The initial step in identification of cholestasis are the finding that of the significantly elevated level of total bilirubin, more than 20% is conjugated bilirubin. The next step is prompt recognition of any specific or treatable primary causes of cholestasis, such as *sepsis*, an *endocrinopathy* (hypothyroidism or panhypopituitarism), *nutritional hepatotoxicity* caused by a specific metabolic illness (galactosemia), or other *metabolic diseases* (tyrosinemia). Recognition of such entities allows institution of appropriate therapy and may possibly prevent further injury.

Hepatobiliary disease may be the initial manifestation of homozygous α-antitrypsin deficiency or of cystic fibrosis. Neonatal liver disease may also be associated with congenital syphilis and speific viral infections, notably echo virus and herpesviruses. The hepatitis viruses (A, B, C) rarely cause neonatal cholestasis.

The final step in evaluating neonates with cholestasis is to differentiate extrahepatic biliary atresia from neonatal hepatitis.

NEONATAL HEPATITIS SYNDROME (INTRAHEPATIC CHOLESTASIS). The term *neonatal hepatitis* implies intrahepatic cholestasis (Fig. 356–1), which has various forms:

1. **Idiopathic neonatal hepatitis**, which can occur in either a sporadic or a familial form, is a disease of unknown cause; most cases are idiopathic. These patients presumably are afflicted with a specific yet undefined metabolic or viral disease. In the past, patients with α_1-antitrypsin deficiency were included in this category; however, after characterization of this metabolic disease, it is possible to define this group of patients precisely.
2. **Infectious hepatitis in a neonate** may be shown to be due to a specific virus, such as herpes simplex, enteroviruses, cytomegalovirus, or, rarely, hepatitis B. This accounts for a small percentage of cases of neonatal hepatitis syndrome.
3. Cases of **intrahepatic bile duct paucity** form a heterogeneous subset of cholestatic diseases that may present as neonatal cholestasis.

INTRAHEPATIC BILE DUCT PAUCITY. Some syndromes characterized morphologically by intrahepatic cholestasis may be clinically manifested either as neonatal hepatitis or as cholestasis in an older child. As patients mature, clinical and histologic features may suggest a specific syndrome. Many such cases are associated with bile duct "paucity" (often erroneously called intrahepatic biliary atresia), which designates an absence or marked reduction in the number of interlobular bile ducts in the portal triads, with normal-sized branches of portal vein and hepatic arteriole. This unusual histologic feature represents congenital bile duct absence, partial failure of bile duct development, progressive bile duct atrophy, or disappearance of the bile ducts due to segmental destructive processes. Biopsy in early life often reveals an inflammatory process involving the bile ducts; subsequent biopsy specimens then show subsidence of the inflammation with residual reduction in the number and diameter of bile ducts, analogous to the "disappearing bile duct syndrome" noted in adults with immune-mediated disorders.

Observations suggest that it is possible to identify distinctive syndromes of isolated intrahepatic bile duct paucity and an intact extrahepatic biliary tree.

Alagille syndrome (arteriohepatic dysplasia) is the most common syndrome incorporating intrahepatic bile duct paucity. Serial assessment of hepatic histology often suggests progressive destruction of bile ducts. Clinical manifestations are expressed in various degrees and may be nonspecific; they include in some patients unusual *facial characteristics* (broad forehead; deep-set, widely spaced eyes; long, straight nose; and an underdeveloped mandible). There may also be *ocular* abnormalities (posterior embryotoxon), *cardiovascular* abnormalities (usually peripheral pulmonic stenosis, sometimes tetralogy of Fallot), *vertebral* arch defects and failure of anterior vertebral arch fusion (butterfly vertebrae), and tubulointerstitial *nephropathy*. Other findings such as growth retardation and defective spermatogenesis may reflect nutritional deficiency. The prognosis for prolonged survival is good, but patients are likely to have pruritus, xanthomas with markedly elevated serum cholesterol levels, and neurologic complications of vitamin E deficiency if untreated. Mutations in human Jagged 1 (*JAG1*), which encodes a ligand for the notch receptor, have been linked to Alagille syndrome.

Byler disease is a rare familial form of *progressive intrahepatic cholestasis* (PFIC) characterized by unique structural abnormalities in the bile canalicular membrane. Affected patients present with failure to thrive, steatorrhea, pruritus, rickets, and low γ-glutamyl transpeptidase levels. Cirrhosis gradually develops.

PFIC type 1 (Byler disease) is mapped to chromosome 18q12, has low serum levels of γ-glutamyltransferase, normal cholesterol, and high serum bile salt levels with low bile chenodeoxycholic acid levels. A mutation in P-type membrane adenosine triphosphatase is the responsible mechanism in Amish families.

PFIC type 2 is like Byler disease but is present in non-Amish families (Middle Eastern Europeans) and has a gene locus at chromosome 2q24. Mutations of the sister of the P glycoprotein gene, which codes for a bile canalicular adenosine triphosphate–dependent bile acid transporter, may be responsible.

PFIC type 3 has high serum levels of γ-glutamyltransferase and histologically has portal bile duct inflammation and proliferation. There is complete absence of the multidrug resistance 3 P glycoprotein, with deficient translocation of phosphatidylcholine across the canalicular membrane.

In **Aagenaes syndrome**, a form of idiopathic familial intrahepatic cholestasis, recurrent cholestasis is associated with lymphedema of the lower extremities.

Zellweger (cerebrohepatorenal) syndrome is a rare autosomal recessive genetic disorder marked by progressive degeneration of the liver and kidneys. The incidence is estimated to be 1/100,000 births; the disease is usually fatal within 6–12 mo. Affected infants have severe, generalized hypotonia and markedly impaired neurologic function with psychomotor retardation. Patients have an abnormal head shape and unusual facies, hepatomegaly, renal cortical cysts, stippled calcifications of the patellas and greater trochanter, and ocular abnormalities. Hepatic cells on ultrastructural examination show an absence of peroxisomes (Chapter 83.2).

Additional cholestatic disorders include neonatal iron storage disease and inborn errors of bile acid biosynthesis. Defective bile acid biosynthesis has been postulated to be an initiating or perpetuating factor in neonatal cholestatic disorders; the hypothesis is that inborn errors in bile acid biosynthesis lead to absence of normal trophic or choleretic primary bile acids and accumulation of primitive (hepatotoxic) metabolities. A new category of metabolic liver disease, **inborn errors of bile acid biosynthesis**, is now a recognizable cause of acute and chronic liver disease; early recognition allows institution of targeted bile acid replacement, which reverses the hepatic injury.

Deficiency of Δ^4-3-oxosteriod-5β reductase, the fourth step in the pathway of cholesterol degradation to the primary bile acids, was first described in a family of four consecutive boys. This disorder is manifested as significant cholestasis and liver failure developing shortly after birth with coagulopathy and metabolic liver injury resembling tyrosinemia. Hepatic histology is characterized by lobular disarray with giant cells, pseudoacinar transformation, and canalicular bile stasis. Mass spectrometry is required to document increased bile acid excretion and the predominance of oxo-hydroxy and oxo-dihydroxy cholenoci acids. Treatment with cholic acid and ursodeoxycholic acid is associated with normalization of biochemical, histologic, and clinical features.

Deficiency of **3β-hydroxy C_{27}-steroid dehydrogenase (3-HSD) isomerase,** the second step in bile acid biosynthesis, causes progressive familial intrahepatic cholestasis. Affected patients usually have jaundice with increased aminotransferase levels and hepatomegaly; however, γ-glutamyl transpeptidase levels and serum cholyglycine levels are normal. The histology is variable, ranging from giant cell hepatitis to chronic active hepatitis. The diagnosis, suggested by mass spectrometry detection of C^{24} bile acids, which retain the 3β-hydroxy-Δ^5 structure, can be confirmed by determination of 3-HSD activity in cultured fibroblasts using 7α-hydroxy-Δ^5 cholesterol as a substrate. Primary bile acid therapy, administered orally to downregulate cholesterol 7α-hydroxylase activity, limit the production of 3β-hydroxy-Δ^5 bile acids, and facilitate hepatic clearance, has been effective in reversing hepatic injury.

BILIARY ATRESIA

The term *biliary atresia* is imprecise because the anatomy of abnormal extrahepatic bile ducts in affected patients varies markedly. A more appropriate terminology would reflect the pathophysiology—namely, *progressive obliterative cholangiopathy.* Patients may have distal segmental bile duct obliteration with patent extrahepatic ducts up to the porta hepatis. This is a surgically correctable lesion, but it is uncommon. The most common form of biliary atresia, accounting for approximately 85% of the cases, is obliteration of the entire extrahepatic biliary tree at or above the porta hepatis. This presents a much more difficult problem in surgical management.

INCIDENCE. Biliary atresia has been detected in 1/10,000–15,000 live births, idiopathic neonatal hepatitis in 1/5,000–10,000. Intrahepatic bile duct paucity appears much less commonly, in about 1/50,000–75,000 live births.

DIFFERENTIATION OF IDIOPATHIC NEONATAL HEPATITIS FROM BILIARY ATRESIA. It may be difficult to differentiate clearly infants with biliary atresia, who require surgical correction, from those with intrahepatic disease (neonatal hepatitis) and patent bile ducts. No single biochemical test or imaging procedure is entirely satisfactory. Diagnostic schemas incorporate clinical, historical, biochemical, and radiologic features.

Idiopathic neonatal hepatitis has a familial incidence of approximately 20%, whereas extrahepatic biliary atresia is unlikely to recur within the same family. Some infants with biliary atresia have an increased incidence of other abnormalities, such as the polysplenia syndrome with abdominal heterotaxia, malrotation, levocardia, and intra-abdominal vascular anomalies. Neonatal hepatitis appears to be more common in premature or small for gestational age infants. Persistently acholic stools suggest biliary obstruction (biliary atresia), but patients with severe idiopathic neonatal hepatitis may have a transient severe impairment of bile excretion. On the other hand, consistently pigmented stools rule against biliary atresia. The finding of bile-stained fluid on duodenal intubaion also excludes biliary atresia. Palpation of the liver may find an abnormal size or consistency in patients with extrahepatic biliary atresia; this is less common with neonatal hepatitis.

Imaging techniques are generally not helpful, but ultrasonography should be carried out early because it may detect a choledochal cyst or another unsuspected cause of cholestasis associated with dilatation of the biliary tract.

Hepatobiliary scintigraphy using imidodiacetic acid analogs has been used by some clinicians to differentiate biliary atresia from neonatal hepatitis. In biliary atresia, hepatocyte function is intact and uptake of the agent is unimpaired, but excretion into the intestine is absent. In patients with neonatal hepatitis, uptake is sluggish, but excretion into the biliary tract and intestine eventually occurs. Oral administration of phenobarbital (5 mg/kg/24 hr) for 5 days before the study enchances biliary excretion of the isotope in patients with neonatal hepatitis.

Liver biopsy provides the most reliable discriminatory evidence. **Biliary atresia** is characterized by bile ductular proliferation, the presence of bile plugs, and portal or perilobular edema and fibrosis, with the basic hepatic lobular architecture intact. In **neonatal hepatitis**, on the other hand, there is severe, diffuse hepatocellular disease, with distortion of lobular architecture, marked infiltration with inflammatory cells, and focal hepatocellular necrosis; the bile ductules show little alteration. Giant cell transformation is found in infants with either condition and has no diagnostic specificity.

Histologic changes similar to those in idiopathic neonatal hepatitis occur in various diseases, including α_1-antitrypsin deficiency, galactosemia, and, various forms of intrahepatic cholestasis. Although paucity of intrahepatic bile ductules may be detected on liver biopsy even within the first few weeks of life, later biopsies in such patients reveal a more characteristic pattern.

MANAGEMENT OF PATIENTS WITH SUSPECTED BILIARY ATRESIA. In infants in whom clinical features and liver biopsy suggest biliary obstruction, exploratory laparotomy and direct cholangiography should be performed to determine the presence and site of obstruction. For patients with **correctable lesion**, direct drainage can be accomplished. When no correctable lesion is found, an examination of frozen sections obtained from the transected porta hepatis can detect the presence of biliary epithelium and determine the size and patency of the residual bile ducts. In some cases, the cholangiogram indicates that the biliary tree is patent but of diminished caliber, suggesting that the cholestasis is not due to biliary tract obliteration but to bile duct paucity or markedly diminished flow in the presence of intrahepatic disease. In these cases, transection of or further dissection into the porta hepatis shoud be *avoided*.

For patients in whom **no correctable lesion** is found, the hepatoportoenterostomy procedure of Kasai can be carried out. The rationale for this operation is that minute bile duct remnants, representing residual channels, may be present in the fibrous tissue of the porta hepatis; such channels may be in direct continuity with the intrahepatic ductule system. In such cases, transection of the porta hepatis with anastomosis of bowel mucosa to the proximal surface of the transection may allow bile drainage. If flow is not rapidly established within the first months of life, progressive obliteration and cirrhosis ensue. If microscopic channels of patency greater than 150 μm in diameter are found, postoperative establishment of bile flow is likely. The Kasai operation is most successful (90%) if performed before 8 wk of life.

Some patients with biliary atresia, even of the "noncorrectable" type, derive long-term benefits from interventions such as the Kasai procedure. In most, however, a degree of hepatic dysfunction persists. Patients with biliary atresia usually have persistent inflammation of the intrahepatic biliary tree, which suggests that biliary atresia reflects a dynamic process involving the entire hepatobiliary system. This may account for the ultimate development of complications such as portal hypertension. The short-term benefit of hepatoportoenterostomy is decompression and drainage sufficient to forestall the onset of cirrhosis and sustain growth until a successful liver transplantation can be done (Chapter 367).

MANAGEMENT OF CHRONIC CHOLESTASIS

With any form of neonatal cholestasis, whether the primary disease is idiopathic neonatal hepatitis, intrahepatic bile duct paucity, or biliary atresia, affected patients are at increased risk for chronic complications. These reflect various degrees of residual hepatic functional capacity and are due directly or indirectly to diminished bile flow:

1. Any substance normally excreted into bile is retained in the liver, with subsequent accumulation in tissue and in serum. Involved substances include bile acids, bilirubin, cholesterol, and trace elements.
2. Decreased delivery of bile acids to the proximal intestine leads to inadequate digestion and absorption of dietary long-chain triglycerides and fat-soluble vitamins.
3. Impairment of hepatic metabolic function may alter hormonal balance and utilization of nutrients.
4. Progressive liver damage may lead to biliary cirrhosis, portal hypertension, and liver failure.

Treatment of such patients (Table 356–2) is empirical, and the best guide is careful monitoring. At present, no therapy is known to be effective in halting the progression of cholestasis or in preventing further hepatocellular damage and cirrhosis.

A major concern is growth failure, which is related in part to malabsorption and malnutrition resulting from ineffective digestion and absorption of dietary fat. Use of a medium-chain triglyceride-containing formula may improve caloric balance.

TABLE 356–2 Suggested Medical Management of Persistent Cholestasis

Clinical Impairment	Management
Malnutrition resulting from malabsorption of dietary long-chain triglyceride	Replace with dietary formula or supplements containing medium-chain triglycerides
Fat-soluble vitamin malabsorption:	
Vitamin A deficiency (night blindness, thick skin)	Replace with 10,000–15,000 IU/day as Aquasol A
Vitamin E deficiency (neuromuscular degeneration)	Replace with 50–400 IU/day as oral α-tocopherol or TPGS
Vitamin D deficiency (metabolic bone disease)	Replace with 5,000–8,000 IU/day of D_2 or 3–5 μg/kg/day of 25-hydroxycholecalciferol
Vitamin K deficiency (hypoprothrombinemia)	Replace with 2.5–5.0 mg every other day as water-soluble derivative of menadione
Micronutrient deficiency	Calcium, phosphate, or zinc supplementation
Deficiency of water-soluble vitamins	Supplement with twice the recommended daily allowance
Retention of biliary constituents such as bile acids and cholesterol (itch or xanthomas)	Administer choleretics (Ursodeoxycholic acid, 15–20 mg/kg/day) or bile acid binders (cholestyramine 8–16 g/day)
Progressive liver disease	
Portal hypertension (variceal bleeding, ascites, hypersplenism)	Interim management (control bleeding; salt restriction; spironolactone)
End-stage liver disease (liver failure)	Transplantation

TPGS = D-tocopherol polyethylene glycol-1000 succinate.

With chronic cholestasis and prolonged survival, children with hepatobiliary disease may experience deficiencies of the fat-soluble vitamins (A, D, E, and K). Inadequate absorption of fat and fat-soluble vitamins may be exacerbated by administration of the bile acid binder cholestyramine. Metabolic bone disease is common.

A degenerative neuromuscular syndrome is found with chronic cholestasis caused by malabsorption and therefore deficiency of vitamin E; affected children experience progressive areflexia, cerebellar ataxia, ophthalmoplegia, and decreased vibratory sensation. Specific morphologic lesions have been found in the central nervous system, peripheral nerves, and muscles. These lesions resemble those found in animals with vitamin E deficiency and are potentially reversible in young children (i.e., those <3–4 yr old). The deficiency may be prevented by oral administration of large doses (up to 1,000 IU/day) of vitamin E; patients unable to absorb sufficient quantities may require administration of D-tocopherol polyethylene glycol-1000 succinate orally. Serum levels may be monitored as a guide to efficacy; affected children have low serum vitamin E concentrations, increased hydrogen peroxide hemolysis, and low ratios of serum vitamin E to total serum lipids (<0.6 mg/g for children younger than 12 yr and <0.8 mg/g for older patients).

Serum vitamin A concentration can usually be maintained at normal levels in patients who have chronic cholestasis and who received oral supplementation of vitamin A esters. It is essential to monitor the vitamin A status in such patients.

Pruritus is a particularly troublesome complication of chronic cholestasis, often with the appearance of xanthomas. Both features seem to be related to the accumulation of cholesterol and bile acids in serum and in tissues. Elimination of these retained compounds is difficult when bile ducts are obstructed, but if there is any degree of bile duct patency, administration of ursodeoxycholic acid may increase bile flow or interrupt the enterohepatic circulation of bile acids and thus decrease the xanthomas and ameliorate the pruritus (see Table 356–2). Ursodeoxycholic acid therapy may also lower serum cholesterol levels. The recommended dose is 15 mg/kg/24 hr.

In patients with portal hypertension, variceal hemorrhage and the development of hypersplenism are common. However, episodes of gastrointestinal hemorrhage in patients who have chronic liver disease may be due not to esophageal varices but to gastritis or peptic ulcer disease. Because the management of these various complications differ, differentiation perhaps via endoscopy is necessary before treatment is initiated (Chapter 366).

In patients with **ascites**, initial management consists of dietary salt restriction; sodium intake is limited to 0.5 g (~1–2 mEq/kg/24 hr). It is not necessary to restrict fluid intake in patients with adequate renal output. Diuresis may be maintained by the use of agents such as furosemide, alone or in combination with spironolactone (3–5 mg/kg/24 hr in four doses). Patients with ascites but without peripheral edema are at risk for reduced plasma volume and decreased urine output during diuretic therapy. Tense ascites alters renal blood flow and systemic hemodynamics. Paracentesis and intravenous albumin infusion may improve hemodynamics, renal perfusion, and symptoms. Follow-up includes dietary counseling and monitoring of serum and urinary electrolyte concentrations (Chapters 366 and 369).

In patients with advanced liver disease, hepatic transplantation may have a success rate greater than 85% (Chapter 367). If the operation is technically feasible, it will prolong life and may correct the metabolic error in diseases such as α_1-antitrypsin deficiency, tyrosinemia, or Wilson disease. Success depends on adequate intraoperative, preoperative, and postoperative care and on cautious use of immunosuppressive agents. Scarcity of donors of small livers severely limits the application of liver transplantation for infants and children. However, the use of *reduced*-size transplants and living donors has increased the ability to treat small children successfully.

PROGNOSIS

The prognosis for infants with biliary atresia was discussed earlier. For patients with idiopathic neonatal hepatitis, the variable prognosis may reflect the heterogeneity of the disease. In **sporadic** cases, 60–70% recover with no evidence of hepatic structural or functional impairment. Approximately 5–10% have persistent fibrosis or inflammation, and a smaller percentage have more severe liver disease, such as cirrhosis. Death of infants usually occurs early in the course of the illness, owing to hemorrhage or sepsis. Of infants with idiopathic neonatal hepatitis of the **familial** variety, only 20–30% recover; 10–15% acquire chronic liver disease with cirrhosis. Liver transplantation may be required.

356.2 Cholestasis in the Older Child

Acute viral hepatitis accounts for most cases of cholestasis with onset after the neonatal period. Many of the conditions causing neonatal cholestasis may also cause chronic cholestasis in older patients. An adolescent with conjugated hyperbilirubinemia should be evaluated for acute and chronic hepatitis, α_1-antitrypsin deficiency, Wilson disease, liver disease associated with inflammatory bowel disease, and the syndromes of intrahepatic cholestasis (with or without bile duct paucity). Other causes include obstruction caused by cholelithiasis, abdominal tumors or enlarged lymph nodes, or hepatic inflammation resulting from drug ingestion. Management is similar to that proposed for neonatal cholestasis (see Table 356–2).

356.3 Hepatic Rickets

Russell W. Chesney

Rickets is common in children with chronic hepatic disorders, particularly in extrahepatic biliary atresia, when failure of bile salt secretion prevents adequate absorption of vitamin D and other fat-soluble vitamins. Rickets may also occur in neonatal hepatitis or chronic hepatic failure and after hepatocellular damage induced by total parenteral nutrition. Reduced absorption of vitamin D accounts for hepatic rickets. The usual findings of nutritional rickets are noted—reduced serum 25 (OH) D values, hypocalcemia, roentgenographic evidence, and elevated serum alkaline phosphatase activity (bone and hepatic isoenzyme levels are raised). Because rickets mainly relates to vitamin D malabsorption, this form can be treated with high enough doses to overcome malabsorption. Thus, 4,000–10,000 IU of vitamin D_2 (100–250 μg), 50 μg of 25 (OH) D, or 0.2 μg/kg of 1,25 $(OH)_2D$ should be given daily, along with oral calcium. Calcium supplements are particularly indicated in infants who have chronic liver disease with ascites and who are receiving loop diuretics, such as furosemide, which result in excessive urinary calcium losses.

Aagenaes O: Hereditary recurrent cholestasis with lymphoedema: Two new families. Acta Pediatr Scand 63:465, 1974.

Alagille D, Estrada A, Hadchovel M, et al: Syndromic paucity of interlobular bile ducts (Alagille syndrome or arteriohepatic dysplasia): Review of 80 cases. J Pediatr 110:195, 1987.

Arrese M, Ananthananarayanan M, Suchy FJ: Hepatobiliary transport: Mechanisms of development and cholestasis. Pediatr Res 44:141, 1998.

Balistreri WF: Neonatal cholestasis. J Pediatr 106:171, 1985.

Bull LN, van Eijk MJT, Pawlikowska L, et al: A gene encoding a P-type ATPase mutated in two forms of hereditary cholestasis. Nature Genet 18:219, 1998.

Danks DM, Campbell PE, Smith AL, et al. Prognosis of babies with neonatal hepatitis. Arch Dis Child 52:368, 1977.

Debray D, Pariente D, Gauthier F, et al: Cholelithiasis in infancy: A study of 40 cases. J Pediatr 122:385, 1993.

Kasai M, Mochizuki I, Ohkohchi N, et al: Surgical limitations for biliary atresia: Indications for liver transplantation. J Pediatr Surg 24:851, 1989.

Hoffenberg EJ, Narkewicz MR, Sondheimer JM, et al: Outcome of syndromic paucity of interlobular bile ducts (Alagille syndrome) with onset of cholestasis in infancy. J Pediatr 127:220, 1995.

Laurent J, Gauthier F, Bernard O, et al: Long-term outcome after surgery for biliary atresia: Study of 40 patients surviving for more than 10 years. Gastroenterology 99:1793, 1990.

Mowat AP, Psacharopoulos HT, Williams R: Extrahepatic biliary atresia versus neonatal hepatitis: Review of 137 prospectively investigated infants. Arch Dis Child 51:763, 1976.

Oda T, Elkahloun AG, Pike BL, et al: Mutations in the human *Jagged1* gene are responsible for Alagille syndrome. Nature Genet 16:235, 1997.

Ryckman FC, Fisher RA, Pedersen SH, et al: Improved survival in biliary atresia patients in the present era of liver transplantation. J Pediatr Surg 28:382, 1993.

Sokol RJ, Heubi JE, Butler-Simon N, et al: Treatment of vitamin E deficiency during chronic childhood cholestasis with oral D-tocopheryl polyethylene glycol-1000 succinate. Gastroenterology 93:975, 1987.

Stringer MD, Dhawan A, Davenport M, et al: Choledochal cysts: Lessons from a 20 year experience. Arch Dis Child 73:528, 1995.

Whitington PF, Balistreri WF: Liver transplantation in pediatrics: Indications, contraindications, and pre-transplant management. J Pediatr 118:169, 1991.

Trauner M, Meier PJ, Boyer JL: Molecular pathogenesis of cholestasis. N Engl J Med 339:1217, 1998.

Yoon PW, Bresee JS, Olney RS, et al: Epidemiology of biliary atresia: A population-based study. Pediatrics 99:376, 1997.

CHAPTER 357
Metabolic Diseases of the Liver

William F. Balistreri

See also Chapters 81 and 98.3.

Because the liver has a central role in synthetic, degradative, and regulatory pathways involving carbohydrate, protein, lipid, trace element, and vitamin metabolism, many metabolic abnormalities or specific enzyme deficiencies affect the liver primarily or secondarily (Table 357–1). Liver disease may arise when absence of an enzyme produces a block in a metabolic pathway, when unmetabolized substrate accumulates proximal

TABLE 357–1 Inborn Errors of Metabolism Manifested as Hepatobiliary Dysfunction

Disorders of Carbohydrate Metabolism

- Disorders of **galactose** metabolism
  - Galactosemia
- Disorders of **fructose** metabolism
  - Hereditary fructose intolerance (aldolase deficiency)
  - Fructose-1,6 diphosphatase deficiency
- **Glycogen storage** diseases
  - Type I
    - Von Gierke (Ia)
    - Type Ib
  - Type III (Cori/Forbes)
  - Type IV (Andersen)
  - Type VI (Hers)

Disorders of Amino Acid and Protein Metabolism

- Disorders of **tyrosine** metabolism
  - Transient
    - Neonatal
    - Associated with severe liver disease (e.g., cirrhosis)
  - Nontransient
    - Hereditary tyrosinemia (type I)
    - Tyrosinemia, type II
- Inherited **urea cycle** enzyme defects
  - CPS deficiency
  - OTC deficiency (X-linked dominant)
  - Citrullinemia
  - Argininosuccinic aciduria
  - Argininemia
  - N-AGS deficiency

Disorders of Lipid Metabolism

- Wolman disease
- Cholesteryl ester storage disease
- Gaucher disease
- Niemann-Pick type C

Disorders of Bile Acid Metabolism

- Isomerase deficiency
- Reductase deficiency
- Zellweger syndrome (cerebrohepatorenal)

Disorders of Metal Metabolism

- Wilson's disease
- Hepatic copper overload
- Indian childhood cirrhosis
- Neonatal iron storage disease (perinatal hemochromatosis)

Disorders of Bilirubin Metabolism

- Crigler-Najjar
  - Type I
  - Type II—Arias
  - Gilbert disease
  - Dubin-Johnson
  - Rotor

Miscellaneous

- α_1-Antitrypsin deficiency
- Cystic fibrosis
- Erythropoietic protoporphyria

CPS = Carbamoyl phosphate synthetase; OTC = ornithine transcarbamoylase; N-AGS = N-*acetylglutamate synthetase.*

to a block, when deficiency of an essential substance produced distal to an aberrant chemical reaction develops, or when synthesis of an abnormal metabolite occurs. The spectrum of pathologic changes includes (1) *hepatocyte injury,* with subsequent failure of other metabolic functions, often eventuating in cirrhosis or liver tumors or both; (2) *storage* of lipid, glycogen, or other products manifested as hepatomegaly, often with complications specific to deranged metabolism (e.g., decreased blood glucose in patients with glycogen storage disease); and (3) absence of structural change despite profound metabolic effects, as with urea cycle defects. The clinical manifestations of metabolic diseases of the liver mimic infections, intoxications, and hematologic and immunologic diseases (Table 357–2). Further clues are provided by family history of a similar

TABLE 357–2 Clinical Manifestations That Suggest the Possibility of Metabolic Disease

- Jaundice, hepatomegaly (± splenomegaly), fulminant hepatic failure
- Hypoglycemia, organic acidemia, lactic acidemia, hyperammonemia, bleeding (coagulopathy)
- Recurrent vomiting, failure to thrive, short stature, dysmorphic features
- Developmental delay/psychomotor retardation, hypotonia, progressive neuromuscular deterioration, seizures
- Cardiac dysfunction/failure, unusual odors, rickets, cataracts

illness or by the observation that the onset of symptoms is closely associated with a change in dietary habits (e.g., initiation of ingestion of fructose). In most cases, clinical and laboratory evidence guide the evaluation. Liver biopsy offers morphologic study and permits enzyme assays, as well as quantitative and qualitative assays of various other constituents. Such studies require cooperation of experienced laboratories and careful attention to collection and handling of specimens.

357.1 Inherited Deficient Conjugation of Bilirubin

(Familial Nonhemolytic Unconjugated Hyperbilirubinemia)

Hepatic glucuronyl transferase activity (Chapter 98.3) is deficient in two genetically and functionally distinct disorders (Crigler-Najjar syndrome) producing congenital nonobstructive, nonhemolytic, unconjugated hyperbilirubinemia. The molecular mechanism of the various Crigler-Najjar syndromes is complex. This is partly because the activity of multiple glucuronyl transferase isoforms is deficient in various phenotypes of the Crigler-Najjar syndrome. Low enzyme levels with unconjugated hyperbilirubinemia also occur in **Gilbert syndrome,** a benign disorder, owing to a missense mutation in the transferase **(UGTI)** gene.

CRIGLER-NAJJAR SYNDROME (TYPE I GLUCURONYL TRANSFERASE DEFICIENCY). This form is inherited as an autosomal recessive trait and is due to mutations in the UDP(B)-GT gene. Parents of affected children have partial defects in conjugation as determined by hepatic enzyme assay or by measurement of glucuronide formation, but their serum bilirubin concentrations are normal.

Clinical Manifestations. Severe unconjugated hyperbilirubinemia develops in homozygous infants during the first 3 days of life, and without treatment, serum concentrations of 25–35 mg/dL are reached during the 1st mo. Kernicterus, an almost universal complication of this disorder, is usually first noted in the early neonatal period, but some treated infants have survived childhood without clinical sequelae. Stools are pale yellow. Persistence of unconjugated hyperbilirubinemia at levels above 20 mg/dL after the 1st wk of life in the absence of hemolysis should suggest the syndrome.

Diagnosis. The diagnosis of Crigler-Najjar syndrome is based on the early age of onset and the extreme level of bilirubin elevation in the absence of hemolysis. In the bile, bilirubin concentration is less than 10 mg/dL compared with normal concentrations of 50–100 mg/dL, and there is no bilirubin glucuronide. Definitive diagnosis is established by measuring hepatic glucuronyl transferase activity in a liver specimen obtained by a closed biopsy; open biopsy should be avoided because surgery and anesthesia may precipitate kernicterus. DNA diagnosis is also available. Identification of the heterozygous state in the parents is also strongly suggestive of the diagnosis. Differential diagnosis is discussed in Chapter 98.3. Type II disease may be distinguished from type I by the marked decline in serum bilirubin level that occurs in type II disease after 1 wk of treatment with phenobarbital.

Treatment. Serum bilirubin concentration should be kept below 20 mg/dL for at least the first 2–4 wk of life; in low birthweight infants, the levels should be kept lower. This usually requires repeated exchange transfusions and phototherapy. Because the risk of kernicterus persists into adult life, although the serum bilirubin levels required to produce brain injury beyond the neonatal period are considerably higher (usually >35 mg/dL), phototherapy is generally continued throughout the early years of life. In older infants and children, phototherapy is used mainly during sleep in order not to interfere with normal activities. However, despite the administration of increasing intensities of light for longer periods, the serum bilirubin decrement response to phototherapy decreases with age. Cholestyramine or agar may be used to bind photobilirubin products, thus interfering with the enterohepatic recirculation of bilirubin. Prompt treatment of intercurrent infections, febrile episodes, and other types of illness may help prevent the later development of kernicterus, which may occur at bilirubin levels of 45–55 mg/dL. All patients with type I have eventually experienced severe kernicterus by young adulthood, despite vigorous continuous management that maintained neurologic normality during childhood. Orthotopic hepatic transplantation cures the disease and has been successful in a small number of patients. Other therapeutic modalities have included plasmapheresis and limitation of bilirubin production. The latter option, inhibiting bilirubin generation, is possible via inhibition of heme oxygenase using metalloporphyrin therapy. Genetically engineered enzymatic replacement therapy, liver-directed gene therapy, and hepatocyte transplantation remain potential therapeutic options in the future.

CRIGLER-NAJJAR SYNDROME. GLUCURONYL TRANSFERASE DEFICIENCY TYPE II. This autosomal dominant disease with marked variability of penetrance may present in a manner similar to type I syndrome, or it may be a less severe disorder, occasionally even without neonatal manifestations. Studies have suggested that Crigler-Najjar syndrome type II is caused by homozygous mutation in glucuronyl transferase isoform I activity.

Clinical Manifestations. When this disorder presents in the neonatal period, unconjugated hyperbilirubinemia usually occurs during the first 3 days of life; serum bilirubin concentrations may be in a range compatible with physiologic jaundice or may be at pathologic levels. The concentrations characteristically remain elevated into and after the 3rd wk of life, persisting in a range of 1.5–22 mg/dL; concentrations in the lower part of this range may create uncertainty about whether chronic hyperbilirubinemia is present. The onset of kernicterus is unusual. Stool color is normal, and the infants are without clinical signs or symptoms of disease. There is no evidence of hemolysis.

Diagnosis. Concentration of bilirubin in bile is nearly normal in type II syndrome. Jaundiced infants and young children having type II syndrome respond readily to 5 mg/kg/24 hr of oral phenobarbital with a decrease in serum bilirubin concentration to 2–3 mg/dL within 7–10 days. Those with type I syndrome do not respond.

Treatment. Long-term reduction in serum bilirubin levels can be achieved with continued administration of phenobarbital at 5 mg/kg/24 hr. The cosmetic and psychosocial benefit should be weighed against the risks of an effective dose of the drug because there is a small long-term risk of kernicterus in the absence of hemolytic disease.

INHERITED CONJUGATED HYPERBILIRUBINEMIA

In inherited conjugated hyperbilirubinemias, which are autosomal recessive disorders characterized by mild jaundice, the transfer of bilirubin and other organic anions from liver to bile is defective. Chronic mild conjugated hyperbilirubinemia is usually detected during adolescence or early adulthood but may occur as early as the 2nd year of life. The results of routine liver function tests are normal. Jaundice may be exacerbated with infection, pregnancy, oral contraceptives, alcohol consumption, or surgery. There is usually no morbidity, and life expectancy is normal; but these disorders may initially present difficult problems in the differential diagnosis of more serious diseases.

DUBIN-JOHNSON SYNDROME. Dubin-Johnson syndrome is considered to be an autosomal recessive inherited defect in hepatocyte secretion of bilirubin glucuronide. The defect in hepatic excretory function is not limited to conjugated bilirubin excretion but also involves several organic anions normally excreted from the liver cell into bile. Absent function of multiple drug-resistant protein (MRPZ), an adenosine triphosphate (ATP)–dependent canicular transporter, is the responsible defect. Bile acid excretion is normal, and serum bile acid levels are normal. Urinary coproporphyrin excretion is normal in quantity; however, coproporphyrin I constitutes 80% of the total. Coproporphyrin III is normally greater than 75% of the total. Oral and intravenous cholangiography fails to visualize the biliary tract. The defect is in porphyrin metabolism or excretion, with more than 90% of the normal total urinary coproporphyrin excretion occurring as a coproporphyrin I isomer. Roentgenography of the gallbladder is also abnormal. The liver cells contain black pigment similar to melanin.

ROTOR SYNDROME. These patients have an additional deficiency in organic anion uptake. Total urinary coproporphyrin excretion is elevated, with a relative increase in the amount of the coproporphyrin I isomer. The gallbladder is normal by roentgenography, and liver cells contain no black pigment. Sulfobromophthalein excretion is often abnormal.

357.2 Wilson Disease

Wilson disease (hepatolenticular degeneration) is an autosomal recessive disorder characterized by degenerative changes in the brain, liver disease, and Kayser-Fleischer rings in the cornea (Chapter 634). The incidence is 1/500,000–100,000 births. It is fatal if untreated; however, specific effective treatment is available. Rapid diagnostic investigation of the possibility of Wilson disease in a patient presenting with any form of liver disease, particularly if older than 5 yr, not only facilitates early institution of management of Wilson disease and related genetic counseling but also allows appropriate treatment of non-Wilson liver disease once copper toxicosis is ruled out.

PATHOGENESIS. Defective mobilization of copper from lysosomes in liver cells for excretion into bile is the basis for the multiorgan damage in patients with Wilson disease. Relentless accumulation of copper in the liver reaches the point at which the retention capacity is exceeded. Copper then escapes the liver to damage other organs, particularly the brain and kidneys, and accumulates in the cornea, visible as Kayser-Fleischer rings. The underlying mechanism of liver damage in Wilson disease is presumably oxidant injury to the hepatocyte mitochondria, which is the target organelle in copper-induced toxicity. Lipid peroxidation of the mitochondria resulting from copper overload leads to functional alterations.

The abnormal gene for Wilson disease is on chromosome 13; linkage studies have assigned the Wilson disease locus to chromosome 13 at q14–q21. The gene encodes amino acid structural motifs consistent with a role in copper transport. The Wilson disease gene, like the Menkes disease gene, is predicted to encode a copper-binding, cation-transporting P-type ATPase and acts as a copper pump with ATP as an energy source. Markers close to the Wilson disease gene allow accurate diagnosis in presymptomatic siblings. More than 80 mutations in the gene have been identified, and one of these is found predominantly in patients with a later age of onset. Mutations that completely destroy gene function are associated with an onset of disease symptoms as early as 2–3 yr of age, when WD may not typically be considered in the differential diagnosis. Milder mutations can be associated with neurologic symptoms or liver disease as late as 50 yr of age. Cloning of the gene for Wilson disease raises the prospect of precise presymptomatic detection of Wilson disease, timely initiation of therapy, and ultimately gene therapy.

Fetal and neonatal liver normally contains relatively high concentrations of sulfur-rich copper-binding protein (metallothionein) and of copper; serum ceruloplasmin and copper levels are relatively low. The mechanisms responsible for copper homeostasis in older children reach maturity by 2 yr of age. The wilsonian trait may be expressed after this time, but Wilson disease is not clinically manifested before age 5 yr.

Altered incorporation of copper into hepatic proteins such as ceruloplasmin is associated with diffuse accumulation of copper in the cytosol of hepatocytes. Later, as liver cells are overloaded, copper is distributed to other tissues, to which it is toxic, primarily as a potent inhibitor of enzymatic processes. Ionic copper inhibits pyruvate oxidase in brain and ATPase in membranes, leading to decreased ATP-phosphocreatine and potassium content of tissue. The glycolytic pathway and microsomal membrane ATPases are inhibited.

CLINICAL MANIFESTATIONS. Copper enters the circulation in a non–ceruloplasmin-bound form and accumulates in many organs. The symptoms of Wilson disease are due to copper-induced injury in these various organs. Manifestations are variable, with a tendency to familial patterns. The younger the patient, the more likely hepatic involvement will be the predominant manifestation. After age 20 yr, neurologic symptoms predominate. Forms of hepatic disease include asymptomatic hepatomegaly (with or without splenomegaly), subacute or chronic hepatitis, or fulminant hepatic failure. Cryptogenic cirrhosis, portal hypertension, ascites, edema, esophageal bleeding, or other effects of hepatic dysfunction (delayed puberty, amenorrhea, or coagulation defect) may be manifestations of Wilson disease.

Neurologic and psychiatric disorders may develop insidiously or precipitously, with intention tremor, dysarthria, dystonia, deterioration in school performance, or behavioral changes. Kayser-Fleischer rings may be absent in young patients with liver disease but are always present in patients with neurologic symptoms. Hemolysis may be an initial manifestation, possibly related to the release of large amounts of copper from damaged hepatocytes; this form of Wilson disease is usually fatal without transplantation. During hemolytic episodes, urinary copper excretion and serum copper levels (non–ceruloplasmin bound) are markedly elevated. Manifestations of Fanconi syndrome and progressive renal failure with alterations in tubular transport of amino acids, glucose, and uric acid may be present. Unusual manifestations include arthritis and endocrinopathies, such as hypoparathyroidism.

PATHOLOGY. All grades of hepatic injury occur, with fatty change, ballooned hepatocytes, glycogen granules, minimal inflammation, and enlarged Kupffer cells. The lesion may be indistinguishable from that of chronic hepatitis. Ultrastructural changes include large, dense mitochondria with altered smooth endoplasmic reticulum.

DIAGNOSIS. The clinical suspicion is confirmed by study of indices of copper metabolism. Wilson disease should be considered in children and teenagers with unexplained acute or chronic liver disease, neurologic symptoms of unknown cause, acute hemolysis, psychiatric illnesses, behavioral changes, Fanconi syndrome, or unexplained bone disease.

The best screening test is to measure the serum ceruloplasmin level. Most patients with Wilson disease have decreased ceruloplasmin levels. Serum copper level may be elevated in early Wilson disease, and urinary copper excretion (usually <40 μg/day) is increased to greater than 100 μg/day and often up to 1,000 μg or more per day. In equivocal cases, the response of urinary copper output to chelation may be of diagnostic help; after a 1-g oral dose of D-penicillamine, affected patients excrete 1,200–2,000 μg/24 hr.

Liver biopsy is of value for examination of the histology and for measurement of the hepatic copper content (normally <10 μg/g dry weight). In Wilson disease, hepatic copper content exceeds 250 μg/g dry weight. In healthy heterozygotes, levels may be intermediate.

Family members of patients with proven cases require screening for presymptomatic Wilson disease. Such screening should include determination of the serum ceruloplasmin level and urinary copper excretion. If these results are abnormal or equivocal, liver biopsy should be carried out to determine morphology and hepatic copper content. Genetic testing will be possible in the near future.

TREATMENT. Administration of copper-chelating agents leads to rapid excretion of excess deposited copper in patients with Wilson disease. A major attempt should be made to restrict copper intake to less than 1 mg/day. Foods such as liver, shellfish, nuts, and chocolate should be avoided. If the copper content of the water exceeds 0.1 mg/L, it may be necessary to demineralize the water. Chelation therapy is currently best managed with oral administration of penicillamine (β, β-dimethylcysteine) in a dose of 1 g/day in two doses before meals for adults and 0.5–0.75 g/day for patients younger than 10 yr. In response to D-penicillamine, urinary copper excretion markedly increases and there may be slow clinical improvement. Urinary copper levels may become normal with continued administration of D-penicillamine, with marked improvement in hepatic and neurologic function and the disappearance of Kayser-Fleischer rings. Toxic effects of penicillamine are uncommon and consist of hypersensitivity reactions (Goodpasture syndrome, systemic lupus erythematosus, polymyositis), interaction with collagen and elastin, deficiency of other elements such as zinc, as well as aplastic anemia and nephrosis. Because penicillamine is an antimetabolite of vitamin B_6, additional amounts of this vitamin are necessary. For those patients who are unable to tolerate penicillamine, triethylene tetramine dihydrochloride Trien, TETA, trientine) at a dose of 0.5–2 g/24 hr is an acceptable alternative.

Prognosis. Untreated patients with Wilson disease die of the hepatic, neurologic, renal, or hematologic complications. The prognosis for patients receiving prompt and continuous D-penicillamine is variable and depends on the time of initiation of and the individual responsiveness to chelation. Liver transplantation should be considered for patients with fulminant liver disease, decompensated cirrhosis, or progressive neurologic disease; the latter indication remains controversial. In asymptomatic siblings of affected patients, expression of the disease can be prevented by early institution of chelation therapy.

357.3 Hepatic Copper Overload Syndrome

Another form of childhood cirrhosis apparently associated with a genetic disturbance in copper metabolism has been described. This syndrome differs from Wilson disease in its earlier onset. Affected children experience progressive lethargy, abdominal distention, and jaundice and die before 6 yr of age. The hepatic histopathology resembles that of Indian childhood cirrhosis.

357.4 Indian Childhood Cirrhosis

Indian childhood cirrhosis is a fatal familial disorder that occurs predominantly in rural India in middle income Hindu families. It has been reported also in the Middle East, in West Africa, and in Central America. It affects children of both sexes, with onset usually at 1–3 yr of age. Hepatomegaly is often the 1st sign; fever, anorexia, and jaundice occur. There is in most cases rapid evolution to cirrhosis and liver failure. Serum immunoglobulin levels and hepatic copper concentrations are markedly elevated. No effective therapy is known.

It has been suggested that excessive dietary copper may have a role in the cause, owing to the use of copper and brass in cooking and for storage of water and milk. Early introduction of copper-contaminated milk into infant diets may explain the epidemiologic features. There may be a predisposing inherited susceptibility.

357.5 Neonatal Iron Storage Disease (NISD)

NISD is a rare form of fulminant liver disease of unknown cause characterized by diffuse increased iron deposition in the liver, pancreas, heart, and endocrine organs without evidence of increased iron intake (ingestion or transfusion). Inheritance is autosomal recessive. Affected infants may be born prematurely, or with intrauterine growth retardation. A large placenta is found, and a rapidly fatal progressive illness characterized by hepatomegaly, hypoglycemia, hypoprothrombinemia, hypoalbuminemia, and hyperbilirubinemia follows. Symptoms begin in utero or in the 1st wk of life. The coagulopathy is refractory to therapy with vitamin K. The diagnosis can be confirmed through documentation of extrahepatic siderosis (biopsy material of buccal mucosal glands is laden with iron) or MRI determination of iron storage in organs such as the pancreas.

The hepatic pathology reveals fibrosis, regenerative nodules, giant cell formation, necrosis, and hepatocellular hemosiderin deposits not unlike those in adult-type hereditary hemochromatosis. Hyperferritinemia is present.

Treatment with chelating agents (deferoxamine) alone is ineffective. Preliminary studies suggest that aggressive antioxidant therapy, combined with iron chelation, may be effective if initiated very early. Liver transplantation should also be an early consideration.

357.6 α-Antitrypsin Deficiency

See also Chapter 407.4

A small percentage of individuals homozygous for deficiency of the major serum protease inhibitor, α_1-antitrypsin, have neonatal cholestasis and later childhood cirrhosis. α_1-Antitrypsin, a glycoprotein synthesized by the liver, accounts for 80% of the serum α_1-globulin fraction. α_1-Antitrypsin is present in more than 20 different codominant alleles, only a few of which are associated with defective protease inhibitors. The most common allele of the protease inhibitor (Pi) system is M, and the normal phenotype is PiMM. The 2 allele predisposes to clinical deficiency; patients with liver disease are usually PiZZ and have serum α_1-antitrypsin levels less than 2 mg/mL (approximately 10–20% of normal). The incidence of the PiZZ genotype in the white population is estimated at 1/2,000–4,000. Intermediate phenotypes PiMS, PiMZ, and PiSZ are not definitively associated with liver disease. The null genotype has no periodic acid–Schiff (PAS)-positive inclusions and is not associated with liver disease. Of all PiZZ persons, fewer than 20% develop neonatal cholestasis. These patients are indistinguishable from other infants with "idiopathic" neonatal hepatitis, of whom they constitute approximately 5–10%.

In affected patients, the course of liver disease is highly variable. Jaundice, acholic stools, and hepatomegaly are present during the 1st week of life, but the jaundice usually clears during the 2nd–4th mo. Complete resolution, persistent liver disease, or the development of cirrhosis may follow. Older children may present with manifestations of chronic liver disease or cirrhosis, with evidence of portal hypertension.

The fact that liver disease is not universal suggests a complex pathogenesis. The liver disease may be secondary to retention of α_1-antitrypsin in the liver.

The diagnosis is best made by determination of a α_1-antitrypsin (Pi) phenotype and confirmed by liver biopsy. PAS-positive disease-resistant intracytoplasmic globules are seen in periportal hepatocytes. Immunofluorescence and immunocytochemical studies have shown this material to be antigenically related to α_1-antitrypsin. It has been suggested that abnormal biosynthesis of the protein or defective glycosylation may interfere with excretion of the product from the rough endoplasmic reticulum into the extracellular space. Electron microscopy shows amorphous deposits (glycoprotein) within dilated rough endoplasmic reticulum.

The pattern of neonatal liver injury may be highly variable. Hepatocellular damage with giant cell transformation, minimal inflammation, and bile stasis may be noted. Various degrees of portal fibrosis with biliary duct proliferation occur.

Liver transplantation has been curative. There is no other effective therapy for liver disease yet, but in the future, gene therapy will be possible.

Abno S, Yamada Y, Keino H, et al: A new type of defect in the gene for bilirubin uridine 5′-diphosphate-glucuronosyltransferase in a patient with Crigler-Najjar syndrome type I. Pediatr Res 35:629, 1994.

Adamson M, Reiner B, Olson JL, et al: Indian childhood cirrhosis in an American child. Gastroenterology 102:1771, 1992.

Arias IM: New genetics of inheritable jaundice and cholestatic liver disease. Lancet 352:82, 1998.

Balistreri WF: Fetal and neonatal bile acid synthesis and metabolism: Clinical implications. J Inherit Metab Dis 14:459, 1991.

Balistreri WF: Nontransplant options for the treatment of metabolic liver disease: Saving livers while saving lives. Hepatology 19:782, 1994.

Balistreri WF: Inborn errors of bile acid biosynthesis: Clinical and therapeutic aspects. *In:* AF Hofmann, G Paumgartner, A Stiehl (eds): Bile Acids in Gastroenterology: Basic and Clinical Advances. London, Kluwer Academic Publishers, 1995, pp 333–353.

Bavdekar AR, Bhave SA, Pradhan AM, et al: Long term survival in Indian childhood cirrhosis treated with D-penicillamine. Arch Dis Child 74:32, 1996.

Bowcock AM, Farrer LA, Hebert JM, et al: Eight closely linked loci place the Wilson disease locus within 13q14–q21. Am J Hum Genet 43:664, 1988.

Brusilow SW, Maestri NE: Urea cycle disorders: Diagnosis, pathophysiology, and therapy. Adv Pediatr 43:127, 1996.

Bull PC, Thomas GR, Rommens JM, et al: The Wilson disease gene is a putative copper transporting P-type ATPase similar to the Menkes gene. Nature Genet 5:327, 1993.

Burchell A: Molecular pathology of glucose-6-phosphatase. FASEB J 4:2978, 1990.

Clayton PT, Leonard JV, Lawson AM, et al: Familial giant cell hepatitis associated with synthesis of 3β, 7α, 12α-trihydroxy-5-cholenoic acids. J Clin Invest 79:1031, 1987.

Crystal RG: α_1-Antitrypsin deficiency, emphysema, and liver disease: Genetic basis and strategies for therapy. J Clin Invest 85:1343, 1990.

Daugherty CC, Setchell KDR, Heubi JE: Resolution of hepatic biopsy alterations in three siblings with bile acid treatment of an inborn error of bile acid metabolism (δ^4-3-oxosteroid 5β-reductase deficiency). Hepatology 18:1096, 1993.

Fox IJ, Chowdhury JR, Kaufman SS, et al: Treatment of the Crigler-Najjar syndrome type I with hepatocyte transplantation. N Engl J Med 338:1422, 1998.

Frydman M, Bonne-Tamir B, Farrer LA, et al: Assignment of the gene for Wilson disease to chromosome 13: Linkage to the esterase D locus. Proc Natl Acad Sci USA 82:1819, 1985.

Hoogstraten J, deSha DJ, Knisely AS: Fetal and liver disease may precede extrahepatic siderosis in neonatal hemochromatosis. Gastroenterology 98:1699, 1990.

Knisely AS, Magid MS, Dische MR, Cutz E: Neonatal hemochromatosis. Birth Defects 23:75, 1987.

Knisely AS, O'Shea PA, Stocks JF, et al: Oropharyngeal and upper respiratory tract mucosal gland siderosis in neonatal hemochromatosis: An approach to biopsy diagnosis. J Pediatr 113:871, 1988.
Lake JR: Hepatocyte transplantation. N Engl J Med 338:1463, 1998.
Lefkowitch JH, Honig CL, King ME, et al: Hepatic copper overload and features of Indian childhood cirrhosis in an American sibship. N Engl J Med 307:271, 1982.
Lindstedt S, Holme E, Lock EA, et al: Treatment of hereditary tyrosinemia type 1 by inhibition of 4-hydroxyphenylpyruvate dioxygenase. Lancet 340:813, 1992.
Maestri NE, Brusilow SW, Clissold DB, et al: Long-term treatment of girls with ornithine transcarbamylase deficiency. N Engl J Med 335:855, 1996.
McCullough AJ, Fleming CR, Thistle JL, et al: Diagnosis of Wilson disease presenting as fulminant hepatic failure. Gastroenterology 84:161, 1983.
Perlmutter DH: The cellular basis for liver injury in α_1-antitrypsin inhibitor deficiency. Hepatology 13:172, 1991.
Persico M, Ramano M, Muraca M, et al: Responsiveness to phenobarbital in an adult with Crigler-Najjar disease associated with neurological involvement and skin hyperextensibility. Hepatology 13:213, 1991.
Sato H, Adachi Y, Koiwai O: The genetic basis of Gilbert's syndrome. Lancet 347:557, 1996.
Scheinberg IH, Sternlieb I: Is non-Indian childhood cirrhosis caused by excess dietary copper? Lancet 344:1002, 1994.
Schilsky ML, Scheinberg H, Sternlieb I: Prognosis of Wilsonian chronic active hepatitis. Gastroenterology 100:762, 1991.
Setchell KDR, Street JM: Inborn errors of bile acid synthesis. Semin Liver Dis 7:85, 1987.
Setchell KDR, Suchy FJ, Welsh MS, et al: 3-Oxosteroid 5β-reductase deficiency described in identical twins with neonatal hepatitis a new inborn error in bile acid synthesis. J Clin Invest 82:2148, 1988.
Singh I: Biochemistry of peroxisomes in health and disease. Mol Cell Biochem 167:1, 1997.
Sternlieb I: Perspective on Wilson disease. Hepatology 12:1234, 1990.
Sveger T: Liver diseases in alpha-1 antitrypsin deficiency detected by screening of 200,000 infants. N Engl J Med 294:1316, 1976.
Sveger T, Eriksson S: The liver in adolescents with α_1-antitrypsin deficiency. Hepatology 22:514, 1995.
Teckman JH, Qu DF, Perlmutter DH: Molecular pathogenesis of liver disease in alpha(1)-antitrypsin deficiency. Hepatology 24:1504, 1996.
van der Veere CN, Sinaasappel M, McDonagh AF, et al: Current therapy for Crigler-Najjar syndrome type 1: Report of a world registry. Hepatology 24:311, 1996.
van der Veere CN, Jansen PLM, Sinaasappel M, et al: Oral calcium phosphate: A new therapy for Crigler-Najjar disease? Gastroenterology 112:455, 1997.
Vanspronsen FJ, Smit GPA, Wijburg FA, et al: Tyrosinemia type I: Considerations of treatment strategy and experiences with risk assessment, diet and transplantation. J Inherit Metab Dis 18:111, 1995.
Vennarecci G, Gunson BK, Ismail T, et al: Transplantation for end stage liver disease related to alpha$_1$-antitrypsin. Transplantation 61:1488, 1996.
Walshe JM: Treatment of Wilson disease: The historical background. Q J Med 89:553, 1996.

CHAPTER 358
Liver Abscess

William F. Balistreri

LIVER ABSCESS. Hepatic abscesses occur in infants in association with sepsis, umbilical vein infection, or vessel cannulation. Beyond infancy, hepatic abscesses occur most commonly in immunosuppressed patients. Of a large series of hepatic abscesses, 40% were found in patients with chronic granulomatous disease, and 20% in otherwise immunosuppressed patients (e.g., leukemia). Pyogenic hepatic abscesses may arise from (1) the portal circulation in patients with pylephlebitis or intra-abdominal sepsis (appendicitis, inflammatory bowel disease); (2) generalized sepsis; (3) cholangitis associated with biliary tract obstruction, such as by gallstones, in inflammatory bowel disease, after a Kasai procedure, and with choledochal cysts; (4) systemic spread from an intra-abdominal infection or contiguous spread (which usually produces large abscesses); and (5) cryptogenic biliary tract infections. Small abscesses (microabscesses) are most commonly secondary to bacteremia, candidemia, or cat-scratch disease. Implicated organisms include predominantly *Staphylococcus aureus, Escherichia coli, Salmonella,* and anaerobic organisms. Symptoms are nonspecific and may suggest systemic infection. Patients may have fever and pain in the right upper quadrant, and the liver is enlarged and may be tender to percussion. Jaundice is uncommon; serum aminotransferase and alkaline phosphatase activities may be mildly elevated. The erythrocyte sedimentation rate is high, and leukocytosis is noted. The results of blood cultures may be positive. Roentgenographic study of the chest may show elevation of the right hemidiaphragm with decreased mobility. Ultrasound or gallium scans or both may indicate the site of the abscess. In most cases, treatment requires percutaneous ultrasonogram- or CT-guided needle aspiration or surgical drainage. Antibiotic therapy is based on the culture results and Gram stain of the abscess fluid. *Entamoeba histolytica* may also cause hepatic abscesses in symptomatic or asymptomatic patients with amebic infection of the gastrointestinal tract (Chapter 271). Multiple infectious hepatic (and/or splenic) granulomas may be seen with cat scratch disease or fungi.

Chambon M, Delage C, Bailly JL, et al: Fatal hepatic necrosis in a neonate with echovirus 20 infection: Use of the polymerase chain reaction to detect enterovirus in liver tissue. Clin Infect Dis 24:523, 1997.
Pineiro-Carrero VM, Andres JM: Morbidity and mortality in children with pyogenic liver abscess. Am J Dis Child 143:1424, 1989.

CHAPTER 359
Liver Disease Associated with Systemic Disorders

William F. Balistreri

INFLAMMATORY BOWEL DISEASE. Hepatobiliary disease may complicate ulcerative colitis and Crohn disease (see Chapter 337). Both the manifestations and the severity vary. Fatty liver, cholangitis, drug-induced injury, chronic hepatitis, portal fibrosis, cirrhosis, hepatic abscesses, infarction, portal vein thrombosis, sclerosing cholangitis, carcinoma of the biliary tract, and cholelithiasis all have been associated. These complications are more likely to occur in patients with other extraintestinal complications, but there is no correlation with the severity of the inflammatory bowel disease. The cause of abnormalities in liver function in patients with ulcerative colitis or Crohn disease is unknown. Total colectomy has not been beneficial in preventing or managing hepatobiliary complications in patients with ulcerative colitis.

Extensive fatty change in the liver has been found, especially in malnourished or chronically incapacitated patients with inflammatory bowel disease. Most patients have no symptoms; they have only hepatomegaly as a sign. The chemical abnormalities are mild. The fatty infiltration usually subsides with therapy.

Primary sclerosing cholangitis may be difficult to distinguish from chronic hepatitis in patients with inflammatory bowel disease. Patients may be asymptomatic or may have jaundice, pruritus, or abdominal pain. Elevation of alkaline phosphatase (ALP), 5′-nucleotidase, or γ-glutamyltransferase activities is almost universal. This complication can occur any time in the course of inflammatory bowel disease.

Sclerosing cholangitis (fibrosing inflammation of various segments of the bile ducts) may lead to obliteration of the duct lumen. The clinical and biochemical picture is that of cholestasis, often with intermittent attacks of acute cholangitis (fever, jaundice, right upper quadrant pain, anorexia, weight loss, and pruritus), followed by portal hypertension. This complication is associated with ulcerative colitis and rarely with Crohn disease.

Primary sclerosing cholangitis (*not* associated with inflammatory bowel disease) is uncommon in children. Cholangiography reveals beading and irregularity of the intrahepatic and extrahepatic bile ducts. Treatment is aimed at improving biliary drainage and attempting to halt progression of the obliterative process. Symptomatic treatment is required for such complications as pruritus, malnutrition, and infection. There is no definitive treatment. Ursodeoxycholic acid, in a dose of 15 mg/kg/24 hr, may lead to amelioration of pruritus and a decrease in abnormal biochemical values. The course is usually slowly progressive to a fatal outcome if liver transplantation is not carried out.

BACTERIAL SEPSIS. (See Chapters 106 and 173.) This may be complicated by liver disease. The most frequently associated organisms are *Escherichia coli, Klebsiella pneumoniae,* and *Pseudomonas aeruginosa.* It is postulated that bacterial endotoxin directly inhibits bile formation by altering the bile canalicular membrane. Clinical manifestations may be subtle and difficult to differentiate from other causes of cholestasis. Serum bilirubin level is elevated, usually predominantly in the conjugated fraction. Serum ALP and aminotransferase activities may be elevated. Liver biopsy shows intrahepatic cholestasis with little or no hepatocyte necrosis. Kupffer cell hyperplasia and an increase in inflammatory cells are also common. Similar findings may occur with urosepsis.

CARDIAC DISEASE. Hepatic congestion and injury may occur as a complication of severe *chronic* or *acute congestive heart failure* (Chapter 448) or *cyanotic heart disease* (Chapters 436 to 438). Hepatic dysfunction derives from hypoxemia, systemic venous congestion, and low cardiac output. Hepatic manifestations of left- and right-sided heart failure are similar. With decreased cardiac output, there is decreased hepatic blood flow and centrizonal hypoxia. Hepatic necrosis leads to lactic acidosis, elevated aminotransferase activities, jaundice, prolonged partial thromboplastin time, and possibly hypoglycemia. With right-sided heart failure, increases in right atrial and hepatic venous pressures lead to centrizonal sinusoidal distention that presents a barrier to oxygen diffusion. Hemorrhage, pressure atrophy, and necrosis follow. Jaundice and tender hepatomegaly occur. Ascites may also occur with chronic right-sided congestive heart failure. In patients with shock liver, elevated aminotransferase activities may return rapidly to normal when perfusion and cardiac function improve. A syndrome of fulminant hepatic failure may occur, particularly in patients with aortic coarctation. Hepatic necrosis may be found in patients with hypoplastic left-sided heart syndrome.

HEMOGLOBINOPATHIES. Patients with *sickle cell anemia* (Chapter 468.1) or *sickle cell thalassemia* (Chapter 468.1) may have hepatic dysfunction owing to acute or chronic virus-associated hepatitis, iron overload, hepatic crises related to severe intrahepatic cholestasis, and ischemic necrosis. In addition, cholelithiasis and a benign form of extreme hyperbilirubinemia have been noted. Hepatic sickle cell crisis or "sickle hepatopathy" may produce intense right upper quadrant pain, fever, leukocytosis, right upper quadrant tenderness, and jaundice. Bilirubin levels may be markedly elevated; ALP activities may be only moderately elevated.

On occasion, children with sickle cell disease experience bilirubin levels exceeding 20 mg/dL; these levels are unaccompanied by severe pain or fever. There is no change in hematocrit or reticulocyte count nor any association with a hemolytic crisis. The clinical course is benign.

CHOLESTASIS ASSOCIATED WITH TOTAL PARENTERAL NUTRITION. The most common metabolic complication of *total parenteral nutrition* (TPN) in premature infants is the development of various degrees of liver dysfunction. Cholestasis is the most severe form and is potentially fatal. It is the major factor limiting effective long-term use of TPN (Chapter 93).

In *low birthweight infants,* the incidence of TPN-associated cholestasis is inversely correlated with birthweight. It develops with TPN in almost half of infants with birthweights less than 1,000 g, in 20% of those 1,000–1,500 g, and in 5–10% of those 1,500–2,000 g. The incidence of cholestasis also correlates with the duration of TPN, with onset usually after 2 wk. Respiratory distress, acidosis, hypoxia, necrotizing enterocolitis, short-bowel syndrome, and sepsis seem to enhance the likelihood and severity of cholestasis. Associated illness, the exclusion of enteral intake, and the nature of the underlying disorder that necessitates TPN may also affect the incidence.

The onset is usually insidious, with progressive jaundice and hepatic enlargement or splenomegaly. In low birthweight infants, the onset of jaundice may overlap the phase of physiologic unconjugated hyperbilirubinemia. Any icteric infant who has received TPN for more than 1 wk should have all bilirubin determinations fractionated. Cholestasis is frequently first detected through routine monitoring of infants receiving TPN. A slow progression of abnormalities is found in biochemical measurements of hepatic function. Serum bile acid concentrations may increase. Rises in serum aminotransferase activities may be a late finding. An elevation in serum ALP activity may be due to rickets, a common complication of TPN in low birthweight infants.

In addition to cholestasis, biliary complications of intravenous nutrition include cholelithiasis and the development of biliary sludge, associated with thick, inspissated gallbladder contents. These may be asymptomatic.

An effort must be made to differentiate TPN-associated hepatic dysfunction from benign causes of hepatomegaly, such as the deposition of glycogen or fat, which is common with TPN. Serum bilirubin and bile acid levels remain within the normal range in the latter situation. Consideration of other causes of cholestasis is also appropriate. The group in which TPN-associated cholestasis most frequently occurs (i.e., infants in a neonatal intensive care unit) often receives blood products or drugs. Therefore, hepatic disease related to drug-induced liver disease is a consideration.

The most striking histologic finding in TPN-associated liver disease is canalicular cholestasis, which may begin after less than 2 wk of TPN. Bile duct proliferation may resemble that in biliary atresia. Portal fibrosis is a late finding. Progression of injury to cirrhosis is possible. Milder changes may be reversible with discontinuation of TPN and initiation of oral feedings.

The pathogenesis of TPN-associated cholestasis is most likely multifactorial. Infants are of low birthweight, are receiving nothing by mouth, may have significant gastrointestinal disease, and often have other systemic complications. The administered nutrient solution has potential toxicity and may induce specific deficiencies. The omission of oral feedings and the absence of intraluminal nutrients blunt the output of the gastrointestinal hormones, which are normal stimulants to bile flow and to development of the hepatobiliary system. Potential hepatotoxins include bacterial endotoxins, specific amino acids or metabolic or degradation products, aluminum, copper, or manganese; the last two are particularly hepatotoxic.

The goal in treatment of infants with TPN-associated cholestasis is to avoid progressive liver injury. It has been shown that with the administration of oral feedings, gradual resolution of the liver disease occurs. Initiation of oral feedings of small volume or infusion of nutrients by continuous nasogastric drip may enhance biliary flow and intestinal motility. This effect may occur even when the enteral intake does not provide the total caloric needs. Improved solutions that meet the specific needs of neonates may prevent deficiencies and avoid toxicities. In the decision to continue TPN, one must weigh the risk of further hepatic injury against the risk of malnutrition.

In *older children,* TPN-associated cholestasis is less common and less severe than in infants. Hepatic steatosis without cholestasis is often the only abnormality. However, biochemical abnormalities are not uncommon in older patients who are maintained on TPN for prolonged periods, either at home or in the hospital. Patients with chronic intestinal disease, which may be complicated by infection or bacterial overgrowth, are particularly susceptible to hepatic dysfunction. In most such patients, partial enteral alimentation reverses the abnormalities. It may be necessary at any age, when ALP or aminotransferase activities are elevated, to evaluate the underlying liver disease by liver biopsy.

BONE MARROW TRANSPLANTATION. Hepatic dysfunction is common in patients who have undergone *bone marrow transplantation.* Its genesis is multifactorial and may be related to (1) infections (viral, bacterial, or fungal), drugs, parenteral nutrition, chemotherapy, or radiation; (2) veno-occlusive disease (VOD); or (3) graft versus host disease (GVHD); or any combination of these. Candidates for bone marrow transplantation have often had pre-existing liver disease, such as viral hepatitis, drug-related injury, or malignant infiltration. Percutaneous liver biopsy in such patients may show extensive bile duct injury in GVHD, viral inclusions in cytomegalovirus disease, or the characteristic endothelial lesion in VOD, but the histologic distinction is often unclear. This presents a dilemma because treatment of one suspected complication (e.g., initiation of immunosuppressive therapy for GVHD) may have a deleterious effect if the symptoms are due to another (e.g., fungal or viral infection).

VOD of the liver usually has its onset 1–3 wk after bone marrow transplantation but may appear up to 6 wk afterward. The most characteristic presentation is onset of rapid weight gain, with ascites, hepatomegaly, right upper quadrant pain, jaundice, and oliguria. Hepatic encephalopathy and fulminant hepatic failure may follow. Less severe forms may be characterized by jaundice and ascites with a slow resolution; a mild form of VOD has histologic changes as the sole manifestation. The diagnosis rests on the exclusion of other diseases, such as congestive cardiomyopathy, constrictive pericarditis, and venous thrombosis (Budd-Chiari syndrome).

Pathologic changes in patients with VOD are best demonstrated using special (trichrome) stains to highlight the central veins. An early lesion is concentric narrowing of the lumina of small central veins, owing to edema in the subendothelial zone. There is a dense, wavy continuous band of collagen in the central veins and centrilobular hemorrhagic necrosis. The lesions may be patchy. The venular changes may progress to complete obliteration. The cause of VOD following bone marrow transplantation is not clear; it may be related to radiation, antineoplastic drugs, or both. Risk factors for VOD include high-dose conditioning regimens, leukemia, advanced age, and pre-existing liver disease.

Budd-Chiari syndrome involves occlusion of the inferior vena cava or hepatic veins and tributaries; it may be caused by obstruction resulting from a web, mass, or thrombus. The disease has rarely been noted in children; however, a number of associated diseases may increase the risk. These include trauma, coagulopathies, sickle cell anemia, leukemia, polycythemia vera, hepatic abscesses, irradiation, and GVHD. The syndrome is to be regarded as distinct from VOD, which affects the centrilobular and sublobular hepatic veins, sparing the larger veins; it is not associated with thrombosis.

GVHD of the liver may be acute or chronic and is generally concomitant with GVHD in other target organs (Chapter 137). Cholestasis and hepatic injury of various degrees occur; there may be hepatic tenderness, dark urine, acholic stools, itching, and anorexia. There are parallel rises in serum bilirubin level and ALP activity; aspartate aminotransaminase elevation is less striking. GVHD is characterized histologically by degeneration and loss of small bile ducts and sparse inflammation, along with cholestasis.

COLLAGEN VASCULAR DISEASE. Hepatic involvement in patients with *collagen vascular disease* is uncommon. It has been noted especially in patients with systemic lupus erythematosus. Reactive hepatitis, chronic hepatitis, steatosis, and hepatic infarction have also been described. The association of hepatic injury with drug therapy, such as salicylate use, must be differentiated.

Balistreri WF: The liver—the next frontier in the treatment of patients with cystic fibrosis. *In:* Reyes HB, Leuschner U, Arias I (eds): Pregnancy, Sex Hormones, and the Liver. Proceedings of the 89th Falk Symposium: Lancaster, UK, Kluwer Academic Publishers, 1996, pp 114–135.

Buchanan GR, Glader BE: Benign course of extreme hyperbilirubinemia in sickle cell anemia: Analysis of six cases. J Pediatr 91:21, 1977.

Cohen JA, Kaplan MM: Left sided heart failure presenting as hepatitis. Gastroenterology 74:583, 1978.

Colombo C, Battezzati PM, Podda M, et al: Ursodeoxycholic acid for liver disease associated with cystic fibrosis: A double-blind multicenter trial. Hepatology 23:1484, 1996.

Duthie A, Doherty DG, Donaldson PT, et al: The major histocompatibility complex influences the development of chronic liver disease in male children and young adults with cystic fibrosis. J Hepatol 23:532, 1995.

El-Shabrawi M, Wilkinson ML, Portmann B, et al: Primary sclerosing cholangitis in childhood. Gastroenterology 92:1226, 1987.

Gentile-Kocher S, Bernard O, Brunnelle F, et al: Budd Chiari syndrome in children: Report of 22 cases. J Pediatr 113:30, 1988.

Hofmann AF: Defective biliary secretion during total parenteral nutrition: Probable mechanisms and possible solutions. J Pediatr Gastroenterol Nutr 20:376, 1995.

McDonald GB, Sharma P, Matthews DE, et al: Veno-occlusive disease of the liver after bone marrow transplantation: Diagnosis, incidence, and predisposing factors. Hepatology 4:116, 1984.

Moseley RH: Sepsis-associated cholestasis. Gastroenterology 112:302, 1997.

Mullick FG, Moran CA, Ishak KG: Total parenteral nutrition: A histopathologic analysis of the liver changes in 20 children. Mod Pathol 7:190, 1994.

Narkewicz MR, Sokol RJ, Beckwith B, et al: Liver involvement in Alpers disease. J Pediatr 119:260, 1991.

Nemeth A, Ejderhamm J, Glaumann H, et al: Liver damage in juvenile inflammatory bowel disease. Liver 10:239, 1990.

Sale GE, Shulman HM: Liver disease after marrow transplantation. *In:* Sale GE, Shulman HM (eds): The Pathology of Bone Marrow Transplantation. Chicago, Year Book Medical Publishers, 1984.

Sisto A, Feldman P, Garel L, et al: Primary sclerosing cholangitis in children: Study of five cases and review of the literature. Pediatrics 80:818, 1987.

Snover DC, Weisdorf SA, Ramsay NK, et al: Hepatic graft-versus-host disease: A study of the predictive value of the liver biopsy in diagnosis. Hepatology 4:123, 1984.

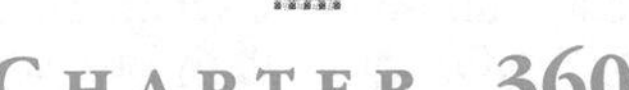

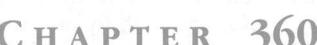

CHAPTER 360

Reye Syndrome and "Reye-like" Diseases

(The Mitochondrial Hepatopathies)

William F. Balistreri

The previously high incidence of this syndrome of acute encephalopathy and fatty degeneration of the liver has decreased markedly. This decline has been attributed to an increased awareness of the highly significant association between this disorder and ingestion of aspirin-containing medications by children with influenza-like illness or varicella. However, investigations of Reye syndrome uncovered a wide variety of previously undefined metabolic diseases whose clinical picture is similar and that need to be considered in the differential diagnosis of acute liver injury mimicking Reye syndrome (Table 360–1).

TABLE 360–1 Diseases That Present a Clinical/Pathologic Picture Resembling Reye Syndrome

Metabolic disease
- Organic acidurias
- Disorders of oxidative phosphorylation
- Urea cycle defects (carbamoyl phosphate synthetase, ornithine transcarbamylase)
- Fructosemia
- Defects in fatty acid oxidation metabolism
  - Acyl-CoA dehydrogenase deficiencies
  - Systemic carnitine deficiency
  - Hepatic carnitine palmitoyltransferase deficiency
  - 3-OH, 3-methylglutaryl-CoA lyase deficiency

Central nervous system infections or intoxications (meningitis, encephalitis, toxic encephalopathy)
Hemorrhagic shock with encephalopathy
Drug ingestion (salicylate, valproate)
Toxin (hypoglycin A, valproate)

CoA = coenzyme A.

The pathophysiology of Reye syndrome involves generalized loss of mitochondrial function, leading to disturbances in fatty acid and carnitine metabolism. Detailed studies have now delineated an entire class of mitochondrial hepatopathies—inherited disorders that are characterized by episodes of illness resembling Reye syndrome.

"CLASSIC" REYE SYNDROME

Despite the markedly decreased incidence, it is important to remember the lessons taught by the Reye syndrome experience.

EPIDEMIOLOGY. Case reports of Reye syndrome were sporadic until 1974, when almost 400 cases were reported in the United States, with a mortality rate of more than 40%. The incidence was increased in direct temporal and geographic relationship to viral epidemics, especially those caused by influenza B and varicella. By 1988, the incidence had declined dramatically; only 20 cases were reported; today this disorder is rare.

Reye syndrome was most commonly at approximately 6 yr of age, with most cases in the 4–12 yr age range. There was no gender difference in incidence, but rural and suburban populations appeared to be more frequently affected than urban populations. It is very likely that mild cases were missed and that patients recovered without event. In any case, in the late 1970s, Reye syndrome was the most common potentially lethal virus-associated encephalopathy in the United States.

CLINICAL MANIFESTATIONS. Classic Reye syndrome exhibits a stereotypic, biphasic course. It usually occurs in a previously healthy child. A prodromal febrile illness, an upper respiratory tract infection (in 90% of the cases), or chickenpox (in 5–7%) is followed by an interval in which the child has seemingly recovered. The abrupt onset of protracted vomiting then occurs, usually within 5–7 days after the onset of the viral illness. Delirium, combative behavior, and stupor may occur simultaneously or within a few hours after the onset of vomiting. Neurologic symptoms may rapidly progress to seizures, coma, and death; focal neurologic signs are absent. There is a slight to moderate liver enlargement with abnormalities of hepatic function; patients remains anicteric. Cerebrospinal fluid (CSF) is normal except for elevated pressure.

DIAGNOSIS. The clinical features are best reflected in the system of clinical staging that has been proposed (Table 360–2); grades I through III represent mild to moderate illness; grades IV and V represent severe illness. The majority of affected children have mild illness without progression. The CSF is normal.

There is explosive release from liver and muscle of such enzymes as aminotransferases, creatine kinase, and lactic dehydrogenase. The activity of the mitochondrial enzyme serum glutamate dehydrogenase is greatly increased. Patients who are not in coma and who have a threefold or higher elevation in serum ammonia level are more likely to progress to coma, as are patients who have hypoprothrombinemia unresponsive to vitamin K. Younger patients may have hypoglycemia; however, these patients should be carefully screened for the presence of metabolic disease. (see Table 360–1).

Pathology. The striking and characteristic gross pathologic feature of Reye syndrome is a yellow to white liver, reflective of a high content of triglyceride. Light microscopy shows a uniform foaminess of liver cell cytoplasm with microvesicular fatty accumulation, which may be concealed in routine preparations. Electron microscopic changes include a unique alteration of mitochondrial morphology. At present, biopsy should be carried out to rule out metabolic or toxic liver disease, especially in patients younger than 1–2 yr. Histologic examination of brain tissue reveals a similar pattern of injury. Grossly, marked edema is noted.

Pathogenesis. The major site of injury is the mitochondria. The activities of hepatic intramitochondrial enzymes, including ornithine transcarbamylase (OTC), carbamoylphosphate synthetase (CPS), and pyruvate dehydrogenase, are reduced, often to less than half of their normal values. Hyperammonemia may result from acquired decreases in the activities of OTC and CPS.

The reasons for mitochondrial dysfunction are unknown. No toxic factor has yet been conclusively identified, but studies have suggested an etiologic link among Reye syndrome, use of aspirin, and viral infections. **It is prudent to avoid the use of aspirin as an antipyretic in patients with influenza or varicella.**

TREATMENT. Successful management of Reye syndrome requires (1) precise diagnostic evaluation to preclude disorders resembling Reye syndrome; those disorders, which are more likely to be encountered, include defects in fatty acid oxidation, oxidative phosphorylation, and other metabolic injuries presenting as acute liver failure; and (2) control of increased intracranial pressure (ICP) secondary to cerebral edema, which is the major lethal factor.

Early diagnosis may be aided by a high level of clinical suspicion and by assessment of hepatic function in suspected cases. Marked elevation of aminotransferase activities, prolongation of prothrombin time, and elevation of the serum ammonia level above 125–150 μg/dL suggest the diagnosis. It is imperative that cerebral edema be identified and counteracted and that aerobic metabolism be maintained.

Management varies with the severity of the illness. Whereas observation alone may suffice in patients with grade 1 severity, more aggressive therapy is needed in patients with more severe neurologic deterioration. All patients should initially receive glucose (10–15%) intravenously, because glycogen depletion is common. In patients with cerebral edema, the amount of fluid administered should be restricted to approximately 1500 mL/m^2 day. Hyperthermia should be avoided. Coagulopathy is managed with vitamin K, fresh frozen plasma, and platelet transfusions.

TABLE 360–2 Clinical Staging of Reye Syndrome

Grade	Symptoms at Time of Admission
I	Usually quiet, **lethargic** and sleepy, vomiting, laboratory evidence of liver dysfunction
II	Deep lethargy, **confusion,** delirium, combative, hyperventilation, hyper-reflexic
III	Obtunded, **light coma** ± seizures, decorticate rigidity, intact pupillary light reaction
IV	Seizures, deepening coma, **decerebrate rigidity,** loss of oculocephalic reflexes, fixed pupils
V	Coma, loss of deep tendon reflexes, respiratory arrest, fixed dilated pupils, **flaccidity/decerebrate** (intermittent); isoelectric electroencephalogram

In more severely ill, comatose patients, endotracheal intubation permits adequate oxygenation; hyperventilation induces hypocarbia, which decreases cerebral blood flow by cerebral vasoconstriction. Close monitoring of ICP assists in decisions about management. Stimulation of patients should be minimized because procedures such as suctioning may generate increases in ICP.

An indwelling arterial catheter permits continuous assessment of cerebral perfusion pressure. The ICP should be held to less than 20 mm Hg and the cerebral perfusion pressure to greater than 50 mm Hg. Pressure (CSF) monitoring provides an effective guide to therapy. Pentobarbital (2.5 mg/kg) to maintain a serum barbiturate level of 20–30 μg/mL may have a protective effect on the central nervous system by decreasing cerebral metabolic demands, decreasing cerebral blood flow, and causing cerebral vasoconstriction. Excessive pentobarbital may reduce cardiac function, lowering blood pressure and, therefore, cerebral perfusion pressure.

PROGNOSIS. The duration of disordered cerebral function during the acute stage of illness is the best predictor of eventual outcome. In patients with grade 1 disease, recovery is rapid and complete. In patients with more severe disease there may be subsequent subtle neuropsychologic defects noted (in intelligence, school achievement, visuomotor integration, and concept formation).

DISORDERS OF OXIDATIVE PHOSPHORYLATION

Oxidative phosphorylation (OXPHOS) includes the oxidation of fuel molecules by oxygen and the concomitant energy transduction into adenosine triphosphate. During the oxidation process, reducing equivalents are transferred from respiratory substrates to oxygen via four multienzyme complexes: reduced nicotinamide-adenine dinucleotide (NAD) coenzyme Q reductase ***(complex I)***, succinate coenzyme Q reductase ***(complex II)***, coenzyme Q H_2-cytochrome *c* reductase ***(complex III)***, and cytochrome *c* oxidase ***(complex IV)***. Genetic defects of OXPHOS are a cause of rapidly fatal hepatic failure in neonates. There may also be a delayed-onset from defective OXPHOS; affected children present later in life with hepatomegaly and jaundice, often with neurologic involvement.

Belay E, Bresee JS, Holman RC, et al: Reye's syndrome in the United States from 1981 through 1997. N Engl J Med 340:1377, 1999.
Bougneres PF, Rocchiccioli F, Koluraa S, et al: Medium-chain acyl-CoA dehydrogenase deficiency in two siblings with a Reye-like syndrome. J Pediatr 106:918, 1985.
Cormier-Daire V, Chretien D, Rustin P, et al: Neonatal and delayed-onset liver involvement in disorders of oxidative phosphorylation. J Pediatr 130:817, 1997.
Greene CL, Blitzer MG, Shapira E: Inborn errors of metabolism and Reye syndrome: Differential diagnosis. J Pediatr 113:156, 1988.
Hardie RM, Newton LH, Bruce JC, et al: The changing clinical pattern of Reye syndrome 1982–1990. Arch Dis Child 74:400, 1996.
Hurwitz ES, Barrett MJ, Bergman D, et al: Public health service study of Reye syndrome and medications: Report of the main study. JAMA 257:1905, 1987.
Lichtenstein PK, Heubi JE, Daugherty CC, et al: Grade I Reye syndrome: A frequent cause of vomiting and liver dysfunction after varicella and upper-respiratory-tract infection. N Engl J Med 309:133, 1983.
Mazzella M, Cerone R, Bonacci W, et al: Severe complex I deficiency in a case of neonatal-onset lactic acidosis and fatal liver failure. Acta Pediatr 86:326, 1997.
Pollitt RJ: Disorders of mitochondrial B-oxidation: Prenatal and early postnatal diagnosis and the irrelevance to Reye syndrome and sudden infant death. J Inherit Metab Dis 12:215, 1989.
Rowe PC, Valle D, Brusilow SW: Inborn errors of metabolism in children referred with Reye syndrome: A changing pattern. JAMA 260:3167, 1988.
Shoffner JM, Wallace DC: Oxidative phosphorylation diseases and mitochondrial DNA mutations: Diagnosis and treatment. Annu Rev Nutr 14:535, 1994.
Stanley CA, Hale DE: Genetic disorders of mitochondrial fatty acid oxidation. Curr Opin Pediatr 6:476, 1994.

CHAPTER 361
Autoimmune (Chronic) Hepatitis

Benjamin L. Shneider and Frederick J. Suchy

Autoimmune hepatitis is a continuing hepatic inflammatory process manifested by elevated serum aminotransaminase concentrations and liver-associated serum autoantibodies. Older definitions required chronicity specifying the duration of liver disease for at least 6 mo. Current criteria emphasize that in the presence of either severe liver disease or physical stigmata of chronic liver disease (clubbing, spider telangiectasia, hepatosplenomegaly) a shorter time may be employed. The severity is variable; the affected child may have only biochemical evidence of liver dysfunction, may have stigmata of chronic liver disease, or may present in hepatic failure.

Chronic hepatitis can also be caused by persistent viral infection, drugs, metabolic diseases, or unknown factors (Table 361–1). Approximately 15–20% of cases are associated with hepatitis B infection (Chapter 177); unusually severe disease may be caused by superimposed infection with hepatitis D (a defective RNA virus that is dependent on replicating hepatitis B virus). Over 90% of hepatitis B infections in the 1st yr of life become chronic compared with 5–10% among older children and adults. Chronic hepatitis develops in over 50% of acute hepatitis C virus infections. Patients receiving blood products or who have had massive transfusions are at increased risk. Hepatitis A or E viruses do not cause chronic hepatitis. Drugs commonly used in children that may cause chronic liver injury include isoniazid, methyldopa, pemoline, nitrofurantoin, dantrolene, minocycline, pemoline, and the sulfonamides. Metabolic diseases can lead to chronic hepatitis including α_1-antitrypsin deficiency, inborn errors of bile acid biosynthesis, and Wilson disease. Steatohepatitis, usually associated with obesity, is another common cause of chronic hepatitis; it is relatively benign and responds to weight reduction. However, progression to cirrhosis has been described in adults. In most cases, the cause of chronic hepatitis is unknown; in many, an autoimmune mechanism is suggested by the finding of serum antinuclear and anti–smooth muscle antibodies and by multisystem involvement (arthropathy, thyroiditis, rashes, and Coombs-positive hemolytic anemia).

TABLE 361–1 Disorders Producing a Chronic Hepatitis

Chronic Viral Hepatitis

- Hepatitis B
- Hepatitis C
- Hepatitis D

Autoimmune Hepatitis

- Antiactin antibody positive
- Anti–liver-kidney microsomal antibody positive
- Antisoluble liver antigen antibody positive
- Others (includes antibodies to liver-specific lipoproteins or asialoglycoprotein)
- Overlap syndrome with sclerosing cholangitis and autoantibodies
- Systemic lupus erythematosus

Drug-Induced Hepatitis

Metabolic Disorders Associated with Chronic Liver Disease

- Wilson disease
- α_1-Antitrypsin deficiency
- Tyrosinemia
- Niemann-Pick disease type 2
- Glycogen storage disease type IV
- Cystic fibrosis
- Galactosemia
- Bile acid biosynthetic abnormalitics

Histologic features help characterize chronic hepatitis. Subdivision of chronic hepatitis into a persistent vs active form on the basis of histologic findings is not as useful as once thought. The finding of inflammation contained within the limiting plate of the portal tract (chronic persistent hepatitis) and an absence of fibrosis/cirrhosis suggest a more benign course. The finding of activity on biopsy may be predictive of response to antiviral therapy if hepatitis B infection is present and is a criterion used in the diagnosis of autoimmune hepatitis. Histologic features help identify the etiology; characteristic PAS-positive, diastase-resistant granules are seen in α_1-antitrypsin deficiency, while macrovesicular and microvesicular neutral fat accumulation within hepatocytes is a feature of steatohepatitis.

Autoimmune hepatitis is a clinical constellation that suggests an immune-mediated disease process; it is responsive to immunosuppressive therapy. Past terminologies such as lupoid hepatitis and chronic active autoimmune hepatitis have been replaced by the more accurate designation autoimmune hepatitis.

ETIOLOGY. The etiology of autoimmune hepatitis is unknown. It may be the result of an imbalance between CD4 and CD8 T-lymphocyte activity. Genetic predisposition may play an important role in the development of autoimmune hepatitis, although viral infection or drug exposure may initiate the process.

PATHOLOGY. The histologic features common to untreated cases include (1) inflammatory infiltrates, consisting of lymphocytes and plasma cells that expand portal areas and often penetrate the lobule; (2) moderate to severe piecemeal necrosis of hepatocytes extending outward from the limiting plate; and (3) variable necrosis, fibrosis, and zones of parenchymal collapse spanning neighboring portal triads or between a portal triad and central vein (bridging necrosis). Distortion of hepatic architecture may be severe; cirrhosis may be present in children at the time of diagnosis.

CLINICAL MANIFESTATIONS. The clinical features and course of autoimmune hepatitis are extremely variable. Signs and symptoms at the time of presentation include a wide spectrum of disease including a substantial number of asymptomatic patients and some who have an acute, even fulminant, onset. In 25–30% of patients with autoimmune hepatitis, particularly children, the illness may mimic acute viral hepatitis. In most, the onset is insidious. Patients may be asymptomatic or have fatigue, malaise, behavioral changes, anorexia, and amenorrhea, sometimes for many months before jaundice or stigmata of chronic liver disease are recognized. Extrahepatic manifestations may include arthritis, vasculitis, nephritis, thyroiditis, Coombs-positive anemia, and rash. Some patients' initial clinical features may reflect cirrhosis (ascites, bleeding esophageal varices, or hepatic encephalopathy).

There is usually mild to moderate jaundice. Spider telangiectasias and palmar erythema may be present. The liver is often tender and slightly enlarged but may not be felt in patients with cirrhosis. The spleen is commonly enlarged. Edema and ascites may be present in advanced cases. Evidence of involvement of other organ systems may be found.

LABORATORY FINDINGS. There is a moderate elevation (usually less than 1,000 IU/L) of serum aminotransferase activities. Serum bilirubin concentrations (predominantly the direct reacting fraction) are commonly 2–10 mg/dL. Serum alkaline phosphatase activity is normal to slightly increased. Serum γ-globulin levels may show marked polyclonal elevations. Hypoalbuminemia is common. The prothrombin time is prolonged, most often as a result of vitamin K deficiency but also as a reflection of impaired hepatocellular function. A normochromic normocytic anemia, leukopenia, and thrombocytopenia are present and become more severe with the development of portal hypertension and hypersplenism.

Most patients with autoimmune hepatitis have hypergammaglobulinemia. Serum IgG levels usually exceed 16 g/L. Characteristic patterns of serum autoantibodies define several subgroups of autoimmune hepatitis. The most common pattern is the formation of non–organ specific antibodies, such as antiactin (smooth muscle), antinuclear, and antimitochondrial antibodies. Approximately 50% of these patients are 10–20 yr of age. High titers of a liver-kidney microsomal (LKM) antibody are detected in another form that usually affects children 2–14 yr of age. A subgroup of primarily young women may demonstrate autoantibodies against a soluble liver antigen but not against nuclear or microsomal proteins. Some patients demonstrate only anti–smooth muscle or antinuclear antibodies. Autoantibodies are rare in healthy children so that titers as low as 1:40 should be considered significant. Up to 20% of patients with apparent autoimmune hepatitis may not have autoantibodies at presentation. Antibodies to a cytochrome P450 component of LKM are commonly found in adult patients with chronic hepatitis C infection. Homologies in antigenic peptide epitopes between the hepatitis C virus and cytochrome P450 may explain this. Other less common autoantibodies include rheumatoid factor, anti–parietal cell antibodies, and antithyroid antibodies. A Coombs-positive hemolytic anemia may be present.

DIAGNOSIS. Autoimmune hepatitis is a clinical diagnosis based upon certain diagnostic criteria; no single test will make this diagnosis. Diagnostic criteria with scoring systems have been developed for adults and modified slightly for children. Important positive features include female gender, primary elevation in transaminases and not alkaline phosphatase, elevated γ-globulin levels, the presence of autoantibodies (most commonly antinuclear, smooth muscle, or liver kidney microsome), and characteristic histologic findings. Important negative features include the absence of viral markers (hepatitis B, C, D) of infection, absence of a history of drug or blood product exposure, and negligible alcohol consumption.

All other conditions that might lead to chronic hepatitis should be excluded. The differential diagnosis includes α_1-antitrypsin deficiency (Chapter 357.6) and Wilson disease (Chapter 357.2). The former disorder must be excluded by performing α_1-antitrypsin phenotyping and the latter by measuring serum ceruloplasmin and 24-hr urinary copper excretion. Other inherited causes of chronic liver disease include tyrosinemia, Niemann-Pick disease type 2, glycogen storage disease type IV, and cystic fibrosis. Chronic active hepatitis may occur in patients with inflammatory bowel disease, but liver dysfunction in such patients is more commonly due to pericholangitis or sclerosing cholangitis. Endoscopic retrograde cholangiography may be required to exclude autoimmune primary sclerosing cholangitis. An ultrasonogram should be done to identify a choledochal cyst or other structural disorders of the biliary system. Dilated or obliterated veins on ultrasonography suggest the possibility of the Budd-Chiari syndrome. The differential diagnosis is noted in Table 361–1.

TREATMENT. Corticosteroid therapy, with or without low doses of azathioprine, improves the clinical, biochemical, and histologic features in most patients with autoimmune hepatitis and prolongs survival in most patients with severe disease.

The goal is to suppress or eliminate hepatic inflammation with minimal side effects. Prednisone at an initial dose of 1–2 mg/kg/24 hr is continued until aminotransferase values return to less than twice the upper limit of normal. The dose should then be lowered in 5-mg decrements over 4 to 6 wk until a maintenance dose of less than 20 mg/24 hr is achieved. In patients who respond poorly, who experience severe side effects, or who cannot be maintained on low-dose steroids, azathioprine (1.5 mg/kg/24 hr, up to 100 mg/24 hr) may be added, with frequent monitoring for bone marrow suppression. Alternate-day corticosteroid therapy should be used with great caution. This form of treatment may produce improvement or even normalization of serum aminotransferase activities, but histologic resolution may not occur. In patients with a mild and relatively asymptomatic presentation, some favor a lower starting dose of prednisone (10–20 mg) coupled with the simultaneous early administration of either 6-mercaptopurine (1–1.5 mg/kg/24 hr) or azathioprine (1.5–2.0 mg/kg/24 hr). Anecdotal reports have shown a potential for cyclosporine and tacrolimus in the management of cases refractory to standard therapy. Use of these agents should be reserved for practitioners with extensive experience in their administration, because they have a poor therapeutic to toxic ratio.

Histologic progress should be assessed by liver biopsy 6 mo to 1 yr after the initiation of treatment, because normal results of biochemical tests during therapy do not ensure histologic resolution. Disappearance of symptoms and biochemical abnormalities and either resolution of the necroinflammatory process on biopsy (remission) or at least improvement to a pattern of chronic persistent hepatitis justify an attempt to gradually discontinue medication. There is a high rate of relapse after discontinuation of therapy.

The therapy of chronic viral hepatitis differs from that for autoimmune disease (also see Chapter 177). Chronic hepatitis B infection is defined by persistently elevated serum levels of HBV DNA and HbsAg, with or without HbeAg. In addition, there is persistent elevated serum aminotransferases and histologic evidence of chronic hepatitis. Therapy with interferon-α (6 million U/m^2 body surface area subcutaneously, 3 × wk) for 4–6 mo will induce a remission (defined as undetectable HBV DNA and HBeAg) in 25–40%. Side effects of interferon-α include systemic flu-like episodes, anxiety, poor mental concentration, development of autoantibodies, and increased susceptibility to bacterial infection. Lamivudine, an oral nucleoside analog, also holds promise alone or in combination with interferon.

Chronic hepatitis C virus is defined by the presence of serum anti-HCV antibodies and HCV RNA in addition to elevated aminotransferases and histologic evidence of chronic hepatitis. Therapy includes interferon-α (3 million U/m^2 body surface area, 3 × wk) for 6 mo. Remission is induced in 40–50%; however, 50% will relapse after therapy is stopped. The combination of interferon and oral ribavirin may improve the outcome.

PROGNOSIS. The initial response to therapy in autoimmune hepatitis is generally prompt, with a greater than 75% rate of remission. Transaminases and bilirubin fall to near-normal levels often within the first 1–3 mo. When present, abnormalities in serum albumin and prothrombin time also respond over a longer period (3–9 mo). In patients meeting the criteria for tapering and then withdrawal of treatment (25 to 40% of children), 50% are weaned from all medication; in the other 50%, relapse occurs after a variable period. Relapse usually responds to retreatment. Many children will not meet the criteria for an attempt at discontinuation of immunosuppression and should be maintained on the smallest dose of prednisone that minimizes biochemical activity of the disease. A careful balance of the risks of continued immunosuppression and ongoing hepatitis must be continually evaluated. This may require sequential liver biopsies and continual screening for complications of medical therapy (ophthalmologic examination, bone density measurement, blood pressure monitoring). Intermittent flares of hepatitis can occur and may require restarting of prednisone therapy. Some children have a relatively steroid-resistant form of hepatitis. Progression to cirrhosis may occur in autoimmune hepatitis despite a good response to drug therapy and prolongation of life.

Orthotopic liver transplantation has been successful in patients with end-stage liver disease associated with autoimmune hepatitis (Chapter 367). Nonetheless, disease may recur after transplantation. Thus, indication for transplantation should include evidence of hepatic decompensation and not resistance to standard immunosuppressive regimens.

Baldridge AD, Perez-Atayde AR, Graeme-Cook F, et al: Idiopathic steatohepatitis in childhood: A multicenter retrospective study. J Pediatr 127:700, 1995.

Birnbaum AH, Benkov KJ, Pittman NS, et al: Recurrence of autoimmune hepatitis in children after liver transplantation. J Pediatr Gastroenterol Nutr 25:20, 1997.

Brown JL: Efficacy of combined interferon and ribavirin for treatment of hepatitis C. Lancet 351:78, 1998.

Czaja A: The variant forms of autoimmune hepatitis. Ann Intern Med 125:588, 1996.

Gregorio GV, Portmann B, Reid F, et al: Autoimmune hepatitis in childhood: A 20 year experience. Hepatology 25:541, 1997.

Herzog D, Rasquin-Weber AM, Debray D, et al: Subfulminant hepatic failure in autoimmune hepatitis type 1: An unusual form of presentation. J Hepatol 27:578, 1997.

Hochman JA, Woodard SA, Cohen MB, et al: Exacerbation of autoimmune hepatitis: Another hepatotoxic effect of pemoline therapy. Pediatrics 101:106, 1998.

Hoofnagle JH, Di Bisceglie AM: The treatment of chronic viral hepatitis. N Engl J Med 336:347, 1997.

Krawitt EL: Autoimmune hepatitis. N Engl J Med 334:897, 1996.

Lai CL, Chien RN, Leung NWY, et al: A one-year trial of lamivudine for chronic hepatitis B. N Engl J Med 339:61, 1998.

Maggiore G: Chronic hepatitis in children. Curr Opin Pediatr 7:539, 1995.

Neuberger J: Primary biliary cirrhosis. Lancet 350:875, 1997.

Poynard T, Marcellin P, Lee SS, et al: Randomised trial of interferon α2b ribavirin for 48 weeks or for 24 weeks versus interferon α2b plus placebo for 48 weeks for treatment of chronic infection with hepatitis C virus. Lancet 352:1426, 1998.

Teitelbaum JE, Perez-Atayde AR, Cohen M, et al: Minocycline-related autoimmune hepatitis. Arch Pediatr Adolesc Med 152:1132, 1998.

CHAPTER 362
Drug- and Toxin-Induced Liver Injury

Frederick J. Suchy

The liver is the main site of drug metabolism and is particularly susceptible to structural and functional injury after ingestion, parenteral administration, or inhalation of chemical agents, drugs, plant derivatives (home remedies), or environmental toxins. The possibility of drug use or toxin exposure at home or in the parental workplace should be explored for every child with liver dysfunction. The clinical spectrum of illness may vary from asymptomatic biochemical abnormalities of liver function to fulminant failure.

Hepatic metabolism of drugs and toxins is mediated by a sequence of enzymatic reactions that, in large part, transform hydrophobic, less excretable molecules into more nontoxic, hydrophilic compounds that can be readily excreted in urine or bile. *Phase 1* of the process involves enzymatic activation of the substrate to reactive intermediates containing a carboxyl, phenol, epoxide, or hydroxyl group. Mixed-function monooxygenase, cytochrome C-reductase, various hydrolases, and the cytochrome P450 system are involved in this process. Nonspecific induction of these enzymatic pathways, which commonly occurs with administration of certain drugs such as anticonvulsants, may alter the metabolism of other drugs and increase the potential for hepatotoxicity. A single agent may be metabolized by more than one biochemical reaction. The reactive intermediates that are potentially damaging to the cell are enzymatically conjugated in *phase 2* reactions with glucuronic acid, sulfate, or glutathione. Some drugs may be directly metabolized by these conjugating reactions without first undergoing *phase 1* activation. Pathways for biotransformation develop early in life, with the possible exception of enzymes for oxidizing polycyclic aromatic hydrocarbons and for forming glucuronide conjugates. Mechanisms for the uptake and excretion of organic ions may also be deficient early in life. Some cases of idiosyncratic hepatotoxicity may occur as a result of aberrations in *phase 1* drug metabolism producing intermediates of unusual hepatotoxic potential combined with developmental, acquired, or relative inefficiency of *phase 2* conjugating reactions. Therefore, children may be more or less susceptible than adults to hepatotoxic reactions; for example, liver injury after the use of the anesthetic halothane is rare in children, and acetaminophen toxicity is unusual in infants compared with adolescents, whereas most cases of fatal hepatotoxicity associated with sodium valproate use have been reported in children. Excess or prolonged therapeutic administration of acetaminophen combined with reductions in caloric or protein intake may produce hepatotoxicity in children. It is proposed that in this setting, acetaminophen metabolism may be impaired by reduced synthesis of sulfated and glucuronated metabolites and reduced stores of glutathione. In some cases, immaturity of hepatic drug metabolic pathways may prevent degradation of a toxic agent; under other circumstances, the same immaturity might limit the formation of toxic metabolites.

Chemical hepatotoxicity may be (1) *predictable* or (2) *idiosyncratic. Predictable* hepatotoxicity implies a high incidence of hepatic injury in exposed individuals, with dose dependence. The agents involved may damage the hepatocyte directly through alteration of membrane lipids (peroxidation) or through denaturation of proteins; such agents include carbon tetrachloride and trichloroethylene. Indirect injury may occur through interference with metabolic pathways essential for cell integrity or through distortion of cellular constituents by covalent binding of a reactive metabolite; examples include the liver injury produced by acetaminophen or by antimetabolites such as methotrexate or 6-mercaptopurine.

Idiosyncratic hepatotoxicity is infrequent and unpredictable. The likelihood of injury is not dose dependent and may occur at any time during exposure to the agent. An idiosyncratic reaction may be immunologically mediated as a result of prior sensitization (hypersensitivity); extrahepatic manifestations of hypersensitivity may include fever, rash, arthralgia, and eosinophilia. Duration of exposure before reaction is generally 1–4 wk, with prompt recurrence of injury on re-exposure.

Studies indicate that arene oxides, generated through oxidative (cytochrome P450) metabolism of aromatic anticonvulsants (phenytoin, phenobarbital, carbamazepine), may initiate the pathogenesis of hypersensitivity reactions. Arene oxides, formed in vivo, may bind to cellular macromolecules, thus perturbing cell function and possibly initiating immunologic mechanisms of liver injury. Idiosyncratic drug reactions in certain patients may reflect aberrant pathways for drug metabolism, with production of toxic intermediates (isoniazid and sodium valproate may cause liver damage through this mechanism). Duration of drug use before liver injury varies (weeks to 1 yr or more), and the response to re-exposure may be delayed.

The *pathologic* spectrum of drug-induced liver disease is extremely wide, is rarely specific, and may mimic other liver diseases (Table 362–1). Predictable hepatoxins such as acetaminophen produce centrilobular necrosis of hepatocytes. Steatosis is an important feature of tetracycline (microvesicular) and ethanol (macrovesicular) toxicities. A cholestatic hepatitis can be observed with injury caused by erythromycin estolate and chlorpromazine. Cholestasis without inflammation may be a toxic effect of estrogens and anabolic steroids. Use of oral contraceptives and androgens has also been associated with benign and malignant liver tumors. Some idiosyncratic drug reactions may produce mixed patterns of injury with diffuse cholestasis and cell necrosis. Several antineoplastic drugs and some herbal remedies have produced hepatic veno-occlusive disease. Chronic hepatitis has been associated with the use of methyldopa and nitrofurantoin.

TABLE 362–1 Patterns of Hepatic Drug Injury

Disease	Drug
Centrilobular necrosis	Acetaminophen
	Halothane
Microvesicular steatosis	Valproic acid
Acute hepatitis	Isoniazid
General hypersensitivity	Sulfonamides
	Phenytoin
Fibrosis	Methotrexate
Cholestasis	Chlorpromazine
	Erythromycin
	Estrogens
Veno-occlusive disease	Irradiation plus busulfan
	Cyclophosphamide
Portal and hepatic vein thrombosis	Estrogens
	Androgens
Biliary sludge	Ceftriaxone
Hepatic adenoma or hepatocellular carcinoma	Oral contraceptives
	Anabolic steroids

Clinical manifestations may be mild and nonspecific, such as fever and malaise. Fever, rash, and arthralgia may be prominent in cases of hypersensitivity. In ill, hospitalized patients, the signs and symptoms of hepatic drug toxicity may be difficult to separate from the underlying illness. The differential diagnosis should include acute and chronic viral hepatitis, biliary tract disease, septicemia, ischemic and hypoxic liver injury, malignant infiltration, and inherited metabolic liver disease.

The *laboratory features* of drug- or toxin-related liver disease are extremely variable. Hepatocyte damage may lead to elevations of serum aminotransferase activities and serum bilirubin levels and to impaired synthetic function as evidenced by decreased serum coagulation factors and albumin. Hyperammonemia may occur with liver failure or with selective inhibition of the urea cycle (sodium valproate). Toxicologic screening of blood and urine specimens may aid in the detection of drug or toxin exposure. Percutaneous liver biopsy may be necessary to distinguish drug injury from complications of an underlying disorder or from intercurrent infection.

Slight elevation of serum aminotransferase activities (generally less than two to three times normal) may occur during therapy with drugs, particularly anticonvulsants, capable of inducing microsomal pathways for drug metabolism. Liver biopsy reveals proliferation of smooth endoplasmic reticulum but no significant liver injury. Liver test abnormalities often resolve with continued drug therapy.

Treatment of drug- or toxin-related liver injury is mainly supportive. Contact with the offending agent should be avoided. Corticosteroids may have a role in immune-mediated disease. *N*-acetylcysteine therapy, by stimulating glutathione synthesis, is effective in preventing hepatotoxicity when administered within 16 hr after an acute overdose of acetaminophen and appears to improve survival in patients with severe liver injury even up to 36 hr after ingestion (also see Chapter 722.2). Orthotopic liver transplantation may be required for treatment of drug- or toxin-induced hepatic failure.

The *prognosis* of drug- or toxin-induced liver injury depends on its type and severity. Injury is usually completely reversible when the hepatotoxic factor is withdrawn. The mortality of submassive hepatic necrosis with fulminant liver failure may, however, exceed 50%. With continued use of certain drugs, such as methotrexate, effects of hepatotoxicity may proceed insidiously to cirrhosis. Neoplasia may follow long-term androgen therapy. Rechallenge with a drug suspected of having caused previous liver injury is rarely justified and may result in fatal hepatic necrosis.

Drug-Induced Liver Disease

Farrell GC: Drug-induced hepatic injury. J Gastroenterol Hepatol 12:S242, 1997.
Heubi JE, Baracci MB, Zimmerman HJ: Therapeutic misadventures with acet-

aminophen: Hepatotoxicity after multiple doses in children. J Pediatr 132:22, 1998.
Kearns GL: Pharmacogenetics and development: Are infants and children at increased risk for adverse outcomes? Curr Opin Pediatr 7:220, 1995.
Larrey D, Pageaux GP: Genetic predisposition to drug-induced hepatotoxicity. J Hepatol 2:12, 1997.
Lee WM: Drug-induced hepatotoxicity. N Engl J Med 333:1118, 1995.
Rivera-Penera T, Gugig R, Davis J, et al: Outcome of acetaminophen overdose in pediatric patients and factors contributing to hepatotoxicity. J Pediatr 130:300, 1997.
Roberts EA: Drug-induced liver disease in children. *In:* Suchy FJ (ed): Liver Disease in Children. St. Louis, CV Mosby 1994, pp 523–549.
Rosh J, Dellert S, Narkewicz M, et al: Four cases of severe hepatotoxicity associated with pemoline: Possible autoimmune pathogenesis. Pediatrics 101:921, 1998.

CHAPTER 363
Fulminant Hepatic Failure

Frederick J. Suchy

Fulminant hepatic failure is strictly defined as a clinical syndrome resulting from massive necrosis of hepatocytes or from severe functional impairment of hepatocytes in a patient who does not have a pre-existing liver disease. The disorder usually evolves over a period of fewer than 8 wk. Synthetic, excretory, and detoxifying functions of the liver all are severely impaired, with hepatic encephalopathy an essential diagnostic criterion. This narrow definition may be problematic in infants because liver failure in the perinatal period may associated with prenatal liver injury and even cirrhosis. Examples include neonatal iron storage disease, tyrosinemia, and some cases of congenital viral infection. In these disorders, liver disease may be noticed at birth or after several days of apparent well-being. Fulminant Wilson disease also occurs in children who were previously asymptomatic but by definition have pre-existing liver disease. Moreover, in some cases of liver failure, particularly in so-called non-A, non-B, non-C hepatitis, the onset of encephalopathy may occur later, from 8–28 wk after the onset of jaundice.

ETIOLOGY. Fulminant hepatic failure is most commonly a complication of viral hepatitis (A, B, D, E, possibly C, and others). An unusually high risk of fulminant hepatic failure occurs in young people who have combined infections with the hepatitis B virus (HBV) and hepatitis D. Mutations in the precore region of HBV DNA have been associated with fulminant and severe hepatitis. HBV is also responsible for some cases of fulminant liver failure in the absence of serological markers of HBV infection but with HBV DNA found in the liver. Hepatitis C and E viruses are uncommon causes of fulminant hepatic failure in the United States. Patients with chronic HCV are at risk if they have superinfection with HAV. An additional, unidentified virus accounts for the majority of what in the past has been termed fulminant non-A, non-B, non-C hepatitis. This form may be the most common cause of fulminant hepatic failure in children. The disease occurs sporadically and usually without the parenteral risk factors of HBV or HCV Epstein-Barr virus, herpes simplex virus, adenovirus, enterovirus, cytomegalovirus, parvovirus B19, and varicella-zoster infections may produce fulminant hepatitis in children.

Various hepatotoxic drugs and chemicals may also cause fulminant hepatic failure. Predictable liver injury may occur after exposure to carbon tetrachloride and *Amanita phalloides* mushroom or after acetaminophen overdose. Idiosyncratic damage may follow the use of drugs such as halothane or sodium valproate. Ischemia and hypoxia resulting from hepatic vascular occlusion, congestive heart failure, cyanotic congenital heart disease, or circulatory shock may produce liver failure. Metabolic disorders associated with hepatic failure include Wilson disease, acute fatty liver of pregnancy, galactosemia, hereditary tryosinemia, hereditary fructose intolerance, neonatal iron storage disease, defects in β-oxidation of fatty acids, and deficiencies of mitochondrial electron transport.

PATHOLOGY. Liver biopsy usually reveals patchy or confluent massive necrosis of hepatocytes. Multilobular or bridging necrosis may be associated with collapse of the reticulin framework of the liver. There may be little or no regeneration of hepatocytes. A zonal pattern of necrosis may be observed with certain insults (e.g., centrilobular damage is associated with acetaminophen hepatotoxicity or with circulatory shock). Evidence of severe hepatocyte dysfunction rather than cell necrosis may occasionally be the predominant histologic finding (e.g., microvesicular fatty infiltrate of hepatocytes is observed in Reye syndrome, β-oxidation defects, and tetracycline toxicity).

PATHOGENESIS. The mechanisms that lead to fulminant hepatic failure are poorly understood. It is unknown why only about 1–2% of patients with viral hepatitis experience liver failure. Massive destruction of hepatocytes may represent both a direct cytotoxic effect of the virus and an immune response to the viral antigens. One third to one half of patients with HBV-induced liver failure become negative for serum hepatitis B surface antigen within a few days of presentation and often have no detectable HBV antigen or HBV DNA in serum. These findings suggest a hyperimmune response to the virus that underlies the massive liver necrosis. Formation of hepatotoxic metabolites that bind covalently to macromolecular cell constituents is involved in the liver injury produced by drugs such as acetaminophen and isoniazid; fulminant hepatic failure may follow depletion of intracellular substrates involved in detoxification, particularly glutathione. Whatever the initial cause of hepatocyte injury, various factors may contribute to the pathogenesis of liver failure, including impaired hepatocyte regeneration, altered parenchymal perfusion, endotoxemia, and decreased hepatic reticuloendothelial function.

The pathogenesis of hepatic encephalopathy may relate to increased serum levels of ammonia, false neurotransmitters, amines, increased γ-aminobutyric acid receptor activity, or increased circulating levels of endogenous benzodiazepine-like compounds. Decreased hepatic clearance of these substances may produce marked central nervous system dysfunction.

CLINICAL MANIFESTATIONS. Fulminant hepatic failure may complicate previously known acute liver disease or be the presenting feature of liver disease. A child with fulminant hepatic failure has usually been previously healthy and most often has no risk factors for liver disease such as hepatitis or blood product exposure. Progressive jaundice, fetor hepaticus, fever, anorexia, vomiting, and abdominal pain are common. A rapid decrease in liver size without clinical improvement is an ominous sign. A hemorrhagic diathesis and ascites may develop. Patients should be closely observed for hepatic encephalopathy, which is initially characterized by minor disturbances of consciousness or motor function. Irritability, poor feeding, and a change in sleep rhythm may be the only findings in infants; asterixis may be demonstrable in older children. Patients are often somnolent or confused or combative on arousal and eventually may become responsive only to painful stimuli. Patients may rapidly progress to deeper stages of coma in which extensor responses and decerebrate and decorticate posturing appear. Respirations are usually increased early, but respiratory failure may occur in stage IV coma (Table 363–1).

LABORATORY FINDINGS. Serum direct and indirect bilirubin levels and serum aminotransferase activities may be markedly elevated. However, serum aminotransferase activities do not correlate well with the severity of the illness and may actually decrease as a patient deteriorates. The blood ammonia concentration is usually increased. Prothrombin time is always pro-

TABLE 363–1 Stages of Hepatic Encephalopathy

	Stages			
	I	*II*	*III*	*IV*
Symptoms	Periods of lethargy, euphoria; reversal of day–night sleeping; may be alert	Drowsiness, inappropriate behavior, agitation, wide mood swings, disorientation	Stupor but arousable, confused, incoherent speech	Coma IVa responds to noxious stimuli IVb no response
Signs	Trouble drawing figures, performing mental tasks	Asterixis, fetor hepaticus, incontinence	Asterixis, hyperreflexia, extensor reflexes, rigidity	Areflexia, no asterixis, flaccidity
Electroencephalogram	Normal	Generalized slowing, θ waves	Markedly abnormal, triphasic waves	Markedly abnormal bilateral slowing, δ waves, electric-cortical silence

longed and often does not improve after parenteral administration of vitamin K. Hypoglycemia can occur, particularly in infants. Hypokalemia, hyponatremia, metabolic acidosis, or respiratory alkalosis may develop.

TREATMENT. Management of fulminant hepatic failure is supportive. No therapy is known to reverse hepatocyte injury or to promote hepatic regeneration.

An infant or child with advanced hepatic coma should be treated in an intensive care unit where continuous monitoring of vital functions is possible. Endotracheal intubation may be required to prevent aspiration, to reduce cerebral edema by hyperventilation, and to facilitate pulmonary toilet. Mechanical ventilation and supplemental oxygen are often necessary in advanced coma. Electrolyte and glucose solutions should be administered intravenously to maintain urine output, to correct or prevent hypoglycemia, and to maintain normal serum potassium concentrations. Hyponatremia is common but is usually dilutional and not a result of sodium depletion. Parenteral supplementation with calcium, phosphorus, and magnesium may be required. Coagulopathy should be treated with parenteral administration of vitamin K and may require fresh frozen plasma; disseminated intravascular coagulation may also occur. Plasmapheresis may permit temporary correction of the bleeding diathesis without resulting in volume overload. Continuous hemofiltration is useful for management of fluid overload and acute renal failure. Prophylactic use of antacids or H_2 receptor blockers or both should be considered because of the high risk of gastrointestinal bleeding. Hypovolemia should be avoided and treated with cautious infusions of fluids and blood products. Renal dysfunction may result from dehydration, acute tubular necrosis, or functional renal failure (hepatorenal syndrome). Patients should be monitored closely for infection, including sepsis, pneumonia, peritonitis, and urinary tract infections. At least 50% of patients experience serious infection. Gram-positive organisms *(Staphylococcus aureus, Staphylococcus epidermidis)* are the most common pathogens, but gram-negative and fungal infections are also observed. Cerebral edema is an extremely serious complication that responds poorly to measures such as corticosteroid administration and osmotic diuresis. Monitoring intracranial pressure may be useful in preventing severe cerebral edema, in maintaining cerebral perfusion pressure, and in establishing the suitability of a patient for liver transplantation.

Gastrointestinal hemorrhage, infection, constipation, sedatives, electrolyte imbalance, and hypovolemia may precipitate encephalopathy and should be identified and corrected. Protein intake should be restricted or eliminated. The gut should be purged with several enemas. Lactulose should be given every 2–4 hr orally or by nasogastric tube in doses (10–50 mL) sufficient to cause diarrhea. The dose is then adjusted to produce several acidic, loose bowel movements daily. Lactulose syrup diluted with 1–3 volumes of water may also be given as a retention enema every 6 hr. Lactulose, a nonabsorbable disaccharide, is metabolized to organic acids by colonic bacteria; it probably lowers blood ammonia levels through decreasing microbial ammonia production and through trapping of ammonia in acidic intestinal contents. Oral or rectal administration of a nonabsorbable antibiotic such as neomycin may reduce enteric bacteria responsible for ammonia production. Flumazenil, a benzodiazepine antagonist, may reverse early hepatic encephalopathy.

Controlled trials have shown a worsened outcome of fulminant hepatic failure in patients treated with corticosteroids. Various approaches have been used to assist the liver in removing neuroactive toxins, such as plasmapheresis or perfusion of the patient's plasma through a column of charcoal or other binding resins. Although patients may experience an improvement in encephalopathy, little evidence shows that these treatments improve survival. Several liver assist devices containing cultured hepatocytes are also being used experimentally in an effort to allow regeneration of a patient's liver or to temporize until a suitable organ donor becomes available. Orthotopic liver transplantation may be life saving in patients who reach advanced stages of hepatic coma. Reduced-size allografts and living donor transplantation have been important advances in the treatment of infants with hepatic failure. Partial auxiliary orthotopic or heterotopic liver transplantation is successful in a small number of children and in some cases has allowed regeneration of the native liver and eventual withdrawal of immunosupression (Chapter 367).

PROGNOSIS. Children with hepatic failure may fare somewhat better than adults, but overall mortality exceeds 70%. The prognosis may vary considerably with the cause of liver failure and stage of hepatic encephalopathy. With intensive medical support, survival rates of 50–60% occur with hepatic failure complicating acetaminophen overdose and with fulminant HAV or HBV infection. In contrast, recovery can be expected in only 10–20% of patients with liver failure caused by non-A, non-B, non-C hepatitis or an acute onset of Wilson's disease. In patients who progress to stage IV coma (see Table 363–1), the prognosis is extremely poor. Major complications such as sepsis, severe hemorrhage, or renal failure increase the mortality. The prognosis is particularly poor in patients with liver necrosis and multiorgan failure. Studies indicate that jaundice for more than 7 days before the onset of encephalopathy, a prothrombin time more than 50 sec, and a serum bilirubin level more than 17.5 mg/dL (300 μmol/L) indicate a poor prognosis irrespective of the initial stage of hepatic coma. Survival of 50–75% is being achieved in patients with the poorest prognosis after orthotopic liver transplantation. Patients who recover from fulminant hepatic failure with only supportive care do not usually experience cirrhosis or chronic liver disease. Aplastic anemia is a common and usually fatal complication of fulminant hepatic failure secondary to sporadic non-A, non-B, non-C hepatitis.

Anand AC, Nightengale P, Neuberger JM: Early indicators of prognosis in fulminant hepatic failure: An assessment of the King's criteria. J Hepatol 26:62, 1997.

Bonatti H, Muiesan P, Connolly S, et al: Liver transplantation for acute liver failure in children under 1 year of age. Transplant Proc 29:434, 1997.

Cade R, Wagemaker H, Vogel S, et al: Hepatorenal syndrome: Studies of the effect of vascular volume and intraperitoneal pressure on renal and hepatic function. Am J Med 82:427, 1987.

Daas M, Plevak DJ, Wijdicks EF, et al: Acute liver failure: Results of a 5-year clinical protocol. Liver Transplant Surg 1:210, 1995.
Dasarathy S, Mullen KD: Benzodiazepines in hepatic encephalopathy: Sleeping with the enemy. Gut 42:764, 1998.
Jalan R, Hayes PC: Hepatic encephalopathy and ascites. Lancet 350:1309, 1997.
Lee WM: Management of acute liver failure. Semin Liver Dis 16:369, 1996.
Liang TJ, Jeffers L, Reddy RK, et al: Fulminant or subfulminant non-A, non-B viral hepatitis: The role of hepatitis C and E viruses. Gastroenterology 104:556, 1993.
Mas A, Rodés J: Fulminant hepatic failure. Lancet 349:1081, 1997.
Rivera-Penera T, Moreno J, Skaff C, et al: Delayed encephalopathy in fulminant hepatic failure in the pediatric population and the role of liver transplantation. J Pediatr Gastroenterol Nutr 24:128, 1997.
Vento S, Garofano T, Renzini C, et al: Fulminant hepatitis associated with hepatitis A virus superinfection in patients with chronic hepatitis C. N Engl J Med 338:286, 1998.

CHAPTER 364

Cystic Diseases of the Biliary Tract and Liver

Frederick J. Suchy

Cystic lesions of liver parenchyma or of the biliary system may be recognized initially during infancy and childhood. Their classification is not yet satisfactory. Pathologic features may be found in common among several of these disorders, but different patterns of inheritance indicate that their etiology is heterogeneous.

CHOLEDOCHAL CYSTS. These are congenital dilatations of the common bile duct that may cause progressive biliary obstruction and biliary cirrhosis. Cylindrical and spherical cysts of the extrahepatic ducts are the most common types. Segmental or diffuse dilatation can be observed. A diverticulum of the common bile duct or dilatation of the intraduodenal portion of the common duct (choledochocele) is a variant. Cystic dilatation of the intrahepatic bile ducts may be associated with a choledochal cyst.

The pathogenesis of choledochal cysts remains uncertain. Some reports have suggested that junction of the common bile duct and the pancreatic duct before their entry into the sphincter of Oddi may allow reflux of pancreatic enzymes into the common bile duct, causing inflammation, localized weakness, and dilatation of the duct. Other possibilities are that choledochal cysts represent malformations of the common duct or that they occur as part of the disease spectrum that includes neonatal hepatitis and biliary atresia.

Approximately 75% of cases appear during childhood. The infant typically presents with cholestatic jaundice; severe liver dysfunction including ascites and coagulopathy can rapidly evolve if biliary obstruction is not relieved. An abdominal mass is rarely palpable. In an older child, the classic triad of abdominal pain, jaundice, and mass occurs in fewer than 33% of patients. Features of acute cholangitis (fever, right upper quadrant tenderness, jaundice, leukocytosis) may be present. The diagnosis is made by ultrasonography; choledochal cysts have been identified prenatally using this technique.

The treatment of choice is primary excision of the cyst and a Roux-en-Y choledochojejunostomy. Simple drainage into the small bowel is less satisfactory owing to a risk for development of carcinoma in the residual cystic tissue. The postoperative course may be complicated by recurrent cholangitis or stricture at the anastomotic site.

CYSTIC DILATATION OF THE INTRAHEPATIC BILE DUCTS (CAROLI DISEASE). Congenital, saccular dilatation may affect several segments of the intrahepatic bile ducts; the dilated ducts are lined by cuboidal epithelium and are in continuity with the main duct system, which is usually normal. Caroli actually described two variants: *Caroli disease,* characterized by ectasias of the intrahepatic bile ducts without other abnormalities, and *Caroli syndrome,* in which congenital ductal dilatation is associated with features of congenital hepatic fibrosis and the renal lesion of autosomal recessive polycystic renal disease. Caroli syndrome is more common, but both varieties may occur in the same family and are inherited in an autosomal recessive fashion. Choledochal cysts have also been associated with Caroli disease. There is a marked predisposition to ascending cholangitis and calculus formation within the abnormal bile ducts.

Affected patients usually experience symptoms of acute cholangitis as children or young adults. Fever, abdominal pain, mild jaundice, and pruritus occur; and a slightly enlarged, tender liver is palpable. Elevated alkaline phosphatase (ALP) activity, direct-reacting bilirubin levels, and leukocytosis may be observed during episodes of acute infection. In patients with Caroli syndrome, clinical features may be due to a combination of recurring bouts of cholangitis reflecting the intrahepatic ductal abnormalities and portal hypertensive bleeding resulting from hepatic fibrosis. Ultrasonography shows the dilated intrahepatic ducts, but definitive diagnosis and extent of disease must be determined by percutaneous transhepatic or endoscopic cholangiography. Magnetic resonance cholangiography is a noninvasive alternative to direct cholangiography.

Cholangitis and sepsis are treated with appropriate antibiotics. Calculi may require surgery. Partial hepatectomy may be curative in rare cases when disease is confined to a single lobe. The prognosis is otherwise guarded, largely owing to difficulties in controlling cholangitis and biliary lithiasis and to a significant risk for developing cholangiocarcinoma.

CONGENITAL HEPATIC FIBROSIS. This is an autosomal recessive disorder characterized pathologically by diffuse periportal and perilobular fibrosis in broad bands that contain distorted bile ductlike structures and that often compress or incorporate central or sublobular veins. The ductlike structures may become dilated to the point of microcyst formation but do not communicate with the biliary tract. Irregularly shaped islands of liver parenchyma contain normal-appearing hepatocytes. Caroli disease and choledochal cysts have been associated (see earlier discussion). About 75% of patients have renal disease, such as renal tubular ectasia, nephronophthisis, or autosomal recessive polycystic renal disease. Congenital hepatic fibrosis also occurs as part of the COACH syndrome (*C*erebellar vermis hypoplasia, *O*ligophrenia, congenital *A*taxia, *C*oloboma, and *H*epatic fibrosis).

The disorder usually has its clinical onset in childhood, with hepatosplenomegaly or with bleeding secondary to portal hypertension. Cholangitis may occur in patients who have associated abnormalities of bile ducts.

Hepatocellular function is well preserved. Serum aminotransferase activities and bilirubin levels are usually normal; serum ALP activity may be slightly elevated. The serum albumin level and prothrombin time are normal. Liver biopsy is usually required for diagnosis.

Treatment of this disorder should focus on control of bleeding from esophageal varices. Infrequent mild bleeding episodes may be managed by endoscopic sclerotherapy or band ligation of the varices. After more severe hemorrhage, portacaval anastomosis may bring relief of portal hypertension. The prognosis may be greatly improved by a shunting procedure, but survival in some patients may be limited by renal failure.

A **solitary liver cyst** (nonparasitic) rarely occurs in childhood. Abdominal distention and pain may be present, and a poorly defined right upper quadrant mass may be palpable. These benign lesions are best left undisturbed unless they compress adjacent structures or a complication occurs, such as hemorrhage into the cyst.

AUTOSOMAL DOMINANT POLYCYSTIC KIDNEY DISEASE (ADPKD) (Chapter 529.2). ADPKD, a common inherited disease, affects 1/1,000 live births. It is characterized by progressive renal cyst development and enlargement and an array of extrarenal manifestations. There is a high degree of intrafamilial and interfamilial variability in the clinical expression of the disease.

At least three genetic loci are seen in ADPKD. The PKD 1 gene (accounting for 85% of cases) is on chromosome 16p13.3 and encodes for a novel protein called *polycystin,* which may have a potential role in cell-cell and cell-matrix interactions. The PKD 2 gene (~15% of cases) is on chromosome 4q13–23 and encodes for a protein thought to interact in some fashion with polycystin. A third locus is unmapped but has been demonstrated in some reported families.

Multiple hepatic lesions have been associated with ADPKD and include the ductal plate malformation with cystic communicating duct elements, dilated and apparently noncommunicating cysts, and biliary microhamartomas (the so-called von Meyenburg complexes). Segmental dilatation of the intrahepatic ducts (Caroli disease) and congenital hepatic fibrosis have been reported. Approximately 50% of patients with renal failure have demonstrable hepatic cysts that are not in continuity with the biliary tract. The hepatic cysts increase with age but are extremely uncommon before the age of 16 yr. Hepatic cystogenesis appears to be influenced by estrogens. Although the frequency of cysts is similar in males and females, the development of large hepatic cysts is largely a complication in females. Hepatic cysts are often asymptomatic but may cause pain and are occasionally complicated by hemorrhage, infection, or hepatic venous outflow obstruction from mechanical compression of hepatic veins, resulting in tender hepatomegaly and exudative ascites. Selected patients with severe symptomatic polycystic liver disease and favorable anatomy benefit from liver resection or fenestration.

Subarachnoid hemorrhage may result from the associated cerebral arterial aneurysms.

AUTOSOMAL RECESSIVE POLYCYSTIC KIDNEY DISEASE (ARPKD) (Chapter 529.1). ARPKD presents predominantly in childhood. Bilateral enlargement of the kidneys is caused by a generalized dilatation of the collecting tubules. The disorder is invariably associated with congenital hepatic fibrosis and various degrees of biliary ductal ectasia. The gene responsible for ARPKD has been localized to chromosome 6p21, with no evidence for genetic heterogeneity among the different clinical phenotypes.

ARPKD normally presents in early life, often shortly after birth, and is generally more severe than ADPKD. Patients with ARPKD may die in the perinatal period owing to renal failure or lung dysgenesis. The kidneys in these patients are usually markedly enlarged and dysfunctional. Respiratory failure may result from compression of the chest by grossly enlarged kidneys, from fluid retention, or from concomitant pulmonary hypoplasia. The clinical pathologic findings within a family tend to breed true, although there has been some variability in the severity of the disease and the time for presentation within the same family.

The liver in patients with ARPKD demonstrates various degrees of periportal fibrosis, bile ductular hyperplasia, and biliary dysgenesis. Liver disease and complications from hepatic fibrosis are most likely to be clinically significant in patients whose kidney disease allows prolonged survival. The most prominent clinical problem in older patients with ARPKD and congenital hepatic fibrosis is portal hypertension. Although portal hypertensive bleeding may occur during the first year of life, it more commonly presents in older children with hematemesis or melena. Firm or hard hepatomegaly is usually present. Splenomegaly is a frequent finding accompanied by hypersplenism. Owing to dilatation of the intrahepatic bile ducts, these patients are at increased risk of bacterial cholangitis. Caroli disease or a congenital, segmental, sacular dilatation of the intrahepatic bile ducts may coexist with congenital hepatic fibrosis and ARPKD.

Hemorrhage from esophagial varicies may be initially managed by using endoscopic sclerotherapy or banding. Some patients with well-preserved hepatic function may benefit from a selective portacaval shunt. Biliary sepsis should be aggressively treated. Recurrent bouts of bacterial cholangitis can lead to progressive loss of hepatic function. Rare patients may have unilateral involvement that can be treated by hepatic resection. Hepatic transplantation may be required for patients with hepatic failure.

Variable abnormalities of bile ducts (irregular dilatation, proliferation, cysts) and portal fibrosis may be associated with Meckel's syndrome, 17–18 trisomy, tuberous sclerosis, and asphyxiating thoracic dystrophy.

Choledochal Cysts

Miyano T, Yamataka, A: Choledochal cysts. Curr Opin Pediatr 9:283, 1997.
Stringer MD, Dhawan A, Davenport M, et al: Choledochal cysts: Lessons from a 20 year experience. Arch Dis Child 73:528, 1995.

Caroli Disease

Asselah T, Ernst O, Sergent G, et al: Caroli's disease: A magnetic resonance cholangiopancreatography diagnosis. Am J Gastroenterol 93:109, 1998.
Desmet VJ: Ludwig symposium on biliary disorders—part I. Pathogenesis of ductal plate abnormalities. Mayo Clin Proc 73:80, 1998.
Keane F, Hadzic N, Wilkinson ML, et al: Neonatal presentation of Caroli's disease. Arch Dis Child Fetal Neonatal Ed 77:F145, 1997.

Congenital Hepatic Fibrosis

Desmet VJ: What is congenital hepatic fibrosis? Histopathology 20:465–77, 1992.
Gentile M, Di Carlo A, Susca F, et al: COACH syndrome: report of two brothers with congenital hepatic fibrosis, cerebellar vermis hypoplasia, oligophrenia, ataxia, and mental retardation. Am J Med Genet 64:514, 1996.
Perisic VN. Long-term studies on congenital hepatic fibrosis in children. Acta Paediatr 84:695, 1995.

Polycystic Diseases of the Liver and Kidney

D'Agata ID, Jonas MM, Perez-Atayde AR, et al: Combined cystic disease of the liver and kidney. Semin Liver Dis 14:215, 1994.
Griffin MD, Torres VE, Kumar R: Cystic kidney diseases. Curr Opin Nephrol Hypertens 6:276, 1997.
Martinez JR, Grantham JJ: Polycystic kidney disease: Etiology, pathogenesis, and treatment. Dis Mon 41:693, 1995.
Zerres K, Rudnik-Schoneborn S, Deget F, et al: Autosomal recessive polycystic kidney disease in 115 children: Clinical presentation, course and influence of gender. Arbeitsgemeinschaft fur Padiatrische, Nephrologie. Acta Paediatr 85:437, 1996.

Chapter 365
Diseases of the Gallbladder

Frederick J. Suchy

ANOMALIES. The gallbladder is congenitally absent in about 0.1% of the population. Hypoplasia or absence of the gallbladder may be associated with extrahepatic biliary atresia or cystic fibrosis. Duplication of the gallbladder occurs rarely.

ACUTE HYDROPS (Table 365–1). Acute noncalculous, noninflammatory distention of the gallbladder may occur in infants and children. It is defined by the absence of calculi, bacterial infection, or congenital anomalies of the biliary system. The disorder may complicate acute infections, but the cause is often not identified. Hydrops of the gallbladder may also develop in patients receiving long-term parenteral nutrition, presumably as a result of gallbladder stasis during the period of enteral fasting. Hydrops is distinguished from acalculous cholecystitis

TABLE 365–1 Conditions Associated with Hydrops of the Gallbladder

Kawasaki disease	Thalassemia
Streptococcal pharyngitis	Total parenteral nutrition
Staphylococcal infection	Prolonged fasting
Leptospirosis	Viral hepatitis
Ascariasis	Sepsis
Threadworm	Henoch-Schönlein purpura
Sickle cell crisis	Mesenteric adenitis
Typhoid fever	Necrotizing enterocolitis

by the absence of a significant inflammatory process and a generally benign prognosis.

Affected patients usually have right upper quadrant pain with a palpable mass. Fever, vomiting, and jaundice may be present and are usually associated with a systemic illness such as streptococcal infection. Ultrasonography shows a markedly distended, echo-free gallbladder, without dilatation of the biliary tree. Acute hydrops is usually treated conservatively and rarely needs cholecystostomy and drainage. At laparotomy, a large, edematous gallbladder is found to contain white, yellow, or green bile. Obstruction of the cystic duct by mesenteric adenopathy is occasionally observed. Cholecystectomy is required if the gallbladder is gangrenous. Pathologic examination of the gallbladder wall shows edema and mild inflammation. Cultures of bile are usually sterile. Treatment of gallbladder hydrops is usually nonsurgical, with a focus on supportive care and managing the intercurrent illness. Spontaneous resolution and return of normal gallbladder function usually occur over a period of several weeks.

CHOLECYSTITIS AND CHOLELITHIASIS. *Acute acalculous cholecystitis* is uncommon in children and is usually caused by infection. Reported pathogens include streptococci (groups A and B), gram-negative organisms, particularly *Salmonella*, and *Leptospira interrogans*. Parasitic infestation with ascaris or *Giardia lamblia* may be found. Acalculous cholecystitis may rarely follow abdominal trauma or burn injury or may be associated with a systemic vasculitis, such as periarteritis nodosa.

Clinical features include right upper quadrant or epigastric pain, nausea, vomiting, fever, and jaundice. Right upper quadrant guarding and tenderness are present. Ultrasonography discloses an enlarged, thick-walled gallbladder, without calculi. Serum alkaline phosphatase activity and direct-reacting bilirubin levels are elevated. Leukocytosis is usual.

The diagnosis is confirmed at laparotomy. Cholecystectomy and treatment of the systemic infection are required.

Cholelithiasis is relatively rare in otherwise healthy children, occurring more commonly in patients with various predisposing disorders (Table 365–2). Gallstones, composed of a mixture of cholesterol, bile pigment, calcium, and inorganic matrix, are common. In children, more than 70% of gallstones are the pigment type, 15–20% are cholesterol stones, and the remainder are of unknown composition. Stones of pure cholesterol or bile pigment may also occur. Biliary dyskinesia, a disorder of impaired gallbladder contractility, is an abnormality predisposing to gallstones in late childhood and teenage years.

The most important clinical feature is recurrent abdominal pain, which is often colicky and localized to the right upper quadrant. An older child may have intolerance for fatty foods. Acute cholecystitis may be the first manifestation, with fever, pain in the right upper quadrant, and often a palpable mass. Pain may radiate to an area just below the right scapula. A plain roentgenogram of the abdomen may reveal opaque calculi, but radiolucent (cholesterol) stones are not visualized. Accordingly, ultrasonography is the method of choice for gallstone detection. Cholecystectomy is usually curative; operative cholangiography should be done at the time of surgery to preclude common duct calculi. Dissolution of cholesterol gallstones with oral ursodeoxycholic acid is ineffective in the treatment of gallstones in children, except in terms of relieving symptoms while on treatment.

TABLE 365–2 Conditions Associated with Cholelithiasis

Chronic hemolytic disease (sickle cell anemia, spherocytosis)
Obesity
Ileal resection or disease
Cystic fibrosis
Chronic liver disease
Prolonged parenteral nutrition
Prematurity with complicated medical or surgical course
Prolonged fasting or rapid weight reduction
Treatment of childhood cancer
Abdominal surgery
Pregnancy

Laparoscopic cholecystectomy is commonly performed in symptomatic children with cholelithiasis. Common bile duct stones are unusual in children, occurring in 2–6% of cases with cholelithiasis, often in association with obstructive jaundice and pancreatitis. Endoscopic retrograde cholangiography with stone extraction performed before or after laparoscopic cholecystectomy is the procedure of choice in this setting.

Patients with hemolytic disease (including sickle cell anemia, the thalassemias, and red blood cell enzymopathies) and Wilson disease are at increased risk for black pigment cholelithiasis. Cirrhosis and chronic cholestasis also increase the risk for pigment gallstones. Increasing numbers of sick premature infants are being found to have gallstones; their treatment is often complicated by such factors as bowel resection, necrotizing enterocolitis, prolonged parenteral nutrition without enteral feeding, cholestasis, frequent blood transfusions, and use of diuretics. Cholelithiasis in premature infants is often asymptomatic and may resolve spontaneously. Brown pigment stones have been found in patients with obstructive jaundice and infected intra- and extrahepatic bile ducts. These stones are usually radiolucent, owing to a lower content of calcium phosphate and carbonate and a higher amount of cholesterol than in black pigment stones.

Cholesterol cholelithiasis in children most frequently affects obese adolescent girls. Cholesterol gallstones are found also in children with disturbances of the enterohepatic circulation of bile acids, including patients with ileal disease and bile acid malabsorption, such as those with ileal resection, ileal Crohn disease, and cystic fibrosis. Pigment stones may also occur in these patients.

Cholesterol gallstone formation seems to result from an excess of cholesterol in relation to the cholesterol-carrying capacity of micelles in bile. Supersaturation of bile with cholesterol leading to crystal and stone formation could result from decreased bile acid or from an increased cholesterol concentration in bile. Other initiating factors that may be important in stone formation include gallbladder stasis or the presence in bile of abnormal mucoproteins or bile pigments that may serve as a nidus for cholesterol crystallization.

Barton LL, Luisiri A, Dawson JE: Hydrops of the gallbladder in childhood infections. Pediatr Infect Dis J 14:163, 1995.

McEvoy CF, Suchy FJ: Biliary tract disease in children. Pediatr Clin North Am 43:75, 1996.

Newman KD, Powell DM, Holcomb GW: The management of choledocholithiasis in children in the era of laparoscopic cholecystectomy. J Pediatr Surg 32:1116, 1997.

Rescorla FJ: Cholelithiasis, cholecystitis, and common bile duct stones. Curr Opin Pediatr 9:276, 1997.

Suchy FJ: Anatomy, anomalies and pediatric disorders of the biliary tract. *In:* Feldman M, Scharschmidt BF, Sleisenger MH (eds): Gastrointestinal and Liver Disorders, 6th ed. Philadelphia, WB Saunders, 1998, pp 905–928.

CHAPTER 366
Portal Hypertension and Varices

Frederick J. Suchy

Portal hypertension—defined as an elevation of portal pressure above 10–12 mm Hg—is a major cause of morbidity and mortality in children with liver disease. The normal portal venous pressure is approximately 7 mm Hg. The clinical features of the various forms of portal hypertension may be similar, but the associated complications, management, and prognosis can vary significantly and depend on whether the process is complicated by hepatic insufficiency.

ETIOLOGY. Numerous causes of portal hypertension result from obstruction to portal blood flow anywhere along the course of the portal venous system. The various disorders associated with portal hypertension are outlined in Table 366–1. Portal hypertension may occur as a result of prehepatic, intrahepatic, or posthepatic obstruction to the flow of portal blood.

Extrahepatic portal vein obstruction is an important cause of portal hypertension in childhood. The obstruction may occur at any level of the portal vein. Umbilical infection with or without a history of catheterization of the umbilical vein may be causal in neonates. The infection can spread potentially from the umbilical vein to the left branch of the portal vein and eventually to the main portal venous channel. Intra-abdominal infections including acute appendicitis and primary peritonitis can be causal in older children. Portal vein thrombosis has also been associated with neonatal dehydration and systemic infection. In older children, inflammatory bowel disease can be associated with a hypercoagulable state and portal venous obstruction. Thrombosis of the portal vein has also occurred in association with biliary tract infections and primary sclerosing cholangitis. Portal vein thrombosis has also been associated with hypercoagulable states such as factor V Leiden deficiency or protein C and protein S deficiencies. The portal vein can be replaced by a fibrous remnant or contain an organized thrombus. Obstruction by a web or diaphragm can also occur. At least half of reported cases have no defined cause.

TABLE 366–1 Causes of Portal Hypertension

Extrahepatic Portal Hypertension
Portal Vein Obstruction
Portal vein thrombosis or cavernous transformation
Splenic vein thrombosis
Increased Portal Flow
Arteriovenous fistula
Intrahepatic Portal Hypertension
Hepatocellular Disease
Acute and chronic viral hepatitis
Cirrhosis
Congenital hepatic fibrosis
Wilson disease
α_1-Antitrypsin deficiency
Glycogen storage disease type IV
Hepatotoxicity
Methotrexate
Parenteral nutrition
Biliary Tract Disease
Extrahepatic biliary atresia
Cystic fibrosis
Choledochal cyst
Sclerosing cholangitis
Intrahepatic bile duct paucity
Idiopathic Portal Hypertension
Postsinusoidal Obstruction
Budd-Chiari syndrome
Veno-occlusive disease

Uncommonly, presinusoidal hypertension can be caused by increased flow through the portal system as a result of a congenital or acquired arteriovenous fistula.

The intrahepatic causes of portal hypertension are numerous. Obstruction to flow can occur on the basis of a presinusoidal process including acute and chronic hepatitis, congenital hepatic fibrosis, or schistosomiasis. Portal infiltration with malignant cells or granulomas can also contribute. An idiopathic form of portal hypertension characterized by splenomegaly, hypersplenism, and portal hypertension without occlusion of portal or splenic veins and with no obvious disease in the liver has been described. In some patients, noncirrhotic portal fibrosis has been observed.

Cirrhosis is the predominant cause of portal hypertension and is related to obstruction of blood through the portal vein. The numerous causes of cirrhosis include recognized disorders such as extrahepatic biliary atresia, metabolic liver disease such as α_1-antitrypsin deficiency, Wilson's disease, glycogen storage disease type IV, hereditary fructose intolerance, and cystic fibrosis.

Postsinusoidal causes of portal hypertension are also observed during childhood. The Budd-Chiari syndrome occurs with obstruction to hepatic veins anywhere between the efferent hepatic veins and the entry of the inferior vena cava into the right atrium. In most cases, no specific cause can be found, but the thrombosis can complicate neoplasms, collagen vascular disease, infection, and trauma. Veno-occlusive disease is the most frequent cause of hepatic vein obstruction in children. In this disorder, occlusion of the centrilobular venules or sublobular hepatic veins occurs. The disorder occurs after total body irradiation with or without cytotoxic drug therapy that is commonly used before bone marrow transplantation. The disease has also occurred after ingestion of herbal remedies containing the pyrrolizidine alkaloids, which are sometimes taken as medicinal teas.

PATHOPHYSIOLOGY. The primary hemodynamic abnormality in portal hypertension is increased resistance to portal blood flow. This is the case whether the resistance to portal flow has an intrahepatic cause such as cirrhosis or is due to portal vein obstruction. Portosystemic shunting should decompress the portal system and thus significantly lower portal pressures. However, despite the development of significant collaterals deviating portal blood into systemic veins, portal hypertension is maintained by an overall increase in portal venous flow and thus maintenance of portal hypertension. A hyperdynamic circulation is achieved by tachycardia, an increase in cardiac output, and decreased systemic vascular resistance. Splanchnic dilatation also occurs. Overall, the increase in portal flow likely contributes to an increase in variceal transmural pressure. The increase in portal blood flow is related to the contribution of hepatic and collateral flow; the actual portal blood flow reaching the liver is reduced. It is also likely that hepatocellular dysfunction and portosystemic shunting lead to the generation of various humoral factors that cause vasodilatation and an increase in plasma volume.

Many of the portal hypertension complications can be accounted for by the development of a remarkable collateral circulation. Collateral vessels may form prominently in areas in which absorptive epithelium joins stratified epithelium, particularly in the esophagus or anorectal region. The superficial submucosal collaterals, especially those in the esophagus and stomach and to a lesser extent those in the duodenum, colon, or rectum, are prone to rupture and bleeding under increased pressure. In portal hypertension, the vascularity of the stomach is also abnormal and demonstrates prominent submucosal arteriovenous communications between the muscularis mucosa and dilated precapillaries and veins. The resulting lesion—a vascular ectasia—has been called *congestive gastropathy* and contributes to a significant risk of bleeding from the stomach.

CLINICAL MANIFESTATIONS. Bleeding from esophageal varices is the most common presentation. In patients with underlying hepatic disease, physical examination may show jaundice and stigmas of cirrhosis such as palmar erythema and vascular telangiectasias. Ascites may be present in patients with intrahepatic causes of portal hypertension but is uncommon with portal vein obstruction. Dilated cutaneous collateral vessels carrying blood from the portal to systemic circulation may be apparent in the periumbilical region. In the absence of clinical or biochemical features of liver disease and a liver of normal size, portal vein obstruction is most likely. However, well-compensated cirrhosis cannot be completely ruled out under these conditions. An enlarged, hard liver with minimal disturbance of hepatic function suggests the possibility of congenital hepatic fibrosis. Hemorrhage, particularly in children with portal vein obstruction, may be precipitated by minor febrile, intercurrent illness. The mechanism is often unclear; aspirin or other nonsteroidal anti-inflammatory drugs may be a contributing factor by damaging the integrity of a congested gastric mucosa or interfering with platelet function. Coughing during a respiratory illness can also increase intravariceal pressure. The bleeding may become apparent with hematemesis or with melena. Gastrointestinal hemorrhage can also originate from portal hypertensive gastropathy or from gastric, duodenal, peristomal, or rectal varices. Splenomegaly, sometimes with hypersplenism, is the next most common presenting feature in portal vein obstruction and may be discovered first on routine physical examination. Because more than half of patients in many series with portal vein obstruction do not experience bleeding until after age 6 yr, the diagnosis should be suggested in a child without hepatocellular disease who had a complicated neonatal course and in whom asymptomatic splenomegaly later developed.

Children with portal hypertension, regardless of the underlying cause, may have recurrent bouts of life-threatening hemorrhage. In patients with portal vein obstruction and normal hepatic function, the bleeding usually stops spontaneously. In patients with intrahepatic disease, the combination of portal hypertension and poor liver synthetic ability (coagulopathy) can make bleeding much more difficult to control. Moreover, esophageal hemorrhage and cirrhosis may have injurious effects on the liver, further impairing hepatic function and sometimes precipitating jaundice, ascites, and encephalopathy.

DIAGNOSIS. In patients with established chronic liver disease or in those in whom portal vein obstruction is suspected, an experienced ultrasonographer should be able to demonstrate the patency of the portal vein. In addition, the use of Doppler flow ultrasonography may demonstrate the direction of flow within the portal system. The pattern of flow correlates with the severity of cirrhosis and encephalopathy. Hepatopetal flow is more likely to be associated with variceal bleeding. Ultrasonography is also effective in detecting the presence of esophageal varices. Another important feature of extrahepatic portal vein obstruction is so-called cavernous transformation of the portal vein in which an extensive complex of small collateral vessels have formed to bypass the obstruction. Various other imaging techniques also contribute to further definition of the portal vein anatomy but are required less often; CT and MRI provide similar information to ultrasonography. Selective arteriography of the celiac axis, superior mesenteric artery, and splenic vein may be useful in precise mapping of the extrahepatic vascular anatomy. This is not required to establish a diagnosis but may prove valuable in planning surgical decompression of portal hypertension.

Endoscopy is the most reliable method for detecting esophageal varices and for identifying the source of gastrointestinal bleeding. Although bleeding from esophageal or gastric varices is most common in children with portal hypertension, up to one third of patients, particularly those with cirrhosis, may have bleeding from some other source such as portal hypertensive gastropathy or gastric or duodenal ulcerations. Once a diagnosis of portal hypertension has been established, several endoscopic features of esophageal varices may predict a risk for hemorrhage. There is a strong correlation between variceal size as assessed endoscopically and the probability of hemorrhage. Red spots apparent over varices at the time of endoscopy are a strong predictor of eminent hemorrhage.

TREATMENT. The therapy of portal hypertension can be divided into emergency treatment of potentially life-threatening hemorrhage and prophylaxis directed at prevention of initial or subsequent bleeding. It must be emphasized that many trials of therapy are based on experience with adults with portal hypertension.

Treatment of patients with variceal hemorrhage must focus on fluid resuscitation initially in the form of crystalloid infusion followed by the replacement of red blood cells. Correction of coagulopathy by administration of vitamin K or the infusion of platelets or fresh frozen plasma, or both therapies, may be required. A nasogastric tube should be placed to document the presence of blood within the stomach and to monitor for ongoing bleeding. An H_2 receptor blocker such as ranitidine should be given intravenously to reduce the risk of bleeding from gastric erosions. In most patients, particularly those with extrahepatic portal hypertension and with normal hepatic synthetic function, bleeding usually stops spontaneously. Care should be taken in fluid resuscitation of children after bleeding to avoid producing an excessively high venous pressure and an increased risk for further bleeding.

Pharmacologic therapy to decrease portal pressure may be considered in patients with continued bleeding. Vasopressin or one of its analogs has been commonly used and is thought to act by increasing splanchnic vascular tone and thus decreasing portal blood flow. Vasopressin is administered initially with a bolus of 0.33 U/kg over 20 min followed by a continued infusion of the same dose on an hourly basis or a continuous infusion of 0.2 U/1.73 m^2/min. The drug has a half-life of approximately 30 min. Its use may be limited by the side effects of vasoconstriction, which can impair cardiac function and perfusion to the heart, bowel, and kidneys and may also, as a result, exacerbate fluid retention. Nitroglycerin, usually given as a portion of a skin patch, has also been used to decrease portal pressure and, when used in conjunction with vasopressin, may ameliorate some of its untoward effects. The somatostatin analog octreotide decreases splanchnic blood flow with fewer side effects. Although studies in adults are promising, its use and efficacy in children have not been well evaluated.

After an episode of variceal hemorrhage or in patients in whom bleeding cannot be controlled, endoscopic sclerosis of esophageal varices is an important option. In this technique, sclerosants are injected either intravariceally or paravariceally until bleeding has stopped. Although bleeding may be controlled acutely in most cases, further sessions of sclerotherapy are required to achieve temporary obliteration of the varices. Treatments may be associated with further bleeding, bacteremia, esophageal ulceration, and stricture formation. Most centers do not perform endoscopic sclerotherapy of varices prophylactically but use the procedure as a bridge to the time of liver transplantation or until collateral circulation develops in extrahepatic portal vein obstruction. Endoscopic elastic band ligation of varices has been introduced as a safer and potentially as effective therapy for obliteration of varices. Experience with the technique in children is limited.

In patients who continue to bleed despite pharmacologic and endoscopic methods to control hemorrhage, a Sengstaken-Blakemore tube may be placed to stop hemorrhage by mechanically compressing esophageal and gastric varices. The device may be the only option to control life-threatening hemorrhage but carries a significant rate of complications and a high rate of bleeding when the device is removed. It poses a particularly high risk for pulmonary aspiration, and the tube is not well tolerated in children without significant sedation.

Various surgical procedures have been devised to divert portal blood flow and to decrease portal pressure. A portacaval shunt diverts nearly all of the portal blood flow into the subhepatic inferior right vena cava. Although portal pressure is significantly reduced, because of the significant diversion of blood from the liver, patients with parenchymal liver disease have a marked risk for hepatic encephalopathy. More selective shunting procedures, such as mesocaval or distal splenorenal shunt, may effectively decompress the portal system while allowing a greater amount of portal blood flow to the liver. The small size of the vessels makes these operations technically challenging in infants and small children, and there is a significant risk of failure as a result of shunt thrombosis. Therefore, orthotopic liver transplantation represents a much better therapy for portal hypertension resulting from intrahepatic disease. A prior portosystemic shunting operation does not preclude a successful liver transplantation but makes the operation technically more difficult. Portosystemic shunting may remain an option in children with extrahepatic portal hypertension, particularly in those patients who are suffering from potentially life-threatening hemorrhage not effectively controlled by other measures and who reside a great distance from emergency medical care. A transjugular intrahepatic portosystemic shunt (TIPS), in which a stent is placed by an interventional radiologist between the right hepatic vein and the right or left branch of the portal vein, can aid in the management of portal hypertension in children, especially in those needing temporary relief before liver transplantation. However, the TIPS procedure may precipitate hepatic encephalopathy and is prone to thrombosis.

Long-term treatment with nonspecific β-blockers such as propranolol has been used extensively in adults with portal hypertension. These agents may act by lowering cardiac output and portal perfusion. Evidence in adult patients shows that β-blockers may reduce the incidence of variceal hemorrhage and improve long-term survival. A therapeutic effect is thought to result when the pulse rate is reduced by at least 25%. There is limited published experience with the use of this therapy in children.

PROGNOSIS. Portal hypertension secondary to intrahepatic disease has a poor prognosis. Portal hypertension is usually progressive in these patients and is often associated with deteriorating liver function. Efforts should be directed toward prompt treatment of acute bleeding and prevention of recurrent hemorrhage with available methods. Patients with progressive liver disease and significant esophageal varices ultimately require orthotopic liver transplantation. Liver transplantation might also be considered for patients with portal hypertension secondary to hepatic vein obstruction or resulting from severe veno-occlusive disease.

In patients with portal vein obstruction, episodes of bleeding may become less frequent and severe with age as a collateral circulation develops. Most patients can be treated conservatively with endoscopic sclerotherapy when necessary. Portosystemic shunting procedures may be required in some patients.

Alvarez F, Bernard O, Brunelle F, et al: Portal obstruction in children: I. Clinical investigation and hemorrhage risk. J Pediatr 103:696, 1983.

Alvarez F, Bernard O, Brunelle F, et al: Portal obstruction in children: II. Results of surgical portosystemic shunts. J Pediatr 103:703, 1983.

Avgerinos A, Nevens F, Raptis, et al: Early administration of somatostatin and efficacy of sclerotherapy in acute oesophageal variceal bleeds: the European acute bleeding oesophageal variceal episodes (ABOVE) randomised trials. Lancet 350:1495, 1997.

Gentil-Kocher S, Bernard O, Brunelle F, et al: Budd-Chiari syndrome in children: Report of 22 cases. J Pediatr 113:30, 1988.

Hackworth CA, Leef JA, Rosenblum JD, et al: Transjugular intrahepatic portosystemic shunt creation in children: Initial clinical experience. Radiology 206:109, 1998.

Heyman MB, LaBerge JM, Somberg KA, et al: Transjugular intrahepatic portosystemic shunts (TIPS) in children. J Pediatr 131:914, 1997.

Maksoud JG, Goncalves EP: Treatment of portal hypertension in children. World J Surg 18:251, 1994.

Saran S, Lomba G, Kumar M, et al: Comparison of endoscopic ligation and propranolol for the primary prevention of variceal bleeding. N Engl J Med 340:988, 1999.

Shun A, Delaney DP, Martin HC, et al: Portosystemic shunting for paediatric portal hypertension. J Pediatr Surg 32:489, 1997.

Sokal E, Van Hoorebeeck N, Van Obbergh L, et al: Upper gastrointestinal tract bleeding in cirrhotic children candidates for liver transplantation. Eur J Pediatr 151:326, 1992.

Stringer MD, McClean P: Treatment of oesophageal varices. Arch Dis Child 77:476, 1997.

CHAPTER 367

Liver Transplantation

Kenneth L. Cox

With current immunosuppression and surgical techniques, 1- and 5-yr survival rates for children after orthotopic liver transplantation are 81% and 77%, respectively. Orthotopic liver transplantation is standard therapy for end-stage pediatric liver disease. Approximately 500 children in the United States undergo this procedure each year. The most frequent indication is extrahepatic biliary atresia after a failed portoenterostomy (Kasai) procedure. Metabolic liver disease and acute hepatic necrosis are next in frequency (Table 367–1).

Early referral to a transplant center is important so that patients and their families may be evaluated and treated in a timely fashion. Medical and psychosocial issues are assessed to determine the appropriateness of transplant, optimal management, and urgency. Hyperbilirubinemia, variceal bleeding, encephalopathy, coagulopathy, hypoalbuminemia, ascites, and

TABLE 367–1 Indications for Pediatric Liver Transplantation

Indication	% of Cases
Biliary atresia	43
Metabolic liver disease	13
α_1-Antitrypsin deficiency	6
Tyrosinemia	2
Wilson disease	1
Other	4
Acute hepatic necrosis (idiopathic)*	11 (63%)*
Idiopathic cirrhosis	6
Biliary hypoplasia (Alagille)	5 (79%)
Neonatal hepatitis	3
Hyperalimentation	3
Autoimmune hepatitis	2
Tumors (hepatoblastoma)	2 (54%)
Cystic fibrosis	2
Primary sclerosing cholangitis	1
Congenital hepatic fibrosis	1
Familial cholestasis	1
Miscellaneous	7

**The most common indication and percentage of cases in the category.*

Data from United Network for Organ Sharing Data Base for 3,595 pediatric liver transplants performed on children who were 0–17 yrs. of age.

poor growth are predictive of increased morbidity and mortality from liver disease and are used to determine the urgency for liver transplantation. Early evaluation allows sufficient time to find a donor and for families to learn about liver transplantation. Prompt referral of patients with fulminant hepatic failure is critical because a majority quickly die without liver transplantation. Counseling families about the special needs of children with chronic illness improves the psychosocial outcome.

Pretransplantation management is critical to the success of the procedure and to limiting morbidity from liver disease. Areas of major importance are nutrition (including vitamins) and immunizations. Patients with liver disease have malabsorption as well as anorexia. Formula containing medium-chain triglycerides is helpful because bile salts are not necessary for their absorption. Caloric requirements may be as high as 150 kcal/kg/24 hr; nocturnal nasogastric tube drip feedings may be required because of anorexia. Fat-soluble vitamin deficiencies must be prevented. Vitamin E deficiency (ataxia, peripheral neuropathy, gross motor delay) is best avoided by using a well-absorbed preparation containing D-α-tocopherol polyethylene glycol succinate. Vitamin D deficiency–associated bone disease is prevented by oral preparations of 25-hydroxyvitamin D_3. Early changes of vitamin A deficiency appear in the conjunctiva and cornea; they are prevented by using an oral, water-soluble preparation of vitamin A. Vitamin K deficiency is commonly encountered as a prolonged prothrombin time, which may respond to oral supplementation but often requires parenteral vitamin K. Prothrombin time and serum levels of vitamins E, D, and A should be monitored. Iron deficiency due to occult blood loss and zinc deficiency associated with chronic diarrhea may occur. Immunizations, especially those containing live viruses (measles-mumps-rubella, varicella, oral polio), should be given on schedule because immunosuppression after transplantation may prevent administration.

Medical management should also be directed toward control of variceal bleeding, ascites, encephalopathy, coagulopathy, and sepsis.

The success of *transplantation* has been enhanced by better preservation of the organ (up to 18 hr ex vivo with <2% primary nonfunction), refinements in surgical technique, and advances in immunosuppressive therapy. In pediatrics, the donor pool size has been expanded by using a lobe or segment of the liver from a cadaver or living donor and by using ABO blood type mismatch. Most frequently, the biliary tract is connected to a Roux-en-Y loop of jejunum, and direct vascular connections are made. Donor venous grafts are occasionally used if pretransplant portal vein thrombosis is present. Steroids and either cyclosporine (Sandimmune or Neoral) or tacrolimus (FK506, Prograf) are standard therapy to prevent rejection. Compared with cyclosporine (Sandimmune), tacrolimus is associated with lower rates of acute and chronic rejection and reduced use of corticosteroids. Cyclosporine has been reformulated from a bile salt–dependent, fat-soluble form (Sandimmune) to a better absorbed, water-soluble microemulsion (Neoral). Hirsutism and gingival hyperplasia are specific side effect of cyclosporine, whereas post-transplant lymphoproliferative disease (PTLD), cardiomyopathy, disturbances of glucose metabolism, and neurologic complications are more common with tacrolimus, especially with high blood levels (>20 ng/mL). OKT3 and azathioprine are also used occasionally.

Early *complications* include fluid shifts, electrolyte imbalance, renal dysfunction, and hypertension. Vascular complications, such as thrombosis of graft vessels, also may be an ominous early problem. After this early phase, infection and organ rejection are the most frequent problems. Bacterial infections are most common, followed by viral (especially cytomegalovirus and adenovirus), fungal, and rarely parasitic *(Pneumocystis carinii)* infections. Hospital stays are usually 2–3 wk but may be several months. Late complications may arise (rejection, cyclosporine- or FK506-induced renal dysfunction, lymphoproliferative disease). The latter is related to Epstein-Barr virus and may resolve if diagnosed early and if immunosuppression is stopped or markedly reduced. Progression to lymphoma may occur.

The prognosis for survivors is very encouraging. Growth improves, and stigmas of chronic liver disease resolve. Children and their families resume more normal lives. Close follow-up of medical and psychosocial issues is necessary. If chimerism between host and graft cells is present, some patients may completely stop immunosuppressive therapy. There has been limited success in creating and detecting chimerism.

Burdelski M: Liver transplantation in children. Acta Pediatr Suppl 395:27, 1994.

Cao S, Cox KL: Epstein-Barr virus lymphoproliferative disorders after liver transplantation. Clin Liver Dis 1:453, 1997.

Codoner-Franch P, Bernard O, Alvarez F: Long term follow-up of growth in height after successful liver transplantation. J Pediatr 124:368, 1994.

Cox KL, Freese DK: Tacrolimus (FK506): The pros and cons of its use as an immunosuppressant in pediatric liver transplantation. Clin Invest Med 19:389, 1996.

Starzl TE, Demetris AJ, Murase N, et al: Cell migration, chimerism, and graft acceptance. Lancet 339:1579, 1992.

United Network for Organ Sharing (UNOS) Scientific Registry data as of January 1998.

Wayman KI, Cox KL, Esquivel CO: Neurodevelopmental outcome of young children with extrahepatic biliary atresia 1 year after liver transplantation. J Pediatr 131:894, 1997.

Whittington PF, Balistreri WF: Liver transplantation in pediatrics: Indications, contraindications, and pretransplant management. J Pediatr 118:667, 1991.

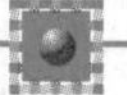

SECTION 7

Peritoneum

CHAPTER 368
Malformations

Jeffrey S. Hyams

Congenital peritoneal bands may be responsible for intestinal obstruction; numerous other anomalies may occur in the course of the development of the peritoneum but are rarely of clinical importance. Intra-abdominal herniations infrequently occur through ringlike formations produced by anomalous peritoneal bands. Absence of the omentum or its duplication occurs rarely. Omental cysts arise in obstructed lymphatic channels within the omentum. They may be congenital or may result from trauma and are usually asymptomatic. Abdominal pain or partial small bowel obstruction may result from compression or torsion of the small bowel from traction on the omentum.

CHAPTER 369
Ascites

Jeffrey S. Hyams

Ascites is an accumulation of serous fluid within the peritoneal cavity. Multiple causes of ascites have been described (Table 369–1). In children, hepatic, renal, and cardiac disease are the most common causes.

The clinical hallmark of ascites is abdominal distention, but this may also be caused by other conditions, including gaseous distention, fecal retention, tumor masses, peritoneal hemorrhage, extreme bladder distention, pregnancy, and obesity. Considerable intraperitoneal fluid may accumulate before ascites is detectable by the five classic physical signs: bulging flanks, flank dullness, shifting dullness, fluid wave, and the "puddle sign" (decreased auscultation of high-frequency vibrations in central abdomen when flicking side of abdomen with patient on hands and knees). Umbilical herniation may be associated with tense ascites. Ultrasound examination can detect small amounts of ascites.

The course, prognosis, and treatment of ascites depend entirely on the cause. Patients with any type of ascites are at increased risk for spontaneous bacterial peritonitis.

TABLE 369–1 Causes of Ascites

Hepatic	**Gastrointestinal**
Cirrhosis	Infarcted bowel
Congenital hepatic fibrosis	Perforation
Portal vein obstruction	**Neoplastic**
Fulminant hepatic failure	Lymphoma
Budd-Chiari syndrome	Neuroblastoma
Lysosomal storage disease	**Gynecologic**
Renal	Ovarian tumors
Nephrotic syndrome	Ovarian torsion, rupture
Obstructive uropathy	**Pancreatic**
Perforation of urinary tract	Pancreatitis
Peritoneal dialysis	Ruptured pancreatic duct
Cardiac	**Miscellaneous**
Heart failure	Systemic lupus erythematosus
Constrictive pericarditis	Ventriculoperitoneal shunt
Inferior vena cava web	Eosinophilic ascites
Infectious	Chylous ascites
Abscess	Hypothyroidism
Tuberculosis	
Chlamydia	
Schistosomiasis	

369.1 Chylous Ascites

Chylous ascites can result from an anomaly, injury, or obstruction of the intra-abdominal portion of the thoracic duct. Although uncommon, it can occur at any age. Causes include congenital malformations, peritoneal bands, generalized lymphangiomatosis, chronic inflammatory processes of the bowel, tumors, enlarged lymph nodes, previous abdominal surgery, and trauma.

In neonates, rapidly progressing abdominal distention is noted along with poor weight gain and loose stools. Peripheral edema is common. Massive chylous ascites may result in scrotal edema, inguinal and umbilical herniation, and respiratory embarrassment.

Diagnosis of chylous ascites depends on the demonstration of milky ascitic fluid obtained via paracentesis after a fat-containing feeding. Fluid analysis will reveal a high protein content, elevated triglycerides, and lymphocytosis. If the patient has had nothing by mouth, the fluid will appear serous. Hypoalbuminemia, hypogammaglobulinemia, and lymphopenia are common.

Treatment includes the provision of a high-protein, low-fat diet supplemented with medium-chain triglycerides that are absorbed directly into the portal circulation. Parenteral alimentation may be necessary if nutrition remains impaired on oral feedings and also in order to decrease lymph flow to facilitate sealing at the point of lymph leakage. Paracentesis should be repeated only if abdominal distention causes respiratory distress. Laparotomy may be indicated to search for the site of the leak if a trial of dietary management has been unsuccessful.

Browse NL, Wilson NM, Russo F, et al: Aetiology and treatment of chylous ascites. Br J Surg 79:1145, 1992.

Griscom NT, Colodny AH, Rosenberg HK, et al: Diagnostic aspects of neonatal ascites: Report of 27 cases. AJR 128:961, 1977.

Unger SW, Chandler JG: Chylous ascites in infants and children. Surgery 93:455, 1983.

CHAPTER 370
Peritonitis

Jeffrey S. Hyams

Inflammation of the peritoneal lining of the abdominal cavity may result from infectious, autoimmune, and chemical processes. Infectious peritonitis is usually defined as primary (spontaneous) or secondary. In primary peritonitis, the source of infection originates outside the abdomen and seeds the peritoneal cavity via hematogenous or lymphatic spread. Secondary peritonitis arises from the abdominal cavity itself through either extension from or rupture of an intra-abdominal viscus or an abscess within an organ.

Peritonitis in the neonatal period may arise from a transplacental in utero infection; more frequently, it is the result of infection acquired during or shortly after birth. It may be a manifestation of septicemia, a direct extension from an umbilical infection or from perforation of the intestine, necrotizing enterocolitis, or, rarely, the sequela of a ruptured appendix or Meckel diverticulum. Meconium peritonitis is described in Chapter 330.2.

370.1 Acute Primary Peritonitis

ETIOLOGY AND EPIDEMIOLOGY. Primary peritonitis usually refers to bacterial infection of the peritoneal cavity without a demonstrable intra-abdominal source. Most cases occur in children with ascites resulting from nephrotic syndrome or cirrhosis. Rarely, it may occur in previously healthy children. Most frequently, isolated bacteria include pneumococci, group A streptococci, enterococci, staphylococci, and gram-negative enteric bacteria, especially *Escherichia coli* and *Klebsiella pneumoniae.* The genders are affected equally; most cases occur before 6 yr of age. *Mycobacterium tuberculosis* and *M. bovis* are rare causes of peritonitis.

CLINICAL MANIFESTATIONS. Onset may be insidious or rapid and is characterized by fever, abdominal pain, vomiting, diarrhea, and a "toxic appearance." Hypotension and tachycardia are common along with shallow, rapid respirations because of discomfort associated with breathing. Abdominal palpation may demonstrate rebound tenderness and rigidity. Bowel sounds are hypoactive or absent. The prior use of corticosteroids may diminish the clinical expression of peritonitis.

DIAGNOSIS AND TREATMENT. Leukocytosis (on complete blood count) with a marked predominance of polymorphonuclear cells is common, although the level of the white cell count may be affected by pre-existing hypersplenism in patients with cirrhosis. Proteinuria is present in subjects with nephrotic syndrome. Roentgenographic examination of the abdomen reveals dilatation of the large and small intestines, with increased separation of loops secondary to bowel wall thickening. Distinguishing primary peritonitis from appendicitis may be impossible in patients without a history of nephrotic syndrome or cirrhosis; accordingly, the diagnosis of primary peritonitis is made only at laparotomy. In a child with known renal or hepatic disease and ascites, the presence of peritoneal signs should prompt a diagnostic paracentesis. Infected fluid usually reveals a white cell count of 250 cells/mm_3 or greater, with more than 50% polymorphonuclear cells.

Other peritoneal fluid findings suggestive of primary peritonitis include a pH less than 7.35, arterial-ascitic fluid pH gradient greater than 0.1, and elevated lactate. Gram stain of the ascitic fluid characteristically reveals a single species of gram-positive or, less often, gram-negative bacteria. The presence of mixed bacterial flora on ascitic fluid examination or free air on abdominal roentgenogram in children with presumed primary peritonitis mandates laparotomy to localize a perforation as a likely intra-abdominal source of the infection. Inoculation of ascitic fluid obtained at paracentesis directly into blood culture bottles will increase the yield of positive cultures. Parenteral antibiotic therapy with cefotaxime and an aminoglycoside should be started promptly, with subsequent changes dependent on sensitivity testing (vancomycin for resistant pneumococci). Therapy should be continued for 10–14 days.

Culture-negative neutrocytic ascites is a variant of primary peritonitis with a cell count of 500 cells/mm^3, a negative culture, no intra-abdominal source of infection, and no prior treatment with antibiotic. It should be treated in a similar manner as primary peritonitis.

Bhuva M, Ganger D, Jensen D: Spontaneous bacterial peritonitis: An update on evaluation, management and prevention. Am J Med 97:169, 1994.
Gorensek MJ, Lebel MH, Nelson JD: Peritonitis in children with nephrotic syndrome. Pediatrics 81:849, 1988.
Nohr CW, Marshall BG: Primary peritonitis in children. Can J Surg 27:179, 1984.
Veeragandham RS, Lynch FP, Canty TG, et al: Abdominal tuberculosis in children: Review of 26 cases. J Pediatr Surg 31:170, 1996.

370.2 Acute Secondary Peritonitis

This is most often due to the entry of enteric bacteria into the peritoneal cavity through a necrotic defect in the wall of the intestines or other viscus as a result of obstruction or infarction or after rupture of an intra-abdominal visceral abscess. It commonly follows perforation of the appendix. Other gastrointestinal causes include incarcerated hernias, rupture of a Meckel diverticulum, midgut volvulus, intussusception, hemolytic-uremic syndrome, peptic ulceration, inflammatory bowel disease, necrotizing cholecystitis, necrotizing enterocolitis, typhlitis, and traumatic perforation. Peritonitis in the neonatal period most often occurs as a complication of necrotizing enterocolitis but may be associated with meconium ileus or spontaneous (or indomethacin-induced) rupture of the stomach or intestines. In postpubertal females, bacteria from the genital tract *(Neisseria gonorrhoeae, Chlamydia trachomatis)* may gain access to the peritoneal cavity via the fallopian tubes, causing secondary peritonitis. The presence of a foreign body, such as a ventriculoperitoneal catheter or peritoneal dialysis catheter, can predispose to peritonitis, with skin microorganisms, such as *Staphylococcus epidermidis, S. aureus,* and *Candida albicans,* contaminating the shunt.

CLINICAL MANIFESTATIONS. Similar to primary peritonitis, characteristic symptoms include fever (39.5°C or more), diffuse abdominal pain, nausea, and vomiting. Physical findings of peritoneal inflammation include rebound tenderness, abdominal wall rigidity, a paucity of body motion (lying still), and decreased or absent bowel sounds from a paralytic ileus. Massive exudation of fluid into the peritoneal cavity, along with the systemic release of vasodilatory substances, can lead to the rapid development of shock. A "toxic appearance," irritability, and restlessness are common. Basilar atelectasis as well as intrapulmonary shunting may develop with progression to acute respiratory distress syndrome.

Laboratory studies reveal a peripheral white cell count greater than 12,000 cells/mm^3 with a marked predominance of polymorphonuclear forms. Roentgenograms of the abdomen may reveal free air in the peritoneal cavity, evidence of ileus or obstruction, peritoneal fluid, and obliteration of the psoas shadow.

TREATMENT. Aggressive fluid resuscitation and support of cardiovascular function should begin immediately. Stabilization of the patient before surgical intervention is mandatory. Antibiotic therapy must provide coverage for those organisms that predominate at the site of presumed origin of the infection. For perforation of the lower gastrointestinal tract, a regimen of ampicillin, gentamicin, and clindamycin will adequately address infection by *E. coli, Klebsiella, Bacteriodes* species, and enterococci. Alternative therapy could include ticarcillin–clavulanic acid and an aminoglycoside. Surgery to repair a perforated viscus should proceed after the patient is stabilized and antibiotic therapy initiated. Intraoperative peritoneal fluid cultures will indicate whether a change in the antibiotic regimen is warranted.

370.3 Acute Secondary Localized Peritonitis (Peritoneal Abscess)

ETIOLOGY. Intra-abdominal abscesses may develop within visceral intra-abdominal organs (hepatic, splenic, renal, pancreatic, tubo-ovarian abscesses) or in the interintestinal, periappendiceal, subdiaphragmatic, subhepatic, pelvic, and retroperitoneal spaces. Most commonly, periappendiceal and pelvic abscesses arise from a perforation of the appendix. Transmural inflammation with fistula formation may result in intra-abdominal abscess formation in children with Crohn disease.

CLINICAL MANIFESTATIONS. Prolonged fever, anorexia, vomiting, and lassitude are suggestive of the development of an intra-abdominal abscess. The peripheral white cell count is elevated, as is the erythrocyte sedimentation rate. With an appendiceal abscess, there is localized tenderness and a palpable mass in the right lower quadrant.

A pelvic abscess is suggested by abdominal distention, rectal tenesmus with or without the passage of small-volume mucous stools, and bladder irritability. Rectal examination may reveal a tender mass anteriorly. Subphrenic gas collection, basal atelectasis, elevated hemidiaphragm, and pleural effusion may be present with a subdiaphragmatic abscess. Psoas abscess can develop from extension of infection from a retroperitoneal appendicitis, Crohn disease, or a perirenal or intrarenal abscess. Abdominal findings may be minimal, and presentation may include a limp, hip pain, and fever. Both ultrasound examination as well as CT scanning can be used to localize intra-abdominal abscesses. Gallium scanning is usually not needed.

TREATMENT. An abscess should be drained and appropriate antibiotic therapy provided. Drainage may be performed under radiologic control (ultrasonogram or CT guidance) and an indwelling drainage catheter left in place. Initial broad-spectrum antibiotic coverage with ampicillin, gentamicin, and clindamycin should be started and can be modified depending on the results of sensitivity testing. The treatment of appendiceal rupture complicated by abscess formation may be problematic, because intestinal phlegmon formation can make surgical resection more difficult. Intensive antibiotic therapy for 4–6 wk followed by an interval appendectomy is often the treatment course followed.

Schwartz MZ, Tapper D, Solenberger RI: Management of perforated appendicitis in children: The controversy continues. Ann Surg 197:407, 1983.

Wilson-Storey D, Scobie WG: Appendix masses—A 15 year review. Pediatr Surg Int 4:165, 1989.

CHAPTER 371
Diaphragmatic Hernia

Gary E. Hartman

Herniation of abdominal contents into the thoracic cavity may occur as a result of a congenital or traumatic defect in the diaphragm. Symptomatology and prognosis depend on the location of the defect and associated anomalies. The defect may be at the esophageal hiatus (hiatal), adjacent to the hiatus (paraesophageal), retrosternal (Morgagni), or posterolateral (Bochdalek). Although all these defects are congenital, the term *congenital diaphragmatic hernia* (CDH) has become synonymous with herniation through the posterolateral foramen of Bochdalek. These lesions usually present with profound respiratory distress in the neonatal period, may be associated with anomalies of other organ systems, and have a significant (40–50%) mortality.

EPIDEMIOLOGY. Reports of the incidence of CDH vary from 1 in 5,000 live births to 1 in 2,000 if stillbirths are included. Defects are more common on the left (70–85%) and are occasionally (5%) bilateral. Malrotation of the intestine and some degree of pulmonary hypoplasia occur in virtually all cases and are considered components of the lesion and not associated anomalies. True associated anomalies have been recognized in 20–30% and include central nervous system lesions, esophageal atresia, omphalocele, cardiovascular lesions, and recognized syndromes. In addition to trisomy 21, the lethal syndromes of trisomy 13, trisomy 18, Fryn, Brachmann–de Lange, and Pallister-Killian have been described. Tetrasomy 12p mosaicism (Pallister-Killian syndrome) may have a normal peripheral blood karyotype as a result of infrequent involvement of lymphocytes. This lethal syndrome can be diagnosed by karyotype from amniocentesis or neonatal bone marrow or fibroblasts. Reports of occurrence of CDH in twins, siblings, and offspring are sporadic. An autosomal recessive inheritance mode has been suggested in families with complete agenesis of the diaphragm.

ETIOLOGY. Separation of the developing thoracic and abdominal cavities is accomplished by closure of the posterolateral pleuroperitoneal canals during the 8th wk of gestation. Failure of this canal to close has been the postulated mechanism for the development of congenital posterolateral diaphragmatic hernia. This may be the mechanism in patients with a small diaphragmatic defect. Production of unilateral or bilateral diaphragmatic defects in experimental animals by in utero drug exposure suggests an additional mechanism that may explain larger defects. Portions of the diaphragm and the pulmonary parenchyma arise from the developing thoracic mesenchyme, which, if disrupted, may explain the absence of the major portion of a hemidiaphragm and the severe pulmonary hypoplasia that usually accompanies such a large defect.

PATHOLOGY. The pathologic changes in infants with congenital diaphragmatic hernia are not limited to the diaphragm. The diaphragmatic defect may be small and slitlike or include the entire hemidiaphragm. Both lungs are small compared with those of age- and weight-matched controls, with the lung on the side of the defect more severely affected. There is a decrease in the number of alveoli and bronchial generations. The pulmonary vasculature is abnormal, with a decrease in volume and marked increase in muscular mass in the arterioles. Although there is some evidence that the pulmonary abnormalities are due to compression by the intrathoracic abdominal viscera, it is not accepted that physical compression is the sole or primary cause.

CLINICAL MANIFESTATIONS. Although many cases are identified by prenatal ultrasonography, the majority of infants with CDH experience severe respiratory distress within the first hours of life. A small group will present beyond the neonatal period. Patients with a delayed presentation may experience vomiting as a result of intestinal obstruction or mild respiratory symptoms. Delayed presentation of right diaphragmatic hernia after a documented episode of group B streptococcal sepsis is a well-described sequence. Occasionally, incarceration of the intestine will proceed to ischemia with sepsis and cardiorespiratory collapse. Unrecognized diaphragmatic hernia has been the cause of sudden death in infants and toddlers.

DIAGNOSIS. Prenatal diagnosis by ultrasonography is common. Careful evaluation for other anomalies should include echocardiography and amniocentesis. Occasionally, a fetus with ultrasonographic diagnosis in utero will have no abnormality on postnatal x-ray film. Parents with the ultrasonographic diagnosis of diaphragmatic hernia must be counseled carefully by a multidisciplinary group with significant experience with this condition if unnecessary terminations and unrealistic expectations are to be avoided.

After birth most infants with diaphragmatic hernia will experience severe respiratory collapse within the first 24 hr. The absence of breath sounds and shift of heart sounds common to CDH and pneumothorax will be accompanied by a scaphoid abdomen in the infants with CDH. Thoracentesis or tube thoracostomy should be withheld if CDH is considered a possibility. Chest roentgenogram is usually diagnostic (Fig. 371–1). The lateral view frequently demonstrates the intestine passing through the posterior portion of the diaphragm. Occasionally, congenital cystic lesions of the lung may produce a similar radiographic appearance. Differentiation from diaphragmatic hernia may be accomplished by postnatal ultrasonography or injection of contrast into the stomach or umbilical artery catheter to identify intestine above the diaphragm. In older children with atypical symptoms, contrast studies of the gastrointestinal tract are usually required. Ultrasonography and fluoroscopy are helpful in distinguishing eventration from true hernia, and computed tomography may be necessary to exclude pneumatoceles or complicated effusions.

TREATMENT. The availability of extracorporeal membrane oxygenation (ECMO) and the utility of preoperative stabilization have been the major stimuli to aggressive therapy (Chapter 97.7). Diaphragmatic hernia was once considered a surgical emergency, with urgent operative reduction offering these infants the optimal outcome. Recognition of the role of pulmonary hypertension in addition to pulmonary hypoplasia and the adverse effects of operative repair on pulmonary function prompted critical re-evaluation of that strategy. It is also clear that the postnatal mass effect of the herniated viscera is a minor factor in the cardiorespiratory compromise compared with the pulmonary hypertension and hypoplasia.

Initial resuscitation has traditionally consisted of attempted stabilization with sedation and paralysis and modest hyperventilation (partial pressure of carbon dioxide of 25–30 mm Hg). Permissive hypercapnia with gentle ventilation has been proposed by a number of centers with reports of equal or improved survival and decreased incidence of need for ECMO. Volume resuscitation, dopamine, and bicarbonate (to maintain pH >7.50) may also be helpful. If the infant stabilizes and demonstrates stable pulmonary vascular resistance without significant right-to-left shunting, repair of the diaphragm is performed at 24–72 hr of age. If stabilization is not possible or significant shunting persists, most infants will require ECMO support. Vasoactive drugs (dopamine, nitric oxide) may provide some improvement but have been disappointing as definitive therapy for the pulmonary hypertension associated with diaphragmatic hernia. Surfactant administration has also been shown to produce a transient improvement in oxygenation in some infants with CDH.

ECMO with paralysis and nasogastric suction may produce a dramatic reduction of the volume of herniated viscera. The duration of ECMO for neonates with diaphragmatic hernia is significantly longer than for those with persistent fetal circulation or meconium aspiration and may last up to 3–4 wk. Timing of repair of the diaphragm on ECMO is controversial;

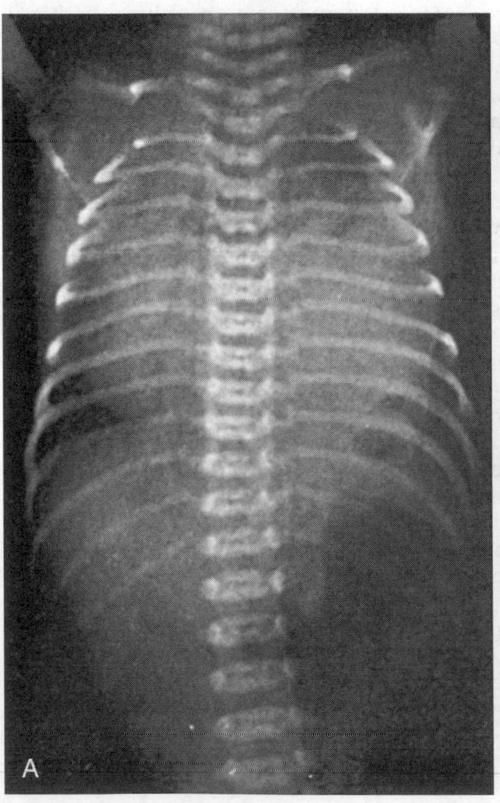

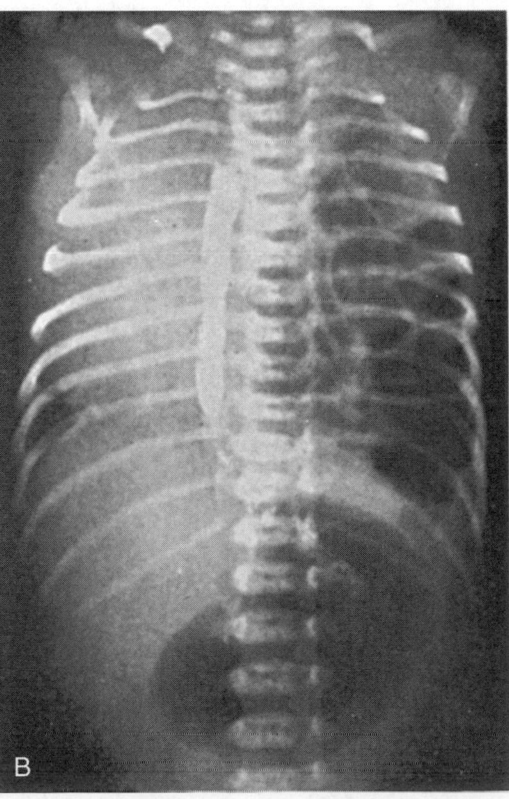

Figure 371–1 Congenital diaphragmatic hernia. *A,* Film exposed shortly after birth: distortion of shadow of the left leaf of the diaphragm with huge, masslike density in left hemithorax displacing the heart to the right. *B,* Film exposed about 20 min after *A.* As the result of swallowed air, coils of air-filled small bowel are now demonstrated in the left hemithorax. The esophagus is outlined by swallowed contrast material. Operative correction was attempted because of extreme dyspnea. Infant died 5.5 hr after birth.

some centers prefer early repair to allow a greater duration of postrepair ECMO, whereas many centers defer repair until the infant has demonstrated the ability to tolerate weaning from ECMO. In either case, recurrence of pulmonary hypertension carries a high mortality, and weaning from ECMO support should be cautious. If the patient cannot be weaned from ECMO after repair, options include discontinuing support or therapies such as nitric oxide or single-lung transplantation. High-frequency jet ventilation and oscillatory ventilation have had limited success in newborns with CDH.

The abdominal surgical approach is favored because the accompanying malrotation may be addressed if necessary, and the abdominal wall may be left open with skin only closed or a Silastic pouch applied if abdominal pressure is considered excessive. Synthetic patch (polytetrafluoroethylene) is now preferred over autologous muscle transfer or tight primary closure for large defects.

The appreciation of the compressive effects of the herniated viscera and the availability of prenatal diagnosis suggested the utility of in utero measures directed at potentially reversing the pulmonary hypoplasia and, it is hoped, the pulmonary vascular changes. Prenatal treatment with glucocorticoids has stimulated pulmonary maturity in experimental animals with diaphragmatic hernia. In utero reduction of the herniated viscera also has been successsfully performed. The randomized trial comparing in utero repair with standard postnatal therapy has been discontinued, since there was no difference in mortality or morbidity between treatment groups. In experimental animals, occluding the trachea in utero enhances lung growth by preventing lung fluid egress. Trials of tracheal ligation are in progress in humans at the fetal treatment centers in San Francisco and Philadelphia. To be considered for in utero tracheal ligation, the fetus must be single, must be diagnosed before 24 wk of gestation, and have a normal karyotype and intra-abdominal liver. Ligation is attempted between 24 and 28 wk of gestation in appropriate candidates. A second operative procedure is required near term to allow removal of the tracheal clips and intubation or reconstruction of the trachea.

PROGNOSIS. Studies of infants with CDH identified in utero (27–55%) report lower survival than noted in reports limited to live births (42 66%). It appears that the majority of fetuses with the diagnosis of CDH who do not survive pregnancy die as a result of elective termination. The incidence of spontaneous fetal demise among fetuses diagnosed as having CDH appears to be 7–10%. Of those surviving to delivery, survival appears to range from 42–66% despite current modalities including ECMO. Factors associated with a poor prognosis include associated major anomaly, symptoms before 24 hr of age, distress severe enough to require ECMO, and delivery in a nontertiary center. Initial attempts at intrauterine repair were associated with a low survival (29%), although current results are more encouraging.

In the past, survivors of CDH repair were clinically normal, although some abnormalities could be detected by pulmonary function testing. With current treatment modalities, a significant number of survivors are being identified with serious sequelae, primarily pulmonary, neurologic, and growth retardation. These long-term sequelae are probably the result of survival of infants with more severe pulmonary compromise than was previously possible. Ten to 20% of CDH survivors now require oxygen therapy at discharge.

Studies have documented abnormalities of pulmonary function in the perioperative period and years after repair. Survivors of CDH repair studied at 6–11 yr of age demonstrate significant decreases in forced expiratory flow at 50% of vital capacity and peak expiratory flow. The lung on the affected side is larger than predicted, suggesting hyperinflation, and has reduced perfusion. These patients had undergone repair before the availability of ECMO. In studies of neonatal pulmonary function, neonates with CDH requiring ECMO demonstrate significantly decreased compliance, dynamic compliance, and tidal volume when compared with those not requiring ECMO. After repair, infants with CDH also have evidence of reactive airway disease. Survivors of CDH have evidence of restrictive lung disease and airway reactivity, which are related to the severity of their initial respiratory failure.

Significant neurologic abnormalities have been identified in survivors of CDH. The incidence of neurologic abnormalities is higher in those infants requiring ECMO (67% vs 24%). The abnormalities are similar to those seen in neonates treated with ECMO for other diagnoses and include developmental delay, abnormal hearing or vision, seizures, and abnormal CT. The majority of neurologic abnormalities are classified as mild or moderate.

Growth and nutrition are compromised in CDH survivors who require ECMO. Forty to 50% are at less than the 5th percentile for weight at 2 yr of age. Weight:length ratio is less than the 5th percentile in 40% of survivors at 1 yr and at the 21st percentile at 2 yr. Nearly all ECMO survivors demonstrate clinical evidence of gastroesophageal reflux, and 20% or more have required fundoplication. Dilation of the esophagus with altered motility that resolves during the 1 yr of life has been correlated with a prenatal history of polyhydramnios.

Other long-term problems occurring in this population include pectus excavatum, scoliosis, fixed pulmonary hypertension, and recurrent herniation. Recurrent hernia formation is common in newborns with large defects requiring synthetic patch repair. Reherniation has been reported in 20–40% of those requiring patch repair and occurs within the 1st yr.

Survivors of CDH repair, particularly those requiring ECMO support, have a variety of long-term abnormalities that appear to improve with time but require close monitoring and multidisciplinary support.

371.1 Foramen of Morgagni Hernia

The anteromedial diaphragmatic defect through the foramen of Morgagni accounts for 2% or less of diaphragmatic hernias. The transverse colon or small intestine is usually contained in the hernia sac. Symptoms are gastrointestinal and typically occur beyond the neonatal period. Repair is recommended for all patients and can be accomplished by laparotomy.

371.2 Paraesophageal Hernia

Paraesophageal hernia is differentiated from hiatal hernia in that the gastroesophageal junction is in the normal location. The herniation of the stomach alongside or adjacent to the gastroesophageal junction is prone to incarceration with strangulation and perforation. This unusual diaphragmatic hernia should be repaired promptly after identification.

371.3 Eventration

Eventration of the diaphragm consists of a thinned diaphragmatic muscle producing elevation of the entire hemidiaphragm or, more commonly, the anterior aspect of the hemidiaphragm. Most eventrations are asymptomatic and do not require repair. Large or symptomatic eventrations may be repaired by plication through an abdominal or a thoracic approach.

Breaux CW, Rouse TM, Cain WS, et al: Improvement in survival of patients with congenital diaphragmatic hernia utilizing a strategy of delayed repair after medical and/or extracorporeal membrane oxygenation stabilization. J Pediatr Surg 26:333, 1991.

Harrison MR, Adzick NS, Estes JM, et al: A prospective study of the outcome for fetuses with diaphragmatic hernia. JAMA 271:382, 1994.
Harrison MR, Adzick NS, Flake AW, et al: Correction of congenital diaphragmatic hernia in utero: VI. Hard-earned lessons. J Pediatr Surg 28:1411, 1993.
Hedrick HL, Kaban JM, Pacheco BA, et al: Prenatal glucocorticoids improve pulmonary morphometrics in fetal sheep with congenital diaphragmatic hernia. J Pediatr Surg 32:217, 1997.
McGahren ED, Mallik K, Rodgers BM: Neurological outcome is diminished in survivors of congenital diaphragmatic hernia requiring extracorporeal membrane oxygenation. J Pediatr Surg 32:1216, 1997.
Nakayama DK, Motomyama EK, Mutich RL, et al: Pulmonary function in newborns after repair of congenital diaphragmatic hernia. Pediatr Pulmonol 11:49, 1991.
Sweed Y, Puri P: Congenital diaphragmatic hernia: Influence of associated malformations on survival. Arch Dis Child 69:68, 1993.
Thibeault DW, Haney B: Lung volume, pulmonary vasculature, and factors affecting survival in congenital diaphragmatic hernia. Pediatrics 101:289, 1998.
Van Meurs KP, Robbins ST, Reed VL, et al: Congenital diaphragmatic hernia: Long-term outcome in neonates treated with extracorporeal membrane oxygenation. J Pediatr 122:893, 1993.

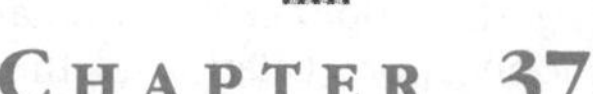

CHAPTER 372
Epigastric Hernia

Gary E. Hartman

Epigastric hernias are defects in the linea alba between the xyphoid and the umbilicus. They are uncommon in childhood, constituting less than 1% of hernias requiring operation. Similar defects below the umbilicus are even more uncommon. These hernias usually contain preperitoneal fat and rarely cause symptoms. They may appear as an intermittent bulge or a midline mass if the fat is incarcerated. Herniation of intestine or other viscera is extremely rare. Repair is indicated for symptomatic hernias or for diagnosis in the case of a mass. Treatment of asymptomatic hernias of the linea alba is less clear. Some believe that many will resolve spontaneously and discourage elective repair. Others believe that they never resolve and will eventually require repair. Abdominal symptoms other than local pain and tenderness should prompt further diagnostic study rather than repair of the epigastric hernia.

372.1 Incisional Hernia

Hernia formation at the site of a previous laparotomy is uncommon in childhood. Factors associated with an increased risk of incisional hernia include increased intra-abdominal pressure, wound infection, and midline incision. Transverse abdominal incisions are favored because of their increased strength and blood supply, which reduce the likelihood of wound infection and incisional hernia. Although most incisional hernias will require repair, operation should be deferred until the child is in optimal medical condition. Some incisional hernias will resolve, especially those occurring in infants. Some recommend elastic bandaging to discourage enlargement of the hernia and to promote spontaneous healing. Newborns with abdominal wall defects represent the largest group of children with incisional hernias. Initial management should be conservative, with repair deferred until about 1 yr of age. Incarceration is very uncommon but is an indication for prompt repair.

Neblett KW, Holcomb TM: Umbilical and other abdominal wall hernias. *In:* Ashcraft KW, Holder TM (eds): Pediatric Surgery. Philadelphia, WB Saunders, 1993, pp 557–561.
Robin AP: Epigastric hernia. *In:* Nyhus LM, Condon RE (eds): Hernia. Philadelphia, JB Lippincott, 1989, pp 360–366.

PART XVIII

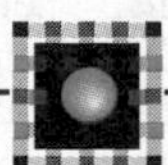

The Respiratory System

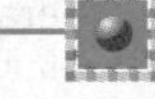

SECTION 1

Development and Function

CHAPTER 373

Development of the Respiratory System

Gabriel G. Haddad and J. Julio Pérez Fontán

In terrestrial animals, the gas-exchanging apparatus is invaginated into alveolar (reptiles, amphibia, mammals) or parabronchial (birds) lungs. Such a design maximizes the contact surface with the atmosphere while limiting excessive water and heat losses through evaporation. Gas-exchanging surfaces in invaginated lungs depend on two important factors. First, to be mechanically stable, gas-exchanging surfaces are coated with a surface-active material, the pulmonary surfactant, which prevents them from sticking to each other or collapsing (see Chapter 97.3). Second, invaginated lungs also depend on an external mechanism to force air in and out of the gas-exchanging spaces. In mammals and other higher vertebrates, this mechanism resembles a bellows pump operated by muscles. The function of these respiratory muscles is regulated by a network of sensors, which relay information from the blood (e.g., gases), the airways (e.g., stretch), and the pump itself to a control center in the brain. The pump can in this manner generate large and rapid changes in force and hence lung ventilation, providing the adaptability demanded by the fast metabolic pace of warm-blooded animals.

The development of the respiratory system encompasses three distinct processes: morphogenesis or formation of all the necessary structures, adaptation to postnatal atmospheric breathing, and dimensional growth. In most mammalian species, the first two processes take place primarily before or shortly after birth. Growth, in contrast, continues after birth at a pace that is generally dictated by the functional needs of the other growing organs and metabolic activity of the animal. The effects of an injury to the respiratory system depend, therefore, not only on the severity and chronicity of the injury but also on the timing of the injury in relation to the developmental timetable of the lungs. Insults occurring during morphogenesis, for instance, tend to produce severe and irreversible disruptions of respiratory structure and function, often incompatible with survival. In contrast, injuries that take place during later stages of lung growth are frequently reversible and, if not, can be compensated for by the growth process itself.

PRENATAL DEVELOPMENT: MORPHOGENESIS. In humans and other mammals, the morphogenesis of the respiratory system is divided into five periods (Fig. 373–1). The first, or *embryonic period,* begins at approximately 4 wk of gestation, when the primitive airways appear as a ventral outpouching on the endodermal epithelium of the foregut. This outpouching divides almost immediately into two main stem bronchial buds, which burrow rapidly into the mesenchyme separating the foregut from the coelomic cavity. The bronchial buds start to branch, first by monopodal outgrowth (secondary branches grow out of a main branch) and then by asymmetric dichotomy (two secondary branches originate from one main branch).

The peribronchial mesenchyme or *splanchnopleura* plays an essential role in shaping the lungs during the embryonic period. Close contact between this mesenchyme and the epithelium of the bronchial buds is essential for the continued branching of the airways. Although the factors that promote bronchial division are not fully identified, steroid-induced secretion of growth factors by the mesenchymal fibroblasts, specific interactions with acellular components of the mesenchyme, and even direct molecular communications between fibroblasts and endodermal cells across gaps in the basal membrane have been proposed as signaling mechanisms. The interactions between mesenchyme and the bronchial bud endoderm are organ-specific.

The pulmonary vasculature is a mesenchymal derivative. Soon after their appearance, the bronchial buds are surrounded by a vascular plexus, which originates from the aorta and drains into the major somatic veins. This vascular plexus connects with the pulmonary artery and veins to complete the pulmonary circulation at the 7th wk of gestation but retains some aortic connections that form the bronchial arteries. All the supporting structures of the lungs, including the pleura, the septal network of the lungs, and the smooth muscle, cartilage, and connective covers of the airways, originate from the mesenchyme.

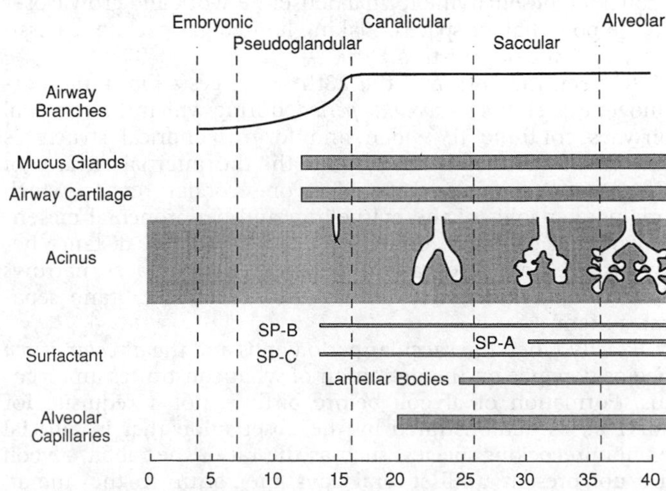

Figure 373–1 Development of various pulmonary structures during the five stages of prenatal lung development (see text).

Toward the 6th wk of gestation, at the beginning of the second or *pseudoglandular period,* the lungs resemble an exocrine gland with a thick stroma crossed by narrow ducts lined by an epithelium of tall cells that almost fill the lumen. The major airways are already present and are in close association with pulmonary arteries and veins. The trachea and the foregut are now separated after the progressive fusion of epithelial ridges growing from the primitive airway. The incomplete fusion of these ridges results in a **tracheoesophageal fistula**, a common congenital malformation. During the pseudoglandular period, the airways continue to branch until the entire conducting airway system is formed, including the primitive bronchioles that eventually give rise to the air-exchanging portions of the lungs. Simultaneously, the pluripotential cells that line the airways differentiate, starting from the trachea and main bronchi, in a process that also appears to be under some degree of mesenchymal control. They soon form a thinner, pseudostratified epithelium containing ciliated, secretory (Clara), globular, and neuroendocrine (Kulchitsky) cells of neuroectodermal origin. Mucous glands, cartilage, and smooth muscle can be easily distinguished by the 16th wk of gestation.

The diaphragm is formed during this period. Its central tendon originates from the transverse septum, a plate of mesodermal tissue located between the pericardium and the stalk of the yolk sac. Its lateral portions are formed by the pleuroperitoneal folds, which grow from the body wall until they fuse with the esophageal mesentery and the transverse septum. The fusion eliminates the communication between thorax and abdomen and establishes a barrier to the caudal growth of the lungs. Its failure, usually on the left side, causes the **congenital diaphragmatic hernia of Bochdalek**. This defect, which is the most frequent type of diaphragmatic hernia, allows the abdominal organs to enter the primitive pleural cavity and interferes with airway and pulmonary vascular branching. The result is severe hypoplasia of the lung, particularly on the side of the hernia (see Chapter 371). Initially membranous, the normal diaphragm is eventually invaded by striated muscle derived from cervical myotomes.

During the third or *canalicular period,* between the 16th and 26–28th wk of gestation, epithelial growth predominates over mesenchymal growth. As a result, the bronchial tree develops a more tubular appearance, whereas its distal regions subdivide further to lay the structural foundations of the pulmonary acinus. The epithelial cells in these regions become more cuboidal and start to express some of the antigen markers that characterize cells as type II pneumocytes. Some cells become flatter and can be identified as potential type I pneumocytes by the presence of a sparse endoplasmic reticulum and abundant cytoplasmic glycogen. The capillaries contained in the distal bronchial mesenchyme form a denser network and grow closer to the potential air spaces, making limited gas exchange possibly by 22 wk of gestation.

Between the 26th and the 28th wk of gestation, lung morphogenesis enters its *saccular period,* during which the terminal airways continue to widen and form cylindrical structures known as saccules. Initially smooth, the internal surface of the saccules soon develops ridges or secondary crests, which originate as folds of the epithelium and peribronchial mesenchyme and contain a double capillary layer. The distance between the capillaries and the potential air spaces narrows further until eventually only a thin basal membrane separates them.

Exactly when the saccular period ends and the *alveolar period* begins depends on the definition of what constitutes an alveolus. Formation of alveoli before birth is not a requisite for survival, as demonstrated by the observation that in altricial or nonprecocious species, such as the rat or the rabbit, alveoli are not present until several days after birth. In the human fetus, the saccular septation initiated with the appearance of the secondary crests continues at a rapid rate so that multifaceted structures analogous to the alveoli of the mature lung can be seen at 32 wk of gestation. In more precocious species such as the sheep and the horse, the lungs contain even more alveoli at birth than are present in humans. There is substantial evidence that the timing and progression of alveolar septation is under endocrine regulation. Thyroid hormones stimulate septation, whereas glucocorticoids impair it in a fashion that, at least in the rat, can be irrevocable (even though they accelerate the thinning of the alveolar capillary membranes). Alveolarization is also influenced by physical stimuli. Both the stretch by the liquid contained in the fetal lung and the periodic distention provided by the action of the respiratory muscles during fetal breathing, for instance, appear to be necessary for the development of the acini. Their absence when the lungs or chest are compressed (as in the case of a diaphragmatic hernia or oligohydramnios) or when fetal breathing is abolished (e.g., by spinal cord lesions) results in **pulmonary hypoplasia** with reduced numbers of alveoli.

A number of gene families have been identified as being essential for development. The homeo-domain or homeo-box (hox) gene family was discovered first in *Drosophila* and was later shown to be well preserved in mammals and critical in mammalian organ development, including that of the respiratory system. Hoxa-1,2,3,5, and Hoxb-3,4,6,7,8 mRNA transcripts have been identified using molecular biologic techniques in branching regions of the developing mouse lung. These Hox genes were differentially expressed in time and space in early lung development, indicating that they play a role in the differentiation, maturation, and proliferation of various lung cells throughout the various phases of lung development. Furthermore, some of these genes seem to be important in distal versus proximal branching and differentiation. Hoxa-2 seems to be tied to a proximal role, whereas Hoxb-6 is involved in distal airway branching. Also of importance is the fact that the expression of some of these genes is controlled by retinoic acid. This may be related to a possible therapeutic role of retinoic acid at later stages of lung development or in injured lungs.

ADAPTATION TO AIR-BREATHING. The transition from placental dependence to autonomous gas exchange requires adaptive changes in the lungs. These changes include the production of surfactant in the alveoli, the transformation of the lung from a secretory to a gas-exchanging organ, and the establishment of parallel pulmonary and systemic circulations.

As soon as the newborn takes the first breath of air, an air-liquid interface becomes established inside the lungs. Unless the surface tension generated at this interface is reduced, the walls of the air spaces would tend to stick together and collapse, threatening the geometric stability of the lungs. The pulmonary surfactant makes such a reduction possible by forming a hydrophobic lipid monolayer at the very surface of the liquid film that lines the air spaces (see Chapter 97.3). Pulmonary surfactant is a heterogeneous mixture of phospholipids and proteins secreted into the saccular or alveolar subphase by the type II pneumocytes. Its presence is first recognized in characteristic secretory organelles known as lamellar bodies as early as the 24th wk of gestation. However, surfactant lipids, of which the most abundant is phosphatidylcholine, are not detectable in the amniotic fluid until the 30th wk of gestation, suggesting that there is a chronologic gap between surfactant synthesis and secretion. Labor probably shortens this gap because phospholipids are consistently found in the air spaces of infants born before the 30th wk of gestation. Three apoproteins (SP-A, SP-B, SP-C) identified in pulmonary surfactant (a fourth lectin-like glycoprotein, SP-D, has been isolated, but its function and regulation are still poorly understood) promote the spreading of the surfactant layer and are therefore essential for the effective reduction of surface tension. Apoproteins also appear to be important for the reuptake and recycling of surfactant products and for the formation of tubular myelin (the structures in which surfactant is stored in the liquid subphase).

Surfactant apoproteins and phospholipids share some, but not all, of their regulatory influences. Glucocorticoids, for instance, increase the synthesis of both apoproteins and lipids; accordingly, their prenatal administration has been used to prevent the respiratory distress syndrome associated with prematurity. Because many actions of the steroids involve direct stimulation of response elements in apoprotein and phospholipid enzyme genes and therefore require messenger RNA production, sufficient time must elapse between steroid administration and birth. Thyroid hormones also enhance the synthesis of phospholipids by a receptor-mediated mechanism, but, unlike the glucocorticoids, have little or no effect on surfactant apoprotein synthesis. Conversely, β-adrenergic agonists and other agents that raise cellular cyclic adenosine monophosphate content increase apoprotein synthesis and phosphatidylcholine secretion into the air spaces but have no effect on phospholipid synthesis. Insulin, hyperglycemia, ketosis, and androgens may have negative effects on the production of surfactant proteins and phospholipids, thus explaining the high incidence of respiratory distress syndrome in infants of diabetic mothers and the slight maturational delay of the lungs of male fetuses compared with female fetuses.

Surfactant proteins and lipids also may play an important role in lung immunity, although the molecular details are not known. Surfactant proteins A and D are lectins (bind to carbohydrates) and belong to the collectins family of genes. These proteins, present in the serum and lungs, stimulate phagocytosis and chemotaxis, produce reactive oxygen species, and regulate the production and release of cytokines by immune cells. Alternatively, surfactant lipids can suppress immunity. It is possible that the ratio between surfactant lipids and proteins is important in regulating the immune status of the lungs. This may be critical in premature infants and in newborns who lack surfactant proteins; knock-out mice with SP-A deficiency have a major problem with infections.

The fetal lung is a secretory organ. Throughout gestation, a Cl^--, K^+-, and H^+-enriched fluid is produced in its peripheral air spaces with the help of a Cl^- pump. The presence of this fluid appears to be important for the development of the acinus because chronic drainage of the trachea in experimental animals results in lung hypoplasia. Fluid secretion, however, is incompatible with air-breathing. Accordingly, and in preparation for birth, lung fluid production decreases slowly at the end of gestation. This decrease, which is accelerated by the beginning of labor, denotes a transformation in the ion transfer activities of the pulmonary epithelium from Cl^- (and water) secretion to Na^+ (and water) absorption. In experimental animals, such a transformation can be precipitated by the administration of β-adrenergic agonists at doses that result in serum levels comparable to those found during labor. Stimulation of β-receptors is not the only labor-related signal because fluid clearance in the fetal lung is delayed by the Na^+ channel blocker amiloride but not by β-blockers. After birth, the still substantial amount of fluid left in the lungs is absorbed over several hours into the circulation either directly through pulmonary vessels or indirectly through an already very effective lymphatic system. The cellular elements responsible for fluid secretion and absorption in the lungs are not fully identified. It is obvious that a mature alveolar epithelium is not essential for fluid secretion, which is already taking place before alveoli or even saccules exist. Alveolar cells, in contrast, probably play a protagonistic role in fluid absorption. Type II pneumocytes may be involved because they cover a larger portion of the air space surface in the newborn than in the adult and their metabolic machinery appears to be particularly well adapted to active ion transport.

A number of transporters and channels that have importance on water and solute transport in early life have been cloned and identified in the past decade. Most prominent has been the epithelial sodium channel or ENaC. It is the amiloride-sensitive and apical channel that is responsible for sodium and water absorption in the luminal surface of the airways and renal tubular cells. This channel is made up of three types of subunits, α, β, and γ. This channel seems to be critical in early life; knock-out mice for this channel develop pulmonary edema and die soon after birth.

At birth, the pulmonary circulation changes from a high-resistance to a low-resistance system and, as a consequence, pulmonary blood flow becomes capable of accommodating systemic venous return. The change in resistance is brought about by the combined effects of the mechanical forces applied on the pulmonary vascular walls by the expanding lung tissue and the relaxation of the pulmonary arterial smooth muscle caused by the increased alveolar concentrations of oxygen and probably by endogenous release of vasodilators. The subsequent closure of the foramen ovale and the ductus arteriosus completely separates the pulmonary from the systemic circulation. Arterial oxygen tension then rises sharply and becomes homogeneous throughout the body. Pulmonary vascular resistance continues to decrease gradually during the first few weeks after birth through a process of structural remodeling of the pulmonary vessel musculature.

POSTNATAL DEVELOPMENT. The postnatal development of the lungs can be divided into two phases depending on the relative rates of development of the various components of the lungs. During the first phase, which extends to the first 18 mo after birth, there is a disproportionate increase in the surface and volume of the compartments involved in gas exchange. Capillary volume increases more rapidly than air space volume, which, in turn, increases more rapidly than solid tissue volume. These changes are accomplished primarily through a process of alveolar septation. This process is particularly active during early infancy and, contrary to previous belief, may reach completion within the first 2 yr instead of the first 8 yr of life. The configuration of the air spaces becomes progressively more complex, not only because of the development of new septa but also because of the lengthening and folding of the existing alveolar structures. Soon after birth, the double capillary system contained in the alveolar septa of the fetus fuses into one single, denser system. At the same time, new arterial and venous branches develop within the circulatory system of the acinus and muscle starts to appear in the medial layer of the intra-acinar arteries.

During the second phase, all compartments grow more proportionately to each other. Although there is little question that new alveoli can still be formed, the majority of the growth occurs through an increase in the volume of existing alveoli. Alveolar and capillary surfaces expand in parallel with somatic growth. As a result, taller individuals tend to have larger lungs. However, the final size of the lungs and, ultimately, the dimensions of the individual constituents of the acinus are also influenced by factors such as the subject's level of activity and prevailing state of oxygenation (altitude), which allow for a better adaptation of lung structure and function. The same factors are probably operative in the compensatory responses to pulmonary disease and injury.

Bucher U, Reid L: Development of the intrasegmental bronchial tree: The pattern of branching and development of cartilage at various stages of intrauterine life. Thorax 16:207, 1961.

Gross I: Regulation of fetal lung maturation. Am J Physiol 259:L337, 1990.

Langston C, Kida K, Reed M, et al: Human lung growth in late gestation and in the neonate. Am Rev Respir Dis 129:607, 1984.

O'Brodovich H: Epithelial ion transport in the fetal and perinatal lung. Am J Physiol 261:C555, 1991.

Tchepichev S, Ueda J, Canessa C, et al: Lung epithelial Na channel subunits are differentially regulated during development and by steroids. Am J Physiol 269:C805, 1995.

CHAPTER 374
Regulation of Respiration

Gabriel G. Haddad

Pediatricians need to be familiar with the general principles of the regulation of respiration because (1) clinical situations involving one or more elements of the respiratory control system are prevalent, especially in critically ill patients (e.g., apnea, upper airway obstruction, severe asthma, hypoventilation, and heart failure, or hypoxemia from various causes); (2) transition from fetal to neonatal life is an extremely complex process during which there are major changes in almost every aspect of respiratory control; and (3) understanding of the neural control of respiration is likely to increase significantly in the next 1–2 decades because of the explosive advances in understanding brain function in general.

THE RESPIRATORY CONTROL SYSTEM IS A NEGATIVE FEEDBACK SYSTEM WITH A CENTRAL CONTROLLER. The overall aim of the respiratory feedback system is to keep blood gas homeostasis in a normal range in the most economical way, from an energy consumption and mechanical standpoint. The term *negative* in this concept refers to the fact that the controller attempts to rectify the deviation from normality. If CO_2 increases, for example as a result of airway obstruction, the output of the controller is increased in an attempt to increase alveolar ventilation and decrease CO_2. To accomplish this, the feedback system makes use of both an afferent limb and an efferent limb. The afferent limb is made up of tissues (e.g., the airways) that have receptor endings and can send information to the central controller about certain functional parameters, such as the magnitude of stretch of the airways. The carotid bodies that inform the central controller of the status of O_2 and pH represent another important part of the afferent system. Both airway and carotid body sensors have a way to compare signals, the inherent set point signal and the real actual one, note differences, and translate these differences into information (e.g., a decrease or increase in action potential volleys) to the central nervous system. The efferent loop is the part of the feedback system that is responsible for the execution of the decision made centrally to increase or decrease central respiratory output (i.e., increase or decrease respiratory muscle output). There are many muscles of respiration, the intercostal muscles and the diaphragm being only two of them. Activity and timing of the airway muscles, as is seen later, are crucial in determining airway resistance and, therefore, the magnitude of ventilation.

THE CENTRAL CONTROLLER INTEGRATES INCOMING AFFERENT INFORMATION AND GENERATES AND MAINTAINS RESPIRATION. It is not known in precise mechanistic and cellular terms how and where integration and generation of breathing takes place. A number of ideas have emerged regarding the nature and location of the "respiratory center or centers." Two groups of medullary neurons have been considered as potential sites for the initiation of respiration, namely, the nucleus tractus solitarius and the nucleus ambiguus (and retroambiguus). At present there is more support for the latter than the former, although the evidence is not strong for either. Another area in the medulla (pre-Bötzinger) has been implicated as a major site for the generation of respiration. In addition, the nature of the central respiratory rhythm generator is not clear. Indeed, the respiratory controller may be a group of neurons that either form an *emergent network* or are *endogenous* or *conditional bursters*. In the first case, respiratory neurons would not have special properties (e.g., bursting properties) that would make their membrane potential oscillate. This type of a respiratory rhythm generator would *not* be like the sinus node cells of the heart. Rather, the output of the network that they form would oscillate because of the special *interconnections* and synaptic interactions among these respiratory neurons. In the second case, in a manner similar to that of the heart, the respiratory neurons would have special properties that make *individual neurons* "burst" or oscillate (pacemaker), even if they are disconnected from any other neurons (endogenous burster) and placed in a culture dish. A conditional burster neuron is a neuron that oscillates only when exposed to certain chemicals (e.g., neurotransmitters). From evidence thus far, it is likely that, independent of the location of the central pattern generator, a respiratory oscillatory output takes place by virtue of the synaptic and cellular-molecular properties of the neurons in these locations. This oscillatory output from the brain stem then drives the phrenic motor neurons in the spinal cord which, in turn, stimulate the diaphragm and other respiratory muscles to contract and move air in the lungs. Understanding the endowment of these cells in terms of properties and their communications is important to appreciate fully the intricacies of respiratory generation and maintenance. One issue regarding the activation (or inactivation of various respiratory muscles) is how the central output gets "distributed" on various muscles to ensure patency of airways and contraction of the appropriate muscles in order to optimize the work of breathing and lessen the energy needed to move a certain volume of air and ensure alveolar ventilation. This issue becomes important in some pathologic states during which airway muscle activation may not be well coordinated with chest wall muscle activation, leading to lack of airway patency and inefficient gas exchange.

AFFERENT INFORMATION IS NOT NECESSARY FOR INITIATING RESPIRATION BUT PLAYS AN IMPORTANT ROLE IN MODULATING BREATHING. A multitude of afferent messages converge on the brain stem at any one time. Chemoreceptors and mechanoreceptors in the larynx and upper airways sense stretch, air temperature, and chemical changes over the mucosa and relay this information to the brain stem. Afferent impulses from these areas travel through the superior laryngeal nerve and the 10th cranial nerve (vagus). The superior laryngeal nerve joins and becomes part of the vagal trunk at the nodose ganglion. Changes in O_2 or CO_2 tensions are sensed at the carotid and aortic bodies, and afferent impulses travel through the carotid and aortic sinus nerves. Thermal or metabolic changes are sensed by skin or mucosal receptors or by hypothalamic neurons and are carried through spinal or central tracts to the brain stem for integrative purposes. Furthermore, afferent information to the brain stem need not be only formulated and sensed by the peripheral nervous system. For example: (1) Sensors of CO_2 lie on the ventral surface of the medulla oblongata and therefore feedback about CO_2 levels comes from the brain stem itself, and (2) emotions and changes in mood that result from central nervous system processing in the limbic system influence respiration through pathways connecting higher brain centers to the brain stem.

Afferent information from the peripheral or central nervous system is not a prerequisite for generating and maintaining respiration. When the brain stem and spinal cord are removed from the body and maintained in vitro, rhythmic phrenic activity can be detected and measured for hours. Other experiments in vivo in which several sensory systems are blocked simultaneously (with local anesthesia to block vagal afferents, 100% O_2 to eliminate carotid discharges, sleep to eliminate wakeful stimuli, and chronic administration of diuretics to alkalinize the blood) indicate that afferent information is not necessary to initiate an inherent respiratory rhythm in brain stem respiratory networks. However, both in vitro and in vivo studies demonstrate that in the absence or elimination of afferent information regarding CO_2 levels, O_2 levels, a wakeful stimulus, and so on, the inherent rhythm of the central generator (respiratory frequency) is slow. Hence, chemoreceptors, temperature receptors, mechanoreceptors, and laryngeal receptors and their afferents play an important part in *modulating* respiration and rhythmic behavior.

The neonate is more exquisitely sensitive to afferent input than is the adult. Laryngeal reflexes are extremely potent in inhibiting respiration in the newborn. Aspiration and stimulation of laryngeal chemoreceptors in premature infants (who lack the ability of a strong cough), especially when these infants are anemic or hypoglycemic or even during normal sleep, can cause life-threatening respiratory events. Similarly, when neonatal animals are deprived of carotid bodies, prolonged and severe apneic episodes are induced, which can prove fatal in a large percentage of these animals.

CENTRAL INTEGRATION AND PROCESSING IN THE BRAIN STEM IS HIERARCHICAL. Respiratory muscles can be recruited to perform different tasks at different times. For example, the diaphragm and some abdominal muscles are activated not only during tidal breathing but also during expulsive maneuvers such as coughing and straining. In other conditions, respiratory muscles can be totally inhibited. For example, when delivering a speech, CO_2 responsiveness is decreased substantially because speech muscles are recruited mostly at the expense of other respiratory muscles. Bottle- or breast-feeding in the young is often associated with a reduction in ventilation and a drop in arterial PO_2 because of partial inhibition of respiratory muscles and breathing efforts. Presented with a number of neurophysiologic signals (representing options about various needs), the central controller responds differently to various stimuli and can enhance or reduce the effect of certain stimuli. Therefore, there is a hierarchy that is used by brain stem networks for determining the response of the respiratory system at any one time.

Changes in the state of consciousness modulate the ability of the brain stem to respond to afferent stimuli. For example, trigeminal afferent impulses are less inhibited by cortical influences during quiet sleep than during rapid eye movement (REM) sleep or wakefulness. Thus, the effect of trigeminal stimulation on respiration is more pronounced in quiet sleep. Similarly, age is important. The response of the brain stem to stimuli varies with maturation and thus with cortical input to brain stem structures.

RESPIRATORY MUSCLES AND CHEST WALL PROPERTIES—FOR EXAMPLE, EFFERENT ORGAN—UNDERGO POSTNATAL MATURATION AND CAN FATIGUE. Effective ventilation requires *coordinated interaction* between the respiratory muscles of the chest wall (including the diaphragm and intercostals) and those of the upper airway (including the pharynx and the larynx) under various conditions of altered respiratory drive. In infants, a specific sequential pattern of nerve and muscle activation occurs so that some upper airway muscles contract prior to and during the early part of inspiratory flow: the genioglossus muscle contracts, moving the tongue forward, which prevents pharyngeal obstruction and the vocal cords abduct, reducing inspiratory laryngeal resistance. Laryngeal muscles also modulate expiratory flow and thus may influence lung volume. Imbalance of pharyngeal and diaphragmatic activities or their responses to chemoreceptor or mechanoreceptor stimulation may contribute to obstructive apnea in infants and children.

Because the *respiratory muscles* are responsible for executing central neural responses and because muscle and chest wall properties change with age in early life, it is likely that neural responses can be influenced by pump properties. Thus, it is important to consider the maturational changes of respiratory muscles and the chest wall. For example, one of the important maturational aspects of of respiratory muscles (e.g., in skeletal muscles) is their pattern of innervation. In the adult, one muscle fiber is innervated by one motoneuron. Therefore, if a motoneuron innervates certain muscle fibers (e.g., about 200 muscle fibers in the case of the diaphragm), these fibers do not receive innervation from any other motoneuron. In the newborn, however, each fiber is innervated by two or more motoneurons, and the axons of different motoneurons can synapse on the same muscle fiber—thus the term *polyneuronal innervation*. Synapse elimination takes place postnatally and, in the case of the diaphragm, the adult type of innervation is reached by several weeks of age depending on the animal species. The time course of polyneuronal innervation of the diaphragm in the human newborn is not known.

The neuromuscular junctional folds, postsynaptic membranes, and acetylcholine receptors and metabolism undergo major postnatal maturational changes. The acetylcholine quantal content per end plate potential is lower in the newborn than in the adult rat diaphragm. The newborn diaphragm is also more susceptible to neuromuscular transmission failure than is that of the adult, especially at higher frequencies of stimulation. Whether this is the result of differences in acetylcholine metabolism between the newborn and the adult or whether this is related to the neuromuscular junction itself is not known.

In addition to an increase in cross-sectional area and muscle mass, *muscle fiber types* in the diaphragm change as a function of gestational and postnatal age. However, there are conflicting reports about the composition of fiber types in young muscle, and it is not known whether human newborn muscles are more oxidative- or fatigue-resistant than those of the adult. The sarcoplasmic reticulum of the premature diaphragm is, however, underdeveloped compared with that of the adult. This is one major reason for the delay in the release and uptake of Ca^{2+}, which may have functional significance. The poorly developed sarcoplasmic reticulum in the newborn causes increased contraction and relaxation time in neonatal muscle fibers. This increased relaxation time may be an important factor in impeding blood flow and limiting oxidative metabolism when the muscle is under a load.

The *chest wall* in newborn infants is highly compliant. Because of this and because young infants spend a large proportion of time in REM sleep, during which the intercostal muscles are inhibited, there is little splinting of the chest wall for diaphragmatic action. Therefore, with every breath in supine infants (especially in REM sleep), the chest wall is sucked in paradoxically at a time when the abdomen expands. This creates an additional load on the respiratory system and results in a higher work of breathing per minute ventilation in the infant than in the adult. Some believe that this may be an important reason for the newborn's susceptibility to muscle fatigue and respiratory failure.

THE NEWBORN AND YOUNG RESPOND DIFFERENTLY TO STIMULI COMPARED WITH THE MATURE INDIVIDUAL. The young child and neonate respond to various stimuli in a different way than does the adult. In response to low O_2, the newborn does not sustain an increase in ventilation, and often ventilation decreases to below baseline levels. CO_2 levels do not increase at a time when ventilation is decreasing, suggesting that ventilation is matching metabolic needs. This neonatal response to low O_2 can be considered an intermediate response between those of the fetus and the adult; the fetus shuts off all respiratory efforts in response to O_2 deprivation, and the adult hyperventilates as long as the stimulus is present. The mechanism or mechanisms for the lack of sustained increase in ventilation during hypoxia in the newborn is not well understood. In addition to differences in metabolic rate during hypoxemia among neonates and adults, changes in the mechanical properties of the lung and airways, maturation of carotid chemoreceptors, and alterations in the cellular and membrane properties of central neurons have all been proposed as potential individual or combined mechanisms. It is clinically important that neonatal tissues resist O_2 deprivation and do not injure as easily as those of the adult. This is true for the heart, brain, and kidneys, organs known to be sensitive to hypoxia and ischemia in the mature animal or human. These differences between newborn and adult sensitivity to anoxic injury are not well understood but possibly relate to the ability of the newborn cell to metabolize lactate and ketone, to downregulate metabolism during severe O_2 deprivation, and to regulate certain protein synthesis (e.g., heat-shock proteins) differently from the adult.

CO_2 response is also reduced in the young. Whether this is a reflection of an inherent difference in sensitivity or the result of differences in mechanical function is not known and, presumably, is related to both mechanical and central differences.

Although alterations in responsiveness can be secondary to a number of differences between the young and the mature organism, the central neuronal changes with maturation seem especially important. For example, the soma of lumbar and phrenic motoneurons increases with age, and their input resistance (or inverse of membrane conductance) decreases with age. The decrease in input resistance results in major part from the increase in soma size, but other mechanisms, such as a change in the geometry of the dendrites and their outgrowth, a change in the number of ion channels per surface area, and an increase in the number of synapses onto motoneurons, cannot be ruled out. Axonal velocity also increases with age, and action potentials of phrenic and hypoglossal motoneurons decrease in duration. There are also major maturational changes in active cellular properties in some motoneurons or premotor neurons. For example, with increasing postnatal age, neurons in the area of the nucleus tractus solitarius develop cellular properties important for repetitive firing. Changes in neuronal properties could play an important role in the integrative abilities of neuronal cells and, therefore, in their response to stimulation.

CLINICAL IMPLICATIONS

Apnea (See Chapter 97.2). Although there are numerous studies on apnea in the newborn and adult human, there are also a number of controversies. Further, the length of the respiratory pause that has been defined as apnea has varied. Apnea can be defined statistically as a respiratory pause that exceeds 3 SD of the mean breath time for an infant or a child at any particular age. This definition requires data from a population of infants at that age, lacks physiologic value, and does not differentiate between relatively shorter or longer respiratory pauses. Alternatively, the definition of apnea may be based on the fact that respiratory pauses are associated with cardiovascular or neurophysiologic changes. Such definition relies completely on the functional assessment of pauses and is, therefore, more relevant clinically. Because infants have higher O_2 consumption (per unit weight) than the adult and relatively smaller lung volume and O_2 stores, it is possible that short (e.g., seconds) respiratory pauses that may not be clinically important in the adult can present serious consequences in the very young or premature infant.

Independent of age group, respiratory pauses are more prevalent during sleep than during the waking state. The frequency and duration of respiratory pauses depend on the sleep state in human infants. Respiratory pauses are more frequent and shorter in REM than in quiet sleep and are more frequent in younger than in older infants.

Although there is controversy regarding the pathogenesis of respiratory pauses, there is a consensus about certain observations. Normal full-term infants, children, and adult humans exhibit respiratory pauses during sleep. Paradoxically, some believe that the presence of respiratory pauses and breathing irregularity is a "healthy" sign and that the complete absence of such pauses may be indicative of abnormalities. However, prolonged apnea can be life-threatening. The pathogenesis of these apneas may relate to the clinical condition of the patient at the time of the apnea, associated cardiovascular (systemic or pulmonary) changes, the chronicity of the clinical condition, the perinatal history, and whether the cause is central or peripheral. Prolonged apneic spells require therapy and, optimally, treatment should be targeted to the underlying pathophysiology. A septic infant should be treated for the infection and a seizing infant with antiepileptic medication. The child with **congenital hypoventilation syndrome** (or **Ondine's curse**), in the absence of pharmacologic therapy, should be placed on mechanical ventilation until properly paced with phrenic stimulators (Chapter 375.2).

Upper Airway Obstruction (see Chapter 383). Upper airway obstruction (UAO) during sleep is recognized with increasing frequency in children. In contrast to adults with UAO, in whom the cause of obstruction often remains obscure, many children have anatomic abnormalities. A common cause of UAO in children is tonsillar and adenoidal hypertrophy due to repeated upper respiratory infections. Other associated abnormalities include craniofacial malformations, micrognathia, and muscular hypotonia. The usual site of obstruction in UAO in both infants and adults is the oropharynx, between the posterior pharyngeal wall, the soft palate, and the genioglossus. During sleep (especially REM sleep), upper airway muscles, including those of the oropharynx, lose tone and trigger an episode of UAO.

Snoring with recurrent periods of respiratory pauses commonly occurs during sleep in children. Parents frequently describe periods of increasing chest wall movement without air flow and with cyanosis. In older children, the syndrome may include failure to thrive, developmental delay, and poor school performance. Hypertension and daytime hypersomnolence are less common abnormalities in children than in adults. Children with long-standing signs and symptoms of UAO during sleep can present with right ventricular failure and cor pulmonale. The treatment, therefore, varies but should be targeted primarily at the underlying cause of obstruction. Some of these infants benefit from tonsillectomy and adenoidectomy or, if obese, by a reduction in weight. In some refractory cases, successful treatment has included continuous positive airway pressure applied through the nose.

Haddad GG: Control of breathing in children. *In*: Edelman NH, Santiago T (eds): Contemporary Issues in Pulmonary Disease. New York, Churchill Livingstone, 1986, pp 57–80.

Haddad GG: Cellular and membrane properties of brainstem neurons in early life. *In*: Haddad GG, Farber J (eds): Developmental Neurobiology of Breathing. Lung Biology in Health and Disease, Vol 53. New York, Marcel Dekker, 1991, pp 591–614.

Haddad GG, Donnelly DF, Bazzy AR: Developmental Control of Respiration: Neurobiologic Basis. *In:* Dempsey JA, Pack AI (eds): Regulation of breathing. Lung Biology in Health and Disease, Vol 79. New York, Marcel Dekker, 1994, pp 743–785.

CHAPTER 375

Respiratory Pathophysiology

J. Julio Pérez Fontán and Gabriel G. Haddad

Through evolution, terrestrial organisms have developed a dedicated system that combines the abilities to extract from the atmosphere the oxygen needed for oxidation of metabolic substrates and to remove from their bodies the carbon dioxide generated in the process. In humans, this respiratory system consists of a pumping mechanism (the respiratory muscles, the chest wall, and the conducting airways), a membrane gas exchanger (the gas-exchanging portions of the lungs), and a central neural control connected to a network of chemical and mechanical sensors distributed throughout the circulation and the respiratory system itself. Basic to this arrangement is the close integration of respiratory and circulatory functions, which assures not only the efficiency of gas exchange but also the ability to adapt to the variable demands of life. Alterations in the components of the respiratory system or its interaction with the circulatory system give rises to a variety of clinical manifestations. The most severe of these manifestations is the development of abnormal partial pressures of oxygen and carbon dioxide, a situation known as respiratory failure.

MECHANICAL DYSFUNCTION OF THE RESPIRATORY SYSTEM. The mechanical processes that move gas and blood in and out of the lungs are more easily disrupted by disease than those involved in the diffusion of gases across membranes or in the neural control of breathing. Consequently, even before respiratory failure occurs respiratory disease is usually detected either as an apparent or subjective increase in the effort that the individual makes during breathing (respiratory distress and dyspnea) or as a limitation in the respiratory system's ability to accommodate increased demands for gas exchange such as those created by exercise or fever. The presence of respiratory distress or exercise intolerance provides the clinician with a reasonable indication that the problem is mechanical in nature and most likely caused by dysfunction of the respiratory pump or the pulmonary circulation.

WORK AND ENERGY COST OF BREATHING. Clinically the most prominent effect of respiratory pump dysfunction is an increase in the work that the respiratory muscles do to keep up with the body's demands for gas exchange. The increased work is frequently accommodated through an increase in the neural drive to the respiratory muscles, which may be perceived by the patient as shortness of breath (dyspnea) or by an observer as *respiratory distress.* On occasion, however, the work load demands cannot be met by the contractile machinery of the respiratory muscles and *respiratory failure* ensues.

In physical terms, work is a discrete quantity obtained by multiplying the force needed to move an object by the distance over which the object is moved. In the case of breathing movements, which take place in three dimensions, work is defined as the product of lung volume change by the pressure that the respiratory muscles must generate to produce that volume change. This product is graphically represented by the area enclosed between the volume-pressure relationships of the lungs and chest wall and the volume axis (Figs. 375–1 and 375–2).

Volume-pressure relationships are determined by properties such as the ease with which the lung tissue is stretched or the amount of resistance that the airways oppose to the passage of air. Thus the work of breathing describes in one single value the overall mechanical behavior of the respiratory system, providing in the process a valuable account of the energy cost of the breathing activity.

RESTRICTIVE AND OBSTRUCTIVE RESPIRATORY DYSFUNCTIONS. Although it has the same units as work and indeed can be converted into work, energy is an attribute of objects or systems. The respiratory muscles extract energy from the metabolic substrates that are brought to them by the blood. Energy is then transformed into physical work or is otherwise dissipated as heat. Depending on how energy is handled after its transformation into work, it is possible to divide the work of breathing into two components.

First, an important portion of the work of breathing produces reversible rearrangements of the alveolar gas-liquid interface and tissue molecular structures as the lungs and chest wall are stretched during inflation. As a result of their reversible nature, the energy stored in such rearrangements remains available to be used during deflation. These types of processes are responsible for the *elastic* properties of lung tissue. They are exemplified by the behavior of a rubber band, which stores energy when stretched and returns it when allowed to recover its original shape.

Another large portion of the work of breathing produces

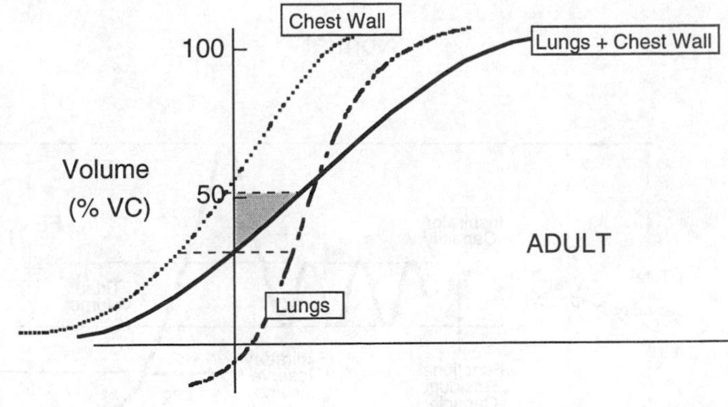

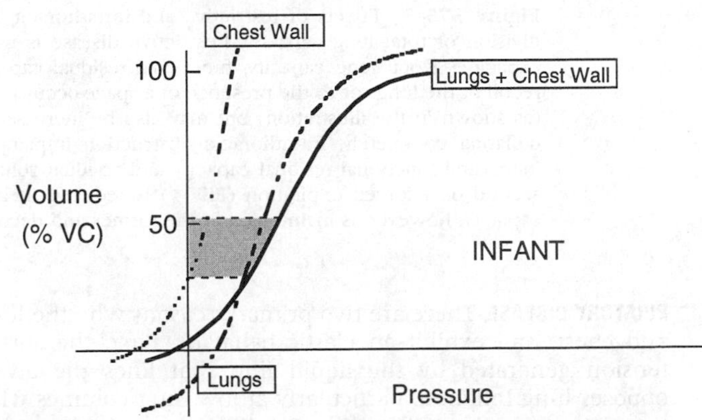

Figure 375–1 Idealized elastic volume-pressure relationships of the lungs, chest wall, and respiratory system in the adult and the infant. Volume is expressed as a proportion of vital capacity (VC). At any volume, the pressure that the respiratory muscles generate to oppose the elastic recoil of the respiratory system is equivalent to the sum of the recoil pressures of lungs and chest wall. The intersection of each relationship with the volume axis corresponds to the relaxation volume of each component (the volume at which the elastic recoil is zero). The volume elastic pressure relationships of the lungs are similar in the adult and infant. The volume–elastic pressure relationship of the chest wall is steeper in the infant, causing the relaxation volume of the respiratory system to be lower than in the adult. The shaded area represents the elastic work done by the respiratory muscles for a characteristic tidal volume. Note that this work is greater in the infant because the recoil of the chest wall does not contribute to inflate the lungs as it does in the adult. (From Pérez Fontán JJ: Mechanics of breathing. *In*: Gluckman PD, Heymann MA [eds]: Perinatal and Pediatric Pathophysiology: A Clinical Perspective. London, Edward Arnold, 1993.)

nonreversible molecular rearrangements or interactions. The energy so spent is permanently lost, usually by being converted into heat, which is then dissipated into the atmosphere or carried away by the circulating blood. All the mechanical processes that result in energy dissipation take place only in the presence of movement. As a result, the magnitude of the work done in connection with these processes bears a strong relationship to the rate at which gas flows in and out of the lungs. In this regard, the respiratory system exhibits a *resistive* behavior analogous to that of a household pipe, for which the pressure at the water main determines the flow of water.

Establishing a diagnosis and formulating a therapy for children with respiratory disease is greatly aided by the clinician distinguishing between conditions that alter primarily the *elastic (restrictive respiratory disease)* and *resistive (obstructive respiratory disease)* properties of the respiratory system. This distinction is facilitated by an understanding of the physiologic bases of these properties.

ELASTIC PROPERTIES OF THE RESPIRATORY SYSTEM: RESTRICTIVE RES-

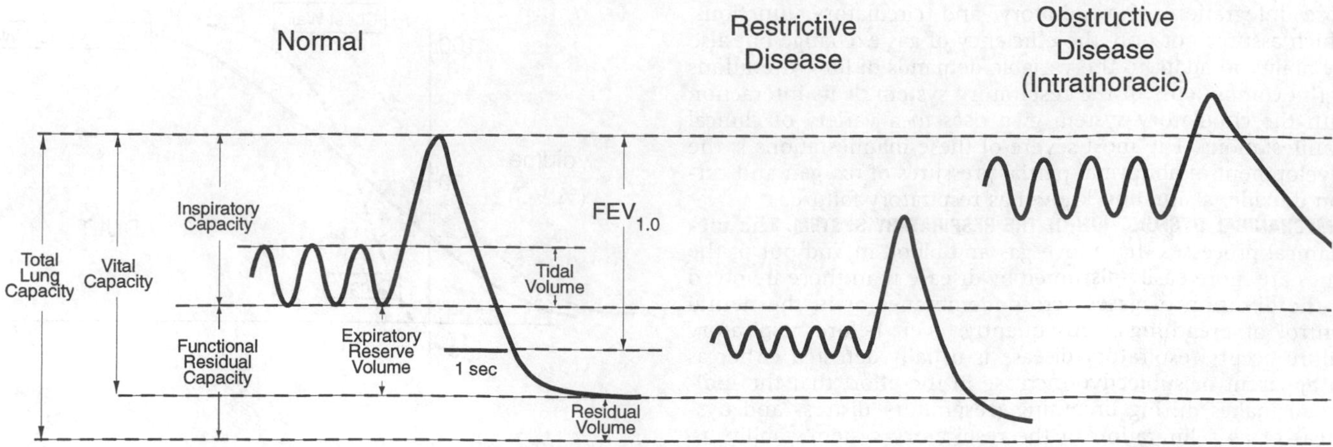

Figure 375–2 Effects of restrictive and intrathoracic obstruction on the divisions of total lung capacity. *Left,* Functional division of total lung capacity. Restrictive disease is usually characterized by a pattern of shallow, rapid breaths All lung capacities (total lung capacity, functional residual capacity, and vital capacity) are reduced owing either to the increased recoil of the lungs or to the presence of a space-occupying lesion that limits lung inflation. Residual volume is often decreased (as shown in the illustration) but may also be increased if an abnormal configuration of the chest prevents the lungs from deflating completely. Intrathoracic obstruction impairs the ability of the lungs to deflate and thus causes gas trapping, increasing functional residual capacity and residual volume at the expense of vital capacity. The volume exhaled in the first second of a forced expiration ($FEV_{1.0}$) is reduced in both restrictive and obstructive disease. The ratio of $FEV_{1.0}$ to vital capacity, however, is maintained in the former and decreased in the latter.

PIRATORY DISEASE. There are two primary reasons why the lungs and chest wall exhibit an elastic behavior. First, the surface tension generated by the liquid film that lines the alveoli opposes lung inflation, particularly at low lung volumes when the air spaces are smaller and, in fulfillment of Laplace's law, the same surface tension causes the inward-acting pressure to be greater. By coating the surface of the alveolar film with a monolayer of hydrophobic molecules, alveolar surfactant diminishes or neutralizes this pressure in a volume-dependent manner. Conveniently, surfactant is less spread out when the surface area of the alveolar film contracts, and therefore it is more effective at low than at high lung volumes. Even in the presence of normal amounts of surfactant in the air spaces, surface tension is responsible for approximately 65% of the elastic recoil of the lungs. When surfactant is absent or dysfunctional *(respiratory distress syndrome of the newborn)* (see Chapter 97.3) elastic recoil becomes markedly increased and alveolar collapse ensues.

The second reason explaining the elastic behavior of the respiratory system is that the solid components of the lungs and chest wall have elastic properties themselves. These elastic properties can be traced to the presence of a specialized fibrous scaffolding in these tissues. Particularly in the lungs, collagen and elastin fibers form a supportive web embedded in the alveolar walls and the septa that separate the individual constituents of the lung. Together with the pulmonary surfactant, this web preserves alveolar and airway stability. By anchoring different intrapulmonary structures to each other, septal fibers assure that the recoil forces generated within the lungs by the action of the respiratory muscles are evenly transmitted to alveolar walls, airways, and vessels. The resulting *mechanical interdependence* is responsible for the increase in the caliber of airways and vessels as the lungs inflate. It is also critical to keep lung inflation homogeneous within the constraints imposed by the shape of the chest wall.

Both surface tension and elastic forces generated by lung fibers depend on the dimensions of the air spaces. Thus, it is not surprising that the overall elastic recoil of the lungs is highly dependent on lung volume just like, in the example of the rubber band, tension depends on the extent to which the rubber band is stretched. The relationship between volume and elastic pressure can be obtained easily for the lungs and the chest wall together or independently by measuring the corresponding pressure changes while the lungs are passively inflated and deflated in a stepwise manner. All three relationships are sigmoid (see Fig. 375–1). Volume therefore increases much less for a given pressure change at low and high volumes than at the intermediate volumes at which normal breathing takes place. In this range, the relationship is steeper and relatively linear and can therefore be described accurately by a fixed ratio of volume to pressure changes, which defines the concept of *compliance.*

A graphic analysis of the volume-pressure relationships of the lungs and the chest wall clarifies how the mechanical behaviors of these two components interact to shape the volume-pressure relationship of the respiratory system as a whole (see Fig. 375–1). Two premises define these interactions: First, at any volume the elastic recoil of the respiratory system is equal to the sums of the individual elastic recoils of the lungs and chest wall. Second, the volume changes experienced by the lungs, the chest wall, and the respiratory system are identical. Based on these premises, it becomes easy to understand, for instance, how pleural pressure (which, when the respiratory muscles are relaxed, represents the elastic recoil of the chest wall) may be high in a patient with asthma who has no intrinsic chest wall anomalies but whose lung volume is markedly increased by gas trapping. Because the heart and vessels inside the thorax are exposed to pleural pressure, cardiac output and arterial blood pressure often undergo an exaggerated decrease during inspiration as lung volume increases even further *(pulsus paradoxus).*

A similar analysis also demonstrates some other principles that regulate lung volume. Each relationship crosses the volume axis at a different point, regardless of age (see Fig. 375–1). This point defines the *relaxation volume,* which is the volume at which no elastic recoil is generated. Under normal conditions, the relaxation volume of the lungs is considerably smaller than that of the chest wall, a discrepancy that has several important consequences. First, it forces the respiratory system as a whole to adopt a relaxation volume intermediate between that of the lungs and that of the chest wall. After the newborn period, this volume coincides with the *functional residual capacity,* the gas volume of the lungs at the end of a tidal expiration (see Fig. 375–2). In addition, the opposing recoils of the lungs and the chest wall at the relaxation volume of the respiratory system create a negative pleural pressure; this pressure promotes the return of venous blood into the heart and keeps the lung and chest wall attached to each other. If the pleural space was open to the atmosphere and the lungs and the chest wall were allowed to change volume freely, the lungs would collapse and the chest wall would expand. This happens when a *pneumothorax* develops. Finally, for at least a portion of the volume range, the outward-acting recoil of the chest wall helps the expansion of the lungs, thereby reducing energy expenditure during inspiration.

Restrictive lung disease occurs when surface tension is abnormally high (respiratory distress syndrome of the newborn) (see Chapter 97.3), when the structure or composition of the solid constituents of the lung is altered (interstitial edema, pneumonitis, fibrosis), or when the alveolar spaces are filled with liquid or inflammatory cells that limit inflation (alveolar edema, pneumonia). *Restrictive chest wall disease,* in contrast, is usually caused by structural anomalies of the chest wall itself (scoliosis or rib cage dystrophy), neuromuscular disease, or abdominal distention. Whether originating in the lungs or the chest wall, restrictive respiratory disease has common clinical characteristics. First, only the work performed during inspiration increases, and thus the increased load is carried almost exclusively by the inspiratory muscles, the diaphragm in particular. Second, the subject typically tries to minimize energy demands by adopting a pattern of rapid and shallow breathing, which, when present, almost always indicates a restrictive derangement. Last, the increased elastic recoil of the lungs or the chest wall lowers the relaxation volume of the respiratory system as a whole. Consequently, the functional residual capacity and, to a more variable extent, the forced vital capacity are reduced in all forms of restrictive disease (see Fig. 375–2). Because the recoil forces transmitted through the fibrous network of the lungs are minimal at low lung volumes, alveoli become unstable and alveolar collapse tends to complicate the situation by further decreasing ventilation-perfusion ratios and causing hypoxemia.

RESISTIVE PROPERTIES OF THE RESPIRATORY SYSTEM: OBSTRUCTIVE RESPIRATORY DISEASE. The resistive behavior of the respiratory system results from molecular rearrangements and interactions initiated by motion. Under normal conditions, the most important of these interactions is the friction of the air against the airway walls. When friction is the only factor, Poiseuille's law predicts that the pressure losses are directly proportional to the viscosity of the gas, the length of the pipe, and the rate of airflow, and inversely proportional to the fourth power of the airway's radius. Just on this basis, it is easy to understand how airway diseases such as *croup* or *viral bronchiolitis* increase the work of breathing more in newborns and small infants, who have smaller radius airways, than in older children. However, friction is not the only source of resistive work. Molecular interactions and velocity changes within the breathing gas itself, particularly when the flow becomes turbulent in pathologically narrow portions of the airways, can result in considerable energy dissipation. Unlike wall friction, the pressure needed to overcome turbulence depends on the density and not on the viscosity of the gas. This is the reason why children with *croup* have less respiratory difficulty and stridor when the air they breathe is replaced with a mixture of oxygen and helium, which has a lower density than air or oxygen. Finally, nonreversible molecular rearrangements within the tissue or the gas-liquid interface play an important role in the resistive properties of the lungs and the respiratory system as a whole.

The resistive behavior of the respiratory system can also be analyzed graphically (Fig. 375–3). The volume-pressure relationships of the lungs, chest wall, and respiratory system as a whole form characteristic loops; they show *hysteresis,* which means that the relationships have different courses during inspiration and expiration. The presence of hysteresis always denotes that there is an energy loss from the system. Moreover, the greater the hysteresis, the larger is this energy loss. Accordingly, the width of the loop formed by the pressure-volume relationships of the respiratory system or its components (which has the units of pressure) can be used as a quantitative estimate of resistive behavior. When divided by the rate of gas flow, it yields the *resistance* of each component, a measurement that summarizes various properties that cause resistive energy dissipation. The graphic analysis of the volume-pressure relationships of the respiratory system also reveals that, even though resistive work is done during inspiration and expiration, usually the inspiratory portion of the work alone represents an energy burden. Under normal circumstances, expiration does not require the contraction of any muscles; it is passive, and all expiratory resistive work is performed by the elastic recoil accumulated during inspiration in the lungs and chest wall. However, when expiratory resistance is elevated by disease (asthma, bronchiolitis) or when the individual needs to accelerate the emptying of the lungs to increase ventilation (exercise), abdominal and other accessory muscles of expiration become engaged. This engagement in a resting child is a good indication of the presence of obstructive respiratory disease.

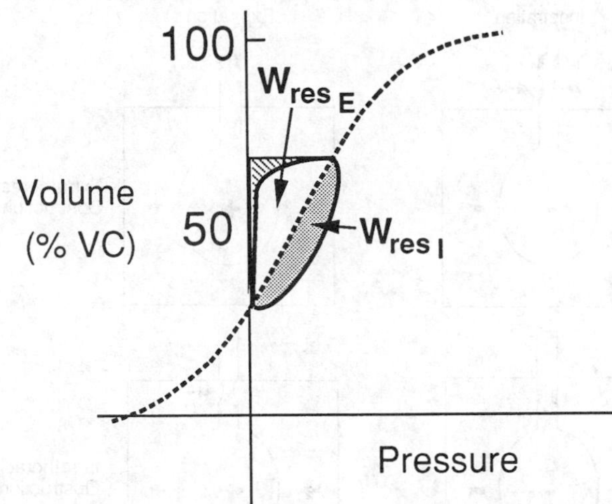

Figure 375–3 Graphic analysis of the resistive behavior of the respiratory system during a tidal breath. In the presence of airway flow, energy dissipation causes the relationship between lung volume (expressed as a proportion of vital capacity) and the pressure that the respiratory muscles must generate to form a loop (hysteresis). The area enclosed by this loop represents the work done to overcome resistive pressures such as those caused by the friction of the air against the airway walls. Only the inspiratory portion of this work (W_{resI}), however, is performed by the respiratory muscles. The expiratory portion (W_{resE}) is done by the energy accumulated in elastic elements of the respiratory system during inspiration. (From Pérez Fontán JJ: Mechanics of breathing. *In*: Gluckman PD, Heymann MA [eds]: Perinatal and Pediatric Pathophysiology: A Clinical Perspective. London, Edward Arnold, 1993.)

Proper diagnosis and evaluation of airway obstruction require additional understanding of the relationships between airway caliber and lung volume. Airway caliber is determined by the coupling of airway wall elasticity and airway transmural pressure. The former depends on the state of health and maturity of the airway tissue (immature airways tend to collapse more easily) and is influenced by the tone of the muscles contained in the airway wall. This tone is, in turn, regulated by neural efferents, which are activated by the central nervous system to stiffen the airway walls during inspiration, particularly under conditions in which breathing activity must increase (during exercise, hypoxia, or hypercarbia).

Airway transmural pressure is the difference between the pressures acting on the inside and outside surfaces of the

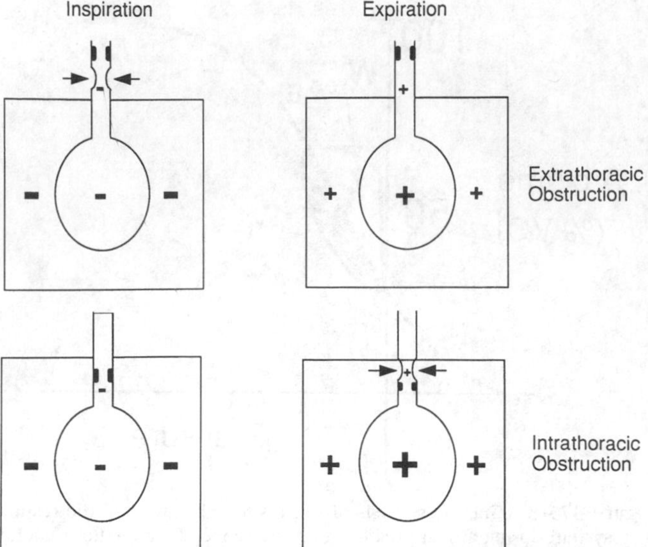

Figure 375–4 Effect of inspiration and expiration on the caliber of the airways during extrathoracic and intrathoracic airway obstruction. Extrathoracic obstruction is exacerbated during inspiration because the pressure inside the airway becomes very negative with respect to the atmospheric pressure outside, causing the airway to collapse (*arrows*). Intrathoracic obstruction, in contrast, is exacerbated during expiration because the pressure outside the airways (which is similar to pleural pressure) rapidly exceeds the pressure inside, causing the airways downstream from the obstruction point to collapse (*arrows*). (From Pérez Fontán JJ, Lister G: Respiratory failure. *In*: Toulukian RJ [ed]: Pediatric Trauma, 2nd ed. St. Louis, CV Mosby, 1990.)

airway wall. It varies during the respiratory cycle in a fashion that depends on whether the airways are intrathoracic or extrathoracic (Fig. 375–4). Extrathoracic airways (nose, pharynx, larynx, the extrathoracic portion of the trachea) are exposed to atmospheric pressure on the outside. Because the pressure acting on the inside surface is subatmospheric during inspiration and supra-atmospheric during expiration, the transmural pressure in this portion of the airway is always negative (narrowing or even collapsing the airway) during inspiration and always positive (dilating the airway) during expiration. The outside surface of the intrathoracic airways is exposed either to pleural pressure (trachea and main bronchi) or to the stresses generated by lung inflation within the lung tissue (intrapulmonary bronchi, bronchioles, and alveolar ducts). These stresses are transmitted to the airway walls by their tissue attachments to the alveolar septa and, when averaged, they add up to a value close to the pleural pressure. During inspiration, the pressure inside the airways is greater than the pressure inside the alveoli. Alveolar pressure, in turn, is always greater than pleural pressure (otherwise, the lungs would have a negative elastic recoil). Consequently, the transmural pressure of the intrathoracic airways always becomes more positive (dilating the airways) as the lungs inflate. During expiration, in contrast, the pressure at all points inside the airways must be lower than alveolar pressure. Whether the pressure inside a certain point in the airways is higher or lower than pleural pressure, however, depends on how much pressure has been lost upstream from the point in question. If the loss is large, the pressure inside the intrathoracic airways can become lower than pleural pressure. The transmural pressure then becomes negative and the airway tends to collapse, a problem that is compounded further if the airway wall is abnormally soft (as in the premature infant or in *bronchomalacia*). The more the subject tries to overcome the resultant increase in expiratory resistance by making use of the expiratory muscles, the more the pleural pressure increases and the more the airway collapses, leading to a situation in which outward airflow cannot increase any more regardless of the effort. The expiratory flow at which such *flow limitation* occurs is reproducible for a given lung volume. Determinations of maximal expiratory flow during respiratory function testing take advantage of this reproducibility to evaluate and follow the function of the intrathoracic airways over time or in response to specific therapies.

Airway obstruction causes an exaggeration of the normal changes in airway caliber (see Fig. 375–4). When the extrathoracic airway is obstructed (croup, foreign body), the pressure inside the airways distal to the narrowing becomes more negative during inspiration through the actions of the diaphragm and other inspiratory muscles to overcome the increased resistance at the point of obstruction. Therefore, the extrathoracic airway collapses downstream from the level of the obstruction, usually causing an audible vibration or inspiratory *stridor* as the gas rushes through the obstruction. When the intrathoracic airway is obstructed (asthma, tracheobronchomalacia), the pleural pressure must become more positive during expiration. Because the inside pressure beyond the obstruction decreases, the intrathoracic airways downstream from the obstruction tend to collapse, producing an exacerbation of the obstruction, audible expiratory *wheezes,* and flow limitation at low expiratory flows.

DISTINCTION BETWEEN RESTRICTIVE AND OBSTRUCTIVE RESPIRATORY DYSFUNCTION: PULMONARY FUNCTION TESTING. A careful physical examination frequently yields sufficient information to establish whether an infant or child is suffering from a predominantly restrictive or obstructive ailment (Table 375–1). However, complicated diagnostic problems and the follow-up of those patients for whom a diagnosis has already been made are aided greatly by the performance of pulmonary function tests. These tests combine gas flow and lung volume measurements to characterize in detail each patient's physiologic derangement. Gas flows rates are most informative if measured during a forced expiratory maneuver generated either voluntarily, if the patient is old enough to cooperate, or by the application of an inflatable jacket to the chest surface, when the patient is too young or uncooperative. In addition to being

TABLE 375–1 Characteristic Clinical Findings of Restrictive and Obstructive Lung Disease in Infants and Children

		Obstructive Disease	
	Restrictive Disease	*Extrathoracic*	*Intrathoracic*
Breathing rate	Increased	Decreased	Normal or increased
Duration of inspiration	Reduced	Prolonged	Unchanged
Duration of expiration	Reduced	Unchanged	Prolonged
Accessory respiratory muscles	Inspiratory	Inspiratory	Inspiratory and expiratory (abdominal)
Rib cage distortion (retractions)	Present	Present	Often present
Amplitude of breathing movements	Shallow	Normal or reduced	Normal or reduced
Auscultatory findings	Crackles Grunting	Inspiratory stridor	Expiratory wheezing
Radiographic appearance of lungs	Decreased lung volume Alveolar densities	Normal	Increased lung volume

relatively simple to determine, gas flow rates obtained under conditions of flow limitation in the airways are highly reproducible and thus can be compared over time.

Expiratory flow measurements are easier to interpret if flow is plotted against lung volume, forming characteristic flow-volume loops (Fig. 375–5). As a basic principle in the interpretation of these loops, restrictive disease causes proportional decreases in flow rate and lung volume; obstructive disease decreases flow rate but not lung volume. Extrathoracic airway obstruction reduces inspiratory flow, frequently causing the inspiratory limb of the flow-volume loop to become flat. Expiratory flow is unaltered, unless the airway narrowing is severe or rigid enough (intraluminal masses, long segment tracheal stenosis) to obliterate the normal dilatation of the upper airway during expiration. Intrathoracic obstruction reduces expiratory flow more than inspiratory flow. Expiratory flow limitation is reached at lower expiratory flow rates as the lungs deflate. This phenomenon is responsible for the characteristic "scoop" in the expiratory limb of the flow-volume loop found in patients with intrathoracic airway obstruction (see Fig. 375–5). It is also the reason why the maximal flow measured at functional residual capacity is a more sensitive indicator of intrathoracic airway obstruction than is the peak expiratory flow.

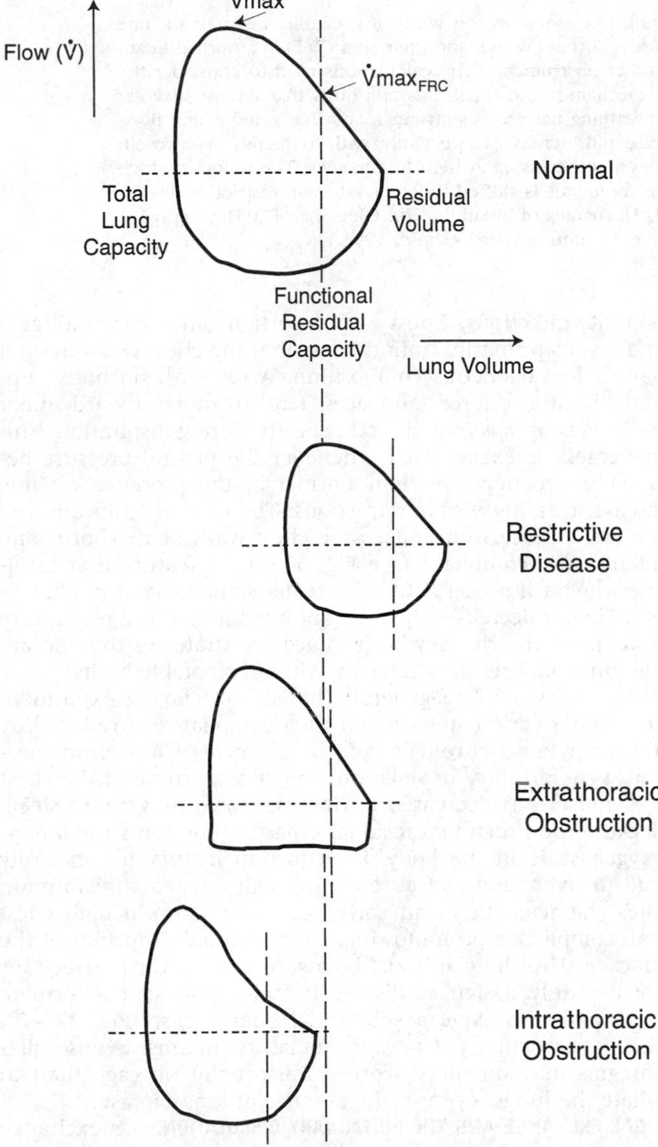

Figure 375–5 Flow volume loops obtained by plotting the gas flow generated during a forced vital capacity maneuver in which, after a forced exhalation, the subject inhales to vital capacity and exhales to residual volume. The direction of the loops is clockwise. Inspiration is downward; expiration is upward. $\dot{V}_{max}$ represents peak expiratory flow. $\dot{V}max_{FRC}$ is the maximal flow recorded at functional residual capacity. Restrictive disease reduces lung volumes and both inspiratory and expiratory flow rates without changing the shape of the loop. Extrathoracic obstruction is exacerbated during inspiration and thus flattens the inspiratory limb of the loop without altering the expiratory limb. Intrathoracic obstruction increases functional residual capacity and reduces all expiratory flows. The flow reduction becomes more severe as lung volume decreases, creating a characteristic concavity or "scoop" in the expiratory limb of the loop.

Lung volume measurements can be obtained either with a body plethysmograph or by combining spirometry and gas dilution or washout techniques. Typically, both intrathoracic airway obstruction and restrictive respiratory disease reduce vital capacity. However, intrathoracic obstruction almost always increases residual volume and functional residual capacity, whereas restrictive disease tends to decrease both measurements, causing the ratio of residual volume to vital capacity to remain relatively unaltered. Although both obstructive and restrictive disease may decrease the volume expelled from the lungs in the first second of a forced expiratory maneuver (FEV_1), only obstructive disease diminishes the ratio of this volume to vital capacity. Combinations of restrictive and obstructive disease are not uncommon and, when present, are difficult to diagnose by pulmonary function testing alone. The presence of restrictive disease should be suspected whenever gas flow rates are decreased out of proportion with the FEV_1: vital capacity ratio or when the total lung capacity is reduced.

RESPONSE TO RESPIRATORY DISEASE: EFFICIENCY OF THE DEVELOPING RESPIRATORY SYSTEM. When the respiratory workload increases in the course of an illness, the respiratory system initiates two types of responses. The most immediate is to increase the output of the respiratory muscles at the cost of increased energy expenditure. This response is limited not only by substrate availability but also by the ability of the muscles to generate a maximal contraction force. The second response is usually an attempt to improve the efficiency of respiration by changing the respiratory pattern.

The respiratory system is inherently an inefficient machine. Efficiency values as low as 8% (indicating that only 8% of the energy consumed by the muscles is transformed into actual volume-pressure work) have been reported in resting adults. Even lower values have been suggested in term newborn and premature infants. Because the baseline values are so low, disease-induced changes in efficiency usually have a large effect on the energy required for breathing. Factors that determine respiratory system efficiency include the breathing pattern; the configuration, length, and functional state of the diaphragm; and the degree of chest wall distortion that occurs with each breath.

Each breathing pattern is a unique combination of breathing frequency and tidal volume. Different breathing patterns can yield the same minute ventilation, but there is only one specific respiratory pattern that results in minimal energy expenditure at any time. This optimal pattern varies predictably depending on the mechanical characteristics of the respiratory system (Fig. 375–6). Breathing frequency, for instance, increases when elastic recoil becomes greater in the course of a restrictive derangement. In contrast, the frequency decreases when the resistive properties of the respiratory system become exaggerated by airway obstruction. It is therefore possible to categorize respiratory disease as primarily restrictive or obstructive, depending on whether the patient breathes rapidly and shallowly or slowly and more deeply. It is important to remember, however, that breathing pattern is regulated by influences other than energetic considerations. It is common for children with respiratory disease to breathe transiently at

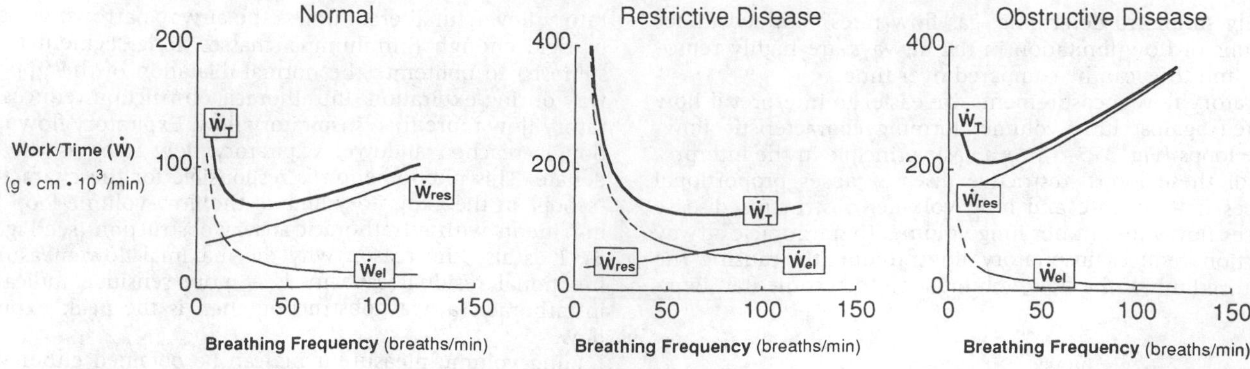

Figure 375–6 Schematic representation of the effects of breathing frequency on the work of breathing per unit of time (W-breathing power) needed to overcome elastic forces (Ẇel), resistive forces (Ẇres), and their sum (ẆT) in a normal infant and two infants with respiratory disease (one restrictive and the other obstructive). The calculations used to construct the representation are based on typical measurements of respiratory mechanics and on the assumptions that minute alveolar ventilation is constant regardless of the breathing frequency, that breathing pattern is sinusoidal, and that volume- and flow-pressure relationships are linear. Elastic and resistive power decrease and increase, respectively, with frequency. As a result, total power follows a bimodal course, decreasing at low frequencies and increasing at high frequencies. The point at which total power reaches a minimum defines the optimal frequency. This frequency is shifted to lower values in restrictive disease and to higher values in obstructive disease. (From Pérez Fontán JJ: Mechanics of breathing. *In*: Gluckman PD, Heymann MA [eds]: Perinatal and Pediatric Pathophysiology: A Clinical Perspective. London, Edward Arnold, 1993.)

frequencies that depart substantially from optimum. Crying and agitation can in this manner reduce the efficiency of the respiratory system and precipitate respiratory failure.

Like other skeletal muscles, the diaphragm can develop its maximal force only if it starts from an optimal length. This length is attained when the lungs approximate their functional residual capacity (see Fig. 375–2). At this volume, the diaphragm adopts the shape of a dome-capped cylinder (Fig. 375–7). In addition to increasing the volume displaced for a given fiber shortening, this shape allows for an area of the diaphragmatic muscle to be in direct apposition to the rib cage. This *area of apposition* serves an important function during inspiration. It allows the abdominal contents to push the lower ribs forward and laterally, increasing the volume of the lungs. The shape of the diaphragm in the infant, particularly in the newborn, may not take advantage of these features (see Fig. 375–7). The lower portion of the rib cage has large anteroposterior and lateral diameters. As a result, the diaphragmatic insertions are spread out, limiting the range of lengths of the diaphragmatic fibers.

Until now, this discussion has assumed that the chest wall expands uniformly during lung inflation. In reality, different portions of the rib cage and abdomen not only can change volume independently of one another but also can do it in

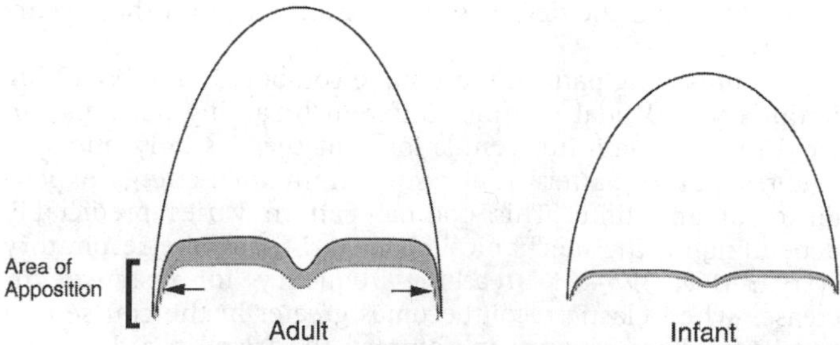

Figure 375–7 Schematic representations of the differences in the geometric shapes of the diaphragm of the adult and infant. The diaphragm of the adult (*left*) has the shape of a dome-capped cylinder. A portion of the cylinder's is side apposed to the rib cage, providing a way of transforming the vertical movement of the diaphragm into the anterior and lateral movement of the rib cage in inspiration (see text). The diaphragm of the infant (*right*) is flatter and less capable of displacing large volumes in the vertical direction. In addition, it lacks a substantial area of apposition and thus has limited expanding action on the rib cage.

opposite directions. Chest wall distortion can occur at all ages and results primarily from the fact that the chest wall does not have a homogeneous composition. Areas with no bony support, like the intercostal spaces, tend to move inward under the effects of negative pleural pressure during inspiration. This movement is exaggerated whenever the pleural pressure becomes more negative than normal in the presence of lung disease, creating visible retractions. The limited ossification of the ribs and sternum makes the chest walls of newborns and infants very compliant (see Fig. 375–1), a feature that facilitates the birth process but also creates some mechanical liabilities. First, it decreases the relaxation volume of the respiratory system, forcing the newborn to acquire strategies to maintain the functional residual capacity within acceptable limits. These strategies, which are generally based on delaying expiration, are easily overwhelmed when lung compliance is reduced by disease, when neurologic control is impaired by central nervous system injury or sedation, or when the tone of the chest wall muscles is decreased during rapid eye movement sleep. Because the functional residual capacity represents the largest oxygen store in the body, its reduction in infants can easily lead to hypoxemia because of the high oxygen consumption rates characteristic at an early age. In addition, a high chest wall compliance promotes increased regional distortion of the rib cage. The clinician must be aware that rib cage retractions are not only a sign of disease but also represent a form of work and may have a substantial energy cost (Fig. 375–8). This is particularly true in premature infants, whose diaphragms may do more work to distort the rib cage than to inflate the lungs, even in the absence of lung disease.

GAS EXCHANGE AND THE PULMONARY CIRCULATION. Gas exchange in the lungs takes place in millions of small units, each consisting of a pulmonary capillary and the neighboring portion of the air space. Before arriving there, the venous blood returning to the heart is propelled by the right ventricle into a branching network of pulmonary vessels.

SPECIAL CHARACTERISTICS OF THE PULMONARY CIRCULATION. After the adaptations that take place during the newborn period (see Chapter 97.1), the pulmonary circulation offers a much lower resistance to the passage of blood than does the systemic circulation. As a result, the pulmonary blood flow can be accommodated with relatively low blood pressures in the pulmonary artery, allowing the right ventricle to lose part of its muscle mass to become a chamber more adapted to handle volume than pressure loads. Reversal of this situation occurs

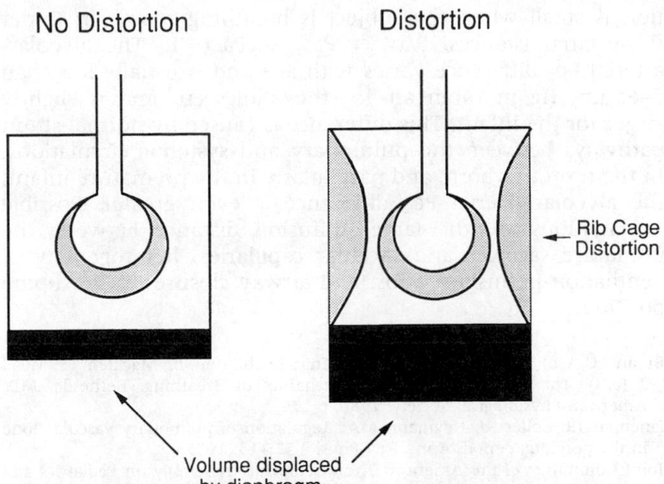

Figure 375–8 Schematic representation of the effects of rib cage distortion on the volume displaced by the diaphragm during inspiration. During a nondistorted inspiration, the volume displaced by the diaphragm is analogous to the tidal volume that enters the lungs. However, during a distorted inspiration, the volume displaced by the diaphragm must increase in proportion to the inward movement of the rib cage to maintain tidal volume unchanged. (From Pérez Fontán JJ: Mechanical dysfunction of the respiratory system. *In*: Fuhrman BP, Zimmerman JJ [eds]: Pediatric Critical Care. St. Louis, Mosby-Yearbook, 1992.)

in a variety of clinical situations, which, as a common denominator, cause *pulmonary arterial hypertension*. Physiologic stimuli such as chronic hypoxemia and increased shear stress or tension in the vascular walls can produce smooth muscle hypertrophy and deposition of elastin and type I collagen, leading eventually to the obliteration of pulmonary vessels in experimental animals. Similar stimuli and possibly a failure to curtail the proliferative vascular response that they induce are probably the origin of many cases of pulmonary hypertension complicating parenchymal lung disease or left-to-right shunts in childhood.

Pulmonary arterioles (the resistance vessels in the pulmonary circulation) are considerably more reactive to changes in partial pressures of oxygen and carbon dioxide in their environment than are systemic arterioles. Even small fluctuations in these partial pressures can cause marked changes in pulmonary vascular tone. Alveolar hypoxemia is a particularly powerful vasoconstrictive stimulus, which provides the lungs with a local regulatory system to minimize arterial hypoxemia by directing nonoxygenated blood away from areas where ventilation is poor. Hypercarbia produces pulmonary vasoconstriction; hypocarbia causes pulmonary vasodilation. The effect of carbon dioxide on the pulmonary vasculature is not the same as on other vascular beds. For example the carbon dioxide effect on the cerebral vasculature is exactly the opposite.

Pulmonary vessels are for the most part intrapulmonary structures and, as such, they are subjected to the forces generated inside the lungs during breathing. Alveolar vessels, which are contained entirely in the alveolar walls, become compressed as the lungs inflate and the alveolar pressure raises relative to pleural pressure (which is the pressure to which the heart and major vessels are exposed). Conversely, extra-alveolar vessels, arterial or venous, become dilatated during inflation by virtue of their mechanical linkages to the surrounding lung tissue (mechanical interdependence). Because the effect of inflation over the extra-alveolar vessels predominates at low lung volumes and the effect over the alveolar vessels predominates at high lung volumes, the total resistance of the pulmonary circulation follows a biphasic, U-shaped relationship with respect to lung volume, decreasing at low lung volumes and increasing at higher lung volumes. The inflection point of the relationship, where resistance is minimal, coincides with the functional residual capacity, which therefore represents the point at which pulmonary blood flow is maximal for any given pulmonary arterial pressure.

Finally, the pulmonary circulation is the site of an active exchange of water and solutes between the vascular space and the interstitium of the lung (the continuous space that exists between alveolar epithelium and endothelium and around airways and pulmonary vessels). The exchange occurs across the endothelial cells or the inter-endothelial cell junctions and is regulated by a balance of hydrostatic and protein osmotic (oncotic) forces. Increases in fluid filtration, leading to pulmonary edema, occur either when the microvascular pressures increase relative to the protein osmotic pressures (left ventricular failure, pulmonary venous obstruction) or when the water and solute permeability of the endothelium is increased (in virtually any form of lung injury). Confined initially to the pulmonary interstitium, edematous fluid is removed by an effective system of lymphatic vessels. When the capacity of these vessels is exceeded, however, fluid can penetrate the gas spaces, interfering even further with both the mechanical function of the lungs and gas exchange.

FACTORS DETERMINING THE EFFICIENCY OF GAS EXCHANGE IN THE LUNGS. Because the arterial blood is a weighted mixture of the blood that passes through these units, the arterial concentrations or contents of oxygen and carbon dioxide depend fundamentally on the way in which blood flow and ventilation are matched within the lungs (Fig. 375–9). On one extreme, nonperfused units, which continue to receive ventilation, do not contribute directly to the composition of the arterial blood but waste a portion of the ventilatory effort. In this regard,

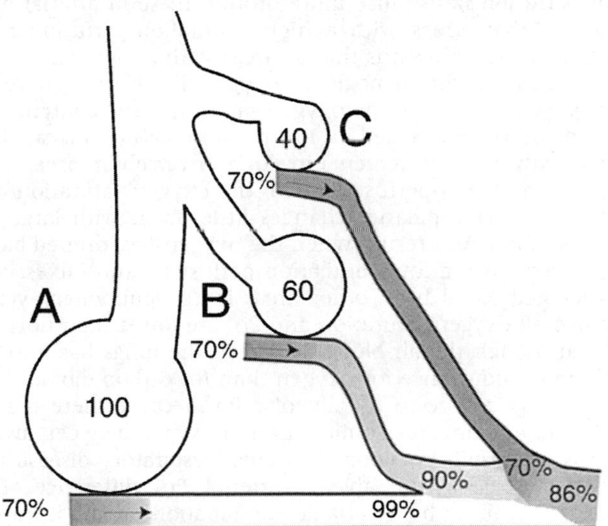

Figure 375–9 Diagram demonstrating the effects of decreased ventilation: perfusion ratios on arterial oxygenation in the lungs. Three alveolar-capillary units are illustrated. Unit A has normal ventilation and an alveolar Po_2 of 100 mm Hg (shown by the number in the middle of the air space). The blood that circulates through this unit raises its oxygen saturation from 70% (the saturation of mixed venous blood) to 99%. Unit B has a lower ventilation: perfusion ratio and a lower alveolar Po_2 of 60 mm Hg. The blood that circulates through this unit reaches a saturation of only 90%. Finally, unit C is not ventilated at all. Its alveolar Po_2 is equivalent to that of the venous blood, which travels through the unit unaltered. The oxygen saturation of the arterial blood reflects the weighted contributions of these three units. If it is assumed that each unit has the same blood flow, the arterial blood would have a saturation of only 86%. Ventilation-perfusion mismatch is the most common mechanism of arterial hypoxemia in lung disease. Supplemental oxygen increases the arterial Po_2 by raising the alveolar Po_2 in lung units that, like B, have a ventilation: perfusion ratio greater than zero.

they act as dead space. On the other extreme, nonventilated units, which continue to receive blood flow, contaminate the arterial blood with venous blood. They act as a shunt (or promote venous admixture). Between these two extremes, there is usually a wide spectrum of ventilation-perfusion ratios that define the final composition of the arterial blood. The factors that determine this composition are different for carbon dioxide and oxygen.

The partial pressure of carbon dioxide (P_{CO_2}) in the arterial blood is directly proportional to carbon dioxide production and inversely proportional to alveolar ventilation. The latter can be calculated as the difference of minute ventilation (the amount of gas that enters and leaves the lungs in 1 minute) and dead space ventilation (the portion of the minute ventilation that does not contribute to alveolar gas exchange). Dead space ventilation is usually increased by respiratory disease because of the presence of a large number of gas exchange units with high ventilation-perfusion ratios. If the individual is unable to compensate with a sufficient increase in minute ventilation, the arterial P_{CO_2} rises to greater than its normal values of 33–45 mm Hg.

The partial pressure of oxygen (P_{O_2}) in the arterial blood is influenced by several variables, including the P_{O_2} or fractional oxygen concentration (F_{IO_2}) of the inspired gas, the P_{O_2} of the venous blood, the hemoglobin oxygen capacity, and the respective alveolar gas and capillary blood flows in the lungs. With other factors being constant, increases in gas flow (ventilation) with respect to blood flow (perfusion) augment pulmonary capillary and arterial P_{O_2}. Conversely, decreases in the ventilation-perfusion ratio decrease pulmonary capillary and arterial P_{O_2} (see Fig. 375–9). Regional differences in ventilation-perfusion ratios exist in normal lungs. When exaggerated, these differences cause hypoxemia. To understand the mechanism, it is important to recognize that areas with a low ventilation-perfusion ratio cause more of a decrease in arterial oxygenation than areas with a high ventilation-perfusion ratio increase it. The reason is that in areas with a low ventilation-perfusion ratio, the hemoglobin-oxygen dissociation curve favors large decreases in the oxygen saturation and content (the volume of oxygen carried by 100 mL of blood) of the capillary blood with small decrements in P_{O_2}. Conversely in areas with a high ventilation-perfusion ratio, the oxygen saturation and content in the capillaries changes little, even with large increases in P_{O_2}. As a result, when the oxygen-desaturated blood from areas with a low ventilation-perfusion ratio mixes with oxygenated blood from other areas in the pulmonary veins, the overall oxygen saturation and P_{O_2} are lower than normal.

Even though the air-blood barrier in the lungs has a lower diffusion conductance for oxygen than for carbon dioxide, the arterial P_{O_2} is close to the alveolar P_{O_2} because there is normally enough time for equilibration of oxygen between alveolar gas and capillary blood. However, respiratory disease frequently increases the alveolar-arterial P_{O_2} difference. This increase is caused by a variable combination of true intrapulmonary shunting in areas where the ventilation-perfusion ratio is zero (alveolar collapse) and ventilation-perfusion mismatch. Diffusion impairment may contribute to hypoxemia in interstitial lung disease in adults, but its contribution is questionable in childhood diseases. The alveolar-arterial P_{O_2} difference can be calculated at the bedside to quantify the amount of gas exchange impairment by measuring the arterial P_{O_2} and calculating the alveolar P_{O_2} (P_{AO_2}) as

$$P_{AO_2} = P_{IO_2} - P_{aCO_2}/R + F_{IO_2}\,P_{aCO_2}\,(1 - R)$$

where P_{IO_2} represents the partial pressure of inspired oxygen [(F_{IO_2} (P_B − 47)], P_{aCO_2} is the arterial partial pressure of carbon dioxide (considered equivalent to the alveolar partial pressure), and R is the respiratory quotient (carbon dioxide production/oxygen consumption). The last term of this equation is small when the subject is breathing room air; under those circumstances, $P_{AO_2} \cong P_{IO_2} - P_{aCO_2}/R$. The alveolar-arterial P_{O_2} difference varies with age and is usually less than 5–6 mm Hg in room air for the adolescent and is slightly larger for the infant. This difference is caused by normal shunt pathways between the pulmonary and systemic circulations. In the term newborn, and particularly in the premature infant, the alveolar-arterial P_{O_2} difference is even greater. Possible explanations are the larger diffusion distance between the immature saccules and saccular capillaries, heterogeneity of ventilation-perfusion ratios, and airway closure in the supine position.

Bryan AC, Wohl MEB: Respiratory mechanics in children. *In*: Macklem PT, Mead J (eds): The Respiratory System: Mechanics of Breathing. Bethesda, MD, American Physiological Society, 1986, p 179.

Fineman JR, Soifer SJ, Heymann MA: Regulation of pulmonary vascular tone in the perinatal period. Annu Rev Physiol 57:115, 1995.

Joint Committee of the American Thoracic Society Assembly on Pediatrics and the European Respiratory Society Pediatrics Assembly: Respiratory mechanics in infants: Physiologic evaluation in health and disease. Am Rev Respir Dis 147:474, 1993.

Rysconi F, Castagneto M, Gagliardi L, et al: Reference values for respiratory rate in the first 3 years of life. Pediatrics 94:350, 1994.

Staub NC: Pulmonary edema. Physiol Rev 54:678, 1974.

Weibel ER: The Pathway for Oxygen: Structure and Function of the Mammalian Respiratory System. Cambridge, MA, Harvard University Press, 1984.

West JB: Ventilation/Blood Flow and Gas Exchange. Oxford, Blackwell Scientific, 1990.

375.1 Respiratory Failure

Gabriel G. Haddad and J. Julio Pérez Fontán

Respiratory failure is defined by significant alterations in the arterial P_{O_2} and P_{CO_2} (also see Chapter 64.3). This definition is convenient because blood gas analysis is readily available and easy to interpret. In addition, arterial P_{O_2} and P_{CO_2} are tightly regulated by the central nervous system based on the information provided by a complex system of sensors and effector organs, for example muscle; consequently alterations in their values usually indicate that the mechanisms that execute the regulation are either overwhelmed by disease or have failed. Defining respiratory failure on the basis of gas exchange alone also has disadvantages. Blood gas tensions can easily be misinterpreted. Arterial P_{O_2} may be normal if the individual is breathing increased inspired oxygen concentrations or decreased without alterations in respiratory function if there is an intracardiac right-to-left shunt. Arterial P_{CO_2} can also be elevated as a compensatory mechanism in patients with chronic metabolic alkalosis as well as in the absence of intrinsic respiratory impairment. Blood gas analysis requires time and should not delay the initiation of lifesaving therapy.

PATHOPHYSIOLOGY. Gas exchange alterations in respiratory failure result from abnormalities in the mechanical properties of the lungs and chest wall, the function of the respiratory muscles or their innervation, or respiratory control. Distinguishing among these three possibilities is usually easy. Mechanical abnormalities typically increase both the ventilatory requirements and the physical effort required to fulfill these requirements. The patient acquires tachypnea and rib cage distortion (retractions), recruits accessory muscles of respiration (scalene, sternocleidomastoid, abdominal muscles), and offers an overall impression of air hunger (dyspnea), all of which are manifestations of an increased respiratory drive. Abnormalities of the respiratory muscles or their innervation are also associated with an increased central drive, but this drive is not translated into effective respiratory movements. Tachypnea with shallow respiratory efforts and profound dyspnea are characteristic, but retractions may be absent. Alterations in the respiratory control are almost always associated with decreased respiratory drive and therefore produce few or no signs of respiratory difficulty, even in the presence of considerable derangement in gas exchange.

Respiratory failure in children is caused more frequently by abnormalities in the mechanical function of the lungs and the chest wall than by neuromuscular or control abnormalities. Both restrictive and obstructive disease increase the work of breathing and therefore raise the energy demands of the respiratory muscles. If these demands are met, the mechanical abnormality remains compensated. If the demands exceed the capabilities of the respiratory muscles, respiratory failure develops. It is useful to conceptualize the interplay between work and energy demands as a balance, with the work of breathing on one side and the energy available to the contractile machinery of the respiratory muscles on the other side (Fig. 375–10). The position of the fulcrum depends on the efficiency of the system. Under normal circumstances, energy availability greatly exceeds energy demands, and even substantial increases in the work of breathing can be compensated. However, when efficiency is reduced by rib cage distortion, overinflation of the lungs, or respiratory muscle fatigue, insufficient energy is transformed into work and the balance moves in the direction of respiratory failure.

Recognizing the mechanisms that compensate for the increases in the work of breathing is just as important as blood gas analysis for the diagnosis and management of respiratory failure. These mechanisms involve an increased effort on the part of the respiratory muscles. The diaphragm, intercostal, and other respiratory muscles are skeletal muscles, and they can fatigue for example; the diaphragm can fail and stop generating the alveolar ventilation needed to keep up with carbon dioxide production. Newborns appear to have an increased propensity for respiratory muscle fatigue. This probably relates to decreased breathing efficiency caused by mechanical factors such as the high compliance of the chest wall and the small surface of apposition of the diaphragm to the rib cage, rather than to maturational changes in the intrinsic properties of the respiratory muscles themselves.

Respiratory muscles can generate enormous pressures and sustain large increases in work for a prolonged period; nonetheless, failure of respiratory muscles can occur. In addition to immaturity, factors such as malnutrition, decreased perfusion, electrolyte disorders, and hypophosphatemia increase the vulnerability of the respiratory muscles to failure. Reversing malnutrition, improving blood flow and substrate delivery, and correcting electrolyte abnormalities are therefore important steps to maintain the force-generating ability of the respiratory muscles and to delay respiratory failure. Such considerations are critical in chronic diseases, such as asthma, cystic fibrosis, and bronchopulmonary dysplasia, and in patients being weaned from prolonged ventilatory support.

ETIOLOGY. Acute respiratory failure may occur de novo as a complication of diseases as varied as pneumonia, pulmonary edema caused by congestive heart failure, or airway obstruction (epiglottitis, asthma). It also frequently occurs as a complication of a chronic respiratory disease. Intercurrent illnesses such as those caused by the respiratory syncytial virus or influenza frequently overcome the ability of an infant or child with bronchopulmonary dysplasia or cystic fibrosis to compensate for a pre-existing respiratory dysfunction. In some patients, even the relatively small increase in ventilatory demands created by an increase in temperature may be sufficient to precipitate worsening hypoxemia and hypercarbia.

CLINICAL MANIFESTATIONS AND DIAGNOSIS. The limited ability of the developing respiratory system to compensate for disease-induced mechanical abnormalities makes the early recognition of respiratory failure critical. Respiratory failure should be anticipated rather than recognized so that alterations in gas exchange can be prevented (see Chapter 64.3).

During physical examination, the clinician should avoid interfering with the patient's own mechanisms of compensation.

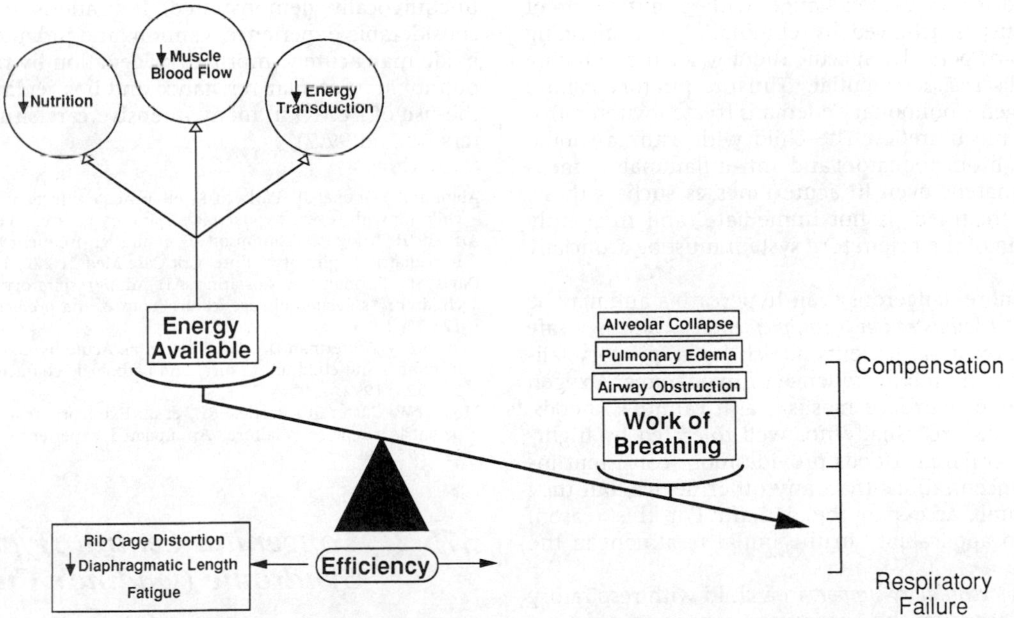

Figure 375–10 Schematic representation of the factors that determine the development of respiratory failure in the presence of abnormalities in the mechanical function of the respiratory system. The balance between the energy available for conversion into work by the respiratory muscles and the work that these muscles must perform depends on the efficiency with which the work is performed. Disease-related abnormalities, such as alveolar collapse, pulmonary edema, and airway obstruction, increase the work of breathing. Similarly, decreased availability of nutrients in malnutrition or when muscle blood flow is limited as well as intrinsic alterations in the transduction of energy by the muscles reduce the energy available. Under these circumstances, decreases in the efficiency of the system caused by rib cage distortion, lung overinflation (which decreases the length of the diaphragmatic fibers), or fatigue can easily displace the fulcrum to the left, precipitating respiratory failure. (From Lister G, Pérez Fontán JJ: Congenital heart disease. *In:* Loughlin GM. Eigen H [eds]: Respiratory Disease in Children: Diagnosis and Management, Baltimore. Williams & Wilkins. 1994,)

An awake child with upper airway obstruction caused by croup or epiglottitis, for instance, may be more stable in a mother's arms because the increased gas flows generated during crying make breathing mechanically inefficient and can precipitate failure. Similarly, most patients with severe restrictive and obstructive disease tolerate the supine position poorly because the weight of the abdominal organs imposes an additional burden on the diaphragm.

The physical examination is useful in the evaluation of children with respiratory disease (see Chapters 64.3 and 377). In a child suspected of respiratory failure, this evaluation should always start with a rapid assessment of the adequacy of ventilation, including the presence and vigor of the respiratory movements, breathing rate, extent of the respiratory movements, the presence of cyanosis, and the presence of signs of upper airway obstruction. A child with grossly inadequate respiratory efforts or complete airway obstruction will not survive long unless ventilation of the lungs is restored immediately. In addition, special attention must be paid to the patient's state of consciousness. Hypoxemia and hypercarbia frequently cause lethargy and confusion alternating with agitation. Whether resulting from these or other concurrent mechanisms, central nervous system depression requires immediate attention because it further limits the ability of the respiratory system to deal with mechanical loads and leaves the airway unprotected against obstruction and aspiration of foreign materials.

Acute hypoxemia and hypercapnia result in dilatation of the cerebral blood vessels and increased blood flow, often accompanied by severe headache. The sudden increased work of the accessory muscles of breathing may result in severe lower back pain. Although moderate to severe hypercapnia can cause peripheral vasodilation, mild to moderate hypoxemia can cause peripheral vasoconstriction, and the patient may complain of cold extremities. Other symptoms of hypoxia include restlessness, dizziness, and impaired thought.

TREATMENT. The goal of treatment of respiratory failure is the restoration of adequate gas exchange with a minimum of complications. This is achieved by eliminating the initiating factors as quickly as possible. Specific therapy for the initiating or underlying disease is essential. Thus respiratory failure caused by cardiogenic pulmonary edema is treated with inotropic medications and diuretics. The child with asthma should be managed with bronchodilators and anti-inflammatory medications. Unfortunately, even in acute illnesses such as these, the response to treatment is not immediate, and frequently the entire function of the respiratory system must be artificially supported.

Hypoxemia is more dangerous than hypercarbia and may be easier to correct. *Administration of supplemental oxygen* is a safe and wise precaution in all patients at risk for respiratory failure, even if there is no initial evidence of hypoxemia. Oxygen can be administered with face masks, nasal cannulas, hoods, or tents. Face masks are usually not well tolerated by frightened infants and children. Hoods provide more consistent inspired oxygen concentrations than any other device, but they are bulky and limit access to the patient. For this reason, they have limited applicability in the initial treatment in the emergency room.

The *indication for ventilatory support* in a child with respiratory failure is usually based on the persistence or worsening of gas exchange abnormalities(see Chapters 64.3 and 64.4). Mechanical ventilation is necessary in a child with pneumonia in whom severe hypoxemia and hypercarbia develops because even the most effective antibiotic therapy requires time. On occasion, ventilatory support must be instituted in the absence of alterations in the $Pa{CO_2}$ when the dysfunction of other systems places gas exchange at jeopardy by severely limiting the compensatory ability of the respiratory system. Cardiovascular shock is a typical example. In this condition, decreased blood flow and substrate delivery to the respiratory muscles may reduce the force that these muscles can develop and can precipitate respiratory failure, even in the absence of substantial mechanical abnormalities of the respiratory system.

Ventilatory support usually (but not always) requires intubation of the trachea with an endotracheal tube or less often a tracheostomy cannula (see Chapters 64.3 and 64.4). Regardless of the type of ventilator, the objective of mechanical ventilation is not to normalize arterial blood gas tensions but rather to provide "adequate" gas exchange. The definition of what is "adequate" has changed substantially. At present, there is reasonable consensus among those treating critically ill children that some degree of hypercarbia and hypoxemia is acceptable in order to minimize oxygen- and stretch-induced lung injury and barotrauma. Moderate (permissive) hypercarbia ($Pa{CO_2}$ 60–80 mm Hg) has no detectable negative consequences over short periods, especially if the rise in $Pa{CO_2}$ is not very acute, in part because its effects on the arterial pH are reduced through renal retention of bicarbonate. Moderate hypoxemia (oxygen saturation 85–90%) is similarly well tolerated in otherwise stable patients, particularly if the hemoglobin concentration and the cardiac output are maintained at physiologic values and conditions such as fever and agitation, which increase tissue oxygen demands, are avoided. Artificial-mechanical ventilation is usually initiated with conventional volume-driven ventilators; high-frequency jet or oscillator ventilators are often used as rescue therapy if conventional ventilators fail to improve oxygenation (See Chapters 64.3 and 64.4).

Extracorporeal membrane oxygenation (ECMO) or carbon dioxide removal, or both, are employed in the treatment of newborns and small infants with life-threatening, refractory respiratory failure that is unresponsive to mechanical ventilation and is expected to resolve in a short time (see Chapters 66 and 97.7). Because of its risks (from vascular cannulation and anticoagulation) and the fact that its benefits over conventional management in non-neonatal patients have not been unequivocally demonstrated, indications for ECMO require considerable experience, caution, and judgment. Inhaled nitric oxide may acutely improve oxygenation by reducing increased pulmonary vascular resistance and has replaced, by and large, the use of ECMO in many intensive care situations (see Chapters 66 and 97.7).

Abman SH, Griebel JL, Parker DK, et al: Acute effects of inhaled nitric oxide in children with severe hypoxemic respiratory failure. J Pediatr 124:881, 1994.

Arnold JH, Truog RD, Thompson JE, et al: High-frequency oscillatory ventilation in pediatric respiratory failure. Crit Care Med 21:272, 1993.

Davis SL, Furman DP, Costarino AT: Adult respiratory distress syndrome in children: Associated disease, clinical course, and predictors of death. J Pediatr 123:35, 1993.

DeBruin W, Notterman DA, Magid M, et al: Acute hypoxemic respiratory failure in infants and children: Clinical and pathologic characteristics. Crit Care Med 20:1223, 1992.

Moler FW, Custer JR, Bartlett RH, et al: Extracorporeal life support for severe pediatric respiratory failure: An updated experience 1991–1993. J Pediatr 124:875, 1994.

375.2 Congenital Central Hypoventilation Syndrome (Ondine's Curse)

Gabriel G. Haddad

In children having congenital central hypoventilation syndrome (CCHS), there are usually no detectable *gross* anatomic abnormalities, although brain stem tumors and arteriovenous malformations have been described and other neurologic diseases must be considered. The primary defect is in the central nervous system, but there may also be abnormalities in other elements of the respiratory feedback loop (e.g., carotid bodies, peripheral chemosensitivity).

PATHOGENESIS AND PATHOPHYSIOLOGY. The cause and pathogenesis of CCHS are unknown. Although there are reports of familial cases, the specific mode of inheritance is unknown. There is a rare association of CCHS with Hirschprung's disease (Ondine-Hirschprung syndrome or neurocristopathy or Haddad's syndrome). In one such case, a missense mutation in exon 12 of the RET proto-oncogene has been reported, suggesting a genetic basis for these abnormalities.

Patients with CCHS or CCHS with Hirschsprung's disease have no carbon dioxide sensitivity and no ventilatory response to carbon dioxide during sleep. During wakefulness, the carbon dioxide set point is much lower, and they respond to it, unless the condition is severe enough for hypoventilation to occur even in the awake state. These children also have been shown to have no sensitivity to hypoxia. This lack of sensitivity to carbon dioxide and the respiratory failure do not improve with time, and the oldest patients with CCHS still show the same failures. Older children with CCHS show an increase in ventilation when they are exercised at various work rates, and the increase in ventilation they exhibit may not be related to anaerobic stimuli (lactate or pH) but rather to neural reflexes (e.g., limb movements) or hormonal cues.

Although the pathogenesis of this disease is not clear, certain pathophysiology mechanisms play an important role. There are at least two main pathways that regulate respiration in animals and humans. One is an automatic or metabolic pathway, during which the subject's consciousness or sensorium does not play a major role, such as during sleep (except to some degree in rapid eye movement sleep). The other is more dependent on sensory feedback and on a voluntary pathway. In CCHS, the condition expresses itself best during sleep in which time sensory feedback plays a relatively minor role. The defect may be in the automatic control system, which resides mostly in the brain stem anatomically. Physiologic evidence indicates that the respiratory failure in these children is mostly based on defects in central mechanisms rather than on peripheral (carotid) mechanisms, although contribution from the interactions between peripheral and central mechanisms also may be important. It is also important that premotor neurons, those that communicate with phrenic or intercostal motoneurons, can be excited enough to drive the respiratory musculature in certain instances (e.g., wakefulness). Although searches for pharmacologic stimulation have failed, the fact that functional stimulation of the respiratory system is achievable in CCHS (e.g., during wakefulness and during exercise) suggests that pharmacologic or other interventional strategies are potentially important for devising future therapies.

On postmortem examination of some CCHS patients, absence of the arcuate nucleus has been seen, but the relation of this anomaly to the disease is not clear. Gliosis in brain stem structures has also been noted, but this could be part of a more generalized response of the central nervous system to hypoxia and ischemia resulting from long-term and intermittent respiratory failure.

CLINICAL MANIFESTATIONS. Patients with CCHS usually present early in life, often in the first few hours after delivery. Most children are the products of uneventful pregnancies and are term infants with appropriate weight for gestational age; Apgar scores have been variable. Symptoms of respiratory failure, with slow and irregular respiratory efforts, long respiratory pauses (lasting up to 40 sec), and cyanosis, appear in the first day of life. Cardiac, respiratory, infectious, and metabolic diseases, including intrautrine drug exposure, should be ruled out. One hallmark of this condition is that patients *fail* to respire adequately during sleep, not during wakefulness, although children with the most severe respiratory failure may hypoventilate in the waking state as well. In most neonates with CCHS, the $Paco_2$ accumulates to very high levels, sometimes up to 80–90 mm Hg, during sleep and drops to normal levels soon after the infants awaken. Infants in the first few weeks of life have been shown to have long respiratory pauses, a relatively normal tidal volume, and a very low respiratory rate (dropping to as low a level as 8–10 breaths/min during sleep) with interspersed respiratory pauses. Respiratory rates are generally normal during wakefulness, and the lowest respiratory rates have been found in non–rapid eye movement or quiet sleep. This suggests "persistence of fetal respiration."

Because respiratory failure in these infants has a central cause, the hypoxemia that ensues is commensurate with hypoventilation with little or no abnormality in the arterial-alveolar (A-a) gradient. However, in some children, the hypoventilation may be severe enough to produce airway closure, microatelectasis, and an increase in the A-a gradient.

In a sizable subset of these infants, abdominal distention, constipation, or complete failure to pass meconium occurs. Rarely, a child with CCHS also has diagnosed Hirschsprung's disease with variable aganglionosis of the colon and small intestine. Whether all patients with congenital CCHS have some degree of aganglionosis of the large bowel is unknown.

Patients with CCHS also have a faster heart rate than normal for their age and slow heart rate variability, an almost fixed heart rate with little sinus arrhythmia. This raises the question of whether these infants have generalized abnormalities in the autonomic regulation of vital functions. Other anomalies suggesting this possibility, found on autopsy, include multiple ganglioneuroblastomas of the sympathetic chain and the adrenal medulla.

DIFFERENTIAL DIAGNOSIS. Other neurologic diseases or conditions have to be excluded before this diagnosis is made. Brain stem infarction, tumors, arteriovenous malformations, syringomyelia, Leigh's necrotizing encephalomyelopathy, olivopontocerebellar degeneration, and Mobius syndrome should be considered.

TREATMENT. Management should include general and nutritional care, ventilatory support, and prevention of acidosis, cerebral hypoxia, and ischemia. Some of these infants can grow and gain developmental and neurologic milestones that are close to normal for age, although hypoventilation abnormalities persist. These abnormalities may be a result of episodes of hypoxia or part of the spectrum of CCHS.

Phrenic nerve pacing has been used in patients after the age of 2 yr. Although there are complications related to pacing, including phrenic nerve fibrosis, infections, and multiple surgeries, a number of these patients have eventually become independent of mechanical ventilators.

Bogousslavsky J, Khurana R, Deruaz JP, et al: Respiratory failure and unilateral caudal brainstem infarction. Ann Neurol 28:668, 1990.

Bolk S, Angrist M, Schwartz S, et al: Congenital central hypoventilation syndrome: mutation analysis of the receptor tyrosine kinase RET. Am J Med Genet 63:603, 1996.

Haddad GG, Mazza NM, Defendini R, et al: Congenital failure of automatic control of ventilation, gastrointestinal motility and heart rate. Medicine (Baltimore) 57:517, 1978.

Mellins RB, Balfour HH, Turino GM, et al: Failure of automatic control of ventilation (Ondine's curse). Medicine (Baltimore) 49:487, 1990.

Mukhopadhyay S, Wilkinson PW: Cerebral arteriovenous malformation, Ondine's curse and Hirschsprung's disease. Dev Med Child Neurol 32:1087, 1990.

Sakai T, Wakizakas A, Matsuda H, et al: Point mutation in exon 12 of the receptor tyrosine kinase proto-oncogene RET in Ondine-Hirschsprung syndrome. Pediatrics 101:924, 1998.

Shea SA, Andres LP, Shannon DC, et al: Ventilatory responses to exercise in humans lacking ventilatory chemosensitivity. J Physiol (Lond) 468:623, 1993.

Verloes A, Elmer C, Lacombe D, et al: Ondine-Hirschsprung syndrome (Haddad syndrome). Further delineation in two cases and review of the literature. Eur J Pediatr 152:75, 1993.

Weese-Mayer DE, Silvestri JM, Menzies LJ, et al: Congenital central hypoventilation syndrome: Diagnosis, management, and long-term outcome in thirty-two children. J Pediatr 120:381, 1992.

CHAPTER 376

Defense Mechanisms and Metabolic Functions of the Lung

Gabriel G. Haddad and J. Julio Pérez Fontán

376.1 Defense Mechanisms

GENERAL OVERVIEW. There are a number of defense mechanisms in the lungs. Effective and multiple defense mechanisms are especially important because the respiratory system, unlike other organs, is constantly exposed to the changing and often "polluted" environment containing irritants, pathogens, and allergens. The defense system of the respiratory system is composed of three limbs. The cough reflex, which relies on the integrity of the airways, the respiratory muscles, and the central nervous system control centers. The cilia and mucociliary apparatus rely on the morphologic and functional integrity of the cilia and the respiratory epithelium (see Chapter 417). The mechanical defenses of the respiratory system that protect the lung include the filtering of particles, the warming and humidification of inspired air, and the absorption of noxious fumes and gases by the vascular upper airway. The temporary cessation of breathing, reflexly shallow breathing, laryngospasm, or even bronchospasm limits the depth and amount of penetration of foreign matter. Spasm or decreased breathing can provide only brief protection. Cough also is another important mechanism. Aspiration of food, secretions, and foreign bodies is prevented by swallowing and closure of the epiglottis. The respiratory tract distal to the larynx is normally sterile. The immune system is important in determining the propensity of individuals to lung infections.

The *upper airway* includes the nose, paranasal sinuses, and pharynx; the *lower airway* consists of the remainder of the system from the larynx peripherally. The nose has a relatively large surface area lined with a richly vascular, ciliated epithelium, and by the time the air column reaches the bifurcation of the trachea, up to 75% of the warming and humidification of the inspired air has occurred. During exhalation, heat and moisture are removed from the air stream. Gross filtering of particles larger than 10–15 mm is achieved by the coarse hairs at the nasal orifices, and most inhaled particles larger than 5 mm are impacted on the nasal surface.

Because the larynx is relatively narrow and ringed with cartilage, it is relatively susceptible to obstruction in young children, particularly by inflammation, because the resultant swelling of tissues rapidly encroaches on the lumen and produces inspiratory stridor.

The trachea and bronchi are lined with pseudostratified, ciliated, columnar epithelium and occasional goblet cells. Mucous glands occupy approximately one third of the thickness of the airway wall and for the most part lie between the epithelial surface and the cartilage. The trachea is supported by incomplete rings of cartilage with a muscular membrane posteriorly. Irregular plates of cartilage support the bronchi, especially at bifurcations. These diminish and finally disappear in the smallest bronchi. The goblet cells and principally the submucosal glands secrete the mucous layer, which is 2–5 mm in depth and rests on the tips of the cilia. Each ciliated cell has about 275 cilia; movement results from action by microtubules within each cilium. The cilia beat within a periciliary fluid layer at about 1,000 beats/min, moving the mucous blanket toward the pharynx at a rate of approximately 10 mm/min in the trachea. In the respiratory portion of the lung, the surface cells gradually become cuboidal and then flat; ciliated cells and goblet cells are usually absent.

The final 25% of the warming and humidifying of the inspired air stream occurs in the trachea and large bronchi. Failure of humidification permits dry air to reach more distal airways. Particles 1–5 mm in size precipitate out on the tracheobronchial mucous blanket so that only particles of 1 mm or less reach the respiratory bronchioles and air spaces, where some may deposit and many will be exhaled.

Respiratory tract secretions are derived primarily from mucous (glycoproteins) and serous cells of the submucosal glands that empty onto the surface epithelium; from goblet cells and Clara cells, the special secreting cells in the surface epithelium of bronchi and bronchioles, respectively; from transudation from the vascular space; and from alveolar fluid, which contributes most of the phospholipid found in tracheobronchial mucus. This mucus is about 95% water.

Beyond infancy, collateral alveolar ventilation can occur increasingly with development of the *pores of Kohn* between alveoli, which provide a means for gas to pass from one lobule to another, perhaps even between segments of lung. Bronchiolar-alveolar communications, known as the *canals of Lambert,* are also found. These anatomic connections may be helpful in preventing or delaying atelectasis.

CLEARANCE OF PARTICLES. Particles deposited in conducting airways are cleared within hours by the mucociliary mechanism, whereas clearance of those reaching the alveoli may take several days to months. The latter may be phagocytized by alveolar macrophages and removed from lungs by the mucociliary system or carried into the interstitium for clearance by the lymphocytes into regional nodes or the blood. Some particles penetrate into the interstitium without phagocytosis. Mucociliary clearance may be aided by cough, which propels excess mucus up the airways at pressures of up to 300 mm Hg and at flows of up to 5–6 L/sec. Mucus raised by the cough mechanism is usually swallowed by young children but may be expectorated.

DEFENSE AGAINST MICROBIAL AGENTS. Phagocytosis and mucociliary clearance may not be sufficient protection from living agents, such as bacteria and viruses. Additional factors include cellular killing of organisms and immune responses to assist in the phagocytosis-killing process. Alveolar and interstitial macrophages, derived from monocytes, are an essential component of the defense system of the lung. The engulfment and killing of living particles by these macrophages may be enhanced by opsonins or by small lymphocytes. The principal antibody in respiratory secretions is secretory IgA, which is produced by plasma cells in the submucosa of the airways (see Chapter 124.3). Two molecules of IgA combine with a polypeptide (secretory component) produced by the respiratory epithelium to yield secretory IgA, which is highly resistant to digestion by proteolytic enzymes released after lysis of bacteria and dead cells. IgA can neutralize certain viruses and toxins and helps in the lysis of bacteria. IgA may also prevent antigenic substances from penetrating the epithelial surfaces. Pulmonary secretory IgA reaches adult levels in the first month of life. IgG and IgM are also found in the secretions when lung inflammation occurs.

Lysozyme, lactoferrin, and interferon may also play a defensive role in respiratory secretions. In addition, a small fraction of the antibodies of the respiratory surface is made up of IgE, which plays an important role in allergic reactions (Chapter 141).

IMPAIRED DEFENSE MECHANISMS. The phagocytic ability of alveolar macrophages and, in most cases, the mucociliary mechanism can be impaired by ethanol ingestion, cigarette smoke, hypoxemia, starvation, chilling, corticosteroids, nitrogen dioxide, ozone, increased oxygen concentration, narcotics, and some anesthetic gases. The antibacterial killing capacity of the macrophages can be decreased by acidosis, azotemia, and recent acute viral infections, especially rubeola and influenza. Beryllium and asbestos, organic dust from cotton and sugar cane, and gases such as sulfur, nitrogen dioxide, ozone, chlorine, ammonia, and cigarette smoke, are toxic to epithelial cells.

Mucociliary clearance can be reduced by hypothermia, hyperthermia, morphine, codeine, and hypothyroidism. Inhalation of dry gas by mouth breathing during periods of nasal obstruction, after performance of a tracheostomy, or during use of poorly humidified oxygen results in drying of the mucous membranes and slowing of the ciliary beat. Cold air may irritate the tracheobronchial tree.

Damage to the respiratory epithelium may be reversible with rhinitis, sinusitis, bronchitis, bronchiolitis, acute respiratory infections associated with high levels of air pollution, and the epithelial shedding that can occur in asthma, or with some irritants, bronchospasm, edema, congestion, and perhaps mild surface ulceration. However, severe ulceration, bronchiectasis, bronchiolectasis, squamous cell metaplasia, and fibrosis represent serious injury and permanent impairment of the normal clearance mechanism. Other events that can adversely affect the lung include hyperventilation, alveolar hypoxia, pulmonary thromboembolism, pulmonary edema, hypersensitivity reactions, and certain drugs such as salicylates.

Newhouse MT, Bienenstock J: Respiratory tract defense mechanisms. *In:* Baum GL, Wolinsky E (eds): Textbook of Pulmonary Diseases. Boston, Little, Brown, 1989, pp 21–47.

Proctor DF: The upper airways. I: Nasal physiology and defense of the lungs. Am Rev Respir Dis 115:97, 1977.

Wilmott RW, Fiedler MA, Stark JM: Host defense mechanisms. *In:* Chernick V, Boat T (eds): Kendig's Textbook on Disorders of the Respiratory Tract in Children, 6th ed. Philadelphia, WB Saunders, 1998, pp 238–264.

376.2 Metabolic Functions

The lung contains more than 40 separate cell types. Among these heterogeneous cells, the type I and II pneumocytes, alveolar macrophages, and Clara cells are unique to the lung. The lung can synthesize lipids and proteins, including glycoproteins, secretory antibodies, interferon, proteolytic and fibrinolytic enzymes and activators, collagen, and elastin. Tissue factors such as thromboplastin are found in higher concentration in the lung than in any other organ. Megakaryocytes are concentrated in the lung.

The large alveolar type II pneumocyte synthesizes and releases lung surfactant. Injury to this cell or deficiency in this surfactant pathway results in neonatal respiratory distress syndrome (Chapter 97.3). A major function of surfactant is to stabilize alveolar air spaces by attenuating surface forces and decreasing their unevenness. Another cell type, the neuroepithelial cell, is present at the airway bifurcation and is found in larger proportion in early life. These cells are serotonin-rich and have transmitter vesicles that are depleted when exposed to low inhaled oxygen concentration. These cells sense oxygen in the airways through plasma membrane K^+ channels. How they affect respiratory output is not clear at present, although they can send afferent information to the central nervous system via the vagus nerve.

Because the lung has the only capillary bed through which the entire blood flow must pass in the normal state, the pulmonary capillary circulation is ideally positioned to control circulating vasoactive hormones. Angiotensin II, up to 50 times more active than its precursor, is converted from angiotensin I during one passage through the pulmonary circulation. Some vasoactive materials, including serotonin, bradykinin, adenosine triphosphate, and prostaglandins E_1, E_2, and F_2, are almost completely removed or inactivated by one passage through the pulmonary circulation, whereas others, such as epinephrine, prostaglandins A_1 and A_2, angiotensin II, and vasopressin, may be minimally affected. Norepinephrine and histamine are taken up to a moderate degree. Failure of inactivation or periodic release of substances such as serotonin, bradykinin, histamine, slow-reacting substance of anaphylaxis (SRS-A), eosinophil chemotactic factor, platelet aggregation factor, endocrine substances, and so forth, may be important in the pathogenesis of some pulmonary disease or as a mediator of secondary effects. These chemicals can contribute to systemic and pulmonary hypertension, systemic hypotension, and pulmonary edema.

Fishman AP: Non-respiratory functions of the lung. Chest 72:84, 1977.

Said S: Metabolic and Endocrine Functions of the lung. *In:* Chernick V, Boat T (eds): Kendig's Textbook on Disorders of the Respiratory Tract in Children, 6th ed. Philadelphia, WB Saunders, 1998, pp 74–85.

CHAPTER 377
Diagnostic Approach to Respiratory Disease

Gabriel G. Haddad and Regina M. Palazzo

The history and physical examination are the most important first steps in diagnosing respiratory disease. The observed signs and symptoms significantly influence the direction of the subsequent investigations.

HISTORY. Family and personal histories are essential for interpreting physical findings and diagnosing respiratory system disease. A pertinent history should include questions about respiratory symptoms, their chronicity, and their timing during day or night, and whether they are associated with any activity such as exercise or food intake. Further, the respiratory system interacts with a number of other systems, and questions related to cardiac, gastrointestinal, central nervous system, hematologic, and immune systems may be relevant. For example, questions related to gastrointestinal reflux or immune status may be important in a patient with repeated cases of pneumonia.

PHYSICAL EXAMINATION. Respiratory dysfunction usually produces detectable alterations in the pattern of breathing. Values for normal respiratory rates are presented in Table 64–5. As can be seen in this table, respiratory rates depend on many factors, including age. It is important at the bedside not to be satisfied with one respiratory rate measurement because respiratory rates, especially in the young, are exquisitely sensitive to extraneous stimuli. These rates vary among infants but average 40–50 breaths/min in the first weeks of life and usually less than 60 breaths/min in the first few days of life. Respiratory control abnormalities may cause the child to breathe at a low rate or periodically. Mechanical abnormalities produce compensatory changes that are generally directed at maintaining or increasing ventilation. These changes include variable increases in the breathing rate, chest wall retractions, and nasal flaring. Children with restrictive disease breathe at faster rates, and their respiratory excursions are shallow. An expiratory grunt is common as the child attempts to raise the functional residual capacity by closing the glottis at the end of expiration. Children with obstructive disease take slower, deeper breaths. When the obstruction is extrathoracic (from the nose to the midtrachea), inspiration is more prolonged than is expiration, and an inspiratory stridor can usually be heard. When the obstruction is intrathoracic, expiration is more prolonged than is inspiration, and the patient often has to make use of accessory expiratory muscles. Lung percussion is usually dull in restrictive lung disease and tympanitic in obstructive disease but has limited value in small infants because it cannot discriminate between noises originating from tissues that are close to each other. Auscultation confirms the presence of inspiratory or expiratory prolongation and provides information about the symmetry and quality of air movement. In addition, it often detects abnormal or adventitious sounds such as *stridor* (a predominant inspiratory monophonic noise), *rales* or *crackles* (high pitch, interrupted sounds found during inspiration and more rarely during early expiration, which denote opening of previously closed air spaces), or *wheezes* (musical, continuous sounds usually caused by the development of turbulent flow in narrow airways).

BLOOD GAS ANALYSIS. An arterial blood gas analysis is probably the single most useful test of pulmonary function. Since cyanosis is influenced by skin perfusion and blood hemoglobin concentration, it is an unreliable sign of hypoxemia. Arterial hypertension, tachycardia, and diaphoresis are late, and by no means exclusive, signs of hypoventilation. Blood gas exchange is evaluated most accurately by the *direct* measurement of arterial Po_2, Pco_2, and pH (see Chapters 62 and 97.3). The blood specimen is best collected *anaerobically* in a heparinized syringe containing only enough heparin solution to displace the air from the syringe. The syringe should be sealed, placed in ice, and carried to the laboratory for immediate analysis. Although these measurements have no substitute in many conditions, they require arterial puncture and have been replaced to a great extent by noninvasive monitoring (see Chapters 62 and 97.3).

The age and clinical condition of the patient need to be taken into account when interpreting blood gas tensions. With the exception of neonates, values of arterial Po_2 lower than 85 mm Hg are usually abnormal for a child breathing room air at sea level. Calculation of the alveolar-arterial oxygen gradient is useful in the analysis of arterial oxygenation, particularly when the patient is not breathing room air or in the presence of hypercarbia. Values of arterial Pco_2 exceeding 45 mm Hg usually indicate hypoventilation or a severe ventilation-perfusion mismatch, unless they reflect respiratory compensation for metabolic alkalosis (see Chapter 52).

TRANSILLUMINATION OF THE CHEST. In infants up to at least 6 mo of age, a pneumothorax may often be diagnosed by transillumination of the chest wall using a fiberoptic light probe. Free air in the pleural space often results in an unusually large halo of light in the skin surrounding the probe. This test is unreliable in older patients or in those with subcutaneous emphysema or atelectasis.

RADIOGRAPHIC TECHNIQUES

CHEST ROENTGENOGRAMS. Whenever possible, a posteroanterior and a lateral view (upright and in full inspiration), should be obtained. Portable films, although useful, may give a somewhat distorted image. Expiratory films may easily be misinterpreted, although a comparison of expiratory and inspiratory films may be useful in the evaluation of a child with suspected foreign body (localized failure of the lung to empty reflects bronchial obstruction). If pleural fluid is suspected, decubitus films are indicated. Films taken in a recumbent position are difficult to interpret if there is fluid within the pleural space or a cavity.

UPPER AIRWAY FILMS. A lateral view of the neck can yield invaluable information about upper airway obstruction and particularly about the condition of the retropharyngeal space, supraglottic area, and subglottic space (the latter should also be viewed in a posteroanterior projection). Knowing the phase of respiration during which the film was taken is often essential for accurate interpretation. Magnified airway films are often helpful in delineating the upper airways. Patients with suspected obstruction should not be sent unattended to the radiology department.

SINUS AND NASAL FILMS. Roentgenographic examination of the sinuses is indicated when sinus disease is suspected. A computed tomographic scan gives the most information. Because of the small size and slow development of the frontal and maxillary sinus cavities in children, transillumination is not as successful in documenting sinus disease as are roentgenograms. Sinus roentgenograms are particularly useful in patients with suspected continuous sinus infection. The need for examining the nasal passages in children is unusual and occurs most often when the neonate presents with obstruction or when a tumor or occult foreign body is suspected.

COMPUTED TOMOGRAPHY AND MAGNETIC RESONANCE IMAGING. Computed tomography (CT) delineates the internal structure of the thorax in much greater detail than is possible with plain roentgenograms. Technical advances have greatly enhanced the utility of this diagnostic modality (even three-dimensional reconstruction is often feasible), whereas scan times and radiation exposure have been markedly reduced. Computed tomographic scans are of particular importance in the evaluation of mediastinal and pleural lesions, solid or cystic parenchymal lesions, and suspected bronchiectasis. Intravenous contrast material can be infused during the scan to enhance vascular structures.

Magnetic resonance imaging (MRI) may be useful for the same disease entities as CT. MRI is an excellent procedure to delineate hilar and vascular anatomy associated with vascular rings or slings.

FLUOROSCOPY. Fluoroscopy is especially useful for evaluating stridor and abnormal movement of the diaphragm or mediastinum. Many procedures, such as needle aspiration or biopsy of a peripheral lesion, are also best accomplished with the aid of fluoroscopy. Videotape recording, which does not increase radiation exposure, may allow detailed study through "replay" capability during a brief exposure to fluoroscopy.

CONTRAST STUDIES

Barium Swallow. This study, performed with fluoroscopy and spot films, is indicated in the evaluation of patients with recurrent pneumonia, persistent cough of undetermined cause, stridor, or persistent wheezing. The technique may be modified by using barium of different textures and thicknesses, ranging from thin liquid to solids, to evaluate swallowing mechanics, the presence of vascular rings, and tracheoesophageal fistulas, especially when aspiration is suspected. A contrast esophagram has been used in the evaluation of newborns with suspected esophageal atresia, but this procedure entails a high risk of pulmonary aspiration and is not usually recommended. Barium swallows are useful in the evaluation of suspected gastroesophageal reflux, but the interpretation may not be straightforward.

Bronchograms. The details of smaller bronchi that cannot be easily evaluated by plain films or even bronchoscopy may be delineated by instilling contrast material directly into the airway. This is indicated in patients with suspected bronchiectasis or airway anomalies who are potential surgical candidates, although computed tomographic scanning and MRI have supplanted bronchography. Sedation and topical anesthesia, or even general anesthesia, are required.

Pulmonary Arteriograms. These studies allow detailed evaluation of the pulmonary vasculature and are helpful in assessing pulmonary blood flow and in diagnosing congenital anomalies, such as lobar agenesis, unilateral hyperlucent lung, vascular rings, and arteriovenous malformations and are sometimes useful in evaluating solid or cystic lesions. Real time and Doppler echocardiography are noninvasive methods that often reveal similar information and are performed prior to arteriography.

Aortograms. Thoracic aortograms demonstrate the aortic arch and its major vessels, and the systemic (bronchial) pulmonary circulation. They are useful in evaluating vascular rings and suspected pulmonary sequestration. Although most hemoptysis is from the bronchial arteries, bronchial arteriography is seldom helpful in diagnosing or treating intrapulmonary bleeding in children. Echocardiography with or without CT or MRI is helpful in delineating some of these lesions and should be performed before aortography.

Pneumoperitoneum and Pneumothorax. In selected situations, such as in the evaluation of diaphragmatic eventration, it may be advantageous to inject a small amount of air into the pleural or peritoneal cavity, outlining the limits of the diaphragm or pleural surfaces by air contrast. Rapidly absorbed, the air causes no functional impairment.

Radionuclide Lung Scans. The usual scan uses intravenous injection of material (macroaggregated human serum albumin labeled with ^{99m}Tc) that will be trapped in the pulmonary capillary bed. The distribution of radioactivity, proportional to pulmonary capillary blood flow, is useful in evaluating pulmonary embolism and congenital cardiovascular and pulmonary defects. Acute changes in the distribution of pulmonary perfusion may reflect alterations of pulmonary ventilation.

The distribution of pulmonary ventilation also may be determined by scanning following the inhalation of a radioactive gas such as ^{133}Xe. After the intravenous injection of ^{133}Xe dissolved in saline, both pulmonary perfusion and ventilation can be evaluated by continuous recording of the rate of appearance and disappearance of the xenon over the lung. Appearance of xenon early after injection is a measure of perfusion, whereas the rate of washout during breathing is a measure of ventilation in the pediatric population. The most important indication for this test is to demonstrate defects in the pulmonary arterial distribution that may occur with congenital malformations or pulmonary embolism. Abnormalities in regional ventilation are also easily demonstrable in congenital lobar emphysema, cystic fibrosis, and asthma.

RESPIRATORY FUNCTION TESTING

OVERVIEW. The measurement of respiratory function in infants and young children may be difficult because of the lack of cooperation. Attempts have been made to overcome this limitation by creating standard tests that do not require the patient's active participation. Respiratory function tests still provide only a partial insight into the mechanisms of respiratory disease at early ages.

Whether restrictive or obstructive, most forms of respiratory disease cause alterations in lung volume and its subdivision (see Fig. 375–2). Restrictive diseases typically decrease total lung capacity (TLC), which is the total volume of gas contained in the lungs at the end of a maximal inspiration. TLC includes residual volume (the volume of gas contained in the lungs at the end of a forced expiration), which is not accessible to direct determinations. It must therefore be measured indirectly by gas dilution methods or, preferably, by plethysmography. Restrictive disease also decreases vital capacity (VC), which is the total amount of gas that can be inhaled after a forced expiration. VC can be measured by spirometry and is commonly used at the bedside to assess the progression of neuromuscular disorders. Obstructive diseases produce gas trapping and thus increase residual volume and functional residual capacity (the volume contained in the lungs at the end of a tidal expiration), particularly when these measurements are considered with respect to TLC.

Measurements of elastic recoil and respiratory compliance require knowledge of the lung volume at which the measurements were made in order to be properly interpreted. Similarly, measurements of airway and total respiratory resistance are technically cumbersome and difficult to interpret because of the large and variable contribution of the upper airway (nose, pharynx, and larynx) and lung and chest wall tissues to these resistances.

Airway obstruction is most frequently evaluated from determinations of gas flow in the course of a forced expiratory maneuver. The peak expiratory flow is reduced in advanced obstructive disease. The wide availability of simple devices that perform this measurement at the bedside makes it useful for assessing children with airway obstruction. Evaluation of peak flows requires a voluntary effort, and peak flows may not be altered when the obstruction is moderate or mild. Other gas flow measurements require that the child inhale to TLC and then exhale as far and as fast as possible for several seconds. Cooperation and good muscle strength are therefore necessary for the measurements to be reproducible. The forced expiratory volume in 1 sec (FEV_1) correlates well with the severity of obstructive diseases. The maximal midexpiratory flow rate, the average flow greater than the middle 50% of the forced vital capacity, is a more reliable indicator of mild airway obstruction. Its sensitivity to changes in residual volume and vital capacity, however, limits its use in children with more severe disease. The construction of flow-volume relationships during the forced vital capacity maneuvers overcomes some of these limitations by expressing the expiratory flows as a function of lung volume.

PRACTICAL ISSUES AND SPECIFIC PULMONARY FUNCTION TESTS. A *spirometer* is used to measure VC and its subdivisions and expiratory (or inspiratory) flow rates (see Fig. 375–2). A simple *manometer* can measure the maximal inspiratory and expiratory force a subject generates, normally at least 30 cm H_2O, which is useful in evaluating the neuromuscular component of ventilation. Expected normal values for VC, functional residual capacity, TLC, and residual volume are obtained from prediction equations based on body height.

Flow rates measured by spirometry usually include the volume expired in the 1st sec (FEV_1) and the maximal midexpiratory flow rate. More information results from a maximal expir atory flow-volume curve, in which expiratory flow rate is plotted against expired lung volume (expressed in terms of either VC or TLC). Flow rates at lung volumes less than about 75% VC are relatively independent of effort. Expiratory flow rates at low lung volumes (less than 50% VC) are influenced much more by small airways than are flow rates at high lung volumes (FEV_1). The flow rate at 25% VC (V_{25}) is a useful index of small airway function. Low flow rates at high lung volumes associated with normal flow at low lung volumes suggest upper airway obstruction (see Chapters 374 and 375).

Airway resistance (R_{AW}) is measured in a plethysmograph and is expressed as centimeters of water/liter/second. Alternatively, the reciprocal of R_{AW}, *airway conductance* (G_{AW}), may be used. Because airway resistance measurements vary with the lung volume at which they are taken, it is convenient to use specific airway resistance, SR_{AW} (SR_{AW} = R_{AW} H lung volume), which is nearly constant in subjects older than 6 yr (normally less than 7 sec/cm H_2O).

The *diffusing capacity for carbon monoxide* is related to oxygen diffusion and is measured by rebreathing from a container having a known initial concentration of carbon monoxide or by using a single breath technique. Decreases in diffusing capacity for carbon monoxide reflect decreases in effective alveolar capillary surface area or decreases in diffusibility of the gas across the alveolar-capillary membrane. This test is rarely used in pediatrics because primary diffusion abnormalities are unusual in children. *Regional gas exchange* may be conveniently estimated with the perfusion-ventilation xenon scan. Determining *arterial blood gas* levels also disclose the effectiveness of alveolar gas exchange (see earlier).

CLINICAL USES. Pulmonary function testing, although rarely resulting in a diagnosis, is helpful in *defining the type of process* (e.g., obstruction, restriction) and the *degree of functional impairment* in following the course and treatment of disease, and in *estimating the prognosis.* It is also useful in *preoperative evaluation* and in confirmation of functional impairment in patients having subjective complaints but a normal physical examination. In most patients with obstructive disease, a repeat test after administering a bronchodilator is warranted.

Most tests require some cooperation and understanding by the patient, and interpretation is greatly facilitated if the test conditions and the patient's behavior during the test are known. Accurate testing of children aged 3–6 yr requires great patience by the physician and training of the patient, whereas most children aged 6 yr or older can be tested reliably without excessive difficulty. Infants and young children who cannot or will not cooperate with test procedures can be studied in a limited number of ways, which often require sedation. Flow rates and pressures during tidal breathing, with or without transient interruption of the flow, may be useful to assess some aspects of airway resistance or obstruction and to measure compliance of the lungs and thorax. Expiratory flow rates may be studied in sedated infants with passive compression of the chest and abdomen with a rapidly inflatable jacket. Gas dilution or plethysmographic methods may also be used in sedated infants to measure functional residual capacity and R_{AW}.

MICROBIOLOGY: EXAMINATION OF SECRETIONS

The specific diagnosis of infection in the lower respiratory tract depends on the proper handling of an adequate specimen obtained in an appropriate fashion. Nasopharyngeal or throat cultures are often used but may not correlate with cultures obtained by more direct techniques from the lower airways. Sputum specimens are preferred and are often obtained from patients who do not expectorate by deep throat swab immediately after coughing. Specimens may also be obtained directly from the tracheobronchial tree by nasotracheal aspiration (usually heavily contaminated), by transtracheal aspiration through the cricothyroid membrane (useful in adults and adolescents but hazardous in children), and in infants and children by a sterile catheter inserted into the trachea either during direct laryngoscopy or through an endotracheal tube. A specimen also may be obtained at bronchoscopy. A percutaneous lung tap or an open biopsy is the only way to obtain a specimen that may be absolutely free of oral flora.

A specimen obtained by direct expectoration is usually assumed to be of tracheobronchial origin, but often, especially in children, it is not from this source. The presence of alveolar macrophages—large, mononuclear cells—is the hallmark of tracheobronchial secretions. Both nasopharyngeal and tracheobronchial secretions may contain ciliated epithelial cells, which are more commonly found in sputum. Nasopharyngeal and oral secretions often contain large numbers of squamous epithelial cells. Sputum may contain both ciliated and squamous epithelial cells.

During sleep, mucociliary transport continually brings tracheobronchial secretions to the pharynx, where they are swallowed. An early morning fasting gastric aspirate often contains material from the tracheobronchial tract that is suitable for culture for acid-fast bacilli.

The absence of polymorphonuclear leukocytes in a Wright-stained smear of sputum or bronchoalveolar lavage (BAL) fluid containing adequate numbers of macrophages may be significant evidence against a bacterial infectious process in the lower respiratory tract, assuming that the patient has normal neutrophil counts and function. Eosinophils suggest allergic disease. Iron stains may reveal hemosiderin granules within macrophages, suggesting pulmonary hemosiderosis. Specimens should also be examined by Gram stain. Bacteria within or near macrophages and neutrophils can be significant. Viral pneumonia may be accompanied by intranuclear or cytoplasmic inclusion bodies visible on Wright-stained smears, and fungal forms may be identifiable on Gram or silver stains.

EXERCISE TESTING

Exercise testing (also see Chapter 430.5) is a more direct approach for detecting diffusion impairment as well as other forms of respiratory disease. Measurements of heart and respiratory rate, minute ventilation, oxygen consumption, carbon dioxide production, and arterial blood gases during incremental exercise loads often provide invaluable information about the functional nature of the disease. Often a simple assessment of the patient's exercise tolerance in conjunction with other more static forms of respiratory function testing may allow a distinction between respiratory and nonrespiratory disease in children.

SLEEP STUDIES

The sleep state has an important influence on respiratory function, particularly in the newborn and young infant. Polysomnographic studies are often helpful when abnormalities of central respiratory control, muscular disorders, or respiratory complications from gastroesophageal reflux are suspected. For the latter condition, pH probe studies are indicated in which a pH probe is placed in the esophagus and prolonged (usually over several hours) monitoring is undertaken (see Chapter 323). These studies, which usually include the simultaneous assessment of ventilatory effort, airway gas flow, gas exchange, and sleep state, are also useful in the diagnosis and management of nocturnal hypoxemia and hypercarbia in children with chronic respiratory disease (see Chapter 375.2).

LUNG VISUALIZATION AND LUNG SPECIMEN-BASED DIAGNOSTIC TESTS

ENDOSCOPY

Laryngoscopy. The evaluation of stridor, problems with vocalization, and other upper airway abnormalities usually require direct inspection. Although indirect (mirror) laryngoscopy may be reasonable in older children and adults, it is rarely feasible in infants and small children. Direct laryngoscopy may be performed with either a rigid or a flexible instrument. The safe use of the rigid scope for examination of the upper airway requires topical anesthesia and either sedation or general anesthesia, whereas the flexible laryngoscope can often be used in the office setting with or without sedation. Further advantages to the flexible scope include the ability to assess the airway without the distortion that may be introduced by the use of the rigid scope and the ability to assess airway dynamics more accurately. Since there is a relatively high incidence of concomitant lesions in the upper and lower airways, it is often prudent to examine the airways above and below the glottis, even when the primary indication is in the upper airway (stridor).

Bronchoscopy and Bronchoalveolar Lavage. Bronchoscopy is the inspection of the airways. BAL is a method used to obtain a representative specimen of fluid and secretions from the lower respiratory tract, which is useful for the cytologic and microbiologic diagnosis of lung diseases, especially in those who are unable to expectorate sputum. Commonly, BAL is performed after the general inspection of the airways and prior to tissue sampling with a brush or biopsy forceps. BAL is accomplished by gently wedging the scope into a lobar, segmental, or subsegmental bronchus and sequentially instilling and withdrawing sterile nonbacteriostatic saline in a volume sufficient to ensure that some of the aspirated fluid contains material that originated from the alveolar space. Nonbronchoscopic BAL can be performed in intubated patients by instilling and withdrawing saline through a catheter passed though the artificial airway and blindly wedged into a distal airway. In either case, the presence of alveolar macrophages documents that an alveolar sample has been obtained. Because the methods used to perform BAL involve passage of the equipment through the upper airway, there is a risk of contamination of the specimen by upper airway secretions. Careful cytologic examination and quantitative microbiologic cultures are important for correct interpretation of the data. BAL can often obviate the need for more invasive procedures such as open lung biopsy, especially in immunocompromised individuals.

Indications for diagnostic bronchoscopy and BAL include recurrent or persistent pneumonia or atelectasis, unexplained or localized and persistent wheeze, the suspected presence of a foreign body, hemoptysis, suspected congenital anomalies, mass lesions, interstitial disease, and pneumonia in the immunocompromised host. Indications for therapeutic bronchoscopy and BAL include bronchial obstuction by mass lesions, foreign bodies or mucus plugs, and general bronchial toilet and bronchopulmonary lavage. The individual undergoing bronchoscopy ventilates around the flexible scope, whereas with the rigid scope ventilation is accomplished through the scope. Rigid bronchoscopy is preferentially indicated for the extraction of foreign bodies and the removal of tissue masses and in patients with massive hemoptysis. In other cases, the flexible scope offers the advantages that it can be passed through endotracheal or tracheostomy tubes, can be introduced into bronchi that come off the airway at acute angles, and can be safely and effectively inserted with topical anesthesia and conscious sedation.

Regardless of the instrument used, the procedure performed, or its indications, the most common *complications* are sedation-related. The relatively more common complications include transient hypoxemia, laryngospasm, bronchospasm, and cardiac arrythmias. Iatrogenic infection, bleeding, pneumothorax, and pneumomediastinum are rare but reported complications of bronchoscopy or BAL. Subglottic edema is a more common complication of rigid bronchoscopy than of flexible procedures in which the scopes are smaller and less likely to traumatize the mucosa. Postbronchoscopy croup is treated with oxygen, mist, vasoconstrictor aerosols, and corticosteroids as necessary.

Thoracoscopy. The pleural cavity may be examined through a thoracoscope, which is similar to a rigid bronchoscope. The thoracoscope is inserted through an intercostal space and the lung is partially deflated, thus allowing the operator to view the surface of the lung, the pleural surface of the mediastinum and diaphragm, and the parietal pleura. Multiple thoracoscopic instruments can be inserted, allowing endoscopic lung or pleural biopsy, bleb resection, pleural abrasion, and ligation of vascular rings.

PERCUTANEOUS TAPS

Thoracentesis. For diagnostic or therapeutic purposes, fluid may be removed from the pleural space by needle puncture (see Chapter 418). Generally, as much fluid as possible should be withdrawn, and an *upright* chest roentgenogram should be obtained following the procedure. Complications of thoracentesis include infection, pneumothorax, and bleeding. Thoracentesis on the right may be complicated by puncture or laceration of the capsule of the liver, and on the left, by puncture of lacteration of the capsule of the spleen. Specimens obtained should always be cultured, examined microscopically for evidence of bacterial infection, and evaluated for total protein and total differential cell counts. Lactic acid dehydrogenase, glucose, cholesterol, triglyceride (chylous), and amylase determinations may also be useful. If malignancy is suspected, cytologic examination is imperative.

Transudates result from mechanical factors influencing the rate of formation or reabsorption of pleural fluid and generally require no further diagnostic evaluation. *Exudates* result from inflammation or other disease of the pleural surface and underlying lung and require a more complete diagnostic evaluation. In general, transudates have a total protein of less than 3 g/dL or a ratio of pleural protein to serum protein less than 0.5, a total leukocyte count of fewer than 2,000/mm^3 with a predominance of mononuclear cells, and low lactate dehydrogenase levels. Exudates have high protein levels and a predominance of polymorphonuclear cells (although malignant or tuberculous effusions may have a higher percentage of mononuclear cells). Complicated exudates often require continuous chest tube drainage and have a pH less than 7.20. Tuberculous effusions may have low glucose and high cholesterol content.

Lung Tap. Using a technique similar to that used for thoracentesis (see Chapter 418), a percutaneous lung tap is the most direct method of obtaining bacteriologic specimens from the pulmonary parenchyma and is the only technique other than open lung biopsy not associated with at least some risk of contamination by oral flora. After local anesthesia, a needle attached to a syringe containing nonbacteriostatic sterile saline is inserted using aseptic technique through the inferior aspect of an intercostal space in the area of interest. The needle is rapidly advanced into the lung; the saline is injected and reaspirated, and the needle is withdrawn. These actions are performed as quickly as possible. This procedure usually yields a few drops of fluid from the lung, which should be cultured and examined microscopically.

Major indications for a lung tap are roentgenographic infiltrates of undetermined cause, especially those unresponsive to therapy in immunosuppressed patients who are susceptible to unusual organisms. Complications are the same as for thoracentesis, but the incidence of pneumothorax is higher and somewhat dependent on the nature of the underlying disease process. In patients with poor pulmonary compliance, such as children with *Pneumocystis* pneumonia, the rate may approach 30%, with 5% requiring chest tubes. Bronchopulmonary lavage has replaced lung taps for most purposes.

LUNG BIOPSY. Lung biopsy may be the only way to establish a diagnosis, especially in protracted, noninfectious disease. In infants and small children, thoracoscopic or open surgical biopsies are the procedures of choice, and in expert hands there is low morbidity. Biopsy through the 3.5 mm diameter pediatric bronchoscopes limits the sample's size and diagnostic abilities. As well as ensuring that an adequate specimen is obtained, the surgeon can inspect the lung surface and choose the site of biopsy. In older children, transbronchial biopsies can be performed using flexible forceps through a bronchoscope, an endotracheal tube, a rigid bronchoscope, or an endotracheal tube, usually with fluoroscopic guidance. This technique is most appropriately used when the disease is diffuse such as *Pneumocystis* pneumonia or after rejection of a transplanted lung. The diagnostic limitations related to the small size of the biopsy specimens can be mitigated by the ability to obtain several samples. The risk of pneumothorax related to bronchoscopy is increased when transbronchial biopsies are part of the procedure; however, the ability to obtain biopsy specimens in a procedure performed with topical anesthesia and conscious sedation offers advantages to the select population for whom this procedure offers a reasonable diagnostic yield.

SWEAT TESTING. See Chapter 416.

Baughman RP (ed): Bronchoalveolar Lavage. St. Louis, MO, Mosby–Year Book, 1992.

Dailey RH, Simon B, Young GP, et al: The Airway: Emergency Management. St. Louis, MO, Mosby–Year Book, 1992.

Haddad GG, Lai TL, Epstein MA, et al: Breath-to-breath variations in rate and depth of ventilation in sleeping infants. Am J Physiol 243:R164, 1982.

Haddad GG, Leistner HL, Lai TL, Mellins RB: Ventilation and ventilatory pattern during sleep in aborted sudden infant death syndrome. Pediatr Res 15:879, 1981.

Holcomb GW III (ed): Pediatric Endoscopic Surgery. Norwalk, CT, Appleton & Lange, 1994.

Hughes WT, Buescher ES: Pediatric Procedures, 2nd ed. Philadelphia, WB Saunders, 1980.

Margolis P, Ferkol T, Marsocci S, et al: Accuracy of the clinical examination in detecting hypoxemia in infants with respiratory illness. J Pediatr 124:552, 1994.

Morse M, Cassels DE: Cardiopulmonary data for children and young adults. Springfield, Ill, Charles C Thomas, 1962.

Morse M, Schultz FW, Cassels DE: The lung volume and its subdivision in normal boys 10 to 17 years of age. J Clin Invest 31:380, 1952.
Prakash UBS: Bronchoscopy. New York, Raven Press, 1994.
Putnam CE: Diagnostic Imaging of the Lung. New York, Marcel Dekker, 1990.
Saccomanno G: Diagnostic Pulmonary Cytology. Chicago, American Society of Clinical Pathologists Press, 1986.

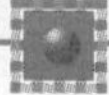

SECTION 2

Upper Respiratory Tract

Margaret A. Kenna

Children and adults preferentially breathe through their nose unless nasal obstruction interferes. However, most newborns are obligate nasal breathers, and significant nasal obstruction presenting at birth, such as choanal atresia, may be a life-threatening situation for the infant unless an alternate to the nasal airway is established.

PHYSIOLOGY. In addition to olfaction, the nose provides initial warming and humidification of inspired air. In the anterior nasal cavity, turbulent airflow and coarse hairs enhance the deposition of large particulate matter; the remaining nasal airways filter out particles as small as 6 μm in diameter. In the turbinate region, the airflow becomes laminar and the air stream is narrowed and directed superiorly, enhancing particle deposition, warming, and humidification. Nasal passages contribute as much as 50% of the total resistance of normal breathing. *Nasal flaring,* a sign of respiratory distress, reduces the resistance to inspiratory airflow through the nose and may improve ventilation.

The nasal mucosa is more vascular, especially in the turbinate region, than in the lower airways; however, the surface epithelium is similar, with ciliated cells, goblet cells, submucosal glands, and a covering blanket of mucus. In addition to mucous glycoproteins, which provide viscoelastic properties, the nasal secretions contain lysozyme and secretory IgA, both of which have antimicrobial activity, and IgG, IgE, albumin, histamine, bacteria, lactoferrin, and cellular debris. Aided by the ciliated cells, mucus flows toward the nasopharynx, where the air stream widens, the epithelium becomes squamous, and secretions are wiped away by swallowing; replacement of the mucous layers occurs about every 10–20 min. Flow of mucus anterior to the inferior turbinate is anterior. Estimates of daily mucus production vary from 0.1–0.3 mg/kg/24 hr, with most of the mucus being produced by the submucosal glands.

ANATOMY. The *paranasal sinuses* develop in the facial bones as air cells lined with ciliated, mucus-secreting epithelium. The frontal, maxillary and anterior ethmoid sinuses drain into the middle meatus, whereas the posterior ethmoid cells and sphenoid sinus drain into the superior meatus of the nose. Development of the sinuses begins at 3–5 mo of gestation but occurs mostly after birth, with the maxillary and ethmoid sinuses being the earliest to form. They are seen on plain radiographs by 1–2 yr of age but can be identified on fine-cut computed topography (CT) in the neonate. The frontal sinuses usually begin their ascent into the frontal bone by the 2nd yr but, along with the sphenoid sinuses, are not readily visible on plain radiographs until 5–6 yr of age or later. Growth of the sinuses continues through adolescence, with the frontal and sphenoid sinuses often being somewhat asymmetric; up to 5% of the population has no significant frontal sinus development. Hypoplasia of the maxillary sinuses, or the septa within the maxillary sinuses, is seen occasionally.

The adenoids on the posterior nasopharyngeal wall and the tonsils at the base of the tongue are directly in line with the mucociliary flow and the air stream, enhancing the protective function of this lymphoid tissue. The eustachian tubes, also lined with mucus-secreting, ciliated epithelium, enter the lateral walls of the nasopharynx and connect the nasopharynx to the middle ear.

Acquired anatomic abnormalities suggestive of sinusitis seen on plain sinus radiographs include mucosal thickening greater than 4 mm, air-fluid levels, or opacification. High-resolution CT of the paranasal sinuses, the current "gold-standard" for evaluation of disease of the paranasal sinuses, often reveals abnormalities, either congenital or acquired, that are not seen on plain films.

CHAPTER 378

Congenital Disorders of the Nose

Margaret A. Kenna

Congenital *structural nasal malformations* are uncommon compared with acquired abnormalities. Occasionally, the nasal bones are congenitally absent so that the bridge of the nose fails to develop, resulting in nasal hypoplasia. Congenital absence of the nose (arrhinia), complete or partial duplication, or a single centrally placed nostril may occur in isolation but are usually a part of malformation syndromes. Rarely, supernumerary teeth may be found in the nose, or teeth may grow into it from the maxilla.

On occasion, nasal bones are sufficiently malformed to produce severe narrowing of the nasal passages. Often such narrowing is associated with a high and narrow hard palate. Children with these defects may have more severe obstruction to airflow during infections of the upper airways and are more susceptible to the development of chronic or recurrent hypoventilation (see Chapter 383). Rarely, the alae nasi may be sufficiently thin and poorly supported to result in inspiratory obstruction or there may be congenital nasolacrimal duct obstruction with cystic extension into the nasopharynx causing respiratory distress.

A wide variety of nasal and midface abnormalities exist that may be part of more extensive craniofacial anomalies. These children are best treated by a team consisting of experienced pediatric, surgical, dental, and rehabilitation specialists.

CHOANAL ATRESIA. This is the most common congenital anomaly of the nose and has a frequency of approximately 1/7,000 live births. It consists of a unilateral or bilateral bony (90%) or membranous (10%) septum between the nose and the pharynx. Nearly 50% of affected infants have other congenital anomalies, with the anomalies occurring more frequently in bilateral cases. The CHARGE syndrome—*c*oloboma; *h*eart disease; *a*tresia choanae; *r*etarded growth and development or CNS anomalies, or both; *g*enital anomalies or hypogonadism, or both; and *e*ar anomalies or deafness, or both—is one of the more common anomalies associated with choanal atresia.

CLINICAL MANIFESTATIONS. Because newborn infants have a variable ability to breathe through their mouths, nasal obstruction does not produce the same symptoms in every infant. When only one side is affected, the infant usually does not have severe symptoms at birth and may be asymptomatic for a prolonged period, often until the 1st respiratory infection, when the diagnosis may be suggested by unilateral nasal discharge or disproportionately severe nasal obstruction. Infants with bilateral choanal atresia who have difficulty with mouth breathing make vigorous attempts to inspire, often suck in their lips, and develop cyanosis. Distressed children then cry (which relieves the cyanosis) and become more calm, only to repeat the cycle after closing their mouths. Those who are able to breathe through their mouths at once experience difficulty when sucking and swallowing, becoming cyanotic when they attempt to feed.

DIAGNOSIS. This is established by the inability to pass a firm catheter through each nostril 3–4 cm into the nasopharynx. The atresia plate may be seen directly with fiberoptic rhinoscopy. The anatomy is best visualized by using high-resolution CT.

TREATMENT. Initially, this consists of promptly providing an oral airway, maintaining the mouth in an open position, or intubation. Passage of an orogastric tube is often sufficient to prevent the complete opposition of tongue and soft palate and to ensure an open airway. Other techniques use a feeding nipple with large holes at the tip or an oral airway (such as those used in anesthesia). Once an oral airway is established, the infant can be fed by gavage until breathing and eating without the assisted airway is possible. In bilateral cases, intubation or tracheotomy may be indicated. If the child is free of other serious medical problems, operative intervention can be considered in the neonate, with transnasal repair becoming more common because of the advent of small magnifying endoscopes and smaller surgical instruments and drills. Tracheotomy should be considered in cases (especially bilateral cases) in which the child has other potentially life-threatening problems and in whom early surgical repair of the choanal atresia may not be appropriate or feasible. Operative correction of unilateral obstruction may be deferred for several years. In both unilateral and bilateral cases, restenosis necessitating dilation or reoperation, or both, is common.

Congenital defects of the nasal septum, such as *perforation* or *deviation,* are rare. Perforation can be developmental (very rare) but, more commonly, is acquired after birth secondary to infection, such as syphilis or tuberculosis, or trauma. The most common cause of septal deviation noted at birth is that due to birth trauma. If recognized during the first few days of life, it may be corrected with immediate realignment using blunt probes, cotton applicators, and topical anesthesia. Formal surgical correction may eventually be required but is usually postponed to avoid disturbance of midface growth. Although mild septal deviations are common (and usually asymptomatic), significantly abnormal formation of the septum is infrequent unless other malformations are also present, such as cleft lip or palate.

Pyriform aperture stenosis is a bony abnormality of the anterior nasal aperture. These children may present with severe nasal obstruction at birth or shortly thereafter. Diagnosis is made by CT of the nose. Surgical repair via an anterior approach may be needed if the child cannot feed or breathe without difficulty.

Congenital midline nasal masses include *dermoids, gliomas,* and *encephaloceles* (in descending order of frequency). They present intranasally or extranasally and may have intracranial connections. Nasal dermoids often have a dimple or pit on the nasal dorsum, sometimes with hair being present, and may predispose to intracranial infections if an intracranial connection is present. Recurrent infection of the dermoid itself is common. Gliomas or heterotopic brain tissue is firm, whereas encephaloceles are soft and enlarge with crying or the Valsalva maneuver. Diagnosis is based on physical examination findings and results from imaging studies. CT provides the best bony detail, but magnetic resonance imaging may be needed to further define intracranial extention. Surgical excision of these masses is generally required, with the extent and surgical approach based on the type and size of the mass.

Other nasal masses include hemangiomas, congenital nasolacrimal duct obstruction (which may present as a nasal mass), nasal polyps, and tumors such as rhabdomyosarcoma. Nasal polyps are rarely present at birth, but the others often present at birth or in early infancy. Diagnosis is based on physical examination and imaging studies. Treatment depends on the type and location of the mass but may involve surgical removal or biopsy.

Poor development of the paranasal sinuses is associated with recurrent or chronic upper airway infection in Down syndrome.

Brown OE, Myer CM, Manning SC: Congenital nasal pyriform aperture stenosis. Laryngoscope 99:86, 1989.

Hughes GB, Sharpino G, Hunt W, Tucker HM: Management of the midline nasal mass: A review. Head Neck Surg 2:222, 1980.

Maniglia AJ, Goodwin WJ, Arnold JE, et al: Intracranial abscesses secondary to nasal sinus and orbital infections in adults and children. Arch Otolaryngol Head Neck Surg 115:1424, 1989.

Richardson M, Osguthorpe JD: Surgical management of choanal atresia. Laryngoscope 98:915, 1988.

Schwartz DA, Lieberman SA, Viles PH, et al: An unusual cause of respiratory distress in a neonate. Pediatrics 101:479, 1998.

Stankiewicz JA: The endoscopic repair of choanal atresia. Otolaryngol Head Neck Surg 103:931, 1990.

CHAPTER 379
Acquired Disorders of the Nose

Margaret A. Kenna

379.1 Foreign Body

Food, crayons, small toys, erasers, paper wads, beads, beans, stones, pieces of sponge, and other foreign bodies are frequently introduced into the nose by children. Initial symptoms are local obstruction, sneezing, relatively mild discomfort and, rarely, pain. Irritation results in mucosal swelling and, because some foreign bodies are hygroscopic and increase in size as water is absorbed, signs of local obstruction and discomfort may increase with time. Infection usually follows and gives rise to a purulent, malodorous, or bloody discharge. The patient may also present with a generalized body odor—bromhidrosis.

DIAGNOSIS. Unilateral nasal discharge and obstruction should suggest the presence of a foreign body, which can often be seen on examination with a nasal speculum or otoscope placed in the nose. Purulent secretions must often be removed so that the foreign object can actually be seen; often a headlight, suction, and topical decongestants may be needed. The object is usually situated anteriorly at first, but through unskilled attempts at removal it may be forced deeper into the nose.

TREATMENT. Removal should be carried out promptly to minimize the danger of aspiration and prevent local tissue necrosis. This can usually be performed with topical anesthesia, using either forceps or nasal suction. If there is marked swelling or bleeding, general anesthesia may be needed to remove the object. Infection usually clears promptly after the removal of the object, and generally no further therapy is necessary.

COMPLICATIONS. Tetanus is a rare complication of long-standing nasal foreign bodies in nonimmunized children. Toxic shock syndrome is also rare and most commonly occurs from nasal surgical packing (Chapter 182.2).

379.2 Epistaxis

Nosebleeds are rare in infancy and common in childhood; their incidence decreases after puberty. Diagnosis and treatment depend on the location and cause of the bleeding.

ANATOMY. The most common location for bleeding is in the area of Kiesselbach's plexus, an area in the anterior septum where vessels from both the internal and external carotid arteries converge. The thin mucosa in this area, as well as the anterior location, make it prone to exposure to dry air and trauma. Other blood supply to the nose is from the internal carotid artery, through the anterior and posterior ethmoid arteries, as well as the sphenopalatine and terminal branchs of the internal maxillary arteries from the external carotid system.

ETIOLOGY. Common causes of nosebleeds from the anterior septum include digital trauma, foreign bodies, dry air, and inflammation, including upper respiratory tract infections, sinusitis, and allergic rhinitis. Young infants with significant gastroesophageal reflux into the nose may occasionally present with epistaxis secondary to mucosal inflammation. In many children, there is frequently a family history of childhood epistaxis. Susceptibility is increased during respiratory infections and in the winter when dry air irritates the nasal mucosa, resulting in formation of fissures and crusting. Severe bleeding may be encountered with congenital vascular abnormalities, such as hereditary hemorrhagic telangiectasias, varicosities, hemangiomas, and in children with thrombocytopenia, deficiency of clotting factors, hypertension, renal failure, or venous congestion. Nasal polyps or other intranasal growths may be associated with epistaxis. Recurrent, and frequently severe, nosebleeds may be the initial presenting symptom in juvenile nasal angiofibromas, most commonly seen in adolescent males. The incidence of Kiesselbach's plexus bleeding seems to decrease with adolescence.

CLINICAL MANIFESTATIONS. Epistaxis usually occurs without warning, with blood flowing slowly but freely from one nostril or occasionally from both. In children with nasal lesions, bleeding may follow physical exercise. When bleeding occurs at night, the blood may be swallowed and may become apparent only when the child vomits or passes blood in the stools. Posterior epistaxis may manifest as anterior nasal bleeding or, if copious, the patient may vomit blood as the initial symptom.

TREATMENT. Most nosebleeds stop spontaneously in a few minutes. The nares should be compressed and the child kept as quiet as possible, in an upright position with the head tilted forward to avoid blood trickling posteriorly into the pharynx. Cold compresses applied to the nose may also help. If these measures do not stop the bleeding, local application of a solution of oxymetazoline (Afrin) or neosynephrine (0.25–1%) may be useful. If bleeding persists, an anterior nasal pack may need to be inserted; if bleeding originates in the posterior nasal cavity, combined anterior and posterior packing is necessary. After bleeding has been controlled, and if a bleeding site is identified, its obliteration by cautery with silver nitrate may prevent further difficulties. As the septal cartilage derives its nutrition from the overlying mucoperichondrium, only one side of the septum should be cauterized at a time to reduce the chance of a septal perforation. If a patient lives in a dry environment, a room humidifier may prevent epistaxis.

In patients with severe or repeated epistaxis, blood transfusions may be necessary. Otolaryngologic evaluation is indicated for these children and for those with bilateral bleeding or with hemorrhage that does not arise from Kiesselbach's plexus. Hematologic evaluation (for coagulopathy and anemia), along with nasal endoscopy and diagnostic imaging, may be needed to make a definitive diagnosis in some cases of severe recurrent epistaxis. Replacement of deficient clotting factors may be required for patients who have an underlying hematologic disorder (see Chapter 482). Profuse epistaxis associated with a nasal mass in a boy near puberty may signal a **juvenile nasopharyngeal angiofibroma.** This unusual tumor has been reported in a 2-yr-old and in 30- to 40-yr-olds, but the incidence peaks in adolescent and preadolescent boys. Computed tomography with contrast is the best initial evaluation. Arteriography, embolization, and extensive surgery may be needed.

Surgical intervention may also be needed for bleeding from the internal maxillary artery or other vessels that may cause bleeding in the posterior nasal cavity.

OTHER ACQUIRED ABNORMALITIES OF THE NOSE. Many acquired abnormalities of the nose and paranasal sinuses, such as trauma (including nasal and midface fractures) and tumors, present with epistaxis. Other abnormalities that may cause change in the shape of the nose and paranasal sinuses but few other symptoms include fibro-osseus lesions (ossifying fibroma, fibrous dysplasia, and cementifying fibroma) and mucoceles of the paranasal sinuses. These conditions can be suspected on physical examination, with further definition obtained by radiography (usually computed tomography) and biopsy. Although these are considered benign lesions, they may all greatly change the architecture of the surrounding bony structures and often require surgical intervention for management.

Wurman LH: Epistaxis. *In:* Gates GA (ed): Current Therapy in Otolaryngology Head and Neck Surgery, 5th ed. St Louis, CV Mosby, 1994, p 354.

CHAPTER 380
Nasal Polyps

Margaret A. Kenna

ETIOLOGY. Nasal polyps are benign pedunculated tumors formed from edematous, usually chronically inflamed nasal mucosa. They usually originate from the ethmoid sinus and present in the middle meatus. Occasionally, they appear within the maxillary antrum and can extend to the nasopharynx (antrochoanal polyp). Large or multiple polyps may completely obstruct the nasal passage. The polyps originating from the ethmoid sinus are usually smaller and multiple, as compared with the large and usually single antral choanal polyp.

Cystic fibrosis is the most common childhood cause of nasal polyposis and should be suspected in any child less than 12 yr with nasal polyps, even in the absence of typical respiratory and digestive symptoms; up to 25% of children with cystic fibrosis acquire nasal polyps. Nasal polyposis is also associated with chronic sinusitis and allergic rhinitis. In the uncommon "aspirin triad," nasal polyps are associated with aspirin sensitivity and asthma.

CLINICAL MANIFESTATIONS. Obstruction of nasal passages with hyponasal speech and mouth breathing is prominent. Profuse mucoid or mucopurulent rhinorrhea may also be present. An examination of the nasal passages shows glistening, gray, grapelike masses squeezed between the nasal turbinates and the septum. Polyps can be readily distinguished from the well-vascularized turbinate tissue, which is pink or red. Prolonged presence of polyps may widen the bridge of the nose and erode adjacent osseous structures.

TREATMENT. Local or systemic decongestants are not usually effective in shrinking the polyps, although they may provide symptomatic relief from the associated mucosal edema. Intranasal steroid sprays, and sometimes systemic steroids, may provide dramatic shrinkage of nasal polyps and have proved useful in children with cystic fibrosis. Polyps should be removed surgically if complete obstruction, uncontrolled rhinorrhea, or deformity of the nose appears. If the underlying pathogenic mechanism cannot be eliminated (e.g., cystic fibrosis), the polyps may soon return. Functional endoscopic sinus surgery may provide more complete polyp removal and treatment of other associated nasal disease; in some cases this has reduced the need for frequent surgeries.

Antral choanal polyps must be surgically removed and do not respond to medical measures. Since these types of polyps are not generally associated with any other underlying disease process, the recurrence rate is much less than for other types of polyps.

Magit AE: Tumors of the nose, paranasal sinuses, and nasopharynx. *In:* Bluestone CD, Stool SE, Kenna MA (eds): Pediatric Otolaryngology, 3rd ed. Philadelphia, WB Saunders, 1996, pp 893–904.

CHAPTER 381

Infections of the Upper Respiratory Tract

Neil E. Herendeen and Peter G. Szilagy

381.1 Upper Respiratory Infections or "Colds" or Nasopharyngitis

Upper respiratory infections (URIs) are the most frequently occurring illness in childhood. On average, children acquire three to eight URIs/year, whereas their parents experience two to four/year. URIs are the most common medical reason for school or work absenteeism, causing more than 25 million lost school days and 21 million lost work days/year and accounting for nearly 7% of all visits to pediatricians and family physicians. Americans now spend more than $2 billion dollars each year on medications to treat the symptoms of the common cold. A national survey found that more than one third of 3-yr-old children were given an over-the-counter cold medication during the prior month.

Although URIs are encountered more frequently during the fall and winter months, there is no evidence that low temperatures or "cold air" per se either promote the spread of viruses or decrease our resistance to them. There is little difference in the incidence of colds by sex, race, or geographic region. Environmental factors that increase the likelihood of acquiring colds include attendance at child care facilities, smoking, passive exposure to smoke, low income, crowding and, perhaps, psychologic stress.

ETIOLOGY. More than 200 viruses can cause URIs (Table 381–1). Rhinoviruses compose more than one third of all these viruses. Patients acquire lifelong immunity to individual serotypes but, unfortunately, more than 100 rhinovirus serotypes have been characterized. Thus, developing immunity to all rhinoviruses takes a long time. Parainfluenza viruses (types 1–4) often produce lower respiratory disease but, particularly in reinfections, the symptoms may present as uncomplicated URIs. Respiratory syncytial virus (RSV) often begins in infants as a URI but then spreads to the lower respiratory tract. Older children and adults with naturally acquired RSV usually have typical upper respiratory symptoms that may last for 2 wk. Other less common causes are listed in Table 381–1. Although all these viruses may produce systemic symptoms, including fever and malaise, actual viremia does not occur with the common cold. Viral shedding usually peaks 2–7 days after the start, continuing for up to 2 wk. (See Part XVI, Section 12 for chapters on specific viruses.)

TABLE 381–1 Infectious Agents Associated with the Common Cold

Category	Agents
Common viruses that usually cause common colds	Rhinoviruses Parainfluenza viruses Respiratory syncytial virus Coronaviruses
Common agents that occasionally cause symptoms of the common cold	Adenoviruses Enteroviruses Influenza viruses Parainfluenza viruses Reoviruses *Mycoplasma pneumoniae*
Agents that rarely cause symptoms of the common cold	*Coccidioides immitis* *Histoplasma capsulatum* *Bordetella pertussis* *Chlamydia psittaci* *Coxiella burnetii*

Adapted from Cherry JD: The common cold. In: *Feigin RD, Cherry JD (eds): Textbook of Pediatric Infectious Diseases. Philadelphia, WB Saunders, 1998.*

EPIDEMIOLOGY. Children are the major reservoir of cold viruses, often acquiring a new virus from another child in school or in child care. The secondary attack rate within schools depends on the age of children and on their prior immunity. When a new serotype of rhinovirus or RSV is introduced into a school or child care setting, up to two thirds of children can become infected. The incubation period for cold viruses is usually 2 to 5 days but may last as long as 8 days. Children who acquire a new URI frequently introduce the virus into the home. Fortunately, a brief exposure in the same room (such as in a pediatrician's waiting room) to a person with a URI produces a low incidence of transmission.

Cold viruses may be transmitted by three routes: large-particle droplets, which can travel a short distance (from a cough or a sneeze) to directly inoculate another person; small-particle aerosols, which can travel longer distances and deposit directly in alveoli of other individuals; and secretions (on contaminated hands or on fomites), which are transmitted by direct physical contact. Most cold viruses require close contact for transmission.

PATHOGENESIS AND IMMUNOLOGY. The pathophysiology is not well understood owing in part to the multiple viral agents involved. The most likely progression of the disease is shown in Figure 381–1. The offending virus invades the epithelial cells of the upper respiratory tract. Inflammatory mediators (probably not histamine) are released, altering vascular permeability and causing edema and nasal stuffiness. Stimulation of cholinergic nerves in the nose and upper respiratory tract leads to increased mucus production (rhinorrhea) and occasionally to bronchoconstriction, resulting in a cough. Cellular damage to the nasopharynx is probably the mechanism that causes the sore and scratchy throat. Injury to cilia in the nasal epithelial cells may decrease ciliary function and impair clearance of nasal secretions.

The immune response to different cold viruses is variable. Within 1 day of infection by rhinovirus, specific neutralizing IgA is found in nasal secretions. Within days the nasal secretions contain IgG, which presumably participates in the fight against the virus. About 1 wk after infection, specific serum IgG (and also IgM) is detectable in up to 80% of individuals and persists for years. Most adults have serum antibody to

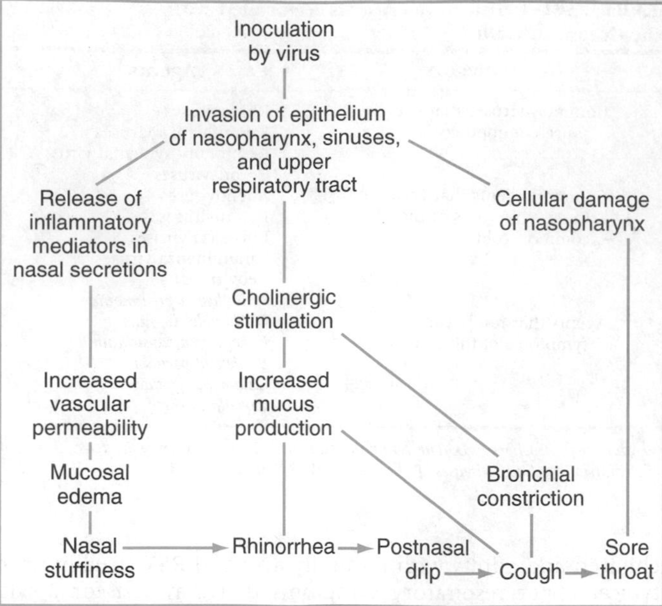

Figure 381–1 Pathophysiology of the common cold.

many rhinovirus serotypes, suggesting long-term immunity. Both secretory and serum antibodies thus play a role in fighting rhinovirus infections and in preventing reinfections. This defense, however, falters in two instances: First, some individuals (up to 20%, for reasons not well understood) do not acquire serum neutralizing antibody to a specific rhinovirus infection; second, a large viral challenge can overcome a beleaguered antibody system, leading to reinfection with rhinovirus.

Children and adults frequently become reinfected with parainfluenza virus or RSV, leading to the common cold. The risk of reinfection is inversely related to the existing level of serum neutralizing antibody; however, the exact role of either secretory (primarily IGA) antibody or serum neutralizing antibody in reinfections with parainfluenza virus or RSV is unclear. Cell-mediated immunity and interferon production do not appear to play an important immunologic role in RSV infections; their role in URIs caused by other viruses is not yet understood.

CLINICAL MANIFESTATIONS. In older children and adults, the initial symptoms are usually nasal irritation and a scratchy throat. Most individuals can usually sense a cold that is about to start. Within hours, a thin nasal discharge and sneezing are present. A sore throat is noted, partly due to postnasal drip and mouth-breathing. Myalgia, a feeling of "being cold," headache, malaise, and decreased appetite are often present. Children may complain of headache and eye irritation and may have a low-grade fever. By the 2nd to 3rd day, the nasal discharge becomes thicker and is often purulent. Although the child usually feels better, sneezing, sore throat, and nighttime cough (the latter two symptoms due to postnasal drip) are common. The nose may become tender and excoriated. The nasal secretions become progressively more purulent due to shedding of epithelial and white blood cells. Most systemic symptoms subside within 5–7 days. However, rhinitis and a hacky cough may persist for another week, until the nasal epithelial cells have regenerated.

Infants have a more variable presentation, frequently with a fever. Nasal symptoms follow a similar course as in older children. Infants with URIs are often irritable and restless. Nasal congestion may make feeding and sleeping difficult, and cough may lead to vomiting. Some infants have mild diarrhea. Although some infants appear quite ill, others do not suffer much from URIs and may have three to four colds during a winter with virtually no difficulty except for rhinorrhea.

Complications can occur. The most common bacterial complication is otitis media, in which new symptoms appear, such as earache, fever, and irritability (see Chapter 646). Parents often recognize that the character and severity of the illness has somehow changed. Less common bacterial complications include sinusitis, which follows obstruction of paranasal sinuses ostia and lower respiratory tract disease (pneumonia). Asthma in infants and children can be triggered by any of the viruses causing URIs because of allergy-mediated airway hyperactivity. The thick, purulent, nasal drainage that occurs after a few days of an URI does not usually imply a bacterial infection but is generally due to the resolving inflammatory process.

History. The most important component of the evaluation of a child with a URI is a careful history. The physician should determine if systemic symptoms are present, if the course of the child's illness is consistent with a common cold, if the rhinorrhea is bilateral, and if the patient has a history of allergic conditions. Other important issues concern whether there is exposure to cigarette smoke, whether the child been essentially healthy, and whether this illness appears similar to previous URIs. It is useful to ask parents how ill their child appears to them, how they have managed prior URIs, whether they have attempted any treatment or medications, and whether they believe the treatment is helping.

Physical Examination. Most infants or children with a URI appear relatively healthy. The color and thickness of the nasal secretions do not help differentiate a bacterial, viral, or allergic cause. In allergic rhinitis, the nasal turbinates are edematous, although not always pale or violaceous. Examination of the pharynx may reveal one of the three patterns of viral nasopharyngitis described further on. The presence of associated signs should be noted, including otitis media, facial or sinus tenderness, enlarged cervical lymph nodes, respiratory findings (tachypnea, retractions, wheezes, rales or rhonchi), and allergic facies.

LABORATORY FINDINGS. Laboratory tests rarely add anything useful to the information from a careful history and physical examination. Cultures of the throat or nasopharynx are rarely indicated. Obtaining a white blood cell count or sedimentation rate is not helpful. If clinical findings suggest sinusitis, a roentgenogram of the sinuses may confirm the diagnosis. If allergic rhinitis is suspected, examination of nasal secretions under the microscope using a Wright's or Hansel's stain may reveal eosinophils. However, the absence of eosinophils does not rule out the diagnosis of allergic rhinitis. Determining a specific viral diagnosis does not affect management and is expensive. If the clinical picture is consistent with pertussis, a nasopharyngeal culture or fluorescent antibody study can confirm the diagnosis (see Chapter 195).

DIAGNOSIS AND DIFFERENTIAL DIAGNOSIS. A key decision in evaluating children with URIs is to determine whether the illness is just a common cold or whether a secondary infection or complication is present. The diagnosis is based on a judgment that the typical progression of symptoms has occurred, that there has been a history of contacts, and that a knowledge of community outbreaks exists. Frequently children present with nasopharyngitis (both nasal congestion and pharyngitis). The pharyngeal lesions tend to have one of three patterns: erythema alone, usually due to infection with rhinoviruses, parainfluenza, RSV, influenza, or rotavirus; cobblestone or follicular, frequently produced by adenovirus and certain enteroviruses; or vesicular or ulcerative, usually due to enterovirus or herpes simplex virus.

Objective evidence of pharyngitis, allergic signs, otitis media, or respiratory abnormalities such as tachypnea, retractions, or wheezing suggest other diagnoses. The differential diagnosis is

TABLE 381–2 Differential Diagnosis of the Common Cold

Etiology	Key Points on History or Physical Examination
Infections	
Sinusitis	Age (>2 yr), duration (>10 days), high fever, unilateral headache, or facial tenderness, nasal discharge
Pharyngitis (streptococcal)	Exudate, petechiae, tender cervical lymph nodes, minimal congestion
Pneumonia (viral or bacterial)	Respiratory signs
Allergy	
Allergic rhinitis	History of atopy, itchy and watery eyes, allergic facies, nasal eosinophilia
Structural	
Foreign body	Unilateral, foul-smelling
Anatomic (polyp, adenoids)	Duration (>2 mo), often unilateral
Systemic Disease	
Cystic fibrosis or immune deficiency	Failure to thrive, duration (>2 mo), diarrhea, pneumonia, and other infections

listed in Table 381–2. Allergy is suggested by a history of atopic symptoms in the patient and family.

In adolescents, two additional entities may produce nasal congestion. Overuse of cocaine or other drugs, including topical decongestants, may cause chronic rhinitis known as "rhinitis medicamentosa." Emotional stress or exposure to cold temperatures may produce a vasomotor response and watery nasal discharge.

Although most cases of URI are straightforward, a cause other than viruses should be sought if colds are chronic, more frequent than 8/yr, or associated with a patient who is failing to thrive or has persistent systemic signs and symptoms.

TREATMENT. Parents and older children understandably want the physician to "do something" about a child's URI, and it is tempting for physicians to turn to medications. There are more than 800 over-the-counter medications available to treat the common cold and dozens of prescription medications.

For most URIs the best treatment is no pharmacologic treatment. If the child is not very ill, it is best to avoid most medications; they usually do not work, and they all have potential side effects that are worse than the usual cold symptoms. It is also important to teach parents (and physicians) that giving medications is not synonymous with giving treatment. Education about the natural history of URIs, instruction about when to call if the child worsens or fails to improve, and suggestions about supportive measures are all important therapies. Written instructions and handouts are useful.

When children with URIs *are* uncomfortable, the most bothersome symptoms are fever and malaise, rhinorrhea or nasal congestion, and a persistent cough. Therapy should be directed toward a specific symptom that is causing discomfort. Acetaminophen (10–15 mg/kg/dose) or ibuprofen (10 mg/kg/dose) is often helpful in relieving the constitutional symptoms and the fever that may be present during the 1st day or two. Aspirin should be avoided because of the association with Reye's syndrome and because influenza can mimic the common cold in children.

Management of URIs include nonpharmacologic therapy and medications. Nonpharmacologic therapy (Table 381–3) may ameliorate the rhinorrhea and cough. For infants, saline nose drops, either purchased or made by parents (1/4 tsp of salt mixed with 8 oz of warm water), can loosen the secretions and induce sneezing. Gentle use of a bulb syringe following the adminstration of saline drops can temporarily relieve nasal obstruction and may be particularly helpful prior to feedings. Many parents feel that a water vaporizer placed in the room helps infants to sleep better and facilitates bulb suctioning. Although a possible mechanism is that humidified air dilutes nasal secretions, there is little scientific evidence for benefit from water vaporizers for URIs in infants. Elevating the head of the bed may help for older children. Frequent intake of fluids is important. Fluid intake, throat lozenges, and cough drops may help a scratchy throat and cough by increasing hydration and swallowing. Home remedies are used throughout the world to treat URIs. Remedies such as tea with lemon and honey, and chicken soup increase hydration and are pleasant, readily available at home, safe, and inexpensive.

TABLE 381–3 Nonpharmacologic Therapy for Cold Symptoms in Infants

Good hydration	Elevating head (older children)
Saline nose drops	Parents ceasing smoking
Bulb syringe	Educational handout
Water vaporizer	

Pharmacotherapy for URIs includes four types of medications in addition to antipyretics: antihistamines, decongestants (sympathomimetics), expectorants, and cough suppressants. Unfortunately, most preparations contain at least two types. A review of clinical trials of over-the-counter cold medications found only four scientifically valid studies on children: Two performed on preschool children found no benefits, whereas two performed on older children found some improvements in cold symptoms. A greater number of studies have been performed on adults. Table 381–4 summarizes the effectiveness of the different medications commonly used to treat URI symptoms. The clinician and parents must weigh the small potential benefits of these medications against the potential side effects. In infants especially, serious side effects can occur and include extreme lethargy or irritability and unusual central nervous system or cardiovascular effects; thus, medications other than acetaminophen or ibuprofen should not be given to infants with URIs.

Many parents ask physicians for antibiotics to treat URIs. Antibiotics do not shorten the duration of cold symptoms and do not reduce the risk of complications.

Although there have been multiple studies evaluating the ability of vitamin C to either prevent or treat URIs in adults, there is no clear benefit, and ascorbic acid can be toxic in high doses. Thus, it is not recommended that children with URIs be given high doses of vitamin C. There is no evidence for the effectiveness of multivitamins, rare elements such as zinc, or chest rubs in children. The effect of chicken soup has not been scientifically studied.

PREVENTION. Since URIs are transmitted by contaminated hands or by sneezes, frequent hand washing after contact with an infected person reduces the risk of secondary infection. Avoidance, such as keeping children out of child care, is usually impractical. Neither ascorbic acid nor multivitamins are effective as preventive agents. Although breast-feeding offers theoretical hope, evidence is lacking for its effectiveness in preventing URIs.

The most promising area for prevention of colds includes

TABLE 381–4 Pharmacologic Treatment of Cold Symptoms

Category	Medication	Effectiveness
Fever	Acetaminophen	+ +
	Ibuprofen	+ +
Rhinorrhea and stuffiness	Antihistamine	0
	Decongestant	+
Cough	Expectorant	0
	Suppressant (codeine or dextromethorphan)	+
Duration	Antibiotics	0
	Vitamin C	0
	Multivitamins	0
	Zinc, heavy metals	0

0 = not effective; + = somewhat effective; + + = effective.

specific antiviral measures. Vaccines, unfortunately, have been difficult to produce. The number of antigenic types is large, nasal IgA production responds poorly to inactivated antigens, and immunity has been short-lived. Under study conditions, the use of nasal tissues impregnated with virucidal agents has shown modest reductions in the incidence of newly acquired colds. However, in everyday family life the effectiveness of this approach seems doubtful. Immunoglobulin therapy against RSV is indicated in high-risk patients for serious lower respiratory infection (Chapter 253).

Cherry JD: The common cold. *In:* Feigin RD, Cherry JD (eds): Textbook of Pediatric Infectious Diseases. Philadelphia, WB Saunders, 1998, pp 128–133.

Gadomski A, Horton L: The need for rational therapeutics in the use of cough and cold medicine in infants. Pediatrics 89:774, 1992.

Smith MBH, Feldman W: Over-the-counter cold medications: A critical review of clinical trials between 1950 and 1991. JAMA 269:2258, 1993.

Szilagyi PG: What can we do about the common cold? Contemp Pediatr 7:23, 1990.

381.2 Sinusitis

Childhood sinusitis occurs commonly but is not easily recognized. Each case of viral rhinitis is also a viral rhinosinusitis. The spectrum of disease includes self-limited viral rhinosinusitis, acute bacterial sinusitis, subacute bacterial sinusitis, and chronic sinusitis. The true prevalence of sinus infection is unknown, as is the natural history of the disease if left untreated. Many of the management strategies invoked for the treatment of otitis media are used for sinusitis because the organisms are frequently the same, and the rate of comorbidity is as high as 50%.

ETIOLOGY. Paranasal sinuses form as evaginations of the mucous membranes of the nasal meatus. The mucous lining of each paranasal sinus is identical to the mucosal lining of the nose. Maxillary and ethmoid sinuses are anatomically present in utero; frontal sinuses begin to develop by age 1–2 yr but, along with the sphenoid sinuses, are not usually seen radiographically until 5–6 yr of age. The anatomic position of the ostia draining each sinus cavity makes ciliary motility the most important aspect of preventing sinus infection. Factors that impair normal mucociliary transport may increase the risk of sinusitis and include cigarette smoke exposure, cold and dry inspired air, viral URI, allergic rhinitis, swimming, gastroesophageal reflux, cystic fibrosis, immunodeficiency, and ciliary dyskinesia. Any factor causing nasal obstruction can also predispose to sinusitis, including foreign bodies, polyps, enlarged adenoids, extreme septal deviation, tumors, or trauma.

In the absence of effective pulsatile movement of mucus by the cilia, stagnation of secretions occurs within the sinuses, which then become a culture medium for bacteria. The inflammatory response of the respiratory epithelium increases secretory activity and further impairs ciliary function.

Organisms recovered in children with acute sinusitis are usually the same as those seen in acute otitis media: *Streptococcus pneumoniae, Moraxella catarrhalis,* and nontypable *Haemophilus influenzae.* In chronic sinusitis, α-hemolytic streptococci, *Staphylococcus aureus,* and anaerobes are seen, and frequently multiple types of bacteria are present.

CLINICAL MANIFESTATIONS. Sinusitis in children does not have the same cluster of symptoms as it does in adults. Headaches, facial pain, tenderness, and facial edema occur in adolescents and adults but are not common in preadolescents. Cough and nasal discharge are the most common clinical manifestations of acute sinusitis in children. The cough occurs in the daytime and frequently is worse when lying supine during naps or bedtime. The nasal discharge may be clear or purulent. Sore throat secondary to postnasal drip may be present, and the child may sniff or snort to clear the drainage. Older children may complain of malodorous breath, decreased sense of smell, facial or frontal pressure, or fever.

Most upper respiratory tract infections improve by 7 to 10 days. If symptoms persist without improvement for more than 10 days, a diagnosis of acute sinusitis should be considered. A less common but more severe form of acute sinusitis can occur with symptoms for less than 10 days in the child with fever higher than 39°C, purulent nasal discharge, headache, and eye swelling. Subacute or chronic sinusitis is defined by symptoms such as cough and nasal discharge for more than 30 days.

On physical examination, the nasal mucosa is usually erythematous and swollen. If allergic rhinitis is a contributing factor, the turbinates may be pale and boggy. Mucopurulent material sometimes can be seen draining into the posterior nasopharynx. Palpation of the bones overlying the sinuses may elicit pain, particularly in older children. Transillumination of the maxillary and frontal sinuses is rarely helpful, in part because of asymmetrical sinus development. Evidence of otitis media is a common finding as well. A careful eye examination is important to rule out the complications of periorbital and orbital cellulitis, orbital abscess, and optic neuritis. Other physical findings can be seen with the infrequent complications of meningitis, epidural or subdural abscess, cavernous or saggital sinus thrombosis, and osteomyelitis.

The value of sinus roentgenograms and computed tomography is controversial. The diagnostic features of mucosal thickening, air-fluid levels, and sinus opacification seen on roentgenogram are not always helpful in distinguishing viral rhinosinusitis from acute or chronic bacterial sinusitis. Microscopic examination of nasal secretions usually reveals cellular debris and neutrophils but may suggest an allergic component if many eosinophils are present. Nasal swab cultures do not correlate well with cultures of sinus aspirates and therefore are not recommended. Sinus aspiration by direct antral puncture is the only reliable method of obtaining a bacterial culture but should be reserved for life-threatening conditions, immunocompromised hosts, or illness unresponsive to therapy.

TREATMENT. This consists primarily of effective antimicrobial therapy. Amoxicillin is a reasonable initial choice. In areas in which *H. influenzae* and *M. catarrhalis* producing β-lactamase are common, or for treatment failures, oral amoxicillin with potassium clavulanate, macrolides, and 2nd- and 3rd-generation cephalosporins may be prescribed (see chapters on specific agents). Trimethoprim-sulfamethoxazole is ineffective against group A β-hemolytic streptococci. Treatment should last until 7 days after symptom resolution, usually 14–21 days. Decongestants may provide some symptomatic relief but do not clear the infection faster. Antihistamines are not helpful and may interfere with sinus drainage because of thickened secretions. Nasal irrigation with saline solution can be taught to children in order to promote drainage and reduce swelling.

Clement PA, Bluestone CD, Gordts F, et al: Management of rhinosinusitis in children: Consensus meeting, Brussels, Belgium, September 13, 1996. Arch Otolaryngol Head Neck Surg 124:31, 1998.

O'Brien KL, Dowell SF, Schwartz B, et al: Acute sinusitis-principals of judicious use of antimicrobial agents. Pediatrics 101:174, 1998.

Wald ER: Diagnosis and management of sinusitis in children. Adv Pediatr Infect Dis 12:1, 1996.

381.3 Acute Pharyngitis

Pharyngitis is part of most upper respiratory tract infections; however, in the strict sense, *acute pharyngitis* refers to conditions in which the principal involvement is in the throat. The presence or absence of tonsils does not affect the susceptibility, the frequency, or the course or complications of the illness. The disease is uncommon in children less than 1 yr of age. The incidence then increases to a peak at 4–7 yr but continues throughout later childhood and adult life.

ETIOLOGY. Acute pharyngitis is generally caused by viruses. Group A β-hemolytic *Streptococcus* (see Chapter 184) is the only common bacterial causative agent and, except during epidemics, it accounts for probably fewer than 15% of cases. *Mycoplasma* and *Arcanobacterium haemolyticum* may also produce pharyngitis. Other bacteria may proliferate during acute viral infections and may therefore be cultured in large numbers from the pharynx of an affected person but are not usually the causitive agent of symptoms. Pharyngeal gonococcal infection should be considered in sexually active adolescents or victims of sexual abuse.

CLINICAL MANIFESTATIONS. Viral and streptococcal pharyngitis have many overlapping signs and symptoms. **Viral pharyngitis** is generally considered a disease of relatively gradual onset with early signs of fever, malaise, and anorexia with moderate throat pain. Frequently, a close contact has a common cold. Conjunctivitis, rhinitis, cough, hoarseness, coryza, anterior stomatitis, discrete ulcerative lesions, viral exanthems, and diarrhea strongly suggest that a viral agent rather than *Streptococcus* is the cause. Small ulcers may form on the soft palate and the posterior pharyngeal wall. Exudates may appear on lymphoid follicles of the palate and tonsils and may be indistinguishable from exudates encountered with streptococcal disease. The cervical lymph nodes are often moderately enlarged and firm and may or may not be tender. Leukocyte counts have little value in differentiating viral from bacterial disease. The entire illness may last less than 24 hr and does not usually persist for more than 5 days. Significant complications are rare.

Streptococcal pharyngitis in a child older than 2 yr may begin with nonspecific complaints of headache, abdominal pain, and vomiting. These symptoms may be associated with a fever as high as 40°C (104°F). Hours after the initial complaints, the throat may become sore; however, only one third of patients demonstrate the classic tonsillar enlargement, exudates, and pharyngeal erythema. The degree of pharyngeal pain is inconstant and may vary from slight to severe cases in which swallowing is difficult. Anterior cervical lymphadenopathy usually occurs early, and the nodes are often tender. Fever may continue for 1–4 days; in severe disease, the child may remain ill for as long as 2 wk. The physical findings most suggestive of streptococcal disease are diffuse redness of the tonsils and tonsillar pillars, with a petechial mottling of the soft palate, whether or not lymphadenitis or follicular exudates are found. Clinical scoring systems have been devised to predict the probability of group A β-hemolytic streptococcal infection. The positive predictive value of these streptococcal scorecards range from 70–80%. The features most strongly suggestive of streptococcal pharyngitis are age between 5 and 15 yr, clinical evidence of acute pharyngitis, fever, and the absence of URI symptoms.

Group A β-hemolytic streptococcal infection is uncommon in children less than 2 yr. When it does occur, it may produce a more persistent illness. This form of illness, streptococcosis, is characterized by coryza with postnasal discharge, variable fever (sometimes lasting for 4–8 wk) pharyngitis, anorexia, and tender cervical lymphadenitis.

DIAGNOSIS AND DIFFERENTIAL DIAGNOSIS. Diagnosis can be made by the rapid detection method for streptococcal antigens or by culture after pharyngeal swabbing. Rapid detection has advanced from latex agglutination to optical immunoassay and chemiluminescent DNA probes, which offer sensitivity equal to standard throat culture.

A syndrome of purulent nasal discharge, pharyngitis, and fever may also be associated with positive pharyngeal cultures for pneumococci or *H. influenzae*. Although this syndrome is probably a complication of viral pharyngitis, some of these patients respond to antibiotics.

When a membranous exudate is present on the tonsils, diphtheria should be considered, especially in the underimmunized child. Infectious mononucleosis may also cause a membranous exudate resembling that found in diptheria or streptococcal pharyngitis. Mononucleosis with a secondary streptococcal infection is well recognized. Herpangina (Chapter 243) is not usually associated with tonsillar exudates but rather with many vesiculoulcerative lesions on the anterior pillars and soft palate.

Children and adolescents who smoke tobacco or marijuana excessively may acquire pharyngeal inflammation and sore throat. Allergic rhinitis with a nonpurulent postnasal drip may also cause a sore throat. Gonococcal pharyngeal infections are usually asymptomatic.

COMPLICATIONS. With viral infections, the complication rate is low, although purulent bacterial otitis media may occur. In debilitated children, both viral and streptococcal infections may lead to large, chronic ulcers in the pharynx. With bacterial disease, the spectrum of illness can extend from pharyngitis to tonsillitis to abscess formation in the retrophayngeal, lateral pharyngeal, or peritonsillar spaces. Sinusitis and otitis media are commonly associated with pharyngitis; rarely, meningitis can occur. Acute glomerulonephritis and rheumatic fever may follow streptococcal infections and are a leading reason we spend so much time and effort in promptly treating streptococcal pharyngitis (see Chapters 184.1 and 519.1).

TREATMENT. Since even exudative tonsillitis is usually of viral origin, for which there is no specific therapy, the use of antibiotics should be guided by the results of antigen detection tests or cultures, unless there are strong clinical and epidemiologic grounds to suspect a streptococcal infection. Treatment within the first 9 days after onset of symptoms is effective in preventing the long-term sequelae of rheumatic fever. Streptococcal pharyngitis is best treated orally with penicillin (125 mg for children <60 lb; 250 mg for older children and adults; three times daily for 10 days). This usually produces prompt clinical response with defervescence within 24 hr and shortens the course of illness by an average of 1.5 days. Once-daily amoxicillin (750 mg PO × 10 days) is also effective. Newer cephalosporins and macrolides are also effective, but their use should be discouraged because they are more expensive and promote development of antibiotic resistance.

Most children prefer to remain in bed during the acute phase of the disease. When throat pain is severe, acetaminophen or ibuprofen is often helpful. Gargling with warm saline solution offers some symptomatic relief for throat pain in children old enough to cooperate; in younger children the inhalation of steam occasionally produces similar effects. Because of pain on swallowing, cool bland liquids such as ginger ale are usually more acceptable than solids or hot foods. No attempt should be made to force the child to eat as long as hydration is maintained.

The child with a streptococcal infection is noninfectious to others within a few hours after penicillin therapy has begun. Reculturing is not necessary if symptoms abate. A streptococcal carrier is not at risk for rheumatic fever, is unlikely to transmit infection, and does not require treatment unless there is a history of rheumatic fever in the patient or a sibling. The carrier state does make the differentiation of subsequent pharyngitis more difficult. A few children require antibiotic prophylaxis against streptococcal disease, such as those with past history of rheumatic fever (see Chapter 184.1).

Feder H, Gerber M, Randolph M, et al: Once daily therapy for streptococcal pharyngitis with amoxicillin. Pediatrics 103:47, 1999.

Gerber MA: Strep pharyngitis: Update on management. Contemp Pediatr 14:156, 1997.

Pichichero ME, Cohen R: Shortened course of antibiotic therapy for acute otitis media, sinusitis and tonsillopharyngitis. Pediatr Infect Dis J 16:680, 1997.

Schwartz B, Marcy SM, Phillips WR, et al: Pharyngitis—principles of judicious use of antimicrobial agents. Pediatrics 101:171, 1998.

Wald ER, Green MD, Schwartz B, et al: A streptococcal score card revisited. Pediatr Emerg Care 14:109, 1998.

381.4 Acute Uvulitis

Infections of the uvula are infrequent. They are characterized by fever, pain with swallowing, and drooling. Occasionally there are no symptoms or signs referable to the pharynx. Most cases are due to group A *Streptococcus* or *H. influenzae* type b, often in association with tonsillitis or acute epiglottis. However, isolated uvulitis occurs. In general, streptococcal uvulitis tends to occur in older children (>5 yr), whereas that caused by *H. influenzae* occurs before 5 yr of age. The latter has become rare owing to the widespread use of conjugate Hib vaccine. In suspected cases blood cultures as well as cultures of the uvula and pharynx are indicated. Young children should be examined carefully for evidence of airway obstruction and treated, initially with an intravenous antibiotic that covers ampicillin-resistant *H. influenzae*. Older children can be treated as indicated for streptococcal pharyngitis.

381.5 Retropharyngeal Abscess

During early childhood, the potential space between the posterior pharyngeal wall and the prevertebral fascia contains several small lymph nodes that usually disappear during the 3rd to 4th yr of life. The lymphatic channels that communicate with these nodes drain portions of the nasopharynx as well as the posterior nasal passages. With purulent infections of these areas, the nodes may become infected; this may, in turn, progress to breakdown of the nodes and to suppuration.

ETIOLOGY. Retropharyngeal abscess is usually a complication of bacterial pharyngitis. Less frequently, it occurs after extension of infection from vertebral osteomyelitis or by wound infection following a penetrating injury of the posterior pharynx. Group A hemolytic streptococci, oral anaerobes, and *S. aureus*, in descending order of occurrence, are the most common pathogens.

CLINICAL MANIFESTATIONS. The child usually has a recent or current history of an acute nasopharyngitis or pharyngitis. There is generally an abrupt onset of high fever with difficulty in swallowing, refusal of feeding, severe distress with throat pain, hyperextension of the head, and noisy, often gurgling respirations. The respirations become increasingly labored, and secretions accumulate in the mouth and cause drooling caused by the difficulty in swallowing.

A bulge in the posterior pharyngeal wall is usually apparent. The abscess is sometimes located in an area of the nasopharynx where it may cause nasal obstruction and a bulging forward of the soft palate. Retropharyngeal abscesses may not be detectable by simple inspection. A lateral roentgenogram of the nasopharynx and neck in mild extension reveals the retropharyngeal mass. When an abscess is present, the retropharyngeal soft tissue is more than one half of the width of the adjacent vertebral body. Occasionally, air may be seen in the retropharynx.

If left untreated, the abscess may rupture into the pharynx spontaneously, resulting in aspiration of pus. It may also extend laterally and present externally on the side of the neck or dissect along fascial planes into the mediastinum. Death may occur with aspiration, airway obstruction, erosion into major blood vessels, or mediastinitis.

DIFFERENTIAL DIAGNOSIS. Pressure on the larynx may result in stridor, making retropharyngeal abscess one of the differential diagnostic possibilities in patients with high fever and croup. Many patients have limited neck motion, which may be mistaken for meningismus. Nonfluctuant lymphadenitis may produce a tender bulge in the retropharyngeal space. Tuberculosis of the cervical spine may occasionally produce a lateral retropharyngeal abscess; considerable rigidity of the neck and other signs of spinal involvement are usually present. A computed tomographic scan with contrast may differentiate an underlying pathologic condition or identify an early abscess, allowing early incision and drainage.

TREATMENT. If the abscess is recognized in the prefluctuant stage, intensive treatment with a semisynthetic penicillin (to cover penicillinase-producing *S. aureus*) may prevent suppuration and further abscess development. Single-agent treatment with clindamycin or ampicillin-sulbactam should also be effective. Analgesic drugs may be needed for pain. Because of the risk of airway obstruction, narcotics should be used with great care. When fluctuance is present, the abscess should be incised and antibiotics started; the operation is best performed under general anesthesia.

381.6 Lateral Pharyngeal Abscess

Lateral pharyngeal abscess occurs in the space lateral to the pharynx that extends from the hyoid bone to the base of the skull. The carotid vessels and jugular vein may be intimately associated with the abscess.

The patient usually has high fever and trismus, appears acutely ill, and has severe pain and difficulty when swallowing. The bulge in the lateral pharyngeal wall is obvious. Cervical adenitis is usually present, and torticollis toward the side of the abscess due to muscular spasm is common. Microbiologic features are identical to those of retropharyngeal abscess. Treatment usually requires lateral neck drainage.

381.7 Peritonsillar Abscess

Peritonsillar abscess occurs in the potential space between the superior constrictor muscle and the tonsil (usually at the superior pole). It is almost always caused by group A β-hemolytic streptococci or oral anaerobes in preadolescent or adolescent patients.

CLINICAL MANIFESTATIONS. The abscess is usually preceded by acute pharyngotonsillitis. There may be an afebrile interval of several days, or the fever of the primary infection may not subside. The patient has severe throat pain and trismus because of spasm of the pterygoid muscles and often refuses to swallow or speak. Speech may be characterized as "hot potato" voice. Occasionally, there is sufficient spasm of the homolateral muscles of the neck to produce torticollis. The fever may be septic and reach 40.5°C (105°F). The affected tonsillar area is markedly swollen and inflamed; the uvula is displaced to the opposite side. In untreated patients, the abscess becomes fluctuant within a few days and usually points in the region of the anterior faucial pillar. If the abscess is not incised, spontaneous rupture occurs.

TREATMENT. Antibiotics (usually penicillin) and incision and drainage or aspiration of purulence are required. Outpatient treatment is possible; however, young children usually require general anesthesia and hospitalization. If there is no history of chronic tonsillitis, the chance of recurrence is approximately 10%, and tonsillectomy is not required. If there is a prior history of tonsillitis or a previous abscess, a tonsillectomy should be considered.

CHAPTER 382
Tonsils and Adenoids

Margaret A. Kenna

The term *tonsils* is used in its commonly accepted sense of indicating the two faucial tonsils; the term *adenoids* refers to the nasopharyngeal tonsil. The tonsils and adenoids are part of the lymphoid tissues that circle the pharynx and are known collectively as *Waldeyer's ring*. This consists of the lymphoid tissue on the base of the tongue (lingual tonsil), the two faucial tonsils, the adenoids, and the lymphoid tissue on the posterior pharyngeal wall. This tissue serves as a defense against infection, but it may become a site of acute or chronic infection.

The principal disease processes affecting the tonsils and adenoids are infection and hypertrophy. The latter is often temporary and secondary to infection. Although both tonsils and adenoids are often removed at the same operation, separate tonsillectomy or adenoidectomy may be indicated, especially in children less than 4–5 yr of age. Other abnormalities of the tonsils and adenoids are uncommon in infancy and childhood.

Neoplasms of the tonsils are rare, although 7% of non-Hodgkin lymphomas present in Waldeyer's ring. Rhabdomyosarcomas are the most common malignant nasal tumor in children, and the nasopharynx is a common presenting site (see Chapter 506.1). Adenoid hypertrophy may thus be clinically confused with rhabdomyosarcoma presenting in the nasopharynx.

Acute infections of the tonsils are considered as acute pharyngitis and are discussed in Chapter 381.3.

382.1 Chronic Tonsillitis (Chronically Hypertrophic and Infected Tonsils)

The management of chronic tonsillitis is of special concern because of its frequency and because tonsils are potentially important to the normal development of the immune system.

CLINICAL MANIFESTATIONS. These vary considerably; the significant features are recurrent or persistent sore throat, pain with swallowing, and obstruction to swallowing or breathing. There may be a sense of dryness and irritation in the throat, and the breath may be offensive; these symptoms may be more common with chronic mouth breathing. Constitutional symptoms of chronic tonsillitis are not well defined; children and parents may complain of enlarged cervical lymph nodes, fatigue, decreased appetite, and poor weight gain. Some of these symptoms may be seen in other chronic illnesses as well. Children with chronic tonsillitis may also have adenotonsillar hypertrophy causing symptoms of airway obstruction. Symptoms of adenotonsillar hypertrophy include snoring, mouth breathing, gasping and pausing during sleep, and apnea. Children with severe obstruction may fall asleep during the day, experience enuresis when they were formerly dry at night, and lose (or fail to gain) weight because of the increased calories used for breathing. Rarely, hypertrophied tonsils and adenoids obstructing the upper airway are associated with respiratory distress, chronic hypoxemia, and the development of pulmonary hypertension and cor pulmonale(see Chapter 383).

INDICATIONS FOR TONSILLECTOMY

Chronic Tonsillitis. For children with recurrent throat infections (seven in the past year, five in each of the past 2 yr, or 3 in each of the past 3 yr, or more than any of these), tonsillectomy decreases the number of throat infections in the subsequent 2 yr, compared with no tonsillectomy. However, many children meeting these criteria who have not had tonsillectomy also have a decline in the number of throat infections. Similarly, children with chronic, but fewer incidences of, sore throat illness than described also benefit from tonsillectomy; many of these children do get better without surgery, however. Factors such as severity of illness, the frequency of missing school or child care, any associated complications, or the presence of other medical issues all need to be considered.

Hypertrophic Tonsil and Adenoids. Many children who are referred with the diagnosis of hypertrophied tonsils actually have tonsils that are normal in size for a child of that particular age. Large size alone, without symptoms of obstruction or infection, is not an indication to remove the tonsils. These inappropriate referrals result from the failure to appreciate that it is normal for tonsils to be relatively larger during childhood than in later years, and unless the tonsils are causing medical problems, there is no need for removal.

Tonsils may virtually meet in the midline in some children who are asymptomatic; tonsils of average size are projected toward the midline when the child is gagged and may be interpreted as being hypertrophic. Alternatively, infection does not always produce hypertrophy, and chronically infected tonsils may be small and embedded behind the faucial pillars. There is no certain way to demonstrate directly whether tonsils are harboring chronic infection. Swabs of the tonsil that are then cultured may not grow any pathogenic bacteria, yet if that same tonsil is removed and the core cultured, bacteria may be obtained. The consistency or size of the tonsils and the presence of cheesy material within the crypts are also not reliable guides. Persistent hyperemia of the anterior pillars is a more reliable sign, and enlargement of the cervical lymph nodes is supporting evidence. Persistent enlargement of the node just below and slightly in front of the angle of the jaw is especially significant. Hypertrophy sufficient to obstruct swallowing or breathing is often detectable; such tonsils practically meet in the midline when the throat is examined. However, before tonsillectomy is recommended, it should be ascertained that the hypertrophy is chronic and not the result of a recent acute infection. Tonsils can increase in size greatly during an acute infection and recede after its subsidence, either on their own or in response to a course of antibiotics.

Although chronic or recurrent tonsillitis or adenotonsillar hypertrophy are the usual reasons for tonsillectomy, the only absolute indications for tonsillectomy are the exclusion of tumor and severe aerodigestive tract obstruction (usually severe sleep apnea). Tonsillectomy is of no value in the prevention or treatment of acute or chronic sinusitis, chronic otitis media, and middle ear deafness. There is also no evidence to indicate that the removal of tonsils is justified for infections in the lower respiratory tract. No systemic disturbance in itself is an indication for tonsillectomy. Neither tonsillectomy nor adenoidectomy should be performed as prophylaxis against the "common cold" at any age.

Tonsillectomy in Relation to the Age of the Child. Tonsillectomy in children less than 2–3 yr is generally performed for obstructive sleep symptoms rather than tonsillitis, which is more common in older children. When tonsillectomy is recommended for a child 2–3 yr of age, an overnight stay in the hospital is usually also recommended. In the first few years of life, the indications for adenoidectomy, usually hypertrophy with airway obstruction or otitis media, are present more often than are those for tonsillectomy.

Tonsillectomy in Relation to Active Infection. Tonsillectomy should be postponed until 2–3 wk after subsidence of an infection, except in rare cases of acute respiratory obstruction with pulmonary artery hypertension and cor pulmonale. The other exception to delaying treatment is tonsillectomy for treatment of a peritonsillar abscess; tonsillectomy with drainage of the abscess is often the treatment of choice (see Chapter 381.7).

COMPLICATIONS OF TONSILLECTOMY. The mean duration of postoperative sore throat is 5 days. Referred ear pain and halitosis are common. Minor hemorrhage, postoperative throat infection, or anesthetic complications occur in more than 10% of procedures. Severe hemorrhage or life-threatening complications occur occasionally and are another reason for carefully assessing the indications for surgical intervention. Pulmonary edema, although uncommon, may occur after relief of upper airway obstruction with tonsillectomy or adenoidectomy. Therefore, this therapy should be reserved for settings in which postsurgical respiratory failure can be dealt with effectively. In patients older than 3 yr, outpatient tonsil and adenoid surgery can be performed safely and may be mandated by insurance carriers; however, surgery for airway obstruction and other conditions requires inpatient surgery and intensive postoperative monitoring.

382.2 Adenoidal Hypertrophy (Hypertrophy of Pharyngeal Tonsil; "Adenoids")

Disease of the nasopharyngeal lymphoid tissue (adenoids) tends to parallel that of the faucial tonsils. Hypertrophy and infection may occur separately but often occur together; infection is usually primary. The soft adenoid structure, which occupies most of the posterior superior pharyngeal wall in children, often undergoes hypertrophy, and masses of lymphoid tissue of varying size are formed. These masses may almost fill the vault of the nasopharynx, interfere with the passage of air through the nose, obstruct the eustachian tubes, and block the clearance of nasal mucus.

CLINICAL MANIFESTATIONS. Mouth breathing and persistent rhinitis and nasal drainage are the most characteristic symptoms. Mouth breathing may be present only during sleep, especially when the child lies supine, when snoring is also likely to occur. With severe adenoid hypertrophy, the mouth is kept open during the day as well, and the mucous membranes of the mouth and lips are dry. Chronic nasopharyngitis may be constantly present or recur frequently. The voice is altered with a nasal, muffled quality. The breath is offensive, and taste and smell are impaired. A harassing cough may be present, especially at night, resulting from drainage of pus into the lower pharynx or irritation of the larynx by inspired air that has not been warmed and moistened by passage through the nose. Chronic otitis media may be associated with infected, hypertrophied adenoids and blockage of the eustachian tube orifices; hearing loss is often present secondary to middle ear fluid. Chronic mouth breathing may predispose to a narrow, high-arched palate and an elongated mandible with a characteristic anterior open bite. Referrals from orthodontists for evaluation of nasal obstruction and adenoidectomy are frequent.

A small number of young children with marked adenoidal (also tonsillar) enlargement are unable to breathe through the mouth during sleep. They snort and snore loudly and often display signs of respiratory distress, such as intercostal retractions and nasal flaring. These children are at risk for respiratory insufficiency (hypoxemia, hypercapnia, acidosis) during sleep. Obstructive sleep apnea may result, and some of these children acquire pulmonary arterial hypertension and, ultimately, cor pulmonale (see Chapter 383). Very obese children (e.g., those with Prader-Willi syndrome) and children with a large or posteriorly placed tongue (e.g., those with Pierre Robin syndrome) may also develop experience airway obstruction in sleep, mimicking or complicating the symptoms of adenoid (and tonsillar) hypertrophy. Patients with Down syndrome commonly have macroglossia, tonsillar enlargement, and skull base anomalies, which make them susceptible to obstruction.

DIAGNOSIS. During the first few years of life, the size of adenoids can be assessed by digital palpation. Indirect visualization with a pharyngeal mirror is possible in older, cooperative children. Alternatively, the fiberoptic nasopharyngoscope can be used for visualization of the nasopharynx. Lateral pharyngeal soft tissue radiographs are also helpful for detecting nasopharyngeal air column obliteration. The presence of adenoid hypertrophy can be suspected from such manifestations as mouth breathing, snoring, persistent rhinitis, and recurrent sinusitis.

TREATMENT. Adenoidectomy may be indicated for symptoms such as persistent mouth breathing, hyponasal speech, adenoid facies, repeated or chronic otitis media with effusion, and persistent or recurring nasopharyngitis when these seem to be related to infected hypertrophied adenoid tissue. Tonsillectomy should not be performed routinely for such problems unless separate indications for tonsillectomy exist. Chronic serous otitis media may improve after adenoidectomy in some patients. The same precautions for the complete removal and control of bleeding points, such as in tonsillectomy, should be observed.

Coulthard M, Isaacs D: Retropharyngeal abscess. Arch Dis Child 66:1227, 1991.
Gates GA, Avery CA, Prihoda TJ: Effectiveness of adenoidectomy and tympanostomy tubes in the treatment of chronic otitis media with effusion. N Engl J Med 317:1444, 1987.
Paradise JL: Adenoidectomy and adenotonsillectomy for recurrent or persistent otitis media: Still commonly performed and still controversial (abstract). Pediatr Res 31:99A, 1992.
Paradise JL, Bernard BS, Colborn K, et al: Assessment of adenoidal obstruction in children: Clinical signs versus roentgenographic findings. Pediatrics 101:979, 1998.
Paradise JL, Bluestone CD, Backman RZ, et al: Efficacy of tonsillectomy for recurrent throat infection in severely affected children. N Engl J Med 310:674, 1984. (An older article but the classic one for tonsillectomy.)
Paradise JL, Bluestone CD, Backman RZ, et al: History of recurrent sore throat as an indication for tonsillectomy. N Engl J Med 298:410, 1978.
Rosenfeld RM, Tonsillectomy and adenoidectomy: Changing trends. Ann Otol Rhinol Laryngol 99:187, 1990.
Sclafani AP, Ginsburg J, Shah MK, et al: Treatment of symptomatic chronic adenotonsillar hypertrophy with amoxicillin/clavulanate potassium: Short and long term results. Pediatrics 101:675, 1998.
Spires JR: Treatment of peritonsillar abscess: A prospective study of aspiration vs incision and drainage. Arch Otolaryngol Head Neck Surg 113:984, 1987.
Wiatrak BJ, Myer CM III, Andrews TM: Complications of adenotonsillectomy in children under three years of age. Otolaryngol Head Neck Surg 104:509, 1991.

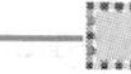

CHAPTER 383 Obstructive Sleep Apnea and Hypoventilation in Children

Carol L. Rosen and Gabriel G. Haddad

Obstructive sleep apnea/hypoventilation (OSA/H) (also see Chapters 64.3 and 382) is a common problem in children that is characterized by a combination of prolonged partial upper airway obstruction and intermittent complete obstruction (obstructive apnea) that disrupts sleep and breathing patterns. It can lead to impaired daytime performance as well as more serious complications such as heart failure, developmental delay, poor growth, and death. Habitual snoring, the most common symptom, occurs in 8–10% of young school children. Although there are no rigorous epidemiologic studies, severe OSA/H is estimated to occur in 1% of children. The OSA/H peak age of 2–5 yr coincides with normal lymphoid hyperplasia and frequent upper respiratory infections. In prepubertal children, the incidence in males and females is similar, which contrasts with the male predominance seen in adults.

PATHOGENESIS. OSA/H occurs when there is a failure to maintain upper airway patency during sleep, which, in turn, affects blood gas homeostasis. Decreased patency can be complete or incomplete and usually occurs during sleep. In severe cases, obstruction is present in both wakefulness and sleep. Normally, airway patency is actively maintained by the dilator muscles of the upper airway. These muscles counterbalance the forces that tend to collapse the upper airway, such as the intraluminal negative pressure generated by the diaphragm and mucosal adhesion forces. Under normal conditions, upper airway patency is maintained despite the fact that the pharyngeal airway is a collapsible tube and the upper airway muscle tone decreases remarkably during sleep, especially during rapid eye movement (REM) sleep. In normal children, arterial oxygen decreases and carbon dioxide increases only slightly during sleep. Conditions that decrease caliber, increase collapsibility, or alter neural control of the upper airway contribute to the development of obstruction. This cascade of events is depicted in Figure 383–1; as upper airway muscle activity decreases, the upper airway narrows and upper airway resistance increases in the presence of anatomic or neurologic factors. Episodes of partial or complete airway obstruction result in impaired gas exchange with hypoxemia and hypercapnia. Decreased airflow, hypercapnia, and hypoxemia are potent stimuli for increased ventilatory effort and upper airway muscle activity. Increased effort and airway muscle tone lead to resumption of airway patency. Arousal from sleep (in the form of electroencephalographic changes, increased muscle tone, or movement) also helps in restoring blood gases. When airflow is restored, oxygen and carbon dioxide levels return to normal. Sleep is re-established, upper airway muscle activity decreases, and the cycle starts again. This cyclicity occurs in the adult population with OSA, and such patients can have up to 400 arousals per night. In the pediatric population with OSA/H, this cyclicity is not well established: Arousals are much rarer in spite of continued hypoventilation and blood gas disturbances throughout the night.

The development of OSA/H can have serious cardiorespiratory and neurobehavioral consequences. Chronic hypoxemia can lead to polycythemia, growth failure, increased pulmonary artery pressure and pulmonary hypertension, right-sided heart failure, arrhythmias, or even death. Recurrent arousals can lead to sleep fragmentation, loss of normal sleep patterns, and excessive daytime sleepiness. OSA/H has been associated with other daytime sequelae including behavioral problems, impaired school performance, and accidents. Finally, sleep fragmentation itself can suppress arousal responses and further impair the ability to re-establish upper airway patency and restore gas exchange.

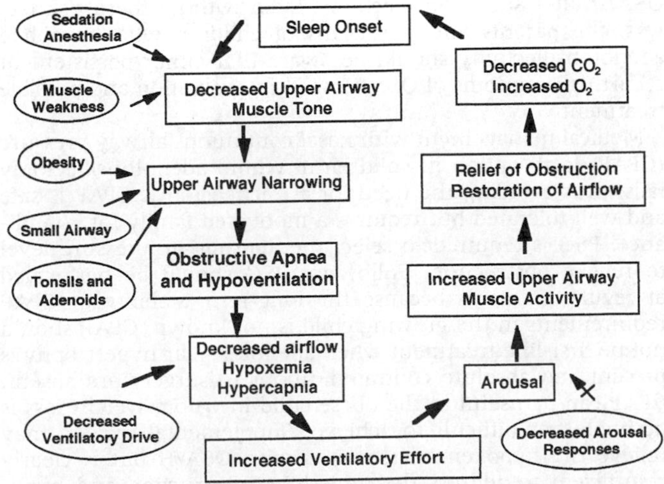

Figure 383–1 Pathophysiology of OSA/H in children.

TABLE 383–1 Predisposing Factors to Obstructive Sleep-Apnea and Hypoventilation

Anatomic factors that narrow the upper airway
Adenotonsillar hypertrophy
Trisomy 21
Other genetic or craniofacial syndromes associated with
Midface hypoplasia
Small nasopharynx
Micrognathia or retrognathia
Choanal atresia or stenosis
Macroglossia
Cleft palate
Obesity
Nasal obstruction
Laryngomalacia
Sickle cell disease
Velopharyngeal flap repair
Neurologic factors that decrease pharyngeal muscular dilator activity
Medications—sedatives or general anesthesia
Brain stem disorders—Chiari malformation, birth asphyxia
Neuromuscular disease

Several medical conditions are major risk factors for OSA/H (Table 383–1). In children, the most common anatomic factor associated with obstruction is adenotonsillar hypertrophy. Other anatomic factors, such as micrognathia, retrognathia, or macroglossia, may force the tongue into the oropharyngeal portion of the airway and occlude it. Fat deposition from morbid obesity or a congenitally small airway also narrows the nasopharynx. Increased resistance from swollen nasal turbinates or choanal stenosis places a greater negative collapsing pressure on the pharyngeal airway. Diminished ventilatory responses to hypoxemia and hypercapnia can attenuate the increase in ventilatory effort and impair an adequate response. Diminished arousal responses can impair the ability to restore upper airway patency (see Fig. 383–1). Finally, sedative medication or general anesthesia can further compromise neural control of the upper airway.

CLINICAL MANIFESTATIONS. Primary snoring, upper airway resistance syndrome, obstructive hypoventilation, and obstructive sleep apnea represent a spectrum of clinical manifestations accompanying increasing severity of upper airway obstruction. However, the majority of children with OSA/H do not present with dramatic, repetitive obstructive apneas. Instead, obstruction is partial and tonic. When phasic obstructive apnea is rare, arousals are infrequent and sleep architecture may not be disturbed. For this reason, daytime hypersomnolence, the most common presenting symptom of OSA/H in adults, is rare in children. Because of this more subtle presentation, children often have an unexpected degree of airway obstruction, impairment of gas exchange, and sleep disturbance that is difficult to predict from the clinical history and physical examination alone.

Common clinical manifestations of OSA/H include chronic mouth breathing, snoring, and restlessness during sleep with or without frequent awakenings. Children may sleep in unusual positions to help maintain a patent upper airway, for example, with the neck hyperextended or prone with the bottom up in the air. Typically, loud snoring is the symptom that most disturbs, and therefore alerts, the parents. Most children with OSA/H breathe normally while awake, but children with the more severe presentation also have noisy, mildly labored awake breathing that clearly worsens with sleep. Parents describe that cyclically, the snoring becomes very loud, followed by silence, a snort, an arousal, and resumption of snoring. When snoring is associated with nocturnal breathing difficulties and witnessed respiratory pauses, this triad of symptoms is highly suggestive of OSA/H in children. However, clinical experience suggests that some infants with serious OSA/H have little or no snoring, and their diagnosis depends on the physician's high index of suspicion.

Less common symptoms include daytime hypersomnolence

resulting from sleep fragmentation that occurs when obstructive apnea is repeatedly terminated by arousals. Behavioral problems and poor school performance have been described, but the incidence of these problems in OSA/H is unknown. However, it is difficult to recognize excessive sleepiness in young children, who normally have daytime naps and early bedtimes. Secondary enuresis that disappears after surgical relief of the upper airway obstruction is occasionally seen, but the mechanisms are poorly understood. In contrast to adults, most children with OSA/H are not obese. In fact, some children are underweight or present with failure to thrive. Several factors can contribute to this growth retardation: dysphagia from large tonsils, chronic hypoxemia, higher metabolic expenditure from increased work of breathing, and insufficient growth hormone release in the absence of deep REM sleep. Children can also present with unexplained right-sided heart failure, but other cardiovascular complications, such as systemic hypertension or life-threatening cardiac arrhythmias, are rarely seen, except in the most long-standing and neglected cases. Finally, in the more severe cases, a relatively minor respiratory illness or infection can trigger an acute episode of respiratory failure.

DIAGNOSIS AND ASSESSMENT. The diagnosis of OSA/H in children is often delayed, despite years of symptoms, for several reasons: (1) absence of awake symptoms, (2) failure to obtain a sleep history, (3) symptoms of snoring or restless sleep are considered inconsequential, (4) parents may be unaware of the problem because the child's most severe symptoms appear during REM sleep in the last 3rd of the night when parents are asleep, and (5) young children may not generate the loud, disruptive snoring noises of an adult. The diagnosis should be suggested by the clinical presentation. A sleep history should be part of every well child examination, and parental reports of habitual snoring should not be dismissed without further investigation. A sleep and breathing history is also important for any child with a medical condition that is a risk factor for OSA/H, especially trisomy 21, craniofacial anomalies, or neuromuscular disorders.

OSA/H cannot be diagnosed from clinical history alone. The physical examination performed during wakefulness may be entirely normal but should not be used to exclude OSA/H when the clinical history suggests otherwise. Features associated with OSA/H include dysmorphic facies, mouth breathing, hyponasal speech, macroglossia, cleft palate, or enlarged tonsils. However, snoring, reports of difficulty breathing, and enlarged tonsils are unreliable predictors of the presence or severity of OSA/H in children. Specific craniofacial anomalies may be apparent. A pectus excavatum deformity can develop in long-standing upper airway obstruction. Morbid obesity mechanically loads the chest wall and narrows the upper airway, but OSA/H is not a consistent feature of obesity. The presence of excessive somnolence during the examination requires urgent evaluation. The presence of stridor or hoarse voice can indicate cranial nerve dysfunction and should prompt a meticulous neurologic examination. In particular, cranial nerve dysfunction, weakness, hyperreflexia, and loss of position and vibratory sense point to brain stem and spinal cord abnormalities. The evaluation would include polysomnography (PSG) or magnetic resonance imaging, or both, with attention to the brain stem, cervicomedullary junction, and spinal cord.

Laboratory findings such as polycythemia or respiratory acidosis with a metabolic alkalosis support the diagnosis of OSA/H when present, but these findings are absent in the majority of pediatric patients. Right ventricular hypertrophy on electrocardiography and dysfunction on echocardiography are seen only in severe cases of OSA/H. A lateral soft tissue radiograph of the neck can identify adenoidal tissue but fails to give a three-dimensional, supine view of the airway during sleep. Although computed tomography or magnetic resonance imaging of the nasopharynx displays airway dimensions and fluoroscopy or endoscopy shows airway dynamics, these imaging techniques are only "snapshots" of the disorder. When procedures require sedation or anesthesia, extreme caution is required if OSA/H is suspected. Such medications have profound effects on upper airway muscle tone, and sudden respiratory decompensation can occur in these children.

PSG, an overnight recording of multiple physiologic sensors during sleep, is the "gold standard" for the diagnosis of OSA/H (see Chapter 377). PSG provides a powerful, quantitative, noninvasive assessment of gas exchange impairment, respiratory pattern, thoracoabdominal movement, and sleep disruption. PSG is especially useful in confirming the diagnosis, in determining the severity of OSA/H, and in documenting the efficacy of treatment. PSG may not be required for diagnostic purposes in all patients. For example, PSG may not be necessary when a child has noisy, awake mouth breathing and tonsils that occlude most of the pharyngeal space; is excessively sleepy; and is observed by skilled personnel to have signs of airway obstruction (apnea and retractions) and hypoxemia. However, in the majority of cases, the clinical presentation is not so obvious. Even though PSG may not be required for diagnosis before treatment, it can provide an important clinical baseline to assess the severity and efficacy of treatment, especially in children who are at increased risk for either failure of adenotonsillectomy or operative and postoperative complications. This group includes very young children and children with complex medical problems or craniofacial anomalies.

Several other disorders should be considered in the differential diagnosis of OSA/H or may coexist with this problem. Occasionally, breathing difficulty associated with nocturnal asthma or upper airway obstruction from gastroesophageal reflux may be confused with OSA/H. New-onset dysphagia and swallowing difficulties associated with an esophageal foreign body that compresses the airway can masquerade as OSA/H. Stridor due to anatomic airway problems, such as laryngomalacia, vascular ring, intraluminal masses, and vocal cord dysfunction, should be considered. Parasomnia events, such as night terrors or even nocturnal seizures, may be mistaken for arousals associated with OSA/H. Narcolepsy and restless leg syndrome should be considered when PSG fails to document OSA/H in a child with daytime hypersomnolence.

TREATMENT. Because adenotonsillar hyperplasia is the most common condition associated with pediatric OSA/H, adenotonsillectomy provides definitive relief of obstruction in the majority of patients. Children with severe OSA/H who benefit from surgery often demonstrate "catch-up" growth. However, children with underlying problems, such as trisomy 21, craniofacial disorders, extreme obesity, neuromuscular disorders such as cerebral palsy or Chiari malformation, or who present before 2 yr of age are at risk for incomplete resolution of OSA/H after adenotonsillectomy. Even without these risk factors, the parents and physicians of children who have had adenotonsillectomy should be aware that either persistent or recurring symptoms of OSA/H need re-evaluation and possible treatment.

Medical management with nasal continuous airway pressure (CPAP) is an option in children in whom adenotonsillectomy fails, thus avoiding the need for a tracheostomy. CPAP is safe and well tolerated but requires a motivated family for compliance. PSG is required to select the appropriate pressure level to relieve obstruction. Follow-up PSG should be performed at regular intervals because the long-term stability of CPAP requirements in the growing child is not known. CPAP should not be first-line treatment when adenotonsillar hypertrophy is present and absolute contraindications to surgery are absent. CPAP can be useful in the obese child in whom weight loss is desirable but difficult to achieve. Supplemental oxygen may relieve the hypoxemia associated with OSA/H but is clearly insufficient to address the underlying obstruction and hypoventilation.

Pharmacologic management has only a limited role in pediatric OSA/H patients. Snoring associated with nasal obstruction can be treated with nasal decongestants and topical steroids, but this management is rarely sufficient to reverse significant OSA/H. Medroxyprogesterone acetate augments ventilatory drive and has been used in the management of the daytime hypoventilation associated with the obesity-hypoventilation syndrome. However, this drug fails to improve nocturnal obstructive symptoms and has adverse effects on growth and pubertal development. Protriptyline is a nonsedating antidepressant with REM suppressant activity that has been tried in adult OSA/H patients. Although it reduces the number of more severe obstructive apnea episodes by decreasing the amount of sleep time spent in REM, it fails to treat the obstructive process and is not recommended.

If serious upper airway obstruction is present in both wakefulness and sleep, tracheostomy is the treatment of choice for vocal cord dysfunction, impaired swallowing, and absent laryngeal protective reflexes. Definitive maxillomandibular reconstructive surgery for children with craniofacial disorders is another therapeutic option but is usually postponed until facial growth is complete. Uvulopalatopharyngoplasty, the resection of redundant pharyngeal tissue, has been used to eliminate snoring in adults, but the failure rate is high. Pediatric experience with this surgery has been limited to children with muscular hypotonia and oropharyngeal tissue redundancy, but no controlled studies using objective measures of efficacy have been performed.

Brooks LJ, Stephens BM, Bacerice AM: Adenoid size is related to severity but not the number of episodes of obstructive apnea in children. J Pediatr 132:682, 1998.

Carroll J: Sleep-related upper-airway obstruction in children and adolescents. Child Adolesc Psychiatry Clin North Am 5:617, 1996.

Gaultier C: Sleep-related breathing disorders: 6. Obstructive sleep apnoea syndrome in infants and children: Established facts and unsettled issues. Thorax 50:1204, 1995.

Gozal D: Sleep-disordered breathing and school performance in children. Pediatrics 102:616, 1998.

Guilleminault C, Korobkin R, Winkle R: A review of 50 children with obstructive sleep apnea syndrome. Lung 159:275, 1981.

Rosen CL, D'Andrea L, Haddad GG: Adult criteria for obstructive sleep apnea do not identify children with serious obstruction. Am Rev Respir Dis 146:1231, 1992.

Ward SL, Marcus CL: Obstructive sleep apnea in infants and young children. J Clin Neurophysiol 13:198, 1996.

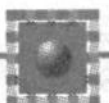

SECTION 3

Lower Respiratory Tract

CHAPTER 384

Congenital Anomalies

Robert C. Stern

384.1 Laryngeal Anomalies

Complete **atresia of the larynx** is incompatible with life; only rarely can an infant found to have this anomaly at birth be saved by immediate needle tracheostomy and high-pressure transtracheal ventilation. A formal tracheostomy is then performed. Subsequent successful surgical restoration of an adequate upper airway has not been reported. Patients with laryngeal atresia often have other congenital defects that also may be incompatible with life. **Laryngeal webs** are uncommon, occasionally familial, defects resulting from incomplete separation of the fetal mesenchyme between the two sides of the larynx. Most webs occur between the vocal cords. Immediate diagnosis of a complete or nearly complete web is essential to prevent asphyxiation of the newborn. The child may have respiratory distress with severe stridor, and the cry is weak and abnormal in character. The obstruction is often incomplete, with only mild stridor and dyspnea. Direct laryngoscopy is required for prompt diagnosis and treatment. Lysis with a carbon dioxide laser is frequently successful, but surgery is occasionally necessary. Thin supraglottic webs can also be incised, but infants with thicker subglottic or intralaryngeal webs require initial incision, excision, and subsequent dilations, which may be unsuccessful because of reformation of the web. An external approach to divide and excise the web with insertion of silicone or metal is often required. Many surgically treated patients need a tracheostomy for a prolonged period thereafter.

Laryngotracheoesophageal cleft is a rare congenital lesion in which there is a long connection between the airway and the esophagus, sometimes extending to the level of the carina. The lesion is caused by failure of dorsal fusion of the cricoid, which normally is completed by the 8th wk of gestation. Several subtypes have been reported. Type 1 lesions are those above the superior portion of the posterior cricoid plate; type 2 lesions extend to the inferior aspect of the posterior cricoid plate; type 3 includes those that involve the "cervical trachea," and type 4 extend into the thoracic trachea and below. Other anomalies, including unilateral pulmonary hypoplasia, may be present. Gestational polyhydramnios is a common association. Symptoms of chronic aspiration, gagging during feeding, and pneumonia suggest H-type tracheoesophageal fistula, but the clinical manifestations are usually more severe and associated with abnormalities in voice. Diagnosis is extremely difficult, but careful roentgenographic studies of swallowing may show aspiration of contrast material into the trachea, indicating the need for endoscopic examination of the airway and perhaps the esophagus. The prognosis depends on the severity of the lesion. Some type 1 lesions can be repaired endoscopically. Successful repair of more severe lesions has been reported but always requires many procedures and prolonged tracheostomy.

384.2 Congenital Laryngeal Stridor

(Including Laryngomalacia and Tracheomalacia)

Stridor persisting or appearing after the first few days of life usually results from disturbances in or adjacent to the larynx. The most common of these, **laryngomalacia** and **tracheomalacia,** are congenital deformities or flabbiness of the epiglottis and supraglottic aperture and weakness of the airway walls, leading to collapse and some airway obstruction with inspiration. Laryngomalacia is the most common congenital laryngeal abnormality. The dominant feature in more than half the cases is floppy arytenoid cartilages; the remainder are equally divided between a floppy epiglottis and short aryepiglottic folds. In about 35% of infants with laryngomalacia, an additional anatomic finding (e.g., tracheomalacia, subglottic stenosis, vocal cord paralysis) is also present. Tracheomalacia is occasionally accompanied by bronchomalacia. Primary bronchomalacia without tracheomalacia is discussed in Chapter 384.3. The embryologic origin of the defect is unknown.

CLINICAL MANIFESTATIONS. Noisy, crowing respiratory sounds, usually associated with inspiration, are relatively common during the neonatal period and the first year of life. Stridor, usually present from birth, may not appear until 2 mo in some patients. In symptomatic patients with laryngomalacia, the male:female ratio may be 2.5:1. Symptoms can be intermittent and are worse when affected infants lie on their backs. Some infants merely have noisy breathing, but others have a laryngeal "crow," hoarseness or aphonia, dyspnea, and inspiratory retractions in the supraclavicular, intercostal, and subcostal space. When retractions are severe, thoracic deformity may result. Infants with severe dyspnea may have difficulty nursing, resulting in undernutrition and poor weight gain. Substantial stridor may persist for several months to 1 yr after birth, occasionally becoming slightly worse in the first few months of life and then gradually disappearing with growth and development of the airway.

DIAGNOSIS. Laryngomalacia can usually be diagnosed by direct laryngoscopy. In the first few days of life, differentiating a congenital laryngeal disturbance from neonatal tetany or laryngeal edema secondary to trauma or aspiration at birth may be difficult. The differential diagnosis includes malformations of the laryngeal cartilages or vocal cords, intraluminal webs, generalized severe chondromalacia of the larynx and trachea, tumors of the larynx, mucus retention cysts, branchial cleft cysts, thyroglossal duct remnants, hypoplasia of the mandible, macroglossia, hemangioma, lymphangioma, Pierre Robin syndrome, congenital goiters, compression of an airway by an innominate artery, subglottic hemangioma, and other vascular anomalies. Other respiratory tract anomalies may be common in patients with laryngomalacia, especially those who are older than 4 mo at presentation. This suggests that full bronchoscopy, rather than laryngoscopy alone, is indicated in these patients.

TREATMENT. Usually no specific therapy is indicated for laryngomalacia; the condition resolves spontaneously, although there may be difficulty in feeding. In one review, only 4/1,415 patients required tracheostomy. Parents should be reassured about the ultimate resolution and counseled to provide slow, careful feedings. A small nipple or dropper or, infrequently, gavage may be required. Most patients seem more comfortable or less noisy lying in a prone position. Severe symptoms may require nasotracheal intubation or, rarely, tracheostomy. Other anatomic laryngeal abnormalities may require surgical intervention or laser treatment. Aortopexy has occasionally been performed for innominate artery compression of an airway.

PROGNOSIS. Although laryngomalacia usually resolves clinically by 18 mo of age, some degree of inspiratory obstruction may persist a little longer. Sophisticated pulmonary function testing reveals that minor abnormalities persist into the teenage years in some patients, but these do not pose any clinically important problems and do not require treatment. However, some patients may develop stridor with respiratory infection, exertion, or crying throughout childhood.

OTHER ANOMALIES. Bifid epiglottis, resulting from cleavage of two thirds or more of the epiglottis, is a rare condition that may not compromise swallowing. It usually does require treatment, however, and is associated with other laryngeal anomalies and with polydactyly. Total absence of the epiglottis is extremely rare. Laryngeal cysts and laryngoceles are occasionally seen; treatment with endoscopic "unroofing" is usually successful.

DuBois JJ, Pokorny WJ, Harberg FJ, et al: Current management of laryngeal and laryngotracheoesophageal clefts. J Pediatr Surg 25:855, 1990.

Fang SH, Ocejo R, Sin M, et al: Congenital laryngeal atresia. Am J Dis Child 143:625, 1989.

Filston HC, Ferguson TB, Oldham HN: Airway obstruction by vascular anomalies. Ann Surg 205:541, 1984.

Lis G, Szczerbinski T, Cichocka-Jarosz E: Congenital stridor. Pediatr Pulmonol 20:220, 1995.

Macfarlane PI, Olinsky A, Phelan PD: Proximal airway function 8–16 years after laryngomalacia: Follow-up using flow-volume loop studies. J Pediatr 107:216, 1985.

Mancuso RF: Stridor in neonates. Pediatr Clin North Am 6:1339, 1996.

Marcus CL, Crockett DM, Ward SLD: Evaluation of epiglottoplasty as treatment for severe laryngomalacia. J Pediatr 117:706, 1990.

Nussbaum E, Maggi JC: Laryngomalacia in children. Chest 98:942, 1990.

Smith RJH, Catlin FI: Congenital anomalies of the larynx. Am J Dis Child 138:35, 1984.

TRACHEOESOPHAGEAL FISTULA

See Chapter 319.

VASCULAR RING

See Chapter 439.

384.3 Bronchomalacia

Bronchomalacia may accompany laryngotracheomalacia or tracheomalacia, or it may occur as an isolated congenital lesion (see also Chapter 384.2).

CLINICAL MANIFESTATIONS. The dominant finding, low-pitched wheezing, is often prominent centrally. When the lesion involves only one mainstem bronchus (usually the left), the wheezing is louder on that side, and delayed air entry can be detected with a double-headed stethoscope. Otherwise, air entry is monophonic (uniform). Hyperinflation does not occur unless the patient also has reactive airways. Thus, most patients do not improve with use of bronchodilators, and β-adrenergic agents may cause worsening.

DIAGNOSIS. Pulmonary function testing may show flattening of the flow-volume loop, but this is not a constant feature. The lesion is difficult to detect on plain radiographs. Definitive diagnosis is by bronchoscopy.

TREATMENT. Gravitational drainage may help with clearance of secretions. Cromolyn may be helpful. β-Adrenergic agents should be avoided, but ipratropium bromide may be useful. Surgically inserted stents may be necessary in severely affected patients, but long-term results of this treatment have not been reported in children.

PROGNOSIS. Bronchomalacia in the absence of reactive airways has a good prognosis, because airflow improves as the airways grow. Wheezing at rest is usually gone by age 5 yr. Patients with reactive airways need considerable supportive treatment, including cromolyn and intermittent systemic corticosteroid. Despite the good prognosis for survival and for a patient's ability to perform the functions of daily living, the prognosis for achieving normal exercise tolerance is limited.

Finder JD: Primary bronchomalacia in infants and children. J Pediatr 130:59, 1997.

384.4 Agenesis or Hypoplasia of the Lung

Bilateral pulmonary agenesis or significant hypoplasia is incompatible with life, presenting with severe respiratory distress and failure; hypoplasia is usually associated with anencephaly, diaphragmatic hernias, urinary tract abnormalities, abnormalities of the thumb, deformities of the thoracic spine and rib cage (thoracic dystrophy), renal anomalies (oligohydramnios), right-sided heart malformations, and congenital pleural effusions. Bilateral hypoplasia is found in 10% of all neonatal autopsies (30% of babies younger than 1 wk); it has an important role in the death of many patients with the conditions previously listed (Chapter 97.7). Unilateral agenesis or hypoplasia may have few symptoms and nonspecific findings, resulting in only one third of the cases being diagnosed during life. Left-sided lesions are more common. In unilateral agenesis, the entire pulmonary parenchyma and supporting structures and airways are absent below the level of the carina.

Pulmonary hypoplasia involves a decrease in both the number of alveoli (up to 67%) and the number of airway generations (up to 50%). The hypoplasia is almost always secondary to another congenital abnormality (e.g., diaphragmatic hernia; asphyxiating thoracic dystrophy; oligohydramnios; cardiovascular anomalies, including tetralogy of Fallot; and others). A child with unilateral pulmonary hypoplasia usually has a small unexpandable lung. Persistent pulmonary hypertension is often present when pulmonary hypoplasia presents in the newborn period (see Chapter 97.7). Occasional reports of parental consanguinity suggest a genetic basis for at least some of these cases.

There is no specific treatment. Supportive measures including mechanical ventilation and supplemental oxygen may allow sufficient pulmonary parenchymal development to permit survival (25% of the infants in one series). Older patients should be given antibiotics for pulmonary infection and should receive annual influenza vaccine. Prognoses for the patients who survive infancy are extremely variable and largely depend on the presence of associated anomalies. The contralateral lung is often larger than normal. The prognosis is worse for right-sided agenesis owing to a higher incidence of associated life-threatening malformations and a higher rate of infection due to spillage into the contralateral lung. Death may also result from complications of pulmonary hypertension associated with congenital heart disease.

Husain AN, Hessel RG: Neonatal pulmonary hypoplasia: An autopsy study of 25 cases. Pediatr Pathol 13:475, 1993.

Kravitz RM: Congenital malformations of the lung. Pediatr Clin North Am 41:453, 1994.

Kresch MJ, Markowitz RI, Smith GJW: Respiratory distress and cyanosis in a term newborn infant. J Pediatr 113:937, 1988.

LOBAR EMPHYSEMA

See Chapter 407.

384.5 Pulmonary Sequestration

A mass of nonfunctioning embryonic and cystic pulmonary tissue that receives its entire blood supply from the systemic circulation is known as a sequestration. Because its venous drainage is to the systemic circulation, these lesions produce a left-to-right shunt. Although most sequestrations do not communicate with functional airways, this is not always the case. Intralobar and extralobar sequestrations may arise through the same pathoembryologic mechanism as a remnant of a diverticular outgrowth of the esophagus. However, some propose that intralobar sequestration is an acquired lesion primarily caused by infection and inflammation, which lead to cystic changes and hypertrophy of a feeding systemic artery. This is consistent with the rarity of this lesion in autopsy series of newborns. Others propose that it is a form of cystadenomatoid malformation. Gastric or pancreatic tissue may be found within the sequestration. Cysts may also be present. Other congenital anomalies, including diaphragmatic hernia and esophageal cysts, are not uncommon. Some believe that intralobar sequestration is often a manifestation of cystadenomatoid malformation and have questioned the existence of intralobar sequestration as a separate entity.

Intralobar sequestration is generally found in a lower lobe and does not have its own pleura. Patients usually present with infection. In older patients, hemoptysis is fairly common. A chest roentgenogram during a period when there is no active infection reveals a mass lesion; an air-fluid level may be present. During infection, the margins of the lesion may be blurred. There is no difference in the incidence of this lesion in each lung. Treatment is surgical removal of the lesion, a procedure that usually requires excision of the entire involved lobe. Segmental resection occasionally suffices.

Extralobar sequestration is much more common in males and almost always involves the left lung. This lesion is enveloped by a pleural covering and is associated strongly with diaphragmatic hernia. Patients may also have other associated abnormalities, such as colonic duplication, vertebral abnormalities, and pulmonary hypoplasia. Many of these patients are asymptomatic when the mass is discovered by routine chest roentgenogram taken for another reason. Other patients present with respiratory symptoms or heart failure. Surgical resection of the involved area is recommended.

Physical findings in patients with sequestration include an area of dullness to percussion and decreased breath sounds over the lesion. During infection, rales may also be present. A continuous or purely systolic murmur may be heard over the back. If findings on routine chest roentgenograms are consistent with the diagnosis, other procedures are indicated before surgical intervention. Bronchography reveals a mass of intrathoracic tissue without connection to the airways. Ultrasonography can help rule out a diaphragmatic hernia. Surgical removal is recommended. Preoperative aortography is recommended to confirm the diagnosis and to delineate the blood supply of the lesion. However, some now believe that Doppler ultrasonography and MRI are sufficient in most cases. Identifying the blood supply before surgery avoids inadvertently severing this systemic artery, a casualty that has accounted for much of the intraoperative mortality in the past.

Case Records of the Massachusetts General Hospital: Case 14–1991. N Engl J Med 324:980, 1991.

Hernanz-Schulman M: Cysts and cystlike lesions of the lung. Radiol Clin North Am 31:631, 1993.

Kravitz RM: Congenital malformations of the lung. Pediatr Clin North Am 41:453, 1994.

Nicolette LA, Kosloske AM, Bartow SA, et al: Intralobar pulmonary sequestration: A clinical and pathological spectrum. J Pediatr Surg 28:802, 1993.

384.6 Bronchogenic Cysts

Bronchogenic cysts arise from abnormal budding of the tracheal diverticulum of the foregut before the 16th wk of gestation and are originally lined with ciliated epithelium. They are most commonly found on the right and near a midline structure (e.g., trachea, esophagus, carina), but peripheral lower lobe and perihilar intrapulmonary cysts are not infrequent. Diagnosis may be precipitated by enlargement of the cyst, which causes symptoms by pressure on an adjacent airway. When the diagnosis is delayed until infection occurs, the ciliated epithelium may be lost, and accurate pathologic diagnosis is then impossible. Cysts are rarely demonstrable at birth. Later, some cysts become symptomatic by becoming infected or by enlarging in size and compromising the function of an adjacent airway. Fever, chest pain, and productive cough are the most common presenting symptoms. A chest roentgenogram reveals the cyst, which may contain an air-fluid level.

Additional information can be obtained by CT scan or barium esophagogram. Treatment for symptomatic cysts is surgical excision after appropriate antibiotic management. Even asymptomatic cysts discovered incidentally by chest roentgenogram taken for another reason should probably be treated by surgical excision, in view of the 75–90% rate of infection.

Hernanz-Schulman M: Cysts and cystlike lesions of the lung. Radiol Clin North Am 31:631, 1993.
Kravitz RM: Congenital malformations of the lung. Pediatr Clin North Am 41:453, 1994.

384.7 Bronchobiliary Fistula

This rare anomaly usually presents life-threatening problems during early infancy, but diagnosis occasionally has been delayed until adulthood. Females are more commonly affected. The bronchobiliary fistula consists of a fistulous connection between the right middle lobe bronchus and the left hepatic ductal system. All patients have recurrent severe bronchopulmonary infection starting in early infancy. Definitive diagnosis requires endoscopy and bronchography or exploratory surgery. Treatment includes surgical excision of the entire intrathoracic portion of the fistula. If the hepatic portion of the fistula does not communicate with the biliary system or duodenum, the involved segment may also have to be resected. Bronchobiliary communications also occur as acquired lesions resulting from hepatic disease complicated by infection.

Gauderer MWL, Oiticica C, Bishop HC: Congenital bronchobiliary fistula: Management of the involved hepatic segment. J Pediatr Surg 28:452, 1993.
Pappas SC, Sasaki A, Minuk GY: Bronchobiliary fistula presenting as cough with yellow sputum. N Engl J Med 307:1027, 1982.
Yamaguchi M, Kanamori K, Fujimura M, et al: Congenital bronchobiliary fistula in adults. South Med J 83:851, 1990.

384.8 Congenital Pulmonary Lymphangiectasis

This disease, characterized by greatly dilated lymphatic ducts throughout the lung, is usually symptomatic with dyspnea and cyanosis in the newborn. Chest roentgenograms reveal punctate and reticular densities or, occasionally, a unilateral hyperlucent lung. Respiration is compromised because of the space-occupying nature of the lesion and possibly because pulmonary compliance is reduced, increasing the work of breathing. Two forms of the disease—one in which the abnormality is limited to the lung and one in which the pulmonary lymphangiectasis is secondary to pulmonary venous obstruction—are always symptomatic in the neonatal period. Familial occurrence of the first type has been reported. Survival beyond infancy is rare. A third form, in which the pulmonary lymphangiectasis is part of a generalized disease involving other organ systems (e.g., intestine), is associated with milder pulmonary disease and survival to midchildhood and beyond. Definitive diagnosis requires lung biopsy. There is no specific treatment.

Case Records of the Massachusetts General Hospital: Case 31–1989. N Engl J Med 321:309, 1989.
Huber A, Schranz D, Blaha I, et al: Congenital pulmonary lymphangiectasia. Pediatr Pulmonol 10:310, 1991.
Verlaat CWM, Peters HM, Semmekrot BA, et al: Congenital pulmonary lymphangiectasis presenting as a unilateral hyperlucent lung. Eur J Pediatr 153:202, 1994.

384.9 Cystic Adenomatoid Malformation

This is the second most common congenital lung lesion; lobar emphysema is the most common. A single lobe of one lung is enlarged and often cystic, compressing the remainder of the ipsilateral lung and frequently causing a mediastinum shift with compression of the contralateral lung. The remaining ipsilateral lung may be hypoplastic as a result of the space-occupying nature of the lesion. Although a slight male preponderance has been reported, in other series 75% were female. The lesion probably results from an embryologic insult, usually before the 35th day of gestation, and seems to involve maldevelopment of terminal bronchiolar structures. Histologic examination reveals little normal lung and many glandular elements. Cysts are very common; cartilage is rare. The presence of cartilage may indicate a somewhat later embryologic insult, perhaps extending into the 10th–24th wk.

Cystic adenomatoid malformations can be diagnosed in utero by ultrasonography. In one series of 16 such cases, the diagnosis was almost always made at 21–23 wk of gestation (range, 18–36 wk). Polyhydramnios was common (25%). In three cases the malformation resolved spontaneously before birth. Each of the three patients who died after neonatal surgery had hypoplasia of the remaining ipsilateral lung.

The common types of postnatal clinical manifestations include neonatal respiratory distress, recurrent respiratory infection, and pneumothorax. Most patients become symptomatic and die in the newborn period, although a few survive after emergency surgery. Rarely, patients are asymptomatic until midchildhood, when brief episodes of recurrent or persistent pulmonary infection or relatively acute chest pain occur. Breath sounds may be diminished with mediastinal shift away from the lesion on physical examination. Chest roentgenograms reveal a cystic mass with mediastinal shift. Occasionally, an air-fluid level suggests a lung abscess. The lesion may be confused with diaphragmatic hernia in a newborn. Surgical excision of the affected lobe (occasionally a segment) is indicated. After surgery, long-term survival into infancy and even later into childhood has been reported, but these patients may be at increased risk for developing primary pulmonary neoplasms.

Cacciari A, Ceccarelli PL, Pilu GL, et al: A series of 17 cases of congenital cystic adenomatoid malformation of the lung: Management and outcome. Eur J Pediatr Surg 7:84, 1997.
Heij HA, Ekkelkamp S, Vos A: Diagnosis of congenital cystic adenomatoid malformation of the lung in newborn infants and children. Thorax 45:122, 1990.
Kravitz RM: Congenital malformations of the lung. Pediatr Clin North Am 41:453, 1994.
Neilson IR, Russo P, Laberge JM, et al: Congenital adenomatoid malformation of the lung: Current management and prognosis. J Pediatr Surg 26:975, 1991.

Chapter 385
Acute Inflammatory Upper Airway Obstruction

David M. Orenstein

GENERAL CONSIDERATIONS. Acute inflammation of the upper airway is of greater importance in infants and small children than in older children because the airway is smaller, predisposing young children to a relatively greater narrowing than is produced by the same degree of inflammation in an older child. The larynx is composed of four cartilages (i.e., thyroid, cricoid, arytenoid, epiglottic) and the soft tissues joining them. The cricoid cartilage encircles the airway just below the vocal cords and defines the narrowest portion of the pediatric upper airway.

Inflammation involving the vocal cords and structures inferior to the cords is called laryngitis, laryngotracheitis, or laryngotracheobronchitis, and inflammation of the structures superior to the cords (i.e., arytenoids, aryepiglottic folds ["false cords"], epiglottis) is called supraglottitis. *Croup* is a generic term encompassing a heterogeneous group of relatively acute conditions (mostly infectious) characterized by a peculiarly brassy or "croupy" cough, which may or may not be accompanied by inspiratory stridor, hoarseness, and signs of respiratory distress due to various degrees of laryngeal obstruction. Such infection in infants and small children is rarely limited to a single area of the respiratory tract; it usually affects, to some degree, the larynx, trachea, and bronchi. When there is sufficient involvement of the larynx to produce symptoms, the laryngeal part of the clinical picture is likely to overshadow tracheal or bronchial signs.

385.1 Infectious Upper Airway Obstruction

ETIOLOGY AND EPIDEMIOLOGY. Viral agents account for most acute infectious upper airway obstructions except those associated with diphtheria, bacterial tracheitis, and acute epiglottitis. The parainfluenza viruses account for approximately 75% of cases; adenoviruses, respiratory syncytial, influenza, and measles viruses cause the remaining viral cases. In one study, *Mycoplasma pneumoniae* was recovered from 3.6% of patients who had acute upper airway obstruction. Although *Haemophilus influenzae* type b is the usual cause of acute epiglottitis, *Streptococcus pyogenes, S. pneumoniae,* and *Staphylococcus aureus* are occasionally implicated. The occurrence of epiglottitis has been dramatically reduced because infections caused by *H. influenzae* type b have been nearly eliminated by the use of the HiB vaccine. Accordingly, other agents have begun to represent a larger proportion of cases of epiglottitis. Viral epiglottitis is a rare and milder illness. Most patients who have viral croup are between the ages of 3 mo and 5 yr, but disease due to *H. influenzae* and *Corynebacterium diphtheriae* is more common from 3–7 yr of age. The incidence of croup is higher in males, and it occurs most commonly during the cold season of the year. Approximately 15% of patients have a strong family history of croup, and laryngitis tends to recur in the same child.

CLINICAL MANIFESTATIONS

Croup (Laryngotracheobronchitis). Croup, the most common form of acute upper airway obstruction, is caused primarily by viruses. The opportunity for pathologic study is rare; the primary findings appear to be inflammatory edema, destruction of ciliated epithelium, and exudate. Secondary bacterial infection is rare. Most patients have an upper respiratory tract infection for several days before cough becomes apparent. With progressive compromise of the upper airway, a characteristic sequence of symptoms and signs occurs. At first, there is only a mild, brassy cough with intermittent inspiratory stridor. As obstruction increases, stridor becomes continuous and is associated with worsening cough, nasal flaring, and suprasternal, infrasternal, and intercostal retractions. As inflammation extends to the bronchi and bronchioles, respiratory difficulty increases, and the expiratory phase of respiration also becomes labored and prolonged. Various degrees of lower respiratory involvement occur. The temperature may be only slightly elevated; it rarely reaches 39–40°C (102–104°F). Symptoms are characteristically worse at night and often recur with decreasing intensity for several days. Older children usually are not seriously ill. Other family members may have mild respiratory illness. The duration of illness ranges from several days to, rarely, several weeks; recurrences are frequent from 3–6 yr of age, decreasing with growth of the airway. Most patients with croup progress only as far as stridor and slight dyspnea before they start to recover. In some, there is worse obstruction. Agitation and crying greatly aggravate the symptoms and signs, and the child prefers to sit up in bed or be held upright.

There may be diminished breath sounds, rhonchi, and scattered crackles. With further compromise of the airway, air hunger and restlessness occur and are then superseded by severe hypoxemia, hypercapnia, and weakness, accompanied by decreased air exchange and stridor, tachycardia, and eventual death from hypoventilation. In the hypoxemic child who may be cyanotic, pale, or obtunded, any manipulation of the pharynx, including use of a tongue depressor, may result in sudden cardiorespiratory arrest. This examination therefore should be deferred, and oxygen should be administered until the patient is transferred to a place in the hospital where optimal management of the airway and shock is possible. Occasionally, the pattern of severe laryngotracheobronchitis may be difficult to differentiate from epiglottitis despite the usually more explosive onset and rapid course of the latter; it also requires similar precautions. Roentgenographic examination of the nasopharynx and upper airway may be helpful (Fig. 385–1).

Acute Epiglottitis (Supraglottitis). This dramatic, potentially lethal condition usually occurs in children 2–7 yr old; the peak incidence occurs at about 3.5 yr. It is seen much less commonly since the widespread use of immunization against *H. influenzae* type b. Epiglottitis is characterized by a fulminating course of high fever, sore throat, dyspnea, rapidly progressive respiratory obstruction, and prostration, although respiratory distress is frequently the first manifestation. Within a matter of hours, it may progress to complete obstruction of the airway and death unless adequate treatment is provided. With adequate treatment, the illness rarely lasts for more than 2–3 days. Often the child, particularly the younger patient, is apparently well at bedtime but awakens later in the evening with high fever, aphonia, drooling, and moderate or severe respiratory distress with stridor. Usually no other family members are ill with acute upper respiratory disease. The older child often complains initially of sore throat and dysphagia. Severe respiratory distress may ensue within minutes or hours of the onset, with inspiratory stridor, hoarseness, brassy cough (less commonly), irritability, and restlessness. Drooling and dysphagia are com-

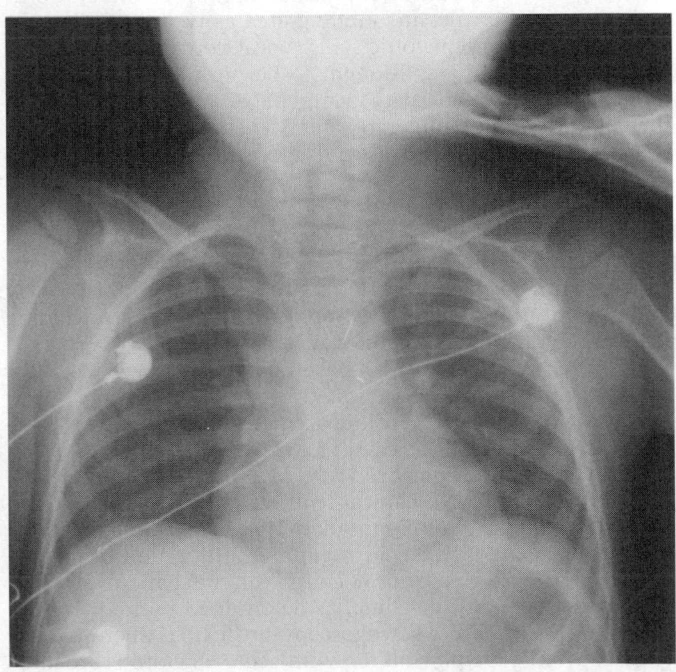

Figure 385–1 Radiograph of an airway of a patient with croup, showing typical subglottic narrowing ("steeple sign").

mon. The neck may be hyperextended, although other signs of meningeal irritation are absent. The older child may prefer a sitting position, leaning forward, with the mouth open and the tongue somewhat protruding. Some children may progress rapidly to a shocklike state characterized by pallor, cyanosis, and impaired consciousness.

The physical examination may disclose moderate or severe respiratory distress with inspiratory and sometimes expiratory stridor, flaring of the alae nasi, and inspiratory retractions of the suprasternal notch, supraclavicular and intercostal spaces, and subcostal area. The pharynx may be inflamed, and there may be an abundance of mucus and saliva, which may also result in rhonchi. With progression, stridor and breath sounds may be diminished as the patient tires. A brief period of air hunger with restlessness and agitation may be followed by rapidly increasing cyanosis, coma, and death. Alternatively, the child may have only mild hoarseness and a large, shiny, cherry-red epiglottis brought into view when the posterior portion of the tongue is depressed. Occasionally, an older cooperative child may voluntarily open the mouth wide enough for a direct view of the inflamed epiglottis.

The diagnosis requires visualization of a large, swollen cherry-red epiglottis by direct examination or laryngoscopy. Occasionally, the other supraglottic structures, especially the aryepiglottic folds, may be more involved than the epiglottis itself. Some patients may have reflex laryngospasm and acute complete obstruction, aspiration of secretions, and cardiorespiratory arrest during or immediately after examination of the pharynx with the use of a tongue blade. These examinations should never be undertaken in a child in whom epiglottitis is thought possible without full preparation for immediate endotracheal intubation under controlled conditions. Children with suspected epiglottitis should not be placed in the supine position because of the risk of increased agitation and gravity-induced change in the position of the epiglottis with increased airway obstruction. Arterial blood gas samples should not be obtained before a definitive diagnosis and the establishment of an artificial airway. If the diagnosis is probable on clinical grounds, preparation should be made immediately for examining and controlling the airway, often in the operating room, by physicians skilled in endotracheal intubation or tracheostomy, or both.

Laryngoscopy reveals intense inflammation of the epiglottis and sometimes of the surrounding area as well, including the arytenoids and aryepiglottic folds, vocal cords, and subglottic regions. If epiglottitis is thought to be possible, although not probable, in a patient with acute upper airway obstruction, the patient should undergo lateral roentgenography of the nasopharynx and upper airway before physical examination of the pharynx (Fig. 385–2). If a roentgenogram shows a normal epiglottis, examination of the epiglottis may be performed while appropriate equipment and personnel are available to control the airway and provide ventilatory support. Patients with suspected epiglottitis should be accompanied by a physician and intubation equipment at all times, including the trip to and from the radiology department.

Establishing an airway by nasotracheal intubation or, less often, by tracheostomy is indicated in patients with epiglottitis, regardless of the degree of apparent respiratory distress, because as many as 6% of children with epiglottitis without an artificial airway die, compared with less than 1% of those with an artificial airway. No clinical features have been recognized that predict fatality. Fulminant pulmonary edema may be associated with acute airway obstruction. The duration of intubation depends on the clinical course of the patient and the duration of epiglottic swelling, as determined by frequent examination using direct laryngoscopy or flexible fiberoptic laryngoscopy. In general, children with acute epiglottitis are intubated for 2–3 days. Because most patients have bacteremia, parenteral antibiotic therapy with cefotaxime, ceftriaxone, or

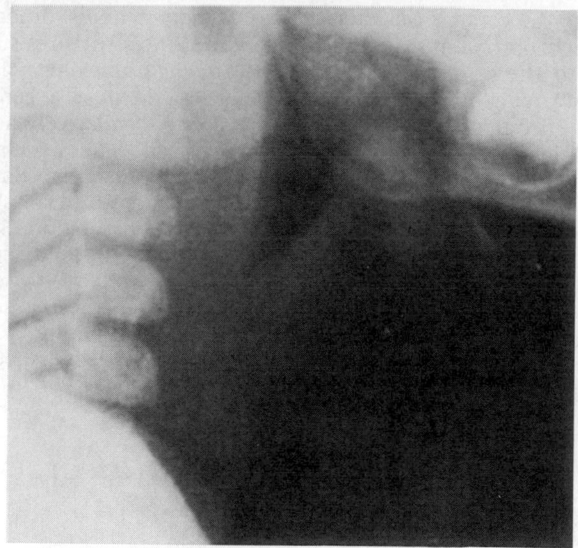

Figure 385–2 Epiglottitis. Lateral roentgenogram of the upper airway reveals the swollen epiglottis.

ampicillin with sulbactam (Unasyn) should be instituted promptly. Concomitant infection is unusual, but meningitis, pneumonia, cervical adenopathy, or otitis media rarely occur.

Acute Infectious Laryngitis. Laryngitis is a common illness; except for diphtheria, most cases are caused by viruses. The onset is usually characterized by an upper respiratory tract infection during which sore throat, cough, and hoarseness appear. The illness is generally mild; respiratory distress is unusual except in the young infant. Hoarseness and loss of voice may be out of proportion to systemic signs and symptoms. In the rare severe case, the patient may present with severe inspiratory stridor, retractions, dyspnea, and restlessness. As the process progresses, air hunger and fatigue become evident, and the child alternates between periods of agitation and exhaustion. The physical examination is usually not remarkable except for evidence of pharyngeal inflammation and, with respiratory distress, evidence of high respiratory obstruction. Inflammatory edema of the vocal cords and subglottic tissue may be demonstrated laryngoscopically. The principal site of obstruction is usually the subglottic area.

Acute Spasmodic Laryngitis (Spasmodic Croup). Spasmodic croup occurs most often in children 1–3 yr of age and is clinically similar to acute laryngotracheobronchitis, except that findings of infection in the patient and family are frequently absent. The cause is viral in some cases, but allergic and psychologic factors may be important in others. Gastroesophageal reflux may play an important role in triggering spasmodic croup, and children with this syndrome deserve careful laryngoscopic examination. The endoscopic documentation of posterior laryngitis (i.e., edema or inflammation of the arytenoid cartilages) suggests reflux. The opportunity for pathologic study is rare; the primary findings appear to be preservation of the epithelium (unlike acute infectious laryngotracheobronchitis) and pale, watery edema. In some cases, there is a familial predisposition to this syndrome.

Occurring most frequently in the evening or nighttime, spasmodic croup begins with a sudden onset that may be preceded by mild to moderate coryza and hoarseness. The child awakens with a characteristic barking, metallic cough, noisy inspiration, and respiratory distress and appears anxious and frightened. Breathing is slow and labored, the pulse is accelerated, and the skin is cool and moist. The patient is usually afebrile. Dyspnea is aggravated by excitement; intermittent episodes of cyanosis are rare. Usually, the severity of the symptoms diminishes within several hours, and the following day, the patient often appears well except for slight hoarseness and cough. Similar, but usually less severe, attacks without extreme respiratory distress may occur for another night or two, eventually concluding in complete recovery. Such episodes often recur several times.

DIFFERENTIAL DIAGNOSIS. These four syndromes must be differentiated from one another and from a variety of other entities that may present upper airway obstruction. *Bacterial tracheitis* is the most important differential diagnostic consideration. *Diphtheritic croup* is rare in North America (see Chapter 187). It is usually preceded by an upper respiratory tract infection for several days. Symptoms usually develop slowly, although respiratory obstruction may occur suddenly; a serous or serosanguineous nasal discharge may occur. Pharyngeal examination reveals the typical gray-white membrane. *Measles croup* almost always coincides with the full manifestations of systemic disease and the course may be fulminant (see Chapter 240).

Sudden onset of respiratory obstruction may be caused by *aspiration of a foreign body* (see Chapter 386). The child is usually 6 mo–2 yr of age. Choking and coughing occur suddenly, usually without prodromal signs of infection, although children with a viral infection can also aspirate a foreign body. A *retropharyngeal* or *peritonsillar abscess* may mimic respiratory obstruction (see Chapters 381.5 and 381.7). Roentgenographic examination of the upper airway and chest is essential in evaluating these possibilities and possible causes of *extrinsic compression* of the airway, such as a hematoma from trauma and *intraluminal obstruction* from masses (e.g., cysts, tumors).

Upper airway obstruction is occasionally associated with *angioedema* of the subglottic areas as part of anaphylaxis and generalized allergic reactions, edema following *endotracheal intubation* for general anesthesia or respiratory failure, *hypocalcemic tetany, infectious mononucleosis,* trauma, and tumors or malformations of the larynx. A croupy cough may be an early sign of *asthma.* Psychogenic stridor (vocal cord dysfunction) can also occur. Epiglottitis, with the characteristic manifestations of drooling or dysphagia and stridor can also result from the accidental ingestion of very hot liquid.

COMPLICATIONS. Complications occur in approximately 15% of patients with viral croup. The most common is extension of the infectious process to involve other regions of the respiratory tract, such as the middle ear, the terminal bronchioles, or the pulmonary parenchyma. Bacterial tracheitis may be a complication of viral croup rather than a distinct disease. Interstitial pneumonia may occur, but it is difficult to differentiate on roentgenograms from the patchy areas of atelectasis secondary to obstruction. Bronchopneumonia is unusual unless aspiration of stomach contents has occurred during a period of severe respiratory distress. Although secondary bacterial pneumonia is unusual, suppurative tracheobronchitis is an occasional complication of laryngotracheobronchitis. Pneumonia, cervical lymphadenitis, otitis or, rarely, meningitis or septic arthritis may occur during the course of epiglottitis. Mediastinal emphysema and pneumothorax are the most common complications of tracheotomy.

PROGNOSIS. In general, the length of hospitalization and the mortality rate for cases of acute infectious upper airway obstruction increase as the infection extends to involve a greater portion of the respiratory tract, except in epiglottitis, in which the localized infection itself may prove fatal. Most deaths from croup are caused by a laryngeal obstruction or by the complications of tracheotomy. Untreated epiglottitis has a mortality rate of 6% in some series, but if the diagnosis is made and appropriate treatment is initiated before the patient is moribund, the prognosis is excellent. The outcome of acute laryngotracheobronchitis, laryngitis, and spasmodic croup is also excellent. As a group, children who need to be hospitalized for croup have somewhat increased bronchial reactivity compared with normal children when tested several years later. The differences are small, and their functional importance is unclear.

TREATMENT. Therapy for *infectious croup* consists primarily of maintaining or providing for adequate respiratory exchange and depends, in part, on the primary location of the disease and its cause. In the bacterial forms, antibiotic therapy is also important.

Most afebrile children with *acute spasmodic croup* or febrile patients with mild *laryngotracheobronchitis* can usually be managed safely and effectively at home. Treatment of underlying and often unsuspected gastroesophageal reflux may prevent spasmodic croup in children known to be susceptible to it.

The use of steam from a shower or bath in a closed bathroom, steam from a vaporizer, or "cold steam" from a nebulizer (which has a safety and perhaps efficacy advantage) often terminates acute laryngeal spasm and respiratory distress within minutes. The same effect has been observed by many parents as they take their child out into the cold night air on the way to the physician's office. This long-recognized phenomenon may be explained by the upper airway's serving as a heat and humidity exchange organ; inspired air that is cooler than body temperature and less than 100% saturated with water vapor results in mucosal cooling, leading to vasoconstriction and lessened edema.

Induction of vomiting by coughing or by syrup of ipecac may also decrease laryngeal spasm. Although vomiting occasionally appears to break the laryngeal spasm, there is no objective evidence for the effectiveness of ipecac, and respiratory distress may be complicated by vomiting, particularly if the patient aspirates gastric contents.

After the laryngeal spasm has diminished, its return may be prevented by the use of warm or cool humidification near the child's bed for the ensuing 2–3 days.

Children with croup should be hospitalized for any of the following: actual or suspected epiglottitis, progressive stridor, severe stridor at rest, respiratory distress, hypoxemia, restlessness, cyanosis, pallor, depressed sensorium, or high fever in a toxic-appearing child. In all cases, the decision for hospitalization is made because of the need for reliable observation and relatively safe tracheotomy or more often nasotracheal intubation, if either of these becomes necessary.

At home or in the hospital, the patient with croup should be watched carefully for intensification of symptoms of respiratory obstruction. The hospitalized child is usually placed in an atmosphere of cool humidity to lessen irritation and drying of secretions and perhaps to lessen edema. Frequent or continuous monitoring of the respiratory rate is essential because increasing tachypnea may be the first sign of hypoxemia and approaching total respiratory obstruction. The patient should be disturbed as little as possible. In cases of moderate to severe respiratory distress, parenteral fluids should be given to make up for insensible and respiratory water loss and decrease the risk of vomiting, with its potential for aspiration. Sedatives are usually contraindicated because restlessness is used as one of the principal clinical indices of the severity of obstruction and the need for tracheotomy or nasotracheal intubation. Opiates, in particular, are contraindicated because they may depress respiration and dry secretions. Oxygen should be used to alleviate hypoxemia and apprehension, but because the oxygen reduces cyanosis, which is an indication for tracheotomy or nasotracheal intubation, these patients must be observed particularly closely. Expectorants, bronchodilating agents, and antihistamines are not helpful.

Laryngotracheobronchitis and *spasmodic croup* do not respond to antibiotics, and antibiotics are not indicated to prevent suprainfection. Nonurgent tests should be delayed to prevent increased symptoms associated with agitation and anxiety. Racemic epinephrine by aerosol (2.25% solution diluted 1:8 with water in doses of 2–4 mL for 15 min) often results in transient relief of symptoms; close observation and repeated treatments usually are necessary. A child sick enough for hospitalization before administering an aerosol should be hospitalized even if there is a dramatic response to the aerosol because the obstruction is likely to return after the aerosol's effects have waned. Racemic epinephrine does not cause rebound worsening of obstruction. However, if the aerosol is administered during the worsening phase of the natural history of the child's illness, the obstruction may be worse after the effects have worn off. If the aerosol is administered at what would have been the peak of the obstruction, the child will be better after the aerosol effects have waned. Frequent treatments help all but the sickest children through this illness. Rarely, there is sufficient obstruction to warrant nasotracheal intubation or tracheotomy.

The use of corticosteroids is probably indicated for the hospitalized child with croup. The theoretical basis for corticosteroid treatment in laryngotracheobronchitis is to reduce inflammatory edema and prevent destruction of ciliated epithelium. A meta-analysis and another review of 10–13 English language studies suggest some beneficial effect of systemic corticosteroids, particularly if doses of dexamethasone phosphate greater than 0.3 mg/kg are employed. There is no substantial evidence suggesting any adverse effect of corticosteroid treatment. The topical, nonabsorbed, inhaled corticosteroid budesonide has benefit in treating children with croup and may be as effective as epinephrine. In the very ill child in the intensive care unit, breathing a helium-oxygen mixture, with its lower density and the resultant improved turbulent airflow, may decrease the work of breathing.

Epiglottitis is a **medical emergency.** If diagnosed by inspection of the epiglottis or by roentgenographic examination or if strongly suspected clinically in a severely ill child, it should be treated immediately with an artificial airway inserted under controlled conditions, usually in an operating room. All patients should receive oxygen en route to the operating room unless it is contraindicated by the increased agitation caused by the mask. Racemic epinephrine and corticosteroids are ineffective; they do not avert the need for an artificial airway and may dangerously delay definitive treatment. Cultures of blood, epiglottic surface, and, in selected cases, cerebrospinal fluid, should be collected at the time of airway stabilization. Ceftriaxone, cefotaxime, or a combination of ampicillin and sulbactam should be given parenterally pending culture and susceptibility reports because of the increasing possibility of ampicillin-resistant strains of *H. influenzae* type b. After insertion of the artificial airway, the patient should improve immediately, respiratory distress and cyanosis should disappear, and normal or near-normal blood gas levels should return. Patients usually fall asleep. The epiglottitis resolves after a few days of antibiotics, and the patient can be weaned from the tracheostomy or nasotracheal tube; antibiotics should be continued for 7–10 days.

Acute laryngeal swelling on an allergic basis responds to epinephrine (1:1,000 dilution in dosage of 0.01 mL/kg to a maximum of 0.3 mL/dose) administered subcutaneously or racemic epinephrine (2.25% solution diluted 1:8 with water in doses of 2–4 mL for 15 min) administered by aerosol. After recovery, the patient and parents should be instructed in emergency administration of these drugs at home. Corticosteroids are frequently required (1–2 mg/kg/24 hr of prednisone every 6 hr).

Reactive mucosal swelling, severe stridor, and respiratory distress unresponsive to mist therapy may follow *endotracheal intubation* for general anesthesia in children. Intermittent use of racemic epinephrine aerosols or occasional use of corticosteroids may be helpful.

Tracheotomy and Endotracheal Intubation (see Chapter 64.1). With the introduction of routine nasotracheal intubation or tracheotomy for epiglottitis, the mortality rate has dropped to almost zero. Both procedures should always be performed in an operating room if time permits; prior intubation and general anesthesia greatly facilitate performing a tracheotomy without complications. The choice of procedure should be based on the local expertise and experience with the procedure and the postoperative care involved with each.

Endotracheal intubation or tracheotomy is required for all patients with epiglottitis, but for patients with laryngotracheobronchitis, spasmodic croup, or laryngitis, it is required only for those rare individuals who have increasing signs of respiratory failure secondary to obstruction despite appropriate treatment. Severe forms of laryngotracheobronchitis that require tracheotomy in a high proportion of patients have been reported during severe measles and influenza A virus epidemics. Assessing the need for these procedures requires experience and judgment because they should not be delayed until cyanosis and extreme restlessness have developed; a pulse rate greater than 150 beats/min and rising, and an elevated P_{CO_2}, especially in a tiring child, are indications of impending respiratory failure (see Chapters 62, 64.3, and 65).

The endotracheal tube or tracheostomy must remain in place until edema and spasm have subsided and the patient is able to handle secretions satisfactorily. It should always be removed as soon as possible, usually within a few days. Adequate resolution of epiglottic inflammation that has been accurately confirmed by fiberoptic laryngoscopy, permitting much more rapid extubation, often occurs within 24 hr. There is some evidence that hydrocortisone (50–100 mg/24 hr) or dexamethasone (0.25–0.5 mg/kg/dose every 6 hr as needed) and racemic epinephrine may be useful to facilitate extubation or to treat croup associated with extubation.

Laryngotracheobronchitis

Denny FW, Murphy TF, Clyde WA Jr, et al: Croup: An 11 year study in a pediatric practice. Pediatrics 71:871, 1984.

Fitzgerald D, Messis C, Johnson M, et al: Nebulized budesonide is as effective as nebulized adrenaline in moderately severe croup. Pediatrics 97:722, 1996.

Johnson DW, Jacobson S, Edney PC, et al: A comparison of nebulized budesonide, intramuscular dexamethasone, and placebo for moderately severe croup. N Engl J Med 339:498, 1998.

Gurwitz D, Corey M, Levison H: Pulmonary function and bronchial reactivity in children after croup. Am Rev Respir Dis 122:95, 1980.

Kairys SW, Olmstead EM, O'Connor GT: Steroid treatment of laryngotracheitis: A meta-analysis of the evidence from randomized trials. Pediatrics 83:683, 1989.

Klassen T, Craig WR, Moher D, et al: Nebulized budesonide and oral dexamethasone for treatment of croup. JAMA 279:1629, 1998.

Singer OP, Wilson WJ: Laryngotracheobronchitis: 2 years' experience with racemic epinephrine. Can Med Assoc J 115:132, 1976.

Skolnik JS: Treatment of croup: A critical review. Am J Dis Child 143:1045, 1989.

Smith MS: Acute psychogenic stridor in an adolescent athlete treated with hypnosis. Pediatrics 72:247, 1983.

Super DM, Cartelli NA, Brooks LJ, et al: A prospective double-blind study to evaluate the effect of dexamethasone in acute laryngotracheitis. J Pediatr 115:323, 1989.

Spasmodic Croup

Contencin P, Narcy P: Gastropharyngeal reflux in infants and children: A pharyngeal monitoring study. Arch Otolaryngol Head Neck Surg 118:1028, 1992.

Epiglottitis

Adams WG, Deaver KA, Cochi SL, et al: Decline in childhood *Haemophilus influenzae* type b (HiB) in the HiB vaccine era. JAMA 269:221, 1993.

Ashcraft CK, Steele RW: Epiglottitis: A pediatric emergency. J Respir Dis 9:48, 1988.

Battaglia JD, Lockhart CH: Management of acute epiglottitis by nasotracheal intubation. Am J Dis Child 120:334, 1975.

Cohen SR, Chai J: Epiglottitis: Twenty-year study with tracheostomy. Ann Otol Rhinol Laryngol 87:1, 1978.

Gonzales Valdepena H, Wald ER, Rose E, et al: Epiglottitis and *Haemophilus influenzae* immunization: the Pittsburgh experience—a five-year review. Pediatrics 96:424, 1995.

Kulick RM, Selbst SM, Baker MD, et al: Thermal epiglottitis after swallowing hot beverages. Pediatrics 81:441, 1988.

Molteni RA: Epiglottitis: Incidence of extraepiglottic infection: Report of 72 cases and review of the literature. Pediatrics 58:526, 1976.

Rapkin RH: The diagnosis of epiglottitis: Simplicity and reliability of radiographs of the neck in differential diagnosis of the croup syndrome. J Pediatr 80:96, 1975.

385.2 Bacterial Tracheitis

Bacterial tracheitis, an acute bacterial infection of the upper airway, does not involve the epiglottis but, like epiglottitis and croup, is capable of causing life-threatening airway obstruction. *Staphylococcus aureus* is the most commonly isolated pathogen. Parainfluenza virus type 1, *Moraxella catarrhalis,* nontypable *H. influenzae,* and anaerobic organisms have also been implicated. Most patients are younger than 3 yr of age, although older children have occasionally been affected. There are no clear sex differences in incidence or severity. Bacterial tracheitis usually follows an apparently viral respiratory infection (especially laryngotracheitis). The tracheitis may be a bacterial complication of a viral disease, rather than a primary bacterial illness. This life-threatening entity is now probably more common than epiglottitis.

CLINICAL MANIFESTATIONS. Typically, the child has a brassy cough, apparently as part of a viral laryngotracheobronchitis. High fever and "toxicity" with respiratory distress may occur immediately or after a few days of apparent improvement. Usual treatment for croup (e.g., mist, intravenous fluid, aerosolized racemic epinephrine) is ineffective. Intubation or tracheostomy is usually necessary. The major pathologic feature appears to be mucosal swelling at the level of the cricoid cartilage, complicated by copious thick, purulent secretions. Suctioning these secretions, although occasionally affording temporary relief, usually does not sufficiently obviate the need for an artificial airway.

DIAGNOSIS. The diagnosis is based on evidence of bacterial upper airway disease, which includes moderate leukocytosis with many band forms, high fever, and purulent airway secretions, and an absence of the classic findings of epiglottitis.

TREATMENT. Appropriate antimicrobial therapy, which usually includes antistaphylococcal agents, should be instituted in any patient with croup whose course suggests secondary bacterial tracheitis. When bacterial tracheitis is diagnosed by direct laryngoscopy or is strongly suspected on clinical grounds, an artificial airway is usually indicated. Supplemental oxygen may be necessary.

COMPLICATIONS. Chest roentgenograms often show patchy infiltrates and may show focal densities. Subglottic narrowing and a rough and ragged tracheal air column can often be demonstrated roentgenographically. If airway management is not optimal, cardiorespiratory arrest can occur. Toxic shock syndrome has been associated with tracheitis (see Chapter 182.2).

PROGNOSIS. The prognosis for most patients is excellent. Patients usually become afebrile within 2–3 days of the institution of appropriate antimicrobial therapy, but prolonged hospitalization may be necessary. With a decrease in mucosal edema and purulent secretions, extubation can be accomplished safely, and the patient can be observed carefully while antibiotics and oxygen therapy are continued. The mean duration of hospitalization was 12 days in one series.

Brook I: Aerobic and anaerobic microbiology of bacterial tracheitis in children. Pediatr Emerg Care 13:16, 1997.

Denneny JC III, Handler SD: Membranous laryngotracheobronchitis. Pediatrics 70:705, 1982.

Nelson WE: Bacterial croup: A historical perspective. J Pediatr 105:52, 1984.

CHAPTER 386

Foreign Bodies in the Larynx, Trachea, and Bronchi

David M. Orenstein

The air passages of children are common sites for foreign bodies to lodge; poor supervision by adults or older siblings is occasionally a contributing factor. The symptoms, physical findings, and complications produced by foreign bodies depend on their nature, location, and the degree of obstruction. For example, a sharp or irritating object lodged in the larynx produces severe local edema and, later, suppurative perichondritis. An obstructing object in a bronchus produces distal atelectasis and later produces bronchiectasis, pulmonary abscess, or empyema.

Most foreign bodies aspirated into the respiratory tract are expelled immediately by reflex cough and never require medical attention. If an object too large to be eliminated by mucociliary clearance is aspirated and is not expelled by coughing, respiratory symptoms inevitably result. A large foreign body that can occlude the upper airway is an immediate threat to life. Smaller objects that lodge in one of the main stem or lobar bronchi cause more chronic and usually less severe symptoms.

After the initial symptoms, which may have been forgotten, there is often a symptom-free interval that may last from hours to weeks. On occasion, dysphagia may occur from the swelling that results from a foreign body in the region of the larynx. Foreign bodies in the upper esophagus may cause symptoms referable to the air passages by compression or by the overflow of food or secretions into the larynx. Occasionally, an airway foreign body is not diagnosed until it is revealed by pathologic examination of a lobe that has been removed because of chronic bronchiectasis.

386.1 Laryngeal Foreign Bodies

CLINICAL MANIFESTATIONS. A laryngeal foreign body causes a cough that soon becomes croupy and hoarse and, with profound obstruction, aphonia is seen. Hemoptysis, dyspnea with wheezing, and cyanosis may occur. Obstruction resulting from the foreign body alone or its inflammatory reaction may prove fatal if the signs of high respiratory tract obstruction are not promptly recognized and appropriate treatment given. Hot dogs and bread are two of the most common causes of fatal aspiration. Peanut butter is particularly difficult to remove by cough or instrumentation.

DIAGNOSIS. Roentgenographic and direct laryngoscopic examinations usually reveal or suggest the presence of a foreign body in the larynx (Fig. 386–1). A radiopaque foreign body in the neck is clearly demonstrated on a lateral roentgenogram. When it is lodged anteriorly, it is in the larynx; when it is behind the soft tissue shadows of the larynx, it is in the hypopharynx or the cervical esophagus. The plane in which the foreign body lies is another differential factor in its localization. If it lies in the sagittal plane, it is probably in the larynx. If it is in the coronal plane, it is probably in the esophagus. Even if the foreign body is not radiopaque, high-kilovoltage airway films may suggest its presence. Films should always be taken from the lateral and the anteroposterior projections. In some cases, administering a small amount of opaque contrast material orally may be helpful. Direct laryngoscopy with a rigid open-tube endoscope, usually performed by an otolaryn-

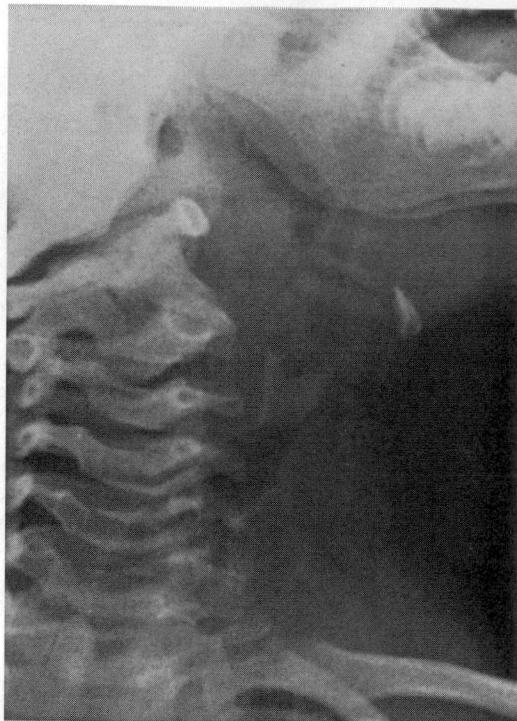

Figure 386–1 Foreign body (fragment of sea shell) in the larynx of a 2-yr-old child treated for "croup" 6 days before the object was suspected. Fortunately, a tracheotomy was not required despite the presence of moderately severe laryngeal edema.

gologist, confirms the diagnosis and provides access for removal of the foreign body. When there is a severe degree of dyspnea, tracheotomy may be advisable before the laryngoscopic examination.

386.2 Tracheal Foreign Bodies

Although a tracheal foreign body may be responsible for cough, hoarseness, dyspnea, and cyanosis, the characteristic signs are wheeze and the audible slap and palpable thud produced by momentary expiratory impaction at the subglottic level. The diagnosis may occasionally be made from the symptoms, physical signs, and roentgenogram of the chest, but in most cases, a definite diagnosis can be made only by bronchoscopy.

386.3 Bronchial Foreign Bodies

CLINICAL MANIFESTATIONS. The initial symptoms of a bronchial foreign body are usually similar to those of foreign bodies in the larynx or trachea. Cough, wheeze, blood-streaked sputum, and metallic taste with metallic foreign bodies also may be produced by bronchial foreign bodies. The degree of obstruction and the stage at which the patient is seen determine the observed symptoms and pathologic changes. A nonobstructing, nonirritating foreign body may produce few symptoms, even after a prolonged time. An obstructing foreign body quickly produces symptoms and signs and pathologic changes. If there is only slight obstruction (e.g., bypass valve), the passage of air in both directions with only slight interference may produce a wheeze. If the obstruction is greater, one of two pathologic conditions may develop. If the obstruction allows air entry but not exit (i.e., check valve or ball valve obstruction), obstructive overinflation ensues. In the case of complete obstruction, which allows neither air entry nor exit, obstructive atelectasis is produced as the air distal to the obstruction is absorbed. If either condition is allowed to persist, chronic bronchopulmonary disease may develop.

Right and left main stem bronchial foreign body aspiration occur with roughly equal frequency. There is usually an immediate episode of choking, gagging, and paroxysmal coughing, which may lead to medical consultation. If this acute episode does not occur or is missed or if its importance is underestimated by the parents, a latent period of minutes to months may pass with only occasional cough or slight wheezing; the patient may acquire recurrent lobar pneumonia or intractable "asthma," often with bilateral wheezing and many episodes of status asthmaticus. Occasionally, chronic wheezing starts immediately after the aspiration. Rarely, the patient with a foreign body presents with hemoptysis, occasionally months or years after aspiration. History may reveal a forgotten episode of choking while eating or while playing with small objects. Older siblings (3–6 yr of age) may have supplied the aspirated object. The physical examination may reveal a tracheal shift. Breath sounds are decreased on the side of the obstruction, but this sign may not be obvious if there is diffuse wheezing. There may be delayed air entry or exit on the obstructed side, detectable with a two-headed differential stethoscope.

Obstruction of both main bronchi may produce severe dyspnea and even asphyxia. If the foreign body is a vegetable (e.g., peanut), a severe condition known as *vegetal* or *arachidic bronchitis* results, characterized by cough, a septic type of fever, and dyspnea. Chronic suppuration may occur when a bronchial foreign body has been present for a long time.

DIAGNOSIS. Most patients with an airway foreign body have a suggestive history. The possibility of a foreign body must be considered in acute or chronic pulmonary lesions regardless of the history of an aspiration event.

If an object causes complete obstruction in the expiratory phase but allows air to pass in the inspiratory phase, air enters the distal portion of the lung on inspiration but little or none escapes during expiration (i.e., *check or ball valve*). This produces obstructive overinflation (Fig. 386–2). Complete blockage of the bronchus by the object itself or in combination with the inflammatory swelling of the bronchial mucosa results in a *stop valve* obstruction, and the air in the distal portion of the lung is soon absorbed, leaving an area of atelectasis (Fig. 386–3). The physical signs of these results of bronchial obstruction from foreign bodies include limited chest expansion, decreased vocal fremitus, dull (i.e., atelectasis) or hyperresonant (i.e., overinflation) percussion note, and diminished breath sounds distal to the foreign body. If there is complete obstruction, with a "drowned lung" or with atelectasis, there is absence of vocal fremitus, which may lead to an erroneous diagnosis of empyema. Various degrees of tympany may bc dcmonstrated over areas of obstructive emphysema. Crackles are more likely on the uninvolved side than on the involved one.

In check valve obstruction, the obstructive overinflation makes it possible to localize a bronchial foreign body by fluoroscopy. The obstructed lung remains expanded during expiration, but the heart and the mediastinum shift to the opposite side as the unobstructed lung empties. The diaphragm is low, flattened, and fixed on the obstructed side; its excursion is free and exaggerated on the unobstructed side. These roentgenographic differences between the lungs are more evident on expiration than on inspiration. With complete obstruction of the bronchus producing obstructive atelectasis, the heart and the mediastinum are drawn toward the obstructed side and remain there during both phases of respiration. The diaphragm on the obstructed side remains high, but that on the unobstructed side moves normally. Films taken at the end of inspiration and expiration show only a slight difference resulting from the filling and emptying of the unobstructed lung. Even

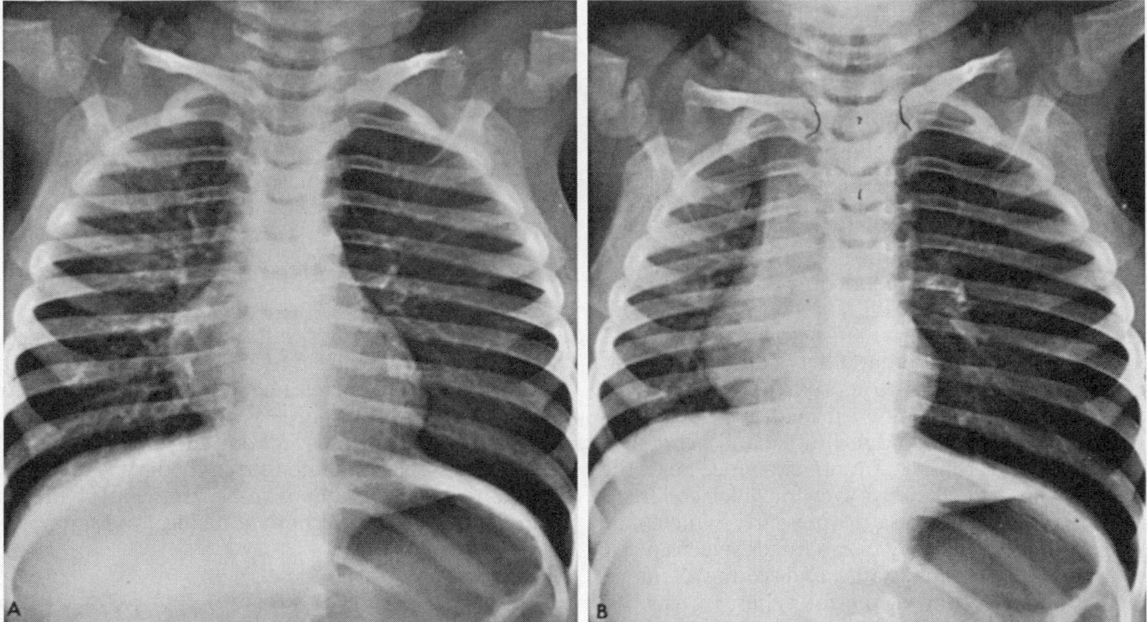

Figure 386–2 Obstructive overinflation due to a peanut fragment in the left mainstem bronchus. *A*, The inspiratory film appears relatively normal except for a slight mediastinal shift to the right. *B*, In expiration, the left lung remains overaerated (i.e., ball-valve mechanism), and the mediastinum moves far to the right.

extensive roentgenographic procedures may not completely rule out the presence of a foreign body. The definitive diagnosis of bronchial foreign body is made by direct bronchoscopic visualization (see Chapter 377). Flexible fiberoptic bronchoscopy may be employed, particularly if the history and physical examination are equivocal. However, the flexible instrument is generally not useful for foreign body removal because it does not permit adequate airway control or instrumentation. Therefore, if the history, physical examination, and roentgenograms strongly suggest a bronchial foreign body, the diagnostic instrument of choice is the rigid or open-tube bronchoscope.

PROGNOSIS. Foreign bodies lodged in the air passages almost invariably cause serious problems if they are not removed.

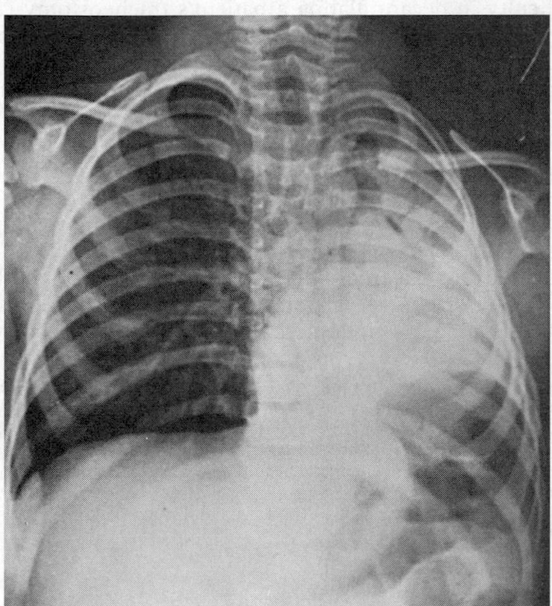

Figure 386–3 Obstructive atelectasis of the left lung caused by a foreign body lodged in the left mainstem bronchus. Notice that the heart is drawn completely into the left side of the chest.

Fortunately, most can be removed safely by a skilled bronchoscopist. Most patients who are diagnosed and treated quickly recover completely after removal. The incidence of complications, including aspiration pneumonia and airway trauma, and the need for tracheostomy because of subglottic edema rises significantly if the diagnosis is delayed longer than 24 hr.

PREVENTION. Foreign body aspiration can be prevented. Small objects should be kept out of the reach of children who are too young to obey restrictions. Children too young to chew and swallow carefully should not be given small pieces of candy, nuts, or similar food. Similarly, toys containing small or loosely attached parts should not be given to children who are still putting such objects into their mouths. Nuts, which account for more than half of airway foreign bodies, and popcorn are particularly appealing to children, and parents should resist the urge to indulge their young child. Beads, button boxes, and coins should not be given to toddlers as playthings. Safety pins should always be closed and should not be left near a baby or in reach of small children. Balloons are underestimated as potential foreign bodies.

TREATMENT. Endoscopy and removal of the foreign body with a rigid open-tube bronchoscope under direct visualization should be performed as soon as possible. Rarely, a thoracotomy is necessary to "milk" the object into position for removal by bronchoscopy. Occasionally, especially when a vegetal foreign body has been in place for a long time, lobectomy may be necessary. Biplane fluoroscopy may be helpful when opaque foreign bodies are lodged in peripheral bronchi. Treatment with pulmonary physiotherapy and bronchodilators is not recommended because of the risk of dislodging a distal foreign body, allowing it to move to and obstruct a larger airway, such as a main stem bronchus, the trachea, or larynx. A delay in performing endoscopy may increase morbidity by allowing more inflammation to develop around the object.

Treating complications is important to obtaining a good outcome. Secondary infections should be treated with appropriate antibiotics. The outcome of the aspiration of a large foreign body that may be immediately life-threatening depends on proper and prompt action taken at the scene of the aspiration.

Emergency treatment of local upper airway obstruction is part of the basic rescuer course in cardiopulmonary resuscitation of the American Heart Association (see Chapters 58 and 64.1). These procedures are used only for children who are aphonic and not breathing. The recommendations for treating infants and young children differ slightly from those for treating teenagers and adults. If the patient can breathe and is able to cough or speak, none of the maneuvers described should be undertaken. For patients who are genuinely choking, the recommendations of the Committee on Accident and Poison Prevention of the American Academy of Pediatrics are as follows: For infants (<1 yr), the repetitive use of four back blows and four chest thrusts is recommended. Abdominal thrusts should not be used. The back blows are delivered while holding the infant with the head lower than the trunk. Four blows are delivered with the heel of the hand between the scapulas. The purpose of this maneuver is to loosen the foreign body. After the back blows, the patient is turned, and four chest thrusts are delivered using the same technique and hand positioning as used for closed cardiac compression (i.e., over the midsternum for infants and slightly lower for older children). This maneuver increases intrathoracic pressure, which may cause expulsion of the foreign body. Blind finger sweeps of the mouth should not be used in infants and young children. Instead, after the administration of the four chest thrusts, the mouth should be opened and a visualized foreign body should be grasped and removed. After each sequence of back blows, chest thrusts, and visual attempts to remove the foreign body, rescue breathing should be attempted for the unconscious patient. If unsuccessful, the sequence is repeated.

A young child (>1 yr) should be placed on his or her back. The rescuer kneels next to the patient and, using the heel of one hand, performs 6 to 10 abdominal thrusts (Chapter 64.1) by pushing upward and inward from the midabdomen, midway between the umbilicus and the rib cage. If this is unsuccessful, the victim's mouth is opened by using the tongue-jaw lift, and a visualized foreign body is removed (see Chapter 64.1). Blind sweeps of the mouth should not be made. Rescue breathing should then be attempted before the entire sequence is repeated. Although there is controversy concerning the precise technique to be used in total upper airway obstruction by a foreign body, pediatricians should provide up-to-date information on these techniques to parents and should urge parents to expect their baby sitters (including teenagers) to be familiar with the symptoms and emergency treatment of foreign body aspiration.

Baker SP, Fisher RS: Childhood asphyxiation by choking or suffocation. JAMA 244:1343, 1980.

Blazer S, Naveh Y, Friedman A: Foreign body in the airway: A review of 200 cases. Am Rev Dis Child 134:68, 1980.

Blumhagen JD, Weisenberg RL, Brooks JG, et al: Endotracheal foreign bodies: Difficulties in diagnosis. Clin Pediatr 19:480, 1980.

Committee on Accident and Poison Prevention: Revised first aid for the choking child. Pediatrics 78:177, 1986.

Esclamado RM, Richardson MA: Laryngotracheal foreign bodies in children. Am J Dis Child 141:259, 1987.

Kloske AM: Respiratory foreign body. *In:* Hilman BH (ed): Pediatric Respiratory Disease: Diagnosis and Treatment. Philadelphia, WB Saunders, 1993, p 513.

Rothman BF, Boeckman CR: Foreign bodies in the larynx and tracheobronchial tree in children. Ann Otol Rhinol Laryngol 89:434, 1980.

CHAPTER 387
Subglottic Stenosis

David M. Orenstein

387.1 Acute Subglottic Stenosis

Acute stenosis may result from an acute infection producing edema of the subglottic region or epiglottis and arytenoiditis; from inflammation secondary to the inspiration of a vegetal foreign body and, especially, after instrumentation for the removal of such an object; from edema of an allergic reaction; or from a foreign body lodged in the larynx. Treatment consists of immediate provision of an airway by intubation or tracheotomy, followed by appropriate medical therapy.

387.2 Chronic Subglottic Stenosis

Chronic subglottic stenosis is a frequent sequela of tracheotomy in which damage of the first tracheal ring or cricoid cartilage results in perichondritis and subsequent overgrowth of cartilage or fibrous tissue. Chronic stenosis may also result from laryngeal diphtheria, syphilis, tuberculosis, radiation burns, or external trauma. The most common cause is neonatal endotracheal intubation. Congenital laryngeal stenosis may be transmitted as an autosomal dominant trait in some patients. "Silent" gastroesophageal reflux with aspiration of gastric acid into the subglottic region may be responsible for many cases.

CLINICAL MANIFESTATIONS. The clinical manifestations of chronic laryngeal stenosis may include dyspnea with audible stridor and suprasternal, supraclavicular, and intercostal retractions, or they may be limited to an inability to decannulate a patient's tracheostomy or remove an endotracheal tube. The diagnosis is made by direct laryngoscopy and roentgenographic examination. Scarring and stenosis usually develop in the subglottic region, occasionally with necrosis of cartilage.

TREATMENT. Milder cases may not need treatment. Mild cases of difficulty in decannulating a patient's tracheostomy can be treated by replacing the tracheostomy cannula with a smaller one and closure of this tube, at first partial and then complete, with a cork, which re-educates the patient to breathe through the mouth and permits the removal of the cannula. If this method is unsuccessful, dilation through a direct laryngoscope may help but should not be performed too frequently. For some children, external surgery with or without the use of an indwelling mold may be necessary. A cricoid-split operation is successful in severe cases. In all cases, children should be investigated for gastroesophageal reflux, which should be treated aggressively (see Chapter 323). The prognosis for eventual cure is good, but treatment may require months or years.

Landing BH: State of the art: Congenital malformations and genetic diseases of the respiratory tract. Am Rev Respir Dis 120:151, 1979.

Little FB, Kohut RI, Koufman JA, et al: Effect of gastric acid on the pathogenesis of subglottic stenosis. Ann Otol Rhinol Laryngol 94:516, 1985.

McGill TJI, Healy GB: Congenital and acquired lesions of the infant larynx. Clin Pediatr 17:584, 1978.

Proctor DF: The upper airways: 11. The larynx and trachea. Am Rev Respir Dis 115:315, 1977.

CHAPTER 388
Trauma to the Larynx

Robert C. Stern

BIRTH TRAUMA. Laryngeal injury during birth is not uncommon and may result in *dislocation of the cricothyroid* or *cricoarytenoid articulations*. Hoarseness and, at times, wheezing or fluttering respiratory sounds are heard. The diagnosis is made by direct laryngoscopic examination. Treatment by direct laryngoscopic manipulations, using a laryngeal dilator, may occasionally be effective, but tracheotomy should be performed if there is evidence of hypoxia.

Unilateral or bilateral *recurrent laryngeal nerve paralysis* may also be produced by birth trauma, especially during forceps delivery. Bilateral paralysis is often associated with central nervous system disease (Chiari's malformation). Paralysis of one cord may produce only hoarseness and slight stridor without dyspnea. Unilateral paralysis is usually on the left. Bilateral paralysis produces dyspnea with stridor. In unilateral and bilateral vocal cord paralysis, chronic aspiration can lead to recurrent pneumonia. Direct laryngoscopic examination establishes the diagnosis. Tracheotomy is usually necessary for bilateral paralysis. An older child may wear a valvular cannula, or a laryngoplasty with lateral fixation of one vocal cord may be performed to improve the airway and permit decannulation if breathing through the larynx does not improve spontaneously.

POSTNATAL TRAUMA. Any trauma, such as that brought about by a fall against a hard object, may produce acute or chronic stenosis of the larynx, as may high tracheotomy and prolonged intubation. Serious laryngotracheal trauma is rare; of 30,000 trauma cases in one series, only 12 involved the larynx and only one patient thus affected was a child. In children, the flexibility and motility of the larynx protect against serious nonpenetrating injury. Penetrating injuries are usually obvious and require treatment by an otolaryngologic surgeon. Serious nonpenetrating injuries may be deceptive because substantial edema and even a compressing hematoma may give surprisingly few external clues. Laryngeal fracture should be suspected in patients who have hoarseness, hemoptysis, or subcutaneous emphysema after neck trauma. Laryngoscopy and, occasionally, surgical exploration may be indicated in patients who have relatively normal physical findings but whose history is compatible with substantial blunt neck trauma. Most patients with serious laryngeal or upper tracheal injuries require tracheostomy as part of their treatment; if there are signs of high obstruction, the need may be urgent. The normal voice is frequently not recovered. Similarly, severe thermal injury (after accidental inhalation of steam or smoke) is often best managed with tracheostomy. Ingestion of caustic substances has also been associated with laryngeal lesions.

Acute *overuse of the voice* (e.g., prolonged screaming at a concert or athletic event) may cause transient hoarseness. With cessation of this stress, the voice returns to normal without other treatment. The roles of resting the voice (i.e., minimal or no use of speech at all) or misting in accelerating recovery are not clear. Acute laryngitis is fairly common in older children during mild viral respiratory infections; spontaneous recovery is the rule, and the importance of steam and other therapeutic maneuvers is unknown. Occasionally, a teenager may develop chronic laryngitis from heavy cigarette smoking. The differential diagnosis of persistent hoarse voice includes vocal ("singer's" or "screamer's") nodules, papillomas, and serious tumors such as rhabdomyosarcoma. A laryngeal abscess is a rare cause of persistent hoarseness. These masses are diagnosed by laryngoscopy and may require surgical treatment, which may be followed by voice training. Otolaryngologic consultation is indicated for any child with unexplained continuous hoarseness persisting longer than 1 wk.

Benjamin B: Prolonged intubation injuries of the larynx: Endoscopic diagnosis, classification, and treatment. Ann Otol Rhinol Laryngol 102(Suppl 160): 1, 1990.
Jurkovich G, Luterman A: Laryngotracheal trauma: A protocol approach to a rare injury. Laryngoscope 96:660, 1986.
Kadish H, Schunk J, Woodward GA: Blunt pediatric laryngotracheal trauma: Case reports and review of the literature. Am J Emerg Med 12:207, 1994.
Moulin D, Bertrand JM, Buts JP, et al: Upper airway lesions in children after accidental ingestion of caustic substances. J Pediatr 106:408, 1985.

CHAPTER 389
Neoplasms of the Larynx and Trachea

Robert C. Stern

Papilloma is the most common tumor of the larynx in childhood; it rarely becomes malignant and often disappears after puberty. The pink, warty tumors may grow profusely from any portion of the larynx, although usually from the vocal cords. This disease is caused by the human papillomavirus (see Chapter 257). When maternal vaginal condyloma is present, material containing this virus may be aspirated during delivery, producing disease in a small fraction of exposed infants.

The initial symptom is hoarseness, but dyspnea is likely if the condition is allowed to persist. Asphyxia may occur. Direct laryngoscopy accomplishes diagnosis (confirmed histologically) and treatment, because the papilloma can be easily removed with forceps. Care should be taken not to damage normal tissue. Cure usually occurs, although rapid recurrence is common at first. Tracheostomy may be required because of recurrences and the threat of aspiration. Cryosurgery and laser surgery have been advocated as alternative or adjuvant therapy. Radical excision and radiation are contraindicated.

Extension of the disease into the lower airways and lungs can occur. The factors that predispose to this complication are unknown. *Respiratory papillomatosis* is a much more serious disease and carries a high mortality rate. Patients with laryngobronchial papillomatosis that fails to respond to usual treatment may improve after receiving systemic bleomycin. Human leukocyte interferon has been reported to be beneficial for patients with recurrent severe disease. However, in one controlled study, the patients in the treatment group had a better course for 6 mo, but this was not sustained for the next 6 mo. Some success with ribavirin was reported in one 3-yr-old patient. Papilloma may recur many years, even decades, after apparent cure. Malignant degeneration into squamous cell carcinoma has been reported in young children. This complication is more likely after radiation treatment.

Vocal nodules or small tumors may occur in children at the junction of the anterior and middle thirds of the cords. They are usually bilateral and produce slight hoarseness. Spontaneous regression may occur if strenuous use of the voice is avoided. They may be removed under direct laryngoscopic view or treated with laser.

Primary tracheal tumors are much less frequent. Although they may have been symptomatic (wheezing, cough, or pneumonia), because of their rarity and the absence of hoarseness as a presenting symptom, they are not usually diagnosed until 75% of the tracheal lumen has been occluded. At that point, patients can present with respiratory arrest. The usual laboratory evaluation for wheezing/asthma (e.g., standard radiograph, standard pulmonary function testing) is not sufficient. Pulmonary function technicians usually emphasize the expiratory portion of the flow-volume loop (a valid inspiratory portion would be needed to detect tracheal obstruction), and plain chest radiographs usually do not show tracheal soft tissue very well, especially in the upper trachea. Tracheal tumors should be considered in patients with "monophonic" (same in all lung fields) wheezing and lack of response to bronchodilators, but even in those patients, other diagnoses (e.g., vocal cord adduction) would be more likely. Most tracheal tumors in childhood are benign. Treatment varies with the exact diagnosis.

Chaput M, Ninane J, Gosseye S, et al: Juvenile laryngeal papillomatosis and epidermoid carcinoma. J Pediatr 114:269, 1989.
Gjonaj ST, Lowenthal DB, Dozor AJ, et al: Pneumonias, asthma, pneumothorax, and respiratory arrest caused by a tracheal mass. J Pediatr 99:604, 1997.
Healy GB, Gelber RD, Trowbridge AL, et al: Treatment of recurrent respiratory papillomatosis with human leukocyte interferon. N Engl J Med 319:401, 1988.
Mehta P, Herold N: Regression of juvenile laryngobronchial papillomatosis with systemic bleomycin therapy. J Pediatr 97:479, 1980.
Morrison GAJ, Kotecha B, Evans NG: Ribavirin treatment for juvenile respiratory papillomatosis. J Laryngol Otol 107:423, 1993.

CHAPTER 390
Bronchitis

David M. Orenstein

390.1 Acute Bronchitis

Although the diagnosis of acute bronchitis is frequently made, this condition may not exist in children as an isolated clinical entity. Bronchitis is associated with several other conditions of the upper and lower respiratory tracts, and the trachea is usually involved. Bronchiolitis is an entirely different illness (see Chapter 391).

Asthmatic bronchitis is a commonly used term that may no longer serve a useful purpose, as bronchial inflammation ("*bronchitis*") is an integral part of asthma. Asthma exacerbations are commonly triggered by upper respiratory tract infections. Calling such exacerbations "asthmatic bronchitis," although technically correct, may obscure the patient's and family's understanding that this is *asthma*.

Acute tracheobronchitis is commonly associated with an upper respiratory tract infection such as nasopharyngitis but is also associated with influenza, pertussis, measles, typhoid fever (and other salmonelloses), diphtheria, and scarlet fever. An acute, primary, undifferentiated tracheobronchitis also occurs, most commonly in older children and adolescents. It is likely that, except for the bacterial diseases mentioned, acute tracheobronchitis is of viral origin. Pneumococci, staphylococci, *Haemophilus influenzae,* and various hemolytic streptococci may be isolated from the sputum, but their presence does not imply a bacterial cause, and antibiotic therapy does not appreciably alter the course of the illness. Some children appear to be far more susceptible to acute tracheobronchitis than others. The reasons are unknown, but allergy, climate, air pollution, and chronic infections of the upper respiratory tract, particularly sinusitis, may be contributing factors.

CLINICAL MANIFESTATIONS. Acute bronchitis is usually preceded by a viral upper respiratory infection. Secondary bacterial infection with *Streptococcus pneumoniae, Moraxella catarrhalis,* or *H. influenzae* may occur. Typically, the child presents a frequent, dry, hacking, unproductive cough of relatively gradual onset, beginning 3–4 days after the appearance of rhinitis. Low substernal discomfort or burning anterior chest pain is often present and may be aggravated by coughing. As the illness progresses, the patient may be bothered by whistling sounds during respiration (probably rhonchi), soreness of the chest, and occasionally by shortness of breath. Coughing paroxysms or gagging on secretions is associated occasionally with vomiting. Within several days, the cough becomes productive, and the sputum changes from clear to purulent. Usually within 5–10 days, the mucus thins, and the cough gradually disappears. The considerable malaise often associated with the illness may continue for 1 wk or more after acute symptoms have subsided.

Physical findings vary with the age of the patient and the stage of the disease. Initially, the child is usually afebrile or has low-grade fever, and there are signs of nasopharyngitis, conjunctival infection, and rhinitis. Later, auscultation reveals roughening of breath sounds, coarse and fine moist rales, and rhonchi that may be high-pitched, resembling the wheezing of asthma.

In otherwise healthy children, complications are few, but in undernourished children or those in poor health, otitis media, sinusitis, and pneumonia are common. Children with repeated attacks of acute bronchitis should be carefully evaluated for the possibility of respiratory tract anomalies, including ciliary disorders, foreign bodies, bronchiectasis, immune deficiency, tuberculosis, allergy, sinusitis, tonsillitis, adenoiditis, and cystic fibrosis.

TREATMENT. There is no specific therapy; most patients recover uneventfully without any treatment. In small infants, pulmonary drainage is facilitated by frequent shifts in position. Older children are more comfortable in high humidity, but there is no evidence that this shortens the duration of illness. Irritating and paroxysmal coughing may cause considerable distress and interfere with sleep. Although suppression of cough may increase the possibility of suppuration, judicious use of cough suppressants (including codeine) may be appropriate for symptomatic relief. Antihistamines, which dry secretions, should not be used, and expectorants are not helpful. Antibiotics do not shorten the duration of the viral illness or decrease the incidence of bacterial complications. However, patients with recurrent episodes may occasionally improve with such treatment, suggesting that some secondary bacterial infection is present.

390.2 Chronic Bronchitis

Although adult chronic bronchitis is defined as 3 mo or more of productive cough each year for 2 or more consecutive years, there is no such accepted standard for children. Its very existence as a separate entity has been questioned, which emphasizes the importance of searching for an underlying immunologic or mucosal abnormality. A chronic or frequently recurring productive cough usually indicates an underlying pulmonary or systemic disease; affected patients should be evaluated for asthma, immune deficiencies, cigarette smoke (primary or second-hand) exposure, anatomic abnormalities, environmental disease, upper airway infection with postnasal discharge, cystic fibrosis, ciliary dyskinesis, and bronchiectasis. Cough and wheezing are common, and in one study, all 22 reported patients with chronic bronchitis had evidence of allergic disease. Rarely, bronchial irritation may be secondary to the chronic inhalation of dust or noxious fumes. Tobacco or marijuana smoking is obviously pertinent historical information. Teenagers should be similarly questioned about industrial fumes or automobile exhaust exposure at school or work.

390.3 Air Pollution and Cigarette Smoking

Correlation of a specific *pollutant* (e.g., NO_2, particulate matter) with a specific childhood respiratory disease or pulmonary symptom is difficult to establish. Any one substance for which such an association is demonstrated may be a marker for one or more other pollutants that are really responsible. However, this does not invalidate the large number of studies indicating that high levels of overall air pollution cause or aggravate lung disease in children. Air pollutants also impair pulmonary function in exercising children and teenagers. Children and parents should be advised of these relationships.

An increased incidence and exacerbations of bronchitis and other forms of acute and chronic lung disease are associated with *cigarette smoking*. The increased morbidity from respiratory infections in teenagers who smoke is reflected in school and work absences and in functional and pathologic evidence of small airway abnormalities. For example, cigarette smoking is a risk factor for the severity of influenza in young men. Smoking parents, especially those whose children have chronic lung disease, should be advised that they are subjecting their children's lungs to significant amounts of second-hand cigarette smoke in the home; they should be urged to stop smoking.

The Committee on Genetics and Environmental Hazards of the American Academy of Pediatrics has reported that tobacco smoking is one of the most important "sources of environmental contamination and a significant threat to the health of children." It urges physicians to support legislation that would prohibit smoking in public places frequented by children, "particularly in hospitals and other health facilities."

The use of *wood-burning stoves* also has been associated with a variety of pediatric pulmonary problems. Indoor wood burning results in exposure to particulate matter and polycyclic hydrocarbons. Wheezing and episodic pneumonia have been described in exposed children. In one study, 84% of children exposed to wood-burning stoves (compared with 3% of controls) were reported to have at least one severe respiratory symptom. Systemic problems can also occur if the wood has been treated with toxic materials (e.g., arsenic poisoning has been reported in one family).

CLINICAL MANIFESTATIONS. The chief symptom is cough, with or without expectoration. The child usually complains of chest soreness, and characteristically these signs and symptoms are worse at night. Wheezing may also be prominent, and physical findings are similar to those of acute bronchitis. Some patients with bronchitis cough up large, solid, hypereosinophilic mucoid "casts" of the airways, giving rise to the term *plastic bronchitis*. These casts may be related to metaplastic bronchial epithelium, elements of which, together with inflammatory cells with or without an infectious agent and noncellular material, can be found on histologic examination.

COURSE AND PROGNOSIS. The course and prognosis depend on appropriate management or eradication of any underlying illness. Complications are those of the underlying illness.

TREATMENT. When an underlying cause for chronic bronchitis is found, appropriate management should be started. Anti-inflammatory or allergy management may be helpful even when no underlying cause can be discovered. Autogenous vaccines or inhalation of antibiotics is not effective.

Bartecchi CE, MacKenzie TD, Schrier RW: The human cost of tobacco use. N Engl J Med 330:907, 1994.

Braun-Fahrlander C, Ackermann-Liebrich U, Schwartz J, et al: Air pollution and respiratory symptoms in preschool children. Am Rev Respir Dis 145:42, 1992.

Chilmonczyk BA, Salmun LM, Megathlin KN, et al: Association between exposure to environmental tobacco smoke and exacerbations of asthma in children. N Engl J Med 328:1665, 1993.

Gergen PJ, Fowler JA, Maurer KR, et al: The burden of environmental tobacco smoke exposure on the respiratory health of children 2 months through 5 years of age in the United States: Third National Health and Nutrition Examination Survey, 1988–1994. Pediatrics 101:E8, 1998. Internet site: Pediatrics.org/cgi/content/full/101/2/e8.

Gold DR, Wang X, Wypij D, et al: Effects of cigarette smoking on lung function in adolescent boys and girls. N Engl J Med 335:931, 1996.

Koenig JQ, Covert DS, Hanley QS, et al: Prior exposure to ozone potentiates subsequent response to sulfur dioxide in adolescent asthmatic subjects. Am Rev Respir Dis 141:377, 1990.

Morris K, Morganlander M, Coulehan JL, et al: Wood-burning stoves and lower respiratory tract infection in American Indian children. Am J Dis Child 144:105, 1990.

Perez-Soler A: Cast bronchitis in infants and children. Am J Dis Child 143:1024, 1989.

Samet JM, Marbury MC, Spengler JD: Health effects and sources of indoor air pollution. Parts 1 and 2. Am J Respir Dis 136:1486; 137:221, 1988.

Smith TF, Ireland TA, Zaatari GS, et al: Characteristics of children with endoscopically proved chronic bronchitis. Am J Dis Child 139:1039, 1985.

Taussig LM, Smith SM, Blumenfield R: Chronic bronchitis in childhood: What is it? Pediatrics 67:1, 1981.

CHAPTER 391
Bronchiolitis

David M. Orenstein

Acute bronchiolitis, a common disease of the lower respiratory tract of infants, results from inflammatory obstruction of the small airways. It occurs during the first 2 yr of life, with a peak incidence at approximately 6 mo of age, and in many localities it is the most frequent cause of hospitalization of infants. The incidence is highest during the winter and early spring. The illness occurs sporadically and epidemically.

ETIOLOGY AND EPIDEMIOLOGY. Acute bronchiolitis is predominantly a viral illness. The respiratory syncytial virus (RSV) is the causative agent in more than 50% of cases (see Chapter 253); parainfluenza 3 virus, mycoplasma, some adenoviruses, and occasionally other viruses produce most of the remaining cases. Adenovirus may be associated with long-term complications, including bronchiolitis obliterans (see Chapter 392) and unilateral hyperlucent lung syndrome (Swyer-James syndrome). There is no firm evidence that bacteria cause bronchiolitis. Occasionally, bacterial bronchopneumonia may be confused clinically with bronchiolitis.

Bronchiolitis occurs most commonly in male infants between 3 and 6 mo of age who have not been breast-fed and who live in crowded conditions. The source of the viral infection is usually a family member with minor respiratory illness. Older children and adults tolerate bronchiolar edema better than infants and do not acquire the clinical picture of bronchiolitis even when the smaller airways of the respiratory tract are infected by a virus.

In one report, sophisticated pulmonary function studies were performed on a large population of normal infants. The follow-up analysis revealed that wheezy respiratory illnesses were significantly more common among infants whose initial total respiratory conductance was in the lowest third of those tested. Diminished lung function may play a role in determining which infants with viral infection acquire bronchiolitis.

Infants whose mothers smoke cigarettes are more likely to acquire bronchiolitis than are infants of nonsmoking mothers. Despite the known risks of respiratory infections in children who attend child care, bronchiolitis is more likely to develop in infants who stay home with mothers who are heavy smokers than in infants who attend day care centers.

PATHOPHYSIOLOGY. Acute bronchiolitis is characterized by bronchiolar obstruction due to edema and accumulation of mucus and cellular debris and by invasion of the smaller bronchial radicles by virus. Because resistance to airflow in a tube is inversely related to the fourth power of the radius, even minor thickening of the bronchiolar wall in infants may profoundly affect airflow. Resistance in the small air passages is increased during the inspiratory and expiratory phases, but because the radius of an airway is smaller during expiration, the resultant ball valve respiratory obstruction leads to early air trapping and overinflation. Atelectasis may occur when an obstruction becomes complete and trapped air is absorbed (see Chapter 406).

The pathologic process impairs the normal exchange of gases in the lung. Ventilation-perfusion mismatch results in hypoxemia early in the course. Carbon dioxide retention (hypercapnia) does not usually occur except in severely affected patients. The higher the respiratory rate, the lower the arterial oxygen tension. Hypercapnia usually does not occur until respirations exceed 60 breaths/min; it then increases in proportion to the tachypnea.

CLINICAL MANIFESTATIONS. Most affected infants have a history of exposure to older children or adults with minor respiratory diseases within the week preceding the onset of illness. The infant first has a mild upper respiratory tract infection with serous nasal discharge and sneezing. These symptoms usually last several days and may be accompanied by diminished appetite and fever of 38.5–39°C (101–102°F), although the temperature may range from subnormal to markedly elevated. The gradual development of respiratory distress is characterized by paroxysmal wheezy cough, dyspnea, and irritability. Breast- or bottle-feeding may be particularly difficult because the rapid respiratory rate may not permit time for sucking and swallowing. In mild cases, symptoms disappear in 1–3 days. In more severely affected patients, symptoms may develop within several hours, and the course is protracted. Other systemic manifestations, such as vomiting and diarrhea, are usually absent.

An examination reveals a tachypneic infant, with a hyperexpanded chest and often in extreme distress. Respirations range from 60–80 breaths/min; severe air hunger and cyanosis may occur. The alae nasi flare, and use of the accessory muscles of respiration results in intercostal and subcostal retractions, which are shallow because of the persistent distention of the lungs by the trapped air. The depression of the liver and spleen by the overinflated lungs may result in their being palpable below the costal margin. Widespread fine crackles may be heard at the end of inspiration and in early expiration. The expiratory phase of breathing is prolonged, and wheezes are usually audible. In the most severe cases, breath sounds are barely audible when bronchiolar obstruction is almost complete.

Roentgenographic examination reveals hyperinflation of the lungs and an increased anteroposterior diameter on lateral view. Scattered areas of consolidation are found in about 30% of patients and are caused by atelectasis secondary to obstruction or by inflammation of the alveoli. Early bacterial pneumonia cannot be excluded on radiographic grounds alone.

The white blood cell and differential cell counts are usually within normal limits. Lymphopenia, commonly associated with many viral illnesses, is usually not found. Nasopharyngeal cultures reveal normal bacterial flora. Virus may be demonstrated in nasopharyngeal secretions by antigen detection (e.g., by enzyme immunoassay), by PCR, or culture.

DIFFERENTIAL DIAGNOSIS. The condition most commonly confused with acute bronchiolitis is asthma. One or more of the following favors the diagnosis of asthma: a family history of asthma, repeated episodes in the same infant, sudden onset without preceding infection, eosinophilia, and an immediate favorable response to the administration of a single dose of aerosolized albuterol. Repeated attacks represent an important differential point: Fewer than 5% of recurrent attacks of clinical bronchiolitis have viral infections as a cause. Other entities that may be confused with acute bronchiolitis are cystic fibrosis, heart failure, a foreign body in the trachea, pertussis, organophosphate poisoning, and bacterial bronchopneumonias associated with generalized obstructive pulmonary overinflation.

COURSE AND PROGNOSIS. The most critical phase of illness occurs during the first 48–72 hr after the onset of cough and dyspnea. During this period, the infant appears desperately ill, apneic spells occur in the very young infant, and respiratory acidosis is likely to be noticed. After the critical period, improvement occurs rapidly and often dramatically. Recovery is complete in a few days. The case fatality rate is less than 1%; death may result from prolonged apneic spells, severe uncompensated respiratory acidosis, or profound dehydration secondary to the loss of water vapor from tachypnea and the inability to drink fluids. Infants with conditions such as congenital heart disease, bronchopulmonary dysplasia, immunodeficiency diseases, or cystic fibrosis have a greater morbidity rate and a slightly increased mortality rate. Estimates of mortality among infants with these high-risk conditions who contract RSV bronchiolitis decreased from 37% in 1982 to 3.5% in 1988. Bacterial complications, such as bronchopneumonia or sepsis, are uncommon. Otitis media may occur. Cardiac failure during bronchiolitis is rare, except in children with underlying heart disease.

A significant proportion of infants with bronchiolitis have hyperreactive airways during later childhood, but the relation of these two entities, if any, is not understood. The suggestion that a single episode of bronchiolitis may result in long-term small airway abnormality requires further investigation. These abnormalities may be partially explained by the finding that infants with low total respiratory conductance are more likely to acquire bronchiolitis in response to viral respiratory infection. The infants with bronchiolitis in whom reactive airways develop are more likely to have a family history of asthma and allergy, a prolonged acute episode of bronchiolitis, and exposure to cigarette smoke.

PREVENTION. RSV immune globulin intravenous (RSV-IGIV) or intramuscularly administered monoclonal antibody to RSV (Palivizumab) given just prior to and during RSV season is effective in preventing severe RSV disease in at-risk infants (see Chapter 253). It is recommended for infants less than 2 yr with chronic lung disease (bronchopulmonary dysplasia) or prematurity but should not be given to those with symptomatic cyanotic congenital heart disease because of increased complications, including increased mortality.

TREATMENT. Infants with respiratory distress should be hospitalized, but only supportive treatment is indicated. The child is commonly placed in an atmosphere of cool, humidified oxygen to relieve hypoxemia and reduce insensible water loss from tachypnea; this treatment usually relieves the dyspnea and cyanosis and allays anxiety and restlessness. Sedatives should be avoided whenever possible because of potential depression of respiration. The infant is usually more comfortable sitting at a 30 to 40 degree angle or with the head and chest slightly elevated so that the neck is somewhat extended. Oral intake must often be supplemented or replaced by parenteral fluids to offset the dehydrating effect of tachypnea. Electrolyte balance and pH should be adjusted by suitable intravenous solutions.

Ribavirin (Vibrazole), an antiviral agent administered by aerosol, may be considered for infants with congenital heart disease or bronchopulmonary dysplasia. There is no convincing evidence of ribavirin's impact on the duration of hospitalization, requirement for supportive therapies such as oxygen or mechanical ventilation, or mortality. Some high-risk infants not treated with ribavirin have a good prognosis.

Antibiotics have no therapeutic value unless there is secondary bacterial pneumonia. The low incidence of bacterial complications is not reduced further by antibiotic therapy. Corticosteroids are not beneficial and may be harmful under certain conditions. However, corticosteroids have not been evaluated in patients with severe adenovirus bronchiolitis in whom long-term severe sequelae (e.g., necrotizing lesions) might be more likely. Studies that have shown apparent benefit from corticosteroids have failed to exclude infants with asthma. Bronchodilating aerosolized drugs (e.g., albuterol) are frequently used empirically; studies are divided between those that demonstrate benefit and those that demonstrate no benefit or even harm. If improvement is documented after a trial of inhaled albuterol, it should be continued. Epinephrine or other adrenergic agents have a theoretical basis for use in that they might be expected to decrease venous engorgement and mucosal swelling by causing vasoconstriction, and in two studies, aerosolized epinephrine provided some benefit to infants with bronchiolitis. Chinese herbs were shown in one study to decrease symptom duration by 2.6 days. Some patients may progress rapidly to respiratory failure, requiring ventilatory assistance.

Andrade MA, Hoberman A, Glustein J, et al: Acute otitis media in children with bronchiolitis. Pediatrics 101:617, 1998.
Committee on Infectious Diseases (American Academy of Pediatrics): Reassessment of the indications for ribavirin therapy in respiratory syncytial virus infections. Pediatrics 97:137, 1996.
Dobson JV, Stephens-Groff SM, McMahon SR, et al: The use of albuterol in hospitalized infants with bronchiolitis. Pediatrics 101:361, 1998.
Englund J, Piedra P, Ahn Y-M, et al: High-dose, short-duration ribavirin aerosol therapy compared with standard ribavirin therapy in children with suspected respiratory syncytial virus infection. J Pediatr 125:635, 1994.
Gadomski A, Lichenstein R, Horton L, et al: Efficacy of albuterol in the management of bronchiolitis. Pediatrics 93:907, 1994.
Hall CB, McBride JT, Walsh EE, et al: Aerosolized ribavirin treatment of infants with respiratory syncytial viral infection: A randomized double blind study. N Engl J Med 308:1443, 1983.
Klassen TP, Sutcliffe T, Watters LK, et al: Dexamethasone in salbutamol-treated inpatients with acute bronchiolitis: A randomized, controlled trial. J Pediatr 130:191, 1997.
Kong XT, Fang HT, Jiang GQ, et al: Treatment of acute bronchiolitis with Chinese herbs. Arch Dis Child 68:468, 1993.
Kritjansson S, Lodrup Carlsen KC, Wennergren G, et al: Nebulised racemic adrenalin in the treatment of acute bronchiolitis in infants and toddlers. Arch Dis Child 69:650, 1993.
Martinez FD, Morgan WJ, Wright AL, et al: Diminished lung function as a predisposing factor for wheezing respiratory illness in infants. N Engl J Med 319:112, 1988.
McConnochie KM, Roghmann KJ: Predicting clinically significant lower respiratory tract illness in childhood following mild bronchiolitis. Am J Dis Child 139:625, 1985.
Richter H, Seddon P: Early nebulized budesonide in the treatment of bronchiolitis and the prevention of postbronchiolitic wheezing. J Pediatr 132:849, 1998.
Schuh S, Canny G, Reisman JJ, et al: Nebulized albuterol in acute bronchiolitis. J Pediatr 117:633, 1990.
Wald ER, Dashefsky B: Ribavirin. Red book committee recommendation questioned. Pediatrics 93:672, 1994.

CHAPTER 392
Bronchiolitis Obliterans

David M. Orenstein

In *bronchiolitis obliterans,* the bronchioles and smaller airways are injured, and the attempted repair produces large amounts of granulation tissue that causes airway obstruction. Eventually, the airway lumens are obliterated with nodular masses of granulation and fibrosis. The precipitating injury commonly cannot be identified, particularly in children. Some adult cases are related to the inhalation of the oxides of nitrogen or other chemicals. The syndrome has also been associated with connective tissue diseases and some drugs (e.g., penicillamine). Most pediatric cases can be temporally related to pulmonary infection, such as measles, influenza, adenovirus, mycoplasmal infection, and pertussis. Obliterative bronchiolitis is a common and ominous complication of lung transplantation and is also seen as part of chronic graft-versus-host disease after bone marrow transplantation (see Chapters 137 and 449.2).

CLINICAL MANIFESTATIONS. Initially, cough, respiratory distress, and cyanosis may occur and may be followed by a brief period of apparent improvement. Progressive disease is reflected by increasing dyspnea, cough, sputum production, and wheezing. The pattern may resemble bronchitis, bronchiolitis, or pneumonia. The chest roentgenographic findings range from normal to a pattern that suggests miliary tuberculosis. *Swyer-James syndrome* may develop with unilateral hyperlucency and a decrease in pulmonary vascular markings in about 10% of cases. Bronchography shows obstruction of the bronchioles, with little or no contrast material reaching the periphery of the lung. In many patients, computed tomography reveals bronchiectasis. Pulmonary function test findings are variable, with severe obstruction being most common, but restriction or a combination of obstruction and restriction is seen. The diagnosis may be confirmed by lung biopsy.

TREATMENT AND PROGNOSIS. There is no specific treatment. In lung transplant recipients, immune suppression with tacrolimus may be associated with a lower incidence of bronchiolitis obliterans than is suppression with cyclosporine. The pathologic features suggests a progressive fibrotic picture that could theoretically be delayed by corticosteroid treatment. Some forms of bronchiolitis obliterans in adults, especially bronchiolitis obliterans organizing pneumonia, respond well to corticosteroid treatment. No definitive data about corticosteroid efficacy exist for children. Some patients deteriorate rapidly and die within weeks of the onset of the initial symptoms, but most in the nontransplant population survive, some with chronic disability.

Epler GR, Colby TV, McLoud TC, et al: Bronchiolitis obliterans organizing pneumonia. N Engl J Med 312:152, 1985.
Hardy KA: Obliterative bronchiolitis. *In:* Hilman BC (ed): Pediatric Respiratory Disease. Diagnosis and Treatment. Philadelphia, WB Saunders, 1993, p 218.
Keenan RJ, Konishi H, Kawai A, et al: Clinical trial of tacrolimus versus cyclosporine in lung transplantation. Ann Thorac Surg 60:580, 1995.

392.1 Follicular Bronchitis

Follicular bronchitis is a rare problem in children. The cause is unknown. Most affected children have tachypnea and cough by 6 wk of age. Diffuse crackles are heard on auscultation of the lung fields. Roentgenograms usually reveal a diffuse interstitial pattern, but the picture may be relatively normal. Computed tomography may show subtle interstitial nodules, even in children with normal plain films. The diagnosis is made by lung biopsy. Most children gradually improve, although in some the disorder is life-threatening, with a single or recurrent episodes of respiratory failure. Some affected children seem to respond to corticosteroid treatment.

Kinane BT, Mansell AL, Zwerdling RG, et al: Follicular bronchitis in the pediatric population. Chest 104:1183, 1993.

CHAPTER 393
Aspiration Pneumonias and Gastroesophageal Reflux–Related Respiratory Disease

David M. Orenstein

Despite mechanisms for keeping the contents of the gastrointestinal tract out of the respiratory tract (Table 393–1), there are many instances in which dysfunctional swallowing or gastroesophageal reflux can cause or worsen respiratory disease (see Chapter 323). The numerous mechanisms for reflux-associated respiratory disease (Fig. 393–1) include aspiration, with direct mechanical and chemical effects (e.g., obstruction of laryngeal or bronchial lumen, pneumonitis); neurally mediated effects from the airway; and neurally mediated effects from the esophagus.

Respiratory disorders and their therapy can also cause or worsen reflux. The most common mechanism is increasing the gastroesophageal pressure gradient by increasing intragastric pressure, as occurs when the abdominal muscles are tensed with coughing and forced expiratory maneuvers, for example, in cystic fibrosis, bronchopulmonary dysplasia, or asthma. Much of the increased intra-abdominal pressure is also transmitted to the diaphragm and then to the lower esophageal sphincter, augmenting its antireflux action. Hyperinflation also may predispose to reflux by flattening the diaphragm, rendering it less effective in augmenting the lower esophageal sphincter. Intrapleural pressure is more negative than normal with inspiration against an obstructed airway, as occurs in laryngospasm and asthma, favoring movement of gastric contents into the esophagus.

Theophylline and orally administered β-agonist drugs may relax the lower esophageal sphincter pressure and increase gastric acid secretion. Nasogastric tubes used for nutritional supplementation in many children with chronic respiratory disorders predispose the child to gastroesophageal reflux. Mechanical ventilation with tracheal intubation impairs airway protective mechanisms and may predispose the child to aspiration. Mechanically ventilated patients are usually kept supine, a position that is provocative for reflux. Chest physical therapy and postural drainage increases reflux in children with cystic fibrosis, probably in part because of gravity.

Johannesson N, Andersson K, Joelsson B, Persson C: Relaxation of the lower esophageal sphincter and stimulation of gastric secretion and diuresis by antiasthmatic xanthines. Am Rev Respir Dis 131:26, 1985.

Orenstein DM, Orenstein SR: Gastroesophageal reflux and dysfunctional swallowing. *In:* Loughlin GM, Eigen H (eds): Respiratory Disease in Children. Baltimore, Williams & Wilkins, 1994, p 563.

Schindlbeck N, Heinrich, Clueller-Lissner S: Effects of albuterol (salbutamol) on esophageal motility and gastroesophageal reflux in healthy volunteers. JAMA 260:3156, 1988.

393.1 Aspiration Pneumonia

ASPIRATION OF FOOD AND VOMITUS. Infants with obstructive lesions such as esophageal atresia or duodenal obstruction; hypotonic, weak, and debilitated infants and children with no obstructive lesions; patients with familial dysautonomia; and patients with impaired consciousness may aspirate, or regurgitate and then aspirate, food and vomitus, causing a chemical pneumonia. Aspiration, rarely, may be an immediate cause of death by asphyxiation. Hydrochloric acid is an important determinant of lung injury. After aspiration of gastric contents, there frequently is a relatively brief latent period before the onset of signs and symptoms of pneumonia. More than 90% of patients have symptoms within 1 hr, and almost all patients have symptoms within 2 hr. Fever, tachypnea, and cough are common. Apnea and shock may also occur.

Physical examination reveals diffuse crackles, wheezing, and possibly cyanosis. Chest roentgenograms reveal alveolar and, occasionally, reticular infiltrates that may be localized but often are more extensive and are frequently bilateral. The irritated mucous membrane may also subsequently become the site for bacterial invasion and pneumonia. Aspiration from gastroesophageal reflux occasionally can be demonstrated by barium swallow roentgenography, but radionuclide milk scanning is more sensitive, particularly if images are collected repeatedly over many hours. Bronchoalveolar lavage fluid may be examined for lipid-filled macrophages, lactose, or dyes that had been administered orally to support the diagnosis of reflux-related aspiration, but false-positive and false-negative results limit the usefulness of these methods.

Prophylaxis is essential. Care should be taken to avoid feedings in amounts that overdistend the stomach, especially in infants who are fed by gavage. After being fed, the infant should be placed on the right side. When the infant is supine, the head should be elevated. Critically ill patients may benefit from reduction of gastric acidity with cimetidine or ranitidine.

Treatment by immediate suctioning of the airway and administering oxygen are indicated for aspiration. Endotracheal intubation with suctioning and mechanical ventilation is often required for severe cases. Although the prophylactic use of antibiotics and corticosteroids is advocated by some for patients who have aspirated gastric contents, evidence of their benefit is lacking. Some data suggest that corticosteroid treatment may predispose the patient to pneumonia caused by gram-negative organisms. Previously healthy nonhospitalized patients may become infected with mouth flora (predominantly anaerobes); clindamycin or penicillin is effective therapy. Chronically ill hospitalized patients may be colonized with gram-negative flora (e.g., *Pseudomonas, Escherichia coli, Klebsiella*); additional coverage with an aminoglycoside may be indicated.

Prognosis depends partly on the severity of aspiration and partly on the underlying disease. Most patients demonstrate clearing of infiltrates within 2 wk; the mortality rate for patients with massive aspiration is about 25%.

Brook I, Finegold SM: Bacteriology of aspiration pneumonia in children. Pediatrics 65:1115, 1980.

TABLE 393–1 Prevention of Respiratory Sequelae due to Reflux

Structure	Protective Functions	Dysfunctions
Stomach	Antegrade emptying	Delayed gastric emptying
Esophagus and associated structures	Diaphragmatic hiatal tone	Hiatal hernia
Lower esophageal sphincter (LES)	LES tone; differentiates gas from liquid	Hypotensive LES; transient LES relaxations to liquid
Body	Secondary peristalsis	Impaired esophageal clearance
Upper esophageal sphincter (UES)	UES tone; differentiates gas from liquid	Hypotensive UES; transient UES relaxations to liquid
Larynx, pharynx, mouth	Swallow reflex; cord closure; arytenoid-epiglottic approximation	Impaired swallow reflex; impaired cord closure; impaired arytenoid-epiglottic approximation

From Putnam PE, Ricker DH, Orenstein SR: Gastroesophageal reflux. In: *Beckerman RC, Brouillette RT, Hunt CE (eds): Respiratory Control Disorders in Infants and Children. Baltimore, Williams & Wilkins, 1992, p 323.*

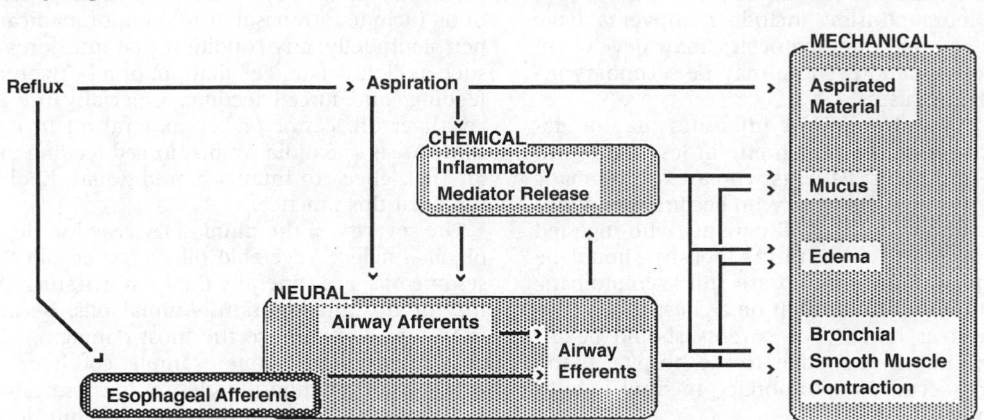

Figure 393–1 Mechanisms of reflux-associated respiratory dysfunction. Reflux may lead to direct pulmonary aspiration of refluxed material, producing mechanical obstruction of the airway lumen. Pulmonary aspiration also leads to the release of chemical mediators of inflammation, which leads to obstruction of the lumen by mucus, mucosal edema, and bronchial smooth muscle contraction. Aspiration stimulates the airway's neural afferents, which influence airway efferents, inducing the release of chemical inflammatory mediators and leading to mucus secretion, edema formation, and bronchial smooth muscle contraction. Reflux can stimulate esophageal afferents, which also influence airway efferents.

Colombo J, Hallbert T: Recurrent aspiration in children: Lipid-laden alveolar macrophage quantitation. Pediatr Pulmonol 3:86, 1987.
DeePaso WJ: Aspiration pneumonia. Clin Chest Med 12:269, 1991.
McVeagh P, Howman-Giles R, Kemp A: Pulmonary aspiration studied by radionuclide milk scanning and barium swallow roentgenography. Am J Dis Child 141:917, 1987.
Stagus R, Martin A, Binns S, et al: The significance of fat-filled macrophages in the diagnosis of aspiration associated with gastrooesophageal reflux. Aust Paediatr J 21:275, 1985.
Wolfe JE, Bone RC, Ruth WE: Effects of corticosteroids in the treatment of patients with gastric aspiration. Am J Med 83:719, 1977.

ASPIRATION OF BABY POWDER. Aspiration pneumonia resulting from inhalation of zinc stearate baby powder is rare because the use of baby powder has decreased and the containers still being used control the outflow of powder. However, catastrophic aspirations still occur. Severe respiratory distress almost immediately follows inhalation. Generalized obstructive overinflation with an expiratory type of dyspnea occurs as a result of an inflammatory reaction caused by the zinc stearate powder. After inhalation, the powder is almost immediately drawn into the finer bronchioles because of its extreme lightness; for this reason, suctioning with a bronchoscope is useful to remove the secretions that may subsequently accumulate in the larger air passages. Immediate treatment is oxygen therapy in an atmosphere of high humidity.

The commonly used dusting (i.e., baby) powders today contain magnesium silicate and other silicates; some contain calcium undecylenate. Although not as dangerous as zinc stearate, these powders can also cause serious aspiration pneumonitis. Talc is chemically related to asbestos, and "talcum powder" may contain microscopic asbestos particles, which have the potential to cause malignancy. Systemic corticosteroid treatment appeared to be useful in one patient who had severe dyspnea after aspirating talc.

Cotton WH, Davidson PJ: Aspiration of baby powder. N Engl J Med 313:1662, 1985.
Mofenson HC, Caraccio TR, Okun S, et al: Hazards of baby powder. Pediatrics 78:546, 1986.

PNEUMONITIS FROM OTHER CHEMICALS. Many chemicals, particularly if inhaled in high concentrations, may cause an inflammatory reaction consisting of edema, cellular infiltration, and acute respiratory distress. Prolonged exposure to lower concentrations of these same agents or other chemicals may cause chronic interstitial pneumonitis, characterized by granuloma formation. For example, shellac, polyvinylpyrrolidone (found in hair spray), gum arabic, beryllium, mercury vapors, and chlorine may cause this reaction. Corticosteroids may reduce the inflammatory reaction and prevent fibrosis.

393.2 *Hydrocarbon Pneumonia*

ETIOLOGY. Hydrocarbons, such as furniture polish, kerosene, charcoal lighter fluid, and gasoline, occasionally are accidentally ingested by young children, causing a secondary pneumonitis. Also see Chapter 722.9. Gasoline may be aspirated by teenagers attempting to siphon gasoline. In general, the lower the viscosity and the higher the volatility of the hydrocarbon compound, the greater is the pulmonary toxicity. In 1990, there were 30,000 hydrocarbon ingestions reported to poison control centers, with four deaths.

PATHOGENESIS. Hydrocarbons are probably aspirated during swallowing, vomiting, or gastric lavage. The low viscosity of hydrocarbons allows them to flow from the hypopharynx into the larynx. Ingestion of large quantities of these bad-tasting liquids is unusual, and gastric lavage is contraindicated unless the hydrocarbon contains poison, such as a potent insecticide for example, organophosphate. Hydrocarbons may interact with pulmonary surfactant, resulting in alveolar collapse. Alveolar macrophages may also be injured. The pulmonary changes observed in animals after hydrocarbon aspiration are edema, inflammation, and hemorrhage.

CLINICAL MANIFESTATIONS. Coughing and vomiting follow ingestion almost immediately. Within hours, there may be temperature elevation (38–40°C). However, with less extensive aspiration, the onset of pulmonary symptoms and inflammation may be delayed 12–24 hr. The pulmonary findings may include dyspnea, diminished resonance on percussion, suppressed or tubular breath sounds, and crackles. Hypoxemia and cyanosis, caused by inflammation and edema, may be aggravated by the displacement of alveolar gas with vaporized hydrocarbon. Pneumonic involvement is disclosed more frequently by roentgenographic examination than by physical findings. Roentgenograms may occasionally show minimal changes a few hours after ingestion, only to progress rapidly after that time with extensive infiltrates. Despite what may be a stormy clinical course, which averages 2–5 days, recovery occurs in most cases. Systemic symptoms of hydrocarbon ingestion, including somnolence, convulsions, and coma, may occur and sometimes dominate the course (see Chapter 722.9).

COMPLICATIONS. Pneumothorax, subcutaneous emphysema of the chest wall, and pleural effusion, including empyema, have occurred. After the 1st wk, pneumatoceles may develop in areas of extensive consolidation. There may be secondary infection with bacteria or viruses.

TREATMENT. Symptoms and radiologic infiltrates may be delayed, and no patient should be sent home in less than 6 hr, even if there are no symptoms. Patients who are symptomatic when they are first examined, patients who become symptomatic during 6 hr of observation, and all patients who ingested a particularly toxic agent (e.g., furniture polish) should be admitted to the hospital. Patients who are still asymptomatic after 6 hr and who have a normal result on a chest roentgenogram can be observed at home, but parents should be instructed to return the infant or toddler to the hospital if any respiratory symptoms occur. No pulmonary therapy is indicated before symptoms develop.

After ingestion of small to moderate amounts of hydrocarbons, induction of vomiting or gastric lavage is contraindicated because of the risk of aspiration, especially if several hours have elapsed. If a large volume of hydrocarbon is thought to be in the stomach, nasogastric suction performed with great care to avoid aspiration rarely may be necessary to reduce the other dangers of hydrocarbon poisoning, including central nervous system toxicity. The risk of aspiration during gastric lavage or suctioning can be minimized if an endotracheal tube with a balloon cuff can be inserted without inducing vomiting before lavage. For dyspnea, cyanosis, or chemical pneumonitis, supportive measures, including oxygen, physiotherapy and, if necessary, continuous positive airway pressure or other forms of ventilatory assistance, are important components of therapy. A prokinetic agent is usually indicated for intestinal motility.

The routine use of antibiotics is not recommended; the occurrence of secondary infection of the affected lung can usually be readily detected by the reappearance of fever on the 3rd–5th day after ingestion and can then be suitably treated with penicillin G and tobramycin. Corticosteroids have no beneficial effect on the course of the illness and may be harmful. Pneumatoceles, when they occur, rarely rupture and do not require treatment. Parents must be reminded to keep cleaning fluids and kerosene in locked cabinets out of reach of children and out of the home.

PROGNOSIS. Although most children survive without complications or sequelae, some progress rapidly to respiratory failure and death.

The prognosis depends on a variety of factors, including the volume of the ingestion or aspiration, the specific agent involved, and the adequacy of medical care. In one series, only 39 of 950 patients had symptoms; 4 required assisted ventilation, and 2 died. Long-term pulmonary function studies several years later are inconclusive, but if lasting damage does occur, the small airways seem to be at greatest risk.

Bergeson PS, Hales SW, Lustgarten MD, et al: Pneumatoceles following hydrocarbon ingestion. Report of three cases and review of the literature. Am J Dis Child 129:49, 1975.

Brown J III, Burke B, Dajani AS: Experimental kerosene pneumonia: Evaluation of some therapeutic regimens. J Pediatr 84:396, 1974.

Guruntz D, Kattan M, Levison H, et al: Pulmonary function abnormalities in asymptotic children after hydrocarbon pneumonitis. Pediatrics 62:789, 1978.

Klein BL, Simon JE: Hydrocarbon poisonings. Pediatr Clin North Am 33:411, 1986.

Litovits T, Bailery K, Schmitz B, et al: 1990 Annual report of the American Association of Poison Control Centers National Data Collection System. Am J Emerg Med 9:461, 1991.

393.3 Lipoid Pneumonia

Lipoid pneumonia is a chronic, interstitial, proliferative inflammation resulting from aspiration of lipoid material; it occurs principally in debilitated infants.

PATHOGENESIS. Factors that may be responsible for aspiration of oil include intranasal instillation of medicated oils, including petroleum jelly; any condition that interferes with swallowing, such as cleft palate, debilitation, or a horizontal position during feeding; and forced feeding, especially the administration of cod liver oil, castor oil, or mineral oil to crying children. In some areas of Saudia Arabia, forced feeding of rendered animal fat (i.e., ghee) to infants is traditional; lipoid pneumonia has followed this practice.

The severity of the pulmonary reaction depends on the kind of oil inhaled. Vegetable oils, such as olive, cottonseed, and sesame oils, are generally the least irritating and produce minimal or no inflammation. Animal oils, because of their high fatty acid content, are the most damaging. Milk aspirated by debilitated infants is one example; cod liver oil also belongs in this category. Liquid petrolatum is chemically inert and is not as irritative as some of the other oils but does act as a foreign body. Excessive use of lip gloss can also cause pneumonitis in teenagers.

The reaction begins as an interstitial proliferative inflammation, and there may be an exudative pneumonia. In the second stage, there is diffuse, chronic, proliferative fibrosis and sometimes superimposed acute infectious bronchopneumonia. In the third stage, there are multiple localized nodules, tumorlike paraffinomas. There are numerous macrophages in the involved areas, with giant cell formation of the foreign body type. The lipoid substance is found in intracellular and extracellular areas. The oil-laden cells may be carried to the hilar lymph nodes.

CLINICAL MANIFESTATIONS. There are no characteristic signs or symptoms; a cough is common, and severe cases may include dyspnea. Unless there is superimposed infection, the physical examination may be normal, although with extensive involvement, there may be some impairment to percussion and a change in voice and breath sounds. Secondary bronchopneumonic infections are common.

The roentgenographic appearance is characteristic (Fig. 393–2). Mild involvement is manifested by an increase in the density and extent of the hilar shadows. With increasing involvement, there is greater density of the perihilar shadows, which widen in all directions. Pulmonary changes may be limited to the right lung, and in the infant who is recumbent most of the time, the changes may be mainly in the right upper lobe.

PROGNOSIS. The prognosis is guarded. It depends on the general condition of the patient, the extent of pulmonary damage, the discontinuation of oil inhalation, and the avoidance of intercurrent infections.

PREVENTION. Intranasal medications in an oily vehicle should not be used. Administration of mineral oil, cod liver oil, and castor oil should be avoided, if possible. Infants who regurgi-

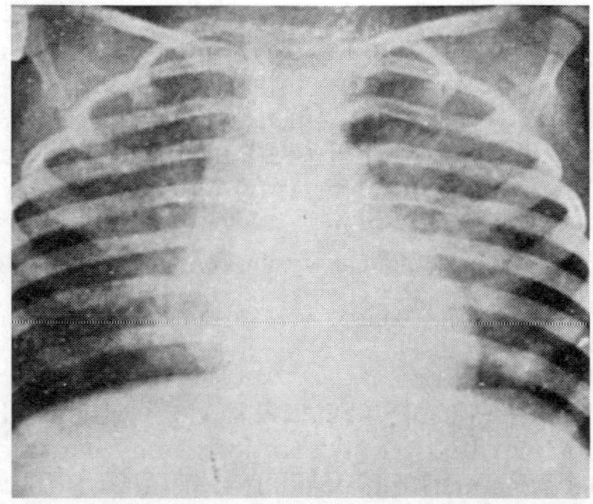

Figure 393–2 Lipoid pneumonia. The roentgenogram shows an increased density radiating from the hilus of each lung in an infant 13 mo of age after intranasal application of liquid petrolatum three times daily for 5 mo.

tate or vomit frequently should be placed prone to reduce the likelihood of aspiration.

TREATMENT. There is no specific therapy other than elimination of further exposure.

Annobil SH, Ogunbiyi AO, Benjamin B: Chest radiographic findings in childhood lipoid pneumonia following aspiration of animal fat. Eur J Radiol 16:217, 1993.

Bection DL, Lowe JE, Falleta JM: Lipoid pneumonia in an adolescent girl secondary to use of lip gloss. J Pediatr 105:421, 1984.

Berg BW, Saenger JS: Exogenous lipoid pneumonia. N Engl J Med 338:512, 1998.

Brown AC, Slocum PC, Putthoff SL, et al: Exogenous lipoid pneumonia due to intranasal application of petroleum jelly. Chest 105:968, 1994.

393.4 Respiratory Disorders Caused or Worsened by Gastroesophageal Reflux or Its Treatment

ASPIRATION PNEUMONIA. Direct aspiration of refluxed materials can cause pneumonia, particularly in children with depressed consciousness (e.g., sleep, general anesthesia, severe mental retardation). Microaspiration may also cause a chemical pneumonitis or asthma-like symptoms, or both.

ASTHMA. Many more children with asthma have abnormal amounts of reflux than do healthy control children. Patients with nocturnal asthma are particularly likely to have reflux. Reflux seems to cause or worsen asthma through vagal pathways originating with acid stimulation of esophageal receptors. Esophageal acidification may not cause bronchospasm directly but may heighten airway responsiveness to other stimuli.

BRONCHOPULMONARY DYSPLASIA. There is some suggestion that reflux may prolong the course of bronchopulmonary dysplasia and that treatment of reflux improves pulmonary function in some infants. Physicians should be alert to the possibility of reflux in infants with bronchopulmonary dysplasia who are slow to respond to standard treatment or who have prominent nocturnal symptoms.

CYSTIC FIBROSIS. A high proportion of patients with cystic fibrosis may have gastroesophageal reflux. How much of this is related to hyperinflation or to treatment (e.g., postural drainage, bronchodilator drugs) is unclear. There is some suggestion that respiratory disease may improve with treatment of the reflux.

TRACHEOESOPHAGEAL FISTULA. All patients born with tracheoesophageal fistula have esophageal dysmotility and most have reflux. Some may experience aspiration.

OBSTRUCTIVE APNEA. Obstructive apnea can occur in sleeping or awake infants. In a specific clinical syndrome described in awake infants, shortly after a feeding, the seated or supine infant suddenly stops breathing. These infants are staring, plethoric, and often have rigid posturing. Subsequently, they become pale or cyanotic and perhaps hypotonic. Coughing, choking, and gagging are absent.

CENTRAL APNEA AND APPARENT LIFE-THREATENING EVENTS. Many infants with apparent life-threatening events have reflux, and several studies have shown that some infants with recurrent respiratory arrest become free of such episodes after treatment for reflux.

STRIDOR. Some infants, particularly those with mild airway compromise from some other cause, such as laryngomalacia, have stridor during episodes of reflux and lessened stridor after antireflux therapy.

Reflux-induced laryngeal inflammation may cause recurrent or spasmodic croup.

HOARSENESS. In adults, inflammation and edema of the larynx, particularly its posterior aspects, is associated with reflux, and their laryngeal symptoms respond to acid suppression therapy. This association probably exists for children.

COUGH. In some adults, cough has been identified as the sole manifestation of reflux and has responded to antireflux therapy. Cough is also associated with reflux in some infants.

HICCUPS. Hiccups have been associated with reflux in adults and children.

RESPIRATORY SIDE EFFECTS OF ANTIREFLUX TREATMENT. Bethanechol, a cholinergic agent that promotes gastric motility and augments lower esophageal pressure, can provoke bronchospasm.

Irwin R, Zawacki J, Curley F, et al: Chronic cough as the sole presenting manifestation of gastroesophageal reflux. Am Rev Respir Dis 140:1294, 1989.

Lew C, Keens T, O'Neal M, et al: Gastroesophageal reflux recovery from bronchopulmonary dysplasia. Clin Res 29:149A, 1981.

Martin M, Grunstein M, Larsen G: The relationship of gastroesophageal reflux to nocturnal wheezing in children with asthma. Ann Allergy 49:318, 1982.

Nielson D, Heldt G, Tooley W: Stridor and gastroesophageal reflux in infants. Pediatrics 85:1034, 1990.

Orenstein DM, Orenstein SR: Gastroesophageal reflux and dysfunctional swallowing. *In:* Loughlin GM, Eigen H (eds): Respiratory Disease in Children. Baltimore, Williams & Wilkins, 1994, p 563.

Putnam P, Orenstein S: Hoarseness in a child with gastroesophageal reflux. Acta Paediatr Scand 81:635, 1992.

Vinocur CD, Marmon L, Schidlow DV, Weintraub WH: Gastroesophageal reflux in the infant with cystic fibrosis. Am J Surg 149:182, 1985.

CHAPTER 394
Silo Filler's Disease

Robert C. Stern

The acute or subacute interstitial pneumonia of silo filler's disease is caused by inhalation of the oxides of nitrogen, gases most commonly encountered in freshly filled silos, especially corn silos. Nitric and nitrous acids, formed when these gases dissolve, can produce severe burns throughout the respiratory epithelium. A chemical pneumonitis is also involved.

Diagnosis requires a history of entering a silo within 4 wk (usually within 24–100 hr) of its being filled and two or more of the following symptoms at exposure: dyspnea, wheezing, cough, nausea, "choking," or "fatigue." At presentation, which is rarely days or weeks later, one or more of the following should be observed: infiltrates or edema on the chest film; hypoxemia; methemoglobinemia; biopsy or autopsy findings consistent with chemical pneumonitis, including hyperplastic epithelium, widened and edematous interalveolar septa, or alveoli filled with mononuclear cells and fibroblasts. The chest examination reveals rales in about one third of cases. Intravenous corticosteroids are usually given, but no controlled data on their efficacy are available. The death rate in patients who present for medical care is 10–20%. This disease is preventable; no one should enter a freshly filled silo for at least 14 days.

Zwemer FL, Pratt DS, May JJ: Silo filler's disease in New York State. Am Rev Respir Dis 146:650, 1992.

CHAPTER 395
Paraquat Lung

Robert C. Stern

Paraquat, a dipyridylium compound used as a weed killer, accumulates selectively in the lungs and is highly toxic. The mechanism of toxicity is thought to involve production of a superoxide anion. Death is very likely in patients showing radiologic findings. The pulmonary lesion is secondary to systemic absorption through the gastrointestinal tract, skin, or lungs (e.g., smoking contaminated marijuana) and consists of proliferative bronchiolitis, alveolitis, hemorrhage causing intra-alveolar hyaline membranes, and fibrosis. Gas exchange is impaired. Some of these patients probably have adult respiratory distress syndrome (see Chapter 64.3). Paraquat is a corrosive that also causes painful lesions of the mouth and esophagus, renal tubular damage, azotemia, and hematuria. Renal damage may result in prolongation of toxic blood levels, during which time fibroblasts proliferate, filling the terminal air spaces. Except for general supportive measures, no specific treatment (e.g., infused superoxide dismutase; *N*-acetylcysteine) is effective. Oxygen may increase pulmonary toxicity. Lung transplantation was unsuccessful in one patient who died 2 wk later after changes typical of paraquat toxicity had occurred in the transplanted lung. Increased incidence may reflect the large-scale use of paraquat in attempts to kill marijuana plants. Survivors have restrictive pulmonary disease initially but then may show substantial recovery within a few years.

Bismuth C, Hall AH, Baud FJ, et al:, Pulmonary dysfunction in survivors of acute paraquat poisoning. Vet Hum Toxicol 38:220, 1996.

Copland GM, Kolin A, Shulman HS: Fatal pulmonary intra-alveolar fibrosis after paraquat ingestion. N Engl Med 291:290, 1974.

Hudson M, Patel SB, Ewen SWB, et al: Paraquat induced pulmonary fibrosis in three survivors. Thorax 46:201, 1991.

CHAPTER 396
Hypersensitivity to Inhaled Materials

Robert C. Stern

Repeated inhalation of organic antigens may result in chronic pneumonitis that progressively worsens with continued exposure. Although the syndrome is most common in adults, it has been reported frequently in children and rarely in infants. Unlike those of asthma, the symptoms of this hypersensitivity syndrome are almost entirely unrelated to bronchospasm (see Chapter 145). Symptoms may result from inhalation of small particles from moldy hay (farmer's lung), maple bark (maple bark stripper's disease), sugar cane fiber (bagassosis), redwood tree bark, pigeon or other bird droppings and feathers (bird fancier's disease), cheese, desiccated pituitary powder, dusty output from air conditioners, and a fungus or mold associated with the specific material to which the patient is exposed.

CLINICAL MANIFESTATIONS. The signs and symptoms are similar in all of these diseases. Within several hours after exposure, cough, dyspnea, chest pain, and sometimes fever occur with few physical findings, although occasional wheezes and moist rales may be audible. Roentgenograms may show minimal emphysema, but findings are usually normal. If no further exposure occurs, the symptoms abate over a period of several days; if contact with the responsible antigen continues, symptoms progress to severe dyspnea and cyanosis associated with diffuse, fine, interstitial or nodular densities and peripheral alveolar infiltrates on chest roentgenogram and occasionally irreversible loss of pulmonary function. The disease should be suspected in children with relatively mild symptoms including cough, fever, and occasional dyspnea, particularly if bronchopneumonia persists despite appropriate treatment with antibiotics.

PATHOLOGY. Histologically, the infiltrate consists of subacute granulomatous inflammation with accumulation of plasma cells, lymphocytes, epithelioid cells, and giant cells of the Langhans type. With continued exposure, inflammatory lesions may be replaced by fibrosis.

DIAGNOSIS. Patients may have moderate to marked leukocytosis, particularly with acute attacks, elevated serum levels of immunoglobulins (IgG, IgM, and IgA fractions), and a primary restrictive pattern on pulmonary function tests. Arterial blood gas analysis reveals moderate or marked hypoxemia, usually without hypercapnia. Skin testing with the suspected antigen may cause a vigorous delayed hypersensitivity response and is especially useful if an Arthus reaction can be demonstrated histologically by skin biopsy of the test site. Demonstration of a serum precipitin to a given antigen, although characteristic of the disease, is frequently encountered in apparently well persons and is not diagnostic. If the disease is strongly suspected on the basis of clinical findings and environmental history but serum precipitins are not found by a commercial laboratory, repeat analysis by a specialized laboratory should be considered. Empirical treatment with corticosteroids may be reasonable. Lung biopsy reveals a diffuse fibrotic or granulomatous response. If the antigen is available in purified form, an inhalation challenge may be diagnostic.

TREATMENT. Optimal therapy requires complete elimination of exposure to the suspected or proven antigen, which includes thoroughly cleaning the home after the source of antigen has been eliminated. Administration of adrenal corticosteroids (e.g., prednisone in initial dosage of 1–1.5 mg/kg/24 hr) usually results in prompt remission of symptoms; continued use for 1–6 mo may prevent subsequent development of pulmonary fibrosis in cases of chronic exposure. Corticosteroid therapy may be slowly tapered after evidence of recovery of lung function or after several weeks without exposure to a known antigen. If hypersensitivity pneumonitis is strongly suspected but the antigen remains unknown, long-term use of corticosteroid therapy, perhaps on an alternate-day regimen, may be indicated. Patients should be cautioned that re-exposure to the antigen is extremely dangerous even long after apparent complete recovery. Even if treatment is optimal and the exposure is eliminated, some fatalities occur, and a substantial percentage of patients do not completely regain their previous pulmonary status.

Cunningham AS, Fink JN, Schlueter DP: Childhood hypersensitivity pneumonitis due to dove antigen. Pediatrics 58:436, 1976.

Eisenberg JD, Montanero A, Lee RG: Hypersensitivity pneumonitis in an infant. Pediatr Pulmonol 12:186, 1992.

Keith HH, Holsclaw DS, Donsky EH: Pigeon breeder's disease in children: A family study. Chest 79:107, 1981.

O'Connell EJ, Zora JA, Gillespie DN, et al: Childhood hypersensitivity pneumonitis (farmer's lung): Four cases in siblings with long-term follow-up. J Pediatr 114:995, 1989.

Yee WFH, Castile RG, Cooper A, et al: Diagnosing bird fancier's disease in children. Pediatrics 85:848, 1990.

CHAPTER 397
Pulmonary Aspergillosis

Robert C. Stern

Several species of the genus *Aspergillus* (especially *Aspergillus fumigatus*) are potentially pathogenic. A spectrum of pulmonary manifestations may ensue, depending on the type of exposure and condition of the host (see Chapter 233).

All *Aspergillus* pulmonary disease begins with inhalation of spores. If neither colonization nor allergy to the organism occurs, there is no disease. If colonization does not occur but a patient becomes allergic to the organism and has ongoing exposure, an allergic alveolitis may develop. If colonization and infection occur (even without allergy), *Aspergillus* pneumonia develops. Profoundly neutropenic or immunosuppressed patients (as a result of either disease or drugs) have a greatly increased chance of invasive disease or necrotizing pneumonia. Hematogenous spread to other organs may occur particularly in low birthweight infants. Local spread to contiguous structures (muscles, ribs, pericardium, and heart) can also occur. However, parenchymal invasion in previously normal children is rare. Infection of an extant cavity results in an *Aspergillus* mycetoma (aspergilloma).

If colonization with or without infection occurs and the patient develops an allergy to the organism, allergic bronchopulmonary aspergillosis (ABPA) may ensue. ABPA without infection or tissue invasion is the most common *Aspergillus*-related disease in children. Most cases occur in patients with chronic pulmonary disease (e.g., asthma, cystic fibrosis). In some, the immunologic response that leads to ABPA appears to be genetically determined.

CLINICAL MANIFESTATIONS. ABPA should be suspected in an immunosuppressed or chronically ill child who presents with a relatively acute onset of cough, wheezing, and low-grade fever. The cough may be productive, and occasionally, brown plugs are expectorated and on microscopic examination contain hyphae. *Aspergillus* can be recovered from this material by culture. Hemoptysis is a common feature of invasive aspergillosis and aspergillomas and may be the presenting symptom.

Many patients have multiple precipitin lines on diffusion of serum against *Aspergillus* antigen. The immediate skin test reaction is often strongly positive, and a type III hypersenitivity (Arthus) reaction can usually be demonstrated after skin testing. Chest roentgenograms show transient, occasionally extensive infiltrates. *Aspergillus* (ABPA) can be strongly suspected in a child with precipitating antibody to *Aspergillus* antigen, a positive result on a skin test, and elevated serum IgE levels. A definite *diagnosis* should be made if there also is substantial eosinophilia or if *Aspergillus*-specific IgE or IgG is found in the patient's serum. Some believe that central bronchiectasis is always present in aspergillosis. However, *Aspergillus* organisms are frequently recovered from cultures of respiratory tract secretions of patients with chronic pulmonary disease without symptoms of ABPA. Recovery of these organisms without typical symptoms and serologic evidence of hypersensitivity is not an indication for treatment. Identification of circulating carbohydrates (e.g., galactomannan) by analysis of blood or urine may prove to be a valuable diagnostic test for invasive disease.

TREATMENT. The best approach to treatment of ABPA is not clear. Aerosolized amphotericin or direct instillation of amphotericin into the trachea has been recommended, but the correct dosage has not been established. Systemic amphotericin B (0.5–1.0 mg/kg/24 hr, intravenously) with or without flucytosine (50–150 mg/kg/24 hr) may be effective. Although aerosolized corticosteroids have been recommended, only systemic corticosteroid (e.g., prednisone, 0.5 mg/kg/24 hr for 2 wk followed by the same dose on alternate days for 3 mo) is effective and remains the treatment of choice. Itraconazole may be useful when given with systemic corticosteroid. A reasonable goal is reduction of IgE levels to a range consistent with those in asthmatics (without ABPA) who live in the same geographic area. In any case, IgE levels should be obtained immediately after corticosteroid treatment. If, on follow-up, the IgE rises to twice this level or higher, serious consideration should be given to reinstitution of the same regimen described earlier. In patients with underlying asthma, aerosolized bronchodilators, β-agonists, and cromolyn may be helpful.

Aspergillomas may respond to specific antifungal chemotherapy or occasionally resolve spontaneously. However, surgical resection with local instillation of amphotericin is considered the treatment of choice. The prognosis, whatever the treatment, depends heavily on the underlying chronic illness. Invasive aspergillosis may be so fulminant that antifungal chemotherapy is not efficacious. Treatment generally consists of amphotericin B combined with 5-fluorocytosine. Itraconazole may also be useful. Treatment should be continued for 2–3 wk.

Controlled trials of cytokines (including interferon-γ) as a preventive agent in patients at high risk for invasive aspergillosis are under way. Similarly, granulocyte colony-stimulating factor and granulocyte–macrophage colony-stimulating factor by shortening the duration of neutropenia, may also decrease the risk of invasive disease.

Bardana EJ, Sobti KL, Cianciulli FD, et al: Aspergillus antibody in patients with cystic fibrosis. Am J Dis Child 129:1164, 1975.

Case Records of the Massachusetts General Hospital: Case 45–1993. N Engl J Med 329:1484, 1993.

Greenberger PA, Petterson R: Diagnosis and management of allergic bronchopulmonary aspergillosis. Ann Allergy 56:444, 1986.

Walsh TJ, Gonzalez C, Lyman CA, et al: Invasive fungal infections in children: Recent advances in diagnosis and treatment. Adv Pediatr Infect Dis 11:187, 1966.

Yamada H, Kohno S, Koga H, et al: Topical treatment of pulmonary aspergilloma by antifungals. Chest 103:1421, 1993.

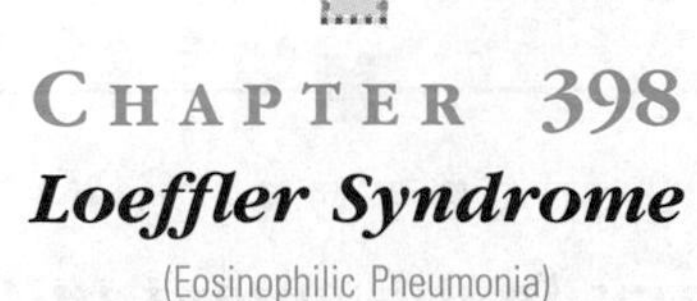

CHAPTER 398
Loeffler Syndrome

(Eosinophilic Pneumonia)

Robert C. Stern

Loeffler syndrome is characterized by widespread transitory pulmonary infiltrations, which roentgenographically vary in size but may resemble those of miliary tuberculosis, and by a blood eosinophilia level that may be as high as 70%. The clinical course is usually not severe and ranges from a few days to several months. Patients usually have paroxysmal attacks of coughing, dyspnea, pleurisy, and little or no fever. There may be associated hepatomegaly, especially in infants and young children, and biopsy sections of the liver have revealed multiple focal areas of necrosis, granuloma formation, and eosinophilic infiltration. These children have hyperglobulinemia, presumably as a result of hepatic dysfunction and in response to parasitic invasion of tissue. Localized pneumonic consolidation with associated eosinophilia may occur. Autopsy studies have revealed evidence of eosinophilic infiltrations in the lungs and in other organs.

Loeffler syndrome may be an unusual allergic manifestation of various antigens and not a distinct clinical entity. Although certain toxic reactions to drugs (e.g., antibiotics, L-tryptophan, crack cocaine) are included in Loeffler syndrome, in children they are usually manifestations of helminthic infections. Perhaps the most common pathogen in this country is the larva of the dog ascarid, *Toxocara canis,* and less often of the cat ascarid, *Toxocara cati* (see Chapter 285). Other roundworms may be responsible for the syndrome; these include *Ascaris lumbricoides* (usually responsible for transient pulmonary lesions), *Strongyloides stercoralis,* and hookworms (see Chapter 283). So-called tropical eosinophilia may manifest as Loeffler's syndrome and is probably caused by a number of different helminths. Paragonimiasis, caused by a lung fluke (see Chapter 297), may produce the syndrome and extrapulmonary manifestations. A drug reaction may also result in this syndrome; aspirin, penicillin, sulfonamides, and imipramine are among those implicated.

The hypereosinophilic syndrome, rare in children, is characterized by eosinophilia for more than 6 mo and may be an early manifestation of eosinophilic or acute lymphoblastic leukemia. Also see Chapter 129.

One variant of eosinophilic pneumonia is characterized by an acute course of fever and rapid progression to severe hypoxemia, in addition to the eosinophilia and diffuse pulmonary infiltrates. These young adult patients responded quickly to oral corticosteroids, and none relapsed after the dose was tapered and discontinued.

The differential diagnosis of Loeffler syndrome includes bronchiolitis obliterans, eosinophilic pneumonia with vasculitis (polyarteritis and other collagen diseases); pulmonary eosinophilia with asthma, including allergic bronchopulmonary aspergillosis; tropical pulmonary eosinophilia secondary to infection with filaria; acute (adult) respiratory distress syndrome; and nonleukemic prolonged pulmonary eosinophilia (i.e., chronic eosinophilic pneumonia). The latter entity is unusual in childhood but has been reported in an infant.

Allen JN, Pacht ER, Gadek JE, et al: Acute eosinophilic pneumonia as a reversible cause of noninfectious respiratory failure. N Engl J Med 321:569, 1989.
Alp H, Daum RS, Abrahams C, et al: Acute eosinophilic pneumonia: A cause of reversible, severe, nonimfectious respiratory failure. J Pediat 132: 540,1998.
O'Sullivan BP, Nimkin K, Gang DL: A fifteen-year-old boy with eosinophilia and pulmonary infiltrates. J Pediatr 123:660, 1993.

CHAPTER 399
Pulmonary Involvement in Collagen Diseases

Robert C. Stern

Rheumatic pneumonia is a rare complication of acute rheumatic fever, rheumatoid arthritis, or other connective tissue diseases, characterized clinically by extensive pulmonary consolidation and rapidly progressive functional deterioration and pathologically by alveolar exudate, inflammatory interstitial infiltrates, and necrotizing arteritis. Physical findings are unexpectedly minimal; often there are no rales. Chest roentgenograms reveal transient areas of infiltrate that resemble pulmonary edema. There is no specific treatment; patients may respond to corticosteroids. If the lesion is diagnosed by lung biopsy, treatment with immunosuppressive agents (e.g., cyclophosphamide [Cytoxan]) may be valuable.

Lovell D, Lindsley C, Langston C: Lymphoid interstitial pneumonia in juvenile rheumatoid arthritis. J Pediatr 105:947, 1984.
Oetgen WJ, Boice, JA, Lawless OJ: Mixed connective tissue disease in children and adolescents. Pediatrics 67:333, 1981.
Park S, Nyhan WL: Fatal pulmonary involvement in dermatomyositis. Am J Dis Child 129:723, 1975.
Rajani KB, Aschbacher LV, Kinney TR: Pulmonary hemorrhage and systemic lupus erythematosus. J Pediatr 93:810, 1978.
Serlin SP, Rmisza ME, Gay JH: Rheumatic pneumonia: The need for a new approach. Pediatrics 56:1075, 1975.
Winterbauer RH, De Paso W, Lammert J: Pulmonary disease in rheumatoid arthritis patients. J Respir Dis 10:35, 1989.

CHAPTER 400
Desquamative Interstitial Pneumonitis

Robert C. Stern

The cause of desquamative interstitial pneumonitis is usually unknown but can occasionally be traced to adenovirus, congenital rubella infection, organic dust (antigen) inhalation, or drugs (e.g., nitrofurantoin). The disease is characterized pathologically by massive proliferation of alveolar cells and thickening of the alveolar walls. The presence of many alveolar macrophages, some of which fuse to form giant cells, also contributes to filling the alveolar air spaces. The degree of desquamation is far greater than the degree of alveolar wall thickening. Long-standing desquamative interstitial pneumonitis may progress to chronic interstitial fibrosis, but fibrosis is less marked than in usual interstitial pneumonitis. Occasional families have more than one affected child. Most children have a history of preceding upper respiratory infection, although the relationship of the desquamative pneumonitis to these infections of probable viral origin has not been firmly established. In two infants, desquamative interstitial pneumonitis and congenital rubella were associated. Circulating immune complexes and alveolar deposition of IgG and complement suggest an immune basis for the disease.

CLINICAL MANIFESTATIONS. Symptoms usually develop slowly. As alveolar function is compromised, tachypnea and dyspnea occur; as the disease progresses, nonproductive cough, anorexia, and weight loss ensue. Cyanosis eventually results; clubbing is not a constant feature, and fever is unusual. Physical findings include tachypnea, nasal flaring, and occasionally fine rales. The use of the accessory muscles of respiration is not as prominent as one would expect in obstructive diseases exhibiting an equal amount of hypoxemia.

LABORATORY MANIFESTATIONS. Chest roentgenograms reveal a diffuse, hazy, ground-glass appearance, particularly at the lung bases, along with poorly defined hilar densities. Viral and bacteriologic cultures and acute and convalescent sera analyses are not helpful diagnostically. Arterial blood samples show hypoxemia; most patients seek medical care before the advent of hypercapnia. Hypoxia at rest is most likely the result of a ventilation-perfusion abnormality, but a diffusion defect eventually occurs, resulting in severe exercise intolerance. Bronchoalveolar lavage abnormalities have not been sufficiently defined to allow diagnosis. Definitive diagnosis requires open lung biopsy.

TREATMENT. Some patients with desquamative interstitial pneumonitis recover without specific treatment. However, the prognosis is guarded when the diagnosis is made before 1 yr of age (8 of 14 died within 4 yr in one report). With worsening pulmonary status or rapid deterioration shown on the chest roentgenogram, an open lung biopsy is important to establish a definitive diagnosis. These patients usually respond to corticosteroid therapy with rapid resolution of symptoms and gradual improvement on roentgenogram. A few corticosteroid-resistant patients are reported, and various other treatments, including immunosuppression, have been proposed; corticosteroid therapy may be less effective in familial cases. Chloroquine phosphate (10 mg/kg/24 hr) has been effective in some corticosteroid-resistant patients, including those with a family history of the disease. Supportive treatment including supplemental oxygen is often necessary. Corticosteroid therapy without a lung biopsy diagnosis is hazardous; chronic viral pneumonitis can present with a similar clinical picture and may be worsened by corticosteriod depression of host defenses. Relapses are reported when therapy is prematurely stopped. A patient treated with lung transplantation developed an unusual alveolar fibrinous exudate, associated with the presence of histiocytes and lymphocytes. These findings suggest an abnormal response to rejection.

Avital A, Godfrey S, Maayan CH, et al: Chloroquine treatment of interstitial lung disease in children. Pediatr Pulmonol 18:356, 1994.

Bokulic RE, Hilman BC: Interstitial lung disease in children. Respir Med 41:543, 1994.

Case Records of the Massachusetts General Hospital: Case 49–1993. N Engl J Med 329:1797, 1993.

Fan LL, Kozinetz CA, Deterding RR, et al: Evaluation of a diagnostic approach to pediatric interstitial lung disease. Pediatrics 101:82, 1998.

Farrell PM, Gilbert EF, Zimmerman JJ, et al: Familial lung disease associated with proliferation and desquamation of type II pneumocytes. Am J Dis Child 140:262, 1986.

Stillwell PC, Norris DG, O'Connell EJ, et al: Desquamative interstitial pneumonitis in children. Chest 77:155, 1980.

Tal A, Maer E, Bar-Ziv J, et al: Fatal desquamative interstitial pneumonitis in three infant siblings. J Pediatr 104:873, 1984.

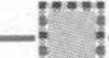

CHAPTER 401
Hypostatic Pneumonia

Robert C. Stern

Hypostatic pneumonia occurs after prolonged passive pulmonary congestion and may occur postoperatively or in any marasmic state. Lying for a long time in one position favors its development. Patients have dependent congestion, edema, and pneumonia. The symptoms are not characteristic. Neither dyspnea nor fever develops unless these symptoms are secondary to another disorder such as infection or congestive heart failure. The physical signs are principally slight dullness on percussion, feeble respiratory sounds, and the presence of moist rales. Hypostatic congestion is usually a terminal event. There is no specific treatment. Prophylaxis is of the greatest importance; the position of any immobile patient should be changed frequently.

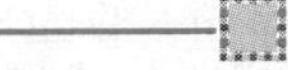

CHAPTER 402
Pulmonary Hemosiderosis (Pulmonary Hemorrhage)

Dorr G. Dearborn

Bleeding in the lower respiratory tract in children is unusual but can be life-threatening. During infancy and prepubertal childhood, infections, trauma, and foreign bodies are probably the most common causes of pulmonary hemorrhage. More extensive hemorrhage in this age range can arise from any of the remaining secondary and primary causes listed in Table 402–1, although the rare immune-related vascular diseases are limited to older children and adolescents. Following a hemorrhage, macrophages convert the iron of hemoglobin into hemosiderin, hence the term *hemosiderosis.* Since it takes the macrophage 36 to 48 hr to form hemosiderin, and hemosiderin-laden macrophages are resident in the alveoli for only about 2 wk, alveolar hemosiderosis is an indicator of previous bleeding, and its persistence is an indication of continued bleeding. The term *pulmonary hemosiderosis* should be reserved for persistent or chronic bleeding.

TABLE 402–1 Causes of Pulmonary Hemorrhage

Infection (extensive)
Bacterial, fungal, parasitic
Chronic with bronchiectasis*
Trauma
Crush injury, suffocation, foreign body
Cardiovascular
Increased pulmonary venous pressure
Arteriovenous malformations
Pulmonary emboli, infarcts
Vasculitis
Autoimmune disorders*
Immune complex disorders*
Anti–glomerular basement membrane antibodies*
Toxic (penicillamine, cocaine)
Neoplasia (carcinoid)
Associated with antibodies to cow milk proteins
Idiopathic

**Limited to school-age children and older.*

Pulmonary hemorrhage can be either focal or diffuse. Focal hemorrhage is usually an acute process in the conducting airways, whereas diffuse hemorrhage results from abnormalities of alveolar capillaries with a continuing, sometimes exacerbating, course. Notably, alveolar hemorrhage can occur without sufficient blood reaching the central airways to produce hemoptysis and may not produce visible infiltrates on chest roentgenographs. Acute pulmonary hemorrhage that does produce alveolar infiltrates can show rapid clearing in 1 to 2 days, distinguishing these infiltrates from infectious infiltrates. An acute hemorrhage is usually accompanied by a drop in hematocrit, an increase in reticulocyte count, and a stool that tests positive for occult blood. The accompanying respiratory distress, including cough, wheeze, and tachypnea, may be mild and transient or may be sufficiently severe to cause respiratory failure depending on the quantity of blood in the alveoli and airways. A more insidious onset may occur with only fatigue, mild dyspnea, and anemia. Diagnosis is most readily confirmed with the use of Prussian blue staining for hemosiderin within alveolar macrophages obtained by bronchoalveolar lavage (BAL) or by examination of sputum or gastric aspirates. Even overt pulmonary hemorrhage requiring ventilator support should be followed by alveolar macrophage cytologic studies several (>3) wk after the acute hemorrhage to demonstrate continued hemosiderosis denoting a chronic process. Significant alveolar hemorrhage can be ongoing and clinically undetectable except by iron stain cytologic studies of BAL samples.

SECONDARY PULMONARY HEMOSIDEROSIS. Heart disease that causes a chronic increase in pulmonary venous pressure, such as mitral stenosis, can lead to intrapulmonary hemorrhage and secondary hemosiderosis. Pulmonary arteriovenous malformations can be a component of hereditary hemorrhagic telangiectasia (Osler-Weber-Rendu syndrome) but are seldom accompanied by hemoptysis and hemosiderosis in infancy and childhood. Although pulmonary embolism is not often considered in infants and children, it is a well-known complication of central venous catheters and may result in local bleeding. Rarely, pulmonary hemorrhage is seen with hemolytic-uremic syndrome, anaphylactoid purpura, or thrombocytopenic purpura. It can also result from graft-versus-host disease and is a concern especially during the early neutropenic phase after bone marrow transplant, when endogenous bacterial endotoxin from the intestine can be an inflammatory stimulant in the lung.

VASCULAR DISEASES. The entire spectrum of the pulmonary vasculature, including capillaries, can be involved in vascular inflammatory disorders and, in some cases, the inflammatory lesions of the capillaries may be the only pulmonary vascular manifestation of a systemic disorder. Capillary inflammation (capillaritis) may arise from immune processes in which immune complex deposition or formation can be demonstrated (e.g., systemic lupus erythematosus and *Goodpasture syndrome*). The role of an immune mechanism can be less clear, as in the necrotizing vasculitis of Wegener granulomatosis. Nephritis or other systemic manifestations are usually evident, but the initial presentation of Goodpasture syndrome (pulmonary hemosiderosis with glomerulonephritis) can be similar to idiopathic pulmonary hemosiderosis, with only hemoptysis and iron-deficient anemia. Adolescents who present with hemoptysis should be evaluated for vascular diseases, including testing for circulating anti–glomerular basement membrane antibodies and antibodies to cytoplasmic components to neutrophils (ANCA). Histopathologic confirmation by biopsy of kidney, lung, or other tissue may be necessary for definitive diagnosis. The severity of pulmonary involvement is highly variable but can be devastating. Corticosteriod immunosuppression may need to be intensified with cyclophosphamide or azathioprine. The successful use of plasmapheresis during acute massive pulmonary hemorrhage has been limited to Goodpasture syndrome.

PRIMARY PULMONARY HEMOSIDEROSIS WITH HYPERSENSITIVITY TO COW MILK (HEINER SYNDROME). Although the pathophysiology is not understood, some infants and children with pulmonary hemosiderosis have circulating IgG antibodies against cow milk proteins. Heiner originally detected these "milk precipitins" by immunodiffusion. Antibody levels against cow milk proteins in excess of 200 μg/mL may be comparable. These children have the typical picture of idiopathic hemosiderosis often accompanied by chronic rhinitis, recurrent otitis media, gastrointestinal symptoms, and growth retardation. The symptoms improve when cow milk is removed from the diet and return with its reintroduction. Some patients fail to improve at all on a milk-free diet, and others without multiple milk precipitins have improved. Hypertrophied nasopharyngeal lymphoid tissue can be sufficiently obstructive to lead to secondary cor pulmonale. In general, patients with hemosiderosis and precipitins to cow milk have a better prognosis than do those with other forms of hemosiderosis, and the former individuals may eventually lose their sensitivity to milk. Corticosteroids may be useful, at least during acute bleeding episodes.

IDIOPATHIC PULMONARY HEMOSIDEROSIS. The cause of idiopathic pulmonary hemosiderosis remains unknown, although environmental toxins have been suggested. Onset usually occurs in early childhood and rarely later than early adult life. It is a rare disorder with a reported yearly incidence of 0.24 (Sweden) and 1.23 (Japan) cases per million children. Most of the clinical manifestations are related to blood in the alveoli and to the effects of chronic blood loss. Symptoms are those of recurrent or chronic pulmonary disease and include cough, hemoptysis, dyspnea, wheezing, and occasional cyanosis associated with fatigue and pallor. The cough may be productive of bloody sputum, or the infant or child may simply vomit large quantities of swallowed blood. During acute attacks, which usually last 2–4 days, the child may be febrile. Digital clubbing is often present.

The usual clinical features of fever, tachycardia, tachypnea, leukocytosis, respiratory distress, and abnormal roentgenographic findings may suggest bacterial pneumonia, but accompanying anemia and rapid clearing of the chest roentgenogram should lead to the correct diagnosis. In some children, the early manifestations of illness are related to chronic iron deficiency anemia and the characteristic pulmonary symptoms do not appear until much later. Although the child may have severe pulmonary manifestations without roentgenographic abnormalities, seldom is the roentgenographic picture abnormal before pulmonary symptoms have occurred.

The anemia is typically microcytic and hypochromic; serum iron concentration is low, and there may be elevations in bilirubin, urobilinogen, and reticulocyte count. The stool usually contains occult blood, which presumably is swallowed. By definition, hemosiderin is found in alveolar macrophages obtained by BAL or biopsy and provisionally in smears of sputum or gastric aspirates. Roentgenographic changes range from minimal infiltrates resembling pneumonia to massive pulmonary involvement with secondary atelectasis. Hilar lymphadenopathy can occur with long-standing disease.

Diagnosis is by the exclusion of known causes for pulmonary hemorrhage and the persistence of hemosiderosis beyond the acute 2–3 wk period after a documented pulmonary hemorrhage. Significant hemosiderosis is indicated by iron stain cytologic studies on bronchoalveolar lavage samples showing greater than 10% of the macrophages containing hemosiderin or an iron index greater than 25 (scoring 100 macrophages for amount of hemosiderin 0 to 3+ with a maximal score of 300). Culturing of bronchoalveolar lavage samples for bacteria, viruses, and fungi helps exclude various infectious processes producing hemosiderosis. Although no longer required for diagnosis, open lung biopsy demonstrates intra-alveolar hemorrhage, large numbers of hemosiderin-laden macrophages, alveolar epithelial hyperplasia, and eventually interstitial fibrosis and small artery hypertensive changes. Absence of immunoglobulin or complement deposition on the alveolar basement membrane virtually excludes immune-based vascular disease, and all biopsy specimens should be subjected to this test.

Approximately one half of the patients die within 1–5 yr, usually from acute pulmonary hemorrhage and progressive respiratory failure. A milk-free diet may be worth trying in severe cases even if antibodies against cow milk proteins are at low titers. Corticosteroids (prednisone, 1 mg/kg/24 hr) produce remission in some patients and are of no benefit in others. Maintenance corticosteroid therapy has been used between attacks with variable results. More extensive immune suppression with the addition of azathioprine or cyclophosphamide can be helpful.

IDIOPATHIC PULMONARY HEMORRHAGE AND HEMOSIDEROSIS IN INFANTS. Acute idiopathic pulmonary hemorrhage in young infants has been reported in clusters in Cleveland, Chicago, Milwaukee, and Detroit, and sporadic cases have occurred elsewhere in the United States. In Cleveland, a case-control study of the epidemiology led by the Centers for Disease Control and Prevention found an association with chronic water damage in the homes along with growth of a fungus, *Stachybotrys chartarum.* Aerosolized spores from this fungus are sufficiently small to be inhaled out to the distal airways and contain several classes of toxins including trichothecenes, which are potent protein synthesis inhibitors. Conceptually, local release of these toxins during rapid endothelial basement membrane formation in young infants could lead to fragile capillaries, which would be at risk for stress hemorrhage. The Centers for Disease Control study also suggested that environmental tobacco smoke is one of the stresses leading to hemorrhage.

With the inclusion of cases found at postmortem examination, the mortality rate in the Cleveland area has exceeded 30%, and for the years 1993–1995, the incidence in the limited geographic cluster area reached 1.5 cases/thousand live births. Most of the infants present with acute respiratory distress and overt pulmonary hemorrhage, many requiring ventilator support and blood transfusions. Some infants presenting without frank hemoptysis but with unexplained respiratory failure were found to have pulmonary hemorrhage on tracheal intubation. The subtle presentation of some infants and the similarity of prodromal symptoms to acute life-threatening events has led to inclusion of this disorder in the differential diagnosis and evaluation for acute life-threatening events (see Chapter 714). In young infants who breath through the nose, hemoptysis may present as an atraumatic epistaxis. Most of the infants have had repeat BAL more than 3 wk after the initial hemorrhage and were uniformly found to have continued low-grade bleeding. This hemosiderosis continues for 3 to 12 mo, during which time the infants are at risk for a massive, stress-related hemorrhage. Other manifestations observed in some infants include neurologic problems (e.g., seizures and developmental delay), concomittant infection, and hemolysis with hemoglobinuria. Fever and leukocytosis are not usually present.

Treatment for these infants beyond the initial supportive measures has included removing them from their original fungal and smoke environment. In the Cleveland infants, this has led to a fivefold decrease in the rebleeding frequency. In addition, high-dose corticosteroids (methylprednisolone, 1 mg/kg, intravenously every 6–12 hr) have been used at the time of the acute hemorrhage followed by oral prednisone (1 to 2 mg/kg/day) for a few weeks. Daily or every-other-day prednisone (0.5 to 1 mg/kg) is maintained until the iron-stained BAL cytologic results have returned to nearly normal. Although the use of corticosteroids here is empirical, they may be suppressing inflammation, a major component in animal studies of pulmonary stachybotryomycotoxicosis. Anecdotally, several of the Cleveland deaths occurred in infants who either did not receive corticosteroids or in whom they were discontinued early. Reticulocyte counts and frequent stool guaiac testing help guide the corticosteroid therapy and scheduling of repeat bronchoscopies. Some infants have received corticosteroids for longer than 12 mo. One patient in whom corticosteroids were discontinued for 4 mo had a subsequent massive pulmonary hemorrhage at 22 mo of age following the return of tobacco smoke to his environment. Vulnerability to stress hemorrhage appears to persist for 1 to 2 yr, whereupon surviving children seem normal. The potential causative overlap of this disorder with other forms of pulmonary hemosiderosis has yet to be determined.

American Academy of Pediatrics: Toxic effects of indoor molds. Pediatrics 101:712, 1998.

Boat TF: Pulmonary Hemorrhage and Hemoptysis. *In:* Chernick V, Boat TF (eds): Kendig's Disorders of the Respiratory Tract in Children, 6th ed. Philadelphia, WB Saunders, 1998, pp 623–633.

Centers for Disease Control: Update: Pulmonary Hemorrhage/Hemosiderosis Among Infants—Cleveland, Ohio, 1993–1996. Morbid Mortal Week Rep 46:33, 1997.

Dearborn DG: Pulmonary hemorrhage in infants and children. Curr Opin Pediatr 9:219, 1997.

Dearborn DG, Infeld MD, Smith PG, Allan TM: Pulmonary hemorrhage and hemosiderosis in infants. http://gcrc.meds.cwru.edu/stachy.htm

Etzel RA, Montaña E, Sorenson WG, et al: Acute pulmonary hemorrhage in infants associated with exposure to Stachybotrys atra and other fungi. Arch Pediatr Adolesc Med 152:757, 1998.

Green RJ, Ruoss SJ, Kraft SA, et al: Pulmonary capillaritis and alveolar hemorrhage. Chest 110:1305, 1996.

Montana E, Etzel RA, Allan TM, et al: Environmental risk factors associated with pediatric idiopathic pulmonary hemosiderosis in a Cleveland community. Pediatrics 99:E5, 1997. (http://www.pediatrics.org/cgi/content/full/99/1/e5)

Sherman JM, Winnie G, Thomassen MJ, et al: Time course of hemosiderin production and clearance by human pulmonary macrophages. Chest 86:409, 1984.

West JB, Mathieu-Costello O: Vulnerability of pulmonary capillaries in heart disease. Circulation 92:622, 1995.

CHAPTER 403
Pulmonary Alveolar Proteinosis

Harvey R. Colten and Aaron Hamvas

Pulmonary alveolar proteinosis (PAP) is a clinical disorder characterized histopathologically by the accumulation of periodic acid Schiff–positive, diastase-resistant lipid-rich proteinoaceous fluid in alveolar spaces. Two clinical childhood forms of PAP have been described: a fatal congenital form and an acquired type, similar to that described in adults.

The *congenital form* of the disorder is immediately apparent in the newborn period and rapidly leads to respiratory failure. The disorder is often clinically and radiographically indistinguishable from other pulmonary and cardiac disorders of the newborn, such as neonatal pneumonia, generalized bacterial infection, persistent pulmonary hypertension, meconium aspiration, infantile respiratory distress syndrome, alveolar capillary dysplasia, and congenital heart disease, especially total anomalous pulmonary venous return. The incidence of congenital PAP is unknown.

Although the mechanisms that contribute to the congenital form of alveolar proteinosis are largely undefined, an inherited deficiency in surfactant protein B (SP-B) has been associated with a small proportion of the cases (see next section). Additional insights into other possible mechanisms have been gained from murine strains with targeted disruption of macrophage colony-stimulating factor or granulocyte-macrophage colony stimulating factor (GM-CSF) and its receptor. These mice have no overt hematologic abnormalities but exhibit alveolar proteinosis apparently due to an inability to clear otherwise normal pulmonary surfactant from the air space. A deficiency in expression of the β subunit of the GM-CSF receptor has been described in four human infants with alveolar proteinosis; deficiencies of GM-CSF ligand have not been identified in humans. No mechanism has been delineated for most of the currently identified cases of congenital alveolar proteinosis.

An *acquired* or *"adult" form* of alveolar proteinosis has also been described, but it is rare in children. It affects males three times as often as females and may be primary (i.e., idiopathic, with no identifiable causative factor) or secondary to a variety of inciting agents, including dust, noxious chemicals, and infection, particularly in the setting of systemic immunosuppression. The chief difference between the primary and secondary forms of adult PAP is the distribution of the pathologic process, that is, diffuse in primary PAP and patchy in secondary PAP. Patients with acquired PAP present with dyspnea, fatigue, cough, weight loss, chest pain, or hemoptysis. In the later stages, cyanosis and digital clubbing may be seen. Pulmonary function testing reveals a restrictive pattern, and arterial blood gas determinations show marked hypoxemia and a chronic respiratory alkalosis.

DIAGNOSIS. The presence of alveolar proteinosis can be ascertained by lung biopsy. In cases of congenital alveolar proteinosis due to mechanisms other than SP-B deficiency (see next section), immunohistochemical staining reveals abundant quantities of alveolar and intracellular surfactant proteins A and B. Examination of peripheral blood and bone marrow for clonogenic stimulation of monocyte-macrophage precursors, GM-CSF receptor and ligand expression, and GM-CSF binding determines whether a deficiency in GM-CSF ligand or receptor is a contributing mechanism.

TREATMENT. Untreated idiopathic congenital alveolar proteinosis is fatal, and thus far medical therapy has not been successful. Lung transplantation therefore is the only currently available therapeutic option. Bone marrow transplantation reverses the alveolar proteinosis in GM-CSF receptor–deficient mice and should be considered an experimental therapy for infants with congenital alveolar proteinosis due to this genetic abnormality.

Repeated bronchoalveolar lavage is therapeutic for patients with the acquired form of PAP. Administration of recombinant GM-CSF may improve pulmonary function in adults with acquired idiopathic alveolar proteinosis; clinical trials are in progress.

403.1 Surfactant Protein B Deficiency

Inherited deficiency of surfactant apoprotein protein B (SP-B) presents in the immediate neonatal period with pulmonary failure. This autosomal recessive disorder is fatal in homozygous SP-B–deficient patients and typically affects full-term newborns. It is clinically and radiographically similar to the respiratory distress syndrome of premature infants but is refractory to conventional interventions, including mechanical ventilation, surfactant replacement therapy, glucocorticoid administration, and extracorporeal membrane oxygenation. SP-B deficiency has been recognized in diverse racial and ethnic groups. Heterozygous SP-B–deficient patients are clinically normal and as adults have normal pulmonary function.

MOLECULAR GENETICS. At least 10 molecular defects in the SP-B gene have been identified in patients with SP-B deficiency. The most common among these is a net two base-pair insertion (121ins2) in codon 121 that generates a frame shift and interruption of SP-B protein translation. The insertion generates a restriction fragment polymorphism that is useful for diagnosis (Fig. 403–1). This mutation accounts for 75% of the alleles found in the approximately 60 patients from 30 families identified with SP-B deficiency to date. The other mutations have been identified in one family each.

PATHOLOGY. Although SP-B deficiency was first described in the context of the congenital form of alveolar proteinosis, this

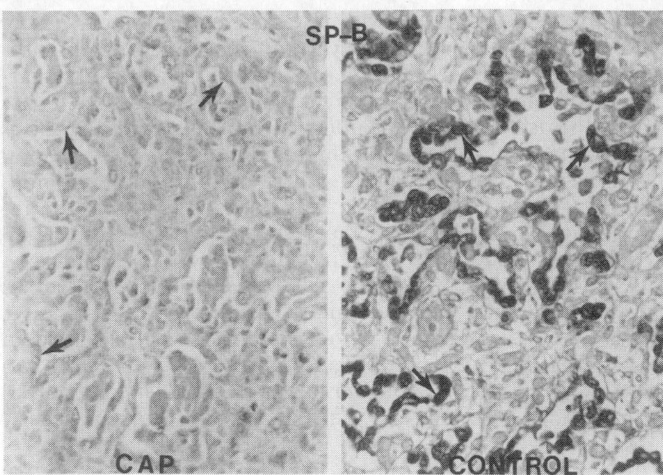

Figure 403–2 Immunostaining of a lung section for surfactant protein B (SP-B). Type II pneumocytes (*arrows*) are negative for SP-B in an infant with congenital alveolar proteinosis (CAP). Intense immunoreactivity for SP-B is present in an age-matched control.

histologic description is neither necessary nor sufficient for the diagnosis of SP-B deficiency. The lungs of several homozygous 121ins2 SP-B–deficient patients had histologic features of desquamative interstitial pneumonitis with little detectable alveolar proteinosis at the time of lung transplantation. The absence of SP-B protein assayed immunohistochemically definitively establishes a diagnosis of SP-B deficiency (Fig. 403–2). Associated findings include an increased amount and abnormal tissue distribution of the surfactant proteins SP-A and SP-C and expression of an incompletely processed SP-C peptide. Ultrastructural findings suggest abnormal surfactant lipid structure and function, including disorganized lamellar bodies, a lack of tubular myelin, and an accumulation of lipid and SP-A between the alveolar epithelium and basement membrane.

DIAGNOSIS. Concurrent analyses of the infant's peripheral blood for the 121ins2 mutation (using restriction fragment polymorphism analysis of polymerase chain reaction–amplified genomic DNA) and of tracheal effluent for the presence or absence of SP-B protein are the first steps in establishing the diagnosis of SP-B deficiency. Definitive diagnosis is established by immunostaining of lung biopsy tissue for the surfactant proteins. In affected families, an antenatal diagnosis can be established by molecular assays of a chorionic villus biopsy or amniocytes or, late in gestation, by measuring surfactant proteins in amniotic fluid, permitting advanced planning of a therapeutic regimen.

TREATMENT. Because virtually all patients with SP-B deficiency die within 3 mo, prompt recognition is critical to provide treatment options for the affected infant and family. Conventional neonatal intensive care interventions only temporize, and replacement therapy with commercially available surfactants is ineffective. Thus, the only therapy is lung transplantation. Such transplantation has been successful. The oldest living SP-B–deficient survivor following lung transplantation is 4 yr old, but this may not be an option a family wishes to pursue. This therapy has succeeded in five of seven patients who have survived to undergo transplantation, but the medical and surgical care is highly specialized and available only at a few institutions. The relative scarcity of available infants' lungs for transplantation suggests that gene therapy may be the treatment of choice in the future. Genetic counseling is also important to convey the risks for future pregnancies and the availability of antenatal diagnosis and therapeutic options.

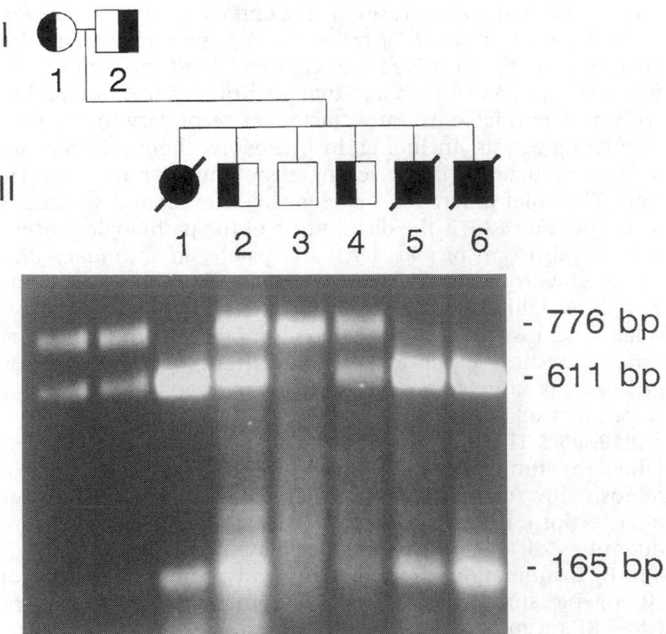

Figure 403–1 Restriction fragment length polymorphism of a 6-base pair fragment of the SP-B gene in a family with three homozygous deficient patients. (From Nogee LM, Garnier G, Dietz HC, et al: A mutation in the surfactant protein B gene as the basis for a fatal neonatal respiratory disease in multiple kindreds. J Clin Invest 93:1860, 1994.)

Dranoff G, Crawford AD, Sadelain M, et al: Involvement of granulocyte-macrophage colony-stimulating factor in pulmonary homeostasis. Science 264:713, 1994.

Hamvas A: Inherited surfactant protein-B deficiency. Adv Pedatr 44:369, 1997.
Hamvas A, Nogee, LM, Mallory G-B, et al: Lung transplantation for treatment of infants with sufactant protein B deficiency. J Pediatr 130:231, 1997.
Ikegami M, Ueda T, Hull WM, et al: Surfactant metabolism in transgenic mice after granulocyte macrophage-colony stimulating factor ablation. Am J Physiol 270:l650, 1996.
Klein JM, Thompson MW, Snyder JM, et al: Transient surfactant protein deficiency in a term infant with severe respiratory failure. J Pediatr 132:244, 1998.
Mahut B, Delacourt C, Scheinmann P, et al: Pulmonary alveolar proteinosis: Experience with eight pediatric cases and a review. Pediatrics 97:117, 1996.
Nogee LM, deMello DE, Dehner LP, Colten HR: Pulmonary surfactant protein B deficiency in congenital pulmonary alveolar proteinosis. N Engl J Med 328:406, 1993.
Nogee LM, Garnier G, Singer L, et al: A mutation in the surfactant protein B gene responsible for fatal neonatal respiratory disease in multiple kindreds. J Clin Invest 93:1860, 1994.

CHAPTER 404
Idiopathic Diffuse Interstitial Fibrosis of the Lung
(Hamman-Rich Syndrome)

Robert C. Stern

Diffuse interstitial pulmonary fibrosis is a chronic, usually fatal disorder of unknown origin, ordinarily observed in adults but occasionally in infants and children. Although idiopathic pulmonary fibrosis is clearly a group of diseases, its separation into various subgroups, based on histologic characteristics, is controversial. One type, desquamative interstitial pneumonitis, is discussed elsewhere (Chapter 400). The clinical characteristics of the others (in one scheme: usual interstitial pneumonitis, acute interstitial pneumonitis, and nonspecific interstitial pneumonitis) are summarized here. All are very rare in childhood. The occurrence of several affected individuals in certain families suggests an autosomal dominant genetic basis of inheritance for some of these patients.

The disease has been hypothesized to result from an uncontrolled inflammatory process following an otherwise minor insult to the lower respiratory tract. A chronic inflammatory state occurs and eventually leads to progressive fibrosis. Alveolar macrophages, perhaps stimulated by immune complexes, may have a pivotal role by releasing chemotactic factors and stimulants of fibrosis, including fibronectin and alveolar macrophage–derived growth factor.

The clinical pattern is characterized by progressive pulmonary insufficiency resulting from interstitial fibrosis and alveolar-capillary block. The onset is usually insidious, with dyspnea initially occurring only with exercise but later present even at rest. A dry cough is common and may produce blood. Patients are usually afebrile. As the disease progresses, anorexia, weight loss, and fatigability occur, followed by cyanosis, clubbing, cor pulmonale, and right-sided cardiac failure. The lungs are usually clear on auscultation, but rales are occasionally detected. Most children die of respiratory failure, often after one of the frequent intercurrent pulmonary infections. Serial roentgenograms show progressive widespread granular or reticular mottling or small nodular densities. Hypoxemia may be present and increases dramatically with exercise. Airway resistance is not increased, and vital capacity, compliance, and diffusion capacity are decreased. Bronchoalveolar lavage fluid contains many inflammatory cells and relatively large numbers of mast cells.[67] Ga scans usually have positive results, with the abnormality restricted to the lungs. Idiopathic diffuse interstitial fibrosis must be distinguished from desquamative interstitial pneumonitis (Chapter 400) and lymphoid interstitial pneumonitis (usually AIDS; see Chapter 268). These diseases vary greatly in prognosis, and although some features of treatment overlap, others do not. Lung biopsy is needed for definitive diagnosis. Open biopsy is favored, but adequate tissue for diagnosis has also been obtained during fiberoptic bronchoscopy or thoracoscopy. If the disease is non-uniform, several tissue samples are desirable.

The pulmonary pathology is variable. During the early stage of the disease, fibrosis is usually not present, but there is cellular infiltration of the walls of the alveoli, alveolar ducts, and peribronchial tissue by lymphocytes, plasma cells, and occasionally eosinophils. This usually progresses to extensive and diffuse proliferation of fibrous tissue throughout all the lobes of the lung and is associated with organization of intra-alveolar exudate.

Corticosteroids may give some symptomatic relief but do not alter the progression of the disease or improve pulmonary function. Other therapy is also symptomatic. Immunosuppressant drugs and antimalarials (e.g., chloroquine) have been used with benefit in some adults and children. A chronic inflammatory state has been demonstrated in the lungs of 50% of first-degree relatives of persons with the autosomal recessive form of the disease. If this finding proves to be predictive of subsequent clinical disease, strategies for preventive treatment might be devised.

Avital A, Godfrey S, Maayan Ch, et al: Chloroquine treatment of interstitial lung disease in children. Pediatric Pulmonology 18:356, 1994.
Bitterman PB, Rennard SI, Keogh BA, et al: Familial idiopathic pulmonary fibrosis: Evidence of lung inflammation in unaffected family members. N Engl J Med 314:1343, 1986.
Bokulic RE, Hilman BC: Interstitial lung disease in children. Respir Med 41:543, 1994.
Crystal RG, Bitterman PB, Rennard SI, et al: Interstitial lung disease of unknown cause: Disorders characterized by inflammation of the lower respiratory tract. N Engl J Med 310:154, 1984.
Katzenstein A-LA, Myers JL: Idiopathic pulmonary fibrosis. Clinical relevance of pathologic classification. Am J Respir Crit Care Med 157:1301, 1998.

CHAPTER 405
Pulmonary Alveolar Microlithiasis

Robert C. Stern

This rare disease of unknown cause often has its onset during childhood, but the clinical manifestations may be delayed until later years. Pulmonary alveolar microlithiasis is characterized by widely disseminated intra-alveolar calculi (primarily calcium and phosphorus salts), which create a characteristic pattern on the roentgenogram (Fig. 405–1). The disease is frequently recognized when the roentgenogram is taken for an unrelated illness or when symptoms are still minimal. Definitive diagnosis requires lung biopsy, but characteristic bronchoalveolar lavage analysis and high resolution CT findings can be extremely suggestive.

The frequent familial incidence (50% of families) and the large percentage (52 [23%] of the 225 reported patients) with Turkish ancestry strongly suggest a genetic basis (probably autosomal recessive), at least for some patients. No specific metabolic abnormalities have been identified. Serum calcium and phosphorus levels are normal. No treatment is available, and patients eventually die, usually during the middle years of adulthood, of slowly progressive cardiorespiratory failure, often with superimposed infection. Bronchopulmonary lavage is ineffective. After the patient's diagnosis, other family members should be screened by chest roentgenograms, and parents should be counseled that future children also risk developing

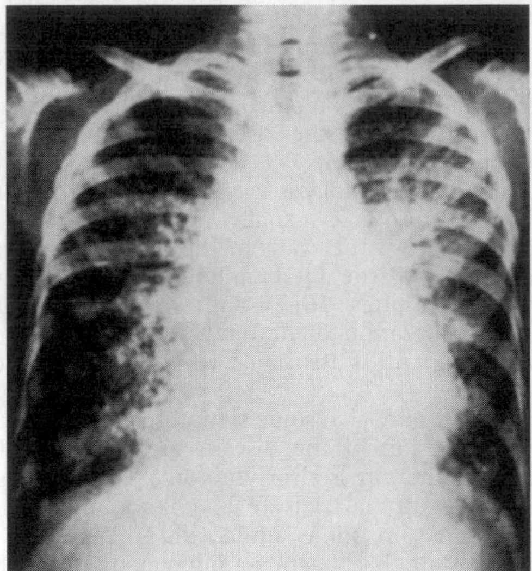

Figure 405–1 Roentgenogram of the chest of a 7-yr-old boy with pulmonary alveolar microlithiasis. (From Clark RB III. Johnson FC: Idiopathic pulmonary alveolar microlithiasis: A case report and brief review of the literature. Pediatrics 28:650, 1961.)

the disease. These children require prompt treatment of respiratory infection and should be advised about the dangers of smoking and exposure to industrial fumes. Immunization to measles and pertussis should be completed and yearly influenza vaccine given.

Moran CA, Hochholzer L, Hasleton PS et al:, Pulmonary alveolar microlithiasis. A clinicopathologic and chemical analysis of seven cases. Arch Pathol Lab Med 121:607, 1997.

Prakash UBS, Barham SS, Rosenow EC III, et al: Pulmonary alveolar microlithiasis: A review including ultrastructural and pulmonary function studies. Mayo Clin Proc 58:290, 1983.

Schmidt H, Lorcher U, Kitz R, et al:, Pulmonary alveolar microlithiasis in children. Pediatr Radiol 26:33, 1996.

Ucan ES, Keyf AI, Aydilek R, et al: Pulmonary alveolar microlithiasis: Review of Turkish reports. Thorax 48:171, 1993.

Wallis C, Whitehead B, Malone M, et al:, Pulmonary alveolar microlithiasis in childhood: Diagnosis by transbronchial biopsy. Pediatr Pulmonol 21:62, 1996.

CHAPTER 406
Atelectasis

Robert C. Stern

Congenital atelectasis and hyaline membrane disease are discussed in Chapter 97.3.

ACQUIRED ATELECTASIS

ETIOLOGY. Atelectasis, the imperfect expansion or collapse of air-bearing tissue, is not uncommon in infants and children. Collapse results from complete obstruction of air intake into the alveolar sacs; the obstruction usually persists sufficiently long to permit absorption of alveolar air into the blood. In general, the causes may be divided into three groups: external pressure directly on the pulmonary parenchyma or a bronchus or bronchiole; intrabronchial or intrabronchiolar obstruction; and any factor responsible for a continuously decreased amplitude of respiratory excursion or for respiratory paralysis. Bronchoconstriction and increased bronchosecretion due to allergy or other stimuli including embolus and chest wall trauma may also be contributing factors. Exudate formation may be responsible for atelectasis, as in patients with cystic fibrosis.

External Pressure. External factors may operate by direct interference with expansion of lungs (e.g., pleural effusion, pneumothorax, intrathoracic tumors, diaphragmatic hernia) or by external compression of a bronchus, completely obstructing ingress of air (e.g., enlarged lymph node, tumors, cardiac enlargement). The right middle lobe is especially likely to become atelectatic because of extrinsic compression from lymph nodes that encircle its bronchus and drain both the middle and upper lobe. Tuberculosis, although it should be considered in any patient with atelectasis, has been replaced by allergic disease or asthma as the most common cause of right middle lobe atelectasis. In the *right middle lobe syndrome,* intermittent collapse of this lobe occurs in association with exacerbations of asthmatic disease (see Chapter 145).

Intrabronchial or Intrabronchiolar Obstruction. See also Chapter 386. Complete intraluminal obstruction of a bronchus may be produced by a foreign body; by a neoplasm; by granulomatous tissue, as in tuberculosis; or by secretions (including mucus plugs), such as with cystic fibrosis, bronchiectasis, pulmonary abscess, asthma, chronic bronchitis, or acute laryngotracheobronchitis.

Obstruction of one or more bronchioles in a given area may be produced by any of the conditions mentioned, but widespread bronchiolar obstruction is most often produced by bronchiolitis or interstitial pneumonitis and by asthma. Generalized obstructive overinflation is the initial result of such bronchiolar obstructions, but as the pathologic changes progress, some of the bronchioles may become completely obstructed, and small areas of atelectasis and emphysema are then interspersed. Patchy atelectasis is relatively common in acute bronchiolitis or asthma and is probably always present in advanced chronic diffuse infections, such as the pulmonary infection associated with cystic fibrosis.

Reduced Amplitude of Respiratory Excursion or Respiratory Paralysis. Respiratory compromise may result from interference with the movements of the thoracic cage (e.g., neuromuscular abnormalities as in cerebral palsy, poliomyelitis, spinal muscular atrophy, myasthenia gravis; osseous deformities caused by rickets, scoliosis, kyphosis, scleroderma, overly restrictive casts, and surgical dressings); defective movement of the diaphragm (e.g., paralysis of phrenic nerve, increased abdominal pressure); or restriction of respiratory effort because of postoperative pain.

PATHOLOGY. Atelectatic (airless) areas are firm in consistency and deep red.

CLINICAL MANIFESTATIONS. Symptoms vary with the cause and extent of the atelectasis. A small area is likely to be asymptomatic. When a large area of previously normal lung becomes atelectatic, especially when it does so suddenly, dyspnea accompanied by rapid shallow respirations, tachycardia, and often cyanosis occurs. If the obstruction is removed, the symptoms disappear rapidly. Even atelectasis of an entire lobe may not result in changes in the percussion note because of compensatory expansion of adjacent lung tissue. However, when atelectasis occurs in an area of severe pre-existing disease, the patient may have transient pain but often does not complain of increased dyspnea. No new physical findings may be detected in these patients. However, after partial or complete re-expansion, physical findings of the underlying lung disease, including rales and wheeze, may become evident. Breath sounds are decreased or absent over extensive atelectatic areas.

DIAGNOSIS. The diagnosis can usually be established by roentgenographic examination (Fig. 406–1). Small areas may be indistinguishable from pneumonic consolidations, but those that involve several lobules can usually be identified by the contraction of the area. Bronchoscopic examination reveals a collapsed main bronchus when the obstruction is at the

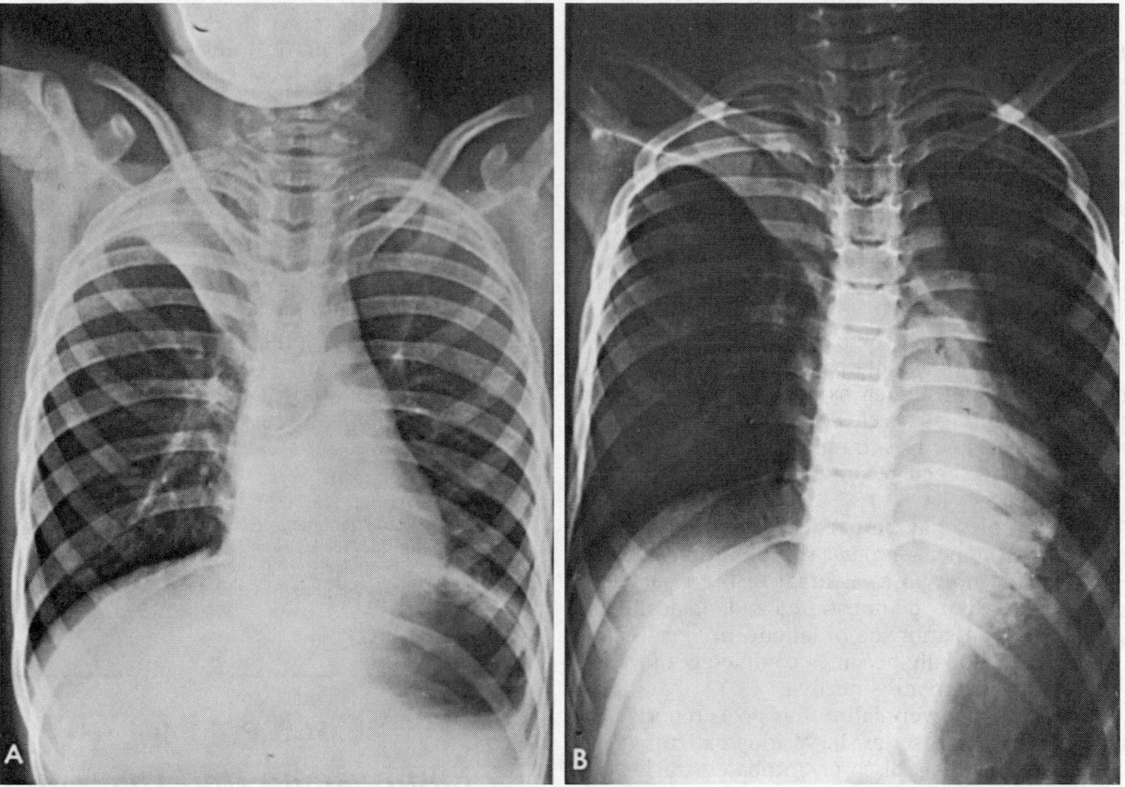

Figure 406–1 Atelectasis that occurred postoperatively and disappeared spontaneously. *A*. The right upper lobe and the left lower lobe are collapsed. *B*. The atelectasis of the left lower lobe is demonstrated on the overpenetrated film.

tracheobronchial junction and may also disclose the nature of the obstruction.

PROGNOSIS. If the obstruction disappears spontaneously or is removed, the atelectasis usually disappears unless secondary infection has occurred. The atelectatic area is more susceptible to infection because mucociliary clearance is impaired and cough is ineffective. In persistent cases, bronchiectasis is a frequent complication, and pulmonary abscess is occasionally a complication.

TREATMENT. *Bronchoscopic examination* is immediately indicated if atelectasis is the result of a foreign body or any other bronchial obstruction that may be relieved. It is also indicated when

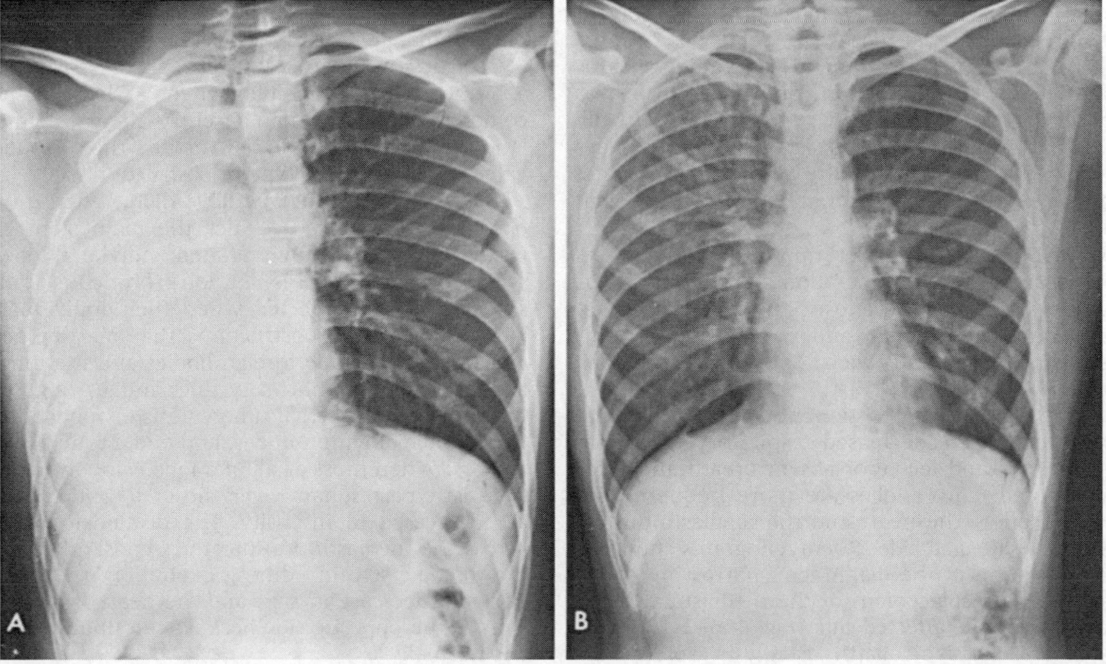

Figure 406–2 *A*. Massive atelectasis of the right lung. The patient has asthma. The heart and the other mediastinal structures are shifted to the right during the atelectatic phase. *B*. Comparison study after reaeration following bronchoscopic removal of a mucus plug from the right mainstem bronchus.

an isolated area of atelectasis persists for several weeks. It is usually advisable to suction the orifice of the involved bronchus; a **mucous plug** can occasionally be removed, with prompt re-expansion. If no anatomic basis for atelectasis is found and no material can be obtained by suctioning, the introduction of a small amount of saline followed by suctioning allows recovery of bronchial secretions for culture and, possibly, for cytologic examination. Frequent *changes in the child's position and deep breathing* may be beneficial. *Oxygen* therapy is indicated when there is dyspnea or substantial hemoglobin desaturation. Morphine and atropine should be avoided if possible.

If the atelectasis is unchanged or only partially helped by bronchoscopy, *postural drainage* and, occasionally, *antibiotics* are indicated. In some conditions, such as asthma, *bronchodilator* and *corticosteroid* treatment may accelerate atelectasis clearance. Intermittent positive pressure breathing, incentive inspirometry, and blow bottles have been recommended, but their efficacy remains unproved.

Repeated bronchoscopies may be needed. Postural drainage should be continued at home. *Lobectomy* should not be considered unless chronic infection poses a threat to the remainder of the lung, bronchiectasis is demonstrated radiologically, or systemic symptoms, such as anorexia or fatigue, are persistent. The atelectatic area occasionally becomes completely fibrosed; in this case, no further treatment is needed.

Intrapulmonary percussive ventilation has been reported to be successful, in uncontrolled series, in various patients (e.g., patients with neuromuscular disease, intubated/tracheotomized patients). Patients with neuromuscular disease, in whom rapid mobilization of secretions may be dangerous, often require some form of cough assistance (inexsufflator and/or chest compression [i.e., artificial cough]). Aerosolized recombinant human DNase, which is approved only for the treatment of cystic fibrosis, has occasionally been proposed for patients without cystic fibrosis but with persistent atelectasis. No published data support its use for this indication.

MASSIVE PULMONARY ATELECTASIS

Massive collapse of one or both lungs is most often a postoperative complication but occasionally results from other causes, such as trauma, asthma, pneumonia, tension pneumothorax, aspiration of foreign material (either a solid object large enough to obstruct a mainstem bronchus or liquids such as water or blood), following extubation, or paralysis, such as in diphtheria or poliomyelitis. Massive atelectasis is usually produced by a combination of factors: immobilization or decreased use of the diaphragm and the respiratory muscles, obstruction of the bronchial tree, and abolition of the cough reflex.

CLINICAL MANIFESTATIONS. The onset in postoperative cases usually occurs within 24 hr after operation but may not occur for several days, with dyspnea, cyanosis, and tachycardia. An affected child is extremely anxious and, if old enough, complains of chest pain. Prostration is likely. The temperature may be as high as 39.5–40°C (103–104°F).

The physical signs are characteristic. The chest appears flat on the affected side, where decreased respiratory excursion, dullness to percussion, and feeble or absent breath and voice sounds are also noted. Lower lobes are more frequently involved than upper ones. The heart and the mediastinum are displaced toward the affected side. Roentgenograms show the collapsed lung, elevation of the diaphragm, narrowing of the intercostal spaces, and displacement of the mediastinal structures and heart toward the affected side (Fig. 406–2).

PROGNOSIS. Bilateral massive collapse usually is rapidly fatal, although prompt bronchoscopic aspiration and mechanical ventilation may be lifesaving. In unilateral cases, the prognosis is usually good.

PREVENTION. Prophylaxis is of the greatest importance. The incidence of postoperative atelectasis can be reduced by adequate ventilation during anesthesia. After operation, the child's position in bed should be changed frequently and collections of secretions in the oropharynx should be aspirated; when consciousness returns, the child should be encouraged to breathe deeply. Incentive inspirometers may be useful. Tight thoracic or abdominal binders should be avoided.

TREATMENT. For bilateral atelectasis, bronchoscopic aspiration should be performed immediately. For only unilateral atelectasis, the child should be placed on the unaffected side; forced coughing or crying while the child is lying on the unaffected side may also be helpful, as is positive pressure ventilation, but when these measures are unsuccessful, bronchoscopic aspiration should be performed.

Relapses are not infrequent, and the child should be kept under constant observation.

Birnkrant DJ, Pope JF, Lewarski J, et al: Persistent pulmonary consolidation treated with intrapulmonary percussive ventilation: A preliminary report. Pediatr Pulmonol 21:246, 1996.

Stiller K, Geake T, Taylor J, et al: Acute lobar atelectasis: A comparison of two chest physiotherapy regimens. Chest 98:1336, 1990.

CHAPTER 407
Emphysema and Overinflation

David M. Orenstein

Pulmonary emphysema is distention of air spaces with irreversible disruption of the alveolar septa. It may be generalized or localized, involving part or all of a lung. Overinflation is distention with or without alveolar rupture. Overinflation is often reversible.

Compensatory overinflation may be acute or chronic and occurs in normally functioning pulmonary tissue when, for any reason, a sizable portion of the lung is removed or becomes partially or completely airless, which may occur with pneumonia, atelectasis, empyema, and pneumothorax.

Obstructive overinflation results from partial obstruction of a bronchus or bronchiole, when air leaving the alveoli becomes more difficult than air entry; there is a gradual accumulation of air distal to the obstruction, the so-called bypass, ball valve, or check valve type of obstruction (see Chapter 386).

LOCALIZED OBSTRUCTIVE OVERINFLATION. When a bypass type of obstruction partially occludes the main stem bronchus, the entire lung becomes overinflated; individual lobes are affected when the obstruction is in a lobar bronchus, and segments or subsegments are affected when their individual bronchi are blocked. Localized obstructions that may be responsible for overinflation include foreign bodies and the inflammatory reaction to them, abnormally thick mucus (e.g., asthma, cystic fibrosis), endobronchial tuberculosis or tuberculosis of the tracheobronchial lymph nodes, and endobronchial or mediastinal tumors. When most or all of a lobe is involved, the percussion note is hyperresonant over the area, and the breath sounds are decreased in intensity. The distended lung may extend across the mediastinum into the opposite hemithorax. Under fluoroscopic scrutiny during expiration, the overinflated area does not decrease in size, and the heart and the mediastinum shift to the opposite side because the unobstructed lung empties normally.

Unilateral hyperlucent lung may be associated with a variety of cardiac and pulmonary diseases of children, but in some patients, it occurs without easily demonstrable underlying active disease. More than one half the cases follow one or more episodes of pneumonia; a rising titer to adenovirus has been documented in several children. This condition may follow obliterative bronchiolitis and may include obliterative vasculitis as well, accounting for the greatly diminished perfusion and vascular marking on the affected side.

Patients may present with signs and symptoms of pneumonia, but some are discovered only when a chest roentgenogram is obtained for an unrelated reason. A few patients have hemoptysis. Physical findings may include hyperresonance and decreased breath sounds over the involved area. The chest roentgenogram reveals unilateral hyperlucency and a small lung with the mediastinum shifted toward the more abnormal lung. This condition has been labeled *Swyer-James* or *Macleod syndrome.* Some patients show a mediastinal shift away from the lesion with expiration. Bronchiectasis may be demonstrated by computed tomography or bronchography. In some patients, previous chest roentgenograms have been normal or have shown only an acute pneumonia, suggesting that a hyperlucent lung is an acquired lesion. No specific treatment is known; it may become less symptomatic with time.

Congenital lobar emphysema may result in severe respiratory distress in early infancy and may be caused by localized obstruction. Familial occurrence has been reported. Symptoms usually become apparent in the neonatal period but may be delayed for as long as 5–6 mo in 5% of patients. Some patients remain undiagnosed until school age or beyond. A part, but more often all, of a lobe may be involved; the left upper lobe is most often affected. In many cases, obstruction is not demonstrable, but it is assumed to be produced by a check valve type of mechanism.

Such obstructions have been attributed to defective or overly compliant cartilage in the bronchi, mucosal folds that create a valvelike obstruction, bronchial stenosis, and external compression by aberrant vessels or tumors. A radiolucent lobe and a mediastinal shift are often revealed by roentgenographic examination. If the distention is considerable, the emphysematous lung compresses the unaffected portion of lung below or above it and the opposite lung by extending across the mediastinum (Fig. 407–1). Immediate surgery and excision of the lobe may be lifesaving when cyanosis and severe respiratory distress are present, but some patients respond to medical treatment. Some children with apparent congenital lobar emphysema have reversible overinflation, without the classic alveolar septal rupture implied in the term *emphysema.*

Overinflation of all three lobes of the right lung has been produced by anomalous location of the left pulmonary artery, which impinges on the right main stem bronchus. Hyperinflation also occurs in patients with the absent pulmonary valve type of tetralogy of Fallot and secondary aneurysmal dilatation of the pulmonary artery, which partially compresses the main stem bronchi. A number of neonates have acquired lobar overinflation while being treated for hyaline membrane disease with assisted ventilation, suggesting an acquired cause. Medical management, sometimes with selective intubation of the unaffected bronchus or high-frequency ventilation, has occasionally been successful and lobectomy avoided.

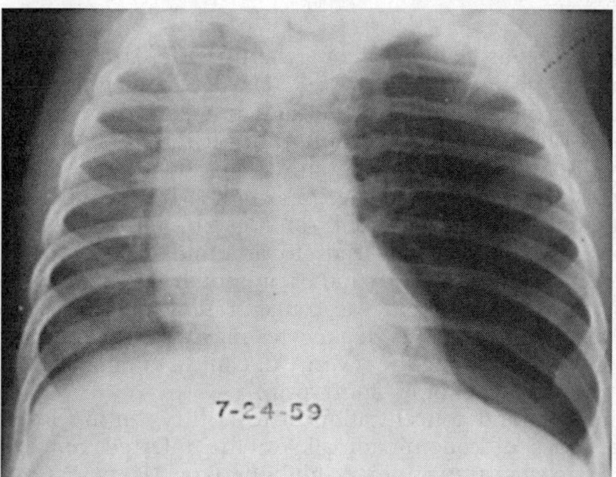

Figure 407–1 Congenital left upper lobe emphysema. Notice the extension of the emphysematous lobe into the left lower lobe and its displacement of the mediastinum toward the right.

Becroft DM: Bronchiolitis obliterans, bronchiectasis, and other sequelae of adenovirus type 21 infection in young children. J Clin Pathol 24:72, 1971.

Cumming GR, Macpherson RI, Chernick V: Unilateral hyperlucent lung syndrome in children. J Pediatr 78:250, 1971.

Dickman GL, Short BL, Krauss DR: Selective bronchial intubation in the management of unilateral pulmonary interstitial emphysema. Am J Dis Child 131:365, 1977.

Eigen H, Lemen RJ, Waring WW: Congenital lobar emphysema: Long-term evaluation of surgically and conservatively treated children. Am Rev Respir Dis 116:823, 1976.

McBride JT, Wohl MEB, Strieder D, et al: Lung growth and airway function after lobectomy in infancy for congenital lobar emphysema. J Clin Invest 66:962, 1980.

McKenzie SA, Allison DJ, Singh MP, et al: Unilateral hyperlucent lung: The case for investigation. Thorax 35:745, 1980.

Shannon DC, Todres ID, Moylan FMB: Infantile lobar hyperinflation: Expectant treatment. Pediatrics 59:1012, 1977.

Wall MA, Eisenberg JD, Campbell JR: Congenital lobar emphysema in a mother and daughter. Pediatrics 70:131, 1982.

407.1 Generalized Obstructive Overinflation

Acute overinflation of the lung depends on widespread involvement of the bronchioles and is reversible. It occurs more commonly in infants than in children and may be secondary to a number of clinical conditions, including asthma, cystic fibrosis, acute bronchiolitis, interstitial pneumonitis, atypical forms of acute laryngotracheobronchitis, aspiration of zinc stearate powder, chronic passive congestion secondary to a congenital cardiac lesion, and miliary tuberculosis.

PATHOLOGY. In chronic overinflation, many of the alveoli are ruptured and communicate with one another, producing distended saccules. Air may also enter the interstitial tissue (i.e., interstitial emphysema), resulting in pneumomediastinum and pneumothorax (see Chapters 419 and 420).

CLINICAL MANIFESTATIONS. Generalized obstructive overinflation is characterized by dyspnea, with difficulty in exhaling. The lungs become increasingly overdistended, and the chest remains expanded during expiration. An increased respiratory rate and decreased respiratory excursions result from the overdistention of the alveoli and their inability to be emptied normally through the narrowed bronchioles. Air hunger is responsible for forced respiratory movements. Overaction of the accessory muscles of respiration results in retractions at the suprasternal notch, the supraclavicular spaces, the lower margin of the thorax, and the intercostal spaces. There is scarcely any reduction in size of the overdistended chest during expiration, unlike the flattened chest during inspiration and expiration in cases of laryngeal obstruction. Hoarseness and stridor do not occur as they do with laryngeal obstruction. Cyanosis is common in the severe cases. The percussion note is hyperresonant, and on auscultation the inspiratory phase is usually less prominent than the expiratory phase, which is prolonged and roughened. Fine or medium crackles may be heard.

DIAGNOSIS. Roentgenographic and fluoroscopic examinations of the chest are a great help in establishing the diagnosis. Both leaves of the diaphragm are low and flattened, the ribs are farther apart than usual, and the lung fields are less dense (Fig. 407–2). The movement of the diaphragm is restricted;

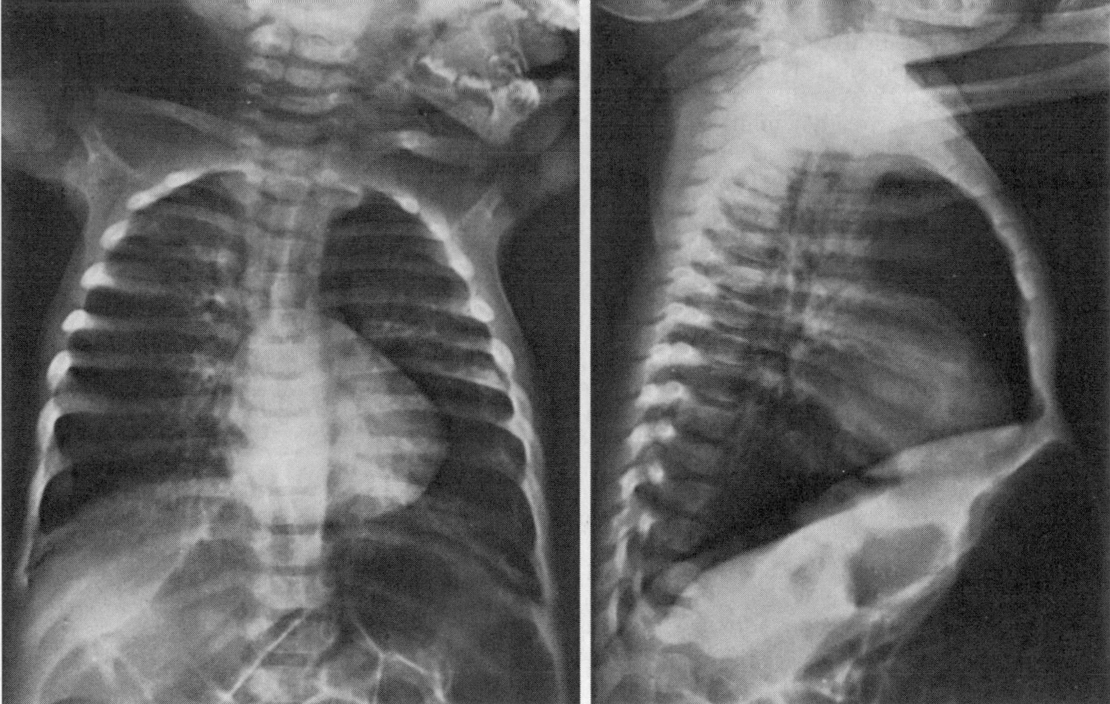

Figure 407–2 Generalized obstructive emphysema (overinflation): frontal and lateral projections of the thorax. Notice the flattened diaphragms, the sternal bowing, and the increased retrosternal airspace.

this is best demonstrated by fluoroscopic or ultrasonographic examination. The normal doming of the diaphragm during expiration is decreased, and the excursion of the low, flattened diaphragm in severe cases is barely discernible. The anteroposterior diameter of the chest is increased, and the sternum may be bowed outward.

407.2 Bullous Emphysema

Bullous emphysematous blebs or cysts (*pneumatoceles*) result from overdistention and rupture of alveoli during birth or shortly thereafter, or they may be sequelae of pneumonia and other infections. They have been observed in tuberculous lesions while the patient was being treated with specific antibacterial therapy. These emphysematous areas presumably result from rupture of distended alveoli, forming a single or multiloculated cavity. The cysts may become large and may contain some fluid; an air-fluid level may be demonstrated on the roentgenogram. They must be differentiated from pulmonary abscesses. In most cases, the cysts disappear spontaneously within a few months, although they may persist for a year or more. Aspiration or surgery is not indicated except in cases of severe respiratory and cardiac embarrassment.

407.3 Subcutaneous Emphysema

Whenever free air finds its way into the subcutaneous tissue, most commonly as a result of pneumomediastinum or pneumothorax, subcutaneous emphysema occurs. It may be a complication of fracture of the orbit permitting free air to escape from the nasal sinuses. In the neck and thorax, subcutaneous emphysema may follow tracheotomy, deep ulcerations in the pharyngeal region, esophageal wounds, or any perforating lesion of the larynx or trachea. It is occasionally a complication of thoracentesis, asthma, or abdominal surgery. Air rarely may be formed in the subcutaneous tissues by gas-producing bacteria.

If the cause is an air leak from the respiratory system, the problem is usually self-limited and, although it can be uncomfortable, requires no specific treatment. Resolution occurs by resorption of subcutaneous air after elimination of its source. Rarely, dangerous compression of the trachea by air in the surrounding soft tissue requires surgical intervention.

Kress MB, Finklestein AH: Giant bullous emphysema occurring in tuberculosis in childhood. Pediatrics 30:269, 1962.

Nelson WE, Smith LW: Generalized obstructive emphysema in infants. J Pediatr 26:36, 1945.

Victoria MS, Steiner P, Rao M: Persistent pneumatoceles in children. Chest 79:359, 1981.

407.4 α_1-Antitrypsin Deficiency and Emphysema

Homozygous deficiency of α_1-antitrypsin is an important cause of the early onset of severe panacinar emphysema in adults in the 3rd and 4th decades of life and an important cause of liver disease in children, but it rarely causes pulmonary disease in children. α_1-Antitrypsin and other serum antiproteases are thought to be important in the inactivation of proteolytic enzymes released from dead bacteria or leukocytes in the lung. Deficiency leads to accumulation of these enzymes, proteolytic destruction of pulmonary tissue, and development of emphysema. The concentration of proteases (e.g., elastase) in the patients' leukocytes may also be an important factor in determining the severity of clinical pulmonary disease with a given level of α_1-antitrypsin.

The type and concentration of α_1-antitrypsin are inherited as a series of codominant alleles; the inferred genotype is referred to as the protease inhibitor type (Pi type). Normal persons are classified as Pi type MM. Types null/null and ZZ and, to a lesser extent, other abnormal Pi types, such as SZ, have been associated with early adult-onset emphysema. Some

Pi types are associated with a characteristic form of infantile cirrhosis (see Chapter 357.6), which is considerably more common than childhood-onset pulmonary disease.

Most patients who have the Pi-type ZZ defect have little or no detectable pulmonary disease during childhood. A few have very early onset of chronic pulmonary symptoms, including dyspnea, wheezing, and cough, and panacinar emphysema has been documented by lung biopsy results. Smoking greatly increases the risk of emphysema developing in most Pi types.

Physical examination may reveal growth failure, an increased anteroposterior diameter of the chest with a hyperresonant percussion note, crackles if there is active infection, and clubbing. Severe emphysema may depress the diaphragm, making the liver and spleen more easily palpable. Chest roentgenograms reveal overinflation with depressed diaphragms. Serum has a low trypsin inhibitory capacity, and immunoassay confirms the low level of α_1-antitrypsin.

Danazol, an analog of testosterone, increases hepatic α_1-antitrypsin synthesis, but masculinizing effects make this drug unacceptable for women, and the overall toxicity prevents long-term administration in men. Enzyme replacement appears to be a more promising approach to treatment. α_1-Antitrypsin can be readily purified from pooled human blood and, because it is relatively heat-resistant, inactivation of hepatitis and other viruses is easily accomplished. Intravenous administration raises the blood antiprotease level into an acceptable range and results in the appearance of the transfused antiprotease in pulmonary lavage fluid. Severe toxicity has not been reported. The Food and Drug Administration has approved the use of purified blood-derived human enzyme for ZZ and null/null patients. Pure α_1-antitrypsin, produced by recombinant DNA technology, is also available. The aerosolized form appears to be effective, but it is extremely expensive ($20,000–$30,000/yr), and controversy continues over its clinical use. The possibility of more direct therapy with gene insertion has also been suggested.

Nonspecific therapy includes aggressive treatment of pulmonary infection, routine use of pneumococcal and influenza vaccines, bronchodilators, and advice about the risks of smoking.

Treatment is also indicated for other members of the family found to have Pi ZZ phenotypes or null/null, even if they are asymptomatic. Persons with the MZ Pi type do not have an increased risk for the development of pulmonary disease. The clinical significance of the SZ Pi type is unknown, but nonspecific treatment seems reasonable. All persons with low levels of serum antiprotease should be warned that the eventual development of emphysema is partially related to environmental factors, including exposure to industrial fumes and particularly cigarette smoking.

Ad Hoc Committee on Alpha 1-Antitrypsin Replacement Therapy of the Standards Committee, Canadian Thoracic Society: Current status of alpha-1-antitrypsin replacement therapy: Recommendations for the management of patients with severe hereditary deficiency. Can Med Assoc J 146:841, 1992.

Cox DW, Levison H: Emphysema of early onset associated with a complete deficiency of alpha-1-antitrypsin (null homozygotes). Am Rev Respir Dis 137:371, 1988.

Gadek JE, Crystal RG: Experience with replacement therapy in the destructive lung disease associated with severe alpha-1-antitrypsin deficiency. Am Rev Respir Dis 127(Pt 2):545, 1983.

Hubbard RC, Crystal RG: Strategies for aerosol therapy of alpha 1-antitrypsin deficiency by the aerosol route. Lung 168(Suppl):565, 1990.

Setoguchi Y, Jaffe HA, Chu CS, Crystal RG: Intraperitoneal in vivo gene therapy to deliver alpha 1-antitrypsin to the systemic circulation. Am J Respir Cell Mol Biol 10:369, 1994.

Sveger T: Prospective study of children with α_1-antitrypsin deficiency: Eight-year-old follow-up. J Pediatr 104:91, 1984.

Talamo RC, Levison H, Lynch MJ, et al: Symptomatic pulmonary emphysema in childhood associated with hereditary α_1-antitrypsin and elastase inhibitor deficiency. J Pediatr 79:20, 1971.

CHAPTER 408
Pulmonary Edema

David M. Orenstein

ETIOLOGY. Pulmonary edema results from the transudation of fluid from the pulmonary capillaries into the alveolar spaces and the bronchioles. It is usually associated with circulatory or neurocirculatory collapse and is often a terminal event in a variety of diseases. Although pulmonary edema may vary in severity, it is an ominous finding even in its mildest stages. It is a common manifestation of left ventricular failure, with the edema resulting from a rise in pulmonary venous pressure, or it may be caused by hypervolemia from intravenous infusion that is either too rapid or too large. It may also be a manifestation of acute or chronic nephritis or, rarely, of upper airway obstruction or pneumonic and other infections with substantial degrees of toxicity. Poisoning by substances such as barbiturates, morphine, epinephrine, and alcohol may be responsible for the development of pulmonary edema, as may the inhalation of toxic gases, such as illuminating gas, ammonia, and nitrogen dioxide, or the ingestion and consequent aspiration of highly volatile hydrocarbons, such as lighter fluid (see Chapter 393.2).

CLINICAL MANIFESTATIONS. The onset is variable, but it is rapid in most cases. The child often complains of difficulty in breathing or a sense of oppression or pain in the chest. Cough is common and often produces a frothy, pink-tinged sputum. There is tachypnea, and the pulse is rapid and weak. The child is usually pale and may be cyanotic. On physical examination, dullness to percussion and moist, bubbly crackles are heard in the lower portions of the chest. There may be wheezing due to peribronchiolar edema early in the course. Chest roentgenograms may show a diffuse perihilar infiltrate (butterfly distribution). Engorged lymphatics in intralobular septa, demonstrated as peripheral and horizontal lines (Kerley B), may be evident. Occasionally, one lung is affected more than the other. If the pulmonary edema is superimposed on another pulmonary process (e.g., pneumococcal pneumonia, left-sided heart failure, cystic fibrosis), the clinical and roentgenographic findings of the primary illness may obscure those of the pulmonary edema.

TREATMENT. Treatment is directed at the primary disease causing the pulmonary edema. Administering oxygen relieves some of the dyspnea and chest pain; when possible, it is best accomplished by intermittent positive pressure. Dyspnea can often be relieved by morphine sulfate (0.1 mg/kg). If pulmonary edema is secondary to excessive parenteral administration of fluids or blood or to heart failure; administration of diuretics such as furosemide (1 mg/kg), digitalis, or bronchodilators; rarely, the application of tourniquets or inflated blood pressure cuffs to the extremities or the withdrawal of blood may be lifesaving.

408.1 High-Altitude Pulmonary Edema

High-altitude pulmonary edema (HAPE) occurs at altitudes above 2,700 m (8,860 ft). Patients with an absent or hypoplastic right pulmonary artery appear particularly vulnerable. The pathogenesis is not fully understood; studies have shown large amounts of high molecular weight proteins, erythrocytes, and leukocytes in bronchoalveolar lavage fluid from mountain climbers with HAPE, suggesting that there is a "large-pore" leak. Total protein concentrations in lung fluid are the same as serum concentrations, also suggesting increased pulmonary capillary permeability. The extreme neutrophil invasion characteristic of other acute pulmonary injuries is not present. Microhemorrhages may also play a role.

The altitude achieved and the rapidity of ascent affect the incidence of HAPE. Cough, shortness of breath, restlessness, vomiting, headache, and chest pain are the most common symptoms and occur within hours of high-altitude exposure. Not all persons are affected, and even affected persons may not have symptoms with every exposure. Children have an incidence of HAPE two to three times that of adults. Chest roentgenography reveals bilateral, patchy pulmonary infiltrates.

Administration of oxygen and a return to lower altitudes are indicated. Bed rest, diuretics, antibiotics, and corticosteroids have been used, but their efficacy has not been established. Recovery usually occurs within 48 hr, and further residence at a high altitude usually is tolerated without symptoms, but the disease may recur after returning to a high altitude after even a brief visit to lower levels. HAPE may be prevented by the administration of the calcium channel blocker nifedipine prior to ascent.

Bartsch P, Maggiorini M, Ritter, et al: Prevention of high-altitude pulmonary edema by nifedipine. N Engl J Med 325:1284, 1991.
Kurland G: Adaptation to high altitude. *In:* Hilman BC (ed): Pediatric Respiratory Disease: Diagnosis and Treatment. Philadelphia, WB Saunders, 1993, p 406.
Rios B, Driscoll DJ, McNamara DG: High-altitude pulmonary edema with absent right pulmonary artery. Pediatrics 75:314, 1985.
Schoene RB, Hackett PH, Henderson WR, et al: High-altitude pulmonary edema: Characteristics of lung lavage fluid. JAMA 256:63, 1986.
Spring CL, Rackow EC, Fein IA, et al: The spectrum of pulmonary edema; differentiation of cardiogenic, intermediate, and no cardiogenic forms of pulmonary edema. Am Rev Respir Dis 124:716, 1981.
Yarrow M, Waldman N, Niermeyer S, et al: The diagnosis of acute mountain sickness in preverbal children. Arch Pediatr Adolesc Med 152:683, 1998.

CHAPTER 409
Pulmonary Embolism and Infarction

Robert C. Stern

Pulmonary embolism is uncommon in infants and children. However, in one series, pulmonary emboli were found in 3.7% of children at autopsy and had contributed to death in about 1%. Although they often arise from thrombi in the femoral and pelvic veins (often in postoperative patients), emboli in children and adolescents can also arise from abdominal and head veins. Scoliosis surgery, in particular, may predispose to deep vein thrombosis and pulmonary embolization. Emboli are not uncommon after spinal cord injury, severe burns, or prolonged inactivity or as a complication of intravenous infusions. Pulmonary embolism may be common in sick neonates. The most frequent underlying cause is a medical device, such as an intravenous line, arteriovenous fistula, or other implanted device; however, emboli also occur in newborns with congenital heart disease and in infants of diabetic mothers. The original source of the embolus may be an infarcted placenta or a thrombus in the umbilical vein, perhaps dislodged by the insertion of a catheter. Asphyxia and subsequent respiratory distress may also predispose to pulmonary embolization in neonates. Fortunately, pulmonary hypoxic injury often does not occur after pulmonary artery embolism because the lung normally has two arterial sources for oxygen (pulmonary and bronchial arteries) and may derive some oxygen from retrograde flow from the pulmonary veins.

In adolescents, recent abortion, drug abuse, hypercoagulation disorders (deficiency of protein C or S, antithrombin III; presence of lupus anticoagulant; factor V Leiden; see Chapter 484), or oral contraceptives may be the predisposing problem. As indwelling central venous catheters for home treatment of malignancies and infection have become more common, the incidence of associated embolization, including air and clotted blood, has increased. Urokinase, a thrombolytic drug frequently used to clear these lines, may rarely have a role in embolization if the clots are not totally lysed before the line is flushed.

Intrapulmonary thrombosis may also occur in sickle cell anemia; the subsequent infarction is often difficult to differentiate from pneumonia. Fat emboli are most likely to be derived from fractured bones; they also arise from necrotic tissue in the bone marrow of patients with sickle cell disease. Numerous pulmonary infarcts resulting from small emboli may be associated with severe dehydration in diarrheal disease, cyanotic heart disease, bacterial endocarditis, ventriculoatrial shunts for the treatment of hydrocephalus, and long-standing nutritional deficiencies.

Pulmonary thomboembolism occasionally is responsible for sudden and unexpected death of pediatric patients with various chronic diseases. In one series, a source of the embolus was a central venous catheter. Other patients with chronic heart disease were found to have an intracardiac thrombus at autopsy.

CLINICAL MANIFESTATIONS AND DIAGNOSIS. Embolism of the pulmonary artery or its larger branches produces a variable clinical picture. The clinical pattern often suggests pneumonia, and the diagnosis may not be made until autopsy. Dyspnea is common, although often transient; pain and collapse are often absent. If present, pain is usually substernal, but it may be pleural and may radiate to the shoulder. Tachypnea is the most consistent physical finding. Although there are often no physical signs, if the infarct is sufficiently large, resonance may be impaired and a pleural friction rub may be detected. Breath sounds may be distant or absent, and moist rales may be heard. Expectorated material, which may be profuse, often contains blood. Large emboli can cause acute right-sided heart failure by raising pulmonary arterial pressure. However, infarction often does not occur, and the classic infarction triad of pleuritic chest pain, hemoptysis, and infiltrate is usually absent in patients with pulmonary emboli. The case fatality rate is high, but recovery may occur even when the area of infarction is relatively large. Secondary infection may result in abscess formation. Emboli carrying bacteria (e.g., right-sided endocarditis) may also be responsible for numerous pulmonary abscesses.

Chest roentgenograms, although useful in ruling out other treatable causes of a patient's symptoms (e.g., pneumothorax), often appear normal and rarely are diagnostic. Pulmonary angiography is the gold standard diagnostic test for pulmonary embolism and is usually reasonably safe in patients who do not have pulmonary hypertension and right ventricular end-diastolic pressure greater than 20 mm Hg. Helical CT scanning is emerging as a safe alternative and is very accurate. In critically ill patients in whom definitive diagnosis is urgent, pulmonary perfusion studies, ventilation scintiphotography, and pulmonary angiogram should be considered; only angiography gives unequivocal evidence of embolism, but its risk must be weighed against the risk of therapy. In addition to the classic physical findings of thrombophlebitis, impedance plethysmography can provide definitive, noninvasive demonstration of lower extremity deep vein thrombosis and assessment of its extent. Radiolabeled fibrinogen, Doppler ultrasonography, and contrast venography are also used. Other laboratory findings that may be diagnostically helpful are the presence of D-dimers. D-Dimers are found in 89% of patients with confirmed embolism, but they are also found in patients with many other entities. Therefore, the absence of D-dimers may be helpful in ruling out embolism. In children who are not gravely ill, empirical low-dose heparin therapy when scans are highly probable for pulmonary embolism may be preferable to angiography.

Exchange transfusion should precede arteriography in patients with sickle cell anemia; otherwise, massive, potentially fatal pulmonary thrombosis may occur.

Chronic showers of emboli from ventriculoatrial shunts may cause gradual obliteration of the pulmonary vascular bed and eventually produce pulmonary hypertension. The clinical findings are those of pulmonary hypertension and may include accentuation of the pulmonic component of the second heart sound and the development of pulmonary or tricuspid insufficiency. In severe cases, exercise intolerance and right-sided heart failure occur, indicating that substantial compromise of lung function has already taken place. Serial electrocardiograms that show increasing right ventricular hypertrophy may give an early clue to continuing chronic embolization. Diagnosis may be confirmed by right-sided heart catheterization and determination of pulmonary arterial blood pressure. If chronic embolization is suspected, the shunts should be removed.

The diagnosis of pulmonary embolism is often missed in children, especially if the source of the emboli is not a lower extremity. Pediatricians often wrongly think that embolism is almost exclusively an adult disease. Furthermore, children often have serious underlying diseases whose symptoms and physical findings dominate a patient's course even after embolization has occurred.

TREATMENT. Massive embolization of the larger branches of the pulmonary artery is a medical emergency. The initial treatment objective is cardiovascular support and prevention of circulatory collapse and pulmonary insufficiency by cardiotonic drugs, oxygen, and mechanical ventilation. Surgical removal of pulmonary emboli is unlikely to be successful and should be considered a desperation measure. However, if initial treatment, including heparinization, is unsuccessful and the source of the emboli is a lower extremity, a surgical attempt to prevent their access to the inferior vena cava may be worthwhile.

After stabilization and definitive diagnosis, efforts should be made to prevent further embolization. Intravenous heparin (loading dose: 50–75 units/kg; maintenance dose: 18 units/kg/hr) should be given by continuous infusion; the dose should be adjusted to maintain the clotting time at about twice the control value (or the APTT at 1.5 times the control). After 7–10 days of intravenous heparin, 3–6 mo of oral coumarin therapy usually is indicated, unless the source of the emboli has been definitively eliminated. Low molecular weight heparin may be more effective and safer than standard unfractionated heparin. In some patients, it may be prudent to reinstitute coumarin if the situation that led to the original embolus recurs (e.g., surgery, trauma, obesity). Initiation and maintenance of heparin treatment is difficult and potentially dangerous. If the hospital has a rigid algorithm for heparin treatment in adults, pediatricians and house officers may want to consult it when faced with an older child or teenager with probable deep vein thrombosis and pulmonary embolism.

Thrombolytic treatment (various agents including urokinase, streptokinase, anisoylated streptokinase–plasminogen activator complex, and recombinant tissue plasminogen activator) may add therapeutic benefit to heparinization, but this may prove to be economically feasible/justifiable only in patients with massive embolism. This therapy is contraindicated in patients with recent bleeding (e.g., intracranial or gastrointestinal) or trauma. The use of this therapy in pulmonary embolism is an area of intense investigation.

PROGNOSIS. Prognosis depends largely on the severity of the obstruction. In previously normal patients, pulmonary hypertension occurs at about 60% occlusion, and death is likely with 85% occlusion. Hypercapnia is an ominous finding.

Arnold J, O'Brodovich H, Whyte R, et al: Pulmonary thromboembolic after neonatal asphyxia. J Pediatr 106:806, 1985.

Bernstein D, Coupey S, Schonberg SK: Pulmonary embolism in adolescence. Am J Dis Child 140:667, 1986.

Byard RW, Cutz E: Sudden and unexpected death in infancy and childhood due to pulmonary thromboembolism. Arch Pathol Lab Med 114:142, 1990.

David M, Andrew M: Venous thromboembolic complications in children. J Pediatr 123:337, 1993.

Evans DA, Wilmott RW: Pulmonary embolism in children. Pediatr Clin North Am 41:569, 1994.

Leizorovicz A, Simonneau G, Decousus H, et al: Comparison of efficacy and safety of low molecular weight heparins and unfractionated heparin in initial treatment of deep venous thrombosis: A meta-analysis. Br Med J 309:299, 1994.

Uden A; Thromboembolic complications following scoliosis surgery in Scandinavia. Acta Orthrop Scand 50:175, 1979.

409.1 Hemoptysis

Hemoptysis, the sudden coughing or expectoration of blood or blood-tinged sputum, is a frightening secondary symptom that may result from many possible primary disorders (Table 409–1). The cause can be determined by historical data, physical examination findings, and specific laboratory tests, including a chest roentgenogram and possibly bronchoscopy, depending on the potential primary causes. Hemoptysis must be differentiated from epistaxis (e.g., blood in nares, dripping in the posterior nasopharynx) and hematemesis (e.g., nausea, emesis, abdominal pain, and tenderness). Patients with he-

TABLE 409–1 Differential Diagnosis of Hemoptysis

Primary Disorder	Differential Diagnoses
Infection	Lung abscess
	Pneumonia*
	Tuberculosis
	Bronchiectasis* (cystic fibrosis,* ciliary dyskinesia)
	Necrotizing pneumonia
	Fungus (especially allergic bronchopulmonary aspergillosis or mucormycosis)
	Parasite
	Herpes simplex
Foreign body	Retained object
Congenital defect	Heart defects
	Eisenmenger syndrome
	Abnormal arteriovenous connections
	Arteriovenous malformation
	Telangiectasia (Osler-Weber-Rendu)
	Pulmonary sequestration
	Bronchogenic cyst
Inflammatory autoimmunity	Henoch-Schönlein purpura
	Goodpasture syndrome
	Wegener granulomatosis
	Systemic lupus erythematosus
	Sarcoidosis
Pulmonary hemosiderosis	Idiopathic
	Infections
	With milk allergy (Heiner syndrome)
Trauma	Contusion*
	Fracture trachea, bronchus
	Gunshot wound
Iatrogenic problem	Postsurgical
	Post-transbronchial lung biopsy*
	Post-diagnostic lung puncture*
Tumors	Benign tumor (e.g., neurogenic, hamartoma, hemangioma, carcinoid)
	Malignant tumor (e.g., adenoma, bronchogenic carcinoma)
Pulmonary embolus	
Other	Factitious
	Endometriosis
	Coagulopathy*
	Heart failure
	Postsurfactant therapy in neonates
	Kernicterus
	Hyperammonemia
	Intracranial hemorrhage
	Epistaxis*

**Common cause of hemoptysis.*

moptysis often present with cough, gurgling sounds in the lung, crackles, and signs of the underlying primary disease. Other features that help differentiate hemoptysis from hematemesis include color (bright red/frothy vs dark red/brown), pH (alkaline vs acid), associate material (sputum vs food remnants), and associated symptoms (coughing vs nausea). However, none of these is diagnostic. In addition, patients with hemoptysis have characteristic historical and physical findings (e.g., previous diagnosis of chronic pulmonary disease, chronic cough and sputum production, clubbing).

Treatment includes maintaining a patent airway, providing oxygen, correcting coagulation disorders, bronchoscopy, and arteriographic embolization of the bleeding vessel. Bleeding severity and duration may be greatly affected by body position, and patients often know the optimal position from experience. Massive hemoptysis can be slowed or stopped by intratracheal epinephrine or intravenous pitressin, and this can be lifesaving. However, pitressin is a temporizing measure, and these patients almost always require additional treatment (e.g., bronchial artery embolization).

Fabian MC, Smitheringale A: Hemoptysis in children: the Hospital for Sick Children experience. J Otolaryngol 25:44, 1996.
Jones D, Davies R: Massive hemoptysis. Br Med J 300:889, 1990.
Panitch H, Schidlow D: Pathogenesis and management of hemoptysis in children. Int Pediatr 4:241, 1989.
Pianosi P, Al-sadoon H: Hemoptysis in children. Pediatr Rev 17:344, 1996.

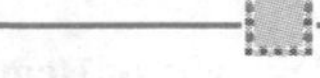

CHAPTER 410
Bronchiectasis

Robert C. Stern

Bronchiectasis is characterized by permanent dilatation of the subsegmental airways associated with inflammatory destruction of bronchial and peribronchial tissue, accumulation of exudative material in dependent bronchi, and in some cases, distention of dependent bronchi.

ETIOLOGY. Some patients may have *congenital bronchiectasis* (including Williams-Campbell syndrome), possibly caused by an arrest in bronchial development leading to cyst formation and destruction of the bronchial wall when the cysts become infected. Alternatively, development of the bronchial cartilaginous supports may be defective. Tracheobronchomegaly is a rare congenital condition in which the distal trachea and main bronchi are grossly dilated; a similar condition may be associated with recurrent pneumonia.

Most cases of bronchiectasis are acquired after birth, usually resulting from chronic pulmonary infection, but the mechanisms involved are poorly understood. Obstruction of the bronchial tree followed by infection is one likely cause. Measles, pertussis, and pneumonia are rare causes of bronchiectasis. Cystic fibrosis is the most common underlying disease in children with generalized bronchial involvement. HIV disease is another important cause of childhood bronchiectasis. Other predisposing factors include aspiration of a foreign body, often a nonopaque one, enlarged bronchopulmonary nodes owing to tuberculosis, recurrent and chronic lung infections, sarcoidosis, neoplasm, lung abscess, localized cysts, emphysema with compression of the other lung, allergy (including allergic bronchopulmonary aspergillosis), and asthma. Patients with immunodeficiency syndromes, especially panhypogammaglobulinemia, may have bronchiectasis, usually after repeated attacks of bacterial pneumonia and bronchitis. Recurrent aspiration pneumonitis in familial dysautonomia can lead to bronchiectasis. Primary ciliary dyskinesis (see Chapter 417) results in chronic pulmonary infection, which eventually leads to bronchiectasis. Gastroesophageal reflux with chronic aspiration may be a cause of bronchiectasis. Patients with congenital heart disease may develop bronchiectasis secondary to infection related to compression of an airway by an abnormally positioned or very large blood vessel, including those used in shunting procedures.

Reversible bronchiectasis or pseudobronchiectasis occurs commonly after pertussis. Shortly after or during these illnesses, the bronchi may appear cylindrically dilated on bronchography, but if these studies are repeated months later, the changes will have disappeared.

PATHOLOGY. The first destructive change is a loss of ciliated epithelium, which is regenerated as cuboidal and squamous epithelium. Concurrently, the elastic tissue within the bronchial walls disappears and thickening occurs because of interstitial edema, fibrosis, and round cell infiltration. In adjacent parenchymal and peribronchial tissue, multiple abscesses may develop, and obstructive endarteritis of the small pulmonary vessels is usually characteristic. Generally, bronchiectasis follows a segmental distribution, except in cystic fibrosis. The right middle lobe segments, the basal segments of the lower lobes, and the lingular segments of the left upper lobe are most frequently affected. The right lower lobe is commonly involved in aspiration of a foreign body, and the right middle lobe is most frequently affected by hilar lymphadenopathy.

CLINICAL MANIFESTATIONS. In symptomatic cases, cough is invariably present and produces copious mucopurulent sputum during acute respiratory infections. The sputum usually is swallowed by young children. Physical activity or change in position, particularly while reclining, often initiates a bout of coughing.

Recurrent infections of the lower respiratory tract are common; they tend to persist and are difficult to control. Anorexia, irritability, and poor weight gain are also common. Fever is much less common. Later in the course, during acute exacerbations, hemoptysis may occur, varying in severity from blood-streaked sputum to exsanguinating hemorrhage. Bronchiectasis characteristically follows an intermittently improving and relapsing course.

Physical findings are absent or few. Clubbing of the fingers may affect patients with symptoms persisting for more than 1 yr. Moist or musical rales may be heard or elicited by cough; during acute exacerbations, physical signs of atelectasis or diffuse pneumonitis are often present. Extensive bronchiectasis is attended by persistent dyspnea and retarded physical development.

DIAGNOSIS. Although there are no pathognomonic findings for bronchiectasis on standard chest radiographs, marked linear streaking ("railroad tracks") with loss of volume ("crowding") is highly suggestive. Bronchography, the previous gold standard for diagnosing bronchiectasis, has been largely replaced by CT. This imaging technique is not quite as sensitive as bronchography but is considerably safer and can be done sequentially to follow the patient's course. Thin-section high-resolution CT may be needed. A CT scan after inhalation of xenon may prove even more sensitive. Ventilatory and diffusion studies may reveal more widespread or severe pulmonary involvement than suspected otherwise.

DIFFERENTIAL DIAGNOSIS. Every patient with suspected or proven bronchiectasis should be evaluated for sinusitis, ciliary dyskinesis, immune deficiency diseases, tuberculosis, asthma or other respiratory allergy, and cystic fibrosis. If such a diagnosis cannot be made, these patients should have bronchoscopy to exclude bronchial stenosis, strictures, tumors, and foreign bodies, and they should possibly have bronchography to document the bronchiectasis and determine its extent and severity. A familial deficiency of bronchial cartilage has been proposed as an explanation of some cases of bronchiectasis in childhood and may be suggested by marked dilatation of the 2nd–4th-order bronchi during inspiration and apparent collapse during expiration. Bronchoscopic washings and sputum samples should be cultured for routine pathogens, mycobacteria, and fungi, and a tuberculin skin test should be done.

The *right middle lobe syndrome* consists of subacute or chronic pneumonitis, bronchial obstruction, and atelectasis, and it is generally caused by extrinsic compression of the middle lobe bronchus by hilar nodes, followed by peribronchitis and chronic infection. Bronchiectasis may result. On occasion, this syndrome is related to asthma or congenital anomalies of the bronchi.

Young's syndrome is characterized by sinusitis and bronchiectasis, often symptomatic in childhood, and by azoospermia, not detectable until later, when semen analysis can be done. Clubbing is rarely seen. Some patients develop azoospermia after a period of fertility. Urologic procedures to re-establish fertility later have been disappointing. The severity of pulmonary symptoms seems to ameliorate during adolescence or young adult life. Cystic fibrosis should be considered and tested for by DNA analysis because the sweat test may be negative.

Yellow nail syndrome consists of pleural effusion and lymphedema, associated with discolored nails. Bronchiectasis occurred in 5 of 12 patients in one report.

TREATMENT. Therapy includes elimination of all foci of respiratory infection, effective mucus clearance (e.g., postural drainage), and when indicated, antibiotic therapy. Postural drainage must be carried out intensively as long as secretions are being formed and is one of the most important aspects of management.

Systemic antibiotic therapy should be administered during acute exacerbations in courses of 2–3 wk. Patients with cystic fibrosis often require more prolonged therapy (see Chapter 416). Prolonged treatment for most other patients increases the risks of acquiring resistant flora and of drug reactions. The appropriate drug is selected on the basis of the antibiotic susceptibility of bacteria isolated from sputum or at bronchoscopy. If no potential pulmonary pathogens are recovered, antibiotics should not be used. Administering antibiotics by aerosol inhalation immediately after appropriate mucus clearance may also be helpful but should not be continued for excessively long periods, because this encourages the establishment of a drug-resistant bacterial flora. *Pseudomonas* can be particularly troublesome. Patients with proven bronchiectasis should be given influenza vaccine every year.

When localized severe disease progresses despite adequate medical management, segmental or lobar resection should be considered, even though the long-term results are often discouraging. Some patients with lobar bronchiectasis, especially those with the right middle lobe syndrome, do very well after lobectomy. Surgery may also be indicated when an intrinsic anatomic obstruction of the bronchus is found or when suppurative lesions result from aspiration of fragmented foreign bodies, especially such vegetal objects as grass fibers or fragments of peanut that elude bronchoscopic removal.

Barker AF, Bardana EJ Jr: Bronchiectasis: Update of an orphan disease. Am Rev Respir Dis 137:969, 1988.
Davis PB, Hubbard VS, McCoy K, et al: Familial bronchiectasis. J Pediatr 102:177, 1983.
Dees SC, Spock A: Right middle lobe syndrome in children. JAMA 197:8, 1966.
Handelsman DJ, Conway AJ, Boylan LM, et al: Young's syndrome: Obstructive azoospermia and chronic sinopulmonary infections. N Engl J Med 310:3, 1984.
Kornreich L, Horev G, Ziv N, Grunebaum M: Bronchiectasis in children: Assessment by CT. Pediatr Radiol 23:120, 1993.
Mitchell RE, Bury RG: Congenital bronchiectasis due to deficiency of bronchial cartilage (Williams-Campbell syndrome): Case report. J Pediatr 87:230, 1975.

Chapter 411
Pulmonary Abscess

Robert C. Stern

A lung abscess is a suppurative process resulting in destruction of the pulmonary parenchyma and formation of a cavity containing purulent material. In children, they most often result from *aspiration of infected material* when the local defense mechanisms are overwhelmed by a large number of virulent microorganisms or are compromised by factors such as alcohol, drug abuse, recent surgery (particularly tonsillectomy or adenoidectomy), or systemic disease. Aspirated material containing bacteria that are normal inhabitants of the nasopharynx and oropharynx reaches the most dependent portions of the lung. The posterior segments of the upper lobes and the superior segments of the lower lobes are most frequently involved when aspiration occurs in the recumbent position, and anaerobic bacteria, including *Bacteroides, Fusobacterium,* and anaerobic streptococci, are commonly isolated. The basilar segments of the lower lobes are the most likely to be affected when aspiration occurs in the erect position (e.g., during dental procedures). *Pneumonia* caused by aerobic pyogenic microorganisms (*Staphylococcus aureus* and *Klebsiella*) or *bronchial obstruction* due to a tumor or foreign body may occasionally be complicated by abscess formation. *Metastatic lung abscess* secondary to bacteremia or to septic emboli from right-sided bacterial endocarditis and septic thrombophlebitis is uncommon in children. Rare causes also include amebic abscess of the lung and infections with *Nocardia, Actinomyces,* and mycobacteria.

PATHOLOGY. Lung abscesses occur when pulmonary parenchyma becomes obstructed, infected, and then suppurative and necrotic. Initial inflammatory changes are followed by suppuration and thrombosis of the local blood vessels, which result in necrosis and liquefaction. Granulation tissue forms around the periphery of the abscess and may succeed in walling off the area, but more commonly, the abscess ruptures into a bronchus. Contents of the abscess may then be coughed up or aspirated into other parts of the pulmonary tree, causing additional abscess formation. Sputum is usually fetid. Peripheral abscesses may involve the adjacent pleura, with development of an associated pleural effusion. Abscesses may rupture into the pleural cavity and produce empyema.

CLINICAL MANIFESTATIONS. The onset is generally insidious, with fever, malaise, anorexia, and weight loss. Cough, often associated with hemoptysis and producing copious amounts of foul-smelling or purulent sputum, is characteristic about 10 days after the onset in untreated patients. Lung abscess secondary to staphylococcal and *Klebsiella* pneumonia produces the acute signs and symptoms described for bacterial pneumonia. There may be respiratory distress, spiking fevers, chest pain, and marked leukocytosis.

The *diagnosis* is generally made by roentgenographic examination when a cavity with or without a fluid level surrounded by alveolar infiltration is demonstrated (Fig. 411–1). Gram stain of the sputum may reveal numerous polymorphonuclear leukocytes and findings consistent with anaerobic microorganisms, such as pleomorphic, slender, gram-negative bacilli (*Bacteroides, Fusobacterium*); gram-negative rods with tapered ends (*Fusobacterium*); large gram-positive bacilli (*Clostridium*); and tiny to small cocci (anaerobic streptococci). Sputum cultures characteristically yield a mixture of anaerobic bacteria. If the abscess is adjacent to the chest wall, particularly if the pathogen is unknown, percutaneous drainage guided by ultrasonog-

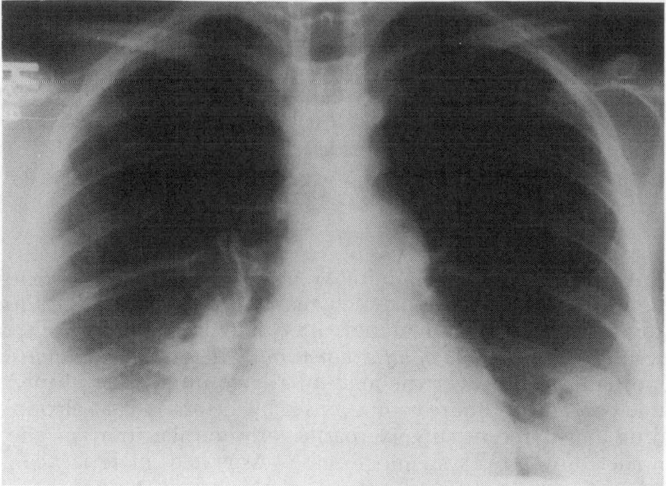

Figure 411–1 Bilateral lower lobe abscesses in an adolescent with *Fusobacterium* sepsis. A cavity with surrounding infiltrate is visible in the left lower lobe.

raphy or CT can be done as a primary diagnostic procedure. This procedure may also be indicated for patients who are not responding to empirical antibiotic treatment.

TREATMENT. If a predominant aerobic organism is identified, optimally from blood or pleural fluid, appropriate antibiotic therapy is initiated. Transtracheal aspirations may yield valuable microbiologic data in selected patients. The procedure should be performed by an experienced physician and the aspirated material Gram stained as well as cultured. CT-guided aspiration may also be feasible. However, if lung abscess is secondary to aspiration and the Gram stain result is compatible with anaerobic bacteria, treatment with clindamycin or piperacillin for 4–6 wk is the treatment of choice pending the results of anaerobic sputum culture. Alternative treatment in children allergic to penicillin is chloramphenicol or metronidazole. Many consider clindamycin the agent of choice. Antibiotics should be given parenterally for at least 2–3 wk. Appropriate investigation for dental disease should be done in older children and adolescents.

Serial chest roentgenograms show gradual diminution in the size of the abscess cavity over a period of several weeks or months. Most patients are afebrile within 1 wk of institution of appropriate antibiotic therapy. Delayed response is common. Bronchoscopy is indicated only to identify and remove a foreign body. Routine use of bronchoscopy to facilitate drainage or to obtain culture material is controversial. Chest tube drainage is necessary if empyema occurs. Surgical drainage of a lung abscess is almost never indicated, and resection should be considered only in children with recurrent hemoptysis, necrosis, a bronchopleural fistula, repeated episodes of infection, or suspicion of malignancy. However, percutaneous drainage may be appropriate, especially for seriously ill children, in whom it can be lifesaving.

The overall prognosis for complete recovery from primary lung abscess is excellent. In patients with secondary lung abscess, the prognosis depends heavily on the underlying disease.

Brook I: Lung abscesses and pleural empyema in children. Adv Pediatr Infect Dis 8:159, 1993.

De Boeck K, Van Cauter A, Fivez H, et al: Percutaneous drainage of lung abscess in a malnourished child. Pediatr Infect Dis J 10:163, 1991.

Levine MM, Ashman R, Heald F: Anaerobic (putrid) lung abscess in adolescence. Am J Dis Child 130:77, 1976.

CHAPTER 412
Lung Hernia

Robert C. Stern

Protrusion of the lung beyond its normal thoracic boundaries may be seen after chest trauma or thoracic surgery, as a congenital abnormality, or in patients with pulmonary diseases such as cystic fibrosis and asthma, which cause frequent cough and generate high intrathoracic pressure. It may also result from a congenital weakness of the suprapleural membranes or musculature of the neck. More than half of congenital lung hernias and almost all acquired hernias are cervical. Congenital cervical hernias usually occur anteriorly through a gap between the scalenus anterior and sternocleidomastoid muscles. Elsewhere, cervical herniation is prevented by the trapezius muscle (posteriorly, at the thoracic inlet) and the three scalene muscles (laterally).

The presenting symptom of a cervical hernia is usually a neck mass noticed while straining or coughing. Some are asymptomatic and detected only when a chest film is taken for another reason. Findings on physical examination are normal except during a Valsalva's maneuver, when a soft bulge may be noticed in the neck. In most cases, no treatment is necessary. However, these hernias may cause problems during attempts to place a central venous catheter through the jugular or subclavian veins. Spontaneous resolution can occur.

Paravertebral or parasternal hernias are usually associated with rib anomalies. Intercostal hernias usually occur parasternally, where the external intercostal muscle is absent. Posteriorly, despite the seemingly inadequate internal intercostal muscle, the paraspinal muscles usually prevent herniation. Straining, coughing, or playing a musical instrument may have a role in causing intercostal hernias, but in most cases, there is probably a pre-existing defect in the thoracic wall.

Surgical treatment for lung hernia is occasionally justified for cosmetic reasons. In patients with severe chronic pulmonary disease and chronic cough and for whom cough suppression is contraindicated, permanent correction may not be achieved.

Bhalla M, Leitman BS, Forcade C, et al: Lung hernia: Radiographic features. Am J Roentgenol 154:51, 1990.

Bronsther B, Coryllos E, Epstein B, et al: Lung hernias in children. J Pediatr Surg 3:544, 1968.

Glenn C, Bonekat W, Cua A, et al: Lung hernia. Am J Emerg Med 15:260, 1997.

CHAPTER 413
Pulmonary Tumors

Robert C. Stern

True carcinoma of the lung is rare in children and adolescents. The six youngest reported patients range from 1–15 yr of age in case reports. Other reported patients were 19, 20, and 25 yr of age. Heavy and long-duration smoking appears to be the most important risk factor even in these older patients. Various primary tumors have been reported, but all are extremely rare. Fewer than 380 cases, including 291 malignancies, have been reported. Bronchial adenoma and carcinoid are the most common primary tumors. Metastatic lesions, such as Wilms tumor, osteogenic sarcoma, and hepatoblastoma, are the most common forms of pulmonary malignancy in children (see Part XXI). A high incidence of "inflammatory pseudotumors" clouds the statistics. Patients with symptoms or with roentgenographic or other laboratory findings suggesting pulmonary malignancy should be searched carefully for a tumor at another site before surgical excision is carried out. Pulmonary tumors may present with fever, hemoptysis, wheezing, cough, pleural effusion, chest pain, dyspnea, or recurrent or persistent pneumonia or atelectasis. Isolated primary lesions and isolated metastatic lesions discovered long after the primary tumor has been removed are best treated by excision. The prognosis varies and depends on the type of tumor involved.

Eggli KD, Newman B: Nodules, masses, and pseudomasses in the pediatric lung. Radiol Clin North Am 31:651, 1993.
Hancock BJ, Di Lorenzo M, Youssef S, et al: Childhood primary pulmonary neoplasms. J Pediatr Surg 28:1133, 1993.
Keita O, Lagrange J-L, Michiels J-F, et al: Primary bronchogenic squamous cell carcinoma in children: Report of a case and review of the literature. Med Pediatr Oncol 24:50, 1995.
Roviaro Gc, Varoli F, Zannini P, et al: Lung cancer in the young. Chest 87:456, 1985.

413.1 Pulmonary Hemangiomatosis

In this rare and ultimately fatal disease, uncontrolled vascular proliferation causes progressive dyspnea and eventually leads to death due to massive hemoptysis or pulmonary hypertension. Its cause is unknown, although infection may have a role. The vascular abnormality involves the smallest (capillary size) vessels in some patients and slightly larger vessels in others. The pathologic angiogenic process may also extend into other intrathoracic tissues (e.g., mediastinum, pericardium, thymus) or the spleen. Patients usually present with hemoptysis or with right-sided heart failure secondary to pulmonary hypertension. Routine chest films are often similar to those seen in interstitial lung disease. The diagnosis is made by pulmonary angiography (which helps to preclude other forms of veno-occlusive disease) and open lung biopsy. The disease can be locally invasive but is not known to metastasize. The primary process appears to be angiogenesis. Most patients die within 1–5 yr from the onset of symptoms.

A substantial and sustained clinical improvement in a 12-yr-old boy treated with recombinant interferon-α-2a (initial dose: 1 million units/m^2/24 hr and then raised rapidly to 3 million units/m^2/24 hr) has been reported. Although some hemoptysis was still present, the patient tolerated the treatment well and was still clinically stable 14 mo later. The success of this treatment is additional evidence that the primary lesion is angiogenesis.

Faber CN, Yousem SA, Dauber JH, et al: Pulmonary capillary hemangiomatosis: A report of three cases and a review of the literature. Am Rev Respir Dis 140:808, 1989.
White CW, Sondheimer HM, Crouch EC, et al: Treatment of pulmonary hemangiomatosis with recombinant interferon α-2a. N Engl J Med 320:1197, 1989.

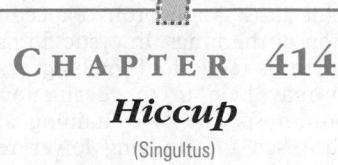

CHAPTER 414
Hiccup
(Singultus)

Robert C. Stern

Hiccup (frequent or rhythmic clonic contraction of the diaphragm) is usually a transient nuisance. Prolonged hiccup, however, can be a diagnostic and therapeutic challenge and can be life threatening. Hiccup can result from various central nervous system diseases (e.g., posterior fossa tumors, brain injury, encephalitis), local irritation along the route of the phrenic nerve or at the diaphragm (e.g., tumor, pleurisy, pneumonia, intrathoracic adenopathy, pericarditis, gastroesophageal reflux, esophagitis, or surgical trauma), and systemic causes (e.g., alcohol intoxication, uremia). Transient hiccup is a benign, acute toxicity associated with many drugs, especially sedatives. Unusual causes of hiccup include a foreign body or insect in the ear (perhaps by stimulation of the vagus nerve). Hiccups occur frequently in young infants, in whom they may be associated with apnea or hyperventilation.

A great many folklore remedies have been used for hiccup. Many of these involve maneuvers that result in aerophagia, breath-holding, or pharyngeal stimulation; others use distraction. For intractable hiccup, various drugs are said to be effective (e.g., haloperidol, metoclopramide, baclofen, and diverse anesthetic agents).

Brouillette RT, Thach BT, Abu-Osba YK, et al: Hiccups in infants: Characteristics and effects on ventilation. J Pediatr 96:219, 1980.
Howard RS: Persistent hiccups. Br Med J 305: 1237, 1992.
Johnson BR, Kriel RL: Baclofen for chronic hiccups. Pediatr Neurol 15:66, 1996.

CHAPTER 415
Chronic or Recurrent Respiratory Symptoms

Thomas F. Boat and David M. Orenstein

Respiratory tract symptoms such as cough, wheeze, and stridor may occur frequently or persist for long periods in a substantial number of children, others may have persistent or recurring lung infiltrates with or without symptoms. Determining the cause of these chronic findings can be difficult because symptoms may be caused by a rapid succession of unrelated acute respiratory tract infections or by a single pathophysiologic process, and there is a paucity of easily performed, specific diagnostic tests for many acute and chronic respiratory conditions. Pressure from the affected child's family for a quick remedy because of concern over symptoms related to breathing may complicate diagnostic and therapeutic efforts.

A systematic approach to the diagnosis and treatment of these children consists of assessing whether the symptoms are the manifestation of a minor problem or a life-threatening process; determining the most likely underlying pathogenic mechanism; selecting the simplest effective therapy for the underlying process, which may often be only symptomatic therapy; and carefully evaluating the effect of therapy. Failure of this approach to identify the process responsible or to effect improvement signals the need for more extensive and perhaps invasive diagnostic efforts, including bronchoscopy.

JUDGING THE SERIOUSNESS OF CHRONIC RESPIRATORY COMPLAINTS. Clinical manifestations suggesting that a respiratory tract illness may be life-threatening or associated with the potential for chronic disability are listed in Table 415–1. If none of these signs are detected, the chronic respiratory process is usually benign. For example, active, well-nourished, and appropriately growing infants who present with intermittent noisy breathing but no other physical or laboratory abnormalities require only symptomatic treatment and parental reassurance. However, benign-appearing but persistent symptoms occasionally may be the harbinger of a serious lower respiratory tract problem

TABLE 415–1 Indicators of Serious Chronic Lower Respiratory Tract Disease in Children

- Persistent fever
- Ongoing limitation of activity
- Failure to grow
- Failure to gain weight appropriately
- Clubbing of the digits
- Persistent tachypnea and labored ventilation
- Chronic purulent sputum
- Persistent hyperinflation
- Substantial and sustained hypoxemia
- Refractory roentgenographic infiltrates
- Persistent pulmonary function abnormalities
- Family history of heritable lung disease
- Cyanosis and hypercarbia

and, conversely, a few children (e.g., those with infection-related asthma) may have recurrent life-threatening episodes but few or no symptoms in the interval. Repeated examinations over an extended period, both when the child appears healthy and when the child is symptomatic, are often helpful in sorting out the severity and chronicity of lung disease.

RECURRENT OR PERSISTENT COUGH. Cough is a reflex response of the lower respiratory tract to stimulation of irritant or cough receptors in the airways' mucosa. The most common cause in children is reactive airways (asthma). Because cough receptors also reside in the pharynx, paranasal sinuses, stomach, and external auditory canal, the source of a persistent cough may need to be sought beyond the lungs. Specific lower respiratory stimuli include excessive secretions, aspirated foreign material, inhaled dust particles or noxious gases, and an inflammatory response to infectious agents or allergic processes. Some of the conditions responsible for chronic cough are listed in Table 415–2.

Characteristics of cough that may aid in distinguishing its origin are presented in Table 415–3. Additional useful information may include a history of atopic conditions (e.g., asthma, eczema, urticaria, allergic rhinitis), a seasonal or environmental variation in frequency or intensity of cough, and a strong family history of atopic conditions, all suggesting an allergic cause; symptoms of malabsorption or family history indicative

TABLE 415–2 Differential Diagnosis of Recurrent and Persistent Cough in Children

Recurrent Cough

- Bronchial reactivity, including allergic asthma
- Drainage from upper airways
- Aspiration syndromes
- Frequently recurring respiratory tract infections
- Idiopathic pulmonary hemosiderosis

Persistent Cough

- Hypersensitivity of cough receptors following infection
- Reactive airways disease (asthma)
- Chronic sinusitis
- Bronchitis, tracheitis owing to chronic infection, smoking (in older children)
- Bronchiectasis, including cystic fibrosis, primary ciliary dyskinesia, immunodeficiency
- Foreign body aspiration
- Recurrent aspiration owing to pharyngeal incompetence, tracheolaryngoesophageal cleft, tracheoesophageal fistula
- Gastroesophageal reflux, with or without aspiration
- Pertussis syndrome
- Extrinsic compression of the tracheobronchial tract (vascular ring, neoplasm, lymph node, lung cyst)
- Tracheomalacia, bronchomalacia
- Endobronchial or endotracheal tumors
- Endobronchial tuberculosis
- Habit cough
- Hypersensitivity pneumonitis
- Fungal infections
- Inhaled irritants, including tobacco smoke
- Irritation of external auditory canal

TABLE 415–3 Characteristics of a Chronic Cough and Their Etiologic Significance

Type of Cough	Likely Responsible Condition
Loose (discontinuous), productive	Bronchitis, asthmatic bronchitis, cystic fibrosis, bronchiectasis
Brassy	Tracheitis, habit cough
With stridor	Laryngeal obstruction, pertussis
Paroxysmal (with or without gagging and vomiting)	Cystic fibrosis, pertussis syndrome, foreign body
Staccato	Chlamydial pneumonitis
Nocturnal	Upper or lower respiratory tract allergic reaction, or both, sinusitis
Most severe on awakening in morning	Cystic fibrosis, bronchiectasis, chronic bronchitis
With vigorous exercise	Exercise-induced asthma, cystic fibrosis, bronchiectasis
Disappears with sleep	Habit cough, mild hypersecretory states such as in cystic fibrosis and asthma
Tight (wheezy)	Reactive airways

of cystic fibrosis; symptoms related to feeding, suggesting aspiration; a choking episode, suggesting foreign body aspiration; headache or facial edema associated with sinusitis; and a smoking history in older children and adolescents or the presence of a smoker in the house.

Considerable information pertaining to the cause of chronic cough can be obtained during the *physical examination.* Posterior pharyngeal drainage combined with a nighttime cough suggests chronic upper airway disease such as sinusitis. An overinflated chest suggests chronic airway obstruction, as in asthma or cystic fibrosis. An expiratory wheeze, with or without diminished intensity of breath sounds, strongly suggests asthma or asthmatic bronchitis but may also be consistent with a diagnosis of cystic fibrosis, vascular ring, aspiration of foreign material, or pulmonary hemosiderosis. Careful auscultation during forced expiration may reveal expiratory wheezes that are otherwise undetectable and that are the only indication of underlying reactive airways. Coarse crackles suggest bronchiectasis, including cystic fibrosis, but may also attend an acute or subacute exacerbation of asthma. Clubbing of the digits is seen in most patients with bronchiectasis but in only a few other respiratory conditions with chronic cough. Tracheal deviation suggests foreign body aspiration or a mediastinal mass.

It is essential to allow sufficient examination time to detect a spontaneous cough. If not spontaneous, most children by 4–5 yr of age can cough on request. Asking the child to take a maximal breath and forcefully exhale repeatedly usually induces a cough reflex. Children who cough as often as several times a minute with regularity are likely to have a habit (tic) cough. If the cough is loose, every effort should be made to obtain sputum; most older children can comply. It is sometimes possible to pick up small bits of sputum with a throat swab quickly inserted into the lower pharynx while the child coughs with the tongue protruding. Clear mucoid sputum is most often associated with an allergic reaction or asthmatic bronchitis. Cloudy (purulent) sputum suggests a respiratory tract infection but may also reflect increased cellularity (eosinophilia) due to an asthmatic process. Very purulent sputum is characteristic of bronchiectasis. Malodorous expectorations suggest anaerobic infection of the lungs. In cystic fibrosis the sputum, even when purulent, is rarely foul smelling.

Laboratory tests may help in the evaluation of a chronic cough. Only sputum specimens containing alveolar macrophages should be used for studying lower respiratory tract processes. Sputum eosinophilia suggests asthma, asthmatic bronchitis, or hypersensitivity reactions of the lung, but a polymorphonuclear cell response suggests infection; if sputum is unavailable, the presence of eosinophilia in nasal secretions also suggests atopic disease. If most of the cells in sputum are macrophages, postinfectious hypersensitivity of cough receptors should be suspected. Sputum macrophages can be stained for hemosiderin content, which is diagnostic of pulmonary hemosiderosis, or for lipid content, which in large amounts suggests, but is not specific for, repeated aspiration. Children whose coughs persist longer than 6 wk should be tested for cystic fibrosis. Sputum culture is helpful but not specific because throat flora may contaminate the sample.

Hematologic assessment may reveal anemia that is the result of pulmonary hemosiderosis or eosinophilia that accompanies asthma and other hypersensitivity reactions of the lung. Infiltrates on the chest roentgenogram suggest cystic fibrosis, bronchiectasis, foreign body, hypersensitivity pneumonitis, or tuberculosis. When asthma equivalent cough is suspected, a trial of bronchodilator therapy may be diagnostic. After the initial evaluation, especially if the cough does not respond to initial therapeutic efforts, more specific diagnostic procedures may be indicated, including an immunologic or allergic evaluation, chest and paranasal sinus imaging, esophagograms, tests for gastroesophageal reflux, special microbiologic studies, evaluation of ciliary morphologic features, and bronchoscopy.

Habit cough ("psychogenic cough tic") must be considered in any child with a cough that has lasted for weeks or months, that has been refractory to treatment, that disappears with sleep, and that typically has a harsh, "barking" quality. This cough may be absent if the physician listens outside the examination room, but will reliably appear immediately on direct attention to the child and the symptom. It typically begins with an upper respiratory infection, but then lingers. The child misses many days of school because the cough disrupts the classroom. This disorder accounts for many unnecessary medical procedures and courses of medication. It is treatable with assurance that a lung pathologic condition is absent and that the child should resume full activity, including school. This assurance, together with speech therapy techniques that allow the child to reduce musculoskeletal tension in the neck and chest and that increase the child's awareness of the initial sensations that trigger cough, has been very successful, often within minutes. This approach does not depend on deception, unlike a reportedly successful technique that involves wrapping the child's chest with a bedsheet to "strengthen weakened muscles" until the coughing stops. The designation "habit cough" is preferable to "psychogenic cough" because it carries no stigma and because most of these children do not have significant emotional problems. When the cough disappears, it does not re-emerge as another symptom.

RECURRENT OR PERSISTENT WHEEZE. Wheezing is a relatively frequent and particularly troublesome manifestation of obstructive lower respiratory tract disease in children. The site of obstruction may be anywhere from the intrathoracic trachea to the small bronchi or large bronchioles, but the sound is generated by turbulence in larger airways that collapse with forced expiration. Children younger than 2–3 yr of age are especially prone to wheezing, because bronchospasm, mucosal edema, and accumulation of excessive secretions have a relatively greater obstructive effect on their smaller airways. In addition, the compliant airways in young children collapse more readily with active expiration. Isolated episodes of acute wheezing, such as may occur with bronchiolitis, are not uncommon, but wheezing that recurs or persists for longer than 4 wk suggests other diagnoses (Table 415–4). Most recurrent or persistent wheezing in children is the result of reactive airways disease. Nonspecific environmental factors such as cigarette smoke may be important contributors.

Frequently recurring or persistent wheezing starting at or soon after birth suggests a variety of other diagnoses, including congenital structural abnormalities involving the lower respiratory tract or tracheobronchomalacia. Wheezing that attends cystic fibrosis is most common in the first year of life. Sudden onset of severe wheezing in a previously healthy child should suggest foreign body aspiration.

TABLE 415–4 Causes of Recurrent or Persistent Wheezing in Children

- Reactive airways disease
  - Atopic asthma
  - Infection-associated airway reactivity
  - Exercise-induced asthma
  - Salicylate-induced asthma and nasal polyposis
  - Asthmatic bronchitis
  - Other hypersensitivity reactions
    - Hypersensitivity pneumonitis
    - Tropical eosinophilia
    - Visceral larva migrans
    - Allergic bronchopulmonary aspergillosis
- Aspiration
  - Foreign body
  - Food, saliva, gastric contents
  - Laryngotracheoesophageal cleft
  - Tracheoesophageal fistula, H-type
  - Pharyngeal incoordination or neuromuscular weakness
- Cystic fibrosis
- Primary ciliary dyskinesia
- Cardiac failure
- Bronchiolitis obliterans
- Extrinsic compression of airways
  - Vascular ring
  - Enlarged lymph node
  - Mediastinal tumor
  - Lung cysts
- Tracheobronchomalacia
- Endobronchial masses
- Gastroesophageal reflux
- Pulmonary hemosiderosis
- Sequelae of bronchopulmonary dysplasia
- "Hysterical" glottic closure
- Cigarette smoke, other environmental insults

Repeated examination may be required to verify a history of wheezing in a child with episodic symptoms and should be directed toward assessing air movement, ventilatory adequacy, and evidence of chronic lung disease, such as fixed overinflation of the chest, growth failure, and digital clubbing. Clubbing suggests chronic lung infection and is rarely prominent in uncomplicated asthma. Tracheal deviation from foreign body aspiration should be sought. It is essential to rule out wheezing secondary to congestive heart failure. Allergic rhinitis, urticaria, eczema, or evidence of ichthyosis vulgaris suggests asthma or asthmatic bronchitis. The nose should be examined for polyps, which may exist with allergic conditions or cystic fibrosis.

Sputum eosinophilia and elevated serum IgE levels suggest allergic reactions. An FEV_1 increase of 15% in response to bronchodilators is confirmatory of reactive airways. Specific microbiologic studies, special imaging studies of the airways and cardiovascular structures, diagnostic studies for cystic fibrosis, and bronchoscopy should be considered if the response is unsatisfactory.

FREQUENTLY RECURRING OR PERSISTENT STRIDOR. Stridor, a harsh, medium-pitched, inspiratory sound associated with obstruction of the laryngeal area or the extrathoracic trachea, is often accompanied by a croupy cough and hoarse voice. Stridor is most commonly observed in children with croup; foreign bodies and trauma may also cause acute stridor. However, a small number of children acquire recurrent stridor or have persistent stridor from the first days or weeks of life (Table 415–5). Most congenital anomalies of large airways that produce stridor become symptomatic soon after birth. Increase of stridor when a child is supine suggests laryngomalacia or tracheomalacia. An accompanying history of hoarseness or aphonia suggests involvement of the vocal cords.

Physical examination for recurrent or persistent stridor is usually unrewarding, although changes in its severity and intensity due to changes of body position should be assessed. Anteroposterior and lateral roentgenograms, contrast esophagography, fluoroscopy, computed tomography, and magnetic

TABLE 415–5 Causes of Recurrent or Persistent Stridor in Children

Recurrent	Persistent
Allergic (spasmodic) croup	Laryngeal obstruction
Respiratory infections in a child with otherwise asymptomatic anatomic narrowing of the large airways	Laryngomalacia
Laryngomalacia	Papillomas, other tumors
	Cysts and laryngoceles
	Laryngeal webs
	Bilateral abductor paralysis of the cords
	Foreign body
	Tracheobronchial disease
	Tracheomalacia
	Subglottic tracheal webs
	Endotracheal, endobronchial tumors
	Subglottic tracheal stenosis
	Congenital
	Acquired
	Extrinsic masses
	Mediastinal masses
	Vascular ring
	Lobar emphysema
	Bronchogenic cysts
	Thyroid enlargement
	Esophageal foreign body
	Tracheoesophageal fistulas
	Other
	Gastroesophageal reflux
	Macroglossia, Pierre Robin syndrome
	Cri du chat syndrome
	Hysterical stridor
	Hypocalcemia

resonance imaging are potentially useful diagnostic tools. In most cases, direct observation is necessary for diagnosis. Undistorted views of the larynx are best obtained with fiberoptic laryngoscopy.

RECURRENT AND PERSISTENT LUNG INFILTRATES. Roentgenographic lung infiltrates due to acute pneumonia usually resolve within 1–3 wk, but a substantial number of children, particularly infants, fail to completely clear infiltrates within a 4-wk period. They may be febrile or afebrile and may display a wide range of respiratory symptoms and signs. Persistent or recurring infiltrates present a diagnostic challenge (Table 415–6).

Symptoms associated with chronic lung infiltrates during the first several weeks of life (but not related to neonatal respiratory distress syndrome) suggest infection acquired in utero or during descent through the birth canal. Early appearance of chronic infiltrates may also be associated with cystic fibrosis or congenital anomalies, which result in aspiration or airway obstruction. A history of recurrent infiltrates, wheezing, and cough may reflect asthma, even in the first year of life.

One uncommon but characteristic syndrome appearing in the first year of life with recurrent lung infiltrates is pulmonary hemosiderosis related to cow milk hypersensitivity. Children with a history of bronchopulmonary dysplasia frequently have episodes of respiratory distress attended by wheezing and new lung infiltrates. Recurrent pneumonia in a child with frequent otitis media, nasopharyngitis, adenitis, or dermatologic manifestations suggests an immunodeficiency state, complement deficiency, or phagocytic defect. Particular attention must be directed to the possibility that the infiltrates represent lymphocytic interstitial pneumonitis or opportunistic infection associated with human immunodeficiency virus infection. A history of paroxysmal coughing in an infant suggests pertussis syndrome or cystic fibrosis. Persistent infiltrates, especially with loss of volume, in a toddler should suggest foreign body aspiration.

Overinflation and infiltrates suggest cystic fibrosis or chronic asthma. A "silent chest" with infiltrates should arouse suspicion of alveolar proteinosis, *Pneumocystis carinii* infection, desquamative interstitial pneumonitis, or tumors. Growth should be carefully assessed to determine whether the lung process has had systemic effects, indicating substantial severity and chronicity as in cystic fibrosis or alveolar proteinosis. Cataracts, retinopathy, or microcephaly suggest in utero infection. Chronic rhinorrhea may be associated with atopic disease, cow milk intolerance, cystic fibrosis, or congenital syphilis. The absence of tonsils and cervical lymph nodes suggests a combined immunodeficiency state.

Diagnostic studies should be performed selectively, based on information obtained from history and physical examination and on a thorough understanding of the conditions listed in Table 415–6. Cytologic evaluation of sputum, if available, may be helpful. Chest computed tomography often provides more precise anatomic detail concerning the infiltrate. Bronchoscopy is indicated for detecting foreign bodies, congenital or acquired anomalies of the tracheobronchial tract, and obstruction by

TABLE 415–6 Diseases Associated with Recurrent or Persistent Lung Infiltrates Beyond the Neonatal Period

- Recurrent or migrating infiltrates
  - Asthma*
  - Repeated aspiration*
  - Hypersensitivity pneumonitis
  - Pulmonary hemosiderosis*
  - Foreign body
  - Sickle cell disease
  - Cystic fibrosis*
  - Congenital infection*
    - Cytomegalovirus
    - Rubella
    - Syphilis
  - Acquired infection
    - Cytomegalovirus*
    - Tuberculosis*
    - HIV
    - Other viruses*
    - *Chlamydia**
    - *Mycoplasma, Ureaplasma**
    - Pertussis*
    - Fungal organisms
    - *Pneumocystis carinii**
- Inadequately treated bacterial infection
- Congenital anomalies
  - Lung cysts*
  - Pulmonary sequestration
  - Bronchial stenosis
  - Vascular ring
  - Congenital heart disease with large left to right shunt
- Aspiration
  - Pharyngeal incompetence (e.g., cleft palate)*
  - Laryngotracheoesophageal cleft*
  - Tracheoesophageal fistula*
  - Gastroesophageal reflux*
  - Foreign body
  - Lipid aspiration
- Immunodeficiency, phagocytic deficiency*
  - Humoral, cellular, combined immunodeficiency states*
  - Chronic granulomatous disease and related phagocytic defects*
  - Complement deficiency states*
- Allergy-hypersensitivity
  - Pulmonary hemosiderosis (cow milk–related, other*)
  - Asthma
  - Hypersensitivity pneumonitis (allergic alveolitis)
- Cystic fibrosis*
- Primary ciliary dyskinesia (Kartagener syndrome)
- Other bronchiectases
- Sarcoidosis
- Neoplasms (primary, metastatic)
- Interstitial pneumonitis and fibrosis*
  - Usual (Hamman-Rich)
  - Desquamative
  - Lymphoid (acquired immunodeficiency syndrome)
- Alveolar proteinosis
- Pulmonary lymphangiectasia*
- α_1-Antitrypsin deficiency
- Drug-induced, radiation-induced inflammation and fibrosis
- Collagen-vascular diseases
- Eosinophilic pneumonias
- Visceral larva migrans
- Histiocytosis
- Leukemia

**Conditions likely to cause chronic lung infiltrates in infants.*

endobronchial or extrinsic masses. Bronchoscopy provides access to secretions that can be studied cytologically and microbiologically. Alveolar lavage fluid is diagnostic for alveolar proteinosis and persistent pulmonary hemosiderosis and may suggest aspiration syndromes. If all appropriate studies have been completed and the condition remains undiagnosed, lung biopsy may yield a definitive diagnosis.

Optimal medical or surgical treatment of chronic lung infiltrates frequently depends on a specific diagnosis, but chronic conditions may be self-limiting (e.g., severe and prolonged viral infections in infants); in these cases, symptomatic therapy may maintain adequate lung function until spontaneous improvement occurs. Helpful measures include inhalation and physical therapy for excessive secretions, antibiotics for secondary bacterial infections, supplementary oxygen for hypoxemia, and maintenance of adequate nutrition. Because the lung of a young child has remarkable recuperative potential, normal lung function may ultimately be achieved with treatment despite the severity of pulmonary insult occurring during infancy or early childhood.

Anderson VM, Haesoon L: Lymphocytic interstitial pneumonitis in pediatric AIDS. Pediatr Pathol 8:417, 1988.
Blager F, Gay M, Wood R: Voice therapy techniques adapted to treatment of habit cough: A pilot study. J Communication Disord 21:393, 1988.
Cloutier MM, Loughlin GM: Chronic cough in children: A manifestation of airway hyperreactivity. Pediatrics 67:6, 1981.
Holberg CJ, Wright AL, Martinez FD, et al: Child day care, smoking by caregivers, and lower respiratory tract illness in the first 3 years of life. Pediatrics 91:885, 1993.
Lokshin B, Lindgren S, Weinberger M, et al: Outcome of habit cough in children treated with a brief session of suggestion therapy. Ann Allergy 67:579, 1991.
Mamlock R: A cost-effective approach to the diagnosis and treatment of the wheezing infant. Allergy Asthma Proc 18:149, 1997.
Mancuso RF: Stridor in neonates. Pediatr Clin North Am 43:1339, 1996.
Martinez FD, Wright AL, Taussig LM, et al: Asthma and wheezing in the first six years of life. N Engl J Med 332:133, 1995.
Morgan WJ, Taussig LM: The child with persistent cough. Pediatr Rev 8:249, 1987.
Orenstein SR, Orenstein DM: Gastroesophageal reflux and respiratory disease in children. J Pediatr 112:847, 1988.
Skoner D, Caliquiri L: The wheezing infant. Pediatr Clin North Am 35:1011, 1988.
Stagno S, Brasfield DM, Brown MB, et al: Infant pneumonitis associated with cytomegalovirus, chlamydia, pneumocystis, and ureaplasma: A prospective study. Pediatrics 68:322, 1981.

CHAPTER 416
Cystic Fibrosis

Thomas F. Boat

Cystic fibrosis (CF) is an inherited multisystem disorder of children and adults, characterized chiefly by obstruction and infection of airways and by maldigestion and its consequences. It is the most common life-limiting recessive genetic trait among whites. A dysfunction of epithelial surfaces is the predominant pathogenetic feature and is responsible for a broad, variable, and sometimes confusing array of presenting manifestations and complications.

CF is the major cause of severe chronic lung disease in children and is responsible for most exocrine pancreatic insufficiency during early life. It is also responsible for many cases of salt depletion, nasal polyposis, pansinusitis, rectal prolapse, pancreatitis, cholelithiasis, and insulin-dependent hyperglycemia. CF may present as failure to thrive and occasionally as cirrhosis or other forms of hepatic dysfunction. Therefore, this disorder enters into the differential diagnosis of many pediatric conditions.

GENETICS. CF occurs in approximately 1/3,500 white live births and 1/17,000 black infants in the United States. The estimated incidence worldwide varies from 1/377 live births in parts of Brittany to 1/90,000 Asian infants in Hawaii. Generally, the CF gene is most prevalent among Northern and Central Europeans and in individuals who come from these areas.

CF is inherited as an autosomal recessive trait. All of the more than 700 gene mutations that contribute to the CF syndrome occur at a single locus on the long arm of chromosome 7. The CF gene codes for a protein of 1,480 amino acids called the *CF transmembrane regulator* (CFTR). CFTR is expressed largely in epithelial cells of airways, the gastrointestinal tract (including pancreas and biliary system), the sweat glands, and the genitourinary system. CFTR has ion channel and regulatory functions that are perturbed variably by the different mutations. The most prevalent mutation of CFTR is the deletion of a single phenylalanine residue at amino acid 508 (ΔF508). This mutation is responsible for the high incidence of CF in northern European populations and is considerably less frequent in other populations, such as those in southern Europe and Israel. Approximately 50% of individuals with CF and Northern European ancestry are homozygous for ΔF508. The remainder of patients have an extensive array of mutations, none of which has a prevalence of more than several per cent (Table 416–1), except in circumscribed populations. For example, the W1282X mutation occurs in 60% of the Ashkenazi Jews with CF. The relationship between genotype and phenotype is highly complex. Mutations categorized as "severe" (e.g., ΔF508) are associated almost uniformly with pancreatic insufficiency. Several mutations (e.g., 3849 + 10 Kb C>T) are found in patients with normal sweat chloride concentrations. Severity of lung disease and presence of liver disease cannot be predicted by genotype. This suggests a major environmental (acquired) component of organ system dysfunction, or perhaps the presence of as yet unidentified modifying genes that contribute to the CF phenotype.

Using probes for 30 of the most frequent mutations, the genotype of 80–90% of Americans with CF can be ascertained. Increasing the number of probes to 70 improves mutation ascertainment by only a few per cent. Thus, not all children with CF can be identified by DNA testing as currently performed. Furthermore, the presence of modifications in both CFTR genes does not always cause CF manifestations.

The high frequency of the CF gene has been hypothetically ascribed to resistance to the morbidity and mortality associated with cholera through the ages. Cultured CF intestinal epithelial cells homozygous for the ΔF508 mutation are unresponsive to the secretory effects of cholera toxin.

PATHOGENESIS. Four long-standing observations are of funda-

TABLE 416–1 Prevalent Cystic Fibrosis Mutations in the Caucasian Population*

Mutation	%
ΔF508	66.0
G542X	2.4
G551D	1.6
N1303K	1.3
W1282X	1.2
R533X	0.7
621 + 1G>T	0.7
1717 − 1G>T	0.6
R117H	0.3
R1162X	0.3
G85E	0.2
R347P	0.2
Δ1507	0.2
3849 + 10kbC>T	0.2

**CF mutations meet one or more of the following criteria: (1) cause CFTR dysfunction; (2) introduce a premature termination signal; (3) alter "invariant" nucleotides of splice sites; (4) change the amino acid sequence, not found in normal genes from 100 carriers of CF mutations within the same ethnic group.*

From Rosenstein BJ, Cutting GR: The diagnosis of cystic fibrosis: A consensus statement. J Pediatr 132:589, 1998.

mental pathophysiologic importance: failure to clear mucous secretions, a paucity of water in mucous secretions, an elevated salt content of sweat and other serous secretions, and chronic infection limited to the respiratory tract. The relationships among these findings were unclear until the early 1980s when it was demonstrated that there is a greater negative potential difference across the respiratory epithelia of CF patients than across the respiratory epithelia of control subjects. Aberrant electrical properties were also demonstrated for CF sweat gland duct epithelium. Subsequent studies demonstrated that the membranes of CF epithelial cells are unable to secrete chloride ions in response to cyclic adenosine monophosphate–mediated signals, and that, at least in the respiratory tract, excessive amounts of sodium are absorbed through these membranes (Fig. 416–1). These defects can be traced to a dysfunction of CFTR (Fig. 416–2).

After isolation of the CFTR gene and its characterization, it became clear that cyclic adenosine monophosphate–stimulated chloride conductance was a function of CFTR itself and that this function was absent in epithelial cells with many different mutations of the CFTR gene. CFTR mutations appear to fall into five classes, albeit with some overlap: I, defective CFTR production due to premature transcription termination signals; II, defective CFTR processing and trafficking to the apical membrane (e.g., ΔF508); III, defective regulation of chloride channel function due to mutations in CFTR phosphorylation or adenosine triphosphate–binding sites; IV, defective chloride conductance due to missense mutations in the membrane-spanning domains of CFTR that line the channel; and V, abnormal splicing of CFTR. The importance of these functional categories is not clear, as categories do not correlate with specific clinical features or their severity.

The postulated epithelial pathophysiology in airways involves an inability to secrete salt and secondarily secrete water in the face of excessive reabsorption of salt and water. The proposed outcome is insufficient water on the airway surface to hydrate secretions. Desiccated secretions become more viscous and elastic (rubbery) and are harder to clear by mucociliary and other mechanisms. These secretions are retained and obstruct airways, starting with those of the smallest caliber, the bronchioles. Airflow obstruction at the level of small airways is the earliest observable physiologic abnormality of the respiratory system. Although this hypothesis is appealing, physiologic evidence for alteration of surface liquid composition in CF airways has been elusive.

CFTR: A cAMP-Regulated Chloride Channel

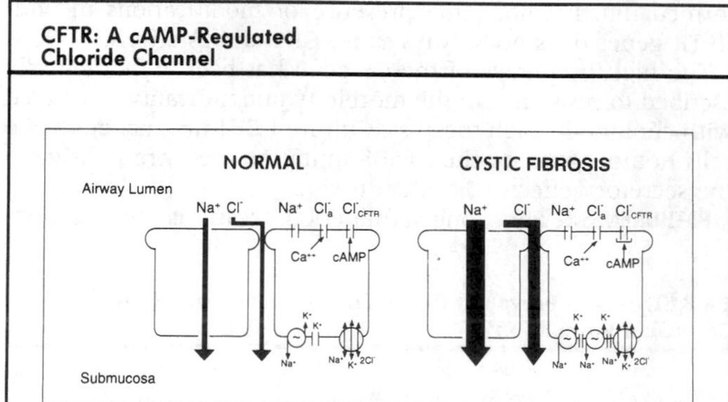

Figure 416–1 The net ion flow across normal and cystic fibrosis (CF) airway epithelia under basal conditions (*large arrows*). Because water follows salt movement, the predicted net flux of water would be from the airway lumen to the submucosa and would be greater across CF epithelia. The increased Na^+ absorption by CF cells is associated with an increased amiloride-sensitive Na^+ conductance across the apical (luminal) membrane and increased Na^+, K^+-ATPase sites at the basolateral membrane. The cAMP-mediated apical membrane conductance of Cl^- associated with the CF transmembrane regulator (CFTR) does not function in CF epithelia, but an alternative, calcium-activated Cl^- conductance is present in normal and CF cells. It is postulated that CF cells have a limited ability to secrete Cl^- and absorb Na^+ in excessive amounts, limiting the water available to hydrate secretions and allow them to be cleared from the airways lumen. (From Knowles MR: Contemporary perspectives on the pathogenesis of cystic fibrosis. New Insights into Cystic Fibrosis 1:1, 1993.)

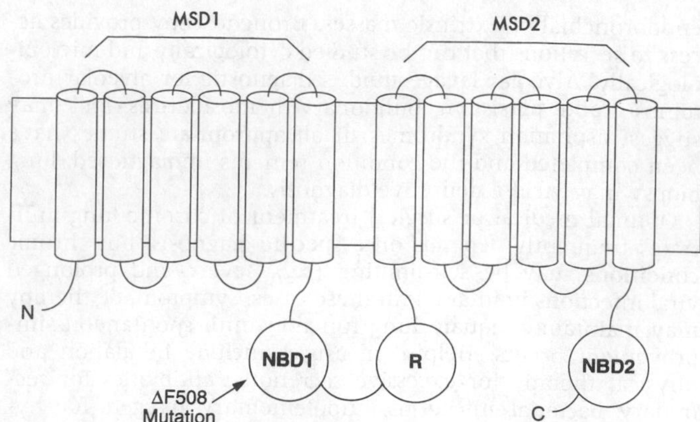

Figure 416–2 The predicted structure of a cystic fibrosis transmembrane regulator (CFTR) shows that the molecule is anchored in the cell membrane by two membrane-spanning domains (MSD1, MSD2). These domains form a channel through which chloride and probably water can pass. Two nucleotide-binding domains (NBD1, NBD2) interact with ATP to provide energy for CFTR functions. The R domain has many sites for phosphorylation by cAMP-dependent kinases. This domain is involved in the regulation of CFTR functions such as chloride conductance. The most common CFTR mutation, ΔF508, is localized to the NBD1 region. This region and the NBD2 site are particularly susceptible to mutation. However, mutations associated with typical manifestations of CF occur in all domains. (From Welsh MJ, Anderson MP, Rich DP, et al: Cystic fibrosis transmembrane conductance regulator. Neuron 8:821, 1992.)

It is plausible that similar pathophysiologic events take place in the pancreatic and biliary ducts (and in the vas deferens), leading to desiccation of proteinaceous secretions and obstruction. Because the function of sweat gland duct cells is to absorb rather than secrete chloride, salt is not retrieved from the isotonic primary sweat as it is transported to the skin surface; chloride and sodium levels consequently are elevated.

Chronic infection in CF is limited to the endobronchial spaces of the airways. The most likely explanation for infection is a sequence of events starting with failure to clear inhaled bacteria promptly and then proceeding to persistent colonization and an inflammatory response in airway walls. An alternative hypothesis, that abnormal CFTR creates an inflammatory state prior to first infection or amplifies the inflammatory response to initial viral infection, is based on lung lavage evidence for cytokines such as interleukin-8 and neutrophiles in the absence of recovered bacteria within the first months of life. These events occur first in small airways, perhaps because clearance of altered secretions is more difficult from these regions. Chronic bronchiolitis and bronchitis are the initial lung manifestations, but after months to years, structural changes in airway walls produce bronchiolectasis and bronchiectasis.

The agents of airway injury include neutrophil products, such as oxidative radicals and proteases, and immune reaction products. With advanced lung disease, infection may extend to peribronchial lung parenchyma. Several inflammatory products, including proteases, are responsible for the mucus hypersecretion that is characteristic of chronic airways disease.

A finding that is not readily explained is the high prevalence of airways colonization with *Staphylococcus aureus* and *Pseudomonas aeruginosa,* two organisms that rarely infect the lungs of other individuals. There is evidence that the CF airway epithelial cells or surface liquids provide a favorable environment for attachment or induce adherence properties of these organisms. Furthermore, CF airways epithelium may be compromised in its innate defenses against the organisms, through either acquired or genetic alterations. Another puzzle is the propensity for *P. aeruginosa* to undergo mucoid transformation in the CF airways.

Although functional deficits may occur in cellular immunity, mucosal immune function, and the alternate pathway for complement as lung infection progresses to an advanced stage, the immune system in CF appears to be fundamentally intact. Nutritional deficits, including fatty acid deficiency, have been implicated as predisposing factors for respiratory tract infection. The 10–15% of individuals who retain substantial exocrine pancreatic function have statistically lower sweat chloride values, delayed onset of colonization with *P. aeruginosa*, and slower deterioration of lung function. However, nutritional factors are only contributory in part because preservation of pancreatic function does not preclude development of typical lung disease.

PATHOLOGY. Striking changes are characteristically observed in the organs that secrete mucus. Eccrine sweat glands and parotid salivary glands, including ducts, are not involved pathologically despite abnormalities in the electrolyte content of their secretory product.

The earliest pathologic lesion in the *lung* is that of bronchiolitis (i.e., mucous plugging and an inflammatory response in the walls of the small airways). With time, mucus accumulation and inflammation extend to the larger airways (bronchitis). Goblet cell hyperplasia and submucosal gland hypertrophy become prominent pathologic expressions of a hypersecretory state, which is most likely a response to chronic airways infection. Organisms appear to be confined to the endobronchial space; invasive bacterial infection is not characteristic. With long-standing disease, evidence of airway destruction such as bronchiolar obliteration, bronchiolectasis, and bronchiectasis becomes prominent. Scanning electron microscopy of the airway surface appears normal, except for scattered areas of squamous cell metaplasia, although freeze-fracture studies have found alterations of tight junctions and apical membrane changes that are probably caused by chronic inflammation. Bronchiectatic cysts and emphysematous bullae or subpleural blebs are frequent with advanced lung disease, the upper lobes being most commonly involved. These enlarged air spaces may rupture and cause pneumothorax. Interstitial disease is not a prominent (common) feature, although areas of fibrosis appear eventually. True emphysema occurs but is not a general pathologic finding. Bronchial arteries are enlarged and tortuous, contributing to a propensity for hemoptysis in bronchiectatic airways. Small pulmonary arteries eventually display medial hypertrophy, which would be expected in secondary pulmonary hypertension.

The *paranasal sinuses* are uniformly filled with secretions, and the lining contains hyperplastic and hypertrophied secretory elements. Polypoid lesions within the sinuses, mucopyocele, and erosion of bone have been reported. The nasal mucosa may contain inflammatory cells, be edematous, and form large or multiple polyps, usually from a base surrounding the ostia of the maxillary and ethmoid sinuses.

The *pancreas* is usually small, occasionally cystic, and often difficult to find at postmortem examination. The extent of involvement varies at birth. In infants, the acini and ducts are often distended and filled with eosinophilic material. In 85–90% of patients, the lesion progresses to complete or almost complete disruption of acini and replacement with fibrous tissue and fat. Infrequently, foci of calcification may be seen on roentgenograms of the abdomen. The islets of Langerhans contain a normal number of β cells, although they may begin to show architectural disruption by fibrous tissue during the 2nd decade of life.

The *intestinal tract* shows only minimal changes. Esophageal and duodenal glands are often distended with mucous secretions. Concretions may form in the appendiceal lumen or cecum. Crypts of the appendix and rectum may be dilatated and filled with secretions.

Focal biliary cirrhosis secondary to blockage of intrahepatic bile ducts is uncommon in early life, although it is responsible for occasional cases of prolonged neonatal jaundice. This lesion becomes more prevalent and extensive with age and is found in 25% or more of patients at postmortem examination. Infrequently, this process proceeds to symptomatic multilobular biliary cirrhosis that has a distinctive pattern of large irregular parenchymal nodules and interspersed bands of fibrous tissue. In addition, approximately 30% of patients have fatty infiltration of the liver, in some cases despite apparently adequate nutrition. At autopsy, hepatic congestion secondary to cor pulmonale is frequently observed. The gallbladder may be hypoplastic and filled with mucoid material and not infrequently contains stones. The epithelial lining often displays extensive mucous metaplasia. Atresia of the cystic duct and stenosis of the distal common bile duct have been observed.

Mucus-secreting *salivary glands* are usually enlarged and display focal plugging and dilatation of ducts.

Glands of the uterine cervix are distended with mucus, and copious amounts of mucus collect in the cervical canal. Endocervicitis may be prevalent in teenagers and young women. In more than 95% of males, the body and tail of the epididymis, the vas deferens, and the seminal vesicles are obliterated or atretic.

Generalized amyloidosis has been reported rarely (see Chapter 165).

CLINICAL MANIFESTATIONS. Mutational heterogeneity and environmental factors appear responsible for highly variable involvement of the lung, pancreas, and other organs. A list of presenting manifestations is lengthy, although pulmonary and gastrointestinal presentations predominate (Table 416–2).

Respiratory Tract. Cough is the most constant symptom of pulmonary involvement. At first, the cough may be dry and hacking, but eventually it becomes loose and productive. In older patients, the cough is most prominent on arising in the morning or after activity. Expectorated mucus is usually purulent. Some patients remain asymptomatic for long periods or seem to have only prolonged acute respiratory infections. Others acquire a chronic cough within the first weeks of life or they repeatedly have pneumonia. Extensive bronchiolitis is attended by wheezing, which is a frequent symptom during the 1st years of life. As lung disease progresses, exercise intolerance, shortness of breath, and failure to gain weight or grow are noted. Exacerbations of lung symptoms eventually require hospitalization for effective treatment. Finally, cor pulmonale, respiratory failure, and death supervene. Colonization with *Burkholderia cepacia* may be associated with particularly rapid pulmonary deterioration and death.

TABLE 416–2 Presenting Features of More Than 20,000 Cystic Fibrosis Patients in the United States*

Feature	Percent
Acute or persistent respiratory symptoms	50.5
Failure to thrive, malnutrition	42.9
Abnormal stools	35.0
Meconium ileus, intestinal obstruction	18.8
Family history	16.8
Electrolyte, acid-base abnormality	5.4
Rectal prolapse	3.4
Nasal polyps, sinus disease	2.0
Hepatobiliary disease	0.9
Other†	1.0–2.0

**Data from the Patient Registry, Cystic Fibrosis Foundation, Bethesda, MD.*

†Includes pseudotumor cerebri, azoospermia, acrodermatitis-like rash, vitamin deficiency states, hypoproteinemic edema, hypoprothrombinemia with bleeding, meconium plug syndrome.

The rate of progression of lung disease is the chief determinant of morbidity and mortality. The course of lung disease, however, is largely independent of genotype. A few mutations (e.g., R117H) may substantially or even fully spare the lungs. Male gender and exocrine pancreatic sufficiency also are associated with a slower rate of pulmonary function decline. However, early insults to the lungs (e.g., severe viral infections) are likely to be the major determinant of pulmonary outcome.

Early physical findings include increased anteroposterior diameter of the chest, generalized hyperresonance, scattered or localized coarse crackles, and digital clubbing. Expiratory wheezes may be heard, especially in young children. Cyanosis is a late sign. Common pulmonary complications include atelectasis, hemoptysis, pneumothorax, and cor pulmonale and usually appear beyond the 1st decade of life.

Even though roentgenographically the paranasal sinuses are virtually always opacified, acute sinusitis is infrequent. Nasal obstruction and rhinorrhea are common, caused by inflamed, swollen mucous membranes or, in some cases, nasal polyposis. Nasal polyps are most troublesome between 5 and 20 yr of age.

Intestinal Tract. In 15–20% of newborn infants with CF, the ileum is completely obstructed by meconium (meconium ileus). The frequency is greater (~30%) among siblings born subsequent to a child with meconium ileus, reflecting a higher prevalence in certain genotypes. Abdominal distention, emesis, and failure to pass meconium appear within the first 24–48 hr of life (see Chapter 98.1). Abdominal roentgenograms (Fig. 416–3) show dilatated loops of bowel with air-fluid levels and frequently a collection of granular, "ground glass" material in the lower central abdomen. Rarely, meconium peritonitis results from intrauterine rupture of the bowel wall and can be detected roentgenographically by the presence of peritoneal or scrotal calcifications. Meconium plug syndrome occurs with increased frequency in infants with CF but is less specific than meconium ileus for this condition. Ileal obstruction with fecal material *(distal intestinal obstruction syndrome or meconium ileus equivalent)* occurs in older patients, causing cramping abdominal pain and abdominal distention.

More than 85% of affected children show evidence of maldigestion due to exocrine pancreatic insufficiency. Symptoms include frequent, bulky, greasy stools and failure to gain weight even when food intake appears to be large. Characteristically, stools contain readily visible droplets of fat. A protuberant abdomen, decreased muscle mass, poor growth, and delayed maturation are typical physical signs. Excessive flatus may be a problem. A number of mutations are associated with preservation of some exocrine pancreatic function, including R117H and 3849+10kbC→T. Individuals homozygous for ΔF508 virtually all have pancreatic insufficiency.

Less common gastrointestinal manifestations include intussusception, fecal impaction of the cecum with an asymptomatic right lower quadrant mass, and epigastric pain owing to duodenal inflammation. Acid or bile reflux with esophagitis symptoms is common in older children and adults. Subacute appendicitis and periappendiceal abscess have been encountered. Rectal prolapse is relatively frequent. Occasionally, hypoproteinemia with anasarca appears in malnourished infants, especially if children are fed soy-based preparations. Neurologic dysfunction (dementia, peripheral neuropathy) and hemolytic anemia may occur because of vitamin E deficiency. Deficiency of other fat-soluble vitamins is occasionally symptomatic. For example, hypoprothrombinemia owing to vitamin K deficiency may result in a bleeding diathesis. Clinical manifestations of other fat-soluble vitamin deficiencies, such as decreased bone density and night blindness, have been noted. Rickets is rare.

Biliary Tract. Biliary cirrhosis becomes symptomatic in only 2–3% of patients. Manifestations may include icterus, ascites, hematemesis from esophageal varices, and evidence of hypersplenism. A neonatal hepatitis-like picture and massive hepatomegaly owing to steatosis have been reported. Biliary colic

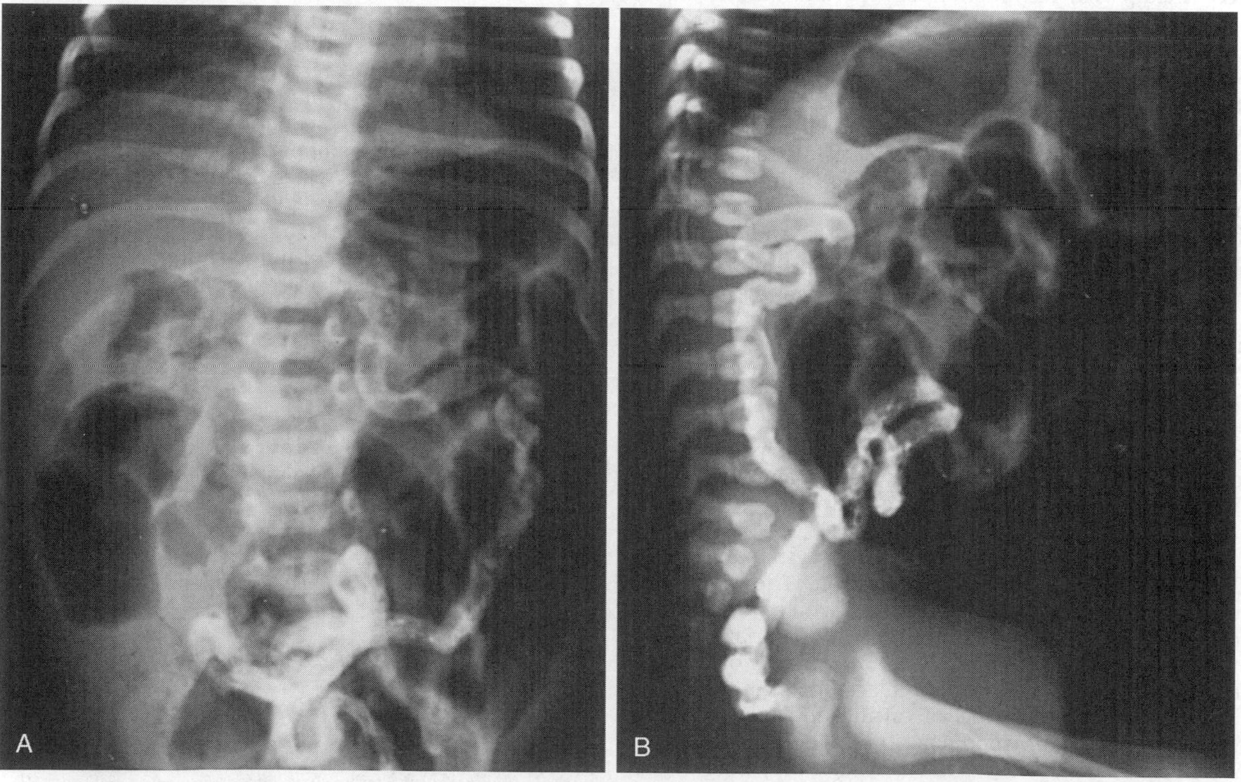

Figure 416–3 *A* and *B*, Contrast enema in a newborn infant with abdominal distention and failure to pass meconium. Notice the small diameter of the sigmoid and ascending colon and dilated, air-filled loops of small intestine. Several air-fluid levels in the small bowel are seen on the upright lateral view.

secondary to cholelithiasis may occur in the 2nd decade of life. Liver disease occurs independent of genotype.

Pancreas. In addition to exocrine pancreatic insufficiency, evidence for hyperglycemia and glycosuria including polyuria and weight loss may appear, especially after 10 yr of age when 8% of individuals acquire diabetes. In most cases, ketoacidosis does not occur, but eye, kidney, and other vascular complications have been noted in patients living 10 yr or more after the onset of hyperglycemia. Recurrent, acute pancreatitis occurs occasionally in individuals who have residual exocrine pancreatic function.

Genitourinary Tract. Sexual development is often delayed, but only by an average of 2 yr. More than 95% of males are azoospermic because of failure of development of wolffian duct structures, but sexual function is generally unimpaired. The incidence of inguinal hernia, hydrocele, and undescended testicle is higher than expected. Adolescent females may experience secondary amenorrhea, especially with exacerbations of pulmonary disease. Cervicitis and accumulation of tenacious mucus in the cervical canal have been noted. The female fertility rate is diminished. Pregnancy is generally tolerated well by women with good pulmonary function but may cause a progression of pulmonary disease and even death in those with moderate or advanced lung problems.

Sweat Glands. Excessive loss of salt in the sweat predisposes young children to salt depletion episodes, especially during the time of gastroenteritis and during warm weather. These children present with hypochloremic alkalosis. Frequently, parents notice salt "frosting" of the skin or a salty taste when they kiss the child. A few genotypes (e.g., 3849 + 10kbC>T) are associated with normal sweat chloride values.

DIAGNOSIS AND ASSESSMENT. The diagnosis of CF has been based for many years on a positive quantitative sweat test ($Cl^- \geq 60$ mEq/L) in conjunction with one or more of the following: typical chronic obstructive pulmonary disease, documented exocrine pancreatic insufficiency, or a positive family history. New diagnostic criteria have been recommended to include additional testing procedures (Table 416–3).

Sweat Testing. The sweat test, using pilocarpine iontophoresis to collect sweat and chemical analysis of its chloride content, remains the standard approach to diagnosis. The procedure requires care and accuracy. A 3 mA electric current is used to carry pilocarpine into the skin of the forearm and locally stimulate the sweat glands. After washing the arm with distilled water, sweat is collected on filter paper or gauze (or with a capillary tube) that has been placed on the stimulated skin and covered to prevent evaporation. After 30–60 min, the filter paper is removed, weighed, and eluted in distilled water. A chloridometer is recommended for the analysis of chloride in these samples. The amount of sweat collected should be measured and reported. For reliable results, at least 50 mg and preferably 100 mg of sweat should be collected. In infants, it may be necessary to use the upper back to obtain enough sweat. Reliable testing may be difficult in the first few weeks of life because of low sweat rates. Positive results should be confirmed; a negative result should be repeated if suspicion of the diagnosis remains.

TABLE 416–3 Diagnostic Criteria for Cystic Fibrosis

Presence of typical clinical features (respiratory, gastrointestinal, or genitourinary)

OR

A history of CF in a sibling

OR

A positive newborn screening test

PLUS

Laboratory evidence for CFTR dysfunction:

Two elevated sweat chloride concentrations obtained on separate days

OR

Identification of two CF mutations

OR

An abnormal nasal potential difference measurement

More than 60 mEq/L of chloride in sweat is diagnostic of CF when one or more other criteria are present. Threshold levels of 40 mEq/L for infants have been suggested. Values between 40 and 60 mEq/L suggest CF at all ages and have been reported in cases with typical involvement. In healthy adults, the sweat chloride values increase slightly, but a value of 60 mEq/L still adequately differentiates CF from other conditions. Chloride concentrations in sweat are somewhat lower in individuals who retain exocrine pancreatic function but remain within the diagnostic range. False-negative test results may be encountered in children with hypoproteinemic edema.

Non-CF conditions associated with elevated concentrations of sweat electrolytes include untreated adrenal insufficiency, ectodermal dysplasia, hereditary nephrogenic diabetes insipidus, glucose-6-phosphatase deficiency, hypothyroidism, hypoparathyroidism, familial cholestasis, pancreatitis, mucopolysaccharidoses, fucosidosis, and malnutrition. Most of these conditions can be easily distinguished from CF by clinical criteria.

Other Diagnostic Tests. The finding of increased potential differences across nasal epithelium, the loss of this difference with topical amiloride application, and the absence of a voltage response to a β-adrenergic agonist have been used to confirm the diagnosis in patients with equivocal or frankly normal sweat chloride values. Failure to sweat when a combination of isoproterenol and atropine is injected into the skin has also been used to characterize CF variants.

Pancreatic Function. Exocrine pancreatic dysfunction is clinically apparent in many patients. However, documentation is desirable if there are questions about the functional status of the pancreas. Measurement of fat balance with a 3-day stool collection or direct documentation of enzyme secretion after duodenal intubation and pancreozymin-secretin stimulation are reliable measures but are excessively cumbersome or invasive for children and are not used routinely. Quantitation of trypsin and chymotrypsin activity in a fresh stool sample is a useful screening test but is not definitive. Measurement of immunoreactive trypsinogen in serum reliably distinguishes patients with CF, with and without pancreatic insufficiency, after 7 yr of age but not before that time. Other indirect measures of pancreatic enzyme secretion are available but have limited or unproven clinical value. Endocrine pancreatic dysfunction may be more prevalent than previously recognized. Some have advocated yearly monitoring of glycosylated hemoglobin levels after 10 yr of age. This approach is more sensitive than spot checks of blood and urine glucose levels.

Radiology. Pulmonary radiologic findings suggest the diagnosis but are not specific. Hyperinflation of lungs occurs early and may be overlooked in the absence of infiltrates or streaky densities. Bronchial thickening and plugging and ring shadows suggesting bronchiectasis usually appear first in the upper lobes. Nodular densities, patchy atelectasis, and confluent infiltrates follow. Hilar lymph nodes may be prominent. With advanced disease, impressive hyperinflation with markedly depressed diaphragms, anterior bowing of the sternum, and a narrow cardiac shadow are noted. Cyst formation, extensive bronchiectasis, dilatated pulmonary artery segments, and segmental or lobar atelectasis are often apparent. Typical progression of lung disease is seen in Figure 416–4. Computed tomography of the chest can be used to detect and localize thickening of bronchial airway walls, mucus plugging, focal hyperinflation, and early bronchiectasis (Fig. 416–5). In general, computed tomography of the chest is not used for routine evaluation of chest disease.

Roentgenograms of paranasal sinuses reveal panopacification and often failure of frontal sinus development. Fetal ultrasonography may suggest ileal obstruction with meconium early

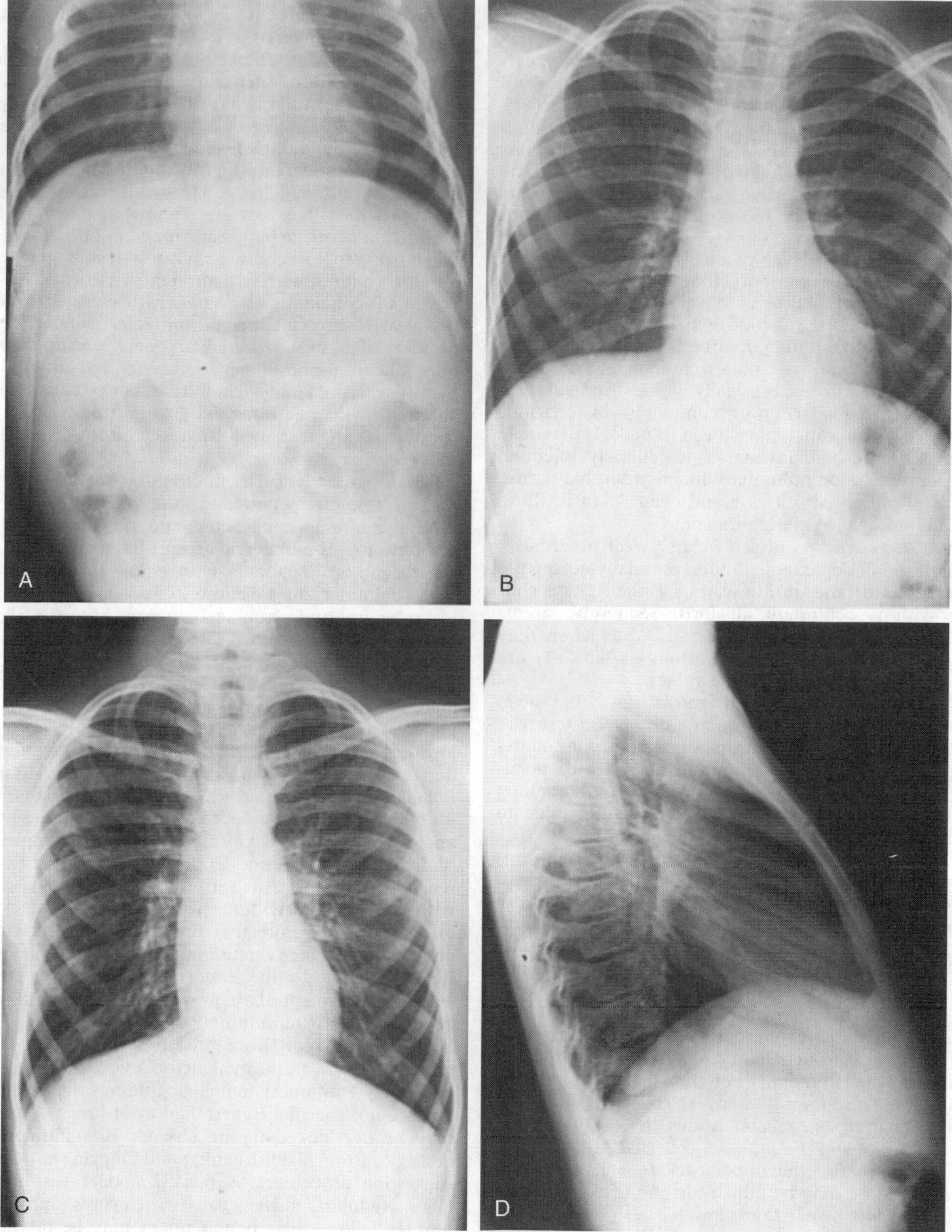

Figure 416–4 Roentgenographic progression of cystic fibrosis lung disease from the diagnosis in an infant to 17 yr of age. *A*, Admitted with cough and wheezing at 2 mo of age. Notice the mild increase in bronchovascular markings, especially in the upper lobe areas. *B*, At age 4 yr, cough was minimal. Bronchovascular markings were mildly increased, and there was some improvement in the upper lobes. The wheeze never recurred. *C* and *D*, At age 13 yr, there was minimal cough and occasional sputum production. The bronchovascular markings were generally further increased, with early bronchiectatic changes in the right upper lobe. The lateral view does not suggest overinflation.

in the 2nd trimester, but this finding is not predictive of meconium ileus at birth.

Pulmonary Function. Pulmonary function studies are not obtained until 5–6 yr of age, by which time most patients show the typical pattern of obstructive pulmonary involvement (see Chapters 375 and 377). Decrease in the midmaximal flow rate is an early functional change, reflecting small airways obstruction. This lesion also affects the distribution of ventilation and increases the alveolar-arterial oxygen difference. The findings of obstructive airway disease and modest responses to a bronchodilator are consistent with the diagnosis of CF at all ages. Residual volume and functional residual capacity are

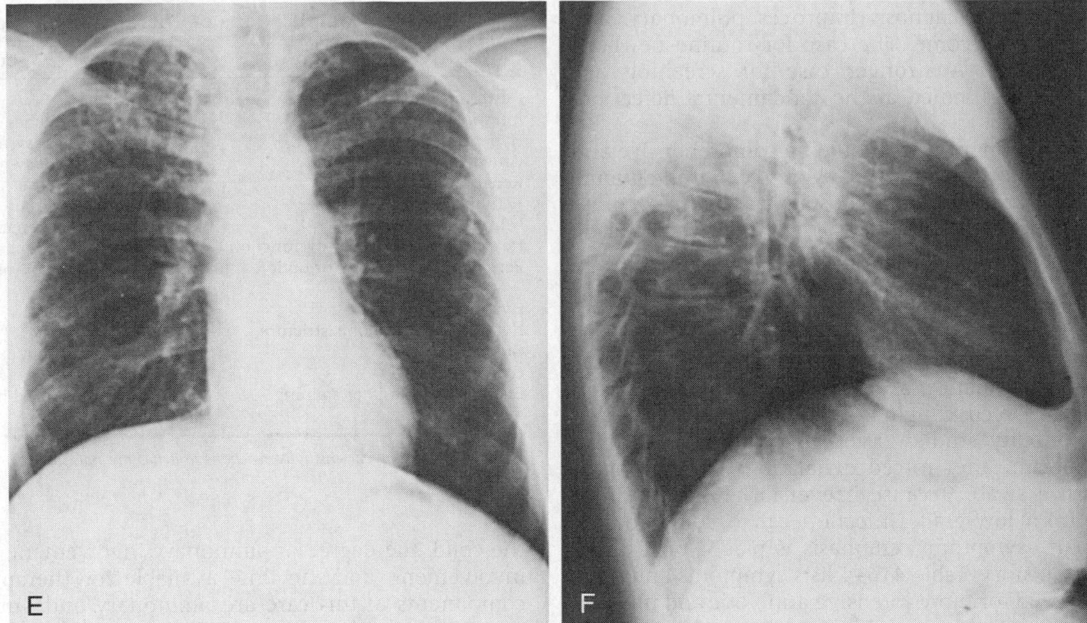

Figure 416–4 *Continued* *E* and *F*, Age 18 yr. During adolescence, cough and sputum production increased even though outpatient antibiotic therapy was intensified. Small-volume hemoptysis, occasional paroxysms of cough, and weight loss as well as increased nodular infiltrates (especially in the right upper lobe) and hyperinflation (as seen on the lateral view) led to the first hospitalization since infancy. Height and weight were maintained in the 25th–50th percentile.

increased early in the course of lung disease. Restrictive changes, characterized by declining total lung capacity and vital capacity, correlate with extensive lung injury and fibrosis and are a late finding. Testing several times a year can be used to evaluate the course of the pulmonary involvement. A few patients reach adolescent or adult life with normal pulmonary function and without evidence of overinflation.

Microbiologic Studies. The finding of *S. aureus* or *P. aeruginosa* on culture of the lower airways (e.g., sputum) strongly suggests a diagnosis of CF. In particular, mucoid forms of *Pseudomonas* are virtually diagnostic of CF in children. *B. cepacia* recovery also suggests CF.

Heterozygote Detection and Prenatal Diagnosis. Mutation analysis should be fully informative when testing potential carriers or a fetus provided that mutations within the family have been previously identified. Testing a spouse of a carrier with a standard panel of probes is approximately 90% sensitive. The rationale for prenatal detection of risk and termination of pregnancy is currently a matter of considerable discussion. A 1977 National Institutes of Health Consensus Conference recommendation to offer prenatal testing to all couples planning to have children as well as individuals with a family history of CF and partners of CF women has been reconsidered because of the medicolegal implications. In addition, termination of pregnancy is a less popular option because expected longevity is approximately 3 decades on average, with promise for an even better prognosis in the future.

Newborn Screening. Most newborns with CF can be identified by determination of immunoreactive trypsinogen in blood spots, coupled with confirmatory sweat or DNA testing. This screening test is at best only 95% sensitive. Although newborn diagnoses can prevent early nutritional deficiencies, there is

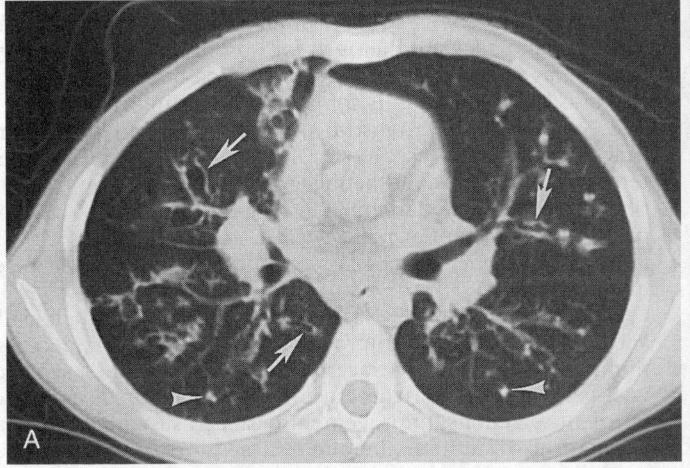

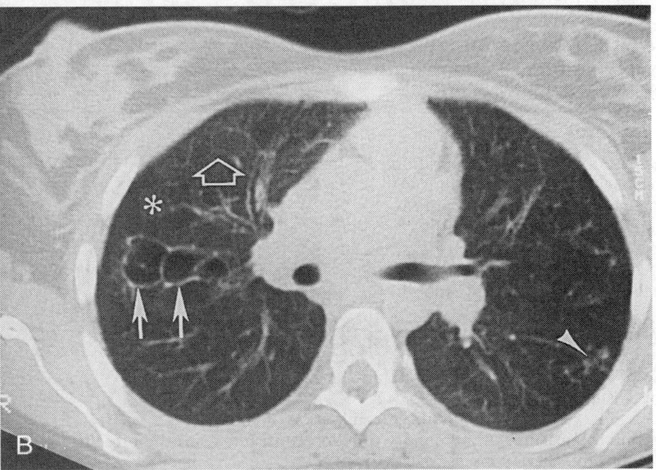

Figure 416–5 CT images of the chest in CF. *A*, A 12-yr-old boy with moderate lung disease. Airway and parenchymal changes are present throughout both lungs. Multiple areas of bronchiectasis (*arrows*) and mucous plugging (*arrowheads*) are seen. *B*, A 19-yr-old girl has mostly normal lung with one area of saccular bronchiectasis in the right upper lobe (*arrows*) and a focal area of peripheral mucous plugging in the right lower lobe (*arrowhead*). Lung density is heterogeneous with areas of normal lung (*open arrow*) and areas of low attenuation reflecting segmental and subsegmental air trapping (*asterisk*).

no evidence that early diagnosis improves pulmonary, and therefore long-term, outcome. The case for routine newborn screening is debatable. A stronger case for screening will emerge when therapies aimed at the fundamental defect are available.

TREATMENT. The treatment plan should be comprehensive and linked to close monitoring and early, aggressive intervention.

General Approach to Care. A period of hospitalization for accurate diagnosis, baseline assessment, initiation of treatment, clearing of pulmonary involvement, and education of the patient and parents is recommended. Follow-up outpatient visits are scheduled every 2–3 mo because many aspects of the condition require careful monitoring. An interval history and physical examination should be obtained at each visit. A sputum sample or, if that is not available, a lower pharyngeal swab taken during or after a forced cough is obtained for culture and antibiotic susceptibility studies. Even asymptomatic patients may produce sputum after forced exhalations or pharyngeal stimulation with a swab. Because irreversible loss of pulmonary function from low-grade infection can occur gradually and without acute symptoms, emphasis is placed on a thorough pulmonary history. Table 416–4 lists symptoms and signs that suggest the need for more intensive antibiotic and physical therapy. Immunoprophylaxis specifically against rubeola, pertussis, and influenza is essential. A nurse, respiratory therapist, social worker, dietitian, and psychologist should participate in the care program as needed. Considerable education and encouragement are required if the patient and parent are to maintain an adequate level of home care.

Because secretions of CF patients are not adequately hydrated, attention in early childhood to oral hydration, especially during warm weather or with acute gastroenteritis, may prevent exacerbation of problems with clearance of mucus from airways. For the same reason, intravenous therapy for dehydration should be initiated early.

The goal of therapy is to maintain a stable condition for prolonged periods. This can be accomplished for most patients by interval evaluation and adjustments of the home treatment program. However, some children have episodic acute or low-grade chronic lung infection that progresses. For these patients, 2 wk or more of intensive inhalation and physical therapy and intravenous antibiotics is indicated. Intravenous antibiotics may be required infrequently or as often as every 2–3 mo. Significant improvement in pulmonary function and the child's well-being is usually achieved.

The basic daily care program varies depending on the age of the child, the degree of pulmonary involvement, other system involvement, and the time available for therapy. The major components of this care are pulmonary and nutritional therapy. Because therapy is medication-intensive, iatrogenic problems arise frequently. Monitoring for these complications is also an important part of management (Table 416–5).

TABLE 416–4 Symptoms and Signs Associated with Exacerbation of Pulmonary Infection in Patients with Cystic Fibrosis

Symptoms

Increased frequency and duration of cough
Increased sputum production
Change in appearance of sputum
Increased shortness of breath
Decreased exercise tolerance
Decreased appetite
Feeling of increased congestion in the chest

Signs

Increased respiratory rate
Use of accessory muscles for breathing
Intercostal retractions
Change in results of auscultatory examination of chest
Decline in measures of pulmonary function consistent with the presence of obstructive airway disease
Fever and leukocytosis
Weight loss
New infiltrate on chest radiograph

From Ramsey B: Management of pulmonary disease in patients with cystic fibrosis. N Engl J Med 335:179, 1996.

TABLE 416–5 Complications of Therapy for Cystic Fibrosis

Complication	Agent
Gastrointestinal bleeding	Ibuprofen
Intestinal obstruction	High-dose enzymes
Hyperglycemia	Corticosteroids (systemic)
Growth retardation	Corticosteroids (systemic, inhaled)
Renal dysfunction	
Tubular	Aminoglycosides
Interstitial nephritis	Semisynthetic penicillins
Hearing loss, vestibular dysfunction	Aminoglycosides
Peripheral neuropathy or optic atrophy, or both	Chloramphenicol (prolonged course)
Hypomagnesemia	Aminoglycosides
Hyperuricemia, colonic stricture	Pancreatic extracts (very large doses)
Goiter	Iodine-containing expectorants
Gynecomastia	Spironolactone
Enamel hypoplasia or staining	Tetracyclines (used in first 8 yr of life)

Note: Common hypersensitivity reactions to drugs are not included.

Pulmonary Therapy. The object is to clear secretions from airways and to control infection. There is a divergence of opinion about specific aspects of therapy. However, the effectiveness of the overall approach, including close supervision, continuity of care, aggressive intervention, and an optimistic outlook, is more important than minor variations in the use of individual measures. When a child is not doing well, every potentially useful aspect of therapy should be considered.

Inhalation Therapy. Aerosol therapy is used to deliver medications and water to the lower respiratory tract, usually before or after segmental postural drainage. Some agents such as bronchodilators can be delivered by metered-dose inhaler with or without a spacer. The mainstay is intermittent delivery using a small compressor that drives a hand-held nebulizer. The basic aerosol solution is 0.45–0.9% saline. In patients with reactive airways, albuterol or other β-agonists can be added. Alternatively, or in addition, cromolyn sodium can be administered by this route. β-Agonists may decrease Pao_2 by increasing ventilation-perfusion mismatch, which is not a problem unless the Pao_2 is marginal.

When the airway pathogens are resistant to oral antibiotics or when the infection is difficult to control at home, aerosolized antibiotics may reduce symptoms, improve pulmonary function, and alleviate the need for hospitalization. Aminoglycosides have been used up to four times daily in home therapy and also in the hospital in conjunction with intravenous therapy. Studies have demonstrated improvement of pulmonary function with large doses of tobramycin, 600 mg/dose administered with an ultrasonic nebulizer or 300 mg bid by conventional nebulization. Carbenicillin (1 g), ticarcillin (0.5 g), and colistin (20–40 mg) have also been used. Sensitization or resistance to antibiotics may occur, but both are surprisingly infrequent.

Human recombinant DNase (2.5 mg), given as a single daily aerosol dose appears to improve pulmonary function, decrease numbers of pulmonary exacerbations, and promote a sense of well-being in patients who have mild to moderate disease and purulent secretions. Improvement has been sustained for 6 mo or more of continuous therapy. Efficacy for patients with severe disease, (e.g., forced vital capacity <40% of predicted) has been difficult to document. Another mucolytic agent, *N*-acetylcysteine, is toxic to ciliated epithelium, and repeated administration should be avoided.

Chest Physical Therapy. This treatment usually consists of chest percussion combined with postural drainage and derives its rationale from the idea that cough clears mucus from large airways, but chest vibrations are required to move secretions from small airways where expiratory flow rates are low. Chest physical therapy (PT) may be particularly useful for patients with CF because they accumulate secretions in small airways first, even before the onset of symptoms. Improvement of pulmonary function generally cannot be demonstrated immediately after this therapy. However, cessation of chest PT in older children with mild to moderate air flow limitation results in deterioration of lung function within 3 wk and prompt improvement of function when therapy is resumed. Chest PT is recommended one to four times a day, depending on the severity of lung dysfunction. Cough or forced expirations are encouraged after each lung segment is "drained." Mechanical percussors have been designed to assist with therapy and may be useful, especially for adolescents. Voluntary coughing, repeated forced expiratory maneuvers with and without positive expiratory pressure, patterned breathing, use of a hand-held flutter device, and vigorous exercise have all been suggested as additional aids to clearance of mucus.

Antibiotic Therapy. Antibiotics are the mainstay of therapy designed to control progression of lung infection. The goal is to reduce the intensity of endobronchial infection and to delay progressive lung damage. The usual guidelines for acute chest infections, such as fever, tachypnea, or chest pain, are often absent. Consequently, all aspects of the patient's history and examination, including anorexia, weight loss, and diminished activity, must be used to guide the frequency and duration of therapy. Antibiotic treatment varies from intermittent short courses of one antibiotic to continuous treatment with one or more antibiotics. Dosages are often two to three times the amount recommended for minor infections because patients with CF have proportionately more lean body mass and higher clearance rates for many antibiotics than do other individuals. Also, it is difficult to achieve effective drug levels of many antimicrobials in respiratory tract secretions.

ORAL ANTIBIOTIC THERAPY. Indications include the presence of respiratory tract symptoms and identification of pathogenic organisms in respiratory tract cultures. Whenever possible, the choice of antibiotics should be guided by in vitro sensitivity testing. Common organisms include *S. aureus*, nontypeable *Haemophilus influenzae*, and *P. aeruginosa*. *B. cepacia* is encountered with increasing frequency. The first two can be eradicated from the respiratory tract in CF, but *Pseudomonas* is more difficult to treat and rarely is eradicated. The usual course of therapy is 2 wk or more, and maximal doses are recommended. Low-dose, continuous antibiotic therapy is not recommended because organisms tend to develop resistance. Useful oral antibiotics are listed in Table 416–6. Use of tetracycline should be avoided in children younger than 9 yr of age. The quinolones are the only broadly effective oral antibiotics for *Pseudomonas* infection, but resistance emerges rapidly. Infection with mycoplasmal or chlamydial organisms has been documented, providing a rationale for the use of macrolides on an empirical basis for flare of symptoms.

INTRAVENOUS ANTIBIOTIC THERAPY. For the patient who has progressive or unrelenting symptoms and signs despite intensive home measures, intravenous antibiotic therapy is indicated. This therapy is usually initiated in the hospital, but often is completed on an ambulatory basis. Although many patients improve within 7 days, it is usually advisable to extend the period of treatment to at least 14 days. Permanent intravenous access can now be provided for long-term therapy in the hospital or at home.

Intravenous antibiotics commonly used are listed in Table 416–6. In general, treatment of *Pseudomonas* infection requires two-drug therapy. A third agent may be required for optimal *S. aureus* coverage. Simultaneous administration of aerosolized antimicrobial agents can increase endobronchial concentrations. The aminoglycosides have a relatively short half-life in many patients with CF. The initial parenteral dose, noted in Table 416–6, is generally given every 8 hr. After blood levels have been determined, the total daily dose should be adjusted. Peak levels of 10 mg/L are desirable, and trough levels should be kept at less than 2 mg/L to minimize the risk of ototoxicity and nephrotoxicity. Once or twice a day aminoglycoside dosing may have advantages over every 8 hr dosing. Changes in therapy should be guided by culture results and by lack of improvement. If patients do not improve, heart failure, reactive airways, and infection with viruses, *Aspergillus fumigatus*, mycobacteria, or other unusual organisms should be consid-

TABLE 416–6 Antimicrobial Agents for Cystic Fibrosis Lung Infection

Route	Organisms	Agents	Dosage (mg/kg/24 hr)	Doses/24 hr
Oral	*Staphylococcus aureus*	Dicloxacillin	25–50	4
		Cephalexin	50	4
		Clindamycin	20	3–4
		Amoxicillin-clavulanate	40	3
	Haemophilus influenzae	Amoxicillin	50–100	3
		Trimethoprim-sulfamethoxazole	20*	2–4
	Pseudomonas aeruginosa	Ciprofloxacin	15–30	2–3
	Empirical	Tetracycline	50–100	3–4
		Erythromycin	50–100	3–4
Intravenous	*S. aureus*	Nafcillin	100–200	4–6
		Vancomycin	40	4
	P aeruginosa	Tobramycin	8–20	1–3
		Amikacin	15–30	2–3
		Netilmicin	6–12	2–3
		Carbenicillin	400	4
		Ticarcillin	400	4
		Piperacillin	300	4
		Ticarcillin-clavulanate	400†	4
		Imipenem-cilastatin	45–90	3–4
		Ceftazidime	150	3
		Aztreonam	150	4
Aerosol	*Burkholderia cepacia*	Chloramphenicol	50–100	4
		Trimethoprim-sulfamethoxazole	20*	4

*Quantity of trimethoprim.
†Quantity of ticarcillin.*

ered. *B. cepacia* may be particularly refractory to antimicrobial therapy.

Bronchodilator Therapy. Reversible airway obstruction occurs in many children with CF, sometimes in conjunction with frank asthma or acute bronchopulmonary aspergillosis. Reversible obstruction is suggested by improvement of 15% or more in flow rates after inhalation of a bronchodilator. Treatment may include use of β-adrenergic agonists by aerosol. Cromolyn sodium or ipratropium hydrochloride are alternative agents, but their efficacy has not been studied systematically.

Anti-inflammatory Agents. Corticosteroids are useful for the treatment of allergic bronchopulmonary aspergillosis and other severe reactive airways disease occasionally encountered in children with CF. Prolonged treatment of standard CF lung disease using an alternate-day regimen initially appeared to improve pulmonary function and diminish hospitalization rates. However, a 4-yr double-blind, multicenter study of this regimen for patients with mild to moderate lung disease found only modest efficacy and prohibitive side effects, including growth retardation, cataracts, and abnormalities of glucose tolerance at a dose of 2 mg/kg and growth retardation at 1 mg/kg. Inhaled corticosteroids have theoretical appeal, but they also slow growth because of systemic absorption. Ibuprofen, given chronically (dose adjusted to achieve a peak serum concentration of 50–100 mg/mL) over 4 yr, is associated with an impressive slowing of disease progression, particularly in younger patients with mild lung disease. Side effects of nonsteroidal antiiflammatory drugs have been encountered infrequently.

Endoscopy and Lavage. Treatment of obstructed airways sometimes includes tracheobronchial suctioning or lavage, especially if atelectasis or mucoid impaction is present. Bronchopulmonary lavage may be performed by the instillation of saline or by a mucolytic agent through a fiberoptic bronchoscope. Antibiotics (usually gentamicin or tobramycin) may also be instilled directly at lavage, transiently achieving a much higher endobronchial concentration than can be obtained by using intravenous therapy. There is no evidence for sustained benefit from repeated endoscopic or lavage procedures.

Expectorants. Systemic drugs, such as iodides and guaiphenesin, do not effectively assist with the removal of secretions from the respiratory tract.

Treatment of Pulmonary Complications. A number of pulmonary complications require extra attention or special measures.

Atelectasis. Lobar atelectasis occurs relatively infrequently; it may be asymptomatic and noted only at the time of a routine chest roentgenogram. Aggressive intravenous therapy with antibiotics and increased chest PT directed at the affected lobe may be effective. If there is no improvement in 5–7 days, bronchoscopic examination of the airways may be indicated. If the atelectasis does not resolve, continued intensive home therapy is indicated, since atelectasis may resolve during a period of weeks or months. Persistent atelectasis may be asymptomatic. Lobectomy should be considered only if expansion is not achieved and the patient has progressive difficulty from fever, anorexia, and unrelenting cough (see Chapter 406).

Hemoptysis. Endobronchial bleeding usually reflects airway wall erosion secondary to infection. With increasing numbers of older patients, hemoptysis has become a relatively frequent complication. Blood streaking of sputum is particularly common. Small volume hemoptysis (<20 mL) should not trigger panic and is usually viewed as a need for intensified antimicrobial and chest PT. When the hemoptysis is persistent or increases in severity, hospital admission is indicated. Massive hemoptysis, defined as total blood loss of 250 mL or more within a 24-hr period, is rare in the first decade and occurs in less than 1% of adolescents, but requires close monitoring and the capability to replace blood losses rapidly. Chest PT is often discontinued until 12–24 hr after the last brisk bleeding episode and is then reinstituted gradually. Patients should receive vitamin K for an abnormal prothrombin time. During brisk hemoptysis, the child and parents require a great deal of reassurance that the bleeding will stop. Blood transfusion is not indicated unless there is hypotension or the hematocrit is significantly reduced. Ticarcillin may interfere with platelet function and aggravate hemoptysis. Bronchoscopy has been used in an effort to localize the site of bleeding. However, usually no bleeding site is found. Lobectomy should be avoided, if possible, because functioning lung should be preserved and because it is difficult to be certain of the bleeding site. Bronchial artery embolization can be useful to control persistent, significant hemoptysis.

Pneumothorax. Pneumothorax (also see Chapter 419) is encountered in less than 1% of children and teenagers, but it is more frequently encountered in older patients and may be life-threatening. The episode may be asymptomatic but is often attended by chest and shoulder pain, shortness of breath, or hemoptysis. If the pneumothorax is smaller than 5–10%, the patient is admitted to the hospital and observed. A pneumothorax greater than 10% or under tension requires rapid, definitive treatment. Because of frequent delayed closure of the air leak and a high rate of recurrence with closed thoracotomy, an open thoracotomy through a small incision with plication of blebs, apical pleural stripping, and basal pleural abrasion is recommended after the first occurrence and within 24 hr of the diagnosis. This procedure is well tolerated even in cases of advanced lung disease. Intravenous antibiotics are begun on admission. The thoracotomy tube is removed as soon as possible, usually on the 2nd or 3rd postoperative day. The patient can then be mobilized and full postural drainage therapy resumed. Recurrences, intraoperative complications, and deaths are rare as a result of this procedure. Closed thoracotomy in conjunction with a sclerosing agent is an alternative approach. Rarely, bilateral simultaneous pneumothorax is encountered; in this case, control of the air leak must be achieved immediately, at least on one side.

Allergic Aspergillosis. This complication may present with wheezing, increased cough, shortness of breath, or marked hyperinflation (see Chapters 233 and 397). In some patients there are new, focal infiltrates on the chest roentgenogram. The presence of rust-colored sputum, the recovery of *Aspergillus* organisms from the sputum, the demonstration of serum antibodies against *A. fumigatus*, or the presence of eosinophils in a fresh sputum sample support the diagnosis. The serum IgE level may be high. Treatment is directed at controlling the inflammatory reaction with corticosteroids. For refractory cases, aerosolized amphotericin B or systemic itraconazole may be required.

Hypertrophic Osteoarthropathy. This complication causes elevation of the periosteum over the distal portions of long bones and bone pain, overlying edema, and joint effusions. Acetaminophen or ibuprofen may provide relief. Control of lung infection usually reduces symptoms. Intermittent arthropathy unrelated to other rheumatologic disorders occurs occasionally, has no recognized pathogenesis, and usually responds to nonsteroidal anti-inflammatory agents.

Acute Respiratory Failure. Acute respiratory failure (see Chapters 64.3 and 375.1) in patients with mild to moderate lung disease rarely occurs and is usually the result of a severe viral illness such as influenza. Because patients with this complication can regain their previous status, intensive therapy is indicated. In addition to aerosol, postural drainage, and intravenous antibiotic treatment, oxygen is required to raise the arterial P_{O_2} to greater than 50 mm Hg. A rising P_{CO_2} may require ventilatory assistance. Endotracheal or bronchoscopic suction may be necessary and can be repeated daily. Right-sided heart failure may occur and should be treated vigorously. Recovery is often slow. Intensive intravenous antibiotic therapy and postural drainage should be continued for 1–2 wk after the patient has regained baseline status.

Chronic Respiratory Failure. Patients eventually acquire chronic respiratory failure from slow deterioration of lung function. Although this can occur at any age, it is seen most frequently in adult patients. Because a long-standing arterial Pao_2 less than 50 mm Hg promotes the development of right-sided heart failure, they usually benefit from low-flow oxygen to raise arterial Po_2 to 55 mm Hg or greater. Increasing hypercapnia may prevent the use of optimal Fio_2. These patients do not benefit substantially from continuous ventilator assistance or tracheostomy. Most patients improve somewhat with intensive antibiotic and pulmonary therapy measures and can be discharged from the hospital. Low-flow oxygen therapy at home is needed, especially with sleep. These patients almost always display cor pulmonale and should be maintained on a reduced salt intake and diuretics. Caution should be exercised to avoid alkalosis that results from diuretic-induced bicarbonate retention. Chronic pain (headache, chest pain, abdominal pain, and limb pain) are frequent at the end of life and respond to judicious use of analgesics, including opioids.

Lung transplantation is an option for increasing numbers of individuals with end-stage lung disease (see Chapter 449.2). Criteria for referral include an FEV1 <30% predicted. Fifty per cent are now surviving 5 yr or more, and lung function as well as quality of life generally improve remarkably. Because of bronchiolitis obliterans and other complications, transplanted lungs cannot be expected to function for the lifetime of a recipient. Individuals with chronic respiratory failure who are on a lung transplant waiting list may be candidates for ventilatory assistance. To date, the demand for donor lungs exceeds the supply and waiting lists continue to grow.

Right-Sided Heart Failure. Some patients experience reversible right-sided heart failure (see Chapter 375.1) as the result of an acute event such as an viral infection or pneumothorax. Individuals with long-standing, advanced pulmonary disease, especially those with severe hypoxemia (Pao_2 <50 mm Hg), often acquire chronic right-sided heart failure. The mechanisms include hypoxemic pulmonary arterial constriction and loss of the pulmonary vascular bed. Pulmonary artery wall changes contribute to increased vascular resistance with time. Cyanosis, increased shortness of breath, increased liver size with a tender margin, ankle edema, jugular venous distention, an unusual weight gain, increased heart size seen on chest roentgenogram, or evidence for right-sided heart enlargement seen on electrocardiogram or echocardiogram help to confirm the diagnosis. Furosemide (1 mg/kg administered intravenously) may result in a good diuresis and confirm the suspicion of fluid retention. Repeated doses are often required at 24–48 hr intervals to reduce fluid accumulation and accompanying symptoms. Concomitant use of spironolactone may protect against potassium depletion and facilitate long-term diuresis. Hypochloremic alkalosis may complicate the chronic use of loop diuretics. Digitalis is not effective in pure right-sided failure, but it may be useful when there is an associated left-sided dysfunction. The arterial Po_2 should be maintained at greater than 50 mm Hg if at all possible. Intensive pulmonary therapy including intravenous antibiotics is most important. Initially, the salt intake should be limited to 2 g sodium/24 hr. Fluid overload and antibiotics with high sodium content should be avoided. No clear-cut long-term benefit from pulmonary vasodilators has been demonstrated. In the past, heart failure usually meant death within several months. However, the prognosis has been improving, and a number of patients survive for 5 yr or more after the appearance of heart failure. Lung transplantation is the best option for reversal (see Chapter 449.2).

Nutritional Therapy. Up to 90% of patients have complete loss of exocrine pancreatic function and inadequate digestion of fats and proteins. They require diet adjustment, pancreatic enzyme replacement, and supplementary vitamins.

Diet. Many infants at the time of diagnosis have nutritional deficits. Young infants who present with wheezy breathing and are fed soy protein formulas do not use this protein well and may acquire hypoproteinemia with anasarca. Infants do not routinely need formulas containing predigested protein and medium-chain triglycerides. A low-fat, high-protein, high-calorie diet was generally recommended in the past for older children. Some children on this diet are deficient in essential fatty acids. With the advent of improved pancreatic enzyme products, normal amounts of fat in the diet are usually tolerated and preferred. Not infrequently, parent-child interactions at feeding time are maladaptive, and behavioral interventions can improve caloric intake.

Most individuals have a higher than normal caloric need because of increased work of breathing and perhaps because of increased metabolic activity related to the basic defect. When anorexia of chronic infection supervenes, weight loss occurs. Further encouragement to eat high-calorie foods may be useful, but weight gain generally is not realized unless lung infection is controlled. With advanced lung disease, weight stabilization or gain has been achieved by nocturnal feeding via nasogastric tube or percutaneous enterostomy or by intravenous hyperalimentation. Long-term benefits of these interventions for lung function, quality of life, and psychologic well-being are less clearly substantiated.

Pancreatic Enzyme Replacement. Extracts of animal pancreas given with ingested food reduce but do not fully correct stool fat and nitrogen losses. Enzyme dosage and product should be individualized for each patient. Enteric-coated, pH-sensitive enzyme microspheres are most often prescribed. Several strengths, up to 20,000 IU of lipase units/capsule are available. Administration of large doses has been linked to colonic strictures requiring surgery. Consequently, enzyme replacement should not exceed 10,000 lipase units/kg/24 hr. One to three capsules/meal is sufficient for most patients; infants may need only one-half capsule or may prefer pancreatin powder. Snacks should be covered. The microsphere preparations usually are sufficiently effective to permit a liberal diet, which may include homogenized milk. Although children with CF display bile salt malabsorption, enzyme preparations containing bile salts are infrequently needed. The dose of enzymes required usually increases with age, but some teenagers and young adults may later have a decrease in their requirement.

Vitamin and Mineral Supplements. Because pancreatic insufficiency results in malabsorption of fat-soluble vitamins (A, D, E, and K), vitamin supplementation is recommended. Capsules containing adequate amounts of all four vitamins for CF patients are now available. Infants with zinc deficiency and rash have been reported. In addition, attention should be paid to iron status; in one study almost one third of children with CF had a low serum ferritin concentration.

Treatment of Intestinal Complications

Meconium Ileus. When meconium ileus (see Chapter 98.1) is suspected, a nasogastric tube is placed for suction, and the infant is hydrated. In some cases diatrizoate (Gastrografin) enemas with reflux of contrast material into the ileum have resulted in the passage of a meconium plug and clearing of the obstruction. Use of this hypertonic solution requires careful replacement of water losses into the bowel. Children in whom this procedure fails require operative intervention. Children who are successfully treated generally have a prognosis similar to that of other patients. Infants with meconium ileus should be treated as having CF until adequate sweat testing can be carried out.

Distal Intestinal Obstruction Syndrome (Meconium Ileus Equivalent) and Other Causes of Abdominal Pain. Despite appropriate pancreatic enzyme replacement, 2–5% of patients accumulate fecal material in the terminal portion of the ileum and in the cecum, which may result in partial or complete obstruction. For intermittent symptoms, pancreatic enzyme replacement should be continued or even increased and laxatives or stool softeners (milk of magnesia, docusate sodium [Colace], mineral oil) given. Increased fluid intake is also recommended. Failure to relieve symptoms signals the need for large-volume bowel lavage with a balanced salt solution containing polyethyleneglycol taken by mouth or by nasogastric tube. When there is complete obstruction, a diatrizoate enema, accompanied by large amounts of intravenous fluids, can be therapeutic. Intussusception, and volvulus must also be considered in the differential diagnosis. Intussusception, usually ileocolic, occurs at any age and often follows a 1–2 day history of "constipation." It can often be diagnosed and reduced by a diatrizoate enema. If a nonreducible intussusception or a volvulus is present, laparotomy is required. Repeated episodes of intussusception may be an indication for cecectomy.

Chronic appendicitis with or without periappendiceal abscess may present with recurrent or persistent abdominal pain, raising the question of need for a laparotomy. A lack of acid buffering in the duodenum appears to promote duodenitis and ulcer formation in some children. Bile reflux is seen in older patients.

Gastroesophageal Reflux. Because several factors raise intra-abdominal pressure, including cough and obstructed airways, pathologic gastroesophageal reflux is not uncommon and may exacerbate lung disease secondary to reflex wheezing and repeated aspiration. Dietary, positional, and medication therapy should be considered. Cholinergic agonists are contraindicated because they trigger mucus secretion and progressive respiratory difficulty. Reduction of stomach acid secretion can help, omeprazole being the most effective agent. Fundoplication is a procedure of last resort.

Rectal Prolapse. This occurs frequently in infants with CF and less commonly in older children. It is usually related to steatorrhea, malnutrition, and repetitive cough. The prolapsed rectum can usually be replaced manually by continuous gentle pressure with the patient in the knee-chest position. Sedation may be helpful. To prevent an immediate recurrence, the buttocks can be taped closed. Adequate pancreatic enzyme replacement, decreased fat and roughage in the diet, and control of pulmonary infection result in improvement. An occasional patient may continue to have rectal prolapse and require surgery.

Liver Disease. Liver function abnormalities associated with biliary cirrhosis can be improved by treatment with ursodeoxycholic acid. The ability of bile acids to prevent progression of cirrhosis has not been clearly documented. Portal hypertension with esophageal varices, hypersplenism, or ascites occurs in 2% or fewer of children with CF (see Chapter 366). The acute management of bleeding esophageal varices includes nasogastric suction and cold saline lavage. Sclerotherapy is recommended after an initial bleed. In the past, significant bleeding has also been treated successfully with portosystemic shunting. Splenorenal anastomosis has been the most effective. Pronounced hypersplenism may require splenectomy. The management of ascites is discussed in Chapter 369.

Obstructive jaundice in newborns with CF requires no specific therapy. Hepatomegaly with steatosis requires careful attention to nutrition and may respond to carnitine repletion. Rarely, biliary cirrhosis proceeds to hepatocellular failure, which should be treated as in other patients with hepatic failure (see Chapters 363 and 366). End-stage liver disease is an indication for liver transplantation in children with CF, especially if pulmonary function is good.

Pancreatitis. Pancreatitis may be precipitated by fatty meals, alcohol ingestion, or tetracycline therapy. Serum amylase and lipase levels may remain elevated for long periods. Treatment is discussed in Chapter 351.

Hyperglycemia. Onset occurs most frequently after the 1st decade; ketoacidosis is rarely encountered. The pathogenesis includes both impaired insulin secretion and insulin resistance. Glucose intolerance without urine glucose losses is usually not treated; glycosylated hemoglobin levels should be followed at least annually. With persistent glycosuria and symptoms, insulin treatment should be instituted. Oral hypoglycemic agents, with or without drugs that reduce insulin resistance, may be effective. Exocrine pancreatic insufficiency and malabsorption make strict dietary control of hyperglycemia difficult. The development of significant hyperglycemia may adversely affect prognosis.

Other Therapy

Nasal Polyps. Nasal polyps (see Chapter 380) occur in 15–20% of patients with CF and are most prevalent in the 2nd decade of life. Local corticosteroids and nasal decongestants occasionally provide some relief. When the polyps completely obstruct the nasal airway, rhinorrhea becomes constant, or widening of the nasal bridge is noticed, surgical removal is indicated; polyps may recur promptly or following a symptom-free interval of months to years. Polyps inexplicably stop developing in many adults.

Salt Depletion. Sweat salt losses can be high, especially in warm arid climates. Children should have free access to salt, and precautions against overdressing infants should be observed. Regimented salt supplements are no longer prescribed. Hypochloremic alkalosis should be suspected in any infant who has had gastroenteritis symptoms, and prompt fluid and electrolyte therapy should be instituted as needed.

Maturation. Delayed sexual maturation, often associated with short stature, occurs fairly frequently. Although many have severe pulmonary infection or poor nutrition, delayed puberty also occurs in patients with otherwise mild disease and is not well explained. Adolescents with CF should receive specific counseling through their developing years concerning sexual maturation and reproductive potential.

Surgery. Minor surgical procedures, including dental work, should be performed under local anesthesia if possible. Patients with good or excellent pulmonary status can tolerate general anesthesia without any intensive pulmonary measures prior to the surgery. Those with moderate or severe pulmonary infection are usually better off with a 1–2 wk course of intensive antibiotic treatment before surgery. If this is impossible, prompt intravenous antibiotic therapy is indicated once it is recognized that major surgery is required. The total time of anesthesia should be kept to a minimum. After induction, tracheal suctioning is useful and should be repeated at least at the end of the operation. Patients with severe disease require monitoring of their blood gases and may require ventilatory assistance in the immediate postoperative period.

After major surgery, cough should be encouraged and postural drainage treatments should be reinstituted as soon as possible, usually within 24 hr. Adequate analgesia is important if early effective therapy is to be achieved. For those with significant pulmonary involvement, intravenous antibiotics are continued for 7–14 postoperative days. Early ambulation and intermittent deep breathing are important; an incentive spirometer can also be helpful. After open thoracotomy for treatment of pneumothorax or lobectomy, the chest tube is the greatest single obstacle to effective pulmonary therapy and should be removed as soon as possible so that full postural drainage therapy can resume.

New Therapies. Several innovative therapies are under investigation. Approaches include stimulation of alternative chloride transport mechanisms, pharmacologic upregulation of mutated CFTR, and gene therapy. Earlier and more effective control of airways infection and inflammation is another experimental therapeutic goal.

PROGNOSIS. CF remains a life-limiting disorder, although survival has improved dramatically during the last 30–40 yr. Infants with severe lung disease occasionally succumb, but most children survive this difficult period and are relatively healthy into adolescence or adulthood. However, the slow progression of lung disease eventually reaches disabling proportions. Life table data now indicate a median cumulative survival of 30 yr.

Male survival is somewhat better than female survival for reasons that are not readily apparent.

For the most part, children with CF have good school attendance records and do not need to be restricted in their activities. A high percentage eventually attend and graduate from college. Most find satisfactory employment, and an increasing number marry.

With increasing life span, a new set of psychosocial considerations has emerged, including dependence-independence issues, self-care, peer relationships, sexuality, sterility, substance abuse, educational and vocational planning, financial burdens, and anxiety concerning health and prognosis. Many of these issues are best addressed in an anticipatory fashion, prior to the onset of psychosocial dysfunction. With appropriate medical and psychosocial support, children and adolescents with CF generally cope well. Achievement of an independent and productive adulthood is a realistic goal for many.

Collins FS: Cystic fibrosis: Molecular biology and therapeutic implications. Science 256:774, 1992.

Colombo C, Apostolo M, Ferrari M, et al: Analysis of risk factors for the development of liver disease associated with cystic fibrosis. J Pediatr 124:393, 1994.

Corey M, Edwards L, Levison H, Knowles M: Longitudinal analysis of pulmonary function decline in patients with cystic fibrosis. J Pediatr 131:809, 1997.

Desmond KJ, Schwenk F, Thomas E, et al: Immediate and long-term effects of chest physiotherapy in patients with cystic fibrosis. J Pediatr 103:538, 1983.

Fitzsimmons SC: The changing epidemiology of cystic fibrosis. J Pediatr 122:1, 1993.

Fitzsimmons SC, Burkhart GA, Borowitz D, et al: High-dose pancreatic-enzyme supplements and fibrosing colonopathy in children with cystic fibrosis. N Engl J Med 336:1283, 1997.

Fuchs JR, Langer JC: Long term outcome after neonatal meconium obstruction. Pediatrics 101:E7, 1998.

Fuchs JR, Borowitz DS, Christiansen PH, et al: Effect of aerosolized recombinant human DNase on exacerbations of respiratory symptoms and on pulmonary function in patients with cystic fibrosis. N Engl J Med 331:637, 1994.

Haeusler G, Frisch H, Waldhor T, et al: Perspectives of longitudinal growth in cystic fibrosis from birth to adult age. Eur J Pediatr 153:158, 1994.

Hamosh A, Fitzsimmons SC, Macek M, et al: Comparison of the clinical manifestations of cystic fibrosis in black and white patients. J Pediatr 132:255, 1998.

Knowles MR, Hohneker KW, Zhou Z, et al: A controlled study of adenoviral-vector-mediated gene transfer in the nasal epithelium of patients with cystic fibrosis. N Engl J Med 333:823, 1995.

Knowles MR: Contemporary perspectives on the pathogenesis of cystic fibrosis: From molecular aspects to clinical manifestations. New Insight Cystic Fibrosis 1:1, 1993.

Knowles M, Gatzy J, Boucher R: Increased bioelectric potential difference across respiratory epithelia in cystic fibrosis. N Engl J Med 305:1489, 1981.

Konstan M, Byard P, Hoppel C, Davis P: Effect of high-dose ibuprofen in patients with cystic fibrosis. N Engl J Med 332:848, 1995.

Lemna WK, Feldman FL, Kerem B, et al: Mutation analysis for heterozygote detection and the prenatal diagnosis of cystic fibrosis. N Engl J Med 322:291, 1990.

Ramsey B: Management of pulmonary disease in patients with cystic fibrosis. N Engl J Med 335:179, 1996.

Ramsey BW, Dorkin HL, Eisenberg JD, et al: Aerosolized tobramycin in patients with cystic fibrosis. N Engl J Med 328:1740, 1993.

Rosenstein BJ, Cutting GR: The diagnosis of cystic fibrosis: A consensus statement. J Pediatr 132:589, 1998.

The CF Genotype-Phenotype Consortium: Correlation between genotype and phenotype in patients with cystic fibrosis. N Engl J Med 329:1308, 1993.

Thomassen MJ, Demko AC, Klinger JD, et al: *Pseudomonas cepacia* colonization among patients with cystic fibrosis. Am Rev Respir Dis 131:791, 1985.

Welsh MJ, Anderson MP, Rich DP, et al: Cystic fibrosis transmembrane conductance regulator: A chloride channel with novel regulation. Neuron 8:821, 1992.

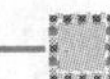

CHAPTER 417
Primary Ciliary Dyskinesia (Immotile Cilia Syndrome)

Gabriel G. Haddad

The group of respiratory disorders making up primary ciliary dyskinesia (PCD) have in common the malfunction of airway cilia. The ciliary abnormality is a result of various inherited primary structural defects in the cilia that lead to repeated and chronic lung infections. However, the ciliary malfunction in these diseases is *not* a result of acquired repeated pulmonary infections.

CHARACTERISTICS OF CILIA

Location and Structure. Airway cilia are located on epithelial surfaces in almost a ubiquitous fashion. They are present in the nose, sinuses, ears, and airways. They are also present in places other than the respiratory epithelium, such as in the fallopian tubes and in sperm. The density of cilia varies, with the majority of cells (50–80%) in the large airways having cilia, far fewer cells in the lower airways having cilia, and no cells in air sacs and alveoli having cilia. The frequency of ciliary beating, or *beatquency,* is about 1–20 Hz, with the higher beatquency occurring in the larger airways, correlating with the mucus velocity in various parts of the tracheobronchial tree.

Cilia are finger-like structures that extend from the surface of cells into the lumen of airways. They have a diameter of 0.25 μm and a length of 306 μm. Each cell usually has about 200 cilia on its surface. Each cilia has a trunk, a basal body (where the cilia attaches to the cell), and a crown, which is a specialized structure presumed to be important in cilia attachment to mucus. The trunk is made of an outer cell membrane and axonemes or cytoskeletal protein structures. The latter form a circular array of nine microtubules in pairs with an additional central pair. Each peripheral pair can attach to the other via bridges or dynein arms. Spokes are also cytoskeletal proteins that join peripheral and central microtubules.

Function. Cilia beat and move by a sliding motion of microtubules. At the outset of the beating cycle, they bend at the base and move backward, perpendicular to the surface. Subsequently, they extend ("slide") as they are rotating in a forward motion. These bending and rotating movements, which are clockwise, three-dimensional rotations, are made possible by adenosine triphosphate hydrolysis and the dynein arms, which are adenosine triphosphatases. When visualized under microscopy, airway cilia are seen to coordinate their activity regionally, and waves of ciliary movements (many cilia together) occur. How this is coordinated and how effective and important such coordination is to ciliary function is not well understood.

The main function of cilia is to transport, through its beating movements, mucus toward the mouth. The effectiveness of this function depends on the beatquency, the composition and thickness of the periciliary fluid and mucus layer above it, and the coordination of ciliary movements. In addition, there are a number of neurochemicals that modulate ciliary beating by increasing beatquency such as β-adrenergic compounds, acetylcholine, bradykinins, and serotonin. Alternatively, lowering airway humidity significantly lowers the frequency of ciliary beating. In addition, increasing bacterial loads decreases its beatquency.

PATHOLOGY. The structural abnormalities of these disorders can be seen with electron microscopy. Defects in both inner and outer dynein arms, radial spoke microtubular assembly, and central core cytoskeletal proteins have been described. It is estimated that there are more than 200 polypeptides in the ciliary structure, and primary ciliary dyskinesia is most likely based on the absence of one or several ciliary cytoskeletal proteins. All these structural defects result in ciliary malfunction characterized by either abnormal beating or immotility of cilia and defective mucociliary clearance of airway secretions. The most likely pathogenic sequence is airway mucus retention and failure to clear pathogenic organisms, followed by chronic or frequently recurring respiratory tract infections and, ultimately, injury to airway walls.

GENETICS. PCD occurs in about 1/20,000 whites and has been reported in Japanese patients. It is probably the 3rd most common form of inherited chronic airway disease of white children, following cystic fibrosis (CF) and genetic immunodeficiency states. The inheritance pattern of PCD has not been established. There is conflicting evidence for autosomal recessive or autosomal dominant inheritance with the mother having a new mutation, mitochondrial inheritance, or an X-linked mutation.

CLINICAL MANIFESTATIONS. About 50% of patients with PCD have Kartegener's syndrome: situs inversus, chronic sinusitis and otitis, and airways disease leading to bronchiectasis. However, only about 25% of patients with situs inversus also have PCD. Situs inversus does not establish or exclude the presence of PCD. Investigators have hypothesized that normal rotation of viscera depends on the motion of ciliated gut cells early in development. The absence of ciliary motility allows random rotation; a dynein defect is at the basis of left-right asymmetry in the inversus viscerum (iv/iv) mouse model.

The course is variable. Individuals with PCD may have respiratory distress during the newborn period or may survive to adulthood without overt chronic sinusitis and airway disease symptoms. However, in one study of PCD, 100% of children had productive cough, sinusitis, and otitis. A feature that is helpful in differentiating PCD from CF is repeated bouts of acute otitis media or chronic serous otitis. Children diagnosed after several years of life often have been treated with tympanostomy tubes; conductive hearing loss is common. Nasal polyps or clubbing is present in about 20% of patients. Many children with PCD experience frequent wheezing and may have an initial diagnosis of asthma. The hallmark symptom is a chronic, often loose or productive cough. Pneumonia may supervene and lower respiratory tract disease can progress to weight loss, diminished exercise tolerance, and bronchiectasis. Respiratory failure in childhood is uncommon, as are lung complications such as pneumothorax and hemoptysis. Lobar atelectasis occurs frequently. Males are frequently infertile and display absent or poor sperm motility.

DIAGNOSIS. PCD should be suspected in children with chronic or recurring upper and lower respiratory tract symptoms, especially in the presence of substantial middle ear disease. Radiographic or computed tomographic imaging shows involvement of the paranasal sinuses. Chest roentgenograms may demonstrate overinflation, bronchial wall thickening, and peribronchial infiltrates. Often, atelectasis and consolidation are present. Bronchiectasis is best detected by computed tomographic scanning. The presence of a right-sided heart in a child with chronic respiratory tract symptoms is virtually diagnostic, but this configuration occurs in only 50% of these patients. Pulmonary function testing of older children yields a typical obstructive pattern.

Mucociliary clearance can be assessed in cooperative children by ascertaining the time to taste perception of a saccharin particle placed on the inferior nasal turbinate. Scrapings or brushings of nasal mucosa can be examined directly by light or, preferably, by phase-contrast microscopy for evidence of motility. In most PCD tissue specimens, little or no ciliary motion is seen. However, because substantial motility has been documented in scrapings of several individuals with absent dynein arms, light microscopic examination of living tissue can be used as a screening tool only. The gold standard is quantitative documentation of abnormal structural elements, such as missing dynein arms or random orientation of cilia in nasal or bronchial biopsies or scrapings on electron microscopic examination. Concordance of ultrastructural abnormalities in cilia and sperm is not complete. To avoid acquired ciliary changes, mucosal specimens should not be obtained until 2 wk after an acute respiratory tract infection. Ultrastructural evaluation should be reserved for highly suspicious cases. However, some of the reported structural abnormalities are also observed after injury to ciliated epithelial cells by viral infection or sulfur dioxide exposure. Therefore, definitive evidence that any structural alteration represents a discrete form of PCD awaits the identification of specific gene mutations.

TREATMENT. Therapy is symptomatic. Cough should be encouraged. Chest physiotherapy assists the clearance of mucus. Antibiotics should be prescribed for evidence of infection of sinuses or lower airways. The choice of antibiotics is best dictated by identification and sensitivity testing of pathogenic organisms, often pneumococcus or untypable *Haemophilus influenzae.* Oral antibiotic administration is usually effective. Bronchodilators can be used for symptomatic wheezing or documentation of reversible airway obstruction. Children should be examined several times each year and followed by periodic chest radiographs and serial pulmonary function testing. Sinus and middle ear symptoms refractory to medical therapy deserve consultation with an otolaryngologist. Surgical intervention may be helpful in selected cases. Prevention of lung infection by measles, pertussis, influenza, and possibly pneumococcal vaccines is highly desirable. Additional preventive measures include avoidance of cigarette smoke and other airway irritants.

PROGNOSIS. Progression of lung disease appears to be much slower for patients with PCD than for those with CF. With proper treatment, disabling lung disease often can be avoided for long periods. A normal life span is possible.

Afzelius BA: A human syndrome caused by immotile cilia. Science 193:317, 1976.

Barlocco EG, Valletta EA, Canciani M, et al: Ultrastructural ciliary defects in children with recurrent infections of the lower respiratory tract. Pediatr Pulmonol 10:11, 1991.

Boat TF, Carson JL: Ciliary dysmorphology and dysfunction—primary or acquired? N Engl J Med 323:1700, 1990.

Carson JL, Collier AM, Hu SS: Acquired ciliary defects in nasal epithelium of children with acute viral upper respiratory infections. N Engl J 312:463, 1985.

Narayan D, Krishnan SN, Upender M, et al: Unusual inheritance of primary ciliary dyskinesia (Kartagener's syndrome). J Med Genet 31:493, 1994.

Pedersen H, Mygind N: Absence of axonemal arms in nasal mucosal cilia in Kartagener's syndrome. Nature 262:494, 1976.

Rutland J, deIongh RU: Random ciliary orientation: A cause of respiratory tract disease. N Engl J Med 323:1681, 1990.

Supp DM, Witte DP, Potter SS, Brueckner M: Mutation of an axonemal dynein affects left-right asymmetry in inversus viscerum mice. Nature 389:963, 1997.

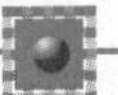

SECTION 4

Diseases of the Pleura

David M. Orenstein

CHAPTER 418
Pleurisy

The most common cause of pleural effusion in children is bacterial pneumonia (see Chapter 175); heart failure, rheumatologic causes, and metastatic intrathoracic malignancy are the next most common causes. Tuberculous effusion has become much less common with improved screening and antituberculous therapy. A variety of other diseases, including lupus erythematosus, aspiration pneumonitis, uremia, pancreatitis, subdiaphragmatic abscess, and rheumatoid arthritis, account for the remainder of the cases. Males and females are affected equally.

Inflammatory processes in the pleura are usually divided into three types: dry or plastic, serofibrinous or serosanguineous, and purulent pleurisy or empyema.

418.1 Dry or Plastic Pleurisy

Dry or plastic pleurisy may be associated with acute bacterial pulmonary infections or may develop during the course of an acute upper respiratory tract illness. The condition is also associated with tuberculosis and connective tissue diseases, such as rheumatic fever.

PATHOLOGY. The process is usually limited to the visceral pleura, with small amounts of yellow serous fluid and adhesions between the pleural surfaces. In tuberculosis, the adhesions develop rapidly, and the pleura is often thickened. Occasionally, fibrin deposition and adhesions may be severe enough to produce a fibrothorax that markedly inhibits the excursions of the lung.

CLINICAL MANIFESTATIONS. Signs and symptoms are often overshadowed by the primary disease. The principal symptom is pain, which is exaggerated by deep breathing, coughing, and straining. Occasionally, pleural pain is described as a dull ache, which is less likely to vary with breathing. The pain is often localized over the chest wall and is referred to the shoulder or the back. Pain with breathing is responsible for grunting and guarding of respirations, the child often lying on the affected side in an attempt to decrease respiratory excursions. Early in the illness, a leathery, rough, to-and-fro friction rub may be audible, but this usually disappears rapidly. Occasionally, increased dullness on percussion and suppressed breath sounds are heard if the layer of exudate is thick. Pleurisy may also be asymptomatic and detected only on roentgenograms, showing a diffuse haziness at the pleural surface or a dense, sharply demarcated shadow. The latter finding may be indistinguishable from small amounts of pleural exudate. Chronic pleurisy is occasionally encountered with conditions such as atelectasis, pulmonary abscess, connective tissue diseases, and tuberculosis.

DIFFERENTIAL DIAGNOSIS. Plastic pleurisy must be distinguished from other diseases, such as epidemic pleurodynia or trauma to the rib cage (particularly fracture of a rib) and from lesions of the dorsal root ganglia, tumors of the spinal cord, herpes zoster, gallbladder disease, and trichinosis. Even if evidence of pleural fluid is not found on physical or roentgenographic examination, a pleural tap in suspected cases often results in the recovery of a small amount of exudate, which, when cultured, usually reveals the underlying bacterial cause in cases associated with an acute pneumonia. Patients with pleurisy and pneumonia should always be screened for tuberculosis.

TREATMENT. Therapy should be aimed at the underlying disease. When pneumonia is present, neither immobilization of the chest with adhesive plaster nor therapy with drugs capable of suppressing the cough reflex is indicated. If pneumonia is not present or is under good therapeutic control, strapping of the chest to restrict expansion may afford relief from pain.

418.2 Serofibrinous Pleurisy

Serofibrinous pleurisy is most commonly associated with infections of the lung or with inflammatory conditions of the abdomen or mediastinum. Less commonly, it is found with connective tissue diseases such as lupus erythematosus, periarteritis, or rheumatic fever. On occasion, it is seen with primary or metastatic neoplasms of the lung, pleura, or mediastinum; tumors are commonly associated with a hemorrhagic pleurisy.

CLINICAL MANIFESTATIONS. Because serofibrinous pleurisy is often preceded by the plastic type, the early signs and symptoms may be those of plastic pleurisy. As fluid accumulates, pleuritic pain may disappear, and the patient may become asymptomatic if the effusion remains small, or there may be only signs and symptoms of the underlying disease. Large fluid collections may produce cough, dyspnea, retractions, tachypnea, orthopnea, or cyanosis. Physical findings depend to some degree on the amount of effusion. Dullness to flatness may be found on percussion. There is a decrease or absence of breath sounds, a diminution in tactile fremitus, a shift of the mediastinum away from the affected side, and occasionally fullness of the intercostal spaces. If the fluid is not loculated, these signs may shift with changes in position. In infants, the physical signs are less definite. Instead of decreased or absent breath sounds, bronchial breathing may be heard. If extensive pneumonia is present, crackles and rhonchi may also be audible. Friction rubs are usually detected only during the early or late plastic stage. The process is usually unilateral.

Roentgenographic examination shows a more or less homogeneous density obliterating the normal markings of the underlying lung. Small effusions may cause obliteration of only the costophrenic or cardiophrenic angles or a widening of the interlobar septa. Examinations should be performed with the patient in the supine and upright positions to demonstrate a shift of the effusion with a change in position; the decubitus position may also be helpful. Ultrasonographic examinations are useful.

DIFFERENTIAL DIAGNOSIS. Thoracentesis should be performed when pleural fluid is present or is suspected, unless the effusion is small and the patient has a classic lobar pneumococcal pneumonia. Examination of fluid is essential to identify acute bacterial infections, and it may disclose tubercle bacilli. Thoracentesis can differentiate serofibrinous pleurisy, empyema, hydrothorax, hemothorax, and chylothorax. In hydrothorax, the fluid has a specific gravity less than 1.015, and evaluation reveals only a few mesothelial cells rather than leukocytes. Chylothorax and hemothorax usually have fluid with a distinctive appearance; differentiating serofibrinous from purulent pleurisy is impossible without microscopic examination of the fluid. The fluid of serofibrinous pleurisy is clear or slightly cloudy and contains relatively few leukocytes and, occasionally, some erythrocytes. Cytologic examination may reveal malignant cells. Protein levels greater than 3 g/dL indicate an exudate and are likely to be associated with an infectious process. Similarly, pleural fluid lactic dehydrogenase values higher than 200 IU/L suggest an exudate. Serofibrinous fluid may rapidly become purulent. A pH less than 7.20 suggests an exudate.

COURSE. Unless the fluid becomes purulent, it usually disappears relatively rapidly, particularly with appropriate treatment of bacterial pneumonias. It persists somewhat longer with tuberculosis and connective tissue diseases and may remain or recur for a long time with neoplasms. As the effusion is absorbed, adhesions often develop between the two layers of the pleura, but little or no functional impairment usually results. Pleural thickening may develop and is occasionally mistaken for small quantities of fluid or for persistent pulmonary infiltrates. Pleural thickening may persist for a long time, but the process usually disappears, leaving no residua.

TREATMENT. Therapy addresses the underlying disease, although with large effusions, draining the fluid makes the patient more comfortable. When a diagnostic thoracentesis is performed, as much fluid as possible, up to about 1 L, should be removed for therapeutic purposes. Rapid removal of 1 L or more of pleural fluid occasionally has been associated with the ensuing development of re-expansion pulmonary edema. If the underlying disease is adequately treated, further drainage is usually unnecessary, but if sufficient fluid reaccumulates to cause respiratory embarrassment, repeated thoracentesis or chest tube drainage should be performed. In older children with parapneumonic effusion, tube thoracostomy is considered necessary if the pleural fluid pH is less than 7.20 or the pleural fluid glucose level is less than 50 mg/dL. If the fluid is clearly purulent, tube drainage is usually indicated. Systemic acidosis reduces the usefulness of pleural fluid pH measurements. Patients with pleural effusions may need analgesia, particularly after thoracentesis or insertion of a chest tube. Those with acute pneumonia often need supplemental oxygen in addition to specific antibiotic treatment.

Ben-Ami TE, O'Donovan JC, Yousefzadeh DK: Sonography of the chest in children. Radiol Clin North Am 31:517, 1993.

Light RW, Girard WM, Jenkinson SG, et al: Parapneumonic effusions. Am J Med 69:507, 1980.

Wolfe WG, Spock A, Bradford WD: Pleural fluids in infants and children. Am Rev Respir Dis 98:1027, 1968.

418.3 Purulent Pleurisy (Empyema)

An accumulation of pus in the pleural spaces is most often associated with pneumonia due to staphylococci and less frequently with pneumococci (especially types 1 and 3) and *Haemophilus influenzae.* The relative incidence of *H. influenzae* empyema has decreased since the introduction of Hib vaccination. In pediatric practice, empyema is most frequently encountered in infants and preschool children. The disease may also be produced by rupture of a lung abscess into the pleural space, by contamination introduced from trauma or thoracic surgery or, rarely, by mediastinitis or the extension of intra-abdominal abscesses.

PATHOLOGY. Most commonly, purulent pleurisy is an extensive process consisting of a series of loculated areas involving a large portion of one or both pleural cavities. Thickening of the parietal pleura occurs. If the pus is not drained, it may dissect through the pleura into lung parenchyma, producing bronchopleural fistulas and pyopneumothorax, or into the abdominal cavity. Rarely, the pus may dissect through the chest wall (i.e., *empyema necessitatis*). Pockets of loculated pus may eventually develop into thick-walled abscess cavities or as the exudate organizes, the lung may collapse and become surrounded by a thick, inelastic envelope (i.e., peel).

CLINICAL MANIFESTATIONS. The initial signs and symptoms are primarily those of bacterial pneumonia. Children treated inadequately or with inappropriate antibiotic agents may have an interval of a few days between the clinical pneumonia phase and the evidence of empyema. Most patients are febrile. In infants, there may be only a moderate exacerbation of respiratory distress. The older child is likely to appear more ill and have greater respiratory difficulty. Physical and roentgenographic findings may be identical to those described for serofibrinous pleurisy, and the two conditions are differentiated only by thoracentesis, which should always be performed when empyema is suspected (see Chapter 418.2). Roentgenographically, finding no shift of fluid with a change of position indicates a loculated empyema. The maximal amount of pus obtainable should be withdrawn by thoracentesis. The appearance of pus produced by different organisms is not distinctive; cultures must always be obtained, and Gram-stained smears should be examined for the presence of microorganisms. Blood cultures have a high yield (62% in one series), but latex agglutination may also be useful. Leukocytosis and an elevated sedimentation rate may be found.

COMPLICATIONS. With staphylococcal infections, bronchopleural fistulas and pyopneumothorax commonly develop. Other local complications include purulent pericarditis, pulmonary abscesses, peritonitis secondary to rupture through the diaphragm, and osteomyelitis of the ribs. Septic complications such as meningitis, arthritis, and osteomyelitis may also occur. With staphylococcal empyema, septicemia occurs infrequently; it is often encountered in *H. influenzae* and pneumococcal infections.

TREATMENT. Most experts advise that if pus is obtained by thoracentesis, closed drainage should be instituted immediately and controlled by an underwater seal or continuous suction. A catheter with the largest possible internal diameter should be inserted into the site where accumulation of pus is suspected; sometimes several tubes are required to drain loculated areas. Closed drainage is usually continued for about 1 wk, even though small amounts of material continue to drain after this time, probably in response to the presence of the tube in the pleural cavity. Chest tubes that are no longer draining should be removed.

Instilling fibrinolytic agents or proteolytic enzymes into the pleural cavity commonly produces severe systemic reactions in small children and does not promote drainage. Antibiotics should not be instilled into the pleural cavity because they do not improve results obtained with systemic antibiotic therapy alone and are associated with local reactions. Controlling empyema by multiple aspirations of the pleural cavity rather than by closed continuous drainage should not be attempted. If the condition is diagnosed early, thoracentesis and antibiotic treatment alone can bring about complete cure.

Systemic antibiotic therapy is required; the selection of the antibiotic should be based on the in vitro sensitivities of the responsible organism. Infant staphylococcal empyema is best treated by parenteral routes with nafcillin or, when applicable, with penicillin G or vancomycin. Pneumococcal infection usually responds to penicillin, ceftriaxone, or cefotaxime but may need vancomycin if penicillin resistance develops; *H. influenzae* responds to cefuroxime, cefotaxime, ceftriaxone, or azithromycin (see Chapter 175). With staphylococcal infections, resolution of the process is slow, and systemic antibiotic therapy is required for 3–4 wk. Clinical response in nonstaphylococcal empyema is also slow, even with optimal treatment; little improvement may occur for as long as 2 wk. In patients with inadequately treated empyema, extensive fibrinous changes may take place over the surface of the collapsed lungs, but surgical decortication procedures are rarely indicated. In the child who remains febrile and dyspneic longer than 72 hr after initiation of therapy with intravenous antibiotics and thoracostomy tube drainage, surgical decortication, via thoracoscopy or open thoracotomy, may speed recovery. If pneumatoceles form, no attempt should be made to treat them surgically or by aspiration, unless they reach sufficient size to cause respiratory embarrassment or become secondarily infected. The long-term clinical prognosis for adequately treated empyema is excellent, and follow-up pulmonary function studies suggest that residual restrictive disease is uncommon, with or without surgical intervention.

McLaughlin FJ, Goldmann DA, Rosenbaum DM, et al: Empyema in children: Clinical course and long-term follow-up. Pediatrics 73:587, 1984.

Murphy D, Lockhart CH, Todd JK: Pneumococcal empyema. Am J Dis Child 134:659, 1980.

Redding GJ, Walund L, Walund D, et al: Lung function in children following empyema. Am J Dis Child 144:1337, 1990.

Siegel JD, Gartner JC, Michaels RH: Pneumococcal empyema in childhood. Am J Dis Child 132:1094, 1978.

CHAPTER 419
Pneumothorax

Pneumothorax is the accumulation of extrapulmonary air within the chest. Pneumothorax is uncommon during childhood. It most often results from leakage of air from within the lung. Air leaks can be primary or secondary and can be spontaneous, traumatic, iatrogenic, or catamenial. Pneumothorax in the neonatal period is also discussed in Chapter 97.8.

EPIDEMIOLOGY AND ETIOLOGY. A primary spontaneous pneumothorax occurs in someone without trauma or underlying lung disease. Spontaneous pneumothorax with or without exertion (valsalva) occurs occasionally in teenagers and young adults, most frequently in males who are tall and thin. Families have been described in which many members have had spontaneous pneumothoraces, with the onset ranging from birth to adulthood. Patients with collagen synthesis defects such as Ehlers-Danlos disease and Marfan's syndrome are unusually prone to the development of pneumothorax.

A pneumothorax arising as a complication of an underlying lung disorder, but without trauma, is a secondary spontaneous pneumothorax. Pneumothorax may occur in pneumonia, usually in connection with empyema; it may also be secondary to pulmonary abscess, gangrene, infarct, rupture of a cyst or an emphysematous bleb (e.g., in asthma), or foreign bodies in the lung. In infant staphylococcal pneumonia, the incidence of pneumothorax is relatively high. It is found in about 5% of hospitalized asthmatic children and usually resolves without treatment. Pneumothorax is a serious complication in cystic fibrosis (CF) (see Chapter 416), occurring in 10–25% of patients older than 10 yr. Pneumothorax also occurs in patients with lymphoma or other malignancies.

External chest or abdominal blunt or penetrating trauma can tear a bronchus or abdominal viscus, with leakage of air into the pleural space.

Iatrogenic pneumothorax can complicate tracheotomy, subclavian line placement, thoracentesis, transbronchial biopsy, or other diagnostic or therapeutic procedures. Pneumothorax may also occur after acupuncture treatment and is classified as iatrogenic or traumatic.

Catamenial pneumothorax, an unusual condition that is by definition associated with menses, results from passage of intra-abdominal air through diaphragmatic defects. When thoracotomy is performed for recurrent pneumothorax of unknown cause in a young woman, an examination of the diaphragm may be appropriate.

Pneumothorax may be associated with a serous effusion (i.e., hydropneumothorax) or a purulent effusion (i.e., pyopneumothorax). Bilateral pneumothorax is rare beyond the neonatal period.

CLINICAL MANIFESTATIONS AND DIAGNOSIS. The onset is usually abrupt, and the severity of symptoms depends on the extent of the lung collapse and on the amount of pre-existing lung disease. Extensive pneumothorax may involve pain, dyspnea, and cyanosis. In infancy, symptoms and physical signs may be difficult to recognize. Moderate pneumothorax may cause little displacement of the intrathoracic organs and few or no symptoms. The severity of pain usually does not directly reflect the extent of the collapse.

Usually, there is respiratory distress, retractions, and markedly decreased breath sounds over the involved lung. The percussion note over the involved area is tympanitic. The larynx, trachea, and heart may be shifted toward the unaffected side. When fluid is present, there is usually a sharply limited area of tympany above a level of flatness to percussion. The presence of amphoric breathing or, when fluid is present in the pleural cavity, of gurgling sounds synchronous with respirations suggests an open fistula connecting with air-containing tissues. Confirmatory evidence is provided when the pneumothorax fills rapidly after it has been aspirated.

The diagnosis can usually be established by roentgenographic examination (Fig. 419–1). Scores are often assigned to pneumothoraces, based on the proportion of a hemithorax filled

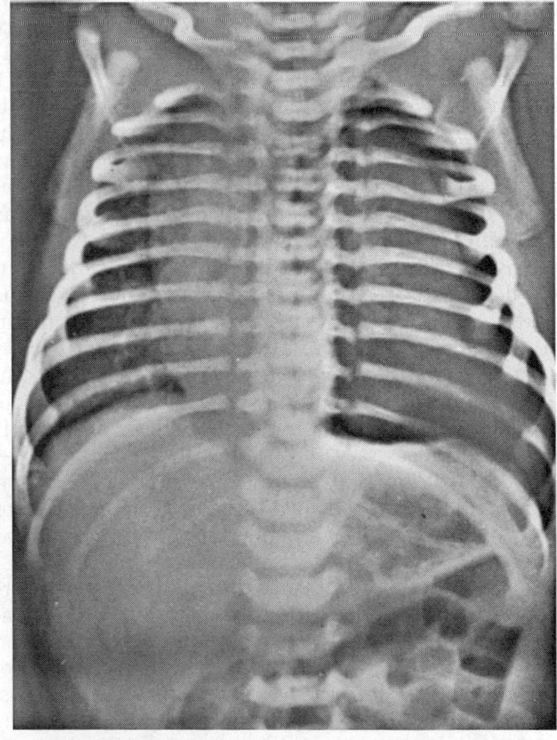

Figure 419–1 Pneumothorax in a newborn infant. The air in the left pleural cavity has partially collapsed the left lung, shifting the heart and mediastinal structures to the right.

with extrapulmonary air. A "25% pneumothorax" is one in which the lung occupies only 75% of the hemithorax. Although this provides a rough idea of the extent of leak and collection of extrapulmonary air, it is often misleading. In conditions like CF, in which the lung is relatively noncompliant, a great deal of air can accumulate under tension without much lung collapse. The amount of air outside the lung also varies with time. A roentgenogram taken early shows less lung collapse than one taken later if the leak continues. Expiratory views accentuate the contrast between lung markings and the clear area of the pneumothorax. When considering the possibility of diaphragmatic hernia, a small amount of barium may be necessary to demonstrate that it is not free air but is a portion of the gastrointestinal tract that is in the thoracic cavity.

It is important to determine whether the pneumothorax is under tension (i.e., tension pneumothorax) because this condition limits expansion of the contralateral lung and may compromise venous return. It may be difficult to determine if a pneumothorax is under tension. Evidence of tension includes shift of mediastinal structures away from the side of air leak. A shift may be absent, as in situations in which the other hemithorax resists the shift, such as in the case of bilateral pneumothorax. When the lungs are both stiff, the unaffected lung may not collapse easily, and shift may not occur. On occasion, the diagnosis of tension pneumothorax is made only on the basis of evidence of circulatory compromise or on hearing a "hiss" of rapid exit of air under tension with the insertion of the thoracostomy tube.

DIFFERENTIAL DIAGNOSIS. Pneumothorax must be differentiated from localized or generalized emphysema, an extensive emphysematous bleb, large pulmonary cavities or other cystic formations, diaphragmatic hernia, compensatory overexpansion with contralateral atelectasis, and gaseous distention of the stomach; in most cases, a chest roentgenogram differentiates among these conditions.

TREATMENT. Therapy varies with the extent of the collapse and the nature and severity of the underlying disease. A small or even moderate-sized pneumothorax in an otherwise normal child may resolve without specific treatment, usually within about 1 wk. A small (<5%) pneumothorax complicating asthma may also resolve spontaneously. Administering 100% oxygen may hasten resolution by increasing the nitrogen pressure gradient between the pleural air and the blood. Patients with chronic hypoxemia should be monitored closely during the administration of supplemental oxygen. Pleural pain deserves analgesic treatment. Codeine may be justified, but its respiratory depressant effect should be considered. Occasionally, morphine or meperidine is needed. If there is more than 5% collapse or if the pneumothorax is recurrent or under tension, definitive treatment is necessary. Pneumothoraces complicating CF frequently recur, and definitive treatment may be justified with the first episode, even with less than 5% collapse (see Chapter 416). Similarly, if pneumothorax complicating malignancy and its treatment does not improve rapidly with observation, chemical pleurodesis or open thoracotomy is often necesssary.

Closed thoracotomy (i.e., simple insertion of a chest tube) and drainage of the trapped air through a catheter, the external opening of which is kept in a dependent position under water, is adequate to re-expand the lung in most patients (see Chapter 97.8). To prevent recurrences when there have already been pneumothoraces, inducing the formation of strong adhesions between the lung and chest wall by a sclerosing procedure may be indicated. This can be carried out by the introduction of tetracycline, talc, or silver nitrate into the pleural space (i.e., chemical pleurodesis). Open thoracotomy through a limited incision, with plication of blebs, closure of fistula, stripping of the pleura (usually in the apical lung where the surgeon has direct vision), and basilar pleural abrasion is also an effective treatment for recurring pneumothorax. Stripping and abrading the pleura leaves raw, inflamed surfaces that heal with sealing adhesions. Postoperative pain is comparable to chemical pleurodesis with silver nitrate, but the chest tube can usually be removed within 24–48 hr, compared with the usual 72-hr minimum for closed thoracotomy and pleurodesis. The thoracoscope has permitted a successful surgical approach to blebectomy, pleural stripping, and instillation of sclerosing agents with somewhat less morbidity than occurs with traditional open thoracotomy.

Extensive pleural adhesions help to prevent recurrent pneumothorax, but they also make thoracic surgery, including lung transplantation, difficult. For conditions in which lung transplantation may be a future consideration (e.g., CF), a stepwise approach to treatment of pneumothorax has been proposed. If the patient is comfortable and the pneumothorax is small, no intervention is warranted. For a larger leak or one that does not resolve, simple thoracostomy tube drainage can be attempted. For continuing leak, or recurrence, the next step could be thoracoscopic blebectomy without pleurabrasion. Only after these steps have failed should the full aggressive pleural stripping and abrasion be undertaken. At any step during this approach, the patient and family should be given the option of the definitive procedure if they understand it may make lung transplantation difficult or impossible. It should also be kept in mind that the longer a chest tube is in place, the greater the chance of pulmonary deterioration, particularly in a patient with CF, in whom strong coughing, deep breathing, and postural drainage are important. These are all difficult to accomplish with a chest tube in place.

Treatment of the underlying pulmonary disease should begin on admission and should be continued throughout the course of treatment directed at the air leak.

Bernhard WF, Malcolm IA, Berry RW, et al: A study of the pathogenesis and management of spontaneous pneumothorax. Dis Chest 42:403, 1962.
Noyes BE, Orenstein DM: Treatment of pneumothorax in cystic fibrosis in the era of lung transplantation. Chest 101:1187, 1992.
Stem H, Toole AL, Merino M: Catamenial pneumothorax. Chest 78:480, 1980.
Wilson WG, Aylsworth AS: Familial spontaneous pneumothorax. Pediatrics 64:172, 1979.
Yellin A, Benfield IR: Pneumothorax associated with lymphoma. Am Rev Respir Dis 134:590, 1986.

CHAPTER 420
Pneumomediastinum

Pneumomediastinum usually results from alveolar rupture during an acute or chronic pulmonary disease. However, a diverse group of nonrespiratory entities can also cause pneumomediastinum, and in some of these, the lung is not the source of the air. For example, pneumomediastinum has been reported after dental extractions, normal menses, obstetric delivery, diabetes mellitus with ketoacidosis, acupuncture, and acute gastroenteritis. Pneumomediastinum can also result from esophageal perforation or penetrating chest trauma. Occasionally, no underlying cause is found; in an apparently normal child, the pneumomediastinum can present as chest pain associated with subcutaneous air.

After intrapulmonary alveolar rupture, air can dissect through the perivascular sheaths and other soft tissue planes toward the hilum and enter the mediastinum. Pneumomediastinum is rarely a major problem in older children because the mediastinum can be depressurized by escape of air into the neck or abdomen. In the newborn, however, the rate at which air can leave the mediastinum is limited, and pneumomediastinum can lead to dangerous cardiovascular compromise or pneumothorax (see Chapter 419). Acute asthma is the most common cause of pneumomediastinum in older children and teenagers. Simultaneous pneumothorax is unusual in these patients.

The principal *clinical manifestations* of pneumomediastinum are transient stabbing pains in the chest that may radiate to the neck. Isolated abdominal pain and sore throat also occur. The patient may have dyspnea, but it is difficult to know if this is really a separate symptom or if it is related to the chest pain. Pneumomediastinum is often difficult to detect by physical examination alone. Subcutaneous emphysema, if present, is diagnostic (see Chapter 407.3). Although cardiac dullness to percussion may be decreased, many of these patients' chests are chronically overinflated, and it is unlikely that the clinician can be sure of this finding. A mediastinal "crunch" is occasionally heard but is easily confused with a friction rub. On chest roentgenogram, the cardiac border, highlighted by the mediastinal air, is more distinct than normal, and on the lateral projection, the posterior mediastinal structures are also clearly defined. Subcutaneous air, seen roentgenographically, confirms the pneumomediastinum.

Treatment is directed primarily at the underlying obstructive pulmonary disease. Analgesics are needed occasionally for chest pain. Rarely, subcutaneous emphysema can cause sufficient tracheal compression to justify tracheotomy; the tracheotomy also decompresses the mediastinum.

Church IA, Richards W: Air leak syndromes as complications of respiratory disease in infancy and childhood. Ann Allergy 39:393, 1977.
Sandler CM, Libshitz HI, Marks G: Pneumoperitoneum, pneumomediastinum and pneumopericardium following dental extraction. Radiology 115:539, 1975.
Shahar I, Angelillo VA: Catamenial pneumomediastinum. Chest 90:776, 1986.
Sturtz GS: Spontaneous mediastinal emphysema. Pediatrics 74:431, 1984.

CHAPTER 421
Hydrothorax

In hydrothorax, the fluid is noninflammatory and has a lower specific gravity (<1.015) than that of a serofibrinous exudate. It contains less protein and fewer cells and is usually associated with an accumulation of fluid in other parts of the body, such as the peritoneal cavity and the subcutaneous tissues. Hydrothorax is most often associated with cardiac or renal disease, although it may be a manifestation of severe nutritional edema, and it rarely results from venous obstruction by neoplasms, enlarged lymph nodes, or adhesions. Hydrothorax is usually bilateral in cases of renal disease and those of nutritional edema; in myocardial disease, it may be bilateral, limited to the right side, or greater on the right than on the left side. The physical signs are the same as those described for serofibrinous pleurisy (see Chapter 418.2), but in hydrothorax, there is more rapid shifting of the level of dullness with changes of position. Treatment is for the primary disorder; aspiration may be necessary when pressure symptoms are notable.

Berger HW, Rammohan G, Neff MS, et al: Uremic pleural effusion. A study in 14 patients on chronic dialysis. Ann Intern Med 82:362, 1975.

CHAPTER 422
Hemothorax

Extensive bleeding into the pleural cavity is rare in children but may result from erosion of a blood vessel in association with inflammatory processes such as tuberculosis and empyema. Hemothorax may complicate a variety of congenital anomalies, including sequestration, patent ductus arteriosus, and pulmonary arteriovenous malformation. It is also an occasional manifestation of intrathoracic neoplasms, blood dyscrasias, and bleeding diatheses, and it may be the result of thoracic trauma, including surgical procedures. Rupture of an aneurysm is unlikely during childhood. Hemothorax also occurs after blunt chest trauma and spontaneously in neonates and older children. A pleural hemorrhage associated with a pneumothorax is called *hemopneumothorax.*

The diagnosis of a hemothorax can be made only by thoracentesis. In every case, an effort must be made to determine and treat the cause. Surgical intervention may be required to control active bleeding, and transfusion is necessary if blood loss is excessive. Inadequate removal of blood in extensive hemothorax may lead to substantial restrictive disease secondary to deposition and organization of fibrin. A decortication procedure may then be necessary.

Berry RB, Light R: When thoracentesis yields bloody pleural fluid. J Respir Dis 7:18, 1986.
Fleisher GR, Fichman KR, Honig PJ: Hemothorax in a child: An unusual cause of chest pain. Clin Pediatr 17:300, 1978.
Wilimas JA, Presbury G, Orenstein D, et al: Hemothorax and hemomediastinum in patients with hemophilia. Acta Haematol 73:176, 1985.

CHAPTER 423
Chylothorax

Chylothorax results from the escape of chyle from the thoracic duct into the thoracic cavity. The incidence has increased as cardiac surgery is performed on more complex congenital abnormalities; about 50% of these cases are now operative complications resulting from rupture of the thoracic duct. Most of the remainder are associated with chest injury or with primary or metastatic intrathoracic malignancy as a result of the pressure of enlarged lymph nodes or tumor. Less common causes include lymphangiomatosis, restrictive pulmonary diseases, thrombosis of the duct or the subclavian vein, and congenital anomalies of the duct system. Chylothorax can occur in child abuse. In some patients, especially newborns, no specific cause is identified. Chylothorax is rarely bilateral and usually occurs on the left side.

The *clinical manifestations* are those related to the presence of fluid in the thoracic cavity. The diagnosis is established when thoracentesis demonstrates a chylous effusion, a milky fluid containing fat, protein, lymphocytes, and other constituents of chyle. In newborn infants who have not yet been fed, the fluid may be clear. A **pseudochylous milky fluid** has been reported in cases of serous effusion, in which the fatty material was thought to arise from degenerative changes within the fluid and not from the presence of lymph. This type of fluid may be differentiated from one containing chyle by shaking it with alkalis or ether; the fluid containing chyle tends to become clear. A more definitive test is the quantitation of fluid triglyceride, which is elevated in chylous fluid, and fluid cholesterol, which may be elevated in chronic serous effusions.

Spontaneous recovery has occurred in more than 50% of the reported cases in infants younger than 1 yr of age. Repeated aspirations may be required to relieve the symptoms of pressure. However, chyle reaccumulates quickly, and repeated thoracenteses may cause considerable loss of calories, protein, and lymphocytes. Immunodeficiencies, including hypogammaglobulinemia, and abnormal cell-mediated immune responses have been associated with repeated thoracenteses for chylothorax. Attempts to prevent these problems by intravenous infusion of pleural contents are technically difficult, dangerous, and of doubtful benefit. Despite large losses of T lymphocytes, clinical problems of infection are uncommon, but these patients should be protected from potentially dangerous viruses, including cytomegalovirus and live virus vaccines.

Treatment should begin in most cases with a brief period of observation on a low-fat (or medium-chain triglyceride), high-protein diet. For most patients, salt restriction and diuresis are also indicated. The total caloric intake should be greater than the average requirement, and several times the daily requirements of the various vitamins, especially the fat-soluble vitamins A and D, should be added. If fluid continues to reaccumulate over 1–2 wk, total parenteral nutrition should be instituted and, if unsuccessful, a more aggressive attempt to locate and ligate the thoracic duct may be indicated. Although even a leaking thoracic duct is difficult to locate, many successful ligations have now been reported for patients with nontraumatic chylothoraces.

Dunkelman H, Sharief N, Berman L, et al: Generalized lymphangiomatosis with chylothorax. Arch Dis Child 64:1058, 1989.
Green HG: Child abuse presenting as chylothorax. Pediatrics 66:620, 1980.
Macfarlane JR, Holman CW: Chylothorax. Am Rev Respir Dis 105:287, 1972.
McWilliams BC, Fan LL, Murphy SA: Transient T-cell depression in post-operative chylothorax. J Pediatr 99:595, 1981.
Van Aerde J, Campbell AN, Smyth JA, et al: Spontaneous chylothorax in newborns. Am J Dis Child 138:961, 1984.

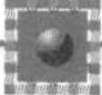

SECTION 5

Neuromuscular and Skeletal Diseases Affecting Pulmonary Function

David M. Orenstein

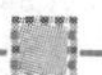

CHAPTER 424

Skeletal Diseases Affecting Pulmonary Function

424.1 Pectus Excavatum

Midline narrowing of the thoracic cavity, called *pectus excavatum* or *funnel chest,* is usually an isolated congenital skeletal abnormality but may be a manifestation of a connective tissue disorder, such as Marfan's syndrome. The condition may also be acquired. Rarely, it is associated with rickets. It is occasionally associated with upper or lower airway obstruction, and when this condition is successfully treated or resolves spontaneously, the pectus deformity may lessen or disappear. There have been reports of the coexistence of pectus excavatum and segmental bronchomalacia, particularly in the left main stem bronchus. Substantial pectus deformity rarely results in demonstrable restrictive pulmonary disease but usually has little or no functional effect.

Exercise testing has suggested an occasional link between pectus excavatum and exercise limitation. More commonly, exercise intolerance in children with pectus excavatum can be explained by limited habitual activity, related to the parents' fears.

In many children, the heart is shifted leftward, and in the rare patient, cardiac function may be adversely affected. Mitral valve prolapse (which may no longer be demonstrable by echocardiography after surgical correction of the pectus) and Wolff-Parkinson-White syndrome appear to be associated abnormalities. The clinical significance of these usually mild cardiac abnormalities is not clear.

Surgical correction of the pectus is not physiologically beneficial for most patients. However, improved exercise capability and normalization of lung perfusion scans and maximal voluntary ventilation have been reported. The functional importance of these findings is not clear. Some patients with severe deformities may seek repair for cosmetic or psychologic reasons.

Fissure of the sternum is the term used when the halves of the sternum remain separated. *Pigeon breast* (i.e., *pectus carinatum*) displays a prominence of the sternum and the cartilaginous parts of the ribs, with lateral depressions of the thorax. A short sternum is a common manifestation of trisomies 18 and 21.

Beiser GD, Epstein SE, Stampfer M, et al: Impairment of cardiac function in patients with pectus excavatum, with improvement after operative correction. N Engl J Med 287:267, 1972.
Castile RG, Staats BA, Westbrook PR: Symptomatic pectus deformities of the chest. Am Rev Respir Dis 126:564, 1982.
Fan L, Murphy S: Pectus excavatum from chronic upper airway obstruction. Am J Dis Child 135:550, 1981.
Godfrey S: Association between pectus excavatum and segmental bronchomalacia. J Pediatr 96:649, 1980.
Park JM, Farmer AF: Wolff-Parkinson-White syndrome in children with pectus excavatum. J Pediatr 112:926, 1988.
Quigley PM, Haller JA, Jelus KL, et al: Cardiorespiratory function before and after corrective surgery in pectus excavatum. J Pediatr 128:638, 1996.
Shamberger RC, Welch KJ, Sanders SP: Mitral valve prolapse associated with pectus excavatum. J Pediatr 111:404, 1987.

424.2 Asphyxiating Thoracic Dystrophy (Jeune Syndrome) (Also see Chapter 697)

Thoracic dystrophy is one manifestation of an autosomal recessive disease that involves a generalized abnormality of skeletal growth. It usually causes life-threatening respiratory difficulties in the newborn period or early infancy. A variety of associated congenital malformations have been reported. Most patients have respiratory distress or infection before 1 yr of age. Older children are occasionally diagnosed when their parents notice an abnormality in the appearance of the chest. A physical examination reveals constriction of the thorax and, usually, short extremities. There is no specific treatment. Surgery to expand the restrictive chest has not been rewarding. However, long-term continuous positive airway pressure was used successfully in one patient. Progressive renal failure occurs frequently among older patients. Respiratory infections should be treated promptly with antibiotics and perhaps with physical therapy. Influenza vaccine should be administered yearly.

Herdman RC, Langer LO: Thoracic asphyxiant dystrophy and renal disease. Am J Dis Child 116:192, 1968.
Oberklaid F, Dantes DM, Mayne V, et al: Asphyxiating thoracic dysplasia: Clinical, radiological, and pathological information on 10 patients. Arch Dis Child 52:758, 1977.
Wiebicke W, Pasterkamp H: Long-term continuous positive airway pressure in a child with asphyxiating thoracic dystrophy. Pediatr Pulmonol 4:54, 1988.

424.3 Achondroplasia

Achondroplasia has been associated with several respiratory abnormalities, including recurrent pneumonia, hypoxemia, cor pulmonale, apnea, and sudden unexplained deaths (see Chapter 697). The incidence apneas and sudden deaths may be related to compression of the medulla and upper cervical spinal cord. The chronic and recurrent respiratory problems may be related to constricted middle and upper airways and to relatively small lungs. Children younger than 2 yr of age with achondroplasia are more likely to have reduced thoracic dimensions compared with normal or older children and adults. However, even older patients have smaller vital capacities than their sitting height would predict.

Stokes DC, Pyeritz RE, Wise RA, et al.: Spirometry and chest wall dimensions in achondroplasia. Chest 93:364, 1988.

424.4 Kyphoscoliosis

Scoliosis, including idiopathic adolescent scoliosis, is discussed in Chapter 685. Mild or moderately severe scoliosis does not usually restrict the chest cage enough to affect pulmonary function seriously. Severe scoliosis, however, can dangerously impair function and may be associated with respiratory failure or cor pulmonale, or both. In addition to the restrictive lesion, children may also have a diffusion abnormality that aggravates hypoxemia. Minor respiratory infections may be life-threatening. Pulmonary function worsens with age. Acute respiratory failure, although rare, does occur before 20 yr of age.

Many patients can be managed without mechanical ventilation, and the intermediate-term prognosis is good. However, even patients with moderate scoliosis may have unexpectedly severe pulmonary problems immediately after a spinal fusion procedure because pain and a body cast restrict breathing and interfere with coughing. The magnitude of the postoperative impairment of pulmonary function correlates with the site and magnitude of the surgery and with the preoperative pulmonary abnormality.

Children with severe scoliosis, especially males, may have abnormalities of breathing during sleep, and the resultant periods of hypoxemia may contribute to the eventual development of pulmonary hypertension. These patients should be treated as if they had life-threatening pulmonary disease. Influenza vaccine should be given yearly. Careful pulmonary function evaluation is essential before elective surgical procedures, especially before fusion. If pulmonary function is marginal (e.g., vital capacity of less than 40–50% of predicted or less than three times the tidal volume), the child should receive instruction in and get experience with positive-pressure breathing before surgery. The possibility that the patient may awaken on assisted ventilation with an endotracheal tube should be discussed before surgery. If possible, the child should actually see the mechanical ventilator and understand how and why it may be used. For patients with marginal pulmonary function, careful postoperative monitoring of blood gases is essential. An occasional child with extremely severe restrictive disease should have a tracheostomy before surgery. Scoliosis surgery may predispose to deep venous thrombosis and pulmonary embolus.

Leech JA, Ernst P, Rogala EJ, et al: Cardiorespiratory status in relation to mild deformity in adolescent idiopathic scoliosis. J Pediatr 106:143, 1985.
Libby DM, Briscoe WA, Boyce B, et al: Acute respiratory failure in scoliosis or kyphosis: Prolonged survival and treatment. Am J Med 73:532, 1982.
Mezon BL, West P, Israels J, et al: Sleep breathing abnormalities in kyphoscoliosis. Am Rev Respir Dis 1222:617, 1980.
Schur MS, Brown JT, Kafer ER, et al: Postoperative pulmonary function in children: Comparison of scoliosis with peripheral surgery. Am Rev Respir Dis 130:46, 1984.

424.5 Rib Anomalies

The absence or malformation of one to two ribs usually has no substantial effect on pulmonary function and does not require treatment. An absence of multiple ribs is associated with vertebral anomalies and, ultimately, with scoliosis. A portion of lung can herniate through the defect in the chest wall; these hernias are most frequent at the level of the 1st–5th ribs and are usually anterior (see Chapter 412). The lung may appear as a soft, easily reducible, usually nontender swelling. Minor abnormalities of muscles caused by a loss of their normal attachments are also associated with this lesion. Most rib anomalies are discovered as incidental findings on chest roentgenograms obtained as part of a work-up for another illness. When the defect is large and associated with lung hernia, rib splitting and strutting techniques can provide functional and cosmetic improvement.

CHAPTER 425
Neuromuscular Diseases with Hypoventilation

A variety of acute (poliomyelitis, Guillain-Barré syndrome, botulism, spinal cord injury) and chronic (muscular dystrophy, progressive spinal muscular atrophy, myasthenia gravis) neuromuscular diseases can cause respiratory problems (see Chapters 615, 616, 622, and 623).

CLINICAL MANIFESTATIONS. Alveolar hypoventilation with hypoxemia and respiratory failure is easily recognized, and the need for emergency measures, including mechanical ventilation, is obvious (see Chapters 64.3 and 375.1). Arterial blood gas determinations and lung volume measurements confirm its presence and are helpful for proper management. The noninvasive measurement of oxyhemoglobin saturation (pulse oximetry) and end-tidal carbon dioxide can substitute for the painful arterial blood gas test (see Chapter 377). The vital capacity, which allows assessment of the inspiratory and expiratory muscles, is particularly useful and should be carefully followed. The difference between the vital capacity obtained with the patient lying down and that obtained with the patient sitting offers a rough guide to the strength of the diaphragm. Maximal inspiratory pressure is another easily obtained and valuable measure of the strength of the respiratory muscles.

Chronic, slowly progressive neuromuscular weakness is most likely to cause the insidious onset of respiratory abnormalities that may ultimately become incapacitating or life-limiting. With progression of weakness, the patient cannot generate sufficient intrathoracic pressure for effective coughing or cannot hold the glottis closed well enough to allow sufficient pressure to build up in the lung. Although tidal volumes may continue to be normal, the progressive decrease in vital capacity also compromises the effectiveness of the cough. Multiple minor episodes of aspiration occur as laryngeal muscles become weaker. With the loss of adequate sigh and a decreased ability of the diaphragm to prevent compromise of the thoracic volume by the abdominal organs, patchy microatelectasis occurs, accompanied by a ventilation-perfusion abnormality and hypoxemia. Microatelectasis also appear to be the major cause of decreased lung compliance in these patients. Recurrent or chronic infection then results and further restricts vital capacity. The increased viscosity of infected secretions aggravates the already impaired mucociliary clearance. Progressive loss of pulmonary tissue from the fibrosis associated with chronic infection and the chronic and worsening hypoxemia may eventually lead to pulmonary arterial hypertension and, ultimately, to right-sided heart failure. Weakness of the pharyngeal and laryngeal muscles may result in obstruction when soft tissue, normally retracted during inspiration, partially occludes the upper airway.

TREATMENT. All children with chronic or progressive muscular weakness require close surveillance for and early treatment of respiratory complications. Prompt antibiotic treatment of upper respiratory infections is indicated. Most patients intermittently require physical therapy, including postural drainage with chest percussion, and parents should be instructed in these techniques. Postural drainage is often effective when used throughout each acute respiratory illness. In some patients, an artificial cough can be accomplished by application of sudden external pressure to the thorax. Some children have been helped in airway clearance by a mechanical vibrating vest. The usefulness of respiratory muscle training in patients with Duchenne muscular dystrophy has not been demonstrated conclusively. In some patients with advanced neuromuscular disease, however, training of specific muscle groups, such as neck muscles or the pectoralis major, may help with the effectiveness of cough and may permit more sustained periods without mechanical ventilation that could be lifesaving during an electrical failure. Influenza vaccine should be administered annually. However, influenza vaccine should be omitted in the extremely rare instances in which it is suspected of playing a role in the causation of the primary disease (e.g., Guillain-Barré syndrome). A pneumococcal vaccine may be indicated. Theophylline has been shown to increase diaphragm strength and endurance, but its clinical application in patients with dystrophic muscles has not been studied.

A permanent tracheostomy to allow better access to the airway for suctioning can be helpful. Some children cannot handle secretions and may need a cuffed endotracheal tube or tracheostomy. A small tracheostomy can be plugged when suctioning is not being performed, allowing the patient to breathe and talk around the tube. A standard tracheostomy may alleviate upper airway obstruction and is useful in carefully selected patients. Children with substantial diaphragmatic weakness may benefit from a mechanical rocking bed to reduce alveolar collapse. Intermittent positive-pressure breathing has also been proposed for this purpose. After pulmonary hypertension and overt right-sided heart failure develop, the prognosis is grave, and treatment with supplemental oxygen and other symptomatic measures allows only temporary improvement.

Ventilator management is indicated for patients whose respiratory failure is likely to be brief (e.g., myasthenia gravis). There is controversy about long-term mechanical ventilation for children with muscular dystrophy (see Chapter 616). Such management is routinely employed by many centers and is well accepted by many patients and families. Those who oppose such treatment point to the fact that these patients have no potential for independent functioning after mechanical ventilation is initiated. Those who support this approach point out that because the diaphragm is among the last muscles to lose strength, these youngsters had no independent functioning for years before the onset of respiratory failure. However, many such patients and families have had acceptable life quality. The addition of the mechanical ventilator makes little difference to their degree of functioning, but it extends their lives. With exquisite attention to details of management, including the use of mechanical devices to aid in cough effectiveness, at least one program has been able to decrease respiratory failure, hospital admissions, and ventilator use for these children.

Bach JR, Ishikawa Y, Kim H: Prevention of pulmonary morbidity for patients with Duchenne muscular dystropy. Chest 105:475, 1994.

Bergofsky EH: State of the art: Respiratory failure in disorders of the thoracic cage. Am Rev Respir Dis 119:643, 1979.

De Troyer A, Deisser P: The effects of intermittent positive pressure breathing on patients with respiratory muscle weakness. Am Rev Respir Dis 124:132, 1981.

Gilgoff IS, Barras DM, Jones MS, et al: Neck breathing: A form of voluntary respiration for the spine-injured ventilator-dependent quadriplegic child. Pediatrics 82:741, 1988.

Greenberg M, Edmonds J: Chronic respiratory problems in neuromyopathic disorders: The nature and management. Pediatr Clin North Am 21:927, 1974.

Macklem PT: Muscular weakness and respiratory function. N Engl J Med 314:775, 1986.

CHAPTER 426
Cough Syncope

Cough syncope has been infrequently reported in children. During a coughing paroxysm in which high intrathoracic pressures are generated, venous obstruction, characterized by redness of the face, is followed by decreased venous return and, ultimately, decreased cardiac output, which results in transient cerebral hypoxia and syncope. Recovery generally occurs within 10 sec to 2 min. Muscular movements and incontinence occur rarely. Although these events may simulate seizures, the underlying neuronal discharges originate in the reticular formation, unlike involvement of the cerebral cortex in true epilepsy. Asthma is the most common precipitating disease. There is no specific treatment.

Katz RM: Cough syncope in children with asthma. J Pediatr 77:48, 1970.

PART XIX

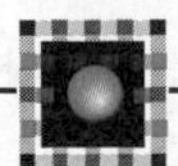

The Cardiovascular System

Daniel Bernstein

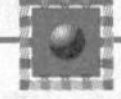

SECTION 1

Developmental Biology of the Cardiovascular System

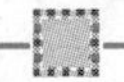

CHAPTER 427
Cardiac Development

Knowledge of the cellular and molecular mechanisms of cardiac development is necessary to understand congenital heart defects and develop strategies for prevention. Developmental cardiologists traditionally grouped defects based on common morphologic patterns, for example, abnormalities of the outflow tracts (the conotruncal lesions such as tetralogy of Fallot and truncus arteriosus) or abnormalities of atrioventricular septation (primum atrial septal defect, complete atrioventricular canal defect). These morphologic categories do not provide an understanding of the mechanisms of heart malformations and their linkage to genetic alterations.

427.1 Early Cardiac Morphogenesis

In the early presomite embryo, the first identifiable cardiac precursors are angiogenetic cell clusters arranged on both sides of the embryo's central axis, which form paired cardiac tubes by 18 days of gestation. These tubes fuse in the midline on the ventral surface of the embryo to form the primitive heart tube by 22 days. Premyocardial cells continue their migration into the region of the heart tube, including epicardial cells and cells derived from the neural crest. The regulation of this early phase of cardiac morphogenesis is controlled in part by the interaction of specific signaling molecules or ligands, usually expressed by one cell type, with specific receptors, usually expressed by another cell type. For example, positional information is conveyed to the developing cardiac mesoderm by the retinoids, isoforms of vitamin A, which bind to specific nuclear receptors and regulate gene transcription. Migration of epithelial cells into the developing heart tube is directed by extracellular matrix proteins, such as fibronectin, interacting with cell surface receptors such as the integrins. The importance of ligands is noted clinically by the spectrum of human cardiac teratogenic effects caused by the retinoid-like drug isotretinoin.

As early as 20–22 days, prior to cardiac looping, the embryonic heart begins to contract, exhibiting phases of the cardiac cycle that are surprisingly similar to those in the mature heart. Morphologists identified segments of the heart tube that were believed to correspond to structures in the mature heart (Fig. 427–1): the sinus venosus and atrium (right and left atria), the primitive ventricle (left ventricle), the bulbus cordis (right ventricle), and the truncus arteriosus (aorta and pulmonary artery). Studies that carefully map the fate of individual heart tube cells demonstrate that this model is oversimplified. Only the trabecular (most heavily muscularized) portions of the left ventricular myocardium are present in the early cardiac tube; the cells that will become the inlet portion of the left ventricle migrate into the cardiac tube at a later stage (after looping is initiated). Even later to appear are the primordial cells that give rise to the great arteries (truncus arteriosus), including cells derived from the neural crest, which are not present until after cardiac looping is complete.

427.2 Cardiac Looping

At approximately 22–24 days, the heart tube begins to bend ventrally and toward the right (see Fig. 427–1) through unknown biomechanical forces. Looping brings the future left ventricle leftward and in continuity with the sinus venosus (future left and right atria), whereas the future right ventricle is shifted rightward and in continuity with the truncus arteriosus (future aorta and pulmonary artery). This pattern of development explains the relatively common occurrence of the cardiac anomalies double-outlet right ventricle and double-inlet left ventricle, and the extreme rarity of double-outlet left ventricle and double-inlet right ventricle (see Chapter 437.5). Cardiac looping, one of the first manifestations of right-left asymmetry in the developing embryo, is critical for the successful completion of cardiac morphogenesis. When cardiac looping is abnormal, there is a high incidence of serious cardiac malformations.

Potential mechanisms for cardiac looping include differential growth rates for myocytes on the convex vs the concave surface of the curve, differential rates of cell death, and mechanical forces generated within myocardial cells via their actin cytoskeleton. The signal for this directionality may be contained in a concentration gradient between the right and left sides of the embryo by the expression of critical signaling molecules, (e.g., members of the TGF [tumor growth factor]-β family of peptide growth factors, and signaling peptides such as *Sonic hedgehog*). In murine models of abnormal looping, the specific defect resides in the dynein gene.

427.3 Cardiac Septation

When looping is complete, the external appearance of the heart is similar to that of the mature heart; internally the structure resembles a single tube, although now it has several

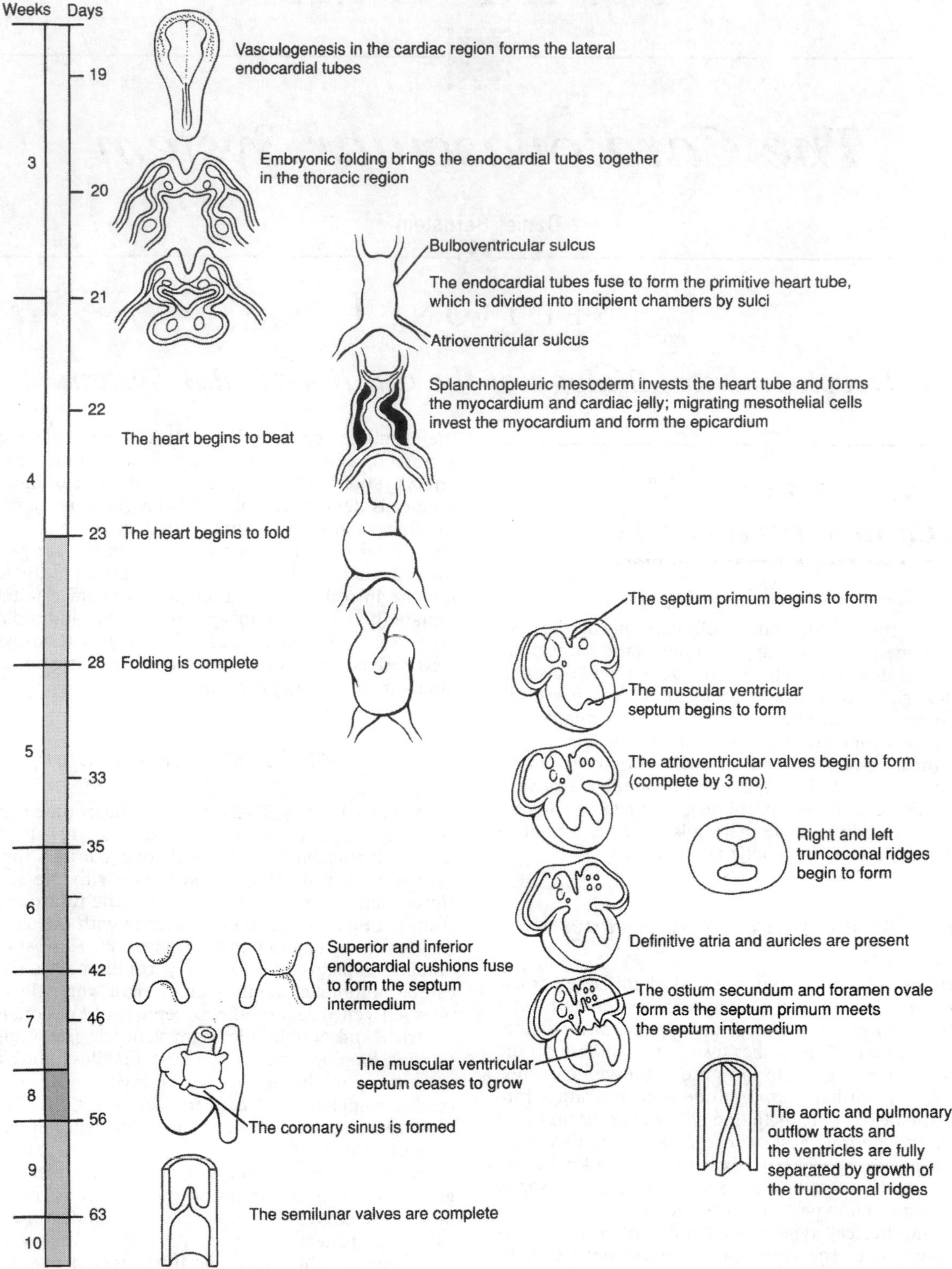

Timeline. Formation of the heart.

Figure 427–1 Timeline of cardiac morphogenesis. (From Larsen WJ: Essentials of Human Embryology. New York, Churchill Livingstone, 1998.)

bulges resulting in the appearance of primitive chambers. The common atrium (comprising both right and left atria) is connected to the primitive ventricle (future left ventricle) via the atrioventricular canal. The primitive ventricle is connected to the bulbus cordis (future right ventricle) via the bulboventricular foramen. The distal portion of the bulbus cordis is connected to the truncus arteriosus via an outlet segment (the conus).

The heart tube now consists of several layers of myocardium and a single layer of endocardium separated by the cardiac jelly, an acellular extracellular matrix secreted by the myocardium. Septation of the heart begins at approximately day 26 with the ingrowth of large tissue masses, the endocardial cushions, at both the atrioventricular and conotruncal junctions (see Fig. 427–1). These cushions consist of protrusions of cardiac jelly, which, in addition to their role in development, also serve a physiologic function as primitive heart valves. Endocardial cells dedifferentiate and migrate into the cardiac jelly in the region of the endocardial cushions, eventually becoming mesenchymal cells that will form part of the atrioventricular valves.

Complete septation of the atrioventricular canal occurs with fusion of the endocardial cushions. Most of the atrioventricular valve tissue is derived from the ventricular myocardium, resulting from an undermining of the ventricular walls. As this process occurs asymmetrically, the tricuspid valve annulus sits closer to the apex of the heart than does the mitral valve annulus. The physical separation of these two valves produces the atrioventricular septum, the absence of which is the primary common defect in patients with atrioventricular canal defects (see Chapter 433.5). If the process of undermining is incomplete, one of the atrioventricular valves may not separate normally from the ventricular myocardium, a possible cause of Ebstein's anomaly (see Chapter 437.7).

The septation of the atria begins at approximately 30 days, with the growth of the septum primum downward toward the endocardial cushions (see Fig. 427–1). The orifice that remains is the ostium primum. The endocardial cushions then fuse and, together with the completed septum primum, divide the atrioventricular canal into right and left segments. A second opening appears in the posterior portion of the septum primum, the ostium secundum, which allows a portion of the fetal venous return to the right atrium to pass across to the left atrium. Finally, the septum secundum grows downward, just to the right of the septum primum. Together with a flap of the septum primum, the ostium secundum forms the foramen ovale, through which fetal blood passes from the inferior vena cava to the left atrium (see Chapter 428).

Septation of the ventricles begins at about day 25 with protrusions of endocardium in both the inlet (primitive ventricle) and outlet (bulbus cordis) segments of the heart. The inlet protrusions fuse into the bulboventricular septum and extend posteriorly toward the inferior endocardial cushion, giving rise to the inlet and trabecular portions of the interventricular septum. Ventricular septal defects can occur in any portion of the developing interventricular septum (see Chapter 433.6). The outlet or conotruncal septum develops from ridges of cardiac jelly, similar to the atrioventricular cushions. These ridges fuse to form a spiral septum, bringing the future pulmonary artery into communication with the anterior and rightward right ventricle, and the future aorta into communication with the posterior and leftward left ventricle. Differences in cell growth of the outlet septum lead to a lengthening of the segment of smooth muscle beneath the pulmonary valve (conus), which separates the tricuspid and pulmonary valves. In contrast, the segment beneath the aortic valve disappears, leading to fibrous continuity of the mitral and aortic valves. Defects in these processes are responsible for conotruncal and aortic arch defects (truncus arteriosus, tetralogy of Fallot, pulmonary atresia, double-outlet right ventricle, interrupted aortic arch), a group of cardiac anomalies often associated with deletions of the DiGeorge critical region of chromosome 22q11 (see Chapters 437 and 438).

427.4 *Aortic Arch Development*

The aortic arch, head and neck vessels, proximal pulmonary arteries, and ductus arteriosus develop from the aortic sac, arterial arches, and dorsal aortae. When the straight heart tube develops, the distal outflow portion bifurcates into the right and left first aortic arches, which join the paired dorsal aortae (Fig. 427–2). The dorsal aortae will fuse to form the descending aorta. The proximal aorta from the aortic valve to the left carotid artery arises from the aortic sac. The 1st and 2nd arches largely regress by about 22 days, with the 1st aortic arch giving rise to the maxillary artery and the 2nd to the stapedial and hyoid arteries. The 3rd arches participate in the formation of the innominate artery and the common and internal carotid arteries. The right 4th arch gives rise to the innominate and right subclavian arteries, and the left 4th arch participates in the formation of the segment of the aortic arch between the left carotid artery and the ductus arteriosus. The 5th arch does not persist as a major structure in the mature circulation. The 6th arches join the more distal pulmonary arteries, with the right 6th arch giving rise to a portion of the proximal right pulmonary artery and the left 6th arch giving rise to the ductus

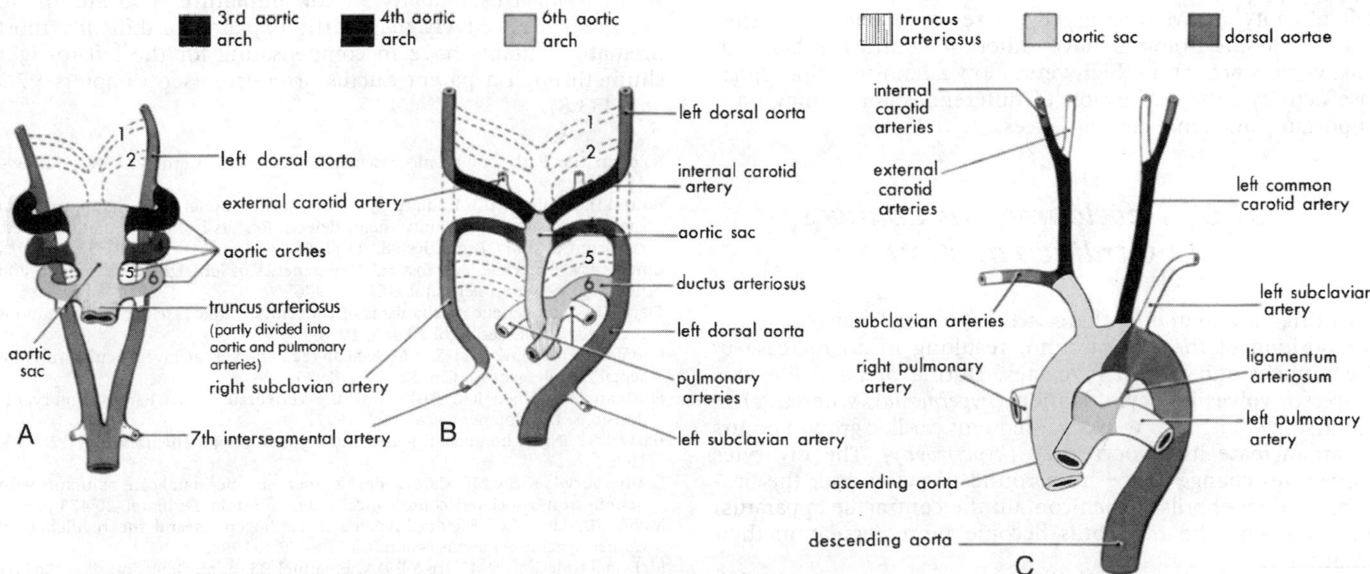

Figure 427–2 Schematic drawings illustrating the changes that result during transformation of the truncus arteriosus, aortic sac, aortic arches, and dorsal aortae into the adult arterial pattern. The vessels that are not shaded or colored are not derived from these structures. *A*, Aortic arches at six weeks; by this stage the first two pairs of aortic arches have largely disappeared. *B*, Aortic arches at seven weeks; the parts of the dorsal aortae and aortic arches that normally disappear are indicated by broken lines. *C*, The arterial vessels of a six-mo-old infant. (From Moore KL, Persaud TVN: The Developing Human. Philadelphia, W.B. Saunders, 1993.)

arteriosus. The aortic arch between the ductus arteriosus and the left subclavian artery is derived from the left-sided dorsal aorta, whereas the aortic arch distal to the left subclavian artery is derived from the fused right and left dorsal aortae. Abnormalities in development of the paired aortic arches are responsible for right aortic arch, double aortic arch, and vascular rings (see Chapter 439.1).

427.5 Cardiac Differentiation

The process by which the totipotential cells of the early embryo become committed to specific cell lineages is called *differentiation*. Precardiac mesodermal cells differentiate into mature cardiac muscle cells, developing an appropriate complement of cardiac-specific contractile elements, regulatory proteins, receptors, and ion channels. Expression of the contractile protein myosin occurs at an early stage of cardiac development, even before fusion of the bilateral heart primordia. Differentiation in these early mesodermal cells is regulated by signals from the anterior endoderm, a process known as *induction*. Several putative early signaling molecules include fibroblast growth factor, activin, and insulin. Signaling molecules interact with receptors on the cell surface that activate second messengers that activate specific *nuclear transcription factors*, (GATA-4, MEF2, Nkx, bHLH and the retinoic acid receptor family), which induce the expression of specific gene products to regulate cardiac differentiation. Some of the primary disorders of cardiac muscle, the cardiomyopathies, may be related to defects in some of these signaling molecules (see Chapter 445).

Developmental processes are chamber-specific. Early in development, ventricular myocytes express both ventricular and atrial *isoforms* of several proteins, for example, atrial natriuretic peptide (ANP) and myosin light chain (MLC). Mature ventricular myocytes do not express ANP and express only a ventricular-specific MLC 2v isoform, whereas mature atrial myocytes express atrial natriuretic peptide (ANP) and an atrial-specific MLC 2a isoform. Many pathologic cardiac conditions, for example, heart failure (see Chapter 445), volume overload (see Chapters 433 and 435), and pressure overload hypertrophy (see Chapter 434), are associated with a recapitulation of fetal cell phenotypes: Mature myocytes re-express fetal proteins. Since different isoforms have different contractile behavior (fast vs slow activation, high versus low adenosine triphosphatase activity), the expression of different isoforms may have important functional consequences.

427.6 Developmental Changes in Cardiac Function

During development, there are profound changes in the composition of the myocardium, resulting in an increase in the number and size of myocytes. During prenatal life, this process involves myocyte division (*hyperplasia*), whereas after the first few postnatal weeks subsequent cardiac growth occurs by an increase in myocyte size (*hypertrophy*). The myocytes themselves change shape from round to cylindrical, the proportion of myofibrils (which contain the contractile apparatus) increases, and the myofibrils become more regular in their orientation.

The plasma membrane (known as the *sarcolemma* in myocytes) is the location of ion channels and transmembrane receptors that regulate the exchange of chemical information from the cell surface to the cell interior. Ion fluxes through these channels control the processes of depolarization and repolarization. Developmental changes have been described for the sodium-potassium pump, the sodium-hydrogen exchanger, and voltage-dependent calcium channels. As the myocyte matures, extensions of the sarcolemma develop toward the interior of the cell (the t-tubule system), which dramatically increases its surface area, and enhances rapid activation of the myocyte. The membrane's α- and β-adrenergic receptors are regulated with development, enhancing the ability of the sympathetic nervous system to control cardiac function as the heart matures.

The *sarcoplasmic reticulum (SR)*, a series of tubules surrounding the myofibrils, controls the intracellular calcium concentration. A series of pumps regulate calcium release to the myofibrils, initiating contraction (ryanodine-sensitive calcium channel), and calcium uptake, initiating relaxation (adenosine triphosphate–dependent SR calcium pump). In immature hearts, this SR calcium transport system is less well developed, resulting in an increased dependency on transport of calcium from outside the cell for contraction. In the mature heart, the majority of calcium activating contraction comes from the SR. This developmental phenomenon may explain the sensitivity of the infant heart to sarcolemmal calcium channel blockers such as verapamil, often resulting in a marked depression of contractility and cardiac arrest (see Chapter 442).

The major contractile proteins (myosin, actin, tropomyosin, and troponin) are organized into the functional unit of cardiac contraction, the sarcomere. Each has several isoforms, which are expressed differentially by location (atrium vs ventricle) and by developmental stage (embryo, fetus, newborn, adult).

Changes in myocardial structure and myocyte biochemistry result in easily quantifiable differences in cardiac function with development. In isolated cardiac muscle strips, force of contraction increases with maturation from fetus to adult. Fetal cardiac function is poorly responsive to changes in both preload (filling volume) and afterload (systemic resistance). The most effective means of increasing ventricular function in the fetus is through increasing heart rate. After birth and with further maturation, preload and afterload play an increasing role in regulating cardiac function. The rate of cardiac relaxation is also developmentally regulated. Decreased ability of the immature SR calcium pump to remove calcium from the contractile apparatus is manifested as a decreased ability of the fetal heart to enhance relaxation in response to sympathetic stimulation. This inability of the immature myocardium to use preload effectively may partly explain the difficulty most premature infants have in compensating for the left-to-right shunt through a patent ductus arteriosus (see Chapters 97.3 and 433.8).

Baldwin HS: Early embryonic vascular development. Cardiovasc Res 31:E34–45, 1996.

Botto LD, Khoury MJ, Mulinare J, et al: Periconceptional multivitamin use and the occurrence of conotruncal heart defects: Results from a population-based, case-control study. Pediatrics 98:911, 1996.

Bowers PN, Brueckner M, Yost HJ: The genetics of left-right development and heterotaxia. Semin Perinatol 20:577, 1996.

Clark EB: Pathogenetic mechanisms of congenital cardiovascular malformations revisited. Semin Perinatol 20:465, 1996.

Eisenberg LM, Markwald RR: Molecular regulation of atrioventricular valvuloseptal morphogenesis. Circ Res 77:1, 1995.

Fishman MC, Chien KR: Fashioning the vertebrate heart: Earliest embryonic decisions. Development 124:2099, 1997.

Harvey RP: NK-2 homeobox genes and heart development. Dev Biol 178:203, 1996.

Leatherbury L, Kirby ML: Cardiac development and perinatal care of infants with neural crest-associated contotruncal defects. Semin Perinatol 20:473, 1996.

Mably JD, Liew CC: Factors involved in cardiogenesis and the regulation of cardiac-specific gene expression. Circ Res 79:4, 1996.

McDonald-McGinn DM, Driscoll DA, Emanuel BS, et al: Detection of a 22q11.2 deletion in cardiac patients suggests a risk for velopharyngeal incompetence. Pediatrics 99:1, 1997.

Smith SM, Dickman ED, Power SC, Lancman J: Retinoids and their receptors in vertebrate embryogenesis. J Nutr 128(Suppl):467S, 1998.

Wilson DI, Burn J, Scambler P, Goodship J: DiGeorge syndrome: Part of CATCH 22. J Med Genet 30:852, 1993.

CHAPTER 428
The Fetal to Neonatal Circulatory Transition

428.1 The Fetal Circulation

Much of the information concerning the fetal circulation has been derived from studies in fetal sheep. The human fetal circulation and its adjustments after birth are probably similar to those of other large mammals.

In the fetal circulation, the right and left ventricles exist in a parallel circuit as opposed to the series circuit of the newborn or adult (Fig. 428–1*A*). In the fetus, gas and metabolite exchange are provided for by the placenta. The lungs do not provide gas exchange, and vessels in the pulmonary circulation are vasoconstricted. There are three cardiovascular structures unique to the fetus that are important for maintaining this parallel circulation: the ductus venosus, foramen ovale, and ductus arteriosus.

Oxygenated blood returning from the placenta, with a Po_2 of about 30–35 mm Hg, flows to the fetus through the umbilical vein. Approximately 50% of umbilical venous blood enters the hepatic circulation, whereas the rest bypasses the liver and joins the inferior vena cava via the *ductus venosus,* where it partially mixes with poorly oxygenated inferior vena cava blood derived from the fetal lower body. This combined lower body plus umbilical venous blood flow (Po_2 of about 26–28 mm Hg) enters the right atrium and is directed preferentially across the *foramen ovale* to the left atrium (see Fig. 428–1*B*). This blood then flows into the left ventricle and is ejected into the ascending aorta. Fetal superior vena cava blood, which is considerably less oxygenated (Po_2 of 12–14 mm Hg), enters the right atrium and preferentially traverses the tricuspid valve, rather than the foramen ovale, and flows primarily to the right ventricle.

From the right ventricle, this blood is ejected into the pulmonary artery. Because the pulmonary arterial circulation is vasoconstricted, only about 10% of right ventricular outflow enters the lungs. The major portion of this blood (which has a Po_2 of about 18–22 mm Hg) bypasses the lungs and flows through the *ductus arteriosus* into the descending aorta to perfuse the lower part of the fetal body as well as to return to the placenta via the two umbilical arteries. Thus, the fetal upper body (including the coronary and cerebral arteries and those to the upper extremities) is perfused exclusively from the left ventricle with blood having a slightly higher Po_2 than the blood perfusing the lower fetal body, which is derived mostly from the right ventricle. Only a small volume of blood from the ascending aorta (10% of fetal cardiac output) flows across the aortic isthmus to the descending aorta.

The total fetal cardiac output—the combined ventricular output of both the left and right ventricles—amounts to about 450 mL/kg/min. Approximately 65% of descending aortic blood flow returns to the placenta; the remaining 35% perfuses the fetal organs and tissues. In the sheep fetus, right ventricular output is approximately two times that of the left ventricle. In the human fetus, with a larger percentage of

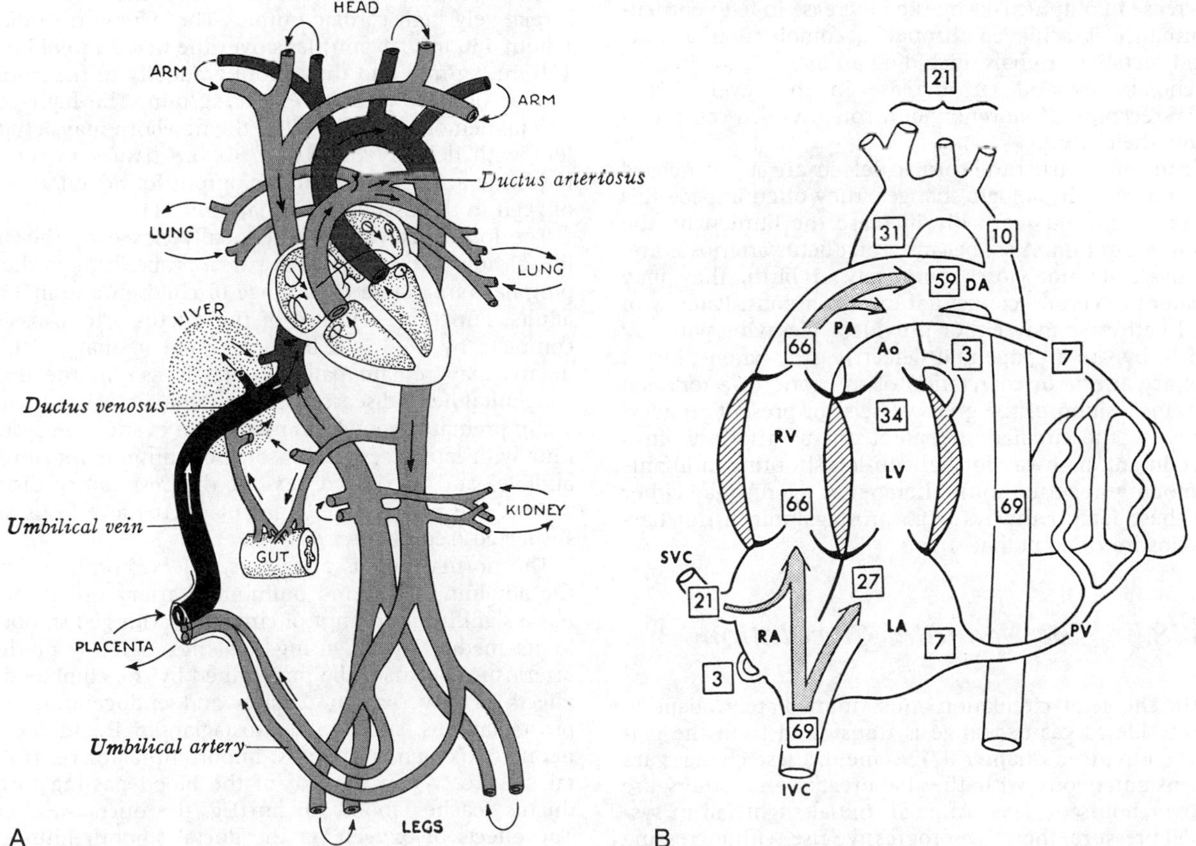

Figure 428–1 *A*, The human circulation before birth (partly after Dawes). Black shading indicates more oxygenated blood, and arrows indicate the direction of flow. *B*, Percentages of combined ventricular output that return to the fetal heart, that are ejected by each ventricle, and that flow through the main vascular channels. Figures are those obtained from study of late-gestation lambs. (From Rudolph AM: Congenital Diseases of the Heart. Chicago, Year Book Medical Publishers, 1974.)

blood flow going to the brain, right ventricular output is probably closer to 1.3 times left ventricular flow. Thus, during fetal life the right ventricle is not only pumping against systemic blood pressure but also is performing a greater volume of work than the left ventricle.

428.2 The Transitional Circulation

At birth, the mechanical expansion of the lungs and increase in arterial Po_2 results in a rapid decrease in pulmonary vascular resistance. Concomitantly, the removal of the low resistance placental circulation results in an increase in systemic vascular resistance. The output from the right ventricle now flows entirely into the pulmonary circulation, and because pulmonary vascular resistance becomes lower than systemic vascular resistance, the shunt through the ductus arteriosus reverses and becomes left to right. Over the course of several days, the high arterial Po_2 constricts the ductus arteriosus and it closes, eventually becoming the ligamentum arteriosum. The increased volume of pulmonary blood flow returning to the left atrium increases left atrial volume and pressure sufficiently to close the foramen ovale functionally, although the foramen may remain probe-patent.

The removal of the placenta from the circulation also leads to closure gof the ductus venosus. The left ventricle is now coupled to the high-resistance systemic circulation, and its wall thickness and mass begin to increase. In contrast, the right ventricle is now coupled to the low-resistance pulmonary circulation, and its wall thickness and mass decrease slightly. The left ventricle, which in the fetus pumped blood only to the upper body and brain, must now deliver the entire systemic cardiac output (approximately 350 mL/kg/min), an almost 200% increase in output. This marked increase in left ventricular performance is achieved through a combination of hormonal and metabolic signals, including an increase in circulating catecholamines and an increase in the level of the myocardial receptors (β-adrenergic) through which catecholamines have their effect.

When congenital structural cardiac defects are superimposed on these dramatic physiologic changes, they often impede this smooth transition and markedly increase the burden on the newborn myocardium. Also, because the ductus arteriosus and foramen ovale do not close completely at birth, they may remain patent in certain congenital cardiac lesions. Patency of these fetal pathways may either provide a lifesaving pathway for blood to bypass a congenital defect (e.g., a patent ductus in pulmonary atresia or coarctation of the aorta or a foramen ovale in transposition of the great vessels) or present an additional stress to the circulation (patent ductus arteriosus in a premature infant, pathway for right-to-left shunting in infants with pulmonary hypertension). Therapeutic agents may either maintain these fetal pathways (e.g., prostaglandin E_1) or hasten their closure (indomethacin).

428.3 The Neonatal Circulation

At birth, the fetal circulation must immediately adapt to extrauterine life as gas exchange is transferred from the placenta to the lung (see Chapter 97). Some of these changes are virtually instantaneous with the 1st breath, and others are effected over hours or days. After an initial slight fall in systemic blood pressure, there is a progressive rise with increasing age. The heart rate slows as a result of a baroreceptor response to an increase in systemic vascular resistance when the placental circulation is eliminated. The average central aortic pressure in the term neonate is 75/50 mm Hg.

With the onset of ventilation, a marked decrease in pulmonary vascular resistance occurs resulting from both active (Po_2-related) and passive (mechanical-related) vasodilation. In the normal neonate, closure of the ductus arteriosus and the fall of pulmonary vascular resistance result in a fall of pulmonary arterial and right ventricular pressures. The major decline of pulmonary resistance from the high fetal levels to the low "adult" levels in the human infant at sea level usually occurs within the first 2–3 days but may be prolonged for 7 days or more. Over the 1st several weeks of life, pulmonary vascular resistance decreases even further secondary to remodeling of the pulmonary vasculature, including thinning of the vascular smooth muscle and recruitment of new vessels. This decrease in pulmonary vascular resistance significantly influences the timing of the clinical presentation of many congenital heart lesions that are dependent on the relative systemic and pulmonary vascular resistances. For example, the left-to-right shunt through a ventricular septal defect may be minimal during the 1st wk after birth when pulmonary vascular resistance is still somewhat high. As pulmonary resistance decreases over the next week or two, the volume of the left-to-right shunt through the ventricular septal defect increases, eventually leading to symptoms of congestive heart failure.

Significant differences between the neonatal circulation and that of older infants may be summarized as follows: (1) Right-to-left or left-to-right shunting may persist across the patent foramen ovale; (2) in the presence of cardiopulmonary disease, continued patency of the ductus arteriosus may allow left-to-right, right-to-left, or bidirectional shunting; (3) the neonatal pulmonary vasculature constricts more vigorously in response to hypoxemia, hypercapnia, and acidosis; (4) the wall thickness and muscle mass of the neonatal left and right ventricles are almost equal; and (5) newborn infants at rest have a relatively high oxygen consumption, which is associated with a relatively high cardiac output. The newborn cardiac output (about 350 mL/kg/min) falls over the first 2 mo of life to about 150 mL/kg/min and then more gradually to the normal adult cardiac output of about 75 mL/kg/min. The high percentage of fetal hemoglobin present in the newborn may actually interfere with delivery of oxygen to the tissues in the neonate, requiring an increased cardiac output for adequate delivery of oxygen to the tissues (see Chapter 97.1).

The foramen ovale is functionally closed by the 3rd mo of life, although it is possible to pass a probe through the overlapping flaps in a large percentage of children and in 15–25% of adults. Functional closure of the ductus arteriosus is usually complete by 10–15 hr in the normal neonate, although the ductus may remain patent much longer in the presence of congenital heart disease, especially that associated with cyanosis. In premature newborn infants, an evanescent systolic murmur with late accentuation or a continuous murmur may be audible, and in the context of the respiratory distress syndrome, the presence of a patent ductus arteriosus should be suspected (see Chapter 97.3).

The normal ductus arteriosus differs morphologically from the adjoining aorta and pulmonary artery in that the ductus has a significant amount of circularly arranged smooth muscle in its medial layer. During fetal life, patency of the ductus arteriosus appears to be maintained by the combined relaxant effects of low oxygen tension and endogenously produced prostaglandins, specifically prostaglandin E_2. In the full-term neonate, oxygen is the most important factor controlling ductal closure. When the Po_2 of the blood passing through the ductus reaches about 50 mm Hg, the ductal wall constricts. The effects of oxygen on the ductal smooth muscle may be direct or mediated by its effects on prostaglandin synthesis. Gestational age also appears to play an important role; the ductus of the premature infant is less responsive to oxygen, even though its musculature is developed.

428.4 *Persistent Pulmonary Hypertension of the Neonate (Persistence of Fetal Circulatory Pathways)*

(See also Chapter 97.7)

Pulmonary hypertension may persist in the newborn under a variety of circumstances and as a result of a number of underlying mechanisms. Pulmonary vasoconstriction following perinatal hypoxia can result in right-to-left shunting via a patent foramen ovale or ductus arteriosus. Persistent pulmonary hypertension of the neonate is also known as *persistent fetal circulation* and may be associated pathologically with increased muscularization of the pulmonary arterial bed. In addition, pulmonary hypertension may be a secondary feature of a variety of primary cardiac and pulmonary diseases.

The numerous disease entities that result in pulmonary hypertension can be classified on the basis of anatomic and physiologic causes in order to formulate a rational approach to diagnosis and management. The term *persistent pulmonary hypertension of the newborn* is applied to all these causes but is not a specific diagnosis.

Pulmonary venous hypertension may occur in infants having a variety of congenital defects that cause pulmonary venous obstruction in the 1st few days of life. These include stenosis of the pulmonary veins, total anomalous pulmonary venous return with obstruction, cor triatriatum, congenital mitral stenosis, and supravalvular mitral membrane. Infants with left ventricular failure caused by a well-defined cardiac lesion can also have pulmonary arterial hypertension. Severe forms of coarctation of the aorta, aortic valve disease, and cardiomyopathy are included in this group. Infants with transient left ventricular dysfunction secondary to hypoxia can also present with both congestive heart failure and pulmonary arterial hypertension.

Hyperviscosity syndrome occurs in patients with polycythemia, which may be secondary to maternal-fetal or fetal-fetal transfusion or due to perinatal hypoxemia (see Chapter 99.3).

Persistence of the fetal circulation occurs in patients with pulmonary vascular constriction (with or without increased pulmonary vascular smooth muscle) but who have no evidence of parenchymal pulmonary disease or a cardiac lesion. Some infants have both a pulmonary vascular constrictive component and pulmonary parenchymal disease. These infants should be classified according to the primary disease entity, for example, meconium aspiration syndrome with secondary pulmonary vascular constriction and right-to-left shunting (see Chapter 97.7).

An anatomically *hypoplastic pulmonary vascular bed* leads to elevated pulmonary resistance and is another cause of persistent pulmonary hypertension of the newborn. This may occur with congenital pulmonary hypoplasia but is also seen secondary to diaphragmatic hernia or other space-occupying intrathoracic masses, and other diseases. Once hypoxia occurs in these patients, the resulting pulmonary vascular constriction may add to the increased pulmonary resistance and exacerbate the cyanosis.

Infants with *congenital heart lesions* in whom there is nonrestrictive communication between the systemic and pulmonary sides of the circulation have pulmonary hypertension. These patients include those with large ventricular septal defects and double-outlet or single ventricles without associated pulmonic stenosis. Such infants acquire medial muscular hypertrophy of small pulmonary vessels and are at risk for the development of pulmonary vascular disease (see Chapter 440).

Perinatal hypoxemia associated with anatomic and physiologic abnormalities results in persistent pulmonary hypertension of mixed causes. For example, infants with diaphragmatic hernia have ipsilateral pulmonary hypoplasia and contralateral pulmonary vasoconstriction, both of which contribute to high pulmonary resistance, hypertension, and right-to-left shunting. Some preterm infants with severe respiratory distress syndrome may also be cyanotic on the basis of pulmonary vasoconstriction, pulmonary hypertension, and right-to-left shunting at the ductus arteriosus and foramen ovale in the 1st few days of life.

Barst RJ, Gersony WM: The pharmacological treatment of patent ductus arteriosus: A review of the evidence. Drugs 38:250, 1989.

Freed MD, Heymann MA, Lewis AB, et al: Prostaglandin E in infants with ductus arteriosus–dependent congenital heart disease. Circulation 64:899, 1981.

Gersony WM: Neonatal pulmonary hypertension: Pathophysiology, classification, and etiology. Clin Perinatol 11:517, 1984.

Gersony WM, Peckham GH, Ellison RC, et al: Effects of indomethacin in premature infants with patent ductus arteriosus: Results of a national collaborative study. J Pediatr 102:895, 1983.

Rudolph AM: Distribution and regulation of blood flow in the fetal and neonatal lamb. Circ Res 57:811, 1985.

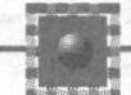

SECTION 2

Evaluation of the Cardiovascular System

CHAPTER 429
History and Physical Examination

The importance of the history and physical examination cannot be overemphasized in the evaluation of infants and children with suspected cardiovascular disorders. After this assessment, patients may require further laboratory evaluation and eventual treatment, or the family may be reassured that no significant problem exists. Although the ready availability of echocardiography may entice the clinician to skip over these preliminary steps, there are several reasons why an initial evaluation by a skilled cardiologist is preferred: (1) The cardiac examination allows the cardiologist to guide the echocardiographic evaluation toward confirming or eliminating specific diagnoses, increasing its accuracy; (2) because the majority of childhood murmurs are innocent, evaluation by a pediatric cardiologist can eliminate unnecessary and expensive laboratory tests; and (3) the cardiologist's knowledge and experience are important in reassuring the patient's family and preventing unnecessary restrictions on healthy physical activity.

HISTORY. A comprehensive cardiac history should start with details of the perinatal period, inquiring as to the presence of cyanosis, respiratory distress, or prematurity. Maternal complications, such as gestational diabetes, medications, systemic lupus erythematosus, or substance abuse, can be associated with cardiac problems. If cardiac symptoms began during infancy, the timing of 1st presentation should be noted; this provides important clues to the specific cardiac condition.

Many of the symptoms of congestive heart failure in infants and children are age-specific. In infants, *feeding difficulties* are common. Inquiry should be made into the frequency of feeding and either the volume of each feed or the time spent on each breast. The infant with heart failure often takes less volume per feeding and become dyspneic or diaphoretic while sucking. After falling asleep exhausted, the baby, inadequately fed, will awaken for the next feeding after a brief time. This cycle continues around the clock and must be carefully differentiated from colic or other feeding disorders. Additional symptoms and signs include those of *respiratory distress*, rapid breathing, nasal flaring, and chest retractions. In older children, heart failure may initially be manifested by *exercise intolerance*, for example, difficulty in keeping up with peers during sports or the need for a nap after coming home from school or by poor growth. Eliciting a history of fatigue in an older child requires questions about age-specific activities, including stair climbing, walking, bicycle riding, physical education class, and competitive sports; information should be obtained regarding more severe manifestations, such as orthopnea and nocturnal dyspnea.

Cyanosis at rest is often overlooked by parents; it may be mistaken for a normal individual variation in coloration. Cyanosis during crying or exercise is more often noted as an abnormal finding by observant parents. However, as many infants and toddlers turn "blue around the lips" when crying vigorously or during breath-holding spells, this must be carefully differentiated from cyanotic heart disease by inquiring as to the inciting factors, length of episodes, and whether the tongue and mucous membranes also appear cyanotic. Newborns have cyanotic extremities **(acrocyanosis)** when undressed and cold, and this must be carefully differentiated from true cyanosis.

Chest pain is an unusual manifestation of cardiac disease in the pediatric patient, although it is a frequent cause for referral to the pediatric cardiologist, especially in adolescents. Nonetheless, a careful history, physical examination and, if indicated, laboratory or imaging tests will assist in identifying the cause of chest pain (Table 429–1).

Cardiac disease may be a manifestation of a known congenital malformation syndrome with typical physical findings (Table 429–2) or of a generalized disorder affecting the heart and other organ systems (Table 429–3). *Extracardiac malformations* may be noted in 20–45% of infants with congenital heart disease. Between 5 and 10% of patients have a known chromosomal abnormality, although this percentage will likely increase dramatically as our knowledge of specific gene defects linked to congenital heart disease increases. A careful family history may also reveal early coronary artery disease or stroke (familial hypercholesterolemia or thrombophilia), generalized muscle disease (muscular dystrophy, dermatomyositis, familial or metabolic cardiomyopathy), or relatives with congenital heart disease.

GENERAL PHYSICAL EXAMINATION. This should begin with a general assessment of the patient, with specific attention to the presence of cyanosis, abnormalities of growth, and any evidence of respiratory distress. It is not uncommon for the beginning examiner to place undue emphasis on cardiac murmurs to the exclusion of the rest of the examination. Evaluation of a murmur must always be performed in the context of other physical findings. Often these associated findings, such as the quality of the pulses or the presence of a ventricular heave, provide important clues to a specific cardiac diagnosis.

Accurate measurement of *height and weight* and plotting on a standard growth chart are important because both cardiac failure and chronic cyanosis result in failure to thrive. Growth failure is usually manifested predominantly by poor weight gain; if length or head circumference is also affected, additional congenital malformations or metabolic disorders may be present.

TABLE 429–1 Differential Diagnosis of Chest Pain in Pediatric Patients

Musculoskeletal (common)

Trauma (accidental, abuse)
Exercise, overuse injury (strain, bursitis)
Costochondritis (Tietze's syndrome)
Herpes zoster (cutaneous)
Pleurodynia
Fibrositis
Slipping rib
Sickle cell anemia vaso-occlusive crisis
Osteomyelitis (rare)
Primary or metastatic tumor (rare)

Pulmonary (common)

Pneumonia
Pleurisy
Asthma
Chronic cough
Pneumothorax
Infarction (sickle cell anemia)
Foreign body
Embolism (rare)
Pulmonary hypertension (rare)
Tumor (rare)

Gastrointestinal (less common)

Esophagitis (gastroesophageal reflux)
Esophageal foreign body
Esophageal spasm
Cholecystitis
Subdiaphragmatic abscess
Perihepatitis (Fitz-Hugh-Curtis syndrome)
Peptic ulcer disease

Cardiac (less common)

Pericarditis
Postpericardiotomy syndrome
Endocarditis
Mitral valve prolapse
Aortic or subaortic stenosis
Arrhythmias
Marfan's syndrome (dissecting aortic aneurysm)
Anomalous coronary artery
Kawasaki's disease
Cocaine, sympathomimetic ingestion
Angina (familial hypercholesterolemia)

Idiopathic (common)

Anxiety, hyperventilation
Panic disorder

Other (less common)

Spinal cord or nerve root compression
Breast-related pathologic condition
Castleman's disease (lymph node neoplasm)

Mild *cyanosis* may be too subtle for early detection, and clubbing of the fingers and toes is not usually manifested until late in the 1st yr of life, even in the presence of severe arterial oxygen desaturation. Cyanosis is best observed over the nail beds, lips, tongue, and mucous membranes. **Differential cyanosis,** manifested by blue lower extremities and pink upper extremities (usually right arm), is seen with right-to-left shunting across a ductus arteriosus in the presence of a coarctation or interrupted aortic arch. Circumoral cyanosis or blueness around the forehead may be the result of prominent venous plexuses in these areas rather than decreased arterial oxygen saturation. The extremities of infants often turn blue when the infant is unwrapped and cold (**acrocyanosis**), and this can be distinguished from central cyanosis by examination of the tongue and mucous membranes.

Heart failure in infants and children usually results in some degree of hepatomegaly and occasionally splenomegaly. The sites of peripheral edema are age-dependent. In infants, edema

TABLE 429–2 Congenital Malformation Syndromes Associated with Congenital Heart Disease

Syndrome	Features
Chromosomal Disorders	
21-Trisomy (Down syndrome)	Endocardial cushion defect, VSD, ASD
22p-Trisomy (cat eye syndrome)	Miscellaneous, total anomalous pulmonary venous return
18-Trisomy	VSD, ASD, PDA, coarctation of aorta, bicuspid aortic or pulmonary valve
13-Trisomy	VSD, ASD, PDA, coarctation of aorta, bicuspid aortic or pulmonary valve
9-Trisomy	Miscellaneous
XXXXY	PDA, ASD
Penta X	PDA, VSD
Triploidy	VSD, ASD, PDA
XO (Turner's syndrome)	Bicuspid aortic valve, coarctation of aorta
Fragile X	Mitral valve prolapse, aortic root dilatation
Duplication 3q2	Miscellaneous
Deletion 4p	VSD, PDA, aortic stenosis
Deletion 9p	Miscellaneous
Deletion 5p (cri du chat syndrome)	VSD, PDA, ASD
Deletion 10q	VSD, TOF, conotruncal lesions*
Deletion 13q	VSD
Deletion 18q	VSD
Syndrome Complexes	
CHARGE association (*c*oloboma, *h*eart, *a*tresia choanae, *r*etardation, *g*enital and *e*ar anomalies)	VSD, ASD, PDA, TOF, endocardial cushion defect
DiGeorge's sequence, CATCH 22	Aortic arch anomalies, conotruncal anomalies
Alagille's syndrome (arteriohepatic dysplasia)	Peripheral pulmonic stenosis
VATER association (*v*ertebral, *a*nal, *t*racheoesophageal, *r*adial, and *r*enal anomalies)	VSD, TOF, ASD, PDA
FAVS (*f*acio-*a*uriculo-*v*ertebral *s*pectrum)	TOF, VSD
CHILD (*c*ongenital *h*emidysplasia with *i*chthyosiform erythroderma, *l*imb *d*efects)	Miscellaneous
Mulibrey nanism (*mu*scle, *li*ver, *br*ain, *ey*e)	Pericardial thickening, constrictive pericarditis
Asplenia syndrome	Complex cyanotic heart lesions with decreased pulmonary blood flow, transposition of great arteries, anomalous pulmonary venous return, dextrocardia, single ventricle, single atrioventricular valve
Polysplenia syndrome	Acyanotic lesions with increased pulmonary blood flow, azygos continuation of inferior vena cava, partial anomalous pulmonary venous return, dextrocardia, single ventricle, common atrioventricular valve
Teratogenic Agents	
Congenital rubella	PDA, peripheral pulmonic stenosis
Fetal hydantoin syndrome	VSD, ASD, coarctation of aorta, PDA
Fetal alcohol syndrome	ASD, VSD
Fetal valproate effects	Coarctation of aorta, hypoplastic left side of the heart, aortic stenosis, pulmonary atresia, VSD
Maternal phenylketonuria	VSD, ASD, PDA, coarctation of aorta
Retinoic acid embryopathy	Conotruncal anomalies
Others	
Apert's syndrome	VSD
Autosomal dominant polycystic kidney disease	Mitral valve prolapse
Carpenter	PDA
Conradi	VSD, PDA
Crouzon	PDA, coarctation of aorta
Cutis laxa	Pulmonary hypertension, pulmonic stenosis
de Lange	VSD
Ellis-van Creveld	Single atrium, VSD
Holt-Oram	ASD, VSD; 1st-degree heart block
Infant of diabetic mother	Hypertrophic cardiomyopathy, VSD, conotruncal anomalies
Kartagener	Dextrocardia
Meckel-Gruber	ASD, VSD
Noonan	Pulmonic stenosis, ASD, cardiomyopathy
Pallister-Hall	Endocardial cushion defect
Rubinstein-Taybi	VSD
Scimitar	Hypoplasia of the right lung, anomalous pulmonary venous return to the inferior vena cava
Smith-Lemli-Opitz	VSD, PDA
Thrombocytopenia and absent radius (TAR)	ASD, TOF
Treacher Collins	VSD, ASD, PDA
Williams' syndrome	Supravalvular aortic stenosis, peripheral pulmonic stenosis

**Conotruncal = TOF, pulmonary atresia, truncus arteriosus, transposition of the great arteries.*
VSD = ventricular septal defect; ASD = atrial septal defect; PDA = patent ductus arteriosus; TOF = tetralogy of Fallot.

is usually seen around the eyes and over the flanks, especially after first waking in the morning. Older children and teenagers manifest both periorbital edema and pedal edema. A frequent first complaint for these older patients is that their clothes no longer fit.

The *heart rate* of newborn infants is rapid and subject to wide fluctuations (Table 429–4). The average rate ranges from 120 to 140 beats/min and may increase to 170+ beats/min during crying and activity, or drop to 70–90 beats/min during sleep. As the child grows older, the average pulse rate decreases and may be as low as 40 beats/min in athletic adolescents. Persistent tachycardia (>200 beats/min in neonates, 150 beats/min in infants, or 120 beats/min in older children), bradycardia, or irregular heart beat other than sinus arrhythmia require

TABLE 429–3 Cardiac Manifestations of Systemic Diseases

Systemic Disease	Cardiac Complications
Inflammatory Disorders	
Sepsis	Hypotension, myocardial dysfunction, pericardial effusion, pulmonary hypertension
Juvenile rheumatoid arthritis	Pericarditis, rarely myocarditis
Systemic lupus erythematosus	Pericarditis, Libman-Sacks endocarditis, coronary arteritis, coronary atherosclerosis (with steroids), congenital heart block
Scleroderma	Pulmonary hypertension, myocardial fibrosis, cardiomyopathy
Dermatomyositis	Cardiomyopathy, arrhythmias, heart block
Kawasaki's disease	Coronary artery aneurysm and thrombosis, myocardial infarction, myocarditis, valvular insufficiency
Sarcoidosis	Granuloma, fibrosis, amyloidosis, biventricular hypertrophy, arrhythmias
Lyme disease	Arrhythmias, myocarditis
Löffler hypereosinophilic syndrome	Endomyocardial disease
Inborn Errors of Metabolism	
Refsum	Arrhythmia, sudden death
Hunter-Hurler	Valvular insufficiency, heart failure, hypertension
Fabry	Mitral insufficiency, coronary artery disease with myocardial infarction
Glycogen storage disease IIa (Pompe's disease)	Short PR interval, cardiomegaly, heart failure, arrhythmias
Carnitine deficiency	Heart failure, cardiomyopathy
Gaucher	Pericarditis
Homocystinuria	Coronary thrombosis
Alkaptonuria	Atherosclerosis, valvular disease
Morquio-Ullrich	Aortic incompetence
Scheie	Aortic incompetence
Connective Tissue Disorders	
Arterial calcification of infancy	Calcinosis of coronary arteries, aorta
Marfan	Aortic and mitral insufficiency, dissecting aortic aneurysm, mitral valve prolapse
Congenital contractural arachnodactyly	Mitral insufficiency or prolapse
Ehlers-Danlos	Mitral valve prolapse, dilatated aortic root
Osteogenesis imperfecta	Aortic incompetence
Pseudoxanthoma elasticum	Peripheral arterial disease
Neuromuscular Disorders	
Friedreich's ataxia	Cardiomyopathy
Duchenne's dystrophy	Cardiomyopathy, heart failure
Tuberous sclerosis	Cardiac rhabdomyoma
Familial deafness	Occasionally arrhythmia, sudden death
Neurofibromatosis	Pulmonic stenosis, pheochromocytoma, coarctation of aorta
Riley-Day	Episodic hypertension, postural hypotension
Von Hippel-Lindau	Hemangiomas, pheochromocytomas
Endocrine-Metabolic Disorders	
Graves	Tachycardia, arrhythmias, heart failure
Hypothyroidism	Bradycardia, pericardial effusion, cardiomyopathy, low-voltage ECG
Pheochromocytoma	Hypertension, myocardial ischemia, myocardial fibrosis, cardiomyopathy
Carcinoid	Right-sided endocardial fibrosis
Hematologic Disorders	
Sickle cell anemia	High-output heart failure, cardiomyopathy, cor pulmonale
Thalassemia major	High-output heart failure, hemochromatosis
Hemochromatosis (1st or 2nd degree)	Cardiomyopathy
Others	
Appetite suppressants (flenfluramine and dexflenfluramine)	Cardiac valvulopathy
Cockayne	Atherosclerosis
Familial dwarfism and nevi	Cardiomyopathy
Jervell and Lange-Nielsen	Prolonged QT interval, sudden death
Kearns-Sayre	Heart block
Leopard (lentiginosis)	Pulmonic stenosis, prolonged QT interval
Progeria	Accelerated atherosclerosis
Rendu-Osler-Weber	Arteriovenous fistula (lung, liver, mucous membrane)
Romano-Ward	Prolonged QT interval, sudden death
Weill-Marchesani	Patent ductus arteriosus
Werner	Vascular sclerosis, cardiomyopathy

investigation to exclude pathologic arrhythmias (see Chapter 442).

Careful evaluation of the *character of the pulses* is an important early step in the physical diagnosis of congenital heart disease. A wide pulse pressure with bounding pulses may suggest an aortic runoff lesion, such as patent ductus arteriosus, aortic insufficiency, an arterial-venous communication, or increased cardiac output secondary to anemia, anxiety, or conditions associated with increased catecholamine secretion. Diminished pulses in all extremities are associated with pericardial tamponade, left ventricular outflow obstruction, or cardiomyopathy. The radial and femoral pulses should always be palpated simultaneously. Normally the femoral pulse should be appreciated immediately before the radial pulse. In older children with coarctation of the aorta, blood flow to the descending aorta may channel through collateral vessels, resulting in the femoral pulse being delayed until after the radial pulse (*radial-femoral delay*).

The *blood pressure* should be measured in the arms as well as in the legs, the latter on at least one occasion to be certain that coarctation of the aorta is not overlooked. Palpation of the femoral or dorsalis pedis pulse, or both, is not reliable

TABLE 429–4 Pulse Rates at Rest

Age	Lower Limits of Normal		Average		Upper Limits of Normal	
Newborn	70/min		125/min		190/min	
1–11 mo	80		120		160	
2 yr	80		110		130	
4 yr	80		100		120	
6 yr	75		100		115	
8 yr	70		90		110	
10 yr	70		90		110	
	Girls	*Boys*	*Girls*	*Boys*	*Girls*	*Boys*
12 yr	70	65	90	85	110	105
14 yr	65	60	85	80	105	100
16 yr	60	55	80	75	100	95
18 yr	55	50	75	70	95	90

alone to exclude a coarctation. In older children, a mercury sphygmomanometer with a cuff that covers approximately two thirds of the upper arm or leg may be used for blood pressure measurement. A cuff that is too small results in falsely high readings, whereas a cuff that is too large records slightly decreased pressures. Pediatric clinical facilities should be equipped with 3-, 5-, 7-, 12-, and 18-cm cuffs to accommodate the large spectrum of pediatric patient sizes. The 1st Korotkoff sounds indicate the systolic pressure. As the cuff pressure is slowly decreased, the sounds usually become muffled before they disappear. The diastolic pressure may be recorded when the sounds become muffled (preferred) or when they disappear altogether; the former is usually slightly higher and the latter slightly lower than the true diastolic pressure. For lower extremity blood pressure determination, the stethoscope is placed over the popliteal artery. Ordinarily, the pressure recorded in the legs with the cuff technique is about 10 mm Hg higher than in the arms.

In infants, the blood pressure can be obtained by auscultation, palpation, or by the oscillometric (Dinamap) device, which, if used properly, provides accurate measurements in infants as well as in older children.

Blood pressure varies with the age of the child and is closely related to height and weight. Significant increases occur during adolescence, and there are many temporary variations before the more stable levels of adult life are attained. Exercise, excitement, coughing, crying, and struggling may raise the systolic pressures of infants and children as much as 40–50 mm Hg greater than their usual levels. Variability of blood pressure among children of approximately the same age and body build should be expected, and serial measurements should always be obtained in the evaluation of a patient with hypertension (Figs. 429–1 and 429–2).

Although of little use in infants, in cooperative older children, inspection of the *jugular venous pulse* wave provides information about the *central venous pressure* and right atrial pressure. The neck veins should be inspected with the patient sitting at a 90-degree angle. Under these conditions, the external jugular vein should not be visible above the clavicles unless the central venous pressure is elevated. Increased venous pressure transmitted to the internal jugular vein may appear as venous pulsations without visible distention; such pulsation is not seen in normal children reclining at an angle of 45 degrees. Because the great veins are in direct communication with the right atrium, changes of pressure and volume of this chamber are also transmitted to the veins. The one exception occurs in superior vena cava obstruction, in which venous pulsatility is lost.

CARDIAC EXAMINATION. The heart should be examined in a systematic manner starting with *inspection and palpation.* A **precordial bulge** to the left of the sternum with increased precordial activity suggests cardiac enlargement. This can often best be appreciated by having the child lay supine with the examiner looking up from the childs feet. A **substernal thrust** indicates the presence of right ventricular enlargement; an **apical heave** is noted with left ventricular hypertrophy. A **hyperdynamic precordium** suggests a volume load such as that found with a large left-to-right shunt, although it may be normal in a thin patient. A **silent precordium** with a barely detectable apical impulse suggests a pericardial effusion or severe cardiomyopathy; it may be normal in an obese patient.

The relationship of the apical impulse to the midclavicular line is also helpful in the estimation of cardiac size: The apical impulse moves laterally and inferiorly with enlargement of the left ventricle. Right-sided apical impulses signify dextrocardia, tension pneumothorax, or left-sided thoracic space-occupying lesions (e.g., diaphragmatic hernia).

Thrills are the palpable equivalent of murmurs and correlate with the area of maximal auscultatory intensity of the murmur. It is important to palpate the suprasternal notch and neck for **aortic bruits,** which may indicate the presence of aortic stenosis or, when faint, pulmonary stenosis. Right lower sternal border and apical systolic thrills are characteristic of ventricular septal defect and mitral insufficiency, respectively. Diastolic thrills are occasionally palpable in the presence of atrioventricular valve stenosis. The timing and localization of thrills should be carefully noted.

Auscultation is an art that can be improved on with practice. The diaphragm of the stethoscope is placed firmly on the chest for high-pitched sounds; a lightly placed bell is optimal for low-pitched sounds. The physician should initially concentrate on the characteristics of the individual heart sounds and their variation with respirations, and later on murmurs. The patient should be supine, lying quietly, and breathing normally. The 1st heart sound is best heard at the apex, whereas the 2nd heart sound should be evaluated at the upper left and right sternal borders. The 1st heart sound is caused by the closure of the atrioventricular valves (mitral and tricuspid); the 2nd sound is caused by the closure of the semilunar valves (aortic and pulmonary; Fig. 429–3). During inspiration, the decrease in intrathoracic pressure results in increased filling of the right side of the heart, increasing right ventricular ejection time and thus delaying pulmonary valve closure; thus the splitting of the 2nd heart sound increases during inspiration and decreases during expiration.

Often the 2nd heart sound appears to be single during expiration. The presence of a normally split 2nd sound is strong evidence against the diagnosis of an atrial septal defect, defects associated with pulmonary arterial hypertension, severe pulmonary valve stenosis, aortic and pulmonary atresia, and truncus arteriosus. Wide splitting is noted in atrial septal defect, pulmonary stenosis, Ebstein's anomaly, total anomalous pulmonary venous return, and right bundle branch block. An accentuated pulmonic component of the 2nd sound with narrow splitting is a sign of pulmonary hypertension. A single 2nd sound occurs in pulmonary or aortic atresia or severe stenosis, truncus arteriosus, and often in transposition of the great arteries.

A 3rd heart sound is best heard with the bell at the apex in mid-diastole. A 4th sound, occurring in conjunction with atrial contraction, may be heard just prior to the 1st heart sound in late diastole. The 3rd sound may be normal in an adolescent with a relatively slow heart rate, but in a patient with the clinical signs of heart failure and tachycardia, it may be heard as a gallop rhythm and may merge with a 4th heart sound, known as a *summation gallop.* A **gallop** rhythm is attributed to poor compliance of the ventricle with an exaggeration of the normal 3rd sound associated with ventricular filling.

Ejection clicks, which are heard in early systole, may be related to dilatation of the aorta or pulmonary artery or to a mildly to moderately stenotic semilunar valve. They are heard so close to the 1st heart sound that they may be mistaken for a split 1st sound. Aortic ejection clicks are best heard at the

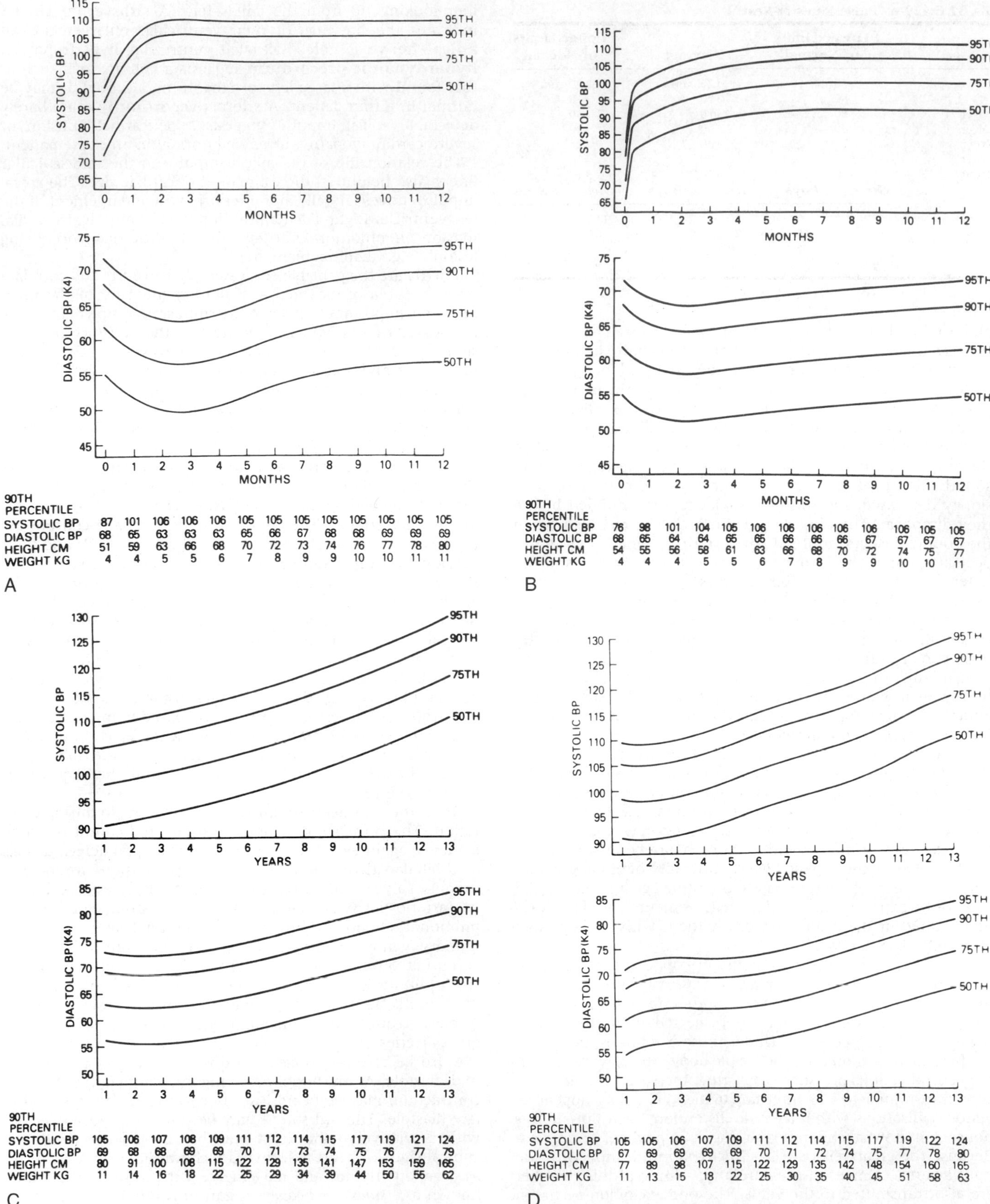

A

90TH PERCENTILE	0	1	2	3	4	5	6	7	8	9	10	11	12
SYSTOLIC BP	87	101	106	106	106	105	105	105	105	105	105	105	105
DIASTOLIC BP	68	65	63	63	63	65	66	67	68	68	69	69	69
HEIGHT CM	51	59	63	66	68	70	72	73	74	76	77	78	80
WEIGHT KG	4	4	5	5	6	7	8	9	9	10	10	11	11

B

90TH PERCENTILE	0	1	2	3	4	5	6	7	8	9	10	11	12
SYSTOLIC BP	76	98	101	104	105	106	106	106	106	106	106	105	105
DIASTOLIC BP	68	65	64	64	65	65	66	66	66	67	67	67	67
HEIGHT CM	54	55	56	58	61	63	66	68	70	72	74	75	77
WEIGHT KG	4	4	4	5	5	6	7	8	9	9	10	10	11

C

90TH PERCENTILE	1	2	3	4	5	6	7	8	9	10	11	12	13
SYSTOLIC BP	105	106	107	108	109	111	112	114	115	117	119	121	124
DIASTOLIC BP	69	68	68	69	69	70	71	73	74	75	76	77	79
HEIGHT CM	80	91	100	108	115	122	129	135	141	147	153	159	165
WEIGHT KG	11	14	16	18	22	25	29	34	39	44	50	55	62

D

90TH PERCENTILE	1	2	3	4	5	6	7	8	9	10	11	12	13
SYSTOLIC BP	105	105	106	107	109	111	112	114	115	117	119	122	124
DIASTOLIC BP	67	69	69	69	69	70	71	72	74	75	77	78	80
HEIGHT CM	77	89	98	107	115	122	129	135	142	148	154	160	165
WEIGHT KG	11	13	15	18	22	25	30	35	40	45	51	58	63

Figure 429–1 *A*, Age-specific percentiles of BP measurements in boys—birth to 12 mo of age. *B*, Age-specific percentiles of BP measurements in girls—birth to 12 mo of age. *C*, Age-specific percentiles for BP measurements in boys—1–13 yr of age. *D*, Age-specific percentiles of BP measurements in girls—1–13 yr of age; Korotkoff phase IV (K4) used for diastolic BP. (From National Heart, Lung, and Blood Institute, Bethesda, MD: Report of the second task force on blood pressure control in children—1987. Reproduced by permission of Pediatrics. Vol. 79, p. 1. Copyright 1987.)

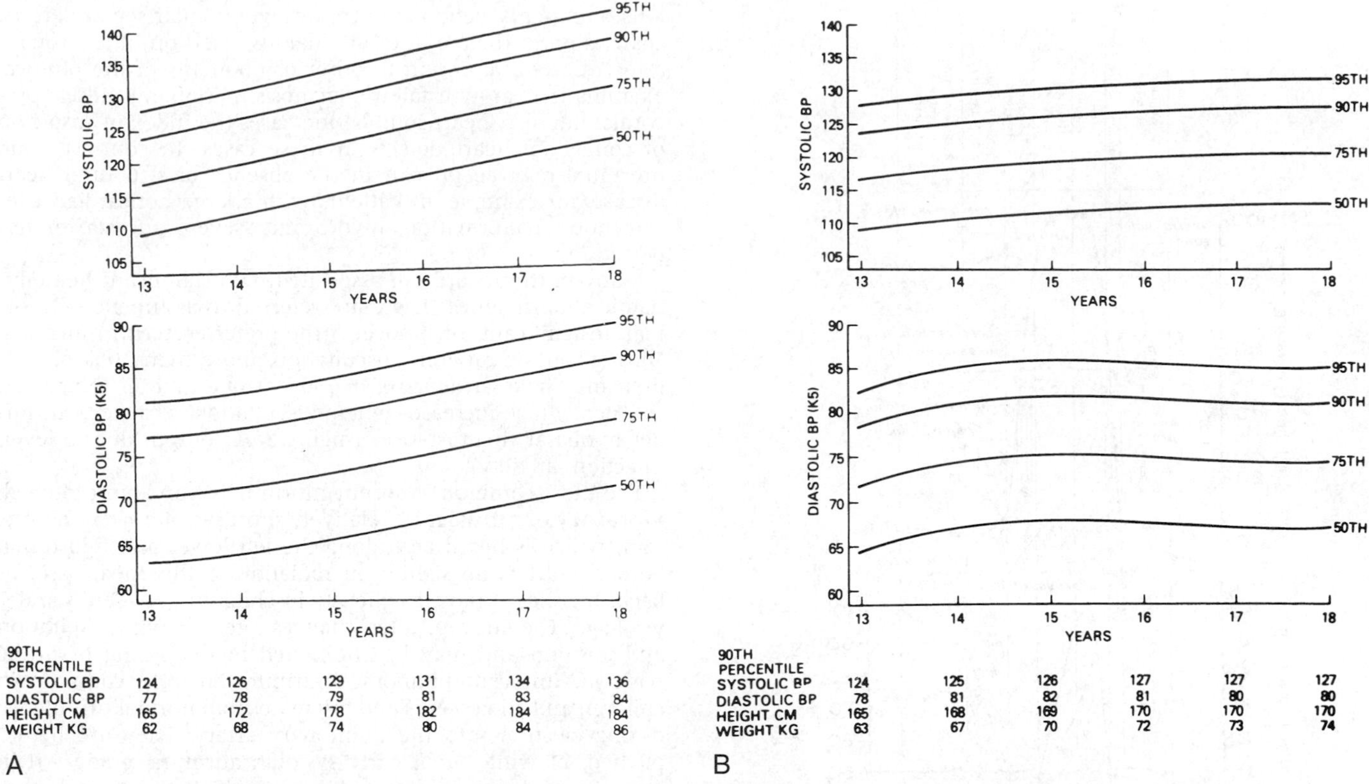

Figure 429–2 *A*, Age-specific percentiles of BP measurements in boys—13–18 yr of age. *B*, Age-specific percentiles of BP measurements in girls—13–18 yr of age; Korotkoff phase V (K5) used for diastolic BP. (From National Heart, Lung, and Blood Institute, Bethesda, MD: Report of the second task force on blood pressure control in children—1987. Reproduced by permission of Pediatrics. Vol. 79, p. 1, Copyright 1987.)

left middle to right upper sternal border and are constant in intensity. They occur in conditions in which the aortic valve is stenotic or the aorta is dilatated (tetralogy of Fallot, truncus arteriosus). Pulmonary ejection clicks, associated with mild to moderate pulmonary stenosis, are best heard at the left middle to upper sternal border and vary with respirations, often disappearing with inspiration. Split 1st heart sounds are usually heard best at the lower left sternal border. A midsystolic click heard at the apex, often preceding a late systolic murmur, suggests mitral valve prolapse.

Murmurs should be described according to their intensity, pitch, timing (systolic or diastolic), variation in intensity, time to peak intensity, area of maximal intensity, and radiation to other areas. Auscultation for murmurs should be carried out across the upper precordium, down the left or right sternal border, and out to the apex and left axilla. Auscultation should also always be performed in the right axilla and over the back. **Systolic murmurs** are classified as ejection, pansystolic, or late systolic according to the timing of the murmur in relation to the 1st and 2nd heart sounds. The intensity of systolic murmurs is graded from I to VI: I, barely audible; II, medium intensity; III, loud but no thrill; IV, loud with a thrill; V, very loud but still requires positioning of the stethoscope at least partly on the chest; and VI, so loud that the murmur can be heard with the stethoscope off the chest.

Systolic ejection murmurs start a short time after a well-heard 1st heart sound, increase in intensity, peak, and then decrease in intensity; they usually end before the 2nd sound. However, in patients with severe aortic or pulmonary stenosis, the murmur may extend beyond the 1st component of the 2nd sound, thus obscuring it. *Pansystolic or holosystolic murmurs* begin almost simultaneously with the 1st heart sound and continue throughout systole, on occasion becoming gradually decrescendo. It is helpful to remember that after the closure of the atrioventricular valves (the 1st heart sound), there is a brief period during which ventricular pressure increases but the semilunar valves remain closed (isovolumic contraction; see Fig. 429–3). Thus, pansystolic murmurs (heard during both isovolumic contraction and the ejection phases of systole) cannot be caused by flow across the semilunar valves because these valves are closed during isovolumic contraction. Pansystolic murmurs are thus related to blood exiting the contracting ventricle via either an abnormal opening (a ventricular septal defect) or atrioventricular (mitral or tricuspid) valve insufficiency. Systolic ejection murmurs usually imply increased flow or stenosis across one of the ventricular outflow tracts (aortic or pulmonic). In infants with rapid heart rates, it is often difficult to distinguish between ejection and pansystolic murmurs. If a clear and distinct 1st heart sound can be appreciated, the murmur is most likely ejection in nature.

A **continuous murmur** is a systolic murmur that continues or "spills" into diastole and indicates continuous flow, such as in the presence of a patent ductus arteriosus or other aortopulmonary communication. This should be differentiated from a **to-and-fro murmur**, which indicates that the systolic component of the murmur ends at or before the 2nd sound and the diastolic murmur begins after semilunar valve closure (e.g., aortic or pulmonary stenosis combined with insufficiency). A late systolic murmur begins well beyond the 1st heart sound and continues until the end of systole. Such murmurs may be heard after a midsystolic click in patients with mitral valve prolapse and insufficiency.

Several types of **diastolic murmurs** (also graded I–VI) can be identified. A **decrescendo diastolic murmur** is a blowing murmur along the left sternal border, beginning with S2 and diminishing toward mid-diastole. When high-pitched, this murmur is associated with aortic valve insufficiency or with pulmonary insufficiency associated with pulmonary hypertension. When low-pitched, this murmur is associated with pulmonary valve insufficiency in the absence of pulmonary hy-

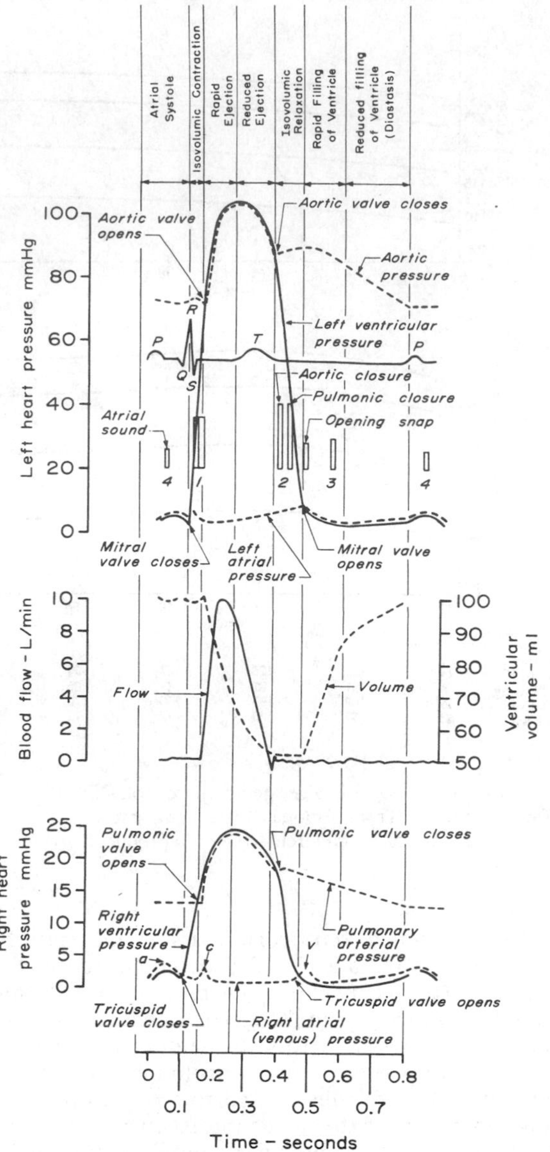

Figure 429–3 Idealized diagram of temporal events of a cardiac cycle.

pertension. A low-pitched decrescendo diastolic murmur is typically noted after surgical repair of the pulmonary outflow tract in defects such as tetralogy of Fallot or in patients with absent pulmonary valves. A **rumbling mid-diastolic murmur** at the left middle and lower sternal border may be due to increased blood flow across the tricuspid valve, such as occurs with atrial septal defect or, less often, because of actual stenosis of this valve. When this murmur is heard at the apex, it is caused by increased flow across the mitral valve, such as occurs with large left-to-right shunts at the ventricular level (ventricular septal defects), at the great vessel level (patent ductus arteriosus, aortopulmonary shunts), or with increased flow because of mitral insufficiency. When an apical diastolic rumbling murmur is longer and is accentuated at the end of diastole (presystolic), it usually indicates anatomic mitral valve stenosis.

The absence of a precordial murmur does not rule out significant congenital or acquired heart disease. Congenital heart defects, some of which are ductal-dependent, may not demonstrate a murmur if the ductus arteriosus closes. These lesions include pulmonary or tricuspid valve atresia and transposition of the great arteries. Murmurs may seem insignificant in patients with severe aortic stenosis, atrial septal defect, anomalous pulmonary venous return, atrioventricular septal defects, coarctation of the aorta, or anomalous insertion of a coronary artery. Careful attention to other components of the physical examination (growth failure, cyanosis, peripheral pulses, precordial impulse, heart sounds) increases the index of suspicion of congenital heart defects in these cases. In contrast, loud murmurs may be present in the absence of structural heart disease, for example, in patients with a large noncardiac arteriovenous malformation, myocarditis, severe anemia, or hypertension.

Many murmurs are not associated with significant hemodynamic abnormalities. These are referred to as functional, normal, insignificant, or innocent (the preferred term) murmurs. During routine random auscultation, more than 30% of children may have an *innocent murmur* at one time in their lives; this percentage increases when auscultation is carried out under nonbasal circumstances (high cardiac output due to fever, infection, anxiety).

The most common innocent murmur is a medium-pitched, **vibratory or "musical,"** relatively short systolic ejection murmur, which is heard best along the left lower and midsternal border and has no significant radiation to the apex, base, or back. It is heard most frequently in children between 3 and 7 yr of age. The murmur often changes intensity with respiration and position and may be attenuated in the sitting or prone position. Innocent pulmonic murmurs are also common in children and adolescents and originate from normal turbulence during ejection into the pulmonary artery. They are higher pitched, blowing, brief, early systolic murmurs, grade I–II in intensity, and are best detected in the 2nd left parasternal space with the patient in the supine position. Features suggestive of heart disease include murmurs that are pansystolic, greater than or equal to grade III, harsh, at the left upper sternal border, and associated with an early or midsystolic click, or an abnormal 2nd heart sound.

The **venous hum** is another example of a common innocent murmur heard during childhood. This is produced by turbulence of blood in the jugular venous system; it has no pathologic significance and may be heard in the neck or anterior portion of the upper chest. It consists of a soft humming sound heard in both systole and diastole and can be exaggerated or made to disappear by varying the position of the head or can be decreased by lightly compressing the jugular venous system in the neck. These simple maneuvers are sufficient to differentiate a venous hum from the murmurs produced by organic cardiovascular disease, particularly a patent ductus arteriosus.

The lack of significance of an innocent murmur should be discussed with the child's parents. It is important to offer complete reassurance because lingering doubts about the importance of a cardiac murmur may have profound effects on child-rearing practices, most often in the form of overprotectiveness. An underlying fear that a cardiac abnormality is present may negatively affect a child's self-image and subtly influence personality development. The physician should explain that the innocent murmur is simply a "noise" and does not indicate the presence of a significant cardiac defect. When asked, "Will it go away?" the best response is to state that because the murmur has no meaning, it does not matter whether it "goes away" or not. Parents should be warned that the intensity of the murmur may increase during febrile illnesses. However, with growth, innocent murmurs are less well heard and often disappear completely. At times, additional studies may be indicated to rule out a congenital heart defect, but "routine" electrocardiographic, chest roentgenographic, and echocardiographic examinations for well children with innocent murmurs should be avoided.

Hansen LK, Birkebaek NH, Oxhøj H: Initial evaluation of children with heart murmurs by the non-specialized paediatrician. Eur J Pediatr 154:15, 1995.

Hohn AR, Dwyer KM, Dwyer JH: Blood pressure in youth from four ethnic groups: The Pasadena Prevention Project. J Pediatr 125:386, 1994.

McCrindle BW, Shaffer KM, Kan JS, et al: Cardinal clinical signs in the differentiation of heart murmurs in children. Arch Pediatr Adolesc Med 150:169, 1996.
Rosner B, Prineas RJ, Loggie MH, et al: Blood pressure nonograms for children and adolescents, by height, sex, and age, in the United States. J Pediatr 123:871, 1993.
Selbst SM: Chest pain in children. Pediatrics 75:1068, 1985.
Swenson JM, Fischer DR, Miller SA, et al: Are chest radiographs and electrocardiograms still valuable in evaluating new pediatric patients with heart murmurs or chest pain? Pediatrics 99:1, 1997.

CHAPTER 430
Laboratory Evaluation

430.1 Radiologic Assessment

The chest roentgenogram may provide information about cardiac size and shape, pulmonary blood flow (vascularity), pulmonary edema, and associated lung and thoracic anomalies that may be associated with congenital syndromes (skeletal dysplasias, extra or deficient numbers of ribs, previous cardiac surgery). Variations are due to differences in body build, the phase of respiration or of the cardiac cycle, abnormalities of the thoracic cage, position of the diaphragm, or pulmonary disease.

The most frequently used measurement of cardiac size is the maximal width of the cardiac shadow in a posteroanterior chest film taken during midinspiration. A vertical line is drawn down the middle of the sternal shadow, and perpendicular lines are drawn from the sternal line to the extreme right and left borders of the heart; the sum of the lengths of these lines is the *maximal cardiac width.* The *maximal chest width* is obtained by drawing a horizontal line between the right and left inner borders of the rib cage at the level of the top of the right diaphragm. When the maximal cardiac width is more than half the maximal chest width (**cardiothoracic ratio** >50%), the heart is usually enlarged. Cardiac size should be evaluated only when the film is taken during inspiration with the patient in an upright position. Diagnosis of "cardiac enlargement" on expiratory or prone films is a common cause of unnecessary referrals and laboratory studies.

The cardiothoracic ratio is a less useful index of cardiac enlargement in infancy than in older children because the horizontal position of the heart may increase the ratio to more than 50% in the absence of true enlargement. Furthermore, the thymus may overlap not only the base of the heart but also virtually the entire mediastinum, thus obscuring the true cardiac silhouette.

The lateral chest roentgenogram may be helpful in infants as well as in older children with pectus excavatum or other conditions that result in a narrow anteroposterior chest dimension. In these situations, the heart may appear small in the lateral view, suggesting that the apparent enlargement in the posteroanterior projection was due to either the thymic image (anterior mediastinum only) or flattening of the cardiac chambers as a result of a structural chest abnormality.

In the posteroanterior view, the left border of the cardiac shadow consists of three convex shadows produced, from above downward, by the aortic knob, the main and left pulmonary arteries, and the left ventricle (Fig. 430–1). In cases of moderate to marked left atrial enlargement, the atrium may project between the pulmonary artery and the left ventricle. The outflow tract of the right ventricle does not contribute to the shadows formed by the left border of the heart. The aortic knob is not as easily seen in infants and children as in adults.

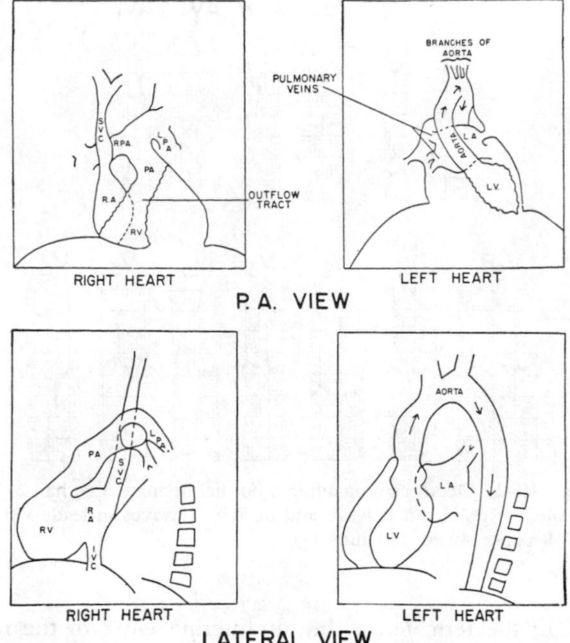

Figure 430–1 Idealized diagrams showing normal position of the cardiac chambers and great blood vessels. P.A. = posteroanterior; SVC = superior vena cava; RA = right atrium; RV = right ventricle; PA = pulmonary artery; RPA = right pulmonary artery; LPA = left pulmonary artery; LA = left atrium; LV = left ventricle; IVC = inferior vena cava. (Adapted and redrawn from Dotter and Steinberg: Radiology 53:513, 1949.)

However, the side of the aortic arch (left or right) often can be inferred as being opposite to the side of the midline from which the air-filled trachea is visualized. This is an important observation because a right-sided aortic arch is often present in cyanotic congenital heart disease, particularly in tetralogy of Fallot. Three structures contribute to the right border of the cardiac silhouette: From above downward they are the superior vena cava, the ascending aorta, and the right atrium.

Enlargement of cardiac chambers or major arteries and veins results in prominence of areas in in which these structures are normally outlined on the chest roentgenogram. In contrast, the electrocardiogram is a more sensitive and accurate index of ventricular *hypertrophy.*

It is also important to assess the degree of *pulmonary vascularity.* Angiocardiographic studies have shown that the hilar shadows are mainly vascular. Pulmonary overcirculation is usually associated with left-to-right shunt lesions, whereas pulmonary undercirculation is associated with obstruction of the outflow tract of the right ventricle.

The esophagus is closely related to the great vessels, and a barium esophagogram can help delineate these structures in the initial evaluation of suspected vascular rings. However, echocardiographic examination best defines intracardiac chamber morphologic features and computed tomography CT and magnetic resonance imaging (MRI) best define extracardiac vascular morphology.

430.2 Electrocardiography

DEVELOPMENTAL CHANGES

The marked changes that occur in cardiac physiology and chamber dominance during the perinatal transition (see Chapter 428) are reflected in the evolution of the electrocardiogram (ECG) during the neonatal time period. Because vascular resistances in the pulmonary and systemic circulations are nearly

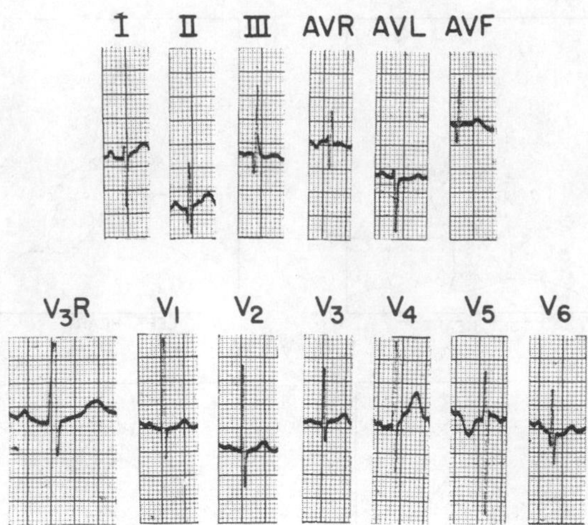

Figure 430–2 Electrocardiogram in a normal neonate less than 24 hr of age. Note the dominant R wave and upright T waves in leads V3R and V1. (V3R paper speed = 50 mm/sec.)

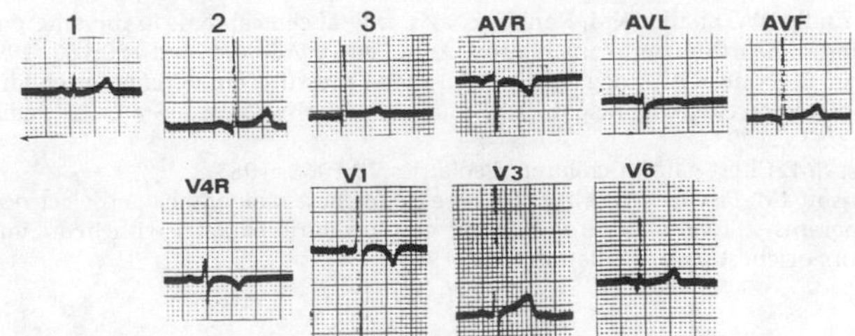

Figure 430–4 Electrocardiogram of a normal child. Note the relatively tall R waves and inversion of the T waves in V4R and V1.

equal in the term fetus, the intrauterine work of the heart results in an equal mass of both the right and left ventricles. After birth, systemic vascular resistance rises when the placental circulation is eliminated, and pulmonary vascular resistance falls when the lungs expand. These changes are reflected in the ECG as the right ventricular wall begins to thin.

The ECG demonstrates these anatomic and hemodynamic features principally by changes in QRS and T-wave morphologic features. It is recommended that a 13-lead ECG be carried out in pediatric patients, including either lead V_3R or V_4R, which are important in the evaluation of right ventricular hypertrophy. On occasion, lead V_1 is positioned too far leftward to reflect right ventricular forces accurately. This problem is present particularly in premature infants in whom the electrocardiographic electrode gel may produce contact among all the precordial leads.

During the 1st days of life, *right axis deviation,* large R waves, and upright T waves in the right precordial leads (V_3R or V_4R and V_1) are the norm (Fig. 430–2). As pulmonary vascular resistance decreases in the 1st few days after birth, the right precordial T waves become negative. In the great majority of instances, this occurs within the 1st 48 hr of life. Upright T waves that persist in leads V_3R, V_4R, or V_1 beyond 1 wk of life are an abnormal finding, indicating right ventricular hypertrophy or strain, even in the absence of QRS voltage criteria. The T wave in V_1 should never be positive before 6 yr of age and may remain negative into adolescence. This finding represents one of the most important yet subtle differences between the pediatric and adult ECG and is a common source of error when adult cardiologists interpret pediatric ECGs.

In the newborn, the mean QRS frontal plane axis normally lies in the range of +110 to +180 degrees. The right-sided chest leads reveal a larger positive (R) than negative (S) wave and may do so for months or years because the right ventricle remains relatively thick throughout infancy. Left-sided leads (V_5 and V_6) also reflect *right-sided dominance* in the early neonatal period when the RS ratio in these leads may be less than 1. A dominant R wave reflecting left ventricular forces quickly becomes evident within the 1st few days of life (Fig. 430–3). Over the years, the QRS axis gradually shifts leftward, and right ventricular forces slowly regress. Leads V_1, V_3R, and V_4R display a prominent R wave until 6 mo to 8 yr of age. The majority of children have an RS ratio greater than 1 in lead V_4R until they are 4 yr of age. The T waves are inverted in V_4R, V_1, V_2, and V_3 during infancy and may remain so into the middle of the 2nd decade of life and beyond. The processes of right ventricular thinning and left ventricular growth are best reflected in the QRS-T pattern over the right precordial leads. The diagnosis of right or left ventricular hypertrophy in the pediatric patient can be made only with an understanding of the normal developmental physiology of these chambers at various ages until adulthood is reached. As the left ventricle becomes dominant, the ECG evolves to the characteristic pattern of the older child (Fig. 430–4) and adult (Fig. 430–5).

Ventricular hypertrophy may result in increased voltage in the R and S waves in the chest leads. The height of these deflections is governed by the proximity of the specific electrode to the surface of the heart; by the sequence of electrical activation through the ventricles, resulting in variable degrees of cancellation of forces; and by hypertrophy of the myocardium. Because the chest wall in infants and children, as well as in

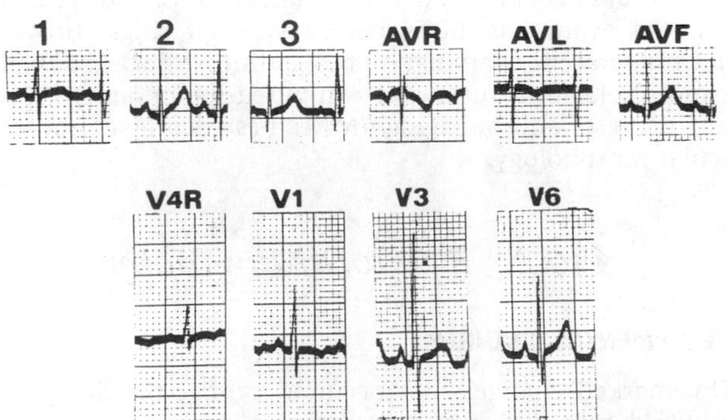

Figure 430–3 Electrocardiogram of a normal infant. Note the tall R and small S waves in V4R and V1 and the inverted T wave in these leads. There is also a dominant R wave in V6.

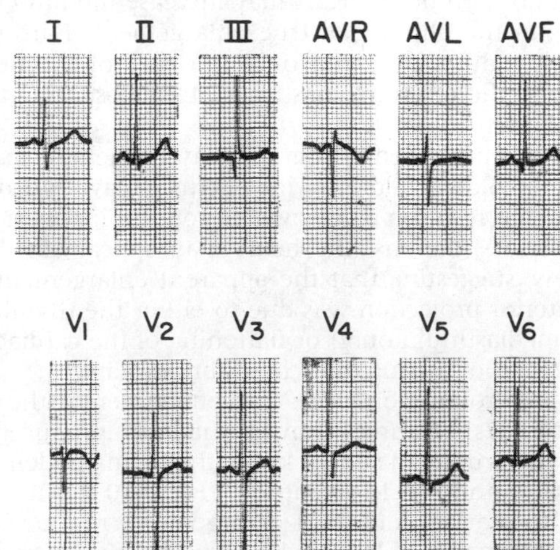

Figure 430–5 Normal adult electrocardiogram. Note the dominant S wave in lead V1. This pattern in an infant would indicate the presence of left ventricular hypertrophy.

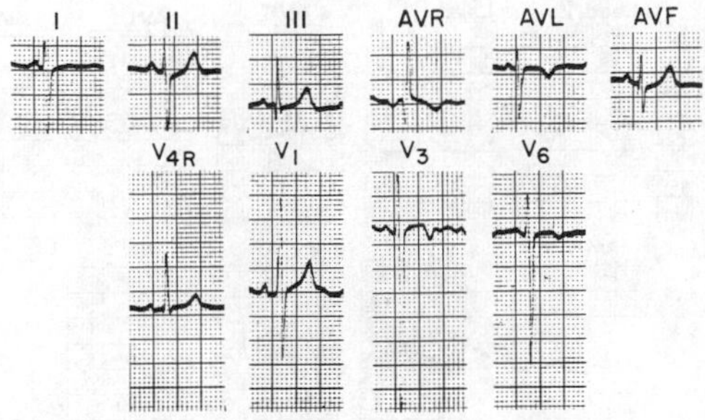

Figure 430–6 Electrocardiogram of an infant with right ventricular hypertrophy (tetralogy of Fallot). Note the tall R waves in the right precordium and deep S waves in V6. The positive T waves in V4R and V1 are also characteristic of right ventricular hypertrophy.

adolescents, may be relatively thin, the diagnosis of ventricular hypertrophy should not be based on voltage changes alone.

The diagnosis of pathologic right ventricular hypertrophy is difficult in the 1st week of life, as physiologic right ventricular hypertrophy is a normal finding. Serial tracings are often necessary to determine whether marked right axis deviation and potentially abnormal right precordial forces or T waves, or both, will persist beyond the neonatal period (Fig. 430–6). In contrast, an adult electrocardiographic pattern seen in a neonate suggests left ventricular enlargement (see Fig. 430–5). The exception is the premature infant, who may display a more "mature" ECG than a full-term infant (Fig. 430–7) as a result of lower pulmonary vascular resistance secondary to underdevelopment of the medial muscular layer of the pulmonary arterioles. Some premature infants display a pattern of generalized low voltage across the precordium.

The electrocardiogram should always be evaluated systematically, avoiding the possibility of overlooking a minor but important abnormality. One approach is to begin with an assessment of the rate and rhythm, followed by a calculation of the mean frontal plane QRS axis, measurements of segment intervals, assessment of voltages, and finally assessment of ST- and T-wave abnormalities.

RATE AND RHYTHM

A brief rhythm strip should be examined to assess whether a P wave always precedes each QRS complex. The P-wave axis should then be estimated as an indication of whether the rhythm is originating from the sinus node. If the atria are situated normally in the chest, the P wave should be upright in leads I and aVF and inverted in lead aVR. With atrial inversion (situs inversus), the P wave may be inverted in lead I. Inverted P waves in leads II and aVF are seen in nodal or junctional rhythms regardless of atrial position. The absence of P waves indicates a rhythm originating more distally in the conduction system. In this case, the morphologic features of the QRS complexes are important in differentiating a junctional (usually a narrow QRS complex) from a ventricular (usually a wide QRS complex) rhythm.

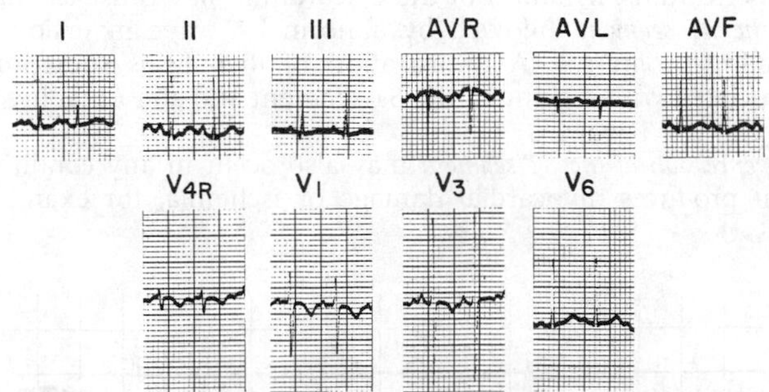

Figure 430–7 Electrocardiogram of a premature infant (weight 2 kg and age 5 wk at the time of tracing). The cardiovascular system was clinically normal. Left ventricular dominance is manifest by R-wave progression across the chest, simulating tracings obtained from older children. Compare with the tracing from a normal full-term infant (Fig. 430–3).

P WAVES

Tall (>2.5 mm), narrow, and spiked P waves are indicative of right atrial enlargement and are seen in congenital pulmonary stenosis, Ebstein's anomaly of the tricuspid valve, tricuspid atresia, and sometimes cor pulmonale. These abnormal waves are most obvious in leads II, V_3R, and V_1 (Fig. 430–8*A*). Similar waves are sometimes seen in thyrotoxicosis. Broad P waves, commonly bifid and sometimes biphasic, are indicative of left atrial enlargement (see Fig. 430–8*B*). They are seen in some patients with large left-to-right shunts (ventricular septal defect [VSD], patent ductus arteriosus [PDA]) and with severe mitral stenosis or regurgitation. Flat P waves may be encountered in hyperkalemia.

QRS COMPLEX

RIGHT VENTRICULAR HYPERTROPHY. For the most accurate assessment of ventricular hypertrophy, pediatric ECGs should include the right precordial lead V_3R or V_4R, or both. Diagnosis of right ventricular hypertrophy depends on the demonstration of the following changes (see Fig. 430–6): (1) a qR pattern in the right ventricular surface leads; (2) a positive T wave in leads $V_{3-4}R$ and V_1–V_3 between the ages of 6 days and 6 yr; (3) a monophasic R wave in V_3R, V_4R, or V_1; (4) an rsR′ pattern in the right precordial leads with the second R wave taller than the initial one; (5) age-corrected increased voltage of the R wave in leads $V_{3-4}R$ or of the S wave in leads V_{6-7}, or both; (6) marked right axis deviation (>120 degrees in patients beyond the newborn period); (7) a complete reversal of the normal adult precordial RS pattern; and (8) right atrial enlargement. At least two of these changes should be present to support a diagnosis of right ventricular hypertrophy.

Abnormal ventricular loading can be characterized as either systolic (due to obstruction of the right ventricular outflow tract, as in pulmonic stenosis) or diastolic (due to increased volume load, as in atrial septal defects). These two types of abnormal loads result in distinct electrocardiographic patterns. The *systolic overload pattern* is characterized by tall, pure R waves in the right precordial leads. In older children, the T waves in these leads are initially upright and later become inverted. In infants and children less than 6 yr of age, the T waves in $V_{3-4}R$ and V_1 are abnormally upright. The *diastolic overload pattern* is characterized by an rsR′ pattern (Fig. 430–9) and slightly increased QRS duration (minor right ventricular conduction de-

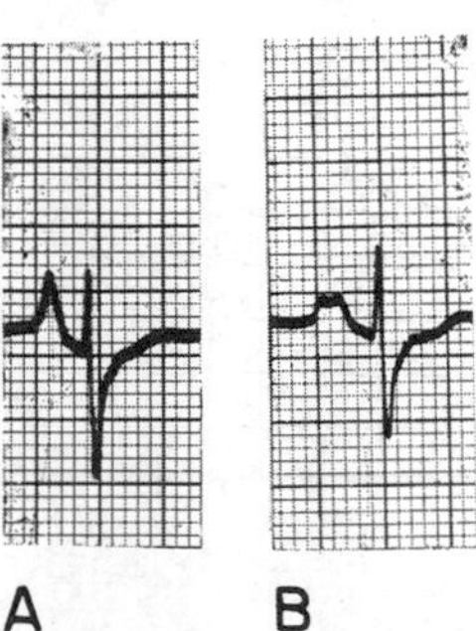

Figure 430–8 Atrial enlargement. *A*, Peaked narrow P waves characteristic of right atrial enlargement. *B*, Wide bifid M-shaped P waves typical of left atrial enlargement.

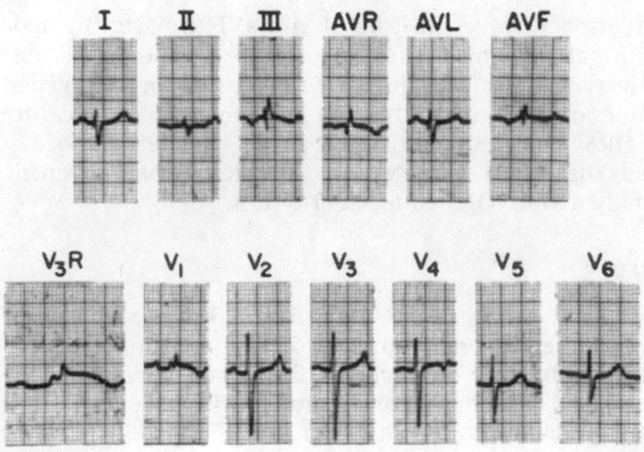

Figure 430–9 Electrocardiogram showing right ventricular conduction delay characterized by an rsR′ pattern in V1 and a deep S wave in V6. (V3R paper speed = 50 mm/sec.)

lay). Patients with mild to moderate pulmonary stenosis may also exhibit an rsR in the right precordial leads.

LEFT VENTRICULAR HYPERTROPHY. The following features indicate the presence of left ventricular hypertrophy (Fig. 430–10): (1) depression of the ST segments and inversion of the T waves in the left precordial leads (V_5, V_6, and V_7), known as a left ventricular strain pattern—these findings suggest the presence of a severe lesion; (2) a deep Q wave in the left precordial leads; and (3) increased voltage of the S wave in V_3R and V_1 or the R wave in V_{6-7}, or both. It is important to emphasize that evaluation of left ventricular hypertrophy should not be based on voltage criteria alone. The concepts of systolic and diastolic overload, although not always consistent, are also useful in evaluating left ventricular enlargement. Severe *systolic overload* of the left ventricle is suggested by straightening of the ST segments and inverted T waves over the left precordial leads; *diastolic overload* may result in tall R waves, a large Q wave, and normal T waves over the left precordium. Finally, the infant with an electrocardiogram that would be considered "normal" for an older child may in fact have left ventricular hypertrophy.

BUNDLE BRANCH BLOCK. Complete right bundle branch block

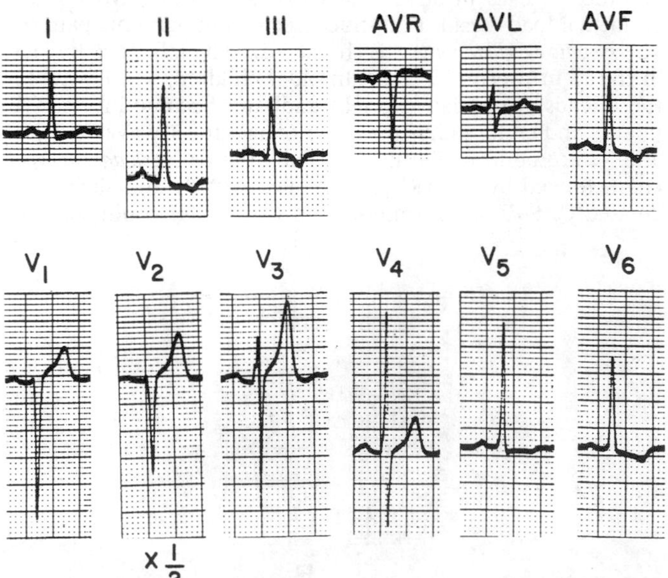

Figure 430–10 Electrocardiogram showing left ventricular hypertrophy in a 12-yr-old child with aortic stenosis. Note the deep S wave in V1-V3 and tall R in V5. Also, T-wave inversion is present in II, III, AVE, and V6.

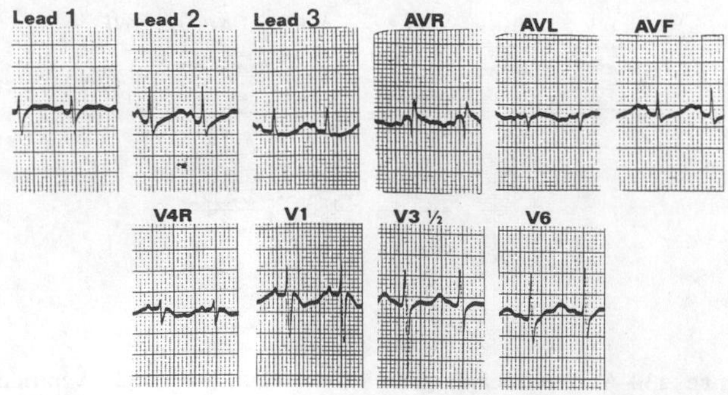

Figure 430–11 Electrocardiogram in hypokalemia (serum potassium 2.7 mEq/L; serum calcium 4.8 mEq/L at time of tracing). Note the prolongation of electrical systole as evidenced by a widened TU wave; also the depression of the ST segment in V4R, V1, and V6.

may be congenital or acquired after surgery for congenital heart disease, especially when a right ventriculotomy has been performed as in repair of tetralogy of Fallot. Congenital left bundle branch block is rare; this pattern is occasionally seen with cardiomyopathy. A bundle branch block pattern may be indicative of a bypass tract associated with one of the pre-excitation syndromes (see Chapter 442).

PR AND QT INTERVALS

The duration of the PR interval shortens with increasing heart rate; thus, assessment of this interval should be based on age- and rate-corrected nomograms. A long PR interval is diagnostic of 1st-degree heart block, the cause of which may be congenital, postoperative, inflammatory (myocarditis, pericarditis, rheumatic fever), or pharmacologic (digitalis).

The duration of the QT interval varies with the cardiac rate; a corrected QT interval (QT_c) can be calculated by dividing the measured QT interval by the square root of the preceding R-R interval. The normal QT_c should be less than 0.45. It is often lengthened with hypokalemia and hypocalcemia; in the former instance, a U wave may be noted at the end of the T wave (Fig. 430–11). A congenitally prolonged QT interval (Fig. 430–12) may be also be seen in children with one of the long QT syndromes. These patients are at high risk for ventricular arrhythmias, including a form of ventricular tachycardia known as *torsade de pointes,* and sudden death (see Chapter 442.4).

ST SEGMENT AND T-WAVE ABNORMALITIES

A slight elevation of the ST segment may occur in normal teenagers and is attributed to early repolarization of the heart. In pericarditis, irritation of the epicardium may cause *elevation of the ST segment* followed by abnormal T-wave inversion as healing progresses. Administration of digitalis is sometimes associated with sagging of the ST segment and abnormal inversion of the T wave.

Depression of the ST segment may also occur in any condition that produces myocardial damage or ischemia, for example,

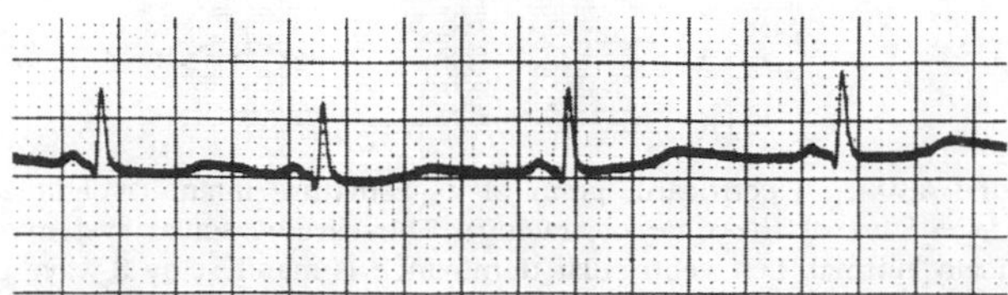

Figure 430–12 Prolonged Q-T interval in a patient with long QT syndrome (LQTS).

severe anemia, carbon monoxide poisoning, aberrant origin of the left coronary artery from the pulmonary artery, glycogen storage disease of the heart, myocardial tumors, and mucopolysaccharidoses. Aberrant origin of the left coronary artery from the pulmonary artery may lead to changes indistinguishable from those of acute myocardial infarction in adults. Similar changes may occur in patients with other rare abnormalities of the coronary arteries and with cardiomyopathy even in the presence of normal coronary arteries. These patterns are often misread in young infants because of the unfamiliarity of pediatricians with this "infarct" pattern, and thus a high index of suspicion must be maintained in infants with symptoms compatible with coronary ischemia.

T-wave inversion may occur in myocarditis and pericarditis, or it may be a sign of either right or left ventricular hypertrophy and strain. Hypothyroidism may produce flat or inverted T waves in association with generalized low voltage. In hyperkalemia, the T waves are commonly of high voltage and are tent-shaped (Fig. 430–13).

430.3 Hematologic Data

In acyanotic infants with large left-to-right shunts, the onset of heart failure often coincides with the nadir of the normal *physiologic anemia* of infancy. Increasing the hematocrit in these patients to greater than 40% can decrease the shunt volume and result in an improvement in symptoms; however, this form of treatment is reserved only for those infants who are not otherwise surgical candidates (extremely premature infants or those with extremely complex congenital heart disease for whom only palliative surgery is possible). In these selected infants, regular evaluation of the hematocrit and booster transfusions when appropriate may be helpful in improving growth.

Polycythemia is frequently noted in cyanotic patients with right-to-left shunts. Patients with severe polycythemia are in a delicate balance between the risks of intravascular thrombosis and a bleeding diathesis. The most frequent abnormalities include accelerated fibrinolysis, thrombocytopenia, abnormal clot retraction, hypofibrinogenemia, prolonged prothrombin time, and prolonged partial thromboplastin time. The preparation of cyanotic patients who are polycythemic for elective surgery, such as dental extraction, includes evaluation for and treatment of abnormal coagulation.

Because of the high viscosity of polycythemic blood (hematocrit >65%), patients with cyanotic congenital heart disease are at risk for the development of vascular thromboses, especially of cerebral veins. Dehydration increases the risk of thrombosis, and thus adequate fluid intake must be maintained during hot weather or intercurrent gastrointestinal illnesses. Diuretics should be used with caution in these patients and may need to be decreased if there is concern over fluid intake. Polycythemic infants with concomitant iron deficiency are at even greater risk for cerebrovascular accidents, probably because of the decreased deformability of microcytic red blood cells. Iron therapy produces improvement, but surgical treatment of the cardiac anomaly is the best therapy.

Severely cyanotic patients should have periodic hemoglobin and hematocrit determinations. Increasing polycythemia, often associated with headache, fatigue, or dyspnea, or a combination of these conditions, is one indication for palliative or corrective surgical intervention. Among cyanotic patients with inoperable conditions, phlebotomy may be required to treat individuals whose hematocrit has risen to the 65–70% level, usually when the polycythemia is associated with symptoms, for example, headache. This procedure is not without risk, especially in patients with extreme elevation of pulmonary vascular resistance. Because these patients do not tolerate wide fluctuations in circulating blood volume, blood should be replaced with fresh frozen plasma or albumin. Whether or not to perform routine phlebotomies for polycythemic patients who are asymptomatic is controversial.

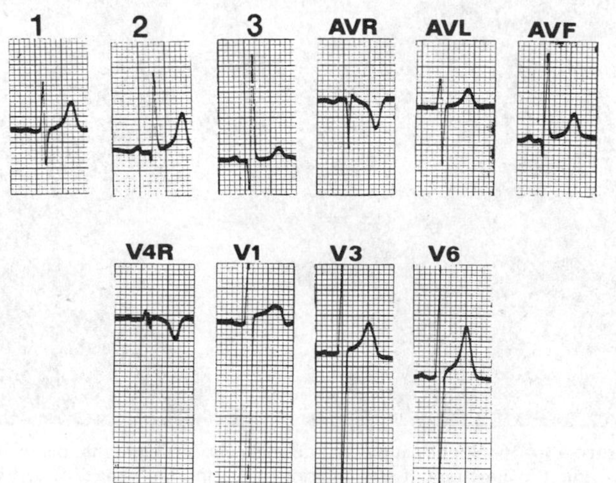

Figure 430–13 Electrocardiogram in hyperkalemia (serum potassium 6.5 mEqL; serum calcium 5.1 mEqL). Note the tall, tent-shaped T waves, especially in leads I, II, and V6.

430.4 Echocardiography

Echocardiography has dramatically reduced the requirement for invasive studies such as cardiac catheterization. The echocardiographic examination can be used to evaluate cardiac structure in congenital heart lesions, estimate intracardiac pressures and gradients across stenotic valves and vessels, quantitate cardiac contractile function (both systolic and diastolic), determine the direction of flow across a defect, examine the integrity of the coronary arteries, evaluate the presence of vegetations due to endocarditis, and the presence of pericardial fluid, cardiac tumors, or chamber thrombi. Echocardiography may also be used to assist in the performance of pericardiocentesis, balloon atrial septostomy (see Chapter 438.2), and endocardial biopsy, and in the placement of flow-directed pulmonary arterial (Swan-Ganz) monitoring catheters. *Transesophageal echocardiography* is used to monitor ventricular function in patients during difficult surgical procedures and can provide an immediate assessment of the results of surgical repair of congenital heart lesions. *Fetal echocardiography* can determine the presence of many congenital heart lesions, often as early as 17–19 wk of gestation, and is especially valuable in evaluating fetal cardiac arrhythmias. A complete echocardiographic examination usually employs a combination of M-mode and two-dimensional imaging as well as pulsed, continuous, and color Doppler flow studies.

M-MODE ECHOCARDIOGRAPHY

M-mode echocardiography displays a one-dimensional slice of cardiac structure varying over time. M-mode echocardiography is mostly used for the measurement of cardiac dimensions (wall thickness and chamber sizes) and cardiac function (fractional shortening, wall thickening). M-mode echocardiography is also useful for assessing the motion of intracardiac structures (opening and closing of valves, movement of free walls and septa) and the anatomy of valves (Fig. 430–14). The most frequently used index of cardiac function in children is the *per cent fractional shortening*, which is calculated as (LVED-LVES)/LVED where LVED = left ventricular (LV) dimension at end-diastole; LVES = LV dimension at end-systole. A normal frac-

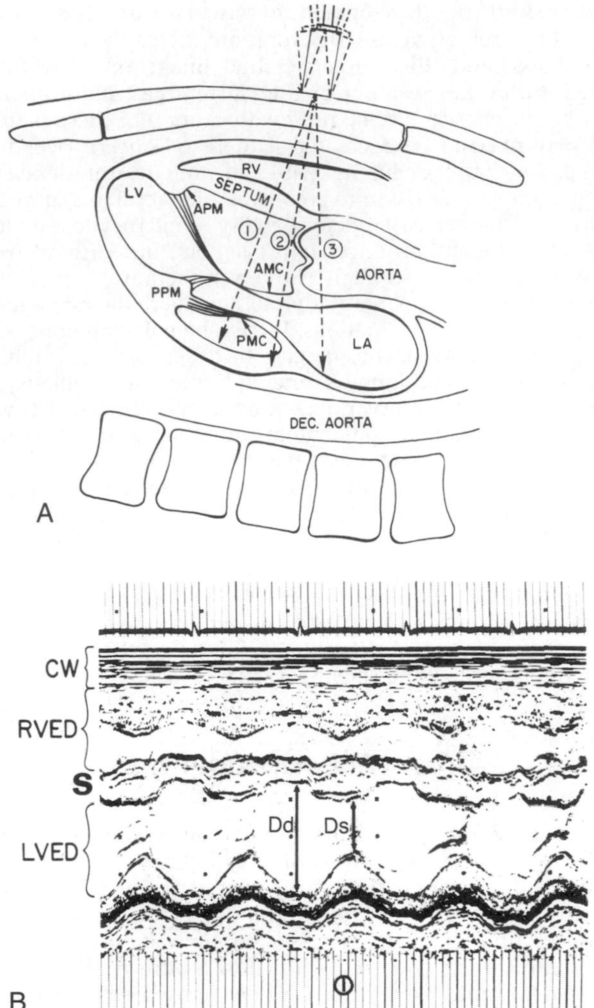

Figure 430–14 The M-mode echocardiogram. *A*, Diagram of sagittal section of heart showing structures traversed by echo beam as it is moved superiorly positions (1), (2), and (3). AMC = anterior mitral cusp; APM = anterior papillary muscle; Dec. aorta = descending aorta; LA = left atrium; LV = left ventricle; PMC = posterior mitral cusp; PPM = posterior papillary muscle; RV = right ventricle. *B*, Echocardiogram from transducer position (1); this is the best view to measure cardiac dimensions and fractional shortening. RVED = RV dimension at end-diastole; LVED = LV dimension at end-diastole (Dd); Ds = LV dimension in systole. CW = chest wall. Fractional shortening is calculated as (LVED-LVES) LVED.

tional shortening is 28–40%. Other M-mode indices of cardiac function include the mean velocity of fiber shortening (Mean V_{CF}), systolic time intervals (LVPEP = LV pre-ejection period, LVET = LV ejection time), and isovolemic contraction time. More sophisticated indices of cardiac function can be derived noninvasively with the assistance of echocardiography (pressure-volume relationship, end-systolic wall stress-strain relationship); however, their accuracy is limited when compared with similar measurements in the catheterization laboratory.

TWO-DIMENSIONAL ECHOCARDIOGRAPHY

Two-dimensional echocardiography provides a real-time image of cardiac structures. With two-dimensional echocardiography the contracting heart is imaged in several standard views (subxiphoid, Fig. 430–15; parasagittal, Fig. 430–16; parasternal, Fig. 430–17; and suprasternal, Fig. 430–18) that emphasize specific structures. Two-dimensional echocardiography has replaced cardiac angiography for the preoperative diagnosis of many, but not all, congenital heart lesions and exceeds angiog-

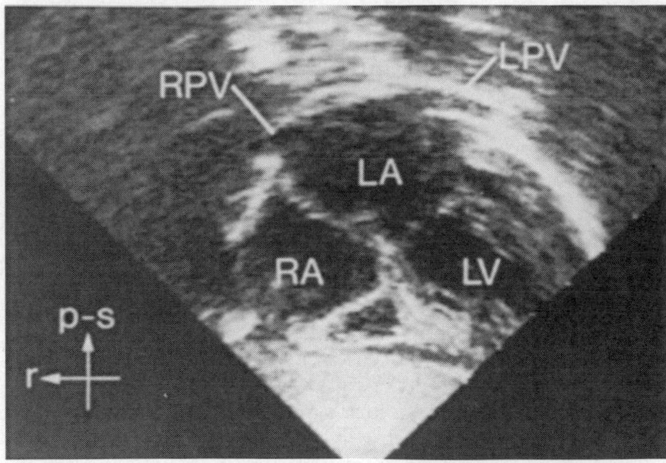

Figure 430–15 Subxiphoid normal echocardiographic view. The anterior angulation shows the mitral valve and the left ventricular inflow tract. Note the pulmonary veins connecting with the left atrium. LA = left atrium; LPV = left pulmonary vein; RPV = right pulmonary vein; LV = left ventricle; p-s = posterior-superior; r = right; RA = right atrium. (From Sanders SP: Echocardiography. *In*: Long WA [ed]: Fetal and Neonatal Cardiology. Philadelphia, WB Saunders, 1990.)

raphy in several areas, for example, in imaging the atrioventricular valves and their chordal attachments. When information from the cardiac examination is not consistent with the echocardiogram, cardiac catheterization is an important tool to confirm the anatomic diagnosis and evaluate the degree of physiologic derangement.

DOPPLER ECHOCARDIOGRAPHY

Doppler echocardiography displays blood flow in cardiac chambers and vascular channels based on the change in frequency imparted to a sound wave by the movement of erythrocytes. In *pulsed Doppler* and *continuous wave Doppler,* the speed and direction of blood flow in the line of the echo beam change the transducer's reference frequency. This frequency change can be translated into volumetric flow (liters/min) data used to estimate systemic or pulmonary blood flow and into pressure (millimeters of mercury) data used to estimate gradients across semilunar or atrioventricular valves, or across sep-

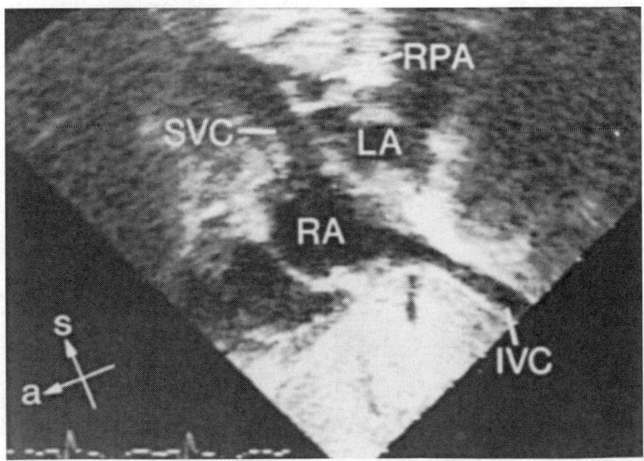

Figure 430–16 Right parasagittal normal echocardiographic plane view showing the junction of the inferior and superior venae cavae with the right atrium. a = anterior; IVC = inferior vena cava; LA = left atrium; RA = right atrium; RPA = right pulmonary artery; s = superior; SVC = superior vena cava. (From Sanders SP: Echocardiography. *In*: Long WA [ed]: Fetal and Neonatal Cardiology. Philadelphia, WB Saunders, 1990.)

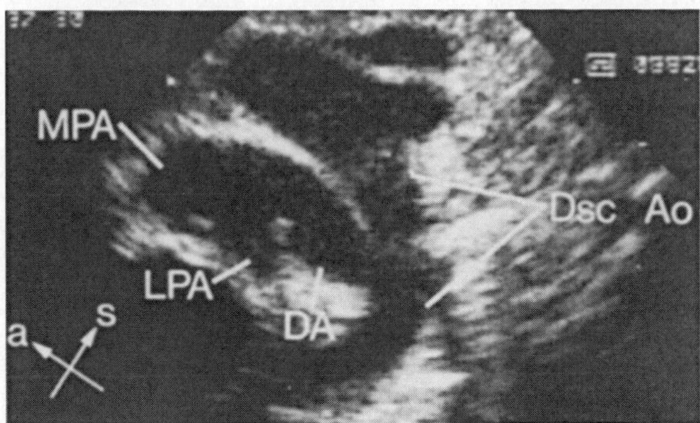

Figure 430–17 Normal high parasternal, parasagittal echocardiographic plane view for imaging the ductus arteriosus. a = anterior; DA = ductus arteriosus; Dsc Ao = descending aorta; LPA = left pulmonary artery; MPA-= main pulmonary artery; s = superior. (From Sanders SP: Echocardiography. *In*: Long WA [ed]: Fetal and Neonatal Cardiology. Philadelphia, WB Saunders, 1990.)

tal defects or vascular communications such as shunts (Fig. 430–19). *Color Doppler* permits a highly accurate assessment of the presence and direction of intracardiac shunts and allows identification of small or multiple left-to-right or right-to-left shunts. The severity of valvular insufficiency is also more accurately evaluated with color Doppler.

TRANSESOPHAGEAL ECHOCARDIOGRAPHY

Transesophageal echocardiography is an extremely sensitive imaging technique that produces a clearer view of smaller lesions, such as vegetations in endocarditis. It is useful in visualizing posteriorly located structures such as the atria, aortic root, and atrioventricular valves. Transesophageal echo has been extremely useful as an intraoperative technique for monitoring cardiac function during both cardiac and noncardiac surgery and for screening for residual cardiac defects after cardiopulmonary bypass. This technique has been especially helpful in evaluating the degree of residual regurgitation in atrioventricular septal defect repairs and in searching for small muscular ventricular septal defects that may have been missed during the closure of larger defects.

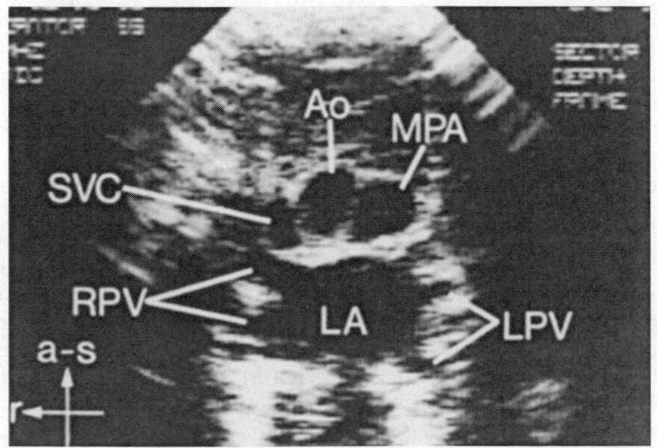

Figure 430–18 Suprasternal notch normal echocardiographic view. Pulmonary veins connecting with the left atrium. Ao = aorta; a-s = anterior-superior; LA = left atrium; LPV = left pulmonary vein; MPA = main pulmonary artery; RPV = right pulmonary vein; r = right; SVC = superior vena cava. (From Sanders SP: Echocardiography. *In*: Long WA [ed]: Fetal and Neonatal Cardiology. Philadelphia, WB Saunders, 1990.)

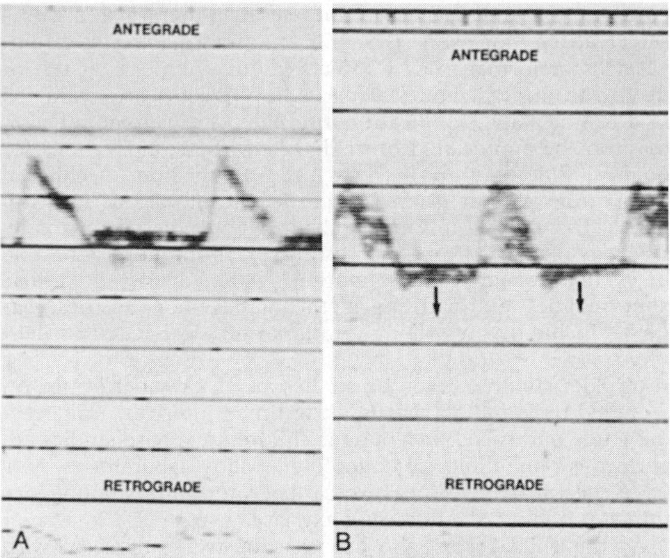

Figure 430–19 Patent ductus arteriosus. *A*, Doppler flow in the proximal descending aorta of normal infant demonstrating the normal antegrade systolic and diastolic flow. *B*, Doppler flow configuration in an infant with patent ductus arteriosus reveals antegrade systolic but retrograde diastolic flow (*arrows*).

FETAL ECHOCARDIOGRAPHY

Fetal echocardiography can be used to evaluate cardiac structures or disturbances of cardiac rhythm. Obstetricians often detect gross abnormalities of cardiac structure on routine obstetric ultrasonography or may refer the patient because of unexplained hydrops fetalis. Fetal echocardiography may be capable of diagnosing congenital heart lesions as early as 17–19 wk of gestation; however, accuracy at this early stage is limited. Serial fetal echos have also demonstrated the importance of flow disturbance in the pathogenesis of congenital heart disease, showing the intrauterine progression of a moderate lesion, for example, aortic stenosis, into a more severe lesion, for example, hypoplastic left heart syndrome. M-mode echocardiography can diagnose rhythm disturbances in the fetus and can determine the success of antiarrhythmic therapy administered to the mother. A screening fetal echocardiogram is recommended for patients with a previous child or 1st-degree relative with congenital heart disease and for patients who are at higher risk of having a child with cardiac disease (e.g., insulin-dependent diabetics, patients with exposure to teratogenic drugs during early pregnancy), and in any fetus in which a chromosomal abnormality is suspected or confirmed.

VENTRICULAR FUNCTION

Sophisticated M-mode and two-dimensional echocardiographic methods of assessing left ventricular systolic and diastolic function, for example, end-systolic wall stress and dobutamine stress echocardiography, have proved useful in the serial assessment of patients at risk for development of ventricular dysfunction. These patients include those receiving anthracycline drugs for cancer chemotherapy, patients at risk for iron overload, and patients being monitored for rejection or coronary artery disease after heart transplantation.

430.5 Exercise Testing

The normal cardiorespiratory system adapts to the extensive demands of exercise with a several fold increase in oxygen consumption and cardiac output. Because there is a large reserve capacity for exercise, significant abnormalities of cardiovascular performance may exist without symptoms at rest or during ordinary activities. Thus, when patients are evaluated in a resting state, significant abnormalities of cardiac function may not be appreciated or, if detected, their implications for quality of life may not be recognized. Permission for children with cardiovascular disease to participate in various forms of physical activity is unfortunately frequently based on totally subjective criteria. Exercise testing plays an important role in evaluating symptoms, quantitating the severity of cardiac abnormalities, and assisting in the management of these patients, including prescribing a rational physical activity schedule.

In older children, exercise studies are usually performed on a graded treadmill apparatus using timed intervals of increasing grade and speed. In younger children, exercise studies are performed on a bicycle ergometer. Many laboratories now have the capacity to measure cardiac output and pulmonary function noninvasively during exercise.

As the child grows, the capacity for work increases with body size and skeletal muscle mass. However, all indices of cardiopulmonary function do not increase in a uniform manner. A major response to exercise is an increase in cardiac output, principally as a result of increased heart rate, but stroke volume, systemic venous return, and pulse pressure are also increased. Systemic vascular resistance is greatly decreased as the blood vessels in working muscle dilate as a response to increasing metabolic demands. As the child becomes older and larger, the response of the heart rate to exercise remains prominent, but the cardiac output increases because of growing cardiac volume capacity and hence stroke volume. The responses to dynamic exercise are not dependent only on age. For any given body surface area, boys have a larger stroke volume than size-matched girls. This increase is also mediated by posture. Augmentation of stroke volume with upright, dynamic exercise is facilitated by the pumping action of working muscles, which overcomes the static effect of gravity and increases systemic venous return.

Dynamic exercise testing defines not only endurance and exercise capacity but also the effect of such exercise on myocardial blood flow and cardiac rhythm. Significant ST-segment depression reflects abnormalities in myocardial perfusion, for example, the subendocardial ischemia that commonly occurs during exercise in children with hypertrophied left ventricles. The exercise electrocardiogram is considered abnormal if ST-segment depression is greater than 2 mm and extends for at least 0.06 sec after the J point (onset of the ST segment) in conjunction with a horizontal-, upward-, or downward-sloping ST segment. Provocation of rhythm disturbances during an exercise study is an important method of evaluating selected patients with known or suspected rhythm disorders. The effect of pharmacologic management can also be tested in this manner.

430.6 Magnetic Resonance Imaging, Electron Beam Computed Tomography, and Radionuclide Studies

MRI is helpful in the diagnosis and management of patients with congenital heart disease. It produces tomographic images of the heart in any projection (Fig. 430–20) with excellent contrast resolution of fat, myocardium, and lung, as well as moving blood from blood vessel walls. MRI has been particularly useful in evaluating areas that are less well visualized by echocardiography, for example, distal branch pulmonary artery anatomy and anomalies of systemic and pulmonary venous return.

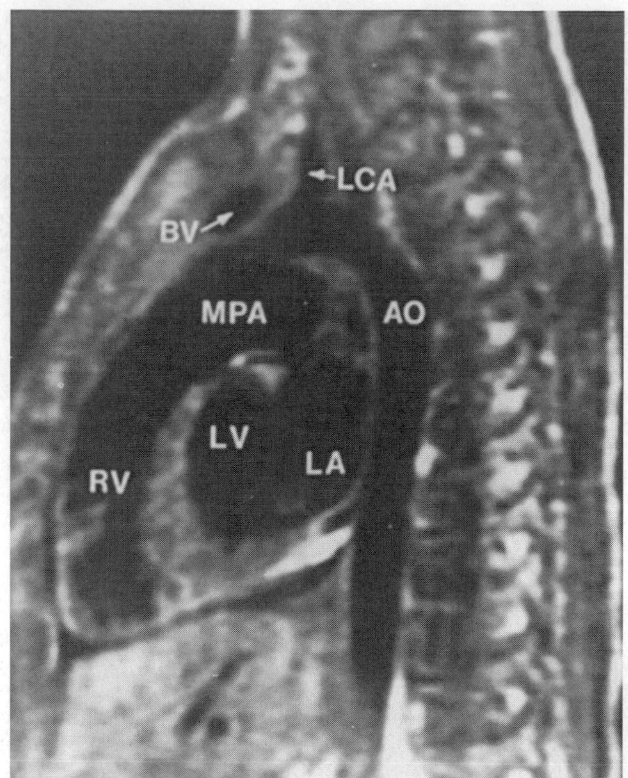

Figure 430–20 Sagittal normal MRI image. AO = aorta; BV = brachiocephalic vein; LA = left atrium; LCA = left coronary artery; LV = left ventricle; MPA = main pulmonary artery; RV = right ventricle. (From Bisset GS III: Cardiac and great vessel anatomy. *In*: El-khoury GY, Bergman RA, Montgomery WJ [eds]: Sectional Anatomy by MR/CT. New York, Churchill Livingstone, 1990.)

Magnetic resonance angiography allows acquisition of images in several tomographic planes. Within each plane, images are obtained at different phases of the cardiac cycle. Thus, when displayed in a dynamic "cine" format, changes in wall thickening, chamber volume, and valve function can be displayed and analyzed. Blood flow velocity and blood flow volume can be approximated. Phosphorus *magnetic resonance spectroscopy* provides a means of demonstrating relative concentrations of high-energy metabolites, for example, adenosine triphosphate, adenosine diphosphate, inorganic phosphate, and phosphocreatine, within regions of the working myocardium.

Electron beam computed tomography (EBCT) scanning is used to perform rapid, respiration-gated cardiac imaging in children with a resolution down to 0.5 mm. Three-dimensional reconstruction of EBCT images (Fig. 430–21) is especially useful in evaluating branch pulmonary arteries, anomalies of systemic and pulmonary venous return, and great vessel anomalies such as coarctation of the aorta.

Radionuclide angiography may be used to detect and quantify shunts and to analyze the distribution of blood flow to each lung. This technique is particularly useful in quantifying the volume of blood flow distribution between the two lungs in patients with abnormalities of the pulmonary vascular tree, after a shunt (Blalock-Taussig or Glenn) operation, or to quantify the success of balloon angioplasty and intravascular stenting procedures. *Gated blood pool scanning* can be used to calculate hemodynamic measurements, to quantify valvular regurgitation, and to detect regional wall motion abnormalities. *Thallium imaging* can be used to evaluate cardiac muscle perfusion. These methods can be used at the bedside of the seriously ill child and can be employed serially, with minimal discomfort and low radiation exposure.

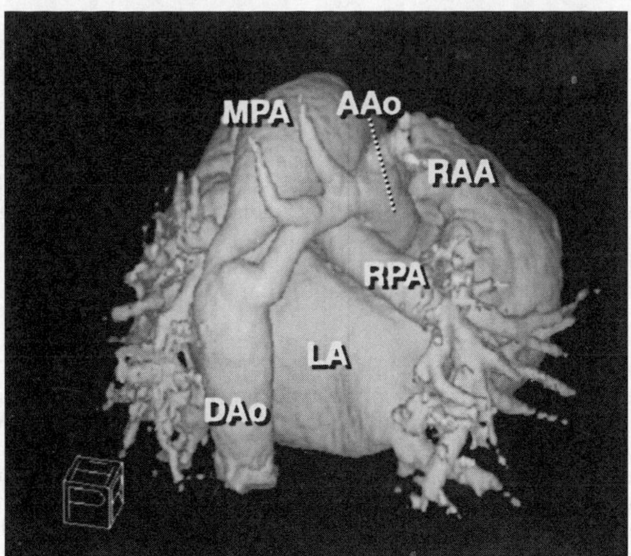

Figure 430–21 Three-dimensional reconstruction of electron beam computer tomographic (EBCT) images from a neonate with severe coarctation of the aorta. The patent ductus arteriosus can be seen toward the left leading from the main pulmonary artery to the descending aorta. The tortuous and narrow coarctated segment is just to the right of the ductus. The transverse aorta is hypoplastic as well. MPA = main pulmonary artery; AAo = ascending aorta; DAo = descending aorta; RAA = right atrial appendage; RPA = right pulmonary artery; LA = left atrium. (Image courtesy of Dr. Paul Pitlick, Stanford University, Stanford, CA.)

430.7 Cardiac Catheterization

Cardiac catheterization is an important tool in the diagnosis of congenital heart disease. During catheterization, blood samples are obtained for measuring oxygen saturation and calculating shunt volumes, pressures are measured for calculating gradients and valve areas, and contrast is injected to delineate structures. Major indications for cardiac catheterization include (1) presurgical evaluation of cardiac anatomy or shunt size, or both, in congenital cardiac lesions when echocardiographic evaluation is incomplete, (2) evaluation of pulmonary vascular resistance and its reactivity to vasodilators or oxygen, (3) follow-up after surgical repair or palliation of complex congenital heart lesions, (4) myocardial biopsy for diagnosis of cardiomyopathy or screening for cardiac rejection after transplantation, (5) interventional cardiac catheterization, and (6) electrophysiologic study or transcatheter ablation, or both (see Chapter 442).

Although the risks are low, cardiac catheterization involves potential complications for the patient and should not be used without an opportunity for benefit. Echocardiography, MRI, EBCT, or radionuclide studies may be used in lieu of multiple cardiac catheterizations in individual patients who require careful monitoring of their hemodynamic status. The number of postoperative catheterizations has increased with the advent of palliative surgical procedures to repair complex congenital heart lesions. Interventional cardiac catheterization has replaced surgical repair in many cases (e.g., pulmonary or aortic valve stenosis, recoarctation of the aorta, closure of small PDA), is competing with it in others (atrial septal defects [ASD], muscular VSD, large PDA), and in others is used as an adjunct to complex surgical repairs (branch pulmonary artery stenosis, closure of a fenestrated Fontan palliation [see Chapter 437.4]).

Cardiac catheterization should be performed with the patient in as close to a basal state as possible. Conscious sedation is routinely used for the majority of these studies; however, if general anesthesia is required, careful choice of an anesthetic agent is warranted to avoid depression of cardiovascular function and subsequent distortion of the calculations of cardiac output, pulmonary and systemic vascular resistances, and shunt ratios.

Cardiac catheterization in critically ill infants with congenital heart disease should be performed in a center where a pediatric cardiovascular surgical team is available in the event that an operation is required immediately afterward. The complication rate of cardiac catheterization and angiography is greatest among critically ill infants; they must be studied in a thermally neutral environment and treated quickly for hypothermia, hypoglycemia, acidosis, or excessive blood loss. The development of soft, flow-directed balloon-tipped catheters has greatly decreased the frequency of complications from catheter manipulation (severe arrhythmias, cardiac perforation, intramyocardial injection of contrast material).

Catheterization usually includes both the right and left sides of the heart. The catheter is passed into the heart under fluoroscopic guidance through a percutaneous entry point in a femoral vein, although occasionally jugular access is used. In infants and in a large number of older children, the left side of the heart can be accessed by passing the catheter across a patent foramen ovale to the left atrium and left ventricle. If the foramen is closed, the left side of the heart can also be catheterized by passing the catheter retrograde via a percutaneous entry into the femoral artery. The catheter can be manipulated through abnormal intracardiac defects (ASDs, VSDs). Complete hemodynamics can be calculated (Table 430–1), including cardiac output, intracardiac left-to-right and right-to-left shunts, and systemic and pulmonary vascular resistances. The normal circulatory dynamics are depicted in Figure 430–22.

TABLE 430–1 Normal Values and Formulas for Determination of Hemodynamics in Cardiac Catheterization

1. Cardiac index 3.0–5.0 $L/min/m^2$
2. Arteriovenous oxygen difference 4.5 ± 0.7 mL/dL
3. Oxygen consumption 140–160 $mL/m^2/min$
4. Arterial oxygen saturation 94–100%
5. Pulmonary arteriolar resistance 50–150 dyn sec cm^{-5} (1 unit = 80 dynes)
6. Cardiac output (Qs) mL/min = systemic flow =

$$\frac{O_2 \text{ intake (mL/min)}}{\left\{\begin{array}{l}O_2 \text{ content of arterial blood (mL/dL)}\\ \text{minus } O_2 \text{ content of mixed venous blood (mL/dL)}\end{array}\right.} \times 100$$

7. Cardiac index = cardiac output (L/min)/m^2 of body surface area
8. Pulmonary artery flow (Qp) =

$$\frac{O_2 \text{ intake (mL/min)}}{\left\{\begin{array}{l}O_2 \text{ content of pulmonary venous blood (mL/dL)}\\ \text{minus } O_2 \text{ content of pulmonary arterial blood (mL/dL)}\end{array}\right.} \times 100$$

If a pulmonary venous sample is not available, it is assumed to be saturated to 95% of capacity

9. Effective pulmonary artery flow (Qep) =

$$\frac{O_2 \text{ intake (mL/min)}}{\left\{\begin{array}{l}\text{pulmonary venous } O_2 \text{ content (100 mL/dL)}\\ \text{minus mixed venous } O_2 \text{ content (100 mL/dL)}\end{array}\right.} \times 100$$

10. Total left to right shunt = pulmonary artery flow minus effective pulmonary artery flow
11. Total right to left shunt = systemic flow minus effective pulmonary artery flow
12. Pulmonary arteriolar resistance $Rp = \frac{PA - PC}{Qp}$

Where R = pulmonary arteriolar resistance (resistance units)
PA = mean pulmonary artery pressure in mm Hg
PC = mean pulmonary "capillary" pressure in mm Hg
Qp = pulmonary flow in $L/min/m^2$

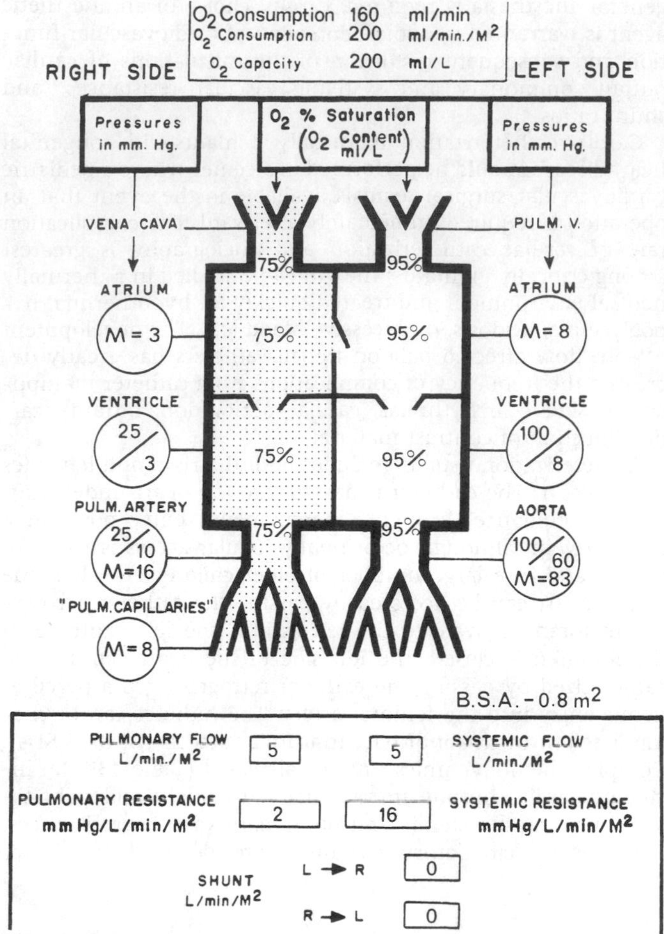

Figure 430–22 Diagram of normal circulatory dynamics with pressures, oxygen contents, and percentage of saturations. (Modified from Nadas AS, Fyler DC: Pediatric Cardiology, 3rd ed. Philadelphia, WB Saunders, 1972.)

THERMODILUTION MEASUREMENT OF CARDIAC OUTPUT

The *thermodilution method* for measuring cardiac output is performed using a flow-directed thermistor-tipped pulmonary arterial (Swan-Ganz) catheter. A known change in heat content of the blood is induced at one point in the circulation (usually the right atrium or inferior vena cava), and the resultant change in temperature is detected at a point downstream (usually the pulmonary artery). The injectate is usually room temperature saline. This method is used to measure cardiac output in the catheterization laboratory in patients without shunts. Monitoring the cardiac output by the thermodilution method can also be useful in managing critically ill infants and children in an intensive care setting after cardiac surgery or in the presence of shock. In this case, a triple-lumen catheter is used for both cardiac output determinations and measurement of pulmonary arterial and pulmonary capillary wedge pressures.

ANGIOCARDIOGRAPHY

The major blood vessels and individual cardiac chambers may be visualized by selective angiocardiography, that is, injection of contrast material into specific chambers or great vessels. This method allows identification of structural abnormalities without interference from the superimposed shadows of normal chambers. *Fluoroscopy* is used to visualize the catheter as it passes through the various heart chambers. After the cardiac catheter is properly placed in the chamber to be studied, a small amount of contrast medium is injected with a power injector and cineangiograms are exposed at rates ranging from 15–90 frames/sec. *Biplane cineangiocardiography* allows detailed evaluation of specific cardiac chambers and blood vessels in two planes simultaneously with the injection of a single bolus of contrast material. This technique is now standard in pediatric cardiac catheterization laboratories and allows one to minimize the volume of contrast material used, which is safer for the patient. Various angled views (e.g., left anterior oblique, cranial angulation) are used to display specific anatomic features best in individual lesions. Digital imaging is beginning to replace standard roentgenographic film for both diagnostic and archival purposes.

The rapid injection of contrast medium under pressure into the circulation is not without risks, and each injection should be carefully planned. Contrast agents consist of hypertonic solutions, some containing organic iodides, which can cause complications, including nausea, a generalized burning sensation, central nervous system symptoms, and allergic reactions. Intramyocardial injection is generally avoided by careful placement of the catheter prior to injection. Hypertonicity of the contrast medium may result in transient myocardial depression and a drop in blood pressure, followed soon afterward by tachycardia, an increase in cardiac output, and a shift of interstitial fluid into the circulation. This shift can transiently increase the symptoms of heart failure in critically ill patients.

INTERVENTIONAL CATHETERIZATION

Nonsurgical treatment of certain cardiac defects is routine with interventional cardiac catheterization. Interventional techniques include balloon dilation of stenotic valves and arteries, embolization of abnormal vascular connections, and catheter closure of both intra- and extracardiac defects. The procedure most often used is *balloon valvuloplasty.* A special catheter with a sausage-shaped balloon at the distal end is passed through an obstructed valve. The balloon is rapidly filled with a mixture of contrast material and saline solution, resulting in tearing of the stenotic valve tissue, usually at the site of inappropriately fused raphe. Valvular pulmonary stenosis can be treated successfully by balloon angioplasty, and in most patients angioplasty has replaced surgical repair as the initial procedure of choice. The clinical results of this procedure are similar to those obtained by open heart surgery without the need for a sternotomy or prolonged hospitalization. Balloon valvuloplasty for aortic stenosis has also yielded excellent results, although as with surgery, aortic stenosis often recurs as the child grows and may require multiple procedures. One complication of both valvuloplasty and surgery is the creation of valvular insufficiency. This complication has more serious implications when it occurs on the aortic as compared with the pulmonary side of the circulation because regurgitation is less well tolerated at systemic arterial pressures.

Balloon angioplasty represents the procedure of choice for patients with restenosis of a coarctation of the aorta after earlier surgery. There is controversy as to whether angioplasty is the best procedure for native (unoperated) coarctation of the aorta because of reports of later aneurysm formation. The risk of angioplasty and valvuloplasty procedures on the left side of the heart are higher in younger patients, especially infants less than 1 yr of age, because of complications at the site of femoral artery catheterization. Low-profile catheters have significantly reduced, although not totally eliminated, these complications. Other applications of the balloon angioplasty technique include amelioration of mitral stenosis, dilation of surgical conduits (Mustard or Senning atrial baffles), relief of branch pulmonary arterial narrowing, dilation of venous obstructions, and the long-used balloon atrial septostomy (Rashkind procedure) for transposition of the great arteries (see Chapter 438.2).

Interventional cardiac catheterization techniques using *metal coils* have been developed for obliteration of arteriovenous shunts and pulmonary collateral vessels, which may be detrimental after surgical repair of pulmonary atresia and VSD. Coils have been used to close small and medium-sized PDAs with excellent results. In patients with branch pulmonary arterial stenoses, previously mixed results with balloon angioplasty alone have been supplanted with the use of *intravascular stents*, which are delivered over a balloon catheter and expanded within the vessel lumen. Once placed, they can often be dilated to successively greater sizes as the patient grows. Placement of stents in small infants and children remains problematic because of the problems of subsequent growth.

There is also increasing experience with catheter-introduced devices to close congenital cardiac defects. There are currently several devices (clamshell, umbrella, button) undergoing clinical trials for closure of small to moderate-sized ASDs. Umbrella devices may also be introduced to close a large PDA not amenable to coil closure. High-risk patients undergoing the Fontan operation (see Chapter 437.4) often have a small fenestration created in the baffle between the right and left sides of the circulation to serve as a "pop-off" for high right-sided pressures in the early surgical period. Patients with these "fenestrated Fontans" are ideal candidates for subsequent closure with a catheter-delivered device. Patients with apical muscular VSDs, especially those associated with other cardiac defects, may be candidates for catheter closure with a clamshell-type device because of the higher risk of standard surgery. Many of these applications remain experimental but are likely to become generally available in the near future.

Cardiac Sounds and Phonocardiography

McNamara DG: Value and limitations of auscultation in the management of congenital heart disease. Pediatr Clin North Am 37:93, 1990.

Mills P, Craige E: Echophonocardiography. Prog Cardiovasc Dis 20:337, 1989.

Newburger JW, Rosenthal A, Williams RG, et al: Noninvasive tests in the initial evaluation of heart murmurs in children. N Engl J Med 308:61, 1983.

Electrocardiogram and Vectorcardiogram

Garson A: The Electrocardiogram in Infants and Children: A Systematic Approach. Philadelphia, Lea & Febiger, 1983.

Garson A, Dick M, Fournier A, et al: The long QT syndrome in children: An international study of 287 patients. Circulation 87:1866, 1993.

Lipman BF, Massey EF: Clinical Scalar Electrocardiography. Chicago, Year Book Medical, 1984.

Marriott H: Rhythm Quizlets Self Assessment. Philadelphia, Lea & Febiger, 1987.

Schwartz PJ, Moss AJ, Vincent GM, et al: Diagnostic criteria for the long QT syndrome: An update. Circulation 88:782, 1993.

Echocardiography

Hatle L, Angelsen B: Doppler Ultrasound in Cardiology, Physical Principles and Clinical Applications. Philadelphia, Lea & Febiger, 1985.

Popp RL: Echocardiography. N Engl J Med 323:101, 1990.

Seward JB, Tajik AJ, Edwards WD, et al: Two-Dimensional Echocardiographic Atlas. I: Congenital Heart Disease. New York, Springer-Verlag, 1987.

Sherman FS, Sahn DJ: Pediatric Doppler echocardiography 1987: Major advances in technology. J Pediatr 110:333, 1987.

Silverman NH: Pediatric Echocardiography. Baltimore, Williams & Wilkins, 1993.

Stümpflen I, Stümpflen A, Wimmer M, et al: Effect of detailed fetal echocardiography as part of routine prenatal ultrasonographic screening on detection of congenital heart disease. Lancet 348:854, 1996.

Wiles HB: Imaging congenital heart disease. Pediatr Clin North Am 37:115, 1990.

Exercise Testing

Braden DS, Strong WF: Cardiovascular responses to exercise in children. Am J Dis Child 144:1255, 1990.

James FW, Blomqvist CG, Freed MD, et al: Standards for exercise testing in the pediatric age group: American Heart Association Council on Cardiovascular Disease in the Young. Circulation 66:1377A, 1982.

Washington RL, van Gundy JC, Cohen C, et al: Normal aerobic and anaerobic exercise data for North American school-age children. J Pediatr 112:223, 1988.

Magnetic Resonance Imaging and Nuclear Medicine

Didier D, Higgins CB, Fisher MR, et al: Congenital heart disease: Gated MR imaging in 72 patients. Radiology 158:227, 1986.

Dilworth LR, Aisen AM, Mancini GB: Determination of left ventricular volumes and ejection fraction by nuclear magnetic resonance imaging. Am Heart J 113:24, 1987.

Hurwitz RA: Quantitation of aortic and mitral regurgitation in the pediatric population: Evaluation by radionuclide angiography. Am J Cardiol 51:252, 1983.

Cardiac Catheterization

Allen HD, Mullins CE: Results of the Valvuloplasty and Angioplasty of Congenital Anomalies Registry. Am J Cardiol 65:772, 1990.

Bridges ND, Perry SB, Keane JF, et al: Preoperative transcatheter closure of congenital muscular ventricular septal defects. N Engl J Med 324:1312, 1991.

Gray DT, Fyler DC, Walker AM, et al: Clinical outcomes and costs of transcatheter as compared with surgical closure of patent ductus arteriosus. N Engl J Med 329:1517, 1993.

Kan JS, White RI, Mitchell SE, et al: Treatment of restenosis of coarctation by percutaneous transluminal angioplasty. Circulation 68:1087, 1983.

Lock JE, Keane JF, Fellows KE: Diagnostic and Interventional Catheterization in Congenital Heart Disease. Dordrecht, The Netherlands, Martinus Nijhoff, 1987.

Mullins CE, Nihill MR, Vick GW, et al: Double balloon technique for dilatation of valvular or vessel stenosis in congenital and acquired heart disease. J Am Coll Cardiol 10:107, 1987.

Nixon PA, Joswiak ML, Fricker FJ: A six-minute walk test for assessing exercise tolerance in severely ill children. J Pediatr 129:362, 1996.

O'Laughlin MP, Slack MC, Grifka RG, et al: Implantation and intermediate-term follow-up of stents in congenital heart disease. Circulation 88:605, 1993.

Radtke W, Lick J: Balloon dilation. Pediatr Clin North Am 37:193, 1990.

Rao PS, Thapar MK, Galal O, et al: Follow-up results of balloon angioplasty of native coarctation in neonates and infants. Am Heart J 120:1310, 1990.

Stanger P, Heymann MA, Tarnoff H, et al: Complications of cardiac catheterization of neonates, infants, and children: A three year study. Circulation 50:595, 1974.

Suarez J, Pan M, Sancho M, et al: Percutaneous transluminal balloon dilatation for discrete subaortic stenosis. Am J Cardiol 58:619, 1986.

Waldman JD, Karp RB: How should we treat coarctation of the aorta? Circulation 87:1043, 1993.

Walsh KP: Interventional cardiology. Arch Dis Child 76:6, 1997.

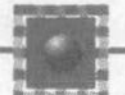

SECTION 3

Congenital Heart Disease

CHAPTER 431

Epidemiology of Congenital Heart Disease

PREVALENCE. Congenital heart disease occurs in 0.5–0.8% of live births. The incidence is higher among stillborns (3–4%), abortuses (10–25%), and premature infants (about 2% excluding patent ductus arteriosus [PDA]). This overall incidence does not include mitral valve prolapse, PDA of the preterm infant, and bicuspid aortic valves (present in 1–2% of adult series). There is a wide spectrum of severity in infants with congenital cardiac defects: About 2–3 in 1,000 newborn infants will be symptomatic with heart disease in the 1st yr of life. The diagnosis is established by 1 wk of age in 40–50% of patients with congenital heart disease and by 1 mo of age in 50–60% of patients. With the advances in both palliative and corrective surgery of the last 20 years, the number of children with congenital heart disease surviving to adulthood has increased dramatically. Despite these advances, congenital heart disease remains the leading cause of death in children with congenital malformations. Table 431–1 summarizes the relative frequency of the most common congenital cardiac lesions.

Most congenital defects are well tolerated in the fetus because of the parallel nature of the fetal circulation. Even the most severe cardiac defects (hypoplastic left heart syndrome) can usually be well compensated for by the fetal circulation. In this example, the entire fetal cardiac output would be ejected by the right ventricle via the ductus arteriosus into both the descending and ascending aorta (the latter filling in a retrograde fashion). It is only after birth when the fetal pathways (ductus arteriosus and foramen ovale) are closed that the full hemodynamic impact of an anatomic abnormality becomes apparent (see Chapter 428). One notable exception is the case of severe regurgitant lesions, most commonly of the tricuspid valve. In these lesions (Ebstein's anomaly [see Chapter 437.7]), the parallel fetal circulation cannot compensate for the volume load imposed on the right side of the heart. In utero heart failure, often with fetal pleural and pericardial effusions, and generalized ascites (nonimmune hydrops fetalis) may occur.

TABLE 431–1 Relative Frequency of Major Congenital Heart Lesions*

Lesions	% of All Lesions
Ventricular septal defect	25–30
Atrial septal defect (secundum)	6–8
Patent ductus arteriosus	6–8
Coarctation of aorta	5–7
Tetralogy of Fallot	5–7
Pulmonary valve stenosis	5–7
Aortic valve stenosis	4–7
d-Transposition of great arteries	3–5
Hypoplastic left ventricle	1–3
Hypoplastic right ventricle	1–3
Truncus arteriosus	1–2
Total anomalous pulmonary venous return	1–2
Tricuspid atresia	1–2
Single ventricle	1–2
Double-outlet right ventricle	1–2
Others	5–10

**Excluding patent ductus arteriosus in preterm neonate, bicuspid aortic valve, physiologic peripheral pulmonic stenosis, and mitral valve prolapse.*

Although the immediate perinatal period marks the time of the most significant transitions in the circulation, the circulation continues to undergo changes after birth, and these later changes may also have a hemodynamic impact on cardiac lesions and their apparent incidence. For example, as pulmonary vascular resistance falls over the 1st several weeks of life, left-to-right shunting through intracardiac defects increases and symptoms become more apparent. Thus, in patients with a ventricular septal defect (VSD), the time of presentation of heart failure is often between 1 and 3 mo of age (see Chapter 433.6). The severity of various defects can also change dramatically with growth; some VSDs may become smaller and even close as the child ages. Alternatively, stenosis of the aortic or pulmonary valve, which may be mild in the newborn period, may become worse if valve orifice growth does not keep pace with patient growth (see Chapter 434). The physician should always be alert for associated congenital malformations, which can adversely affect the patient's prognosis (see Table 429–2).

ETIOLOGY. The cause of most congenital heart defects is unknown. Genetic factors play some role in congenital heart disease; for example, certain types of VSDs (supracristal) are more common in children of Asian background. Furthermore, the recurrence risk of congenital heart disease increases if a 1st-degree relative (parent or sibling) is affected. Approximately 3% of patients with congenital heart disease have an identifiable single gene defect, such as Marfan's or Noonan's syndrome. Thirteen per cent of patients with congenital heart disease have an associated chromosomal abnormality: Heart disease is found in greater than 90% of patients with trisomy 18, 50% of patients with trisomy 21, and 40% of those with Turner's syndrome.

The conotruncal defects represent the best example of a group of cardiac lesions with a genetic basis. These anomalies include tetralogy of Fallot, double-outlet right ventricle, truncus arteriosus, pulmonary atresia, and interrupted aortic arch. Many of these patients also have evidence of *DiGeorge syndrome* (hypocalcemia, thymic hypoplasia, mild facial anomalies) or *Sprintzen velocardiofacial syndrome* (abnormal facies, cleft palate). Cytogenetic analysis using fluorescence in situ hybridiziaton demonstrates that up to 85% of patients with conotruncal lesions have deletions of a segment of chromosome 22q11 known as the DiGeorge critical region. These patients have been grouped into a syndrome known by the mnemonic *CATCH 22* (Cardiac, *A*bnormal facies, *T*hymic hypoplasia, *C*left palate, *H*ypocalcemia).

Two to 4% of cases of congenital heart disease are associated with known environmental or adverse maternal conditions and teratogenic influences, including maternal diabetes mellitus, phenylketonuria, systemic lupus erythematosus, congenital rubella syndrome, and drugs (lithium, ethanol, warfarin, thalidomide, antimetabolites, anticonvulsant agents) (see Table 429–3). Associated noncardiac malformations noted in identifiable syndromes may be seen in as many as 25% of patients with congenital heart disease (see Table 429–2).

There are gender differences in the occurrence of specific cardiac lesions. Transposition of the great arteries and left-sided obstructive lesions are slightly more common in boys (approximately 65%), whereas atrial septal defect, VSD, PDA, and pulmonic stenosis are more common in girls. There are no racial differences in the occurrence of congenital heart lesions as a whole; however, for specific lesions such as transposition of the great arteries, a higher occurrence may be seen in white than in black infants.

GENETIC COUNSELING. Parents who have a child with congenital heart disease require genetic counseling regarding the probability of a cardiac malformation occurring in subsequent children (see Chapter 80). With the exception of syndromes known to be due to a single gene mutation, most congenital heart disease is the result of a multifactorial inheritance pattern, which results in a low risk of recurrence. There is approximately an 0.8% incidence of congenital heart disease in the normal population, and this incidence increases to 2–6% for a 2nd pregnancy following the birth of a child with congenital heart disease or if a parent is affected. This recurrence risk is highly dependent on the type of lesion in the 1st child, being much higher in patients with anomalous pulmonary venous return and left-sided obstructive lesions. When two 1st-degree relatives have congenital heart disease, the risk for a subsequent child may reach 20–30%. In general, when a 2nd child is found to have congenital heart disease, it will tend to be of a similar class as the lesion in their 1st-degree relative (e.g., conotruncal lesions, left-sided obstructive lesions, atrioventricular septation defects). The degree of severity may be variable, as is the presence of associated defects. Certain cardiac lesions, for example, left-sided obstructive lesions, may be associated with a much higher rate of recurrence because of the presence of mild and clinically silent defects, for example, a bicuspid aortic valve in other family members.

Fetal echocardiography improves the rate of detection of congenital heart lesions in high-risk patients (see Chapter 92.5). The resolution and accuracy of fetal echocardiography is not perfect. Congenital heart lesions may also evolve during the course of the pregnancy, for example, moderate aortic stenosis with a normal-sized left ventricle at 18 wk of gestation may evolve into aortic atresia with a hypoplastic left ventricle by 34 wk because of decreased flow through the atria, ventricle, and aorta during the latter half of gestation.

The major factor in determining whether a woman with congenital heart disease, either unoperated or operated, will be able to carry a fetus to term is the mother's cardiovascular status. In the presence of a mild congenital heart defect, or after successful repair of a more severe lesion, normal childbearing is likely. However, in a woman with poor cardiac function, the increased hemodynamic burden imposed by pregnancy may result in significantly increased risk to both mother and fetus. The incidence of spontaneous abortion in the presence of severe congenital heart disease is high, especially when the mother is cyanotic. The maternal risk in these situations is also high. Therefore, it is important to discuss various methods of birth control with young women with repaired or palliated congenital heart lesions. Antibiotic prophylaxis against endocarditis is also indicated at the time of delivery.

Clark EB: Pathogenetic mechanisms of congenital cardiovascular malformations revisited. Semin Perinatol 20:465, 1996.
Crawford DC, Chita SK, Allan LD: Prenatal detection of congenital heart disease: Factors affecting obstetric management and survival. Am J Obstet Gynecol 159:352, 1988.
Ferencz C, Rubin JD, McCarter RJ, et al: Congenital heart disease: Prevalence at live-birth. The Baltimore-Washington Infant Study. Am J Epidemiol 121:31, 1985.
Fyler DC, Buckley DP, Hellenbrand WE, Cohn HE: Report of the New England Regional Infant Cardiac Program. Pediatrics 65(Suppl):376, 1980.
Gillum RF: Epidemiology of congenital heart disease in the United States. Am Heart J 127:919, 1994.
Harvey RP: NK-2 homeobox genes and heart development. Dev Biol 178:203, 1996.
Payne RM, Johnson MC, Grant JW, Strauss AW: Toward a molecular understanding of congenital heart disease. Circulation 91:494, 1995.
Strauss AW, Johnson MC: The genetic basis of pediatric cardiovascular disease. Semin Perinatol 20:564, 1996.
Whittemore R, Wells JA, Castellsague X. A second-generation study of 427 probands with congenital heart defects and their 837 children. J Am Coll Cardiol. 23: 1459–1467, 1994.
Wilson DI, Burn J, Scambler P, Goodship J: DiGeorge syndrome: Part of CATCH 22. J Med Genet 30:852, 1993.

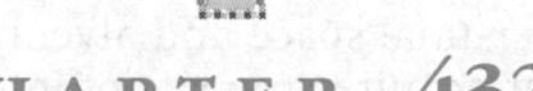

CHAPTER 432
Evaluation of the Infant or Child with Congenital Heart Disease

The initial evaluation of the infant or child with suspected congenital heart disease involves a systematic approach with three major components. First, congenital cardiac defects can be divided into two major groups based on the presence or absence of cyanosis, which can be determined by physical examination aided by pulse oximetry. Second, these two groups can be further subdivided based on whether the chest radiograph shows evidence of increased, normal, or decreased pulmonary vascular markings. Finally, the electrocardiogram can be used to determine whether right, left, or biventricular hypertrophy exists. The character of the heart sounds and the presence and character of any murmurs further narrows the differential diagnosis. The final diagnosis is then confirmed by echocardiography or cardiac catheterization, or both.

ACYANOTIC CONGENITAL HEART LESIONS

Acyanotic congenital heart lesions can be classified according to the predominant physiologic load they place on the heart. Although many congenital heart lesions induce more than one physiologic disturbance, it is helpful to focus on the primary load abnormality for purposes of classification. The most common lesions are those that produce a *volume load,* and the most common of these are the left-to-right shunt lesions. Atrioventricular valve regurgitation and some of the cardiomyopathies are other causes of increased volume load. The second major class of lesions causes an increase in *pressure load,* most commonly secondary to ventricular outflow obstruction (e.g., pulmonic or aortic valve stenosis) or narrowing of one of the great vessels (e.g., coarctation of the aorta). The chest radiograph and electrocardiogram are useful tools for differentiating between these major classes of volume and pressure overload lesions.

LESIONS RESULTING IN INCREASED VOLUME LOAD. The most common lesions in this group are those that cause left-to-right shunting (see Chapter 433): atrial septal defect, ventricular septal defect (VSD), atrioventricular septal defects (AV canal), and patent ductus arteriosus. The pathophysiologic common denominator in this group is a communication between the systemic and pulmonary sides of the circulation, resulting in the shunting of fully oxygenated blood back into the lungs. This shunt can be quantitated by calculating the ratio of pulmonary to systemic blood flow, or Q_p:Q_s. Thus, a 2:1 shunt implies that there is twice the normal pulmonary blood flow.

The direction and magnitude of the shunt across such a communication depends on the size of the defect and the relative pulmonary and systemic pressures and vascular resistances. These factors are dynamic and may change dramatically with age: Intracardiac defects may grow smaller with time;

pulmonary vascular resistance, which is high in the immediate newborn period, decreases to normal adult levels by several weeks of life; chronic exposure of the pulmonary circulation to high pressure and blood flow results in a gradual increase in pulmonary vascular resistance (Eisenmenger physiology, see Chapter 440.2). Thus, in a lesion such as a large VSD, there may be little shunting and few symptoms during the first weeks of life. When the pulmonary vascular resistance declines over the next several weeks, the volume of the left-to-right shunt increases, and symptoms begin to appear.

The increased volume of blood in the lungs decreases pulmonary compliance and increases the work of breathing. Fluid leaks into the interstitial space and alveoli, causing pulmonary edema. The infant acquires the symptoms we refer to as *heart failure,* such as tachypnea, chest retractions, nasal flaring, and wheezing. The term *heart failure* is a misnomer; total left ventricular output is actually several times greater than normal, although much of this output is ineffective because it returns directly to the lungs. To maintain this high level of left ventricular output, heart rate and stroke volume are increased, mediated by an increase in sympathetic nervous system activity. The increase in circulating catecholamines, combined with the increased work of breathing, result in an elevation in total body oxygen consumption, often beyond the oxygen transport ability of the circulation. This leads to the additional symptoms of sweating, irritability, and failure to thrive. Remodeling of the heart occurs, with predominant dilatation and a lesser degree of hypertrophy. If left untreated, pulmonary vascular resistance eventually begins to rise, and by several years of age the shunt volume will decrease and eventually reverse to right-to-left (Eisenmenger physiology, Chapter 440.2).

Additional lesions that impose a volume load on the heart include the regurgitant lesions (see Chapter 435) and the cardiomyopathies (see Chapter 445). Regurgitation of the atrioventricular valves is most commonly encountered in patients with partial or complete atrioventricular septal defects (atrioseptal defects, atrioventricular canal). In these lesions, the combination of a left-to-right shunt with atrioventricular valve regurgitation increases the volume load on the heart and leads to more severe symptoms. Isolated regurgitation of the tricuspid valve is seen in Ebstein's anomaly (see Chapter 437.7). Regurgitation of one of the semilunar valves is usually also associated with stenosis; however, aortic regurgitation may be encountered in patients with a VSD directly under the aortic valve (supracristal VSD).

In contrast to the left-to-right shunts, in which intrinsic cardiac muscle function is usually either normal or increased, heart muscle function is decreased in the cardiomyopathies. Cardiomyopathies may affect systolic contractility or diastolic relaxation, or both. Decreased cardiac function results in increased atrial and ventricular filling pressures, and pulmonary edema occurs secondary to increased capillary pressure. The major causes of cardiomyopathy in infants and children include viral myocarditis, metabolic disorders, and genetic defects (see Chapter 445).

LESIONS RESULTING IN INCREASED PRESSURE LOAD. The pathophysiologic common denominator of these lesions is an obstruction to normal blood flow. The most common are obstructions to ventricular outflow: valvar pulmonic stenosis, valvar aortic stenosis, and coarctation of the aorta (see Chapter 434). Less common are obstruction to ventricular inflow: tricuspid or mitral stenosis and cor triatriatum. Ventricular outflow obstruction can occur at the valve, below the valve (e.g., double-chambered right ventricle, subaortic membrane), or above it (e.g., branch pulmonary stenosis or supravalvar aortic stenosis). Unless the obstruction is severe, cardiac output will be maintained and clinical symptoms of heart failure will be either subtle or absent. This compensation predominantly involves an increase in cardiac wall thickness (hypertrophy) but in later stages also involves dilatation.

The clinical picture is different when obstruction to outflow is severe, usually encountered in the immediate newborn period. The infant may become critically ill within several hours of birth. Severe pulmonic stenosis in the newborn period *(critical PS)* results in signs of right-sided heart failure (hepatomegaly, peripheral edema) as well as cyanosis due to right-to-left shunting across the foramen ovale. Severe aortic stenosis in the newborn period *(critical AS)* presents with signs of left-sided heart failure (pulmonary edema, poor perfusion), right-sided failure (hepatomegaly, peripheral edema), and may progress rapidly to total circulatory collapse. In older children, severe pulmonic stenosis leads to symptoms of right-sided heart failure but not to cyanosis unless a pathway persists for right-to-left shunting (e.g., patency of the foramen ovale).

Coarctation of the aorta usually presents in older children and adolescents with upper body hypertension and diminished pulses in the lower extremities. In the immediate newborn period, however, the presentation of coarctation may be delayed because of the presence of a patent ductus arteriosus. In these patients, the open aortic end of the ductus may serve as a conduit for blood flow to bypass the obstruction partially. These infants then become symptomatic, often dramatically, when the ductus finally closes.

CYANOTIC CONGENITAL HEART LESIONS

This group of congenital heart lesions can also be further divided based on pathophysiology: whether pulmonary blood flow is decreased (tetralogy of Fallot, pulmonary atresia with intact septum, tricuspid atresia, total anomalous pulmonary venous return with obstruction) or increased (transposition of the great vessels, single ventricle, truncus arteriosus, total anomalous pulmonary venous return without obstruction). The chest radiograph is a valuable tool for initial differentiation between these two categories.

CYANOTIC LESIONS WITH DECREASED PULMONARY BLOOD FLOW. These lesions must include both an obstruction to pulmonary blood flow (at the tricuspid valve or right ventricular or pulmonary valve level) and a pathway by which systemic venous blood can shunt from right to left and enter the systemic circulation (via a patent foramen ovale, atrial septal defect, or VSD). Common lesions in this group include tricuspid atresia, tetralogy of Fallot, and various forms of single ventricle with pulmonary stenosis (see Chapter 437). In these lesions, the degree of cyanosis depends on the degree of obstruction to pulmonary blood flow. If the obstruction is mild, cyanosis may be absent at rest. These patients may acquire hypercyanotic ("tet") spells during conditions of stress. In contrast, if the obstruction is severe, pulmonary blood flow may be dependent on the patency of the ductus arteriosus. When the ductus closes during the 1st few days of life, the neonate presents with profound hypoxemia and shock.

CYANOTIC LESIONS WITH INCREASED PULMONARY BLOOD FLOW. In this group of lesions, there is no obstruction to pulmonary blood flow. Cyanosis is caused by either abnormal ventricular-arterial connections or by total mixing of systemic venous and pulmonary venous blood within the heart (see Chapter 438). Transposition of the great vessels is the most common of the former group of lesions. In transposition of the great vessels, the aorta arises from the right ventricle and the pulmonary artery arises from the left ventricle. Systemic venous blood returning to the right atrium is pumped directly back to the body, and oxygenated blood returning from the lungs to the left atrium is pumped back into the lungs. The persistence of fetal pathways (foramen ovale and ductus arteriosus) allows for a small degree of mixing in the immediate newborn period; when the ductus begins to close, these infants acquire extreme cyanosis.

The total mixing lesions include those cardiac defects with a common atrium or ventricle, total anomalous pulmonary venous return, and truncus arteriosus (see Chapter 438). In this group, deoxygenated systemic venous blood and oxygenated pulmonary venous blood mix completely in the heart, resulting in equal oxygen saturations in the pulmonary artery and aorta. If there is no obstruction to pulmonary blood flow, these infants present with a combination of cyanosis and heart failure. In contrast, if pulmonary stenosis is present, these infants present with cyanosis alone, similar to patients with tetralogy of Fallot.

Lister G, Pitt BR: Cardiopulmonary interactions in the infant with congenital heart disease. Clin Chest Med 4:219, 1983.
Lister G, Moreau G, Moss M, Talner NS: Effect of alteration of oxygen transport on the neonate. Semin Perinatol 8:192, 1984.
Mair DD, Ritter DG: Factors influencing systemic oxygen saturation in complete transposition of the great arteries. Am J Cardiol 31:742, 1973.
Talner NS: The physiology of congenital heart disease. *In:* Garson A, Bricker TJ, Fisher, DJ, Neish SR (eds): The Science and Practice of Pediatric Cardiology. Baltimore, Williams & Wilkins, 1998, pp 1107–1118.

CHAPTER 433
Acyanotic Congenital Heart Disease: The Left-to-Right Shunt Lesions

433.1 Atrial Septal Defect

Atrial septal defects (ASDs) can occur in any portion of the atrial septum (secundum, primum, or sinus venosus), depending on which embryonic septal structure has failed to develop normally (see Chapter 427). Less commonly there may be near absence of the atrial septum, creating a functional single atrium. Isolated secundum ASDs account for approximately 7% of congenital heart defects. The majority of cases of ASD are sporadic; however, autosomal dominant inheritance does occur as part of the Holt-Oram syndrome (hypoplastic or absent radii, 1st-degree heart block, ASD).

An isolated valve-incompetent patent foramen ovale (PFO) is a common echocardiographic finding during infancy. An isolated PFO is usually of no hemodynamic significance and is not considered an ASD. A PFO may play an important role if other structural heart defects are present. If right atrial pressure is increased secondary to another cardiac anomaly (e.g., pulmonary stenosis or atresia, tricuspid valve abnormalities, right ventricular dysfunction), venous blood may shunt across the PFO into the left atrium with resultant cyanosis. Because of the anatomic structure of the PFO, left-to-right shunting is unusual outside of the immediate newborn period. In the presence of a large volume load or a hypertensive left atrium (e.g., due to mitral stenosis) there may be enough dilatation of the foramen ovale to result in a significant atrial left-to-right shunt. A valve-competent but probe-patent foramen ovale may be present in 15–30% of adults. An isolated PFO does not require surgical treatment, although it may be a risk for paradoxical systemic embolization.

433.2 Ostium Secundum Defect

Ostium secundum defect, in the region of the fossa ovalis, is the most common form of ASD and is associated with structurally normal atrioventricular (AV) valves. Mitral valve prolapse has been described in association; however, this is rarely an important clinical consideration. Secundum ASDs may be single or multiple (fenestrated atrial septum), and openings of 2 cm or more in diameter are not unusual in symptomatic older children. Large defects may extend inferiorly toward the inferior vena cava and ostium of the coronary sinus, superiorly toward the superior vena cava, or posteriorly. Females outnumber males 3:1 in incidence. Partial anomalous pulmonary venous return, most commonly of the right upper pulmonary vein, may be an associated lesion.

PATHOPHYSIOLOGY. The degree of left-to-right shunting is dependent on the size of the defect, the relative compliances of the right and left ventricles, and the relative vascular resistances in the pulmonary and systemic circulations. In large defects, a considerable shunt of oxygenated blood flows from the left to the right atrium (Fig. 433–1). This blood is added to the usual venous return to the right atrium and is pumped by the right ventricle to the lungs. In large defects, the ratio of pulmonary to systemic blood flow (Qp:Qs) is usually between 2 and 4:1. The paucity of symptoms in infants with ASDs is related to the structure of the right ventricle in early life when its muscular wall is thick and less compliant, thus limiting the left-to-right shunt. As the infant becomes older, and pulmonary vascular resistance drops, the right ventricular wall becomes thinner, and the left-to-right shunt across the ASD increases. The large blood flow through the right side of the heart results in enlargement of the right atrium and ventricle and dilatation of the pulmonary artery. The left atrium may be enlarged; however, the left ventricle and aorta are normal in size. Despite the large pulmonary blood flow, the pulmonary arterial pressure is usually normal because of the absence of a high-pressure communication between the pulmonary and systemic circulations. Pulmonary vascular resistance remains low throughout childhood, although it may begin to increase

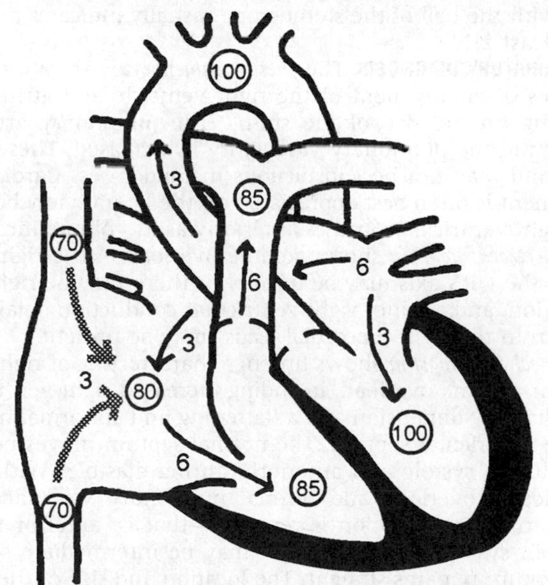

Figure 433–1 Physiology of atrial septal defect (ASD). The circled numbers represent oxygen saturations. The numbers next to the arrows represent volumes of blood flow (in L/min/m²). This illustration shows a hypothetical patient with a pulmonary to systemic blood flow ratio (Qp:Qs) of 2:1. Three L/min/m² of desaturated blood enter the right atrium from the vena cavae, mixing with an additional 3 L of fully saturated blood shunting left to right across the atrial septal defect, resulting in an increase in oxygen saturation in the right atrium. Six liters of blood flow through the tricuspid valve, causing a mid-diastolic flow rumble. The oxygen saturation may be slightly higher in the right ventricle owing to incomplete mixing at the atrial level. The full 6 L flow across the right ventricular outflow tract, causing a systolic ejection flow murmur. Six liters return to the left atrium, with 3 L shunting left to right across the defect and 3 L crossing the mitral valve, to be ejected by the left ventricle into the ascending aorta (a normal cardiac output).

in adulthood, and eventually may result in reversal of the shunt and clinical cyanosis.

CLINICAL MANIFESTATIONS. A child with an ostium secundum defect is most often asymptomatic; the lesion may be discovered inadvertently during a physical examination. Even an extremely large secundum ASD rarely produces clinically evident heart failure in childhood. In younger children, subtle failure to thrive may be present; in older children varying degrees of exercise intolerance may be noted. Often the degree of limitation may go unnoticed by the family until after surgical repair, when the child's growth or activity level increases markedly.

The physical findings of an ASD are usually characteristic but fairly subtle and require careful examination of the heart, with special attention to the heart sounds. Examination of the chest may reveal a mild left precordial bulge. A right ventricular systolic lift is usually palpable at the left sternal border. There is a loud 1st heart sound and sometimes a pulmonic ejection click. In most patients, the 2nd heart sound is characteristically widely split and fixed in its splitting in all phases of respiration. Normally the duration of right ventricular ejection varies with respiration, with inspiration increasing right ventricular volume and delaying the closure of the pulmonary valve. With an ASD, right ventricular diastolic volume is constantly increased and ejection time is prolonged throughout all phases of respiration. A systolic ejection murmur is heard; it is medium pitched, without harsh qualities, seldom accompanied by a thrill, and is best heard at the left middle and upper sternal border. It is produced by the increased flow across the right ventricular outflow tract into the pulmonary artery, not by low-pressure flow across the ASD. A short, rumbling mid-diastolic murmur produced by the increased volume of blood flow across the tricuspid valve is often audible at the lower left sternal border. This finding, which may be subtle and is heard best with the bell of the stethoscope, usually indicates a Qp:Qs of at least 2:1.

LABORATORY DIAGNOSIS. The *chest roentgenogram* shows varying degrees of enlargement of the right ventricle and atrium depending on the size of the shunt. The pulmonary artery is large, and the pulmonary vascularity is increased. These signs vary and may not be conspicuous in mild cases. Cardiac enlargement is often best appreciated on the lateral view because the right ventricle protrudes anteriorly as its volume increases. The *electrocardiogram* shows volume overload of the right ventricle: the QRS axis may be normal or there may be right axis deviation, and a minor right ventricular conduction delay (rsR′ pattern in the right precordial leads) may be present.

The *echocardiogram* shows findings characteristic of right ventricular volume overload, including increased right ventricular end-diastolic dimension and a flattening and abnormal motion of the ventricular septum. The normal septum moves posteriorly during systole and anteriorly during diastole. With right ventricular overload and normal pulmonary vascular resistance, the septal motion is reversed—that is, anterior movement in systole—or the motion may be intermediate so that the septum remains straight. The location and size of the atrial defect are readily appreciated by two-dimensional scanning, with a characteristic brightening of the echo image at the edge of the defect (T-artifact). The shunt is confirmed by pulsed and color flow Doppler. Patients with classic features of a hemodynamically significant ASD on physical examination and chest radiography in whom echocardiographic identification of an isolated secundum ASD is made need not be catheterized prior to surgical closure, with the exception of the older patient in whom there may be a concern regarding pulmonary vascular resistance.

In cases in which the diagnosis is suspect, the shunt size cannot be determined reliably from noninvasive tests, or pulmonary vascular disease is suspected, *cardiac catheterization* confirms the presence of the defect and allows measurement of the shunt ratio and pulmonary pressures. The oxygen content of blood from the right atrium will be much higher than that from the superior vena cava. This feature is not specifically diagnostic because it may occur with partial anomalous pulmonary venous return to the right atrium, with a ventricular septal defect (VSD) in the presence of tricuspid insufficiency, with AV septal defects associated with left ventricular–to–right atrial shunts, and with aorta–to–right atrial communications (e.g., ruptured sinus of Valsalva aneurysm). The pressures in the right side of the heart are usually normal, but small to moderate pressure gradients (<25 mm Hg) may be measured across the right ventricular outflow tract because of functional stenosis related to excessive blood flow. The pulmonary vascular resistance is almost always normal. The shunt is variable depending on the size of the defect, but it may be of considerable volume (as high as 20 L/min/m^2). *Cineangiography,* performed with the catheter through the defect and in the right upper pulmonary vein, demonstrates the defect and the location of the right upper pulmonary venous drainage. Alternatively, pulmonary angiography demonstrates the defect on the levophase (return of contrast to the left side of the heart after passing through the lungs).

PROGNOSIS AND COMPLICATIONS. Secundum ASDs are well tolerated during childhood; symptoms usually do not appear until the 3rd decade or later. Pulmonary hypertension, atrial dysrhythmias, tricuspid or mitral insufficiency, and heart failure are late manifestations; these symptoms may first appear during the increased volume load of pregnancy. Infective endocarditis is extremely rare and antibiotic prophylaxis for isolated secundum ASDs is not recommended. Postoperative complications, such as late heart failure and atrial fibrillation, are more common in patients who undergo operation after 20 yr of age.

Secundum ASDs are usually isolated, although they may be associated with partial anomalous pulmonary venous return, pulmonary valvular stenosis, VSD, pulmonary arterial branch stenosis, and persistent left superior vena cava, as well as mitral valve prolapse and insufficiency. Secundum ASDs are associated with the autosomal dominant **Holt-Oram syndrome.**

TREATMENT. Surgery is advised for all symptomatic patients and also for asymptomatic patients with a Qp:Qs ratio of at least 2:1. The timing for elective closure is usually some time after the 1st year and before entry into school. Closure is carried out at open heart surgery, and the mortality rate is less than 1%. Repair is preferred during early childhood because the surgical mortality and morbidity are significantly greater in adulthood; the long-term risk of arrhythmia is also greater after ASD repair in adults. Occlusion devices, implanted transvenously at cardiac catheterization, are in clinical trials. In patients with small secundum ASDs with minimal left-to-right shunts, the consensus is that closure is not required. It is unclear at present whether the persistence of a small ASD into adulthood increases the risk for stroke enough to warrant prophylactic closure of all these defects.

The results after operation in children with large shunts are excellent. Symptoms disappear rapidly, and physical development frequently appears enhanced. The heart size decreases to normal, and the electrocardiogram shows decreased right ventricular forces. Late arrhythmias are less frequent in patients who have had early repair.

433.3 Sinus Venosus Atrial Septal Defect

Sinus venosus ASD is situated in the upper part of the atrial septum in close relation to the entry of the superior vena cava. Often, one or more pulmonary veins (usually from the right lung) drain anomalously into the superior vena cava. Sometimes the superior vena cava straddles the defect; in this case some systemic venous blood enters the left atrium, but only rarely does this cause clinically evident cyanosis. The hemodynamic disturbance, clinical picture, electrocardiogram, and roentgenogram are similar to those seen in secundum ASD. The diagnosis can usually be made by two-dimensional echocardiography. If cardiac catheterization is carried out to better define the venous drainage, the catheter may enter a right pulmonary vein directly from the superior vena cava. Anatomic correction usually requires the insertion of a patch to close the defect while incorporating the entry of anomalous veins into the left atrium; surgical results are generally excellent. Rarely, sinus venosus defects involve the inferior vena cava.

433.4 Partial Anomalous Pulmonary Venous Return

One or several pulmonary veins may return anomalously to the superior or inferior vena cava, the right atrium, or the coronary sinus and produce a left-to-right shunt of oxygenated blood. Partial anomalous pulmonary venous return usually involves some or all of the veins from only one lung, more often the right one. When there is an associated ASD, it is usually of the sinus venosus type (see Chapter 433.3). Thus, when the finding of a sinus venosus ASD is made by echocardiography, a careful search for associated partial anomalous pulmonary venous return should be made. The history, physical signs, and electrocardiographic and roentgenographic findings are indistinguishable from those of an isolated ostium secundum ASD. Occasionally, an anomalous vein draining into the inferior vena cava is visible on chest radiography as a crescentic shadow of vascular density along the right border of the cardiac silhouette (*scimitar syndrome*); in these cases an ASD usually is not present, but pulmonary sequestration and anomalous arterial supply to that lobe are common findings. Total anomalous pulmonary venous return is a cyanotic lesion and is discussed in Chapter 438.7. Echocardiography usually confirms the diagnosis. Magnetic resonance imaging and electron beam computed tomography are also useful for defining pulmonary venous drainage. At cardiac catheterization, the presence of anomalous pulmonary veins may be demonstrated by selective pulmonary arteriography.

The prognosis is excellent, similar to that for ostium secundum ASDs. When a large left-to-right shunt is present, surgical repair is performed. The associated ASD should be closed in such a way as to direct the pulmonary venous return to the left atrium. A single anomalous pulmonary vein without an atrial communication may be difficult to redirect to the left atrium and, if the shunt is small, may be left unoperated.

433.5 Atrioventricular Septal Defects (Ostium Primum and Atrioventricular Canal or Endocardial Cushion Defects)

The abnormalities encompassed by AV septal defects are grouped together because they represent a spectrum of a basic embryologic abnormality, a deficiency of the AV septum. The *ostium primum defect* is situated in the lower portion of the atrial septum and overlies the mitral and tricuspid valves. In most instances, there is also a cleft in the anterior leaflet of the mitral valve. The tricuspid valve is usually functionally normal, although some anatomic abnormality of the septal leaflet is usually present. The ventricular septum is intact.

AV septal defect, also known as AV canal defect or endocardial cushion defect, consists of contiguous atrial and ventricular septal defects with markedly abnormal AV valves. The severity of the valve abnormalities varies considerably; in the complete form of AV septal defect there is a single AV valve, common to both ventricles, and consisting of an anterior and a posterior bridging leaflet related to the ventricular septum, with a lateral leaflet in each ventricle. The lesion is common among children with Down syndrome and may occasionally occur with pulmonary stenosis.

Transitional varieties of these defects also occur. They include ostium primum defects with clefts in the anterior mitral and septal tricuspid valve leaflets, minor ventricular septal deficiencies and, less commonly, ostium primum defects with normal AV valves. In some patients, the atrial septum is intact, but the inlet VSD simulates that found in the full AV septal defect. These defects are also commonly associated with deformities of the AV valves.

PATHOPHYSIOLOGY. The basic abnormality in patients with *ostium primum defects* is the combination of a left-to-right shunt across the atrial defect with mitral (or occasionally tricuspid) insufficiency. The shunt is usually moderate to large. The degree of mitral insufficiency is usually mild to moderate. Pulmonary arterial pressures are usually normal or only mildly increased. The physiology of this lesion is, therefore, similar to that of an ostium secundum ASD.

In *AV septal defects,* the left-to-right shunt is at both atrial and ventricular levels (Fig. 433–2). Additional shunting may occur directly from the left ventricle to the right atrium because of the absence of the AV septum. Pulmonary hypertension and an early tendency to increase pulmonary vascular resistance are common. AV valvular insufficiency increases the volume load on one or both ventricles. Some right-to-left shunting

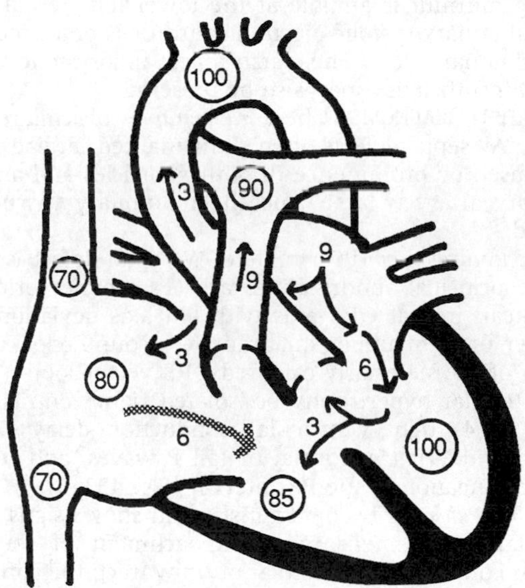

Figure 433–2 Physiology of atrioventricular septal defect (AVSD). The circled numbers represent oxygen saturations. The numbers next to the arrows represent volumes of blood flow (in L/min/m^2). This illustration shows a hypothetical patient with a pulmonary to systemic blood flow ratio (Qp:Qs) of 3:1. Three L/min/m^2 of desaturated blood enter the right atrium from the vena cavae, mixing with 3 L of fully saturated blood shunting left to right across the atrial septal defect, resulting in an increase in oxygen saturation in the right atrium. Six liters of blood flow through the right side of the common AV valve, joined by an additional 3 L of saturated blood shunting left to right at the ventricular level, further increasing the oxygen saturation in the right ventricle. The full 9 L flow across the right ventricular outflow tract into the lungs. Nine liters return to the left atrium, with 3 L shunting left to right across the defect and 6 L crossing the left side of the common AV valve, causing a mid-diastolic flow rumble. Three liters of this volume shunt left to right across the VSD, and 3 L are ejected into the ascending aorta (a normal cardiac output).

may also occur at both the atrial and ventricular levels and lead to mild but significant arterial desaturation. With time, progressive pulmonary vascular disease increases the right-to-left shunt so that clinical cyanosis develops (Eisenmenger physiology, see Chapter 440.2).

CLINICAL PRESENTATION. Many children with *ostium primum defect* are asymptomatic, and the anomaly is discovered during a general physical examination. In patients with moderate shunts and mild mitral insufficiency, the physical signs are similar to those of the secundum ASD, but with an additional apical murmur due to mitral insufficiency.

A history of exercise intolerance, easy fatigability, and recurrent pneumonias may be obtained, especially in infants with large left-to-right shunts and severe mitral insufficiency. In these patients, cardiac enlargement is moderate or marked, and the precordium is hyperdynamic. The auscultatory signs produced by the left-to-right shunt include a normal or accentuated 1st sound; wide, fixed splitting of the 2nd sound; a pulmonary systolic ejection murmur sometimes preceded by a click; and a low-pitched mid-diastolic rumbling murmur at the lower left sternal edge or apex, or both, due to increased flow through the AV valves. Mitral insufficiency may be manifested by an apical harsh (occasionally very high-pitched) holosystolic murmur that radiates to the left axilla.

With *complete AV septal defects,* congestive heart failure and intercurrent pulmonary infection usually appear in infancy. During these episodes, minimal cyanosis may be evident. The liver is enlarged and the infant shows signs of failure to thrive. Cardiac enlargement is moderate to marked, and a systolic thrill is frequently palpable at the lower left sternal border. A precordial bulge and lift may be present as well. The 1st heart sound is normal or accentuated. The 2nd heart sound is widely split if pulmonary flow is massive. A low-pitched, mid-diastolic rumbling murmur is audible at the lower left sternal border, and a pulmonary systolic ejection murmur is produced by the large pulmonary flow. The harsh apical holosystolic murmur of mitral insufficiency may also be present.

LABORATORY DIAGNOSIS. Chest *radiographs* of children with complete AV septal defects often show marked cardiac enlargement caused by prominence of both ventricles and atria. The pulmonary artery is large, and the pulmonary vascularity is increased.

The *electrocardiogram* in complete AV septal defect is distinctive. The principal abnormalities are (1) superior orientation of the mean frontal QRS axis with left axis deviation to the left upper or right upper quadrant, (2) counterclockwise inscription of the superiorly oriented QRS vector loop, (3) signs of biventricular hypertrophy or isolated right ventricular hypertrophy, (4) right ventricular conduction delay (RSR′ in leads V_{3R} and V_1), (5) normal or tall P waves, and (6) occasional prolongation of the PR interval (Fig. 433–3).

The *echocardiogram* is characteristic and shows signs of right ventricular enlargement with encroachment of the mitral valve echo on the left ventricular outflow tract; the abnormally low position of the AV valves results in a "goose-neck" deformity of the left ventricular outflow tract on both echocardiography and angiography. In normal hearts, the tricuspid valve inserts slightly more toward the apex than the mitral valve. In AV septal defects, both valves insert at the same level because of the absence of the AV septum. In complete AV septal defects, the ventricular septal echo is also deficient and the common AV valve is readily appreciated (Fig. 433–4). Pulsed and color flow Doppler echo will demonstrate left-to-right shunting at atrial, ventricular, or ventricular-to-atrial levels and semiquantitate the degree of AV valve insufficiency. Echocardiography is useful for determining the insertion points of the chordae of the common AV valve and for evaluating the presence of associated lesions such as patent ductus arteriosus (PDA) or coarctation of the aorta.

Cardiac catheterization and *angiocardiography* may be required

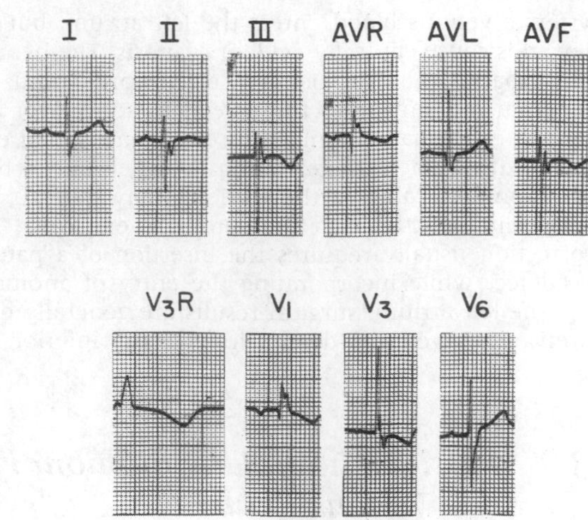

Figure 433–3 Electrocardiogram from a child with an atrioventricular canal. Note the QRS axis of −60 degrees, and the RV conduction delay; RSR′ in V_1 and V_3R. (V_3R paper speed = 50 mm/sec.)

to confirm the diagnosis, although the majority of patients can be operated on without catheterization. These studies demonstrate the magnitude of the left-to-right shunt, the severity of pulmonary hypertension, the degree of elevation of pulmonary vascular resistance, and the severity of insufficiency of the common AV valve. By oximetry, the shunt is usually demonstrable at both the atrial and ventricular levels. The arterial oxygen saturation is normal or only mildly reduced unless severe pulmonary vascular disease is present. Children with ostium primum defects usually have normal or only moderate elevation of pulmonary arterial pressure. Conversely, complete AV septal defects are associated with right ventricular and pulmonary hypertension and in older patients with increased pulmonary vascular resistance (see Chapter 440.2).

Selective left ventriculography is extremely helpful in the diagnosis of AV septal defects. The deformity of the mitral or common AV valve and the distortion of the outflow tract of the left ventricle causes a "gooseneck"-appearing deformity of the left ventricular outflow tract. The abnormal anterior leaflet of the mitral valve is serrated, and mitral insufficiency is noted, usually with regurgitation of blood into both the left and right atria. Direct shunting of blood from the left ventricle to the right atrium may also be demonstrated.

PROGNOSIS AND COMPLICATIONS. The prognosis for complete AV septal defects depends on the magnitude of the left-to-right shunt, the degree of elevation of pulmonary vascular resistance, and the severity of AV valve insufficiency. Death from cardiac failure during infancy used to be frequent before the advent of early corrective surgery. Patients who survived without surgery usually acquired pulmonary vascular obstructive disease or, more rarely, pulmonic stenosis. Most patients with ostium primum defects and minimal AV valve involvement are asymptomatic or have only minor, nonprogressive symptoms until they reach the 3rd to 4th decade of life, similar to the course of patients with secundum ASDs.

TREATMENT. Ostium primum defects are approached surgically from an incision in the right atrium. The cleft in the mitral valve is located through the atrial defect and is repaired by direct suture. The defect in the atrial septum is usually closed by insertion of a patch prosthesis. The surgical mortality rate for ostium primum defects is low. Surgical treatment for complete AV septal defects is more difficult, especially in infants with cardiac failure and pulmonary hypertension. However, because of the risk of pulmonary vascular disease developing as early as 6 to 12 mo of age, surgical intervention must be performed during infancy. Correction of these defects can be accomplished in infancy, relegating palliation with pulmonary

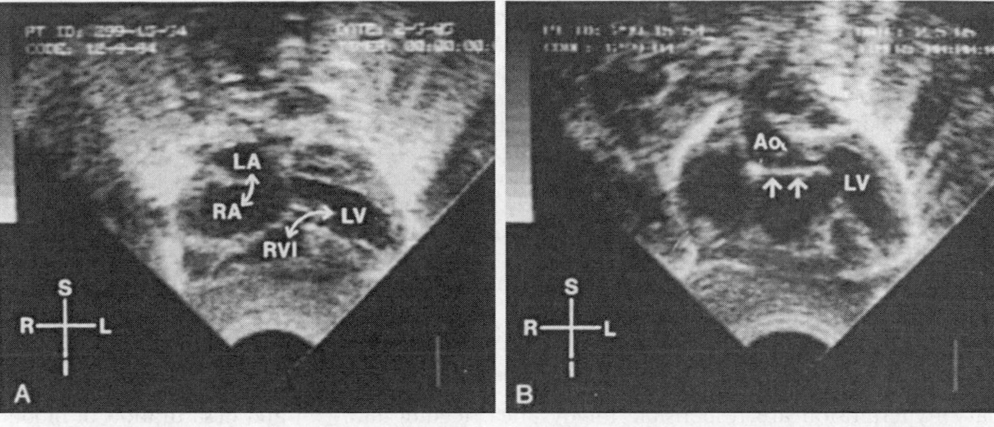

Figure 433–4 Echocardiogram of an atrioventricular septal defect. *A*, Four-chamber view demonstrating both an interatrial and an interventricular septal defect contributing to the large central communication of this lesion (*arrows*). *B*, Left ventricular long axis projection demonstrating the typical goose-neck deformity created by the anterior leaflet of the mitral valve (*arrows*). RA = right atrium; LA = left atrium; RVI = right ventricular inflow; LV = left ventricle; R = right; L = left; S = superior; I = inferior; Ao = aorta.

arterial banding for the subset of patients who are either too small or have other associated lesions making early corrective surgery too risky. The atrial and ventricular defects are patched and the AV valves reconstructed. Complications include surgically induced heart block requiring placement of a permanent pacemaker, excessive narrowing of the left ventricular outflow tract requiring surgical revision, and eventual worsening of mitral regurgitation requiring replacement with a prosthetic valve.

433.6 Ventricular Septal Defect

VSD is the most common cardiac malformation, accounting for 25% of congenital heart disease. Defects may occur in any portion of the ventricular septum; the majority are of the membranous type. These defects are in a posteroinferior position, anterior to the septal leaflet of the tricuspid valve. VSDs between the crista supraventricularis and the papillary muscle of the conus may be associated with pulmonary stenosis and the other manifestations of tetralogy of Fallot (see Chapter 437.1). VSDs superior to the crista supraventricularis (supracristal) are less common; they are found just beneath the pulmonary valve and may impinge on an aortic sinus, causing aortic insufficiency. VSDs in the midportion or apical region of the ventricular septum are muscular in type and may be single or multiple (Swiss cheese septum).

PATHOPHYSIOLOGY. The physical size of the VSD is a major, but not the only, determinant of the size of the left-to-right shunt. The shunt magnitude is also determined by the level of pulmonary vascular resistance compared with systemic vascular resistance. When a small communication is present (usually <0.5 cm^2), the VSD is called *restrictive* and right ventricular pressure is normal. The higher pressure in the left ventricle drives the shunt left to right; the size of the defect limits the magnitude of the shunt. In large *nonrestrictive* VSDs (usually >1.0 cm^2), right and left ventricular pressures are equalized. In these defects, the direction of shunting and the shunt magnitude are determined by the ratio of pulmonary to systemic vascular resistances (Fig. 433–5).

After birth in patients with a large VSD, the pulmonary vascular resistance may remain higher than normal, and thus the size of the left-to-right shunt may initially be limited. As pulmonary vascular resistance continues to fall in the 1st few weeks after birth because of the normal involution of the media of small pulmonary arterioles, the size of the left-to-right shunt increases. Eventually, a large left-to-right shunt ensues, and clinical symptoms become apparent. In most cases during early infancy, the pulmonary vascular resistance is only slightly elevated, and the major contribution to pulmonary hypertension is the extremely large pulmonary blood flow. However, in some infants with a large VSD, pulmonary arteriolar medial thickness never decreases. With continued exposure of the pulmonary vascular bed to high systolic pressure and high flow, pulmonary vascular obstructive disease develops. When the ratio of pulmonary to systemic resistance approaches 1:1, the shunt becomes bidirectional, signs of heart failure abate, and the patient becomes cyanotic (Eisenmenger physiology, see Chapter 440.2).

The magnitude of intracardiac shunts is usually described by the Qp:Qs. If the left-to-right shunt is small (Qp:Qs <1.75:1), the cardiac chambers are not appreciably enlarged and the pulmonary vascular bed is likely normal. If the shunt is large (Qp:Qs >2:1), left atrial and ventricular volume overload occurs, as does right ventricular and pulmonary arterial hypertension. The main pulmonary artery, left atrium, and left ventricle are enlarged.

CLINICAL MANIFESTATIONS. The clinical presentation of patients with a VSD varies according to the size of the defect and the pulmonary blood flow and pressure. *Small VSDs* with trivial left-to-right shunts and normal pulmonary arterial pressures

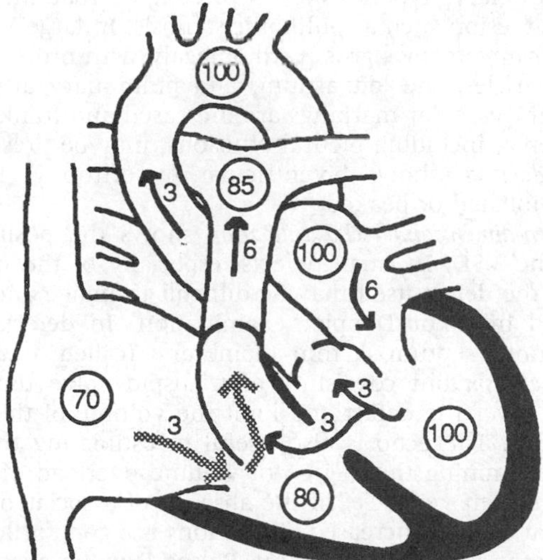

Figure 433–5 Physiology of a large ventricular septal defect (VSD). The circled numbers represent oxygen saturations. The numbers next to the arrows represent volumes of blood flow (in L/min/m^2). This illustration shows a hypothetical patient with a pulmonary to systemic blood flow ratio (Qp:Qs) of 2:1. Three L/min/m^2 of desaturated blood enter the right atrium from the vena cava and flows across the tricuspid valve. An additional 3 L of blood shunt left to right across the VSD, resulting in an increase in oxygen saturation in the right ventricle. Six liters of blood are ejected into the lungs. The pulmonary arterial saturation may be further increased owing to incomplete mixing at right ventricular level. Six liters return to the left atrium and cross the mitral valve, causing a mid-diastolic flow rumble. Three liters of this volume shunt left to right across the VSD, and 3 L are ejected into the ascending aorta (a normal cardiac output).

are the most common. These patients are asymptomatic, and the cardiac lesion is usually found during a routine physical examination. Characteristically, there is a loud, harsh, or blowing holosystolic murmur, heard best over the lower left sternal border and frequently accompanied by a thrill. In a few instances the murmur ends before the 2nd sound, presumably because of closure of the defect during late systole. A short, harsh systolic murmur localized to the apex in a neonate is often a sign of a tiny muscular VSD. In the immediate neonatal period, the left-to-right shunt may be minimal because of higher right-sided pressures, and therefore the systolic murmur may not be audible during the 1st few days of life. In premature infants, the murmur may be heard early because pulmonary vascular resistance decreases more rapidly.

Large VSDs with excessive pulmonary blood flow and pulmonary hypertension are responsible for dyspnea, feeding difficulties, poor growth, profuse perspiration, recurrent pulmonary infections, and cardiac failure in early infancy. Cyanosis is usually absent, but duskiness is sometimes noted during infections or crying. Prominence of the left precordium is common, as are a palpable parasternal lift, a laterally displaced apical impulse and apical thrust, and a systolic thrill. The holosystolic murmur of a large VSD is usually less harsh than that of a small VSD and more blowing in nature because of the absence of a significant pressure gradient across the defect. It is even less likely to be audible in the newborn period. The pulmonic component of the 2nd heart sound may be increased, indicating pulmonary hypertension. The presence of a mid-diastolic, low-pitched rumble at the apex is caused by increased blood flow across the mitral valve and indicates a Qp:Qs of 2:1 or greater. This murmur is best appreciated with the bell of the stethoscope.

LABORATORY DIAGNOSIS. In patients with small VSDs, the *chest radiograph* is usually normal, although minimal cardiomegaly and a borderline increase in pulmonary vasculature may be observed. The *electrocardiogram* is usually normal but may suggest left ventricular hypertrophy. The presence of right ventricular hypertrophy is a warning that the defect is not small and that pulmonary hypertension is present or that there is an associated lesion such as pulmonic stenosis. In large VSDs, the *chest radiograph* shows gross cardiomegaly with prominence of both ventricles, the left atrium, and pulmonary artery. The pulmonary vascular markings are increased and frank pulmonary edema, including pleural effusions, may be present. The *electrocardiogram* shows biventricular hypertrophy; P waves may be notched or peaked.

The *two-dimensional echocardiogram* shows the position and size of the VSD. In small defects, especially of the muscular septum, the defect itself may be difficult to image and is only visualized by color Doppler examination. In defects of the membranous septum, a thin membrane (called a *ventricular septal aneurysm* but consisting of tricuspid valve tissue) can partially cover the defect and limit the volume of the left-to-right shunt. The echo is also useful in estimating the shunt size by examining the degree of volume overload of the left atrium and left ventricle; in the absence of associated lesions, the extent of their increased dimensions is a good reflection of the size of the left-to-right shunt. Pulsed Doppler examination shows if the VSD is pressure-restrictive by calculating the pressure gradient across the defect. This allows estimation of right ventricular pressure and helps determine whether the patient is at risk for the development of early pulmonary vascular disease. The echo can also be useful to determine the presence of aortic valve insufficiency or leaflet prolapse in the case of supracristal VSDs.

The hemodynamics of a VSD can also be demonstrated by *cardiac catheterization*. Catheterization is usually performed only when a comprehensive clinical evaluation leaves continued uncertainty regarding the size of the shunt, when laboratory data do not fit well with the clinical findings, or when pulmonary vascular disease is suspected. Oximetry demonstrates an increase in oxygen content in the right ventricle; because some defects eject blood almost directly into the pulmonary artery (streaming), this increase is occasionally apparent only when pulmonary arterial blood is sampled. Small, restrictive VSDs are associated with normal right-sided heart pressures and pulmonary vascular resistance. Large, nonrestrictive VSDs are associated with equal or near-equal pulmonary and systemic systolic pressures. Pulmonary blood flow may be two to four times systemic blood flow. In these patients with "hyperdynamic pulmonary hypertension," the pulmonary vascular resistance is only minimally elevated because resistance is equal to the pressure divided by the flow. If Eisenmenger syndrome is present, pulmonary artery systolic and diastolic pressures are elevated, the degree of left-to-right shunting is minimal, and desaturation of blood in the left ventricle is encountered. The size, location, and number of ventricular defects are demonstrated by left ventriculography. Contrast medium passes across the defect or defects to opacify the right ventricle and pulmonary artery.

PROGNOSIS AND COMPLICATIONS. The natural course of a VSD depends to a large degree on the size of the defect. A significant number (30–50%) of small defects close spontaneously, most frequently during the 1st 2 years of life. Small muscular VSDs are more likely to close (up to 80%) than membranous VSDs (up to 35%). The vast majority of defects that close do so before age 4 yr, although spontaneous closure has been reported in adults. These VSDs often have ventricular septal aneurysms limiting the magnitude of the shunt. Most children with small defects remain asymptomatic, without evidence of an increase in heart size, pulmonary arterial pressure, or resistance. One of the long-term risks for these patients is infective endocarditis. Some long-term studies of adults with unoperated small VSDs show an increased incidence of arrhythmia, subaortic stenosis, and exercise intolerance. The Council on Cardiovascular Disease in the Young of the American Heart Association states that an isolated, small, hemodynamically insignificant VSD is not an indication for surgery. The declining risk of open heart surgery has led some to suggest that all VSDs be closed electively by mid-childhood.

It is less common for moderate or large VSDs to close spontaneously, although even defects large enough to result in heart failure may become smaller, and up to 8% may close completely. More commonly, infants with large defects have repeated episodes of respiratory infection and heart failure despite optimal medical management. Heart failure may be manifested in many of these infants primarily by failure to thrive. Pulmonary hypertension occurs as a result of high pulmonary blood flow. These patients are at risk for the development of pulmonary vascular disease with time if the defect is not repaired.

Patients with VSD are also at risk for the development of aortic valve regurgitation, the greatest risk occurring in patients with supracristal VSD (see Chapter 433.7). A small number of patients with VSD have acquired infundibular pulmonary stenosis, which then protects the pulmonary circulation from the short-term effects of pulmonary overcirculation and the long-term effects of pulmonary vascular disease. In these patients, the clinical picture changes from that of a VSD with a large left-to-right shunt to a VSD with pulmonary stenosis. The shunt may diminish in size, become balanced, or even become a net right-to-left shunt (see Chapter 437). These patients must be distinguished from those who are acquiring an Eisenmenger physiology (see Chapter 440.2).

TREATMENT. In patients with small VSDs, parents should be reassured of the relatively benign nature of the lesion, and the child should be encouraged to live a normal life, with no restrictions on physical activity. Surgical repair is currently not recommended. As a protection against infective endocarditis, the integrity of primary and permanent teeth should be carefully maintained; antibiotic prophylaxis should be provided for dental visits (including cleanings), tonsillectomy, adenoidectomy, and other oropharyngeal surgical procedures as well as for instrumentation of the genitourinary and lower intestinal tracts (see Chapter 443). These patients can be followed by a combination of clinical examinations and noninvasive laboratory tests until the VSD has closed spontaneously. The electrocardiogram is an excellent means of screening these patients for possible pulmonary hypertension or pulmonic stenosis indicated by right ventricular hypertrophy. Echocardiography is used to screen for the development of left ventricular outflow tract pathology (subaortic membrane or aortic regurgitation) and to confirm spontaneous closure.

In infants with a large VSD, medical management has two aims: to control heart failure and to prevent the development of pulmonary vascular disease. Therapeutic measures are aimed at the control of heart failure symptoms and the maintenance of normal growth (see Chapter 448). If early treatment is successful, the shunt may diminish in size, with spontaneous improvement, especially during the 1st yr of life. The clinician must be alert not to confuse clinical improvement caused by a decrease in defect size with clinical changes caused by the development of Eisenmenger physiology. Because surgical closure can be carried out at low risk in most infants, medical management should not be pursued in symptomatic infants after an initial unsuccessful trial. Pulmonary vascular disease can be prevented when surgery is performed within the 1st yr of life.

Indications for surgical closure of VSD include patients at any age with large defects in whom clinical symptoms and failure to thrive cannot be controlled medically; infants between 6 and 12 mo of age with large defects associated with pulmonary hypertension, even if symptoms are controlled by medication; and patients older than 24 mo of age with a Qp:Qs greater than 2:1. Patients with supracristal VSD of any size are usually referred for surgery because of the high risk of development of aortic valve regurgitation (see Chapter 433.7). Severe pulmonary vascular disease is a contraindication to closure of a VSD.

Results of primary surgical repair are excellent, and complications resulting in long-term problems (e.g., residual ventricular shunts requiring reoperation or heart block requiring a pacemaker) are rare. Pulmonary arterial palliative banding with repair in later childhood is reserved for complicated cases or very premature infants. Surgical risks are higher for defects in the muscular septum, particularly apical defects and multiple (Swiss cheese–type) VSDs. These patients may require pulmonary arterial banding if symptomatic, with subsequent debanding and repair of multiple VSDs at an older age. Clamshell-type catheter occlusion devices are being tested as a means of closing apical muscular VSDs.

After obliteration of the left-to-right shunt, the hyperdynamic heart becomes quiet, cardiac size decreases toward normal (Fig. 433–6), thrills and murmurs are abolished, and pulmonary artery hypertension regresses. The patient's clinical status improves markedly. Most infants begin to thrive, and cardiac medications are no longer required. Catch-up growth occurs in the majority of patients over the next 1–2 yr. In some instances after successful operation, systolic ejection murmurs of low intensity may persist for months. The long-term prognosis after surgery is excellent. Patients with a small VSD and those who have undergone surgical closure without residua are considered to be at standard risk for the purposes of insurability.

433.7 Supracristal Ventricular Septal Defect with Aortic Insufficiency

In this syndrome, the VSD is complicated by prolapse of the aortic valve into the defect and aortic insufficiency, which may eventually occur in 50 to 90% of patients. Although it accounts for approximately 5% of all patients with VSD, a considerably larger incidence is reported among Asian children. The VSD, which may be small or moderate in size, is located anterior to and directly below the pulmonary valve in the outlet septum, superior to the crista supraventricularis. In occasional cases, aortic insufficiency is associated with VSDs located in the membranous septum. The right, or less often the noncoronary, aortic cusp prolapses into the defect and may partially or even completely occlude it. This may limit the amount of left-to-right shunting and give the false impression that the defect is not large. Aortic insufficiency is most often not recognized until late in the 1st decade of life or beyond.

Early heart failure secondary to a large left-to-right shunt

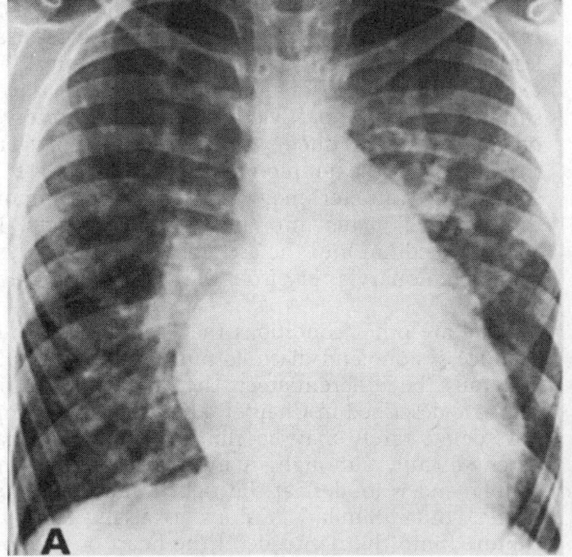

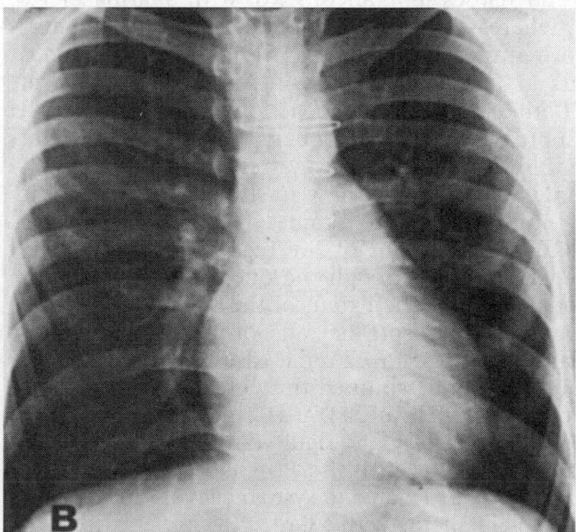

Figure 433–6 *A*, Preoperative roentgenogram in a ventricular septal defect with a large left-to-right shunt and pulmonary hypertension. Significant cardiomegaly, prominence of the pulmonary arterial trunk, and pulmonary overcirculation are evident. *B*, Three years after surgical closure of the defect. There is a marked decrease in the heart size, and the pulmonary vasculature is normal.

rarely occurs, but without operation severe aortic insufficiency and left ventricular failure may ensue. The murmur of a supracristal VSD is usually heard at the middle to upper left sternal border, as opposed to the lower left sternal border, and sometimes is confused with that of pulmonic stenosis. The physical signs of aortic insufficiency (diastolic murmur and wide pulse pressure), when present, are added to those of the VSD. This clinical presentation must be distinguished from PDA or other defects associated with aortic runoff.

The *clinical manifestations* vary widely from trivial aortic regurgitation and small left-to-right shunt in the asymptomatic child to the symptomatic adolescent with florid aortic incompetence and massive cardiomegaly. Most authors recommend closure of all supracristal ventricular VSDs at the time of diagnosis, even in the asymptomatic child, in an attempt to prevent the development of aortic regurgitation. Patients already having significant aortic incompetence require surgical intervention to prevent irreversible left ventricular dysfunction. Surgical options depend on the degree of damage to the valve and include valvuloplasty for mild involvement, and replacement with a prosthesis or homograft, or aortopulmonary translocation (see Chapter 434.5) for severe involvement.

433.8 Patent Ductus Arteriosus

During fetal life, most of the pulmonary arterial blood is shunted through the ductus arteriosus into the aorta (see Chapter 428). Functional closure of the ductus normally occurs soon after birth, but if the ductus remains patent when pulmonary vascular resistance falls, aortic blood is shunted into the pulmonary artery. The aortic end of the ductus is just distal to the origin of the left subclavian artery, and the ductus enters the pulmonary artery at its bifurcation. Female patients with PDA outnumber males 2:1. PDA is also associated with maternal rubella infection during early pregnancy. It is a common problem in the premature infant, where it can cause severe hemodynamic derangements and several major sequelae (see Chapter 97.3).

When a term infant is found to have PDA, the wall of the ductus is deficient in both the mucoid endothelial layer and the muscular media. In contrast, in the premature infant, the patent ductus usually has a normal structural anatomy; in these infants patency is the result of hypoxia and immaturity. Thus a PDA persisting beyond the 1st few weeks of life in a term infant rarely closes spontaneously or with pharmacologic intervention, whereas if early pharmacologic or surgical intervention is not required in the premature infant, spontaneous closure occurs in most instances. A PDA is seen in 10% of patients with other congenital heart lesions and often plays a critical role in providing pulmonary blood flow when the right ventricular outflow tract is stenotic or atretic (see Chapter 437) or in providing systemic blood flow in the presence of aortic coarctation or interruption (see Chapter 434).

PATHOPHYSIOLOGY. As a result of the higher aortic pressure, blood shunts left to right through the ductus, from the aorta to the pulmonary artery. The extent of the shunt depends on the size of the ductus and on the ratio of pulmonary to systemic vascular resistances. In extreme cases, 70% of the left ventricular output may be shunted through the ductus to the pulmonary circulation. If the PDA is small, the pressures within the pulmonary artery, the right ventricle, and the right atrium are normal. However, if the PDA is large, pulmonary artery pressures may be elevated to systemic levels during both systole and diastole. Patients with a large PDA are at extremely high risk for the development of pulmonary vascular disease if left unoperated. There is a wide pulse pressure due to runoff of blood into the pulmonary artery during diastole.

CLINICAL MANIFESTATIONS. There are usually no symptoms associated with a small patent ductus. A large PDA will result in heart failure similar to that encountered in infants with a large VSD. Retardation of physical growth may be a major manifestation in infants with large shunts.

A large PDA will result in striking physical signs attributable to the wide pulse pressure, most prominently bounding arterial pulses. The heart is normal in size when the ductus is small but moderately or grossly enlarged in cases with a large communication. The apical impulse is prominent and, with cardiac enlargement, is heaving. A thrill, maximal in the 2nd left interspace, is often present and may radiate toward the left clavicle, down the left sternal border, or toward the apex. It is usually systolic but also may be palpated throughout the cardiac cycle. The classic continuous murmur has been variously described as being like machinery or rolling thunder in quality. It begins soon after onset of the 1st sound, reaches maximal intensity at the end of systole, and wanes in late diastole. It may be localized to the 2nd left intercostal space or radiate down the left sternal border or to the left clavicle. When there is increased pulmonary vascular resistance, the diastolic component of the murmur may be less prominent or absent. In patients with a large left-to-right shunt, a low-pitched mitral mid-diastolic murmur may be audible at the apex, owing to the increased volume of blood flow across the mitral valve.

LABORATORY DIAGNOSIS. If the left-to-right shunt is small, the *electrocardiogram* is normal; if the ductus is large, left ventricular or biventricular hypertrophy is present. The diagnosis of an isolated, uncomplicated PDA is untenable when right ventricular hypertrophy is noted.

Radiographic studies in a large PDA show a prominent pulmonary artery with increased intrapulmonary vascular markings. The cardiac size depends on the degree of left-to-right shunting; it may be normal or moderately to markedly enlarged. The chambers involved are the left atrium and ventricle. The aortic knob is normal or prominent.

The *echocardiographic* view of the cardiac chambers is normal if the ductus is small. With large shunts, left atrial and left ventricular dimensions are increased. The size of the left atrium is usually quantitated by comparison to the size of the aortic root, known as the LA:Ao ratio. Scanning from the suprasternal notch allows direct visualization of the ductus. Color and pulsed Doppler examination demonstrate systolic or diastolic (or both) retrograde turbulent flow in the pulmonary artery and aortic retrograde flow in diastole.

The clinical pattern is sufficiently distinctive to allow an accurate diagnosis by noninvasive methods in most patients. In patients with atypical findings, or when associated cardiac lesions are suspected, cardiac catheterization may be indicated. *Cardiac catheterization* demonstrates normal or increased pressures in the right ventricle and pulmonary artery, depending on the size of the ductus. The presence of oxygenated blood shunting into the pulmonary artery confirms a left-to-right shunt. The catheter may pass from the pulmonary artery through the ductus into the descending aorta. Injection of contrast medium into the ascending aorta shows opacification of the pulmonary artery from the aorta and identifies the ductus.

There are other conditions that, in the absence of cyanosis, produce systolic and diastolic murmurs in the pulmonic area and must be differentiated. The characteristics of a venous hum are described in Chapter 429. An aorticopulmonary window defect rarely may be clinically indistinguishable from a patent ductus, although in most cases the murmur is only systolic and is loudest at the right rather than the left upper sternal border. Similarly, a sinus of Valsalva aneurysm that has ruptured into the right side of the heart or pulmonary artery, coronary arteriovenous fistulas, and an aberrant left coronary artery with massive collaterals from the right coronary display dynamics similar to that of the PDA with a continuous murmur and a wide pulse pressure. Truncus arteriosus with torrential pulmonary flow also has an "aortic runoff" physiology. Pulmonary branch stenosis can be associated with systolic and diastolic murmurs, but the pulse pressure will be normal. A peripheral arteriovenous fistula also results in a wide pulse pressure, but the distinctive murmur of a PDA is not present. VSD with aortic insufficiency and combined rheumatic aortic and mitral insufficiency may be confused with a PDA, but the murmurs should be differentiated by their to-and-fro rather than continuous nature. The combination of a large VSD and a PDA results in findings more like those in isolated VSD. Echocardiography should be able to eliminate these other diagnostic possibilities. If a PDA is suspected clinically but not visualized on echocardiography, cardiac catheterization is usually indicated.

PROGNOSIS AND COMPLICATIONS. Patients with a small PDA may live a normal span with few or no cardiac symptoms; however, late manifestations may occur. Spontaneous closure of the ductus after infancy is extremely rare. *Cardiac failure* most often occurs in early infancy in the presence of a large ductus but may occur late in life even with a moderate-sized communication. The chronic left ventricular volume load is less well tolerated with aging.

Infective endarteritis may be seen at any age. Pulmonary or systemic emboli may occur. Rare complications include aneurysmal dilatation of the pulmonary artery or the ductus, calcification of the ductus, noninfective thrombosis of the ductus with embolization, and paradoxical emboli. Pulmonary hypertension (Eisenmenger's syndrome) usually occurs in patients with a large PDA who do not undergo surgical treatment (see Chapter 440.2).

TREATMENT. Irrespective of age, patients with PDA require surgical or catheter closure. In patients with a small PDA, the rationale for closure is prevention of endarteritis or other late complications. In patients with a moderate to large PDA, closure is accomplished to treat heart failure or prevent the development of pulmonary vascular disease, or both. Once the diagnosis of moderate to large PDA is made, treatment should not be unduly postponed after adequate medical therapy of cardiac failure has been instituted.

Because the case fatality rate with surgical treatment is considerably less than 1% and the risk without it is greater, ligation and division of the ductus are indicated in the asymptomatic patient, preferably before 1 yr of age. Pulmonary hypertension is not a contraindication to operation at any age if it can be demonstrated at cardiac catheterization that the shunt flow is still predominantly left to right and that severe pulmonary vascular disease is not present. After closure, symptoms of frank or incipient cardiac failure rapidly disappear. There is usually immediate improvement in physical development in the infant who had failed to thrive. The pulse and blood pressure return to normal, and the machinery-like murmur disappears. A functional systolic murmur over the pulmonary area may persist; it may represent turbulence in a persistently dilated pulmonary artery. The radiographic signs of cardiac enlargement and pulmonary overcirculation disappear over several months and the electrocardiogram becomes normal.

Transcatheter closure of a PDA is possible in the cardiac catheterization laboratory. Small PDAs are routinely closed using intravascular coils. Moderate to large PDAs may be closed with a catheter-introduced sac into which several coils are released or with an umbrella-like device, although both of these are still investigational. Another approach involves the use of thoracoscopic surgical techniques to ligate the ductus without the need for a large lateral thoracotomy.

PATENT DUCTUS ARTERIOSUS IN LOW BIRTHWEIGHT INFANTS (see Chapters 92.2 and 97.3)

433.9 Aorticopulmonary Window Defect

The aorticopulmonary window defect consists of a communication between the ascending aorta and the main pulmonary artery. The presence of pulmonary and aortic valves and an intact ventricular septum distinguishes this anomaly from truncus arteriosus (see Chapter 438.8). Symptoms of heart failure appear during early infancy; occasionally there is minimal cyanosis. The defect is usually large and the cardiac murmur is systolic with a mid-diastolic rumble, reflecting the increased blood flow across the mitral valve. In the rare instance when the communication is somewhat smaller and pulmonary hypertension is absent, the examination can mimic a PDA (wide pulse pressure and a continuous murmur at the upper sternal borders). The electrocardiogram shows either left ventricular or biventricular hypertrophy. Radiographic studies demonstrate cardiac enlargement and prominence of the pulmonary artery and intrapulmonary vasculature. The echocardiogram shows enlarged left-sided heart chambers; the window defect can best be delineated with color flow Doppler.

Cardiac catheterization reveals a left-to-right shunt at the level of the pulmonary artery, as well as hyperkinetic pulmonary hypertension, because the defect is almost always large. Selective aortography with injection of contrast medium into the ascending aorta demonstrates the lesion, and manipulation of the catheter from the main pulmonary artery directly to the ascending aorta is also diagnostic.

The aorticopulmonary window defect is surgically corrected during infancy using cardiopulmonary bypass. If surgery is not carried out in infancy, survivors carry the risk of progressive pulmonary vascular obstructive disease, similar to that of other patients who have large intracardiac or great vessel communications.

433.10 Coronary-Arteriovenous Fistula (Coronary-Cameral Fistula)

A congenital fistula may exist between a coronary artery and an atrium, ventricle (especially the right), or pulmonary artery. Sometimes multiple fistulas exist. Regardless of the recipient chamber, the clinical signs are similar to those of PDA, although the machinery-like murmur may be more diffuse. If the flow is substantial, the involved coronary artery may be dilatated or aneurysmal. The anatomic abnormality is usually demonstrable by color flow Doppler echocardiography and, during catheterization, by injection of contrast medium into the ascending aorta. Small fistulas may be hemodynamically insignificant and may even close spontaneously. If the shunt is large, treatment consists either of surgical closure of the fistula or transcatheter coil embolization.

433.11 Ruptured Sinus of Valsalva Aneurysm

When one of the sinuses of Valsalva of the aorta is weakened by congenital or acquired disease, an aneurysm may form and eventually may rupture, usually into the right atrium or ventricle. This condition is extremely rare in childhood. The onset is usually sudden. The diagnosis is suspected in a patient in whom symptoms of acute heart failure develop, associated with a new loud to-and-fro murmur. Color Doppler echocardiography and cardiac catheterization demonstrate the left-to-right shunt at the atrial or ventricular level. Urgent surgical repair is usually required. This condition is often associated with infective endocarditis of the aortic valve.

Atrial Septal Defect

Boutin C, Musewe NN, Smallhorn JF, et al: Echocardiographic follow-up of atrial septal defect after catheter closure by double-umbrella device. Circulation 88:621, 1993.

Makoney L, Truesdell SC, Krzmarzick TR, et al: Atrial septal defects that present in infancy. Am J Dis Child 140:1115, 1986.
Murphy JG, Gersh BJ, McGoon MD, et al: Long-term outcome after surgical repair of isolated atrial septal defect: Follow-up at 27–32 years. N Engl J Med 323:1645, 1990.
Radzik D, Davignon A, van Doesburg N, et al: Predictive factors for spontaneous closure of atrial septal defects diagnosed in the first 3 months of life. J Am Coll Cardiol 22:851, 1993.

Ventricular Septal Defect

Beerman LB, Park SC, Fischer DR, et al: Ventricular septal defect associated with aneurysm of the membranous septum. J Am Coll Cardiol 5:118, 1985.
Bridges ND, Perry SB, Keane JF, et al: Preoperative transcatheter closure of congenital musuclar ventricular septal defects. N Engl J Med 19:1312, 1991.
Hornberger LK, Sahn DJ, Krabill KA, et al: Elucidation of the natural history of ventricular septal defects by serial Doppler color flow mapping studies. J Am Coll Cardiol 13:1111, 1989.
Leung MP, Beerman LB, Siewers RD, et al: Long term follow-up after aortic valvuloplasty and defect closure in ventricular septal defect with aortic regurgitation. Am J Cardiol 60:890, 1987.
Moller JH, Patton C, Varco RL, et al: Late results (30 to 35 years) after operative closure of isolated ventricular septal defect from 1954 to 1960. Am J Cardiol 68:1491, 1991.
Ramaciotti C, Keren A, Silverman NH: Importance of pseudoaneurysms of the ventricular septum in the natural history of isolated perimembranous ventricular septal defects. Am J Cardiol 57:268, 1986.
Weidman WH, Blount SG Jr, DuShane JW, et al: Clinical course in ventricular septal defect. Circulation 56:156, 1977.

Atrioventricular Septal Defect

Becker AE, Anderson RH: Atrioventricular septal defects: What's in a name? J Thorac Cardiovasc Surg 83:461, 1982.
Clapp SK, Perry BL, Farooki ZQ, et al: Surgical and medical results of complete atrioventricular canal: A ten-year review. Am J Cardiol 59:454, 1987.
Marino B, Vairo U, Corno A, et al: Atrioventricular canal in Down syndrome. Am J Dis Child 144:1120, 1990.
Santon E: Repair of atrioventricular septal defects in infancy. J Thorac Cardiovasc Surg 91:505, 1986.

Patent Ductus Arteriosus

Clyman RI, Mauray F, Roman C, et al: Factors determining the loss of ductus arteriosus responsiveness to prostaglandin E. Circulation 68:433, 1983.
Gittenberger-De Groot AC, Van Ertbruggen I, Moulaert A, et al: The ductus arteriosus in the preterm infant: Histologic and clinical observations. J Pediatr 96:88, 1980.
Rothman A, Lucas VW, Sklansky, et al: Percutaneous coil occlusion of patent ductus arteriosus. J Pediatr 130:447, 1997.
Sommer RJ, Gutierrez A, Lai WW, Parness IA: Use of preformed nitinol snare to improve transcatheter coil delivery in occlusion of patent ductus arteriosus. Am J Cardiol 74:836, 1994.

Coronary Arteriovenous Fistula

Velvis H, Schmidt KG, Silverman NH, Turley K: Diagnosis of coronary artery fistula by two-dimensional echocardiography, pulsed Doppler ultrasound and color flow imaging. J Am Coll Cardiol 14:968, 1989.

CHAPTER 434

Acyanotic Congenital Heart Disease: The Obstructive Lesions

434.1 Pulmonary Valve Stenosis with Intact Ventricular Septum

There are various forms of right ventricular outflow obstruction with intact ventricular septum. The most common is isolated valvular pulmonary stenosis, accounting for between 7 and 10% of all congenital heart defects. In this entity, the valve cusps are deformed to various degrees, resulting in incomplete opening during systole. The valve may be bicuspid or tricuspid, with the leaflets partially fused together and with an eccentric outlet. This fusion may be so severe as to leave only a pinhole central opening. If the valve is not severely thickened, it produces a domelike obstruction to right ventricular outflow during systole. Isolated infundibular stenosis, supravalvular pulmonary stenosis, and branch pulmonary artery stenosis are less commonly encountered. In some instances when pulmonary valve stenosis is the dominant lesion, a small associated ventricular septal defect (VSD) is present, and this condition is better classified as pulmonary stenosis with VSD than as tetralogy of Fallot. Pulmonary stenosis and atrial septal defect (ASD) are occasionally seen as associated defects. The clinical and laboratory findings reflect the dominant lesion, but it is important to rule out these associated anomalies. Pulmonary stenosis as a result of valve dysplasia is the common cardiac abnormality of *Noonan's syndrome* (see Chapters 593–596). The mechanism for pulmonic stenosis is unknown, although maldevelopment of the distal portion of the bulbus cordis and the sequelae of fetal endocarditis have been suggested as causes.

PATHOPHYSIOLOGY. The obstruction to outflow from the right ventricle to the pulmonary artery results in increased systolic pressure and wall stress, leading to hypertrophy of the right ventricle (Fig. 434–1). The severity of these abnormalities depends on the size of the restricted valve opening. In severe cases, right ventricular pressure may be higher than systemic arterial systolic pressure, whereas in milder obstruction right ventricular pressure is only mildly or moderately elevated. Pulmonary artery pressure is normal or decreased. It is important to remember that arterial oxygen saturation will be normal even in cases of severe stenosis unless there is an intracardiac communication, such as a VSD or ASD, to allow blood to shunt from right to left. When severe pulmonic stenosis occurs in the neonate, markedly decreased right ventricular compliance may lead to right-to-left shunting through a patent foramen ovale; this is referred to as **critical pulmonic stenosis**.

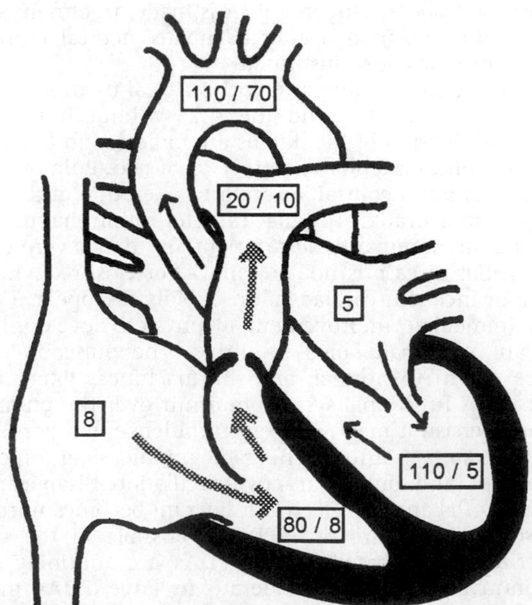

Figure 434–1 Physiology of valvular pulmonary stenosis (PS). The boxed numbers represent pressures in mm Hg. There is no right-to-left or left-to-right shunting, so blood flow through all cardiac chambers is normal at 3 L/min/m^2. The pulmonary to systemic blood flow ratio (Qp:Qs) is 1:1. The right atrial pressure is increased slightly owing to decreased right ventricular compliance. The right ventricle is hypertrophied, and the systolic and diastolic pressures are increased. There is a 60 mm Hg gradient across the thickened pulmonary valve. The main pulmonary artery pressure is slightly low and there is poststenotic dilatation. The left heart pressures are normal. Unless there is right-to-left shunting via a foramen ovale, the patient's systemic oxygen saturation will be normal.

CLINICAL MANIFESTATIONS. With mild or moderate stenosis, there are usually no symptoms. Growth and development are most often normal; older infants and children appear to be well developed and healthy. If the stenosis is severe, there may be signs of right ventricular failure such as hepatomegaly, peripheral edema, and exercise intolerance. In the neonate or young infant with critical pulmonic stenosis, signs of right ventricular failure may be more prominent, and cyanosis is often present because of shunting at the foramen ovale.

With **mild pulmonary stenosis,** the venous pressure and pulse are normal. The heart is not enlarged, the apical impulse is normal, and the right ventricular impulse is not palpable. A sharp pulmonic ejection click, immediately following the 1st heart sound, is heard at the left upper sternal border during expiration. The 2nd heart sound is split, with a pulmonary component of normal intensity that may be slightly delayed. A relatively short low- or medium-pitched systolic ejection murmur is maximally audible over the pulmonic area and radiates minimally to the lung fields bilaterally. The *electrocardiogram* is normal or characteristic of mild right ventricular hypertrophy; there may be inversion of the T waves in the right precordial leads. The only abnormality demonstrable *radiographically* is poststenotic dilatation of the pulmonary artery. *Two-dimensional echocardiography* shows right ventricular hypertrophy and a slightly thickened and domed pulmonic valve; Doppler studies demonstrate a right ventricle-to-pulmonary artery gradient of 30 mm Hg or less.

In **moderate pulmonic stenosis,** the venous pressure may be slightly elevated; in older children a prominent a wave may be noted in the jugular pulse. A right ventricular lift may be palpable at the lower left sternal border. The 2nd heart sound is split, with a delayed and diminished pulmonary component. As the valve motion becomes more limited with more severe degrees of stenosis, both the pulmonic ejection click and the pulmonic second sound may become inaudible. With increasing degrees of stenosis, the peak of the systolic ejection murmur is prolonged later into systole, and its quality becomes louder and harsher (higher frequency). The murmur radiates more prominently to both lung fields.

The *electrocardiogram* reveals varying degrees of right ventricular hypertrophy, sometimes with a prominent spiked P wave. *Radiographically,* the heart can vary from normal size to mildly enlarged because of prominence of the right ventricle; intrapulmonary vascularity may be normal or slightly decreased. The *echocardiogram* shows a thickened pulmonic valve with restricted systolic motion. The Doppler examination shows a ventricular–pulmonary artery pressure gradient in the 30–60 mm Hg range. Mild tricuspid regurgitation may be present and allows Doppler confirmation of the right ventricular systolic pressure.

In **severe stenosis,** mild to moderate cyanosis may be noted if there is an interatrial communication. If hepatic enlargement and peripheral edema are present, they are an indication of right ventricular failure. Elevation of the venous pressure is common and is caused by a large presystolic jugular "a" wave. The heart is moderately or greatly enlarged, and there is a conspicuous parasternal right ventricular lift that frequently extends to the midclavicular line. The pulmonary element of the 2nd sound is usually inaudible. A loud and long harsh systolic ejection murmur, frequently accompanied by a thrill, is maximally audible in the pulmonic area and may radiate widely over the entire precordium, to both lung fields, into the neck, and to the back. The peak of the murmur occurs later in systole as valve opening becomes more restricted. The murmur frequently encompasses the aortic component of the 2nd sound but is not preceded by an ejection click.

The *electrocardiogram* shows gross right ventricular hypertrophy, frequently accompanied by a tall, spiked P wave. *Radiographic studies* confirm the cardiac enlargement and prominence of the right ventricle and atrium. Prominence of the pulmonary artery segment is due to poststenotic dilatation (Fig. 434–2). The intrapulmonary vascularity is decreased. The *two-dimensional echocardiogram* shows severe deformity of the pulmonary valve and right ventricular hypertrophy. In the late stages of the disease, dysfunction of the right ventricle is seen, and the ventricle may become dilated. Doppler studies demonstrate a large gradient (>60 mm Hg) across the pulmonary valve. Tricuspid regurgitation may also be prominent. Fortunately, the classic findings of severe pulmonary stenosis in older children are now rarely seen because of early intervention. The signs of critical pulmonic stenosis are usually encountered in the neonatal period.

Cardiac catheterization is usually not required for diagnostic purposes, but is undertaken as part of a balloon valvuloplasty procedure. Catheterization demonstrates an abrupt pressure gradient across the pulmonary valve. The pulmonary artery pressure is either normal or low. The severity is graded based on the right ventricular systolic pressure or the pressure gradient: a gradient of 10–30 mm Hg in mild cases, 30–60 mm Hg in moderate cases, and greater than 60 mm Hg or with right ventricular pressure greater than systemic pressure in severe cases. If the cardiac output is low or a significant right-to-left shunt exists across the atrial septum, the pressure gradient may underestimate the degree of valve stenosis. *Selective right ventriculography* demonstrates the thickened, poorly mobile valve. In mild to moderate stenosis, the doming of the valve in systole is readily seen. The flow of contrast medium through the stenotic valve in ventricular systole produces a narrow jet of dye that fills the dilatated main pulmonary artery. Subvalvular hypertrophy that may intensify the obstruction may occasionally be present. The angiogram also indicates whether the ventricular septum is intact.

PROGNOSIS AND COMPLICATIONS. Heart failure occurs only in severe cases and most often during the 1st mo of life. The development of cyanosis from a right-to-left shunt across a foramen ovale is most often seen in infancy when the stenosis is severe. Infective endocarditis is a risk but not common in childhood.

Children with mild stenosis can lead a normal life, but their progress should be evaluated at regular intervals. Patients who have small gradients rarely show progression and do not need intervention, but children having moderate stenosis are more likely to acquire a more significant gradient as they grow older. Worsening of obstruction may also be due to the development

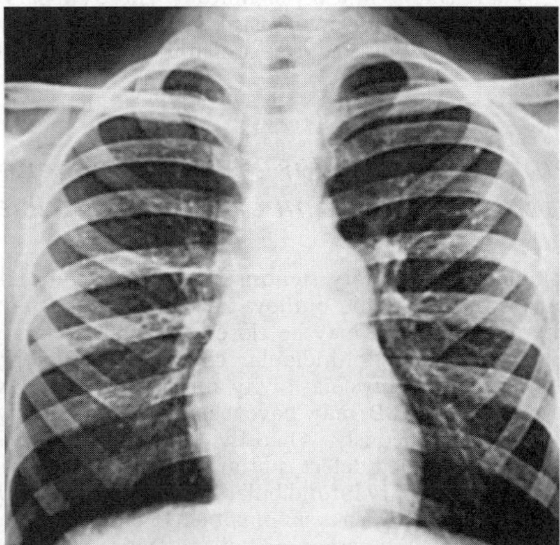

Figure 434–2 Roentgenogram in valvular pulmonary stenosis with a normal aortic root. The heart size is within normal limits, but there is poststenotic dilatation of the pulmonary artery.

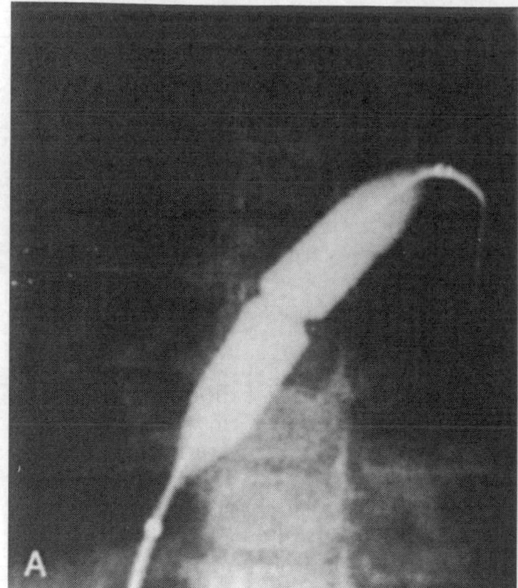

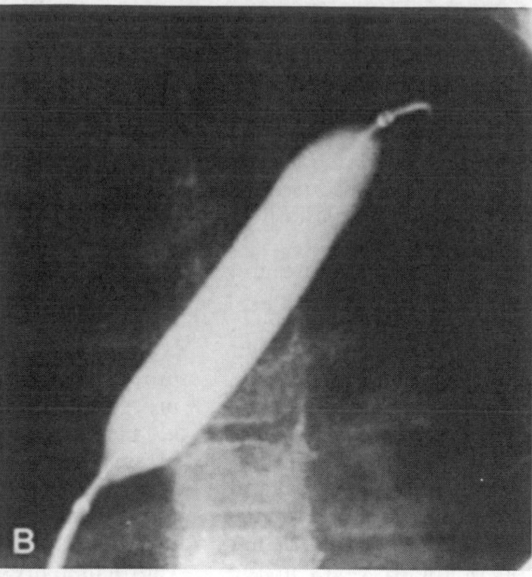

Figure 434–3 Balloon pulmonary valvuloplasty. *A*, Hourglass shape of the balloon at the start of inflation. *B*, Full balloon inflation. The left pulmonary artery is protected from the sharp tip of the catheter with a flexible-tip guide wire. (From Lababidi Z: Neonatal catheter palliations. *In*: Long WA [ed]: Fetal and Neonatal Cardiology. Philadelphia, WB Saunders, 1990.)

of secondary subvalvular muscular and fibrous tissue hypertrophy. In untreated severe stenosis, the course may abruptly worsen with the development of right ventricular dysfunction and cardiac failure. Infants with critical pulmonic stenosis require urgent catheter balloon valvuloplasty or surgical valvotomy.

TREATMENT. Patients with moderate or severe isolated pulmonary stenosis require relief of the obstruction. Balloon valvuloplasty is the initial treatment of choice for the vast majority of patients (Fig. 434–3). Patients with severely thickened pulmonic valves, especially common in those with Noonan's syndrome, may require surgical intervention instead. In the neonate with critical pulmonic stenosis, urgent treatment with either balloon valvuloplasty or surgical valvotomy is warranted.

Excellent results are obtained in the majority of instances. The gradient across the pulmonary valve is markedly reduced or abolished. In the early period after balloon valvuloplasty, a small to moderate residual gradient may remain because of muscular infundibular narrowing; it nearly always resolves with time. A short early decrescendo diastolic murmur at the middle to upper left sternal border resulting from pulmonary valvular insufficiency may be heard. The degree of insufficiency usually is not clinically significant. There appears to be no difference between valvuloplasty and surgery in patient status at late follow-up; recurrence is unusual after successful treatment.

434.2 Infundibular Pulmonary Stenosis and Double-Chamber Right Ventricle

Infundibular pulmonary stenosis is caused by muscular or fibrous obstruction in the outflow tract of the right ventricle. The site of obstruction may be close to the pulmonary valve or well below it; an infundibular chamber may be present between the right ventricular cavity and the pulmonary valve. In many cases, a VSD may have been present initially and later closed spontaneously. When the pulmonary valve is also stenotic, the combined defect is primarily classified as valvular stenosis with secondary infundibular hypertrophy. The *hemodynamics* and *clinical manifestations* of patients with isolated infundibular pulmonary stenosis are similar, for the most part, to those described in the discussion of isolated valvular pulmonary stenosis (see Chapter 434.1).

A more common variation of right ventricular outflow obstruction below the pulmonary valve is that of double-chambered right ventricle. In this condition, there is a muscular band in the midright ventricular region, which divides the chamber into two parts and creates obstruction between the inlet and outlet portions. There is often an associated VSD that may close spontaneously. Obstruction usually is not seen early in life but may progress rapidly in a similar manner to the progressive infundibular obstruction observed with tetralogy of Fallot (see Chapter 437.1).

The *diagnosis* of isolated right ventricular infundibular stenosis or double-chamber right ventricle can be made by echocardiography or cardiac catheterization and angiography, or both. The ventricular septum must be evaluated carefully to determine whether an associated VSD is present. The prognosis for untreated cases of severe right ventricular outflow obstruction is similar to that for valvular pulmonary stenosis. When obstruction is moderate to severe, surgery is indicated. After operation, the pressure gradient is abolished or markedly reduced and the long-term outlook is excellent.

434.3 Pulmonary Stenosis in Combination with an Intracardiac Shunt

Valvular or infundibular pulmonary stenosis, or both, may be associated with either an ASD or a VSD. In these patients, the clinical features depend on the degree of pulmonary stenosis, which determines whether the net shunt is from left to right or from right to left.

The presence of a large left-to-right shunt at the atrial or ventricular level is evidence that the pulmonary stenosis is mild. These patients present with symptoms similar to those of patients with an isolated ASD or VSD. However, with increasing age, worsening of the obstruction may limit the shunt, resulting in a gradual improvement in symptoms. Eventually, particularly in patients with pulmonary stenosis and VSD, further increase in the obstruction may lead to right-to-left shunting and clinical cyanosis. When a patient being followed with a VSD has evidence of decreasing heart failure and increased right ventricular forces on the electrocardiogram, the clinician must differentiate between the development of increasing pulmonary stenosis and the onset of pulmonary vascular disease (Eisenmenger's syndrome).

These anomalies are readily repaired surgically. Defects in the atrial or ventricular septum are closed, and the pulmonary stenosis is relieved by resection of infundibular muscle or pulmonary valvotomy, or both, as indicated. Patients with a predominant right-to-left shunt present with symptoms similar to those of patients with tetralogy of Fallot (see Chapter 437.1).

434.4 Peripheral Pulmonary Stenosis

Single or multiple constrictions may occur anywhere along the major branches of the pulmonary arteries and may range from mild to severe and from localized to extensive. Frequently, these defects are associated with other types of congenital heart disease, including valvular pulmonic stenosis, tetralogy of Fallot, PDA, VSD, ASD, and supravalvular aortic stenosis. A familial tendency has been recognized in some patients with peripheral pulmonic stenosis. A high incidence is found in infants with the congenital rubella syndrome. The combination of supravalvular aortic stenosis with pulmonary arterial branch stenosis, idiopathic hypercalcemia of infancy, elfin facies, and mental retardation is known as Williams syndrome.

With a mild constriction, there is little effect on the pulmonary circulation. With multiple severe constrictions, there is an increase in pressure in the right ventricle and in the pulmonary artery proximal to the site of obstruction. When the anomaly is isolated, the *diagnosis* is suspected by the presence of murmurs in widespread locations over the chest, either anteriorly or posteriorly. These murmurs are usually systolic but may be continuous. Most often, the physical signs are dominated by the associated anomaly, such as tetralogy of Fallot.

In the immediate newborn period, a mild and transient form of peripheral pulmonic stenosis may be present. Physical findings are usually limited to a soft systolic ejection murmur, which can be heard over either or both lung fields. It is the absence of other physical findings of valvular pulmonic stenosis (right ventricular lift, soft pulmonic 2nd sound, systolic ejection click, murmur loudest at the upper left sternal border) that supports this diagnosis. This murmur usually disappears by 1–2 mo.

If the stenosis is severe, the electrocardiogram shows evidence of right ventricular and right atrial hypertrophy, and the *chest radiograph* shows cardiomegaly and prominence of the main pulmonary artery. Generally, the pulmonary vasculature is normal; in some cases small intrapulmonary vascular shadows are seen, which represent areas of poststenotic dilatation. Echocardiography is limited in its ability to visualize the distal branch pulmonary arteries; however, Doppler examination demonstrates the acceleration of blood flow through the stenoses and, if tricuspid regurgitation is present, allows estimation of right ventricular systolic pressure. Magnetic resonance imaging and computed tomography are helpful in delineating distal obstructions; if moderate to severe disease is suspected, the diagnosis is usually confirmed by *cardiac catheterization*.

Severe obstruction of the main pulmonary artery and its primary branches can be relieved during corrective surgery for associated lesions such as tetralogy of Fallot or valvular pulmonary stenosis. If peripheral pulmonic stenosis is isolated, it may be treated by catheter balloon dilation. When peripheral obstruction occurs distally in the intrapulmonary vessels, it is usually not amenable to surgical repair. These obstructions are often multiple and are best treated with repeat balloon angioplasty, although there is a high rate of recurrence. The introduction of expandable intravascular stents, placed by catheter in the distal pulmonary arteries and then dilated with a balloon to the appropriate size, may prevent restenosis.

434.5 Aortic Stenosis

PATHOPHYSIOLOGY. Congenital aortic stenosis accounts for about 5% of cardiac malformations recognized in childhood; a bicuspid aortic valve is one of the most common congenital heart lesions overall, identified in up to 2% of adults. Aortic stenosis is more common in males (3:1). In the most common form, *valvular aortic stenosis*, the leaflets are thickened, and the commissures are fused to varying degrees. The left ventricular systolic pressure is increased as a result of the obstruction to outflow. The ventricular wall hypertrophies in compensation; as its compliance decreases, the end-diastolic pressure increases as well.

Subvalvular (*subaortic*) *stenosis* with a discrete fibromuscular shelf below the aortic valve is also an important form of left ventricular outflow tract obstruction. This lesion is frequently associated with other forms of congenital heart disease and may progress rapidly in severity. It is rarely diagnosed during early infancy and may develop despite prior documentation of no left ventricular outflow tract obstruction. Subvalvular aortic stenosis may become apparent after successful surgery for other congenital heart defects (e.g., coarctation of the aorta, PDA, VSD), may develop in association with mild lesions that have not been surgically repaired, or may occur as an isolated abnormality. Subvalvular aortic stenosis may also be due to a markedly hypertrophied ventricular septum, known as *idiopathic hypertrophic subaortic stenosis* or *hypertrophic cardiomyopathy* (see Chapter 445.2).

Supravalvular aortic stenosis, the least common type, may be sporadic, familial, or associated with Williams syndrome, which includes mental retardation, elfin facies (full face, broad forehead, flattened bridge of nose, long upper lip, and rounded cheeks), and idiopathic hypercalcemia of infancy (see Chapter 78). Stenoses of other arteries, in particular the branch pulmonary arteries, may also be present. Williams syndrome has been shown to be due to a deletion involving the elastin gene on chromosome 7q11.23.

CLINICAL MANIFESTATIONS. Symptoms in patients with aortic stenosis depend on the severity of the obstruction. Severe aortic stenosis that presents in early infancy is termed *critical aortic stenosis* and is associated with left ventricular failure and signs of low cardiac output. Heart failure, cardiomegaly, and pulmonary edema are severe; the pulses are weak in all extremities; and the skin may be pale or grayish. Urine output may be diminished. If the cardiac output is significantly decreased, the intensity of the murmur at the right upper sternal border may be minimal. In contrast, the majority of children with less severe forms of aortic stenosis remain asymptomatic and display normal growth and development. The murmur is usually discovered during routine physical examination. Rarely, an older child with previously undiagnosed severe obstruction to left ventricular outflow will present with fatigue, angina, dizziness, or syncope. Sudden death has been reported with aortic stenosis but usually occurs in patients with severe left ventricular outflow obstruction in whom surgical relief has been delayed.

The physical findings are dependent on the degree of obstruction to left ventricular outflow. In mild stenosis, the pulses, heart size, and apical impulse are all normal. With increasing degrees of severity, the pulses become diminished in intensity and the heart may be enlarged, with a left ventricular apical thrust. In mild to moderate valvular aortic stenosis, there is usually an early systolic ejection click, best heard at the apex and left sternal edge. Unlike the click associated with pulmonic stenosis, its intensity does not vary with respirations. Clicks are unusual in more severe aortic stenosis or in discrete subaortic stenosis. If the stenosis is severe, the 1st heart sound may be diminished because of decreased compliance of the thickened left ventricle. Normal splitting of the 2nd heart sound is present in mild to moderate obstruction. In patients with severe obstruction, the intensity of aortic valve closure is diminished and, rarely in children, the 2nd sound may be split paradoxically (becoming wider in expiration). A 4th heart sound may be audible when the obstruction is severe.

The intensity, pitch, and duration of the systolic ejection murmur is another indication of severity. Generally, the louder, harsher (higher pitch), and longer the murmur, the greater the degree of obstruction. The typical murmur is audible maximally at the right upper sternal border and radiates to the neck and to the left midsternal border. It is usually accompanied by a thrill in the suprasternal notch. In patients with subvalvular aortic stenosis, the murmur may be maximal along the left sternal border or even at the apex. A soft decrescendo diastolic murmur indicative of aortic insufficiency is often present when the obstruction is subvalvular or in patients with a bicuspid aortic valve. Occasionally, an apical short mid-diastolic rumbling murmur is audible, even in the presence of a normal mitral valve; however, this should always raise the suspicion of associated mitral stenosis.

LABORATORY DIAGNOSIS. The diagnosis can usually be made on the basis of the physical examination and the severity of obstruction confirmed by laboratory tests. If the pressure gradient across the aortic valve is mild, the *electrocardiogram* is likely to be normal. The electrocardiogram may occasionally be normal even with more severe obstruction, but evidence of left ventricular hypertrophy and strain (inverted T waves in the left precordial leads) is usually present if severe stenosis is long-standing. The *chest radiograph* frequently shows a prominent ascending aorta, but the aortic knob is normal. The heart size is usually normal. Valvular calcification has been noted only in older children and adults. *Echocardiography* identifies both the site and the severity of the obstruction. Two-dimensional imaging shows left ventricular hypertrophy, the thickened and domed aortic valve, the number of valve leaflets, and a subaortic or supra-aortic membrane, if present. Associated anomalies of the mitral valve or aortic arch or a VSD or PDA are present in up to 20% of cases. In the absence of left ventricular failure, the shortening fraction of the left ventricle may be increased because the ventricle is hypercontractile. In infants with critical aortic stenosis, the left ventricular shortening fraction is usually decreased and the endocardium may be bright, indicating the development of endocardial fibrous scarring, known as **endocardial fibroelastosis**. Doppler studies show the specific site of obstruction and determine the peak and mean systolic left ventricular outflow tract gradients. When severe aortic obstruction is associated with left ventricular dysfunction, the Doppler-derived valve gradient may markedly underestimate the severity of the obstruction due to the low cardiac output.

Graded exercise testing is useful in evaluating the severity of left ventricular outflow tract obstruction in older children. As the severity of the gradient increases, working capacity decreases, systolic blood pressure fails to rise adequately, diastolic blood pressure may rise, and ST segment depression can occur. Because patients with severe aortic stenosis may deny symptoms and have normal electrocardiograms and chest roentgenograms, serial echocardiograms and graded exercise tests may be valuable in determining the timing of cardiac catheterization and surgical or balloon catheter valvuloplasty.

Left heart catheterization demonstrates the magnitude of the pressure gradient from the left ventricle to the aorta. The aortic pressure curve is abnormal if obstruction is severe. In patients with severe obstruction and decreased left ventricular compliance, the left atrial pressure is increased and there may be pulmonary hypertension. The site of obstruction is best identified by selective left ventriculography. Most infants with critical aortic stenosis do not require diagnostic cardiac catheterization but may undergo the procedure for a balloon valvuloplasty. When a critically ill infant with left ventricular outflow tract obstruction undergoes cardiac catheterization, left ventricular function is often markedly decreased. As with the echocardiogram, the gradient measured across the stenotic aortic valve may underestimate the degree of obstruction because of low cardiac output. Actual measurement of the cardiac output by thermodilution and calculation of the aortic valve area is helpful in these cases.

PROGNOSIS. Neonates with critical aortic stenosis may have severe heart failure and deteriorate rapidly to a low-output shock state. Emergency surgery or balloon valvuloplasty is lifesaving, but the mortality risk is not trivial. Neonates who die of critical aortic stenosis frequently have significant endocardial fibroelastosis of the left ventricle.

In older infants and children with mild to moderate aortic stenosis, the prognosis is reasonably good, although disease progression over 5 to 10 yr is common. Patients with aortic valve gradients less than 40–50 mm Hg are considered to have mild disease; those with gradients of 40–70 mm Hg have moderate disease. These patients usually respond well to treatment (either surgery or valvuloplasty), although reoperations on the aortic valve are often required later in childhood or in adult life, and many patients eventually require valve replacement. In unoperated patients with severe obstruction, sudden death is a significant risk, often occurring during or immediately following exercise. Aortic stenosis is one of the more common causes of sudden cardiac death in the pediatric age group.

Patients with moderate to severe degrees of aortic stenosis should not participate in active competitive sports. In patients with milder disease, sports participation is less severely restricted; however, patients should be encouraged to pursue less physically demanding activities. The status of each patient should be reviewed at least annually and intervention advised if progression of signs or symptoms occurs. Lifetime prophylaxis against infective endocarditis is required.

TREATMENT. Balloon valvuloplasty is indicated for children having moderate to severe valvular aortic stenosis to prevent progressive left ventricular dysfunction and the risks of syncope and sudden death. It is generally agreed that valvuloplasty should be advised when the peak-to-peak systolic gradient between the left ventricle and aorta exceeds 60–70 mm Hg at rest, assuming a normal cardiac output, or for lesser gradients when symptoms or electrocardiographic changes are present. For the more rapidly progressive subaortic obstructive lesions, a gradient of 40–50 mm Hg is considered operable. Outside of the neonatal period, surgical treatment is usually reserved for valves that are not amenable to balloon therapy, usually those that are extremely thickened.

In the neonatal period, balloon valvuloplasty is made somewhat more difficult by problems of arterial access. The risk of femoral arterial complications is much higher than in older children, although the development of low-profile balloons has reduced this risk substantially. Currently, both surgical and catheter approaches are being used at different centers for critical aortic stenosis in the newborn period.

Discrete subaortic stenosis can be resected without damage to the aortic valve, the anterior leaflet of the mitral valve, or the conduction system. This type of obstruction usually is not amenable to catheter treatment. Relief of supravalvular stenosis is also achieved surgically, and the results are excellent if the area of obstruction is discrete and is not associated with a hypoplastic aorta. Rarely, one or both coronary arteries may be stenotic at their origins because of a thick supra-aortic fibrous ridge.

Whether surgical or catheter treatment has been carried out, aortic insufficiency or calcification with restenosis is likely to occur years or even decades later, eventually requiring reoperation and often aortic valve replacement. When recurrence occurs, it may not be associated with early symptoms. Signs of recurrent stenosis include electrocardiographic signs of left ventricular hypertrophy, increase in echo Doppler gradient, deterioration of echocardiographic indices of left ventricular function, and recurrence of signs or symptoms during graded treadmill exercise. Evidence of significant aortic regurgitation includes symptoms of heart failure, cardiac enlargement on roentgenogram, and left ventricular dilatation on echocardiogram. The choice of reparative procedure depends on the relative degree of stenosis and regurgitation.

When aortic valve replacement is necessary, the choice of procedure often depends on the age of the patient. Homograft valves tend to calcify more rapidly in younger children; they do not require chronic anticoagulation. Mechanical prosthetic valves are much longer lasting, yet require anticoagulation, which can be difficult to manage in young children. In adolescent girls who are nearing childbearing age, consideration of the teratogenic effects of warfarin may warrant the use of a homograft valve. None of these options is perfect for the younger child who requires valve replacement because neither homograft nor mechanical valves grow with the patient. An alternative operation is aortopulmonary translocation, also known as the Ross procedure. This involves removing the patient's own pulmonary valve and using it to replace the abnormal aortic valve. A homograft is then placed in the pulmonary position. The advantage of this procedure is the potential for growth of the translocated living "neoaortic" valve and the longer longevity of the homograft valve when placed in the lower pressure pulmonary circulation. The long-term success of this operation is being investigated.

434.6 Coarctation of the Aorta

Constrictions of the aorta of varying degrees may occur at any point from the transverse arch to the iliac bifurcation, but 98% occur just below the origin of the left subclavian artery at the origin of the ductus arteriosus (juxtaductal coarctation). The anomaly occurs twice as often in males as in females. Coarctation of the aorta may be a feature of Turner's syndrome (see Chapter 596.2) and is associated with a bicuspid aortic valve in more than 70% of patients. Mitral valve abnormalities (a supravalvular mitral ring or parachute mitral valve) and subaortic stenosis are potential associated lesions. When this group of left-sided obstructive lesions occurs together, they are referred to as the Shone complex.

PATHOPHYSIOLOGY. Coarctation of the aorta can occur as a discrete juxtaductal obstruction or as tubular hypoplasia of the transverse aorta starting at one of the head or neck vessels and extending to the ductal area (preductal or infantile-type coarctation; Fig. 434–4). Often, both components are present. It is postulated that coarctation may be initiated in fetal life by the presence of a cardiac abnormality that results in decreased blood flow anterograde through the aortic valve (e.g., bicuspid aortic valve, VSD).

In patients with a discrete juxtaductal coarctation, ascending aortic blood flows through the narrowed segment to reach the descending aorta, although left ventricular hypertension and hypertrophy result. In the 1st few days of life, the patent ductus arteriosus may serve to widen the juxtaductal area of the aorta and provide temporary relief from the obstruction. In these acyanotic infants, net left-to-right ductal shunting occurs. In contrast, with more severe juxtaductal coarctation or in the presence of transverse arch hypoplasia, right ventricular blood is ejected through the ductus to supply the descending aorta, as it does during fetal life. Perfusion of the lower body is then dependent on right ventricular output (see Fig. 434–4). In this situation, the femoral pulses are palpable, and differential blood pressures may not be helpful in making the diagnosis. The ductal right-to-left shunting is manifested as differential cyanosis, with the upper extremities being pink and the lower extremities being blue.

Such infants may have severe pulmonary hypertension and high pulmonary vascular resistance. Signs of heart failure are prominent. Occasionally, severely hypoplastic segments of the aortic isthmus may become completely atretic, resulting in an

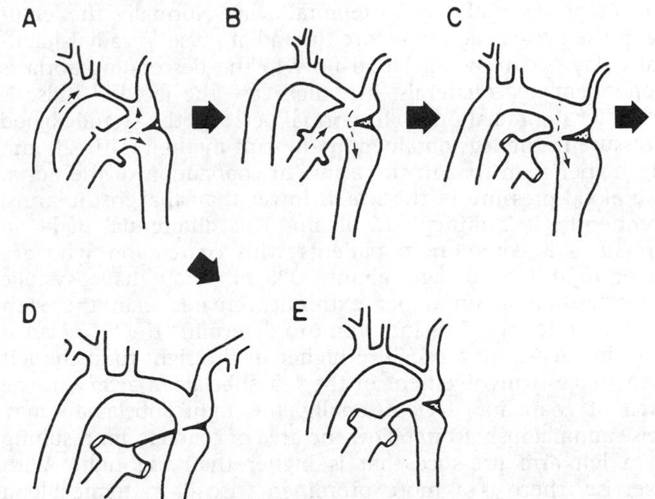

Figure 434–4 Metamorphosis of coarctation. *A*, Fetal prototype. No flow obstruction. *B*, Late gestation. The aortic ventricle increases the output and dilates the hypoplastic segment. Antegrade aortic flow bypasses the shelf via the ductal orifice. *C*, Neonate. Ductal constriction initiates the obstruction by removing the bypass and by increasing antegrade arch flow. *D*, Mature juxtaductal stenosis. Bypass completely obliterated; intimal hypoplasia on the edge of the shelf aggravates stenosis. Collaterals develop. *E*, Infantile-type fetal prototype persists. An intracardiac left-sided heart obstruction precludes an increase in antegrade aortic flow before or after birth. Both isthmal hypoplasia and contraductal shelf are present. Lower body flow often depends on patency of the ductus. (From Gersony WM: Coarctation of the aorta. *In*: Adams FH, Emmanouilides GC, Riemenschneider T [eds]: Moss Heart Disease in Infants, Children, and Adolescents, 4th ed. Baltimore, Williams & Wilkins, 1989.)

interrupted aortic arch, with the left subclavian artery arising either proximal or distal to the interruption. Coarctation associated with arch hypoplasia was referred to as *infantile type* because it usually presented in early infancy due to its severity. *Adult type* referred to the isolated juxtaductal coarctation, which, if mild, usually did not present until later childhood. These terms have been replaced with the more accurate anatomic terms mentioned earlier describing the location and severity of the defect.

The blood pressure is elevated in the vessels that arise proximal to the coarctation; the blood pressure as well as pulse pressure below the constriction are lower. Hypertension is not due to the mechanical obstruction alone but also involves neurohumoral mechanisms. Unless operated on in infancy, coarctation of the aorta usually results in the development of an extensive collateral circulation, chiefly from the branches of the subclavian, the superior intercostal, and the internal mammary arteries to create channels for arterial blood to bypass the area of coarctation. The vessels contributing to the collateral circulation may become markedly enlarged and tortuous by early adulthood.

CLINICAL MANIFESTATIONS. Coarctation of the aorta recognized after infancy is rarely associated with significant symptoms. Some children or adolescents complain about weakness or pain (or both) in the legs after exercise, but in many instances even patients with severe coarctation are asymptomatic. Older children are frequently brought to the cardiologist's attention when they are found to be hypertensive on routine physical examination.

The classic sign of coarctation of the aorta is a disparity in pulsations and blood pressures of the arms and legs. The femoral, popliteal, posterior tibial, and dorsalis pedis pulses are weak (or absent in up to 40% of patients), in contrast to the bounding pulses of the arms and carotid vessels. The radial and femoral pulses should always be palpated simultaneously for the presence of a radial-femoral delay. Normally, the femoral pulse occurs slightly before the radial pulse. A radial-femoral delay occurs when blood flow to the descending aorta is dependent on collaterals, in which case the femoral pulse is felt after the radial pulse. In normal persons, the systolic blood pressure in the legs obtained by the cuff method is 10–20 mm Hg higher than that in the arms. In coarctation of the aorta, the blood pressure in the legs is lower than that in the arms; frequently, it is difficult to obtain. This differential in blood pressures is common in patients with coarctation who are older than 1 yr of age, about 90% of whom have systolic hypertension in an upper extremity greater than the 95th percentile for age. It is important to determine the blood pressure in each arm; a pressure higher in the right than the left arm suggests involvement of the left subclavian artery in the area of coarctation. Occasionally, the right subclavian may arise anomalously from below the area of coarctation, resulting in a left arm pressure that is higher than the right. With exercise, there is a more prominent rise of systemic blood pressure and the upper-to-lower extremity pressure gradient will increase.

The precordial impulse and heart sounds are usually normal; the presence of a systolic ejection click or thrill in the suprasternal notch suggests the presence of a bicuspid aortic valve (present in 70% of cases). A short systolic murmur is often heard along the left sternal border at the 3rd and 4th intercostal spaces. The murmur is well transmitted to the left infrascapular area and occasionally to the neck. Often, the typical murmur of mild aortic stenosis can be heard in the 3rd right intercostal space. Occasionally more significant degrees of obstruction across the aortic valve are present. The presence of a low-pitched mid-diastolic murmur at the apex suggests the presence of mitral valve stenosis. Among older patients with well-developed collateral blood flow, systolic or continuous murmurs may be heard over the left and right sides of the chest laterally and posteriorly. In these patients, a palpable thrill can occasionally be appreciated in the intercostal spaces on the back.

Neonates or infants with more severe coarctation, usually including some degree of transverse arch hypoplasia, present with signs of lower body hypoperfusion, acidosis, and severe heart failure. This presentation may be delayed days or weeks until after closure of the ductus arteriosus. If detected before ductal closure, patients may exhibit differential cyanosis, best demonstrated by simultaneous oximetry of the upper and lower extremities. On physical examination, the heart is large, and there is a systolic murmur heard along the left sternal border with a loud 2nd heart sound.

LABORATORY DIAGNOSIS. The findings on *roentgenographic examination* depend on the age of the patient and on the effects of hypertension and collateral circulation. In infants with severe coarctation, there is cardiac enlargement and pulmonary congestion. During childhood the findings are not striking until after the 1st decade, when the heart tends to be mildly or moderately enlarged because of left ventricular prominence. The enlarged left subclavian artery commonly produces a prominent shadow in the left superior mediastinum. Notching of the inferior border of the ribs from pressure erosion by enlarged collateral vessels is common by late childhood. In most instances, there is an area of poststenotic dilatation of the descending aorta.

The *electrocardiogram* is usually normal in young children but reveals evidence of left ventricular hypertrophy in older patients. Neonates and young infants display right or biventricular hypertrophy. The diagnosis can be made by a careful evaluation of the pulses in all major accessible peripheral arteries and by comparative blood pressure determinations in the arms and legs. The segment of coarctation can usually be visualized by two-dimensional *echocardiography;* associated anomalies of the mitral and aortic valve can also be demonstrated. The descending aorta is hypopulsatile. Color Doppler is useful for demonstrating the specific site of the obstruction. Pulsed and continuous wave Doppler determine the pressure gradient directly at the area of coarctation. However, in the presence of a patent ductus arteriosus, the severity of the narrowing may be underestimated. *Cardiac catheterization* with selective left ventriculography and aortography is useful in selected patients with additional anomalies and as a means of visualizing collateral blood flow. In cases that are well defined by echocardiography, diagnostic catheterization is usually not required prior to surgery.

PROGNOSIS AND COMPLICATIONS. Abnormalities of the aortic valve are present in most patients. Bicuspid aortic valves are common but usually do not produce clinical signs unless the stenosis is significant. The association of a PDA and coarctation of the aorta is also common. Ventricular and ASDs may be suspected by signs of a left-to-right shunt, which are worsened by the increased resistance to flow through the left side of the heart. Mitral valve abnormalities are also occasionally seen, as is subvalvular aortic stenosis.

Severe neurologic damage or even death rarely may occur from associated cerebrovascular disease. Subarachnoid or intracerebral hemorrhage may result from rupture of congenital aneurysms in the circle of Willis, of other vessels with defective elastic and medial tissue, or of normal vessels; these accidents are secondary to hypertension. Abnormalities of the subclavian arteries may include involvement of the left subclavian artery in the area of coarctation, stenosis of the orifice of the left subclavian artery, and anomalous origin of the right subclavian artery.

Untreated, the great majority of older patients with coarctation of the aorta would succumb between the ages of 20 and 40 yr; some live well into middle life without serious disability. The common serious complications are related to systemic hypertension, which may result in premature coronary artery disease, heart failure, hypertensive encephalopathy, or intracranial hemorrhage. Heart failure may be worsened by associated anomalies. Infective endocarditis or endarteritis is a significant complication in adults. Aneurysms of the descending aorta or of the enlarged collateral vessels may develop. In infants with severe coarctation, heart failure and hypoperfusion may be life-threatening and require immediate medical intervention.

TREATMENT. In neonates with severe coarctation of the aorta, closure of the ductus often results in hypoperfusion, acidosis, and rapid deterioration. These patients should be given an infusion of prostaglandin E_1 to reopen the ductus and reestablish adequate lower extremity blood flow. Once a diagnosis has been confirmed and the patient stabilized, surgical repair should be performed. Older infants who present with heart failure but with good perfusion should be managed with anticongestive measures to improve their clinical status prior to surgical intervention.

Older children with significant coarctation of the aorta should be treated relatively soon after diagnosis. Delay is unwarranted, especially after the 2nd decade of life, when the operation may be less successful because of decreased left ventricular function and degenerative changes in the aortic wall. Nevertheless, if cardiac reserve is sufficient, satisfactory repair is possible well into midadult life. Associated valvular lesions increase the hazards of late surgery.

The procedure of choice for isolated juxtaductal coarctation of the aorta is controversial. Operation remains the procedure of choice, and several surgical techniques are used. The area of coarctation can be excised and a primary reanastomosis performed. Often the transverse aorta is splayed open and an "extended end-to-end" anastomosis performed to increase the effective cross-sectional area of the repair. The subclavian flap procedure, which involves division of the left subclavian artery and its incorporation into the wall of the repaired coarctation, is used by some, often in the younger age group. Others favor a patch aortoplasty, in which the area of coarctation is enlarged with a roof of prosthetic material.

After operation there is a striking increase in the amplitude of pulsations in the lower extremities. In the immediate postoperative course, "rebound" hypertension is common and requires medical management. This exaggerated hypertension gradually subsides and in most patients antihypertensive medications can be discontinued. Residual murmurs are common and may be due to associated cardiac anomalies, to a residual flow disturbance across the repaired area, or to collateral blood flow. Rare additional operative problems include spinal cord injury due to aortic cross-clamping if there are poorly developed collaterals, chylothorax, diaphragm injury, and laryngeal nerve injury. If a left subclavian flap is employed, the radial pulse and blood pressure in the left arm are diminished or absent.

In some centers, balloon angioplasty has been used for treatment of "native" or unoperated coarctation. Early reports of results in these patients indicate good relief of the obstruction; however, several have reported the subsequent development of aortic aneurysms. Revised techniques have reduced the incidence of this complication, although the use of angioplasty in native coarctation remains controversial.

Repair of coarctation in the 2nd decade of life or beyond may be associated with a higher incidence of premature cardiovascular disease, even in the absence of residual cardiac abnormalities. There may be early onset of adult hypertension, which has occurred even in patients with adequately resected coarctation.

Although restenosis in older patients after coarctectomy is rare, a significant number of infants operated on before 1 yr of age require revision later in childhood. All patients should be followed carefully for the development of recoarctation and aortic aneurysm. Should recoarctation occur, balloon angioplasty is the procedure of choice. In these patients, scar tissue from prior surgery makes reoperation more difficult, yet makes balloon angioplasty safer because of the lower incidence of aneurysm formation. Relief of obstruction with this technique is usually excellent. Intravascular stents have been utilized in some patients.

POSTCOARCTECTOMY SYNDROME. Postoperative mesenteric arteritis may be associated with hypertension and abdominal pain in the immediate postoperative period. The pain varies in severity and may be associated with anorexia, nausea, vomiting, leukocytosis, intestinal hemorrhage, bowel necrosis, and small bowel obstruction. Relief is usually obtained with antihypertensive drugs (nitroprusside, esmolol, captopril) and intestinal decompression; rarely, surgical exploration is required for bowel obstruction.

434.7 Coarctation with Ventricular Septal Defect

Coarctation in the presence of VSD results in both increased preload and afterload on the left ventricle, and patients with this combination of defects will present either at birth or in the 1st mo of life, often with intractable cardiac failure. The magnitude of a left-to-right shunt through a VSD is dependent on the ratio of pulmonary to systemic vascular resistance. In the presence of a coarctation, the resistance to systemic outflow is elevated by the obstruction, markedly increasing the volume of the shunt. The clinical presentation is that of a seriously ill infant with tachypnea, failure to thrive, and typical findings of heart failure. Often there is not a marked difference in blood pressures between the upper and lower extremities because the cardiac output may be low. Although medical management may be helpful initially, early surgical repair is necessary.

In most cases, coarctation is the major anomaly causing the severe symptoms, and resection of the coarctated segment results in marked improvement. Some repair the coarctation through a left lateral thoracotomy and at the same time place a pulmonary artery band to decrease the ventricular level shunt. Some do not band the pulmonary artery initially, as a number of patients improve sufficiently so that further surgery is not required during early infancy. However, if heart failure makes it difficult to manage these infants after surgery, open repair of the VSD is then performed soon thereafter. Others routinely repair both the VSD and coarctation at the same surgery through a midline sternotomy. When it is determined that a complicated VSD is present (multiple VSDs, apical muscular VSD), pulmonary arterial banding may be performed at the time of coarctation repair to avoid open heart surgery during infancy for these complex ventricular septum abnormalities.

434.8 Coarctation with Other Cardiac Anomalies

Coarctation often occurs in infancy associated with other major cardiovascular anomalies, including hypoplastic left heart, severe mitral or aortic valve disease, transposition of the great arteries, and variations of double-outlet or single ventricle. Severe coarctation may also be associated with endocardial fibroelastosis. The clinical manifestations depend on the effects of the associated malformations as well as on the coarctation itself.

Coarctation of the aorta associated with severe mitral and aortic valve disease may have to be treated within the context of the hypoplastic left heart syndrome (see Chapter 438.10), even if the left ventricular chamber is not severely hypoplastic. Such patients usually have a long segment of narrow transverse aortic arch with or without an isolated coarctation at the site of the ductus arteriosus. Coarctation of the aorta with transposition of the great arteries or single ventricle may be repaired alone or in combination with other palliative measures.

434.9 Congenital Mitral Stenosis

Congenital mitral stenosis is a rare anomaly that can be isolated or associated with other defects, the most common being aortic stenosis and coarctation of the aorta. The mitral valve may be funnel-shaped, with thickened leaflets and chordae tendineae that are shortened and deformed. Other mitral valve anomalies associated with stenosis include *parachute mitral valve* due to a single papillary muscle and *double-orifice mitral valve.*

Symptoms usually appear within the first 2 yr of life. These infants are underdeveloped and usually have obvious dyspnea secondary to heart failure; cyanosis and pallor are common. Some patients, whose symptoms are mainly wheezing, may have been followed with a diagnosis of reactive airway disease. Heart enlargement due to dilatation and hypertrophy of the right ventricle and left atrium is common. Most patients have rumbling apical diastolic murmurs followed by a loud 1st sound, but the auscultatory findings may be relatively obscure. The 2nd sound is loud and split. An opening snap of the mitral valve may be present. The *electrocardiogram* reveals right ventricular hypertrophy with normal, bifid, or spiked P waves, indicating left atrial enlargement. *Roentgenograms* usually show left atrial and right ventricular enlargement and pulmonary congestion. The *echocardiogram* is characteristic, showing thickened mitral valve leaflets, a diminished E-F slope on the M-mode mitral echogram, and an enlarged left atrium with a normal or small left ventricle. Two-dimensional echocardiography examination shows a significant reduction of the mitral valve orifice in diastole. Doppler studies demonstrate a mean pressure gradient across the mitral orifice. At *cardiac catheterization* there is an increase in right ventricular, pulmonary arterial, and pulmonary capillary wedge pressures. Associated anomalies, such as aortic stenosis and coarctation, are demonstrated. *Angiocardiography* shows delayed emptying of the left atrium and the small mitral orifice.

The prognosis for untreated patients is poor. The results of surgical treatment have been mixed; a mitral valve prosthesis is usually required, which requires replacement as the child grows. These patients must be anticoagulated with warfarin, and complications of over- and underanticoagulation are fairly common in infancy. Transcatheter balloon valvuloplasty has been used by several centers as a palliative procedure with mixed results, depending on the anatomy of the valve and the papillary muscles.

434.10 Pulmonary Venous Hypertension

A variety of lesions may result in chronic pulmonary venous hypertension, which when extreme may result in pulmonary arterial hypertension and right-sided heart failure. These lesions include congenital mitral stenosis, mitral insufficiency, total anomalous pulmonary venous return with obstruction, left atrial myxomas, cor triatriatum (stenosis of the common pulmonary vein), individual pulmonary vein stenosis, and supravalvular mitral ring or web. In these conditions, early symptoms can be confused with chronic pulmonary disease such as asthma, as there may be no specific cardiac findings on physical examination. Subtle signs of pulmonary hypertension may be present. The *electrocardiogram* shows right ventricular hypertrophy with spiked P waves. *Roentgenographic studies* reveal cardiac enlargement and prominence of the pulmonary veins in the hilar region, the right ventricle and atrium, and the main pulmonary artery; the left atrium is normal in size or only slightly enlarged.

The *echocardiogram* may demonstrate a left atrial myxoma, cor triatriatum, or a mitral valve abnormality. *Cardiac catheterization* excludes the presence of a shunt and demonstrates pulmonary hypertension with an elevated pulmonary arterial wedge pressure. The left atrial pressure is normal if the lesion is at the level of the pulmonary veins but is elevated if the lesion is at the level of the mitral valve. Selective pulmonary arteriography usually delineates the anatomic lesion. Cor triatriatum, left atrial myxoma, and supravalvular mitral webs can all be successfully managed surgically.

The differential diagnosis includes *pulmonary veno-occlusive disease*, an idiopathic process that produces obstructive lesions in the pulmonary veins of children and young adults. The cause is uncertain. The patient is initially thought to have left-sided heart failure on the basis of congested lungs with apparent pulmonary edema. Dyspnea, fatigue, and pleural effusions are common; cyanosis, digital clubbing, syncope, and hemoptysis are variable findings. The left atrial pressure is normal, but the pulmonary arterial wedge pressure is usually elevated. A normal wedge pressure may be encountered because of the formation of collaterals or if the wedge recording is performed in an uninvolved segment. Angiographically, the pulmonary veins return normally to the left atrium, but one or more pulmonary veins are narrowed, either focally or diffusely.

Lung biopsy demonstrates pulmonary venous and, occasionally, arterial involvement. Pulmonary veins and venules demonstrate fibrous narrowing or occlusion, and there may be pulmonary artery thrombi. Therapy is disappointing, and survival ranges from weeks to months in infants and from months to years in adults. Attempts at surgical repair, balloon dilation, and transcatheter stenting have not significantly improved the prognosis of these patients. Combined heart-lung transplantation (see Chapter 449.2) remains the only moderately successful therapeutic option.

Pulmonary Stenosis

Benson LN, Freedom RM: Interventional cardiac catheterization. Curr Opin Pediatr 1:106, 1989.

Moller JH: Exercise responses in pulmonary stenosis. Prog Pediatr Cardiol 2:8, 1993.

Aortic Stenosis

Donner R, Black I, Spann JF, Carabello BA: Improved prediction of peak left ventricular pressure by echocardiography in children with aortic stenosis. J Am Coll Cardiol 3:349, 1984.

Doyle EF, Arumugham P, Lara E, et al: Sudden death in young patients with congenital aortic stenosis. Pediatrics 53:481, 1974.

Ewart AK, Morris CA, Atkinson D, et al: Hemizygosity at the elastin locus in developmental disorder, Williams syndrome. Nat Genet. 5:11, 1993.

Freed MD: Recreational and sports recommendations for the child with heart disease. Pediatr Clin North Am 31:1307, 1984.

Gerosa G, McKay R, Davies J, Ross DN: Comparison of the aortic homograft and the pulmonary autograft for aortic valve replacement in children. J Thorac Cardiovasc Surg 102:51, 1991.

Keane JF, Driscoll DJ, Gersony WM, et al: Second natural history study of congenital heart defects: Results of treatment of patients with aortic valvar stenosis. Circulation 87(Suppl 2):I16, 1993.

Leichter DA, Sullivan I, Gersony WM: "Acquired" discrete subvalvular aortic stenosis: Natural history and hemodynamics. J Am Coll Cardiol 14:1539, 1989.

Radtke W, Lock J: Balloon dilation. Pediatr Clin North Am 37:193, 1990.

Rocchini A, Beekman RH, Ben Shachar G, et al: Balloon aortic valvuloplasty: Results of the valvuloplasty and angioplasty of congenital anomalies registry. Am J Cardiol 65:784, 1990.

Williams JCP, Barrat-Boyes BG, Lowe JB: Supravalvar aortic stenosis. Circulation 24:1311, 1961.

Zeevi B, Keane JF, Castaneda AR, et al: Neonatal critical valvar aortic stenosis: A comparison of surgical and balloon dilation therapy. Circulation 80:831, 1989.

Coarctation of the Aorta

Ing FF, Starc TJ, Griffiths SP, et al: Early diagnosis of coarctation of the aorta in children: A continuing dilemma. Pediatrics 98:378, 1996.

Rothman A: Coarctation of the aorta: An update. Curr Probl Pediatr 28:37, 1998.

Shaddy RE, Boucek MM, Sturtevant JE, et al: Comparison of angioplasty and surgery for unoperated coarctation of the aorta. Circulation 87:793, 1993.

Shone JD, Sellers RD, Anderson RC, et al: The developmental complex of "parachute mitral valve," supravalvar ring of left atrium, subaortic stenosis, and coarctation of the aorta. Am J Cardiol 11:714, 1963.

Simsolo R, Grunfeld B, Gimenez M, et al: Long-term systemic hypertension in children after successful repair of coarctation of the aorta. Am Heart J 115:1268, 1988.

Mitral Stenosis

Moore P, Adatia I, Spevak PJ, et al: Severe congenital mitral stenosis in infants. Circulation 89:2099, 1994.

Spevak PJ, Bass JL, Ben-Shachar G, et al: Balloon angioplasty for congenital mitral stenosis. Am J Cardiol 66:472, 1990.

Chapter 435

Acyanotic Congenital Heart Disease: Regurgitant Lesions

435.1 Pulmonary Valvular Insufficiency and Congenital Absence of the Pulmonary Valve

Pulmonary valvular insufficiency most often accompanies other cardiovascular diseases or may be secondary to severe pulmonary hypertension. Incompetence of the valve is an expected result after surgery for right ventricular outflow tract obstruction—for example, pulmonary valvotomy in patients with valvular pulmonic stenosis or valvotomy with infundibular resection in patients with tetralogy of Fallot. Isolated congenital insufficiency of the pulmonary valve is rare. These patients are usually asymptomatic because the insufficiency is usually mild.

The prominent physical sign is a decrescendo diastolic murmur at the upper and midleft sternal border, which has a lower pitch than the murmur of aortic insufficiency because of the lower pressures involved. Roentgenograms of the chest show prominence of the main pulmonary artery and, if the insufficiency is severe, right ventricular enlargement. The electrocardiogram is normal or shows minimal right ventricular hypertrophy. Pulsed and color Doppler studies demonstrate retrograde flow from the pulmonary artery to the right ventricle during diastole. The diagnosis can be made at cardiac catheterization if necessary. There is a low pulmonary arterial diastolic pressure. Selective pulmonary arteriography shows the incompetent valve, but this is difficult to evaluate in mild cases because the catheter crossing the valve usually results in some iatrogenic insufficiency during the injection. Isolated pulmonary valvular incompetence is usually well tolerated and does not require surgical treatment. When pulmonary insufficiency is severe, especially if there is also significant tricuspid insufficiency, replacement with a homograft may become necessary to preserve right ventricular function.

Congenital absence of the pulmonary valve is usually associated with a ventricular septal defect, often in the context of tetralogy of Fallot (see Chapter 437.1). In many of these neonates, the pulmonary arteries become widely dilated and compress the bronchi, causing recurrent episodes of wheezing, pulmonary collapse, and pneumonitis. The presence and degree of cyanosis is variable. Florid pulmonary valvular incompetence may not be well tolerated, and death may occur from a combination of bronchial compression, hypoxemia, and heart failure. Correction involves plication of the massively dilated pulmonary arteries, closure of the ventricular septal defect, and placement of a homograft across the right ventricular outflow tract.

435.2 Congenital Mitral Insufficiency

Congenital mitral insufficiency may be isolated but is more often associated with other anomalies, including patent ductus arteriosus, coarctation of the aorta, ventricular septal defect, corrected transposition of the great vessels, anomalous origin of the left coronary artery from the pulmonary artery, or Marfan's syndrome. Mitral insufficiency is common in patients with atrioventricular septal defects (see Chapter 433.5). Mitral insufficiency can also be seen in patients with cardiomyopathy and severe left ventricular dysfunction secondary to dilatation of the valve ring.

In isolated mitral insufficiency, the mitral valve annulus is usually dilatated, the chordae tendineae are short and may insert anomalously, and the valve leaflets are deformed. When mitral insufficiency is severe enough to cause clinical symptoms, the left atrium enlarges as a result of the regurgitant flow and the left ventricle becomes hypertrophied and dilatated. Pulmonary venous pressure is increased and ultimately results in pulmonary hypertension and right ventricular hypertrophy and dilatation. Mild lesions produce no symptoms; the only abnormal sign is the holosystolic murmur of mitral incompetence. Severe regurgitation results in symptoms that can appear at any age. These include poor physical development, frequent respiratory infections, fatigue on exertion, and episodes of pulmonary edema or congestive heart failure. Often these patients will have been followed with a diagnosis of reactive airway disease because of the similarity in pulmonary symptoms.

The typical murmur of mitral insufficiency is a high-pitched (often referred to as a "cooing dove") apical holosystolic murmur. If the insufficiency is moderate to severe, it is usually associated with an apical low-pitched, mid-diastolic rumbling murmur, indicating increased diastolic flow across the mitral valve. The pulmonary component of the 2nd heart sound will be accentuated in the presence of pulmonary hypertension. The *electrocardiogram* usually shows bifid P waves, signs of left ventricular hypertrophy, and sometimes signs of right ventricular hypertrophy. *Roentgenographic examination* shows enlargement of the left atrium, which at times is massive. The left ventricle is prominent, and the pulmonary vascularity is normal or prominent. The *echocardiogram* demonstrates the enlarged left atrium and ventricle. Color Doppler demonstrates the extent of insufficiency, and pulsed Doppler of the pulmonary veins detects retrograde flow when mitral insufficiency is severe. *Cardiac catheterization* shows an elevated left atrial pressure. Pulmonary artery hypertension of varying severity may be present. Selective left ventriculography reveals the severity of mitral regurgitation.

Mitral valvuloplasty can result in striking improvement in symptoms and heart size, but in some patients installation of a prosthetic mechanical mitral valve may be necessary. Prior to surgery, associated anomalies must be identified. In children beyond 3–4 yr, it may be difficult to exclude rheumatic fever as the cause of mitral insufficiency.

435.3 Mitral Valve Prolapse

Mitral valve prolapse results from an abnormal mitral valve mechanism that causes billowing of one or both mitral leaflets, especially the posterior cusp, into the left atrium toward the end of systole. The abnormality is predominantly congenital but may not be recognized until adolescence or adulthood. Mitral valve prolapse is more common in girls, may be inherited as an autosomal dominant trait with variable expression, and thus may affect siblings. It is common in patients with Marfan's syndrome, straight back syndrome, pectus excavatum, and scoliosis. The dominant abnormal signs are auscultatory, although occasional patients may present with chest pain or palpitations. The apical murmur is late systolic and may be preceded by a click, but these signs vary in the same patient so that at times only the click is audible. In the standing or sitting position the click may appear earlier in systole, and the murmur may be more prominent in late systole. Arrhythmias may occur and are primarily unifocal or multifocal premature ventricular contractions.

The *electrocardiogram* is usually normal but may show biphasic T waves, especially in leads II, III, AVF, and V_6; the T-wave abnormalities may vary at different times in the same patient. The *chest roentgenogram* is normal. The *echocardiogram* shows a characteristic posterior movement of the posterior mitral leaflet during mid- or late systole, or pansystolic prolapse of both anterior and posterior mitral leaflets. These M-mode echocardiographic findings must be interpreted cautiously because the appearance of minimal mitral prolapse may be a normal variant. Two-dimensional real-time echocardiography shows that both the free edge and the body of the mitral leaflets move posteriorly in systole toward the left atrium. The presence and severity of mitral regurgitation can be assessed by Doppler.

This lesion is not progressive in childhood, and specific therapy is not indicated. The patient may be at risk for the development of infective endocarditis. Antibiotic prophylaxis is recommended during surgery and dental procedures (see Chapter 443).

Adults (males more often than females) with mitral valve prolapse are at increased risk for cardiovascular complications (sudden death, arrhythmia, cerebrovascular accidents, progressive valve dilatation, heart failure, and endocarditis) in the presence of thickened and redundant mitral valve leaflets.

Often, confusion exists concerning the diagnosis of mitral valve prolapse. The high frequency of mild prolapse on the echocardiogram in the absence of clinical findings suggests that in these cases true *mitral valve prolapse syndrome* is not present. These patients and their parents should be reassured of this, and no special recommendations should be made regarding management or frequent laboratory studies. Otherwise, 15–20% of the general population would be labeled as having a significant, albeit mild, lesion. Endocarditis prophylaxis is indicated only in substantiated cases, usually those with mitral insufficiency.

435.4 Tricuspid Regurgitation

Isolated tricuspid regurgitation is usually associated with Ebstein's anomaly of the tricuspid valve. Ebstein's anomaly may present either without cyanosis or with varying degrees of cyanosis depending on the severity of the tricuspid regurgitation and the presence of an atrial level communication (patent foramen ovale or atrial septal defect). In general, older children tend to present with the acyanotic form, whereas, if detected in the newborn period, Ebstein's anomaly is usually associated with severe cyanosis (see Chapter 437.7).

Tricuspid regurgitation often accompanies right ventricular dysfunction. When the right ventricle becomes dilated because of volume overload or intrinsic myocardial disease, or both, the tricuspid annulus also enlarges, resulting in valve insufficiency. This form of regurgitation may improve if the cause of the right ventricular dilatation is corrected, or it may require surgical plication of the valve annulus. Tricuspid regurgitation is also encountered in newborns with perinatal asphyxia. The cause is thought to be related to an increased susceptibility of the papillary muscles to ischemic damage, leading to transient papillary muscle dysfunction.

Absent Pulmonary Valve

Macartney FJ, Miller GAH: Congenital absence of the pulmonary valve. Br Heart J 32:483, 1970.

Pinsky WW: Absent pulmonary valve syndrome. *In:* Garson A, Bricker JT, Fisher DJ, Neish SR: The Science and Practice of Pediatric Cardiology. Baltimore, Williams & Wilkins, 1998, pp 1413–1419.

Mitral Valve Anomalies

American Academy of Pediatrics: Mitral valve prolapse and athletic competition of children and adolescents. Pediatrics 95:789, 1995.

Glesby MJ, Pyeritz RE: Association of mitral valve prolapse and systemic abnormalities of connective tissue: A phenotypic continuum. JAMA 262:523, 1989.

Marks AR, Choong CY, Sanfilippo AJ, et al: Identification of high-risk and low-risk subgroups of patients with mitral-valve prolapse. N Engl J Med 320:1031, 1989.

CHAPTER 436

Cyanotic Congenital Heart Disease: Evaluation of the Critically Ill Neonate with Cyanosis and Respiratory Distress (see also Chapter 94)

The severely ill neonate with cardiorespiratory distress and cyanosis is a diagnostic challenge. The clinician must perform a rapid evaluation to determine whether congenital heart disease is a cause so that potentially lifesaving measures can be instituted. The differential diagnosis of neonatal cyanosis is noted in Table 94–1.

CARDIAC DISEASE. Congenital heart disease produces cyanosis when obstruction to right ventricular outflow causes intracardiac right-to-left shunting or when complex anatomic defects, unassociated with pulmonary stenosis, cause an admixture of pulmonary and systemic venous return in the heart. Cyanosis from pulmonary edema may also develop in patients with heart failure due to left-to-right shunts, although the degree is usually less severe. In addition, cyanosis may be caused by persistence of fetal pathways, for example, right-to-left shunting across the foramen ovale and ductus arteriosus in the presence of pulmonary outflow tract obstruction or persistent pulmonary hypertension of the newborn (see Chapter 97.7).

DIFFERENTIAL DIAGNOSIS. The initial evaluation of the cyanotic infant begins with observation of the breathing pattern. Weak or irregular respiration is often associated with a weak suck reflex and a central nervous system (CNS) problem. Convulsions and general depression strongly suggest a CNS cause. The infant with primary cardiac or pulmonary disease, in contrast, displays vigorous or labored respirations with tachypnea.

The *hyperoxia test* is one method of distinguishing cyanotic congenital heart disease from pulmonary disease. Neonates with cyanotic congenital heart disease usually do not have significantly raised arterial Pa_{O_2} during administration of 100% oxygen. If the Pa_{O_2} rises above 150 mm Hg during 100% oxygen administration, an intracardiac shunt can usually be excluded, although the Pa_{O_2} of some patients with cyanotic congenital heart lesions may be transiently increased to greater than 150 mm Hg because of intracardiac streaming patterns. In contrast, the Pa_{O_2} in patients with pulmonary disease generally increases significantly as ventilation-perfusion inequalities are overcome by oxygen administration. In infants with a CNS disorder, the Pa_{O_2} completely normalizes during artificial ventilation.

Although a significant heart murmur usually suggests a cardiac basis for cyanosis, several of the more severe cardiac defects (e.g., simple transposition of the great vessels) may not initially be associated with a murmur. The chest roentgenogram may be helpful in the differentiation of pulmonary and cardiac disease; in the latter, it indicates whether pulmonary blood flow is increased, normal, or decreased.

Two-dimensional echocardiography is the definitive noninvasive test to determine the presence of congenital heart disease. The information obtained is essential in avoiding unnecessary cardiac catheterization and angiography in the absence of a cardiac defect as well as in making a specific diagnosis. If echocardiography is not immediately available, the clinician caring for a newborn with possible cyanotic heart disease should not hesitate to start a prostaglandin infusion (for a possible ductal-dependent lesion). Because of the risk of hypoventilation associated with prostaglandins, a practitioner skilled in neonatal endotracheal intubation must be available.

CHAPTER 437

Cyanotic Congenital Heart Lesions: Lesions Associated with Decreased Pulmonary Blood Flow

437.1 Tetralogy of Fallot

Tetralogy of Fallot consists of (1) obstruction to right ventricular outflow (pulmonary stenosis), (2) ventricular septal defect (VSD), (3) dextroposition of the aorta with septal override, and (4) right ventricular hypertrophy (Fig. 437–1). Obstruction to pulmonary arterial blood flow is usually at both the right ventricular infundibulum (subpulmonic area) and pulmonary valve. The main pulmonary artery is often small, and there may be various degrees of branch pulmonary artery stenoses. Complete obstruction of right ventricular outflow (*pulmonary atresia with VSD*) is classified as an extreme form of tetralogy of Fallot.

PATHOPHYSIOLOGY. The pulmonary valve annulus may be of nearly normal size or may be quite small. The valve itself is often bicuspid and, occasionally, is the only site of stenosis. More commonly, there is hypertrophy of the subpulmonic muscle, the crista supraventricularis, which contributes to the infundibular stenosis and results in an infundibular chamber of variable size and contour. When the right ventricular outflow tract is completely obstructed (pulmonary atresia), the anatomy of the branch pulmonary arteries is extremely variable; there may be a main pulmonary artery segment in continuity with the right ventricular outflow, separated by a fibrous but imperforate pulmonary valve, or the entire main pulmonary artery segment may be absent. Occasionally the branch pulmonary arteries may be discontinuous. In these more severe cases, pulmonary blood flow may be supplied by a patent ductus arteriosus (PDA) and by *major aortopulmonary collateral arteries (MAPCAs)* arising from the aorta.

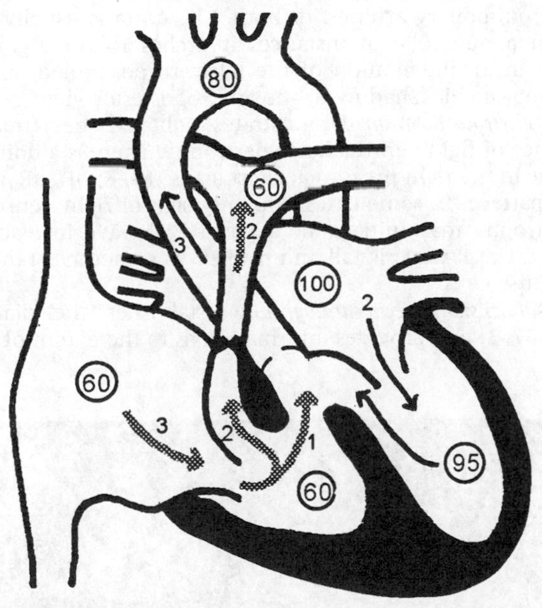

Figure 437–1 Physiology of tetralogy of Fallot (TOF). The circled numbers represent oxygen saturations. The numbers next to the arrows represent volumes of blood flow (in L/min/m²). The atrial (mixed venous) oxygen saturation is decreased secondary to the systemic hypoxemia. Three L/min/m² of desaturated blood enter the right atrium and traverse the tricuspid valve. Two liters flow through the right ventricular outflow tract into the lungs, whereas 1 L shunts right to left through the VSD into the ascending aorta. Thus the pulmonary blood flow is two-thirds normal (Qp:Qs of 0.7:1). Blood returning to the left atrium is fully saturated. Only 2 L of blood flow across the mitral valve. The oxygen saturation in the left ventricle may be slightly decreased owing to right-to-left shunting across the VSD. Two liters of saturated left ventricular blood, mixing with 1 L of desaturated right ventricular blood, are ejected into the ascending aorta. The aortic saturation is decreased, and the cardiac output is normal.

The VSD is usually nonrestrictive and large, is located just below the aortic valve, and is related to the posterior and right aortic cusps. Rarely the VSD may be in the inlet portion of the ventricular septum (atrioventricular septal defect). The normal fibrous continuity of the mitral and aortic valves is usually maintained. The aortic arch is right-sided in 20%; the aortic root is usually large and overrides the VSD to a varying degree. When the aorta overrides the VSD more than 50%, and if there is a significant muscular separation between the aortic valve and the mitral annulus (subaortic conus), this defect is usually classified as a form of *double-outlet right ventricle;* the pathophysiology is the same as that for tetralogy of Fallot.

Systemic venous return to the right atrium and right ventricle is normal. When the right ventricle contracts in the presence of marked pulmonary stenosis, blood is shunted across the VSD into the aorta. Persistent arterial desaturation and cyanosis result. Pulmonary blood flow, when severely restricted by the obstruction to right ventricular outflow, may be supplemented by the bronchial collateral circulation (MAPCAs) and, in the newborn, by a PDA. The peak systolic and diastolic pressures in each ventricle are similar and at systemic level. A large pressure gradient occurs across the obstructed right ventricular outflow tract, and the pulmonary arterial pressure is normal or lower than normal. The degree of right ventricular outflow obstruction determines the timing of onset of symptoms, the severity of cyanosis, and the degree of right ventricular hypertrophy. When obstruction to right ventricular outflow is mild to moderate and there is a balanced shunt across the VSD, the patient may not be visibly cyanotic *(acyanotic or "pink" tetralogy of Fallot).*

CLINICAL MANIFESTATIONS. Infants with mild degrees of right ventricular outflow obstruction may initially present with heart failure caused by a ventricular level left-to-right shunt. Often cyanosis is not present at birth, but with increasing hypertrophy of the right ventricular infundibulum and patient growth, cyanosis occurs later in the 1st yr of life. It is most prominent in the mucous membranes of the lips and mouth and in the fingernails and toenails. In infants with severe degrees of right ventricular outflow obstruction, neonatal cyanosis is noted immediately. In these infants, pulmonary blood flow may be dependent on flow through the ductus arteriosus. When the ductus begins to close in the 1st few hours or days of life, severe cyanosis and circulatory collapse may occur. Older children with long-standing cyanosis who have not undergone operation may have a dusky blue skin surface, gray sclerae with engorged blood vessels, and marked *clubbing* of the fingers and toes. The extracardiac manifestations of long-standing cyanotic congenital heart disease are described in Chapter 441.

Dyspnea occurs on exertion. Infants and toddlers play actively for a short time and then sit or lie down. Older children may be able to walk a block or so before stopping to rest. Characteristically, children assume a *squatting* position for the relief of dyspnea due to physical effort; the child is usually able to resume physical activity within a few minutes. These findings occur most often in patients with significant cyanosis at rest.

Paroxysmal hypercyanotic attacks (*hypoxic, "blue," or "tet" spells*) are a particular problem during the first 2 yr of life. The infant becomes hyperpneic and restless, cyanosis increases, gasping respirations ensue, and syncope may follow. The spell occurs most frequently in the morning on first awakening or following episodes of vigorous crying. Temporary disappearance or decrease in intensity of the systolic murmur is usual as flow across the right ventricular outflow tract diminishes. The spells may last from a few minutes to a few hours but are rarely fatal. Short episodes are followed by generalized weakness and sleep. Severe spells may progress to unconsciousness and, occasionally, to convulsions or hemiparesis. The onset is usually spontaneous and unpredictable. Spells are associated with a reduction of an already compromised pulmonary blood flow, which when prolonged results in severe systemic hypoxia and metabolic acidosis. Infants who are only mildly cyanotic at rest are often more prone to the development of hypoxic spells because they have not acquired the homeostatic mechanisms to tolerate rapid lowering of arterial oxygen saturation such as polycythemia.

Depending on the frequency and severity of hypercyanotic attacks, one or more of the following procedures should be instituted in sequence: (1) placement of the infant on the abdomen in the knee-chest position, making certain that there is no constricting clothing; (2) administration of oxygen (although increasing inspired oxygen will not reverse cyanosis due to intracardiac shunting); and (3) injection of morphine subcutaneously in a dose not in excess of 0.2 mg/kg. Calming the infant, while holding the child in a knee-chest position, may abort progression of an early spell. Premature attempts to obtain blood samples may cause further agitation and be counterproductive.

Since metabolic acidosis develops when the arterial Po_2 is less than 40 mm Hg, rapid correction (within several minutes) with intravenous administration of sodium bicarbonate is necessary if the spell is unusually severe and there is a lack of response to the foregoing therapy. Recovery from the spell is usually rapid once the pH has returned to normal. Repeated blood pH measurements may be necessary because rapid recurrence of acidosis may occur. For spells that are resistant to this therapy, drugs that increase systemic vascular resistance, such as intravenous methoxamine or phenylephrine, improve right ventricular outflow, decrease the right-to-left shunt, and thus improve the symptoms. β-Adrenergic blockade by intravenous administration of propranolol (0.1 mg/kg given slowly to a maximum of 0.2 mg/kg) has also been successful.

Growth and development may be delayed in patients with severe untreated tetralogy of Fallot, particularly when the oxygen saturation is chronically less than 70%. Puberty may also be delayed in patients who do not undergo operation.

The pulse is usually normal, as are the venous and arterial pressures. The left anterior hemithorax may bulge anteriorly because of right ventricular hypertrophy. The heart is usually normal in size, and there is a *substernal right ventricular impulse*. In about half of cases, a *systolic thrill* is felt along the left sternal border in the 3rd and 4th parasternal spaces. The *systolic murmur* is usually loud and harsh; it may be transmitted widely, especially to the lungs, but is most intense at the left sternal border. The murmur is usually ejection in quality at the upper sternal border, but may sound more holosystolic toward the lower sternal border. It may be preceded by a click. The murmur is caused by turbulence through the right ventricular outflow tract. It tends to become louder, longer, and harsher as the severity of pulmonary stenosis increases from mild to moderate; however, it can actually become less prominent with severe obstruction, especially during a hypercyanotic spell. The 2nd heart sound either is single or the pulmonic component is soft. Infrequently, a continuous murmur may be audible, especially if prominent collaterals are present.

LABORATORY DIAGNOSIS. *Roentgenographically,* the typical configuration as seen in the anteroposterior view consists of a narrow base, concavity of the left heart border in the area usually occupied by the pulmonary artery, and normal heart size. The hypertrophied right ventricle causes the rounded apical shadow to be uptilted so that it is situated higher above the diaphragm than normal. The cardiac silhouette has been likened to that of a boot or wooden shoe *(coeur en sabot)* (Fig. 437–2). The hilar areas and lung fields are relatively clear because of diminished pulmonary blood flow or the small size of the pulmonary arteries, or both. The aorta is usually large, and in about 20% of instances it arches to the right; this results in an indentation of the leftward-positioned air-filled tracheobronchial shadow in the anteroposterior view.

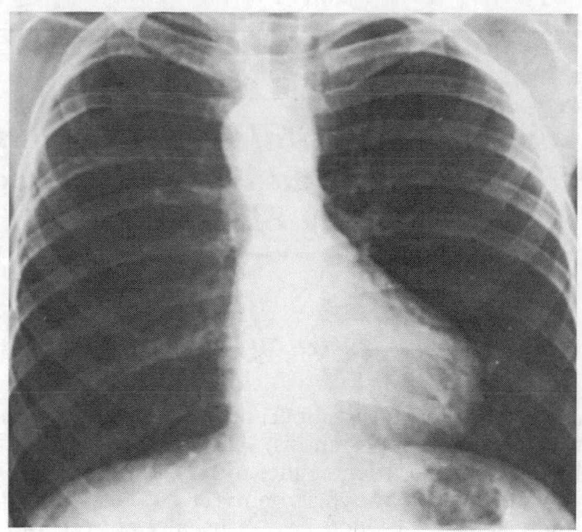

Figure 437–2 Roentgenogram of an 8-yr-old boy with TOF. Note the normal heart size, some elevation of the cardiac apex, concavity in the region of the main pulmonary artery, right sided aortic arch, and diminished pulmonary vascularity.

The *electrocardiogram* demonstrates right axis deviation and evidence of right ventricular hypertrophy. There is a dominant R wave in the right precordial chest leads (Rs, R, qR, qRs) or an RSR′ pattern. In some cases, the only sign of right ventricular hypertrophy may initially be a positive T wave in leads V_3R and V_1. The P wave is tall and peaked or sometimes bifid (see Fig. 430–6).

Two-dimensional echocardiography establishes the diagnosis (Fig. 437–3) and provides information as to the extent of aortic

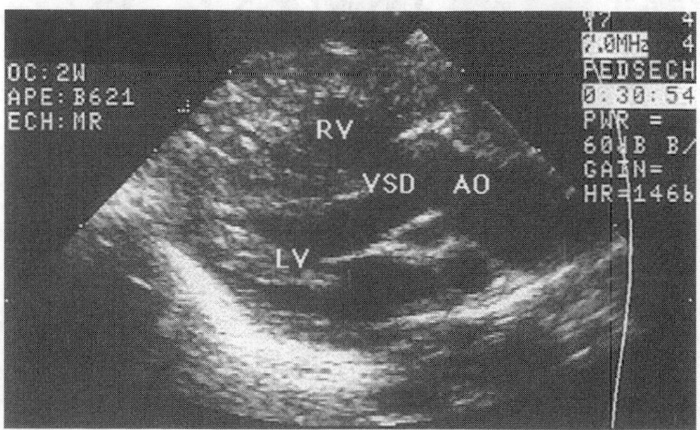

Figure 437–3 Echocardiogram in TOF. This short axis subxiphoid two-dimensional echocardiographic projection demonstrates the anterior/superior displacement of the outflow ventricular septum resulting in stenosis of the subpulmonic right ventricular outflow tract and associated anterior ventricular septal defect. LV = left ventricle; Ao = overriding aortic valve; RV = right ventricle; VSD = ventricular septal defect.

override of the septum, the location and degree of the right ventricular outflow tract obstruction, the size of the proximal branch pulmonary arteries, and the side of the aortic arch. The echo is also useful in determining whether a patent ductus arteriosus is supplying a portion of the pulmonary blood flow. It may obviate the need for catheterization.

Cardiac catheterization demonstrates a systolic pressure in the right ventricle equal to systemic pressure. If the pulmonary artery is entered, there is a marked decrease in pressure, although crossing the right ventricular outflow tract, especially in severe cases, may precipitate a tet spell. The pulmonary arterial pressures are usually lower than normal, in the range of 5 to 10 mm Hg. The level of arterial oxygen saturation depends on the magnitude of the right-to-left shunt; in "pink tets" the systemic saturation may be normal, whereas in a moderately cyanotic patient at rest, it is usually 75–85%.

Selective right ventriculography best demonstrates the anatomy of tetralogy of Fallot. The contrast medium outlines the heavily trabeculated right ventricle. The infundibular stenosis varies in length, width, contour, and distensibility (Fig. 437–4). The pulmonary valve is usually thickened, and the annulus may be small. In patients with pulmonary atresia and VSD, the anatomy of the pulmonary vessels may be extremely complex, for example, discontinuity between the right and left pulmonary arteries. Complete and accurate information regarding the anatomy of the pulmonary arteries is important in evaluating these children as surgical candidates.

Left ventriculography demonstrates the size of the left ventricle, the position of the VSD, and the overriding aorta; it also confirms mitral-aortic continuity, ruling out double-outlet right ventricle. *Aortography* or *coronary arteriography* outlines the course of the coronary arteries. In 5–10% of patients with tetralogy of Fallot, an aberrant major coronary artery crosses over the right ventricular outflow tract; this artery must not be cut during surgical repair. Delineation of normal coronary arteries is important when considering surgery in young infants who may need a patch across the pulmonary valve annulus. Echocardiography may delineate the coronary artery anatomy; angiography is reserved for cases in which there is a question.

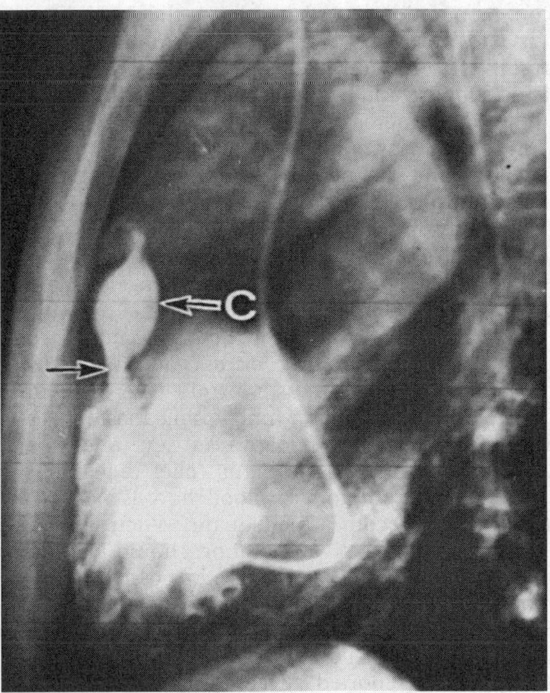

Figure 437–4 Lateral view of a selective right ventriculogram in a patient with TOF. The arrow points to infundibular stenosis that is below the infundibular chamber (C). The narrowed pulmonary valve orifice is seen at the distal end of the infundibular chamber.

PROGNOSIS AND COMPLICATIONS. Prior to correction, patients with tetralogy of Fallot are susceptible to several serious complications. Fortunately, most children have palliation or repair in infancy, and these complications are rare. *Cerebral thromboses,* usually occurring in the cerebral veins or dural sinuses and occasionally in the cerebral arteries, are common in the presence of extreme polycythemia and dehydration. Thromboses occur most often in patients less than 2 yr of age. These patients may have iron deficiency anemia, frequently with hemoglobin and hematocrit levels in the normal range. Therapy consists of adequate hydration and supportive measures. Phlebotomy and volume replacement with fresh frozen plasma are indicated in the extremely polycythemic patient. Heparin is of little value and is contraindicated in hemorrhagic cerebral infarction. Physical therapy should be instituted as early as possible.

Brain abscess is less common than cerebral vascular events. Patients are usually older than 2 yr of age. The onset of the illness is often insidious with low-grade fever or a gradual change in behavior, or both. In some patients there is an acute onset of symptoms, which may develop after a recent history of headache, nausea, and vomiting. Seizures may occur; localized neurologic signs depend on the site and size of the abscess and the presence of increased intracranial pressure. Computed tomography or magnetic resonance imaging confirms the diagnosis. Antibiotic therapy may help to keep the infection localized, but surgical drainage of the abscess is usually necessary (see Chapter 610).

Bacterial endocarditis may occur in the right ventricular infundibulum or on the pulmonic, aortic or, rarely, tricuspid valves. Endocarditis may complicate palliative shunts or, in patients with corrective surgery, any residual pulmonic stenosis or residual VSD. Antibiotic prophylaxis is essential prior to and after dental and certain surgical procedures associated with a high incidence of bacteremia (see Chapter 443).

Heart failure is not a usual feature in patients with tetralogy of Fallot. It may occur in the young infant with "pink" or acyanotic tetralogy of Fallot. As the degree of pulmonary obstruction worsens with age, the symptoms of heart failure resolve and eventually the patient experiences cyanosis, often by 6–12 mo of age. These patients are at increased risk for hypercyanotic spells at this time.

ASSOCIATED CARDIOVASCULAR ANOMALIES. An associated PDA may be present and defects in the atrial septum are occasionally seen. A right aortic arch occurs in approximately 20% of cases of tetralogy of Fallot, and other anomalies of the pulmonary arteries and aortic arch may also be seen. Persistence of a left superior vena cava draining into the coronary sinus may be noted. Multiple VSDs occasionally are present and must be diagnosed prior to corrective surgery. Tetralogy may also occur with an atrioventricular septal defect, often associated with Down syndrome.

Congenital absence of the pulmonary valve produces a distinct syndrome, usually marked by signs of upper airway obstruction (see also Chapter 435.1); cyanosis may be absent, mild, or moderate; the heart is large and hyperdynamic; and a loud to-and-fro murmur is present. Marked aneurysmal dilatation of the main and branch pulmonary arteries results in compression of the bronchi and produces stridorous or wheezing respirations and recurrent pneumonias. If the airway obstruction is severe, reconstruction of the trachea at the time of corrective cardiac surgery may be required to alleviate symptoms.

Absence of a branch pulmonary artery, most often the left, should be suspected if the roentgenographic appearance of the pulmonary vasculature differs on the two sides; absence of a pulmonary artery is often associated with hypoplasia of the affected lung. It is important to recognize the absence of a pulmonary artery, as occlusion of the remaining pulmonary artery during operation seriously compromises the already reduced pulmonary blood flow.

TREATMENT. The treatment of tetralogy of Fallot depends on the severity of the right ventricular outflow tract obstruction. Infants with severe tetralogy require medical treatment and surgical intervention in the neonatal period. Therapy is aimed at providing an immediate increase in pulmonary blood flow to prevent the sequelae of severe hypoxia. The infant should be transported to a medical center adequately equipped to evaluate and treat neonates with congenital heart disease under optimal conditions. It is critical that oxygenation and normal body temperature be maintained during the transfer. Prolonged, severe hypoxia may lead to shock, respiratory failure, and intractable acidosis, and will significantly reduce the chances of survival, even when surgically amenable lesions are present. Cold increases oxygen consumption, which places a further stress on the cyanotic infant, whose oxygen delivery is already limited. Finally, blood glucose levels should be monitored, as infants with cyanotic heart disease are more likely to acquire hypoglycemia.

Infants with marked right ventricular outflow tract obstruction may deteriorate rapidly because as the ductus arteriosus begins to close, pulmonary blood flow is further compromised. The intravenous administration of prostaglandin E_1 (0.05–0.20 μg/kg/min), a potent and specific relaxant of ductal smooth muscle, causes dilatation of the ductus arteriosus and usually provides adequate pulmonary blood flow until a surgical procedure can be performed. This agent should be administered intravenously as soon as the clinical suspicion of cyanotic congenital heart disease is made and continued through the preoperative period and during cardiac catheterization. Postoperatively, the infusion may be continued briefly as a pulmonary vasodilator to augment flow through a palliative shunt or through a surgical valvulotomy.

Infants with less severe right ventricular outflow tract obstruction who are stable and awaiting surgical intervention require careful observation. Prevention or prompt treatment of dehydration is important to avoid hemoconcentration and possible thrombotic episodes. Paroxysmal dyspneic attacks in infancy or early childhood may be precipitated by a relative iron deficiency; iron therapy may decrease their frequency and also improve exercise tolerance and general well-being. Red blood cell indices should be maintained in the normocytic range. Oral propranolol (1 mg/kg every 6 hr) had been used to decrease the frequency and severity of hypercyanotic spells, but with the excellent surgery available, it is preferable to refer the patient for surgical treatment as soon as spells begin.

In general, infants presenting with symptoms and severe cyanosis in the 1st mo of life have marked obstruction of the right ventricular outflow tract or pulmonary atresia. In these infants there are two options: The first is a palliative systemic-to-pulmonary artery shunt, performed to augment pulmonary artery blood flow. The rationale of this surgery is to decrease the amount of hypoxia and to improve linear growth as well as to augment the growth of the branch pulmonary arteries. The second option, in many centers, is corrective open heart surgery performed in early infancy and even in the newborn period in critically ill infants. The advantages of corrective surgery in early infancy versus a palliative shunt and correction in later infancy are controversial. In infants with less severe cyanosis who can be maintained with good growth and absence of hypercyanotic spells, primary repair is performed electively at 6–12 mo of age.

The modified *Blalock-Taussig shunt* is currently the most common aortopulmonary shunt procedure and consists of a Gore-Tex conduit anastomosed side to side from the subclavian artery to the homolateral branch of the pulmonary artery (Fig. 437–5). Sometimes the conduit is brought directly from the ascending aorta to the main pulmonary artery and is called a *central shunt*. The Blalock-Taussig operation can be successfully performed in the newborn period using 3–5 mm diameter shunts and has also been used successfully in premature infants.

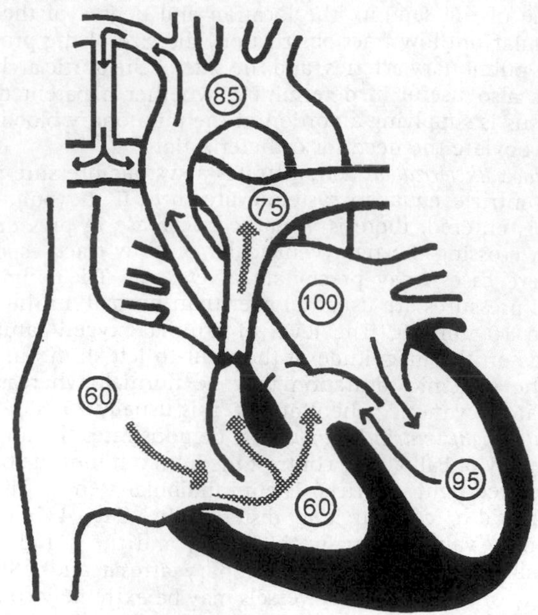

Figure 437–5 Physiology of a Blalock-Taussig shunt in a patient with TOF. The circled numbers represent oxygen saturations. The intracardiac shunting pattern is as described for Figure 437–1. Blood shunts left to right across the shunt from the right subclavian artery to the right pulmonary artery, increasing the total pulmonary blood flow and resulting in a higher oxygen saturation than would exist without the shunt (see Fig. 437–1).

The postoperative course of patients with a successful shunt procedure is relatively uneventful. Postoperative complications following a lateral thoracotomy, such as chylothorax, diaphragmatic paralysis, and Horner's syndrome, may occur. **Chylothorax** may require repeated thoracocentesis and, on occasion, reoperation in order to ligate the thoracic duct. **Diaphragmatic paralysis** due to injury to the phrenic nerve may result in a more difficult postoperative course. Prolonged ventilator support and vigorous physical therapy may be required, but diaphragmatic function usually returns in 1–2 mo unless the nerve was completely divided. Surgical plication of the diaphragm may be indicated. **Horner syndrome** is usually temporary and does not require treatment. Postoperative *cardiac failure* may be caused by a large shunt; its treatment is described in Chapter 448. Vascular problems, other than a diminished radial pulse and occasional long-term arm length discrepancy, are rarely seen in the upper extremity supplied by the subclavian artery used for the anastomosis.

After a successful shunt procedure, cyanosis diminishes. The development of a continuous murmur over the lung fields after the operation indicates a functioning anastomosis. A good shunt murmur may not be heard until several days after surgery. The duration of symptomatic relief is variable. As the child grows, more pulmonary blood flow is needed and the shunt eventually becomes inadequate. When increasing cyanosis develops, a corrective operation should be performed if the anatomy is favorable. If this is not possible (e.g., because of hypoplastic branch pulmonary arteries) or if the 1st shunt lasts only a brief period in a small infant, a second aortopulmonary anastomosis may be required on the opposite side. Several groups have reported success in palliating infants with tetralogy of Fallot using balloon pulmonary valvuloplasty.

Corrective surgical therapy consists of relief of the obstruction of the right ventricular outflow tract by removing obstructive muscle bundles and patch closure of the VSD. If the pulmonary valve is stenotic, a valvotomy is performed. If the pulmonary valve annulus is small or the valve is extremely thickened, a valvectomy may be performed, the pulmonary valve annulus split open, and a *transannular patch* placed across the pulmonary valve ring. When there is a previously established systemic-to-pulmonary shunt, it must be obliterated prior to full repair. The surgical risk of total correction is less than 5%. A right ventriculotomy is performed in many patients, although a transatrial-transpulmonary approach has been used to reduce the long-term risks of a ventriculotomy. Increased bleeding in the immediate postoperative period is common in polycythemic patients. The operative risks may be somewhat higher in small infants because they usually have more severe forms of right ventricular outflow tract obstruction.

After successful total correction, patients are generally asymptomatic and are able to lead unrestricted lives. Immediate postoperative problems include right ventricular failure, transient heart block, residual VSD with left-to-right shunting, myocardial infarction from interruption of an aberrant coronary artery, and disproportionately increased left atrial pressure due to residual collaterals. Postoperative heart failure (particularly in patients with a transannular outflow patch) requires a positive inotropic agent such as digoxin. The long-term effects of isolated, surgically induced pulmonary valvular insufficiency are unknown, but insufficiency is generally well tolerated. The majority of patients after tetralogy repair, and all of those with transannular patch repairs, have a to-and-fro murmur at the left sternal border, usually indicative of mild outflow obstruction and mild to moderate pulmonary insufficiency. Patients with more marked pulmonary valve insufficiency also have moderate to marked heart enlargement. Patients with a severe residual gradient across the right ventricular outflow tract may require reoperation, but mild to moderate obstruction is virtually always present and does not require reintervention.

Follow-up of patients 5–20 yr after operation indicates that the marked improvement in symptoms is generally maintained. Asymptomatic patients have exercise capacities, maximal heart rates, and cardiac outputs that are lower than those of controls. These abnormal findings are more common in patients who had placement of a transannular outflow tract patch and may be less frequent when surgery is undertaken at an early age.

Conduction disturbances are also frequent after operation. The atrioventricular node and the bundle of His and its divisions are in close proximity to the VSD and may be injured during surgery. Permanent complete heart block following surgery is rare. When present, it should be treated by placement of a permanently implanted pacemaker. Even transient complete heart block in the immediate postoperative period is rare in tetralogy patients; it may be associated with an increased incidence of late-onset complete heart block and sudden death. Bifascicular block occurs in about 10% of patients; the long-term significance is uncertain, but in most instances there are no clinical manifestations.

A number of children display premature ventricular beats following repair of tetralogy of Fallot. These are of concern in patients with residual hemodynamic abnormalities; 24-hr electrocardiographic (Holter) monitoring studies should be performed to be certain that occult short episodes of ventricular tachycardia are not occurring. Exercise studies may be useful in provoking cardiac arrhythmias that are not apparent at rest. In the presence of complex ventricular arrhythmias or severe residual hemodynamic abnormalities, prophylactic antiarrhythmia therapy is warranted. Re-repair is indicated if significant residual right ventricular outflow obstruction or severe pulmonary insufficiency is present.

437.2 Pulmonary Atresia with Ventricular Septal Defect

PATHOPHYSIOLOGY. Pulmonary atresia with VSD is an extreme form of tetralogy of Fallot. The pulmonary valve is atretic, rudimentary, or absent, and the pulmonary trunk is atretic or hypoplastic. The entire right ventricular output is ejected into the aorta. Pulmonary blood flow is then dependent on a PDA or on bronchial collateral vessels. The ultimate prognosis depends on the degree of development of the branch pulmonary arteries, which needs to be assessed by cardiac catheterization. If these arteries are well developed, surgical repair with a homograft conduit between the right ventricle and pulmonary arteries is feasible. If the pulmonary arteries are moderately hypoplastic, the prognosis is more guarded, and extensive reconstruction may be required. In these cases, multiple *MAPCAs* may be present and can be incorporated into the repair along with the native pulmonary arteries. If the pulmonary arteries are severely hypoplastic, heart-lung transplantation may be the only therapy (see Chapter 449.2).

CLINICAL MANIFESTATIONS. Patients with pulmonary atresia and VSD present with findings similar to those in patients with severe tetralogy of Fallot. Cyanosis usually appears within the 1st few hours or days after birth; the prominent systolic murmur of tetralogy is usually absent; the 1st heart sound is frequently followed by an ejection click caused by the enlarged aortic root; the 2nd sound is moderately loud and single; and continuous murmurs of a PDA or bronchial collateral flow may be heard over the entire precordium, both anteriorly and posteriorly. Most patients are severely cyanotic and require urgent prostaglandin E_1 infusion and palliative surgical intervention; some patients have heart failure caused by increased pulmonary blood flow via bronchial collateral vessels (MAPCAs); and some infants have adequate pulmonary blood flow and can be managed like patients with uncomplicated tetralogy of Fallot.

LABORATORY DIAGNOSIS. The chest *roentgenogram* demonstrates a small or enlarged heart (depending on the degree of pulmonary blood flow), a concavity at the position of the pulmonary arterial segment, and often the reticular pattern of bronchial collateral flow. The *electrocardiogram* shows right ventricular hypertrophy. The *echocardiogram* identifies aortic override, a thick right ventricular wall, and atresia of the pulmonary valve. Pulsed and color Doppler echocardiography show absence of forward flow through the pulmonary valve, with pulmonary blood flow being supplied by the ductus arteriosus or by MAPCAs. At cardiac catheterization, *right ventriculography* reveals a large aorta, opacified immediately by passage of the contrast medium through the VSD, with no dye entering the lungs through the right ventricular outflow tract. The pathway of pulmonary blood flow from the aorta to the lungs (ductus or collaterals) is demonstrated. Careful delineation of both native pulmonary arteries and MAPCAs by selective contrast injection is required in order to determine the feasibility of surgical correction.

TREATMENT. The surgical procedure of choice depends on whether there is an adequate main pulmonary artery segment and on the size of the branch pulmonary arteries. In patients with small branch pulmonary arteries, surgical intervention is directed toward increasing pulmonary blood flow in the hope that this will stimulate pulmonary artery growth. Two options are currently considered: an aortopulmonary (*Blalock-Taussig* or central) shunt; or the establishment of a connection from the right ventricle directly to the pulmonary artery, either by patch "unroofing" of the outflow tract or by implanting a homograft conduit. There is controversy as to whether this type of bypass stimulates the growth of the pulmonary arteries better than a standard shunt operation.

To be a candidate for full repair, the pulmonary arteries must be of adequate size to accept the full volume of right ventricular output. Complete repair includes closure of the VSD and placement of a homograft conduit from the right ventricle to the pulmonary artery. At the time of reparative surgery, any previous shunts are ligated. Because of intimal tissue proliferation, conduit replacement is usually required in later life; sometimes multiple conduit replacements are required. Patients often have malformations of the primary divisions of the pulmonary arteries in the form of hypoplasia, multiple branch stenoses, absence of a pulmonary artery, and large bronchial collaterals. These vessels are difficult to reconstruct surgically. Some of these patients require repeated transcatheter balloon dilations and eventual stenting of multiple branch pulmonary arterial stenoses.

Acquired total atresia of the right ventricular outflow tract may occur after an aortopulmonary shunt anastomosis for tetralogy of Fallot. In this case, the systolic murmur due to pulmonary stenosis becomes attenuated and then disappears. The completeness of obstruction can be confirmed by echocardiography or by right ventriculography. Corrective surgery of the right ventricular outflow tract can be performed in a manner similar to that used for congenital pulmonary atresia.

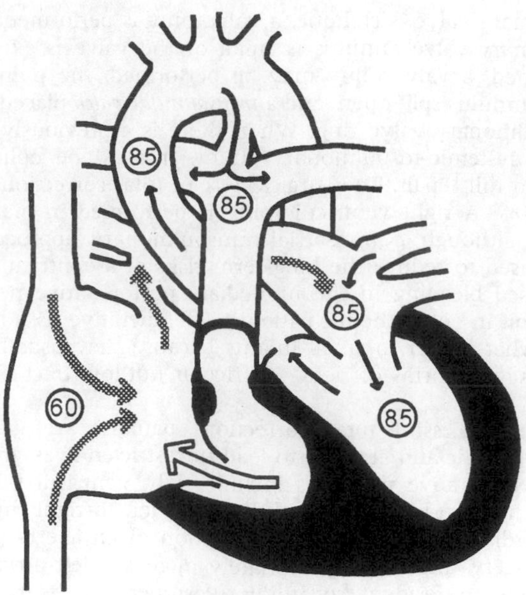

Figure 437–6 Physiology of pulmonary atresia with intact ventricular septum (PA/IVS). The circled numbers represent oxygen saturations. The right atrial (mixed venous) oxygen saturation is decreased secondary to systemic hypoxemia. A small amount of the blood entering the right atrium may cross the tricuspid valve, which is often stenotic as well. The right ventricular cavity is hypertrophied and may be hypoplastic. There is no outlet from the right ventricle owing to the atretic pulmonary valve; thus any blood entering the right ventricle returns to the right atrium via tricuspid regurgitation. Most of the desaturated blood shunts right to left via the foramen ovale into the left atrium, where it mixes with fully saturated blood returning from the lungs. The only source of pulmonary blood flow is via the patent ductus arteriosus. The aortic and pulmonary arterial oxygen saturations will be identical (definition of a total mixing lesion).

437.3 Pulmonary Atresia with Intact Ventricular Septum

PATHOPHYSIOLOGY. In pulmonary atresia with intact ventriculr septum, the pulmonary valve leaflets are completely fused to form a membrane and the right ventricular outflow tract is atretic. Because there is no VSD, there is no egress of blood from the right ventricle. Right atrial pressures increase and blood shunts via the foramen ovale into the left atrium, where it mixes with pulmonary venous blood and enters the left ventricle (Fig. 437–6). The combined left and right ventricular output is pumped solely by the left ventricle into the aorta. In the newborn with pulmonary atresia, the only source of pulmonary blood flow occurs via a PDA. The right ventricle is usually hypoplastic, although the degree of hypoplasia varies considerably. Patients who have a small right ventricular cavity also have a small tricuspid valve annulus, limiting right ventricular inflow. These patients may have sinusoidal channels within the right ventricular wall that communicate directly with the coronary arterial circulation. The high right ventricular pressure results in desaturated blood flowing retrograde via collaterals into the coronary arteries and to the aorta. The prognosis in patients with these sinusoids is guarded. Patients with intermediate-sized or large ventricular cavities may have tricuspid insufficiency, which serves to decompress the right ventricle.

CLINICAL MANIFESTATIONS. As the ductus arteriosus closes in the 1st hours or days of life, infants with pulmonary atresia and intact ventricular septum become markedly cyanotic. Untreated, most patients die within the 1st wk of life. Physical examination reveals severe cyanosis and respiratory distress. The 2nd heart sound is single and loud. Often there are no murmurs; sometimes a systolic or continuous murmur can be heard secondary to ductal blood flow.

LABORATORY DIAGNOSIS. The *electrocardiogram* shows a frontal QRS axis between 0 and +90 degrees, the amount of leftward shift reflecting the degree of hypoplasia of the right ventricle. Tall, spiked P waves indicate right atrial enlargement. QRS voltages are consistent with left ventricular dominance or hypertrophy; right ventricular forces are decreased in proportion to the decreased size of the right ventricular cavity. Most patients with small right ventricles have decreased right ventricular forces; occasionally, patients with larger, thickened right ventricular cavities may show evidence of right ventricular hypertrophy. The chest *roentgenogram* shows decreased pulmonary vascularity, the degree depending on the size of the branch pulmonary arteries and the patency of the ductus or size of bronchial collaterals. The heart may be variable in size. The two-dimensional *echocardiogram* is useful in estimating the right ventricular dimensions and the size of the tricuspid valve annulus, which are of prognostic value. Echocardiography can often demonstrate sinusoidal channels if they are large. *Cardiac catheterization* demonstrates right atrial and right ventricular hypertension. Ventriculography demonstrates the size of the right ventricular cavity, the atretic right ventricular outflow tract, the degree of tricuspid regurgitation, and the intramyocardial sinusoids filling the coronary vessels. Aortography demonstrates filling of the pulmonary arteries via the PDA and is helpful in determining the size and branching patterns of the pulmonary arterial bed.

TREATMENT. Infusion of prostaglandin E_1 is usually effective in keeping the ductus arteriosus open prior to intervention, thus reducing hypoxemia and acidemia prior to surgery. A surgical pulmonary valvotomy is carried out to relieve outflow obstruction whenever possible. To preserve adequate pulmonary blood flow, an aortopulmonary shunt is often performed during the same procedure. Some groups have reported success by performing a surgical unroofing of the right ventricular outflow tract and patch grafting. Several centers have reported success using interventional catheterization, in which the imperforate pulmonary valve is first punctured with a wire or radiofrequency ablation catheter, followed by a balloon valvuloplasty. The aim of surgery or interventional catheterization is to encourage growth of the right ventricular chamber by allowing some forward flow through the pulmonary valve while using the shunt to ensure adequate pulmonary blood flow. Later, if the tricuspid valve annulus and right ventricular chamber are of adequate size, a more extensive valvotomy is carried out and the shunt is taken down. If the right ventricular chamber remains hypoplastic, a modified Fontan procedure (see Chapter 437.4) allows blood to flow to the pulmonary arteries directly from the venae cavae, bypassing the hypoplastic right ventricle. When retrograde coronary perfusion occurs from the right ventricle via myocardial sinusoids, the prognosis may be grave because arrhythmias, coronary ischemia, and sudden death are common. Associated coronary artery abnormalities may be expected. Some infants have benefited from heart transplantation.

437.4 Tricuspid Atresia

PATHOPHYSIOLOGY. In tricuspid atresia there is no outlet from the right atrium to the right ventricle; the entire systemic venous return enters the left side of the heart by means of the foramen ovale or an associated atrial septal defect (Fig. 437–7). Left ventricular blood usually flows into the right ventricle via a VSD. Pulmonary blood flow (and thus the degree of cyanosis) depends on the size of the VSD and the presence and severity of pulmonic stenosis. Pulmonary blood flow may be augmented by, or totally dependent on, a PDA. The inflow portion of the right ventricle is always missing in these patients, but the outflow portion is of variable size. If the ventricular septum is intact, the right ventricle is completely hypoplastic and pulmonary atresia is present (see Chapter 437.3). Most patients with tricuspid atresia present in the early months of life with decreased pulmonary blood flow and cyanosis. Less often, a large VSD in the absence of right ventricular outflow obstruction can lead to high pulmonary flow; patients present

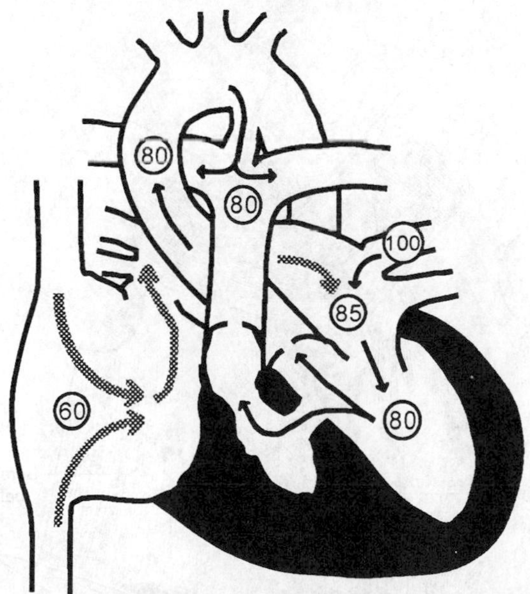

Figure 437–7 Physiology of tricuspid atresia with normally related great vessels. The circled numbers represent oxygen saturations. The right atrial (mixed venous) oxygen saturation is decreased secondary to systemic hypoxemia. The tricuspid valve is nonpatent, and the right ventricle may manifest varying degrees of hypoplasia. The only outlet from the right atrium is to shunt right to left across an atrial septal defect or patent foramen ovale to the left atrium. There, desaturated blood mixes with saturated pulmonary venous return. Blood enters the left ventricle and is ejected either through the aorta or via a ventricular septal defect (VSD) into the right ventricle. In this example, some pulmonary blood flow is derived from the right ventricle, the rest from a patent ductus arteriosus (PDA). In patients with tricuspid atresia, the PDA may close or the VSD may grow smaller, resulting in a marked decrease in systemic oxygen saturation.

with mild cyanosis and heart failure. One variant of tricuspid atresia is associated with transposition of the great arteries. In this case, left ventricular blood flow enters directly into the pulmonary artery, whereas systemic blood flow must traverse the VSD and right ventricle to reach the aorta. In these patients, pulmonary blood flow is usually massively increased and heart failure develops early. If the VSD is restrictive, aortic blood flow may be compromised.

CLINICAL MANIFESTATIONS. Cyanosis is usually evident at birth, with the extent depending on the degree of limitation to pulmonary blood flow. There may be an increased left ventricular impulse, in contrast to the majority of other causes of cyanotic heart disease, in which there is usually an increased right ventricular impulse. The majority of patients have holosystolic murmurs audible along the left sternal border; the 2nd heart sound is usually single. The diagnosis is suspected in 85% of patients before 2 mo of age. In older patients, cyanosis, polycythemia, easy fatigability, exertional dyspnea, and occasional hypoxic episodes occur as a result of compromised pulmonary blood flow. Patients with tricuspid atresia are at risk for spontaneous closure of the VSD, which can occur fairly rapidly, leading to a marked increase in cyanosis.

LABORATORY DIAGNOSIS. *Roentgenographic studies* show either pulmonary undercirculation (usually in patients with normally related great vessels) or overcirculation (usually in patients with transposed great vessels). Left axis deviation and left ventricular hypertrophy are usually present on the *electrocardiogram* (except when there is transposition of the great arteries), distinguishing tricuspid atresia from most other cyanotic heart lesions. The combination of cyanosis and left axis deviation is highly suggestive of tricuspid atresia. In the right precordial leads, the normally prominent R wave is replaced by an rS complex. The left precordial leads show a qR complex, followed by a normal, flat, biphasic or inverted T wave. RV_6 is normal or tall, and SV_1 is generally deep. The P waves are usually biphasic, with the initial component tall and spiked in lead II. The *two-dimensional echocardiogram* reveals the presence of a fibromuscular membrane in place of a tricuspid valve, the variably small right ventricle, VSD, and the large left ventricle and aorta. The degree of obstruction at the level of the VSD or right ventricular outflow tract can be determined by direct measurement and by Doppler examination. The relationship of the great vessels (normal or transposed) can be determined. Blood flow through a patent ductus can be determined by color flow and pulsed Doppler examination.

Cardiac catheterization, indicated if questions remain after echocardiography, shows normal or slightly elevated right atrial pressure with a prominent "a" wave. If the right ventricle is entered through the VSD, the pressure may be lower than the left, reflecting the restrictive nature of the VSD. With right atrial angiography there is immediate opacification of the left atrium from the right atrium followed by left ventricular filling and visualization of the aorta. Absence of direct flow to the right ventricle results in an angiographic filling defect between the right atrium and the left ventricle.

TREATMENT. The management of patients with tricuspid atresia depends on the adequacy of pulmonary blood flow. Severely cyanotic neonates should be maintained on an infusion of prostaglandin E_1 until a surgical aortopulmonary shunt procedure can be performed to increase pulmonary blood flow. The Blalock-Taussig procedure (see Chapter 437.1) or a variation is the preferred anastomosis. Some patients with restrictive atrial level communications are also benefited by a Rashkind balloon atrial septostomy (see Chapter 438.2) or surgical septectomy.

Infants with increased pulmonary blood flow due to an unobstructed pulmonary outflow tract (most often patients with aortopulmonary transposition) require pulmonary arterial banding to decrease the symptoms of heart failure and to protect the pulmonary bed from development of pulmonary vascular disease. Infants with just adequate pulmonary blood flow, who are well *balanced* between cyanosis and pulmonary overcirculation, can be watched closely for the development of increasing cyanosis. This may occur as the VSD begins to get smaller, indicating the need for surgery.

The next stage of palliation for patients with tricuspid atresia involves the creation of an anastomosis between the superior vena cava and the pulmonary arteries (*bidirectional Glenn shunt*; Fig. 437–8*A*). This procedure is performed after the patient has shown signs of outgrowing a previous aortopulmonary shunt, usually between 4 and 12 mo of age. The benefit of the Glenn shunt is that it reduces the volume work on the left ventricle and may lessen the chances of the patient acquiring left ventricular dysfunction later in life. Some centers advocate performing the Glenn anastomosis at an even earlier age (2–4 mo); the benefit of this approach has not yet been confirmed.

The modified Fontan operation is the preferred approach to later surgical management. It is often performed between 1.5 and 3 yr of age, usually after the patient is ambulatory. This procedure was performed by anastomosing the right atrium or atrial appendage directly to the pulmonary artery. Currently, a modification, known as a *cavopulmonary isolation procedure*, is performed. This involves anastomosing the inferior vena cava to the pulmonary arteries, either via a baffle that runs along the lateral wall of the right atrium (see Fig. 437–8B) or via a homograft or Gore-Tex tube running outside the heart. The advantage of this approach is that blood flows by a more direct route into the pulmonary arteries, decreasing the possibility of right atrial dilatation and markedly reducing the incidence of postoperative pleural effusions, which were common with the earlier method. In this completed repair, desaturated blood flows from both venae cavae directly into the pulmonary arteries. Oxygenated blood returns to the left atrium, enters the left ventricle, and is ejected into the systemic circulation. The volume load is completely removed from the left ventricle and the right-to-left shunt is abolished. Because of the reliance on passive filling of the pulmonary circulation, the Fontan procedure is contraindicated in patients with elevated pulmonary vascular resistance, in those with pulmonary artery hypoplasia, and in patients with left ventricular dysfunction. The patient must be in sinus rhythm and not have significant mitral insufficiency.

Postoperative problems after the Fontan procedure include marked elevation of systemic venous pressure, fluid retention, and pleural or pericardial effusions. Pleural effusions used to be a problem in 30–40% of patients; development of the cavopulmonary isolation procedure has reduced this risk to 5%. Late complications include baffle obstruction, causing superior or inferior vena cava syndrome, vena cava or pulmonary artery thromboembolism, protein-losing enteropathy, and supraventricular arrhythmias (atrial flutter, paroxysmal atrial tachycardia), occasionally associated with sudden death. Left ventricular dysfunction may be a late occurrence, often in the teenage or young adult years. Heart transplantation is successful in patients with "failed" Fontan circuits.

437.5 Double-Outlet Right Ventricle with Pulmonary Stenosis

Double-outlet right ventricle with pulmonary stenosis is characterized by both the aorta and pulmonary artery arising

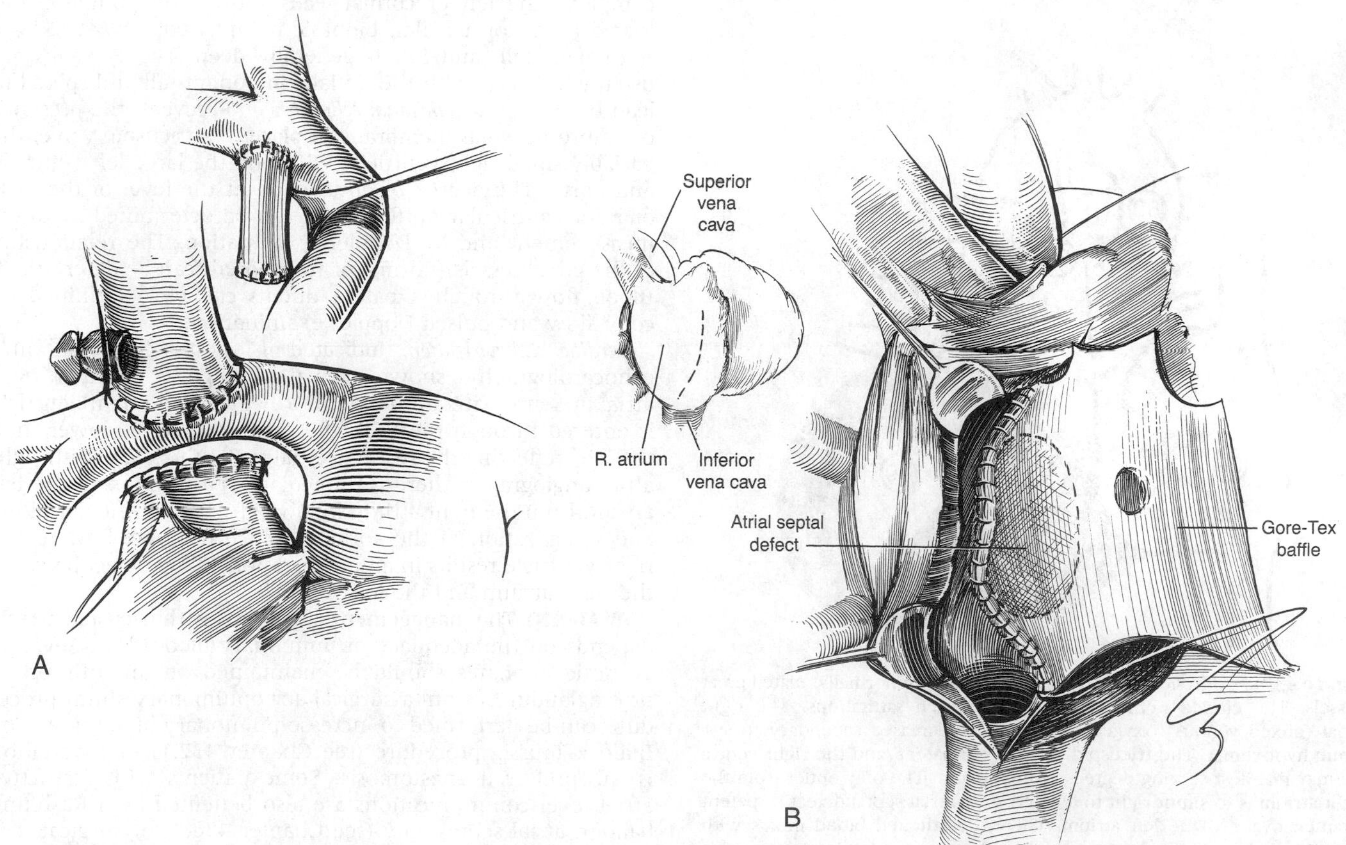

Figure 437–8 *A*, Bidirectional Glenn shunt showing the superior vena cava-right pulmonary anastomosis. *B*, Modified Fontan (cavopulmonary isolation) is completed with placement of baffle to convey inferior vena caval blood along the lateral wall of the right atrium to the superior vena caval orifice. A 4 mm fenestration is sometimes made on the medial aspect of the polytetrafluoroethylene baffle. (From Castaneda AR, Jonas RA, Mayer Jr JE, Hanley FL: Single-ventricle tricuspid atresia. *In*: Cardiac Surgery of the Neonate and Infant. Philadelphia, WB Saunders, 1994.)

from the right ventricle; the outlet from the left ventricle is a VSD into the right ventricle. The aortic and mitral valves are separated by a smooth muscular conus, similar to that seen under the normal pulmonary valve. The aorta may override the VSD by a variable amount but is at least 50% committed to the right ventricle. This defect may be viewed as part of a continuum with tetralogy of Fallot, depending on the degree of aortic override. The physiology is similar to that in tetralogy of Fallot (see Chapter 437.1). The history, physical examination, electrocardiogram, and roentgenograms are as described for tetralogy. The two-dimensional *echocardiogram* demonstrates both great vessels arising from the right ventricle and mitral-aortic valve discontinuity. At *cardiac catheterization*, angiography shows that the aortic and pulmonary valves lie in the same horizontal plane and that the anteriorly displaced aorta arises predominantly or exclusively from the right ventricle. Surgical correction consists of creating an intraventricular tunnel so that the left ventricle ejects blood through the VSD, through the tunnel, and into the aorta. The pulmonary obstruction is relieved either with an outflow patch or with a pulmonary or aortic homograft conduit (*Rastelli operation*). In small infants, palliation with an aortopulmonary shunt provides symptomatic improvement and allows for adequate growth before corrective surgery is performed.

437.6 Transposition of the Great Arteries with Ventricular Septal Defect and Pulmonary Stenosis

This combination of anomalies may mimic tetralogy of Fallot in its clinical presentation (see Chapter 437.1). However, because of the transposition, the site of obstruction is in the left as opposed to the right ventricle. The obstruction can be either valvular or subvalvular; the latter type may be dynamic, related to the interventricular septum or atrioventricular valve tissue, or acquired, as in patients with transposition and VSD after pulmonary arterial banding.

Clinical manifestations vary in age of onset from soon after birth to later infancy, depending on the degree of pulmonic stenosis, and include cyanosis, decreased exercise tolerance, and poor physical development. These manifestations are similar to those described for tetralogy of Fallot; however, the heart may be more enlarged. The pulmonary vasculature as seen on the *roentgenogram* is dependent on the degree of pulmonary obstruction but is often normal. The *electrocardiogram* usually shows right axis deviation, right and left ventricular hypertrophy, and sometimes tall, spiked P waves. *Echocardiography* confirms the diagnosis and is useful in sequential evaluation of the degree and progression of the left ventricular outflow tract obstruction. *Cardiac catheterization* shows that the pulmonary arterial pressure is low and the oxygen saturation in the pulmonary artery exceeds that of the aorta. Selective right and left ventriculography demonstrates the origin of the aorta from the right ventricle, the origin of the pulmonary artery from the left ventricle, the VSD, and the site and severity of the pulmonary stenosis.

Neonates presenting with cyanosis should be started on an infusion of prostaglandin E_1. The preferred surgical *treatment* in hypoxemic infants is an aortopulmonary shunt (see Chapter 437.1). When necessary, balloon atrial septostomy is performed to improve atrial-level mixing and to decompress the left atrium (see Chapter 438.2). The patient can then be followed clinically until older, when a Rastelli operation is the preferred corrective procedure. The Rastelli procedure achieves physiologic and anatomic correction by (1) patch closure of the VSD, directing left ventricular flow to the aorta and (2) connection of the right ventricle to the pulmonary artery by ligating the proximal pulmonary artery and placing an extracardiac homograft conduit between the right ventricle and the distal pulmonary artery (Fig. 437–9). The conduit may eventually become stenotic or functionally restrictive with growth of the patient and require revision. Surgical correction by the Mustard operation (see Chapter 438.2) with simultaneous closure of the VSD and relief of left ventricular outflow obstruction may be an alternative when the position of the VSD is not suitable for a Rastelli operation. Patients with milder degrees of pulmonary stenosis amenable to simple valvotomy may be able to undergo complete correction with an arterial switch procedure (see Chapter 438.2).

437.7 Ebstein Anomaly of the Tricuspid Valve

PATHOPHYSIOLOGY. Ebstein anomaly consists of downward displacement of an abnormal tricuspid valve into the right ventricle. The defect may arise from a failure of the normal process by which the tricuspid valve is separated from the right ventricular myocardium (see Chapter 427). The anterior cusp of the valve retains some attachment to the valve ring, but the other leaflets are adherent to the wall of the right ventricle. The right ventricle is thus divided into two parts by the abnormal tricuspid valve: the 1st, a thin-walled *"atrialized"* portion, is continuous with the cavity of the right atrium; the 2nd, often smaller portion, consists of normal ventricular myocardium. The right atrium is huge, and the tricuspid valve is usually regurgitant, although the degree is extremely variable. The effective output from the right side of the heart is decreased because of the poorly functioning small right ventricle, tricuspid valve regurgitation, and variable degrees of obstruction of the right ventricular outflow tract produced by the large, sail-like, anterior tricuspid valve leaflet. Sometimes right ventricular function is so compromised that it is unable to generate enough force to open the pulmonary valve in systole, producing "functional" pulmonary atresia. Some infants have true anatomic pulmonary atresia. The increased volume of right atrial blood shunts through the foramen ovale to the left atrium, producing cyanosis (Fig. 437–10).

CLINICAL MANIFESTATIONS. The severity of symptoms and the degree of cyanosis is highly variable and depends on the degree of displacement of the tricuspid valve and the severity of right ventricular outflow tract obstruction. In many patients, symptoms are mild and do not occur until the teenage years or young adult life; the patient may present with fatigue or palpitations due to cardiac dysrhythmias. A right-to-left shunt through the foramen ovale is responsible for cyanosis and polycythemia. The central venous pressure may be normal or increased if there is tricuspid insufficiency. On palpation, the precordium is quiet. A holosystolic murmur is audible over most of the anterior left side of the chest resulting from tricuspid regurgitation. A gallop rhythm is common, often associated with multiple clicks at the lower left sternal border. A scratchy diastolic murmur may also be heard at the left sternal border. This murmur is superficial and may mimic a pericardial friction rub.

Newborn infants with severe forms of Ebstein anomaly present with marked cyanosis, massive cardiomegaly, and long systolic murmurs. Death may occur as a result of cardiac failure and hypoxemia. In some of these neonates, spontaneous improvement will occur as pulmonary vascular resistance falls normally, improving the ability of the right ventricle to provide pulmonary blood flow. The majority, however, are dependent on a PDA for pulmonary blood flow.

LABORATORY DIAGNOSIS. The *electrocardiogram* usually shows right bundle branch block without increased right precordial voltage, normal or tall and broad P waves, and a normal or

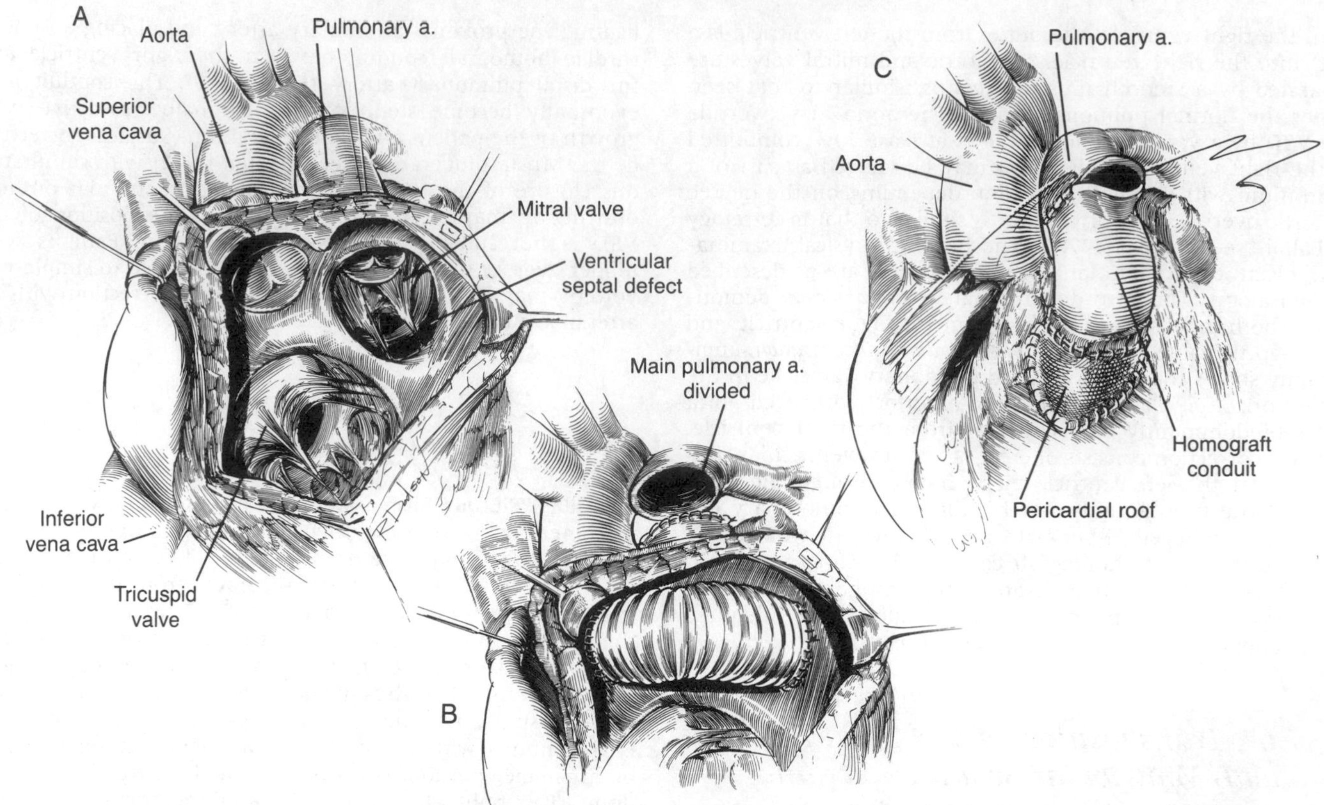

Figure 437–9 *A*, Taussig-Bing type of DORV with subpulmonary stenosis necessitating repair by the Rastelli technique. *B*, Main pulmonary artery is divided and oversewn proximally. The pulmonary valve lies within the baffle pathway. *C*, Completion of the Rastelli repair with a right ventricle–pulmonary artery allograft conduit. (From Castaneda AR, Jonas RA, Mayer Jr JE, Hanley FL: Single-ventricle tricuspid atresia. *In*: Cardiac Surgery of the Neonate and Infant. Philadelphia, WB Saunders, 1994.)

prolonged PR interval. Wolff-Parkinson-White syndrome (see Chapter 442) may be present; patients may have episodes of supraventricular tachycardia. On *roentgenographic examination,* the heart size varies from normal to massive, box-shaped cardiomegaly due to enlargement of the right atrium and ventricle. The pulmonary vasculature can be normal or decreased. *Echocardiography* shows the degree of displacement of the tricuspid valve leaflets, a dilated right atrium, and any right ventricular outflow tract obstruction. Pulsed and color Doppler examination demonstrates the degree of tricuspid regurgitation. In severe cases, the pulmonary valve may appear immobile and pulmonary blood flow may come solely from the ductus arteriosus. It may be difficult to distinguish true from functional pulmonary valve atresia. *Cardiac catheterization,* which is not always necessary, confirms the presence of a large right atrium and abnormal tricuspid valve and any right-to-left shunt at the atrial level. There is a significant risk of arrhythmia during catheterization and angiographic studies.

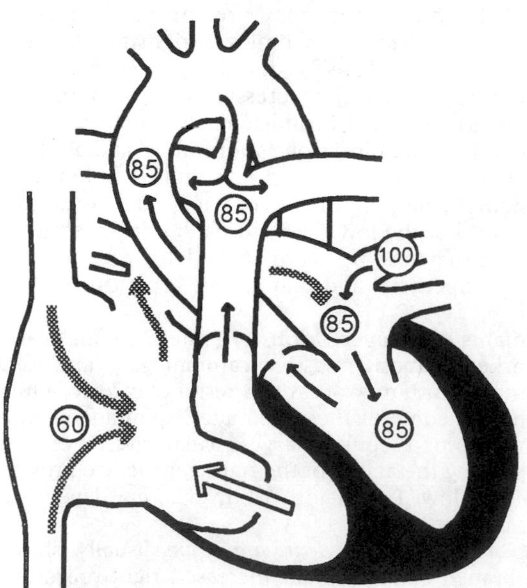

Figure 437–10 Physiology of Ebstein anomaly of the tricuspid valve. The circled numbers represent oxygen saturations. The tricuspid valve leaflets are displaced inferiorly into the right ventricle, resulting in a thin-walled, low-pressure "atrialized" segment of right ventricle. The tricuspid valve is grossly insufficient (*clear arrow*). Right atrial blood flow is shunted right to left across an atrial septal defect or patent foramen ovale, into the left atrium. Some blood may cross the right ventricular outflow tract and enter the pulmonary artery; however, in severe cases the right ventricle may generate insufficient force to open the pulmonary valve, resulting in "functional pulmonary atresia." In the left atrium, desaturated blood mixes with saturated pulmonary venous return. Blood enters the left ventricle and is ejected via the aorta. In this example, some pulmonary blood flow is derived from the right ventricle, the rest from a patent ductus arteriosus (PDA). Neonates with severe Ebstein anomaly will develop severe cyanosis when the PDA closes.

PROGNOSIS AND COMPLICATIONS. The prognosis in Ebstein's anomaly is extremely variable, depending on the spectrum of severity seen. The prognosis is usually poor for the neonate or infant with intractable symptoms and cyanosis. Patients with milder degrees of Ebstein's anomaly usually survive well into adult life.

TREATMENT. Neonates with severe hypoxia who are prostaglandin-dependent have been treated by surgical patch closure of the tricuspid valve, atrial septectomy, and placement of an aortopulmonary shunt (Starnes procedure). This operation creates a functional tricuspid atresia, which can then be further repaired with first a Glenn and then a Fontan operation (see Chapter 437.4). In older children with mild or moderate disease, control of supraventricular dysrhythmias is of primary importance; surgical treatment may not be necessary until adolescence or young adulthood. Repair or replacement of the abnormal tricuspid valve with closure of the atrial septal defect is then carried out.

Tetralogy of Fallot, Pulmonary Atresia with Ventricular Septal Defect and Double-Outlet Right Ventricle

Dabizzi RP, Caprioli G, Aiazzi L, et al: Distribution and anomalies of coronary arteries in tetralogy of Fallot. Circulation 61:95, 1980.

Garson A: Ventricular arrhythmias after repair of congenital heart disease: Who needs treatment? Cardiol Young 1:177, 1991.

Kirklin JW, Pacifico AD, Blackstone EH, et al: Current risks and protocols for operations for double-outlet right ventricle: Derivation from an 18 year experience. J Thorac Cardiovasc Surg 92:913, 1986.

McCaughan BC, Danielson GK, Driscoll DJ, et al: Tetralogy of Fallot with absent pulmonary valve: Early and late results of surgical treatment. J Thorac Cardiovasc Surg 89:280, 1985.

Oku H, Shirotani H, Sunakawa A, et al: Postoperative long term results in total correction of tetralogy of Fallot: Hemodynamics and cardiac function. Ann Thorac Surg 41:413, 1986.

Pacifico AO, Saro ME, Bargeron LM Jr, et al: Transatrial-transpulmonary repair of tetralogy of Fallot. J Thorac Cardiovasc Surg 74:382, 1987.

Sluysmans T, Neven B, Rubay J, et al: Early balloon dilatation of the pulmonary valve in infants with tetralogy of Fallot. Risks and benefits. Circulation 91: 1506, 1995.

Touati GD, Vouhe PR, Amodeo A, et al: Primary repair of tetralogy of Fallot in infancy. J Thorac Cardiovasc Surg 99:396, 1990.

Pulmonary Atresia with Intact Septum

Hanley FL, Sade RM, Blackstone EH, et al: Outcomes in neonatal pulmonary atresia with intact ventricular septum. A multiinstitutional study. J Thorac Cardiovasc Surg. 105:406, 1993.

Latson LA: Nonsurgical treatment of a neonate with pulmonary atresia and intact ventricular septum by transcatheter puncture and balloon dilatation of the atretic valve membrane. Am J Cardiol 68:277, 1991.

Tricuspid Atresia

Donnelly JP, Rosenthal A, Castle VP, et al: Reversal of protein-losing enteropathy with heparin therapy in three patients with univentricular hearts and Fontan palliation. J Pediatr 130:474, 1997.

Gelatt M, Hamilton R, McCrindle W, et al: Risk factors for atrial tachyarrhythmias after the Fontan operation. J Am Coll Cardiol 24:1735, 1994.

Girod DA, Fontan F, Deville C, et al: Long-term results after the Fontan operation for tricuspid atresia. Circulation 75:605, 1987.

Mair DD: The Fontan procedure: The first 20 years. Curr Opin Pediatr 1:94, 1989.

Marino B, Marcelletti C: The cavopulmonary anastomosis in congenital heart disease: A consideration of the classic and bidirectional palliations. Curr Opin Pediatr 2:973, 1990.

Sade RM, Fyfe DA: Tricuspid atresia: Current concepts in diagnosis and treatment. Pediatr Clin North Am 37:151, 1990.

Ebstein's Anomaly

Mair DD, Seward JB, Driscoll DJ, et al: Surgical repair of Ebstein's anomaly: Selection of patients and early and later operative results. Circulation 72:70, 1985.

Starnes VA, Pitlick PT, Bernstein D, et al: Ebstein's anomaly appearing in the neonate. J Thorac Cardiovasc Surg 101:1082, 1991.

Zuberbuhler JR, Allwork SP, Anderson RH: The spectrum of Ebstein's anomaly of the tricuspid valve. J Thorac Cardiovasc Surg 77:202, 1979.

CHAPTER 438

Cyanotic Congenital Heart Disease: Lesions Associated with Increased Pulmonary Blood Flow

438.1 d-Transposition of the Great Arteries

Transposition of the great vessels, a common cyanotic congenital anomaly, accounts for approximately 5% of all congenital heart disease. In this anomaly, the systemic veins return normally to the right atrium and the pulmonary veins return to the left atrium. The connections between the atria and ventricles are also normal *(atrioventricular concordance)*. However, the aorta arises from the right ventricle and the pulmonary artery from the left ventricle (Fig. 438–1). In normally related great vessels, the aorta is *posterior* and to the right of the pulmonary artery; in d-transposition of the great arteries (d-TGA), the aorta is *anterior* and to the right of the pulmonary artery (the "d" indicates a dextropositioned aorta). Desaturated blood returning from the body to the right side of the heart inappropriately goes right out the aorta and back to the body

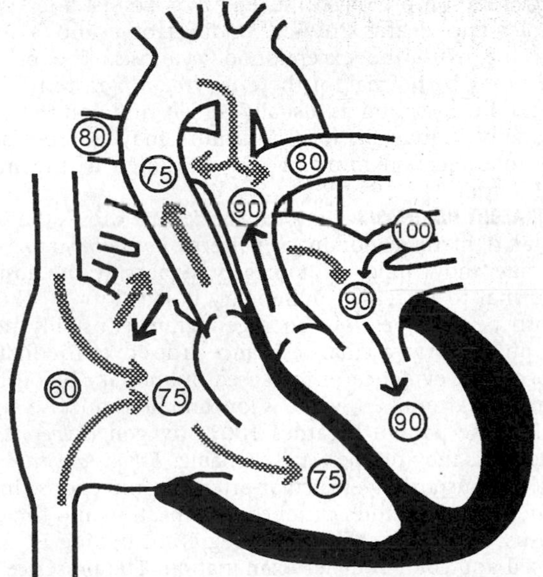

Figure 438–1 Physiology of d-transposition of the great arteries (d-TGA). The circled numbers represent oxygen saturations. The right atrial (mixed venous) oxygen saturation is decreased secondary to systemic hypoxemia. Desaturated blood enters the right atrium, flows through the tricuspid valve into the right ventricle, and is ejected into the transposed aorta, resulting in severe aortic desaturation. Fully saturated pulmonary venous blood flows into the left atrium, across the mitral valve into the left ventricle, and across the transposed pulmonary artery into the lungs. The pulmonary arterial oxygen saturation is thus increased. This lesion would not be compatible with life were it not for the ability of blood to shunt via two fetal pathways: the patent foramen ovale (PFO) and patent ductus arteriosus (PDA). Blood may shunt left to right or bidirectionally at the PFO. Because systemic vascular resistance tends to be higher than pulmonary vascular resistance, blood tends to shunt across the PDA mostly from the aorta to the pulmonary artery. As pulmonary resistance drops in the first few weeks of life, patients with d-TGA will gradually develop increased pulmonary blood flow.

again, whereas oxygenated pulmonary venous blood returning to the left side of the heart is returned directly to the lungs. The systemic and pulmonary circulations consist of two parallel circuits. Survival in these newborns is provided by the foramen ovale and the ductus arteriosus, which permit some mixture of oxygenated and deoxygenated blood. About half of patients with TGA also have a ventricular septal defect (VSD), which provides for better mixing. The clinical presentation and hemodynamics vary in relation to the presence or absence of associated defects. TGA is more common in infants of diabetic mothers and in males (3:1). Prior to the modern era of corrective or palliative surgery, the mortality was greater than 90% in the 1st yr of life.

438.2 d-Transposition of the Great Arteries with Intact Ventricular Septum

d-TGA with intact ventricular septum is also referred to as *simple TGA* or *isolated TGA*. Prior to birth, oxygenation of the fetus is nearly normal, but after birth, once the ductus begins to close, the minimal mixing of the systemic and pulmonary blood via the patent foramen ovale is usually insufficient and severe hypoxemia ensues, usually within the 1st few days of life.

CLINICAL MANIFESTATIONS. Cyanosis and tachypnea are most often recognized within the 1st hours or days of life. Untreated, the vast majority of these infants would not survive the neonatal period. Hypoxemia is usually severe; heart failure is less common. This condition is a medical emergency; only early diagnosis and appropriate intervention can avert the development of prolonged severe hypoxemia and acidosis, which lead to death. Physical findings of cyanosis may be nonspecific, with the exception of cyanosis. The precordial impulse may be normal, or there may be a parasternal heave. The 2nd heart sound is usually single and loud, although occasionally it may be split. Murmurs may be absent, or a soft systolic ejection murmur may be noted at the mid left sternal border.

LABORATORY DIAGNOSIS. The *electrocardiogram* shows the normal neonatal right-sided dominant pattern. *Roentgenograms* of the chest may show mild cardiomegaly, a narrow mediastinum, and normal to increased pulmonary blood flow. In the early newborn period, the chest roentgenogram is usually normal. As the pulmonary vascular resistance drops over the first week or two of life, evidence of increased pulmonary blood flow is evident. The arterial Po_2 value is low and does not rise appreciably after the patient breathes 100% oxygen (*hyperoxia test*), although this may not be totally reliable. *Echocardiography* confirms the transposed ventricular-arterial connections. In addition, the size of the inter-atrial communication and the ductus arteriosus can be visualized; the degree of mixing is assessed by pulsed and color Doppler examination. The presence of left ventricular outflow tract obstruction or a VSD can also be assessed. If echocardiography is not fully diagnostic, *cardiac catheterization* will show right ventricular pressure to be systemic, as this ventricle is supporting the systemic circulation. The blood in the left ventricle and pulmonary artery has a higher oxygen saturation than that in the aorta. Depending on the age at catheterization, the left ventricular and pulmonary arterial pressures can vary from systemic level to less than 50% of systemic level pressures. *Right ventriculography* demonstrates the anterior and rightward aorta originating from the right ventricle as well as the intact ventricular septum. Anomalous coronary arteries are noted in 10–15% of patients. *Left ventriculography* shows that the pulmonary artery arises exclusively from the left ventricle.

TREATMENT. When transposition is suspected, an *infusion of prostaglandin E_1* should be initiated immediately to maintain the patency of the ductus arteriosus and to improve oxygenation (dosage, 0.05–0.20 μg/kg/min). Because of the risk of apnea associated with prostaglandin infusion, an individual skilled at neonatal endotracheal intubation should be available. Hypothermia intensifies the metabolic acidosis resulting from hypoxemia and thus the patient should be kept warm. Prompt correction of acidosis and hypoglycemia is essential.

Infants who remain severely hypoxic or acidotic despite prostaglandin infusion should undergo *Rashkind balloon atrial septostomy* (Fig. 438–2). A Rashkind atrial septostomy is usually performed in all patients in whom any significant delay in operation is necessary. At most centers the arterial switch (Jatene) operation is performed within the first 2 wk of life. If the arterial switch is planned immediately, catheterization and atrial septostomy may often be avoided.

A successful Rashkind atrial septostomy should result in a rise in Pao_2 to 35–50 mm Hg and the elimination of any pressure gradient across the atrial septum. Some patients with TGA and VSD may require balloon atrial septostomy because of poor mixing, even though the VSD is large. Others may benefit from decompression of the left atrium to alleviate the symptoms of increased pulmonary blood flow and left-sided heart failure.

The *arterial switch (Jatene) procedure* is the surgical treatment of choice for neonates with d-TGA and an intact ventricular septum and is usually performed within the first 2 wk of life. The reason for this urgency is that as pulmonary vascular resistance declines after birth, the pressure in the left ventricle (connected to the pulmonary vascular bed) also declines. This results in a decrease in left ventricular mass over the 1st few weeks of life. If the arterial switch operation is attempted after the left ventricular pressure has dropped too far, the left ventricle will be unable to generate adequate pressure to pump to the systemic circulation. The operation involves dividing the aorta and pulmonary artery just above the sinuses and reanastomosing them in their correct anatomic positions. The coronary arteries are then removed from the old aortic root along with a button of aortic wall and reimplanted in the old pulmonary root (the "neoaorta"). By using a button of great

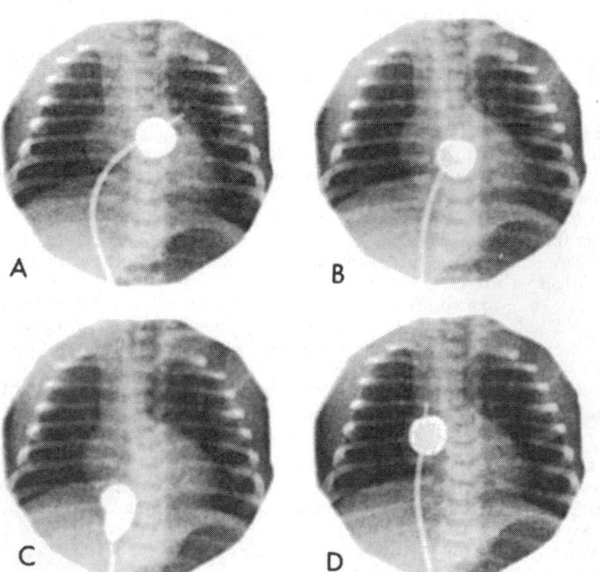

Figure 438–2 Rashkind balloon atrial septostomy. Four frames from a continuous cineangiogram show the creation of an atrial septal defect in a hypoxemic newborn infant with transposition of the great arteries and intact ventricular septum. *A*, Balloon inflated in the left atrium. *B*, The catheter is jerked suddenly so that the balloon ruptures the foramen ovale. *C*, Balloon in the inferior vena cava. *D*, Catheter advanced to the right atrium to deflate the balloon. The time from *A* to *C* is less than 1 sec.

vessel tissue, the surgeon avoids having to suture directly onto the coronary artery (Fig. 438–3). Rarely, a two-stage arterial switch procedure, with initial placement of a pulmonary artery band, may be employed in patients older than 3–4 wk of age who already have a reduction of left ventricular muscle mass and pressure.

The arterial switch procedure has a survival rate of 90–95% for uncomplicated d-TGA. The arterial switch restores the normal physiologic relationships of systemic and pulmonary arterial blood flow and eliminates the long-term complications of the atrial switch procedure (see next paragraph).

Previous operations for d-TGA consisted of some form of *atrial switch procedure* (Mustard or Senning operation). In older infants these procedures produced excellent early survival (about 85–90%) but significant long-term morbidity. Atrial switch procedures reverse blood flow patterns at the atrial level by the surgical formation of an intra-atrial baffle, allowing systemic venous blood to be directed to the left atrium and the left ventricle and then, via the pulmonary artery, into the lungs. The same baffle also permits oxygenated pulmonary venous blood to cross over to the right atrium, right ventricle, and aorta. The atrial switch procedures involve significant atrial surgery and may result in the late development of atrial conduction disturbances, sick-sinus syndrome with brady- and tachyarrhythmias, atrial flutter, sudden death, superior or inferior vena cava syndrome, edema, ascites, and protein-losing enteropathy. Atrial switch operations are now reserved for patients who are not candidates for the arterial switch operation (TGA and severe pulmonic stenosis).

438.3 Transposition of the Great Arteries with Ventricular Septal Defect

If the VSD associated with TGA is small, the clinical manifestations, laboratory findings, and treatment are similar to those described previously for transposition with intact ventricular septum. There is a harsh systolic murmur at the lower left sternal border resulting from flow through the defect. Many of these small defects eventually close spontaneously and often are not addressed at the time of surgery.

When the VSD is large and not restrictive to ventricular ejection, significant mixing of oxygenated and deoxygenated blood usually occurs and *clinical manifestations* of cardiac failure are seen. The onset of cyanosis may be subtle and frequently delayed, and its intensity is variable. Cyanosis can usually be recognized within the 1st mo of life, but some infants may remain undiagnosed for several months. The murmur is holosystolic and generally indistinguishable from that produced by a large VSD in patients with normally related great arteries. The heart is usually significantly enlarged.

Cardiomegaly, narrow mediastinal waist, and increased pulmonary vascularity are demonstrated on the *chest roentgenogram*. The *electrocardiogram* shows prominent P waves and isolated right ventricular hypertrophy or biventricular hypertrophy. Occasionally, dominance of the left ventricle is present. Usually, the QRS axis is to the right, but sometimes it is normal or even to the left. The diagnosis can be confirmed by *echocardiography*, and the extent of pulmonary blood flow can also be assessed by the degree of enlargement of the left atrium and ventricle. In equivocal cases, the diagnosis can be confirmed by *cardiac catheterization*. Right and left ventriculography indicate the presence of arterial transposition and demonstrate the site and size of the ventricular septal defect. Peak systolic pressures are equal in the two ventricles, the aorta, and the pulmonary artery. The left atrial pressure may be much higher than right atrial pressure, indicating a restrictive communication at the atrial level. At the time of cardiac catheterization, a Rashkind balloon atrial septostomy may be performed, even when adequate mixing is occurring at the ventricular level, to decompress the left atrium.

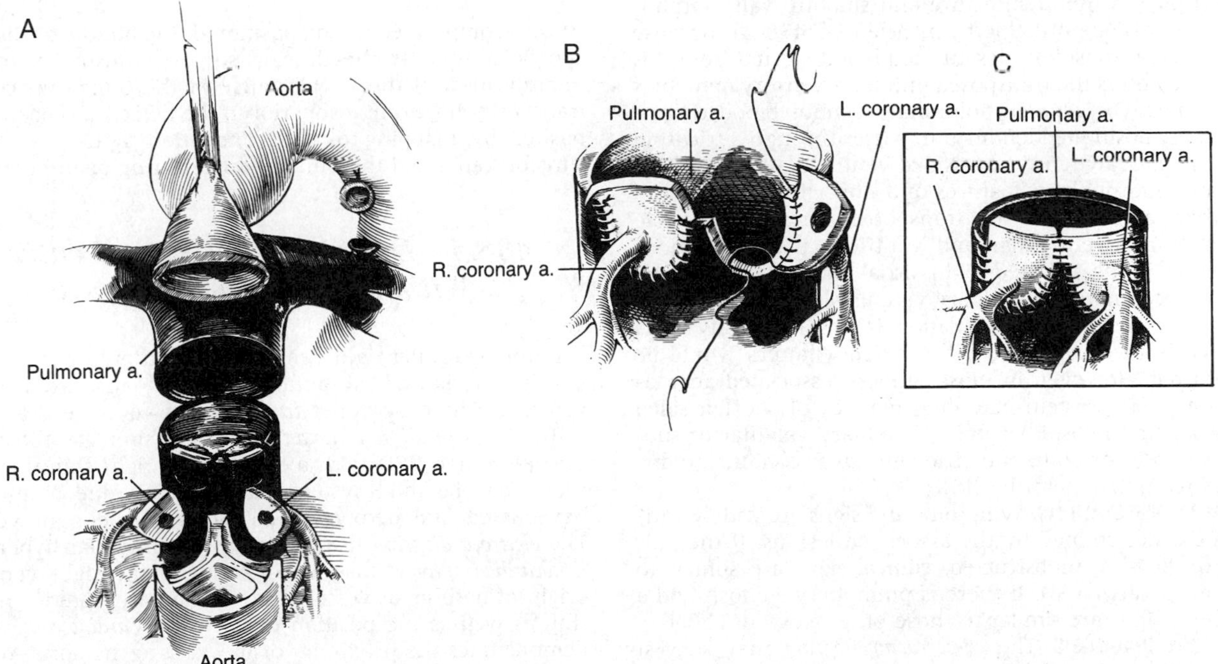

Figure 438–3 Method for translocating the coronary arteries in the arterial switch (Jatene) procedure. *A*, The aorta (anterior) and the pulmonary artery (posterior) have been transected, allowing visualization of the left and right coronary arteries. The coronaries have been excised from their respective sinuses, including a large flap (button) of arterial wall. Equivalent segments of the wall of the pulmonary artery (which will become the neoaorta) are also removed. *B*, The aortocoronary buttons are sutured into the proximal neoaorta. With this technique all sutures are placed in the button of aortic wall, rather than directly on the coronary arteries. *C*, Completed anastomosis of the left and right coronary arteries to the neoaorta. (Adapted from Castañeda AR, Jonas RA, Mayer JE Jr, Hanley FL: Cardiac Surgery of the Neonate and Infant. Philadelphia, WB Saunders, 1994.)

Surgical treatment is advised soon after diagnosis, usually within the first months of life, as heart failure and failure to thrive are difficult to manage and pulmonary vascular disease can develop unusually rapidly. Management includes digitalis and diuretics to lessen the symptoms of heart failure while awaiting surgical repair.

The patient with TGA and a VSD without pulmonic stenosis can be managed with an arterial switch procedure combined with VSD closure. The arterial switch operation can be safely performed after the first 2 wk of life because the VSD results in equal pressures in both ventricles and prevents the regression of the left ventricular muscle mass.

Without treatment, the *prognosis* is poor; the majority of patients succumb in the 1st yr of life because of heart failure, hypoxemia, and pulmonary hypertension. In the past, some survived infancy with medical therapy alone but often acquired pulmonary vascular disease. The clinical picture and treatment of these patients are similar to those described with Eisenmenger's syndrome secondary to an isolated large VSD (see Chapter 440.2).

438.4 l-Transposition of the Great Arteries (Corrected Transposition)

In l-transposition, the atrioventricular relationships are discordant, with the right atrium connected to the left ventricle and the left atrium to the right ventricle *(ventricular inversion)*. The great arteries are also transposed, with the aorta arising from the right ventricle and the pulmonary artery from the left. The aorta arises to the left of the pulmonary artery (hence the designation "l" for levo-transposition). The aorta may be anterior to the pulmonary artery; usually they are nearly side by side. Desaturated systemic venous blood is returned to a normally positioned right atrium, from which it passes through a bicuspid atrioventricular (mitral) valve into a right-sided ventricle that has the architecture and smooth wall morphologic features of the normal left ventricle (Fig. 438–4). Because there is also transposition, desaturated blood ejected from this left ventricle enters the transposed pulmonary artery and flows into the lungs. Oxygenated pulmonary venous blood returns to a normally positioned left atrium, passes through a tricuspid atrioventricular valve into a left-sided ventricle, which has the trabeculated morphologic features of a normal right ventricle, and is then ejected into the transposed aorta. The double inversion of atrioventricular and ventriculoarterial relationships results in desaturated right atrial blood reaching the lungs, and oxygenated pulmonary venous blood appropriately flowing to the aorta. The circulation is physiologically "corrected." Without other defects, the hemodynamics would be nearly normal. However, in most patients, associated anomalies coexist: VSD, Ebstein-like abnormalities of the left-sided atrioventricular (tricuspid) valve, pulmonary valvular or subvalvular stenosis, or both, and atrioventricular conduction disturbances (complete heart block).

CLINICAL MANIFESTATIONS. Symptoms and signs are widely variable and are determined by the associated lesions. If the pulmonary outflow is unobstructed, clinical signs are similar to those of an isolated VSD. If there is pulmonary stenosis and a VSD, clinical signs are similar to those of tetralogy of Fallot.

LABORATORY DIAGNOSIS. The *chest roentgenogram* may suggest the abnormal position of the great arteries; the ascending aorta occupies the upper left border of the cardiac silhouette and has a straight profile. In addition to atrioventricular conduction disturbances, the *electrocardiogram* may show abnormal P waves; absent Q waves in V_6; abnormally present Q waves in leads III, aVR, aVF, and V_1; and upright T waves across the precordium.

Surgical treatment of the associated anomalies, most often the VSD, is complicated by the position of the bundle of His, which can be injured at the time of surgery, causing heart block. Identification of the usual course of the bundle in corrected transposition (running superior to the defect) has been accomplished by mapping of the conduction system so that the surgeon can avoid the bundle of His during open heart repair.

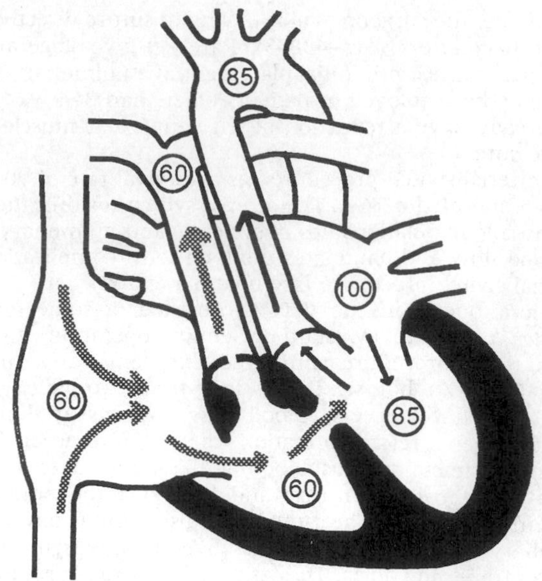

Figure 438–4 Physiology of l- or corrected transposition of the great arteries (l-TGA) with a ventricular septal defect and pulmonic stenosis (VSD + PS). The circled numbers represent oxygen saturation values. The right atrial (mixed venous) oxygen saturation is decreased secondary to systemic hypoxemia. Blood from the right atrium flows through the mitral valve into the "inverted" left ventricle. However, the left ventricle is attached to the transposed pulmonary artery. Therefore, despite the anomalies, desaturated blood still winds up in the pulmonary circulation. Saturated blood returns to the left atrium, traverses the tricuspid valve into the "inverted" right ventricle, and is pumped into the transposed aorta. This circulation would be totally "corrected" were it not for the frequent association of other congenital anomalies, in this case, VSD + PS. Because of the stenotic pulmonary valve, some left ventricular blood flow crosses the VSD and into the right ventricle and the ascending aorta, resulting in systemic desaturation.

438.5 Double-Outlet Right Ventricle Without Pulmonary Stenosis

In double-outlet right ventricle without pulmonary stenosis, both the aorta and the pulmonary artery arise from the right ventricle. The only outlet from the left ventricle is through a VSD. The *clinical manifestations* closely simulate those of an uncomplicated VSD with a large left-to-right shunt, although there may be mild systemic desaturation due to mixing of oxygenated and deoxygenated blood in the right ventricle. The *electrocardiogram* usually shows biventricular hypertrophy. *Echocardiography* is diagnostic, showing the right ventricular origin of both great vessels and their anteroposterior relationship as well as the position of the VSD. *Cardiac catheterization* demonstrates the proximity of the VSD to the aorta, resulting in most of the left ventricular blood being ejected directly into the systemic circulation. The angiogram also confirms the lack of mitral-aortic fibrous continuity and shows the aortic valve displaced superiorly and at the same level as the pulmonary valve. It is important to differentiate this condition from a simple VSD.

Surgical correction is accomplished by creation of an intracardiac tunnel. Blood is then ejected from the left ventricle via the VSD into the aorta. Pulmonary arterial banding may be required in infancy, followed by surgical correction when the child is bigger. When there is associated pulmonary stenosis, there is more marked cyanosis and decreased pulmonary blood flow (see Chapter 437).

438.6 Double-Outlet Right Ventricle with Transposition of the Great Arteries (Taussig-Bing Anomaly)

In double-outlet right ventricle with TGA, the VSD is located above the crista supraventricularis (subarterial VSD) and is either directly subpulmonary or related to both pulmonary and aortic valves (doubly committed VSD). Patients experience cardiac failure early in infancy and are at risk for the development of pulmonary vascular disease and cyanosis. Cardiomegaly is usual, and there is a parasternal systolic ejection murmur, sometimes preceded by an ejection click and a loud closure of the pulmonary valve. Left-sided obstructive lesions are frequent, including coarctation of the aorta, interruption of the aortic arch, and a restrictive VSD, which obstructs left ventricular ejection. The *electrocardiogram* shows right axis deviation and right, left, or biventricular hypertrophy. The *roentgenogram* documents cardiomegaly, a large left atrium, and prominence of the pulmonary artery and pulmonary vasculature. The anatomic features of the anomaly and associated abnormalities are best demonstrated by a combination of echocardiography and selective right and left ventriculography. Palliation may be accomplished by pulmonary arterial banding in infancy with surgical correction at a later age, which may be accomplished by a Rastelli procedure (see Chapter 437) or by an arterial switch procedure (see Chapter 438.2).

438.7 Total Anomalous Pulmonary Venous Return

PATHOPHYSIOLOGY. Abnormal development of the pulmonary veins may result in either partial or complete anomalous drainage into the systemic venous circulation. Partial anomalous pulmonary venous return is usually an acyanotic lesion (see Chapter 433.4). Total anomalous pulmonary venous return (TAPVR) allows total mixing of systemic venous and pulmonary venous blood flow within the heart and thus produces cyanosis.

In TAPVR there is no direct pulmonary venous connection into the left atrium. The pulmonary veins may drain *above the diaphragm* into the right atrium directly, into the coronary sinus, or into the superior vena cava via a "vertical vein" or may drain *below the diaphragm*, joining into a "descending vein" that enters into the inferior vena cava or one of its major tributaries, often via the ductus venosus. This latter form of anomalous venous drainage is most commonly associated with obstruction, usually as the ductus venosus closes soon after birth, although supracardiac anomalous veins may also become obstructed. Occasionally, the drainage may be mixed, with some veins draining above and others below the diaphragm.

In all forms of TAPVR there is mixing of oxygenated and deoxygenated blood before or at the level of the right atrium. Right atrial blood either passes into the right ventricle and pulmonary artery or passes through an atrial septal defect (ASD) or patent foramen ovale into the left atrium. The right atrium and ventricle and the pulmonary artery are usually enlarged, whereas the left atrium and ventricle may be normal or small. The presentation of TAPVR depends on the presence or absence of obstruction of the venous channels (Table 438–1). If the pulmonary venous return is obstructed, severe pulmonary congestion and pulmonary hypertension occur; rapid deterioration occurs without surgical intervention. Obstructed TAPVR is a pediatric cardiac surgical emergency, as prostaglandin therapy may not be helpful.

TABLE 438–1 Anomalous Pulmonary Venous Return

% and Site of Connection	% with Severe Obstruction
Supracardiac (50)	
Left superior vena cava (40)	40
Right superior vena cava (10)	75
Cardiac (25)	
Coronary sinus (20)	10
Right atrium (5)	5
Infracardiac (20)	95–100
Mixed (5)	

CLINICAL MANIFESTATIONS. Three major clinical patterns of TAPVR are seen. Some present in the neonatal period with severe obstruction to pulmonary venous return. This is most prevalent in the infracardiac group (see Table 438–1). Cyanosis and severe tachypnea are prominent. There may be no murmurs. Infants are severely ill and fail to respond to mechanical ventilation. Rapid diagnosis and surgical correction are necessary for survival. Another group presents with heart failure in early life, but there is only mild or moderate obstruction to pulmonary venous return and a large left-to-right shunt. Because pulmonary artery hypertension is present, these infants are severely ill. Systolic murmurs are audible along the left sternal border, and there may be a gallop rhythm. A continuous murmur is occasionally heard along the upper left sternal border over the pulmonary area. Cyanosis is mild. The third group of patients with TAPVR are those in whom pulmonary venous obstruction is not present; there is total mixing of systemic venous and pulmonary venous blood and a large left-to-right shunt. Pulmonary hypertension is absent, and these patients are less likely to be severely symptomatic during infancy. Clinical cyanosis is usually mild or absent.

LABORATORY DIAGNOSIS. The *electrocardiogram* demonstrates right ventricular hypertrophy (usually a qR pattern in V_3R and V_1, and the P waves are frequently tall and spiked). *Roentgenograms* are pathognomonic in older children if the anomalous pulmonary veins enter the innominate vein and persistent left superior vena cava (Fig. 438–5). There is a large supracardiac shadow that together with the normal cardiac shadow forms a "snowman" appearance. This appearance is not helpful for diagnosis in early infancy because of the thymus. In most cases without obstruction, the heart is enlarged, the pulmonary artery and right ventricle are prominent, and the pulmonary vascularity is increased. In neonates with marked pulmonary venous obstruction, the chest roentgenogram demonstrates a perihilar pattern of pulmonary edema and a small heart. This appearance can be confused with primary pulmonary disease. The differential diagnosis includes persistent pulmonary hypertension of the newborn, respiratory distress syndrome, pneumonia (bacterial, meconium aspiration), pulmonary lymphangiectasia, and other heart defects (hypoplastic left heart syndrome).

The *echocardiogram* demonstrates a large right ventricle and usually identifies the pattern of abnormal pulmonary venous connections. The demonstration of a vessel in the abdomen with Doppler venous flow away from the heart is pathognomonic of TAPVR below the diaphragm. Shunting occurs almost exclusively from right to left at the atrial level.

Cardiac catheterization shows that the oxygen saturations of blood in both atria, both ventricles, and the aorta are more or less similar, indicative of a *total mixing lesion*. An increase in systemic venous saturation occurs at the site of entry of the abnormal pulmonary venous channel. In older patients, the pulmonary arterial and right ventricular pressures may be only

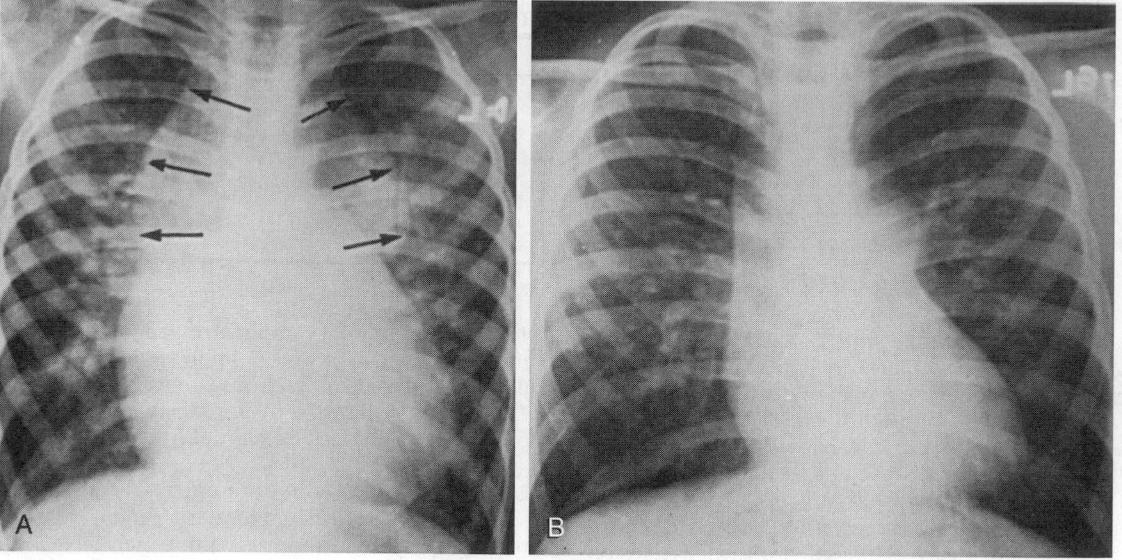

Figure 438–5 Roentgenograms of total anomalous pulmonary venous return to the left superior vena cava. *A*, Preoperative: Arrows point to the supracardiac shadow, which produces the snowman or figure 8 configuration. Cardiomegaly and increased pulmonary vascularity are evident. *B*, Postoperative: showing decrease in size of the heart and supracardiac shadow.

moderately elevated, but in infants who present with pulmonary venous obstruction, pulmonary hypertension is usual. *Selective pulmonary arteriography* shows the anatomy of the pulmonary veins and their point of entry into the systemic venous circulation. Magnetic resonance imaging and computed tomography may be alternative methods of confirming the diagnosis.

TREATMENT. Surgical correction of total anomalous pulmonary venous return during infancy is indicated. Prior to surgery, infants may be stabilized with prostaglandin E_1 to dilate the ductus venosus and the ductus arteriosus. Some may require balloon atrial septostomy; however, this is of little or no benefit in the presence of pulmonary venous obstruction. Surgically, the common pulmonary venous trunk is anastomosed directly to the left atrium, the atrial septal defect is closed, and the connection to the systemic venous circuit is interrupted. Results have been generally good, even for critically ill neonates. If the postoperative hemodynamics are normal, the prognosis is excellent. The postoperative period may be complicated by pulmonary vascular hypertensive crises. In some patients, especially those in whom the diagnosis was delayed, persistent pulmonary hypertension may occur, and the long-term prognosis in these patients is poor. Inhaled nitric oxide or extracorporeal membrane oxygenation may be necessary. Long-term complications include restenosis of the pulmonary venous channel–to–left atrial communication. In patients with stenosis or hypoplasia of the individual pulmonary veins, the prognosis is poor.

438.8 Truncus Arteriosus

PATHOPHYSIOLOGY. In truncus arteriosus, a single arterial trunk (truncus arteriosus) arises from the heart and supplies the systemic, pulmonary, and coronary circulations. A VSD is always present, with the truncus overriding the defect, receiving blood from both right and left ventricles (Fig. 438–6). The number of truncal valve cusps varies from two to as many as six. The pulmonary arteries may arise together from the posterior left side of the persistent truncus arteriosus and then divide into left and right pulmonary arteries (type I truncus arteriosus). In types II and III truncus arteriosus, there is no main pulmonary artery and the right and left pulmonary arteries arise from separate orifices in the posterior (type II) or lateral (type III) aspects of the truncus arteriosus. Type IV truncus has no identifiable connection between the heart and pulmonary arteries, and pulmonary blood flow derives from *major aortopulmonary collateral arteries* arising from the transverse or descending aorta; this form has also been called *pseudotruncus* but is essentially a form of pulmonary atresia with a VSD (see Chapter 437.2).

Both ventricles are at systemic pressure and both eject blood

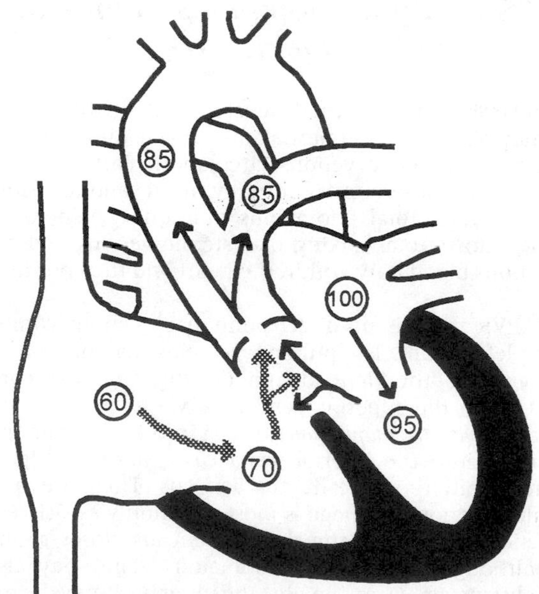

Figure 438–6 Physiology of truncus arteriosus. The circled numbers represent oxygen saturations. The right atrial (mixed venous) oxygen saturation is decreased secondary to systemic hypoxemia. Desaturated blood enters the right atrium, flows through the tricuspid valve into the right ventricle, and is ejected into the truncus. Saturated blood returning from the left atrium enters the left ventricle and is also ejected into the truncus. The common aortopulmonary trunk gives rise to the ascending aorta and to the main or branch pulmonary arteries. The oxygen saturation in the aorta and pulmonary arteries is usually the same (definition of a total mixing lesion). As pulmonary vascular resistance decreases over the first few weeks of life, pulmonary blood flow increases dramatically, resulting in mild cyanosis and congestive heart failure.

into the truncus. When the pulmonary vascular resistance is relatively high immediately after birth, pulmonary blood flow may be normal; as pulmonary resistance drops over the 1st mo of life, blood flow to the lungs is greatly increased and heart failure ensues. Truncus arteriosus is a *total mixing lesion;* there is total admixture of pulmonary and systemic venous returns. Because of the large volume of pulmonary blood flow, clinical cyanosis is usually minimal. If the lesion is left untreated, the pulmonary resistance eventually increases, pulmonary blood flow decreases, and cyanosis becomes more apparent (Eisenmenger's physiology; see Chapter 440.2). The truncal valve is occasionally incompetent, significantly complicating medical and surgical management.

CLINICAL MANIFESTATIONS. The clinical signs of truncus arteriosus vary with age, depending on the level of the pulmonary vascular resistance. In the immediate newborn period, signs of heart failure are usually absent; a murmur and minimal cyanosis are the presenting signs. In the majority of older infants, pulmonary blood flow is torrential and the clinical picture is dominated by heart failure. Cyanosis is minimal. The runoff of blood from the truncus to the pulmonary circulation may result in a wide pulse pressure and bounding pulses. This may be further exaggerated if there is truncal valve insufficiency. The heart is usually enlarged, and the precordium is hyperdynamic. The 2nd heart sound is loud and single. A systolic ejection murmur, sometimes accompanied by a thrill, is usually audible along the left sternal border. The murmur is frequently preceded by an early systolic ejection click. In the presence of truncal valve insufficiency, a high-pitched early diastolic decrescendo murmur is heard at the mid left sternal border. An apical mid-diastolic rumbling murmur, caused by increased flow through the mitral valve, is audible with the bell of the stethoscope. In older children with restricted pulmonary blood flow secondary to the development of pulmonary vascular obstructive disease, progressive cyanosis, polycythemia, and clubbing develop. Truncus arteriosus may be associated with DiGeorge syndrome (Chapter 125.1).

LABORATORY DIAGNOSIS. The *electrocardiogram* shows right, left, or combined ventricular hypertrophy. There is also considerable variation in the *chest roentgenogram.* Cardiac enlargement is due to prominence of both ventricles. The truncus may produce a prominent shadow that follows the normal course of the ascending aorta and aortic knob; the aortic arch is to the right in 50% of patients. Sometimes a high bulge, left of the aortic knob, is produced by the main or left pulmonary artery. The pulmonary vascularity is increased after the 1st few weeks of life. *Echocardiography* demonstrates the large truncal artery overriding the VSD and the pattern of origin of the branch pulmonary arteries. Associated anomalies, such as an interrupted aortic arch, may be noted. Pulsed and color Doppler studies are used to evaluate truncal valve regurgitation. If required, *cardiac catheterization* shows a left-to-right shunt at the ventricular level, with right-to-left shunting into the truncus. Systolic pressures in both ventricles and the truncus are similar. Angiography reveals the large truncus arteriosus and defines more precisely the origin of the pulmonary arteries.

PROGNOSIS AND COMPLICATIONS. Without surgery, many of these patients succumb during infancy or by the 1st or 2nd yr of life. If pulmonary blood flow is restricted by the development of pulmonary vascular disease, the patient may survive into early adulthood.

TREATMENT. In the first few weeks of life, many of these infants can be managed with anticongestive medications; however, as pulmonary vascular resistance falls, heart failure symptoms worsen and surgery is indicated, usually at 4–8 wk of life. Delay of surgery much beyond this period may increase the likelihood of the development of pulmonary vascular disease. At surgery, the VSD is closed, the pulmonary arteries are separated from the truncus, and continuity is established between the right ventricle and the pulmonary arteries with a homograft conduit (Rastelli repair). Immediate surgical results are excellent, but after repair the conduit must be replaced, often several times, as the child grows. In older patients who have already acquired pulmonary vascular obstruction, routine surgical treatment is contraindicated and heart-lung transplantation is the only option.

438.9 Single Ventricle (Double-Inlet Ventricle, Univentricular Heart)

PATHOPHYSIOLOGY. With a single ventricle, both atria empty through a common atrioventricular valve or via two separate valves into a single ventricular chamber, with *total mixing* of systemic and pulmonary venous returns. This chamber may have left, right, or indeterminate ventricular anatomic characteristics. The aorta and pulmonary artery both arise from this single chamber, although one of the great vessels may arise from a rudimentary outflow chamber. The aorta may be posterior, anterior (*malposition*), or side by side with the pulmonary artery, and either to the right or to the left. Pulmonary stenosis or atresia is common.

CLINICAL MANIFESTATIONS. The clinical picture is variable, depending on the associated intracardiac anomalies. If pulmonary outflow is obstructed, the presentation may be similar to that of tetralogy of Fallot: marked cyanosis without heart failure. If pulmonary outflow is unobstructed, the presentation is similar to that of transposition with VSD: minimal cyanosis with marked heart failure.

In patients with pulmonary stenosis, cyanosis is present in infancy and increases in intensity during childhood, when clubbing and polycythemia appear. Dyspnea and fatigue are frequent, cardiomegaly is mild or moderate, a left parasternal lift is palpable, and a systolic thrill is common. The systolic ejection murmur is usually loud; an ejection click may be audible, and the 2nd heart sound is single and loud.

Patients with unobstructed pulmonary outflow have torrential pulmonary blood flow and present in early infancy with tachypnea, dyspnea, failure to thrive, and recurrent pulmonary infections. Cyanosis is only mild or moderate. Cardiomegaly is generally marked, and a left parasternal lift is palpable. The systolic ejection murmur is generally not intense, and the 2nd heart sound is loud and closely split. A 3rd heart sound is common and may be followed by a short mid-diastolic rumbling murmur caused by increased flow through the atrioventricular valves. The eventual development of pulmonary vascular disease reduces pulmonary blood flow so that cyanosis increases and signs of cardiac failure appear to improve (Eisenmenger's physiology; see Chapter 440.2).

LABORATORY DIAGNOSIS. Findings on the *electrocardiogram* are nonspecific. P waves are normal, spiked, or bifid. The precordial lead pattern suggests right ventricular hypertrophy, combined ventricular hypertrophy, or sometimes left ventricular dominance. The initial QRS forces are usually to the left and anterior. *Roentgenographic examination* confirms the degree of cardiomegaly. If present, a rudimentary outflow chamber may produce a bulge on the upper left border of the cardiac silhouette in the posteroanterior projection. In the absence of pulmonary stenosis, the pulmonary vasculature is increased. In the presence of pulmonary stenosis, the pulmonary vasculature is diminished. Absence or near absence of the ventricular septum is the principal *echocardiographic* sign. The echocardiogram can usually determine whether the single ventricle has right, left, or mixed morphologic features. The presence of a rudimentary outflow chamber under one of the great vessels can be identified, and pulsed Doppler can be used to determine whether there is any obstruction to flow through this communication (*bulboventricular foramen*).

If *cardiac catheterization* is performed, the arterial oxygen saturation is seen to be decreased in the presence of severe pulmonary stenosis or obstructive pulmonary hypertension but may be near normal when pulmonary blood flow is unimpeded. The pressure in the ventricular chamber is at systemic level; a gradient may be demonstrated across the entrance to a rudimentary outflow chamber. Pressure measurements and angiography demonstrate whether pulmonary stenosis is present. Severe pulmonary hypertension may be demonstrated in older patients in the absence of pulmonary stenosis.

PROGNOSIS AND COMPLICATIONS. Unoperated, some patients succumb during infancy from heart failure. Others may survive to adolescence and early adult life but finally succumb to the effects of chronic hypoxemia or, in the absence of pulmonary stenosis, to those of pulmonary vascular disease. Patients with moderate pulmonary stenosis have the best prognosis because pulmonary blood flow, although restricted, is still adequate.

TREATMENT. If pulmonary stenosis is severe, an aortopulmonary shunt is indicated. If pulmonary blood flow is unrestricted, pulmonary arterial banding is used to control heart failure and to prevent progressive pulmonary vascular disease. The *Glenn shunt* followed by a modified *Fontan* operation (cavopulmonary isolation procedure, see Chapter 437.4) is the ultimate treatment of choice. If subaortic stenosis is present secondary to a restrictive connection to a rudimentary outflow chamber, surgical relief can be provided by anastomosing the proximal pulmonary artery to the side of the ascending aorta (*Damus-Stansyl-Kaye operation*).

438.10 Hypoplastic Left Heart Syndrome

PATHOPHYSIOLOGY. The term *hypoplastic left heart* is used to describe a related group of anomalies that include underdevelopment of the left side of the heart (e.g., atresia of the aortic or mitral orifice) and hypoplasia of the ascending aorta. The left ventricle may be small and nonfunctional or totally atretic; the right ventricle maintains both pulmonary and systemic circulations (Fig. 438–7). Pulmonary venous blood passes through an atrial defect or dilated foramen ovale from the left to the right side of the heart, where it mixes with systemic venous blood (*total mixing lesion*). When the ventricular septum is intact, which is usually the case, all the right ventricular blood is ejected into the main pulmonary artery; the descending aorta is supplied via the ductus arteriosus, with flow from the ductus also filling the ascending aorta and coronary arteries in a retrograde fashion. In the presence of a VSD and a patent but small aortic orifice, right ventricular blood is ejected to the small left ventricle and ascending aorta, as well as to the pulmonary artery. The major hemodynamic abnormalities are inadequate maintenance of the systemic circulation and, depending on the size of the atrial level communication, either pulmonary venous hypertension (restrictive foramen ovale) or pulmonary overcirculation (moderate or large ASD).

CLINICAL MANIFESTATIONS. Although cyanosis may not always be obvious in the first 48 hr of life, a grayish blue color of the skin is soon apparent, denoting a mix of cyanosis and hypoperfusion. Most infants are diagnosed in the 1st few hours or days of life. If the ductus arteriosus partially closes, signs of systemic hypoperfusion and shock predominate. Signs of heart failure usually appear within the 1st few days or weeks of life and include dyspnea, hepatomegaly, and low cardiac output. The peripheral pulses may be weak or absent. Cardiac enlargement is usual, with a palpable right ventricular parasternal lift. A nondescript systolic murmur is usually present. Extracardiac anomalies, particularly of the kidney and central nervous system, may be present.

LABORATORY DIAGNOSIS. On the *chest roentgenogram*, the heart is variable in size in the 1st days of life, but cardiomegaly develops rapidly and is associated with increased pulmonary

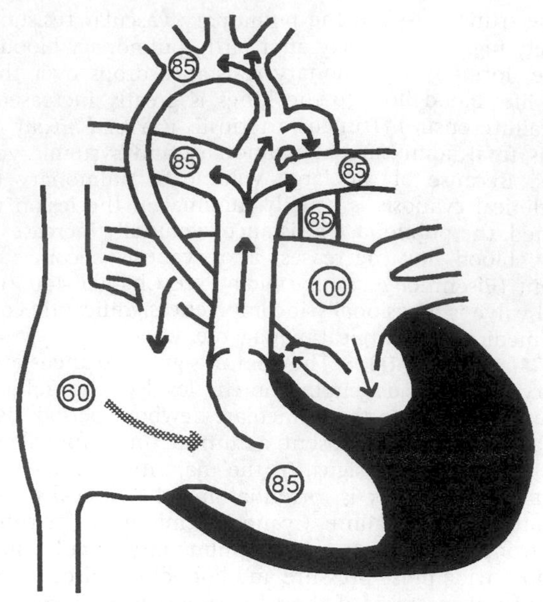

Figure 438–7 Physiology of hypoplastic left heart syndrome (HLHS). The circled numbers represent oxygen saturation values. HLHS is not a single lesion but a constellation of different degrees of hypoplasia of left-sided heart structures. In this example, there is a patent mitral valve, a small left ventricular cavity, and a diminutive ascending aorta. The right atrial (mixed venous) oxygen saturation is decreased secondary to systemic hypoxemia. Desaturated blood enters the right atrium, flows through the tricuspid valve into the right ventricle, and is ejected into the pulmonary artery. Owing to the markedly decreased left ventricular compliance, most of the pulmonary venous blood returning to the left atrium shunts left to right at the atrial level. A small amount of left atrial blood will cross the mitral valve and be ejected into the tiny ascending aorta. The right ventricular oxygen saturation represents a mixing of desaturated systemic venous blood and saturated pulmonary venous blood. Pulmonary artery blood flows into the pulmonary arteries as well as right to left across the patent ductus arteriosus (PDA) into the aorta. Ductal blood flows prograde to the descending aorta as well as retrograde to the ascending aorta, supplying the head and neck vessels as well as the coronary arteries (which arise off the small ascending aorta). Closure of the PDA results in profound hypoxia as well as circulatory collapse.

vascularity. The *electrocardiogram* may show only the normal right ventricular dominance initially, but later P waves become prominent and right ventricular hypertrophy is usual. The *echocardiogram* is diagnostic. There is absence or hypoplasia of the mitral valve and aortic root, a variably small left atrium and left ventricle, and a large right atrium and right ventricle. The size of the atrial communication, by which pulmonary venous blood leaves the left atrium, can be assessed directly and by pulsed and color flow Doppler studies. Suprasternal notch views identify the small ascending aorta and transverse aortic arch and may also demonstrate a discrete coarctation of the aorta in the juxtaductal area. Doppler echocardiography demonstrates the absence of anterograde flow in the ascending aorta and retrograde flow via the ductus arteriosus. These findings are so characteristic that the diagnosis of hypoplastic left heart syndrome can usually be made without the need for *cardiac catheterization*. If a catheterization is necessary, the hypoplastic ascending aorta can be demonstrated by angiography.

PROGNOSIS AND COMPLICATIONS. Patients most often succumb during the 1st months of life, usually during the first week or two. Occasionally, unoperated patients may live for months or rarely years. One third of infants with hypoplastic left heart syndrome have evidence of either a major or minor central nervous system abnormality. Other dysmorphic features may be found in up to 40% of patients. Thus, careful preoperative evaluation (genetic, neurologic, and ophthalmologic) should be performed in patients being considered for either standard surgical therapy or cardiac transplantation.

TREATMENT. There is variable success in the surgical therapy of hypoplastic left heart syndrome. Management options include palliation (the Norwood procedure; Fig. 438–8), heart transplantation and, in some patients, supportive expectant care. There is considerable controversy as to which of the two surgical options is optimal, as well as disagreement over whether a "do nothing" option should be offered to parents.

If a **Norwood procedure** is to be performed, preoperative medical management includes correction of acidosis and hypoglycemia, maintenance of the patency of the ductus arteriosus with prostaglandin E_1 to support systemic blood flow, and prevention of hypothermia. Dilatation of the atrial septum may be indicated if surgery is delayed.

The Norwood procedure is usually performed in three stages. The first stage (see Fig. 438–8) includes an atrial septectomy and transection and ligation of the distal main pulmonary

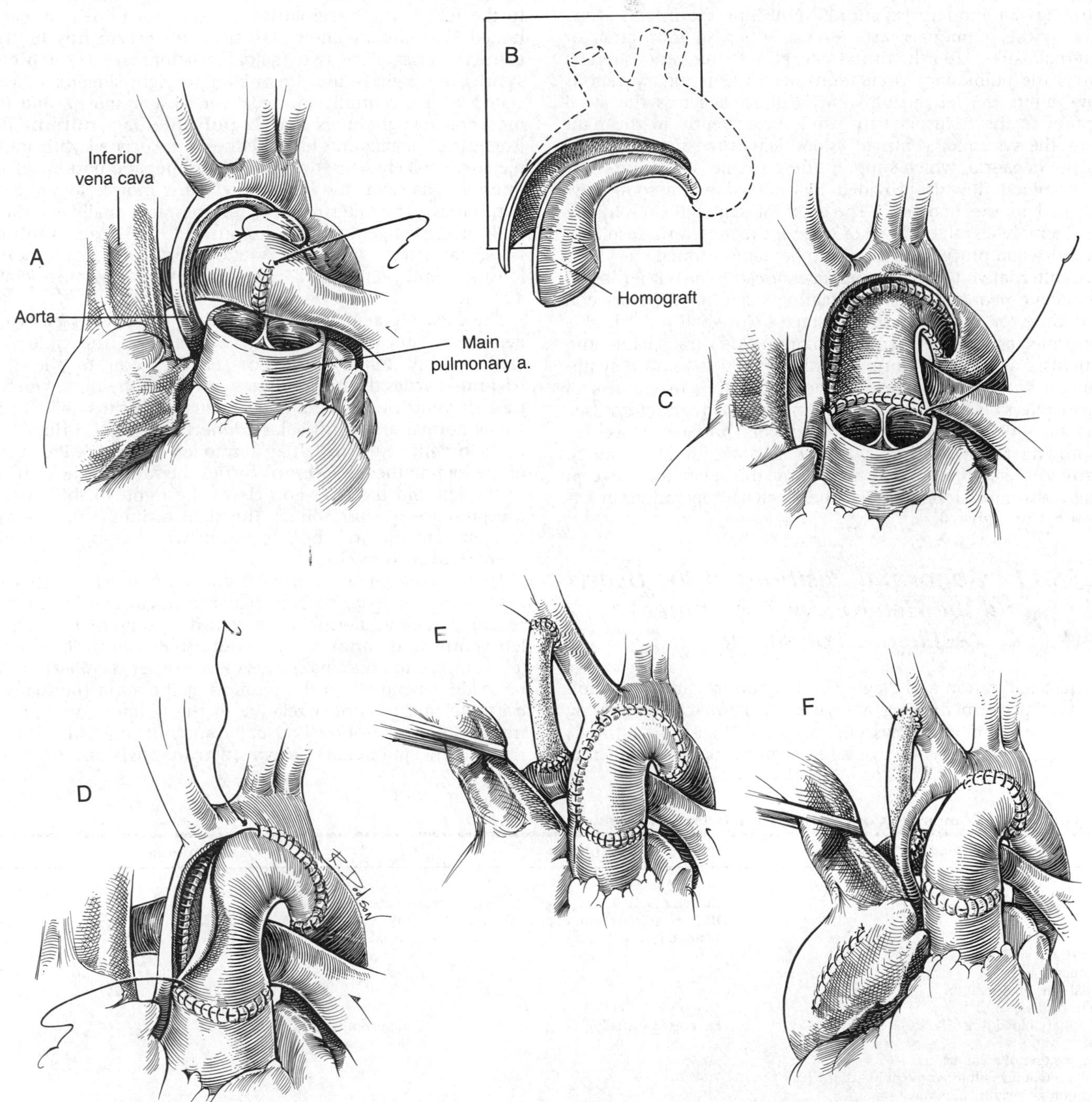

Figure 438–8 Current technique for first-stage palliation of the hypoplastic left heart syndrome. *A*, Incisions used for the procedure, incorporating a cuff of arterial wall allograft. The distal divided main pulmonary artery may be closed by direct suture or with a patch. *B*, Dimensions of the cuff of the arterial wall allograft. *C*, The arterial wall allograft is used to supplement the anastomosis between the proximal divided main pulmonary artery and the ascending aorta, aortic arch, and proximal descending aorta. *D* and *E*, The procedure is completed by an atrial septectomy and a 3.5 mm modified right Blalock shunt. *F*, When the ascending aorta is particularly small, an alternative procedure involves placement of a complete tube of arterial allograft. The tiny ascending aorta may be left in situ, as indicated, or implanted into the side of the neoaorta. (From Castañeda AR, Jonas RA, Mayer Jr JE, Hanley FL: Single-ventricle tricuspid atresia. *In*: Cardiac Surgery of the Neonate and Infant. Philadelphia, WB Saunders, 1994.)

artery; the proximal pulmonary artery is then connected to the transversely opened hypoplastic aortic arch, forming a neoaorta, and the coarcted segment of the aorta is repaired. A synthetic aortopulmonary shunt connects the aorta to the main pulmonary artery to provide controlled pulmonary blood flow. The operative risk for the first-stage Norwood procedure is high and varies greatly among centers, although the best reported results demonstrate a better than 75% survival.

The second stage consists of a Glenn anastomosis, connecting the superior vena cava to the pulmonary arteries (see Chapter 437.4). This is followed by a modified Fontan procedure (cavopulmonary isolation) connecting the inferior vena cava to the pulmonary arteries via either an intra-atrial or external baffle. After the third stage, all systemic venous return enters the pulmonary circulation directly. Pulmonary venous flow enters the left atrium and is directed across the atrial septum to the tricuspid valve and subsequently to the right (now the systemic) ventricle. Blood leaves the right ventricle via the neoaorta, which supplies the systemic circulation. Coronary blood flow is provided by the old aortic root, now attached to the neoaorta. The risks of stages II and III are considerably less than those of stage I; the long-term results of the Norwood procedure remain to be demonstrated.

An alternative therapy is *cardiac transplantation*, either in the immediate neonatal period, obviating stage I of the Norwood procedure, or after a successful stage I Norwood procedure is performed as a bridge to transplantation. After transplantation, patients usually have normal cardiac function and no symptoms of heart failure; these patients have the chronic risk of organ rejection and lifelong immunosuppressive therapy (see Chapter 449). A combination of donor shortage as well as improving results with the Norwood procedure has caused many centers to stop recommending transplantation except when associated lesions make the Norwood operation an exceptionally high risk.

438.11 Abnormal Positions of the Heart and the Heterotaxy Syndromes (Asplenia, Polysplenia)

The classification and diagnosis of abnormal cardiac position are best performed using a segmental approach, identifying first the position of the viscera and atria, then the ventricles, followed by the great vessels. Determination of *visceroatrial situs* can be made by roentgenographic demonstration of the position of the abdominal organs and of the tracheal bifurcation for recognition of the right and left bronchi, and by *echocardiography*. The atrial situs is related to the situs of the viscera and lungs. In **situs solitus**, the viscera are in their normal positions (stomach and spleen on the left, liver on the right), the three-lobed right lung is on the right, and the two-lobed left lung on the left; the right atrium is on the right, whereas the left atrium is on the left. When the abdominal organs and lungs are reversed, an arrangement known as **situs inversus**, the left atrium is to the right and the right atrium to the left. If the visceroatrial situs cannot be readily determined, a condition known as **situs indeterminus** or **heterotaxia** exists. The two major variations are (1) **asplenia syndrome** (right isomerism or bilateral right-sidedness), associated with a centrally located liver, absent spleen, and two morphologic right lungs; and (2) **polysplenia syndrome** (left isomerism, or bilateral left-sidedness), associated with multiple small spleens, absence of the intrahepatic portion of the inferior vena cava, and bilateral left lung morphology (i.e., in both lungs). The heterotaxia syndromes are usually associated with severe congenital heart lesions: ASD, VSD, atrioventricular septal defect, pulmonary stenosis or atresia, and anomalous systemic venous or pulmonary venous return (Table 438–2).

The next segment is the *localization of the ventricles*, which depends on the direction of development of the embryonic cardiac loop. Initial protrusion of the loop to the right (**d-loop**) carries the future right ventricle to the right, whereas the left ventricle remains on the left. With situs solitus, this yields normal atrioventricular connections (right atrium connects to right ventricle, left atrium to left ventricle). Protrusion of the loop to the left (**l-loop**) carries the future right ventricle to the left and the left ventricle to the right. In this case, in the presence of situs solitus, the right atrium connects with the left ventricle and the left atrium with the right ventricle (**ventricular inversion**).

The final segment is that of the *great vessels*. With each type of cardiac loop, the ventricular-arterial relations may be regarded as either normal (right ventricle to pulmonary artery, left ventricle to aorta) or transposed (right ventricle to aorta, left ventricle to pulmonary artery). A further classification can be made depending on the position of the aorta (normally to the right and posterior) relative to the pulmonary artery. In transposition, the aorta is usually anterior and either to the right of the pulmonary artery (**d-transposition**) or to the

TABLE 438–2 Comparison of Cardiosplenic Heterotaxy Syndromes

Feature	Asplenia	Polysplenia
Spleen	Absent	Multiple
Sidedness (isomerism)	Bilateral right	Bilateral left
Lungs	Bilateral trilobar with eparterial bronchi	Bilateral bilobar with hyparterial bronchi
Sex	Male (65%)	Female ≥ male
Right-sided stomach	Yes	Less common
Symmetric liver	Yes	Yes
Partial intestinal rotation	Yes	Yes
Dextrocardia (%)	30–40	30–40
Pulmonary blood flow	Decreased (usually)	Increased (usually)
Severe cyanosis	Yes	No
Transposition of great arteries (%)	60–75	15
Total anomalous pulmonary venous return (%)	70–80	Rare
Common atrioventricular valve (%)	80–90	20–40
Single ventricle (%)	40–50	10–15
Absent inferior vena cava with azygos continuation	No	Characteristic
Bilateral superior vena cava	Yes	Yes
Other common defects	PA, PS	Partial anomalous pulmonary venous return, ventricular septal defect, double-outlet right ventricle
Risk of sepsis	Yes	No
Howell-Jolly and Heinz bodies, pitted erythrocytes	Yes	No
Absent gallbladder; biliary atresia	No	Yes
Mortality	High	Moderately high if symptomatic

PA = pulmonary atresia; PS = pulmonary stenosis.

left (**l-transposition**). These segmental relationships can be determined by *echocardiographic* and *angiographic* studies demonstrating both atrioventricular and ventriculoarterial relationships. The clinical manifestations of these syndromes of abnormal cardiac position are determined primarily by their associated cardiovascular anomalies.

Dextrocardia occurs when the heart is in the right chest; **levocardia** (the normal situation) is present when the heart is in the left chest. *Dextrocardia without associated situs inversus* and *levocardia in the presence of situs inversus* are most often complicated by severe malformations that include various combinations of single ventricle, arterial transposition, pulmonary stenosis, ASDs and VSDs, atrioventricular septal defect, anomalous pulmonary venous return, tricuspid atresia, and pulmonary arterial hypoplasia or atresia. Surveys of older children and adults indicate that dextrocardia with situs inversus and with normally related great arteries (so-called *mirror-image dextrocardia*) is often associated with a functionally normal heart, although congenital heart disease of a less severe nature is common.

Anatomic or functional abnormalities of the lung, diaphragm, and thoracic cage may result in displacement of the heart to the right (**dextroposition**). However, in this case the *cardiac apex* is pointed normally to the left. This is less often associated with congenital heart lesions, although hypoplasia of a lung may be accompanied by anomalous pulmonary venous return from that lung (scimitar syndrome).

The *electrocardiogram* is difficult to interpret in the presence of lesions with discordant atrial, ventricular, and great vessel anatomy. Diagnosis usually requires detailed *echocardiographic* and *cardiac catheterization* studies. Prognosis and treatment of patients with one of the cardiac positional anomalies are determined by the underlying defects. Asplenia increases the risk of serious infections such as bacterial sepsis and requires daily antibiotic prophylaxis.

Transposition of the Great Arteries

Hayes CJ, Gersony WM: Arrhythmias after the Mustard operation for transposition of the great arteries: A long term study. J Am Coll Cardiol 7:133, 1986.

Kirklin JW, Blackstone EH, Tchervenkov CI, et al: Clinical outcomes after the arterial switch operation for transposition: Patient, support, procedural, and institutional risk factors. Circulation 86:1501, 1992.

Newburger JW, Sibert AR, Buckley LP, et al: Cognitive function and age at repair of transpositon of the great arteries in children. N Engl J Med 310:1495, 1984.

Quaegebeur JM, Rohmer J, Ottenkamp J, et al: The arterial switch operation. J Thorac Cardiovasc Surg 92:361, 1986.

Rashkind WJ, Miller WW: Creation of an atrial septal defect without thoracotomy: A palliative approach to complete transposition of the great vessels. JAMA 196:991, 1966.

Rastelli GC, McGoon DC, Wallace RB: Anatomic correction of transposition of the great arteries with ventricular septal defect and subpulmonary stenosis. J Thorac Cardiovasc Surg 58:545, 1969.

Truncus Arteriosus

Bove EL, Lupinetti FM, Pridjian AK, et al: Results of a policy of primary repair of truncus arteriosus in the neonate. J Thorac Cardiovasc Surg 105:1057, 1993.

Heinemann MK, Hanley FL, Fenton KN, et al: Fate of small homograft conduits after early repair of truncus arteriosus. Ann Thorac Surg 55:1409, 1993.

Kirby ML: Cellular and molecular contributions of the cardiac neural crest to cardiovascular development. Trends Cardiovasc Med 3:18, 1993.

Wilson DI, Burn J, Scambler P, et al: DiGeorge syndrome: Part of CATCH 22. J Med Genet 30:852, 1993.

Total Anomalous Pulmonary Venous Return

Choe YH, Lee HJ, Kim HS, et al: MRI of total anomalous pulmonary venous connections. J Comput Assist Tomogr 18:243, 1994.

Duff DG, Nihill MR, McNamara DG: Infradiaphragmatic total anomalous pulmonary venous return. Review of clinical and pathological findings and results of operation in 28 cases. Br Heart J 39:619, 1977.

Huhta J, Gutgesell HP, Nihill MR: Cross sectional echocardiographic diagnosis of total anomalous pulmonary venous connection. Br Heart J 53:525, 1985.

Hypoplastic Left Heart Syndrome

Chiavarelli M, Gundry SR, Razzouk AJ, et al: Cardiac transplantation for infants with hypoplastic left heart syndrome. JAMA 270:2944, 1993.

Glauser TA, Rorke LB, Weinberg PM: Congenital brain abnormalities associated with the hypoplastic left heart syndrome. Pediatrics 85:984, 1990.

OKelly S, Bove E: Hypoplastic left heart syndrome. Br Med J 314:87, 1997.

Starnes VA, Griffin ML, Pitlick PT, et al: Current approach to hypoplastic left heart syndrome: Palliation, transplantation or both? J Thorac Cardiovasc Surg 104:189, 1992.

Dextrocardia and Levocardia

Britz-Cunningham SH, Shah MM, Zuppan CW, et al: Mutation of the connexin 43 gap-junction gene in patients with heart malformations and defects of laterality. N Engl J Med 332:1323, 1995.

Rose V, Izukawa T, Moes CAF: Syndromes of asplenia and polysplenia: A review of cardiac and non-cardiac malformations in 60 cases with special reference to diagnosis and prognosis. Br Heart J 37:840, 1975.

CHAPTER 439
Other Congenital Heart and Vascular Malformations

439.1 Anomalies of the Aortic Arch

RIGHT AORTIC ARCH. In this abnormality, the aorta curves to the right and, if it descends on the right side of the vertebral column, is usually associated with other cardiac malformations. It is found in 20% of cases of tetralogy of Fallot and is common in truncus arteriosus. A right aortic arch without other cardiac anomalies is not associated with symptoms. It can often be visualized on the chest roentgenogram. The trachea is deviated to the left of the midline rather than to the right, as in the presence of a normal left arch. On a barium esophagram, the esophagus is indented on its right border at the level of the aortic arch.

VASCULAR RINGS. Congenital abnormalities of the aortic arch and its major branches result in the formation of vascular rings around the trachea and esophagus with varying degrees of compression. Common anomalies include (1) double aortic arch (Fig. 439–1*A*), (2) right aortic arch with left ligamentum arteriosum, (3) anomalous innominate artery arising further to the left on the arch than usual, (4) anomalous left carotid artery arising further to the right than usual and passing anterior to the trachea, and (5) anomalous left pulmonary artery (vascular sling). In the latter anomaly, the abnormal vessel arises from an elongated main pulmonary artery or from the right pulmonary artery. It courses between and compresses the trachea and the esophagus. Associated congenital heart disease may be present in 5–50% of patients, depending on the vascular anomaly.

CLINICAL MANIFESTATIONS. If the vascular ring produces compression of the trachea and esophagus, symptoms are frequently present during infancy. Chronic wheezing is exacerbated by crying, feeding, and flexion of the neck. Extension of the neck tends to relieve the noisy respiration. Vomiting is frequent. There may be a brassy cough, pneumonia, or sudden death from aspiration.

LABORATORY DIAGNOSIS. Roentgenographic examination of the barium-filled esophagus (Fig. 439–2) and aortography identify the anomaly. An aberrant right subclavian artery is commonly seen but does not cause compression of the trachea. Diagnosis is confirmed by two-dimensional echocardiography, magnetic resonance imaging, computed tomography, or angiography during cardiac catheterization. Bronchoscopy may be used to determine the extent of airway narrowing.

TREATMENT. Surgery is advised for symptomatic patients who have roentgenographic evidence of tracheal compression. The anterior vessel is usually divided in patients with double aortic

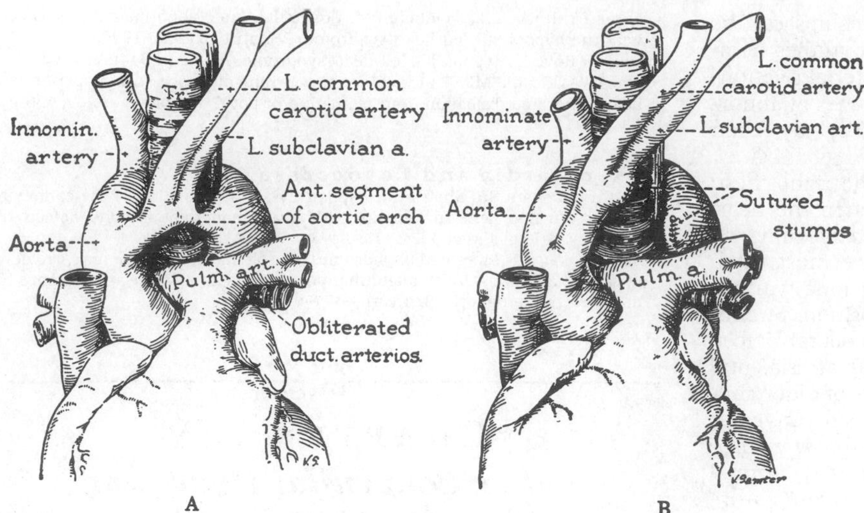

Figure 439–1 Double aortic arch. *A*, Small anterior segment of the double aortic arch (most common type). *B*, Operative procedure for the release of the vascular ring.

arch (see Fig. 439–1*B*). Compression produced by a right aortic arch and left ligamentum arteriosum is relieved by division of the latter. Anomalous innominate or carotid arteries cannot be divided; the tracheal compression is usually relieved by attaching the adventitia of these vessels to the sternum. An anomalous left pulmonary artery is corrected during cardiopulmonary bypass by division at its origin and reanastomosis to the main pulmonary artery after it has been brought in front of the trachea. In this condition, severe tracheomalacia may be present and may require reconstruction of the trachea as well.

439.2 Anomalous Origin of the Coronary Arteries

ANOMALOUS ORIGIN OF THE LEFT CORONARY ARTERY FROM THE PULMONARY ARTERY

In anomalous origin of the left coronary artery from the pulmonary artery, the blood supply to the left ventricular myocardium is severely compromised. Soon after birth, as the pulmonary arterial pressure falls, the perfusion pressure to the left coronary artery becomes inadequate; myocardial ischemia, infarction, and fibrosis result. In some cases, interarterial collateral anastomoses develop between the right and left coronary arteries. Blood flow in the left coronary artery is then reversed, and it empties into the pulmonary artery, resulting in a "myocardial steal" syndrome. The left ventricle becomes dilated, and performance is decreased. Mitral insufficiency is a frequent complication secondary to infarction of a papillary muscle or to a dilated valve ring. Localized aneurysms may also develop in the left ventricular free wall. Occasional patients have adequate myocardial blood flow during childhood and present later in life with a continuous murmur and a small left-to-right shunt via the dilated coronary system (aorta to right coronary to left coronary to pulmonary artery).

CLINICAL MANIFESTATIONS. Evidence of heart failure becomes apparent within the 1st few months of life and is often precipitated by respiratory infection. Recurrent attacks of discomfort, restlessness, irritability, sweating, dyspnea, and pallor with or without mild cyanosis occur and could be interpreted as angina

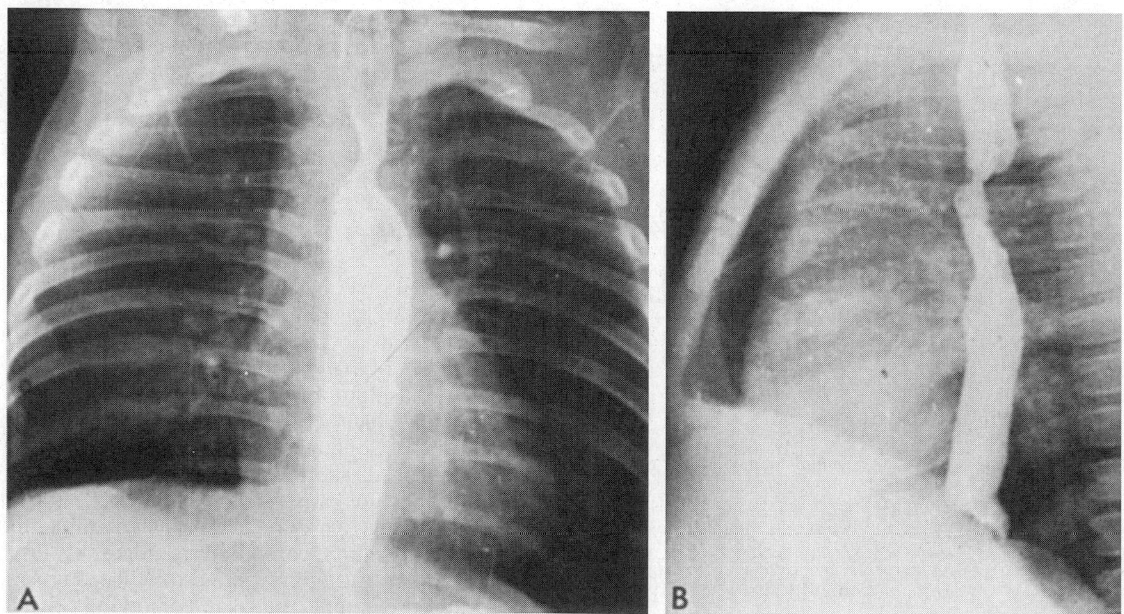

Figure 439–2 Double aortic arch in an infant aged 5 mo. *A*, Anteroposterior view. The barium-filled esophagus is constricted on both sides. *B*, Lateral view. The esophagus is displaced forward. The anterior arch was the smaller and was divided at operation.

pectoris. Cardiac enlargement is moderate to massive. A gallop rhythm is common. If a gallop is present, murmurs may be of the nonspecific, ejection type or may be holosystolic resulting from mitral insufficiency. Older patients with abundant intercoronary anastomoses may have continuous murmurs and minimal left ventricular dysfunction. During adolescence, they may present with angina during exercise. Rare patients with anomalous right coronary artery may present in this manner.

LABORATORY DIAGNOSIS. *Roentgenographic examination* confirms the cardiomegaly. The *electrocardiogram* resembles the pattern described in lateral wall myocardial infarction in adults. A QR pattern followed by inverted T waves is seen in leads I and aVL. The left ventricular surface leads (V_5 and V_6) may also show deep Q waves and exhibit elevated ST segments and inverted T waves (Fig. 439–3). In older patients, an exercise study may be helpful, as ST-T wave changes or symptoms occur. *Two-dimensional echocardiography* may suggest the diagnosis; echo is not always reliable in diagnosing this condition. On two-dimensional imaging alone, the left coronary artery can appear as if it were arising from the aorta. Color Doppler ultrasound examination has improved the accuracy of diagnosis of this lesion and may demonstrate retrograde flow in the left coronary artery. *Cardiac catheterization* is diagnostic; on *aortography* there is immediate opacification of the right coronary artery only. Generally, this vessel is large and tortuous. After filling of the intercoronary anastomoses, the left coronary artery is opacified, and contrast can be seen to enter the pulmonary artery. Pulmonary arteriography may also opacify the origin of the anomalous left coronary artery. Selective left ventriculography usually demonstrates a dilatated left ventricle that empties poorly.

TREATMENT AND PROGNOSIS. Usually death from heart failure occurs within the first 6 mo. Those who survive usually have abundant intercoronary collateral anastomoses. Medical management includes standard therapy for heart failure (diuretics, digoxin, captopril) and for controlling ischemia (nitrates, beta-blocking agents).

Surgical treatment consists of detaching the anomalous coronary artery from the pulmonary artery and anastomosing it to the aorta to establish normal myocardial perfusion. The seriously ill infant with a tiny left coronary artery may present a difficult technical problem. Ligation of the anomalous left coronary artery at its origin was once carried out to prevent runoff from the coronary circuit and possibly to increase myocardial perfusion by the collateral circulation. This operation may occasionally be required. In patients who have already sustained a significant myocardial infarction, cardiac transplantation is the surgical option.

ANOMALOUS ORIGIN OF THE RIGHT CORONARY ARTERY FROM THE PULMONARY ARTERY

Anomalous origin of the right coronary artery from the pulmonary artery rarely manifests in infancy or early childhood. The left coronary artery is enlarged, whereas the right is thin-walled and mildly enlarged. In early infancy, perfusion of the right coronary artery is from the pulmonary artery, whereas later, perfusion is from collaterals of the left coronary vessels. Angina and sudden death can occur in adolescence or adulthood. When recognized, this anomaly should be repaired by reanastomosis of the right coronary artery to the aorta.

ECTOPIC ORIGIN OF THE CORONARY ARTERY FROM THE AORTA WITH ABERRANT PROXIMAL COURSE

In ectopic origin of the coronary artery from the aorta with aberrant proximal course, the aberrant artery may be a left, right, or major branch coronary artery. The site of origin may be the wrong sinus of Valsalva or a proximal coronary artery. The ostium may be hypoplastic, slitlike, or of normal caliber. The aberrant vessel may pass anteriorly, posteriorly, or between the aorta and right ventricular outflow tract; it may tunnel in the conal or interventricular septal tissue. Obstruction due to hypoplasia of the ostia, tunneling between the aorta and right ventricular outflow tract or interventricular septum, and acute angulation produces focal myocardial fibrosis or myocardial infarction. Unobstructive vessels produce no symptoms. Patients with this extremely rare abnormality may manifest myocardial infarction, ventricular arrhythmias, angina pectoris, or syncope; sudden death may occur in young adult or adolescent athletes.

Laboratory diagnosis should include an electrocardiogram, stress testing, two-dimensional echocardiography, and cardiac catheterization with selective coronary angiography.

Treatment is indicated for obstructed vessels and consists of aortoplasty with reanastomosis of the aberrant vessel or, more often, coronary artery bypass grafting using the internal mammary artery.

439.3 Pulmonary Arteriovenous Fistula

Fistulous vascular communications in the lungs may be large and localized, or multiple, scattered, and small. The most com-

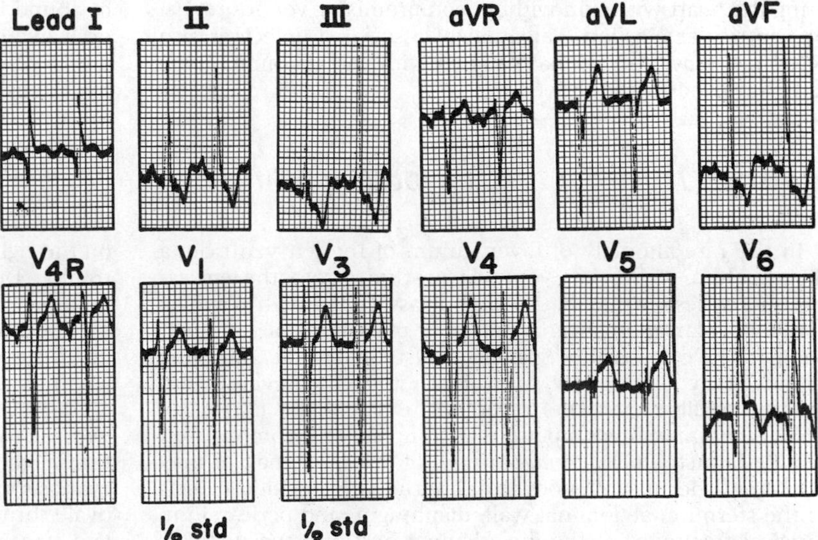

Figure 439–3 Electrocardiogram of 3-mo-old child with anomalous origin of the left coronary artery from the pulmonary artery. Lateral myocardial infarction is present as evidenced by abnormally large and wide Q waves in leads I, V5, and V6; elevated ST segment in V5 and V6; and inversion of TV6.

mon form of this unusual condition is the **Osler-Weber-Rendu syndrome** (hereditary hemorrhagic telangiectasia), which is also manifested by angiomas of the nasal and buccal mucous membranes, gastrointestinal tract, or liver. The usual communication is between the pulmonary artery and pulmonary vein; direct communication between the pulmonary artery and left atrium is extremely rare. Desaturated blood in the pulmonary artery is shunted through the fistula into the pulmonary vein, bypassing the lungs, and enters the left side of the heart; this results in systemic arterial desaturation and sometimes clinical cyanosis. The shunt across the fistula is at low pressure and resistance so that pulmonary arterial pressure is normal; cardiomegaly and heart failure are not present.

The *clinical manifestations* depend on the magnitude of the shunt. Large fistulas are associated with dyspnea, cyanosis, clubbing, a continuous murmur, and polycythemia. Hemoptysis is rare, but when it occurs it may be massive. Features of the Osler-Weber-Rendu syndrome occur in about 50% of patients (or other family members) and include recurrent epistaxis and gastrointestinal tract bleeding. Transitory dizziness, diplopia, aphasia, motor weakness, or convulsions may result from cerebral thrombosis, abscess, or paradoxical emboli. Soft systolic or continuous murmurs may be audible over the site of the fistula. The electrocardiogram is normal. Roentgenographic examination of the chest may show opacities produced by large fistulas; multiple small fistulas may be visualized by fluoroscopy (as abnormal pulsations), magnetic resonance imaging, or computed tomography. Selective pulmonary arteriography demonstrates the site, extent, and distribution of the fistulas.

Treatment by excision of solitary or localized lesions by lobectomy or wedge resection results in complete disappearance of symptoms. In most instances, fistulas are so widespread that surgery is not possible. If there is a direct communication between the pulmonary artery and the left atrium, it can be obliterated by division and suture.

439.4 Ectopia Cordis

In the most common thoracic form of ectopia cordis, the sternum is split and the heart protrudes outside the chest. In other forms, the heart protrudes through the diaphragm into the abdominal cavity or may be situated in the neck. Associated intracardiac anomalies are common. Death occurs in the 1st days of life in most instances, usually from infection, cardiac failure, or hypoxemia. Surgical therapy for neonates without overwhelmingly severe cardiac anomalies consists of covering the heart with skin without compromising venous return or ventricular ejection. Palliation of associated defects is also often necessary. Occasional patients with the abdominal type have survived to adulthood.

439.5 Diverticulum of the Left Ventricle

In the rare anomaly of diverticulum of the left ventricle, a diverticulum of the left ventricle protrudes into the epigastrium. The lesion may be isolated or associated with complex cardiovascular anomalies. A pulsating mass is visible and palpable in the epigastrium. Systolic or systolic-diastolic murmurs produced by blood flow into and out of the diverticulum may be audible over the lower sternum and the mass. The *electrocardiogram* shows a pattern of complete or incomplete left bundle branch block. *Roentgenograms* of the chest may or may not show the mass. Associated abnormalities include defects of the sternum, abdominal wall, diaphragm, and pericardium. Surgical treatment of the diverticulum and of associated cardiac defects can be used in selected cases. Occasionally a diverticulum may be small and not associated with clinical signs or symptoms. These small diverticula are diagnosed at the time of echocardiographic examination for other indications.

Vascular Rings

Azarow KS, Pearl RH, Hoffman MA, et al: Vascular ring: Does magnetic resonance imaging replace angiography? Ann Thorac Surg 53:882, 1992.

Bertrand J-M, Chartrand C, Lamarre A, et al: Vascular ring: Clinical and physiological assessment of pulmonary function following surgical correction. Pediatr Pulmonol 2:378, 1986.

Murdison KA, Andrews BA, Chin AJ: Ultrasonographic display of complex vascular rings. J Am Coll Cardiol 15:1645, 1990.

Anomalous Coronary Artery

Johnsrude CL, Perry JC, Cecchin F, et al: Differentiating anomalous left main coronary artery originating from the pulmonary artery in infants from myocarditis and dilated cardiomyopathy by electrocardiogram. Am J Cardiol 75:71, 1995.

Schmidt KG, Cooper MJ, Silverman NH, Stanger P: Pulmonary artery origin of the left coronary artery: Diagnosis by two-dimensional echocardiography, pulsed Doppler ultrasound and color flow mapping. J Am Coll Cardiol 11:396, 1988.

Vouh PR, Tamisier D, Sidi D, et al: Anomalous left coronary artery from the pulmonary artery: Results of isolated aortic reimplantation. Ann Thorac Surg 54:621, 1992.

Chapter 440 Pulmonary Hypertension

440.1 Primary Pulmonary Hypertension

PATHOPHYSIOLOGY. Primary pulmonary hypertension, of unknown origin, is characterized by pulmonary vascular obstructive disease and right-sided heart failure. It may occur at any age, although most pediatric patients present in the teenage years. In older patients, females outnumber males 1.7:1; however, in younger patients, both genders are represented equally. A genetic component may be present, and there is evidence in some cases of an immunologic disorder. Diet pills, particularly fenfluramines, have also been implicated. Pulmonary hypertension is associated with precapillary obstruction of the pulmonary vascular bed due to hyperplasia of the muscular and elastic tissues and to a thickened intima of the small pulmonary arteries and arterioles. Atherosclerotic changes may be found in the larger pulmonary arteries. In children, venoocclusive disease may account for some cases of primary pulmonary hypertension. For the diagnosis of primary pulmonary hypertension, other causes of elevated pulmonary pressures must be eliminated (chronic pulmonary parenchymal disease, persistent obstruction of the upper airway, congenital cardiac malformations, recurrent pulmonary emboli, alveolar capillary dysplasia, liver disease, autoimmune disease, and moyamoya disease). Pulmonary hypertension places an afterload burden on the right ventricle, which results in right ventricular hypertrophy. Dilatation of the pulmonary artery is present, and pulmonary valve insufficiency may occur. In the later stages of the disease, the right ventricle begins to dilate, tricuspid insufficiency develops, and cardiac output is decreased. Arrhythmias, syncope, and sudden death are common.

CLINICAL MANIFESTATIONS. The predominant symptoms include exercise intolerance and fatigability; occasionally, there is precordial chest pain, dizziness, syncope, or headaches. Peripheral cyanosis may be present, especially if there is a patent foramen ovale through which blood can shunt from right to left; in the late stages of disease, the patient may have cold extremities and a gray appearance associated with low cardiac output. Arterial oxygen saturation is usually normal. If right-sided heart failure has supervened, the jugular venous pressure is elevated, and hepatomegaly and edema are present. Jugular venous "a" waves are present, and when there is functional tricuspid insufficiency, a conspicuous jugular "cv" wave and systolic hepatic pulsations are manifested. The heart is moderately enlarged, and there is a right ventricular heave. The 1st heart sound is often followed by an ejection click emanating from the dilated pulmonary artery. The 2nd heart sound is closely split, loud, and sometimes booming; it is frequently palpable at the upper left sternal border. A presystolic gallop rhythm may be audible at the lower left sternal border. The systolic murmur is soft and short and is sometimes followed by a blowing decrescendo diastolic murmur due to pulmonary insufficiency. In later stages, a holosystolic murmur of tricuspid insufficiency is appreciated at the lower left sternal border.

LABORATORY DIAGNOSIS. *Chest roentgenograms* reveal a prominent pulmonary artery and right ventricle (Fig. 440–1). The pulmonary vascularity in the hilar areas may be prominent, in contrast with the peripheral lung fields, which are clear. The *electrocardiogram* shows right ventricular hypertrophy with spiked P waves.

At *cardiac catheterization* this condition must be differentiated from **Eisenmenger syndrome** (see Chapter 440.2), which is associated with a communication between the left and right sides of the heart or great arteries, as well as from left-sided obstructive lesions that result in pulmonary venous hypertension (see Chapter 434). The presence of pulmonary artery hypertension with a normal pulmonary capillary wedge pressure is diagnostic of primary pulmonary hypertension. If the wedge pressure is elevated and left ventricular pressure end-diastolic pressure is normal, obstruction at the level of the pulmonary veins, left atrium, or mitral valve should be suspected. The risks of cardiac catheterization may be high in severely ill patients with primary pulmonary hypertension.

PROGNOSIS AND TREATMENT. Primary pulmonary hypertension is progressive, and often there is no specific treatment. Some success has been reported using oral calcium channel blocking agents such as nifedipine in children who demonstrate pulmonary vasoreactivity when these agents are administered during catheterization. Continuous intravenous or possibly nebulized prostacyclin (prostaglandin I_2) may also provide temporary relief. Continuous administration of nitric oxide via nasal cannula is being investigated. Anticoagulation may be of value, especially in patients with previous pulmonary thromboemboli. The definitive therapy is heart-lung or lung transplantation (see Chapter 449). In patients with severe pulmonary hypertension and low cardiac output, the terminal event is sudden and related to a lethal arrhythmia. Patients presenting in infancy often have rapid progression and high mortality.

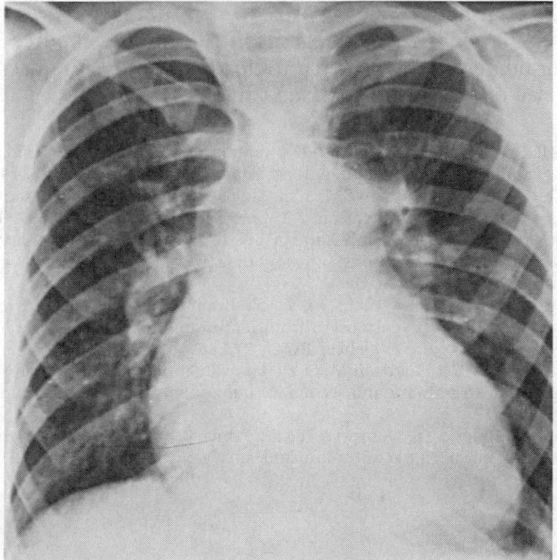

Figure 440–1 Roentgenogram in primary pulmonary hypertension. Note the moderate cardiac enlargement, dilatation of the pulmonary artery, and relative pulmonary undervascularity in the outer two thirds of the lung fields.

440.2 Pulmonary Vascular Disease (Eisenmenger Syndrome)

PATHOPHYSIOLOGY. The term *Eisenmenger syndrome* refers to patients with a ventricular septal defect (VSD) whose shunts have become partially or totally from right to left as a result of the development of pulmonary vascular disease. This physiologic abnormality also can occur with atrial septal defect, atrioventricular septal defect, patent ductus arteriosus, or any other communication between the aorta and pulmonary artery. Pulmonary vascular disease with isolated atrial septal defect is less common and does not occur until late in adulthood.

In Eisenmenger syndrome, the pulmonary vascular resistance after birth either remains high or, after having decreased during early infancy, rises thereafter because of increased shear stress on pulmonary arterioles. Factors playing a role in the rapidity of the development of pulmonary vascular disease include increased pulmonary arterial pressure, increased pulmonary blood flow, and the presence of hypoxia or hypercarbia. Early in the course of disease, pulmonary hypertension (elevated pressure in the pulmonary arteries) is the result of markedly increased pulmonary blood flow (*hyperkinetic pulmonary hypertension*). This form of pulmonary hypertension decreases with pulmonary vasodilators or oxygen, or both. With the development of Eisenmenger syndrome, pulmonary hypertension is the result of *pulmonary vascular disease* (obstructive pathologic changes in the pulmonary vessels). This form of pulmonary hypertension is usually only minimally responsive to pulmonary vasodilators or oxygen or not at all.

PATHOLOGY AND PATHOPHYSIOLOGY. The pathologic changes of Eisenmenger's syndrome occur in the small pulmonary arterioles and muscular arteries (<300 mm) and are graded on the basis of histologic characteristics (*Heath-Edwards classification*): Grade I changes involve medial hypertrophy alone, grade II consists of medial hypertrophy and intimal hyperplasia, grade III involves near obliteration of the vessel lumen, grade IV includes arterial dilatation, and grades V and VI include plexiform lesions, angiomatoid formation, and fibrinoid necrosis. Grades IV–VI indicate irreversible pulmonary vascular obstructive disease. Eisenmenger physiology is defined by an absolute elevation of pulmonary arterial resistance to greater than 12 Wood units (resistance units indexed to body surface area) or by a ratio of pulmonary to systemic vascular resistance greater than or equal to 1.0.

Pulmonary vascular disease occurs more rapidly in patients with trisomy 21 who have left-to-right shunts. It also complicates the natural history in patients with elevated pulmonary venous pressure due to mitral stenosis or left ventricular dysfunction, any patient with transmission of systemic pressure to the pulmonary circulation via an interventricular or great vessel level shunt, and those patients chronically exposed to low P_{O_2} (due to high altitude). Patients with cyanotic congenital heart lesions associated with unrestricted pulmonary blood flow are at particularly high risk.

CLINICAL MANIFESTATIONS. Symptoms usually do not occur until the 2nd or 3rd decade of life, although a more fulminant course may occur. Many patients survive for decades with minimal symptoms. Intracardiac or extracardiac communica-

TABLE 440–1 Extracardiac Complications of Cyanotic Congenital Heart Disease and Eisenmenger Physiology

Problem	Etiology	Therapy
Polycythemia	Persistent hypoxia	Phlebotomy
Relative anemia	Nutritional deficiency	Iron replacement
CNS abscess	Right-to-left shunting	Antibiotics, drainage
CNS thromboembolic stroke	Right-to-left shunting or polycythemia	Phlebotomy
Low-grade DIC, thrombocytopenia	Polycythemia	None for DIC unless bleeding, then phlebotomy
Hemoptysis	Pulmonary infarct, thrombosis, or rupture of pulmonary artery plexiform lesion	Embolization
Gum disease	Polycythemia, gingivitis, bleeding	Dental hygiene
Gout	Polycythemia, diuretic agent	Allopurinol
Arthritis, clubbing	Hypoxic arthropathy	None
Pregnancy complications: abortion, fetal growth retardation, prematurity, maternal illness	Poor placental perfusion, poor ability to increase cardiac output	Bed rest, pregnancy prevention counseling
Infections	Associated asplenia, DiGeorge syndrome, endocarditis	Antibiotics
	Fatal RSV pneumonia with pulmonary hypertension	Ribavirin; RSV immunoglobulin (prevention)
Failure to thrive	Increased oxygen consumption, decreased nutrient intake	Treat heart failure; correct defect early; increase caloric intake
Psychosocial adjustment	Limited activity, cyanotic appearance, chronic disease, multiple hospitalizations	Counseling

CNS = central nervous system; DIC = disseminated intravascular coagulation; RSV = respiratory syncytial virus.

tions that normally would shunt from left to right develop right-to-left shunting as pulmonary vascular resistance exceeds systemic vascular resistance. Cyanosis becomes apparent, and dyspnea, fatigue, and a tendency toward dysrhythmias begin to occur. In the late stages of the disease, heart failure, chest pain, headaches, syncope, and hemoptysis may be seen. Physical examination reveals a right ventricular heave and a narrowly split 2nd heart sound with a loud pulmonic component. A palpable pulmonary artery pulsation may be present at the left upper sternal border. A holosystolic murmur of tricuspid regurgitation may be audible along the left sternal border. An early decrescendo diastolic murmur of pulmonary insufficiency may also be heard along the left sternal border. The degree of cyanosis depends on the stage of the disease.

LABORATORY DIAGNOSIS. Cyanotic patients have various degrees of polycythemia depending on the severity and duration of hypoxia. *Roentgenographically,* the heart varies in size from normal to greatly enlarged; the latter occurs usually late in the course of the disease. The main pulmonary artery is usually prominent, similar to primary pulmonary hypertension (see Fig. 440–1). The pulmonary vessels are enlarged in the hilar areas and taper rapidly in caliber in the peripheral branches. The right ventricle and atrium are prominent. The *electrocardiogram* shows marked right ventricular hypertrophy. The P wave may be tall and spiked.

The *echocardiogram* shows a thick-walled right ventricle and demonstrates the underlying congenital heart lesion. Two-dimensional echocardiography assists in eliminating from consideration lesions such as obstructed pulmonary veins, supramitral membrane, and mitral stenosis. The pulmonary valve echocardiogram shows a characteristic early midsystolic closure, the "W sign." Doppler studies demonstrate the direction of the shunt and the presence of a typical hypertension wave form in the main pulmonary artery. Tricuspid and pulmonary regurgitation can be used in the Doppler examination to estimate the pulmonary arterial pressure.

Cardiac catheterization usually shows a bidirectional shunt at the site of the defect. The systolic pressures are usually equal in the systemic and pulmonary circulations. The pulmonary capillary wedge pressure is normal unless a left-sided heart obstructive lesion or left ventricular failure is the cause of the pulmonary artery hypertension. The arterial oxygen saturation is decreased, reflecting the magnitude of the right-to-left shunt. Response to vasodilator therapy (oxygen, nitroprusside, calcium channel blockers, prostacyclin, nitric oxide) may identify patients with hyperdynamic pulmonary hypertension. Selective angiocardiography can locate the site of the shunt, but these studies are usually avoided in these patients because of increased risk and the accuracy of echocardiography. Selective pulmonary artery injections may be necessary if pulmonary venous obstruction is suspected because of a high wedge pressure and low left ventricular end-diastolic pressure.

TREATMENT. The best management for patients who are at risk for the development of late pulmonary vascular disease is prevention by surgical elimination of large intracardiac or great vessel communications during infancy. Some patients may be missed because they have not shown early clinical manifestations. Pulmonary vascular resistance never decreases substantially at birth in some of these infants and therefore they never acquire enough left-to-right shunting to become clinically apparent. This is a particular risk in patients with congenital heart disease who live at high altitude. It is also a risk in infants with trisomy 21, who are at risk for earlier development of pulmonary vascular disease. Because of the high incidence of congenital heart disease associated with trisomy 21, many physicians recommend routine echocardiography at the time of initial diagnosis, even in the absence of other clinical findings.

Medical treatment of Eisenmenger syndrome is entirely symptomatic (Table 440–1). Older children and adolescents with symptomatic polycythemia may be improved by cautious, repeated phlebotomies with volume replacement. Clinical trials in adults have described short-term benefits from chronic calcium channel blocker or prostacyclin therapy; there is minimal experience with these agents in children. Combined heart-lung or bilateral lung transplantation is the only surgical option for many of these patients (see Chapter 449).

Barst RJ: Pharmacologically induced pulmonary vasodilation in children and young adults with primary pulmonary hypertension. Chest 89:497, 1986.

Gammie JS, Keenan RJ, Pham SM, et al: Single- versus double-lung transplantation for pulmonary hypertension. J Thorac Cardiovasc Surg 115:397, 1998.

Higenbottam TW, Butt AY, Dinh-Xaun AT, et al: Treatment of pulmonary hypertension with the continuous infusion of a prostacyclin analogue, iloprost. Heart 79:175, 1998.

McCann UD, Seiden LS, Rubin LJ, et al: Brain serotonin neurotoxicity and primary pulmonary hypertension from fenfluramine and dexfenfluramine. A systemic review of the evidence. JAMA 278:666, 1997.

Mikhail G, Gibbs J, Richardson M, et al: An evaluation of nebulized prostacyclin in patients with primary and secondary pulmonary hypertension. Eur Heart J 18:1499, 1997.

Sandoval J, Bauerle O, Gomez A, et al: Primary pulmonary hypertension in children: Clinical characterization and survival. J Am Coll Cardiol 25:466, 1995.

Chapter 441
General Principles of Treatment of Congenital Heart Disease

Most patients who have mild congenital heart disease require no treatment. The parents and child should be made aware that a normal life is expected and that no restriction of the child's activities is necessary. Overprotective parents may use the presence of a mild congenital heart lesion or even a functional heart murmur as a means to exert excessive control over their child's activities. Although he or she may not express fears overtly, the child may become anxious regarding early death or debilitation, especially when an adult member of the family acquires symptomatic heart disease. The family may have an unexpressed fear of sudden death, and the rarity of this manifestation should be emphasized in discussions directed at improving their understanding of the child's congenital heart defect. The difference between congenital heart disease and degenerative coronary disease in adults should be emphasized. General health maintenance, including a well-balanced, "heart-healthy" diet, aerobic exercise, and avoidance of smoking, should be encouraged.

Even patients with moderate to severe heart disease need not be markedly restricted in physical activities. Physical education should be modified appropriately to the child's capacity to participate. This can usually be accomplished best by exercise testing. Competitive sports for most of these patients should be discouraged. Patients with severe heart disease and decreased exercise tolerance usually tend to limit their own activities. Dyspnea, headache, and fatigability in cyanotic patients may be a sign of increasing hypoxemia and may require some limitation of activities among those for whom specific medical or surgical treatment is not available. Routine immunizations should be given, with the inclusion of influenza vaccine; patients who might be considered candidates for heart or heart-lung transplantation should not receive live virus vaccinations.

Bacterial infections should be treated vigorously, but the presence of congenital heart disease is not an appropriate reason to use antibiotics indiscriminately. Prophylaxis against infective endocarditis should be carried out during dental procedures, during instrumentation of the urinary tract, and prior to lower gastrointestinal tract manipulation (see Table 443–4).

Cyanotic patients need to be monitored for a multitude of noncardiac manifestations of oxygen deficiency (Table 441–1). Treatment of iron deficiency anemia is important in cyanotic patients who show improved exercise tolerance and general well-being with adequate hemoglobin levels. These patients should also be carefully observed for excessive polycythemia. Cyanotic patients should avoid situations in which dehydration may occur, which leads to increased viscosity and increases the risk of stroke. Diuretics may need to be decreased or temporarily discontinued during episodes of acute gastroenteritis. High altitudes and sudden changes in thermal environment should also be avoided. Phlebotomy with volume replacement should be carried out in symptomatic patients with severe polycythemia (hematocrit >65%); the use of routine phlebotomy in the absence of symptoms is controversial. Patients with severe congenital heart disease or a history of rhythm disturbance should be carefully monitored during anesthesia for even routine surgical procedures. Women with nonrepaired severe congenital heart disease should be counseled on the risks associated with childbearing and on the use of contraceptives and tubal ligation. Pregnancy may be extremely dangerous for patients with chronic cyanosis or pulmonary artery hypertension, or both. Women with mild to moderate heart disease and many of those who have had corrective surgery can have normal pregnancies.

POSTOPERATIVE MANAGEMENT. After successful open heart surgery, the severity of the congenital heart defect, the age and condition (nutritional status) of the patient prior to surgery, the events in the operating room, and the quality of the postoperative care influence the patient's course. Intraoperative factors that influence survival and that should be noted when a patient returns from the operating room include the duration of cardiopulmonary bypass, the duration of aortic cross-clamping (the period of time during which the heart is not being perfused), and the duration of profound hypothermia (usually used in infants: the period of time during which the entire body is not being perfused).

Immediate postoperative care should be provided in an intensive care unit staffed by a team of physicians, nurses, and technicians experienced with the unique problems encountered after open heart surgery. The preparation for postoperative monitoring begins in the operating room, where the anesthesiologist or the surgeon places an arterial catheter to allow direct arterial pressure measurements and arterial sampling for blood gas determination. A central venous catheter is also placed for measuring central venous pressure and for infusions of cardioactive medications. In more complex cases, left atrial or pulmonary artery catheters may be inserted directly into these cardiac structures and used for pressure monitoring purposes. Flow-directed thermodilution monitoring (Swan-Ganz) catheters are sometimes used for monitoring pulmonary capillary wedge pressure and cardiac index. Temporary pacing wires are placed on the atrium or ventricle, or both, in case temporary heart block occurs. Transcutaneous oximetry provides for continuous monitoring of arterial oxygen saturation.

Functional failure of one organ system may cause profound physiologic and biochemical changes in another (see Table 440–1). Respiratory insufficiency, for example, leads to hypoxia, acidosis, and hypercarbia, which, in turn, compromises cardiac, vascular, and renal function. The latter problems cannot be managed successfully until adequate ventilation is reestablished. Thus, it is essential that the primary source of each postoperative problem be identified and treated.

Respiratory failure is a major postoperative complication encountered after open heart surgery. Cardiopulmonary bypass carried out in the presence of pulmonary congestion results in decreased lung compliance, copious tracheal and bronchial secretions, atelectasis, and increased breathing effort. Because fatigue and subsequently hypoventilation and acidosis may rapidly ensue, mechanical positive-pressure endotracheal ventilation may be continued following open heart surgery for a minimum of several hours in relatively stable patients and up to 2–3 days or more in severely ill patients, especially infants. Patients with certain congenital heart lesions may also have airway abnormalities, which could make extubation more difficult.

The electrocardiogram should be monitored continuously during the postoperative period. A change in the heart rate may be the 1st indication of a serious complication, such as hemorrhage, hypothermia, hypoventilation, or heart failure. *Cardiac rhythm disorders* must be diagnosed quickly because a prolonged untreated arrhythmia may add a severe hemodynamic burden to the heart in the critical early postoperative period (see Chapter 442). Injury to the heart's conduction system during surgery can cause postoperative *complete heart block*. This complication is usually temporary and is treated with surgically placed pacing wires that can later be removed. Occasionally, complete heart block is permanent. If heart block persists beyond 10–14 days postoperatively, it requires the insertion of a permanent pacemaker. Tachyarrhythmias are a more common problem in postoperative patients. Junctional

TABLE 441–1 Systems Approach to Postoperative Care Following Surgery for Congenital Heart Disease

System and Problem	Etiology	Treatment or Prevention
Nervous System		
Coma	Global ischemia	Monitor and treat increased intracranial pressure
	Prolonged anesthetic effect	Reverse anesthesia
	Hypoglycemia	Glucose
Focal lesions	Emboli (air, thrombi)	
Seizures	Metabolic (hyponatremia, hypoglycemia), ischemic, embolic disturbances	Phenytoin, correct metabolic disturbances
Diaphragm paralysis	Phrenic nerve injury	Respiratory care
Vocal cord paralysis	Traction on recurrent laryngeal nerve	Respiratory care
Horner's syndrome	Dissection of subclavian artery with sympathetic chain injury	None
Paraplegia	Postcoarctation repair with spinal artery ischemia	Avoid ischemia
Pain	Surgical trauma	Fentanyl, morphine
Anxiety	Stress	Versed, Valium
Respiratory System		
ARDS postpump syndrome	Unknown; possible release of vasoactive substances by cardiopulmonary bypass	PEEP, mechanical ventilation, oxygen
Pulmonary edema	Heart failure, left-sided obstructions, fluid overload	Diuresis, PEEP, mechanical ventilation, inotropic agents
Pleural effusions	Hemothorax	Thoracocentesis
	Early serous effusion	Thoracocentesis
	Delayed postpericardiotomy syndrome	Anti-inflammatory agents
Chylothorax	Injury to thoracic duct	NPO, or medium-chain triglyceride diet Rarely surgical ligation of thoracic duct
Atelectasis	Hypoventilation, poor cough	Chest physiotherapy, PEEP
Pneumonia	Aspiration, nosocomial, bacteremia	Identify bacterial-viral (respiratory syncytial virus) cause; specific antimicrobial therapy
Pulmonary hypertension	Repair of TAPVR, Norwood 1st stage, trisomy 21; prior preoperative pulmonary hypertension	Hyperventilation, hyperoxia, nitroprusside, prostaglandins, nitric oxide, ECMO
Stridor	Vocal cord edema, paralysis	Steroids, rarely tracheotomy
Cardiovascular System		
Bradycardia, sick sinus, atrioventricular block	Injury to interatrial or interventricular conduction system	Atropine, isoproterenol, pacemaker
Right bundle branch block	Right ventriculotomy	Atrial approach to ventricular septal defect repair or tetralogy of Fallot
Tachyarrhythmias	Supraventricular, junctional tachycardia	Antiarrhythmic agents
	Ventricular tachycardia	Defibrillation, antiarrhythmic agents
Poor cardiac output	Cardiogenic—right ventriculotomy or cardiac "stun" (prolonged pump and cross-clamp time) or infarction	Inotropic agents, support preload, reduce afterload, LVAD, ECMO
	Hypocalcemia	Calcium
	Hypovolemia	Support preload with fluids
Pericardial tamponade	Pericardial effusion, acute hemorrhage	Pericardiocentesis
	Serous postpericardiotomy syndrome	Anti-inflammatory agents
Hypertension	Stress or pain	Analgesia
	Postcoarctectomy syndrome	Nitroprusside
Mesenteric arteritis	Postcoarctectomy syndrome	NPO, nitroprusside
Renal-Metabolic System		
Prerenal oliguria	Hypovolemia	Fluid administration
	Poor cardiac output	Inotropic agents
Renal failure	Hypotension, prolonged pump–cross-clamp time, acute tubular necrosis	Improve blood pressure, diuretics, dialysis
Edema	Fluid resuscitation, capillary leak, poor cardiac output, elevated systemic venous pressure	Diuresis, inotropic agents
Hyponatremia	Dilutional, SIADH	Fluid restriction
	Diuretics	Fluid restriction
Hyperglycemia	Hypothermia, inhibition of insulin	None needed (usually), insulin
Hypoglycemia	Rebound following hyperglycemia, hepatic failure	Glucose infusion
Hematologic System		
Hemorrhage	Abnormal PT, PTT, thrombocytopenia	Correct coagulopathy
	Surgical leak	Reoperation, suture
Shunt thrombosis	Poor cardiac output, hypovolemia	Fluids, heparin, reoperation
Anemia (usually reflecting reduced blood volume)	Hemorrhage, hemolysis	Transfuse packed red blood cells
Graft-versus-host disease	Infusion of viable leukocytes to patients with DiGeorge syndrome	Irradiate blood products
Infectious Diseases		
Wound infection (cutaneous, costochondral, sternotomy, mediastinitis, vascular lines, chest tubes)	Contamination in operating room	Antibiotics
Endocarditis	*Staphylococcus epidermidis, Corynebacterium,* contamination in operating room	Antibiotics
Cystitis, pyelonephritis	Contamination of indwelling urinary catheter	Antibiotics, remove catheter
Hepatitis	Blood-borne: cytomegalovirus, Epstein-Barr virus, hepatitis B and hepatitis C viruses	Screen blood products
Postperfusion syndrome (fever, hepatosplenomegaly, atypical lymphocytes, lymphadenopathy, transient rash)	Cytomegalovirus, Epstein-Barr virus	Screen blood products
Psychosocial Conditions		
Anxiety, separation	Age-related, fears, etc.	Preparedness (videotape, play acting); parent visitation, sedation

ARDS = Acute respiratory distress syndrome; TAPVR = total anomalous pulmonary venous return; PEEP = positive end-expiratory pressure; NPO = nothing per os (by mouth); SIADH = syndrome of inappropriate antidiuretic hormone; PT = prothrombin time; PTT = partial thromboplastin time; LVAD = left ventricular assist device; ECMO = extracorporeal membrane oxygenation.

ectopic tachycardia can be a particularly troublesome rhythm to manage (see Chapter 442).

Heart failure with poor cardiac output (see Table 441–1) following cardiac surgery may be secondary to respiratory failure, serious arrhythmias, myocardial injury, blood loss, hypervolemia or hypovolemia, or a significant residual hemodynamic abnormality. Treatment specific to the cause should be instituted. Catecholamines, phosphodiesterase inhibitors, digoxin, nitroprusside and other afterload-reducing agents, and diuretics are the cardioactive agents most often used in patients with myocardial dysfunction in the early postoperative period (see Chapter 448). Postoperative pulmonary hypertension can be managed with inhaled nitric oxide. In patients who are unresponsive to standard pharmacologic treatment, various ventricular assist devices are available, depending on the patient's size. If pulmonary function is adequate, an intra-aortic balloon counterpulsation pump or an external or implantable left ventricular assist device (LVAD) may be used. If pulmonary function is inadequate, extracorporeal membrane oxygenation (ECMO) may be used. These extraordinary measures are useful in maintaining the circulation until cardiac function improves, usually within 2–3 days. They have also been used with some success as a bridge to transplantation in patients with severe nonremitting postoperative cardiac failure.

Acidosis secondary to low cardiac output, renal failure, or hypovolemia must be prevented or promptly corrected. An arterial pH less than 7.3 may result in a decrease in cardiac output with an increase in lactic acid production and may be the forerunner of a series of arrhythmias or cardiac arrest.

Kidney function may be compromised by congestive heart failure and further impaired by prolonged cardiopulmonary bypass (see Table 441–1). Blood and fluid replacement, cardiac inotropic agents, and sometimes vasodilators will usually reestablish normal urine flow in patients with hypovolemia or cardiac failure. Dopamine is a useful inotropic agent because it also increases renal blood flow directly. Renal failure secondary to tubular injury may require temporary peritoneal dialysis or hemofiltration.

Neurologic abnormalities can occur after cardiopulmonary bypass, especially in the neonatal period. Seizures may occur when the patient awakens from sedation and usually can be controlled with phenytoin (Dilantin) or phenobarbital. In the absence of other neurologic signs, isolated seizures in the immediate postoperative period usually carry a good prognosis. Thromboembolism and stroke are rare but serious complications of open heart surgery. Over the long term, both subtle and more substantial learning disabilities may develop.

The *postpericardiotomy syndrome* may occur toward the end of the 1st postoperative week or sometimes be delayed until weeks or months after operation. This febrile illness is characterized by pericarditis and pleurisy, decreased appetite, nausea, and vomiting. In most instances it is self-limiting and associated with a benign course. When pericardial fluid accumulates, the potential danger of cardiac tamponade should be recognized (see Chapter 446). Rarely, arrhythmias may also occur. Symptomatic patients usually respond to salicylates or indomethacin and bed rest. Occasionally steroid therapy or pericardiocentesis is required. A prolonged illness or late recurrences are less usual.

Hemolysis of mechanical origin is seen rarely after repair of certain cardiac defects, for example, atrioventricular septal defects or after the insertion of a mechanical prosthetic valve. It occurs secondary to unusual turbulence of blood at increased pressure. Reoperation may be necessary in rare patients with severe and progressive hemolysis who require frequent blood transfusions, but in most instances the problem slowly regresses.

Infection is another potential postoperative problem. Patients usually receive a broad-spectrum antibiotic for the initial postoperative period. Potential sites of infection include the lungs (usually related to postoperative atelectasis), the subcutaneous tissues at the incision site, the sternum, and the urinary tract (especially after an indwelling catheter has been in place). Sepsis with infective endocarditis is an infrequent complication but can be difficult to manage (see Chapter 443).

Galioto FM: Physical activity for children with cardiac disease. In: Garson A, Bricker JT, Fisher DJ, Neish SR (eds): The Science and Practice of Pediatric Cardiology. Baltimore: Williams & Wilkins, 1998, pp 2585–2592.

Newburger JW, Sibert AR, Buckley LP, Fyler DC: Cognitive function and age at repair of transposition of the great arteries in children. N Engl J Med 310:1495, 1984.

Rithel SC, Pennington G, Boegner R, et al: Extracorporeal membrane oxygenation in children after cardiac surgery. Circulation 86:II-305, 1992.

Todd JL, Todd NW: Conotruncal cardiac anomalies and otitis media. J Pediatr 131:215, 1997.

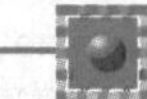

SECTION 4

Cardiac Arrhythmias

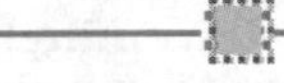

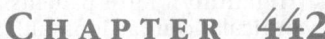

CHAPTER 442

Disturbances of Rate and Rhythm of the Heart

Pediatric arrhythmias may be transient or permanent; congenital (in a structurally normal or abnormal heart) or acquired (rheumatic fever, myocarditis); or caused by a toxin (diphtheria), cocaine, or theophylline or by proarrhythmic or antiarrhythmic drugs; or they may be a sequela of surgical correction of congenital heart disease. The major risk of any arrhythmia is either severe tachycardia or bradycardia leading to decreased cardiac output or degeneration into a more severe arrhythmia, for example, ventricular fibrillation. These complications may lead to syncope, which itself can be dangerous under certain circumstances (e.g., swimming, driving), or to sudden death. When a patient has an arrhythmia, one of the major management issues is to determine whether the particular rhythm is prone to deteriorate into a life-threatening tachyarrhythmia or bradyarrhythmia. Some rhythm abnormalities, such as single premature atrial and ventricular beats, are common among children without heart disease and in the great majority of instances do not pose a risk to the patient.

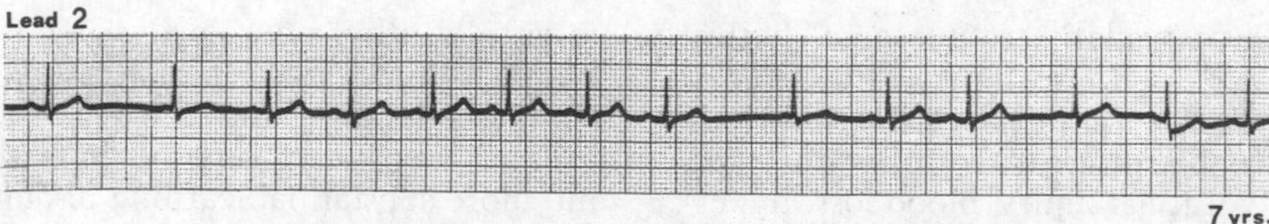

Figure 442–1 Sinus arrhythmia with junctional escape beat. Note the variation in P-P interval with little change in P morphology or P-R interval. When the sinus rate is slow enough, the atrioventricular junction takes over and produces escape beats. This rhythm is normal.

An increasing number of powerful pharmacologic agents are available for treating dysrhythmias in adults, but many have not been studied extensively in children. Problems with frequency of administration, compliance, side effects, and variable responses remain, and selection of an appropriate agent involves empiricism. Fortunately, the majority of rhythm disturbances in children can be reliably controlled with a single agent (Table 442–1). For patients with tachyarrhythmias that are resistant to medical therapy, transcatheter radiofrequency ablation or surgical intervention is available. For patients with bradyarrhythmias, implantable pacemakers are small enough for use in premature infants. Automatic implantable cardioverter-defibrillators (AICDs) are available for use in high-risk patients with malignant ventricular arrhythmias.

442.1 Sinus Arrhythmias and Extrasystoles

Sinus arrhythmia represents a normal physiologic variation in impulse discharges from the sinus node related to respirations. There is a slowing of heart rate during expiration and an acceleration during inspiration. Occasionally, if the sinus rate becomes slow enough, there is an escape beat from the atrioventricular junction region (Fig. 442–1). Irregularities of sinus rhythm are commonly seen in premature infants, especially bradycardia associated with periodic apnea. Sinus arrhythmia is exaggerated during febrile illnesses and by drugs that increase vagal tone, such as digitalis; it is usually abolished by exercise.

Sinus bradycardia is due to slow discharge of impulses from the sinus node. In general, a sinus rate less than 90 beats/min in neonates and less than 60 beats/min thereafter is considered to be sinus bradycardia. It is commonly seen in athletes; in healthy individuals it is without significance. Sinus bradycardia may occur in systemic disease, for example, myxedema, and resolves when the disorder is under control. Sinus bradycardia must be differentiated from sinoatrial and atrioventricular (AV) block. Children with sinus bradycardia are able to increase their heart rate with exercise to much higher than 100 beats/min, whereas patients with AV block are usually unable to do so. Low-birthweight infants display great variation in sinus rate. Sinus bradycardia is common in these infants and may be associated with junctional escape beats. Premature atrial contractions are also frequent. These rhythm changes, especially bradycardia, appear more commonly during sleep and are not associated with symptoms. No therapy is usually necessary.

Wandering atrial pacemaker (Fig. 442–2) is defined as an intermittent shift in the pacemaker of the heart from the sinus node to another part of the atrium. This is not uncommon in childhood and usually represents a normal variant. It may also be seen in patients with central nervous system disturbances, for example, subarachnoid hemorrhage.

Extrasystoles are produced by the discharge of an ectopic focus that may be situated anywhere in atrial, junctional, or ventricular tissue. Usually, isolated extrasystoles are of no clinical or prognostic significance. Under certain circumstances, premature beats may be due to organic heart disease (inflammatory, ischemic, fibrotic, and so on) or to drug toxicity, especially from digitalis.

Premature atrial complexes are common in childhood, even in the absence of cardiac disease. Depending on the degree of prematurity of the beat (coupling interval) and the preceding R-R interval (cycle length), premature atrial complexes may result in a normal, a prolonged (*aberrancy*), or an absent (*blocked premature atrial complex*) QRS complex. The last occurs when the premature impulse is conducted to the ventricle while the specialized ventricular conducting system is partially refractory (Fig. 442–3). Atrial extrasystoles must be distinguished from premature ventricular complexes (PVCs). Careful scrutiny of the electrocardiogram for a premature P wave preceding the QRS that has a different contour from that of the other sinus P waves is essential for diagnosis. Atrial premature complexes often reset the sinus node pacemaker (lack of a compensatory pause); this is not regarded as a reliable means of differentiating atrial from ventricular premature complexes.

PVCs may arise in any region of the ventricles. They are characterized by premature, widened, bizarre QRS complexes that are not preceded by a P wave (Fig. 442–4). When all premature beats have identical contours, they are classified as unifocal in origin. When PVCs vary in contour, they are designated as multifocal. Ventricular extrasystoles are often, but not always, followed by a compensatory pause. The presence of fusion beats, that is, complexes with morphologic features that are intermediate between those of normal sinus beats and those of PVCs, is a clue to the ventricular origin of the extrasystole. Extrasystoles produce a smaller stroke and pulse volume than normal and, if quite premature, may not be audible with a stethoscope or palpable at the radial pulse. When frequent, extrasystoles may assume a definite rhythm, for example, alternating with normal beats (**bigeminy**) or occurring after two normal beats (**trigeminy**). Most patients are unaware of single premature ventricular contractions, although some may

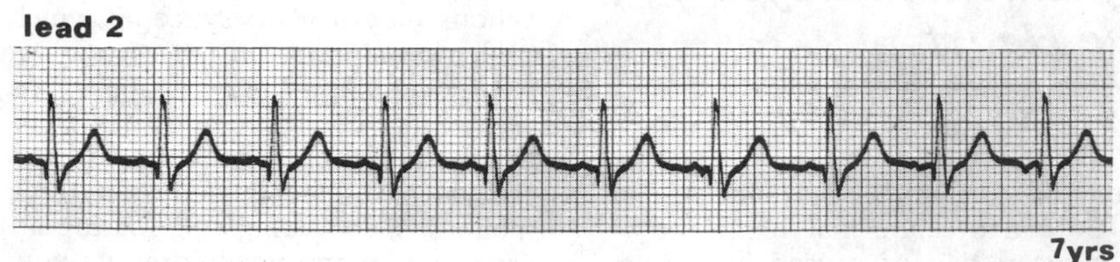

Figure 442–2 Wandering atrial pacemaker. Note the change in P wave configuration in the 7th, 9th, and 10th beats. The 7th P wave may represent a fusion between the sinus P and the ectopic atrial pacemaker seen in the 10th beat.

TABLE 442–1 Antiarrhythmic Drugs Commonly Used in Pediatric Patients, by Class

		Oral Administration		Intravenous Administration*						
Drug	**Indications**	***Maintenance Dose***	***Maximal Maintenance Dose***	***Loading Dose***	***Maximal Dose***	**Comments**	**Side Effects**	**Drug Interactions**	**Proarrhythmias**	**Drug Level**
Class IA: Inhibit Na+ Fast Channel, Prolong Repolarization										
Quinidine sulfate	SVT,† atrial fibrillation, atrial flutter, VPC Digoxin, verapamil, or propranolol must be given first to prevent 1:1 conduction and fast ventricular rate in atrial flutter	20–60 mg/kg/24 hr q 6 hr	2.4 g/24 hr	—	—	—	Nausea, vomiting, diarrhea, fever, cinchonism, QRS and Q-T prolongation, AV node block, asystole, syncope, thrombocytopenia, hemolytic anemia, SLE, blurred vision, convulsions, allergic reactions, exacerbation of periodic paralysis	Enhances digoxin effects	Yes, torsades de pointes	2–7 μg/mL
Quinidine gluconate	Digoxin, verapamil, or propranolol must be given first to prevent 1 : 1 conduction and fast ventricular rate in atrial flutter	20–60 mg/kg/24 hr q 8–12 hr	2.0 g/24 hr	—	—	Oral test dose 2 mg/kg	Same as above	Same as above	Same as above	Same as above
Procainamide	SVT,† atrial fibrillation, atrial flutter; VPC, ventricular tachycardia‡	15–50 mg/kg/24 hr q 4 hr or q 6 hr§	4.0 g/24 hr	3–6 mg/kg over 5 min	20 mg/min to 1.0 g	Intravenous maintenance 20–80 μg/kg/min	P-R, QRS, Q-T interval prolongation, anorexia, nausea, vomiting, rash, fever, agranulocytosis, thrombocytopenia, Coombs'-positive hemolytic anemia, SLE, hypotension, exacerbation of periodic paralysis	Toxicity increased by amiodarone, cimetidine	Yes, torsades de pointes	4–10 μg/mL
Disopyramide	SVT,† atrial fibrillation, atrial flutter, VPC	4–12 mg/kg/24 hr q 6 hr or q 12 hr§	1.2 g/24 hr	—	—	—	Anticholinergic effects, urinary retention, blurred vision, dry mouth, Q-T and QRS prolongation, hepatic toxicity, negative inotropic effects, agranulocytosis, psychosis, hypoglycemia	—	Yes, torsades de pointes	2–4 μg/mL

Table continued on following page

TABLE 442–1 Antiarrhythmic Drugs Commonly Used in Pediatric Patients, by Class

		Oral Administration		Intravenous Administration*						
Drug	**Indications**	***Maintenance Dose***	***Maximal Maintenance Dose***	***Loading Dose***	***Maximal Dose***	**Comments**	**Side Effects**	**Drug Interactions**	**Proarrhythmias**	**Drug Level**
Class IB: Inhibit Na⁻ Fast Channel, Shorten Repolarization										
Lidocaine (class IB)	VPC, ventricular tachycardia,‡ ventricular fibrillation‖	—	—	1 mg/kg; repeat q 5 min 3 times	50–75 mg	Intravenous maintenance 30–50 μg/kg/min	CNS effects, confusion, convulsions, high-degree AV block, asystole, coma, paresthesias, respiratory failure	Propranolol, cimetidine, tocainide increase toxicity	No	1–5 μg/mL
Phenytoin (class IB)	Digoxin-induced arrhythmias with heart block	3–6 mg/kg/24 hr q 12 hr	600 mg	10–15 mg/kg over 1 hr	20 mg/min to 1.0 g	—	Rash, gingival hyperplasia, ataxia, lethargy, vertigo, tremor, macrocytic anemia, bradycardia with rapid push	Amiodarone, oral anticoagulants, cimetidine, nifedipine, disopyramide increase toxicity Phenytoin decreases effect of quinidine, mexiletine, furosemide, disopyramide	No	10–20 μg/mL
Class II: β-Blockers										
Propranolol	SVT,† PVCs, LQTS	1–4 mg/kg/24 hr q 6 hr	16 mg/kg/24 hr or 60 mg/24 hr	0.1–0.15 mg/kg	1 mg/min to 10 mg	Long-acting β-blocking agents (nadolol, atenolol) are preferred for long-term therapy (less frequent administration and fewer CNS side effects)	Bradycardia, loss of concentration or memory, bronchospasm, hypoglycemia, hypotension, heart block, CHF	Use with disopyramide or verapamil exacerbates or precipitates CHF	No	—
Class III: Prolong Repolarization										
Amiodarone	Drug-resistant SVT, JET (congenital or postoperative), VT	Loading dose: 10 mg/kg/24 hr in 1–2 divided doses for 4–14 days; reduce to 5 mg/kg/24 hr for several weeks; if no recurrence, reduce to 2.5 mg/kg/24 hr; may be given for 5 of 7 days/wk	Adult doses: loading = 800–1600 mg/24 hr for 2 wk; then 600–800 mg/24 hr for 1 mo; then 400 mg/24 hr	Loading dose: 2.5–5 mg/kg over 30–60 min, may repeat 2 times; then 2–10 mg/kg/24 hr q 24 hr		Contraindicated in severe sinus node disease or in AV block without pacemaker	Hypo- or hyperthyroidism, elevated triglycerides, hepatic toxicity, pulmonary fibrosis	Digoxin (increases levels), flecainide, procainamide, quinidine, warfarin, phenytoin	Torsades de pointes, bradycardia	0.5–2.5 mg/L
Bretylium	Ventricular tachycardia,‡ ventricular fibrillation‖	—	—	5 mg/kg, then 5–10 mg/kg q 6 hr	30 mg/kg	—	Hypotension, sinus bradycardia, increased sensitivity to catecholamines with transient arrhythmias	Possible hypertension with concurrent sympathomimetic amines	No	—

Class IV: Miscellaneous										
Digoxin (digitalis glycoside)	SVT† (non-WPW), atrial flutter, atrial fibrillation	10 μg/kg/24 hr q 12 hr	0.5 mg	IV dose = ¾ p.o. dose	0.5 mg	Oral total loading dose: Premature: 20 μg/kg Term newborn: 30 μg/kg >6 mo infant: 40 μg/kg give ½ total dose followed by ¼ q 8–12 hr × 2	APC, VPC, bradycardia, AV block, nausea, vomiting, anorexia; prolongs P-R interval	Quinidine, amiodarone, verapamil increase digoxin levels Diuretic, amphotericin-induced hypokalemia increases digoxin arrhythmia	Induces APC, VPC, accelerated AV junctional tachycardia	1–2 ng/mL (>6 mo old) 1.5–3 ng/mL (<6 mo old)
Verapamil (Ca^{2+} channel blocker)	SVT†	2–7 mg/kg/24 hr q 8 hr	480 mg	0.1–0.2 mg/kg q 20 min 2 times (have IV $CaCl_2$ ready)	5–10 mg	Not for use in infants Contraindicated in VT, severe CHF, and atrial fibrillation with WPW	Bradycardia, asystole, high-degree AV block, P-R prolongation, hypotension, CHF	Use with β-blocking agent or disopyramide exacerbates or precipitates CHF; increases digoxin levels and toxicity	No, but may increase AV block	—
Adenosine (purinergic agonist)	SVT†	—	—	50–300 μg/kg; begin with 50 μg/kg and increase by 50–100 μg/kg/dose if no effect; 6–12 mg in adolescents	Must be given as rapid IV (not arterial) push, repeat at higher dose if no effect	Because of short half-life, adverse effects (chest pain, dyspnea, facial flushing) last <1 min; may see transient bradycardia, rarely transient asystole, VPC	May be less effective in patients receiving theophylline; increased heart block with carbamazepine	—	—	—

IV administration of antiarrhythmic drugs should always be at a slow rate, with constant monitoring of blood pressure and an electrocardiogram, particularly in patients with compromised cardiac, renal, or hepatic function. The dose must be modified in patients with abnormal renal or hepatic function. The exception is adenosine, which must be given by rapid IV push, usually followed by a saline flush. It is usually ineffective if given intra-arterially.

†Vagotonic maneuvers (placing face in iced saline or ice bag over the face) may be attempted first. If the patient is severely compromised and critically ill, synchronized DC cardioversion is the treatment of choice for SVT, atrial flutter, and atrial fibrillation.

‡Cardioversion is the treatment of choice for sustained VT with significant hemodynamic compromise. Some cardiologists try chest thump or IV lidocaine, or both. If heart block is present, a temporary ventricular pacemaker may be needed.

§Sustained-release preparations available for clinical use.

‖Defibrillation is treatment of choice.

APC = atrial premature contraction; AV = atrioventricular; CHF = congestive heart failure; CNS = central nervous system; IV = intravenous; JET = junctional ectopic tachycardia; LQTS = long Q-T syndrome; SLE = systemic lupus erythematosus–like illness, antinuclear antibody–positive; SVT = supraventricular tachycardia; VPC = ventricular premature contraction; VT = ventricular tachycardia; WPW = Wolff-Parkinson-White (pre-excitation) syndrome.

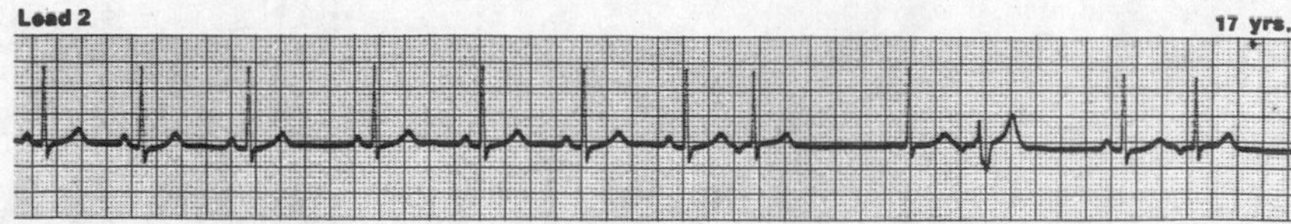

Figure 442–3 Premature atrial contraction (PAC). QRS complexes—the 8th, 10th, and final—in this strip are preceded by a P wave that is inverted, denoting an ectopic origin of atrial depolarization. Note that the 8th and final QRS complexes resemble those of sinus origin, whereas the 10th is aberrantly conducted. This is a function of the preceding cycle length that influences the refractory period of the bundle branches. Note that the pause after the PAC is longer than two P-P intervals, implying that the premature atrial depolarization has invaded and discharged the sinus node, and reset it, so that it fires later.

be aware of a "skipped beat" over the precordium. This sensation is due to the increased stroke volume of the normal beat following a compensatory pause. Anxiety, a febrile illness, or ingestion of various drugs or stimulants may cause premature ventricular beats.

It is important to distinguish PVCs that are benign from those that are likely to degenerate into more severe dysrhythmias. The former usually disappear during the tachycardia of exercise. If they persist or become more frequent during exercise, the arrhythmia may have greater significance. The following criteria are indications for further investigation of PVCs that could require suppressive therapy: (1) two or more ventricular premature beats in a row, (2) multifocal origin, (3) increased ventricular ectopic activity with exercise, (4) R on T phenomenon (premature ventricular depolarization occurs on the T wave of the preceding beat), and (5) presence of underlying heart disease. The basis of therapy for benign PVCs is reassurance that the arrhythmia is not life-threatening. Malignant PVCs are usually secondary to another medical problem, for example, electrolyte imbalance, hypoxia, drug toxicity, cardiac injury, or an intraventricular catheter. Successful treatment includes correction of the underlying abnormality. An intravenous lidocaine bolus and drip is the first line of therapy, with more powerful drugs such as amiodarone reserved for refractory cases or for patients with hemodynamic compromise. The choice of a maintenance oral antiarrhythmic agent is determined empirically or during an electrophysiologic study in the catheterization lab.

442.2 Supraventricular Tachycardia

Supraventricular tachycardias (SVTs) involve components of the conduction system within or above the bundle of His and can be divided into three major categories: *re-entrant tachycardias using an accessory pathway, re-entrant tachycardias without an accessory pathway,* and *ectopic or automatic tachycardias*. Re-entry using an accessory pathway is the most common mechanism of SVT in infants, with an increasing incidence of AV nodal re-entry in childhood. The tachycardia is initiated by a premature atrial beat that is most often conducted to the ventricle through the normal AV nodal pathway (*orthodromic conduction*). The ventricular response finds the AV nodal pathway refractory, but the bypass tract, readily able to conduct in a retrograde fashion, returns to the atrium as an echo beat, which, in turn, transmits back to the ventricle and so on (Fig. 442–5). Atrial and junctional ectopic tachycardias are more commonly associated with abnormal hearts (e.g., cardiomyopathy) or with postoperative congenital heart disease.

CLINICAL MANIFESTATIONS. Re-entrant SVT is characterized by an abrupt onset and cessation; it may be precipitated by an acute infection and usually occurs when the patient is at rest. Attacks may last only a few seconds or may persist for hours. The heart rate usually exceeds 180 beats/min and occasionally may be as rapid as 300 beats/min (Fig. 442–6). The only complaint may be awareness of the rapid heart rate. Many children tolerate these episodes extremely well, and it is unlikely that short paroxysms are a danger to life. If the rate is exceptionally rapid or if the attack is prolonged, precordial discomfort and heart failure may supervene.

In *young infants*, the diagnosis may be more obscure because of the inability to communicate their symptoms. The heart rate at this age is normally rapid, and even in the absence of tachyarrhythmia it increases greatly with crying. Infants with SVT often present with heart failure because the tachycardia goes unrecognized for a long time. The heart rate during paroxysms is frequently in the range of 200–300 beats/min. If the attack lasts 6–24 hr or more with an extremely fast heart rate, the infant may become acutely ill, have an ashen color, and be restless and irritable. Tachypnea and hepatomegaly are the prominent signs of cardiac failure, and there may be fever and leukocytosis. When tachycardia occurs in the fetus, it can cause severe heart failure and hydrops fetalis.

In neonates, SVT usually presents with a narrow QRS complex (<0.08 sec). The P wave is visible on a standard electrocardiogram in only 50–60% of neonates with SVT but is visible with a transesophageal lead in most patients. Differentiation from sinus tachycardia may be difficult; if the rate is greater than 230 beats/min and there is an abnormal P wave axis (the normal P wave is positive in leads I and aVF), SVT is more likely. The heart rate in SVT also tends to be unvarying, whereas in sinus tachycardia the heart rate varies with changes in vagal and sympathetic tone. Differentiation from ventricular tachycardia is critical because digoxin can precipitate ventricular fibrillation in patients with ventricular tachycardia. The absence of P waves and the presence of wide QRS complexes

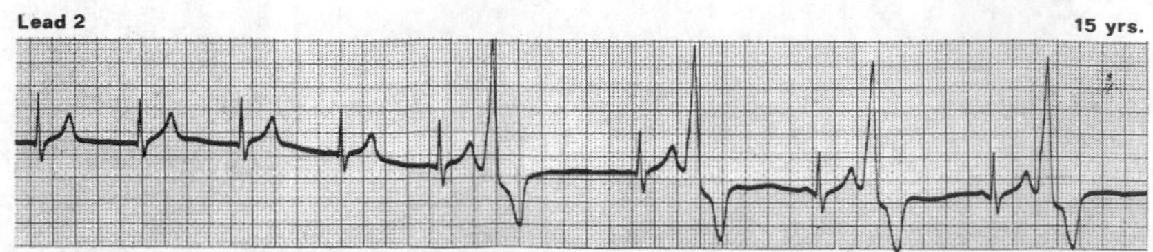

Figure 442–4 Premature ventricular contractions (PVCs) induced by hyperventilation. Note that the premature beat is wide and has a completely different morphology from that of the sinus beat. The premature beat is not preceded by a P wave, and the pause following it is fully compensatory (i.e., the P-P interval containing the PVC equals two sinus cycles); this indicates that the sinus mechanism has not been disturbed by the premature beats.

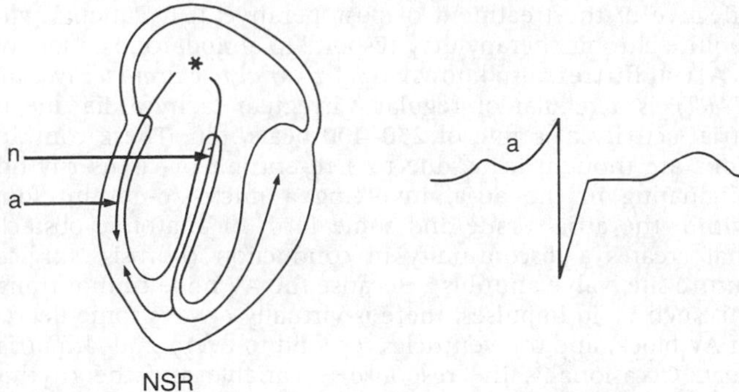

Figure 442–5 Schematic representation of the heart with a right-sided anomalous pathway. The *asterisk* indicates the initiation of the sinus beat. The *arrows* indicate the direction and spread of excitation. The electrocardiograpic complex shown represents a fusion beat that combines activation over the normal (n) and accessory (a) pathways. The latter inscribes the δ wave.

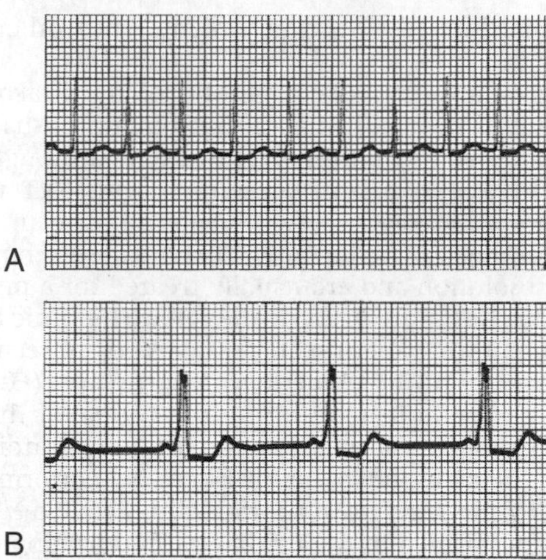

Figure 442–7 *A*, SVT in a child with Wolff-Parkinson-White (WPW) syndrome. Note the normal QRS complexes during the tachycardia. *B*. Later the typical features of WPW syndrome are apparent (short P-R interval, δ wave, and wide QRS).

that are dissimilar to the QRS complex during sinus rhythm are more diagnostic of ventricular tachycardia.

SVT may be associated with a bypass tract, either a concealed accessory pathway (*AV nodal re-entry tachycardia*) or an antegrade conducting pathway (*Wolff-Parkinson-White syndrome*, also known as *pre-excitation syndrome*). SVT may also occur without a bypass tract, in which case re-entry occurs within the sinus node or within the atrium. SVT may occur in the presence of unoperated congenital heart disease (Ebstein's anomaly). In children, SVT may be precipitated by exposure to sympathomimetic amines contained in over-the-counter decongestants.

The typical electrocardiographic features of the **Wolff-Parkinson-White** *syndrome* are usually seen when the patient is not having the tachycardia. These include a short PR interval and slow upstroke of the QRS (delta wave) (Fig. 442–7). Although most often present in patients with a normal heart, this syndrome may also be associated with Ebstein's anomaly and other congenital heart lesions. The anatomic substrates comprising the re-entrant circuit are the AV node and an accessory pre-excitation pathway, consisting of a muscular bridge connecting atrium to ventricle on either the right or the left side of the AV ring (see Fig. 442–5). During sinus rhythm, the impulse is carried over both the AV node and the accessory pathway; it produces some degree of fusion of the two depolarization fronts that results in an abnormal QRS.

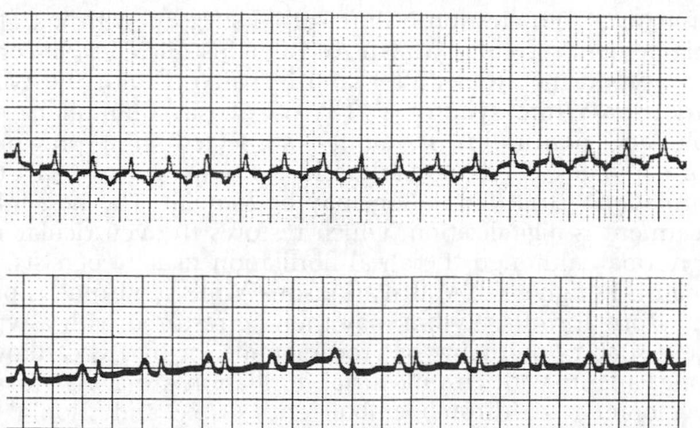

Figure 442–6 The upper tracing shows paroxysmal supraventricular or atrial tachycardia (PAT) with a ventricular rate of 230/min. The lower tracing shows sinus rhythm after DC cardioversion. Note that during the tachycardia, the T wave is deformed by an inverted, presumably retrograde, P wave. The QRS morphology is unchanged during the tachycardia. Low voltage is due to peripheral edema in a 1-day-old infant who had intrauterine tachycardia and hydrops fetalis.

During tachycardia an impulse is usually carried in anterograde fashion through the AV node (*orthodromic conduction*), resulting in a normal QRS complex, and in retrograde fashion through the accessory pathway, reaching the atrium and perpetuating the tachycardia. In these cases, only after cessation of the tachycardia are the typical features of Wolff-Parkinson-White syndrome recognized (see Fig. 442–7). When rapid anterograde conduction occurs through the pre-excitation pathway during tachycardia and the retrograde re-entry pathway to the atrium is via the AV node (*antidromic conduction*), the tachycardiac complexes are wide and the potential for more serious arrhythmias is greater, especially if atrial fibrillation occurs.

TREATMENT. Vagal stimulation by submersion of the face in iced saline (in older children) or an ice bag over the face (in infants) may abort the attack. To abolish the paroxysm, older children may be taught **vagotonic maneuvers** such as the Valsalva maneuver, straining, breath-holding, drinking ice water, or adopting a particular posture. When these measures fail, several pharmacologic alternatives are available (see Table 442–1). In stable patients, adenosine by rapid intravenous push is the treatment of choice because of its rapid onset of action and minimal effects on cardiac contractility. Other drugs that have been used for initial treatment of SVT include infusions of phenylephrine (Neo-Synephrine) or edrophonium (Tensilon), which increase vagal tone through the baroreflex, as well as the antiarrhythmic agents quinidine, procainamide, and propranolol. Calcium channel blockers such as verapamil have also been used in the initial treatment of SVT in older children. Verapamil may reduce cardiac output and produce hypotension and cardiac arrest in infants younger than 1 yr of age; it is contraindicated in this age group. In urgent situations when symptoms of severe heart failure have already occurred, **synchronized DC cardioversion** (0.5–2 watt-sec/kg) is recommended as the initial management.

Once the patient has been converted to sinus rhythm, a longer acting agent is selected for maintenance therapy. In patients without an antegrade accessory pathway, digoxin or propranolol is the mainstay of therapy. In children with evidence of pre-excitation (e.g., Wolff-Parkinson-White syndrome), digoxin or calcium channel blockers may increase the rate of anterograde conduction of impulses through the bypass tract and should be avoided. These patients are usually managed in the long term with propranolol. In patients with resistant tachycardias, procainamide, quinidine, flecainide, propafenone, sotalol, and amiodarone have all been used. It should be recognized that most antiarrhythmic agents can have proarrhythmic and negative inotropic effects. Flecainide in particular should be limited to use in patients with otherwise normal hearts.

If cardiac failure occurs because of prolonged tachycardia in an infant with a normal heart, cardiac function usually returns to normal after sinus rhythm is reinstituted, although this may take days to weeks. Infants presenting with SVT within the first 3–4 mo of life have a lower incidence of recurrence than those presenting at a later age. These patients have a 40% chance of resolution and are usually treated for a minimum of 1 yr after diagnosis, after which the antiarrhythmic agents can be tapered and the patient watched for signs of recurrence.

Twenty-four hour electrocardiographic (Holter) recordings are useful in monitoring the course of therapy and in detecting brief runs of asymptomatic tachycardia. A brief assessment of arrhythmia control can be performed at the bedside using *transesophageal pacing*. More detailed *electrophysiologic studies* performed in the cardiac catheterization laboratory are often indicated in patients with refractory SVTs. During an electrophysiologic study, multiple electrode catheters are placed in different locations in the heart. By comparing the timing of premature beats in different leads, the location of an ectopic focus or bypass tract can be identified. The tachyarrhythmia can be induced by pacing, and different pharmacologic agents can be tested for their ability to inhibit the arrhythmia. These studies are necessary prerequisites to radiofrequency ablation.

Radiofrequency ablation of an accessory pathway is another treatment option for patients in whom multiple agents are required or drug side effects are intolerable or when arrhythmia control is poor. The overall initial success rate ranges from approximately 80% to 95%, depending on the location of the bypass tract or tracts. Surgical ablation of bypass tracts can also be successful in selected patients.

Atrial ectopic tachycardia is an uncommon tachycardia in childhood. It is characterized by a variable rate (seldom greater than 200 beats/min), identifiable P waves with an abnormal axis, and chronicity in either a sustained or intermittent tachycardia. In this form of atrial tachycardia, there is a single automatic focus rather than the more usual re-entry mechanism. Identification of this mechanism is aided by monitoring the electrocardiogram while initiating vagal or pharmacologic therapy. Re-entry tachycardias "break" suddenly, whereas automatic tachycardias gradually slow down and then gradually speed up again. Atrial ectopic tachycardias are usually more difficult to control pharmacologically than are the more common re-entrant tachycardias. If pharmacologic therapy with a single agent is unsuccessful, catheter ablation is suggested and has a greater than 90% success rate.

Chaotic or multifocal atrial tachycardia is characterized by three or more ectopic P waves with three or more different ectopic P-P cycles, frequent blocked P waves, and varying P-R intervals of conducted beats. This arrhythmia occurs most often in infants less than 1 yr of age, usually without cardiac disease, although there is some evidence suggesting an association with viral myocarditis. Drug treatment may not be effective, and multiple agents are often required. Fortunately, when this arrhythmia occurs in infancy, it usually terminates spontaneously by 3 yr of age.

Accelerated junctional ectopic tachycardia (JET) is an automatic (non–re-entry) arrhythmia in which the junctional rate exceeds that of the sinus node so that AV dissociation results. This arrhythmia is most often recognized in the early postoperative period following cardiac surgery and may be extremely difficult to control. Reduction of the infusion rate of catecholamines and control of fever are important adjuncts to management. JET in these patients often disappears spontaneously without specific treatment; JET in the absence of surgery carries a more guarded prognosis. Junctional tachycardia may also be a sign of digitalis intoxication; when this occurs the drug should be discontinued. Intravenous amiodarone is effective in the treatment of postoperative JET. Patients who require chronic therapy may respond to amiodarone or sotalol.

Atrial flutter, also known as *intra-atrial re-entrant tachycardia (IART)*, is a regular or regularly irregular tachycardia due to atrial activity at a rate of 250–400 beats/min. These contractions are thought to be due to a re-entrant or circus rhythm originating in the atria, involving a micro–re-entrant loop within the atrial tissue and some form of anatomic obstacle that creates a discontinuity in conduction (fibrosis, surgical suture site, valve annulus). Because the AV node cannot transmit such rapid impulses, there is virtually always some degree of AV block, and the ventricles respond to every 2nd–4th atrial beat. Occasionally, the response is variable and the rhythm appears irregular.

In older children, atrial flutter usually occurs in the setting of congenital heart disease; neonates with atrial flutter frequently have normal hearts. Atrial flutter may occur during acute infectious illnesses but is most often seen in patients with large stretched atria, such as those associated with long-standing mitral or tricuspid insufficiency, tricuspid atresia, Ebstein's anomaly, or rheumatic mitral stenosis. Atrial flutter can also occur after palliative or corrective intra-atrial surgery. Uncontrolled atrial flutter may precipitate heart failure. Vagal maneuvers (such as carotid sinus pressure or iced saline submersion) or adenosine usually produce a temporary slowing of the heart rate. The diagnosis is confirmed by electrocardiography, which demonstrates the rapid and regular atrial saw-toothed flutter waves. Atrial flutter usually converts immediately to sinus rhythm by DC cardioversion, and this is most often the treatment of choice. Patients with chronic atrial flutter in the setting of congenital heart disease may be at increased risk of thromboembolism and stroke and thus should undergo anticoagulation prior to elective cardioversion. Digitalis slows the ventricular response in atrial flutter by prolonging conduction time through the AV node. After digitalization, a type I agent such as quinidine or procainamide is usually needed to maintain adequate control. Type III agents such as amiodarone and sotalol have shown promise and may be useful in patients refractory to type I agents. Other therapies currently under investigation include radiofrequency ablation and surgical ablation. Neonates with normal hearts who respond to digoxin may be treated for 6–12 mo, after which the medication can often be discontinued.

Atrial fibrillation is much less common in children and rare in infants. The atrial excitation is chaotic and more rapid (300–700 beats/min) and produces an irregularly irregular ventricular response and pulse (Fig. 442–8). This rhythm disorder is most often the result of a chronically stretched atrial myocardium. Atrial fibrillation occurs most frequently in older children with rheumatic mitral valve disease. It is also seen rarely as a complication of intra-atrial surgery, with left atrial enlargement secondary to left AV valve insufficiency, in conditions producing atrial flutter, and in patients with the Wolff-Parkinson-White syndrome. Thyrotoxicosis, pulmonary emboli, and pericarditis should be suspected in a previously normal older child or adolescent who presents with atrial fibrillation. Atrial fibrillation may be familial. The best initial treatment is digitalization, which restores the ventricular rate to normal, although the atrial fibrillation usually persists. Digoxin is not given if Wolff-Parkinson-White syndrome is present. Normal sinus rhythm may then be restored with a type I agent such as quinidine or procainamide, or by DC cardioversion. Patients with chronic atrial fibrillation are at risk for the development of thromboemboli and stroke and should undergo anticoagulation with warfarin. Patients undergoing elective cardioversion should also undergo anticoagulation.

442.3 Ventricular Tachyarrhythmias

Ventricular tachycardia (VT) is less common than SVT in pediatric patients. VT is defined as at least three PVCs at greater

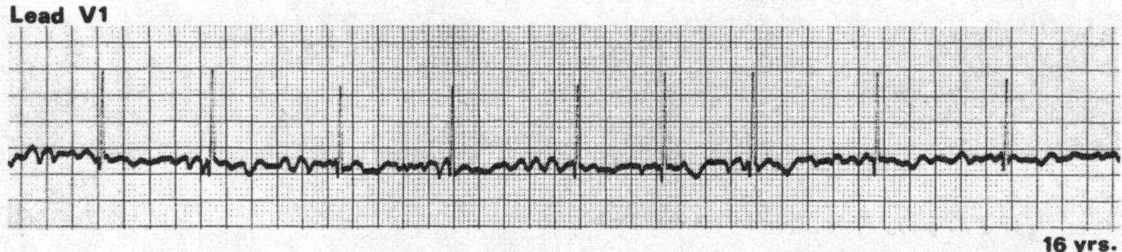

Figure 442–8 Atrial fibrillation, characterized by absence of P waves; presence of fibrillatory waves, which are grossly irregular, rapid undulations; and an irregular ventricular response. Fibrillatory waves may not be visible in all leads and should be carefully sought in every tracing with irregular R-R intervals. (The coexisting qR in V_1 is diagnostic of right ventricular hypertrophy in this patient with Eisenmenger syndrome.)

than 120 beats/min. It may be paroxysmal or incessant. VT may be associated with myocarditis, anomalous origin of a coronary artery, arrhythmogenic right ventricular dysplasia, mitral valve prolapse, primary cardiac tumors, cardiomyopathy, prolonged Q-T interval of either congenital or acquired (proarrhythmic drugs) cause, Wolff-Parkinson-White syndrome, or drugs (cocaine, amphetamines); it may develop many years after intraventricular surgery (tetralogy of Fallot, ventricular septal defect) or occur without obvious organic heart disease. VT must be distinguished from SVT with aberrancy or rapid conduction over an accessory pathway (Table 442–2). The presence of capture and fusion beats helps confirm the diagnosis. Although some children tolerate rapid ventricular rates for many hours, this arrhythmia should be promptly treated because hypotension and degeneration into ventricular fibrillation may result. For patients who are hemodynamically stable, intravenous lidocaine is the initial drug of choice. If treatment is to be successful, it is critical to search for and correct any underlying abnormalities such as electrolyte imbalance, hypoxia, or drug toxicity. Alternative drugs include procainamide, propranolol, and amiodarone (see Table 442–1). Overdrive ventricular pacing may also be effective, although this may occasionally cause the arrhythmia to deteriorate into ventricular fibrillation. In the neonatal period, ventricular tachycardia may be associated with anomalous left coronary artery (see Chapter 439.2) or with a myocardial tumor.

Unless a clearly reversible cause is identified, electrophysiologic study is usually indicated for patients in whom VT has developed.

Ventricular fibrillation is a chaotic dysrhythmia that results in death unless an effective ventricular beat is rapidly restored. A thump on the chest sometimes restores sinus rhythm. Usually external cardiac massage with artificial ventilation and DC defibrillation are necessary. If defibrillation is ineffective or fibrillation recurs, bretylium tosylate may be given intravenously and defibrillation repeated. Isoproterenol may be used as a last resort. After recovery from ventricular fibrillation, a search should be made for the underlying cause. The Q-T interval should be measured to rule out long Q-T syndrome (LQTS). Electrophysiologic study is usually indicated for patients in whom ventricular fibrillation has developed unless a clearly reversible cause is identified. If the Wolff-Parkinson-White syndrome is found, ablation should be performed. For patients in whom no correctable abnormality can be found, an AICD should be strongly considered because of the high risk of sudden death.

442.4 Long Q-T Syndrome

A particularly malignant form of ventricular arrhythmia called *torsades de pointes* occurs in patients with LQTS and is a cause of syncope and sudden death. About 50% of cases are familial: **Romano-Ward syndrome** has autosomal dominant transmission and may be associated with congenital deafness; **Jervell-Lange-Nielsen syndrome** has autosomal recessive transmission. The remainder of cases are sporadic. Genetic studies have identified mutations in cardiac potassium and sodium channels. Drugs may prolong the Q-T interval directly (terfenadine, astemizole) or, more often, when their metabolism is inhibited by drugs such as erythromycin or ketoconazole.

The clinical presentation of LQTS in children is most often a syncopal episode often brought on by exercise, fright, or a sudden startle. Patients can present with seizures, presyncope, and palpitations, and about 10% present initially with cardiac arrest. Diagnosis is based on electrocardiographic and clinical criteria. Not all patients with long Q-T intervals have LQTS, and there are rare patients with normal Q-T intervals on a resting electrocardiogram who may have LQTS syndrome. A heart rate–corrected Q-T interval of greater than 0.47 sec is highly indicative, whereas a Q-T interval of greater than 0.44 sec is suspicious. Other features include notched T waves, T-wave alternans, a low heart rate for age, a history of syncope (especially with stress), and a familial history of either LQTS or unexplained sudden death. Twenty-four hour Holter monitoring and exercise testing are adjuncts to the diagnosis.

Treatment of LQTS includes the use of β-blocking agents at doses that blunt the heart rate response to exercise. Some patients may require a pacemaker because of drug-induced

TABLE 442–2 Diagnosis of Tachyarrhythmias

	Electrocardiographic Findings			
	Heart Rate (beats/min)	***P Wave***	***QRS Duration***	***Regularity***
Sinus tachycardia	<225	Always present Normal axis	Normal	Rate varies with respiration
Atrial tachycardia	180–320	Present—50% Superior axis common	Normal or prolonged (RBBB pattern)	Regular
Atrial fibrillation	120–180	Fibrillatory waves	Normal or prolonged (RBBB pattern)	Irregularly irregular
Atrial flutter	Atrial: 250–400 Ventricular response variable: 100–320	Saw-toothed flutter waves	Normal or prolonged (RBBB pattern)	Regular ventricular response (e.g., 2 : 1, 3 : 1, 3 : 2, and so on)
Ventricular tachycardia	120–240	Absent or atrioventricular dissociation	Usually prolonged	Slightly irregular

RBBB = right bundle branch block.

profound bradycardia. In patients with continued syncope despite treatment and for those who have experienced cardiac arrest, many authorities recommend an AICD.

442.5 Bradyarrhythmias

Sinus arrest and *sinoatrial block* may cause a sudden pause in the heart beat. The former is presumed to be caused by failure of impulse formation within the sinus node and the latter by a block between the sinus impulse and the surrounding atrium. These arrhythmias are rare in childhood except as manifestations of digitalis intoxication or in patients who have had extensive atrial surgery.

AV block may be divided into three forms. In **1st-degree block**, the P-R interval is prolonged, but all the atrial impulses are conducted to the ventricle. In **2nd-degree block**, some impulses are not conducted to the ventricle. In one variant of *2nd-degree block* known as the **Wenckebach type** (also called *Mobitz type I*), the P-P interval remains constant and the P-R interval increases progressively until a P wave is not conducted. In the cycle following the dropped beat, the P-R interval is again shorter (Fig. 442–9). In *Mobitz type II*, occasional atrial beats are not conducted to the ventricle; this conduction defect has more potential to cause syncope and may be progressive. In **3rd-degree block** (complete heart block), no impulses from the atria reach the ventricles.

Congenital complete AV block in children is most often caused by autoimmune injury of the fetal conduction system by maternally derived IgG antibodies (anti-SSA/Ro, anti-SSB/La) in a mother with overt or, more often, asymptomatic systemic lupus erythematosus. Rheumatoid arthritis, dermatomyositis, or Sjögren's syndrome is rarely the primary autoimmune process. Autoimmune disease accounts for 60–70% of all cases of congenital complete heart block and about 80% of cases in which there is a structurally normal heart. Complete heart block is also seen in patients with complex congenital heart disease, abnormal embryonic development of the conduction system, myocardial tumors, myocarditis, myocardial abscess due to endocarditis, LQTS, postsurgical repair of congenital heart disease involving the ventricular septum, and Kearns-Sayre syndrome. The incidence of congenital complete heart block is 1 in 20,000–25,000 live births; a high fetal wastage rate may cause an underestimation of its true incidence. In some infants of mothers with systemic lupus erythematosus, complete heart block is not present at birth but develops within the first 3–6 mo after birth. The arrhythmia is occasionally suspected in the fetus and may produce hydrops fetalis. The dissociation between atrial and ventricular contractions can be diagnosed by fetal echocardiography. Infants with associated congenital heart disease who experience heart failure in the 1st wk of life are at greatest risk for serious illness.

In older children with otherwise normal hearts, the condition is commonly asymptomatic, although syncope may occur. Older infants may have night terrors, tiredness with frequent naps, and irritability. The peripheral pulse is prominent as a result of the compensatory large ventricular stroke volume and peripheral vasodilation; the systolic blood pressure is elevated. Jugular venous pulsations occur irregularly and may be large when the atrium contracts against a closed tricuspid valve (cannon wave). Exercise and atropine may produce an acceleration of 10–20 beats/min or more. Systolic murmurs are frequently audible along the left sternal border, and apical mid-diastolic murmurs are not unusual. Heart block results in enlargement of the heart on the basis of increased diastolic ventricular filling.

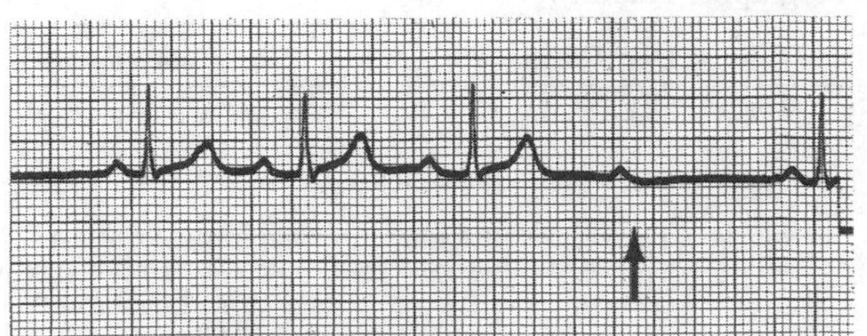

Figure 442–9 Wenckebach phenomenon (Mobitz I). The P-R interval gradually lengthens until the 4th P wave in the cycle is not conducted to the ventricle (*arrow*). The ensuing P-R interval is once again normal.

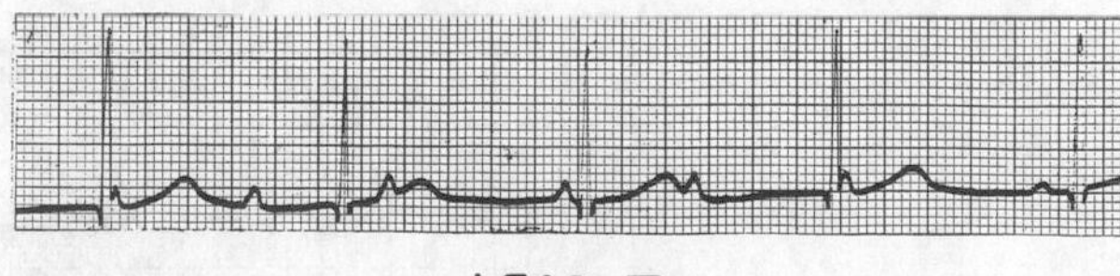

Figure 442–10 Complete atrioventricular block. The ventricular rate is regular at 53/min. The atrial rate varied from 65 to 95/min. The QRS morphology is normal, which is usual in congenital A-V block.

The *diagnosis* is confirmed by electrocardiography; the P waves and QRS complexes have no constant relation (Fig. 442–10). The QRS duration may be prolonged, or it may be normal if the heart beat is initiated high in the bundle of His.

The *prognosis* for congenital complete heart block is usually favorable; patients who have been observed to the age of 30–40 yr have lived normal, active lives. Some patients have episodes of dizziness with or without syncope **(Stokes-Adams attacks)**; this complication requires the implantation of a permanent cardiac pacemaker. Pacemaker implantation should be considered in patients who acquire symptoms such as progressive cardiac enlargement, prolonged pauses, or awake heart rates less than or equal to 40 beats/min.

Cardiac pacing is required in neonates with ventricular rates less than or equal to 50 beats/min who show evidence of hydrops or experience heart failure after birth. Isoproterenol, atropine, or epinephrine may be used to try to increase the heart rate temporarily until pacemaker placement can be arranged. Patients with complete heart block and congenital heart disease should also receive a pacemaker. Transthoracic epicardial pacemaker implants have been traditionally used in infants; transvenous placement of pacemaker leads is available for older infants and young children.

Postsurgical complete AV block can occur after any open heart procedure requiring suturing near the AV valves or crest of the ventricular septum. Because postoperative heart block may be transient, the patient should be maintained with temporary pacing wires inserted at the time of surgery until at least 10–14 days, after which it is much less likely that sinus rhythm will return.

442.6 Sick Sinus Syndrome

The sick sinus syndrome is the result of abnormalities in the sinus node or atrial conduction pathways, or both. This syndrome may occur in the absence of congenital heart disease and has been reported in siblings, but it is most commonly seen after surgical correction of congenital heart defects, especially the atrial switch (Mustard or Senning) operation for transposition of the great arteries. The *clinical manifestations* depend on the heart rate. Most patients remain asymptomatic without treatment. Dizziness and syncope can occur during periods of marked sinus slowing with failure of junctional escape (Fig. 442–11). SVT may alternate with bradycardia *(bradycardia-tachycardia syndrome)*, causing palpitations, exercise intolerance, or dizziness. Treatment must be individualized.

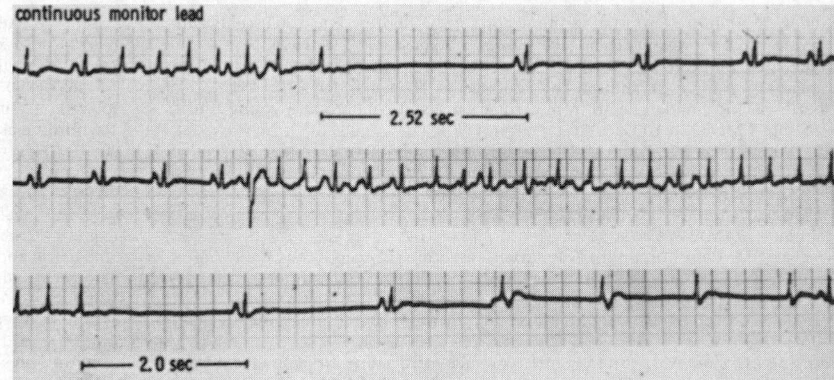

Figure 442–11 Sick sinus syndrome with bradytachycardia. Note the bursts of supraventricular tachycardia, probably multifocal in origin, followed by long periods of sinus arrest and by sinus bradycardia.

Drug therapy to control tachyarrhythmias (e.g., propranolol, quinidine, procainamide) may suppress sinus and AV node function to the degree that symptomatic bradycardia may be produced. Therefore, insertion of a demand ventricular pacemaker in conjunction with drug therapy is usually necessary for symptomatic patients.

442.7 Sudden Death

Sudden death other than sudden infant death syndrome (see Chapter 714) is rare in children less than 18 yr of age. Potential causes are noted in Table 442–3. Approximately 65% of sudden deaths are due to heart-related problems in patients with normal or congenitally (corrected, palliated, or unoperated) abnormal hearts. Symptoms may be absent prior to the event but if present include syncope, chest pain, dyspnea, and palpitations. There may be a family history (dilated or hypertrophic cardiomyopathy, long Q-T interval, right ventricular dysplasia, mitral valve prolapse, Marfan's syndrome) of heart disease or sudden death. Death often follows exertion or exercise.

TABLE 442–3 Potential Causes of Sudden Death in Infants, Children, and Adolescents

SIDS and SIDS "Mimics"
- SIDS
- Long Q-T syndromes
- Inborn errors of metabolism
- Child abuse
- Myocarditis
- Duct-dependent congenital heart disease

Corrected or Unoperated Congenital Heart Disease
- Aortic stenosis
- Tetralogy of Fallot
- Transposition of great vessels (postoperative atrial switch)
- Mitral valve prolapse
- Hypoplastic left heart syndrome
- Eisenmenger's syndrome

Coronary Arterial Disease
- Anomalous origin
- Anomalous tract
- Kawasaki disease
- Periarteritis
- Arterial dissection
- Marfan syndrome
- Myocardial infarction

Myocardial Disease
- Myocarditis
- Hypertrophic cardiomyopathy
- Dilated cardiomyopathy
- Arrhythmogenic right ventricular dysplasia

Conduction System Abnormality/Arrhythmia
- Long Q-T syndromes
- Proarrhythmic drugs
- Pre-excitation syndromes
- Heart block
- Commotio cordis
- Idiopathic ventricular fibrillation
- Heart tumor

Miscellaneous
- Pulmonary hypertension
- Pulmonary embolism
- Heat stroke
- Cocaine
- Anorexia nervosa
- Electrolyte disturbances

SIDS = sudden infant death syndrome.

Commotio cordis is a nearly universally fatal condition that follows blunt trauma to the chest (e.g., from a baseball or hockey puck). Patients experience immediate ventricular fibrillation in the absence of identifiable cardiac trauma (contusion, hematoma, lacerated coronary artery). Death results from ventricular fibrillation that is unresponsive to all resuscitative efforts.

PREVENTION OF SUDDEN DEATH. Many of the more common causes of sudden death in children and adolescents can be identified from the patient's history (prodromal symptoms), the family history, and physical examination.

Avoiding high-risk behavior (cocaine, anorexia nervosa) and knowledge of drug side effects (tricyclic antidepressants) or drug interactions (seldane-erythromycin) is critical. Chest-protecting equipment and softer baseballs may prevent *commotio cordis.*

Benson DW Jr, Smith WM, Dunnigan A, et al: Mechanisms of regular, wide QRS tachycardia in infants and children. Am J Cardiol 49:1778, 1982.

Brugada R, Tapscott T, Czernuszewicz GZ, et al: Identification of a genetic locus for familial atrial fibrillation. N Engl J Med 336:905, 1997.

Case C, Crawford F, Gillette P: Surgical treatment of dysrhythmias. Pediatr Clin North Am 37:79, 1990.

Dick M: Complete heart block in children. Curr Opin Pediatr 2:957, 1990.

Dungan WT, Garson A Jr, Gillette PC: Arrhythmogenic right ventricular dysplasia: A cause of ventricular tachycardia in children with apparently normal hearts. Am Heart J 102:745, 1981.

Dunnigan A, Benson DW Jr, Banditt DG: Atrial flutter in infancy: Diagnosis, clinical features, and treatment. Pediatrics 75:725, 1985.

Fenrich AL, Perry JC, Friedman RA: Flecainide and amiodarone: Combined therapy for refractory tachyarrhythmias in infancy. J Am Coll Cardiol 25:1195, 1995.

Fried MD: Advances in the diagnosis and therapy of syncopy and palpitations in children. Curr Opin Pediatr 6:368, 1994.

Garson A Jr: How to measure the QT interval—what is normal? Am J Cardiol 72:14B, 1993.

Goodwin JF: Sudden cardiac death in the young. Br Med J 314:843, 1997.

Gow R: Ventricular arrhythmias in infants and children. Curr Opin Pediatr 2:963, 1990.

Griffith MJ, Linker NJ, Garratt CJ, et al: Relative efficacy and safety of intravenous drugs for termination of sustained ventricular tachycardia. Lancet 336:670, 1990.

Johnson WH, Dunnigan A, Fehr P, et al: Association of atrial flutter with orthodromic reciprocating fetal tachycardia. Ann J Cardiol 59:374, 1987.

Josephson ME: Antiarrhythmic agents and the danger of proarrhythmic events. Ann Intern Med 111:101, 1989.

Kaminer SJ, Pickoff AS, Dunnigan A, et al: Cardiomyopathy and the use of implanted cardio-defibrillators in children. PACE 13:593, 1990.

Kirk CR, Gibbs JL, Thomas R: Cardiovascular collapse after verapamil in supraventricular tachycardia. Arch Dis Child 62:1265, 1987.

Kugler JD, Danford DA: Management of infants, children, and adolescents with paroxysmal supraventricular tachycardia. J Pediatr 129:324, 1996.
Kugler JD, Danford DA, Deal BJ, et al: Radiofrequency catheter ablation for tachyarrhythmias in children and adolescents. N Engl J Med 330:1481, 1994.
Liberthson RR: Sudden death from cardiac causes in children and young adults. N Engl J Med 334:1039, 1996.
Link MS, Wang PJ, Pandian NG, et al: An experimental model of sudden death due to low-energy chest-wall impact (commotio cordis). N Engl J Med 338:1805, 1998.
Maron BJ, Shirani J, Poliac LC, et al: Sudden death in young competitive athletes. JAMA 276:199, 1996.
Narayan SM, Cain ME, Smith JM: Atrial fibrillation. Lancet 350:943, 1997.
Ommen SR, Odell JA, Stanton MS: Atrial arrhythmias after cardiothoracic surgery. N Engl J Med 336:1429, 1997.
Perry JC, Garson A Jr: Diagnosis and treatment of arrhythmias. Adv Pediatr 36:177, 1989.
Perry JC, Garson A Jr: Supraventricular tachycardia due to Wolff-Parkinson-White syndrome in children: Early disappearance and late recurrence. J Am Coll Cardiol 16:1215, 1990.
Pongiglione G: The role of the pediatric electrophysiologist in the diagnosis and treatment of supraventricular tachydysrhythmias. Curr Opin Pediatr 1:124, 1989.
Ralston MA, Knilans TK, Hannon DW, et al: Use of adenosine for diagnosis and treatment of tachyarrhythmias in pediatric patients. J Pediatr 124:139, 1994.
Rankin AC: Non-sedating antihistamines and cardiac arrhythmia. Lancet 350:1115, 1997.
Risser WL, Anderson SJ, Bolduc SP, et al: Cardiac dysrhythmias and sports. Pediatrics 95:786, 1995.
Ross B: Congenital complete atrioventricular block. Pediatr Clin North Am 37:69, 1990.
Splawski I, Timothy KW, Vincent GM, et al: Molecular basis of the long-QT syndrome associated with deafness. N Engl J Med 336:1562, 1997.
Tan HL, Hou CJY, Lauer MR, et al: Electrophysiologic mechanisms of the long QT interval syndromes and torsade de pointes. Ann Intern Med 122:701, 1995.
Tanel RE, Walsh EP, Triedman JK, et al: Five-year experience with radiofrequency catheter ablation: Implications for management of arrhythmias in pediatric and young adult patients. J Pediatr 131:878, 1997.
Tchou PJ, Kadri N, Anderson J, et al: Automatic implantable cardioverter defibrillators and survival of patients with left ventricular dysfunction and malignant ventricular arrhythmias. Ann Intern Med 109:529, 1988.
Van Hare GF, Stanger P: Ventricular tachycardia and accelerated ventricular rhythm presenting in the first month of life. Am J Cardiol 67:42, 1991.
Van Hare GF, Lesh MD, Scheinman M, et al: Percutaneous radiofrequency catheter ablation for supraventricular tachycardia in children. J Am Coll Cardiol 17:1613, 1991.
Wellens HJJ, Brugada P, Penn OC: The management of preexcitation syndromes. JAMA 257:2325, 1987.
Zimetbaum P, Josephson ME: Evaluation of patients with palpitations. N Engl J Med 338:1369, 1998.
Zipes DP: Guidelines for clinical intracardiac electrophysiologic studies. J Am Coll Cardiol 14:1827, 1989.

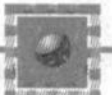

SECTION 5

Acquired Heart Disease

CHAPTER 443
Infective Endocarditis

Infective endocarditis includes acute and subacute bacterial endocarditis as well as nonbacterial endocarditis caused by viruses, fungi, and other microbiologic agents. It is a significant cause of morbidity and mortality among children and adolescents despite advances in the management and prophylaxis of the disease with antimicrobial agents. The inability to eradicate infective endocarditis by prevention or early treatment stems from several factors: The nature of the infecting organisms has changed; physicians, dentists, and the public are not sufficiently aware of the threat of infective endocarditis and the preventive measures available; diagnosis may be difficult when delayed; and special risk groups have emerged, which include an increasing number of intravenous narcotics users, survivors of cardiac surgery, patients taking immunosuppressant medications, and patients who require chronic intravascular catheters.

ETIOLOGY. Previously, *Streptococcus viridans* was the agent most commonly responsible for endocarditis in pediatric patients. *Staphylococcus aureus* is now the leading causative agent in some series, accounting for approximately 39% of episodes. Other organisms cause endocarditis less frequently, and in approximately 10% of cases blood culture results are negative for these organisms (Table 443–1). No relationship exists between the infecting organism and the type of congenital defect, duration of illness, or age of the child. Staphylococcal endocarditis is more common in patients with no underlying heart disease; *S. viridans* is more common after dental procedures, group D enterococci are seen more often after lower bowel or genitourinary manipulation, *Pseudomonas aeruginosa* or *Serratia marcescens* is seen more often among intravenous drug users, and fungal organisms are encountered after open heart surgery.

EPIDEMIOLOGY. Infective endocarditis is most often a complication of congenital or rheumatic heart disease but can also occur in children without a cardiac malformation. In developed countries, congenital heart disease is the overwhelming predisposing factor. Endocarditis is rare in infancy; in this age group it usually follows open heart surgery.

Patients with congenital heart lesions in which a high velocity of blood is ejected through a hole or stenotic orifice are most susceptible to endocarditis. Vegetations are usually formed at the site of the endocardial or intimal erosion that results from the turbulent flow. Children with ventricular septal defects (VSDs), left-sided valvular disease, and systemic-pulmonary arterial communications (including palliative shunts) are at the highest risk. Thus, tetralogy of Fallot, VSD, aortic stenosis, patent ductus arteriosus, transposition of the great arteries, and Blalock-Taussig shunts are the most frequent structural lesions associated with endocarditis. In older patients, congenital bicuspid aortic valves and mitral valve prolapse pose additional risks for endocarditis. Surgical correction of congenital heart disease may reduce but does not eliminate the risk of endocarditis, with the exception of repair of a simple atrial septal defect or patent ductus arteriosus. Children who have had a valve replacement or valved conduit repair are at particularly high risk.

In approximately 30% of patients with infective endocarditis, a predisposing factor is recognized. A surgical or dental procedure can be implicated in approximately 65% of these cases in which the potential source of bacteremia is identified. Poor dental hygiene in children with cyanotic heart disease results in a greater risk for endocarditis. The occurrence of endocarditis directly following heart surgery is relatively low, but it is frequently an antecedent event.

CLINICAL MANIFESTATIONS (Table 443–2). The early symptoms and signs are usually mild, especially when *S. viridans* is the infecting organism. Prolonged fever, without other manifestations (except occasionally weight loss) and persisting for as long as several months, may often be the only medical history.

Alternatively, the onset may be acute and severe, with high, intermittent fever and prostration. Usually the onset and course vary between these two extremes. The symptoms are often nonspecific, consisting of low-grade fever with afternoon elevations, fatigue, myalgia, arthralgia, headache, and at times chills, nausea, and vomiting. New or changing heart murmurs are common, particularly when there is associated heart failure. Splenomegaly and petechiae are relatively common. Serious neurologic complications, such as emboli, cerebral abscesses, mycotic aneurysms, and hemorrhage, are most often associated with staphylococcal disease and may be late manifestations. These complications are manifested by meningismus, increased intracranial pressure, altered sensorium, and focal neurologic signs. Myocardial abscesses may occur with staphylococcal disease and may rupture into the pericardium, producing purulent pericarditis. Pulmonary and other systemic emboli are infrequent, except with fungal disease. Many of the classic skin manifestations develop late in the course of the disease; they are seldom seen in the appropriately treated patient. These manifestations include *Osler nodes* (tender, pea-sized intradermal nodules in the pads of the fingers and toes), *Janeway lesions* (painless small erythematous or hemorrhagic lesions on the palms and soles), and *splinter hemorrhages* (linear lesions beneath the nails). These lesions may represent vasculitis produced by circulating antigen-antibody complexes.

The identification of infective endocarditis is most often based on a high index of suspicion in the evaluation of an infection in a child with an underlying contributory factor.

LABORATORY DIAGNOSIS. The critical information for appropriate treatment of infective endocarditis is obtained from blood cultures. All other laboratory data are secondary in importance (see Table 443–2). Blood specimens for culture should be obtained as promptly as possible, even if the child feels well and has no other physical findings. Three to five separate blood collections should be obtained after careful preparation of the phlebotomy site. Contamination presents a special problem, as bacteria found on the skin may themselves cause infective endocarditis. The timing of collections is not important because bacteremia can be expected to be relatively constant. In 90% of cases of endocarditis, the causative agent is recovered from the 1st two blood cultures. The laboratory should be notified that endocarditis is suspected, as the blood may need to be cultured on enriched media for a longer time than usual (>7 days) to detect nutritionally deficient and fastidious bacteria or fungi. Antimicrobial pretreatment of the patient reduces the yield of blood cultures to 50–60%. The microbiology laboratory should be notified if the patient has received antibiotics so that more sophisticated methods can be used to recover the offending agent. Other specimens that may be cultured include scrapings from cutaneous lesions, urine, synovial fluid, abscesses and, in the presence of manifestations of meningitis, the cerebrospinal fluid. Serologic diagnosis is necessary in patients with unusual or fastidious microorganisms (see Table 443–1).

There should be a high index of suspicion in evaluating infection in a child with an underlying contributing factor. The combination of M-mode, two-dimensional, and transesophageal echocardiography has enhanced the ability to diagnose

TABLE 443–1 Bacterial Agents in Pediatric Infective Endocarditis

Common: Native Valve or Other Cardiac Lesions

Streptococcus viridans group (*S. mutans, S. sanguis, S. mitis*)
Staphylococcus aureus
Group D streptococcus (enterococcus) (*S. bovis, S. faecalis*)

Uncommon: Native Valve or Other Cardiac Lesions

Streptococcus pneumoniae
Haemophilus influenzae
Staphylococcus epidermidis
Coxiella burnetii (Q fever)*
Neisseria gonorrhoeae
*Brucella**
*Chlamydia psittaci**
*Chlamydia trachomatis**
*Chlamydia pneumoniae**
HACEK group†
*Streptobacillus moniliformis**
*Pasteurella multocida**
Campylobacter fetus
Culture negative (10% of cases)

Prosthetic Valve

Staphylococcus epidermidis
Staphylococcus aureus
Streptococcus viridans
Pseudomonas aeruginosa
Serratia marcescens
Diphtheroids
Legionella species*
HACEK group†
Fungi‡

*These fastidious bacteria plus some fungi may produce culture-negative endocarditis. Detection may require special media, incubation for more than 7 days, or serologic tests.

†*HACEK group includes* Haemophilus *species (*H. paraphrophilus, H. parainfluenzae, H. aphrophilus*)*, Actinobacillus actinomycetemcomitans, Cardiobacterium hominis, Eikenella corrodens, *and* Kingella *species.*

‡Candida *species,* Aspergillus *species,* Pseudallescheria boydii, Histoplasma capsulatum.

TABLE 443–2 Manifestations of Infective Endocarditis

History

Prior congenital or rheumatic heart disease
Preceding dental, urinary tract, or intestinal procedure
Intravenous drug use
Central venous catheter
Prosthetic heart valve

Symptoms

Fever
Chills
Chest and abdominal pain
Arthralgia, myalgia
Dyspnea
Malaise
Night sweats
Weight loss
CNS manifestations (stroke, seizures, headache)

Signs

Elevated temperature
Tachycardia
Embolic phenomena (Roth spots, petechiae, splinter nailbed hemorrhages, Osler nodes, CNS or ocular lesions)
Janeway lesions
New or changing murmur
Splenomegaly
Arthritis
Heart failure
Arrhythmias
Metastatic infection (arthritis, meningitis, mycotic arterial aneurysm, pericarditis, abscesses, septic pulmonary emboli)
Clubbing

Laboratory

Positive blood culture result
Elevated erythrocyte sedimentation rate; may be low with heart or renal failure
Elevated C-reactive protein
Anemia
Leukocytosis
Immune complexes
Hypergammaglobulinemia
Hypocomplementemia
Cryoglobulinemia
Rheumatoid factor
Hematuria
Renal failure: azotemia, high creatinine (glomerulonephritis)
Echocardiographic evidence of valve vegetations, prosthetic valve dysfunction or leak, or myocardial abscess

CNS = central nervous system.

endocarditis. M-mode echocardiography can detect valvular vegetations larger than 2–3 mm. Two-dimensional echocardiography can identify the size, shape, location, and mobility of the lesion; when this is combined with Doppler studies, the presence of valve dysfunction (regurgitation, obstruction) can be determined and its effect on left ventricular performance quantified. Echocardiography may also be helpful in predicting embolic complications, as lesions greater than 1 cm and fungating masses are at greatest risk for embolization. The absence of vegetations does not exclude endocarditis, and vegetations are often not visualized in the early phases of the disease or in patients with complex congenital heart lesions.

PROGNOSIS AND COMPLICATIONS. In the preantibiotic era, infective endocarditis was a fatal disease. Despite the use of antibiotic agents, the mortality remains at 20–25%. Serious morbidity occurs in 50–60% of children with documented infective endocarditis; the most common is heart failure caused by vegetations involving the aortic or mitral valve. Myocardial abscesses and toxic myocarditis may also lead to heart failure without characteristic changes in auscultatory findings. Systemic emboli, often with central nervous system manifestations, are a major threat. Pulmonary emboli may occur in children with VSD or tetralogy of Fallot, although massive life-threatening pulmonary embolization is rare. Other complications include mycotic aneurysms, rupture of a sinus of Valsalva, obstruction of a valve secondary to large vegetations, acquired VSD, and heart block as a result of involvement (abscess) of the conduction system. Additional complications include meningitis, osteomyelitis, arthritis, renal abscess, and immune complex–mediated glomerulonephritis.

TREATMENT. Antibiotic therapy should be instituted immediately on diagnosis. When virulent organisms are responsible, small delays may result in progressive endocardial damage and are associated with a greater likelihood of severe complications. The choice of antibiotics, method of administration, and length of treatment are outlined in Table 443–3. High serum bactericidal levels must be maintained long enough to eradicate organisms that are growing in relatively inaccessible avascular vegetations. Between 5 and 20 times the minimum in vitro inhibiting concentration must be produced at the site of infection to destroy bacteria growing at the core of these lesions. Several weeks are required for a vegetation to organize completely; therapy must be continued through this period so that recrudescence can be avoided. A total of 4–6 wk of treatment is recommended, with serumcidal levels by tube dilution of at least 1:8 after a dose of antibiotic. Depending on the

TABLE 443–3 Treatment of Infective Endocarditis

Etiologic Agent	Drug	Dose	Route	Duration of Therapy (wk)
Streptococcus viridans, S. bovis (minimal inhibitory concentration [MIC] ≤0.1 μg/mL)	(1) Penicillin G *or*	200,000–300,000 U/kg/24 hr q 4 hr not to exceed 20 million U/24 hr	IV	4–6
	(2) Penicillin G plus	As above No. 1	IV	2–4
	gentamicin	3–7.5 mg/kg/24 hr q 8 hr not to exceed 240 mg/24 hr	IV	2
S. viridans, S. bovis (MIC ≥0.1 μg/mL)	(3) Penicillin G plus	As above No. 2	IV	4–6
	gentamicin	As above No. 2	IV	2
S. viridans or enterococci (*S. bovis* or *S. faecalis*) (MIC >0.5 μg/mL)	(4) Penicillin G *or*	As above No. 2	IV	4–6
	ampicillin plus	300 mg/kg 24 hr q 4–6 hr not to exceed 12 g/24 hr	IV	4–6
	gentamicin	As above No. 2	IV	4–6
*S. viridans, S. bovis** (penicillin allergy†)	(5) Vancomycin	40–60 mg/kg/24 hr q 8–12 hr not to exceed 2 g/24 hr	IV	4–6
	plus			
	(6) gentamicin if resistant*	As above No. 2	IV	4–6
Staphylococcus aureus	(7) Nafcillin *or*	200 mg/kg/24 hr q 4–6 hr not to exceed 12 g/24 hr	IV	6–8
	oxacillin	As above No. 2		
	plus optional gentamicin		IV	1–2
S. aureus (methicillin resistant) (penicillin allergy)	(8) Vancomycin	As above No. 5	IV	6–8
	plus optional trimethoprim-sulfamethoxazole	12 mg/kg/24 hr trimethoprim q 8 hr not to exceed 1 g/24 hr	IV, PO	4–8
S. aureus (with prosthetic device, methicillin-sensitive)‡	(9) Nafcillin	As above No. 7	IV	6–8
	plus gentamicin	As above No. 2	IV	2
	plus optional rifampin	10–20 mg/kg/24 hr q 12 hr not to exceed 600 mg/24 hr	PO	≥6
S. aureus (with prosthetic device, methicillin-resistant)	(10) Vancomycin	As above No. 5	IV	6–8
	plus gentamicin	As above No. 9	IV	2
	plus optional rifampin	As above No. 9	PO	≥6
S. epidermidis	(11) Vancomycin	As above No. 5	IV	6–8
	plus optional rifampin	As above No. 9	PO	6–8
Haemophilus species	(12) Ampicillin	As above No. 4	IV	4–6
	plus optional gentamicin	As above No. 2	IV	2–4
Unknown				
Postoperative	(13) Vancomycin	As above No. 5	IV	6–8
	plus gentamicin	As above No. 2	IV	2–4
Nonoperative	(14) Nafcillin *or*	As above No. 7	IV	6–8
	vancomycin	As above No. 5	IV	6–8
	plus gentamicin	As above No. 2	IV	2–4
	plus optional ampicillin	As above No. 4	IV	6–8

**Add gentamicin for relatively resistant organisms. Monitor vancomycin peaks 1 hr after infusion (30–45 μg/mL). Adjust dose according to vancomycin levels.*
†Desensitization should be considered for patients who are allergic to penicillin. Cephalosporins are not recommended.
‡May require valve (device) replacement.
IV = intravenous; PO = oral.

TABLE 443–4 Recommendations of the American Heart Association for Prophylaxis Against Bacterial Endocarditis

Dental and Oral Procedures or Surgery of the Upper Respiratory Tract or Esophagus	
For most patients	Oral amoxicillin Adults: 2.0 g Children: 50 mg/kg 1 hr before the procedure
For patients unable to take oral medication	IM or IV ampicillin Adults: 2.0 g Children: 50 mg/kg given within 30 min before the procedure
Ampicillin- and amoxicillin-allergic patients	Oral clindamycin Adults: 600 mg Children: 20 mg/kg 1 hr before the procedure *or* Oral cephalexin* or cefadroxil* Adults: 2.0 g Children: 50 mg/kg 1 hr before the procedure *or* Oral azithromycin *or* clarithromycin Adults: 500 mg Children: 15 mg/kg 1 hr before the procedure
Ampicillin- and amoxicillin-allergic patients unable to take oral medications	IV clindamycin Adults: 600 mg Children: 20 mg/kg Given within 30 min before the procedure *or* IV cefazolin Adults: 1.0 g Children: 25 mg/kg Given within 30 min before the procedure

Gastrointestinal and Genitourinary Tract Surgery and Instrumentation	
High-risk patients	IM or IV ampicillin Adults: 2.0 g Children: 50 mg/kg *plus* IM or IV gentamicin 1.5 mg/kg (maximum dose 120 mg) Given within 30 min before the procedure *plus 6 hr later:* IM or IV ampicillin or oral amoxicillin Adults: 1 g Children: 25 mg/kg
High-risk patients allergic to ampicillin and amoxicillin	IV vancomycin Adults: 1.0 g Children: 20 mg/kg Given over 1–2 hr *plus* IM or IV gentamicin 1.5 mg/kg (maximum dose 120 mg) Complete injection/infusion within 30 min before starting the procedure
Moderate-risk patients	Oral amoxicillin Adults: 2.0 g Children: 50 mg/kg 1 hr before the procedure *or* IM or IV ampicillin Adults: 2.0 g Children: 50 mg/kg Given within 30 min before the procedure
Moderate-risk patients who are allergic to ampicillin and amoxicillin	IV vancomycin Adults: 1.0 g Children: 20 mg/kg Given over 1–2 hr. Complete infusion within 30 min of starting the procedure

**Cephalosporines should not be used in patients with immediate-type hypersensitivity reaction to penicillins.*

High-risk patients: *Prosthetic heart valves (including homografts), previous endocarditis, complex cyanotic congenital heart disease (e.g., transposition of the great vessels, tetralogy of Fallot, single ventricle), systemic-to-pulmonary artery shunts or conduits.*

Moderate-risk patients: *Most other congenital heart diseases (other than those specifically listed previously or further on), acquired valve dysfunction (e.g., rheumatic heart disease), hypertrophic cardiomyopathy.*

Negligible-risk patients (prophylaxis not recommended): *Isolated secundum ASD, surgical repair of ASD, VSD, or PDA (without residua and beyond 6 mo after repair), previous coronary artery bypass surgery, functional heart murmurs, previous Kawasaki disease or rheumatic fever without valve dysfunction, cardiac pacemakers, implantable defibrillators.*

The risk for mitral valve prolapse is controversial. The latest American Heart Association recommendations categorize mitral valve prolapse with regurgitation or thickened leaflets, or both, as a moderate risk; mitral valve prolapse without regurgitation is categorized as a negligible risk (for further details see the reference).

IM = intramuscularly; IV = intravenously; ASD = atrial septal defect; VSD = ventricular septal defect; PDA = patent ductus arteriosus.

Adapted from Dajani AS, Taubert KA, Wilson W, et al: Prevention of bacterial endocarditis. Recommendations by the American Heart Association. JAMA 277:1794, 1997.

TABLE 443–5 Procedures and Endocarditis Prophylaxis

Endocarditis Prophylaxis Recommended*

Dental

Tooth extractions
Periodontal procedures including surgery, scaling and root planing, probing and recall maintenance
Dental implant placement and reimplantation of avulsed teeth
Endodontic (root canal) instrumentation or surgery only beyond the apex
Subgingival placement of antibiotic fibers or strips
Initial placement of orthodontic bands but not brackets
Intraligamentary local anesthesia injections
Prophylactic cleaning of teeth or implants when bleeding is anticipated

Respiratory Tract

Tonsillectomy or adenoidectomy, or both
Surgical operations that involve respiratory mucosa
Bronchoscopy with a rigid broncoscope

Gastrointestinal Tract†

Sclerotherapy for esophageal varices
Esophageal stricture dilation
Endoscopic retrograde cholangiography with biliary obstruction
Biliary tract surgery
Surgical operations that involve intestinal mucosa

Genitourinary Tract

Cystoscopy

Endocarditis Prophylaxis Not Recommended

Dental

Restorative dentistry‡ (operative and prosthodontic) with or without retraction cord§
Local anesthesia injections (nonintraligamentary)
Intracanal endodontic treatment; after placement and build-up
Placement of rubber dams
Postoperative suture removal
Placement of removable prosthodontic or orthodontic appliances
Taking of oral impressions
Fluoride treatments
Taking of oral radiographs
Orthodontic appliance adjustment
Shedding of primary teeth

Respiratory Tract

Endotracheal intubation
Bronchoscopy with a flexible bronchoscope, with or without biopsy§
Tympanostomy tube insertion

Gastrointestinal Tract

Transesophageal echocardiography§
Endoscopy with or without gastrointestinal biopsy§

Genitourinary Tract

Vaginal delivery§
Cesarean section
In uninfected tissue:
- Urethral catheterization
- Uterine dilation and curettage
- Therapeutic abortion
- Sterilization procedures
- Insertion or removal of intrauterine devices

Other

Cardiac catheterization, including balloon angioplasty
Implanted cardiac pacemakers, implanted defibrillators, and coronary stents
Incision or biopsy of surgically scrubbed skin
Circumcision

**Prophylaxis is recommended for patients with high- or moderate-risk heart conditions.*
†Prophylaxis is recommended for high-risk patients; optional for medium-risk patients.
‡This includes restoration of decayed teeth (filling cavities) and replacement of missing teeth.
§Prophylaxis is optional for high-risk patient.
‖Clinical judgment may indicate antibiotic use in selected circumstances that may create significant bleeding.

clinical and laboratory responses, antibiotic therapy may require modification, and in some instances more prolonged treatment is required. With highly sensitive *S. viridans* infections, shortened regimens, including oral penicillin for some portion, have been recommended. In nonstaphylococcal disease, bacteremia usually resolves in 24–48 hr, whereas fever resolves in 5–6 days with appropriate antibiotic therapy. Resolution in staphylococcal disease takes longer.

Digitalis, salt restriction, and diuretic therapy should be used for the treatment of heart failure. Surgical intervention for infective endocarditis is indicated for severe aortic or mitral valve involvement with intractable heart failure. Rarely, a mycotic aneurysm, rupture of an aortic sinus, or dehiscence of an intracardiac patch requires an emergency operation. Other surgical indications include failure to sterilize the blood despite adequate antibiotic levels, a myocardial abscess, recurrent emboli, and failure of medical management. Although antibiotic therapy should be administered for as long as possible prior to surgical intervention, active infection is not a contraindication if the patient is critically ill as a result of severe hemodynamic deterioration from infective endocarditis. Removal of vegetations and, in some instances, valve replacement may be lifesaving, and sustained antibiotic administration will most often prevent reinfection. Replacement of infected prosthetic valves carries a higher risk.

Fungal endocarditis is difficult to manage and has a poor prognosis regardless of treatment. It has been encountered after cardiac surgery, especially in severely debilitated or immunosuppressed patients. The drugs of choice are amphotericin B and 5-fluorocytosine. Surgery to excise infected tissue is occasionally attempted, usually with limited success.

PREVENTION. Antimicrobial prophylaxis prior to various procedures, including dental cleaning and other forms of dental manipulation, reduces the incidence of infective endocarditis in susceptible patients (Tables 443–4 and 443–5). Continuing education regarding prophylaxis is important, especially in teenagers and young adults, who often have poor knowledge of their own congenital heart lesion. Proper general dental care and oral hygiene are most important in decreasing the risk of infective endocarditis in susceptible individuals. Vigorous treatment of sepsis and local infections and careful asepsis during heart surgery and catheterization reduce the incidence of infective endocarditis.

Bisno AL, Dismukes WE, Durack DT, et al: Antimicrobial treatment of infective endocarditis due to viridans streptococci, enterococci, and staphylococci. JAMA 261:1471, 1989.

Cetta F, Warnes CA: Adults with congenital heart disease: Patient knowledge of endocarditis prophylaxis. Mayo Clin Proc 70:50, 1995.

Dajani AS, Taubert KA, Wilson W, et al: Prevention of bacterial endocarditis. Recommendations by the American Heart Association. JAMA 277:1794, 1997.

Geva T, Frand M: Infective endocarditis in children with congenital heart disease: The changing spectrum, 1965–1985. Eur Heart J 9:1244, 1988.

Martin JM, Neches WH, Wald ER: Infective endocarditis: 35 years of experience at a children's hospital. Infect Dis 24:669, 1997.

Morris CD, Reller MD, Menashe VD: Thirty-year incidence of infective endocarditis after surgery for congenital heart disease. JAMA 279:599, 1998.

O'Callaghan C, McDougall P: Infective endocarditis in neonates. Arch Dis Child 63:53, 1988.

Saiman L, Prince A, Gersony WM: Pediatric infective endocarditis in the modern era. J Pediatr 122:847, 1993.

Walterspiel JN, Kaplan SL: Incidence and clinical characteristics of "culture-negative" infective endocarditis in a pediatric population. Pediatr Infect Dis 5:328, 1986.

Weinstein MP, Stratton CW, Ackley A, et al: Multicenter collaborative evaluation of a standardized serum bactericidal test as a prognostic indicator of infective endocarditis. Am J Med 78:262, 1985.

Wilson WR, Karchmer AW, Dajani AS, et al: Antibiotic treatment of adults with infective endocarditis due to streptococci, enterococci, staphylococci and HACEK microorganisms. JAMA 274:1706, 1995.

CHAPTER 444
Rheumatic Heart Disease

Rheumatic involvement of the valves and endocardium is the most important manifestation of rheumatic fever (see Chapter 184.1). The valvular lesions begin as small verrucae composed of fibrin and blood cells along the borders of one or more of the heart valves. The mitral valve is affected most often, followed in frequency by the aortic valve; right-sided heart manifestations are rare. As the inflammation subsides, the verrucae tend to disappear and leave scar tissue. With repeated attacks of rheumatic fever, new verrucae form near the previous ones, and the mural endocardium and chordae tendineae become involved.

PATTERNS OF VALVULAR DISEASE

Mitral Insufficiency

PATHOPHYSIOLOGY. Mitral insufficiency is the result of structural changes that usually include some loss of valvular substance and shortening and thickening of the chordae tendineae. During acute rheumatic fever with severe cardiac involvement, heart failure is caused by a combination of mitral insufficiency coupled with inflammatory disease of the pericardium, myocardium, endocardium, and epicardium. Because of the high volume load and inflammatory process, the left ventricle becomes enlarged. The left atrium dilates as blood regurgitates into this chamber. Increased left atrial pressure results in pulmonary congestion and symptoms of left-sided heart failure. There is usually spontaneous improvement with time, even in patients in whom mitral insufficiency is severe at the onset. The resultant chronic lesion is most often mild or moderate in severity, and the patient is asymptomatic. More than half of patients with acute mitral insufficiency no longer have the mitral murmur 1 yr later. In patients with severe chronic mitral insufficiency, the pulmonary arterial pressure becomes elevated, the right ventricle and atrium become enlarged, and subsequent right-sided heart failure occurs.

CLINICAL MANIFESTATIONS. The physical signs of mitral insufficiency depend on its severity. With mild disease, signs of heart failure are not present, the precordium is quiet, and auscultation reveals a high-pitched holosystolic murmur at the apex, radiating to the axilla. With severe mitral insufficiency, signs of chronic heart failure may be noted. The heart is enlarged, with a heaving apical left ventricular impulse and often an apical systolic thrill. The 2nd heart sound may be accentuated if pulmonary hypertension is present. A 3rd heart sound is usually prominent. A holosystolic murmur is heard at the apex radiating to the axilla. A short mid-diastolic rumbling murmur is caused by increased blood flow across the mitral valve as a result of the insufficiency. The presence of a diastolic murmur does not necessarily mean that mitral stenosis is present. The latter lesion takes many years to develop and is characterized by a diastolic murmur of greater length with presystolic accentuation.

The electrocardiogram and roentgenograms are normal if the lesion is mild. With more severe insufficiency, the *electrocardiogram* shows prominent bifid P waves, signs of left ventricular hypertrophy, and associated right ventricular hypertrophy if pulmonary hypertension is present. *Roentgenographically,* there is prominence of the left atrium and ventricle. Congestion of perihilar vessels, a sign of pulmonary venous hypertension, may also be evident. Calcification of the mitral valve is rare in children. *Echocardiography* shows enlargement of the left atrium and ventricle, and Doppler study demonstrates the severity of the mitral regurgitation. *Heart catheterization* and left ventriculography are considered only if diagnostic questions are not totally resolved on the basis of noninvasive assessment. The degree of opacification of the left atrium during left ventriculography is used as a qualitative assessment of the severity of mitral insufficiency.

COMPLICATIONS. Severe mitral insufficiency may result in cardiac failure that may be precipitated by progression of the rheumatic process, the onset of atrial fibrillation, or infective endocarditis. After many years, the effects of chronic mitral insufficiency may become manifested, including right ventricular failure and atrial and ventricular arrhythmias.

TREATMENT. In patients with mild mitral insufficiency, prophylaxis against recurrences of rheumatic fever is all that is required. The treatment of complicating heart failure (see Chapter 448), arrhythmias (see Chapter 442), and infective endocarditis (see Chapter 443) is described elsewhere. Afterload-reducing agents (hydralazine, captopril) may reduce the regurgitant volume and preserve left ventricular function. Surgical treatment is indicated in patients who, despite adequate medical therapy, have recurrent episodes of heart failure, dyspnea with moderate activity, and progressive cardiomegaly, often with pulmonary hypertension. Although annuloplasty provides good results in some children and adolescents, valve replacement may be required. Prophylaxis against bacterial endocarditis is warranted in these patients for dental or other surgical procedures. The routine antibiotics taken by these patients for rheumatic fever prophylaxis are insufficient to prevent endocarditis.

Mitral Stenosis

PATHOPHYSIOLOGY. Mitral stenosis of rheumatic origin results from fibrosis of the mitral ring, commissural adhesions, and contracture of the valve leaflets, chordae, and papillary muscles over time. It takes 10 yr or more for the lesion to become fully established, although the process may occasionally be accelerated. Rheumatic mitral stenosis is seldom encountered prior to adolescence and usually is not recognized until adult life. Significant mitral stenosis results in increased pressure and enlargement and hypertrophy of the left atrium, pulmonary venous hypertension, increased pulmonary vascular resistance, and pulmonary hypertension. Right ventricular and atrial dilatation and hypertrophy ensue and are followed by right-sided heart failure.

CLINICAL MANIFESTATIONS. Generally, there is a good correlation between symptoms and the severity of obstruction. Patients with mild lesions are asymptomatic. More severe degrees of obstruction are associated with exercise intolerance and dyspnea. Critical lesions can result in orthopnea, paroxysmal nocturnal dyspnea, and overt pulmonary edema as well as atrial arrhythmias. When pulmonary hypertension has developed, right ventricular dilatation may result in functional tricuspid insufficiency, hepatomegaly, ascites, and edema. Hemoptysis due to ruptured bronchial or pleurohilar veins and, occasionally, pulmonary infarction may occur.

The jugular venous pressure is increased in severe disease with heart failure, tricuspid valve disease, or severe pulmonary hypertension. In mild disease, the heart size is normal; however, moderate cardiomegaly is usual with severe mitral stenosis. Cardiac enlargement can be massive when atrial fibrillation and heart failure supervene. A parasternal right ventricular lift is palpable when pulmonary pressure is high. The principal auscultatory findings are a loud 1st heart sound, an opening snap of the mitral valve, and a long, low-pitched, rumbling mitral diastolic murmur with presystolic accentuation at the apex. The mitral diastolic murmur may be virtually absent in patients who are in heart failure. A holosystolic murmur owing to tricuspid insufficiency may be audible. In the presence of pulmonary hypertension, the pulmonic component of the 2nd heart sound is accentuated. An early diastolic murmur may be caused by associated aortic insufficiency or secondary pulmonary valvular insufficiency.

Electrocardiograms and *roentgenograms* are normal if the lesion is mild; as the severity increases, there are prominent and notched P waves and varying degrees of right ventricular hypertrophy. Atrial fibrillation is a common late manifestation. Moderate or severe lesions are associated with roentgenographic signs of left atrial enlargement and prominence of the pulmonary artery and right-sided heart chambers; there may be calcifications noted in the region of the mitral valve. Severe obstruction is associated with a redistribution of pulmonary blood flow so that the apices of the lung have a greater perfusion (the reverse of normal). *Echocardiography* shows distinct narrowing of the mitral orifice during diastole and left atrial enlargement, and Doppler can estimate the transmitral pressure gradient. *Cardiac catheterization* quantitates the diastolic gradient across the mitral valve and the degree of elevation of pulmonary arterial pressure.

TREATMENT. Intervention is indicated when there are clinical signs and hemodynamic evidence of severe obstruction but prior to the severe manifestations outlined earlier. Surgical or balloon catheter mitral valvotomy generally yields good results; valve replacement is avoided unless absolutely necessary. Balloon valvuloplasty is indicated in symptomatic, stenotic, pliable, noncalcified valves of patients without atrial arrhythmias or thrombi.

Aortic Insufficiency

In chronic rheumatic aortic insufficiency, sclerosis of the aortic valve results in distortion and retraction of the cusps. Regurgitation of blood results in a volume overload with dilatation and hypertrophy of the left ventricle. Combined mitral and aortic insufficiency are more common than aortic involvement alone.

CLINICAL MANIFESTATIONS. Symptoms are unusual except in severe aortic insufficiency. The large stroke volume and forceful left ventricular contractions may result in palpitations. Excessive sweating and heat intolerance are related to vasodilation. Dyspnea on exertion can progress to orthopnea and pulmonary edema; angina may occur during heavy exercise. Nocturnal attacks with sweating, tachycardia, chest pain, and hypertension may occur.

The pulse pressure is wide with bounding peripheral pulses. The systolic blood pressure is elevated, and the diastolic pressure is lowered. In severe aortic insufficiency, the heart is enlarged, and there is a left ventricular apical heave. There may be a diastolic thrill. The typical murmur begins immediately with the 2nd heart sound and continues until late in diastole. The murmur is heard over the upper and middle left sternal border with radiation to the apex and to the aortic area. Characteristically, it has a high-pitched blowing quality and is easily audible in full expiration, with the diaphragm of the stethoscope placed firmly on the chest and the patient leaning forward. A systolic ejection murmur is frequent because of the increased stroke volume. An apical presystolic murmur (Austin Flint) resembling that of mitral stenosis is sometimes heard and is the result of the large regurgitant aortic flow in diastole that prevents the mitral valve from opening fully.

Roentgenograms show enlargement of the left ventricle and aorta. The *electrocardiogram* may be normal but in advanced cases reveals signs of left ventricular hypertrophy and strain with prominent P waves. The *echocardiogram* shows a large left ventricle and diastolic mitral valve flutter or oscillation caused by regurgitant flow hitting the valve leaflets. Doppler studies demonstrate the degree of aortic runoff into the left ventricle.

Cardiac catheterization is necessary only when the echocardiographic data are equivocal.

PROGNOSIS AND TREATMENT. Mild and moderate lesions are well tolerated. Many adolescents with severe regurgitation are symptom-free and tolerate advanced lesions into the 3rd–4th decades. Unlike mitral insufficiency, aortic insufficiency does not regress. Patients with combined lesions during the episode of acute rheumatic fever may have only aortic involvement 1–2 yr later. Treatment in most cases consists of prophylaxis against the recurrence of acute rheumatic fever and occurrence of infective endocarditis. Surgical intervention (valve replacement) should be carried out well in advance of the onset of heart failure, pulmonary edema, or angina, when there are signs of decreasing myocardial performance as manifested by increasing left ventricular dimensions on the echocardiogram. Surgery is considered when early symptoms are present, there are ST-T wave changes on the electrocardiogram, or there is evidence of decreasing left ventricular ejection fraction.

Tricuspid Valve Disease

Primary tricuspid involvement is rare following rheumatic fever. *Tricuspid insufficiency* is more common secondary to right ventricular dilatation resulting from unrepaired left-sided lesions. The signs produced by tricuspid insufficiency include prominent pulsations of the jugular veins, systolic pulsations of the liver, and a blowing holosystolic murmur at the lower left sternal border that increases in intensity during inspiration. Concomitant signs of mitral or aortic valve disease, with or without atrial fibrillation, are frequent. Signs of tricuspid insufficiency decrease or disappear when heart failure produced by the left-sided lesions is successfully treated. Tricuspid valvuloplasty may be required in rare cases.

Pulmonary Valve Disease

Pulmonary insufficiency usually occurs on a functional basis secondary to pulmonary hypertension. This is a late finding with severe mitral stenosis. The murmur (Graham Steell murmur) is similar to that of aortic insufficiency, but the peripheral arterial signs (bounding pulses) are absent. The correct diagnosis is confirmed by two-dimensional echocardiography and Doppler studies.

Anonymous: Acute rheumatic fever at a Navy training center, San Diego, California. MMWR 37:101, 1988.

Barnett LA, Cunningham MW: A new heart-cross-reactive antigen in *Streptococcus pyogenes* is not M protein. J Infect Dis 162:875, 1990.

Dajani AS, Bisno AL, Chung KJ, et al: Prevention of rheumatic fever: A statement for health professionals by the Committee on Rheumatic Fever, Endocarditis and Kawasaki Disease of the Council on Cardiovascular Disease in the Young, the American Heart Association. Pediatr Infect Dis J 8:263, 1989.

Griffiths SP, Gersony WM: Acute rheumatic fever in New York City (1969 to 1988): A comparative study of two decades. J Pediatr 116:882, 1990.

Guilherme L, Weidebach W, Kiss MH, et al: Association of human leukocyte class II antigens with rheumatic fever or rheumatic heart disease in Brazilian population. Circulation 83:1995, 1991.

Holmes DR, Nishimura RA, Reeder GS: Aortic and mitral balloon valvuloplasty: Emergence of a new percutaneous technique. Int J Cardiol 16:227, 1987.

Markowitz M, Kaplan EL: Reappearance of rheumatic fever. Adv Pediatr 36:39, 1989.

Westlake RM, Graham TP, Edwards KM: An outbreak of acute rheumatic fever in Tennessee. Pediatr Infect Dis J 9:97, 1990.

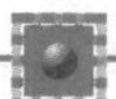

SECTION 6

Diseases of the Myocardium and Pericardium

CHAPTER 445

Diseases of the Myocardium

In adults, ischemic myocardial damage is a prominent component of cardiac disease; in children, myocardial function is relatively unimpaired in the majority of congenital heart lesions. In some congenital lesions (left-to-right shunts), the myocardium may even be functioning at a supranormal level (high-output state). Children with unoperated congenital heart disease, long-standing volume, pressure overload, or chronic hypoxia may eventually experience myocardial dysfunction. In the majority of children with diseases of the myocardium, causes other than congenital heart disease are predominant (see Table 445–1).

In the past, cardiomyopathies were divided into primary or idiopathic (those with unknown cause) and secondary (those resulting from a wide range of diseases, including infections, endocrine disorders, metabolic and nutritional diseases, neuromuscular diseases, blood diseases, and tumors). More recently, molecular biologic methods have identified specific causes in many patients who had been classified as having "idiopathic" cardiomyopathy. In some, specific gene defects have been identified; in others, the polymerase chain reaction (PCR) has detected evidence of prior viral myocarditis. Perhaps a more useful scheme for classifying cardiomyopathies is based on the structural and functional abnormalities that predominate: *dilated cardiomyopathy, hypertrophic cardiomyopathy,* and *restrictive cardiomyopathy.* The prevalence of cardiomyopathy in the newborn period is 10 in 100,000 live births, whereas for all children the prevalence is 36 in 100,000 for dilated cardiomyopathy and 2 in 100,000 for hypertrophic and restrictive cardiomyopathies.

445.1 Dilated Cardiomyopathy

PATHOPHYSIOLOGY. Dilated cardiomyopathy is characterized by massive cardiomegaly as a result of the extensive dilatation of the ventricles, most prominently the left. Varying degrees of ventricular hypertrophy are also present. The cause in the vast majority of pediatric cases is unknown (*idiopathic dilated cardiomyopathy*); a remote history of viral illness in many patients suggests that the disease may be a sequela of a previous myocarditis. Active myocarditis is identified in 2–15% of patients. In 20% of cases, the disease is familial, with autosomal dominant, autosomal recessive, X-linked, and mitochondrial inheritance patterns. Potential gene loci include the dystrophin-associated glycoprotein complex (anchoring of myocytes) and the cyclic adenosine monophosphate response element binding protein, a basic leucine zipper nuclear transcription factor that regulates gene expression. Patients with

TABLE 445–1 Etiology of Myocardial Disease

Familial-Hereditary

Mitochondrial myopathy syndromes*
Hypertrophic cardiomyopathy*
Duchenne muscular dystrophy*
Other muscular dystrophies (Becker's, limb girdle)
Myotonic dystrophy
Kearns-Sayre (progressive external ophthalmoplegia)
Friedreich's ataxia
Hemochromatosis
Fabry's disease
Primary endocardial fibroelastosis
Idiopathic dilatated cardiomyopathy (familial, enteroviral, autoimmune)
Arrhythmogenic right ventricular dysplasia (familial and nonfamilial)

Infection

Virus: coxsackievirus A and B,* adenovirus,* human immunodeficiency virus (HIV), echovirus, rubella, varicella, influenza, mumps, Epstein-Barr, measles, poliomyelitis
Rickettsiae: psittacosis, *Coxiella,* Rocky Mountain spotted fever
Bacteria: diphtheria, *Mycoplasma,* meningococcus, leptospirosis, Lyme disease, typhoid fever, tuberculosis, *Streptococcus,* listeriosis
Parasites: Chagas disease, toxoplasmosis, Loa loa, *Toxocara canis,* schistosomiasis, cysticercosis, *Echinococcus,* trichinosis
Fungi: histoplasmosis, coccidioidomycosis, actinomycosis

Metabolic, Nutritional, Endocrine

Pompe's disease
Carnitine deficiency syndromes*
Mucopolysaccharidosis
Beriberi (thiamine deficiency)
Keshan's disease (selenium deficiency)
Kwashiorkor
Hypothyroidism
Hyperthyroidism
Carcinoid
Pheochromocytoma
Hypercholesterolemia
Infant of diabetic mother*
Sphingolipidoses

Connective Tissue–Granulomatous Disease–Infiltrative

Systemic lupus erythematosus
Infant of mother with SLE
Scleroderma
Churg-Strauss vasculitis
Rheumatoid arthritis
Rheumatic fever
Sarcoidosis
Amyloidosis
Dermatomyositis
Periarteritis nodosa
Leukemia

Drugs–Toxins

Adriamycin*
Cyclophosphamide
Chloroquine
Ipecac (emetine)
Iron overload (hemosiderosis)
Sulfonamides
Mesalezine
Chloramphenicol
Hypersensitivity reaction
Alcohol
Irradiation
Herbal remedy (blue cohosh)

Coronary Arteries

Kawasaki's disease*
Medial necrosis
Anomalous left coronary artery

Other

Anemia*
Sickle cell anemia (sickling)*
Hypereosinophilic syndrome (Löffler's syndrome)
Endomyocardial fibrosis
Ischemia-hypoxia
Peripartum cardiomyopathy
Uhl right ventricular anomaly
Histiocytoid (oncocytic, lipidotic) cardiomyopathy
Acute eosinophilic necrotizing myocarditis
Restrictive cardiomyopathy
Chronic tachyarrhythmias

**Relatively common etiology of myocarditis-cardiomyopathy.*

dilatated cardiomyopathy may have infectious causes other than viral infection as well as endocrine-metabolic disorders, exposure to cardiotoxic agents such as doxorubicin, systemic disorders such as connective tissue disease, and familial muscular or neuromuscular disorders. Cardiac causes include congenital and acquired abnormalities of the coronary arteries, tachyarrhythmias, and familial hypercholesterolemia.

Myocardial biopsy early in the disease process may be useful; a specific cause is rarely found when biopsies are obtained after long-standing disease, in which case histologic findings consist mainly of areas of fibrosis and compensatory hypertrophy. The viral cause of many of these "idiopathic" cases may be uncovered with PCR. If a family history suggests one of the familial myopathies, DNA studies on both affected and nonaffected family members may help to determine the specific gene defect.

CLINICAL MANIFESTATIONS. All age groups may be affected. Usually the onset is insidious, but sometimes symptoms of heart failure occur suddenly. Irritability, anorexia, abdominal pain, cough due to pulmonary congestion, and dyspnea with exertion are common. When the disease is fully established, the skin is cool and pale, the arterial pulse is decreased, the pulse pressure is narrow, and tachycardia is present. The jugular venous pressure is increased, and hepatomegaly and edema are common. The heart is enlarged, and holosystolic murmurs of mitral and tricuspid insufficiency may be present. A summation gallop rhythm is usually audible.

LABORATORY DIAGNOSIS. The *electrocardiogram* shows a combination of atrial enlargement, varying degrees of left ventricular hypertrophy, and nonspecific T-wave abnormalities. The *roentgenogram* confirms the cardiomegaly. Pulmonary congestion and pleural effusions may also be present. The *echocardiogram* shows dilatation of the left atrium and ventricle and poor contractility. The right ventricle may also be affected. Doppler studies show decreased flow velocity through the aortic valve and mitral regurgitation. In long-standing cases, evidence of pulmonary hypertension may exist.

PROGNOSIS AND MANAGEMENT. The course of the disease is usually progressively downhill, although some patients may remain stable for years. Vigorous treatment of heart failure (see Chapter 448) may result in a temporary remission, but relapses are common, and in time patients tend to become resistant to therapy. At this point, the prognosis for survival beyond a year is poor. Serious complications include ventricular arrhythmias leading to syncope and sudden death as well as pulmonary or systemic emboli from intracardiac thrombi. Patients with severely depressed myocardial function should be monitored closely for arrhythmia and, if present, treated aggressively with antiarrhythmic agents or an automatic implantable cardioverter-defibrillator. They should also receive systemic anticoagulation with warfarin. β-Adrenergic blocking agents such as metoprolol and carvedilol have been used in adults with cardiomyopathy, resulting in improvement in exercise capacity and, in some studies, a reduction in hospitalization and mortality. Experience with these drugs in children is currently limited. When medical therapy fails, heart transplantation has been used in infants and children with dilatated cardiomyopathy (see Chapter 449). Because of the scarcity of pediatric donor organs, patients with cardiomyopathy should be referred to a pediatric heart transplant center for an initial evaluation early in the course of disease.

GENETIC CARDIOMYOPATHIES. Several familial cardiomyopathies have been mapped to specific chromosomes and some to specific genes. The most progress has been made in the X-linked cardiomyopathies, several of which have been linked to abnormalities of the dystrophin gene, which is responsible for Duchenne muscular dystrophy.

NEUROMUSCULAR DISEASES. Heart disease is common in *Friedreich's ataxia* (see Chapter 606.1), chiefly affecting the left ventricle and resulting in a dilatated or restrictive cardiomyopathy. In some patients, exercise intolerance, chest pain, and heart failure have been the presenting symptoms. Arrhythmias may also occur and consist of atrial tachycardia, fibrillation, or extrasystoles. In *Duchenne muscular dystrophy* (see Chapter 616.1), 50% of children have post mortem evidence of myocardial involvement similar to that of the striated muscle. Most often the cardiac symptoms are overshadowed by peripheral muscular and pulmonary complications. The electrocardiogram may reveal tachycardia, abnormalities of the P waves, a short PR interval, and abnormal Q and T waves. Minimal evidence of right or left ventricular hypertrophy may also be noted. Some patients experience heart failure, although these symptoms must be distinguished from those caused by pulmonary failure. In the less severe forms of muscular dystrophy, for example, *Becker's dystrophy,* cardiac involvement may be more prominent and the primary cause of exercise intolerance and respiratory symptoms. Other X chromosome–linked dilatated cardiomyopathies have been described without associated skeletal muscle involvement. Some limited experience with heart transplantation exists in patients with the milder Becker's dystrophy.

KAWASAKI'S DISEASE (See Chapter 166). The arteritis associated with Kawasaki's disease initially involves small arterioles, but in the 2nd and 3rd wk of illness, medium-sized arteries become inflamed and aneurysmal dilatation of the coronary arteries may occur. During the healing phase, areas of both coronary dilatation and stenosis may result and can lead to myocardial infarction and death. Myocarditis is a less common manifestation of Kawasaki's disease but, when present, manifests as heart failure early in the course.

AUTOIMMUNE DISEASES. *Rheumatic carditis* is described in Chapter 184.1. The cardiovascular manifestations of juvenile rheumatoid arthritis, systemic lupus erythematosus, periarteritis nodosa, dermatomyositis, and scleroderma are described in Part XV.

ENDOCRINE DISORDERS. Hyperthyroidism (see Chapter 578) produces tachycardia, vasodilation, a wide pulse pressure, cardiac enlargement and, occasionally, atrial fibrillation. Hypothyroidism can produce cardiac dysfunction in adults, but seldom produces gross cardiac involvement in children. The electrocardiogram is characterized by bradycardia, low voltage of all complexes (especially of the P and T waves), left axis deviation, and prolonged electrical systole. These signs usually disappear within 1 mo after initiation of adequate thyroid therapy. Diabetic cardiomyopathy is rare in children; however, infants of diabetic mothers can experience cardiac hypertrophy and dilatation. Cardiomyopathy may be caused by chronic exposure to elevated catecholamines in patients with pheochromocytoma.

METABOLIC AND NUTRITIONAL DISEASES. Among vitamin deficiency diseases, *beriberi* (see Chapter 44.2) causes the most conspicuous cardiac damage. In patients with malnutrition such as kwashiorkor, the deficiencies are often multiple, and it may be difficult to separate the cardiac lesion of one nutritional disease from that of another (see Chapters 42.1 and 42.2). Other nutritional and metabolic causes of cardiac dysfunction include selenium (see Chapter 41.6) and taurine deficiency and carnitine deficiency (Chapter 83.1).

HEMATOLOGIC DISEASES. In infants and children, severe anemia may be associated with cardiac involvement. Although the cardiac output increases when the hemoglobin is less than about 7 g/dL, significant cardiac enlargement occurs with an extreme reduction in hemoglobin (3–4 g or less). The heart rate is rapid, the pulse pressure widened, and the venous pressure increased. A systolic flow murmur at the apex or along the left sternal border is usual; diastolic murmurs may occur in the same areas, and a gallop rhythm is also common. Electrocardiographic changes include depressed ST segments and flat T waves. In patients with congenital heart lesions, anemia can place extra stress on the heart's ability to maintain adequate oxygen delivery and can result in considerable worsening of heart failure symptoms. *Treatment* is directed toward the cause of the anemia. If blood transfusions are indicated in the presence of cardiomegaly or heart failure, only small volumes (5 mL/kg) of packed red blood cells should be administered at any one time (see Chapter 476). Sometimes it is more prudent to use exchange transfusion to avoid an acute increase in blood volume.

DISORDERS OF THE CORONARY ARTERIES. Anomalous origin of the left coronary artery from the pulmonary artery is one of the major causes of myocardial ischemia in infants (see Chapter 439.2). Coronary calcinosis is a rare disorder in infants and children in which the coronary arteries are tortuous and calcareous. Other blood vessels may be similarly involved. The onset of cardiac failure is sudden; death usually occurs in infancy. Rare coronary artery malformations include coronary ostial stenosis and coronary artery stenosis in the setting of supravalvar aortic stenosis (see Chapter 434.5). Patients with homozygous familial hypercholesterolemia may acquire coronary atherosclerosis at an early age. Patients who have undergone heart transplantation are at risk for the development of graft coronary artery disease (see Chapter 449).

DOXORUBICIN (ADRIAMYCIN) CARDIOTOXICITY. This chemotherapeutic agent can cause acute myocarditis and a chronic cardiomyopathy. The most common manifestation is a severe, chronic, dose-dependent cardiomyopathy, which occurs in about 30% of patients when the total cumulative dose exceeds 550 mg/m^2 but may be seen occasionally, even in patients with doses as low as 200 mg/m^2. One study has shown abnormalities of echocardiographic indices of left ventricular function (wall stress) in as many as 65% of children receiving doses greater than 220 mg/m^2. When radiation therapy is combined with doxorubicin, the risk of cardiac damage is even greater.

Cardiomyopathy may become manifested months or even years after doxorubicin treatment. Cardiomegaly is principally due to left ventricular and left atrial enlargement. T-wave flattening or inversion is nonspecific evidence of cardiac involvement. Acute electrocardiographic changes, including long Q-T interval, may be present in 40% of patients immediately following a single dose. Early changes in cardiac function, even in the absence of symptoms, may be detected by serial echocardiograms or radionuclide (MUGA) scans, but no method is totally able to predict which patients are at risk. The child's condition may remain clinically stable for many years even with a decreased fractional shortening. Once symptoms of heart failure develop, the case fatality rate is as high as 30–50%. Cardiac transplantation has been used with success in these patients (see Chapter 449).

Acute myocarditis is less common and usually occurs during the course of administration of the drug. It is frequently reversible, and the long-term prognosis may be somewhat better. Supportive treatment consists of anticongestive medications such as digoxin, diuretics, and afterload-reducing agents.

IPECAC CARDIAC TOXICITY. This occurs with chronic intentional ipecac abuse secondary to anorexia nervosa or bulimia nervosa. Manifestations include chest pain, tachycardia, dyspnea, hypotension, arrhythmias, flattening and inversion of T waves, ST segment abnormalities, prolongation of Q-T and P-R intervals, cardiac failure, and potentially death. Differentiating the cardiac abnormalities caused by ipecac from those of chronic starvation, abnormal diets, and electrolyte abnormalities may be difficult.

445.2 Hypertrophic Cardiomyopathy

PATHOPHYSIOLOGY. Hypertrophic cardiomyopathies in children may be secondary to obstructive congenital heart disease (critical aortic stenosis, coarctation of the aorta), to an inborn error of metabolism (glycogen storage disease or mucopolysaccharidosis), or may be idiopathic. This latter condition is known variably as *hypertrophic cardiomyopathy, idiopathic hypertrophic subaortic stenosis,* or *asymmetric septal hypertrophy,* although subaortic obstruction is present in only about 25% of cases. Massive ventricular hypertrophy with principal involvement of the ventricular septum characterizes the disease, but all portions of the left ventricle, and sometimes of the right ventricle, are affected. Varying degrees of myocardial fibrosis are also present. The mitral valve is displaced anteriorly by hypertrophy of the papillary muscles, and the left ventricular cavity is distorted by the massive generalized hypertrophy. Microscopically, patchy areas of abnormally thick and short muscle fibers are arranged in circular collections and interspersed among normal as well as hypertrophied muscle fibers. Electron microscopy shows a disarray of myofibrils and myofilaments.

The hypertrophic and fibrosed muscle has a decreased distensibility (compliance) so that there is resistance to left ventricular filling; systolic pumping function remains intact (or even hyperdynamic) until late in the course of the disease. Obstruction to left ventricular outflow develops in 25% of patients owing to apposition of the abnormally placed anterior mitral leaflet against the hypertrophied septum. Varying degrees of mitral valve insufficiency are also common.

EPIDEMIOLOGY. Hypertrophic cardiomyopathy is most often inherited in an autosomal dominant pattern with a wide variability in penetrance. Siblings of the proband may not be affected as children but may show evidence of the disease as they reach adolescence and adulthood. Mutations of the cardiac myosin heavy-chain gene are responsible for 30–40% of familial hypertrophic cardiomyopathies. Other mutations involve the troponin T, α-tropomyosin, and myosin-binding protein genes. Genetic testing may eventually make it possible to predict which patients are likely to suffer from arrhythmias and sudden death. Other gene alterations associated with hypertrophic cardiomyopathy include those of the mitochondrial respiratory chain enzymes, which give rise to a maternal pattern of inheritance.

In childhood, hypertrophic cardiomyopathy may be somewhat different from the disease in adults: There is a greater tendency for right ventricular outflow obstruction to occur. The left ventricular wall may be diffusely thickened as opposed to only the septal portion being thickened.

CLINICAL MANIFESTATIONS. Many children are asymptomatic, and about 50% of cases are first evaluated because of either a heart murmur or an affected family member. In others, the clinical pattern is dominated by weakness, fatigue, dyspnea on effort, palpitations, angina pectoris, dizziness, and syncope. There is risk of sudden death even in asymptomatic children. The pulse is brisk because of the early systolic ejection of blood from the ventricle. There is a prominent left ventricular lift and double apical impulse. The 1st and 2nd heart sounds are usually normal. The rarity of systolic ejection clicks helps to differentiate hypertrophic obstructive cardiomyopathy from valvular aortic stenosis. The systolic murmur is ejection in type and of medium intensity; it is heard maximally at the left sternal edge and apex. The murmur may increase shortly after exercise is discontinued, during the Valsalva maneuver, or during assumption of the erect position.

LABORATORY DIAGNOSIS. The *electrocardiogram* shows left ventricular hypertrophy with or without ST segment depression and T-wave inversion. Signs of the Wolff-Parkinson-White syndrome and other intraventricular conduction defects may be present. *Roentgenograms* show mild cardiomegaly with prominence of the left ventricle. The *echocardiogram* shows left ventricular hypertrophy predominantly affecting the interventricular septum, systolic anterior motion of the anterior leaflet of the mitral valve, and premature closure of the aortic valve. Doppler studies demonstrate the presence of a left ventricular outflow tract gradient, which usually occurs in mid- to late systole, when the muscular obstruction to the outflow is maximal.

Echocardiography has largely replaced *cardiac catheterization* for initial diagnosis, although catheterization can be useful in assessing a patient's candidacy for surgery. Many patients who do not have a left ventricular outflow tract gradient at rest may acquire a significant gradient after administration of isoproterenol, amyl nitrite, or nitroglycerin. Left ventriculography shows encroachment on the left ventricular cavity by the hypertrophied muscle, especially by the interventricular septum. Midsystolic cavity obliteration occurs in more severe cases. Mitral insufficiency is common. A discrete obstruction with secondary muscular hypertrophy should be ruled out, as surgical management of discrete subaortic stenosis is effective (see Chapter 434.5). The *prognosis* of hypertrophic cardiomyopathy is unpredictable, especially in the asymptomatic patient, who may remain stable for years. Some patients progress to chronic heart failure, and others are at risk for sudden death caused by arrhythmia.

TREATMENT. There is no standardized therapy. Competitive sports and strenuous physical activity should be discouraged because most sudden deaths occur after physical exertion. Digitalis or aggressive diuresis is contraindicated in most patients. Infusion of isoproterenol or other inotropic agents should also be avoided other than for diagnostic purposes in the controlled environment of the catheterization laboratory. β-Adrenergic blocking agents (propranolol) and calcium channel blocking agents (verapamil, nifedipine) have been used with some success in decreasing the degree of outflow obstruction and slowing the development of hypertrophy; these drugs do not necessarily affect the long-term prognosis and do not reduce the incidence of sudden death. Calcium channel blockers should not be used during infancy. Patients with arrhythmias should be treated aggressively. A pacemaker has been used to alter septal depolarization in some older patients. Surgery involving ventricular septal myotomy has been successfully accomplished in some patients, especially in those with disabling angina or syncope associated with left ventricular outflow tract obstruction (resting or provoked gradient of ≥50 mm Hg). Mitral valve replacement may be needed if obstruction cannot be alleviated.

HYPERTROPHIC CARDIOMYOPATHY IN INFANTS OF DIABETIC MOTHERS. In *infants of diabetic mothers,* a transient form of hypertrophic cardiomyopathy may be encountered with or without left ventricular outflow tract obstruction. The increased left ventricular mass usually regresses within several months.

CORTICOSTEROIDS IN PREMATURE INFANTS. Premature infants who are receiving *corticosteroids* for chronic lung disease may also experience a transient hypertrophic cardiomyopathy, which usually resolves rapidly with cessation of steroid therapy.

GLYCOGEN STORAGE DISEASE. Cardiac as well as skeletal muscles are affected in the generalized form of glycogen storage disease known as type II or *Pompe's disease* (see Chapter 84.1). Cardiomegaly is massive; murmurs are insignificant. Pulmonary atelectasis with secondary infection is common and is related to compression by the enlarged heart. The *electrocardiogram* is characteristic and shows prominent P waves, a short PR interval, massive QRS voltage, signs of isolated left or biventricular hypertrophy, and intraventricular conduction delays. *Roent-*

genograms confirm the striking cardiomegaly with prominence of the left ventricle. The echocardiogram shows severe ventricular hypertrophy. The prognosis is poor.

445.3 Restrictive Cardiomyopathies

Poor ventricular compliance is the major abnormality in restrictive cardiomyopathies, and inadequate filling of the ventricular cavities occurs during diastole. This results in *clinical manifestations* that closely simulate those of constrictive pericarditis (see Chapter 446.1). In its full-blown form, restrictive cardiomyopathy results in dyspnea, edema, ascites, hepatomegaly, increased venous pressure, and pulmonary congestion. The heart is mildly or moderately enlarged, and murmurs are nonspecific. The electrocardiogram shows prominent P waves, often normal QRS voltage, ST segment depression, and T-wave inversion. Roentgenographic examination shows mild to moderate cardiomegaly. *Differential diagnosis* from constrictive pericarditis is critical, although difficult, as the latter can be treated surgically. Restrictive cardiomyopathy may be idiopathic, associated with a systemic disease such as scleroderma, amyloidosis, or sarcoidosis, an inborn error of metabolism (mucopolysaccharidosis), hypereosinophilic syndrome, malignancies, or radiation therapy; or may result from a congenital abnormality such as isolated noncompaction of the left ventricular myocardium. The *prognosis* for restrictive cardiomyopathy is generally poor. Treatment is directed toward relief of heart failure (see Chapter 448); calcium channel blocking agents may be used to increase diastolic compliance. Antiarrhythmic agents are used as required, and anticoagulation with warfarin is indicated in those lesions with increased risk of mural thrombosis and stroke. Cardiac transplantation has been used effectively in some of these patients as long as multiple organ involvement from systemic disease is not present.

LÖFFLER'S HYPEREOSINOPHILIC SYNDROME. This disorder produces severe multisystem dysfunction (skin, lung, nervous system, liver), and the predominant cause of death is restrictive cardiomyopathy with endocardial fibrosis of the mitral and tricuspid valves and of the right and left ventricles. Subsequent formation of endocardial thrombi results in embolization. Löffler's syndrome should be distinguished from nonrestrictive, nonfibrotic acute *eosinophilic necrotizing myocarditis*, an acute rapidly fatal illness, and from *hypersensitivity myocarditis* (characterized by fever, rash, tachycardia, eosinophilia, drug allergy, and arrhythmias). Steroids and cytotoxic agents may be beneficial in the hypereosinophilic syndromes. Anticoagulant therapy may reduce the incidence of thromboembolism.

MUCOPOLYSACCHARIDOSIS. In this disorder, most commonly *Hurler's syndrome*, mucopolysaccharides accumulate in many organs, including the heart and great vessels (see Chapter 85). The most pronounced lesions are found in the valves and coronary arteries, but abnormalities in the pericardium and aorta are not uncommon. The heart may be moderately enlarged, with electrocardiographic signs of left ventricular hypertrophy. Cardiac murmurs may result from insufficiency and stenosis of the mitral and aortic valves. Sometimes the pulmonary and tricuspid valves are also involved. Coronary arterial disease may result in angina and perhaps explain the frequent occurrence of sudden death. The prognosis is poor.

ISOLATED NONCOMPACTION OF THE LEFT VENTRICLE. This cardiomyopathy of unknown cause results in elements of both left ventricular restriction and dilatation. Patients may present at any age, from infancy to young adulthood, with varying severity of congestive heart failure. The echocardiogram is diagnostic and shows a specific pattern of left ventricular hypertrophy with deep muscular crypts. Patients may be at risk for ventricular arrhythmias and sudden death, as well as mural thromboses and stroke. Although some patients may remain stable for years, others may deteriorate rapidly. Cardiac transplantation has been used successfully in this group of patients.

445.4 Myocarditis

Myocarditis refers to inflammation, necrosis, or myocytolysis that may be caused by many infectious, connective tissue, granulomatous, toxic, or idiopathic processes affecting the myocardium with or without associated systemic manifestations of the disease process or involvement of the endocardium or pericardium (see Table 445–1). Coronary pathology is uniformly absent. The most common manifestation is heart failure, although arrhythmias and sudden death may be the first detectable signs. Viral infections are the most common cause.

ETIOLOGY AND EPIDEMIOLOGY. The true incidence of viral myocarditis in children is unknown, as many mild cases go undetected. Viral myocarditis is typically a sporadic but occasionally epidemic illness. Its manifestations are to some degree age-dependent: In early infancy, viral myocarditis often occurs as an acute, fulminant disease; in toddlers and young children, it occurs as an acute but less fulminant myopericarditis; and in older children and adolescents, it is often asymptomatic and comes to clinical attention primarily as a precursor to idiopathic dilatated cardiomyopathy. The most common causative agents are adenovirus and coxsackievirus B, although many known viral agents have been implicated.

PATHOPHYSIOLOGY. Acute viral myocarditis may produce a fulminant inflammatory process characterized by cellular infiltrates, cell degeneration and necrosis, and subsequent fibrosis. Viral myocarditis may also become a chronic process with persistence of viral RNA or DNA (but not infectious virus particles) in the myocardium. Chronic inflammation is then perpetuated by the host immune response, which includes T lymphocytes activated against viral-host antigenic alterations. Such cytotoxic lymphocytes and natural killer cells, together with persistent and possibly defective viral replication, may impair myocyte function without obvious cytolysis. Alternatively, the persistent viral infection may alter major histocompatibility complex antigen expression, with resultant exposure of neoantigens to the immune system. In addition, some viral proteins may share antigenic epitopes with host cells, resulting in autoimmune damage to the antigenically related myocyte. Release of cytokines such as tumor necrosis factor-α and interleukin 1 may participate in the initiation of the altered immune response. The net final result of chronic viral-associated inflammation is often dilatated cardiomyopathy.

CLINICAL MANIFESTATIONS. The presentation depends on the patient's age and the acute or chronic nature of the infection. The *neonate* may present with fever, severe heart failure, respiratory distress, cyanosis, distant heart sounds, weak pulses, tachycardia out of proportion to the fever, mitral insufficiency caused by dilatation of the valve annulus, a gallop rhythm, acidosis, and shock. There may be evidence of viral hepatitis, aseptic meningitis, and an associated rash. In the most fulminant form, death may occur within 1–7 days of the onset of symptoms. The chest roentgenogram demonstrates an enormously enlarged heart and pulmonary edema; the electrocardiogram reveals sinus tachycardia, reduced QRS complex voltage, and ST segment and T-wave abnormalities. Arrhythmias may be the first clinical manifestation and in the presence of fever and a large heart strongly suggest acute myocarditis.

The *older patient* with acute myocarditis may also present with acute congestive heart failure; however, more commonly patients present with the gradual onset of congestive heart failure or the sudden onset of ventricular arrhythmias. In these patients, the acute infectious phase has usually passed and an idiopathic dilatated cardiomyopathy is present (see Chapter 445.1).

LABORATORY DIAGNOSIS. The sedimentation rate and heart enzymes (creatine phosphokinase, lactate dehydrogenase) may be elevated in acute or chronic myocarditis. If positive, serum viral titers are helpful; negative titers do not eliminate the diagnosis. Paired studies of ventricular biopsies and serum samples using the polymerase chain reaction (PCR) have shown viral genome present routinely in cardiac samples yet absent in peripheral blood. *Echocardiography* demonstrates poor ventricular function and often a pericardial effusion, mitral valve regurgitation, and the absence of coronary artery or other congenital heart lesions. Myocarditis can be confirmed by endomyocardial biopsy. This is performed during cardiac catheterization and can also detect other causes of cardiomyopathy (storage disease, mitochondrial defects). The PCR has been used to identify specific viral RNA or DNA.

DIFFERENTIAL DIAGNOSIS. The predominant diseases mimicking acute myocarditis include carnitine deficiency, hereditary mitochondrial defects, idiopathic dilatated cardiomyopathy, pericarditis, endocardial fibroelastosis, and anomalous origin of the left coronary artery (see Table 445–1).

TREATMENT. The approach to treating acute myocarditis involves supportive measures for severe congestive heart failure (see Chapter 448). Dopamine or epinephrine may be helpful if there is poor cardiac output with systemic hypotension. However, all inotropic agents, including digoxin, should be used with caution, as patients with myocarditis may be more susceptible to the arrhythmogenic properties of these agents. Digoxin is often started at half the normal dosage. Pericardiocentesis should be performed if there is evidence of cardiac tamponade, and culture of the pericardial fluid may yield the offending viral agent. Arrhythmias should be treated aggressively and may require the use of intravenous amiodarone to achieve adequate control. For infants and children having cardiogenic shock, extracorporeal membrane oxygenation may be indicated. In larger children and adolescents, implantation of a left ventricular assist device has been performed, usually as a bridge to heart transplantation, which is the treatment of choice in patients with refractory heart failure (see Chapter 449). The role of corticosteroids in the treatment of acute viral myocarditis is controversial. In a small series of pediatric patients, treatment with prednisone (2 mg/kg daily, tapered to 0.3 mg/kg daily over 3 mo) was effective in reducing myocardial inflammation and in improving cardiac function. Relapse was noted to occur when immunosuppression was discontinued. Trials in adult patients have shown mixed results. Trials are evaluating the use of intravenous gamma globulin.

PROGNOSIS. The outcome of the symptomatic neonate with acute viral myocarditis remains poor, with a mortality as high as 75%. Patients with lesser symptoms may have a somewhat better prognosis, and complete resolution has been described. The outcome of older patients with chronic dilatated cardiomyopathy associated with prior viral infection is also poor without therapy. These patients continue to have dilatation, fibrosis, and deteriorating cardiac function. Spontaneous resolution has occurred in various adult studies in 10–50% of patients. However, as many as 50% of untreated older patients die within 2 yr of presentation and 80% within 8 yr without heart transplantation.

445.5 Nonviral Causes of Myocarditis

BACTERIAL INFECTIONS. In *diphtheria* (see Chapter 187) the toxin of the bacillus may produce peripheral circulatory failure or toxic myocarditis within the first 2 wk of the disease. In addition to therapy for diphtheria, treatment for cardiogenic shock is essential. Diphtheritic toxic myocarditis is characterized by the development of atrioventricular block, bundle branch block, or extrasystoles. Heart failure occurs later and is associated with cardiac enlargement and a gallop rhythm. In addition to the arrhythmia, the electrocardiogram shows ST segment depression and T-wave inversion in most leads. The immediate prognosis is grave (about 50% mortality). Treatment includes strict bed rest until all signs of myocarditis have disappeared as well as management of arrhythmias, including cardiac pacing. Digitalis is reserved for patients with frank congestive heart failure, but this drug must be used with care because of the possibility of increased myocardial sensitivity.

In many *systemic bacterial infections,* circulatory involvement is manifested as peripheral circulatory collapse or toxic myocarditis. Toxic myocarditis, as evidenced by tachycardia, a gallop rhythm, and cardiac enlargement, may complicate pneumonia, infective endocarditis, and septicemia. A myocardial depressant factor may produce an acute toxic cardiomyopathy. The prognosis depends on the ability to control the primary infection.

RICKETTSIAL DISEASES. *Rocky Mountain spotted fever* (see Chapter 225.1) may be complicated by hypotension and peripheral vascular collapse. This complication has been attributed to the general vasculitis characteristic of the disease, but acute myocarditis may be a contributing factor.

PARASITIC AND FUNGAL INFECTIONS. Lesions in the myocardium have been described in association with *histoplasmosis, coccidioidomycosis, toxoplasmosis,* and *trichinosis.* In these conditions, the cardiac lesion seldom produces clinical signs of myocarditis. *Actinomycosis* may involve the pericardium and myocardium by direct contiguity to a pulmonary abscess. *Hydatid cysts* of the pericardium may be found on routine roentgenograms of the chest and usually produce symptoms only when they rupture. *Schistosomiasis* may produce pulmonary hypertension and cor pulmonale. *Cruz trypanosomiasis* (Chagas disease) may produce either acute or subacute myocarditis and can lead to sudden death.

445.6 Endocardial Fibroelastosis

Endocardial fibroelastosis (EFE) has been called *fetal endocarditis, endocardial fibrosis, prenatal fibroelastosis, elastic tissue hyperplasia,* and *endocardial sclerosis.* In *primary* EFE, there is no apparent predisposing valvular lesion or other congenital heart abnormality. In *secondary* EFE, severe congenital heart disease of the left-sided obstructive type (e.g., aortic stenosis or atresia, forms of hypoplastic left heart syndrome, or severe coarctation of the aorta) is present. In *secondary* EFE, the ventricular cavity is often contracted, whereas in the primary disease a dilatated left ventricular chamber is seen, usually during infancy. However, in young adults, a contracted form of primary EFE has been observed. No cause for primary EFE has been firmly established, although an association with mumps infection has been implied through analysis of affected myocardial specimens with the PCR.

Pathologically, there is a white, opaque fibroelastic thickening of the endocardium, usually in the left ventricle, which frequently obscures the trabeculation of the inner surfaces of the cardiac chamber. The lesion may spread to involve the valves. Microscopically, the lesion consists of a fibroelastic thickening of the endocardium and may result in subendocardial degeneration or necrosis of muscle with vacuolation of muscle fibers. The involved valve leaflets are characterized by a myxomatous proliferation with an increase in collagenous elements.

The *clinical manifestations* are variable. Infants, usually younger than 6 mo of age, who apparently had been in good health, experience severe congestive heart failure, often precipitated by a respiratory infection. Affected infants may manifest dyspnea, cough, anorexia, hepatomegaly, edema, failure to thrive, and recurrent pulmonary infections. Chronic heart failure can be controlled for some time by digitalis and diuret-

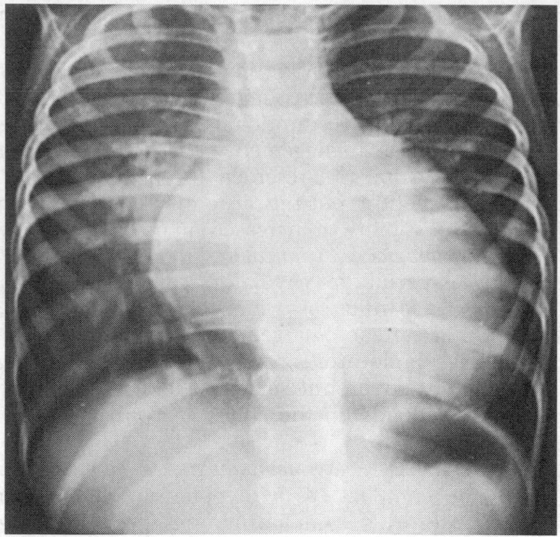

Figure 445–1 Roentgenogram of a 7-mo-old girl with endocardial fibroelastosis. Note the enlargement of the heart, without a distinctive contour and clear lung fields.

ics; however, most patients eventually succumb. Infants in whom valvular lesions or associated congenital cardiovascular defects are predominant usually expire in the 1st mo of life. *Roentgenograms* confirm significant cardiac enlargement (Fig. 445–1). The electrocardiogram is abnormal with changes indicative of left atrial and left ventricular hypertrophy with strain. The echocardiogram shows a bright-appearing endocardial surface and a dilatated, poorly functioning left ventricle.

Treatment is directed toward alleviation of congestive heart failure and prevention of intercurrent infections. End-stage EFE, with signs of heart failure despite a maximal medical regimen, is an indication for heart transplantation (see Chapter 449).

Dilated Cardiomyopathy

Brown CA, OConnell JB: Myocarditis and idiopathic dilated cardiomyopathy. Am J Med 99:309, 1995.

Burch M, Runciman M: Dilated cardiomyopathy. Arch Dis Child 74:479, 1996.

Imperato-McGinley J, Gautier T, Ehlers K, et al: Reversibility of catecholamine-induced dilated cardiomyopathy in a child with a pheochromocytoma. N Engl J Med 316:793, 1987.

Katz AM: Cardiomyopathy of overload: A major determinant of prognosis in congestive heart failure. N Engl J Med 322:100, 1990.

Kelly DP, Strauss AW: Inherited cardiomyopathies. N Engl J Med 330:913, 1994.

Leiden JM: The genetics of dilated cardiomyopathy—emerging clues to the puzzle. N Engl J Med 337:1080, 1997.

Lipshultz SE, Colan SD, Gelber RD, et al: Late cardiac effects of doxorubicin therapy for acute lymphoblastic leukemia in childhood. N Engl J Med 324:808, 1991.

Muntoni F, Cau M, Ganau A, et al.: Brief report: Deletion of the dystrophin muscle-promoter region associated with X-linked dilated cardiomyopathy. N Engl J Med 329:921, 1993.

Parrillo JE: Heart disease and the eosinophil. N Engl J Med 323:1560, 1990.

Parrillo JE, Cunnion RE, Epstein SE, et al: A prospective, randomized, controlled trial of prednisone for dilated cardiomyopathy. N Engl J Med 321:1061, 1989.

Spirito P, Seidman CE, McKenna WJ, Maron BJ: The management of hypertrophic cardiomyopathy. N Engl J Med 336:775, 1997.

Towbin JA, Hejtmancik JF, Brink P, et al: X-linked dilated cardiomyopathy: Molecular genetic evidence of linkage to the Duchenne muscular dystrophy (dystrophin) gene at the Xp21 locus. Circulation 87:1954, 1993.

Watkins H, McKenna WJ, Thierfelder L, et al: Mutations in the genes for cardiac troponin T and alpha-tropomyosin in hypertrophic cardiomyopathy. N Engl J Med 332:1058, 1995.

Hypertrophic Cardiomyopathy

Bonow RO, Dilsizian V, Rosing DR, et al: Verapamil-induced improvement in left ventricular diastolic filling and increased exercise tolerance in patients with hypertrophic cardiomyopathy: Short- and long-term effects. Circulation 72:853, 1985.

Maron BJ: Hypertrophic cardiomyopathy. Lancet 350:127, 1997.

Niimura H, Bachinski LL, Sangwatanaroj S, et al: Mutations in the gene for cardiac myosin-binding protein C and late-onset familial hypertrophic cardiomyopathy. N Engl J Med 338:1248, 1998.

Oakley C: Aetiology, diagnosis, investigation, and management of the cardiomyopathies. Br Med J 315:1520, 1997.

Rosenzweig A, Watkins H, Hwang D-S, et al: Preclinical diagnosis of familial hypertrophic cardiomyopathy by genetic analysis of blood lymphocytes. N Engl J Med 325:1753, 1991.

Restrictive Cardiomyopathy

Cetta F, O'Leary PW, Seward JB, Driscoll DJ: Idiopathic restrictive cardiomyopathy in childhood: Diagnostic features and clinical course. Mayo Clin Proc 70:634, 1995.

Denfield SW, Rosenthal G, Gajarski RJ, et al: Restrictive cardiomyopathies in childhood. Tex Heart J 24:38, 1997.

Guenthard J, Wyler F, Fowler B, et al: Cardiomyopathy in respiratory chain disorders. Arch Dis Child 72:223, 1995.

Kushwaha SS, Fallon JT, Fuster V: Restrictive cardiomyopathy. N Engl J Med 336:267, 1997.

Myocarditis

Anonymous: Cardiac biopsy in myocarditis. Lancet 336:283, 1990.

Anonymous: Dilated cardiomyopathy and enteroviruses. Lancet 336:971, 1990.

Bowles NE, Richardson PJ, Olsen EGJ, et al: Detection of coxsackie-B-virus-specific RNA sequences in myocardial biopsy samples from patients with myocarditis and dilated cardiomyopathy. Lancet 1:1120, 1986.

Chan KY, Iwahara M, Benson LN, et al: Immunosuppressive therapy in the management of acute myocarditis in children: A clinical trial. J Am Coll Cardiol 17:458, 1991.

Lange LG, Schreiner GF: Immune mechanisms of cardiac disease. N Engl J Med 330:1129, 1994.

Scott GB, Hutto C, Makuch RW, et al: Survival in children with perinatally acquired human immunodeficiency virus type 1 infection. N Engl J Med 321:1791, 1989.

Young LHY, Joag SV, Zheng L-M, et al: Perforin-mediated myocardial damage in acute myocarditis. Lancet 336:1019, 1990.

CHAPTER 446
Diseases of the Pericardium

Major diseases that involve the pericardium are noted in Table 446–1. In some diseases pericardial involvement is one manifestation of a generalized illness; the prominence of the pericardial component varies depending on the disease.

PATHOPHYSIOLOGY. Pericardial inflammation results in an accumulation of fluid in the pericardial space. The fluid varies according to the cause of the pericarditis and may be serous, fibrinous, purulent, or hemorrhagic. **Cardiac tamponade** occurs when the amount of pericardial fluid reaches a level that compromises cardiac function. In a healthy child, there is normally 10–15 mL of fluid in the pericardial space, whereas in an adolescent with pericarditis, an excess of 1,000 mL of fluid may accumulate. For every small increment of fluid, the pericardial pressure rises slowly; once a critical level is reached, there is a rapid rise in pressure, culminating in severe cardiac compression. Inhibition of ventricular filling during diastole, elevated systemic and pulmonary venous pressures and, if untreated, eventual compromised cardiac output and shock occur.

CLINICAL MANIFESTATIONS. The first symptom of pericardial disease is often precordial pain. The major complaint is a sharp, stabbing sensation over the precordium and often the left shoulder and back; the pain may be exaggerated by lying supine and relieved by sitting, especially leaning forward. Because there is no sensory innervation of the pericardium, the pain is probably referred pain from diaphragmatic and pleural irritation. Cough, dyspnea, abdominal pain, vomiting, and fever may also occur. The presence of symptoms or signs associated with other organs depends on the cause of the pericarditis.

Many of the findings on physical examination relate to the

TABLE 446–1 Etiology of Pericardial Disease

Congenital Anomalies
Absence (partial, complete)
Cysts
Mulibrey nanism (*mu*scle, *li*ver, *br*ain, *ey*e) with congenital pericardial thickening and constriction

Infectious
Viral (coxsackievirus B, Epstein-Barr virus influenza, adenovirus)
Bacterial (*Streptococcus, Pneumococcus, Staphylococcus, Meningococcus, Mycoplasma,* tularemia)
Immune complex (*Meningococcus, H. influenzae*)
Tuberculosis
Fungal (histoplasmosis, actinomycosis)
Parasitic (toxoplasmosis, echinococcus)

Connective Tissue Diseases
Rheumatoid arthritis
Rheumatic fever
Systemic lupus erythematosus
Systemic sclerosis
Sarcoidosis

Metabolic-Endocrine
Uremia
Hypothyroidism
Chylopericardium

Hematology-Oncology
Bleeding diathesis
Malignancy (primary, metastatic)
Radiotherapy-induced

Other
Trauma (penetrating or blunt injury)
Iatrogenic (catheter-related)
Postpericardiotomy (cardiac surgery)
Aortic dissection
Idiopathic
Familial Mediterranean fever

degree of fluid accumulation in the pericardial sac. The presence of a friction rub is helpful but is a variable sign in acute pericarditis, becoming apparent usually when the effusion is small. When the effusion is larger, muffled heart sounds may be the only auscultatory finding. Narrow pulses, tachycardia, neck vein distention, and an increased **pulsus paradoxus** suggest significant fluid accumulation.

The pulsus paradoxus is caused by the normal slight decrease in systolic arterial pressure during inspiration. With cardiac tamponade, this normal phenomenon is exaggerated probably because of decreased filling of the left side of the heart with the inspiratory phase of respiration. The degree of the pulsus paradoxus is determined with a mercury manometer. The patient is told to breathe normally without exaggeration. Allowing the manometer to fall slowly, the first Korotkov sound will initially be heard intermittently (varying with respirations). This first point is noted, and the manometer is then allowed to fall until the first Korotkov sound is heard continuously. The difference between these two systolic pressures is the pulsus paradoxus. A pulsus paradoxus of greater than 20 mm Hg in a child with pericarditis is an indicator of the presence of cardiac tamponade; a 10–20 mm Hg change is equivocal. An increased pulsus paradoxus may also be seen in patients with severe dyspnea of any cause, with pulmonary disease (emphysema or asthma), in obese individuals, or in patients being ventilated with a positive-pressure respirator. In these patients, the paradoxical pulse is due to a marked increase in intrathoracic pressure. The cause of a paradoxical pulse in a child on a ventilator after heart surgery may therefore be difficult to assess.

LABORATORY DIAGNOSIS. The specific findings depend on the underlying disease. The effects of pericarditis on the *electrocardiogram* are multiple. Low voltage of the QRS complexes results from a damping effect of the pericardial fluid. Pressure on the myocardium by fluid or exudate produces a current of injury that results in mild elevation of ST segments. Generalized T-wave inversion occurs as a consequence of associated myocardial inflammation. The ST segment and T-wave changes with pericarditis are more generalized than those seen with myocardial infarction, and the ST segment elevations tend to precede the T-wave changes. *Electrical alternans,* demonstrated by a variable QRS complex amplitude, may be present. There may be an interval when the electrocardiogram is in a transitional phase and appears to be normal. This may occur during the acute phase of the illness prior to diagnosis. In some instances, clear-cut abnormalities are never identified.

A relatively large pericardial effusion must be present to cause an enlarged cardiac shadow with the usual "water-bottle" configuration on *chest roentgenogram* (Fig. 446–1). In most instances, the lung fields are clear. With constrictive pericardial disease, the heart is relatively small and calcification may be present.

The *echocardiogram* is a sensitive technique for evaluating the size and progression of pericardial effusions. Normally, the pericardium is closely adherent to the epicardium, and the two layers can only be narrowly separated by the ultrasound beam. In patients with pericardial effusion, a clear, echo-free space is recorded between the epicardium and pericardium. A posterior effusion is recorded behind the left ventricular epicardium and ends at the junction of the left ventricle and left atrium. An anterior effusion will be recorded between the chest wall and the anterior right ventricular wall. The presence of both an anterior and posterior effusion generally indicates a large col-

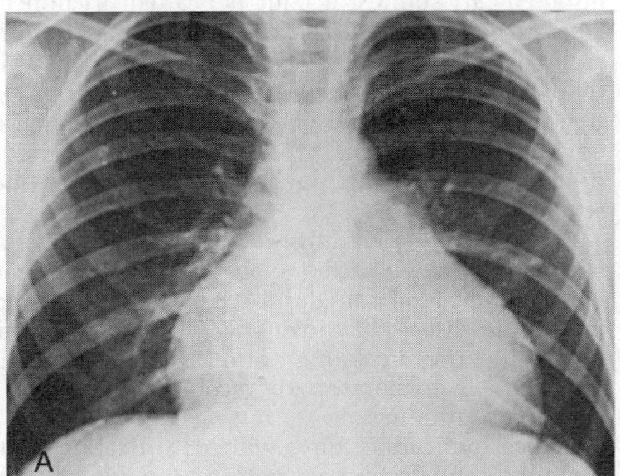

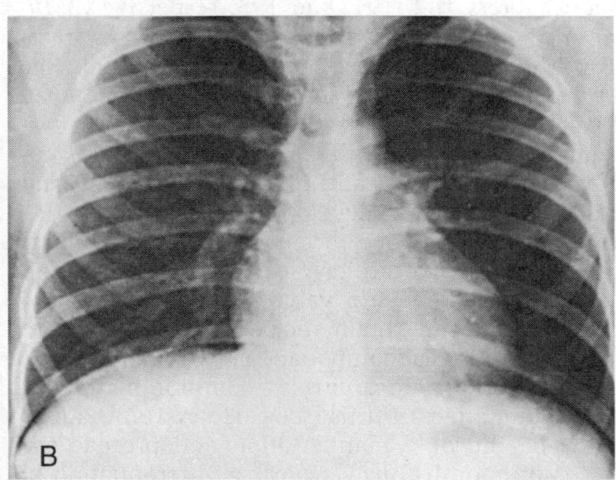

Figure 446–1 Roentgenograms in acute nonspecific perticarditis. *A.* Increase in cardiopericardial shadow caused by pericardial effusion. *B.* One month later after complete recovery.

lection of fluid. Flattening of septal motion and collapse of the right ventricular outflow during diastole are signs of pericardial tamponade.

DIFFERENTIAL DIAGNOSIS

Viral and Acute Benign Pericarditis. These entities are considered synonymous because most episodes of acute benign pericarditis follow or coincide with viral illness. Viruses recognized to cause pericarditis include coxsackievirus B, influenza, echovirus, and adenovirus. The pathogenesis is unclear but may be related to a hypersensitivity reaction to the viral disease. Pericardial inflammation is not necessarily the precursor of a generalized inflammatory process. Most cases are mild, and recovery occurs within several weeks. Only symptomatic treatment, usually with nonsteroidal anti-inflammatory agents such as indomethacin, is indicated. In rare instances, the patient is severely ill, and cardiac tamponade may ensue. There are also patients in whom a chronic relapsing illness occurs. The differential diagnosis between these patients and those with collagen vascular disease may be difficult. The latter patients respond dramatically to corticosteriods or nonsteroidal anti-inflammatory agents; milder forms may be controlled with aspirin. The clinical course may vary from months to 1–2 yr, during which time patients are dependent on drug therapy for suppression of the pericarditis. Ultimately, these patients improve, and the prognosis is good.

The clinical differential diagnosis between acute pericarditis and myocarditis may be difficult; usually each includes a component of the other. Management of these conditions is quite different; anti-inflammatory treatment and urgent response to cardiac tamponade are appropriate in the former, and therapy for heart failure is required in the latter. The echocardiogram can demonstrate the size of the pericardial effusion and also indicate the presence of myocardial dysfunction.

Purulent Pericarditis. This is most often associated with bacterial infections such as pneumonia, epiglottitis, meningitis, or osteomyelitis. Usually there are signs and symptoms of the primary infection. Once the purulent process is established, if untreated the course is fulminant, terminated by acute cardiac tamponade and death. Open pericardial drainage is required along with appropriate intravenous antibiotics. Although closed pericardial aspiration provides a sample of the exudate for diagnostic purposes and may be lifesaving in the face of severe cardiac compression, without open drainage and removal of adhesions, tamponade almost invariably recurs. Open pericardial drainage has significantly increased survival. Rarely, with infections that are identified extremely early and with pericardial fluid that is more of a transudate than an exudate, multiple pericardial taps with placement of a drain and antibiotic therapy have been successful. The most common organisms implicated in purulent pericarditis are *Staphylococcus aureus, Haemophilus influenzae* type b, and *Neisseria meningitidis.* (For treatment, see Chapters 182, 191, and 193, respectively.) *Tuberculous pericarditis* rarely occurs in children. Extensive treatment with antituberculous chemotherapy is required (see Chapter 212). *Immune complex–mediated pericarditis* (sterile) may occur 5–7 days after the initiation of therapy for severe systemic or meningeal infection with meningococcus or *H. influenzae* type b. Therapy includes anti-inflammatory agents and pericardiocentesis if tamponade develops.

Acute Rheumatic Fever. Pericarditis occurs in acute rheumatic fever as a component of pancarditis (see Chapters 184.1 and 444). It is associated with acute valvulitis. Pericarditis and other manifestations of acute rheumatic pancarditis respond to therapy with steroids. Cardiac tamponade is extremely rare.

Juvenile Rheumatoid Arthritis. Pericarditis is a common manifestation of juvenile rheumatoid arthritis (see Chapter 156). Rarely, pericarditis may be the only manifestation and precede the onset of arthritis by months or even years. Differentiation of rheumatoid pericarditis from that seen with other collagen vascular disease, particularly lupus erythematosus, may be difficult. Treatment consists of steroids or salicylates, which may be needed on a long-term basis.

Uremia. Uremic pericarditis occurs only in the presence of prolonged severe renal failure and results from chemical irritation of the pericardium secondary to the metabolic abnormalities. It may culminate in cardiac tamponade or cause recurrent hypotension during hemodialysis. If adequate relief of uremic pericarditis does not occur with hemodialysis, pericardiectomy is recommended.

Neoplastic Disease. Neoplastic pericardial effusion is seen in patients with Hodgkin's disease, lymphosarcoma, and leukemia, and results from direct neoplastic invasion of the pericardium. Cardiac tamponade may occur late in the course of the illness. Rarely, pericardial infiltration is the initial manifestation of neoplastic disease. Patients with malignancy may also acquire pericarditis as a result of radiation therapy to the mediastinum.

Postpericardiotomy Syndrome (Chapter 441). Pericardial effusions may be seen 1–2 wk or longer following open heart surgery and in some echocardiographic series are diagnosed in 15–23% of postoperative patients. The syndrome is a nonspecific hypersensitivity reaction to trauma to the pericardium and the epicardial surface of the heart. High titers of antiheart antibodies have been reported to correlate with clinical signs of the syndrome. Patients may present with low-grade fever, lethargy, loss of appetite, abdominal pain, and precordial or pleural chest pain. In most children, the syndrome is a relatively short illness and responds well to therapy with aspirin or other nonsteroidal anti-inflammatory agents. Corticosteroids are rarely needed and are reserved for the more severe cases. Treatment is maintained for 1–3 mo, but recurrences may be seen as long as 1 yr postoperatively and require reinstitution of therapy.

446.1 Constrictive Pericarditis

In most instances, constriction occurs months or years after the initial pericarditis, but occasionally it may be an acute, rapidly progressive process. Constrictive pericarditis most often occurs without an immediate preceding illness or generalized systemic disease.

The *clinical manifestations* occur as a result of impairment of diastolic ventricular filling, compromise of myocardial contractility, and resultant depression of cardiac function. Hepatomegaly and ascites may be out of proportion to the other signs and symptoms, thus suggesting chronic liver disease. Liver function studies are only mildly abnormal; careful physical examination reveals other subtle findings of constriction, including neck vein distention, narrow pulses, quiet precordium, distant heart sounds, a faint pericardial friction rub, and increased pulsus paradoxus. Typical findings become apparent gradually and may be overlooked. The auscultatory presence of an early pericardial knock and the appearance of calcification of the pericardium on chest roentgenogram are the more obvious manifestations. Protein-losing enteropathy with hypoproteinemia and lymphopenia may be seen in association with severe constriction.

Constrictive pericarditis may be difficult to distinguish from chronic restrictive cardiomyopathy (see Chapter 445.3). Impaired myocardial function occurs with both conditions. The myocardial disease of constrictive pericarditis is usually reversible with pericardiectomy. At times, a definite diagnosis can be made only by exploratory thoracotomy and direct examination of the pericardium.

Radical pericardiectomy with decortication of the pericardium over a wide area of the heart, including the systemic and pulmonary veins, is the only effective treatment for constrictive pericarditis. In most patients, surgical intervention elicits a rapid response characterized by increased cardiac output and prompt diuresis. The long-term prognosis is usually excellent.

Fowler NO: Cardiac tamponade: A clinical or an echocardiographic diagnosis? Circulation 87:1738, 1993.
Gersony WM, Hordof AH: Infective endocarditis and diseases of the pericardium. Pediatr Clin North Am 25:831, 1978.
Hara KS, Ballard DJ, Ilstrup DM, et al: Rheumatoid pericarditis: Clinical features and survival. Medicine 69:81, 1990.
Nishimura RA, Connolly DC, Parkin TW, et al: Constrictive pericarditis: Assessment of current diagnostic procedures. Mayo Clin Proc 60:397, 1985.
Sinzobahamvya N, Ikeogu MO: Purulent pericarditis. Arch Dis Child 62:696, 1987.

CHAPTER 447
Tumors of the Heart

Primary tumors of the heart are rare in infancy and childhood and are most often benign. Clinical manifestations depend primarily on the location of the tumor and, to a lesser extent, on the histologic type.

The most common benign cardiac tumors in children are rhabdomyomas, fibromas, and myxomas. *Rhabdomyomas* occur as single or, usually, multiple nodules embedded in chamber walls. They often remain clinically unimportant and regress with age but may cause mechanical obstruction, heart failure, or arrhythmias. They may be familial and are often found in association with **tuberous sclerosis**. Most rhabdomyomas are seen in infants younger than 1 yr of age. Incessant ventricular tachycardia in a child younger than 2 yr of age should raise the suspicion of a small endocardial or epicardial *rhabdomyoma* or *Purkinje cell tumor. Fibromas* are usually solitary nonencapsulated nodules, located in the ventricles; they can be massive. The treatment of rhabdomyomas and fibromas depends on their location and size. Small asymptomatic tumors in the myocardial wall or ventricular septum may be observed for growth or regression. Rhabdomyomas associated with tuberous sclerosis often resolve as the child grows older. Large tumors that show signs of obstructing blood flow and those producing ventricular arrhythmias should be removed. Large and diffuse tumors may interfere with cardiac performance. Removal of large lesions is often difficult because insufficient normal myocardium may remain. Heart transplantation may be the only recourse for patients with extensive tumors.

Myxomas develop in intracavitary locations, most frequently (75%) in the left atrium and most often in females (75%). These tumors are solid, smooth, pedunculated masses (1–8 cm) that attach to the interatrial septum, protrude into the atrial chamber, and, by their position relative to the mitral or tricuspid valve, cause intermittent obstruction and a clinical picture consistent with stenosis (syncope, heart failure, atrial fibrillation). A myxoma should be considered in the presence of fainting spells, a positional character (supine vs erect) to the murmur, or evidence of systemic or pulmonary embolization. Atrial myxomas can also cause fever, malaise, arthralgias, and systemic emboli mimicking endocarditis, rheumatic fever, or systemic lupus erythematosus. Laboratory features include a high sedimentation rate, hematuria, and echocardiographic evidence of the tumor. Atrial myxomas may be associated with multiple pigmented skin lesions (lentiginosis), myxoid fibroadenomas of the breast, cutaneous myxomas, and adrenal pigmented nodules. Some are associated with various cutaneous and connective tissue lesions and testicular tumors or pituitary adenomas (Carney syndrome). Treatment consists of surgical excision, which must include all the base of the tumor to prevent recurrence.

Other benign tumors include *papillomas,* which are attached to valve leaflets and may present in the neonate; *lipomas,* which are situated in ventricular walls; and *mesotheliomas,* which may involve the atrioventricular node and cause abnormalities of electrical conduction, including complete heart block.

Primary malignant cardiac tumors in children are almost exclusively *sarcomas.* These tumors are usually located in the right side of the heart, atrial septum, right atrial wall, or root of the pulmonary artery. They may extend either into the adjacent chamber to cause obstruction to blood flow or into the pericardial cavity to produce effusion or tamponade. The heart also may be involved in the metastatic dissemination of a noncardiac malignancy, such as leukemia or lymphoma, or in Wilms' tumor by direct extension of the tumor into the right atrium via the inferior vena cava. Physical examination reflects the location and size of the tumor if it interferes with blood flow. Conduction system involvement can be assessed by electrocardiography. Two-dimensional echocardiography is diagnostic and allows excellent visualization of the location and extent of the tumor. Doppler studies evaluate the extent of blood flow obstruction caused by the tumor. Cardiac catheterization may provide further information about the anatomy of the tumor and the hemodynamic effects. When indicated, surgical intervention is directed toward complete removal of the tumor, relief of obstruction, and control of any arrhythmias. Long-term outcome depends on the type of tumor, completeness of surgical removal, and the postsurgical integrity of the normal heart structures and myocardium. For tumors that are unresectable because of their inability to be separated from normal heart tissue, heart transplantation is an effective treatment.

Bini RM, Westaby S, Bargeron LM, et al: Investigation and management of primary cardiac tumors in infants and children. J Am Coll Cardiol 2:351, 1983.
Birnbaum S, McGahan JP, Janos GG, et al: Fetal tachycardia and intramyocardial tumors. J Am Coll Cardiol 6:1358, 1985.
Coltart DJ, Billingham ME, Popp RL, et al: Left atrial myxoma: Diagnosis, treatment and cytological observations. JAMA 234:950, 1975.
Felner JM, Knopf WD: Echocardiographic recognition of intracardiac and extracardiac masses. Echocardiography 2:1, 1985.
Garson A Jr, Gillette PC, Titus JL, et al: Surgical treatment of ventricular tachycardia in infants. N Engl J Med 310:1443, 1984.

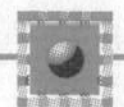

SECTION 7

Cardiac Therapeutics

CHAPTER 448

Heart Failure

Heart failure is defined as a state in which the heart cannot deliver an adequate cardiac output to meet the metabolic needs of the body. In early stages of heart failure, various compensatory mechanisms are evoked to maintain normal metabolic function (cardiac reserve). As these mechanisms become ineffective, increasingly severe clinical manifestations result.

PATHOPHYSIOLOGY. The heart can be viewed as a pump with an output proportional to its filling volume and inversely proportional to the resistance against which it pumps. As the ventricular end-diastolic volume increases, the healthy heart increases cardiac output until a maximum is reached and cardiac output can no longer be augmented (the Frank-Starling principle; Fig. 448–1). The increased stroke volume obtained in this manner is due to the stretching of myocardial fibers but also results in increased wall tension, which increases myocardial oxygen consumption. Hearts working under various types of stress function along different Frank-Starling curves. Cardiac muscle with a compromised intrinsic contractility requires a greater degree of dilatation to produce an increased stroke volume and does not achieve the same maximal cardiac output as normal myocardium. If a cardiac chamber is already dilatated because of a lesion causing an increased preload (e.g., a left-to-right shunt or valvular insufficiency), there is little room for further dilatation and augmentation of cardiac output. The presence of lesions that result in increased afterload to the ventricle (aortic or pulmonic stenosis, coarctation of the aorta) decreases cardiac performance, resulting in a depressed Frank-Starling relationship. The ability of the immature heart to increase cardiac output in response to increased preload is less than that of the mature heart. Thus, premature infants are more compromised by a left-to-right shunt than is a full-term infant.

Systemic oxygen transport is calculated as the product of the cardiac output and the systemic oxygen content. The cardiac output can be calculated as the product of heart rate and stroke volume. The primary determinants of stroke volume are the *afterload* (pressure work), *preload* (volume work), and *contractility* (intrinsic myocardial function). Abnormalities of heart rate can also compromise cardiac output, producing both bradyarrhythmias and tachyarrhythmias; the latter shorten the diastolic time interval for ventricular filling. Alterations in the oxygen carrying capacity of the blood (e.g., anemia or hypoxemia) also lead to a decrease in systemic oxygen transport, and if compensatory mechanisms are inadequate can also result in decreased delivery of substrate to the tissues.

In some cases of heart failure, the cardiac output is normal or increased, yet because of decreased systemic oxygen content (secondary to anemia) or increased oxygen demands (secondary to hyperventilation, hyperthyroidism, or hypermetabolism), there is an inadequate amount of oxygen delivered to meet the body's needs. This condition, **high-output failure**, results in the development of signs and symptoms of heart failure when there is no basic abnormality in myocardial function and the cardiac output is greater than normal. It is also seen with large systemic arteriovenous fistulas. These conditions reduce peripheral vascular resistance and cardiac afterload and increase myocardial contractility. Heart "failure" results when the demand for cardiac output exceeds the ability of the heart to respond. Chronic severe high-output failure may eventually result in a decrease in myocardial performance as the metabolic requirements of the myocardium are not met.

One major compensatory mechanism for increasing cardiac output is an increase in sympathetic tone, secondary to increased adrenal secretion of circulating epinephrine and increased neural release of norepinephrine. The initial beneficial effects of sympathetic stimulation include increased heart rate and myocardial contractility; both serve to increase cardiac output. Because of localized vasoconstriction, blood flow may be redistributed from the cutaneous, visceral, and renal beds to the heart and brain. Prolonged increases in sympathetic stimulation can have deleterious effects as well, including hypermetabolism, increased afterload, arrhythmogenesis, increased myocardial oxygen requirements, and direct myocar-

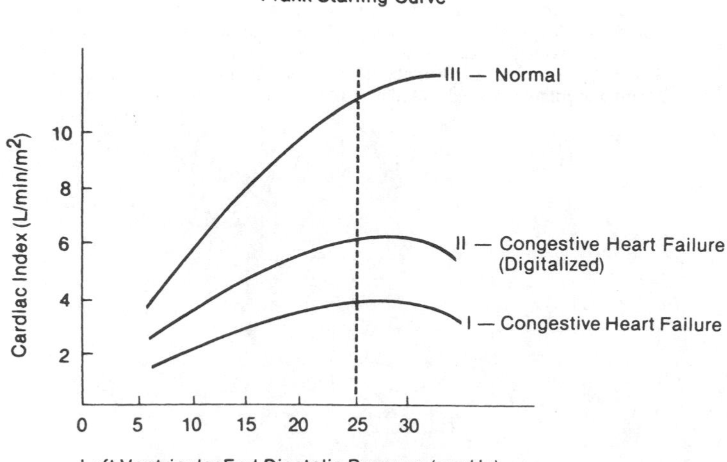

Figure 448–1 The Frank-Starling relationship. As the left ventricular end-diastolic pressure (LVED) increases, cardiac index increases, even in the presence of congestive heart failure, until a critical level of LVED is reached. Adding an inotropic agent (digoxin) shifts the curve from I and II. (From Gersony WM, Steep CN: *In*: Dickerman JD, Lucey JF [eds]: Smith's The Critically Ill Child: Diagnosis and Medical Management, 3rd ed. Philadelphia, WB Saunders, 1984.)

dial toxicity. Peripheral vasoconstriction can result in decreased renal, hepatic, and gastrointestinal tract function.

CLINICAL MANIFESTATIONS. The clinical manifestations depend on the degree of cardiac reserve under various conditions. A critically ill infant or child who has exhausted the compensatory mechanisms to the point that cardiac output is no longer sufficient to meet the basal metabolic needs of the body is symptomatic at rest. Other patients may be comfortable when quiet but are incapable of increasing cardiac output in response to even mild activity without experiencing significant symptoms. Conversely, it may take rather vigorous exercise to compromise cardiac function in children who have less severe heart disease. A thorough history is extremely important in making the diagnosis of heart failure and in evaluating the possible causes. Parents who observe their infant on a daily basis may not recognize subtle changes that have occurred over the course of days or weeks. Cyanosis may be considered merely "a deep coloring" and not recognized as an abnormal finding. The history of a young infant should also focus on feeding (see Chapter 429). The infant with heart failure often takes less volume per feeding, becomes dyspneic while sucking, and may perspire profusely. Eliciting a history of fatigue in an older child requires specific questions about activity.

In children, the signs and symptoms of heart failure are similar to those in adults and include fatigue, effort intolerance, anorexia, abdominal pain, and cough. Dyspnea is a reflection of pulmonary congestion. Elevation of systemic venous pressure may be gauged by clinical assessment of the jugular venous pressure and liver enlargement. Orthopnea and basilar rales may be present; edema is usually discernible in dependent portions of the body, or anasarca may be present. Cardiomegaly is invariably noted. A gallop rhythm is common; other auscultatory findings are specific to the basic cardiac lesion.

In infants, heart failure may be more difficult to identify. Prominent manifestations include tachypnea, feeding difficulties, poor weight gain, excessive perspiration, irritability, weak cry, and noisy, labored respirations with intercostal and subcostal retractions as well as flaring of the alae nasi. The signs of cardiac pulmonary congestion may be indistinguishable from those of bronchiolitis; wheezing is the most prominent finding. Pneumonitis with or without atelectasis is common, especially of the right middle and lower lobes; it is due to bronchial compression by the enlarged heart. Hepatomegaly usually occurs, and cardiomegaly is invariably present. In spite of pronounced tachycardia, a gallop rhythm can frequently be recognized. The other auscultatory signs are those produced by the underlying cardiac lesion. Clinical assessment of the jugular venous pressure in infants may be difficult because of the shortness of the neck and the difficulty of observing a relaxed state. Edema may be generalized, usually involving the eyelids as well as the sacrum, and less often the legs and feet. The differential diagnosis is age-dependent (Table 448–1).

LABORATORY DIAGNOSIS. *Roentgenograms of the chest* show cardiac enlargement. The pulmonary vascularity is variable depending on the cause of the heart failure. Infants and children with large left-to-right shunts have exaggeration of the pulmonary arterial vessels to the periphery of the lung fields, whereas patients with cardiomyopathy may have a relatively normal pulmonary vascular bed early in the course of disease. Fluffy perihilar pulmonary markings suggestive of venous congestion and acute pulmonary edema are seen only with more severe degrees of heart failure.

Chamber hypertrophy by *electrocardiography* may be helpful in assessing the cause of heart failure but does not establish the diagnosis. In cardiomyopathies, left or right ventricular ischemic changes may correlate well with clinical and other noninvasive parameters of ventricular function. Low-voltage QRS morphologic characteristics with ST-T wave abnormalities may also suggest myocardial inflammatory disease but can also be seen with pericarditis. The electrocardiogram is the best tool for evaluating rhythm disorders as a potential cause of heart failure.

TABLE 448–1 Etiology of Heart Failure

Fetal
Severe anemia (hemolysis, fetal-maternal transfusion, parvovirus B19–induced anemia, hypoplastic anemia)
Supraventricular tachycardia
Ventricular tachycardia
Complete heart block
Premature Neonate
Fluid overload
Patent ductus arteriosus
Ventricular septal defect
Cor pulmonale (bronchopulmonary dysplasia)
Hypertension
Full-Term Neonate
Asphyxial cardiomyopathy
Arteriovenous malformation (vein of Galen, hepatic)
Left-sided obstructive lesions (coarctation of aorta, hypoplastic left side of the heart)
Large mixing cardiac defects (single ventricle, truncus arteriosus)
Viral myocarditis
Infant-Toddler
Left-to-right cardiac shunts (ventricular septal defect)
Hemangioma (arteriovenous malformation)
Anomalous left coronary artery
Metabolic cardiomyopathy
Acute hypertension (hemolytic-uremic syndrome)
Supraventricular tachycardia
Kawasaki's disease
Child-Adolescent
Rheumatic fever
Acute hypertension (glomerulonephritis)
Viral myocarditis
Thyrotoxicosis
Hemochromatosis-hemosiderosis
Cancer therapy (radiation, doxorubicin)
Sickle cell anemia
Endocarditis
Cor pulmonale (cystic fibrosis)
Cardiomyopathy (hypertrophic, dilatated)

Echocardiographic techniques are useful in assessing ventricular function. The most commonly used parameter is the fractional shortening, determined as the difference between end-systolic and end-diastolic diameters divided by the end-diastolic diameter. The normal fractional shortening is between 28 and 40%, compared with the normal ejection fraction (which measures volume) of 55–65% measured by angiography. The pre-ejection:ejection period ratio measured by M-mode echocardiography should be less than 40%. A long pre-ejection time with a short ejection time usually denotes myocardial failure. Doppler studies can be used to calculate cardiac output. *Arterial oxygen levels* may be decreased when ventilation-perfusion inequalities occur secondary to pulmonary edema. When heart failure is severe, respiratory or metabolic *acidosis,* or both, may be present. Infants with heart failure often display *hyponatremia* caused by renal water retention. Total body sodium may actually be increased. Chronic diuretic treatment can decrease serum sodium levels further.

TREATMENT. The underlying cause of cardiac failure must be removed or alleviated if possible. If the cause is a congenital cardiac anomaly amenable to surgery, medical treatment is indicated to prepare the patient for operation and in the immediate postoperative period while the heart is recovering from the effects of cardiopulmonary bypass. If the cause is a cardiomyopathy, medical management provides temporary relief from symptoms and allows the patient time to wait for a heart donor if heart transplantation is indicated.

General Measures. Strict bed rest is rarely necessary except in extreme cases, but it is important that the child rest often and sleep adequately. Most older patients feel better sleeping in a semiupright position. For infants with heart failure, an infant chair may be advisable. After patients begin to respond to treatment, restrictions on activities can often be modified within the context of the specific diagnosis and the patient's ability. For patients with severe pulmonary edema, positive-pressure ventilation may be required along with other drug therapy. β-Adrenergic agonists, such as dopamine, epinephrine, and dobutamine, along with afterload-reducing agents (e.g., nitroprusside, captopril), may be required in an intensive care setting.

Diet. Infants with heart failure may fail to thrive because of increased metabolic requirements and decreased caloric intake. Increasing daily calories is an important aspect of their management. Increasing the number of calories per ounce of infant formula (or supplementing breast feedings) may be beneficial. Many infants do not tolerate an increase beyond 24 calories per oz because of diarrhea or because these formulas provide too large a solute load for compromised kidneys.

Severely ill infants may lack sufficient strength for effective sucking because of extreme fatigue, rapid respirations, and generalized weakness. In these circumstances, nasogastric feedings may be helpful. In many children with cardiac enlargement, gastroesophageal reflux is a major problem. The use of continuous drip nasogastric feedings at night, administered by pump, may improve caloric intake while decreasing the problems with reflux. Occasionally, medical or surgical intervention to correct reflux is necessary (Nissen's fundoplication). Continued malnutrition may be an important factor in the decision to undertake earlier surgical intervention in patients who have an operable congenital heart lesion.

The use of low-sodium formulas in the routine management of infants with heart failure is not recommended because these preparations are often poorly tolerated. The use of more potent diuretic agents allows more palatable standard formulas to be used for nutrition while controlling salt and water balance by chronic diuretic administration. Most older children can be managed with "no added salt" diets and abstinence from foods containing large amounts of sodium. A strict extremely low sodium diet is rarely required.

Digitalis. Digoxin is the digitalis glycoside used most often in the pediatric patient. Its half-life of 36 hr is long enough to allow daily or twice daily administration and short enough to limit toxic effects from overdosage. It is absorbed well by the gastrointestinal tract (60–85%), even in infants. When taken with or after meals, the rate of absorption may be somewhat retarded, but the amount of digoxin absorbed is usually unchanged. Absorption is greater with the elixir than with tablets. An initial effect can be seen as early as 30 min after administration, and the peak effect for oral digoxin is at approximately 2–6 hr. When the drug is administered intravenously, the initial effect is seen in 15–30 min, and the peak effect occurs at 1–4 hr. The drug crosses the placenta, and therefore the fetus with heart failure (secondary to arrhythmia) can be treated by administering digoxin to the mother. Digoxin is eliminated by the kidney, and dosing must be adjusted based on the patient's renal function. The rate of excretion is proportional to the glomerular filtration rate. After intravenous administration, 50–70% is excreted unchanged in the urine. The half-life of digoxin may be up to 6 days in patients with anuria, in whom slower hepatic excretion pathways are utilized.

Rapid digitalization of infants and children in heart failure may be carried out intravenously. The dose depends on the patient's age (Table 448–2). The recommended schedule is to give one half of the total digitalizing dose immediately and the succeeding two one-quarter doses at 12-hr intervals later. The electrocardiogram must be closely monitored and rhythm strips obtained prior to each of the three digitalizing doses.

TABLE 448–2 Dosage of Drugs Commonly Used for the Treatment of Congestive Heart Failure

Drug	Dosage
Digoxin Digitalization PO (1/2 initially, followed by 1/4 every 8–12 hr × 2)	Premature: 20 μg/kg Full-term neonate (up to 1 mo): 20–30 μg/kg Infant or child: 25–40 μg/kg Adolescent or adult: 0.5–1 mg in divided doses IV dose is 75% of PO dose
Digoxin maintenance	5–10 μg/kg/day, divided q 12 hr Trough serum level: 1.5–3.0 ng/mL <6 mo old 1–2 ng/mL >6 mo old IV dose is 75% of PO dose
Furosemide (Lasix)	
IV	1–2 mg/dose, prn
PO	1–4 mg/kg/day, divided qd to qid
Bumetanide (Bumex)	
IV	0.01–0.1 mg/kg/dose
PO	0.05–0.1 mg/kg/day, divided q 6–8 hr
Chlorothiazide (Diuril) PO	20–50 mg/kg/day, divided bid or tid
Spironolactone (Aldactone) PO	1–3 mg/kg/day, divided bid or tid
β-adrenergic agonists IV	
Dobutamine	2–20 μg/kg/min
Dopamine	2–30 μg/kg/min
Isoproterenol	0.01–0.5 μg/kg/min
Epinephrine	0.05–1.0 μg/kg/min
Norepinephrine	0.1–2.0 μg/kg/min
Phosphodiesterase inhibitors IV	
Amrinone	3–10 μg/kg/min
Milrinone	0.25–1.0 μg/kg/min
Afterload-reducing agents	
Captopril (Capoten) PO	
Infants	0.1–0.5 mg/kg/dose, q 8–12 hr (maximum 4 mg/kg/day) Prematures: start at 0.01 mg/kg/dose
Children	0.1–2 mg/kg/day, q 8–12 hr (adult dose is 6.25–25 mg/dose)
Enalapril (Vasotec) PO	0.08–0.5 mg/kg/dose q 12–24 hr (maximum 1 mg/kg/day)
Hydralazine (Apresoline) PO	
IV or IM	0.1–0.5 mg/kg/dose (maximum 20 mg)
PO	0.25–1.0 mg/kg/dose, q 6–8 hr (maximum 200 mg/day)
Nitroglycerin	0.25–5 μg/kg/min
Nitroprusside (Nipride) IV	0.5–8 μg/kg/min
Prazosin	0.005–0.05 mg/kg/dose q 6–8 hr, maximum 0.1 mg/kg/dose

Note: Pediatric doses based on weight should not exceed adult doses. As recommendations may change, these doses should always be double checked. Doses may also need to be modified in any patient with renal or hepatic dysfunction.

PO = by mouth; IV = intravenously; prn = as necessary; qd = every day; qid = three times per day; bid = twice daily.

Digoxin should be discontinued if a new rhythm disturbance is noted. A prolongation of the PR interval is not necessarily an indication to withhold digitalis, but a delay in administering the next dose or a reduction in the dosage should be considered depending on the patient's clinical status. Serum digoxin determination is helpful when digitalis toxicity is suspected, although it may be less reliable in infants. ST segment or T-wave changes are commonly noted with digitalis administration and should not affect the digitalization regimen. Baseline serum electrolyte levels should be measured prior to and after digitalization. Hypokalemia and hypercalcemia exacerbate digitalis toxicity. Because hypokalemia is relatively common in patients receiving diuretics, the potassium level should be followed closely in patients receiving a potassium-wasting diuretic (e.g., furosemide) in combination with digitalis.

Maintenance digitalis therapy is started approximately 12 hr after full digitalization. The daily dosage is divided in two and given at 12-hr intervals for more consistent blood levels and more flexibility in case of toxicity. The dosage is one quarter of the total digitalizing dose. For patients who are initially given digitalis intravenously, maintenance digoxin can be given orally once oral feedings are tolerated. Because absorption from the gastrointestinal tract is less certain, the oral maintenance dose is usually 20–25% higher than when digoxin is used parenterally (see Table 448–2). The normal daily dose of digoxin for older children (>5 yr of age) calculated by body weight should not exceed the usual adult dose of 0.2–0.5 mg/24 hr.

Patients who are not critically ill may be given digitalis initially by the oral route, and in most instances digitalization is completed within 24 hr. When slow digitalization is desirable, for example, in the immediate postoperative period, initiation of a maintenance digoxin schedule without a prior loading dose achieves full digitalization in 7–10 days. Often, this can be carried out on an outpatient basis.

If an infant improves significantly when receiving digitalis over a period of a few months and the need for the drug appears to be lessening (e.g., a ventricular septal defect that is becoming smaller), the dosage is not increased as the child gains weight. If the clinical status warrants, the drug is discontinued.

Measurement of a *serum digoxin level* is useful under several circumstances: (1) when a standard dose of digoxin is not having beneficial therapeutic effects, (2) when an unknown amount of digoxin has been administered or ingested accidentally, (3) when renal function is impaired or if drug interactions are possible (e.g., quinidine), (4) when there is a question regarding compliance, and (5) when a toxic response is suspected. Blood is usually drawn immediately prior to a dose but at minimum 4 hr after the last dose so that tissue-plasma equilibration has occurred. A normal blood level in an infant is approximately 2–4 ng/mL and in older children 1–2 ng/mL. Exceeding these levels does not generally add to the management of heart failure significantly and only increases the risk of toxicity. In suspected toxicity, elevated serum digoxin levels are not in themselves diagnostic of toxicity but must be interpreted as an adjunct to other clinical and electrocardiographic findings (rhythm and conduction disturbances). Nausea and vomiting are less frequent in pediatric patients. Hypokalemia, hypomagnesemia, hypercalcemia, cardiac inflammation due to myocarditis, and prematurity may all potentiate digitalis toxicity. A cardiac arrhythmia that develops in a child who is taking digitalis also may be related to the primary cardiac disease rather than to the drug. Any form of arrhythmia occurring after the institution of digitalis therapy must be considered to be drug-related until proved otherwise. Succeeding doses should be withheld until the issue is resolved.

Diuretics. These agents interfere with reabsorption of water and sodium by the kidneys, which results in the reduction of circulating blood volume and thereby reduces pulmonary fluid overload and ventricular filling pressures. They are most often used in conjunction with digitalis therapy in patients with severe congestive heart failure.

Furosemide is the most commonly used diuretic in patients with heart failure. It inhibits the reabsorption of sodium and chloride in the distal tubules and the loop of Henle. Patients requiring acute diuresis should be given intravenous or intramuscular furosemide at an initial dose of 1–2 mg/kg. This usually results in rapid diuresis and prompt improvement in clinical status, particularly if symptoms of pulmonary congestion are present. Chronic furosemide therapy is then prescribed at a dose of 1–4 mg/kg/24 hr given between one and four times a day. Careful monitoring of electrolytes is necessary with long-term furosemide therapy because there may be significant loss of potassium. Potassium chloride supplementation is usually required unless the potassium-sparing diuretic spironolactone is given concomitantly. When furosemide is administered every other day, dietary potassium supplementation may be adequate to maintain normal serum potassium levels. Chronic administration of furosemide may cause contraction of the extracellular fluid compartment, resulting in a "contraction alkalosis" (see Chapter 55.8).

Spironolactone is an inhibitor of aldosterone and enhances potassium retention. It is usually given orally in two to three divided doses of 2–3 mg/kg/24 hr. Combinations of spironolactone and chlorothiazide are commonly used for convenience and because they eliminate the need for potassium supplementation, which is often poorly tolerated.

Chlorothiazide is used occasionally for diuresis in children with less severe chronic heart failure. It is less immediate in action and less potent than furosemide, and it affects the reabsorption of electrolytes in the renal tubules only. The usual dose is 20–40 mg/kg/24 hr in divided doses. Potassium supplementation is often required if this agent is used alone.

Afterload-Reducing Agents. This group of drugs reduces ventricular afterload by decreasing peripheral vascular resistance thereby improving myocardial performance. Some of these agents also decrease systemic venous tone, significantly reducing preload. Afterload reducers are especially useful in children with heart failure secondary to cardiomyopathy and in patients with severe mitral or aortic insufficiency. They may also be effective in patients with heart failure secondary to left-to-right shunts. They are usually not used in the presence of stenotic lesions of the left ventricular outflow tract. Afterload-reducing agents are most often used in conjunction with other anticongestive drugs such as digoxin and diuretics.

Nitroprusside should be administered only in an intensive care setting and for as short a time as possible. Its short intravenous half-life makes it ideal for titrating the dose in critically ill patients. Peripheral arterial vasodilation and afterload reduction are the major effects, but venodilation causing a decrease in venous return to the heart may also be beneficial. Blood pressure must be continuously monitored because sudden hypotension can occur. Nitroprusside is contraindicated when there is pre-existing hypotension. As the drug is metabolized, small amounts of circulating cyanide are produced, which are detoxified in the liver to thiocyanate, which is excreted in the urine. When high doses of nitroprusside are administered for several days, toxic symptoms related to thiocyanate poisoning may occur (fatigue, nausea, disorientation, acidosis, and muscular spasm). If nitroprusside use is prolonged, blood thiocyanate levels should be monitored; values greater than 10 g/dL are consistent with clinical symptoms of toxicity.

Captopril is an orally active angiotensin-converting enzyme inhibitor that produces arterial dilatation by blocking the production of angiotensin II, resulting in significant afterload reduction. Venodilation and consequent preload reduction have also been reported. This agent also interferes with aldosterone production and thereby also helps control salt and water retention. The oral dose is 0.3–6 mg/kg/24 hr given in two to three divided doses. The adverse reactions to captopril include hypotension and its sequelae (e.g., syncope, weakness, and dizziness). A maculopapular pruritic rash is encountered in 5–8% of patients, but the drug may be continued because the rash often disappears spontaneously with time. Neutropenia, renal toxicity, and chronic cough also occur. Enalapril is a longer acting angiotensin-converting enzyme inhibitor.

Hydralazine is a direct arteriolar smooth muscle relaxant and has virtually no effects on preload. It is occasionally administered together with a venodilating agent, such as one of the nitrate derivatives. The usual oral dose of hydralazine is 0.5–7.5 mg/kg/24 hr in three divided doses. Many patients require increasing dosages with time in order to maintain the peripheral dilating effects (tachyphylaxis). Adverse reactions with hydralazine include headache, palpitations, nausea, and vomiting. In addition, systemic lupus erythematosus occasionally occurs after administration of large doses of hydralazine over prolonged periods; these manifestations are reversible when the drug is discontinued.

Adrenergic Agonists. *Dopamine* has fewer chronotropic and arrhythmogenic effects than does isoproterenol. In addition, it results in selective renal vasodilation, which is particularly useful in patients with the compromised kidney function that is often associated with low cardiac output. At a dose of 2–10 μg/kg/min, dopamine results in increased contractility with little peripheral vasoconstrictive effects. However, if the dose is increased beyond 15 μg/kg/min, its peripheral α-adrenergic effects may result in vasoconstriction. At high doses, dopamine may potentially cause an increase in pulmonary vascular resistance.

Dobutamine, a derivative of dopamine, is useful in treating low cardiac output. It causes direct inotropic effects with a moderate (albeit less than isoproterenol) reduction in peripheral vascular resistance. Dobutamine can be used as an adjunct to dopamine therapy in order to avoid the vasoconstrictive effects of high-dose dopamine. Dobutamine is also less likely to cause cardiac rhythm disturbances. The usual dose is 2–20 μg/kg/min.

Isoproterenol, an intravenous preparation used for treating low cardiac output, has both central and peripheral β-adrenergic effects and therefore enhances myocardial contractility and also reduces cardiac afterload. The drug is administered in an intensive care setting, where the dose is titrated between 0.01 and 1.5 μg/kg/min. Continuous determinations of arterial blood pressure and heart rate are mandatory, and measuring cardiac output at the bedside with a pulmonary thermodilution catheter may also be helpful in assessing drug efficacy. Because isoproterenol has a marked chronotropic effect, it should not be used in patients who already have significant tachycardia. Children receiving isoproterenol must be carefully monitored for atrial or ventricular premature depolarizations. Often, as isoproterenol or other β-adrenergic agonist treatment is withdrawn, digoxin therapy is added for continued inotropic effect.

Phosphodiesterase Inhibitors. Milrinone is useful in treating patients with low cardiac output who are refractory to standard therapy. It works by inhibition of phosphodiesterase, preventing the degradation of intracellular cyclic adenosine monophosphate. Milrinone has both positive inotropic effects on the heart and significant peripheral vasodilatory effects and has generally been used as an adjunct to dopamine or dobutamine therapy in the intensive care unit. It is given at an initial loading dose of 50 μg/kg intravenously followed by an intravenous infusion of 0.25–1 μg/kg/min. A major side effect is hypotension secondary to peripheral vasodilation. The hypotension can usually be managed by the administration of intravenous fluids to restore adequate intravascular volume. Amrinone, another phosphodiesterase inhibitor, can cause thrombocytopenia; the severity appears to be related to both the rate of infusion and the duration of therapy. It is reversible when the drug is discontinued.

Chronic Treatment with β-Blockers. Studies in adult patients with dilatated cardiomyopathy have shown that β-adrenergic blocking agents, introduced gradually as part of a comprehensive heart failure treatment program, are capable of improving exercise tolerance, decreasing hospitalizations, and reducing overall mortality. The agents most often used are metoprolol, a β_1-receptor selective antagonist, and carvedilol, an agent with both α- and β-receptor blocking as well as free radical scavenging effects.

448.1 Cardiogenic Shock (See also Chapter 64.2)

Cardiogenic shock may occur as a complication of (1) severe cardiac dysfunction, often following surgery; (2) septicemia; (3) severe burns; (4) immunologic disease (anaphylaxis); (5) hemorrhage or dehydration; (6) severe debilitation; and (7) acute central nervous system disorders. It is characterized by low cardiac output and hypotension, resulting in inadequate tissue perfusion.

Treatment is aimed at reinstitution of adequate cardiac output and peripheral perfusion to prevent the untoward effects of prolonged ischemia to vital organs as well as management of the underlying cause. Under physiologic conditions, the cardiac output is increased as a result of sympathetic discharge, which increases heart rate. However, in the presence of cardiogenic shock with marked tachycardia, heart rate will not increase further and may reduce cardiac output by decreasing diastolic filling time. Cardiac output must be increased by increasing stroke volume. If the rate of fluid administration is increased, the central venous pressure and ventricular filling pressure (preload) increase and the Frank-Starling mechanism results in an increased stroke volume. Optimal filling pressure is variable and depends on a number of extracardiac factors, including ventilatory support with high positive end-expiratory pressure, peak inspiratory pressure, and intra-abdominal pressure. The increased pressure necessary to fill a relatively noncompliant ventricle should also be considered, particularly after open heart surgery. If incremental fluid administration does not result in improved cardiac output, abnormal myocardial contractility or an abnormally high afterload, or both, must be implicated as the cause of the low cardiac output.

Myocardial contractility improves when treatment of the basic cause of shock is instituted, hypoxia is eliminated, and acidosis is corrected. However, dopamine, epinephrine, and dobutamine improve cardiac contractility, increase heart rate, and ultimately increase cardiac output.

The use of cardiac glycosides to treat acute low cardiac output states should be avoided. Digoxin has a slower effect than do catecholamines, even with intravenous administration. In addition, adverse effects may result from larger doses and toxicity is less predictable, depending on myocardial and serum potassium and calcium levels. Because it is common for

TABLE 448–3 Treatment of Cardiogenic Shock*

	Determinants of Stroke Volume		
	Preload	***Contractility***	***Afterload***
Parameters measured	CVP, PCWP, LAP, cardiac chamber size on echocardiography	CO, BP, fractional shortening on echocardiography, MV O_2 saturation	BP, peripheral perfusion, SVR
Abnormal physiologic manifestations	Low CVP, PCWP, or LAP ↓ CO ↓ BP	High CVP, PCWP, or LAP; low MV O_2 saturation ↓ CO ↓ BP	High CVP, PCWP, LAP, or SVR ↓ CO → or ↑ BP
Treatment to improve cardiac output	Volume expansion, crystalloid, colloid, blood	β-Adrenergic agonists, phosphodiesterase inhibitors	Afterload-reducing agents

**The goal is to improve peripheral perfusion by increasing cardiac output: cardiac output = heart rate × stroke volume.*
CVP = central venous pressure; PCWP = pulmonary capillary wedge pressure; LAP = left atrial pressure (measured with an indwelling LA line); CO = cardiac output (measured with a thermodilution catheter); BP = blood pressure; SVR = systemic vascular resistance (calculated from CO and mean BP); MV O_2 saturation = mixed venous oxygen saturation (measured with a central venous catheter); ↓ = decreased; → = normal; ↑ = increased.

patients with cardiovascular shock to have compromised renal perfusion, the administration of digoxin may result in high persistent blood levels because it is excreted in the kidneys. When digoxin is required for these patients, a lower and less frequent dosage should be used, and serum digoxin levels must be monitored frequently.

Patients with cardiogenic shock may have a marked increase in systemic vascular resistance, resulting in high afterload and poor peripheral perfusion. If increased systemic vascular resistance is persistent and the administration of positive inotropic agents alone does not improve tissue perfusion, the use of afterload-reducing agents may be appropriate, for example, nitroprusside used in combination with dopamine. In these patients, use of a pulmonary thermodilution catheter to measure cardiac index and to calculate systemic vascular resistance can be indispensable in guiding therapeutic decisions.

Some patients with cardiogenic shock may benefit from intra-aortic balloon counterpulsation, which reduces afterload by mechanical means and also increases diastolic coronary perfusion. Patients with reversible ventricular failure, for example, those in the immediate postoperative state, may also benefit from extracorporeal membrane oxygenation.

Sequential evaluation and management of cardiovascular shock is mandatory (see Chapter 64.2). Table 448–3 outlines general *treatment principles* for acute cardiac circulatory failure under most circumstances. The treatment of infants and children with low cardiac output following cardiac surgery depends on the nature of the operative procedure and the patient's status after surgery (see Chapter 441).

Artman M, Graham T: Guidelines for vasodilator therapy of congestive heart failure in infants and children. Am Heart J 113:121, 1987.
Bristow MR, Gilbert EM, Abraham WT, et al: Carvedilol produces dose-related improvements in left ventricular function and survival in subjects with chronic heart failure. MOCHA Investigators. Circulation 94:2807, 1996.
Cohn JN: The management of chronic heart failure. N Engl J Med 335:490, 1996.
Friedman WF, George BL: Medical progress: Treatment of congestive heart failure by altering loading conditions of the heart. J Pediatr 106:697, 1985.
Gilbert EM, Abraham WT, Olsen S, et al: Comparative hemodynamic, left ventricular functional, and antiadrenergic effects of chronic treatment with metoprolol versus carvedilol in the failing heart. Circulation 94:2817, 1996.
Harrison DG, Bates JN: The nitrovasodilators. New ideas about old drugs. Circulation 87:1461, 1993.
Hayes CJ, Butler VP Jr, Gersony WM: Serum digoxin studies in infants and children. Pediatrics 52:561, 1973.
Lang D, von Bernuth G: Serum concentration and serum half-life of digoxin in premature and mature infants. Pediatrics 59:902, 1977.
Loggie JMH, Kleinman LI, VanMaanen EF: Renal function and diuretic therapy in infants and children. J Pediatr 86:485, 657, 825, 1975.
Perkin RM, Levin DL: Shock in the pediatric patient. Part I: Clinical pathophysiology. J Pediatr 101:163, 1982.
Perkin RM, Levin DL: Shock in the pediatric patient. Part II: Therapy. J Pediatr 101:319, 1982.
Steeds RP, Channer KS: Drug treatment in heart failure. Br Med J 316:567, 1998.

CHAPTER 449
Pediatric Heart and Heart-Lung Transplantation

449.1 Pediatric Heart Transplantation

As of 1997, 3400 heart transplants had been performed on children at 201 centers worldwide. Survival in children compares favorably with that in adults: 75% at 1 yr and 65% at 5 yr (Fig. 449–1). Greater than 50% of patients are alive at 10 yr. As new therapeutic regimens are introduced, the long-term outlook for pediatric heart transplant recipients continues to improve. A small but growing number of children are surpassing 15- and 20-yr survival.

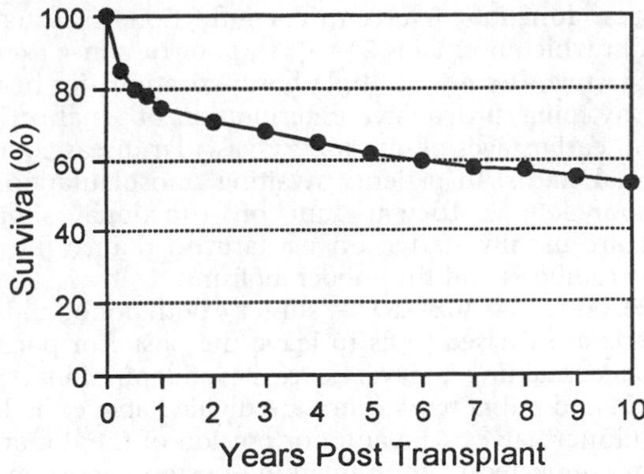

Figure 449–1 Survival after pediatric heart transplantation. Data based on over 3,000 patients transplanted worldwide from 1982 through 1996 as listed with the Registry of the International Society for Heart and Lung Transplantation.

INDICATIONS. Heart transplantation is performed in infants and children with end-stage cardiomyopathies who have become refractory to medical therapy and in patients with some forms of complex congenital heart disease for whom standard surgical procedures are extremely high risk (e.g., hypoplastic left heart syndrome). The cardiomyopathies account for 65% of heart transplants in the pediatric age group, although the percentage of patients with congenital lesions (currently 24%) is gradually increasing. As a secondary procedure, heart transplantation is used in children who have previously undergone conventional surgery for congenital heart disease and who later acquire myocardial dysfunction.

RECIPIENT AND DONOR SELECTION. Potential heart transplant recipients must be free of serious noncardiac medical problems, such as neurologic disease, systemic infection, severe hepatic or renal disease, or severe malnutrition. Many children with ventricular dysfunction may acquire pulmonary hypertension and even pulmonary vascular disease, which would preclude heart transplantation. For this reason, pulmonary vascular resistance is measured at cardiac catheterization, both at rest and in response to vasodilators. Patients with fixed elevated pulmonary vascular resistance (>6–8 Wood units) are at higher risk for heart transplantation and may be considered candidates for heart-lung transplantation (see Chapter 449.2). A comprehensive social service consultation is an important component of the recipient evaluation. Because of the complex post-transplantation medical regimen, the family must have a history of compliance. Detailed informed consent must be obtained.

Donor shortage is a serious problem for both adults and children. There is a national registry of transplant recipients in the United States (UNOS—the United Network for Organ Sharing), and allografts are matched by ABO blood group and body weight. HLA matching is not currently feasible for heart transplantation; with modern immunosuppression, it may offer only minimal advantage. Physicians caring for a patient who may be a potential donor should contact the organ donor coordinator at a transplanting institution, who can best judge the appropriateness of organ donation and has experience in interacting with donor families. Contraindications for *organ donation* include prolonged cardiac arrest with moderate to severe cardiac dysfunction, ongoing systemic illness or infection, and pre-existing severe cardiac disease. A history of resuscitation alone or reparable congenital heart disease is not an automatic exclusion for donation.

The decision of when to place a patient on the transplant waiting list is based on many factors, including extremely poor ventricular function (left ventricular fractional shortening of <10%, in which normal is 28–40%), poor response to medical anticongestive therapy, multiple hospitalizations for heart failure, arrhythmia, progressive deterioration of renal or hepatic function, early stages of pulmonary vascular disease, and poor nutritional status. In patients awaiting transplantation, those with poor left ventricular function (fractional shortening <15%) are usually started on warfarin to reduce the risk of mural thrombosis and thromboembolism.

PERIOPERATIVE MANAGEMENT. At surgery, both donor and recipient hearts are excised so as to leave the posterior portions of the atria containing the venae cavae and pulmonary veins. The aorta and pulmonary artery are divided above the level of the semilunar valves. The anterior portion of the donor's atria are then connected to the remaining posterior portion of the recipient's atria, avoiding the need for delicate suturing of the venae cavae or pulmonary veins. The donor and recipient great vessels are connected via end-to-end anastomoses.

In the immediate postoperative period, immunosuppression is achieved using a triple-drug regimen. One common protocol calls for cyclosporine, 10 mg/kg/24 hr; azathioprine, 2 mg/kg/24 hr; and prednisone, started at 0.6–1.0 mg/kg/24 hr and tapered to 0.2 mg/kg/24 hr over the first 6–12 wk, although in children, a wide range of cyclosporine doses are required to achieve therapeutic serum levels. In many centers an antilymphocyte preparation is added in the 1st week, either antithymocyte globulin or the monoclonal murine antihuman T lymphocyte antibody (OKT3). In children who do not experience significant graft rejection, steroids can be tapered to an alternate-day regimen after the first 6–12 mo; in many patients steroids can be totally eliminated. In some centers, steroids are not routinely included as part of maintenance immunosuppression but are added later for the treatment of acute rejection episodes. Some centers prefer tacrolimus (FK506, Prograf) as part of the initial regimen instead of cyclosporine. Agents such as mycophenolate mofetil (MMF, CellCept) and rapamycin may be used as a substitute for azathioprine; their enhanced efficacy in children remains to be tested.

Most pediatric heart transplant recipients can be extubated within the first 48 hr after transplantation and are out of bed within 3–4 days. These patients are often discharged within the first 2 wk after transplantation. In patients with pre-existing high-risk factors, postoperative care is considerably prolonged.

DIAGNOSIS AND MANAGEMENT OF ACUTE GRAFT REJECTION. Posttransplantation management consists of adjusting medications to maintain a balance between the risk of rejection and the side effects of overimmunosuppression. Along with infection, acute graft rejection is a leading cause of death in adult and pediatric heart transplant recipients. The incidence of acute rejection is greatest within the first 3 mo after transplantation and decreases considerably thereafter. Most pediatric patients experience at least one episode of acute rejection within the 1st yr after transplantation, usually at the time of weaning of one of their immunosuppressive medications.

Clinical manifestations of acute rejection may include fatigue, fluid retention, fever, diaphoresis, abdominal symptoms, and a gallop rhythm. The *electrocardiogram* may show reduced voltage, atrial or ventricular arrhythmias, or heart block. *Roentgenographic* examination may show an enlarged heart, effusions, or pulmonary edema. Cyclosporine modifies the clinical course of rejection; most rejection episodes occur without any detectable clinical symptoms. On *echocardiography,* indices of systolic left ventricular function usually do not deteriorate until rejection is severe. Techniques evaluating wall thickening and left ventricular diastolic function have not fulfilled their promise as predictors of early rejection. Most transplant centers do not rely on echocardiography alone in rejection surveillance.

Myocardial biopsy is the most reliable method of monitoring patients for rejection. Biopsy specimens are taken from the right ventricular side of the interventricular septum and can be performed relatively safely in small infants and children. In older children, myocardial biopsies may be performed as often as every 1–4 wk during the first 3–6 mo after transplantation. The frequency is then reduced to two or four biopsies per year unless the patient has an episode of rejection. In infants, surveillance biopsies are usually performed less often and may be as infrequent as once or twice per year. Children may have clinically unsuspected rejection episodes even 5–10 years after transplantation; most centers continue routine surveillance biopsies, albeit at less frequent intervals (every 6–12 mo).

Criteria for grading cardiac rejection are based on a system developed by the International Society for Heart and Lung Transplantation (ISHLT), taking into account the degree of cellular infiltration and whether myocyte necrosis is present. ISHLT grades 1 and 2 rejection are usually mild enough not to warrant immediate treatment, and more than 50% of these episodes may resolve spontaneously. A repeat biopsy specimen is usually obtained within several weeks. For patients with ISHLT grade 3 or 4 rejection, treatment is instituted with either intravenous methylprednisolone or a "bump and taper" of oral prednisone. For rejection episodes resistant to steroid therapy, additional therapeutic regimens include a repeat course of an antilymphocyte preparation (OKT3 or antithymocyte globulin), methotrexate, or total lymphoid irradiation. Patients with repeated episodes of rejection may also benefit from being switched from cyclosporine to tacrolimus (or vice versa) and from azathioprine to mycophenolate. Rare patients with refractory rejection require retransplantation.

COMPLICATIONS OF IMMUNOSUPPRESSION

Infection. This is one of the two leading causes of death in pediatric transplant patients (Fig. 449–2). The incidence of infection is greatest in the first 3 mo after transplantation when immunosuppressive doses are highest. Viral infections are the most common, especially cytomegalovirus, which accounts for as many as 25% of infectious episodes. Cytomegalovirus infection may occur as a primary infection in patients without prior exposure to the virus or as a reactivation. Severe cytomegalovirus infection can be disseminated, associated with pneumonitis, and may provoke an episode of acute graft rejection or graft coronary disease (see later). Many centers use intravenous gancyclovir or cytomegalovirus immune globulin (CytoGam), or both, as prophylaxis in any patient receiving a heart from a donor who is positive for cytomegalovirus, or in any recipient who has serologic evidence of prior cytomegalovirus disease.

Most normal childhood viral illnesses are well tolerated and usually do not require special treatment. Otitis media and routine upper respiratory tract infections can be treated in the outpatient setting, although fever or symptoms that last beyond the usual course require further investigation. Varicella exposure is treated with varicella immune globulin, and if the patient acquires clinical varicella infection, treatment with intravenous acyclovir attenuates the illness.

Bacterial infections are the next most frequent, with the lung being the most common site of infection (35%), followed

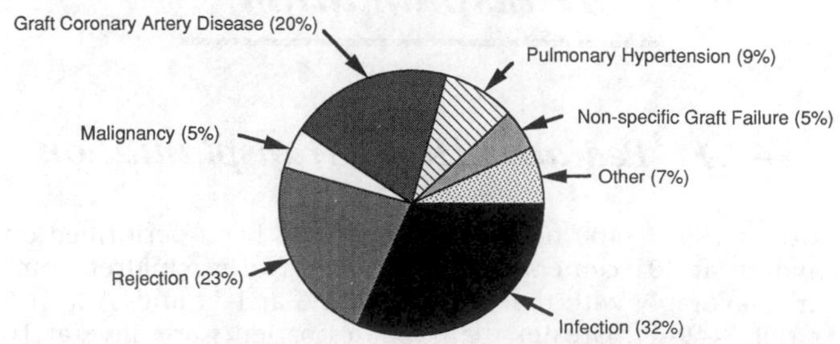

Figure 449–2 Major causes of death after pediatric heart transplantation. (Data from Stanford University.)

by the blood, urinary tract, and, less commonly, the sternotomy site. Other sources of post-transplantation infection include fungi (14%) and protozoa (6%). The incidence of serious infections is lower in children who can be managed without steroids.

Growth Retardation. Patients requiring chronic steroid administration usually manifest decreased linear growth. Alternate-day steroid regimens usually result in improved linear growth. In patients who experience rejection when steroids are weaned, other immunosuppressants (methotrexate, total lymphoid irradiation) have shown promise as steroid-sparing agents. In children surviving greater than 5 yr after transplantation, growth is normal in 75%.

Hypertension. This is common in patients treated with cyclosporine. It is due to a combination of plasma volume expansion and defective renal sodium excretion. Corticosteroids usually potentiate cyclosporine-induced hypertension. Patients are usually managed with a combination of a diuretic and a vasodilator. Agents that work via calcium channel blockade have the additional advantage of possibly attenuating graft coronary disease (see later). The incidence of hypertension may be slightly lower in patients treated with tacrolimus.

Renal Function. Chronic administration of cyclosporine can lead to a tubulointerstitial nephropathy in adults, but severe renal dysfunction is rare in children. Most pediatric patients gradually increase their serum creatinine during the 1st year after transplantation; if renal dysfunction occurs, it usually responds to a decrease in cyclosporine dosage. Long-term patients rarely require renal transplantation.

Neurologic Complications. Neurologic side effects of cyclosporine and tacrolimus include tremor, myalgias, paresthesias, and rarely seizures. These complications can be treated with reduced doses of medication and occasionally with oral magnesium supplementation. Intracranial infections pose a significant risk, especially because some of the more common signs (nuchal rigidity) may be absent in immunosuppressed patients. The most common organisms are *Aspergillus, Cryptococcus neoformans,* and *Listeria monocytogenes.* Aseptic meningitis can be seen days or weeks after OKT3 administration and is usually self-limiting.

Tumors. One of the serious complications limiting long-term survival in pediatric heart transplant patients is the risk of neoplastic disease. The most common is post-transplant lymphoproliferative disease (PTLD). This condition is associated with Epstein-Barr virus. It usually responds to reduction in immunosuppression and acyclovir and only occasionally requires chemotherapy. An increased risk of skin cancer requires that children use appropriate precautions when exposed to sunlight.

Chronic Rejection. Graft coronary artery disease (CAD) is a manifestation of chronic graft rejection and occurs in 10–20% of children. The cause is still unclear, although it is thought to be a form of immunologically mediated vessel injury. Hypercholesterolemia and hyperglycemia increase the risk of this disease. Unlike native coronary atherosclerosis, graft CAD is a diffuse process with a high degree of distal vessel involvement. Because the transplanted heart has been denervated, patients do not experience symptoms such as angina pectoris during ischemic episodes, and thus most centers perform coronary angiography annually to screen for coronary abnormalities. Several reports have suggested that dobutamine stress echocardiography is useful as a screening tool. Standard coronary artery bypass procedures are usually not helpful because of the diffuse nature of the process, and repeat heart transplantation has been the only effective treatment. Calcium channel blockers, such as diltiazem, have been shown to either prevent or delay the onset of graft coronary disease in adult transplant patients. One class of cholesterol-lowering agents, the HMG-CoA reductase inhibitors (pravastatin, atorvastatin), reduce the risk of both graft CAD and rejection.

Other Complications. Corticosteroids usually result in cushingoid facies, steroid acne, and striae. Cyclosporine can cause a subtle change in facial features with hypertrichosis and gingival hyperplasia. These cosmetic features can be particularly disturbing to adolescents and may be the motivation for noncompliance. Many of these complications are dose-related and improve as immunosuppressive medications are weaned. Osteoporosis and aseptic necrosis are additional reasons for reducing steroid dosage as soon as possible. Diabetes and pancreatitis are rare but serious complications.

Rehabilitation. Despite the potential risks of immunosuppression, the prospect for rehabilitation in pediatric heart transplant recipients is excellent. Almost 95% of pediatric heart transplant recipients have no functional limitations in their daily lives. At 2 yr follow-up, almost 70% of patients do not require rehospitalization for transplant-related problems.

Pediatric heart transplant recipients can attend day care or school and participate in noncontact competitive sports and other age-appropriate activities. Standardized measurements of ventricular function are close to normal. Because the transplanted heart is denervated, the increase in heart rate and cardiac output during exercise is slower in transplant recipients, and maximal heart rate and cardiac output responses are mildly attenuated. These subtle abnormalities are rarely noticeable by the patient.

Growth of the transplanted heart is excellent, although a mild degree of ventricular and septal hypertrophy is commonly seen even years after transplantation. The sites of the atrial and great vessel anastomoses grow without developing obstruction. However, in neonates who undergo transplantation for the hypoplastic left heart syndrome, juxtaductal aortic coarctation may recur.

As assessed by standardized psychological testing, the psychological adjustment to heart transplantation in children is usually good. There is sometimes a problem with noncompliance once patients reach adolescence, resulting in life-threatening rejection. Early intervention by social service counselors may be able to reduce this risk.

449.2 Heart-Lung and Lung Transplantation

More than 370 heart-lung and greater than 350 lung (single or double) transplants have been performed in children at approximately 60 institutions worldwide. The primary indications for heart-lung transplantation include complex congenital heart disease with pulmonary hypoplasia or Eisenmenger's syndrome, primary pulmonary hypertension, congenital lung abnormalities, α_1-antitrypsin deficiency, and end-stage parenchymal lung disease (bronchopulmonary dysplasia, chronic lung disease, interstitial fibrosis, and cystic fibrosis). Many of these patients with normal hearts may also be candidates for single- or double-lung transplantation if right ventricular function is preserved. In some patients with Eisenmenger's physiology, double-lung transplantation can be performed in combination with repair of intracardiac defects. Patients with cystic fibrosis are not candidates for single-lung grafts because of the risk of infection from the diseased contralateral lung. Patients are selected using many of the same criteria as for heart transplant recipients (see Chapter 449.1).

Post-transplant immunosuppression is achieved with a triple-drug regimen, similar to that used for heart transplantation; many groups avoid steroids during the early postoperative period to promote better airway healing. Unlike patients with isolated heart transplants, few patients with lung transplants can be weaned off steroids. Prophylaxis against infection is achieved with trimethoprim-sulfamethoxazole or aerosolized pentamidine. Gancyclovir and cytomegalovirus immune globulin prophylaxis are used as in heart transplant recipients (see Chapter 449.1).

Pulmonary rejection is common in heart-lung transplant recipients, whereas heart rejection is encountered less often than in those patients with isolated heart transplants. Symptoms of lung rejection may include fever and fatigue, although many episodes are minimally symptomatic. Surveillance for rejection is performed by following pulmonary functions (forced vital capacity, forced expiratory volume in 1 second [FEV_1], forced expiratory flow, mid–expiratory phase [$FEV_{25\%-75\%}$]), systemic arterial oxygen tension, chest roentgenograms, and by serial transbronchial biopsy. Routine biopsies are performed frequently in the first 3 mo and then quarterly thereafter. Because of technical limitations, biopsies are not performed in infants, who are followed with clinical criteria alone.

Actuarial *survival* after heart-lung or lung transplantation in children is currently 65–70% at 1 yr and 40–45% at 5 yr; improved patient selection and postoperative management are continually improving these survival statistics. As in isolated heart transplantation, infection remains the leading cause of early death, accounting for nearly 50% of all mortality in the 1st yr after transplantation. Other causes of early morbidity and mortality include tracheal complications, pulmonary venous obstruction, donor lung dysfunction, bleeding, and acute rejection. *Obliterative bronchiolitis* (OB), a form of chronic rejection, remains a major limitation to long-term survival in a significant number of patients. Between 10 and 50% of long-term survivors of lung transplantation develop OB. Increasing immunosuppression has markedly reduced the incidence of OB. Additional late complications include the development of airway stenosis, accelerated graft coronary artery disease (although less common than in isolated heart transplantation), and other side effects of chronic immunosuppression (see Chapter 449.1).

Postoperative indices of *cardiopulmonary function* and exercise capacity show significant improvement. More than 95% of patients are without activity limitations at 2-yr follow-up. Problems of donor availability are even more severe with lung transplantation. Living-related lung transplantation, in which a lobe from a parent is transplanted into a child, may partially alleviate this problem.

Heart Transplantation

Baum D, Bernstein D, Starnes VA, et al: Pediatric heart transplantation at Stanford: Results of a 15 year experience. Pediatrics 88:203, 1991.

Bernstein D, Baum D, Berry G, et al: Neoplastic disorders after pediatric heart transplantation. Circulation 88(part 2):230, 1993.

Billingham M, Cary N, Hammond M, et al: A working formulation for the standardization of nomenclature in the diagnosis of heart and lung rejection: Heart rejection study group. J Heart Transplant 9:587, 1990.

Boucek MM, Novick RJ, Bennett LE, et al: The Registry of the International Society of Heart and Lung Transplantation: First official pediatric report—1997. J Heart Lung Transplant 16:1189, 1997.

Canter C, Naftel D, Caldwell R, et al: Survival and risk factors for death after cardiac transplantation in infants. A multi-institutional study. The Pediatric Heart Transplant Study. Circulation 96:227, 1997.

Gao SZ, Schroeder JS, Alderman EL, et al: Clinical and laboratory correlates of accelerated coronary artery disease in the cardiac transplant patient. Circulation 76(Suppl 5):56, 1987.

Grattan MT, Moreno-Cabral CE, Starnes VA, et al: Cytomegalovirus infection is associated with cardiac allograft rejection and atherosclerosis. JAMA 261:3561, 1989.

Green M, Wald ER, Fricker FJ, et al: Infections in pediatric orthotopic heart transplant recipients. Pediatr Infect Dis 8:87, 1989.

Hotson JR, Enzmann DR: Neurologic complications of cardiac transplantation. Neurol Clin 6:346, 1988.

Pahl E, Zales VR, Fricker FJ, Addonizio LJ: Posttransplant coronary artery disease in children. A multicenter national survey. Circulation 90(5 Pt 2):II56, 1994.

Schowengerdt KO, Naftel DC, Seib PM, et al: Infection after pediatric heart transplantation: Results of a multiinstitutional study. The Pediatric Heart Transplant Study Group. J Heart Lung Transplant 16:1207, 1997.

Schroeder JS, Gao SZ, Alderman EL: A preliminary study of diltiazem in the prevention of coronary artery disease in heart transplant recipients. N Engl J Med 3:164, 1993.

Shaddy RE, Naftel DC, Kirklin JK, et al: Outcome of cardiac transplantation in children. Survival in a contemporary multi-institutional experience. Pediatric Heart Transplant Study. Circulation 94(9 Suppl):II69, 1996.

Sigfusson G, Fricker FJ, Bernstein D, et al: Long term survivors of pediatric heart transplantation: A multicenter report of 68 children who have survived greater than five years. J Pediatr 130:862, 1997.

Starnes VA, Griffin ML, Pitlick PT, et al: Current approach to hypoplastic left heart syndrome: Palliation, transplantation or both? J Thorac Cardiovasc Surg 104:189, 1992.

Wood AJ, Maurer G, Niederberger W, et al: Cyclosporine: Pharmacokinetics, metabolism, and drug interactions. Transplant Proc 15(Suppl 1):2409, 1983.

Lung Transplantation

Boucek MM, Novick RJ, Bennett LE, et al: The Registry of the International Society of Heart and Lung Transplantation: First official pediatric report—1997. J Heart Lung Transplant 16:1189, 1997.

Conte JV, Robbins RC, Reichenspurner H, et al: Pediatric heart-lung transplantation: Intermediate-term results. J Heart Lung Transplant 15:692, 1996.

Mendeloff EN, Huddleston CB, Mallory GB, et al: Pediatric and adult lung transplantation for cystic fibrosis. J Thorac Cardiovasc Surg 115:404, 1998.

Spray TL, Mallory GB, Canter CE, et al: Pediatric lung transplantation for pulmonary hypertension and congenital heart disease. Ann Thorac Surg 54:216, 1992.

Starnes VA, Oyer PE, Bernstein D, et al: Heart, heart-lung, and lung transplantation in the first year of life. Ann Thorac Surg 53:306, 1992.

Sweet SC, Spray TL, Huddleston CB, et al: Pediatric lung transplantation at St. Louis Children's Hospital, 1990–1995. Am J Respir Crit Care Med 155:1027, 1997.

Theodore J, Starnes VA, Lewiston NJ: Obliterative bronchiolitis. Clin Chest Med 11:309, 1990.

Watson TJ, Starnes VA: Pediatric lobar lung transplantation. Semin Thorac Cardiovasc Surg 8:313, 1996.

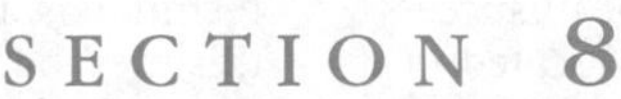

SECTION 8

Diseases of the Peripheral Vascular System

CHAPTER 450

Disease of the Blood Vessels (Aneurysms and Fistulas)

450.1. Kawasaki's Disease

(see also Chapters 166 and 445.5)

Aneurysms of the coronary or systemic arteries may complicate Kawasaki's disease and are the leading cause of morbidity in this disease (Fig. 450–1). Other than in Kawasaki's disease, aneurysms are not common in children and occur most frequently in the aorta in association with coarctation of the aorta, patent ductus arteriosus, and Marfan's syndrome, and in intracranial vessels (see Chapter 609). They may also occur secondary to an infected embolus; infection contiguous to a blood vessel; trauma; congenital abnormalities of vessel structure, especially of the medial wall; and arteritis, for example, polyarteritis nodosa and Takayasu's arteritis (see Chapter 167).

450.2 Arteriovenous Fistulas

Arteriovenous fistulas may be limited to small cavernous hemangiomas or may be extensive (see Chapters 514.2 and 656). The most common sites in infants and children are within the cranium, in the liver, in the lung, in the extremities, and in vessels in or near the thoracic wall. These fistulas, although usually congenital, may follow trauma or be a manifestation of hereditary hemorrhagic telangiectasia (Osler-Weber-Rendu syndrome). Femoral arteriovenous fistulas are a rare complication of percutaneous femoral catheterization.

CLINICAL MANIFESTATIONS. Clinical symptoms occur only in association with large arteriovenous communications when arterial blood flows into a low-pressure venous system, increasing local venous pressure and decreasing arterial flow distal to the fistula. Systemic arterial resistance falls because of the runoff of blood through the fistula. Compensatory mechanisms include tachycardia and increased stroke volume so that cardiac output rises. The total blood volume is also increased. In large fistulas, left ventricular dilatation, a widened pulse pressure, and heart failure occur. Injection of contrast material into an artery proximal to the fistula confirms the diagnosis.

Large *intracranial arteriovenous fistulas* most often occur in the newborn infant in association with a *vein of Galen malformation.* The large intracranial left-to-right shunt results in heart failure secondary to the demand for high cardiac output. Patients with smaller communications may not have cardiovascular manifestations but later acquire hydrocephalus (see Chapter 601.11) or seizure disorders. The newborn infant with a large symptomatic intracranial arteriovenous fistula has a grave prognosis; some survive with medical management but are subject to later complications caused by the intracranial mass. The diagnosis can often be made by auscultation of a continuous murmur over the cranium. Older children with more diffuse intracranial arteriovenous malformations may be recognized on the basis of intracranial calcification and a high cardiac output, without cardiac failure.

Hepatic arteriovenous fistulas may be generalized or localized in the liver and may be hemangioendotheliomas or cavernous hemangiomas. The fistula may be located between the hepatic artery and the ductus venosus or portal vein. Congenital hemorrhagic telangiectasia may also be associated. Large arteriovenous fistulas are associated with an increased cardiac output and heart failure. Hepatomegaly is usual, and systolic or continuous murmurs may be audible over the liver.

Peripheral arteriovenous fistulas usually involve the extremities and are associated with disfigurement, swelling of the extremity, and visible hemangiomas. Some are located in areas that result in upper airway obstruction. Because only a small minority result in large arterial runoff, cardiac failure is uncommon.

TREATMENT. Medical management of heart failure is initially helpful in the neonate with these conditions; with time the size of the shunt may diminish and symptoms spontaneously regress. Hemangiomas of the liver often disappear completely with time. Large liver hemangiomas have been treated with steroids, ε-aminocaproic acid, interferon, local compression, embolization, or local radiation; the beneficial effects of these management options are not firmly established, as individual patients display marked variations in clinical course without treatment. *Catheter embolization* is rapidly becoming the treatment of choice for many patients with a symptomatic arteriovenous fistula. Embolic agents that have been used include detachable balloons, steel (Gianturco) coils, and liquid tissue adhesives (cyanoacrylate). Often, multiple procedures are necessary before the flow is significantly reduced. *Surgical removal*

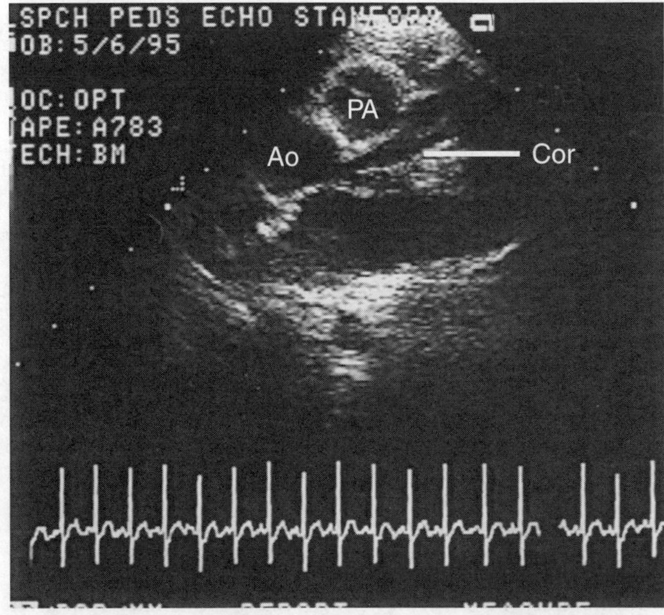

Figure 450–1 Two-dimensional echocardiogram showing giant coronary artery aneurysms in a patient with Kawasaki disease. Cor = coronary artery; PA = pulmonary artery; Ao = aorta.

of a large fistula may be attempted in the presence of severe cardiac failure and lack of improvement with medical treatment. Surgical treatment may be contraindicated or unsuccessful when the lesion is extensive and diffuse or is located in a position where adjoining tissue may be injured during the surgery or related procedures.

Fong LV, Lee SH, Salmon AP: Diagnosis of cerebral arteriovenous malformations by colour Doppler examination. Eur Heart J 13:415, 1992.

Ford EG, Stanley P, Tolo V, et al: Peripheral congenital arteriovenous fistulae: Observe, operate, or obturate? J Pediatr Surg 27:714, 1992.

Friedman DM, Verma R, Madrid M, et al: Recent improvement in outcome using transcatheter embolization techniques for neonatal aneurysmal malformations of the vein of Galen. Pediatrics 91:583, 1993.

Grifka RG, Mullins CE, Gianturco C, et al: New Gianturco-Grifka vascular occlusion device. Initial studies in a canine model. Circulation 91:1840, 1995.

CHAPTER 451
Systemic Hypertension

Systemic hypertension occurs commonly in adults and if untreated is a major risk factor for myocardial infarction, stroke, and renal failure. It is estimated that 60 million Americans have hypertension, and that only 10% are being treated adequately. The prevalence of hypertension increases with age: ranging from 15% of young adults to 60% of individuals older than 65 yr of age. In infants and younger children, systemic hypertension is uncommon, and when present it is usually indicative of an underlying disease process (*secondary hypertension*). Older children and particularly adolescents may acquire *primary or essential hypertension* (with no underlying cause); hypertension may track into adulthood. To increase early detection of hypertension, accurate blood pressure measurements should be part of the routine annual physical examination of all children. A careful family history of hypertension should be identified.

Accurate measurement of blood pressure requires careful attention to the comfort of the patient and is highly dependent on proper use of the equipment, whether a simple sphygmomanometer or a state of the art automated device. Obtaining an accurate blood pressure measurement in infants is often the most difficult and time-consuming part of the physical examination. Patients of any age have some level of anxiety associated with measurement of blood pressure, which may lead to a false diagnosis of hypertension. The blood pressure can be measured with the patient either seated or supine; infants may be held in the lap of a parent. Subsequent measurements taken for comparison should be obtained with the patient in the same position. Careful attention to cuff size is necessary to avoid overdiagnosis. A wide variety of bladder sizes should be available in any medical office where children are routinely cared for. The cuff should completely encircle the upper arm to ensure uniform compression; the inflatable bladder should cover at least two thirds of the length of the upper arm and three quarters of its circumference. A cuff that is too short or narrow artificially increases the blood pressure readings. Blood pressure should be obtained in all four extremities to detect coarctation of the aorta (see Chapter 434.6).

Systolic pressure is indicated by the appearance of the 1st Korotkov sound. The true diastolic pressure probably lies between the muffling and the disappearance of Korotkov sounds; muffling may be difficult to appreciate in smaller children. Palpation is useful for a rapid assessment of the systolic blood pressure, although the palpated pressure is usually about 10 mm Hg less than that obtained via auscultation. Doppler is an extremely accurate method of measuring the systolic blood pressure; it is less so for the diastolic pressure. Oscillometric techniques are used frequently in infants and young children; this method is susceptible to artifacts and is best for measuring the mean blood pressure.

Blood pressure increases gradually with age; therefore, standard nomograms are necessary for interpretation of blood pressure values (see Figs. 429–1 and 429–2). If mild hypertension is found, it is imperative that the measurement be repeated twice more over a period of 6 wk. Anxiety usually decreases as the patient becomes more comfortable with the procedure; thus, repeated measurements are necessary to avoid inappropriately labeling a patient as hypertensive. A blood pressure that is consistently above the 95th percentile for age requires further evaluation. Ambulatory blood pressure monitoring may be especially useful in adolescents who have borderline hypertension in the office setting.

ETIOLOGY AND PATHOPHYSIOLOGY. Blood pressure is the product of the cardiac output and the peripheral vascular resistance. An increase in either cardiac output or peripheral resistance results in an increase in blood pressure; if one of these factors increases while the other decreases, blood pressure may not increase. When hypertension is the result of another disease process, it is referred to as *secondary hypertension*. When there is no identifiable cause, it is referred to as *primary* or *essential hypertension*. Many factors, including heredity, diet, stress, and obesity, may play a role in the development of essential hypertension.

Secondary hypertension is most common in infants and younger children. Many childhood diseases may be responsible for both acute and chronic elevation of blood pressure (Tables 451–1 and 451–2). The most likely cause varies with age. Hypertension in the newborn is most often associated with umbilical artery catheterization and renal artery thrombosis. Hypertension during early childhood may be due to renal disease, coarctation of the aorta, endocrine disorders, or medications. In adolescents, essential hypertension becomes increasingly common. The severity of hypertension is also helpful in distinguishing secondary from primary hypertension; in general, children and adolescents with essential hypertension have blood pressures at or only slightly above the 95th percentile for age.

Renal and renovascular hypertension accounts for the majority of children with secondary hypertension. A history of urinary tract infection is present in 25–50% of these patients and is often related to an obstructive lesion of the urinary tract. Renovascular hypertension may be associated with sodium retention and increased renin secretion. Other renal parenchymal lesions associated with hypertension are detailed in Tables 451–1 and 451–2. The reduced glomerular filtration rate in patients with nephritis results in salt and water retention, whereas mass lesions (cysts, solid tumors, hematoma) may impair renal perfusion and stimulate renin production by the juxtaglomerular apparatus. Both Wilms' tumor and juxtaglomerular cell tumor (hemangiopericytoma) may secrete renin or other pressors without feedback control.

Lesions such as renal artery stenosis cause hypertension through stimulation of the *renin-angiotensin-aldosterone system*. Renin is a proteolytic enzyme secreted by the juxtaglomerular cells that converts angiotensinogen to angiotensin I. Renin secretion is affected by afferent arteriolar perfusion pressure in the kidney, sodium concentration in plasma and tubular urine, sympathetic nervous system activation, and other factors, such as prostaglandins, potassium intake, and atrial natriuretic peptides. Angiotensin I possesses little physiologic activity and is rapidly converted to angiotensin II by angiotensin-converting enzyme (ACE). This converting enzyme is also responsible for the metabolic degradation of vasodilating kinins. Angiotensin II is a potent vasoconstrictor and also stimulates aldosterone secretion, leading to salt and water retention.

Several *endocrinopathies* are associated with hypertension, usually those involving the thyroid, parathyroid, and adrenal glands. Systolic hypertension and tachycardia are common in hyperthyroidism; however, diastolic pressure is usually not elevated. Hypercalcemia, whether secondary to hyperparathyroidism or other causes, often results in mild elevation in blood pressure because of an increase in vascular tone. Adrenocortical disorders (aldosterone-secreting tumors, adrenal hyperplasia, Cushing's syndrome) may produce hypertension if there is an increase in mineralocorticoid secretion. **Pheochromocytomas** are catecholamine-secreting tumors that give rise to hypertension because of the cardiac and peripheral vascular effects of epinephrine and norepinephrine. Children with pheochromocytoma usually have sustained rather than intermittent hypertension (see Chapter 590). Approximately 5% of patients with neurofibromatosis acquire pheochromocytoma. Altered sympathetic tone can be responsible for acute or intermittent elevation of blood pressure in children with Guillain-Barré syndrome, poliomyelitis, burns, and Stevens-Johnson syndrome. Sympathetic outflow from the central nervous system is also affected by intracranial lesions.

In adolescents, a number of *drugs of abuse, therapeutic agents,* and *toxins* may cause hypertension. Cocaine may provoke a rapid increase in blood pressure and can result in seizures or intracranial hemorrhage. Phencyclidine causes transient hypertension that may become persistent in chronic abusers. Tobacco use may also increase blood pressure. Sympathomimetic agents used as nasal decongestants, appetite suppressants, and stimulants for attention deficit disorder produce peripheral vasoconstriction and varying degrees of cardiac stimulation. Individuals vary in their susceptibility to these effects. Oral contraceptives should be suspected as a cause of hypertension in adolescent females, although the incidence is low with the use of low-estrogen preparations. Immunosuppressant agents such as cyclosporine and tacrolimus cause hypertension in organ transplant recipients, which is exacerbated by the coadministration of steroids. Blood pressure may be elevated in patients with poisoning by a heavy metal.

Essential hypertension is more commonly recognized in adolescents than in younger children and is often accompanied by a strong family history. The cause of essential hypertension is likely to be multifactorial; however, genetic alterations of calcium and sodium transport, the renin-angiotensin system, and insulin sensitivity have been implicated in this disorder. Normotensive children of hypertensive parents may show abnormal physiologic responses that are similar to those of their parents. When subjected to stress or competitive tasks, the offspring of hypertensive adults, as a group, respond with greater increases in heart rate and blood pressure than do children of normotensive parents. Similarly, some children of hypertensive parents may excrete higher levels of urinary

TABLE 451–1 Conditions Associated with Transient or Intermittent Hypertension in Children

Renal

Acute postinfectious glomerulonephritis
Anaphylactoid (Henoch-Schönlein) purpura with nephritis
Hemolytic-uremic syndrome
Acute tubular necrosis
After renal transplant (immediate and during episodes of rejection)
After blood transfusion in patients with azotemia
Hypervolemia
After surgical procedures on genitourinary tract
Pyelonephritis
Renal trauma
Leukemic infiltration of kidney
Obstructive uropathy associated with Crohn's disease

Drugs and Poisons

Cocaine
Oral contraceptives
Sympathomimetic agents
Amphetamines
Phencyclidine
Corticosteroids and adrenocorticotropic hormone
Cyclosporine treatment post-transplantation
Licorice (glycyrrhizic acid)
Lead, mercury, cadmium, thallium
Antihypertensive withdrawal (clonidine, methyldopa, propranolol)
Vitamin D intoxication

Central and Autonomic Nervous System

Increased intracranial pressure
Guillain-Barré syndrome
Burns
Familial dysautonomia
Stevens-Johnson syndrome
Posterior fossa lesions
Porphyria
Poliomyelitis
Encephalitis

Miscellaneous

Preeclampsia
Fractures of long bones
Hypercalcemia
After coarctation repair
White cell transfusion
Extracorporeal membrane oxygenation
Chronic upper airway obstruction

TABLE 451–2 Conditions Associated with Chronic Hypertension in Children

Renal

Chronic pyelonephritis
Chronic glomerulonephritis
Hydronephrosis
Congenital dysplastic kidney
Multicystic kidney
Solitary renal cyst
Vesicoureteral reflux nephropathy
Segmental hypoplasia (Ask-Upmark kidney)
Ureteral obstruction
Renal tumors
Renal trauma
Rejection damage following transplantation
Postirradiation damage
Systemic lupus erythematosus (other connective tissue diseases)

Vascular

Coarctation of thoracic or abdominal aorta
Renal artery lesions (stenosis, fibromuscular dysplasia, thrombosis, aneurysm)
Umbilical artery catheterization with thrombus formation
Neurofibromatosis (intrinsic or extrinsic narrowing of vascular lumen)
Renal vein thrombosis
Vasculitis
Arteriovenous shunt
Williams-Beuren syndrome
Moyamoya disease

Endocrine

Hyperthyroidism
Hyperparathyroidism
Congenital adrenal hyperplasia (11β-hydroxylase and 17-hydroxylase defect)
Cushing's syndrome
Primary aldosteronism
Dexamethasone-suppressible hyperaldosteronism
Pheochromocytoma
Other neural crest tumors (neuroblastoma, ganglioneuroblastoma, ganglioneuroma)
Diabetic nephropathy
Liddle's syndrome

Central Nervous System

Intracranial mass
Hemorrhage
Residual following brain injury
Quadriplegia

Essential Hypertension

Low renin
Normal renin
High renin

catecholamine metabolites or may respond to sodium loading with greater weight gain and increases in blood pressure than do those without a family history of hypertension. The abnormal responses in children with affected parents tend to be greater in the black population than in white individuals. Erythrocyte sodium transport, free calcium concentration in platelets and leukocytes, urine kallikrein excretion, and sympathetic nervous system receptors have been investigated as other possible markers for the development of subsequent hypertension.

Categorization of essential hypertension according to the level of plasma renin activity (high, normal, low) has been useful in understanding the pathophysiology and in developing treatment regimens in adults; similar large studies have not been conducted in adolescents with primary hypertension. A large number of adult patients with essential hypertension appear to be especially sensitive to salt intake. The mechanism of salt sensitivity is not clear and may involve the chloride ion rather than sodium. A subgroup of salt-sensitive individuals appear to have impaired ability for urinary excretion of a sodium load. Atrial natriuretic peptides stimulate sodium excretion by the kidneys; their role in the maintenance of normal blood pressure and the development of hypertension is being investigated.

Tracking of blood pressure is the process by which, over time, individuals maintain their relative ranking of blood pressure with respect to their peers. Children and young adolescents with blood pressure greater than the 90th percentile for age are threefold more likely to become adults with hypertension than are children with blood pressure at the 50th percentile. Adolescents with essential hypertension may progress from a high cardiac output and normal systemic vascular resistance state to the adult pattern of normal cardiac output with elevated systemic vascular resistance. There are racial differences, however: Black adults with hypertension have greater elevations in peripheral resistance, whereas hypertensive white adults predominantly show an increase in cardiac output.

CLINICAL MANIFESTATIONS. Children and adolescents with essential hypertension are usually asymptomatic; the blood pressure elevation is usually mild and is detected during a routine examination or evaluation prior to athletic participation. These children may have mild to moderate obesity.

Children with secondary hypertension can have blood pressure elevations ranging from mild to severe. Unless the pressure has been sustained or is rising rapidly, hypertension does not usually produce symptoms. Therefore clinical manifestations of the underlying disease, such as growth failure in children with chronic renal disease, are the most frequent reasons for detecting the hypertension. With substantial hypertension, however, headache, dizziness, epistaxis, anorexia, visual changes, and seizures may occur. Hypertensive encephalopathy is suggested by the presence of vomiting, temperature elevation, ataxia, stupor, and seizures. Regardless of the cause, end organ (cardiac and renal) dysfunction occurs in the face of marked hypertension.

Young children and infants with unexplained heart failure or seizures should have their blood pressure measured. Such patients often cannot communicate symptoms such as headache, and their behavior may not be considered abnormal until the complications of hypertension are present. After blood pressure has been lowered, parents of hypertensive infants often comment in retrospect that their child had been increasingly irritable before the hypertension was recognized.

LABORATORY DIAGNOSIS. The diagnosis of essential hypertension is suggested by the patient's age (usually adolescent), level of blood pressure elevation (usually mild), weight (mild to moderate obesity), positive family history, and the paucity of signs and symptoms of underlying disease. It is uncommon to make this diagnosis in children younger than 10 yr of age. Obesity is associated with essential hypertension; except with disorders of the adrenal cortex, patients with secondary hypertension are rarely obese. Heredity is also a strong determinant of blood pressure; therefore, an adolescent with mild elevation of pressure and a strong family history of essential hypertension is less likely to have an underlying disease. Adolescents suspected of having essential hypertension require regular measurement of blood pressure to determine the course of the evaluation over time. If the pressure continues to rise over several weeks or months of observation, additional diagnostic studies to eliminate secondary hypertension are indicated.

The diagnosis of secondary hypertension is also suggested by the patient's age (younger), level of blood pressure elevation (varying from mild to extreme), or presence of symptoms. The history may include intermittent febrile illnesses, which might suggest recurring infection of the urinary tract (reflux nephropathy). A family history of renal disease or premature cardiovascular disease should be elicited. Careful measurement of height and weight are important because they are often less than normal in children with chronic disease. Physical examination should determine the presence of flank masses or abdominal bruits. Blood pressure should be measured in all four extremities to rule out coarctation of the aorta. Generally, the systolic blood pressure in the lower limbs should be 10–20 mm Hg higher than that in the upper limbs. Screening tests should include a complete blood count, urinalysis, and determination of serum electrolyte, blood urea nitrogen, serum creatinine, and uric acid levels. Urine culture should be performed even if the sediment is unremarkable. Echocardiography and electrocardiography are helpful in assessing the chronicity of the hypertension, which, if long-standing, should lead to left ventricular hypertrophy.

Renal imaging is discussed in Chapters 545–549. Although renal ultrasonography provides a comparison of kidney size and a view of the anatomy of the collecting system, an intravenous pyelogram is not adequate for detecting differences in renal perfusion. A radionuclide scan is helpful in distinguishing variation in perfusion or scarring of the two kidneys. Renal Doppler ultrasonography and angiography can demonstrate lesions in the main arteries or in the segmental branches; at angiography, venous blood samples should be collected from both renal veins and the inferior vena cava for assay of plasma renin activity. Doppler ultrasonography may demonstrate abnormal arterial and venous blood flow.

Peripheral plasma renin activity is a useful screening test for both renovascular and renal parenchymal disease. Normal values gradually decrease with age and vary among laboratories. A suppressed value suggests excess mineralocorticoid effect, and an elevated value is associated with renal or renovascular involvement. One approach to the adolescent with hypertension is summarized in Figure 451–1. A pregnancy test may be useful in the sexually active female who is noted to be hypertensive (preeclampsia).

COURSE AND PROGNOSIS. The natural history of essential hypertension that is first detected during childhood or adolescence is under investigation in several large long-term population studies. Many of these children continue to have essential hypertension as adults, although the correlation is not perfect. In adults with essential hypertension, drug therapy has been shown to be beneficial in reducing the incidence of congestive heart failure, renal failure, and stroke.

The prognosis of the child with secondary hypertension is primarily determined by the nature of the underlying disease and its responsiveness to specific therapy. Survival in patients with underlying chronic renal diseases is determined by the patient's response to dialysis and the success of renal transplantation. In patients with renovascular disease, the degree of evaluation of renal vein renin activity may help predict response to therapy. A discrepancy in renin secretion between the two kidneys of more than 1.5:1 suggests that the kidney

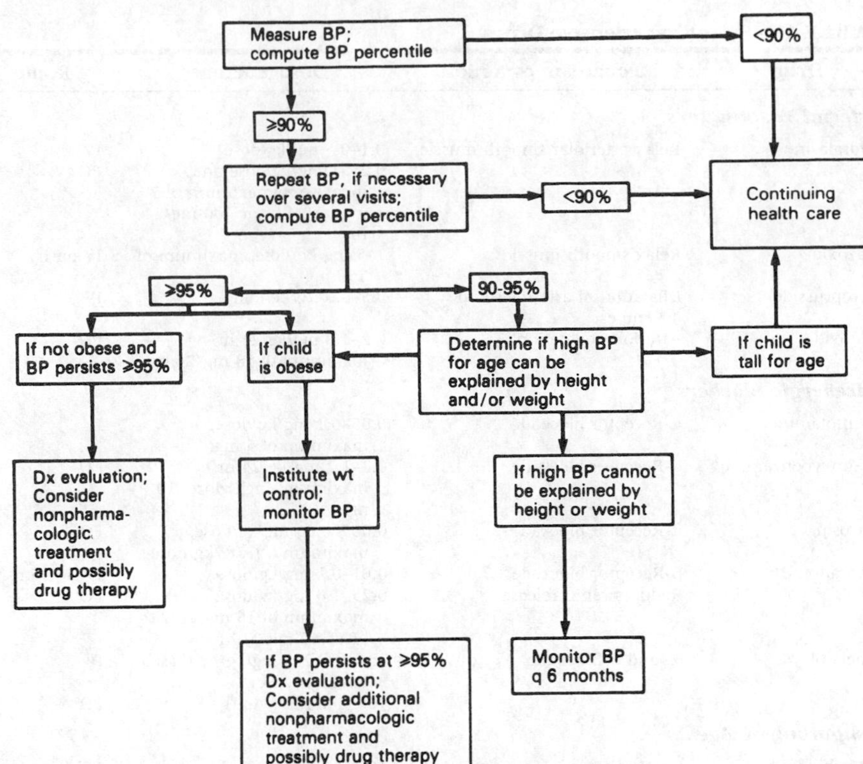

Figure 451–1 Algorithm for identifying children with high BP. Note that whenever BP measurement is stipulated, the average of at least two measurements should be used. (From National Heart, Lung, and Blood Institute, Bethesda, MD: Report of the second task force on blood pressure control in children—1987. Reproduced by permission of Pediatrics 79:1, 1987.)

producing the higher level is primarily responsible for the hypertension. In this case, surgical correction yields a high probability of marked improvement or resolution of the hypertension. The prognosis after surgical repair of coarctation of the aorta is variable and is partly dependent on the age at which correction is performed. The majority of patients operated on during infancy and childhood establish normal systemic blood pressure following surgery unless recoarctation occurs; patients diagnosed during adolescence, however, are at risk for persistently elevated pressure. The long-term outcome is favorable for neonates who experience hypertension as a complication of umbilical artery catheterization. Few of these infants require therapy beyond 12 mo of age, and most show marked improvement in renal perfusion.

PREVENTION. The prevention of high blood pressure may be viewed as part of the prevention of cardiovascular disease and stroke, the leading cause of death in adults in the United States. Other risk factors for cardiovascular disease include obesity, elevated serum cholesterol levels, high dietary sodium intake, a sedentary lifestyle, and alcohol and tobacco use. Beginning in childhood and continuing through adolescence, it is especially important to discourage cigarette smoking because of the pulmonary and cardiovascular consequences. The increase in arterial wall rigidity and blood viscosity that are associated with exposure to the components of tobacco may cause or exacerbate hypertension. Population approaches to prevention of essential hypertension include reduction in sodium intake and increase in physical activity through school-based programs.

TREATMENT. Both nonpharmacologic and pharmacologic approaches to treatment are useful in managing children with elevated blood pressure. Adolescents with essential hypertension are usually best managed initially with *nonpharmacologic* therapy. Intervention should focus on the risk factors that were cited as important in prevention. Because many patients with mild elevation of pressure are obese, weight reduction may result in a 5–10 mm Hg reduction in systolic pressure. A reduction in sodium intake often lowers pressure by a similar amount. A consistent program of aerobic exercise also has been noted to reduce blood pressure in patients with mild essential hypertension. In view of these benefits and the undesirable effects of many antihypertensive drugs, a well-supervised program of nonpharmacologic therapy should be enthusiastically prescribed for most young patients with essential hypertension. Adolescents should be counseled about the adverse effects of tobacco and alcohol on blood pressure. When the patient is unable to cooperate with the nonpharmacologic approach or the reduction of blood pressure is insufficient, antihypertensive agents should be prescribed. However, adolescents who are poorly compliant with changes in lifestyle are also unlikely to be compliant with a long-term drug regimen.

For many children with secondary hypertension and for selected patients with essential hypertension, *pharmacologic* therapy is required. A number of antihypertensive drugs are available for both hypertensive emergencies and chronic therapy (Table 451–3). In response to a *hypertensive crisis,* it is important to select an agent with a rapid and predictable onset of action and to monitor the blood pressure carefully as it is being reduced. Because hypertensive encephalopathy is a possible complication of hypertensive emergencies, antihypertensive agents with minimal central nervous system side effects should be chosen to avoid confusion between symptoms of disease and adverse effects of the drug. Intravenous administration is often preferred in order to carefully titrate the fall in blood pressure. Because too rapid reduction in blood pressure may interfere with adequate organ perfusion, a stepwise reduction of pressure should be planned. In general, the pressure should be reduced by about one third of the total planned reduction during the 1st 6 hr and the remaining amount over the following 48–72 hr.

In most *hypertensive emergencies,* the drugs of choice are intravenous labetalol or nitroprusside or sublingual nifedipine. Labetalol blocks both α- and β-adrenergic receptors; with a single dose followed by continuous infusion, controlled reduction in blood pressure can be achieved. Similar control is possible with an infusion of nitroprusside. Nifedipine has a rapid onset of action, but its short duration of action must be anticipated. Because nifedipine is available only as a liquid within a cap-

TABLE 451–3 Antihypertensive Drugs

Drug	Mechanism of Action	Dosage Range	Route	Duration	Side Effects
Arterial Vasodilators					
Hydralazine	Relax arteriolar smooth muscle	0.1–0.5 mg/kg/dose 0.25–1 mg/kg/dose and increase to maximum of 7 mg/kg/24 hr or 200 mg/24 hr	IV PO	2–4 hr 6–8 hr	Tachycardia, nausea Drug-induced lupus
Diazoxide	Relax smooth muscle	1–5 mg/kg/dose, maximum of 150 mg	IV push	6–24 hr	Tachycardia, hypotension, hyperglycemia
Nitroprusside	Dilatation of arterioles and venules	0.5–8.0 μg/kg/min	IV	With infusion	Thiocyanate production, rarely hypothyroidism
Minoxidil	Arteriolar dilatation	0.2–1.0 mg/kg/24 hr, maximum of 50 mg/24 hr	PO	12–24 hr	Hypertrichosis, fluid retention
Adrenergic Blockers					
Phentolamine	α-Receptor blockade	0.05–0.1 mg/kg/dose, maximum of 5 mg	IV	1–2 hr	Reflex tachycardia
Phenoxybenzamine	α-Receptor blockade	0.2–1.2 mg/kg/24 hr, maximum single dose, 10 mg	PO	6–12 hr	Tachycardia may progress to arrhythmia
Prazosin	α-Receptor blockade	0.005–0.05 mg/kg/dose, maximum 0.1 mg/kg/dose	PO	6–12 hr	First-dose orthostatic hypotension
Propranolol	β-Receptor blockade Reduces renin release	0.01–0.1 mg/kg/dose 0.25–1.0 mg/kg/dose, maximum of 16 mg/kg/24 hr or 60 mg/24 hr	IV slow push PO	6–8 hr	Bronchospasm, bradycardia, vivid dreams
Labetalol	α- and β-Blockade	Titrate 0.2–2 mg/kg/hr (based on adult dose) 100–400 mg (adult)	IV PO	With infusion 12 hr	Orthostasis, dizziness, bronchospasm
Sympatholytic Agents					
α-Methyldopa	Decreases sympathetic tone	10 mg/kg/24 hr and increase to maximum of 65 mg/kg/24 hr or 3 g/24 hr	PO	6–12 hr	Sedation, hepatic dysfunction, positive Coombs' reaction
Clonidine	CNS α_2-agonist	3–5 μg/kg/dose, maximum of 0.9 mg/24 hr	PO	6–8 hr	Sedation, constipation, rebound withdrawal, hypertension
Renin-Angiotensin Inhibitors					
Captopril	ACE inhibition	0.1–0.5 mg/kg/dose and increase to maximum of 4 mg/kg/24 hr	PO	8–12 hr	Proteinuria, neutropenia, rash, dysgeusia
Enalaprilat	ACE inhibition	0.005–0.010 mg/kg/dose Adult dose 1.25 mg	IV over 5 min	8–12 hr	Transient hypotension
Enalapril	ACE inhibition	0.08–0.1 mg/kg/dose, increase to maximum of 1 mg/kg/24 hr	PO	12–24 hr	Hypotension
Calcium Channel Blockers					
Nifedipine	Calcium channel blocker	0.2–0.5 mg/kg/dose, maximum of 10 mg	PO SL	Repeat q 4–6 hr	Facial flushing, tachycardia
Verapamil	Calcium channel blocker	4–8 mg/kg/24 hr (dose not well established) Not used in patients <1 yr	PO	8 hr	Limited pediatric experience
Diuretic Agents					
Hydrochlorothiazide	Diuresis	1–4 mg/kg/24 hr	PO	12–24 hr	Hypokalemia, hyperuricemia, hypercalcemia
Furosemide	Diuresis	1 mg/kg/dose 1–2 mg/kg/dose	IV PO	4–6 hr 4–6 hr	Hypokalemia, alkalosis

Note: *Pediatric doses based on weight should not exceed adult doses. Because recommendations may change, these doses should always be double checked. Doses may also need to be modified in any patient with renal or hepatic dysfunction.*

IV = intravenously; PO = by mouth; CNS = central nervous system; ACE = angiotensin-converting enzyme; SL = sublingual.

sule, administration to younger children has presented some difficulty. Although the drug has often been placed in the sublingual space in order to achieve rapid absorption, gastrointestinal absorption is also sufficiently rapid to be effective in a hypertensive crisis. Intravenous hydralazine and diazoxide, when given at intervals, are alternative agents for the management of acute hypertensive crises, but such an approach may not provide the desired gradual reduction in blood pressure. Most children with hypertensive crisis have chronic or acute renal disease; in these patients, management of blood pressure also requires careful attention to fluid balance and requires diuresis. Intravenous furosemide is usually effective, even though glomerular filtration may be impaired.

In selecting a drug regimen for *long-term use*, an understanding of the underlying pathophysiology is helpful. Drugs with different sites and mechanisms of action are available so that therapy can be tailored to the specific pathologic condition. For example, excessive activity of the renin-angiotensin-aldosterone system may be treated effectively by a β-blocking drug (e.g., propranolol) for suppression of renin secretion, an ACE inhibitor (e.g., captopril), or, rarely, an aldosterone antagonist (e.g., spironolactone). ACE inhibitors are useful, not only in patients with high renin hypertension that is secondary to renovascular or renal parenchymal disease but also in patients with high-renin essential hypertension. Excess angiotensin production is the likely cause of most hypertension in the neonate following partial occlusion of a renal vessel by thrombus. Captopril is an effective agent in most of these patients, but it must be used with careful attention to renal function. α-Adrenergic blocking agents (phentolamine, phenoxybenzamine) are beneficial in patients with neural crest tumors who have high circulating levels of catecholamines. In such patients, β-blocking drugs are also needed to control heart rate, or an agent with dual blocking action (labetalol) may be used. Sympathetic blockade with labetalol is also efficacious in patients who experience marked stimulation of the cardiovascular system from high doses of cocaine.

Young patients with essential hypertension who require drug therapy may be treated initially with a diuretic or a β-blocking agent. Patients with volume-dependent hypertension usually have an adequate response to diuretics; those with high-renin, high cardiac output physiology respond best to β-blockers. If the pressure is not lowered adequately, a calcium channel blocker may be added to the diuretic and an ACE inhibitor may replace the β-blocker. Chronic use of diuretics may result in elevation of serum lipids, which may increase the risk of ischemic heart disease in adults with hypertension. Long-term investigations of this side effect in children are not available. β-Blocking agents have also been associated with changes in serum lipids, and some studies suggest a mild reduction in exercise tolerance in patients treated with propranolol. Patients with reactive airway disease are not able to tolerate a β-blocking agent.

Because of these side effects, the ACE inhibitors and calcium channel blockers may be considered for initial therapy in the adolescent with significant hypertension. Although captopril has been used more often in the pediatric and adolescent populations, newer ACE inhibitors such as enalapril have a longer duration of action and require less frequent administration of drug.

In patients with long-standing or poorly controlled hypertension, the underlying pathophysiology is often complex. Such patients frequently require trials of combinations of antihypertensive agents in order to gain control of markedly elevated or labile pressure. The basic principle of combination antihypertensive therapy is the coadministration of drugs with different sites or mechanisms of action. Because compliance may become a problem, the drug regimen should be as simple as possible and should take advantage of longer acting agents that can be administered once or twice daily, when available. Drug calendars, parental supervision, and close patient-physician communication also help ensure compliance.

In patients with renal artery stenosis due to fibromuscular dysplasia, percutaneous balloon angioplasty may cure as many as 50%. Angioplasty is not successful for renal artery stenosis because of atherosclerotic plaques. If angioplasty is unsuccessful, placement of an intravascular stent or surgery may be indicated.

Anonymous: Fenoldopam—a new drug for parenteral treatment of severe hypertension. Med Lett 40:57, 1998.

Arroll B, Beaglehole R: Does physical activity lower blood pressure: A critical review of the clinical trials. J Clin Epidemiol 45:439, 1992.

Capolan MS, Cohn RA, Langman CB, et al: Favorable outcome of neonatal aortic thrombosis and renovascular hypertension. J Pediatr 115:291, 1989.

Choi Y, Kang BC, Kim KJ, et al: Renovascular hypertension in children with moyamoya disease. J Pediatr 131:258, 1997.

Dimsdale JE: Reflections on the impact of antihypertensive medications on mood, sedation, and neuropsychologic functioning. Arch Intern Med 152:35, 1992.

Farine M, Arbus GS: Management of hypertensive emergencies in children. Pediatr Emerg Care 5:51, 1989.

Gillman MW, Ellison RC: Childhood prevention of essential hypertension. Pediatr Clin North Am 40:179, 1993.

Greydanus DE, Rowlett JD: Hypertension in adolescence. Adolesc Health Update 6:1, 1993.

Harshfield GA, Alpert BS, Pullman DA, et al: Ambulatory blood pressure readings in children and adults. Pediatrics 94:180, 1994.

Houtman PN, Dillon MJ: Screening for hypertension in fit children. J Hum Hypertens 5:345, 1991.

Ingelfinger JR: Pediatric hypertension. Curr Opin Pediatr 6:198, 1994.

Jung FF, Ingelfinger JR: Hypertension in childhood and adolescence. Pediatr Rev 14:169, 1993.

Medical Letter: Drugs for hypertension. Med Lett Drugs Ther 41:23, 1999.

National High Blood Pressure Education Program Working Group: Update on the 1987 task force report on high blood pressure in children and adolescents: A working group report from the National High Blood Pressure Education Program. Pediatrics 98:649, 1996.

Schneeweiss A: Cardiovascular drugs in children. II: Angiotensin-converting enzyme inhibitors in pediatric patients. Pediatr Cardiol 11:199, 1990.

Sinaiko AR: Hypertension in children. N Engl J Med 335:1968, 1996.

Stanley JC: Surgical intervention in pediatric renovascular hypertension. Child Nephrol Urol 12:167, 1992.

Task Force on Blood Pressure Control in Children: Report of the second task force on blood pressure control in children—1987. Pediatrics 79:1, 1987.

Tyagi S, Kaul UA, Satsangi DK, Arora R: Percutaneous transluminal angioplasty for renovascular hypertension in children: Initial and long-term results. Pediatrics 99:44, 1997.

Weir MR: Impact of age, race, and obesity on hypertensive mechanisms and therapy. Am J Med 90:3S, 1991.

Wolfish NM, Delbrouck NF, Shanon A, et al: Prevalence of hypertension in children with primary vesicoureteral reflux. J Pediatr 123:559, 1993.

Zerin JM, Hernandez RJ: Renal imaging in children with persistent hypertension. Pediatr Clin North Am 40:165, 1993.

PART XX

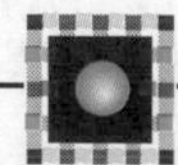

Diseases of the Blood

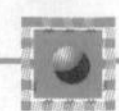

SECTION 1

The Hematopoietic System

CHAPTER 452

Development of the Hematopoietic System

Robin K. Ohls and Robert D. Christensen

Hematopoietic regulation in the human fetus differs markedly from that in an adult. In an adult, homeostatic maintenance is a prime function of hematopoietic regulation, whereas in the embryo and fetus, constant changes characterize all phases of hematopoiesis. During developmental erythropoiesis, the constant growth of the fetus and the resultant need to increase the red blood cell (RBC) mass necessitates an extraordinary erythropoietic effort. In addition, the relatively low oxygen tensions but high metabolic rates of fetal tissues demand a system of oxygen delivery distinct from that present in adults. During developmental granulopoiesis, the sterile intra-amniotic environment results in a low demand for neutrophils and obviates the need for maintenance of a large neutrophil reserve in the embryo and early fetus. Knowledge of developmental hematopoietic regulation helps clinicians to interpret postnatal hematologic data and to appreciate the erythropoietic and granulocytopoietic capacities and limitations of prematurely delivered neonates.

Developmental hematopoiesis occurs in three anatomic stages—mesoblastic, hepatic, and myeloid. Mesoblastic hematopoiesis occurs in extra embryonic structures, principally in the yolk sac, and begins between the 10th and 14th day of gestation. By 6–8 wk gestation, the liver replaces the yolk sac as the primary site of blood cell production, and by 10–12 wk gestation, extraembryonic hematopoiesis has essentially ceased. Hematopoiesis occurs in the liver throughout the remainder of gestation, although production begins to diminish during the second trimester as bone marrow hematopoiesis increases. The liver, however, remains the predominant hematopoietic organ through wk 20–24 of gestation.

Each hematopoietic organ houses distinct hematopoietic populations. For example, at 18–20 wk of gestation, more than 85% of the cells in the fetal liver are erythroid and virtually no neutrophils are present. In contrast, at this same time, fewer than 40% of the cells within the bone marrow are erythroid and as many as 15% are neutrophils. Moreover, the subpopulations of leukocytes present in the liver and marrow differ during gestation. Macrophages precede granulocytes in both the liver and marrow, and the ratio of macrophages to granulocytes decreases with increasing gestation. Thus, not only does the anatomic site of hematopoiesis change during gestation, but the populations of cells generated at those sites are distinct. The mechanisms responsible for the changing anatomic sites of hematopoiesis and for the differences in blood cells produced in the yolk sac, liver, and marrow have not been determined. Regardless of gestational age or anatomic location, production of all hematopoietic tissues begins with pluripotent stem cells that are capable of both self-renewal and of clonal maturation into all blood cell lineages. Progenitor cells differentiate under the influence of hematopoietic growth factors (Table 452–1) produced by the fetus.

Erythroid and granulocytic blood cell indices change during gestation and continue to change through the 1st year of life. Circulating RBC and granulocyte concentrations gradually increase during the 2nd and 3rd trimester (Table 452–2). In parallel with increasing RBC concentrations, hematocrit values increase from 30–40% during the 2nd trimester and continue to increase to term values during the latter part of the 3rd trimester. Term hematocrit values range from 50–63% (variability related to delayed clamping of the umbilical cord and to the sampling site). Unlike the blood concentrations of RBCs and neutrophils, platelet concentrations remain constant from 18 wk gestation through term, with a range of 150,000–450,000/μL.

Mean cell volumes generally are inversely proportional to gestation and inversely proportional to the life span of the cell. The mean cell volume (MCV) of RBCs is more than 180 femtoliters (fL) in an embryo, falls to the 130s by midgestation, then decreases to 115 fL by 40 wk gestation (Table 452–2). Mean platelet volumes (MPV) are 10–12 fL at birth and can sometimes be helpful in determining whether diminished platelet counts are primarily due to decreased production (small MPV) or increased destruction (normal to large MPV).

GRANULOCYTOPOIESIS

Mesenchymal cells with some of the properties of macrophages are present in the 1st mo of gestation. Some aspects of embryonic tissue remodeling take place by the actions of such cells. Whether these early phagocyte-like cells are derived from the same lineage as macrophages and neutrophils (by way of progenitors termed colony-forming unit granulocyte-macrophages [CFU-GM]) is not known. Thus, although some cells with phagocytic properties may be present in an embryo, essentially no neutrophils are observed until the midtrimester, and blood obtained from human fetuses in utero during the midtrimester contains very low concentrations of neutrophils. In fetuses of 20 wk gestation, Forrester reported a mean absolute blood neutrophil concentration of only 190/μL, a range of 0–490/μL, and a mode concentration of zero. Concordant with the low circulating concentrations of neutrophils, no mature neutrophils were present in the liver of normal human fetuses electively aborted at 14–24 wk gestation. Similarly, neutrophils were not observed in the liver or bone marrow of human abortuses until 16–18 wk gestation, and thereafter there were

TABLE 452–1 Characteristics of Hematopoietic Growth Factors

Growth Factors	Molecular Mass (kD)	Chromosomal Location	Principal Target Cell
I. Erythropoietin	30–39	7q11–22	CFU-E, fetal BFU-E
II. Colony-Stimulating Factors			
G-CSF	18–22	17q11.2–21	CFU-G, CFU-MIX, mature neutrophil
GM-CSF	18–30	5q23–31	CFU-MIX, CFU-GM, BFU-E, monocyte, mature neutrophil
M-CSF	45–70 Dimer of 2 subunits	5q33.1	CFU-M, macrophage
SCF	36	12	CFU-Mix, BFU-E, CFU-GM, mast cell
III. Interleukins			
IL-1	17	Alpha 2q13 Beta 2q13–21	Hepatocyte, macrophage, lymphocyte
IL-2	15–20	4q26–27	T cell, cytotoxic lymphocyte
IL-3	14–30	5q23–31	CFU-MIX, CFU-Meg, CFU-GM, BFU-E, macrophage
IL-4	16–20	5q23–31	T cell, B cell
IL-5	46 Dimer of 2 subunits	5q23–31	CFU-Eo, B cell
IL-6	19–26	7p21–24	CFU-MIX, CFU-GM, BFU-E, monocyte, B cell, T cell, cytotoxic lymphocyte
IL-7	25	8q12–13	B cell
IL-8	8–10	4	Neutrophil, endothelial cell, T cell
IL-9	16	5q31–32	BFU-E, CFU-MIX
IL-10	18.7	1	Macrophage, lymphocyte
IL-11	23	19q13	CFU-Meg, B cell, keratinocyte
IL-12	70–75 Dimer of 2 subunits	?	T cell, NK cell, macrophage
IL-13	9	5q23–31	Pre-B lymphocyte, macrophage
IL-14	53	—	B lymphocyte
IL-15	14–15	—	B lymphocyte, T lymphocyte, cytotoxic lymphocyte
IL-16	12–14	—	T lymphocyte
IV. Thrombopoietin	35–38	3q27–28	Megakaryocyte progenitor, megakaryocyte

G-CSF, granulocyte colony-stimulating factor; GM-CSF, granulocyte-macrophage colony-stimulating factor; M-CSF, macrophage colony-stimulating factor; SCF, stem cell factor.

significantly lower concentrations of mature neutrophils in the bone marrow of human fetuses (up to 22 wk gestation) than in the marrow of term neonates or adults.

Despite the near absence of neutrophils in 1st and 2nd trimester fetuses, CFU-GM are abundant in fetal liver, bone marrow, and blood. In rodents, the number of CFU-GM per gram of body weight is far fewer in animals delivered prematurely than in those delivered at term and is lower in term animals than in adults. The quantity of CFU-GM per gram of body weight in a developing human fetus has not been reported. Thus, it is not clear whether, as in experimental animals, preterm human infants have a relatively small supply of granulocytic progenitors. The venous blood of adults contains about 20–300 CFU-GM/mL. In contrast, the blood of term infants contains about 2,000 CFU-GM/mL, and even higher concentrations are noted in the blood of infants delivered prematurely. The high concentrations of CFU-GM in fetal blood do not indicate a large total body quantity of CFU-GM. It is likely that a significant percentage of the fetal CFU-GM are in the circulation, whereas the liver and marrow contain relatively low concentrations.

When fetal CFU-GM are cultured in vitro in the presence of recombinant granulocyte colony-stimulating Factor (G-CSF) they undergo maturation into colonies of neutrophils. CFU-GM of fetal origin often clonally mature into larger colonies, containing more cells, than do CFU-GM obtained from the bone marrow of adults. The physiologic role of G-CSF includes upregulation of neutrophil production, and this appears to be the case for fetuses and neonates as well as for adults. Thus, the low quantities of circulating and storage neutrophils in a midtrimester human fetus may in part be due to low production of G-CSF. Supporting this hypothesis are observations of poor production of G-CSF by cells of human fetal origin. Monocytes isolated from the blood of adults produce G-CSF when stimulated with various inflammatory mediators such as bacterial lipopolysaccharide (LPS) or interleukin-1 (IL-1). In contrast, monocytes isolated from the umbilical cord blood of preterm infants and from the liver and bone marrow of aborted fetuses up to 24 wk gestation generate only small quantities (10–100 times less per cell) of G-CSF protein and mRNA after LPS or IL-1 stimulation. Despite the poor capacity to generate G-CSF, receptors for G-CSF on the surface of fetal and neonatal neutrophils are equal in number and affinity to those on adult neutrophils.

Thus, granulocytopoiesis appears to be virtually absent in the human embryo, and granulocyte production is a very minor component of hematopoiesis in a fetus even up through the 22–24th wk of gestation. This is not because of absence of

TABLE 452–2 Blood Cell Indices During Gestation and at Birth

Week of Gestation	Total WBC Counts* (×10⁹/L)	Corrected WBC Counts (×10⁹/L)	Platelets (×10⁹/L)	RBC (×10¹²/L)	Hb (g/dL)	Hct (%)	MCV (fL)
18–21 (n = 760)	4.68 ± 2.96	2.57 ± 0.42	234 ± 57	2.85 ± 0.36	11.69 ± 1.27	37.3 ± 4.3	131.1 ± 11.0
22–25 (n = 1,200)	4.72 ± 2.82	3.73 ± 2.17	247 ± 59	3.09 ± 0.34	12.2 ± 1.6	38.6 ± 3.9	125.1 ± 7.8
26–29 (n = 460)	5.16 ± 2.53	4.08 ± 0.84	242 ± 69	3.46 ± 0.41	12.91 ± 1.38	40.9 ± 4.4	118.5 ± 8.0
>30 (n = 440)	7.71 ± 4.99	6.40 ± 2.99	232 ± 87	3.82 ± 0.64	13.64 ± 2.21	43.6 ± 7.2	114.4 ± 9.3
Term		18.1 (9.0–30.0)	290 ± 100	4.70 ± 0.40	16.5 ± 1.5	51.0 ± 4.5	108 ± 5.0

**Including normoblasts.*
RBC = red blood cells; Hb = hemoglobin; Hct = hematocrit.
Adapted from Forestier F, Daffos F, Catherine N, et al: Developmental hematopoiesis in normal human fetal blood. Blood 77:2361, 1991.

neutrophil progenitor cells but rather a relative lack of the major neutrophil regulatory growth factor, G-CSF. On this basis, one might anticipate that newborns who are delivered extremely prematurely would be at significant risk for serious bacterial infection. Indeed, of all the risk factors for neonatal infection analyzed by the national collaborative study on neonatal infections, premature birth showed the strongest correlation.

THROMBOPOIESIS

Like other blood cells, megakaryocytes are produced after clonal maturation of committed progenitors, termed colony-forming unit–megakaryocyte (CFU-Meg), into megakaryoblasts. This blast cell is similar in appearance to other primitive committed cells, but DNA synthesis is generally more rapid and occurs without cell division, a process referred to as *endomitosis*. Megakaryoblasts grow considerably in size within a few days, with a single nucleus that may have 4–16 times the normal DNA content. The cytoplasm also increases in volume, and cellular organelles appear. Long strips of cytoplasm are peeled off the body of the cell and ultimately break up into platelets. Erythropoietin (EPO), IL-6, and IL-11 induce platelet formation. Thrombopoietin (TPO), a 353 amino acid protein with some homology to EPO and interferons (alpha, beta), induces megakaryocyte proliferation from immature precursors, promotes the development of mature megakaryocytes, and increases overall platelet counts. TPO stimulates CFU-Meg production of cord blood progenitors, but such studies have not been performed on neonatal infants.

ERYTHROPOIESIS

Erythropoiesis in utero is controlled by erythroid growth factors produced solely by the fetus. EPO does not cross the placenta in humans, monkeys, or sheep; therefore, stimulation of maternal EPO production does not result in stimulation of fetal RBC production. Moreover, suppression of maternal erythropoiesis by hypertransfusion does not suppress fetal erythropoiesis.

Although the mechanism of erythropoietic regulation in adults is known to a significant degree, it is unclear if the same mechanism of erythropoietic regulation exists in fetuses or in infants born prematurely. Production of RBCs is governed by various growth factors produced by accessory cells such as macrophages, lymphocytes, and stromal cells. These factors stimulate maturation, growth, and differentiation at various stages of RBC production. Of all the factors stimulating erythropoiesis, none has a more important regulatory role than EPO. EPO is a 30–39-kD glycoprotein that binds to specific receptors on the surface of erythroid precursors and stimulates their differentiation and clonal maturation into mature RBCs. The regulation of EPO gene expression involves an oxygen-sensing mechanism, and both hypoxia and anemia stimulate erythropoiesis by stimulating mRNA transcription and EPO production. EPO mRNA production is regulated by *cis*-acting elements in the promoter and 3′ enhancer regions that are responsive to hypoxia. Two factors, hepatic nuclear factor 4 (HNF-4) and hypoxic inducible factor (HIF), exhibit specific transcriptional activation for EPO. The precise development of HNF-4, HIF, and other transcriptional activators in fetuses and premature infants remain to be determined.

EPO is produced by the fetal liver during the 1st and 2nd trimester, principally by cells of monocyte/macrophage origin. Sometime during the 3rd trimester and the 1st few weeks of life, the anatomic site of EPO production shifts from the liver to the kidneys. The specific stimulus for the shift of EPO production from liver to kidneys is unknown but might involve the significant changes in arterial oxygen tension that occur at birth. In animal models, the sensitivity of the hepatic hypoxia-sensing mechanism is decreased compared with renal sensitivity. The liver also appears to require more prolonged hypoxia to achieve an EPO response. Although EPO mRNA and protein can be found in the human fetal kidneys, it is not known whether this production is biologically relevant. However, renal production of EPO is not essential for normal fetal erythropoiesis, as evidenced by the normal serum EPO concentrations and normal hematocrit values of anephric fetuses.

Studies of bone marrow cells in tissue culture have added to our understanding of how erythroid precursors respond to growth factors. When bone marrow cells are placed in semi-solid media culture systems for 5–7 days, the EPO-sensitive precursors, termed colony-forming units–erythroid (CFU-E), clonally mature into clusters containing 30–100 normoblasts. Erythroid-specific progenitors that are less well differentiated than CFU-E, hence more primitive cells, are termed burst-forming units–erythroid (BFU-E). Twelve to 14 days after bone marrow cells are placed in semi-solid culture systems, BFU-E develop into large clusters of normoblasts, each containing 200–10,000 normoblasts. BFU-E from human fetuses respond in a slightly different fashion from BFU-E isolated from adults. BFU-E of fetal origin generally develop into erythroid clones more rapidly and generally develop substantially more normoblasts than do BFU-E of adult origin. Moreover, BFU-E from adult bone marrow require a combination of EPO plus another factor such as IL-3 or GM-CSF in order to clonally mature, whereas many fetal BFU-E mature in the presence of EPO alone.

HEMOGLOBIN. The combustion that is essential to life requires that tissues receive a constant supply of oxygen. The evolutionary development of oxygen-carrying proteins, the hemoglobins, increased the ability of blood to transport oxygen. Furthermore, the combination of oxygen with hemoglobin and its dissociation from it are accomplished without expenditure of metabolic energy.

Hemoglobin is a complex protein consisting of iron-containing heme groups and the protein moiety globin. A dynamic interaction between heme and globin gives hemoglobin its unique properties in the reversible transport of oxygen. The hemoglobin molecule is a tetramer made up of two pairs of polypeptide chains, each chain having a heme group attached. The polypeptide chains of various hemoglobins are of chemically different types. The major hemoglobin of a normal adult (Hb A) is made up of one pair of alpha (α) and one pair of beta (β) polypeptide chains and represented as $\alpha_2\beta_2$. The major hemoglobin in the fetus (HbF) is represented by $\alpha_2\gamma_2$.

The various globin chains differ in both the number and sequence of amino acids, and their synthesis is directed by separate genes (Fig. 452–1). Two sets of genes for the α chains are located on human chromosome 16. Two pairs of alleles provide the genetic information for the structure of the α chain. β, γ, δ genes are closely linked on chromosome 11.

Within the RBCs of an embryo, fetus, child, and adult, six different hemoglobins may normally be detected: the embryonic hemoglobins, Gower-1, Gower-2, and Portland; the fetal hemoglobin, HbF; and the adult hemoglobins, Hb A and A_2. The electrophoretic mobilities of hemoglobins vary with their chemical structures. The time of appearance and quantitative relationships among the hemoglobins are determined by complex developmental processes (Fig. 452–2).

EMBRYONIC HEMOGLOBINS. The blood of early human embryos contains two slowly migrating hemoglobins, Gower-1 and Gower-2, and Hb Portland, which has HbF–like mobility. The zeta (ζ) chains of Hb Portland and Gower-1 are structurally quite similar to α chains. Both Gower hemoglobins contain a unique type of polypeptide chain, the epsilon (ϵ) chain. Hb Gower-1 has the structure $\zeta_2\epsilon_2$, and Gower-2, $\alpha_2\epsilon_2$. Hb Portland has the structure $\zeta_2\gamma_2$. In embryos of 4–8 wk gestation, the Gower hemoglobins predominate, but by the 3rd mo they have disappeared.

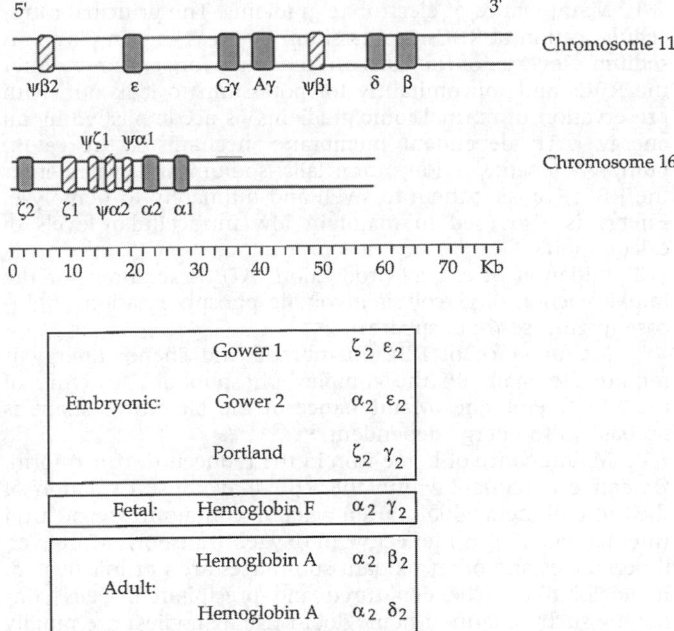

Figure 452–1 Organization of the globin genes. The bottom line reflects the scale in kilobases. Transcription of mRNA takes place from the 5′ to the 3′ end. The upper segment represents the beta-like globin genes on chromosome 11 and the lower segment the alpha-like genes on chromosome 16. Regions of the gene that code for primary globin proteins are shown as shaded segments, and regions that code for pseudogenes ("ψ", nonexpressed remnants) are shown as hatched segments. The composition of embryonic, fetal, and adult hemoglobins is listed. α = alpha; β = beta; γ = gamma; δ = delta; ϵ = epsilon; ζ = zeta.

FETAL HEMOGLOBIN. HbF contains γ polypeptide chains in place of the β chains of Hb A. Its resistance to denaturation by strong alkali is the basis for determining the presence of fetal RBCs in the maternal circulation (the Kleihauer-Betke test). After the 8th gestational wk, HbF is the predominant hemoglobin; at 24 wk gestations it constitutes 90% of the total hemoglobin. During the 3rd trimester, a gradual decline occurs, so that at birth HbF averages 70% of the total. Synthesis of HbF decreases rapidly postnatally, and by 6–12 mo of age only a trace is present. Less than 2.0% can be detected by alkali denaturation in older children and adults. HbF is heterogeneous because of two types of γ chains, whose synthesis is directed by two sets of genes. The chains differ at position 136 in the presence of either a glycine (Gγ) or an alanine (Aγ) residue. In newborns, the relative proportion or ratio of Gγ to Aγ chain is 3:1.

ADULT HEMOGLOBINS. Some Hb A ($\alpha_2\beta_2$) can be detected in even the smallest embryos. Accordingly, it is possible as early as 16–20 wk gestation to make a prenatal diagnosis of major β-chain hemoglobinopathies, such as thalassemia major. Prenatal diagnosis is based on techniques that examine the rates of synthesis of β chains or the structure of newly synthesized β chains. Earlier diagnosis is possible using molecular biology techniques and sampling of chorionic villus tissue or amniotic fluid if DNA structural defects are a cause of the hemoglobinopathies. Similarly, gene deletion disorders such as the α-thalassemias are detectable by the same method.

By the 24th wk of gestation, approximately 5–10% of Hb A is present. A steady increase follows, so that at term, Hb A averages 30%. By 6–12 mo of age, the normal Hb A pattern appears. The minor Hb A component Hb A_2 contains delta (δ) chains and has the structure $\alpha_2\delta_2$. It is seen only when significant amounts of Hb A are also present. At birth, less than 1.0% of Hb A_2 is seen, but by 12 mo of age the normal level of 2.0–3.4% is attained. Throughout life, the normal ratio of Hb A to A_2 is about 30:1.

NORMAL RELATIONSHIPS AMONG THE HEMOGLOBINS. During fetal life and early childhood, the rates of synthesis of γ and β chains and the amounts of Hb A and HbF are inversely related. This relationship has been attributed to a "switch mechanism" similar to genetic regulatory mechanisms in bacteria, but the genetic, biologic, and developmental processes that direct a switchover from predominantly γ-chain synthesis in utero to predominantly β-chain synthesis after birth are unclear. It is not certain whether the mechanisms involve selective genetic inhibition or facilitation. The increase in the α_1/α_2 globin ratio occurring after 36 wk gestation corresponds with a rapid decline in γ-globin synthesis, suggesting that these changes could be regulated by a coordinated molecular mechanism. It has been shown that differential selection and amplified production of RBC precursors derived from BFU-E result in considerable HbF production. This may be the basis for the increased levels of HbF that occur in many hypoproliferative or hemolytic anemias. Alternative explanations involve more basic genetic regulators in the DNA sequences that flank the hemoglobin gene complexes.

ALTERATIONS OF THE HEMOGLOBINS BY DISEASE. Because hemoglobins containing ϵ chains are normally present only very early in intrauterine life, they are largely of theoretical interest. Small amounts of the Gower hemoglobins have been detectable in a few newborn infants with 13/15-trisomy. Increased levels of Hb Portland have been found in cord blood of stillborn infants with homozygous α-thalassemia.

HbF levels may be influenced by various factors. Because the HbF level is elevated during the 1st year of life, knowledge of its normal decline is important (Fig. 452–3). In persons heterozygous for β-thalassemia (β-thalassemia trait), postpartum decrease of HbF is retarded; about 50% of such persons have elevated levels of HbF (>2.0%) in later life. In homozygous thalassemia (Cooley anemia) and in hereditary persis-

Figure 452–2 Proportions of the various human hemoglobin polypeptide chains through early life. The hemoglobin electrophoretic pattern typical for each period is also shown. (Modified from Pearson HA: Recent advances in hematology. J Pediatr 69:466, 1966.)

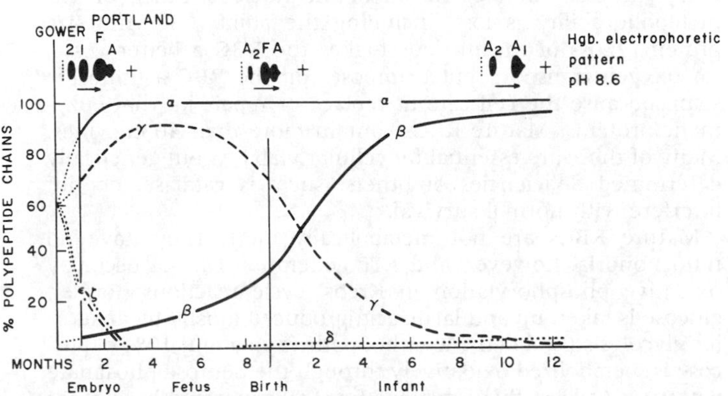

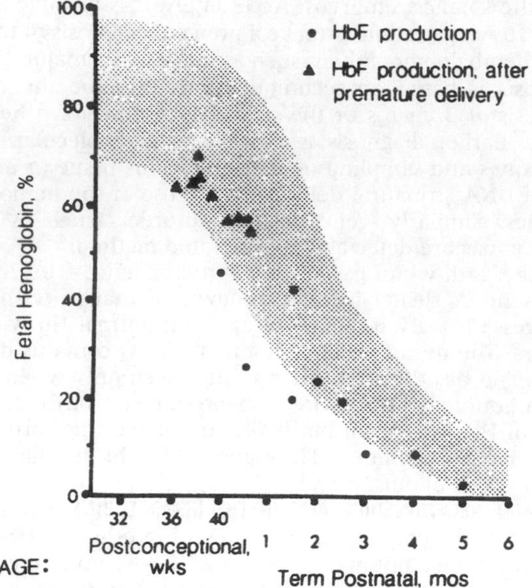

Figure 452–3 Pre- and postnatal changes in the percentage of total hemoglobin represented by fetal hemoglobin (HbF) *(shaded area)*. The triangles represent postnatal production by reticulocytes in premature infants, and the dots represent cord blood and postnatal reticulocyte production in term infants. (From Brown MS: Fetal and neonatal erythropoiesis, In: Stockman JA, Pochedly C (eds): Developmental and Neonatal Hematology, New York, Raven Press, 1988.)

tence of HbF, large amounts of HbF are characteristically found. In patients with major β-chain hemoglobinopathies (e.g., Hb SS, SC), HbF is usually increased, particularly during childhood. Preterm infants treated with human recombinant EPO may increase HbF production during active erythropoiesis. Finally, moderate elevations of HbF may occur in many diseases accompanied by hematologic stress, such as hemolytic anemias, leukemia, and aplastic anemia, because of a minor population of RBCs that contains increased amounts of HbF, as can be demonstrated by the acid-elution staining technique of Kleihauer and Betke. Tetramers of γ chains (γ_4 or Hb Barts) or β chains (β_4, Hb H) may be found in α-thalassemia syndromes.

The normal adult level of Hb A_2 (2.0–3.4%) is seldom altered. Levels of Hb A_2 exceeding 3.4% are found in most persons with the β-thalassemia trait and in those with megaloblastic anemias secondary to vitamin B_{12} and folic acid deficiency. Decreased HbA_2 levels are found in those with iron deficiency anemia and α-thalassemia.

METABOLISM OF THE RBC. The nucleated RBCs in bone marrow participate in various metabolic functions, including active protein synthesis. After extrusion of the nucleus, much of this metabolic ability is lost, including the ability to synthesize proteins. Loss of the nucleus makes the RBC a better vessel for oxygen transport, but it imposes on the RBC a finite life span, because the cell cannot replace or repair its vital enzymatic proteins. Mature RBCs contain more than 40 enzymes. Many of these are essential for cellular viability, but genetically determined deficiencies of others, such as catalase, do not interfere with normal survival.

Mature RBCs are not metabolically inert. They have no mitochondria, however, and ATP generation cannot occur by oxidative phosphorylation in Krebs' cycle reactions. Rather, glucose is taken up and lactic acid produced mostly by anaerobic glycolysis (Embden-Meyerhof pathway); about 10% of glucose is metabolized oxidatively through the pentose phosphate pathway. At least five functions for ATP generated by glucose metabolism are essential to normal cell viability:

1. Maintenance of electrolyte gradients. The principal intracellular cation of RBCs is potassium, whereas that in plasma is sodium. Reversal of the constant tendency for sodium to enter the RBCs and concomitantly for potassium to leak out, with preservation of normal ionic gradients, is accomplished by an energy (ATP)-dependent membrane mechanism, the cation pump. When the cation pump fails, sodium and water enter the RBCs, causing them to swell and ultimately to hemolyze. Energy is also used to maintain low intracellular levels of calcium ion.

2. Initiation of energy production. ATP is required for the initial reaction of glycolysis involving phosphorylation of glucose to glucose-6-phosphate.

3. Maintenance of RBC membrane and shape. Energy is required to maintain the complex phospholipid structure of the RBC membrane. Maintenance of the biconcave shape is probably also energy dependent.

4. Maintenance of heme iron in the reduced (ferrous) form. Oxidative potentials within the RBC may cause oxidation of the iron of hemoglobin. Hemoglobin containing ferric iron (methemoglobin) is ineffective in oxygen transport. Moreover, if perioxides and other oxidant substances are not inactivated, hemoglobin may be denatured and precipitated. Cells containing such denatured hemoglobin (Heinz bodies) are rapidly removed from the circulation. Protection of RBCs from the effects of oxidation ultimately depends on NADPH and NADH. These compounds are continually regenerated by activities of the glycolytic pathway and pentose shunt. In many genetically determined deficiencies of glycolytic and pentose pathway enzymes, hemolytic states occur because the energy necessary to perform these vital functions cannot be generated.

5. Maintenance of the levels of organic phosphates such as 2,3-diphosphoglycerate and ATP within the RBCs. These compounds interact with hemoglobin and have profound effects on oxygen affinity.

Bailie KEM, Irvine AD, Bridges JM, et al: Granulocyte and granulocyte–macrophage colony stimulating factors in cord and maternal serum at delivery. Pediatr Res 35:164, 1994.

Brugnara C, Platt OS: The neonatal erythrocyte and its disorders. *In*: Nathan DG, Orkin SH (eds): Nathan and Oski's Hematology of Infancy and Childhood. 5th ed. Philadelphia, WB Saunders, 1998, pp 17–52.

Cairo MS: Therapeutic implications for dysregulated colony-stimulating factor expression in neonates. Blood 82:2269, 1993.

Carbonell F, Calvo W, Fliedner TM: Cellular composition of human fetal bone marrow. Acta Anat 113:371, 1982.

Forestier F, Daffos F, Catherine N, et al: Developmental hematopoiesis in normal human fetal blood. Blood 77:2360, 1991.

Goldberg MA, Dunning SP, Bunn HF: Regulation of the erythropoietin gene: Evidence that the oxygen sensor is a heme protein. Science 242:524, 1998.

Holbrook ST, Christensen RD: Hematopoietic growth factors. Adv Pediatr 39:23, 1991.

Keleman E, Calvo W, Fliedner TM: Atlas of Human Hematopoietic Development. Berlin, Springer-Verlag, 1979.

Keleman E, Janossa M: Macrophages are the first differentiated blood cells formed in human embryonic liver. Exp Hematol 8:996, 1980.

Liechty KW, Schibler KR, Ohls RK, et al: The failure of newborn mice infected with *Escherichia coli* to accelerate neutrophil production correlates with their failure to increase transcripts for granulocyte colony-stimulating factor and interleukin-6. Biol Neonate 64:31, 1993.

Lok S, Kaushansky K, Holly R, et al: Cloning and expression of murine thrombopoietin cDNA and stimulation of platelet production in vivo. Nature 369:565, 1994.

Metcalf D: Hematopoietic regulators: Redundance or subtlety? Blood 82:3515, 1993.

Nathan DG: The beneficence of neonatal hematopoiesis. [Editorial.] N Engl J Med 321:1190, 1989.

Nathan DG: Regulation of hematopoiesis. Pediatr Res 27:423, 1990.

Ohls RK, Li Y, Abdel-Mageed A, et al: Neutrophil pool sizes and granulocyte colony-stimulating factor production in human mid-trimester fetuses. Pediatr Res 37:806, 1995.

Schibler KR, Christensen RD: Defective production of interleukin-6 by monocytes: A possible mechanism underlying several host defense deficencies of neonates. Pediatr Res 31:18, 1992.

Slayton WB, Juul S, Calhoun DA, et al: Hematopoiesis in the liver and marrow of human fetuses at 5 to 16 weeks postconception: Quantitative assessment of macrophage and neutrophil populations. Pediatr Res 43:774, 1998.

CHAPTER 453
The Anemias

Elias Schwartz*

Anemia is defined as a reduction of the red blood cell (RBC) volume or hemoglobin concentration below the range of values occurring in healthy persons. Table 453–1 lists the means and ranges for hemoglobin and hematocrit values by age groups of well-nourished children. There may be racial differences in hemoglobin levels. Black children have levels about 0.5 g/dL lower than those of white and Asian children of comparable age and socioeconomic status, possibly in part because of the high incidence of alpha thalassemia in blacks. Alternatively, higher levels of RBC 2,3-diphosphoglycerate (2,3-DPG) have been found in black children, which would permit better oxygen delivery and a lower hemoglobin.

Although a reduction in the amount of circulating hemoglobin deceases the oxygen-carrying capacity of the blood, few clinical disturbances occur until the hemoglobin level falls below 7–8 g/dL. Below this level, pallor becomes evident in the skin and mucous membranes. Physiologic adjustments to anemia include increased cardiac output, increased oxygen extraction (increased arteriovenous oxygen difference), and a shunting of blood flow toward vital organs and tissues. In addition, the concentration of 2,3-DPG increases within the RBC. The resultant "shift to the right" of the oxygen dissociation curve, reducing the affinity of hemoglobin for oxygen, results in more complete transfer of oxygen to the tissues. The same shift may also occur at high altitude. When moderately severe anemia develops slowly, surprisingly few symptoms or objective findings may be evident, but weakness, tachypnea, shortness of breath on exertion, tachycardia, cardiac dilatation, and congestive heart failure ultimately result from increasingly severe anemia, regardless of its cause.

Anemia is not a specific entity but results from many underlying pathologic processes. A useful classification of the anemias of childhood divides them into three groups by the RBC mean corpuscular volume (MCV): microcytic, macrocytic, or normocytic. RBC size changes with age, and before an anemia can be specifically characterized with respect to RBC size, normal developmental changes in the MCV should be understood (see Table 453–1). Table 453–2 classifies the important anemias of childhood by the MCV. Anemias in childhood may also be classified by variations in cell size, as reflected by alterations in the RBC distribution width (RDW). The RDW, as determined by the use of electronic cell counting, is the coefficient of variation of RBC size (standard deviation of the MCV $\div$ mean MCV $\times$ 100). Knowledge of both the MCV and the RDW can be helpful in the initial classification of anemias of childhood (Table 453–3). In every case of significant anemia, it is essential to review the appearance of RBCs on a peripheral blood smear (Fig. 453–1). Specific morphologic features may point to the underlying diagnosis. In addition, the presence of polychromatophilia, which correlates roughly with the degree of reticulocytosis, indicates that the marrow is able to respond to RBC loss or destruction.

When oxygen delivery by red blood cells (RBCs) to tissues is decreased, various mechanisms, including expanded cardiac output, increased production of 2,3-diphosphoglycerate (2,3-DPG) in RBCs, and higher levels of erythropoietin (EPO) help the body to modify the deficiency. RBC production by the bone marrow in response to EPO may expand severalfold and may compensate for mild to moderate reductions in RBC life span. In various anemias, the bone marrow loses its usual capacity for sustained production and expansion of the RBC mass. In these instances, absolute reticulocyte numbers in the peripheral blood are decreased. If the normal reticulocyte percentage of total RBCs during most of childhood is about 1.0% and the expected RBC count is approximately $4.0 \times 10^6/mm^3$, then the normal absolute reticulocyte number should be about $40,000/mm^3$. In the presence of anemia, EPO production and the absolute number of reticulocytes should rise. A normal or low absolute number or percentage of reticulocytes in response to anemia indicates relative bone marrow failure or ineffective erythropoiesis (e.g., megaloblastic anemia, thalassemia). Measurement of the serum transferrin receptor (TfR) level or examination of the bone marrow distinguishes between these possibilities, because TfR is elevated in ineffective erythropoiesis (or in iron deficiency) and is decreased in marrow RBC hypoproliferation.

Koerper MA, Mentzer WC, Brecher G, Dallman PR: Developmental change in red blood cell volume: Implication in screening infants and children for iron deficiency and thalassemia trait. J Pediatr 89:580, 1976.

*Modified from original in 15th edition by Bruce M. Camitta.

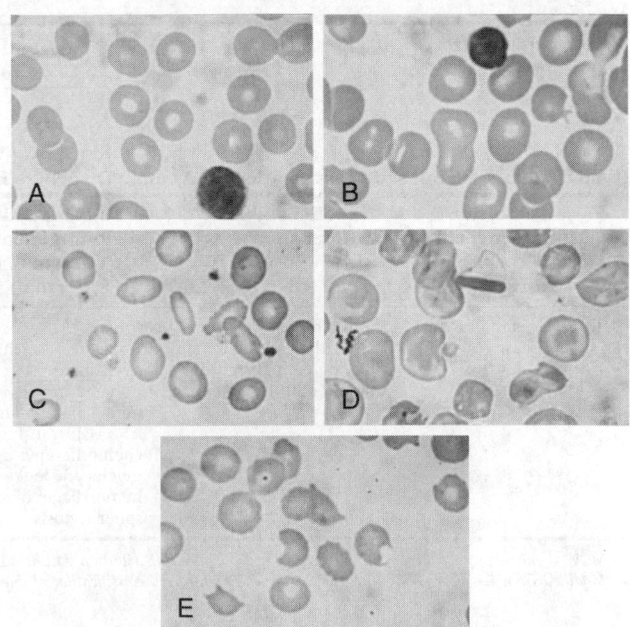

Figure 453–1 Morphologic abnormalities of the red blood cell. *A,* Normal. *B,* Macrocytes (folic acid or vitamin B_{12} deficiency). *C,* Hypochromic microcytes (iron deficiency). *D,* Target cells (Hb CC disease). *E,* Schizocytes (hemolytic-uremic syndrome). (Provided by Dr. E. Schwartz.) See also color section.

TABLE 453–1 Hematologic Values During Infancy and Childhood

	Hemoglobin (g/dL)		Hematocrit (%)		Reticulocytes (%)	MCV (fL)	Leukocytes (WBC/mm³)		Neutrophils (%)		Lymphocytes (%)	Eosinophils (%)	Monocytes (%)
Age	***Mean***	***Range***	***Mean***	***Range***	***Mean***	***Lowest***	***Mean***	***Range***	***Mean***	***Range***	***Mean****	***Mean***	***Mean***
Cord blood	16.8	13.7–20.1	55	45–65	5.0	110	18,000	(9,000–30,000)	61	(40–80)	31	2	6
2 wk	16.5	13.0–20.0	50	42–66	1.0		12,000	(5,000–21,000)	40		63	3	9
3 mo	12.0	9.5–14.5	36	31–41	1.0		12,000	(6,000–18,000)	30		48	2	5
6 mo–6 yr	12.0	10.5–14.0	37	33–42	1.0	70–74	10,000	(6,000–15,000)	45		48	2	5
7–12 yr	13.0	11.0–16.0	38	34–40	1.0	76–80	8,000	(4,500–13,500)	55		38	2	5
Adult													
Female	14	12.0–16.0	42	37–47	1.6	80	7,500	(5,000–10,000)	55	(35–70)	35	3	7
Male	16	14.0–18.0	47	42–52		80							

**Relatively wide range.*
fL = femtoliters; MCV = mean corpuscular volume; WBC = white blood cells.

TABLE 453–2 Classification of Anemia

Microcytic
- Iron deficiency
- Thalassemias
- Lead poisoning
- Chronic disease
  - Infection
  - Cancer
  - Inflammation
  - Renal disease
- Vitamin B_6 responsive
- Copper deficiency
- Sideroblastic (some)

Normocytic
- Decreased production
  - Aplastic anemia
    - Congenital
    - Acquired
  - Pure RBC aplasia
    - Congenital (Diamond-Blackfan)
    - Acquired (transient erythroblastopenia)
  - Bone marrow replacement
    - Leukemia
    - Tumors
    - Storage diseases
    - Osteopetrosis
    - Myelofibrosis
- Blood loss
  - Internal or external
- Sequestration
- Hemolysis: Intrinsic RBC abnormalities
  - Hemoglobinopathies
  - Enzymopathies
  - Membrane disorders
    - Hereditary spherocytosis
    - Acquired: paroxysmal nocturnal hemoglobinuria
- Hemolysis: Extrinsic RBC abnormalities
  - Immunologic
    - Passive (hemolytic disease of the newborn)
    - Active: Autoimmune
  - Toxins
  - Infections
  - Microangiopathic
    - Disseminated intravascular coagulation (DIC)
    - Hemolytic uremic syndrome
    - Hypertension
    - Cardiac disease

Macrocytic
- Normal newborn (spurious)
- Reticulocytosis (spurious)
- Vitamin B_{12} deficiency
- Folate deficiency
- Oroticaciduria
- Myelodysplasia
- Liver disease
- Hypothyroidism (some)
- Vitamin B_6 deficiency (some)
- Thiamine deficiency

RBC = red blood cell.

TABLE 453–3 Proposed Classification of Anemic Disorders Based on Red Blood Cell Mean (MCV) and Heterogeneity (RDW)

Microcytic Homogeneous (MCV low, RDW normal)	Microcytic Heterogeneous (MCV low, RDW high)	Normocytic Homogeneous (MCV normal, RDW normal)	Normocytic Heterogeneous (MCV normal, RDW high)	Macrocytic Homogeneous (MCV high, RDW normal)	Macrocytic Heterogeneous (MCV high, RDW high)
Heterozygous thalassemia Chronic disease	Iron deficiency Hb S–β-thalassemia; hemoglobin H; red cell fragmentation	Normal Chronic disease, chronic liver disease; nonanemic hemoglobinopathy (e.g., AS, AC); transfusion; chemotherapy; chronic myelocytic leukemia; hemorrhage; hereditary spherocytosis	Mixed deficiency Early iron deficiency anemia; anemic hemoglobinopathy (e.g., SS, SC); myelofibrosis; sideroblastic	Aplastic anemia Preleukemia	Folate deficiency Vitamin B_{12} deficiency; immune hemolytic anemia; cold agglutinin; high count

MCV = mean corpuscular volume; RDW = red blood cell distribution width; AS = sickle cell trait, AC = hemoglobin C trait; SS = sickle cell anemia; SC = hemoglobin SC disease.
Modified from Bessman JD, Gilmer P, Gardener F: Improved classification of anemias by MCV and RDW. Am J Clin Pathol 80:322, 1983.

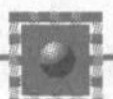

SECTION 2

Anemias of Inadequate Production[*]

Elias Schwartz

CHAPTER 454

Congenital Hypoplastic Anemia

(Diamond-Blackfan Syndrome)

This rare condition usually becomes symptomatic in early infancy, frequently with pallor in the neonatal period, but may first be noted later in childhood. About 75% of cases are diagnosed by 3 mo of age. The most characteristic features are macrocytic anemia, reticulocytopenia, and a deficiency or absence of red blood cell (RBC) precursors in an otherwise normally cellular bone marrow.

ETIOLOGY. Dominant or recessive patterns of inheritance are indicated by familial occurrence in about 15% of patients. In about 25% of patients, there are mutations in the gene for ribosomal protein S19 (one of 79 ribosomal proteins), mapped to chromosome 19q13. The patients were heterozygous for deficiency of the protein and were sporadic or familial cases. Most evidence indicates that the primary defects are in the erythroid precursor and are not due to immunologic damage to normal stem cells. High levels of EPO are present in serum and urine. A search for mutations in the EPO receptor gene has been negative. In patients, no defects have been found in the genes for mast/stem cell growth factor (MGF) or its receptor, c-*kit*, nor does prednisone correct the anemias in mice with deficiencies of MGF or c-*kit*. Erythroid progenitors in this disorder have an unusual sensitivity to withdrawal of EPO, with resultant increased apoptosis (programmed cell death).

CLINICAL MANIFESTATIONS. Although hematopoiesis is generally adequate in fetal life, some affected infants appear pale in the first days after birth; rarely, hydrops fetalis occurs. Profound anemia usually becomes evident by 2–6 mo of age, occasionally somewhat later. The liver and spleen are not enlarged initially. About one third of affected children have congenital anomalies, most commonly craniofacial deformities or defects of the upper extremities, including triphalangeal thumbs. The abnormalities are diverse, with no specific pattern emerging in the majority of those affected.

LABORATORY FINDINGS. The RBCs are usually macrocytic, with elevated levels of folic acid and vitamin B_{12}. Assay of RBCs reveals a pattern characteristic of a "young" RBC population, including elevated fetal hemoglobin (Hb F) and increased expression of "i" antigen. Adenosine deaminase activity is increased in RBCs of patients with this disorder. These findings may help distinguish congenital RBC aplasia from acquired transient erythroblastopenia of childhood (Chapter 456). Thrombocytosis or thrombocytopenia and occasionally neutropenia may also be present initially. Reticulocytes are diminished, even when the anemia is severe. RBC precursors are markedly reduced in the marrow in most patients, but other marrow elements are usually normal. Serum iron levels are elevated.

DIFFERENTIAL DIAGNOSIS. Congenital hypoplastic anemia must be differentiated from other anemias with low reticulocyte counts. The anemia of the convalescent phase of hemolytic disease of the newborn may, on occasion, be associated with markedly reduced erythropoiesis. This terminates spontaneously at 5–8 wk of age. Aplastic crises characterized by reticulocytopenia and by decreased numbers of RBC precursors, frequently caused by parvovirus B19 infections, may complicate various types of hemolytic disease, but usually after the first several months of life. Infection with this virus in utero may also cause pure RBC aplasia in infancy, even with hydrops fetalis at birth. The syndrome of transient erythroblastopenia of childhood (Chapter 456) may be differentiated from Diamond-Blackfan syndrome by its relatively late onset (although it may occasionally develop in infants younger than 6 mo) and by biochemical differences in RBCs.

PROGNOSIS. Median survival is more than 40 yr of age. The outlook is best in those who respond to corticosteroid therapy. About half of the patients are long-term responders. In the others, survival depends on transfusions. Some children in each group may eventually have spontaneous remissions (about 14%). By late childhood, children who do not respond to corticosteroids may have had 100 or more transfusions, and hemosiderosis may result unless chelation therapy for excess iron is carried out appropriately. The liver and spleen enlarge, and secondary hypersplenism with leukopenia and thrombocytopenia may occur in children who do not receive adequate chelation or in those with chronic hepatitis acquired from transfusions. The complications of chronic transfusions are similar to those in β-thalassemia major, and prevention and treatment of iron overload should be equally aggressive in both groups of transfused patients (see Chapter 468.9).

TREATMENT. Corticosteroid therapy is frequently beneficial if begun early; three fourths of patients respond initially. The mechanism of its effect is unknown.

Prednisone in three or four divided doses totaling 2 mg/kg/24 hr is used as an initial trial. RBC precursors appear in bone marrow 1–3 wk after therapy is begun, and then normoblastosis and a brisk peripheral reticulocytosis occur. The hemoglobin may reach normal levels in 4–6 wk. The dose of corticosteroid may then be reduced gradually by tapering divided doses and then by eliminating all except a single, lowest effective daily dose. This dose should then be doubled, used on alternate days, and tapered still further while maintaining the hemoglobin level at 10 g/dL or above. In some patients, very small amounts of prednisone, as low as 2.5 mg, may be sufficient to sustain adequate erythropoiesis.

In patients who do not respond to corticosteroid therapy, transfusions at intervals of 4–8 wk are necessary to sustain life. Chelation therapy for iron overload with deferoxamine administered subcutaneously via a battery-powered portable pump should be begun when excess iron accumulation is reflected by serum ferritin levels exceeding 1,000 mg/dL, but preferably after 5 yr of age, because the medication may interfere with normal growth. An oral iron chelator, deferiprone

*Drs. Howard Pearson and James A. Stockman were authors of these sections in earlier editions. Their contributions are gratefully acknowledged.

(L1), is in clinical trials and may offer an alternative if it is shown to be effective and to have acceptable toxicity. Other therapies, including androgens, cyclosporine, cyclophosphamide, antithymocyte globulin (ATG), high-dose intravenous immunoglobulin, EPO, and interleukin-3 have not had a consistent beneficial effect and may have a high incidence of side effects. High-dose methylprednisolone (30–100 mg/kg/24 hr; tapered after 3 days) has been beneficial in some patients. Splenectomy may decrease the need for transfusion if hypersplenism or isoimmunization has developed. Bone marrow transplantation has a role in children who do not respond to corticosteroids and who have a histocompatible donor. The rate of engraftment is high, providing further evidence that immunosuppression is not the primary cause of this disorder. Transplantation of umbilical cord cells from an HLA-compatible newborn sibling has resulted in successful hematopoietic reconstitution.

454.1. Pearson Marrow-Pancreas Syndrome

This form of congenital hypoplastic anemia may be initially confused with Diamond-Blackfan syndrome or transient erythroblastopenia of childhood. The marrow failure usually appears in the neonatal period and is characterized by a macrocytic anemia, elevated Hb F and RBC adenosine deaminase, vacuolated erythroblasts and myeloblasts in the marrow, and occasional neutropenia and thrombocytopenia. Filgrastim (G-CSF) may reverse episodes of severe neutropenia. Other features are failure to thrive, insulin-dependent diabetes mellitus, and exocrine dysfunction due to fibrosis of the pancreas, lactic acidosis, renal Fanconi syndrome with vacuolated tubular cells, muscle and neurologic impairment, and, frequently, early death. This multiorgan disorder is due to mitochondrial DNA (mtDNA) deletions, with heterogeneity in different tissues and between patients. The heterogeneity accounts for the variable clinical picture, and a change in proportions of mtDNA types in tissues over time may result in spontaneous improvement of RBC hypoproliferation.

CHAPTER 455
Acquired Pure Red Blood Cell Anemias

A number of forms of acquired anemia with reticulocytopenia and reduced red blood cell (RBC) precursors in the marrow have been described. Most of these are rare in childhood, and the causes of most of them are uncertain. In some cases in adults, remission has followed removal of a tumor of the thymus. Association with thymoma has been reported in a child. Autoantibodies against erythropoietin (EPO) have been described. The acquired pure RBC anemias may respond to therapy with corticosteroids, and a trial is indicated in any chronic case. High-dose intravenous immunoglobulin (IVIG) or antilymphocyte globulin has been used effectively in some adults and children. The presence of a complement-dependent antibody cytotoxic for erythroblasts in some adults, and rarely in children, has led to the use of other immunosuppressive therapy in some patients.

Large doses of chloramphenicol may inhibit erythropoiesis. Reticulocytopenia, erythroid hypoplasia, and vacuolated pronormoblasts in the marrow are reversible effects of this drug. This effect differs from the idiosyncratic and rare development of severe aplastic anemia in recipients of the drug.

Episodes of acute failure of erythropoiesis may follow various viral infections. Parvovirus B19 is the best documented viral cause of RBC aplasia (Chapter 244). This small, single-stranded DNA virus is the cause of fifth disease (erythema infectiosum), usually manifested in children by facial erythema and a maculopapular rash on the trunk and, occasionally, by joint pains or arthritis. It may also be associated with systemic necrotizing vasculitis in some children. The virus is particularly infective and cytotoxic for erythroid progenitor cells in the marrow, interacting specifically with the RBC P antigen as a receptor. Characteristic nuclear inclusions in erythroblasts and giant pronormoblasts can be seen with light microscopy of bone marrow. Hemophagocytosis may also be seen in the marrow, perhaps accounting for the occasional granulocytopenia and thrombocytopenia. Because infection with this virus is usually transient, with recovery usually occurring in less than 2 wk, anemia is not present or not noticed in otherwise normal children, in whom the life span of peripheral RBCs is 110–120 days. In patients with hemolysis, such as that due to hereditary spherocytosis or sickle cell disease, in whom RBC life span is much shorter, a cessation of erythropoiesis due to parvovirus infection may cause severe anemia, the "aplastic crisis" occurring in these diseases. Recovery from moderate to severe anemia is usually spontaneous, heralded by a wave of nucleated RBCs and subsequent reticulocytosis in the peripheral blood. An RBC transfusion may occasionally be necessary for marked symptoms due to anemia. Rarely, persistence of parvovirus infection may occur in patients unable to mount an adequate antibody response to the virus, as in children with congenital immunodeficiency diseases, those being treated with immunosuppressive agents, and those with AIDS. The resultant pure RBC aplasia may be severe. The viral infection in these chronically infected patients may be treated with high-dose IVIG, which contains neutralizing antibody to the virus. Different clinical manifestations of infection with this virus and destruction of erythroid precursors occur with infections in utero, in which there is increased fetal wastage in the first and second trimesters, and infants may be born with hydrops fetalis and viremia. Congenital infection may also cause congenital pure RBC aplasia due to induction of tolerance. The presence of persistent congenital parvovirus infection needs to be detected by examination of bone marrow DNA because immunologic tolerance to the virus may prevent the usual development of specific antibodies (Chapter 244).

Other viruses causing suppression of erythropoiesis usually affect the production of at least one other hematopoietic cell as well and may also cause increased destruction of peripheral blood cells by immunologic mechanisms. These include hepatitis virus (non-A, non-B, non-C), Epstein-Barr virus, cytomegalovirus, and HIV.

CHAPTER 456
Transient Erythroblastopenia of Childhood (TEC)

This syndrome of severe, transient hypoplastic anemia occurs mainly in previously healthy children between 6 mo and 3 yr of age, with most older than 12 mo at onset; it is more common than congenital hypoplastic anemia. The cause of this acquired decrease in red blood cell (RBC) production is not clear, although it frequently follows a viral illness. Parvovirus B19 infections, which may cause hypoplasia in children with hemolytic anemia, do not appear to be commonly associated with TEC. Human herpesvirus type 6 has been detected in some affected children. Reticulocytes and bone marrow erythroid precursors are markedly decreased, but neutropenia may occur and platelet numbers are usually normal. Mean corpuscular volume is usually normal for age, and fetal hemoglobin (HbF) levels are normal before the recovery phase. RBC adenosine deaminase (ADA) levels are normal in this disorder, whereas they may be elevated in congenital hypoplastic anemia. Differentiation from the latter disease may be difficult, but differences in age of onset and in age-related MCV, HbF, and ADA may be helpful.

Most children recover within 1–2 mo, and recurrence is rare. RBC transfusions may be necessary for severe anemia in the absence of signs of early recovery. The anemia develops slowly, and marked symptoms usually develop only with severe anemia. Corticosteroid therapy does not appear to be of any value in this disorder.

CHAPTER 457

Anemia of Chronic Disorders and Renal Disease

Anemia complicates a number of chronic systemic diseases associated with infection, inflammation, or tissue breakdown. Examples of such conditions include chronic pyogenic infections, such as bronchiectasis and osteomyelitis; chronic inflammatory processes, such as rheumatoid arthritis, systemic lupus erythematosus, and ulcerative colitis; malignancies; and advanced renal disease. In the latter, an additional major component is decreased production of erythropoietin (EPO) due to damage of the cells producing this cytokine. Despite diverse underlying causes, the erythroid abnormalities are similar. Red blood cell (RBC) life span is moderately decreased, reflecting increased RBC destruction by a hyperactive reticuloendothelial system. The increased hemolysis is less important, however, than a relative failure of bone marrow response, reflecting both hypoactivity of marrow and an EPO production inadequate for the degree of anemia. Another finding is abnormalities of iron metabolism, including defective iron release from tissues into the plasma. Suppression of the erythroid response in the marrow appears to result primarily from an increase in tumor necrosis factor (TNF), which acts on bone marrow stromal cells to produce interferon (IFN)-β as a primary mediator, and an increase in interleukin-1 (IL-1), which acts on T cells to produce IFN-γ as a primary mediator. IL-6 levels may also be elevated. Recombinant human EPO can overcome this effect if the EPO level in a patient is less than 500 mU/mL. TNF and IL-1 decrease EPO production in perfused kidneys and hepatoma cells, corresponding to the two sites of EPO production, accounting for the inadequate EPO response in this type of anemia. The specific stimulant of increased TNF and IL-1 production in these patients has not been identified.

CLINICAL MANIFESTATIONS. Although the important symptoms and signs are those of the underlying disease, the quality of life may be affected by the mild to moderate anemia present.

LABORATORY FINDINGS. Hemoglobin concentrations usually range from 6 to 9 g/dL. The anemia is usually normochromic and normocytic; about one third of patients may have modest hypochromia and microcytosis. Absolute reticulocyte counts are normal or low, and leukocytosis is common. Free erythrocyte protoporphyrin (FEP) levels are frequently elevated and provide a sensitive reflection of derangements of iron metabolism. They return to normal after successful treatment of the primary disease. The serum iron level is low, without the increase in total iron-binding capacity that occurs in iron deficiency. This pattern of low serum iron and low to normal iron-binding protein is a regular and valuable diagnostic feature. Serum ferritin level may be elevated. Serum transferrin receptor (TfR) level is normal, unless iron deficiency is present. The bone marrow has normal cellularity; the RBC precursors are low to adequate, marrow hemosiderin may be increased, and granulocytic hyperplasia may be present. A frequent clinical challenge is to identify concomitant iron deficiency in patients with an inflammatory disease. Measurement of TfR/ferritin ratio may be useful, because it is elevated when iron deficiency is present. A trial of iron therapy may resolve the issue, although there may be no response when inflammation due to the primary disease persists. Intravenous iron saccharate is effective in iron deficiency associated with juvenile rheumatoid arthritis.

TREATMENT AND PROGNOSIS. Because these anemias are secondary to other disease processes, they do not respond to iron or hematinics unless there is concomitant deficiency. Transfusions raise the hemoglobin concentration only temporarily and are rarely indicated. If the underlying systemic disease can be controlled, the anemia is corrected spontaneously. Recombinant human EPO can increase the hemoglobin level and improve activity and the sense of well-being in patients with cancer and end-stage renal failure and in those with anemia of chronic inflammation. Treatment with iron is usually necessary for an optimal EPO effect.

CHAPTER 458

Congenital Dyserythropoietic Anemias

These rare inherited normocytic or macrocytic anemias display multinuclearity and abnormal chromatin patterns in red blood cell (RBC) precursors. Three major types have been distinguished, with considerable variation within each type and overlap among them. Type I (about 15% of cases) is defined by binuclearity of erythroblast (<10%), thin internuclear chromatin bridges between separate erythroblasts, and megaloblastic morphology. RBCs are macrocytic. The genetic defect maps to chromosome 15q15.1–15.3. Type II (>60% of cases) has erythroblastic, multinuclearity (15–30%) and a positive acidified serum (Ham) test result, but only to 30% of normal sera. The sugar water test, frequently positive in paroxysmal nocturnal hemoglobinuria, when the Ham test is also positive, is negative in this disorder. RBCs in type II (HEMPAS: *h*ereditary *e*rythroblastic *m*ultinuclearity associated with a *p*ositive *a*cidified *s*erum lysis test) are strongly agglutinated by anti-i antibody. The defects in this variant involve abnormalities of glycosylation, including deficiencies of α-mannosidase II and *N*-acetyl-glucosaminyltransferase II, leading to abnormal oligosaccharides on RBC surface proteins. Types I and II appear to be inherited as autosomal recessive traits. Type III (<15% of cases) has pronounced erythroid multinuclearity. Linkage analysis of one large family suggests the defective gene is on chromosome 15q21–q25. It appears to be inherited as an autosomal dominant trait in some families. In each type there are variable degrees of anemia (occasionally presenting as hydrops fetalis, more commonly as neonatal anemia, or even as late as adolescence or adult life), ineffective erythropoiesis, and increased intestinal uptake of iron. Findings of chronic hemolysis, such as intermittent jaundice, gallstones, and splenomegaly, are common. Blood transfusions may occasionally be needed for severe anemia. Splenectomy may help patients with anemia severe enough to require chronic transfusions. Restriction of iron intake and iron chelation therapy should be of value in patients with iron overload.

CHAPTER 459
Physiologic Anemia of Infancy

Normal newborns have higher hemoglobin and hematocrit levels with larger red blood cells (RBCs) than older children and adults. Within the first week of life, a progressive decline in hemoglobin level begins and persists for approximately 6–8 wk. The result of this decline is generally referred to as *physiologic anemia of infancy.* Several factors are operative. First, erythropoiesis abruptly ceases with onset of respiration at birth, when the arterial oxygen saturation rises toward 95%. Concomitantly, levels of erythropoietin (EPO) are low, perhaps because the liver is the major site of EPO production in the neonatal period, rather than the kidneys, and because of the relative insensitivity of the liver to EPO release with tissue hypoxia. In addition, EPO has a decreased half-life and an increased volume of distribution in newborns. A shortened survival of the fetal RBCs also contributes to the development of physiologic anemia. Furthermore, the sizable expansion of blood volume that accompanies rapid weight gain during the first 3 mo of life adds to the need for increased RBC production. In addition, RBC function is influenced by the higher levels of serum phosphate in newborns than later on in infancy. RBC phosphate and 2,3-diphosphoglycerate (2,3-DPG) increase, facilitating release of oxygen from the normal adult hemoglobin (Hb A) that is present and decreasing tissue hypoxia. When the hemoglobin level has fallen to 9–11 g/dL at 2–3 mo of age in full-term infants, erythropoiesis resumes. This "anemia" should be viewed as a physiologic adaptation to extrauterine life.

Premature infants also develop a physiologic anemia. The same factors are operative as in term infants, but they are exaggerated. The decline in hemoglobin level is both more extreme and more rapid. Minimal hemoglobin levels of 7–9 g/dL commonly occur by 3–6 wk of age, and in very small premature infants levels may be even lower (Chapter 99).

In preterm infants, the inability to produce compensatory amounts of EPO accounts in part for the greater decline in hemoglobin concentrations, but frequent phlebotomies in sick infants for diagnostic and monitoring purposes, particularly in very small infants, are a major cause of anemia and the need for repeated transfusions. When premature infants are transfused with adult blood containing Hb A, the shift of the oxygen dissociation curve as a result of the presence of Hb A facilitates delivery of oxygen to the tissues. Accordingly, the definition of anemia and the need for transfusion in premature infants must be based not only on hemoglobin level but also on oxygen requirements and the ability of an infant's circulating hemoglobin to release oxygen.

The marginal erythropoietic equilibrium responsible for physiologic anemia can add to anemia accompanying processes with increased hemolysis, such as congenital hemolytic states, which may be associated with severe anemia in the early weeks of life. Late hyporegenerative anemia, with absence of reticulocytes, may occur in infants with rhesus factor (Rh) hemolytic disease, perhaps because of low serum EPO levels. Bone marrow hypoplasia may also follow intrauterine transfusions, also accompanied by low EPO levels. Some infants with bronchopulmonary dysplasia may develop anemia associated with deficient production of EPO, and a trial of EPO in such patients may be warranted.

Dietary factors may also aggravate physiologic anemia. Deficiency of folic acid superimposed on the physiologic process may result in more severe anemia. Vitamin E deficiency and therapy do not appear to have a role in anemia of prematurity, despite early suggestions to the contrary. A controlled and blinded study of oral vitamin E administration (25 IU/dL-α-tocopherol, colloidal aqueous solution) to infants less than 1,500 g showed no difference in hemoglobin levels, reticulocytes, RBC morphology, or platelet counts. Breast milk and modern formulas appear to provide adequate vitamin E. Oral vitamin C supplementation (50 mg/24 hr) does not cause hemolysis in premature infants. Supplemental iron starting at approximately 4 mg/kg/24 hr for preterm babies 4–8 wk old and by 4 mo in full-term infants should not cause significant hemolysis due to oxidation.

Unless perinatal blood loss has been significant, iron deficiency should not be considered as a cause of anemia in the first 3 mo of life. Assuming an infant is born with adequate iron stores, dietary iron deficiency cannot be a cause of anemia until these iron stores have been exhausted. In the absence of blood loss, this does not occur until the birthweight has approximately doubled.

TREATMENT. As a developmental process, physiologic anemia usually requires no therapy other than ensuring that the diet of the infant contains essential nutrients for normal hematopoiesis, especially folic acid and iron. Premature infants who are feeding well and growing normally rarely need transfusion unless iatrogenic blood loss has been significant. In otherwise healthy premature infants, hemoglobin levels as low as 6.5 g/dL are usually well tolerated. However, the optimal level of hematocrit for premature infants is not settled. Assessment of the overall clinical condition, including growth rate, and monitoring of hematocrit are the best guides to transfusion of RBCs. RBC transfusions do not appear to affect the course of apneic spells and bradycardia. When transfusions are necessary, a volume of RBCs about 10–15 mL/kg is recommended. The number of donors for an infant should be minimized. In early preterm infants (<1,250 g), the half-life of transfused RBCs is about 30 days. Anemia in very low birthweight preterm infants may be related to a relative deficiency of EPO, and clinical trials indicate that premature infants who do not have severe illnesses and are treated with recombinant human EPO and iron during the first 6 wk of life, at doses about 250 IU/kg three times per week subcutaneously and intravenous iron sucrose (6 mg/kg) weekly or oral iron sulphate (6 mg/kg/24 hr in 3 divided doses), require fewer transfusions. However, the cost of EPO treatment is higher than that of RBC transfusion.

CHAPTER 460
Megaloblastic Anemias

The megaloblastic anemias have in common certain abnormalities of red blood cell (RBC) morphology and maturation. The RBCs at every stage of development are larger than normal and have an open, finely dispersed nuclear chromatin and an asynchrony between maturation of nucleus and cytoplasm, with the delay in nuclear progression being more evident with further cell divisions. Megaloblastic morphology may be seen in a number of conditions; almost all cases in children result from a deficiency of folic acid, vitamin B_{12}, or both. Both substances are cofactors required in the synthesis of nucleoproteins, and deficiencies result in defective synthesis of DNA and, to a lesser extent, RNA and protein. Ineffective erythropoiesis results from arrest in development or premature death of cells in the marrow. In the peripheral blood, RBCs are large (increased mean corpuscular volume [MCV]) and frequently oval, hypersegmented neutrophils appear, and giant platelets may also be found. In the marrow, the late nucleated megaloblastic RBC may appear well hemoglobinized but still retains an immature nucleus rather than the usual clumped chromatin. Giant metamyelocytes and bands are also present in the marrow. Megaloblastic anemias due to malnutrition are relatively uncommon in the United States.

460.1 Folic Acid Deficiencies

MEGALOBLASTIC ANEMIA OF INFANCY

This disease is caused by a deficient intake or absorption of folic acid (see also Chapters 40 and 44.8). Folates are abundant in many foods, including green vegetables, fruits, and animal organs (liver, kidney). Folic acid is absorbed throughout the small intestine, after pteroylglutamate reacts with membrane-associated folate-binding proteins. Pteroylpolyglutamates, found in cabbage, lettuce, and other foods, are absorbed less efficiently than pteroylmonoglutamate (folic acid). Pteroly polyglutamate hydrolase activity in the brush border aids the conversion to the monoglutamate. Surgical removal or disorders of the small intestine may lead to folate deficiency. There is an active enterohepatic circulation. Much of the folate in the plasma is loosely bound to albumin. Pteroylglutamate is not biologically active. It is reduced by dihydrofolate reductase to tetrahydropteroylglutamate (tetrahydrofolate), which is transported into tissue cells and polyglutamated. Dietary deficiency is usually compounded by rapid growth or infection, which may increase folic acid requirements. The normal adult daily requirement is about 100 μg/24 hr, which rises to 350 μg/24 hr in pregnancy. The requirements on a weight basis are higher in the pediatric age range in comparison with adults owing to the increased needs of growth. The needs are also increased with accelerated tissue turnover, as in hemolytic anemia. Human and cow's milk provide adequate amounts of folic acid. Goat's milk is clearly deficient; folic acid supplementation must be given when it is the main food. Unless supplemented, powered milk may also be a poor source of folic acid.

CLINICAL MANIFESTATIONS. Mild megaloblastic anemia has been reported in very low birthweight infants, and routine folic acid supplementation is advised. Megaloblastic anemia has its peak incidence at 4–7 mo of age, somewhat earlier than iron deficiency anemia, although the two may be present concomitantly in infants with poor nutrition. Besides having the usual clinical features of anemia, affected infants with folate deficieny are irritable, fail to gain weight adequately, and have chronic diarrhea. Hemorrhages due to thrombocytopenia occur in advanced cases. Folic acid deficiency may accompany kwashiorkor, marasmus, or sprue.

LABORATORY FINDINGS. The anemia is macrocytic (MCV >100 fl). Variations in RBC shape and size are common (see Fig. 453-1*B*). The reticulocyte count is low, and nucleated RBCs demonstrating megaloblastic morphology are often seen in the blood. Neutropenia and thrombocytopenia may be present, particularly in long-standing deficiencies. The neutrophils are large, some with hypersegmented nuclei; more than 5% of neutrophils have five or more nuclear segments. Normal serum folic acid levels are 5–20 ng/mL; deficiency is accompanied by levels less than 3 ng/mL. Levels of RBC folate are a better indicator of chronic deficiency. The normal RBC folate level is 150–600 ng/mL of packed cells. Levels of iron and vitamin B_{12} in serum are usually normal or elevated. Serum activity of lactic acid dehydrogenase (LDH) is markedly elevated. The bone marrow is hypercellular because of erythroid hyperplasia. Megaloblastic changes are prominent, although some normal RBC precursors may also be found. Large, abnormal neutrophilic forms (giant metamyelocytes) with cytoplasmic vacuolation are seen, as well as hypersegmentation of the nuclei of megakaryocytes.

TREATMENT. When the diagnosis is established or in severely ill children, folic acid may be administered orally or parenterally in a dose of 1–5 mg/24 hr. If the specific diagnosis is in doubt, 50–100 μg/24 hr of folate may be used for a week as a diagnostic test, or 1 μg/24 hr of cyanocobalamin parenterally for suspected vitamin B_{12} dificiency. Because a hematologic response can be expected within 72 hr, transfusions are indicated only when the anemia is severe or the child is very ill. Folic acid therapy should be continued for 3–4 wk. If juvenile pernicious anemia is present or if the anemia recurs after therapy, the prolonged use of folic acid should be avoided, because in pernicious anemia folic acid may produce a partial response to the anemia without decreasing the neurologic abnormalities.

MEGALOBLASTIC ANEMIA OF PREGNANCY

Folate requirements increase markedly during pregnancy, in part to meet fetal needs. Decreases in serum and RBC folate levels occur in as many as 25% of pregnant women at term and may be aggravated by infection. Folate supplementation of at least 400 μg/24 hr is recommended from the start of pregnancy to prevent neural tube defects and to meet growth needs. Mothers with folate deficiency may have babies with normal folate stores owing to selective transfer of folate to the fetus via placental folate receptors.

FOLIC ACID DEFICIENCY IN MALABSORPTION SYNDROMES

Diffuse inflammatory or degenerative disease of the intestine may reduce intestinal pteroylpolyglutamate hydrolase activity as well as markedly impair absorption of folate. Celiac disease, chronic infectious enteritis, and enteroenteric fistulas may lead to folic acid dificiency and megaloblastic anemia. Measurement of serum folate is used to assess small intestinal absorptive functions in malabsorptive disorders. Oral folic acid supplements of 1 mg/24 hr may be indicated in these states (see Chapter 340).

CONGENITAL FOLATE MALABSORPTION

An autosomal recessive defect in the intestinal absorption of folic acid and an associated inability to transfer folate from the plasma to the central nervous system has been associated with megaloblastic anemia, convulsions, mental retardation, and cerebral calcifications. Infants present at 2–3 mo of age with severe megaloblastic anemia. Early and intensive treatment with intramuscular folinic acid (5-formyltetrahydrofolate) is important to correct the hematologic defect and to try to prevent neurologic deterioration.

FOLIC ACID DEFICIENCY ASSOCIATED WITH ANTICONVULSANTS AND OTHER DRUGS

Many patients have low serum levels of folic acid during therapy with certain anticonvulsant drugs (e.g., phenytoin, primidone, phenobarbital), but they usually do not develop anemia. Frank megaloblastic anemia is rare and responds to folic acid therapy, even if administration of the offending drug is continued. Absorption of folic acid is impaired by anticonvulsant drugs, but increased use of folate also occurs. Megaloblastic anemia has occurred in users of oral contraceptives, but the cause is not clear.

A number of drugs have antifolic acid activity as their primary pharmacologic effect and regularly produce megaloblastic anemia. Methotrexate binds to dihydrofolate reductase and prevents formation of tetrahydrofolate, the active form. Pyrimethamine, used in the therapy of toxoplasmosis, and trimethoprim, used for treatment of various infections, may induce folic acid deficiency and, occasionally, megaloblastic anemia. Therapy with folinic acid (5-formyltetrahydrofolate) is usually beneficial.

CONGENITAL DIHYDROFOLATE REDUCTASE DEFICIENCY

This has been reported in several patients who were unable to form biologically active tetrahydrofolate and who developed severe megaloblastic anemia in early infancy. These patients were successfully treated with large doses of folic acid or folinic acid. Deficiency of methylene tetrahydrofolate reductase has been described in some patients with homocystinuria without hematologic abnormalities.

460.2 Vitamin B_{12} (Cobalamin) Deficiency

Vitamin B_{12} is derived from cobalamin in food, mainly animal sources, secondary to production by microorganisms. Humans cannot synthesize vitamin B_{12}. The cobalamins are released in the acidity of the stomach and combine there with R proteins and intrinsic factor (IF), traverse the duodenum, where pancreatic proteases break down the R proteins, and are absorbed in the distal ileum via specific receptors for IF-cobalamin. In addition, some vitamin B_{12} from large doses may diffuse through mucosa in the intestine and mouth. In plasma, vitamin B_{12} is bound to transcobalamin (TC) II, the physiologically important transporter, as well as to TCI and TCIII. TCII-cobalamin enters cells by receptor-mediated endocytosis, and cobalamin is converted to active forms (methylcobalamin and adenosylcobalamin) important in the transfer of methyl groups and DNA synthesis.

Vitamin B_{12} deficiency may therefore result from inadequate intake, surgery involving the stomach or terminal ileum, lack of secretion of IF by the stomach, consumption or inhibition of the B_{12}-IF complex, abnormalities involving the receptor sites in the terminal ileum, or abnormalities of TCII. Although TCI binds 80% of serum cobalamin, a deficiency of this protein results in low serum B_{12} levels but not in megaloblastic anemia (see Chapter 44.2).

Because vitamin B_{12} is present in many foods, dietary deficiency is rare. It may occur in cases of extreme dietary restriction (strict vegetarians: "vegans") in which no animal products are consumed. Vitamin B_{12} dificiency is not common in kwashiorkor or infantile marasmus. Cases occur in breast-fed infants whose mothers have deficient diets or pernicious anemia.

JUVENILE PERNICIOUS ANEMIA

This rare autosomal recessive disorder results from an inability to secrete gastric IF or secretion of a functionally abnormal IF. It differs from the typical disease in adults in that the stomach secretes acid normally and is histologically normal.

CLINICAL MANIFESTATIONS. The symptoms of juvenile pernicious anemia become prominent at 9 mo–11 yr of age. This interval is consistent with exhaustion of the stores of vitamin B_{12} acquired in utero. As the anemia becomes severe, weakness, irritability, anorexia, and listlessness occur. The tongue is smooth, red, and painful. Neurologic manifestations include ataxia, paresthesias, hyporeflexia, Babinski responses, clonus, and coma.

LABORATORY FINDINGS. The anemia is macrocytic, with prominent macro-ovalocytosis of the RBCs (see Fig. 453–1*B*). The neutrophils may be large and hypersegmented. In advanced cases, neutropenia and thrombocytopenia, simulating aplastic anemia or leukemia, occur. Serum vitamin B_{12} levels are less than 100 pg/mL. Concentrations of serum iron and serum folic acid are normal or elevated. Serum LDH activity is markedly increased. Moderate elevations (2–3 mg/dL) of serum bilirubin levels may be found. Excessive excretion of methylmalonic acid in the urine (normal amount, 0–3.5 mg/24 hr) is a reliable and sensitive index of vitamin B_{12} deficiency. In contrast to many adult cases with pernicious anemia, serum antibodies directed against parietal cells or intrinsic factor cannot be detected in children with this disorder. Gastric acidity may be reduced initially but returns to normal when vitamin B_{12} therapy is instituted if activity is absent in gastric secretion.

Absorption of vitamin B_{12} is usually assessed by the Schilling test. When a normal person ingests a small amount of vitamin B_{12} into which ^{57}Co has been incorporated, the radioactive vitamin combines with the IF in stomach secretions and passes to the terminal ileum, where absorption occurs. Because the absorbed vitamin is bound to TCII and incorporated into tissues, little or none is normally excreted in the urine. If a large dose (1 mg) of nonradioactive vitamin B_{12} is injected parenterally after 2 hr ("flushing dose"), 10–30% of the previously absorbed radioactive vitamin appears in the urine in 24 hr. Children with pernicious anemia usually excrete 2% or less under these conditions. To confirm that absence of IF is the basis of the B_{12} malabsorption, 30 mg of IF is given with a second dose of radioactive vitamin B_{12}. Normal amounts of radioactive vitamin should now be absorbed and flushed out in the urine. On the other hand, when vitamin B_{12} malabsorption results from absence of ileal receptor sites or other intestinal causes, no improvement in absorption occurs with IF. The Schilling test result remains abnormal in pernicious anemia, even when therapy has completely reversed the hematologic and neurologic manifestations of the disease.

TREATMENT. A prompt hematologic response follows parenteral administration of vitamin B_{12} (1 mg), usually with reticulocytosis in 2–4 days, unless there is concurrent inflammatory disease. The physiologic requirement for vitamin B_{12} is 1–5 μg/24 hr, and hematologic responses have been observed with these small doses, indicating that administration of a minidose may be used as a therapeutic test when the diagnosis of vitamin B_{12} deficiency is in doubt. If there is evidence of neurologic involvement, 1 mg should be injected intramuscularly daily for at least 2 wk. Maintenance therapy is necessary throughout a patient's life; monthly intramuscular administration of 1 mg of vitamin B_{12} is sufficient. Oral therapy may succeed because of mucosal diffusion with high doses, but it is not generally advisable owing to uncertainty of absorption.

TRANSCOBALAMIN DEFICIENCY

TCII is the principal physiologic transport vehicle for vitamin B_{12}. The role of TCII in B_{12} transport is similar to that of transferrin (Tf) for iron; specific receptors for TCII and Tf exist on cells needing vitamin B_{12} or iron. A congenital deficiency is inherited as an autosomal recessive condition, with failure to absorb and transport vitamin B_{12}. Most patients lack TCII, but some have functionally defective forms. Severe megaloblastic anemia occurs in early infancy. Therapy requires massive parenteral doses of vitamin B_{12}.

VITAMIN B_{12} MALABSORPTION DUE TO INTESTINAL CAUSES

Cases have been reported of familial occurrence of absence or defect of the receptor for IF-B_{12} in the terminal ileum, in some instances associated with proteinuria *(Imerslund-Grasbeck syndrome)*. Decreased receptor activity may be detected in the urine of affected patients by a radioisotope binding assay. Histology of the stomach is normal, and IF and acid are present in gastric secretions. This autosomal recessive disorder is due to defects in the CUBN gene on chromosome 10p12.1, resulting in decreased expression of the IF-B_{12} receptor, cubilin. Parenteral treatment with vitamin B_{12} monthly corrects the deficiency.

Surgical resection of the terminal ileum, inflammatory diseases such as regional enteritis, neonatal necrotizing enterocolitis, and tuberculosis may also impair absorption of vitamin B_{12}. When the terminal ileum has been removed, lifelong parenteral administration should be used if the Schilling test indicates that vitamin B_{12} is not absorbed.

An overgrowth of intestinal bacteria within diverticula or duplications of the small intestine may cause vitamin B_{12} deficiency by consumption of or competition for the vitamin or by splitting of its complex with IF. In these cases, hematologic response may follow appropriate antibiotic therapy. Similar mechanisms may operate when the fish tapeworm *Diphyllobothrium latum* infests the upper small intestine. When megaloblastic anemia occurs in these situations, the serum vitamin B_{12} level is low, the gastric juice contains intrinsic factor, and the abnormal Schilling test result is not corrected by addition of exogenous IF.

VITAMIN B_{12} DEFICIENCY IN OLDER CHILDREN

In some cases of vitamin B_{12} malabsorption in adolescence, atrophy of the gastric mucosa and achlorhydria have been noted. These cases may be related to the syndrome of malabsorption of vitamin B_{12} occurring in combination with cutaneous candidiasis, hypoparathyroidism, and other endocrine deficiencies. The serum contains antibodies against IF and parietal cells. An abnormal Schilling result is corrected by addition of exogenous IF. Parenteral vitamin B_{12} should be administered regularly to these patients.

460.3 Rare Megaloblastic Anemias

Oroticaciduria is a rare genetically determined defect in pyrimidine biosynthesis associated with severe megaloblastic anemia, neutropenia, failure to thrive, and crystalluria, caused by excretion of orotic acid (Chapter 86). Physical and mental retardation are frequently present. The anemia is refractory to vitamin B_{12} or folic acid but responds promptly to administration of the pyrimidine uridine (100–150 μg/kg/24 hr). The basic defects, which involve many tissues, include deficiencies of orotate phosphoribosyltransferase and orotidine-5-phosphate decarboxylase, enzymes essential for formation of uridine-5′-phosphate. Inheritance is autosomal recessive. Megaloblastic anemia can also occur in the *Lesch-Nyhan syndrome*, in which regeneration of purine nucleotides is blocked (Chapter 86).

Cases of *thiamine-responsive* and *thiamine-dependent megaloblastic anemia* have been reported. Administration of thiamine, 100 mg/24 hr, produced a brisk reticulocyte response and a sustained increase in hemoglobin level. Sensorineural deafness and diabetes mellitus were associated.

Megaloblastic anemia has also been encountered in a group of children with inability to convert cobalamin to its biologically active metabolites, adenosylcobalamin and methylocabalamin, perhaps because of a deficiency in a cobalamin reductase. There are seven types of cobalamin (cbl) defects; cbl A to cbl G are based on complemention groups. The methionine synthase gene appears to have mutations in cbl G. These disorders are characterized by neurologic abnormalities and either methylmalonic aciduria, homocystinuria, or both. Abnormalities are usually noted in the early weeks of life and include failure to thrive, lethargy, hypotonia, macrocytosis with megaloblastic bone marrow changes and anemia or pancytopenia, and hepatic dysfunction. The megaloblastic changes may reverse and other symptoms may improve with hydroxycobalamin treatment, 1 mg/24 hr IM initially, gradually changed to a dose 2 to 3 times per wk up to once a month.

CHAPTER 461
Iron Deficiency Anemia

Anemia resulting from lack of sufficient iron for synthesis of hemoglobin is the most common hematologic disease of infancy and childhood. Its frequency is related to certain basic aspects of iron metabolism and nutrition. The body of a newborn infant contains about 0.5 g of iron, whereas the adult content is estimated at 5 g. To make up for this discrepancy, an average of 0.8 mg of iron must be absorbed each day during the first 15 yr of life. In addition to this growth requirement, a small amount is necessary to balance normal losses of iron by shedding of cells. Accordingly, to maintain positive iron balance in childhood, about 1 mg of iron must be absorbed each day.

Iron is absorbed in the proximal small intestine, mediated in part by duodenal proteins (HFE, hephaestin, Nramp[2], and mobilferrin). Because absorption of dietary iron is assumed to be about 10%, a diet containing 8–10 mg of iron daily is necessary for optimal nutrition. Iron is absorbed two to three times more efficiently from human milk than from cow's milk, perhaps partly because of differences in calcium content. Breast-fed infants may, therefore, require less iron from other foods. During the first years of life, because relatively small quantities of iron-rich foods are eaten, it is often difficult to attain sufficient iron. For this reason, the diet should include such foods as infant cereals or formulas that have been fortified with iron; both of these are very effective in preventing iron deficiency. Formulas with 7–12 mg Fe/L for full-term infants and premature infant formulas with 15 mg/L for infants less than 1,800 g at birth are effective. Infants breast-fed exclusively should receive iron supplementation from 4 mo of age. At best, an infant is in a precarious situation with respect to iron. Should the diet become inadequate or external blood loss occur, anemia ensues rapidly.

Adolescents are also susceptible to iron deficiency because of high requirements due to the growth spurt, dietary deficiencies, and menstrual blood loss. In the United States, about 9% of 1–2 yr-olds are iron deficient; 3% have anemia. Of adolescent girls, 9% are iron deficient and 2% have anemia. In boys, a 50% decrease in stored iron occurs as puberty progresses.

ETIOLOGY. Low birthweight and unusual perinatal hemorrhage are associated with decreases in neonatal hemoglobin mass and stores of iron. As the high hemoglobin concentration of the newborn falls during the first 2–3 mo of life, considerable iron is reclaimed and stored (Chapter 99). These reclaimed stores are usually sufficient for blood formation in the first 6–9 mo of life in term infants. In low birthweight infants or those with perinatal blood loss, stored iron may be depleted earlier, and dietary sources become of paramount importance. Anemia caused solely by inadequate dietary iron is unusual before 4–6 mo but becomes common at 9–24 mo of age. Thereafter, it is relatively infrequent. The usual dietary pattern observed in infants with iron deficiency anemia is consumption of large amounts of cow's milk and of foods not supplemented with iron.

Blood loss must be considered a possible cause in every case of iron deficiency anemia, particularly in older children. Chronic iron deficiency anemia from occult bleeding may be caused by a lesion of the gastrointestinal (GI) tract, such as a peptic ulcer, Meckel's diverticulum, a polyp, or hemangioma, or by inflammatory bowel disease. In some geographic areas, hookworm infestation is an important cause of iron deficiency. Pulmonary hemosiderosis may be associated with unrecognized bleeding in the lungs and recurrent iron deficiency after treatment with iron. Chronic diarrhea in early childhood may be associated with considerable unrecognized blood loss. Some infants with severe iron deficiency in the United States have chronic intestinal blood loss induced by exposure to a heat-labile protein in whole cow's milk. Loss of blood in the stools each day can be prevented either by reducing the quantity of whole cow's milk to 1 pint/24 hr or less, by using heated or evaporated milk, or by feeding a milk substitute. This GI reaction is not related to enzymatic abnormalities in the mucosa, such as lactase deficiency, or to typical "milk allergy." Involved infants characteristically develop anemia that is more severe and occurs earlier than would be expected simply from an inadequate intake of iron.

Histologic abnormalities of the mucosa of the GI tract, such as blunting of the villi, are present in advanced iron deficiency anemia and may cause leakage of blood and decreased absorption of iron, further compounding the problem.

Intense exercise conditioning, as occurs in competitive athletics in high school, may result in iron depletion in girls; this occurs less commonly in boys.

CLINICAL MANIFESTATIONS. Pallor is the most important clue to iron deficiency. Blue scleras are also common, although also found in normal infants. In mild to moderate iron deficiency (hemoglobin levels of 6–10 g/dL), compensatory mechanisms, including increased levels of 2,3-diphosphoglycerate (2,3-DPG) and a shift of the oxygen dissociation curve, may be so effective that few symptoms of anemia are noted, although affected children may be irritable. Pagophagia, the desire to ingest unusual substances such as ice or dirt, may be present. In some children, ingestion of lead-containing substances may lead to concomitant plumbism. When the hemoglobin level falls below 5 g/dL, irritability and anorexia are prominent. Tachycardia and cardiac dilation occur, and systolic murmurs are often present.

The spleen is enlarged to palpation in 10–15% of patients. In long-standing cases, widening of the diploë of the skull similar to that in congenital hemolytic anemias may occur. These changes resolve slowly with adequate replacement therapy. Children with iron deficiency anemia may be obese or may be underweight, with other evidence of poor nutrition. The irritability and anorexia characteristic of advanced cases may reflect deficiency in tissue iron, because with iron therapy striking improvement in behavior frequently occurs before significant hematologic improvement.

Iron deficiency may have effects on neurologic and intellectual function. A number of reports suggest that iron deficiency anemia, and even iron deficiency without significant anemia, affects attention span, alertness, and learning of both infants and adolescents. In a controlled trial, adolescent girls with serum ferritin levels of 12 ng/L or less but without anemia improved verbal learning and memory after taking iron for 8 wk.

Monoamine oxidase (MAO), an iron-dependent enzyme, has a crucial role in neurochemical reactions in the central nervous system. Iron deficiency produces decreases in the activities of enzymes such as catalase and cytochromes. Catalase and peroxidase contain iron, but their biologic essentiality is not well established. Iron deficiency causes rigidity of red blood cells (RBCs) and may be associated with stroke in young children. Administration of iron may decrease the frequency of breath-holding spells, suggesting a role for iron deficiency or anemia.

LABORATORY FINDINGS. In progressive iron deficiency, a sequence of biochemical and hematologic events occurs. First, the tissue iron stores represented by bone marrow hemosiderin disappear. The level of serum ferritin, an iron-storage protein, provides a relatively accurate estimate of body iron stores in the absence of inflammatory disease. Normal ranges are age dependent, and decreased levels accompany iron deficiency. Next, serum iron level decreases (also age dependent), the iron-binding capacity of the serum increases, and the percent saturation falls below normal (also varies with age). When the availability of iron becomes rate limiting for hemoglobin synthesis, a moderate accumulation of heme precursors, free erythrocyte protoporphyrins (FEP), results.

As the deficiency progresses, the RBCs become smaller than normal and their hemoglobin content decreases. The morphologic characteristics of RBCs are best quantified by the determination of mean corpuscular hemoglobin (MCH) and mean corpuscular volume (MCV). Developmental changes in MCV require the use of age-related standards for diagnosis of microcytosis (see Table 453–1). With increasing deficiency, the RBCs become deformed and misshapen and present characteristic microcytosis, hypochromia, poikilocytosis, and increased RBC distribution width (RDW); see Fig. 453–1*C*). The reticulocyte percentage may be normal or moderately elevated, but absolute reticulocyte counts indicate an insufficient response to anemia. Nucleated RBCs may occasionally be seen in the peripheral blood. White blood cell counts are normal. Thrombocytosis, sometimes of a striking degree (600,000–1,000,000/mm^3), may occur or, in a few cases, thrombocytopenia. The mechanisms of these platelet abnormalities are not clear. They appear to be a direct consequence of iron deficiency, perhaps with associated GI blood loss or associated folate deficiency, and they return to normal with iron therapy and dietary change. The bone marrow is hypercellular, with erythroid hyperplasia. The normoblasts may have scanty, fragmented cytoplasm with poor hemoglobinization. Leukocytes and megakaryocytes are normal. Hemosiderin cannot be demonstrated in marrow specimens by Prussian blue staining. In about a third of cases, occult blood can be detected in the stools.

DIFFERENTIAL DIAGNOSIS (see Table 453–2). Iron deficiency must be differentiated from other hypochromic microcytic anemias. In lead poisoning associated with iron deficiency, the RBCs are morphologically similar, but coarse basophilic stippling of the RBCs, an artifact of drying the slide, is frequently prominent. Elevations of blood lead, FEP, and urinary coproporphyrin levels are seen (Chapter 721). The blood changes of β-thalassemia trait resemble those of iron deficiency (Chapter 468.9), but RDW is usually normal or only slightly elevated. α-Thalassemia trait occurs in about 3% of blacks in the United States and in many Southeast Asian peoples. The diagnosis requires direct identification of DNA defects or difficult globin synthesis studies after the newborn period. The diagnosis can be assumed when a patient having familial hypochromic microcytic anemia with normal iron studies, including ferritin, has normal levels of Hb A2 and Hb F and normal hemoglobin electrophoresis. In the newborn period, infants with α-thalassemia trait have 3–10% Bart hemoglobin and the MCV is decreased (Chapter 468.9). Thalassemia major, with its pronounced erythroblastosis and hemolytic component, should present no diagnostic confusion. Hb H disease, a form of α-thalassemia with hypochromia and microcytosis, also has a hemolytic component due to instability of the β-chain tetramers resulting from a deficiency of α globin. The RBC morphology of chronic inflammation and infection, though usually normocytic, may be microcytic, but in these conditions both the serum iron level and iron-binding ability are reduced and serum ferritin levels are normal or elevated. The serum transferrin receptor (TfR) level is useful in the distinction between iron deficiency anemia and anemia of chronic disease, because it is not affected by inflammation. The concentration is elevated in iron deficiency and within the normal range in anemia of chronic disease. An elevation of the TfR/log ferritin ratio is especially sensitive in detecting iron deficiency anemia. Elevations of FEP are not specific to iron deficiency and are observed in patients with lead poisoning, chronic hemolytic anemia, anemia associated with chronic disorders, and some of the porphyrias.

TREATMENT. The regular response of iron deficiency anemia to adequate amounts of iron is an important diagnostic and therapeutic feature. Oral administration of simple ferrous salts (sulfate, gluconate, fumarate) provides inexpensive and satisfactory therapy. No evidence shows that addition of any trace metal, vitamin, or other hematinic substance significantly increases the response to simple ferrous salts. For routine clinical use, physicians should be familiar with an inexpensive preparation of one of the simple ferrous compounds. The therapeutic dose should be calculated in terms of elemental iron; ferrous sulfate is 20% elemental iron by weight. A daily total of 6 mg/kg of elemental iron in three divided doses provides an optimal amount of iron for the stimulated bone marrow to use. Intolerance to oral iron is uncommon in children. A parenteral iron preparation (iron dextran) is an effective form of iron and is usually safe when given in a properly calculated dose, but the response to parenteral iron is no more rapid or complete than that obtained with proper oral administration of iron, unless malabsorption is a factor.

While adequate iron medication is given, the family must be educated about the patient's diet, and the consumption of milk should be limited to a reasonable quantity, preferably 500 mL (1 pint)/24 hr or less. This reduction has a dual effect: The amount of iron-rich foods is increased, and blood loss from intolerance to cow's milk proteins is reduced. When the reeducation of child and parent is not successful, parenteral iron medication may be indicated. Iron deficiency can be prevented in high-risk populations by providing iron-fortified formula or cereals during infancy.

The expected clinical and hematologic responses to iron therapy are described in Table 461–1.

Within 72–96 hr after administration of iron to an anemic child, peripheral reticulocytosis is noted. The height of this response is inversely proportional to the severity of the anemia. Reticulocytosis is followed by a rise in the hemoglobin level, which may increase as much as 0.5 g/dL/24 hr. Iron medication should be continued for 8 wk after blood values are normal. Failures of iron therapy occur when a child does not receive the prescribed medication, when iron is given in a form that is poorly absorbed, or when there is continuing unrecognized blood loss, such as intestinal or pulmonary loss, or with menstrual periods. An incorrect original diagnosis of nutritional iron deficiency may be revealed by therapeutic failure of iron medication.

TABLE 461–1 Responses to Iron Therapy in Iron Deficiency Anemia

Time After Iron Administration	Response
12–24 hr	Replacement of intracellular iron enzymes; subjective improvement; decreased irritability; increased appetite
36–48 hr	Initial bone marrow response; erythroid hyperplasia
48–72 hr	Reticulocytosis, peaking at 5–7 days
4–30 days	Increase in hemoglobin level
1–3 mo	Repletion of stores

Because a rapid hematologic response can be confidently predicted in typical iron deficiency, blood transfusion is indicated only when the anemia is very severe or when superimposed infection may interfere with the response. It is not necessary to attempt rapid correction of severe anemia by transfusion; the procedure may be dangerous because of associated hypervolemia and cardiac dilatation. Packed or sedimented RBCs should be administered slowly in an amount sufficient to raise the hemoglobin to a safe level at which the response to iron therapy can be awaited. In general, severely anemic children with hemoglobin values less than 4 g/dL should be given only 2–3 mL/kg of packed cells at any one time (furosemide may also be administered as a diuretic). If there is evidence of frank congestive heart failure, a modified exchange transfusion using fresh-packed RBCs should be considered, although diuretics followed by slow infusion of packed RBCs may suffice.

CHAPTER 462
Other Microcytic Anemias

SIDEROBLASTIC ANEMIAS

The sideroblastic anemias are a heterogeneous group of hypochromic microcytic anemias whose basic defects may be abnormalities of heme metabolism. Serum iron levels are increased. In the bone marrow, ringed sideroblasts are found; these are nucleated red blood cells (RBCs) with a perinuclear collar of coarse hemosiderin granules that represent iron-laden mitochondria.

Pearson syndrome, a combination of refractory sideroblastic anemia with vacuolation of marrow precursor cells and exocrine pancreatic dysfunction, is caused by various deletions in mitochondrial DNA (Chapter 454.1). Acquired sideroblastic anemias occur in adults with various inflammatory and malignant processes or with alcoholism, but some of these anemias that first appear in adults may be due to a genetic defect in erythroid 5-aminolevulinate synthase (ALS2). In two adult patients, different point mutations were found in mitochondrial subunit I of cytochrome C oxidase.

A form of sideroblastic anemia transmitted as an X-linked recessive trait usually becomes symptomatic by late childhood. Splenomegaly is usually present. Free erythrocyte protoporphyrin (FEP) levels are not elevated. Some cases of sideroblastic anemia are responsive to pyridoxine (vitamin B_6) given in doses of 200–300 mg/24 hr, although other findings of vitamin B_6 deficiency are not observed. In one kindred with *X-linked pyridoxine-responsive sideroblastic anemia*, a thr-to-ser substitution was identified at amino acid residue 388 of ALS2, near the pyridoxal phosphate cofactor binding site, affecting heme precursor synthesis. Other pyridoxine-responsive kindreds had amino acid substitutions at positions 125, 172, 299, and 426, with decreased enzyme activity. In a pyridoxine-refractory patient, a position 190 asp-to-val mutation affecting proteolytic processing of the ALS2 precursor was found. In another kindred, with a son and daughter with *pyridoxine-refractory sideroblastic anemia*, the children each received a different X chromosome, indicating an autosomal defect.

LEAD POISONING (See Chapter 721)

RARE TYPES OF HYPOCHROMIC MICROCYTIC ANEMIA

Isolated cases of hypochromic microcytic anemia with other abnormalities of iron metabolism are known; some cases have had defects in iron mobilization or reutilization. *Congenital absence of iron-binding protein* (atransferrinemia) is associated with severe hypochromic anemia despite iron overload and requires infusions of apo-transferrin and iron chelation therapy, although the latter may be avoided if the transferrin infusions are started early. Iron is absorbed normally and is deposited in the visceral organs rather than in bone marrow.

Several patients have had refractory hypochromic anemia associated with lymphatic tumors or lymphoid hyperplasia. Correction of the anemia followed removal of the abnormal lymphatic tissue in these patients. (See also Chapter 455.)

Families with several siblings having hypochromic microcytic anemia and deficient iron absorption have been described. These families resemble the mK/mK defect in mice, who have defects in iron absorption and erythroid iron utilization. The abnormalities in mice are due to a missence mutation in $Nramp^2$, which may be a major cellular iron transporter.

General

Hoffman R, Benz EJ, Shattil SJ, et al: Hematology: Basic Principles and Practices, 3rd ed. New York, Churchill Livingstone, 1999.

Miller DR, Baehner RL: Blood Diseases of Infancy and Childhood, 7th ed. St. Louis, CV Mosby, 1995.

Nathan DG, Orkin SH: Nathan and Oski's Hematology of Infancy and Childhood, 5th ed. Philadelphia, WB Saunders, 1998.

Williams WJ, Beutler E, Erslev AJ, Lichtman MA: Hematology, 4th ed. New York, McGraw-Hill, 1990.

Pure RBC Anemias

Ball SE, McGuckin, CP, Jenkins, G, et al: Diamond-Blackfan anaemia in the U.K.: Analysis of 80 cases from a 20-year birth cohort. Br J Haematol 94:645, 1996.

Bernini JC, Carrillo JM, Buchanan GR: High-dose intravenous methylprednisolone therapy for patients with Diamond-Blackfan anemia refractory to conventional doses of prednisone. J Pediatr 127:654, 1995.

Cherrick I, Karayalcin G, Lanzkowsky P: Transient erythroblastopenia of childhood. Am J Pediatr Hematol Oncol 16:320, 1994.

Gustavsson P, Willig TN, van Haeringen A, et al: Diamond-Blackfan anaemia: Genetic homogeneity for a gene on chromosome 19q13 restricted to 1.8 Mb. Nature Genet 16:368, 1997.

Özsoylu S: High-dose intravenous corticosteroid treatment for patients with Diamond-Blackfan syndrome resistant or refractory to conventional treatment. Am J Pediatr Hematol Oncol 10:217, 1988.

Marks PW, Mitus AJ: Congenital dyserythropoietic anemias. Am J Hematol 51:55, 1996.

Anemia of Chronic Disease

Cazzola M, Ponchio L, de Benedetti F, et al: Defective iron supply for erythropoiesis and adequate endogenous erythropoietin production in the anemia associated with systemic-onset juvenile chronic arthritis. Blood 87:4824, 1996.

Means RT, Krantz SB: Progress in understanding the pathogenesis of the anemia of chronic disease. Blood 80:1639, 1992.

Physiologic Anemia of Infancy

Bednarek FJ, Weisberger S, Richardson DK, et al: Variations in blood transfusions among newborn intensive care units. J Pediatr 133:601, 1998.

Fain J, Hilsenrath P, Widness JA, et al: A cost analysis comparing erythropoietin and red cell transfusions in the treatment of anemia of prematurity. Transfusion 35:936, 1995.

Lachance C, Chessex P, Fouron JC, et al: Myocardial, erythropoietic, and metabolic adaptations to anemia of prematurity. J Pediatr 125:278, 1994.

Meyer MP, Haworth C, Meyer JH: A comparison of oral and intravenous iron supplementation in preterm infants receiving recombinant erythropoietin. J Pediatr 129:258, 1996.

Zipursky A, Brown EJ, Watts J, et al: Oral vitamin E supplementation for the prevention of anemia in premature infants: A controlled trial. Pediatrics 79:61, 1987.

Megaloblastic Anemias

Beck WS: Diagnosis of megaloblastic anemia. Annu Rev Med 42:311, 1991.

Monagle PT, Tauro GP: Infantile Megaloblastosis secondary to maternal vitamin B_{12} deficiency. Clin Lab Haematol 19:23, 1997.

Poncz M, Colman N, Herbert V, et al: Therapy of congenital folate malabsorption. J Pediatr 98:76, 1981.

Microcytic Anemia

Booth IW, Aukett MA: Iron deficiency anaemia in infancy and early childhood. Arch Dis Child 76:549, 1997.

Bruner AB, Joffe A, Duggan AK, et al: Randomised study of cognitive effects of iron supplementation in non-anaemic iron-deficient adolescent girls. Lancet 348:992, 1996.

Centers for Disease Control and Prevention: Recommendations to prevent and control iron deficiency in the United States. MMWR 47:1, 1998.

Fleming MD, Trenor CC III, Su MA, et al: Microcytic anaemia mice have a mutation in Nramp2, a candidate iron transporter gene. Nature Genet 16:383, 1997.

Hall RT, Wheeler RE, Benson J, et al: Feeding iron-fortified premature formula during initial hospitalization to infants less than 1800 grams birth weight. Pediatrics 92:409, 1993.

Looker AC, Dallman PR, Caroll MD, et al: Prevalence of iron deficiency in the United States. JAMA 277:973, 1997.

Lozoff B, Wolf AW, Jimenez E: Iron-deficiency anemia and infant development: Effects of extended oral iron therapy. J Pediatr 129:382, 1996.

Pearson HA: The naming of a syndrome. J Pediatr Hematol Oncol 19:271, 1997.

Punnonen K, Irjala K, Rajamaki A: Serum transferrin receptor and its ratio to serum ferritin in the diagnosis of iron deficiency. Blood 89:1052, 1997.

Walter T, Pino P, Pizarro F, et al: Prevention of iron-deficiency anemia: comparison of high- and low-iron formulas in healthy infants after 6 months of life. J Pediatr 132:635, 1998.

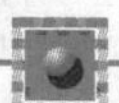

SECTION 3

Hemolytic Anemias

CHAPTER 463

Definitions and Classification of Hemolytic Anemias

George B. Segel

Hemolysis is defined as the premature destruction of red blood cells (RBCs). If the rate of destruction exceeds the capacity of the marrow to produce RBCs, anemia results. Normal RBC survival time is 110–120 days, and approximately 1% of RBCs (the senescent ones) are removed each day and replaced by the marrow to maintain the RBC count. During hemolysis, RBC survival is shortened, and increased marrow activity results in a heightened reticulocyte percentage and number. Hemolysis should be suspected as a cause of anemia if an elevated reticulocyte count is present in the absence of bleeding or administration of hematinic therapy. The marrow can increase its output two- to threefold acutely, with a maximum of six- to eightfold if hemolysis is long standing. The reticulocyte percentage can be corrected to measure the magnitude of the marrow production in response to hemolysis as follows:

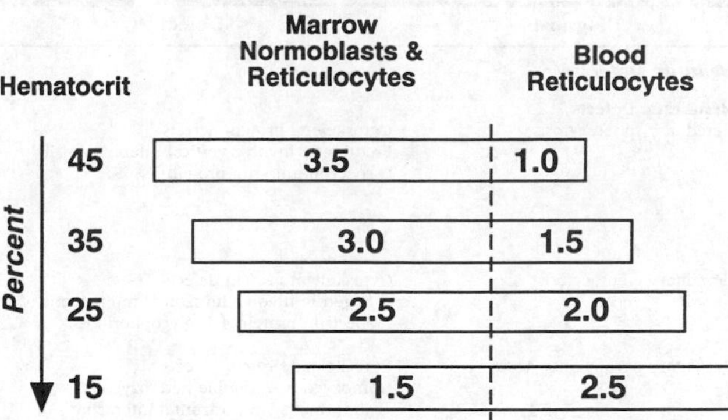

Figure 463–1 Number of days for maturation of reticulocytes in the marrow and blood. (Modified from Hillman RS, Finch CA: Red Cell Manual. Philadelphia, FA Davis, 1983.) The duration of maturation as blood reticulocytes is taken as μ.

$$\text{Reticulocyte index} = \text{reticulocyte \%} \times \frac{\text{observed hematocrit}}{\text{normal hematocrit}} \times \frac{1}{\mu}$$

where μ is a maturation factor related to the severity of the anemia (Fig. 463–1). In the absence of hemolysis, the reticulocyte index is 1.0, representing normal marrow activity.

As anemia becomes more severe, there is more erythropoietin stimulation of erythropoiesis, and *reticulocytes* are released from the marrow earlier, spending more than 1 day as reticulocytes in the blood. In terms of measuring the marrow response, it is inappropriate to count reticulocytes produced yesterday in today's calculation of the reticulocyte index. The maturation factor, μ, provides this correction (Fig. 463–1). The usual marrow response in a chronic hemolytic anemia is reflected by a reticulocyte index of 3–4, with a maximum of 6–8 corresponding to maximal marrow output.

The *erythroid hyperplasia* resulting from chronic hemolytic anemia in children, especially thalassemia, may be so extensive that the medullary spaces expand at the expense of the cortical bone. These changes may be evident on physical examination or on x-rays of the skull and long bones (see Fig. 468–3). A propensity to fracture long bones can occur also.

Direct assessment of the severity of hemolysis requires measurement of the RBC survival time using RBCs tagged with the radioisotope $Na_2{}^{51}CrO_4$. The normal value for the ^{51}Cr half-life is 25–35 days. This value is less than the expected half-life of 50–60 days because of the elution of ^{51}Cr from the labeled RBCs at the rate of about 1% per day.

Several other plasma, urinary, or fecal chemical alterations reflect the presence of hemolysis. The *degradation of hemoglobin* results in the biliary excretion of heme pigments and increased fecal urobilinogen (Fig. 463–2). Elevations of serum unconjugated bilirubin also may accompany hemolysis.

Gallstones composed of calcium bilirubinate may be formed in children as young as 4 yr of age. Three heme-binding proteins in the plasma are altered during hemolysis (Fig. 463–2). Hemoglobin binds to haptoglobin and hemopexin, both of which are reduced. Oxidized heme binds to albumin to form methemalbumin, which is increased. When the capacity of these binding molecules is exceeded, free hemoglobin appears in the plasma and can be seen easily if the RBCs are sedimented in a capillary hematocrit tube. If present, free hemoglobin in the plasma is prima facie evidence of intravascular hemolysis. When the tubular reabsorptive capacity of the kidneys for hemoglobin is exceeded, free hemoglobin appears in the urine. Even in the absence of hemoglobinuria, iron loss may result from reabsorbed hemoglobin and the shedding of renal epithelial cells containing hemosiderin. This may lead to secondary iron deficiency during chronic intravascular hemolysis. When hemoglobin is degraded, an α-methene bridge is broken in the cyclic tetrapyrrole of the heme moiety, with release of carbon monoxide (CO) (Fig. 463–2). The amount of CO in the blood or expired air provides a dynamic measure of the hemolytic rate. End-tidal CO is being evaluated in several research laboratories but is not used in clinical laboratories to measure hemolysis.

The hematocrit during hemolysis is dependent on the severity of the hemolysis and on the marrow response in producing

Figure 463–2 Red cell destruction and the catabolism of hemoglobin (Hb) based on the description by Hillman and Finch. (From Hillman RS, Finch CA: Red Cell Manual. Philadelphia, FA Davis, 1983.)

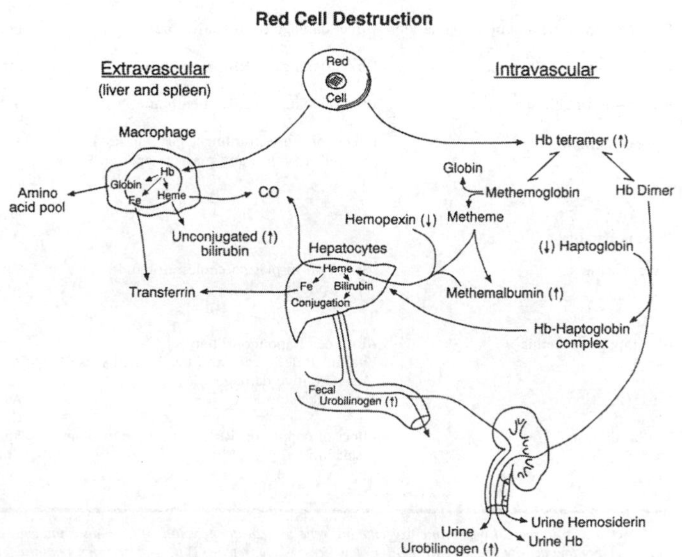

TABLE 463–1 Hemolytic Anemias and Their Treatment

Diagnosis	Defect	Laboratory Tests	Treatment
Cellular Defects			
Membrane Defects			
Hereditary spherocytosis	Cytoskeletal protein defects Frequently involve vertical interactions of spectrin ankyrin, protein 3	Spherocytes on blood film Negative Coombs test eliminates immune hemolysis Increased incubated osmotic fragility Abnormal cytoskeletal protein analysis	If Hb > 10 g/dl and retic. < 10%—none If severe anemia, poor growth, aplastic crises and age < 2 years—transfusion If Hb < 10 g/dl and retic. > 10% or massive spleen-splenectomy, preferably > age 6 but earlier if necessary Folic acid 1 mg qd
Hereditary elliptocytosis	Cytoskeletal protein defects Frequently involve horizontal interactions of spectrin, protein 4.1, glycophorin C	Elliptocytes on blood film RBCs mildly heat sensitive Abnormal cytoskeletal protein analysis	Mild types—no treatment Chronic hemolysis–transfusion and splenectomy as recommended for spherocytosis (above) Folic acid 1 mg qd
Hereditary pyropoikilocytosis	Cytoskeletal protein defects Homozygous or double heterozygous abnormality in horizontal interactions of α spectrin	Extreme variation in RBC size and shape on blood film Thermal sensitivity-fragmentation at 45°C for 15 min	Transfusion and splenectomy as recommended for spherocytosis (above) Folic acid 1 mg qd
Hereditary stomatocytosis	Cytoskeletal protein defects Decreased protein 7.2b (one subset) Abnormal RBC cation and water content	Stomatocytes on blood film	Splenectomy should be avoided (see text) Folic acid 1 mg qd
Paroxysmal nocturnal hemoglobinuria	Primary acquired marrow disorder RBCs unusually sensitive to complement-mediated lysis	Ham's test, sucrosis lysis test Marrow aspirate and biopsy to assess cellularity Decreased decay accelerating factor Decreased WBC, CD55, and CD59 or decreased RBC CD59 by flow cytometry	Folic acid 1 mg qd Mild cytopenias—no treatment Chronic hemolysis and other cytopenias—Prednisone 60 mg qd initially, then taper if possible; chronic 15–40 mg qod Iron for secondary iron deficiency Androgens—Halotestin, danazol Anticoagulation Marrow transplant for pancytopenia
Enzyme Deficiencies			
Pyruvate kinase deficiency	Decreased or abnormal enzyme	PK assay-decreased Vmax or rarely high Km variant	If severe anemia with symptoms, poor growth and age < 2 years—transfusion Splenectomy > age 6 but earlier if necessary Folic acid 1 mg qd
G6PD deficiency	A type: age-labile enzyme Mediterranean type: no enzyme activity in circulating RBCs	Glucose-6-phosphate dehydrogenase	Avoid oxidant stress to RBCs Transfusion if acute anemia is symptomatic
Hemoglobin Abnormalities (For discussion of hemoglobinopathies, see sections on these topics)			
Extracellular Defects			
Autoimmune			
Autoimmune hemolytic anemia "warm" antibody	Alteration in membrane surface antigen (Rh) or abnormal response of B lymphocytes, causing autoantibody formation	Spherocytes on blood film Positive direct Coombs test to IgG "warm" antibody directed against RBCs Positive indirect Coombs test and antibody detectable in plasma Thermal amplitude 35–40° C Some complement (C3b) may be detected on RBCs Tests for underlying disease	If Hb >10 g/dL + retic <10%—none Severe anemia may require transfusion Prednisone 2 mg/kg/24 hr IVIG Danazol Splenectomy Immunosuppressives Folic acid 1 mg/24 hr if chronic
"Cold" antibody	"Cold" or IgM autoantibody directed against I/i antigen system	Agglutination or rouleaux on blood film Positive direct Coombs' test to complement (C3b) Tests for underlying disease Serology for infectious mononucleosis; anti-i present Serology for *Mycoplasma pneumoniae;* anti-I present	If Hb >10 g/dL + retic <10%—none Severe anemia may require transfusion Avoid exposure to cold If severe: immunosuppressives and plasmapheresis Prednisone—*less* effective Splenectomy—*not* useful Folic acid 1 mg/24 hr if chronic
Fragmentation Hemolysis			
DIC, TTP, HUS	Direct damage to RBC membrane	Fragments on blood film	Treat underlying condition Transfusion: but transfused cells also will have shortened life span
Extracorporeal membrane oxygenation	Direct damage to RBC membrane	Fragments on blood film	Supportive Transfusion until ECMO discontinued
Prosthetic heart valve	Direct damage to RBC membrane	Fragments on blood film	Folic acid 1 mg/24 hr Iron for secondary iron deficiency
Burns—thermal injury	Direct damage to RBC membrane	Spherocytes on blood film	Supportive Transfusion
Hypersplenism	Effects of sequestration, ↓ pH, lipases and other enzymes, and macrophages on RBCs	Thrombocytopenia and neutropenia	Treat underlying condition—cytopenias usually mild Splenectomy if complicating other anemia, e.g., thalassemia major Folic acid 1 mg/24 hr
Plasma Factors			
Liver disease	Alteration in plasma cholesterol and phospholipids	Target cells or spiculated RBCs on blood film Abnormal liver function tests	Treat underlying condition Transfusion: but transfused cells also will have shortened life span Folic acid 1 mg/24 hr
Abetalipoproteinemia	Absence of apolipoprotein β Vitamin E deficiency and heightened sensitivity to oxidative damage	Acanthocytes on blood film Absent chylomicrons, VLDL and LDL	Vitamin E (A, K, and D) Folic acid 1 mg/24 hr Dietary restriction of triglycerides
Infections	Toxic effects on RBCs	Associated symptoms and signs Cultures	Antibiotics Supportive
Wilson disease	Effect of copper on RBC membrane, usually self-limited	Spherocytes on blood film Copper, ceruloplasmin Penicillamine challenge and urine copper excretion	Penicillamine Supportive Transfusion if acute anemia is symptomatic

ECMO = extracorporeal membrane oxygenation; retic = reticulocyte count; DIC = disseminated intravascular coagulation; TTP = thrombotic thrombocytopenic purpura; HUS = hemolytic uremic syndrome; VLDL = very low density lipoproteins; LDL = low density lipoproteins; IVIG = intravenous immunoglobin; RBC = red blood cell; Hb = hemoglobin.
Modified from Asselin BL, Segel GB: In: Rakel R (ed): Conn's Current Therapy. Philadelphia, WB Saunders, 1994, pp 338–339.

RBCs. The shortened RBC life span and heightened RBC production result in a marked susceptibility to *aplastic or hypoplastic crises*, characterized by erythroid marrow failure and reticulocytopenia, accompanied by a rapid reduction in hemoglobin and hematocrit. The most common cause of aplastic crises is parvovirus B19, which is erythrocytotropic in marrow culture in vitro (see Chapters 244 and 468). Aplastic crises may produce a precipitous and life-threatening decline in the hematocrit, which usually lasts 10–14 days. Such transient erythroid marrow failure has little effect on persons with a normal RBC life span but has a proportionately greater effect as the RBC life span is shortened by hemolysis. A second infection with parvovirus is uncommon, but other infections may compromise the erythroid marrow output, resulting in various degrees of hypoplasia or hypoplastic crises.

The hemolytic anemias may be classified as either (1) cellular, resulting from intrinsic abnormalities of the membrane, enzymes, or hemoglobin; or (2) extracellular, resulting from antibodies, mechanical factors, or plasma factors. Most of the cellular defects are inherited (paroxysmal nocturnal hemoglobinuria is acquired), and most of the extracellular defects are acquired (abetalipoproteinemia with acanthocytosis is inherited). Table 463–1 shows the most common hemolytic anemias, their underlying defects, the diagnostic laboratory tests, and the current recommendations for treatment.

CHAPTER 464
Hereditary Spherocytosis

George B. Segel

Hereditary spherocytosis is a common cause of hemolysis and hemolytic anemia, with a prevalence of approximately 1/5,000 in people of Northern European extraction. It is the most common familial and congenital abnormality of the red blood cell (RBC) membrane. Affected individuals may be asymptomatic without anemia and with minimal hemolysis or may have a severe hemolytic anemia. Hereditary spherocytosis has been described in most ethnic groups but is most common among persons of Northern European origin.

ETIOLOGY. Hereditary spherocytosis usually is transmitted as an autosomal dominant and, less frequently, as an autosomal recessive disorder. As many as 25% of patients have no previous family history. Of these patients, most represent new mutations, and a few result from recessive inheritance. The most common molecular defects are abnormalities of spectrin or ankyrin, which are major components of the cytoskeleton responsible for RBC shape. A recessive defect has been described in α-spectrin; dominant defects, in β-spectrin and in protein 3; and dominant and recessive defects, in ankyrin. A deficiency in spectrin, protein 3, or ankyrin results in uncoupling in the "vertical" interactions of the lipid bilayer skeleton and the loss of membrane microvesicles (Fig. 464–1). The loss of membrane without a proportional loss of volume causes sphering of the RBCs and an associated increase in cation permeability, cation transport, adenosine triphosphate utilization, and glycolytic metabolism. The decreased deformability of the spherocytic RBCs impairs cell passage from the splenic cords to the splenic sinuses, and the spherocytic RBCs are destroyed prematurely in the spleen. Splenectomy markedly improves the RBC life span and cures the anemia.

CLINICAL MANIFESTATIONS. Hereditary spherocytosis may be a cause of hemolytic disease in the newborn and may present with anemia and hyperbilirubinemia sufficiently severe to require phototherapy or exchange transfusions. The severity in infants and children is variable. Some children remain asymptomatic into adulthood, but others may have severe anemia with pallor, jaundice, fatigue, and exercise intolerance. Severe cases may be marked by expansion of the diploë of the skull and the medullary region of other bones, but to a lesser extent than in thalassemia major. After infancy, the spleen is usually enlarged, and pigmentary (bilirubin) gallstones may form as early as age 4–5 yr. At least 50% of unsplenectomized patients ultimately form gallstones, although for the most part, they remain asymptomatic. Because of the high RBC turnover and heightened erythroid marrow activity, children with hereditary spherocytosis are susceptible to aplastic crisis, primarily as a result of parvovirus, and to hypoplastic crises associated with various other infections. Such erythroid marrow failure may result rapidly in profound anemia (hematocrit <10%), high-output heart failure, hypoxia, cardiovascular collapse, and death.

LABORATORY FINDINGS. Evidence for hemolysis includes reticulocytosis and hyperbilirubinemia. The hemoglobin level usually is 6–10 g/dL, but it can be in the normal range. The reticulocyte count often is heightened to 6–20%, with a mean of approximately 10%. The mean corpuscular volume is normal, whereas the mean corpuscular hemoglobin concentration often is increased (36–38 g/dL RBCs). The RBCs on the blood film vary in size and include polychromatophilic reticulocytes and spherocytes (Fig. 464–2*A*). The spherocytes are smaller in diameter and on the blood film are hyperchromic as a result of the high hemoglobin concentration. The central pallor is less conspicuous than in normal cells. Spherocytes may be the predominant cell or may be relatively sparse, depending on severity of the disease, but they usually account for more than 15–20% of the cells when hemolytic anemia is present. Erythroid hyperplasia is evident in the marrow aspirate or biopsy. The marrow expansion may be evident on routine roentgenographic examination. Evidence of hemolysis may include elevated indirect bilirubin, decreased haptoglobin, and the presence of gallstones by ultrasonography.

The *diagnosis* of hereditary spherocytosis usually is established clinically from the blood film, showing many spherocytes and reticulocytes, from the family history, and from splenomegaly. The presence of spherocytes in the blood can be confirmed with an osmotic fragility test. The RBCs are incubated in progressive dilutions of an iso-osmotic buffered salt solution. Exposure to hypotonic saline causes RBCs to swell, and the spherocytes lyse more readily than biconcave cells in hypotonic solutions. This feature is accentuated by depriving the cells of glucose for 24 hr at 37°C, a so-called incubated osmotic fragility test.

As a research tool, the specific protein abnormality can be established in 80% of these patients by RBC membrane protein analysis using gel electrophoresis and densitometric quantitation. The protein abnormalities are more evident in patients who have had a splenectomy. Studies to define the underlying defects in the cytoskeleton may require assessment of protein synthesis, stability, assembly, and binding to the other membrane proteins.

DIFFERENTIAL DIAGNOSIS. The major alternative consideration when large numbers of spherocytes are seen on the blood film is immune hemolysis. Isoimmune hemolytic disease of the newborn, particularly due to ABO incompatibility, mimics hereditary spherocytosis. The detection of antibody on an infant's RBCs using a direct Coombs test should establish the diagnosis of immune hemolysis. Other autoimmune hemolytic anemias also are characterized by spherocytes, and there may be evidence of a previously normal hemoglobin, hematocrit, and reticulocyte count. Rare causes of spherocytosis include thermal injury, clostridia septicemia with exotoxemia, and Wilson disease, each of which may present with a transient hemolytic anemia (see Table 463–1).

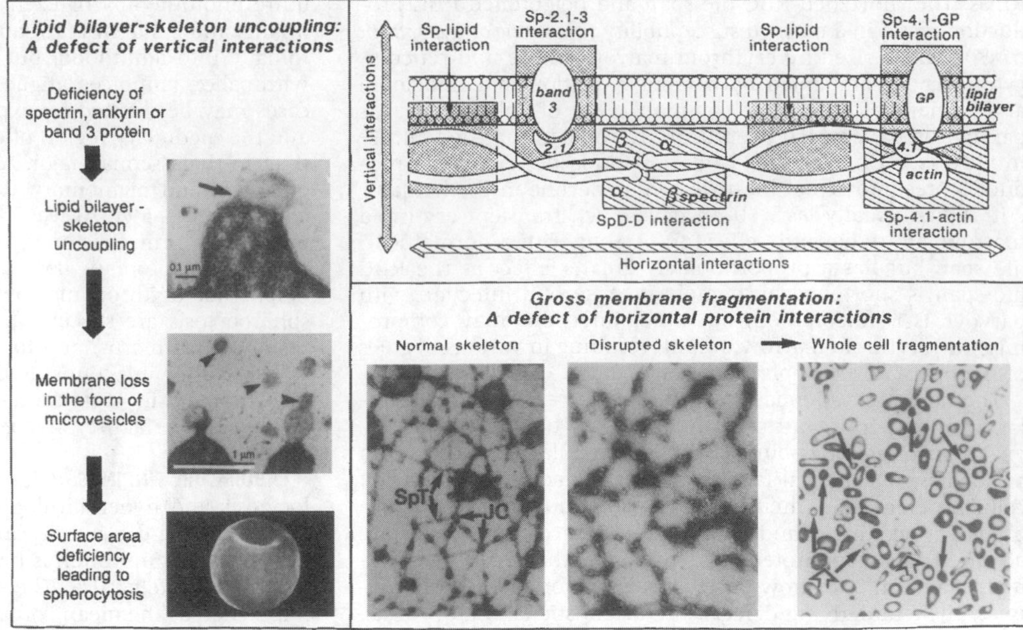

Figure 464–1 Vertical and horizontal interactions of membrane proteins and the pathobiology of the red cell lesion in hereditary spherocytosis (HS) and hereditary elliptocytosis/hereditary pyropoikilocytosis (HE/HPP). *Left*: A defect of vertical or transverse interactions as exemplified by the red cell membrane lesion in HS. Partial deficiencies of spectrin, ankyrin (band 2.1), or band 3 protein lead to uncoupling of the membrane lipid bilayer from the underlying skeleton *(arrow)* followed by a formation of spectrin-free microvesicles of approximately 0.2–0.5 μm in diameter *(arrowheads)*. These vesicles can be visualized by transmission electron microscopy, but they are not seen during examination of blood films. The subsequent loss of cell surface and a decrease in the surface/volume ratio leads to spherocytosis. *Right*: Defect of horizontal or parallel interactions of skeletal proteins as exemplified by the membrane lesion in hemolytic forms of HE associated with a defect of spectrin heterodimer self-association. The molecular lesion involving a weakened self-association of spectrin heterodimers to tetramers represents a horizontal defect of the stress-supporting protein interactions. It leads to a disruption of the membrane skeletal lattice and, consequently, whole cell destabilization followed by red cell fragmentation and poikilocytosis. Such fragments are readily seen on stained blood films. (Modified from Palek J, Jarolim P: Clinical expression and laboratory detection of red blood cell membrane protein mutations. Semin Hematol 30:249, 1993.)

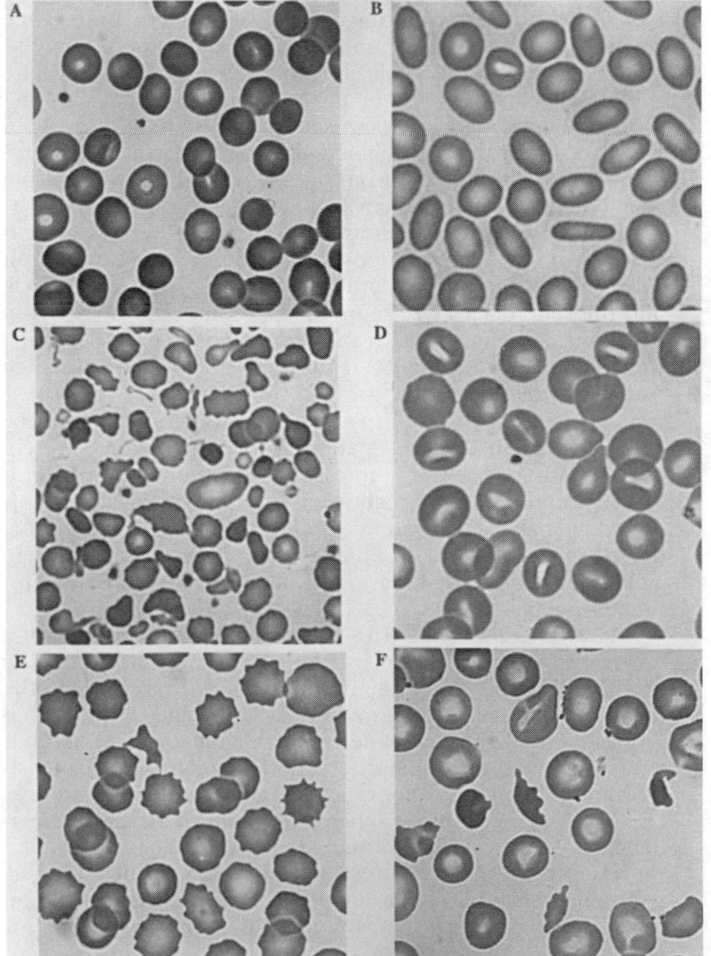

Figure 464–2 Morphology of abnormal red cells. *A*, Hereditary spherocytosis; *B*, hereditary elliptocytosis; *C*, hereditary pyropoikilocytosis; *D*, hereditary stomatocytosis; *E*, acanthocytosis; *F*, fragmentation hemolysis. See also color section.

TREATMENT. Because the spherocytes in hereditary spherocytosis are destroyed almost exclusively in the spleen, splenectomy eliminates most of the hemolysis associated with this disorder. After splenectomy, osmotic fragility often improves with loss of the abnormal "tail" because of diminished splenic conditioning and less RBC membrane loss, and the anemia, reticulocytosis, and hyperbilirubinemia resolve. Whether all patients with hereditary spherocytosis should undergo splenectomy is controversial. Some hematologists do not recommend splenectomy for those patients whose hemoglobin values exceed 10 g/dL and whose reticulocyte counts are less than 10%. Folic acid, 1 mg/24 hr, should be administered to prevent secondary folic acid deficiency. For patients with more severe anemia and reticulocytosis or those with hypoplastic or aplastic crises, poor growth, or cardiomegaly, splenectomy is recommended after age 5–6 yr to avoid the heightened risk of postsplenectomy sepsis in younger children. The introduction of laporoscopic splenectomy decreases the length of hospital stay and may replace open splenectomy. Vaccines for encapsulated organisms such as pneumococcus, meningococcus, and *Haemophilus influenzae* type b should be administered before splenectomy, and oral prophylactic penicillin V (age <5 yr: 125 mg/12 hr; age ≥5 yr through adulthood: 250 mg/12 hr) administered thereafter. Postsplenectomy thrombocytosis is commonly observed but needs no treatment and usually resolves spontaneously. In one report, partial splenectomy provided substantial increases in hemoglobin and reductions in the reticulocyte count, with potential maintenance of splenic phagocytic and immune function. This technique, if substantiated, would be particularly useful for those children younger than 5 yr with severe disease and could be used in older patients with mild disease.

CHAPTER 465
Hereditary Elliptocytosis

George B. Segel

Hereditary elliptocytosis is an uncommon disorder that varies markedly in severity. Mild hereditary elliptocytosis produces no symptoms, but more severe varieties may result in neonatal poikilocytosis and hemolysis, chronic or sporadic hemolytic anemias, or hereditary pyropoikilocytosis (HPP), which is a severe disorder with microspherocytosis and poikilocytosis. Although hereditary elliptocytosis is rare in Western populations, it is more commonly found in West Africa, where the abnormalities (spectrin mutations) may provide resistance to malarial infection.

ETIOLOGY. Hereditary elliptocytosis is inherited as a dominant disorder. In the rare instances when two abnormal alleles are inherited (HPP), the patient exhibits a particularly severe hemolytic anemia. Various molecular defects have been described in hereditary elliptocytosis; these produce abnormalities of α- and β-spectrin and defective spectrin heterodimer self-association (see Fig. 464–1). Such defects in the horizontal protein interactions result in gross membrane fragmentation, particularly in homozygous HPP. Less commonly, mutations in protein 4.1 and glycophorin C may produce elliptocytosis.

CLINICAL MANIFESTATIONS. Elliptocytosis may be noted as an incidental finding on a routine blood film and may not be associated with clinically significant hemolysis (see Fig. 464–2*B*). The diagnosis of hereditary elliptocytosis is established by the findings on the blood film, the autosomal dominant inheritance pattern, and the absence of other causes of elliptocytosis, such as deficiencies of iron, folic acid, or B_{12}. Hemolytic elliptocytosis may produce neonatal jaundice, even though characteristic elliptocytosis may not be evident at that time. The blood of the affected newborn may show bizarre poikilocytes and pyknocytes. The usual features of a chronic hemolytic process with elliptocytosis are manifested later as anemia, jaundice, splenomegaly, and osseous changes. Cholelithiasis may occur in later childhood, and aplastic crises have been reported. The most severe form is HPP, which is characterized by extreme microcytosis (mean corpuscular volume 50–60 fL), extraordinary variation in the cell size and shape, and primarily microspherocytic rather than elliptocytic cells (see Fig. 464–2*C*). These patients inherit a mutant spectrin from one parent, who has mild or no elliptocytosis, and a partial spectrin deficiency from the other parent, who is hematologically normal.

LABORATORY FINDINGS. The blood film is the most important test to establish hereditary elliptocytosis (see Fig. 464–2*B*). The red blood cells (RBCs) show various degrees of elongation and may actually be rod shaped. Ovalocytes, in contrast to elliptocytes, are less elongated and may reflect a condition termed *Southeast Asian ovalocytosis*, which is associated with a mutant protein 3 but does not cause hemolysis. In hereditary elliptocytosis, other abnormal RBC shapes may be present, depending on the severity of hemolysis. They include microcytes, spherocytes, and other poikilocytes. The reticulocyte count reflects the severity of hemolysis, and erythroid hyperplasia and indirect hyperbilirubinemia may be present. Increased thermal instability is characteristic of HPP; the abnormal spectrin denatures and the cells lyse at 45–46°C instead of the usual 49–50°C. The specific protein abnormality can be established by protein separation and analysis techniques.

TREATMENT. If hereditary elliptocytosis represents a morphologic abnormality on the blood film without hemolysis, no treatment is necessary. Patients with chronic hemolysis should receive folic acid 1 mg/24 hr to prevent secondary folic acid deficiency. Splenectomy decreases the hemolysis and should be considered if the hemoglobin is less than 10 g/dL and the reticulocyte count is greater than 10%. The RBCs on the blood film may be more abnormal after splenectomy even though hemoglobin increases and the reticulocytes decrease.

CHAPTER 466
Hereditary Stomatocytosis

George B. Segel

Hereditary stomatocytosis is a rare condition in which the red blood cells (RBCs) are cup shaped. On stained blood film, they present a mouthlike slit in place of the usual circular area of central pallor (Fig. 464–2*D*). Acquired stomatocytosis may be seen in several conditions, especially liver disease. Hereditary stomatocytosis may be associated with alterations in RBC hydration status or with deficiency in Rh antigens. The hydrocytic or overhydrated variety is associated with abnormalities within the region of protein 7.2, or "stomatin," which has been mapped to chromosome 9. A defective transcription promoter results in stomatin reduction, which may impair regulation of cation tranport. Hemolytic anemia may be associated with hereditary stomatocytosis, but splenectomy is not consistently effective as treatment. Symptomatic thrombocytosis may complicate splenectomy if the hemolysis is not decreased. Furthermore, patients have developed the life-threatening tendency toward in situ thrombosis after splenectomy. This may be related to abnormal adherence of the stomatocytic RBCs to vascular endothelium as well as to the thrombocytosis.

CHAPTER 467
Other Membrane Defects

George B. Segel

PAROXYSMAL NOCTURNAL HEMOGLOBINURIA

ETIOLOGY. Paroxysmal nocturnal hemoglobinuria (PNH) reflects an abnormality of marrow stem cells that affects many blood cell lines. The disease is not inherited; it is an acquired disorder of hematopoiesis characterized by a defect in proteins of the cell membrane that renders the red blood cells (RBCs) (and other cells) susceptible to damage by serum complement. The deficient membrane-associated proteins include decay-accelerating factor, the C8 binding protein, and other proteins that normally impede complement lysis at various steps. The underlying defect involves the glycolipid anchor that maintains these proteins on the cell surface. Various mutations in the *PIG-A* gene involved in glycosylphosphatidylinositol biosynthesis have been identified in patients with PNH. More than one PIG-A mutation often occurs in an individual patient, suggesting multiclonality. Furthermore, glycophosphatidylinositol-deficient cells are found at low frequency in normal persons. This suggests that injury to thc normal marrow stem cells provides a selective advantage to the PNH clones in the genesis of this disease.

CLINICAL MANIFESTATIONS. PNH is a rare disorder, particularly in children, but 26 patients with a mean age of 13 yr (0.8–21.4 yr) were diagnosed at Duke University Medical Center between 1966 and 1991. Approximately 60% of these patients presented with marrow failure, and the remainder had either intermittent or chronic anemia, often with prominent intravascular hemolysis. Nocturnal and morning hemoglobinuria is a classic finding in adults if hemolysis is worse during sleep. However, chronic hemolysis is more common in PNH despite its name. In addition to chronic hemolysis, thrombocytopenia and leukopenia are often characteristic. Thrombosis and thromboembolic phenomena are serious complications that may be related to altered glycoproteins on the platelet surface and resultant platelet activation. Abdominal, back, and head pain may be prominent complaints. Hypoplastic or aplastic pancytopenia may precede or follow the onset of PNH, and rarely PNH progresses to acute myelogenous leukemia. The mortality in PNH is related primarily to the development of aplastic anemia or thrombotic complications. The predicted survival for children is 80% for 5 yr, 60% for 10 yr, and 28% for 20 yr.

LABORATORY FINDINGS. The diagnosis of PNH is established classically by a positive result in the acid serum (Ham) or the sucrose lysis test, which activate the alternate and classic pathways of complement lysis, respectively. Hemosiderinuria is common and reflects the intravascular hemolysis. Markedly reduced levels of RBC acetylcholinesterase activity and reduced levels of *decay-accelerating factor* also are found. Flow cytometry now is the best diagnostic test for PNH. Using anti-CD59 for RBCs and anti-CD55 and anti-CD59 for granulocytes, flow cytometry is more sensitive than the classic RBC lysis tests in detecting the reduced glycolipid-bound membrane proteins.

TREATMENT. Splenectomy is not indicated. Glucocorticoids such as prednisone (2 mg/kg/24 hr) have been used to treat acute hemolytic episodes and should be tapered as soon as the hemolysis abates. Prolonged anticoagulation therapy may be of benefit when thromboses occur. Because of chronic loss of iron as hemosiderin in the urine, iron therapy may be necessary. Androgens, such as halotestin and danazol, antithymocyte globulin, cyclosporin, and growth factors such as erythropoietin and G-CSF have been used to treat marrow failure. Bone marrow transplantation has been successful in treating some cases.

ACANTHOCYTOSIS

Acanthocytosis is characterized by RBCs with irregular circumferential pointed projections (Fig. 464–2*E*). This morphologic finding is seen with alterations in the cholesterol/phospholipid ratio in some patients with liver disease and in congenital abetalipoproteinemia associated with malabsorption, neuromuscular abnormalities, and retinitis pigmentosa (Chapters 84.4, 340.12). It also is associated with the rare X-linked *McLeod syndrome*: absence of the Kx (Kell) antigen, late-onset myopathy, neurologic abnormalities, splenomegaly, and hemolysis with acanthocytosis.

General

Nathan DG, Orkin SH: Nathan and Oski's Hematology of Infancy and Childhood, 5th ed. Philadelphia, WB Saunders, 1998.

Oski FA, Naiman JL: Hematologic Problems of the Newborn, 3rd ed. Philadelphia, WB Saunders, 1982.

Stockman JA III, Pochedly C: Developmental and Neonatal Hematology. New York, Raven Press, 1988.

Hemolytic Anemias

Asselin BL, Segel GB: Nonimmune Hemolytic Anemia. *In:* Rakel R (ed): Conn's Current Therapy. Philadelphia, WB Saunders, 1994, p 336.

Dacie JV: The Haemolytic Anemias, 3rd ed. New York, Grune & Stratton, 1985.

Hillman RS, Finch CA: Red Cell Manual. Philadelphia, FA Davis, 1974.

Hereditary Spherocytosis and Other Membrane Proteins

Eber SW, Armbrust R, Schroter W: Variable clinical severity of hereditary spherocytosis: Relation to erythrocytic spectrin concentration, osmotic fragility, and autohemolysis. J Pediatr 117:409, 1990.

Gallagher PG, Forget BG: Structure, organization and expression of the human band 7.2b gene, a candidate gene for hereditary hydrocytosis. J Biol Chem 270:26358, 1995.

Kelleher JH, Lerban NLC, Mortimer PP: Human serum "parvovirus": A specific cause of aplastic crisis in children with hereditary spherocytosis. J Pediatr 102:722, 1983.

Manno CS, Cohen AR: Splenectomy in mild hereditary spherocytosis: Is it worth the risk? Am J Pediatr Hematol Oncol 11:300, 1989.

Michaels LA, Cohen AR, Zhao H, et al: Screening for hereditary spherocytoses by use of automated erythrocyte indexes. J Pediatr 130:957, 1997.

Miragha del Guidice E, Francese M, Nobili B, et al: High frequency of de novo mutations in anthyrin gene (ANK1) in children with hereditary spherocytoses. J Pediatr 132:117, 1998.

Palek J, Jarolim P: Clinical expression and laboratory detection of red blood cell membrane protein mutations. Semin Hematol 30:249, 1993.

Stewart GW, Amess JA, Eber SW, et al: Thromboembolic disease after splenectomy for hereditary stomatocytosis. British J Haematol 93:303, 1996.

Tchernia G, Gauthier F, Mielot F, et al: Initial assessment of the beneficial effect of partial splenectomy in hereditary spherocytosis. Blood 81:2014, 1993.

Paroxysmal Nocturnal Hemoglobinuria

Hall SE, Rosse WF: The use of monoclonal antibodies and flow cytometry in the diagnosis of paroxysmal nocturnal hemoglobinuria. Blood 87:5332, 1996.

Hillmen P, Lewis SM, Bessler M, et al: Natural history of paroxysmal nocturnal hemoglobinuria. N Engl J Med 333:1253, 1995.

Miyata T, Yamada N, Irda Y, et al: Abnormalities in PIG-A transcripts in granulocytes from patients with paroxysmal nocturnal hemoglobinuria. N Engl J Med 330:249, 1994.

Ware RE, Hall SE, Rosse WF: Paroxysmal nocturnal hemoglobinuria with onset in childhood and adolescence. N Engl J Med 325:991, 1991.

CHAPTER 468
Hemoglobin Disorders

George R. Honig

The clinical disorders that result from abnormalities of the globin genes comprise a diverse group of hematologic diseases.

Normal hemoglobins are tetrameric molecules containing pairs of α or α-like and β or β-like globin-heme subunits. The normal postnatal hemoglobins include hemoglobin (Hb) A ($\alpha_2\beta_2$), Hb F ($\alpha_2\gamma_2$), and Hb A_2 ($\alpha_2\delta_2$). The embryonic hemoglobins, which usually disappear before birth, include Hb Gower-1 ($\zeta_2\epsilon_2$), Hb Gower-2 ($\alpha_2\epsilon_2$), and Hb Portland ($\zeta_2\gamma_2$) (see also Chapter 468). The genes for the α and ζ chains are encoded on chromosome 16; those for the β group have been localized to chromosome 11. The nucleotide sequences of all these genes have been determined, and many globin-gene abnormalities have been characterized at the molecular level.

The hemoglobin disorders are subdivided into three major groups. The *structural abnormalities,* including the hemoglobinopathies, result from changes in the amino acid sequences of the globin chains. Most have a single amino acid substitution; in others, however, amino acids may be deleted or inserted, or other, more complex structural changes may be present. The *thalassemias* are expressed as quantitative defects, in which the synthesis of one or more of the globin chains is decreased or, in the most severe forms, is totally suppressed. The *hereditary persistence of fetal hemoglobin (HPFH) syndromes* are characterized by elevated levels of Hb F continuing throughout adult life. Almost all these abnormalities result from the same types of molecular defects: Nucleotides may be substituted, deleted, or inserted into globin-gene DNA.

HEMOGLOBIN STRUCTURAL ABNORMALITIES
(Hemoglobinopathies)

More than 700 structural variants of hemoglobin have been identified. Most are rare, but a few, including some severely pathologic forms, occur with high frequency in certain populations. Many abnormal hemoglobins are readily identified by electrophoresis, but some are electrophoretically "silent" and require other laboratory studies for identification. Numerous hemoglobin variants that have abnormal electrophoretic mobility, including both benign and pathologic forms, exhibit very similar electrophoresis findings and cannot be specifically identified by this means alone.

468.1 Sickle Cell Hemoglobinopathies

Sickle hemoglobin (Hb S) differs from normal adult hemoglobin by a substitution of glutamic acid at the 6th position of its β chains by valine. In the oxygenated state, Hb S functions normally. When this hemoglobin is deoxygenated, an interaction between the β6 valine and complementary regions on the β chains of an adjacent molecule results in formation of highly ordered molecular polymers; these elongate to form filamentous structures, which aggregate into rigid, crystal-like rods. This process of molecular polymerization is responsible for the spiny, brittle character of sickle erythrocytes (RBCs) under conditions of decreased oxygenation. Certain other abnormal hemoglobins, notably Hb C, Hb D Los Angeles, and Hb O Arab, participate in the molecular polymerization of deoxy-Hb S. Hb A does so to a smaller degree, but Hb F is totally excluded from the deoxy-Hb S polymer.

RBCs of heterozygous (sickle cell trait) individuals have been shown to resist invasion by malarial parasites, and this resistance appears to have provided protection against the frequently lethal *falciparum* form of the disease. The β^S gene is found in high frequency in those living in regions in which *Plasmodium falciparum* malaria has been endemic, including many parts of Africa, the Mediterranean area, and parts of Turkey, the Middle East, and India. In individuals from several geographic areas, the sickle mutation has been shown to exist in genetic linkage with discrete sets of closely associated markers. Some of these Hb S "haplotypes" appear to be predictive of the degree of severity of the sickle cell disease. Those associated with particularly mild disease are accompanied by significantly higher levels of Hb F. Patients who have sickle cell disease and who co-inherit genes for α-thalassemia may also have disease of modified severity.

Hb S is readily identified by electrophoresis. A confirmatory solubility test excludes other abnormal hemoglobins with similar electrophoretic mobility. Although affected newborns express only small quantities of Hb S, because of the predominance of Hb F at birth, the sickle cell syndromes can nevertheless be identified reliably in neonates by various laboratory methods. Neonatal screening programs for detecting infants with sickle cell disease are widely established in the United States. These disorders can also be determined antenatally using amniocyte or chorionic villus DNA by methods that identify the specific β^S nucleotide substitution.

SICKLE CELL ANEMIA
(Homozygous Hb S)

This disorder is characterized by severe chronic hemolytic disease resulting from premature destruction of the brittle, poorly deformable RBCs. Other manifestations of sickle cell anemia are attributable to ischemic changes resulting from vascular occlusion by masses of sickled cells. The clinical course of affected children is typically associated with intermittent episodic events, often referred to as "crises."

CLINICAL MANIFESTATIONS. Affected newborns seldom exhibit clinical features of sickle cell disease; hemolytic anemia gradually develops over the 1st 2–4 mo, parallelling the replacement of much of the fetal hemoglobin by Hb S. Other clinical manifestations are uncommon before 5–6 mo of age. Acute sickle dactylitis, presenting as the *hand-foot syndrome,* is frequently the 1st overt evidence that sickle cell disease is present in an infant. Its associated findings include painful, usually symmetric swelling of the hands and feet. The underlying abnormality is ischemic necrosis of the small bones, believed to be caused by a choking off of the blood supply as a result of the rapidly expanding bone marrow. Roentgenograms are not informative in the acute phase but later show evidence of extensive bony destruction and repair (Fig. 468–1).

Acute painful episodes represent the most frequent and prominent manifestation of sickle cell disease. Most patients experience some pain on a nearly daily basis. Episodes of severe pain that require hospitalization and parenteral analgesic administration average about 1/yr in children with Hb SS, but this interval varies considerably. Some patients never experience severe pain, and others require hospital admission with such frequency that they become seriously disabled. In young children, pain often involves the extremities; in older patients, head, chest, abdominal, and back pain occur more commonly. In an individual patient, pain tends to recur in a limited number of sites. Intercurrent illnesses accompanied by fever, hypoxia, and acidosis, all of which promote the deoxygenation of Hb S, may precipitate sickle pain episodes, but acute pain also develops frequently without an apparent antecedent event. Sickle-related abdominal pain may mimic that of an acute surgical condition.

More extensive vaso-occlusive events in these patients can produce gross ischemic damage. Acute pain episodes may progress to infarction of bone marrow or bone. Splenic infarcts are common in children, causing pain and contributing to the process of "autosplenectomy." Pulmonary infarction, often occurring in association with pneumonitis or microscopic fat emboli (from bone marrow infarction) may produce the severe clinical picture of *acute chest syndrome*. Strokes caused by cerebrovascular occlusion are among the most catastrophic acute events and are a frequent cause of hemiplegia. As many as 10% of children with sickle cell anemia, mainly preadolescent

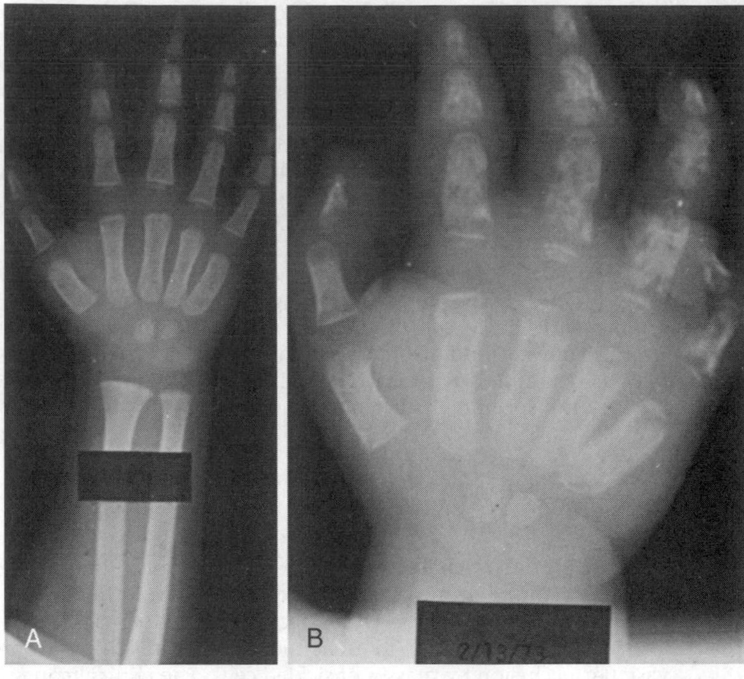

Figure 468–1 Roentgenograms of an infant with sickle cell anemia and acute dactylitis. *A*, The bones appear normal at the onset of the episode. *B*, Destructive changes and periosteal reaction are evident 2 wk later.

and older patients, exhibit sequelae of cerebrovascular occlusion. Findings of increased blood flow velocity by transcranial Doppler studies have been shown to be predictive of increased risk of stroke in these patients, and this may help to identify children who will benefit from preventive therapy. Ischemic damage may also affect the myocardium, liver, and kidneys. Renal function is progressively impaired by diffuse glomerular and tubular fibrosis, and hyposthenuria accompanied by polyuria is a characteristic finding in patients older than 5 yr. Renal papillary necrosis and nephrotic syndrome also develop occasionally. *Priapism* is a relatively frequent complication that results from the pooling of blood in the corpora cavernosa, causing obstruction of the venous outflow.

Young children with Hb SS may have splenic enlargement associated with their hemolytic disease, with progression to the syndrome of *hypersplenism* accompanied by worsening anemia and sometimes thrombocytopenia. *Acute splenic sequestration* is a distinct and episodic event that occurs in infants and young children with sickle cell anemia, often following an acute febrile illness. For unknown reasons, large amounts of blood become acutely pooled in the spleen, which becomes massively enlarged, and signs of circulatory collapse rapidly develop. Blood transfusions in the acute phase may be lifesaving.

Altered splenic function in young children with sickle cell disease is a significant factor leading to their increased susceptibility to meningitis, sepsis, and other serious infections, mainly caused by pneumococci and *Haemophilus influenzae*. In the absence of specific antibody to the polysaccharide capsular antigens of these organisms, splenic activity is essential for removing these bacteria when they invade the blood. Despite frequent enlargement of the spleen in young patients with Hb SS, its phagocytic and reticuloendothelial functions have been shown to be markedly reduced. As an additional risk factor, children with sickle cell disease have also been shown to have deficient levels of serum opsonins, of the alternate complement pathway, against pneumococci. Children with sickle cell disease also have increased susceptibility to *Salmonella* osteomyelitis (partly because of bone necrosis).

In common with patients having other forms of chronic hemolytic anemia, children with Hb SS are at risk of developing a rapid, potentially life-threatening decrease in their hemoglobin level (aplastic episodes) in association with parvovirus B19 infection (see Chapter 244).

An additional group of sickle cell sequelae is attributable primarily to the hemolytic anemia that accompanies this disorder. Cardiomegaly is invariably present in older children, often caused partly by sickle-related cardiomyopathy. Increased iron absorption contributes to parenchymal damage of the liver, pancreas, and heart. Symptomatic gallstone formation is common in adolescent and older patients, occasionally occurring in children as young as 5 yr.

By midchildhood, most patients are underweight, and puberty is frequently delayed. Zinc deficiency, which is prevalent in children with sickle cell disease, may contribute to their poor growth and delayed maturation. Chronic leg ulcers are relatively uncommon in children, seldom occurring before late adolescence.

LABORATORY FINDINGS. Hemoglobin concentrations usually range from 5–9 g/dL. The peripheral blood smear typically contains target cells, poikilocytes, and irreversibly sickled cells (Fig. 468–2*A*). These findings allow Hb SS and most of the other forms of sickle cell disease to be readily distinguished from sickle cell trait and other clinically benign conditions. Reticulocyte counts usually range from 5–15%, and nucleated RBCs and Howell-Jolly bodies may be present. The total white blood cell count is elevated to 12,000–20,000/mm^3, with a predominance of neutrophils. The platelet count is usually increased; the sedimentation rate is slow. Other changes include abnormal liver function test results, hyperbilirubinemia, and diffuse hypergammaglobulinemia. The bone marrow is markedly hyperplastic and shows erythroid predominance. Roentgenograms show expanded marrow spaces and osteoporosis.

DIAGNOSIS. The diagnosis is normally established by hemoglobin studies. Electrophoresis at an alkaline pH demonstrates a characteristic mobility, intermediate between those of Hb A and Hb A_2. To distinguish Hb S from other hemoglobins with similar electrophoretic properties, another (confirmatory) test is required, such as electrophoresis at an acidic pH, a sickle cell preparation in which sickling is observed when the cells are deoxygenated, or, most commonly, a hemoglobin solubility test. In the Hb S solubility test, a measured amount of hemoglobin is added to a concentrated buffer that contains a reduc-

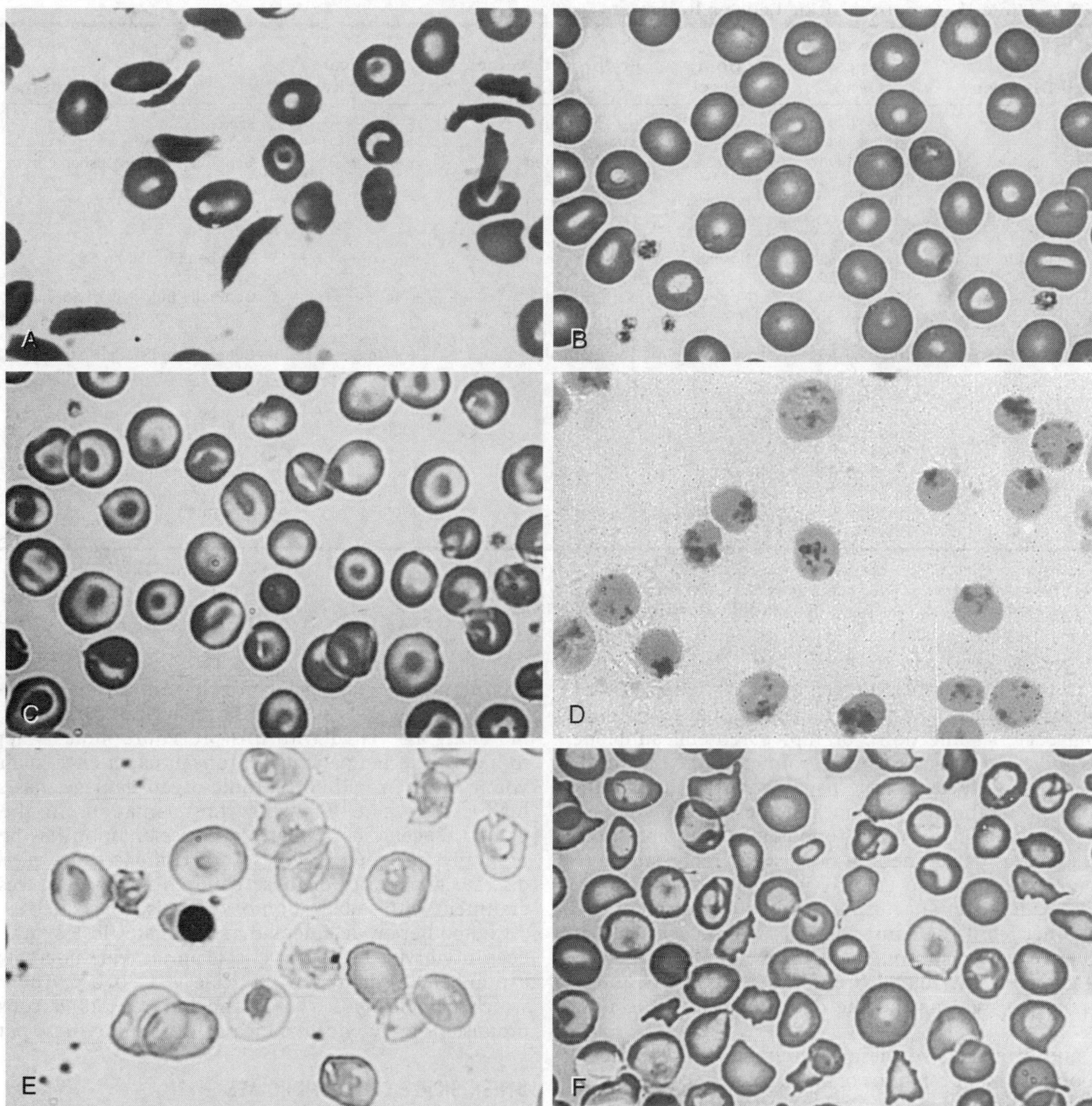

Figure 468–2 Red blood cell (RBC) morphology associated with hemoglobin disorders. *A*, Sickle cell anemia (Hb SS): target cells and fixed (irreversibly sickled) cells. *B*, Sickle cell trait (Hb AS): normal RBC morphology. *C*, Hemoglobin CC: target cells and occasional spherocytes. *D*, Congenital Heinz body anemia (unstable hemoglobin): RBCs stained with supravital stain (brilliant cresyl blue) reveal intracellular inclusions. *E*, Homozygous β^0-thalassemia: severe hypochromia with deformed RBCs and normoblasts. *F*, Hemoglobin H disease (α-thalassemia): anisopoikilocytosis with target cells. (Courtesy of Dr. John Bolles, The ASH Collection, University of Washington, Seattle, WA.)

ing agent; a turbid precipitate forms when more than about 15% Hb S is present. Beyond infancy, RBCs from patients with Hb SS contain between 2% and 20% Hb F with normal level of Hb A_2. Hb A is notably absent. The identification of Hb S in each parent provides supportive evidence for the diagnosis of sickle cell anemia.

DIFFERENTIAL DIAGNOSIS. The various clinical manifestations of sickle cell disease, including limb pain, heart murmurs, hepatosplenomegaly, and anemia, may suggest a number of other diagnoses, including rheumatic fever or rheumatoid arthritis, osteomyelitis, and leukemia. In patients who have a Hb SS electophoresis pattern and concomitant microcytosis (mean corpuscular volume [MCV] $<$78 fL), possibilities that require consideration include iron deficiency or a combination of Hb S with α- or β^0-thalassemia (Table 468–1).

TREATMENT. Measures directed toward preventing serious complications of sickle cell disease are among the most important elements of treatment. Maintaining full immunization status is particularly important. Administration of a polyvalent pneumococcal vaccine may be beneficial, but unfortunately, the forms of these vaccines currently available appear to be poorly immunogenic in children who have Hb SS and who are younger than 5 yr. *H. influenzae* immunization has been shown to be efficacious in infants with sickle cell disease, and this as well as hepatitis B immunizations are indicated. Prophylactic penicillin is highly effective in preventing serious pneumococcal infections and should be administered to all young children with sickle cell disease. Oral penicillin V (age $<$5 yr: 125 mg/12 hr; age $\geq$5 yr: 250 mg/12 hr) is given starting by 4 mo of age. By 5 yr of age, except in children who have had a severe pneumococcal infection or splenectomy, penicillin prophylaxis usually can be discontinued. Parents of children with Hb SS also need to be aware of the need to bring the child promptly to medical attention for acute illness,

TABLE 468–1 Clinically Important Sickle Cell Syndromes

Sickle Cell Disorder	Hemoglobin Composition (%)	Hb A_2 Level	Erythrocyte Volume (MCV)	Clinical Severity	Clinical Features
Hb SS	Hb S: 80–95 Hb F: 2–20	Normal	Normal	+ + to + + + +	See text
Hb S–β⁰-thalassemia	Hb S: 75–90 Hb F: 5–25	Increased	Decreased	+ + to + + + +	Generally indistinguishable from SS
Hb S–β⁺-thalassemia	Hb S: 5–85 Hb A: 10–30 Hb F: 5–10	Increased	Decreased	+ to + + +	Generally milder than SS
Hb SS with α-thalassemia trait (−,α/−,α)	Hb S: 78–88 Hb F: 10–20	Normal	Decreased	+ + to + + + +	May be milder than SS
Hb SC	Hb S: 45–50 Hb C: 45–50 Hb F: 2–5	Normal	Normal	+ to + + +	Generally milder than SS; higher frequency of bone infarcts and proliferative retinal disease
Hb SO Arab	Hb S: 50–55 Hb O: 40–45 Hb F: 2–15	Normal	Normal	+ + to + + + +	Generally indistinguishable from SS
Hb SD Los Angeles	Hb S: 45–50 Hb D: 30–40 Hb F: 5–20	Normal	Normal	+ + to + + + +	May be as severe as SS
Hb S/HPFH*	Hb S: 65–80 Hb F: 15–30	Normal	Normal	0 to +	Usually asymptomatic
Hb AS*	Hb S: 32–45 Hb A: 52–65	Normal	Normal	0 to +	Asymptomatic

**These conditions do not ordinarily produce sickle cell disease.*
MCV = mean corpuscular volume; HPFH = the African type of hereditary persistence of fetal hemoglobin.
Adapted from Honig GR, Adams JG III: Human Hemoglobin Genetics. Vienna, Springer-Verlag, 1986.

especially with a temperature exceeding 38.5°C regardless of the use of prophylaxis. Because of the substantial risk of life-threatening bacterial infections, prompt parenteral antibiotic therapy is indicated for infants and young children with an acute onset of high fever. Febrile patients with temperatures greater than 40°C, those who appear toxic or with findings suggestive of meningitis or other serious infection, and those who have previously had pneumococcal sepsis represent acute medical emergencies. Blood culture, intravenous ceftriaxone, and hospital admission for further antibiotic treatment are indicated. Other febrile patients older than 6 mo generally can be treated effectively on an outpatient basis. In low-risk, well-appearing children, after blood cultures are obtained, intravenous ceftriaxone is given, and the dose is repeated the next day.

Parents and caretakers of these children should also be informed about the manifestations of acute splenic sequestration and the need for immediate medical attention for a child with rapid splenic enlargement and pallor.

Painful episodes can frequently be managed with oral acetaminophen, alone or with codeine. More severe episodes may require hospitalization and parenteral administration of narcotics. Anti-inflammatory agents, especially ketorolac, may decrease or eliminate the need for narcotic analgesics. Dehydration or acidosis should be rapidly corrected by the intravenous route, but overhydration should be avoided. Blood transfusions are seldom indicated for painful episodes, and it is doubtful whether transfusion can ameliorate the course of a pain crisis. For patients with disabling chronic pain, for those with ischemic organ damage (acute chest, priapism) or stroke, or in preparation for major surgery, however, transfusions of normal RBCs can provide symptomatic relief and prevent further ischemic complications. A first stroke may be prevented by transfusion of children with sickle cell disease and abnormal transcranial Doppler ultrasonography. For children with stroke, cardiomyopathy, and other severe complications, chronic long-term transfusion regimens are a mainstay of therapy. These patients also may require iron chelation treatment to prevent the development of hemosiderosis. Packed RBC transfusions are specifically indicated for acute splenic sequestration and aplastic episodes. Repeated episodes of splenic sequestration are an indication for splenectomy.

Bone marrow transplantation from a normal donor can be curative in patients with sickle cell disease, but the risks and morbidity associated with this procedure limit its application to highly selected patients. European experience, mainly from young children without chronic organ damage, has shown a high success rate following transplantation. In the United States, allogenic bone marrow transplantation has been used primarily in patients with severe complications of sickle cell disease. A majority of these children achieved successful engraftment with stabilization of their disease sequelae.

Chemotherapy regimens that stimulate Hb F synthesis have been used with beneficial effect, on an experimental basis, in a number of children with sickle cell disease. These agents, which include hydroxyurea and butyrate, offer considerable promise of more effective means for treating these patients.

OTHER SICKLE CELL SYNDROMES

Sickling disorders of various degrees of severity result from Hb S existing in combination with other abnormal hemoglobins or thalassemias (see Table 468–1). Several of these syndromes, including Hb SD Los Angeles, Hb SO Arab, and Hb S–β⁰-thalassemia, present a clinical picture virtually indistinguishable from that of sickle cell anemia. Most of the others produce less severe manifestations.

Hb SC disease results from the concurrence of genes for Hb S and Hb C. Painful episodes and other vaso-occlusive manifestations are usually less severe in this condition than those associated with Hb SS. Most affected children have persistent splenomegaly, and bone infarcts occur more frequently than in those with Hb SS. Septicemia may also occur. Retinal vascular changes, predominantly in adolescents and adults, may lead to hemorrhage with retinal detachment. The hemoglobin concentration averages 9–10 g/dL, with the blood smear showing target cells and characteristic spindle-shaped RBCs.

468.2 Sickle Cell Trait

(Heterozygous Hb S; Hb AS)

Heterozygous expression of the gene for Hb S is usually associated with a totally benign clinical course. About 8%

of African-Americans have sickle cell trait; 35–45% of their hemoglobin is Hb S. This low level of Hb S is insufficient to produce sickling manifestations under usual circumstances, but under conditions of severe hypoxia, vaso-occlusive complications may occur. Splenic infarcts and other ischemic sequelae may occur in individuals with Hb AS as a result of hypoxia associated with general anesthesia. Hyposthenuria is usually present in older children and adults. Gross hematuria occasionally develops in otherwise well individuals. The hematologic findings in sickle cell trait are indistinguishable from normal (Fig. 468–2*B*). The diagnosis is established by hemoglobin electrophoresis, with confirmatory sickle testing.

468.3 Other Hemoglobinopathies

HEMOGLOBIN C

Hemoglobin C ($\alpha_2\beta_2{}^6$lysine) occurs in about 2% of African-Americans. In the heterozygous state (Hb AC), no anemia or disease is present, but increased numbers of target cells are seen in the peripheral blood. In homozygous individuals (Hb CC disease), a moderately severe hemolytic anemia with hemoglobin levels from 8–11 g/dL, a reticulocytosis of 5–10%, and splenomegaly is typically observed. The peripheral blood contains striking numbers of target cells and occasional spherocytes (Fig. 468–2*C*).

HEMOGLOBIN E

Hemoglobin E ($\alpha_2\beta_2{}^{26}$lysine) is prevalent in populations from Southeast Asia, particularly Thailand and Cambodia. Homozygous Hb E is a clinically mild hemolytic disorder, often accompanied by splenomegaly. The blood smear shows prominent target cells and microcytosis. The syndrome of Hb E–β^0-thalassemia, which is quite prevalent in Southeast Asian populations, ranges in expression from a relatively mild hemolytic anemia to a very severe Cooley anemia-like disorder with profound anemia and hepatosplenomegaly. At least in part, the variability in the expression of this syndrome is attributed to a moderating effect of co-inherited genes for α-thalassemia. Electrophoresis shows the presence of only Hb E and Hb F.

468.4 Unstable Hemoglobin Disorders

(Congenital Heinz Body Anemia)

A substantial group of abnormal hemoglobins, most of which are uncommon or rare, are characterized by molecular instability, leading to denaturation and precipitation of hemoglobin within the RBCs. In the more severe forms of these disorders, amorphous masses of the denatured hemoglobin, known as Heinz bodies, attach to the RBC membrane, damaging the cell and shortening its survival. The Heinz bodies, which are particularly prominent after splenectomy, can be visualized by supravital staining of the RBCs with brillliant cresyl blue (Fig. 468–2*D*). These hemolytic anemias are inherited in an autosomal dominant mode, but many of the severe forms apparently occur as new mutations.

Most of the severe types involve the hemoglobin β chains, and hemolysis first becomes apparent 3–6 mo after birth, when Hb F is replaced by adult hemoglobin. Anemia with increased reticulocytes, jaundice, and splenomegaly is characteristically present, becoming more pronounced with infections or after exposure to oxidant drugs or chemicals. With some of the unstable β-chain abnormalities, hemolysis is accompanied by excretion of darkly pigmented dipyrrolic compounds in the urine. In contrast to the clinical picture of chronic hemolytic disease typically associated with the highly unstable hemoglobins, some of the less severe abnormalities (e.g., Hb Zürich and Hb Hasharon) produce mild and usually inapparent anemia. With fever, infections, or exposure to oxidant conditions, however, affected individuals may experience acute hemolytic episodes similar to those associated with glucose-6-phosphate dehydrogenase (G6PD) deficiency.

Some unstable hemoglobins can be detected by electrophoresis, but many of them comigrate with Hb A. Heating at 50°C or treating the hemolysate with a 17% buffered solutions of isopropanol produces a precipitate of the unstable hemoglobin, and screening tests based on these methods are used to detect these abnormalities. Examples include Hb Köln, Hb Hammersmith, and Hb Abraham Lincoln. Splenectomy is sometimes of benefit in these patients, particularly those with severe splenomegaly.

468.5 Abnormal Hemoglobins with Increased Oxygen Affinity

More than 100 different rare, abnormal hemoglobins have been identified as having increased oxygen affinity, as indicated by a leftward displacement of their oxygen dissociation curves. Because of their increased oxygen affinity, these hemoglobins release oxygen inefficiently to the tissues, resulting in a relative degree of hypoxia. The hypoxic stimulus increases erythropoietin production, with the development of secondary erythrocytosis. Hemoglobin levels in affected individuals typically range from 16–19 g/dL. Some of these variants can be demonstrated by electrophoresis, but many of them have normal electrophoretic properties (e.g., Hb Chesapeake, Hb Malmö, Hb Kempsey).

468.6 Abnormal Hemoglobins Causing Cyanosis

Several rare hemoglobin variants exhibit markedly decreased oxygen affinity. The oxygen dissociation curves of blood from affected individuals are significantly displaced to the right. Examples of these abnormalities, which produce benign cyanosis, include Hb Kansas and Hb Beth Israel.

An additional group of abnormal hemoglobins that cause cyanosis is the Hb M group. These variants all have amino acid substitutions at positions in the molecule that are close to the heme groups. The structural changes in these hemoglobins have the effect of stabilizing the heme iron atoms in the ferric (Fe^{3+}) state, rendering them incapable of binding oxygen. The Hb M syndromes are characterized by a brown blood, even when fully oxygenated, and by cyanosis. Two of the Hb M variants, Hb M Saskatoon and Hb M Hyde Park, are also unstable and produce chronic hemolytic anemia. The Hb M variants that result from β-chain substitutions, such as Hb M Saskatoon, have an onset of cyanosis beginning at 4–6 mo of age, whereas the α-chain variants, such as Hb M Iwate, produce cyanosis that is apparent at birth. The autosomal dominant mode of inheritance of these abnormalities helps distinguish them from other causes of congenital cyanosis.

Methemoglobinemias resulting from Hb M can be differentiated from other forms of methemoglobinemia by characteristic changes in the spectral absorption patterns of hemoglobin solutions and by the presence of normal levels of NADH cytochrome b5 reductase (see Chapter 468.7). Electrophoresis can demonstrate some (but not all) of the Hb M variants. These are clinically benign abnormalities, except for the hemolytic disease that accompanies two of the Hb M group, and no treatment is required.

468.7 Hereditary Methemoglobinemia

The iron of both oxygenated and deoxygenated hemoglobin is normally in the ferrous (Fe^{2+}) state, which is essential for its oxygen-transporting function. Oxidation of hemoglobin iron to the ferric state yields methemoglobin, which is nonfunctional and colors the blood brown; in sufficient concentration, it causes cyanosis. The blood of healthy persons contains methemoglobin, but the intraerythrocytic methemoglobin-reducing system maintains its concentration at less than 2% of the total hemoglobin.

HEREDITARY METHEMOGLOBINEMIA WITH DEFICIENCY OF NADH CYTOCHROME b5 REDUCTASE. Four types of enzymopenic hereditary methemoglobinemia have been identified. All have a recessive mode of inheritance. In type I, the most frequent of these rare disorders, a deficiency of cytochrome b5 reductase is limited to RBCs, and cyanosis is the only consequence. Type II is a severe, progressive disorder that accounts for approximately 10% of patients with hereditary methemoglobinemia. In this disorder, the deficiency of cytochrome b5 reductase is generalized to all tissues. Affected individuals present with methemoglobinemia and severe encephalopathy, appearing before 1 yr of age, and with mental retardation, microcephaly, retarded growth, attacks of bilateral athetoid movements, strabismus, opisthotonos, and generalized hypertonia. In type III disease, the enzyme deficiency is demonstrable in RBCs, platelets, lymphocytes, and granulocytes. Clinically, cyanosis is the only manifestation. Type IV disease results from a deficiency of RBC cytochrome b5 and is associated with chronic cyanosis.

Clinically, cyanosis may vary in intensity with season and diet. The time of onset of cyanosis also varies; in some patients it appears at birth, in others as late as adolescence. Although as much as 50% of the total circulating hemoglobin may be in the form of nonfunctional methemoglobin, little or no cardiorespiratory distress occurs in these patients, except on exertion.

Daily oral *treatment* with ascorbic acid (200–500 mg in divided doses) gradually reduces the quantity of methemoglobin to about 10% of the total pigment and alleviates the cyanosis as long as therapy is continued. Chronic high doses of ascorbic acid have been associated with hyperoxaluria and renal stone formation. Methylene blue given intravenously (1–2 mg/kg) promptly eliminates both methemoglobin and cyanosis, and this effect can be maintained by daily oral administration of methylene blue (3–5 mg/kg).

468.8 Syndromes of Hereditary Persistence of Fetal Hemoglobin

These disorders are characterized by the production of elevated levels of Hb F beyond the neonatal period. At least 20 distinct forms of HPFH have been identified, affecting many different ethnic groups. Various molecular abnormalities have been determined as the cause of these conditions; for example, the common African forms result from extensive DNA deletions that encompass the entire β-globin gene. The normal changeover from γ-globin synthesis to β-chain synthesis consequently cannot take place in individuals with these affected chromosomes. In heterozygotes for the common African types, the level of Hb F is 15–30%. These types are characterized by a uniform distribution of Hb F in the RBCs (pancellular HPFH) as compared with some of the other forms, in which the Hb F is unevenly distributed (heterocellular HPFH). Rare homozygotes for the African deletion HPFH forms have 100% Hb F in their RBCs. Except for mild microcytosis, they have normal hematologic findings. Individuals who have genes for both sickle hemoglobin and African pancellular HPFH have levels of Hb S in their RBCs that are similar to those in patients with sickle cell anemia (see Table 468–1). This combination, however, is clinically benign, presumably because the elevated Hb F in all the RBCs inhibits the sickling process.

468.9 Thalassemia Syndromes

The thalassemias are a heterogeneous group of heritable hypochromic anemias of various degrees of severity. Underlying genetic defects include total or partial deletions of globin chain genes and nucleotide substitutions, deletions, or insertions. The consequences of these various changes are a decrease or absence of mRNA for one or more of the globin chains or the formation of functionally defective mRNA. The result is a decrease or total suppression of hemoglobin polypeptide chain synthesis. More than 200 distinct mutations are known to produce thalassemia phenotypes; many of these mutations are unique to localized geographic regions. In general, the globin chains synthesized in thalassemic RBCs are structurally normal. In severe forms of α-thalassemia, abnormal homotetramer hemoglobins (β_4 or γ_4) are formed, but their component globin polypeptides have normal structure. Conversely, a number of structurally abnormal hemoglobins also produce thalassemia-like hematologic changes. In characterizing the expression of the various thalassemia genes, superscript designations are used to distinguish those that produce a demonstrable globin chain product, although at decreased levels (e.g., β^+-thalassemia) from those in which the synthesis of the affected globin chain is totally suppressed (e.g., β^0-thalassemia).

Thalassemia genes are remarkably widespread, and these abnormalities are believed to be the most prevalent of all human genetic diseases. Their main distribution includes areas bordering the Mediterranean Sea, much of Africa, the Middle East, the Indian subcontinent, and Southeast Asia. From 3–8% of Americans of Italian or Greek ancestry and 0.5% of black Americans carry a gene for β-thalassemia. In some regions of Southeast Asia, as many as 40% of the population have one or more thalassemia genes. The geographic areas in which thalassemia is prevalent closely parallel the regions in which *P. falciparum* malaria was formerly endemic. Resistance to lethal malarial infections by carriers of thalassemia genes apparently represented a strong selective force that favored their survival in these areas of endemic disease.

HOMOZYGOUS β^0-THALASSEMIA

(Cooley Anemia; Thalassemia Major)

CLINICAL MANIFESTATIONS. Homozygous β^0-thalassemia usually becomes symptomatic as a severe, progressive hemolytic anemia during the 2nd 6 mo of life. Regular blood transfusions are necessary in these patients to prevent the profound weakness and cardiac decompensation caused by the anemia. Without transfusion, life expectancy is no more than a few years. In untreated cases or in those receiving infrequent tranfusions at times of severe anemia, hypertrophy of erythropoietic tissue occurs in medullary and extramedullary locations. The bones become thin, and pathologic fractures may occur. Massive expansion of the marrow of the face and skull (Fig. 468–3) produces characteristic facies. Pallor, hemosiderosis, and jaundice combine to produce a greenish-brown complexion. The spleen and liver are enlarged by extramedullary hematopoiesis and hemosiderosis. In older patients, the spleen may become so enlarged that it causes mechanical discomfort and secondary hypersplenism. Growth is impaired in older children; puberty is delayed or absent because of secondary endocrine abnormalities. Diabetes mellitus resulting from pancreatic siderosis may also occur. Cardiac complications, including intractable arrhythmias and chronic congestive failure caused by myocardial

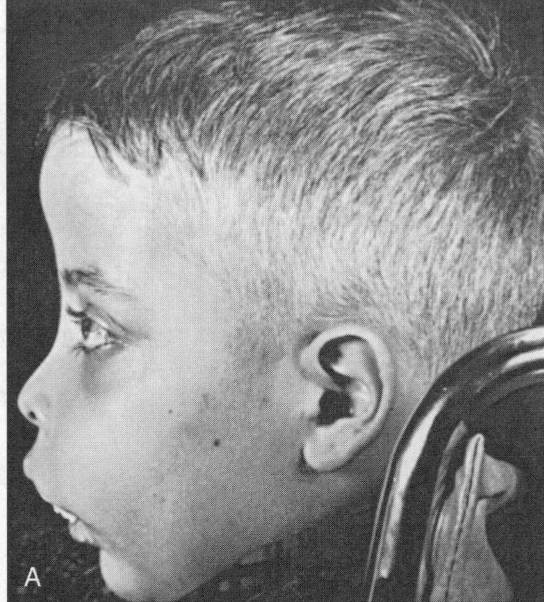

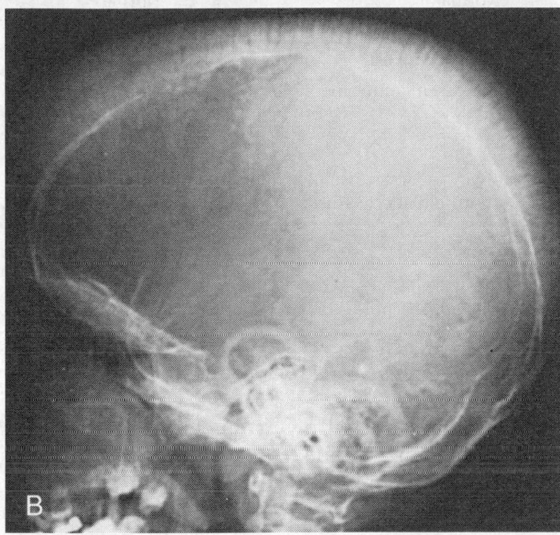

Figure 468–3 *A*, Facial deformities in an inadequately transfused patient with thalassemia major (Cooley anemia). Severe maxillary hyperplasia and malocclusion are present. *B*, Roentgenogram of the skull demonstrates the maxillary overgrowth and shows prominent widening of the diploic spaces, with the "hair-on-end" appearance caused by vertical trabeculae. These changes can usually be prevented by an appropriate transfusion regimen.

siderosis, have been common terminal events. With modern regimens of comprehensive care for these patients, many of these complications can be prevented and others ameliorated and delayed in their onset.

LABORATORY FINDINGS. The RBC morphologic abnormalities in untransfused patients with homozygous β^0-thalassemia are extreme. In addition to severe hypochromia and microcytosis (see Fig. 468–2*E*), many bizarre, fragmented poikilocytes and target cells are present. Large numbers of nucleated RBCs circulate, especially after splenectomy. Intraerythrocytic inclusions, which represent precipitated excess α chains, are also seen after splenectomy. The hemoglobin level falls progressively to lower than 5 g/dL unless transfusions are given. The unconjugated serum bilirubin level is elevated. The serum iron level is high, with saturation of the transferrin. A striking biochemical feature is the presence of very high levels of Hb F in the RBCs (Table 468–2). Dipyrrolic compounds render the urine dark brown, especially after splenectomy.

TREATMENT. Transfusions are given on a regular basis to maintain the hemoglobin level above 10 g/dL. This "hypertransfusion" regimen has striking clinical benefits; it permits normal activity with comfort, prevents progressive marrow expansion and cosmetic problems associated with facial bone changes, and minimizes cardiac dilatation and osteoporosis. Transfusions of 15–20 mL/kg of packed cells are usually necessary every 4–5 wk.

Hemosiderosis is an inevitable consequence of prolonged transfusion therapy, because each 500 mL of blood delivers to the tissues about 200 mg of iron that cannot be excreted by physiologic means. Myocardial siderosis has been a significant contributing factor in the early death of these patients. Hemosiderosis can be decreased or even prevented with parenteral administration of the iron-chelating drug deferoxamine, which forms an iron complex that can be excreted in the urine. A sustained high blood level of deferoxamine is needed for adequate iron excretion. The drug is usually administered subcutaneously over an 8- to 12-hr period using a small portable pump (during sleep), 5 or 6 nights/wk. Patients who adhere to this regimen are able to control the accumulation of excessive body iron. Lethal complications of hepatic and myocardial siderosis can thus be prevented or significantly delayed. An orally active iron chelating agent, deferiprone, has been studied in a number of clinical trials and has been shown to promote iron excretion from patients with transfusion-related siderosis. A significant percentage of patients treated with deferiprone, however, have been shown to have progressive increases in their hepatic iron stores. This agent alone does not therefore appear to be sufficient for preventing long-term iron toxicity in these patients.

Hypertransfusion in these patients effectively prevents massive splenomegaly resulting from extramedullary erythropoiesis. Splenectomy eventually becomes necessary, however, because of the size of the organ or because of secondary hypersplenism. Splenectomy increases the risk of severe, overwhelming sepsis; therefore, the operation should be performed only for significant indications (see Chapter 493) and should be deferred as long as possible. The most frequent indication for splenectomy is an increased need for transfusion. A transfusion requirement exceeding 240 mL/kg of packed RBCs/yr is usually evidence of hypersplenism and is an indication for considering splenectomy. Immunization of these patients with hepatitis B, *H. influenzae* type b, pneumococcal, and meningococcal vaccines is desirable, and prophylactic penicillin therapy is also recommended.

Bone marrow transplantation is curative in these patients and has been performed with increasing success, even in patients who have been transfused extensively. This procedure, however, carries considerable risks of morbidity and mortality and generally can be used only for patients who have nonaffected histocompatible siblings.

OTHER β-THALASSEMIA SYNDROMES

The homozygous expression of milder (β^+) thalassemia genes produces a Cooley's anemia-like syndrome of lesser severity ("thalassemia intermedia"; see Table 468–2). Skeletal deformities and hepatosplenomegaly develop in these patients, but their hemoglobin levels are usually maintained at 6–8 g/dL without transfusion. Nevertheless, they may develop severe hemosiderosis, attributable to their greatly increased gastrointestinal iron absorption. For such patients, who do not receive deferoxamine chelation therapy, a low-iron diet is indicated.

Several structurally abnormal hemoglobins produce β-thalassemia–like hematologic changes and, when present in combination with a gene for β-thalassemia, also result in a thalassemia intermedia syndrome. Among these are the Hb Lepore variants, which are composed of α chains in combination with hybrid δβ fusion globin chains. The Lepore hemoglo-

TABLE 468–2 Clinical and Hematologic Features of the Principal Forms of Thalassemias

Type of Thalassemia	Globin Genotype*	Hematologic Features	Clinical Expression	Hemoglobin Findings
β-Thalassemias				
β^0 homozygous	β^0/β^0	Severe anemia; nomoblastemia (see Fig. 461–2*E*)	Cooley's anemia	Hb F >90% No Hb A Hb A_2 increased
β^+ homozygous	β^+/β^+	Anisocytosis, poikilocytosis; moderately severe anemia	Thalassemia intermedia	Hb A: 20–40% Hb F: 60–80%
β^0 heterozygous	β/β^0	Microcytosis, hypochromia, mild to moderate anemia	May have splenomegaly, jaundice	Increased Hb A_2 and Hb F
β^+ heterozygous	β/β^+	Microcytosis, hypochromia, mild anemia	Normal	Increased Hb A_2 and Hb F
β silent carrier, heterozygous	β/β^+	Normal	Normal	Normal
δβ heterozygous	$\delta\beta/(\delta\beta)^0$	Microcytosis, hypochromia, mild anemia	Usually normal	Hb F: 5–20% Hb A_2: normal or low
γδβ heterozygous	$\gamma\delta\beta/(\gamma\delta\beta)^0$	Newborn: microcytosis, hemolytic anemia, normoblastemia Adult: similar to heterozygous δβ	Newborn: hemolytic disease with splenomegaly Adult: similar to heterozygous δβ	Normal
α-Thalassemias				
α Silent carrier	−,α/α,α	Mild microcytosis or normal	Normal	Normal
α Trait	−,α/−,α or −,−/α,α	Microcytosis, hypochromia, mild anemia	Usually normal	Newborn: Hb Bart's (γ_4), 5–10% Child or adult: normal
Hb H disease	−,α/−,−	Microcytosis, inclusion bodies by supravital staining; moderately severe anemia (see Fig. 461–2*F*)	Thalassemia intermedia	Newborn: Hb Bart's (γ_4), 20–30% Child or adult: Hb H (γ_4), 4–20%
α-Hydrops fetalis	−,−/−,−	Anisocytosis, poikilocytosis; severe anemia	Hydrops fetalis; usually stillborn or neonatal death	Hb Bart's (γ_4), 80–90%; no Hb A or Hb F

β: Normal β-globin gene; B^0 and β^+: β-thalassemia genes.
Adapted from Honig GR, Adams JG III: Human Hemoglobin Genetics. Vienna, Springer-Verlag, 1986.

bins are identified by electrophoresis, in which they exhibit Hb S–like mobility.

Most forms of *heterozygous β-thalassemia* are associated with mild anemia. The hemoglobin concentration typically averages 2–3 g/dL lower than age-related normal values. The RBCs are hypochromic and microcytic, with poikilocytosis, ovalocytosis, and often basophilic stippling. Target cells may be present but usually are not prominent and are not specific for thalassemia. The MCV is low, averaging 65 fL, and the mean corpuscular hemoglobin (MCH) values are also low (<26 pg). A mild decrease in RBC survival can be shown, but overt signs of hemolysis are usually absent. The serum iron level is normal or elevated.

Individuals with thalassemia trait are often misdiagnosed as having iron deficiency anemia and may be inappropriately treated with iron for extended periods. More than 90% of persons with β-thalassemia trait have diagnostic elevations of Hb A_2 of 3.4–7%. About 50% of these individuals also have slight elevations of Hb F, about 2–6%. In a small number of otherwise typical cases, normal levels of Hb A_2 with Hb F levels ranging from 5–15% are found, representing the δβ type of thalassemia (see Table 468–2). The silent carrier form of β-thalassemia produces no demonstrable abnormality in heterozygous individuals (see Table 468–2), but the gene for this condition, when inherited together with a gene for β^0-thalassemia, results in a thalassemia intermedia syndrome.

A rare type of deletion defect, which involves the γ-, δ-, and β-globin genes, produces a clinical picture similar to that of δβ-thalassemia trait in heterozygous individuals. In the newborn period, however, this defect is accompanied by significant hemolytic disease with microcytosis, normoblastemia, and splenomegaly (see Table 468–2). The hemolytic process is self-limited, but supportive transfusions may be required.

α-THALASSEMIA

Microcytic anemias resulting from deficient synthesis of α-globin chains are prevalent in Africa, Mediterranean area countries, and much of Asia. Deletions of α-globin genes account for most of these abnormalities. Four α-globin genes are present in normal individuals, and four distinct forms of α-thalassemia have been identified as corresponding to deletions of one, two, three, or all four of these genes (see Table 468–2).

Deletion of a single α-globin gene produces the silent carrier α-thalassemia phenotype. No hematologic abnormality is usually evident, except for mild microcytosis. Approximately 25% of black Americans have this form of α-thalassemia.

Individuals *lacking two α-globin genes* exhibit the feature of α-thalassemia trait, with mild microcytic anemia. In affected newborns, small quantities of Hb Bart's (γ_4) can be identified by hemoglobin electrophoresis. Beyond about 1 mo of age, Hb Bart's is no longer detectable, and the levels of Hb A_2 and F are characteristically normal. Inclusions of precipitated hemoglobin may be visualized in RBC smears, however, after supravital staining.

Deletion of three of the four α-globin genes is associated with a thalassemia intermedia–like syndrome, Hb H disease. Microcytic anemia in this condition is accompanied by abnormal RBC morphology (see Fig. 468–2*F*), with prominent intracellular inclusions present in the RBCs after supravital staining. Hb H (β_4) is highly unstable; it can be readily identified by electrophoresis, but unless special measures are taken to prevent its precipitation during sample preparation, it may escape detection.

The most severe form of α-thalassemia, resulting from *deletion of all of the α-globin genes,* is accompanied by a total absence of α-chain synthesis. Because Hb F, A, and A_2 all contain α chains, none of these hemoglobins is produced. Hb Bart's (γ_4)

accounts for most of the hemoglobin in affected infants, and because γ_4 has a high oxygen affinity and therefore cannot transport oxygen to the tissues, these infants are severely hypoxic. Their RBCs also contain small quantities of the normal embryonic Hb Portland ($\zeta_2\gamma_2$), which functions as an effective oxygen transporter. Most of these infants are stillborn, and most who are born alive die within a few hours. These infants are severely hydropic, with congestive heart failure and massive generalized edema. Those that survive with aggressive neonatal management are also transfusion dependent.

The *types of α-thalassemia genes vary among affected populations*, and these differences account for the α-thalassemia syndromes that predominate in specific population groups. In black Americans, α-thalassemia genes are prevalent, with almost all affected individuals having the deletion arrangement (−, α) that produces a single α-locus chromosome. In this population, therefore, α-thalassemia occurs mainly as the silent carrier phenotype (−, α/α, α) or as α-thalassemia trait (−, α/−, α). Chromosomes with deletions of both of the α loci (−, −) are prevalent in both Mediterranean and Asian populations, and Hb H disease (−, α/−, −) therefore occurs with significant frequency in both groups. The two α-locus deletion defects in Asians are often accompanied by retention of the ζ-globin genes (i.e., ζ−, −), whereas those from Mediterranean countries usually are not (−, −). The latter type of defect, therefore, cannot support the synthesis of Hb Portland ($\zeta_2\gamma_2$), which appears to be essential for intrauterine survival of fetuses with the hydrops fetalis form of α-thalassemia. Accordingly, the hydrops fetalis form almost exclusively affects infants of Asian ancestry. An *acquired α-thalassemia* syndrome, which may be associated with a large deletion involving the α-globin genes, includes Hb H disease accompanied by mental retardation, microcephaly, and hypogonadism.

A number of abnormal hemoglobins also produce α-thalassemia–like changes. The α-chain variant Hb Constant Spring occurs commonly in Far Eastern populations and is frequently observed in patients with Hb H disease who have the genotype (α^A, $\alpha^{Co\ Sp}$/−, −). The gene for Hb G Philadelphia, which is the most prevalent α-chain abnormality of black Americans, usually occurs on a single-locus chromosome (−, α^G). Individuals who express this abnormal hemoglobin therefore may also exhibit α-thalassemia–like hematologic changes.

468.10 Hemochromatosis

Excessive storage of iron, primarily in the form of hemosiderin in parenchymal cells, can result in impairment of the structure and function of the liver, heart, gonads, skin, and joints. *Hereditary hemochromatosis*, which results from homozygosity for the HLA-linked hemochromatosis allele, usually does not become clinically apparent until adult life. The underlying metabolic defect in this disorder is unknown. Symptomatic individuals exhibit massive iron stores with the classic clinical triad of cirrhosis, bronzing of the skin, and diabetes mellitus. Serum ferritin levels are characteristically greatly elevated, with increased transferrin saturation. The gene for this disorder is frequently linked to HLA types A-3, B-7, and B-14, and in families with an affected individual, this association provides an opportunity for screening siblings and children before the onset of symptomatic iron storage. With treatment by repeated phlebotomy, organ damage can be prevented.

Neonatal hemochromatosis is an acquired syndrome resulting from severe liver disease arising prenatally. Various forms of fetal hepatopathy can give rise to this clinical entity, which consists of severe liver dysfunction or liver failure, accompanied by massive iron stores and siderosis. Most of these infants have had a fatal outcome, although some have survived.

Transfusion-induced hemosiderosis, in patients repeatedly transfused for congenital or acquired anemia, can produce clinical and pathologic features quite similar to those in patients with transfusion-dependent thalassemia (see Chapter 468.9).

Hemoglobin Disorders

Bunn HF, Forget BG: Hemoglobin: Molecular, Genetic, and Clinical Aspects. Philadelphia, WB Saunders, 1986.

Honig GR, Adams JG III: Human Hemoglobin Genetics. Vienna, Springer-Verlag, 1986.

Weatherall DJ, Clegg JB, Higgs DR, Wood WG: The hemoglobinopathies. *In:* Scriver CR, Beaudet AL, Sly WS, Valle D (eds): The Metabolic Basis of Inherited Disease, 7th ed. New York, McGraw-Hill, 1995.

Sickle Cell Disease

Adams RJ, McKie VC, Carl EM, et al: Long-term stroke risk in children with sickle cell disease screened with transcranical Doppler. Ann Neurol 42:699, 1997.

Adams RJ, McKie VC, Hsu L, et al: Prevention of a first stroke by transfusion in children with sickle cell anemia and abnormal results on transcranial Doppler ultrasonography. N Engl J Med 339:5, 1998.

Bjornson AB, Falletta JM, Verter JI, et al: Serotype-specific immunoglobulin G antibody responses to pneumococcal polysaccharide vaccine in children with sickle cell anemia: Effects of continued penicillin prophylaxis. J Pediatr 129:828, 1996.

Bunn HF: Pathogenesis and treatment of sickle cell disease. N Engl J Med 337:762, 1997.

Charache S, Terrin ML, Moore RD, et al: Effect of hydroxyurea on the frequency of painful crises in sickle cell anemia. N Engl J Med 332:1317, 1995.

Falletta JM, Woods GM, Verter JI, et al: Discontinuing penicillin prophylaxis in children with sickle cell anemia. J Pediatr 127:685, 1995.

Gaston MH, Verter JI, Woods G, et al: Prophylaxis with oral penicillin in children with sickle cell anemia: A randomized trial. N Engl J Med 314:1593, 1986.

Hongeng S, Wilimas JA, Harris S, et al: Recurrent *Streptococcus pneumoniae* sepsis in children with sickle cell disease. J Pediatr 130:814, 1997.

Kinney TR, Ware RE: The adolescent with sickle cell anemia. Hematol Oncol Clin North Am 10:1255, 1996.

Koshy M, Weiner SJ, Miller ST, et al: Surgery and anesthesia in sickle cell disease. Blood 86:3676, 1995.

Leonard MB, Zemel BS, Kawchak DA, et al: Plasma zinc status, growth, and maturation in children with sickle cell disease. J Pediatr 132:467, 1998.

Marcinak JF, Frank AL, Labotka RL, et al: *Haemophilus influenzae* type B vaccine in children with sickle cell disease: Antibody persistence after vaccination at age one and one-half to six years. Pediatr Infect Dis J 10:157, 1991.

Newborn screening for sickle cell disease and other hemoglobinopathies. Pediatrics 83:813, 1989.

Ohene-Frempong K, Weiner SJ, Sleeper LA, et al: Cerebrovascular accidents in sickle cell disease: Rates and risk factors. Blood 91:288, 1998.

Olivieri NF, Vichinsky EP: Hydroxyurea in children with sickle cell disease: Impact on splenic function and compliance with therapy. J Pediatr Hematol Oncol 20:26, 1998.

Pearson HA, Spencer RP, Cornelius EA: Functional asplenia in sickle cell anemia. N Engl J Med 281;293, 1969.

Powars D: Natural history of sickle cell disease—the first ten years. Semin Hematol 12:267, 1975.

Powars D, Hiti A: Sickle cell anemia. β_s gene cluster haplotypes as genetic markers for severe disease expression. Am J Dis Child 147:1197, 1993.

Rana S, Houston PE, Surana N, et al: Discontinuation of long-term transfusion therapy in patients with sickle cell disease and stroke. J Pediatr 131:757, 1997.

Reid CD, Charache S, Lubin B (eds): Management and Therapy of Sickle Cell Disease. NIH Publication no. 95-2117. Washington, DC, U.S. Dept. of Health and Human Services, 1995.

Serjeant GR, Serjeant BE, Thomas PW, et al: Human parvovirus infection in homozygous sickle cell disease. Lancet 341:1237, 1993.

Sickle Cell Disease Guideline Panel: Sickle Cell Disease: Screening, Diagnosis, Management, and Counseling in Newborns and Infants. Clinical Practice Guideline No. 6. Publication no. 93-0562. Rockville, MD, Agency for Health Care Policy and Research, 1993.

Vermylen C, Cornu G: Bone marrow transplantation for sickle cell disease. The European experience. Am J Pediatr Hematol Oncol 16:18, 1994.

Wang WC, Langston JW, Steen G, et al: Abnormalilties of intra central nervous system in very young children with sickle cell anemia. J Pediatr 132:994, 1998.

Wilimas JA, Flynn PM, Harris S, et al: A randomized study of outpatient treatment with ceftriaxone for selected febrile children with sickle cell disease. N Engl J Med 329:472, 1993.

Wong W-Y, Overturf GD, Powars DR: Infection caused by *Streptococcus pneumoniae* in children with sickle cell disease: Epidemiology, immunologic mechanisms, prophylaxis, and vaccination. Clin Infect Dis 14:1124, 1992.

Methemoglobinemia

Jaffe ER, Hultquist DE: Cytochrome b_5 reductase deficiency and enzymopenic hereditary methemoglobinemia. *In:* Scriver CR, Beaudet AL, Sly WS, Valle D (eds): The Metabolic Basis of Inherited Disease, 7th ed. New York, McGraw-Hill, 1995.

Thalassemia

Brittenham GM, Griffith PM, Nienhuis AW, et al: Efficacy of deferoxamine in preventing complications of iron overload in patients with thalassemia major. N Engl J Med 331:567, 1994.

Chik K, Shing MMK, Lick, et al: Treatment of hemoglobin Bart's hydrops with bone marrow transplantation. J Pediatr 132:1039, 1998.

Hoffbrand AV, AL-Refaie F, Davis B, et al: Long-term trial of deferiprone in 51 transfusion-dependent iron overloaded patients. Blood 91:295, 1998.

Honig GR, Sharon BI: Globin synthesis-thalassemia syndromes. *In*: Gross S, Roath S (eds): Hematology—A Problem-Oriented Approach. Baltimore, Williams & Wilkins, 1996.

Lucarelli G, Galimberti M, Polchi P, et al: Marrow transplantation in patients with thalassemia responsive to iron chelation therapy. N Engl J Med 329:840, 1993.

Modell B, Berdouks V: The Clinical Approach to Thalassaemia. London, Grune & Stratton, 1984.

Nathan D: An orally active iron chelator. N Engl J Med 332:953 1995.

Olivieri NF, Brittman GM, McLaren CE, et al: Long-term safety and effectiveness of iron-chelation therapy with deferiprone for thalassemia major. N Engl J Med 339:417, 1998.

Piomelli S, Hart D, Graziano J, et al: Current strategies in the management of Cooley's anemia. Ann N Y Acad Sci 445:256, 1985.

Sharon BI, Honig GR: Management of congenital hemolytic anemia. *In*: Rossi EC, Simon TL, Moss GS (eds): Principles of Transfusion Medicine. Baltimore, Williams & Wilkins, 1991.

Weatherall DJ: Hemoglobin E β-thalassemia: An increasingly common disease with some diagnostic pitfalls. J Pediatr 132:765, 1998.

Weatherall DJ: The thalassemias. *In:* Stamatoyannopoulos G, Nienhuis AW, Majerus PW, Varmus H (eds): The Molecular Basis of Blood Diseases. Philadelphia, WB Saunders, 1994.

Wilkie AOM, Buckle VJ, Harris PC, et al: Clinical features and molecular analysis of the α thalassemia/mental retardation syndromes. I. Cases due to deletions involving chromosome band 16p13.3. Am J Hum Genet 46:1112, 1990.

Hemochromatosis

Bothwell TH, Charlton RW, Motulsky AG: Hemochromatosis. *In*: Scriver CR, Beaudet AL, Sly WS, Valle D (eds): The Metabolic Basis of Inherited Disease, 7th ed. New York, McGraw-Hill, 1995.

Burke W, Thomson E, Khoury MJ, et al: Hereditary hemochromatosis gene discovery and its implications for population-based screening, JAMA 280:172, 1998.

Knisely AS: Neonatal hemochromatosis. Adv Pediatr 39:383, 1992.

Oliviera MG, Fermandes A, Silva AC, et al: A case of neonatal haemochromatosis. Acta Pediatr 87:102, 1998.

Saddi R, Schapira G: Hemochromatosis, idiopathic. *In*: Buyse ML (ed): Birth Defects Encyclopedia. Cambridge, MA, Blackwell, 1990.

CHAPTER 469
Enzymatic Defects

George B. Segel

DEFICIENCIES OF ENZYMES OF THE GLYCOLYTIC PATHWAY

Various red blood cell (RBC) enzymatic defects produce hemolytic anemias, characterized by a lack of spherocytes and few distinguishing features on the blood film. Deficiencies of most of the enzymes in both the anaerobic Embden-Meyerhof pathway and the oxidative hexose monophosphate (pentose) shunt have been described (Fig. 469–1). The most common glycolytic enzyme defect as a cause of hemolytic anemia is pyruvate kinase (PK) deficiency, although it is rare disorder, with only 300–400 cases reported.

469.1 Pyruvate Kinase Deficiency

A congenital hemolytic anemia occurs in persons homozygous for an autosomal recessive gene that causes either a marked reduction in RBC PK or production of an abnormal enzyme with decreased activity. Generation of adenosine triphosphate (ATP) within RBCs is impaired, and low levels of ATP, pyruvate, and the reduced form of nicotinamide-adenine dinucleotide (NAD^+) are found (Fig. 469–1). The concentration of 2,3-diphosphoglycerate (2,3-DPG) is increased, and this increase is beneficial in facilitating oxygen release from hemoglobin but detrimental in inhibiting hexokinase as well as enzymes of the hexose monophosphate shunt. In addition, an unexplained decrease occurs in the sum of the adenine (ATP, adenosine diphosphate [ADP], and adenosine monophosphate [AMP]) and pyridine (NAD^+ and NADH) nucleotides, and this further impairs glycolysis. As a consequence of decreased ATP, RBCs cannot maintain the potassium and water content; the cells become rigid, and the RBC life span is considerably reduced.

ETIOLOGY. The human PK gene has been mapped to chromosome 1q21, and various mutations occur in this structural gene, which codes for a protein with 543 amino acids and forms a functional tetramer. Most affected patients are compound heterozygotes for two diffrent PK gene defects. The many possible combinations likely account for the variability in clinical severity.

CLINICAL MANIFESTATIONS AND LABORATORY FINDINGS. The clinical manifestations vary from a severe neonatal hemolytic anemia to mild, well-compensated hemolysis noted first in adulthood. Severe jaundice and anemia may occur in the neonatal period, and kernicterus has been reported. The hemolysis in older children and adults varies in severity, with hemoglobin values from 8–12 g/dL associated with some pallor, jaundice, and splenomegaly. These patients usually do not require transfusion. A severe form of the disease has a relatively high incidence among the Amish of the midwestern United States.

Polychromatophilia and mild macrocytosis reflect the elevated reticulocyte count. Spherocytes are uncommon, but a few spiculated pyknocytes are usually found. Nonincubated osmotic fragility is normal. Autohemolysis is moderately or markedly increased, but the addition of glucose does not regularly correct the abnormality as it does in hereditary spherocytosis.

Diagnosis relies on demonstration of a marked reduction of PK activity or an increase in the Michaelis-Menten dissociation constant (Km) for its substrate, phosphoenolpyruvate, in the RBCs. Other RBC enzyme activities are normal or elevated. No abnormalities of hemoglobin are noted. The white cells have normal PK activity and must be excluded from hemolysates used to measure PK activity. Heterozygous carriers usually have moderately reduced levels of PK activity.

TREATMENT. Exchange transfusions may be indicated for hyperbilirubinemia in newborns. Transfusions of packed RBCs are necessary for severe anemia or for aplastic crises. If the anemia is consistently severe or if frequent transfusions are required, splenectomy should be performed after 5–6 yr of age. Although not curative, the operation may be followed by higher hemoglobin levels and by strikingly high (30–60%) reticulocyte counts. Deaths resulting from overwhelming pneumococcal sepsis have followed splenectomy; thus, immunization with vaccines for encapsulated organisms should be given before splenectomy, and prophylactic penicillin should be administered after splenectomy.

469.2 Other Glycolytic Enzyme Deficiencies

Chronic nonspherocytic hemolytic anemias of varying severity have been associated with deficiencies of other enzymes in the glycolytic pathway, including hexokinase, glucose phosphate isomerase, and aldolase, which are inherited as autosomal recessive disorders. *Phosphofructokinase (PFK) deficiency* occurs primarily in Ashkenazi Jews in the United States and results in hemolysis associated with a myopathy classified as glycogen storage disease type VII (see Chapter 84.1). Clinically,

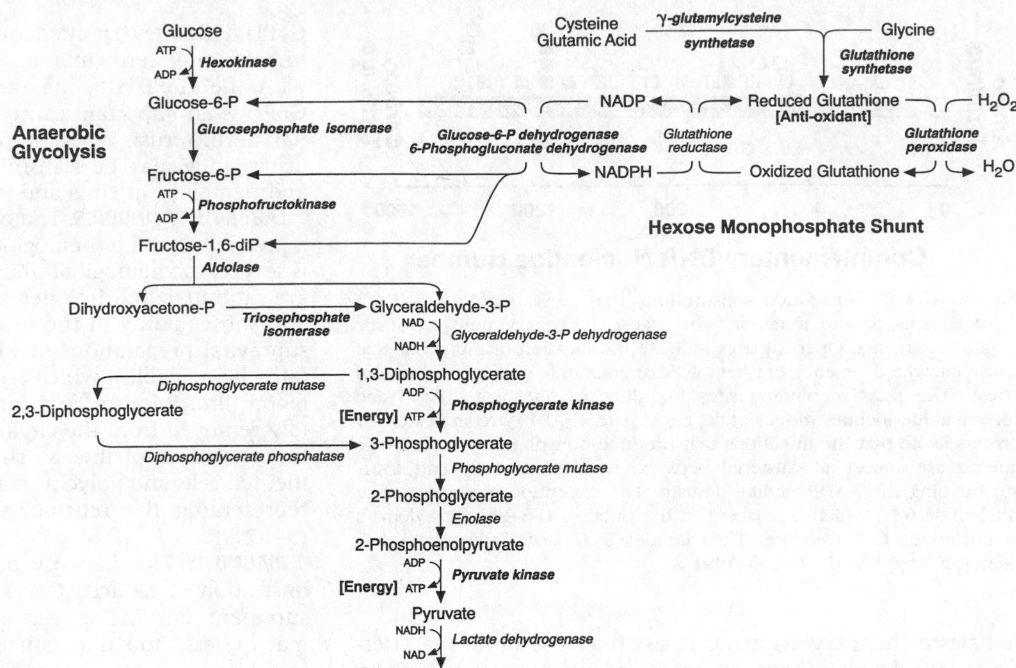

Figure 469–1 Red cell metabolism. Glycolysis and the hexose monophosphate pathway. The enzyme deficiencies clearly associated with hemolysis are shown in bold type.

a hemolytic anemia is complicated by muscle weakness, exercise intolerance, cramps, and possibly myoglobinuria. Enzyme assays for PFK are low in RBCs and muscle.

Triose phosphate isomerase (TPI) deficiency is an autosomal recessive disorder affecting many systems. Affected patients have hemolytic anemia, cardiac abnormalities, and lower motor neuron and pyramidal tract impairment without mental retardation. They usually die in early childhood. The TPI gene has been cloned and sequenced and is localized on chromosome 12.

Phosphoglycerate kinase (PGK) is the first ATP-generating step in glycolysis. At least 12 kindreds with PGK deficiency now have been described. PGK is the only glycolytic enzyme inherited on the X chromosome. Affected males have progressive extrapyramidal disease, seizures, and variable mental retardation in conjunction with hemolytic anemia. The gene for PGK is particularly large, spanning 23 kb, and various mutations producing single amino acid substitutions result in PGK deficiency.

DEFICIENCIES OF ENZYMES OF THE HEXOSE MONOPHOSPHATE PATHWAY AND RELATED COMPOUNDS

The most important function of the hexose monophosphate pathway is to maintain glutathione in its reduced state (GSH) as protection against oxidation of RBCs (Fig. 469–1). About 10% of the glucose taken up by RBCs passes through this pathway to provide the NADPH necessary for conversion of oxidized glutathione (GSSG) to GSH. Maintenance of GSH is essential for the physiologic inactivation of oxidant compounds, such as hydrogen peroxide, that accumulate within RBCs. If glutathione, or any compound or enzyme necessary for maintaining it in the reduced state, is decreased, the SH groups of the RBC membrane are oxidized and the hemoglobin becomes denatured and may precipitate into RBC inclusions called *Heinz bodies*. Once Heinz bodies have formed, an acute hemolytic process results from damage to the RBC membrane by the precipitated hemoglobin, the oxidant agent, and the action of the spleen. The damaged RBCs then are rapidly removed from the circulation.

469.3 Glucose-6-Phosphate Dehydrogenase (G6PD) and Related Deficiencies

G6PD deficiency is the most important disease of the hexose monophosphate pathway and is responsible for two clinical syndromes, an episodic hemolytic anemia induced by infections or certain drugs and a spontaneous chronic nonspherocytic hemolytic anemia. This X-linked enzyme deficiency affects more than 200 million people, and it represents an example of "balanced polymorphism" in which there is an evolutionary advantage of resistance to *Falciparum* malaria in heterozygous females that outweighs the small negative effect of affected hemizygous males.

The deficiency is caused by inheritance of any of a large number of abnormal alleles of the gene responsible for the synthesis of the G6PD molecule. The G6PD gene has been cloned and sequenced, and at least 90 mutations have been identified. Some of these mutations that cause episodic versus chronic hemolysis are shown in Fig. 469–2. Milder disease is associated with mutations near the N-terminus of the G6PD molecule, and chronic nonspherocytic hemolytic anemia with mutations clustered near the C-terminus. The normal enzyme found in most populations is designated G6PD B^+. A normal variant designated G6PD A^+ is common in the African-American population. More than 100 distinct enzyme variants of G6PD are associated with a wide spectrum of hemolytic disease.

EPISODIC OR INDUCED HEMOLYTIC ANEMIA

ETIOLOGY. Synthesis of RBC G6PD is determined by a gene on the X chromosome. Diseases involving this enzyme therefore occur more frequently in males than in females. About 13% of male African-Americans have a mutant enzyme (G6PD A^-) that results in a deficiency of RBC G6PD activity to 5–15% or less of normal. Italians, Greeks, and other Mediterranean, Middle Eastern, African, and Asian ethnic groups also have a high incidence, ranging from 5–40%, of a variant designated G6PD B^- (G6PD Mediterranean). The G6PD activity of homozygous

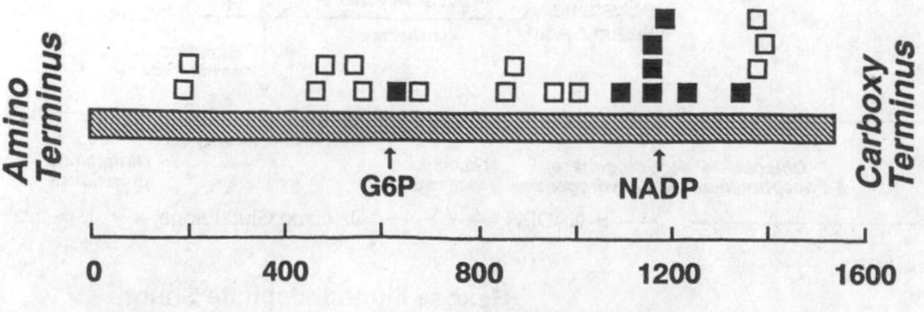

Figure 469–2 Nucleotide substitutions that cause G6PD deficiency. Solid squares denote mutations that cause hereditary nonspherocytic hemolytic anemia. Open squares indicate the location of mutations that cause enzyme deficiency but hemolytic anemia only under conditions of stress. The putative binding sites for glucose-6-phosphate (G6P) and nicotinamide-adenine dinucleotide phosphate (NADP) are indicated by arrows. Note that the mutations that produce nonspherocytic hemolytic anemia are almost all clustered between nucleotides 1089 and 1361, surrounding the NADP-binding domain. The exception is a mutation at nucleotide 637, which is adjacent to the putative G-6-P binding domain at nucleotide 605. (Modified from Beutler E: Glucose-6-phosphate deficiency. N Engl J Med 324:169, 1991.)

females or hemizygous males is less than 5% of normal. Heterozygous females have an intermediate enzymatic activity and, as an example of random X chromosome inactivation (Lyon's hypothesis), have two populations of RBCs: One is normal, and the other is deficient in G6PD activity. Most heterozygous females do not have clinical hemolysis after exposure to oxidant drugs. Rarely, the majority of the RBCs are G6PD deficient in heterozygous females because of random inactivation of the normal X chromosome.

Considerable variation in the defect among various racial groups is noted. For example, the defect in black Americans is less severe than in affected whites. In black Americans, the electrophoretically distinct enzyme variant is unstable in vivo, and its activity is decreased primarily in the older RBCs in the circulation. The enzyme activity of RBCs containing the variant enzyme (G6PD B^-) in whites is very low, often less than 1% of normal in the entire RBC population. A third common mutant enzyme with markedly reduced activity (G6PD Canton) occurs in about 5% of Chinese. A large number of other rare enzyme variants have been associated with drug-induced hemolysis.

CLINICAL MANIFESTATIONS. In the usual pattern of G6PD deficiency, symptoms develop 24–48 hr after a patient has ingested a substance that has oxidant properties. Drugs that have these properties include aspirin, sulfonamides, and antimalarials such as primaquine (Table 469–1). In some patients, ingestion of fava beans, a Mediterranean dietary staple, may also produce an acute and severe hemolytic syndrome called *favism*. This results from oxidative products derived from two glucosidic compounds, vicine and convicine, which are hydrolyzed to divicine and isouramil, ultimately producing hydrogen peroxide and other reactive oxygen products.

The degree of hemolysis varies with the inciting agent, the amount ingested, and the severity of the enzyme deficiency in the patient. In severe cases, hemoglobinuria and jaundice result, and the hemoglobin concentration may fall precipitously and be life threatening. In the A^- variety (black Americans), the stability of the folded protein dimer is impaired, and this defect is accentuated as RBCs age. Thus, some spontaneous recovery of the hemolysis may be observed even if administration of the drug is continued. This recovery is a result of the age-labile enzyme, which is abundant and more stable in younger RBCs. The associated reticulocytosis produces a compensated hemolytic process. Infection also may result in hemolysis, and significant hemolysis may occur even when no exposure to drugs can be documented (see Chronic Hemolytic Anemias Associated with Deficiencies of G6PD, later). In A^- G6PD deficiency, spontaneous hemolysis may occur in premature but not term infants. In Greek and Chinese newborns with the G6PD B^- and Canton varieties, the deficiency of G6PD is an important cause of hyperbilirubinemia and potential kernicterus. When a pregnant woman ingests oxidant drugs, they may be transmitted to her G6PD-deficient fetus, and hemolytic anemia and jaundice may be apparent at birth.

LABORATORY FINDINGS. The onset of acute hemolysis results in a precipitous fall in hemoglobin and hematocrit. If the episode is severe, the hemoglobin-binding proteins such as haptoglobin are saturated, and free hemoglobin may appear in the plasma and subsequently in the urine (see Fig. 463–2). Unstained or supravital preparations of RBCs reveal Heinz bodies (precipitated hemoglobin), which are not visible on the Wright-stained blood film. Because cells containing these inclusions are rapidly removed from the circulation, they are not seen after the first 3–4 days of illness. The blood film reveals a few fragmented cells and polychromatophilic cells (bluish, large RBCs), representing the reticulocytosis, which often is substantial (5–15%).

DIAGNOSIS. The diagnosis depends on direct or indirect demonstration of reduced G6PD activity in RBCs. By direct measurement, enzyme activity in affected persons is 10% of normal or less, and the reduction of enzyme is more extreme in whites and Asians than in African-Americans. Satisfactory screening tests are based on decoloration of methylene blue, on the reduction of methemoglobin, or on the fluorescence of NADPH. Immediately after a hemolytic episode, reticulocytes and young RBCs predominate. These young cells have significantly higher enzyme activity than do older cells in the A^- variety. Testing may therefore have to be deferred for a few weeks before a diagnostically low level of enzyme can be shown. The diagnosis can be suspected when the G6PD activity is within the low normal range in the presence of a high reticulocyte count. G6PD variants also can be detected by electrophoretic analysis.

PREVENTION AND TREATMENT. Prevention of hemolysis constitutes the most important therapeutic measure. When possible, males belonging to ethnic groups with a significant incidence of G6PD deficiency (e.g., Greeks, southern Italians, Sephardic Jews, Filipinos, southern Chinese, African-Americans, and Thais) should be tested for the defect before known oxidant drugs are given. The usual doses of aspirin and trimethoprim sulfamethoxazole do not cause clinically relevant hemolysis in the A^- variety. However, aspirin administered for acute

TABLE 469–1 Agents Precipitating Hemolysis in Glucose-6-Phosphate Dehydrogenase Deficiency

Medications	Chemicals
Antibacterials	Phenylhydrazine
Sulfonamides	Benzene
Trimethoprim-sulfamethoxazole	Naphthalene
Nalidixic acid	**Illness**
Chloramphenicol	Diabetic acidosis
Nitrofurantoin	Hepatitis
Antimalarials	
Primaquine	
Pamaquine	
Chloroquine	
Quinacrine	
Others	
Phenacetin	
Vitamin K analogs	
Methylene blue	
Probenecid	
Acetylsalicylic acid	
Phenazopyridine	

Reproduced from Asselin BL, Segel GB. In: *Rakel R (ed): Conn's Current Therapy. Philadelphia, WB Saunders, 1994, p 341.*

rheumatic fever (60–100 mg/kg/24 hr) may produce a severe hemolytic episode. When hemolysis has occurred, supportive therapy may require blood transfusions, although recovery is the rule when the oxidant agent is removed.

CHRONIC HEMOLYTIC ANEMIAS ASSOCIATED WITH DEFICIENCIES OF G6PD OR RELATED FACTORS

Chronic nonspherocytic hemolytic anemia has been associated with profound deficiency of G6PD caused by enzyme variants, particularly those defective in quantity, activity, or stability. The gene defects leading to chronic hemolysis are located primarily in the region of the NADP binding site near the C-terminus of the protein (see Fig. 469–2). These include the Loma Linda, Tomah, Iowa, Beverly Hills, Nashville, Riverside, Santiago de Cuba, and Andalus variants. Persons with G6PD B^- (Mediterranean) enzyme deficiency occasionally have chronic hemolysis, and the hemolytic process may worsen after ingestion of oxidant drugs. The location of the gene defect in these patients has not been defined. Splenectomy is of little value in these types of chronic hemolysis.

Other enzyme defects may impair the regeneration of GSH as an oxidant "sump" (see Fig. 469–1). A mild, chronic nonspherocytic anemia has been reported in association with decreased RBC GSH, resulting from γ-glutamylcysteine synthetase or glutathione synthetase deficiencies. 6-Phosphogluconate dehydrogenase deficiency has been associated primarily with drug-induced hemolysis, and hemolysis with hyperbilirubinemia has been related to a deficiency of glutathione peroxidase in newborn infants.

CHAPTER 470

Hemolytic Anemias Resulting from Extracellular Factors

George B. Segel

AUTOIMMUNE HEMOLYTIC ANEMIAS

A number of extrinsic agents and disorders may lead to premature destruction of red blood cells (RBCs) (see Table 463–2). Among the most clearly defined are antibodies associated with immune hemolytic anemias. The hallmark of this group of diseases is a positive result of a direct Coombs test, which detects a coating of immunoglobulin or components of complement on the RBC surface. The most important immune hemolytic disorder in pediatric practice is hemolytic disease of the newborn (erythroblastosis fetalis), caused by transplacental transfer of maternal antibody active against the RBCs of the fetus, that is, isoimmune hemolytic anemia (Chapter 99.2). Various other immune hemolytic anemias are autoimmune (Table 470–1) and may be idiopathic or related to various infections (Epstein-Barr virus, rarely HIV, cytomegalovirus, and Mycoplasma), immunologic diseases (systemic lupus erythematosus [SLE], rheumatoid arthritis), immunodeficiency diseases (agammaglobulinemia and dysgammaglobulinemias), neoplasms (lymphoma, leukemia, and Hodgkin disease), or drugs (methyldopa, levodopa). Other drugs (penicillins, cephalosporins) cause immune hemolysis that is not autoimmune. The antibodies are "drug dependent" and usually (though not always) have no "specificity" for RBC membrane antigens.

TABLE 470–1 Diseases Characterized by Immune-Mediated Red Blood Cell Destruction

Autoimmune Hemolytic Anemia due to Warm Reactive Autoantibodies

- Primary (idiopathic)
- Secondary
  - Lymphoproliferative disorders
  - Connective tissue disorders (especially systemic lupus erythematosus)
  - Nonlymphoid neoplasms (e.g., ovarian tumors)
  - Chronic inflammatory diseases (e.g., ulcerative colitis)

Autoimmune Hemolytic Anemia Due to Cold Reactive Autoantibodies (Cryopathic Hemolytic Syndromes)

- Primary (idiopathic) cold agglutinin disease
- Secondary cold agglutinin disease
  - Lymphoproliferative disorders
  - Infections (*Mycoplasma pneumoniae,* Epstein-Barr virus)
- Paroxysmal cold hemoglobinuria
  - Primary (idiopathic)
  - Congenital or tertiary syphilis
  - Viral syndromes (most common)

Drug-Induced Immune Hemolytic Anemia

- Hapten/drug adsorption (e.g., penicillin)
- Ternary (immune) complex (e.g., quinine or quinidine)
- True autoantibody induction (e.g., methyldopa)

Modified from Packman CH: Autoimmune hemolytic anemias. In: *Rakel R (ed): Conn's Current Therapy. Philadelphia, WB Saunders, 1995, p 305.*

AUTOIMMUNE HEMOLYTIC ANEMIAS ASSOCIATED WITH "WARM" ANTIBODIES

ETIOLOGY. In the autoimmune hemolytic anemias, abnormal antibodies are directed against RBCs, but the pathogenetic mechanisms are uncertain. The autoantibody may be produced as an inappropriate immune response to a RBC antigen or to another antigenic epitope similar to a RBC antigen. Alternatively, an infectious agent may in some way alter the RBC membrane so that it becomes "foreign" or antigenic to the host.

In most instances of warm antibody hemolysis, no underlying cause can be found, and it is called *primary* or *idiopathic* (Table 470–1). If the autoimmune hemolysis is associated with an underlying disease such as a lymphoproliferative disorder, SLE, or immunodeficiency, it is called *secondary.* In as many as 20% of cases of immune hemolysis, drugs may be implicated.

Drugs (e.g., penicillin or sometimes cephalosporins) that cause hemolysis via the "hapten" mechanism (immune but not autoimmune) bind tightly to the RBC membrane (Table 470–1). Antibodies to the drug, either newly or previously formed, bind to the drug molecules on RBCs, mediating their destruction in the spleen. In other cases, certain drugs, such as quinine and quinidine, do not bind to RBCs but rather form part of a "ternary complex," consisting of the drug, a RBC membrane antigen, and an antibody that recognizes both (see Table 470–1). Methyldopa may by unknown mechanisms incite true autoantibodies to RBC membrane antigens.

CLINICAL MANIFESTATIONS. Autoimmune hemolytic anemias may occur in either of two general clinical patterns. The first, an acute transient type lasting 3–6 mo and occurring predominantly in children ages 2–12 yr, accounts for 70–80% of patients. It is frequently preceded by an infection, usually respiratory. The onset may be acute, with prostration, pallor, jaundice, pyrexia, and hemoglobinuria, or may be more gradual in onset, with primarily fatigue and pallor. The spleen is usually enlarged and is the primary site for destruction of IgG-coated RBCs. Underlying systemic disorders are unusual in this group. A consistent response to glucocorticoid therapy, low mortality, and full recovery are characteristic of the acute form. The other clinical pattern involves a prolonged and chronic course, which is more frequent in infants and in children older than 12 yr. Hemolysis may continue for many months or years. Abnormalities involving other blood elements are common, and the response to glucocorticoids is variable and inconsistent. Mortality is about 10%, often attributable to an underlying systemic disease.

LABORATORY FINDINGS. In many cases, the anemia is profound, with hemoglobin levels less than 6 g/dL. Considerable spherocytosis and polychromasia are present. More than 50% of the circulating RBCs may be reticulocytes, and nucleated RBCs usually are present. In some cases, a low reticulocyte count may be present, particularly early in the episode. Leukocytosis is common. The platelet count is usually normal, but immune thrombocytopenic purpura *(Evans' syndrome)* is an occasional concomitant. The prognosis for patients with Evans' syndrome is poor, because many develop chronic disease, including some with SLE.

Results of the direct test are strongly positive, and free antibody can sometimes be demonstrated in the serum (indirect Coombs test). These antibodies are active between 35°C and 40°C ("warm" antibodies) and most often belong to the immunoglobulin G (IgG) class. They do not require complement for activity and usually do not produce agglutination in vitro; they are "incomplete." Antibodies from the serum and those eluted from the RBCs react with RBCs of many persons, in addition to those of the patient. They often have been regarded as nonspecific panagglutinins, but careful studies have revealed specificity for RBC antigens of the Rh system in 70% (~50% adults) of patients. Complement, particularly C3b, may be detected on the RBCs in conjunction with IgG. The Coombs test result is occasionally negative because of the limited sensitivity of the Coombs reaction. A minimum of 260–500 molecules of IgG is necessary on the RBC membrane to produce a positive reaction. Special tests are required to detect the antibody in cases of "Coombs-negative" autoimmune hemolytic anemia.

TREATMENT. Transfusions usually are only of transient benefit but may be required initially because of the severity of the anemia until the effect of other treatment is observed. It may be extremely difficult to find compatible blood; blood in which the RBCs give the least positive in vitro reaction by Coombs technique should be chosen. It is sometimes necessary to give blood that is "incompatible" as judged by cross matching. Failure to transfuse a profoundly anemic infant or child may lead to serious morbidity and even death.

Those patients with mild disease and compensated hemolysis may not require any treatment. If the hemolysis is severe and results in significant anemia or symptoms, treatment with glucocorticoids is initiated. Glucocorticoids decrease the rate of hemolysis by blocking macrophage function, decreasing the production of the autoantibody, and perhaps by enhancing the elution of antibody from the RBCs. Prednisone or its equivalent is administered in a dose of 2 mg/kg/24 hr. In some patients with severe hemolysis, doses up to 6 mg/kg/24 hr of prednisone may be required to reduce the rate of hemolysis. Treatment should be continued until the rate of hemolysis decreases, and then the dose is gradually reduced. If relapse occurs, resumption of full dosage may be necessary. The disease tends to remit spontaneously within a few weeks or months. The Coombs test result may remain positive, even after hemolysis has subsided. When hemolytic anemia remains severe despite glucocorticoid therapy, or if very large doses are necessary to maintain a reasonable hemoglobin level, intravenous immunoglobulin and danazol may be tried. Splenectomy may be beneficial but is complicated by a heightened risk of infection with encapsulated organisms, particularly in patients younger than 2 yr. Prophylaxis is indicated with appropriate vaccines (pneumoccocal, meningococcal, and *Haemophilus influenzae* type b) before splenectomy and with oral penicillin after splenectomy. Immunosuppressive agents have been of some benefit in chronic cases refractory to conventional therapy. Various plasmapheresis techniques may be used in refractory cases but generally are not helpful.

COURSE AND PROGNOSIS. The acute variety of idiopathic autoimmune hemolytic disease in childhood varies in severity but is self-limited, and mortality from untreatable anemia is rare. Approximately 30% of patients develop chronic hemolysis, often associated with an underlying disease, such as SLE, lymphoma, or leukemia. Mortality in the chronic cases depends on the primary disorder.

AUTOIMMUNE HEMOLYTIC ANEMIAS ASSOCIATED WITH "COLD" ANTIBODIES

RBC antibodies that are more active at low temperatures and agglutinate RBCs at temperatures below 37°C have been called "cold" antibodies. They are primarily of the IgM class and require complement for activity. The highest temperature associated with RBC agglutination is called the *thermal amplitude*. A higher thermal amplitude results in hemolysis with less severe exposure to a cold environment. High antibody titers are associated with high thermal amplitude.

COLD AGGLUTININ DISEASE. Cold antibodies usually have specificity for the oligosaccharide antigens of the I/i system. They may occur in primary or idiopathic cold agglutinin disease, secondary to infections such as *Mycoplasma pneumoniae* and Epstein-Barr virus, or secondary to lymphoproliferative disorders. After *Mycoplasma* infection, the anti-I levels may increase considerably, and occasionally, enormous increases may occur to titers of 1:30,000 or greater. The antibody has specificity for the I antigen and reacts poorly with human cord blood cells, which possess the i antigen but exhibit low levels of I. Patients with infectious mononucleosis occasionally develop cold agglutinin disease, and the antibodies in these patients often have anti-i specificity. Spontaneous RBC agglutination is observed in the cold, and RBC aggregates are seen on the blood film. The mean corpuscular volume may be spuriously elevated because of cell agglutination. The severity of the hemolysis is related to the thermal amplitude of the antibody, which itself is partly dependent on the IgM antibody titer.

When very high titers of cold antibodies are present and active near body temperature, severe intravascular hemolysis with hemoglobinemia and hemoglobinuria may occur and be heightened on a patient's exposure to cold. Each IgM molecule has the potential to active a C1 molecule so that large amounts of complement are found on the RBCs in cold agglutinin disease. These sensitized RBCs may undergo intravascular complement lysis or be destroyed in both the liver and spleen.

Cold agglutinin disease is less common in children than in adults, and it more frequently results in an acute, self-limited episode of hemolysis. Glucocorticoids are much less effective in cold agglutinin disease and are not particularly useful. Patients should avoid exposure to cold and should be treated for any underlying disease. In the infrequent patients with severe hemolytic disease, the treatment includes immunosuppression and plasmapheresis. Splenectomy is not useful in cold agglutinin disease.

PAROXYSMAL COLD HEMOGLOBINURIA. This form of hemolytic anemia is mediated by the Donath-Landsteiner hemolysin, which is an IgG cold-reactive autoantibody with anti-P specificity. This antibody fixes large amounts of complement in the cold, and the RBCs lyse as the temperature is increased. Most reported cases are self-limited and usually are associated with nonspecific viral infections. They are now rarely found in association with congenital or acquired syphilis. This disorder may account for 30% of immune hemolytic episodes among children. Treatment includes transfusions for severe anemia and avoidance of cold ambient temperatures.

CHAPTER 471

Hemolytic Anemias Secondary to Other Extracellular Factors

(See Table 463–1)

George B. Segel

FRAGMENTATION HEMOLYSIS. Red blood cell (RBC) destruction occurs in this group of diseases because of mechanical injury as the cells traverse a damaged vascular bed. This may be microvascular when RBCs are sheared by fibrin in the capillaries during intravascular coagulation or when renovascular disease accompanies the hemolytic-uremic syndrome (Chapter 526) or thrombotic thrombocytopenic purpura. Larger vessels may he involved in the Kasabach-Merritt syndrome (giant hemangioma and thrombocytopenia) or when a replacement heart valve is poorly epithelialized. The blood film shows many "schistocytes" or fragmented cells as well as polychromatophilia, reflecting the reticulocytosis (see Fig. 464–2*F*). Secondary iron deficiency may complicate the intravascular hemolysis because of urinary iron loss (see Fig. 463–2). Treatment should be directed toward the underlying condition, and the prognosis depends on the effectiveness of this treatment. The benefit from transfusion is transient because the transfused cells are destroyed as quickly as those produced by the patient.

THERMAL INJURY. Extensive burns may directly damage the RBCs and result in hemolysis with spherocytosis. Blood loss and marrow suppression may contribute to anemia and require blood transfusion. More recently, erythropoietin (EPO) has been used as treatment for diminished RBC production.

RENAL DISEASE. The anemia of uremia is multifactorial in origin. EPO production may be decreased and the marrow suppressed by toxic metabolites. Furthermore, the RBC life span often is shortened owing to retention of metabolites and organic acidemia. The use of EPO in chronic renal disease has markedly decreased the need for blood transfusion.

LIVER DISEASE. Change in the ratio of cholesterol to phospholipids in the plasma may result in changes in the composition of the RBC membrane and shortening of the RBC life span. Some patients with liver disease have many target RBCs on the blood film, whereas others have a preponderance of spiculated cells.

TOXINS AND VENOMS. Bacterial sepsis due to *Haemophilus influenzae*, staphylococci, and streptococci may be complicated by accompanying hemolysis. A particularly severe hemolytic anemia has been observed in clostridial infections and results from a hemolytic clostridial toxin. Large numbers of spherocytes may be seen on the blood film in this condition. Spherocytic hemolysis also may be noted after bites by various snakes, including cobras, vipers, and rattlesnakes, which have phospholipases in their venom. Large numbers of bites by insects such as bees, wasps, and yellow jackets also may cause spherocytic hemolysis by a similar mechanism (see Chapter 724).

WILSON DISEASE. An acute and self-limited episode of hemolytic anemia may precede by years the onset of hepatic or neurologic symptoms in Wilson disease. This appears to result from the toxic effects of free copper on the RBC membrane. The blood film often (but not always) shows large numbers of spherocytes, and the Coombs test result is negative. Because early diagnosis of Wilson's disease permits prophylactic treatment with penicillamine and prevention of hepatic and neurologic disease, correct assessment of this rare type of hemolysis is most important.

Enzymatic Defects of Red Cells

Arese P, De Flora A: Pathophysiology of hemolysis in glucose-6-phosphate dehydrogenase deficiency. Semin Hematol 27:1, 1990.

Beutler E: Glucose-6-phosphate dehydrogenase deficiency. N Engl J Med 324:169, 1994.

Kaplan M, Muraca M, Hammerman C, et al: Bilirubin conjugation, reflected by conjugated bilirubin fractions, in glucose-6-phosphate dehydrogenase–deficient neonates: A determining factor in the pathogenesis of hyperbilirubinemia. Pediatrics 102(3):E37, 1998.

Mason PJ: Annotation: New insights into G6PD deficiency. Br J Haematol 94:585, 1996.

Tanaka KR, Zerez CR: Red cell enzymopathies of the glycolytic pathway. Semin Hematol 27:165, 1990.

Zimmerman SA, Ware RE, Forman L, et al: Glucose-6-phosphate dehydrogenase Durham: A de novo mutation associated with chronic hemolytic anemia. J Pediatr 131:284, 1997.

Autoimmune Hemolytic Anemia

Buchanan GR, Boxer LA, Nathan DG: The acute and transient nature of idiopathic immune hemolytic anemia in childhood. J Pediatr 88:780, 1976.

Flores G, Cunningham-Rundles C, Newland AC, Bussel JB: Efficacy of intravenous immunoglobulin in the treatment of autoimmune hemolytic anemia: Results in 73 patients. Am J Hematol 44:237, 1993.

Packman CH: Autoimmune hemolytic anemia. *In:* Rakel R (ed): Conn's Current Therapy. Philadelphia, WB Saunders, 1995, pp 305–312.

Packman CH, Leddy JP: Acquired hemolytic anemia due to warm-reacting antibodies. *In:* Beutler E, Lichtman MA, Coller BS, Kipps TC (eds): Hematology. New York, McGraw-Hill, 1995, pp 677–685.

SECTION 4

Polycythemia (Erythrocytosis)

CHAPTER 472

Primary Polycythemia

(Polycythemia Rubra Vera)

Bruce M. Camitta

Polycythemia exists when the red blood cell (RBC) count, the hemoglobin level, and the total RBC volume all exceed the upper limits of normal. In postpubertal children, a hemoglobin greater than 16 g/dL and a total RBC mass greater than 35 mL/kg (males) or greater than 31 mL/kg (females) indicate polycythemia. Measurement of the total RBC volume by radioisotopic techniques is essential in the differential diagnosis of polycythemia. True polycythemia is characterized by increases of both the RBC and total blood volumes. A decrease in plasma volume, such as occurs in acute dehydration and burns, may result in a high hemoglobin value. However, these situations are more accurately designated hemoconcentration because the RBC mass is not increased and normalization of the plasma volume restores the hemoglobin to normal levels.

Primary polycythemia vera, a myeloproliferative disorder, has been reported in only a few children. In vitro cultures of erythroid precursors of affected persons do not require added erythropoietin to stimulate growth. Diagnostic criteria are increased total RBC volume, arterial oxygen saturation of 92% or greater, and splenomegaly. Supportive laboratory abnormalities include thrombocytosis (>400,000/μL), leukocytosis (>12,000/μL), increased leukocyte alkaline phosphatase (>100 U/L), and increased vitamin B_{12} (>900 pg/mL) or increased unsaturated B_{12} binding capacity. (>2,200 pg/mL). Erythropoietin levels are normal or low. Treatment includes phlebotomy and (if necessary) antiproliferative chemotherapy. The disease may be complicated by bleeding or thrombosis. It may evolve into myelofibrosis or acute leukemia. Prolonged survival is not unusual.

Berlin N (ed): Polycythemia vera. Semin Hematol 34:1, 1997.
Danish EH, Rasch CA, Harris JW: Polycythemia vera in childhood: Case report and review of the literature. Am J Hematol 9:421, 1980.

CHAPTER 473
Secondary Polycythemia

Bruce M. Camitta

The differential diagnosis of secondary polycythemia is shown in Table 473–1. Polycythemia may be present in any clinical situation associated with chronic arterial oxygen desaturation. Cardiovascular defects involving right-to-left shunts and pulmonary diseases interfering with proper oxygenation are the most common causes of hypoxic polycythemia. Clinical findings usually include cyanosis, hyperemia of the sclerae and mucous membranes, and clubbing of the fingers. As the hematocrit rises above 65%, clinical manifestations of hyperviscosity, such as headache and hypertension, may require phlebotomy (also see Chapter 99.3). On the other hand, the increased demand for red blood cell (RBC) production may cause iron deficiency. Iron-deficient RBCs are more rigid, further increasing the risk of intracranial thrombosis in these patients. Because microcytosis may occur only as a late manifestation of iron deficiency in children with hypoxic polycythemia, routine periodic assessment of iron status, with treatment of iron deficiency, should be performed in these children. Living at high altitudes also causes hypoxic polycythemia; the hemoglobin level increases about 4% for each rise of 1,000 m in altitude. Partial obstruction of a renal artery rarely results in polycythemia.

TABLE 473–1 Differential Diagnosis of Polycythemia

Primary (Polycythemia Vera)

Secondary

- Neonatal
  - Normal intrauterine environment
  - Twin-twin or maternal-fetal hemorrhage
  - Infants of diabetic mothers
  - Intrauterine growth retardation
  - Trisomies 13, 18, or 21
  - Adrenal hyperplasia
  - Thyrotoxicosis
- Hypoxia
  - Altitude
  - Cardiac disease
  - Lung disease
  - Central hypoventilation
- Hemoglobinopathy
  - High oxygen affinity variants
  - Methemoglobin reductase deficiency
  - Chronic carbon monoxide exposure
- Hormonal
  - Malignant tumors
    - Renal, hepatic, adrenal, cerebellar, other
  - Renal disease
    - Cysts, hydronephrosis
  - Adrenal disease
    - Virilizing hyperplasia, Cushing's syndrome
  - Anabolic steroid therapy
- Familial

Spurious (Plasma Volume Decrease)

TABLE 473–2 Sequential Evaluation of Polycythemia

1. Complete blood count including differential white blood count
2. Rule out plasma volume decrease
3. Diagnose secondary polycythemia
   - Arterial oxygen saturation
   - Carboxyhemoglobin
   - Renal ultrasonography
   - Abdominal/cranial CT
4. Special studies for polycythemia vera
   - Leukocyte alkaline phosphatase
   - B_{12}/B_{12} binding capacity
   - Erythropoietin level
   - Red blood cell colony formation

More subtle forms of hypoxia may also cause polycythemia. Congenital methemoglobinemia resulting from a deficiency of cytochrome b5 reductase may cause cyanosis and polycythemia (see Chapter 468.7). This condition is transmitted as an autosomal recessive trait. Most affected individuals are asymptomatic. Neurologic abnormalities may be present in patients whose enzyme deficit is not limited to hematopoietic cells. Dominantly transmitted polycythemia is caused by hemoglobins that have increased oxygen affinity. Cyanosis may occur in the presence of as little as 1.5 g/dL of methemoglobin but is uncommon in other hemoglobin variants unless hyperviscosity results in localized hypoxemia. See Chapter 99.3.

Polycythemia has also been associated with benign and malignant lesions that secrete erythropoietin. Exogenous or endogenous excess of anabolic steroids also may cause polycythemia. In several families, benign polycythemias have been transmitted as dominant or recessive conditions, the bases of which are not known.

Sequential studies to evaluate polycythemia are outlined in Table 473–2. For mild disease, observation is sufficient. When the hematocrit exceeds 65–70% (hemoglobin >23 g/dL), blood viscosity markedly increases. Periodic phlebotomies may prevent or decrease symptoms. Apheresed blood should be replaced with plasma or saline to prevent hypovolemia in patients accustomed to a chronically elevated total blood volume.

Oh W: Neonatal polycythemia and hyperviscosity. Pediatr Clin North Am 33:523, 1986.
Spivak JL: Erythrocytosis. *In*: Hoffman R, Benz EJ, Shattil SJ, et al (eds): Hematology: Basic Principles and Practice, 2nd ed. New York, Churchill Livingstone, 1995, p 484.

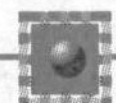

SECTION 5

The Pancytopenias

Philip A. Pizzo ■ Alan D. D'Andrea

Pancytopenia can result from either a failure of production of hematopoietic progenitors, their destruction, or replacement of the bone marrow by tumor or fibrosis. Although selective cytopenias are important clinical entities (see Chapters 131.1, 454–458, 490), pancytopenia is a loss of all marrow elements. The clinical consequences include anemia, neutropenia, and thrombocytopenia and, depending on the degree and duration of their impairment, can lead to serious illness and death. Pancytopenia can be constitutional, arising as a consequence of an inherited genetic defect affecting hematopoietic progenitors, or can be acquired as a consequence of either direct destruction of progenitors, immune-mediated damage to either hematopoietic progenitors or their nurturing microenvironment, or suppression of or crowding out of progenitors by tumor cells or fibrosis. In this section, the constitutional and acquired pancytopenias are considered separately. Because the principles of supportive care are generally independent of the etiology of the pancytopenia, they are presented in Chapters 476–480. ■

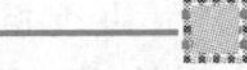

CHAPTER 474

The Constitutional Pancytopenias

ETIOLOGY. Although Fanconi anemia is the best-recognized constitutional pancytopenia, a number of other infrequent genetic disorders have also been implicated. These genetic syndromes (Table 474–1) include various modes of inheritance and may be associated with a number of congenital abnormalities, especially of the bones, kidneys, and heart. Because the hematologic manifestations of the congenital pancytopenias may not become manifested until the first years to even decades of life, a genetic predisposition to bone marrow failure should be considered in all cases of aplastic anemia in children (see later). These disorders can be autosomal recessive (e.g., Fanconi anemia, dyskeratosis congenita), X linked, or autosomal dominant (e.g., dyskeratosis congenita). Several of these genetic disorders may present initially with a single cytopenia and subsequently progress to pancytopenia (e.g., Shwachman-Diamond syndrome, amegakaryocytic thrombocytopenia, reticular dysgenesis). In addition, a number of inheritable familial marrow dysfunction syndromes have been associated with pancytopenia (which can also be autosomal recessive, autosomal dominant, or X linked), and aplastic anemia also occurs in association with other genetic disorders (e.g., Down, Dubowitz, and Seckel syndromes). Thus, pancytopenia can be either the primary disease manifestation or can emerge as a rare complication during the course of another illness. Because of the chromosomal fragility or defective repair mechanisms that may be associated, several of these disorders can also be complicated by cancer or other organ dysfunction(s).

EPIDEMIOLOGY. Although the true incidence of these disorders is unknown, the constitutional pancytopenias are rare. The most common disorder is Fanconi anemia, of which approximately 1,000 cases have been described, in contrast to only about 45 cases of amegakaryocytic thrombocytopenia. Depending on geography, the heterozygote frequency of Fanconi

TABLE 474–1 Inherited Bone Marrow Failure Syndromes

Feature	Fanconi Anemia	Dyskeratosis Congenita	Shwachman-Diamond Syndrome	Amegakaryocytic Thrombocytopenia
Cases reported	1,000	225	200	45
Male/female	1.3	4.3	1.7	1.6
Genetics	Autosomal recessive	X linked; autosomal recessive, dominant	Autosomal recessive	X linked, or autosomal recessive
Physical abnormalities (%)	80	100	40	60
Hand/arm anomalies (%)	48	15	<2	0
Median age (yr) at diagnosis of initial hematologic disease	7.5	16	4 mo	<1 wk
First hematologic manifestation	Pancytopenia	Pancytopenia	Neutropenia	Thrombocytopenia
Bone marrow	Aplastic	Aplastic	Hypocellular or myeloid arrest	Absent or small megakaryocytes
Aplastic anemia (%)	>95	50	20	45
Leukemia (%)	12	0.4	5	5
Liver disease (%)	4	0	0	0
Cancer	5	10	0	0
Hb F	Increased	Increased	Increased	Increased
Chromosomes	Breaks increased with clastogens	Bleomycin sensitive	Normal	Normal
Spontaneous remissions	Very rare	None	Rare	BMT
Treatment, responses	BMT, androgens, 50%, transient	Androgens, 50%, transient	G-CSF, BMT, 80%	None
Prognosis	Poor	Poor	Fair	Poor
Prenatal diagnosis	Chromosome breaks, FAC	Xq28 RFLP	Neutropenia	Thrombocytopenia
Predicted median survival age (yr)	30	33	35	3

RFLP = restriction fragment length polymorphism; BMT = bone marrow transplantation; G-CSF = granulocyte colony-stimulating factor.
Modified from Alter BP, Young NS: The bone marrow failure syndromes. In: *Nathan DG, Orkin FA (eds): Nathan and Oski's Hematology of Infancy and Children, 5th ed. Philadelphia, WB Saunders, 1998.*

anemia ranges from 1/100 to 1/300. The familial aplastic anemias are much less common.

PATHOLOGY AND PATHOGENESIS. One of the hallmarks of Fanconi anemia is evidence of spontaneous or clastogen-induced chromosome breaks. Lymphoid, hematopoietic (including progenitors), and fibroblast cells from patients with Fanconi anemia demonstrate a number of cytogenetic abnormalities, including defective DNA repair, increased susceptibility of hematopoietic cells to oxidant stress, and decreased cell survival. Eight genetic complementation groups of Fanconi anemia have been identified. Two genes, corresponding to complementation groups A and C, have been cloned, but the functions of these genes or gene products are mostly unknown. It is likely that the absence of these gene products contributes directly to the poor growth of hematopoietic progenitor cells and the heightened risk of malignancies. Depressed levels of granulocyte-macrophage colony-stimulating factor (GM-CSF), stem cell factor, and interleukin 6 (IL-6) also have been observed in children with Fanconi syndrome, suggesting that an abnormal cytokine network contributes to the pathogenesis of the bone marrow failure in these patients. Increased cellular sensitivity to γ-interferon may account, at least in part, for the pancytopenia of Fanconi anemia.

Chromosome breakage has also been observed in approximately 10% of patients with dyskeratosis congenita, and decreased hematopoietic cytokines have been found in some patients with the Shwachman-Diamond syndrome. However, the pathogenesis of these disorders and that of the familial marrow dysfunction syndromes remain undefined.

CLINICAL MANIFESTATIONS. Various physical abnormalities accompany most of the congenital pancytopenias, particularly Fanconi anemia and dyskeratosis congenita. Patients having Fanconi anemia are characterized by hyperpigmentation and café-au-lait spots, skeletal abnormalities (especially absent or hypoplastic thumbs), short stature, and a wide array of integumentary and organ abnormalities. *Dyskeratosis congenita* is also very commonly associated with hyperpigmentation as well as nail dystrophy of both the hands and feet, leukoplakia, and a number of ocular abnormalities, including epiphora, blepharitis, and cataracts. The relative frequencies of these abnormalities are compared in Table 474–1. Approximately 14–25% of patients with the cytogenetic abnormalities of Fanconi anemia lack the major physical stigmas of Fanconi syndrome and have been designated as having the "Estren-Damashek" subtype. A diversity of cutaneous, skeletal, growth, and organ abnormalities can also be found in 30–40% of the other congenital and familial pancytopenias, although they do not follow any uniform pattern.

LABORATORY FINDINGS. Depending on the specific disorder, thrombocytopenia, leukopenia, lymphopenia, or anemia generally precedes the onset of pancytopenia. Further, hematologic abnormalities may precede or follow elucidation of other physical defects. As noted earlier, chromosomal breaks occur in most patients with Fanconi anemia compared with 10% of those with dyskeratosis congenita. Children with Fanconi anemia and dyskeratosis congenita generally have macrocytosis as well as mild poikilocytosis and anisocytosis, and their red blood cells (RBCs) contain higher levels of i antigen and hemoglobin F than are found in acquired aplasia. The age of onset of hematologic abnormalities ranges from infancy to adolescence. Once peripheral pancytopenia is evident, bone marrow examination generally confirms a hypoplastic or aplastic state comparable to that in acquired aplastic anemias.

Additional laboratory examination should include skeletal radiographs as well as examination of the genitourinary tract and, depending on the diagnosis, more detailed examination of the eyes, gastrointestinal tract, heart, teeth, and gonads (in males).

DIAGNOSIS. The presence of characteristic skeletal and cutaneous abnormalities coupled with short stature should suggest the diagnosis of congenital pancytopenia even in the absence of hematologic problems. In contrast, when a child presents with evidence of bone marrow failure, a genetic or familial defect should always be considered and evaluated by cytogenetic examination, including chromosomal breakage studies. This is particularly important because approximately 20% of individuals with congenital pancytopenias may occasionally not have any of the physical abnormalities that are considered characteristic of these syndromes (see Table 474–1).

COMPLICATIONS. The major complications related to the congenital pancytopenias include the consequences of bone marrow failure, a heightened risk for leukemia and other cancers, and organ complications that are specific to the primary defect (e.g., liver problems in Fanconi syndrome, malabsorption in Shwachman-Diamond syndrome). Infection and bleeding represent the major hematologic manifestations leading to life-threatening complications (see Chapter 476). Depending on their degree and duration, the hematologic abnormalities may respond to supportive care initially, but when pancytopenia ensues (depending on the syndrome, this occurs in 20–90% of patients), more aggressive therapies are required. As more knowledge is gained about the molecular and cellular pathogenesis of these syndromes, it may be possible to delay some of the hematologic complications (see later).

TREATMENT. The traditional backbone of therapy for patients with congenital anemias has been steroids and androgens (especially oxymetholone or nandrolone), alone or in combination. Although 50–75% of patients show some evidence of improvement with androgens, relapse is common and complications (especially hepatic tumors or obstructive liver disease) occur. Improvements in RBCs generally precede those in white blood cells, and it may take months to achieve a maximum benefit. These therapies have been shown to prolong life by approximately 2 yr and hence can be considered palliative only.

The only "curative" therapy to date has been bone marrow transplantation. However, patients with congenital pancytopenias also have an increased predisposition to malignancy, and the preparative regimens generally used during bone marrow transplantation can adversely affect this susceptibility. Accordingly, lower doses of alkylating agents in the preparative regimens appear to be appropriate. Furthermore, most patients with Fanconi anemia do not have histocompatible donors. Transplantation from unmatched donors results in considerable morbidity, owing to the increased intensity of graft versus host disease in these children. Encouraging results have been reported when GM-CSF was administered subcutaneously to children with Fanconi anemia and pancytopenia. A significant increase in the neutrophil count was observed in six of seven patients who were treated at the Children's Hospital (Boston) and this was sustained for more than a year without any evidence of leukemia. More transient responses have been observed with G-CSF. Additional follow-up is important, and it is possible that treatment of these patients with multiple cytokines (erythropoietin, IL-3, IL-6) may offer additional benefits. Ultimately, the best hope for these children will emerge from an understanding of the molecular defects that produce the syndromes; once these are identified, gene therapy may become a feasible consideration.

PROGNOSIS. When marrow failure develops, the prognosis is guarded. Although bone marrow transplantation and hematopoietic growth factor reconstitution offer some hope, neither overcomes the risks for subsequent cancer or other organ complications.

GENETIC COUNSELING. Once an index case has been identified, genetic counseling is important and must be oriented to the patterns of inheritance and the prospect for prenatal diagnosis. Based on the presence of cytogenetic and chromosomal breakage or, in the case of amegakaryocytic thrombocytopenia, fetal blood platelet counts, a diagnosis can be suspected or confirmed.

CHAPTER 475
The Acquired Pancytopenias

ETIOLOGY AND EPIDEMIOLOGY. Various drugs, chemicals, toxins, infectious agents, radiation, or immune disorders can result in pancytopenia, either by direct destruction of hematopoietic progenitors, by disruption or destruction of the supporting marrow microenvironment and its necessary growth factors, or by direct or indirect (e.g., virus-related) immune-mediated destruction of marrow elements (Table 475–1). Whenever a child presents with pancytopenia, a careful history of exposure to known risk factors should be obtained. The possibility of a genetic predisposition to bone marrow failure should always be considered, even in the absence of the classic physical findings associated with Fanconi anemia and the other congenital pancytopenias (see Chapter 474). The overall incidence of acquired aplastic anemia is relatively low, with an approximate cumulative annual incidence in both children and adults, in the United States and Europe, of 2–6 cases per million per year.

A number of drugs can result in transient (albeit severe) and predictable bone marrow depression. Most notable, of course, are antineoplastic agents (e.g., anthracyclines, alkylators, antimetabolites) as well as certain antibiotics (e.g., chloramphenicol). Permanent damage can also be done if sufficient doses of these agents are administered and is more likely with certain agents (e.g., benzene). Aplastic anemia or pancytopenia can follow administration of a great many different kinds of drugs and chemicals (including certain insecticides, antibiotics, anticonvulsants, nonsteroidal anti-inflammatory agents, antihistamines, sedatives, and metals). The relative frequency of aplastic anemias ranges from approximately 1/25,000–40,000 for chloramphenicol to 1/350,000 for cimetidine, and it is even less frequent for other agents. A genetic predisposition may exist and may increase the likelihood of pancytopenia after exposure to the drug or chemical.

TABLE 475–1 A Classification of the Aplastic Anemias

Acquired

Secondary
- Radiation
- Drugs and chemicals
  - Predictable: cytotoxic agents, benzene
  - Idiosyncratic: chloramphenicol, anti-inflammatory drugs, antiepileptics, gold
- Viruses
  - Epstein-Barr virus (infectious mononucleosis)
  - Hepatitis
  - Parvovirus B19
  - Human immunodeficiency virus (HIV)
- Immune diseases
  - Eosinophilic fasciitis
  - Hypoimmunoglobulinemia
- Thymoma
- Pregnancy
- Paroxysmal nocturnal hemoglobinuria
- Preleukemia

Idiopathic

Inherited

- Fanconi anemia
- Dyskeratosis congenita
- Shwachman-Diamond syndrome
- Reticular dysgenesis
- Amegakaryocytic thrombocytopenia
- Familial aplastic anemias
- Preleukemia, myelodysplasia, monosomy 7
- Nonhematologic syndromes (e.g., Down, Dubowitz, and Seckel syndromes)

Modified from Alter BP, Young NS: The bone marrow failure syndromes. In: *Nathan DG, Orkin SH (eds): Nathan and Oski's Hematology of Infancy and Childhood, 5th ed. Philadelphia, WB Saunders, 1998.*

A number of viruses can either directly or indirectly result in bone marrow failure. Parvovirus B19 is classically associated with pure red blood cell (RBC) aplasia, but in patients with sickle cell disease or in other compromised hosts (e.g., with cancer or AIDS), it can result in a transient aplastic crisis (Chapters 244 and 468). Pancytopenia can also be associated with hepatitis virus (both hepatitis B virus and hepatitis C virus), as well as with dengue virus, presumably consequent to the immune activation that accompanies these virus infections. Herpes viruses, particularly Epstein-Barr virus (EBV) and cytomegalovirus (CMV), can result in bone marrow failure, either in genetically predisposed patients (e.g., those with the X-linked lymphoproliferative syndromes with EBV) or caused by bone marrow graft rejection with CMV. HIV has also been associated with a number of hematologic abnormalities, including anemia, neutropenia, thrombocytopenia, and pancytopenia.

Patients with evidence of bone marrow failure should also be evaluated for paroxysmal nocturnal hemoglobinuria (PNH) and collagen vascular diseases, although these are very uncommon complications of these diseases in childhood. Pancytopenia without peripheral blasts may be due to bone marrow replacement by leukemic or neuroblastoma malignant cells.

PATHOLOGY AND PATHOGENESIS. The hallmark of aplastic anemia is peripheral pancytopenia coupled with hypoplastic or aplastic bone marrow. The severity of the disease is related to the degree of myelosuppression. Severe aplastic anemia is defined as a condition in which two or more cell components have become seriously compromised (i.e., an absolute neutrophil count $<500/mm^3$, a platelet count $<20,000/mm^3$, a reticulocyte count $<1\%$ after correction for the hematocrit) in a patient whose bone marrow biopsy material is hypocellular. As noted earlier, bone marrow failure can result from various etiologies and mechanisms. For example, it can be a consequence of stem cell failure that is either related to a drug, toxin, or virus or that has resulted from either cell-mediated or antibody-dependent cytotoxicity. Abnormalities of the supporting microenvironment resulting from drugs, toxins, viruses, or immune-mediated mechanisms can also cause bone marrow failure. A loss of critical hematopoietic growth factors can contribute to the marrow failure state.

CLINICAL MANIFESTATIONS, LABORATORY FINDINGS, AND DIFFERENTIAL DIAGNOSIS. Acquired pancytopenia is usually characterized by anemia, leukopenia, and thrombocytopenia, in the setting of elevated serum cytokine levels. The pancytopenia results in increased risks of fatigue, cardiac failure, infection, and bleeding. Other treatable disorders, such as cancer, collagen vascular disorders, PNH, or infections that may respond to specific therapies (e.g., intravenous immune globulin for parvovirus) should be considered in the differential diagnosis. Careful examination of the peripheral blood smear for RBC, leukocyte, and platelet morphology is important. In children, the possibility of a congenital pancytopenia must always be considered and chromosomal breakage should be evaluated (see earlier). The presence of fetal hemoglobin suggests a congenital pancytopenia but is not diagnostic. To rule out PNH, a Ham's test should be performed. Bone marrow examination should include both aspiration and a biopsy, and the marrow should be carefully evaluated for cellularity and morphology. The presence of more than 70% lymphocytes has a poor prognosis.

COMPLICATIONS. The major complications of severe pancytopenia are predominantly related to the risk of life-threatening bleeding due to prolonged thrombocytopenia or to infection secondary to protracted neutropenia. Patients with protracted neutropenia due to bone marrow failure are at risk not only for serious bacterial infections but also for invasive mycoses. The general principles of supportive care that have evolved from the treatment of cancer victims suffering malignancy or chemotherapy-related myelosuppression should be fully extended to the care of patients with acquired pancytopenias (Chapter 179).

TREATMENT. As with the congenital pancytopenias, the treatment of the children with acquired pancytopenia requires comprehensive supportive care coupled with an attempt to treat the underlying marrow failure. The major therapies include the use of antithymocyte globulin (ATG), either alone or with corticosteroids, cyclosporine, bone marrow transplantation, and the use of one or more hematopoietic colony-stimulating factors. For patients with a matched sibling donor, allogeneic bone marrow transplantation offers a 45–70% chance of long-term survival. The risks associated with this approach include the immediate complications of the transplantation, graft versus host disease (which increases with patients' age), and the increased risk for subsequent cancers (Chapters 135 and 139). Because only a quarter to a third of patients have a matched donor, the use of bone marrow registries for unrelated donors and unmatched donors has also been successfully pursued. Alternatively, ATG (without transplantation) has had a response rate of 45%, and the survival rate of these patients (60%) is not significantly different from that of patients who have undergone bone marrow transplantation. The use of hematopoietic growth factors, though successful in some patients, has not had a major impact to date, although it remains possible that combinations of cytokines will have a greater effect, at least in patients who do not have significant stem cell depletion. Other therapies that have been used in the past with inconsistent results include androgens, cyclophosphamide, and plasmapheresis.

PROGNOSIS. Although spontaneous recovery rarely occurs, patients with severe pancytopenia have an extremely poor prognosis unless they respond to treatment.

PANCYTOPENIAS CAUSED BY MARROW REPLACEMENT

Processes that either infiltrate or replace the bone marrow can also present as or result in an acquired pancytopenia. This can occur either before or during malignancy (classically either neuroblastoma or leukemia in children) or as a consequence of osteoporosis (marble bone disease), myelofibrosis, or myelodysplasia. Although uncommon, evidence of a hypoplastic anemia can precede, generally by months (and only rarely by a year), the onset of acute leukemia. This is important to appreciate in evaluating and monitoring children who present with what appears to be an acquired aplastic anemia. Similarly, it is important to consider the prospect that the apparent bone marrow failure may be due to a collagen vascular disease (e.g., rheumatoid arthritis) or an underlying myelodysplastic syndrome, making morphologic examination of the peripheral blood and the bone marrow critically important. Chromosomal analysis, which, in the case of certain myelodysplastic syndromes, might reveal clonality, can be particularly helpful. The treatment and prognosis of these children are dictated by the appropriate diagnosis and management of the true underlying disease.

Alter BP, Young NS: The bone marrow failure syndromes. *In*: Nathan DG, Orkin SH (eds): Hematology of Infancy and Childhood, 5th ed. Philadelphia, WB Saunders, 1998, pp 237–335.

Brown KE, Tisdale J, Barrett J, et al: Hepatitis-associated aplastic anemia. N Engl J Med 336:1059, 1997.

DiBartolomeo P, Digirolama G, Olioso P, et al: Allogenic bone marrow transplantation for Fanconi anemia. Bone Marrow Transplant 16:53, 1992.

Guinan EC, Lopez KD, Huhn RD, et al: Evaluation of granulocyte-macrophage colony-stimulating factor for the treatment of pancytopenia in children with Fanconi anemia. J Pediatr 124:144, 1994.

Lipton JM: The hematologic garden: How does it grow? J Pediatr 132:565, 1998.

Socie G, Henry-anar M, Bacigalupo A, et al: Malignant tumor occurring after treatment of aplastic anemia. N Engl J Med 329:1152, 1993.

Young NS, Maciejewski J: The pathophysiology of acquired aplastic anemia. N Engl J Med 336:1365, 1997.

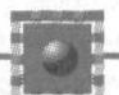

SECTION 6

Blood and Blood Component Transfusions

Ronald G. Strauss

Blood transfusions frequently are lifesaving, and modern intensive care of premature neonates, children with cancer, and transplant recipients would be impossible without them. However, transfusions are not without risks, and they should be given only when true benefits are likely, for example, to correct a deficiency or functional defect of a blood component that has caused a clinically significant problem. The principles of transfusion support for children and adolescents are similar to those for adults, but infants have many special needs. Accordingly, each of these two age groups is discussed separately within each section. Many of the transfusion guidelines provided are updated versions of those formulated originally by the Pediatric Hemotherapy Committee of the American Association of Blood Banks. However, it is important that they be adapted to fit local standards of practice. In particular, terms such as "severe" and "symptomatic" must be defined by local physicians. ■

CHAPTER 476

Red Blood Cell Transfusions and Erythropoietin Therapy

Red blood cells (RBCs) are the most frequently transfused blood component. They are given to increase the oxygen-carrying capacity of the blood and to maintain satisfactory tissue oxygenation. Guidelines for RBC transfusions in *children and adolescents* are similar to those for adults (Table 476–1). However, transfusions may be given more stringently to children because hemoglobin levels are lower in normal children than in adults and, except in defined circumstances, children do not usually have the underlying cardiorespiratory diseases that develop with aging in adults. Thus, children should have less-impaired abilities to compensate for RBC loss. In the perioperative period, for example, it is unnecessary for children to maintain hemoglobin levels of 80 g/L or greater, a level frequently desired for adults. There should be a compelling reason to administer any postoperative RBC transfusion, because most children (without continued bleeding) can quickly restore their RBC mass if given iron therapy. As is true for adults, the most important measures in the treatment of acute hemorrhage, occurring with surgery or injury in children, are first to control the hemorrhage and to restore tissue perfusion, with crystalloid and /or colloid solutions. Then, if the estimated blood loss is greater than 25% of the circulating blood volume (i.e., >17 mL/kg body weight) and the patient's condition remains unstable, RBC transfusions may be indicated. In acutely ill children with severe pulmonary disease requiring assisted ventilation, it is common practice to maintain the hemoglobin level close to the normal range. Although this recommendation seems logical, its efficacy has not been documented by controlled scientific studies.

TABLE 476–1 Guidelines for Pediatric RBC Transfusions

Children and Adolescents
Acute loss >25% circulating blood volume
Hemoglobin <8.0 g/dL* in perioperative period
Hemoglobin <13.0 g/dL and severe cardiopulmonary disease
Hemoglobin <8.0 g/dL and symptomatic chronic anemia
Hemoglobin <8.0 g/dL and marrow failure
Infants Within First 4 Mo of Life
Hemoglobin <13.0 g/dL and severe pulmonary disease
Hemoglobin <10.0 g/dL and moderate pulmonary disease
Hemoglobin <13.0 g/dL and severe cardiac disease
Hemoglobin <10.0 g/dL and major surgery
Hemoglobin <8.0 g/dL and symptomatic anemia

*Hematocrit estimated by Hb g/dL × 3.

With anemias that develop slowly, the decision to transfuse RBCs should not be based solely on blood hemoglobin levels, because children with chronic anemias may be asymptomatic despite very low hemoglobin levels. Patients with iron deficiency anemia, for example, often are treated successfully with oral iron alone, even at hemoglobin levels below 50 g/L. Factors other than hemoglobin concentration that should be considered in the decision to transfuse RBCs include (1) the patient's symptoms, signs, and functional capacities; (2) the presence or absence of cardiorespiratory and central nervous system disease; (3) the cause and anticipated course of the anemia; and (4) alternative therapies such as recombinant human erythropoietin (EPO) therapy, which has been demonstrated to reduce the need for RBC transfusions and to improve the overall condition of children with chronic renal insufficiency (see Chapter 543.2). In anemias that are likely to be permanent, one must also consider the effects of anemia on growth and development and the potential toxicity of repeated transfusion. RBC transfusions for disorders such as sickle cell anemia and thalassemia are discussed in Chapters 468.1 and 468.9.

For *neonates*, clearly established indications for RBC transfusions, based on controlled scientific studies, do not exist. Generally, RBCs are given to maintain a hemoglobin value believed to be most desirable for each neonate's clinical status (Table 476–1). This clinical approach is imprecise, but more physiologic indications, such as RBC mass, available oxygen, and measurements of oxygen delivery and tissue extraction, are not usually available in clinical practice. Because definitive data are limited, it is important that pediatricians critically evaluate the need for neonatal RBC transfusions in light of the pathophysiology involved.

During the first weeks of life, all neonates experience a decline in circulating RBC mass caused by both physiologic factors and, in sick premature infants, by phlebotomy blood losses. In healthy term infants, the nadir hemoglobin value rarely falls below 9 g/dL at an age of approximately 10–12 wk. This "physiologic" drop in RBCs does not require transfusions. In contrast, this decline occurs earlier and is more pronounced in premature infants, even in those without complicating illnesses, in whom the mean hemoglobin concentration falls to approximately 8 g/dL in infants of 1.0–1.5 kg birthweight and to 7 g/dL in infants less than 1.0 kg. A key reason the nadir hemoglobin values of premature infants are lower than those of term infants is the former group's relatively diminished EPO output in response to anemia (see Chapters 99.1, 452, and 476). The mechanisms responsible for low EPO levels in neonatal plasma are only partially defined. One factor is reliance of preterm infants on the liver as the primary site of EPO production during the first weeks of life. This is important because the liver is less responsive than are the kidneys to anemia and tissue hypoxia. Thus, preterm infants exhibit a sluggish EPO response to falling hematocrit values. Low plasma EPO levels provide a rationale to use recombinant EPO in the treatment of the anemia of prematurity, and more than 20 controlled trials have been reported. Unquestionably, proper doses of EPO and iron effectively stimulate neonatal erythropoiesis. However, the efficacy of EPO therapy to substantially diminish RBC transfusions has not been convincingly demonstrated—particularly, for sick, extremely premature neonates. The role of recombinant EPO as treatment for the anemia of prematurity remains only partially defined (see Chapter 99.1).

Despite the promise of EPO therapy, many low birthweight preterm infants need RBC transfusions (Table 476–1). In neonatal patients with severe respiratory disease, defined as those requiring relatively large quantities of oxygen and ventilator support, it is customary to maintain the blood hemoglobin above 130 g/L (hematocrit >40%). Proponents believe that transfused RBCs containing adult hemoglobin, with their superior interaction with 2,3-diphosphoglycerate (2,3-DPG), leading to better oxygen offloading than that of fetal hemoglobin, are likely to provide optimal oxygen delivery throughout the period of diminished pulmonary function. Although this practice is widely recommended, little evidence is available to establish its efficacy or to define its optimal use (i.e., the best hemoglobin level for each degree of pulmonary dysfunction). It seems logical to presume that infants with less severe cardiopulmonary disease require less vigorous support, hence, the lower hemoglobin level suggested for those with only moderate disease. Consistent with the rationale for optimal oxygen delivery in neonates with severe respiratory disease, it seems logical to maintain the hemoglobin value above 130 g/L (hematocrit >40%) in neonates with severe cardiac disease leading to either cyanosis or congestive heart failure.

The optimal hemoglobin level for neonates facing *major surgery* has not been established by definitive studies. However, it seems reasonable to maintain the hemoglobin above 100 g/dL (hematocrit >30%) because of limited ability of a neonate's heart, lungs, and vasculature to compensate for anemia; the inferior offloading of oxygen due to the diminished interaction between fetal hemoglobin and 2,3-DPG; and the developmental impairment of neonatal renal, hepatic, and neurologic function. This transfusion guideline is simply a recommendation and should be applied with flexibility to individual infants facing different kinds of surgery.

Stable neonates do not require RBC transfusions unless they exhibit clinical problems attributable to anemia. Proponents of RBC transfusions for symptomatic anemia believe that the low RBC mass contributes to tachypnea, dyspnea, apnea, tachycardia, bradycardia, feeding difficulties, and lethargy and that these problems can be alleviated by transfusing RBCs. However, it is important to remember that anemia is only one of several possible causes of these problems, and RBC transfusions should be given only when clinical problems seem to be manifestations of anemia (i.e., not otherwise explained).

The *RBC product of choice* for children and adolescents is the standared suspension of RBCs isolated from whole blood by centrifugation and stored in an anticoagulant/preservative medium at a hematocrit value of about 60%. The usual dose is 10–15 mL/kg, but transfusion volumes vary greatly depending on clinical circumstances (e.g., continued vs arrested bleeding, hemolysis, etc.). For neonates, many centers transfuse the same RBC product as selected for older children, whereas others prefer a packed RBC concentrate (hematocrit of 70–90%) infused slowly (2–4 hr) at a dose of about 15 mL/kg body weight. Because of the small quantity of extracellular fluid given at these high hematocrit values and the slow rate of transfusion, the type of anticoagulant/preservative medium selected is believed not to pose risks for the majority of premature infants. In addition, packing by centrifugation at the time the aliquot is issued for transfusion ensures a consistent RBC dose with each transfusion. Of note, the traditional use of relatively fresh RBCs (<7 days of storage) is being challenged in hopes that donor exposure can be diminished by using a single unit of RBCs for each infant, regardless of the duration of RBC storage. Neonatologists who object to this practice and insist on transfusing fresh RBCs generally are fearful of the rise in plasma potassium (K^+) level that occurs in banked RBCs during extended storage. After 42 days of storage, plasma K^+ levels are ≅50 mEq/L (0.05 mEq/mL), a value that at first glance seems alarmingly high. However, the dose of bioavailable K^+ transfused (i.e., that in the extracellular fluid) is quite small. An infant weighing 1.0 kg, given a 15 mL/kg transfusion of packed RBCs (hematocrit 80%), will receive 3 mL of extracellular fluid that contains only 0.15 mEq of K^+, and it will be transfused slowly. Several clinical studies have documented the safety of this approach for small volume (15 mL/kg) transfusions. However, this does not apply to large volume (>25 mL/kg) transfusions, in which greater doses of K^+ may be harmful, especially if infused rapidly.

Chapter 477
Platelet Transfusions

Guidelines for platelet (PLT) support of *children and adolescents* with quantitative and qualitative PLT disorders are similar to those for adults (Table 477–1), in which the risk of life-threatening bleeding following injury or occurring spontaneously can be related to the severity of thrombocytopenia. PLT transfusions should be given to patients with PLT counts less than 50×10^9/L when they are bleeding or are scheduled for an invasive procedure. Studies of thrombocytopenic patients with serious complications (e.g., infection, anemia) due to bone marrow failure indicate that spontaneous bleeding increases markedly when PLT levels fall below 20×10^9/L. For this reason, many pediatricians recommend prophylactic PLT transfusions to maintain a PLT count above 20×10^9/L in children with thrombocytopenia due to bone marrow failure. This threshold has been challenged, and some favor a PLT transfusion trigger of $5–10 \times 10^9$/L for uncomplicated cases. However,

TABLE 477–1 Guidelines for Pediatric Platelet Transfusions

Children and Adolescents
PLTs <50 × 10^9/L and bleeding
PLTs <50 × 10^9/L and invasive procedure
PLTs <20 × 10^9/L and marrow failure with additional hemorrhagic risk factors
PLTs normal with qualitative PLT defect and bleeding or invasive procedure
Infants Within First 4 Mo of Life
PLTs <100 × 10^9/L and bleeding
PLTs <50 × 10^9/L and invasive procedure
PLTs <20 × 10^9/L and clinically stable
PLTs <100 × 10^9/L and clinically unstable

PLTs = platelets.

severe thrombocytopenia commonly occurs in association with fever, antimicrobial therapy, active bleeding, need for an invasive procedure, disseminated intravascular coagulation, and other severe clotting abnormalities, situations in which the PLT count at which transfusions are given needs to be raised to levels suggested by Table 477–1.

Qualitative PLT disorders may be inherited or acquired (e.g., in advanced hepatic or renal insufficiency or after cardiopulmonary bypass). In such patients, PLT transfusions are justified only if significant bleeding occurs. Because PLT dysfunction may be present long-term and repeated transfusions may lead to alloimmunization and refractoriness, prophylactic PLT transfusions are rarely justified unless an invasive procedure is planned. In these cases, a bleeding time of greater than twice the upper limit of laboratory normal may be taken as diagnostic evidence that PLT dysfunction exists, but this test is poorly predictive of hemorrhagic risk or the need to transfuse PLTs. In these patients, alternative therapies, particularly desmopressin acetate, should be considered to avoid PLT transfusions.

In *neonates*, hemostasis is quantitatively and qualitatively different from that of older children, and the potential exists for either serious hemorrhage or thrombosis. About 25% of neonates treated in intensive care units exhibit blood PLT counts less than 150×10^9/L at some time during admission. Although many pathogenetic mechanisms are involved in these sick neonates, the predominant one is accelerated PLT destruction. In addition, diminished PLT production is present, as evidenced by decreased numbers of megakaryocyte progenitors and relatively low levels of thrombopoietin in neonates, when compared with children and adults.

Blood PLT counts less than 100×10^9/L pose significant clinical risks for premature neonates. In one study, infants with birthweight less than 1.5 kg and a blood PLT count less than 100×10^9/L were compared with nonthrombocytopenic infants of similar birthweight. The bleeding time was prolonged at PLT counts less than 100×10^9/L, and PLT dysfunction was suggested by bleeding times that were disproportionately long for the degree of thrombocytopenia present. Hemorrhage was greater in thrombocytopenic infants than in controls. Of particular importance, the incidence of intracranial hemorrhage in thrombocytopenic infants with birthweight less than 1.5 kg was 78% vs 48% for nonthrombocytopenic infants of similar size. Moreover, the extent of hemorrhage and neurologic morbidity was greater in the thrombocytopenic group. However, in a randomized trial, transfusing PLTs whenever the PLT count fell below 150×10^9/L and maintaining the average PLT count above 200×10^9/L versus transfusing PLTs only when the PLT count fell below 50×10^9/L to maintain the average PLT count at about 100×10^9/L did not diminish the incidence of intracranial hemorrhage (28% vs 26%). Thus, there is no documented benefit to transfusing PLTs for mild thrombocytopenia (i.e., PLT counts $>100\times10^9$/L). Although basic questions about the relative risks of different degrees of thrombocytopenia in various clinical settings are only partially answered, guidelines acceptable to many neonatologists are listed in Table 477–1.

The ideal goal of most PLT transfusions is to raise the PLT count to greater than 50×10^9/L, and for neonates greater than 100×10^9/L. This can be achieved consistently by the infusion of 10 mL/kg of standard PLT concentrates, prepared either by centrifugation of fresh units of whole blood or by automated plateletpheresis, for infants and children weighing up to 30 kg. For larger children, the appropriate dose is four to six pooled concentrates from whole blood units or one apheresis unit. PLT concentrates should be transfused as rapidly as a patient's overall condition permits, certainly within 2 hr. Patients requiring repeated PLT transfusions should receive filtered (leukocyte-reduced) blood products, including PLT concentrates, to diminish alloimmunization and PLT refractoriness.

Routinely reducing the volume of platelet concentrates for infants and small children by additional centrifugation steps is both unnecessary and unwise. Transfusion of 10 mL/kg PLT concentrate adds 10×10^9 PLTs to 70 mL of blood (the blood volume of a 1 kg neonate), a number calculated to increase the PLT count by 143×10^9/L. This calculated increment is consistent with the increment reported in clinical studies. Generally, 10 mL/kg is not an excessive transfusion volume, providing the intake of other intravenous fluids, medications, and nutrients is monitored and adjusted. It is important to minimize repeated transfusion of group O PLTs to group A or B recipients, because passive anti-A or -B can lead to hemolysis. Although proven methods exist to reduce the volume of PLT concentrates when truly warranted (i.e., many transfusions anticipated, in which the quantity of passive anti-A or -B might lead to hemolysis or failure to respond to 10 mL/kg of unmodified PLT concentrate), additional processing should be performed with great care because of probable PLT loss, clumping, and dysfunction caused by the additional handling.

CHAPTER 478
Neutrophil (Granulocyte) Transfusions

Guidelines for granulocyte transfusions (GTX) are listed in Table 478–1. Although GTX have been used sparingly, the ability to collect markedly higher numbers of neutrophils from donors stimulated with recombinant granulocyte colony-stimulating factor (G-CSF) has led to renewed interest, particularly for marrow or peripheral blood progenitor cell transplantation. GTX should be reconsidered at institutions where neutropenic patients continue to die of progressive bacterial and fungal infections despite the optimal use of antimicrobial agents and recombinant myeloid growth factors.

The role of GTX added to antibiotics for patients with severe neutropenia ($<0.5\times10^9$/L) due to bone marrow failure is similar for both adults and children. Infected neutropenic patients usually respond to antibiotics alone, provided bone marrow function recovers early in infection. Because children with newly diagnosed leukemia respond rapidly to induction chemotherapy, only rarely are they candidates for GTX. In contrast, infected children with sustained bone marrow failure (i.e., malignant neoplasms resistant to treatment, aplastic anemia, and bone marrow transplant recipients) may benefit when GTX are added to antibiotics. The use of GTX for bacterial sepsis that is unresponsive to antibiotics in patients with severe neutropenia ($<0.5\times10^9$/L) is supported by most of the controlled studies (see Chapter 179).

Children with qualitative neutrophil defects (neutrophil dysfunction) usually have adequate numbers of blood neutrophils but are susceptible to serious infections because their cells kill pathogenic microorganisms inefficiently. Neutrophil dysfunction syndromes are rare, and no definitive studies have estab-

TABLE 478–1 Guidelines for Pediatric Granulocyte Transfusions

Children and Adolescents
Neutrophils $<0.5\times10^9$/L and bacterial infection unresponsive to appropriate antimicrobial therapy
Qualitative neutrophil defect and infection (bacterial or fungal) unresponsive to appropriate antimicrobial therapy
Infants Within First 4 Mo of Life
Neutrophils $<3.0\times10^9$/L (1st wk of life) or $<1.0\times10^9$/L (thereafter) and fulminant bacterial infection

lished the efficacy of GTX. However, several patients with progressive life-threatening infections have improved strikingly with the addition of GTX to antimicrobial therapy. These disorders are chronic, and because of the risk of inducing alloimmunization, GTX are recommended only when infections are clearly unresponsive to antimicrobial drugs.

Neonates are unusually susceptible to severe bacterial infections, and a number of defects of neonatal body defenses may be contributing factors (see Chapter 105). These abnormalities are accentuated in sick premature neonates, and it is logical to consider GTX. Neonates exhibiting fulminant sepsis, relative neutropenia ($<3.0 \times 10^9$/L during the first week of life; $<1.0 \times 10^9$/L thereafter), and a severely diminished neutrophil marrow storage pool ($<10\%$ of nucleated marrow cells being postmitotic neutrophils) are at particularly great risk of dying if treated with antibiotics only. Although some studies have shown a significant benefit from GTX, it is rarely used. Instead, some neonatologists consider alternative therapies that include intravenous immunoglobulin (IVIG) and recombinant myeloid growth factors. Results of studies evaluating IVIG have been mixed, but a meta-analysis found significant benefit for neonates with proven sepsis. Current data are insufficient to determine whether recombinant myeloid growth factors should have a role in treating these neonates, although both granulocyte colony and granulocyte-macrophage colony stimulating factors have been demonstrated to enhance myelopoiesis and to increase neutrophil blood counts in infants.

Once the decision to provide GTX has been made, an adequate dose of fresh leukapheresis cells must be transfused. Neonates and infants weighing less than 10 kg should receive $1\text{–}2 \times 10^9$/kg neutrophils per GTX. Larger infants and children should receive a total dose of at least 1×10^{10} neutrophils per each GTX; the preferred dose for adolescents is $5\text{–}8 \times 10^{10}$ per GTX—a dose requiring donors to be stimulated with G-CSF. GTX should be given daily until either the infection resolves or the blood neutrophil count persistently exceeds 0.5×10^9/L in the absence of the post-transfusion increment that follows GTX from G-CSF stimulated donors.

CHAPTER 479
Transfusions of Fresh Frozen Plasma

Guidelines for fresh frozen plasma (FFP) transfusions in children (Table 479–1) are similar to those for adults. FFP is transfused to replace clinically significant deficiencies of plasma proteins for which more highly purified concentrates are not available. Transfusion of FFP is efficacious for the treatment of deficiencies of clotting factors II, V, VII, X, and Xl. Factor XIII and fibrinogen deficiencies are treated with cryoprecipitate. Requirements for FFP vary with the specific factor being replaced, but a starting dose of 15 mL/kg is usually satisfactory. Transfusion of FFP is no longer recommended for treatment of patients with severe hemophilia A or B, because safer factor VIII and IX concentrates are available. Moreover, mild to moderate hemophilia A and certain types of von Willebrand's disease can be treated with I-deamino-(8-D-arginine)-vasopressin (DDAVP) (see Chapter 482). An important use of FFP, albeit rare in children, is for rapid reversal of warfarin effects in patients who are actively bleeding or who require emergency surgery (i.e., in whom functional deficiencies of factors II, VII, IX, and X cannot be rapidly reversed by vitamin K). Results of screening coagulation tests (prothrombin, activated partial thromboplastin, and thrombin times) should not be assumed, by themselves, to reflect the integrity of the coagulation system. To justify FFP transfusions, coagulation test results must be related to the clinical condition of the patient. Transfusion of FFP in patients with chronic liver disease and prolonged clotting times is not recommended unless bleeding is present or an invasive procedure is planned.

TABLE 479–1 Guidelines for Pediatric FFP Transfusions

Infants, Children, Adolescents
Severe clotting factor deficiency and bleeding
Severe clotting factor deficiency and invasive procedure
Emergency reversal of warfarin effects
Dilutional coagulopathy and bleeding
Anticoagulant protein (AT-III, protein C and S) replacement
Plasma exchange replacement fluid for thrombotic thrombocytopenic purpura

AT-III = Antithrombin III.

Although its major benefit has been in the treatment of bleeding associated with clotting factor deficiencies, FFP also contains several anticoagulant proteins (antithrombin III, protein C, and protein S), whose deficiencies have been associated with thrombosis. In selected situations, FFP may be appropriate as replacement therapy in patients with these disorders. However, when available, purified concentrates are preferred. Other indications for FFP include replacement fluid during plasma exchange in patients with thrombotic thrombocytopenic purpura or other disorders for which FFP is likely to be beneficial (e.g., plasma exchange in a patient with bleeding and a severe coagulopathy). FFP is not indicated for correction of hypovolemia or as immunoglobulin replacement therapy, because safer alternatives exist (e.g., albumin solutions and intravenous immunoglobulin, respectively).

In *neonates*, FFP transfusions merit special considerations. Clotting times are prolonged owing to developmental deficiency of clotting proteins, and FFP should be transfused only after reference to normal values expected for the birthweight and age of the infant in question. The indications for FFP in neonates include (1) reconstitution of red blood cell (RBC) concentrates to simulate whole blood for use in massive transfusions (e.g., exchange transfusion or cardiovascular surgery), (2) hemorrhage secondary to vitamin K deficiency, (3) disseminated intravascular coagulation with bleeding, and (4) bleeding in congenital coagulation factor deficiency when more specific treatment is either unavailable or inappropriate. The use of prophylactic FFP transfusions to prevent intraventricular hemorrhage in premature infants is not recommended. Although still used occasionally as a suspending agent to adjust the hematocrit values of RBC concentrates before use for small-volume RBC transfusions to neonates, FFP offers no apparent medical benefit over the use of sterile solutions for this purpose. This practice should be discouraged. In addition, the use of FFP in partial exchange transfusion for the treatment of neonatal hyperviscosity syndrome is unnecessary, because safer colloid solutions are available.

When treating bleeding infants, cryoprecipitate is often considered because of its small volume. However, cryoprecipitate contains only fibrinogen and factors VIII and XIII. Thus, it is not effective for treating other clotting factor deficiencies—despite the convenience of a small infusion volume.

CHAPTER 480
Risks of Blood Transfusions

Although the risks of allogeneic blood transfusions are extraordinarily low, transfusions must be given judiciously. A current estimate for risk of transfusion-associated HIV is 1/800,000 with estimates ranging from 1/300,000 to 1/2,000,000 donor exposures. The risk of viral hepatitis C is about 1/100,000 donor exposures. Transfusion-associated cytomegalovirus can be eliminated by transfusing cellular blood products, filtered with leukocyte-reduction filters, or by selecting blood from donors seronegative for antibody to cytomegalovirus. Additional infectious risks include syphilis, parvovirus B19, Epstein-Barr virus, and Chagas disease. Other transfusion-associated risks of a noninfectious nature that may occur in infants include fluid overload, graft versus host disease, electrolyte and acid-base imbalances, iron overload, increased susceptibility to oxidant damage, exposure to plasticizers, hemolysis when T-antigen activation of red blood cells (RBCs) has occurred, immunosuppression, and alloimmunization, although alloimmunization to RBC and leukocyte antigens seems to be very uncommon in infants. Some adverse effects are seen only in massive transfusion settings such as exchange transfusions, when relatively large quantities of blood are needed, and are rare in the small-volume transfusions usually given.

Premature infants are known to have immune dysfunction, but their risk of post-transfusion graft versus host disease is not well established. The postnatal age of the infant, the number of immunocompetent lymphocytes in the transfusion product, the degree of human leukocyte antigen (HLA) compatibility between donor and recipient, and other poorly described phenomena may determine which infants are truly at risk. Regardless, many centers caring for very preterm infants transfuse *gamma-irradiated cellular products*. For all patients, directed donations with blood from first-degree relatives should be irradiated because of the risk of engraftment with HLA haploidentical lymphocytes. Cellular blood products given as intrauterine and exchange transfusions are irradiated, as are transfusions for patients with severe congenital immunodeficiency disorders and recipients of bone marrow transplants. Other groups potentially at risk, but for whom no conclusive data are available, are patients receiving T-cell antibody therapy (antithymocyte globulin or OKT3), recipients of organ allografts, patients infected with HIV, and cancer patients receiving immunosuppressive drug regimens. Current practice uses gamma irradiation from a cesium, cobalt, or linear acceleration source at doses ranging from 2,500–5,000 cGy; a minimum dose of 2,500 cGy is required. All cellular blood components should be irradiated, but frozen "acellular" products such as fresh frozen plasma and cryoprecipitated antihemophilic factor do not require it. Leukocyte reduction cannot be substituted for gamma irradiation to prevent graft versus host disease.

Andrew M, Castle V, Saigal S, et al: Clinical impact of neonatal thrombocytopenia. J Pediatr 110:457, 1987.

Andrew M, Vegh P, Caco C, et al: A randomized, controlled trial of platelet transfusions in thrombocytopenic premature infants. J Pediatr 123:285, 1993.

AuBuchon JP, Birkmeyer JD, Busch MP: Safety of the blood supply in the United States: Opportunities and controversies. Ann Intern Med 127:904, 1997.

Blanchette VS, Hume HA, Levy GJ, et al: Guidelines for auditing pediatric blood transfusion practices. Am J Dis Child 145:787, 1991.

College of American Pathologists Task Force: Practice parameter for the use of fresh-frozen plasma, cryoprecipitate, and platelets. JAMA 271:777, 1994.

Liu EA, Mannino FL, Lane TA: Prospective, randomized trial of the safety and efficacy of a limited exposure transfusion program for premature neonates. J Pediatr 125:92, 1994.

Murray NA, Watts TL, Roberts IA: Endogenous thrombopoietin levels and effect of recombinant human thrombopoietin on megakaryocyte precursors in term and preterm babies. Pediatr Res 43:148, 1998.

Strauss RG: Current status of granulocyte transfusions to treat neonatal sepsis. J Clin Apheresis 5:25, 1989.

Strauss RG: Perinatal platelet and granulocyte transfusions. *In:* Kennedy MS, Wilson SM, Kelton JG (eds): Perinatal Transfusion Medicine. Arlington, VA, American Association of Blood Banks, 1990, p 123.

Strauss RG: Transfusion therapy in neonates. Am J Dis Child 145:904, 1991.

Strauss RG: Therapeutic granulocyte transfusions in 1993. Blood 81:1675, 1993.

Strauss RG: Selection of white cell-reduced blood components for transfusions in early infancy. Transfusion 33:352, 1993.

Strauss RG: Granulocyte transfusions. *In:* Rossi EC, Simon TL, Moss GS (eds): Principles of Transfusion Medicine, 2nd ed. Baltimore, Williams & Wilkins, 1996, p 321.

Strauss RG: Recombinant erythropoietin for the anemia of prematurity: Still a promise, not yet a panacea. J Pediatr 131:653, 1997.

Strauss RG, Burmeister LF, Johnson K, et al: AS-1 red blood cells for neonatal transfusions: A randomized trial assessing donor exposure and safety. Transfusion 36:873, 1996.

Strauss RG, Levy GJ, Sotelo-Avila C, et al: National survey of neonatal transfusion practices: II Blood component therapy. Pediatrics 91:530, 1993.

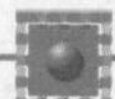

SECTION 7

Hemorrhagic and Thrombotic Diseases

Robert R. Montgomery ■ J. Paul Scott

When blood vessels are injured, the clotting process maintains vascular integrity or causes blood flow to cease through the injured vessel. If clotting is impaired, hemorrhage occurs. If clotting is excessive, thrombosis and its complications occur. The response needs to be rapid and regulated to assure hemostasis. Trivial trauma should not initiate a systemic reaction but must initiate a localized response. Once clotting is initiated, anticoagulants must confine the clotting process to the site of injury to stop hemorrhage. The clot must then be physiologically lysed to re-establish blood vessel patency. These hemostatic mechanisms are very complex and involve local reactions of the blood vessel, the multiple activities of the platelet, the interaction of specific coagulation factors both with each other and with platelets, the regulation of clotting by anticoagulant factors and their inhibitors, and the factors that initiate and regulate the fibrinolytic process.

The vascular endothelium is the primary barrier against hemorrhage. When small vessels are transected, active vasoconstriction minimizes the local hemorrhage even without activation of clotting. Platelets are essential for the control of hemorrhage from small blood vessels. More extensive injury (involvement of large blood vessels) requires the participation and coordination of the full hemostatic process to provide a firm, stable, fibrin clot. The extent of this clotting is localized by the anticoagulation system; the removal of the clot requires appropriate fibrinolysis.

Isolated deficiencies of individual anticoagulants (clotting factor inhibitors) predispose the patient to excessive thrombosis. In acquired hemostatic disorders there are frequently multiple problems with homeostasis that complicate our understanding of the patient's dysregulated hemostasis. The primary illness (sepsis) and its secondary effect (shock) activate coagulation and fibrinolysis and impair the host's ability to restore normal hemostatic function. In disseminated intravascular coagulation, procoagulant clotting factors and anticoagulant proteins are consumed, leaving the hemostatic system dysregulated. Similarly, newborn infants or patients with severe liver disease have synthetic deficiencies of both procoagulant and anticoagulant proteins. Such dysregulation causes the patient to be predisposed to both hemorrhage and thrombosis with mild or moderate triggers that result in major alterations in the hemostatic process. Acquired hemostatic disorders may be the result of a secondary or tertiary response to another stimulus. ■

CHAPTER 481

Hemostasis

481.1 Hemostatic Mechanism

The classic hemostatic mechanism includes the vascular response, platelet adhesion, platelet aggregation, clot formation, clot stabilization, limitation of clotting to the site of injury by regulatory anticoagulants, and re-establishment of vascular patency through fibrinolysis and vascular healing. The laboratory study of this mechanism requires the isolated study of this response as a series of independent events; however, in vivo, these events are tightly integrated. For example, fibrinogen serves as the ligand between platelets during platelet aggregation and also serves as the end protein resulting in the fibrin clot. von Willebrand factor (vWf) provides another example of a single protein with multiple functions. It circulates in a complex with factor VIII, with vWf serving as the adhesive ligand for platelet adhesion and factor VIII serving as one of the major regulating cofactors controlling clotting. The hemostatic mechanism is further complicated by the fact that in vivo the interactions may occur through different pathways than are studied through clinical laboratory testing. In vitro clotting is characterized by using the activated partial thromboplastin time (PTT) and the prothrombin time (PT). The PT measures the clotting process through the addition of tissue factor, which, together with factor VII, activates factor X (Fig. 481–1). In vivo factor VII activates factor X and factor XI, but as routinely studied in the clinical laboratory, this step is not evaluated. If tissue factor and factor VII activated only factor X, it is difficult to understand why the most severe bleeding disorders are factor VIII (hemophilia A) and factor IX (hemophilia B) deficiency. Nevertheless, the mechanisms studied by the PTT and the PT permit us to evaluate clotting factor deficiencies even though these pathways may not be the same as those occurring physiologically.

Following vascular injury, vasoconstriction occurs and flowing blood is subjected to exposure to the subendothelial matrix (Fig. 481–2). The initial event following injury involves platelet adhesion to vWf when the vWf is modified through interaction with subendothelial matrix. Following adherence, platelets become activated and release storage granules containing adenosine diphosphate (ADP), thromboxane A_2, and other stored proteins. These result in the aggregation and recruitment of other platelets to the platelet plug. Aggregation involves the interaction of specific receptors on the platelet surface with plasma hemostatic proteins—primarily fibrinogen. During the process of platelet activation, internalized platelet phospholipids (primarily phosphotidylserine) become externalized and interact at two specific, rate-limiting steps in the clotting process—those involving the cofactors factor VIII and factor V. Vascular injury also releases tissue factor and an altered vascular surface that initiates the clotting cascade and results in the generation of the fibrin clot. The stable fibrin-platelet plug is ultimately formed through clot retraction and cross linking of the fibrin clot by factor XIII.

Examination of the interaction of clotting factors shown in Fig. 481–1 discloses what has been termed the waterfall cascade. Inactive clotting factors denoted by roman numerals become activated. The activated clotting factor then initiates the activation of the next sequential clotting factor in a systematic manner. This results in the amplification of the process to give a burst of clotting where it is physiologically needed. In the clinical laboratory, factor XII is activated using a surface (silica or glass) or contact activators, such as ellagic acid. Factor VII is activated and interacts with tissue factor through a similar cascade. The former is the pathway measured by the PTT and the latter by the PT. This process is accelerated by the

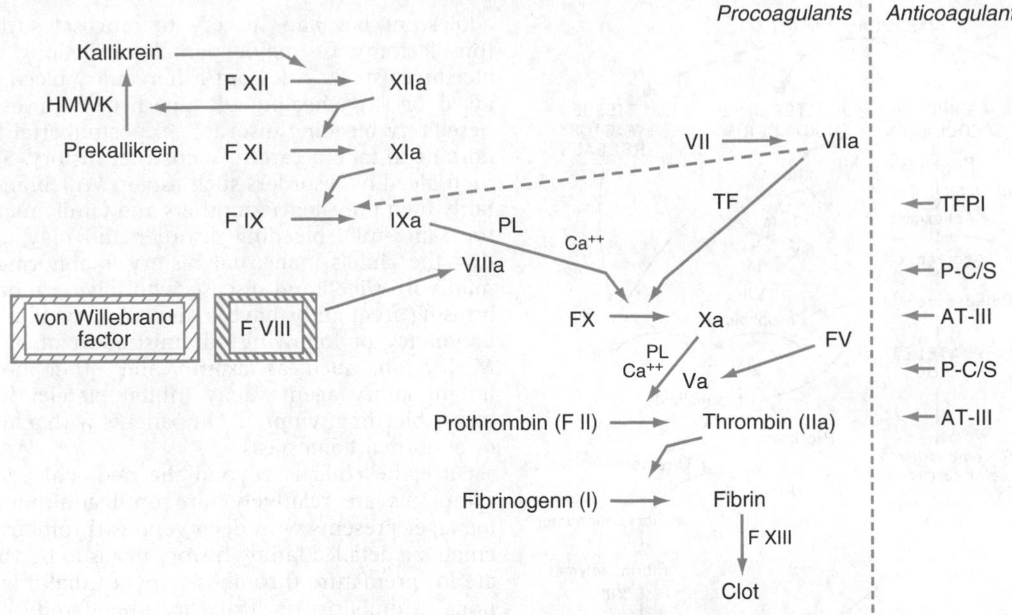

Figure 481–1 Clotting cascade with sequential activation and amplification of clot formation. Many of the factors are activated by the clotting factor above them in the cascade. The activated factors are designated by the addition of an "a." *Right side*, The major anticoagulants and the sites that they regulate (TFPI regulates TF and VIIa; protein C and S regulate factors VIII and V; and AT-III regulates Xa and thrombin [Xa]). The dotted line illustrates that in vivo TF and VIIa activate both IX and X, but in vitro we measure only the activation of factor X. Unactivated factor VIII, when bound to its carrier protein, von Willebrand factor, is protected from protein C inactivation. When thrombin or Xa activates factor VIII, it becomes unbound to von Willebrand factor, where it can participate with IXa in the activation of factor X in the presence of phospholipid and calcium. Factor XIII cross links the fibrin clot and thereby makes it more stable. HMWK = high molecular weight kininogen; PL = phospholipid; Ca^{++} = calcium; TF = tissue factor; TFPI = tissue factor pathway inhibitor; P-C/S = protein C and protein S; AT-III = antithrombin III.

interaction with phospholipid and calcium at the steps involving factor VIII and factor V. Deficiencies of clotting factors result in either isolated prolongations of the PTT or PT or an alteration in both. This is useful in determining hereditary clotting factor deficiencies; in acquired hemostatic disorders encountered in clinical practice, however, more than one clotting factor is frequently deficient so that the relative prolongation of the PTT and PT must be assessed.

Since clotting factors were named in the order of discovery they do not necessarily reflect the sequential order of activation (Table 481–1). In fact, factors III, IV, and VI were not subsequently found to be independent proteins, and thus these terms are no longer used. The dual mechanisms of activating clotting have been termed the intrinsic (surface activation) and extrinsic (tissue factor–mediated) pathways. The intrinsic pathway involves the initial activation of factor XII, which is accelerated by two other plasma proteins, prekallikrein and high molecular weight kininogen. When factor XII is activated, it produces XIIa, which activates XI to XIa and then IX to IXa. The factor IXa complexes with factor VIII, platelet phospholipid, and calcium to activate factor X. The extrinsic system is measured by the prothrombin time and is initiated by a complex between tissue factor and factor VII to activate factor X. This is the in vitro pathway, but in vivo the complex between tissue factor and factor VII triggers activation of factor IX. Whether factor X is activated by the intrinsic or the extrinsic pathway, Xa is generated, which complexes with factor V, platelet phospholipid, and calcium to activate prothrombin to thrombin (also referred to as IIa). Once thrombin is generated, fibrinogen is converted to a fibrin clot. This loose fibrin clot is then cross linked by factor XIII (transglutaminase). Figure 481–1 is an oversimplified diagram, since Xa can activate both factor VIII and factor V, and thrombin can activate factor V, factor VIII, factor XI, and platelets. After thrombin activates the procoagulant system, thrombin binds to thrombomodulin on the endothelial cell surface, where it activates the anticoagulant system. Thrombomodulin modulates thrombin from being a procoagulant to being an anticoagulant that activates protein C. Activated protein C inactivates factor V and factor VIII, which, in turn, limits further thrombin generation.

Virtually all procoagulant proteins are balanced by an anticoagulant protein that regulates or inhibits procoagulant function. There are four clinically important, naturally occurring anticoagulants that regulate the extension of the clotting process. These include antithrombin III (ATIII), protein C, protein S, and tissue factor pathway inhibitor (TFPI). The primary action of antithrombin IIII is to regulate factor Xa and thrombin. It may also serve to regulate IXa, XIa, and XIIa, but this

TABLE 481–1 The Coagulation Factors

Clotting Factors	Synonym	Disorder
I	Fibrinogen	Congenital deficiency (afibrinogenemia) and dysfunction (dysfibrogenemia)
II	Prothrombin	Congenital deficiency or dysfunction
V	Labile factor, proaccelerin	Congenital deficiency (parahemophilia)
VII	Stable factor or proconvertin	Congenital deficiency
VIII	Antihemophilic factor (AHF)	Congenital deficiency is hemophilia A (classic hemophilia)
IX	Christmas factor	Congenital deficiency is hemophilia B
X	Stuart-Prower factor	Congenital deficiency
XI	Plasma thromboplastin antecedent	Congenital deficiency, sometimes referred to as hemophilia C
XII	Hageman factor	Congenital deficiency is not associated with clinical symptoms
XIII	Fibrin-stabilizing factor	Congenital deficiency

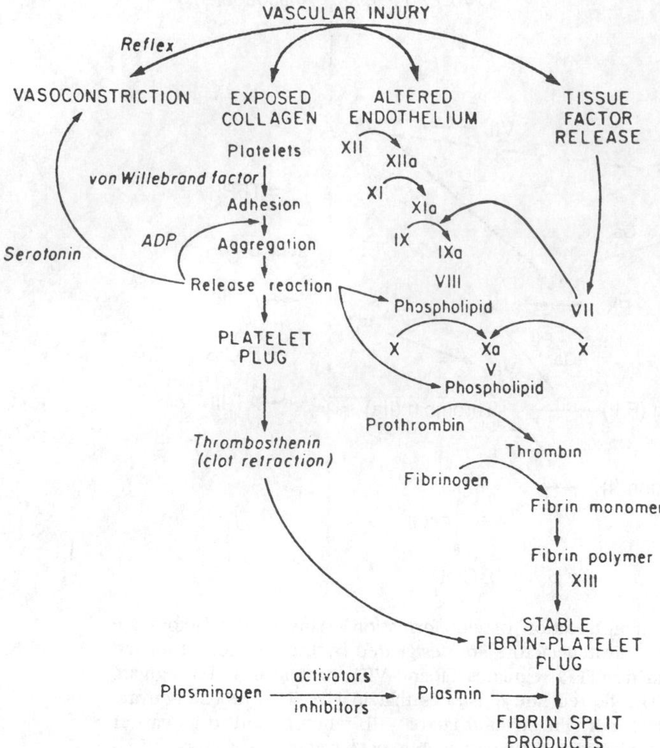

Figure 481–2 Diagrammatic representation of the hemostatic mechanism. (From Nathan DG, Oski FA: Hematology of Infancy and Childhood, 3rd ed. Philadelphia, WB Saunders, 1987.)

activity is less important. Protein C, in the presence of thrombin bound to thrombomodulin, becomes activated protein C (APC). In the presence of the cofactor protein S, activated protein C serves as the primary mechanism of regulating activated factor V and activated factor VIII. The final inhibitor is TFPI, which quickly shuts down the activation of factor X by factor VII and tissue factor and shifts the activation site of tissue factor and factor VII to that of factor IX and XI (see Fig. 481–1).

Once a stable fibrin-platelet plug is formed, the fibrinolytic system limits its extension and also lyses the clot to re-establish vascular integrity. Plasmin is generated from plasminogen by either urokinase-like or tissue-type plasminogen activator. Plasmin serves to degrade the fibrin clot (fibrinolysis). In the process of dissolving the fibrin clot, fibrin degradation products are produced. This pathway is regulated by plasminogen activator inhibitors (PAI-1) and α_2-antiplasmin.

481.2 The Clinical and Laboratory Evaluation

HISTORY. For most hemostatic disorders, whether they be hemorrhagic or thrombotic, the clinical history provides the most useful information. For a hemorrhagic condition the history should determine the site or sites of bleeding, the severity and duration of hemorrhage, and the age of symptom onset. Was the bleeding spontaneous or after trauma? Was there a previous personal or family history of similar problems? One should determine if symptoms correlate with the degree of injury or trauma. Does bruising occur spontaneously? Are there lumps with bruises for which there is minimal trauma? If there has been previous surgery or significant dental procedures, was there any increased bleeding? If a child or adolescent has had surgery to mucosal surfaces, such as a tonsillectomy or major dental extractions, the absence of bleeding usually rules out a hereditary bleeding disorder. Delayed or slow healing of superficial injuries may suggest a hereditary bleeding disorder. In postpubertal females it is important to take a careful menstrual history. Since some common bleeding disorders such as von Willebrand disease have a fairly high prevalence, mothers and family members may have the same mild bleeding disorder and may not be cognizant that the child's menstrual history is abnormal. Women with mild von Willebrand disease who have a moderate history of bruising frequently have a reduction of that bruising during pregnancy or following administration of birth control pills. Medication, such as aspirin and other nonsteroidal anti-inflammatory agents, may inhibit platelet function and increase bleeding symptoms in patients with a low platelet count or abnormal hemostasis.

Once the child is beyond the neonatal period, thrombotic symptoms are relatively rare until adulthood. If a child or teenager presents with deep venous thrombosis or pulmonary emboli, a detailed family history needs to be obtained to evaluate for premature thrombosis, myocardial infarction, deep venous thrombosis, or stroke in other family members. In the neonate, physiologic deficiencies of procoagulants and anticoagulants cause the hemostatic mechanism to be dysregulated, and clinical events can be in the direction of hemorrhage or thrombosis. Even in the absence of a family history, the presence of thrombosis in the child or teenager is sufficient to initiate the evaluation of the individual for hereditary or acquired predisposition to thrombosis.

PHYSICAL EXAMINATION. The physical examination should focus on whether symptoms are primarily associated with the mucous membranes or skin (mucocutaneous bleeding) or the muscles and joints (deep bleeding). The examination should determine the presence of petechiae, ecchymoses, hematomas, hemarthroses, or mucous membrane bleeding. Patients with defects in platelet-blood vessel wall interaction (von Willebrand disease or platelet function defects) usually have mucous membrane bleeding (epistaxis, menorrhagia, hematuria, gastrointestinal bleeding); petechiae on the skin and mucous membranes; and small, ecchymotic lesions of the skin sometimes associated with hematomas. Individuals with a clotting factor deficiency such as factor VIII or factor IX deficiency have symptoms of deep bleeding into muscles and joints with much more extensive ecchymoses and hematoma formation. Patients with mild von Willebrand disease or other mild bleeding disorders may have no abnormal findings on physical examination.

LABORATORY TESTS. Patients who have a positive bleeding history or are actively hemorrhaging should have a platelet count, bleeding time, PTT, and PT. If these are normal, a thrombin time and vWf testing should be considered. In individuals with abnormal screening tests, further specific factor work-up should be undertaken. In a patient with an abnormal bleeding history and a positive family history, normal screening tests should not preclude further laboratory evaluation.

There are no effective routine screening tests for hereditary thrombotic disorders. If the family history is positive or the clinical thrombosis is unexplained, specific anticoagulant assays should be undertaken. Thrombosis is rare in children, and, when present, the possibility of a hereditary predisposition must be considered and evaluated in the laboratory.

Bleeding Time. The bleeding time assesses the function of platelets and their interaction with the vascular wall. Disposable standardized devices have been developed that control the length and depth of the skin incision. A blood pressure cuff is applied to the upper arm and inflated to 40 mm Hg for children and adults. In term newborns and younger children a modified device has been developed and used with a lower blood pressure cuff pressure. The bleeding time is a difficult laboratory test to standardize, and there is much interlaboratory and interindividual variation. Although platelet counts less than 100,000/mm³ are associated with prolonged bleeding times, disproportionate prolongations of the bleeding times may suggest a qualitative platelet defect or von Willebrand disease. Following the incision with the bleeding time device, blood is blotted from the margin of the incision at 30 sec intervals until bleeding ceases. While each laboratory must establish its own normal range, bleeding usually stops within 4–8 min.

Platelet Count. The platelet count is essential in the evaluation of the child with a positive bleeding history because thrombocytopenia is the most common acquired cause of a bleeding diathesis in children. Patients with a platelet count above 50,000/mm³ rarely have significant clinical bleeding. Although adults with elevated platelet counts (thrombocythemia, >1,000,000/mm³) may have thrombotic complications, pediatric patients rarely are symptomatic with isolated thrombocythemia.

"Activated" Partial Thromboplastin Time (PTT). The PTT as performed in the clinical laboratory is actually an "activated" PTT (or APTT); most refer to it as the PTT. This test measures the initiation of clotting at the level of factor XII through sequential steps to the final clot end point. It does not measure factor VII, factor XIII, or anticoagulants. The PTT employs a contact activator (silica, kaolin, or ellagic acid) in the presence of calcium and phospholipid. Because of different reagents and laboratory instruments the normal range for the PTT varies between one hospital laboratory and another. Normal ranges are much more variable from laboratory to laboratory than with the PT.

Prothrombin Time (PT). The PT measures the extrinsic clotting system following the activation of clotting by tissue factor (thromboplastin) in the presence of calcium. It is not prolonged with deficiencies of factors VIII, IX, XI, or XII. In most laboratories the normal PT ranges between 10 and 13 sec. The PT has been standardized using the International Normalized Ratio (INR) so that values can be compared from one laboratory or instrument to another. The INR is used to determine similar degrees of anticoagulation with coumadin-like medications and is not intended as a screening test for clotting factor deficiencies.

Thrombin Time. The thrombin time measures the final step of the clotting cascade in which fibrinogen is converted to fibrin. The normal thrombin time varies between laboratories but is usually between 11 and 15 sec. Prolongation of the thrombin time occurs with reduced fibrinogen levels (hypofibrinogenemia or afibrinogenemia), with dysfunctional fibrinogen (dysfibrinogenemia), or by substances that interfere with fibrin polymerization such as heparin or fibrin split products. If heparin contamination is a potential cause for a long thrombin time, a reptilase time is usually ordered.

Reptilase Time. The reptilase time uses a snake venom to clot fibrinogen. Unlike the thrombin time, the reptilase time is not sensitive to heparin and is prolonged only by reduced or dysfunctional fibrinogen and fibrin split products. Therefore, if the thrombin time is prolonged but the reptilase time is normal, the prolonged thrombin time is due to heparin and does not indicate the presence of fibrin split products or reduced concentration or function of fibrinogen.

Mixing Studies. If there is prolongation of the PT or PTT, a mixing study is usually performed. Normal plasma is added to the patient's plasma, and the PTT or PT is repeated. Correction of the PT or PTT by 1:1 mixing with normal plasma suggests the deficiencies of a clotting factor, since a 50% level of individual clotting proteins is sufficient to produce a normal PT or PTT. If the clotting time is not corrected or only partially corrected, an inhibitor is usually present. If the mixing study does not correct or becomes more prolonged and the patient has clinical bleeding, an inhibitor against factor VIII, IX, or XI may be present. If the patient has no bleeding symptoms and both the PTT and the mixing study are prolonged, a lupus-like anticoagulant is often present. These patients usually have a long PTT, do not bleed, and may have a clinical predisposition to excessive clotting.

Clotting Factor Assays. Each of the clotting factors can be measured in the clinical laboratory using individual factor-deficient plasmas. In general, severe deficiency of factor VIII or factor IX is less than 1% of normal plasma (< 1 U/dL or <1%), moderate deficiency between 1 and 5% of normal, and mild deficiencies greater than 5% and below the normal range. For most clotting factors the normal range is between 50 and 150 U/dL (50–150%).

In patients with hemophilia A or hemophilia B, inhibitors of factor VIII or factor IX may develop after exposure to replacement therapy. To quantitate the amount of inhibitor present, the standardized clinical assay of these clotting inhibitors is termed the Bethesda assay. One Bethesda Unit is defined as the amount that will inhibit 50% of the clotting factor in normal plasma.

Platelet Aggregation. When a qualitative platelet function defect is suspected, platelet aggregation testing is usually ordered. Platelet-rich plasma from the patient is activated with one of a series of agonists (ADP, epinephrine, collagen, thrombin or thrombin-receptor peptide, and ristocetin). Repeat testing or testing of other symptomatic family members can help determine the hereditary nature of the defect.

Testing for Thrombotic Predisposition. Hereditary predisposition to thrombosis is associated with a reduction of anticoagulant function (protein C, protein S, AT-III); presence of a factor V molecule that is resistant to inactivation by protein C (factor V Leiden); elevated procoagulants (a mutation of the prothrombin gene); or deficiency of fibrinolysis (plasminogen deficiency). If warranted by the clinical severity and history of thrombosis, specific tests of the natural anticoagulants are ordered. While both immunologic and functional tests are usually available, a functional assay of protein C, protein S, and antithrombin III is usually measured.

Factor V Leiden is a common mutation in factor V that is associated with significant risk of thrombosis. A point mutation in the factor V molecule prevents the inactivation of activated factor V by protein C. This defect has also been termed APC resistance and is easily be diagnosed by DNA testing.

The *prothrombin gene mutation (G20210A)* is a mutation in the noncoding portion of the prothrombin gene with a G at position 20210 being replaced by an A. This mutation increases the amount of prothrombin mRNA, is associated with elevated levels of prothrombin, and causes a thrombotic predisposition. This abnormality is easily identified using molecular (DNA) diagnostic testing.

Elevated Homocysteine. If homocysteine levels are increased as a result of genetic mutations, patients have a predisposition to both arterial and venous thrombosis as well as an increase in arteriosclerosis. Elevated homocysteine may be reduced by the administration of folic acid in some patients with genetic abnormalities.

Tests of the Fibrinolytic System. The euglobulin clot lysis time (ELT) is used to assess a reduction of fibrinolysis. More specific tests are available in most laboratories to determine the levels of plasminogen, plasminogen activator, and inhibitors of fibrinolysis. An increase in fibrinolysis may be associated with hemorrhagic symptoms, and a delay in fibrinolysis is associated with thrombosis.

HEMOSTASIS IN THE NEWBORN. The normal newborn infant has a reduced level of most procoagulants and anticoagulants. This renders the newborn at simultaneous increased risk for both hemorrhage and thrombosis. Table 481–2 lists the levels of hemostatic proteins in the newborn and older children. In general, there is a more marked abnormality in the preterm

TABLE 481–2 Reference Values for Coagulation Tests in Healthy Children*

Tests	28–31 Weeks' Gestation	30–36 Weeks' Gestation	Full Term	1–5 Years	6–10 Years	11–18 Years	Adult
Screening Tests							
PT (sec)	15.4 (14.6–16.9)	13.0 (10.6–16.2)	13.0 (10.1–15.9)	11 (10.6–11.4)	11.1 (10.1–12.0)	11.2 (10.2–12.0)	12 (11.0–14.0)
APTT (sec)	108 (80–168)	53.6 (27.5–79.4)‡§	42.9 (31.3–54.3)‡	30 (24–36)	31 (26–36)	32 (26–37)	33 (27–40)
BT (min)	—	—	—	6 (2.5–10)‡	7 (2.5–13)‡	5 (3–8)‡	4 (1–7)
Procoagulants							
Fibrinogen	256 (160–550)	243 (150–373)‡§	283 (167–399)	276 (170–405)	279 (157–40)	30 (154–448)	278 (156–40)
II	31 (19–54)	45 (20–77)‡	48 (26–70)‡	94 (71–116)‡	88 (67–107)‡	83 (61–104)‡	108 (70–146)
V	65 (43–80)	88 (41–144)§	72 (34–108)‡	103 (79–127)	90 (63–116)‡	77 (55–99)‡	106 (62–150)
VII	37 (24–76)	67 (21–113)‡	66 (28–104)‡	82 (55–116)‡	86 (52–120)‡	83 (58–115)‡	105 (67–143)
VII procoagulant	79 (37–126)	111 (5–213)	100 (50–178)	90 (59–142)	95 (58–132)	92 (53–131)	99 (50–149)
vWF	141 (83–223)	136 (78–210)	153 (50–287)	82 (60–120)	95 (44–144)	100 (46–153)	92 (50–158)
IX	18 (17–20)	35 (19–65)§‡	53 (15–91)†‡	73 (47–104)‡	75 (63–89)‡	82 (59–122)‡	109 (55–163)
X	36 (25–64)	41 (11–71)‡	40 (12–68)‡	88 (58–116)‡	75 (55–101)‡	79 (50–117)	106 (70–152)
XI	23 (11–33)	30 (08–52)‡§	38 ± (40–66)‡	30 (08–52)‡	38 (10–66)	74 (50–97)‡	97 (56–150)
XII	25 (05–35)	38 (10–66)‡§	53 (13–93)‡	93 (64–129)	92 (60–140)	81 (34–137)‡	108 (52–164)
PK	26 (15–32)	33 (09–89)‡	37 (18–69)‡	95 (65–130)	99 (66–131)	99 (53–145)	112 (62–162)
HMWK	32 (19–52)	49 (09–89)‡	54 (06–102)‡	98 (64–132)	93 (60–130)	91 (63–119)	92 (50–136)
XIIIa‖	—	70 (32–108)‡	79 (27–131)‡	108 (72–143)	109 (65–151)	99 (57–140)	105 (55–155)
XIIIb‖	—	81 (35–127)‡	76 (30–122)‡	113 (69–156)‡	116 (77–154)‡	102 (60–143)	98 (057–137)
Anticoagulants							
ATIII	28 (20–38)	38 (14–62)‡§	63 (39–87)‡	111 (82–139)	111 (90–131)	106 (77–132)	100 (74–126)
Protein C	—	28 (12–44)‡§	35 (17–53)‡	66 (40–92)‡	69 (45–93)‡	83 (55–111)‡	96 (64–128)
Protein S	—	—	—	—	—	—	—
Total (U/mL)	—	26 (14–38)‡§	36 (12–60)‡	86 (54–118)	78 (41–114)	72 (52–92)	81 (61–113)
Free (U/mL)	—	—	—	45 (21–69)	42 (22–62)	38 (26–55)	45 (27–061)
Plasminogen (U/mL)	—	170 (112–248)‖	195 (125–265)‖	98 (78–118)	92 (75–108)	86 (68–103)	99 (77–122)
TPA (ng/mL)	—	8.48 (3.00–16.70)	9.6 (5.0–18.9)	2.15 (1.0–4.5)‡	2.42 (1.0–5.0)‡	2.16 (1.0–4.0)‡	1.02 (.68–1.36)
a_2AP (U/mL)	—	78 (40–116)	85 (55–115)	105 (93–117)	99 (89–110)	98 (78–118)	102 (68–136)
PAI-1	—	5.4 (0.0–12.2)‡	6.4 (2.0–15.1)	5.42 (1.0–10.0)	6.79 (2.0–12.0)‡	6.07 (2.0–10.0)‡	3.60 (0–11.0)

Data from Andrew M, Paes B, Johnston M: Development of the hemostatic system in the neonate and young infant. Am J Pediatr Hematol Oncol 12:95, 1990; and Andrew M, Vegh P, Johnston M, et al: Maturation of the hemostatic system during childhood. Blood 80:1998, 1992.

**All factors except fibrinogen are presented as units/mL (fibrinogen in mg/mL), where pooled normal plasma contains 1 unit/mL. All data are expressed as the mean followed by the upper and lower boundary encompassing 95% of the normal population.*

†Levels for 19–27 weeks and 28–31 weeks are from multiple sources and cannot be analyzed statistically.

‡Values are significantly different from those of adults.

§Values are significantly different from those of full-term infants.

‖Value given as CTA units/mL.

Abbreviations: PT = prothrombin time; INR = international normalized ratio; APTT = activated partial thromboplastin time; VIII = factor VIII procoagulant activity; vWf = von Willebrand factor; PK = prekallikrein; HMWK = high molecular-weight kininogen.

infant. While major differences exist in the normal ranges for newborn and preterm infants, these ranges vary greatly between laboratories. During gestation there is progressive maturation and increase of the clotting factors synthesized by the liver. The extremely premature infant will have a prolonged PTT and PT as well as a marked reduction in anticoagulant proteins (proteins C, S, and AT-III). Note that fibrinogen, factor V, factor VIII, vWf, and platelets are near-normal throughout the later stages of gestation (see Chapter 99.4).

Andrew M, Montgomery RR: Acquired disorders of hemostasis. *In:* Nathan DG, Orkin SH (eds): Hematology of Infancy and Childhood, 5th ed. Philadelphia, WB Saunders, 1998, pp 1677–1717.

Andrew M, Booker L: Hemostatic disorders in newborns. *In:* Polin RA, Fox WW (eds): Fetal and Neonatal Physiology, 2nd ed. Philadelphia, WB Saunders, 1998, p 1368.

Grabowski EF, Corrigan JJ Jr: Hemostasis: General considerations. *In:* Miller DR, Baehner RL (eds): Blood Diseases of Infancy and Childhood, 7th ed. St. Louis, CV Mosby, 1995, pp 849–865.

Handin RI: Blood platelets and the vessel wall. *In:* Nathan DG, Orkin SH (eds): Hematology of Infancy and Childhood, 5th ed. Philadelphia, WB Saunders, 1998, pp 1511–1529.

Hathaway WE, Goodnight SH Jr: Disorders of Hemostasis and Thrombosis. A Clinical Guide. New York, McGraw-Hill, 1993.

Lusher JM: Approach to the bleeding patient. *In:* Nathan DG, Orkin SH (eds): Hematology of Infancy and Childhood, 5th ed. Philadelphia, WB Saunders, 1998, pp 1574–1584.

Montgomery RR, Scott JP: Hemostasis: Diseases of the fluid phase. *In:* Nathan DG, Orkin SH (eds): Hematology of Infancy and Childhood, 4th ed. Philadelphia, WB Saunders, 1993, pp 1605–1650.

Stuart MF, Graeber JE: Normal hemostasis in the fetus and newborn: vessels and platelets. *In:* Polin RA, Fox WW (eds): Fetal and Neonatal Physiology, 2nd ed. Philadelphia, WB Saunders, 1998, p 1834.

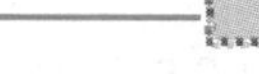

CHAPTER 482
Hereditary Clotting Factor Deficiencies (Bleeding Disorders)

Hemophilia A (factor VIII deficiency) and hemophilia B (factor IX deficiency) are the most common and serious congenital coagulation factor deficiencies. The symptoms of hemophilia A and B are virtually identical. Hemophilia C refers to the bleeding disorder associated with reduced levels of factor XI and is discussed separately in subchapter 482.2. The contact factors (factor XII, high molecular weight kininogen, and prekallikrein), which are associated with significant prolongation of the APTT but are not associated with hemorrhage are discussed in subchapter 482.3. Subsequent subchapters briefly discuss other coagulation factor deficiencies that are less common.

482.1 Factor VIII or Factor IX Deficiency (Hemophilia A or B)

Factor VIII and factor IX deficiencies are the most common severe inherited bleeding disorders. Hemophilia has been recognized as a clinical entity since biblical times, when Talmudic writings permitted the avoidance of circumcision when there was a repeated history of death from circumcisional bleeding in male siblings. Whole blood or plasma was used during the mid–twentieth century for treatment of hemophilia. The "concentrate" era of treatment began in 1964 with the discovery that cryoprecipitate, a fraction of plasma that contained factor VIII, could be used to treat hemophilia A. Shortly thereafter, concentrates for both factor VIII and factor IX were commercially developed. In 1985 the genes for both factor VIII and factor IX were cloned. This has resulted in the development of recombinant factor VIII and factor IX for treating patients with hemophilia and avoids the infection risk of plasma-derived transfusion-transmitted diseases.

PATHOPHYSIOLOGY. Factor VIII and factor IX participate in a complex required for the activation of factor X. Together with phospholipid and calcium, they form the "tenase," or factor X-activating, complex. Figure 481–1 illustrates the clotting process as it occurs in the test tube, with factor X being activated by either the complex of factor VIII and factor IX or the complex of tissue factor and factor VII. In vivo factor VII and tissue factor can also activate factor IX. This may be one reason that deficiencies of factor VIII and factor IX are the severest bleeding disorders. In the laboratory, however, the prothrombin time (PT) measures the activation of factor X by factor VII and is therefore normal in patients with factor VIII or factor IX deficiency.

Following injury, the initial hemostatic event is the formation of the platelet plug together with the generation of the fibrin clot that prevents further hemorrhage. In hemophilia A or hemophilia B, clot formation is delayed and is not robust. Thus, patients with hemophilia do not bleed more rapidly. There is, instead, a slowing of the rate of clot formation. When untreated bleeding occurs in a closed space such as a joint, cessation of bleeding may be the result of tamponade. With open wounds, in which tamponade cannot occur, profuse bleeding may result in significant blood loss. The clot that is formed may be friable, and rebleeding occurs during the physiologic lysis of clots or with minimal trauma.

CLINICAL MANIFESTATIONS. Neither factor VIII nor factor IX crosses the placenta; thus, bleeding symptoms may be present from birth or occur in the fetus. Occasionally, neonates with hemophilia may sustain intracranial hemorrhage. Surprisingly, only about 30% of affected male infants with hemophilia bleed with circumcision. Thus, if the family history does not alert the physician to be suspicious for its presence, hemophilia may go undiagnosed in the newborn. It is only when a child begins to crawl and walk that mobility causes the initiation of easy bruising, intramuscular hematomas, and hemarthroses. Bleeding from minor traumatic lacerations of the mouth may persist for hours or days and may cause the parents to seek medical evaluation. Even in patients with severe hemophilia, only 90% have evidence of increased bleeding by 1 yr of age. Although bleeding may occur in any area of the body, the hallmark of hemophilia is the hemarthrosis. Bleeding into joints may be induced by minor trauma; nonetheless, many hemarthroses are spontaneous. The earliest joint bleeds appear most commonly in the ankle, because of the lack of stability of this joint as the toddler assumes an upright posture. In the older child and adolescent, hemarthroses of the knees and elbows are the most debilitating. While the child's early joint bleeds are recognized only following major swelling and fluid accumulation in the joint space, older children are frequently able to recognize bleeding earlier than the physician.

While most muscular hemorrhages are visible, iliopsoas bleeding requires specific mention. Patients may lose large volumes of blood into the iliopsoas muscle and verge on hypovolemic shock with only a vague area of referred pain in the groin. The diagnosis is made clinically by the inability to extend the hip but demands confirmation with ultrasonography or CT scan together with aggressive replacement therapy.

Life-threatening bleeding in the hemophilic patient is caused by bleeding into vital structures (CNS, upper airway) or by exsanguination (external, gastrointestinal, or iliopsoas hemorrhage). Prompt treatment with clotting factor concentrate for these life-threatening hemorrhages is imperative. If head trauma is of sufficient concern so as to suggest radiologic evaluation, factor replacement should precede radiologic evaluation. Life-threatening hemorrhages require replacement therapy to achieve a level equal to that of normal plasma (100 U/dL or 100%).

Patients with mild hemophilia who have factor VIII activities greater than 5% usually do not have spontaneous hemorrhaging. These patients may experience prolonged bleeding following dental work, surgery, or injuries following moderate trauma. If they develop a "target" joint site of bleeding, recurrent bleeding may then become spontaneous because of the underlying pathology in the joint.

LABORATORY FINDINGS. The laboratory screening test that is affected by a reduced level of factor VIII or factor IX is the APTT. In severe hemophilia, this APTT is usually (2) to (3) times the upper limits of normal of the APTT. The other screening tests of the hemostatic mechanism (platelet count, bleeding time, prothrombin time, and thrombin time) are normal. Unless the patient has an inhibitor to factor VIII, the mixing of normal plasma with patient plasma results in correction of the PTT. The specific assay for factor VIII and factor IX will confirm the diagnosis of hemophilia. If correction does not occur on mixing, an inhibitor may be present. In 14–25% of patients who receive infusions of factor VIII or factor IX, a factor-specific antibody may develop. These antibodies are directed against the active clotting site and are termed inhibitors. In such patients the quantitative Bethesda assay for inhibitor should be performed.

GENETICS AND CLASSIFICATION. Hemophilia occurs in approximately 1:5,000 males, with 85% having factor VIII deficiency and 10–15% having factor IX deficiency. Hemophilia shows no apparent racial predilection, appearing in all ethnic groups. The severity of hemophilia is classified on the basis of the patient's baseline level of factor VIII or factor IX with 1 unit of each factor defined as the amount in 1 mL of normal plasma. Severe hemophilia is characterized by having <1.0 U/dL (<1%) of the specific clotting factor. Moderate hemophilia patients have 1–5 U/dL, and mild hemophilia patients have levels >5 U/dL. The hemostatic level for factor VIII is >30–40 U/dL and >25–30 U/dL for factor IX.

The genes for both factor VIII and factor IX are carried near the terminus of the long arm of the X chromosome and are therefore X-linked traits. The majority of patients have reduction in the amount of clotting factor protein; however, 5–10% of hemophilia A and 40–50% of hemophilia B patients make a dysfunctional protein. One specific genetic mutation in hemophilia A warrants further discussion. Approximately 45–50% of patients with severe hemophilia A have the same mutation, in which there is an internal inversion within the factor VIII gene that results in no protein being produced. This mutation can be detected in the blood of patients or carriers and in the amniotic fluid by molecular techniques. Because of the multiple genetic causes of either factor VIII or factor IX deficiency, however, most patients are classified based upon the amount of factor VIII or factor IX clotting activity. In the newborn, factor VIII levels may be artificially elevated because of the acute-phase response elicited by the birth process. This may cause a mildly affected patient to have normal or near-normal levels of factor VIII. Patients with severe hemophilia will not have detectable levels. In contrast, factor IX levels are physiologically low in the newborn. If severe hemophilia is present in the family, an undetectable level of factor IX is diagnostic of severe hemophilia B. Sometimes with mild factor

IX deficiency, the presence of hemophilia can be confirmed only after several weeks of life.

Some female carriers of hemophilia A or hemophilia B will have sufficient reduction of their factor VIII or factor IX through lionization of the X chromosome to produce mild bleeding disorders in carriers. Factor VIII or factor IX levels should be determined in all known carriers to assess the need for treatment in the event of surgery or clinical bleeding.

Because factor VIII is carried in plasma by von Willebrand factor (vWf), the ratio of factor VIII to vWf is sometimes used to diagnose carriers of hemophilia. When possible, specific genetic mutations should be identified in the propositus and used to test other family members at risk for either having hemophilia or being carriers.

TREATMENT. The prevention of trauma is important to the care of the child with hemophilia, but bleeds may occur in the absence of trauma. Early psychosocial intervention helps the family achieve a balance between overprotection and permissiveness. Aspirin and other nonsteroidal anti-inflammatory drugs that affect platelet function should be avoided by patients with hemophilia. Although recombinant products may avoid exposure to transfusion-transmitted diseases, the infant should be immunized against hepatitis B virus in the neonatal period in case plasma-derived products are used with future bleeds. Patients should be periodically screened for hepatitis and abnormalities in liver function. Calculation of the dose of factor VIII (FVIII) or factor IX (FIX) is as follows:

$$\begin{matrix}\text{Dose of FVIII}\\ \text{(units, U)}\end{matrix} = \left(\begin{matrix}\text{u/dL (\%) desired}\\ \text{rise in plasma FVIII}\end{matrix}\right) \times \begin{matrix}\text{Body Weight}\\ \text{(kg)}\end{matrix} \times 0.5$$

$$\begin{matrix}\text{Dose of FIX}\\ \text{(units, U)}\end{matrix} = \left(\begin{matrix}\text{u/dL (\%) desired}\\ \text{rise in plasma FIX}\end{matrix}\right) \times \begin{matrix}\text{Body Weight}\\ \text{(kg)}\end{matrix} \times 1.0^*$$

REPLACEMENT THERAPY. When bleeding occurs, the factor VIII level must be raised to hemostatic levels (35–40%) or for life-threatening or major bleeds to 100% (100 U/dL). Table 482–1 summarizes the treatment of some common types of hemorrhage in a patient with hemophilia.

With the availability of recombinant replacement products, prophylaxis has been recommended for many young children to prevent spontaneous bleeding and early joint deformities.

With mild factor VIII hemophilia, the patient's endogenously produced factor VIII can be released by the administration of desmopressin acetate (DDAVP). In moderate or severe factor VIII deficient patients, the stored levels of factor VIII in the body are inadequate, and the DDAVP is ineffective. On the other hand, exposing the mildly hemophilic patient to transfusion-transmitted diseases or the cost of recombinant products warrants the use of DDAVP if it is effective. Most centers administer a trial of DDAVP to determine the level of factor VIII achieved following its infusion. DDAVP is not effective in the treatment of factor IX–deficient hemophilia B.

CHRONIC COMPLICATIONS. The long-term complications of hemophilia A and B include chronic joint destruction, the risk of transfusion-transmitted infectious diseases, and the development of an inhibitor to either factor VIII or factor IX. While the aggressive or prophylactic approach to treatment has reduced the problems of chronic joint arthropathy, these problems have not been eliminated. Furthermore, while transfusion-transmitted diseases are minimized or negated by using highly purified or recombinant products, many older patients, however, have been exposed to plasma-derived products. As a result, transfusion-transmitted diseases, including HIV and hepatitis C or B, may be the major long-term cause of morbidity and mortality. The incidence of inhibitors appears similar in patients using either recombinant or plasma-derived products for factor VIII replacement. Highly purified factor IX or recombinant factor IX seems to increase the incidence of factor IX inhibitors.

Historically, chronic arthropathy is the major long-term disability of hemophilia. The natural history of untreated hemophilia is one of cyclical recurrent hemorrhages into specific joints. As further hemorrhages occur into the same joint, the patient is said to have developed a "target" joint for future bleeds. After joint hemorrhage, proteolytic enzymes are released by white blood cells into the joint space and heme iron induces macrophage proliferation—all of which contribute to inflammation in the synovium. The synovium thickens and develops frondlike projections into the joint that are susceptible to being pinched and may induce further hemorrhage. The cartilaginous surface becomes eroded and ultimately may even expose raw bone, leaving the joint susceptible to articular fusion. When the first bleeds occur in a child's joints, the joint has not been previously damaged. The synovium is therefore elastic and can accommodate a large amount of blood. Frequently the swelling is much greater than the pain. In contrast, the older patient with advanced arthropathy may have such a scarred joint that there is little space for bleeding. In these patients the pain is much greater than the physical findings. Once a target joint is seen to be developing, modern treatment usually requires placing the patient on short- or long-term prophylaxis to prevent progression of the arthropathy and to reduce inflammation.

Many patients are now placed on lifelong prophylaxis programs to prevent spontaneous joint bleeding. Such programs, while expensive, are highly effective at preventing or greatly modulating the degree of joint pathology. Since gene therapy may be available within the lifetime of pediatric patients, keeping joints normal through prophylaxis is a logical path. If moderate joint arthropathy develops, prevention of future bleeding will require higher plasma levels of clotting factors, and the individual will be less amenable to gene therapy.

While infection from transfusion-transmitted diseases has been dramatically reduced by using plasma-derived products that are heat treated, immunopurified, and chemically treated, most hemophilia centers recommend the use of recombinant products, because they are free from known human transmitted viruses. Although some of these products have been produced or even reformulated in human albumin, the risk of viral infection is theoretical. While HIV infection devastated the adult hemophilic population, alteration in manufacturing practices in the early to mid-1980s has eliminated this risk today. However, many adults remain with HIV infection. The experience with this "epidemic" requires that great vigilance be exercised to prevent similar unexpected infections in the future. Chronic hepatitis C and even hepatitis B remain as problems for many older patients with hemophilia, but the use of recombinant products has virtually eliminated this risk in younger patients. Parvovirus and hepatitis A are nonenveloped viruses that may escape solvent detergent treatment and heat treatment. Thus, plasma-derived products may continue to transmit these infectious agents. The potential for Creutzfeldt-Jakob disease to be transmitted through blood remains controversial but unsubstantiated.

Infusion of the deficient clotting factor may initiate an immune response in patients with either factor VIII or factor IX deficiency. The antibody to factor VIII or factor IX is usually an antibody that blocks the clotting activity and is therefore defined as an inhibitor. Inhibitors are suspected clinically when patients who have responded well to replacement therapy suddenly become less responsive or are identified during routine follow-up testing. Inhibitors develop in approximately 25% of patients with hemophilia A; the percentage is somewhat lower in patients with hemophilia B, many of whom make an inactive dysfunctional protein that renders them less susceptible to an immune response. Many patients who develop an inhibitor lose this inhibitor with continued regular

*With recombinant FIX this number should be 1.4.

TABLE 482–1 Treatment of Hemophilia

Type of Hemorrhage	Hemophilia A	Hemophilia B
Hemarthrosis*	20 units/kg factor VIII concentrate†; 15 units/kg if treated early. If hemorrhage is severe, repeat the dose the following day and consider additional treatment every other day until the joint "normalizes"	30 units/kg factor IX concentrate; 20 units/kg if treated early
Muscle or significant subcutaneous hematoma	20 units/kg factor VIII concentrate; may need every-other-day treatment until well resolved	30 units/kg factor IX concentrate; may need treatment every 2–3 days until well controlled
Mouth, deciduous tooth, or tooth extraction	20 units/kg factor VIII concentrate; antifibrinolytic therapy; remove loose deciduous tooth	30 units/kg factor IX concentrate: antifibrinolytic therapy§; remove loose deciduous tooth
Epistaxis	Apply pressure for 15–20 min; pack with petrolatum gauze; antifibrinolytic therapy; 20 units/kg factor VIII concentrate if above fails	Apply pressure for 15–20 min; pack with petrolatum gauze; antifibrinolytic therapy; 30 units/kg factor IX concentrate if above fails (4 hr after antifibrinolytic dose)
Major surgery, life-threatening hemorrhage (e.g., CNS, GI, airway)	50 units/kg factor VIII concentrate, then initiate continuous infusion of 2–3 units/kg/hr to maintain factor VIII >100 U/dL for 24 hr, then given 2–3 units/kg/hr continuously for 5–7 days to maintain the level >50 U/dL and an additional 5–7 days at a level >30 U/dL	80 units/kg factor IX concentrate, then 20–40 units/kg every 12–24 hr to maintain factor IX >40 U/dL for 5–7 days and then >30 U/dL for 5 days‡
Iliopsoas hemorrhage	50 units/kg factor VIII concentrate, then 25 units/kg every 12 hr until asymptomatic, then 20 units/kg every other day for total 10–14 days‖	80 units/kg factor IX concentrate, then 20–40 units/kg every 12–24 hr to maintain factor IX >40 U/dL until asymptomatic, then 30 U every other day for total 10–14 days‡‖
Hematuria	Bed rest; 1½ × maintenance fluids; if not controlled in 1–2 days, 20 units/kg factor VIII concentrate; if not controlled, give prednisone (unless HIV-infected)	Bed rest: 1½ × maintenance fluids; if not controlled in 1–2 days 30 units/kg factor IX concentrate; if not controlled, give prednisone (unless HIV-infected)

**For hip hemarthrosis, orthopedic evaluation for possible aspiration is advisable.*

†For mild or moderate hemophilia, desmopressin, 0.3 μg/kg should be used instead of factor VIII concentrate if patient is known to respond with a hemostatic level of factor VIII; if repeated doses are given, monitor factor VIII levels for tachyphylaxis.

‡If repeated doses of factor IX concentrate are required, use highly purified, specific, factor IX concentrate.

§*Do not give antifibrinolytic therapy until 4 to 6 hr after a dose of prothrombin complex concentrate.*

‖*Repeat radiologic assessment should be performed before discontinuation of therapy.*

From Montgomery RR, Gill JC, Scott JP: Hemophilia and von Willerbrand disease. In: *Nathan DG, Orkin SH (eds): Nathan and Oski's Hematology of Infancy and Childhood, 5th ed. Philadelphia, WB Saunders, 1998.*

infusions. Others develop a higher titer with subsequent infusions and may need to go through desensitization programs, in which high doses of factor VIII or factor IX are infused in an attempt to saturate the antibody and to permit the body to develop tolerance. If desensitization fails, these patients are treated with either activated prothrombin complex concentrates or factor VIIa. The use of these products bypasses the inhibitor in many instances but increases the risk for thrombosis. Inhibitor patients require referral to a hospital that cares for many such patients and has a comprehensive hemophilia program.

COMPREHENSIVE CARE. Hemophilia patients today are managed through large hemophilia comprehensive care centers. Such centers are dedicated to identifying early signs of chronic debilitation and take a modern approach to replacement therapy and treatment of complications such as hepatitis C and HIV. Such centers involve physicians, nurses, orthopedists, physical therapists, psychosocial workers, and comprehensive nurses.

482.2 Factor XI Deficiency (Hemophilia C)

Factor XI deficiency is an autosomal deficiency associated with mild to moderate bleeding symptoms. It is frequently encountered in Ashkenazi Jews but has been found in many other ethnic groups. In Israel, 1–3:1,000 are homozygous for this deficiency. Sephardic Jews are rarely affected. While the condition is referred to as hemophilia C, the bleeding tendency is not as great as in factor VIII or factor IX deficiency. The bleeding associated with factor XI deficiency is not correlated with the amount of factor XI. Some patients with severe deficiency may have minimal or no symptoms at the time of major surgery. Unless the patient previously had surgery without bleeding, treatment is usually undertaken. There is no licensed concentrate of factor XI available in the United States; therefore, the physician must use fresh frozen plasma (FFP) or enroll the patient in a clinical trial of factor XI concentrate. Minor surgeries can be controlled with local pressure; dental extractions can be monitored closely and the patient treated only if hemorrhage occurs. Major surgery should probably be approached with replacement therapy unless the patient has had prior surgery with no treatment and without bleeding. In a patient with homozygous deficiency of factor XI, the PTT is often longer than it is in patients with either severe factor VIII or factor IX deficiency. The paradox of fewer clinical symptoms with a longer PTT is surprising, but this is the result of factor VII being able to activate factor IX in vivo. The deficiency of factor XI can be confirmed by specific factor XI assays. Plasma infusions of 1 U/kg usually increase the plasma concentration by 2 U/dL. Thus, the infusion of 10–15 mL of plasma/kg will result in a plasma level of 20–30 U/dL (20–30%), a level usually sufficient to control moderate hemorrhage. Frequent infusions of plasma would be necessary to achieve higher levels of factor XI. Because the factor XI half-life is usually 48 hr or greater, maintaining adequate levels of factor XI is not usually difficult. Chronic joint bleeding is rarely a problem, and, for most patients, factor XI deficiency is a concern only at the time of major surgery.

482.3 Deficiencies of the Contact Factors (Nonbleeding Disorders)

Deficiencies of factor VIII, factor IX, and factor XI all cause isolated prolongation of PTT. Deficiencies of the contact factors also prolong the PTT but are not causes of clinical bleeding. These factors include factor XII, prekallikrein, and high molecular weight kininogen. Because these contact factors function at the step of initiation of the intrinsic clotting system, the PTT is markedly prolonged when these factors are absent. Thus one encounters the paradoxical situation in which there is an extremely prolonged PTT but no evidence of clinical bleeding. It is important that these individuals be well informed about the meaning of their clotting factor deficiency, since they do not need treatment even if major surgery is undertaken. On rare occasions, factor XII deficiency is associated with von Willebrand disease and has been termed von Willebrand San Diego. Thus, if a patient with reduced factor XII is identified who has bleeding symptoms, it is advisable to carry out von Willebrand screening.

482.4 Factor VII Deficiency

Factor VII deficiency is a rare bleeding disorder that is usually detected only in the homozygous state. Individuals with this deficiency may have spontaneous intracranial hemorrhage and frequent mucocutaneous bleeding. They will have a markedly prolonged PT but a normal PTT. Factor VII assays demonstrate a marked reduction of factor VII. Since the plasma half-life of factor VII is 2–4 hr, therapy with FFP is difficult and often complicated by fluid overload. Commercial concentrates of factor VII are becoming available, but even these concentrates may need to be given continuously during a major intracranial hemorrhage to achieve adequate hemostasis.

482.5 Factor X Deficiency

This is a rare autosomal disorder that results in mucocutaneous and post-traumatic bleeding. This deficiency is the result of either a quantitative deficiency or a dysfunctional molecule. A reduced factor X level is associated with a prolongation of both the PT and the PTT. In patients with hereditary deficiency of factor X, factor X levels can be increased using either FFP or prothrombin complex concentrate. The half-life of factor X is approximately 30 hr, and its volume of distribution is similar to factor IX. Thus, 1 U/kg will increase the plasma level of factor X 1 U/dL.

Although rarely a problem in pediatric patients, systemic amyloidosis may be associated with factor X deficiency due to the adsorption of factor X on the amyloid. Transfusion therapy is often not successful because of the rapid clearance.

482.6 Prothrombin (Factor II) Deficiency

This deficiency is caused either by a markedly reduced prothrombin level (hypoprothrombinemia) or by a functionally abnormal prothrombin (dysprothrombinemia). Laboratory testing in homozygous patients demonstrates a prolonged PT and PTT. Factor II or prothrombin assays demonstrate the markedly reduced prothrombin level. Treatment can be achieved using either prothrombin complex concentrates or FFP. In prothrombin deficiency, FFP is useful, because the half-life of prothrombin is 3.5 days. One unit/kg of prothrombin will increase the plasma concentration by 1 U/dL.

482.7 Fibrinogen Deficiency

Congenital afibrinogenemia is a rare autosomal recessive disorder in which there is an absence of fibrinogen. Interestingly, these patients do not bleed as frequently as hemophilia patients and rarely have hemarthroses. Affected patients may present in the neonatal period with gastrointestinal hemorrhage or hematomas following vaginal delivery. Laboratory testing demonstrates a marked prolongation of the PTT, PT, and thrombin time. In the absence of a consumptive coagulopathy, absent fibrinogen is diagnostic. In addition to the quantitative deficiency of fibrinogen, a number of dysfunctional fibrinogens have been reported (dysfibrinogenemia). Currently, no fibrinogen concentrates are commercially available. Since the plasma half-life of fibrinogen is between 2 and 4 days, treatment with either FFP or cryoprecipitate is effective. The hemostatic level of fibrinogen is above 60 mg/dL. Each bag of cryoprecipitate contains 100–150 mg of fibrinogen. Some clinical assays for fibrinogen are inhibited by high doses of heparin. Thus, a markedly prolonged thrombin time should be confirmed with a reptilase time.

482.8 Factor V Deficiency

The deficiency of factor V, also known as labile factor, is an autosomal recessive, mild to moderate bleeding disorder that has also been termed parahemophilia. Hemarthroses occur rarely; mucocutaneous bleeding and hematomas are the most common symptoms. Severe menorrhagia is a frequent symptom in women. Laboratory evaluation demonstrates a prolonged PTT and PT. Specific assays for factor V demonstrate a reduction in factor V levels. The only currently available therapeutic product that contains factor V is FFP. Factor V is lost rapidly from FFP. It is therefore important to use FFP that is less than 2 mo old. Infusing 6 mL/kg of FFP every 12 hr can treat patients with severe factor V deficiency. Rarely, one encounters the patient with a negative family history of bleeding who has an acquired antibody to factor V. Often, these patients do not bleed because the factor V in platelets prevents excessive bleeding.

482.9 Combined Deficiency of Factor V and Factor VIII

Combined deficiency of factor V and factor VIII has been demonstrated to be secondary to the absence of an intracellular transport protein, ERGIC-53, which is responsible for transporting factor V and factor VIII from the endoplasmic reticulum to the Golgi compartments. ERGIC-53 is encoded on chromosome 18. The deficiency of factor VIII and factor V is not related to defective genes for those proteins but is secondary to a deficiency of a transport protein. This explains the paradoxical deficiency of two factors, one encoded on chromosome 1 and the other on the X chromosome.

482.10 Factor XIII Deficiency (Fibrin-Stabilizing Factor or Transglutaminase Deficiency)

Since factor XIII is responsible for the cross linking of fibrin or the stabilization of fibrin clot, symptoms of delayed hemorrhage are secondary to poor maintenance of hemostasis. Typically, patients will have trauma one day and then develop a bruise or hematoma on the following day. Clinical symptoms include mild bruising, delayed separation of the umbilical stump beyond 4 wk, poor wound healing, and, in women, recurrent spontaneous abortions. The usual screening tests for hemostasis are normal in patients with factor XIII deficiency. Screening tests for factor XIII deficiency are based on the observation that there is an increased solubility of the clot owing to the lack of cross linking. The normal clot remains insoluble in the presence of 5 M urea, whereas the clot formed from a patient with factor XIII deficiency is solubilized. More specific assays for factor XIII are immunologic. Since the half-life of factor XIII is 5–7 days and the hemostatic level is 2–3 U/dL, infusion of FFP or cryoprecipitate will correct the deficiency in these patients. Plasma contains 1 U/dL, and cryoprecipitate contains 75 U/bag. In patients with significant bleeding symptoms, prophylaxis can be achieved with infusion of cryoprecipitate every 3–4 wk.

482.11 Antiplasmin or Plasminogen Activator Inhibitor (PAI) Deficiency

Deficiency of either of these two antifibrinolytic proteins results in increased plasmin generation and the premature lysis of fibrin clots. Patients have mucocutaneous bleeding but rarely have joint hemorrhages. Since the usual hemostatic tests are normal, further work-up of a patient with a positive bleeding history should include the euglobulin clot lysis time that measures fibrinolytic activity and is shortened in the presence of these deficiencies. Specific assays for α_2 antiplasmin and PAI are available. Treatment can be accomplished using FFP.

Bauer KA: Rare hereditary coagulation factor abnormalities. *In*: Nathan DG, Orkin SH (eds): Hematology of Infancy and Childhood, 5th ed. Philadelphia, WB Saunders, 1998, pp 1660–1675.

Gill JC, Montgomery RR: Principles of therapy for hemostasis factor deficiencies. *In*: Nathan DG, Orkin SH (eds): Hematology of Infancy and Childhood, 4th ed. Philadelphia, WB Saunders, 1993, pp 1796–1818.

Hedner U, Glazer S, Pingel K, et al: Successful use of recombinant factor VIIa in patients with severe haemophilia A during synovectomy. Lancet 2:1193, 1988.

Hilgartner MW, Corrigan JJ Jr: Coagulation disorders. *In*: Miller DR, Baehner RL (eds): Blood Diseases of Infancy and Childhood, 7th ed. St. Louis, CV Mosby, 1995, pp 924–986.

Manco-Johnson MJ, Nuss R, Geraghty S, et al: Results of secondary prophylaxis in children with severe hemophilia. Am J Hematol 47:113, 1994.

Mannucci PM, Canciani MJ, Rota L, Donoran BS: Response of factor vIII/vWf to DDAVP in healthy subjects and patients with haemophilia A and von Willebrand's disease. Br J Haematol 47:283, 1981.

Menitove JE, Gill JC, Montgomery RR: Preparation and clinical use of plasma and plasma fractions. *In*: Hematology, 5th ed. New York, McGraw-Hill, 1994.

Montgomery RR, Scott JP: Hemostasis: Diseases of the fluid phase. *In*: Nathan DG, Orkin SH (eds): Hematology of Infancy and Childhood, 4th ed. Philadelphia, WB Saunders, 1993, pp 1605–1650.

Montgomery RR, Gill JC, Scott JP: Hemophilia and von Willebrand disease. *In*: Nathan DG, Orkin SH (eds): Hematology of Infancy and Childhood, 5th ed. Philadelphia, WB Saunders, 1998, pp 1631–1659.

White GC, McMillan CW, Kingdom HS, Shoemaker CB: Use of recombinant antihemophilic factor in treatment of two patients with classic hemophilia. N Engl J Med 320:166, 1989.

CHAPTER 483
von Willebrand Disease

von Willebrand disease is the most common hereditary bleeding disorder, with some reports suggesting that it is present in 1–2% of the general population. von Willebrand disease is inherited autosomally, but most centers report more women than men. Since menorrhagia is a major symptom, it may cause more women to seek diagnosis. von Willebrand disease is classified on the basis of whether the protein is quantitatively reduced but not absent (type 1), qualitatively abnormal (type 2), or absent (type 3) (Fig. 483–1).

PATHOPHYSIOLOGY. von Willebrand factor (vWf) is a large multimeric glycoprotein that is synthesized in megakaryocytes and endothelial cells and stored in α granules and Weibel-Palade bodies, respectively. During normal hemostasis, vWf adheres to the subendothelial matrix following vascular damage. When vWf binds to the subendothelial matrix, the conformation of vWf is changed so that it causes platelets to adhere to vWf through their glycoprotein IB (GPIB) receptor. These platelets are then activated, causing the recruitment of additional platelets and exposing phosphatidylserine, which is an important regulatory step for factor V– and factor VIII–dependent steps in the clotting cascade. vWf also serves as the carrier protein for plasma factor VIII. Deficiency of vWf may cause a secondary deficiency in factor VIII, even though the gene for factor VIII is normal. This is the cause of autosomal deficiency of factor VIII, now known to be a molecular abnormality of vWf.

CLINICAL MANIFESTATIONS. Patients with von Willebrand disease usually have symptoms of mucocutaneous hemorrhage, including excessive bruising, epistaxis, menorrhagia, and postoperative hemorrhage, particularly after mucosal surgery such as tonsillectomy or wisdom tooth extraction. Since a teenager's menstrual history is usually put in the context of other family members, excessive menstrual bleeding is not always recognized as being abnormal, because others in the family may be affected with the same disorder. If a menstruating female presents with iron deficiency, a detailed history of bruising and other bleeding should be elicited and further evaluation undertaken, if indicated.

Since vWf is an acute-phase protein, stress will increase its level. Thus patients may not bleed with procedures that incur major stress, such as appendectomy and childbirth, but may bleed excessively at the time of cosmetic or mucosal surgery. Bruising symptoms may diminish during pregnancy, since the vWf levels may double or triple during pregnancy. Rarely, patients with von Willebrand disease may have gastrointestinal telangiectasias. This combination results in major bleeding and accounts for numerous hospital admissions for patients with severe disease. In patients with type 3 or homozygous von Willebrand disease, bleeding symptoms are much more profound. These patients are usually diagnosed early in life and may have severe epistaxis or menorrhagia that results in major blood loss and possibly shock. Rarely, patients with severe type 3 von Willebrand disease may have joint hemorrhages or spontaneous central nervous system hemorrhages.

LABORATORY FINDINGS. Patients with von Willebrand disease are said to have a long bleeding time and a long PTT. These tests are not universally prolonged except in patients with type 3 von Willebrand disease. Therefore, normal screening tests do not preclude the diagnosis of von Willebrand disease. If the history is suggestive of a bleeding disorder, von Willebrand testing must be undertaken, including a quantitative assay for vWf antigen, vWf activity (ristocetin cofactor activity, or vWf R:Co), plasma factor VIII activity, determination of vWf structure (vWf multimers), and a platelet count. While the platelet count is usually normal in most patients, those with type 2B disease or platelet-type (pseudo-) von Willebrand disease may have lifelong thrombocytopenia. Figure 483–1 lists the variants of von Willebrand disease and summarizes their laboratory findings.

GENETICS. Chromosome 12 contains the gene for vWf. Each of the type 2 variants listed in Figure 483–1 has specific areas of the molecule affected. The phenotype can guide the genetic diagnosis of the specific mutation.

TREATMENT. Treatment of von Willebrand disease is directed toward increasing the plasma level of vWf and factor VIII. Since the gene for factor VIII is normal in patients with von Willebrand disease, elevating the plasma concentration of vWf will permit the normal recovery and survival of the endogenously produced factor VIII. The most common form of von Willebrand disease is type 1. In these patients the synthetic von Willebrand Disease Variants

Lab test	Type 1	Type 2A	Type 2B	Type 2M	Type 2N	Type 3
BT	N or ↑	↑↑	N or ↑	↑↑	N	↑↑↑↑
PTT	N or ↑	N or ↑	N or ↑	N	↑	↑↑↑
FVIII	N or ↓	N or ↓	N or ↓	N	↓↓↓	↓↓↓
vWF:Ag	↓	↓	↓	↓	↓	↓↓↓↓
vWFR:Co	↓	↓↓↓	↓↓	↓↓↓	↓	↓↓↓↓
vWF multimers	N but ↓	Abnormal	Abnormal	N but ↓	N but ↓	Absent
						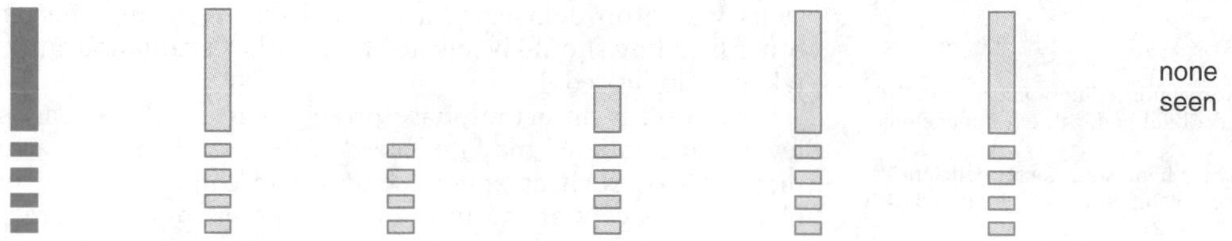 none seen

Figure 483–1 This figure summarizes the more common variants of von Willebrand disease. Laboratory testing is listed on the left and the results most commonly found with each of the variants. N is normal, ↑→↑ ↑ ↑ ↑ is degree of increase, and ↓→↓ ↓ ↓ ↓ is degree of decrease. A graphic representation of von Willebrand factor multimers is presented at the bottom of each column. Normal is shown in the first column; light gray illustrates a reduction in staining intensity; figure illustrates the size multimers that are present.

BT = bleeding time; PTT = partial thromboplastin time; FVIII = factor VIII; vWF:Ag = von Willebrand factor antigen; vWF R:Co = von Willebrand factor activity as measured by the ristocetin cofactor assay.

drug DDAVP induces the release of vWf from the endothelial cells. In some patients with type 2 variants, DDAVP may similarly be effective, but in other circumstances the released vWf is dysfunctional. In patients who are unresponsive to DDAVP, who have a variant in which DDAVP release of vWf is not effective, or who have type 3 disease in which there is no vWf to be released, replacement therapy must be used. Until recently, no products were licensed to treat von Willebrand disease; intermediate-purity factor VIII concentrates contain vWf in addition to factor VIII. Improved production of these intermediate-purity factor VIII concentrates has resulted in better preservation of von Willebrand structure and function and a marked reduction in risk of transfusion-transmitted infections. vWf distributes only to the intravascular space, because it is so large. Therefore, 1 U/kg will increase the plasma level by 2 U/dL (2%). The plasma half-life of both factor VIII and vWf is 12 hr. Purified vWf concentrates or recombinant vWf concentrates may become available in the near future. These will be useful in presurgical management or in prophylaxis. When used for acute bleeding, however, these vWf concentrates may need to be supplemented by an infusion of recombinant factor VIII. Both vWf and factor VIII are required for normal hemostasis. If only vWf is replaced, the endogenous correction of the factor VIII level takes 12–24 hr. Dental extractions and sometimes nosebleeds can be managed with both DDAVP and an antifibrinolytic agent such as epsilon amino caproic acid (amicar).

von Willebrand Variants

Type 1 von Willebrand disease is the most common form and accounts for 85% of cases. Bleeding symptoms include epistaxis, bruising, and menorrhagia. If bleeding is excessive, DDAVP administration at a dose of 0.3 μg/kg given intravenously will increase the level of vWf and factor VIII by three to five fold. Intranasal DDAVP (Stimate) is particularly helpful for the outpatient treatment of bleeding episodes.

Type 2A von Willebrand disease is due to the abnormal proteolysis of vWf, with only the smallest vWf multimers being present. This results in a reduction in vWf antigen with a much greater reduction in vWf activity. While DDAVP is safe in these patients, it is not always effective, because normal multimers are not maintained in plasma. Significant bleeding should be treated with vWf replacement therapy.

Type 2B von Willebrand disease may be caused by one of several mutations resulting in "hyperactive" vWf. The abnormal vWf binds spontaneously to platelets, causing platelet activation and clumping. The larger molecular weight multimers of vWf are cleared from the circulation, and moderate to severe thrombocytopenia is common. The laboratory diagnosis is based on demonstration that the "hyperactive" 2B vWf binds to platelets and agglutinates them at low concentrations of ristocetin—a concentration that would not agglutinate normal platelets. If one administers DDAVP to these patients, the abnormal "hyperactive" 2B vWf would be released, and thrombocytopenia might occur. These patients usually respond to the infusion of vWf.

Type 2M von Willebrand disease is caused by mutations that result in the loss of the platelet-binding function of vWf. The binding of this protein to factor VIII is normal, so that the factor VIII levels will be equal to the vWf levels, but the platelet-dependent interaction of vWf is reduced significantly. DDAVP will increase vWf and factor VIII levels, but the released type 2M vWf may not have sufficient activity to cause cessation of bleeding. Thus, vWf replacement therapy may need to be employed.

Type 2N von Willebrand disease is due to the loss of factor VIII binding by vWf. This has also been termed autosomal hemophilia. With this variant, platelet interaction with vWf is normal, but the 2N vWf binds weakly (or not at all) to factor VIII, resulting in rapid clearance of normal factor VIII. Thus, the factor VIII level is reduced much more than the vWf levels. Commonly, patients who have symptomatic bleeding are compound heterozygotes who have inherited a gene for type 1 von Willebrand disease from one parent and one for type 2N von Willebrand disease from the other. Rarely, 2N mutations are inherited from both parents and the vWf levels are normal. In the patient who is compound heterozygous of type 1 and type 2N, the one allele makes no protein and the other allele makes a functionally abnormal protein, resulting in all of the vWf being dysfunctional. While DDAVP will release the 2N vWf, the sustained factor VIII levels occasionally may be inadequate for normal hemostasis. von Willebrand factor replacement therapy is usually effective.

Platelet type (pseudo-) von Willebrand disease is actually an abnormality of the GPIB receptor on platelets. This can be considered the converse abnormality of type 2B, in that the GPIB receptor on platelets is hyperfunctional and binds plasma vWf spontaneously. This results in thrombocytopenia and a loss of high molecular weight multimers that are indistinguishable from 2B type von Willebrand disease. Specific testing, however, will demonstrate that this is a platelet abnormality rather than a plasma abnormality.

Type 3 von Willebrand disease is the homozygous or compound heterozygous inheritance of vWf deficiency. Patients exhibit undetectable plama levels of vWf and only low, but measurable, levels of factor VIII. These patients will have major hemorrhage, but interestingly, only rarely have joint hemorrhages. This severe form occurs in approximately 1:500,000 individuals, so it is quite rare. Intracranial hemorrhage, major epistaxis, and menorrhagia in women are the major features. Treatment must be with vWf-containing concentrates. DDAVP is not effective.

Ginsburg D, Konkle BA, Gill JC, et al: Molecular basis of human von Willebrand disease: analysis of von Willebrand factor mRNA. Proc Natl Acad Sci USA 86:3723, 1989.

Hillery CA, Mancuso DJ, Sadler JE, et al: Type 2M von Willebrand disease: F606I and I662F, mutations in the glycoprotein Ib binding domain selectively impair ristocetin, but not botrocetin-mediated binding of von Willebrand factor to platelets. Blood 91:1011, 1998.

Kroner PA, Kluesendorf KL, Montgomery RR: Expressed full-length von Willebrand factor containing missense mutations linked to type IIb von Willebrand's disease shows enhanced binding to platelets. Blood 79:2048, 1991.

Kroner PA, Friedman KD, Fahs SA, et al: Abnormal binding of factor VIII is linked with the substitution of Gln for Arg[91] in von Willebrand factor in a variant form on von Willebrand disease. J Biol Chem 266:10146, 1991.

Mannucci PM, Canciani MT, Rota L, Donoran BS: Response of factor VIII/vWf to DDAVP in healthy subjects and patients with haemophilia A and von Willebrand's disease. Br J Haematol 47:283, 1981.

Montgomery RR, Gill JC, Scott JP: Hemophilia and von Willebrand disease. *In:* Nathan DG, Orkin SH (eds): Hematology of Infancy and Childhood, 5th ed. Philadelphia, WB Saunders, 1998, pp 1631–1659.

Montgomery RR, Coller BS: von Willebrand disease. *In:* Colman RW, Hirsh J, Marder VJ, Salzman E (eds): Hemostasis and Thrombosis, Basic Principles and Clinical Practice. Philadelphia, Lippincott, 1994, pp 134–168.

Scott JP, Montgomery RR: Therapy of von Willebrand disease. Semin Thromb Hemost 19:37, 1993.

White GC, Montgomery RR: Clinical aspects and therapy of von Willebrand disease. *In:* Hematology: Basic Principles and Practice, 3rd ed. New York, Churchill Livingstone, 1999.

CHAPTER 484
Hereditary Predisposition to Thrombosis

Hereditary causes of thrombosis are well recognized in pediatrics. In addition, the newborn is predisposed to both hemorrhage and thrombosis because of the physiologic deficiency of various regulatory proteins. The more premature the infant, the greater the deficiency. In the first few days to weeks of life the normal newborn is physiologically predisposed to thrombosis. Those with hereditary deficiencies of anticoagulants may have major symptoms. Following the neonatal period, young children have resistance to clinical thrombosis even if they have a heterozygous hereditary deficiency of an anticoagulant protein. It is not until the teenage years or during periods of major clinical disease or inflammation that thrombotic symptoms surface and become more prominent with age.

PATHOPHYSIOLOGY AND CLINICAL MANIFESTATIONS. The predominant anticoagulants are illustrated in Figure 481–1. The major causes of hereditary predisposition to thrombosis include deficiencies of protein C, protein S, plasminogen and AT-III, and, more commonly, mutations of the genes for factor V and prothrombin.

The hereditary mutation of factor V, termed *factor V Leiden*, results in a factor V molecule that, when activated, is not subsequently inactivated by activated protein C. This leaves the patient with unregulated "active" factor V. Another mechanism, the *prothrombin mutation (G20210A)*, is observed in patients with a mutation in the 3′-untranslated end of the mRNA for prothrombin that results in increased levels of prothrombin synthesis. Children with these hereditary mutations have an increased frequency of venous thrombosis. Adolescents may have recurrent abortions. If one evaluates young adults with thrombosis, factor V Leiden and the prothrombin mutation (G20210A) are the most common associated abnormalities.

While patients with heterozygous deficiencies may be predisposed to thrombosis, those with *homozygous protein C deficiency* have fatal purpura fulminans in the neonatal period if untreated. Such infants were probably overlooked in the past because the symptoms were thought to be secondary to sepsis and disseminated intravascular coagulation. Since the newborn is physiologically deficient in protein C, its absence is difficult to determine except in a laboratory that has established normal ranges for neonates and preterm infants. If an individual has undetectable levels of protein C, this is most likely a hereditary disorder. The physiologic deficiency of protein C in the newborn coupled with true sepsis may also lead to nearly undetectable levels of protein C.

LABORATORY FINDINGS. There are no screening tests for hereditary deficiencies of anticoagulants such as protein C, protein S, antithrombin III, or factor V Leiden and prothrombin 20210; thus, specific testing is required. A careful family history is perhaps the most productive investigation and often reveals thromboembolic diseases in family members at a young age. If hereditary deficiency of anticoagulant or regulatory proteins is suspected, specific assays should be undertaken. Techniques that quantitate the amount and function of antithrombin III, protein C, and free protein S are well established. Genetic DNA testing for factor V Leiden and the prothrombin mutation (G20210A) are more sensitive and specific than clotting-based tests.

TREATMENT. Homozygous deficiency of protein C presents with purpura fulminans in the first few hours of life. Since no licensed protein C concentrate is currently available, fresh frozen plasma (FFP) is the only immediately available source of protein C. Amelioration of symptoms usually requires 10–15 mL/kg of FFP every 8–12 hr. Clinical trials are in progress using a plasma protein C concentrate, which eliminates the need for large amounts of FFP. After the infant's symptoms are reduced, the amount of FFP or protein C concentrate is adjusted and monitored by frequent protein C levels. When the infant is beyond the neonatal period, high-dose warfarin (to achieve an INR 4–5) may prevent most of the thrombotic problems but acute intermittent thromboses require additional FFP or protein C concentrate (see also Chapter 485).

Andrew M, Montgomery RR: Acquired disorders of hemostasis. *In:* Nathan DG, Orkin SH (eds): Nathan and Oski's Hematology of Infancy and Childhood, 5th ed. Philadelphia, WB Saunders, 1998, pp 1677–1717.

Esmon CT: Blood coagulation. *In:* Nathan DG, Orkin SH (eds): Hematology of Infancy and Childhood, 5th ed. Philadelphia, WB Saunders, 1998, pp 1531–1556.

Hilgartner MW, Corrigan JJ Jr: Coagulation disorders. *In:* Miller DR, Baehner RL (eds): Blood Diseases of Infancy and Childhood, 7th ed. St. Louis, CV Mosby, 1995, pp 924–986.

Hogstrom JN, Walter J, Bluebond-Langner R, et al: Prevalence of the factor V Leiden mutation in children and neonates with thromboembolic disease. J Pediatr 133:777, 1998.

CHAPTER 485
Acquired Thrombotic Disorders

The occlusion of a blood vessel with a platelet plug or fibrin clot may occur in vessels of any size. Capillary and small vessel occlusion are seen in vasculitic diseases and as complications of disseminated intravascular coagulation (DIC); medium-sized vessel occlusions are seen in homocystinuria, cyanotic congenital heart disease, dehydration, and polyarteritis nodosa; and in larger vessels, in aortic thrombosis, superior vena cava thrombosis in the newborn, deep venous thrombosis (DVT), sickle cell anemia, and pulmonary embolism. The mechanism leading to thrombosis is vessel injury, in addition to one or all of the following: abnormal platelet adhesiveness-aggregation, an activated coagulation mechanism, an inactive inhibitor system, an inactive fibrinolytic mechanisms and reduced blood flow. Arterial thrombosis appears to depend on vascular injury and platelet activation under high shear, whereas venous thrombosis generally occurs in low-flow (low-shear) conditions associated with activation of the coagulation mechanism or with an impaired inhibitor-fibrinolytic system.

The clinical manifestations reflect organ or tissue injury resulting from a severe reduction in blood perfusion or distention due to occlusion of venous outflow. In general, vascular occlusive events in children have an acute or sudden onset. The diagnosis is made by Doppler ultrasound or MRI. Other laboratory studies are rarely helpful in diagnosing a thromboembolic event except in two settings: when the event is a result of DIC (in which case the patient demonstrates thrombocytopenia; hypofibrinogenemia; reduced factors II, V, and VIII; and positive D-dimers) and, in rare patients, when caused by congenital deficiencies of natural inhibitors (Chapter 484).

Acquired thrombotic and embolic events are uncommon in otherwise healthy children. Nevertheless, there are increasing reports of thromboembolism (TE) in newborns and in patients with specific diseases (Table 485–1). Arterial events usually present as stroke (at any age), a cold and pulseless lower extremity with or without renal involvement (aortic thrombosis in the newborn), and, rarely, myocardial infarction, although any arterialized organ can be affected. Venous events usually present as DVT with or without phlebitis, pulmonary embolism, and renal vein thrombosis.

The *lupus anticoagulant* (antiphospholipid antibody) *syndrome* may be primary (idiopathic) or associated with systemic lupus erythematosus, infections, drug reactions, or other autoimmune diseases. Associated features include livedo reticularis, thrombocytopenia, recurrent fetal loss, and thrombosis (arterial or venous, or both). The activated partial thromboplastin time (PTT or APTT) may be prolonged, but specific assays are needed to detect the antiphospholipid antibody. Treatment includes warfarin with or without aspirin.

Treatment of TE is designed to remove the thrombus or embolus (e.g., by thrombectomy or thrombolytic agents) or to inhibit the formation and propagation of a thrombus with drugs (anticoagulants), thereby allowing physiologic lysis.

TABLE 485–1 Causes of Disseminated Intravascular Coagulation

Infectious
Meningococcemia (purpura fulminans)
Other gram-negative bacteria (*Haemophilus, Salmonella, Escherichia coli*)
Gram-positive bacteria (group B streptococci, staphylococci)
Rickettsia (Rocky Mountain spotted fever)
Virus (cytomegalovirus, herpes simplex, hemorrhagic fevers)
Malaria
Fungus
Tissue Injury
Central nervous system trauma (massive head injury)
Multiple fractures with fat emboli
Crush injury
Profound shock or asphyxia
Hypothermia or hyperthermia
Massive burns
Malignancy
Acute promyelocytic leukemia
Acute monoblastic or myelocytic leukemia
Widespread malignancies (neuroblastoma)
Venom or Toxin
Snake bites
Insect bites
Microangiopathic Disorders
"Severe" thrombotic thrombocytopenic purpura or hemolytic-uremic syndrome
Giant hemangioma (Kasabach-Merritt syndrome)
Gastrointestinal Disorders
Fulminant hepatitis
Severe inflammatory bowel disease
Reye syndrome
Hereditary Thrombotic Disorders
Antithrombin III deficiency
Homozygous protein C deficiency
Newborn
Maternal toxemia
Group B streptococcal infections
Abruptio placentae
Severe respiratory distress syndrome
Necrotizing enterocolitis
Congenital viral disease (cytomegalovirus, herpes simplex)
Erythroblastosis fetalis
Miscellaneous
Severe acute graft rejection
Acute hemolytic transfusion reaction
Severe collagen-vascular disease
Kawasaki disease
Heparin-induced thrombosis
Infusion of "activated" prothrombin complex concentrates
Hyperpyrexia/encephalopathy, hemorrhagic shock syndrome

Modified from Montgomery RR, Scott IP. Hemostasis: Diseases of the fluid phase. In: *Nathan DG, Oski FA (eds). Hematology of Infancy and Childhood, 4th ed. Vol 2. Philadelphia: WB Saunders, 1993.*

VENOUS THROMBOSIS AND THROMBOPHLEBITIS. Superficial thrombophlebitis is treated by anti-inflammatory drugs (nonsteroidal agents), heat compresses, rest, and elevation of the affected part. Patients with DVT or thrombophlebitis are treated with anticoagulation and sometimes with thrombolytic agents. Heparin anticoagulation should be used in a full dose for 3–5 days, with warfarin added for an additional 6 mo in those patients with proximal (above the knee) venous thrombosis. Patients with calf vein thrombosis may not require treatment, but thrombosis above the knee should be treated with heparin for 3–5 days and then with warfarin or subcutaneous heparin for an additional 6 mo. Acute iliofemoral venous thrombosis may also be treated with thrombolytic agents followed by anticoagulation with heparin and warfarin. Experience with thrombolytic therapy in children is limited, but its efficacy is probably similar to that seen in adults.

PULMONARY EMBOLISM. The patient with acute pulmonary embolism (PE) can be treated with heparin or thrombolytic drugs. Thrombolytic therapy produces a more rapid clinical improvement than heparin therapy, but the overall survival and long-term pulmonary function abnormalities appear to be the same in both treatment groups. Rarely, embolectomy is used when there is a large embolism and no benefit from thrombolytic or anticoagulant therapy.

ARTERIAL THROMBOSIS. The primary approach to arterial thrombosis is with fibrinolytic therapy with either recombinant tPA (rtPA) or urokinase. Rarely, surgical removal of the clot is performed if lytic therapy is not successful or if the thrombosis affects a major organ or limb. Thrombolytic therapy cannot be employed if there has been recent surgery or CNS thrombosis/hemorrhage.

STROKE. Arterial occlusion in the brain occurs when there is a vascular injury or anomaly or embolization from the heart; often these strokes are idiopathic. Venous thrombosis of cerebral vessels can be seen in those with cyanotic heart disease, inflammatory lesions of the brain, hyperviscosity states, or congenital thrombophilia. The therapeutic approach is directed toward the cause of the occlusion. Anticoagulation and/or platelet inhibitor drugs may be used. The presence of a hemorrhagic infarct is a contraindication for anticoagulant therapy. It is not known whether thrombolytic therapy is effective or safe in children with nonhemorrhagic strokes. Heparin therapy of strokes appears to improve outcome in adults, with some reports of similar success in children.

485.1 Anticoagulant and Thrombolytic Therapy

STANDARD UNFRACTIONATED HEPARIN. Heparin enhances the rate by which antithrombin III neutralizes the activities of several of the activated clotting proteins, especially thrombin. The average half-life of intravenously administered heparin is about 60 min in adults and can be as short as 30 min in the newborn. Heparin does not cross the placenta. The half-life of heparin is dose dependent; that is, the higher the dose, the longer the circulating half-life. In thrombotic disease the half-life may be shorter than normal in patients with significant TE (such as pulmonary embolism) and longer than normal in patients with cirrhosis and uremia.

Anticoagulation with heparin is contraindicated in the following circumstances: a pre-existing coagulation defect or bleeding abnormality; a recent CNS hemorrhage; bleeding from inaccessible sites; malignant hypertension; bacterial endocarditis; recent surgery of the eye, brain, or spinal cord; and current administration of regional or lumbar block anesthesia. Despite these precautions, the frequency of bleeding in patients given heparin anticoagulation is about 0.2–1%.

Heparin can be given as an intravenous or subcutaneous injection. It should not be given as an intramuscular injection. While heparin can be administered by intermittent bolus injections of 75–100 U/kg every 4 hr, continuous administration is associated with a lower risk of secondary hemorrhage. The current recommendation for continuous heparin is to give a bolus injection of 75 U/kg, followed by a continuous infusion of 28 U/kg/hr in infants under 1 yr of age or 20 U/kg/hr in children older than 1 yr. The goal is a PTT between 60 and 85 sec, which should correlate with a heparin level of 0.35–0.7 antifactor Xa U/mL. If the PTT is <60 sec, increase the heparin dose rate by 10%. If it is <50 sec, re-administer a bolus of 50 U/kg, and then increase the dose rate by 10%. If the PTT is >90 sec, stop the heparin dose for 30 min and then decrease the dose rate by 10%. If the dose must be adjusted, repeat the PTT in 4 hr. Once a stable therapeutic level has been reached, recheck the PTT daily. In newborns with low clotting factors, in patients with a lupus inhibitor, or in patients with elevated factor VIII (stress or surgery), the PTT may not reflect the correct degree of anticoagulation, and specific heparin levels should be performed so that the heparin level is 0.35–0.07 U/mL by anti-Xa assay or 0.2–0.4 U/mL by protamine sulfate assay.

Heparin can be neutralized immediately by using protamine sulfate. Because of the rapid clearance rate of heparin, however, most patients can be treated by stopping the infusion. One mg of protamine sulfate neutralizes between 90 and 110 units of heparin. Because heparin has a rapid in vivo metabolic decay, only half the total dose of protamine should be administered. A clotting test is performed to determine whether adequate neutralization has occurred; if not, the additional protamine can be given. Protamine itself is an anticoagulant; thus, if too much is given the clotting time may be prolonged. Although excess protamine has an anticoagulant effect, it rarely (if ever) is a cause of clinical bleeding. Once heparin is neutralized, the patient is returned to the original "prothrombotic" state.

Low Molecular Weight Heparin. Low molecular weight (LMW) heparins or heparinoids are either currently in use or undergoing clinical trials. Adult patients rarely need to have heparin levels monitored, but in pediatric patients there is more diversity in response. Thus, monitoring should be performed to be sure that a therapeutic level is achieved. For therapeutic treatment, 1 mg/kg of enoxaparin every 12 hr subcutaneously is usually effective. The PTT cannot be used to monitor LMW heparin; only a factor Xa assay can be used. The therapeutic level is >0.6 units/mL at 3 hr post injection. Prophylaxis is achieved with doses of 0.5 mg/kg every 12 hr subcutaneously. Prophylaxis levels demonstrate an anti-Xa assay of >0.3 units. Once a therapeutic range is achieved, routine monitoring is not required or required only infrequently.

WARFARIN. The coumarin derivatives are oral anticoagulant drugs that act by decreasing the rate of synthesis and gamma carboxylation of the vitamin K–dependent coagulation factors II, VII, IX, and X. In addition, protein C and protein S (the vitamin K–dependent anticoagulants) are affected. These drugs inhibit vitamin K–dependent carboxylation of the precursor coagulation proteins. Warfarin probably acts by competitively inhibiting vitamin K metabolism. Following the administration of warfarin, the levels of factors II, VII, IX, and X decrease gradually, according to their respective plasma half-life. Because factor VII has the shortest half-life, its level is the first to decrease, followed by factors IX and X, and finally factor II. It generally takes about 4–5 days to reduce levels of all four coagulation factors consistent with effective anticoagulation.

The prothrombin time (PT) is the clotting test used to assess warfarin anticoagulation. Current recommendations are based on the International Normalized Ratio (INR), which permits comparison of PTs using a wide variety of reagents or instrument. The INR for standard treatment of thrombosis is 2.0–3.0. For mechanical heart valves, treatment of homozygous protein C deficiency, and DVTs associated with the lupus anticoagulant, the INR should be between 3.0 and 4.0.

The dose of warfarin in children is 0.2 mg/kg/24 hr orally. After 48 hr the dose is adjusted based upon the INR. If the INR is 1.1–1.4, increase the dose by 20%; if it is 1.5–1.9, increase by 10%. If the INR is 3.2–3.5, decrease the dose by 20%. If the INR is >3.5, hold the dose until the INR is <3.5, then restart at 20% less than the previous dose. If the INR is 2.0–3.0, continue the same dose.

The most serious side effect of warfarin is hemorrhage. This is often related to changes in the dose or metabolism of the drug. The addition or removal of certain drugs in the patient's therapeutic regimen can have significant effects on oral anticoagulation. For example, warfarin's effect can be enhanced by the administration of antibiotics, salicylates, anabolic steroids, chloral hydrate, laxatives, allopurinol, vitamin E, and methylphenidate HCl; its effect can be diminished by barbiturates, vitamin K, oral contraceptives, phenytoin, and others. Warfarin-induced bleeding is treated by discontinuation of the drug and the administration of vitamin K. Generally, the amount of vitamin K given is equal to the amount of the daily warfarin dose. The vitamin can be administered orally, subcutaneously, or intravenously (not intramuscularly). Correction of the coagulopathy begins within 6–8 hr and should be complete in 24–48 hr. If the patient is having a significant bleeding problem, fresh frozen plasma (15 ml/kg) should be given at the same time as the vitamin K is administered.

Coumarin anticoagulants are contraindicated in essentially the same circumstances as those for heparin therapy. The oral anticoagulants are teratogenic, cross the placenta, and should not be given during pregnancy. Although breast milk contains warfarin, the quantity is insignificant and the drug can be used in the lactating mother.

THROMBOLYTIC THERAPY. Thrombolytic therapy involves the removal of blood clots by enzymatic digestion. It is accomplished by the in vivo generation of plasmin through the administration of plasminogen activators such as streptokinase, urokinase, and tissue-type plasminogen activator (rtPA). Urokinase and rtPA act as direct activators, whereas streptokinase acts by binding to plasminogen, and the streptokinase-plasminogen complex becomes the plasminogen activator. For this therapy to be effective, the patient must have a relatively fresh clot (<3–5 days old) the clot must be accessible to the lytic agent; and there must be an adequate amount of plasminogen. Once plasmin has been formed, it lyses fibrin. The plasmin generated by urokinase and streptokinase can produce a systemic hyperfibrinolytic state; when this occurs, the plasmin can degrade other plasma proteins, including fibrinogen, and factors V and VIII, resulting in a hemorrhagic disorder. rtPA is relatively more fibrin specific than urokinase; it serves as an activator within or on a fibrin clot. Clinical trials with rtPA suggest that a systemic hyperfibrinolytic state is rarely produced. The initial dose of rtPA is 0.1 mg/kg/hr with therapeutic effect determined by an increase in concentration of D-dimers or fibrin degradation products (FDP). With urokinase, a loading dose of 4400 U/kg is administered and then followed by 4400 U/kg/hr with therapeutic effectiveness monitored by a moderate drop in fibrinogen and the presence of detectable D-dimers.

Thrombolytic therapy has been reported to be beneficial in those with pulmonary embolism, DVT, certain arterial occlusive events, and occluded access shunts. However, there are no controlled trials on its use in the pediatric group.

Andrew M, Vegh P, Johnston M, et al: Maturation of the hemostatic system during childhood. Blood 80:1998, 1992.

Andrew M, Montgomery RR: Acquired disorders of hemostasis. *In*: Nathan DG, Orkin SH (eds): Nathan and Oski's Hematology of Infancy and Childhood, 5th ed. Philadelphia, WB Saunders, 1998, pp 1677–1717.

Andrew M, Mitchell L, Vegh P, Ofosu F: Thrombin regulation in children differs from adults in the absence and presence of heparin. Thromb Haemost 72:836, 1994.

Hathaway WE, Bonnar J: Hemostatic disorders of the pregnant woman and newborn infant. New York, Elsevier Science, 1987.

Hilgartner MW, Corrigan JJ Jr: Coagulation disorders. *In*: Miller DR, Baehner RL (eds): Blood Diseases of Infancy and Childhood, 7th ed. St. Louis, CV Mosby, 1995, pp 924–986.

CHAPTER 486
Postneonatal Vitamin K Deficiency

Although "late" hemorrhagic disease has been reported in breast-fed children, vitamin K deficiency occurring after the neonatal period is usually secondary to a lack of oral intake or the long-term use of broad-spectrum antibiotics. Intestinal malabsorption of fats may accompany cystic fibrosis or biliary atresia and result in a deficiency of fat-soluble, dietary vitamin K with a reduced synthesis of the vitamin K–dependent clotting factors (factors II, VII, IX, X, protein C, and protein S). Prophylactic administration of water-soluble vitamin K orally is indicated in these cholestatic situations (2–3 mg/24 hr for children and 5–10 mg/24 hr for adolescents and adults) or administering vitamin K 1–2 mg intravenously. In patients with advanced cirrhosis, synthesis of many of the clotting factors may be reduced because of hepatocellular damage. In these patients, vitamin K may be ineffective. The anticoagulant properties of warfarin (coumadin) and related anticoagulants depend on interference with vitamin K with a concomitant reduction of factors II, VII, IX, and X. Rat poison (superwarfarin) produces a similar deficiency; vitamin K is a specific antidote.

Andrew M, Montgomery RR: Acquired disorders of hemostasis. *In*: Nathan DG, Orkin SH (eds): Hematology of Infancy and Childhood, 5th ed. Philadelphia, WB Saunders, 1998, pp 1677–1717.

Hilgartner MW, Corrigan JJ Jr: Coagulation disorders. *In*: Miller DR, Baehner RL (eds): Blood Diseases of Infancy and Childhood, 7th ed. St. Louis, CV Mosby, 1995, pp 924–986.

CHAPTER 487
Liver Disease

Coagulation abnormalities are common in patients with severe liver disease and are estimated to be as high as 85%. Only 15% of patients, however, have significant clinical bleeding states. The severity of the coagulation abnormality appears to be directly proportional to the extent of hepatocellular damage. The most common mechanism causing the defect is decreased synthesis of the coagulation factors. Almost all the coagulation factors are produced exclusively in the liver except factor VIII. Severe liver disease characteristically has normal to increased (not reduced) levels of factor VIII activity in plasma. In some instances, disseminated intravascular coagulation (DIC) or hyperfibrinolysis may complicate liver diseases, making the differentiation of severe liver disease from DIC difficult.

The treatment of the coagulopathy of liver disease consists of replacement with fresh frozen plasma (FFP) or cryoprecipitate. FFP (10–15 mL/kg) contains all clotting factors, but replacement of fibrinogen may require cryoprecipitate. For severe hypofibrinogenemia, cryoprecipitate is recommended to replace fibrinogen at a dose of 4 to 5 bags/10 kg. Because a reduction in the vitamin K–dependent coagulation factors is common in those with acute and chronic liver disease, vitamin K therapy can be given as a trial. The vitamin K can be given orally, subcutaneously, or intravenously (not intramuscularly) in a dose of 1 mg/24 hr for infants, 2–3 mg for children, and 5–10 mg for adolescents and adults. An inability to correct the coagulopathy indicates that the coagulopathy may be caused by a reduction in one or more of the non–vitamin K dependent proteins or because the liver is severely impaired and cannot produce the precursor vitamin K proteins.

Frequently, severe liver disease is associated with moderate prolongation of the bleeding time that is not corrected by either vitamin K or plasma replacement. DDAVP (0.3 μg/kg IV) has been found to be effective in shortening the bleeding time and can be used prior to liver biopsy.

Andrew M, Montgomery RR: Acquired disorders of hemostasis. *In:* Nathan DG, Orkin SH (eds): Hematology of Infancy and Childhood, 5th ed. Philadelphia, WB Saunders, 1998, pp 1677–1717.

Hilgartner MW, Corrigan JJ Jr: Coagulation disorders. *In:* Miller DR, Baehner RL (eds): Blood Diseases of Infancy and Childhood, 7th ed. St. Louis, CV Mosby, 1995, pp 924–986.

CHAPTER 488
Acquired Inhibitors of Coagulation

Acquired circulating anticoagulants (inhibitors) are antibodies that react or cross react with clotting proteins, causing screening tests such as the PTT and PT to be prolonged. Many of these anticoagulants are autoantibodies that react with phospholipid and thereby interfere with clotting in vitro. These antibodies have been referred to as the lupus inhibitor. These circulating anticoagulants are uncommon in otherwise normal children. They are found in patients with systemic lupus erythematosus (SLE) or lymphomas or in those with penicillin or other drug reactions. Spontaneous inhibitors have been reported in children following incidental viral infections. Paradoxically, these lupus-like inhibitors are rarely associated with bleeding symptoms and the true lupus inhibitor is commonly associated with thrombosis. Occasionally, a patient with lupus will have a specific autoantibody against prothrombin (factor II). This antibody does not inactivate prothrombin but causes accelerated clearance of the factor II complex, resulting in a deficiency of prothrombin. These patients may bleed and require treatment.

Rarely, antibodies may spontaneously arise against a specific clotting factor, such as factor VIII or von Willebrand factor, similar to those seen more frequently in elderly patients. These patients are prone to excessive hemorrhage and may require specific treatment. In patients with hereditary deficiency of clotting factors (factor VIII or factor IX), antibodies may develop following exposure to transfused factor replacement concentrates. These hemophilic inhibitory antibodies are discussed in Chapter 482.

LABORATORY FINDINGS. Inhibitors against specific coagulation factors usually affect factors VIII, IX, and XI or, rarely prothrombin. The partial thromboplastin time (PTT) or the prothrombin time (PT) may be prolonged and is not corrected in vitro with the addition of normal plasma, unless the antibody is a non-inhibitory antibody that promotes rapid clearance of the protein. Specific factor assays determine which factor is involved.

The most common inhibitor is the "lupus inhibitor" that is found in patients with SLE, other collagen vascular diseases, or, most often, common viral infections, including HIV. It produces a prolonged PTT and, if severe, a prolonged PT. The addition of normal, platelet-poor plasma in a 1:1 ratio with the test plasma does not correct the abnormal tests, but the addition of platelets neutralizes the anticoagulant. More specific assays are available to identify the lupus inhibitor.

TREATMENT. Management of the patient with an inhibitor against a coagulation factor is the same as for the hemophilia patient who develops an alloantibody against factor VIII or IX. Infusions of a prothrombin complex concentrate, activated prothrombin complex concentrate (FEIBA or Autoplex), porcine factor VIII, or activated factor VII concentrate may be needed to control significant bleeding. Spontaneous inhibitors, usually following a viral infection, tend to disappear within a few weeks to months. Inhibitors seen with an underlying disease disappear when the primary disease is treated. The classic lupus inhibitor will often disappear following appropriate treatment of SLE. If thrombosis arises, this should be treated as any other thrombosis, although monitoring treatment with the PTT or PT is complicated by the lupus inhibitor and may require specific assays such as a heparin assay rather than the PTT or a factor X level rather than a PT. Maintenance of an INR of 3–4, higher than for other patients with deep venous thrombosis, is recommended when thrombosis occurs with lupus inhibitors.

Andrew M, Montgomery RR: Acquired disorders of hemostasis. *In:* Nathan DC, Orkin SH (eds): Hematology of Infancy and Childhood, 5th ed. Philadelphia, WB Saunders, 1998, pp 1677–1717.

Hilgartner MW, Corrigan JJ Jr: Coagulation disorders. *In:* Miller DR, Baehner RL (eds): Blood Diseases of Infancy and childhood, 7th ed. St. Louis, CV Mosby, 1995, pp 924–986.

CHAPTER 489
Disseminated Intravascular Coagulation (Consumptive Coagulopathy)

Consumption coagulopathy refers to a large group of conditions, including disseminated intravascular coagulation (DIC). Consequences of this process include widespread intravascular deposition of fibrin, which may lead to tissue ischemia and necrosis, a generalized hemorrhagic state, and hemolytic anemia.

ETIOLOGY. A number of pathologic life-threatening processes, including hypoxia, acidosis, tissue necrosis, shock, and endothelial damage, may incite episodes of DIC (Fig. 489–1). Accordingly, it is not surprising that a large number of conditions have been reported to be associated with DIC, including septic shock (especially meningococcemia), incompatible blood transfusions, rickettsial infections, snakebite, purpura fulminans, giant hemangioma, and malignancies, especially acute promyelocytic leukemia. While the clinical symptoms are primarily hemorrhagic, the initiating event is usually excessive activation of clotting, which consumes the physiologic anticoagulants (protein C, protein S, AT-III) and then consumes procoagulants, resulting in a deficiency of factor VIII, factor V, prothrombin, fibrinogen, and platelets. The end result of this sequence of events is usually hemorrhage.

CLINICAL MANIFESTATIONS. Most frequently, DIC accompanies a severe systemic disease process. Bleeding frequently first oc-

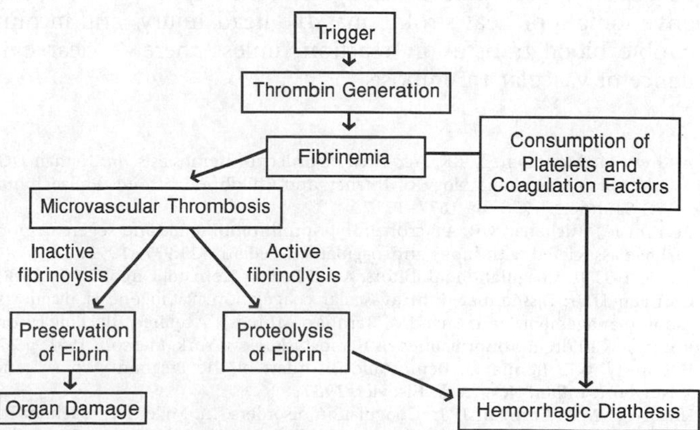

Figure 489–1 Disseminated intravascular coagulation.

curs from sites of venipuncture or surgical incision. The skin may show petechiae and ecchymoses. Tissue necrosis may involve many organs and can be most spectacularly seen as infarction of large areas of skin, subcutaneous tissue, or kidneys. Anemia caused by hemolysis may develop rapidly owing to microangiopathic hemolytic anemia.

LABORATORY FINDINGS. There is no well-defined sequence of events. The consumption coagulation factors (II, V, VIII, and fibrinogen) and platelets may be consumed by the ongoing intravascular clotting process, with prolongation of the prothrombin, partial thromboplastin, and thrombin times. Platelet counts may be profoundly depressed. The blood smear may contain fragmented, burr, and helmet-shaped red blood cells (schizocytes). In addition, because the fibrinolytic mechanism is activated, fibrinogin degradation products (FDPs) appear in the blood. The D-dimer assay is equally sensitive and more specific for DIC than the FDP test. The D-dimer is a formed by fibrinolysis of a cross-linked fibrin clot.

TREATMENT. The most important component of therapy is control or reversal of the process that initiated the DIC. Infection, shock, acidosis, and hypoxia must be treated promptly and vigorously. If the underlying problem can be controlled, bleeding quickly ceases, and there is improvement of the abnormal laboratory findings. Blood components are used for replacement therapy in patients who have hemorrhage. This may consist of platelet infusions (for thrombocytopenia), cryoprecipitate (for hypofibrinogenemia), and/or fresh frozen plasma (for replacement of other coagulation factors and natural inhibitors).

In some patients the treatment of the primary disease may be inadequate or incomplete, or the replacement therapy may not be effective in controlling the hemorrhage. When this occurs the DIC may be treated with heparin to prevent ongoing consumption of factors. Since administering heparin to patients with a deficiency of both clotting factors and platelets rnay result in profound hemorrhage, the heparin is usually started together with clotting factor and platelet replacement. Heparin is usually administered continuously starting with a low dose of 5–10 U/kg/hr. Since anticoagulants may be low because of consumption, treatment with AT-III concentrates may be helpful and will potentiate the antithrombotic effect of heparin. The duration and effectiveness of heparin therapy can be judged by serial measurements of the platelet count, fibrinogen level, and D-dimer assay. Early trials of a protein C concentrate in patients with DIC appear promising, especially for purpura fulminans.

Heparin has been found occasionally to be effective in children with DIC associated with purpura fulminans and promyelocytic leukemia. Administration of continuous heparin at a dose of 10–15 U/kg/hr without a loading dose is used for those with progranulocytic leukemia. Heparin is not indicated and has been reported to be ineffective in septic shock, snake envenomation, heat stroke, massive head injury, and incompatible blood transfusion reaction, unless there is clear evidence of vascular thrombosis.

Andrew M, Montgomery RR: Acquired disorders of hemostasis. *In:* Nathan DG, Orkin SH (eds): Hematology of Infancy and Childhood, 5th ed. Philadelphia, WB Saunders, 1998, pp 1677–1717.

Bernini JC, Buchanan GR, Ashcroft J: Hypoprothrombinemia and severe hemorrhage associated with lupus anticoagulant. J Pediatr 123:937, 1993.

Corrigan JJ Jr: Coagulation inhibitors. Am J Pediatr Hematol Oncol 2:281, 1980.

Corrigan JJ Jr: Disseminated intravascular coagulation: Pathogenesis, diagnosis, and management. *In:* Lusher JM, Barnhart MI (eds): Acquired Bleeding Disorders in Children: Abnormalities of Hemostasis. New York, Masson, 1981, p 27.

Hathaway WE, Bonnar J: Hemostatic Disorders of the Pregnant Woman and Newborn Infant. New York, Elsevier, 1987.

Hilgartner MW, Corrigan JJ Jr: Coagulation disorders. In: Miller DR, Baehner RL (eds): Blood Diseases of Infancy and Childhood, 7th ed. St. Louis, CV Mosby, 1995, pp 924–986.

CHAPTER 490
Disorders of the Platelets and the Blood Vessels

MEGAKARYOPOIESIS. Platelets are non-nucleated cellular fragments produced by megakaryocytes within the bone marrow and other tissues. Megakaryocytes are large polyploid cells. When the megakaryocyte approaches maturity, budding of the cytoplasm occurs and large numbers of platelets are liberated. Platelets circulate with a life span of 7 to 10 days. Thrombopoietin (TPO) is the major hormone that controls platelet production. Levels of TPO appear to correlate inversely with platelet number and with megakaryocyte mass. Thus, levels of TPO are highest in thrombocytopenic states associated with decreased marrow megakaryopoiesis and may be variable in states of increased platelet production.

The platelet plays multiple hemostatic roles. The platelet surface possesses a number of important receptors for adhesive proteins, including von Willebrand factor (vWf) and fibrinogen as well as receptors for agonists that trigger platelet aggregation, such as thrombin and collagen. Following injury to the blood vessel wall, subendothelial collagen binds vWf. Von Willebrand factor undergoes a conformational change that induces binding of the platelet glycoprotein Ib complex (the vWf receptor). This process is called platelet adhesion. Platelets then undergo activation. During the process of activation, the platelets generate thromboxane A_2 from arachidonic acid via the enzyme cyclooxygenase. After activation they release agonists such as ADP, ATP, Ca^{2+}, serotonin, and coagulation factors into the surrounding milieu. Circulating fibrinogen binds to its receptor on the activated platelets, the GPIIb-IIIa complex, linking platelets together in a process called aggregation. This series of events forms a hemostatic plug at the site of vascular injury. The serotonin and histamine liberated during activation increase local vasoconstriction. In addition to acting in concert with the vessel wall to form the platelet plug, the platelet provides the catalytic surface upon which coagulation factors assemble and eventually generate thrombin through a sequential series of enzymatic cleavages. Lastly, the platelet contractile apparatus mediates clot retraction.

THROMBOCYTOPENIA. The normal platelet count is 150 to 450 $\times$ 10^9/L. Thrombocytopenia refers to a reduction in platelet count below 150,000. Causes of thrombocytopenia include (1) decreased production on either a congenital or an acquired basis, (2) sequestration of the platelets within an enlarged spleen or other organ, and (3) increased destruction of normally synthesized platelets either on an immune or a nonimmune basis. Also see Chapters 474, 475, and 489.

490.1 Idiopathic Thrombocytopenic Purpura

The most common cause for acute onset of thrombocytopenia in an otherwise well child is (autoimmune) idiopathic thrombocytopenic purpura (ITP).

ETIOLOGY. One to four weeks following exposure to a common viral infection, a small number of children develop an autoantibody directed against the platelet surface. The exact antigenic target for most such antibodies in acute ITP remains undetermined. Following binding of the antibody to the platelet surface, circulating antibody-coated platelets are recognized by the Fc receptor on the splenic macrophages, ingested, and destroyed. A preceding history of a viral illness is described in about 50–65% of cases of childhood ITP. The reason why some children respond to a common infection with an autoimmune disease remains unknown. Virtually every common infectious virus has been described in association with ITP, including Epstein-Barr (EBV) and HIV. EBV-related ITP is usually of short duration and follows the course of infectious mononucleosis. HIV-associated ITP is usually chronic.

CLINICAL MANIFESTATIONS. The classic presentation of ITP is that of a perfectly healthy 1- to 4-yr-old child who has the sudden onset of generalized petechiae and purpura. The parents often state that the child was fine yesterday and now is covered with bruises and purple dots. Often there is bleeding from the gums and mucous membrane, particularly with profound thrombocytopenia (platelet count $<10 \times 10^9$/L). There is a history of a preceding viral infection 1 to 4 wk before onset of the thrombocytopenia. The physical examination is normal other than the finding of petechiae and purpura. Splenomegaly is rare. The presence of abnormal findings such as hepatosplenomegaly or remarkable lymphadenopathy suggests other diagnoses. When the onset is insidious, especially in an adolescent, the possibility of chronic ITP or that thrombocytopenia is a manifestation of a systemic illness (systemic lupus erythematosus [SLE]) is more likely.

Seventy to eighty percent of children who present with acute ITP will have spontaneous resolution of their ITP within 6 mo. Therapy does not appear to affect the natural history of the illness. Less than 1% of cases develop intracranial hemorrhage. Nevertheless, the objective of early therapy is to raise the platelet count to $>20 \times 10^9$/L and prevent the rare development of intracranial hemorrhage. About 10–20% of children who present with acute ITP go on to develop chronic ITP.

LABORATORY FINDINGS. Severe thrombocytopenia (platelet count $<20 \times 10^9$/L) is common, and platelet size is normal or increased, reflective of increased platelet turnover. In acute ITP, the hemoglobin, white count, and differential should be normal. The hemoglobin may be decreased if there have been profuse nosebleeds or menorrhagia. The bone marrow examination, when done, reveals normal granulocytic and erythrocytic series with characteristically normal or increased numbers of megakaryocytes. Some of the megakaryocytes may appear to be immature and are reflective of increased platelet turnover. Indications for a bone marrow aspiration include an abnormal WBC count or differential or unexplained anemia as well as findings suggestive of bone marrow disease on history and physical examination. Other laboratory tests should be done as indicated by history and physical examination. An antinuclear antibody (ANA) test is more often positive in adolescents with ITP and may indicate a higher likelihood of eventual chronic ITP. HIV studies should be done in at-risk populations, especially sexually active teens. Platelet antibody testing is seldom useful in acute ITP. A Coombs test should be done if there is unexplained anemia to rule out Evans syndrome (autoimmune hemolytic anemia and thrombocytopenia).

DIFFERENTIAL DIAGNOSIS. The well-appearing child with moderate to severe thrombocytopenia and otherwise normal CBC has a limited differential diagnosis that includes exposure to medication that induces drug-dependent antibodies, splenic sequestration due to previously unappreciated portal hypertension, and, rarely, early aplastic processes such as Fanconi anemia. Other than congenital syndromes such as amegakaryocytic thrombocytopenia and thrombocytopenia-absent radius syndrome, most marrow processes that interfere with platelet production will also cause abnormal synthesis of red blood cells and leukocytes and therefore will manifest abnormalities in the CBC. Disorders that cause increased platelet destruction on a nonimmune basis are usually serious systemic illnesses with obvious clinical findings (hemolytic-uremic syndrome, disseminated intravascular coagulation). Isolated enlargement of the spleen suggests the potential for hypersplenism due to either liver disease or portal vein thrombosis. Autoimmune thrombocytopenia may be an initial manifestation of SLE, HIV infection, or rarely, lymphoma. Wiskott-Aldrich syndrome must be considered in young males found to have low platelet counts, particularly if there is a history of eczema and recurrent infections.

TREATMENT. There are no data that treatment affects either short- or long-term clinical outcome of ITP. When compared with untreated controls, treatment appears to be capable of inducing a more rapid rise in platelet count to the theoretically safe level of 20×10^9/L. Initial treatment options include the following:

1. *Intravenous immunoglobulin* (IVIG) in a dose of 0.8 to 1 g/kg/day × 1–2 day induces a rapid rise in platelet count (usually $>20 \times 10^9$/L) in 95% of patients within 48 hr. IVIG therapy is both expensive and time-consuming to administer. Additionally, there is a high frequency of headaches and vomiting suggestive of aseptic meningitis following IVIG infusions.
2. *Prednisone.* Corticosteroid therapy has been used for many years to treat acute and chronic ITP in adults and children. Doses of 1–4 mg/kg/24 hr of prednisone appear to induce a more rapid rise in platelet counts than in untreated patients with ITP. It is often suggested that a bone marrow examination be performed to rule out other causes for thrombocytopenia, especially acute lymphoblastic leukemia, prior to institution of prednisone therapy in acute ITP. Corticosteroid therapy is usually continued for 2 to 3 wk or until a rise in platelet count above 20,000 has been achieved with a rapid taper to avoid the long-term side effects of corticosteroid therapy, especially growth failure, diabetes mellitus, and osteoporosis.
3. *IV Anti-D Therapy.* The role of IV anti-D in initial therapy of acute ITP is under investigation. When given to Rh-positive individuals, IV anti-D induces a mild hemolytic anemia. RBC-antibody complexes bind to Fc receptors and interfere with platelet destruction, thereby causing a rise in platelet count. This increase appears to be somewhat slower than after IVIG. Whether this is a biologically relevant delay remains unclear, as 80–85% of patients receiving anti-D in a dose of 50 μg/kg have demonstrated a rise in platelet count to levels above 20×10^9/L within 2 days. Each of these three medications may be used to treat exacerbations of ITP, which commonly occur several weeks after an initial course of therapy.

At the present time, there is no consensus regarding the management of acute ITP. Treatment guidelines have been published by the American Society of Hematology, but there is significant disagreement within the field. Intracranial hemorrhage remains rare, and there are no data that treatment actually reduces the incidence of intracranial hemorrhage in ITP because of the rarity of the event.

The role of splenectomy in ITP should be reserved for one of two circumstances. The older child (≥4 yr) with severe ITP that has lasted longer than 1 yr (chronic ITP) and whose symptoms are not easily controlled with therapy is a candidate for splenectomy. Splenectomy is associated with a lifelong risk of overwhelming postsplenectomy infection caused by encapsulated organisms. Splenectomy must also be considered when life-threatening hemorrhage (intracranial hemorrhage) complicates acute ITP if the platelet count cannot rapidly be corrected with transfusion of platelets and administration of IVIG and corticosteroids.

CHRONIC ITP. Those 10–20% of patients who present with acute ITP who have persistent thrombocytopenia for >6 mo have chronic ITP. At that time a careful re-evaluation for associated disorders should be performed, especially for autoimmune disease such as SLE and chronic infectious disorders such as HIV as well as nonimmune causes of chronic thrombocytopenia such as type 2B von Willebrand disease, X-linked thrombocytopenia, and Wiskott-Aldrich syndrome. Therapy should be aimed at controlling symptoms and preventing serious bleeding. In ITP the spleen is the primary site of antiplatelet antibody synthesis as well as the primary site of platelet destruction. Splenectomy is successful in inducing a complete remission in 64–88% of children with chronic ITP. This must be balanced against the lifelong risk of overwhelming postsplenectomy infection. This decision is often affected by lifestyle issues as well as the ease with which the child can be managed using medical therapy such as IVIG, corticosteroids, or IV anti-D. Prior to splenectomy the child should receive pneumococcal vaccine, and after splenectomy he or she should receive penicillin prophylaxis for some time.

490.2 Drug-Induced Thrombocytopenia

A number of drugs are associated with immune thrombocytopenia as the result of either an immune process or a megakaryocyte injury. Some common drugs used in pediatrics that cause thrombocytopenia include valproic acid, phenytoin, sulfonamides, and trimethoprim-sulfamethoxazole. Heparin-induced thrombocytopenia (and rarely thrombosis) is seldom seen in pediatrics but occurs when, after exposure to heparin, the patient develops an antibody directed against the heparin-platelet factor 4 complex.

490.3 Nonimmune Platelet Destruction

The syndromes of DIC, hemolytic-uremic syndrome, and thrombotic thrombocytopenic purpura share the hematologic picture of a *microangiopathic hemolytic anemia* in which there is red cell destruction evidenced by the presence of RBC fragments, including helmet cells, schistocytes, spherocytes, and burr cells, and a consumptive thrombocytopenia.

490.4 Hemolytic-Uremic Syndrome (HUS)

(See Chapter 526.)

This acute disease of infancy and early childhood usually follows an episode of acute gastroenteritis, often triggered by *E. coli* 0157H7. Shortly thereafter, signs and symptoms of hemolytic anemia, thrombocytopenia, and acute renal failure ensue. Sometimes neurologic symptoms are associated with these findings.

Hemolytic anemia is characterized by abnormal red cell morphology with the presence of helmet cells, spherocytes, schistocytes, burr cells, and other distorted forms. Thrombocytopenia despite normal numbers of megakaryocytes in the marrow indicates excessive platelet destruction. Tests for DIC are usually normal except for elevated fibrin(ogen) degradation products. Evaluation of the urine shows the presence of protein, red blood cells, and casts indicating renal damage. The presence of anuria and severe azotemia indicates grave renal damage. Treatment for most cases of hemolytic-uremic syndrome involves institution of careful fluid management and prompt appropriate dialysis. Treatment using plasmapheresis is usually reserved for patients with hemolytic-uremic syndrome associated with major neurologic complications.

490.5 Thrombotic Thrombocytopenic Purpura (TTP)

This rare pentad of fever, microangiopathic hemolytic anemia, thrombocytopenia, abnormal renal function, and CNS changes is clinically similar to hemolytic-uremic syndrome, though TTP usually presents in adults and occasionally in adolescents. Microvascular thrombi within the CNS cause subtle, shifting neurologic signs that vary from changes in affect and orientation to aphasia, blindness, and convulsions. Prompt recognition of this disorder is critical. Laboratory findings demonstrate a microangiopathic hemolytic anemia characterized by abnormal red cell morphology with schistocytes, spherocytes, helmet cells, and an elevated reticulocyte count in association with thrombocytopenia. Coagulation studies are usually nondiagnostic. The treatment of TTP is plasmapheresis, which is effective in 80–95% of cases. Corticosteroids and splenectomy are reserved for refractory cases. TTP appears to be caused by an acquired deficiency of a metalloproteinase enzyme responsible for cleaving the high molecular weight multimers of vWf, which appear to play a pivotal role in the evolution of the microangiopathy. The role of this enzyme in childhood HUS is uncertain, but a deficiency of the metalloproteinase may be causative in some rare familial cases of HUS or TTP.

490.6 Kasabach-Merritt Syndrome

(also see Chapter 656)

The association of a giant hemangioma with localized intravascular coagulation causing thrombocytopenia and hypofibrinogenemia is called the Kasabach-Merritt syndrome. In most patients the site of the hemangiomas is obvious, but retroperitoneal and intra-abdominal hemangiomas may require body imaging for detection. Inside the hemangioma there is platelet trapping and activation of coagulation with fibrinogen consumption and generation of fibrin(ogen) degradation products. Arteriovenous malformation within the lesions can cause heart failure. The pathology of these lesions is undergoing scrutiny, as some authors contend that Kasabach-Merritt syndrome is really a kaposiform hemangioendothelioma rather than a simple hemangioma. The peripheral blood smear shows microangiopathic changes. Multiple modalities have been used to treat Kasabach-Merritt syndrome, including surgical excision (if possible), local x-ray therapy, laser photocoagulation, corticosteroids in high doses, and antiangiogenic factors such as interferon $\alpha 2$. Over time most patients who present in infancy have regression of the hemangioma. Treatment of the associated coagulopathy may benefit from a trial of antifibrinolytic therapy with ϵ-aminocaproic acid (Amicar).

490.7 Sequestration

Individuals with massive splenomegaly develop thrombocytopenia, since the spleen acts as a sponge for platelets and sequesters large numbers. Most such patients will also have mild leukopenia and anemia on the CBC. Individuals who have thrombocytopenia caused by splenic sequestration should undergo a work-up to diagnose the etiology of splenomegaly, including infectious, infiltrative, neoplastic, obstructive, and hemolytic causes.

490.8 Congenital Thrombocytopenic Syndromes

Congenital amegakaryocytic thrombocytopenia is caused by a rare defect in hematopoiesis that usually manifests within the first few days to weeks of life, when the child presents with petechiae and purpura caused by profound thrombocytopenia.

Other than skin and mucous membrane findings, the physical examination is normal. Examination of the bone marrow shows an absence of megakaryocytes. These patients often progress to marrow failure (aplasia) over time. Bone marrow transplantation is curative.

Thrombocytopenia–absent radius (TAR) syndrome consists of thrombocytopenia that presents in early infancy and radial anomalies of variable severity from mild changes to marked limb shortening. In many such individuals there are also other skeletal abnormalities of the lower extremities. Intolerance to formula may complicate management by triggering gastrointestinal bleeding. The thrombocytopenia of TAR syndrome is puzzling, as it frequently remits over the first few years of life. The molecular basis for amegakaryocytic thrombocytopenia and TAR syndrome is undefined at present.

The *Wiskott-Aldrich syndrome (WAS)* is characterized by thrombocytopenia with tiny platelets, eczema, and recurrent infections due to immune deficiency (Chapter 126.11). WAS is inherited as an X-linked disorder, and the gene for WAS has been sequenced. The WAS protein may play an integral role in regulating the cytoskeletal architecture of both platelets and T lymphocytes in response to receptor-mediated cell signaling. The WAS protein is common to all cells of hematopoietic lineage. Molecular analysis of families with *X-linked thrombocytopenia* has shown that many have a point mutation within the WAS gene, whereas individuals with the full manifestation of WAS have large gene deletions. Examination of the bone marrow in WAS shows normal number of megakaryocytes, although the megakaryocytes may have bizarre morphology. Transfused platelets have a normal life span. Splenectomy often corrects the thrombocytopenia, suggesting that the platelets formed in WAS have accelerated destruction. After splenectomy, these patients are at increased risk of overwhelming infection and require lifelong antibiotic prophylaxis against encapsulated organisms. About 5% of WAS patients develop lymphoreticular malignancies. Successful bone marrow transplantation cures WAS.

490.9 Neonatal Thrombocytopenia

(See Chapter 99.4)

Thrombocytopenia in the newborn rarely is indicative of a primary disorder of megakaryopoiesis but more often is the result of either systemic illness or transfer of maternal antibodies directed against fetal platelets.

Thrombocytopenia may occur in various fetal and neonatal infections and be responsible for severe spontaneous bleeding. Neonatal thrombocytopenia often occurs in association with congenital viral infections, especially rubella and CMV; protozoal infections such as toxoplasmosis; syphilis; and bacterial infections, especially those caused by gram-negative bacilli. The constellation of marked thrombocytopenia and abnormal abdominal findings is common in necrotizing enterocolitis and other causes of necrotic bowel. The presence of thrombocytopenia in an ill child requires a prompt search for viral and bacterial pathogens.

Antibody-mediated thrombocytopenia in the newborn occurs because of transplacental transfer of maternal antibodies directed against fetal platelets.

Neonatal alloimmune thrombocytopenic purpura (NATP) is caused by the development of maternal antibodies against antigens present on fetal platelets that are shared with the father and recognized as foreign by the maternal immune system. This is the platelet equivalent of Rh disease of the newborn (Chapter 99.2). The incidence of NATP is 1 in 4,000–5,000 live births. The clinical picture in NATP is that of an apparently well child who, within the first few days after delivery, develops generalized petechiae and purpura. Laboratory studies show a normal maternal platelet count, yet moderate to severe thrombocytopenia in the newborn. Detailed historical review should show no evidence of maternal thrombocytopenia in the past. Up to 30% of infants with severe NATP may develop intracranial hemorrhage, either prenatally or in the perinatal period. Unlike Rh disease, first pregnancies may develop severe thrombocytopenia, and subsequent pregnancies may be more severely affected than the first pregnancy.

The diagnosis of NATP is made by checking for the presence of maternal alloantibodies directed against the father's platelets. Specific studies can be done to identify the target alloantigen. The most common cause is incompatibility for $P1^{A1}$. Specific DNA sequence polymorphisms have been identified that permit informative prenatal testing to identify at-risk pregnancies. The differential diagnosis of NATP includes transplacental transfer of maternal antiplatelet autoantibodies (maternal ITP) and, more commonly, viral or bacterial infection.

Therapy of NATP is the administration of intravenous immunoglobulin (IVIG) prenatally to the mother. Treatment usually begins in the second trimester and is continued throughout the pregnancy. Fetal platelet counts can be monitored by percutaneous umbilical blood sampling (PUBS). Delivery should be performed by cesarean section. Following delivery, if severe thrombocytopenia persists, transfusion of one unit of phenotypically matched platelets (washed maternal platelets) will cause a rise in platelet counts to provide effective hemostasis. After there has been one affected child, genetic counseling is critical to inform the parents of the high risk of thrombocytopenia in subsequent pregnancies.

Children born to mothers with ITP (maternal ITP) appear to have a lower risk of serious hemorrhage, although severe thrombocytopenia occurs. The mother's pre-existing platelet count may have some predictive value, in that severe maternal thrombocytopenia prior to delivery appears to predict a higher risk of fetal thrombocytopenia. Nevertheless, in mothers who have had splenectomy for ITP, the maternal platelet count may be normal and is not predictive of fetal thrombocytopenia.

Treatment may include prenatal administration of corticosteroids to the mother and, post delivery, administration of IVIG and sometimes corticosteroids to the infant. The thrombocytopenia in an infant, whether due to NATP or maternal ITP, usually resolves within 2 to 4 mo following delivery. The highest risk period remains in the immediate perinatal period.

490.10 Thrombocytopenia Due to Acquired Decreased Production

Disorders of the bone marrow that inhibit megakaryopoiesis usually affect red cell and white cell production. Infiltrative disorders, including malignancies such as ALL, histiocytosis, lymphomas, and storage disease, usually cause either abnormalities on physical examination (lymphadenopathy, hepatosplenomegaly, masses) or abnormalities of the white cell count, or anemia. Aplastic processes may present with isolated thrombocytopenia, although there are usually clues on the CBC (leukopenia, neutropenia, anemia or macrocytosis). Children with constitutional aplastic anemia (Fanconi anemia) often have abnormalities on examination, including radial anomalies, other skeletal anomalies, short stature, microcephaly, and hyperpigmentation. A bone marrow examination should be done when thrombocytopenia is associated with abnormalities found on physical examination or on examination of the other blood cell lines.

490.11 Platelet Function Disorders

In the clinical laboratory, abnormal platelet function is screened using the bleeding time, which measures indirectly the platelet count, platelet function, and interaction of platelets with the blood vessel wall. Unfortunately, the bleeding time is dependent upon a number of other factors, including the skill of the technician and the cooperation of the patient. Therefore, its predictive value is often problematic. A normal bleeding time does not rule out a mild platelet function defect in a clinically symptomatic individual. Platelet function in the clinical laboratory is currently measured using platelet aggregometry. In the aggregometer, agonists such as collagen, ADP, ristocetin, arachidonic acid, and thrombin are added to platelet-rich plasma, and the clumping of platelets over time is measured by an automated machine. At the same time, modern instruments measure the release of granular contents such as ATP from the platelets following activation. In this manner, the ability of platelets to aggregate and their metabolic activity can be assessed simultaneously.

490.12 Acquired Disorders of Platelet Function

A number of systemic illnesses are associated with platelet dysfunction, most commonly liver disease, kidney disease (uremia), and those disorders that trigger increased amounts of fibrin degradation products. These disorders frequently cause a prolonged bleeding time and are often associated with other abnormalities of the coagulation mechanism. The most important element of treatment is to treat the primary illness. If treatment of the primary process is not feasible, infusions of DDAVP have been helpful in augmenting hemostasis and correcting the bleeding time. In some patients, transfusions of platelets and/or cryoprecipitate have also been helpful in improving hemostasis.

Many drugs alter platelet function. The most commonly used drug that alters platelet function in adults is acetylsalicylic acid (aspirin). Aspirin irreversibly acetylates the enzyme cyclooxygenase, which is critical in the formation of thromboxane A_2. Aspirin usually causes moderate platelet dysfunction, which becomes more prominent if there is some other abnormality of the hemostatic mechanism. Other commonly used drugs that affect platelet function include other nonsteroidal anti-inflammatory drugs, valproic acid, and high-dose penicillin. Therefore, when evaluating a patient for a possible platelet dysfunction, it is critically important to exclude the presence of other exogenous agents and to study the patient, if possible, off all medications for 2 wk.

490.13 Congenital Abnormalities of Platelet Function

Severe platelet function defects usually present with petechiae and purpura shortly after birth, especially after vaginal delivery. Defects in the receptor for vWf, the GPIb complex, or fibrinogen, GPIIb-IIIa, cause severe congenital platelet dysfunction.

Bernard-Soulier syndrome, a congenital bleeding disorder, is characterized by thrombocytopenia with giant platelets and a markedly prolonged bleeding time. Platelet aggregation tests show absent ristocetin-induced platelet aggregation but normal aggregation to all other agonists. von Willebrand factor studies are normal. Ristocetin induces the binding of vWf to platelets. The cause for this severe platelet dysfunction is the absence or severe deficiency of the vWf receptor (GPIb complex) on the platelet membrane. This complex interacts with the platelet cytoskeleton; the defect in this interaction is thought to be the cause for the large platelet size.

Glanzmann thrombasthenia is a congenital disorder associated with severe platelet dysfunction that yields a prolonged bleeding time and a normal platelet count. The platelet morphology and size are normal on the peripheral blood smear. The mean platelet volume bleeding time is markedly prolonged. Aggregation studies show abnormality of aggregation with all agonists used except ristocetin, because ristocetin agglutinates platelets and does not require a metabolically active platelet. This disorder is caused by deficiency of the platelet fibrinogen receptor, GPIIb/IIIa, an integrin complex on the platelet surface that undergoes conformational changes when platelets are activated. Fibrinogen binds this complex and causes platelets to aggregate. This disorder is inherited in an autosomal recessive manner.

Hereditary deficiency of platelet storage granules occurs in two well-characterized but rare syndromes that involve deficiency of intracytoplasmic granules. **Dense body deficiency** is characterized by the absence of the granules that contain ADP, ATP, Ca^{2+}, and serotonin. This disorder is diagnosed by absent release of ATP on platelet aggregation studies and ideally characterized by electron microscopic (EM) studies. **Gray platelet syndrome** is caused by the absence of platelet α granules resulting in platelets that appear gray on Wright stain of peripheral blood. This rare syndrome has absent aggregation and release with most agonists other than thrombin and ristocetin. EM studies are diagnostic.

OTHER HEREDITARY DISORDERS OF PLATELET FUNCTION. Abnormalities in the pathways of platelet activation and release of granular contents cause a heterogeneous group of platelet function defects that are usually manifested as increased bruising, epistaxis, and/or menorrhagia. Symptoms may be subtle and are often made more obvious by high-risk surgery, such as tonsillectomy/adenoidectomy, or by administration of nonsteroidal anti-inflammatory drugs. In the laboratory, the bleeding time is variable, although it is frequently but not always prolonged. Platelet aggregation studies show deficient aggregation with one or two agonists and/or abnormal release of granular contents.

Formation of thromboxane from arachidonic acid after activation of phospholipase is critical to normal platelet function. Deficiency or dysfunction of enzymes such as cyclooxygenase and thromboxane synthase, which metabolize arachidonic acid, causes abnormal platelet function. In the aggregometer, platelets from such patients fail to aggregate in response to arachidonic acid.

The most common platelet function defects may be those characterized by a variable bleeding time and abnormal aggregation with one or two agonists, including collagen and ADP. These patients have normal aggregation with thrombin. Some of these individuals have only decreased release of ATP from intracytoplasmic granules. This selective release defect is a common cause of a mild platelet function defect.

The treatment of platelet function defects depends on the severity of the diagnosis and of the hemorrhagic event. In all but the severe platelet function defects, DDAVP 0.3 μg/kg IV in 50 cc saline may be used for mild to moderate bleeding episodes. In addition to its effect on stimulating levels of vWF and factor VIII, DDAVP corrects the bleeding time and provides normal hemostasis in many individuals with mild to moderate platelet function defects. For individuals with Bernard-Soulier syndrome or Glanzmann thrombasthenia, platelet transfusions, 1 unit/5–10 kg body weight, will correct the defect in hemostasis and may be life-saving.

490.14 Disorders of the Blood Vessels

HENOCH-SCHÖNLEIN PURPURA (HSP). This syndrome is characterized by the sudden development of a purpuric skin rash, arthritis, abdominal pain, and renal involvement (see Chapter 167.1). The characteristic skin rash, consisting of petechiae and often palpable purpura, usually involves the lower extremities and buttocks. Coagulation studies are normal. The pathologic lesions in the skin, intestines, and synovium are a leukocytoclastic angiitis—inflammatory damage to the endothelium of the capillary and postcapillary venules mediated by white cells and macrophages. The trigger for HSP is unknown. In the kidney the lesion is focal glomerulonephritis with deposition of IgA.

EHLERS-DANLOS SYNDROME. This disorder of collagen structure causes easy bruising and poor wound healing (see Chapter 665). Suggestive findings on physical examination include soft, velvety skin that is hyperelastic and lax joints that are easily subluxed. More than 10 variants of Ehlers-Danlos syndrome have been described. The most serious forms have been associated with sudden rupture of visceral organs. Coagulation screening tests are usually normal, other than the bleeding time, which may be mildly prolonged. Platelet aggregation studies are either normal or mildly abnormal with deficient aggregation to collagen.

ACQUIRED DISORDERS. Scurvy, chronic corticosteroid therapy, and severe malnutrition are associated with "weakening" of the collagen matrix that supports the blood vessels and therefore are associated with easy bruising and, particularly in the case of scurvy, bleeding gums and loosening of the teeth. Lesions of the skin that initially look like petechiae and purpura may be seen in vasculitic syndromes such as SLE.

Athreya B: Vasculitis in children. Pediatr Clin North Am 42:1239, 1995.

Beardsley DS, Nathan DG: Platelet abnormalities in infancy and childhood. *In:* Nathan DG, Orkin SH (eds): Hematology of Infancy and Childhood, 5th ed. Philadelphia, WB Saunders, 1998, pp 1585–1630.

Beighton P, De Paepe A, Steinmann B, et al: Ehlers-Danlos syndromes: Revised nosology, Am J Med Genet 77:31, 1998.

Blanchette V, Imbach P, Andrew M, et al: Randomised trial of intravenous immunoglobulin G, intravenous anti-D, and oral prednisone in childhood acute immune thrombocytopenic purpura. Lancet 344:703, 1994.

Brickell PM, Katz DR, Thrasher AJ: Wiskott-Aldrich syndrome: Current research concepts. Br J Haematol 101:603, 1998.

Bussel JB, Corrigan JJ Jr: Platelet and vascular disorders. *In:* Miller DR, Baehner RL (eds): Blood Diseases of Infancy and Childhood, 7th ed. St. Louis, CV Mosby, 1995, pp 866–923.

Bussel JB, Berkowitz RL, Lynch L, et al: Antenatal management of alloimmune thrombocytopenia with intravenous gamma-globulin: A randomized trial of the addition of low-dose steroid to intravenous gamma-globulin. Am J Obstet Gynecol 174:1414, 1996.

Bussel JB, Zabusky MR, Berkowitz RL, et al: Fetal alloimmune thrombocytopenia. N Engl J Med 337:22, 1997.

Dubansky AS, Boyett JM, Faletta J, et al: Isolated thrombocytopenia in children with acute lymphoblastic leukemia: A rare event in a pediatric oncology group study. Pediatrics 84:1068, 1989.

George JN, Woolf SH, Raskob GE, et al: Idiopathic thrombocytopenic purpura: A practice guideline developed by explicit methods for The American Society of Hematology. Blood 88:3, 1996.

Lilleyman JS: Intracranial haemorrhage in idiopathic thrombocytopenic purpura. Arch Dis Child 71:251, 1994.

Sarkar M, Mulliken JB, Kozakewich HP, et al: Thrombocytopenic coagulopathy (Kasabach-Merritt phenomenon) is associated with kaposiform hemangioendothelioma and not with common infantile hemangioma. Plast Reconstr Surg 100:1377, 1997.

Sullivan KA, et al: A multiinstitutional survey of the Wiskott-Aldrich syndrome. J Pediatr 125:876, 1994.

Sutor AH: Thrombocytosis in childhood. Semin Thrombos Hemost 21:330, 1995.

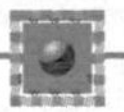

SECTION 8

The Spleen

James French ■ Bruce M. Camitta

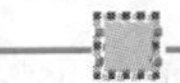

CHAPTER 491

Anatomy and Function of the Spleen

ANATOMY. The splenic precursor is recognizable by 5 wk of gestation. At birth, the spleen weighs approximately 11 g. Thereafter, it enlarges until puberty, reaching an average weight of 135 g before diminishing in size during adulthood. The major splenic components are a lymphoid compartment (white pulp) and a filtering system (red pulp). The white pulp consists of periarterial lymphatic sheaths of T cells with embedded germinal centers containing B cells. The red pulp has a skeleton of fixed reticular cells, mobile macrophages, partially collapsed endothelial passages (cords of Billroth), and splenic sinuses. A marginal zone rich in dendritic (antigen-presenting) cells separates the red pulp from the white. The splenic capsule contains smooth muscle and contracts in response to epinephrine. Approximately 10% of the blood delivered to the spleen flows rapidly through a closed vascular network. The other 90% flows more slowly through an open system (the splenic cords) where it is filtered through 1–5-μm slits before entering the splenic sinuses.

FUNCTION. Unique anatomy and blood flow enable the spleen to perform reservoir, filtering, and immunologic functions more effectively. The spleen receives 5–6% of the cardiac output but normally contains only 25 mL of blood. It can retain much more when it enlarges. Hematopoiesis is a major splenic function from 3–6 mo of fetal life. Splenic blood formation can be resumed in patients with myelofibrosis or severe hemolytic anemia. Factor VIII and platelets are stored in the spleen and can be released by stress or an epinephrine injection.

The spleen removes excess membrane from young red blood cells (RBCs), and loss of this function is characterized by target cells, poikilocytosis, and decreased osmotic fragility. It is also the primary site for destruction of old RBCs; this function is assumed by other reticuloendothelial cells after splenectomy. The spleen also removes damaged and abnormal RBCs. Spherocytes and antibody-coated RBCs and platelets are detained in the marginal zone and red pulp, where they are then phagocytosed or lysed. In addition, the spleen removes intracytoplasmic inclusions from RBCs without cell lysis. Functional or anatomic hyposplenia is characterized by continued circulation of cells containing these nuclear remnants (Howell-Jolly bodies) and other debris in the RBC. The latter may appear as "pits" on indirect microscopy.

Immunoglobulin, properdin, and tuftsin are produced in the spleen. The spleen has a minor role in antibody responses to intramuscularly or subcutaneously injected antigens but is required for early antibody production after exposure to intravenous antigens. Thus, young (nonimmune) or hyposplenic individuals are at increased risk for sepsis caused by pneumococci and other encapsulated bacteria. The spleen can also use phagocytosis to trap and destroy bacteria or parasitized RBCs.

Shurin SB: Disorders of the spleen. *In:* Handin RI, Lux SE, Stossel TP(eds): Blood: Principles and Practice of Hematology. Philadelphia, JB Lippincott, 1995, p 1359.

CHAPTER 492
Splenomegaly

CLINICAL MANIFESTATIONS. A soft, thin spleen may be palpable in 15% of neonates, 10% of normal children, and 5% of adolescents. However, in most individuals, the spleen must be two to three times its normal size before it is palpable. The spleen is best examined in a supine patient by palpating across the abdomen toward the left costal margin from below as the patient inspires deeply. One should remember that an enlarged spleen may descend into the pelvis; thus, when splenomegaly is suspected, the abdominal examination should begin at a lower starting point. Superficial abdominal venous distention may be present when splenomegaly is a result of portal hypertension. Radiologic detection or confirmation of splenic enlargement is done with ultrasonography, CT, or a technetium-99m sulfur colloid scan. The latter also assesses splenic function.

DIFFERENTIAL DIAGNOSIS. Specific causes of splenomegaly are listed in Table 492–1. Unique problems are discussed next.

TABLE 492–1 Common Causes of Splenomegaly

Infection	
Bacterial:	Typhoid fever, endocarditis, septicemia, abscess
Viral:	Epstein-Barr, cytomegalovirus, and others
Protozoal:	Malaria, toxoplasmosis
Hematologic Processes	
Hemolytic anemia:	Congenital, acquired
Extramedullary hematopoiesis:	Thalassemia, osteopetrosis, myelofibrosis
Neoplasms	
Malignant:	Leukemia, lymphoma, metastatic disease
Benign:	Hemangioma, hamartoma
Infiltration and Storage Diseases	
Lipidoses:	Niemann-Pick, Gaucher diseases
Mucopolysaccharidosis infiltration:	Histiocytosis
Congestion	
Cirrhosis or hepatic fibrosis	
Hepatic portal or splenic vein obstruction	
Congestive heart failure	
Cysts	
Congenital (true cysts)	
Acquired (pseudocysts)	
Miscellaneous	
Lupus erythematosus, sarcoidosis, rheumatoid arthritis	

PSEUDOSPLENOMEGALY. Abnormally elongated mesenteric connections may produce a wandering or proptotic spleen. An enlarged left lobe of the liver, a left upper quadrant mass, or a splenic hematoma may be mistaken for splenomegaly. Splenic cysts may contribute to splenomegaly or mimic it; these may be congenital (epidermoid) or acquired (pseudocyst) after trauma or infarction. Cysts are usually asymptomatic and are found on radiologic evaluation. Splenosis after splenic rupture or an accessory spleen (present in 10% of normal individuals) may also mimic splenomegaly. Most, however, are not palpable. The syndrome of *congenital polysplenism* includes cardiac defects, left-sided organ anomalies, bilobed lungs, biliary atresia, and pseudosplenomegaly (see Chapter 438.4)

HYPERSPLENISM. Hypersplenism is characterized by increased splenic function (sequestration or destruction of circulating cells), which results in peripheral blood cytopenias, increased bone marrow activity, and splenomegaly. It is usually secondary to another disease and may be cured by treatment of the underlying condition or, if absolutely necessary, by splenectomy.

CONGESTIVE SPLENOMEGALY (BANTI'S SYNDROME). Splenomegaly may result from obstruction in the hepatic, portal, or splenic veins. Wilson disease, galactosemia, biliary atresia, and α-antitrypsin deficiency result in hepatic inflammation, fibrosis, and vascular obstruction. Congenital abnormalities of the portal or splenic veins may cause vascular obstruction. Septic omphalitis or umbilical venous catheterization in neonates may also result in secondary obliteration of these vessels. Splenic venous flow may be obstructed by masses of sickled erythrocytes. When the spleen is the site of vascular obstruction, splenectomy cures hypersplenism. However, the obstruction usually is in the hepatic or portal systems, and portocaval shunting may be more helpful, because both portal hypertension and thrombocytopenia contribute to variceal bleeding.

CHAPTER 493
Hyposplenism, Splenic Trauma, Splenectomy

Congenital absence of the spleen is associated with complex cyanotic heart defects, dextrocardia, bilateral trilobed lungs, and heterotopic abdominal organs (Ivemark syndrome; see Chapter 438.11). *Functional hyposplenism* may occur in normal neonates, especially premature infants. Children with sickle cell hemoglobinopathies may develop splenic hypofunction as early as 6 mo of age. Initially, this is due to vascular obstruction that can be reversed with red blood cell (RBC) transfusions. The spleen eventually autoinfarcts, resulting in a fibrotic, permanently nonfunctioning spleen. Functional hyposplenism may also occur in malaria, after irradiation to the left upper quadrant, and when the reticuloendothelial function of the spleen is overwhelmed (as in severe hemolytic anemias or metabolic storage diseases). Splenic hypofunction is characterized by RBC inclusions in peripheral blood smears, "pits" on interference microscopy, and poor uptake of technetium on spleen scan. Patients with functional hyposplenism or asplenia are at increased risk of sepsis from encapsulated organisms.

TRAUMA. Injury to the spleen may occur with left flank or abdominal trauma. Small splenic capsular tears may cause abdominal or referred left shoulder pain as a result of peritoneal irritation by blood. Larger tears result in more severe blood loss with similar pain and signs of hypovolemia. Previously enlarged spleens (as in infectious mononucleosis) are more likely to rupture with minor trauma.

Treatment of a small capsular injury should include careful observation with attention to changes in vital signs or abdominal findings, serial hemoglobin determinations, and the availability of prompt surgical intervention should a patient's condition deteriorate. RBC transfusion requirements should be minimal (<25 mL/kg/48 hr). These patients are usually hospitalized 10–14 days and have their activities restricted for months. A laparotomy with or without splenectomy is indicated for more marked abdominal bleeding, for clinical instability or deterioration, or when other organ damage is suspected. Partial splenectomy and splenic repairs should be substituted for total splenectomy when feasible.

SPLENECTOMY. Because of the risk of postoperative sepsis, splenectomy (open or laparoscopic) should be limited to specific indications. These include splenic rupture, anatomic defects, severe hemolytic anemias, immune cytopenias, metabolic storage diseases, secondary hypersplenism, and (rarely) surgical indications, including exposure of the left upper quadrant. The major long term risk of splenectomy is sudden overwhelming infection (sepsis or meningitis). This risk is especially high in children younger than 5 yr at the time of surgery. The risk of sepsis is slightly less following splenectomies performed for trauma, RBC membrane defects, and immune thrombocytopenia (2–4%) than when there is pre-existing immune deficiency (Wiskott-Aldrich syndrome, Hodgkin disease) or reticuloendothelial blockade (storage diseases, severe hemolytic anemias) (8–30%).

Encapsulated bacteria such as *Streptococcus pneumoniae* (>60% of cases), *Haemophilus influenzae,* and *Neisseria meningitides* are the most common organisms associated with postsplenectomy sepsis. Streptococci and staphylococci are encountered less frequently. Because the spleen is responsible for filtering the blood and early antibody responses, sepsis (with or without meningitis) can progress rapidly, leading to death within 12–24 hr of onset. Febrile splenectomized patients should be treated promptly with antibiotics. A broad-spectrum cephalosporin (cefotaxime: 50 mg/kg q 8 hr) or vancomycin (10 mg/kg q 6 hr) to cover penicillin-resistant pneumococci is recommended until specific antibiotic susceptibility is known. Splenectomized patients are also at increased risk for contracting protozoal infections such as malaria and babesiosis.

Preoperative, intraoperative, and postoperative management may decrease the risk of postsplenectomy infection. It is important to be certain of the need for splenectomy and, if possible, to postpone the operation until the patient is 5 yr of age or older. Vaccination with pneumococcal, *H. influenzae,* and meningococcal vaccines before splenectomy may be helpful to reduce postsplenectomy sepsis. However, vaccine efficacy is lower in children younger than 2 yr. In trauma cases, splenic repair or partial splenectomy should be considered in an attempt to preserve splenic function. Partial splenectomy or partial splenic embolization may also be sufficient to ameliorate some forms of hemolytic anemia. Surgical splenosis (distributing small pieces of spleen throughout the abdomen) has been suggested as a way to decrease the risk of sepsis in patients whose splenectomy is necessitated by trauma. However, the splenic tissue that regrows frequently has inadequate function. Prophylaxis with oral penicillin V (125 mg twice daily for children <5 yr; 250 mg twice daily for children ≥ 5 yr) should be given for at least 2 yr after splenectomy (to at least 6 yr of age). Prophylaxis may be continued into adulthood for high-risk patients. Penicillin reduces the risk of pneumococcal sepsis in patients with hemoglobin SS, but other populations have not been well studied. Although the greatest risk is in the immediate postoperative period, reports of deaths occurring many years after splenectomy suggest that the risk (and need for prophylaxis) may be lifelong. Other postoperative measures include patient and family education, wearing a medical information bracelet, and prompt evaluation and treatment of fevers.

Cesko I, Hajdu J, Toth T, et al: Ivemark syndrome with asplenia in siblings. J Pediatr 130:822, 1997.

Deodhar HA, Marshall RS: Increased risk of sepsis after splenectomy. Br Med J 307:1408, 1993.

Eraklis AJ, Filler RM: Splenectomy in childhood: A review of 1413 cases. J Pediatr Surg 7:382, 1972.

Farah RA, Rogers ZR, Thompson WR, et al: Comparison of laparoscopic and open splenectomy in children with hematologic disorders. J Pediatr 131:41, 1997.

Gorse DJ: The relationship of the spleen to infection. *In:* Bowlder AJ (ed): The spleen: Structure, Function and Clinical Significance. New York, von Nostrand Reinhold, 1990, p 269.

Hayes TC, Britton HA, Mewborne EB, et al: Symptomatic splenic hamartoma: Case report and literature review. Pediatrics 101(5):E10, 1998.

Israel DM, Hassal E: Partial splenic embolization in children with hypersplenism. J Pediatr 124:95, 1993.

Shapiro ED, Berg AT. The protective efficacy of polyvalent pneumococcal polysaccharide vaccine. N Engl J Med 325:1453, 1991.

Sherman R: Perspective in management of trauma to the spleen. J Trauma 20:1, 1980.

Tchernia G, Gauthier F: Initial assessment of the beneficial effect of partial splenectomy in hereditary spherocytosis. Blood 81:2014, 1993.

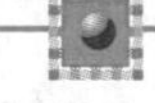

SECTION 9

The Lymphatic System

Alice Rock ■ Bruce M. Camitta

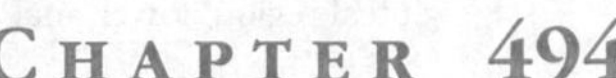

CHAPTER 494

Anatomy and Functions of the Lymphatic System

The lymphatic system includes circulating lymphocytes, lymphatic vessels, lymph nodes, spleen, tonsils, adenoids, Peyer patches, and thymus. Lymph, an ultrafiltrate of blood, is collected by lymphatic capillaries that are present in all organs except the brain and the heart. These join to form progressively larger vessels that drain regions of the body. During their course, the lymphatic vessels carry lymph to the lymph nodes. In the nodes, lymph is filtered through sinuses where particulate matter and infectious organisms are phagocytosed, processed, and presented as antigens to surrounding lymphocytes. This results in stimulation of antibody production, T-cell responses, and cytokine secretion (Chapter 123).

Lymph composition can vary with the site of lymph drainage. It is usually clear, but drainage of lymph from the intestinal tract may be milky (chylous) because of the presence of fats. The protein content is intermediate between an exudate and transudate. The protein level may be increased with inflammation or in lymph from the liver or intestines. Lymph also contains variable numbers of lymphocytes.

CHAPTER 495
Abnormalities of Lymphatic Vessels

Abnormalities of the lymph vessels may be congenital or acquired. Signs and symptoms may result from increased lymphatic tissue mass or from leakage of lymph. *Lymphangiectasia* is a dilation of the lymphatics. Pulmonary lymphangiectasia causes respiratory distress (Chapter 384.8). Involvement of the intestinal lymphatics causes hypoproteinemia and lymphocytopenia secondary to loss of lymph into the intestines (Chapter 340.10). *Lymphangioma* (cystic hygroma) is a mass of dilated lymphatics. Some of these lesions also have a hemangiomatous component (see Chapter 514.2). *Lymphatic dysplasia* may cause multisystem problems. These include lymphedema, chylous ascites, chylothorax, and lymphangiomas of bone, lung, or other locations. *Lymphedema* is caused by obstruction of lymph flow. Congenital lymphedema may be found in Turner syndrome, Noonan syndrome, and the autosomal dominantly inherited Milroy disease. Lymphedema praecox causes progressive lower extremity edema, usually in females 10–25 yr old. Lymphedema has also been found in association with intestinal lymphangiectasia, cerebrovascular malformation, ptosis, yellow dystrophic nails, distichiasis, and cholestasis. Acquired obstruction of the lymphatics can result from tumor, postirradiation fibrosis, filariasis, and postinflammatory scarring. Injury to the major lymphatic vessels can cause collection of lymph fluid in the abdomen (chylous ascites) and chest (chylothorax). *Lymphangitis* is an inflammation of the lymphatics draining an area of infection. On examination, tender red streaks extend proximally from the infected site. Regional nodes may also be enlarged and tender. *Staphylococcus aureus* and group A streptococci are the most frequent pathogens.

Halliard RI, McKenobey JBJ, Phillips MJ: Congenital abnormalities of the lymphatic system. A new clinical classification. Pediatrics 86:988, 1990.

CHAPTER 496
Lymphadenopathy

Most lymph nodes are not palpable in a newborn infant. With varied antigenic exposure, lymphoid tissue increases in volume so that cervical, axillary, and inguinal nodes are often palpable during childhood. They are not considered enlarged until their diameter exceeds 1 cm for cervical or axillary nodes and 1.5 cm for inguinal nodes. Other lymph nodes usually are not palpable or visualized with usual radiologic procedures.

Lymph node enlargement is due to proliferation of normal lymphoid elements or to infiltration by malignant or phagocytic cells. In most patients, a careful history and a complete physical examination suggest the proper diagnosis (Table 496–1). Nonlymphoid masses (cervical rib, thyroglossal cyst, branchial sinus or cyst, cystic hygroma, goiter, sternomastoid muscle tumor, neurofibroma) occur frequently in the neck, less often in other areas. Acutely infected nodes are usually tender. Erythema and warmth of the overlying skin, may also be noted. Fluctuance suggests abscess formation. Tuberculous nodes may be matted. With chronic infection, most of these signs are not present. Tumor-bearing nodes are usually firm and nontender and may be matted or fixed to the skin or underlying structures.

Generalized adenopathy (enlargement of more than two noncontiguous node regions) is due to systemic disease (Table 496–2) and is often accompanied by abnormal physical findings in other systems. In contrast, localized adenopathy is most frequently due to infection in the involved node or its drainage area (Tables 496–3 and 496–4). Regional lymphadenitis as a result of infectious agents other than bacteria may be characterized by atypical anatomic locations, a prolonged course, a draining sinus, lack of prior pyogenic infection, and unusual clues in the history (cat scratches, tuberculosis exposure, vene-

TABLE 496–1 Evaluation of Possible Adenopathy

Is the swelling a lymph node?
Is the node enlarged?
What are the characteristics of the node?
Is the adenopathy local or generalized?

TABLE 496–2 Common Causes of Generalized Lymphadenopathy

Infections

Typhoid fever, tuberculosis, AIDS, mononucleosis, cytomegalovirus, rubella, varicella, rubeola, histoplasmosis, toxoplasmosis, other

Autoimmune Diseases

Rheumatoid arthritis, lupus erythematosus, dermatomyositis

Malignancies

Primary: Hodgkin disease, non-Hodgkin lymphoma, histiocytic disorders
Metastatic: Leukemia, neuroblastoma, rhabdomyosarcoma, other

Lipid Storage Diseases

Gaucher disease, Niemann-Pick disease

Drug Reactions

Other

Sarcoidosis, serum sickness

TABLE 496–3 Drainage Areas of Regional Nodes

Node	Drainage area
Abdominal and pelvic:	Lower extremity, abdomen, pelvic organs
Axillary:	Hand, arm, chest wall, upper and lateral abdominal wall, breast
Cervical:	Tongue, external ear, parotid, superficial tissues of the head and neck, larynx, trachea, thyroid
Epitrochlear:	Hand, forearm
Iliac:	Lower abdomen, part of the genitals, urethra, bladder
Inguinal:	Scrotum and penis in males, vulva and vagina in females; skin of the lower abdomen, perineum, gluteal region, lower anal canal, lower extremity
Mediastinal:	Thoracic viscera
Occipital:	Posterior scalp
Popliteal:	Knee joint, skin of the lateral lower leg and foot
Preauricular:	Eyelid, conjunctivas, cheek, temporal scalp
Submaxillary/submental:	Teeth, gums, tongue, buccal mucosa
Supraclavicular:	Head, neck, arms, superficial thorax, lungs, mediastinum, abdomen. Right supraclavicular adenopathy is usually due to an intrathoracic problem. Left supraclavicular adenopathy is usually due to an intra-abdominal problem

TABLE 496–4 Common Causes of Regional Node Enlargement

Occipital	
Roseola, rubella, scalp infections	
Periauricular	
Cat-scratch disease, eye infections	
Cervical	
Streptococcal/staphylococcal adenitis or tonsillitis, mononucleosis, toxoplasmosis, malignancies, Kawasaki disease	
Submaxillary	
Hodgkin or non-Hodgkin lymphoma, tuberculosis, histoplasmosis	
Axillary	
Infections of the arm/chest wall, cat-scratch disease, malignancies	
Mediastinal	
Malignancies (T-cell lymphoma/leukemia, thymoma, teratoma, other), tuberculosis, histoplasmosis, coccidioidomycosis, sarcoidosis	
Abdominal	
Malignancies, mesenteric adenitis	
Ilioinguinal	
Infections of the leg, groin	

real disease). A firm, fixed node should always suggest the possibility of malignancy, regardless of the presence or absence of systemic symptoms or other abnormal physical findings.

Evaluation and treatment of lymphadenopathy are guided by the probable etiologic factor, as determined from the history and physical examination. Many patients have a viral infection and need no intervention. If a bacterial infection is suspected, antibiotic treatment covering at least streptococci and staphylococci is indicated. Surgical drainage is required if an abscess forms. The size of involved nodes should be documented before treatment. Failure to decrease in size within 10–14 days suggests the need for further evaluation. In a minority of cases, the cause of lymphadenopathy is not initially evident, and further evaluation may include complete blood count with differential; evaluation for Epstein-Barr virus, cytomegalovirus, *Toxoplasma*, cat-scratch disease *(Bartonella henselae)*, and sexually transmitted diseases; antistreptolysin O or anti-DNAase serologic tests; tuberculosis skin test; and chest radiograph. Consultation with infectious disease or oncology specialists may be helpful. Biopsy should be considered in patients with persistent or unexplained fever, weight loss, night sweats, hard nodes, fixation of the nodes to surrounding tissues, supraclavicular adenopathy, or mediastinal adenopathy. Biopsy may also be indicated if there is an increase in size over baseline in 2 wk, no decrease in size in 4–6 wk, no regression to "normal" in 8–12 wk, or the development of new signs and symptoms.

Bedros AA, Mann JP: Lymphadenopathy in children. Adv Pediatr 28:341, 1981.
Knight PJ, Mulne AF, Vassay LE: When is lymph node biopsy indicated in children with enlarged peripheral nodes? Pediatrics 69:391, 1982.
Tuerlinckx D, Bodart E, Delos M, et al: Unifocal cervical Castleman disease in two children. Eur J Pediatr 156:701, 1997.

PART XXI

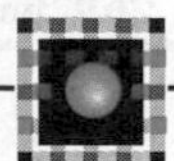

Neoplastic Diseases and Tumors

CHAPTER 497
Introduction to Pediatric Neoplastic Diseases and Tumors

William M. Crist

Only about 1% of new cases of cancer in the United States occur in children (6,500 annual cases), yet malignancy remains the major cause of death due to disease between the ages of 1 and 15 yr. Pediatric cancers differ markedly from adult malignancy in their nature, distribution, and prognosis. Acute lymphoblastic leukemia, central nervous system tumors (described in Chapter 611), and sarcomas predominate in children (Table 497–1), whereas acute and chronic forms of myeloid leukemias, chronic lymphoid leukemia, and carcinomas are more common in adults. Further, the distribution of cases by tumor site of origin varies with age during childhood (Fig. 497–1).

Pediatric oncologists face unique challenges because treatment with irradiation, surgery, and chemotherapy can adversely affect growth and development. Given the relative

< 5 Yr
Lymphoma (10%)
Brain (13%)
Acute Leukemia (36%)
Other (9%)
Ovary/Testis (2%)
Soft Tissue (7%)
Eye (6%)
Kidney (10%)
Neuroblastoma (7%)
5-9 Yr
Lymphoma (16%)
Acute Leukemia (31%)
Brain (25%)
Neuroblastoma (3%)
Other (10%)
Soft Tissue (5%)
Kidney (5%)
Eye (2%)
Bone (3%)
10-14 Yr
Acute Leukemia (18%)
Lymphoma (25 %)
Soft Tissue (5%)
Ovary/Testis (3%)
Bone (11%)
Brain (18%)
Other (16%)
Thyroid (4%)
15-19 Yr
Acute Leukemia (12%)
Eye (4%)
Soft Tissue (5%)
Lymphoma (27 %)
Ovary/Testis (11%)
Brain (10%)
Bone (7%)
Other (10%)
Thyroid (8%)
Melanoma (6%)

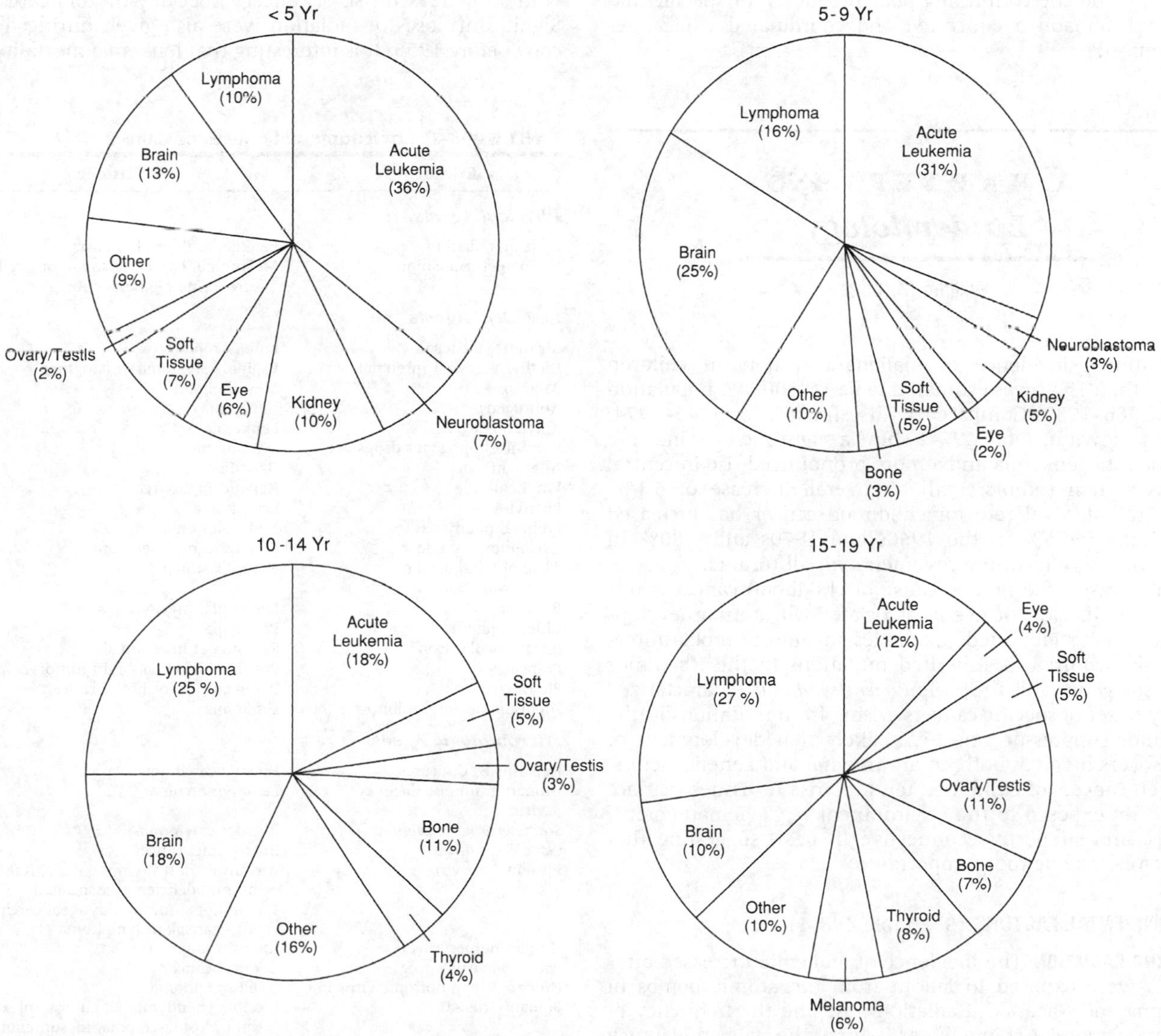

Figure 497–1 Percentage of primary tumors by site of origin for different age groups. (Adapted from National Cancer Institute Monograph No. 57, SEER Program.)

TABLE 497–1 Incidence and Survival Rates of Some Common Childhood Cancers: Summary of Trends by Site*

Site	Average Rate 1973–1974	1986–1987	% Change	Five-Year Survival Rate (%)/Year of Diagnosis 1960–1963	1974–1976	1986–1993
Acute lymphocytic leukemia	2.9	3.3	14.4†	4	53	80
Brain and nervous system	2.5	3.2	29.4†	35	54	61
Bone	0.7	0.8	12.5†	20	54	64
Hodgkin's disease	0.8	0.6	−17.5	52	49	94
Non-Hodgkin's disease	0.8	1.1	31.7	18	45	73
Kidney	0.7	0.8	7.5	33	74	92
Soft tissue	0.7	0.8	5.2	38	60	73
All sites	13.2	14.0	6.1†	28	56	72

**Rates are per 100,000 whites, ages 0–14 yr, and are age adjusted to the 1970 standard population in the United States.*
†The estimated annual percentage change over the 15-yr interval is significantly different from 0 ($p < .05$).
From Ries LAG, Hankey BF, Edwards BK (eds): Cancer Statistics Review 1973–1987. The Surveillance Program Division of Cancer Prevention and Control. NIH publication no. 90-2789. Bethesda, MD, Department of Health and Human Services, 1988; and Parker SL, Tong T, Bolden S, Wingo PA: Cancer Statistics, 1997. CA Cancer J Clin 47:1, 1997.

rarity of specific types of childhood cancer and the sophisticated technology and expertise required for diagnosis, treatment, and monitoring of late effects, it is important that all children with cancer be treated on standard clinical protocols in clinical research settings. These centers have the required facilities and expertise and are committed to learning more about the optimal treatment of pediatric malignancy through participation in national clinical trials. Such treatment has substantially decreased mortality; nonetheless, the late effects of therapy and the continuing poor prognosis for specific malignancies demand a concerted and coordinated clinical research effort.

CHAPTER 498
Epidemiology

William M. Crist

The annual incidence of malignant tumors in children younger than 15 yr was estimated to be 14/100,000 population during 1986–1987. Compared with estimates for 1973–1974, the rates shown in Table 497–1 show a slight increase in acute lymphoblastic leukemia and a more pronounced rise in central nervous system tumors, with an overall increase of 6.1%. The overall survival rate for childhood cancer has increased dramatically (~25% in the 1960s and 1970s and ~80% in 1997), with significant improvements for all tumors.

In most cases, the precise cause of childhood cancer is unknown. Specific genetic events associated with tumor development are being identified. Examples include retinoblastoma, caused by acquired or inherited mutations in the Rb tumor suppressor gene, and the *Li-Fraumeni syndrome*, characterized by early onset of specific cancers arising from mutations in the p53 tumor suppressor gene. It is likely that development of most cancers involves both environmental and genetic factors. However, cancers of childhood tend to arise in tissues that are not directly exposed to the environment (e.g., hematopoietic, nervous, and supportive connective tissues), suggesting that host factors may be more important.

ENVIRONMENTAL FACTORS (See Table 498–1)

IONIZING RADIATION. The incidence of leukemia increased after children were exposed to fallout from the atomic bombs in Hiroshima and Nagasaki. Radiation dose and the frequency of leukemia were related in a linear fashion; the type and latency of leukemia were related to age at exposure. Increases in acute lymphoblastic and chronic myeloid leukemias were noted in younger children, whereas acute myeloid leukemia was noted with increased frequency among older children. These leukemias developed quickly, with a peak rate of occurrence 5 yr after exposure. The incidence of breast cancer is also increased among middle-aged women who were younger than 10 yr when they were exposed. Critical environmental events can cause cancers with varying latency periods. The earlier use of radiation therapy for nonmalignant conditions including enlarged thymus, large tonsils, or tinea capitis was associated with an increased risk of cancer, especially thyroid carcinoma. Significant doses of radiation were also given during fluoroscopy before 1955. It is interesting that leukemia mortality rates

TABLE 498–1 Environmental Causes of Cancer

Etiology	Cancer
Physical Agents	
Ionizing radiation	Leukemia, thyroid, breast
Ultraviolet irradiation	Melanoma, basal and squamous cell in xeroderma pigmentosum
Chemical Agents	
Cigarette, tobacco	Lung, oropharynx, larynx
Diethylstilbestrol (prenatal)	Vaginal carcinoma in daughter
Asbestos	Mesothelioma
Androgens	Hepatoma
Alkylating agents	Leukemia
Immunosuppressant drugs	Lymphoma
Aflatoxin	Hepatic carcinoma
Vinyl chloride	Hepatic angiosarcoma
Phenytoin	Lymphoma
Prenatal phenytoin	Neuroblastoma
Cyclophosphamide	Bladder cancer, leukemia
Alcohol (fetal alcohol syndrome)	Neuroblastoma
Benzene	Leukemia, myelodysplasia
Chloramphenicol	Leukemia
Intramuscular iron	Sarcoma at injection site
Pesticides	Possible leukemia, brain tumors
Phytoestrogens	Reduced risk for breast cancer
Topoisomerase II inhibitors	Leukemia
Microbiologic Agents	
Hepatitis B, C viruses	Hepatic carcinoma
Human immunodeficiency virus	Leiomyosarcoma
Schistosoma haematobium	Bladder carcinoma
Clonorchis sinensis	Biliary tract cancer
Epstein-Barr virus	African Burkitt's lymphoma, X-linked immunodeficiency–associated lymphoma, nasopharyngeal carcinoma, post-transplant lymphoma
Human herpesvirus 8	Kaposi's sarcoma
Papillomavirus	Cervical cancer
Human T-lymphotropic virus I	T-cell lymphoma
Simian virus 40	Possible ependymoma, choroid plexus tumor, osteosarcoma, mesothelioma

From Behrman R, Kliegman R (eds): Nelson Essentials of Pediatrics, 2nd ed. Philadelphia, WB Saunders, 1994.

for children younger than 5 yr declined substantially during the early 1960s, before chemotherapy significantly affected cure rates but after these questionable uses of radiation were curtailed.

Exposure of a fetus to diagnostic x-rays in utero has been associated with a risk ratio of about 1.5 for development of a childhood tumor, but a causal relationship has not been proved. Second malignancies are a risk in patients who have received substantial doses of therapeutic radiation (brain tumors in patients treated with cranial radiation for leukemia). Also see Chapter 718.

ULTRAVIOLET RADIATION. Excessive exposure to sunlight during childhood and adolescence can cause skin cancer later in life (see Chapter 662). Children who have a genetic predisposition such as xeroderma pigmentosum or other congenital defects in DNA repair are at increased risk of developing neoplasms associated with ultraviolet radiation (Chapter 662).

DRUGS. Intrauterine exposure to *diethylstilbestrol* (DES) confers an increased risk of clear cell adenocarcinoma of the vagina in daughters of women given this drug. Also, exposed children of both sexes commonly have malformations of the genital tract (see also Chapter 561). DES is currently the only proven human transplacental carcinogen, although two cases of neuroblastoma have been reported in infants with fetal hydantoin syndrome and another has been reported in a child with fetal alcohol syndrome.

Immunosuppressive agents administered after renal or other transplantation have been associated with an increased incidence of malignancy (particularly non-Hodgkin's lymphoma). The distribution of tumor types in immunosuppressed individuals differs from that in other children, suggesting that immune surveillance may be more effective against some cancers than others.

Treatment of aplastic anemia (especially of the Fanconi type) with *anabolic androgenic steroids* can cause liver tumors, including hepatocellular carcinoma, hepatoma, and hepatic adenoma. The underlying condition may contribute to tumorigenesis, because similar tumors have not been reported in athletes who use anabolic steroids to produce muscle hypertrophy. Such athletes may well be at risk (Chapter 695). Cancer chemotherapies, especially alkylating agents and epipodophyllotoxins, can cause second neoplasms, with a cumulative risk as high as 12% 25 yr after treatment.

DIET. An unexplained association between high fat intake, obesity, and the incidence of cancers of the breast, colon, and uterus has been noted in adults. Data to support preventive dietary modifications in children are lacking.

VIRUSES

RNA VIRUSES. Convincing evidence supports both vertical and horizontal transmission of leukemia and lymphoma associated with type C RNA viruses in animals. Retroviruses also cause leukemia/lymphoma in cats and cows via horizontal transmission. A type of T-cell leukemia affecting adults and, occasionally, adolescents has been associated with a retrovirus (human T-cell leukemia virus, or HTLV-1). See Chapter 269. This form of leukemia is endemic on two islands in southern Japan and occurs in the Caribbean and sporadically elsewhere, including the United States and Israel. The latency period can be longer than 20 yr.

DNA VIRUSES. Epstein-Barr virus (EBV), which causes infectious mononucleosis, is also implicated in Burkitt's lymphoma, lymphoepithelioma, and Hodgkin's disease. The association is geographic: 90–95% of Burkitt's lymphomas in Africa are EBV related, vs only 20–30% in the United States. It is thought that chronic stimulation of B lymphocytes by EBV can set the stage for specific chromosomal translocations that contribute to malignant transformation (see Chapter 499). Chronic malarial infection appears to increase the risk of Burkitt's lymphoma by decreasing immune surveillance of genetically altered cells.

PAPOVA VIRUSES. This family of viruses causes warts and papillomas in various tissues. Subtypes of the virus appear to have strong tissue tropisms. Types 6 and 11 are found in lesions of laryngeal papillomatosis as well as condylomata acuminata. Although these viral lesions rarely undergo spontaneous malignant transformation, malignant conversion to squamous cell carcinomas is frequent after exposure to a secondary carcinogen, such as cigarette smoke or therapeutic irradiation. Subtypes 16 and 18 appear to be etiologic factors in carcinoma of the uterine cervix.

Daniels JL, Olshan AF, Savitz DA: Pesticides and childhood cancers. Environ Health Perspect 105:1068, 1997.

Kony SJ, de Vathaire F, Chompret A, et al: Radiation and genetic factors in the risk of second malignant neoplasms after a first cancer in childhood. Lancet 350:91, 1997.

Preston-Martin S, Navidi W, Thomas D, et al: Los Angeles study of residential magnetic fields and childhood brain tumors. Am J Epidemiol 143:105, 1996.

Robison LL: General Principles of the Epidemiology of Childhood Cancer. *In*: Pizzo PA, Poplack DG (eds): Principles and Practice of Pediatric Oncology. Philadelphia, JB Lippincott, 1997, p 1.

Sankila R, Olsen JH, Anderson H, et al: Risk of cancer among offspring of childhood cancer survivors. N Engl J Med 338:1339, 1998.

Stenton SC: Simian virus 40 and human maligancy. Br Med J 316:877, 1998.

Swerdlow AJ, De Stavola BL, Swanwick MA, et al: Risks of breast and testicular cancers in young adult twins in England and Wales: Evidence on prenatal and genetic aetiology. Lancet 350:1723, 1997.

CHAPTER 499
Molecular Pathogenesis

Richard J. Bram and Michael J. McManus

Specific genetic mutations in key genes within tumor cells can cause or contribute to their aberrant behavior.

ACTIVATION OF PROTO-ONCOGENES. Proto-oncogenes are normal progenitors of animal tumor retroviral oncogenes. These genes encode various proteins including growth factors, growth factor receptors, tyrosine kinases, and transcription factors. These proteins are vital components in the network of signal transduction that regulates cell growth, division, and differentiation. The proto-oncogenes can be abnormally activated by various molecular mechanisms. Chromosomal translocations can result in deregulation of the gene's expression by juxtaposing the gene with immunoglobulin or T-cell receptor gene sequences, as seen in leukemias and lymphomas. Proto-oncogenes can also be activated by amplification of their DNA sequences, up to hundreds of copies, as part of a longer amplified DNA sequence called an *amplicon*. Amplicons can exist as extrachromosomal elements, such as double-minute chromosomes. An example of gene amplification in pediatric oncology is the amplification of the MYCN gene in poor-prognosis neuroblastoma. Proto-oncogenes can be activated by point mutations that alter protein function. The N-ras proto-oncogene is mutated in 25–30% of acute nonlymphocytic leukemias. The *ret* gene encodes a receptor tyrosine kinase that is activated by a point mutation. These mutations in the Ret kinase are associated with multiple endocrine neoplasia syndromes and familial thyroid carcinoma.

CREATION OF FUSION GENES. The fusion of fragments from two genes via chromosomal translocations or inversions is a common mechanism of leukemogenesis. Targets of these translocations include genes that encode transcription factors (see Table 499–1). Formation of a fusion gene may result in the production of a chimeric protein with new and potentially oncogenic

TABLE 499–1 Oncogene Activation in Pediatric Tumors

Mechanism	Chromosome	Genes	Protein Function	Tumor
Chromosomal translocation	t(9;22)	bcr-abl	Chimeric tyrosine kinase	CML, ALL
	t(1;19)	E2A-pbx1	Chimeric transcription factor	Pre-B ALL
	t(14;18)	c-myc	Transcription factor	Burkitt's lymphoma
	t(15;17)	APL-RARα	Chimeric transcription factor	APL
Gene amplification	Amplicon	N-myc	Transcription factor	Neuroblastoma
	Amplicon	EGFR gene	Growth factor receptor, tyrosine kinase	Glioblastoma
Point mutation	1p	N-ras	GTPase	AML
	10q	Ret	Tyrosine kinase	MEN2

ALL = acute lymphocytic anemia; AML = acute myelocytic leukemia; APL = acute promyelocytic leukemia; CML = chronic myelocytic leukemia; MEN2 = multiple endocrine neoplasia type 2.

properties. The downstream effects of these aberrant transcription factors are poorly understood; therefore, the mechanism of leukemogenesis is unknown. Emerging evidence suggests that the aberrant transcriptional regulation of homeobox-containing genes has a vital role in hematopoietic cell differentiation and leukemogenesis. Alternatively, the normal pathways of programmed cell death (apoptosis) that are active in B- and T-cell precursors may be defective. In this case, lymphoid cells that contain damaged DNA and/or improperly rearranged antigen receptor genes are not destroyed but rather may accumulate additional genetic mutations that establish a malignant state. Aberrant fusion genes have also been detected in childhood solid tumors. Ewing's sarcoma has a t(11:22), and frequently the alveolar histologic subtype of rhabdomyosarcomas has a t(2;13) or t(1;13). These genetic abnormalities in pediatric solid tumors have been useful as molecular diagnostic markers and in combination with histopathologic and clinical information help subclassify childhood sarcomas.

DISRUPTION OF TUMOR SUPPRESSOR GENES. In contrast to the proto-oncogenes, tumor suppressor genes (antioncogenes) normally act to suppress cell growth or induce programmed cell death (apoptosis). These functions give a level of protection against the development of malignant transformation. Induction of DNA damage by radiation, for example, activates the p53 tumor suppressor protein, which in turn stops the cell from dividing until its DNA has been repaired. An additional property of p53 is its ability to initiate apoptosis (the "suicide" pathway) when the DNA of a cell is damaged beyond the point of repair. As such, p53 is regarded as an important "guardian of the genome," and loss of its function through mutation tends to facilitate tumor development or progression.

Other tumor suppressors include the retinoblastoma gene product Rb, an important cell cycle regulatory protein, loss of which leads to retinoblastoma and osteosarcoma; the neurofibromatosis genes (NF1 and NF2), which are also associated with sarcomas and brain tumors; and WT1, associated with Wilms' tumor. The p16/INK4a gene, which is deleted in many different types of cancer, has been shown to be a potent inhibitor of growth through its effects on the cyclin class of cell cycle regulatory proteins. Both copies of the p16 gene are deleted in about 60–80% of childhood T-ALL and 20–30% of B-precursor ALL. The physically overlapping p19/ARF gene, which has an independent ability to block progression of the cell cycle, may also contribute to the potency of p16 as a tumor suppressor locus.

CANCER PREDISPOSITION SYNDROMES (Table 499–2). Tumor suppressor genes are also known as *recessive oncogenes* because both copies must be inactivated to allow development of neoplastic transformation, a process described in Knudson's two-hit model of cancer development. This model explains the difference in age of onset between *sporadic and familial retinoblastoma*. In the former, both copies of the Rb gene must randomly acquire inactivating mutations, whereas in familial retinoblastoma, development of cancer is accelerated by inheritance of one dysfunctional Rb gene from an affected parent. Patients with familial retinoblastoma frequently develop several tumors in both eyes at an early age and are at increased risk of developing osteosarcomas as adolescents. Although the effects of tumor suppressor genes at the cellular level are recessive (i.e., both alleles mutated), their clinical pattern of inheritance is autosomal dominant (i.e., one allele inherited). Thus, 50% of offspring from couples with one affected parent carry the mutant (cancer-prone) gene. *The Li-Fraumeni syndrome*, characterized by frequent development of sarcomas, cancers of the breast, bone, lung, and brain, as well as leukemias, is caused by inheritance of one defective copy of the p53 gene. Similarly, neurofibromatosis is frequently inherited in an autosomal dominant fashion, although 50% of cases present without a family history owing to the high rate of spontaneous mutation of the NF1 gene.

A second mechanism responsible for inherited predisposition to develop cancer involves defects in DNA repair. Syndromes associated with excessive numbers of broken chromosomes due to repair defects include *Bloom's syndrome, ataxia-telangiectasia*, and *Fanconi's pancytopenia*; patients have significantly increased rates of cancer, especially leukemia. *Xeroderma pigmentosum* likewise increases the risk of skin cancer, owing to defects in repair to DNA damaged by ultraviolet light. These disorders display a pattern of autosomal recessive inheritance.

A third category of inherited cancer predisposition is characterized by defects in immune surveillance, a process that has an important role in removing transformed cells that escape apoptosis. This group includes patients with *Wiskott-Aldrich syndrome, severe combined immunodeficiency, common variable immunodeficiency*, and the *X-linked lymphoproliferative syndrome*. The most common types of malignancy in these patients are lymphoma and leukemia. Cure rates for immunodeficient children with cancer are much poorer than for nonimmunodeficient patients with similar malignancies, suggesting a role for the immune system in cancer treatment as well as in cancer prevention.

It is important to minimize the mutagen exposure of children with a familial cancer-prone syndrome. Parents and patients must be reminded to avoid excessive direct sunlight and tobacco smoke.

TABLE 499–2 Familial or Genetic Susceptibility to Malignancy

Disorder	Tumor/Cancer	Comment
Chromosomal Syndromes		
Chromosome 11p—(deletion) with sporadic aniridia	Wilms tumor	Associated with genitourinary anomalies, mental retardation, WT1 gene
Chromosome 13q—(deletion)	Retinoblastoma, sarcoma	Associated with mental retardation, skeletal malformations: autosomal dominant (bilateral) or sporadic new mutation, RB1 gene
Trisomy 21	Lymphocytic or nonlymphocytic leukemia	Risk is 15 times normal
Klinefelter's syndrome (47, XXY)	Breast cancer, extragonadal germ cell tumors	
Gonadal dysgenesis XO/XY	Gonadoblastoma	Gonads must be removed; 25% chance of gonadal malignancy
Trisomy 8	Preleukemia	
Noonan's syndrome	Schwannoma, myelodysplasia	
Monosomy 5 or 7	Myelodysplastic syndromes	Recurrent infections may precede neoplasia
DNA Fragility		
Xeroderma pigmentosum	Basal, squamous cell skin cancers	Autosomal recessive; failure to repair solar-damaged DNA
Fanconi's anemia	Leukemia	Autosomal recessive; 10% risk for acute myelogenous leukemia; chromosome fragility, positive diepoxybutane test result
Bloom's syndrome	Leukemia, lymphoma	Autosomal recessive; chromosome fragility; high risk for malignancy
Ataxia-telangiectasia	Lymphoma, leukemia	Autosomal recessive; sensitive to x-radiation, radiomimetic drugs; chromosome fragility
Dysplastic nevus syndrome	Melanoma	Autosomal dominant
Immunodeficiency Syndromes		
Wiskott-Aldrich syndrome	Lymphoma, leukemia	Immunodeficiency; X-linked recessive
X-linked immunodeficiency (Duncan's syndrome)	Lymphoma	Epstein-Barr virus is inciting agent
X-linked agammaglobulinemia	Lymphoma, leukemia	Immunodeficiency
Severe combined immunodeficiency	Leukemia, lymphoma	Immunodeficiency; X-linked recessive
Others		
Neurofibromatosis 1	Neurofibroma, optic glioma, acoustic neuroma, astrocytoma, meningioma, pheochromocytoma, sarcoma	Autosomal dominant; NF1 gene
Neurofibromatosis 2	Bilateral acoustic neuromas, meningioma	Autosomal dominant; NF2 gene
Tuberous sclerosis	Fibroangiomatous nevi, myocardial rhabdomyoma	Autosomal dominant
Hemochromatosis	Hepatoma	Cirrhosis; autosomal dominant/recessive
Retinoblastoma	Sarcoma	Increased risk of secondary malignancy 10–20 yr later, RB1 gene
Glycogen storage disease I	Hepatic adenoma	Usually with cirrhosis, autosomal recessive
Familial adenomatous polyposis coli	Adenocarcinoma of colon	Autosomal dominant, APC gene
Gardner syndrome	Adenocarcinoma of colon; skull and soft tissue tumors	Autosomal dominant, APC gene
Peutz-Jeghers syndrome	Gastrointestinal carcinoma, ovarian neoplasia	Autosomal dominant
Hemihypertrophy ± Beckwith's syndrome	Wilms tumor, hepatoblastoma, adrenal carcinoma	25% develop tumor, most in first 5 yr of life
Tyrosinemia, galactosemia	Hepatic carcinoma	Nodular cirrhosis; autosomal recessive
Multiple endocrine neoplasia syndrome I (Wermer's syndrome)	Parathyroid adenoma, pancreatic islet tumor, pituitary adenoma carcinoid	Autosomal dominant; Zollinger-Ellison syndrome
Multiple endocrine neoplasia syndrome II (Sipple's syndrome)	Medullary carcinoma of the thyroid, hyperparathyroidism, pheochromocytoma	Autosomal dominant; monitor calcitonin and calcium levels
Multiple endocrine neoplasia III (multiple mucosal neuroma syndrome)	Mucosal neuroma, pheochromocytoma, medullary thyroid carcinoma; Marfan habitus; neuropathy	Autosomal dominant
Rendu-Osler-Weber syndrome	Angioma	Autosomal dominant
von Hippel-Lindau disease	Hemangioblastoma of the cerebellum and retina, pheochromocytoma, renal cancer	Autosomal dominant, mutation of tumor-suppressor gene, VHL gene
Cancer family syndrome	Colonic, uterine carcinoma	Autosomal dominant
Li-Fraumeni syndrome	Bone, soft tissue sarcoma, breast	Mutation of p53 tumor-suppressor gene, autosomal dominant
BRCA1 and 2	Breast, ovarian	DNA repair defect

From Behrman R, Kliegman R (eds): Nelson Essentials of Pediatrics, 2nd ed. Philadelphia, WB Saunders, 1994.

CHAPTER 500
Principles of Diagnosis

William M. Crist

PRINCIPLES OF DIAGNOSIS. The majority of childhood cancers are curable. The prognosis relates most strongly to tumor type, extent of disease at diagnosis, and effectiveness of the treatment. Rapid diagnosis helps to ensure that appropriate therapy is given in a timely fashion and, hence, optimizes the chances of cure. Because most physicians in general practice rarely encounter children with cancer, they should be alert for an atypical course of a common childhood condition (Table 500–1).

Delays in diagnosis are particularly likely in certain clinical situations. The cardinal symptom of both osteosarcoma and Ewing's sarcoma is localized, usually persistent pain. Because these tumors occur during the 2nd decade of life, a time of increased physical activity, patients often associate the pain with an episode of trauma. Prompt radiologic evaluation can help ensure the diagnosis. Tumors of the nasopharynx or middle ear may mimic infection. Prolonged unexplained ear pain, nasal discharge, retropharyngeal swelling, or trismus should be investigated as possible signs of malignancy. Cervical lymph node enlargement is common in children with infection, as in patients with lymphoma. Persistent or progressively enlarging nodes (often painless) are suggestive of lymphoma and indicate the need for biopsy.

The early symptoms of leukemia may be limited to low-grade fever or bone and joint pain. Blood counts, with particular attention to normocytic anemia or mild thrombocytopenia, may indicate the need for bone marrow examination, even when leukemic blast cells are not seen in the blood smear. Malignancy can also occur in neonates and should be consid-

TABLE 500–1 Common Manifestations of Childhood Malignancy

Sign/Symptom	Nonmalignant Condition Mimicked	Significance	Example
Hematologic			
Pallor, anemia	Iron-deficiency anemia, blood loss	Bone marrow infiltration	Leukemia, neuroblastoma
Petechiae, thrombocytopenia	Idiopathic thrombocytopenic purpura	Bone marrow infiltration	Leukemia, neuroblastoma
Fever, pharyngitis, neutropenia	Streptococcal/viral pharyngitis	Bone marrow infiltration	Leukemia, neuroblastoma
Systemic			
Bone pain, limp, arthralgia	Osteomyelitis, rheumatologic disease, trauma	Primary bone tumor, metastasis to bone	Osteosarcoma, Ewing's sarcoma, leukemia, neuroblastoma
Fever of unknown origin, weight loss, night sweats	Collagen vascular disease, chronic infection	Lymphoreticular malignancy	Hodgkin's disease, non-Hodgkin's lymphoma
Painless lymphadenopathy	Epstein-Barr virus, cytomegalovirus	Lymphoreticular malignancy	Leukemia, Hodgkin's disease, non-Hodgkin's lymphoma, Burkitt's lymphoma
Cutaneous lesion	Abscess, trauma	Primary or metastatic disease	Neuroblastoma, leukemia, histiocytosis X, melanoma
Abdominal mass	Organomegaly, hydronephrosis, constipation	Adrenal-renal tumor	Neuroblastoma, Wilms' tumor, hepatoblastoma
Hypertension	Renovascular disease, nephritis	Sympathetic nervous system tumor	Neuroblastoma, pheochromocytoma, Wilms' tumor
Diarrhea	Inflammatory bowel disease	Vasoactive intestinal polypeptide	Neuroblastoma, ganglioneuroma
Soft tissue mass	Abscess	Local or metastatic tumor	Ewing's sarcoma, osteosarcoma, neuroblastoma, rhabdomyosarcoma, eosinophilic granuloma, Askin's tumor
Vaginal bleeding	Foreign body, coagulopathy	Uterine tumor	Yolk sac tumor, rhabdomyosarcoma
Emesis, visual disturbances, ataxia, headache, papilledema	Migraine	Increased intracranial pressure	Primary brain tumor; metastasis
Chronic ear discharge	Otitis media	Middle or inner ear mass	Rhabdomyosarcoma
Ophthalmologic Signs			
Leukocoria	Cataract, glaucoma	White pupil	Retinoblastoma
Periorbital ecchymosis	Trauma	Metastasis	Neuroblastoma
Miosis, ptosis, heterochromia	Third nerve paresis	Horner's syndrome: compression of cervical sympathetic nerves	Neuroblastoma
Opsoclonus/ataxia	Drug reaction	Neurotransmitters? Autoimmunity?	Neuroblastoma
Exophthalmos, proptosis	Graves' disease	Orbital tumor	Rhabdomyosarcoma
Thoracic Mass			
Anterior mediastinal	Infection (tuberculosis), lymphadenopathy, sarcoidosis	Cough, stridor, pneumonia, tracheal-bronchial compression	Thymoma, teratoma, T-cell lymphoma, thyroid
Posterior mediastinal	Esophageal disease	Vertebral or nerve root compression; dysphagia	Neuroblastoma, neuroenteric cyst

Modified from Behrman R, Kliegman R (eds): Nelson Essentials of Pediatrics, 2nd ed. Philadelphia, WB Saunders, 1994.

ered in children with masses or "blueberry muffin" spots on their skin.

When a malignant neoplasm is suspected, the immediate goal is to determine its nature and extent. A tentative diagnosis can often be inferred from the patient's presenting symptoms, age, and tumor location. An abdominal mass is much more likely to be a neuroblastoma or Wilms' tumor in a young child than in a child older than 10 yr.

A thorough search for metastatic disease usually precedes biopsy of a suspicious lesion. The surgeon can make a more informed choice between an attempt at complete resection and a more limited procedure when the presence or likelihood of disseminated disease is known. The appropriate preoperative studies depend on the tentative diagnosis. Several noninvasive techniques (computed tomography, magnetic resonance imaging) are useful in evaluating for metastatic lesions; also, bone marrow aspiration, biopsy, or both may be needed. These studies are also used in assessing the disease stage, which is critical in determining the prognosis and developing a treatment plan.

Central to the diagnosis of any tumor is histologic examination. The initial specimen of tumor tissue should be obtained under conditions that allow for a full range of pathologic studies. In some cases, such as suspected lymphomas, fresh tissue may be needed for special studies. These studies may take time; thus, it is often impossible to discuss the specific diagnosis with a family immediately after surgery. The surgeon must search carefully at biopsy, excision, or exploration for evidence of regional dissemination to lymph node groups or to adjacent organs. If total resection is attempted, the pathologist must carefully examine the margins for microscopic residual tumor because subsequent treatment depends on this information. The treatment plan must be carefully explained to parents and, if possible, to the patient. An honest discussion of the facts is the best policy. Children should be told all that they can understand and would find useful or wish to know. Special concerns, such as the possible need to amputate a limb, the loss of hair during chemotherapy, and possible temporary or permanent functional impairment must be anticipated and fully discussed. It may be necessary to repeat explanations several times before distraught family members truly understand what is being said. Throughout treatment, parents, patients, siblings, and medical staff will need help in expressing feelings of anxiety, depression, guilt, and anger.

CHAPTER 501
Principles of Treatment

William M. Crist

Treatment of children with cancer is complex, requiring the expertise of teams of specialized health care providers (i.e., pediatric pathologists, oncologists, radiotherapists, surgeons, radiologists, and various support staff including nutritionists, social workers, psychologists, and nurses). The best chance for cure exists during the initial course of treatment; patients should be referred to an appropriate specialized center as soon as possible when the diagnosis of cancer is suspected. The remarkable increases in cure rates for childhood malignancies would not have occurred without the participation of patients and their physicians in clinical research programs at these centers.

Whenever possible, treatment is given on an outpatient basis. Children should remain at home and in school as much as possible throughout treatment. The intensity of many treatment regimens is such that some patients miss a considerable amount of school in the 1st year after diagnosis. Tutoring should be encouraged so children do not fall behind; counseling should be provided as appropriate.

Development of selective, highly effective therapy for cancer has been hindered by lack of understanding of ways to modify the molecular mechanisms underlying malignant transformation. Also, de novo or acquired resistance to chemotherapy and irradiation remains an obstacle. Therapy, therefore, continues to be largely empirical. Further, because of the lack of selectivity of available therapy for malignant versus nonmalignant cells, toxicity remains a troublesome issue that is especially problematic in children.

Local therapy with surgery or irradiation or both is an important component of treatment for most solid tumors, but systemic multiagent chemotherapy is usually necessary because tumor dissemination is generally present, even if undetectable. Chemotherapy alone is generally insufficient to eradicate gross residual tumors. Hence, children with malignant tumors may require treatment with all three modalities. Unfortunately, most effective treatments have a narrow therapeutic index (i.e., ratio of efficacy to toxicity). Therefore, acute and chronic toxicity can be minimized but not entirely avoided.

501.1 Chemotherapy

Traditional drugs for treatment of cancer are selected from several classes of agents, including hormones, antimetabolites, antibiotics, plant alkaloids, and alkylating agents (Table 501–1). Most of these agents can produce cytotoxicity to both malignant and normal cells. The increased metabolic and cell cycle activity of malignant cells makes them more susceptible to the cytotoxic effects of chemotherapy. Specific tumor-directed therapies include antisense messenger RNA, tumor antigen–specific monoclonal antibodies, and antiangiogenic agents. *Angiostatin* and *endostatin* inhibit the angiogenesis associated with the development of metastatic disease. Results of human studies are not available, but results of animal studies are encouraging.

501.2 Acute Complications and Supportive Care

Early complications of therapy include metabolic disorders, bone marrow suppression, and immunosuppression. Patients with a large tumor burden may have had substantial breakdown of tumor cells; renal function can be impaired by tubular precipitates of uric acid crystals (Table 501–2). This occurs most often with leukemia and lymphoma, particularly Burkitt's lymphoma, but can occur with large solid tumors (e.g., hepatoblastoma, germ cell tumors, and neuroblastoma). Before therapy is initiated, the serum levels of uric acid and creatinine should be measured and adequate hydration ensured; allopurinol (a xanthine oxidase inhibitor) can be given, if necessary, to lower uric acid levels to within the normal range. In the metabolic *tumor lysis syndrome*, phosphates and potassium are released into the circulation in large quantities as cells are lysed by treatment. Symptomatic hyperkalemia and hyperphosphatemia with subsequent hypocalcemia develop in the setting of inadequate renal function.

Tumors that invade and replace bone marrow can cause pancytopenia; all chemotherapy regimens can produce *myelosuppression*. Anemia can be corrected by transfusions of packed red blood cells, and thrombocytopenia by platelet infusions. Patients receiving immunosuppressive therapy should receive

TABLE 501–1 Cancer Chemotherapy

Drug*	Action	Metabolism	Excretion	Indication	Toxicity
Antimetabolites					
Methotrexate	Folic acid antagonist; inhibits dihydrofolate reductase	Hepatic	Renal, 50–90% excreted unchanged; biliary	ALL, lymphoma, medulloblastoma, osteosarcoma	Myelosuppression (nadir 7–10 days), mucositis, stomatitis, dermatitis, hepatitis; renal and CNS with high-dose administration; prevent with leucovorin, monitor levels
6-Mercaptopurine (Purinethol)	Purine analog, inhibits purine synthesis	Hepatic; allopurinol inhibits metabolism	Renal	ALL	Myelosuppression, hepatic necrosis, mucositis; allopurinal increases toxicity
Cytarabine (Ara-C)	Pyrimidine analog; inhibits DNA polymerase	Hepatic	Renal	ALL, lymphoma	Myelosuppression, conjunctivitis, mucositis, CNS dysfunction
Alkylating Agents					
Cyclophosphamide (Cytoxan)	Alkylates guanine; inhibits DNA synthesis	Hepatic	Renal	ALL, lymphoma, sarcoma	Myelosuppression, hemorrhagic cystitis, pulmonary fibrosis, inappropriate ADH secretion, bladder cancer, anaphylaxis
Ifosfamide (Ifex)	Similar to cyclophosphamide	Hepatic	Renal	Lymphoma, Wilms' tumor, sarcoma, germ cell and testicular tumors	Similar to cyclophosphamide; CNS dysfunction, cardiac toxicity
Antibiotics					
Doxorubicin (Adriamycin) and daunorubicin (Cerubidine)	Binds to DNA, intercalation	Hepatic	Biliary, renal	ALL, AML, osteosarcoma, Ewing's sarcoma, lymphoma, neuroblastoma	Cardiomyopathy, red urine, tissue necrosis on extravasation, myelosuppression, conjunctivitis, radiation dermatitis, arrhythmia
Dactinomycin	Binds to DNA, inhibits transcription	—	Renal, stool; 30% excreted unchanged drug	Wilms' tumor, rhabdomyosarcoma, Ewing's sarcoma	Tissue necrosis on extravasation, myelosuppression, radiosensitizer, mucosal ulceration
Bleomycin (Blenoxane)	Binds to DNA, cuts DNA	Hepatic	Renal	Hodgkin's disease, lymphoma, germ cell tumors	Pneumonitis, stomatitis, Raynaud's phenomenon, pulmonary fibrosis, dermatitis
Vinca Alkaloids					
Vincristine (Oncovin)	Inhibits microtubule formation	Hepatic	Biliary	ALL, lymphoma, Wilms' tumor, Hodgkin's disease, Ewing's sarcoma, neuroblastoma, rhabdomyosarcoma	Local cellulitis, peripheral neuropathy, constipation, ileus, jaw pain, inappropriate ADH secretion, seizures, ptosis, minimal myelosuppression
Vinblastine (Velban)	Inhibits microtubule formation	Hepatic	Biliary	Hodgkin's disease; Langerhans cell histiocytosis	Local cellulitis, leukopenia
Enzymes					
L-Asparaginase	Depletion of L-asparagine	—	Reticuloendothelial system	ALL	Allergic reaction, pancreatitis, hyperglycemia, platelet dysfunction and coagulopathy, encephalopathy
Pegaspargase	Polyethylene glycol conjugate of L-asparagine	—	As above	As above	Indicated for patients with allergy to L-asparaginase
Hormones					
Prednisone	Unknown; lymphocyte modification?	Hepatic	Renal	ALL; Hodgkin's disease, lymphoma	Cushing's syndrome, cataracts, diabetes, hypertension, myopathy, osteoporosis, infection, peptic ulceration, psychosis
Miscellaneous					
Carmustine (nitrosourea)	Carbamylation of DNA; inhibits DNA synthesis	Hepatic; phenobarbital increases metabolism, decreases activity	Renal	CNS tumors, lymphoma, Hodgkin's disease	Delayed myelosuppression (4–6 wk); pulmonary fibrosis, carcinogenic, stomatitis
Cisplatin (Platinol)	Inhibits DNA synthesis	—	Renal	Gonadal tumors; osteosarcoma, neuroblastoma, CNS tumors, germ cell tumors	Nephrotoxic; aminoglycosides may increase nephrotoxicity, myelosuppression, ototoxicity, tetany, neurotoxicity, hemolytic-uremic syndrome; anaphylaxis
Etoposide (VePesid)	Topoisomerase inhibitor	—	Renal	ALL, lymphoma, germ cell tumor	Myelosuppression, secondary leukemia
Etretinate (Tegison) (vitamin A analog) and tretinoin	Enhances normal differentiation	Liver	Liver	Some leukemias; neuroblastoma	Dry mouth, hair loss, pseudotumor cerebri, premature epiphyseal closure

**Many drugs produce nausea and vomiting during administration, and many cause alopecia with repeated doses.*
ADH = antidiuretic hormone; ALL = acute lymphocytic leukemia; AML = acute myelogenous leukemia; CNS = central nervous system.
From Behrman R, Kliegman R (eds): Nelson Essentials of Pediatrics, 2nd ed. Philadelphia, WB Saunders, 1994.

TABLE 501–2 Oncologic Emergencies

Condition	Manifestations	Etiology	Malignancy	Treatment
Metabolic				
Hyperuricemia	Uric acid nephropathy, gout	Tumor lysis syndrome	Lymphoma, leukemia	Allopurinol; alkalize urine; hydration and diuresis
Hyperkalemia	Arrhythmias, cardiac arrest	Tumor lysis syndrome	Lymphoma, leukemia	Polystyrene resin (Kayexalate); sodium bicarbonate, glucose and insulin; check for pseudohyperkalemia from leukemic cell lysis in test tube
Hyperphosphatemia	Hypocalcemic tetany; metastatic calcification, photophobia, pruritus	Tumor lysis syndrome	Lymphoma, leukemia	Hydration, forced diuresis; stop alkalization; oral aluminum hydroxide to bind phosphate
Hyponatremia	Seizure, lethargy; asymptomatic	SIADH; fluid, sodium losses in vomiting, diarrhea, diuresis	Leukemia; CNS tumor	Restrict free water for SIADH; replace sodium if depleted
Hypercalcemia	Anorexia, nausea, polyuria, pancreatitis, gastric ulcers; prolonged PR, shortened QT interval	Bone resorption; ectopic parathormone, vitamin D, or prostaglandins	Hodgkin's disease; metastasis to bone	Hydration and furosemide diuresis; corticosteroids; plicamycin; calcitonin; diphosphonates
Hematologic				
Anemia	Pallor, weakness, heart failure	Bone marrow suppression or infiltration; blood loss	Any with chemotherapy	Packed red blood cell transfusion
Thrombocytopenia	Petechiae, hemorrhage	Bone marrow suppression or infiltration	Any with chemotherapy	Platelet transfusion
Disseminated intravascular coagulation	Shock, hemorrhage	Sepsis, hypotension, tumor factors	Promyelocytic leukemia; others	Fresh frozen plasma; platelets, correct infection, etc
Neutropenia	Infection	Bone marrow suppression or infiltration	Any with chemotherapy	If febrile, give broad-spectrum antibiotics and G-CSF if appropriate
Hyperleukocytosis (>50,000/mm³)	Hemorrhage, thrombosis; pulmonary infiltrates, hypoxia; tumor lysis syndrome; visual disturbances	Leukostasis; vascular occlusion	Leukemia	Leukapheresis; chemotherapy
Graft versus host disease	Dermatitis, diarrhea, hepatitis	Immunosuppression and nonirradiated blood products; bone marrow transplantation	Any with immunosuppression	Corticosteroids; cyclosporine; antithymocyte globulin
Space-Occupying Lesions				
Spinal cord compression	Back pain ± radicular *Cord above T10:* Symmetric weakness, increased DTR; sensory level present; toes up; bowel, bladder signs *Conus medullaris* (T10–12): Symmetric weakness, increased knee reflexes, decreased ankle reflexes; saddle sensory loss; toes up or down *Cauda equina* (below L2): Asymmetric weakness, loss of DTR and sensory deficit; toes down	Metastasis to vertebra and extramedullary space	Neuroblastoma; medulloblastoma	MRI or myelography for diagnosis; corticosteroids; radiotherapy; laminectomy; chemotherapy
Increased intracranial pressure	Confusion, coma, emesis, headache, hypertension, bradycardia, seizures, papilledema, hydrocephalus; III and VI nerve palsies	Primary or metastatic brain tumor	Neuroblastoma, astrocytoma; glioma	Computed tomography or MRI for diagnosis; corticosteroids; phenytoin; ventricular-peritoneal shunt; radiotherapy; chemotherapy
Superior vena cava syndrome	Distended neck veins, plethora, edema of head and neck, cyanosis; proptosis; Horner's syndrome	Superior mediastinal mass	Lymphoma	Chemotherapy; radiotherapy

SIADH = inappropriate antidiuretic hormone secretion; CNS = central nervous system; G-CSF = granulocyte colony-stimulating factor; DTR = deep tendon reflex; MRI = magnetic resonance imaging.

From Behrman R, Kliegman R (eds): Nelson Essentials of Pediatrics, 2nd ed. Philadelphia, WB Saunders, 1994.

irradiated blood products to prevent graft versus host disease. Granulocytopenia (counts $< 500/mm^3$) poses the risk of life-threatening infections (Table 501–3). Febrile granulocytopenic patients should be hospitalized and treated with empirical broad-spectrum intravenous antimicrobial therapy pending the results of appropriate cultures of blood, urine, or any obvious sites of infection (see Chapter 179). Treatment is continued until fever resolves and the granulocyte count rises. If fever persists beyond 1 wk while on broad-spectrum antibiotics, consideration must be given to a possible fungal infection. Fungal infections caused by *Candida* and *Aspergillus* species are common in immunosuppressed patients. Opportunistic organisms such as *Pneumocystis carinii* can produce fatal pneumonia. Prophylactic treatment with trimethoprim/sulfamethoxazole is given when severe or chronic immunosuppression is anticipated (see also Chapter 179).

Viruses of low pathogenicity can produce serious disease in the setting of immunosuppression caused by malignancy or its treatment. Patients should not be given live virus vaccines. Children who are receiving chemotherapy and who are exposed to chickenpox should receive varicella zoster immunoglobulin and, if clinical disease develops, should be hospitalized and treated with intravenous acyclovir.

It is common for patients undergoing cancer therapy to lose 10% or more of their body weight. Patients may reduce their food intake because of temporary treatment-associated nausea, stomatitis, and vomiting. Appetite loss is not a cause for alarm. *Malnutrition* is a particular risk in patients receiving radiotherapy of the abdomen or head and neck, intensive chemotherapy, or total body irradiation and high-dose chemotherapy for marrow transplantation. If oral supplementation proves inadequate, such patients may require enteral tube feedings or parenteral hyperalimentation. No conclusive evidence, however, shows that total parenteral nutrition improves the response to therapy.

501.3 *Late Sequelae* (Table 501–4)

Late consequences of therapy can cause significant morbidity. Successful surgical resection may require the sacrifice of important functional structures. Irradiation can produce irreversible organ damage, with symptoms and functional limitations depending on the organ involved and the severity of the damage. Many radiation-related problems do not become obvious until a patient is fully grown—for example, when asymmetry of irradiated and nonirradiated areas or extremities becomes noticeable. Irradiation of fields that include endocrine organs can cause hypothyroidism, pituitary dysfunction, or sterility. Cranial and spinal irradiation, in sufficient doses, can produce neurologic dysfunction and growth retardation, respectively.

TABLE 501–4 Long-Term Sequelae of Cancer Therapy

Problem	Etiology
Infertility	Alkylating agents; radiation
Second cancers	Genetic predisposition; radiation, alkylating agents
Sepsis	Splenectomy
Hepatotoxicity	Methotrexate, 6-mercaptopurine, radiation
Amputation	Surgery for osteogenic sarcoma
Scoliosis	Radiation, surgery
Pulmonary (pneumonia, fibrosis)	Radiation, bleomycin, busulfan, nitrosoureas
Cardiomyopathy	Doxorubicin, daunomycin; radiation
Leukoencephalopathy	Cranial irradiation ± methotrexate
Impaired cognition/intelligence	Cranial irradiation ± methotrexate
Pituitary dysfunction (isolated growth hormone deficiency, panhypopituitary)	Cranial irradiation
Hypothyroidism	Neck irradiation

Chemotherapy also carries the risk of long-lasting organ damage. Of particular concern are leukoencephalopathy following high-dose methotrexate therapy, sterility in male patients treated with alkylating agents (e.g., cyclophosphamide), myocardial damage from anthracyclines, pulmonary fibrosis after bleomycin, pancreatitis after asparaginase, and hearing loss associated with cisplatin. Development of these sequelae may be dose related and are usually irreversible. Appropriate baseline and intermittent testing while on therapy should be done before these drugs are administered to ensure that there is no pre-existing damage to the organs likely to be affected and to permit monitoring of treatment-induced changes.

Perhaps the most serious late effect is the occurrence of *second cancers* in patients successfully cured of a first malignancy. The risk appears to be cumulative, increasing by about 0.5%/yr to 12% at 25 yr after treatment. Patients who have been treated for childhood cancer should be examined annually, with particular attention to possible late effects of therapy, including second malignancies.

501.4 *Bone Marrow Transplant*

(See also Chapters 135–140)

Peter M. Anderson

Toxic agents and ionizing radiation may cause permanent damage to bone marrow progenitor cells; neoplastic diseases

TABLE 501–3 Infectious Complications of Malignancy

Predisposing Factor	Etiology	Site of Infection	Infectious Agents
Neutropenia	Chemotherapy, bone marrow infiltration	Sepsis, shock, pneumonia, soft tissue, proctitis, mucositis	*Staphylococcus aureus, Staphylococcus epidermidis; Escherichia coli, Pseudomonas aeruginosa, Candida, Aspergillus;* anaerobic oral and rectal bacteria
Immunosuppression, lymphopenia, lymphocyte-monocyte dysfunction	Chemotherapy, prednisone	Pneumonia, meningitis, disseminated viral infection	*Pneumocystis carinii, Cryptococcus neoformans, Mycobacterium; Nocardia, Listeria monocytogenes, Candida, Aspergillus, Strongyloides; Toxoplasma,* varicella-zoster, cytomegalovirus, herpes simplex
Splenectomy	Staging of Hodgkin's disease	Sepsis, shock, meningitis	Pneumococcus, *Haemophilus influenzae*
Indwelling central venous catheter	Nutrition, administration of chemotherapy	Line sepsis, tract or tunnel infection, exit site infection	*S. aureus, S. epidermidis, Candida albicans; P. aeruginosa; Aspergillus; Corynebacterium JK, Streptococcus faecalis, Mycobacterium fortuitum, Propionibacterium acnes*

From Behrman R, Kliegman R (eds): Nelson Essentials of Pediatrics, 2nd ed. Philadelphia, WB Saunders, 1994.

often disseminate widely and may be difficult to eradicate with surgery, chemotherapy, and irradiation. In some malignancies and certain other disease states, use of bone marrow or peripheral blood stem cells (PBSC) together with chemotherapy given at very high doses, with or without irradiation, may provide lifesaving treatment. Stem cells are capable of repopulating a patient's failed bone marrow and shortening the duration of pancytopenia after high-dose chemotherapy. Although bone marrow was the most widely used source of stems cells for many years, PBSC are being increasingly used because they are effective in reconstituting hematopoiesis and are easily obtained by apheresis.

Bone marrow is harvested by numerous aspirations of small aliquots of marrow from the iliac bones of the donor. Liquid marrow is then filtered through devices resembling fine mesh screens to remove bone spicules, and the marrow is placed into a plastic bag similar to those used for blood transfusion. Marrow is infused intravenously into the recipient in a manner that is similar to a red blood cell transfusion.

If the source of stem cells used is the patient, the transplant is termed *autologous. Syngeneic* stem cells are obtained from an identical twin. If the stem cells are from a nonidentical individual, the transplant is termed *allogeneic*. The best donors for allogeneic transplantation are siblings who inherit identical HLA haplotypes (i.e., chromosome 6, which encodes HLA) from each parent. On average, siblings have a 25% chance of being HLA identical. If an allogeneic source of stem cells is needed and no HLA identical sibling is available, alternative donors include unrelated donors who are phenotypically matched at HLA (i.e., at least five of six HLA loci matched) and umbilical cord blood. Registries of donors whose HLA types are known and who are willing to donate marrow have expanded dramatically. More than 2 million individuals are in the National Marrow Donor Program in the United States.

For neoplastic diseases that can be effectively treated with high-dose chemotherapy followed by autologous transplantation, autologous PBSC have become the most widely used source of hematopoietic stem cells. PBSC are obtained after the host is recovered from chemotherapy or a human protein that stimulates white blood cell production (granulocyte or granulocyte/macrophage colony-stimulating factor [G- or GM-CSF]). The increased number of stem cells that are released into the blood can be harvested using apheresis. Apheresis generally takes 3 to 4 hr per session, and it requires intravenous access capable of high flow rates. A cryoprotectant is added to harvested PBSC before controlled rate freezing to maintain viability when and after the cells are frozen for convenient storage. Cryopreserved PBSC are rapidly thawed and infused into the patient after high-dose chemotherapy, with or without radiation. When infused in adequate numbers, PBSC can be used in allogeneic or autologous transplants to promote rapid recovery of hematopoiesis.

Autologous stem cell transplantation is used for various high-risk chemotherapy-responsive neoplastic diseases, including many of the common childhood cancers that are known to be at high risk of treatment failure with standard therapy because of previous relapse or initial extent of disease. Results are best if patients can achieve a state of minimal residual disease with other forms of therapy before transplantation. Although a major limitation of the procedure is the relatively high incidence of recurrent disease, durable remissions and cures have been obtained in situations where conventional chemotherapy or radiotherapy or both did not produce durable responses.

Allogeneic transplantation remains a high morbidity and mortality procedure. Common side effects include sterility, severe mucositis, pancytopenia, early and late susceptibility to opportunistic infections, difficulty eating, and veno-occlusive disease of the liver. Allogenic transplantation can also be complicated by *graft versus host disease (GVHD)*, a process mediated by reactivity of the donor T cells against host tissues (see Chapter 137). Prevention of GVHD requires depletion of T cells from the hematopoietic stem cell graft or pharmacologic immunosuppression in the early phases of the transplant.

Commonly used regimens to prevent GVHD include cyclosporine with or without methotrexate and/or steroids. Acute GVHD may comprise macular rash, diarrhea, or liver function abnormalities (i.e., elevation of alkaline phosphatase and 5′ nucleotidase). Accurate diagnosis of GVHD generally requires biopsy of skin, intestine, rectum, or liver. Treatment of acute GVHD is with corticosteroids with or without antithymocyte globulin. Some patients also develop chronic GVHD manifested by dry eyes, dry mouth, skin changes, or liver abnormalities. For GVHD to be considered chronic, symptoms must be present at least 3 mo after transplant.

Because of the high risks associated with allogeneic transplantation, it is generally reserved for life-threatening or lethal conditions such as cancer and primary disorders of the marrow or immune system in which other therapy including autologous transplantation would not be as effective. Examples include juvenile myelomonocytic leukemia, acute lymphoblastic leukemia (ALL) in second or greater remission, ALL at very high risk of relapse because of specific chromosomal abnormalities, acute myeloid leukemia in first or second remission, chronic myelogenous leukemia, severe combined immunodeficiency, hemophagocytic lymphohistiocytosis, aplastic anemia, Diamond-Blackfan anemia, severe β thalassemia, and some inborn errors of metabolism.

501.5 Palliative Care (also see Chapter 38)

For a minority of children with cancer, the disease is lethal. At all stages of caring for children with cancer, particularly dying patients, principles of palliative care should be applied to relieve pain and suffering and to provide comfort (Fig. 501–1).

Pain is a serious cause of suffering among patients with cancer and may be due to organ obstruction or compression and bone metastasis; pain may also be neuropathic. Pain should be managed in a stepwise manner (Fig. 501–2) in accordance with the principles of selecting the appropriate analgesic, prescribing the appropriate dose, administering the drug by the appropriate route, and choosing an appropriate drug dosing schedule to prevent persistent pain and relieve breakthrough pain. In addition, the dose should be aggressively titrated while attempts are made to prevent, anticipate, and manage side effects. Adjuvant drugs and sequential trials of analgesic drugs should be considered.

Additional palliative care issues are noted in Table 501–5. The goals in the care of dying patients are to avoid distress for the patient, family, and caregivers; to be in general accord with the patient's and family's wishes; and to be consistent with clinical, cultural, and ethical standards.

Treatment and Bone Marrow Transplantation

Armitage JO: Bone marrow transplantation. N Engl J Med 330:827, 1994.

Curtis RE, Rowlings PA, Geeg J, et al: Solid cancers after bone marrow transplantation. N Engl J Med 336:897, 1997.

Falk S, Fallon M: Emergencies. Br Med J 315:1525, 1997.

Frewin R, Henson A, Provan D: Haematological emergencies. Br Med J 314:1333, 1997.

Harris AL: Are angiostatin and endostatin cures for cancer? Lancet 351:1598, 1998.

Hartmann LC, Tschetter LK, Habermann TM, et al: Granulocyte colony-stimulating factor in severe chemotherapy-induced afebrile neutropenia. N Engl J Med 336:1776, 1997.

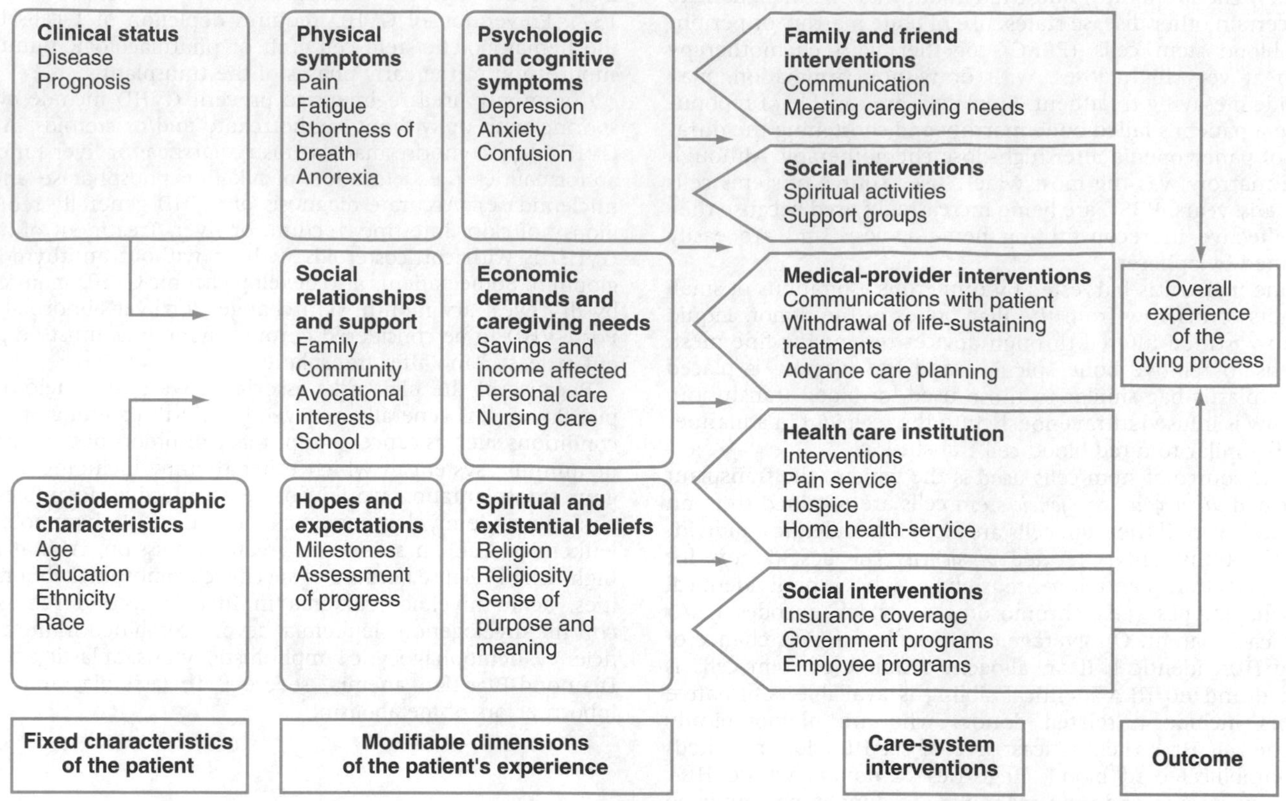

Figure 501–1 Framework for palliative care of cancer patients. (From Emanuel E, Emanuel L: The promise of a good death. Lancet 351:SII21, 1998.)

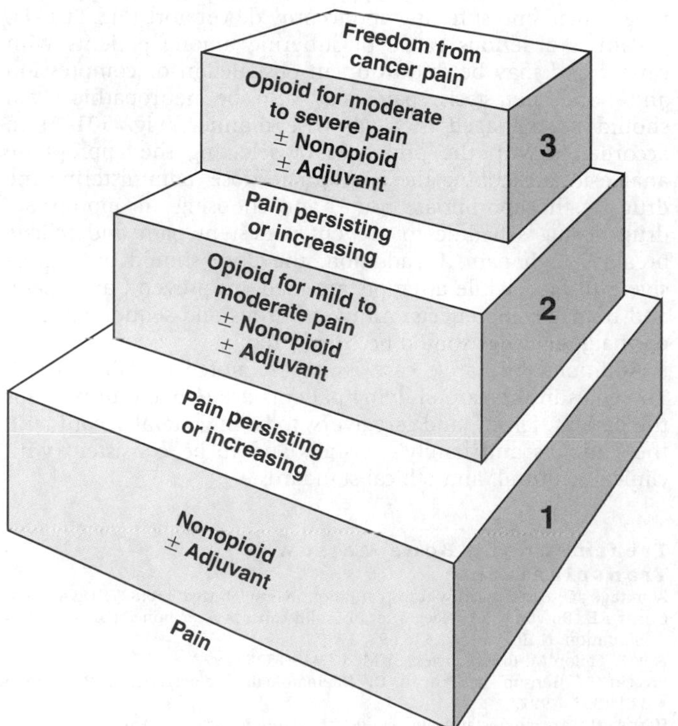

Figure 501–2 Stepwise approach to pain management. (Reproduced by permission from WHO from Cancer Pain Relief, 2nd ed. Geneva, World Health Organization, 1996.)

TABLE 501–5 Suggested Assessment Questions for Palliative Cancer Care

Modifiable Dimension of Patient's Experience	Specific Area	Suggested Assessment Questions	Potential Follow-up Questions
Physical symptoms	General Pain	• What symptom bothers you most? • Aside from everyday kinds of pain like minor headaches, sprains, or toothaches, how much pain have you had during the past week?	• Are you taking your pain medication as prescribed? • Would you like more treatment for your pain, have the same treatment, or have less treatment for your pain?
Psychologic and cognitive symptoms	Depression	• During the past 4 weeks, how much of the time have you felt downhearted and blue?	• Do you know what is bothering you? • Would you like to see someone to talk about your feelings?
Economic demands and caregiving needs	Economic demands	• How much of an economic or financial hardship is the cost of your illness and medical care for you and your family? • Has your illness meant having to use all or most of your family's savings?	• What is costing you and your family so much?
	Caregiving needs	• How much help do you need with personal care, such as help with bathing or eating? • How much help have you needed from someone in your family?	• How much additional help do you need with personal care? • Would having a home-health aide be of help?
Social relationships and supports	Social support	• How often is there someone to confide in and talk to about yourself or your problems? • How often is there someone to have a good time with?	
Spiritual and existential beliefs	Spiritual beliefs	• Since your illness, have you become more spiritual or religious? • Do you pray?	• Do you have a spiritual or religious community that helps in your personal spiritual journey? • What have you been praying for?
Hopes and expectations	Milestones	• Is there a special event that would add a great deal of meaning to your life?	• What do we have to do to make sure that event takes place?
Advance-care planning	Advance-care directive	• Have you filled out a living will stating your preferences for medical care in case of a life-threatening situation? • Have you talked to your family about your plans regarding your medical care at the end of your life?	

From Emanuel EJ, Emanuel LL: The promise of a good death. Lancet 351: SII21, 1998.

Lane D: The promise of molecular oncology. Lancet 351:SII17, 1998.
Sanders JE: Bone marrow transplantation for pediatric malignancies. Pediatr Clin North Am 44:1005, 1997
Sarafoglou K, Boulad F, Gillio A, et al: Gonadal function after bone marrow transplantation for acute leukemia during childhood. J Pediatr 130:210, 1997.
Tannock IF: Conventional cancer therapy: Promise broken or promise delayed. Lancet 351:SII9, 1998.

Palliative Care

Emanuel EJ, Emanuel LL: The promise of good death. Lancet 351:SII21, 1998.
Levy MH: Pharmacologic treatment of cancer pain. N Engl J Med 335:1124, 1996.

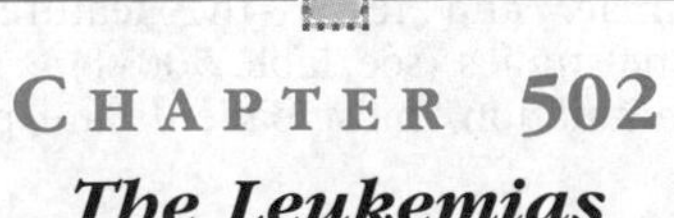

CHAPTER 502
The Leukemias

William M. Crist and William A. Smithson

Leukemias, the most common childhood cancers, account for about one third of pediatric malignancies. Acute lymphoblastic leukemia (ALL) represents about 75% of all cases in children and has a peak incidence at age 4 yr. Acute myeloid leukemia (AML) accounts for about 20% of leukemias, with an incidence that is stable from birth through age 10 and increases slightly during the teenage years. Most of the remaining leukemias are of the chronic myeloid form; chronic lymphoid leukemia rarely affects children. The overall annual incidence of leukemia in white children is 43.7 per million population and in black children, 24.3 per million children age 0 to 14 yr. The clinical features of the leukemias are similar, because all involve severe disruption of bone marrow function. Specific clinical and laboratory features differ, however, and there is marked variability in responses to therapy and in prognosis.

502.1 Acute Lymphoblastic Leukemia

Childhood ALL was the first form of disseminated cancer shown to be curable with chemotherapy and irradiation. ALL occurs slightly more frequently in boys than girls. Reports of geographic clusters of childhood leukemia have suggested some shared environmental factor. Some studies suggest an in utero origin for leukemias presenting between 5 mo and 2 yr of age. Investigations to date have not discovered the cause. Lymphoid leukemias occur more often than expected in patients with Down and Bloom's syndromes and in immunodeficiency diseases (e.g., congenital hypogammaglobulinemia, ataxia-telangiectasia). Epstein-Barr virus has been implicated in the pathogenesis of some cases of B-cell leukemia.

PATHOLOGY. ALL is subclassified according to the morphologic, immunologic, cytogenetic, and molecular genetic features of the leukemic cells. Definitive diagnosis is generally based on examination of a bone marrow aspirate. The cytologic appearance of the blast cells is so variable, even within a single

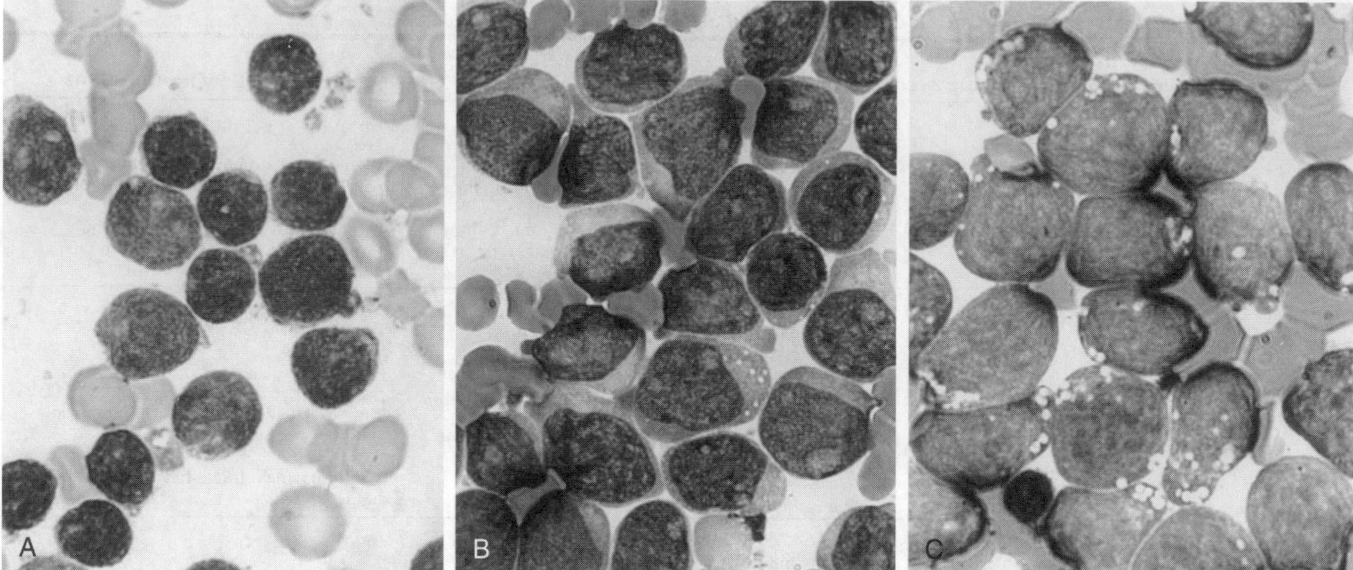

Figure 502–1 Examples of FAB morphologic subtypes of ALL. *A,* L1 blasts are small with scanty cytoplasm; *B,* L2 blasts are larger with more cytoplasm, irregular nuclear membranes, and prominent nucleoli; *C,* L3 blasts have basophilic cytoplasm with vacuolization. See also color section.

specimen, that no completely satisfactory morphologic classification has been devised. The French-American-British (FAB) system distinguishes three morphologic subtypes, L1 to L3. L1 lymphoblasts are predominantly small, with little cytoplasm; L2 cells are larger and pleomorphic with increased cytoplasm, irregular nuclear shape, and prominent nucleoli; and L3 cells have finely stippled and homogeneous nuclear chromatin, prominent nucleoli, and deep blue cytoplasm with prominent vacuolation (Fig. 502–1). Because of the essentially subjective distinction between L1 and L2 blasts and a poor correlation with immunologic and genetic findings, only the L3 subtype appears clinically meaningful.

Classification of ALL therefore depends on a combination of cytologic, immunologic, and karyotypic features. Monoclonal antibodies that recognize lineage-associated cell surface antigens can determine the immunophenotype in most cases. The majority are derived from B-progenitor cells; about 15% derive from T-progenitor cells, and 1% from relatively mature B cells. These immunophenotypes have both prognostic and therapeutic implications. The subtypes of ALL and their relative incidences are shown in Table 502–1, along with certain clinical characteristics. A minority of cases cannot be readily classified because they demonstrate antigen expression associated with several different cell lineages (i.e., mixed lineage or biphenotypic ALL).

Chromosomal abnormalities can be identified in at least 80% of childhood ALL. The karyotypes of leukemic cells have diagnostic, prognostic, and therapeutic significance. Further, they pinpoint sites for molecular studies to detect genes that may be involved in leukemic transformation and proliferation. Childhood ALL can also be classified by the number of chromosomes per leukemic cell (ploidy) and by structural chromosomal rearrangements such as translocations.

Another biologic marker with potential usefulness is terminal deoxynucleotidyltransferase (TdT) activity, which is present in B-progenitor-cell and T-cell ALL. Because this enzyme is absent in normal lymphocytes, it can be useful in identifying leukemic cells in difficult diagnostic situations. For example, TdT activity in cells from cerebrospinal fluid (CSF) may help to distinguish early central nervous system (CNS) relapse from aseptic meningitis.

Most patients with leukemia have disseminated disease at diagnosis, with widespread bone marrow involvement and the presence of leukemic blast cells in circulating blood. Spleen, liver, and lymph nodes are usually involved. Hence, there is no anatomic staging system for ALL. However, other features are used to assign children to groups with better and worse prognosis.

CLINICAL MANIFESTATIONS. About two thirds of children with ALL have had signs and symptoms of their disease for less than 4 wk at the time of diagnosis. The first symptoms are usually nonspecific and may include anorexia, irritability, and lethargy. Patients may have a history of viral respiratory infection or exanthem from which they have not appeared to recover fully. Progressive bone marrow failure leads to pallor, bleeding, petechiae, and fever—the features that usually prompt diagnostic studies (see Table 500–1).

On initial examination, most patients are pale, and about

TABLE 502–1 Incidence of the Subtypes of Acute Lymphoblastic Leukemia in a Single Study, with Incidence of Some Clinical Features at the Time of Diagnosis

Subtype	No. of Patients	%	Age (Median)	Leukocyte Count (× 10^3) (Median)	% Male	% with a Mediastinal Mass	Associated Chromosomal Abnormalities
T (T +)	44	14	7.4 yr	61.2	67.1	38.2	t(11;14)
B (slg +)	2	0.6					t(8;14)
PreB (clg +)	56	18	4.7 yr	12.2	54.8	1.2	t(1;19)
Early preB (T−, slg −, clg−)	209	67	4.4 yr	12.4	56.5	1.0	t(9;22)
Infant early preB	33	NA	< 1 yr	50.0	55	None	t(4;11)

Adapted from Pullen JD, Boyett JM, Crist WM, et al: Pediatric Oncology Group utilization of immunologic markers in the designation of acute lymphoblastic leukemia subgroups. Influence on treatment response. Ann N Y Acad Sci 428:26, 1983.

50% have petechiae or mucous membrane bleeding. About 25% have fever, which may be falsely ascribed to an upper respiratory infection or otitis media. Lymphadenopathy is occasionally prominent; splenomegaly is found in about 60% of patients, whereas hepatomegaly is less common. About 25% of patients present with significant bone pain and arthralgias caused by leukemic infiltration of the perichondral bone or joint or by leukemic expansion of the marrow cavity. Rarely, signs of increased intracranial pressure, such as headache and vomiting, indicate leukemic meningeal involvement. Children with T-cell ALL are likely to be older and are more often male; many have an anterior mediastinal mass, a feature that is strongly associated with this subtype of the disease (see Table 500–1).

DIAGNOSIS. On initial examination, most patients have anemia, although only about 25% have hemoglobin levels below 6 g/dL. Most patients also have thrombocytopenia, but as many as 25% have platelet counts greater than 100,000/mm^3. About half of the patients have white blood cell (WBC) counts less than 10,000/mm^3, and about 20% have counts greater than 50,000/mm^3. The diagnosis of leukemia is suggested by the presence of blast cells on a peripheral blood smear but is confirmed by examination of bone marrow, which is usually completely replaced by leukemic lymphoblasts. The marrow occasionally is initially hypocellular. Cytogenetic studies in these cases may be useful in identifying specific abnormalities associated with preleukemic syndromes. If the marrow cannot be aspirated or the specimen is hypocellular, bone marrow biopsy provides the needed material for study. Cytogenetic studies can be performed on biopsy specimens if they are placed in tissue culture medium.

A chest radiograph is necessary to search for a mediastinal mass. Bone radiographs may show altered medullary trabeculae, cortical defects, or subepiphyseal bone resorption. These findings lack clinical or prognostic significance, and a skeletal survey is usually unnecessary. CSF should be examined for leukemic cells, as early involvement of the CNS has important prognostic and therapeutic implications. Uric acid level and renal function should be determined before treatment is started (see Chapter 501.2).

DIFFERENTIAL DIAGNOSIS. The diagnosis of ALL is usually straightforward once the possibility has been considered. Inclusion of ALL in the differential diagnosis may be delayed if a child has been sick and febrile with adenopathy for several weeks. The differential diagnosis includes bone marrow failure due to aplastic anemia and myelofibrosis. Infectious mononucleosis produces a somewhat similar clinical picture, but careful examination of the blood smear should identify atypical lymphocytes. If doubt remains, a bone marrow aspirate demonstrates a normal cell population. Some patients have unexplained fever and joint pain that has been diagnosed as rheumatoid arthritis for months. Mature lymphocytosis secondary to pertussis or benign lymphocytosis is easily distinguished from ALL by morphology alone. Infiltration of the marrow by other types of malignant cells (neuroblastoma, rhabdomyosarcoma, Ewing's sarcoma, and retinoblastoma) can occasionally produce pancytopenia. These tumor cells are usually found in clumps scattered throughout normal marrow tissue but may occasionally replace the marrow completely. Evidence of a primary tumor is usually found in some other site.

TREATMENT. Contemporary treatment of ALL is based on clinical risk, although there is no universal definition of risk groups. In general, patients with a standard or average risk of relapse are between the ages of 1 and 10 yr, have a WBC count under 100,000/mm^3, lack evidence of a mediastinal mass or CNS leukemia, and have a B-progenitor cell immunophenotype. The presence of certain specific chromosomal translocations (as discussed later) should be ruled out. The treatment program for standard-risk patients includes administration of induction chemotherapy until the bone marrow no longer shows morphologically identifiable leukemic cells, "prophylactic" treatment of the CNS, and continuation chemotherapy. A sample treatment plan is outlined in Table 502–2.

A combination of prednisone, vincristine, and asparaginase produces remission in about 98% of children with standard-risk ALL within 4 wk. Fewer than 5% of patients require another 2 wk of induction therapy. Consolidation and intensification phases of therapy using several chemotherapeutic agents are often given after the induction of remission to produce further rapid reduction in leukemic cell number and improve ultimate outcome. Systemic continuation therapy includes the antimetabolites methotrexate and 6-mercaptopurine plus vincristine and prednisone, which should be given for 2 to 3 yr.

In the absence of prophylactic treatment, the CNS was the initial site of relapse in more than 50% of patients. Leukemic cells are usually present in the meninges at diagnosis even if they are not identifiable in the CSF. These cells survive systemic chemotherapy because of poor drug penetration of the blood-brain barrier. Cranial irradiation prevents overt CNS leukemia in most patients but produces late neuropsychologic effects, particularly in younger children. Therefore, standard-risk patients typically receive intrathecal chemotherapy to prevent clinical CNS involvement.

Patients with T-cell ALL often suffer a relapse within 3 to 4 yr if treated with a standard-risk regimen. With more intensive multidrug regimens, 50% or more achieve long-term remission. One goal is to develop targeted therapy that exploits the unique characteristics of leukemic T cells. As an example of this approach, monoclonal antibodies to T-cell-associated surface antigens can be conjugated to immunotoxins. The antibody-immunotoxin complex would then attach to T lymphoblasts, undergo endocytosis, and kill the cells.

B-cell cases with L3 morphology and surface immunoglobulin expression have had a poor prognosis. These patients are now best treated with short (3–6 mo) but very intensive regimens developed for advanced B-cell lymphoma. With this approach, cure rates have improved dramatically, from 20% a decade ago to over 70% or more.

RELAPSE. The bone marrow is the most common site of relapse, although any site can be affected. In most centers, bone

TABLE 502–2 An Effective Treatment Regimen for Low-Risk Acute Lymphoblastic Leukemia

Remission Induction (4–6 wk)

Vincristine 1.5 mg/m^2 (max. 2 mg) IV/wk
Prednisone 40 mg/m^2 (max. 60 mg) po/day
Asparaginase 10,000 U/m^2/day biweekly IM

Intrathecal Treatment

Triple therapy: MTX*
HC*
Ara-C*
Wkly × 6 during induction and then every 8 wk for 2 yr

Systemic Continuation Treatment

6-MP 50 mg/m^2/day PO
MTX 20 mg/m^2/wk PO, IV, IM
Pulse of MTX ± 6-MP given at higher doses

With Reinforcement

Vincristine 1.5 mg/m^2 (max. 2 mg) IV every 4 wks
Prednisone 40 mg/m^2/day PO × 7 days every 4 wks

MTX = methotrexate; HC = hydrocortisone; Ara-C = cytarabine; IV = intravenous; PO = oral; IM = intramuscular; 6-MP = 6-mercaptopurine.
**The dose of intrathecal medication is age adjusted.*

Age*	MTX	HC	Ara-C
≤1 yr	10 mg	10 mg	20 mg
2–8 yr	12.5 mg	12.5 mg	25 mg
≥ 9 yr	15 mg	16 mg	30 mg

marrow is examined at infrequent intervals to confirm continued remission. If bone marrow relapse is detected, intensive retrieval therapy that includes drugs not used previously may achieve cures in 15–20% of patients, especially those who have had a long first remission (≥18 mo). For patients who experience bone marrow relapse during treatment, intensive chemotherapy followed by bone marrow transplantation from a matched sibling or related donor offers a better chance of cure. Autologous, haploidentical, or matched unrelated donor transplants are options for those without histocompatible sibling donors (Chapter 501.4).

The most important extramedullary sites of relapse are the CNS and the testes. The early manifestations of CNS leukemia are due to increased intracranial pressure and include vomiting, headache, papilledema, and lethargy. Chemical meningitis secondary to intrathecal therapy can produce the same symptoms and must be considered in the differential diagnosis. Convulsions and isolated cranial nerve palsies may occur with CNS leukemia or as side effects of methotrexate or vincristine. Hypothalamic involvement is rare but must be suspected in the presence of excessive weight gain or behavioral disturbances. CSF pressure is usually elevated, and the fluid shows a pleocytosis due to leukemic cells. If the cell count is normal, leukemic cells may be identified in smears of CSF specimens after centrifugation (i.e., cytospin).

Patients with CNS relapse should be given intrathecal chemotherapy weekly for 4 to 6 wk until lymphoblasts have disappeared from the CSF. Doses should be age adjusted because CSF volume is not proportional to body surface area (see Table 502–2). Cranial irradiation is the only treatment that completely eradicates overt CNS leukemia and should be given after intrathecal therapy. Systemic treatment should also be intensified, because these patients are at high risk of subsequent bone marrow relapse. Finally, preventive CNS therapy should be repeated in any patient whose disease has reoccurred in the bone marrow or in any extramedullary site.

Testicular relapse generally produces painless swelling of one or both testicles. Patients are often unaware of the abnormality, mandating careful attention to testicular size at diagnosis and during follow-up. The diagnosis is confirmed by biopsy. Treatment should include irradiation of the gonads. Because a testicular relapse usually signals impending bone marrow relapse, systemic therapy should be reinforced for patients who are still on treatment or reinstituted for those who have a relapse after treatment. CNS-directed therapy should also be repeated.

PROGNOSIS. The overall cure rate for childhood ALL is estimated at about 80%. Thus, parents can generally be assured at the time of diagnosis that the possibility of cure is very good. Numerous clinical features have emerged as prognostic indicators, only to lose their significance as treatment improves. For example, immunophenotype is important in assigning risk-directed therapy, but its prognostic significance has largely been eliminated by contemporary treatment regimens. Hence, appropriate risk-directed treatment is the single most important prognostic factor. The initial WBC count has a consistent inverse linear relationship to the likelihood of cure. Age at diagnosis is also a reliable predictor. Patients who are older than 10 yr and those younger than 12 mo and who have a chromosomal rearrangement involving the 11q23 region fare much worse than children in the intermediate age group. Several other chromosomal abnormalities influence treatment outcome. Hyperdiploidy with more than 50 chromosomes is associated with a favorable outcome and responds well to antimetabolite-based therapy. Two chromosomal translocations—the t(9;22), or Philadelphia chromosome, and the t(4;11)—confer a poor prognosis. Some advocate bone marrow transplantation during initial remission in patients with these translocations. B-progenitor-cell ALL with the t(1;19) has a somewhat less promising prognosis than other cases with this immunophenotype; only 60% of patients will still be in remission after 5 yr unless intensive therapy is used. Rearrangement of TEL/AML1 genes in B-progenitor ALL appears to confer an exceptionally favorable prognosis, regardless of WBC count or age, and is present in 25% of this phenotype of ALL.

502.2 Acute Myeloid Leukemia

Carola A. S. Arndt and Peter A. Anderson

AML accounts for 15–20% of the approximately 2,500 cases of pediatric leukemia diagnosed in the United States annually. Certain genetic conditions, such as trisomy 21, Diamond-Blackfan syndrome, Fanconi's aplastic anemia, Bloom's syndrome, Kostmann's syndrome, paroxysmal nocturnal hemoglobinuria, Li-Fraumeni syndrome, and neurofibromatosis are associated with a predisposition to development of AML. Exposure to drugs such as alkylating agents, epipodophyllotoxins, and nitrosoureas and to ionizing radiation are also associated with an increased risk of developing AML.

CLINICAL MANIFESTATIONS. AML may present with signs and symptoms related to anemia, thrombocytopenia, or neutropenia (see Table 500–1). Children may present with fatigue and pallor or heart failure secondary to anemia. Bruising, petechiae, epistaxis, or gum bleeding secondary to thrombocytopenia may be presenting manifestations, as may fever secondary to infection associated with neutropenia. Patients sometimes have hepatic or splenic enlargement, lymphadenopathy, or gum hypertrophy. A localized mass of leukemic cells, known as a *chloroma,* may herald the onset of AML. Orbital or epidural locations are common sites of chloromas. At diagnosis, anemia and thrombocytopenia are usually profound. The WBC may be normal, high, or low. With extremely high WBC count (>100,000/mm³), sludging of blood due to increased viscosity and stickiness of the WBCs may occur, resulting in cerebrovascular symptoms (see Table 501–2).

DIAGNOSIS. The diagnosis of AML requires demonstration of greater than 25% myeloblasts in the bone marrow. Characterization of the blasts morphologically, immunophenotypically, and immunohistochemically distinguishes ALL from AML. Within AML, the most commonly used classification system is the FAB, which separates AML into seven subtypes according to morphologic appearance and histochemical staining properties (Table 502–3). Certain karyotypic abnormalities are associated with specific subtypes of AML. For example, t(15;17) is found in most cases of acute promyelocytic leukemia (APL). APL is often associated with a life-threatening form of disseminated intravascular coagulation at presentation owing to release of procoagulant substances from the leukemic blast cells.

TABLE 502–3 Subtypes of Nonlymphoid Leukemia

Type	FAB Classification
Acute myeloid leukemia (AML)	
Myeloblastic, no maturation	M0 and M1
Myeloblastic, some maturation	M2
Hypergranular promyelocytic	M3
Myelomonocytic	M4
Monocytic	M5
Erythroleukemia	M6
Megakaryocytic	M7
Chronic myelocytic leukemia (CML)	
Adult form	
Chronic phase	
Accelerated phase	
Blast crisis	
Juvenile myelomonocytic leukemia (JMML)	

Inversion of chromosome 16 is often associated with eosinophilia and the FAB M4 subtype.

Secondary leukemia is often associated with chromosomal abnormalities, which affect 11q23 or with monosomy 7. Myelodysplastic syndrome, which often evolves into AML, may have associated chromosomal changes such as trisomy 8 or deletion of chromosome 5 or 7 (monosomy).

TREATMENT. With aggressive initial induction regimens containing an anthracycline and cytosine arabinoside with or without other agents, remission can be achieved in 80% or more of patients. About 10% of patients die early (i.e., during induction therapy) as a result of induction failure, overwhelming infection, or hemorrhage. Vigorous supportive care with broad-spectrum antibiotics, antifungals, blood products, and nutritional support must be provided. Up to 6 wk or longer may be required to induce remission and for the marrow to recover from the effects of chemotherapy. During this time, most patients are critically ill. CNS prophylaxis with intrathecal chemotherapy is also required to minimize the likelihood of CNS relapse. After initial induction of remission, children who have an HLA-matched related stem cell donor should undergo stem cell transplantation. Either bone marrow or peripheral blood stem cells can be used. About 70% of patients who can receive a matched sibling transplant are cured. Optimal therapy for patients who do not have a matched donor is yet to be defined. The use of interleukin 2 to produce immune modulation with an antileukemic effect is under study during remission after completion of chemotherapy.

Patients with APL benefit from retinoic acid in addition to chemotherapy including anthracycline. Such patients should not receive marrow transplants in first remission. For reasons that are not understood, children with Down syndrome and AML have a particularly good cure rate (⩾80%) with chemotherapy alone.

PROGNOSIS. For patients with an HLA-matched family donor, the cure rate is about 70% using chemotherapy followed by bone marrow transplantation. For those without a suitable donor, chemotherapy alone cures about 50%. Myelodysplastic syndrome or secondary AML does not usually respond in a durable manner to chemotherapy. Children with AML who relapse have an extremely poor prognosis. If they do not have an HLA identical donor, they should be considered for alternative types of bone marrow transplantation such as HLA-matched unrelated donor, cord blood transplants, or haploidentical transplants, although such transplants are associated with a very high risk of complications including infection and graft versus host disease.

502.3 Juvenile Chronic Myelogenous Leukemia (JCML) or Juvenile Myelomonocytic Leukemia (JMML)

JMML is a clonal condition involving the pluripotent stem cell, usually presenting in children younger than 2 yr.

CLINICAL MANIFESTATIONS. Frequent presenting clinical features include skin lesions (e.g., eczema, xanthoma, café au lait spots), lymphadenopathy, and hepatosplenomegaly which may be massive and cause respiratory embarrassment. Patients with type I neurofibromatosis have an increased incidence of JMML.

DIAGNOSIS. JMML is characterized by peripheral blood monocytosis, increased marrow monocyte precursors, peripheral blood blast count of less than 5%, marrow blast count of less than 30%, thrombocytopenia, anemia, and leukocytosis. Erythrocytes have fetal characteristics including increased fetal hemoglobin and i antigen score. The Philadelphia chromosome is absent. Most cases have normal cytogenetics; cytogenetic abnormalities, when found, usually involve chromosome 7 or 8.

TREATMENT. The treatment of choice for JMML is bone marrow transplantation. Unfortunately, up to 50% of patients suffer relapse even after transplantation. Treatment with chemotherapy has limited effectiveness, although durable remissions have been observed occasionally.

502.4 Leukemia and Down Syndrome

Patients with Down syndrome have a risk of developing leukemia that is 10 to 30 times that of the general population.

Neonates and infants with Down syndrome may have a condition known as *transient myeloproliferative syndrome*, which mimics congenital leukemia. Such patients may have hepatosplenomegaly, anemia, thrombocytopenia, and a significant leukemoid reaction. These abnormalities usually resolve spontaneously. Close follow-up is indicated because these children have a higher incidence of subsequent development of leukemia, especially the acute megakaryocytic subtype of AML (FAB M7). Children who have Down syndrome and who develop AML have a much better prognosis than do other children; the reason for the superior outcome is unknown.

502.5 Chronic Myelogenous Leukemia

William M. Crist

Chronic myelogenous leukemia (CML) is a clonal disorder of the hematopoietic stem cell characterized by a specific translocation, the t(9;22)(q34;q11), known as the Philadelphia chromosome. This translocation juxtaposes the *bcr* gene on chromosome 22 with the *abl* gene on chromosome 9, producing a fusion gene that encodes the bcr-abl fusion protein. CML accounts for only 3–5% of cases of leukemia in children. In most cases there are no predisposing features.

CML has a biphasic or triphasic course. During the chronic phase, which usually lasts for 3–4 yr, WBC counts are easily controlled with low-dose chemotherapy such as hydroxyurea or with interferon. Progression to a myeloid or lymphoid blast crisis resembling acute leukemia may occur rapidly or may follow an accelerated phase of the disease. In the accelerated phase or blast crisis, the blood counts become difficult to control and additional cytogenetic abnormalities often develop.

PATHOLOGY. CML is characterized by myeloid hyperplasia with increased numbers of differentiating myeloid cells in blood and bone marrow. The Philadelphia chromosome is easily detectable by cytogenetic analysis in most cases; in most other patients, Southern blot analysis or polymerase chain reaction techniques reveals the *bcr-abl* rearrangement.

CLINICAL FEATURES. The onset of symptoms is generally insidious, and the diagnosis is made when a blood count is performed for another reason. Patients may present with splenomegaly (which can be massive) or with symptoms of hypermetabolism, including weight loss, anorexia, and night sweats. Symptoms of leukostasis, such as visual disturbance or priapism, rarely occur.

DIAGNOSIS. Laboratory abnormalities are usually confined initially to elevated WBC counts, which may exceed 100,000/mm^3, with all forms of myeloid cells seen in the blood smear. Platelet counts may also be abnormally high. Other laboratory abnormalities include elevated serum levels of vitamin B_{12} and uric acid and reduced or absent WBC alkaline phosphatase activity. The bone marrow is hypercellular, with normal myeloid cells in all stages of differentiation; megakaryocytes may be increased in number. Eosinophilia or basophilia or both are common. Cytogenetic or molecular studies showing the Philadelphia chromosome confirm the diagnosis.

TREATMENT. In the chronic phase, leukocytosis and symptoms can be controlled by chemotherapy with hydroxyurea, but the Philadelphia chromosome will not be suppressed. In addition to controlling the leukocytosis, α interferon produces cytogenetic remission in about 20% of cases; it appears to lengthen the chronic phase. The best treatment for children is allogenic bone marrow transplant. The long-term survival rate of children who receive an allograft from an HLA-identical sibling in early chronic phase is about 80%. When the donor is a partially matched family member or a matched unrelated individual, transplant-related mortality is higher and survival is around 50–60%. Lymphoid blast crisis can usually be reverted to the chronic phase with standard ALL therapy, whereas myeloid crisis is generally refractory to standard AML chemotherapy, and the median survival is only 3–4 mo. If bone marrow transplant is delayed until the accelerated phase or until blast crisis occurs, survival is reduced.

Molecular Pathogenesis

Caldas C: Molecular assessment of cancer. Br Med J 316:1360, 1998.
Fearon ER: Human cancer syndromes: Clues to the origin and nature of cancer. Science 278:1043, 1997.
Haber DA, Fearon ER: The promise of cancer genetics. Lancet 351:SII1, 1998.
Look AT: Oncogenic transcription factors in the human acute leukemias. Science 278:1059, 1998.
Nichols KE, Li FP, Haber DA, et al: Childhood cancer predisposition: Applications of molecular testing and future implications. J Pediatr 132:389, 1998.
Rubnitz JE, Crist WM: Molecular genetics of childhood cancer: Implications for pathogenesis, diagnosis, and treatment. Pediatrics 100:101,1997.
Wong FL, Boice JD, Abramson DH, et al: Cancer incidence after retinoblastoma. JAMA 278:1261, 1997.

Acute Lymphoblastic Leukemia

Evans WE, Relling MV, Rodman JH, et al: Conventional compared with individualized chemotherapy for childhood acute lymphoblastic leukemia. N Engl J Med 338:499, 1998.
Gale KB, Ford AM, Repp R, et al: Backtracking leukemia to birth: Identification of clonotypic gene fusion sequences in neonatal blood spots. Proc Natl Acad Sci U S A 94:13950, 1997.
Gorlick R, Goker E, Trippett T, et al: Intrinsic and acquired resistance to methotrexate in acute leukemia. N Engl J Med 14:1041, 1996.
Grundy RG, Leiper AD, Stanhope R, et al: Survival and endocrine outcome after testicular relapse in acute lymphoblastic leukaemia. Arch Dis Child 76:190, 1997.
Hongeng S, Krance RA, Bowman LC, et al: Outcomes of transplantation with matched-sibling and unrelated donor bone marrow in children with leukaemia. Lancet 350:767, 1997.
Liesner RJ, Goldstone AH: The acute leukaemias. Br Med J 314:733, 1997.
Linet MS, Hatch EE, Kleinerman RA: Residential exposure to magnetic fileds and acute lymphoblastic leukemia in children. N Engl J Med 337:1, 1997.
Nachman JB, Sather HN, Sensel MG, et al: Augumented post-induction therapy for children with high-risk acute lymphoblastic leukemia and a slow response to initial therapy. N Engl J Med 338:1663, 1998.
Pui CH: Acute lymphoblastic leukemia. Pediatr Clin North Am 44:831, 1997.
Roberts WM, Estrov Z, Ouspenskaia MV: Measurement of residual leukemia during remission in childhood acute lymphoblastic leukemia. N Engl J Med 336:317, 1997.

Down Syndrome and Leukemia

Lange B, Kobrinsky N, Barnard D, et al: Distinctive demography, biology and outcome of acute myeloid leukemia and myelodysplastic syndrome in children with Down syndrome: Children's cancer group studies 2861 and 2891. Blood 91:608, 1998.
Ragab A, Abdel-Mageed A, Shuster J, et al: Clinical characteristics and treatment outcome of children with acute lymphoblastic leukemia and Down's syndrome. A pediatric oncology group study. Cancer 67:1057, 1991.
Ravindranath Y, Abella E, Krischer J, et al: Acute myeloid leukemia in Down's syndrome is highly responsive to chemotherapy: Experience on pediatric oncology group AML study 8498. Blood 80:2210, 1992.

Acute and Chronic Myelogenous Leukemia

Arico M, Brandi A, Pui C-H: Juvenile myelomonocytic leukemia. Blood 90:479, 1997.
Ebb DH, Weinstein HJ: Diagnosis and treatment of childhood acute myelogenous leukemia. Pediatr Clin North Am 44:847, 1997.
Grier HE, Civin CI: Myeloid leukemias, myelodysplasia, and myeloproliferative diseases in children. *In*: Nathan DG, Orkin SH (eds): Nathan and Oski's Hematology of Infancy and Childhood, 5th ed. Philadelphia, WB Saunders, 1998, p 1286.
Kantajarian HM, Deisseroth A, Kurzrock R, et al: Chronic myelogenous leukemia: a concise update. Blood 82:691, 1993.
Liang D-C, Ma S W, Lu T H, et al: Transient myeloproliferative disorder and acute myeloid leukemia: Study of six neonatal cases with long-term follow-up. Leukemia 7:1521, 1993.
Tallman MS, Anderson JW, Schiffer CA, et al: All-*trans*-retinoic acid in acute promyelocytic leukemia. N Engl J Med 337:1021, 1997.

CHAPTER 503 Lymphoma

(See Chapters 494 to 496 for related discussion of the immune and lymphatic systems.)

Gerald S. Gilchrist

Lymphoma is the third most common cancer in children in the United States, with an annual incidence of 13.2 per million children. The two broad categories of lymphoma, Hodgkin's disease and non-Hodgkin's lymphoma (NHL) have such different clinical manifestations and treatments that they are considered separately.

503.1 Hodgkin's Disease

Hodgkin's disease accounts for about 5% of cancers in children and adolescents younger than 15 yr in the United States. This does not include the older adolescents who account for a substantial proportion of newly diagnosed patients. Although in industrialized countries the highest rate is in adolescents and young adults, in developing countries younger children are more frequently diagnosed.

Three forms of Hodgkin's disease have been identified in epidemiologic studies: a childhood form (≤ 14 yr old), a young adult form (15–34 yr old), and an older adult form (55–74 yr old). The epidemiologic similarities of Hodgkin's disease in young patients to paralytic polio in the 1940s and 1950s suggest an infectious cause. The possible role of Epstein-Barr virus (EBV) is further supported by serologic studies and the frequent presence of EBV genome in biopsy material. Males predominate in patients younger than 10 yr at diagnosis, with roughly equal gender incidence in adolescence. Pre-existing immunodeficiency, either congenital or acquired, increases the risk of developing Hodgkin's disease. A genetic predisposition or a common exposure to the same etiologic agent could account for an apparent increased risk in twins and first-degree relatives ranging from three to seven-fold.

PATHOLOGY. The Reed-Sternberg cell, a large (15 to 45 μm in diameter) cell with multiple or multilobulated nuclei, is considered the hallmark of Hodgkin's disease, although similar cells are seen in infectious mononucleosis, NHL, and other conditions. The cellular origin of the Reed-Sternberg cell remains in dispute. An infiltrate of apparently normal lymphocytes, plasma cells, and eosinophils surround the Reed-Sternberg cell and vary with the histologic subtype. Other features that distinguish the histologic subtypes include various degrees of fibrosis and the presence of collagen bands, necrosis, or malignant reticular cells. The four major histologic subtypes are *lymphocyte predominant, nodular sclerosing, mixed cellularity,* and *lymphocyte depleted*. Historically, prognosis was linked to histologic subtype, with lymphocyte predominant most favorable and lymphocyte depleted least favorable. Since the advent of curative therapy, their prognostic significance has diminished.

Hodgkin's disease appears to arise in lymphoid tissue and spreads to adjacent lymph node areas in a relatively orderly fashion. Hematogenous spread also occurs, leading to involve-

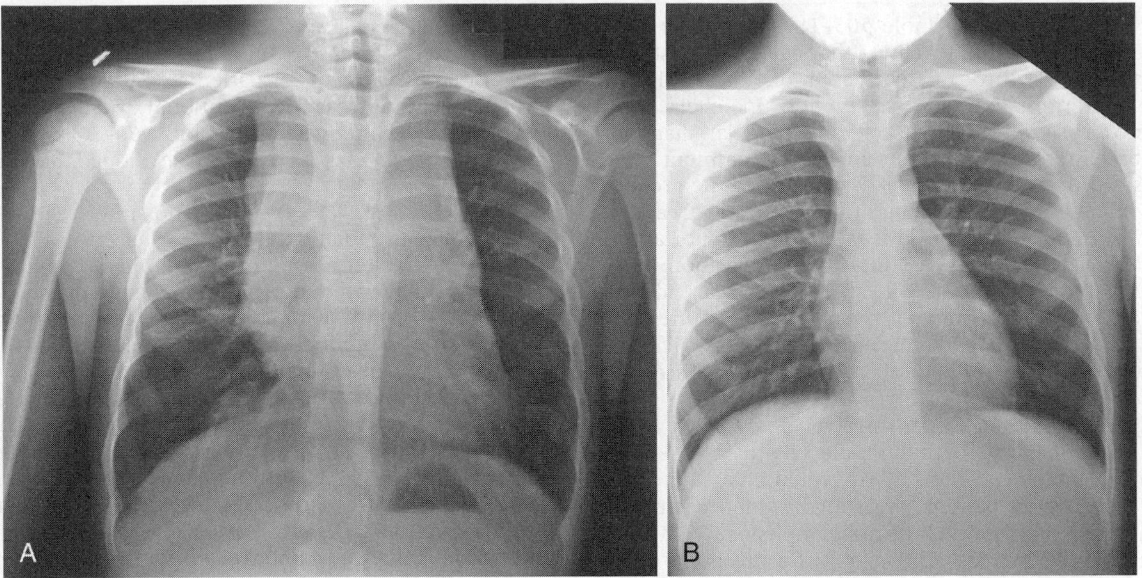

Figure 503–1 *A*, Anterior mediastinal mass in a patient with Hodgkin's disease prior to therapy. *B*, Complete disappearance of mediastinal mass in same patient 2 months following therapy.

ment of the liver, spleen, bone, bone marrow, or brain, and is usually associated with systemic symptoms. Levels of various cytokines have been shown to be elevated in patient sera or are produced by cultured cell lines or Hodgkin's disease tissue. They may well be responsible for the systemic symptoms of fever and night sweats (interleukin 1 or 2) and weight loss (tissue necrosis factor [TNF]).

Various degrees of cellular immune impairment can be identified in the majority of newly diagnosed Hodgkin's disease cases. The severity of the immune defect varies with the extent of disease and persists even after successful curative therapy. Whether it predisposes to the disease or results from it is unknown.

CLINICAL MANIFESTATIONS. Painless, firm, cervical or supraclavicular adenopathy is the most common presenting sign. Inguinal or axillary adenopathy sites are uncommon areas of presentation. An anterior mediastinal mass is often present and can disappear quickly with therapy (Fig. 503–1*A* and *B*). Clinically detectable hepatosplenomegaly is rarely encountered. Depending on the extent and location of nodal and extranodal disease, patients might present with symptoms and signs of airway obstruction, pleural or pericardial effusion, hepatocellular dysfunction, or bone marrow infiltration (anemia, neutropenia, or thrombocytopenia). Nephrotic syndrome is a rare but recognized presenting feature of Hodgkin's disease.

Systemic symptoms considered important in staging are unexplained fever, weight loss, or drenching night sweats (Table 503–1). Less common and not considered of prognostic significance are symptoms of pruritus, lethargy, anorexia, or pain that worsens after ingestion of alcohol.

Because of the impaired cellular immunity, concomitant tuberculous or fungal infections may complicate Hodgkin's disease and predispose to complications during immunosuppressive therapy. Varicella-zoster infections occur at some time during the course of the disease in about 30%.

DIAGNOSIS. Any patient with persistent, unexplained adenopathy unassociated with an obvious underlying inflammatory or infectious process should have a chest radiograph to identify the presence of a mediastinal mass before undergoing node biopsy. Unless signs or symptoms dictate otherwise, additional laboratory studies can be delayed until the biopsy results are available. Patients who have persistently enlarged lymph nodes, even after serologically proven infectious mononucleosis, should also be considered for biopsy.

Formal excisional biopsy is preferred over needle biopsy to ensure that adequate tissue is obtained, both for light microscopy and for appropriate immunocytochemical studies, culture, and cytogenetic analysis if routine studies fail to provide a firm diagnosis. Hodgkin's disease is rarely diagnosed with certainty on frozen section. Ideally, a portion of the biopsy specimen should be frozen and stored to allow for other studies.

Once the diagnosis of Hodgkin's disease is established, extent of disease (i.e., stage) should be determined. Table 503–2 documents the diagnostic work-up once the histologic diagnosis has been established. These studies should provide all the information needed to clinically stage the disease based on the

TABLE 503–1 Ann Arbor Staging System for Hodgkin's Disease*

Stage I	Involvement of a single lymph node region or of a single extralymphatic organ or site
Stage II	Involvement of two or more lymphoid regions on the same side of the diaphragm; or localized involvement of an extralymphatic organ or site and of one or more lymph node regions on the same side of the diaphragm
Stage III	Involvement of lymph node regions on both sides of the diaphragm, which may be accompanied by localized involvement of an extralymphatic organ or site or by splenic involvement
Stage IV	Diffuse or disseminated involvement of one or more extralymphatic organs or tissues, with or without associated lymph node enlargement

**Stages are further categorized as A or B, based on the absence or presence, respectively, of systemic symptoms of fever and/or weight loss.*

TABLE 503–2 Studies Necessary for Clinical Staging of Hodgkin's Disease

Complete blood count
Erythrocyte sedimentation rate, serum ferritin, serum copper
Liver function tests
Chest radiograph
Chest CT with contrast
Abdominal CT with contrast
Gallium scan
Bone marrow biopsy

Ann Arbor classification (see Table 503–1). A complete blood count (CBC) identifies abnormalities that might suggest marrow involvement. Erythrocyte sedimentation rate (ESR), serum copper determination, and serum ferritin levels are of some prognostic significance and, if abnormal at diagnosis, serve as a baseline to evaluate the effects of treatment. Liver function tests, though not particularly sensitive to the presence of liver involvement, can influence treatment and treatment complications. A chest radiograph is particularly important for measuring the size of the mediastinal mass in relation to the maximal diameter of the thorax. Chest CT more clearly defines the extent of a mediastinal mass if present and identifies hilar nodes and pulmonary parenchymal involvement, which may not be evident on chest radiographs. Abdominal CT scan can identify gross subdiaphragmatic involvement of nodes together with enlargement and defects in the liver and spleen. A gallium scan is particularly helpful in identifying areas of increased uptake, which can then be re-evaluated at the end of treatment, especially in patients with mediastinal masses that do not completely resolve on chest radiographs or CT. MRI has not been shown to increase the diagnostic precision of the evaluation. Lymphangiography, although unique in its ability to demonstrate intrinsic abnormalities in lymph nodes, is not without risk, is labor intensive and uncomfortable, and fails to visualize upper para-aortic nodes. It is rarely performed in pediatric practice, where systemic therapy has become the cornerstone of treatment and would be expected to eliminate relatively small foci of disease.

Surgical staging is no longer routinely performed and should be considered only if findings will significantly influence therapy. Bone marrow biopsy is necessary in only those patients with advanced (stage III or IV) disease or with "B" symptoms. Table 503–1 lists the separate lymph node regions as they are applied to the staging process for Hodgkin's disease.

TREATMENT. Because of concern about late effects, treatment of children in North America has evolved from primary treatment with extended-field radiation therapy to use of multiagent chemotherapy as the cornerstone of treatment, supplemented in selected cases, by relatively low-dose involved-field irradiation (2,000–2,500 cGy). Treatment is largely determined by disease stage, patient's age at diagnosis, the presence or absence of B "symptoms," and the presence of bulky nodal disease.

Early Stage Disease (Stages I, II, and IIIA). Cure rates with radiation alone (3,500–4,500cGy) in *surgically staged* early stage disease range from 40–80%, and the overwhelming majority of those who suffer relapse can be salvaged with a combination of multiagent chemotherapy or additional irradiation or both, resulting in cure rates of 90% or more. Unfortunately, this approach produces growth retardation in skeletally immature children and in some fully grown individuals and is associated with significant long-term morbidity, including thyroid failure, cardiac and pulmonary dysfunction, and an increased risk of breast cancer. For these reasons, many centers treating children and adolescents used combined modality therapy or even chemotherapy alone.

The chemotherapy regimens in current use are based on MOPP* (nitrogen mustard [Mustargen], vincristine [Oncovin], procarbazine, and prednisone), or ABVD* (doxorubicin [Adriamycin], bleomycin, vinblastine, and dacarbazine), or combinations of the two. As originally conceived, a minimum of six cycles of chemotherapy were given with significant cumulative toxicity, including second malignancies, sterility, and cardiac and pulmonary dysfunction. The long-term toxicity is determined by the total dose of the offending agents. Newly developed programs are aimed at reducing total drug doses and treatment duration and even elimination of radiation therapy.

Advanced Disease (Stages IIIB and IV). Chemotherapy, based on the same regimens as used in early stage disease, is considered the primary treatment for patients with advanced disease. Because the cure rate with conventional drug combinations, with or without radiation therapy, is only 60–70%, new and more aggressive regimens have been developed and are now in clinical trials.

TREATMENT OF RELAPSE. Patients who suffer relapse after initial treatment with radiation alone, or after an initial remission of at least 12 mo after chemotherapy alone or combined modality therapy usually respond to additional chemotherapy or irradiation or both. Those who never achieve remission or who suffer relapse after an initial remission of less than 12 mo after chemotherapy or combined modality therapy have a poorer prognosis and are candidates for myeloablative chemotherapy and autologous stem cell or bone marrow transplant rescue.

PROGNOSIS. Most treatment programs result in disease-free survival rates of 60% or more, with overall cure rates above 90% in those with early stage disease and exceeding 70% in more advanced cases. All newly diagnosed cases in children and adolescents should be treated with curative intent; this is consistently and effectively achieved with combined modality therapy. The choice of program is then largely selected on the basis of observed or anticipated long-term complications. Elimination of routine staging laparotomy and splenectomy avoids concerns about surgical morbidity and postsplenectomy infections.

503.2 Non-Hodgkin's Lymphoma (NHL)

NHL results from malignant clonal proliferation of lymphocytes of T-, or B-, or indeterminate cell origin. NHL occurs with an annual incidence of 9.1 per million white and 4.6 per million black children younger than 15 yr in the United States. In equatorial Africa, 50% of childhood cancers are lymphomas, a result of the very high incidence of Burkitt's lymphoma. Unlike Hodgkin's disease, the incidence of NHL increases steadily throughout life. In some situations there is overlap with acute lymphoblastic leukemia. Patients with lymphoblastic NHL and more than 25% lymphoblasts in the bone marrow are arbitrarily classified and treated as if they had ALL, whereas patients with B-cell ALL are treated similarly to patients with Burkitt's lymphoma even if no extramedullary disease is present.

PATHOLOGY AND PATHOGENESIS. EBV infection has a major role in the pathogenesis of Burkitt's lymphoma. The EBV genome is present in tumor cells in 95% of "endemic" cases in equatorial Africa compared to 20% in "sporadic" cases in the United States. How EBV contributes to the pathogenesis of Burkitt's lymphoma remains unclear. Pre-existing immunodeficiency (congenital or acquired) also predisposes to the development of NHL.

Although elaborate classifications of NHL have been developed, they have little application to the pediatric disease. Most cases of NHL in children are high-grade, diffuse neoplasms. Three histologic subtypes are recognized: *lymphoblastic* (usually of T-cell origin), *large cell* (of T-, or B-, or indeterminate cell origin), and *small noncleaved cell lymphoma* (SNCCL, Burkitt's and non-Burkitt's subtypes, B-cell origin). The diagnosis and classification of childhood NHL requires considerable hematopathologic expertise and adequate diagnostic tissue, both fresh and frozen.

Chromosomal translocation involving proto-oncogenes (e.g., *tall, rhomb2, rhombi, hox11, lyl1, myc, lck*) and T-cell receptor genes on chromosomes 7 or 14 results in activation of the proto-oncogene, contributing to malignant transformation in some cases of lymphoblastic lymphoma. In a subset of large-

*For information about acute drug toxicity, see Table 501–1.

cell lymphomas with anaplastic histology, a t(2;5) results in rearrangement and fusion of the *npm* gene on chromosome 5 with the *ALK* gene on chromosome 2, leading to formation of a chimeric protein that may cause inappropriate phosphorylation of substrates involved in cell growth and proliferation. In SNCCL, one of three chromosomal translocations [i.e., t(8;14), t(8;22), t(2;8)] results in approximation of the *myc* proto-oncogene on chromosome 8 to a regulatory region of either the kappa, lambda, or mu chain genes, resulting in dysregulation of *myc*, thus contributing to transformation.

CLINICAL MANIFESTATIONS. Presenting signs and symptoms vary with disease site and extent, and these in turn correlate with histologic subtype.

Lymphoblastic lymphoma often presents with intrathoracic tumor (usually a mediastinal mass) and associated dyspnea, chest pain, dysphagia, pleural effusion, or superior vena cava syndrome. Cervical or axillary adenopathy is present in up to 80% of patients at diagnosis. Primary involvement of bone, bone marrow, testis, or skin is not uncommon. The central nervous system (CNS) may also be involved.

SNCCL presents as an abdominal tumor in 80% of U.S. cases with abdominal pain or distention, bowel obstruction, change in bowel habits, intestinal bleeding, or rarely intestinal perforation. Other sites include CNS, bone marrow, and peripheral lymph nodes. Jaw involvement occurs in less than 20% of U.S. cases, compared with 70% of younger patients in equatorial Africa.

Large cell lymphomas (LCL) occur in many sites, including the abdomen and mediastinum. Extramedullary sites include skin, bone, and soft tissues. CNS involvement is rare, in contrast to SNCCL and lymphoblastic NHL.

LABORATORY FINDINGS. Laboratory findings vary, depending on sites or organs involved. Elevated serum uric acid levels and other features of tumor lysis syndrome often complicate the presentation of SNCCL. Elevated serum level of lactate dehydrogenase is a measure of tumor burden and may occur with any NHL subtype. A normal CBC does not preclude marrow involvement. CT or MRI of the chest or abdomen or both provides key information on disease extent. Surgical staging is not necessary.

DIAGNOSIS AND STAGING. Prompt tissue diagnosis and staging is important because of the rapid growth rate of lymphomas, especially SNCCL. To ensure adequate tissue for accurate diagnosis and subtyping, multiple needle biopsy specimens or a large wedge of tumor should be obtained. Table 503–3 lists the studies necessary to accurately stage the disease and provides baseline measurements of organ function needed before treatment is instituted. In cases with airway compromise and associated anesthesia risk and no easily accessible tissue to sample, empirical therapy may be started.

The St. Jude staging system defines tumor extent, which is important for treatment (Table 503–4). Stage I applies to localized disease, stage II regional (except for mediastinal tumors, which are designated stage III), stage III extensive, and stage IV disseminated (CNS and/or bone marrow).

TABLE 503–3 Pretreatment Studies for Staging Pediatric Non-Hodgkin's Lymphoma

- Complete blood count
- Serum electrolytes, uric acid, lactate dehydrogenase, creatinine, calcium, phosphorus
- Liver function tests
- Chest radiograph and chest CT if abnormal
- Abdominal and pelvic ultrasonography and/or CT scan
- Gallium scan and/or bone scan
- Bilateral bone marrow aspirate and biopsy
- Spinal fluid cytology

TABLE 503–4 A Staging System for Non-Hodgkin's Lymphoma in Childhood

Stage I

A single tumor (extranodal) or single anatomic area (nodal), with the exclusion of mediastinum or abdomen.

Stage II

A single tumor (extranodal) with regional node involvement.
Two or more nodal areas on the same side of the diaphragm.
Two single (extranodal) tumors with or without regional node involvement on the same side of the diaphragm.
A primary gastrointestinal tract tumor, usually in the ileocecal area, with or without involvement of associated mesenteric nodes only, which must be grossly (>90%) resected.

Stage III

Two single tumors (extranodal) on opposite sides of the diaphragm.
Two or more nodal areas above and below the diaphragm.
Any primary intrathoracic tumor (mediastinal, pleural, thymic).
Any extensive primary intra-abdominal disease.

Stage IV

Any of the above, with initial involvement of central nervous system and/or bone marrow at time of diagnosis.

From Murphy SB: Classification, staging, and end results of treatment of childhood non-Hodgkin's lymphomas: Dissimilarities from lymphomas in adults. Semin Oncol 7:332, 1980.

TREATMENT AND PROGNOSIS. Surgical excision of localized intra-abdominal tumors often precedes the diagnosis of NHL. In this and other situations, multiagent chemotherapy is the primary treatment. Tumor lysis syndrome (ie., high serum potassium, uric acid, and high phosphorus with low calcium levels) frequently complicates initial treatment of disseminated disease. Appropriate hydration with addition of sodium bicarbonate to produce dilute alkaline urine, administration of allopurinol, and correction of electrolyte abnormalities are essential to minimize this life-threatening complication.

NHL, unlike Hodgkin's disease, is considered a disseminated disease from the time of diagnosis. Even patients with limited stage disease require chemotherapy. Patients with limited stage NHL, regardless of histologic subgroup, are effectively treated with 6 cycles of CHOP (cyclophosphamide, vincristine, methotrexate, and prednisone) or chemotherapy for three cycles, followed by 6 mo of mercaptopurine and methotrexate. About 90% are cured with this regimen. Other effective regimens are available but appear to offer no advantage. The emphasis now is on decreasing morbidity of therapy for these children while maintaining the high cure rate.

TREATMENT OF ADVANCED NHL. Patients with advanced NHL are best treated with different therapy, depending on histologic subtype.

Lymphoblastic. The chemotherapy regimens for nonlocalized lymphoblastic lymphoma are intensive, of moderate duration, and include several chemotherapeutic agents given in cycles. CNS therapy using cranial irradiation or intrathecal chemotherapy or both is important for prevention of CNS disease. These intensive treatment programs are continued for 15–18 mo.

SNCCL. Relatively short-duration (3–6 mo) intensive chemotherapy including an alkylating agent coupled with other active agents produces survival rates of 70–80% in those with disseminated disease. If relapse occurs, it becomes evident in the 1st yr after diagnosis.

LCL. Treatment for patients with this rather heterogeneous group of tumors is controversial. Intensive multiagent chemotherapy regimens similar to those used for lymphoblastic lymphoma have produced long-term survival rates of 50–70%, as have short, intensive regimens designed for Burkitt's NHL (used only for the B-cell subset of large-cell cases). Event-free survival as high as 80% has been reported for this subset. In France, immunophenotype-directed therapy is used for these cases.

Hodgkin's Disease

Bhatia S, Robison LL, Oberlin O, et al: Breast cancer and other second neoplasms after childhood Hodgkin's disease. N Engl J Med 334:745, 1996.

Hudson MM, Donalson SS: Hodgkin's disease. *In*: Pizzo PA, Poplack DG (eds): Principles and Practice of Pediatric Oncology. Philadelphia, JB Lippincott, 1997, p 523.

Hudson MM, Donaldson SS: Hodgkin's disease. Pediatr Clin North Am 44:891, 1997.

Hudson MM, Pratt CB: Risk of delayed second primary neoplasms after treatment of malignant lymphoma. Surg Oncol Clin North Am 2:319, 1993.

Schwartz RS: Hodgkin's disease—time for a change. N Engl J Med 337:495, 1997.

Non-Hodgkin's Lymphoma

Liebowitz D: Epstein-Barr virus and a cellular signaling pathway in lymphoma from immunosuppressed patients. N Engl J Med 338:1413, 1998.

Link MP, Shuster JJ, Donaldson SS, et al: Treatment of children and young adults with early-stage non-Hodgkin's lymphoma. N Engl J Med 331:1259, 1997.

Reiter A, Schrappe M, Parwaresch R, et al: Non-Hodgkin's lymphomas of childhood and adolescence: Results of a treatment stratified for biologic subtypes and stage-A report of the Berlin-Frankfurt-Munster group. J Clin Oncol 13:359, 1995.

Sandlund JT, Downing JR, Crist WM: Non-Hodgin's lymphoma in childhood. N Engl J Med 334:1238, 1996.

Shad A, Magrath I: Non-Hodgkin's lymphoma. Pediatr Clin North Am 44:863, 1997.

Tugergen DG, Krailo MD, Meadows AT, et al: Comparison of treatment regimens for pediatric lymphoblastic non-Hodgkin's lymphoma: A children's cancer group study. J Clin Oncol 13:1368, 1995.

Webb A, Cunningham D, Cotter F, et al: BCL-2 antisense therapy in patients with non-Hodgkin lymphoma. Lancet 349:1137, 1997.

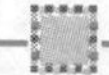

CHAPTER 504
Neuroblastoma

Michael J. McManus and Gerald S. Gilchrist

Neuroblastoma (NB), a common tumor of neural crest origin, demonstrates an extremely variable clinical presentation and biologic behavior. NB may undergo spontaneous regression or differentiation into benign ganglioneuromas; NB in older children with regional or distant metastatic disease is extremely aggressive and resistant to treatment. NB accounts for about 8% of childhood cancers and is the most common solid tumor of childhood outside of the central nervous system. The annual incidence of NB is 10/1 million children. About 500 new cases are diagnosed each year in the United States. NB is the most frequently diagnosed neoplasm in infants. The median age at diagnosis is 2 yr; 90% of cases are diagnosed before the age of 5 yr. The incidence is slightly higher in males and in whites. There may be an association with Beckwith-Wiedemann syndrome.

PATHOLOGY, PATHOGENESIS, AND PROGNOSIS. NB is a small round cell tumor with variable degrees of neural differentiation (ganglioneuroma, ganglioneuroblastoma, and neuroblastoma). Prognosis has been shown to vary with histologic definition of tissue pattern (i.e., Shimada's classification). A favorable prognosis NB subtype is based on the amount of stroma, degree of tumor cell differentiation, and number of tumor cell mitoses. The tumors may resemble other small round cell tumors: rhabdomyosarcoma, Ewing's sarcoma, and non-Hodgkin's lymphoma.

Genetic analysis of NB has led to molecular classification. Genetic characteristics of NB of prognostic importance include loss of heterozygosity for the short arm of chromosome 1, amplification of the *mycn* (*n-myc*) proto-oncogene, hyperdiploidy of tumor cell DNA content, and defects in the nerve growth factor receptor. *Mycn* is amplified in about 25% of NB; amplification is strongly associated with advanced tumor stage, rapid tumor progression, and poor outcome. It has prognostic importance, independent of stage and age. The prognosis for children with NB can be best determined by combined clinical features of the patient (age, extent of tumor) and biologic features (*mycn* copy number, ploidy of the tumor—hyperdiploidy confers better outcome if < 1 yr of age), and chromosome 1p deletion. Thus, therapy can be reduced for patients predicted to fare well with minimal therapy and intensified in those predicted to be at high risk of relapse.

CLINICAL PRESENTATION. NB may develop at any site of sympathetic nervous system tissue. Most NB arises in the abdomen, either in the adrenal gland or in retroperitoneal sympathetic ganglia. About 30% of tumors arise in the cervical, thoracic, or pelvic ganglia. Cervical involvement may produce a Horner's syndrome. Distant sites of metastasis commonly include the bone marrow, bone, liver, and skin. Infants more commonly have localized disease, usually in the cervical or thoracic region. NB may be incidentally noted on a chest radiograph. Older children commonly have abdominal neuroblastoma and disseminated disease. The signs and symptoms of NB reflect the tumor site and extent of disease. Abdominal NB commonly presents as a hard, fixed abdominal mass that is producing discomfort. Massive involvement of the liver may occur especially in infants with widespread disease and may cause significant respiratory compromise. NB also extends into neural formina, producing spinal cord and nerve root compression. Metastatic disease can be associated with myriad signs and symptoms including fever, irritability, failure to thrive, bone pain, bluish subcutaneous nodules, orbital proptosis, and periorbital ecchymoses (Fig. 504–1). Opsoclonus-myoclonus is a rare paraneoplastic syndrome seen in children with NB; it may be a presenting sign of the disease. An affected child presents with chaotic eye movements, myoclonus, and ataxia—hence the description "dancing eyes, dancing feet syndrome." Children with NB and this syndrome may have a better prognosis; the neurologic deficits may persist even after successful treatment for the malignancy. Autoantibodies against neural tissue may be responsible for this syndrome.

Catecholamine production may cause hypertension, whereas other vasoactive substances may produce a secretory diarrhea.

DIAGNOSIS AND STAGING. NB is generally discovered as a mass or multiple masses on plain radiographs, CT, or MRI (Fig. 504–2). Tumor markers are elevated in 95% of cases and help to confirm the diagnosis (i.e., elevated homovanillic acid [HVA] and vanillylmandelic acid [VMA] in urine). A pathologic diagnosis is made from tumor tissue obtained by biopsy. NB can be diagnosed in a typical presentation without a primary tumor biopsy if the patient has neuroblasts observed in bone marrow (Fig. 504–3) and elevated VMA or HVA in the urine.

Evaluation for metastatic disease should include bone scan to detect cortical bone involvement and bone marrow aspirates and biopsies to detect marrow disease. The clinical extent of

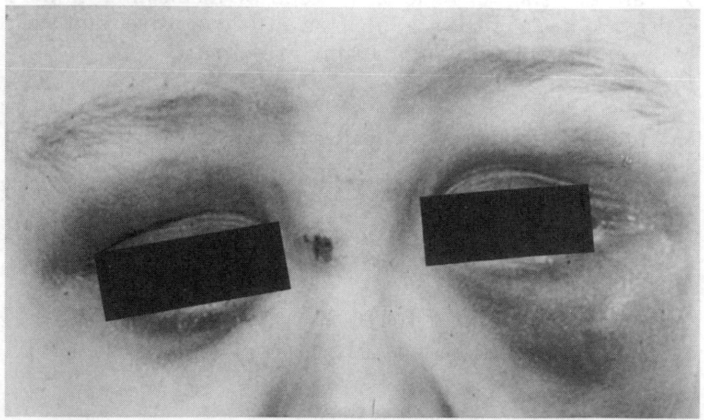

Figure 504–1 Periorbital metastases of neuroblastoma, with proptosis and ecchymoses.

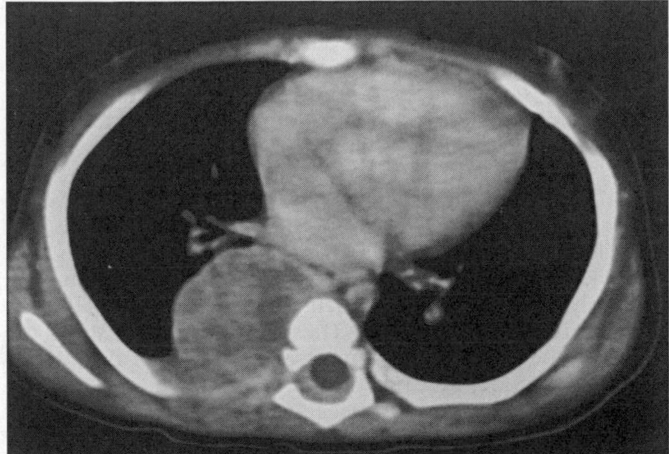

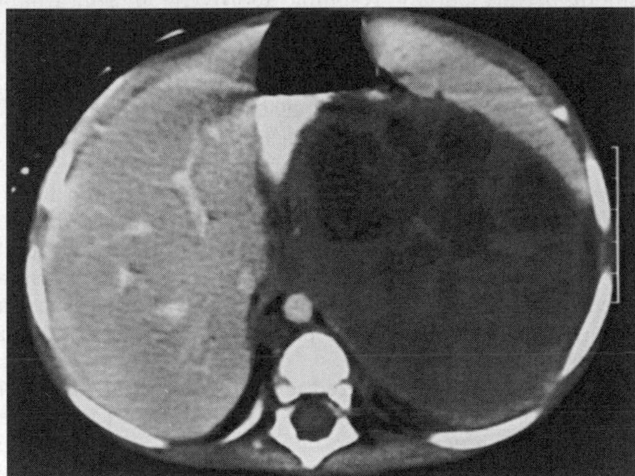

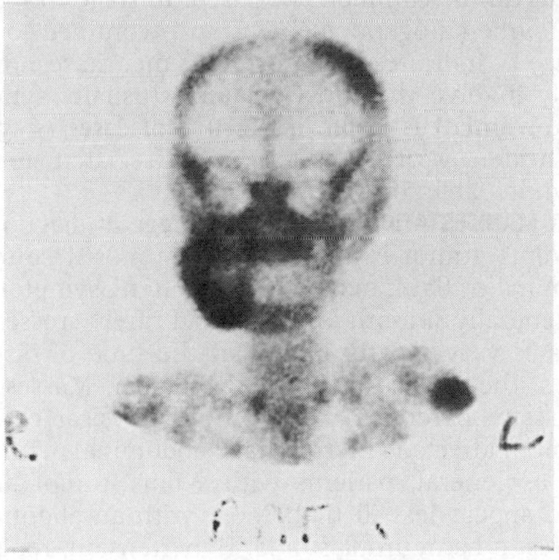

Figure 504–2 *Top,* CT scan of a thoracic neuroblastoma with intraspinal extension at diagnosis. *Middle,* CT scan of an adrenal primary with extensive lymph node involvement. *Bottom,* Bone scintigraphy with technetium diphosphonate demonstrating diffuse skeletal involvement.

disease and age, together with cytogenetic and molecular markers performed on the tumor tissue, are used to estimate the prognosis and for determination of risk-directed therapy. Although several staging systems have been used, the International Neuroblastoma Staging System (INSS) is universally used. In the INSS, stage 1 includes tumors confined to the organ or structure of origin. Stage 2 tumors extend beyond the structure of origin but not across the midline, with (stage 2B) or without (stage 2A) ipsilateral lymph node involvement. Stage 3 tumors extend beyond the midline, with or without bilateral lymph node involvement. Stage 4 tumors are disseminated to distant sites (e.g., bone, bone marrow, liver, distant lymph nodes, other organs). Stage 4S refers to age less than 1 yr with dissemination to liver, skin, or bone marrow without bone involvement and with a primary tumor that would otherwise be stage 1 or 2.

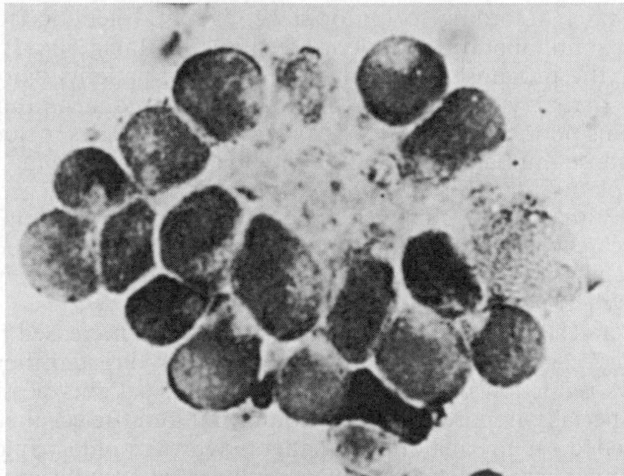

Figure 504–3 Neuroblastoma cells aspirated from the bone marrow. Clumps of cells often contain three or more cells with or without evidence of rosette formation. Rosettes of cells surrounding an inner mass of fibrillary material are characteristic of neuroblastoma.

The most important clinical and biologic prognostic factors are the age of the patient at diagnosis, extent of tumor, *mycn* status, and presence of 1p deletions in the tumor (Table 504–1). The overall disease-free survival of patients with stage 1 or 2 disease is between 75 and 95%. Patients with stage 4 disease who are older than 1 yr have a disease-free survival of only about 25%.

TREATMENT. The respective role of surgery, radiation, or chemotherapy is dependent on stage. Surgical excision should always be considered, taking into account tumor location, tumor extent determined by imaging studies (plain radiographs, CT, or MRI), and relationship of tumor to major organs or other vital structures. Emergency surgery may be necessary when organ function is compromised. Patients with paraspinal tumors that are compressing the spinal cord represent a surgical emergency. Chemotherapy (e.g., cisplatin, doxorubicin, vincristine, and cyclophosphamide) often converts a tumor that was unresectable to one that can be completely resected. Surgical exploration is often useful in refining staging by directly addressing the question of resectability and by identifying and taking biopsy samples of lymph nodes and other organs or structures that might have tumor involvement. Treatment is risk directed. In general, infants and children with early stage disease without *mycn* amplification or 1p deletion can often be cured by surgery alone. Infants with more advanced disease require addition of chemotherapy (i.e., cisplatin, etoposide, vincristine, cyclophosphamide), as do older children. Addition of radiation therapy to four-agent chemotherapy may benefit children with stage 3 tumors. Estimated

TABLE 504–1 Prognostic Factors in Neuroblastoma

	Three-Yr Survival		
	95%	*25–50%*	*<5%*
Age	<1 yr	>1 yr	1–5 yr
International Neuroblastoma Staging System	1, 2, 4S	3, 4	3, 4
MYCN	Normal	Normal	Amplified
Chromosome 1p deletion	<5%	25–50%	80–90%

Adapted from Brodeur GM, Maris JM, Yamashiro DJ, et al: Biology and genetics of human neuroblastomas. J Pediatr Hematol Oncol 19:93, 1997.

cure rates according to tumor stage, age, and genetic factors using contemporary treatment are shown in Table 504–1. Because the prognosis for the large number of patients who are older than 1 yr at diagnosis and have advanced stage tumors remains poor, a number of experimental approaches including high-dose multiagent chemotherapy followed by bone marrow transplant and ^{131}I-methyiodobenzylguanidine therapy are being evaluated. Full supportive therapy (blood products, intensive care with management of infectious complications, and availability of irradiation for all blood products) must be available when patients receive intensive therapy.

Overall, the cure rate for neuroblastoma has increased from about 25% in the 1960s to about 55%. Risk-directed therapy makes reduction of side effects for low-risk patients possible, an especially important goal in young children. Better therapy is needed for the majority of patients who are older children with advanced disease or patients with *mycn* amplification or 1p deletion in their tumors.

Acharya S, Jayabose S, Kogan SJ, et al: Prenatally diagnosed neuroblastoma. Cancer 80:304, 1997.

Ambros IM, Zellner A, Roald B, et al: Role of ploidy: Chromosome 1p, and Schwann cells in the maturation of neuroblastoma. N Engl J Med 334:1505, 1996.

Caron H, Van Sluis P, De Kraker J, et al: Allelic loss of chromosome 1p as a predictor of unfavorable outcome in patients with neuroblastoma. N Engl J Med 334:225, 1996.

Castleberry RP: Biology and treatment of neuroblastoma. Pediatr Clin North Am 44:919, 1997.

Posner JB: Autoantibodies in childhood opsoclonus-mycoclonus syndrome. J Pediatr 130:855, 1997.

Woods WG, Tuchman M, Robison LL, et al: A population-based study of the usefulness of screening for neuroblastoma. Lancet 348:1682, 1996.

CHAPTER 505
Neoplasms of the Kidney

Peter M. Anderson

505.1 Wilms' Tumor

Wilms' tumor accounts for most renal neoplasms in childhood and occurs with approximately equal frequency in both sexes and in all races, with an annual incidence of 7.8 per million children younger than 15 yr. An important feature of Wilms' tumor is its association with congenital anomalies, the most common being genitourinary anomalies (4.4%), hemihypertrophy (2.9%), and sporadic aniridia (1.1%) (Table 505–1).

Deletions involving one of at least two loci on chromosome 11 have been noted in cells of about 30% of Wilms' tumors. Hemizygous constitutional deletions of one of these loci, 11p13, are also associated with two rare syndromes that include Wilms' tumor: the WAGR syndrome (Wilms' tumor, aniridia, genitourinary malformations, and mental retardation) and the Denys-Drash syndrome (Wilms' tumor, nephropathy, and genital abnormalities). The existence of a second locus, 11p15, may explain the association of Wilms' tumor with Beckwith-Wiedemann syndrome, a congenital syndrome characterized by several types of embryonal neoplasms, hemihypertrophy, macroglossia, and visceromegaly. A third locus may be involved in familial Wilms' tumor. More than 85% of Wilms' tumors with anaplasia have a mutation in the p53 tumor suppressor gene, which is a rare event in the Wilms' tumor without anaplasia (i.e., more favorable histology).

PATHOLOGY. Wilms' tumor is usually a solitary growth that may occur in any part of either kidney. In gross appearance, it is sharply demarcated and variably encapsulated. Small areas of hemorrhage are common. The tumor usually distorts the renal outline and often compresses residual normal kidney into a surrounding thin rim (Fig. 505–1).

The classic microscopic appearance of favorable-histology Wilms' tumor is triphasic: Epithelial, blastemal, and stromal elements are present and resemble abortive glomeruli. Anaplasia is found in only about 10% of cases, but these cases account for 60% of deaths due to Wilms' tumor. This unfavorable histologic subtype, which tends to occur in older, nonwhite patients, features cells three times the normal size, with hyperchromatic nuclei and abnormal mitoses.

Two renal tumors that were previously considered to be unfavorable subtypes of Wilms' tumor have been reclassified. *Rhabdoid tumor,* a highly malignant neoplasm composed of cells with fibrillar eosinophilic inclusions, is found most often in very young patients. *Clear cell sarcoma* of the kidney is characterized by a spindle cell pattern with a striking vasocentric arrangement; it shows a male predominance and a tendency to metastasize to bone.

The staging system most frequently used is that of the National Wilms Tumor Study (NWTS) Group. Stage I tumors are limited to the kidney and can be completely excised with the capsular surface intact. The stage II tumor extends beyond the kidney but can be completely excised. In stage III, postsurgical residual nonhematogenous extension is confined to the abdomen. Stage IV indicates hematogenous metastases, which most frequently involve the lung. Bilateral (usually synchronous) renal involvement is noted in 5–10% of cases (stage V). The relative incidences of stages I–IV and associated survival rates are shown in Table 505–2.

CLINICAL MANIFESTATIONS. The median age at diagnosis of unilateral Wilms' tumor is about 3 yr. The most frequent sign is an abdominal or flank mass, which is often asymptomatic. The mass is generally smooth and firm and rarely crosses the midline. Masses vary greatly in size at the time of discovery. In one series, the mean diameter was 11 cm. Masses are often discovered by parents or on routine physical examination. About half of affected children have abdominal pain, vomiting, or both. In general, patients with Wilms' tumor are slightly older and appear less ill than those with an abdominal mass that proves to be neuroblastoma. Hypertension, reported in as many as 60% of patients, results from renal ischemia due to pressure on the renal artery.

DIAGNOSIS. Wilms' tumor must be suspected in any young child with an abdominal mass. In 10–25% of cases, microscopic or gross hematuria suggests a renal tumor. Ultrasonography (the initial imaging modality) may indicate that the mass

TABLE 505–1 Syndromes and Their Associated Clinical and Genetic Characteristics

Syndrome	Clinical Characteristics	Chromosome Location
WAGR syndrome	*W*ilms', *a*niridia, *g*enitourniary abnormalities, and mental *r*etardation	del 11p13 (WT1 locus)
Beckwith-Wiedemann syndrome	Organomegaly (liver, kidney, adrenal, pancreas), macroglossia, omphalocele, hemihypertrophy	del 11p15.5 (WT2 locus) (may also involve IGF2 and/or H19 genes)
Wilms' tumor	Favorable histology	Germ line p53 (99.2%)
Wilms' tumor	Anaplastic (unfavorable) histology	Mutant p53 (86%)

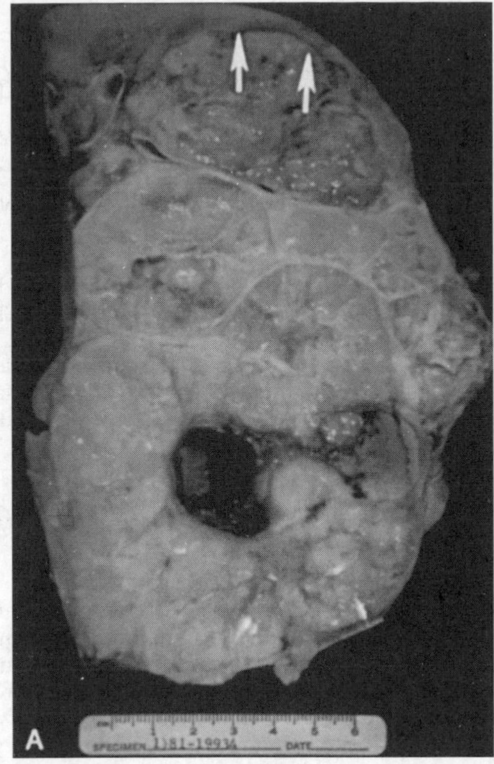

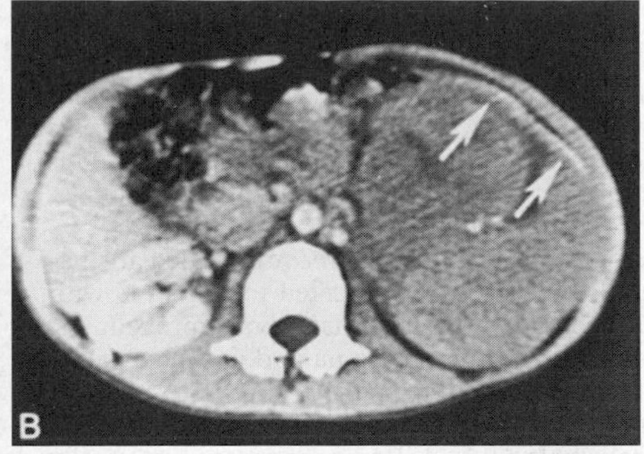

Figure 505–1 Wilms' tumor. *A,* Gross specimen shows a large mass compressing a small rim of normal renal tissue *(arrows). B,* CT scan of kidney. A rim of compressed normal tissue represents the residual normal renal parenchyma *(arrows).*

is intrarenal. The major differential diagnostic consideration is neuroblastoma.

CT offers several advantages in evaluating a possible Wilms' tumor. These include confirmation of intrarenal tumor origin, which usually rules out neuroblastoma; detection of multiple masses; determination of the extent of tumor, including vena cava involvement; and evaluation of the opposite kidney. The typical Wilms' tumor arises from the kidney as an inhomogeneous mass with areas of low density indicating necrosis on CT studies without contrast enhancement. Areas of hemorrhage and small focal calcifications are generally less common and less prominent than in neuroblastoma. Tumors enhance slightly after injection of contrast medium. There is often a sharp demarcation between the tumor and normal parenchyma, correlated with a pseudocapsule, and persistent ellipsoid areas of increased attenuation corresponding to the compressed uninvolved renal parenchyma (see Fig. 505–1). Once neuroblastoma is considered less likely, other considerations in the differential diagnosis are hydronephrosis, renal cysts, and mesoblastic nephroma (most common in neonates, in whom Wilms' tumor does not occur) or other renal malignancies, such as renal cell carcinoma, soft tissue sarcoma, and lymphoma.

Pulmonary metastases are evident on chest radiographs in 10–15% of patients at the time of diagnosis. CT scan of the chest is useful, particularly to visualize portions of the lung below the level of the dome of the diaphragm (Fig. 505–2). Evaluation of bone and bone marrow should be considered only if the patient has a clear cell sarcoma or rhabdoid tumor or has persistent bone pain.

Certain rare paraneoplastic syndromes may be associated with Wilms' tumor; the tumor may produce erythropoietin, leading to polycythemia.

TREATMENT. The immediate treatment for unilateral tumors is surgical removal of the affected kidney through a flank incision even if pulmonary metastases are present. At the time of nephrectomy, careful inspection of the other kidney is needed to preclude the possibility of bilateral tumor, and the liver should be evaluated for possible metastases. The retroperitoneal lymph nodes and renal vein stump should be examined. Every attempt should be made to remove the tumor without spillage, but because postoperative chemotherapy and radiation are capable of destroying residual tumor, complete resection should not be attempted if the procedure would pose serious risks.

The NWTS group has shown that combination chemotherapy with vincristine and actinomycin is superior to single-

TABLE 505–2 Wilms' Tumor: Survival by Stage and Histology

Histology/Stage	No. of Patients	2 yr %	4 yr %
FH/I	546	98	97
II	281	96	94
III	290	91	88
IV	126	88	82
Anaplastic I	20	89	89
Anaplastic II–IV	40	56	54

Unfavorable histology (UH) refers to cases with anaplasia (focal or diffuse); all other cases are referred to as favorable histology (FH).
From D'Angro GJ: Wilms' tumor status report. J Clinic Oncol 9:877, 1990.
Data from NWTS-3.

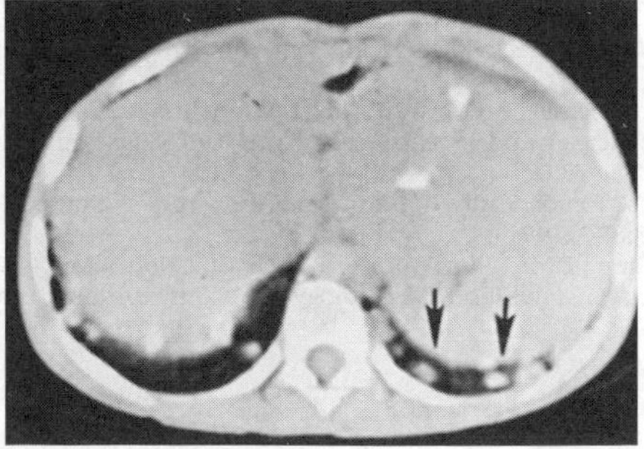

Figure 505–2 Wilms' tumor on CT scan of the chest showing metastatic lesions below the dome of the diaphragm *(arrows),* which would be difficult to visualize on plain radiograph.

agent therapy in localized disease and that doxorubicin is a significant addition to the treatment of advanced disease. For patients with advanced-stage disease, who require radiation in addition to surgery and chemotherapy, the dosage and fields have been modified to reduce the incidence of scoliosis. Pulmonary irradiation and three-drug combination chemotherapy are now recommended for patients with stage IV disease.

Preoperative therapy is not generally recommended for patients with unilateral disease but is indicated for patients with bilateral tumors to facilitate eventual renal salvage procedures. This approach preserves renal parenchyma and optimizes renal function without compromising survival.

PROGNOSIS. The most significant prognostic variables are histology and stage (see Table 505–2). Recurrence has historically carried a poor prognosis, although addition of newer agents and salvage regimens may improve outcome for the small group of patients who have a recurrence.

505.2 Other Renal Neoplasms

NEPHROBLASTOMATOSIS. Immature renal elements called *nephrogenic rests* occur in approximately 30% of unilateral Wilms' tumors and in most, if not all, bilateral tumors. These Wilms' tumor precursor lesions may be unifocal and deep within the renal parenchyma (intralobar rest) or multifocal (perilobar rest). Subsequent (asynchronous) development of Wilms' tumor in the other kidney is more likely in patients with this feature (particularly intralobar rests) at presentation. The finding of nephrogenic rests in one kidney should prompt a careful inspection of the contralateral kidney at the time of surgery, as well as radiographic follow-up with CT scanning.

MESOBLASTIC NEPHROMA. Congenital mesoblastic nephroma is a massive, firm, infiltrative, solitary renal mass, grossly and microscopically resembling a leiomyoma or a low-grade leiomyosarcoma with trapped nephrons. The infiltrative margins are difficult to distinguish histologically from normal or dysplastic renal stroma. Electron microscopy shows the cells to be fibroblasts or myofibroblasts. This tumor accounts for the majority of congenital renal tumors. It occurs more often in males and has been noted to produce renin. The tumor is generally thought to be benign, and resection is adequate therapy. An occasional patient has a very cellular tumor that resembles a clear cell sarcoma. Such tumors may recur locally and even metastasize and would then benefit from chemotherapy and irradiation.

RENAL CELL CARCINOMA. This tumor is rare in the 1st decade of life but occurs occasionally in teenagers. The initial findings are an abdominal mass and hematuria. Complete resection may result in cure, but the prognosis is poor for patients with postoperative residual disease.

DeBaun MR, Siegel MJ, Choyke PL: Nephromegaly in infancy and early childhood: A risk factor for Wilms' tumor in Beckwith-Wiedemann syndrome. J Pediatr 132:401, 1998.

DeBaun MR, Tucker MA: Risk of cancer during the first four years of life in children from the Beck-Wiedemann syndrome registry. J Pediatr 132:398, 1998.

Green DM, Coppes MJ, Breslow NE, et al: Wilms tumor. *In*: Pizzo PA, Poplack DG (eds): Principles and Practice of Pediatric Oncology. Philadelphia, JB Lippincott, 1997, p 831.

National Wilms' Tumor Study Committee: Wilms' tumor: Status report, 1990. J Clin Oncol 9:877, 1991.

Petruzzi MJ, Green DM: Wilms' tumor. Pediatr Clin North Am 44:939, 1997.

Pritchard-Jones K, Hawkins MM: Biology of Wilms' tumour. Lancet 349:663, 1997.

CHAPTER 506
Soft Tissue Sarcomas

William M. Crist and Carola A. S. Arndt

Soft tissue sarcomas have an annual incidence of 8.4 per million white children younger than 15 yr. The incidence in black children is 50% that for white children. Rhabdomyosarcoma accounts for more than half of these tumors (Table 506–1). The prognosis is most strongly associated with extent of disease at diagnosis, primary tumor site, and treatment used.

506.1 Rhabdomyosarcoma

The most common pediatric soft tissue sarcoma, rhabdomyosarcoma accounts for 5–8% of childhood cancers. These tumors occur at virtually any anatomic site but are most often found in the head and neck (40%), genitourinary tract (20%), extremities (20%), and trunk (10%); retroperitoneal and "other" account for the remainder of primary sites. Both age and tumor histology appear related to primary site. Extremity lesions are more likely to occur in older children and to have alveolar histology.

Rhabdomyosarcoma occurs with increased frequency in patients with neurofibromatosis and has been associated with maternal breast cancer in the Li-Fraumeni syndrome, suggesting a genetic influence.

PATHOLOGY. Rhabdomyosarcoma is thought to arise from the same embryonic mesenchyme as striated skeletal muscle. On the basis of light microscopic appearance, it belongs to the group of small round cell tumors, which includes Ewing's sarcoma, neuroblastoma, and non-Hodgkin's lymphoma. Definitive diagnosis of a pathologic specimen may require immunohistochemical studies using antibodies to skeletal muscle (e.g., desmin, muscle-specific actin, and Myo-D) and electron microscopy.

Determination of the specific histiotype is important in treatment planning and assessment of prognosis. There are four recognized histologic subtypes. The *embryonal type* accounts for about 60% of all cases and has an intermediate prognosis. The *botryoid type*, a variant of the embryonal form in which tumor cells and an edematous stroma project into a body cavity like a bunch of grapes, accounts for 6% of cases and is most often found in the vagina, uterus, bladder, nasopharynx, and middle ear (see Chapter 649). *Alveolar tumors*, which account for about 15% of cases, are often characterized by 2;13 or 1;13 chromosomal translocations. The tumor cells tend to grow in cores that often have cleftlike spaces resembling alveoli. Alveolar tumors occur most often in the trunk and extremities and carry the poorest prognosis. The *pleomorphic type* (adult form) is rare in childhood (1% of cases). About 20% of patients are considered to have *undifferentiated sarcomas*.

CLINICAL MANIFESTATIONS. The most common presenting feature is a mass that may or may not be painful. Symptoms are due to displacement or obstruction of normal structures. Origin in the nasopharynx may be associated with nasal congestion, mouth breathing, epistaxis, and difficulty with swallowing and chewing. Regional extension into the cranium can produce cranial nerve paralysis, blindness, and signs of increased intracranial pressure with headache and vomiting. When the tumor develops in the face or cheek, there may be swelling, pain, trismus, and, as extension occurs, paralysis of cranial nerves. Tumors in the neck can produce progressive swelling with

TABLE 506–1 Nonrhabdomyosarcoma Soft Tissue Sarcomas

Tissue Type	Tumor	Natural History and Biology
Adipose	Liposarcoma	A very rare tumor. Usually arises in the extremities or retroperitoneum; associated with a nonrandom translocation, t(12;16)(q13;p11). Tends to be locally invasive and rarely metastasizes; wide local excision is the treatment of choice. The role of radiation therapy and chemotherapy in treating gross residual or metastatic disease is not established.
Fibrous	Fibrosarcoma	The most common soft tissue sarcoma in children younger than 1 yr. Congenital fibrosarcoma is a low-grade malignancy that commonly arises in the extremities or trunk and rarely metastasizes. Surgical excision is the treatment of choice; dramatic responses to preoperative chemotherapy may occur. In children older than 4 yr, the natural history is similar to that in adults (a 5-yr survival rate of 60%); wide surgical excision and preoperative chemotherapy are commonly used.
	Malignant fibrous histiocytoma	Most commonly arises in the trunk and extremities, deep in the subcutaneous layer. Histologically subdivided into storiform, giant cell, myxoid, and angiomatoid variants. The angiomatoid type tends to affect younger patients and is curable with surgical resection alone. Wide surgical excision is the treatment of choice. Chemotherapy has produced objective tumor regressions.
Vascular	Hemangiopericytoma	Often arises in the lower extremities or retroperitoneum; may present with hypoglycemia and hypophosphatemic rickets. Both benign and malignant histology. Nonrandom translocations t(12;19)(q13;q13) and t(13;22)(q22;q11) have been described. Complete surgical excision is the treatment of choice. Chemotherapy and radiotherapy may produce responses.
	Angiosarcoma	Rare in children; 33% arise in skin, 25% in soft tissue, and 25% in liver, breast or bone. Associated with chronic lymphedema and exposure to vinyl chloride in adults. Survival rate is poor (12% at 5 yr) despite some responses to chemotherapy/radiotherapy.
	Hemangioendothelioma	Can occur in soft tissue, liver, and lung. Localized lesions have a favorable outcome; lesions in lung and liver are often multifocal and have a poor prognosis.
Peripheral nerves	Neurofibrosarcoma	Also known as the malignant peripheral nerve sheath tumor. Develops in up to 16% of patients with NF1; almost 50% occur in patients with NF1. Deletions of chromosome 22q11-q13 or 17q11 and p53 mutations have been reported. Commonly arises in trunk and extremities and is usually locally invasive. Complete surgical excision is necessary for survival; response to chemotherapy is suboptimal.
Synovium	Synovial sarcoma	The most common NRSTS in some series. Often presenting in the 3rd decade, but 33% of patients are younger than 20 yr. Typically arises around the knee or thigh and is characterized by a nonrandom translocation t(X;18)(p11;q11). Wide surgical excision is necessary. Radiotherapy is effective in microscopic residual disease, and ifosfamide-based therapy is active in advanced disease.
Unknown	Alveolar soft part sarcoma	Slow-growing tumor; tends to recur or metastasize to lung and brain years after diagnosis. Often arises in the extremities and head and neck. A myogenic origin has been recently proposed. Resection of primary and metastatic sites, when possible, is recommended.
Smooth muscle	Leiomyosarcoma	The most common pediatric retroperitoneal soft tissue tumor. Often arises in the gastrointestinal tract and may be associated with a t(12;14)(q14;q23) translocation. Can occur with acquired immunodeficiency syndrome and during immunosuppression for renal transplantation. Complete surgical excision is the treatment of choice.

NF = Neurofibromatosis; NRSTS = nonrhabdomyosarcoma soft tissue sarcoma.

neurologic symptoms following regional extension. Orbital primaries are usually diagnosed early in their course because of associated proptosis, periorbital edema, ptosis, change in visual acuity, and local pain. When the tumor arises in the middle ear, the most common early signs are pain, hearing loss, chronic otorrhea, or a mass in the ear canal; extensions of tumor produce cranial nerve paralysis and signs of an intracranial mass on the involved side. An unremitting croupy cough and progressive stridor can accompany rhabdomyosarcoma of the larynx. Because most of these signs and symptoms are also associated with common childhood conditions, clinicians must be alert to the possibility of tumor.

Rhabdomyosarcoma of the trunk or extremities is often first noticed after trauma and may be regarded initially as a hematoma. When the swelling does not resolve or increases, malignancy should be suspected. Involvement of the genitourinary tract can produce hematuria, obstruction of the lower urinary tract, recurrent urinary tract infections, incontinence, or a mass detectable on abdominal or rectal examination. Paratesticular tumors usually present as a painless, rapidly growing mass in the scrotum. Vaginal rhabdomyosarcoma may present as a grapelike mass of tumor tissue bulging through the vaginal orifice (sarcoma botryoides) and can cause urinary tract or large bowel symptoms. Vaginal bleeding or obstruction of the urethra or rectum may occur. Similar findings can be noted with uterine primaries.

Tumors in any location may disseminate early, with presenting symptoms of pain or respiratory distress associated with pulmonary metastases. Extensive bone involvement can produce symptomatic hypercalcemia. In such cases, it may be difficult to identify the primary lesion.

DIAGNOSIS. Early diagnosis of rhabdomyosarcoma requires a high index of suspicion. Unfortunately, several months often elapse between the initial symptoms and biopsy. Diagnostic procedures are determined mainly by the area of involvement. With signs and symptoms in the head and neck area, radiographs should be examined for evidence of a tumor mass and for indications of bony erosion. CT scans should be performed to identify intracranial extension and may also reveal bony involvement at the base of the skull; this may be difficult to visualize. For abdominal and pelvic tumors, ultrasound examination and CT with oral and intravenous contrast media can help delineate the tumor. Cystourethrograms are useful for tumors in the bladder. A radionuclide scan and a full skeletal metastatic survey should be performed before definitive surgery. A chest radiograph and CT scan should be obtained, and bone marrow (aspirate and needle biopsy) should be examined. The results of these studies are used to plan the nature and extent of surgery. The most essential element of the diagnostic workup is examination of tumor tissue.

TREATMENT. Patients with completely resected tumors have the best prognosis. Unfortunately, most rhabdomyosarcomas are not completely resectable. At the initial surgery, tumor margins should be carefully defined, and an appropriate search for regional or metastatic disease (e.g., to regional lymph nodes or adjacent structures) should be completed even if the procedure is limited to biopsy. Treatment is based on the primary tumor location and disease stage ("clinical group"). Some patients are given preoperative chemotherapy in an attempt to reduce the extent of surgery required and to preserve vital organs, particularly in the genitourinary tract. In group I tumors, complete local excision is followed by chemotherapy to reduce the likelihood of subsequent metastatic disease. For groups II and III (i.e., microscopic or gross residual tumor, respectively) surgery is followed by local irradiation and systemic multiagent chemotherapy. Children with metastatic (group IV) rhabdomyosarcoma are treated principally with systemic chemotherapy and irradiation.

PROGNOSIS. Among patients with resectable tumor, 80–90% have prolonged, disease-free survival. Unresectable tumor localized to certain "favorable" sites (such as the orbit) also has a high likelihood of cure. About 60% of patients with incompletely resected regional tumor also achieve long-term disease-free survival. Patients with disseminated disease have a poor prognosis; only about half achieve remission, and fewer than half of these are cured. Older children have a poorer prognosis than younger ones.

506.2 Other Soft Tissue Sarcomas

The nonrhabdomyosarcoma soft tissue sarcomas (NRSTS) constitute a heterogeneous group of tumors that account for 3% of all childhood malignancies. Because they are relatively rare in children, much of the information about their natural history and treatment has been derived from studies of adult patients. In children, the median age at diagnosis is 12 yr, and males predominate (male:female ratio 2.3:1). The most common histologic types are synovial sarcoma (42%), fibrosarcoma (13%), malignant fibrous histiocytoma (12%), and neurogenic tumors (10%). Table 506–1 describes the clinical features, treatment, and prognosis of the most common NRSTS. These tumors commonly arise in the trunk or lower extremities. Tumor size, stage (clinical group), invasiveness, and histologic grade correlate with survival.

Surgery remains the mainstay of therapy, but a careful search for lung and bone metastases should be undertaken before surgical excision. Lymph node spread is rare, and routine dissection is not recommended. Adjuvant chemotherapy should be considered for high-grade, completely resected tumors, whereas postoperative radiotherapy is used for patients with microscopic residual disease. Patients with unresectable or metastatic disease are treated with multiagent chemotherapy that includes vincristine, doxorubicin, ifosfamide, cyclophosphamide, imidazole carboxamide (DTIC), and dactinomycin.

CHAPTER 507
Neoplasms of Bone

Carola A. S. Arndt

The annual incidence of malignant bone tumors in the United States is approximately 5.6 cases per million white children younger than 15 yr, with a slightly lower incidence in black children. Osteosarcoma is the most common primary malignant bone tumor in children and adolescents, followed by Ewing's sarcoma. In children younger than 10 yr, Ewing's sarcoma is more common than osteosarcoma. Both tumor types occur most frequently in the 2nd decade of life. Other differences between these tumors are noted in Table 507–1 and Figure 507–1.

TABLE 507–1 Comparison of Osteosarcoma and Ewing's Family of Tumors

Feature	Osteosarcoma	Ewing's Family of Tumors
Age	Second decade	Second decade
Race	All races	Primarily whites
Sex (M:F)	1.5:1	1.5:1
Cell	Spindle cell–producing osteoid	Undifferentiated small round cell, probably of neural origin
Predisposition	Retinoblastoma, Li-Fraumeni syndrome, Paget's disease, radiotherapy	None known
Site	Metaphyses of long bones	Diaphyses of long bones, flat bones
Presentation	Local pain and swelling; often history of injury	Local pain and swelling; fever
Radiographic findings	Sclerotic destruction (less commonly lytic); sunburst pattern	Primarily lytic, multilaminar periosteal reaction ("onion skinning")
Differential diagnosis	Ewing's sarcoma, osteomyelitis	Osteomyelitis, eosinophilic granuloma, lymphoma, neuroblastoma, rhabdomyosarcoma
Metastasis	Lungs, bones	Lung, bones
Treatment	Chemotherapy Ablative surgery of primary tumor	Chemotherapy Radiotherapy and/or surgery of primary tumor
Outcome	Without metastases: 70% cured; with metastases at diagnosis, ≤20% survival	Without metastases: 60% cured; with metastases at diagnosis, 20–30% survival

507.1 Osteosarcoma

The highest risk period for development of osteosarcoma is during the adolescent growth spurt. This suggests an association between rapid bone growth and malignant transformation. Patients with osteosarcoma are taller than their peers of similar age. Although the cause of osteosarcoma is unknown, certain genetic or acquired conditions predispose patients to development of osteosarcoma. Patients with hereditary retinoblastoma have a significantly increased risk of developing osteosarcoma. The sites of osteosarcoma in these patients were initially thought to be in previously irradiated areas; however, they have since been shown to arise in sites far from the radiation field. Predisposition to development of osteosarcoma in these patients is thought to be related to loss of heterozygosity of the Rb gene. Osteosarcoma also occurs in the *Li-Fraumeni syndrome,* which is a familial cancer syndrome associated with germline mutations of the p53 gene. Kindreds with Li-Fraumeni syndrome have a spectrum of malignancies in first-degree relatives including carcinoma of the breast, soft tissue sarcomas, brain tumors, leukemia, adrenal cortical carcinoma, and other malignancies. *Rothmund-Thomson syndrome* is a rare syndrome associated with short stature, skin telangiectasias, small hands and feet, hypoplastic or absent thumbs, and a high risk of osteosarcoma. Osteosarcoma can also be induced by radiation for Ewing's sarcoma, craniospinal radiation for brain tumors, or high-dose radiation for other malignancies. Other benign conditions that can be associated with malignant transformation to osteosarcoma include Paget's disease, enchondromatosis, multiple hereditary exostoses, and fibrous dysplasia.

PATHOLOGY. The pathologic diagnosis of osteosarcoma is made by demonstration of a highly malignant, pleomorphic, spindle cell neoplasm associated with the formation of malignant osteoid and bone. There are four pathologic subtypes of conventional high-grade osteosarcoma: osteoblastic, fibroblastic, chondroblastic, and telangiectatic. No significant differences in outcome are associated the various subtypes, although the chondroblastic component of that subtype may not respond as well to chemotherapy.

Telangiectatic osteosarcoma may be confused with aneurys-

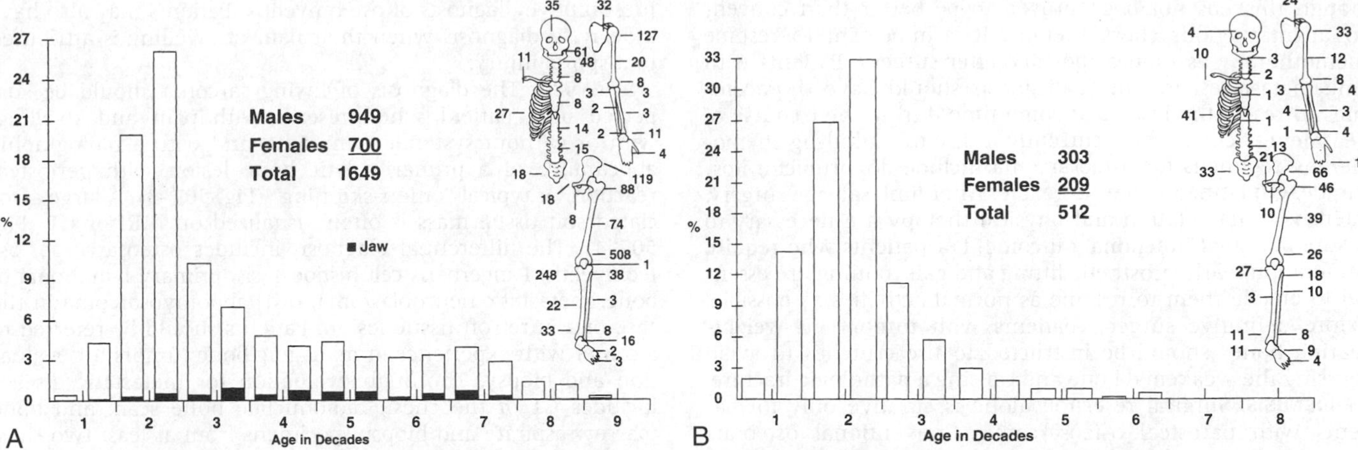

Figure 507–1 *A,* Age and skeletal distribution of 1,649 cases of osteosarcoma in the Mayo Clinic files. *B,* Age and skeletal distribution of 512 cases of Ewing sarcoma in the Mayo Clinic files. (Unni KK [ed]: Dahlin's Bone Tumors: General Aspects and Data on 11,087 Cases, 5th ed., Philadelphia, Lippincott-Raven, 1996. Reprinted by permission of the Mayo Foundation.)

mal bone cyst because of its lytic appearance radiographically. High-grade osteosarcoma typically arises in the diaphyseal region of long bones and invades the medullary cavity. It may also be associated with a soft tissue mass. Two variants of osteosarcoma, parosteal and periosteal osteosarcoma, should be distinguished from conventional osteosarcoma because of their characteristic clinical features. Parosteal osteosarcoma is a low-grade, well-differentiated tumor that does not invade the medullary cavity and is most commonly found in the posterior aspect of the distal femur. Surgical resection alone is often curative in this lesion, which has a low propensity for metastatic spread. Periosteal osteosarcoma is a rare variant, which arises on the surface of the bone but has a higher rate of metastatic spread than the parosteal type and an intermediate prognosis.

CLINICAL MANIFESTATIONS. Pain and swelling are the most common presenting manifestations of osteosarcoma. Because these tumors occur most frequently in active adolescents, initial complaints may be attributed to a sports injury or sprain. Clinicians must be aware that any bone or joint pain not responding to conservative therapy within a reasonable amount of time should be investigated thoroughly. Additional clinical findings may include limitation of motion, joint effusion, tenderness, and warmth. Results of routine blood work, such as a complete blood count and chemistry panel, are usually normal, although alkaline phosphatase or lactic dehydrogenase levels may be elevated.

DIAGNOSIS. The diagnosis of a bone tumor should be suspected in a patient who presents with deep bone pain, often causing nighttime awakening, a palpable mass, and a radiograph demonstrating a lesion. The lesion may be mixed lytic and blastic in appearance, but new bone formation is usually visible; the classic appearance is the sunburst pattern (Fig. 507–2). When osteosarcoma is suspected, the patient should be referred to a center with experience in managing bone tumors. The biopsy should be performed by the surgeon who will ultimately perform the definitive surgery so that the incisional biopsy site can be placed in a manner that will not compromise the ultimate limb salvage procedure. Tissue is usually obtained for molecular and biologic studies at the time of the initial biopsy. Before biopsy, MRI of the primary lesion and the entire bone should be performed to evaluate the tumor for its proximity to nerves and blood vessels, soft tissue and joint extension, as well as for skip lesions. The metastatic work-up should be performed before biopsy and includes CT of the chest and radionuclide bone scan to evaluate for lung and bone metastases, respectively. The differential diagnosis of a lytic bone lesion includes histiocytosis, Ewing's sarcoma, lymphoma, and bone cyst.

TREATMENT. The survival of children with nonmetastatic osteosarcoma was only 20% at 5 yr with surgery alone. It is well established that with chemotherapy and surgery, the 5-yr disease-free survival rate of patients with nonmetastatic extremity osteosarcoma is 65–75%. The current approach is to treat patients with preoperative chemotherapy in an attempt to facilitate limb salvage operations and to immediately treat micrometastatic disease. Up to 80% of patients are able to undergo limb salvage operations after initial chemotherapy. Some institutions use intra-arterial chemotherapy to infuse chemotherapy directly into an artery feeding the tumor, al-

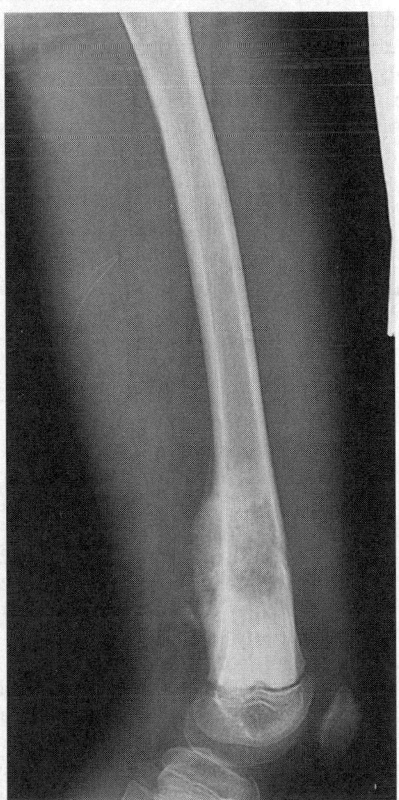

Figure 507–2 Radiograph of an osteosarcoma of the femur with typical "sunburst" appearance of bone formation.

though this has not been proved to be better than conventional intravenous chemotherapy. It is important to resume chemotherapy as soon as possible after surgery. Patients with lung metastases present at diagnosis should have thoracotomies to resect the lesions at some time during their course of treatment. Active agents currently in use in multidrug chemotherapy regimens for osteosarcoma include doxorubicin, ifosfamide, cisplatin, and methotrexate. After limb salvage surgery, intensive rehabilitation and physical therapy are necessary to ensure maximal functional outcome. For patients who require amputation, early prosthetic fitting and gait training are essential to enable them to resume as normal activities as possible. Before definitive surgery, patients with tumors on weight-bearing bones should be instructed to use crutches to avoid stressing the weakened bone and causing a pathologic fracture.

PROGNOSIS. Surgical resection alone is curative only for patients with parosteal osteosarcoma. Conventional osteosarcoma requires multiagent chemotherapy. Up to 75% of patients with nonmetastatic extremity osteosarcoma are cured with current multiagent treatment protocols. Patients with pelvic tumors do not have as favorable a prognosis as those with extremity primaries. Twenty to 30% of patients who have limited numbers of pulmonary metastases can also be cured with aggressive chemotherapy and resection of lung nodules. Patients with bone metastases and those with widespread lung metastases have an extremely poor prognosis. Long-term follow-up of patients with osteosarcoma is important to monitor for late effects of chemotherapy such as cardiotoxicity from anthracycline. Patients who develop late isolated lung metastases may be cured with surgical resection alone.

507.2 Ewing Sarcoma

Ewing sarcoma, an undifferentiated sarcoma of bone, may also arise from soft tissue. The term *Ewing sarcoma family of tumors* refers to a group of small round cell undifferentiated tumors thought to be of neural crest origin; these generally carry the same chromosomal translocation. This family of tumors includes Ewing sarcoma of bone and soft tissue and peripheral primitive neuroectodermal tumor (PPNET). Treatment protocols are the same whether the tumors arise in soft tissue or bone. Tumors arising in bone are evenly distributed between extremity and central axis (pelvis, spine, and chest wall) primary sites. Tumors whose primary site is in the chest wall are often referred to as Askin tumors.

PATHOLOGY. Immunohistochemical staining assists in the diagnosis of Ewing sarcoma in order to differentiate it from other small round blue cell tumors such as lymphoma, rhabdomyosarcoma, and neuroblastoma. Histochemical stains may react positively with certain neural markers on tumor cells (neuron-specific enolase and S-100), especially in PPNET. Reactivity with muscle markers (e.g., desmin, actin) is absent. Additionally, the cell surface glycoprotein MIC-2 is usually positive. A specific chromosomal translocation, t(11;22), or a variant thereof is found in most of the Ewing sarcoma family of tumors. Analysis for the translocation by routine cytogenetics or polymerase chain reaction analysis for the chimeric fusion gene products EWS/FLI1 or EWS/ERG can be helpful in confirming the diagnosis in very undifferentiated tumors.

CLINICAL MANIFESTATIONS. Symptoms of Ewing sarcoma are similar to those of osteosarcoma. Pain, swelling, limitation of motion, and tenderness over the involved bone or soft tissue are common presenting symptoms. In the case of huge chest wall primaries, patients may present with respiratory distress. Patients with paraspinal or vertebral primary tumors may present with symptoms of cord compression. Ewing sarcoma is often associated with systemic manifestations such as fever or weight loss; patients may have undergone treatment for a presumptive diagnosis of osteomyelitis. Patients may also have a delay in diagnosis when their pain or swelling is attributed to a sports injury.

DIAGNOSIS. The diagnosis of Ewing sarcoma should be suspected in a patient who presents with pain and swelling, with or without systemic symptoms, and with a radiographic appearance of a primarily lytic bone lesion with periosteal reaction, or typical "onion-skinning" (Fig. 507–3). A large associated soft tissue mass is often visualized on MRI or CT (Fig. 507–4). The differential diagnosis includes osteosarcoma, osteomyelitis, Langerhans cell histiocytosis, primary lymphoma of bone, metastatic neuroblastoma, or rhabdomyosarcoma in the case of a pure soft tissue lesion. Patients should be referred to a center with experience in managing bone tumors for evaluation and biopsy. Thorough evaluation for metastatic disease includes CT of the chest, radionuclide bone scan, and bone marrow aspirate and biopsy specimens from at least two sites. MRI of the tumor and the entire length of involved bone should be performed to determine the exact extension of the soft tissue and bony mass and the proximity of tumor to neurovascular structures. Biopsy should be performed preferably by the surgeon who will perform the ultimate surgical procedure to avoid compromising an ultimate potential for limb salvage by a poorly planned biopsy incision. CT-guided biopsy of the lesion often provides diagnostic tissue. It is important to obtain adequate tissue for special stains, cytogenetics, and molecular studies.

TREATMENT. Ewing sarcoma family of tumors are best managed with a comprehensive multidisciplinary approach incorporating the surgeon, chemotherapist, and radiation oncologist in planning therapy. Multiagent chemotherapy is important because it can rapidly shrink the tumor and is generally given before attempting local control. The addition of ifosfamide and etoposide to the standard agents of vincristine, doxorubicin, and cyclophosphamide improves the outcome of nonmetastatic Ewing sarcoma. Chemotherapy usually causes dramatic shrinkage of the soft tissue mass and rapid significant pain

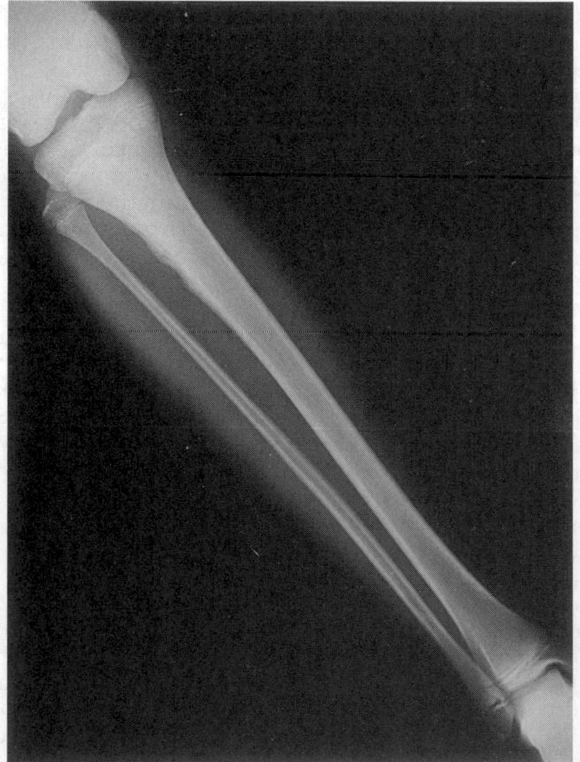

Figure 507–3 Radiograph of a tibial Ewing sarcoma showing periosteal elevation or "onion-skinning."

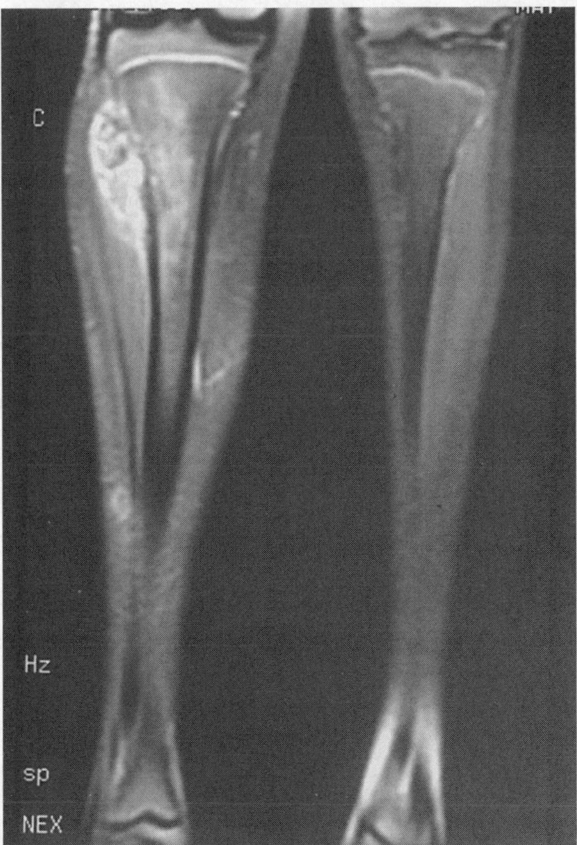

Figure 507–4 MRI of a tibial Ewing sarcoma showing a large associated soft tissue mass.

relief. Ewing's sarcoma is considered a very radiosensitive tumor, and local control may be achieved with radiation or surgery. There is controversy about the potential superiority of surgical resection compared with radiation for local control of the primary tumor. Radiation therapy is associated with a risk of radiation-induced second malignancies, especially osteosarcoma, as well as failure of bone growth in skeletally immature patients. Many centers prefer surgical resection if possible to achieve local control. It is important to provide patients with crutches if the tumor is in a weight-bearing bone to avoid a pathologic fracture before definitive local control. Chemotherapy should be resumed as soon as possible after surgery.

PROGNOSIS. Patients with small, nonmetastatic, distally located extremity tumors have the best prognosis. Such patients enjoy up to a 75% cure rate. Patients with pelvic tumors have, until recently, had a much worse outcome. Patients with metastatic disease at diagnosis, especially bone or bone marrow metastases, have a poor prognosis, with fewer than 30% surviving long term. New approaches, such as very intensive chemotherapy with peripheral blood stem cell rescue, are being investigated in these patients.

Long-term follow-up of patients with Ewing's sarcoma is important because of the potential for late effects of treatment such as anthracycline cardiotoxicity, second malignancies, especially in the radiation field, and late relapses even 10 yr after initial diagnosis.

Osteosarcoma

Link M, Eilber F: Osteosarcoma. *In*: Pizzo PA, Poplack DG (eds): Principles and Practice of Pediatric Oncology. Philadelphia, Lippincott-Raven, 1997, p 889.

Meyers P, Gorlick R: Osteosarcoma. Pediatr Clin North Am 44:973, 1997.

Link MP, Goorin AM, Horowitz M, et al: Adjuvant chemotherapy of high grade osteosarcoma of the extremity. Clin Orthop 270:8, 1991.

Ewing's Sarcoma

Delattre O, Zucman J, Melot T, et al: The Ewing family of tumors—a subgroup of small round cell tumors defined by specific chimeric transcripts. N Engl J Med 331:294, 1994.

Grier H: The Ewing family of tumors. Ewing's sarcoma and primitive neuroectodermal tumors. Pediatr Clin North Am 44:991, 1997.

Horowitz M, Malawer M, Woo S, et al: Ewing's sarcoma family of tumors: Ewing's sarcoma of bone and soft tissue and the peripheral primitive neuroectodermal tumors. *In*: Pizzo PA, Poplack DG (eds): Principles and Practice of Pediatric Oncology. Philadelphia, JB Lippincott, 1997, p 831.

Kretschmar C: Ewing's sarcoma and the "peanut" tumors. N Engl J Med 331:325, 1994

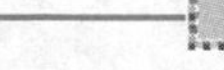

CHAPTER 508
Retinoblastoma

Gerald S. Gilchrist and Dennis M. Robertson

Retinoblastoma occurs in 1/18,000 live births in the United States, with no racial or gender predilection. Bilateral involvement is evident in 20–30% of patients. A small proportion of patients have other associated congenital anomalies. Overall, about 60% of cases are unilateral and nonhereditary, 15% unilateral and hereditary, and 25% bilateral and hereditary.

The retinoblastoma gene (RB1) is located on the long arm of chromosome 13 and acts as a tumor suppressor gene. If both alleles are nonfunctional as a result of either deletion or mutation, absence or dysfunction of the retinoblastoma protein leads to defective intracellular transcription and unchecked cell proliferation resulting in the malignant phenotype.

Familial cases are generally multifocal and bilateral, whereas nonfamilial cases tend to have unilateral, unifocal involvement. According to the "two-hit" model, two mutational events are required for tumor development. In the heritable form, one mutated Rb gene is inherited through the germ line and a second mutation occurs in the somatic retinal cell subsequently. In the noninherited form of retinoblastoma, both mutations occur in retinal cells (see Chapter 499).

PATHOLOGY. Retinoblastoma may arise in any of the nucleated layers of the retina and exhibit various degrees of differentiation; it tends to outgrow its blood supply, resulting in necrosis and calcification.

Endophytic tumors arise from the inner surface of the retina, grow into the vitreous, and tend to seed to other areas of the retina. Exophytic tumors grow from the outer retinal layer and may produce retinal detachment.

Extraocular extension into the orbit may occur through the choroid or optic nerve invasion. Hematogenous or lymphatic spread to more distant sites occasionally occurs.

CLINICAL MANIFESTATIONS. If not detected by routine neonatal ophthalmologic screening in the context of a positive family history, retinoblastoma classically presents with a white pupillary reflex (leukocoria) (Fig. 508–1). This abnormality is often first noticed when a red reflex is not present in a flash photograph of the child's face or at routine newborn or well-child examination. Strabismus is commonly the initial presenting complaint. Orbital inflammation, hyphema, or pupil irregularity occurs with advancing disease. Pain is usually a feature if secondary glaucoma is present.

DIAGNOSIS. The diagnosis is made ophthalmoscopically under general anesthesia by an ophthalmologist. This allows complete visualization of both eyes and facilitates photographing and mapping of the tumors. Retinal detachment or vitreous hemorrhage can complicate the evaluation.

Orbital ultrasonography and CT are used to evaluate intraocular extent and extraocular spread. MRI is not intended for

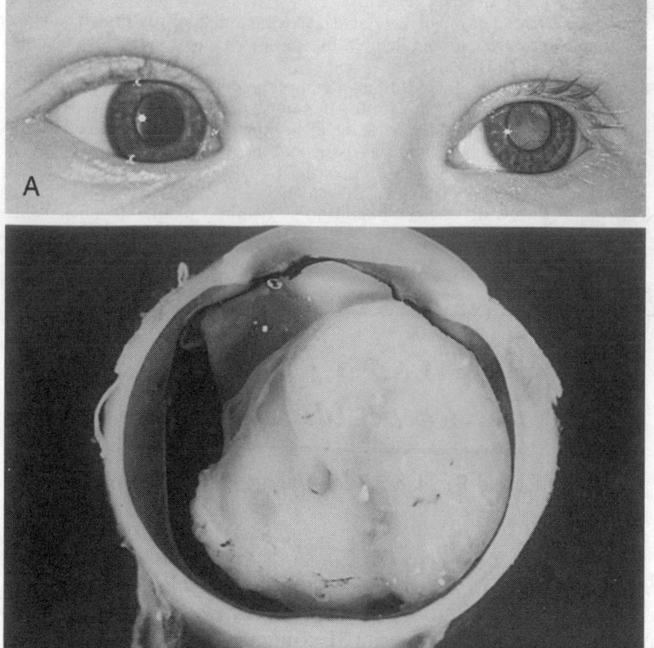

Figure 508–1 *A*, Leukocoria noted in the left eye of a child presenting with retinoblastoma. *B*, A large white tumor mass noted within the posterior chamber of the enucleated eye. (From Shields JA, Shields CL: Current management of retinoblastoma. Mayo Clin Proc 1;69:50, 1994.)

routine examination. Bone scan, cerebrospinal fluid evaluation, and bone marrow sampling are necessary only if indicated by other clinical, laboratory, or imaging studies.

Differential diagnosis of an intraocular tumor includes hyperplastic primary vitreous, Coat disease, cataract, visceral larva migrans, choroidal coloboma, and retinopathy of prematurity.

TREATMENT. The primary aim of treatment is cure with a secondary goal of preserving vision. As newer modalities for local control of intraocular tumor and more effective systemic chemotherapy have been developed, primary enucleation is no longer routinely undertaken.

Unilateral Disease. Enucleation is undertaken if there is no potential for useful vision. If feasible, small tumors can be treated with laser photocoagulation or cryotherapy with careful follow-up for evidence of recurrence or new tumor growth. Larger tumors often respond to multiagent chemotherapy including carboplatin, vincristine, and etoposide, thus facilitating successful focal therapy. If this approach fails, external beam irradiation or brachytherapy should be considered, although this approach may result in significant orbital deformity and a high incidence of second malignancies, particularly in patients with germ line mutations.

Bilateral Disease. The traditional approach involved enucleation of the more severely affected eye and irradiation of the remaining eye in hope of salvaging some useful vision. With the availability of effective chemotherapy, an attempt can be made to salvage both eyes with some degree of functional vision. Depending on the response to chemotherapy, local tumor control is attempted using laser photocoagulation, cryotherapy, or hyperthermia. External beam irradiation or brachytherapy may still be necessary with large residual tumor masses; enucleation may be required for nonresponsive or recurrent tumors.

PROGNOSIS. After primary enucleation of unilateral intraocular tumors, the cure rate exceeds 90%. Early reports of patients treated with local tumor ablation with or without chemotherapy suggest the potential for equally impressive survival but with retention of some degree of vision in most cases. Those with bilateral disease have fared less well, with respect to both survival and salvage of useful vision.

Children with germ line RB1 mutations are at significant risk for developing second malignancies, particularly if they have had radiation therapy. Other radiation-related complications include cataracts, orbital growth deformities, lacrimal dysfunction, and late retinal vascular injury.

Donaldson SS, Egbert PR, Newsham I, et al: Retinoblastoma. *In*: Pizzo PA, Poplack DG (eds): Principles and Practice of Pediatric Oncology. Philadelphia, JB Lippincott, 1997, p 733.

Gallie BL, Budning A, DeBoer G, et al: Chemotherapy and focal therapy can cure intraocular retinoblastoma without radiotherapy. Arch Ophthalmol 114:1321, 1996.

Mohney BG, Robertson DM, Schomberg PJ, et al: Second monocular tumors in survivors of heritable retinoblastoma and prior radiation therapy. Am J Ophthalmol 126:269, 1998.

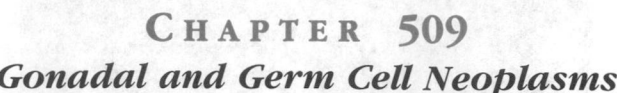

CHAPTER 509
Gonadal and Germ Cell Neoplasms

William A. Smithson

Most malignant tumors of the ovary and testis are of germ cell origin. They occur with an incidence of 4.2 cases per million population per year. In males, germ cell tumors are most common in whites. There are no known environmental causes for gonadal or extragonadal germ cell tumors. In other genetic syndromes with a high risk of cancer, germ cell neoplasms seldom occur.

PATHOLOGY. The germ and nongerm cell tumors arise from primordial germ cells and coelomic epithelium, respectively. Germ cell tumors may contain benign and malignant elements in different areas of the tumor; extensive sectioning is essential to make the correct diagnosis. There are many histologically distinct subtypes. Extragonal germ cell tumors include teratomas (sacral, retroperitoneal, pineal, other), with or without endodermal sinus tumor or embryohal carcinoma (Fig. 509–1). Non–germ cell tumors of the ovary include epithelial (serous and mucinous) and sex cord–stomal tumors; testicular tumors include sex cord–stromal tumors (Leydig's cell, Sertoli's cell).

CLINICAL MANIFESTATIONS, DIAGNOSIS, AND GENERAL APPROACH TO THERAPY. The clinical presentation of *germ cell neoplasms* depends on location. *Gonadal germ cell neoplasms* usually present with painless masses; ovarian tumors are often quite large before diagnosis. *Extragonadal germ cell tumors* occur in the midline, including the suprasellar region, pineal region, neck, mediastinum, and retroperitoneal and sacrococcygeal areas. Symptoms relate to mass effect, but the intracranial germ cell tumors often present with anterior and posterior pituitary deficits.

α-Fetoprotein (AFP) level is elevated in most patients with malignant germ cell tumors. Another marker less often elevated is the β subunit of human chorionic gonadotropin (β-HCG). If its levels are elevated, either hormone provides important confirmation of the diagnosis and serves as a means to monitor the patient for tumor remission and recurrence. Both serum and cerebrospinal fluid should be assayed for these markers in the case of intracranial lesions.

Diagnosis begins with physical examination and imaging studies including plain radiographs of the chest and ultrasonography of the abdomen. CT or MRI scans can further delineate the primary tumor. If germ cell malignancy is strongly suspected, preoperative staging with CT scan of the chest and bone scan are appropriate. Primary surgical resection is indicated for

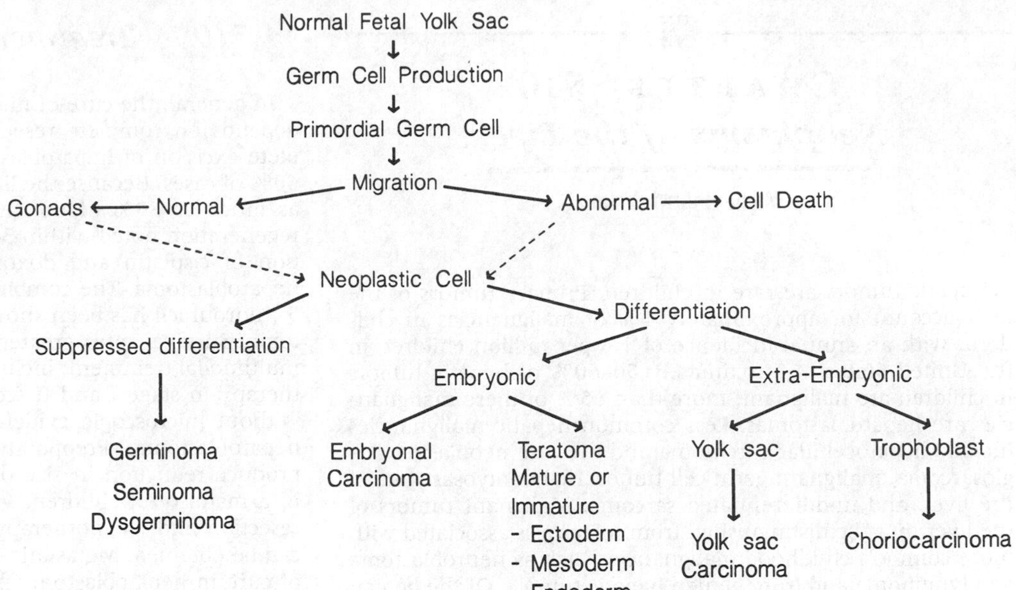

Figure 509–1 Tumors of germ cell origin. (Adapted from Pierce GB, Abeli MR: Embryonal carcinoma of the testis. Pathol Annu 5:27, 1970.)

tumors deemed resectable. The exception is intracranial lesions; in this site, the diagnosis can be made with imaging and AFP or β-HCG determinations. For intracranial lesions, primary therapy comprises radiation and chemotherapy.

Gonadoblastoma frequently occurs in patients with gonadal dysgenesis and a Y chromosome. This syndrome is characterized by failure of full masculinization of external genitalia and the presence of internal urogenital duct structures (often including the presence of a uterus) in association with incomplete organization of the gonad into a normal testicle. If this syndrome is diagnosed, imaging with ultrasonography or CT of the gonad is performed, and surgical resection of the tumor is generally curative. Prophylactic resection of dysgenetic gonads at the time of diagnosis is recommended because gonadoblastomas, some of which contain malignant germ cell tumor elements, frequently develop. Gonadoblastomas may produce abnormal amounts of estrogen. Undescended testicles (cryptorchidism) are at greater risk for germ cell malignancy and may be found as part of more generalized syndromes (Klinfelter's syndrome). Orchiopexy before puberty may reduce the risk, whereas testicular biopsy may increase the risk of malignancy.

Teratomas occur in many locations, present as masses, and if benign are curable by surgery. They are not associated with elevated markers unless malignancy is present. The sacrococcygeal region is the most frequent tumor site of teratomas; this is peculiar to neonates and infants and can be present at birth. The frequency of malignancy in this location varies from less than 10% at under 2 mo to over 50% at over 2 mo. Immature teratomas containing frankly malignant elements require chemotherapy regardless of surgical results.

Germinomas occur intracranially, in the mediastinum, and in the gonads. In the ovary, they are called *dysgerminomas*; in the testis, *seminoma*. They are often tumor marker negative (i.e., AFP and β-HCG) despite being malignant. If located intracranially, they are highly curable with a combination of radiation and chemotherapy. In other extragonadal and gonadal locations, surgical resection followed by chemotherapy is frequently curative.

Embryonal carcinoma most often occurs in the testes. Surgical resection is sufficient if the disease is confined to the testicle and markers (AFP and/or β-HCG) return to normal in the postoperative period. If a tumor is noted outside the testicle on imaging or if tumor markers are elevated, chemotherapy can be given and is generally curative.

Endodermal sinus or *yolk sac tumor* and *choriocarcinoma* appear highly malignant by histologic criteria. Both occur at gonadal and extragonadal sites. If the tumor is intracranial, irradiation and chemotherapy must be used. If the tumor occurs in the testis or ovary or in another location, surgery is used first, followed by chemotherapy. Chemotherapy is frequently used subsequently without irradiation, depending on the age of the child and location. Radiation is used only for chemotherapy refractory tumors.

In addition to germ cell tumors of the ovary, *epithelial carcinomas* (usually an adult tumor), *Sertoli-Leydig cell tumors*, and *granulosa cell tumors* may occur in children. Both of the latter tumors produce hormones that cause virilization or feminization or precocious puberty, depending on pubertal stage and the balance between Sertoli's (estrogen production) and Leydig's cells (androgen production). Diagnostic work-up usually focuses on the chief complaint of inappropriate sex steroid effect and includes hormone measurements, which reflect gonadotropin-independent sex steroid production. Appropriate imaging, to rule out a functioning gonadal tumor, is also performed (i.e., CT or MRI). Surgery is usually curative.

THERAPY. Complete surgical excision of the tumor is generally indicated, except for patients with central nervous system (CNS) primaries. For testicular tumors, an inguinal approach is indicated. Lymph node dissections were used after orchiectomy, but they are seldom performed today because availability of better imaging techniques, tumor markers, and development of highly effective chemotherapy have diminished their importance. Chemotherapy regimens including cisplatin, bleomycin, and either vinblastine or etoposide are generally curative even if metastases are present. Except for germ cell tumors of the CNS, use of irradiation is limited to those tumors that are not amenable to complete excision and are refractory to chemotherapy.

PROGNOSIS. The overall cure rate for children with germ cell tumors is about 80–90%.

Bosl GJ, Motzer RJ: Testicular germ-cell cancer. N Engl J Med 337:242, 1997.
Castleberry RP, Cushing B, Perlman E, et al: Germ cell tumors. *In*: Pizzo PA, Poplack DG (eds): Principles and Practice of Pediatric Oncology. Philadelphia, JB Lippincott, 1997, p 921.
Parker L: Causes of testicular cancer. Lancet 350:827, 1997.

CHAPTER 510
Neoplasms of the Liver

Michael J. McManus

Hepatic tumors are rare in children. Primary tumors of the liver account for approximately 1% of malignancies in children, with an annual incidence of 1.6 per million children in the United States. Approximately 50–60% of hepatic tumors in children are malignant; more than 65% of these malignancies are hepatoblastomas. Less common hepatic malignancies include hepatocellular carcinoma and the rare neoplasms: angiosarcoma, malignant germ cell tumor, rhabdomyosarcoma of the liver, and undifferentiated sarcoma. Malignant tumors of the liver must be distinguished from metastasis associated with more common childhood malignancies such as neuroblastoma and lymphoma and from benign hepatic tumors. Of the benign tumors, which usually present within the first 6 mo of life, the most common are hemangiomas, hamartomas, and hemangioendotheliomas. The cause of malignant hepatic tumors is unknown. Some hepatoblastomas have loss of heterozygosity at chromosome 11p15, suggesting the loss of a tumor suppressor gene. Hepatoblastomas are associated with Beckwith-Wiedemann syndrome and can show a similar loss of genomic imprinting of the insulin-like growth factor–II gene. Hepatocellular carcinoma in children can be associated with hepatitis B viral infection, the chronic form of hereditary tyrosinemia, glycogen storage disease, α_1-antitrypsin deficiency, and biliary cirrhosis.

HISTOLOGY. Hepatoblastoma usually arises from the right lobe of the liver and is unifocal. The two histologic types of hepatoblastoma are the epithelial type containing fetal or embryonal malignant cells (either as a mixture or as pure elements) and the mixed type containing mesenchymal and epithelial elements. The type of epithelial element is a histologic prognostic factor, with pure fetal histology predicting a more favorable outcome. Hepatocellular carcinoma generally presents as a multicentric, invasive tumor consisting of large pleomorphic cells with a lack of underlying cirrhosis.

CLINICAL PRESENTATION. Hepatoblastomas generally present within the first 18 mo of life in a child with a large, asymptomatic abdominal mass. Examination reveals abdominal distention and an enlarged liver. As the disease progresses, weight loss, anorexia, vomiting, and abdominal pain may ensue. Metastatic spread of hepatoblastoma most commonly involves regional lymph nodes and the lungs. In contrast, hepatocellular carcinoma generally presents in older children with a median age of 12 yr at diagnosis. These children have a hepatic mass, abdominal distention, and symptoms of anorexia, weight loss, and abdominal pain. Rarely, hepatic tumors, especially hepatocellular carcinoma, can present as an acute abdominal crisis with rupture of the tumor and hemoperitoneum. A valuable serum tumor marker, α-fetoprotein (AFP), is used in the diagnosis and monitoring of these hepatic tumors. AFP level is elevated in approximately 70% of children with hepatoblastoma and 50% of children with hepatocellular carcinoma. Hepatitis B and C viral serology should be obtained, especially in an older child with a suspected hepatic tumor. Diagnostic imaging should include plain radiographs and ultrasonography of the abdomen to detect the hepatic mass. Ultrasonography can differentiate malignant hepatic masses from benign vascular lesions. CT or MRI scanning is an accurate method of defining the extent of intrahepatic tumor involvement and the potential for surgical resection. Evaluation for metastatic disease should include CT scan of the chest and bone scan.

510.1 Treatment of Hepatoblastoma

In general, the cure of malignant hepatic tumors in children depends on complete resection of the primary tumor. Complete excision of hepatoblastoma can be accomplished in 50–60% of cases. Because the liver retains an ability to regenerate, as much as 85% of the liver can be resected, with hepatic regeneration noted within 3–4 mo after surgery. The combination of cisplatin and doxorubicin is effective treatment for hepatoblastoma. The combination of cisplatin, vincristine, and 5-fluorouracil has been shown to be equally effective and less toxic. Survival rates greater than 90% can be achieved with multimodal treatment, including surgery and adjuvant chemotherapy in stage I and II (complete surgical resection with or without microscopic evidence of tumor cells at the margin) hepatoblastoma. Preoperative chemotherapy regimens can produce reduction in size of an unresectable hepatoblastoma in a majority of children. With subsequent complete surgical resection and chemotherapy, cure rates in the range of 60% can be obtained. Metastatic disease further reduces the chance of cure in hepatoblastoma, but complete regression of disease can often be obtained with chemotherapy and surgical resection of the primary tumor and isolated pulmonary metastatic disease.

510.2 Treatment of Hepatocellular Carcinoma

Because of the multicentric origin of hepatocellular carcinoma, complete resection of this tumor is accomplished in only 30–40% of cases. Even with complete surgical resection, only 30% of children are long-term survivors. The fibrolamellar variant of hepatocellular carcinoma has a somewhat better prognosis. Chemotherapy, including cisplatin, doxorubicin, etoposide, and 5-fluorouracil, has shown some activity against this tumor, but improved long-term outcome has been difficult to achieve. Other techniques such as chemoembolization and liver transplantation are under study as therapy for hepatocellular carcinomas.

Chang MH, Chen CJ, Lai MS, et al: Universal hepatitis B vaccination in Taiwan and the incidence of hepatocellular carcinoma in children. N Engl J Med 336:1855, 1997.

Geiger JD: Surgery for hepatoblastoma in children. Curr Opin Pediatr 8:276, 1996.

Ikeda H, Matsuyama S, Tnaimura M: Association between hepatoblastoma and very low birth weight: A trend or a chance? J Pediatr 130:557, 1997.

Newman KD: Hepatic tumors in children. Semin Pediatr Surg 6:38, 1997.

Raney B: Hepatoblastoma in children: A review. J Pediatr Hematol Oncol 19:418, 1997.

CHAPTER 511
Gastrointestinal Neoplasm

William A. Smithson

511.1 Salivary Gland Tumors

About 60% of salivary gland masses are infectious in origin (Chapter 316). The most common neoplasms are benign hemangiomas and lymphangiomas, which are usually present in infancy. CT with contrast is the most useful imaging modality for distinguishing between these tumors. Surgery may be indicated for lymphangiomas if the facial nerve can be preserved. Hemangiomas eventually involute; surgery is not usually indicated. Therapy with either prednisone or interferon can shrink hemangiomas that need to be treated because of interference with function.

Several salivary gland tumors are of epithelial origin. The most common is the benign mixed tumor, which most commonly occurs in adolescent females and is curable by surgery. *Mucoepidermoid carcinoma, acinic cell carcinoma,* and *adenocarcinomas* account for the majority of malignant epithelioid tumors in children and adolescents. They are managed surgically, with radiation therapy used if there is incomplete resection, high-grade tumors with muscle involvement, or recurrence. Prognosis is generally good; most patients survive after resection but with high risk for local recurrence. No chemotherapy has been established. For tumors recurring after radiation, existing protocols for adults need to be adapted, because the tumors are much more common and histologically similar in adults.

511.2 Nasopharyngeal Carcinoma

This tumor accounts for only about 1% of pediatric malignancies. Nevertheless, it constitutes about 30% of malignant tumors of the nasopharynx in children under 15 yr. The incidence is higher in China. Environmental factors, especially Epstein-Barr virus infection, are etiologically important.

Patients usually present with cervical adenopathy but may have earlier symptoms caused by the primary tumor mass; eustachian tube blockage and nasal obstruction with epistaxis can be early findings. The mass is not usually visible on routine physical examination. Nasopharyngeal carcinoma is one of the tumors associated with *paraneoplastic syndromes* including clubbing (hypertrophic osteoarthropathy), fever of unknown origin, and the syndrome of inappropriate secretion of antidiuretic hormone.

CT and MRI images are helpful in both identifying and defining masses in the head and neck. Diagnosis is made by biopsy of the mass or of a suspicious cervical lymph node. The differential includes rhabdomyosarcoma, lymphoma, and benign juvenile nasopharyngeal angiofibroma. Metastases to the lungs, bones, liver, and bone marrow may be present.

Surgery is important for staging and diagnosis. Radiation therapy is effective for control of the primary tumor and regional nodal metastases. Chemotherapy with 5-fluorouracil, cisplatinum, and methotrexate is effective but not always curative.

Prognosis is good if the tumor is localized. Unfortunately, metastasis to cervical lymph nodes that is often present at diagnosis diminishes the opportunity for cure. Reports of cure in patients with advanced disease with radiation and chemotherapy justify intensive treatment at a cancer center. New agents such as interferon are being evaluated in prospective trials.

Late effects in children cured of this disease are related to relatively high-dose radiation to the nasopharynx and neck. Salivary gland dysfunction, trismus, hypothyroidism, thyroid carcinoma, and other secondary malignancies have been observed. Cisplatinum use can be associated with permanent high-frequency hearing loss, peripheral neuropathy, and loss of renal function.

511.3 Carcinoma of the Stomach

Adenocarcinoma of the stomach was formerly one of the leading causes of death in adults in the United States. It has been reported in children. The decline in incidence in the United States and the persisting higher incidence in Japanese in and outside of Japan are evidence for both environmental and genetic influences. Symptoms are the result of mass effect or bleeding. Diagnosis is usually made by endoscopic biopsy.

Surgery is the only curative modality; prognosis is poor and related to the fact the disease is often beyond surgical boundaries at diagnosis and is not highly sensitive to chemotherapy or irradiation.

511.4 Pancreatic Tumors

Pancreatic tumors may be of either endocrine or nonendocrine origin.

Tumors of endocrine origin include *insulinomas* and *gastrinomas*. These and other functioning tumors occur in the autosomal dominantly inherited multiple endocrine neoplasia type 1 (MEN-1). Hypoglycemia accompanied by higher than expected (for serum glucose) insulin levels or refractory gastric ulcers (Zollinger-Ellison syndrome) indicate the possibility of a pancreatic tumor (see Chapter 353). Peculiar to childhood are *pancreatoblastomas*, which are embryonal tumors that secrete α-fetoprotein and may contain both endocrine and exocrine elements. Their clinical behavior is malignant but not well characterized owing to their rarity. Presurgical chemotherapy should be considered for lesions not primarily resectable. Resection can be curative; adjuvant chemotherapy has been used, but its effectiveness is not established.

Cysts of the pancreas occur in von Hippel–Lindau disease. Solid and cystic papillary tumors mimic pancreatic ontogeny. Their natural history is still being determined. Metastases have been reported, but adjuvant therapy following surgical excision cannot yet be recommended.

Carcinoma of the exocrine pancreas is a major problem in adults, accounting for 2% of diagnoses and 5% of deaths due to cancer. It is very rare in childhood. No definite etiologies are known. Several genetic syndromes including MEN-1 lead to an increased incidence of pancreatic cancer in adult life.

Diagnosis is suggested by CT scanning. Surgery is the only known effective therapy. Prognosis is good for completely resected endocrine tumors but very poor for carcinomas, even with extensive surgery.

Children who survive partial or complete pancreatectomy may have decreased pancreatic exocrine and endocrine reserve.

511.5 Colonic Polyps

Most polyps are isolated (five or fewer) juvenile polyps distinguishable pathologically and endoscopically from the important multiple polyposis syndromes. Solitary polyps are seldom premalignant.

Familial adenomatous polyposis is inherited as an autosomal dominant with a high degree of penetrance. The incidence of colonic cancer is nearly 100%, and colectomy using continent reservoir and endorectal pull-through technique is often recommended. Any condition with adenomatous polyps poses a high risk of cancer and includes Gardner's and Turcot's syndromes.

Generalized juvenile polyposis, also inherited in an autosomal dominant pattern, is precancerous in spite of the fact that most of the polyps have the typical appearance of juvenile polyps.

Because nonpolyposis colon cancer is also heritable and many benign polyps occur in childhood, referral to a pediatric center with expertise in genetics, gastroenterology, pathology, and surgery is recommended before decisions about screening procedures and prophylactic colectomy.

511.6 Adenocarcinoma of the Colon and Rectum

This is a common cancer in adults, accounting for 15% of all cancers. It usually occurs after age 50. The incidence in adolescence is low; nevertheless, suspicious gastrointestinal blood loss or a change in bowel habit requires special barium enema (with meticulous bowel preparation) or endoscopy because of the possibility of colon cancer. No environmental cause has been identified, but diet (i.e., high fat) may be important. Patients with ulcerative colitis and familial adenomatous polyposis have high enough incidence that frequent endoscopies and possible prophylactic colectomy may be recommended. An increase in colonic carcinoma is noted in patients with Crohn's disease as well, and strategies similar to those recommended for ulcerative colitis should be considered.

Hereditary nonpolyposis colorectal cancer (Lynch's syndrome) and various polyposis syndromes make the diagnosis more likely in children and adolescents. Endoscopic screening is recommended in childhood for some syndromes.

Treatment begins with surgery. Radiation and chemotherapy can improve survival. Prognosis is dependent on the stage at diagnosis, confirming the importance of early diagnosis and screening.

Adenocarcinoma of the colon has been reported as a second malignancy in patients treated in childhood for cancer with abdominal radiation.

Alexander HR, Kelsen DG, Tepper JC: Cancer of the stomach. *In:* DeVita VT, Hellman S, Rosenberg SA (eds): Cancer Principles and Practice of Oncology, 5th ed. Philadelphia, Lippincott-Raven, 1997, p 1021.

Cohen AM, Minsky BD, Schilsky RL: Cancer of the colon. *In:* DeVita VT, Hellman S, Rosenberg SA (eds): Cancer Principles and Practice of Oncology, 5th ed. Philadelphia, Lippincott-Raven, 1997, p 1144.

Douglass EC, Pratt CB: Management of infrequent cancers of childhood. *In:* Pizzo PA, Poplack DG (eds): Principles and Practice of Pediatric Oncology, 5th ed. Philadelphia, Lippincott-Raven, 1997, p 977.

Illnow U, Willberg B, Schwamborn D, et al: Pancreatoblastoma in children: Case report and review of the literature. Eur J Pediatr Surg 6:369, 1996.

Lindor NM, Greene MH: The Concise Handbook of Family Cancer Syndromes. J Natl Cancer Inst 90:1040, 1998.

Wunsch LP, Flemming P, Werner U, et al: Diagnosis and treatment of papillary cystic tumor of the pancreas in children. Eur J Pediatr Surg 7:45, 1997.

CHAPTER 512
Carcinomas

William A. Smithson

Clear cell adenocarcinomas of the vagina and cervix were rare until diethylstilbestrol (DES) was widely used to prevent premature delivery (Chapter 561). Girls whose mothers took DES during pregnancy experienced a markedly increased incidence of this rare tumor later in life. The peak incidence is between age 15 and 22 yr, with the youngest patient reported being age 7 yr. DES is now contraindicated in pregnant women.

CARCINOMA OF THE THYROID. (See Chapter 579.) Carcinoma of the thyroid occurs rarely in children. It is usually diagnosed and managed by endocrinologists. It occurs as part of *Gardner's syndrome* and *multiple endocrine neoplasia type* 2 (MEN-2). When one of the triad of pheochromocytoma, medullary thyroid carcinoma, or hyperparathyroidism occurs in a family with MEN-2, the others should also be screened for periodically. Exposure to irradiation, either therapeutic or accidental (such as in the Chernobyl nuclear accident), markedly increases the incidence. Most cases are cured with surgery or ^{131}I.

CARCINOMA OF THE ADRENAL GLAND. These tumors arise from the adrenal cortex and may or may not produce excess hormones. The most common syndromes are Cushing's, virilization, and hyperaldosteronism; mass effects predominate in nonfunctioning tumors. There is a bimodal age incidence at under age 5 and age 30–50 yr. Tumors may be benign or malignant, and clinical behavior can be predicted by histology and tumor size. Diagnosis is suggested by CT or MRI. Endocrine work-up preoperatively is indicated.

Treatment is surgical and is often curative when tumors are small and completely resected. Radiation can delay or prevent local recurrence and is useful for metastatic lesions. No chemotherapy regimen is curative, but the drug mitotane blocks the excess endocrine effects and can provide useful palliation.

Prognosis relates to the degree of malignancy and extent of surgical resection.

Dehner LP: Pediatric Surgical Pathology, 2nd ed. Baltimore, Williams & Wilkins, 1987, p 62.

Lindor NM, Green MH: The Concise Handbook of Family Cancer Syndromes. J Natl Cancer Inst 90:1040, 1998.

Schlumberger MJ: Papillary and follicular thyroid carcinoma. N Engl J Med 338:297, 1998.

CHAPTER 513
Cancer of the Skin

(Also see Chapters 662 and 676)

William A. Smithson

Squamous cell and *basal cell carcinomas* of the skin rarely occur in children. Surgical excision or chemical ablation is generally curative. There is a high incidence of squamous and basal cell carcinoma in *xeroderma pigmentosa. Melanoma* also occurs at low frequency in children. It usually arises in pigmented nevi, which exhibit asymmetry, border irregularity, color variation, and diameter greater than 6 mm. Patients with such lesions should be referred to a dermatologist for evaluation. Bleeding, a subcutaneous mass, and pruritus are other hallmarks of malignant change in a melanocytic nevus. Other pigmented nevi at high risk to become malignant are those in areas irradiated for treatment of cancer earlier in childhood. Pathology of pigmented lesions in children is different from that of adults and may mimic malignancy. Pathologists familiar with pediatric histopathology should be consulted in suspected cases of melanoma in a child.

About 10% of patients with giant hairy nevus develop melanoma; these cases are usually referred to plastic surgeons for resection. Genetic factors are implicated by increased familial incidence and occurrence in the *dysplastic nevus* and *neurocutaneous melanosis syndromes.*

The major environmental factor contributing to skin cancer pathogenesis is sun exposure. Wearing clothing and using sunscreens to avoid excess sun exposure has become an important part of pediatric preventive practice. A family history of melanoma significantly increases risk. Melanoma and basal cell carcinomas are being reported as second malignant neoplasms in survivors of childhood cancer. Pigmented nevi within radiated fields are at higher risk of becoming melanomas.

Diagnosis of malignant melanoma is made by excisional biopsy. Wide excision, lymph node sampling, and removal are indicated if melanoma is diagnosed. Metastasis to lungs, liver, and bones should be sought. Radiation may be useful if regional lymph nodes are involved. No systemic chemotherapy has been effective for metastatic disease. Immunotherapy directed at melanoma antigens and interferon are undergoing clinical trials.

Prognosis is related to the thickness or depth of penetration of the primary lesion and is very poor for deep or metastatic lesions.

Wu SJ, Lambert DR: Melanoma in children and adolescents. Pediatr Dermatol 14:87, 1997.

CHAPTER 514
Benign Tumors

William J. Shaughnessy and Carola A. S. Arndt

Various benign tumors in infants and children present diagnostic challenges (Table 514–1). Many of these tumors require treatment. Some, although histologically benign, can be life threatening.

514.1 Benign Tumors and Tumor-Like Processes of Bone

Benign bone lesions in children are common in comparison with the relatively rare malignant neoplasms of bone. No single history element or diagnostic test is sufficient to rule out malignancies or suggest non-neoplastic conditions. A broad range of diagnostic possibilities must be considered when confronted with an unknown bone lesion. Benign lesions may be painless or painful, especially if a pathologic fracture is impending. Night pain that awakens a child is suggestive of malignancy; relief of such pain with aspirin is common with benign lesions such as **osteoid osteomas**. Rapidly enlarging lesions are usually associated with malignancy, but several benign lesions, such as **aneurysmal bone cysts**, may enlarge faster than most malignancies. Several conditions, such as osteomyelitis, may simulate the appearance of benign bone tumors.

Many benign bone tumors are diagnosed incidentally or after pathologic fracture. Management of these fractures is similar to that of nonpathologic fractures in the same location. It is unusual for benign bone tumors to interfere with fracture healing. Likewise, the fractures rarely result in changes or healing of these tumors, which are usually treated after the fracture has healed.

Radiographs of any suspected bone lesion should always be obtained in two planes. Additional studies may be necessary to help arrive at the correct diagnosis and to guide treatment. Despite the benign nature of these lesions, many require intervention.

Osteochondroma (exostosis) is one of the most common benign bone tumors in children. Many are completely asymptomatic and unrecognized. The true incidence of this lesion is therefore unknown. Most osteochondromas develop in childhood, arising from the metaphysis of long bones, particularly the distal femur, proximal humerus, and proximal tibia. The lesion enlarges with the child until skeletal maturity. Most are discovered between the ages of 5 and 15 yr when the child or parent notices a bony, nonpainful mass. Some are discovered

TABLE 514–1 Benign Bone Tumors and Cysts

Disease	Characteristics	Roentgenography	Treatment	Prognosis
Osteochondroma (osteocartilaginous exostosis)	Common; distal metaphysis of femur, proximal humerus, proximal tibia; painless, hard, nontender mass	Bony outgrowth, sessile or pedunculated	Excision, if symptomatic	Excellent; malignant transformation rare
Multiple hereditary exostoses	Osteochondroma of long bones; bone growth disturbances	As above	As above	Recurrences
Osteoid ostoma	Point tenderness; pain relieved by aspirin; femur and tibia; predominantly found in boys	Osteosclerosis surrounds small radiolucent nidus, 1 cm	As above	Excellent
Giant osteoid osteoma (osteoblastoma)	As above, but more destructive	Osteolytic component; size > 1 cm	As above	Excellent
Enchondroma	Tubular bones of hands and feet; pathologic fractures, swollen bone; Ollier's disease if multiple lesions are present	Radiolucent diaphyseal or metaphyseal lesion; may calcify	Excision or curettage	Excellent; malignant transformation rare
Nonossifying fibroma	Silent; rare pathologic fracture; late childhood adolescence	Incidental roentgenographic finding; thin sclerotic border, radiolucent lesion	None or curettage with fractures	Excellent; heals spontaneously
Eosinophilic granuloma	Age 5–10 yr; skull, jaw, long bones; pathologic fracture; pain	Small, radiolucent without reactive bone; punched-out lytic lesion	Biopsy, excision rare; irradiation	Excellent; may heal spontaneously
Brodie's abscess	Insidious local pain; limp; suspected as malignancy	Circumscribed metaphyseal osteomyelitis; lytic lesions with sclerotic rim	Biopsy; antibiotics	Excellent
Unicameral bone cyst (simple bone cyst)	Metaphysis of long bone (femur, humerus); pain, pathologic fracture	Cyst in medullary canal, expands cortex; fluid-filled unilocular or multilocular cavity	Curettage; steroid injection into lesion	Excellent, some heal spontaneously
Aneurysmal bone cyst	As above; contains blood, fibrous tissue	Expands beyond metaphyseal cartilage	Curettage, bone graft	Excellent

From Behrman R, Kliegman R (eds): Nelson Essentials of Pediatrics, 2nd ed. Philadelphia, WB Saunders, 1994.

when irritated by pressure during athletic or other activities. Radiographically, osteochondromas appear as stalks or broad-based projections from the surface of the bone, usually in a direction away from the adjacent joint. Invariably, the lesion is radiographically smaller than suggested by palpation because the cartilage "cap" covering the lesion is not seen. This cartilage cap may be up to 1 cm thick. Both the cortex of the bone and the marrow space of the involved bone are continuous with the lesion. Malignant degeneration to a chondrosarcoma is rare in children but may occur in as many as 1% of adults. Routine removal is not performed unless the lesion is large enough to cause symptoms or if rapid growth occurs. **Multiple hereditary exostoses** is a related but rare condition characterized by the presence of multiple osteochondromas. Severely involved children may have short stature, limb length inequality, premature partial physeal arrests, and deformity of both the upper and lower extremities. These individuals need to be monitored carefully during growth.

Enchondroma is a benign lesion of hyaline cartilage occurring centrally in the bone. The majority are asymptomatic and occur in the hands. Most are discovered incidentally, although pathologic fractures often lead to the diagnosis. Radiographically, the lesions occupy the medullary canal, are radiolucent, and sharply marginated. Punctate or stippled calcification may be present within the lesion, but this is much more common in adults than children. The vast majority of enchondromas are solitary. Most can be observed, with curettage and bone grafting reserved for those lesions that are symptomatic or large enough to weaken the bone structurally. Multifocal involvement is referred to as **Ollier's disease** and may result in bony dysplasia, short stature, limb length inequality, and joint deformity. Surgery may be necessary to correct or prevent such deformities. When *multiple enchondromas* are associated with angiomas of the soft tissue, the condition is referred to as **Maffucci's syndrome**. A high rate of malignant transformation has been reported in both of these multifocal conditions.

Chondroblastoma is a rare lesion usually found in the epiphysis of long bones. Most patients present in the 2nd decade with complaints of mild to moderate pain in the adjacent joint. Common sites include the hip, shoulder, and knee. Muscle atrophy and local tenderness may be the only clinical findings. Radiographically, the lesion appears as a sharply marginated radiolucency within the epiphysis or apophysis, occasionally with metaphyseal extension across the physis. Proximity to the joint may cause deformity of the subchondral bone, an effusion, or erosion into the joint. Recognition is important because most lesions can be cured with curettage and bone grafting before joint destruction occurs.

Chondromyxoid fibroma is an uncommon benign bone tumor in children. This metaphyseal lesion usually causes pain and local tenderness. The lesion may occasionally be asymptomatic. Radiographically, chondromyxoid fibroma appears as an eccentric, lobular, metaphyseal radiolucency with sharp, sclerotic, and scalloped margins. The lower extremity is most often involved. Treatment usually consists of curettage and bone grafting or en bloc resection.

Osteoid osteoma is a small benign bone tumor; the majority are diagnosed between 5 and 20 yr of age. The clinical pattern is characteristic, consisting of unremitting and gradually increasing pain, often worst at night and relieved by aspirin. Males are affected more commonly than females. Any bone can be involved, but the most common sites are the proximal femur and tibia. Vertebral lesions may cause scoliosis or symptoms that mimic a neurologic disorder. Examination may reveal a limp, atrophy, and weakness when the lower extremity is involved. Palpation and range of motion do not alter the discomfort. Radiographs are distinctive, showing a round or oval metaphyseal or diaphyseal lucency (0.5–1.0 cm diameter) surrounded by sclerotic bone. The central lucency, or nidus, shows intense uptake on bone scan. About 25% of osteoid osteomas are not visualized on plain radiographs but can be identified with tomography or CT. Because of the small size of the lesion and the location adjacent to thick cortical bone, MRI is poor at detecting osteoid osteomas. Treatment is directed at removing the lesion. This may involve en bloc excision, curettage, or percutaneous CT-guided ablation of the nidus. Patients with mild pain may be treated with salicylates. Some lesions spontaneously resolve after skeletal maturity.

Osteoblastoma is a locally destructive, progressively growing lesion of bone with a predilection for the vertebrae, although almost any bone may be involved. Most patients note the insidious onset of dull aching pain, which may be present for months before they seek medical attention. Spinal lesions may cause neurologic symptoms or deficits. The radiographic appearance is variable and less distinctive than that of other benign bone tumors. About 25% show features suggesting a malignant neoplasm, making biopsy necessary in many cases. Expansile spinal lesions often involve the posterior elements. Treatment involves curettage and bone grafting or en bloc excision, taking care to preserve nerve roots when treating spinal lesions. Surgical stabilization of the spine may be necessary.

Fibromas (nonossifying fibroma, fibrous cortical defect, metaphyseal fibrous defect) are fibrous lesions of bone that occur in 40% of children older than 2 yr. They likely represent a defect in ossification rather than a neoplasm. As such, these lesions are usually asymptomatic. Most are discovered incidentally when radiographs are taken for other reasons, usually to rule out a fracture after trauma. Occasional pathologic fractures can occur through rare large lesions. Physical examination is usually unrevealing. Radiographs show a sharply marginated eccentric lucency in the metaphyseal cortex. Lesions may be multilocular and expansile, with extension from the cortex into the medullary bone. The long axis of the lesion is parallel with that of the bone. Approximately 50% are bilateral or multiple. Because of the characteristic radiographic appearance, most lesions do not require biopsy or treatment. Spontaneous regression can be expected after skeletal maturity. Curettage and bone grafting may be recommended for lesions occupying more than 50% of the bone diameter because of the risk of a pathologic fracture.

Unicameral bone cysts can occur at any age in childhood but are rare before 3 yr and after skeletal maturity. The cause of these fluid-filled lesions is unknown. Some resolve spontaneously after skeletal maturity. Most are asymptomatic until diagnosis, which usually follows a pathologic fracture. Such fractures may occur with relatively minor trauma, such as with throwing or catching a ball. Radiographically, unicameral bone cysts are solitary, centrally located lesions within the medullary portion of the bone. These cysts are most common in the proximal humerus or femur. They often extend to (but not through) the physis and are sharply marginated. Thinning and expansion of the cortex occurs but does not exceed the width of the adjacent physis. Treatment involves allowing the pathologic fracture to heal, followed by aspiration and injection with methylprednisolone or bone marrow. Repeat injections, curettage, and bone grafting are occasionally necessary to treat recurrent lesions.

Aneurysmal bone cyst is a reactive lesion of bone seen during the 1st and 2nd decades of life. The lesion is characterized by cavernous spaces filled with blood and solid aggregates of tissue. Although the femur, tibia, and spine are most commonly involved, this progressively growing, expansile lesion develop in any bone. Pain and swelling are common. Spinal involvement may lead to cord or nerve root compression and associated neurologic symptoms including paralysis. Radiographs show eccentric lytic destruction and expansion of the metaphysis surrounded by a thin sclerotic rim of bone. Posterior elements of the spine are more commonly involved than the vertebral body. Unlike most other benign bone tumors, which are usually confined to a single bone, aneurysmal bone cysts may involve adjacent vertebrae. Rapid growth is characteristic and may lead to confusion with malignant neoplasms. Treatment consists of curettage and bone grafting or excision. Spinal lesions may require stabilization after excision. As with other benign tumors, attempts are made to preserve nerve roots and other vital structures. Recurrence after surgical treatment occurs in 20–30%, is more common in younger than older children, and usually occurs in the first 1–2 yr after treatment.

Fibrous dysplasia is a developmental abnormality characterized by fibrous replacement of cancellous bone. Lesions may be solitary or multifocal (polyostotic), relatively stable, or progressively more severe. Most children are asymptomatic, although those with skull involvement may have swelling or exophthalmos. Pain and limp are characteristic of proximal femoral involvement. Limb length discrepancy, bowing of the tibia or femur, and pathologic fractures may be presenting complaints. The triad of polyostotic disease, precocious puberty, and cutaneous pigmentation is known as **Albright's syndrome** (see Chapter 572.6). Radiographic features of fibrous dysplasia include a lytic or ground-glass expansile lesion of the metaphysis or diaphysis. The lesion is sharply marginated and often surrounded by a thick rim of sclerotic bone. Bowing, especially of the proximal femur, may be present. Treatment usually involves observation. Surgery is indicated for patients with progressive deformity, pain, or impending pathologic fractures. Bone grafting is not as successful in the treatment of fibrous dysplasia as with other benign tumors because the lesion often recurs within the grafted bone. Reconstructive surgical techniques are often necessary to provide stability.

Osteofibrous dysplasia is a lesion that affects children 1–10 yr old. This lesion usually involves the tibia. It is clinically, radiographically, and histologically distinct from fibrous dysplasia. Most children present with anterior swelling or enlargement of the leg. Most have no pain unless associated with a pathologic fracture. Progression is unlikely after 10 yr of age. Radiographs show solitary or multiple lucent, cortical, diaphyseal lesions surrounded by sclerosis. Anterior bowing of the tibia is often present. The radiographic appearance closely resembles that of adamantinoma, a malignant neoplasm, making biopsy more common than with other benign bone tumors. Treatment involves observation. Some lesions heal spontaneously. Excision and bone grafting should be delayed until after age 10 yr because of a high recurrence rate until after this age. Pathologic fractures heal with immobilization.

Eosinophilic granuloma is a monostotic or polyostotic disease with no extraskeletal involvement. This latter finding distinguishes eosinophilic granuloma from the other forms of Langerhans' cell histiocytosis (Hand-Schüller-Christian or Letterer-Siwe variants), which may have a less favorable prognosis (see Chapter 515). Eosinophilic granuloma usually occurs during the first 3 decades of life and is most common in boys between 5 and 10 yr of age. The skull is most commonly affected, but any bone may be involved. Patients usually present with local pain and swelling. There is often marked tenderness and warmth in the area of the involved bone. Spinal lesions may cause pain, stiffness, and occasional neurologic symptoms. The radiographic appearance of the skeletal lesions is similar in all forms of Langerhans' cell histiocytosis but is variable enough to mimic many other benign and malignant lesions of bone. The radiolucent lesions have well-defined or irregular margins with expansion of the involved bone and periosteal new bone formation. Spine involvement may cause uniform compression or flattening of the vertebral body. A skeletal survey is warranted because polyostotic involvement and the typical skull lesions strongly suggest the diagnosis of eosinophilic granuloma. Biopsy is often necessary to confirm the diagnosis because of the broad radiographic differential diagnosis. Treatment includes curettage and bone grafting, low-dose radiation therapy, or steroid injection. Observation for symptomatic lesions is reasonable because most osseous lesions heal spontaneously and do not recur. Children with bone lesions should be evaluated for visceral involvement because treatment of *Hand-Schüller-Christian disease* and *Letterer-Siwe disease* is more complex and often systemic (see Chapter 515).

514.2 Hemangiomas

Hemangiomas are the most common benign tumors of infancy and are found in 1% of neonates (see Chapters 653 and 656). Most do not need therapy. The natural history of hemangiomas is rapid growth during the 1st year of life, slowing of growth in the next 5 yr, and involution by age 10–15 yr. Approximately 10% of hemangiomas cause significant impairment, and 1% are life threatening because of their location. Hemangiomas around the airway can cause airway obstruction. Large hemangiomas may cause thrombocytopenia, microangiopathic hemolytic anemia, and coagulopathy as a result of platelet and red blood cell trapping and activation of the clotting system within the vasculature of the hemangioma. This is called the **Kasabach-Merritt syndrome**. Treatment of patients with Kasabach-Merritt usually consists of supportive care while also beginning therapy with steroids or interferon. Heparin therapy is contraindicated in the treatment of this type of consumptive coagulopathy, and platelet transfusions should be avoided in the absence of life-threatening hemorrhage because they may result in massive swelling of the hemangioma and rebound thrombocytopenia. Large hepatic hemangiomas or hemangioendotheliomas may result in hepatomegaly, anemia, thrombocytopenia, and high-output heart failure.

For those hemangiomas that are life threatening or that threaten vital functions such as eyesight, a trial of corticosteroids is warranted. Approximately 30% of hemangiomas respond dramatically and begin to regress within a week, 40% may stabilize or show a minimal response, and the remainder do not respond. Interferon-α is used in the treatment of hemangiomas, in particular those that do not respond to steroid therapy. Surgical therapy of some hemangiomas may be indicated because they are very invasive and never completely resectable. Laser therapy has been used in special situations. A rare variant of hemangioma, the **Kaposi-like form of infantile hemangioma**, does not respond to corticosteroid therapy and may be controlled with interferon. Interferon-α and steroids should not be used simultaneously, because the side effects may be enhanced and they may be antagonistic.

The most common *lymphatic malformation* seen in children is **cystic hygroma** of the neck, which presents as a painless soft tissue swelling. Treatment of simple lymphatic malformations such as this is surgical resection. They usually do not regress spontaneously. Larger lesions in other areas of the body may require staged surgical resection, because they are often quite diffuse.

514.3 Thymic Tumors

The thymus can be involved by a number of malignant lesions including *lymphomas, malignant germ cell tumors, carcinoids, carcinomas,* and *thymomas.* **Thymomas** are extremely rare in adults and children, with fewer than 10% of thymomas occurring in patients younger than 20 yr. The most frequent conditions associated with thymoma are pure red blood cell aplasia, myasthenia gravis, and hypogammaglobulinemia. Thymomas are slowly growing tumors and rarely metastasize.

The primary treatment is surgical excision. Chemotherapy is reserved for those rare patients with widely disseminated disease that does not respond to alternative therapy with radiation or steroids.

514.4 Infantile Fibromatosis

Fibromatosis lesions are rare, benign fibroblastic proliferations that may occur in virtually any location. Their growth rate is unpredictable. They do not metastasize but may become very large and cause symptoms by compression of adjacent structures. The most effective treatment for these lesions is complete surgical resection with wide margins to prevent local recurrence. In rare instances in which tumors are unresectable, radiation therapy, chemotherapy, or treatment with tamoxifen may be effective in promoting slow tumor regression, but the response to these modalities is unpredictable.

Benign Bone Lesions in Children

Ahn JI, Park JS: Pathologic fractures secondary to unicameral bone cysts. Int Orthop 18:20, 1994.

Campanacci M, Capanna R, Picci P: Unicameral and aneurysmal bone cysts. Clin Orthop 204:25, 1986.

Campanacci M, Laus M: Osteofibrous dysplasia of the tibia and fibula. J Bone Joint Surg 63A:367, 1981.

Dahlin DC, Ivins JC: Benign chondroblastoma: A study of 125 cases. Cancer 30:401, 1972.

Freiberg AA, Loder RT, Heidelberger KT: Aneurysmal bone cysts in young children. J Pediatr Orthop 14:86, 1994.

Kneisl JS, Simon MA: Medical management compared with operative treatment for osteoid osteoma. J Bone Joint Surg 74A:179, 1992.

McLeod RA, Dahlin DC, Beabout JW: The spectrum of osteoblastoma. Am J Roentgenol 126:321, 1976.

Schmale GA, Conrad EU III, Raskind WH: The natural history of hereditary multiple exostoses. J Bone Joint Surg 76A:986, 1994.

Benign Tumors

Enjolras O, Riche M, Merland J, et al: Management of alarming hemangiomas in infancy: A review of 25 cases. Pediatrics 85:491, 1990.

Folkman J, Mulliken J, Ezekowitz A: Antiangiogenic therapy of hemangiomas with interferon alpha. *In:* Stuart-Harris R, Penny RD (eds): Clinical Applications of the Interferons. London, Chapman & Hall Medical, 1997, pp 255–265.

Raney B, Evans A, Gramwetter L, et al: Nonsurgical management of children with recurrent or unresectable fibromatosis. Pediatrics 79:394, 1987.

Reinhardt M, Nelson S, Sencer S, et al: Treatment of childhood lymphangiomas with interferon α. J Pediatr Hematol Oncol 19:232, 1997.

Sadan N, Wolach B: Treatment of hemangiomas of infancy with high doses of prednisone. J Pediatr 128:141, 1996.

CHAPTER 515 Histiocytosis Syndromes of Childhood

Stephan Ladisch

The childhood histiocytoses constitute a diverse group of disorders, which, although rare in occurrence, may be severe in their clinical expression. These disorders are grouped together because they have in common a prominent proliferation/accumulation of cells of the monocyte-macrophage system of bone marrow origin. Although these disorders are sometimes difficult to distinguish clinically, accurate diagnosis is nevertheless essential for facilitating progress in treatment. To this end, a systematic classification of the childhood histiocytoses has been developed (Table 515–1). This diagnostic classification rests on histopathologic findings; therefore, a thorough, comprehensive evaluation of a biopsy specimen obtained at the time of diagnosis is essential. This evaluation includes studies (electron microscopy, immunostaining) that may require special sample processing.

CLASSIFICATION AND PATHOLOGY. Three classes of childhood histiocytosis are recognized, based on histopathologic findings. The most well-known childhood histiocytosis, previously known as histiocytosis X, constitutes class I and includes the clinical entities of **eosinophilic granuloma** (also see chapter 514), **Hand-Schüller-Christian disease**, and **Letterer-Siwe disease**. The name Langerhans' cell histiocytosis (LCH) has been applied to the class I histiocytoses. The normal Langerhans' cell is an antigen-presenting cell of the skin. The hallmark of LCH in all forms is the presence of a clonal proliferation of cells of the monocyte lineage containing the characteristic electron microscopic findings of a Langerhans' cell. This is the Birbeck's granule, a tennis racket–shaped bilamellar granule, which when seen in the cytoplasm of lesional cells in LCH is diagnostic of the disease. Alternatively, the definitive diagnosis of LCH can be made by demonstrating CD1 positivity of lesional cells. The lesions may contain various proportions of these Langerhans' granule–containing cells, lymphocytes, granulocytes, monocytes, and eosinophils.

In contrast to a prominence of an antigen-presenting cell (the Langerhans' cell) in the class I histiocytoses, the class II histiocytoses are characterized by accumulation of antigen-processing cells (i.e., macrophages). With the characteristic morphology of normal macrophages by light microscopy, these phagocytic cells lack the two markers (Birbeck's granules and CD1 positivity) characteristic of the cells found in LCH. The two major diseases among the class II histiocytoses have indistinguishable pathologic findings. One is *familial erythrophagocytic lymphohistiocytosis* (FEL, which is the only inherited form of histiocytosis and is autosomal recessive). The other is the *infection-associated hemophagocytic syndrome (IAHS)*. Both diseases are characterized by disseminated lesions that involve many organ systems. The lesions are characterized by infiltration of the involved organ with activated phagocytic macrophages and lymphocytes, leading to the term lymphohistiocytosis.

The mixed cellular lesions of both the class I and class II histiocytoses suggest that these may be disorders of immune regulation, resulting from either an unusual and unidentified antigenic stimulation or an abnormal and somehow defective cellular immune response. In contrast, the class III histiocytoses are unequivocal malignancies of cells of monocyte-macrophage lineage. By this definition, acute monocytic leukemia and true malignant histiocytosis are included among the class III histiocytoses. These malignancies are considered elsewhere (see Chapter 502). The existence of neoplasms of Langerhans cells' is controversial. Some cases of LCH demonstrate clonality.

CLASS I HISTIOCYTOSES

CLINICAL MANIFESTATIONS. LCH has an extremely variable presentation. The skeleton is involved in 80% of patients and may be the only affected site, especially in children older than 5 yr. Bone lesions may be single or numerous and are seen most commonly in the skull (Fig. 515–1). They may be asymptomatic or associated with pain and local swelling. Involvement of the spine may result in collapse of the vertebral body, which can be seen roentgenographically, and may cause secondary compression of the spinal cord. In flat and long bones, osteolytic lesions with sharp borders occur, and no evidence exists of reactive new bone formation (until the lesions begin to heal). Lesions that involve weight-bearing long bones may result in pathologic fractures. Chronically draining, infected ears are commonly associated with destruction in the mastoid area. Bone destruction in the mandible and maxilla may result in teeth that, on roentgenograms, appear to be free floating. With response to therapy, healing may be complete.

TABLE 515–1 Classification of the Childhood Histiocytoses

Class I	Class II	Class III
	Diseases	
Langerhans' cell histiocytosis	Familial erythrophagocytic lymphohistiocytosis (FEL) Infection-associated hemophagocytic syndrome (IAHS)	Malignant histiocytosis Acute monocytic leukemia
	Cellular Characteristics of the Lesions	
Langerhans' cells with Birbeck's granules	Morphologically normal reactive macrophages with prominent erythrophagocytosis	Neoplastic proliferation of cells with characteristics of monocytes/macrophages or their precursors
	Treatment	
Local therapy for isolated lesions; chemotherapy for disseminated disease	Chemotherapy; allogeneic bone marrow transplantation (experimental)	Antineoplastic chemotherapy, including anthracyclines

Skin involvement occurs in about 50% of patients at some time during their course (usually, a seborrheic dermatitis of the scalp or diaper region). The lesions may spread to involve the back, palms, and soles. The exanthem may be petechial or hemorrhagic, even in the absence of thrombocytopenia. Localized or disseminated lymphadenopathy is present in approximately 33% of patients. Hepatosplenomegaly occurs in approximately 20%. Various degrees of hepatic malfunction may occur, including jaundice and ascites.

Exophthalmos, when present, is often bilateral and is caused by retro-orbital accumulation of granulomatous tissue. Gingival mucous membranes may be involved with infiltrative lesions that appear superficially like candidiasis. In 10–15% of patients, pulmonary infiltrates are found on roentgenogram. The lesions may vary from diffuse fibrosis and disseminated nodular infiltrates to diffuse cystic changes. Rarely, pneumothorax may be a complication. If the lungs are severely involved, tachypnea and progressive respiratory failure may result.

Pituitary dysfunction or hypothalamic involvement may result in growth retardation. In addition, patients may have diabetes insipidus; patients suspected of having LCH should demonstrate the ability to concentrate their urine before going to the operating room for a biopsy. Rarely, panhypopituitarism may occur. Primary hypothyroidism due to thyroid gland infiltration may occur.

Patients who are affected more severely may have systemic manifestations, including fever, weight loss, malaise, irritability, and failure to thrive. Bone marrow involvement may cause anemia and thrombocytopenia. Two uncommon but serious and unusual manifestations of LCH are hepatic involvement (leading to cirrhosis) and a peculiar central nervous system (CNS) involvement characterized by ataxia, dysarthria, and other neurologic symptoms. Associated with multisystem disease, hepatic involvement is frequently already present at the time of diagnosis. In contrast, the CNS involvement, which is progressive, histopathologically characterized by gliosis, and for which no treatment is known, may be observed many years after the initial diagnosis of LCH, which may have consisted only of mild bone disease. Striking is that neither of these manifestations evidence Langerhans' cells or Birbeck's granules.

After tissue biopsy, which is diagnostic and easiest to perform on skin or bone lesions, a thorough clinical and laboratory evaluation should be undertaken. This should include a series of studies in all patients (complete blood count, liver function tests, coagulation studies, skeletal survey, chest roentgenogram, and measurement of urine osmolality). In addition, detailed evaluation of any organ system that has been shown to be involved by physical examination or by these studies should be performed to establish the extent of disease before initiation of treatment.

TREATMENT AND PROGNOSIS. The clinical course of single-system disease (usually, bone, lymph node, or skin) is generally benign, with a high chance of spontaneous remission. Therefore, treatment should be minimal and should be directed at arresting the progression of a lesion (such as a bone lesion) that could result in permanent damage before it resolves spontaneously. Curettage or low-dose local radiation therapy (5–6 Gy) may accomplish this goal. Multisystem disease, in contrast, should be treated with systemic multiagent chemotherapy. Several different regimens have been proposed, but a central element is the inclusion of either vinblastine or etoposide. Treatment including the latter agent has been shown to be very effective in LCH. The response rate to therapy, contrary to previous opinion, may be high, especially if the diagnosis is accurately and expeditiously ascertained. Experimental therapies, suggested only for unresponsive disease (frequently very

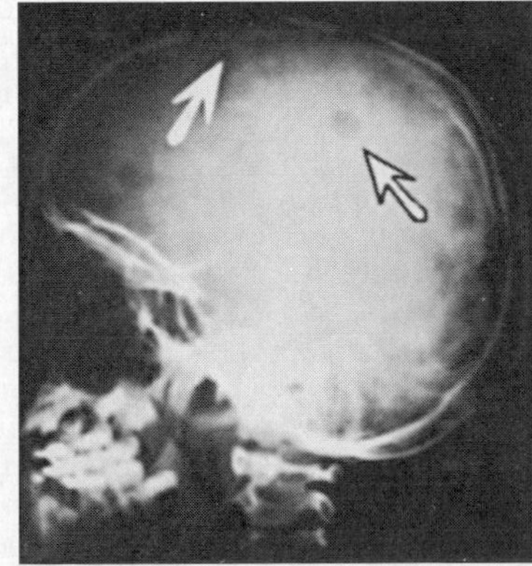
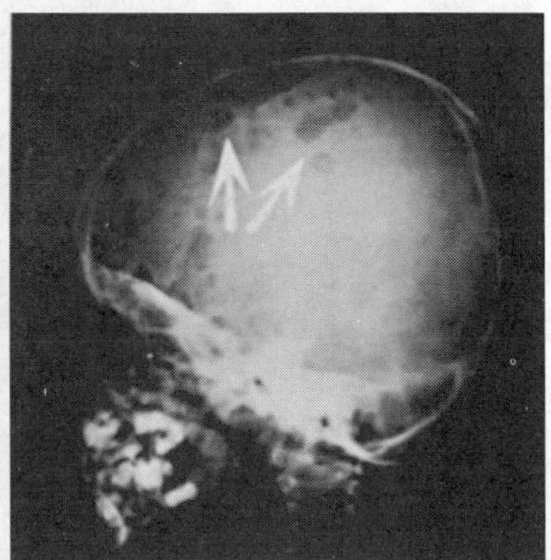

Figure 515–1 Two skull roentgenograms from patients with LCH. The patient on the left was over 2 yr of age and had involvement limited to isolated bone lesions. She had a good recovery. The patient on the right was under 2 yr of age and had extensive bone disease, febrile course, anemia, severe skin eruption, generalized adenopathy, hepatosplenomegaly, pulmonary infiltration, and a fatal outcome despite antitumor chemotherapy. These patients represent opposite ends of the clinical spectrum of LCH.

young children with multisystem disease who have not responded to initial treatment), include immunosuppressive therapy with cyclosporine/antithymocyte globulin and possibly certain new agents and modalities, such as 2-chlorodeoxyadenosine and bone marrow transplantation.

CLASS II HISTIOCYTOSES

CLINICAL MANIFESTATIONS. The major forms of class II histiocytosis, FEL and IAHS, have a remarkably similar presentation, consisting of a generalized disease process, most often with fever, weight loss, and irritability. FEL is also characterized by severe immunodeficiency. Affected children are usually younger than 4 yr (always in FEL); children may present with IAHS at an older age. Physical examination frequently reveals hepatosplenomegaly, symptoms of CNS involvement (with an aseptic meningitis, the cerebrospinal fluid cells are the same phagocytic macrophages as found in the peripheral blood or bone marrow). As in the class I histiocytoses, the *diagnosis* rests on the pathologic findings. Associated laboratory findings in both forms of class II histiocytosis include hyperlipidemia, hypofibrinoginemia, elevated levels of hepatic enzymes, extremely elevated levels of circulating soluble interleukin-2 receptors released by the activated lymphocytes, and sometimes cytopenias. No absolute clinical or laboratory distinction can be made between FEL and IAHS. Without a genetic marker for FEL at present, the distinction can definitively be made only by a positive family history for other affected children in FEL.

TREATMENT AND PROGNOSIS. The diagnostic distinction between FEL and IAHS can sometimes be based on the acute onset of IAHS in the presence of a documented infection. In this case, treatment of the underlying infection, coupled with supportive care, is critical. If the diagnosis is made in a setting of iatrogenic immunodeficiency, immunosuppressive treatment should be withdrawn and supportive care should be instituted along with specific therapy for underlying infection. When FEL is diagnosed or suspected and when an infection cannot be documented, therapy currently includes etoposide or immunosuppressive therapy. Nevertheless, no curative chemotherapy for FEL has been found, and the disease usually is uniformly fatal. Allogeneic bone marrow transplantation may be effective in curing some patients with FEL.

In contrast, in IAHS, when an infection can be documented and effectively treated, the prognosis is good without any other specific treatment. When a treatable infection cannot be documented (as is the case in most patients presumed to have IAHS), the prognosis is as poor as that of FEL and etoposide is also recommended. It is theorized that, by its cytotoxic effect on macrophages, etoposide interrupts cytokine production, the hemophagocytic process, and the accumulation of macrophages, all of which may contribute to the pathogenesis of IAHS. A broad spectrum of infectious agents, viruses (cytomegalovirus, Epstein-Barr virus, human herpesvirus 6), fungi, protozoa, and bacteria may trigger IAHS, usually in the setting of immunodeficiency. A thorough evaluation for infection should be undertaken in immunodeficient patients with hemophagocytosis. Rarely, the same syndrome may be identified in conjunction with a neoplasm (e.g., leukemia); in this case, treatment of the underlying disease causes resolution of the hemophagocytosis. In some patients, interferon and intravenous immunoglobulin have been effective.

Arico M, Janka G, Fischer A, et al: Hemophagocytic lymphohistiocytosis. Report of 122 children from the international registry. FHL study group of the histiocyte society. Leukemia 2:197, 1996.

Bhatia S, Nesbit ME, Egeler RM, et al: Epidemiologic study of Langerhans cell histiocytosis in children. J Pediatr 130:774, 1997.

Estlin EJ, Palmer RD, Windebank KP, et al: Successful treatment of non-familial haemophagocytic lymphohistiocytosis with interferon and gammaglobulin. Arch Dis Child 75:432, 1996.

Filipovich AH: Hemophagocytic lymphohistiocytosis: A lethal disorder of immune regulation. J Pediatr 130:337, 1997.

Gadner H, Heitger A, Grois N, et al: A treatment strategy for disseminated Langerhans cell histiocytosis. Med Pediatr Oncol 23:72, 1994.

Ladisch S, Gadner, Arico M, et al: LCH-I: A randomized trial of etoposide vs. vinblastine in disseminated Langerhans cell histiocytosis. Med Pediatr Oncol 23:107, 1994.

Lahey ME: Histiocytosis X: An analysis of prognostic factors. J Pediatr 87:184, 1975.

Rami B, Schneider U, Wandl-Vergesslich K, et al: Primary hypothyroidism, central diabetes insipidus and growth hormone deficiency in multisystem Langerhans cell histiocytosis: A case report. Acta Paediatr 87:112, 1998.

Ringden O, Lonnqvist B, Holst M: 12-year follow-up of allogenic bone-marrow transplant for Langerhans' cell histiocytosis. Lancet 349:476, 1997.

Willman CL, Busque L, Griffith BB, et al: Langerhans cell histiocytosis (histiocytosis X)—a clonal proliferative disease. N Engl J Med 331:154, 1994.

Writing Group of the Histiocyte Society: Histiocytosis syndromes in childhood. Lancet 1:208, 1987.

PART XXII

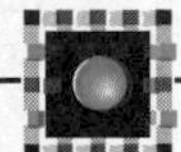

Nephrology

SECTION 1

Glomerular Disease

Jerry M. Bergstein

CHAPTER 516

Introduction to Glomerular Diseases

516.1 Anatomy of the Glomerulus

The kidneys lie in the retroperitoneal space slightly above the level of the umbilicus. They range in length and weight, respectively, from approximately 6 cm and 24 g in a full-term newborn to 12 cm or more and 150 g in an adult. The kidney (Fig. 516–1) has an outer layer, the cortex, which contains the glomeruli, proximal and distal convoluted tubules, and collecting ducts, and an inner layer, the medulla, which contains the straight portions of the tubules, the loops of Henle, the vasa recta, and the terminal collecting ducts (Fig. 516–2).

The blood supply to each kidney usually consists of a main renal artery that arises from the aorta; multiple renal arteries may occur. The main artery divides into segmental branches within the medulla and these into interlobar arteries that pass through the medulla to the junction of the cortex and medulla. At this point, the interlobar arteries branch to form the arcuate arteries, which run parallel to the surface of the kidney. Interlobular arteries originate from the arcuate arteries and give rise to the afferent arterioles of the glomeruli. Specialized muscle cells in the wall of the afferent arteriole, in combination with the lacis cells and that portion of the distal tubule (macula densa) that is adjacent to the glomerulus, form the juxtaglomerular apparatus, which controls the secretion of renin. The afferent arteriole divides into the glomerular capillary network, which then merges into the efferent arteriole (Fig. 516–3). The efferent arterioles of glomeruli next to the medulla (juxtamedullary glomeruli) are larger than those in the outer cortex and provide the blood supply (vasa recta) to the tubules and medulla.

Each kidney contains approximately 1 million nephrons (glomeruli and associated tubules). In humans, formation of nephrons is complete at birth, but functional maturation does not occur until later. Because no new nephrons can be formed after birth, progressive loss of nephrons may lead to renal insufficiency.

The glomerular network of specialized capillaries serves as the filtering mechanism of the kidney. The glomerular capillaries are lined by endothelial cells (Fig. 516–4) having very thin cytoplasm that contains many holes (fenestrations). The glomerular basement membrane (GBM) forms a continuous layer between the endothelial and mesangial cells on one side

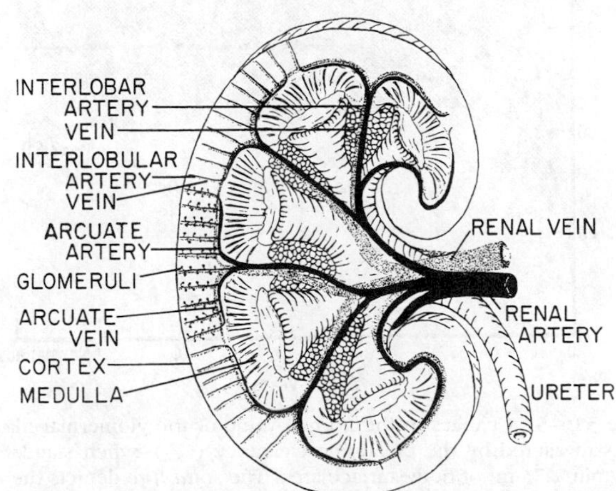

Figure 516–1 Gross morphology of the renal circulation. (From Pitts RF: Physiology of the Kidney and Body Fluids, 3rd ed. Chicago, Year Book Medical Publishers, 1974.)

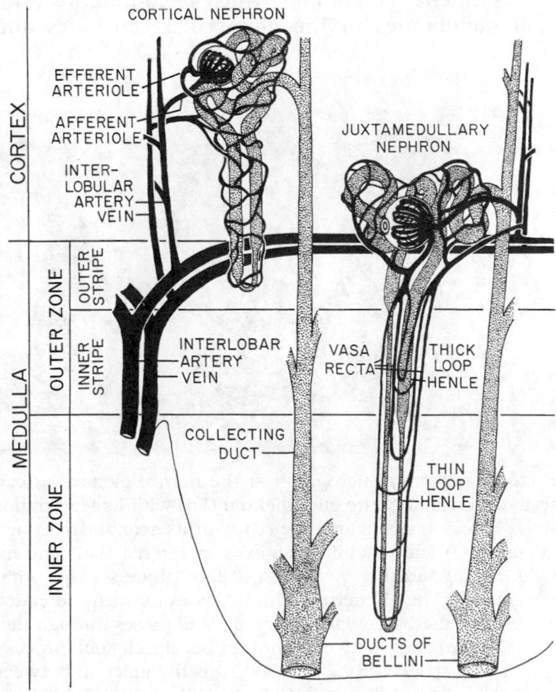

Figure 516–2 Comparison of the blood supplies of cortical and juxtamedullary nephrons. (From Pitts RF: Physiology of the Kidney and Body Fluids, 3rd ed. Chicago, Year Book Medical Publishers, 1974.)

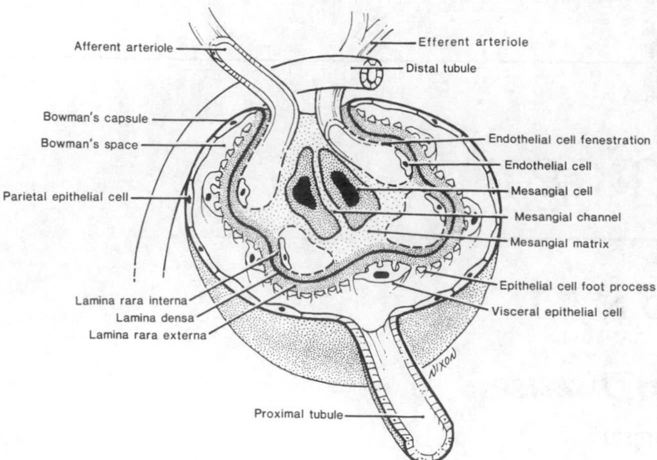

Figure 516–3 Schematic depiction of the glomerulus and surrounding structures.

and the epithelial cells on the other. The membrane has three layers: (1) a central electron-dense lamina densa; (2) the lamina rara interna, which lies between the lamina densa and the endothelial cells; and (3) the lamina rara externa, which lies between the lamina densa and the epithelial cells. The visceral epithelial cells cover the capillary and project cytoplasmic "foot processes," which attach to the lamina rara externa. Between the foot processes are spaces or filtration slits. The mesangium (mesangial cells and matrix) lies between the glomerular capillaries on the endothelial cell side of the basement membrane and forms the medial part of the capillary wall. The mesangium may serve as a supporting structure for the glomerular capillaries and probably has a role in the regulation of glomerular blood flow and filtration and in the removal of macromolecules (such as immune complexes) from the glomerulus, either through intracellular phagocytosis or by transport through intercellular channels to the juxtaglomerular region. The Bowman's capsule, which surrounds the glomerulus, is composed of (1) a basement membrane, which is continuous with the basement membranes of the glomerular capillaries and the proximal tubules, and (2) the parietal epithelial cells, which are continuous with the visceral epithelial cells.

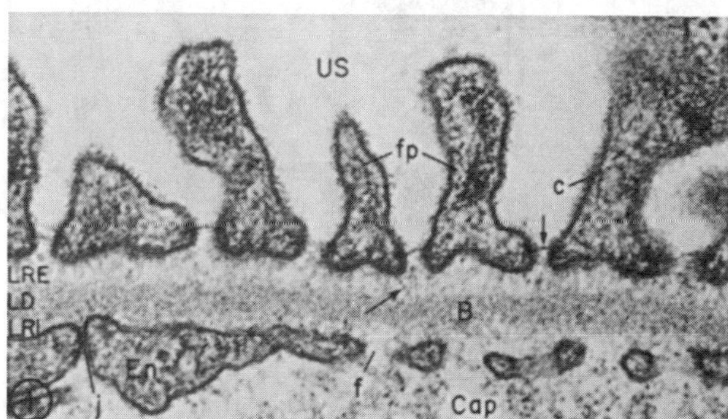

Figure 516–4 Electron micrograph of the normal glomerular capillary (Cap) wall demonstrating the endothelium (En) with its fenestrations (f), the glomerular basement membrane (B) with its central dense layer, the lamina densa (LD) and adjoining lamina rara interna (LRI) and externa (LRE; *long arrow*) and the epithelial cell foot processes (fp) with their thick cell coat (c). The glomerular filtrate passes through the endothelial fenestrae, crosses the basement membrane, and passes through the filtration slits *(short arrow)* between the epithelial cell foot processes to reach the urinary space (US). (×60,000.) J is the junction between two endothelial cells. (From Farquhar MG, Kanwar YS: Functional organization of the glomerulus: State of the science in 1979. *In:* Cummings NB, Michael AF, Wilson CB [eds]: Immune Mechanisms in Renal Disease. New York, Plenum, 1982. Reprinted by permission.)

516.2 Glomerular Filtration

As the blood passes through the glomerular capillaries, the plasma is filtered through the glomerular capillary walls. The ultrafiltrate, which is cell free, contains all the substances in the plasma (electrolytes, glucose, phosphate, urea, creatinine, peptides, low-molecular-weight proteins) except proteins (like albumin and the globulins) having a molecular weight exceeding 68,000. The filtrate is collected in Bowman space and enters the tubules, where its composition is modified in accordance with body needs until it leaves the kidney as urine.

Glomerular filtration is the net result of opposing forces across the capillary wall. The force for ultrafiltration (glomerular capillary hydrostatic pressure) stems from the systemic arterial pressure, as modified by the tone of the afferent and efferent arterioles. The major force opposing ultrafiltration is the glomerular capillary oncotic pressure, which is created by the gradient between the high concentration of plasma proteins within the capillary and the almost protein-free ultrafiltrate in Bowman space. Filtration may be modified by the rate of glomerular plasma flow, the hydrostatic pressure within Bowman space, and the permeability of the glomerular capillary wall.

Although glomerular filtration begins around the 9th wk of fetal life, kidney function does not appear necessary for normal intrauterine homeostasis, the placenta serving as the major excretory organ. After birth, the rate of glomerular filtration increases until growth ceases toward the end of the 2nd decade of life. To facilitate the comparison of the glomerular filtration rates (GFR) of children and adults, the rate is standardized to the surface area (1.73 m^2) of a 70-kg adult. Even after correction for surface area, the GFR of a child does not approximate adult values until the 3rd yr of life (Fig. 516–5).

The GFR may be estimated by measurement of the serum creatinine level (Fig. 516–6). Creatinine is derived from muscle metabolism. Its production is relatively constant, and its excretion is primarily through glomerular filtration (although tubular secretion may become important in renal insufficiency). In contrast to the concentration of blood urea nitrogen, the serum creatinine level is minimally influenced by factors (nitrogen

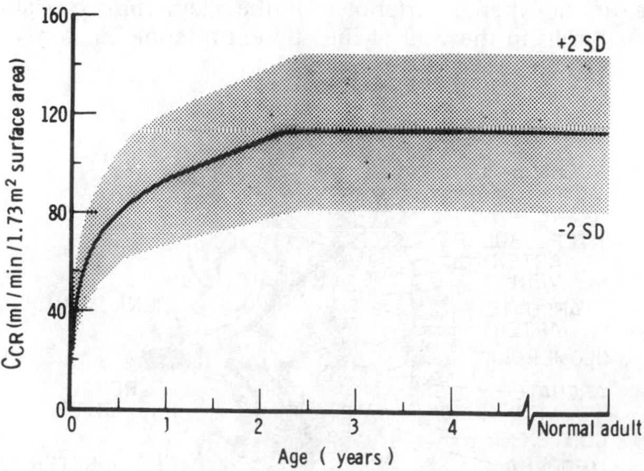

Figure 516–5 Changes in the normal value of the glomerular filtration rate, as measured by the creatinine clearance (C_{CR}), when standardized to mL/min/1.73 m^2 of body surface area. The *solid line* depicts the mean value, and the shaded area includes two standard deviations. (Reprinted by permission of the publishers from McCrory W: Developmental Nephrology. Cambridge, MA, Harvard University Press. Copyright © 1972 by the President and Fellows of Harvard College.)

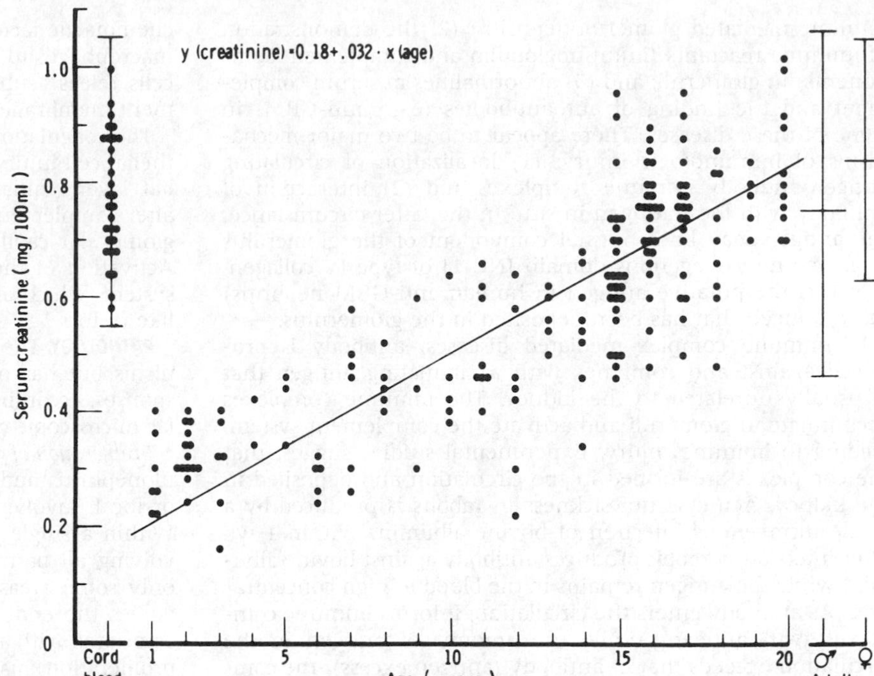

Figure 516–6 The serum creatinine in relation to age. (Reprinted by permission of the publishers from McCrory W: Developmental Nephrology. Cambridge, MA, Harvard University Press. Copyright © 1972 by the President and Fellows of Harvard College.)

balance, state of hydration) other than glomerular function. The serum creatinine is of value only in estimating the GFR in the steady state (e.g., a patient very shortly after the onset of acute renal failure and cessation of urine output may have a normal creatinine level but no effective renal function). The value of the serum creatinine is further compromised by the fact that its level does not rise above normal until the GFR falls below 70% of normal.

The precise measurement of the GFR is accomplished by quantitating the "clearance" of a substance that is freely filtered across the capillary wall and that is neither reabsorbed nor secreted by the tubules. The clearance (C_s) of such a substance is that volume of plasma that, when completely "cleared" of the contained substance, would yield a quantity of that substance equal to that excreted in the urine over a specified time. The clearance is represented by the following formula:

$$C_s(\text{mL/min}) = U_s(\text{mg/mL})V(\text{mL/min})/P_s(\text{mg/mL})$$

where C_s equals the clearance of substance s, U_s reflects the urinary concentration of s, V represents the urinary flow rate, and P_s equals the plasma concentration of s. To correct the clearance for body surface area, the formula is

$$\text{Corrected clearance} = C_s\ (\text{mL/min}) \times 1.73/\text{patient's surface area } (\text{m}^2)$$

The GFR is optimally measured by the clearance of inulin, a fructose polymer having a molecular weight of approximately 5,000. Because the inulin clearance technique is cumbersome, the GFR is commonly estimated by the clearance of endogenous creatinine. When the GFR is relatively normal, the creatinine clearance closely approximates the inulin clearance. However, as the GFR declines, an increasing proportion of the total creatinine in the urine is secreted by tubules, with the result that the creatinine clearance progressively overestimates the actual GFR. There is little merit, therefore, in measuring creatinine clearance when serum creatinine levels exceed 2.0 mg/dL (180 μmol/L); changes in renal function can then be monitored by the serum creatinine concentration.

The absence of plasma proteins larger than the size of albumin from the glomerular filtrate confirms the effectiveness of the glomerular capillary wall as a filtration barrier. Major factors restricting the filtration of these and other macromolecules include their size and their ionic charge.

Clearance studies of macromolecules in animals have shown no restriction to the filtration of molecules up to the size of inulin (molecular weight 5,000). As size increases further, filtration diminishes progressively, approaching zero for substances the size of albumin (molecular weight 68,000). Morphologic studies suggest that the size-selective filtration barrier resides within the GBM.

The endothelial cell, basement membrane, and epithelial cell of the glomerular capillary wall possess strong negative ionic charges. These anionic charges are a consequence of two negatively charged moieties: proteoglycans (heparan sulfate) and glycoproteins containing sialic acid. Proteins in the blood have a relatively low isoelectric point and carry a net negative charge. Consequently, they are repelled by the negatively charged sites in the glomerular capillary wall, thus restricting filtration.

Arant BS Jr: Postnatal development of renal function during the first year of life. Pediatr Nephrol 1:308, 1987.

Brenner BM, Hostetter TH, Humes HD: Glomerular permselectivity: Barrier function based on discrimination of molecular size and charge. Am J Physiol 234:F455, 1978.

Comper WD, Glasgow EF: Charge selectivity in kidney ultrafiltration. Kidney Int 47:1242, 1995.

Latta H: An approach to the structure and function of the glomerular mesangium. J Am Soc Nephrol 2:565, 1992.

Perrone RD, Madias NE, Levey AS: Serum creatinine as an index of renal function: New insights into old concepts. Clin Chem 38:1933, 1992.

Venkatachalam MA, Rennke HG: The structural and molecular basis of glomerular filtration. Circ Res 43:337, 1978.

516.3 Glomerular Diseases

PATHOGENESIS. Glomerular injury may be a result of immunologic, inherited (presumably biochemical), or coagulation disorders. Immunologic injury is the most common cause and results in *glomerulonephritis*, which is both a generic term for several diseases and a histopathologic term signifying inflammation of the glomerular capillaries. Evidence that glomerulonephritis is caused by immunologic injury includes (1) morphologic and immunopathologic similarities to experimental immune-mediated glomerulonephritis; (2) the demonstration of immune reactants (immunoglobulin and complement components) in glomeruli; and (3) abnormalities in serum complement and the finding of autoantibodies (e.g., anti-GBM) in some of these diseases. There appear to be two major mechanisms of immunologic injury: (1) localization of circulating antigen-antibody immune complexes and (2) interaction of antibody with local antigen in situ. In the latter circumstance, the antigen may be a normal component of the glomerulus (e.g., the noncollagenous domain [NC-1] of type IV collagen, which is the putative antigen in human anti-GBM nephritis) or an antigen that has been deposited in the glomerulus.

In immune complex–mediated diseases, antibody is produced against and combines with a circulating antigen that is usually unrelated to the kidney. The immune complexes accumulate in glomeruli and activate the complement system, leading to immune injury. Experimental studies suggest that the complexes are formed in the circulation and deposited in the kidney. Acute serum sickness in rabbits is produced by a single intravenous injection of bovine albumin. Within 1 wk after injection, a rabbit produces antibody against bovine albumin, while the antigen remains in the blood in high concentration. As antibody enters the circulation, it forms immune complexes with antigen. While the amount of antigen in the circulation exceeds that of antibody (antigen excess), the complexes formed are small, remain soluble in the circulation, and are deposited in glomeruli. The processes involved in glomerular localization are not well understood but include attributes of the complex (concentration, charge, size), characteristics of the glomerulus (mesangial trapping, negatively charged capillary wall), hydrodynamic forces, and the influence of various mediators (angiotensin II, prostaglandins).

With deposition of immune complexes in glomeruli, rabbits develop an acute proliferative glomerulonephritis. Immunofluorescence microscopy demonstrates granular ("lumpy-bumpy") deposits containing immunoglobulin and complement in the glomerular capillary wall. Electron microscopic studies show these deposits to be on the epithelial side of the GBM and in the mesangium. For the next few days, as additional antibody enters the circulation, the antigen is ultimately removed from the circulation and the glomerulonephritis subsides. In rabbits, complement does not participate in the capillary injury, which is largely related to influx of macrophages. In other models, complement has a role in capillary injury.

An example of in situ antigen-antibody interaction is anti-GBM antibody disease, in which antibody reacts with antigen(s) of the GBM. Immunopathologic studies reveal linear deposition of immunoglobulin and complement on the GBM, similar to that in Goodpasture disease and certain types of rapidly progressive glomerulonephritis.

The inflammatory reaction that follows immunologic injury results from activation of one or more mediator pathways. The most important of these is the complement system, which has two initiating sequences: (1) the classic pathway, which is activated by antigen-antibody immune complexes; and (2) the alternative or properdin pathway, which is activated by polysaccharides and endotoxin. These pathways converge at C3; from that point on, the same sequence leads to lysis of cell membranes (see Fig. 133–1). The major noxious products of complement activation are produced after activation of C3 and include anaphylatoxin (which stimulates contractile proteins within vascular walls and increases vascular permeability) and chemotactic factors (C5a) that direct neutrophils and perhaps macrophages to the site of complement activation, where the cells release substances that damage vascular cells and basement membranes.

The coagulation system may be activated directly, after endothelial cell injury, which bares the thrombogenic subendothelial layer (initiating the coagulation cascade), or indirectly, after complement activation. Fibrin deposits may occur within glomerular capillaries or within Bowman space in crescents. Activation of the coagulation process may activate the kinin system, which also produces chemotactic and anaphylatoxin-like factors.

PATHOLOGY. The glomerulus may be injured by several mechanisms but has only a limited number of histopathologic responses; accordingly, different disease states may produce similar microscopic changes.

Proliferation of glomerular cells occurs in most forms of glomerulonephritis and may be generalized, involving all glomeruli, or focal, involving only some glomeruli while sparing others. Within a single glomerulus, proliferation may be diffuse, involving all parts of the glomerulus, or segmental, involving only some areas but not others. Proliferation commonly involves the endothelial and mesangial cells and is frequently associated with an increase in the mesangial matrix. Mesangial proliferation may result from immune complex deposition within the mesangium. The resultant increase in cell size and number, and in mesangial matrix, may increase glomerular size and narrow the lumina of glomerular capillaries, leading to renal insufficiency.

Crescent formation in Bowman space (capsule) is a result of proliferation of parietal epithelial cells. Crescents develop in several forms of glomerulonephritis (termed rapidly progressive) and are thought to be a response to fibrin deposited in Bowman's space. New crescents contain fibrin, the proliferating epithelial cells of Bowman space, basement membrane–like material produced by these cells, and macrophages that may have a role in the genesis of glomerular injury. In days to weeks, the crescent is invaded by connective tissue (fibroepithelial crescent); this generally results in glomerular obsolescence. Crescent formation is frequently associated with glomerular cell death. The necrotic glomerulus has a characteristic eosinophilic appearance and usually contains nuclear remnants. Crescent formation is usually associated with generalized proliferation of the mesangial cells and with either immune complex or anti-GBM antibody deposition in the glomerular capillary wall.

In addition to proliferation, certain forms of acute glomerulonephritis show glomerular *exudation of blood cells*, most commonly neutrophils; eosinophils, basophils, and mononuclear cells may be seen in lesser numbers. The thickened appearance of GBM may result from a true *increase in the width of the membrane* (as seen in membranous glomerulopathy), from massive deposition of immune complexes that have staining characteristics similar to the membrane (as seen in systemic lupus erythematosus), or from the interposition of mesangial cells and matrix into the subendothelial space between the endothelial cells and the membrane. The latter may give the basement membrane a split appearance, as seen in type I membranoproliferative glomerulonephritis and other diseases.

Sclerosis refers to the presence of scar tissue within the glomerulus. Occasionally, pathologists use this term to refer to an increase in mesangial matrix.

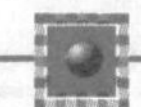

SECTION 2

Conditions Particularly Associated with Hematuria

Jerry M. Bergstein

CHAPTER 517

Clinical Evaluation of the Child with Hematuria

Hematuria may be gross (visible to the naked eye) or microscopic (detected only by dipstick and confirmed by microscopic examination of the urine sediment). Gross hematuria may originate from the kidney, in which case it is generally brown or cola colored and may contain red blood cell (RBC) casts, or from the lower urinary tract (bladder and urethra), in which case the urine is red to pink and may contain clots. Gross hematuria may be associated with edema, hypertension, and renal insufficiency. This constellation of findings is typical of the acute nephritic syndrome and is frequently found in patients with postinfectious (e.g., poststreptococcal) glomerulonephritis, systemic lupus erythematosus (SLE), membranoproliferative glomerulonephritis, anaphylactoid purpura, and rapidly progressive glomerulonephritis. The urine may be colored by pigments other than blood (Table 517–1).

In children, microscopic hematuria is most commonly discovered at periodic health examinations, by dipstick or by microscopic examination of the urine sediment. Because the quantitation of blood (actually hemoglobin) on dipsticks is not precise, results should be interpreted as negative (negative or trace readings) or positive (small, medium, and large readings). A positive result of a dipstick test for blood indicates the need for a urinalysis. Microscopic hematuria is defined as more than 5 RBCs per high power field in the sediment from 10 mL of centrifuged freshly voided urine.

Asymptomatic microscopic hematuria is found in 0.5–2% of school-age children, but whether screening for isolated microscopic hematuria can discover occult renal disease is unclear. Because of this uncertainty and its cost, screening urinalysis with microscopic examination of sediment for hematuria or pyuria is unwarranted in asymptomatic children. On the other hand, a dipstick can detect blood or protein inexpensively.

Causes of hematuria are listed in Table 517–2. Children with gross hematuria should be evaluated carefully because of the increased likelihood of finding hypertension and renal failure.

TABLE 517–1 Urinary Hues

Dark Yellow	Red food coloring
Concentrated urine	Phenolphthalein
Bile pigments	Urates
Red	Pyridium
Blood (red blood cells or hemoglobin)	**Dark Brown or Black**
Myoglobin	Blood
Porphyrins	Homogentisic acid (alcaptonuria)
Beets	Melanin
Blackberries	Tyrosinosis
Deferoxamine	Methemoglobinemia
Chloroquine	
Rifampin	

Children having persistent microscopic hematuria (more than 5 RBCs per high power field on three urinalyses at monthly intervals) should undergo outpatient evaluation. The cost effectiveness of such evaluation remains to be determined.

In the evaluation of a child with hematuria, a thorough history and physical examination and screening laboratory tests may give clues to the cause of hematuria (Table 517–3). For example, a history of recent upper respiratory, skin, or gastrointestinal infection may suggest acute glomerulonephritis, the hemolytic-uremic syndrome, or Henoch-Schönlein purpura. Frequency, dysuria, and unexplained fevers suggest urinary tract infection. A flank mass may signal hydronephrosis, cystic disease, renal vein thrombosis, or tumor. Recurrent episodes of gross hematuria suggest IgA nephropathy, idiopathic hematuria, Alport syndrome, or hypercalciuria. Rash and joint pains point toward Henoch-Schönlein purpura or SLE. A history of trauma, of bleeding difficulties, of drug use, or of kidney disease or high blood pressure in other family members is useful.

Laboratory evaluation of a child with hematuria is done in steps, beginning with the studies most likely to reveal the etiology (see Table 518–1). Depending on the results of the initial group of tests, additional studies may be indicated.

The finding of certain hematologic abnormalities may narrow the differential diagnosis. Anemia may be dilutional (the result of fluid overload in acute renal failure), hemolytic (he-

TABLE 517–2 Causes of Hematuria in Children

Glomerular Diseases
- Recurrent gross hematuria syndrome
  - IgA nephropathy
  - Idiopathic (benign familial) hematuria
  - Alport syndrome
- Acute poststreptococcal glomerulonephritis
- Membranous glomerulopathy
- Systemic lupus erythematosus
- Membranoproliferative glomerulonephritis
- Nephritis of chronic infection
- Rapidly progressive glomerulonephritis
- Goodpasture disease
- Anaphylactoid purpura
- Hemolytic-uremic syndrome

Infection
- Bacterial
- Tuberculosis
- Viral

Hematologic
- Coagulopathies
- Thrombocytopenia
- Sickle cell disease
- Renal vein thrombosis

Stones and Hypercalciuria

Anatomic Abnormalities
- Congenital anomalies
- Trauma
- Polycystic kidneys
- Vascular abnormalities
- Tumors

Exercise

Drugs

TABLE 517–3 Summary of Primary Renal Diseases That Present As Acute Glomerulonephritis

Diseases	Poststreptococcal Glomerulonephritis (PSGN)	IgA Nephropathy	Membranoproliferative Glomerulonephritis	Idiopathic Rapidly Progressive Glomerulonephritis (RPGN)
Clinical manifestations				
Age and sex	All ages, mean 7 yr, 2:1 male	15–35 yr, 2:1 male	15–30 yr, 6:1 male	Mean 58 yr, 2:1 male
Acute nephritic syndrome	90%	50%	90%	90%
Asymptomatic hematuria	Occasionally	50%	Rare	Rare
Nephrotic syndrome	10–20%	Rare	Rare	10–20%
Hypertension	70%	30–50%	Rare	25%
Acute renal failure	50% (transient)	Very rare	50%	60%
Other	Latent period of 1–3 wk	Follows viral syndromes	Pulmonary hemorrhage; iron-deficiency anemia	None
Laboratory findings	↑ ASO titers (70%) Positive streptozyme (95%) ↓ C3–C9 Normal C1, C4	↑ Serum IgA (50%) IgA in dermal capillaries	Positive anti-GBM antibody	Positive ANCA
Immunogenetics	HLA-B12, D "EN" (9)*	HLA-Bw 35, DR4 (4)*	HLA-DR2 (16)*	None established
Renal pathology				
Light microscopy	Diffuse proliferation	Focal proliferation	Focal → diffuse proliferation with crescents	Crescentic GN
Immunofluorescence	Granular IgG, C3	Diffuse mesangial IgA	Linear IgG, C3	No immune deposits
Electron microscopy	Subepithelial humps	Mesangial deposits	No deposits	No deposits
Prognosis	95% resolve spontaneously 5% RPGN or slowly progressive	Slow progression in 25–50%	75% stabilize or improve if treated early	75% stabilize or improve if treated early
Treatment	Supportive	None established	Plasma exchange, steroids, cyclophosphamide	Steroid pulse therapy

**Relative risk.*
ANCA = antineutrophil cytoplasm antibody; GBM = glomerular basement membrane; GN = glomerulonephritis; Ig = immunoglobulin.
Modified from Couser WG. Glomerular disorders. In: *Wyngaarden JB, Smith LH, Bennett JC (eds): Cecil Textbook of Medicine, Vol 1, 19th ed. Philadelphia, WB Saunders, 1992, p 552.*

molytic-uremic syndrome, SLE), due to chronic renal failure, or the result of blood loss (pulmonary hemorrhage in Goodpasture's disease, melena in Henoch-Schönlein purpura, hemolytic-uremic syndrome). Confirmation of a hemolytic state (elevated reticulocyte count and plasma hemoglobin level, with a depressed plasma haptoglobin level) indicates additional studies. Observation of the blood film may reveal a microangiopathic process as seen in the hemolytic-uremic syndrome, renal vein thrombosis, vasculitis, and SLE. In the latter, the presence of autoantibodies may result in a positive Coombs' test result, antinuclear antibody (ANA), leukopenia, and multisystem disease. All black children with hematuria should be screened for sickle hemoglobin, even in the absence of anemia. Thrombocytopenia may result from decreased platelet production (malignancies) or increased platelet consumption (SLE, idiopathic thrombocytopenic purpura, hemolytic-uremic syndrome, renal vein thrombosis). Although urinary RBC morphology may be normal with lower tract bleeding and dysmorphic from glomerular bleeding, cell morphology does not reliably correlate with the site of hematuria. The best screening test for a bleeding diathesis is a thorough history; coagulation studies or platelet counts are not routinely obtained unless personal or family history suggests a bleeding tendency.

Urine culture evaluates the possibility of urinary tract infection. Optimally, a timed urine specimen is also collected to measure the creatinine clearance, as well as protein and calcium excretion. If this is not possible, then determination of the serum creatinine, urine protein by dipstick, and calcium-to-creatinine ratio in a random urine specimen are adequate.

The serum C3 level is determined in all patients, because a low level narrows the differential diagnosis to certain forms of glomerulonephritis: poststreptococcal, lupus, membranoproliferative, and chronic infection. When the hematuria is of less than 6 mo duration, serologic evidence for streptococcal infection should be sought. Throat or skin infections should be cultured for group A streptococci. An ANA titer should be obtained as a test for SLE. If the previously mentioned studies do not yield the diagnosis, ultrasonography or intravenous pyelography should be carried out to preclude structural abnormalities. Cystography is performed is only for patients with infection or for patients in whom a lesion of the lower tract is suspected.

The studies in steps 1 and 2, as presented in Table 518–1, frequently reveal the cause of the hematuria. In some patients, however, results of all these studies are normal and no cause for the hematuria is found. In such patients, despite the lack of a diagnosis, no further studies need be performed. Parents should be reassured that their child does not at that time have evidence of urinary tract disease. Because it remains possible, however, that significant renal disease (e.g., IgA nephropathy, Alport syndrome) may develop, children with persistent microscopic hematuria should have long-term follow-up, with an annual re-evaluation consisting of history, physical examination, blood pressure determination, urinalysis, creatinine clearance, and determination of protein level in a 24-hr specimen.

Renal biopsy may not yield a definitive diagnosis in children with unexplained low-grade microscopic hematuria and no other laboratory abnormalities. Biopsy is indicated for children with persistent microscopic hematuria associated with decreased renal function, proteinuria, or hypertension; for those children having one or more episodes of unexplained gross hematuria; and for those with persistent high-grade microscopic hematuria.

Cystoscopy is not part of the routine evaluation of hematuria in children. Cystoscopy is most helpful in patients having bright red hematuria, dysuria, and sterile urine cultures. In boys, cystoscopy frequently reveals a hemorrhagic lesion in the urethra, probably the result of local trauma. Although neoplasms of the lower urinary tract rarely present as asymptomatic gross hematuria in children, debate persists about the need for cystoscopy to preclude the remote possibility of a tumor.

CHAPTER 518
Recurrent Gross Hematuria

In patients having a syndrome of recurrent gross hematuria (RGH), recurrent episodes of generally painless hematuria occur (mild flank pain may be felt). The gross hematuria usually develops 1–2 days after the onset of a presumably viral upper respiratory tract infection. This short latent period between the onset of infection and the appearance of hematuria contrasts with the 7- to 14-day latent period in children developing acute poststreptococcal glomerulonephritis. Patients with RGH do not have manifestations of the acute nephritic syndrome (edema, hypertension, or renal insufficiency). Diseases causing RGH may also present with persistent microscopic hematuria without episodes of gross hematuria.

Patients having a first episode of gross hematuria are usually hospitalized and evaluated for causes of hematuria (Table 518–1). In patients with RGH, routine radiographic and laboratory studies may fail to reveal a cause of hematuria. The gross hematuria resolves over 1–2 wk, but microscopic hematuria usually persists. Later, with another respiratory infection, gross hematuria recurs. Renal biopsy is indicated after the second episode to determine the nature of any underlying disease, which most frequently is IgA nephropathy, idiopathic hematuria, or familial nephritis (Alport syndrome).

IgA NEPHROPATHY (BERGER NEPHROPATHY). Patients with this disorder have glomerulonephritis with IgA as the predominant immunoglobulin in mesangial deposits, in the absence of any systemic disease such as systemic lupus erythematosus or Henoch-Schönlein purpura.

Pathology and Pathogenesis. On light microscopy, the kidney has focal and segmental mesangial proliferation and increased matrix (Fig. 518–1). Some show generalized mesangial proliferation, occasionally associated with crescent formation and scarring. IgA is the predominant immunoglobulin deposited in the mesangium (Fig. 518–2), but lesser amounts of IgG, IgM, C3, and properdin are common. Electron microscopic studies confirm these findings.

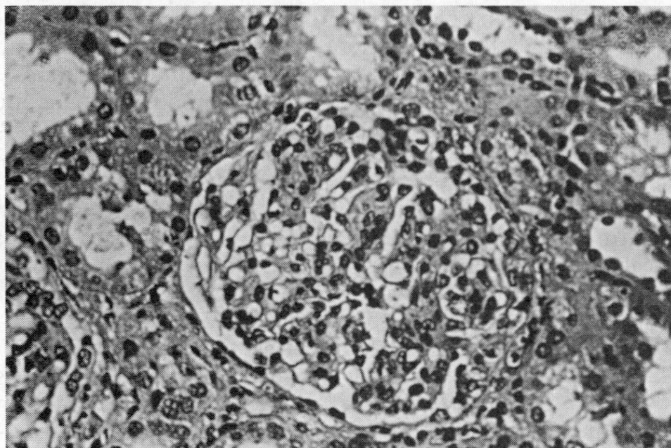

Figure 518–1 Light microscopy of IgA nephropathy demonstrating segmental mesangial proliferation and increased matrix. (×180.)

TABLE 518–1 Evaluation of the Child with Hematuria

Step 1: Studies Performed on All Patients

- Complete blood count
- Urine culture
- Serum creatinine level
- 24-hr urine collection for
  - creatinine
  - protein
  - calcium
- Serum C3 level
- Ultrasonography or intravenous pyelography

Step 2: Studies Performed on Selected Patients

- DNase B titer or Streptozyme test if hematuria is of < 6 mo duration
- Skin or throat cultures when appropriate
- ANA titer
- Urine erythrocyte morphology
- Coagulation studies/platelet count when suggested by history
- Sickle cell screen in all black patients
- Voiding cystourethrography with infection, or when a lower tract lesion is suspected

Step 3: Invasive Procedures

Renal biopsy indicated for
1. Persistent high-grade microscopic hematuria
2. Microscopic hematuria plus any of the following
   a. diminished renal function
   b. proteinuria exceeding 150 mg/24 hr (0.15 g/24 hr)
   c. hypertension
3. Second episode of gross hematuria

Cystoscopy indicated for
  pink to red hematuria, dysuria, and sterile urine culture

Most evidence points to an immune complex cause of IgA nephropathy. If a patient with IgA nephropathy has a transplanted kidney, the nephropathy commonly recurs in the transplanted kidney, indicating the systemic nature of this disorder.

Clinical and Laboratory Manifestations. IgA nephropathy is more common in males than in females (2:1). Patients either present with an episode of gross hematuria or are found to have microscopic hematuria on routine examination. While the gross hematuria lasts, renal function usually remains relatively normal and proteinuria minimal (<1 g/24 hr). Normal serum levels of C3 in IgA nephropathy help to distinguish this disorder from poststreptococcal glomerulonephritis.

Prognosis and Treatment. IgA nephropathy does not lead to significant kidney damage in most patients. Treatment is supportive, and activity need not be restricted. Neither the number of episodes of gross hematuria nor the persistence of microscopic hematuria between episodes correlates with the likelihood of progressive disease. Progressive disease develops in 30% of patients, in whom a poor prognosis is associated with hypertension, diminished renal function, or proteinuria exceeding

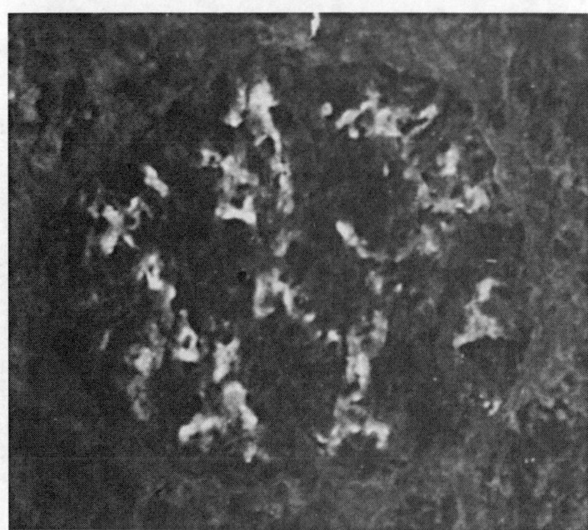

Figure 518–2 Immunofluorescence microscopy of the biopsy from a child having recurrent episodes of gross hematuria demonstrating mesangial deposition of IgA. (×250.)

1 g/24 hr between episodes of gross hematuria, or with histologic evidence of diffuse glomerulonephritis with crescents and scarring, and interstitial inflammation and fibrosis. Although controlled studies are lacking, immunosuppressive therapy may be beneficial in certain patients with progressive IgA nephropathy.

IDIOPATHIC HEMATURIA. Within the clinical spectrum of recurrent episodes of gross hematuria, idiopathic (benign familial) hematuria is defined histologically by normal findings on light and immunofluorescence microscopy. In some patients, electron microscopy demonstrates marked thinning of the glomerular basement membrane (thin basement membrane nephropathy), but the membrane width may be normal in others.

Idiopathic hematuria has a good prognosis, but rare patients may suffer progressive disease after many years. Long-term follow-up is required to preclude Alport syndrome. Both disorders may be familial, and Alport syndrome may have minimal light microscopic changes, negative immunofluorescence, and thin basement membranes. In patients presumed to have idiopathic hematuria, the development of decreased renal function, proteinuria, or hypertension calls for a second renal biopsy.

ALPORT SYNDROME. This is the most common of several types of hereditary nephritis. There is marked variability in clinical presentation, natural history, histologic abnormalities, and genetic patterns.

Pathology. Kidney biopsy specimens during the first decade of life may show few changes on light microscopy. Later, the glomeruli may develop mesangial proliferation and capillary wall thickening, leading to progressive glomerular sclerosis. Tubular atrophy, interstitial inflammation and fibrosis, and foam cells (nonspecific lipid-laden tubular or interstitial cells) develop if the disease progresses. Immunopathologic studies are usually nondiagnostic.

In most patients, electron microscopic studies have revealed thickening, thinning, splitting, and layering of the basement membranes of the glomeruli (Fig. 518–3) and tubules, but these lesions are not specific for Alport syndrome and may be absent in certain families that have the typical clinical manifestations of the syndrome.

Clinical Manifestations. Patients with Alport syndrome most commonly present with asymptomatic microscopic hematuria, but recurrent episodes of gross hematuria are common. In those with microscopic hematuria, the development of proteinuria indicates the need for a kidney biopsy, which establishes the diagnosis.

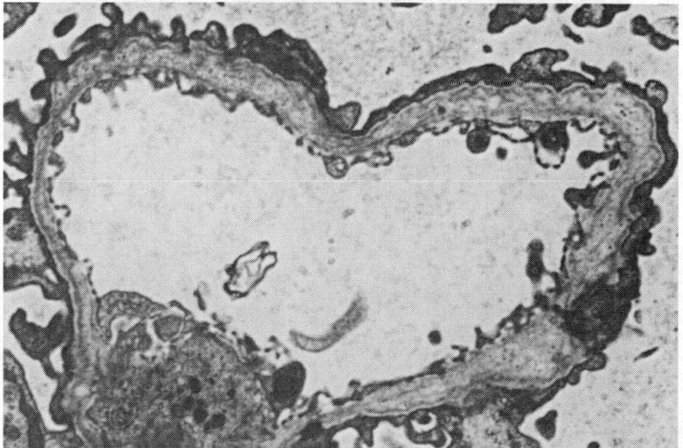

Figure 518–3 Electron micrograph of the biopsy from a child with Alport syndrome, depicting thickening, thinning, splitting, and layering of the glomerular basement membrane. (×16,250.) (From Yum M, Bergstein JM: Basement membrane nephropathy. Hum Pathol 14:996, 1983.)

Besides kidney involvement, a minority of patients have sensorineural hearing loss, which may begin in the high frequency range but progresses to involve the speech range and results in deafness. Approximately 10% of patients have eye abnormalities, the most frequent of which are cataracts, anterior lenticonus, and macular lesions.

Genetics. Alport syndrome is primarily an X-linked dominant disorder. This explains the more severe clinical course in males than females. Autosomal transmission also has been described. Patients with Alport syndrome having no family history may represent a spontaneous mutation of the X-linked form or have the recessive type of the disease. In the X-linked form, the disease results from mutations in the gene that encodes the α5 chain of type 4 collagen. Prenatal testing is available.

Complications. If renal function deteriorates, hypertension, urinary tract infections, and the manifestations of chronic renal failure may appear.

Prevention. Genetic counseling involving the entire family may limit propagation of the genetic abnormality.

Prognosis and Treatment. Males with Alport syndrome commonly develop end-stage renal failure in the 2nd or 3rd decade of life, occasionally in association with hearing loss. There is no specific therapy, but such patients are good candidates for dialysis and kidney transplantation. The development of anti-GBM nephritis in the transplanted kidneys of some patients with Alport syndrome suggests that the GBM of their native kidneys lacks a nephritogenic antigen. Females usually have a normal life span (for this reason, more mothers than fathers transmit the disease to their children) and only subclinical hearing loss.

IDIOPATHIC HYPERCALCIURIA. This possibly autosomal dominant disorder may present as RGH, persistent microscopic hematuria, or dysuria in the absence of stone formation. Hypercalciuria (without hypercalcemia) may result from excessive gastrointestinal absorption of normal dietary calcium intake or a defect in renal tubular calcium reabsorption. The precise mechanisms by which the hypercalciuria causes hematuria or dysuria are unknown. The diagnosis is confirmed by finding a 24-hr urinary calcium excretion exceeding 4 mg/kg. A screening test for hypercalciuria in patients who cannot collect a timed urine specimen may be performed on a random urine specimen by measuring the calcium and creatinine concentrations. A urine calcium to creatinine ratio (mg/mg) exceeding 0.2 suggests hypercalciuria, although normal ratios in infants may be as high as 0.8. Hypercalcemic hypercalciuria due to hyperparathyroidism or vitamin D intoxication must be considered in the differential diagnosis. The presence of proteinuria suggests diseases associated with defects in the renal specific chloride channel (X-linked recessive nephrolithiasis with renal failure, X-linked recessive hypercalciuric hypophosphatemic rickets, and idiopathic low molecular weight proteinuria, hypercalciuria, and nephrocalcinosis in Japanese children).

Hypercalciuria may lead to *nephrolithiasis*. Oral thiazide diuretics can normalize urinary calcium excretion by stimulating calcium reabsorption in the distal tubule. Such therapy may halt the gross hematuria or dysuria and prevent nephrolithiasis. However, the precise indications for thiazide treatment remain controversial. In patients with persistent gross hematuria or dysuria, therapy is initiated with chlorothiazide at a dosage of 10–20 mg/kg/24 hr as a single morning dose. The dosage is titrated upward until the urinary calcium excretion approaches 4 mg/kg/24 hr and the clinical manifestations resolve. After 1 yr of treatment, chlorothiazide is discontinued but may be resumed if gross hematuria, nephrolithiasis, or dysuria recurs. During chlorothiazide therapy, the serum potassium level should be monitored periodically to avoid hypokalemia. Dietary calcium restriction is not recommended because of the obligate requirement for growth. If low urine citrate levels are noted, supplemental citrate may improve hypercalciuria and its symptoms.

IgA Nephropathy

Donadio JV Jr, Grande JP: Immunoglobulin A nephropathy: A clinical perspective. J Am Soc Nephrol 8:1324, 1997.

Galla JH: IgA nephropathy. Kidney Int 47:377, 1995.

Hogg RJ, Silva FG, Wyatt RJ, et al: Prognostic indicators in children with IgA nephropathy—report of the southwest pediatric nephrology study group. Pediatr Nephrol 8:15, 1994.

Idiopathic Hematuria

Feld L, Waz W, Perez L, et al: Hematuria. Pediatr Clin North Am 44:1191, 1997.

Gubler MC, Beaufils H, Noel LH, et al: Significance of thin glomerular basement membranes in hematuric children. Contrib Nephrol 80:147, 1990.

Nieuwhof CMG, de Heer F, de Leeuw P, et al: Thin GBM nephropathy: Premature glomerular obsolescence is associated with hypertension and late onset renal failure. Kidney Int 51:1596, 1997.

Alport Syndrome

Bernstein J: The glomerular basement membrane abnormality in Alport's syndrome. Am J Kidney Dis 10:222, 1987.

Kashtan CE, Michael AF: Alport syndrome. Kidney Int 50:1445, 1996.

Turco AE, Bresin E, Rossetti S, et al: Rapid DNA-based prenatal diagnosis by genetic linkage in three families with Alport's syndrome. Am J Kidney Dis 30:174, 1997.

Idiopathic Hypercalciuria

Alon U, Warady BA, Hellerstein S: Hypercalciuria in the frequency-dysuria syndrome of childhood. J Pediatr 116:103, 1990.

Garcia CD, Miller LA, Stapleton FB: Natural history of hematuria association with hypercalciuria in children. Am J Dis Child 145:1204, 1991.

Matos V, van Melle G, Boulat O, et al: Urinary phosphate/creatinine, calcium/creatinine, and magnesium/creatinine ratios in a healthy pediatric population. J Pediatr 131:252, 1997.

Stapleton FB: Hematuria associated with hypercalciuria and hyperuricosuria: A practical approach. Pediatr Nephrol 8:756, 1994.

Stapleton FB: Making a "dent" in hereditary hypercalciuric nephrolithiasis. J Pediatr 132:764, 1998.

CHAPTER 519
Gross or Microscopic Hematuria

519.1 Acute Poststreptococcal Glomerulonephritis

This disease is the classic example of the acute nephritic syndrome: the sudden onset of gross hematuria, edema, hypertension, and renal insufficiency. It was the most common cause of gross hematuria in children; IgA nephropathy is now the most common cause of gross hematuria.

ETIOLOGY AND EPIDEMIOLOGY. Acute poststreptococcal glomerulonephritis follows infection of the throat or skin with certain "nephritogenic" strains of group A β-hemolytic streptococci. The factors that allow only certain strains of streptococci to be nephritogenic remain unclear. During cold weather, poststreptococcal glomerulonephritis commonly follows streptococcal pharyngitis, whereas during warm weather the glomerulonephritis generally follows streptococcal skin infections or pyoderma. Epidemics of nephritis have been described in association with both throat (serotype 12) and skin (serotype 49) infections; the disease is most commonly sporadic.

PATHOLOGY. As in most forms of acute glomerulonephritis, the kidneys appear symmetrically enlarged. On light microscopy, all glomeruli appear enlarged and relatively bloodless and show diffuse mesangial cell proliferation with an increase in mesangial matrix (Fig. 519–1). Polymorphonuclear leukocytes are common in glomeruli during the early stage of the disease.

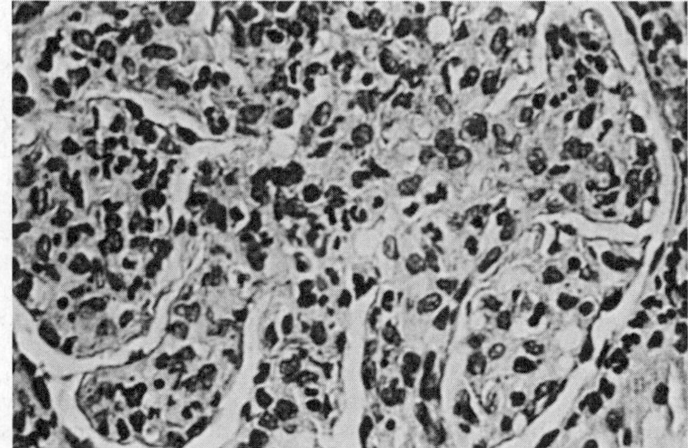

Figure 519–1 Glomerulus from a patient having poststreptococcal glomerulonephritis, appearing enlarged and relatively bloodless and showing mesangial proliferation and exudation of neutrophils. (×400.)

Crescents and interstitial inflammation may be seen in severe cases. These changes are not specific for poststreptococcal glomerulonephritis. Immunofluorescence microscopy reveals lumpy-bumpy deposits of immunoglobulin and complement on the glomerular basement membranes (GBMs) and in the mesangium. On electron microscopy, electron-dense deposits, or "humps," are observed on the epithelial side of the GBM (Fig. 519–2).

PATHOGENESIS. Although morphologic studies and a depression in the serum complement (C3) level strongly suggest that poststreptococcal glomerulonephritis is mediated by immune complexes, the precise mechanisms by which nephritogenic streptococci induce complex formation remain to be determined. Despite clinical and histologic similarities to acute serum sickness in rabbits, the finding of circulating immune complexes in poststreptococcal glomerulonephritis is not uniform and complement activation is primarily through the alter-

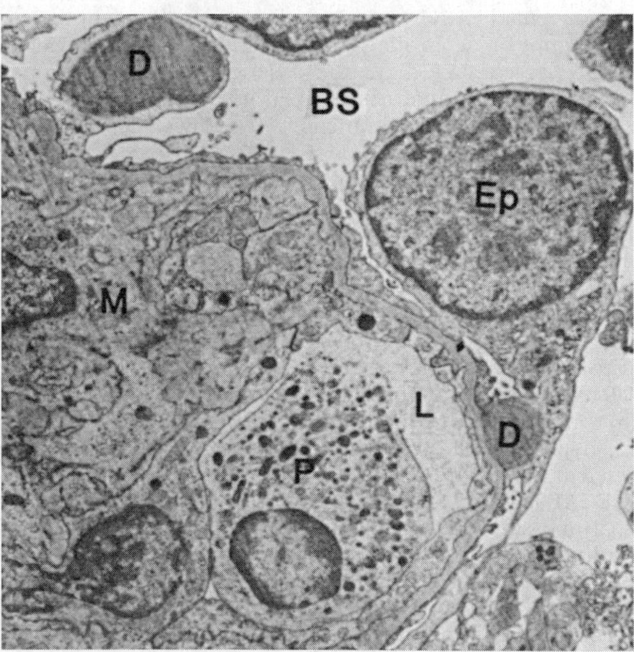

Figure 519–2 Electron micrograph in poststreptococcal glomerulonephritis, demonstrating electron-dense deposits (D) on the epithelial cell (Ep) side of the glomerular basement membrane. A polymorphonuclear leukocyte (P) is present within the lumen (L) of the capillary. BS = Bowman space; M = mesangium.

native rather than the classic (immune complex activated) pathway.

CLINICAL MANIFESTATIONS. Poststreptococcal glomerulonephritis is most common in children but rare before the age of 3 yr. The typical patient develops an acute nephritic syndrome 1–2 wk after an antecedent streptococcal infection. The severity of renal involvement may vary from asymptomatic microscopic hematuria with normal renal function to acute renal failure. Depending on the severity of renal involvement, patients may develop various degrees of edema, hypertension, and oliguria. Encephalopathy or heart failure due to hypertension or both may also develop. The edema is usually a result of salt and water retention, but a nephrotic syndrome may also occur. Nonspecific symptoms such as malaise, lethargy, abdominal or flank pain, and fever are common. The acute phase generally resolves within 2 mo after onset, but urinary abnormalities may persist for more than 1 yr.

DIAGNOSIS. Urinalysis demonstrates red blood cells (RBCs), frequently in association with RBC casts and proteinuria; polymorphonuclear leukocytes are common. A mild normochromic anemia may be present owing to hemodilution and low-grade hemolysis. The serum C3 level is usually reduced.

Confirmation of the diagnosis requires clear evidence of invasive streptococcal infection. A positive result of a throat culture may support the diagnosis or may simply represent the carrier state. To document streptococcal infection properly, an elevated antibody titer to streptococcal antigen(s) should be confirmed. Although most commonly obtained, determination of the ASO titer may not be helpful because it rarely rises after streptococcal skin infections. The best single antibody titer to measure is that to the deoxyribonuclease (DNase) B antigen. An alternative is the Streptozyme test (Wampole Laboratories, Stamford, CT), a slide agglutination procedure that detects antibodies to streptolysin O, DNase B, hyaluronidase, streptokinase, and nicotinamide-adenine dinucleotidase.

In a child with an acute nephritic syndrome, evidence of recent streptococcal infection, and a low C3 level, the clinical diagnosis of poststreptococcal glomerulonephritis is warranted and renal biopsy ordinarily is not indicated. It is important, however, to preclude systemic lupus erythematosus and an acute exacerbation of chronic glomerulonephritis. Considerations for renal biopsy would include the development of acute renal failure or nephrotic syndrome, the absence of evidence for streptococcal infection, the absence of hypocomplementemia, or the persistence of marked hematuria or proteinuria or both, diminished renal function, or a low C3 level for more than 3 mo after onset.

The differential diagnosis of poststreptococcal glomerulonephritis includes many of the causes of hematuria listed in Tables 517–2 and 517–3. Acute glomerulonephritis may also follow infection with coagulase-positive and -negative staphylococci, *Streptococcus pneumoniae*, gram-negative bacteria, and certain fungal, rickettsial, and viral diseases. Bacterial endocarditis may also produce a hypocomplementemic glomerulonephritis with renal failure.

COMPLICATIONS. The complications are those of acute renal failure and include volume overload, heart failure, hypertension, hyperkalemia, hyperphosphatemia, hypocalcemia, acidosis, seizures, and uremia.

PREVENTION. Early systemic antibiotic therapy of streptococcal throat and skin infections does not eliminate the risk of glomerulonephritis. Family members of patients with acute glomerulonephritis should be cultured for group A β-hemolytic streptococci and treated if culture positive.

TREATMENT. Because there is no specific therapy for acute poststreptococcal glomerulonephritis, the management is that of acute renal failure (Chapter 543.1). Although a 10-day course of systemic antibiotic therapy, generally with penicillin, is recommended to limit the spread of the nephritogenic organisms, no evidence shows that antibiotic therapy affects the natural history of glomerulonephritis. Activity need not be restricted, except during the acute phase of the disease when the complications of acute renal failure may be present, because activity has no detrimental effect on healing. Antihypertensive medications (diuretics, angiotensin-converting enzyme inhibitors) are indicated to treat hypertension and to avoid hypertensive complications.

PROGNOSIS. Complete recovery occurs in more than 95% of children with acute poststreptococcal glomerulonephritis. Infrequently, however, the acute phase may be very severe and lead to glomerular hyalinization and chronic renal insufficiency. Mortality in the acute stage can be avoided by appropriate management of the acute renal or cardiac failure and hypertension. Recurrences are extremely rare.

Clark G, White RHR, Glasgow EF, et al: Poststreptococcal glomerulonephritis in children: Clinicopathological correlations and long-term prognosis. Pediatr Nephrol 2:381, 1988.

Lange K, Seligson G, Cronin W: Evidence for the in situ origin of poststreptococcal glomerulonephritis: Glomerular localization of endostreptosin and the clinical significance of the subsequent antibody response. Clin Nephrol 19:3, 1983.

Vogl W, Renke M, Mayer-Eichberger D, et al: Long-term prognosis for endocapillary glomerulonephritis of poststreptococcal type in children and adults. Nephron 44:58, 1986.

CHAPTER 520
Membranous Glomerulopathy
(Glomerulonephritis)

Membranous glomerulopathy is the most common cause of nephrotic syndrome in adults, but it is uncommon in childhood and a rare cause of hematuria.

PATHOLOGY. By light microscopy, the glomeruli show diffuse thickening of the glomerular basement membrane (GBM), without significant proliferative changes (Fig. 520–1). The thickening presumably results from the production of membrane-like material by the visceral epithelial cells in response to immune complexes deposited on the epithelial side of the membrane. This new material may in certain areas resemble spikes on the epithelial side of the GBM. Immunofluorescent microscopy demonstrates granular deposits of IgG and C3, which electron microscopy shows to be located on the epithelial side of the membrane.

PATHOGENESIS. Morphologic studies suggest that membranous

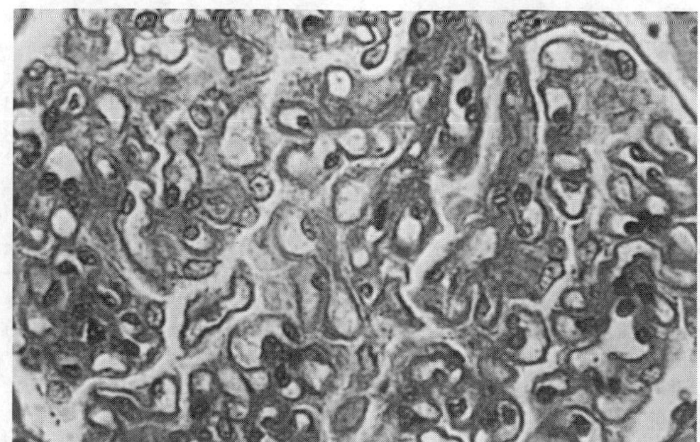

Figure 520–1 Glomerulus from a patient having membranous glomerulopathy, demonstrating diffuse thickening of the glomerular basement membrane in the absence of cellular proliferation. (×400.)

glomerulopathy is an immune complex–mediated disease, but the mechanism of complex formation and the nature of the antigen within the complexes remain unknown.

CLINICAL MANIFESTATIONS. In children, membranous glomerulopathy is most common in the 2nd decade of life. The disease usually presents as nephrotic syndrome. Most patients have microscopic hematuria and occasionally gross hematuria. The blood pressure and C3 levels are normal.

DIAGNOSIS. The diagnosis is confirmed by kidney biopsy. The usual indications for biopsy include the presentation of nephrotic syndrome in a child older than 8 yr or the presence of unexplained hematuria and proteinuria.

Membranous glomerulopathy may occasionally be found in association with systemic lupus erythematosus, cancer, gold or penicillamine therapy, and syphilis and hepatitis B virus infections. These conditions should be considered in patients having membranous disease, because elimination of the presumed stimulus might lead to resolution of the glomerulopathy. Patients with membranous glomerulopathy are at increased risk of renal vein thrombosis.

TREATMENT. Membranous glomerulopathy resolves spontaneously in the majority of children, although some may have persistent proteinuria. The nephrotic state is best controlled with salt restriction and diuretic agents. Studies of adults suggest that immunosuppressive therapy may retard the progressive renal insufficiency observed in some patients.

Hogan SL, Muller KE, Jeannette JC, et al: A review of therapeutic studies of idiopathic membranous glomerulopathy. Am J Kidney Dis 25:862, 1995.

Imperiale TF, Goldfarb S, Berns JS: Are cytotoxic agents beneficial in idiopathic membranous nephropathy? A meta-analysis of the controlled trials. J Am Soc Nephrol 5:1553, 1995.

Latham P, Poucell S, Koresaar A, et al: Idiopathic membranous glomerulopathy in Canadian children: A clinicopathologic study. J Pediatr 101:682, 1982.

Schieppati A, Mosconi L, Perna A, et al: Prognosis of untreated patients with idiopathic membranous nephropathy. N Engl J Med 329:85, 1993.

Wasserstein AG: Membranous glomeruloenphritis. J Am Soc Nephrol 8:663, 1997.

CHAPTER 521
Systemic Lupus Erythematosus

Systemic lupus erythematosus (SLE) is characterized by fever, weight loss, rash, hematologic abnormalities, arthritis, and involvement of the heart, lungs, central nervous system, and kidneys. The nonrenal manifestations are discussed in Chapter 159. Kidney disease, one of the most common manifestions of SLE in childhood, may occasionally be the only manifestation.

PATHOGENESIS AND PATHOLOGY. Studies in a mouse (NZB/NZW) strain and in humans suggest that the clinical manifestations of SLE are mediated by immune complexes. Aberrations in both B-cell and T-cell function are noted.

The classification of lupus nephritis of the World Health Organization (WHO) uses light, immunofluorescent, and electron microscopy. In patients with WHO class I nephritis, no histologic abnormalities are detected. In WHO class II (mesangial lupus nephritis), glomeruli have mesangial deposits containing immunoglobulin and complement; light microscopy may show mild (class II-A) or moderate mesangial hypercellularity and increased matrix (class II-B).

WHO class III (focal segmental lupus glomerulonephritis) shows mesangial deposits in almost all glomeruli and subendothelial deposits (between the endothelial cells and glomerular basement membrane) in some. In addition to focal and segmental mesangial proliferation, occasional glomeruli show capillary wall necrosis, crescent formation, and sclerosis lesions.

WHO class IV (diffuse proliferative lupus nephritis) is the most common and most severe form of lupus nephritis. All glomeruli contain massive mesangial and subendothelial deposits of immunoglobulin and complement. On light microscopy, all glomeruli show mesangial proliferation. The capillary walls are frequently thickened (owing to subendothelial deposits), creating the wire-loop lesion, and they commonly show necrosis, crescent formation, and scarring.

WHO class V (membranous lupus nephritis) is the least common form of lupus nephritis; it resembles idiopathic membranous glomerulopathy histologically, except for mild to moderate mesangial proliferation.

Transformation of the histologic lesion from one class to another (usually to a more severe class) is common, especially in inadequately treated patients.

CLINICAL MANIFESTATIONS. The majority of children with SLE are adolescent females who present with evidence of systemic disease, leading to the ultimate diagnosis. The clinical findings in patients having the milder forms (all class II, some class III) of lupus nephritis include hematuria, normal renal function, and proteinuria of less than 1 g/24 hr. Some patients with class III and all with class IV nephritis have hematuria and proteinuria, with reduced renal function, nephrotic syndrome, or acute renal failure. In some patients with proliferative glomerulonephritis, the finding of normal urinary sediment obscures the renal involvement. Patients with class V nephritis commonly have a nephrotic syndrome.

DIAGNOSIS. The diagnosis of SLE is suggested by the detection of circulating antinuclear antibodies and is confirmed by demonstrating that these antibodies react with native (double-stranded) DNA. In most patients with active disease, C3 and C4 levels are depressed. In view of the lack of clear correlation between the clinical manifestations and the severity of the renal involvement, renal biopsy should be performed on all patients with SLE. The findings guide the selection of immunosuppressive therapy.

TREATMENT. Immunosuppressive therapy in lupus nephritis aims at clinical and serologic remission (normalization of the anti-DNA, C3, and C4 levels). Therapy is initiated in all patients with prednisone, 60 mg/m^2/24 hr, divided into three or four doses. For patients having more severe forms of nephritis (some class III, all class IV), azathioprine is added in a once-daily dose of 2–3 mg/kg. When serologic remission is obtained after 1-2 mo, the schedule of prednisone is reduced to 60 mg/m^2 taken every other day as a single morning dose, being certain that the results of serologic studies remain normal and renal function stable while the schedule is reduced. After a varying period of time, the dose may then be further reduced by 5-mg decrements to 30 mg/m^2, so long as results of serologic studies remain normal and renal function stable. The dose of azathioprine may be reduced gradually while serologic results and renal function are monitored and may be discontinued after 1 yr. Studies of adults suggest that daily oral or monthly intravenous administration of cyclophosphamide may also be effective in corticosteroid-unresponsive or corticosteroid-toxic patients.

PROGNOSIS. Aggressive immunosuppressive therapy has dramatically improved the prognosis of SLE in childhood, but the disease is controlled, not cured. The risk of relapse, as well as the side effects of chronic immunosuppressive therapy, persists; of special concern are the effects of corticosteroids on adolescent girls. Patients with SLE should be treated in conjunction with specialists in medical centers where both medical and psychologic support can be given to both patients and their families.

Austin HA III, Boumpas DT, Vaughan EM, et al: Predicting renal outcomes in severe lupus nephritis: Contributions of clinical and histologic data. Kidney Int 45:544, 1994.

Balow JE, Boumpas DT, Fessler BJ, et al: Management of lupus nephritis. Kidney Int 49(Suppl 53):S-88, 1996.

Bansai VK, Beto JA: Treatment of lupus nephritis: A meta-analysis of clinical trials. Am J Kidney Dis 29:193, 1997.
Baqi N, Moazami S, Singh A, et al: Lupus nephritis in children: A longitudinal study of prognostic factors and therapy. J Am Soc Nephrol 7:924, 1996.
Berden JHM: Lupus nephritis. Kidney Int 52:538, 1997.
Cameron JS: Lupus nephritis. J Am Soc Nephrol 10:413, 1999.

CHAPTER 522
Membranoproliferative (Mesangiocapillary) Glomerulonephritis

The term *chronic glomerulonephritis* implies continuing glomerular injury, such as frequently leads to glomerular destruction and end-stage renal failure. Membranoproliferative glomerulonephritis (MPGN) is the most common cause of chronic glomerulonephritis in older children and young adults.

PATHOLOGY AND PATHOGENESIS. MPGN was initially distinguished from other forms of chronic glomerulonephritis by the finding of hypocomplementemia, in some patients the result of an antibody (called C3 nephritic factor) that activates the alternative complement pathway. Not all patients have hypocomplementemia. Three histologic types are described.

Type I MPGN is the most common form; the glomeruli reveal an accentuation of the lobular pattern, due to a generalized increase in mesangial cells and matrix (Fig. 522–1). The glomerular capillary walls appear thickened and, in some areas, duplicated or split, owing to interposition of mesangial cytoplasm and matrix between the endothelial cells and glomerular basement membrane (GBM) and new basement membrane produced by the endothelial cells. Crescents may be present; when detected in a high percentage of glomeruli, they indicate a poor prognosis. Immunofluorescent microscopy reveals C3 and lesser amounts of immunoglobulin in the mesangium and along the peripheral capillary walls in a lobular pattern (Fig. 522–2), and electron microscopy confirms the presence of immune complex–like deposits in the mesangial and subendothelial regions.

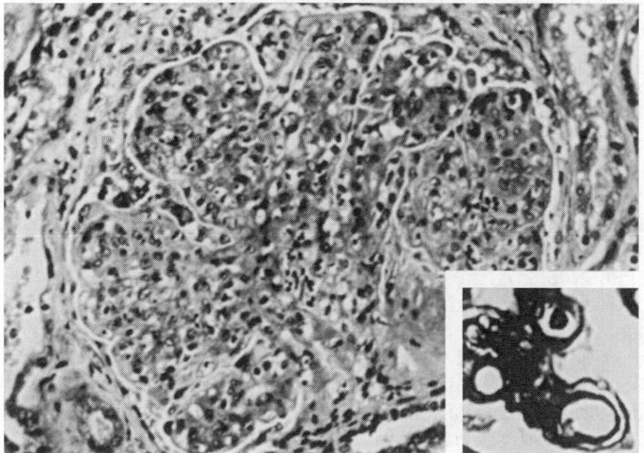

Figure 522–1 Glomerulus from a patient with type I membranoproliferative glomerulonephritis, demonstrating an accentuated lobular pattern, a generalized increase in mesangial cells and matrix, and "splitting" of the glomerular capillary wall *(inset)*. (×250.) (From Kim Y, Michael AF: Idiopathic membranoproliferative glomerulonephritis. Reproduced, with permission, from the Annual Review of Medicine, Vol 31. © 1980 by Annual Reviews, Inc.)

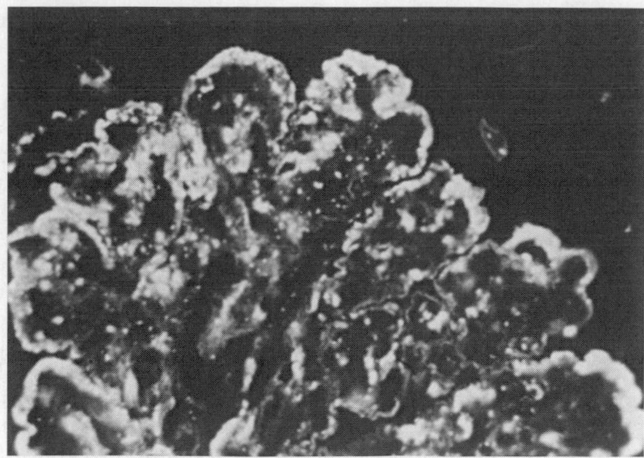

Figure 522–2 Immunofluorescence microscopy in type I membranoproliferative glomerulonephritis, demonstrating granular deposition of C3 along the glomerular basement membranes and in the mesangium. (×610.) (From Kim Y, Michael AF: Idiopathic membranoproliferative glomerulonephritis. Reproduced, with permission, from the Annual Review of Medicine, Vol 31. © 1980 by Annual Reviews, Inc.)

In *type II disease,* the mesangial changes are less prominent than in type I. The capillary walls demonstrate irregular ribbon-like thickening, owing to dense deposits. Splitting of the membrane is rare, but crescents are common. On electron microscopy, the dense deposits are seen as thickenings of GBM in the region of but distinct from the lamina densa. The deposits are also found in Bowman's capsule, mesangium, and tubular basement membranes; their composition is unknown. Immunofluorescent studies show C3, usually with minimal immunoglobulin, along the margin of the dense deposit material.

In *type III disease,* the light and immunofluorescent microscopic findings resemble those found in type I disease. Electron microscopy reveals contiguous subepithelial and subendothelial deposits, associated with disruption and layering of the lamina densa portion of the GBM.

CLINICAL MANIFESTATIONS. MPGN is most common in the 2nd decade of life. The majority of patients present with nephrotic syndrome, and others with gross hematuria or asymptomatic microscopic hematuria and proteinuria. Renal function may be normal to depressed. Hypertension is common. The serum C3 complement level may be decreased.

DIAGNOSIS AND DIFFERENTIAL DIAGNOSIS. The diagnosis of MPGN is made by renal biopsy. Indications for biopsy include onset of nephrotic syndrome in a child older than 8 yr or persistent microscopic hematuria and proteinuria.

Both MPGN and poststreptococcal glomerulonephritis may have gross hematuria, low C3 levels, and elevated antistreptococcal antibody titers as manifestations (coincidental in patients with membranoproliferative disease); their natural histories distinguish between the two. Patients with poststreptococcal glomerulonephritis improve dramatically within 2 mo of onset, whereas in children having MPGN, persistent clinical manifestations lead to kidney biopsy.

PROGNOSIS AND TREATMENT. The outlook for all types of membranoproliferative disease is poor. Complete recovery has been reported, but most cases of type II and many of types I and III progress to end-stage renal failure. Types I and II MPGN may recur in patients with kidney transplants, suggesting the presence of systemic disorder.

No definitive therapy exists, but stabilization of the clinical course has been reported in some patients receiving long-term alternate-day prednisone therapy.

Bergstein JM, Andreoli SP: Response of type I membranoproliferative glomerulonephritis to pulse methylprednisolone and alternate-day prednisone therapy. Pediatr Nephrol 9:268, 1995.

McEnery PT: Membranoproliferative glomerulonephritis: The Cincinnati experience—cumulative renal survival from 1957 to 1989. J Pediatr 116:S109, 1990.

Tarshish P, Bernstein J, Tobin JN, et al: Treatment of mesangio-capillary glomerulonephritis with alternate-day prednisone—a report of The International Study of Kidney Disease in Children. Pediatr Nephrol 6:123, 1992.

CHAPTER 523
Glomerulonephritis of Chronic Infection

Occurrence of glomerulonephritis has been recognized during the course of various chronic infections, including bacterial endocarditis *Streptococcus viridans* and other organisms), infected ventriculoatrial shunts for hydrocephalus *(Staphylococcus epidermidis)*, syphilis, hepatitis B, hepatitis C, candidiasis, and malaria. In each condition, the infecting organism has low virulence and the host is chronically seeded with foreign antigen. In the presence of high levels of circulating antigen, the host's antibody response leads to formation of immune complexes, which deposit in the kidneys and initiate the glomerulonephritis.

The histopathologic findings may resemble poststreptococcal, membranous, or membranoproliferative glomerulonephritis. The clinical manifestations are generally those of an acute nephritic or nephrotic syndrome. The complement C3 level is frequently depressed.

Eradication of the infection before severe glomerular injury occurs usually results in resolution of the glomerulonephritis. Progression to end-stage renal failure has been described.

Chesney RW, O'Regan S, Guyda HJ, et al: Candida endocrinopathy syndrome with membranoproliferative glomerulonephritis: Demonstration of glomerular candida antigen. Clin Nephrol 5:232, 1976.

Hendrickse RG, Adeniyi A: Quartan malarial nephrotic syndrome in children. Kidney Int 16:64, 1979.

Hunte W, Al-Ghraoui F, Cohen RJ: Secondary syphilis and the nephrotic syndrome. J Am Soc Nephrol 3:1351, 1993.

Johnson RJ, Couser WG: Hepatitis B infection and renal disease: Clinical, immunopathogenic and therapeutic considerations. Kidney Int 37:663, 1990.

Johnson RJ, Gretch DR, Yamabe H, et al: Membranoproliferative glomerulonephritis associated with hepatitis C virus infection. N Engl J Med 328:465, 1993.

Neugarten J, Baldwin DS: Glomerulonephritis in bacterial endocarditis. Am J Med 77:297, 1984.

Vella J, Carmody M, Campbell E, et al: Glomerulonephritis after ventriculo-atrial shunt. QJ Med 88:911, 1995.

CHAPTER 524
Rapidly Progressive (Crescentic) Glomerulonephritis

Rapidly progressive describes the clinical course of several forms of glomerulonephritis whose unifying abnormality is the presence of crescents in the majority of glomeruli. The natural history in most forms is rapid progression to end-stage renal failure.

CLASSIFICATION. Crescents may be found in several well-defined types of glomerulonephritis, such as poststreptococcal, lupus, membranoproliferative, and the glomerulonephritides of Goodpasture disease, Henoch-Schönlein purpura, and other forms of vasculitis. The typical findings on light, immunofluorescent, and electron microscopic examinations are maintained despite crescent formation; these histologic findings, in conjunction with appropriate laboratory studies, should reveal the underlying disease. If these recognized forms of glomerulonephritis are excluded, an idiopathic variety of rapidly progressive disease remains.

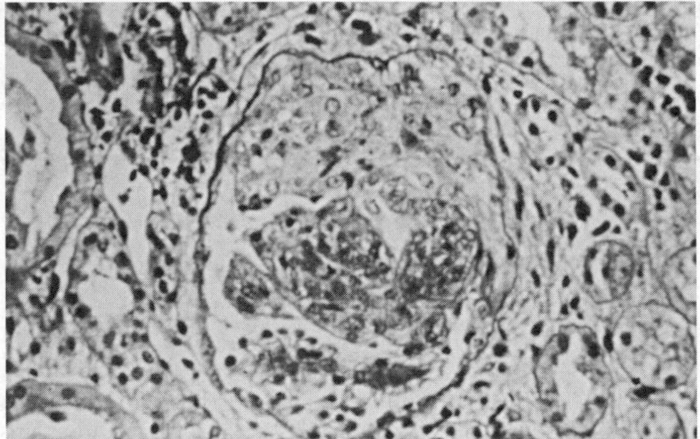

Figure 524–1 Light micrograph of a biopsy specimen from a child with Henoch-Schönlein purpura glomerulonephritis, demonstrating a crescent overlying the glomerulus. (×180.)

PATHOLOGY AND PATHOGENESIS. Crescents are found on the inside of Bowman's capsule and are composed of the proliferating epithelial cells of the capsule and of fibrin, basement membrane–like material, and macrophages (Fig. 524–1). The stimulus for crescent formation is presumed to be the deposition of fibrin in Bowman's space, probably as a result of necrosis or disruption of the glomerular capillary wall. In many patients with the idiopathic variety of rapidly progressive disease, no evidence for immunologic mechanisms can be detected; others have antibodies against glomerular basement membrane or deposits of immune complexes on capillary walls. The complement C3 level is normal.

CLINICAL MANIFESTATIONS. Most patients develop acute renal failure, often after an acute nephritic or nephrotic episode. Progression to end-stage renal failure follows within weeks to months after onset.

DIAGNOSIS AND DIFFERENTIAL DIAGNOSIS. Appropriate serologic studies (antinuclear antibody, C3, anti-deoxyribonucleotidase B titers) should be obtained to search for defined types of glomerulonephritis. Rare forms of vasculitis, such as Wegener granulomatosis and microscopic polyarteritis nodosa, may be suggested by the detection of circulating antineutrophil cytoplasmic antibodies (ANCA). The diagnosis is confirmed by kidney biopsy.

PROGNOSIS AND TREATMENT. Children having rapidly progressive disease associated with poststreptococcal glomerulonephritis may recover spontaneously. Treating the rapidly progressive nephritis of lupus and of Henoch-Schönlein purpura with prednisone and azathioprine has been successful. The prognosis is poor for the remaining types of rapidly progressive glomerulonephritis, although a few patients have been reported to improve with therapy combining pulse methylprednisolone, oral cyclophosphamide, and possibly plasmapheresis or lymphocytapheresis.

Furuta T, Hotta O, Yusa N, et al: Lymphocytapheresis to treat rapidly progressive glomerulonephritis: A randomized comparison with steroid-pulse treatment. Lancet 352:203, 1998.

Jennette JC, Falk RJ: Small vessel vasculitis. N Engl J Med 337:1512, 1997

Roltem M, Fauci AS, Hallahan CW, et al: Wegener granulomatosis in children and adolescents: Clinical presentation and outcome. J Pediatr 122:26, 1993.

Srivastava RN, Moudgil A, Bagga A, et al: Crescentric glomerulonephritis in children: A review of 43 cases. Am J Nephrol 12:155, 1992.

Valentini RP, Smoyer WE, Sedman AB, et al: Outcome of antineutrophil cytoplasmic autoantibodies-positive glomerulonephritis and vasculitis in children: A single-center experience. J Pediatr 132:325, 1998.

CHAPTER 525
Goodpasture Disease

Goodpasture disease (pulmonary hemorrhage and glomerulonephritis associated with antibodies against lung and against glomerular basement membrane [GBM]) should be distinguished from Goodpasture syndrome (a clinical picture of pulmonary hemorrhage and glomerulonephritis that may be seen with several disorders, including systemic lupus erythematosus, Henoch-Schönlein purpura, polyarteritis nodosa, and Wegener granulomatosis). In some patients, anti-GBM nephritis occurs without pulmonary hemorrhage as one form of rapidly progressive glomerulonephritis.

PATHOLOGY. In most patients, the changes on light microscopy resemble those of rapidly progressive glomerulonephritis; immunofluorescent microscopy shows a continuous linear pattern of IgG along the GBM, typical of anti-GBM antibody (Fig. 525–1).

CLINICAL MANIFESTATIONS. Goodpasture disease is rare in childhood. Hemoptysis is usually the presenting complaint, and pulmonary hemorrhage is a potential cause of death. In days to weeks, hematuria, proteinuria, and progressive renal failure develop. The complement C3 level is normal.

DIAGNOSIS. The diagnosis is suggested by kidney biopsy. Other diseases that may show linear GBM staining for IgG are precluded when serum is found to contain anti-GBM antibody.

PROGNOSIS AND TREATMENT. Patients who survive the pulmonary hemorrhage commonly progress to end-stage renal failure. Rates of survival and recovery of renal function have improved with pulse methylprednisolone, oral cyclophosphamide, and plasmapheresis therapy.

Bolton WK: Goodpasture's syndrome: Kidney Int 50:1753, 1996.
Kelly PT, Haponik EF: Goodpasture syndrome: Molecular and clinical advances. Medicine 73:171, 1994.
McCarthy LJ, Cotton J, Danielson C, et al: Goodpasture's syndrome in childhood: Treatment with plasmapheresis and immunosuppression. J Clin Apher 9:116, 1994.

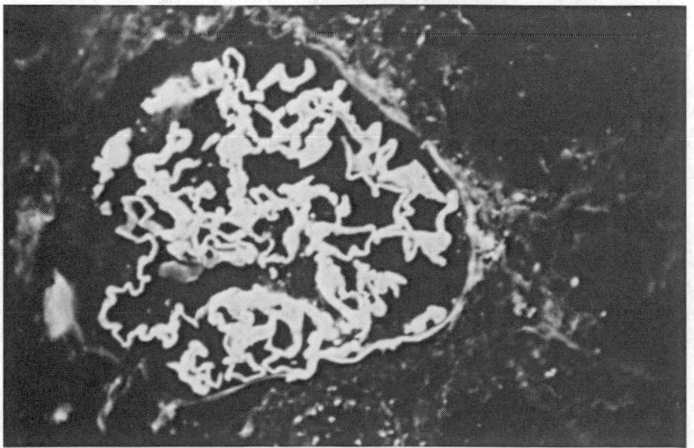

Figure 525–1 Immunofluorescence micrograph demonstrating the continuous linear staining of IgG along the glomerular basement membrane, as found in diseases mediated by antiglomerular basement membrane antibody. (×250.)

CHAPTER 526
Hemolytic-Uremic Syndrome

The hemolytic-uremic syndrome is the most common cause of acute renal failure in young children; the incidence is increasing. It was initially believed to be a renal disorder with secondary hematologic manifestations; however, the syndrome should be regarded as a systemic disease. Hemolytic-uremic syndrome has features common to thrombotic thrombocytopenic purpura, except that the latter tends to occur in young women as a relapsing illness with fever, more dominant central nervous system involvement, thrombocytopenia, and cutaneous signs.

ETIOLOGY. The disease most frequently follows an episode of gastroenteritis caused by an enterohemorrhagic strain of *Escherichia coli* (0157:H7). The reservoir of this organism is the intestinal tract of domestic animals. It is usually transmitted by undercooked meat and unpasteurized milk. Outbreaks have followed ingestion of contaminated apple cider or bathing in a contaminated swimming pool. The organism elaborates a toxin, called verotoxin, which is apparently absorbed from the intestines and initiates endothelial cell injury. It has been less often associated with other bacterial *(Shigella, Salmonella, Campylobacter, Streptococcus pneumoniae), Bartonella,* and viral (coxsackie, ECHO, influenza, varicella, HIV, Epstein-Barr) infections and with endotoxemia. It has been reported also to follow use of oral contraceptives, mitomycin, cyclosporine, and pyran copolymer, an inducer of interferon. In addition, a hemolytic-uremic type of disorder has been reported to be associated with systemic lupus erythematosus, malignant hypertension, pre-eclampsia, postpartum renal failure, and radiation nephritis. There may be an absence of a plasma factor that stimulates endothelial cell prostacyclin production in nondiarrheal and sporadic familial cases. Several reports describe occurrence in more than one member of a family, but the role of genetic factors in predisposition to the disease is unknown.

PATHOLOGY. The initial changes in the glomeruli include thickening of the capillary walls, narrowing of the capillary lumina, and widening of the mesangium. Electron microscopy shows these changes to be the result of subendothelial and mesangial deposition of a granular, amorphous material of unknown origin. Fibrin thrombi can be found in glomerular capillaries and arterioles and may lead to cortical necrosis.

Severely involved glomeruli progress to partial or total sclerosis; severe vascular involvement may render others obsolescent as a result of ischemia. In these severely involved small arteries and arterioles, concentric intimal proliferation leads to vascular occlusion.

PATHOGENESIS. The primary event in pathogenesis of the syndrome appears to be endothelial cell injury. Capillary and arteriolar endothelial injury in the kidney leads to localized clotting. Evidence for disseminated intravascular coagulation is unusual. The microangiopathic anemia results from mechanical damage to the red blood cells (RBCs) as they pass through the altered vasculature. Thrombocytopenia is due to intrarenal platelet adhesion or damage. Damaged RBCs and platelets are removed from circulation by the liver and spleen.

CLINICAL MANIFESTATIONS. The syndrome is most common in children younger than 4 yr. The onset is usually preceded by gastroenteritis (fever, vomiting, abdominal pain, and diarrhea, which is often bloody) or, less commonly, by an upper respiratory tract infection. This is followed in 5–10 days by the sudden onset of pallor, irritability, weakness, lethargy, and oliguria. Physical examination may reveal dehydration, edema, petechiae, hepatosplenomegaly, and marked irritability.

DIAGNOSIS AND DIFFERENTIAL DIAGNOSIS. The diagnosis is supported by the findings of a microangiopathic hemolytic anemia, thrombocytopenia, and acute renal failure. The hemoglobin is commonly in the range of 5–9 g/dL. The blood film reveals helmet cells, burr cells, and fragmented RBCs (Chapter 453). Plasma hemoglobin levels are elevated, and plasma haptoglobin levels diminished. The reticulocyte count is moderately elevated; the Coombs test result is negative. The white blood cell count may rise to 30,000/mm³. Thrombocytopenia (20,000–100,000/mm³; 10^9/L) occurs in more than 90% of patients. Findings on urinalysis are surprisingly mild and usually consist of low-grade microscopic hematuria and proteinuria. Partial thromboplastin time and prothrombin time are usually normal; their prolongation is more commonly due to vitamin K deficiency than to disseminated intravascular coagulation. The severity of the renal involvement, and the complications thereof, vary from mild renal insufficiency to acute renal failure requiring dialysis. Barium contrast roentgenograms (enema) reveal colonic spasm and transient early filling defects. Subsequent intestinal stenosis is a rare sequela.

The sudden onset of acute renal failure in a child should always suggest this entity. The typical history, clinical picture, and laboratory findings confirm the diagnosis in most patients. Other causes of acute renal failure, especially those that can be associated with a microangiopathic anemia (lupus, malignant hypertension), should be precluded. Except in the rare patient who suffers prolonged renal failure (> 2 wk) or who fails to develop thrombocytopenia, a renal biopsy is rarely indicated; it should not be performed in thrombocytopenic patients.

Patients who have bilateral renal vein thrombosis (Chapter 528.3) may be difficult to distinguish from those with the hemolytic-uremic syndrome. Both disorders may be preceded by gastroenteritis, and in both the children may present with dehydration, pallor, and evidence of microangiopathic hemolytic anemia, thrombocytopenia, and acute renal failure. The marked enlargement of kidneys of a child with renal vein thrombosis helps to distinguish the disorders, but angiography may be necessary in obscure cases if renal Doppler ultrasonography is inclusive.

COMPLICATIONS. Complications may include anemia, acidosis, hyperkalemia, fluid overload, heart failure, hypertension, and uremia. In addition, extrarenal involvement may include central nervous system manifestations (irritability, seizures, thrombosis, coma), colitis (melena, perforation), diabetes mellitus, and rhabdomyolysis. The pathogenesis of these complications is unknown; they seem likely to be a result of intravascular thrombosis.

PROGNOSIS AND TREATMENT. With aggressive management of the acute renal failure, more than 90% of patients survive the acute phase, and the majority of these recover normal renal function. Corticosteroids appear to have no value, and experience with platelet inhibitors is so far inconclusive. The treatment has mostly involved anticoagulants, primarily heparin. Analysis of the results fails to demonstrate beneficial effects in most patients, who in any case lack evidence of active hypercoagulation. Fibrinolytic therapy to dissolve intrarenal thrombi would have theoretical benefit, but the risks seem to outweigh the potential gains. Plasmapheresis or administration of fresh frozen plasma, or both, has been recommended, but results do not yet permit interpretation.

Careful medical management of the hematologic and renal manifestations, in conjunction with early and frequent peritoneal dialysis, offers the best chance of recovery from the acute phase. Peritoneal dialysis not only controls the manifestations of the uremic state but also promotes recovery by removing an inhibitor (plasminogen activates inhibitor-1) of fibrinolysis from the circulation, thus allowing endogenous fibrinolytic mechanisms to dissolve vascular thrombi. Long-term observation is necessary to watch for late development of hypertension or chronic kidney disease. Recurrence of the disease is rare.

Bergstein JM, Riley M, Bang NU: Role of plasminogen-activator inhibitor type 1 in the pathogenesis and outcome of the hemolytic-uremic syndrome. N Engl J Med 327:755, 1992.

Boyce TG, Swerdlow DL, Griffin PM: Escherichia coli 0157:H7 and the hemolytic-uremic syndrome. N Engl J Med 333:364, 1995.

Brandt JR, Fouser LS, Watkins SL, et al: Escherichia coli 0157:H7-associated hemolytic-uremic syndrome after ingestion of contaminated hamburgers. J Pediatr 125:519, 1994.

Cabrera GR, Fortenberry JD, Warshaw BL, et al: Hemolytic uremic syndrome associated with invasive Streptococcus pneumoniae infection. Pediatrics 101:699, 1998.

Kelles A, Van Dyck M, Proesmans W: Childhood haemolytic uraemic syndrome: Long-term outcome and prognostic features. Eur J Pediatr 153:38, 1994.

Siegler RL: The hemolytic-uremic syndrome. Pediatr Clin North Am 42:1505, 1995.

Siegler RL: Spectrum of extrarenal involvement in postdiarrheal hemolytic-uremic syndrome. J Pediatr 125:511, 1994.

Spizzirri FD, Rahman RC, Bibiloni N, et al: Childhood hemolytic-uremic syndrome in Argentina: Long-term follow-up and prognostic features. Pediatr Nephrol 11:156, 1997.

CHAPTER 527
Infection as a Cause of Hematuria

Gross or microscopic hematuria may be associated with bacterial, mycobacterial, or viral infections of the urinary tract (Chapter 546). Why the same organism may cause hematuria in one patient with cystitis and not in another is unclear; the occurrence of hematuria may be related to the depth and severity of the inflammatory reaction within the bladder wall.

Urethritis may present with gross or microscopic hematuria, usually in conjunction with urgency and pyuria. Urine cultures occasionally reveal bacteria, *Ureaplasma*, or *Chlamydia* but are usually negative. A history of trauma should be sought. The disorder frequently resolves spontaneously. In children older than 8 yr, treatment can be considered with a 10-day course of doxycycline, with a urinary analgesic (phenazopyridine) given for relief of pain. If conservative management fails, cystoscopy may be required to determine the nature of any underlying abnormality (ulceration, inflammation).

CHAPTER 528
Hematologic Diseases Causing Hematuria

528.1 Coagulopathies and Thrombocytopenia

Gross or microscopic hematuria may be associated with inherited or acquired disorders of coagulation (hemophilias, disseminated intravascular coagulation, thrombocytopenia). In these cases, however, hematuria is not usually the presenting complaint but develops after other manifestations (Part XX, Section 7).

528.2 Sickle Cell Nephropathy

Gross or microscopic hematuria may be seen in children with sickle cell disease or trait. The hematuria presumably results from sickling in the relatively hypoxic, acidic, hypertonic renal medulla, with vascular stasis, diminished blood flow, ischemia, papillary necrosis, and interstitial fibrosis. Additional clinical manifestations of sickle cell nephropathy may include a urinary concentrating defect, renal tubular acidosis, and, rarely, a nephrotic syndrome that morphologically resembles focal sclerosis or membranoproliferative glomerulonephritis. The hematuria resolves spontaneously in the majority of patients (Chapter 468.1).

Falk RJ, Scheinman J, Phillips G, et al: Prevalence and pathologic features of sickle cell nephropathy and response to inhibition of angiotensin-converting enzyme. N Engl J Med 326:910, 1992.

Saborio P, Scheinman JI: Sickle cell nephropathy. J Am Soc Nephrol 10:187, 1999.

528.3 Renal Vein Thrombosis

EPIDEMIOLOGY. Renal vein thrombosis seems to occur in two distinct patterns. In newborns and infants, the disease is commonly associated with asphyxia, dehydration, shock, and sepsis; it occurs rarely in infants of diabetic mothers. After infancy, the disease is more commonly associated with the nephrotic syndrome (most frequently with membranous nephropathy), with cyanotic heart disease, in patients with inherited hypercoagulable states, and with the use of angiographic contrast agents.

PATHOGENESIS. The disease presumably begins in the intrarenal venous radicles, with both antegrade and retrograde spread. The main renal vein may escape involvement. Thrombus formation is presumably mediated by endothelial cell injury (by hypoxia, endotoxin, or contrast media) in conjunction with a hypercoagulable state (hereditary disorder or the nephrotic syndrome) and diminished vascular blood flow, which may be due to hypovolemia (shock, sepsis, dehydration, or nephrotic syndrome) or to the intravascular sludging of blood during neonatal polycythemia.

CLINICAL MANIFESTATIONS. The development of renal vein thrombosis in infants is usually heralded by the sudden onset of gross hematuria and unilateral or bilateral flank masses. Older children commonly present with gross or microscopic hematuria and flank pain. The disease is more frequently unilateral than bilateral; bilateral involvement results in acute renal failure.

DIAGNOSIS. The diagnosis is suggested by the development of hematuria and flank masses in a patient with predisposing clinical factors. Most patients also have a microangiopathic hemolytic anemia and thrombocytopenia. Ultrasonography shows marked enlargement, whereas radionuclide studies reveal little or no renal function in involved kidneys. Doppler flow studies or venacavography of the inferior vena cava may be necessary to confirm the diagnosis, but contrast studies should generally be avoided in order to minimize the risk of further vascular damage.

DIFFERENTIAL DIAGNOSIS. The differential diagnosis includes other causes of hematuria (especially the hemolytic-uremic syndrome) or renal enlargement (hydronephrosis, cystic disease, Wilms tumor, abscess, hematoma).

TREATMENT. For unilateral renal vein thrombosis, treatment is supportive and involves correction of fluid and electrolyte abnormalities and treatment of infection. Prophylactic anticoagulation with heparin is generally recommended but has not been well studied.

Because bilateral renal vein thrombosis frequently leads to chronic renal failure, consideration should be given to use of such measures as thrombectomy or the systemic use of fibrinolytic agents.

PROGNOSIS. In infants, a completely thrombosed kidney undergoes progressive atrophy, ultimately leaving a small, scarred kidney. Nephrectomy should not be performed in the acute phase, and later only if hypertension or chronic infection develops. In older children, the involved kidney may recover function, especially if the thrombosis was associated with nephrotic syndrome or cyanotic heart disease.

Laplante S, Patriquin HB, Robitaille P, et al: Renal vein thrombosis in children: Evidence of early flow recovery with Doppler. US Radiol 189:37, 1993.

Mocan H, Beattie TJ, Murphy AV: Renal venous thrombosis in infancy: Long-term follow-up. Pediatr Nephrol 5:45, 1991.

Ricci MA, Lloyd DA: Renal venous thrombosis in infants and children. Arch Surg 125:1195, 1990.

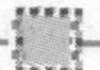

CHAPTER 529
Anatomic Abnormalities Associated with Hematuria

CONGENITAL ANOMALIES. Gross or microscopic hematuria may be associated with most types of malformations of the urinary tract. The sudden onset of usually painless gross hematuria after minor trauma to the flank is frequently associated with ureteropelvic junction obstruction or cystic kidneys.

TRAUMA. Blunt or penetrating injury to the abdomen may injure a kidney. Gross or microscopic hematuria, flank pain, and abdominal rigidity may occur; associated injuries may be present. Urethral trauma may result from crushing-type injury, frequently associated with a fractured pelvis, or from direct injury. The injury is suspected when gross blood appears at the external meatus.

Mirvis SE: Trauma. Radiol Clin North Am 34:1225, 1996.

Taylor GA, Eichelberger MR, Potter BM: Hematuria: A marker of abdominal injury in children after blunt trauma. Ann Surg 208:688, 1988.

Yale-Loehr AJ, Kramer SS, Quinlan DM, et al: CT of severe renal trauma in children: Evaluation and course of healing with conservative therapy. AJR 152:109, 1989.

529.1 Autosomal Recessive Polycystic Kidney Disease

Also known as *infantile polycystic disease*, this rare autosomal recessive disorder (mapped to chromosome 6) may not be detected until after infancy. Besides cysts in the kidneys, cysts may also be found in the liver, with significant liver disease.

PATHOLOGY. Both kidneys are markedly enlarged and grossly show innumerable cysts throughout the cortex and medulla. Microscopic studies show the "cysts" to be dilatations of the collecting ducts. The interstitium and remainder of the tubules may be normal at birth, but development of interstitial fibrosis and tubular atrophy may lead to renal failure.

The majority of patients also have cysts in the liver. In severe cases, the cysts in the liver may be associated with cirrhosis, portal hypertension, and death due to ruptured esophageal varices. When the severity of hepatic manifestations exceeds that of renal involvement, the disorder is called *congenital hepatic fibrosis*. Whether infantile polycystic disease and congenital hepatic fibrosis are the opposite ends of the spectrum of a

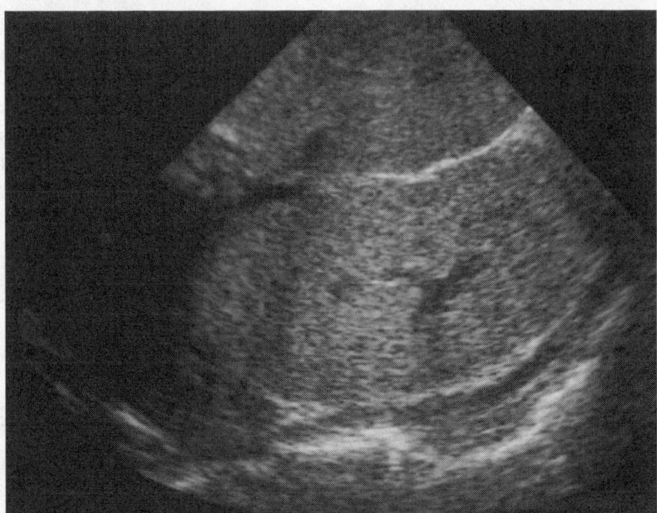

Figure 529–1 Ultrasound examination of a neonate with autosomal recessive polycystic kidney disease demonstrating renal enlargement (9 cm) and increased diffuse echogenicity with complete loss of corticomedullary differentiation due to multiple small cystic interfaces.

single disorder or distinct autosomal recessive disorders with similar manifestations remains to be determined.

CLINICAL MANIFESTATIONS. The typical patient has bilateral flank masses at birth. The disorder may be associated with oligohydramnios, owing to inadequate formation of urine by the fetus. The oligohydramnios may produce Potter syndrome (flat nose, recessed chin, epicanthal folds, low-set abnormal ears, limb abnormalities), as a result of compression of the fetus, as well as pulmonary hypoplasia. The pulmonary hypoplasia may produce neonatal respiratory distress, with spontaneous pneumothorax. The association of developmental disorders of the lungs and kidneys is sufficiently frequent to warrant ultrasonic evaluation of the kidneys in all neonates who have spontaneous pneumothorax. Gross or microscopic hematuria and hypertension (which may be severe) are common. Renal function may be normal or diminished, depending on the severity of the renal malformation. Rarely, patients beyond infancy may first present with a nephrogenic diabetes insipidus–like state, renal insufficiency, or hypertension.

DIAGNOSIS. The diagnosis is suggested by the clinical manifestations and is supported by ultrasonography, which shows markedly enlarged and uniformly hyperechogenic kidneys (Fig. 529–1). Because ultrasonic evaluation of the kidneys may fail to define the cysts, intravenous pyelography may be considered. A satisfactory pyelogram reveals opacification of the dilated collecting ducts. Because these ducts extend from cortex to medulla, they appear as radial streaks similar to the spokes of a wheel. But radiographic studies are rarely able to confirm the diagnosis; therefore, in questionable instances, open surgical biopsy of the liver and right kidney may be performed toward the end of the 1st yr of life to confirm the diagnosis and to permit genetic counseling.

The differential diagnosis includes other causes of bilateral renal enlargement, such as multicystic dysplasia, hydronephrosis, Wilms tumor, and renal vein thrombosis.

TREATMENT. The treatment is supportive, including careful management of the associated hypertension.

PROGNOSIS. Children with severe renal involvement may die in the neonatal period of pulmonary or renal insufficiency. Survivors may live for several years before developing renal insufficiency. During this period, the kidneys shrink in size and the hypertension becomes less severe. When renal failure develops, dialysis and kidney transplantation should be considered. In patients having hepatic fibrosis, cirrhosis may lead to portal hypertension, for which the prognosis is poor.

Roy S, Dillon MJ, Trompeter RS, et al: Autosomal recessive polycystic kidney disease: Long-term outcome of neonatal survivors. Pediatr Nephrol 11:302, 1997.

Shaikewitz ST, Chapman A: Autosomal recessive polycystic kidney disease: Issues regarding the variability of clinical presentation. J Am Soc Nephrol 3:1858, 1993.

Zerres K, Rudnik-Schoneborn S, Deget F, et al: Autosomal recessive polycystic kidney disease in 115 children: Clinical presentation, course and influence of gender. Acta Paediatr 85:437, 1996.

529.2 Autosomal Dominant Polycystic Kidney Disease

Also known as *adult polycystic disease*, this phenotypically variable autosomal dominant disorder is a common cause of end-stage renal failure in adults but is rarely encountered in childhood. At least three different genetic mutations occur: PKD-1 at chromosome 16p13.3 encodes polycystin a membrane glycoprotein; PKD-2 at chromosome 4q13–23, and PKD-3 of unknown locus. In affected adults, both kidneys are enlarged and show cortical and medullary cysts that are primarily dilated tubules. The disease commonly presents in the 4th or 5th decade of life with gross or microscopic hematuria, bilateral flank pain or masses or both, and hypertension. Associated abnormalities may include hepatic cysts, which are commonly asymptomatic but can rarely be associated with congenital hepatic fibrosis, heart valve defects, and aneurysms of the cerebral circulation that may result in intracranial hemorrhage. Children with the disease may present with hematuria, flank or back pain, or unilateral or bilateral flank masses. Hypertension may develop. Prenatal diagnosis by ultrasonography or DNA testing is available. The cysts are frequently demonstrable by ultrasonography (Fig. 529–2), intravenous pyelography, or CT scan. In conjunction with the clinical manifestations and family history, radiographic studies usually confirm the diagnosis. In occult cases, especially those lacking a family history of the disease (the disease has a high spontaneous mutation rate), open renal biopsy may be necessary to confirm the diagnosis. The differential diagnosis includes renal cysts associated with tuberous sclerosis and von Hippel-Lindau disease, both autosomal dominant disorders. Treatment is supportive. End-stage renal failure frequently develops by the 6th or 7th decade but has also been reported with childhood onset.

Fick GM, Duley IT, Johnson AM, et al: The spectrum of autosomal dominant polycystic disease in children. J Am Soc Nephrol 4:1654, 1994.

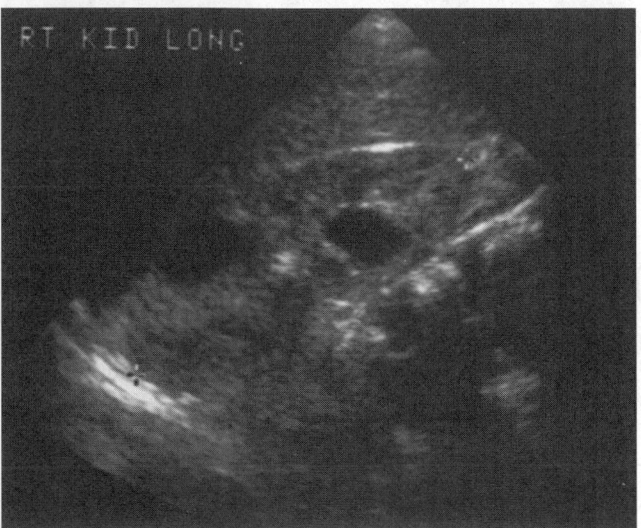

Figure 529–2 Ultrasound examination of an 18-mo-old boy with autosomal dominant polycystic kidney disease demonstrating renal enlargement (10 cm) and two large cysts.

MacDermot KD, Saggar-Malik AK, Economides DL, et al: Prenatal diagnosis of autosomal dominant polycystic kidney disease (PKD1) presenting in utero and prognosis for very early onset disease. J Med Genet 35:13, 1998.
Ong ACM, Harris PC: Molecular basis of renal cyst formation—one hit or two? Lancet 349:1039, 1997.
Perrone RD: Extrarenal manifestations of ADPKD. Kidney Int 51:2022, 1997.
Woolf AS, Winyard PJD: Unraveling the pathogenesis of cystic kidney diseases. Arch Dis Child 72:103, 1995.

529.3 Vascular Abnormalities

Hemangiomas and arteriovenous malformations of the kidneys and lower urinary tract are rare causes of hematuria. They usually present with gross hematuria and the passage of blood clots. Renal colic may develop if the upper tract is involved. The diagnosis is confirmed by angiography.

NEPHROLITHIASIS. (See Chapter 555.)
RENAL TUMORS. (See Chapter 505.)

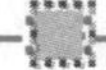

CHAPTER 530 Miscellaneous Etiologies of Hematuria

530.1 Exercise Hematuria

Gross or microscopic hematuria may follow vigorous exercise. Exercise hematuria is rare in females and can be associated with dysuria. The color of the urine may vary from red to black. Blood clots may be present in the urine. Findings on urine culture, intravenous pyelography, voiding cystourethrography, and cystoscopy are normal in most patients. This seems to be a benign condition, and the hematuria generally resolves within 48 hr after cessation of exercise. The absence of red blood cell casts or evidence of renal disease and the presence of dysuria and blood clots in some patients suggest that the source of bleeding lies in the lower urinary tract. Rhabdomyolysis with myoglobinuria or march hemoglobinuria must be considered in the differential diagnosis when associated with exercise.

Abarbanel J, Benet AE, Lask D, et al: Sports hematuria. J Urol 143:887, 1990.
Bailey RR, Dann E, Gillies AHB, et al: What the urine contains following athletic competition. N Z Med J 83:309, 1976.
Siegel AJ, Hennekens CH, Solomon HS, et al: Exercise-related hematuria. JAMA 241:391, 1979.

530.2 Drugs

Gross or microscopic hematuria has been associated with the use of various medications. Mechanisms include alterations in the coagulation system (heparin, warfarin, aspirin), tubular damage (penicillins, sulfonamides), and hemorrhagic cystitis (cyclophosphamide).

Northway JD: Hematuria in children. J Pediatr 78:381, 1971.

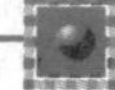

SECTION 3

Conditions Particularly Associated with Proteinuria

Jerry M. Bergstein

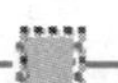

CHAPTER 531 Introduction to the Child with Proteinuria

Protein may be found in the urine of healthy children. A reasonable upper limit of normal protein excretion in healthy children is 150 mg/24 hr (0.15 g/24 hr). Approximately half of this protein derives from the plasma, albumin representing the largest fraction (< 30 mg/24 hr; 0.03 g/24 hr). The remainder of normal urinary protein is Tamm-Horsfall protein, a mucoprotein of unknown function produced in the distal tubule.

Proteinuria is commonly detected by the *dipstick test* and is reported as negative, trace, 1+ (closest to 30 mg/dL), 2+ (closest to 100 mg/dL), 3+ (closest to 300 mg/dL), and 4+ (> 2,000 mg/dL). Dipsticks detect primarily albuminuria and are less sensitive for (and may miss) other forms of proteinuria (e.g., low molecular weight proteins, Bence Jones protein, gamma globulins). The depth of color of the dipstick reaction increases in a semi-quantitative manner with increasing urinary protein concentrations. Owing to their high sensitivity, dipsticks may detect amounts of protein in the urine that are within normal limits. Because the dipstick reaction cannot accurately measure protein excretion, persistent proteinuria should be quantitated by a more precise method (sulfosalicylic acid) in a timed (preferably 24 hr) urine collection. False-positive test results may be found with both the dipstick test (highly concentrated urine, gross hematuria, contamination with chlorhexidine or benzalkonium, pH > 8.0, phenazopyridine therapy) and the sulfosalicylic acid method (radiographic contrast media, penicillin or cephalosporin therapy, tolbutamide, sulfonamides).

In a semi-quantitative fashion, urinary protein excretion can be estimated by measuring the ratio of urinary protein to creatinine concentrations in a random specimen. Urinary creatinine excretion is constant in patients with relatively normal renal function, as is urinary protein excretion in most disease states. Determination of the ratio is especially helpful in quantitating proteinuria when a timed urine collection is not practicable. Ratios (mg/mg) below 0.5 in children younger than 2 yr and less than 0.2 in older children suggest normal protein excretion. A ratio greater than 3 suggests nephrotic-range proteinuria.

Abitbol C, Zilleruelo G, Freundlich M, et al: Quantitation of proteinuria with urinary protein/creatinine ratios and random testing with dipsticks in nephrotic syndrome. J Pediatr 116:243, 1990.

CHAPTER 532

Nonpathologic Proteinuria

Proteinuria in excess of 150 mg/24 hr (0.15 g/24 hr) may be divided into two categories (Table 532–1). In the first category, nonpathologic proteinuria, the excessive protein excretion is apparently not a result of a disease state. The level of proteinuria in this category is generally less than 1,000 mg/24 hr (1.00 g/24 hr) and is never associated with edema.

532.1 Postural (Orthostatic) Proteinuria

Children with this disorder excrete normal or slightly increased amounts of protein in the supine position. In the upright position, the amount of protein in the urine may increase 10-fold or more. The proteinuria is usually discovered at routine urinalysis; its cause is unknown. Hematuria is absent, and the creatinine clearance and C3 complement level are normal. Results of renal biopsy (not part of the evaluation) are normal or show mild nonspecific alterations.

In a child having asymptomatic low-grade proteinuria, a study for postural proteinuria should be performed. At bedtime, the child goes to bed without voiding. After 30 min supine, the child voids in this position. This urine is discarded, but the time of voiding is recorded as the beginning of the supine collection. The child is then given a large glass of liquid and allowed to sleep. In the morning, the child again voids supine before rising; this ends the supine collection and begins the upright collection, which is terminated at bedtime. The child may have normal daily activities, avoiding the supine position. Protein excretion is measured in the two urine collections, and for each collection the result is calculated as milligrams of protein excreted per minute. A finding of essentially normal protein excretion in the supine collection and increased protein excretion in the upright collection establishes the proteinuria as orthostatic.

Studies of adults suggest that postural proteinuria is a benign process, but similar data are not available for children. Accordingly, long-term follow-up of children is necessary (unless the proteinuria resolves) in order to monitor patients for evidence of renal disease (hematuria, hypertension, diminished renal function, or proteinuria exceeding 1 g/24 hr).

Devarajan P: Mechanisms of orthostatic proteinuria: Lessons from a transplant donor. J Am Soc Nephrol 4:36, 1993.
Springberg PD, Garrett LE Jr, Thompson AL, et al: Fixed and reproducible orthostatic proteinuria: Results of a 20-year follow-up study. Ann Intern Med 97:516, 1982.

532.2 Febrile Proteinuria

Transient proteinuria may be found in patients having fever in excess of 38.3°C (101°F). The mechanism of proteinuria associated with fever is unknown. The proteinuria does not exceed +2 on the dipstick and may be considered benign if it resolves when the fever abates. (See Chapter 170.)

Jensen H, Henriksen K: Proteinuria in non-renal infectious disease. Acta Med Scand 196:75, 1974.
Marks MI, McLaine PN, Drummond KN: Proteinuria in children with febrile illnesses. Arch Dis Child 45:250, 1970.

532.3 Exercise Proteinuria

Proteinuria, like hematuria, may follow vigorous exercise. The level rarely exceeds +2 on the dipstick. The disorder can be considered benign if the proteinuria resolves after 48 hr of rest. See Chapter 690.

Campanacci L, Faccini L, Englaro E, et al: Exercise-induced proteinuria. Contrib Nephrol 26:31, 1981.
Poortmans JR: Postexercise proteinuria in humans. JAMA 253:236, 1985.

TABLE 532–1 Classification of Proteinuria

Nonpathologic Proteinuria
- Postural (orthostatic)
- Febrile
- Exercise

Pathologic Proteinuria
- Tubular
  - *Hereditary*
    - Cystinosis
    - Wilson disease
    - Lowe syndrome
    - Proximal renal tubular acidosis
    - Galactosemia
  - *Acquired*
    - Antibiotics
    - Interstitial nephritis
    - Acute tubular necrosis
    - Cystic diseases
    - Heavy metal poisoning (mercury, gold, lead, bismuth, cadmium, chromium, copper)
- Glomerular
  - Persistent asymptomatic
  - Nephrotic syndrome
    - Idiopathic nephrotic syndrome
      - Minimal change
      - Mesangial proliferation
      - Focal sclerosis
    - Glomerulonephritis
    - Tumors
    - Drugs
    - Congenital

CHAPTER 533

Pathologic Proteinuria

The second category of proteinuria may result from glomerular or tubular disorders.

533.1 Tubular Proteinuria

Healthy individuals filter large amounts of proteins of lower molecular weight than albumin (lysozyme, light chains of immunoglobulin, β_2-microglobulin, insulin, growth hormone); these are normally reabsorbed in the proximal tubule. Injury to the proximal tubules results in diminished reabsorptive capacity and the loss of these low molecular weight proteins in the urine; such proteinuria rarely exceeds 1 g/24 hr; it is not associated with edema. Tubular proteinuria (see Table 532–1) may be seen in acquired and inherited disorders and may be associated with other defects of proximal tubular function, such as glucosuria, phosphaturia, bicarbonate wasting, and aminoaciduria. Tubular proteinuria rarely presents a diagnostic dilemma because the underlying disease is usually detected before the proteinuria. Asymptomatic patients having persistent proteinuria generally have glomerular rather than tubular proteinuria. In occult cases, glomerular and tubular proteinuria can be distinguished by electrophoresis of the urine. In tubular proteinuria, the low molecular weight proteins migrate primarily in the α and β regions and little or no albumin is detected, whereas in glomerular proteinuria the major protein is albumin.

Alt JM, Von der Heyde D, Assel E, et al: Characteristics of protein excretion in glomerular and tubular disease. Contrib Nephrol 24:115, 1981.
Waller KV, Ward KM, Mahan JD, et al: Current concepts in proteinuria. Clin Chem 35:755, 1989.

533.2 Glomerular Proteinuria

The most common cause of proteinuria is increased permeability of the glomerular capillary wall. The amount of glomerular proteinuria may range from less than 1 to more than 30 g/24 hr. Glomerular proteinuria may be termed selective (loss of plasma proteins of molecular weight up to and including albumin) or nonselective (loss of albumin and of larger molecular weight proteins such as IgG). Most forms of glomerulonephritis are accompanied by nonselective proteinuria. *Selective proteinuria* occurs primarily in minimal-change nephrosis; the finding of selective proteinuria in that disease increases the likelihood of corticosteroid responsiveness. The determination of urinary protein selectivity is generally of little clinical value, owing to considerable overlap of selectivities among various forms of renal disease.

CHAPTER 534
Persistent Asymptomatic Proteinuria

Persistent asymptomatic proteinuria is defined as proteinuria in an apparently healthy child that occurs without hematuria and persists for 3 mo. The prevalence in school-age children may be as high as 6%. The amount of proteinuria is usually less than 2 g/24 hr; it is never associated with edema. Causes include postural proteinuria, membranous and membranoproliferative glomerulonephritis, pyelonephritis, hereditary nephritis, developmental anomalies, and "benign" proteinuria.

Evaluation of a child having persistent asymptomatic proteinuria should include renal ultrasonography, a urine culture, and measurement of creatinine clearance, 24-hr protein excretion, serum albumin level, and C3 complement level. In patients with low-grade proteinuria (150–1,000 mg/24 hr) in whom other findings are normal, renal biopsy may not be indicated because evidence of a progressive disease is rarely found. Such patients should have an annual re-evaluation consisting of a physical examination and blood pressure determination, urinalysis, and measurement of creatinine clearance and 24-hr protein excretion. Indications for renal biopsy include persistent asymptomatic proteinuria in excess of 1,000 mg/24 or the development of hematuria, hypertension, or diminished renal function.

Dodge WF, West EF, Smith EH, et al: Proteinuria and hematuria in school-age children: Epidemiology and early natural history. J Pediatr 88:327, 1976.
Vehaskari VM, Rapola J: Isolated proteinuria: Analysis of a school-age population. J Pediatr 101:661, 1982.
Yoshikawa N, Kitagawa K, Ohta K, et al: Asymptomatic constant isolated proteinuria in children. J Pediatr 119:375, 1991.

CHAPTER 535
Nephrotic Syndrome

(Nephrosis)

The nephrotic syndrome is characterized by proteinuria, hypoproteinemia, edema, and hyperlipidemia.

ETIOLOGY. Most (90%) children with nephrosis have some form of the idiopathic nephrotic syndrome; minimal-change disease is found in approximately 85%, mesangial proliferation in 5%, and focal sclerosis in 10%. In the remaining 10% of children with nephrosis, the nephrotic syndrome is largely mediated by some form of glomerulonephritis, membranous and membranoproliferative being most common (Table 535–1).

PATHOPHYSIOLOGY. The underlying pathogenetic abnormality in nephrosis is proteinuria, which results from an increase in glomerular capillary wall permeability. The mechanism of this increase in permeability is unknown but may be related, at least in part, to loss of negatively charged glycoproteins within the capillary wall. Focal segmental glomerulosclerosis is characterized by a plasma factor, perhaps produced by lymphocytes, which increases glomerular permeability to proteins. In the nephrotic state, the protein loss generally exceeds 2 g/24 hr and is composed primarily of albumin; the hypoproteinemia is fundamentally a "hypoalbuminemia." In general, edema appears when the serum albumin level falls below 2.5 g/dL (25 g/L).

The mechanism of edema formation in nephrosis is incompletely understood. It seems likely that the edema is initiated by the development of hypoalbuminemia, the result of urinary protein loss. The hypoalbuminemia leads to a decrease in the plasma oncotic pressure, which permits transudation of fluid from the intravascular compartment to the interstitial space. The reduction in intravascular volume decreases renal perfusion pressure, activating the renin-angiotensin-aldosterone system, which stimulates distal tubular reabsorption of sodium. The reduced intravascular volume also stimulates the release of antidiuretic hormone, which enhances the reabsorption of water in the collecting duct. Because of the decreased plasma oncotic pressure, the reabsorbed sodium and water are lost into the interstitial space, exacerbating the edema. That other factors may also have a role in the formation of the edema is indicated by the observations that some patients with nephrotic syndrome have normal or increased intravascular volume and normal to diminished plasma levels of renin and aldosterone. Hypothetical explanations include an intrarenal defect in sodium and water excretion or the presence of a circulating agent that increases capillary wall permeability throughout the body, as well as in the kidneys.

In the nephrotic state, almost all serum lipid (cholesterol, triglycerides) and lipoprotein levels are elevated. Two factors offer at least partial explanation: (1) the hypoproteinemia stimulates generalized protein synthesis in the liver, including the lipoproteins; and (2) lipid catabolism is diminished, owing to reduced plasma levels of lipoprotein lipase, the major enzyme system that removes lipids from the plasma. Whether lipoprotein lipase is lost in the urine is unclear. Lipid abnormalities may contribute to abnormal renal hemodynamics.

TABLE 535–1 Summary of Primary Renal Diseases That Present As Idiopathic Nephrotic Syndrome

	Minimal-Change Nephrotic Syndrome (MCNS)	Focal Segmental Sclerosis	Membranous Nephropathy	Membranoproliferative Glomerulonephritis (MPGN)	
				Type I	*Type II*
Frequency*					
Children	75%	10%	<5%	10%	10%
Adults	15%	15%	50%	10%	10%
Clinical Manifestations					
Age (yr)	2–6, some adults	2–10, some adults	40–50	5–15	5–15
Sex	2:1 male	1.3:1 male	2:1 male	Male-female	Male-female
Nephrotic syndrome	100%	90%	80%	60%	60%
Asymptomatic proteinuria	0	10%	20%	40%	40%
Hematuria	10–20%	60%–80%	60%	80%	80%
Hypertension	10%	20% early	Infrequent	35%	35%
Rate of progression to renal failure	Does not progress	10 years	50% in 10–20 yr	10–20 yr	5–15 yr
Associated conditions	Allergy? Hodgkin's disease, usually none	None	Renal vein thrombosis, cancer, SLE, hepatitis B	None	Partial lipodystrophy
Laboratory Findings	Manifestations of nephrotic syndrome ↑ BUN in 15–30%	Manifestations of nephrotic syndrome ↑ BUN in 20–40%	Manifestations of nephrotic syndrome	Low C1, C4, C3–C9	Normal C1, C4, low C3–C9
Immunogenetics	HLA-B8, B12 (3.5)†	Not established	HLA-DRW3 (12–32)†	Not established	C3 nephritic factor Not established
Renal Pathology					
Light microscopy	Normal	Focal sclerotic lesions	Thickened GBM, spikes	Thickened GBM, proliferation	Lobulation
Immunofluorescence	Negative	IgM, C3 in lesions	Fine granular IgG, C3	Granular IgG, C3	C3 only
Electron microscopy	Foot process fusion	Foot process fusion	Subepithelial deposits	Mesangial and subendothelial deposits	Dense deposits
Response to Steroids	90%	15–20%	May be slow progression	Not established	Not established

**Approximate frequency as a cause of idiopathic nephrotic syndrome. About 10% of adult nephrotic syndrome is due to various diseases that usually present with acute glomerulonephritis.*

†Relative risk.

BUN = blood urea nitrogen; C = complement; GBM = glomerular basement membrane; HLA = human leukocyte antigen; Ig = immunoglobulin; SLE = systemic lupus erythematosus; hepatitis B = hepatitis B virus; ↑ = elevated.

Modified from Couser WG: Glomerular disorders. In: *Wyngaarden JB, Smith LH, Bennett JC (eds.). Cecil Textbook of Medicine, 19th ed. Philadelphia, WB Saunders, 1992, p 560.*

Abrass C: Clinical spectrum and complications of the nephrotic syndrome. J Clin Invest Med 45:143, 1997.

Fuiano G, Esposito C, Sepe V, et al: Effects of hypercholesterolemia on renal hemodynamics: Study in patients with nephrotic syndrome. Nephron 73:430, 1996.

Orth S, Ritz E: The nephrotic syndrome. N Engl J Med 338:1202, 1998.

Palmer BF, Alpern RJ: Pathogenesis of edema formation in the nephrotic syndrome. Kidney Int 51(Suppl 59):S-21, 1997.

535.1 Idiopathic Nephrotic Syndrome

This syndrome accounts for approximately 90% of nephrosis in childhood. Occasional reports that one of the three histologic types has been transformed into another type suggest that this syndrome may be a single disorder with various histologic features. It seems more likely that the syndrome represents several diseases having similar clinical manifestations. Nephrotic syndrome has been reported in certain families with a frequency that appears to be increased over that expected, but it does not appear to be inherited.

ETIOLOGY. The cause remains unknown. Early success in controlling nephrosis with "immunosuppressive" drugs suggested that the disease was mediated by immunologic mechanisms, but evidence for classic mechanisms of immunologic injury has been lacking, and it now seems clear that immunosuppressive drugs have many effects other than suppression of antibody formation. A few patients have evidence supporting IgE mediation of the disease, but increasing evidence suggests that the syndrome may result from an abnormality in thymus-derived (T-cell) lymphocyte function, perhaps through the production of a factor that increases vascular permeability.

PATHOLOGY. Idiopathic nephrotic syndrome occurs in three morphologic patterns. In *minimal-change disease* (85%), the glomeruli appear normal or show a minimal increase in mesangial cells and matrix. Findings on immunofluorescent microscopic studies are typically nondiagnostic. Electron microscopy reveals retraction of the epithelial cell foot processes. More than 95% of children with minimal-change disease respond to corticosteroid therapy.

The *mesangial proliferative group* (5%) is characterized by a diffuse increase in mesangial cells and matrix. The frequency of mesangial deposits containing IgM and C3 by immunofluorescence is not different from that observed in minimal-change disease. Approximately 50–60% of patients with this histologic lesion respond to corticosteroid therapy.

In biopsy specimens from patients having the *focal sclerosis lesion* (10%), the majority of glomeruli appear normal or show mesangial proliferation. Others, especially those close to the medulla (juxtamedullary), show segmental scarring in one or more lobules (Fig. 535–1). A similar lesion may be seen with HIV infection, vesicoureteral reflux, and intravenous heroin abuse. The disease is frequently progressive, ultimately involving all glomeruli, and leads to end-stage renal failure in most patients. Approximately 20% of such patients respond to prednisone or cytotoxic therapy or both. The disease may recur in a transplanted kidney.

CLINICAL MANIFESTATIONS. The idiopathic nephrotic syndrome is more common in boys than in girls (2:1) and most commonly appears between the ages of 2 and 6 yr. It has been reported as early as the last half of the 1st yr of life and in adults. The initial episode and subsequent relapses may follow an apparent viral upper respiratory tract infection. The disease

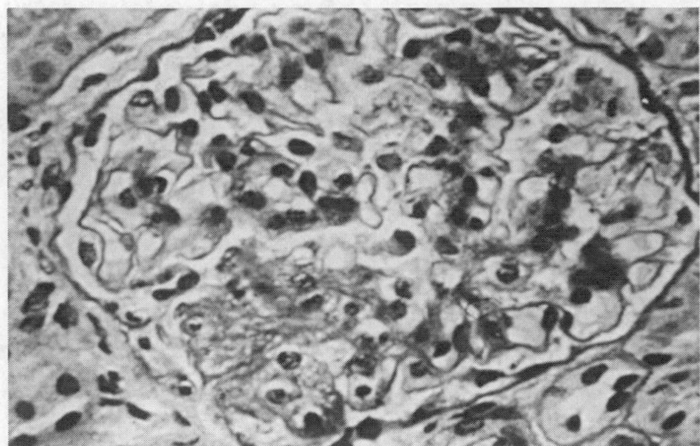

Figure 535–1 Glomerulus from a patient having corticosteroid-resistant nephrotic syndrome, showing mesangial hypercellularity and an area of sclerosis in the lower portion. (×250.)

usually presents as edema, which is initially noted around the eyes and in the lower extremities, where it is "pitting" in nature. With time, the edema becomes generalized and may be associated with weight gain, the development of ascites or pleural effusions, and declining urine output. The edema accumulates in dependent sites and appears to shift from the face and back to the abdomen, perineum, and legs as the day progresses. Anorexia, abdominal pain, and diarrhea are common; hypertension is uncommon.

DIAGNOSIS. Urinalysis reveals +3 or +4 proteinuria; microscopic hematuria may be present, but gross hematuria is rare. Renal function may be normal or reduced. The low creatinine clearance is due to diminished renal perfusion resulting from contraction of the intravascular volume, and it returns to normal when intravascular volume is restored. Protein excretion exceeds 2 g/24 hr. The serum cholesterol and triglyceride levels are elevated, the serum albumin level is generally less than 2 g/dL, and the total serum calcium level is diminished, owing to a reduction in the albumin-bound fraction. The complement C3 level is normal.

Children with onset of nephrotic syndrome between the ages of 1 and 8 yr are likely to have steroid-responsive minimal-change disease; corticosteroid therapy should be initiated without renal biopsy. Minimal-change disease remains common in children who are older than 8 yr and who present with nephrosis, but membranous and membranoproliferative glomerulonephritis become increasingly common; renal biopsy is recommended by some to establish a firm diagnosis before considering therapy.

COMPLICATIONS. Infection is the major complication of nephrosis; it results from increased susceptibility to bacterial infections during relapse. Proposed explanations include decreased immunoglobulin levels, the edema fluid acting as a culture medium, protein deficiency, decreased bactericidal activity of the leukocytes, immunosuppressive therapy, decreased perfusion of the spleen due to hypovolemia, and loss in the urine of a complement factor (properdin factor B) that opsonizes certain bacteria. For reasons that are unclear, **spontaneous peritonitis** is the most frequent type of infection; sepsis, pneumonia, cellulitis, and urinary tract infections may also be noted. Streptococcus pneumoniae is the most common organism causing peritonitis; gram-negative bacteria are also encountered. Fever and physical findings may be minimal in the presence of corticosteroid therapy. Accordingly, a high index of suspicion, prompt evaluation (including cultures of blood and peritoneal fluid), and early initiation of therapy that is effective against both gram-positive and gram-negative organisms are critical to prevention of life-threatening illness. When in remission, all patients having nephrosis should receive polyvalent pneumococcal vaccine.

Additional complications may include an increased tendency to develop arterial and venous thrombosis (owing at least in part to elevated plasma levels of certain coagulation factors and inhibitors of fibrinolysis, decreased plasma level of antithrombin III, and increased platelet aggregation); deficiencies of coagulation factors IX, XI, and XII; and reduced serum levels of vitamin D.

TREATMENT. Children with the first episode of nephrosis may be hospitalized or managed as outpatients for diagnostic, educational, and therapeutic purposes. When edema develops, sodium intake is reduced by the initiation of a "no added salt diet." The family is advised to cook without salt, to hide the salt shaker, and to avoid serving obviously salty foods. Salt restriction is terminated when the edema resolves. Unless the edema is severe, fluid intake is not restricted but need not be encouraged. Affected children may attend school and participate in physical activities as tolerated. Until corticosteroid-induced diuresis begins, mild to moderate edema can be managed at home with chlorothiazide, 10–40 mg/kg/24 hr, in two divided doses. If hypokalemia develops, an oral potassium chloride supplement or spironolactone (3–5 mg/kg/24 hr divided into four doses) may be added.

If the edema becomes severe, resulting in respiratory distress from massive pleural effusions and ascites or in severe scrotal edema, the child should be hospitalized. Sodium restriction should be continued, but further reduction in intake is rarely effective in controlling edema. A swollen scrotum is elevated with pillows to enhance the removal of fluid by gravity. Diuresis may be initiated by oral administration of furosemide (1–2 mg/kg every 4 hr) in conjunction with metolazone (0.2–0.4 mg/kg/24 hr in two divided doses); metolazone may act in both the proximal and distal tubules. When this potent combination is used, electrolyte levels and renal function must be closely monitored. For patients resistant to oral diuretics, intravenous agents may be effective. After a loading dose of 1 mg/kg, furosemide should be given as a constant infusion at the rate of 1 mg/kg/hr in conjunction with chlorothiazide (10 mg/kg every 12 hr). In some instances of severe edema, intravenous administration of 25% human albumin (1 g/kg/24 hr) may be necessary, but the effect is usually transient and volume overload with hypertension and heart failure must be avoided.

After the diagnosis is confirmed by the appropriate laboratory studies, the pathophysiology and treatment of nephrosis are reviewed with the family to enhance their understanding of their child's disease. Remission is then induced by administration of prednisone at a dosage of 60 mg/m²/24 hr (maximum daily dose 60 mg), divided into three or four doses over the day. Divided-dose rather than single-dose therapy is used because some patients who fail to respond to a single daily dose respond to divided doses. The time needed for response to prednisone averages about 2 wk, the response being defined as the point at which urine becomes free of protein. If a child continues to have proteinuria (2+ or greater) after 1 mo of continuous daily divided-dose prednisone, the nephrosis is termed steroid resistant and renal biopsy is indicated to determine the precise cause of the disease.

Five days after the urine becomes protein free (negative, trace, or 1+ on the dipstick), the scheduling of prednisone is changed to 60 mg/m² (maximum dose of 60 mg) taken every other day as a single dose with breakfast. This alternate-day regimen is continued for 3–6 mo. The purpose of alternate-day therapy is to maintain the remission using a relatively nontoxic dose of prednisone, thus avoiding frequent relapses of the disease and the cumulative toxicity of frequent courses of daily administration of corticosteroids. After such a period of alternate-day therapy, prednisone may be discontinued abruptly. Adequate experience indicates sufficient recovery of pituitary-adrenal axis function that patients are not at risk for adrenal insufficiency after abrupt withdrawal of alternate-day prednisone. On the other hand, for up to 1 yr after completing corticosteroid therapy, a child will require stress-related corticosteroid supplementation for severe illness or surgery.

Each relapse of nephrosis is treated in a similar manner. A relapse is defined as the recurrence of edema and not simply of proteinuria, as many children with this condition have intermittent proteinuria that resolves spontaneously. A small number of patients who respond to daily divided-dose therapy have relapses shortly after switching to or after terminating alternate-day therapy. Such patients are termed steroid dependent.

If repeated relapses occur and especially if a child suffers severe corticosteroid toxicity (cushingoid appearance, hypertension, growth failure), then cyclophosphamide therapy should be considered. Cyclophosphamide has been shown to prolong the duration of remission and to prevent relapses in children with frequently relapsing nephrotic syndrome. The potential side effects of the drug (leukopenia, disseminated varicella infection, hemorrhagic cystitis, alopecia, sterility) should be reviewed with the family. The dose of cyclophosphamide is 3 mg/kg/24 hr as a single dose, for a total duration of 12 wk. Alternate-day prednisone therapy is often continued during the course of cyclophosphamide administration. During cyclophosphamide therapy, the white blood count must be monitored weekly and the drug withheld if the count falls below 5,000/mm^3. Steroid-resistant patients may respond to an extended course (3–6 mo) of cyclophosphamide, high-dose pulse methylprednisolone, or cyclosporine.

Renal transplantation is indicated for end-stage renal failure due to steroid-resistant focal and segmental glomerulosclerosis (see Chapter 544). Recurrent nephrotic syndromes develop in 15–55% of transplant recipients. Plasma protein absorption onto protein A–based columns may reduce proteinuria in these patients. Protein absorption removes a fraction (<100,000 MW), which enhances renal protein permeability.

PROGNOSIS. Most children with steroid-responsive nephrosis have repeated relapses until the disease resolves spontaneously toward the end of the 2nd decade of life. It is important to indicate to the family that the child will have no residual renal dysfunction, that the disease is generally not hereditary, and that the child (in the absence of cyclophosphamide or chlorambucil therapy) will remain fertile. To minimize the psychologic effects of the nephrosis, it should be emphasized that when in remission the child is normal and may have unrestricted diet and activity. While a child is in remission, it is generally unnecessary to test the urine for protein.

Arbeitsgemeinschaft für Pädiatrische Nephrologie: Cyclophosphamide treatment of steroid dependent nephrotic syndrome: Comparison of eight week with 12 week course. Arch Dis Child 62:1102, 1987.
Berns JS, Gaudio KM, Krassner LS, et al: Steroid-responsive nephrotic syndrome of childhood: A long-term study of clinical course, histopathology, efficacy of cyclophosphamide therapy and effects on growth. Am J Kidney Dis 9:108, 1987.
Cameron JS: The enigma of focal segmental glomerulosclerosis. Kidney Int 50(Suppl 57):S-119, 1996.
Freundlich M, Bourgoignie JJ, Zilleruelo G, et al: Calcium and vitamin D metabolism in children with nephrotic syndrome. J Pediatr 108:383, 1986.
Gorensek MJ, Lebel MH, Nelson JD: Peritonitis in children with nephrotic syndrome. Pediatrics 81:849, 1988.
Ichikawa I, Fogo A: Focal segmental sclerosis. Pediatr Nephrol 10:374, 1996.
Kaysen G: Nonrenal complications of the nephrotic syndrome. Annu Rev Med 45:201, 1994.
Krensky AM, Ingelfinger JR, Grupe WE: Peritonitis in childhood nephrotic syndrome. Am J Dis Child 136:732, 1982.
Llach F: Hypercoagulability, renal vein thrombosis, and other thrombotic complications of nephrotic syndrome. Kidney Int 28:429, 1985.
Niaudet P, Fuchshuber A, Gagnadoux MF, et al: Cyclosporine in the therapy of steroid-resistant idiopathic nephrotic syndrome. Kidney Int 51(Suppl 58):S-85, 1997.
Savin VJ, Sharma R, Sharma M, et al: Circulating factor associated with increased glomerular permeability to albumin in recurrent focal segmental glomerulosclerosis. N Engl J Med 14:878, 1996.
Tune BM, Mendoza SA: Treatment of idiopathic nephrotic syndrome: Regimens and outcomes in children and adults. J Am Soc Nephrol 8:824, 1997.

535.2 Glomerulonephritis

Nephrotic syndrome may develop during the course of any type of glomerulonephritis but is most common in association with membranous, membranoproliferative, poststreptococcal, lupus, chronic infection (including malaria and schistosomiasis), and Henoch-Schönlein purpura glomerulonephritis. Although the development of a secondary nephrotic syndrome may indicate severe glomerular disease, the nephrotic syndrome frequently resolves if the nephritis improves.

Barsoum RS: Schistosomal glomerulopathies. Kidney Int 44:1, 1993.
Hendrickse RG, Adeniyi A: Quartan malarial nephrotic syndrome in children. Kidney Int 16:64, 1979.
Sitprija V: Nephropathy in falciparum malaria. Kidney Int 34:867, 1988.

535.3 Tumors

See also Chapters 502, 503, and 512.

Nephrotic syndrome has been associated with several extrarenal neoplasms. In patients having solid tumors, such as carcinomas, the glomerular changes resemble membranous glomerulopathy. The renal involvement is presumably mediated by immune complexes composed of tumor antigens and tumor-specific antibodies. In lymphomas (especially Hodgkin's disease), minimal-change disease is most commonly found; proliferative lesions have also been described. In patients having the minimal-change lesion, the nephrosis may develop before or after the malignancy is detected, may resolve as the tumor regresses, and may return if the tumor recurs. The mechanism of the nephrosis is unknown; it has been proposed that the tumor produces a lymphokine that increases glomerular capillary wall permeability.

Alpers CE, Cotran RS: Neoplasia and glomerular injury. Kidney Int 30:465, 1986.
Dabbs DJ, Striker L, Mignon F, et al: Glomerular lesions in lymphomas and leukemias. Am J Med 80:63, 1986.

535.4 Drugs

Nephrotic syndrome has developed during therapy with several types of drugs and chemicals. The histologic picture may resemble membranous glomerulopathy (penicillamine, captopril, gold, nonsteroidal anti-inflammatory drugs, mercury compounds), minimal-change disease (probenecid, ethosuximide, methimazole, lithium), or proliferative glomerulonephritis (procainamide, chlorpropamide, phenytoin, trimethadione, paramethadione).

Radford MG Jr., Holley KE, Grande JP, et al: Reversible membranous nephropathy associated with the use of nonsteroidal anti-inflammatory drugs. JAMA 276:466, 1996.

535.5 Congenital Nephrotic Syndrome

Nephrotic syndrome is rare during the 1st yr of life. Causes of nephrosis developing during the first 6 mo of life include congenital nephrotic syndrome, congenital infection (syphilis, toxoplasmosis, cytomegalovirus), and diffuse mesangial sclerosis of unknown cause (**Drash syndrome**, consisting of nephropathy, Wilms tumor, and genital abnormalities). Nephrosis developing during the last half of the 1st yr is most commonly associated with the idiopathic nephrotic syndrome or drugs. Owing to the diversity of causes of the development of nephrotic syndrome during the 1st year of life, all such patients should have a kidney biopsy to determine the precise cause and severity of the disease.

The *congenital nephrotic syndrome* (Finnish type) is an autosomal recessive disorder that is most common in populations of Scandinavian descent. The gene has been localized to the long arm of chromosome 19. The major pathologic feature in some patients is dilatation of the proximal convoluted tubules (microcystic disease), but this is variable, even within the same kindred. The glomeruli show mesangial proliferation and sclerosis. The pathogenesis of the syndrome is unknown; a reduction in the number of heparan sulfate–rich anionic sites has been demonstrated in the glomerular basement membrane. Although proteinuria is present at birth, the nephrotic syndrome becomes apparent within the first 3 mo of life. Additional clinical features include prematurity, an enlarged placenta, respiratory distress, and separation of the cranial sutures. The clinical course is one of persistent edema and recurrent infections. Death due to infection or renal failure is likely by the age of 5 yr. Corticosteroid and immunosuppressive agents are of no value. Captopril and indomethacin or unilateral nephrectomy may diminish proteinuria and ameliorate the nephrotic state. Otherwise, treatment is supportive, with the ultimate goal of kidney transplantation. In families at risk, antenatal diagnosis is possible by measuring α-fetoprotein level of the amniotic fluid at 16–20 wk of gestation and by chorionic villus haplotype analysis during the first trimester.

Habib R: Nephrotic syndrome in the first year of life. Pediatr Nephrol 7:347, 1993.

Holmberg C, Antikainen M, Ronnholm K, et al: Management of congenital nephrotic syndrome of the Finnish type. Pediatr Nephrol 9:87, 1995.

Jadresic L, Leake J, Gordon I, et al: Clinicopathologic review of twelve children with nephropathy, Wilms tumor, and genital abnormalities (Drash syndrome). J Pediatr 117:717, 1990.

Mannikko M, Kestila M, Lenkkeri U, et al: Improved prenatal diagnosis of the congenital nephrotic syndrome of the Finnish type based on DNA analysis. Kidney Int 51:868, 1997.

Mattoo TK, Al-Sowailem AM, Al-Harbi MS, et al: Nephrotic syndrome in the first year of life and the role of unilateral nephrectomy. Pediatr Nephrol 6:16, 1992.

Pomeranz A, Wolach B, Bernheim J, et al: Successful treatment of Finnish congenital nephrotic syndrome with captopril and indomethacin. J Pediatr 126:140, 1995.

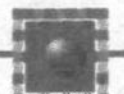

SECTION 4

Tubular Disorders

CHAPTER 536
Tubular Function

Jerry M. Bergstein

Except for reduced protein levels, the ultrafiltrate of blood that enters the proximal tubule is similar to plasma. Body homeostasis is maintained by tubular reabsorption of salts and water.

SODIUM. After the 1st year of life, the tubules have the reabsorptive capacity to lower the urinary sodium concentration to 1 mEq/L (1 mmol/L). Approximately 65% of filtered sodium is isotonically reabsorbed in the proximal tubule. Glucose and amino acids are also reabsorbed in the proximal tubule in conjunction with sodium transport. An additional 25% of filtered sodium is reabsorbed from the ascending limb of the loop of Henle in association with the active transport of chloride. The remainder of sodium reabsorption is accomplished in the distal tubule and collecting duct, mediated in part by aldosterone. Sodium excretion is closely related to the extracellular fluid (ECF) volume and may be modified by factors that regulate the ECF volume.

POTASSIUM. Essentially all of the filtered potassium is reabsorbed, primarily in the proximal tubules. The potassium excreted is derived from distal tubular and collecting duct potassium secretion, as modified by the pH of the ECF, by aldosterone, and by the urinary flow rate and sodium concentration.

CALCIUM. Approximately 98% of filtered calcium is reabsorbed by the tubules. Proximal tubular reabsorption (65% of the filtered load) is linked to sodium reabsorption. Calcium reabsorption is enhanced by parathyroid hormone, thiazide diuretics, and reduction of the ECF volume. Calcium excretion is increased by saline infusion and furosemide.

PHOSPHATE. The majority of the filtered phosphate is reabsorbed in the proximal tubule. Reabsorption is inhibited by parathyroid hormone.

MAGNESIUM. About 25% of filtered magnesium is reabsorbed in the proximal tubule; the major site of magnesium reabsorption and the principal moderator of magnesium excretion is the thick ascending limb of the loop of Henle.

ACIDIFICATION AND CONCENTRATING MECHANISMS. These are discussed in the sections on renal tubular acidosis and nephrogenic diabetes insipidus (Chapters 537 and 538)

MATURATION OF TUBULAR FUNCTION. At birth and for several months thereafter, tubular functional capabilities are at less than adult levels. Tubular function is adequate for healthy infants, but limitations may contribute to fluid and electrolyte abnormalities in sick infants.

Maximal urinary concentrating capacity in a healthy full-term newborn is 600–700 mOsm/kg (mmol/kg) H_2O. This reduction in concentrating capacity in comparison with older children and adults (who can concentrate to more than 1,000 mOsm/kg [mmol/kg] H_2O) is related to reduced glomerular filtration rate (GFR), to tubular cell immaturity, to reduced nephron length, to reduced medullary solute gradient due to increased medullary blood flow and low urea production, and to diminished tubular responsiveness to antidiuretic hormone. Although the ability of newborn infants to dilute the urine is comparable to that of adults, their capacity to excrete a water load is diminished, owing to the reduced GFR. The capacity of neonates to excrete sodium, potassium, hydrogen ion, and phosphate is also limited, owing in part to the low GFR or immaturity of tubular function.

Hogg RJ, Stapleton FB: Renal tubular function. In: Holliday MA, Barratt TM, Vernier RL (eds): Pediatric Nephrology. Baltimore, Williams & Wilkins, 1987, p 59.

CHAPTER 537
Renal Tubular Acidosis

Jerry M. Bergstein

Renal tubular acidosis (RTA) is a clinical state of systemic hyperchloremic acidosis resulting from impaired urinary acidification. Three types exist: distal RTA (type I), proximal RTA (type II), and mineralocorticoid deficiency (type IV). A proposed type III has been found to be a variant of type I. All types are associated with a normal anion gap.

NORMAL URINARY ACIDIFICATION. After the first few months of life, approximately 85% of the filtered bicarbonate is reabsorbed in the proximal tubules, but in premature infants and neonates such reabsorption of bicarbonate is transiently reduced, and bicarbonate wasting results when the serum bicarbonate level exceeds 20–22 mEq/L (mmol/L). Proximal tubular reabsorption of bicarbonate involves the secretion of hydrogen ion into the tubular lumen in exchange for sodium (Chapter 52). The hydrogen ion combines with filtered bicarbonate to form carbonic acid, which, under the influence of carbonic anhydrase, dissociates into carbon dioxide and water. The carbon dioxide diffuses into the proximal tubular cells, where, under the influence of carbonic anhydrase, it is reconverted to carbonic acid. The carbonic acid dissociates to yield a hydrogen ion that is again secreted to absorb additional bicarbonate and to yield a bicarbonate ion that enters the peritubular capillary. The remaining 15% of filtered bicarbonate is reabsorbed in the distal tubule. A normal kidney reabsorbs all filtered bicarbonate, but this does not make the urine acid. Acidification of the urine is mediated by distal tubular and collection duct secretion of hydrogen ion (which is in part mineralocorticoid dependent) and of ammonia (which forms ammonium ion in an acidic urine).

537.1 Proximal Renal Tubular Acidosis

PATHOGENESIS. Proximal RTA results from reduced proximal tubular reabsorption of bicarbonate, presumably owing to deficient carbonic anhydrase production or hydrogen ion secretion. Rather than reabsorbing the normal 85% of filtered bicarbonate, the proximal tubules in this condition may reabsorb only 60%, thus presenting the distal tubules with 40% rather than the usual 15% of the filtered load. Because the distal tubules can, at a maximum, reabsorb only 15% of the normal filtered load of bicarbonate, up to 25% may be lost in the urine. Proximal RTA is generally more severe than distal RTA, because complete loss of the distal bicarbonate recovery mechanism (which is rare) would waste only 15% of filtered bicarbonate. With urinary bicarbonate loss, the serum bicarbonate level falls until it reaches a level (bicarbonate threshold) at which bicarbonate wasting ceases. At this level (15–18 mEq/L [mmol/L]), the quantity of filtered bicarbonate is reduced to an amount that can be totally reabsorbed by the tubules. Because distal tubular acidification mechanisms remain intact, the urine may then be acidified (pH < 5.5). Flooding the distal tubule with sodium bicarbonate stimulates sodium reabsorption in exchange for potassium, leading to hypokalemia. Contraction of the extracellular fluid volume (as a result of the loss of sodium bicarbonate) stimulates chloride reabsorption (resulting in hyperchloremia) and aldosterone secretion (enhancing potassium loss).

Proximal RTA (Table 537–1) may occur as an isolated disorder not associated with other diseases or with other abnormalities of proximal tubular function. Isolated proximal RTA may be transient or persistent, sporadic or inherited (usually autosomal dominant). Proximal RTA may also occur as part of a generalized defect in proximal tubular transport (Fanconi syndrome), characterized by proteinuria, glucosuria, phosphaturia, aminoaciduria, citraturia, and proximal RTA. A primary form of Fanconi syndrome, not associated with other disease states, has been reported to show both autosomal dominant and recessive modes of inheritance. Secondary Fanconi syndrome may develop during the course of several different inherited or acquired disease states (see Table 537–1).

INHERITED FORMS OF FANCONI SYNDROME

Cystinosis (Chapters 537.3 and 82.4).

Lowe Syndrome. See Chapter 537.4.

Galactosemia (see Chapter 84.2). The renal manifestations of this disorder result from prolonged galactose accumulation in the proximal tubules.

Hereditary Fructose Intolerance (see Chapter 84.3). This autoso-

TABLE 537–1 Classification of Renal Tubular Acidosis

Proximal	Distal	Mineralocorticoid Deficiency*
Isolated	Isolated	Adrenal disorders (↓ A, ↑ R)
Sporadic	Sporadic	Addison disease
Hereditary	Hereditary	Congenital hyperplasia
Fanconi syndrome	Secondary	Primary hypoaldosteronism
Primary	Interstitial nephritis	Hyporeninemic hypoaldosteronism (↓ A, ↓ R)
Secondary	Obstructive	Obstruction
Inherited	Reflux	Pyelonephritis
Cystinosis	Pyelonephritis	Interstitial nephritis
Lowe syndrome	Transplant rejection	Diabetes mellitus
Galactosemia	Sickle cell nephropathy	Nephrosclerosis
Hereditary fructose intolerance	Lupus nephritis	Pseudohypoaldosteronism (↑ A, ↑ R)
Tyrosinemia	Ehlers-Danlos syndrome	
Wilson disease	Nephrocalcinosis	
Medullary cystic disease	Hepatic cirrhosis	
Mitochondrial cytopathies	Elliptocytosis	
Acquired	Medullary sponge kidney	
Heavy metals	Toxins	
Outdated tetracycline	Amphotericin B	
Proteinuria	Lithium	
Interstitial nephritis	Toluene	
Hyperparathyroidism		
Vitamin D–deficiency rickets		
Gentamicin		
Cyclosporine		

*A = aldosterone; R = renin.

mal recessive deficiency of fructose-1-phosphate aldolase leads to proximal tubular dysfunction.

Tyrosinemia. Generalized proximal tubular dysfunction is common in hereditary tyrosinemia (see Chapter 82.2).

Wilson Disease. The clinical manifestations of this autosomal recessive disorder include proximal tubular dysfunction; it is discussed in Chapters 357.2 and 606.3.

Medullary Cystic Disease. This disorder is inherited as an autosomal dominant trait, whereas a similar disorder, juvenile nephronophthisis, is inherited as an autosomal recessive trait. Whether these are separate disorders or the same disorder with variable inheritance is uncertain. Children more commonly have the recessive form, whereas the dominant form is more common in adults. The major pathologic finding is cysts in the medulla. Because the "cysts" seem to be dilatations of the distal tubules and collecting ducts, some may also be found in the renal cortex. Progressive interstitial inflammation and fibrosis lead to glomerular sclerosis, cortical atrophy, and renal insufficiency. Some children suffer no clinical problems until reaching end-stage renal failure. Others show manifestations of tubular dysfunction such as polyuria and polydipsia (concentrating defect), sodium wasting, and proximal RTA. Affected children commonly have red or blond hair. Urinalysis may yield normal results or show minimal abnormalities. Radiographic studies show small, poorly functioning kidneys. The diagnosis is confirmed by biopsy or at nephrectomy if either is warranted in preparation for transplantation.

CAUSES OF ACQUIRED FANCONI SYNDROME. These include tubular toxins such as heavy metals (lead, mercury, cadmium, uranium), outdated tetracycline, proteinuric states (myeloma, nephrotic syndrome), and interstitial nephritis. Excessive parathyroid hormone secretion (primary and secondary hyperparathyroidism, vitamin D–deficient rickets) may also cause proximal RTA, presumably by inhibition of carbonic anhydrase.

537.2 Distal Renal Tubular Acidosis

PATHOGENESIS. The genesis of distal RTA is best explained as a deficiency of hydrogen ion secretion by the distal tubule and collecting duct, although other mechanisms may also be involved. Independent of the precise mechanism, the excretion of ammonium ion is also decreased. The lack of secreted hydrogen ion reduces the formation of carbonic acid and then carbon dioxide in the tubular lumen. The loss of bicarbonate in the urine may be 5–15% of the filtered load. Owing to the nature of the defect, the pH of the urine cannot be reduced below 5.8 despite severe systemic acidosis. Loss of sodium bicarbonate results in hyperchloremia and hypokalemia. The hypokalemia is usually less severe than that found in proximal RTA because less bicarbonate is wasted. Hypercalciuria, nephrocalcinosis, and nephrolithiasis may be present.

Distal RTA may occur as an isolated condition not associated with any other disorder; as such it may be sporadic or inherited as an autosomal dominant or recessive trait. Secondary distal RTA may develop during the course of several diseases and intoxications involving the distal tubules and collecting ducts (see Table 537–1).

MEDULLARY SPONGE KIDNEY. This noninherited disorder is characterized by cystic dilatation of the terminal portions of the collecting ducts as they enter the renal pyramids. Although renal function and life span are typically normal, the disorder may be complicated by pyelonephritis, hypercalciuria, nephrocalcinosis (Fig. 537–1), nephrolithiasis, impaired concentrating capacity, and distal RTA.

MINERALOCORTICOID DEFICIENCY

PATHOGENESIS. This form of RTA results from inadequate production of or reduced distal tubular responsiveness to aldosterone. The lack of aldosterone effect impairs the establishment across the tubular cell membrane of an electrochemical gradient (with negative electrical potential in the tubular lumen) favorable to hydrogen ion secretion. In the absence of aldosterone-mediated sodium reabsorption, hyperkalemia develops. Hyperkalemia suppresses renal ammonia production, resulting in a reduction of ammonium ion excretion and, thus, net acid excretion. The net effect is a hyperkalemic, hyperchloremic acidosis. The systemic acidosis may render the urine pH acid (< 5.5).

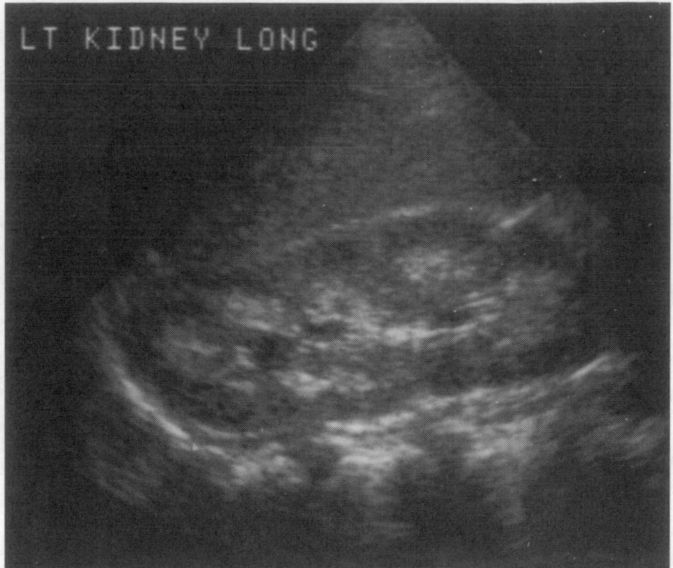

Figure 537–1 Ultrasound examination of a child with distal renal tubular acidosis demonstrating medullary nephrocalcinosis.

Mineralocorticoid-deficiency RTA may result from diseases of the adrenal gland (Addison disease, congenital adrenal hyperplasia, primary hypoaldosteronism) in which aldosterone production is deficient. In these disorders, renal function is normal, urinary sodium wasting is common, and the plasma renin level is elevated. Hyporeninemic hypoaldosteronism is a form of RTA that may result from kidney diseases associated with interstitial damage and destruction of the juxtaglomerular apparatus; it may also be observed with volume expansion and prostaglandin inhibition. In these conditions, plasma levels of renin and, as a result, of aldosterone are reduced; renal function may be compromised. Rarely, type IV RTA may be a result of distal tubular unresponsiveness to aldosterone (pseudohypoaldosteronism); plasma renin and aldosterone levels are elevated, renal function is usually normal, and salt wasting is the rule. In adults, this form of RTA may be observed in patients with medullary disease and renal insufficiency.

CLINICAL MANAGEMENT OF RENAL TUBULAR ACIDOSIS

CLINICAL MANIFESTATIONS. Children having isolated forms of proximal or distal RTA commonly present with growth failure toward the end of the 1st yr of life. Symptoms may include polyuria, dehydration, anorexia, vomiting, constipation, and hypotonia. Children having secondary forms of proximal or distal RTA may present in a similar fashion or with complaints unique to their fundamental disease. Mineralocorticoid deficiency is usually found as an underlying feature of a primary kidney disease.

Distal RTA is complicated by hypercalciuria, which may lead to nephrocalcinosis, nephrolithiasis, and renal parenchymal destruction. The causes of the hypercalciuria are unknown; potential mechanisms include bone breakdown to release calcium carbonate (the carbonate to be converted to bicarbonate in an attempt to control the acidosis) and diminished levels of urinary citrate (which chelates calcium).

Proximal RTA may be complicated by rickets, which may be due to phosphate wasting or insufficient production of 1,25 $(OH)_2D$.

DIAGNOSIS. Before the diagnosis of RTA is considered, other causes of systemic-acidosis, such as diarrhea, inborn errors of metabolism, ingestion, lactic acidosis, diabetes mellitus, and renal failure, should be precluded. The biochemical features of proximal and distal RTA include low serum bicarbonate and potassium levels in association with hyperchloremia. In mineralocorticoid-deficiency RTA, systemic acidosis is associated with hyperkalemia. The anion gap in all forms of RTA is usually normal (see Chapter 52).

Patients suspected of having proximal or distal RTA should be evaluated by comparing the pH (by pH meter) of a first morning urine specimen (collected under mineral oil to prevent the loss of carbon dioxide) with simultaneous measurements of serum electrolytes. In patients who have substantial systemic acidosis (serum bicarbonate level < 18 mEq/L), a urine pH of less than 5.6 supports the diagnosis of proximal RTA, whereas patients with distal RTA have a urine pH of 5.8 or greater. The urinary anion gap (urine concentrations of sodium plus potassium minus chloride) may be an indirect index of ammonium ion excretion that distinguishes proximal from distal RTA. Normal individuals and patients with proximal RTA have a negative gap during metabolic acidosis owing to an increase in ammonium chloride production. Patients with distal RTA have a positive anion gap owing to impaired excretion of hydrogen and ammonium ions.

In patients having mild acidosis (serum bicarbonate level 18–20 mEq/L [mmol/L]), ammonium chloride loading may be required to distinguish between the two types. If proximal RTA is detected, then other defects of proximal tubular function should be sought (glucosuria, phosphaturia, proteinuria, aminoaciduria). When any form of RTA is confirmed, potential underlying causes (see Table 537–1) should be investigated.

TREATMENT. The goals of therapy are correction of the acidosis and maintenance of normal serum bicarbonate and potassium levels. Most patients' conditions can be corrected with oral therapy; in infants having severe acidosis and hypokalemia, intravenous therapy may be required initially. The least expensive and easiest alkalizing solution for oral use is Shohl solution (Bicitra, Willen Drug Company, Baltimore, MD) containing 1 mEq/mL of "bicarbonate equivalent" as sodium citrate. For patients requiring potassium supplementation, potassium citrate can be added (Polycitra, Willen Drug Company, Baltimore, MD) to form a solution that contains 1 mEq/mL each of sodium and potassium, and 2 mEq/mL of bicarbonate equivalent. Sodium bicarbonate tablets (325 and 650 mg) may be used for older patients. Infants may also require oral sodium chloride supplements. Patients with Fanconi syndrome may require phosphate and vitamin D supplements. Patients having mineralocorticoid-deficiency RTA may require diuretics or polystyrene sulfonate resin (Kayexalate, Winthrop Pharmaceuticals, New York, NY) to reduce the serum potassium level to normal.

PROGNOSIS. Isolated proximal RTA, although initially more severe than the distal variety, may resolve during the 1st decade of life. Isolated distal RTA seems to be a lifelong disease; in some instances, renal failure may develop. The prognosis is excellent, however, if the disease is recognized and therapy initiated before the development of nephrocalcinosis. A continuing need for alkali therapy and for lifelong monitoring of clinical status is the rule.

Mineralocorticoid-deficiency RTA most frequently results from obstructive uropathy and usually resolves within 12 mo after correction of the obstruction. In other secondary forms of RTA, the ultimate prognosis may depend on the severity of the primary disorder.

Batlle DC, Hizon M, Cohen E, et al: The use of the urinary anion gap in the diagnosis of hyperchloremic metabolic acidosis. N Engl J Med 318:594, 1988.

Batlle D, Flores G: Underlying defects in distal renal tubular acidosis: New understandings. Am J Kidney Dis 27:869, 1996.

Caldas A, Broyer M, Dechaux M, et al: Primary distal tubular acidosis in childhood: Clinical study and long-term follow-up of 28 patients. J Pediatr 121:233, 1992.

Charnas LR, Bernardina I, Rader D, et al: Clinical and laboratory findings in the oculocerebrorenal syndrome of Lowe, with special reference to growth and renal function. N Engl J Med 324:1318, 1991.

DuBose TD Jr: Hyperkalemic hyperchloremic metabolic acidosis: Pathophysiologic insights. Kidney Int 51:591, 1997.

Haffner D, Weinfurth A, Seidel C, et al: Body growth in primary de Toni-Debre-Fanconi syndrome. Pediatr Nephrol 11:40, 1997.

Hildebrandt F, Strahm B, Nothwang H-G, et al: Molecular genetic identification of families with juvenile nephronophthisis type 1: Rate of progression to renal failure. Kidney Int 51:261, 1997.

Markello TC, Bernardini IM, Gahl WA: Improved renal function in children with cystinosis treated with cysteamine. N Engl J Med 328:1157, 1993.

Niaudet P, Rotig A: The kidney in mitochondrial cytopathies. Kidney Int 51:1000, 1997.

Seikaly M, Browne R, Baum M: Nephrocalcinosis is associated with renal tubular acidosis in children with X-linked hypophosphatemia. Pediatrics 97:91, 1996.

Strisciuglio P, Hu PY, Lim EJ, et al: Clinical and molecular heterogeneity in carbonic anhydrase II deficiency and prenatal diagnosis in an Italian family. J Pediatr 132:717, 1998.

Suchy SF, Olivos-Glander IM, Nussbaum RL: Lowe syndrome, a deficiency of phosphatidyl-inositol 4,5-bisphosphate 5-phosphatase in the Golgi apparatus. Hum Mol Genet 4:2245, 1995.

537.3 Cystinosis

(Lignac Syndrome; Fanconi Syndrome with Cystinosis)

Cystinosis is an autosomal recessive disorder mapped to chromosome 17. The severe form of the disease (*infantile* or *nephropathic cystinosis*) presents in the 1st 2 yr of life and proceeds to renal failure by the end of the 1st decade. Adolescents may be affected by a milder form of the disease characterized by normal growth, minimal renal tubular abnormalities, and slow progression to renal failure. A benign adult form with no renal involvement also exists.

PATHOGENESIS. The disease results from accumulation of cystine within the lysosomes of the bone marrow, liver, spleen, lymph nodes, kidneys, fibroblasts, leukocytes, corneas, conjunctivae, thyroid, pancreas, intestine, and brain. Normally, lysosomal degradation of proteins yields free cysteine, which is transported out of the cell. In cystinosis, a defect in the membrane transport system traps cystine within the lysosome.

CLINICAL MANIFESTATIONS. In the nephropathic variety, initial clinical manifestations may include polyuria and polydipsia (concentrating defect), fever (dehydration, decreased sweat production), growth retardation, rickets, blond hair and fair skin (diminished pigmentation), photophobia, and Fanconi syndrome. Later manifestations may include hypothyroidism, retinopathy leading to decreased visual acuity and occasional blindness, hepatosplenomegaly, and delayed sexual maturation. Intracellular accumulation of cystine in the kidneys leads to chronic nephritis and end-stage renal failure by the end of the 1st decade of life.

DIAGNOSIS. The diagnosis of cystinosis may be suggested by the detection of cystine crystals in the cornea. Because these may be absent, the diagnosis should be confirmed in suspected cases by measurement of leukocyte cystine content. For families at risk, prenatal testing is available.

TREATMENT. Treatment includes correction of the metabolic abnormalities associated with Fanconi syndrome. Specific therapy involves depletion of cystine from tissues with the thiol-containing agent cysteamine. This drug penetrates lysosomal membranes to convert trapped cystine to cysteine, which forms a complex with cysteamine. The complex is then transported out of the lysosome. Early initiation of the drug may prevent or delay deterioration in renal function. Cysteamine eye drops may be helpful in removing corneal cystine crystals.

PROGNOSIS. Patients whose disease progress to end-stage renal failure are satisfactory transplant candidates. After transplantation, which extends survival, patients may develop additional complications of the disease including central nervous system abnormalities, muscle weakness, swallowing dysfunction, and pancreatic endocrine and exocrine insufficiency.

537.4 Oculocerebrorenal Syndrome of Lowe

(Lowe Syndrome)

This rare X-linked recessive disorder is characterized by congenital cataracts, mental retardation, and Fanconi syndrome.

PATHOGENESIS. The gene responsible for this disorder, termed OCRL-1, has been cloned. Gene mutations lead to deficient production of a phosphatase that is important in the transport of vesicles within the Golgi apparatus. Pathologic studies of the kidneys show nonspecific tubulointerstitial changes. Electron microscopy shows thickening of the glomerular basement membranes and changes in the mitochondria of the proximal tubules. At autopsy, brain lesions have been variable and inconsistent. CT and MRI studies show abnormalities in the cerebral white matter.

CLINICAL FEATURES. Promiment initial features of the disease include centrally located congenital cataracts, sometimes associated with glaucoma, moderate to severe mental retardation, hypotonia, and Fanconi syndrome. Although birthweight is usually normal, patients show progressive growth failure over time. Blindness and renal insufficiency may ultimately develop.

TREATMENT. Management includes early removal of the cataracts, adequate nutrition, correction of the biochemical abnormalities, and genetic counseling. Slit-lamp examination of carriers may reveal punctate lenticular opacifications.

537.5 Rickets Associated with Renal Tubular Acidosis

Russell W. Chesney

Rickets may be present in primary renal tubular acidosis (RTA), particularly in type II or proximal RTA. See Chapters 44.10 and 712. Hypophosphatemia and phosphaturia are common in these syndromes, which are characterized by hyperchloremic metabolic acidosis, various degrees of bicarbonaturia, and frequently hypercalciuria and hyperkaliuria. Bone demineralization without overt rickets usually is detected in type I and distal RTA. The metabolic bone disease may be characterized by bone pain, growth retardation, osteopenia, and occasionally pathologic fractures. Although acute metabolic acidosis in vitamin D–deficient animals may impair the conversion of 25(OH)D to $1,25(OH)_2D$, resulting in reduced levels of this active metabolite, the circulating levels of $1,25(OH)_2D$ in patients with either type of RTA are normal. If patients with RTA have azotemia and loss of renal mass, serum $1,25(OH)_2D$ levels are often reduced.

Bone demineralization in distal RTA probably relates to dissolution of bone, because the calcium carbonate in bone may serve as a buffer against the metabolic acidosis that is due to the hydrogen ions retained by patients with RTA.

Administration of sufficient bicarbonate to reverse acidosis stops bone dissolution and the hypercalciuria that is common in distal RTA. Proximal RTA is treated with both bicarbonate and oral phosphate supplements to heal bone disease. Doses of phosphate similar to those used in familial hypophosphatemia should be used (Chapter 711). Vitamin D is needed to offset the secondary hyperparathyroidism that complicates oral phosphate therapy.

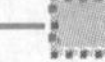

CHAPTER 538 Nephrogenic Diabetes Insipidus

Jerry M. Bergstein

In nephrogenic diabetes insipidus the kidneys fail to respond to antidiuretic hormone (ADH) despite elevated blood levels of ADH.

ETIOLOGY. Primary (congenital) nephrogenic diabetes insipidus is a rare inherited (usually X-linked recessive) disease characterized by complete tubular unresponsiveness to ADH in males and partial unresponsiveness in females. Partial or complete nephrogenic diabetes insipidus (secondary) may also be associated with disorders that (1) result in loss of the medullary concentrating gradient (acute or chronic renal failure, obstructive and postobstructive uropathy, vesicoureteral reflux, cystic diseases, interstitial nephritis, osmotic diuresis, nephrocalcinosis); or (2) diminish the effect of ADH on the tubules (hypokalemia, hypercalcemia, lithium, amphotericin B, and demeclocycline therapy).

PATHOGENESIS. Concentration of the urine depends on the establishment of a hypertonic renal medulla and the permeability of the collecting ducts to water. The hypertonicity of the medulla is established by a countercurrent mechanism linked to reabsorption of sodium and urea. The permeability of the collecting ducts is regulated by ADH, release of which from the neurohypophysis is triggered primarily by osmosensitive neurons located in the hypothalamus and secondarily by monitors of intravascular volume that reside in the heart, large arteries, kidney, liver, and brain. In the kidneys, ADH acts to increase the permeability of the collecting ducts to water by means of a cyclic adenosine monophosphate–dependent mechanism. The activity of ADH is mediated by binding to a type 2 vasopressin (V_2) receptor on the cells of the collecting ducts. Type I receptors are found on platelets and on smooth muscle and liver cells; these receptors are intact in nephrogenic diabetes insipidus. Activation of the V_2 receptor promotes movement of preformed water channels (composed of aquaporin-2 protein) to the luminal membrane of the collecting ducts where it fuses to the membrane, thereby increasing the permeability of the membrane to water. This permits water to flow by passive diffusion from the duct into the hypertonic medullary interstitium of the kidney.

In primary nephrogenic diabetes insipidus, the collecting duct fails to respond normally to ADH, whether endogenous or exogenous, owing to one of several mutations in the V_2 receptor gene. Extrarenal responses (coagulation, fibrinolysis, vasodilatation) to V_2 receptors are also deficient. Rare patients with primary nephrogenic diabetes insipidus showing autosomal recessive inheritance and patients with certain forms of secondary nephrogenic diabetes insipidus (e.g., lithium intoxication) may have ADH resistance due to defective aquaporin-2 expression. Alternatively, secondary forms may result from loss of the hypertonic medullary gradient owing to a solute diuresis or inability of the tubules to reabsorb sodium chloride and urea.

CLINICAL MANIFESTATIONS. Males with primary nephrogenic diabetes insipidus have a dramatic history of polyuria and polydipsia in infancy, often with episodes of hypernatremic dehydration. Females with the primary defect have milder symptoms that may not be detected until later in life. Patients having secondary forms of the disease present with hypernatremia during the course of their primary disorder.

DIAGNOSIS. The diagnosis of primary nephrogenic diabetes insipidus is suspected on clinical history, often with a positive family history in males. Laboratory findings include hypernatremia and dilute urine. If the serum osmolality at initial study exceeds 295 mOsm/kg (mmol/kg) H_2O and concurrent urine osmolality is less than this value, then a dehydration test to establish the diagnosis is unnecessary. The diagnosis is confirmed by administering an intramuscular injection of 0.1–0.2 unit/kg of aqueous vasopressin and measuring the serum and urine osmolality each hour for 4 hr. If the ratio of urine-to-plasma osmolality remains less than 1.0, the patient has nephrogenic diabetes insipidus. If the ratio becomes greater than 1.0, central diabetes insipidus is suggested but psychogenic polydipsia must be precluded. Patients with initial serum osmolality levels less than 295 mOsm/kg (mmol/kg) H_2O should fast (during the day rather than overnight) until serum osmolality exceeds 295 mOsm/kg (mmol/kg) H_2O; vasopressin is then given as before. Withholding of fluids should be terminated if body weight declines by as much as 3%. In patients suspected of having primary nephrogenic diabetes insipidus, appropriate biochemical and cranial imaging studies should be done to preclude secondary causes.

COMPLICATIONS. Primary nephrogenic diabetes insipidus was once thought to be associated with mental retardation. Retardation is more likely the result of repeated episodes of hypertonic dehydration than the consequence of the disease itself. Growth retardation is uniformly present in males with the primary disorder but is usually absent in females. Growth failure was originally thought to result from inadequate caloric intake due to exessive fluid intake, but it now seems that growth failure is intrinsic to the homozygous state. Dilatation of the urinary collecting system may result from excessive urine production. Accordingly, the anatomy of the urinary tract should be examined for evidence of hydronephrosis every few years by renal scan (intravenous pyelography may not visualize the collecting systems when there is rapid flow of large volumes of dilute urine).

TREATMENT. The keys to treatment include the provision of adequate fluid and caloric intake and reduction of the urinary solute load. These are accomplished by limiting the intake of a low-sodium formula (SMA, Wyeth Laboratories, Philadelphia, PA; Similac PM 60/40, Ross Laboratories, Columbus, OH) to only that which is necessary to supply optimal caloric intake for growth. The remainder of the daily fluid requirement (as determined by the maintenance of a normal serum sodium level) is administered as water or fruit juice. The parents should be cautioned that until their child can obtain free access to water, fluids should be offered every 1–2 hr during the day and three times during the night. Once a child becomes old enough to obtain free access to water, the intact thirst mechanism provides the appropriate stimulus for fluid intake.

In patients with the primary disorder, the urinary volume can be dramatically reduced by diuretic therapy. This paradoxical response results because sodium depletion seems to enhance proximal tubular reabsorption of sodium and water. Less water, therefore, is presented to the defective portion of the tubules. Chlorothiazide (20–40 mg/kg/24 hr in divided doses) in conjunction with moderate salt restriction may significantly reduce the need for fluid intake and the frequency of voiding. Patients should be monitored for the development of hypokalemia. Patients who fail to respond to a low-solute diet and diuretics may be candidates for treatment with inhibitors of prostaglandin synthesis (e.g., indomethacin). This type of therapy is of no value for secondary forms of the disease.

PROGNOSIS. Primary nephrogenic diabetes insipidus is a lifelong disease with a good prognosis if hypernatremic dehydration can be avoided. Genetic counseling should be provided for the family; studies to define the precise genetic defect and detect carriers are available. The prognosis for secondary forms of the disease depends on the nature of the primary disorder. The syndrome may resolve after correction of obstructive lesions.

Bichet DG, Oksche A, Rosenthal W: Congenital nephrogenic diabetes insipidus. J Am Soc Nephrol 8:1951, 1997.

Gibbons MD, Koontz WW Jr: Obstructive uropathy and nephrogenic diabetes insipidus in infants. J Urol 122:556, 1979.

Hochberg Z, Van Lieburg A, Even L, et al: Autosomal recessive nephrogenic diabetes insipidus caused by an aquaporin-2 mutation. J Clin Endocrinol Metab 82:686, 1997.

Jakobsson B, Berg U: Effect of hydrochlorothiazide and indomethacin treatment on renal function in nephrogenic diabetes insipidus. Acta Paediatr 83:522, 1994.

Martin P-Y, Schrier RW: Role of aquasporin-2 water channels in urinary concentration and dilution defects. Kidney Int 53(Suppl 65):557, 1998.

CHAPTER 539
Bartter Syndrome

Jerry M. Bergstein

Bartter syndrome is a rare form of renal potassium wasting characterized by hypokalemia, normal blood pressure, vascular insensitivity to pressor agents, and elevated plasma concentrations of renin and aldosterone. In certain families, the disorder may be inherited as an autosomal recessive trait.

PATHOLOGY. Generalized hyperplasia of the juxtaglomerular apparatus, the site of renin production, is observed in most patients. The renal parenchyma is otherwise normal in most patients; a few have shown nonspecific glomerular disease, interstitial disease, or both.

PATHOGENESIS. The cause is unknown. Currently, the disorder is best explained as a primary defect in chloride reabsorption in the ascending limb of the loop of Henle. The resultant decrease in sodium chloride reabsorption in this portion of the loop reduces medullary hypertonicity, perhaps explaining the concentrating defect. The defect in chloride reabsorption presents extra sodium chloride to the distal tubule, where sodium is reabsorbed in exchange for potassium; the result is urinary potassium wasting. The induced hypokalemia stimulates the synthesis of prostaglandins (which may account for the vascular insensitivity to pressor agents and the defect in platelet aggregation); these, in turn, activate the renin-angiotensin-aldosterone system by increasing renin release and by stimulating aldosterone synthesis. The latter exacerbates renal potassium wasting.

CLINICAL MANIFESTATIONS. A severe form of Bartter syndrome (sometimes called hyperprostaglandin E syndrome) may afflict newborns. It is characterized by polyhydramnios, prematurity, dehydration secondary to marked urinary sodium, potassium and water loss, and growth failure; hypercalciuria and nephrocalcinosis are common. Young children typically present with growth failure, muscle weakness, constipation, and polyuria. Older children have muscle weakness or cramps and carpopedal spasms.

DIAGNOSIS. The diagnosis is suggested by the finding of hypokalemia; the serum potassium level is usually less than 2.5 mEq/L. Supportive findings include normal blood pressure;

defective platelet aggregation; hypochloremia; metabolic alkalosis; elevated plasma levels of renin, aldosterone, and prostaglandin E_2; and high urinary levels of potassium and chloride. Some patients may also have hypercalciuria, hyperuricemia, hypomagnesemia, and urinary sodium wasting. The diagnosis may be confirmed by the histologic demonstration of hyperplasia of the juxtaglomerular apparatus, but this abnormality is not found in all patients and is frequently absent in young children.

Bartter syndrome must be differentiated from licorice abuse, laxative or diuretic use, persistent vomiting or diarrhea, pyelonephritis, and diabetes insipidus. Several of these (laxative use, vomiting, diarrhea, diabetes insipidus) are associated with hypovolemia, which results in a low urinary chloride level, whereas Bartter syndrome is associated with an elevated level.

Bartter syndrome may be confused with *Gitelman syndrome.* Both disorders are associated with hypokalemia, renal potassium wasting, activation of the renin-angiotensin-aldosterone axis, and normal blood pressure. Gitelman syndrome commonly presents in older children and young adults with muscle weakness, carpopedal spasms, or tetany. Patients with Bartter syndrome have normal to decreased serum magnesium levels, normal urinary magnesium excretion, and normal to increased calcium excretion; patients with Gitelman syndrome have hypomagnesemia, increased urinary magnesium, and decreased calcium excretion. Gitelman syndrome results from a mutation of the gene for the thiazide-sensitive sodium-chloride co-transporter of the distal tubule located on chromosome 16.

TREATMENT. The goals of therapy are to supply adequate nutrition and to maintain the serum potassium level above 3.5 mEq/L. Therapy is initiated with oral potassium chloride supplementation, increasing the dose until the serum potassium level reaches 3.5 mEq/L or the dosage reaches 250 mEq/24 hr. Reasonably well tolerated potassium preparations include K-Lyte/Cl (Mead Johnson Company, Evansville, IN), flavored effervescent tablets containing 25 or 50 mEq of potassium chloride, and Micro-K 10 Extencaps (A.H. Robins Company, Richmond, VA). Sodium chloride supplementation may also be required in small children. If the serum potassium level remains below 3.5 mEq/L (mmol/L) after reaching a dose of 250 mEq/24 hr of potassium chloride, then triamterene, 5–10 mg/kg/24 hr in divided doses, should be added. If this fails to resolve the hypokalemia, then indomethacin, 3–5 mg/kg/24 hr divided into three doses, should be given. Patients receiving indomethacin should be monitored for signs of gastrointestinal irritation.

PROGNOSIS. The long-term prognosis of Bartter syndrome is uncertain. Many patients remain well, but some cases (especially those with glomerular or interstitial abnormalities) progress to renal insufficiency. Despite severe growth retardation in infancy, normal stature is ultimately obtained. The suggestion that mental retardation occurs in patients who have severe disease in the 1st yr of life remains to be confirmed.

Madrigal G, Saborio P, Mora F, et al: Bartter's syndrome in Costa Rica: A description of 20 cases. Pediatr Nephrol 11:296, 1997.
McCredie DA: Variants of Bartter's syndrome. Pediatr Nephrol 10:419, 1996.
Pollak MR, Delaney VB, Graham RM, et al: Gitelman's syndrome (Bartter's variant) maps to the thiazide-sensitive cotransporter gene locus on chromosome 16q13 in a large kindred. J Am Soc Nephrol 7:2244, 1996.

CHAPTER 540
Interstitial Nephritis

Jerry M. Bergstein

Interstitial nephritis is a histopathologic term signifying inflammation between the glomeruli in the areas surrounding the tubules (the interstitium). Acute and chronic forms are recognized, depending on the nature of the inflammatory infiltrate and the presence or absence of edema and fibrosis. Tubular damage is generally present; glomerular changes may be minimal. Common causes of acute or chronic interstitial nephritis in children are listed in Table 540–1.

ACUTE INTERSTITIAL NEPHRITIS

PATHOLOGY. Whatever the cause of interstitial disease, the interstitial infiltrate is composed of lymphocytes, plasma cells, eosinophils, and occasional neutrophils (Fig. 540–1). The tubules are separated by edema and may show degeneration or frank necrosis. Unless the interstitial nephritis is associated with glomerulonephritis, the glomeruli are normal.

PATHOGENESIS. The genesis of acute interstitial nephritis is poorly understood. When it is due to drug ingestion, failure of the amount of drug administered to correlate with incidence of the syndrome suggests a hypersensitivity reaction. For methicillin, an immunologic mechanism has been suggested in several instances by the finding of anti–tubular basement membrane antibodies. Whether infections cause interstitial inflammation by direct invasion or by other mechanisms remains unclear. In certain forms of glomerulonephritis, tubular basement membrane deposition of immune complexes (lupus, membranoproliferative) or of anti–basement membrane antibodies (Goodpasture, membranous) may initiate the inflam-

TABLE 540–1 Causes of Interstitial Nephritis

Acute	Chronic
Drugs	***Drugs***
Penicillin derivatives	Analgesics
Cephalosporins	Lithium
Sulfonamides	***Infections***
Co-trimoxazole	Pyelonephritis
Rifampin	***Disease-Associated***
Phenytoin	Vesicoureteral reflux
Thiazides	Nephrocalcinosis
Furosemide	Prolonged hypokalemia
Allopurinol	Oxalate nephropathy
Cimetidine	Heavy metals
Amphotericin B	Radiation
Nonsteroidal anti-inflammatory drugs	Obstructive uropathy
Infections	Medullary cystic disease
Streptococcal	Sickle cell disease
Pyelonephritis	
Toxoplasmosis	
Diphtheria	
Brucellosis	
Leptospirosis	
Mononucleosis	
Cytomegalovirus	
Disease-Associated	
Sarcoidosis	
Glomerulonephritis	
Transplant rejection	
Idiopathic	

matory reaction. In sarcoidosis and transplant rejection, cell-mediated mechanisms may have a role.

CLINICAL MANIFESTATIONS. In hospitalized patients, drugs are the most common cause of acute interstitial nephritis. After a week or so of drug therapy, patients develop fever and at times maculopapular skin rash. Urine output may be normal or diminished. Increased numbers of eosinophils may be detected in the blood or urine or both. Acute renal failure or generalized tubular dysfunction or both may result. Other forms of acute interstitial nephritis present a clinical picture resembling acute glomerulonephritis or acute renal failure, along with manifestations of the initiating disorder. The onset may be preceded by anterior uveitis.

DIAGNOSIS. The diagnosis is confirmed by renal biopsy, although acute interstitial nephritis may not be suspected before the biopsy. The differential diagnosis includes other causes of acute nephritis or renal failure.

PREVENTION. The development of drug-related interstitial nephritis may be reduced by using alternative therapeutic agents when possible (substituting nafcillin for methicillin).

TREATMENT AND PROGNOSIS. After appropriate management of the acute renal failure, withdrawal of possible inciting agents, and treatment of precipitating infection, the acute interstitial nephritis may resolve completely, but residual renal dysfunction is common. In patients suffering severe histologic injury and renal failure, high-dose corticosteroid therapy may bring dramatic improvement.

CHRONIC INTERSTITIAL NEPHRITIS

PATHOLOGY. In chronic interstitial nephritis, the inflammatory infiltrate consists of lymphocytes and plasma cells. The edema of the acute form is replaced by interstitial fibrosis. Tubular dilatation and atrophy are widespread. The glomeruli show partial or total sclerosis, presumably as a result of ischemia.

CLINICAL MANIFESTATIONS. In children, chronic interstitial nephritis usually develops in association with an occult structural abnormality of the kidneys or lower urinary tract (cystic disease, obstruction, reflux). The presenting clinical manifestations may be those of chronic renal failure (nausea, vomiting, pallor, headache, fatigue, hypertension, growth failure) or

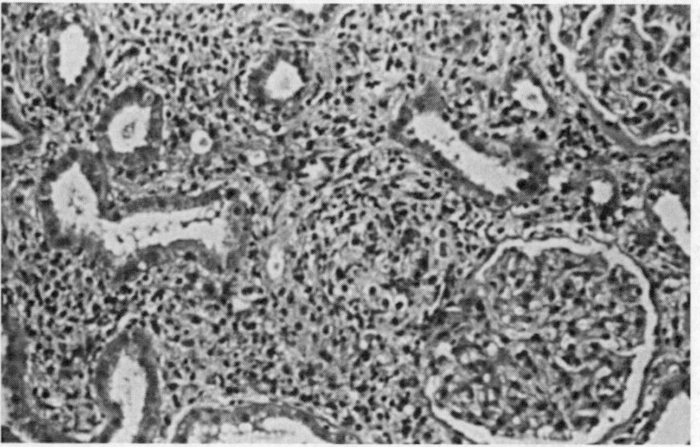

Figure 540–1 Biopsy from a patient having acute interstitial nephritis. The tubules are widely separated by edema and an intense inflammatory infiltrate containing lymphocytes, plasma cells, eosinophils, and neutrophils. The glomeruli are preserved (×80).

manifestations of the underlying disorder (urinary tract infection, flank mass).

DIAGNOSIS. The diagnosis is suggested by the presence of chronic renal insufficiency in association with a known cause of the disorder; renal biopsy is not usually indicated.

TREATMENT AND PROGNOSIS. The natural history of chronic interstitial nephritis is progression to end-stage renal failure. Whether elimination of infection or correction of reflux or obstruction will alter this progression is unclear. In adults, avoidance of analgesics (phenacetin) and lithium before the development of end-stage renal failure may result in improvement in renal function.

Bunchman TE, Bloom JN: A syndrome of acute interstitial nephritis and anterior uveitis. Pediatr Nephrol 7:520, 1993.

Ellis D, Fried WA, Yunis EJ, et al: Acute interstitial nephritis in children: A report of 13 cases and review of the literature. Pediatrics 67:862, 1981.

Jones CL, Eddy AA: Tubulointerstitial nephritis. Pediatr Nephrol 6:572, 1992.

Michel DM, Kelley CJ: Acute interstitial nephritis. J Am Soc Nephrol 9:504, 1998.

Rastegar A, Kashgarian M: The clinical spectrum of tubulointerstitial nephritis. Kidney Int 54:313, 1998.

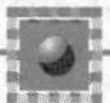

SECTION 5

Toxic Nephropathies—Renal Failure

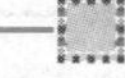

CHAPTER 541

Toxic Nephropathy

Jerry M. Bergstein

Medications, diagnostic agents (iodinated radiographic contrast media), and chemicals may alter the kidneys directly (through reduction of renal blood flow, acute tubular necrosis, intratubular obstruction) or indirectly (through induction of an allergic or hypersensitivity reaction in the vessels or interstitium). Commonly nephrotoxic agents and their clinical manifestations are listed in Table 541–1. Nephrotoxicity is frequently reversible if the noxious agent is removed.

Useful agents should not be withheld because of potential nephrotoxicity, but preventive measures may reduce the risks of nephrotoxicity: (1) in patients with pre-existing renal disease, substitution of ultrasound or isotopic scans for studies using contrast media; (2) substitution of non-nephrotoxic agents for nephrotoxic agents if possible; (3) use of the lowest effective dose of the agent in conjunction with monitoring of the blood level; (4) reduction of the dose in patients with renal insufficiency; (5) avoidance of simultaneous use of several nephrotoxic agents.

TABLE 541–1 Nephrotoxic Compounds*

Nephrotic Syndrome
- Angiotensin-converting enzyme inhibitors
- Gold salts
- Mercurial diuretics
- Mercury compounds
- Nonsteroidal anti-inflammatory drugs
- Paramethadione
- Penicillamine
- Perchlorate
- Probenecid
- Tolbutamide
- Trimethadione

Nephrogenic Diabetes Insipidus
- Amphotericin B
- Demeclocycline
- Lithium carbonate
- Methoxyflurane
- Propoxyphene

Interstitial Nephritis with or Without Papillary Necrosis
- Penicillins (especially methicillin)
- Phenacetin
- Phenylbutazone
- Salicylate
- Sulfonamides
- Nonsteroidal anti-inflammatory agents

Renal Vasculitis with or Without Glomerular Capillary Involvement
- Hydralazine
- Isoniazid
- Sulfonamides
- Any of the numerous other drugs that may cause a hypersensitivity reaction

Nephrocalcinosis or Nephrolithiasis
- Allopurinol
- Ethylene glycol
- Methoxyflurane
- Vitamin D

Miscellaneous Renal Manifestations, Including Proteinuria, Hematuria, Oliguria, Tubular Necrosis, and Renal Failure
- Acyclovir
- Angiotensin-converting enzyme inhibitors
- Arsenic
- Bacitracin
- Cadmium

Fanconi's Syndrome
- Aminoglycosides
- Cadmium
- Ifosfamide
- Lead
- Lysol
- Mercury
- Nitrobenzene
- Outdated tetracycline
- Salicylate
- Uranium

Renal Tubular Acidosis
- Amphotericin B
- Lithium salts
- Toluene sniffing

Interstitial Nephritis with or Without Papillary Necrosis
- Amidopyrine
- *p*-Aminosalicylate
- Bunamiodyl (papillary necrosis only)
- Carbon tetrachloride
- Cephaloridine
- Cephalothin
- Cimetidine
- Cisplatin
- Colistin
- Copper
- Cyclosporine
- Ethylene glycol
- Foscarnet
- Gentamicin
- Gold salts
- Indomethacin
- Interferon-α
- Iron
- Kanamycin
- Mannitol
- Mercury salts
- Mitomycin C
- Neomycin
- Nonsteroidal anti-inflammatory agents
- Pentamidine
- Poisonous mushrooms
- Polymyxin B
- Radiocontrast agents
- Rifampin
- Streptomycin
- Sulfonamides
- Tacrolimus (FK 506)
- Tetrachloroethylene
- Trimethoprim-sulfamethoxazole (hyperkalemia)
- Vancomycin
- Viomycin

**The agents are grouped according to the principal site of injury or manifestations. (Dr. Sean O'Regan assisted in the preparation of this table.)*

Aronoff GR, Berns JS, Brier ME, et al (eds): Drug Prescribing in Renal Failure, 4th ed. Philadelphia, American College of Physicians, 1999.
Becker BN, Fall P, Hall C, et al: Rapidly progressive acute renal failure due to acyclovir: Case report and review of the literature. Am J Kidney Dis 22:611, 1993.
Becker BN, Schulman G: Nephrotoxicity of antiviral therapies. Curr Opin Nephrol Hypertens 5:375, 1996.
Bennett WM: Lead nephropathy. Kidney Int 28:212, 1985.
Bennett WM, Henrich WL, Stoff JS: The renal effects of nonsteroidal anti-inflammatory drugs: Summary and recommendations. Am J Kidney Dis 28:S56, 1996.
Cayco AV, Perazella MA, Hayslett JP: Renal insufficiency after intravenous immune globulin therapy: A report of two cases and an analysis of the literature. J Am Soc Nephrol 8:1788, 1997.
De Vriese AS, Robbrecht DL, Vanholder RC, et al: Rifampicin-associated acute renal failure: Pathophysiologic, immunologic, and clinical features. Am J Kidney Dis 31:108, 1998.
Mendoza SA: Nephrotoxic drugs. Pediatr Nephrol 2:466, 1988.
Meyer KB, Madias NE: Cisplatin nephrotoxicity. Miner Electrolyte Metab 20:201, 1994.
Murgo AJ: Thrombotic microangiopathy in the cancer patient including those induced by chemotherapeutic agents. Semin Hematol 24:161, 1987.
O'Brien KL, Selanikio JD, Hecdivert C, et al: Epidemic of pediatric deaths from acute renal failure caused by diethylene glycol poisoning. JAMA 279:1175, 1998.
Perazella MA, Mahnensmith RL: Trimethoprim-sulfamethoxazole: Hyperkalemia is an important complication regardless of dose. Clin Nephrol 46:187, 1996.
Shah GM, Alvarado P, Kirschenbaum MA, et al: Symptomatic hypocalcemia and hypomagnesemia with renal magnesium wasting associated with pentamidine therapy in a patient with AIDS. Am J Med 89:380, 1990.
Soloman R: Contrast-medium-induced acute renal failure. Kidney Int 53:230, 1998.
Walker RG: Lithium nephrotoxicity. Kidney Int 44:S93, 1993.

CHAPTER 542
Cortical Necrosis

Jerry M. Bergstein

Renal cortical (and frequently medullary) necrosis represents a final common result of several types of renal injury. It usually affects both kidneys and may be patchy or involve the entire cortex.

ETIOLOGY. In newborns, cortical necrosis develops after dehydration, asphyxia, shock, disseminated intravascular coagulation, or renal vein thrombosis or in association with severe congenital heart disease. After the neonatal period, cortical necrosis most commonly develops with the hemolytic-uremic syndrome.

PATHOLOGY. Involved portions of the cortex show infarction, with congestion of the glomeruli, thrombosis of the arterioles, and necrosis of the tubules.

PATHOGENESIS. Cortical necrosis seems to develop when endothelial cell injury occurs in conjunction with diminished renal cortical blood flow. Toxins or other mediators that presumably develop during shock, hemolytic-uremic syndrome, or sepsis (endotoxin) may injure the endothelial cells and initiate intrarenal coagulation, leading to thrombosis and cortical necrosis.

CLINICAL MANIFESTATIONS. Cortical necrosis presents as acute renal failure developing in infants having the previously mentioned predisposing causes. The kidneys are frequently enlarged. Urine output is diminished and may show gross hematuria.

DIAGNOSIS. The diagnosis is supported by ultrasonographic detection of enlarged, nonobstructed kidneys, which on isotopic renal scan show little or no renal blood flow or function. The differential diagnosis includes other causes of renal failure (see Tables 543–1 and 543–2).

TREATMENT AND PROGNOSIS. Therapy is supportive and involves correction of dehydration, asphyxia, and shock and treatment of sepsis. The prognosis depends on the amount of surviving renal cortex.

Chevalier RL, Campbell F, Brenbridge ANAG: Prognostic factors in neonatal acute renal failure. Pediatrics 74:265, 1984.

Lerner GR, Kurnetz R, Bernstein J, et al: Renal cortical and renal medullary necrosis in the first 3 months of life. Pediatr Nephrol 6:516, 1992.

Reimold EW, Don TD, Worthen HG: Renal failure during the first year of life. Pediatrics 59:987, 1977.

Rodriguez-Soriano J, Vallo A, Bilbao F, et al: Different functional characteristics of residual nephrons in infantile vs adult diffuse cortical necrosis. Int J Pediatr Nephrol 3:71, 1982.

CHAPTER 543
Renal Failure

Jerry M. Bergstein

543.1 Acute Renal Failure

Acute renal failure develops when renal function is diminished to the point where body fluid homeostasis can no longer be maintained. Although oliguria (daily urine volume < 400 mL/m^2) is common in renal failure, the urine volume may approximate normal (nonoliguric renal failure) in certain types of acute renal failure (aminoglycoside nephrotoxicity). To monitor renal function, it is important to use biochemical studies (blood urea nitrogen [BUN], creatinine) as well as measurement of urine volume.

ETIOLOGY. The causes of acute failure are listed in Tables 543–1 and 543–2. In the first category (prerenal), decreased perfusion of the kidneys results in decreased renal function; the second category includes direct involvement of the kidneys, and the third (postrenal) is composed primarily of obstructive disorders.

PATHOGENESIS. *Prerenal causes* of acute renal failure produce decreased renal perfusion through decreases in the total or "effective" circulating blood volume. Evidence of kidney damage is absent. Diminished intravascular volume leads to a fall in cardiac output, causing a decline in renal cortical blood flow and glomerular filtration rate (GFR). If, within a certain time, the underlying cause of the hypoperfusion is reversed, then renal function may return to normal. If hypoperfusion persists beyond this critical point, then direct renal parenchymal damage may develop.

TABLE 543–1 Causes of Acute Renal Failure in the Newborn

Renal dysgenesis	Systemic inflammatory response syndrome
Obstructive uropathy	Sepsis
Renovascular accidents	Necrotizing enterocolitis
Congenital heart disease	Anoxia
Dehydration	Shock
Hemorrhage	Renal vein thrombosis

Renal causes of acute renal failure include the rapidly progressive forms of several types of glomerulonephritis (see Table 543–2) that are common causes of acute renal failure in older children. Activation of the coagulation system within the kidneys, resulting in small vessel thrombosis, may lead to acute renal failure. Acute dehydration and the hemolytic-uremic syndrome are the most common causes of acute renal failure in toddlers.

The term **acute tubular necrosis** originally described a syndrome of acute renal failure in the absence of arterial or glomerular lesions. The proposed mechanism of the renal failure was necrosis of the tubular cells. Certain agents (heavy metals, chemicals) may indeed cause renal failure by producing tubular cell necrosis, but significant histologic changes are absent in kidneys from patients having other forms of acute tubular necrosis. The precise mechanism of renal failure in these patients is unknown. Proposed mechanisms include alterations in intrarenal hemodynamics, tubular obstruction, and passive backflow of the glomerular filtrate across injured tubular cells into the peritubular capillaries.

Acute interstitial nephritis is an increasingly common cause of acute renal failure and is usually a result of a hypersensitivity reaction to a therapeutic agent. Tumors may produce acute renal failure by infiltration of the kidneys or by obstruction of the tubules by uric acid crystals (Chapters 502 and 505).

Developmental abnormalities and hereditary nephritis may be associated with acute renal failure. Inability to conserve sodium and water is common in patients having these disorders, but losses are usually compensated by increased oral intake. If oral intake is compromised (vomiting) or extrarenal salt and water loss develops (diarrhea), then these, in conjunction with the obligate urinary salt and water losses, may lead to intravascular volume contraction and renal failure.

Postrenal causes of acute renal failure include obstructions of the urinary tract. With two functioning kidneys, ureteral obstruction must be bilateral to produce renal failure. It is important to recognize that dilatation of the upper collecting system may not occur until several days after acute ureteral obstruction.

CLINICAL MANIFESTATIONS. The presenting signs and symptoms may be dominated or modified by the precipitating disease. Clinical findings related to the renal failure include pallor (anemia), diminished urine output, edema (salt and water overload), hypertension, vomiting, and lethargy (uremic encephalopathy). Complications of acute renal failure include volume overload with heart failure and pulmonary edema, arrhythmias, gastrointestinal bleeding due to stress ulcers or gastritis, seizures, coma, and behavioral changes.

DIAGNOSIS. A carefully taken history may aid in defining the cause of renal failure. Vomiting, diarrhea, and fever suggest dehydration and prerenal azotemia, but these may also precede development of the hemolytic-uremic syndrome or renal

TABLE 543–2 Causes of Acute Renal Failure

Prerenal	Renal	Postrenal
Hypovolemia	Glomerulonephritis	Obstructive uropathy
Hemorrhage	Poststreptococcal	Ureteropelvic junction
Gastrointestinal losses	Lupus erythematosus	Ureterocele
Hypoproteinemia	Membranoproliferative	Urethral valves
Burns	Idiopathic rapidly progressive	Tumor
Renal or adrenal disease with salt wasting	Henoch-Schönlein purpura	Vesicoureteral reflux
Hypotension	Localized intravascular coagulation	Acquired
Septicemia	Renal vein thrombosis	Stones
Disseminated intravascular coagulation	Cortical necrosis	Blood clot
Hypothermia	Hemolytic-uremic syndrome	
Hemorrhage	Acute tubular necrosis	
Heart failure	Heavy metals	
Hypoxia	Chemicals	
Pneumonia	Drugs	
Aortic clamping	Hemoglobin, myoglobin	
Respiratory distress syndrome	Shock	
	Ischemia	
	Acute interstitial nephritis	
	Infection	
	Drugs	
	Tumors	
	Renal parenchymal infiltration	
	Uric acid nephropathy	
	Developmental abnormalities	
	Cystic disease	
	Hypoplasia-dysplasia	
	Hereditary nephritis	

vein thrombosis. Antecedent skin or throat infection suggests poststreptococcal glomerulonephritis. Rash may be found in systemic lupus erythematosus or Henoch-Schönlein purpura. A history of exposure to chemicals and medications should be sought. Flank masses suggest renal vein thrombosis, tumors, cystic disease, or obstruction.

Laboratory abnormalities may include anemia (with the rare exception of blood loss, the anemia is usually dilutional or hemolytic, as in lupus, renal vein thrombosis, and the hemolytic-uremic syndrome); leukopenia (lupus); thrombocytopenia (lupus, renal vein thrombosis, hemolytic-uremic syndrome); hyponatremia (dilutional); hyperkalemia; acidosis; elevated serum concentrations of BUN, creatinine, uric acid, and phosphate (diminished renal function); and hypocalcemia (hyperphosphatemia). The serum C3 level may be depressed (poststreptococcal, lupus, or membranoproliferative glomerulonephritis), and antibodies may be detected in the serum to streptococcal (poststreptococcal glomerulonephritis), nuclear (lupus), neutrophil cytoplasmic antigens (ANCA; Wegener's granulomatosis, microscopic polyarteritis), or to basement membrane (Goodpasture disease) antigens. Chest roentgenography may reveal cardiomegaly and pulmonary congestion (fluid overload). In all patients presenting in acute renal failure, the possibility of obstruction (which, if detected, is quickly reversed by percutaneous nephrostomy) should be immediately assessed by obtaining a plain roentgenogram study of the abdomen, renal ultrasonography, and a radionuclide scan; retrograde pyelography may occasionally be needed to detect occult obstructions. Renal biopsy may ultimately be required to determine the precise cause of renal failure.

TREATMENT. In children with *hypovolemia*, the need for volume replacement may be critical. Initial physical examination of patients should include a careful assessment of the state of hydration. In some oliguric patients it may be impossible to distinguish whether oliguria is due to hypoperfusion (hypovolemia) or impending acute tubular necrosis. Evaluation of the urine may prove helpful in this regard. In patients with hypovolemia, the urine is concentrated (urine osmolality > 500 mOsm/kg), its sodium content is usually less than 20 mEq/L, and the fractional excretion of sodium (urine/plasma sodium concentration divided by the urine/plasma creatinine concentration × 100) is usually less than 1%. By contrast, in patients with acute tubular necrosis, the urine is dilute (osmolality < 350 mOsm/kg), the sodium concentration usually exceeds 40 mEq/L (mmol/L), and the fractional excretion of sodium usually exceeds 1%.

If hypovolemia is detected, intravascular volume should be expanded by intravenous administration of isotonic saline, 20 mL/kg, over 30 min. In the absence of blood loss or hypoproteinemia, colloid-containing solutions are not required for volume expansion. After this infusion, dehydrated patients generally void within 2 hr. Failure to do so mandates a thorough re-evaluation of a patient. Catheterization of the bladder and determination of the central venous pressure may be helpful. Severe dehydration may require additional fluid boluses. If clinical and laboratory evaluations show that the patient is adequately hydrated, then aggressive diuretic therapy may be considered.

In patients with *impending renal failure*, the value of diuretics in preventing development of anuria remains controversial. It seems clear that diuretics have no value in patients with established anuria. In some oliguric patients, furosemide or mannitol or both may increase the rate of urine production. These agents act by altering tubular function, but it should be recognized that the increase in urine flow does not represent an improvement in renal function, nor does it affect the natural history of the disease that precipitated the renal failure. On the other hand, enhancement of urine output may be valuable in the management of hyperkalemia and fluid overload.

The pharmacodynamics of furosemide in renal failure are such that the urinary response (which is a function of the dose and blood level obtained) may be delayed for several hours. In oliguric patients who lack clinical and laboratory evidence of hypovolemia (and who may have already failed to respond to volume expansion), furosemide may be administered as a single intravenous dose of 2 mg/kg at the rate of 4 mg/min (to avoid ototoxicity); if no response occurs, a second dose of 10 mg/kg may be given. Bumetanide may be given (0.1 mg/kg) as an alternative to furosemide. If no increase in urine production is obtained after this dose, then further furosemide therapy is contraindicated. A single intravenous dose of 0.5–1.0 g/kg of mannitol may be given over 30 min in addition to or in place of furosemide. Regardless of the response, no additional mannitol should be given, owing to the risk of toxicity. To increase renal cortical blood flow, dopamine (2 μg/kg/min) may be administered (in the absence of hypertension) in conjunction with diuretic therapy.

Fluid restriction is essential for patients who fail to produce adequate urine output after volume expansion or the administration of diuretics. The degree of fluid restriction depends on the state of hydration. For patients with oliguria or anuria having a relatively normal intravascular volume, fluid administration should initially be limited to 400 mL/m²/24 hr (insensible losses) plus an amount of fluid equal to the urine output for that day. On the other hand, markedly hypervolemic patients may require almost total fluid restriction; omitting the replacement of insensible fluid losses and urine output aids in diminishing the expanded intravascular volume. Access to the vascular space should be maintained; this is best obtained using an infusion pump at the slowest possible rate. In general, glucose-containing solutions (10–30%) without electrolytes are used as maintenance fluids. The composition of the fluid may be modified in accordance with the state of electrolyte balance. Except in overhydrated patients, extrarenal (blood, gastrointestinal tract) fluid losses should be replaced, milliliter for milliliter, with appropriate fluids. Fluid intake, urine and stool output, and body weight should be monitored on a daily basis.

In acute renal failure, rapid development of *hyperkalemia* (serum level > 6 mEq/L) may lead to cardiac arrhythmia and death. Patients should receive no potassium-containing fluid, foods, or medications until adequate renal function is re-established. The earliest electrocardiographic change seen in patients with developing hyperkalemia is the appearance of tall, peaked T waves. This may be followed by ST-segment depression, prolongation of the P-R and widening of the QRS intervals, ventricular fibrillation, and cardiac arrest.

In children with acute renal failure, procedures to deplete body potassium are initiated when the serum potassium value rises to 5.5 mEq/L (mmol/L). To minimize the rate at which the serum potassium rises, all solutions given to patients should contain high concentrations of glucose. Sodium polystyrene sulfonate resin (Kayexalate), 1 g/kg, should be given orally or by retention enema. This material exchanges sodium for potassium. For best results, the resin should be given orally, suspended in 2 mL/kg of 70% sorbitol. Sorbitol produces an osmotic diarrhea, which increases fluid and electrolyte losses (the usual patient in renal failure is hypervolemic, with increased total body sodium and potassium levels) as well as enhances the movement of the resin through the gastrointestinal tract. Because 70% sorbitol is locally irritating to the rectum, the concentration should be reduced to 20% and the volume increased to 10 mL/kg when it is given by enema. Resin therapy may be repeated every 2 hr, the frequency being limited primarily by the risk of sodium overload.

If the serum potassium rises above 7 mEq/L (mmol/L), emergency measures in addition to Kayexalate, must be initiated. The following agents shold be given sequentially:

1. Calcium gluconate 10% solution, 0.5 mL/kg IV, over 10 min. The heart rate must be closely monitored during the infusion; a fall in rate of 20 beats/min requires stopping the infusion until the pulse returns to the preinfusion rate.
2. Sodium bicarbonate 7.5% solution, 3 mEq/kg IV. Possible complications include volume expansion, hypertension, and tetany.
3. Glucose 50% solution, 1 mL/kg, with regular insulin, 1 unit/5 g of glucose, given IV over 1 hr. Patients should be monitored closely for hypoglycemia.

Calcium gluconate does not lower the serum potassium but counteracts the potassium-induced increase in myocardial irritability. Bicarbonate lowers serum potassium level; the mechanism is not clearly defined. The effect of glucose and insulin is to shift potassium from the extracellular to the intracellular compartment. β-Adrenergic receptor agonists given by aerosol also acutely lower potassium levels. The duration of action of these emergency measures is just a few hours. Persistent hyperkalemia, therefore, especially in patients requiring the emergency measures, should be managed by dialysis.

Moderate *acidosis* is common in renal failure as a result of inadequate excretion of hydrogen ion and ammonia, but it rarely requires treatment. Severe acidosis (arterial pH < 7.15, serum bicarbonate < 8 mEq/L [mmol/kg]) may increase myocardial irritability and requires treatment. Because of the risks involved in the rapid infusion of alkali, the acidosis should be corrected only partially by the intravenous route, generally giving enough bicarbonate to raise the arterial pH to 7.20 (which approximates a serum bicarbonate level of 12 mEq/L [mmol/L]). The correction formula is

$$\text{mEq NaHCO}_3\text{ required} = 0.3 \times \text{weight (kg)} \times (12 - \text{serum bicarbonate [mEq/L]})$$

The remainder of the correction, which should be accomplished only after normalization of the serum calcium and phosphorus levels, may be made by oral administration of sodium bicarbonate tablets or sodium citrate solution.

In addition to the risks involved in administration of intravenous bicarbonate that have been noted, correction of acidosis with intravenous bicarbonate may precipitate tetany (Chapter 55.9). In patients with renal failure, an inability to excrete phosphorus leads to hyperphosphatemia and a reciprocal hypocalcemia. Acidosis prevents the development of tetany by increasing the ionized fraction of the total calcium. Rapid correction of acidosis reduces the ionized calcium concentration, resulting in tetany.

Hypocalcemia is treated by lowering the serum phosphorus level. Unless tetany develops, calcium is not given intravenously, in order to avoid reaching a calcium × phosphorus product (mg/dL × mg/dL of 70) in the serum, the point at which calcium salts are deposited in tissue. To lower the serum phosphorus level, a phosphate-binding calcium carbonate antacid is given by mouth, increasing fecal phosphate excretion; common agents include Titralac liquid (3M Company, St. Paul, MN; starting dose 5–15 mL with meals and before bed) and Os-Cal 500 tablets (Marion Laboratories, Kansas City, MO) or regular strength Tums (SmithKline Beecham, Pittsburgh, PA); starting dose one to three tablets with meals and before bed. The total daily dose should be gradually increased until the serum phosphorus level falls to normal.

Hyponatremia is commonly a result of administration of excessive amounts of hypotonic fluids to oliguric-anuric patients. Correction may be accomplished by fluid restriction. Patients whose serum sodium levels acutely fall below 120 mEq/L (mmol/L) are at increased risk for developing cerebral edema and central nervous system hemorrhage. In the absence of dehydration, water restriction is essential. When the serum sodium falls below 120 mEq/L (mmol/L), it may be elevated to 125 mEq/L (mmol/L) by intravenous infusion of hypertonic (3%) sodium chloride, using the following formula:

$$\text{mEq NaCl required} = 0.6 \times \text{weight (kg)} \times (125 - \text{serum sodium [mEq/L]})$$

The risks of administration of hypertonic saline include volume expansion, hypertension, and heart failure; if these occur, they may be treated by dialysis.

Gastrointestinal bleeding may be prevented with calcium carbonate antacids, which also serve to lower the serum phosphorus level. Alternatively, intravenous cimetidine may be administered at a dose of 5–10 mg/kg/12 hr.

Hypertension may result from the primary disease process or expansion of the extracellular fluid volume or both. In patients with renal failure and hypertension, salt and water restriction is critical. Also see Chapter 451.

In children with severe acute symptomatic hypertension,

diazoxide is a useful drug. This potent vasodilator must be given by rapid (< 10 sec) intravenous injection at a dose of 1–3 mg/kg (maximum dose of 150 mg). Blood pressure usually declines within 10–20 min; if the decline following the first injection is insufficient, a second injection may be given 30 min later. Alternatively, nifedipine may be given acutely (0.25–0.5 mg/kg PO). Sodium nitroprusside or labetalol as a continuous intravenous infusion is indicated for hypertensive crises. For less severe hypertension, control of extracellular volume expansion (salt and water restriction, furosemide) and use of β-blockers (propranolol; 1–3 mg/kg/12 hr PO) and vasodilators (Apresoline 0.5–1.5 mg/kg/6 hr IV; minoxidil 0.1–0.5 mg/kg/12 hr PO) are generally effective.

Seizures may be a result of the primary disease process (systemic lupus erythematosus), hyponatremia (water intoxication), hypocalcemia (tetany), hypertension, cerebral hemorrhage, or the uremic state itself. If possible, therapy should be directed toward the precipitating cause. Diazepam is the most effective agent in controlling seizures. It should be remembered that its metabolic products are excreted in the urine and may accumulate in patients with renal insufficiency.

Except in the presence of hemolysis (hemolytic-uremic syndrome, lupus) or bleeding, the *anemia* of acute renal failure is generally mild (hemoglobin 9–10 g/dL), is primarily a result of volume expansion (hemodilution), and does not require transfusion. Blood loss from active bleeding should be replaced appropriately.

In patients with hemolytic anemia or prolonged renal failure, if hemoglobin levels fall below 7 g/dL, blood should be given. In hypervolemic patients, blood transfusion carries the risk of further volume expansion, which may produce hypertension, heart failure, and pulmonary edema. Slow (4–6 hr) transfusion with fresh (to minimize the amount of potassium administered) packed red blood cells (10 mL/kg) diminishes the risk of hypervolemia. In the presence of severe hypervolemia, anemia should be corrected during dialysis.

The *diet* of most previously healthy and well-nourished children who suddenly develop acute renal failure should be restricted initially to fats and carbohydrates, given the likelihood that the acute renal failure will resolve or respond to therapy within a reasonably brief time. Restriction of sodium, potassium, and water administration is important. If renal failure persists beyond 3 days, then an expanded oral diet for renal failure or parenteral hyperalimentation with essential amino acids should be considered.

Indications for *dialysis* in acute renal failure may include various combinations of the following factors: acidosis, electrolyte abnormalities (especially hyperkalemia), central nervous system disturbances, hypertension, fluid overload, and heart failure. Early initiation of dialysis has significantly improved the survival of children with acute renal failure.

Continuous hemofiltration is useful in patients with acute renal failure (especially those with unstable cardiopulmonary dynamics, severe coagulopathies, and unavailability of the peritoneal cavity due to surgery or trauma), fluid overload, and severe electrolyte or acid-base disturbances. Hemofiltration is an extracorporeal therapy in which fluid, electrolytes, and small- and medium-sized solutes are continuously removed from the blood over an extended period by a process called convection or ultrafiltration (Fig. 543–1). In convection, water is moved by pressure through a semipermeable membrane, bringing along other molecules (urea). The blood volume is reconstituted by intravenous infusion of a substitution fluid having a desirable electrolyte composition similar to the blood.

The filter, of which there are several sizes, contains thousands of highly permeable hollow-fiber capillaries that produce a filtrate that is similar to the glomerular filtrate (protein-free, solute concentration similar to the plasma water). The merits of hemofiltration are summarized in Table 543–3.

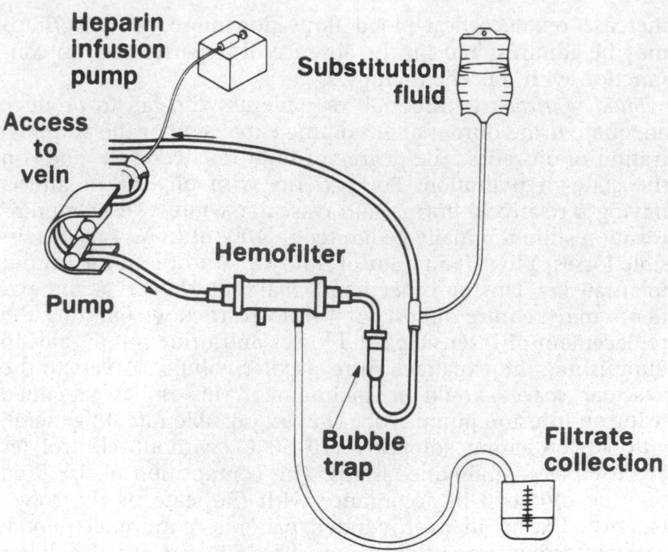

Figure 543–1 Schematic representation of continuous venovenous hemofiltration. (From Amicon, Inc; Diafilter Hemofilters. Beverly, MA, WR Grace, 1990. Used by permission.)

Hemofiltration is performed by two basic configurations. In continuous arteriovenous hemofiltration (CAVH), the blood is pumped through the filter by the patient's heart; the driving force for filtration is the arterial blood pressure. The advantage is that in the absence of a blood pump, filtration decreases or stops if the blood pressure falls. Disadvantages include inadequate production of filtrate in patients with marginal cardiac function and the need for long-term arterial catheterization, which may lead to vascular damage. Vascular access is generally obtained by catheterization of the femoral artery and vein, the brachial artery and jugular vein, or the umbilical vessels. In continuous venovenous hemofiltration (CVVH), blood is moved through the circuit (see Fig. 543–1) by a pump. The rate of filtrate formation is dependent on the pressure generated by the pump speed and is independent of the blood pressure. Because filtration continues despite profound hypotension, a patient's blood pressure must be continuously monitored. Because only venous access is required, double-lumen catheters placed into the subclavian or femoral veins may be used.

In patients who are undergoing CAVH or CVVH and who have inadequate solute removal, dialysate may be circulated through the filter on the ultrafiltrate side of the membrane. This technique, called hemodiafiltration, increases solute removal by adding diffusion to convection.

TABLE 543–3 Merits of Continuous Hemofiltration

Advantages	Disadvantages
Hemodynamic stability	Total body heparinization (bleeding)
Avoids rapid osmolar changes and diminished systemic vascular resistance of hemodialysis	Clotting of filter
Continuous therapy	Inadequate removal of fluid or solutes in certain patients
Around the clock	Infection of access catheter or substitution fluid
Stabilizes volume and composition of body fluids	Leaking from blood lines
Avoids rapid shifts in electrolyte levels	
Controlled fluid and solute removal	
Slow correction of fluid and electrolyte abnormalities	
Can replace ultrafiltrate with large amounts of hyperalimentation fluid	

In certain patients with acute renal failure, careful medical management may minimize complications and delay the need for dialysis; other patients eventually require dialysis for the uremic state itself. The life-threatening complications of uremia are hemorrhage, pericarditis, and central nervous system dysfunction; their precise causes are unknown. The risk of developing these complications correlates more closely with the level of BUN than with that of creatinine.

PROGNOSIS. The prognosis for recovery of renal function depends on the disorder that precipitated the renal failure. In general, recovery of function is likely after renal failure resulting from prerenal causes, the hemolytic-uremic syndrome, acute tubular necrosis, acute interstitial nephritis, or uric acid nephropathy. On the other hand, recovery of renal function is unusual when renal failure results from most types of rapidly progressive glomerulonephritis, bilateral renal vein thrombosis, or bilateral cortical necrosis.

Allgren RL, Marbury TC, Noor Rahman S, et al: Anaritide in acute tubular necrosis. N Engl J Med 336:828, 1997.
Allon M, Shanklin N: Effect of bicarbonate administration on plasma potassium in dialysis patients: Interactions with insulin and albuterol. Am J Kidney Dis 28:508, 1996.
Better OS, Rubinstein I, Winaver JM, et al: Mannitol therapy revisited (1940–1997). Kidney Int 51:886, 1997.
Brater DC: Diuretic therapy. N Engl J Med 339:387, 1998.
Cuthbertson BH: Dopamine in oliguria. Br Med J 314:690, 1997.
Denton MD, Chertow GM, Brady HR: "Renal-dose" dopamine for the treatment of acute renal failure: Scientific rationale, experimental studies and clinical trials. Kidney Int 49:4, 1996.
Ellis EN, Pearson D, Robinson L, et al: Pump-assisted hemofiltration in infants with acute renal failure. Pediatr Nephrol 7:434, 1993.
Forni LG, Hilton PJ: Continuous hemofiltration in the treatment of acute renal failure. N Engl J Med 336:1303, 1997.
Mindell JA, Chertow GM: A practical approach to acute renal failure. Med Clin North Am 81:731, 1997.
Niaudet P, Haj-Ibrahim M, Gagnadoux M-F, et al: Outcome of children with acute renal failure. Kidney Int 17(Suppl):148, 1985.
Thadhani R, Pascual M, Bonventre JV: Acute renal failure. N Engl J Med 334:1448, 1996.

543.2 *Chronic Renal Failure*

ETIOLOGY. The etiology of chronic renal failure in childhood correlates closely with the age of the patient at the time when the renal failure is first detected. Chronic renal failure in children younger than 5 yr is commonly a result of anatomic abnormalities (hypoplasia, dysplasia, obstruction, malformations), whereas after age 5 yr acquired glomerular diseases (glomerulonephritis, hemolytic-uremic syndrome) or hereditary disorders (Alport syndrome, cystic disease) predominate.

PATHOGENESIS. Regardless of the cause of kidney damage, once a critical level of renal functional deterioration is reached, progression to end-stage renal failure is inevitable. The precise mechanisms resulting in progressive functional deterioration are unclear, but factors that may have important roles include ongoing immunologic injury, hemodynamically mediated hyperfiltration in surviving glomeruli, dietary protein and phosphorus intake, persistent proteinuria, and systemic hypertension. Ongoing deposition of immune complexes or anti–glomerular basement membrane (GBM) antibodies in the glomerulus may result in persistent glomerular inflammation that leads to eventual scarring.

Hyperfiltration injury may be an important final common pathway of ultimate glomerular destruction, independent of the initiating mechanism of renal injury. Once nephrons are lost for any reason, the remaining nephrons undergo structural and functional hypertrophy mediated, at least in part, by an increase in glomerular blood flow. The increased blood flow in association with dilatation of the afferent arterioles and angiotensin II–induced constriction of the efferent arterioles increase the driving force for glomerular filtration in the surviving nephrons. This beneficial "hyperfiltration" in surviving glomeruli, which serves to preserve renal function, may also damage these glomeruli by mechanisms that are not understood. Potential mechanisms of damage include the direct effect of the elevated hydrostatic pressure on the integrity of the capillary wall, the resultant increase in the passage of proteins across the capillary wall, or both. Ultimately, this leads to changes in the mesangium and epithelial cells with the development of glomerular sclerosis. As sclerosis advances, the remaining nephrons suffer an increasing excretory burden, resulting in a vicious cycle of increasing glomerular blood flow and hyperfiltration. Angiotensin-converting enzyme inhibition reduces hyperfiltration by inhibiting angiotensin II production, thereby dilating the efferent arteriole, and slows the progression of renal failure.

Experimental models of chronic renal insufficiency have shown that a high-protein diet accelerates the development of renal failure, perhaps by means of afferent arteriolar dilatation and hyperperfusion injury. Studies of humans confirm that in normal individuals, the GFR correlates directly with protein intake; however, dietary protein restriction does not consistently slow the progression of renal failure.

Some controversial studies using animal models suggest that dietary phosphorus restriction preserves renal function in chronic renal insufficiency. Whether this beneficial effect is due to the prevention of calcium-phosphate salt deposition in the blood vessels and tissues or to suppression of secretion of parathyroid hormone, a potential nephrotoxin, is unclear.

Persistent proteinuria or systemic hypertension due to any cause may directly damage the glomerular capillary wall, leading to glomerular sclerosis and initiation of hyperfiltration injury. Proteinuria and hypertension are dominant factors in the progression of renal insufficiency.

As renal function begins to deteriorate, compensatory mechanisms develop in the remaining nephrons to maintain a normal internal environment. When the GFR falls below 20% of normal, a complex constellation of clinical, biochemical, and metabolic abnormalities develops; together, these constitute the uremic state. The pathophysiologic manifestations of the uremic state are listed in Table 543–4.

CLINICAL MANIFESTATIONS. In patients developing chronic renal failure from glomerular or hereditary diseases, the renal disease is usually detected because of clinical manifestations apparent before the onset of renal insufficiency. The development of renal failure may be insidious, however, in patients having anatomic abnormalities, and their presenting complaints may be nonspecific (headache, fatigue, lethargy, anorexia, vomiting, polydipsia, polyuria, growth failure). Physical examination occasionally may be unrevealing, but most patients with chronic renal failure appear pale and weak and have hypertension. Patients having anatomic abnormalities, in whom the renal failure has developed slowly over several years, may also have growth retardation and rickets.

TREATMENT. The management of chronic renal failure requires close monitoring of a patient's clinical (physical examination, growth, and blood pressure) and laboratory status. Blood studies to be followed routinely include the hemoglobin (anemia), electrolytes (hyponatremia, hyperkalemia, acidosis), BUN and creatinine (nitrogen accumulation and level of renal function), calcium and phosphorus levels, and alkaline phosphatase activity (hypocalcemia, hyperphosphatemia, osteodystrophy). Periodic examination of intact parathyroid hormone (PTH) levels and roentgenographic studies of bone may be of value in detecting early evidence of osteodystrophy. Chest roentgenography and echocardiography may be helpful in assessing cardiac function. Nutritional status may be monitored by periodic evaluation of the serum albumin, zinc, transferrin, folic acid, and iron levels. Optimally, patients should be treated in conjunction with a medical center capable of supplying medi-

TABLE 543–4 Pathophysiology of Chronic Renal Failure

Manifestation	Mechanisms
Accumulation of nitrogenous waste products (azotemia)	Decline in glomerular filtration rate
Acidosis	Urinary bicarbonate wasting Decreased ammonia excretion Decreased acid excretion
Sodium wasting	Solute diuresis Tubular damage Functional tubular adaptation for sodium excretion
Sodium retention	Nephrotic syndrome Congestive heart failure Anuria Excessive salt intake
Urinary concentrating defect	Nephron loss Solute diuresis Increased medullary blood flow
Hyperkalemia	Decline in glomerular filtration rate Acidosis Excessive potassium intake Hypoaldosteronism
Renal osteodystrophy	Decreased intestinal calcium absorption Impaired production of 1,25-dihydroxyvitamin D by the kidneys Hypocalcemia and hyperphosphatemia Secondary hyperparathyroidism
Growth retardation	Protein-calorie deficiency Renal osteodystrophy Acidosis Anemia Inhibitors of insulin-like growth factors Unknown factors
Anemia	Decreased erythropoietin production Low grade hemolysis Bleeding Decreased erythrocyte survival Inadequate iron intake Inadequate folic acid intake Inhibitors of erythropoiesis
Bleeding tendency	Thrombocytopenia Defective platelet function
Infection	Defective granulocyte function Impaired cellular immune functions
Neurologic (fatigue, poor concentration, headache, drowsiness, loss of memory, slurred speech, muscle weakness and cramps, seizures, coma, peripheral neuropathy, asterixis)	Uremic factor(s) Aluminum toxicity
Gastrointestinal ulceration	Gastric acid hypersecretion—gastritis Reflux Decreased motility
Hypertension	Sodium and water overload Excessive renin production
Hypertriglyceridemia	Diminished plasma lipoprotein lipase activity
Pericarditis and cardiomyopathy	Unknown
Glucose intolerance	Tissue insulin resistance

cal, nursing, social service, and nutritional support as they progress to end-stage renal failure.

Diet in Chronic Renal Failure. In children with renal insufficiency, the growth rate diminishes when the GFR falls below 50% of normal. The precise cause of growth failure is unknown; a major factor is inadequate caloric intake (<70% of recommended dietary allowance). The optimal caloric intake in renal insufficiency is unknown, but an attempt should be made to equal or exceed (in patients with growth failure) the recommended daily caloric allowance for age. Caloric intake can be enhanced by adding to the diet unrestricted amounts of carbohydrate (sugar, jam, honey, glucose polymers: Polycose, Ross Laboratories, Columbus, OH) and fat (medium-chain triglycerides oil: MCT Oil, Mead Johnson and Company, Evansville, IN) as tolerated by a patient. If oral caloric intake is inadequate, intermittent or overnight nasogastric or gastrostomy tube feedings can be initiated. Recombinant human growth hormone therapy combined with optimal dialysis improves linear growth.

When BUN exceeds approximately 80 mg/dL, patients may develop nausea, vomiting, and anorexia. These symptoms result from accumulation of nitrogenous waste products and can be relieved by restricting dietary protein intake. Because children in renal failure continue to require adequate protein intake for growth, protein is provided at a level of 2.5 g/kg/24 hr and should consist of proteins of high biologic value that are metabolized primarily to usable amino acids rather than to nitrogenous wastes. The proteins of highest biologic value are those of eggs and milk, followed by meat, fish, and fowl. Because cow's milk contains a high concentration of phosphate, moderate restriction or the use of a formula containing a reduced amount of phosphate (Similac PM 60/40, Ross Laboratories, Columbus, OH), sometimes in conjunction with an oral phosphate binder (see renal osteodystrophy), may be indicated.

Owing to inadequate intake or dialysis losses, children with renal insufficiency may become deficient in water-soluble vitamins. These should be routinely supplied, using preparations such as Nephrocaps (Fleming, Fenton, MO). Zinc and iron supplements should be added only after deficiencies are confirmed. Supplementation with fat-soluble vitamins A, E, and K is not required.

Water and Electrolyte Management in Chronic Renal Failure. Until the development of end-stage renal failure requires the initiation of dialysis, water restriction is rarely necessary in children with renal insufficiency, because water needs are regulated by the thirst center in the brain.

Most children with renal insufficiency maintain normal sodium balance with the sodium intake derived from an appropriate diet. Some patients whose renal insufficiency is a consequence of anatomic abnormalities may waste sodium in the urine and require dietary salt supplementation. On the other hand, patients with high blood pressure, edema, or heart failure may require sodium restriction, sometimes in conjunction with aggressive furosemide therapy (1–4 mg/kg/24 hr).

In most children with renal insufficiency, potassium balance is maintained until renal function deteriorates to the level at which dialysis is initiated. Hyperkalemia may develop in patients having only moderate renal insufficiency as a result of excessive dietary potassium intake, the development of severe acidosis, or aldosterone deficiency (destruction of the juxtaglomerular apparatus). Hyperkalemia may be controlled by reducing dietary potassium intake and adding oral alkalizing agents and/or Kayexalate (Winthrop Pharmaceuticals, New York, NY), an oral resin that (in 1 g/kg/dose) binds to and removes potassium from the intestine.

Acidosis in Chronic Renal Failure. Acidosis develops in almost all children with renal insufficiency and need not be treated unless the serum bicarbonate falls below 20 mEq/L (mmol/L). Either Bicitra (1 mL equals 1 mEq of base) or sodium bicarbonate tablets (325 and 650 mg; 325 mg equals 4 mEq of base) may be used to raise the serum bicarbonate above 20 mEq/L (mmol/L).

Renal Osteodystrophy. The term *renal osteodystrophy* is used to indicate a spectrum of bone diseases resulting from defective mineralization due to renal failure. In children, the disease resembles rickets; in adults, osteomalacia. At any age, excessive suppression of PTH release may result in low bone turnover disease.

When the GFR declines to approximately 25% of normal, compensatory mechanisms to enhance phosphate excretion become inadequate, resulting in hyperphosphatemia, which promotes hypocalcemia. Both hypocalcemia and hyperphosphatemia stimulate PTH release, which enhances bone resorption to release calcium in an attempt to correct the hypocalcemia. Continued hypersection of PTH leads to fibrosis of the bone marrow space (*osteitis fibrosis cystica*).

In association with progressive renal damage, the kidneys also cannot convert adequate amounts of 25-hydroxycholecalciferol to the active vitamin D, 1,25-dihydroxycholecalciferol. Deficiency of active vitamin D decreases intestinal calcium absorption and diminishes the responsiveness of bone to PTH, further promoting hypocalcemia. Vitamin D deficiency also promotes PTH secretion, causing additional bone breakdown. Also see Chapters 44.10 and 706.

Clinical manifestations of renal osteodystrophy may include growth retardation, muscle weakness, bone pain, skeletal deformities, and slipped epiphyses.

Laboratory studies may demonstrate normal to decreased serum calcium, normal to increased phosphorus, and increased alkaline phosphatase and intact-PTH levels. Radiographs of the hands, wrists, and knees show subperiosteal resorption of bone with widening of the metaphyses.

The goals of treatment include normalization of the serum calcium and phosphorus levels and maintenance of the intact-PTH level in the range of 200–400 pg/mL. Hyperphosphatemia may be controlled with a low-phosphate formula (Similac PM 60/40) and by enhancing fecal phosphate excretion by using oral calcium carbonate, an antacid that also binds phosphate in the intestinal tract. The usual dose range is 1–4 tsp (Titralac, 3M Company, St. Paul, MN) or tablets (Os-Cal 500 tablets, Marion Laboratories, Kansas City, MO; regular strength Tums, SmithKline Beecham, Pittsburgh, PA) with each meal and before bed. Because aluminum may be absorbed from the gastrointestinal tract, especially in small children, and can lead to aluminum poisoning (dementia, osteomalacia), aluminum antacids should be used rarely, if ever, with periodic monitoring of the serum aluminum level.

Hypocalcemia may result from hyperphosphatemia, inadequate dietary intake, and decreased intestinal calcium absorption caused by a deficiency in the active form (1,25-dihydroxycholecalciferol) of vitamin D. If the serum calcium level remains low after correction of the serum phosphorus, oral calcium supplements (Neo-Calglucon syrup, Dorsey Pharmaceuticals, East Hanover, NJ; Os-Cal tablets, Marion Laboratories, Kansas City, MO; regular strength Tums, SmithKline Beecham, Pittsburgh, PA) at a dose of 500 2,000 mg/24 hr can be administered.

Vitamin D is converted to its active form (1,25-dihydroxycholecalciferol) by 1-hydroxylation in the kidneys. With severe kidney destruction, insufficient conversion results in vitamin D deficiency. Vitamin D therapy is indicated (1) in patients having persistent hypocalcemia despite reduction of the serum phosphorus level below 6 mg/dL and the addition of oral calcium supplements; and (2) in patients with osteodystrophy, as indicated by elevated serum alkaline phosphatase and PTH levels and roentgenographic evidence of rickets. Therapy may be initiated with one capsule (0.25 mg) per day of the active form of dihydroxyvitamin D (Rocaltrol, Roche Laboratories, Nutley, NJ) or 0.05–0.20 mg/24 hr of dihydrotachysterol solution (DHT oral solution, Roxane Laboratories, Columbus, OH), which is metabolized to its active form in the liver. The dose of vitamin D is progressively increased until the serum calcium level and alkaline phosphatase activity are normal, the intact-PTH level is reduced to 200–400 pg/mL, and roentgenographic healing of the rickets is seen. The dose of vitamin D should then be reduced to the initial level. Side effects of vitamin D therapy include reduction of renal function, hypercalcemia, and hyperphosphatemia. Because normal bone requires adequate levels of PTH to promote appropriate bone remodeling, oversuppression of PTH should be avoided because this results in low turnover (aplastic, adynamic) osteodystrophy.

Despite adequate nutritional intake and correction of osteodystrophy, electrolyte abnormalities, acidosis, and anemia, many children with chronic renal failure have marked growth retardation. Growth in these patients may be accelerated with recombinant human growth hormone therapy.

TABLE 543–5 Merits of Recombinant Human Erythropoietin Therapy

Benefits	Potential Complications
Avoid blood transfusions	Iron deficiency
Reduced sensitization to histocompatibility antigens	Most require iron therapy
Reduced exposure to infectious diseases	Hypertension
Improved appetite	Seizures
Enhanced physical fitness	Decreased dialyzer clearance
Increased activity during day	Hyperkalemia
Improved sleep	Clotting of vascular access
Improved well-being	

Anemia in Chronic Renal Failure. Anemia is common in chronic renal failure and is primarily the result of inadequate erythropoietin production by the failing kidneys, but inadequate dietary intake of iron and folic acid should not be overlooked. In most patients, the hemoglobin level stabilizes in the range of 6–9 g/dL; transfusion therapy is not indicated, because this would further suppress erythropoietin production. If the hemoglobin falls below 6 g/dL, 10 mL/kg of packed red blood cells should be administered cautiously (the small volume reduces the risk of circulatory overload). The problem of anemia has been alleviated with the introduction of recombinant human erythropoietin therapy. Erythropoietin can be administered subcutaneously to predialysis and peritoneal dialysis patients, and intravenously to patients on hemodialysis. The goal is to maintain hemoglobin concentration within the range of 11–12 g/dL. The merits of erythropoietin therapy are summarized in Table 543–5.

Hypertension in Chronic Renal Failure. Hypertensive emergencies should be treated with oral nifedipine (0.25–0.5 mg/kg) or intravenous administration of diazoxide (Hyperstat, Schering Corporation, Kenilworth, NJ). The dose of diazoxide is 1–3 mg/kg, up to a maximum of 150 mg; it is given within 10 sec by manual injection. When severe hypertension is associated with circulatory overload, 2–4 mg/kg of furosemide may also be administered at the rate of 4 mg/min (see Chapter 451). Sodium nitroprusside should be used with great caution in renal insufficiency, owing to the possible accumulation of toxic thiocyanate.

Treatment of sustained hypertension may include a combination of salt restriction (2–3 g/24 hr), furosemide (1–4 mg/kg/24 hr), propranolol (Inderal, Ayerst Laboratories, New York, NY; 1–6 mg/kg/24 hr), hydralazine (Apresoline, CIBA Pharmaceutical Company, Summit, NJ; 1–6 mg/kg/24 hr), and nifedipine (Pfizer Labs, New York, NY; 0.2–2.0 mg/kg/24 hr). Minoxidil and captopril should be used only in patients whose blood pressure is inadequately controlled with the previously mentioned measures and should be administered with the guidance of a pediatric nephrologist. Captopril may produce hyperkalemia.

Drug Dosage in Chronic Renal Failure. Because many drugs are excreted by the kidneys, their administration to patients with renal insufficiency must be altered to maximize effectiveness and minimize the risk of toxicity (Chapter 727).

543.3 End-Stage Renal Failure

The incidence of end-stage renal disease in children is 20 per million population. In the treatment of end-stage renal failure in children, the ultimate goal is a successful kidney transplant (Chapter 544).

Dialysis is generally initiated when a patient's creatinine level approaches 10 mg/dL, depending on the patient's clinical status, the results of other laboratory studies, and the availability of a kidney donor. If histocompatibility or other studies reveal that no family donor is available, patients are placed on a waiting list for a cadaver kidney in the hope that one will become available before dialysis is required. Children are usually hospitalized for initiation of dialysis. If, in preparation for transplantation, bilateral nephrectomies are required (for severe hypertension, vesicoureteral reflux, or chronic pyelonephritis), these may be done at this time.

Peritoneal dialysis is the standard technique for the majority of children requiring long-term dialysis. However, some require hemodialysis and the use of long-term indwelling subclavian vein catheters and arteriovenous fistulas created at the wrist.

In **continuous ambulatory peritoneal dialysis** (CAPD), dialysis across the peritoneal membrane removes excess body water through an osmotic gradient created by the glucose concentration in the dialysate; wastes are removed by diffusion from the peritoneal capillaries into the dialysate. CAPD is not as efficient as hemodialysis, but the fact that it is continuous around the clock (compared with 12–18 hr/wk for hemodialysis) permits the maintenance of satisfactory levels of BUN and creatinine. Access to the peritoneal cavity is achieved by inserting a soft Tenckhoff catheter through a midline infraumbilical incision; the catheter is brought out through the skin by means of a subcutaneous tunnel and connected to an extension tube that has a spike for insertion into the dialysis bag.

The parents (and patient, if more than 10–12 yr old) are then taught the techniques of connecting the bags of dialysate, allowing the dialysate to run in and dwell in the peritoneal cavity for the prescribed time, draining the dialysate back into the dialysate bag, and replacing the used bag of dialysate with a fresh one. Such exchanges are performed three to five times per day between arising and bedtime. Because the advantages of CAPD seem to far outweigh the risks (Table 543–6), CAPD is the optimal form of long-term dialysis for most children. Modifications of the procedure include mechanical devices for spiking the bags (with or without ultraviolet sterilization during the connection) and Y-shaped dual bag systems. The latter permits drainage of spent dialysate into an empty bag, followed by instillation of fresh dialysate from the second bag, after which the patient disconnects from the bag system by covering the end of the catheter tubing with a cap containing a povidone-iodine–impregnated sponge. These modifications have decreased the frequency of peritonitis and have improved patients' acceptance of the technique.

An alternative to CAPD is **continuous cyclic peritoneal dialysis** (CCPD). This procedure reverses the schedule of CAPD by providing the exchanges at night rather than during the day. The exchanges are performed automatically during sleep by a simple cycler machine. This permits an uninterrupted day of activities, a reduction in the number of connections and disconnections (which should decrease the risk of peritonitis), and a reduction in the time required by patients and parents to perform dialysis, reducing the risk of fatigue and burnout.

The success rate for kidney transplants in children older than 5 yr approximates that for adults, and successful grafts have been performed in children as small as 5 kg. Ongoing research into better and less toxic means to prevent graft rejection should improve these statistics. Psychologic aspects of care of these children are discussed in Chapters 28.1 and 37.

TABLE 543–6 Value of Continuous Ambulatory Peritoneal Dialysis (CAPD)

Advantages	Disadvantages
Rapid training	Catheter malfunction
Technical simplicity (no machines)	Infection
Greater mobility	Poor appetite
Minimal dietary restriction	Poor body image
Feel better than hemodialysis patients	Parental "burnout" (emotional exhaustion)
Steady state chemistries	
Can live far from medical center	Elevated serum lipid levels
Cheaper than hemodialysis	
Improved growth rate	
Fewer blood transfusions	

Becker N, Brandt JR, Sutherland TA, et al: Improved outcome of young children on nightly automated peritoneal dialysis. Pediatr Nephrol 11:676, 1997.

Bennett WM, Aronoff GR, Golper TA, et al (eds): Drug Prescribing in Acute Renal Failure, 2nd ed. Philadelphia, American College of Physicians, 1991.

Burton C, Harris KPG: The role of proteinuria in the progression of chronic renal failure. Am J Kidney Dis 27:765, 1996.

Eberst ME, Berkowitz LR: Hemostasis in renal disease: Pathophysiology and management. Am J Med 96:168, 1994.

Feld LG, Lieberman E, Mendoza SA, et al: Management of hypertension in the child with chronic renal disease. J Pediatr 129:S18, 1996.

Fine RN: Growth hormone treatment of children with chronic renal insufficiency, end-stage renal disease and following renal transplantation-update 1997. J Pediatr Endocrinol Metabol 10:361, 1997.

Frasier CL, Arieff AI: Nervous system complications in uremia. Ann Intern Med 109:143, 1988.

Harvey E, Secker D, Braj B, et al: The team approach to the management of children on chronic peritoneal dialysis. Adv Renal Replacement Therapy 3:3, 1996.

Hellerstein S, Holliday MA, Grupe WE, et al: Nutritional management of children with chronic renal failure. Pediatr Nephrol 1:195, 1987.

Hercz G, Pei Y, Greenwood C, et al: Aplastic osteodystrophy without aluminum: The role of "suppressed" parathyroid function. Kidney Int 44:860, 1993.

Hruska KA, Teitelbaum SL: Renal osteodystrophy. N Engl J Med 333:166, 1995.

Hulstijn-Dirkmaat GM, Damhuis IHW, Jetten MLJ, et al: The cognitive development of pre-school children treated for chronic renal failure. Pediatr Nephrol 9:464, 1995.

Jabs K, Harmon WE: Recombinant human erythropoietin therapy in children on dialysis. Adv Ren Replace Ther 3:24, 1996.

Kuizon BD, Nelson PA, Salusky IB: Tube feeding in children with end-stage renal disease. Miner Electrolyte Metab 23:306, 1997.

MacKenzie HS, Brenner BM: Current strategies for retarding progression of renal disease. Am J Kid Dis 31:161, 1998.

Maschio G, Alberti D, Janin G, et al: Effect of angiotensin-converting enzyme inhibitor benazepril on the progression of chronic renal insufficiency. N Engl J Med 334:939, 1996.

Matsusaka T, Hymes J, Ichikawa I: Angiotensin in progressive renal diseases: Theory and practice. J Am Soc Nephrol 7:2025, 1996.

Morrison G, Murray TG: Electrolyte, acid-base, and fluid homeostasis in chronic renal failure. Med Clin North Am 65:429, 1981.

Pastan S, Bailey J: Dialysis therapy. N Engl J Med 338:1428, 1998.

Postlethwaite RJ, Eminson DM, Reynolds JM: Growth in renal failure: A longitudinal study of emotional and behavioural changes during trials of growth hormone treatment. Arch Dis Child 78:222, 1998.

Querfeld U: Disturbances of lipid metabolism in children with chronic renal failure. Pediatr Nephrol 7:749, 1993.

Ravelli AM: Gastrointestinal function in chronic renal failure. Pediatr Nephrol 9:756, 1995.

Sanchez CP, Salusky IB: The renal bone disease in children treated with dialysis. Adv Ren Replace Ther 3:14, 1996.

Sedman A, Friedman A, Boineau F, et al: Nutritional management of the child with mild to moderate chronic renal failure. J Pediatr 129:S13, 1996.

Vanholder R, Ringoir S: Infectious morbidity and defects of phagocytic function in end-stage renal disease: A review. J Am Soc Nephrol 3:1541, 1993.

Wingen AM, Fabian-Bach C, Schaefer F, et al: Randomised multicentre study of a low-protein diet on the progression of chronic renal failure in children. Lancet 349:1117, 1997.

CHAPTER 544
Renal Transplantation

Rodrigo E. Urizar

Long-term dialysis therapy for end-stage renal disease (ESRD) is frequently associated with failure to thrive, social maladaptation, lack of sexual maturation, and chronic encephalopathy (in the very young) and explains the reluctance to dialyze children extensively unless more acceptable alternatives are unavailable. Optimal treatment for children with ESRD is early renal transplantation (RT) from a living related

TABLE 544–1 Criteria for Performing Living Related Donor or Cadaveric Renal Transplantation in Pediatric Patients

Renal failure, chronic or end-stage renal disease of any etiology
Age, weight dependent to accommodate adult kidney
Good nutritional condition
Absence of
- Active infection
- Severe mental retardation
- Obstructed urinary tract (ileal loops, colonic diversions and bladder augmentation procedures are helpful in many instances)
- Gastrointestinal, liver, pancreas, or cardiovascular disease
- Serious psychosocial or behavioral problems, and noncompliance with medication and dietary regimen
- Sensitization in recipient
- Massive obesity

From Mauer SM, Nevins TE, Ascher N: Renal transplantation in children. In: *Edelman CM Jr (ed): Pediatric Kidney Disease. Boston, Little, Brown & Co, 1992, pp 941–981.*

donor (LRD-RT). Although less successful than LRD-RT, cadaveric (CAD) grafts are also used in children.

EPIDEMIOLOGY. The United States Renal Data System (USRDS) documents 20 new ESRD cases per million children each year, peaking at about age 11–15 yr. Before 1 yr of age, the incidence is 0.2 patient/million/year. An estimated 43–45% of 2,000 pediatric RTs performed in this country used kidneys donated by parents (37%) and, to a lesser extent, by siblings or other relatives (6%). Preemptive RT (carried out without previous dialysis) constitutes 22% of LRD engraftings. Indications for RT are noted in Table 544–1.

A well-functioning graft (LRD or CAD) may fully rehabilitate the patient. Nonetheless, the expectant graft recipient and relatives must understand that RT is not a permanent cure for ESRD. Furthermore, a poorly functioning transplanted kidney (uncontrollable progressive rejection) is associated with serious morbidity, mortality, and prospective return to long-term dialysis or initiation of it. The transiency of renal grafts has committed transplant programs to many engraftments per patient, a goal seriously hampered by the limited availability of CAD kidneys. The latter may reflect reticence of the lay and professional community (general public, nurses, physicians) toward organ donation.

Causes of ESRD vary with the patient's age and include congenital renal diseases (53%), glomerulonephritides (20%), focal segmental glomerular sclerosis (12%), metabolic diseases (10%), and miscellaneous (5%) (Tables 544–2 and 544–3). Although the glomerulopathies constitute a significant proportion of this population (particularly in 13–17 yr olds), congenital and obstructive processes predominate in the very young (<5 yr).

TREATMENT. Children weighing less than 15–20 kg have a transperitoneal graft via a midline incision; in those weighing more than 20 kg, the kidney is placed retroperitoneally in the right iliac fossa. Renal vessels are anastomosed to the recipient iliac vessels and the ureter is reimplanted in the bladder (ureteroneocystostomy). The extraperitoneal kidney facilitates access for future percutaneous biopsies. The donor and recipient clinical laboratory evaluations before RT are summarized in Table 544–4. Very young age of the recipient may be an obstacle to RT. For both LRD and CAD recipients, age less than 24 mo is associated with decreased graft survival. Nevertheless, some institutions accept patients 5–6 mo old weighing 5–6 kg to be engrafted with adult kidneys. In addition, pediatric patients transplanted with small kidneys do not fare as well as expected. Specifically, for CAD recipients, donor age of less than 6 yr is associated with decreased graft survival. Kidney grafts from LRD have significantly better survival than CAD-

TABLE 544–2 Most Frequent Hereditary-Metabolic Diseases of Childhood That Lead to End-Stage Renal Disease

Nephronophthisis—medullary cystic disease
Congenital nephrotic syndrome
Alport syndrome
Nephropathic and juvenile cystinosis
Primary oxalosis with oxaluria
Polycystic kidney disease (both infantile and adult varieties)
Nail-patella syndrome

TABLE 544–3 Individual Glomerulopathies of Childhood That May Progress to Chronic/End-Stage Renal Disease

Entity	Clinical Manifestation
Idiopathic rapidly progressive GN (crescentic GN, mediated by immune complexes)	Acute progressive renal failure
IgA nephropathies (Berger disease, anaphylactoid or Henoch-Schönlein purpura)	Chronic active GN, nephrotic syndrome, occasionally RPGN
Membranoproliferative glomerulonephritis (idiopathic; types I, II, and III)	Acute and chronic nephritic syndrome, occasionally RPGN
Focal segmental glomerulosclerosis	Nephrotic syndrome, progressive renal failure, acute/chronic active progressive GN, occasionally RPGN
Systemic lupus GN (WHO types 3 & 4)	
Microangiopathic syndromes (hemolytic, uremic, and thrombotic thrombocytopenic purpura syndromes)	Acute, chronic, and occasionally RPGN
Vasculitis (polyarteritis nodosa and Wegener granulomatosis)	Same
Anti–basement membrane antibody diseases (Goodpasture syndrome and idiopathic RPGN)	Acute, progressive renal failure, and RPGN with or without pulmonary renal syndrome

GN = Glomerulonephritis; RPGN = rapidly progressive glomerulonephritis.

TABLE 544–4 Clinical and Laboratory Evaluation of Prospective Living Related Kidney Donor and Recipient

Recipient

Complete history and physical examination—updated immunizations, including pneumococcal and hepatitis B
Transplant orientation session: patient (if old enough), parents, prospective donors, transplant surgeon or representative, nephrologist or representative, social worker
Laboratory data
- Blood group (ABO)
- Tissue typing (HLA-A, -B, -C, -D/DR), MLC
- Hepatitis, cytomegalovirus, varicella, Epstein-Barr virus panel
- CBC, complement (C3, C4), ANA, quantitative Ig
- Serum creatinine, electrolytes, cholesterol, liver function tests, coagulation profile, blood sugar
- Urinalysis, urine and throat cultures
- Chest radiograph (two-position), bone age films (if not previously available)
- Neurologic consult and EEG and CT scan of brain (for infants)
- Dental evaluation
- Cultures: exit site of all catheters and peritoneal fluid in patients undergoing CAPD
- Complete urologic evaluation for those with obstructive or congenital urinary tract problems
- 24-hr protein excretion

Donor

Complete history and physical examination
Chest radiographs
Electrocardiogram
Renal ultrasonography (IVP if necessary)
Laboratory
- CBC, ESR, ABO blood groups, HLA and MLC testing
- Coagulation profile
- Serum creatinine and electrolytes, liver function tests, blood sugar
- Urinalysis, urine culture, 24-hr urine protein and creatinine excretion
- Hepatitis, cytomegalovirus, herpes, Epstein-Barr virus antibody titers
- Renal angiogram

EEG = electroencephalogram; CT = computed tomography; CAPD = continuous ambulatory peritoneal dialysis; IVP = intravenous pyelogram; CBC = complete blood count; ESR = erythrocyte sedimentation rate.

From Mauer SM, Nevins TE, Ascher N: Renal transplantation in children. In: *Edelman CM Jr (ed): Pediatric Kidney Disease. Boston, Little, Brown & Co, 1992, pp 941–981.*

TABLE 544–5 Renal Diseases That May Recur in Pediatric Transplant Recipients

Condition	Results	Graft Damage
FSGS with nephrotic syndrome	Massive proteinuria with nephrosis (20–30%)	About 50% loss within 1 yr
MPGN	Mostly main dense deposit disease in glomeruli	Possibly 50% loss
Goodpasture syndrome and other RPGN Wegener granulomatosis	Rare in children but produce nephritic/nephrotic syndrome	High losses; exact number unknown because of rarity in children
IgA nephropathies	Development of IgA	Graft is seldom lost
HSP and IgA GN	Glomerular deposits	
HUS/TTP	More severe microangiopathy in graft; do not use cyclosporine	Occurs frequently but exact number unknown
Hyperoxalosis/oxaluria	Heavy deposits of Ca oxalate; kidney tissue destruction	High losses
Cystinosis	Cystine deposits in macrophages but not in kidney tissue	Good survival
De novo glomerulonephritis	Membranoproliferative Type I pattern—chronic rejection	Associated with graft loss
Membranous glomerulopathy	Associated with chronic rejection reaction	Graft loss
Alport syndrome	Lack of Goodpasture; antigen may induce production of anti–glomerular basement membrane antibodies by graft	Graft may be lost (lungs are spared)

FSGS = Focal segmental glomerular sclerosis; MPGN = membranoproliferative (or mesangiocapillary) glomerulonephritis; RPGN = crescentic, necrotizing rapidly progressive glomerulonephritis; HUS/TTP = hemolytic uremic thrombotic thrombocytopenic purpura syndromes (microangiopathies); HSP = Henoch-Schönlein purpura.
From Mauer SM, Nevins TE, Ascher N: Renal transplantation in children. In: *Edelman CM Jr (ed): Pediatric Kidney Disease. Boston, Little, Brown & Co, 1992, pp 941–981.*

RT. Approximately 90% of kidneys from LRD function adequately by 1 yr and 80% by the 3rd yr; the figures for CAD-RT are 72% and 65%, respectively. Generally CAD-RT in children is less favorable than in adults. In transplant recipients who are younger than 1 yr, the 2-yr graft survival is less than that of older children. Overall, by 39 mo after RT, 80% of LRD and 58% of CAD-RT were functional. Approximately 50% of graft failure has been due to rejection (RR). In 26%, RR was acute, whereas in 7% recurrence of the original renal disease induced the transplant failure. Although almost any glomerulopathy may redevelop in the graft, focal segmental glomerulosclerosis is observed most frequently (Table 544–5). Thrombosis-related kidney failure occurs in 15% of cases. In patients with LRD-RT, thrombotic episodes developed in very young recipients, presumably because of hemodynamic and/or technical problems. Conversely, graft thrombosis in CAD-RT is unaffected by the recipient age but is proportional to the donor age. In older children, acute renal failure is frequently due to tubular necrosis which may contribute to graft loss. In summary, identified risks for graft loss in the pediatric population include recipient age less than 2 yr, cadaveric donor less than 6 yr, previous renal transplantation, delayed graft function (acute tubular necrosis [ATN]), and lack of antilymphocyte therapy with antithymocyte globulin (ATGAM) or OKT3.

HISTOCOMPATIBILITY. The major histocompatibility complex (MHC) genes, present on the short arm of chromosome 6, encode the human leukocyte antigens (HLA) (Fig. 544–1). These are composed of class I proteins (tissue transplantation antigens) and cell-mediated immunotoxicity; class II proteins that control induction of immune response; and class III proteins, which include tumor necrosis factor (TNF) and complement components (C2 and C4). Each chromosome 6 contains all three classes of proteins: HLA-A, -B, and -C for class I; HLA-DP, -DQ, and -DR for class II; and C2, C4, and TNF for class III. Multiple and co-dominant alleles (polymorphism) exist for each protein: 23(A), 47(B), 8(C), 19(D), 16(DR), 3(DQ), and 6(DP). The A, B, and DR proteins are regarded as the most important in clinical transplantation. The HLA genes concentrated within a defined area of chromosome 6 are inherited as a packet or haplotype. Each individual inherits a haplotype of HLA genes from each parent concurrently, and both contribute to the offspring's HLA profile. The parent donor and child recipient share 50% of the haplotypes; a child typically has one representative antigen from class I, II, and III loci of each parent, whereas among siblings, all, some, or no haplotypes may be shared (2 haplotype, 1 haplotype, or 0 haplotype match). By definition, in the absence of recombination, a child is a 1 haplotype match to each parent and transmission (inheritance) of haplotypes occurs in a co-dominant mendelian fashion (Fig. 544–2). In the genetically related donor/recipient pair, the probability of a good HLA match increases and graft loss decreases.

Cellular expression of class I and II antigens, restricted to B and T lymphocytic cells and macrophages, multiplies with inflammation and by the action of lymphokines (interleukins 2, 4, and 5) secreted by T cells. CD4 (T-helper) and CD8 (T-suppressor) cell surface markers have high affinity for MHC (HLA) I (histocompatibility) antigens. When attached to cells displaying class I antigen, they transmit signals to synthesize cytokines or to lyse cells. In the acute and chronic rejection

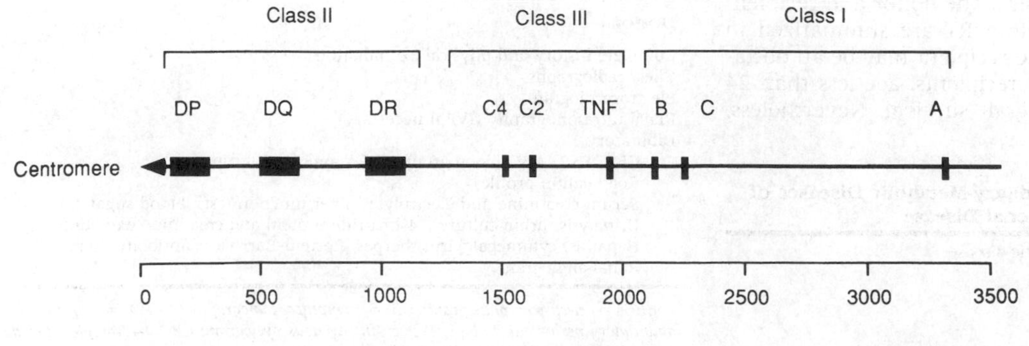

Figure 544–1 Organization of HLA region of chromosome 6. The loci for HLA-A, -B, and -C are found in the class I region. The loci encoding HLA-DR, -DQ, and -DP are found in the class II region, centromeric to class I. In between class I and II are the so-called class III genes, which encode some of the complement proteins as well as some cytokines. (From Grimm PC, Laufer J, Ettenger RB: The immunobiology of renal transplantation. *In:* Edelman CM Jr [ed]: Pediatric Kidney Disease. Boston, Little, Brown, 1992.)

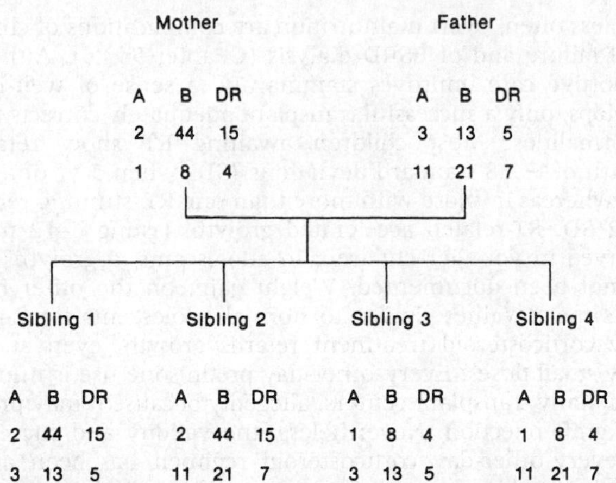

Figure 544–2 Inheritance of haplotypes and HLA profile in four theoretical siblings. Sibling 1 is a 1 haplotype match to siblings 2 and 3, and a 0 haplotype match to sibling 4. (From Terasaki PI, Park MS, Danovitch GM: Histocompatibility testing, crossmatching and allocation of cadaveric kidney transplants. *In:* Danovitch GM [ed]: Handbook of Kidney Transplantation. Boston, Little, Brown, 1992.)

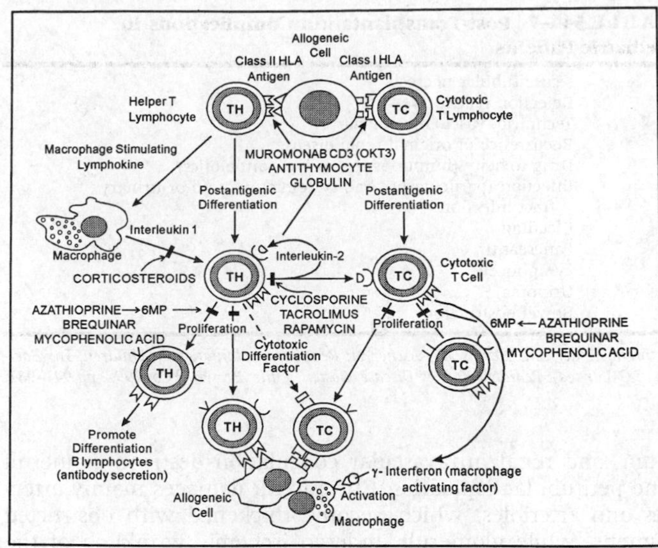

Figure 544–3 A representation of allograft rejection and the proposed sites of action for immunosuppressive medications. (From Shaefer MS, Collier DS: Immunosuppression for solid organ transplantation. Dialysis Transplant 22:542, 1993.)

reaction, both cellular and humoral mechanisms damage the graft, whereas antibodies, preformed or induced by T-helper cells, mediate accelerated (hyperacute) forms of the rejection reaction (Fig. 544–3). In the cellular variety, the graft is infiltrated by lymphocytes—T-helper and suppressor cells, B lymphocytes, macrophages, plasma cells, and monocytes—resulting in hemorrhage, edema, accumulation of polymorphonuclear leukocytes, activated platelets, and clotting.

Clinically, RR is manifested by swelling and tenderness of the graft, fever, oliguria, hypertension, and progressive elevation of serum creatinine level. Renal ultrasonography may reveal an enlarged graft with echogenic cortex, and a renal scan demonstrates decreased blood flow. Graft biopsy material shows signs of rejection with relatively intact glomeruli, mild ultrastructural changes, and negative glomerular immunofluorescence. Differentiation between RR, ATN, cyclosporine toxicity, and de novo occurrence of the original renal disease in the graft requires a kidney biopsy. *Hyperacute* or *accelerated rejections* are seldom observed because pretransplant cross matching (MLC) detects the presence of pre-existing anti-HLA antibodies. In this condition, the kidney becomes dark and soft as it is revascularized. Anti-HLA antibodies bind to endothe-

TABLE 544–6 Immunosuppressive Agents

Drug	Dose	Mechanisms	Side Effect(s)
Azathioprine (Imuran)	1–3 mg/kg/24 hr	Antiproliferative agent, purine analog; specific for T lymphocytes; decreases IgG and IgM antibodies; blocks primary and secondary immune response, both cell and humoral	Bone marrow suppression; hepatotoxicity; pancreatitis
Prednisone and methylprednisolone	5–10 mg/kg/24 hr 10–1,000 mg IV dose	Antilymphocyte action; decrease IL-1; decrease inflammation; decrease fungicidal action; decrease new cell formation; decrease monocyte migration	Psychologic disturbances; NaCl retention; volume expansion, weight gain (increased appetite); arterial hypertension; myopathy; infections; growth retardation
Cyclosporine (Sandimmune)	10 mg/kg/dose 4–6 mg/kg/24 hr (maintenance)	Fungal undecapeptide inhibits helper T-cell, lesser effect on T-suppressors; decreases IL-2	Nephrotoxicity, hepatotoxicity, hypertension, CNS toxicity (tremor, confusion, seizures, coma), IV reaction due to carrier, gingival hyperplasia, hypertrichosis
Tacrolimus (FK506)	0.05–0.1 mg/kg/24 hr continuous IV infusion 0.15–0.3 mg/kg/24 hr bid, PO	As per cyclosporine; used as primary agent or rescue therapy if cyclosporine fails	As per cyclosporine; possible steroid sparing and fewer side effects compared with cyclosporine
Antithymocyte Ig (ATGAM) and antilymphoblast (MALG)	10–30 mg/kg/24 hr 10–30 mg/kg/24 hr	Horse IgG polyclonal antibody to T lymphocytes Horse IgG antibody to T lymphocytes; same as above	Common to both: chills and fever (15–20%), erythema, pruritus, thrombocytopenia, anaphylactoid reaction, leukopenia Opportunistic infections (delayed side effect common to these drugs)
OKT3 (Orthoclone, Muromonab)	2.5–5.0 mg/24 hr	IgG2a binds to CD3 of T cells; removed by RES	Fever (78%), tachycardia (68%), chills (60%), headaches (40%), hypertension, nausea, vomiting, diarrhea, hypotension, and wheezing
Cellcept (Mycophenolate mofetil)	1,000–2,000 mg/24 hr	Antiproliferative agent, purine analog, inhibitor of adhesion molecule functions	Bone marrow suppression, hepatomas, pancreatitis, peptic ulcer, nausea, vomiting, diarrhea
Daclizumab	1 mg/kg (max 100 mg) Before transplant and 2, 4, 6, 8 wk after transplant	Monoclonal antibody Blocks IL-2 receptor	Few

RES = Reticuloendothelial system; CNS = central nervous system.
From Shaefer MS, Collier DS: Immunosuppression for solid organ transplantation. Dialysis Transplant 22:542, 1993.

TABLE 544–7 Post-Transplantation Complications in Pediatric Patients

Acute tubular necrosis
Rejection reaction
Technical: vascular, urologic
Recurrence of original renal disease
Drug toxicity (immunosuppressives, antibiotics)
Infection (particularly viral, systemic); wound or urinary tract infection
Bleeding
Pancreatitis
Lymphocele
Urinoma
Bowel obstruction

From Mauer SM, Nevins TE, Ascher N: Renal transplantation in children. In: Edelman CM Jr (ed): Pediatric Kidney Disease. Boston, Little, Brown & Co, 1992, pp 941–981.

lium, and renal intravascular coagulation destroys glomeruli and peritubular capillaries. Chronic RR damages mainly arteries and arterioles, which become thickened with obstructed lumens, while glomeruli undergo ischemic wrinkling of the basement membrane, Mononuclear cells infiltrate the interstitium, and arteriolar walls may display immunoglobulin deposits.

Histocompatibility testing is considered of paramount importance in prolonging the survival of LRD and CAD-RT. Having HLA-A, -B, -C, and -D/DR identical with an MLC nonstimulatory sibling donor produces the best graft survival results. The second best is the sibling or parent donor who has one haplotype match.

PRINCIPLES OF IMMUNOSUPPRESSION AND THERAPY OF REJECTION REACTION. Immune system stimulation by foreign protein (renal graft) results in activation of cell-mediated and humoral-mediated immune inflammation with cell destruction, or RR (see Fig. 544–3). (See also Chapter 136.) To subdue or control this process, which otherwise results in acute graft loss, the use of immunosuppressive medications is mandatory. The current drugs, doses, mechanism(s) of action, and side effects are listed in Table 544–6 and Figure 544–3. Sequential immunosuppression with azathioprine, cyclosporine, and low-dose corticosteroids is the most frequently used protocol. Fifty per cent of pediatric patients with LRD and 65% of those receiving CAD kidneys develop RR (with one or more acute episodes in most transplants); 62% of first episodes are successfully treated, whereas only 30% can be reversed when four or more crises have occurred. Chronic RR is relentless and unresponsive to therapy. In addition, concurrent RR with complications, particularly infection, places patients at higher risk of graft loss or death. If complications occur as a result of immunosuppression, one should treat the complication and abandon the graft. The use of ATGAM or OKT3 prophylactically in the immediate postoperative period improves the short-term graft outcome in 50% of pediatric CAD recipients. In addition, 6 mo after LRD or CAD transplant, these children have lower mean serum creatinine levels, the interval from transplant to first RR is lengthened, and the 1-yr graft survival is improved.

GROWTH AND RENAL TRANSPLANTATION. Stunted linear growth and, less often, overt malnutrition are complications of chronic renal failure and of ESRD dialysis (Chapter 543.3). Although supportive care improves stamina and a sense of well-being develops, only a successful transplant adequately corrects these abnormalities. Most children awaiting RT show retarded growth of −2.8 standard deviations (SD) when 5 yr of age or less, whereas in those with more than one RT, stunting reaches −3.2 SD. RT-related accelerated growth, lasting 6–12 mo, is observed in younger children; in adolescents, a growth spurt has not been documented. Weight gain, on the other hand, yields mean values similar to normal adolescents for 2–3 yr. Daily corticosteroid treatment retards growth, even at relatively small doses. Every-other-day prednisone use is unpopular in many transplant centers, allegedly because it may precipitate graft rejection. Nevertheless, the validity and success of the every-other-day corticosteroid regimen has been amply demonstrated in children. Steroids may be used daily for 6 mo in decreasing doses, then switched to every other day and tapered to 0.5–0.2 mg/kg given as a single dose every other day.

Judicious use of recombinant human growth hormone before and after RT improves linear growth significantly, although there are contradictory data indicating that graft function may decrease.

COMPLICATIONS. Complications that develop after RT are summarized in Table 544–7. Of these, infection is the most common cause of death during the first year after RT. Cytomegalovirus (CMV) infection is common. CMV antibody titers must be routinely screened in the donor and recipient. CMV infection may be primary, transmitted by the RT itself or by blood transfusions, or reactivated by immunosuppression in a seropositive patient (Table 544–8). The latter disease becomes apparent 1–3 mo after RT. About 90% may be self-limited and asymptomatic, and 5–10% lead to death; direct tissue damage by CMV may also result in graft loss. In addition, CMV disease usually triggers a rejection reaction. This poses a serious therapeutic dilemma: Although immunosuppression may reactivate the disease, it is indispensable for graft retention. Low-dose immunosuppressive agents with the use of antiviral drugs (ganciclovir and anti-CMV immunoglobulin intravenously) control the infection, and kidney biopsy helps monitor the RR. Immunosuppression must be discontinued in systemic (lung, brain, liver) CMV infection. If RR is unresponsive, the kidney should be abandoned. Concomitant infection with other viruses (varicella-zoster, Epstein-Barr, herpes simplex, hepatitis) requires thorough investigation and treatment. *Pneumocystis carinii* has all but disappeared owing to prophylactic use of trimethoprim-sulfamethoxazole, which also prevents bacterial urinary tract infections.

The mortality of pediatric RT recipients is 4–4.5%; in 40–45% of these, mortality is due to infection. The 2-yr patient survivals for LRD and CAD-RT are 95% and 92%, respectively. Renal diseases that recur in the transplanted kidney are listed in Table 544–5. Pediatric RT recipients may develop tumors, mainly lymphomas, sarcomas, and carcinomas, with significant death rates years after the RT.

TABLE 544–8 Types of Cytomegalovirus Infection in the Pediatric Renal Transplant Recipient

Type of Infection	Type of Patient	Symptomatic	Prevention
Primary	Seronegative with seropositive kidney, transfusion of leukocytes, blood products transfusion	60%	Avoidance of CMV infection or use active immunization (live attenuated vaccine: Towne strain; not very effective)
Reactivation	Seropositive before transplantation	<20%	High titer human hyperimmune anti-CMV globulin (CytoGam)
Superinfection	Seropositive patient transplanted with CMV+ kidney	40%	Human IgG concentrates (CMV nonspecific Gammagard or Polygam)

CMV, Cytomegalovirus.
From Snydman DR: Prevention of cytomegalovirus-associated diseases with immunoglobulin. Transplant Proc 23:131, 1991.

Bartosh SM, Aronson AJ, Swanson-Prewitt EE, et al: OKT3 induction in pediatric renal transplantation. Pediatr Nephrol 7:45, 1993.

Briscoe DM, Kim MS, Lillehei C, et al: Outcome of renal transplantation in children less than 2 years of age. Kidney Int 42:657, 1992.

Broyer M: Results and side effects of treating children with growth hormone after kidney transplantation—a preliminary report. Acta Pediatr 417 (suppl): 76, 1996.

Cochat P, Castelo F, Glastre C, et al: Outcome of cadaver kidney transplantation in small children. Acta Paediatr 83:78, 1994.

Ferraresso M, Kahan BD: New immunosuppressive agents for pediatric transplantation. Pediatr Nephrol 7:567, 1993.

First MR: Long-term complications after transplantation. Am J Kidney Dis 22:477, 1993.

Gagnadoux MF, Niaudet P, Broyer M: Non-immunologic risk factors in pediatric renal transplantation. Pediatr Nephrol 7:89, 1993.

Gruber SA, Chavers B, Skjel KL, et al: De novo cancer after pediatric kidney transplantation. Transplant Proc 23:1373, 1991.

Harmon WE: Opportunistic infections in children following renal transplantation. Pediatr Nephrol 5:118, 1991.

Harmon WE, Stablein D, Alexander SR, et al: Graft thrombosis in pediatric renal transplant recipients. Transplantation 51:406, 1991.

Harmon WE, Alexander SR, Tejani A, et al: The effect of donor age on graft survival in pediatric cadaver renal transplant recipients. A report of the North American Pediatric Renal Transplant Cooperative Study. Transplantation 54:232, 1992.

Iragorri S, Pillay D, Scrine M, et al: Prospective cytomegalovirus surveillance in pediatric renal transplant patients. Pediatr Nephrol 7:55, 1993.

Lewis R, Podbielski J, Sprayberry S, et al: Stability of renal allograft glomerular filtration rate associated with long-term use of cyclosporine-A. Transplantation 55:1014, 1993.

McEnery PT, Stablein DM, Arbus G, et al: Renal transplantation in children. A report of the North American Pediatric Renal Transplant Cooperative Study. N Engl J Med 326:1727, 1992.

McEnery PT, Alexander SR, Sullivan K, et al: Renal transplantation in children and adolescents: The 1992 annual report of the North American Pediatric Renal Transplant Cooperative Study. Pediatr Nephrol 7:711, 1993.

Suthanthiran M, Strom T: Renal transplantation. N Engl J Med 331:365, 1994.

Vincenti F, Kirkman R, Light S, et al: Interleukin-2 receptor blockade with daclizumab to prevent acute rejection in renal transplantation. N Engl J Med 338:161, 1998.

Yadim O, Grimm P, Ettenger RB: Renal transplantation in children. Pediatr Ann 20:657, 1991.

PART XXIII

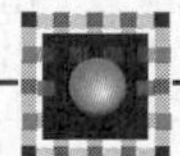

Urologic Disorders in Infants and Children

Jack S. Elder

CHAPTER 545

Congenital Anomalies and Dysgenesis of the Kidneys

The kidney is derived from the ureteral bud and the metanephric blastema. During the 5th wk of gestation, the ureteral bud arises from the mesonephric (wolffian) duct and penetrates the metanephric blastema, which is an area of undifferentiated mesenchyme on the nephrogenic ridge. The ureteral bud undergoes a series of approximately 15 generations of divisions, and by 20 wk of gestation forms the entire collecting system: the ureter, renal pelvis, calyces, papillary ducts, and collecting tubules. Under the inductive influence of the ureteral bud, nephron differentiation begins during the 7th wk of gestation. By 20 wk of gestation, when the collecting system is developed, approximately 30% of the nephrons are present. Nephrogenesis continues at a nearly exponential rate and is complete by 36 wk of gestation.

The fetal kidneys play a minor role in the maintenance of fetal salt and water homeostasis. The rate of urine production increases throughout gestation and at term, volumes have been reported to be 51 mL/hr. The glomerular filtration rate is 25 mL/min/1.73 m^2 at term and thereafter triples by 3 mo of age. The increase in glomerular filtration rate is due to a reduction in intrarenal vascular resistance and redistribution of intrarenal blood flow to the cortex, where more nephrons are located.

Dysgenesis of the kidney includes aplasia, dysplasia, hypoplasia, and cystic disease.

RENAL AGENESIS. Bilateral renal agenesis is incompatible with extrauterine life. Death occurs shortly after birth from pulmonary hypoplasia. This condition is termed *Potter syndrome*. The newborn has a characteristic facial appearance, termed *Potter facies* (Fig. 545–1). The eyes are widely separated and have epicanthic folds, the ears are low set, the nose is broad and compressed flat, the chin is receding, and there are limb anomalies. Bilateral renal agenesis should be suspected when maternal ultrasonography demonstrates oligohydramnios, nonvisualization of the bladder, and absent kidneys. The incidence is 1 in 3,000 births and represents 20% of newborns with the Potter phenotype. Other common causes of neonatal renal failure associated with the Potter phenotype include cystic renal dysplasia and obstructive uropathy. Less common causes are autosomal recessive polycystic kidney disease (infantile), renal hypoplasia, and medullary dysplasia.

Renal agenesis means that the kidney did not form because of an abnormal ureteral bud and is distinguished from aplasia, an extreme form of dysplasia in which a nubbin of nonfunctioning tissue is seen capping a normal or abnormal ureter. Clinically, this distinction may be difficult. *Hereditary renal adysplasia* is used to describe families in which renal agenesis, renal dysplasia, multicystic kidney (dysplasia), or a combination, occurs in a single family. This disorder has an autosomal dominant inheritance pattern with a penetrance of 50–90% and variable expression. Associated anorectal, cardiovascular, and skeletal abnormalities are seen in newborns with both hereditary renal adysplasia and bilateral renal agenesis.

Unilateral renal agenesis is often discovered during the course of an evaluation for other congenital anomalies or for urinary tract symptoms. Its incidence is increased in newborns with a single umbilical artery. With true agenesis, the ureter and the ipsilateral bladder hemitrigone are absent. The contralateral kidney undergoes compensatory hypertrophy, to some degree prenatally, but primarily after birth. Approximately 15% have contralateral vesicoureteral reflux, and most males have an ipsilateral absent vas deferens because the wolffian duct is

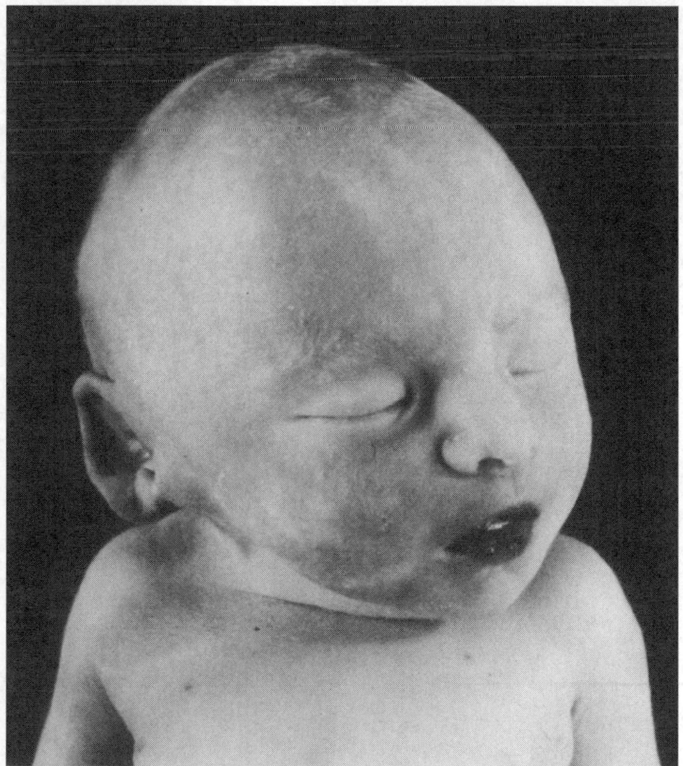

Figure 545–1 Stillborn with renal agenesis exhibiting the characteristic Potter facies. (Courtesy of Barbara Burke, M.D., Department of Laboratory Medicine and Pathology. University of Minnesota Hospital, Minnesota.)

absent. Because the wolffian and müllerian ducts are contiguous, müllerian abnormalities in girls are also common. The *Mayer-Rokitansky-Kuster-Hauser syndrome* refers to a group of associated findings that include unilateral renal agenesis or ectopia, ipsilateral müllerian defects, and vaginal agenesis. Some individuals are diagnosed as having unilateral renal agenesis based on a finding of an absent kidney on ultrasonography or excretory urography. Some of these patients actually were born with a hypoplastic kidney or a multicystic dysplastic kidney that underwent complete cyst regression. The specific diagnosis is not critical. However, if the finding of an absent kidney is based on an ultrasonogram, a functional imaging study such as an excretory urogram or renal scan should be performed because some of these patients may have an ectopic kidney. Individuals with a solitary kidney should avoid contact sports such as football and karate. If there is a normal contralateral kidney, renal function should remain normal over time.

RENAL DYSPLASIA AND HYPOPLASIA. The term *dysplasia* is technically a histologic diagnosis and refers to focal, diffuse, or segmentally arranged primitive structures, specifically primitive ducts, resulting from abnormal metanephric differentiation. Nonrenal elements, such as cartilage, may be present. The condition may affect all or only part of the kidney. If cysts are present, the condition is termed *cystic dysplasia.* If the entire kidney is dysplastic with a preponderance of cysts, the kidney is referred to as a *multicystic dysplastic kidney* (Fig. 545–2). The pathogenesis of dysplasia is multifactorial. The "bud" theory proposes that if the ureteral bud arises in an abnormal location, such as an ectopic ureter, there is inappropriate penetration and induction of the metanephric blastema that causes abnormal kidney differentiation—dysplasia. Renal dysplasia may also occur with severe obstructive uropathy early in gestation, as with the most severe cases of posterior urethral valves, or in a multicystic dysplastic kidney, in which a portion of the ureter is absent.

A multicystic kidney is a congenital condition in which the kidney is replaced by cysts, does not function, and may result from ureteral atresia. Renal size is highly variable. The incidence is approximately 1 in 2,000. Clinicians may incorrectly assume that *multicystic kidney* and *polycystic kidney* are synonymous terms. Polycystic kidney disease is an inherited disorder that may be autosomal recessive or autosomal dominant and affects both kidneys. A multicystic kidney is usually unilateral and is not inherited. Bilateral multicystic kidneys are incompatible with life.

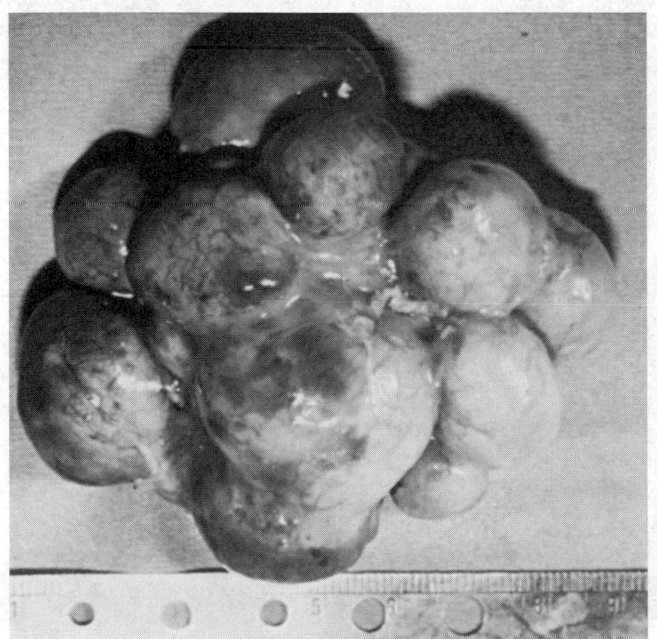

Figure 545–2 Surgical specimen of a multicystic dysplastic kidney associated with ureteral atresia.

Multicystic dysplastic kidney is the most common cause of an abdominal mass in the newborn. In many cases it is discovered incidentally during antenatal sonography. In some individuals, the cysts are identified prenatally and postnatally; no renal tissue is identified because of cyst regression in utero. Contralateral vesicoureteral reflux is identified in 15%, and contralateral hydronephrosis is present in 5–10% of patients. Sonography shows the characteristic appearance of a kidney replaced by multiple cysts of varying sizes that do not communicate, and no identifiable parenchyma is present; the diagnosis should be confirmed with a renal scan, which should demonstrate nonfunction. A voiding cystourethrogram is also advisable because of the high incidence of contralateral reflux. Management is controversial. There have been a few reports of renin-mediated hypertension and Wilms tumor arising in these kidneys. Neoplasms arise from the stromal, not the cystic, component. Consequently, even if the cysts regress completely, the likelihood that the kidney could develop a neoplasm is not altered. Because of the occult nature of these potential problems, annual follow-up with sonography and blood pressure measurements is recommended. If there is an abdominal mass, any cysts enlarge, the stromal core increases in size, or hypertension develops, nephrectomy is recommended. Alternatively, in lieu of follow-up screening, nephrectomy may be performed through a 2.5–3-cm flank incision when the child is 6–12 mo old. The Section on Urology of the American Academy of Pediatrics has an ongoing registry to determine the long-term risk of the nonoperative management of multicystic kidneys.

Renal hypoplasia refers to a small nondysplastic kidney that has less than the normal number of calyces and nephrons. The term refers to a group of conditions with an abnormally small kidney and should be distinguished from aplasia, in which the kidney is rudimentary. If the condition is unilateral, the diagnosis usually is made incidentally during evaluation for another urinary tract problem or hypertension. Bilateral hypoplasia usually presents with the manifestations of chronic renal failure and is a leading cause of end-stage renal disease during the 1st decade of life. A history of polyuria and polydipsia is common. Urinalysis results may be normal. A rare form of bilateral hypoplasia is called *oligomeganephronia,* in which the number of nephrons is markedly reduced but those present are markedly hypertrophied.

The *Ask-Upmark kidney,* also termed *segmental hypoplasia,* refers to small kidneys, usually weighing not more than 35 g, with one or more deep grooves on the lateral convexity, underneath which the parenchyma consists of tubules resembling those in the thyroid gland. It is unclear whether the lesion is congenital or acquired. Most patients are 10 yr or older at diagnosis and have severe hypertension. Nephrectomy usually controls the hypertension.

ANOMALIES IN SHAPE AND POSITION. During renal development the kidneys normally ascend from the pelvis into their normal position behind the ribs. The normal process of ascent and rotation of the kidney may be incomplete, resulting in renal ectopia or nonrotation. The ectopic kidney may be in a pelvic, iliac, thoracic, or contralateral position. If it is contralateral, in 90% of individuals there is fusion of the two kidneys. The incidence of renal ectopia is approximately 1 in 900.

Renal fusion anomalies are common. The lower poles of the kidneys may fuse in the midline, resulting in a *horseshoe kidney* (Fig. 545–3). Horseshoe kidneys occur in 1 in 500 births but are seen in 7% of patients with Turner's syndrome. Horseshoe kidney is one of the many renal anomalies that occur in 30% of these patients. Wilms tumors are four times more frequent in children with horseshoe kidneys than in the general population. In addition, stone disease and hydronephrosis secondary

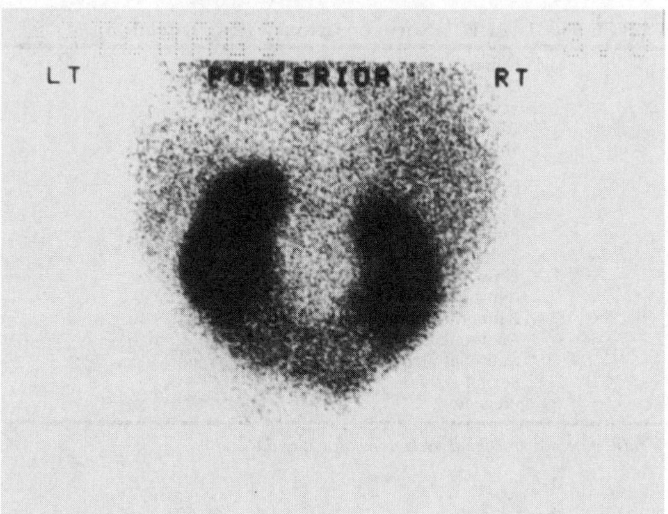

Figure 545–3 Isotopic renogram showing the characteristic configuration of a horseshoe kidney with an isthmus of functioning parenchyma.

to ureteropelvic junction obstruction are potential late complications. There also appears to be a slightly increased incidence of multicystic dysplastic kidney affecting one of the two sides of a horseshoe kidney. With *crossed fused ectopia,* one kidney crosses over to the other side and the parenchyma of the two kidneys fuse. Renal function is generally normal. The most common finding is that the left kidney may cross over and fuse with the lower pole of the right kidney. The insertion of the ureter does not change. In addition, the adrenal glands remain in their normal positions. The clinical significance of this anomaly is that if renal surgery is necessary, the blood supply is variable and may make partial nephrectomy more difficult.

Baudoin P, Provoost AP, Molenaar JC: Renal function up to 50 years after unilateral nephrectomy in childhood. Am J Kidney Dis 21:603, 1993.

Bauer SB: Anomalies of the kidney and ureteropelvic junction. *In:* Walsh PC, Retik AB, Vaughan ED Jr, Wein AJ (eds): Campbell's Urology, 7th ed. Philadelphia, WB Saunders, 1998, pp 1708–1755.

Elder JS, Hladky D, Selzman AA: Outpatient nephrectomy for non-functioning kidneys. J Urol 154:712, 1995.

Glassberg KI: Renal dysplasia and cystic disease of the kidney. *In:* Walsh PC, Retik AB, Vaughan ED Jr, Wein AJ (eds): Campbell's Urology, 7th ed. Philadelphia, WB Saunders, 1998, pp 1757–1813.

Homsy YL, Anderson JH, Oudjhane K, et al: Wilms tumor and multicystic dysplastic kidney disease. J Urol 159:2256, 1997.

Maluf NSR: On the enlargement of the normal congenitally solitary kidney. Br J Urol 79:836, 1997.

Minevich E, Wacksman J, Phipps L, et al: The importance of accurate diagnosis and early close followup in patients with suspected multicystic dysplastic kidney. J Urol 158:1301, 1997.

Selzman AA, Elder JS: Contralateral vesicoureteral reflux in children with a multicystic kidney. J Urol 153:1252, 1995.

Wacksman J, Phipps L: Report of the multicystic kidney registry: Preliminary findings. J Urol 150:1870, 1993.

Webb NJA, Lewis MA, Bruce J, et al: Unilateral multicystic dysplastic kidney: The case for nephrectomy. Arch Dis Child 76:31, 1997.

CHAPTER 546
Urinary Tract Infections

(Also see Chapter 527)

PREVALENCE AND ETIOLOGY. Approximately 3–5% of girls and 1% of boys acquire a urinary tract infection (UTI). In girls, the average age at the first diagnosis is 3 yr, which coincides with the onset of toilet training. In boys, most UTIs occur during the 1st yr of life; UTIs are much more common in uncircumcised boys. The prevalence of UTIs varies with age. During the 1st yr of life, the male:female ratio is 2.8:5.4:1. Beyond 1–2 yr, there is a striking female preponderance, with a male:female ratio of 1:10.

Urinary tract infections are caused mainly by colonic bacteria. In females, 75–90% of all infections are caused by *Escherichia coli,* followed by *Klebsiella* and *Proteus.* Some series report that in males older than 1 yr of age, *Proteus* is as common as *E. coli;* others report a preponderance of gram-positive organisms in males. *Staphylococcus saprophyticus* is a pathogen in both sexes. Viral infections, particularly adenovirus, may also occur, especially as a cause of cystitis.

UTIs have been considered an important risk factor for the development of renal insufficiency or end-stage renal disease. Some have questioned the importance of UTI as a risk factor because only 2% of children with current renal insufficiency report a history of UTI. This paradox is probably secondary to better recognition of the risks of UTI and prompt diagnosis and therapy.

CLASSIFICATION OF URINARY TRACT INFECTION. There are three basic forms of UTI: pyelonephritis, cystitis, and asymptomatic bacteriuria.

Clinical pyelonephritis is characterized by any or all of the following: abdominal or flank pain, fever, malaise, nausea, vomiting, jaundice in neonates, and occasionally diarrhea. Some newborns and infants may show nonspecific symptoms such as poor feeding, irritability, and weight loss. These symptoms are an indication that there is bacterial involvement of the upper urinary tract. Involvement of the renal parenchyma is termed *acute pyelonephritis,* whereas if there is no parenchymal involvement, the condition may be termed *pyelitis.* Acute pyelonephritis may result in renal injury, which is termed *pyelonephritic scarring.*

Cystitis indicates that there is bladder involvement and includes dysuria, urgency, frequency, suprapubic pain, incontinence, and malodorous urine. Cystitis does not cause fever and does not result in renal injury.

Asymptomatic bacteriuria refers to children who have a positive urine culture without any manifestations of infection and occurs almost exclusively in girls. This condition is benign and does not cause renal injury, except in pregnant women, in whom asymptomatic bacteriuria, if left untreated, can result in a symptomatic UTI. Some girls are mistakenly identified as having asymptomatic bacteriuria when they are actually are symptomatic, experiencing day or night incontinence or perineal discomfort.

PATHOGENESIS AND PATHOLOGY. Nearly all UTIs are ascending infections. The bacteria arise from the fecal flora, colonize the perineum, and enter the bladder via the urethra. In uncircumcised boys, the bacterial pathogens arise from the flora beneath the prepuce. In some cases, the bacteria ascend to the kidney to cause pyelonephritis. In rare cases, renal infection may occur by hematogenous spread.

If bacteria ascend from the bladder to the kidney, acute pyelonephritis may occur. Normally the simple and compound papillae in the kidney have an antireflux mechanism that prevents urine from flowing in a retrograde manner into the collecting tubules. Some compound papillae, typically located in the upper and lower poles of the kidney, allow intrarenal reflux. Infected urine then stimulates an immunologic and inflammatory response (Fig. 546–1). The result may cause renal injury and scarring (Fig. 546–2).

It was once assumed that infants were at greatest risk for renal scarring from acute pyelonephritis. Children of any age with a febrile UTI may have acute pyelonephritis with renal scarring. The exception to this observation is that if a child with UTIs has a normal 2,3-dimercaptosuccinic acid (DMSA)

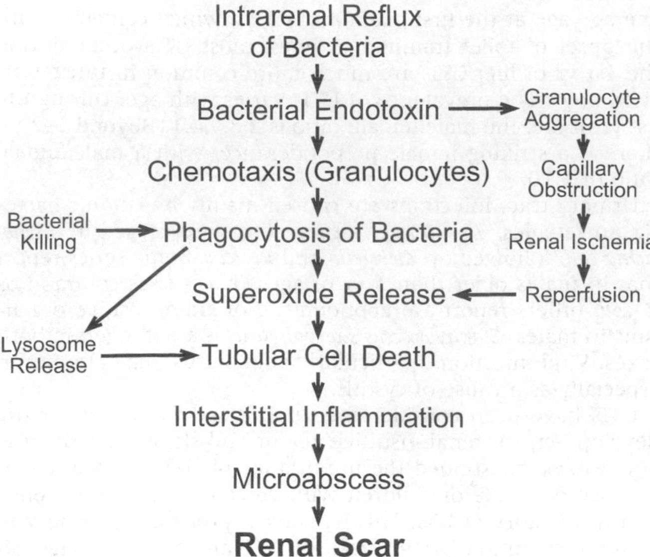

Figure 546–1 Pathogenesis of pyelonephritic scarring following acute pyelonephritis. (Adapted from Roberts JA: Pathogenesis of pyelonephritis. J Urol 129:1102, 1983.)

scan by 4 yr of age, the risk of pyelonephritogenic scarring from future UTIs is low.

Host risk factors for UTI are listed in Table 546–1. Vesicoureteral reflux is reviewed in Chapter 547. In girls, UTIs often occur at the onset of toilet training because of voiding dysfunction that occurs at that age. The child is trying to retain urine to stay dry, yet the bladder may have uninhibited contractions forcing urine out. The result may be high-pressure, turbulent urine flow or incomplete bladder emptying, both of which increase the likelihood of bacteriuria. Voiding dysfunction may occur in the toilet-trained child who voids infrequently. Obstructive uropathy resulting in hydronephrosis increases the risk of UTI because of urinary stasis. Urethral instrumentation during a voiding cystourethrogram or nonsterile catheterization may infect the bladder with a pathogen. Constipation can increase the risk of UTI because it may cause voiding dysfunction.

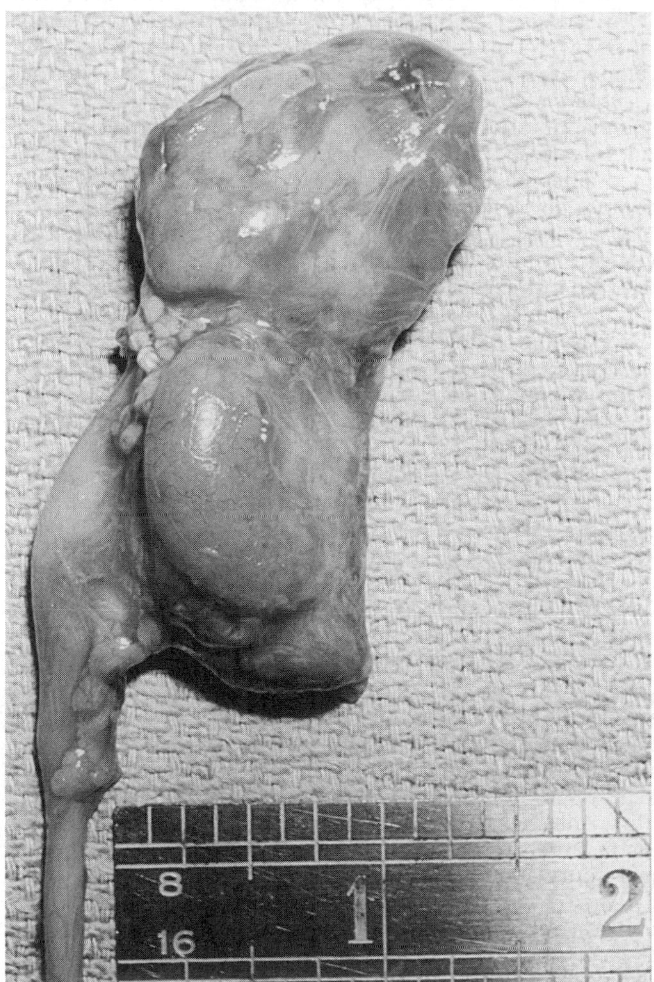

Figure 546–2 Scarred kidney from recurrent pyelonephritis.

TABLE 546–1 Risk Factors for Urinary Tract Infection

Risk Factors
Female
Uncircumcised male
Vesicoureteral reflux*
Toilet training
Voiding dysfunction
Obstructive uropathy
Urethral instrumentation
Wiping from back to front
Bubble bath
Tight clothing—underwear
Pinworm infestation
Constipation
P fimbriated bacteria*
Anatomic abnormality (e.g., labial adhesion)
Neuropathic bladder
Sexual activity
Pregnancy

Risk increased for clinical pyelonephritis, not cystitis.

The pathogenesis of UTI is based in part on the presence of bacterial pili or fimbriae on the bacterial surface. There are two types of fimbriae, type I and type II. Type I fimbriae are found on most strains of *E. coli*. Because attachment to target cells can be blocked by D-mannose, these fimbriae are referred to as "mannose-sensitive." They have no role in pyelonephritis. The attachment of type II fimbriae is not inhibited by mannose, and these are known as "mannose-resistant." These fimbriae are expressed by only certain strains of *E. coli*. The receptor for type II fimbriae is a glycosphingolipid that is present on both the uroepithelial cell membrane and red blood cells. The Gal 1–4 Gal oligosaccharide fraction is the specific receptor. Because these fimbriae can agglutinate by P blood group erythrocytes, they are known as P fimbriae. Bacteria with P fimbriae are more likely to cause pyelonephritis. Between 76 and 94% of pyelonephritogenic strains of *E. coli* have P fimbriae, compared with 19–23% of cystitis strains.

Other host factors for UTI include anatomic abnormalities precluding normal micturition, such as a labial adhesion. This lesion acts as a barrier and causes vaginal voiding. A neuropathic bladder may cause UTIs if there is incomplete bladder emptying or detrusor-sphincter dyssynergia, or both. Sexual activity is associated with UTIs in girls, generally because of incomplete bladder emptying. Finally, during pregnancy 4–7% have asymptomatic bacteriuria, which can result in a symptomatic UTI.

Xanthogranulomatous pyelonephritis is a rare type of renal infection characterized by granulomatous inflammation with giant cells and foamy histiocytes. It may present clinically as a renal mass or an acute or chronic infection. Renal calculi, obstruction, and infection with *Proteus* or *E. coli* contribute to the development of this lesion, which usually requires total or partial nephrectomy.

DIAGNOSIS. To make the diagnosis of a UTI, the urine must be cultured. A UTI may be suspected based on the symptoms or findings on urinalysis, or both, but a culture is necessary for confirmation and appropriate therapy.

The diagnosis of UTI depends on having the proper sample

of urine. There are several ways to obtain a urine sample; some are more accurate than others.

In toilet-trained children, a *midstream urine sample* is usually satisfactory. Most studies have failed to show any benefit to formally cleansing the introitus before obtaining the specimen. If the culture shows greater than 100,000 colonies of a single pathogen, or if there are 10,000 colonies and the child is symptomatic, it is considered a UTI. In uncircumcised males, the prepuce must be retracted; if the prepuce is not retractable, this method of urine collection is not reliable.

In infants, the application of an adhesive, sealed, *sterile collection bag* after disinfection of the skin of the genitals can be useful, particularly if the culture is negative. However, a positive culture may reflect a contaminant, particularly in girls and uncircumcised boys. In such cases, if the urinalysis result is positive, the patient is symptomatic, and there is a single organism cultured with a colony count greater than 100,000, there is a presumed UTI. However, if any of these criteria are not met, confirmation of infection with a catheterized sample is recommended (see next paragraph).

When greater assurance as to the possibility of infection is needed, a *catheterized specimen* must be obtained. Proper skin preparation and good technique of catheterization are important. The use of a No. 5 French polyethylene feeding tube in infants or a No. 8 French tube with proper lubrication in older children minimizes the chance of urethral trauma and contamination. Only a few milliliters need to be aspirated with a syringe to obtain the urine sample. Catheterization shortly after spontaneous voiding produces a measure of the residual urine in the bladder and helps assess problems related to bladder emptying.

Prompt plating of the urine sample is important because if the urine sits at room temperature for more than 60 min, overgrowth of a minor contaminant may suggest a UTI, when in fact the urine is uninfected. Placing the sample in a refrigerator is a reliable method of storing the urine until it can be cultured.

A urinalysis should be obtained from the same specimen as that cultured. Pyuria (leukocytes in the urine) suggests infection, but infection can occur in the absence of pyuria; consequently, this finding is more confirmatory than diagnostic. Conversely, pyuria can be present without UTI. Nitrites and leukocyte esterase are usually positive in infected urine. Microscopic hematuria is common in acute cystitis. White blood cell casts in the urinary sediment suggest renal involvement, but these are rarely seen. If the child is asymptomatic and the urinalysis result is normal, it is highly unlikely that the urine is infected. However, if the child is symptomatic, a UTI is possible, even if the urinalysis result is negative.

With acute renal infection, leukocytosis, neutrophilia, and elevated erythrocyte sedimentation rate and C-reactive protein are common. The latter two are nonspecific markers of bacterial infection, and elevation does not mean than the child has acute pyelonephritis. With a renal abscess, the white blood count is markedly elevated to greater than 20,000 to 25,000. Because sepsis is common in pyelonephritis, particularly in infants and in any child with obstructive uropathy, blood cultures should be considered.

Acute hemorrhagic cystitis is frequently caused by *E. coli*; it has been attributed also to adenovirus types 11 and 21. Adenovirus cystitis is more frequent in males; it is self-limiting, with hematuria lasting approximately 4 days. *Eosinophilic cystitis* is a rare form of cystitis of obscure origin that occasionally has been found in children. The usual symptoms are those of cystitis with hematuria, ureteral dilatation, and filling defects in the bladder caused by masses that consist histologically of inflammatory infiltrates with eosinophils.

TREATMENT. Acute cystitis should be treated promptly to prevent its possible progression to pyelonephritis. If the symptoms are severe, a specimen of bladder urine is obtained for culture and treatment is started immediately. If the symptoms are mild or the diagnosis doubtful, treatment can be delayed until the results of culture are known, and the culture can be repeated if the results are uncertain. For example, if midstream culture grew between 10^4 and 10^5 colonies of a gram-negative organism, a second culture may be obtained by catheterization before treatment is initiated. If treatment is initiated before the results of a culture and sensitivities are available, a 3- to 5-day course of therapy with trimethoprim-sulfamethoxazole (see later) is effective against most strains of *E. coli*. Nitrofurantoin (5–7 mg/kg/24 hr in three to four divided doses) is also effective and has the advantage of being active against *Klebsiella-Enterobacter* organisms. Amoxicillin (50 mg/kg/24 hr) is also effective as initial treatment but has no clear advantages over the sulfonamides or nitrofurantoin.

In acute febrile infections suggestive of pyelonephritis, a 14-day course of broad-spectrum antibiotics capable of reaching significant tissue levels is preferable. If the child is acutely ill, parenteral treatment with ceftriaxone (50–75 mg/kg/24 hr, not to exceed 2 g) or ampicillin (100 mg/kg/24 hr) with an aminoglycoside such as gentamicin (3 to 5 mg/kg/24 hr in three divided doses) is preferable. The potential ototoxicity and nephrotoxicity of aminoglycosides should be considered, and serum creatinine levels must be obtained prior to initiating treatment as well as daily thereafter as long as treatment continues. Treatment with aminoglycosides is particularly effective against *Pseudomonas*, and alkalinization of urine with sodium bicarbonate increases their effectiveness in the urinary tract. The combination of sulfamethoxazole and trimethoprim (Cotrim, Bactrim, Septra), either orally or intravenously, is effective against a variety of gram-negative organisms other than *Pseudomonas* and is considered by some authorities to be the treatment of choice for oral therapy. Nitrofurantoin should not be used in children with a febrile UTI because it does not achieve significant renal tissue levels. Ciprofloxacin is an alternative agent for resistant microorganisms, particularly *Pseudomonas*, in patients older than 17 yr. Children who are dehydrated, are unable to drink fluids, or in whom sepsis is a possibility should be admitted to the hospital for intravenous rehydration and intravenous antibiotic therapy. In some children with a febrile UTI, intramuscular injection of a loading dose of ceftriaxone followed by oral therapy with a broad-spectrum antimicrobial agent is effective.

Children with a renal or perirenal abscess or with infection in obstructed urinary tracts require surgical or percutaneous drainage in addition to antibiotic therapy and other supportive measures.

A urine culture should be performed 1 wk after the termination of treatment of any UTI to ensure that the urine remains sterile. Given the tendency of urinary tract infections to recur even in the absence of predisposing anatomic factors, a follow-up urine culture should be performed periodically for 1–2 yr, even when the child is asymptomatic.

If recurrences are frequent, identifying predisposing factors to UTI is beneficial. Fox example, many school-aged girls have voiding dysfunction, and treatment of this condition often reduces the likelihood of recurrent UTI. Some children with urinary tract infections void infrequently and many also have severe constipation. Counseling of parents and patients to try to establish more normal patterns of voiding and defecation may be helpful in controlling recurrences. In addition, prophylaxis against reinfection, using either the sulfamethoxazole-trimethoprim combination or nitrofurantoin at one third of the normal therapeutic dose once a day, is often effective. Prophylaxis with amoxicillin also may be effective, but the risk of breakthrough UTI is higher because bacterial resistance may be induced. Other indications for long-term prophylaxis (neurogenic bladder, urinary tract stasis and obstruction, reflux, and calculi) are discussed in other chapters.

The main consequences of chronic renal damage caused by

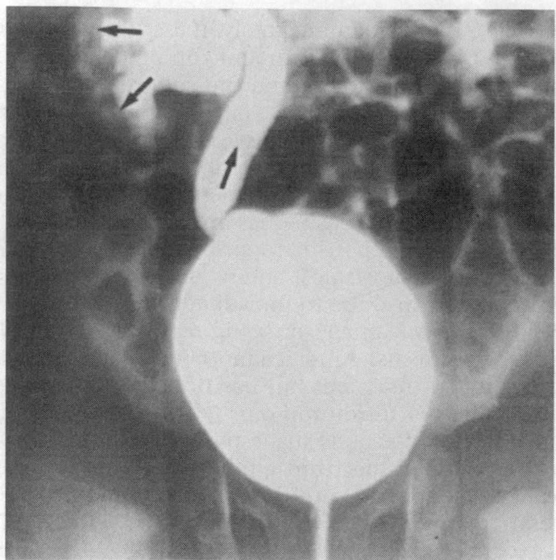

Figure 546–3 Intrarenal reflux. Voiding cystourethrogram in a young infant male with a past history of a urinary tract infection. Note the right vesicoureteral reflux with ureteral dilatation, with opacification of the renal parenchyma representing intrarenal reflux.

pyelonephritis are arterial hypertension and renal insufficiency; when they are found they should be treated appropriately (see Chapters 451 and 543).

IMAGING STUDIES. The goal of imaging studies in children with a UTI is to identify anatomic abnormalities that predispose to infection. A renal ultrasonogram should be obtained to rule out hydronephrosis and renal or perirenal abscesses; ultrasonography also may show acute pyelonephritis (in 30% of cases) by demonstrating an enlarged kidney. Power Doppler ultrasonography has been slightly more sensitive but is unreliable in identifying all cases. Ultrasonography demonstrates 30% of renal scars. Normally, the difference in renal lengths between the two kidneys is less than 1 cm, and a larger disparity may be an indication of impaired renal growth. Renal ultrasonography is also sensitive for detecting pyonephrosis, a condition that may require prompt drainage of the collecting system by percutaneous nephrostomy.

A voiding cystourethrogram (VCUG) is also indicated in all children younger than 5 yr with a UTI, any child with a febrile UTI, school-aged girls who have had two or more UTIs, and any male with a UTI. The most common finding is vesicoureteral reflux, which is identified in approximately 40% of patients (Fig. 546–3). Timing of the VCUG is controversial. The study is often delayed for 2–6 wk to allow inflammation in the bladder to resolve. The incidence of reflux is identical, irrespective of whether the VCUG is obtained during treatment of the UTI or after 6 wk. Consequently, obtaining the VCUG before the child is discharged from the hospital is recommended. If available, radioisotopic voiding cystourethrography instead of a contrast VCUG can be used in girls; this technique causes less radiation exposure to the gonads than does the contrast study. In boys, radiographic definition of the urethra is important; accordingly, contrast VCUG is recommended for the initial work-up.

Some parents question the need for a VCUG if the ultrasonogram is normal, feeling that the cystogram is traumatic to the child. Sonography is insensitive in detecting reflux; indeed, only 40% of children with reflux have any abnormality on sonography. The VCUG should not be performed using general anesthesia, as the study is incomplete without a voiding phase and it subjects the child unnecessarily to the risk and cost of anesthesia. In selected cases, oral or nasal midazolam (0.5 mg/kg oral route, 0.2 mg/kg nasal route), which causes anterograde amnesia and anxiolysis, may be used. We have found that this medication is efficacious and safe and provides an acceptable experience with VCUG. Vital signs are monitored and pulse oximetry is used; no anesthesiologist is present.

When the diagnosis of acute pyelonephritis is uncertain, renal scanning with technetium-labeled DMSA or glucoheptonate is useful. The presence of a parenchymal filling defect on the renal scan supports the diagnosis of pyelonephritis but may not differentiate an acute from a chronic process. The DMSA scan shows a filling defect (i.e., acute pyelonephritis) in approximately 50% of children with a febrile UTI, irrespective of age. In children with grade III, IV, or V reflux, 80–90% of patients with a febrile UTI have a focal defect. In patients with acute pyelonephritis, approximately 50% will acquire a scar in that site over the following 5 mo. If the DMSA scan is normal during a febrile UTI, no scarring results from that particular infection. Computed tomography is another diagnostic tool that can diagnose acute pyelonephritis, but clinical experience with DMSA is much greater. The routine use of DMSA scans during the acute episode in children with clinical manifestations of pyelonephritis and positive urine cultures is unnecessary.

If vesicoureteral reflux is present, a DMSA scan (Fig. 546–4) often is performed to assess whether renal scarring is present. The DMSA is considered the most sensitive and accurate study for demonstrating scarring. In the past, excretory urography often was used, but it is not as sensitive as the DMSA scan in demonstrating renal scarring; in addition, visualization of the collecting system in infants and young children often is suboptimal, there is a slight risk of a contrast allergy, and it can take 1–2 yr for a renal scar to appear on the urogram. Computed tomography also has been used by some to evaluate the upper urinary tract, as it is effective in demonstrating renal scarring (Fig. 546–5).

The frequently performed cystoscopies and measurements

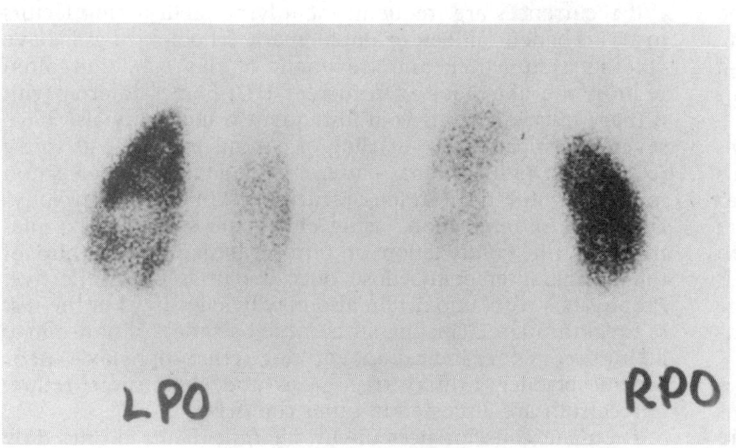

Figure 546–4 DMSA renal scan showing bilateral photopenic areas indicative of renal scarring.

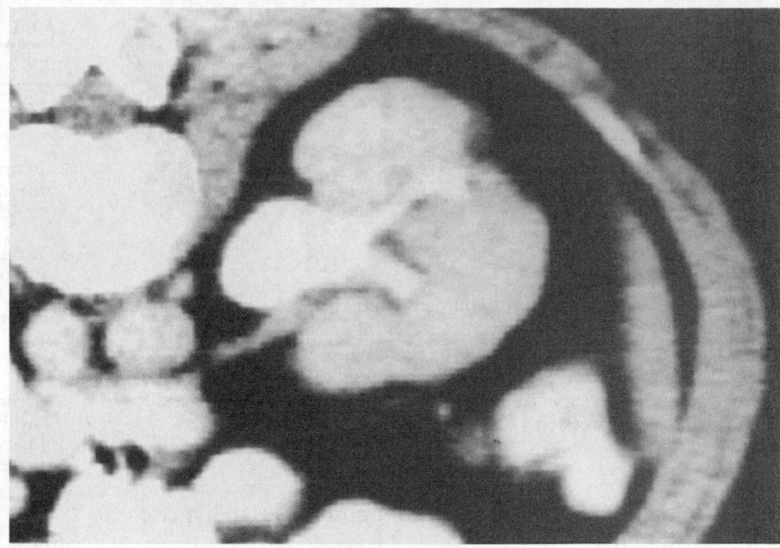

Figure 546–5 CT scan showing an area of parenchymal thinning corresponding to an underlying calyx, characteristic of pyelonephritic scarring or reflux nephropathy.

of urethral caliber advocated for girls in the past contribute nothing to the therapeutic decisions to be made in children with UTIs. Narrowing of the female urethra was once postulated to be a contributing factor in the development of UTIs, but the urethras of girls with recurrent UTIs are not narrower than those of girls without infections.

Benador D, Benador N, Slosman DO, et al: Cortical scintigraphy in the evaluation of renal parenchymal changes in children with pyelonephritis. J Pediatr 124:17, 1994.

Benador D, Benador N, Slosman DO, et al: Are younger children at highest risk of renal sequelae after pyelonephritis? Lancet 349:17, 1997.

Chessare JB: Circumcision: Is the risk of urinary infection really the pivotal issue? Clin Pediatr 31:100, 1992.

Coulthard MB, Lambert HJ, Keir MJ: Occurrence of renal scars in children after their first referral for urinary tract infection. Br Med J 315:918, 1997.

Dacher J-N, Pfister C, Monroc M, et al: Power Doppler sonographic pattern of acute pyelonephritis in children: Comparison with CT. AJR 166:1451, 1996.

Ditchfield MR, de Campo JF, Nolan TM, et al: Risk factors in the development of early renal cortical defects in children with urinary tract infection. AJR 162:1393, 1994.

Elder JS, Longenecker R. Premedication with oral midazolam for voiding cystourethrography in children: Safety and efficacy. AJR 164:1229, 1995.

Hoberman A, Chao HP, Keller DM, et al: Prevalence of urinary tract infections in febrile infants. J Pediatr 123:17, 1993.

Jakobsson B, Berg U, Svensson L: Renal scarring after acute pyelonephritis. Arch Dis Child 70:111, 1994.

Koff SA, Wagner TT, Jayanthi VR: The relationship among dysfunctional elimination syndromes, primary vesicoureteral reflux and urinary tract infections in children. J Urol 160:1019, 1998.

Lee H-J, Pyo J-W, Choi E-H, et al: Isolation of adenovirus type 7 from the urine of children with acute hemorrhagic cystitis. Pediatr Infect Dis J 15:633, 1996.

Loening-Baucke V: Urinary incontinence and urinary tract infection and their resolution with treatment of chronic constipation of childhood. Pediatrics 100:228, 1997.

Roberts JA: Factors predisposing to urinary tract infections in children. Pediatr Nephrol 10:517, 1996.

Rushton HG: The evaluation of acute pyelonephritis and renal scarring with technetium 99m-dimercaptosuccinic acid renal scintigraphy: Evolving concepts and future directions. Pediatr Nephrol 11:108, 1997.

Rushton HG: Urinary tract infections in children. Epidemiology, evaluation and management. Pediatr Clin North Am 44:1133, 1997.

Smellie JM, Poulton A, Prescol NP: Retrospective study of children with renal scarring associated with reflux and urinary infection. Br Med J 308:1193, 1994.

Smith EM, Elder JS: Double antimicrobial prophylaxis for breakthrough urinary tract infections in girls. Urology 43:708, 1994.

Stokland E, Hellstrom M, Jacobsson B, et al: Renal damage one year after first urinary tract infection: Role of dimercaptosuccinic acid scintigraphy. J Pediatr 129:815, 1996.

Uhari M, Nuutinen M, Turtinen J: Adverse reactions in children during long term antimicrobial therapy. Pediatr Infect Dis J 15:404, 1996.

Vernon SJ, Coulthard MG, Lambert HJ, et al: New renal scarring in children who at age 3 and 4 years had had normal scans with dimercaptosuccinic acid: Follow up study. Br Med J 315:905, 1997.

Wan J, Kaplinsky R, Greenfield S: Toilet habits of children evaluated for urinary tract infection. J Urol 154:797, 1995.

CHAPTER 547
Vesicoureteral Reflux

Vesicoureteral reflux is the retrograde flow of urine from the bladder to the ureter and renal pelvis. The ureter is normally attached to the bladder in an oblique direction, perforating the bladder muscle (detrusor) laterally and proceeding between the bladder mucosa and detrusor muscle, creating a flap-valve mechanism that prevents reflux (Fig. 547–1). Reflux occurs when the submucosal tunnel between the mucosa and detrusor muscle is short or absent or there is a weak detrusor muscle, or both. Reflux is usually a birth defect, occurs in families, and affects approximately 1% of children.

Reflux predisposes to renal infection (pyelonephritis) by facilitating the transport of bacteria from the bladder to the upper urinary tract. The inflammatory reaction caused by a pyelonephritic infection may result in renal injury or scarring. Extensive renal scarring impairs renal function and may result in renin-mediated hypertension, reflux nephropathy, renal insufficiency, end-stage renal disease, reduced somatic growth, and morbidity during pregnancy. Reflux nephropathy had once accounted for as much as 15–20% of end-stage renal disease in children and young adults. Currently, with greater attention to the management of urinary tract infections and a better understanding of reflux, it is a less common cause.

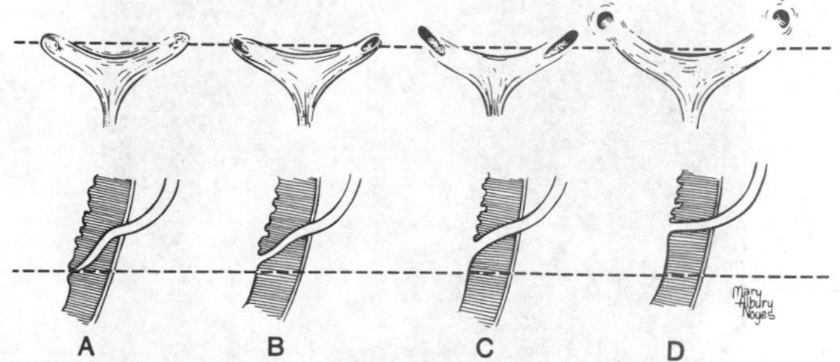

Figure 547–1 Normal and abnormal configuration of the ureteral orifices. Shown from left to right, progressive lateral displacement of the ureteral orifices and shortening of the intramural tunnels. *Top,* Endoscopic appearance. *Bottom,* Sagittal view through the intramural ureter.

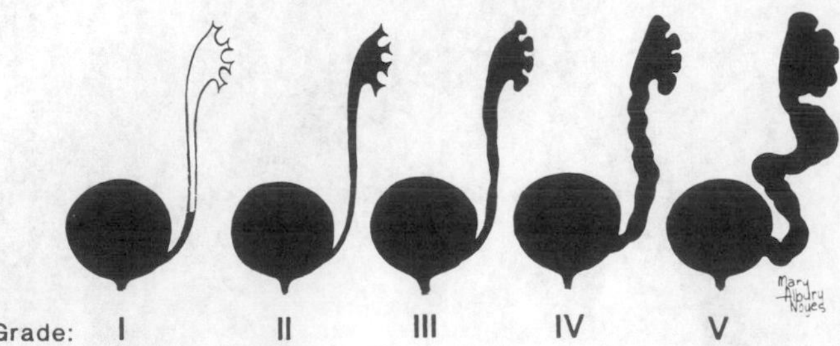

Figure 547–2 Grading of vesicoureteral reflux. Grade I: reflux into a nondilated ureter. Grade II: reflux into the upper collecting system without dilatation. Grade III: reflux into dilated ureter and/or blunting of calyceal fornices. Grade IV: reflux into a grossly dilated ureter. Grade V: massive reflux, with significant ureteral dilatation and tortuosity and loss of the papillary impression.

TABLE 547–1 Classification of Vesicoureteral Reflux

Type	Cause
1. Primary	Congenital incompetence of the valvular mechanism of the vesicoureteral junction
2. Primary associated with other malformations of the ureterovesical junction	Ureteral duplication Ureterocele with duplication Ureteral ectopia Paraureteral diverticula
3. Secondary to increased intravesical pressure	Neuropathic bladder Non-neuropathic bladder dysfunction Bladder outlet obstruction
4. Secondary to inflammatory processes	Severe bacterial cystitis Foreign bodies Vesical calculi Clinical cystitis
5. Secondary to surgical procedures involving the ureterovesical junction	

Nevertheless, it is one of the most common causes of hypertension in children.

CLASSIFICATION. Reflux severity is graded using the International Study Classification of I to V and is based on the appearance of the urinary tract on a contrast voiding cystourethrogram (VCUG) (Figs. 547–2 and 547–3). The more severe the reflux, the higher the rates of renal injury. Reflux severity is an indirect indication of the degree of abnormality of the ureterovesical junction.

Reflux may be primary or secondary (Table 547–1). Primary vesicoureteral reflux results from an anatomic deformity of the ureterovesical junction (see Fig. 547–1). Conditions such as bladder instability or cystitis can precipitate reflux or worsen pre-existing reflux if there is a marginally competent ureterovesical junction. In the most severe cases, there is such massive reflux into the upper tracts that the bladder becomes overdistended. This condition, termed the *megacystic-megaureter syndrome,* occurs primarily in males and may be unilateral or bilateral (Fig. 547–4). In this particular condition, reimplantation of the ureters into the bladder to correct reflux resolves the condition.

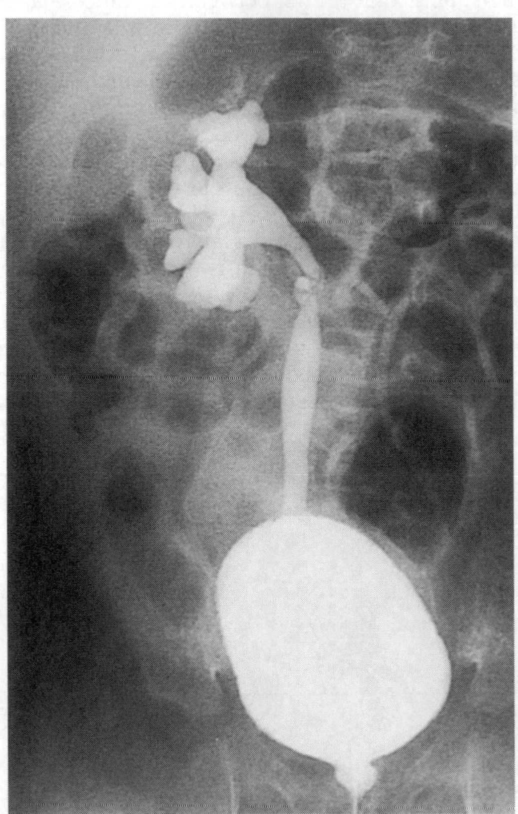

Figure 547–3 Voiding cystourethrogram (VCUG) showing grade IV right vesicoureteral reflux with intrarenal reflux.

Approximately 1 in 125 children has a duplication of the upper urinary tract in which two ureters rather than one drain the kidney. In a duplicated system, the lower pole ureter drains higher and more lateral in the bladder, and the upper pole ureter is typically inferomedial. Reflux occurs in as many as 50% of cases, usually into the lower ureter, which typically has a less competent valve, but in some cases reflux occurs into both the lower and upper systems (Fig. 547–5). With a duplication anomaly, some patients have an ectopic ureter, in which the upper pole ureter drains outside the bladder. If the ectopic ureter drains into the bladder neck, it usually is obstructed and often refluxes. Reflux into the lower pole ureter is also common. Duplication anomalies are common in children with a ureterocele, which is a cystic swelling of the intramural portion of the distal ureter. Often there is reflux into the associated lower pole ureter or the contralateral ureter. Reflux typically is present when the ureter enters a diverticulum (Fig. 547–6).

In children with neuropathic bladder, as occurs in myelomeningocele and sacral agenesis, reflux is present in 25% at

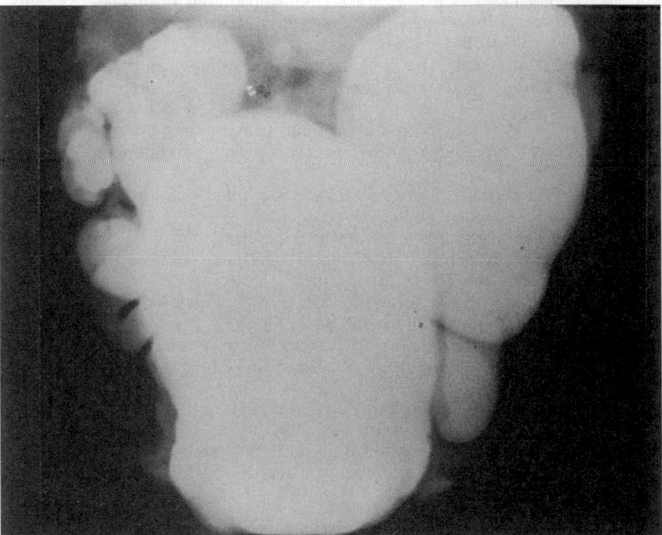

Figure 547–4 VCUG in male newborn with megacystic-megaureter syndrome. Note the massive ureteral dilatation due to high-grade vesicoureteral reflux. The bladder is very distended. There was no urethral obstruction or neuropathic dysfunction.

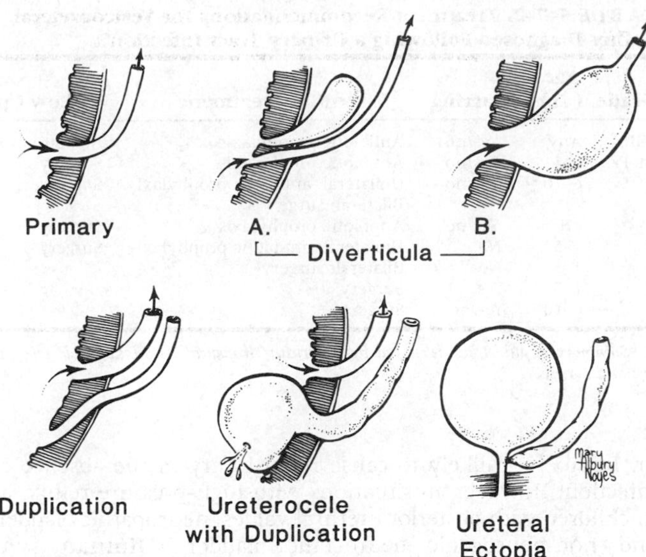

Figure 547–5 Various anatomic defects of the ureterovesical junction associated with vesicoureteral reflux.

birth. Reflux is seen in 50% of boys with posterior urethral valves. Clinically, reflux with increased intravesical pressures (as in detrusor-sphincter dyssynergia or bladder outlet obstruction) can result in renal injury, even in the absence of infection.

Primary reflux is found in association with a number of congenital urinary tract abnormalities. Fifteen per cent of children with a multicystic dysplastic kidney or renal agenesis have reflux into the contralateral kidney, whereas 15% of children with a ureteropelvic junction obstruction have reflux into either the hydronephrotic kidney or the contralateral kidney.

Reflux is an inherited trait. Approximately 35% of siblings of children with reflux also have reflux; the majority are asymptomatic. The likelihood of a sibling having reflux is independent of the grade of reflux or sex of the index child. Approximately 12% of asymptomatic siblings with reflux have evidence of renal scarring. In addition, 50% of offspring of women with reflux have reflux. Consequently, many believe that siblings of children with reflux should be screened even if they have not had a UTI. Screening with a radionuclide cystogram of all siblings 3 yr or younger and any sibling with a UTI is appropriate. Older siblings could undergo renal ultrasonography, and if an abnormality is found, cystography is recommended. Primary reflux is uncommon in African-Americans.

CLINICAL MANIFESTATIONS. Usually reflux is discovered during an evaluation for a urinary tract infection. In these children, 80% with reflux are female, and the average age at diagnosis is 2–3 yr. In other children, voiding cystourethrography is part of an evaluation of voiding dysfunction, renal insufficiency, hypertension, or other suspected pathology of the urinary tract. Primary reflux may be discovered during an evaluation of prenatal hydronephrosis. In this population, 80% of affected children are male, and the reflux grade usually is higher than in females diagnosed with a urinary tract infection.

DIAGNOSIS. Diagnosis of reflux generally requires catheterization of the bladder, instillation of a solution containing iodinated contrast or a radiopharmaceutical, and radiologic imaging of the lower and upper urinary tract—a VCUG or radionuclide cystogram, respectively. The bladder and upper urinary tracts are imaged during bladder filling and voiding. Reflux occurring during bladder filling is termed *low-pressure* or *passive reflux;* reflux occurring during voiding is termed *high-pressure* or *active reflux.* Children with passive reflux are less likely to show spontaneous reflux resolution than are children who exhibit only active reflux. Radiation exposure during radionuclide cystography is significantly less when compared with standard contrast cystography. However, the contrast study provides more anatomic information, such as demonstration of a duplex collecting system, ectopic ureter, paraurethral diverticulum, bladder outlet obstruction in boys, upper urinary tract stasis, and signs of voiding dysfunction. Furthermore, the reflux grading system is based on the appearance on VCUG. Consequently, the VCUG is used in most centers as the initial study. For follow-up evaluation, the radionuclide cystogram is often preferred because of the lower radiation exposure (Fig. 547–7).

Children undergoing cystography may be psychologically or emotionally traumatized by the catheterization, or both. Careful preparation by caregivers or administering oral or nasal midazolam before the study can result in a more acceptable

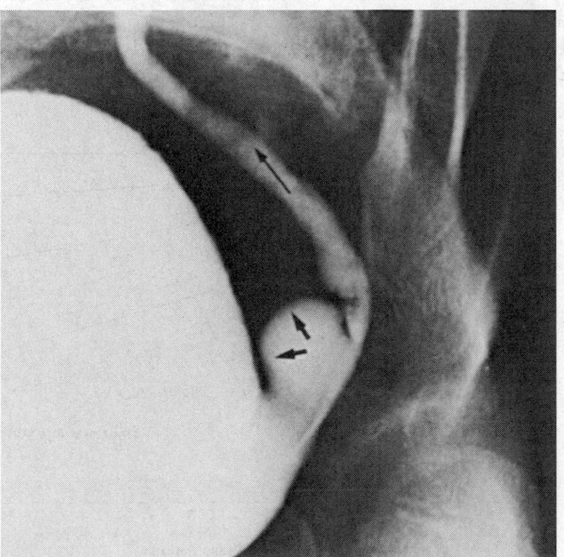

Figure 547–6 Reflux and bladder diverticulum. The voiding cystourethrogram demonstrates left vesicoureteral reflux and a paraureteral diverticulum.

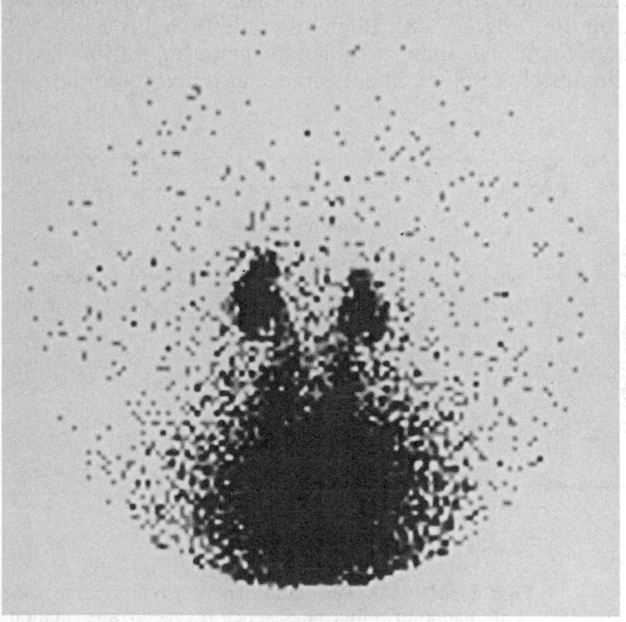

Figure 547–7 Radionuclide cystogram shows bilateral reflux.

experience. A technique of detecting reflux without catheterization is termed *indirect cystography* and involves injecting an intravenous radiopharmaceutical that is excreted by the kidneys, waiting for it to be excreted into the bladder, and imaging the lower urinary tract while the patient voids. This technique detects only 50% of reflux cases.

Once reflux is diagnosed, graded, and determined to be primary or secondary, it is important to assess the upper urinary tract. The goal of upper tract imaging is to assess whether renal scarring and associated urinary tract anomalies are present. Renal imaging can be performed by ultrasonography, excretory urography (intravenous pyelogram), or renal scintigraphy. Ultrasonography is a noninvasive method of evaluating the kidney, as it can demonstrate hydronephrosis, renal duplication with an obstructed upper pole system, and gross renal scars and allows one to monitor renal growth over time. Only 30% of renal scars are demonstrated with this technique. Intravenous pyelography involves injection of an iodinated contrast agent and provides good anatomic detail of the kidneys. Approximately 90% of scars are demonstrated with this technique. Renal scintigraphy usually involves dimercaptosuccinic acid, which demonstrates renal cortical detail well and is reliable in demonstrating nearly all renal scarring. It is less reliable than the other two studies in demonstrating renal anomalies such as hydronephrosis.

It is important to assess whether the child has evidence of voiding dysfunction, including urgency, frequency, diurnal incontinence, infrequent voiding, or a combination of these. In addition, bowel habits should be assessed. Children with bladder instability often require anticholinergic therapy and a voiding routine in addition to antibiotic prophylaxis.

Following diagnosis, the child's height, weight, and blood pressure should be measured. If upper tract imaging shows renal scarring, a serum creatinine measurement should be obtained. The urine should be assessed for infection and proteinuria. Cystoscopy is of no value in determining the prognosis or selecting treatment. Urethral dilatation is not beneficial.

NATURAL HISTORY. The incidence of renal scarring or reflux nephropathy increases with the grade of reflux. With bladder growth and maturation, there is a tendency for reflux to resolve or improve over time. Lower grades of reflux are much more likely to resolve than are higher grades. For grades I and II reflux, the likelihood of resolution is similar irrespective of age at diagnosis and whether it is unilateral or bilateral. For grade III, a younger age at diagnosis and unilateral reflux generally are associated with a higher rate of spontaneous resolution (Fig. 547–8). Bilateral grade IV reflux is much less likely to resolve than is unilateral grade IV reflux. Grade V reflux rarely resolves. The mean age at reflux resolution is 6–7 yr. Reflux is unlikely to cause renal injury in the absence of infection. However, in situations with high-pressure reflux, as in children with posterior urethral valves, neuropathic bladder, and non-neurogenic neurogenic bladder (**Hinman syndrome**), sterile reflux can cause significant renal damage. Children with high-grade reflux who acquire a UTI are at significant risk for pyelonephritis and renal scarring.

TABLE 547–2 Treatment Recommendations for Vesicoureteral Reflux Diagnosed Following a Urinary Tract Infection*

Grade	Age (Yr)	Scarring	Initial Treatment	Follow-Up
I–II	Any	Yes/no	Antibiotic prophylaxis	No consensus
III–IV	0–5	Yes/no	Antibiotic prophylaxis	Surgery
III–IV	6–10	Yes/no	Unilateral: antibiotic prophylaxis Bilateral: surgery	Surgery
V	<1	Yes/no	Antibiotic prophylaxis	Surgery
V	1–5	No	Unilateral: antibiotic prophylaxis	Surgery
V	1–5	No	Bilateral: surgery	
V	1–5	Yes	Surgery	
V	6–10	Yes/no	Surgery	

**Summary of guidelines developed by American Urological Association; age refers to age at diagnosis.*

TREATMENT. The goals of treatment are to prevent pyelonephritis, renal injury, and other complications of reflux. Medical therapy is based on the principle that reflux often resolves over time and that the morbidity or complications of reflux may be prevented nonsurgically. The basis for surgical therapy is that in selected children, ongoing reflux has caused or has a significant potential for causing renal injury or other reflux-related complications and that elimination of reflux minimizes the likelihood of these problems. The International Reflux Study showed that in children with grades III and IV reflux, medical therapy and surgical therapy yielded similar results with regard to new renal scarring and renal function, but that the incidence of clinical pyelonephritis was 2.5 times higher in the children managed medically. At the end of the 5-yr study, less than half of the medically managed children had shown reflux resolution.

Evidence-based guidelines pertaining to the treatment of reflux diagnosed following a UTI were published in 1997 by the American Urological Association (Table 547–2). A guide for parents based on the report is available to assist the physician in discussing treatment options with the parents. The decision about whether to recommend medical or surgical therapy is based on the risk of reflux to the patient, the likelihood of spontaneous resolution, and parental-patient preferences.

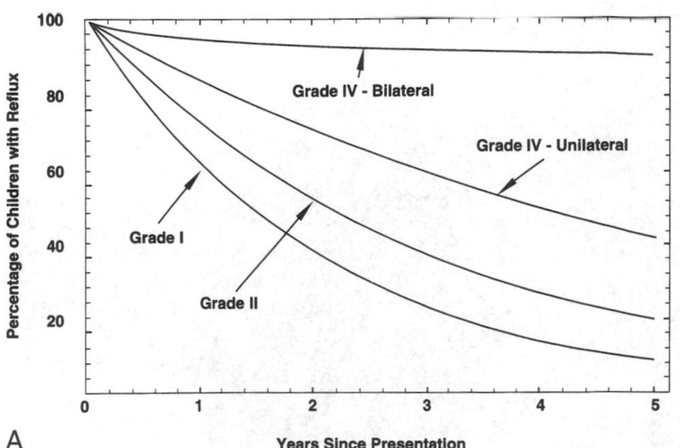

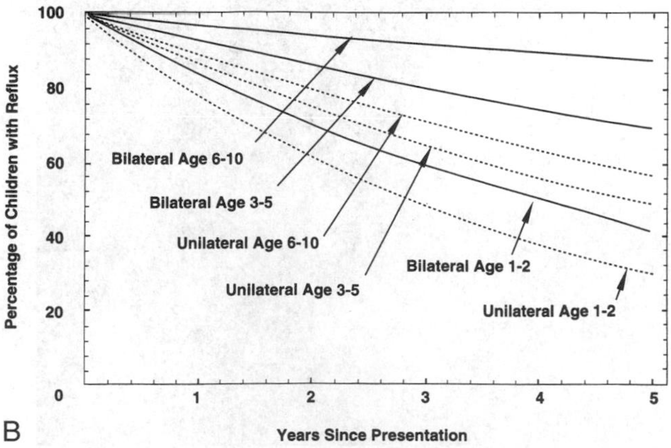

Figure 547–8 *A,* Per cent chance of reflux persistence, grades I, II, and IV, for 1-5 years following presentation. *B,* Per cent chance of reflux persistence by age at presentation, grade III, for 1-5 years following presentation. (From J Urol 157: 1846, 1997.)

Continuous antibiotic prophylaxis is the cornerstone in the initial management of children with reflux. Drugs commonly used for prophylaxis include sulfamethoxazole-trimethoprim, trimethoprim alone, and nitrofurantoin, generally administered once daily at a dose of one quarter to one third of the dose necessary to treat an acute infection. Prophylaxis is usually continued until reflux resolves or until the risk of reflux to the individual is considered to be low. Medical management with antibiotic prophylaxis is considered successful if the child remains free of infection, has no new renal scarring, and the reflux resolves spontaneously. Breakthrough UTI, development of new renal scars, or failure of reflux to resolve would be considered failure of medical management. Noncompliance, allergic reaction, or side effects to the prescribed medication may preclude medical management or lead to its failure.

In children with ongoing reflux, follow-up evaluation should be performed at least annually, at which time the child's height, weight, and blood pressure should be recorded. The child's voiding pattern is assessed, and if voiding dysfunction is present, it should be treated. A urine culture should be performed if there are symptoms or signs of a UTI, or both. Cystography (radionuclide) is generally performed every 12–18 mo. Periodic upper tract imaging should be performed to monitor the status of the upper urinary tracts.

Surgical therapy can be performed either through a suprapubic incision or by endoscopic means. Open surgical management involves modifying the abnormal ureterovesical attachment to create a 4:1 to 5:1 ratio of intramural ureter length:ureteral diameter. Numerous techniques have been described. Some involve opening the bladder (Politano-Leadbetter, Cohen transtrigonal, Glenn-Anderson), whereas others accomplish reflux correction by an extravesical approach (Lich-Gregoire, detrusorrhaphy). If there is a simple duplication anomaly, both ureters are reimplanted together, termed a *common sheath reimplant.* When correcting reflux associated with severe ureteral dilatation, termed a *megaureter,* the ureter must be tapered or narrowed to a more normal size to allow a normal length:width ratio for the intramural tunnel, and a corner of the bladder is attached to the psoas tendon, termed a *psoas hitch.* If the refluxing kidney is poorly functioning, nephrectomy or nephroureterectomy is indicated. Some clinicians are investigating the role of laparoscopic reflux correction via an extravesical approach.

Open surgical repair is generally performed in children with breakthrough UTI, unresolving reflux, and grade IV or V reflux. In general, blood loss is minimal and the hospital stay averages 2–4 days. The success rate in children with primary reflux is approximately 95% for grades I through IV, with 2.5% experiencing persistent reflux and 2.5% having ureteral obstruction that requires correction. For grade V reflux, the success rate is approximately 80%. In lower grades of reflux, a failed reimplantation often occurs in children with undiagnosed voiding dysfunction. In children with secondary reflux, the success rate is slightly lower than that with primary reflux.

The technique of endoscopic repair of reflux involves injection of a bulking agent via a cystoscope under the ureteral orifice, creating an artificial flap-valve. This technique has been termed the *STING (subtrigonal injection).* Collagen has been used with 70–80% initial success, but at 1 yr 30% of those successfully treated have a recurrence. Because collagen is gradually broken down, most centers have not adopted this bulking agent. Another technique, termed *tissue engineering,* harvests a piece of cartilage from the ear, the cells are grown on a scaffold, and 4–6 wk later a suspension of these cells is injected. In preliminary clinical trials this bulking agent appears to be effective in correcting reflux and is stable.

Connolly LP, Treves ST, Connolly SA, et al: Vesicoureteral reflux in children: Incidence and severity in siblings. J Urol 157:2287, 1997.

Ditchfield MR, De Campo JF, Cook DJ, et al: Vesicoureteral reflux: An accurate predictor of acute pyelonephritis in childhood urinary tract infection? Radiology 190:413, 1994.

Elder JS: Commentary: Importance of antenatal diagnosis of vesicoureteral reflux. J Urol 148:1750, 1992.

Elder JS, Longenecker R: Premedication with oral midazolam for voiding cystourethrography in children: safety and efficacy. AJR 164:1229, 1995.

Elder JS, Peters CA, Arant BS Jr, et al: Pediatric Vesicoureteral Reflux Guidelines Panel Summary Report on the management of primary vesicoureteral reflux in children. J Urol 157:1846, 1997.

Elder JS, Peters CA, Arant BS Jr, et al: Report On the Management of Primary Vesicoureteral Reflux in Children. Baltimore, American Urological Association, 1997.

Feather S, Woolf AS, Gordon I, et al: Vesicoureteric reflux: All in the genes? Lancet 348:725, 1996.

Greenfield SP, Ng M, Wan J: Resolution rates of low grade vesicoureteral reflux stratified by patient age at presentation. J Urol 157:1410, 1997.

Hiraoka M, Hori C, Tsukahara H, et al: Congenitally small kidneys with reflux as a common cause of nephropathy in boys. Kidney Int 52:811, 1997.

Koff SA, Wagner TT, Jayanthi VR: The relationship among dysfunctional elimination syndromes, primary vesicoureteral reflux and urinary tract infections in children. J Urol 160:1019, 1998.

Lama G, Salsano ME, Pedulla M, et al: Angiotensin converting enzyme inhibitors and reflux nephropathy: 2-year follow-up. Pediatr Nephrol 11:714, 1997.

Noe HN: The long term results of prospective sibling reflux screening. J Urol 148:1739, 1992.

Phillips DA, Watson AR, MacKinlay D: Distress and the micturating cystourethrogram: Does preparation help? Acta Paediatr 87:175, 1998.

Puri P, Cascio S, Lakshmandass G, et al: Urinary tract infection and renal damage in sibling vesicoureteral reflux. J Urol 160:1028, 1998.

Wan J, Greenfield SP, Ng M, et al: Sibling reflux: A dual center retrospective study. J Urol 156:677, 1996.

CHAPTER 548
Obstructions of the Urinary Tract

Obstructive lesions of the urinary tract occur at any level from the urethral meatus to the calyceal infundibula. Obstruction can be congenital (anatomic) or caused by trauma, neoplasia, calculi, inflammatory processes, or surgical procedures (Table 548–1). The pathophysiologic effects of obstruction depend on its level, extent of involvement, age of onset, and acute or chronic nature. In childhood, most obstructive lesions are congenital and may therefore be present during fetal life.

ETIOLOGY. Severe ureteral obstruction of early onset in fetal life results in renal dysplasia, ranging from the multicystic kidney, usually associated with ureteral or pelvic atresia (see Fig. 545–2), to various degrees of histologic renal cortical dysplasia seen with less severe obstruction. Chronic ureteral obstruction in late fetal life or after birth results in dilatation of the ureter, renal pelvis, and calyces, with alterations of renal parenchyma ranging from minimal tubular changes to dilatation of Bowman's space, glomerular fibrosis, and interstitial fibrosis. After birth, infections often complicate obstruction and may increase renal damage.

CLINICAL MANIFESTATIONS. Urinary tract obstruction generally causes hydronephrosis, which typically is asymptomatic in its early phases. An obstructed kidney secondary to a ureteropelvic junction (UPJ) or ureterovesical junction obstruction may cause upper abdominal or flank pain on the affected side; pyelonephritis may occur because of urinary stasis. Occasionally an upper urinary tract stone occurs, which can cause abdominal and flank pain and hematuria. With bladder outlet obstruction, the urinary stream may be weak; urinary tract infection (UTI) is common. Many of these lesions are identified by antenatal sonography; an abnormality involving the genitourinary tract is suspected in as many as 1 in 100 fetuses.

Obstructive renal insufficiency can manifest itself by failure to thrive, vomiting, diarrhea, or other nonspecific signs and symptoms. In older children, infravesical obstruction can be associated with overflow urinary incontinence or a poor uri-

TABLE 548–1 Types and Causes of Urinary Tract Obstruction

Location	Cause
Infundibula	Congenital Calculi Inflammatory (tuberculosis) Traumatic Postsurgical Neoplastic
Renal pelvis	Congenital (infundibulopelvic stenosis) Inflammatory (tuberculosis) Calculi Neoplasia (Wilms tumor, neuroblastoma)
Ureteropelvic junction	Congenital stenosis Calculi Neoplasia Inflammatory Postsurgical Traumatic
Ureter	Congenital obstructive megaureter Midureteral structure Ureteral ectopia Ureterocele Retrocaval ureter Ureteral fibroepithelial polyps Ureteral valves Calculi Postsurgical Extrinsic compression Neoplasia (neuroblastoma, lymphoma, and other retroperitoneal or pelvic tumors) Inflammatory (Crohn disease, chronic granulomatous disease) Hematoma, urinoma Lymphocele Retroperitoneal fibrosis
Bladder outlet and urethra	Neurogenic bladder dysfunction (functional obstruction) Posterior urethral valves Anterior urethral valves Diverticula Urethral strictures (congenital, traumatic, or iatrogenic) Urethral atresia Ectopic ureterocele Meatal stenosis (males) Calculi Foreign bodies Phimosis Extrinsic compression by tumors Urogenital sinus anomalies

nary stream. Acute ureteral obstruction causes flank or abdominal pain; there may be nausea and vomiting. Chronic ureteral obstruction can be silent or can cause vague abdominal or typical flank pain with increased fluid intake.

DIAGNOSIS. Urinary tract obstruction is often silent. In the newborn, a palpable abdominal mass is most commonly a hydronephrotic or multicystic dysplastic kidney. With infravesical obstructive lesions in boys, a walnut-sized mass, representing the bladder, is palpable just above the pubic symphysis. A patent urachus should suggest urethral obstruction. Urinary ascites in the newborn usually is caused by posterior urethral valves.

Urinary tract obstruction may be diagnosed prenatally by ultrasonography, typically showing hydronephrosis. Further ultrasonography and a more complete evaluation should be undertaken in the neonatal period. Infection and sepsis may be the first indications of an obstructive lesion of the urinary tract. The combination of infection and obstruction poses a serious threat to infants and children and usually requires parenteral administration of antibiotics and drainage of the obstructed kidney. Renal ultrasonography should be performed in all children during the acute stage of febrile urinary tract infections.

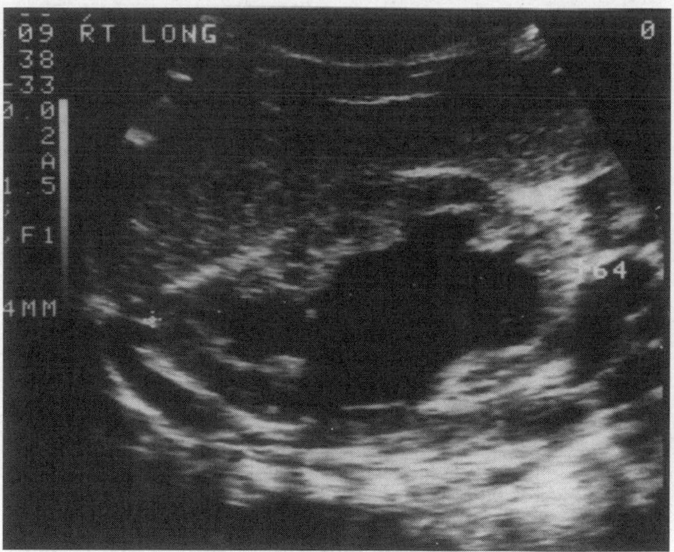

Figure 548–1 Ultrasonographic image of the right kidney with marked pelvic and calyceal dilatation (grade IV hydronephrosis) in an infant with ureteropelvic junction obstruction.

IMAGING STUDIES

Renal Ultrasonography. The common characteristic of obstruction is the presence of a dilated urinary tract. Hydronephrosis is frequently an ultrasonographic finding (Fig. 548–1). Dilatation is not always indicative of obstruction and may persist after surgical correction of an obstructive lesion. Dilatation may result from vesicoureteral reflux, or it may be a manifestation of abnormal development of the urinary tract, even when there is no obstruction. Renal length, degree of caliectasis and parenchymal thickness, and presence or absence of ureteral dilatation should be assessed. Ideally, the severity of hydronephrosis should be graded from 1 to 4 using the Society for Fetal Urology grading scale (Table 548–2). One may ascertain that the contralateral kidney is normal, and the bladder should be imaged to see whether the bladder wall is thickened, the lower ureter is dilated, and whether bladder emptying is complete. In acute or intermittent obstruction, the dilatation of the collecting system may be minimal and ultrasonography may be misleading.

Voiding Cystourethrography. In all cases of congenital hydronephrosis and in any child with ureteral dilatation, a voiding cystourethrogram (VCUG) should be obtained to rule out vesicoureteral reflux as a possible cause of the dilatation. In males, the voiding cystourethrogram also is necessary to rule out

TABLE 548–2 Society for Fetal Urology Grading System for Hydronephrosis

Grade of Hydronephrosis	Renal Image: *Central Renal Complex*	Renal Image: *Renal Parenchymal Thickness*
0	Intact	Normal
1	Slight splitting	Normal
2	Evident splitting, complex confined within renal border	Normal
3	Wide splitting pelvis dilated outside renal border, calyces uniformly dilated	Normal
4	Further dilatation of pelvis and calyces (calyces may appear convex)	Thin

After Maizels M, Mitchell B, Kass E, et al: Outcome of nonspecific hydronephrosis in the infant: A report from the registry of the Society for Fetal Urology. J Urol 152:2324, 1994.

urethral obstruction, particularly in cases of suspected posterior urethral valves. In infravesical obstruction in infants, the bladder may be palpable because of chronic distention and incomplete emptying. In older children, the urinary flow rate can be measured in a simple noninvasive way with a urinary flowmeter, and decreased flow in the presence of normal bladder contraction is suggestive of infravesical obstruction. When the urethra cannot be catheterized to obtain a voiding cystourethrogram, one must suspect a urethral stricture or an obstructive urethral lesion. Retrograde urethrography with contrast injected into the urethral meatus helps delineate the anatomy of the urethral obstruction.

Radioisotope Studies. Renal scintigraphy is used to assess renal anatomy and function. The two most common radiopharmaceuticals are mercaptoacetyl triglycine (MAG-3) and technetium-99m–dimercaptosuccinic acid (DMSA). MAG-3 is excreted by renal tubular secretion; it is used to assess differential renal function and, when furosemide is administered, drainage can also be measured. DMSA is a renal cortical imaging agent and is used to assess differential renal function and to demonstrate whether renal scarring is present. It is used infrequently in children with obstructive uropathy.

In a *MAG-3 diuretic renogram,* a small dose of technetium-labeled MAG-3 is injected intravenously (Fig. 548–2; see Fig. 548–4). During the first 2 to 3 min, renal parenchymal uptake is analyzed and compared, allowing computation of differential renal function. Subsequently, excretion is evaluated. After 20 to 30 min, furosemide is injected intravenously, and the rapidity and pattern of drainage from the kidneys to the bladder are analyzed. If no obstruction is present, half of the radionuclide should be cleared from the renal pelvis within 10 to 15 min, termed the half-life or T 1/2. In the presence of significant upper tract obstruction, the T 1/2 generally is greater than 20 min. A T 1/2 between 15 and 20 min is indeterminate. The images generated usually provide an accurate assessment of the site of obstruction. Numerous variables affect the outcome of the diuretic renogram. For example, newborn kidneys are functionally immature, and in some cases even normal kidneys may not demonstrate normal drainage following diuretic administration. Dehydration prolongs parenchymal transit and can blunt the diuretic response. Giving an insufficient dose of furosemide may result in inadequate drainage. If vesicoureteral reflux is present, continuous catheter drainage is mandatory to prevent radionuclide from refluxing from the bladder into the dilated upper tract, which would prolong the washout phase. Because of the numerous variables, the Society for Fetal Urology and the Pediatric Nuclear Medicine Club jointly developed a standardized method for performing diuretic renography in infants and children, termed the *well-tempered renogram.*

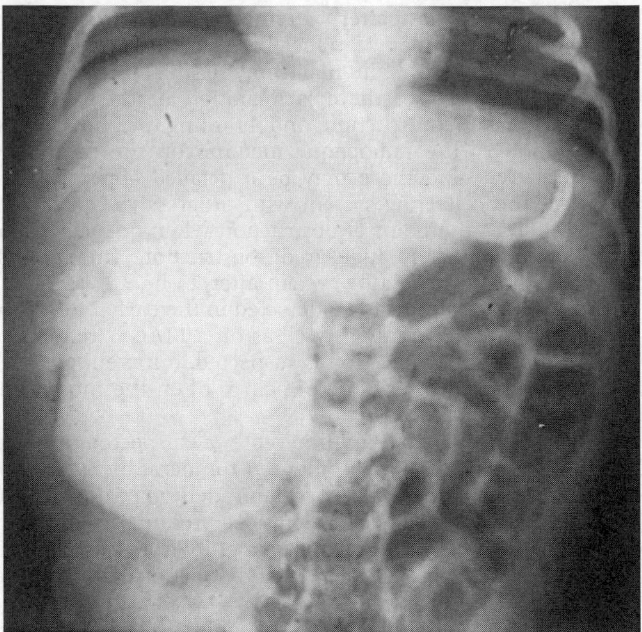

Figure 548–3 Ureteropelvic junction obstruction. Excretory urogram in a newborn, showing dilatation of the right renal pelvis and blunting of the calyces characteristic of a ureteropelvic junction obstruction.

The MAG-3 diuretic renogram is considered superior to the excretory urogram in infants and children with hydronephrosis because bowel gas and immaturity of renal function often cause the intravenous pyelogram (IVP) images to be suboptimal. In addition, the diuretic renogram provides an objective assessment of the relative function of each kidney.

Excretory Urogram (IVP). In older children, the IVP is still useful in selected cases (Fig. 548–3). The plain film of the abdomen should be inspected for calculi, spinal abnormalities, and an

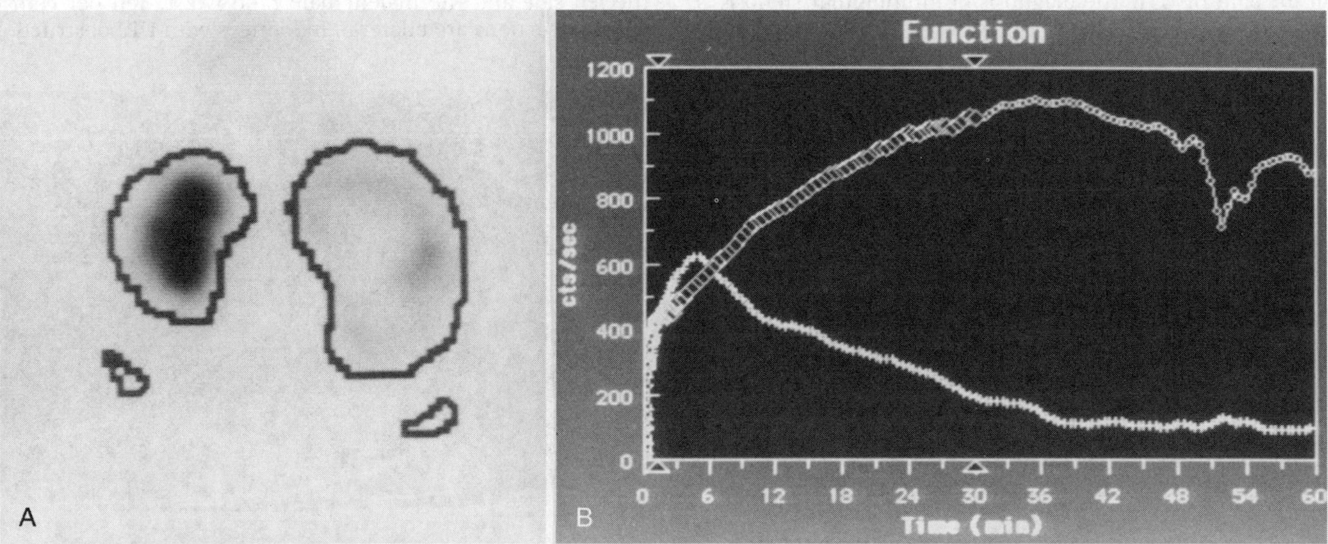

Figure 548–2 MAG-3 diuretic renogram in a 6-wk-old infant with right hydronephrosis detected by prenatal ultrasonography. The right kidney is on the right side of the image. *A,* Differential renal function: left kidney 70%, right kidney 30%. *B,* Following administration of furosemide, drainage from the left kidney was normal, and drainage from the right kidney was slow, consistent with right ureteropelvic junction obstruction. Pyeloplasty was performed on the right kidney (see Fig. 548–4).

abnormal intestinal gas pattern. In infravesical obstruction, the bladder wall is irregular or trabeculated because of detrusor hypertrophy. A postvoid film may show residual bladder urine. In ureteral obstruction, there is dilatation of the collecting system above the obstruction and blunting of the calyces. Concentration of the radiopaque medium on the obstructed side is impaired, and there may be a delayed appearance of contrast in the collecting system with progressive increase in concentration at the point of obstruction when delayed radiographs are obtained. In high-grade obstruction, the contrast may remain in the collecting system after 24 hr.

Urinary extravasation can be detected in the early or delayed films of a urographic study as well as on a MAG-3 renogram. When intermittent obstruction is suspected, intravenous urography during an acute episode of pain is often the most valuable diagnostic study.

Computed Tomography. In children with a suspected ureteral calculus, noncontrast spiral computed tomography of the abdomen and pelvis provides an excellent method of demonstrating whether a calculus (or calculi) is present, its location, and whether there is significant proximal hydronephrosis. This study is replacing IVP as the initial study of choice in these patients.

Ancillary Studies. In equivocal cases, another way to assess whether obstruction is present is by performing an antegrade pressure-perfusion flow study, termed a *Whitaker test.* Percutaneous access to the renal pelvis is obtained; the collecting system is then perfused with radiopaque contrast at a measured flow rate, usually 10 mL/min. The pressures in the renal pelvis and the bladder are monitored during this infusion, and pressure differences exceeding 20 cm H_2O are suggestive of obstruction. Antegrade pyelography is obtained at the same time, which provides excellent delineation of the anatomy of the collecting system. This test usually requires general anesthesia. In other cases, cystoscopy with retrograde pyelography provides excellent images of the upper urinary tract (Fig. 548–5).

SPECIFIC TYPES OF URINARY TRACT OBSTRUCTION AND THEIR TREATMENT

Hydrocalycosis. This term refers to a localized dilatation of the calyx caused by obstruction of its infundibulum, termed *infundibular stenosis.* Such obstruction can be developmental in origin or secondary to inflammatory processes, such as UTI. When the abnormality is not discovered by antenatal ultrasonography or incidentally, it is usually discovered during evaluation for pain or UTI. The diagnosis of infundibular stenosis is usually established by IVP.

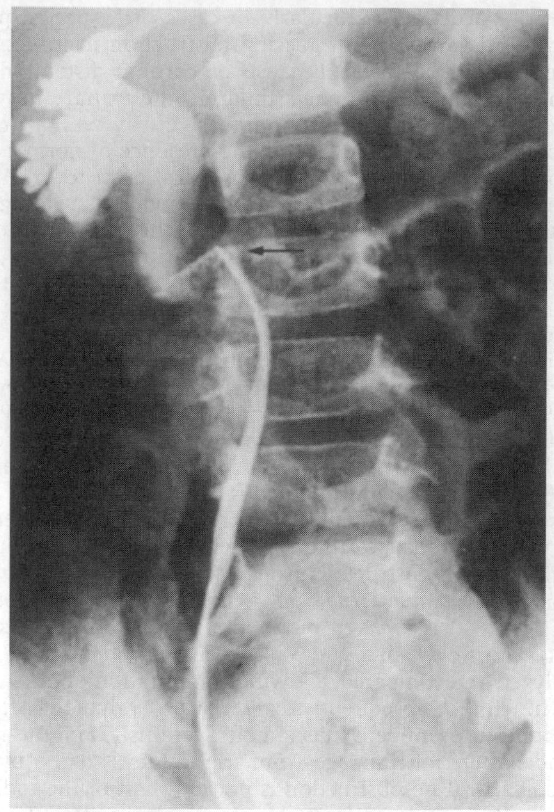

Figure 548–5 Retrocaval ureter. Retrograde pyelogram showing medial deviation of a dilated upper ureter to the level of the 3rd lumbar vertebra, characteristic of a retrocaval ureter.

Ureteropelvic Junction Obstruction. This is the most common obstructive lesion in childhood and is usually caused by intrinsic stenosis (see Figs. 548–1 through 548–4). At times an accessory artery to the lower pole of the kidney also causes extrinsic obstruction. UPJ obstruction most commonly presents (1) on maternal ultrasonography revealing fetal hydronephrosis; (2) as a palpable renal mass in a newborn or infant; (3) as abdominal, flank, or back pain; (4) as a febrile UTI; or (5) as hematuria after minimal trauma. Approximately 60% of cases occur on the left side and the male:female ratio is 2:1. Ten per cent of UPJ obstructions are bilateral. In kidneys with UPJ obstruction,

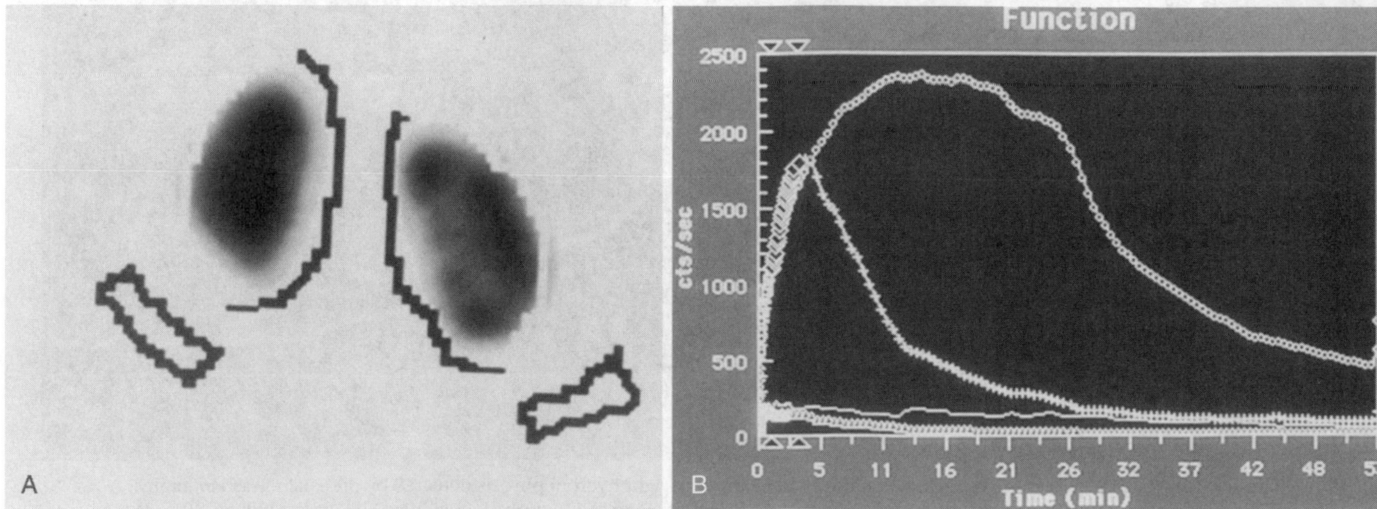

Figure 548–4 Same patient as in Figure 548–2. *A* and *B*, MAG-3 diuretic renogram at 14 mo of age shows equal function in the two kidneys and prompt drainage following the administration of furosemide.

renal function may be significantly impaired from pressure atrophy. The anomaly is corrected by performing a pyeloplasty, in which the stenotic segment is excised and the normal ureter and renal pelvis are reattached. Success rates are 91–98%.

Lesser degrees of UPJ obstruction may cause mild hydronephrosis, which usually is nonobstructive, and typically these kidneys function normally. The spectrum of UPJ abnormalities has been referred to as *anomalous UPJ*. Another cause of mild hydronephrosis is fetal folds of the upper ureter, which also are nonobstructive.

The diagnosis can be difficult to establish in an asymptomatic infant in whom dilatation of the renal pelvis is found incidentally in a prenatal ultrasonogram. After birth, the sonographic study is repeated to confirm the prenatal finding. A VCUG is necessary because 15% of patients have ipsilateral vesicoureteral reflux. If no dilatation is found after birth, a renal sonogram should be repeated at 1 mo of age because the dilatation may be minimal immediately after birth secondary to transient oliguria but may become more evident a few weeks later. Consequently, it is best to perform the 1st postnatal ultrasonographic study after the 3rd day of life because oliguria in the newborn may mask the dilatation. Subsequently, a MAG-3 diuretic renogram is performed. If the kidney shows grade 1 or 2 hydronephrosis, renal function in the involved kidney is good, and drainage is satisfactory, a period of observation is usually appropriate. In many infants, mild to moderate hydronephrosis improves with time. Long-term follow-up is indicated. If the hydronephrosis is grade 3 or 4, spontaneous resolution is less likely. During the period of follow-up, the child should receive antibiotic prophylaxis, usually trimethoprim-sulfamethoxazole. If the differential function on renography is normal, the infant can be followed with serial ultrasonograms. If there is no improvement, a diuretic renogram after 6–12 mo may help in the decision between continued observation or surgical repair. Early surgical repair is indicated in infants with an abdominal mass, bilateral severe hydronephrosis, a solitary kidney, or diminished function in the involved kidney. In older children who present with symptoms, diagnosis usually is established by sonography and diuretic renography or IVP.

In the *differential diagnosis,* the following entities should be considered: (1) megacalycosis, a congenital nonobstructive dilatation of the calyces without pelvic or ureteric dilatation; (2) vesicoureteral reflux with marked dilatation and kinking of the ureter; and (3) midureteral or distal ureteral obstruction when the ureter is not well visualized on the urogram.

Midureteral Obstruction. Congenital ureteral stenosis or a ureteral valve in the midureter is rare and is corrected by excision of the strictured segment and reanastomosing the normal upper and lower ureteral segments. A *retrocaval ureter* is an anomaly in which the upper right ureter travels posterior to the inferior vena cava. In this anomaly, the vena cava may cause extrinsic compression and obstruction. An IVP shows the right ureter to be medially deviated at the level of the 3rd lumbar vertebra. The diagnosis may be confirmed by retrograde pyelography (see Fig. 548–5). Surgical treatment consists of transection of the upper ureter, moving it anterior to the vena cava, and reanastomosing the upper and lower segments. Repair is necessary only when obstruction is present. Retroperitoneal tumors, fibrosis caused by surgical procedures, inflammatory processes (as in chronic granulomatous disease), and radiation therapy can cause acquired midureteral obstruction.

Ectopic Ureter. An ectopic ureter refers to a ureter that drains outside the bladder. They are three times as common in girls as in boys. In girls, the ectopic ureter usually drains the upper pole of a duplex collecting system (i.e., two ureters), whereas in boys there is often only a single system. In girls, approximately 35% enter the urethra at the bladder neck, 35% enter the urethrovaginal septum, 25% enter the vagina, and a few drain into the cervix, uterus, Gartner's duct, or a urethral diverticulum. With the exception of the ectopic ureter entering the bladder neck, all cause continuous urinary incontinence from the affected renal moiety. In addition, UTI is common because of urinary stasis. In boys, ectopic ureters enter the posterior urethra (above the external sphincter) in 47%, prostatic utricle in 10%, seminal vesicle in 33%, the ejaculatory duct in 5%, and the vas deferens in 5%. Consequently, in boys, an ectopic ureter does not cause incontinence, and most patients present with a UTI or epididymitis. Evaluation includes a renal sonogram, VCUG, and IVP or renal scan, preferably the latter. The sonogram shows the affected hydronephrotic kidney or dilated upper pole and ureter down to the bladder (Fig. 548–6). If the ectopic ureter drains into the bladder neck (female), a VCUG usually shows reflux into the ureter. Otherwise, there is no reflux into the ectopic ureter, but there may be reflux into the ipsilateral lower pole ureter or contralateral collecting system. Renal scintigraphy demonstrates whether the affected segment has significant function.

Treatment depends on the status of the renal unit drained by the ectopic ureter. If there is satisfactory function, ureteral reimplantation into the bladder or ureteroureterostomy (anastomosing the ectopic upper pole ureter into the normally inserting lower pole ureter) is indicated. If function is poor, partial or total nephrectomy is indicated.

Ureterocele. A ureterocele is a cystic dilatation of the terminal ureter and is obstructive because of a pinpoint ureteral orifice. Ureteroceles are much more common in females than in males.

Ureteroceles are nearly always associated with ureteral duplication (Fig. 548–7). The ureter involved with the ureterocele drains the upper renal moiety, which frequently functions poorly or is dysplastic because of congenital obstruction. The lower pole ureter drains into the bladder superior and lateral to the upper pole ureter and frequently refluxes. *Ectopic ureteroceles* typically extend submucosally into the urethra. Rarely, large ectopic ureteroceles may cause bladder outlet obstruction and retention of urine; in females, the ureterocele may prolapse from the urethral meatus (see Chapter 552). Affected children often are discovered by prenatal sonography or present with a UTI. Both simple and ectopic ureteroceles can be bilateral. Sonography is effective in demonstrating the ureterocele and whether the associated obstructed system is dupli-

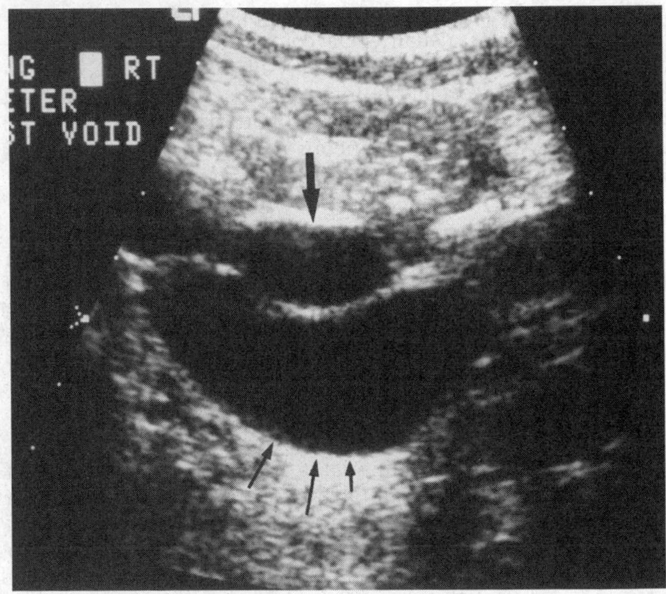

Figure 548–6 Ultrasonographic image of the right dilated ureter *(thin arrows)* extending behind and caudal to a nearly empty bladder *(arrow)* in a girl with urinary incontinence and ectopic ureter draining into the vagina.

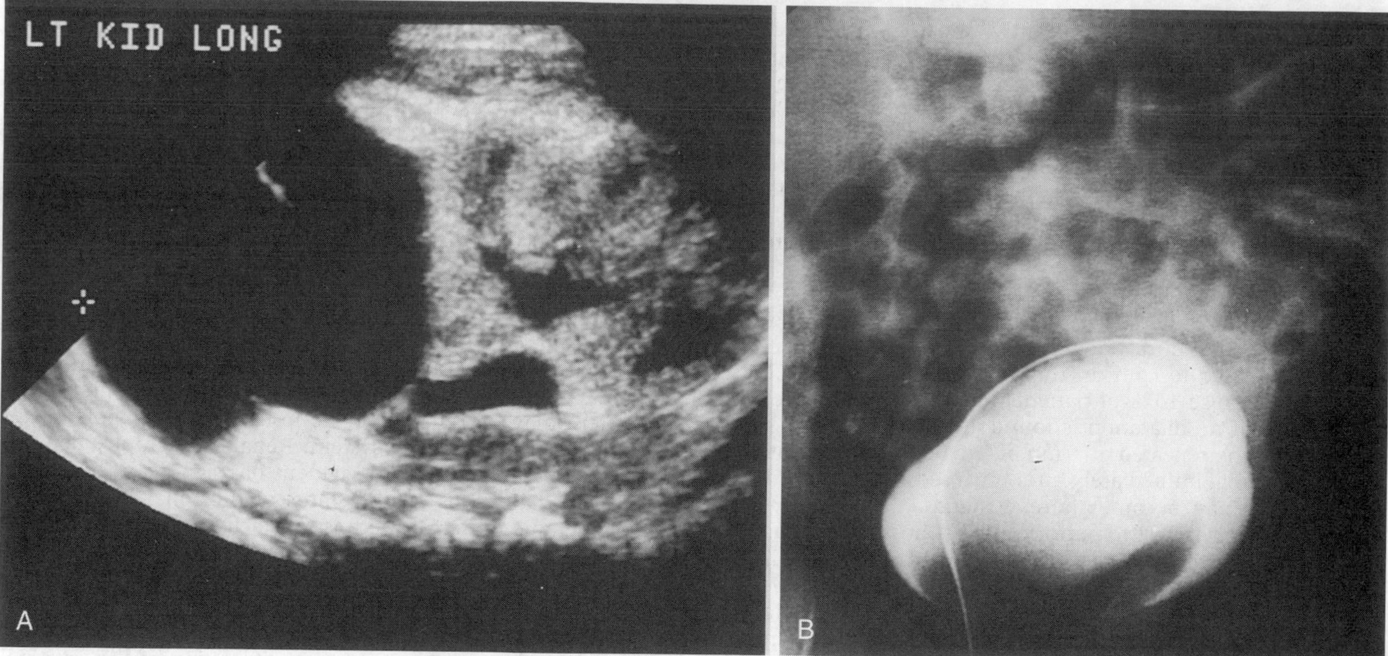

Figure 548–7 *A*, Infant with ectopic ureterocele. Sonogram of left kidney shows massive dilatation of the upper pole and a normal lower pole. *B*, VCUG shows large ureterocele, draining the left upper pole, in the bladder. No reflux is present.

cated or single. IVP usually shows a filling defect, sometimes large, in the bladder corresponding to the ureterocele and characteristic findings of duplication of the collecting systems (poor or absent function of the upper collecting system and caudal displacement of the lower collecting system). Renal scintigraphy is most accurate in demonstrating whether the affected renal moiety has significant function.

Treatment of ectopic ureteroceles usually involves excision of the upper pole of the kidney and most of the associated ureter. When the ectopic ureterocele is small and there is low-grade or no reflux in the ipsilateral duplicated ureter, the decompressed ureterocele need not be excised and usually causes no further problems. Large ureteroceles, however, or those with high-grade reflux to the ipsilateral lower ureter, are best treated by excision of the ureterocele and reimplantation of the remaining ureter, plus partial upper moiety nephroureterectomy. This can usually be accomplished in a single operation. In the treatment of an acutely ill, septic infant with an obstructing ureterocele, drainage of the involved collecting system may be necessary, either by transurethral puncture cystoscopically or by percutaneous nephrostomy of the upper collecting system.

Simple ureteroceles are associated with nonduplicated collecting systems, and the orifice is in the expected location in the bladder (Fig. 548–8). They are usually discovered during an investigation for a UTI. IVP reveals varying degrees of ureteral and calyceal dilatation, and there is a round filling defect in the bladder. In delayed films, the cystic dilatation of the ureter may be clearly visible and full of contrast material. Bladder ultrasonography is sensitive for detecting the ureterocele. Transurethral incision of the ureterocele effectively relieves the obstruction, but it may result in vesicoureteral reflux necessitating ureteral reimplantation later. Some prefer open excision of the ureterocele and reimplantation as the initial form of treatment. Small, simple ureteroceles incidentally discovered without upper tract dilatation may not require treatment. In questionable cases, diuresis renography is useful.

Megaureter. A classification of megaureters (dilated ureter) is given in Table 548–3. There are numerous disorders that can cause ureteral dilatation, and many are nonobstructive.

Megaureters are usually discovered through screening ultrasonography of the kidneys and bladder because of a prenatal diagnosis of hydronephrosis or postnatal UTI, hematuria, or abdominal pain. A careful history, physical examination, and voiding cystourethrography identify causes of secondary mega-

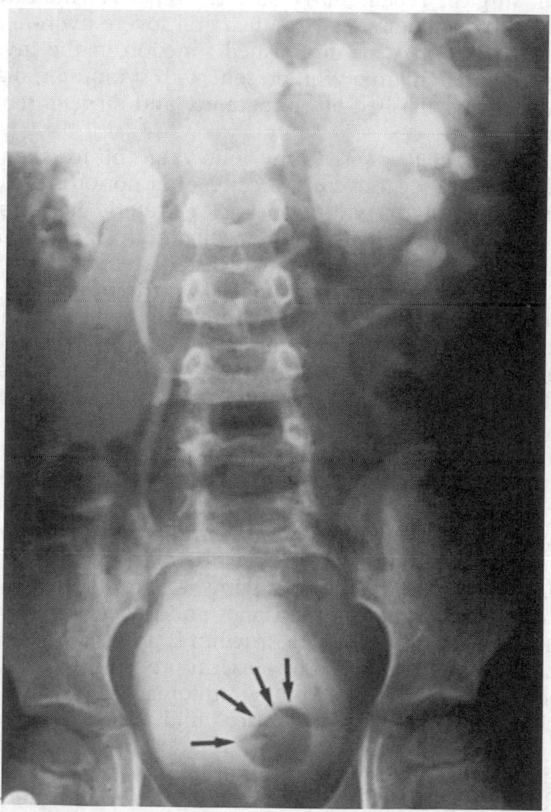

Figure 548–8 Simple intravesical ureterocele. Excretory urogram shows left hydronephrosis and a round filling defect on the left side of the bladder corresponding to a simple ureterocele causing left ureteral obstruction. This lesion was treated by transurethral incision and drainage of the ureterocele.

TABLE 548–3 Classification of Megaureter

Refluxing		Obstructed		Nonrefluxing and Nonobstructed	
Primary	***Secondary***	***Primary***	***Secondary***	***Primary***	***Secondary***
Primary reflux Megacystic-megaureter syndrome Ectopic ureter Prune-belly syndrome	Neuropathic bladder Hinman syndrome Posterior urethral valves Bladder diverticulum Postoperative	Intrinsic (primary obstructed megaureter) Ureteral valve Ectopic ureter Ectopic uretocele	Neuropathic Bladder Hinman syndrome Posterior urethral valves Ureteral calculus Extrinsic Postoperative	Nonrefluxing, Nonobstructive	Diabetes insipidus Infection Persistent after relief of obstruction

ureters and refluxing megaureters as well as the prune-belly syndrome. Primary obstructed megaureters and nonobstructed megaureters probably represent opposite extremes of a spectrum of the same anomaly.

The primary obstructed nonrefluxing megaureter results from abnormal development of the distal ureter, with collagenous tissue replacing the muscle layer. There is disruption of normal ureteral peristalsis, and the proximal ureter widens. Usually there is not a true stricture. On IVP, the distal ureter is more dilated in its distal segment and tapers abruptly at or above the junction of the bladder (Fig. 548–9). The lesion may be unilateral or bilateral. Dilatation of the upper collecting system and calyceal blunting are suggestive of obstruction. Megaureter predisposes to UTI, urinary stones, and flank pain because of urinary stasis. In most cases, diuresis renography, and sequential sonographic studies can reliably differentiate obstructed from nonobstructed megaureters. Generally, most megaureters diminish in size over time. Obstructed megaureters require surgical treatment, with excision of the narrowed segment, ureteral tapering, and reimplantation of the ureter. The results of surgical reconstruction are usually good, but the prognosis depends on pre-existing renal function and whether complications develop.

If differential renal function is normal (>45%) and the child is asymptomatic, it seems safe to follow the patient with serial ultrasonography and diuretic renography to monitor renal function and drainage. If renal function deteriorates, upper urinary tract drainage slows, or UTI occurs, ureteral reimplantation is recommended. These children should receive prophylactic antimicrobial therapy while there is urinary stasis in the upper ureter and kidney.

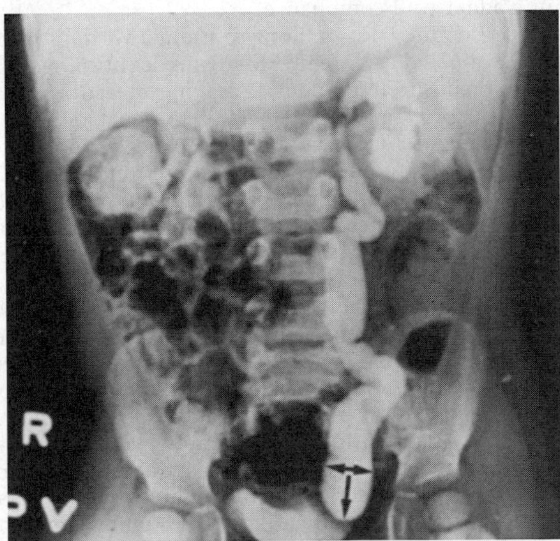

Figure 548–9 Obstructed megaureter. Excretory urogram in a girl with a history of a febrile urinary tract infection. The right side is normal. The left side reveals hydroureteronephrosis with predominant dilatation of the distal ureter. Note the characteristic appearance of the distal ureter. There was no vesicoureteral reflux. The diagnosis of obstruction was confirmed by diuretic renography.

Prune-Belly Syndrome. This syndrome, also called *triad syndrome* or *Eagle-Barrett syndrome,* occurs in approximately 1 in 40,000 births; 95% of affected individuals are male. The characteristic association of deficient abdominal muscles, undescended testes, and urinary tract abnormalities probably results from severe urethral obstruction in fetal life (Fig. 548–10). Oligohydramnios and pulmonary hypoplasia are frequent complications in the perinatal period. Many affected infants are stillborn. Urinary tract abnormalities include massive dilatation of the ureters and upper tracts and a very large bladder, with a patent urachus or a urachal diverticulum. Most patients have vesicoureteral reflux. The prostatic urethra is usually dilated and the prostate is hypoplastic. The anterior urethra may be dilated, resulting in a megalourethra. Rarely, there is urethral stenosis or atresia. The kidneys usually show various degrees of dysplasia, and the testes are usually intra-abdominal. There is often malrotation of the bowel. Cardiac abnormalities occur in 10% of cases; more than 50% have abnormalities of the musculoskeletal system, including limb abnormalities and scoliosis. In females, anomalies of the urethra, uterus, and vagina are usually present.

Many neonates with prune-belly syndrome have difficulty with effective bladder emptying because the bladder musculature is poorly developed and the urethra may be narrowed. When no obstruction is present, the goal of treatment is the prevention of urinary tract infection with antibiotic prophylaxis. When obstruction of the ureters or urethra is demonstrated, temporary drainage procedures, such as a vesicostomy, may help to preserve renal function until the child is old enough for surgery. Some children with prune-belly syndrome have been found to have classic or atypical posterior urethral

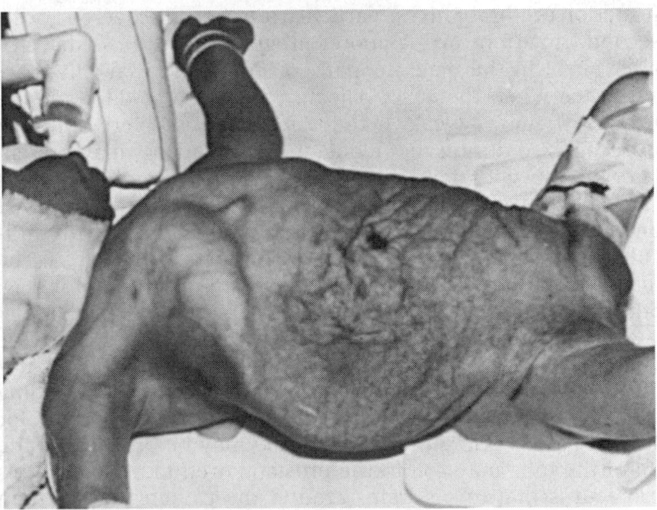

Figure 548–10 Prune-belly syndrome. Photograph of a 1,600-g newborn with the prune-belly syndrome. Note the lack of tonicity of the abdominal wall and the wrinkled appearance of the skin.

valves. Urinary tract infections are frequent and should be treated promptly. Correction of the undescended testes by orchidopexy can be difficult in these children because the testes are located high in the abdomen and is best accomplished in the 1st 6 mo of life. Reconstruction of the abdominal wall offers cosmetic and functional benefits.

The prognosis ultimately depends on the degree of pulmonary hypoplasia and renal dysplasia. One third of children with prune-belly syndrome are stillborn or die in the 1st few months of life because of pulmonary complications. Of the long-term survivors, as many as 30% develop end-stage renal disease from dysplasia or complications of infection or reflux, and eventually require renal transplantation. The results of renal transplantation in these patients are favorable.

Bladder Neck Obstruction. Bladder neck obstruction is usually secondary to ectopic ureterocele, bladder calculi, or a tumor of the prostate (rhabdomyosarcoma). The manifestations include difficulty voiding, urinary retention, urinary tract infection, and bladder distention with overflow incontinence. Apparent bladder neck obstruction is common in cases of posterior urethral valves, but it seldom has any functional significance. Primary bladder neck obstruction may never occur.

Posterior Urethral Valves. The most common cause of severe obstructive uropathy in children is posterior urethral valves, occurring only in boys. This lesion occurs in approximately 1 in 8,000 boys. Urethral valve refers to tissue leaflets fanning distally from the prostatic urethra to the external urinary sphincter. Typically the leaflets are separated by a slitlike opening. Valves are of unclear embryologic origin and cause varying degrees of obstruction. Approximately 30% of patients experience end-stage renal disease or chronic renal insufficiency. The prostatic urethra dilates and the bladder muscle undergoes hypertrophy. Vesicoureteral reflux occurs in 50% of patients and distal ureteral obstruction may result from a chronically distended bladder or bladder muscle hypertrophy. The renal changes range from mild hydronephrosis to severe renal dysplasia; their severity probably depends on the severity of the obstruction and the time of its onset in fetal life. As in other cases of obstruction or renal dysplasia, there may be oligohydramnios and pulmonary hypoplasia.

Affected boys with posterior urethral valves are discovered prenatally when maternal ultrasonography reveals bilateral hydronephrosis, a distended bladder and, if the obstruction is severe, oligohydramnios. Prenatal bladder decompression by percutaneous vesicoamniotic shunt or open fetal surgery has been reported. Experimental and clinical evidence of the possible benefits of fetal intervention is lacking, and these procedures should be considered experimental. Prenatally diagnosed posterior urethral valves, particularly when discovered in the second trimester, carry a poorer prognosis than those detected after birth. In the male neonate, posterior urethral valves are suspected when there is a palpably distended bladder and the urinary stream is weak. If the obstruction is severe and goes unrecognized during the neonatal period, infants may present later in life with failure to thrive due to uremia or sepsis caused by infection in the obstructed urinary tract. With lesser degrees of obstruction, children present later in life with difficulty in achieving diurnal urinary continence or with UTI. The diagnosis is established by voiding cystourethrography (Fig. 548–11) or perineal ultrasonography.

After the diagnosis is established, renal function and the anatomy of the upper urinary tract should be carefully evaluated. In the healthy neonate, a small polyethylene feeding tube (No. 5 or 8 French) is inserted in the bladder and left for several days. Passing the feeding tube may be difficult, as the tip of the tube may coil in the prostatic urethra. A sign of this problem is that urine drains around the catheter rather than through it. A Foley (balloon) catheter should not be used, because the balloon may cause severe bladder spasms, which may produce severe ureteral obstruction.

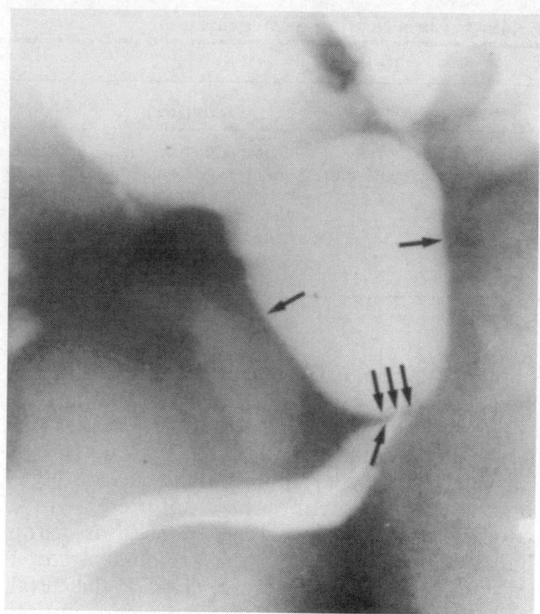

Figure 548–11 Posterior urethral valves. Voiding cystourethrogram in an infant with posterior urethral valves. Note the dilatation of the prostatic urethra and the transverse linear filling defect corresponding to the valves.

If the serum creatinine level remains normal or returns to normal, treatment consists of transurethral ablation of the valve leaflets, which is performed endoscopically under general anesthesia. If the urethra is too small for transurethral ablation, temporary vesicostomy is preferred, in which the dome of the bladder is exteriorized on the lower abdominal wall. When the child is older, the valves may be ablated and the vesicostomy closed.

If the serum creatinine level remains high or increases despite bladder drainage by a small catheter, secondary ureteral obstruction, irreversible renal damage, or renal dysplasia should be suspected. In such cases, a vesicostomy should be performed. Cutaneous pyelostomy rarely affords better drainage when compared with cutaneous vesicostomy, and the latter also allows continued bladder growth and gradual improvement in bladder wall compliance.

Infants presenting later in life with uremia without infection should be evaluated and treated following identical guidelines. In the septic and uremic infant, lifesaving measures must include prompt correction of the electrolyte imbalance and control of the infection by appropriate antibiotics. Drainage of the upper tracts by percutaneous nephrostomy and hemodialysis may be necessary. After the patient's condition becomes stable, step-by-step evaluation and treatment can be undertaken. Most boys presenting with incontinence can be treated by primary valve ablation.

Favorable prognostic factors include having a normal prenatal ultrasonogram between 18 and 24 wk of gestation, a serum creatinine level less than 0.8 to 1.0 mg/dL after bladder decompression, and visualization of the corticomedullary junction on renal sonography. There are several situations in which a "pop-off valve" may occur during urinary tract development, which preserves the integrity of one or both kidneys. For example, 15% of boys with posterior urethral valves have unilateral reflux into a nonfunctioning dysplastic kidney, termed the *VURD syndrome* (valves, unilateral reflux, dysplasia). In these boys, the high bladder pressure is dissipated into the nonfunctioning kidney, allowing normal development of the contralateral kidney. In newborn boys with urinary ascites, the urine generally leaks out from the obstructed collecting system through the renal fornices, allowing normal renal development. Unfavorable prognostic factors include the presence of oligohydramnios in utero, identification of hydronephrosis before 24 wk of gestation, a serum creatinine level greater than 1.0 mg/dL after bladder decompression, identifying cortical cysts in both kidneys, and persistence of diurnal incontinence beyond 5 yr of age.

The prognosis in the newborn is related to the degree of pulmonary hypoplasia and potential for recovery of renal function. Severely affected infants are often stillborn. Of those who survive the neonatal period, approximately 30% retain some degree of renal insufficiency and many eventually require renal transplantation. In some series, renal transplantation in children with posterior urethral valves has a lower success rate than does transplantation in children with normal bladders, presumably because of the adverse influence of altered bladder function on graft function and survival.

Following valve ablation, antimicrobial prophylaxis is beneficial in preventing UTI, as hydronephrosis often persists to some degree for many years. These boys should be evaluated annually with a renal ultrasonogram, and physical examination, including assessment of somatic growth and blood pressure, urinalysis, and serum electrolytes. Many boys have significant polyuria resulting from a concentrating defect secondary to prolonged obstructive uropathy. If these children acquire a systemic illness with vomiting or diarrhea, or both, urine output cannot be used to assess the child's hydration status. They can become dehydrated quickly, and there should be a low threshold for hospital admission for intravenous rehydration. Some of these patients have renal tubular acidosis, requiring oral bicarbonate therapy. If there is any significant degree of renal dysfunction, growth impairment, or hypertension, they should be followed closely by a pediatric nephrologist. When vesicoureteral reflux is present, expectant treatment and prophylactic doses of antibacterial drugs are advisable. If breakthrough UTI occurs, surgical correction should be undertaken.

Following treatment, boys with urethral valves often do not achieve diurnal urinary continence as early as other boys. Incontinence may result from uninhibited bladder contractions, poor bladder compliance, bladder atonia, or polyuria. Often these boys need to undergo urodynamic evaluation with urodynamics or videourodynamics to plan therapy. Boys with noncompliance are at significant risk for ongoing renal damage, even in the absence of infection. Urinary incontinence usually improves with age, particularly after puberty. Meticulous attention to bladder compliance, emptying, and infection may improve results in the future.

Urethral Atresia. The most severe form of obstructive uropathy in boys is urethral atresia. In utero there is a distended bladder, bilateral hydroureteronephrosis, and oligohydramnios. In most cases, these babies are stillborn or succumb to pulmonary hypoplasia. Some boys with prune-belly syndrome also have urethral atresia. If the urachus is patent, oligohydramnios is unlikely and the baby usually survives. Urethral reconstruction is difficult, and most patients are managed with continent urinary diversion.

Urethral Hypoplasia. Urethral hypoplasia is a less severe form of obstructive uropathy than is urethral atresia in boys. In urethral hypoplasia, the urethral lumen is extremely small. This condition is rare. These neonates typically have bilateral hydronephrosis and a distended bladder. Passage of a small pediatric feeding tube through the urethra is difficult or impossible. Usually a cutaneous vesicostomy must be performed to relieve upper urinary tract obstruction, and the severity of renal insufficiency is variable. The most severely affected boys have end-stage renal disease. Treatment includes urethral reconstruction, gradual urethral dilatation, or continent urinary diversion.

Urethral Strictures. Urethral strictures *in males* usually result from urethral trauma, either iatrogenic (catheterization, endoscopic procedures, or previous urethral reconstruction) or accidental (straddle injuries or pelvic fractures). Because these lesions may develop gradually, the decrease in force of the urinary stream is seldom noticed by the child or the parents. More commonly, the obstruction causes symptoms of bladder instability, hematuria, or dysuria. Catheterization of the bladder is usually impossible. The diagnosis is made by a voiding film obtained during intravenous urography or retrograde urethrography. Ultrasonography has also been used to diagnose urethral strictures. Endoscopy is confirmatory. Endoscopic treatment of short strictures by dilatation or internal urethrotomy is usually successful. Longer strictures surrounded by periurethral fibrosis often require urethroplasty. Repeated endoscopic procedures should generally be avoided, as they may cause additional urethral damage. Noninvasive measurement of the urinary flow rate and pattern is useful for diagnosis and follow-up.

In females, true urethral strictures are exceptional because the female urethra is protected from trauma, particularly in childhood. In the past it was thought that a distal urethral ring commonly caused obstruction of the female urethra and urinary tract infection and that affected girls benefited from urethral dilatation. The diagnosis was suspected when a "spinning top" deformity of the urethra was found in the voiding cystourethrogram and was confirmed by urethral calibration. Treatment for this condition invariably included antibiotic therapy, and adequately controlled studies were not performed. Subsequent studies showed no correlation between the radiologic appearance of the urethra in the voiding cystourethrogram and the urethral caliber, and no significant difference in urethral caliber between females with recurrent cystitis and normal age-matched controls. Consequently, urethral dilatation in girls is rarely necessary.

Anterior Urethral Valves and Urethral Diverticula in the Male. *Anterior urethral valves* are rare. The obstruction is not obstructing valve leaflets, as occurs in the posterior urethra. Rather, it is a urethral diverticulum in the penile urethra that expands during voiding. The distal extension of the diverticulum causes extrinsic compression of the distal penile urethra, causing urethral obstruction. Typically there is a soft mass on the ventral surface of the penis at the penoscrotal junction. In addition, the urinary stream often is weak and the physical findings associated with posterior urethral valves often are present. The diverticulum may be small and minimally obstructive or in other cases may be severely obstructive and cause renal insufficiency. The diagnosis is suspected on physical examination and is confirmed during voiding cystourethrography. Treatment involves open excision of the diverticulum or transurethral excision of the distal urethral cusp. *Urethral diverticula* occasionally occur following extensive hypospadias repair.

Fusiform dilatation of the urethra or megalourethra may result from underdevelopment of the corpus spongiosum and support structures of the urethra. This condition is commonly associated with the prune-belly syndrome.

Male Urethral Meatal Stenosis. See Chapter 552.

Baskin LS, Zderic SA, Snyder HM, et al: Primary dilated megaureter: Long-term followup. J Urol 152:618, 1994.

Bogaert GA, Kogan BA, Mevorach RA, et al: Efficacy of retrograde endopyelotomy in children. J Urol 156:734, 1996.

Capolicchio G, Homsy YL, Houle A-M, et al: Long-term results of percutaneous endopyelotomy in the treatment of children with failed open pyeloplasty. J Urol 158:1534, 1997.

Coplen DE, Duckett JW: The modern approach to ureteroceles. J Urol 153:166, 1995.

Cuckow PM, Dinneen MD, Risdon RA, et al: Long-term renal function in the posterior urethral valves, unilateral reflux and renal dysplasia syndrome. J Urol 158:1004, 1997.

Denes ED, Barthold JS, Gonzalez R: Early prognostic value of serum creatinine levels in children with posterior urethral valves. J Urol 157:1441, 1997.

Duel BP, Mogbo K, Barthold JS, et al: Prognostic value of initial renal ultrasound in patients with posterior urethral valves. J Urol 160:1198, 1998.

Elder JS: Antenatal hydronephrosis: Fetal and neonatal management. Pediatr Clin North Am 44:1299, 1997.

Elder JS, Koff SA: The pathophysiology and biological potential of hydronephrosis in the fetus and neonate. *In:* O'Donnell B, Koff SA (eds): Pediatric Urology, 3rd ed. Oxford, Butterworth Heinemann, 1997, pp 380–391.
Elder JS, Hladky D, Selzman AA: Outpatient nephrectomy for non-functioning kidneys. J Urol 154:712, 1995.
Flashner SC, Mesrobian H-G J, Flatt JA, et al: Nonobstructive dilatation of upper urinary tract may later convert to obstruction. Urology 42:569, 1993.
Freedman AL, Bukowski TP, Smith CA, et al: Fetal therapy for obstructive uropathy: Specific outcomes diagnosis. J Urol 156:720, 1996.
Good CD, Vinnicombe SJ, Minty IL, et al: Posterior urethral valves in male infants and newborns: Detection with US of the urethra before and during voiding. Radiology 198:387, 1996.
Hutton KAR, Thomas DFM, Davies BW: Prenatally detected posterior urethral valves: Qualitative assessment of second trimester scans and prediction of outcome. J Urol 158:1022, 1997.
King LR: Hydronephrosis: When is obstruction not obstruction? Urol Clin North Am 22:31, 1995.
Maizels M, Mitchell B, Kass E, et al: Outcome of nospecific hydronephrosis in the infant: A report from the registry of the Society for Fetal Urology. J Urol 152:2324, 1994.
Maizels M, Reisman M, Flom LS, et al: Grading nephroureteral dilatation detected in the first year of life: Correlation with obstruction. J Urol 148:609, 1992.
Manivel JC, Pettmato G, Reinberg Y, et al: Prune belly syndrome: Clinicopathological study of 28 cases. Pediatr Pathol 9:691, 1989.
O'Reilly P, Aurell M, Britton K, et al: Consensus on diuresis renography for investigating the dilated upper urinary tract. J Nucl Med 37:1872, 1996.
Perez-Aytes A, Graham JM, Hersh JH, et al: Urethral obstruction sequence and lower limb deficiency: Evidence for the vascular disruption hypothesis. J Pediatr 123:398, 1993.
Plaire JC, Pope JC IV, Kropp BP, et al: Management of ectopic ureters: Experience with the upper tract approach. J Urol 158:1245, 1997.
Reinberg Y, Chelimsky G, González R: Urethral atresia and the prune belly syndrome. Report of 6 cases. Br J Urol 72:122, 1993.
Salem YH, Majd M, Rushton HG, et al: Outcome analysis of pediatric pyeloplasty as a function of patient age, presentation and differential renal function. J Urol 154:1889, 1995.
Shalaby-Rana E, Lowe LH, Blask AN, et al: Imaging in pediatric urology. Pediatr Clin North Am 44:1065, 1997.
Society for Fetal Urology and Pediatric Nuclear Medicine Council: The "well tempered diuretic renogram": A standard method to examine the asymptomatic neonate with hydronephrosis or hydroureteronephrosis. J Nucl Med 33:2047, 1992.
Tietjen DN, Gloor JM, Husmann DA: Proximal urinary diversion in the management of posterior urethral valves: Is it necessary? J Urol 158:1008, 1997.
Vates TS, Bukowski T, Triest J, et al: Is there a best alternative to treating the obstructed upper pole? J Urol 156:744, 1996.

CHAPTER 549
Anomalies of the Bladder

BLADDER EXSTROPHY

Exstrophy of the urinary bladder occurs about once in every 35,000 to 40,000 births. The male:female ratio is 2:1. The severity ranges from a small vesicocutaneous fistula in the abdominal wall or simple epispadias to complete exstrophy of the cloaca involving exposure of the entire hindgut and the bladder.

CLINICAL MANIFESTATIONS. These anomalies result when the mesoderm fails to invade the cephalad extension of the cloacal membrane; the extent of this failure determines the degree of the anomaly. In classic bladder exstrophy (Fig. 549–1), the bladder protrudes from the abdominal wall, and its mucosa is exposed. The umbilicus is displaced downward, the pubic rami are widely separated in the midline, and the rectus muscles are separated. In males, there is complete epispadias with a wide and shallow scrotum. Undescended testes and inguinal hernias are common. Females also have epispadias, with separation of the two sides of the clitoris and wide separation of the labia. The anus is displaced anteriorly in both sexes, and there may be rectal prolapse. The consequences of untreated bladder exstrophy are total urinary incontinence and an increased incidence of bladder cancer, usually adenocarcinoma.

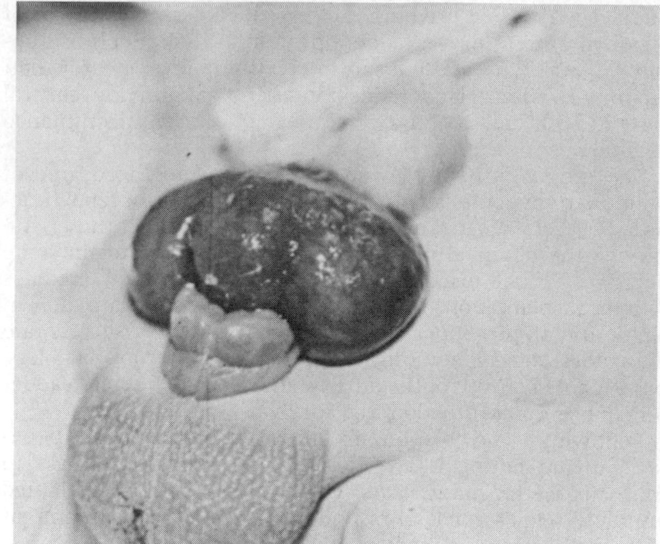

Figure 549–1 Classic bladder exstrophy. The bladder is exposed in the midline; the umbilical cord is displaced caudally; the penis is epispadiac; and the scrotum is broad.

The genital deformities can produce sexual disability in both sexes, particularly in the male. The wide separation of the pubic rami causes a characteristic broad-based gait but no significant disability. In classic bladder exstrophy, the upper urinary tracts usually are normal.

TREATMENT. Management of bladder exstrophy should start at birth. The bladder should be covered with plastic wrap to keep the bladder mucosa moist. Application of gauze or petroleum-gauze to the bladder mucosa should be avoided. The infant should then be promptly transferred to a center equipped for the treatment of such anomalies. Conventional therapy includes a series of three staged reconstructive procedures in boys and two staged procedures in girls. A single stage complete reconstruction in the neonatal infant is being evaluated.

Prompt closure of the exstrophied bladder is the preferred treatment. During this procedure the abdominal wall is mobilized and the pubic rami are brought together in the midline. If the bladder closure is performed during the 1st 48 hr of life, there is sufficient mobility of the pubic rami to allow approximation of the pubic symphysis. If the procedure is delayed, however, the pelvic bone must be broken (pelvic osteotomy) to allow the pubic rami to be brought together. Early bladder closure can be applied to almost all neonatal infants with classic bladder exstrophy. Treatment should be deferred in selected situations when surgery would be excessively risky or complex, such as in a premature baby.

The initial operation is the closure of the bladder, closure of the abdominal wall and, in the male, elongation of the urethral plate and penis. Postoperatively, the infant's upper urinary tract is monitored closely for the possible development of hydronephrosis and infection. The majority of such infants have vesicoureteral reflux and should receive antibiotic prophylaxis. In the male, the second stage is epispadias repair, which is generally performed between 1 and 2 yr of age. At this point the child has total urinary incontinence because there is no external urinary sphincter.

The final stage of reconstruction involves creation of a sphincter muscle for bladder control and correction of the vesicoureteral reflux. In general, the child is at least 3 yr of age, the bladder capacity must be at least 60 to 80 mL, and the child must have gained rectal control.

At puberty, the pubic hair is distributed to the sides of the external genitals. A monsplasty is performed to provide a more normal escutcheon.

PROGNOSIS. This plan of treatment has yielded more than 70% continence in some centers, with less than 15% deterioration of the upper urinary tract. This continence rate reflects not only the successful reconstruction but also the quality and size of the bladder. It appears that children who have reconstructive surgery as newborns have a greater chance of obtaining a normally functioning bladder. Children who remain incontinent for more than 1 yr following bladder neck reconstruction or those who are not eligible for bladder neck reconstruction because of a small bladder capacity are candidates for an alternative reconstructive procedure to achieve dryness. Such procedures include (1) augmentation cystoplasty, in which the bladder is enlarged with a patch of small or large bowel to increase its capacity; (2) creation of a neobladder out of small and large bowel with placement of a continent abdominal stoma through which clean intermittent catheterization can be performed; (3) placement of an artificial urinary sphincter, with possible augmentation cystoplasty; and (4) ureterosigmoidostomy, in which the ureters are detached from the bladder and sutured to the sigmoid colon. Individuals with the latter procedure void from the rectum and rely on their anal sphincter for continence. This operation was popular in the past and is still employed in some centers; it is attractive because it avoids the need for external urinary diversion. However, it carries a significant risk of chronic pyelonephritis, upper urinary tract damage, metabolic acidosis resulting from absorption of hydrogen ions and chloride in the intestine, and a 15% long-term risk of colonic carcinoma.

Late follow-up has shown that most men with exstrophy have a somewhat short penis but satisfactory sexual function. Fertility has been low, probably because of iatrogenic injury to the secondary sexual organs during reconstruction. In women, fertility is not affected, but uterine prolapse during pregnancy is a problem.

OTHER EXSTROPHY ANOMALIES

The more complex cases of *cloacal exstrophy*, with an incidence of 1 in 400,000, have an omphalocele and severe abnormalities of the colon and the rectum, and often have short bowel syndrome. Approximately 50% of patients have an upper urinary tract anomaly, and 50% have spina bifida. Current reconstructive techniques result in a satisfactory outcome in most patients with permanent urinary diversion (either ileal conduit or continent urinary diversion) and a colostomy. Because the penis in these individuals usually is diminutive, genital reconstruction in males with cloacal exstrophy generally has been unsatisfactory, and most authors recommend assigning a female gender to such infants.

Epispadias is in the spectrum of exstrophy anomalies, affecting approximately 1 in 117,000 boys and 1 in 480,000 girls. In boys, the diagnosis is obvious because the prepuce is distributed primarily on the ventral aspect of the penile shaft and the urethral meatus is on the dorsum of the penis. In girls, the clitoris is bifid and the urethra is split dorsally. Distal epispadias in boys usually is associated with normal urinary control and normal upper urinary tracts and should be repaired by 6–12 mo of age. In the more severe cases of epispadias, the sphincter is incompletely formed and these individuals (male and female) have total urinary incontinence and usually separation of the pubic rami. These children require surgical reconstruction procedures analogous to those of the 2nd and 3rd stages of management of patients with classic bladder exstrophy.

BLADDER DIVERTICULA

Bladder diverticula usually occur at the ureterovesical junction and are associated with vesicoureteral reflux (see Fig. 547–6), because the diverticulum interferes with the normal flap-valve attachment between the ureter and bladder. Congenital diverticula occur in other locations also. Bladder diverticula are also commonly associated with distal urethral obstruction or neurogenic bladder dysfunction. Small diverticula require no treatment other than that of the primary disease, whereas large diverticula may contribute to inefficient voiding, residual urine, urinary stasis, and urinary tract infections and should be excised.

URACHAL ANOMALIES

Urachal abnormalities are more common in males than in females. A patent urachus can occur as an isolated anomaly, or it may be associated with prune-belly syndrome. In this condition, there is continuous urinary drainage from the umbilicus. The tract should be excised surgically. Another urachal anomaly is the urachal cyst, which can become infected. Typical symptoms and physical findings include suprapubic pain, fever, irritative voiding symptoms, and an infraumbilical mass, which can be erythematous. Diagnosis is made by ultrasonography or computed tomography. Treatment is intravenous antibiotic therapy and drainage and excision. Other urachal anomalies include the urachal diverticulum, which is a diverticulum of the bladder dome, and external urachal sinus, which is a blind external sinus that opens at the umbilicus. These lesions should be excised.

Cilento BG Jr, Bauer SB, Retik AB, et al: Urachal anomalies: Defining the best diagnostic modality. Urology 52:120, 1998.

Elder JS: Continent appendico-colostomy: A variant of the Mitrofanoff principle for pediatric urinary tract reconstruction. J Urol 148:117, 1992.

Goldman IL, Caldamone AA, Gauderer MWL, et al: Infected urachal cysts; A review of ten cases. J Urol 140:375, 1988.

Hollowell JG, Hill PD, Duffy PG, et al: Evaluation and treatment of incontinence after bladder neck reconstruction in exstrophy and epispadias. Br J Urol 71:743, 1993.

Johnston JH: Vesical diverticula without urinary obstruction in childhood. J Urol 84:535, 1960.

Stein R, Hohenfellner M, Fisch M, et al: Social integration, sexual behaviour and fertility in patients with bladder exstrophy—a long-term follow up. Eur J Pediatr 155:678, 1996.

Zaontz MR, Steckler RE, Shortliffe LMD, et al: Multicenter experience with the Mitchell technique for epispadias repair. J Urol 160:172, 1998.

CHAPTER 550
Neuropathic Bladder

Jack S. Elder

Neuropathic bladder dysfunction in children is usually congenital and may result from myelomeningocele, lipomeningocele, sacral agenesis, or other spinal abnormalities. Acquired diseases and traumatic lesions of the spinal cord are less frequent. Central nervous system tumors, sacrococcygeal teratoma, and spinal abnormalities associated with imperforate anus can also result in abnormal innervation of the bladder or sphincter, or both.

MYELODYSPLASIA. Myelodysplasia (*spina bifida*) describes various abnormal conditions of the vertebral column that affect spinal cord function, including *myelomeningocele*, and *meningocele* (see Chapter 601). The incidence of myelodysplasia is 1 in 1,000 births in the United States, but with antenatal screening and abortion, the incidence is decreasing.

The most important consequences of neurogenic bladder dysfunction are urinary incontinence, urinary tract infections (UTIs), and upper tract deterioration. Hydronephrosis, pyelonephritis, and renal function deterioration were once the most common causes of premature demise of affected individuals.

In the neonate, renal ultrasonography, a random check of postvoid residual urine volumes, and a voiding cystourethrogram are performed following closure of the back. Approximately 10–15% of patients have hydronephrosis and 25% have vesicoureteral reflux. A *urodynamic study* is also performed. This study involves filling the bladder with saline and measuring the bladder volume and pressure, as well as assessing sphincter tone. During bladder filling, the bladder may show (1) uninhibited (premature) contractions at low volumes, (2) normal bladder volume with contraction at an appropriate volume, or (3) atonia (lack of bladder contraction). Bladder compliance or elasticity may also be reduced. The sphincter may show (1) normal tone with relaxation during bladder contraction, (2) reduced or absent tone, or (3) normal or increased tone that increases during bladder contraction (termed *detrusor-sphincter dyssynergia*) (Fig. 550–1).

Renal damage usually results from failure of the sphincter to relax during a bladder contraction. This dyssynergia results in functional obstruction of the bladder outlet, leading to high intravesical pressure, bladder muscle hypertrophy and trabeculation, and transmission of the high pressure into the upper urinary tract, causing hydronephrosis (Fig. 550–2). Vesicoureteral reflux and UTI compound the problem. Treatment includes reduction of bladder pressure with anticholinergic drugs (oxybutynin, 0.2 mg/kg/24 hr in two or three divided doses) and clean intermittent catheterization every 3–4 hr. If there is vesicoureteral reflux or UTIs, antimicrobial prophylaxis is also prescribed. In the newborn or infant, temporary urinary diversion by cutaneous vesicostomy is a satisfactory alternative for severe reflux. Clean intermittent catheterization and anticholinergic therapy cure the reflux in up to 80% of patients without ureteral dilatation (grades I and II). Children with more severe reflux require corrective surgery followed by intermittent catheterization and anticholinergic drugs. When intermittent catheterization is difficult or if anticholinergic agents are not well tolerated, a temporary cutaneous vesicostomy provides effective bladder decompression. Failure of these methods to relieve intravesical pressures is an indication for augmentation enterocystoplasty and intermittent catheterization.

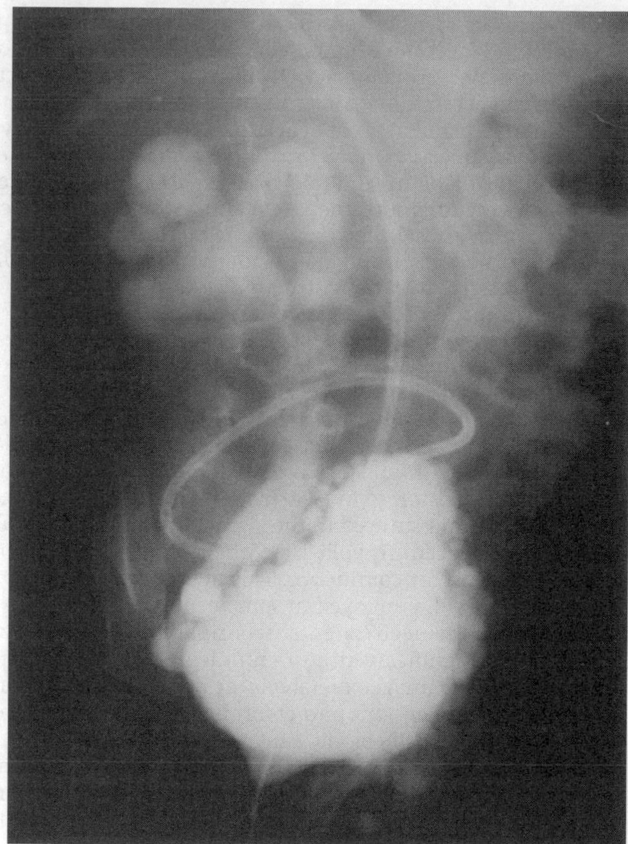

Figure 550–2 Voiding cystourethrogram in an infant with myelodysplasia shows a severely trabeculated bladder with multiple diverticula and grade V (out of V) right vesicoureteral reflux. Evaluation showed severe detrusor-sphincter dyssynergia.

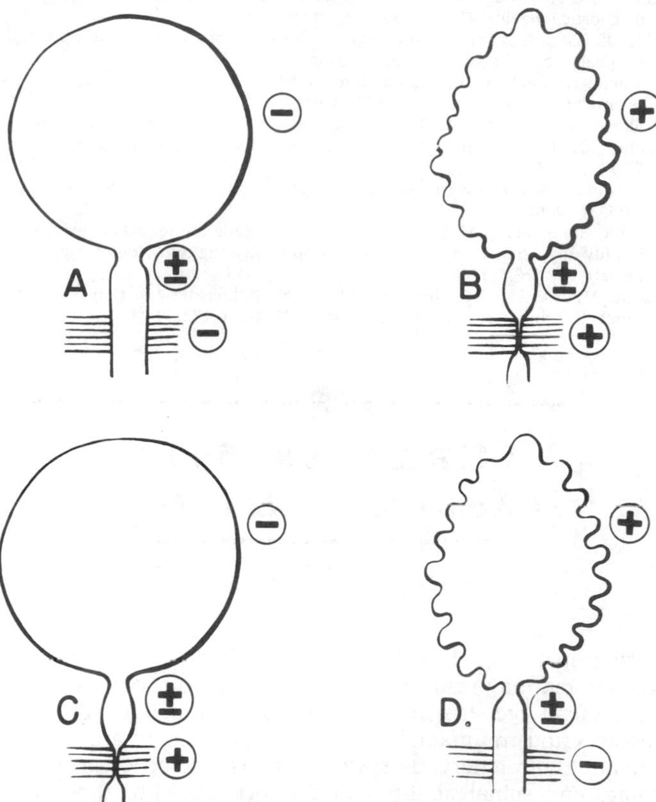

Figure 550–1 Grouping of neurogenic bladder dysfunction according to the innervation, tonicity, and coordination of the detrusor and sphincters described by Guzman. This grouping is based on data from imaging studies, cystometrography, and electromyography of the sphincters. Patients in group *B* are at risk of developing reflux and hydronephrosis. For guidance in the treatment of incontinence, group *A* benefits from procedures that increase outlet resistance, group *B* from anticholinergics or bladder augmentation surgery, and group *C* from intermittent catheterization, and group *D* requires both increased outlet resistance and pharmacologic or surgical bladder enlargement. Most patients require intermittent catheterization to empty. (Modified from Gonzalez R: Urinary incontinence. *In:* Kelalis PK, King LR, Belman AB [eds]: Clinical Pediatric Urology. Philadelphia, WB Saunders, 1992, p 387.)

Urinary incontinence in the child with neuropathic bladder can result from total or partial denervation of the sphincter, bladder hyperreflexia, poor bladder compliance, chronic urinary retention, or a combination of these factors. Less than 5% of children born with myelodysplasia achieve normal continence. Supravesical diversion, commonly performed in the 1970s to prevent incontinence, had a high long-term complication rate and is now seldom employed.

Incontinence often is addressed around 4 yr of age. Nearly all children require clean intermittent catheterization to stay dry. This technique allows efficient bladder emptying with minimal risk of symptomatic UTI. The treatment of incontinence is tailored to the individual case. The urinary tract should be evaluated with renal ultrasonography, a voiding cystourethrogram, and a urodynamic study, including bladder capacity. If the sphincter tone is sufficient and the bladder has adequate compliance, intermittent catheterization every 3–4 hr is usually successful in keeping the child dry. If there are unstable bladder contractions, an anticholinergic medication such as oxybutynin chloride or hyoscyamine is prescribed to increase bladder capacity. If there is sphincter incompetence, α-adrenergic medications are used to try to enhance continence. Bacteriuria is seen in up to 50% of children using intermittent self-catheterization, but it seldom causes symptoms. In the absence of reflux, there seems to be little cause for concern. Antibacterial prophylaxis can often be effective in keeping the urine sterile while intermittent catheterization is used. With this treatment plan, 40–85% of patients are dry, depending on one's definition of continence. Some children wear a pad in their underwear or a diaper but state that they are dry.

If there is persistent incontinence despite these measures, reconstructive urinary tract surgery usually can provide complete or satisfactory continence. If urethral resistance is low, implantation of an artificial sphincter is usually successful. This sphincter consists of an inflatable cuff that is placed around the bladder neck, a pressure-regulating balloon implanted in the extraperitoneal space, and a pumping mechanism that is implanted in the scrotum of males and in the labia of females. Alternatively, bladder neck reconstructive procedures often are successful. If the bladder capacity or bladder compliance is low, or if there are persistent uninhibited contractions despite anticholinergic therapy, enlargement of the bladder with a patch of small or large intestine or stomach, termed *augmentation cystoplasty* or *enterocystoplasty,* is effective. These patients still need to perform clean intermittent catheterization. If urethral catheterization is difficult, a continent stoma may be incorporated into the urinary tract reconstruction. A common method is termed the *Mitrofanoff* procedure, in which the appendix is isolated from the cecum on its vascular pedicle and is interposed between the bladder and abdominal wall to allow intermittent catheterization through a dry stoma. Many of these patients also have bowel problems with constipation, and some benefit from a procedure termed the *antegrade continence enema* procedure, in which the appendix is brought out to the skin to allow a catheter to be inserted for antegrade enema.

There are important potential complications of enterocystoplasty:

1. The urine is usually colonized with gram-negative bacteria, and attempts to sterilize the urine for prolonged periods usually fail. There is no evidence that chronic bacteriuria in these patients is associated with renal damage. Therefore, only symptomatic UTIs should be treated.

2. The enteric mucosal surface in contact with the urine absorbs ammonium, chloride, and hydrogen ions and loses potassium. Hyperchloremic metabolic acidosis can result and may require medical treatment. Chronic acidosis may compromise skeletal growth. This complication is more common in patients with compromised renal function. To overcome this limitation of enterocystoplasty in patients with chronic renal insufficiency, a gastric segment can be used instead of a segment of the small or large intestine. The stomach secretes chloride and hydrogen ions; thus, pre-existing metabolic acidosis remains stable or improves. However, the possibility of intractable metabolic alkalosis and peptic ulceration of the augmentation has diminished the enthusiasm for this procedure.

3. Perforation of the augmented bladder and peritonitis are serious complications that are potentially life-threatening. This complication seems to result from acute or chronic overdistention of the augmented bladder. These patients typically present with severe abdominal pain. Prompt diagnosis and treatment with exploratory laparotomy and bladder closure are necessary. Meticulous adherence to the prescribed program of intermittent catheterization to avoid bladder overdistention is important.

4. Bladder calculi have developed in as many as 70% of children followed for 10 yr after enterocystoplasty. The calculi develop because of mucus that accumulates in the bladder and acts as a nidus for stone formation.

5. The potential for malignancy secondary to enterocystoplasty is unknown but based on past experience with ureterosigmoidostomy and some reported cases, it is prudent to advise yearly endoscopic examinations or urine cytologic studies beginning in the 10th postoperative year.

LATEX ALLERGY. One of the most serious problems encountered by as many as 35% individuals with spina bifida and other urologic conditions that require clean intermittent catheterization and urinary tract reconstructive procedures is latex allergy. This IgE-mediated allergy is acquired and is secondary to repeated exposure to the medically associated latex allergen. Latex allergy may manifest with watery eyes, sneezing, itching, hives, or anaphylaxis when blowing up a balloon or if an examiner is using latex gloves. Intraoperatively, a sensitized individual can experience anaphylactic shock. Routinely providing a latex-free environment for these children is the best policy.

OCCULT SPINAL DYSRAPHISM. Approximately 1 in 4,000 patients have occult spinal dysraphism, which includes lipomeningocele, intradural lipoma, diastematomyelia, tight filum terminale, dermoid cyst-sinus, aberrant nerve roots, anterior sacral meningocele, and cauda equina tumor. More than 90% of patients have a cutaneous abnormality overlying the lower spine, including a small dimple, tuft of hair, dermal vascular malformation, or a subcutaneous lipoma (Fig. 550–3). Often these children have high arched feet, discrepancy in muscle size and strength between the legs, and a gait abnormality. Newborns and young infants usually have a normal neurologic examination. Older children often have absent perineal sensation and back pain. Lower urinary tract function is abnormal in 40% of patients, including incontinence, recurrent UTI, and fecal soiling. The likelihood of a normal examination is inversely related to the age at surgical correction of the spinal

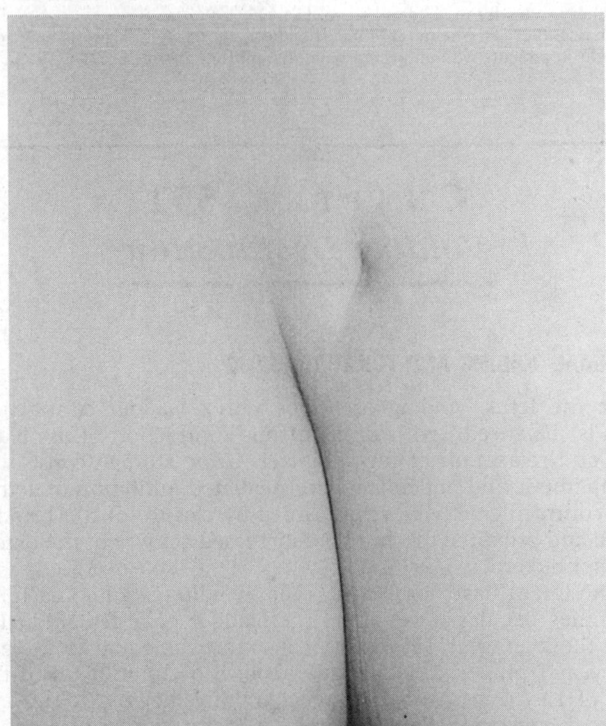

Figure 550–3 Buttocks of teenage boy with tethered cord secondary to lipomeningocele. Note sacral dimple and deviation of gluteal fold to the left.

lesion. In infants with abnormal urodynamics, 60% revert to normal; in older children only 27% become normal. Management of the urinary tract in other children is similar to that described for myelodysplasia.

SACRAL AGENESIS. Sacral agenesis is defined as the absence of part or all of two or more lower vertebral bodies. This condition is more common in the offspring of women with diabetes. These children have flattened buttocks and a low, short gluteal cleft, but usually have no orthopedic deformity, although some have high arched feet. Palpation of the coccygeal area reveals the absent vertebrae. Approximately 20% of cases are undetected until the age of 3–4 yr; many are diagnosed following unsuccessful toilet training. Urodynamic studies in these children show a variety of patterns, and most need clean intermittent catheterization and pharmacotherapy to stay dry.

CEREBRAL PALSY. Children with cerebral palsy have reasonable bladder control. However, continence is achieved at a later age than in unaffected children. Their upper urinary tracts are usually normal. Urodynamic studies have shown that most have uninhibited bladder contractions. Timed voiding and anticholinergic therapy is usually effective. Clean intermittent catheterization rarely is necessary. Also see Chapters 37 and 607.1.

Bomalaski MD, Teague JL, Brooks B: The long-term impact of urologic management on the quality of life in children with spina bifida. J Urol 156:778, 1995.
Bosco PJ, Bauer SB, Colodny AH, et al: The long-term follow-up of artificial urinary sphincters in children. J Urol 146:396, 1991.
Edelstein RA, Bauer SB, Kelly MD, et al: The long-term urologic response of neonates with myelodysplasia treated proactively with intermittent catheterization and anticholinergic therapy. J Urol 154:1500, 1995.
Elder JS: Continent appendico-colostomy: A variant of the Mitrofanoff principle for pediatric urinary tract reconstruction. J Urol 148:117, 1992.
Ewalt DH, Bauer SB: Pediatric neurourology. Urol Clin North Am 23:501, 1996.
Fernandes E, Reinberg Y, Vernier R, et al: Neurogenic bladder in children. Review of pathophysiology and current treatment. J Pediatr 124:1, 1994.
Gibson PJ, Britton J, Hall DMB, et al: Lumbosacral skin markers and identification of occult spinal dysraphism in neonates. Acta Pediatr 84:208, 1995.
Kurzrock EA, Polse S: Renal deterioration in myelodysplastic children: Urodynamic evaluation and clinical correlates. J Urol 159:1657, 1998.
Landwehr LP, Boguniewicz M: Current perspectives on latex allergy. J Pediatr 128:305, 1996.
Levesque PE, Bauer SB, Atala A, et al: Ten-year experience with the artificial urinary sphincter in children. J Urol 156:625, 1996.
Satar N, Bauer SB, Shefner J, et al: The effects of delayed diagnosis and treatment in patients with an occult spinal dysraphism. J Urol 154:754, 1995.

CHAPTER 551
Voiding Dysfunction

NORMAL VOIDING AND TOILET TRAINING

In the fetus, voiding occurs by reflex bladder contraction and is "balanced," with simultaneous contraction of the bladder and relaxation of the sphincter. Urine storage consists of sympathetic and pudendal nerve-mediated inhibition of detrusor contractile activity accompanied by closure of the bladder neck and proximal urethra with increased activity of the external sphincter.

The infant has coordinated, reflex voiding as often as 15 to 20 times per day. Over time, the bladder enlarges gradually, and the average *bladder capacity* in ounces is equal to the age (in years) plus 2. This formula applies to children up to the age of 12–14 yr. At 2–4 yr, toilet training begins. To achieve normal conscious bladder control, several steps must occur: (1) awareness of bladder filling, (2) cortical inhibition (suprapontine modulation) of reflex (unstable) bladder contractions, (3) ability to consciously tighten the external sphincter to prevent incontinence, (4) normal bladder growth, and (5) motivation by the child to stay dry. The *transitional phase of voiding* refers to the period when children are acquiring bladder control. Girls typically acquire bladder control before boys, and bowel control is typically achieved before urinary control. By 5 yr of age, 90–95% are nearly completely continent during the day and 80–85% are continent at night (also see Chapter 20).

NOCTURNAL ENURESIS (See Chapter 20.3)

Nocturnal enuresis is the occurrence of involuntary voiding at night at 5 yr, the age when volitional control of micturition is expected. Enuresis may be primary (75%; nocturnal urinary control never achieved) or secondary (25%; the child was dry at night for at least a few months, and then enuresis occurs). In addition, 75% of children with enuresis are wet only at night, whereas 25% are wet day and night. This distinction is important because the pathogenesis of the two patterns is different. Approximately 60% of children with nocturnal enuresis are boys. Family history is also important and is positive in 50% of cases. Although primary nocturnal enuresis may be polygenetic, candidate genes have been localized to both chromosomes 12 and 13. If one parent was enuretic, each child has a 44% risk of enuresis; if both parents were enuretic, each child has a 77% likelihood of enuresis.

Nocturnal enuresis without overt daytime voiding symptoms affects up to 20% of children at the age of 5 yr; it ceases spontaneously in approximately 15% of involved children every year thereafter. Its frequency among adults is less than 1%.

The *pathogenesis* of primary nocturnal enuresis (normal daytime voiding habits) is multifactorial and includes

- Delayed maturation of the cortical mechanisms that allow voluntary control of the micturition reflex.
- Sleep disorder—enuretic children are classically described as being deep sleepers, although no specific sleep pattern has been described. Enuresis can occur in any stage of sleep. All children are most difficult to arouse in the first third of the night and are easiest to awaken in the last third of the night, but enuretic children are more difficult to arouse than those with normal bladder control.
- Reduced antidiuretic hormone production at night, resulting in an increased urine output, which explains why children with enuresis often are described as "soaking the bed."
- Genetic factors, with chromosomes 12 and 13q the likely sites of the gene for enuresis; family history is often positive in enuretic children, as described earlier.
- Psychologic factors, often implicated in secondary enuresis.
- Organic factors, such as urinary tract infection (UTI) or obstructive uropathy, which is an uncommon cause of enuresis.
- Sleep apnea (snoring) secondary to enlarged adenoids.

A careful history should be obtained, especially with respect to fluid intake at night and pattern of nocturnal enuresis. Children with diabetes insipidus, diabetes mellitus, and chronic renal disease may have a high obligatory urinary output and a compensatory polydipsia. The family should be asked whether the child snores loudly at night. A complete physical examination should include palpation of the abdomen and rectal examination after voiding to assess the possibility of a chronically distended bladder. The child with nocturnal enuresis should be examined carefully for neurologic and spinal abnormalities. There is an increased incidence of bacteriuria in enuretic girls and, if found, should be investigated and treated (see Chapter 546), although this does not always lead to resolution of bed-wetting. Urinalysis should be obtained after an overnight fast and evaluated for specific gravity or osmolality, or both, to exclude polyuria as a cause of frequency and incontinence and to ascertain that the concentrating ability is normal. The absence of glycosuria should be confirmed. If there are no daytime symptoms and if the physical examination and urinalysis are normal, and culture is negative, further evaluation for urinary tract pathology generally is not warranted. A renal ultrasonogram is reasonable in an older child with enuresis or in children who do not respond appropriately to therapy.

The best approach to *treatment* is to reassure parents that the condition is self-limited and to avoid punitive measures that may affect the child's psychologic development adversely (see Chapter 20.3). Fluid intake in the evening should be restricted to 2 oz after 6 or 7 P.M. if the child weighs less than 75 lb, 3 oz if the child weighs 75 to 100 lb, and 4 oz if the child weighs more than 100 lb. In addition, the parents should be certain that the child voids at bedtime. If the child snores and the adenoids are enlarged, referral to an otolaryngologist should be considered, as adenoidectomy may result in cure of the enuresis.

Active treatment should be avoided in children less than 6 yr because enuresis is extremely common in younger children. The simplest initial measure is motivational and includes a star chart for dry nights. Waking the child a few hours after they go to sleep to have them void often allows them to awaken dry, although this measure is not curative. Some have recommended that children try holding their urine for longer periods during the day, but there is no evidence that this approach is beneficial. *Conditioning therapy* involves use of an auditory alarm attached to electrodes in the underwear. The alarm sounds when the child voids and is intended to awaken the child and alert them to void. This form of therapy is considered curative and has a reported success of 30–60%. Often the alarm wakes up other family members and not the enuretic child; persistence for several months is necessary. Conditioning therapy tends to be most effective in older children. The primary role of psychologic therapy is to help the child deal with enuresis psychologically and help motivate them to get up to void at night if they awaken with a full bladder.

Pharmacologic therapy is intended to treat the symptom of enuresis and is not curative. One form of treatment is *desmopressin acetate,* which is a synthetic analog of antidiuretic hormone and reduces urine production overnight. It is available as a tablet, with a dosage of 0.2–0.6 mg at bedtime. In the past it was used as a nasal spray, with a dosage of 10 μg (1 spray) to 40 μg (4 sprays total) at bedtime. The lowest effective dose should be used. It is important to reduce evening fluid intake, and the drug should not be used if the child has a systemic illness with vomiting or diarrhea. Hyponatremia has been reported in a few children, primarily those who were not using the medication properly. In children with rhinorrhea, the nasal spray is not absorbed and consequently is ineffective. Desmopressin acetate is effective in 40–60% of children. If effective, it should be used for 3–6 mo, and then an attempt should be made to taper it. If tapering results in recurrent enuresis, the medication may be started again at the higher dosage. No adverse events have been reported with the long-term use of desmopressin acetate. Another pharmacologic agent is *imipramine,* which is a tricyclic antidepressant. This medication has mild anticholinergic and α-adrenergic effects and may alter the sleep pattern also. The dosage of imipramine is 25 mg in children 6–8 yr, 50 mg in children 9–12 yr, and 75 mg in teenagers. Reported success rates are 30–60%. Side effects include anxiety, insomnia, and dry mouth. In addition, the drug is one of the most common causes of poisoning by prescription medication in younger siblings. Oxybutynin chloride, a pure anticholinergic agent, has been used in some children with primary nocturnal enuresis, but the response rate is low.

DIURNAL INCONTINENCE

Daytime incontinence not secondary to neurologic abnormalities is common in children. At age 5 yr, 95% have been dry during the day at some time and 92% are dry. At 7 yr, 96% are dry, although 15% have significant urgency at times. At 12 yr, 99% are dry during the day. The most common cause of daytime incontinence is a pediatric unstable bladder (also termed *uninhibited bladder, bladder spasms*). Table 551–1 lists this and other causes of diurnal incontinence in children.

TABLE 551–1 Causes of Urinary Incontinence in Childhood

Pediatric unstable bladder (uninhibited bladder)
Infrequent voiding
Detrusor-sphincter dyssynergia
Non-neurogenic neurogenic bladder (Hinman syndrome)
Vaginal voiding
Giggle incontinence
Cystitis
Bladder outlet obstruction (posterior urethral valves)
Ectopic ureter and fistula
Sphincter abnormality (epispadias, exstrophy; urogenital sinus abnormality)
Neurogenic
Overflow incontinence
Traumatic
Iatrogenic
Behavioral
Combination

Important points in the history include the pattern of incontinence, including the frequency, the volume of urine lost during incontinent episodes, whether the incontinence is associated with urgency or giggling, whether it occurs after voiding, and whether the incontinence is continuous. In addition, the frequency of voiding and whether there is nocturnal enuresis, a strong, continuous urinary stream, or sensation of incomplete bladder emptying should be assessed. Other urologic problems such as UTIs, reflux, neurologic disorders, or a family history of duplication anomalies should be assessed. Bowel habits also should be evaluated, as incontinence is common in children with constipation or encopresis, or both. Diurnal incontinence may occur in girls with a history of sexual abuse. Physical examination is directed at identifying signs of organic causes of incontinence: short stature, hypertension, enlarged kidneys or bladder, or both, constipation, labial adhesion, ureteral ectopy (Figs. 551–1 to 551–3), back or sacral anomalies (Fig. 550–3), and neurologic abnormalities. A uri-

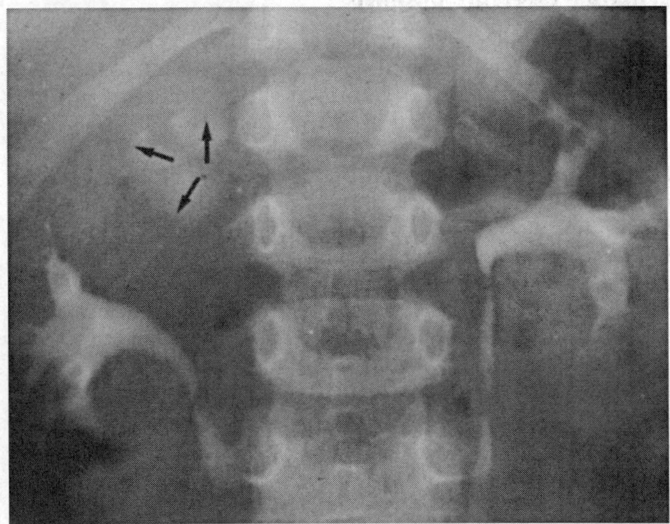

Figure 551–1 Duplication of the right collecting system with ectopic ureter. Excretory urogram in a female presenting with a normal voiding pattern and constant urinary dribbling. The left kidney is normal and the right side, well visualized, is the lower collecting system of a duplicated kidney. On the upper pole opposite the 1st and 2nd vertebral bodies, note the accumulation of contrast material corresponding with a poorly functioning upper pole drained by a ureter opening in the vestibule.

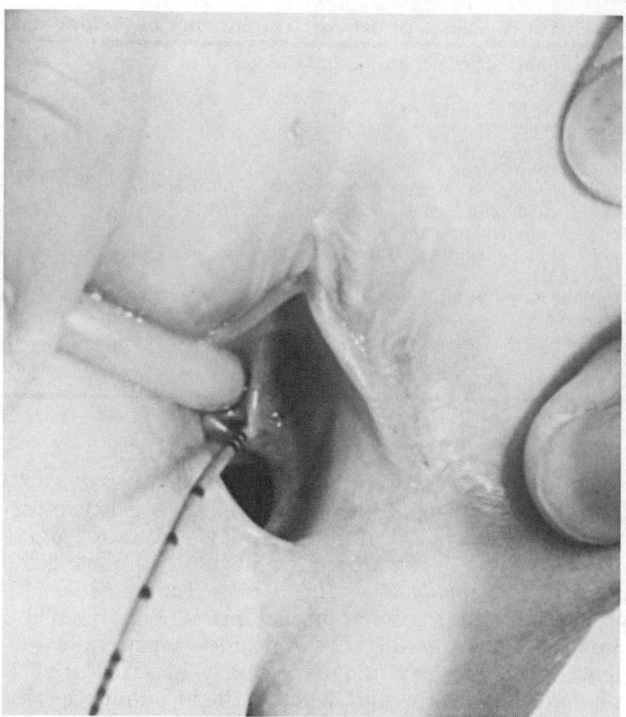

Figure 551–2 Ectopic ureter. The photograph shows an ectopic ureter entering the vestibule next to the urethral meatus. The thin ureteral catheter with transverse marks has been introduced into this ectopic ureter. This girl had a normal voiding pattern and constant urinary dribbling.

nalysis or culture, or both, should be performed to check for infection. In some cases, assessing the postvoid residual urine volume or urinary flow rate is appropriate. Imaging is reserved for children who have significant physical findings, a family history of urinary tract anomalies, UTIs, or those who do not respond to therapy appropriately. A renal ultrasonogram with or without a voiding cystourethrogram is indicated. Cystometrography may be helpful if there is evidence of neurologic disease or if empirical therapy is ineffective.

PEDIATRIC UNSTABLE BLADDER

A pediatric unstable bladder is smaller than normal and exhibits strong uninhibited contractions. These children typically exhibit urinary frequency, urgency, and urge incontinence. Such symptoms are also seen in about 25% of children with nocturnal enuresis. Often girls will squat down on their foot to try to prevent incontinence. Many children indicate they do not feel the need to urinate, even just before they are incontinent. In females, a history of recurrent UTI is common, but incontinence may persist long after infections are brought under control. It is not clear in these cases if the voiding dysfunction is a sequel of the infections or if the voiding dysfunction disposes to recurrent infections. In addition, constipation is common. Initial therapy is timed voiding every 1.5–2 hr and anticholinergic therapy with oxybutynin chloride or hyoscyamine. Constipation and UTIs also should be addressed. This treatment program is usually prolonged and should be interrupted periodically to determine its continued need. Children not responding to this simple treatment should be evaluated endoscopically and urodynamically to rule out other possible forms of bladder or sphincter dysfunction.

NON-NEUROGENIC NEUROGENIC BLADDER (HINMAN SYNDROME)

Hinman syndrome is a more serious but less common disorder involving failure of the external sphincter to relax during voiding in children without neurologic abnormalities. Children with this syndrome, also called *detrusor-sphincter dyssynergia*, typically exhibit a staccato stream, day and night wetting, recurrent UTIs, constipation, and encopresis. Evaluation of affected children often reveals vesicoureteral reflux, a trabeculated bladder, and a decreased urinary flow rate with an intermittent pattern. In severe cases, hydronephrosis, renal insufficiency, and even end-stage renal disease can occur. The pathogenesis of this syndrome is uncertain but usually seems to involve learning abnormal voiding habits during toilet training because the syndrome rarely is seen in infants. Urodynamic studies and magnetic resonance imaging of the spine are indicated to rule out a neurologic cause for the bladder dysfunction. The treatment is usually complex and may include anticholinergic therapy, timed voiding, treatment of constipation, behavioral modification, and encouragement of relaxation during voiding. Biofeedback has been used successfully in older children to teach relaxation of the external sphincter. In severe cases, intermittent catheterization is necessary to ensure bladder emptying. In selected patients, external urinary diversion is necessary to protect the upper urinary tract. These children require long-term treatment and careful follow-up.

INFREQUENT VOIDING

Infrequent voiding is a common disorder of micturition, usually associated with urinary tract infections. Affected children, usually girls, void only twice a day rather than the normal four to seven times. With bladder overdistention and prolonged retention of urine, growth of bacteria can lead to recurrent UTIs. Some of these children are constipated. Some also have occasional episodes of incontinence due to overflow

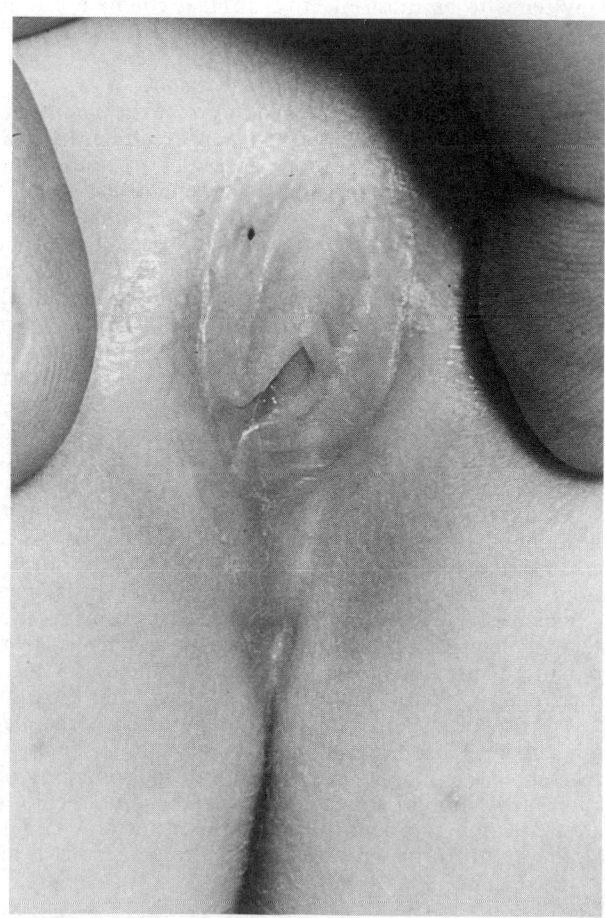

Figure 551–3 Labial adhesion. Note the inability to visualize the urethral meatus and vagina.

or urgency. The disorder is behavioral. When the children have UTIs, the treatment is antibacterial prophylaxis and encouragement of frequent voiding and complete emptying of the bladder by double voiding until a normal pattern of micturition is re-established.

VAGINAL VOIDING

In girls with vaginal voiding, incontinence typically occurs following urination after the girl stands up. Usually the volume of urine is 5–10 mL. One of the most common causes is *labial adhesion* (see Fig. 551–3). This lesion is seen in young girls and can be managed either by topical application of estrogen cream to the adhesion or lysis in the office. Some girls experience vaginal voiding because they do not separate their legs widely during urination. These girls are usually overweight or do not pull their underwear down to their ankles when they urinate. Management involves encouragement of the girl to separate the legs as widely as possible during urination. The most effective way to do this is to have the child sit backward on the toilet seat during micturition.

OTHER CAUSES OF INCONTINENCE IN GIRLS

Ureteral ectopia, usually associated with a duplicated collecting system in girls, can produce urinary incontinence characterized by constant dribbling of urine during day and night, even though they void regularly. Sometimes the urine production from the renal segment drained by the ectopic ureter is small, and urinary drainage is confused with watery vaginal discharge. Children with a history of vaginal discharge or incontinence and an abnormal voiding pattern require careful study. The ectopic orifice is usually difficult to find. On ultrasonography or intravenous urography, one may suspect duplication of the collecting system (see Fig. 551–1), but the upper collecting system drained by the ectopic ureter usually has poor or delayed function. Computed tomography of the kidneys helps rule out subtle duplication that may not be discovered on intravenous urography. Examination under anesthesia for an ectopic ureteral orifice in the vestibule or the vagina is often necessary (see Fig. 551–2). The treatment in these cases is either partial nephrectomy, with removal of the upper pole segment of the duplicated kidney and its ureter down to the pelvic brim, or ipsilateral ureteroureterostomy, in which the upper pole ectopic ureter is anastomosed to the normally positioned lower pole ureter.

Giggle incontinence is a condition that typically affects girls between 7 and 15 yr of age. The incontinence occurs suddenly during giggling, and the entire bladder volume is lost. The pathogenesis is thought to be sudden relaxation of the urinary sphincter. Anticholinergic medication and timed voiding rarely are effective. The most effective treatment is methylphenidate administration.

Total incontinence may be secondary to *epispadias*. This condition, which affects only 1 of 480,000 females, is characterized by separation of the pubic symphysis, separation of the right and left sides of the clitoris, and a patulous urethra. Treatment is bladder neck reconstruction to repair the totally incompetent urethra.

A short, incompetent urethra may be associated with certain urogenital sinus malformations. The diagnosis of these malformations requires a high index of suspicion and a careful physical examination of all incontinent girls. In these cases, urethral and vaginal reconstruction can often restore continence.

VOIDING DISORDERS WITHOUT INCONTINENCE

Some children have the abrupt onset of severe urinary frequency, voiding as often as every 10–15 min during the day, without dysuria, UTI, daytime incontinence, or nocturia. The most common age for these symptoms to occur is 4–6 yr, after the child is toilet-trained. This condition is termed the *daytime frequency syndrome of childhood* or *pollakiuria*. The condition is functional, that is, no anatomic problem is detected. Often the symptoms occur just before a child starts kindergarten or if the child is having emotional family stress–related problems. These children should be checked for UTI, and the clinician should ascertain that the child is emptying the bladder satisfactorily. Occasionally pinworms can cause these symptoms. The condition is self-limited, and symptoms generally resolve within 2–3 mo. Anticholinergic therapy rarely is effective.

Some children have the *dysuria-hematuria syndrome,* in which the child has dysuria without UTI and microscopic or gross hematuria. This condition affects children who are toilet-trained and often is secondary to hypercalciuria. A 24-hr urine sample should be obtained and calcium and creatinine excretion assessed. A 24-hr calcium excretion of more than 4 mg/kg is abnormal and deserves treatment with thiazides because some of these children may be at risk for urolithiasis.

Arnell H, Hjalmas K, Jagervall M, et al: The genetics of primary nocturnal enuresis: Inheritance and suggestion of a second major gene or chromosome 12q. J Med Genet 34:360, 1997.

Bloom DA: Sexual abuse and voiding dysfunction. J Urol 153:777, 1995.

Bloom DA, Faerber G, Bomalaski MD: Urinary incontinence in girls. Evaluation, treatment, and its place in the standard model of voiding dysfunctions in children. Urol Clin North Am 22:521, 1995.

Eggert P, Kuhn B: Antidiuretic hormone regulation in patients with primary nocturnal enuresis. Arch Dis Child 73:508, 1995.

Fernandes E, Vernier R, Gonzalez R: The unstable bladder in children. J Pediatr 118:831, 1991.

Hoebeke P, Walle JV, Theuis M, et al: Outpatient pelvic floor therapy in girls with daytime incontinence and dysfunctional voiding. Urology 48:923, 1997.

Koff SA, Byard MA: The daytime urinary frequency syndrome of childhood. J Urol 140:1280, 1988.

Loening-Baucke V: Urinary incontinence and urinary tract infection and their resolution with treatment of chronic constipation of childhood. Pediatrics 100:228, 1997.

Moffatt MEK: Nocturnal enuresis: A review of the efficacy of treatments and practical advice for clinicians. Dev Behav Pediatr 18:49, 1997.

Moffatt MEK, Harlos S, Kirshen AJ, et al: Desmopressin acetate and nocturnal enuresis: How much do we know? Pediatrics 92:420, 1993.

Monda JM, Husmann DA: Primary nocturnal enuresis: A comparison among observation, imipramine, desmopressin acetate, and bed wetting alarm systems. J Urol 154:745, 1995.

Sher PK, Reinberg Y: Successful treatment of giggle incontinence with methylphenidate. J Urol 156:656, 1996.

Skoog SJ, Stokes A, Turner KL: Oral desmopressin: A randomized double-blind placebo controlled study of effectiveness in children with primary nocturnal enuresis. J Urol 158:1035, 1997.

Varley CK, McClellan L: Case study: Two additional sudden deaths with tricyclic antidepressants. J Am Acad Chil Adolesc Psychiatry 36:390, 1997.

Wan J, Greenfield S: Enuresis and common voiding abnormalities. Pediatr Clin North Am 44:1117, 1997.

Wan J, Kaplinsky R, Greenfield S: Toilet habits of children evaluated for urinary tract infection. J Urol 154:797, 1995.

Wennergren H, Oberg B: Pelvic floor exercises for children: A method of treating dysfunctional voiding. Br J Urol 76:9, 1995.

Wojcik LJ, Caldamone AA: Evaluation and management of pediatric daytime incontinence. *In:* Elder JS (ed): Pediatric Urology for the General Urologist. New York, Igaku-Shoin, 1996, pp 135–158.

Wolfish NM, Pivik RT, Busby KA: Elevated sleep arousal thresholds in enuretic boys: Clinical implications. Acta Pediatr 86:381, 1997.

CHAPTER 552
Anomalies of the Penis and Urethra

HYPOSPADIAS. Hypospadias refers to a urethral opening that is on the ventral surface of the penile shaft and affects 1 in 250 male newborns. There is incomplete development of the prepuce, termed a *dorsal hood,* in which the foreskin is on the sides and dorsal aspect of the penile shaft and absent ventrally.

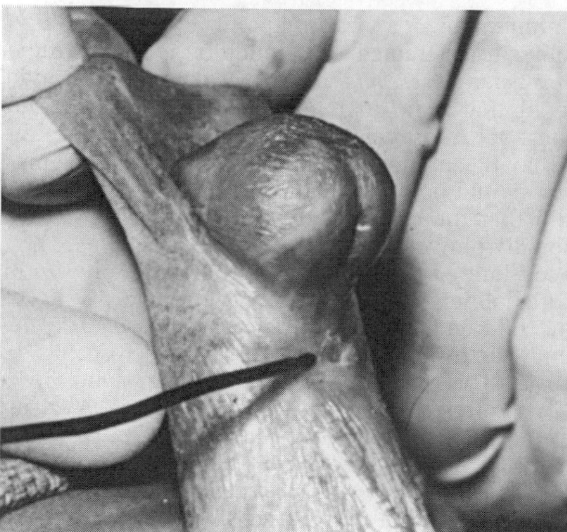

Figure 552–1 Subcoronal hypospadias. Note the urethral meatus in the subcoronal position and the incomplete or hooded prepuce. There was no ventral curvature of the penis in this case.

Some boys, particularly those with proximal hypospadias, have chordee, in which there is ventral penile curvature during erection. The incidence of hypospadias may be increasing, possibly because of in utero exposure to estrogenic or antiandrogenic endocrine disrupting chemicals (polychlorbiphenyls, phytoestrogens).

Hypospadias is classified according to the position of the urethral meatus after taking into account whether chordee is present (Fig. 552–1). The deformity is described as glanular (on the glans penis), coronal, subcoronal, midpenile, penoscrotal, scrotal, and perineal. Approximately 60% of cases are distal, 25% are subcoronal or midpenile, and 15% are proximal. In the more severe cases, the scrotum is bifid and sometimes extends to the dorsal base of the penis (scrotal engulfment) (Fig. 552–2). There is also a *megameatal variant,* in which the foreskin is normal, but there is either coronal or subcoronal hypospadias with a "fish mouth" meatus (Fig. 552–3).

Hypospadias usually is an isolated anomaly. However, hypospadias is common in boys with multiple congenital anomalies. Testes are undescended in 10% of boys with hypospadias,

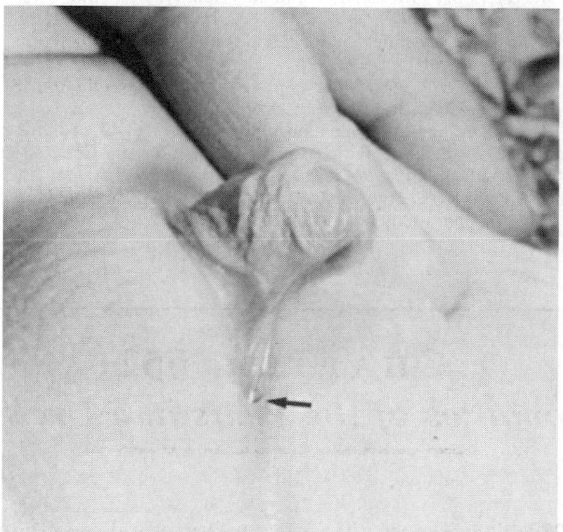

Figure 552–2 Severe perineoscrotal hypospadias. Note the ventral curvature and the underdeveloped ventral surface of the penis, the hooded prepuce, and the urethral meatus in the midline of the bifid scrotum. This child had palpable gonads and a normal chromosome pattern.

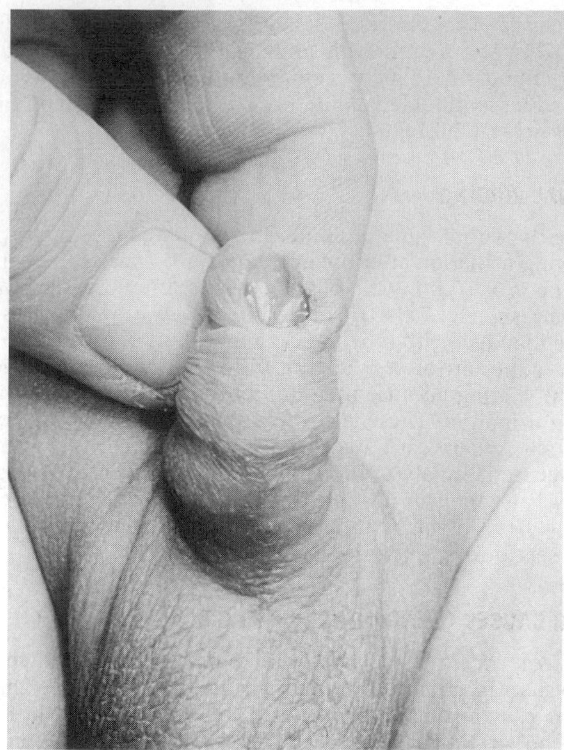

Figure 552–3 Megameatal variant of hypospadias. Note fish-mouth meatus. This boy has been circumcised.

and inguinal hernias are also common. In the newborn, the differential diagnosis of proximal hypospadias with an undescended testis should include forms of ambiguous genitals, particularly masculinization of females (congenital adrenal hyperplasia) and mixed gonadal dysgenesis. A karyotype should be obtained in all patients with midpenile or proximal hypospadias and cryptorchidism (see Chapter 593). Boys with penoscrotal hypospadias should undergo a voiding cystourethrogram, as 5–10% have a dilated prostatic utricle, which is a remnant of the müllerian system. The incidence of other anomalies of the genitourinary tract in boys with hypospadias is low, and with the exception of the more severe cases of perineal hypospadias, radiographic studies of the urinary tract are unnecessary.

Complications of untreated hypospadias include (1) deformity of the urinary stream, either ventral deflection or severe splaying; (2) sexual dysfunction secondary to penile curvature; (3) infertility if the urethral meatus is proximal; and (4) meatal stenosis (congenital), which is extremely rare. The goal of hypospadias surgery is to correct not only the cosmetic but also the functional deformity.

The treatment begins in the newborn period. Circumcision should be avoided, as the foreskin is often essential for the repair. The ideal age for repair in a healthy infant is 6–12 mo. This age is chosen because (1) there is no greater risk of general anesthesia at this age than at 2–3 yr, (2) penile growth over the next several years is slow, (3) the child does not remember the surgical procedure, and (4) analgesic needs may be less than in older children. Most cases are repaired in a single operation on an outpatient basis. Often a skin flap from the penile shaft or foreskin is used, and the remaining foreskin is used for ventral skin coverage. The complication rate is low—less than 5% for distal hypospadias, 5–10% for midpenile hypospadias, and 15% for proximal hypospadias. Complications include urethrocutaneous fistula, hematoma, wound infection, meatal stenosis, urethral diverticulum, and wound dehiscence. Repair of hypospadias is a technically demanding operation and should be performed by surgeons with extensive experience.

CHORDEE WITHOUT HYPOSPADIAS. In some boys there is ventral penile curvature (chordee) and incomplete development of the foreskin (dorsal hood), but the urethral meatus is at the tip of the glans. In most of these boys, the urethra is normal but there is insufficient ventral penile skin or prominent, inelastic ventral bands of dartos fascia that prevent a normal straight erection. In some cases, however, the urethra is short and hypoplastic, and a formal urethroplasty is necessary for repair. The only sign of this anomaly in the neonate may be the dorsal hood deformity, and delayed repair under general anesthesia at 6 mo of age is recommended.

PHIMOSIS AND PARAPHIMOSIS. Phimosis refers to the inability to retract the prepuce. At birth phimosis is physiologic. Over time the adhesions between the prepuce and glans lyse and the distal phimotic ring loosens so that in 90% of uncircumcised males the prepuce becomes retractable by the age of 3 yr. Accumulation of epithelial debris under the infantile prepuce is not pathologic and does not require surgical treatment. In older boys, phimosis may be physiologic, pathologic from inflammation and scarring at the tip of the foreskin, or occur after circumcision (see discussion of trapped penis further on). The prepuce may have been retracted forcefully on one or two occasions in the past, which can result in a cicatricial scar that prevents subsequent foreskin retraction. In boys with persistent phimosis, application of a steroid cream to the foreskin three times daily for 1 mo can loosen the phimotic ring. If there is ballooning of the foreskin during voiding or phimosis beyond 10 yr of age, circumcision is recommended.

Paraphimosis occurs when the foreskin is retracted behind the coronal sulcus and the prepuce cannot be pulled back over the glans (Fig. 552–4). Painful venous stasis in the foreskin distal to the corona results, with edema leading to severe pain and inability to reduce the foreskin. Treatment includes lubrication of the foreskin and glans and then compressing the glans and simultaneously placing distal traction on the foreskin to try to push the phimotic ring beyond the coronal sulcus. In rare cases, emergency circumcision under general anesthesia is necessary.

CIRCUMCISION. Whether the newborn male should undergo circumcision is controversial. In the United States, circumcision is usually performed for social reasons. Reasons given in support of circumcision include prevention of penile cancer, phimosis, and balanitis and reducing the risk of urinary tract infection (UTI) and sexually transmitted diseases.

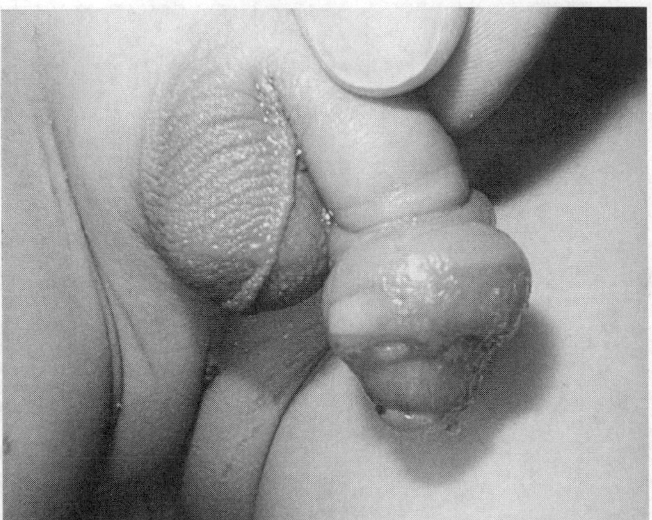

Figure 552–4 Paraphimosis. Foreskin has been retracted proximal to the glans penis and has become markedly swollen secondary to venous congestion.

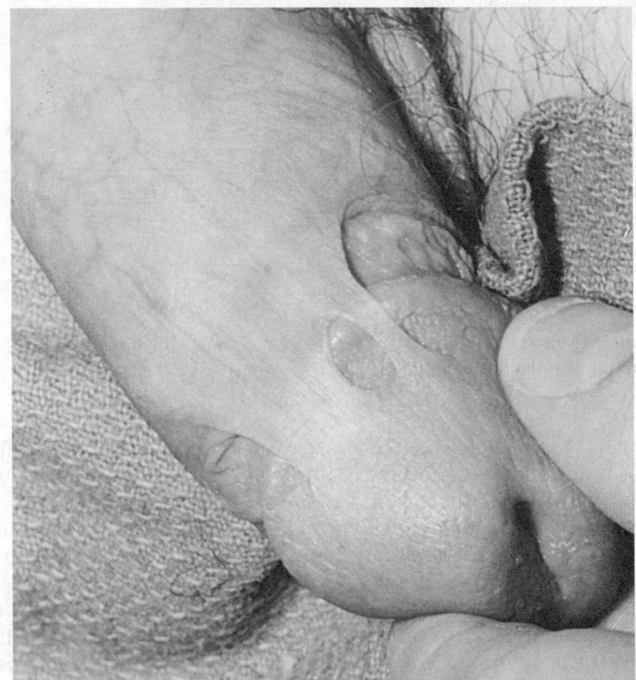

Figure 552–5 Skin bridge between glans and penile shaft resulting from penile adhesions forming after newborn circumcision. Skin bridges cause painful penile curvature during erection and predispose to infection under the adhesion and should be excised.

There have been only a handful of reports of adult men who were circumcised at birth and subsequently acquired penile carcinoma, but in Scandinavian countries, where few men are circumcised and hygiene is good, the incidence of penile cancer is low. UTIs are 10 to 15 times more common in uncircumcised infants than in circumcised infants, the urinary pathogens arising from bacteria that colonize the space between the prepuce and glans. The risk of febrile UTI is primarily between birth and 6 mo, but there is an increased risk of UTI at least through 5 yr of age. Many recommend circumcision in babies who are predisposed to UTI, such as those with congenital hydronephrosis and reflux. Whether circumcision reduces the risk of sexually transmitted diseases, in particular acquired immunodeficiency syndrome, is unresolved, because most of the data have been acquired from countries in which the prevalence of acquired immunodeficiency syndrome is high, and it has been difficult to ascertain whether the sexual practices of the circumcised and uncircumcised subjects were similar.

Complications following neonatal circumcision include bleeding, wound infection, meatal stenosis, secondary phimosis, and removal of insufficient foreskin and dense penile adhesions (skin bridge; Fig. 552–5); 0.2–3% of patients have a subsequent operative procedure. Boys with a large hydrocele or hernia are at particular risk for secondary phimosis (see discussion of trapped penis further on). Potentially serious complications include sepsis, amputation of the distal part of the glans, removal of an excessive amount of foreskin, and urethrocutaneous fistula. Circumcision should not be performed in neonates with hypospadias, chordee without hypospadias, a dorsal hood deformity (relative contraindication), or in those with a small penis.

When performing a neonatal circumcision, local analgesia, such as a dorsal nerve block or application of EMLA cream, is recommended.

PENILE TORSION. Penile torsion is a rotational defect of the penile shaft. It usually occurs in a counterclockwise direction,

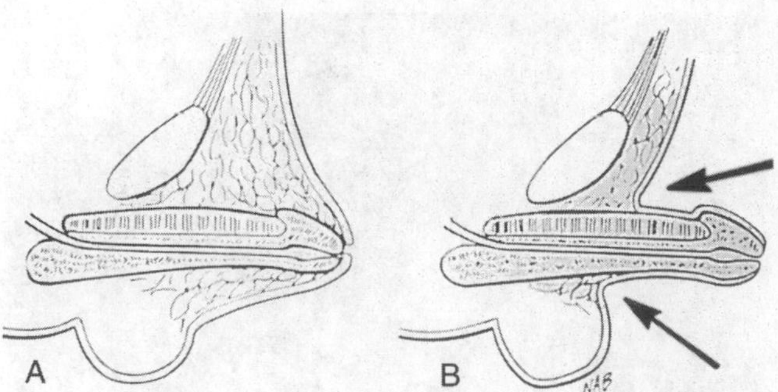

Figure 552–6 Concealed penis *(A)*, which may be visualized by retracting skin lateral to penile shaft *(B)*.

that is, to the left side. In most cases, penile development is normal, and the condition is unrecognized until circumcision is performed or the foreskin is retractable. Penile torsion also occurs in some boys with hypospadias. The defect has primarily cosmetic significance and correction is unnecessary if the rotation is less than 60 degrees from the midline.

INCONSPICUOUS PENIS. The term *inconspicuous penis* refers to a penis that appears to be small. A *webbed penis* is a condition in which the scrotal skin extends onto the ventrum of the penis. This deformity represents an abnormality of the attachment between the penis and scrotum. Although the cosmetic appearance is only mildly abnormal, if a routine circumcision is performed, the penis tends to retract into the scrotum and can result in secondary phimosis. In rare cases, the distal urethra is hypoplastic, necessitating urethral reconstruction. The *concealed (hidden or buried) penis* is a normally developed penis that is camouflaged by the suprapubic fat pad (Fig. 552–6). This anomaly may be congenital or iatrogenic following circumcision. A *trapped penis* is an acquired form of inconspicuous penis and refers to a phallus that becomes embedded in the suprapubic fat pad following circumcision (Fig. 552–7). This deformity may occur after neonatal circumcision in a baby who has significant scrotal swelling from a large hydrocele or inguinal hernia or after routine circumcision in a baby with a webbed penis. This complication can predispose to UTIs and may cause urinary retention.

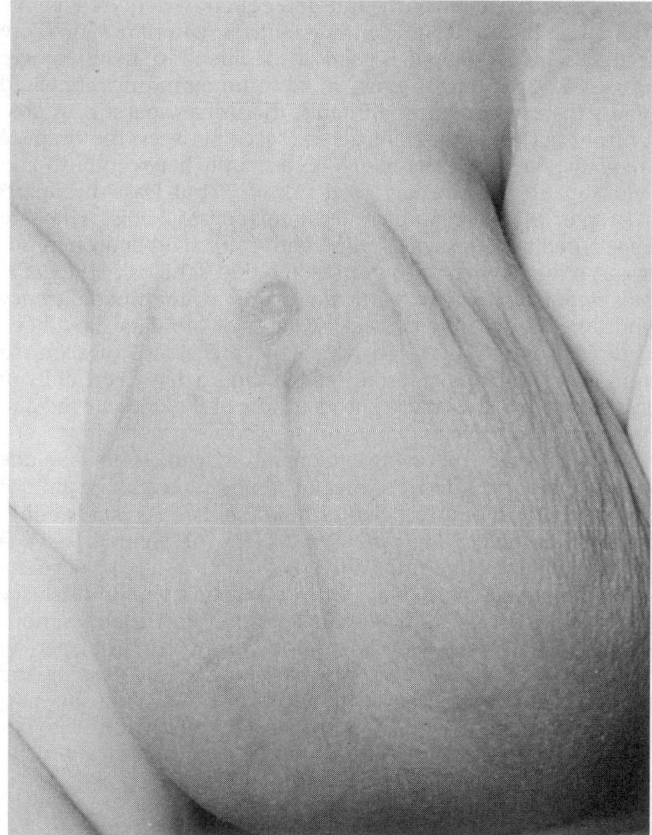

Figure 552–7 Concealed, trapped penis secondary to circumcision. This baby's penis is normal length; large hydroceles predisposed him to this complication.

Micropenis is defined as a normally formed penis that is at least 2.5 standard deviations below the mean in size (Fig. 552–8). Typically, the ratio of the length of the penile shaft to its circumference is normal. The pertinent measurement is the *stretched penile length*, which is measured by gently stretching the penis and measuring the distance from the penile base under the pubic symphysis to the tip of the glans. The mean length of a newborn penis is 3.5 ± 0.7 cm and 1.1 ± 0.2 cm in diameter, and it should be at least 1.9 cm in length. Micropenis results from a hormonal abnormality that occurs after 14 wk of gestation. The most common causes include (1) hypogonadotropic hypogonadism, (2) hypergonadotropic hypogonadism (primary testicular failure), and (3) idiopathic micropenis. The most common cause of micropenis is failure of the hypothalamus to produce an adequate amount of gonadotropin-releasing hormone, and typically occurs in Kallmann syndrome, Prader-Willi syndrome, and Lawrence-Moon-Biedl syndrome. In some cases, there is growth hormone deficiency. Primary testicular failure may result from gonadal dysgenesis or rudimentary testes syndrome and also occurs in Robinow syndrome. All these children should be examined by a pediatric endocrinologist and pediatric urologist. Evaluation includes a karyotype, assessment of anterior pituitary function, testicular function, and magnetic resonance imaging to determine the anatomic integrity of the hypothalamus and the anterior pituitary gland as well as the midline structure of the brain. One of the difficult questions is whether androgen therapy is essential during childhood because stimulation of penile growth in a prepubertal boy may limit the growth potential of the penis in puberty. In addition, studies of small numbers of men with micropenis suggest that many, although not all, have satisfactory sexual function. Consequently, a decision for gender reassignment is made infrequently.

OTHER PENILE ANOMALIES. Agenesis of the penis affects approximately 1 in 10 million boys. The karyotype is almost always 46,XY, and the usual appearance is that of a well-developed

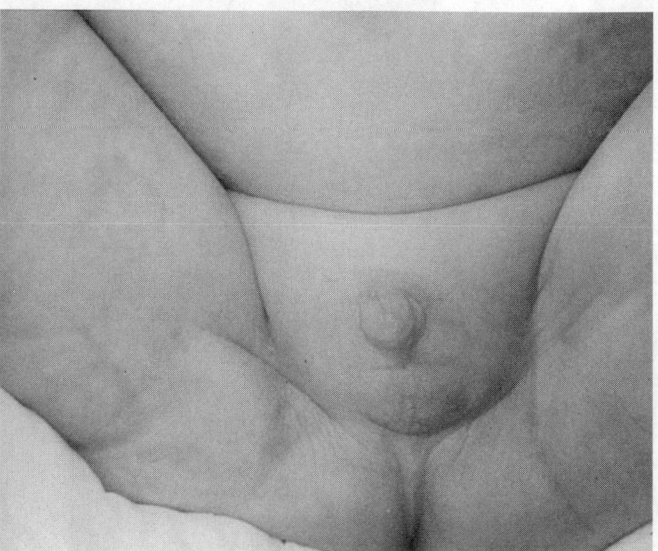

Figure 552–8 Infant with microphallus. Also note the small scrotum, which was empty.

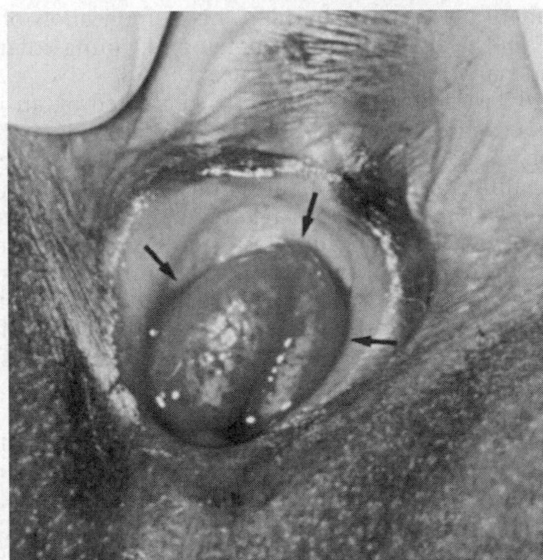

Figure 552–9 Urethral prolapse in a 4-yr-old black girl who had bloody spotting on her underwear.

scrotum with descended testes and an absent penile shaft. Upper urinary tract abnormalities are common. In most cases, gender reassignment is recommended in the newborn period. *Diphallia* ranges from a small accessory penis to complete duplication. *Lateral penile curvature* usually is caused by overgrowth or hypoplasia of a corporal (erectile) body and usually is congenital. Surgical repair is recommended at 6–12 mo.

MEATAL STENOSIS. Meatal stenosis is a condition that is almost always acquired and occurs following neonatal circumcision. It probably results from severe inflammation of the denuded glans. If the meatus is pinpoint, boys void with a forceful, fine stream that goes a great distance. These boys may experience dysuria, frequency, or hematuria, or a combination of these conditions, without UTI between the ages of 3 and 8 yr. Other boys have dorsal deflection of the urinary stream. Although the meatus may be small, hydronephrosis or voiding difficulty is extremely rare unless there is associated balanitis xerotica obliterans. Treatment is meatoplasty, in which the urethral meatus is opened surgically; this procedure can be performed either under anesthesia as an outpatient or in the office using local anesthesia (EMLA cream) with or without sedation. Routine cystoscopy is unnecessary.

OTHER MALE URETHRAL ANOMALIES. Parameatal urethral cyst presents as an asymptomatic small cyst on one side of the urethral meatus. Treatment is excision under anesthesia. *Congenital urethral fistula* is a rare deformity in which a fistula is present from the penile urethra. It is usually an isolated abnormality. Treatment is fistula closure. *Megalourethra* is a large urethra that is usually associated with abnormal development of the corpus spongiosum. This condition is most commonly associated with prune-belly syndrome. *Urethral duplication* is a rare condition in which the two urethral channels lie in the same sagittal plane, and the more normal urethra is the one positioned more ventrally. Some children have significant obstructive uropathy and require major reconstructive surgery. *Urethral hypoplasia* is a rare condition in which the urethra is extremely small but patent. In some cases, a temporary cutaneous vesicostomy is necessary for satisfactory urinary drainage. Either gradual enlargement of the urethra or major urethroplasty is necessary. *Urethral atresia* refers to nondevelopment of the urethra and is nearly always fatal unless the urachus remains patent throughout gestation.

URETHRAL PROLAPSE (FEMALE). Urethral prolapse is encountered predominantly in black females between 1 and 9 yr of age. The most common signs are bloody spotting on the underwear or diaper, although dysuria or perineal discomfort may also occur (Fig. 552–9). An inexperienced examiner may mistake the finding for sexual abuse. The usual therapy consists of application of estrogen cream two to three times daily for 3–4 wk and sitz baths. Surgical excision and reapproximation of the mucosal edges is curative.

OTHER FEMALE URETHRAL LESIONS. Paraurethral cyst results from

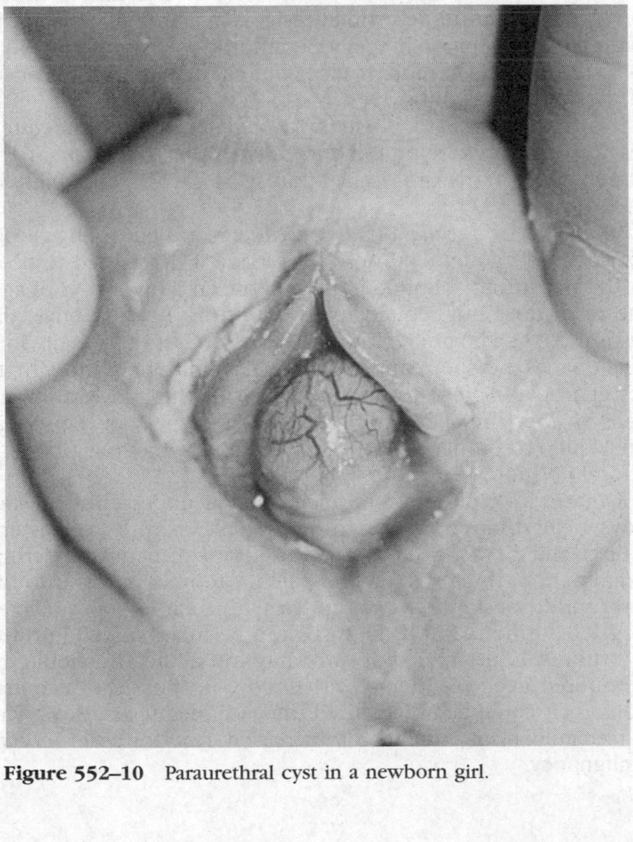

Figure 552–10 Paraurethral cyst in a newborn girl.

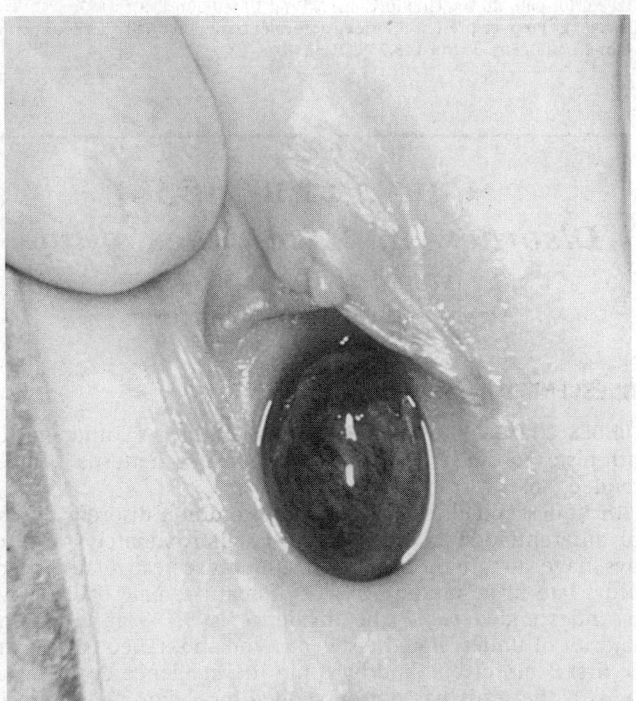

Figure 552–11 Prolapsed ectopic ureterocele in a female infant. She had a nonfunctioning upper pole collecting system connected to the ureterocele.

retained secretions in Skene glands secondary to ductal obstruction (Fig. 552–10). These lesions are present at birth and most regress in size during the first 4–8 wk, although occasionally it is necessary to incise them. A *prolapsed ectopic ureterocele* appears as a cystic mass protruding from the urethra and is a presenting symptom in 10% of girls with a ureterocele, which is a cystic swelling of the terminal ureter (Fig. 552–11). Ultrasonography should be performed to visualize the upper urinary tracts to confirm the diagnosis. Usually the ureterocele is either incised or an upper urinary tract reconstructive procedure is necessary.

Aaronson IA: Micropenis: Medical and surgical implications. J Urol 152:4, 1994.
Albers N, Ulrichs C, Gluer S, et al: Etiologic classification of severe hypospadias: Implications for prognosis and management. J Pediatr 131:386, 1997.
American Academy of Pediatrics, Section on Urology: Timing of elective surgery on the genitalia of male children with particular reference to the risks, benefits, and psychological effects of surgery and anesthesia. Pediatrics 97:590, 1996.
American Academy of Pediatrics Task Force on Circumcision: Circumcision Policy Statement. Pediatrics 103:686, 1999.
Anveden-Hertzberg L, Gauderer MWL, Elder JS: Urethral prolapse: An often misdiagnosed cause of urogenital bleeding in girls. Pediatr Emerg Care 11:212, 1995.
Atilla MK, Dundaroz R, Odabas O, et al: A nonsurgical approach to the treatment of phimosis: Local nonsteroidal anti-inflammatory ointment application. J Urol 158:196, 1997.
Baskin LS, Canning DA, Snyder HM, et al: Treating complications of circumcision. Pediatr Emerg Care 12:62, 1996.
Belman AB: Hypospadias update. Urology 49:166, 1997.
Cartwright PC, Snow BW, McNees DC: Urethral meatotomy in the office using topical EMLA cream for anesthesia. J Urol 156:857, 1996.
Craig JC, Knight JF, Suresh Kumar P, et al: Effect of circumcision on incidence of urinary tract infection in preschool boys. J Pediatr 128:23, 1996.
Golubovic Z, Milanovic D, Vukadinovic V, et al: The conservative treatment of phimosis in boys. Br J Urol 78:786, 1996.
Lander J, Brady-Fryer B, Metcalfe JB, et al: Comparison of ring block, dorsal penile nerve block, and topical anesthesia for neonatal circumcision. A randomized clinical trial. JAMA 278:2157, 1997.
Laumann EO, Masi CM, Zuckerman EQ: Circumcision in the United States. Prevalence, prophylactic effects, and sexual practice. JAMA 277:1052, 1997.
Reilly JM, Woodhouse CRJ: Small penis and the male sexual role. J Urol 142:569, 1989.
Snodgrass W, Koyle M, Manzoni G, et al: Tubularized incised plate hypospadias repair: Results of a multicenter experience. J Urol 156:839, 1996.
Steckler RE, Zaontz MR, Skoog SJ, et al: Cryptorchidism, pediatricians, and family practitioners: Patterns of practice and referral. J Pediatr 127:948, 1995.
Taddio A, Stevens B, Craig K, et al: Efficacy and safety of lidocaine-prilocaine cream for pain during circumcision. N Engl J Med 336:1197, 1997.
Wiswell TE: Prepuce presence portends prevalence of potentially perilous periurethral pathogens. J Urol 148:739, 1992.

CHAPTER 553
Disorders and Anomalies of the Scrotal Contents

UNDESCENDED TESTES

UNDESCENDED AND RETRACTILE TESTES. Failure to find one or both testes in the scrotum may indicate that the testis is undescended, absent, or retractile.

An undescended testis is the most common disorder of sexual differentiation in boys. At birth, approximately 4.5% of boys have an undescended testis. Because testicular descent occurs late in gestation, 30% of premature male babies have an undescended testis; the incidence is 3.4% at term. The majority of undescended testes descend spontaneously during the first 3 mo of life, and by 6 mo the incidence decreases to 0.8%. If the testis has not descended by 6 mo, it will remain undescended. Cryptorchidism is bilateral in 10–20% of cases. There is some evidence that the incidence of cryptorchidism is increasing. Some boys have secondary cryptorchidism following repair of an inguinal hernia. This complication of hernia repair is most common in neonates and young infants and affects as many as 1–2% of patients.

The process of testicular descent is regulated by an interaction between hormonal and mechanical factors, including testosterone, dihydrotestosterone, müllerian-inhibiting factor, the gubernaculum, intra-abdominal pressure, and the genitofemoral nerve. The testis develops at 7–8 wk of gestation. At 10–11 wk, the Leydig cells produce testosterone, which stimulates differentiation of the wolffian (mesonephric) duct into the epididymis, vas deferens, seminal vesicle, and ejaculatory duct. At 32–36 wk, the testis, which is anchored at the internal inguinal ring by the gubernaculum, begins its process of descent. The gubernaculum distends the inguinal canal and guides the testis into the scrotum.

Undescended testes are usually in the inguinal canal. Some boys have an ectopic testis, typically in the superficial inguinal pouch or perineum. Some testes are intra-abdominal; these are nonpalpable. Approximately 15% of patients have a nonpalpable testis; in these the testis is present in 50%. In a newborn with bilateral nonpalpable testes, one should suspect that the child could be a virilized female with congenital adrenal hyperplasia.

The consequences of cryptorchidism include infertility, malignancy, associated hernias, torsion of the cryptorchid testis, and the possible psychologic effects of an empty scrotum.

The undescended testis is histologically normal at birth, but pathologic changes can be demonstrated at 6–12 mo. Delayed germ cell maturation, reduction in germ cell number, hyalinization of the seminiferous tubules, and reduced Leydig cell number are typical; these changes are progressive over time if the testis remains undescended. Similar, although less severe, changes are found in the contralateral descended testis after 4–7 yr. Following treatment for bilateral undescended testes, approximately 50–65% of patients are fertile; 85% of boys treated for a unilateral undescended testis are fertile.

The risk of *malignancy* in the undescended testis is 4 to 10 times higher than that in the general population and is approximately 1 in 80 with a unilateral undescended testis and 1 in 40 to 1 in 50 for bilateral undescended testes. The peak age for this tumor is 15–45 yr. The most common tumor developing in an undescended testis is a seminoma (65%); in contrast, following orchiopexy, seminomas represent only 30% of testis tumors. Orchiopexy does not change the risk of cancer of the testis developing.

Indirect inguinal hernias usually accompany undescended testes but are rarely symptomatic. *Torsion and infarction* of the undescended testis can occur because of excessive mobility of such testes.

"Acquired" or *ascending undescended testes* are becoming recognized more frequently. These boys have a descended testis at birth, but during childhood, often between 4 and 10 yr of age, the testis does not remain in the scrotum. In such boys, the testis often can be pulled into the scrotum, but there is obvious tension on the spermatic cord. This condition is thought to result from incomplete disappearance of the processus vaginalis so that the spermatic cord does not grow as rapidly as the child, resulting in the testis gradually moving out of a scrotal position.

Retractile testes often are misdiagnosed as undescended testes. Boys older than 1 yr of age often have a brisk cremasteric reflex, and if the child is anxious or ticklish during scrotal examination, the testis may be difficult to manipulate into the scrotum. Boys should be examined with their legs in a relaxed frog-leg position, and if the testis can be manipulated into the scrotum comfortably, it is probably retractile. It should be monitored every 6–12 mo with follow-up physical examinations, as it could be an acquired undescended testis. Boys with a retractile testis are not at increased risk for infertility or malignancy.

TABLE 553–1 Differential Diagnosis of Scrotal Masses in Boys and Adolescents

Painful	Painless
Testicular torsion	Hydrocele
Torsion of appendix testis	Inguinal hernia*
Epididymitis	Varicocele*
Trauma: ruptured testis, hematocele	Spermatocele*
Inguinal hernia (incarcerated)	Testicular tumor*
Mumps orchitis	Henoch-Schönlein purpura*
	Idiopathic scrotal edema

**Occasionally associated with discomfort.*

Treatment of the undescended testis is recommended at 9–15 mo. Most testes can be brought down to the scrotum with an operation *(orchiopexy)*. This procedure involves an inguinal incision, mobilization of the testis and spermatic cord, and correction of the indirect inguinal hernia. The procedure is typically performed on an outpatient basis with a success rate of 98%.

If the testis is *nonpalpable*, diagnostic laparoscopy is performed to determine its location. Approximately 50% of patients have an intra-abdominal testis or a testis that is located high in the inguinal canal; in the remaining patients, the testis is absent. When the testis is *absent*, usually an atrophic remnant is found in the scrotum or inguinal canal. The atrophy is thought to result from testicular torsion in utero. These gonads have been termed *vanishing testes*. In the majority of cases, orchiopexy of the intra-abdominal testis located immediately inside the internal inguinal ring is successful, but orchiectomy should be considered in the more difficult cases or when the testis appears to be atrophic. Two-stage orchidopexy is sometimes needed in high abdominal testes. Testicular protheses are available for older children and adolescents when the absence of the gonad in the scrotum may have an undesirable psychologic effect.

Hormonal treatment is used infrequently. The concept is that testicular descent is under androgen regulation, and that human chorionic gonadotropin (which stimulates Leydig cell production of testosterone) or luteinizing hormone–releasing hormone may stimulate testicular descent. Although hormonal treatment has been used in Europe, randomized controlled trials have not shown either hormone to be very effective. There is some evidence that a luteinizing hormone–releasing hormone analog, buserelin, may be helpful in increasing germ cell number and normalizing testicular histologic features, but these findings are preliminary.

SCROTAL SWELLING

Scrotal swelling may be acute or chronic, painful or painless. Abrupt onset of painful scrotal swelling necessitates prompt evaluation, as some conditions, such as testicular torsion and incarcerated inguinal hernia, require emergency surgical management. The differential diagnosis is shown in Tables 553–1 and 553–2.

A detailed history is helpful in determining the cause of the swelling and includes (1) onset of pain—with testicular torsion the pain often is sudden in onset and may be associated with exercise or minor genital trauma, (2) duration of pain, (3) radiation of pain—inguinal discomfort is common with an inguinal hernia or epididymitis and associated flank pain may occur with passage of a ureteral calculus, (4) previous episodes of similar pain are common in boys with intermittent testicular torsion or inguinal hernia, (5) nausea and vomiting are associated with testicular torsion and inguinal hernia, and (6) irritative urinary symptoms, such as dysuria, urgency, and frequency are indicative of a urinary tract infection, which can cause epididymitis. Boys with lower urinary tract pathology may be prone to epididymitis.

TABLE 553–2 Differential Diagnosis of Scrotal Swelling in Newborns

Hydrocele	Scrotal hematoma
Inguinal hernia (reducible)	Testicular tumor
Inguinal hernia (incarcerated)*	Meconium peritonitis
Testicular torsion*	Epididymitis*

**Occasionally associated with discomfort.*

Physical examination in boys with a painful scrotum may be difficult. Some have advocated performing a spermatic cord block or administering intravenous analgesia to facilitate the examination, but such measures are usually unnecessary. Scrotal wall erythema is common in testicular torsion, epididymitis, torsion of the appendix testis, and an incarcerated hernia. In boys with a normal cremasteric reflex, testicular torsion is unlikely. Absence of a cremasteric reflex, however, is nondiagnostic.

Pertinent laboratory studies include a urinalysis and culture. A positive urinalysis is suggestive of epididymitis. Serum studies generally are not helpful in establishing a diagnosis, unless a testis tumor is suspected. Following initial evaluation, *imaging studies* may be helpful in establishing the diagnosis. These studies include a testicular flow scan and color Doppler ultrasonography. Imaging studies are used to assess whether testicular blood flow is normal, reduced, or increased. In addition, if a hydrocele is present and the testis is nonpalpable, or if an abnormality of the testis is found, ultrasonography may be helpful. Imaging studies are not 100% accurate; they should not be used to decide whether a boy with testicular pain should be referred for urologic care.

The ^{99m}Tc-pertechnetate *testicular flow scan* can demonstrate whether there is blood flow to the testis. Following intravenous injection of the radionuclide, flow and static images are obtained. Testicular torsion usually appears as a "cold spot" of absent flow to the affected testis. Inflammatory conditions usually cause hyperemia. Accuracy in demonstrating blood flow is approximately 95%. A false-negative scan may occur in a boy with testicular torsion if the degree of torsion is less than 360 degrees. The test can often be obtained on an emergent basis during the day, but at night, it may take 2–3 hr to perform and interpret the study.

Color Doppler ultrasonography allows assessment of testicular blood flow and testicular morphologic features. Accuracy is 95% if the ultrasonographer is experienced. A false-negative study may occur in a boy with testicular torsion if the degree of torsion is less than 360 degrees. In addition, in prepubertal boys blood flow may be difficult to demonstrate in as many as 30% of normal testes.

TESTICULAR (SPERMATIC CORD) TORSION

Testicular torsion requires prompt diagnosis and treatment to save the testis. Torsion is the most common cause of testicular pain in boys 12 yr and older and is uncommon in those less than 10 yr. It is caused by inadequate fixation of the testis within the scrotum resulting from a redundant tunica vaginalis, allowing excessive mobility of the testis. The abnormal attachment has been termed a *bell clapper deformity* and is often bilateral. Shortly after torsion occurs, venous congestion begins; subsequently arterial flow is interrupted. The likelihood of testis survival depends on the duration and severity of torsion. Within 4 to 6 hr of absent blood flow to the testis, spermatogenesis may be lost.

Testicular torsion produces acute pain and swelling of the scrotum. On examination, the scrotum is swollen, tender, and often difficult to examine. The cremasteric reflex is nearly always absent. The condition can be differentiated from an incarcerated hernia because swelling in the inguinal area is often absent. If the pain has lasted less than 4–6 hr, manual detorsion may be attempted. This maneuver is performed by rotating the testis inward (the left testis is rotated clockwise). Successful manual detorsion results in dramatic pain relief.

Treatment is prompt surgical exploration and detorsion. If the testis is explored within 6 hr of torsion, up to 90% of the gonads will survive. Survival decreases rapidly with a delay of more than 6 hr. If the degree of torsion is 360 degrees or less, the testis may have sufficient arterial flow to allow the gonad to survive, even after 24–48 hr. The testis is then fixed in the scrotum with nonabsorbable sutures, termed *scrotal orchiopexy*, to prevent torsion in the future. The contralateral testis should be fixed in the scrotum because the condition may be bilateral. If the testis appears nonviable, orchiectomy is performed (Fig. 553–1).

Testicular torsion can also occur in the fetus or neonate and results from incomplete attachment of the tunica vaginalis to the scrotal wall and is "extravaginal." When torsion occurs in utero, the baby is usually born with a large, firm, nontender testis. Usually the ipsilateral hemiscrotum is ecchymotic (Fig. 553–2). In these cases, the testis is rarely viable because torsion was a remote event. However, the contralateral testis is at increased risk for torsion until 1 mo beyond term. Many pediatric urologists recommend exploration to establish the diagnosis, remove the necrotic testis, and anchor the contralateral testis. In other cases, the initial examination is normal, and acute scrotal swelling is recognized subsequently. In such cases, the testis occasionally may be saved.

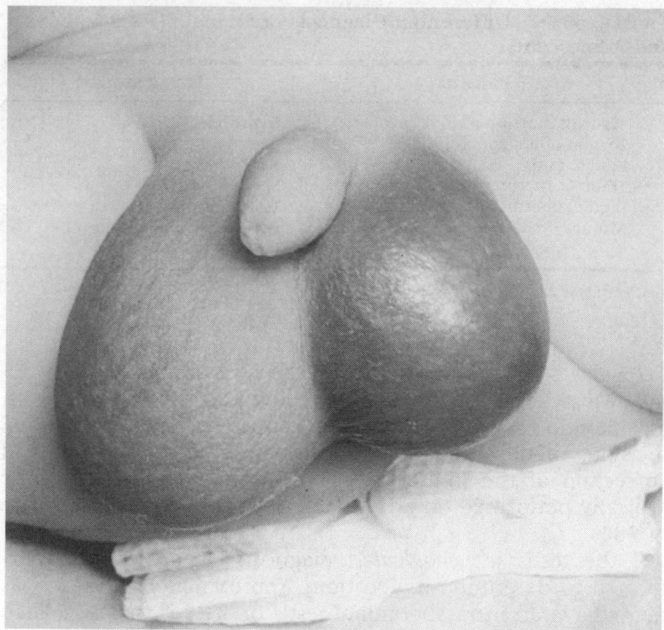

Figure 553–2 Left testicular torsion in a newborn. Left hemiscrotum is ecchymotic, and the testis was slightly enlarged, quite firm, and nontender.

TORSION OF THE APPENDIX TESTIS

Torsion of the appendix testis is the most common cause of testicular pain in boys between 2 and 11 yr but is rare in adolescents. The appendix testis is a stalklike structure that is a vestigial embryonic remnant of the müllerian (paramesonephric) ductal system that is attached to the upper pole of the testis. When it undergoes torsion, progressive inflammation and swelling of the testis and epididymis occurs, resulting in testicular pain and scrotal erythema. The onset of pain is usually gradual. Palpation of the testis usually reveals a 3–5 mm tender indurated mass on the upper pole (Fig. 553–3). In some cases, the appendage that has undergone torsion may be visible through the scrotal skin, termed the *blue dot sign*. In some boys, distinguishing torsion of the appendix from testicular torsion is difficult. In such cases, a testicular flow scan or color Doppler ultrasonography may be helpful.

The natural history of torsion of the appendix testis is for the inflammation to resolve in 3–10 days. Nonoperative treatment is recommended, including bed rest and analgesia with nonsteroidal anti-inflammatory medication for 5 days. If the diagnosis is uncertain, scrotal exploration is recommended.

EPIDIDYMITIS

Acute inflammation of the epididymis is an ascending retrograde infection from the urethra, through the vas into the epididymis. This condition causes acute scrotal pain and swelling. It is rare before puberty and should raise the question of a congenital abnormality of the wolffian duct, such as an ectopic ureter entering the vas. After puberty, epididymitis becomes progressively more common and is the principal cause of acute painful scrotal swelling in young, sexually active adult men. Urinalysis usually reveals pyuria. Epididymitis can

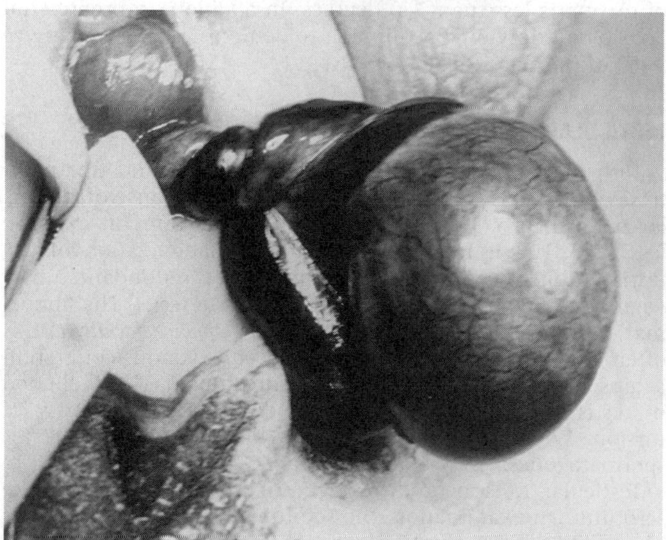

Figure 553–1 Left testicular torsion in an adolescent; the testis is necrotic.

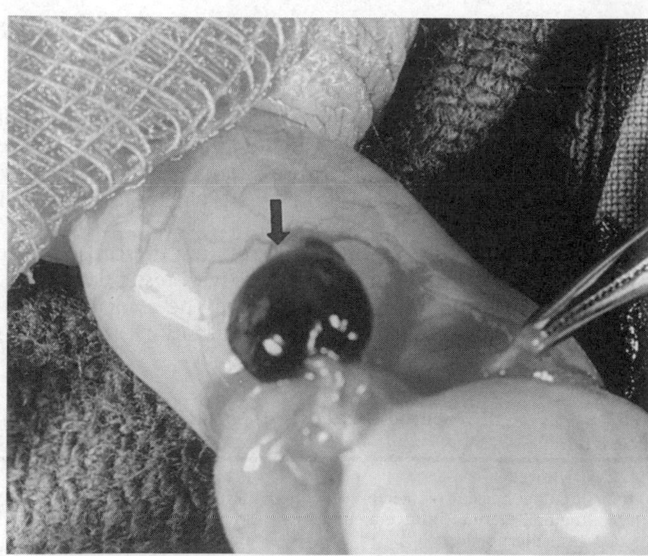

Figure 553–3 Torsion of the appendix testis, which is necrotic *(arrow)*.

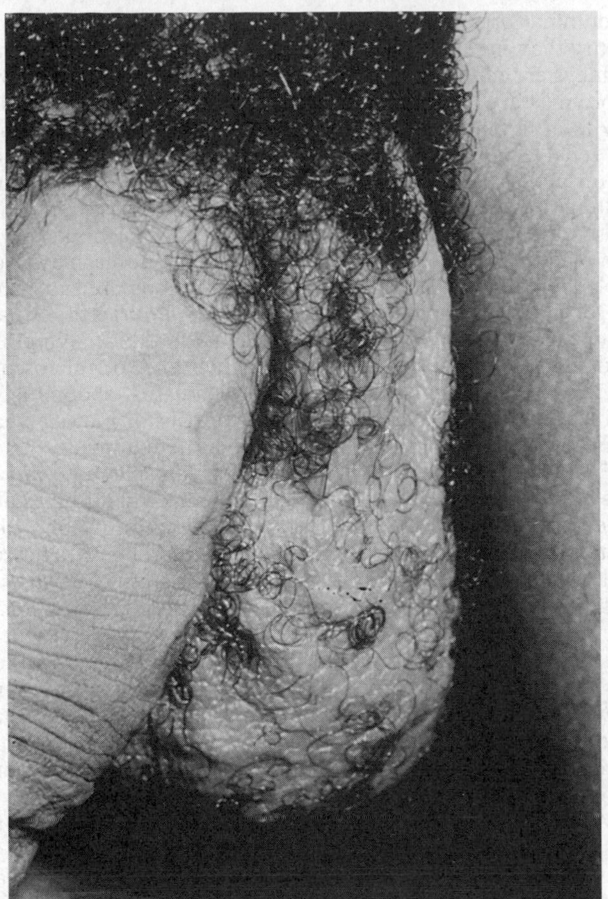

Figure 553–4 Left varicocele in an adolescent boy.

be infectious (usually gonococcus, *Chlamydia*), but often the organism remains undetermined. Treatment consists of bed rest and antibiotics. Differentiation from torsion can be difficult, and in children surgical exploration is usually required.

VARICOCELE

A varicocele is an abnormal dilatation of the pampiniform plexus in the scrotum (Fig. 553–4). Dilatation of the pampiniform venous plexus results from valvular incompetence of the spermatic vein. Approximately 15% of adult men have a varicocele; 15% are subfertile. Varicocele is the most common surgically correctable cause of subfertility in men. A varicocele is found in 5% of adolescent boys, but it is rare in boys less than 10 yr old. Varicoceles occur predominantly on the left side, are bilateral in 10% of cases, and rarely involve the right side only. A varicocele in a boy less than 10 yr or one on the right side may be indicative of an abdominal or retroperitoneal mass; an ultrasonographic scan should be performed.

A varicocele usually is a painless paratesticular mass, often described as a "bag of worms." Occasionally patients describe a dull ache in the affected testis. Usually the varicocele is decompressed when the patient is supine and prominent when standing. Testicular size should be documented because if the affected testis is small, spermatogenesis probably has been adversely affected.

The goal of varicocelectomy is to maximize chances for fertility. Surgical treatment of varicoceles in children and adolescents is indicated in boys with a significant disparity in testicular size or pain in the affected testis, or if the contralateral testis is diseased or absent. Typically the involved testis enlarges and catches up with the normal testis over the following 1–2 yr. Varicocelectomy should also be considered in boys with a large varicocele, even without a disparity in testicular size. Surgical repair is performed by ligation of the veins of the pampiniform plexus through an inguinal incision or by ligating the internal spermatic vein in the retroperitoneum. The operation is carried out on an ambulatory basis.

SPERMATOCELE

A spermatocele is a cystic lesion containing sperm that is attached to the upper pole of the sexually mature testis. Spermatoceles are usually painless and are incidental findings on physical examination. Enlargement of the spermatocele or pain is an indication for removal.

HYDROCELE

A hydrocele is an accumulation of fluid in the tunica vaginalis (Fig. 553–5). Approximately 1–2% of male neonates have a hydrocele. In most cases, the hydrocele is noncommunicating (the processus vaginalis was obliterated during development). In such cases, the hydrocele fluid disappears by 1 yr of age. If there is a persistently patent processus, the hydrocele persists and becomes progressively larger during the day and is small in the morning. A rare variant of a hydrocele is the *abdominoscrotal hydrocele,* in which there is a large, tense hydrocele that extends into the lower abdominal cavity. In some older boys, a noncommunicating hydrocele may result from an inflammatory condition within the scrotum, such as testicular torsion, torsion of the appendix testis, epididymitis, or testicular tumor. The risk of a communicating hydrocele is the development of an inguinal hernia.

On examination, hydroceles are smooth and nontender. Transillumination of the scrotum confirms the fluid-filled nature of the mass. If compression of the fluid-filled mass completely reduces the size of the hydrocele, an inguinal hernia is the likely diagnosis.

Most hydroceles resolve by 12 mo of age following reabsorption of the hydrocele fluid. If the hydrocele is large and tense, however, early surgical correction is recommended because it is difficult to verify that the child does not have a hernia, and large hydroceles rarely disappear spontaneously. Hydroceles persisting beyond 12–18 mo are usually communicating and should be repaired. Surgical correction is similar to a herniorrhaphy. Through an inguinal incision, the spermatic cord is identified, the hydrocele fluid is drained, and a high ligation of the processus vaginalis is performed.

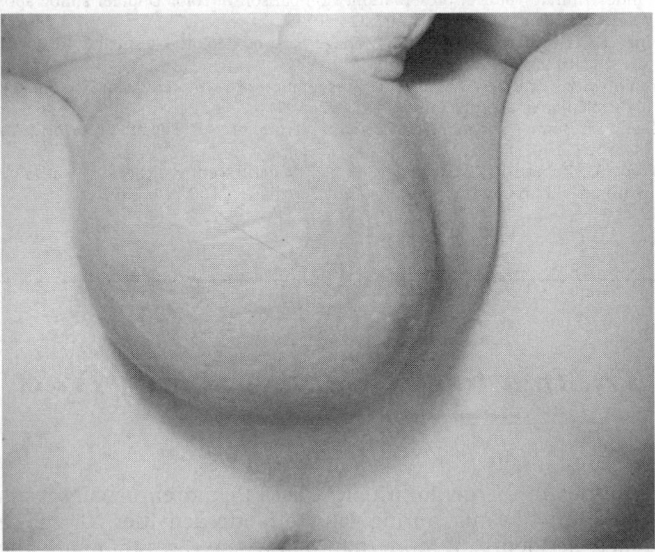

Figure 553–5 Newborn with large right hydrocele.

INGUINAL HERNIA

This condition is similar to hydrocele and is discussed in Chapter 346.

TESTICULAR TUMOR

Testicular and paratesticular tumors can occur at any age, including in the newborn. Approximately 65% are malignant. Most present as a painless, hard testicular mass that does not transilluminate. Scrotal ultrasonography should be performed to confirm the finding of a testicular mass and may help to delineate the type of testis tumor. Serum tumor markers, α-fetoprotein and β-human chorionic gonadotropin, should be determined. Definitive therapy includes surgical exploration through an inguinal incision. In most cases a radical orchiectomy, consisting of removal of the entire testis and spermatic cord, is performed, but if the ultrasonographic study or surgical exploration suggests that the tumor is benign, such as a teratoma or epidermoid cyst, removal of the mass only may be performed.

Allen TD, Elder JS: Shortcomings of color Doppler sonography in the diagnosis of testicular torsion. J Urol 154:1508, 1995.

Clarnette TD, Rowe D, Hasthorpe S, et al: Incomplete disappearance of the processus vaginalis as a cause of ascending testis. J Urol 157:1889, 1997.

Cortes D, Thorup JM, Lindenberg S: Fertility potential after unilateral orchiopexy: An age independent risk of subsequent infertility when biopsies at surgery lack germ cells. J Urol 156:217, 1996.

Elder JS: Laparoscopy for impalpable testes: Significance of the patent processus vaginalis. J Urol 152:776, 1994.

Elder JS: Evaluation and management of boys with a nonpalpable testis. *In:* Elder JS (ed): Pediatric Urology for the General Urologist. New York: Igaku-Shoin, 1996, pp 119–134.

Hadziselimovic F, Herzog B, Jenny P: The chance for fertility in adolescent boys after corrective surgery for varicocele. J Urol 154:731, 1995.

Jefferson RH, Perez LM, Joseph DB: Critical analysis of the clinical presentation of acute scrotum: A 9-year experience at a single institution. J Urol 158:1198, 1997.

Kass EJ, Lundak B: The acute scrotum. Pediatr Clin North Am 44:1251, 1997.

Kirsch AJ, Escala J, Duckett JW, et al: Surgical management of the nonpalpable testis: The Children's Hospital of Philadelphia experience. J Urol 159:1340, 1998.

Lee PA, O'Leary LA, Songer NJ, et al: Paternity after bilateral cryptorchidism: A controlled study. Arch Pediatr Adolesc Med 151:260, 1997.

Lee PA, O'Leary LA, Songer NJ, et al: Paternity after unilateral cryptorchidism: A controlled study. Pediatrics 98:676, 1996.

Lenzi A, Gandini L, Bagolan P, et al: Sperm parameters after early left varicocele treatment. Fertil Steril 69:347, 1998.

Lindgren BW, Darby EC, Faiella L, et al: Laparoscopic orchiopexy: Procedure of choice for the nonpalpable testis? J Urol 159:2132, 1998.

Paduch DA, Niedzielski J: Repair versus observation in adolescent varicocele: A prospective study. J Urol 158:1128, 1997.

Paltiel HJ, Connolly LP, Atala A, et al: Acute scrotal symptoms in boys with an indeterminate clinical presentation: Comparison of color Doppler sonography and scintigraphy. Radiology 207:223, 1998.

Pinto KJ, Noe HN, Jerkins GR: Management of neonatal testicular torsion. J Urol 158:1196, 1997.

Rabinowitz R, Hulbert WC Jr: Late presentation of cryptorchidism: The etiology of testicular re-ascent. J Urol 157:1892, 1997.

Skoog SJ: Benign and malignant pediatric scrotal masses. Pediatr Clin North Am 44:1229, 1997.

Skoog SJ, Roberts KP, Goldstein M, et al: The adolescent varicocele: What's new with an old problem in young patients? Pediatrics 100:112, 1997.

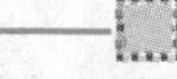

CHAPTER 554
Trauma to the Genitourinary Tract

Injuries to the genitourinary tract in children usually result from blunt trauma during falls, athletic activities, or motor vehicle accidents. In more than half of the cases there are also major injuries to the brain, spinal cord, skeleton, lungs, or abdominal organs. Children are at greater risk of blunt renal injury than are adults because of less body fat and because the kidneys are not located directly behind the ribs. Children with a pre-existing renal anomaly such as hydronephrosis secondary to a ureteropelvic junction obstruction, horseshoe kidney, or renal ectopia are also at increased risk for renal injury. Blunt abdominal or flank trauma often causes a renal injury. Falling may cause a deceleration injury that causes an injury to the renal pedicle, interrupting blood flow to the kidney. If the bladder is full, blunt lower abdominal trauma may cause a bladder rupture. Rupture of the membranous urethra occurs in 30% of cases of pelvic fractures. Straddle injuries are usually associated with trauma to the bulbous urethra. Symptoms and signs of urinary tract injury include gross or microscopic hematuria, bleeding from the urethral meatus, abdominal or flank pain, a flank mass, fractured lower ribs or lumbar transverse processes, and a perineal or scrotal hematoma.

Evaluation of the patient begins after an adequate airway has been established and the patient is hemodynamically stable (see Chapter 64). With significant abdominal injury or with a history of gross hematuria, the bladder should be catheterized, unless blood is dripping from the urethral meatus, which is an indication of potential urethral injury. Passing the catheter in the presence of a urethral injury may increase the extent of the damage and convert a partial membranous urethral tear into a total disruption. In these patients, a retrograde urethrogram should be performed by injecting radiopaque contrast into the urethral meatus. Oblique radiographs demonstrate the extent of the injury and whether urethral continuity is preserved or has been disrupted.

When the bladder can be catheterized, a static cystogram is obtained, infusing a contrast solution through the catheter by gravity, ideally using fluoroscopy. Flat and oblique views are often obtained; a postvoid film also should be obtained because in some cases, extravasation may be hidden by the full bladder. Bladder ruptures can be intraperitoneal or extraperitoneal. All intraperitoneal ruptures require surgical repair. Minor extraperitoneal near-ruptures might be treated by catheter drainage but generally require surgical treatment.

Computed tomography is performed next to evaluate the kidneys, ureters, and bladder. Excretory urography (intravenous pyelography) was once performed, but computed tomography is preferred because associated injuries are also demonstrated. Prompt function of both kidneys without extravasation usually excludes major renal injury. Renal injuries are usually classified as minor and major. Minor renal injuries are most common and include contusion of the renal parenchyma and shallow cortical lacerations not involving the collecting system. Major renal injuries include deep lacerations involving the collecting system, the shattered kidney, and renal pedicle injuries. Complete absence of function of one kidney without contralateral compensatory hypertrophy (indicative of congenital absence) should be regarded as an indication of major injury to the renal pedicle. Renal angiography was once used to evaluate renal injuries further, particularly if a renal pedicle injury is suspected. Currently, these studies are rarely used because such patients are often hemodynamically unstable, and management is not significantly affected by the findings. In some cases, a pre-existing renal anomaly may be demonstrated on the study. A ruptured ureteropelvic junction obstruction may be apparent if the kidney is intact but the distal ureter is not visualized.

Minor renal injuries such as contusions are managed by bed rest and monitoring of vital signs until abdominal or flank discomfort and gross *hematuria* has resolved. Children with a *major renal injury* are usually admitted to an intensive care unit for continuous monitoring of vital signs and urine output. Intravenous antibiotics are also administered. These injuries are also managed nonoperatively, as Gerota's fascia often causes tamponade of bleeding from the kidney, and dramatic healing of the injured parenchyma can occur, even with significant urinary extravasation. During renal exploration shortly after abdominal trauma, it can be difficult to identify normal and devitalized parenchyma, and the likelihood of having to perform a nephrectomy can be significant. Approximately 10% of children with a major renal injury undergo surgical exploration because of hemodynamic instability, persistent extravasation, persistent hematuria, or to correct a congenital renal deformity. If the child is being explored for other abdominal injuries, the injured kidney is examined. If there is persistent extravasation because of intermittent ureteral obstruction from a blood clot, passage of a temporary double-J stent endoscopically between the bladder and kidney may allow resolution. If there is a renal pedicle injury, nephrectomy is necessary. The kidney can be salvaged by emergency renal revascularization only if the kidney is explored within 2–3 hr of the injury. All penetrating injuries of the kidneys should be explored. In addition to loss of renal function, the main long-term complication of renal injury is renin-mediated hypertension. Children who sustain renal injuries must have periodic measurement of blood pressure.

Ureteral injuries are usually iatrogenic. Injuries of the ureter by blunt or penetrating trauma require immediate surgical attention.

Treatment of a *membranous urethral injury* is controversial. There is often a large pelvic hematoma with tamponade, and attempting to repair the injury immediately can be treacherous and result in significant hemorrhage. Many such injuries are initially managed by temporary suprapubic cystostomy, with continuous bladder drainage for 3–6 mo. Subsequently, open or endoscopic urethroplasty can be performed. Alternatively, some try to achieve urethral continuity under anesthesia and leave a urethral catheter for several months. These patients typically require urethroplasty. Erectile dysfunction, urethral stricture, and urinary incontinence are the major complications of rupture of the membranous urethra.

Penile injury is uncommon. Some boys who are in the process of toilet training sustain an injury to the glans penis if the lid of the toilet falls while they are urinating. These boys often have a hematoma covering half the glans. Typically they have no difficulty urinating and do not need extensive evaluation. Adolescent boys who indulge in extremely vigorous sexual intercourse may sustain rupture of one of the corporal bodies. These boys have severe swelling of the penile shaft and require emergency exploration and repair. Boys with penetrating injuries of the penis also require emergency debridement and repair.

Testicular injuries are relatively uncommon in children because of the small size of the testes and their mobility within the scrotum. Such injuries usually result from blunt trauma during athletic activity. Typically they have significant scrotal swelling, testicular pain, and tenderness. Sonography demonstrates rupture of the tunica albuginea, which is the capsule of the testis, and surrounding hemorrhage. Prompt surgical treatment of testicular injuries increases the salvage rate.

Brown SL, Elder JS, Spirnak JP: Are pediatric patients more susceptible to major renal injury from blunt trauma? A comparative study. J Urol 160:138, 1998.
Smith EM, Elder JS, Spirnak JP: Major blunt renal trauma in the pediatric population: Is a non-operative approach indicated? J Urol 149:646, 1993.
Spirnak JP: Lower urinary tract trauma. *In:* Resnick MI, Older RA (eds): Diagnosis of Genitourinary Disease, 2nd ed. New York, Thieme, 1997, pp 438–444.
Wessells H, McAninch JW: Upper urinary tract trauma. *In:* Resnick MI, Older RA (eds): Diagnosis of Genitourinary Disease, 2nd ed. New York, Thieme, 1997, pp 425–437.

CHAPTER 555
Urinary Lithiasis

Urinary lithiasis in children is less common in the United States than in other parts of the world. The wide geographic variation in the incidence of lithiasis in childhood is related to climatic, dietary, and socioeconomic factors. Approximately 7% of urinary calculi occur in children less than 16 yr of age. In the United States, most children with stone disease have a metabolic abnormality. The exceptions are patients with a neuropathic bladder, who are prone to infection-initiated renal stones, and those who have urinary tract reconstruction with intestine, which predisposes to bladder calculi. Metabolic stones are twice as common in boys as in girls and are rare in African-Americans. In Southeast Asia, urinary calculi are endemic and are related to dietary factors.

STONE FORMATION. The composition and site of urinary calculi vary, depending on the pathogenesis. Most stones are composed of calcium, oxalate, uric acid, cystine, ammonium, or phosphate crystals, or a combination of these substances (Table 555–1). The risk of stone formation is increased with increasing concentrations of these crystals and reduced with increasing concentrations of inhibitors. Renal calculi develop from crystals that form on the calyx and aggregate to form a calculus. Bladder calculi may be stones that formed in the kidney and traveled down the ureter, or they may form primarily in the bladder.

Stone formation depends on four factors. *Matrix* is a mixture of protein, nonamino sugars, glucosamine, water, and organic ash. Matrix makes up 2–9% of the dry weight of urinary stones and is arranged within the stones in organized concentric laminations. *Precipitation-crystallization* refers to supersatu-

TABLE 555–1 Classification of Urolithiasis

Calcium Stones (Calcium Oxalate and Calcium Phosphate)
- Hypercalciuria
  - Absorptive
  - Renal leak
  - Resorptive
  - Distal renal tubular acidosis (type 1) (calcium phosphate)
  - Hyperparathyroidism
  - Sarcoidosis
  - Furosemide administration
  - Vitamin D excess
  - Immobilization
  - Corticosteroid administration
  - Cushing disease
- Hyperuricosuria
- Heterozygous cystinuria
- Hyperoxaluria (calcium oxalate)
  - Primary hyperoxaluria, types 1 and 2
  - Secondary hyperoxaluria
  - Enteric hyperoxaluria
- Hypocitruria
- Renal tubular acidosis

Cystine Stones
- Cystinuria

Struvite Stones (Magnesium Ammonium Phosphate)
- Urinary tract infection (urea-splitting organism)
- Foreign body
- Urinary stasis

Uric Acid Stones
- Hyperuricosuria
- Lesch-Nyhan syndrome
- Myeloproliferative disorders
- After chemotherapy
- Inflammatory bowel disease

Indinavir Stones

Nephrocalcinosis

ration of the urine with specific ions comprising the crystal. Once a nucleus of crystal forms, the crystals aggregate by chemical and electrical forces. Increasing the saturation of urine with respect to the ions increases the rate of nucleation, crystal growth, and aggregation and increases the likelihood of stone formation and growth. *Epitaxy* refers to the aggregation of crystals of different composition but similar lattice structure, thus forming stones of a heterogeneous nature. The lattice structures of calcium oxalate and monosodium urate have similar structures, and calcium oxalate crystals can aggregate on a nucleus of monosodium urate crystals. Urine also contains *inhibitors* of stone formation, including citrate, diphosphonate, and magnesium ion.

CLINICAL MANIFESTATIONS. Children with urolithiasis usually have gross or microscopic hematuria. If the calculus is in the renal pelvis, calyx, or ureter and causes obstruction, abdominal or flank pain (renal colic) occurs. Typically the pain radiates anteriorly to the scrotum or labia. Often the pain is intermittent, corresponding to periods of obstruction of urine flow, which increases the pressure in the collecting system. If the calculus is in the distal ureter, the child may have irritative symptoms of dysuria, urgency, and frequency. If the stone has passed into the bladder, the child is usually asymptomatic. If the stone is in the urethra, dysuria and difficulty voiding may result. Some children pass small amounts of gravel-like material.

DIAGNOSIS. Approximately 90% of urinary calculi are calcified to some degree and consequently are radiopaque on a plain abdominal film. Some calculi are only a few millimeters in diameter and may not be obvious, particularly if they are in the ureter. Struvite (magnesium ammonium phosphate) stones are radiopaque. Cystine and uric acid calculi may be radiolucent, but often are slightly opacified. Some children have *nephrocalcinosis,* which is calcification of the renal tissue itself. Nephrocalcinosis is seen most commonly in premature neonates receiving furosemide, which causes hypercalciuria, and in children with medullary sponge kidney.

In a child with suspected renal colic, a *noncontrast spiral computed tomographic scan of the abdomen and pelvis* is performed in many centers. This study takes only a few minutes to perform, delineates the number and location of calculi, and demonstrates whether the involved kidney is hydronephrotic. In the past, an excretory urogram generally was performed. This test demonstrates a delay in visualization of the collecting system compared with the normal side, and if there is a ureteral calculus, there is columnization of contrast down to the stone. If the calculus is radiolucent or small, the urogram may not demonstrate the stone. Consequently, the noncontrast spiral computed tomographic scan is preferred. Another alternative is to obtain a plain radiograph of the abdomen and pelvis plus a renal ultrasonogram. If a small calculus is in the ureter, it may not be imaged by these two studies, and if the calculus is not causing impaired urinary flow at the time of the study, the renal ultrasonogram may not show hydronephrosis. In a child with a calculus that already has been diagnosed, however, serial plain films or renal ultrasonography can be used to follow the status of the calculus, such as whether it has grown or diminished in size, or moved. If a child has a renal pelvic calculus, a ureteropelvic junction obstruction should be suspected. In some cases, it can be difficult to determine whether hydronephrosis in such a child is secondary to an obstructing stone or the ureteropelvic junction obstruction, or both. Finally, even though a ureteral or renal pelvic stone may be obstructive, a MAG-3 diuretic renogram has no role in assessing whether the stone itself is causing significant obstruction.

Any material that resembles a calculus should be sent for analysis by a laboratory that specializes in the identification of the components of urinary calculi.

METABOLIC EVALUATION. A metabolic evaluation for the most common predisposing factors should be undertaken in all children with urolithiasis, bearing in mind that structural, infectious, and metabolic factors often coexist. This evaluation should not be undertaken in a child who is in the process of passing a stone because the altered diet and hydration status, as well as the effect of obstruction on the kidney, may alter the results of the study. The basic laboratory studies required are listed in Table 555–2, and the normal values for 24-hr urine collections are shown in Table 555–3. In children with hypercalciuria, further studies of calcium excretion with dietary calcium restriction and calcium loading are necessary.

TABLE 555–2 Laboratory Tests Suggested to Evaluate Urolithiasis

Serum
- Calcium
- Phosphorus
- Uric acid
- Electrolytes and anion gap
- Creatinine
- Alkaline phosphatase

Urine
- Urinalysis
- Urine culture
- Calcium:creatinine ratio
- Spot test for cystinuria
- 24-hr collection for
  - Creatinine clearance
  - Calcium
  - Phosphate
  - Oxalate
  - Uric acid
  - Dibasic amino acids (if cystine spot test result is positive)

PATHOGENESIS OF SPECIFIC RENAL CALCULI

Calcium Stones. Most urinary calculi in children in the United States are composed of calcium oxalate or calcium phosphate, or both. The most common metabolic abnormality in these individuals is hypercalciuria. Between 30 and 60% of children with calcium stones have hypercalciuria without hypercalcemia. Other metabolic aberrations that predispose to stone disease include hyperoxaluria, hyperuricosuria, hypocitruria, heterozygous cystinuria, hypomagnesuria, hyperparathyroidism, and renal tubular acidosis.

Hypercalciuria may be absorptive, renal, or resorptive. The primary disturbance in *absorptive hypercalciuria* is intestinal hyperabsorption of calcium. In some children, an increase in 1,25-dihydroxyvitamin D is associated with the increased calcium absorption, and in others the process is independent of vitamin D. *Renal hypercalciuria* refers to impaired renal tubular reabsorption of calcium. Renal leak of calcium causes mild hypocalcemia, which triggers an increased production of parathyroid hormone, with increased intestinal absorption of calcium and increased mobilization of calcium stores. *Resorptive hypercalciuria* is uncommon and is found in patients with primary hyperparathyroidism. Excess parathyroid hormone secretion stimulates intestinal absorption of calcium and mobilization of calcium stores. A brief summary of the metabolic evaluation of children with hypercalciuria is shown in Table 555–4.

TABLE 555–3 Normal Values for Urine Chemistries in Children

	Mg/Kg/24 Hr
Calcium	<4.0
Oxalate	<0.57
Uric acid	<10.7
Citrate	>2.0
Cystine	
Heterozygote	1.4–2.8
Homozygote	>5.7
Phosphate	<15.0

TABLE 555–4 Metabolic Evaluation of Children with Hypercalciuria

	Serum Calcium	Restricted Calcium (Urine)	Fasting Calcium (Urine)	Calcium Load (Urine)	Parathyroid Hormone (Serum)
Absorptive	N	N or I	N	I	I
Renal	N	I	I	I	N
Resorptive	I	I	I	I	I

N = Normal; I = increased.

Hyperoxaluria is another potentially important cause of calcium stones. Oxalate increases the solubility product of calcium oxalate crystallization 7 to 10 times more than calcium. Consequently, hyperoxaluria significantly increases the likelihood of calcium oxalate precipitation. Oxalate is found in high concentration in tea, coffee, spinach, and rhubarb. *Primary hyperoxaluria* is a rare autosomal recessive disorder that can be subclassified into glycolic aciduria and L-glyceric aciduria. Most patients with primary hyperoxaluria have glycolic aciduria; oxalic and glycolic acids are increased in the urine of affected individuals. Both defects cause increased endogenous production of oxalate, with hyperoxaluria, urolithiasis, nephrocalcinosis, and renal injury. Death from renal failure occurs by age 20 yr in untreated patients. Oxalosis, defined as extrarenal deposition of calcium oxalate, occurs when renal insufficiency is present with elevated plasma oxalate. Calcium oxalate deposits appear first in blood vessels and bone marrow, and with time appear throughout the body. *Secondary hyperoxaluria* is more common and can occur in patients with increased intake of oxalate and oxalate precursors such as vitamin C, in those with pyridoxine deficiency, and in children with intestinal malabsorption.

Enteric hyperoxaluria refers to disorders such as inflammatory bowel disease, pancreatic insufficiency, and biliary disease, in which there is gastrointestinal malabsorption of fatty acids, which bind intraluminal calcium and form salts that are excreted in the feces. Normally calcium forms a complex with oxalate to reduce oxalate absorption, but if calcium is unavailable, there is increased absorption of unbound oxalate.

Hypocitruria refers to a low excretion of citrate, which is an inhibitor of calcium stone formation. Citrate acts as an inhibitor of calcium urolithiasis by forming complexes with calcium, increasing the solubility of calcium in the urine and inhibiting the aggregation of calcium phosphate and calcium oxalate crystals. Disorders such as chronic diarrhea, intestinal malabsorption, and renal tubular acidosis may cause hypocitruria. It may also be idiopathic.

Renal tubular acidosis (RTA) is a syndrome involving a disturbance of acid-base balance within the kidney that can be classified into three types, one of which predisposes to renal calculi that are typically calcium phosphate. In type 1, the distal nephron does not secrete hydrogen ion into the distal tubule. The urine pH is never less than 5.8, and hyperchloremic hypokalemic acidosis results. Patients acquire nephrolithiasis, nephrocalcinosis, muscle weakness, and osteomalacia. Type 1 RTA can be an autosomal dominant disorder, but more often it is acquired and associated with systemic diseases such as Sjögren's syndrome, Wilson disease, primary biliary cirrhosis, and lymphocytic thyroiditis, or it results from amphotericin B, lithium, or toluene (an organic solvent associated with glue sniffing).

Approximately 5–8% of individuals with *cystic fibrosis* have urolithiasis. Typically the stones are calcium and often become manifested in adolescence or young adulthood. Microscopic nephrocalcinosis also occurs in younger children with the disease. These patients do not have hypercalciuria, and the propensity for urolithiasis has been speculated to result from an inability to excrete a sodium chloride load or from intestinal malabsorption.

Other disorders may play a role in causing calcium stones. *Hyperuricosuria* may be related to the epitactic growth of calcium oxalate crystals around a nucleus of uric acid crystals or to the action of uric acid as a counterinhibitor of urinary mucopolysaccharides, which inhibit calcium oxalate crystallization. *Heterozygous cystinuria* is found in some patients with calcium stones. The mechanism is unknown but may be similar to that of uric acid. *Sarcoidosis* causes an increased sensitivity to vitamin D_3 and thus an increased absorption of calcium from the gastrointestinal tract. In *Lesch-Nyhan syndrome*, there is excessive uric acid synthesis. These patients are more likely to form uric acid stones, but some of these stones may be calcified. *Immobility* may cause hypercalciuria by mobilization of calcium stores. High-dose *corticosteroids* may cause hypercalciuria and calcium oxalate precipitation. *Furosemide*, which is administered in the neonatal intensive care unit to neonates with hyaline membrane disease, also can cause severe hypercalciuria, urolithiasis, and nephrocalcinosis.

In some children, calcium calculi are *idiopathic*. This diagnosis should not be given until a complete metabolic evaluation has been performed.

Cystine Calculi. Cystinuria accounts for 1% of renal calculi in children. The condition is a rare autosomal recessive disorder of the epithelial cells of the renal tubule that prevents absorption of the four dibasic amino acids (cystine, ornithine, arginine, and lysine) and results in excessive urinary excretion of these products. The only known complication of this familial disease is the formation of calculi, owing to the low solubility of cystine. The patients usually have acidic urine, which leads to a higher rate of precipitation. In the homozygous patient, the daily excretion of cystine usually exceeds 500 mg, and stone formation occurs at an early age. Heterozygotes excrete 100 to 300 mg/day and typically do not have clinical urolithiasis. The sulfur content of cystine gives these stones their faint radiopaque appearance.

Struvite Calculi. Urinary tract infections caused by urea-splitting organisms (most often *Proteus*, and occasionally *Klebsiella, Escherichia coli, Pseudomonas*, and others) result in urinary alkalinization and excessive production of ammonia, which can lead to the precipitation of magnesium ammonium phosphate (struvite) and calcium phosphate. In the kidney, often the calculi have a staghorn configuration, filling the calyces. The stones act as foreign bodies, causing obstruction, perpetuating infection, and causing gradual renal damage. Patients with struvite stones may also have metabolic abnormalities that predispose to stone formation. These stones are often seen in children with neuropathic bladder dysfunction, particularly those who have undergone an ileal conduit procedure. In children who have undergone urinary tract reconstruction with augmentation cystoplasty or continent diversion, or both, struvite stones may form in the reconstructed bladder.

Uric Acid Calculi. Calculi containing uric acid represent less than 5% of all cases of lithiasis in children in the United States but are more common in less developed areas of the world. Hyperuricosuria with or without hyperuricemia is the common underlying factor in most cases. The stones are radiolucent. The diagnosis should be suspected when there is a persistently acid urine and urate crystalluria. Hyperuricosuria may result from various inborn errors of purine metabolism that lead to overproduction of uric acid, the end product of purine metabolism in humans. Children with the Lesch-Nyhan syndrome and patients with glucose-6-phosphatase deficiency form urate calculi as well. In children with short-bowel syndrome, and particularly those with ileostomies, chronic dehydration and acidosis are sometimes complicated by uric acid lithiasis. One of the most common causes of uric acid lithiasis is the rapid turnover of purine with some tumors and myeloproliferative diseases. The risk of uric acid lithiasis is especially great when treatment of these diseases causes rapid breakdown of nucleoproteins. Uric acid calculi or "sludge" can fill the entire upper collecting system and cause renal failure and even anuria. Urates are also present within calcium-containing stones. In these cases, more than one predisposing factor for stone formation may exist. A related disorder is *2,8-dihydroxyadenine lithiasis,* which results from a deficiency in adenine phosphoribosyltransferase. The stones are radiolucent and can be differentiated from uric acid calculi by mass spectrometry but not by routine chemical analysis. In contrast to uric acid, which is soluble in alkaline urine, the solubility of 2,8-dihydroxyadenine changes little within physiologic pH ranges.

Indinavir Calculi. Indinavir sulfate is a protease inhibitor approved for the treatment of human immunodeficiency virus infection. As many as 4% of patients acquire symptomatic nephrolithiasis. Most of the calculi are radiolucent and composed of indinavir-based monohydrate, although calcium oxalate or phosphate, or both, have been present in some. After each dose, 12% of the drug is excreted unchanged in the urine. The urine in these patients often contains crystals of characteristic rectangles and fan-shaped or starburst crystals. Indinavir is soluble at a pH of less than 5.5. Consequently, dissolution therapy by urinary acidification with ammonium chloride or ascorbic acid should be considered.

Nephrocalcinosis. Nephrocalcinosis refers to calcium deposition within the renal tissue. Often nephrocalcinosis is associated with urolithiasis. The most common causes are furosemide (administered to premature neonates), distal RTA, hyperparathyroidism, medullary sponge kidney, hypophosphatemic rickets, sarcoidosis, cortical necrosis, hyperoxaluria, prolonged immobilization, Cushing syndrome, hyperuricosuria, and renal candidiasis.

TREATMENT. In a child with a renal or ureteral calculus, the decision whether to remove the stone is dependent on the location, size, composition (if known), and whether obstruction or infection, or both, is present. Small ureteral calculi often pass spontaneously, although the child may experience severe renal colic. The narrow parts of the ureter include the ureteropelvic junction and the midureter where it crosses the common iliac artery; the narrowest segment is the ureterovesical junction. In some cases, passage of a ureteral stent past the stone endoscopically allows relief of pain and dilates the ureter sufficiently to allow the calculus to pass. In cases such as children with a uric acid calculus or infant with a furosemide-associated calculus, dissolution therapy may be effective.

If the calculus does not pass or seems unlikely to pass, or if there is associated urinary tract infection, removal is necessary. Newer modalities of stone removal, both endoscopically and by percutaneous access to the kidney, have been effective in children. Extracorporeal shock wave lithotripsy has been successfully applied to children with renal and ureteral stones at a success rate of more than 75%.

In children with urolithiasis, treatment of the underlying metabolic disorder should be addressed. Because lithiasis results from having too high a concentration of specific substances in the urine, often an effective method of preventing further stones is by maintaining a continuous high urine output by maintaining a high fluid intake. The high fluid intake should be continued at night, and usually it is necessary to get up at least once at night to urinate and drink more water.

In children with hypercalciuria, some reduction in calcium and sodium intake is necessary, but caution is urged in the growing child. Thiazide diuretics also reduce renal calcium excretion. Addition of potassium citrate, an inhibitor of calcium stones, with a dosage of 1–2 mEq/kg/24 hr is beneficial. An excellent source of citrate is lemonade, as 4 ounces of lemon juice contains 84 mEq of citric acid. A daily mixture of 4 ounces of reconstituted lemon juice in 2 L of water, and sweetened to taste should significantly increase the urinary citrate level. In difficult cases, neutral orthophosphate should be given also, although it is poorly tolerated.

In patients with uric acid stones, allopurinol is effective. Allopurinol is an inhibitor of xanthine oxidase and is effective in reducing the production of both uric acid and 2,8-dihydroxyadenine and can help control recurrence of both types of stones. In addition, urinary alkalinization with sodium bicarbonate or sodium citrate is beneficial. The urine pH should be at least 6.5 and can be monitored at home by the family. Maintaining a high urine pH can also prevent recurrence of cystine calculi. Cystine is much more soluble when the urinary pH is greater than 7.5, and alkalinization of urine with sodium bicarbonate or sodium citrate is effective. Another important medication is D-penicillamine, which is a chelating agent that binds to cysteine or hemicystine, increasing the solubility of the product. Although poorly tolerated by many patients, it has been reported to be effective in dissolving cystine stones and in preventing recurrences when hydration and urinary alkalinization fail. *N*-acetylcysteine appears to have low toxicity and may be effective in controlling cystinuria, but long-term experience with it is lacking.

Treatment of type 1 RTA involves correction of the metabolic acidosis and replacement of potassium and sodium loss. Sodium or potassium citrate therapy, or both, is necessary. When the metabolic acidosis is corrected, the urinary citrate excretion returns to normal.

Treatment of primary hyperoxaluria involves hepatic transplantation because the defective enzymes are hepatic. Ideally this procedure should be performed before renal failure occurs. In the most severe cases renal transplantation is also necessary.

Abrams SA, Yergey AL, Schanler RJ, et al: Hypercalciuria in premature infants receiving high mineral content diets. J Pediatr Gastroenterol Nutr 18:20, 1994.
Alon US: Nephrocalcinosis. Curr Opin Pediatr 9:160, 1997.
Alon US, Scagliotti D, Garola RE: Nephrocalcinosis and nephrolithiasis in infants with congestive heart failure treated with furosemide. J Pediatr 125:149, 1994.
Balaji KC, Menon M: Mechanism of stone formation. Urol Clin North Am 24:1, 1997.
Chow GK, Strem SB: Contemporary urological intervention for cystinuric patients: Immediate and long-term impact and implications. J Urol 160:341, 1998.
Dalrymple NC, Verga M, Anderson KR, et al: The value of unenhanced helical computerized tomography in the management of acute flank pain. J Urol 159:735, 1998.
Hoppe B, Hesse A, Neuhaus T, et al: Urinary saturation and nephrocalcinosis in preterm infants: Effect of parenteral nutrition. Arch Dis Child 69:299, 1993.
Jones CA, King S, Shaw NJ, et al: Renal calcification in preterm infants: Follow up at 4–5 years. Arch Dis Child 76:f185–f189, 1997.
Katz SM, Krueger LJ, Falkner B: Microscopic nephrocalcinosis in cystic fibrosis. N Engl J Med 319:263, 1988.
Kronner KM, Casale AJ, Cain MP, et al: Bladder calculi in the pediatric augmented bladder. J Urol 160:1096, 1998.
Kroovand RL: Pediatric urolithiasis. Urol Clin North Am 24:173, 1997.
Lerner LB, Cendron M, Rous SN: Nephrolithiasis from indinavir, a new human immunodeficiency virus drug. J Urol 159:2074, 1998.
Lim DJ, Walker RD III, Ellsworth PI, et al: Treatment of pediatric urolithiasis between 1984 and 1994. J Urol 156:702, 1996.
Losty P, Surana R, O'Donnell B: Limitations of extracorporeal shock wave lithotripsy for urinary tract calculi in young children. J Pediatr Surg 28:1037, 1993.
Matthews LA, Doershuk CF, Stern RC, et al: Urolithiasis and cystic fibrosis. J Urol 155:1563, 1996.
Meyers DA, Mobley TB, Jenkins JM, et al: Pediatric low energy lithotripsy with lithostar. J Urol 153:453, 1995.
Pope JC IV, Trusler LA, Klein AM, et al: The natural history of nephrocalcinosis in premature infants treated with loop diuretics. J Urol 156:709, 1996.
Schurman SJ, Norden AGW, Scheinman SJ: X-linked recessive nephrolithiasis: Presentation and diagnosis in children. J Pediatr 132:859, 1998.
Seltzer MA, Low RK, McDonald M, et al: Dietary manipulation with lemonade to treat hypocitraturic calcium nephrolithiasis. J Urol 156:907, 1996.

PART XXIV

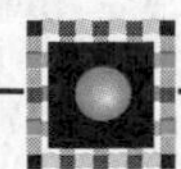

Gynecologic Problems of Childhood

Joseph S. Sanfilippo

CHAPTER 556

History and Physical Examination

NEONATE. The initial gynecologic assessment of newborn infants should begin with the breast examination. Not uncommonly, as a result of maternal endogenous estrogen production, breast tissue is increased in neonates; nipple discharge may be noted (see Chapter 559). The abdomen is gently palpated for evidence of organomegaly, and the external genitalia are assessed for any ambiguity. The labia should be grasped gently and separated, allowing inspection of the introitus-hymenal area. On completion of the inspection segment of the examination, a rectal examination is performed. A midline structure, indicative of the uterus, is usually palpable, but the adnexa should not be apparent at this time. Abducting the hips with the labia gently retracted frequently facilitates inspection of the introital area. A normal protuberant hymen with associated thin white mucoid discharge from the vagina is often perceptible. In the first few weeks of life, a small amount of vaginal bleeding may occur, reflecting the decline in circulating levels of maternal estrogens.

PREPUBERTAL CHILD. A pediatric or adolescent patient undergoing her first gynecologic examination should be treated with particular care, because the initial encounter may well set the tone for all future gynecologic examinations. If the examination is painful or uncomfortable or if there is a significant lack of rapport between the patient and the examiner, the child may suffer lasting psychologic consequences. A gentle, caring attitude by the physican will go far in enabling the patient to relax at the time and during all future gynecologic examinations.

The history is obtained primarily from the parent(s), who should be integrally involved in the physical examination of a child in this age group. In addition, patients should have a sense of control over the examination, be involved, and should experience no discomfort. These goals are facilitated by providing an adequate explanation before the examination.

Much information can be obtained by inspection of the vulvovaginal area. Ideally, a patient is placed in a frog-leg position. If this is not satisfactory, then a knee-chest position with a Valsalva's maneuver allows adequate assessment of the introital (lower-third) vaginal area. Magnification often can be accomplished with use of a colposcope or hand-held magnifying glass; appropriate documentation is also important. Visualizing the vestibule permits assessment of any discharge. Use of an aseptic technique in which an intravenous tubing (butterfly) is passed into a soft number 12 bladder catheter, all of which is then attached to a 1-mL tuberculin syringe, allows aspiration of any fluid in the vagina as well as successful lavage. Wet mounts can be obtained and evaluated as indicated, as well as cultures for further evaluation of vulvovaginitis. Other instrumentation used for the genital examination include an otoscope or Cameron-Myers vaginoscope. Gentle traction on the labia upward and outward further exposes the vaginal introitus and permits assessment. Calcium alginate (Calgi) swabs are also useful, especially for obtaining cultures from the vagina. A number of variations of the normal-appearing hymen occur, and care must be taken to determine if a patient has an imperforate, microperforate, or septate hymen. If an inadequate examination is accomplished in an office-clinic setting, then consideration for sedation or examination under anesthesia is appropriate.

ADOLESCENT. Obtaining a history in this age group may take place initially in the presence of the patient's parents. However, an adolescent should be made aware of the concept of confidentiality and be given the opportunity to provide her own history without the parents being present (see Part XII). This can be accomplished in the examination room before the actual physical examination. Concern for the presence of vaginal discharge, the potential for sexually transmitted disease, pregnancy, or menstrual aberration should be explored. Physicans should win the confidence of the adolescent, provide a relaxed atmosphere for the examination, and communicate to the teenager one's availability for consultation. Indications for the first pelvic examination in adolescents are presented in Table 556–1.

The teenage patient, in a manner similar to that for a pediatric patient, should be involved in the examination. The examination is best performed in the absence of parents, but a chaperone should be present and may serve to neutralize any adverse psychosocial aspects of the situation. Communication should occur between the physician and the patient throughout the examination. The examination should be performed in the dorsal lithotomy position with an effort made to maintain eye contact. Appropriate-sized specula should be available, including the small Pedersen's (8 cm in depth). The 4–5 cm

TABLE 556–1 Suggested Indications for Pelvic Examination in Adolescents

Age 18
Sexually active
Past or current
- Menstrual irregularities
- Severe dysmenorrhea
- Unexplained abdominal pain
- Unexplained dysuria
- Abnormal vaginal discharge

Modified from The adolescent obstetric-gynecologic patient. ACOG Technical Bull 145:3, 1990.

pediatric speculum is best avoided in that it results in inadequate visualization; however, the pediatric-sized Huffman's speculum is appropriate.

Inspection of the vulva is followed by palpation of Bartholin's urethral Skene's glands. The clitoris, which is normally 2–4 mm wide, is then assessed. A clitoris wider than 10 mm, especially in the presence of other signs of virilization, is abnormal. The hymenal configuration should also be evaluated. A patient should be told immediately prior to insertion of the speculum that she will experience a pressure sensation. Before touching the introitus, it is useful to touch the inner thigh with the speculum. Trauma to the urethra should be avoided, and displacement of the fourchette posteriorly further facilitates proper speculum placement. Discussion with the adolescent about techniques to relax the perineal musculature is often helpful.

Once the speculum portion of the examination is complete, a bimanual examination is undertaken. In a virginal female, a single digit examination with an appropriately lubricated, gloved finger allows proper palpation of the vaginal walls and cervix and bimanual assessment of the uterus and the adnexa. The cul-de-sac is assessed, and a rectovaginal examination performed to complete the bimanual exam.

Cavanaugh R: Obtaining a personal and confidential history from adolescents. An opportunity for prevention. J Adolesc Health Care 2:118, 1986.

Greydanus DE: Contraception. *In:* Sanfilippo JS, Lavery JP (eds): Pediatric Adolescent Obstetrics and Gynecology. New York, Springer-Verlag, 1985, p 234.

Phillips S, Bohannon W, Heald F: Teenager's choices regarding the presence of family members during the examination of genitalia. J Adolesc Health Care 7:245, 1986.

Pokorny SF: Pediatric vulvovaginitis. *In:* Kaufman R, Friedrich E, Gardner H (eds): Benign Diseases of the Vulva and Vagina. Chicago, Year Book Medical Publishers, 1989, p 55.

Pokorny SF, Stormer J: Atraumatic removal of secretions from the prepubertal vagina. Am J Obstet Gynecol 156:5, 1987.

Sanders JM Jr, Durant RH, Chastain DO: Pediatricians use of chaperons when performing gynecologic examinations on adolescent females. J Adolesc Health Care 10:110, 1989.

Talbot CW: The gynecologic examination of the pediatric patient. Pediatr Ann 15:501, 1986.

CHAPTER 557

Vulvovaginitis

Vulvovaginitis is the most common childhood or adolescent gynecologic problem (also see Chapter 119). Vulvovaginal irritation results from the lack of labial fat pads and pubic hair for protection of the external genitalia. The labia minora tend to open when a child squats; this, in turn, causes exposure of the more sensitive tissues within the hymenal ring. In addition, the close proximity of the anal orifice to the vagina allows transfer of fecal bacteria to the vulvovaginal area. Masturbation may also be a contributing factor.

The squamous epithelium of the vaginal mucosa is sensitive to steroid hormones. In the relatively low estrogenic environment, the thin atrophic epithelium becomes susceptible to bacterial invasion. Thus, recurrent vulvovaginitis usually ceases once a girl reaches puberty and the pH of the vagina becomes more acidic. In part, this change results from increased production of acetic and lactic acids, a phenomenon accompanied by an increase in superficial cell proliferation and glycogen as well as by enhancement of normal bacterial flora (Table 557–1).

The main clinical manifestations, in order of frequency, include vaginal discharge, erythema, and pruritus. Vaginal culture, cytology, and vaginoscopy may be indicated for evaluation of pediatric patients with vulvovaginitis. Infections are primarily located in the vulva and vagina (57%) in the majority of patients. *Candida* species are very commonly identified, followed by β-hemolytic streptococci group B and enterococci species.

Leukocyte esterase dipsticks are a rapid screening test for vaginitis and cervicitis. The technique has been used to identify trichomonads, *Candida*, and bacterial vaginosis and to evaluate cervical secretions for identification of gonococcal and chlamydial infections.

PATHOLOGIC VAGINAL DISCHARGE. In pediatric patients, vaginal discharge is a common presenting complaint. It is often the primary symptom of vulvitis, vaginitis, or vulvovaginitis. Pruritus, frequent urination, dysuria, or enuresis may be associated signs and symptoms. Vulvitis is manifested primarily by dysuria and pruritus, associated with erythema of the vulva. It commonly has a more protracted course than vaginitis; the latter is characterized by discharge without associated dysuria, pruritus, or erythema. Vulvovaginitis involves a combination of these manifestations. The color, odor, and duration of the discharge should be noted. Although there are a number of causes of vulvovaginitis in pediatric patients, the more common ones include poor perineal hygiene, *Candida* infection, and a foreign body.

NONSPECIFIC VULVOVAGINITIS. Patients with poor perineal hygiene often develop a condition known as nonspecific vulvovaginitis. Overall, nonspecific vulvovaginitis accounts for 70% of all pediatric vulvovaginitis cases. The discharge is characteristically brown or green, has a fetid odor, and is associated with a vaginal pH of 4.7–6.5. In 68% of reported cases, this vaginitis is associated with coliform bacteria secondary to fecal contamination. The next most common bacterial organisms associated with nonspecific vulvovaginitis are hemolytic *Streptococcus* and coagulase-positive *Staphylococcus*. These organisms are often transmitted manually from the nasopharynx. Clothing, chemicals, cosmetics, and soap products or detergents used for bathing or laundry may also cause irritation that leads to nonspecific vulvovaginitis. Tight-fitting clothing, such as jeans, leotards, and tights, as well as rubber pants or plastic-coated paper diapers, have also been implicated.

Nonspecific vulvovaginitis occasionally can result in chronic infection, which may cause significant psychologic consequences for a child and her parents alike. Physicians should emphasize the importance of avoiding "vaginal fixation," while encouraging proper perineal hygiene.

Successful treatment of nonspecific vulvovaginitis should include instruction in perineal hygiene, switching from tight-fitting underwear, the use of sitz baths with mild soap, and air drying the vulva. Patients should be instructed in appropriate bowel and bladder habits, emphasizing the need to wipe fecal material away from the vulvovaginal area. Recurrent vulvovaginitis should be treated with systemic antibiotics such as amoxicillin or cephalosporins. Topical estrogen cream or polysporin ointment is often helpful.

SPECIFIC VULVOVAGINITIS (see Table 557–1). *Gardnerella vaginalis* is the most common organism cultured in pediatric or adolescent patients with vulvovaginitis, followed by *Candida*. Other identified organisms include enterococci and anaerobic bacteria such as *Peptococcus, Peptostreptococcus, Veillonella parvula, Eubacterium, Propionibacterium,* and *Bacteroides* species. Protozoa, helminths, and viruses should also be considered as etiologic agents. *Treatment* depends on the offending organism (see Table 557–1).

LABIAL ADHESIONS. In this disorder, the labia minora have a central line of adherence from an area immediately inferior to the clitoris to the fourchette (Fig. 557–1). Labial adhesions are commonly seen in patients younger than 6 yr, and the condition is often asymptomatic. The lesions usually are associated with local inflammation in association with the hypoestrogenic state of preadolescents. Pooling of urine in the vagina and

TABLE 557–1 Specific Vulvovaginitis

Organism	Presentation	Diagnosis	Treatment
Enterobiasis (pinworms)	Perineal pruritus (nocturnal); gastrointestinal symptoms; variable vulvovaginal contamination from feces	Adult worms in stool or eggs on perianal skin	Mebendazole; repeat in 3 wk if necessary
Giardiasis	Asymptomatic fecal contaminant, vaginal discharge, diarrhea, malabsorption syndrome	Protozoal flagellate (cyst or trophozoites) in feces	Metronidazole or quinacrine
Molluscum contagiosum	Vulvar lesions, nodules with umbilicated area; white core of curdlike material	Isolation of poxvirus	Dermal curettage of papule
Phthirus pubis (pediculosis pubis)	Pruritus, excoriation, sky-blue macules; inner thigh or lower abdomen	Nits on hair shafts, lice—skin or clothing	Lindane lotion (Kwell); also see Chapter 674
Sarcoptes scabiei (scabies)	Nocturnal pruritus, pruritic vesicles, pustules in runs	Mites; ova black, dots of feces (microscopic)	1% lindane
Shigella species (shigellosis)	Fever, malaise, fecal contamination, diarrhea; blood and mucus, cramps, pus in stool	Stools; white blood cells and red blood cells, positive for *Shigella*	Trimethoprim and sulfamethoxazole; chloramphenicol, ampicillin, or tetracycline
Staphylococcus and *Streptococcus*	Vaginal discharge to vulvovaginal area; spread from primary lesion	Positive culture results of appropriate organism	Penicillin or cephalosporin

From Sanfilippo J: *Adolescent girls with vaginal discharge. Pediatr Ann 15:509, 1986.*

recurrent vulvovaginitis appear to provide a continuous nidus for recurrent urinary tract infections. Recurrent urinary tract symptoms occur in 20–40% of patients and should be treated. Once the vaginal pH becomes more acidic, as occurs with adolescence, the recurrent labial adhesions almost always disappear.

Topical estrogen cream applied each evening for 1 wk is the *treatment* of choice and is effective in over 90% of reported cases. Elimination of the agglutination may require 2–8 wk of therapy. Cleansing followed by application of a bland ointment such as petrolatum should continue for 1–2 mo after the adhesions separate. Mechanical separation of the adhesions is advisable only if the adhesions appear to separate easily and if it does not cause significant trauma. Once the adhesions are separated, the patient should be re-examined for any predisposing cause, such as the presence of a vaginal septum.

CANDIDIASIS. *Candida* infection is often associated with a diaper rash (see Chapters 5, 230.1, and 653). *Candida* vulvovaginitis, though rare in children, must be considered, especially for girls with chronic mucocutaneous candidiasis (Chapter 230.4). The presence of *Candida*-infected tissue may be indicative of significant immunosuppression. Underlying factors such as diabetes mellitus should be considered. *Treatment* with an imidazole cream (e.g., clotrimazole) is frequently effective, except in cases of chronic mucocutaneous candidiasis.

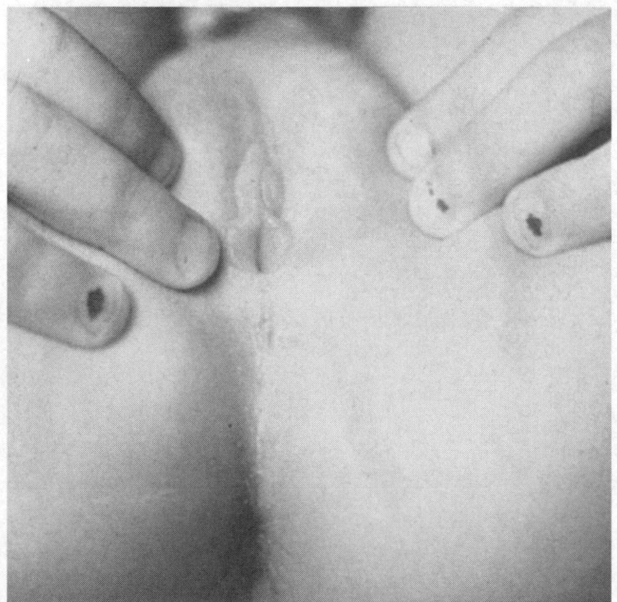

Figure 557–1 Labial adhesions. See also color section.

DIAPER DERMATITIS. This entity is a common problem occurring in the first several weeks of life (see Chapters 5, 146, and 653).

MOLLUSCUM CONTAGIOSUM. This common infection of the skin is caused by molluscum contagiosum virus, or poxvirus (Part XVI, Section 12). Molluscum contagiosum presents as an umbilicated, dome-shaped papule. The central umbilication usually is associated with a pulpy core. Vulvar lesions appear to result from autoinoculation or from close contact (sexual or nonsexual) with an infected individual. The incubation period is 2–7 wk. Diagnosis is confirmed by light microscopic visualization of viral inclusions (molluscum bodies) in the central core. *Treatment* requires elimination of the lesions, usually by gentle curettage; other methods of therapy include cryosurgery or electrocautery.

INTERTRIGO. Intertrigo can occur in the genitocrural areas in association with friction, obesity, and moisture in the area. Miliaria and secondary infection can also occur in association with intertrigo. The affected areas are red and macerated. Careful hygiene, combined with bland emollients and sometimes a mild corticosteroid, is an effective treatment.

IMPETIGO. This entity is commonly identified during the first several weeks of life. It is usually caused by *Staphylococcus aureus*, often phage group II, type 71, which may be acquired from the mother, other relatives, or staff. Impetigo tends to affect the vulva and periumbilical areas, causing lesions or blisters that later become crusted. Extensive spread and complications may ensue if treatment with antibiotics is not promptly instituted (Chapter 182.1).

MALASSEZIA FURFUR (Chapter 232). This condition is caused by *Pityrosporum orbiculare* and is manifested by scaly macules on the trunk in postpubertal patients, but lesions have been reported on the face and genital area. The diagnosis is established by visualization of hyphae and spores on wet preparation with 10% potassium hydroxide. *Treatment* requires application of topical imidazoles (e.g., clotrimazole).

HERPES SIMPLEX VIRUS (see also Chapter 245). Herpes simplex virus (HSV) types 1 and 2 involves the vulvar area. The types are not exclusively site specific, but type 2 is commonly responsible for genital lesions and type 1, in general, for facial-oral lesions. The infection is characterized by papules that become vesicles, with the virus affecting the dorsal root ganglia. Differential diagnoses include any eroded or blistering lesions as well as herpes zoster. A definitive diagnosis is established by culturing the virus or visualizing it via electron mi-

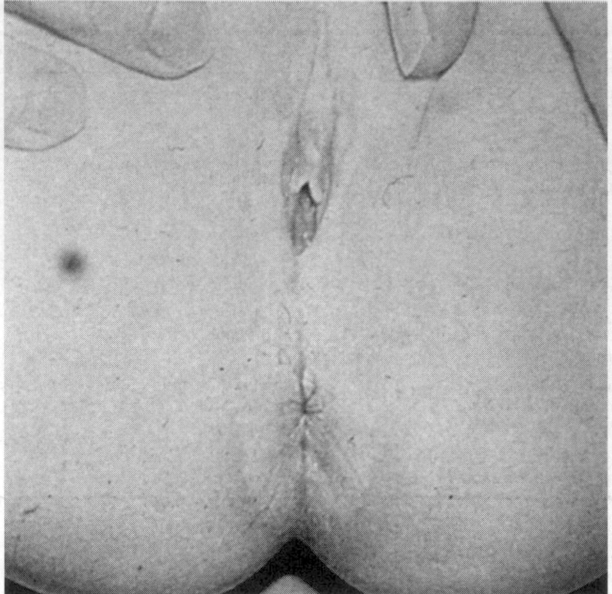

Figure 557–2 Lichen sclerosus.

croscopy. *Treatment* with topical acyclovir reduces viral shedding and accelerates healing.

HUMAN PAPILLOMAVIRUS (HPV). HPV is associated with a number of serotypes, including 6, 11, 16, and 18, which usually are noted in the anogenital region (also see Chapter 257). Types 16 and 18 are particularly associated with malignant and premalignant lesions of the vulva. Differential diagnoses include molluscum contagiosum, condyloma accuminatum, and vulvar intraepithelial neoplasia. The possibility of child sexual abuse must be strongly considered when these lesions are identified. *Treatment* is usually symptomatic and remains a challenge for clinicians.

LICHEN SCLEROSUS. This is a chronic atrophic skin disease characterized by small, pink to ivory, flat-topped papules that are several millimeters in diameter. The papules appear to coalesce into plaques that become wrinkled and atrophic. The anogenital lesions frequently resemble an hourglass or a figure 8 (Fig. 557–2). Vesicles and bullae may spread over the vulva with associated hemorrhage. A biopsy is often required for accurate diagnosis.

The onset of lichen sclerosus in most children usually occurs before 7 yr of age. The youngest reported patient was an infant only several weeks old. The onset of menarche often results in spontaneous improvement of the lesions, but the process usually continues. Patients are often intermittently symptomatic, and there is no relationship between menarche and symptomatic improvement or resolution of the disease. Atrophy of the labia minora and clitoral phimosis, as well as contracture of the introitus, may occur.

The cause of lichen sclerosus is unknown, but it is believed to be related to an autoimmune disorder. Positive immunofluorescence for fibrin, serum complement (C3), or immunoglobulin M (IgM) in involved areas has been demonstrated in 75% of patients.

Treatment is symptomatic; emollients and topical corticosteroids usually provide relief. Corticosteroids are the treatment of choice for lichen sclerosus in adults and have been efficacious in children, as well. Betamethasone dipropionate 0.05% is recommended. Minimal side effects are associated with this treatment. After the initial response, a milder topical corticosteroid may be used to prevent recurrence. Topical estrogens and androgens also have been advocated, but these agents may produce a vaginal discharge as well as other secondary problems, such as breast development and clitoral enlargement. Secondary infections should be treated with antibiotics. Some affected individuals demonstrate Koebner's phenomenon. For relief, these individuals should avoid tight-fitting clothing and genital trauma. Laser vaporization has also been advocated.

LICHEN PLANUS. Vulvar lichen planus is often associated with oral mucosal and subcutaneous lesions. The vulvar lesions, characterized by angular violaceous, flat-topped papules, may simulate leukoplakia. In addition, the oral lesions consist of minute white papules that form a lacy pattern and usually are located on the buccal mucosa. The lesions are intensely pruritic and may become excoriated and macerated; erosions and ulcerations may even occur in severe cases. Diagnosis requires biopsy. Exacerbation or recurrence of the lesions is common.

Treatment consists of topical intralesional corticosteroids and antihistamines to control the pruritus. Squamous cell carcinoma may occur with long-standing, hypertrophic, vulvar lichen planus; therefore, long-term follow-up and histologic examination of any changed or otherwise suspicious area is advisable.

LICHEN SIMPLEX CHRONICUS (NEURODERMATITIS). This is a chronic, lichenified plaque that causes pruritus. Scratching and inflammation may result, causing a vicious cycle. The condition is rare in children. *Treatment* with antihistamines and topical or intralesional corticosteroids is recommended.

SEBORRHEIC DERMATITIS (see Chapter 661). This presents as erythematous, oily, circumscribed patches that can be found on the face, scalp, and chest as well as on intertriginous areas of the body. There may also be fissures and associated secondary infection around the vulva; secondary bacterial or candidal infection is quite common, causing pain, pruritus, dysuria, and vaginal bleeding. Acute episodes are best *treated* with sitz baths or topical aluminum acetate solution (Burow's solution). Exacerbating factors, such as tight clothing or rubber pants, should be eliminated. Systemic antibiotics with appropriate topical antifungal medication should be administered for secondary infection.

ATOPIC DERMATITIS (see Chapter 146). This affects 3% of all children. Patients present with hay fever or asthma or both, and generally a family history is noted. The vulvar lesion is characterized as a chronic condition accompanied by intense pruritus, erythema, papules, and vesicles, with oozing and crusting of the involved areas. Associated circumscribed, lichenified scaly patches may be seen on the vulvar area. Pruri-

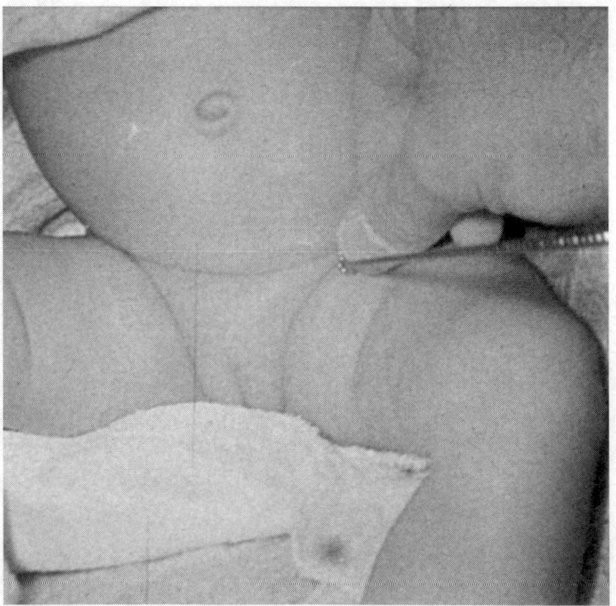

Figure 557–3 Vulvar psoriasis. See also color section.

tus often causes scratching, which results in excoriation of the lesions. Secondary bacterial or candidal infection is common.

Antihistamines are necessary for control of pruritus. Sitz baths with mild soap and lubricants are helpful. Topical corticosteroids such as 1% hydrocortisone are also effective. Secondary bacterial or candidal infections require specific treatment.

CONTACT DERMATITIS (see Chapter 661). In either allergic or irritant contact dermatitis, the vulva may be affected by edematous, erythematous, oozing lesions that are sometimes accompanied by vesicles or pustules. Chronic contact dermatitis is often associated with thickened and lichenified lesions. The clue to correct diagnosis of this condition is the limitation of the dermatitis to the area of contact with the etiologic agent. There may also be a secondary candidal or bacterial infection. Some common etiologic agents are soaps, powders, bubble baths, feminine hygiene sprays, topical medications, toilet paper, rubber, and certain types of clothing. *Treatment* should include avoidance of the offending agents and sitz baths, or compresses with topical aluminum acetate solution (Burow's solution) during acute episodes. Mild topical corticosteroids such as 0.5–1% hydrocortisone cream applied several times daily may further aid healing and alleviate vulvar irritation. Recurrence can be prevented by removal of the offending etiologic agent.

VULVAR PSORIASIS (see Chapter 663). This is frequently associated with lesions of other parts of the body and is characterized by violaceous papules or plaques with a thick, adherent, silvery scale (Fig. 557–3). The intertriginous areas may show "inverse" psoriasis, a variation that does not occur on the extremities. Vulvar lesions usually are poorly demarcated and may present as scaly patches, most commonly on the mons pubis. The vulvar lesions are often resistant to therapy; therefore, a multifaceted approach is essential. A corticosteroid cream (e.g., 1% hydrocortisone) should be used in conjunction with control of secondary infection and pruritus.

ENTEROBIASIS (see Chapter 284). Pinworms *(Enterobius vermicularis)* are helminths that may carry colonic bacteria to the perineum, causing recurrent vulvovaginitis. Female pinworms emerge from the anus to deposit eggs. Vulvovaginitis develops in about 20% of girls infected with *E. vermicularis*. The plastic tape test should be used to search for the organism if it is suspected or in cases of undiagnosed recurrent vulvovaginitis. Victims typically have pruritus and nocturnal episodes of scratching. *Treatment* consists of pyrantel pamoate (see Table 557–1).

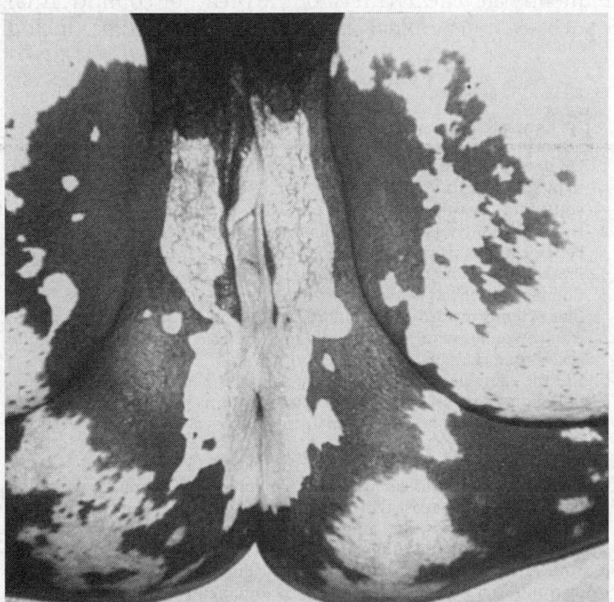

Figure 557–4 Vitiligo. See also color section.

SHIGELLOSIS (see Chapter 197). *Shigella flexneri* and *S. sonnei* cause various gastrointestinal symptoms in association with vaginitis. Forty-seven per cent of patients present with a bloody vaginal discharge and 2% with diarrhea. Systemic antibiotics are the treatment of choice. Bowel colonization with *Shigella* can result in subclinical gastrointestinal symptoms in 10% of household members.

VITILIGO. This presents as sharply demarcated pink to ivory patches that tend to spread and coalesce (Fig. 557–4). The skin on the patch is smooth and shows no palpable changes. It may be differentiated from lichen sclerosus because the hyperpigmented patches are asymptomatic. No treatment is necessary unless cosmetic problems result.

Chacko MR, Kozinetz CA, Hill R, et al: Leukocyte esterase dipstick as a rapid screening test for vaginitis and cervicitis. J Pediatr Adolesc Gynecol 9:185, 1996.

Charles V, Charles SX: A case of vulvo-vaginal diphtheria in a girl of seven years. Indian Pediatr 15:257, 1978.

Clark JA, Muller SA: Lichen sclerosus et atrophicus in children: A report of 24 cases. Arch Dermatol 95:476, 1967.

Davis AJ, Goldstein DP: Treatment of pediatric lichen sclerosus with the CO_2 laser. Adolesc Pediatr Gynecol 2:103, 1989.

Fisher G, Rogers, M: Treatment of childhood vulvar lichen sclerosus with potent topical corticosteroid. Pediatr Dermatol 14:235, 1997.

Gerstner G, Grunberger W, Boschitsch E, et al: Vaginal organisms in prepubertal children with and without vulvovaginitis. Arch Gynecol 231:247, 1982.

Jones R: Childhood vulvovaginitis and vaginal discharge in general practice. Fam Pract 13:369, 1996.

Koumantakis EE, Hassan EA, Deligeoroglou EK, Creatsas GK: Vulvovaginitis during childhood and adolescence. J Pediatr Adolesc Gynecol 10:39, 1997.

Leung AK, Robson WL, Tay Uyboco J: The incidence of labial fusion in children. J Paediatr Child Health 29:235, 1993.

Murphy T, Nelson J: Shigella vaginitis: Report of 38 patients and review of the literature. Pediatrics 63:511, 1979.

Paradise J, Willis E: Probability of vaginal body in girls with genital complaints. Am J Dis Child 139:472, 1985.

Redmond CA, Cowell CA, Krafchik BR: Genital lichen sclerosus in prepubertal girls. Adolesc Pediatr Gynecol 1:177, 1988.

Sobel JD: Vaginitis. N Engl J Med 337:1896, 1997.

Williams T, Callen J, Owen L: Vulvar disorders in the prepubertal female. Pediatr Ann 15:588, 1986.

Young SJ, Wells DL, Ogden EJ: Lichen sclerosus, genital trauma and child sexual abuse. Aust Fam Physician 22:729, 1993.

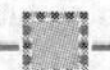

CHAPTER 558
Bleeding

The entities responsible for isolated vaginal bleeding include exposure to exogenous sex steroids; foreign body; hemorrhagic cystitis; hypothyroidism; precocious puberty; the presence of an ovarian cyst; trauma, which may or may not be associated with sexual abuse; urethral prolapse; vulvovaginitis; and neoplasms. See Chapter 116 for discussion of menstrual problems.

FOREIGN BODY. A foreign body is commonly responsible for vaginal bleeding in pediatric patients. The presence of a foul-smelling discharge with associated vaginal bleeding suggests this possibility. Wadded toilet paper is the most common foreign body identified in the vagina. A plain roentgenogram or ultrasonography of the pelvis is often helpful. A vaginal foreign body was found in 18% of preadolescent girls with vaginal bleeding with or without discharge and in 50% of those with bleeding and no discharge.

URETHRAL PROLAPSE. Vulvar bleeding can be associated with urethral prolapse. This uncommon disorder is characterized by the urethral mucosa's protruding through the meatus and forming a hemorrhagic, often sensitive vulvar mass that bleeds easily. The "mass" is separate from the vagina. Patients may have difficulty with urination, depending on the size of the mass and whether or not it occludes the urethral meatus. The entity responds to topical application of estrogens because the distal urethra is estrogen sensitive. Urethral prolapse is often misdiagnosed when there is urogenital bleeding.

GENITAL TRAUMA. Although most injuries to this area are accidental, the possibility of physical or sexual abuse must be considered (see Chapter 35.1). Blunt injury may cause blood vessels beneath the perineal skin to rupture. Blood accumulating under the skin forms a hematoma, which may present as a round, tense, tender mass. Contusion of the vulva usually does not require treatment. A small vulvar hematoma often can be controlled by pressure with an ice pack. Analgesics may be required.

Penetrating injuries to the vaginal area warrant further careful evaluation, including serious considerations of the possibility of sexual abuse. A detailed examination is necessary, especially in the presence of active bleeding. The potential for bowel or bladder trauma must also be considered.

GENITAL TUMORS. Benign and malignant tumors of the vulva should be considered when vaginal bleeding occurs in pediatric patients. A broad spectrum of entities, ranging from capillary hemangiomas through malignancies such as rhabdomyosarcoma, requires appropriate tissue diagnosis and treatment. The most common tumors include endodermal carcinoma, which occurs most often in young children; mesonephric carcinoma, which arises in a remnant of a mesonephric duct and occurs more often in girls age 3 or older; and clear cell adenocarcinoma, which is often associated with a history of antenatal exposure to diethylstilbestrol (see Chapters 509 and 561).

CAPILLARY VENOUS MALFORMATION OF THE LABIA MAJORA. Capillary venous malformation has been reported as a cause of vaginal bleeding in pediatric patients with expansion in volume on response to hormonal changes at puberty. The differential diagnoses include hemangioma and other vascular malformation(s). Diagnosis is based on an evaluation that includes ultrasonography, MRI, and abdominal arteriography. The malformation can be locally excised.

American College of Obstetricians and Gynecologists: Dysfunctional Uterine Bleeding. ACOG Technical Bulletin 134, Washington, DC, 1989.

Anveden-Hertzberg L, Gauderer MW, Elder JS: Urethral prolapse: An often missed diagnosis cause of urogenital bleeding in girls. Pediatr Emerg Care 11:212, 1995.

Gidwani GP: Vaginal bleeding in adolescence. J Reprod Med 29:419, 1984.

Grant DB: Vaginal bleeding in childhood. Pediatr Adolesc Gynecol 1:173, 1983.

Kempinaire A, De Raeve L, Roseeuw D, et al: Capillary-venous malformation in the labia majora of a 12-year-old girl. Dermatology 194:405, 1997.

Kerns DL, Terman DL, Larson CS: The role of physicians in reporting and evaluating child sexual abuse cases. Future Child 4:119, 1994.

Muram D, Sanfilippo JS, Hertweck SP: Vaginal bleeding in childhood and menstrual disorders in adolescence. In: Sanfilippo JS (ed): Pediatric and Adolescent Gynecology. Philadelphia, WB Saunders, 1994, pp 222–231.

CHAPTER 559
Breast Disorders

The mammary glands are derived from the epidermal layer. Beginning at approximately 6 wk of gestation, epidermal cells migrate to the mesenchyme and form the mammary ridges. Breast buds, lactiferous ducts, and fully developed mammary glands eventually form. Breast development normally occurs in girls between the ages of 8½ and 13 yr. The rate of breast growth varies, and development is often asymmetric. Complete development may not occur until a woman is in her early 20s.

BREAST SELF-EXAMINATION. Early diagnosis is central to improving health care for breast abnormalities, including carcinoma. Instruction in breast self-examination should be given to adolescents (Table 559–1).

CONGENITAL ANOMALIES. Complete absence of a breast, *amastia*, is rare; more frequently it is unilateral and often associated with other abnormalities, such as **Poland's syndrome** (aplasia of the pectoralis muscles, rib deformities, webbed fingers, and radial nerve aplasia). Amastia can be iatrogenic, as a result of inadvertent excision of a breast bud. *Athelia* is defined as absence of one or both nipples. This condition is also rare and may not be associated with absent breast tissue. Both abnormalities require surgical correction.

Supernumerary breasts (polymastia) and *supernumerary nipples* (polythelia) are relatively common (Fig. 559–1); they occur along the milk lines and are usually asymptomatic. There is an association between polythelia and anomalies of the urinary and cardiovascular systems. In general, surgical excision of accessory breasts or nipples is not necessary. However, if the aberrant breasts or nipples become symptomatic, excision may be indicated.

Hypoplasia of the breasts varies in degree from a nearly total absence of breast tissue to well-formed breasts that are considered by the patient to be too small. There are three general causes for poor or absent breast development: (1) The onset of breast development may be delayed, and the breasts develop slowly but are normal in all other respects. (2) A patient's family history may include late breast development. (3) Ovarian function may have failed or been suppressed (see Chapter 560). Treatment depends on the underlying cause.

Breast atrophy is seen occasionally in adolescents and is almost uniformly secondary to dietary changes such as occurs with anorexia nervosa. Correction of the underlying problem results in re-establishment of breast tissue.

NEONATAL BREAST ABNORMALITIES. Bilateral breast hypertrophy may occur as a result of elevated circulating endogenous steroid hormones in late gestation. It may be associated with discharge from the nipples known as "witch's milk." Repeated manipulation of the breast can exacerbate the condition. On occasion, the hypertrophy is associated with mastitis caused by a staphylococcal infection; antibiotics should be administered.

MASTODYNIA. Painful breast engorgement (mastodynia) usually is associated with ovulatory cycles; this is uncommon in adolescents until approximately 18 mo after menarche, the time that may be necessary to establish ovulatory cycles. There is frequently a cyclical pattern of the breast discomfort. Analgesics such as nonsteroidal anti-inflammatory drugs, including

TABLE 559–1 How to Do Breast Self-Examination

1. Lie down. Flatten your right breast by placing a pillow under your right shoulder. If your breasts are large, use your right hand to hold your right breast while you do the exam with your left hand.
2. Use the sensitive pads of the middle three fingers on your left hand. Feel for lumps using a rubbing motion.
3. Press firmly enough to feel different breast tissues.
4. Completely feel all of the breast and chest area to cover breast tissue that extends toward the shoulder. Allow enough time for a complete exam. Women with small breasts need at least 2 minutes to examine each breast. Larger breasts take longer.
5. Use the same pattern to feel every part of the breast tissue. Choose the method easiest for you. The three patterns preferred by women and their doctors are the circular, clock, or oval pattern; the vertical strip; and the wedge.
6. After you have completely examined your right breast, then examine your left breast using the same method. Compare what you have felt in one breast with the other.
7. You may also want to examine your breasts while bathing, when your skin is wet and lumps may be easier to feel.
8. You can check your breasts in a mirror; look for any change in size or contour, dimpling of the skin, or spontaneous nipple discharge.

Published with permission of The American Cancer Society.

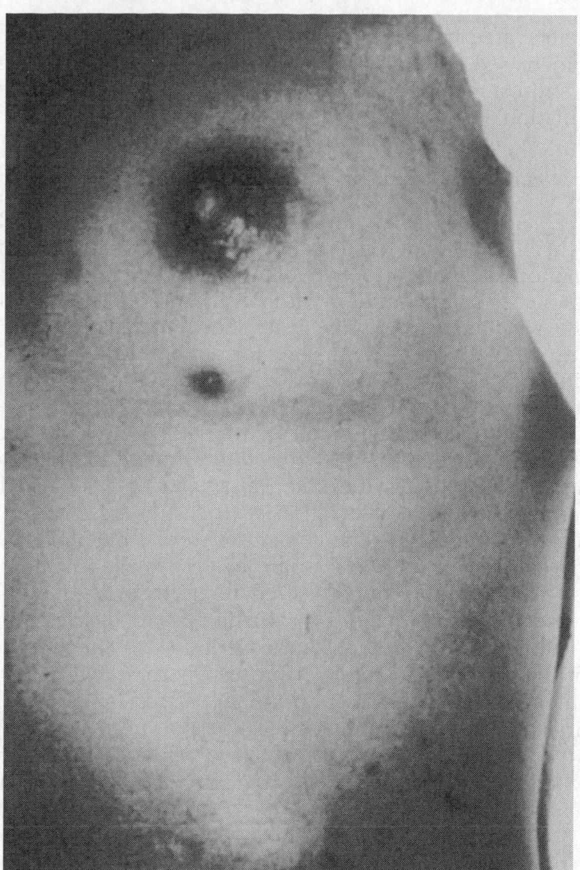

Figure 559–1 Polythelia.

ibuprofen, as well as the use of a good support bra, are often helpful in alleviating discomfort.

BREAST MASSES. A retrospective review of breast disease in adolescent females revealed that about 54% have fibroadenomas and 13% have virginal hypertrophy. Fibrocystic or proliferative breast disease occurs in about 24%. Primary rhabdomyosarcoma, metastatic rhabdomyosarcoma, metastatic neuroblastoma, and non-Hodgkin's lymphoma occur in 2–3% of all breast masses in this age group. Other diagnoses include polythelia, accessory breast tissue, mastitis, hemangioma, fat necrosis, and intramammary lymph nodes.

A thorough history and physical examination are mandatory for any pediatric or adolescent patient who has a breast mass. The clinical problem should be reviewed with a radiologist before initiating any radiologic assessment. Needle aspiration and biopsy are often essential for evaluation of palpable breast abnormalities. Large breast tumors also occur in adolescents. Although malignancy is often suspected because of rapid growth of the mass and skin ulceration, breast tumors can have varied presentations. Giant fibroadenomas in adolescence may be treated by simple enucleation.

Malignant Tumors. Although rare, breast *cancer* does occur in adolescents. Early menarche in association with anovulatory cycles is a risk factor. The estrogen-to-androgen ratio appears to be critical, with androgens having a protective effect.

Cystosarcoma phylloides, an uncommon breast tumor in adults, may occur in adolescents. It is characterized by asymmetric breast enlargement in association with a firm, mobile, circumscribed mass. The tumor often increases rapidly in size and can become quite large. Fixation of the tumor to the skin or chest wall is rare. The majority of these tumors are benign, but malignant cystosarcoma phylloides with metastases has been reported. Excision is the preferred initial therapy in adolescent patients, regardless of the histologic classification of the lesion. Malignant cystosarcoma is more likely to recur than is a benign lesion. Fatal metastatic cystosarcoma phylloides in an adolescent has occurred.

Breast tumors also may be the first manifestation of relapse (extramedullary) in acute lymphoblastic leukemia. Reports in the literature include a case of radiation-induced sarcoma of the breast in a female adolescent and a case of *liposarcoma* in a 17-yr-old black female who previously had a total mastectomy.

MACROMASTIA (VIRGINAL HYPERTROPHY). The cause of massive breast enlargement during puberty and early adolescence is unknown, but the condition probably represents an end-organ increased sensitivity to circulating estrogens. It is bilateral, often occurs over a brief period, and most commonly affects girls 13–17 yr old (see Chapter 115). Physical and psychologic problems may occur in adolescents with macromastia. Posture problems and discomfort often result. Reduction mammoplasty is the *treatment* of choice but should be delayed until late adolescence to allow for complete breast development. Surgical intervention often necessitates relocation of the nipple, which may result in decreased sensation and altered lactation. In addition, strong emotional support should be provided.

MASTITIS AND ABSCESS. Mastitis and breast abscess may require antibiotic therapy as well as incision and drainage. See Chapter 182.

TRAUMA AND INFLAMMATION. Breast trauma in adolescent females is more common because of the increased number of young women participating in contact sports. The trauma usually takes the form of contusion or hematoma and often resolves without incident. Fat necrosis occasionally occurs and results in either late cystic changes in the breast or fibrosis with retraction of skin or the nipple over the injured area. These late changes may mimic those associated with malignancy; biopsy may be the only means of differentiating the two.

MAMMARY DYSPLASIA. This common lesion is characterized by changes associated with the menstrual cycle. Hormonal imbalance associated with exaggerated responses in the breast tissue, especially in the upper and outer quadrants during the premenstrual phase of the cycle, may be etiologic. The extent of *treatment* depends on the degree of symptoms. Ibuprofen is often helpful. In addition, methylxanthines and caffeine (e.g., coffee, tea, carbonated drinks) should be eliminated from the diet.

NIPPLE DISCHARGE. This must be carefully evaluated and a distinction made between the presence of galactorrhea (spontaneous flow of milk) and bloody discharge. Evaluation of *galactorrhea* in children is the same as for adults. Serum prolactin levels are obtained to rule out the presence of a pituitary prolactinoma (see Chapter 570.2). If a pituitary tumor or adenoma is suspected on the basis of markedly elevated serum prolactin levels, with or without headaches and bitemporal hemianopsia, appropriate radiologic (CT, MRI) assessment is necessary. Another cause of galactorrhea is hypothyroidism in association with elevated levels of thyroid-releasing hormone, which also stimulates prolactin release. Treatment of galactorrhea (non–thyroid related) consists primarily of dopamine agonists such as bromocriptine (Parlodel). Surgical intervention, usually in the form of transsphenoidal hypophysectomy, is rarely required. Galactorrhea secondary to chest wall surgery in an adolescent has also been reported. The galactorrhea occurred for 2 mo and was associated with transient amenorrhea.

Bloody nipple discharge can be indicative of duct ectasia. Cytologic assessment and surgical consultation are indicated. Nipple discharge in association with Montgomery's tubercles also has been reported. These secretions can be episodic and vary in color from clear to brown, but they are usually not milky. This discharge evolves over a period of 3–5 wk, may be associated with breast lumps, and is a benign, self-limited problem. Intraductal breast papillomas have occurred in adolescents.

Apter D, Vinko R: Early menarche, a risk factor for breast cancer, indicates early onset of ovulatory cycles. J Clin Endocrinol Metab 57:82, 1983.
Briggs R, Walters M, Rosenthal D: Cystosarcoma phylloides in adolescent female patients. Am J Surg 146:712, 1983.
Cromer B, Frankel M, Kader L: Compliance with breast self-examination and instruction in healthy adolescents. J Adolesc Health Care 10:105, 1989.
Diehl G, Kaplan D: Breast masses in adolescent females. J Adolesc Health Care 6:353, 1985.
Ellegaard J, Bendix-Hanson K, Boesen A, et al: Breast tumor as a first manifestation of extramedullary relapse in acute lymphoblastic leukemia. Scand J Haematol 33:288, 1984.
Heyman R, Rauh J: Areolar gland discharge in adolescent females appears to be benign. J Adolesc Health Care 4:285, 1983.
Letson G, Moore D: Galactorrhea secondary to chest wall surgery in an adolescent. J Adolesc Health Care 5:277, 1984.
Ngala Kenda J: Fatal metastatic cystosarcoma phylloides in a young woman: Report of a case. Arch Surg 118:871, 1983.
Raganoonan C, Fairbairn J, Williams S, et al: Giant breast tumors of adolescence. Aust N Z J Surg 57:243, 1987.
Simmons P, Wold L: Surgically treated breast disease in adolescent females: A retrospective review of 185 cases. Adolesc Pediatr Gynecol 2:95, 1989.
Watkind F, Giacomantonio M, Salisbury S: Nipple discharge and breast lump related to Montgomery's tubercles in adolescent females. J Pediatr Surg 23:718, 1988.

CHAPTER 560
Hirsutism and Polycystic Ovarian Syndrome

Hirsutism (excessive hair growth) must be distinguished from *virilization*. The latter involves increased body hair, acne, deepening of the voice, change in body habitus due to increased muscle mass, and clitoromegaly (see Chapter 586). *Premature pubarche* is defined as the appearance of genital hair or axillary hair or both before age 8 yr (Chapter 572). *Adrenarche*, the output of increased androgen from the adrenal glands, usually occurs between ages 12 and 18 yr and is discussed in Chapter 14.

Polycystic ovarian syndrome is believed to have its origin at the time of puberty. Teenagers usually present with menstrual disturbances or hirsutism. Ultrasonographic assesment identifies multicystic ovaries, a characteristic "pearl necklace." The prevalence of polycystic ovaries increases throughout puberty and has been as high as 26% by age 15 yr.

HIRSUTISM IN ADOLESCENTS. Table 560–1 lists the causes of hirsutism. *Androgen-producing tumors* of adrenal or gonadal origin should be considered when an adolescent presents with excessive hair growth. However, hirsutism is most often *idiopathic*, with normal total circulating androgen levels. Sex hormone–binding globulin (SHBG) levels may be decreased in hirsute patients; thus, a higher fraction of bioactive androgens occurs despite normal serum androgen levels. SHBG levels are affected by a number of factors. Androgens, specifically testosterone, cause a decrease in SHBG levels; estrogens and dexamethasone tend to increase SHBG. Futhermore, a decline in SHBG occurs with increasing age, especially from prepuberty to adolescence. Body weight has an inverse correlation with SHBG levels independent of androgen levels.

HAIR-AN syndrome is the acronym for the association of hirsutism, androgen excess, insulin resistance, and acanthosis nigricans. The pathogenesis of this syndrome is unknown. However, a defect in membrane insulin receptors is noted. Elevated androgen levels contribute to the development of acanthosis.

Hyperprolactinemia, a central nervous system disorder, is an occasional cause of hyperandrogenemia (see Chapter 570). Approximately 40% of patients with hyperprolactinemia exhibit androgenic abnormalities. Laboratory findings may include elevated free testosterone due to decreased SHBG levels and increased adrenal production of 17-hydroxyprogesterone and androstenedione following adrenocorticotropic hormone stimulation.

Polycystic ovary syndrome (PCO, chronic anovulation, Stein-Leventhal syndrome) is the most commonly diagnosed ovarian cause of hirsutism (see Chapter 592). The underlying biochemical cause of PCO is unknown, and controversy exists about whether the basic defect is central (hypothalamic or pituitary regulation of gonadotropins) or ovarian (defect in a peptide hormone, perhaps inhibin, with resultant abnormal feedback to the pituitary gland). The usual hormonal pattern of PCO begins with altered luteinizing hormone release (a ratio of luteinizing hormone [LH] to follicle-stimulating hormone of 2:1 or 3:1, shortened pulse frequency, and slightly increased pulse amplitude of LH). Adolescents with hyperandrogenism display an exaggerated LH pulsatility similar to that found in adults with PCO syndrome. Patients with PCO also have hyperinsulinemia in association with insulin resistance. This results in a metabolic derangement of steroid metabolism, primarily androgens, at the ovarian level. It is the insulin resistance aspect that is hypothesized to be associated with the increase in androstenedione production by the ovaries. Peripheral conversion to testosterone contributes to the commonly identified increase in total serum testosterone levels that are an integral part of the PCO hormonal pattern.

Hirsutism in adolescents can also be due to a heterozygous form of *21-hydroxylase deficiency* (see Chapter 586.1). This has been called adult-onset congenital adrenal hyperplasia

TABLE 560–1 Causes of Hirsutism

Peripheral
Idiopathic
Partial androgen insensitivity (5-α-reductase deficiency)
HAIR-AN syndrome (hirsutism, androgenization, insulin resistance, and acanthosis nigricans)
Hyperprolactinemia
Gonadal
Polycystic ovary syndrome (PCO, chronic anovulation)
Ovarian neoplasm (Sertoli-Leydig cell, granulosa cell, thecoma, gynandroblastoma, lipoid cell, luteoma, hypernephroma, Brenner's tumor)
Gonadal dysgenesis (Turner's mosaic with XY, or H-Y antigen positive)
Adrenal
Cushing's syndrome
Adrenal hyper-responsiveness
Congenital adrenal hyperplasia (classic, cryptic, adult onset)
21-hydroxylase deficiency
11-hydroxylase deficiency
3β-hydroxysteroid deficiency
17α-hydroxylase deficiency
Adrenal neoplasm (adenoma, cortical carcinoma)
Exogenous
Minoxidil
Dilantin
Cyclosporine
Anabolic steroids
Acetazolamide (Diamox)
Penicillamine
Oral contraceptives
Danazol
Androgenic steroids
Psoralens
Hydrochlorothiazide
Phenothiazines
Congenital Anomalies
Trisomy 18 (Edward's syndrome)
Cornelia de Lange's syndrome
Hurler's syndrome
Juvenile hypothyroidism

From Bailey-Pridham DD, Sanfilippo JS: Hirsutism in the adolescent female. Pediatr Clin North Am 36:581, 1989.

TABLE 560–2 Treatment of Hirsutism: Idiopathic and Polycystic Ovary Syndrome

Medication	Dose*	Comments
Oral contraceptives (estrogen dominant)	35 μg	Decrease in plasma testosterone, androstenedione, and DHEA-S
Spironolactone	100 mg bid	Decreased androgen production and androgen receptor competition
Medroxyprogesterone acetate depot (Depo-Provera)	150–250 mg q 2–4 wk	Decreased testosterone production and 17-ketosteroid levels
Cyproterone acetate	Diane, 2 mg Androcur, 100 mg	Decreased plasma testosterone, androstenedione, SHBG, induces "insulinemia"
Dexamethasone	0.25–0.5 mg	Dose adequate if plasma-free testosterone <15 pg/mL
Cimetidine	200–300 mg tid–qid	Decreased serum testosterone, increased serum estradiol
GnRH agonist (Flutamide)	250 mg tid	5α-reductase inhibitor; decreased testosterone and androstenedione

*Dosages given are for a 70-kg female. Daily dosages are indicated unless otherwise specified.
From Bailey-Pridham DD, Sanfilippo JS: Hirsutism in the adolescent female. Pediatr Clin North Am 36:581, 1989; with permission.*

(AOCAH). Various other forms of congenital adrenal hyperplasia and congenital anomalies are also associated with hirsutism. Clinically, it may be difficult to distinguish between PCO and AOCAH.

Ovarian hyperthecosis, which can be familial, may be a variant of PCO. Hyperthecosis is defined as isolated islands of luteinized cells within the ovary, contributing to increased androgen production. Ovarian androgen production and peripheral effects are similar to those associated with PCO.

Medications, radiation, and chronic irritation (e.g., the placement of a cast) can also initiate localized, nonendocrinologic hair growth.

Treatment of Hirsute Patients. Treatment alternatives for idiopathic hirsutism and PCO are outlined in Table 560–2. Hirsutism secondary to hyperprolactinemia is best treated with bromocriptine. In patients with multicystic (polycystic) ovaries and primary hypothyroidism, the polycystic ovaries resolve rapidly with adequate doses of thyroid replacement therapy. If an exogenous cause such as a medication is producing hirsutism, the exogenous agent should be eliminated.

Even when the increased tissue androgen effect is reversed by appropriate treatment, hair follicles converted to terminal hair may still produce that type of hair. Electrolysis may then provide an improved cosmetic appearance, with the assurance that if the underlying abnormality is controlled, no new hair growth should ensue.

Cushing's syndrome or disease, androgen-producing tumors, and congenital adrenal hyperplasia are discussed in Chapters 586 and 587.

Apter D, Siegberg R, Laatikainen T: Pulsatile secretion of luteinizing hormone in adolescents with hyperandrogenism. Adolesc Pediatr Gynecol 1:104, 1988.
Belgorosky A, Rivarola M: Progressive increase in non-sex hormone binding globulin-bound testosterone and estradiol from infancy to late prepuberty in girls. J Clin Endocrinol Metab 67:234, 1988.
Boor JT, Herwig J, Schrezenneir J, et al: Familial insulin resistant diabetes associated with acanthosis nigricans, polycystic ovaries, hypogonadism, pigmentary retinopathy, labrinthine deafness, and mental retardation. Am J Med Genet 45:649, 1993.
Franks S: Polycystic ovary syndrome. Arch Dis Child 77:89, 1997.
Judd H, Scully R, Herbst A, et al: Familial hyperthecosis: Comparison of endocrinologic and histologic findings with polycystic ovarian disease. Am J Obstet Gynecol 117:976, 1973.
Kamilaris T, DeBold C, Manolus K, et al: Testosterone secreting adrenal adenoma in a peripubertal patient. JAMA 258:2558, 1987.
Lindsay A, Voorhess M, MacGillivray M: Multicystic ovaries in primary hypothyroidism. Obstet Gynecol 61:433, 1983.
Parker L, Sack J, Fisher D, et al: The adrenarche: Prolactin, gonadotropins, adrenal androgens and cortisol. J Clin Endocrinol Metab 60:409, 1985.
Rosen G, Kaplan B, Lobo R: Menstrual function and hirsutism in patients with gonadal dysgenesis. Obstet Gynecol 71:677, 1988.
Speroff L, Glass RH, Kase NG: Hirsutism. *In:* Speroff L, Glass RH, Kase NG (eds): Clinical Gynecologic Endocrinology and Infertility, 4th ed. Baltimore, Williams & Wilkins, 1994, pp 483–502.
Zumogg B, Freeman R, Coupa S, et al: A chronobiologic abnormality of luteinizing hormone secretion in teenage girls with the polycystic ovary syndrome. N Engl J Med 309:1206, 1983.

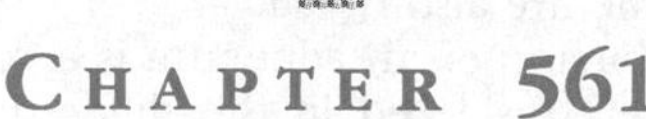

CHAPTER 561
Neoplasms

The most common gynecologic neoplasm found in children is of ovarian origin and usually presents as an abdominal mass. Paraovarian tumors are next in frequency, followed by uterine neoplasms. The vagina or vulva may also be the site of benign or malignant lesions in children (see Chapter 558); cervical dysplasia may occur in adolescents. Breast masses are discussed in Chapter 559.

Chemotherapy, especially with alkalating agents (cyclophosphamide, busulphan, chlorambucil, and nitrogen mustard), is associated with germ cell damage in the postpubertal ovary. The prepubertal ovary, on the other hand, is markedly resistant to chemotherapeutic effects on germ cells. The role of combined oral contraceptive therapy during chemotherapy in adolescents remains controversial.

Survivors of childhood cancer who previously underwent abdominal or gonadal irradiation have a higher rate of spontaneous abortions. However, the incidence of congenital malformations is not increased in comparison with the general population. Patients who have evidence of premature ovarian failure may be candidates for assisted reproductive technology with use of donor ova and appropriate counseling.

OVARIES. Most often, the *clinical manifestations* of ovarian tumors are abdominal pain, a mass, or both. In adolescents, the most common ovarian neoplasm is the **teratoma**. It is usually benign, but malignant teratomas may occur. Calcification on abdominal roentgenogram is often a hallmark of a benign teratoma. During surgery, the opposite ovary should be evaluated, and if there is any question about the possibility of a neoplasm, a biopsy specimen obtained. Ovarian **adenomas** are the second most common benign ovarian tumor.

With respect to **germ cell tumors**, the most common is the dysgerminoma, followed in incidence by malignant teratomas, endodermal sinus tumors, embryonal carcinomas, mixed cell neoplasms, and gonadoblastomas. Immature teratomas and endodermal sinus tumors are more aggressive malignancies than dysgerminomas and occur in a significantly higher proportion of younger girls (< 10 yr of age). In this age group, 10-yr survival rates were 73% for epithelial carcinomas, 44% for sex cord stromal tumors, 73% for dysgerminomas, 33% for malignant teratomas, 39% for endodermal sinus tumors, 25% for embryonal carcinomas, 30% for other germ cell neoplasms, and 100% for gonadoblastomas. Dysgerminomas usually are associated with XY gonadal dysgenesis; Y-DNA probes are important in their diagnosis. Tumor markers such a α-fetoprotein, carcinoembryonic antigen, and the antigen CA-125 are also used to assess ovarian malignancy.

Treatment consists of surgical excision followed by postoperative chemotherapy; radiotherapy is often necessary. Staging at the beginning of therapy is of the utmost importance. In many cases, a second-look procedure is indicated in order to decide about subsequent treatment of these neoplasms.

Sex cord stromal tumors comprise 5% of ovarian neoplasms, of which the granulosa cell tumor is the most common. Isosexual precocity and occasionally virilization may be observed in the juvenile variety. The characteristic histologic features include nodular architecture, follicle formation, microcysts, cell necrosis, and increased mitotic activity.

Ovarian Follicular Cysts. These cysts occur from birth to puberty and usually disappear spontaneously. On ultrasound examination, the cyst usually presents as a nonechogenic area, frequently larger than 20 mm at its greatest diameter; diffuse swelling of the ovarian parenchyma and follicular enlargement of the cortical zone are also noted.

Ovarian Torsion. Torsion of an adnexum is a complication that should always be considered in the differential diagnosis of ovarian tumor, and prompt surgical intervention is necessary. Torsion often presents with intermittent sharp abdominal pain that, in many cases, radiates down the ipsilateral extremity. It should be considered in the differential diagnosis of abdominal pain in the pediatric female patient. Bilateral ovarian torsion also may occur in infancy. When unilateral torsion is diagnosed, oophoropexy (plication) of the contralateral adnexa may be indicated.

Adnexal torsion can often be evaluated and managed with the use of laparoscopy. The underlying cause is usually an associated ovarian cyst or neoplasm. Recovery of ovarian function after laparoscopic detorsion has been reported with identification of normal follicle development on ultrasonography. Therefore, it is recommended that adnexal torsion be managed conservatively.

Autoamputation of the Ovary. This entity presents as a small, calcified, free-floating mass associated with absent adnexa. The child may be asymptomatic, and ultrasonography is often helpful in establishing the diagnosis. It has been hypothesized that antenatal or subclinical ovarian torsion leads to necrosis, calcification, and separation of the adnexa from their blood supply.

Juvenile Granulosa Cell Tumors of the Ovary. Juvenile granulosa cell tumors (JGCT) account for 1–2% of all ovarian tumors. The median age of presentation is 7.6 yr, with a range of 6 mo–17.5 yr. The majority of patients have abdominal distention and sexual precocity. Patients appear to have increasingly better prognosis with the advent of multidrug chemotherapy including cisplatin-based regimens. However, neurotoxicity, especially ototoxicity, and bone marrow depression are serious complications.

CERVIX. *Cervical intraepithelial neoplasia* (CIN), diagnosed in sexually active teenagers and young adults, is associated with abnormal cytologic findings in 2–3% of patients. The prevalence of dysplasia and carcinoma in situ is 18.8/1,000 for those 15–19 yr of age, and biopsy-proven cases of all grades of CIN in the teenage population have a prevalence of 13.3/1,000. The Bethesda Classification System with the Papanicolaou (Pap) smear is widely used for diagnosis (Table 561–1). The overall frequency of abnormal Pap smear results in the adolescent population is 3.8%, and 1% of all abnormal Pap smears are associated with CIN. Papillomavirus infection (Chapter 257) and altered vaginal flora are consistent findings in patients with CIN. Abnormal Pap smear results in adolescents also correlate with significant CIN and should be followed up with a biopsy. Colposcopic examination is essential when CIN is diagnosed in an adolescent. Other pathologic abnormalities of the cervix include cervical polyps and mixed mesodermal tumors. The latter may represent a mixed, heterologous, or homologous sarcoma of the uterine cervix.

TABLE 561–1 The Bethesda System

Specimen Quality	Satisfactory for examination
	Satisfactory but limited by . . . .
	Unsatisfactory owing to . . . .
	too few cells
	obscuring blood and inflammation
	fixation artifact (air-dried)
	broken slide
	lack of clinical information
Diagnosis	Within normal limits
	Benign cell change
	infection due to *Candida, Trichomonas,* herpesvirus, *Actinomyces*
	reactive or reparative change
	Epithelial cell abnormality
	squamous
	ASCUS (abnormal squamous cells of undetermined significance)
	LSIL (low-grade squamous intraepithelial lesion)
	HSIL (high-grade squamous intraepithelial lesion)
	squamous cell carcinoma
	Reactive or reparative change
	Glandular
	endometrial cells in a postmenopausal woman
	AGUS (abnormal glandular cells of undetermined significance)
	endocervical adenocarcinoma
	endometrial adenocarcinoma

UTERUS (BENIGN AND MALIGNANT TUMORS OF THE UTERINE CORPUS). *Adenocarcinoma of the corpus* is rare in children and adolescents. Vaginal bleeding not associated with sexual precocity is a frequent presenting sign. Treatment consists of hysterectomy, with removal of the ovaries, followed by adjunctive radiotherapy or chemotherapy or both, depending on the operative findings. *Mixed mesodermal tumors* and *leiomyomas* of the uterus should be included in the differential diagnosis of a pelvic mass in an adolescent. *Leiomyosarcoma,* although extremely rare, has also been noted in an adolescent; the presentation is variable, but abnormal vaginal bleeding usually is present.

VAGINA. *Gartner's duct (mesonephric) cyst* is a common vaginal wall abnormality. It usually is an incidental finding and requires no specific therapy. In sexually active patients, excision may be necessary if there is associated dyspareunia. *Paramesonephric (müllerian) duct cysts* often become symptomatic at menarche when the cavity fills with menstrual blood. Women who were exposed to **diethylstilbestrol (DES) in utero** have a high incidence of *adenosis of the vagina and cervix.* These patients also have potential reproductive abnormalities, including infertility, habitual abortion, and tubal and uterine cavity abnormalities. Clear cell adenocarcinoma of the vagina and cervix is a rare sequela of DES exposure in utero.

Sarcoma botryoides, a vaginal carcinoma that occurs primarily in pediatric patients, is best treated by surgical excision. Chemotherapy is usually administered postoperatively. Any questionable vulvar lesion should be submitted for histologic examination. *Liposarcoma of the vulva* has been reported in a 15-yr-old girl. *Malignant melanoma of the vulva* has also been described in a 14-yr-old patient.

Ablin A, Issacs H Jr: Germ cell tumors. *In:* Pizzo PA, Poplack DG (eds): Pediatric Oncology. Philadelphia, JB Lippincott, 1989, pp 713–731.

Berenson A, Pokorny S, Dutton R: The autoamputated ovary: A rare cause of abdominal calcification. Adolesc Pediatr Gynecol 2:99, 1989.

Brooks J, Livolsi V: Liposarcoma presenting on the vulva. Am J Obstet Gynecol 156:73, 1987.

Calaminus G, Wessalowski R, Harms D, Gobel U: Juvenile granulosa cell tumors of the ovary in children and adolescents: Results from 33 patients registered in a prospective cooperative study. Gynecol Oncol 64:447, 1997.

Cohen Z, Shinhar D, Kopernik G, Mares AJ: The laparoscopic approach to uterine adnexal torsion in childhood. J Pediat Surg 31:1557, 1996.

Copeland LJ, Gershenson DM, Saul PB, et al: Sarcoma botryoides of the female genital tract. Obstet Gynecol 66:262, 1985.

Fields KR, Neinestein LS: Uterine myomas in adolescents: Case reports and a review of the literature. J Pediatr Adolesc Gynecol 9:195, 1996.
Freedman R, Kopf A, Jones W: Malignant melanoma in association with lichen sclerosus on the vulva of a 14-year-old. Am J Dermatopathol 6:253, 1984.
Graif M, Itzchak Y: Sonographic evaluation of ovarian torsion in childhood and adolescence. AJR 150:647, 1988.
Gribbon M, Ein SH, Mancer K: Pediatric malignant ovarian tumors: A three-year review. J Pediatr Surg 27:480, 1992.
Guijon F, Paraskevas M, Brunham R: The association of sexually transmitted diseases with cervical intraepithelial neoplasia: A case-controlled study. Am J Obstet Gynecol 151:185, 1985.
Hassan E, Relakis C, Maralliotakis I, et al: Cervical cytology in adolescence. Clin Exp Obstet Gynecol 24:28, 1997.
Hicks ML, Piver S: Conservative surgery plus adjuvant therapy for vulvovaginal rhabdomyosarcoma, diethylstilbestrol, clear cell adenocarcinoma of the vagina and unilateral germ cell tumors of the ovary. Obstet Gynecol Clin North Am 19:219, 1992.
Liapi C, Evain-Biron D: Diagnosis of ovarian follicular cyst from birth to puberty: A report of 20 cases. Acta Paediatr Scand 76:91, 1987.
Major T, Borsos A, Lampe L, Juhasz B: Ovarian malignancies in childhood and adolescence. Eur J Obstet Gynecol Reprod Biol 63:65, 1995.
Mangan SA, Legano LA, Rosen CM, et al: Increased prevalence of abnormal Papanicolaou smears in early adolescence. Arch Pediatr Adolesc Med 151:481, 1997.
Nicholson HS, Byrne J: Fertility and pregnancy after treatment for cancer during childhood or adolescence. Cancer 71 (Suppl):3392, 1993.
Parker-Jones K: Gynecologic issues in pediatric oncology. Clin Obstet Gynecol 40:200, 1997.
Powell JL, Otis CN: Management of advanced juvenile granulosa cell tumor of the ovary. Gynecol Oncol 64:282, 1997.
Rosenfeld WD, Kleinhaus S, Kutcher R, et al: Leiomyoma in a 15-year-old girl. Adolesc Pediatr Gynecol 1:109, 1988.
Roye CF: Abnormal cervical cytology in adolescents: A literature review. J Adolesc Health 13:643, 1992.
Sadeghi S, Hsieh E, Gonn S: Prevalence of cervical intraepithelial neoplasia in sexually active teenagers and young adults: Results of data analysis of mass Papanicolaou screening of 796,337 women in the United States in 1981. Am J Obstet Gynecol 148:726, 1984.
Sagot P, Lopes P, Mensier A, et al: Carbon dioxide laser treatment of cervical dysplasia in teenagers. Eur J Obstet Gynecol Reprod Biol 46:143, 1992.
Shalev E, Bustan M, Yarom I, Peleg D: Recovery of ovarian function after laparoscopic detorsion. Hum Reprod 10:2965, 1995.
Starceski P, Lee P, Siever W: Bilateral ovarian pathology and torsion in infancy: Assessment of pubertal and gonadal function. Adolesc Pediatr Gynecol 1:199, 1988.
Young RH, Kozakewich WP, Scully RE: Metastatic ovarian tumors in children: A report of 14 cases and review of the literature. Int J Gynecol Pathol 12:8, 1993.

CHAPTER 562
Developmental Anomalies

EMBRYOLOGY. The uterus is formed by fusion of the cordal elements of the müllerian ducts, a process that occurs at 8 wk of gestation. The fusion begins from the cordal end (Müller's tubercle) and is completed at the upper level of the fundus. A median septum is present until the end of the 1st trimester of gestation.

The vagina is formed from the terminal portion of the utero-vaginal canal (müllerian origin), which is met by the posterior aspect of the urogenital sinus (terminal portion of Müller's tubercle). Further thickening occurs in the portion of the posterior wall of the urogenital sinus that is in contact with Müller's tubercle. The tissue is of combined urogenital and müllerian duct origin and is known as the vaginal epithelial plate. Bilateral evaginations of the vaginal epithelial plate encircle the caudal aspect and form the uterine canal. Canalization of the vaginal plate occurs and proceeds in a caudal direction to form the vagina. The process elongates the vaginal structure, leaving the cranial two thirds of müllerian origin and the caudal one third of urogenital origin.

The paramesonephric system is responsible for müllerian tract development. Failure of lateral fusion or lack of resorption of the vertical midline septum results in a müllerian anomaly. Because of the intimate anatomic and embryologic development of the urinary and genital systems, the urinary tract is often also affected; skeletal defects, including spina bifida occulta, occur as well. Common müllerian duct anomalies and associated heritable disorders are presented in Tables 562–1 and 562–2.

CONGENITAL ABSENCE OF THE VAGINA (MAYER-ROKITANSKY-KÜSTER-HAUSER SYNDROME). This anomaly is often discovered in adolescents who present with primary amenorrhea. Vaginal agenesis is characterized by primary amenorrhea, a normal vulva, a duplication anomaly of the uterus, attenuated fallopian tubes, normal ovaries, normal female karyotype, normal female phenotype, and associated anomalies (most frequently renal and skeletal). Absence of the vagina has significant anatomic, physiologic, and psychologic implications for the patient and family.

INCOMPLETE VERTICAL FUSION OF THE VAGINA. Transverse and longitudinal vaginal septa represent failure of completion of canalization of the vagina. Not uncommonly, the patient presents with amenorrhea and cyclical pain, which is a result of cryptomenorrhea. Müllerian agenesis must be differentiated from androgen insensitivity (testicular feminization); serum testosterone levels are usually in the male range with the latter syndrome.

Müllerian agenesis is associated with renal anomalies in 34% and skeletal anomalies in 12% of patients. Unilateral renal agenesis (15%) is the most common abnormality. The most frequent skeletal anomalies are vertebral. Klippel-Feil syndrome has been associated with müllerian agenesis. Müllerian agenesis, with a reported incidence of 1/5,000 to 1/20,000, is more common than androgen insensitivity and is second in frequency to gonadal dysgenesis as a cause of primary amenorrhea. Patients usually have a normal female karyotypc of 46 XX, but autosomal translocation of chromosomes 12q and 14q occurs. Affected siblings have been reported, as well as families with variable expression of defects in müllerian, renal, and skeletal systems.

An intravenous pyelogram (IVP) is indicated to identify associated renal anomalies. An evaluation for skeletal anomalies is also indicated. A karyotype should be obtained. A pelvic ultrasound examination is helpful in defining the anomaly; CT scanning and MRI provide increased detail. Laparoscopy is usually reserved for evaluating a pelvic mass and associated abnormalities.

Vaginoplasty is best deferred until a patient has matured and should be supported by counseling for both patient and family. The MacIndoe procedure, the usual treatment of choice, involves the use of a skin graft, usually from the buttocks, to create a vagina after appropriate dissection of the vulvovaginal area. Other reconstructive procedures have included fasciocutaneous flaps.The artificial vaginal epithelium changes cytologically to an almost normal appearing vaginal mucosa. Various dilatation procedures result in an increased vaginal size, which ultimately permits intercourse. Squamous cell carcinoma of the reconstructed vagina has been reported and appears to be related to the type of tissue transplanted. Radiotherapy is usually the primary method of treatment for this particular squamous cell carcinoma.

TABLE 562–1 Common Müllerian Anomalies

Hydrocolpos	Accumulation of mucus or nonsanguineous fluid in the vagina
Hemihematometra	Atretic segment of vagina with menstrual fluid accumulation
Hydrosalpinx	Accumulation of serous fluid in the fallopian tube, often an end result of pyosalpinx
Didelphic uterus	Two cervices, each associated with one uterine horn
Bicornuate uterus	One cervix associated with two uterine horns
Unicornuate uterus	Result of failure of one müllerian duct to descend

TABLE 562–2 Heritable Disorders Associated with Müllerian Anomalies

Mode of Inheritance	Disorder	Associated Müllerian Defect
Autosomal dominant	Camptobrachydactyly	Longitudinal vaginal septa
	Hand-foot-genital	Incomplete müllerian fusion
Autosomal recessive	Kaufman-McCusick	Transverse vaginal septa
	Johanson-Blizzard	Longitudinal vaginal septa
	Renal-genital-middle ear anomalies	Vaginal atresia
	Fraser's syndrome	Incomplete müllerian fusion
	Uterine hernia syndrome	Persistent müllerian duct derivatives
Polygenic/multifactorial	Mayer-Rokitansky-Küster-Hauser syndrome	Müllerian aplasia
X linked	Uterine hernia syndrome	Persistent müllerian duct derivatives

From Shulman L, Elias S: Developmental abnormalities of the female reproductive tract: Pathogenesis and nosology. Adolesc Pediatr Gynecol 1:232, 1988.

TRANSVERSE VAGINAL SEPTA. The incidence of transverse vaginal septa is approximately 1/80,000 females. The patient usually presents with amenorrhea, which may be associated with cyclical pelvic pain, a pelvic mass, and cryptomenorrhea. Although usually asymptomatic until puberty, *hydrometrocolpos* may occur in children. Transverse vaginal septa may be associated with other congenital anomalies, although this occurs less often than with müllerian agenesis. The most common site of the septum is between the middle and upper thirds of the vagina. These patients have a functional uterus, although their fertility is often compromised; 47% of affected females in one retrospective series had spontaneous abortions. The prognosis is worse for higher obstructions. There is also an increased incidence of endometriosis secondary to retrograde menstruation.

Evaluation of transverse vaginal septa includes careful pelvic examination and often pelvic imaging to delineate the anatomic abnormalities. Treatment is surgical resection of the obstruction from below. Anastomosis of the upper and lower segments should be attempted, if at all possible, to prevent stenosis. A skin graft may be necessary. A Lucite form is often placed in the vagina to maintain patency.

DISORDERS OF LATERAL FUSION. These include a number of anatomic variations of nonobstructive longitudinal septum as well as the obstructed hemivagina. The latter may be associated with a didelphic uterus and often with a pelvic mass, which represents retrograde menstruation associated with the occluded hemivagina. Menses, often cyclical, represent an unobstructed outflow tract from one of the uterine horns.

UTERINE ABNORMALITIES. The incidence of uterine anomalies ranges from 1/100 to 1/1,000. Anomalous development of the uterine cavity may have varied *clinical manifestations.* Patients may present with primary amenorrhea or with irregular or even regular menses. There may be an asymptomatic pelvic mass or dysmenorrhea. In adolescents and adults, pregnancy wastage and infertility may cause the first suspicion of uterine anomaly.

Diagnosis should include a pelvic ultrasound examination, IVP, and skeletal inspection for anomalies. Karyotyping and diagnostic laparoscopy may be necessary, depending on the presentation and laboratory assessment. A hysterosalpingogram may be helpful.

Treatment depends on the specific anomaly, and surgical repair has included Strassman metroplasty, Jones "wedge" metroplasty, and Tompkins metroplasty. The obstructions to the outflow tract must also be relieved; this may necessitate creation of a vaginal window or excision of a hemivagina. Retrograde menstruation in a uterine horn must also be evaluated and, if present, appropriate surgical correction provided.

CONGENITAL ATRESIA OF THE UTERINE CERVIX. This extremely rare anomaly often presents at puberty with cryptomenorrhea, amenorrhea, and pelvic pain. It is associated with significant renal anomalies in 5–10% of patients. On examination, complete absence of a cervix but a palpable uterus are found. Pelvic imaging is helpful in defining the abnormality. Treatment may include laparotomy to create a uterovaginal fistula. If this is impossible, a hysterectomy may be necessary. Other associated anomalies include mesonephric cysts, which are remnants of the wolffian duct, incomplete reduplication of internal genitalia (e.g., didelphic uterus), and unilateral renal aplasia. In addition, gastrointestinal (42.9%), respiratory (47.6%), central nervous system (28.6%), cardiovascular (38.1%), and musculoskeletal abnormalities (33.3%) have been reported with this lesion.

COMPLETE VULVAR DUPLICATION. This rare congenital anomaly presents in infancy and consists of two vulvas, vaginas, and bladders, a didelphic uterus, a single rectum and anus, and two renal systems.

LABIAL HYPERTROPHY. Elongation of the labia minora may be present at birth. This usually is of no consequence, but surgical revision may be necessary if symptoms develop.

CLITORAL ABNORMALITIES. Agenesis of the clitoris is rare. Clitoral duplication has been reported, often associated with pelvic organ abnormalities, including agenesis of other genital structures and bladder exstrophy.

CLITORAL HYPERTROPHY IN ASSOCIATION WITH AMBIGUOUS GENITALIA. See Chapter 586.

HYMENAL ABNORMALITIES. An imperforate hymen can be present in pediatric patients and is often associated with mucocolpos; it can also be associated with hydrometrocolpos. Other hymenal abnormalities include cribriform or stenotic hymen.

MANAGEMENT OF EMERGENCIES ASSOCIATED WITH CONGENITAL MALFORMATIONS OF THE FEMALE GENITAL TRACT

The *clinical manifestations* of a müllerian anomaly are varied. There may be a pelvic mass, which may or may not be associated with symptoms. A vaginal bulging mass or hemivagina is indicative of complete or partial outflow tract obstruction. An adolescent may present with pelvic pain, either in association with primary amenorrhea or several months after the onset of menarche. Patients may be asymptomatic until there is evidence of repeat pregnancy wastage. When presentation is symptomatic, emergent management may be required.

OUTFLOW TRACT OBSTRUCTION. Obstruction may result from a number of distinct anomalies including the imperforate hymen, transverse vaginal septum, and noncommunicating rudimentary horn. As menstrual fluid accumulates proximal to the obstruction, the resulting hematocolpos, hematometra, or hematocolpometra causes cyclic pain or a pelvic mass. These obstructions are best considered according to the location of the obstruction.

Distal Vagina/Imperforate Hymen. This is the most common obstructive anomaly, and familial occurrences have been reported. In the newborn period and early infancy, it may be diagnosed by a bulging membrane due to a mucocolpos from maternal estrogen stimulation. If not noted at this time, it is not often diagnosed until puberty, when menstrual fluid accumulates. The *clinical manifestations* often are a bulging blue-black membrane, pain, primary amenorrhea, and normal secondary sex characteristics. Depending on the circumstance, patients may have cyclic abdominal pain or a pelvic mass.

Treatment requires incision/resection of the membrane, thus relieving the outflow tract obstruction. Repair should occur at time of diagnosis if a patient is symptomatic. Although the lesion may be repaired anytime during infancy, childhood, or adolescence, surgery is facilitated by estrogen stimulation and thus ideally performed in adolescence.

Proximal or Midvaginal Transverse Septum. Vertical fusion defects can result in a transverse septum, which may be imperforate and associated with hematocolpos or hematometra in adolescents, mucocolpos in children, or a small, pinpoint aperture and cyclic menses. Patients frequently become symptomatic as fluid accumulates in the vagina. As with an imperforate hymen, a mass may be present, and the vagina appears short or blind ended. The approach to resection of the septum depends on the presence or absence of an opening. In the presence of an opening, cannulation should be attempted with resection of the septum. Postoperatively, a vaginal stent may be necessary.

Rudimentary Horns. This emergency results from the presence of a horn with a functional endometrium and outflow tract obstruction. As with other types of outflow tract obstruction, severe lower abdominal pain with a pelvic mass is the primary *clinical manifestation*. In contrast to other forms of outflow tract obstruction, however, primary amenorrhea is usually not present because the opposite horn is unlikely to be obstructed. Asymptomatic rupture of a rudimentary horn in an adult has occurred.

Ultrasonography is instrumental in visualizing the rudimentary horn. An IVP or renal ultrasonography also should be obtained because of associated anomalies. If there is evidence of a functional endometrium, surgical extirpation is recommended.

RUDIMENTARY HORN PREGNANCY. This occurs in 1/40,000–140,000 pregnancies and 1/5,000–15,000 ectopic pregnancies. It may be a result of a fibromuscular or fibrous band connecting the unicornuate uterus and the rudimentary horn, but 80–85% of cases are noncommunicating. The latter is probably the result of transperitoneal migration of either sperm or the fertilized ovum. In contrast to tubal pregnancies, rudimentary horn pregnancies are often not detected until the second trimester. Because of the greater muscle wall thickness of most horns, rupture typically occurs later than in tubal gestation.

Most cases are diagnosed only after rupture occurs, when patients have acute abdominal pain and peritoneal signs and are often in shock. When rupture occurs, intraperitoneal hemorrhage may be massive and life threatening and requires immediate surgical intervention. Maternal mortality is about 5%, with 90% of this occurring within 10–15 min after rupture. Fetal demise occurs in 98%.

Before rupture, diagnosis of a rudimentary horn pregnancy may be difficult. It should be suspected in any gravida with a known rudimentary horn, and these patients should be closely monitored until an intrauterine pregnancy has been documented. In those who have not been previously identified as having a rudimentary horn, findings on early pelvic examination are similar to findings of tubal ectopic pregnancy and include deviation of the cervix to one side with an adnexal mass on the opposite side. Ultrasound findings before rupture include an extrauterine gestational sac and placenta within the horn next to a slightly enlarged uterus.

Treatment consists of surgical resection of the rudimentary horn.

ACUTE URINARY RETENTION. Outflow tract obstruction resulting in accumulation of fluid in the vagina or uterus may cause urinary retention as a result of mucocolpos in the first years of life or hematocolpos, hematometra, or hematocolpometra during the pubertal years. The retained fluid in the vagina compresses the urethra, and this is aggravated when the fluid-filled uterus applies pressure on the posterior wall of the bladder and changes the angle of the urethra. Pressure on the sacral plexus from the distended vagina may also be contributory.

The usual *clinical manifestations* in adolescents are lower abdominal pain and the inability to void. There also may be hesitancy and incomplete voiding for several days before presentation. Adolescents also generally have primary amenorrhea, a history of cyclic lower abdominal pain, and a pelvic mass. However, if the obstruction is unilateral, as with a noncommunicating rudimentary horn or an obstructed hemivagina, the patient may have normal menses.

Temporary but immediate relief can be provided by urethral catheterization. If resistance occurs with an appropriately sized rubber catheter, a pediatric feeding tube may be used, or if necessary, a spinal needle may be passed suprapubically to empty the bladder. Urine should be sent for urinalysis and culture because urinary stasis promotes infection. Once the acute condition has been treated, the underlying problem should be appropriately evaluated and the obstructing mass evaluated. Urinary tract infections also have been associated with müllerian anomalies. This may result from renal anomalies with vesicourethral reflux, or it may precede retention as a result of vaginal outflow obstruction. Antibiotic treatment is indicated.

Achiron R, Tadmor O, Kamar R: Prerupture ultrasound diagnosis of interstitial and rudimentary horn pregnancy in the second trimester. Int J Reprod Med 37:89, 1992.

American Fertility Society: The American Fertility Society classifications of adnexal adhesions, distal tubal occlusion, tubal occlusion secondary to tubal ligation, tubal pregnancies, müllerian anomalies, and intrauterine adhesions. Fertil Steril 49:944, 1988.

Bejanga I: Hematocolpos with imperforate hymen. Int Surg 63:97, 1978.

Bergh P, Breen J, Gregori C: Congenital absence of the vagina—the Mayer-Rokitansky-Küster-Hauser syndrome. Adolesc Pediatr Gynecol 2:73, 1989.

Brevetti L, Brevetti G, Lawrence J, Soper R: Pyocolpos: Diagnosis and treatment. J Pediatr Surg 32:110, 1997.

Fedele L, Bianchi S, Agnoli B, et al: Urinary tract anomalies associated with unicornuate uterus. J Urol 155:847, 1996.

Freedman M: Uterine anomalies. Semin Reprod Endocrinol 4:39, 1986.

Horejsi JA: Incomplete reduplication of internal genitalia and unilateral renal aplasia syndrome. Adolesc Pediatr Gynecol 1:42, 1988.

Joshi N, Sotrel G: Diagnostic laparoscopy in apparent uterine agenesis. J Adolesc Health Care 9:403, 1988.

Lewis V, Money J: Gender-identity/role. Par A:XY (androgen insensitivity) syndrome and XX (Rokitansky) syndrome, vaginal atresia compared. *In:* Dennerstein L, Burroughs G (eds): Handbook of Psychosomatic Obstetrics and Gynecology. New York, Elsevier Biomedical Press, 1983, p 61.

Loong E, Yuen P: Acute urinary retention caused by a unilateral hematometra. Arch Gynecol Obstet 247:211, 1990.

Nagele F, Langle R, Stolzlechner J, et al: Noncommunicating rudimentary horn—obstetric and gynecologic implications. Acta Obstet Gynecol Scand 74:566, 1995.

Nisanian A: Hematocolpometra presenting as urinary retention: A case report. J Reprod Med 38:57, 1993.

Peter J, Steinhardt G: Acute urinary retention in children. Pediatr Emerg Care 9:205, 1993.

Robischon K, Baram D, Phipps WR: Presentation of a müllerian anomaly with outflow obstruction after tubal ligation. Fertil Steril 65:866, 1996.

Rock J, Azziz R: Genital anomalies in childhood. Clin Obstet Gynecol 30:682, 1987.

Rock JA, Horowitz IR: Surgical conditions of the vagina and urethra. *In:* Rock JA, Thompson JD (eds): Te Linde's Operative Gynecology. Philadelphia, Lippincott-Raven, 1997, p 913.

Rolen A, Choquette A, Semmens J: Rudimentary uterine horn: Obstetric and gynecologic implications. Obstet Gynecol 27:806, 1966.

Shulman LP, Elias S: Developmental abnormalities of the female reproductive tract: Pathogenesis and nosology. Adolesc Pediatr Gynecol 1:230, 1987.

Sorenson S: Estimated prevalence of müllerian anomalies. Acta Obstet Gynecol Scand 67:441, 1988.

Usta IM, Awwad JT, et al: Imperforate hymen: Report of an unusual familial occurrence. Obstet Gynecol 82:655, 1993.

Wiermsa A, Peterson L, Justema E: Uterine anomalies associated with unilateral renal agenesis. Obstet Gynecol 47:654, 1976.

Yu T, Lin M: Acute urinary retention in two patients with imperforate hymen. Scand J Urol Nephrol 27:543, 1993.

CHAPTER 563
Athletic Gynecologic Problems

The most common gynecologic problem in female athletes is menstrual aberration, usually manifested as amenorrhea or oligomenorrhea. Female adolescents who participate in strenuous training have low serum estradiol levels and are predisposed to bone demineralization. Puberty and menarche may be delayed.

Endogenous opiates within the hypothalamus may inhibit gonadotropin-releasing hormone neurons and thus affect luteinizing hormone secretion and reproductive function. There is also an increase in corticotropin secretion. A change in body composition and weight loss are involved in the menstrual defect. Amenorrheic runners tend to have less body fat than eumenorrheic runners, and menarche is delayed approximately 3 yr in ballet dancers (in comparison with nonathletic adolescents) preparing for a professional career. Delayed puberty in association with endurance training does not appear to be related to significant alteration in follicle-stimulating hormone and luteinizing hormone levels. It is important to assess nutritional status and other potential causes before delayed puberty is attributed to athletic activities.

Baer JT, Taper LJ, Gwazdauskas FG, et al: Diet, hormonal, and metabolic factors affecting bone mineral density in adolescent amenorrheic and eumenorrheic female runners. J Sports Med Phys Fitness 32:51, 1992.
Ding JH, Sheckter CB, Drinkwater BL, et al: High serum cortisol levels in exercise-associated amenorrhea. Ann Intern Med 108:530, 1988.
Warren MD, Brooks-Gunn J, Hamilton LH, et al: Scoliosis and fractures in young ballet dancers. Relation to delayed menarche and secondary amenorrhea. N Engl J Med 314:1348, 1986.

CHAPTER 564
Gynecologic Needs of Mentally Handicapped Children

Perineal hygiene is a major problem for mentally handicapped pediatric or adolescent patients. Initially, an adequate gynecologic examination and Papanicolaou smear should be provided. A number of medical approaches should then be considered to suppress menses. Depo-medroxyprogesterone acetate, usually prescribed at a dose of 150 mg, may be injected intramuscularly every 3 mo. Alternatively, oral contraceptives do not produce amenorrhea but result in a marked decrease in the quantity of menstrual flow. Before hysterectomy, there should be a thorough discussion with parents or custodians after a trial of medical treatment has not been successful. An ethics advisory committee should be consulted to aid in decisions about sterilizing mentally handicapped patients (see also Chapters 2 and 37).

Elkins T, Hoyle D, Darnton T, et al: The use of a societally based ethics class advisory committee to aid in decisions to sterilize mentally handicapped patients. Adolesc Pediatr Gynecol 1:190, 1988.
Elkins T, McNeeley S, Rosen D, et al: A clinical observation of a program to accomplish pelvic exams in difficult-to-manage patients with mental retardation. Adolesc Pediatr Gynecol 1:195, 1988.
Ortho Pharmaceuticals. 1996 Video presentation. The patient with mental retardation: Issues in gynecologic care.

CHAPTER 565
Gynecologic Imaging

A transabdominal ultrasonic approach with use of a distended bladder to serve as an imaging window allows appropriate identification of the uterus and the ovaries; bladder distention with urine displaces gas-filled bowel loops out of the pelvis, with resultant enhanced imaging. A 7.5 or 5 MHz transducer is usually used, especially with larger children and teenagers. Normal values are listed in Table 565–1.

Pelvic masses can be identified at any age. Ovarian cysts and hydrocolpos or hydrometrocolpos are the most common abnormalities noted in neonates. Hydrocolpos is defined as dilatation of the vagina, which usually is associated with accumulation of serous fluid or urine (if there is a urogenital sinus). Hydrometrocolpos causes dilatation of both the uterus and the vagina. It may also be associated with vaginal or cervical atresia, stenosis, or an imperforate hymen. Most large ovarian cysts (simple cystic) in children may be safely observed with serial pelvic ultrasonography and tend to decrease in size or completely resolve. A solid mass requires a tissue diagnosis.

Ultrasonography is a key screening tool, enabling appropriate diagnosis in patients presenting with ambiguous genitalia, ovarian or uterine masses, primary amenorrhea, and abdominal or pelvic pain. MRI and CT are required when further detailed anatomic assessment is necessary.

Siegel MJ, Surratt JT: Pediatric gynecologic imaging. Obstet Gynecol Clin North Am 19:103, 1992.
Warner BW, Kuhn JC, Barr LL: Conservative management of large ovarian cysts in children: The value of serial pelvic ultrasonography. Surgery 112:749, 1992.

TABLE 565–1 Normal Ovarian and Uterine Dimensions

Ovary

Birth

15 mm long, 3 mm wide, 2.5 mm thick
Ovarian volume 0.7 cm^3*

Post Puberty

22.5–50.0 mm in length
1.5–3 cm in width; 0.6–1.5 cm in thickness
Ovarian volume 1.8–5.7 cm^3*

Uterus

Neonate

Length 2.3–4.6 cm
Anteroposterior diameter 0.8–2.2 cm

Infant to 7 yr of age

Length 2.5–3.3 cm
Anteroposterior diameter 0.4–1.0 cm

Post Puberty

Length 6 cm

Ovarian volume can be determined by using the formula: length × height × width × 0.523.

Sanfilippo JS, Lavery JP: The spectrum of ultrasound: Antenatal to adolescent years. Semin Reprod Endocrinol 6:47, 1988.

PART XXV

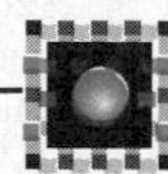

The Endocrine System

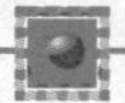

SECTION 1

Disorders of the Hypothalamus and Pituitary Gland

CHAPTER 566

Hormones of the Hypothalamus and Pituitary

John S. Parks

The anterior pituitary gland originates from Rathke's pouch as an invagination of the oral ectoderm. It then detaches from the oral epithelium and becomes an individual structure of rapidly proliferating cells. Persistent remnants of the original connection between Rathke's pouch and the oral cavity can develop into craniopharyngiomas, which are the most common type of tumor in this area. Five cell types in the anterior pituitary produce six peptide hormones. Somatotropes produce growth hormone (GH), lactotropes produce prolactin (PRL), thyrotropes make thyroid-stimulating hormone (TSH), corticotropes express pro-opiomelanocortin (POMC), the precursor of corticotropin (adrenocorticotropic hormone [ACTH]), and gonadotropes express both luteinizing hormone (LH) and follicle-stimulating hormone (FSH).

A series of sequentially expressed transcriptional activation factors direct the differentiation and proliferation of anterior pituitary cell types. These proteins are members of a large family of DNA-binding proteins resembling the homeobox genes originally recognized in *Drosophila*. For the most part, their functions have been defined in the developing mouse pituitary. The consequences of mutations in several of these genes are evident in mouse and human forms of multiple pituitary hormone deficiency.

The Rathke's pouch homeobox (Rpx) mouse genes are expressed in precursors of all five cell types early in development, at embryonic day 8.5 (e8.5), and they are not expressed after day e13.5. Pituitary OTX or Ptx-1 is also expressed early. This protein is capable of activating transcription from the POMC, GH, and PRL promoters as well as the promoter of the α-glycoprotein subunit (α-GSU) that is common to LH, FSH, and TSH. In vitro, it can also activate the β-LH and β-FSH subunits. It acts cooperatively with the transcription factor POU1F1 (formerly termed *Pit-1)* in activation of transcription from the GH and PRL promoters. Ptx-1 appears to be necessary for expression of the next transcription factor in the cascade, termed *P-Lim.* P-Lim protein appears by day e9.5. It activates the α-GSU promoter and acts synergistically with POU1F1 to increase transcription from the PRL, β-TSH, and POU1F1 promoters. Targeted disruption of this gene in the mouse produces a phenotype of hypopituitarism in which Rathke's pouch develops normally, but the anterior and intermediate lobes of the pituitary fail to develop. The Ptx-2 gene, also known as the Riegl gene, is expressed from day e11 into adult life. Its DNA-binding domain differs from that of Ptx-1 by only 2 of 60 amino acids. The Ptx-1 protein is also found in developing eye, tongue, kidney, testis, and umbilicus. Expression of the "Prophet of Pit-1" or PROP1 gene begins at day e10.5 and is over by day e14.5. This protein is found in the nuclei of somatotropes, lactotropes, and thyrotropes. Its role includes turning off Rpx and turning on POU1F1. The gene originally called Pit-1 was recently renamed POU1F1 or POU-homeodomain factor 1. It appears at day e14.5 and is necessary for emergence of somatotropes, lactotropes, and a definitive population of thyrotropes. This protein persists in the mature pituitary and is involved in activation of GH, PRL, and β-TSH expression.

ANTERIOR LOBE HORMONES. The protein hormones produced by the anterior pituitary act on other endocrine glands and on certain body cells to affect almost every organ. Anterior pituitary cells are themselves controlled by neuropeptide-releasing and release-inhibiting hormones that are produced by hypothalamic neurons, secreted into the capillaries of the median eminence, and carried by portal veins to the anterior pituitary. Many conditions formerly classified as pituitary in origin are caused by hypothalamic defects. The identification and availability of hypothalamic hormones permit more precise delineation of these conditions.

Human GH is a protein with 191 amino acids. Its gene (GH1) is the first in a cluster of five closely related genes on the long arm of chromosome 17 (q22–24). The four other genes have greater than 90% sequence identity with the GH1 gene. They consist of the CS1 and CS2 genes, which encode the same human chorionic somatomammotropin (hCS) protein, a placental growth hormone gene (GH2), and a partly disabled pseudogene (CSP). Syncytiotrophoblastic cells of the fetal placenta produce large quantities of hCS, and placental GH replaces pituitary GH in the maternal circulation after 20 wk of gestation. When the fetal genome lacks the CS1, CS2, GH2, and CSP genes, hCS and placental GH are absent, but fetal growth and postpartum lactation are normal.

The GH1 gene is expressed in pituitary somatotropes under the control of two hypothalamic hormones. Growth hormone-releasing hormone (GHRH) stimulates and somatostatin inhibits GH release. Alternating secretion of GHRH and somatostatin accounts for the rhythmic secretion of GH. Peaks of GH occur when peaks of GHRH coincide with troughs of somatostatin. A second stimulatory system, parallel to that involving the GHRH receptor, is stimulated by synthetic growth hormone releasing peptides (GHRPs) and some nonpeptide agonists.

When plasma levels of GH are measured by standard radioimmunoassay (RIA), its secretion appears to be pulsatile, but when measured by an ultrasensitive immunoradiometric assay, which can measure GH in a previously undetectable range, it is observed to be secreted in a rhythmic fashion with a dominant 2-hr periodicity. The highest levels of GH are achieved during sleep when measured by RIA or immunoradiometric assay.

The three molecular species of GHRH contain 37, 40, or 44 amino acids. A fully active 29–amino acid synthetic GHRH is available for diagnostic use. Somatostatin exists in 14– and 28–amino acid forms. Somatostatin production is not limited to the hypothalamus. It also acts through autocrine and paracrine mechanisms in the islets of Langerhans and in the gastrointestinal tract. Somatostatin inhibits secretion of insulin, glucagon, secretin, gastrin, vasoactive intestinal peptide (VIP), GH, and thyrotropin. In the pancreatic islets, it is localized to the D cells. Somatostatin-secreting pancreatic tumors (i.e., somatostatinomas) have been reported in adults. A potent, long-acting somatostatin analog, octreotide, which inhibits GH preferentially over insulin, is available to treat patients with GH-secreting tumors. It is also useful in managing patients with gastrinomas, insulinomas, glucagonomas, VIPomas, and carcinoid tumors (see Chapters 88 and 511.4). ^{123}I-labeled octreotide appears to be useful in localizing somatostatin receptor–positive tumors and their metastases.

GH acts through binding to receptor molecules on the surface of target cells. The GH receptor is a single-chain molecule of 620 amino acids. It has an extracellular domain, a single membrane-spanning domain, and a cytoplasmic domain. Proteolytically cleaved fragments of the extracellular domain circulate in plasma and act as a GH-binding protein. As in other members of the cytokine receptor family, the cytoplasmic domain of the GH receptor lacks intrinsic kinase activity; instead, GH binding induces receptor dimerization and activation of a receptor-associated Janus kinase (Jak2). Phosphorylation of the kinase and other protein substrates initiates a series of events that leads to alterations in nuclear gene transcription.

The mitogenic actions of GH are mediated through increases in the synthesis of insulin-like growth factor-I (IGF-I), formerly named *somatomedin C*, a single-chain peptide with 70 amino acids coded for by a gene on the long arm of chromosome 12. IGF-I has considerable homology to insulin. Circulating IGF-I is synthesized primarily in the liver and formed locally in mesodermal and ectodermal cells, particularly in the growth plate of children, where its effect is exerted by paracrine or autocrine mechanisms. Circulating levels of IGF-I are related to blood levels of GH to a large extent, except in the fetus and during the neonatal period. IGF-I circulates bound to several different binding proteins; the major one is a 150-kd complex (IGF-BP3), which is decreased in GH-deficient children but is in the normal range in children who are short for other reasons. Human recombinant IGF-I is being used experimentally to determine its therapeutic potential in conditions characterized by end organ resistance to GH. IGF-II is a single-chain protein with 67 amino acids that is coded for by a gene on the short arm of chromosome 11. It has homology to IGF-I, but much less is known about its physiologic roles, although it appears to be an important mitogen in bone cells, where it occurs in a concentration many times higher than that of IGF-I.

Several disorders of growth are caused by abnormalities of the genes that code for the GHRH receptor, Pit-1, GH1, the GH receptor, and IGF-I.

Prolactin is composed of 199 amino acids, and its gene is located on chromosome 6. The major prolactin-inhibiting factor is dopamine, and medications that disrupt hypothalamic dopaminergic pathways result in increased serum levels of prolactin. Serum levels of prolactin are increased after administration of thyrotropin-releasing hormone (TRH), in states of primary hypothyroidism, and after disruption of the pituitary stalk, as may occur in children with craniopharyngioma.

The main established role for prolactin is the initiation and maintenance of lactation. Concentrations in amniotic fluid are 10–100 times the levels in maternal or fetal serum. The major source of amniotic prolactin appears to be the decidua. Mean serum levels in children and in fasting adults of both sexes are about 5–20 μg/L, but levels in the fetus and in neonates during the 1st wk of life are usually higher than 200 μg/L.

TSH consists of two glycoprotein chains linked by hydrogen bonding. The α-chain is identical to that found in FSH, LH, and chorionic gonadotropin (hCG). The β-chain is unique in each of these hormones and confers specificity. The gene for the α-chain has been mapped on chromosome 6, that for the α-chain of TSH on chromosome 1, and those for the β-chains for LH and human chorionic gonadotropin on chromosome 19. TSH increases iodine uptake, iodide clearance from the plasma, iodotyrosine and iodothyronine formation, thyroglobulin proteolysis, and release of thyroxine (T_4) and triiodothyronine (T_3) from the thyroid. Most of the effects of TSH are mediated by cyclic adenosine monophosphate. Deficiency of TSH results in inactivity and atrophy of the thyroid, and excess results in hypertrophy and hyperplasia.

TRH was the first hypothalamic hormone to be isolated, characterized, and synthesized. It is a tripeptide ([pyro] Glu-His-Pro-NH2). Thyroxine and triiodothyronine inhibit TSH secretion by blocking the action of TRH on the pituitary cell. TRH also stimulates the release of prolactin in both sexes. Synthetic TRH is useful for testing pituitary reserves of TSH and prolactin.

ACTH is derived by proteolytic cleavage from a large precursor glycoprotein product of the pituitary gland called *POMC*. Cleavage of POMC yields ACTH, a single chain of 39 amino acids, and β-lipotropin (β-LPH), a 91–amino acid glycoprotein. Further cleavage of ACTH and β-LPH in the pituitary yields yet other hormonal products. The α-melanocyte–stimulating hormone is identical to the first 13 amino acids of ACTH but has no corticotropin activity. Cleavage of β-LPH results in neurotropic peptides with morphinomimetic activity (fragment 61-91 is β-endorphin), and β-melanocyte–stimulating hormone consists of a 17–amino acid fragment of β-LPH.

ACTH acts primarily on the adrenal cortex. It produces changes in structure, chemical composition, enzymatic activity, and release of corticosteroid hormones. ACTH release has a diurnal rhythm. The level is lowest between 10 P.M. and 2 A.M., with peak levels reached about 8 A.M. Levels of β-LPH and β-endorphin are elevated in patients with increased levels of ACTH. It appears that ACTH rather than MSH is the principal pigmentary hormone in humans.

POMC peptides are also produced in nonpituitary tissues. In the testis, some peptides act as autocrine regulators of androgen-secreting Leydig cells, and others may potentiate or oppose the action of FSH on Sertoli cells.

Secretion of ACTH, β-endorphin, and other POMC-related peptides is regulated by corticotropin-releasing hormone (CRH). CRH is a 41–amino acid peptide found predominantly in the median eminence but also in other areas of the brain and in tissues outside the brain, particularly the placenta. During pregnancy, levels of CRH rise several hundred–fold, increase further during labor and delivery, and then fall to nonpregnant levels within 24 hr. Its source is probably the placenta, which contains the peptide and its mRNA. Synthetic ovine CRH and human CRH have been used clinically. The ovine CRH is the clinical agent of choice because responses to it are greater and longer lasting than those with human CRH. It is particularly useful in differentiating the different forms of Cushing's syndrome.

Gonadotropic hormones include two glycoproteins: LH and FSH. Each has an α subunit and a β subunit. The α subunits of these two hormones and of TSH are identical; specificity of hormone action resides in the β subunit, which is different for each of the three. Receptors for FSH on the ovarian granulosa cells and on testicular Sertoli cells mediate FSH stimulation of follicular development in the ovary and of gametogenesis in the testis. On binding to specific receptors on ovarian theca cells and testicular Leydig cells, LH promotes luteinization of the ovary and Leydig cell function of the testis. The receptors for LH and FSH belong to a class of receptors with seven membrane-spanning protein domains. Receptor occupancy activates adenylyl cyclase through mediation of G proteins.

Hypothalamic control of gonadotropic hormones has long been known, and separate releasing hormones for FSH and LH were once anticipated. Luteinizing hormone–releasing hormone, a decapeptide, has been isolated, synthesized, and widely used in clinical studies. Because it leads to the release of LH and FSH from the same gonadotropic cells, it appears that there is only one gonadotropin-releasing hormone.

Secretion of LH is inhibited by androgens and estrogens, and secretion of FSH is suppressed by gonadal production of inhibin, a 31-kd glycoprotein produced by the Sertoli cells. Inhibin consists of α and β subunits joined by disulfide bonds. The β-β dimer (activin) also occurs, but its biologic effect is to stimulate FSH secretion. The biologic features of these newer hormones are being delineated. In addition to its endocrine effect, activin has paracrine effects in the testis. It facilitates LH-induced testosterone production, indicating a direct effect of Sertoli cells on Leydig cells analogous to the interaction of these cells through the paracrine effects of POMC.

The posterior lobe of the pituitary is part of a functional unit, the neurohypophysis, that consists of the neurons of the supraoptic and paraventricular nuclei of the hypothalamus; neuronal axons, which form the pituitary stalk; and neuronal terminals in the median eminence or in the posterior lobe.

HORMONES OF THE NEUROHYPOPHYSIS. The neurohypophysis is the source of *arginine vasopressin* (AVP; antidiuretic hormone) and of *oxytocin.* Both are octapeptides, differing in only two amino acids. These hormones are produced by neurosecretion in the hypothalamic nuclei. Vasopressin derives its name from early observations of its pressor and antidiuretic activities; however, the latter is its physiologically important function. At levels 50–1,000 times those found in blood, it affects blood pressure, intestinal contractility, hepatic glycogenolysis, platelet aggregation, and release of factor VIII. AVP and oxytocin are secreted by separate cells of the supraoptic and paraventricular nuclei. Secreted concurrently in equimolar amounts with these hormones are *vasopressin neurophysin* (neurophysin II) and *oxytocin neurophysin* (neurophysin I). Each hormone binds to its respective neurophysin and is transported to the nerve terminals in the posterior pituitary, where it is secreted in the free form. RIAs of the neurophysins provide a direct index of AVP and oxytocin levels in plasma. The concentration of AVP in umbilical cord plasma appears to be a sensitive indicator of fetal stress.

AVP has a short half-life and responds quickly to changes in hydration. The stimuli for AVP release are increased plasma osmolality, perceived by osmoreceptors in the hypothalamus, and decreased blood volume, perceived by baroreceptors in the carotid sinus of the aortic arch. AVP changes the permeability of the renal tubular cell membrane through cyclic adenosine monophosphate. A synthetic analog, desmopressin, combines high potency, selectivity for antidiuretic hormone receptors, and resistance to degradation by proteases. Small amounts administered intranasally are effective therapy for patients with diabetes insipidus.

CHAPTER 567
Hypopituitarism

John S. Parks

This chapter discusses the hypopituitary states associated with a deficiency of growth hormone (GH), with or without a deficiency of other pituitary hormones (Table 567–1). Isolated deficiencies of thyrotropin, corticotropin (adrenocorticotropic hormone [ACTH]), and gonadotropin are also addressed. Affected children have in common a phenotype of growth impairment that is specifically corrected by replacement of GH.

ETIOLOGY

Congenital Defects. Pituitary hypoplasia can occur as an isolated phenomenon or in association with more extensive developmental abnormalities, such as anencephaly, holoprosencephaly (i.e., cyclopia, cebocephaly, orbital hypotelorism), and septo-optic dysplasia (de Morsier's syndrome). In the *Hall-Pallister syndrome,* absence of the pituitary gland is associated with hypothalamic hamartoblastoma, postaxial polydactyly, nail dysplasia, bifid epiglottis, imperforate anus, and anomalies of the heart, lungs, and kidneys. *Rieger's syndrome* represents a complex malformation syndrome that sometimes includes deficiency of several anterior pituitary hormones. In this condition, there are colobomas of the iris, a high risk of glaucoma, and sometimes abnormal development of the kidneys, gastrointestinal tract, and umbilicus. Most cases are sporadic, but some have involved a dominant mode of transmission linked to abnormalities on chromosome 4q25. The disease is caused by deletion or mutation of one copy of the Ptx-2 or Riegl gene. Thus, it represents an example of a complex disorder caused by haploinsufficiency for a single gene.

Hypoplasia of the pituitary with anencephaly has long been known, but recent observations reveal a large residuum of normal pituitary function and suggest that hypoplasia may be secondary to the hypothalamic defect. With hypothalamic-releasing hormones, it is possible to determine whether defects in pituitary function reside in the pituitary or hypothalamus. Deficiency of GH occurs in 4% of all patients with *cleft lip or cleft palate* and in 32% of those who also have *short stature. Midfacial anomalies* or the finding of a *solitary maxillary central incisor* indicate a high likelihood of GH deficiency.

Bilateral or unilateral optic nerve hypoplasia is often associated with hypopituitarism. When it is also associated with absence of the septum pellucidum, the condition is known as *septo-optic dysplasia.* The fundus exhibits hypoplastic disks with typical double rims and sparse retinal vessels. Endocrine abnormalities are extremely variable. Hormonal deficiency most often involves GH alone, but multiple pituitary deficiencies, including diabetes insipidus, may occur. The defect resides primarily in the hypothalamus. Delay in linear growth may begin as early as 3 mo of age or may not be observed before 3–4 yr of age. Affected newborns often have apnea, hypotonia, seizures, prolonged jaundice, hypoglycemia without hyperinsulinism, and (in males) microphallus. The condition is usually sporadic but has been reported in siblings with homozygosity for an inactivating mutation of the Hesx-1 gene. The cause is unknown, but young maternal age and nulliparity are strongly associated factors.

Aplasia of the pituitary without abnormalities of the brain or skull is rare, but affected infants are being increasingly recognized because hypoglycemia occurs early and, in males, there is microphallus. Some infants have shown evidence of the neonatal hepatitis syndrome, but the relationship with hypopituitarism is obscure. The condition has been reported in

TABLE 567–1 Etiologic Classification of Hypopituitarism

- Development defects
  - Anencephaly
  - Holoprosencephaly (i.e., cyclopia, cebocephaly, orbital hypotelorism)
  - Midfacial anomalies (e.g., hypertelorism)
  - Septo-optic dysplasia (de Morsier's syndrome)
  - Cleft lip and palate
  - Solitary maxillary central incisor
  - Hall-Pallister syndrome (i.e., hypothalamic hamartoblastoma, imperforate anus, polydactyly)
  - Rieger's syndrome with mutations in the Ptx-2 or Riegl gene
- Genetic defects of GH or GHRH
  - Isolated GH deficiency
  - Autosomal recessive type I
    - Type IA with deletions of the GH1 gene
    - Type IB with mutations in GH1 or other genes
    - Type IB with mutations in the GHRH-receptor gene
  - Autosomal dominant type II with mutations in GH1 or other genes
  - X-linked type III with or without hypogammaglobulinemia
  - Multiple pituitary deficiencies
    - Autosomal recessive type I
      - GH, TSH, ACTH, LH, and FSH +/− ACTH deficiency with mutations in the PROP1 gene
      - GH, TSH, and PRL deficiencies with mutations in the POU1F1 gene
    - Autosomal dominant type II
      - GH, TSH, and PRL deficiencies with mutations in the POU1F1 gene
    - X-linked type III
      - GH, TSH, ACTH, LH, and FSH deficiency
- Destructive lesions
  - Trauma
    - Perinatal trauma (e.g., trauma, anoxia, hemorrhagic infarction)
    - Basal skull fractures
    - Child abuse
- Infiltrative lesions
  - Tumors
  - Histiocytosis X

GH = growth hormone; GHRH = growth hormone–releasing hormone; TSH = thyroid-stimulating hormone; ACTH = adrenocorticotropic hormone (corticotropin); LH = luteinizing hormone; FSH = follicle-stimulating hormone; PRL = prolactin.

siblings of both sexes, and consanguinity has been observed in two families; autosomal recessive inheritance is suggested. Studies of some children have placed the defect in the hypothalamus. This may be a heterogeneous group of disorders.

In *empty-sella syndrome,* a deficient sellar diaphragm leads to herniation of the suprasellar subarachnoid space into the sella turcica, with remodeling of the sella and flattening of the pituitary gland. It may develop after surgery or radiation therapy, or it may be idiopathic. Of 17 pediatric cases, significant hypopituitarism was found in 5. Empty-sella syndrome with an enlarged sella and hypopituitarism has been observed in siblings.

Other syndromes in which short stature is a prominent feature may be associated with deficiency of GH. For example, some patients with Turner, Fanconi, the Russell-Silver, Rieger, or Williams have hypopituitarism.

Destructive Lesions. Any lesion that damages the hypothalamus, pituitary stalk, or anterior pituitary may cause pituitary hormone deficiency. Because such lesions are not selective, multiple hormonal deficiencies are usually observed. The most common lesion is the craniopharyngioma (see Chapter 611). Central nervous system germinoma, eosinophilic granuloma, tuberculosis, sarcoidosis, toxoplasmosis, and aneurysms may also cause hypothalamic-hypophyseal destruction. These lesions are frequently associated with roentgenographic changes in the skull. Besides diabetes insipidus, a deficiency of GH and other pituitary hormones may occur in children with histiocytosis, especially if they are treated with cranial irradiation. Enlargement of the sella or deformation or destruction of the clinoid processes usually indicates a tumor. Intrasellar or suprasellar calcifications usually indicate a craniopharyngioma. Trauma, including child abuse, traction at delivery, anoxia, and hemorrhagic infarction, may also damage the pituitary, its stalk, or the hypothalamus.

Improved survival of children who receive radiotherapy for malignancies of the central nervous system or other cranial structures has resulted in a substantial group of patients with GH deficiency. Children with acute lymphocytic leukemia who have received prophylactic cranial irradiation also belong in this group. Growth typically slows during radiation therapy or chemotherapy, improves for a year or two, and then declines with the development of hypopituitarism. Spinal irradiation contributes to disproportionately poor growth of the trunk. The dose of radiation and the fractionation schedule used are important determinants of the incidence of hypopituitarism. GH deficiency is almost universal 5 yr after therapy with a total dose of 35–45 Gy. Subtler defects are seen with doses around 20 Gy. Deficiency of GH is the most common defect, but deficiencies of thyroid-stimulating hormone (TSH) and ACTH may also occur. Unlike in other forms of hypopituitarism, puberty is not delayed. A pubertal growth spurt at a normal to early age may lessen clinical suspicion of GH deficiency.

Idiopathic Hypopituitarism. Many patients with early expression of combined pituitary hormone deficiencies have anatomic abnormalities detectable by magnetic resonance imaging. The anterior pituitary and pituitary stalk are often smaller than normal, and a bright spot representing the posterior pituitary is located in the hypothalamus rather than in its normal location. This finding is referred to as an ectopic posterior pituitary. The mechanisms underlying this phenomenon are not known. Association with breech birth, forceps delivery, and intrapartum and maternal bleeding suggests that birth trauma and anoxia may be pathogenic factors in some instances.

Genetic Forms of Hypopituitarism. Genetic forms of hypopituitarism account for more than 5% of cases. With advances in molecular strategies for recognizing specific gene abnormalities, genetic diagnoses are being made in patients without a positive family history of hypopituitarism. As in idiopathic hypopituitarism, the defect may be limited to GH, or it can involve deficiencies of several other anterior pituitary hormones. Roman numerals are used to denote the mode of inheritance. In the McKusick classification of isolated GH deficiency (IGHD), type I is autosomal recessive, type II is autosomal dominant, and type III is X-linked. Similarly, autosomal recessive multiple pituitary hormone deficiency is type I, and the X-linked form is type III.

Isolated Growth Hormone Deficiency. Among families with autosomal recessive IGHD, some have complete deletions of the GH1 gene and are considered to have IGHD type IA. Early reports of this disorder stressed the tendency of these children to form antibodies to human GH during treatment and to experience a lessening of growth response. With more widespread application of Southern blotting and polymerase chain reaction techniques for detecting GH1 gene deletions and with the availability of less antigenic biosynthetic GH preparations, it appears that a minority acquire such antibodies. There are several different sizes of deletions, reflecting nonhomologous crossing over at different sites in the GH and CS gene cluster. The smallest and most common deletions are 6.7 kb in length. Other deletion sizes are 7.0, 7.6, and greater than 45 kb. All cases show extreme postnatal growth failure and fail to release GH after stimulation with growth hormone-releasing hormone (GHRH) or more conventional stimuli to GH release.

Autosomal recessive IGHD type IB is heterogeneous with respect to severity and the sites of mutations. Some children have 1- or 2-base pair deletions in the GH1 gene that introduce a frameshift, followed by an early translational stop signal. Homozygosity for this type of GH1 allele or compound heterozygosity for a small and a large GH1 deletion results in total absence of GH and a clinical picture that is as severe as that of IGHD type IA. Other families have mutations at the beginning of the fourth intron of the GH1 gene. These mutations result in the use of an alternative splice site in exon 4, producing a frameshift and a mutant protein that diverges from normal GH after amino acid 102. In some IGHD IB families, tracking the restriction fragment length polymorphisms shows that transmission of the disease is not linked to transmission of GH1 alleles. Attempts to link IGHD IB to defects in the GHRH gene have been uniformly unsuccessful. The little mouse model of IGHD IB is caused by a mutation in the gene for the GHRH receptor. At least two families have been shown to have GH deficiency as a result of mutations that introduce translation stop codons in the extracellular domain of the GHRH receptor. In these, as in other recessive forms of IGHD IB, the defect resides at the level of the pituitary, and there is no increase in GH release after challenge with GHRH.

Some cases of autosomal dominant IGHD III are caused by mutations in the GH1 gene. They involve single-base substitutions in intron 3 that result in omission of exon 3 from the spliced mRNA. The predicted protein has a molecular weight of 17,000 kd, lacks amino acids 32 to 71, and lacks one of the cysteine residues involved in the formation of intramolecular disulfide bonds. It has been speculated that this mutant protein forms intermolecular bonds with the product of the normal GH1 allele and interferes with secretion of GH from secretory granules.

The gene responsible for X-linked IGHD III has not been identified. In several families, GH deficiency has been transmitted along with immunoglobulin deficiency. The disorder in these families may involve deletion of several contiguous genes, or it may involve inactivation of a gene that is essential for both GH and immunoglobulin synthesis.

The existence of short stature due to biologically inactive GH was first proposed in the 1970s. Some patients with normal to high levels of circulating GH by immunoassay appeared to have lower levels of GH when assessed by receptor binding and cell proliferation assays. The first proof of a biologically inactive GH was provided in 1996 in a child who was heterozygous for a mutation changing arginine to cysteine at position 77. The mutant protein binds to GHBP and to the GH receptor, but it does not result in activation of Jak2 kinase. Its dominant negative mechanism of action reflects a higher than normal binding affinity for the receptor. Interestingly, the patient demonstrated severe intrauterine growth retardation as well as postnatal growth failure. This suggests that a competitive antagonist for receptor binding has a more severe effect on fetal growth than does complete inactivation of the receptor for GH.

Multiple Pituitary Hormone Deficiency. Mutations in the pituitary transcription factors PROP1 and POU1F1 have been implicated as causes of multiple pituitary hormone deficiency in mice and humans. Positional cloning was used to identify the PROP1 gene as the cause of Ames dwarfism in the mouse. Subsequent studies showed that missense mutations and 1- or 2-base pair deletions were responsible for multiple pituitary hormone deficiency in humans. The Ames mouse lacks GH, prolactin (PRL), and TSH but has normal ACTH production and is not totally deficient in LH and FSH. All the patients with PROP1 mutations who have been described to date have had deficiencies of LH and FSH as well as GH, PRL, and TSH. About one third have also been deficient in ACTH. PROP1 defects are emerging as a common cause of hypopituitarism. In a series of 53 Polish cases, more than half were due to PROP1 mutations. Pituitary size is usually small, but patients in some families have demonstrated pathologic enlargement of the anterior pituitary during childhood. With time, there is involution and development of an empty sella turcica. The human mutations have produced greater loss of PROP1 function than the mutation responsible for Ames dwarfism in the mouse. So far, the described mutations have been recessive in nature. Since the PROP1 protein forms homodimers and heterodimers with other transcription factors, there is a strong possibility that dominant negative mutations will be identified.

POU1F1 was originally identified as a nuclear protein that bound to the GH and PRL promoters. Mutations in POU1F1 were found to be responsible for Snell and Jackson dwarfism in the mouse and combined hormone deficiencies in humans. Ten different types of recessive loss of function mutations have been identified in humans. Homozygotes have complete deficiency of GH and PRL and variable degrees of central hypothyroidism. Anterior pituitary size, as assessed by magnetic resonance imaging, may be normal or small. Puberty develops spontaneously. Most of the dominant cases have involved a mutation causing substitution of tryptophan for arginine at position 271. The mutant protein has normal to increased promoter-binding activity but is incapable of activating transcription.

Growth Hormone–Receptor Defects. Children with *Laron's syndrome* have all the clinical findings of those with hypopituitarism, but they have elevated levels of circulating GH. Levels of insulin-like growth factor-I (IGF-I) are low and fail to respond to exogenous human GH (hGH). Serum GH-binding activity, reflecting a circulating form of the extracellular domain of the GH receptor, is low in most patients. A variety of gene defects has been discovered in different families, ranging from the deletion of several exons of the gene, through nonsense mutations, to missense mutations, and to mutations that alter splicing of pre-mRNA. More than 40 affected individuals in two large Ecuadorian kindreds are homozygous for a base substitution that creates a new splice site and results in a protein that lacks 12 of the amino acids normally found in the extracellular domain. A second kindred living in the Bahamas expresses a different mutation that also introduces a new splice site and results in a nonfunctional protein. Most of the mutations responsible for Laron's syndrome produce a loss of GH-binding activity. However, some are associated with normal or increased levels of binding. The mutant protein in at least one family retains normal affinity for GH binding but lacks the ability to form dimers of GH receptor around a single bound GH molecule. In other families, there is increased serum GH binding activity due to overproduction of a receptor that lacks the transmembrane domain and has no capacity for signal transduction.

Insulin-like Growth Factor I Defects. Although mutations in pituitary transcription factor, GHRH receptor, GH, and GH receptor genes have minimal effects on prenatal growth, mutation of the IGF-I gene produces profound intrauterine growth retardation. The patient reported by Woods and colleagues was 5.4 SD below the mean for length at birth and 6.9 SD below the mean for height at age 15 yr. This patient was homozygous for deletion of exons 3 and 4 of the IGF-I gene. There was an absence of circulating IGF-I, but elevated level of GH and IGF-BP3.

CLINICAL MANIFESTATIONS

Patients Without Demonstrable Lesions of the Pituitary. The child with hypopituitarism is usually of normal size and weight at birth. Retrospective studies of children with multiple pituitary hormone deficiencies and those with genetic defects of the GH1 or GHR gene indicate that birth length averages 1 SD below the mean. Children with severe defects in GH production or action fall more than 4 SD below the mean by 1 yr of age. Others with less severe deficiencies may have regular but slow growth in height, with the increments always below the normal percentiles, or periods of lack of growth may alternate with short spurts of growth. Delayed closure of the epiphyses permits growth beyond the age when normal persons cease to grow. Without treatment, adult heights are 4 to 12 SD below the mean.

Infants with congenital defects of the pituitary or hypothalamus usually present neonatal emergencies such as apnea, cyanosis, or severe hypoglycemia. Microphallus in the male provides an additional diagnostic clue. Deficiency of GH may be accompanied by hypoadrenalism and hypothyroidism, and clinical manifestations of hypopituitarism evolve more rapidly than in the usual child with hypopituitarism. Prolonged neonatal jaundice is common. It involves elevation of conjugated and unconjugated bilirubin and may be mistaken for neonatal hepatitis.

The head is round, and the face is short and broad. The frontal bone is prominent, and the bridge of the nose is depressed and saddle-shaped. The nose is small, and the nasolabial folds are well developed. The eyes are somewhat bulging. The mandible and the chin are underdeveloped and infantile, and the teeth, which erupt late, are frequently crowded. The neck is short and the larynx is small. The voice is high-pitched and remains high after puberty. The extremities are well proportioned, with small hands and feet. The genitals are usually underdeveloped for the child's age, and sexual maturation may be delayed or absent. Facial, axillary, and pubic hair usually is lacking, and the scalp hair is fine. Symptomatic hypoglycemia, usually after fasting, occurs in 10–15% of children with panhypopituitarism and those with IGHD. Intelligence is usually normal. Affected children may become shy and retiring.

Patients with Demonstrable Lesions of the Pituitary. The child is normal initially, and manifestations similar to those seen in idiopathic pituitary growth failure gradually appear and progress. When complete or almost complete destruction of the pituitary gland occurs, signs of pituitary insufficiency are present. Atrophy of the adrenal cortex, thyroid, and gonads results in loss of weight, asthenia, sensitivity to cold, mental torpor, and absence of sweating. Sexual maturation fails to take place or regresses if already present; there may be atrophy of the gonads and genital tract with amenorrhea and loss of pubic and axillary hair. There is a tendency to hypoglycemia and coma. Growth ceases. Diabetes insipidus may be present early but tends to improve spontaneously as the anterior pituitary is progressively destroyed.

If the lesion is an expanding tumor, symptoms such as headache, vomiting, visual disturbances, pathologic sleep patterns, decreased school performance, seizures, polyuria, and growth failure may occur. Slowing of growth may antedate neurologic signs and symptoms, especially with craniopharyngiomas, but symptoms of hormonal deficit account for only 10% of presenting complaints. In other patients, the neurologic manifestations may precede the endocrinologic, or evidence of pituitary insufficiency may first appear after surgical intervention. In children with craniopharyngiomas, visual field defects, optic atrophy, papilledema, and cranial nerve palsy are common.

LABORATORY FINDINGS. The diagnosis of classic GH deficiency is suspected in cases of profound postnatal growth failure, with heights more than 3 SD below the mean for age and gender. Acquired GH deficiency can occur at any age. There is dramatic slowing of growth, but when the disorder is of short duration, height may still be within the normal range. A strong clinical suspicion is important in establishing the diagnosis because laboratory measures of GH sufficiency lack specificity. Observation of low serum levels of IGF-I and the GH-dependent IGF-BP3 can be helpful. Values that are in the upper part of the normal range for age effectively exclude GH deficiency. Values for normally growing and children with hypopituitarism overlap during infancy and childhood.

Definitive diagnosis rests on demonstration of absent or low levels of GH in response to stimulation. A variety of provocative tests have been devised that rapidly increase the level of GH in normal children. These include a 20-min period of strenuous exercise or administration of L-dopa, insulin, arginine, clonidine, or glucagon. Peak levels of GH less than 7 μg/L are compatible with GH deficiency. The frequency of false-negative responses in normally growing children with any single test is considered to be approximately 20%. If this were true, about 4% of normal children would fail both tests. One study suggests that a majority of normal prepubertal children fail to achieve GH values greater than 7 μg/L with two pharmacologic tests. The researchers suggest that 3 days of estrogen priming should be used before GH testing to achieve greater diagnostic specificity.

During the 3 decades in which hGH was obtained by extraction from human pituitary glands culled at autopsy, its supply was sharply limited and only patients with classic GH deficiency were treated. With the advent of an unlimited supply of recombinant GH, there has been a marked interest in redefining the criteria for GH deficiency to include children with lesser degrees of deficiency. It has become popular to evaluate the spontaneous secretion of GH by measuring its level every 20 min during a 24- or 12-hr (8 P.M.–8 A.M.) period. Some short children with normal levels of GH when studied by provocative tests show little spontaneous GH secretion. Such children are considered to have GH neurosecretory dysfunction. With the collection of more normative data, it is clear that frequent GH sampling also lacks diagnostic specificity. There is a wide range of spontaneous GH secretion in normally growing prepubertal children and considerable overlap with the values observed in children with classic GH deficiency. Although the clinical and laboratory criteria for GH deficiency in patients with severe (classic) hypopituitarism are well established, the diagnostic criteria are unsettled for short children with lesser degrees of GH deficiency.

In addition to establishing the diagnosis of GH deficiency, it is necessary to examine other pituitary functions. Levels of TSH, thyroxine (T_4), ACTH, cortisol, dehydroepiandrosterone sulfate, gonadotropins, and gonadal steroids may provide evidence of other pituitary hormonal deficiencies. The defect can be localized to the hypothalamus if there is a normal response to the administration of hypothalamic-releasing hormones for GH, TSH, ACTH, or gonadotropins. When there is a deficiency of TSH, serum levels of T_4 and TSH are low. A normal rise in TSH and PRL after stimulation with thyrotropin-releasing hormone places the defect in the hypothalamus, and absence of such a response localizes the defect to the pituitary. An elevated level of plasma PRL taken at random in the patient with hypopituitarism is also strong evidence that the defect is in the hypothalamus rather than in the pituitary. Some children with craniopharyngioma have elevated PRL levels before surgery, but after surgery, PRL deficiency occurs because of pituitary damage. Antidiuretic hormone deficiency may be established by appropriate studies.

ROENTGENOGRAPHIC EXAMINATION. Roentgenograms of the skull are most helpful when there is a destructive or space-occupying lesion causing hypopituitarism. Evidence of increased intracranial pressure may be found in patients with nausea, vomiting, loss of vision, headache, or an increase in circumference of the head. Enlargement of the sella, especially ballooning with erosion and calcifications within or above the sella, may be detected. Magnetic resonance imaging is indicated in all patients with hypopituitarism. In addition to providing detail about space-occupying lesions, it can define the size of the anterior and posterior pituitary lobes and the pituitary stalk. It is superior to computed tomography in differentiating a full from an empty sella turcica. The posterior pituitary is readily recognized as a bright spot. In many cases of idiopathic multiple pituitary hormone deficiency with prenatal or perinatal onset, the posterior pituitary bright spot is ectopic. It appears at the base of the hypothalamus rather than in the pituitary fossa. This diagnostic technique can provide timely confirmation of suspected hypopituitarism in a newborn with hypoglycemia and micropenis.

Skeletal maturation is markedly delayed in patients with long-standing GH deficiency. The bone age tends to be approximately 75% of chronologic age. It may be even more delayed for patients with TSH and GH deficiency. The fontanels may remain open beyond the 2nd yr, and intersutural wormian bones may be found. Long bones are slender and osteopenic. Newer methods of assessing body composition, such as dual photon x-ray absorptiometry, show deficient bone mineralization, deficiencies in lean body mass, and a corresponding increase in adiposity.

DIFFERENTIAL DIAGNOSIS. The causes of growth disorders are legion. *Systemic conditions* such as inflammatory bowel disease, celiac disease, occult renal disease, and anemia must always be considered. A few otherwise normal children are short (i.e., >3 SD below the mean for age) and grow 5 cm/yr or less but have normal levels of GH in response to provocative tests and normal spontaneous episodic secretion. Most of these children show increased rates of growth when treated with GH in doses comparable to those used to treat children with hypopituitarism. Plasma levels of IGF-I in these patients may be normal or low. Several groups of treated children have achieved final or near final adult heights. Different studies have found changes in adult height that range from −2.5 to +7.5 cm compared to pretreatment predictions. There are no methods that can reliably predict which of these children will become taller as adults as a result of GH treatment and which will have compromised adult height. Such treatment of short children without proven hypopituitarism is undergoing experimental trials.

Constitutional growth delay is one of the variants of normal growth commonly encountered by the pediatrician. Length and weight measurements of affected children are normal at birth, and growth is normal for the first 4–12 mo of life. Growth then decelerates to near or below the 3rd percentile for height and weight. By 2–3 yr of age, growth resumes at a normal rate of 5 cm/yr or more. Studies of GH secretion and other studies are within normal limits. Bone age is closer to height age than to chronologic age. Detailed questioning often reveals other family members (frequently one or both parents) with histories of short stature in childhood, delayed puberty, and eventual normal stature. The prognosis for these children to achieve normal adult height is good. Boys with unusual degrees of delayed puberty may benefit from a short course of testosterone therapy to hasten puberty after 14 yr of age. The cause of this variant of normal growth is thought to be persistence of the relatively hypogonadotropic state of childhood (see Chapter 14). Constitutional growth delay can be differentiated from genetic short stature by the level of skeletal maturation, which is consistent with chronologic age in the latter condition. Genetic short stature is usually found in other family members. Results of studies of hormones related to growth, however, are normal.

Primary hypothyroidism is usually easily diagnosed on clinical grounds. Responses to GH provocative tests may be subnormal, and enlargement of the sella may be present. Low T_4 and elevated TSH levels clearly establish the diagnosis. Pituitary hyperplasia recedes during treatment with thyroid hormone. Because thyroid hormone is a necessary prerequisite for normal GH synthesis, its levels must always be assessed before GH studies.

Emotional deprivation is an important cause of retardation of growth and mimics hypopituitarism. The condition is known as psychosocial dwarfism, maternal deprivation dwarfism, or hyperphagic short stature. The mechanisms by which sensory and emotional deprivation interfere with growth are not fully understood. Functional hypopituitarism is indicated by low levels of IGF-I and by inadequate responses of GH to provocative stimuli. Puberty may be normal or even premature in its appearance. Appropriate history and careful observations reveal disturbed mother-child or family relations and provide clues to the diagnosis (see Chapter 35.2). Proof may be difficult to establish because the adults responsible often hide the true family situation from professionals, and the children rarely divulge their plight. Emotionally deprived children frequently have perverted or voracious appetites, enuresis, encopresis, insomnia, crying spasms, and sudden tantrums. The subgroup of children with hyperphagia and a normal body mass index tends to show catch-up growth when placed in a less stressful environment.

The *Silver-Russell syndrome* is characterized by short stature, frontal bossing, small triangular facies, sparse subcutaneous tissue, shortened and incurved 5th fingers, and in many cases, asymmetry (i.e., hemihypertrophy). Affected children have low birthweights for gestational age. Studies have revealed some degree of GH secretory deficiency in very short children with intrauterine growth retardation, whether or not they have Silver-Russell syndrome. Short-term treatment with GH often results in increased rates of growth, but its long-term benefits are unknown.

TREATMENT. The Lawson Wilkins Pediatric Endocrine Society and the Academy of Pediatrics have published guidelines for treatment with recombinant growth hormone. In children with classic GH deficiency, treatment should be started as soon as possible to narrow the gap in height between patients and their classmates during childhood and to have the greatest effect on mature height. The recommended dose of hGH is 0.18–0.3 mg/kg/wk. It is administered subcutaneously in six or seven divided doses. If the effect of therapy wanes, compliance should be evaluated before the dose is increased. Concurrent treatment with GH and a luteinizing hormone–releasing hormone agonist has been used in the hope that interruption of puberty will delay epiphyseal fusion and prolong growth. This strategy may augment final height, but it can also increase the discrepancy in physical maturity between GH-deficient children and their age peers. Therapy should be continuous until near final height is achieved. Criteria for stopping treatment include a growth rate less than 1 inch per yr and a bone age of greater than 14 yr in girls and greater that 16 yr in boys.

Some patients treated with GH have subsequently acquired leukemia. The risk of leukemia in treated patients may be double that in the general population. There is conflicting evidence about whether GH treatment confers an increase in risk or whether the increased incidence reflects the consequences of therapeutic radiation for craniopharyngiomas and brain tumors. Other reported side effects include pseudotumor cerebri, slipped capital femoral epiphysis, gynecomastia, and worsening of scoliosis. There is an increase in total body water during the first 1–2 wk of treatment. Fasting and postprandial insulin levels are characteristically low before treatment, and they normalize during GH replacement. Development of diabetes mellitus is rare. Older GH-deficient patients treated with cadaver pituitary extracts are at risk for Creutzfeldt-Jakob disease for at least 10–15 yr after therapy. Recombinant GH has eliminated this risk.

Maximal response to GH occurs in the first year of treatment. With each successive year of treatment, the response tends to decrease. Some patients receiving GH acquire reversible hypothyroidism. Periodic evaluation of thyroid function is indicated for all patients treated with GH. GHRH is nearly as effective as GH in the treatment of children with hypothalamic causes of hypopituitarism with a deficiency of GHRH, but daily subcutaneous injections are required. When a depot form becomes available, it may provide a practical form of treatment for this group of children. Recombinant IGF-I may prove useful in the treatment of children with Laron's syndrome and possibly those with GH1 gene deletions and high titers of antibodies.

The doses of GH used to treat children with classic GH deficiency usually enhance the growth of many non–GH-deficient children as well. Intensive investigation is in progress to determine the full spectrum of short children who may benefit from treatment with GH. Growth hormone is currently approved for treatment of children with growth failure as a result of Turner syndrome and end-stage renal failure before kidney transplantation. Children with intrauterine growth retardation, Noonan syndrome, skeletal dysplasia, and others experience increases in growth velocity when treated with GH. There are preliminary indications that GH treatment adds an average of 2 inches to adult height in children with the Russell-Silver syndrome. In children with all other causes of short stature, it is unknown whether GH treatment increases their final height, and treatment of such patients should be confined to prospective clinical trials until further data establish the validity of this expensive, long-term form of therapy.

Replacement should also be directed at other hormonal deficiencies. In TSH-deficient subjects, thyroid hormone is given in full replacement doses. In ACTH-deficient patients, the optimal dose of hydrocortisone should not exceed 10 mg/m²/24 hr. Increases are made during illness or in anticipation of surgical procedures. Therapy can often be deferred until growth has been completed if the deficiency is partial. In patients with a deficiency of gonadotropins, gonadal steroids are given when bone age reaches the age at which puberty usually takes place. For infants with microphallus, one or two 3-mo courses of monthly intramuscular injections of 25 mg of testosterone enanthate may bring the penis to normal size without an inordinate effect on osseous maturation.

Allen DB, Fost NC: Growth hormone therapy for short stature: Panacea or Pandora's box. J Pediatr 117:16, 1990.

Amselem S, Duquesnoy P, Goossens M: Molecular basis of Laron dwarfism. Trend Endocrinol Metab 2:35, 1991.

August GP, Gulius JR, Blethen SL: Adult height in children with growth hormone deficiency who are treated with biosynthetic growth hormone: The National Cooperative Growth Study experience. Pediatrics 102:512, 1998.

Berg MA, Guevara-Aguirre J, Rosenbloom AL, et al: Mutation creating a new splice site in the growth hormone receptor genes of 37 Ecuadorian patients with Laron syndrome. Hum Mutat 1:24, 1992.

Cacciari E, Tassoni P, Parisi G, et al: Pitfalls in diagnosing impaired growth hormone (GH) secretion: Retesting after replacement therapy of 63 patients defined as GH deficient. J Clin Endocrinol Metab 74:1284, 1992.

Cara JF, Kreiter ML, Rosenfield RL: Height prognosis of children with true precocious puberty and growth hormone deficiency: Effect of combination therapy with gonadotropin releasing hormone agonist and growth hormone. J Pediatr 120:709, 1992.

Clayton PE, Shalet SM: Dose dependency of time of onset of radiation-induced growth hormone deficiency. J Pediatr 118:226, 1991.

Cogan JC, Phillips JA III, Sakati N, et al: Heterogeneous growth hormone (GH) gene mutations in familial GH deficiency. J Clin Endocrinol Metab 76:1224, 1993.

Committee on Drugs and Committee on Bioethics: Considerations related to the use of recombinant human growth hormone in children. Pediatrics 99:122, 1997.

Costin G, Murphree AL: Hypothalamic-pituitary function in children with optic nerve hypoplasia. Am J Dis Child 139:249, 1985.

Dean HJ, Bishop A, Winter JSD: Growth hormone deficiency in patients with histiocytosis. J Pediatr 109:615, 1986.

de Zegher F, Albertsson-Wikland, Wilton P, et al: Growth hormone treatment of short children born short for gestational age: Metanalysis of four independent, randomized, controlled, multicentre studies. Acta Paediatr Suppl 417:27, 1996.

Donaldson DL, Hallowell JG, Pan E, et al: Growth hormone secretory profiles: Variation on consecutive nights. J Pediatr 115:51, 1989.

Duquesnoy P, Sobrier ML, Duriez B, et al: A single amino acid substitution in the exoplasmic domain of the human growth hormone (GH) receptor confers familial GH resistance (Laron syndrome) with positive GH binding activity by abolishing receptor homodimerization. EMBO J 13:1386, 1994.

Guevara-Aguirre J, Rosenbloom AL, Fielder PJ, et al: Growth hormone receptor deficiency in Ecuador: Clinical and biochemical phenotype in two populations. J Clin Endocrinol Metab 76:417, 1993.

Guidelines for the use of growth hormone in children with short stature. A report by the Drug and Therapeutics Committee of the Lawson Wilkins Pediatric Endocrine Society. J Pediatr 127:857, 1995.

Hall JG, Pallister PD, Carren SK, et al: Congenital hypothalamic hamartoblastoma, hypopituitarism, imperforate anus, and postaxial polydactyly: A new syndrome? Part 1: Clinical, causal and pathogenetic considerations. Am J Med Genet 7:47, 1980.

Hasegawa Y, Hasegawa T, Aso T, et al: Clinical utility of insulin-like growth factor binding protein-3 in the evaluation and treatment of short children with suspected growth hormone deficiency. Eur J Endocrinol 131:27, 1994.

Herman SP, Baggenstoss AM, Clothier MD: Liver dysfunction and histiologic abnormalities in neonatal hypopituitarism. J Pediatr 87:892, 1975.

Kamijo T, Phillips JA III, Ogawa M, et al: Screening for growth hormone gene deletions in patients with isolated growth hormone deficiency. J Pediatr 118:245, 1991.

Kappy M, Blizzard RM, Migeon CJ: Wilkins: The Diagnosis and Treatment of Endocrine Disorders in Childhood and Adolescence, 4th ed. Springfield, IL, Charles C Thomas, 1994.

Kuroiwa T, Okabe Y, Hasuo K, et al: MR imaging of pituitary dwarfism. Am J Neuroradiol 12:161, 1991.

LaFranchi S: Human growth hormone. Who is a candidate for treatment? Postgrad Med 91:367, 1992.

Laron Z, Lilos P, Klinger B: Growth curves for Laron syndrome. Arch Dis Child 68:768, 1993.

Lesage C, Walker J, Landier F, et al: Near normalization of adolescent height with growth hormone therapy in very short children without growth hormone deficiency. J Pediatr 119:29, 1991.

Littley MD, Shalet SM, Beardwell CG, et al: Radiation-induced hypopituitarism is dose-dependent. Clin Endocrinol 31:363, 1989.

Lovinger RD, Kaplan SL, Grumbach MM: Congenital hypopituitarism associated with neonatal hypoglycemia and microphallus: Four cases secondary to hypothalamic hormone deficiencies. J Pediatr 87:1171, 1975.

Low LC: The therapeutic use of growth-hormone-releasing hormone. J Pediatr Endocrinol 6:15, 1993.

MacGillivary MH, Blethen SL, Buchlis JG, et al: Current dosing of growth hormone in children with growth hormone deficiency: How physiologic? Pediatrics 102:527, 1998.

Margalith D, Tze WJ, Jan JE: Congenital optic nerve hypoplasia with hypothalamic-pituitary dysplasia. Am J Dis Child 139:361, 1985.

Marin GM, Domene HM, Barnes KM, et al: The effects of estrogen priming and puberty on the growth hormone response to standardized treadmill exercise and arginine-insulin in normal girls and boys. J Clin Endocrinol Metab 79:537, 1994.

Miller WL, Kaplan SL, Grumbach MM: Child abuse as a cause of post-traumatic hypopituitarism. N Engl J Med 302:724, 1980.

Moell C, Marky I, Hovi L, et al: Cerebral irradiation causes blunted pubertal growth in girls treated for acute leukemia. Med Pediatr Oncol 22:375, 1994.

Neely EK, Rosenfeld RG: Use and abuse of human growth hormone. Annu Rev Med 45:407, 1994.

Parks JS, Abdul-Latif H, Kinoshita E, et al: Genetics of growth hormone gene expression. Horm Res 40:54, 1993.

Parks JS, Adess ME, Brown MR: Genes regulating hypothalamic and pituitary development. Acta Paediatr Suppl 423:28, 1997.

Pfäffle RW, DiMattia GE, Parks JS, et al: Mutation of the POU-specific domain of Pit-1 and hypopituitarism without pituitary hypoplasia. Science 257:1118, 1992.

Radovick S, Nations M, Du Y, et al: A mutation in the POU-homeodomain of Pit-1 responsible for combined pituitary hormone deficiency. Science 257:1115, 1992.

Ranke MB, Lindberg A: Growth hormone treatment of short children born small for gestational age or with Silver-Russell syndrome: results from KIGS (Kabi International Growth Study), including the first report on final height. Acta Paediatr Suppl 417:18, 1996.

Rose SR, Ross JL, Uriarte M, et al: The advantage of measuring stimulated as compared with spontaneous growth hormone levels in the diagnosis of growth hormone deficiency. N Engl J Med 319:201, 1988.

Rosenfeld RG, Rosenbloom AL, Guevara-Aguirre J: Growth hormone (GH) insensitivity due to primary GH receptor deficiency. Endocr Rev 15:369, 1994.

Semina EV, Reiter R, Leysens NJ, et al: Cloning and characterization of a novel bicoid-related homeobox transcription factor gene, RIEG, involved in Rieger syndrome. Nat Genet 14:392, 1996.

Skuse D, Albanese A, Stanhope R, et al: A new stress-related syndrome of growth failure and hyperphagia in children, associated with reversibility of growth hormone inufficiency. Lancet 348:353, 1996.

Stanhope R, Albanese A, Hindmarsh P, Brook CG: The effects of growth hormone therapy on spontaneous sexual development. Horm Res 38(Suppl 1):9, 1992.

Takahashi Y, Kaji H, Okimura Y, et al: Short stature caused by a mutant growth hormone. N Engl J Med 334:432, 1996.

Tanaka T, Satoh M, Yasunaga T, et al: GH and GnRH analog treatment in children who enter puberty at short stature. J Pediatr Endocrinol Metab 10:623, 1997.

Tatsumi K, Miyai K, Notomi T, et al: Cretinism with combined hormone deficiency caused by a mutation in the Pit-1 gene. Nat Genet 1:56, 1992.

Walker JM, Bond SA, Voss LD, et al: Treatment of short normal children with growth hormone: A cautionary tale? Lancet 336:1331, 1990.

White MC, Chahal P, Banks L, et al: Familial hypopituitarism associated with an enlarged pituitary fossa and an empty sella. Clin Endocrinol 24:63, 1986.

Wilson DM, Dotson RJ, Neely EK, et al: Effects of estrogen on growth hormone following clonidine stimulation. Am J Dis Child 147:63, 1993.

Woods KA, Camacho-Hubner C, Savage MO, Clark AJ: Intrauterine growth retardation and postnatal growth failure associated with deletion of the insulin-like growth factor gene. N Engl J Med 35:1363, 1996.

Wu W, Cogan JD, Pfaffle RW, et al: Mutations in PROP1 cause familial combined pituitary hormone deficiency. Nat Genet 18:147, 1998.

Zadik Z, Landau H, Limoni Y, et al: Predictors of growth response to growth hormone in otherwise normal short children. J Pediatr 121:44, 1992.

CHAPTER 568
Diabetes Insipidus

H. William Harris, Jr.

Diabetes insipidus (DI) is a disease characterized by polyuria and excessive thirst. DI may result from either a lack of arginine vasopressin (AVP; antidiuretic hormone), or failure of AVP-sensitive epithelial cells of the kidney collecting duct to respond normally to the hormone. When considering the diagnosis or treatment of DI, it is useful to divide DI into its two major forms. Central DI results from various abnormalities of AVP synthesis or secretion, or both, that result in a lack of circulating AVP to modulate renal water reabsorption. Nephrogenic DI (NDI) results from a lack of a normal response by AVP-sensitive kidney tubules to increase renal water reabsorption in the presence of adequate AVP. Central DI or NDI may be caused by inherited primary forms of the disease or may result from a variety of secondary or acquired causes.

PATHOGENESIS

Normal Physiology. AVP is synthesized by the supraoptic and paraventricular nuclei of the hypothalamus and then transported through axons to the posterior pituitary where the hormone is stored until its release (also see Chapter 566). AVP is synthesized initially as a prohormone (propressophysin or VP-NP) that is subsequently packaged and processed in secretory granules within hypothalamic neurons. AVP is then released to distribute itself in the body's extracellular space where it normally exhibits a half-life of approximately 10–25 min. Although AVP secretion is controlled by multiple factors (e.g., alterations in blood volume and other hormones), AVP release from the posterior pituitary is primarily regulated by alterations in plasma osmolality. Under normal circumstances, control of AVP release is set so that secretion of hormone is very low or undetectable when plasma osmolality falls to less than a threshold value (approximately 280 mOsm/kg in healthy adolescents and adults). As plasma osmolality rises to greater than this osmotic threshold, AVP secretion increases in a manner that closely correlates with the level of plasma osmolality. Thirst is also regulated largely by alterations in plasma osmolality and appears to be mediated by a collection of neurons in the same area of the brain that mediates AVP secretion.

AVP receptors are classified as V_1 and V_2 receptors and are present in multiple organs in the body. The primary site of AVP action in the kidney is a nephron segment called the *collecting duct.* In the absence of AVP stimulation, the apical or urine-facing cell membranes of AVP-responsive collecting duct epithelial cells exhibit an extremely low water permeability. This low water permeability permits the excretion of a large volume of dilute urine (100 mOsm/kg) produced by active solute transport in more proximal nephron segments. In contrast, AVP stimulation of the collecting duct causes rapid increases in its water permeability. When AVP binds to the V_2 receptor present on the basolateral (blood-facing) membrane of collecting duct epithelial cells, the V_2 receptor interacts via G protein coupling with adenylyl cyclase to increase intracellular cyclic adenosine monophosphate levels within collecting duct epithelial cells. Elevations in intracellular cyclic adenosine monophosphate serve as the second messenger to initiate the fusion of subapical vesicles containing a water channel protein into the collecting duct membrane. As shown in Figure 568–1, this water channel protein of approximately 29,000 d is called aquaporin 2 (AQP 2) and possesses an extremely narrow water-filled transmembrane pore that allows for the transport of water but not other small solutes (including urea and sodium) across the apical membrane. Transepithelial water reabsorption occurs in response to the osmotic gradient that exists between the tubular fluid and the surrounding kidney interstitium. When body water stores require maximal conservation under normal circumstances in the presence of AVP, collecting ducts in the kidney cortex reabsorb approximately two thirds of the water presented to the collecting ducts to create iso-osmotic urine (280–300 mOsm/kg). In contrast, collecting ducts located more distally in the hyperosmotic regions of the kidney medulla reabsorb more water to create a hyperosmotic (1,200–2,000 mOsm/kg) concentrated urine. Removal of AVP stimulation produces retrieval of AQP 2 vesicles from the apical membrane and a return to a low water permeability state.

Etiology and Pathophysiology of Central Diabetes Insipidus. Any lesion that damages the neurohypophyseal unit responsible for AVP synthesis and release may result in central DI. The central common lesion in central DI is a lack of adequate circulating AVP necessary to respond to the body's demands for water conservation. Primary inherited forms of central DI are rare. These genetic abnormalities include an autosomal dominant form of central DI characterized by variable onset (birth to several years of age) and severity. Mutations have been localized to the vasopressin-neurophysin (VP-NP) gene on chromosome 20 where disruptions in the processing of this AVP precursor may cause selective death of magnocellular neurons over time. Other inherited diseases associated with central DI include *Wolfram syndrome* (autosomal recessive/mitochondrial disorder, chromosome 4) and *septo-optic dysplasia* (see Chapter 567).

Secondary or acquired causes of central DI are more common. These include tumors of the suprasellular and chiasmatic regions, particularly craniopharyngiomas (Figure 568–2), optic

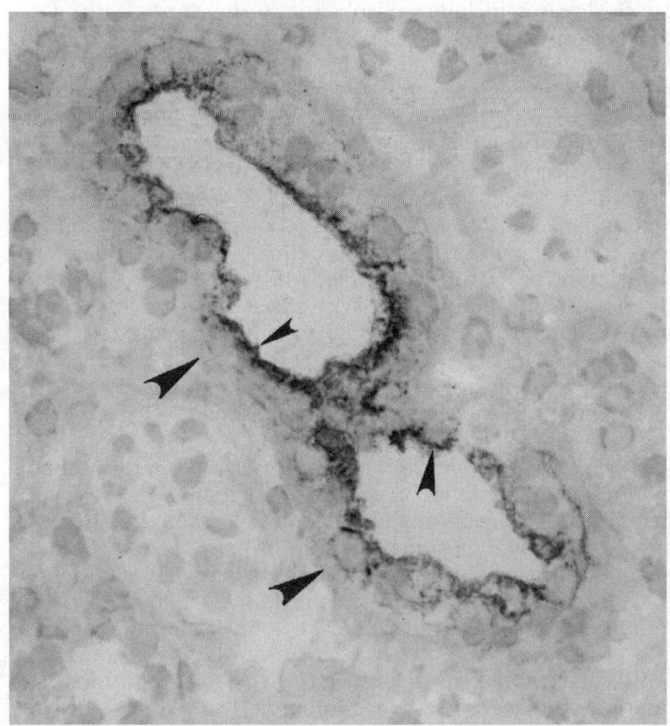

Figure 568–1 Immunolocalization of the AVP-elicited AQP 2 water channel in human collecting duct. The binding of a specific anti–AQP 2 antiserum is indicated by the rose-colored reaction product and localizes AQP 2 to the apical membrane of collecting duct epithelial cells. Note that most of the AQP 2 is present in the apical membrane (small arrowheads) instead of the basolateral membrane (larger arrowheads) where the V_2 receptor is located. Other kidney tubules not expressing AQP 2 are stained light blue in this section from human kidney cortex.

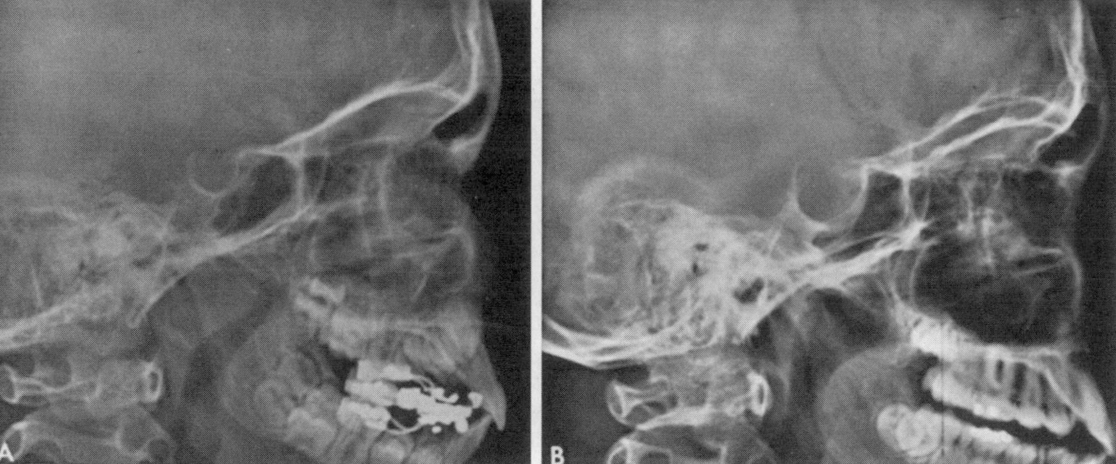

Figure 568–2 Skull roentgenographs of a child with central DI. *A*, Roentgenograph of the skull of a 9-yr-old boy with polydipsia, polyuria, nocturia, and enuresis. Urine specific gravity was 1.010 after water deprivation. Growth was normal. The sella turcica was considered roentgenographically to be at the upper limit of normal but was probably enlarged. *B*, The patient returned at 14 yr of age because of growth failure and delay in sexual maturation. Note the enlargement and thinning of the sella turcica as well as the absence of intrasellar or suprasellar calcification. Neurologic and ophthalmologic examinations were normal. At surgery, a large craniopharyngioma was found.

gliomas, and germinomas. The symptoms of increased intracranial pressure may accompany those of DI or may follow years later. In a similar manner, injuries to the head, especially basal skull fractures, may produce DI either immediately or after a delay of several months. Operative procedures near the pituitary or hypothalamus may result in transitory or permanent DI. Central DI is often present as a terminal event in patients with severely compromised brain function.

Central DI may be associated with many systemic diseases. These diseases include encephalitis, histiocytosis, sarcoidosis, tuberculosis, actinomycosis, and leukemia. Central DI resulting from the presence of autoantibodies to AVP-producing cells has also been reported. In the newborn, DI has been reported in association with asphyxia, intraventricular hemorrhage, intravascular coagulopathy, *Listeria monocytogenes* sepsis, and group B streptococcal meningitis.

In many instances, the exact cause of central DI cannot be determined initially. However, after careful examination and long-term follow-up, only approximately 20% of these patients may be classified as idiopathic. Importantly, in more than one half of all patients with intracranial tumors, clinical or neuroradiological signs (or both) are not manifested until 1 yr after DI has been diagnosed, and in 25% of patients the delay is as long as 4 yr. Thus, periodic evaluation for an interval of at least 4 yr after DI is diagnosed is required before the entity is called idiopathic.

Etiology and Pathophysiology of Nephrogenic Diabetes Insipidus. Abnormalities in kidney function and structure that affect the collecting duct are causes of nephrogenic DI. Abnormalities that affect collecting duct function in both the cortex and medulla of the kidney produce more significant polyuria than lesions that are localized primarily to the kidney medulla. Primary inherited causes of nephrogenic DI result from mutations that affect both the V_2 receptor as well as the AQP 2 water channel. The V_2 receptor gene is localized to the X chromosome and multiple families possessing mutations that either inactivate the function or alter the intracellular processing of the V_2 receptor have been reported. The male members of these families are severely affected, whereas females are asymptomatic carriers of the disease. However, in some pedigrees, females also manifest either mild or severe NDI symptoms presumably via an X chromosomal inactivation mechanism. Cases have also been reported where V_2 receptor mutations appear de novo within a given family. In contrast, detailed examination of individuals manifesting an inherited autosomal recessive form of NDI have revealed these patients are complex heterozygotes possessing mutations in the AQP 2 gene localized to chromosome 12.

Secondary or acquired forms of nephrogenic DI are more common than primary inherited forms and are associated with a variety of disorders or drug administration. A major side effect of lithium therapy is development of NDI, which is often severe and persists despite discontinuation of the drug. NDI is also associated with prolonged intervals of hypercalcemia or hypokalemia and is present in conjunction with inherited disorders of renal development, including polycystic kidney disease, juvenile nephronophthisis, and renal dysplasia. Disease processes that cause injury to collecting ducts and surrounding renal tubules, including sickle cell anemia, chronic pyelonephritis, sarcoidosis, amyloidosis, and urinary tract obstruction, may produce either mild or severe symptoms.

CLINICAL MANIFESTATIONS. Although polyuria and polydipsia are the hallmarks of DI, these symptoms may not be recognized immediately by either family members or caregivers. Often, the clinical features of NDI are dominated by signs and symptoms of chronic dehydration. In infants with NDI, such symptoms include irritability, poor feeding, growth failure, and intermittent high fevers. If unrecognized, intervals of dehydration and hypernatremia may result in brain damage and impairment of mental function, leading to abnormal behavior, including mental retardation, hyperactivity, distractibility, short attention span, and restlessness. In children who have acquired bladder control, enuresis may be the first symptom. Signs and symptoms of central DI depend on the primary lesion. For example, patients with hypothalamic tumors may have disturbances in growth, progressive cachexia or obesity, hyperpyrexia, sleep disturbance, sexual precocity, or emotional disorders. Lesions initially causing DI may eventually destroy the anterior pituitary and its associated endocrine axes. Patients with either central DI or NDI must be distinguished from other individuals who manifest primary polydipsia that is caused either by a defect in thirst (dipsogenic DI, adipsia-hypodipsia—absence or blunting of normal thirst) or by mental illness (psychogenic polydipsia). Because the thirst centers of the brain are immediately adjacent to the neurons responsible for AVP secretion, a combined central DI as well as derangement of the normal thirst mechanism is possible.

Long-standing states of polyuria may cause the development

of megacystis and, more rarely, hydroureter and hydronephrosis that can mimic lower urinary tract obstruction. It is important to emphasize that many patients with DI have compensated for their lack of urinary concentrating ability by drinking large amounts of fluid and thus become extremely vulnerable when deprived of free access to water. This is particularly true during hospitalization during which patients with NDI may be placed on fluid restriction or prevented from ingesting their large oral water intake and given only "maintenance" intravenous fluid regimens.

DIAGNOSIS AND TREATMENT. The daily volume of urine in patients with DI varies widely depending on the specific cause of DI. In general, the urine is pale and colorless, and its specific gravity varies between 1.001 and 1.010 with a corresponding osmolality of 50–300 mOsm/kg. Other renal function studies are normal. Serum osmolality may vary widely depending on the hydration status of the patient, and often DI is first considered in the setting of life-threatening hypernatremia. A careful patient history, including an actual quantitation of how much the patient drinks per day, voiding patterns, and dietary and drug intake, provides important clues as to the diagnosis of DI. Obtaining a serum AVP measurement is often helpful in establishing the diagnosis of DI when the patient initially presents to medical attention and is clearly in a hyperosmolar state voiding hypo-osmotic urine prior to medical therapy. An extremely low or absent serum AVP level under these conditions strongly suggests the diagnosis of central DI. However, often the diagnosis of either central DI or NDI requires either a water deprivation test or administration of 1-desamino-8-D-arginine vasopressin (DDAVP) to test whether the patient is capable of responding to AVP. During a water deprivation test, patients must be monitored closely not only for signs of dehydration but also for surreptitious water intake. In patients with severe DI, a 3 hr interval of water deprivation may result in elevation of serum osmolality, whereas urine osmolality remains at less than plasma values.

In central DI, administration of DDAVP either intranasally or by intravenous infusion raises urine osmolality. In milder cases of central DI, urine osmolality may exceed that of plasma, and the response to DDAVP is attenuated. Patients with primary polydipsia concentrate urine during an 8-hr water deprivation test without DDAVP administration. Radiologic studies including magnetic resonance imaging (MRI) of the skull may reveal evidence of an intracranial tumor in the form of calcifications, enlargement of the sella turcica, erosion of the clinoid processes, or increased width of suture lines. MRI can differentiate the posterior pituitary from the anterior pituitary by a hyperintense signal called the *bright spot*. The bright spot is present in scans of most normal patients but is usually absent in patients with hypothalamic-neurohypophyseal tract lesions.

Although individuals with NDI may also exhibit increases in serum osmolality after 3–8 hr of water deprivation, their corresponding urine osmolality does not increase. Moreover, administration of either intranasal or intravenous DDAVP produces no increase in urine osmolality. In normal individuals, DDAVP administration exerts a vasodilatory response that is manifested in the form of flushing, fall in diastolic blood pressure, and a rise in pulse rates. These cardiovascular effects as well as transient releases of von Willebrand factor antigen, factor VII activity, and tissue-type plasminogen activator are believed to be mediated by extrarenal V_2 receptors. In patients with X-linked V_2 receptor mutations, none of these DDAVP-mediated effects is present. Careful consideration should be taken to eliminate secondary causes of NDI, including appropriate studies of the anatomy of the kidney and lower urinary tract as well as a search for the presence of systemic or metabolic diseases that may cause NDI.

The cornerstone of therapy for central DI is administration of DDAVP, usually via an intranasal route. DDAVP binds almost exclusively to V_2 receptors and is more resistant to degradation by body peptidases than endogenous AVP. Thus, the antidiuretic effects of DDAVP last 8–10 hr as compared with 1–3 hr for AVP. The usual intranasal dose used for treatment of central DI ranges from 5–10 μg, given in single or divided dosages. Children younger than 2 yr of age require smaller doses (0.15–0.5 μg/kg/24 hr). It is important to individualize therapy and allow patients to revert to mild polyuria before the next dose is given. Intravenous therapy is also available for patients who are comatose, undergoing surgery, or are unable to use intranasal therapy optimally.

Therapy for NDI should ensure a sufficient intake of water to replace the large urinary water losses. Because renal water requirements are directly proportional to renal osmolar solute loads, restriction of sodium intake reduces obligatory water losses by the kidney. Thus, a diet containing low sodium (less than 1 mmol/kg/24 hr), adequate protein (2 g/kg/24 hr), and 300–400 mL/kg of water is recommended. Several drugs have been demonstrated to reduce the polyuria of NDI. Thiazide diuretics (hydrochlorothiazide, 2–4 mg/kg/24 hr) may reduce urine output by 50% but may produce hypokalemia. Thiazides appear to act by reducing the amount of water and solute presented to the collecting duct by inducing a state of mild volume depletion. Prostaglandin synthesis inhibitors such as indomethacin (2 mg/kg/24 hr) also reduce polyuria and may be used in combination with hydrochlorothiazide. Prolonged use of indomethacin may result in gastrointestinal, central nervous system, or hematopoietic side effects. Finally, the potassium-sparing diuretic amiloride (20 mg/1.73 m^2/24 hr) also reduces urine output and may also be used in combination with hydrochlorothiazide.

It is important to appreciate the unique intravenous fluid requirements of children with NDI. After episodes of dehydration, these patients usually require replacement of large quantities of water but not sodium. Thus, intravenous rehydration regimens designed for children with normal renal function are not optimal and may even be life-threatening. Judicious use of intravenous fluids (0.45% or 0.25% sodium chloride) together with frequent determinations of serum electrolytes are important in the management of these patients.

PROGNOSIS AND GENETIC COUNSELING. The prognosis of children with central DI is often determined by the underlying process causing the abnormality in AVP secretion. Central DI may be transient or long-standing. Uncomplicated central DI can be managed to permit a high quality of life for patients affected by this disorder.

The prognosis for children with NDI is also good provided that there is careful clinical and laboratory monitoring. Early reports of associated mental retardation of children with inherited X-linked NDI have now been determined to result from brain damage caused by intervals of hypernatremia and dehydration resulting from suboptimal therapy. These data highlight the importance of clinical care in early infancy. However, there are isolated reports of the development of chronic renal failure in patients with NDI. For children suspected of possessing V_2 receptor or AQP 2 water channel protein mutations, the technology is available for determination of specific genetic lesions by DNA sequence analyses. Educational materials for both families and physicians as well as summaries of relevant research efforts in nephrogenic DI are provided by the NDI Foundation, Eastsound, WA, USA (Internet address: www.ndif.org).

CHAPTER 569
Other Abnormalities of Arginine Vasopressin Metabolism and Action

H. William Harris Jr.

569.1 Syndrome of Inappropriate Secretion of Antidiuretic Hormone

Although syndrome of inappropriate secretion of antidiuretic hormone (SIADH) is one of the most common abnormalities in arginine vasopressin (AVP) secretion encountered in adult medicine, its incidence in the pediatric population is rare. In this condition, plasma levels of AVP are inappropriately elevated as compared to normal with respect to concurrent body osmolality, and AVP levels are not suppressed by further decreases in blood osmolality. Thus, the combination of hyponatremia and low serum osmolality together with an inappropriately high urine osmolality and low urine volume are hallmarks of SIADH. Careful studies should eliminate other possible causes of hyponatremia, including cardiac failure, nephrotic syndrome, chronic liver disease, glucocorticoid deficiency, surreptitious diuretic use, or hypothyroidism.

ETIOLOGY AND PATHOGENESIS. SIADH may be caused by either inappropriate secretion of AVP from its normal hypothalamic source or, less often, secretion of peptides that mimic AVP's action by neoplastic tissues. AVP secretion that is not regulated by the normal osmotic feedback mechanisms results in continued water reabsorption by the kidney collecting duct and progressive dilution of body osmolality.

Although its exact pathogenesis is not fully understood, SIADH is often associated with multiple disease processes that alter central nervous system (CNS) and hypothalamic function. These diseases include direct insults to the brain such as meningitis, encephalitis, brain tumors and abscesses, CNS leukemia, subarachnoid hemorrhages, Guillain-Barré syndrome, head trauma, and surgical procedures. Other diseases causing SIADH include pneumonia, tuberculosis, acute intermittent porphyria, cystic fibrosis, infant botulism, perinatal asphyxia, and use of positive pressure ventilatory support. SIADH has also been reported after administration of vincristine or vinblastine.

Malignant tumors, including those of the lung, particularly oat cell carcinoma; Ewing's sarcoma; and tumors of the pancreas, duodenum, or thymus are associated with the development of SIADH. SIADH may disappear on removal of lung carcinoma.

CLINICAL MANIFESTATIONS AND LABORATORY FINDINGS. Often SIADH is first recognized on finding an inappropriately low value for serum sodium in a child without other major symptoms and no evidence of dehydration. Skin turgor and blood pressure are usually normal, particularly if the serum sodium concentration is greater than 120 mEq/L. Overt clinical manifestations of SIADH are generally attributable to the magnitude of hypotonicity of body fluids as well as the rate at which water intoxication develops. Symptoms of the latter include nausea, vomiting, irritability, and personality changes that may manifest themselves as combativeness, confusion, and hallucinations. When serum sodium values are less than 110 mEq/L, a variety of neurologic complications are encountered, including seizures, stupor, or coma.

The classic constellation of laboratory findings consists of low values for serum sodium, potassium, chloride, and osmolality, whereas serum bicarbonate levels may be normal. In contrast, urine osmolality is usually less than maximally dilute, with values ranging from 250–1,400 mOsm/kg, depending on the course of the disease. Hypouricemia is common, whereas renal and adrenal function tests are normal.

TREATMENT. Therapy for SIADH consists of simultaneously treating the underlying disorder causing SIADH and restricting fluids. Sodium replacement for urinary losses of sodium should be provided, but both intravenous and oral water administration should be reduced significantly based on careful calculations of actual insensible and body water losses. Serum as well as urine electrolytes and osmolality should be closely monitored and the patient's status re-evaluated on a frequent basis. In circumstances of severe water intoxication, intravenous administration of a combination of furosemide and 300 mL/m^2 of 1.5% sodium chloride (hypertonic saline) causes rapid increases in serum sodium concentrations and diuresis. In some cases, demeclochlorotetracycline (demeclocycline) has been used as therapy to block AVP's action on the collecting duct. In severe life-threatening situations, hemodialysis has been used to partially normalize serum electrolytes and remove excess body water.

569.2 Cerebral Salt Wasting

Children with acute or chronic CNS damage may acquire a syndrome of cerebral salt wasting. Cerebral salt wasting is distinct from SIADH as already described despite the presence of multiple common clinical and laboratory findings. Cerebral salt wasting has been reported in patients with closed head trauma, CNS surgery, tumors, or meningitis, as well as one case report without apparent CNS abnormalities. In contrast to SIADH, children with cerebral salt wasting exhibit a combination of hypovolemia and hyponatremia, excessive renal sodium losses, and marked elevations of plasma atrial natriuretic hormone (ANP). On the basis of the combination of elevated plasma ANP levels and decreased or normal plasma concentrations of aldosterone and vasopressin, it has been suggested that cerebral salt wasting is due to inappropriate secretion of ANP. Treatment includes volume-for-volume replacement of urine sodium losses and oral sodium supplementation after discharge from the hospital to correct and maintain normal fluid balance.

Barrett TG, Bundley SE: Wolfram (DIDMOAD) syndrome. J Med Genet 34:838, 1997.

Bichet DG, Razi M, Lonergan M, et al: Hemodynamic and coagulation responses to 1-desamino [8-D-arginine] vasopressin in patients with congenital nephrogenic diabetes insipidus. N Engl J Med 383:887, 1988.

Birmbaumer M, Seibold A, Gilbert S, et al: Molecular cloning of the receptor for human antidiuretic hormone. Nature 357:333, 1992.

Crawford JD, Kennedy GC: Chlorothiazide in diabetes insipidus renalis. Nature 193:891, 1959.

Czernichow P, Pomerade R, Basmaciogullari A, et al: Diabetes insipidus in children. III: Anterior pituitary dysfunction in idiopathic types. J Pediatr 106:41, 1985.

Deen PMT, Croes H, van Aubel RAMH, et al: Water channels encoded by mutant aquaporin-2 genes in nephrogenic diabetes insipidus are impaired in their cellular routing. J Clin Invest 95: 2291, 1995.

Deen PMT, Verdijk MAJ, Knoers NVAM, et al: Requirement of human renal water channel aquaporin-2 for vasopressin-dependent concentration of urine. Science 264:92, 1994.

Ganong CA, Kappy MS: Cerebral salt wasting in children. The need for recognition and treatment. Am J Dis Child 147:167, 1993.

Harris HW Jr, Zeidel ML: Cell biology of vasopressin. *In:* Brenner BM (ed): The Kidney, 5th ed. Philadelphia, WB Saunders, 1995, p 516.

Henricks SA, Lippe B, Kaplan SA, et al: Differential diagnosis of diabetes insipidus: Use of DDAVP to terminate the seven hour water deprivation test. J Pediatr 98:224, 1981.

Hofmann S, Bezold R, Jaksch M, et al: Wolfram (DIDMOAD) syndrome and Leber hereditary optic neuropathy (LHON) are associated with distinct mitochondrial DNA haplotypes. Genomics 39:8, 1997.

Knoers N, Monnens LAH: Nephrogenic diabetes insipidus. *In:* Avner E, Barrett M (eds): Pediatric Nephrology, 3rd ed. 1993, p 318.

Kohn B, Norman ME, Feldman H, et al: Hysterical polydypsia (compulsive water drinking) Am J Dis Child 130:210, 1976.

Maghrue M, Villa A, Arico M, et al: Correlation between magnetic resonance imaging of posterior pituitary and neurohypophyseal function in children with diabetes insipidus. J Clin Endocrinol Metab 74:795, 1992.

Miller WL: Molecular genetics of familial central diabetes insipidus. J Clin Endocrinol Metab 77:592, 1993.

Monnens L, Smulders Y, Van Lier H, et al: DDAVP test for assessment of renal concentrating capacity for infants and children. Nephron 29:151, 1991.

Olias G, Richter D, Schmale H: Heterologous expression of human vasopressin-neurophysin percursors in a pituitary cell line: Defective transport of a mutant protein from patients with familial diabetes insipidus. DNA Cell Biol 15:929, 1996.

Rosenthal W, Siebold A, Antaramian A, et al: Molecular identification of the gene responsible for congenital nephrogenic diabetes insipidus. Nature 359:233, 1992.

Sklar C, Fertig A, David R: Chronic syndrome of inappropriate secretion of antidiuretic hormone in childhood. Am J Dis Child 139:733, 1985.

CHAPTER 570

Hyperpituitarism, Tall Stature, and Overgrowth Syndromes

Pinchas Cohen

HYPERPITUITARISM. Primary hyperpituitarism is rare in children, but secondary hypersecretion of pituitary hormones is an expected finding in conditions in which deficiency of a target organ results in decreased hormonal feedback, as in primary hypogonadism or hypoadrenalism. In primary hypothyroidism, pituitary hyperfunction and hyperplasia can enlarge and erode the sella and, on rare occasions, increase intracranial pressure. Such changes should not be confused with primary pituitary tumors; they disappear when the underlying thyroid condition is treated. Pituitary hyperplasia also occurs in response to stimulation by ectopic production of releasing hormones such as that seen occasionally in patients with Cushing's syndrome, secondary to corticotropin–releasing hormone excess, or in children with acromegaly secondary to growth hormone–releasing hormone (GHRH) produced by a variety of systemic tumors.

Primary hypersecretion of pituitary hormones by an adenoma is uncommon in childhood. The most commonly encountered pituitary tumors are those that secrete corticotropin, prolactin, or growth hormone (GH). With rare exceptions, pituitary adenomas that secrete gonadotropins or thyrotropin occur in adults. Hypothalamic hamartomas that secrete gonadotropin-releasing hormone are known to cause precocious puberty. It is suspected that some pituitary tumors may result from stimulation with hypothalamic-releasing hormones and in other instances, as in McCune-Albright syndrome, the tumor is caused by a constitutive activating mutation of the G-protein (G_s) gene.

TALL STATURE. The normal distribution of height predicts that 2.5% of the population will be taller than 2 SD (97%) above the mean. However, the social acceptability and even desirability of tallness (heightism) makes tall stature an uncommon complaint. In North America, it is extremely unusual for males to seek help regarding excessive height, although in Europe it is somewhat more common. Even in females, tall stature has become more socially acceptable, although tall girls may still approach their physician with a desire to curb their growth rate.

Differential Diagnosis of Tall Stature. Table 570–1 lists the causes of tall stature in childhood and adolescence. Of these, the normal variant, familial or constitutional tall stature, is by far the most common cause. Almost invariably, a family history of tallness can be elicited, and no organic pathologic condition is present. The child is often tall throughout childhood and enjoys excellent health. The parent of the constitutionally tall adolescent may reflect unhappily upon his or her own adolescence as a tall teenager. There are no abnormalities in the physical examination and the laboratory studies, if obtained, always produce negative results.

Klinefelter syndrome (XXY syndrome) is a relatively common (1:500–1,000 live male births) abnormality associated with tall stature, mild mental retardation, gynecomastia, and decreased upper body:lower body segment ratio. The testes are invariably small, although androgen production by Leydig cells is often at the low normal range. Spermatogenesis and Sertoli cell function are defective, and infertility results. *XYY syndrome* is associated with tall stature and possible behavioral and mental problems. *Marfan syndrome* is an autosomal dominant connective tissue disorder consisting of tall stature, increased arm span, and decreased upper body:lower body segment ratio. Additional abnormalities include arachnodactyly, ocular abnormalities, and cardiac anomalies (see Chapter 705). *Homocystinuria* is an autosomal recessive inborn error of amino acid metabolism that causes mental retardation when untreated and has many features resembling Marfan syndrome, particularly ocular manifestations. *Hyperthyroidism* in adolescents is associated with rapid growth but normal adult height. It is almost always caused by Grave disease and is much more common in females. Children with *precocious puberty* are often unusually tall but do not grow to be giants because their epiphyses close early and growth ceases prematurely. *Exogenous obesity* is a common condition in adolescence and may be associated with rapid linear growth and early maturation; adult height is typically normal.

The purpose of the diagnostic evaluation of tall stature is to distinguish the commonly occurring normal variant constitutional variety from the rare pathologic conditions. Often, when the history is suggestive of familial tall stature and the physical examination is entirely normal, no laboratory tests are indicated. It is valuable to obtain a bone age roentgenogram to be able to predict adult height, which serves as a basis for discussions with the family and for management decisions. If, however, the history is suggestive of a disorder or the physical examination reveals abnormalities, additional laboratory tests should be obtained. Insulin-like growth factor-1 (IGF-1) and IGF binding protein-3 (IGFBP-3) are excellent screening tests for GH excess and can be verified with a glucose suppression test. Laboratory evidence of GH excess mandates magnetic resonance imaging (MRI) evaluation of the pituitary. Chromosome analysis is useful in males, especially when the upper:lower body segment ratio is decreased or when mental retardation is present. If Marfan syndrome or homocystinuria is suspected from the physical examination, referral to a cardiologist and an ophthalmologist should be made. Thyroid function tests are useful to diagnose or rule out hyperthyroidism when this disorder is suspected.

Treatment of Tall Stature. Reassurance of the family and the patient is central to the management of normal variant tall stature. The use of the bone age to predict adult height may provide some comfort, as will general supportive discussions on the social acceptability of this condition. Although treat-

TABLE 570–1 Differential Diagnosis of Tall Stature

Normal variants
Familial (constitutional) tall stature
Abnormal variants
Pituitary gigantism
Cerebral gigantism (Sotos syndrome)
Klinefelter syndrome
XYY syndrome
Marfan syndrome
Homocystinuria
Hyperthyroidism
Obesity

ment is available for girls and boys with excessive growth, its use should be restricted to patients with (1) a predicted adult height greater than 3 SD above the mean (77 inches in males, 72 inches in females) and (2) evidence of significant psychosocial impairment. For the family that feels strongly about treatment, a trial of sex steroids is possible. Such therapy is designed to accelerate puberty and epiphyseal fusion and is therefore of little benefit when given in late puberty; ideally, therapy is initiated prepubertally or in early puberty. Oral ethinyl estradiol at a dose of 0.15–0.5 mg/24 hr until cessation of growth occurs has been used successfully in girls before the bone age has reached 12 yr, reducing the predicted height by 5 to 10 cm on average. If necessary, a progestational agent can be added after 1 yr of unopposed estrogen. In boys, treatment should begin before the bone age reaches 14 yr; testosterone enanthate is used at a dose of 500 mg intramusculary every 2 wk for 6 mo. Although no long-term complications of sex steroid therapy have been clearly documented, short-term side effects are common. These include lipid abnormalities, thromboembolism, cholelithiasis, hypertension, nausea, menstrual irregularities, and acne fulminans. The lack of extensive experience with this form of therapy and the risks involved should be carefully weighed and discussed with the family before embarking on therapy.

PITUITARY GIGANTISM AND ACROMEGALY. In young persons with open epiphyses, overproduction of GH results in gigantism; in persons with closed epiphyses, the result is acromegaly. Often, some acromegalic features are seen with gigantism, even in children and adolescents; after closure of the epiphyses, the acromegalic features become more prominent. Pituitary gigantism is rare and its cause most often is a pituitary adenoma, but gigantism has been observed in a 2.5-yr-old boy with a hypothalamic tumor that presumably secreted GHRH. Other tumors, particularly in the pancreas, have produced acromegaly by secretion of large amounts of GHRH with resultant hyperplasia of the somatotrophs.

The usual *clinical manifestations* consist of rapid linear growth, coarse facial features, and enlarging hands and feet. In young children, rapid growth of the head may precede linear growth. Some patients have behavioral and visual problems. In most of the recorded cases, the abnormal growth became evident at puberty, but the condition has been established as early as the newborn period in one child and at 21 mo of age in another. Giants may grow to a height of 8 ft or more. Acromegaly consists chiefly of enlargement of the distal parts of the body, but manifestations of abnormal growth involve all portions. The circumference of the skull increases, the nose becomes broad, and the tongue is often enlarged, with coarsening of the facial features. The mandible grows excessively, and the teeth become separated. Visual field defects and neurologic abnormalities are common; signs of increased intracranial pressure appear later. The fingers and toes grow chiefly in thickness. There may be dorsal kyphosis. Fatigue and lassitude are early symptoms. Delayed sexual maturation or hypogonadism may occur. Tufting of the phalanges and increased heel pad thickness are common.

Laboratory findings reveal elevated GH levels, which may occasionally reach 400 ng/mL. There is usually no suppression of GH levels by the hyperglycemia of a glucose tolerance test. IGF-I and IGFBP-3 levels are consistently elevated in acromegaly, whereas other growth factors are not. Most patients also have marked hyperprolactinemia as a result of plurihormonal adenomas that secrete GH and prolactin. Adenomas may compromise other anterior pituitary function through growth or cystic degeneration. Secretion of gonadotropins, thyrotropin, or corticotropin may be impaired. Computed tomography or MRI delineates the tumor. Osseous maturation is normal.

Treatment of adenoma includes surgery, irradiation, and medical therapy; each has advantages and disadvantages. Octreotide, a long-acting analog of somatostatin, is 45 times more active than the native peptide in suppressing GH secretion. Experience in adults with acromegaly indicates that octreotide persistently suppresses GH, IGFBP-3, and IGF-I concentrations and reduces tumor size in a significant number of patients. This agent may be helpful in some patients as primary therapy or when surgery has not been successful.

570.1 Sotos Syndrome (Cerebral Gigantism)

Although it is characterized by rapid growth, there is no evidence that Sotos syndrome is an endocrine disorder. A hypothalamic defect has been suggested as a cause, but none has been demonstrated functionally or at necropsy. Birthweight and length are above the 90th percentile in most affected infants, and macrocrania may be noted. Growth is rapid and by 1 yr of age affected infants are above the 97th percentile in height. Accelerated growth continues for the first 4–5 yr and then returns to a normal rate. Puberty usually occurs at the normal time but may occur slightly early. The hands and feet are large, with thickened subcutaneous tissue. The head is large and dolichocephalic, the jaw is prominent, there is hypertelorism, and the eyes have an antimongoloid slant. Clumsiness and awkward gait are characteristic, and affected children have great difficulty in sports, in learning to ride a bicycle, and in other tasks requiring coordination. Some degree of mental retardation affects most patients; in some children, perceptual deficiencies may predominate. A typical case is seen in Figure 570–1. Osseous maturation is compatible with the patient's height. GH levels and other endocrine studies are usually normal; there are no distinctive laboratory or radio-

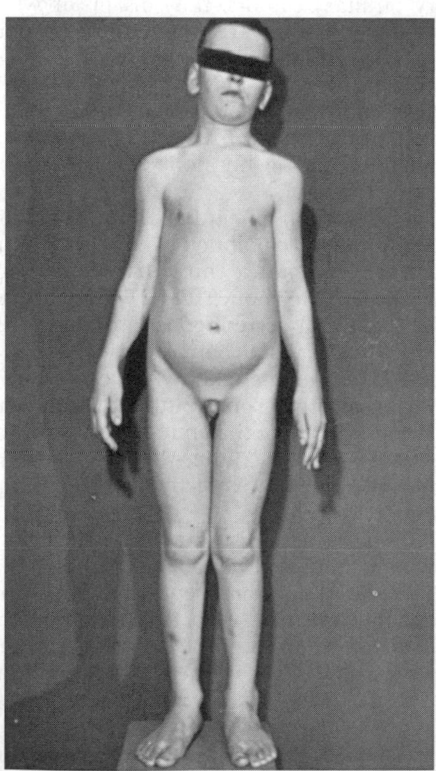

Figure 570–1 Cerebral gigantism in an 8-yr-old boy. The height age was 12 yr; the bone age was 12 yr; IQ was 60; the electroencephalogram had abnormal findings. Notice the prominence of the forehead and the jaw and the large hands and feet. Sexual development was consistent with chronological age. Hormone study results were normal. The adult height was 208 cm (6 ft 10 in); his sexual development was normal. He wears size 18 shoes.

logic markers. Abnormal electroencephalograms are common; other studies frequently reveal a dilatated ventricular system. Most cases are sporadic. Familial cases are usually consistent with autosomal dominant inheritance, occasionally with autosomal recessive inheritance. Affected patients may be at increased risk for neoplasia; hepatic carcinoma and Wilms, ovarian, and parotid tumors have been reported.

570.2 Prolactinoma

Prolactin-secreting pituitary adenomas are the most common tumors of the pituitary in adolescents. With the advent of MRI, more of these tumors, particularly microadenomas (<1 cm) are being detected. The most common presenting manifestations are headache, amenorrhea, and galactorrhea. The disorder affects more than twice as many girls as boys; most have undergone normal puberty before becoming symptomatic. Only a few children have delayed puberty. In some kindreds with type I multiple endocrine neoplasia, prolactinomas are the presenting feature during adolescence.

Prolactin levels may be moderately (40–50 ng/mL) or markedly (10,000–15,000 ng/mL) elevated. Most prolactinomas in children have been large (macroadenomas), have caused the sella to enlarge and, in some cases, have caused visual field defects. Approximately one third of patients with macroadenomas acquire hypopituitarism, particularly GH deficiency.

Prolactinomas should not be confused with the hyperprolactinemia and pituitary hyperplasia that may occur in patients with primary hypothyroidism, which is readily treated with thyroid hormone (see Chapter 575). Moderate elevations (<200 ng/mL) of prolactin are also associated with a variety of medications, with pituitary stalk dysfunction such as may occur with craniopharyngioma, and with other benign conditions.

Treatment for most children has been surgical resection by the transfrontal or transsphenoidal approach. However, most patients can be managed effectively by treatment with bromocriptine, the standard drug for treating hyperprolactinemia. About 80% of adult patients respond with shrinkage of the tumor and marked decreases in serum prolactin levels. New drugs such as the long-acting cabergoline are also available.

570.3 Overgrowth Syndromes

A group of disorders associated with excessive somatic growth and growth of specific organs are collectively referred to as overgrowth syndromes. These disorders appear to be caused by excess availability of insulin-like growth factor-II (IGF-II) encoded by the gene *Igf2.* The best described of these syndromes is the *Beckwith-Wiedemann syndrome* (BWS), which is an overgrowth malformation syndrome that occurs with an incidence of 1/13,700 births. It is manifested as a fetal overgrowth syndrome, in which hypertrophy dominates the clinical picture. Typically macroglossia, hepatosplenomegaly, nephromegaly, and hypoglycemia secondary to pancreatic β cell hyperplasia in a large for gestational age infant compose the clinical picture at birth (see Chapter 103). An additional complication is that these children are predisposed to a specific subset of childhood neoplasms, including Wilms tumor and adrenocortical carcinoma. Overexpression of IGF-II in BWS may be caused by a number of genetic disruptions including gene duplication, loss of heterozygosity, and relaxation or loss of imprinting of the Igf2 gene. Various lines of investigation have localized "imprinted" genes involved in BWS and associated childhood tumors to chromosome 11p. These include, in addition to Igf2, the gene H19, which is involved in Igf2 suppression as well as the gene WT-1 (the Wilms tumor gene). Mutations in GPC3, a glypican gene (which code for an IGF-II neutralizing membrane receptor), cause the related *Simpson-Golabi-Behmel overgrowth syndrome.*

Colao A, Di Sarno A, Landi ML, et al: Long-term and low-dose treatment with cabergoline induces macroprolactinoma shrinkage. J Clin Endocrinol Metab 82:3574, 1997.

Daughaday WH: Pituitary gigantism. Endocrinol Metab Clin North Am 21:633, 1992.

Kane LA, Leinung MC, Scheithaver BW, et al: Pituitary adenomas in childhood and adolescence. J Clin Endocrinol Metab 79:1135, 1994.

Morison IM, Becroft DM, Taniguchi T, et al: Somatic overgrowth associated with overexpression of insulin-like growth factor II. Nat Med 2:311, 1996.

Rajasoorya C, Holdaway IM, Wrightson P, et al: Determinants of clinical outcome and survival in acromegaly. Clin Endocrinol 41:95, 1994.

Serri O: Progress in management of hyperprolactinoma. N Engl J Med 331:942, 1994.

Sorgo W, Scholler K, Heinze E, Teller WM: Critical analysis of height reduction in estrogen treated tall girls. Eur J Pediatr 142:260, 1984.

Sotos JF: Overgrowth. Genetic syndromes and other disorders associated with overgrowth. Clin Pediatr 36:157, 1997.

Weinman E, Bergmann S, Böhls HJ: Oestrogen treatment of constitutional tall stature: A risk-benefit ratio. Arch Dis Child 78:148, 1998.

CHAPTER 571
Physiology of Puberty

Luigi Garibaldi

Between early childhood and approximately 8–9 yr of age (i.e., *prepubertal* stage), the hypothalamic-pituitary-gonadal axis is dormant, as reflected by undetectable serum concentrations of luteinizing hormone (LH) and sex hormones (i.e., estradiol in girls, testosterone in boys). In this phase, the activity of the hypothalamus and pituitary is thought to be suppressed by neuronal restraint pathways and by the negative feedback provided in young children by the minute amounts of circulating gonadal steroids.

One to 3 yr before the onset of puberty becomes clinically evident, low serum levels of LH during sleep become demonstrable (i.e., *peripubertal* period). This sleep-entrained LH secretion occurs in a pulsatile fashion and probably reflects endogenous episodic discharge of hypothalamic gonadotropin-releasing hormone (GnRH). Nocturnal pulses of LH continue to increase in amplitude and, to a lesser extent, in frequency as clinical puberty approaches. This pulsatile secretion of gonadotropins is responsible for the enlargement and maturation of the gonads and the secretion of sex hormones. The appearance of the secondary sex characteristics in *early puberty* is the visible culmination of the sustained, active interaction occurring among hypothalamus, pituitary, and gonads in the peripubertal period. By *midpuberty,* LH pulses become evident even during the daytime and occur at about 90–120 min intervals.

A second critical event occurs in middle or late adolescence in girls, in whom cyclicity and ovulation occur. A positive feedback mechanism develops whereby rising levels of estrogen in midcycle cause a distinct increase of LH.

The factors that normally activate or restrain the hypothalamic neurons responsible for GnRH secretion (i.e., a neurosecretory unit known as *the GnRH pulse generator*) are unknown. It is clear that GnRH is the major, if not the only, hormone responsible for the onset and progression of puberty because pubertal development can be reproduced in sexually immature or gonadotropin-deficient animals and humans by pulsed administration of GnRH.

The interpretation of the hormonal changes of puberty is

complex because of several factors. First, pituitary gonadotropins are heterogeneous and circulate in multiple isoforms: more bioactive isoforms of LH may be preponderant during puberty. Second, LH immunoreactivity is variable in different immunoassays, and the results of LH measurements vary widely among laboratories. Third, the pulsatile secretion of gonadotropins and the synergism of FSH and LH in promoting gonadal maturation make interpretation of single serum gonadotropin concentrations difficult. Measurement of gonadotropins in serially obtained (every 10–20 min for 12–24 hr) serum samples or timed urine collections is more meaningful. Fourth, important sex differences exist in the maturation of the hypothalamus and pituitary gland, and serum LH concentrations rise earlier in the course of the pubertal process in boys than in girls.

The effects of gonadal steroids (i.e., testosterone in boys and estradiol in girls) on bone growth and osseous maturation have become increasingly clear, with the characterization of estrogen deficiency states in males. Both aromatase deficiency and estrogen receptor defects result in delayed epiphyseal fusion and tall stature in affected males. These observations suggest that estrogens, rather than androgens, are responsible for the process of bone maturation that ultimately leads to epiphyseal fusion and cessation of growth. Estrogens also mediate the increased production of growth hormone, which, along with a direct effect of sex steroids on bone growth, is responsible for the pubertal growth spurt.

The age at onset of puberty varies and is more closely correlated with osseous maturation than with chronologic age (see Chapter 14). In girls, the breast bud is usually the first sign of puberty (10–11 yr), followed by the appearance of pubic hair 6–12 mo later. The interval to menarche is usually 2–2.5 yr but may be as long as 6 yr. In the United States, at least one sign of puberty is present in approximately 95% of girls by 12 yr of age and in 99% of girls by 13 yr of age. Peak height velocity occurs early (at breast stage II–III, typically between 11 and 12 yr of age) in girls and always precedes menarche. The mean age of menarche is about 12.75 yr. There are, however, wide variations in the sequence of changes involving growth spurt, breast bud, pubic hair, and maturation of the internal and external genitals.

In boys, growth of the testes (>3 mL in volume or 2.5 cm in longest diameter) and thinning of the scrotum are the first signs of puberty. These are followed by pigmentation of the scrotum and growth of the penis (see Chapter 14). Pubic hair then appears. Appearance of axillary hair usually occurs in midpuberty. In boys, unlike girls, acceleration of growth begins after puberty is well under way and is maximal at genital stage IV–V (typically between 13 and 14 yr of age). In boys, the growth spurt occurs approximately 2 yr later than in girls, and growth may continue beyond 18 yr of age.

Genetic and environmental factors affect the onset of puberty. The drop in menarcheal age in the past century probably reflects better nutrition and improved general health. American black girls are significantly more advanced in the development of secondary sex characteristics than white girls. Ballet dancers, gymnasts, runners, and other girl athletes in whom leanness and strenuous physical activity have coexisted from early childhood frequently exhibit a marked delay in puberty or menarche; the same individuals frequently have oligomenorrhea or amenorrhea as adults. This observation supports the thesis that the energy balance is closely related to the activity of the GnRH pulse generator and the mechanisms initiating and sustaining puberty.

Adrenocortical androgens also play a role in pubertal maturation. Serum levels of dehydroepiandrosterone (DHEA) and its sulfate (DHEAS) begin to rise at approximately 6–8 yr of age, before any increase in LH or sex hormones and before the earliest physical changes of puberty are apparent; this process has been called *adrenarche*. DHEAS is the most abundant adrenal C19 steroid in the blood, and its serum concentration remains fairly stable over 24 hr; a single measurement of this hormone is commonly used as a marker of adrenal androgen secretion. Although adrenarche typically antedates the onset of gonadal activity (i.e., gonadarche) by a few years, the two processes do not seem to be causally related because adrenarche and gonadarche are dissociated in conditions such as central precocious puberty and adrenocortical failure.

CHAPTER 572
Disorders of Pubertal Development

Luigi Garibaldi

Precocious puberty is generally defined as the onset of secondary sexual characteristics before 8 yr of age in girls and 9 yr in boys. This definition is somewhat arbitrary, however, because of the marked variation in the age at which puberty begins in normal children, particularly if they belong to different ethnic groups.

Precocious pubertal development may be classified as gonadotropin-dependent, also called *true* or *central* precocious puberty, or gonadotropin-independent, also called *peripheral* precocious puberty or precocious *pseudopuberty* (Table 572–1). True precocious puberty is always isosexual and stems from hypothalamic-pituitary-gonadal activation. The gonadotropin-mediated increase in the size and activity of the gonads leads to increasing sex hormone secretion and progressive sexual maturation. In precocious pseudopuberty, some of the secondary sex characteristics appear, but there is no activation of the normal hypothalamic-pituitary-gonadal interplay. In this latter group, the sex characteristics may be isosexual or heterosexual ("contrasexual") (see Chapters 14 and 571).

Precocious pseudopuberty may induce maturation of the hypothalamic-pituitary-gonadal axis and eventually trigger the onset of true sexual precocity. This mixed type of precocious puberty occurs commonly in conditions such as congenital adrenal hyperplasia and McCune-Albright syndrome, when the bone age reaches the pubertal range (10.5–12.5 yr).

572.1 Gonadotropin-Dependent Precocious Puberty

Gonadotropin-dependent precocious puberty occurs at least 10-fold more frequently in girls than in boys and is usually sporadic, although some cases are familial. In more than 90% of girls, sexual precocity is idiopathic. A structural central nervous system (CNS) abnormality can, however, be demonstrated by computed tomography (CT) or magnetic resonance imaging (MRI) in 25–75% of boys with central precocious puberty.

CLINICAL MANIFESTATIONS. Sexual development may begin at any age and generally follows the sequence observed in normal puberty. In girls, the first sign is development of the breast; pubic hair may appear simultaneously but more often appears later. Maturation of the external genitals, the appearance of axillary hair, and the onset of menstruation follow. The early menstrual cycles may be more irregular than they are with normal puberty. The initial cycles are usually anovulatory, but pregnancy has been reported as early as 5.5 yr of age (Fig. 572–1).

In boys, enlargement of the testes is followed by enlargement

TABLE 572–1 Conditions Causing Precocious Puberty

- Gonadotropin-dependent puberty (true precocious puberty)
  - Idiopathic (constitutional, functional)
  - Organic brain lesions
    - Hypothalamic hamartoma
    - Brain tumors, hydrocephalus, severe head trauma
  - Hypothyroidism, prolonged and untreated
- Combined gonadotropin-dependent and gonadotropin-independent puberty
  - Treated congenital adrenal hyperplasia
  - McCune-Albright syndrome, late
  - Familial male precocious puberty, late
- Gonadotropin-independent puberty (precocious pseudopuberty)
  - Females
    - Isosexual (feminizing) conditions
      - McCune-Albright syndrome
      - Autonomous ovarian cysts
      - Ovarian tumors
        - Granulosa-theca cell tumor associated with Ollier disease
        - Teratoma, chorionepithelioma
        - Sex-cord tumor with annular tubules (SCTAT) associated with Peutz-Jeghers syndrome
        - Feminizing adrenocortical tumor
        - Exogenous estrogens
      - Heterosexual (masculinizing) conditions
        - Congenital adrenal hyperplasia
        - Adrenal tumors
        - Ovarian tumors
        - Glucocorticoid receptor defect
        - Exogenous androgens
  - Males
    - Isosexual (masculinizing) conditions
      - Congenital adrenal hyperplasia
      - Adrenocortical tumor
      - Leydig cell tumor
      - Familial male precocious puberty
      - Isolated
      - Associated with pseudohypoparathyroidism
      - hCG-secreting tumors
        - Central nervous system
        - Hepatoblastoma
        - Mediastinal tumor associated with Klinefelter syndrome
      - Teratoma
      - Glucocorticoid receptor defect
      - Exogenous androgen
    - Heterosexual (feminizing) conditions
      - Feminizing adrenocortical tumor
      - Sex-cord tumor with annular tubules (SCTAT) associated with Peutz-Jeghers syndrome
      - Exogenous estrogens
- Incomplete (partial) precocious puberty
  - Premature thelarche
  - Premature adrenarche
  - Premature menarche

hCG = human chorionic gonadotropin.

of the penis, appearance of pubic hair, and acne. Erections are common, and nocturnal emissions may occur. The voice deepens, and linear growth is accelerated. Testicular biopsies have shown stimulation of all elements of the testes, and spermatogenesis has been observed as early as 5–6 yr of age.

In affected girls and boys, height, weight, and osseous maturation are advanced. The increased rate of bone maturation results in early closure of the epiphyses, and the ultimate stature is less than it would have been otherwise. Without treatment, approximately one third of girls and an even larger percentage of boys achieve a height below the 5th percentile as adults. Mental development is usually compatible with chronologic age. Emotional behavior and mood swings are not uncommon, but serious psychologic problems are rare.

Although the clinical course is variable, three main patterns of pubertal progression can be identified, at least in girls. Most girls (particularly those younger than 6 yr of age at onset) have *rapidly progressive* sexual precocity, characterized by rapid physical and osseous maturation, leading to a loss of height potential. Other girls (generally older than 6 yr of age at the onset) have a *slowly progressive variant,* characterized by parallel advancement of osseous maturation and linear growth, with preserved height potential. A small percentage of girls have spontaneously regressive or *unsustained* central precocious puberty. This variability in the natural course of sexual precocity underscores the need for longitudinal observation at the onset of sexual development, before treatment is considered.

LABORATORY FINDINGS. Sensitive immunometric (including immunoradiometric, immunofluorimetric, and chemiluminescent) assays for luteinizing hormone (LH) have largely replaced the traditional LH radioimmunoassays and offer greater diagnostic sensitivity using random blood samples. With these new assays, serum LH concentrations are undetectable in prepubertal children, but they become detectable in 50–70% of girls and a higher percentage of boys with central sexual precocity. Measurement of LH in serial blood samples obtained during sleep has greater diagnostic power than measurement in a single random sample and typically reveals a well-defined pulsatile secretion of LH. Intravenous administration of gonadotropin-releasing hormone *(GnRH stimulation test)* is a helpful diagnostic tool, particularly for boys, in whom a brisk LH response (LH peak >5–10 IU/L) with predominance of LH over follicle-stimulating hormone (FSH) occurs in the early phase of precocious puberty. In girls with sexual precocity, however, the nocturnal LH secretion and the LH response to GnRH may be low at breast stage II–early stage III (immunometric-LH peak often <5 IU/L), and the LH:FSH ratio may remain low until midpuberty.

In central precocious puberty, sex hormone concentrations are usually appropriate for the stage of puberty in both sexes. Thus, serum estradiol concentrations in girls are low or undetectable in the early phase of sexual precocity, as they are in normal puberty. In boys, serum testosterone levels are detectable or clearly elevated by the time the parents seek medical attention, particularly if an early morning blood sample is obtained. Osseous maturation is variably advanced, often more than 2–3 SD. Pelvic ultrasonography in girls reveals progressive enlargement of the ovaries, followed by enlargement of the uterus to pubertal size. CT or MRI may demonstrate physiologic enlargement of the pituitary gland, as seen in normal puberty.

DIFFERENTIAL DIAGNOSIS. Organic CNS causes of central sexual precocity should be ruled out by CT or MRI, particularly in girls younger than 6 yr of age and all boys. However, in children presenting without neurologic signs or symptoms, the CNS lesions causing precocious puberty are rarely malignant and seldom require neurosurgical intervention.

Gonadotropin-independent causes of isosexual precocious puberty must be considered in the differential diagnosis (see Table 572–1). For girls, these include tumors of the ovaries, autonomously functioning ovarian cysts, feminizing adrenal tumors, McCune-Albright syndrome, and exogenous sources of estrogens. For boys, congenital adrenal hyperplasia, adrenal tumors, Leydig cell tumors, chorionic gonadotropin-producing tumors, and familial male precocious puberty should be considered.

TREATMENT. The observation that the pituitary gonadotropic cells require pulsatile, rather than continuous, stimulation by GnRH to maintain the ongoing release of gonadotropins provides the rationale for using GnRH agonists for treatment of central precocious puberty. By virtue of being more potent and having a longer duration of action than native GnRH, these GnRH analogs "desensitize" the gonadotropic cells of the pituitary to the stimulatory effect of endogenous GnRH and effectively halt the progression of central sexual precocity. Virtually all boys and the large subgroup of girls with rapidly progressive precocious puberty are candidates for treatment. However, girls with slowly progressive puberty do not seem to benefit in terms of height prognosis from GnRH agonist therapy. Rare patients require treatment for psychologic or social reasons alone.

Depot preparations of long-acting GnRH analogs, which

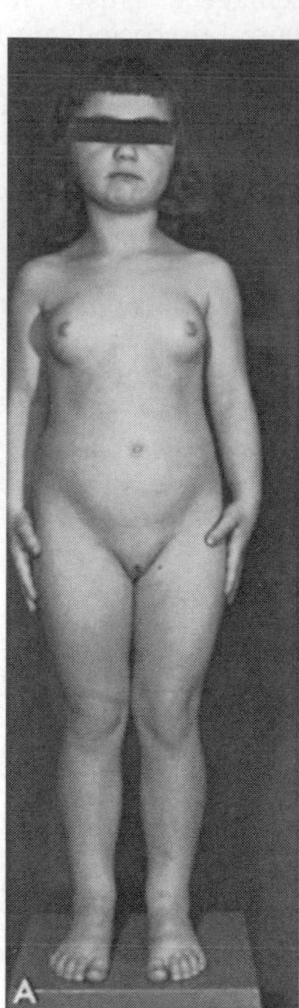

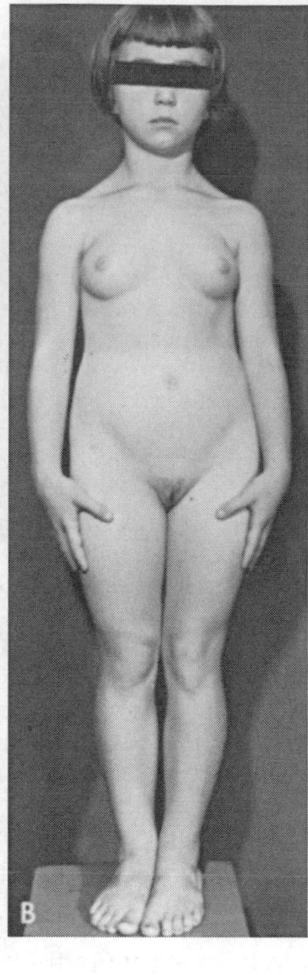

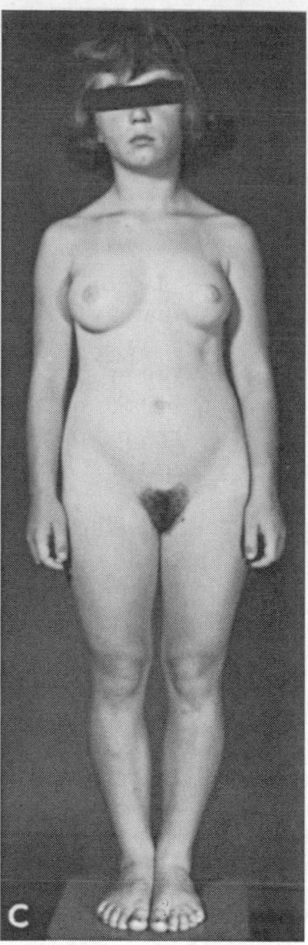

Figure 572–1 Idiopathic precocious puberty. Patient *(A)* at $3\frac{11}{12}$, *(B)* at $5\frac{8}{12}$, and *(C)* at $8\frac{1}{2}$ yr of age. Breast development and vaginal bleeding began at $2\frac{1}{2}$ yr of age. Osseous age was $7\frac{1}{2}$ yr at $3\frac{11}{12}$ and 14 yr at 8 yr of age. Repeated estrogen assays varied between normal prepubertal and adult female levels. Urinary gonadotropins were not demonstrable until the child was 5 yr of age. Intelligence and dental age were normal for chronological age. Growth was completed at 10 yr; ultimate height was 142 cm (56 in).

maintain fairly constant serum concentration of the drug for weeks, constitute the preparations of choice for treatment of central precocious puberty. Leuprolide acetate (Lupron Depot Ped),the only depot preparation approved for this use in the United States, is given in a dose of 0.25–0.3 mg/kg (minimum, 7.5 mg) intramuscularly once every 4 wk. Other long-acting preparations (triptorelin [Decapeptyl]; goserelin acetate [Zoladex]) are approved for treatment of precocious puberty in other countries. Recurrent sterile fluid collections at the sites of injections are the most troublesome local side effect and occurs in less than 5% of treated patients. In children with such local reactions, treatment should be changed to daily subcutaneous injections of an aqueous analog (e.g., Leuprolide, 50 μg/kg/24 hr) or intranasal administration of the GnRH agonist nafarelin [Synarel], 800 μg bid. With regard to the latter, the potential for irregular compliance and the variable absorption of the intranasal route may limit the long-term benefit on adult height.

PROGNOSIS. Treatment results in decrease of the growth rate, generally to age-appropriate values, and an even greater decrease of the rate of osseous maturation. Some children, particularly those with greatly advanced (pubertal) bone age, may show marked deceleration of growth rate and a complete arrest in the rate of osseous maturation. Treatment results in enhancement of the predicted height, although the actual adult height of patients followed to epiphyseal closure is approximately 1 SD below their midparental height. In girls, breast development may regress in those with Tanner stage II–III development. Most commonly, the size of the breasts remains unchanged in girls with stage III–V development or may even increase slightly because of progressive adipose tissue deposition. The amount of glandular tissue decreases. Growth of pubic hair does not progress during treatment. Menses, if present, cease. Pelvic ultrasonography demonstrates a decrease of the ovarian and uterine size. In boys, there is decrease of testicular size, variable regression of pubic hair, and a decrease in the frequency of erections. Except for a decrease in bone density (of uncertain clinical significance), no serious adverse effects of GnRH analogs have been reported in children treated for sexual precocity.

If treatment is effective, the serum sex hormone concentrations decrease to prepubertal levels (testosterone, <20 ng/dL in boys; estradiol, <10 pg/mL in girls), and the serum LH concentration, as measured by sensitive immunometric assays, decreases to less than 1 IU/L. Moreover, the incremental FSH and LH response to GnRH stimulation decreases to less than 1–2 IU/L. Serum LH and sex hormone levels remain suppressed for as long as therapy is continued, but puberty resumes promptly when therapy is discontinued. In girls, menarche and ovulatory cycles generally appear within 6–18 mo of cessation of therapy.

572.2 Precocious Puberty Resulting from Organic Brain Lesions

ETIOLOGY. With the advent of CT and MRI, *hypothalamic hamartoma* has been recognized as one of the most common brain lesions causing true precocious puberty (Fig. 572–2). This congenital malformation consists of ectopically located neural tissue containing GnRH secretory neurons and functions as an accessory GnRH pulse generator. On MRI, it appears as a small pedunculated mass attached to the tuber cinereum or the floor of the third ventricle or, less often, as a sessile mass (Fig. 572–3), which remains static in size over the years. This lesion is infrequently associated with gelastic or psychomotor seizures.

A wide variety of lesions of the CNS, usually involving the hypothalamus by scarring, invasion, or pressure, have been associated with gonadotropin-dependent sexual precocity. These lesions probably induce sexual maturation by interrupting poorly characterized pubertal restraint pathways. They include postencephalitic scars, tuberculous meningoencephalitis, hydrocephalus, tuberous sclerosis, severe head trauma, and neoplasms such as astrocytomas, ependymomas, and optic

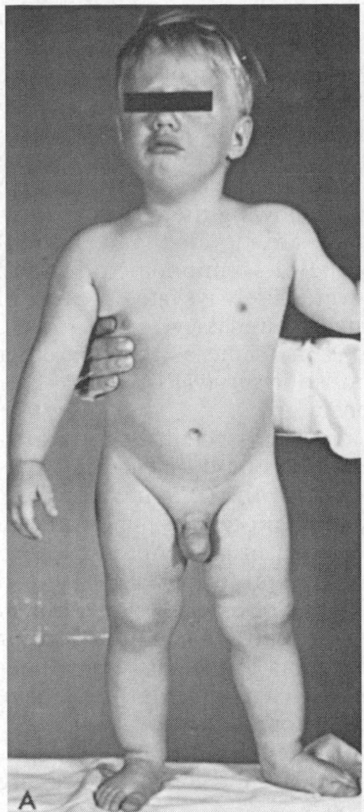

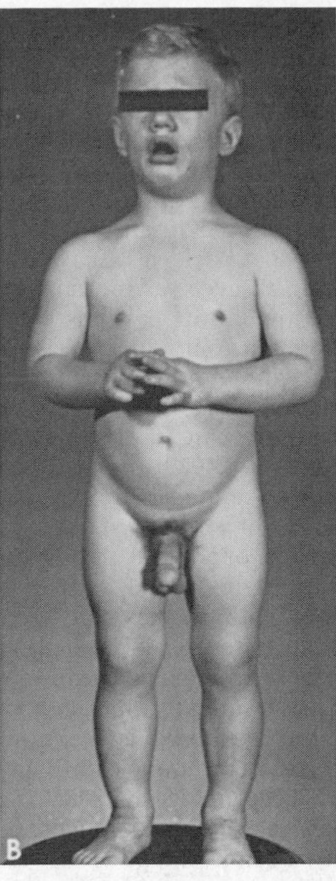

Figure 572–2 Precocious puberty with central nervous system lesion. Photographs at 1.5 *(A)* and 2.5 *(B)* yr of age. Accelerated growth, muscular development, osseous maturation, and testicular development were consistent with the degree of secondary sexual maturation. In early infancy, the patient began having frequent spells of rapid, purposeless motion; later in life, he had episodes of uncontrollable laughing with ocular movements. At 7 yr, he exhibited emotional lability, aggressive behavior, and destructive tendencies. Although a hypothalamic hamartoma had been suspected, it was not established until computed tomographic scanning became available, when the patient was 23 yr of age. Epiphyses fused at 9 yr of age; final height was 142 cm (56 in). At 24 yr of age, he developed an embryonal cell carcinoma of the retroperitoneum.

tract tumors. Tumors of the latter type (typically slowly progressive or indolent optic gliomas) are highly prevalent (15–20%) in children with neurofibromatosis type 1 and are the main, if not the sole, causative factor for central sexual precocity in a small subset (approximately 3%) of children with neurofibromatosis type 1.

About half the tumors in the pineal region are germinomas or astrocytomas; the remainder consist of a wide variety of histologically distinct tumor types. These tumors, too, cause precocious puberty by interrupting CNS inhibitory pathways to the hypothalamus or, in boys, by secreting human chorionic gonadotropin (hCG), which stimulates the Leydig cells of the testes. Intracranial hCG-secreting germinomas usually do not produce precocious puberty in girls, presumably because complete ovarian function cannot occur without FSH priming.

CLINICAL MANIFESTATIONS. Some of these tumors or malformations (e.g., hypothalamic hamartomas) remain static in size or grow slowly, producing no signs other than precocious puberty. For lesions causing neurologic symptoms, the neuroendocrine manifestations may be present for 1–2 yr before the tumor can be detected radiologically. Hypothalamic signs or symptoms such as diabetes insipidus, adipsia, hyperthermia, unnatural crying or laughing (gelastic seizures), obesity, and cachexia should suggest the possibility of an intracranial lesion. Visual signs (e.g., proptosis) may be the first manifestation of an optic glioma.

The sexual precocity is always isosexual, and the endocrine patterns are generally those found in children without demonstrable organic lesions. Rapidly progressive sexual precocity in very young children suggests the likelihood of a hypothalamic hamartoma. In conditions other than hypothalamic hamartoma, growth hormone deficiency may occur and may be masked by the growth-promoting effect of the increased sex hormone levels.

TREATMENT. Neurosurgical intervention is not indicated for hypothalamic hamartomas, except for rare patients with intractable seizures. For other neurologic lesions, therapy depends on the nature and location of the pathologic process. Regardless of the cause, therapy with GnRH analogs is as effective in children with organic brain lesions causing central precocious puberty as it is in children with idiopathic sexual precocity, and the analogs are the therapy of choice to halt premature sexual development. Combined growth hormone therapy should be considered for patients with associated growth hormone deficiency.

572.3 Precocious Puberty Following Irradiation of the Brain

Radiation therapy, generally for leukemia or intracranial tumors, increases the risk of precocious puberty considerably, whether the irradiation is directed to the hypothalamic area or to areas of the brain anatomically distant from the hypothalamus (see Chapter 611). Low-dose radiation (i.e., 18–24 Gy) hastens the onset of puberty almost exclusively in girls. High-dose radiation (25–47 Gy) triggers precocious sexual development in both sexes, and the risk of sexual precocity is inversely

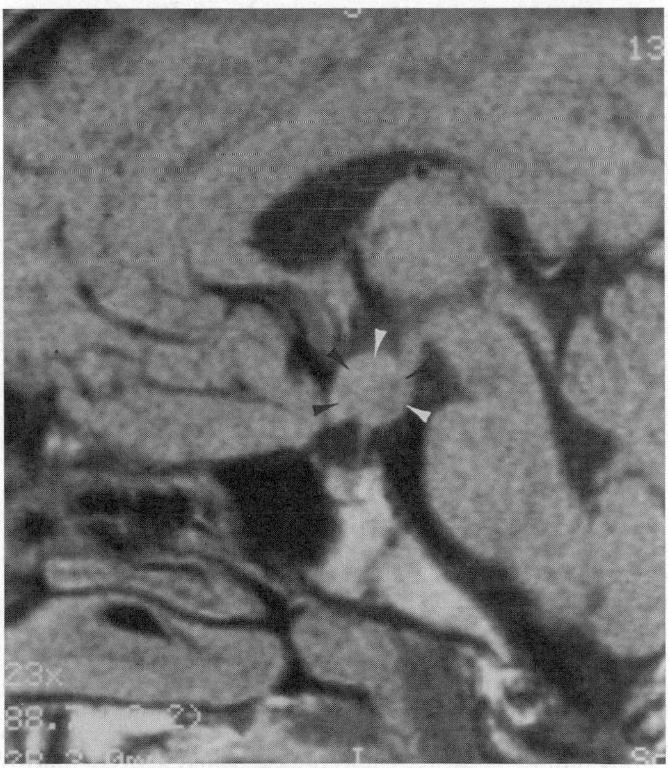

Figure 572–3 Magnetic resonance image of a central nervous system lesion in a child with central precocious puberty. A 6-yr-old girl was referred for stage IV breast development and growth acceleration. Serum luteinizing hormone and estradiol concentrations were in the adult range. The midsagittal T1-weighted image shows an isointense hypothalamic mass (arrowheads), typical of a hamartoma. (From Sharafuddin M, Luisiri A, Garibaldi LR, et al: MR imaging diagnosis of cerebral precocious puberty: Importance of changes in the shape and size of the pituitary gland. Am J Roentgenol 162:1167, 1994.)

proportional to the age of the child at the time radiation was administered.

This type of sexual precocity often occurs in the face of growth hormone deficiency and may be associated with other conditions (i.e., spinal irradiation, hypothyroidism) adversely affecting the prognosis for an acceptable adult height. Unless careful attention is paid to early signs of pubertal development in these children, the combination of growth hormone deficiency and the growth-promoting effect of sex steroids often results in a "normal" growth rate at the expense of a rapidly advancing bone age and impaired adult height potential.

TREATMENT. As in other types of central precocious puberty, GnRH analogs are effective in arresting pubertal progression in this patient population. However, concomitant growth hormone deficiency (or thyroid hormone deficiency, or both) must be diagnosed and treated promptly in order for the adult height prognosis to improve.

Paradoxically, hypopituitarism with gonadotropin deficiency may subsequently develop as a late effect of high-dose CNS irradiation in patients with or without a history of precocious puberty; in this case substitution therapy with sex steroids is required.

572.4 Syndrome of Precocious Puberty and Hypothyroidism

In children with untreated hypothyroidism, the onset of puberty is usually delayed until epiphyseal maturation has reached 12–13 yr of age. Precocious puberty in a child with untreated hypothyroidism and a prepubertal bone age presents a strikingly unphysiologic association, yet it is not uncommon and may occur in as many as 50% of children with severe hypothyroidism of long duration. These children have the usual manifestations of hypothyroidism, including retardation of growth and osseous maturation. The cause of the hypothyroidism is most often undiagnosed lymphocytic thyroiditis and rarely thyroidectomy or overtreatment with antithyroid drugs.

Sexual development in girls consists primarily of breast enlargement and menstrual bleeding; the latter may occur even in girls with minimal breast enlargement. Pelvic ultrasonography may reveal large, multicystic ovaries. Boys have testicular enlargement associated with modest or no penile enlargement and no pubic hair development. Enlargement of the sella, which is typical of long-standing primary hypothyroidism, may be demonstrated by skull films or MRI. Plasma levels of thyroid-stimulating hormone (TSH) are markedly elevated, often greater than 1,000 μU/mL, and those of prolactin are mildly elevated. Although both FSH and LH are low, when measured by specific assays, the massively elevated concentrations of TSH appear to interact with the FSH receptor ("specificity spillover"), thus inducing FSH-like effects in the absence of LH effects on the gonads. As a consequence, unlike in true precocious puberty, testicular enlargement occurs without substantial Leydig cell stimulation and testosterone secretion in affected boys. In affected girls, ovarian estrogen production occurs without a concomitant increase in androgens. Thus, the precocious puberty associated with hypothyroidism behaves as an incomplete form of gonadotropin-dependent puberty. Treatment of the hypothyroidism results in a rapid return to normal of the biochemical and clinical manifestations. Macroorchidism (testicular volume >30 mL) may persist in adult life despite adequate L-thyroxine therapy.

572.5 Gonadotropin-Secreting Tumors

HEPATIC TUMORS. Isosexual precocious puberty may be uncommonly associated with hepatoblastoma. All reported cases have been males, with the age of onset varying from 4 mo–8 yr (average, 2 yr). An enlarged liver or mass in the upper quadrant should suggest the diagnosis. The tumor cells produce hCG, which stimulates the LH receptors in the Leydig cells of the testes. The testicular histologic appearance reveals interstitial cell hyperplasia and absence of spermatogenesis. Plasma levels of hCG and α-fetoprotein are usually markedly elevated; they serve as useful markers for following the effects of therapy. Plasma levels of testosterone are elevated, and the FSH and LH levels, as measured by specific, immunometric assays, are low; in the past, LH levels were falsely elevated because of cross reaction with hCG on radioimmunoassay.

Treatment for these tumors is the same as that for other carcinomas of the liver; prognosis for survival beyond 1–2 yr from the time of diagnosis is poor.

OTHER TUMORS. Chorionic gonadotropin–secreting choriocarcinomas, teratocarcinomas, or teratomas (also called *ectopic pinealomas* or *atypical teratomas),* located in the CNS, mediastinum, gonads, or adrenal glands, may cause precocious puberty, more commonly (10–20-fold) in boys than in girls. About a dozen boys with mediastinal tumors and precocious puberty had small testes, leading to the diagnosis of Klinefelter syndrome. Why extragonadal tumors (particularly mediastinal) occur more frequently than gonadal tumors in patients with Klinefelter syndrome is unknown. Affected patients often have marked elevations of hCG and α-fetoprotein.

PRECOCIOUS PSEUDOPUBERTY. The adrenal causes of pseudopuberty are discussed in Chapter 586, and the gonadal causes are discussed in Chapters 594 and 597.

572.6 McCune-Albright Syndrome (Precocious Puberty with Polyostotic Fibrous Dysplasia and Abnormal Pigmentation)

McCune-Albright syndrome consists of endocrine dysfunction associated with patchy cutaneous pigmentation and fibrous dysplasia of the skeletal system. Although sexual precocity in girls was the major recognized endocrinopathy in the past, associated pituitary, thyroid, and adrenal aberrations have been increasingly recognized. Molecular advances have clearly established it as a prototypical model of autonomous hyperfunction of multiple glands. The disorder is caused by a missense mutation in the gene encoding the α subunit of G_s, the G protein that stimulates cyclic adenosine monophosphate (cAMP) formation, resulting in the formation of the putative *gsp* oncoprotein. Activation of receptors (e.g., corticotropin [adrenocorticotropic hormone—ACTH], TSH, FSH, LH receptors) that operate with a cAMP-dependent mechanism as well as cell proliferation, ensue. Because the mutation is somatic, rather than genomic, it is expressed differently in different glands or tissues; hence, the variability of clinical expression in different patients.

Precocious puberty has been described predominantly in girls (Fig. 572–4). The average age at onset in affected girls is about 3 yr, but vaginal bleeding has occurred as early as 4 mo of age and secondary sex characteristics have occurred as early as 6 mo. Young girls have suppressed levels of LH and FSH, and there is no response to GnRH stimulation. Estradiol levels vary from normal to markedly elevated (>900 pg/ml), are often cyclic, and may correlate with the size of the cysts. In boys, precocious puberty is less common but has been reported in several instances. Unlike ovarian enlargement in girls, testicular enlargement in boys is fairly symmetric. It is followed by the appearance of phallic enlargement and pubic hair, as in normal puberty. Testicular histologic studies have demonstrated large seminiferous tubules and no or minimal Leydig

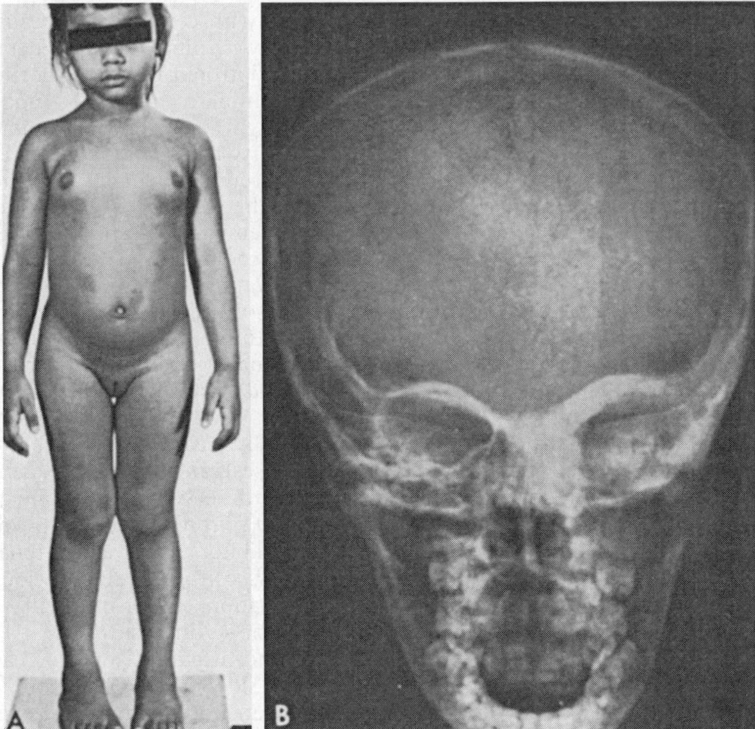

Figure 572–4 Precocious puberty associated with polyostotic fibrous dysplasia (McCune-Albright syndrome) in a girl 4.5 yr of age; at this time, her height age and osseous age were normal. Menarche occurred at 4 yr of age. *A*, Notice the bilateral breast development, the hyperpigmented spots on the abdomen, and the prominence of the left side of the face. *B*, Roentgenograms revealed fibrous dysplasia in the distal end of the left ulna and thickening of the bones about the left orbit and the maxillary portion of the frontal bones shown here.

cell hyperplasia; these findings may simply reflect the fact that biopsy specimens were obtained at an early stage of pubertal development. In both girls and boys, when the bone age reaches the usual pubertal age range, gonadotropin secretion begins, and the response to GnRH becomes pubertal. True (gonadotropin-dependent) precocious puberty overrides the antecedent (gonadotropin-independent) precocious pseudopuberty. In girls, menses become more regular, but often not completely, and fertility has been documented.

The *hyperthyroidism* that occurs in this condition differs from that characteristic of Graves disease. There is an equal distribution among males and females, and the goiters tend to be multinodular. Clinical hyperthyroidism is uncommon in children, but goiters, mildly elevated T_3 levels, suppressed TSH levels, and abnormalities on ultrasonography have been reported.

In patients with associated *Cushing syndrome,* bilateral nodular adrenocortical hyperplasia has occurred in early infancy, antedating the sexual precocity. ACTH levels are low, and adrenal function is not suppressed by large doses of dexamethasone.

Increased secretion of growth hormone occurs uncommonly and is manifested clinically by *gigantism* or *acromegaly* or by *increased rates of growth* even in the absence of precocious puberty. Girls and boys are affected equally. Serum levels of growth hormone are elevated and increase during sleep; they are augmented by thyrotropin-releasing hormone and poorly inhibited by oral glucose. Serum levels of prolactin are increased in most patients, but fewer than half the patients have a demonstrable pituitary tumor.

Of the *extraglandular manifestations,* phosphaturia, leading to rickets or osteomalacia, is probably the most common. Cardiovascular and hepatic involvement are rare but may be life-threatening (e.g., severe neonatal cholestasis).

All patients must be thoroughly investigated. Functioning ovarian cysts often disappear spontaneously; aspiration or surgical excision of cysts is rarely indicated. For girls with persistent estradiol secretion, agents that interfere with the final step of estrogen biosynthesis, that is, aromatase inhibitors such as testolactone, letrozole, or anastrozole, or antiestrogens (such as tamoxifen) may limit, to a variable extent, the estrogen effects on pubertal and osseous maturation. These compounds, however, have not been approved by the United States Food and Drug Administration for this indication and may be hepatotoxic. Associated therapy with long-acting agonists of GnRH is indicated only for patients whose puberty has shifted from a gonadotropin-independent to a predominantly gonadotropin-dependent mechanism. Cushing syndrome requires adrenalectomy. Octreotide, a long-acting somatostatin inhibitor, has been used to treat the hypersomatotropism. The prognosis is favorable for longevity, but deformities, repeated fractures, pain, and occasional cranial nerve compression may result from the bony lesions.

572.7 Familial Male Gonadotropin-Independent Precocious Puberty

Familial male gonadotropin-independent precocious puberty is a rare, autosomal dominant form of sexual precocity that is transmitted from affected males and unaffected female carriers of the gene to their male offsprings. Signs of puberty appear by 2–3 yr of age. The testes are only slightly enlarged. Testicular biopsies show Leydig cell maturation and, in some instances, marked hyperplasia. Maturation of seminiferous tubules may be present. Testosterone levels are markedly elevated to the same range seen in boys with true precocious puberty; however, baseline levels of LH are prepubertal, pulsatile secretion of LH is absent, and LH does not respond to stimulation with GnRH. The cause for activation of Leydig cells independent of gonadotropin stimulation is a missense mutation of the LH receptor leading to constitutive activation of cAMP production.

Osseous maturation may be markedly advanced; when it reaches the pubertal age range, normal gonadotropin secretion intervenes because maturation of the hypothalamus is enhanced by exposure to abnormal levels of sex hormones. Precocious puberty then becomes gonadotropin-dependent. This sequence of events is similar to that occurring in children with McCune-Albright syndrome or in those with congenital adrenal hyperplasia, in whom sexual precocity is initially gonadotropin-independent but becomes gonadotropin-dependent when maturation of the hypothalamus initiates normal gonadotropin secretion.

Gonadotropin-independent precocious puberty has been diagnosed in two unrelated boys with type IA pseudohypoparathyroidism who had a single mutation of the $G_{s\alpha}$ protein. This mutation is inactivating at normal body temperature and causes pseudohypoparathyroidism, but in the cooler temperature of the testes, it is constitutionally activating, resulting in adenyl cyclase stimulation and production of testosterone. Although this mutation differs from the constitutive LH receptor mutation, which usually causes familial male gonadotropin-independent precocious puberty, the end result is the same.

TREATMENT. Young boys have been successfully treated with ketoconazole (600 mg/24 hr in 8-hr divided doses), an antifungal drug that inhibits 17,20-lyase and testosterone synthesis. Other investigators have used a combination of spironolactone (to block androgen action) and aromatase inhibitors (such as testolactone, letrozole, or anastrozole) because estrogens derived from androgens stimulate bone maturation. Unfortunately, these medications are unable to revert the serum testosterone to the normal (prepubertal) concentrations or completely block the testosterone effects. They slow down, but do not halt, the progression of puberty and do not improve the height prognosis. Boys whose GnRH pulse generator has matured become resistant to treatment and require combined therapy with GnRH agonists.

572.8 Incomplete (Partial) Precocious Development

Isolated manifestations of precocity without development of other signs of puberty are not unusual; development of the breasts in girls and growth of sexual hair in both sexes are the two most common forms.

PREMATURE THELARCHE. This term applies to a transient condition of isolated breast development that most often appears in the first 2 yr of life; in some girls breast development is present at birth and persists. Breast development may be unilateral or asymmetric and often fluctuates in degree. Growth and osseous maturation are normal or slightly advanced. The genitals show no evidence of estrogenic stimulation. The condition is usually sporadic and is rarely familial. Breast development may regress after 2 yr, often persists for 3–5 yr, and is rarely progressive. Menarche occurs at the expected age, and reproduction is normal. Basal serum levels of FSH and their responses to GnRH stimulation may be greater than those seen in normal controls. Plasma levels of LH and estradiol are generally below the limits of detection. Ultrasonographic examination of the ovaries reveals normal size, but a few small cysts are not uncommon.

In some girls of the same age group, breast development may be associated with definite evidence of systemic estrogen effects, such as growth acceleration or bone age advancement. Pelvic ultrasonography may reveal enlarged ovaries or uterus. This condition has been referred to as *exaggerated* or *atypical thelarche*. It differs from central sexual precocity because it is spontaneously regressive. GnRH stimulation elicits a robust FSH response and a minimal LH response. The pathogeneses of typical and exaggerated forms of thelarche are unclear, although a delay in the transition from the activated (neonatal-infantile) to the inactive (prepubertal) pituitary-ovarian axis may underlie both conditions.

Premature thelarche is a benign condition but may be the first sign of true or pseudoprecocious puberty, or it may be caused by exogenous exposure to estrogens. In addition to a detailed history, a bone age should be obtained. The serum concentrations of FSH, LH, and estradiol are generally low and not diagnostic. Pelvic ultrasonographic examination is rarely indicated. Continued observation is important because the condition cannot be readily distinguished from true precocious puberty. Regression and recurrence suggest functioning follicular cysts. Occurrence of thelarche in children older than 3 yr of age most often is caused by a condition other than benign precocious thelarche.

PREMATURE ADRENARCHE. This term applies to the appearance of sexual hair before the age of 8 yr in girls or 9 yr in boys without other evidence of maturation. It is much more frequent in girls than in boys and may occur more frequently in American black girls than in others. Hair appears on the mons and labia majora in girls, perineal and scrotal area in boys; axillary hair generally appears later. Adult-type axillary odor is common. Affected children are slightly advanced in height and osseous maturation.

Premature adrenarche is an early maturational event of adrenal androgen production. This event coincides with precocious maturation of the zona reticularis, an associated decrease in 3-β-hydroxysteroid dehydrogenase activity, and an increase in 17,20-lyase activity. These enzymatic changes result in increased basal and ACTH-stimulated serum concentrations of the Δ^5steroids (17hydroxypregnenolone and DHEA) and, to a lesser extent, of the Δ^4steroids (particularly androstenedione) compared with age-matched controls. The levels of these steroids and those of DHEAS are usually comparable to those of children in the early stages of normal puberty.

Premature adrenarche is a benign condition that requires no therapy. However, a subset of patients have one or more features of systemic androgen effect, such as marked growth acceleration, clitoral (girls) or phallic (boys) enlargement, cystic acne, or advanced bone age (>2 SD above the mean for age). In these patients with *atypical premature adrenarche*, an ACTH stimulation test with measurement of serum 17-hydroxyprogesterone is indicated to rule out nonclassic congenital adrenal hyperplasia due to 21-hydroxylase deficiency. Epidemiologic and molecular genetic studies have shown that the prevalence of nonclassic 21-hydroxylase deficiency is approximately 3–6% of unselected children presenting with precocious pubarche; the prevalence of other enzyme defects (i.e., 3-β-hydroxysteroid dehydrogenase or 11-β-hydroxylase deficiencies) is extremely low.

Although premature adrenarche is a benign condition, longitudinal observations suggest that girls with premature adrenarche are at high risk for hyperandrogenism and polycystic ovarian syndrome as adults.

PREMATURE MENARCHE. This is a rare entity, much less frequent than premature thelarche or premature adrenarche. In girls presenting with isolated vaginal bleeding in the absence of other secondary sexual characteristics, more common causes such as vulvovaginitis, foreign body, or sexual abuse, and uncommon causes such as urethral prolapse and sarcoma botryoides must be carefully excluded (see Chapter 506). The majority of girls with idiopathic premature menarche have only one to three episodes of bleeding; puberty occurs at the usual time and menstrual cycles are normal. Plasma levels of gonadotropins are normal, but estradiol levels may be elevated, probably owing to bursts of ovarian activity. Occasional patients are found to have ovarian follicular cysts on ultrasonography.

572.9 Medicational Precocity

A variety of medications can induce the appearance of secondary sexual characteristics that may be confused with precocious puberty. A careful history focused on exploring the possibility of accidental exposure to or ingestion of sex hormones is important. Precocious pseudopuberty has occurred in both boys and girls from the accidental ingestion of estrogens (including contraceptive pills) and from the administration of anabolic steroids. Estrogens in cosmetics, hair creams, and breast augmentation creams have caused breast development in girls and gynecomastia in boys; estrogens are readily absorbed through the skin. Contamination of vitamin tablets by sex hormones has been reported to cause precocious pseudopuberty. An "epidemic" of premature thelarche and precocious pseudopuberty in Puerto Rico has been attributed to contamination of meats, particularly chicken, with estrogens used in animal husbandry but has not been proved. Exogenous estrogens may produce an intense, dark brown color in the areola of the breasts that is not usually seen in endogenous types of precocity. The precocious changes disappear after cessation of exposure to the hormones.

Anasti JN, Flack MR, Froehlich J, et al: A potential novel mechanism for precocious puberty in juvenile hypothyroidism. J Clin Endocrinol Metab 80:276, 1995.

Apter D, Butzow TL, Laughlin GA, et al: Gonadotropin-releasing hormone pulse generator activity during pubertal transition in girls: Pulsatile and diurnal patterns of circulating gonadotropins. J Clin Endocrinol Metab 76:940, 1993.

Balducci R, Boscherini B, Mangiantini A, et al: Isolated precocious pubarche: An approach. J Clin Endocrinol Metab 79:582, 1994.

Boepple PA, Frisch LS, Wierman ME, et al: The natural history of autonomous gonadal function, adrenarche, and central puberty in gonadotropin-independent precocious puberty. J Clin Endocrinol Metab 75:1550, 1992.

Breyer P, Haider A, Pescovitz OH: Gonadotropin-releasing hormone agonists in the treatment of girls with central precocious puberty. Clin Obstet Gynecol 36:764, 1993.

Conn PM, Crowley WR Jr: Gonadotropin-releasing hormone and its analogues. Annu Rev Med 45:391, 1994.

Demir A, Dunkel L, Stenman U, Voutilainen R: Age-related course of urinary gonadotropins in children. J Clin Endocrinol Metab 80:1457, 1995.

DiMeglio L, Hirsch-Pescovitz O: Disorders of puberty: Inactivating and activating molecular mutations. J Pediatr 131(Suppl):S8, 1997.

Feuillan PP: McCune-Albright syndrome. Curr Ther Endocrinol Metab 5:205, 1994.

Fontoura M, Brauner R, Prevot C, et al: Precocious puberty in girls: Early diagnosis of a slowly progressing variant. Arch Dis Child 64:1170, 1989.

Garibaldi LR, Aceto T Jr, Weber C: The pattern of gonadotropin and estradiol secretion in exaggerated thelarche. Acta Endocrinol (Copenh) 128:345, 1993.

Garibaldi LR, Picco P, Magier S, et al: Serum luteinizing hormone concentrations, as measured by a sensitive immunoradiometric assay, in children with normal, precocious or delayed pubertal development. J Clin Endocrinol Metab 72:888, 1991.

Habiby R, Silverman B, Listenick A, et al: Precocious puberty in children with neurofibromatosis type 1. J Pediatr 126:364, 1995.

Holland FJ: Gonadotropin-independent precocious puberty. Endocrinol Metab Clin North Am 20:191, 1991.

Ibanez L, Potau N, Virdis R, et al: Postpubertal outcome in girls diagnosed of premature pubarche during childhood: Increased frequency of functional ovarian hyperandrogenism. J Clin Endocrinol Metab 76:1599, 1993.

Iiri T, Herzmark P, Nakamoto JM, et al: Rapid GDP release from $G_{s\alpha}$ in patients with gain and loss of endocrine function. Nature 371:164, 1994.

Ilicke A, Prager Lewin R, Kauli R, et al: Premature thelarche: Natural history and sex hormone secretion in 68 girls. Acta Paediatr Scand 73:756, 1984.

Jay N, Mansfield MJ, Blizzard RM, et al: Ovulation and menstrual function of adolescent girls with central precocious puberty after therapy with gonadotropin-releasing hormone agonists. J Clin Endocrinol Metab 75:890, 1992.

Jensen AB, Brocks V, Hohn K, et al: Central precocious puberty in girls: Internal genitalia before, during, and after treatment with long-acting gonadotropin-releasing hormone analogues. J Pediatr 132:105, 1998.

Kletter GB, Kelch RP: Disorders of puberty in boys. Endocrinol Metab Clin North Am 22:455, 1993.

Kosugi S, Van Dop C, Geffner ME, et al: Characterization of heterogeneous mutations causing constitutive activation of the LH receptor in familial male precocious puberty. Hum Mol Genet 4:183, 1995.

Kulin HE: The assessment of gonadotropins during childhood and adolescence: An ongoing struggle. Endocrinologist 4:279, 1994.

Laue L, Jones J, Barnes KM, et al: Treatment of familial male precocious puberty with spironolactone, testolactone, and deslorelin. J Clin Endocrinol Metab 76:151, 1993.

Lee PA, Witchel SF: The influence of estrogens on growth. Curr Opin Pediatr 9:431, 1997.

Mahachoklertwattana P, Kaplan SL, Grumbach MM: The luteinizing hormone–releasing hormone–secreting hypothalamic hamartoma is a congenital malformation: Natural history. J Clin Endocrinol Metab 77:118, 1993.

Nakagaware A, Ikeda K, Tsuneyoshi M, et al: Hepatoblastoma producing alpha-fetoprotein and human chorionic gonadotropin. Cancer 56:1636, 1985.

Neely EK, Hintz RL, Wilson DM, et al: Normal ranges for immunochemiluminometric gonadotropin assays. J Pediatr 127:40, 1995.

Oberfield S, Chin D, Uli N, et al: Endocrine late effects of childhood cancers. J Pediatr 131:(Suppl):S37, 1997.

Oerter KE, Manasco P, Barnes KM, et al: Adult height in precocious puberty after long-term treatment with deslorelin. J Clin Endocrinol Metab 73:1235, 1991.

Oerter-Klein K, Marta PM Jr, Blizzard RM, et al: A longitudinal assessment of hormonal and physical alterations during normal puberty in boys. II: Estrogen levels as determined by an ultrasensitive bioassay. J Clin Endocrinol Metab 81:3203, 1996.

Olgivy-Stuart AL, Clayton PE, Shalet SM: Cranial irradiation and early puberty. J Clin Endocrinol Metab 78:1282, 1994.

Pescovitz OH, Hench KD, Barnes KM, et al: Premature thelarche and central precocious puberty: The relationship between clinical presentation and the gonadotropin response to luteinizing hormone–releasing hormone. J Clin Endocrinol Metab 67:474, 1988.

Premawardhana LD, Vora JP, Mills R, et al: Acromegaly and its treatment in the McCune-Albright syndrome. Clin Endocrinol 36:605, 1992.

Rosenfield RL: Selection of children with precocious puberty for treatment with gonadotropin releasing hormone analogs. J Pediatr 124:989, 1994.

Schmidt H, Kiess W: Secondary central precocious puberty in a girl with McCune-Albright syndrome responds to treatment with GnRH analogue. J Pediatr Endocrinol Metab 11:77, 1998.

Sharafuddin MJ, Luisiri A, Garibaldi LR, et al: MR imaging diagnosis of central precocious puberty: Importance of changes in the shape and size of the pituitary gland. Am J Roentgenol 162:1167, 1994.

Shaul PW, Towbin RB, Chernausek SD: Precocious puberty following severe head trauma. Am J Dis Child 139:467, 1985.

Shenker A, Weinstein LS, Moran A, et al: Severe endocrine and nonendocrine manifestations of the McCune-Albright syndrome associated with activating mutations of stimulatory G protein Gs. J Pediatr 123:509, 1993.

Styne DM: New aspects in the diagnosis and treatment of pubertal disorders. Pediatr Clin North Am 44:505, 1997.

Van Winter JT, Noller KL, Zimmerman D, et al: Natural history of premature thelarche in Olmsted County, Minnesota, 1940 to 1984. J Pediatr 116:278, 1990.

SECTION 2

Disorders of the Thyroid Gland

Stephen LaFranchi

CHAPTER 573
Thyroid Development and Physiology

The fetal thyroid bilobed shape is recognized by 7 wk of gestation, and characteristic thyroid follicle cell and colloid formation is seen by 10 wk. Thyroglobulin synthesis occurs from 4 wk, iodine trapping by 8–10 wk, and thyroxine (T_4) and, to a lesser extent, triiodothryonine (T_3) synthesis and secretion occurs from 12 wk of gestation. There is evidence that three transcription factors, TTF-1, TTF-2, and PAX8, are important in thyroid gland morphogenesis and differentiation. These factors also bind to the promotors of thyroglobulin and thyroid peroxidase genes and so also influence thyroid hormone function. Hypothalamic neurons synthesize thyrotropin-releasing hormone (TRH) by 6–8 wk, the pituitary portal vessel system begins development by 8–10 wk, and TSH secretion is seen by 12 wk of gestation. Maturation of the hypothalamic-pituitary-thyroid axis occurs over the second half of gestation, but normal feedback relationships are not mature until 1–2 mo of postnatal life. Another transcription factor, Pit-1, is important for differentiation and growth of thyrotrophs, along with somatotrophs and lactotrophs.

The main function of the thyroid gland is to synthesize T_4 and T_3. The only known physiologic role of iodine is in the synthesis of these hormones; the recommended dietary allowance of iodine is greater than 30 μg/kg/24 hr for infants, 70–120 μg/24 hr for children, and 150 μg/24 hr for adolescents and adults. The daily intake in North America varies from 240 to more than 700 μg. Whatever the chemical form ingested, iodine eventually reaches the thyroid gland as iodide. Thyroid tissue has an avidity for iodine and is able to trap (with a gradient of 100:1), transport, and concentrate it in the follicular lumen for synthesis of thyroid hormone. Iodine transport is carried out by the sodium-iodide symporter, the gene for which has been cloned.

Before trapped iodide can react with tyrosine, it must be oxidized; this reaction is catalyzed by thyroidal peroxidase. The thyroid cells also elaborate a specific thyroprotein, a globulin with approximately 120 tyrosine units. Iodination of tyrosine forms monoiodotyrosine and diiodotyrosine; two molecules of diiodotyrosine then couple to form one molecule of T_4 or one molecule of diiodotyrosine and one of monoiodotyrosine to form T_3. Once formed, hormones are stored as thyroglobulin in the lumen of the follicle (colloid) until ready to be delivered to the body cells. Thyroglobulin is a large globular glycoprotein with a molecular weight of about 660,000 and under normal conditions is detectable in the blood of most individuals at nanogram levels. T_4 and T_3 are liberated from thyroglobulin by activation of proteases and peptidases.

The metabolic potency of T_3 is three to four times that of T_4. In adults, the thyroid produces approximately 100 μg of T_4 and 20 μg of T_3 daily. Only 20% of circulating T_3 is secreted by the thyroid; the remainder is produced by deiodination of T_4 in the liver, kidney, and other peripheral tissues by type I 5′-deiodinase. Selenocysteine has been identified in the active center of the iodothyronine deiodinases. Thus, selenium indirectly plays a role in normal growth and development. In the pituitary and brain, approximately 80% of required T_3 is produced in situ from T_4 by a different enzyme, type II 5′-deiodinase. In the fetal rat, although plasma levels of T_3 are very low, cerebral concentrations increase to almost adult levels. T_3 carries out most of the physiologic actions of the thyroid hormones. T_4 is more abundant, but it binds weakly to nuclear receptors, and most of its physiologic effects occur by conversion to T_3. The level of T_3 in blood is 1/50 that of T_4.

The thyroid hormones increase oxygen consumption, stimulate protein synthesis, influence growth and differentiation, and affect carbohydrate, lipid, and vitamin metabolism. The free hormones enter cells, where T_4 may be converted to T_3 by deiodination. Intracellular T_3 then enters the nucleus, where it binds to thyroid hormone receptors. Thyroid hormone receptors are members of the steroid hormone receptor superfamily that includes glucocorticoids, estrogen, progesterone, vitamin D, and retinoids. Four different isoforms of the thyroid hormone receptor (α_1 and α_2, β_1 and β_2) are expressed in different tissues; the protein product of the formerly designated *c-erb A* proto-oncogene (now called *THRA2*) has been identified as the α_2 thyroid hormone receptor in the brain and hypothalamus. Thyroid hormone receptors consist of a ligand-binding domain (binds T_3), hinge region, and DNA-binding domain (zinc finger). Binding of T_3 activates the thyroid hormone receptor response element, resulting in production of an encoded mRNA and protein synthesis and of secretion specific for the target cell. In this manner, a single hormone, T_4, acting through tissue-specific thyroid hormone receptor isoforms and gene-specific thyroid response elements, can produce multiple effects in various tissues.

About 70% of the circulating T_4 is firmly bound to *thyroxine-binding globulin* (TBG). Less important carriers are thyroxine-binding prealbumin, now named *transthyretin,* and albumin. Only 0.03% of T_4 in serum is not bound and comprises free T_4. Approximately 50% of circulating T_3 is bound to TBG, and 50% is bound to albumin; 0.30% of T_3 is unbound or free T_3. Because the concentration of TBG is altered in many clinical circumstances, its status must be considered when interpreting T_4 or T_3 levels.

The thyroid is regulated by thyroid-stimulating hormone (TSH), a glycoprotein produced and secreted by the anterior pituitary. This hormone activates adenylate cyclase in the thyroid gland to effect release of thyroid hormones. TSH is composed of two noncovalently bound subunits (chains): α and β (hTSH-β). The α subunit is common to luteinizing hormone, follicle-stimulating hormone, and chorionic gonadotropin; the specificity of each hormone is conferred by the β subunit. TSH synthesis and release are stimulated by TSH-releasing hormone (thyrotropin [TRH]), which is synthesized in the hypothalamus and secreted into the pituitary. TRH is found in other parts of the brain besides the hypothalamus and in many other organs; aside from its endocrine function, it seems to serve as a neurotransmitter. TRH, a simple tripeptide, was the first neuropeptide to be identified, synthesized, and used in clinical medicine. In states of decreased production of thyroid hormone, TSH and TRH are increased. Exogenous thyroid hormone or increased thyroid hormone synthesis inhibits TSH and TRH production. Except in the neonate, levels of TRH in serum are very low.

Further control of the level of circulating thyroid hormones occurs in the periphery. In many nonthyroidal illnesses, extrathyroidal production of T_3 decreases; factors that inhibit thyroxine-5′-deiodinase include fasting, chronic malnutrition, acute illness, and certain drugs. Levels of T_3 may be significantly decreased, whereas levels of T_4 and TSH remain normal. Presumably, the decreased levels of T_3 result in decreased rates of oxygen production, of substrate use, and of other catabolic processes.

Burrow GH, Fisher DA, Larsen PR: Maternal and fetal thyroid function. N Engl J Med 331:1072, 1994.
Cavalieri RD: Iodine metabolism and thyroid physiology: Current concepts. [Review] Thyroid 7:177, 1997.

573.1 *Thyroid Hormone Studies*

SERUM THYROID HORMONES. Methods are available to measure all of the thyroid hormones in sera: thyroxine (T_4), free T_4, triiodothyronine (T_3), free T_3, and the diiodothyronines. A metabolically inert T_3 (3,5′,3′-triiodothyronine), called reverse T_3, is also present in sera. Age must be considered in interpreting results, particularly in the neonate.

Thyroglobulin (Tg) is a glycoprotein dimer that is secreted through the apical surface of the thyrocyte into the colloid. Small amounts escape into the circulation and are measurable in serum. Levels increase with thyroid-stimulating hormone (TSH, also called thyrotropin) stimulation and decrease with TSH suppression. Levels are increased in the neonate, in patients with Graves disease, other forms of autoimmune thyroid disease, and in those with endemic goiter. The most marked elevations of Tg occur in patients with differentiated carcinoma of the thyroid. Athyreotic infants may have markedly reduced levels of Tg in serum.

TSH levels in serum are an extremely sensitive indicator of primary hypothyroidism. A 3rd generation of assays (chemiluminescent assays) that can measure complete suppression of TSH below the normal range is now standard. These sensitive TSH assays obviate the need for thyrotropin-releasing hormone (TRH) stimulation in the diagnosis of most patients with thyroid disorders.

After the neonatal period, normal levels of TSH are below 6 μU/mL. TSH secretion can be stimulated by intravenous administration (7 μg/kg) of TRH. In normal subjects, TRH administration increases baseline levels of TSH within 30 min. In hyperthyroidism, there is no rise in serum levels of TSH in response to TRH because the elevated levels of thyroid hormones block the effect of TRH on the pituitary. In patients with even very mild degrees of thyroid failure, administration of TRH results in an exaggerated TSH response. Patients with pituitary or hypothalamic failure have low basal levels of TSH, although it may not be below the lower range of normal; a normal response to TRH localizes the defect in the hypothalamus.

FETAL AND NEWBORN THYROID. Fetal serum T_4 increases progressively from midgestation to approximately 11.5 μg/dL at term. Fetal levels of T_3 are low before 20 wk and then gradually rise to about 45 ng/dL at term. Reverse T_3 levels, however, are very high in the fetus (250 ng/dL at 30 wk) and fall to 150 ng/dL at term. Serum levels of TSH gradually rise to 10 mU/L at term. Approximately one third of maternal T_4 crosses the placenta to the fetus. Maternal T_4 may play a role in fetal development, especially that of the brain, before the synthesis of fetal thyroid hormones begins. The fetus of a hypothyroid mother may be at risk for neurologic damage, and a hypothyroid fetus may be partially protected by maternal T_4 until delivery.

At birth, there is an acute release of TSH; peak serum concentrations reach 60 mU/L in 30 min in full-term infants. A rapid decline occurs in the ensuing 24 hr and a more gradual decline within the next 5 days to below 10 μU/mL. The acute increase in TSH produces a dramatic rise in levels of T_4 to approximately 16 μg/dL and of T_3 to approximately 300 ng/dL in about 4 hr. This T_3 seems largely derived from increased peripheral conversion of T_4 to T_3. T_4 levels gradually fall during the first 2 wk of life to 12 μg/dL. T_3 levels then decline during the 1st wk of life to levels under 200 ng/mL. Serum free T3 concentrations are approximately 540 pg/dL in infancy and decline to 210–440 pg/dL in childhood. Reverse T_3 levels are maintained for 2 wk (200 ng/dL) and fall by 4 wk to around 50 ng/dL. The amount of T_4 that crosses the placenta is not sufficient to interfere with a diagnosis of congenital hypothyroidism in the neonate.

SERUM THYROXINE-BINDING GLOBULIN. The thyroid hormones are transported in plasma bound to TBG, a glycoprotein synthesized in the liver. TBG is now most accurately measured by radioimmunoassay. Estimation of TBG levels is occasionally necessary because TBG is increased or decreased in a variety of clinical situations, with effects on the level of total thyroxine. TBG binds about 70% of T_4 and 50% of T_3. TBG levels increase in pregnancy and in the newborn period, and with administration of estrogens (oral contraceptives), perphenazine, and heroin, and decrease with androgens, anabolic steroids, glucocorticoids, and L-asparaginase. These effects are the results of modulation of hepatic synthesis of TBG. Phenytoin (diphenylhydantoin) is another cause of drug-induced abnormality of thyroid function tests. Phenytoin, an inducer of hepatic enzymes, stimulates hepatic degradation of T_4 and accelerates transport of T_4 into tissues. Phenobarbital and carbamezepine have a similar effect. Some drugs, particularly phenytoin, also inhibit binding of T_4 and T_3 to TBG. Decreased or increased levels of TBG also occur as genetic traits (see later). TBG levels may be markedly decreased owing to decreased production with liver disease or loss in the urine, as in infants with congenital nephrotic syndrome.

IN VIVO RADIONUCLIDE STUDIES. Markedly improved direct tests of thyroid function have made radioiodine uptake studies less useful. The iodine-trapping or concentrating mechanism of the thyroid can be evaluated by measuring the uptake of radioactive isotope ^{123}I (half-life of 13 hr). The technology allows doses of radioiodine (0.1–0.5 mCi) that are only a fraction of those formerly used. Technetium (^{99m}Tc) is a particularly useful radioisotope for children, because in contrast to iodine, it is trapped but not organified by the thyroid and has a half-life of only 6 hr. Thyroid scanning may be indicated to detect ectopic thyroid tissue, to evaluate thyroid nodules, or to assess the presence of thyroid tissue in questions of thyroid agenesis. These studies should be performed with ^{99m}Tc as pertechnetate because it has the advantages of lower radiation exposure and high-quality scintigrams. Use of ^{131}I in children should be limited to those known to have thyroid cancer.

THYROID ULTRASONOGRAPHIC STUDIES. Thyroid ultrasound examinations can determine the location, size, and shape of the thyroid gland, and they can assess the solid or cystic nature of nodules. Ultrasound is not as reliable as radionuclide studies in evaluating infants with suspected thyroid dysgenesis, particularly ectopic glands. Ultrasound examinations are very useful in identifying normal thyroid gland position in children with suspected thyroglossal duct cysts. In children with autoimmune thyroiditis, ultrasound reveals scattered hypoechogenicity. Ultrasound examinations are more accurate than physical examination in estimating goiter size and assessing thyroid nodules.

Fisher DA: Physiological variations in thyroid hormones: Physiological and pathophysiological considerations. Clin Chem 42:135, 1996.

CHAPTER 574
Defects of Thyroxine-Binding Globulin

Abnormalities in levels of thyroxine-binding globulin (TBG) are not associated with clinical disease and do not require treatment. They are usually uncovered by a chance finding of abnormally low or high levels of thyroxine (T_4) and may be a source of confusion in the diagnosis of hypo- or hyperthyroidism.

TBG deficiency occurs as an X-linked dominant disorder. Congenital TBG deficiency is most often discovered through screening programs for neonatal hypothyroidism that use levels of T_4 as the primary screen. Affected patients have low levels of T_4 and elevated resin triiodothyronine uptake (RT_3U), but levels of free T_4 and thyroid-stimulating hormone (TSH) are normal. The diagnosis is confirmed by the finding of absent or low levels of TBG. The disorder is more readily recognized in males because it is caused by a gene on the short arm of the X chromosome. TBG deficiency occurs in 1 in 2,400 newborn males, 36% of whom have TBG levels less than 1 mg/dL. Milder forms of TBG deficiency occur in approximately 1/42,000 heterozygous females. Complete TBG deficiency (<5 μg/dL) occurs much less frequently. Three of eight families with complete TBG deficiency have been found to have a codon mutation (leucine to proline); other patients with reduced affinity of TBG for T_4 have had other point mutations that affect the tertiary structure of the protein. Acquired TBG deficiency occurs with androgen and glucocorticoid treatment, hepatic insufficiency (not hepatitis), and renal disease and proteinuria.

TBG excess is also a harmless X-linked dominant anomaly, occurring in about 1/25,000 persons. It has been recognized primarily in adults, but neonatal screening programs are uncovering the condition in the neonate. The level of T_4 is elevated, T_3 is variably elevated, TSH and free T_4 are normal, and RT_3U is decreased. The elevated levels of TBG confirm the diagnosis. In neonates, levels of T_4 as high as 95 μg/dL have been found, which decrease to 20–30 μg/dL after 2–3 wk. Such high levels of T_4 are thought to be related in part to the normally elevated levels of TBG in neonates during the 1st mo of life, presumably as an effect of maternal estrogens. Affected patients are euthyroid. Family studies may be indicated to alert other affected individuals. Acquired elevations of TBG occur with pregnancy, estrogen treatment, and hepatitis.

Familial dysalbuminemic hyperthyroxinemia is an autosomal dominant disorder that may be confused with hyperthyroidism. Markedly increased binding of T_4 to an abnormal albumin variant leads to increased serum concentrations of T_4. However, the levels of free T_4, free T_3, and TSH are normal. Levels of T_3 are normal or only slightly elevated. Affected patients are euthyroid.

Refetoff S: Inherited thyroxine-binding globulin abnormalities in man. Endocr Rev 10:275, 1989.

CHAPTER 575
Hypothyroidism

Hypothyroidism results from deficient production of thyroid hormone or a defect in thyroid hormonal receptor activity (Table 575–1). The disorder may be manifested from birth. When symptoms appear after a period of apparently normal thyroid function, the disorder may be truly "acquired" or may only appear so as a result of one of a variety of congenital defects in which the manifestation of the deficiency is delayed. The term *cretinism* is often used synonymously with congenital hypothyroidism but should be avoided.

CONGENITAL HYPOTHYROIDISM

Congenital causes of hypothyroidism may be sporadic or familial, goitrous or nongoitrous. In many cases, the deficiency of thyroid hormone is severe, and symptoms develop in the early weeks of life. In others, lesser degrees of deficiency occur, and manifestations may be delayed for months

ETIOLOGY

Thyroid Dysgenesis. Since the establishment of nationwide programs for neonatal screening for congenital hypothyroidism, millions of neonates have been screened. The prevalence of congenital hypothyroidism has been found to be 1/4,000 infants worldwide, lower in black Americans (1/20,000), and higher in Hispanics and Native Americans (1/2,000). Developmental defects (thyroid dysgenesis) account for 90% of infants in whom hypothyroidism is detected; in about one third, even sensitive radionuclide scans can find no remnants of thyroid tissue *(aplasia)*. In the other two thirds of infants, rudiments of thyroid tissue are found in an ectopic location, anywhere from the base of the tongue *(lingual thyroid)* to the normal position in the neck. Most infants with congenital hypothyroidism are asymptomatic at birth, even if there is complete agenesis of the thyroid gland. This situation is attributed to the transplacental passage of moderate amounts of maternal thyroxine (T_4), which provides fetal levels that are 33% of normal at birth. These low serum levels of T_4 and concomitantly elevated levels of thyroid-stimulating hormone (TSH) make it possible to screen and detect most hypothyroid neonates.

Factors important in normal thyroid migration and development are now being discovered. Three transcription factors, TTF-1, TTF-2, and PAX-8, are important for thyroid morphogenesis and differentiation. In an investigation of 98 neonates with congenital hypothyroidism, two were found to have mutations in the PAX-8 gene. One infant had thyroid ectopy, whereas the other had thyroid hypoplasia. Thyroid dysgenesis occurs sporadically, but familial cases have occasionally been reported. Twice as many females as males are affected. The frequent finding of thyroid dysgenesis confined to only one of a pair of monozygotic twins suggests the operation of a deleterious factor during intrauterine life. For years, it had been proposed that maternal antithyroid antibodies might be that factor, especially because antibodies in patients with autoimmune thyroid disease belong predominantly to the IgG class and can cross the placenta. Although thyroid peroxidase (TPO) antibodies have been detected in some mother-infant pairs, there is little evidence of their pathogenicity. The demonstration of thyroid growth-blocking and cytotoxic antibodies in some infants with thyroid dysgenesis, as well as in their mothers, suggests a more likely pathogenetic mechanism.

Ectopic thyroid tissue (lingual, sublingual, subhyoid) may provide adequate amounts of thyroid hormone for many years or

TABLE 575–1 Etiologic Classification of Hypothyroidism

Pit-1 (homeobox protein) mutations
  Deficiency of thyrotropin, growth hormone, and prolactin
Thyrotropin-releasing hormone (TRH) deficiency
  Isolated?
  Multiple hypothalamic deficiencies (e.g., craniopharyngioma)
TRH unresponsiveness
  Mutations in TRH receptor
Thyrotropin (TSH) deficiency
  Mutations in β-chain
  Multiple pituitary deficiencies
Thyrotropin unresponsiveness
  $G_s\alpha$ mutation (e.g., type IA pseudohypoparathyroidism)
  Mutation in TSH receptor
Defect of fetal thyroid development
  Aplasia, ectopia (dysgenesis)
Defect in thyroid hormone synthesis (e.g., goitrous hypothyroidism)
  Iodide transport defect
  Thyroid peroxidase defect
  Thyroglobulin synthesis defect
  Deiodination defect
Iodine deficiency (endemic goiter)
  Neurologic type
  Myxedematous type
Maternal antibodies
  Thyrotropin receptor–blocking antibody (TRBAb)
  (Also termed thyrotropin binding inhibitor immunoglobulin)
Maternal medications
  Radioiodine, iodides
  Propylthiouracil, methimazole
  Amiodarone
Autoimmune (acquired hypothyroidism)
  Hashimoto's thyroiditis
  Polyglandular autoimmune syndrome, types I, II, and III
Iatrogenic
Propylthiouracil, methimazole, iodides, lithium, amiodarone
Irradiation
  Radioiodine
  Radiographs (neck or whole body)
Thyroidectomy
Systemic disease
  Cystinosis
  Histiocytic infiltration
Resistance to thyroid hormone (only occasional clinical manifestations of hypothyroidism)

may fail in early childhood. Affected children come to clinical attention because of a growing mass at the base of the tongue or in the midline of the neck, usually at the level of the hyoid. Occasionally, ectopia is associated with thyroglossal duct cysts. It may occur in siblings. Surgical removal of ectopic thyroid tissue from a euthyroid individual usually results in hypothyroidism, because most such patients have no other thyroid tissue. Newborn screening programs may detect these patients and avoid delayed diagnosis.

Thyrotropin Receptor-Blocking Antibody. Thyrotropin receptor-blocking antibody (TRBAb) is called *thyroid-binding inhibitor immunoglobulin*. An unusual cause of transitory congenital hypothyroidism is the transplacental passage of maternal antibodies that inhibit binding of TSH to its receptor in the neonate. The frequency is approximately 1/50,000–100,000 infants. It should be suspected whenever there is a history of maternal autoimmune thyroid disease, including Hashimoto's thyroiditis, Graves disease, hypothyroidism while the patient is receiving replacement therapy, or recurrent congenital hypothyroidism of a transient nature in subsequent siblings. In these situations, maternal levels of TRBAb should be measured during pregnancy. Affected infants and their mothers often also have thyrotropin receptor–stimulating antibodies and TPO antibodies. Technetium pertechnetate and ^{125}I scans may fail to detect any thyroid tissue, mimicking thyroid agenesis, but after the condition remits, a normal thyroid gland is demonstrable following discontinuation of replacement treatment. The half-life of the antibody is 21 days, and remission of the hypothyroidism occurs in about 3 mo. Correct diagnosis of this cause of congenital hypothyroidism prevents protracted unnecessary treatment, alerts the clinician to possible recurrences in future pregnancies, and allows a favorable prognosis.

Defective Synthesis of Thyroxine. A variety of defects in the biosynthesis of thyroid hormone may result in congenital hypothyroidism; when the defect is incomplete, compensation occurs, and onset of hypothyroidism may be delayed for years. A goiter is almost always present, and the defect is detected in 1/30,000–50,000 live births in neonatal screening programs. These defects are genetically determined and are transmitted in an autosomal recessive manner.

Defect of Iodide Transport. This rare defect has been reported in nine related infants of the Hutterite sect, and about half the cases are from Japan. Consanguinity has occurred in about one third of the families. It almost certainly involves mutations in the gene coding for the sodium-iodine symporter. In the past, clinical hypothyroidism, with or without a goiter, often developed in the first few months of life, but in recent years, the condition has been detected in neonatal screening programs. In Japan, however, untreated patients acquire goiter and hypothyroidism after 10 yr of age, perhaps because of the very high iodine content (often 19 mg/24 hr) of the Japanese diet.

The energy-dependent mechanisms for concentrating iodide are defective in the thyroid and salivary glands. In contrast to other defects of thyroid hormone synthesis, uptake of radioiodine and pertechnetate is low; a saliva:serum ratio of ^{123}I may be required to establish the diagnosis. This condition responds to treatment with large doses of potassium iodide, but treatment with T_4 is preferable.

Thyroid Peroxidase Defects of Organification and Coupling. This is the most common of the T_4 synthetic defects. After iodide is trapped by the thyroid, it is rapidly oxidized to reactive iodine, which is then incorporated into tyrosine units. This process requires generation of H_2O_2, thyroid peroxidase, and hematin (an enzyme cofactor); defects can involve each of these components, and there is considerable clinical and biochemical heterogeneity. In the Dutch neonatal screening program, 23 infants were found with a complete organification defect (1/60,000), but its prevalence in other areas is unknown. A characteristic finding in all patients with this defect is a marked decrease in thyroid radioactivity when perchlorate or thiocyanate is administered 2 hr after administration of a test dose of radioiodine. In these patients, perchlorate discharges 40–90% of radioiodine compared with less than 10% in normal individuals. Several mutations in the TPO gene have been reported in children with congenital hypothyroidism. Patients with **Pendred's syndrome**, a disorder comprising sensorineural deafness and goiter, also have a positive perchlorate discharge. However, the defect involves iodine transport in the thyroid gland and chloride transport in the ear.

Defects of Thyroglobulin Synthesis. This heterogeneous group of disorders, characterized by goiter, elevated TSH, low T_4 levels, and absent or low levels of thyroglobulin (TG), has been reported in approximately 100 patients. Studies in animal models with congenital goiter have disclosed point mutations of the gene for TG in Afrikander cattle and in Dutch goitrous goats. Analogous molecular defects have been described in a few patients.

Defects in Deiodination. Monoiodotyrosine and diiodotyrosine released from thyroglobulin are normally deiodinated within the thyroid or in peripheral tissues by a deiodinase. The liberated iodine is recycled in the synthesis of TG. Patients with a deficiency of this enzyme experience severe iodine loss from the constant urinary excretion of nondeiodinated tyrosines, leading to hormonal deficiency and goiter. The deiodination defect may be limited to thyroid tissue only or to peripheral tissue only, or it may be universal.

Radioiodine. Hypothyroidism has been reported as a result of inadvertent administration of radioiodine during pregnancy for treatment of Graves disease or cancer of the thyroid. Although only a few affected infants have been reported, a 1976 mail survey of endocrinologists uncovered 237 cases of women who had inadvertently received therapeutic doses of ^{131}I during the 1st trimester of pregnancy. The fetal thyroid is capable of trapping iodide by 70–75 days. Whenever radioiodine is administered to a woman of childbearing age, a pregnancy test must be performed before a therapeutic dose of ^{131}I is given, regardless of the menstrual history or putative history of contraception. Administration of radioactive iodine to lactating women is also contraindicated because it is readily excreted in milk.

Thyrotropin Deficiency. Deficiency of TSH and hypothyroidism may occur in any of the conditions associated with developmental defects of the pituitary or hypothalamus (see Chapter 567). More often in these conditions, the deficiency of TSH is secondary to a deficiency of thyrotropin-releasing hormone (TRH). TSH-deficient hypothyroidism is found in 1/30,000–50,000 infants, but only 30–40% of these cases are detected by neonatal thyroid screening. The majority of affected infants have multiple pituitary deficiencies and present with hypoglycemia, persistent jaundice, and micropenis in association with septo-optic dysplasia, midline cleft lip, midface hypoplasia, and other midline facial anomalies.

Pit-1 mutations are a recessive cause of hypothyroidism secondary to TSH deficiency. Affected children also have deficiency of growth hormone and prolactin. Pit-1, a gene transcription factor, is essential to differentiation, maintenance, and proliferation of somatotrophs, lactotrophs, and thyrotrophs. Examination of prolactin and TSH responses to TRH stimulation can detect these patients. Failure of the prolactin response to TRH should prompt examination of the Pit-1 gene.

Isolated deficiency of TSH is a rare autosomal recessive disorder that has been reported in five sibships. DNA studies in two Japanese children and in three children in two related Greek families have revealed different point mutations in the TSH β subunit gene.

A mutation in the TSH-receptor gene has been reported in three siblings with elevated levels of TSH and normal levels of T_4; two of them had been detected during neonatal screening. Despite persistent resistance to TSH through childhood, they remained euthyroid without treatment. Patients in three other reports of presumed TSH-receptor gene mutations had severe hypothyroidism which required treatment. The disorder is inherited in an autosomal recessive fashion. Both homozygous and compound heterozygous mutations in the TSH receptor gene have been reported.

Thyrotropin Hormone Unresponsiveness. Mild congenital hypothyroidism has been detected in newborn infants who subsequently proved to have type Ia pseudohypoparathyroidism. The molecular cause of resistance to TSH in these patients is the generalized impairment of cyclic adenosine monophosphate activation caused by genetic deficiency of the α subunit of the guanine nucleotide regulatory protein, G_s (see Chapter 582).

Several instances of isolated TSH unresponsiveness have been detected. Serum levels of T_4 were low, those of TSH by radioimmunoassay and bioassay were elevated, and there was no response to exogenous TSH administration.

Thyrotropin-Releasing Hormone Abnormality. A patient with a TRH receptor abnormality resulting in isolated TSH deficiency and hypothyroidism has been reported. This condition was suspected because of failure of both TSH and prolactin to respond to TRH stimulation. Investigations disclosed a compound heterozygote mutation in the gene coding for the TRH receptor, resulting in inability of the receptor to bind TRH.

Thyroid Hormone Unresponsiveness. An increasing number of patients are being found with resistance to the actions of endogenous and exogenous T_4 and T_3. Most patients have goiter, and levels of T_4, T_3, free T_4, and free T_3 are elevated. These findings have often led to the erroneous diagnosis of Graves disease, although most affected patients are clinically euthyroid. The unresponsiveness may vary among tissues. There may be subtle clinical features of hypothyroidism, including mild mental retardation, growth retardation, and delayed skeletal maturation. One neurologic manifestation is an increased association of attention-deficit hyperactivity disorder; the converse is not true, however, because individuals with attention-deficit hyperactivity disorder do not have an increased risk of thyroid hormone resistance. It is presumed that these patients have incomplete resistance to thyroid hormone. TSH levels are diagnostic in that they are not suppressed as in Graves disease but instead are moderately elevated or normal but inappropriate for the levels of T_4 and T_3 when measured by a sensitive TSH assay. A TSH response to TRH occurs in these patients, unlike the situation in Graves disease. The failure of TSH suppression indicates that the resistance is generalized and affects the pituitary gland as well as peripheral tissues. The disorder is most often inherited in an autosomal dominant fashion. More than 40 distinct point mutations in the hormone-binding domain of the β-thyroid receptor have been identified. Different phenotypes do not correlate with genotypes. The same mutation has been observed in individuals with generalized or isolated pituitary resistance, even in different individuals of the same family. Individuals heterozygous for a complete deletion of one *hTRb* allele are normal; a child homozygous for the receptor mutation showed unusually severe resistance. These cases support the dominant negative effect of mutant receptors, in which the mutant receptor protein inhibits normal receptor action in heterozygotes. Elevated levels of T_4 on neonatal thyroid screening should suggest the possibility of this diagnosis. No treatment is usually required unless growth and skeletal retardation are present.

Two infants of consanguineous matings are known to have an autosomal recessive form of thyroid resistance. These infants had manifestations of hypothyroidism early in life, and DNA studies revealed a major deletion of the β-thyroid receptor in one individual. The resistance appears to be more severe in this form of the entity.

On rare occasions, resistance to thyroid hormone may selectively affect the pituitary gland. Because the peripheral tissues are not resistant to thyroid hormones, the patient presents with a goiter and manifestations of hyperthyroidism. The laboratory findings are the same as those seen with generalized thyroid hormone resistance. This condition must be differentiated from a pituitary TSH-secreting tumor. At least one young child has been successfully treated with D-thyroxine therapy. Bromocriptine administration, which interferes with TSH secretion, was reported to be successful in another patient.

Iodine Exposure. Congenital hypothyroidism may result from fetal exposure to excessive iodides or antithyroid drugs. Perinatal exposure may occur with the use of iodine antiseptic to prepare the skin for cesarian section or painting of the cervix prior to delivery. These conditions are transitory and must not be mistaken for the other forms of hypothyroidism described. In the neonate, topical iodine-containing antiseptics used in nurseries and by surgeons can also cause transient congenital hypothyroidism, especially in low birthweight infants, and can lead to abnormal results on neonatal screening tests. In older children, the usual sources of iodides are proprietary preparations used to treat asthma. In a few instances, the cause of hypothyroidism was amiodarone, an antiarrhythmic drug with a high iodine content. In most of these instances goiter is present (see Chapter 577.3).

Iodine Deficiency–Endemic Goiter. Essentially unseen in the United States, iodine deficiency or endemic goiter is the most common cause of congenital hypothyroidism worldwide. Borderline iodine deficiency is more likely to cause problems in preterm infants who depend on a maternal source of iodine.

Thyroid Function in Preterm Babies. Postnatal thyroid function in preterm babies is qualitatively similar but quantitatively reduced compared with that of term infants. The cord serum T_4 is decreased in proportion to gestational age and birthweight. The postnatal TSH surge is reduced, and infants with complications of prematurity, such as respiratory distress syndrome, actually experience a fall in serum T_4 in the first week of life. As these complications resolve, the serum T_4 gradually rises so that generally by 6 wk of life it meets the T_4 concentrations seen in term infants. Serum free T_4 concentrations seem less affected, and when measured by equilibrium dialysis, these levels are often normal. Preterm babies also have a higher frequency of transient TSH elevations and apparent transient primary hypothyroidism. Premature infants less than 28 wk of gestation may have problems resulting from a combination of immaturity of the hypothalamic-pituitary-thyroid axis and loss of the maternal contribution of thyroid hormone and so may be candidates of temporary thyroid hormone replacement.

CLINICAL MANIFESTATIONS. The clinician is becoming increasingly dependent on neonatal screening tests for diagnosis of congenital hypothyroidism. Laboratory errors occur, however, and awareness of early symptoms and signs must be maintained. Congenital hypothyroidism is twice as common in girls as in boys. Before neonatal screening programs, congenital hypothyroidism was rarely recognized in the newborn because the signs and symptoms are usually not sufficiently developed. It can be suspected and the diagnosis established during the early weeks of life if the initial but less characteristic manifestations are recognized. Birthweight and length are normal, but head size may be slightly increased because of myxedema of the brain. Prolongation of physiologic icterus, caused by delayed maturation of glucuronide conjugation, may be the earliest sign. Feeding difficulties, especially sluggishness, lack of interest, somnolence, and choking spells during nursing, are often present during the 1st mo of life. Respiratory difficulties, due in part to the large tongue, include apneic episodes, noisy respirations, and nasal obstruction. Typical respiratory distress syndrome may also occur. Affected infants cry little, sleep much, have poor appetites, and are generally sluggish. There may be constipation that does not usually respond to treatment. The abdomen is large, and an umbilical hernia is usually present. The temperature is subnormal, often less than 35°C (95°F), and the skin, particularly that of the extremities, may be cold and mottled. Edema of the genitals and extremities may be present. The pulse is slow, and heart murmurs, cardiomegaly, and asymptomatic pericardial effusion are common. Anemia is often present and is refractory to treatment with hematinics. Since symptoms appear gradually, the diagnosis is often delayed.

These manifestations progress; retardation of physical and mental development becomes greater during the following months, and by 3–6 mo of age, the clinical picture is fully developed (Fig. 575–1). When there is only a partial deficiency of thyroid hormone, the symptoms may be milder, the syndrome incomplete, and the onset delayed. Although breast milk contains significant amounts of thyroid hormones, particularly T_3, it is inadequate to protect the breast-fed infant with congenital hypothyroidism, and it has no effect on neonatal thyroid screening tests.

The child's growth is stunted, the extremities are short, and the head size is normal or even increased. The anterior and posterior fontanels are open widely; observation of this sign at birth may serve as an initial clue to the early recognition of congenital hypothyroidism. Only 3% of normal newborn infants have a posterior fontanel larger than 0.5 cm. The eyes appear far apart, and the bridge of the broad nose is depressed. The palpebral fissures are narrow and the eyelids swollen. The mouth is kept open, and the thick and broad tongue protrudes from it. Dentition is delayed. The neck is short and thick, and there may be deposits of fat above the clavicles and between the neck and shoulders. The hands are broad and the fingers short. The skin is dry and scaly, and there is little perspiration. Myxedema is manifested, particularly in the skin of the eyelids, the back of the hands, and the external genitals. Carotenemia may cause a yellow discoloration of the skin, but the scleras remain white. The scalp is thickened, and the hair is coarse, brittle, and scanty. The hairline reaches far down on the forehead, which usually appears wrinkled, especially when the infant cries.

Development is usually retarded. Hypothyroid infants appear lethargic and are late in learning to sit and stand. The voice is hoarse, and they do not learn to talk. The degree of physical and mental retardation increases with age. Sexual maturation may be delayed or may not take place at all.

The muscles are usually hypotonic, but in rare instances generalized muscular pseudohypertrophy occurs *(Kocher-Debré-Sémélaigne syndrome)*. Affected children may have an athletic appearance because of pseudohypertrophy, particularly in the calf muscles. Its pathogenesis is unknown; nonspecific histochemical and ultrastructural changes seen on muscle biopsy return to normal with treatment. Boys are more prone to development of the syndrome, which has been observed in siblings born to a consanguineous mating. Affected patients have hypothyroidism of longer duration and severity.

LABORATORY FINDINGS. Most newborn screening programs in North America measure levels of T_4, supplemented by mea-

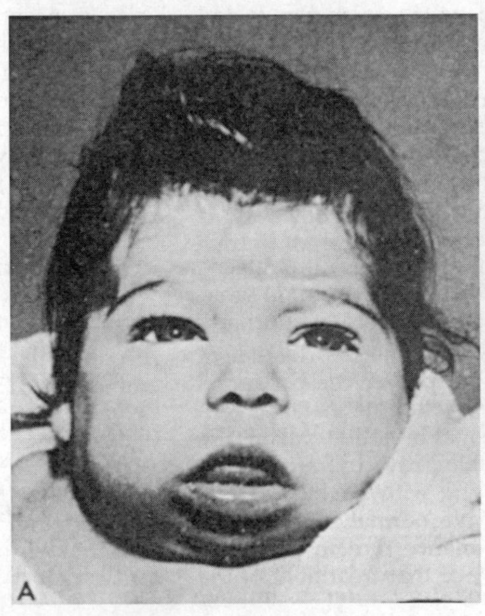

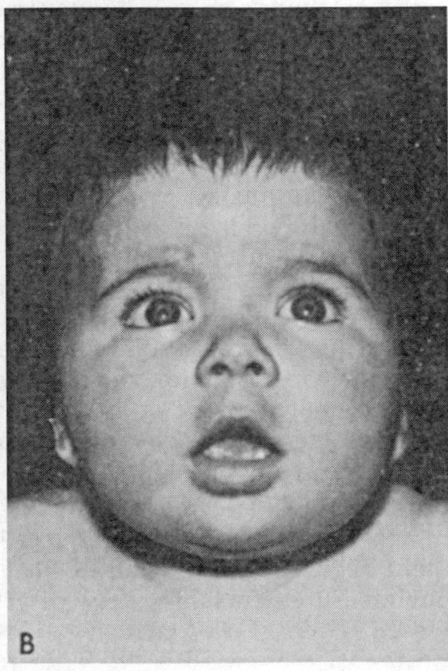

Figure 575–1 Congenital hypothyroidism in an infant 6 mo of age. The infant ate poorly in the neonatal period and was constipated. She had a persistent nasal discharge and a large tongue; she was very lethargic; and she had no social smile and no head control. *A*, Notice the puffy face, dull expression, and hirsute forehead. Tests revealed a negligible uptake of radioiodine. Osseous development was that of a newborn. *B*, Four mo after treatment, notice the decreased puffiness of the face, the decreased hirsutism of the forehead, and the alert appearance.

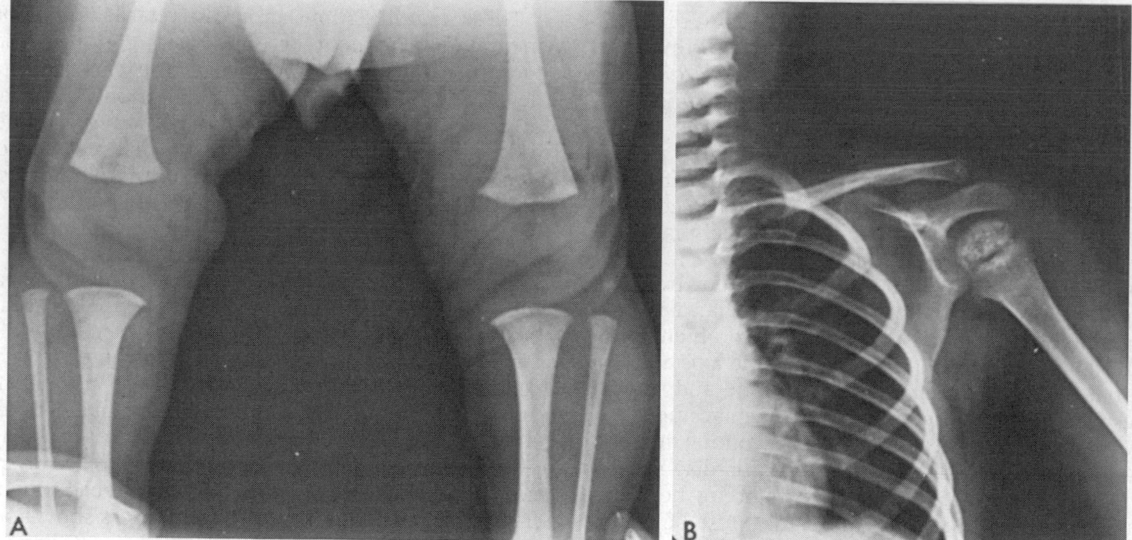

Figure 575–2 Congenital hypothyroidism. *A*, Absence of distal femoral epiphysis in a 3-mo-old infant who was born at term. This is evidence for the onset of the hypothyroid state during fetal life. *B*, Epiphyseal dysgenesis in the head of the humerus in a 9-yr-old girl who had been inadequately treated with thyroid hormone.

surement of TSH when T_4 is low. This approach identifies infants with primary hypothyroidism, those with low levels of thyroxine-binding globulin, some with hypothalamic or pituitary hypothyroidism, and infants with a delayed rise in TSH levels. European and Japanese neonatal screening programs are based on a primary measurement of TSH; this approach misses infants with delayed TSH elevation, low thyroxine-binding globulin levels, and hypothalamic or pituitary hypothyroidism but may detect infants with subclinical hypothyroidism (normal T_4, elevated TSH). With any of these assays, special care should be given to the normal range of values for age of the patient, particularly in the first weeks of life. Regardless of the approach used for screening, some infants escape detection because of technical or human errors; clinicians must maintain their vigilance for clinical manifestations of hypothyroidism.

Serum levels of T_4 are low; serum levels of T_3 may be normal and are not helpful in the diagnosis. If the defect is primarily in the thyroid, levels of TSH are elevated, often to greater than 100 mU/L. Serum levels of prolactin are elevated, correlating with those of TSH. Serum levels of TG are usually low in infants with thyroid agenesis or defects of TG synthesis or secretion, but they may be elevated with ectopic glands and other inborn errors of thyroxine synthesis.

Special attention should be paid to monoamniotic twins, because in at least four cases neonatal screening failed to detect the discordant twin with hypothyroidism, and the diagnosis was not made until the infants were 4–5 mo of age. Apparently, transfusion of euthyroid blood from the unaffected twin normalized the serum level of T_4 and TSH in the affected twin at the initial screening.

Retardation of osseous development can be shown roentgenographically at birth in about 60% of congenitally hypothyroid infants and indicates some deprivation of thyroid hormone during intrauterine life. For example, the distal femoral epiphysis, normally present at birth, is often absent (Fig. 575–2*A*). In untreated patients, the discrepancy between chronological age and osseous development increases. The epiphyses often have multiple foci of ossification (epiphyseal dysgenesis, Fig. 575–2*B*); deformity ("breaking") of the 12th thoracic or 1st or 2nd lumbar vertebra is common. Roentgenograms of the skull show large fontanels and wide sutures; intersutural (wormian) bones are common. The sella turcica is often enlarged and round; in rare instances there may be erosion and thinning. Delays in formation and eruption of teeth may occur. Cardiac enlargement or pericardial effusion may be present.

Scintigraphy can help to pinpoint the underlying cause in infants with congenital hypothyroidism, but treatment should not be unduly delayed for this study. ^{123}I-sodium iodide is superior to ^{99m}Tc-sodium pertechnetate for this purpose. Neither ultrasonographic examination of the thyroid nor serum levels of TG are reliable alternatives to radionuclide scanning. Demonstration of ectopic thyroid tissue is diagnostic of thyroid dysgenesis and establishes the need for lifelong treatment with T_4. Failure to demonstrate any thyroid tissue suggests thyroid aplasia, but this also occurs in neonates with TRBAb and in infants with the iodide-trapping defect. A normally situated thyroid gland with a normal or avid uptake of radionuclide indicates a defect in thyroid hormone biosynthesis. Patients with goitrous hypothyroidism may require extensive evaluation, including radioiodine studies, perchlorate discharge tests, kinetic studies, chromatography, and studies of thyroid tissue, if the biochemical nature of the defect is to be determined.

The electrocardiogram may show low-voltage P and T waves with diminished amplitude of QRS complexes and suggest poor left ventricular function and pericardial effusion. The electroencephalogram frequently shows low voltage. In children older than 2 yr of age, the serum cholesterol level is usually elevated. Brain magnetic resonance imaging prior to treatment is reportedly normal, although proton magnetic resonance spectroscopy shows high levels of choline-containing compounds, which may reflect blocks in myelin maturation.

TREATMENT. Sodium-L-thyroxine given orally is the treatment of choice. Because 80% of circulating T_3 is formed by monodeiodination of T_4, serum levels of T_4 and T_3 in treated infants return to normal. This is also true in the brain, where 80% of required T_3 is produced locally from T_4. In neonates, the initial starting dose is 10–15 μg/kg (37.5 *or* 50 μg/24 hr). Thyroxine tablets should not be mixed with soy protein formulas or iron, because these can bind T_4 and inhibit its absorption. Levels of T_4 and TSH should be monitored at recommended intervals and maintained in the normal range for age. Children with hypothyroidism require about 4 μg/kg/24 hr, and adults require only 2 μg/kg/24 hr.

Later, confirmation of the diagnosis may be necessary for some infants, to rule out the possibility of transient hypothyroidism. This is unnecessary in infants with proven thyroid ectopia or in those who manifest elevated levels of TSH after

6–12 mo of therapy because of poor compliance or an inadequate dose of T_4. Discontinuation of therapy at about 3 yr of age for 3–4 wk results in a marked increase in TSH levels in children with permanent hypothyroidism.

The only untoward effects of sodium-L-thyroxine are related to its dose. Overtreatment may risk craniosynostosis and temperment problems. An occasional older child (8–13 yr) with acquired hypothyroidism may experience pseudotumor cerebri within the first 4 mo of treatment. In older children, after catch-up growth is complete, the growth rate provides an excellent index of the adequacy of therapy. Parents should be forewarned about changes in behavior and activity expected with therapy, and special attention must be given to any developmental or neurologic deficits.

PROGNOSIS. With the advent of neonatal screening programs for detection of congenital hypothyroidism, the prognosis for affected infants has improved dramatically. Early diagnosis and adequate treatment from the first weeks of life result in normal linear growth and intelligence comparable with that of unaffected siblings. Some screening programs report that the most severely affected infants, as judged by the lowest T_4 levels and retarded skeletal maturation, have slightly reduced (5–10 points) IQs and other neuropsychologic sequelae, such as incoordination, hypo- or hypertonia, short attention span, and speech problems. Approximately 20% of children have a neurosensory hearing deficit. Without treatment, affected infants become mentally deficient dwarfs. Thyroid hormone is critical for normal cerebral development in the early postnatal months; biochemical diagnosis must be made soon after birth, and effective treatment must be initiated promptly to prevent irreversible brain damage. Delay in diagnosis, inadequate treatment, and poor compliance in the first 2–3 yr of life result in variable degrees of brain damage. When onset of hypothyroidism occurs after 2 yr of age, the outlook for normal development is much better even if diagnosis and treatment have been delayed, indicating how much more important thyroid hormone is to the rapidly growing brain of the infant.

ACQUIRED HYPOTHYROIDISM

ETIOLOGY. The most common cause of acquired hypothyroidism is lymphocytic thyroiditis. Autoimmune thyroid disease may be part of polyglandular syndromes; children with Down, Turner, and Klinefelter syndromes are at higher risk for associated autoimmune thyroid disease (see Chapter 576). Although typically seen in adolescence, it occurs as early as in the 1st year of life. Some patients with congenital thyroid dysgenesis or with incomplete genetic defects in thyroid hormone synthesis may not display clinical manifestations until childhood and appear to have acquired hypothyroidism; these conditions are now detected by newborn screening programs. Subtotal thyroidectomy for thyrotoxicosis or cancer may result in hypothyroidism, as may removal of ectopic thyroid tissue. For example, *lingual thyroid, subhyoid median thyroid,* or thyroid tissue in a *thyroglossal duct cyst* usually constitutes the only source of thyroid hormone, and excision results in hypothyroidism. Because subhyoid glands usually mimic thyroglossal duct cysts, ultrasonographic examination or a radionuclide scan before surgery is indicated in these patients.

Children with *nephropathic cystinosis,* a disorder characterized by intralysosomal storage of cystine in body tissues, acquire impaired thyroid function. Hypothyroidism may be overt, but compensated forms are more common, and periodic assessment of TSH levels is indicated. By 13 yr of age, two thirds of these patients require T_4 replacement.

Histiocytic infiltration of the thyroid in children with Langerhans cell histiocytoses may result in hypothyroidism.

Irradiation of the area of thyroid that is incidental to the treatment of Hodgkin's disease or other head and neck malignancies or that is administered before bone marrow transplantation often results in thyroid damage. About one third of such children acquire elevated TSH levels within a year after therapy, and 15–20% progress to hypothyroidism within 5–7 yr. Some clinicians recommend periodic TSH measurements, but others recommend treatment of all exposed patients with doses of T_4 to suppress TSH (see Chapter 503.1).

Protracted ingestion of medications containing iodides can cause hypothyroidism, usually accompanied by goiter (see Chapter 577). Amiodarone, a drug used for cardiac arrhythmias and consisting of 37% iodine by weight, causes hypothyroidism in about 20% of treated children. It affects thyroid function directly by its high iodine content as well as by inhibition of 5′-deiodinase, which converts T_4 to T_3. Children treated with this drug should have serial measurements of T_4, T_3, and TSH.

CLINICAL MANIFESTATIONS. Deceleration of growth is usually the first clinical manifestation, but this sign often goes unrecognized (Fig. 575–3). Myxedematous changes of the skin, constipation, cold intolerance, decreased energy, and an increased need for sleep develop insidiously. Surprisingly, schoolwork and grades usually do not suffer, even in severely hypothyroid children. Osseous maturation is delayed, often strikingly,

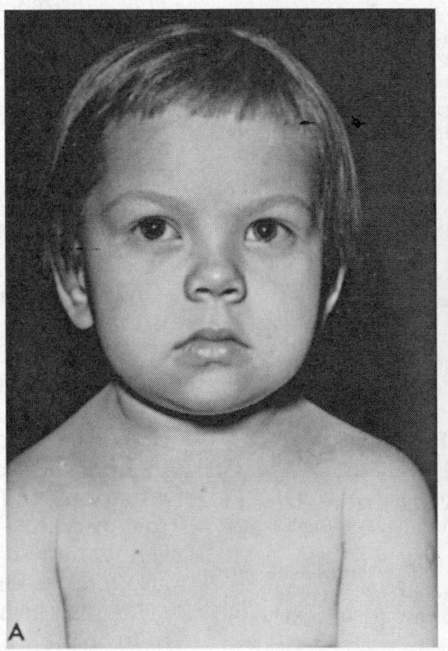

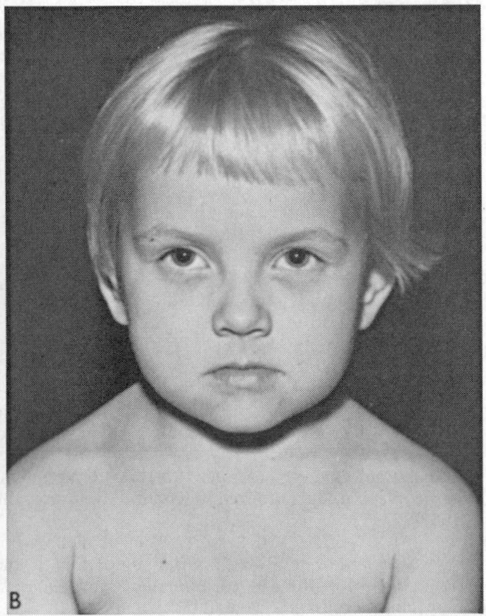

Figure 575–3 *A,* Acquired hypothyroidism in a girl 6 yr of age. She was treated with a wide variety of hematinics for refractory anemia for 3 yr. She had almost complete cessation of growth, constipation, and sluggishness for 3 yr. The height age was 3 yr; the bone age was 4 yr. She had a sallow complexion and immature facies with a poorly developed nasal bridge. Serum cholesterol, 501 mg/dL; radioiodine uptake, 7% at 24 hr; PBI, 2.8 mg/dL. *B,* After therapy for 18 mo, notice the nasal development, the increased luster and decreased pigmentation of hair, and the maturation of face. The height age was 5.5 yr; the bone age was 7 yr. There was a decided improvement in her general condition. Menarche occurred at 14 yr. The ultimate height was 155 cm (61 in). She graduated from high school. The disorder was well controlled with sodium-L-thyroxine daily.

which is an indication of the duration of the hypothyroidism. Adolescents typically have delayed puberty, whereas younger children may present with galactorrhea or pseudoprecocious puberty. Galactorrhea is a result of increased TRH stimulating prolactin secretion. The precocious puberty, characterized by breast development in girls and macro-orchidism in boys, is thought to be the result of abnormally high TSH concentrations binding to the follicle-stimulating hormone receptor with subsequent stimulation.

Some children present with headaches and visual problems; they usually have hyperplastic enlargement of the pituitary gland, often with suprasellar extension, after long-standing hypothyroidism; this condition, believed to be the result of thyrotroph hyperplasia, may be mistaken for a pituitary tumor (see Chapter 567).

All these changes return to normal with adequate replacement of T_4, but in children with long-standing hypothyroidism, catch-up growth may be incomplete. During the first 18 mo of treatment, skeletal maturation often exceeds expected linear growth, resulting in a loss of about 7 cm of predicted adult height. The cause for this is unknown.

Diagnostic studies and treatment are the same as those described for congenital hypothyroidism. Measurement of antithyroglobulin and antiperoxidase (formerly antimicrosomal) antibodies may pinpoint autoimmune thyroiditis as the cause. During the 1st year of treatment, deterioration of schoolwork, poor sleeping habits, restlessness, short attention span, and behavioral problems may ensue, but these are transient; forewarning families about these manifestations enhances appropriate management. These may be partially ameliorated by starting at subreplacement T_4 doses and advancing slowly.

Anasti JN, Flack MR, Froehlich J, et al: A potential novel mechanism for precocious puberty in juvenile hypothyroidism. J Clin Endocrinol Metab 80:276, 1995.

Adams A, Matthews C, Collingwood TH, et al: Genetic analysis of 29 kindreds with generalized and pituitary resistance to thyroid hormone. J Clin Invest 94:506, 1994.

American Academy of Pediatrics: Newborn screening for congenital hypothyroidism: Recommended guidelines. Pediatrics 91:1203, 1993.

Biebermann H, Schoneberg T, Krude H, et al: Mutations in the human thyrotropin receptor gene causing thyroid hyperplasia and persistent congenital hypothyroidism. J Clin Endocrinol Metab 82:3471, 1997.

Brent GA: The molecular basis of thyroid hormone action. N Engl J Med 331:847, 1994.

Brown RS, Bellisario RL, Mitchell E, et al: Detection of thyrotropin binding inhibitory activity in neonatal blood spots. J Clin Endocrinol Metab 77:1005, 1993.

Collu R, Tang J, Castagne J, et al: A novel mechanism for isolated central hypothyroidism: Inactivating mutations in the thyroropin-releasing hormone receptor gene. J Clin Endocrinol Metab 82:1361, 1997.

Cosman BC, Schullmger JN, Bell JJ, et al: Hypothyroidism caused by topical povidone-iodine in a newborn with omphalocele. J Pediatr Surg 23:356, 1988.

Cutler AT, Benezra-Obeiter R, Brink SJ: Thyroid function in young children with Down syndrome. Am J Dis Child 140:479, 1986.

Dacou-Voutetakis C, Felquate DM, Drakopoulou M, et al: Familial hypothyroidism by a nonsense mutation in the thyroid-stimulating hormone β-subunit gene. Am J Hum Genet 46:988, 1990.

Delange F: The disorders induced by iodine deficiency. [Review] Thyroid 4:107, 1994.

Delange F: Neonatal screening for congenital hypothyroidism: Results and perspectives. [Review] Horm Res 48:51, 1997.

Fisher DA: Management of congenital hypothyroidism. J Clin Endocrinol Metab 72:523, 1991.

Germak JA, Foley TP Jr: Longitudinal assessment of L-thyroxine therapy for congenital hypothyroidism. J Pediatr 117:211, 1990.

Glorieux J, Dussault J, Van Vliet G: Intellectual development at age 12 years of children with congenital hypothyroidism diagnosed by newborn screening. J Pediatr 121:581, 1992.

Grant DB, Fuggle P, Tokar S, Smith I: Psychomotor development in infants with congenital hypothyroidism diagnosed by newborn screening. Acta Med Aust 19:54, 1992.

Hauser P, Zametkin AJ, Martinez P, et al: Attention deficit–hyperactivity disorder in people with generalized resistance to thyroid hormone. N Engl J Med 328:997, 1993.

Hunter MK, Mandel SH, Sesser DE, et al: Follow-up of newborns with low thyroxine and nonelevated thyroid-stimulating hormone–secreting concentrations: Results of the 20-year experience in the Northwest Regional Newborn Screeening Program. J Pediatr 132:70, 1998.

LaFranchi SH, Hanna CE, Krainz PL, et al: Screening for congenital hypothyroidism with specimen collection at two time periods: Results of the Northwest Regional Screening Program. Pediatrics 76:734, 1985.

Mandel SH, Hanna CE, Boston BA, et al: Thyroxine binding globulin deficiency detected by newborn screening. J Pediatr 122:227, 1993.

Muir A, Daneman D, Daneman A, et al: Thyroid scanning, ultrasound, and serum thyroglobulin in determining the origin of congenital hypothyroidism. Am J Dis Child 142:214, 1988.

New England Congenital Hypothyroidism Collaborative: Correlation of cognitive test scores and adequacy of treatment in adolescents with congenital hypothyroidism. J Pediatr 124:383, 1994.

Oakley GA, Muir T, Ray M, et al: Increased incidence of congenital malformations in children with transient thyroid-stimulating hormone elevation on neonatal screening. J Pediatr 132:726, 1998.

Parks JS, Kinoshita EI, Pfaffle RW: Pit-1 and hypopituitarism. Trends Endocrinol Metab 4:81, 1993.

Refetoff S, Weiss RE, Usala SJ: The syndromes of resistance to thyroid hormones. Endocr Rev 14:348, 1993.

Rivkees SA, Bode HH, Crawford JD: Long-term growth in juvenile acquired hypothyroidism: The failure to achieve normal adult stature. N Engl J Med 318:519, 1988.

Rovet JF, Ehrlich RM, Sorbara DL: Neurodevelopment in infants and preschool children with congenital hypothyroidism: Etiological and treatment factors affecting outcome. J Pediatr Psychol 17:187, 1992.

Siragusa V, Boffelli S, Weber G, et al: Brain magnetic resonance imaging in congenital hypothyroid infants at diagnosis. Thyroid 7:761, 1997.

Thorpe-Beeston JG, Nicolaides KH, Fetton CV, et al: Maturation of the secretion of thyroid hormone and thyroid-stimulating hormone in the fetus. N Engl J Med 324:532, 1991.

Toft AD: Drug therapy: Thyroxine therapy. N Engl J Med 331:174, 1994.

VanDop C, Conte FA, Koch TK, et al: Pseudotumor cerebri associated with initiation of levothyroxine therapy for juvenile hypothyroidism. N Engl J Med 308:1076, 1983.

CHAPTER 576
Thyroiditis

LYMPHOCYTIC THYROIDITIS (HASHIMOTO'S THYROIDITIS; AUTOIMMUNE THYROIDITIS)

Lymphocytic thyroiditis is the most common cause of thyroid disease in children and adolescents and accounts for many of the enlarged thyroids formerly designated "adolescent" or "simple" goiter. It is also the most common cause of acquired hypothyroidism, with or without goiter. Its incidence may be as high as 1% among schoolchildren.

ETIOLOGY. This typical organ-specific autoimmune disease is characterized histologically by lymphocytic infiltration of the thyroid. Early in the course of the disease, there may be hyperplasia only; this is followed by infiltration of lymphocytes and plasma cells between the follicles and by atrophy of the follicles. Lymphoid follicle formation with germinal centers is almost always present; the degree of atrophy and fibrosis of the follicles varies from mild to moderate.

Intrathyroidal lymphocyte subsets differ from those in blood. About 60% of infiltrating lymphoid cells are T cells, and about 30% express B-cell markers; the T-cell population is represented by helper ($CD4^+$) and cytotoxic ($CD8^+$) cells. The participation of cellular events in the pathogenesis is clear. Certain HLA haplotypes (HLA-DR4, HLA-DR5) are associated with an increased risk of goiter and thyroiditis, and others (HLA-DR3) are associated with the atrophic variant of thyroiditis. Much remains to be discovered about the disturbance in immunoregulation and how it interacts with genetic predisposition and environmental factors in the pathogenesis of autoimmune thyroid disease.

A variety of different thyroid antigen autoantibodies are also involved in the process. Thyroid antiperoxidase antibodies (TPOAbs), formerly called "antimicrosomal antibodies," are demonstrable in the sera of 90% of children with lymphocytic thyroiditis and in many patients with Graves disease. For many years, TPOAbs were considered nonpathogenic, but evidence now shows that TPOAbs inhibit enzyme activity and stimulate natural killer cell cytotoxicity. With the molecular cloning of the TPO gene, a new generation of ultrasensitive tests for the measurement of these antibodies is under development.

Antithyroglobulin antibodies occur in a smaller percentage of affected children but are much more common in adults. Thyrotropin receptor-blocking antibodies are frequently present, especially in patients with hypothyroidism, and it is now believed that they are related to the development of hypothyroidism and thyroid atrophy in patients with autoimmune thyroiditis.

CLINICAL MANIFESTATIONS. The disorder is four to seven times more frequent in girls than in boys. It may occur during the first 3 yr of life but becomes sharply more common after 6 yr of age and reaches a peak incidence during adolescence. The most common clinical manifestations are growth retardation and goiter. The goiter may appear insidiously and may be small or large. In most patients, the thyroid is diffusely enlarged, firm, and nontender. In about one third of patients, the gland is lobular and may seem to be nodular. Most of the affected children are clinically euthyroid and asymptomatic; some may have symptoms of pressure in the neck. Some children have clinical signs of hypothyroidism, but others who appear clinically euthyroid have laboratory evidence of hypothyroidism. A few children have manifestations suggestive of hyperthyroidism, such as nervousness, irritability, increased sweating, or hyperactivity, but results of laboratory studies are not necessarily those of hyperthyroidism. Occasionally, the disorder may coexist with Graves disease. Ophthalmopathy may occur in lymphocytic thyroiditis in the absence of Graves disease.

The clinical course is variable. The goiter may become smaller or may disappear spontaneously, or it may persist unchanged for years while the patient remains euthyroid. Most children who are euthyroid at presentation remain euthyroid, although a percentage of patients acquire hypothyroidism gradually within months or years; thyroiditis is the cause of most cases of nongoitrous (atrophic) hypothyroidism.

Familial clusters of lymphocytic thyroiditis are common; the incidence in siblings or parents of affected children may be as high as 25%. Autoantibodies to thyroglobulin and human thyroid peroxidase in these families appear to be inherited in an autosomal dominant fashion, with reduced penetrance in males. The concurrence within families of patients with lymphocytic thyroiditis, "idiopathic" hypothyroidism, and Graves disease provides cogent evidence for a basic relationship among these three conditions. The disorder has been associated with many of the other autoimmune disorders more often than would be expected by chance alone. Autoimmune thyroiditis occurs in 10% of patients with *type I polyglandular autoimmune syndrome,* which consists of hypoparathyroidism, Addison's disease, and mucocutaneous candidiasis. The association of Addison's disease with insulin-dependent diabetes mellitus or autoimmune thyroid disease, or both, is known as *Schmidt syndrome* or *type II polyglandular autoimmune disease.* Autoimmune thyroid disease also tends to be associated with pernicious anemia, vitiligo, or alopecia. TPOAbs are found in approximately 20% of white and 4% of black children with diabetes mellitus. Autoimmune thyroid disease has an increased incidence in children with congenital rubella. Lymphocytic thyroiditis is also associated with certain chromosomal aberrations, particularly Turner syndrome and Down syndrome. In children with Down syndrome, one study reported that 28% had antithyroid antibodies (predominantly anti-TPOs), 7% had subclinical hypothyroidism, 7% had overt hypothyroidism, and 5% had hyperthyroidism. In a study of girls with Turner syndrome, 41% had antithyroid antibodies (again, predominantly anti-TPOs), 18% had goiter, and 8% had subclinical or overt hypothyroidism. Another study of 75 girls with Turner syndrome found that autoimmune thyroid disease increased from the first (15%) to the third (30%) decade of life. Boys with Klinefelter syndrome are also at risk for autoimmune thyroid disease.

LABORATORY FINDINGS. The definitive diagnosis can be established by biopsy of the thyroid, but this procedure is rarely indicated for clinical purposes alone. Thyroid function tests are often normal, although the level of thyroid-stimulating hormone (TSH) may be slightly or even moderately elevated in some individuals, termed *subclinical hypothyroidism.* The fact that many children with lymphocytic thyroiditis do not have elevated levels of TSH indicates that the goiter may be caused by the lymphocytic infiltrations or by thyroid growth-stimulating immunoglobulins. In 50% of children, thyroid scans reveal irregular and patchy distribution of the radioisotope, and in about 60% or more, the administration of perchlorate results in a greater than 10% discharge of iodide from the thyroid gland. Thyroid ultrasonography shows scattered hypoechogenicity in most patients. Most patients with lymphocytic thyroiditis have serum antibody titers to TPO, but the antithyroglobulin test for thyroid antibodies is positive in fewer than 50%. When both tests are used, approximately 95% of patients with thyroid autoimmunity are detected. In general, levels in children and adolescents are lower than those in adults with lymphocytic thyroiditis, and repeated measurements are indicated in questionable instances because titers may increase later in the course of the disease.

Antithyroid antibodies may also be found in almost half the siblings of affected patients and in a significant percentage of the mothers of children with Down syndrome or Turner syndrome without demonstrable thyroid disease. They are also found in 20% of children with diabetes mellitus and in 23% of children with the congenital rubella syndrome.

TREATMENT. If there is evidence of hypothyroidism, replacement treatment with sodium-L-thyroxine (50–150 μg daily) is indicated. The goiter usually shows some decrease in size but may persist for years. Antibody levels fluctuate in both treated and untreated patients and persist for years. Because the disease may be self-limited in some instances, the need for continued therapy requires periodic re-evaluation. Untreated patients should also be checked periodically. Prominent nodules that persist despite suppressive therapy should be examined histologically because thyroid cancer has occurred in patients with lymphocytic thyroiditis.

OTHER CAUSES OF THYROIDITIS

Specific conditions such as tuberculosis, sarcoidosis, mumps, and cat-scratch disease are rare causes of thyroiditis.

Acute suppurative thyroiditis is uncommon; it is usually preceded by a respiratory infection. The left lower lobe is affected predominantly. Abscess formation may occur. Anaerobic organisms, with or without aerobes, are the most common organisms; *Eikenella corrodens* has been reported. Recurrent episodes or the detection of a mixed bacterial flora suggests that the infection arises from a thyroglossal duct remnant or, more often, from a piriform sinus fistula. Exquisite tenderness of the gland, swelling, erythema, dysphagia, and limitation of head motion are characteristic findings. Systemic manifestations are often absent, and leukocytosis is present. Scintigrams of the thyroid often reveal decreased uptake in the affected areas, and ultrasonography may show a complex echogenic mass. Thyroid function is usually normal, but thyrotoxicosis due to escape of thyroid hormone has been encountered in a child with suppurative thyroiditis resulting from *Aspergillus.* When suppuration occurs, incision and drainage and administration of antibiotics are indicated. After the infection subsides, a barium esophagram is indicated to search for a fistulous tract; if one is found, exteriorization is indicated.

Subacute nonsuppurative thyroiditis (de Quervain disease) is rare in children. It is thought to have a viral cause and remits spontaneously. The disorder becomes manifested by a vague tenderness over the thyroid and low-grade fever or by severe pain in the region of the thyroid and systemic manifestations with chills and high fever. Inflammation results in leakage of preformed thyroid hormone from the gland into the circulation. Serum levels of T_4 and T_3 are elevated, and mild symptoms of hyperthyroidism may be present, but radioiodine uptake is depressed. The erythrocyte sedimentation rate is increased. The course is variable, usually passing through a euthyroid to a hypothyroid phase; remission usually occurs in several months. Occasionally, this condition is superimposed on lymphocytic thyroiditis.

Boyages SC, Halpern JP, Maberly GF, et al: Possible role for thyroid autoimmunity. Lancet 2:529, 1989.

Chiovato L, Vitti P, Santini F, et al: Incidence of antibodies blocking thyrotropin effect in vitro in patients with euthyroid or hypothyroid autoimmune thyroiditis. J Clin Endocrinol Metab 71:40, 1990.

Foley TP Jr, Abbassi V, Copeland KC, et al: Brief report: Hypothyroidism caused by chronic autoimmune thyroiditis in very young infants. N Engl J Med 330:466, 1993.

Gruneiro de Papendieck L, Iorcansky S, Coco R: High incidence of thyroid disturbances in 49 children with Turner syndrome. J Pediatr 111:258, 1987.

Gutekunst R, Hafermann W, Mansky T, Scriba PC: Ultrasonography related to clinical and laboratory findings in lymphocytic thyroiditis. Acta Endocrinol (Copenh) 121:129, 1989.

Hayashi Y, Tamai H, Fukata S, et al: A long-term clinical, immunological, and histological follow-up study of patients with goitrous chronic lymphocytic thyroiditis. J Clin Endocrinol Metab 61:1172, 1985.

Mangklabruks A, Cox N, DeGroot IJ: Genetic factors in autoimmune thyroid disease analyzed by restriction fragment length polymorphisms of candidate genes. J Clin Endocrinol Metab 73:236, 1991.

Matsuura N, Konishi J, Yuri K, et al: Comparison of atrophic and goitrous autoimmune thyroiditis in children: Clinical, laboratory and TSH-receptor antibody studies. Eur J Pediatr 149:529, 1990.

Perheentupa J: Autoimmune polyendocrinopathy–candidiasis–ectodermal dystrophy (APECED). [Review] Horm Metab Res 28:353, 1996.

Phillips D, McLachlan S, Stephenson A, et al: Autosomal dominant transmission of autoantibodies to thyroglobulin and thyroid peroxidase. J Clin Endocrinol Metab 70:742, 1990.

Pueschel SM, Pezzallo JC: Thyroid dysfunction in Down syndrome. Am J Dis Child 139:636, 1985.

Queen JS, Clegg HW, Council JC, et al: Acute suppurative thyroiditis caused by *Eikenella corrodens*. J Pediatr Surg 23:359, 1988.

Rallison ML, Dobyns BM, Keating FR, et al: Occurrence and natural history of chronic lymphocytic thyroiditis in childhood. J Pediatr 86:675, 1975.

Rallison ML, Dobyns BM, Meikle AW, et al: Natural history of thyroid abnormalities: Prevalence, incidence, and regression of thyroid diseases in adolescents and young adults. Am J Med 91:363, 1991.

Rich EJ, Mendelman PM: Acute suppurative thyroiditis in pediatric patients. Pediatr Infect Dis J 6:936, 1987.

Weetman AP: Autoimmune thyroiditis: Predisposition and pathogenesis. Clin Endocrinol 36:307, 1992.

CHAPTER 577

Goiter

A goiter is an enlargement of the thyroid gland. Persons with enlarged thyroids may have normal function of the gland *(euthyroidism)*, thyroid deficiency *(hypothyroidism)*, or overproduction of the hormones *(hyperthyroidism)*. Goiter may be congenital or acquired, endemic or sporadic.

The goiter often results from increased pituitary secretion of thyrotropic hormone in response to decreased circulating levels of thyroid hormones. Thyroid enlargement may also result from infiltrative processes that may be inflammatory or neoplastic. Goiter in patients with thyrotoxicosis is caused by thyrotropin receptor-stimulating antibodies.

577.1 Congenital Goiter

Congenital goiter is usually sporadic and may result from a fetal thyroxine (T_4) synthetic defect or the administration of antithyroid drugs or iodides during pregnancy for the treatment of thyrotoxicosis. Goitrogenic drugs and iodides cross the placenta and at high doses may interfere with synthesis of thyroid hormone, resulting in goiter and hypothyroidism in the fetus. The concomitant administration of thyroid hormone with the goitrogen does not prevent this effect, because insufficient amounts of T_4 cross the placenta. Iodides are included in many proprietary preparations used to treat asthma; these preparations must be avoided during pregnancy because they have often been a cause of unexpected congenital goiter. Amiodarone, an antiarrhythmic drug with a 37% iodine content, has also caused congenital goiter with hypothyroidism. Even when the infant is clinically euthyroid, there may be retardation of osseous maturation, low levels of T_4, and elevated levels of thyroid-stimulating hormone (TSH). Because these effects can occur when the mother takes only 100–200 mg of propylthiouracil/24 hr, all such infants should undergo thyroid studies at birth. Administration of thyroid hormone to affected infants may be indicated to treat clinical hypothyroidism, to hasten the disappearance of the goiter, and to prevent brain damage. Because the condition is rarely permanent, thyroid hormone may be safely discontinued after the antithyroid drug has been excreted by the neonate, usually after a week or so.

Enlargement of the thyroid at birth may occasionally be sufficient to cause respiratory distress that interferes with nursing and may even cause death. The head may be maintained in extreme hyperextension. When respiratory obstruction is severe, partial thyroidectomy rather than tracheostomy is indicated (Fig. 577–1).

Goiter is almost always present in the congenitally hyperthyroid infant. These goiters usually are not large; the infant manifests clinical symptoms of hyperthyroidism, and the mother often has a history of Graves disease (see Chapter 578.1). TSH receptor–activating mutations are also a recognized cause of congenital goiter.

When no causative factor is identifiable, a defect in synthesis of thyroid hormone should be suspected. Neonatal screening programs find congenital hypothyroidism caused by such a defect in 1/30,000–50,000 live births. Study of this group of infants is complex. If the infant is hypothyroid, it is advisable to treat immediately with thyroid hormone and to postpone more detailed studies for later in life. Because these defects are transmitted by recessive genes, a precise diagnosis is important for genetic counseling. Monitoring subsequent pregnancies with ultrasonography can be useful in detecting fetal goiters (see Chapters 575 and 92.4).

Iodine deficiency as a cause of congenital goiters has become rare but persists in isolated endemic areas. More important is the recent recognition that severe iodine deficiency early in pregnancy may cause neurologic damage during fetal development, even in the absence of goiter. The iodine deficiency may result in maternal and fetal hypothyroidism, preventing the partially protective transfer of maternal thyroid hormones.

When the "goiter" is lobulated, asymmetric, firm, or large to an unusual degree, a teratoma within or in the vicinity of the thyroid must be considered in the differential diagnosis (see Chapter 579).

577.2 Endemic Goiter and Cretinism

The association between dietary deficiency of iodine and the prevalence of goiter or cretinism has been recognized for more than half a century. A moderate deficiency of iodine can be

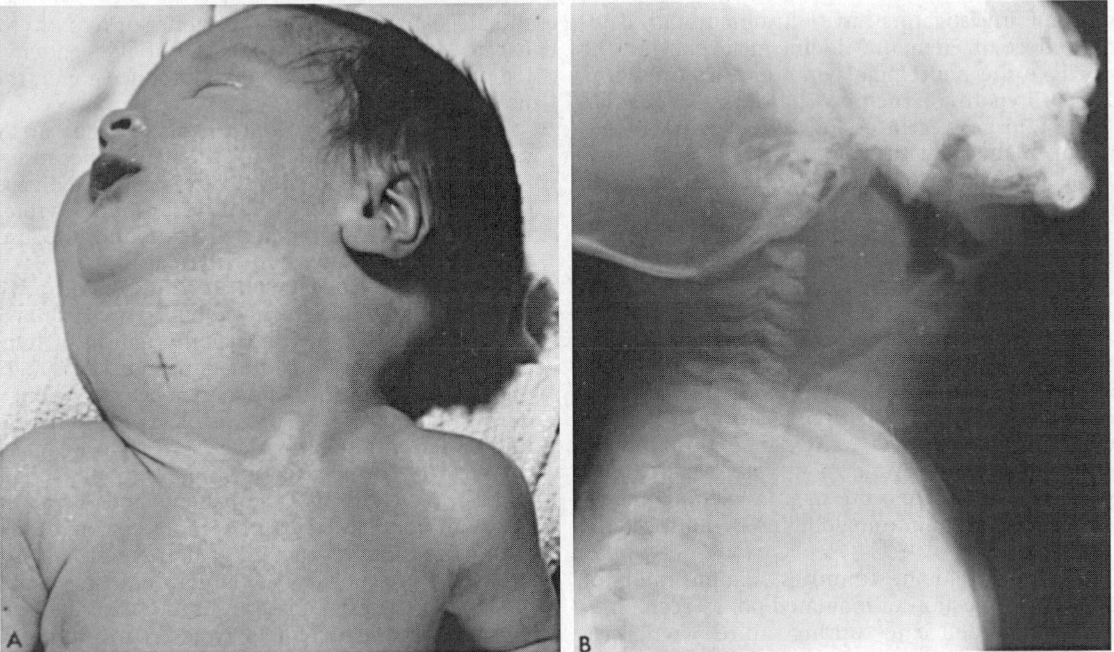

Figure 577–1 Congenital goiter in infancy. *A*, Large congenital goiter in an infant born to a mother with thyrotoxicosis who had been treated with iodides and methimazole during pregnancy. *B*, A 6-wk-old infant with increasing respiratory distress and cervical mass since birth. The operation revealed a large goiter that almost completely encircled the trachea. Notice the anterior deviation and posterior compression of the trachea. Partial thyroidectomy completely relieved the symptoms. It is apparent why a tracheostomy is not adequate treatment for these infants. The cause for the goiter was not found.

overcome by increased efficiency in the synthesis of thyroid hormone. Iodine liberated in the tissues is returned rapidly to the gland, which resynthesizes triiodothyronine (T_3) preferentially at a higher rate than normal. This increased activity is achieved by compensatory hypertrophy and hyperplasia, which satisfy the demands of the tissues for thyroid hormone. In geographic areas where deficiency of iodine is severe, decompensation and hypothyroidism may result. It is estimated that 800 million individuals in developing countries live in areas of iodine deficiency.

Seawater is rich in iodine, and the iodine content of fish and shellfish is also high. Endemic goiter is rare therefore in populations living along the sea. Iodine is deficient in the water and native foods in the Pacific West and the Great Lakes areas of the United States. Deficiency of dietary iodine is even greater in certain Alpine valleys, the Himalayas, the Andes, the Congo, and the highlands of Papua New Guinea. In areas such as the United States, where iodine is provided in foods from other areas and in iodized salt, endemic goiter has disappeared. Iodized salt in the United States contains potassium iodide (100 μg/g) and provides excellent prophylaxis. Further iodine intake in the United States is contributed by iodates used in baking, iodine-containing coloring agents, and iodine-containing disinfectants used in the dairy industry. The recommended daily allowance of iodine for infants is greater than 30 μg/kg/24 hr; this amount is exceeded fourfold in breast-fed infants and 10-fold in infants fed cow's milk in the United States.

CLINICAL MANIFESTATIONS. If the deficiency of iodine is mild, thyroid enlargement does not become noticeable except when there is increased demand for the hormone during periods of rapid growth, as in adolescence and during pregnancy. In regions of moderate iodine deficiency, goiter observed in schoolchildren may disappear with maturity and reappear during pregnancy or lactation. Iodine-deficient goiters are more common in girls than in boys. In areas where iodine deficiency is severe, as in the hyperendemic highlands of Papua New Guinea, nearly half the population has large goiters, and endemic cretinism is common.

Serum T_4 levels are often low in individuals with endemic goiter, although clinical hypothyroidism is rare. This is true in New Guinea, the Congo, the Himalayas, and South America. Despite low serum levels of thyroid hormone, serum TSH concentrations are often only moderately increased. In such patients, circulating levels of T_3 are elevated. Moreover, T_3 levels are also elevated in patients with normal T_4 levels, indicating a preferential secretion of T_3 by the thyroid in this disease.

Endemic cretinism, the most serious consequence of iodine deficiency, has been recognized for centuries; it occurs only in geographic association with endemic goiter. The term *endemic cretinism* includes two different but overlapping syndromes—a neurologic type and a myxedematous type. The frequency of the two types varies among different populations. In Papua New Guinea, the neurologic type occurs almost exclusively, but in Zaire, the myxedematous type predominates. Both types are found in all endemic areas, and some individuals have intermediate or mixed features.

The neurologic syndrome is characterized by mental retardation, deaf-mutism, disturbances in standing and gait, and pyramidal signs such as clonus of the foot, the Babinski sign, and patellar hyperreflexia. Affected individuals are goitrous but euthyroid, have normal pubertal development and adult stature, and have little or no impaired thyroid function. Individuals with the myxedematous syndrome also are mentally retarded and deaf and have neurologic symptoms, delayed sexual development and growth, myxedema, and absence of goiter; serum T_4 levels are low, and TSH levels are markedly elevated. Delayed skeletal maturation may extend into the 3rd decade or later. Ultrasonographic examination shows thyroid atrophy.

PATHOGENESIS. The pathogenesis of the neurologic syndrome has been attributed to iodine deficiency and hypothyroxinemia during pregnancy, leading to fetal and postnatal hypothyroidism. Although some investigators have attributed brain damage to a direct effect of elemental iodine deficiency in the fetus, others believe the neurologic symptoms are caused by fetal and maternal hypothyroxinemia. There is evidence that the human fetal brain has receptors for thyroid hormone before development of the fetal thyroid, and there is also evidence of transplacental passage of maternal thyroid hormone into the fetus, which normally might ameliorate the effects of fetal hypothyroidism on the developing nervous system. The pathogenesis of the myxedematous syndrome leading to thyroid atrophy is more bewildering. Searches for additional environmental factors that may provoke continuing postnatal hypothyroidism have led to incrimination of selenium deficiency, goitrogenic foods, thiocyanates, and *Yersinia*. Studies from Western China suggest that thyroid autoimmunity may play a role. Myxedematous cretins with thyroid atrophy, but not euthyroid cretins, were found to have thyroid growth-blocking immunoglobulins of the kind found in infants with sporadic congenital hypothyroidism. Others are skeptical about any role of thyroid growth-blocking immunoglobulins in goitrogenesis and endemic goiter.

TREATMENT. In many developing countries, administration of a single intramuscular injection of iodinated poppy seed oil to women prevents iodine deficiency during future pregnancies for about 5 yr. This form of therapy given to children less than 4 yr of age with myxedematous cretinism results in a euthyroid state in 5 mo. However, older children respond poorly and adults not at all to iodized oil injections, indicating an inability of the thyroid gland to synthesize hormone; these patients require treatment with T_4. In the Xinjiang province of China, where the usual methods of iodine supplementation had failed, iodination of irrigation water has increased iodine levels in soil, animals, and human beings.

577.3 Sporadic Goiter

The term *sporadic goiter* encompasses goiters developing from a variety of causes; patients are usually euthyroid but may be hypothyroid. The most common cause of sporadic goiter is **lymphocytic thyroiditis** (see Chapter 576). Intrinsic biochemical defects in the synthesis of thyroid hormone are almost always associated with goiter. The occurrence of the disorder in siblings, onset in early life, and possible association with hypothyroidism (goitrous hypothyroidism) are important clues to the diagnosis.

IODIDE GOITER. A small percentage of patients treated with iodide preparations for prolonged periods acquire goiters. Iodides are commonly included for their expectorant effect in cough medicines and in proprietary mixtures for asthma. Goiters resulting from iodine administration are firm and diffusely enlarged, and in some instances hypothyroidism may develop. In normal individuals, acute administration of large doses of iodine inhibits the organification of iodine and the synthesis of thyroid hormone (Wolff-Chaikoff effect). This effect is short-lived and does not lead to hypothyroidism. When iodide administration continues, an autoregulatory mechanism in normal persons limits iodine trapping and permits the level of iodide in the thyroid to fall and organification to proceed normally. In patients with iodide-induced goiter, this escape does not occur because of an underlying abnormality of biosynthesis of thyroid hormone. The persons most susceptible to the development of iodide goiter are those with lymphocytic thyroiditis or with a subclinical inborn error in thyroid hormone synthesis and those who have had a partial thyroidectomy.

Lithium carbonate also causes goiters; it is currently widely used as a psychotropic drug. Lithium competes with iodide; the mechanism producing the goiter or hypothyroidism is similar to that described earlier for iodide goiter. Lithium and iodide also act synergistically to produce goiter; their combined use should be avoided.

Amiodarone, a drug used to treat cardiac arrhythmias, can cause thyroid dysfunction with goiter because it is rich in iodine. It is also a potent inhibitor of 5′-deiodinase, preventing conversion of T_4 to T_3. It can cause hypothyroidism, particularly in patients with underlying autoimmune disease; in other patients, it may cause hyperthyroidism.

SIMPLE GOITER (COLLOID GOITER). A few children with euthyroid nontoxic goiters have simple goiters, a condition of unknown cause not associated with hypothyroidism or hyperthyroidism and not caused by inflammation or neoplasia. The condition predominates in girls and has a peak incidence before and during the pubertal years. Histologic examination of the thyroid either is normal or reveals variable follicular size, dense colloid, and flattened epithelium. The goiter may be small or large. It is firm in half the patients and is occasionally asymmetric or nodular. Levels of TSH are normal or low, scintiscans are normal, and thyroid antibodies are absent. Differentiation from lymphocytic thyroiditis may not be possible without a biopsy, but biopsy ordinarily is not indicated. Therapy with thyroid hormone may help avoid progression to a large multinodular goiter, although it is difficult to separate any treatment effects from the natural history, which is for the goiter to decrease in size. Untreated patients should be re-evaluated periodically. This condition must be differentiated from lymphocytic thyroiditis (see Chapter 576).

MULTINODULAR GOITER. Rarely, a firm goiter with a lobulated surface and single or multiple palpable nodules is encountered. Areas of cystic change, hemorrhage, and fibrosis may be present. The incidence of this condition has decreased markedly with the use of iodine-enriched salt. A mild goitrogenic stimulus, acting over a long time, is thought to be the cause. Ultrasonographic examination may reveal multiple echo-free and echogenic lesions that are nonfunctioning on scintiscans. Thyroid studies are usually normal, but TSH may be elevated and thyroid antibodies may be present. The condition occurs in children with McCune-Albright syndrome (usually resulting in hyperthyroidism) and has been described in three children (including two siblings) with digital anomalies and cystic renal disease. Dominant nodules within a multinodular goiter, particularly those not suppressed by replacement therapy with T_4, may be an indication for evaluation by fine-needle aspiration because malignancy cannot readily be ruled out.

TOXIC GOITER (HYPERTHYROIDISM). See Chapter 578.

577.4 Intratracheal Goiter

One of the many ectopic locations of thyroid tissue is within the trachea. The intraluminal thyroid lies beneath the tracheal mucosa and is frequently continuous with the normally situated extratracheal thyroid. The thyroid tissue is susceptible to goitrous enlargement, which involves the normally situated and the ectopic thyroid. When there is obstruction of the airway associated with a goiter, it must be ascertained whether the obstruction is extratracheal or endotracheal. If obstructive manifestations are mild, administration of sodium-L-thyroxine usually causes the goiter to decrease in size. When symptoms are severe, surgical removal of the endotracheal goiter is indicated (also see Chapter 577.1).

Goiter

Daneman D, Davy T, Mancer K, et al: Association of multinodular goiter, cystic renal disease, and digital anomalies. J Pediatr 107:270, 1985.

Feuillan PP, Shawker T, Rose SR, et al: Thyroid abnormalities in the McCune-

Albright syndrome. Ultrasonography and hormonal studies. J Clin Endocrinol Metab 71:1596, 1990.

Pharoah POD, Buttfield IH, Hetzel BS: Neurological damage to the foetus resulting from severe iodine deficiency during pregnancy. Lancet 1:308, 1971.

Randolph J, Grunt JA, Vawter GF: The medical and surgical aspects of intratracheal goiter. N Engl J Med 268:457, 1963.

Vicens-Calvet E, Potau N, Carreras E, et al: Diagnosis and treatment in utero of goiter with hypothyroidism caused by iodine overload. J Pediatr 133:147, 1998.

Goitrous Cretinism

Abramowicz MJ, Targovnik HM, Cochaux P, et al: Identification of a mutation in the coding sequence of the human thyroid peroxidase gene causing congenital goiter. J Clin Invest 90:1200, 1992.

Benmiloud M, Chaouki ML, Gutekunst R, et al: Oral iodized oil for correcting iodine deficiency: Optimal dosing and outcome indicator selection. J Clin Endocrinol Metab 79:20, 1994.

Bikker H, den Hartog MT, Baas F, et al: A 20-base pair duplication in the human thyroid peroxidase gene results in a total iodide organification defect and congenital hypothyroidism. J Clin Endocrinol Metab 79:248, 1994.

Boyages SC, Halpern JP, Maberly GF, et al: A comparative study of neurological and myxedematous endemic cretinism in western China. J Clin Endocrinol Metab 67:1262, 1988.

Boyages SC, Halpern JP, Maberly GF, et al: Endemic cretinism: Possible role for thyroid autoimmunity. Lancet 2:529, 1989.

Boyages SC, Halpern JP, Maberly GF, et al: Supplementary iodine fails to reverse hypothyroidism in adolescents and adults with endemic cretinism. J Clin Endocrinol Metab 70:336, 1990.

Couch RM, Dean HJ, Winter JSD: Congenital hypothyroidism caused by defective iodide transport. J Pediatr 106:950, 1985.

DeLong GR, Leslie PW, Wang SH, et al: Effect on infant mortality of iodination of irrigated water in a severely iodine-deficient area of China. Lancet 350:771, 1997.

Gattereau A, Bernard B, Bellabarba D, et al: Congenital goiter in four euthyroid siblings with glandular and circulating iodoproteins and defective iodothyronine synthesis. J Clin Endocrinol Metab 37:118, 1973.

Illum P, Kiaer HW, Hvidberg-Hansen J, et al: Fifteen cases of Pendred's syndrome. Congenital deafness and sporadic goiter. Arch Otolaryngol 96:297, 1972.

Medeiros-Neto G, Targovnik HM, Vassart G: Defective thyroglobulin synthesis and secretion causing goiter and hypothyroidism. Endocr Rev 14:165, 1993.

Weetman AP: Is endemic goiter an autoimmune disease? [Editorial] J Clin Endocrinol Metab 78:1017, 1994.

CHAPTER 578
Hyperthyroidism

Hyperthyroidism results from excessive secretion of thyroid hormone and, with few exceptions, is due to diffuse toxic goiter (Graves disease) during childhood. Germ line mutations of the thyroid-stimulating hormone (TSH) receptor resulting in constitutively activating (i.e., gain of function) mutations have been reported in both familial (autosomal dominant) and sporadic cases of nonautoimmune hyperthyroidism. These patients, who may present in the neonatal period or in later childhood, have thyroid hyperplasia with goiters and suppressed levels of TSH. Different activating mutations have been identified in some cases of thyroid adenomas. Hyperthyroidism occurs in some patients with McCune-Albright syndrome, which is associated with autonomous thyroid adenomas. Other rare causes of hyperthyroidism that have been observed in children include toxic uninodular goiter (Plummer disease), hyperfunctioning thyroid carcinoma, thyrotoxicosis factitia, subacute thyroiditis, and acute suppurative thyroiditis. Suppression of plasma TSH indicates that the hyperthyroidism is not pituitary in origin. Hyperthyroidism due to excess thyrotropin secretion is rare and, in most cases, is caused by pituitary unresponsiveness to thyroid hormone. TSH-secreting pituitary tumors have been reported only in adults. In infants born to mothers with Graves disease, hyperthyroidism may occur as a transitory phenomenon or as classic Graves disease during the neonatal period. Choriocarcinoma, hydatidiform mole, and struma ovarii have caused hyperthyroidism in adults but have not been recognized as causes in children.

578.1 Graves Disease

ETIOLOGY. Enlargement of the thymus, splenomegaly, lymphadenopathy, infiltration of the thyroid gland and retro-orbital tissues with lymphocytes and plasma cells, and peripheral lymphocytosis are well-established findings in Graves disease. In the thyroid gland, T helper cells ($CD4^+$) tend to predominate in dense lymphoid aggregates; in areas of lower cell density, cytotoxic T cells ($CD8^+$) predominate. The percentage of activated B lymphocytes infiltrating the thyroid is higher than in peripheral blood. A postulated failure of T suppressor cells allows expression of T helper cells, sensitized to the TSH antigen, which interact with B cells. These cells differentiate into plasma cells, which produce thyrotropin receptor-stimulating antibody (TRSAb). TRSAb binds to the receptor for TSH and stimulates cyclic adenosine monophosphate, analogous to TSH itself. In addition to TRSAb, thyrotropin receptor-blocking antibody (TRBAb) may also be produced, and the clinical course of the disease usually correlates with the ratio between the two antibodies.

The ophthalmopathy occurring in Graves disease appears to be caused by antibodies against antigens shared by the thyroid and eye muscle. TSH receptors have been identified in retro-orbital adipocytes and may represent a target for antibodies. The antibodies that bind to the extraocular muscles and orbital fibroblasts stimulate the synthesis of glycosaminoglycans by orbital fibroblasts and produce cytotoxic effects on muscle cells.

In whites, Graves disease is associated with HLA-B8 and HLA-DR3; the latter carries a sevenfold relative risk for Graves disease. Therefore, it is not surprising that Graves disease is also associated with other HLA-D3–related disorders such as Addison's disease, insulin-dependent diabetes mellitus, myasthenia gravis, and celiac disease. Systemic lupus erythematosus, rheumatoid arthritis, vitiligo, idiopathic thrombocytopenic purpura, and pernicious anemia have been described in children with Graves disease. In family clusters, the conditions associated most frequently with Graves disease are lymphocytic thyroiditis, autoimmune hypothyroidism, and neonatal hyperthyroidism.

CLINICAL MANIFESTATIONS. About 5% of all patients with hyperthyroidism are less than 15 yr of age; the peak incidence in these children occurs during adolescence. Graves disease has begun between 6 wk and 2 yr of age in children born to mothers without a history of hyperthyroidism. The incidence is about five times higher in girls than in boys.

The clinical course in children is highly variable but usually is not as fulminant as it is in many adults. Symptoms develop gradually; the usual interval between onset and diagnosis is 6–12 mo and may be longer in prepubertal children compared with adolescents. The earliest signs in children may be emotional disturbances accompanied by motor hyperactivity. The children become irritable, excitable, and cry easily because of emotional lability. Their schoolwork suffers as a result of a short attention span. Tremor of the fingers can be noticed if the arm is extended. There may be a voracious appetite combined with loss of or no increase in weight. The size of the thyroid is variable. It may be enlarged so little that it escapes detection initially, but with careful examination, a goiter is found in almost all patients. Exophthalmos is noticeable in most patients but is usually mild. Lagging of the upper eyelid as the eye looks downward, impairment of convergence, and retraction of the upper eyelid and infrequent blinking may be present (Fig. 578–1). The skin is smooth and flushed, with excessive sweating. Muscular weakness is uncommon but may be severe enough to result in falling spells. Tachycardia, palpi-

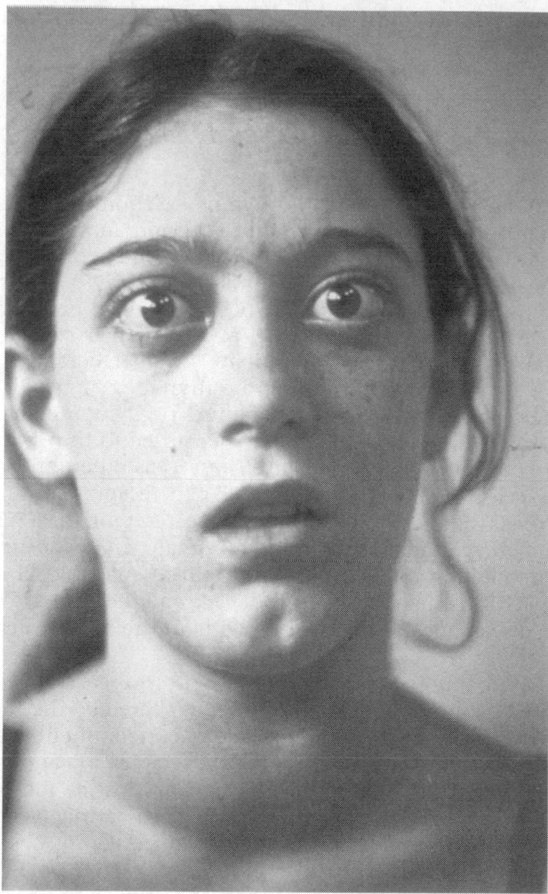

Figure 578–1 A 15-yr-old female with classic Graves disease. Clinical features include a goiter and exophthalmos. She was treated with antithyroid drugs, to which she had a good response.

tations, dyspnea, and cardiac enlargement and insufficiency cause discomfort but rarely endanger the patient's life. Atrial fibrillation is a rare complication. Mitral regurgitation, probably resulting from papillary muscle dysfunction, is the cause of the apical systolic murmur present in some patients. The systolic blood pressure and the pulse pressure are increased. Many of the findings in Graves disease result from hyperactivity of the sympathetic nervous system.

Thyroid "crisis," or "storm," is a form of hyperthyroidism manifested by an acute onset, hyperthermia, and severe tachycardia and restlessness. There may be rapid progression to delirium, coma, and death. "Apathetic," or "masked," hyperthyroidism is another variety of hyperthyroidism characterized by extreme listlessness, apathy, and cachexia. A combination of both forms may also occur. These symptom complexes are rare in children.

LABORATORY FINDINGS. Serum levels of thyroxine (T_4), triiodothyronine (T_3), free T_4, and free T_3 are elevated. In some patients, levels of T_3 may be more elevated than those of T_4. Levels of TSH are suppressed to less than normal levels. Thyroid peroxidase antibodies are often present. Most patients with newly diagnosed Graves disease have measurable TRSAb, and its disappearance predicts remission of the disease. Assays of TSH receptor antibodies are rarely necessary for diagnosis or management of Graves disease. Radioiodine is rapidly and diffusely concentrated in the thyroid, but this study is rarely necessary. Very young children with Graves disease often have advanced skeletal maturation and craniostenosis. Bone density may be reduced at diagnosis but returns to normal with treatment.

DIFFERENTIAL DIAGNOSIS. Diagnosis is rarely difficult once hyperthyroidism is considered. Elevated levels of T_4 and free T_4 in association with suppressed levels of TSH are usually diagnostic. The presence of TRSAb establishes the cause as Graves disease.

Most other causes of hyperthyroxinemia are rare but may result in erroneous diagnosis. Patients with elevated thyroxine-binding globulin levels or familial dysalbuminemic hyperthyroxinemia have normal levels of free T_4 and TSH. If a thyroid nodule is palpable, or if T_3 is preferentially elevated, a functional thyroid nodule must be considered; radionuclide study is diagnostic. If precocious puberty, polyostotic fibrous dysplasia, or café-au-lait pigmentation is present, the autonomous thyroid disorder of McCune-Albright syndrome is likely. Patients with generalized thyroid hormone unresponsiveness have elevated levels of free T_4, but levels of TSH are inappropriately elevated or normal. Patients with pituitary unresponsiveness to thyroid hormone also have clinical hyperthyroidism, but their levels of TSH are elevated or normal, and they must be differentiated from patients with TSH-secreting pituitary tumors, who have elevated serum levels of the TSH α chain.

When hyperthyroxinemia is caused by exogenous thyroid hormone, levels of free T_4 and TSH are the same as those seen in Graves disease, but the level of thyroglobulin is very low, whereas in patients with Graves disease, it is elevated.

TREATMENT. Most pediatric endocrinologists recommend medical therapy rather than radioiodine or subtotal thyroidectomy. The two thionamide drugs in widest use are propylthiouracil (PTU) and methimazole (Tapazole). Both compounds inhibit incorporation of trapped inorganic iodide into organic compounds, and they may also suppress levels of TRSAb by directly affecting intrathyroidal autoimmunity. However, there are important differences between the two drugs. Methimazole is at least 10 times more potent than PTU on a weight basis and has a much longer serum half-life (6–8 hr vs 0.5 hr); PTU generally is administered three times daily, but methimazole can be given once daily. Unlike methimazole, PTU is heavily protein-bound and has a lesser ability to cross the placenta and to pass into breast milk; theoretically, PTU is the preferred drug during pregnancy and for nursing mothers. PTU, more than methimazole, inhibits extrathyroidal conversion of T_4 to T_3; this may be advantageous in the treatment of neonatal thyrotoxicosis.

Toxic reactions occur with both drugs; most are mild, but some are life-threatening. They are unpredictable and can occur after therapy of any duration. There is increasing evidence that these reactions may be fewer in patients treated with methimazole. Transient leukopenia ($<4,000/mm^3$) is common; it is asymptomatic and is not a harbinger of agranulocytosis, and it usually is not a reason to discontinue treatment. Transient urticarial rashes are common. They can be managed by a short period off therapy, restarting the alternate antithyroid drug. The most severe reactions are hypersensitive and include agranulocytosis, hepatitis, hepatic failure, a lupus-like syndrome, glomerulonephritis, and a vasculitis involving the skin and other organs. Although uncommon, these reactions have been reported with both drugs, and it is probably best to treat unusually hypersensitive patients with radioiodine or thyroidectomy. Cases of congenital skin defects (aplasia cutis) have been seen in infants exposed in fetal life to methimazole, but this association does not appear to be a strong one.

The initial dosage of PTU is 5–10 mg/kg/24 hr given three times daily, and that of methimazole is 0.25–1.0 mg/kg/24 hr given once or twice daily. Smaller initial dosages should be used in early childhood. Careful surveillance is required after treatment is initiated. Raising serum levels of TSH to greater than normal indicates overtreatment and leads to increased size of the goiter. Clinical response becomes apparent in 2–3 wk, and adequate control is evident in 1–3 mo. The dose is decreased to the minimal level required to maintain a euthyroid state.

Drug therapy may be necessary for 5 yr or longer because there appears to be a remission rate of about 25% every 2 yr. If a relapse occurs, it usually appears within 3 mo and almost always within 6 mo after therapy has been discontinued. Therapy may be resumed in case of a relapse. Patients older than 13 yr of age, boys, those with a higher body mass index, and those with small goiters and modestly elevated T_3 levels appear to have earlier remissions.

A β-adrenergic blocking agent such as propranolol (0.5–2.0 mg/kg/24 hr, given three times daily) is a useful supplement in the management of severely toxic patients. Thyroid hormones potentiate the actions of catecholamines, which include tachycardia, tremor, excessive sweating, lid lag, and stare. These symptoms abate with the use of propranolol, which does not, however, alter thyroid function or exophthalmos.

Surgery or radioiodine treatment is indicated when adequate cooperation for medical management is not possible or when adequate trial of medical management has failed to result in permanent remission or severe side effects preclude further use of antithyroid drugs. Subtotal thyroidectomy, a rather safe procedure if performed by an experienced team, is performed only after the patient has been brought to a euthyroid state. This may be accomplished with PTU or methimazole over 2–3 mo. After a euthyroid state has been attained, 5 drops of a saturated solution of potassium iodide/24 hr are added to the regimen for 2 wk before surgery to decrease the vascularity of the gland. Complications of surgical treatment are rare and include hypoparathyroidism (transient or permanent) and paralysis of the vocal cords. The incidence of residual or recurrent hyperthyroidism or hypothyroidism depends on the extent of the surgery. Some recommend near-total thyroidectomy. The incidence of recurrence is low, but that of hypothyroidism may exceed 50%.

Radioiodine has proved to be an effective, relatively safe first or alternate therapy for Graves disease in children. Pretreatment with antithyroid drugs is unnecessary; if a patient is taking them, they should be stopped 5 days before radioiodine administration. Most children become euthyroid after one dose (88% in one study), but a few may require a second or third dose. Because the full effects of treatment may not be complete for 2–3 mo, adjunctive therapy with a β-adrenergic antagonist and lower doses of antithyroid drugs are recommended. Although there have been concerns about radiation oncogenesis and genetic damage, follow-up of treated children for as long as 40 yr has not shown this. The risk of benign adenoma may be increased (0.6–1.9% in one study). The major consequence of radioiodine is hypothyroidism, which occurs in 10–20% of patients after the first year and in about 3% per year thereafter.

The ophthalmopathy remits gradually and usually independently of the hyperthyroidism. Severe ophthalmopathy may require treatment with prednisone.

578.2 Congenital Hyperthyroidism

Onset of neonatal hyperthyroidism usually begins prenatally and is present at birth, although it may not be noticed until a few days after birth; occasionally, onset may be delayed for several weeks or more. The mothers of these infants have active Graves disease; Graves disease in remission or, rarely, hypothyroidism; and a history of lymphocytic thyroiditis. The condition is caused by transplacental passage of TRSAb, but the clinical onset, severity, and course may be modified by the concurrent presence of TRBAb and by the transplacental passage of antithyroid drugs taken by the mother. Very high levels of TRSAb usually result in classic neonatal hyperthyroidism, but if the infant has been exposed to the antithyroid drugs, onset of symptoms is delayed 3–4 days to allow degradation of the maternally derived antithyroid drug. If TRBAb is also present, onset of hyperthyroid symptoms may be delayed for several weeks.

Neonatal hyperthyroidism occurs in only about 2% of infants born to mothers with a history of Graves disease. The finding of very high levels of TRSAb in these mothers usually predicts the occurrence of an affected infant. Fetal tachycardia and goiter may allow prenatal diagnosis. Unlike Graves disease at all other ages, neonatal hyperthyroidism affects males as often as females. The disorder usually remits spontaneously within 6–12 wk but may persist longer, depending on the levels of TRSAb. Mild asymptomatic hyperthyroxinemia also occurs. Occasionally, classic neonatal Graves disease does not remit but persists for several years or longer. These children have impressive family histories of Graves disease. In these infants, TRSAb transfer from the mother apparently blends with the infantile onset of autonomous Graves disease.

Many of the infants are premature and appear to have intrauterine growth retardation. Most have goiters. The infant is extremely restless, irritable, and hyperactive and appears anxious and unusually alert. Microcephaly and ventricular enlargement may be present. The eyes are opened widely and appear exophthalmic (Fig. 578–2). There may be extreme tachycardia and tachypnea, and the temperature is elevated. In severely affected infants, there is a progression of symptoms; weight loss occurs despite a ravenous appetite, hepatosplenomegaly increases, and jaundice may become manifested. Cardiac decompensation is common, and severe hypertension may occur. The infant may die if therapy is not instituted promptly. The serum level of T_4 is markedly elevated and TSH is suppressed. Advanced bone age, frontal bossing with triangular facies, and cranial synostosis are common, especially in infants with persistent clinical manifestations of hyperthyroidism. Prognosis for intellectual development is guarded in infants with neonatal Graves disease.

Treatment consists of oral administration of propranolol (2

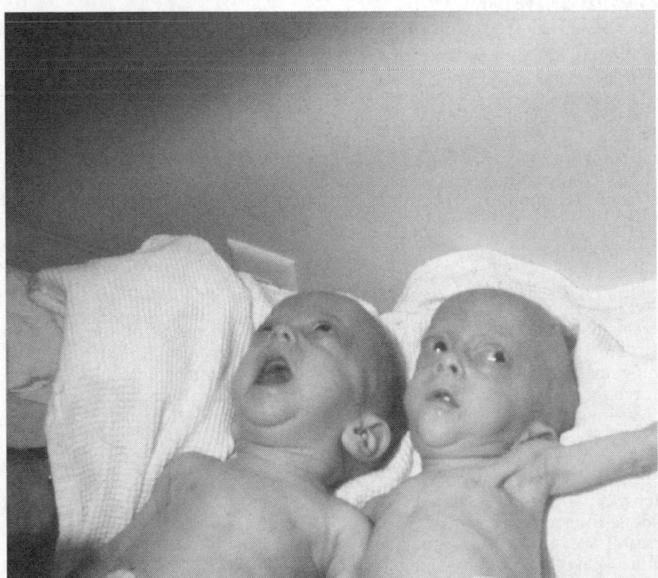

Figure 578–2 Two males (twins) with neonatal hyperthyroidism confirmed by abnormal thyroid function tests. Clinical features include lack of subcutaneous tissue due to a hypermetabolic state and a wide-eyed, anxious stare. They were given the diagnosis of neonatal Graves disease, but, in fact, their mother did not have Graves disease; they had persistent, not transient, hyperthyroidism. At age 8 yr they were treated with radioiodine. They are now believed to have had some other form of neonatal hyperthyroidism, such as a constitutive activation of the TSH receptor.

mg/kg/24 hr, orally in three divided doses) and PTU (5–10 mg/kg/24 hr given every 8 hr); Lugol solution (1 drop every 8 hr) may be added. When propranolol is used during pregnancy to treat thyrotoxicosis, it crosses the placenta and may cause respiratory depression in the newborn infant. If the thyrotoxic state is severe, parenteral fluid therapy and corticosteroids may be indicated. If heart failure occurs, digitalization is indicated. After a euthyroid state is reached, only PTU treatment is necessary. The dose should be gradually tapered to keep the infant euthyroid. Most cases remit by 3–4 mo of age.

Occasionally, neonatal hyperthyroidism does not remit but persists into childhood. These patients may have an impressive family history of hyperthyroidism, but TSH-stimulating antibodies are absent. Advanced osseous maturation, microcephaly, and mental retardation occur when treatment is delayed. Several cases of neonatal hyperthyroidism, without evidence for autoimmune disease in infant or mother, have now been reported due to a mutation in the TSHR gene, which produced constitutive activation of the receptor. Hyperthyroidism recurs when antithyroid drugs are discontinued; these children must be treated with radioiodine or surgery.

Bahn RS, Heufelder AE: Pathogenesis of Graves' ophthalmopathy. N Engl J Med 329:1468, 1993.
Cheron RG, Kaplan MM, Larsen PR, et al: Neonatal thyroid function after propylthiouracil therapy for maternal Graves' disease. N Engl J Med 304:525, 1981.
Clark JD, Gelfand MJ, Elgazzar AH: Iodine-131 therapy of hyperthyroidism in pediatric patients. J Nucl Med 36:442, 1995.
Daneman D, Howard NJ: Neonatal thyrotoxicosis: Intellectual impairment and craniosynostosis in later years. J Pediatr 97:257, 1980.
Darby CP: Three episodes of spontaneous thyroid storm occurring in a nine year-old child. Pediatrics 30:927, 1962.
DeLuca G, Chaussain JL, Job JC: Hyperfunctioning thyroid nodules in children and adolescents. Acta Paediatr Scand 75:118, 1986.
Duprez L, Parma J, Van Sande J, et al: Germline mutations in the thyrotropin receptor gene cause non-autoimmune autosomal dominant hyperthyroidism. Nat Genet 7:396, 1994.
Foley TP, White C, New A: Juvenile Graves disease: Usefulness and limitations of thyrotropin receptor antibody determinations. J Pediatr 110:378, 1987.
Glaser NS, Styne DM: Predictors of early remission of hyperthyroidism in children. J Clin Endocrinol Metab 82:1719, 1997.
Hashizume K, Ichikawa K, Sakurai A, et al: Administration of thyroxine in treated Graves' disease. Effects on the level of antibodies to thyroid stimulating hormone receptors and on the risk of recurrence of hyperthyroidism. N Engl J Med 324:947, 1991.
Kopp P, van Sande J, Parma J, et al: Brief report: Congenital hyperthyroidism caused by a mutation in the thyrotropin-receptor gene. N Engl J Med 332:150, 1995.
Levy WJ, Schumacher P, Gupta M: Treatment of childhood Graves' disease: A review with emphasis on radioiodine treatment. Cleve Clin J Med 55:373, 1988.
Lippe BM, Landow EM, Kaplan SA: Hyperthyroidism in children treated with long-term medical therapy: Twenty-five percent remission rate every two years. J Clin Endocrinol Metab 64:1241, 1987.
Mastorakos G, Mitsiades NS, Doufas AG, et al: Hyperthyroidism in McCune-Albright syndrome with a review of thyroid abnormalities sixty years after the first report. Thyroid 7:433, 1997.
Milham S Jr: Scalp defects in infants of mothers treated for hyperthyroidism with methimazole or carbimazole during pregnancy. Teratology 32:321, 1985.
Perelman AH, Clemons RD: The fetus in maternal hyperthyroidism. Thyroid 2:225, 1992.
Shulman DI, Muhar I, Jorgensen EV, et al: Autoimmune hyperthyroidism in prepubertal children and adolescents: Comparison of clinical and biochemical features at diagnosis and responses to medical therapy. Thyroid 7:755, 1997.
Sills IN: Hyperthyroidism. Pediatr Rev 15:417, 1994.
Soreide JA, van Heerden JA, Lo CY, et al: Surgical treatment of Graves' disease in patients younger than 18 years. World J Surg 20:794, 1996.
Stenszky V, Kozma L, Balazs C, et al: The genetics of Graves disease: HLA and disease susceptibility. J Clin Endocrinol Metab 61:835, 1985.
Viscardi RM, Shea M, Sriwantanakul K, et al: Hyperthyroxinemia in newborns due to excess thyroxine-binding globulin. N Engl J Med 309:897, 1983.
Volpe R, Ehrlich R, Steiner G, et al: Graves' disease in pregnancy years after hypothyroidism with recurrent passive-transfer neonatal Graves' disease in offspring. Therapeutic considerations. Am J Med 77:572, 1984.
Zakarija M, McKenzie JM: Pregnancy-associated changes in the thyroid-stimulating antibody of Graves' disease and the relationship to neonatal hyperthyroidism. J Clin Endocrinol Metab 57:1036, 1983.

CHAPTER 579
Carcinoma of the Thyroid

EPIDEMIOLOGY. Carcinoma of the thyroid is rare in children; the annual incidence in children less than 15 yr of age is approximately 0.5 cases/million, compared with an annual incidence at all ages around the world ranging from 0.5 to 10 cases/million. Unlike other malignancies in childhood, thyroid cancer usually has an indolent course, even after pulmonary metastases have developed.

PATHOGENESIS. Genetic factors and radiation exposure are important factors in the pathogenesis of thyroid cancer. Rearrangements of the RET proto-oncogene are found in 3–33% of papillary carcinomas and 60–80% of those occurring after irradiation, as in children in Belarus exposed to radiation after the nuclear accident at Chernobyl or in those who were exposed to external radiation in childhood. Inactivating point mutations of the p53 tumor-suppressor gene are rare in patients with differentiated thryoid carcinoma but are common in those with anaplastic thyroid cancer. Overall, 5–10% of cases of papillary thyroid carcinoma are familial and are usually inherited in an autosomal dominant manner. The thyroid gland of children is unusually sensitive to exposure to external radiation. There probably is no threshold dose; 1 Gy results in a 7.7 relative risk of thyroid cancer. In the past, about 80% of children with cancer of the thyroid had received irradiation of the neck and adjacent areas during infancy for benign conditions such as "enlarged" thymus, hypertrophied tonsils and adenoids, hemangiomas, nevi, eczema, tinea capitis, and "cervical adenitis." With the disuse of irradiation for benign conditions, this cause of thyroid cancer has vanished. However, the long-term survival of children who have received therapeutic irradiation of areas of the neck for neoplastic disease has now made this cause of thyroid cancer and nodules increasingly prevalent; increased dose, younger age at time of treatment, and female sex are factors that increase the risk of thyroid cancer developing. Long-term risk data for cancer are sparse, but 15–50% of children who have received irradiation and chemotherapy for Hodgkin disease, leukemia, and other malignancies of the head and neck have elevated levels of thyroid-stimulating hormone (TSH) within the 1st yr of therapy, and 5–20% progress to hypothyroidism during the next 5–7 yr. Most large groups of treated children have a 10–30% incidence of benign thyroid nodules and an increased incidence of thyroid cancer. The latter begins to appear within 3–5 yr after radiation treatment and reaches a peak in 15–25 yr. It is unknown whether there is a period after which no more tumors develop. Administration of iodine-131 for diagnostic or therapeutic purposes does not appear to increase the risk of thyroid cancer.

Histologically, the carcinomas are papillary (80%), follicular (17%), medullary (2%), or mixed differentiated tumors. These are usually slow-growing tumors and may remain dormant for years. The type of tumor and the natural course of disease in irradiated and nonirradiated patients are the same, except that multicentricity is more frequent in irradiation-induced cancer. Undifferentiated (anaplastic) thyroid neoplasms are rare in children and usually have a rapidly fatal course.

CLINICAL MANIFESTATIONS. Girls are affected twice as often as boys. The average age at diagnosis is 9 yr, but the onset may be as early as the 1st yr of life. A painless nodule in the thyroid or in the neck is the usual first evidence of disease. Cervical lymph node involvement is often present at the time of initial diagnosis. Any unexplained cervical lymph node enlargement requires examination of the thyroid, which occasionally has a primary tumor too small to be felt; the diagnosis is based on biopsy results of the lymph node. The lungs are the most common site of metastases beyond the neck. There may be no clinical manifestations referable to them; roentgenographically, they appear as diffuse miliary or nodular infiltrations, principally in the basal portions. They may be mistaken for tuberculosis, histoplasmosis, or sarcoidosis. Other sites of metastases include the mediastinum, long bones, skull, and axilla. Almost all children are euthyroid, but rarely, the carcinoma may be functional and produce symptoms of hyperthyroidism.

DIAGNOSIS. In the case of a solitary nodule, an ultrasonographic examination of the thyroid can provide information on the consistency of the nodule (solid vs cystic) and whether other nonpalpable nodules are present. A thyroid scan, preferrably using ^{123}I or ^{99m}Tc-pertechnetate, can provide information on trapping function, and whether the nodule is "cold vs warm vs hot." The majority of cold nodules are benign. There is a developing view that the most helpful diagnostic test in the case of a solitary nodule is fine-needle aspiration (FNA). Experience in adults using FNA generally shows a 5–10% false-negative rate and a 1–2% false-positive rate, with an overall diagnostic accuracy of 90–95%. Other tests of thyroid function are normal, but Hashimoto's thyroiditis has been associated with thyroid cancer.

TREATMENT. Because differentiated thyroid carcinoma is a chronic disease with a long survival, optimal therapy is still evolving. There is increasing evidence that small (<2 cm) papillary carcinoma, the least aggressive type, is effectively treated by subtotal thyroidectomy and suppressive doses of thyroid hormone. Papillary carcinomas tend to be multicentric, and several studies show that half these children have regional lymph node involvement at presentation. For larger papillary carcinomas, follicular carcinoma, or regional lymph node involvement, near-total thyroidectomy with excision of regional lymph nodes appears to be the treatment of choice. There is no role for radical neck dissection. Thyroidectomy is usually followed by an ablative dose (30–100 mCi) of ^{131}I.

After surgery, all patients should be treated with sodium-L-thyroxine in doses sufficient to suppress TSH. Periodic determinations of thyroglobulin (TG) levels should also be performed, because TG is an excellent marker for tumor recurrence in patients taking thyroxine (T_4). If the patient has undergone a total thyroidectomy or iodine-131 ablation, the serum TG level should be less than 5 ng/mL when T_4 suppressive therapy is being received.

PROGNOSIS. For any form of therapy, survival or recurrence does not appear to be different for patients with or without involvement of the cervical nodes. Even patients with cervical or pulmonary metastases have survived many years.

More than 95% of patients are alive 25 yr after initial treatment if the tumor was intrathyroid, less than 2 cm in diameter, and classified as grade 1. Greater tumor size, distant spread, and greater atypia are associated with increased cumulative mortality.

579.1 Solitary Thyroid Nodule

Solitary nodules of the thyroid are uncommon in children. The most common cause is benign follicular adenoma. In the past, it was estimated that as many as half were carcinomas, but later studies have indicated that there is an approximately 15% incidence of malignancy, perhaps because of decreasing exposure of children to radiation. Children exposed to radiation have a high incidence of benign adenoma and carcinoma of the thyroid.

Benign disorders that may present as solitary thyroid nodules include benign adenomas (e.g., follicular, embryonal, Hürthle cell), colloid (adenomatous) nodule, lymphocytic thyroiditis, thyroglossal duct cyst, ectopically located normal thyroid tissue, a single median thyroid, agenesis of one of the lateral thyroid lobes with hypertrophy of the contralateral lobe, thyroid cysts, and abscess. A suddenly appearing or rapidly enlarging thyroid mass may indicate hemorrhage into a benign adenoma. In most cases, the child is euthyroid, and thyroid function studies are normal. When lymphocytic thyroiditis is the cause of the nodule, T_4 may be low, TSH may be elevated, and thyroid antibodies are usually present. Radionuclide imaging, if performed , may reveal a moth-eaten appearance. Rarely, lymphocytic thyroiditis may be associated with carcinoma of the thyroid. Ultrasonography is particularly useful in detecting cystic lesions.

The diagnostic studies to delineate the underlying cause include serum thyroid function tests, antithyroid antibody determinations, ultrasonographic examination of the thyroid, radionuclide uptake and scan, and FNA (see under Diagnosis). Response to a trial of suppressive T_4 treatment to look for shrinkage of nodule size is not reliable. Although thyroid carcinomas generally present as a solid, cold nodule, most cold nodules are benign lesions. FNA is useful in avoiding surgery for benign nodules. However, surgery without delay is indicated when the nodule is hard or has grown rapidly, when there is evidence of tracheal or vocal cord involvement, or when there is enlargement of adjacent lymph nodes. All persons with a history of head or neck irradiation should have careful examinations of the thyroid at least every 2 yr indefinitely.

Rarely, thyroid nodules may be functional, producing hyperthyroidism *(Plummer disease)*. The uptake of radionuclide is concentrated in the nodule ("hot" or "warm" nodule), and thyroid function studies indicate that the nodule is functioning autonomously. Such nodules are usually benign, but a few instances of carcinoma in such cases have been reported. T_4 levels are usually normal, but triiodothyronine (T_3) levels are elevated (T_3 toxicosis), and TSH levels are suppressed. Treatment consists of surgical removal of the nodule.

579.2 Medullary Carcinoma

Medullary carcinoma of the thyroid arises from the parafollicular cells (C cells) of the thyroid and accounts for about 2% of thyroid malignancies. The most common symptom is goiter or a palpable thyroid nodule. Roentgenograms may reveal dense, conglomerate, homogeneous calcification in the thyroid. Metastases to the regional lymph nodes and to the liver are common, and these also may calcify. Death may result, but long survivals are common.

The tumors occur sporadically, as a familial autosomal dominant disorder, and as components of two distinct autosomal dominant syndromes. The susceptibility for all these disorders has been associated with germ line mutations of the RET proto-oncogene, which maps to chromosome 10q11.2. When the tumor occurs sporadically, it is usually unicentric, but in the familial form, it is usually multicentric, and it begins as hyperplasia of parafollicular cells. The tumors are often too small to be found by palpation, scintigraphy, or ultrasonographic examination in at-risk patients in these families. Diagnosis of medullary carcinoma should lead to a careful search for associated tumors, particularly pheochromocytoma. No clinically recognizable manifestations result from the elevated serum levels of calcitonin or from the calcitonin gene-related peptide.

MULTIPLE ENDOCRINE NEOPLASIA, TYPE IIA. When hyperplasia or carcinoma of C cells is associated with adrenal medullary hyperplasia or pheochromocytoma and parathyroid hyperplasia, it is known as multiple endocrine neoplasia (MEN) IIA. The inheritance pattern for MEN IIA is autosomal dominant, with a high degree of penetrance and variable expressivity. At least 19 different specific missense mutations of exon 10 or 11 of the extracellular domain of the RET gene have been described for MEN IIA and for cases of familial medullary thyroid carcinoma. DNA analysis permits unambiguous identification of carriers of the RET proto-oncogene gene. C-cell hyperplasia or tumors usually appear earlier than pheochromocytoma. Pheochromocytomas are frequently bilateral and may be multiple. Adrenal medullary hyperplasia is known to precede pheochromocytoma, but the detectable latent period is short. Hypercalcemia is a late manifestation and indicates hyperparathyroidism. The parathyroid glands may reveal chief-cell hyperplasia or only hypercellularity.

MULTIPLE ENDOCRINE NEOPLASIA, TYPE IIB. The distinguishing feature of MEN IIB, also called the *mucosal neuroma syndrome,* is the occurrence of multiple neuromas and a characteristic phenotype associated with medullary carcinoma and pheochromocytoma. This condition is also autosomal dominant, and 93% of families have a missense mutation of the RET proto-oncogene. However, the mutation is in exon 16, the tyrosine catalytic domain of RET; all patients have had the same point mutation.

The neuromas most often occur on the tongue, buccal mucosa, lips, and conjunctivae. Peripheral neurofibromas and café-au-lait patches may be present, and intestinal ganglioneuromatosis is common. Diffuse proliferation of nerves and ganglion cells is found in mucosal, submucosal, myenteric, and subserosal plexus involving the small and large bowel as well as the esophagus. The patients may be tall, with arachnodactyly and a Marfan-like appearance. Scoliosis, pectus excavatum, pes cavus, and muscular hypotonia are common. The eyelids may be thickened and everted, the lips patulous and blubbery, the jaw prognathic. Feeding difficulties, poor sucking, diarrhea, constipation, and failure to thrive may begin in infancy or early childhood, many years before the appearance of neuromas or endocrine symptoms.

TREATMENT. Total thyroidectomy is indicated for all children who are shown by DNA studies to carry the gene. Recognition of familial forms of this tumor is critical to the early diagnosis in children at risk. Evidence suggests that thyroidectomy must be performed early because medullary carcinoma has been seen in a 6-mo-old child with MEN IIB and in a 3-yr-old child with MEN IIA. Monitoring the levels of calcitonin is useful in following the course of the disease after operation and detecting metastatic lesions. Periodic screening for the development of pheochromocytoma is indicated.

Ashcroft NW, Van Herle AJ: The comparative value of serum thyroglobulin measurements and iodine ^{131}I total body scans in the follow-up of patients treated with differentiated thyroid cancer. Am J Med 71:806, 1981.

Crom DB, Kaste SC, Tubergen DG, et al: Ultrasonography for thyroid screening after head and neck irradiation in childhood cancer survivors. Med Pediatr Oncol 28:15, 1997.

Degnan BM, McClellan DR, Francis GL: An analysis of fine-needle aspiration biopsy of the thyroid in chldren and adolescents. J Pediatr Surg 31:903, 1996.

DeGroot LJ: Diagnostic approach and management of patients exposed to irradiation of the thyroid. J Clin Endocrinol Metab 69:925, 1989.

Eng C, Smith DP, Mulligan LH, et al: Point mutation within the tyrosine kinase domain of the *RET* proto-oncogene in multiple endocrine neoplasia type 2B and related sporadic tumors. Hum Mol Genet 3:237, 1994.

Feinmesser R, Lubin E, Segal K, et al: Carcinoma of the thyroid in children—a review. J Pediatr Endocrinol Metab 10:561, 1997.

Flannery TK, Kirkland JL, Copeland KC, et al: Papillary thyroid cancer: A pediatric perspective. Pediatrics 98:464, 1996.

Fleming ID, Black TL, Thompson EI, et al: Thyroid dysfunction and neoplasia in children receiving neck irradiation for cancer. Cancer 55:1190, 1985.

Heshmati HM, Gharib H, Khosla S, et al: Genetic testing in medullary thyroid carcinoma syndromes: Mutation types and clinical significance. Mayo Clin Proc 72:430, 1997.

Hopwood NJ, Kelch RP: Thyroid masses: Approach to diagnosis and management in childhood and adolescence. Pediatr Rev 14:481, 1993.

Hung W, Anderson KD, Chandra RS, et al: Solitary thyroid nodules in 71 children and adolescents. J Pediatr Surg 27:1407, 1992.

Keiser HR, Beaven MA, Doppham J, et al: Sipple's syndrome: Medullary thyroid carcinoma, pheochromocytoma and parathyroid disease. Ann Intern Med 78:561, 1973.

Kirk JM, Mort C, Grand DB, et al: The usefulness of serum thyroglobulin in the follow-up of differentiated thyroid carcinoma in children. Med Pediatr Oncol 20:201, 1992.

Lafferty AR, Batch JA: Thyroid nodules in childhood and adolescence—thirty years of experience. J Pediatr Endocrinol Metab 10:479, 1997.

Lips CJM, Landsvater RM, Höppener JWM, et al: Clinical screening as compared with DNA analysis in families with multiple endocrine neoplasia type 2A. N Engl J Med 331:828, 1994.

Mazzaferri EL: Management of a solitary thyroid nodule. N Engl J Med 328:553, 1993.

Nikiforov YE, Rowland JM, Bove KE, et al: Distinct pattern of ret oncogene rearrangements in morphological variants of radiation-induced and sporadic thyroid papillary carcinomas in children. Cancer Res 57:1690, 1997.

Raab SS, Silverman JF, Elsheikh TM, et al: Pediatric thyroid nodules: Disease demographics and clinical management as determined by fine needle aspiration biopsy. Pediatrics 95:46, 1995.

Schlumberger MJ: Papillary and follicular thyroid carcinoma. N Engl J Med 338:297, 1998.

Scott MD, Crawford JD: Solitary thyroid nodules in childhood: Is the incidence of thyroid carcinoma declining? Pediatrics 58:521, 1976.

Stjernholm MR, Freudenborrg JC, Mooney HS, et al: Medullary carcinoma of the thyroid before age 2 years. J Clin Endocrinol Metab 51:252, 1980.

Vane D, King DR, Boles ET Jr: Secondary thyroid neoplasm in pediatric cancer patients: Increased risk with improved survival. J Pediatr Surg 19:855, 1984.

Zimmerman D: Thyroid neoplasia in children. Curr Opin Pediatr 9:407, 1997.

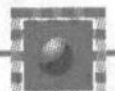

SECTION 3

Disorders of the Parathyroid Glands

Daniel A. Doyle ■ Angelo M. DiGeorge

CHAPTER 580

Hormones and Peptides of Calcium Homeostasis and Bone Metabolism

Parathyroid hormone (PTH) and vitamin D are the principal regulators of calcium homeostasis (Chapters 44, 49, and 706). Calcitonin and PTH-related peptide (PTHrP) appear to be important primarily in the fetus.

PARATHYROID HORMONE. PTH is an 84-amino acid chain (9,500 d), but its biologic activity resides in the first 34 residues. In the parathyroid gland, a pre-pro-PTH (115-amino acid chain) and a proparathyroid hormone (90 amino acids) are synthesized. Pre-pro-PTH is converted to pro-PTH and pro-PTH to PTH. PTH (1–84) is the major secretory product of the gland, but it is rapidly cleaved in the liver and kidney into smaller COOH-terminal, midregion, and NH_2-terminal fragments.

The occurrence of these fragments in serum has led to the development of a variety of assays. The 1–34 amino-terminal (N-terminus) fragments possess biologic activity but are present in low amounts in the circulation; assay of these fragments is most useful for detecting acute secretory changes. The carboxy-terminal (C-terminus) and midregion fragments, although biologically inert, are cleared more slowly from the circulation and represent 80% of plasma immunoreactive PTH; values of the C-terminal fragment are 50–500 times the level of the active hormone. The C-terminal assays are effective in detecting patients with hyperparathyroidism, but because C-terminal fragments are removed from the circulation by glomerular filtration, these assays are less useful for evaluating the secondary hyperparathyroidism characteristic of renal disease. Only certain sensitive radioimmunoassays for PTH can differentiate the subnormal concentrations that occur in hypoparathyroidism from normal levels. A sensitive 15-min immunochemiluminometric assay, developed for intraoperative use, can provide the surgeon with useful information.

When serum levels of calcium fall, the signal is transduced via the calcium-sensing receptor, and secretion of PTH increases. PTH stimulates activity of 1α-hydroxylase in the kidney, enhancing production of 1,25-dihydroxycholecalciferol ($1,25[OH]_2D_3$). The increased level of $1,25[OH]_2D_3$ induces synthesis of a calcium-binding protein *(calbindin-D)* in the intestinal mucosa with resultant absorption of calcium. PTH also mobilizes calcium by directly enhancing bone resorption, an effect that requires $1,25[OH]_2D_3$. The effects of PTH on bone and kidney are mediated through binding to specific receptors on the membranes of target cells and through activation of a transduction pathway involving a G protein coupled to the adenylate cyclase system (also see Chapter 582).

The *calcium-sensing receptor* regulates the secretion of PTH and the reabsorption of calcium by the renal tubules in response to alterations in serum calcium concentrations. The gene for the receptor is located on chromosome 3q13.3–q21 and encodes a cell surface protein of 1,078 amino acids that is expressed in parathyroid glands and kidneys and belongs to the family of G protein–coupled receptors. In the normally functioning calcium-sensing receptor, hypocalcemia induces increased secretion of PTH and hypercalcemia depresses PTH secretion. Loss of function mutations result in an increased set point with respect to serum calcium, resulting in hypercalcemia and in the conditions familial hypocalciuric hypercalcemia and neonatal severe hyperparathyroidism. Gain of function mutations result in depressed secretion of PTH in response to hypocalcemia, leading to the syndrome of familial hypocalcemia with hypercalciuria.

PARATHYROID HORMONE-RELATED PEPTIDE. PTHrP is homologous to PTH only in the first 13 amino acids of its amino terminus, 8 of which are identical to PTH. Its gene is on the short arm of chromosome 12, and that of PTH is on the short arm of chromosome 11.

PTHrP, like PTH, activates PTH receptors in kidney and bone cells and increases urinary cyclic adenosine monophosphate and renal production of $1,25[OH]_2D_3$. It is produced in almost every type of cell of the body, including every tissue of the embryo at some stage of development. PTHrP is critical for normal fetal development. Inactivating mutations of the receptor for PTH/PTHrP result in a lethal bone disorder characterized by short limbs and markedly advanced bone maturation known as *Blomstrand Chondrodysplasia*. It appears to have a paracrine or autocrine role because serum levels are low except in a few clinical situations. Cord blood contains levels of PTHrP that are threefold higher than in serum from adults; it is produced by the fetal parathyroid glands and appears to be the main agent stimulating maternal-fetal calcium transfer. PTHrP appears to be essential for normal skeletal maturation of the fetus, which requires 30 g of calcium. During pregnancy, maternal absorption of calcium increases from about 150 mg daily to 400 mg during the second trimester.

As in cord blood, PTHrP levels are increased during lactation and in patients with benign breast hypertrophy. Breast milk and pasturized bovine milk have levels of PTHrP that are 10,000 times higher than those of normal plasma. Most instances of the hormonal hypercalcemia syndrome of malignancy are caused by elevated concentrations of PTHrP.

VITAMIN D. See Chapters 44 and 49.

CALCITONIN. Calcitonin (CT) is a 32-amino acid polypeptide. Its gene is on chromosome 11p and is tightly linked to that of PTH. The CT gene encodes three peptides: CT, a 21-amino acid carboxy-terminal flanking peptide (katacalcin), and a CT gene–related peptide. Katacalcin and CT are cosecreted in equimolar amounts by the parafollicular cells (C cells) of the thyroid gland. CT appears to be of little consequence in children and adults because very high levels in patients with medullary carcinoma of the thyroid (a tumor arising from the C cells) does not cause hypercalcemia. In the fetus, however, circulating levels are high and appear to augment bone metabolism and skeletal growth; these high levels are probably stimulated by the normally high fetal calcium levels. Unlike the high levels in cord blood and circulating concentrations in young children, levels in older children and adults are low. Infants and children with congenital hypothyroidism (and presumed deficiency of C cells) have lower levels of CT than do normal children.

Its action appears to be independent of PTH and vitamin D. Its main biologic effect appears to be the inhibition of bone resorption by decreasing the number and activity of bone-resorbing osteoclasts. This action of CT is the rationale behind its use in treatment of Paget's disease. CT is synthesized in other organs, such as the gastrointestinal tract, pancreas, brain, and pituitary. In these organs, CT is thought to behave as a neurotransmitter to impose a local inhibitory effect on cell function.

CHAPTER 581
Hypoparathyroidism

ETIOLOGY (Table 581–1). Hypocalcemia is common from 12–72 hr of life, especially in premature infants, in infants with asphyxia at birth, and in infants of diabetic mothers *(early neonatal hypocalcemia)* (see Chapter 102). After the 2nd–3rd day and during the 1st wk of life, the type of feeding is also a determinant of the level of serum calcium *(late neonatal hypocalcemia)*. The role played by the parathyroid glands in these hypocalcemic infants remains to be clarified, although functional immaturity of the parathyroid glands has often been invoked as a pathogenetic factor. In a group of infants with *transient idiopathic hypocalcemia* (1–8 wk of age) serum levels of PTH were significantly lower than those in normal infants. It is possible that the functional immaturity is a manifestation of a delay in development of the enzymes that convert glandular PTH to secreted PTH; other mechanisms are also possible.

Hyperparathyroidism During Pregnancy. This may result in transient hypocalcemia of the newborn infant. It appears that neonatal hypocalcemia results from suppression of the fetal parathyroid glands by exposure to elevated levels of calcium in maternal serum. Tetany usually develops within 3 wk but may be delayed 1 mo or more if the infant is breast-fed. Hypocalcemia may persist for weeks or months. When the cause of hypocalcemia in infants is unknown, their mothers should have measurements of calcium, phosphorus, and PTH. Most affected mothers are asymptomatic, and the cause of their hyperparathyroidism is usually a parathyroid adenoma.

Aplasia or Hypoplasia of the Parathyroid Glands. This is often associated with the *DiGeorge/velocardiofacial syndrome*. This syndrome occurs in 1/10,000 newborns. In 90% of patients the condition is caused by a deletion of *chromosome 22q11.2*. Approximately 25% of these patients inherit the chromosomal abnormality from one of their parents. Neonatal hypocalcemia occurs in 60% of affected patients, but it is transitory in the majority; however, hypocalcemia may recur later or may have its onset later in life. Associated abnormalities of the 3rd and 4th pharyngeal pouches are common; these include conotruncal defects of the heart in 25%, velopharyngeal insufficiency in 32%, cleft palate in 9%, renal anomalies in 35%, and aplasia of the thymus with severe immunodeficiency in 1%. This syndrome has also been reported in a small number of patients with a deletion of chromosome 10p, in infants of diabetic mothers, and in infants born to mothers treated with retinoic acid for acne early in pregnancy.

X-Linked Recessive Hypoparathyroidism. Familial clusters of hypoparathyroidism with various patterns of transmission have been described. In two large North American pedigrees, this disorder appears to be transmitted by an *X-linked recessive gene* located on Xq26-q27. In these families, the onset of afebrile seizures characteristically occurs in infants from 2 wk-6 mo of age. The absence of parathyroid tissue after detailed examination of a boy with this condition suggests it is a defect in embryogenesis.

Autosomal Recessive Hypoparathyroidism with Dysmorphic Features. This syndrome has been described in Middle Eastern children. Parental consanguinity occurred for almost all of several dozen affected patients. Profound hypocalcemia occurs early in life, and dysmorphic features include microcephaly, deep-set eyes, beaked nose, micrognathia, and large floppy ears. Intrauterine and postnatal growth retardation are severe, and mental retardation is common. The putative gene is on chromosome 1q42-43. The autosomal recessive form of hypoparathyroidism that occurs with type I polyglandular autoimmune disease is described subsequently. In a few patients with autosomal recessive inheritance of isolated hypoparathyroidism, mutations of the PTH gene have been found.

Autosomal Dominant Hypoparathyroidism. These patients have an activating mutation of the Ca^{2+}-sensing receptor, forcing the receptor to an "on" state with subsequent depression of PTH secretion even during hypocalcemia. The hypocalcemia is usually mild and may not require treatment beyond childhood.

Hypoparathyroidism Associated with Mitochondrial Disorders. Mitochondrial DNA mutations in Kearnes-Sayre syndrome and in mitochondrial trifunctional protein have been associated with hypoparathyroidism. A diagnosis of mitochondrial cytopathy should be considered in patients with unexplained symptoms such as ophthalmoplegia, sensorineural hearing loss, cardiac conduction disturbances, and tetany.

Surgical Hypoparathyroidism. Removal or damage of the parathyroid glands may complicate thyroidectomy. Hypoparathy-

TABLE 581–1 Etiologic Classification of Hypocalcemia

- Parathyroid hormone (PTH) deficiency
  - Aplasia or hypoplasia of parathyroids
    - With 22q11 deletion
      - DiGeorge syndrome
      - Velocardiofacial syndrome
      - Conotruncal-face syndrome
    - With 10p13 deletion
      - DiGeorge syndrome
    - With maternal diabetes mellitus or retinoic acid treatment during pregnancy
    - With CHARGE syndrome
    - With X-linked isolated hypoparathyroidism
  - Preproparathyroid hormone gene mutation
    - Autosomal dominant
  - Autoimmune parathyroiditis
    - Isolated
    - With type 1 autoimmune polyendocrinopathy
      - Mutation of AIRE* gene
      - Calcium-sensing receptor antibodies
  - Infiltrative lesions
    - Hemosiderosis (treatment of thalassemia)
    - Copper deposition (Wilson disease)
  - Unknown causes of hypoparathyroidism
    - With dysmorphic features in Middle Eastern children
      - Autosomal recessive
    - Kenny-Caffey syndrome
      - Autosomal recessive
- PTH receptor defects (pseudohypoparathyroidism)
  - Type IA (inactivating mutation of $G_{s\alpha}$)
    - With gonadotropin-independent precocious puberty
  - Type IB (normal $G_{s\alpha}$)
  - Type II (normal cyclic adenosine monophosphate response)
- Ca^{2+}-sensing receptor activating mutation
  - Sporadic
  - Autosomal dominant
- Mitochondrial DNA mutations
  - Kearns-Sayre syndrome and other mutations
- Magnesium deficiency
  - Absorption defect
  - Renal tubular defect
  - Aminoglycoside therapy
- Exogenous inorganic phosphate excess
  - Laxatives
  - Soft drinks with phosphoric acid
- Vitamin D deficiency
  - Nutritional
  - Vitamin D deficiency (rickets)
    - Mutation of 1α(OH)ase ($P450^{vdl\alpha}$)

*AIRE = *autoimmune regulator.*

roidism has developed even when the parathyroid glands have been identified and left undisturbed at the time of operation. This presumably is the result of interference with the blood supply or of postoperative edema and fibrosis. Symptoms of tetany may occur abruptly postoperatively and may be temporary or permanent. In some instances, symptoms may develop insidiously and go undetected until months after thyroidectomy. Occasionally, the first evidence of surgical hypoparathyroidism may be the development of cataracts. The status of parathyroid function should be carefully monitored in all patients undergoing thyroidectomy.

Deposition of iron pigment or of copper in the parathyroid glands (e.g., thalassemia) (e.g., Wilson disease) may produce hypoparathyroidism.

Autoimmune Hypoparathyroidism. An autoimmune mechanism for hypoparathyroidism is strongly suggested by the finding of parathyroid antibodies and by its frequent association with other autoimmune disorders or organ-specific antibodies. Autoimmune hypoparathyroidism is often associated with Addison's disease and chronic mucocutaneous candidiasis. The association of at least two of these three conditions has been tentatively classified as *autoimmune polyglandular disease, type I.* It is also known as *autoimmune-polyendocrinopathy-candidiasis-ectodermal dystrophy.* This syndrome is inherited in an autosomal recessive fashion and is not related to any single HLA-associated haplotype. One third of patients with this syndrome have all three components; two thirds have only two of three conditions. The candidiasis almost always precedes the other disorders (70% of cases occur in children younger than 5 yr of age); the hypoparathyroidism (90% after 3 yr of age) usually occurs before Addison disease (90% after 6 yr of age). A variety of other disorders occur at various times and include alopecia areata or totalis, malabsorption disorder, pernicious anemia, gonadal failure, chronic active hepatitis, vitiligo, and insulin-dependent diabetes. Some of these associations may not appear until adult life. Autoimmune thyroid disease is a rare concomitant finding.

Affected siblings may have the same or different constellations of disorders (e.g., hypoparathyroidism and Addison disease). The disorder is exceptionally prevalent among Finns and Iranian Jews. The gene for this disorder is designated AIRE (autoimmune regulator); it is located on chromosome 21q22. It appears to be a transcription factor that plays an essential role in the development of immunologic tolerance. Patients with Addison disease as part of polyendocrinopathy syndrome type I have demonstrated adrenal-specific autoantibody reactivity directed against the side-chain cleavage enzyme.

Idiopathic Hypoparathyroidism. This term should be reserved for the small residuum of children with hypoparathyroidism for whom no causative mechanism can be defined. Most children in whom onset of hypoparathyroidism occurs after the first few years of life have an autoimmune condition. Autoantibodies to the extracellular domain of the calcium-sensing receptor have been identified in some patients with acquired hypoparathyroidism. One should always consider incomplete forms of DiGeorge syndrome or an activating calcium-sensing receptor mutation in the differential diagnosis.

CLINICAL MANIFESTATIONS. There is a spectrum of parathyroid deficiencies with clinical manifestations varying from no symptoms to those of complete and long-standing deficiency. Mild deficiency may be revealed only by appropriate laboratory studies. Muscular pain and cramps are early manifestations; they progress to numbness, stiffness, and tingling of the hands and feet. There may be only a positive Chvostek or Trousseau sign or laryngeal and carpopedal spasms. Convulsions with loss of consciousness may occur at intervals of days, weeks, or months. These episodes may begin with abdominal pain, followed by tonic rigidity, retraction of the head, and cyanosis. Hypoparathyroidism is frequently mistaken for epilepsy. Headache, vomiting, increased intracranial pressure, and papilledema may be associated with convulsions and may suggest a brain tumor.

In patients with long-standing hypocalcemia, the teeth erupt late and irregularly. Enamel formation is irregular, and the teeth may be unusually soft. The skin may be dry and scaly, and the nails of the fingers and toes may have horizontal lines. Mucocutaneous candidiasis, when present, antedates the development of hypoparathyroidism; the candidal infection most often involves the nails, the oral mucosa, the angles of the mouth, and less often, the skin.

Cataracts in patients with long-standing untreated disease are a direct consequence of hypoparathyroidism; other autoimmune ocular disorders such as keratoconjunctivitis may also occur. Manifestations of Addison disease, lymphocytic thyroiditis, pernicious anemia, alopecia areata or totalis, hepatitis, and primary gonadal insufficiency may also be associated with those of hypoparathyroidism.

Permanent physical and mental deterioration occur if initiation of treatment is long delayed.

LABORATORY FINDINGS. The serum calcium level is low (5–7 mg/dL) and the phosphorus elevated (7–12 mg/dL). Blood levels of ionized calcium (usually approximately 45% of the total) more nearly reflect physiologic adequacy but are also low. The serum level of alkaline phosphatase is normal or low, and the level of $1,25[OH]_2D_3$ is usually low, but high levels have been found in some children with severe hypocalcemia. The level of magnesium is normal but should always be checked in hypocalcemic patients. Levels of PTH are low when measured by immunometric assay. Administration of the synthetic 1–34 fragment of human PTH (teriparatide acetate) results in increased urinary levels of cyclic adenosine monophosphate and phosphate. This response differentiates hypoparathyroidism from pseudohypoparathyroidism. With the advent of very sensitive PTH assays, this test is usually not necessary. Roentgenograms of the bones occasionally reveal an increased density limited to the metaphyses, suggestive of heavy metal poisoning, or an increased density of the lamina dura. Roentgenograms or computed tomography of the skull may reveal calcifications in the basal ganglia. There is a prolongation of the QT interval on the electrocardiogram, which disappears when the hypocalcemia is corrected. The electroencephalogram usually reveals widespread slow activity; the tracing returns to normal after the serum calcium has been within the normal range for a few weeks, unless irreversible brain damage has occurred or unless the parathyroid insufficiency is associated with epilepsy. When hypoparathyroidism occurs concurrently with Addison disease, the serum level of calcium may be normal, but hypocalcemia appears after effective treatment of the adrenal insufficiency.

TREATMENT. Emergency treatment for neonatal tetany consists of intravenous injections of 5–10 mL of a 10% solution of calcium gluconate at the rate of 0.5–1 mL/min while heart rate is monitored. Additionally, 1,25-dihydroxycholecalciferol (calcitriol) should be given. The initial dosage is 0.25 μg/24 hr; the maintenance dosage ranges from 0.01–0.10 μg/kg/24 hr, to a maximum of 1–2 μg/24 hr. Calcitriol has a short half-life and should be given in two equal divided doses; it has the advantages of rapid onset of effect (1–4 days) and rapid reversal of hypercalcemia after discontinuation in the event of overdosage (i.e., calcium levels begin to fall in 3–4 days). Calcitriol is now supplied as an oral solution (1μg/mL, Roche Pharmaceuticals).

After normocalcemia has been achieved, one may wish to continue therapy with vitamin D_2 because it is considerably less costly than calcitriol. The usual dosages are 0.1–0.5 mg/24 hr in infants and young children. One milligram of vitamin D_2 has a biologic activity of 40,000 IU. Older children require 1.25–2.50 mg (50,000–100,000 IU) once daily. Vitamin D_2 has a slow onset of effect, and reversal of hypercalcemia after discontinuation of treatment is markedly delayed; its main advantage is its low cost.

An adequate intake of calcium should be ensured. Supplemental calcium can be given in the form of calcium gluconate or calcium glubionate (Neo-Calglucon) to provide 800 mg of elemental calcium daily, but it is rarely essential. Foods with a high phosphorus content such as milk, eggs, and cheese should be reduced in the diet.

Clinical evaluation of the patient and frequent determinations of the serum calcium levels are indicated in the early stages of treatment to determine the requirement for calcitriol or vitamin D_2. If hypercalcemia occurs, therapy should be discontinued and resumed at a lower dose after the serum calcium level has returned to normal. In long-standing cases, repair of cerebral and dental changes is not likely. Pigmentation, lowering of the blood pressure, or weight loss may indicate adrenal insufficiency, which requires specific treatment.

DIFFERENTIAL DIAGNOSIS. Magnesium deficiency must be considered in patients with unexplained hypocalcemia. Concentrations of serum magnesium less than 1.5 mg/dL (1.2 mEq/L) are usually abnormal. *Familial hypomagnesemia* with secondary hypocalcemia has been reported in about 50 patients, most of whom developed tetany and seizures at 2–6 wk of age. Administration of calcium is ineffective, but administration of magnesium promptly corrects both calcium and magnesium levels. Oral supplements of magnesium are necessary to maintain levels of magnesium in the normal range. Two genetic forms have been described. One is caused by an autosomal recessive gene on chromosome 9, resulting in a specific defect in absorption of magnesium. The other is caused by an autosomal dominant gene on chromosome 11q23, resulting in renal loss of magnesium.

Hypomagnesemia also occurs in malabsorption syndromes such as granulomatous colitis and cystic fibrosis. Patients with autoimmune polyglandular disease type I and hypoparathyroidism may also have concurrent steatorrhea and low magnesium levels. Therapy with aminoglycosides causes hypomagnesemia by increasing urinary loses.

It is not clear how low levels of magnesium lead to hypocalcemia. Evidence suggests that hypomagnesemia impairs release of PTH and induces resistance to the effects of the hormone, but other mechanisms also may be operative.

Poisoning with inorganic phosphate leads to hypocalcemia and tetany. Infants administered large doses of inorganic phosphates, either as laxatives or as sodium phosphate enemas, have had sudden onset of tetany, with serum calcium levels less than 5 mg/dL and markedly elevated levels of phosphate. Symptoms are quickly relieved by intravenous administration of calcium. The mechanism of the hypocalcemia is not clear (see Chapter 51).

Hypocalcemia may occur early in the course of treatment of *acute lymphoblastic leukemia*. Hypocalcemia is usually associated with hyperphosphatemia resulting from destruction of lymphoblasts.

Episodic symptomatic hypocalcemia occurs in the *Kenny-Caffey syndrome*, which is characterized by medullary stenosis of the long bones, short stature, delayed closure of the fontanel, delayed bone age, and eye abnormalities. Idiopathic hypoparathyroidism and abnormal PTH levels have been found. Autosomal dominant and autosomal recessive modes of inheritance have been reported.

CHAPTER 582
Pseudohypoparathyroidism (Albright Hereditary Osteodystrophy)

In contrast to the situation in hypoparathyroidism, in pseudohypoparathyroidism (PHP), the parathyroid glands are normal or hyperplastic histologically, and they can synthesize and secrete parathyroid hormone (PTH). Serum levels of immunoreactive PTH are elevated even when the patient is hypocalcemic and may be elevated when the patient is normocalcemic. Neither endogenous nor administered PTH raises the serum levels of calcium or lowers the levels of phosphorus. The genetic defects in the hormone receptor adenylate cyclase system are classified into various types depending on the phenotypic and biochemical findings.

TYPE IA. This type accounts for the majority of patients with PHP. Affected patients have a genetic defect of the α subunit of the stimulatory guanine nucleotide-binding protein ($G_{s\alpha}$). This coupling factor is required for PTH bound to cell surface receptors to activate cyclic adenosine monophosphate (cAMP). Heterogeneous mutations of the $G_{s\alpha}$ gene have been documented; the gene is located on chromosome 20q13.2. Deficiency of the $G_{s\alpha}$ subunit is a generalized cellular defect and accounts for the association of other endocrine disorders with type IA PHP. The defect is inherited as an autosomal dominant trait, and the paucity of father-to-son transmissions is thought to be due to decreased fertility in males.

Tetany is often the presenting sign. Affected children have a short, stocky build and a round face. Brachydactyly with dimpling of the dorsum of the hand is usually present. The 2nd metacarpal is involved least often. As a result, the index finger may occasionally be longer than the middle finger. Likewise, the 2nd metatarsal is only rarely affected. There may be other skeletal abnormalities such as short and wide phalanges, bowing, exostoses, and thickening of the calvaria. These patients frequently have calcium deposits and metaplastic bone formation subcutaneously. Moderate degrees of mental retardation, calcification of the basal ganglia, and lenticular cataracts are common in patients who are diagnosed late.

Some members of affected kindreds may have the usual anatomic stigmata of PHP, but serum levels of calcium and phosphorus are normal despite reduced $G_{s\alpha}$ activity; however, PTH levels may be slightly elevated. Such patients have been labeled as having *pseudopseudohypoparathyroidism*. Transition from normocalcemia to hypocalcemia often occurs with increasing age of the patient. These phenotypically similar but metabolically dissimilar patients may occur in the same family and have the same mutations of $G_{s\alpha}$ protein. It is not known what other factors cause clinically overt hypocalcemia in some affected patients and not in others. There is some evidence to suggest that the $G_{s\alpha}$ mutation is paternally transmitted in pseudopseudohypoparathyroidism and maternally transmitted in patients with type Ia disease. The gene may be imprinted in a tissue specific manner.

In addition to resistance to PTH, resistance to other G protein–coupled receptors for thyroid-stimulating hormone (TSH), gonadotropins, and glucagon may result in various metabolic effects. Clinical hypothyroidism is uncommon, but basal levels of TSH are elevated, and thyrotropin-releasing hormone–stimulated TSH responses are exaggerated. Moderately decreased levels of thyroxine and increased levels of TSH have been detected by newborn thyroid screening programs, leading to the detection of type IA PHP in infancy. In adults, gonadal dysfunction is common, as manifested by sexual immaturity, amenorrhea, oligomenorrhea, and infertility. Each of these abnormalities can be related to deficient synthesis of cAMP secondary to a deficiency of $G_{s\alpha}$, but it is not clear why resistance to other G protein–dependent hormones (e.g., corticotropin, vasopressin) is much less affected.

Serum levels of calcium are low, and those of phosphorus and alkaline phosphatase are elevated. Clinical diagnosis can be confirmed by demonstration of a markedly attenuated response in urinary phosphate and cAMP after intravenous infusion of the synthetic 1–34 fragment of human PTH (teriparatide acetate), but this compound is no longer commercially available in the United States. Definitive diagnosis is established by demonstration of the mutated G protein.

Type IA with Precocious Puberty. Two boys have been reported with both type IA PHP and gonadotropin-independent precocious puberty (see Chapter 572.6). They were found to have a temperature-sensitive mutation of the G_s protein. Thus at normal body temperature (37°C), the G_s is degraded, resulting in PHP, but in the cooler temperature of the testes (33°C), the G_s mutation results in constitutive activation of the luteinizing hormone receptor and precocious puberty.

TYPE IB. Affected patients have normal levels of G protein activity and a normal phenotypic appearance. These patients have resistance to PTH but not to other hormones. Serum levels of calcium, phosphorus, and immunoreactive PTH are the same as those in patients with type IA PHP. These patients also show no rise in cAMP in response to exogenous administration of PTH. Bioactive PTH is not increased. The pathophysiology of the disorder in this group of patients is uncertain. Proposed explanations include production of inhibitory PTH peptides, a defect in PTH receptor expression, or a defect in the catalytic subunit of adenyl cyclase. It is likely that the cause of the abnormality in this group is heterogeneous.

TYPE II. This type of pseudohypoparathyroidism has been detected in only a few patients and differs from type I in that the urinary excretion of cAMP is elevated both in the basal state and after stimulation with PTH, but phosphaturia does not increase. Phenotypically, patients are normal and hypocalcemia is present. The defect appears to be distal to cAMP because it is normally activated, but the cell is unable to respond to the signal.

CHAPTER 583
Hyperparathyroidism

Excessive production of parathyroid hormone (PTH) may result from a primary defect of the parathyroid glands such as an adenoma or hyperplasia *(primary hyperparathyroidism).*

More often, the increased production of PTH is compensatory, usually aimed at correcting hypocalcemic states of diverse origins *(secondary hyperparathyroidism).* In vitamin D–deficient rickets and the malabsorption syndromes, intestinal absorption of calcium is deficient, but hypocalcemia and tetany may be averted by increased activity of the parathyroid glands. In pseudohypoparathyroidism, PTH levels are elevated because a mutation in the $G_{s\alpha}$ protein interferes with response to PTH. Early in chronic renal disease, hyperphosphatemia results in a reciprocal fall in the calcium concentration with a consequent increase in PTH, but in advanced stages of renal failure, production of $1,25[OH]_2D_3$ is also decreased, leading to worsening hypocalcemia and further stimulation of PTH. In some instances, if stimulation of the parathyroid glands has been sufficiently intense and protracted, the glands may continue to secrete increased levels of PTH for months or years after renal transplantation, with resulting hypercalcemia.

ETIOLOGY. Childhood hyperparathyroidism is rare. Onset during childhood is usually the result of a single benign adenoma. It usually becomes manifested after 10 yr of age. There have been a number of kindreds in which multiple members have hyperparathyroidism transmitted in an autosomal dominant fashion. Most of the affected family members are adults, but children have been involved in about a third of the pedigrees. Some affected patients in these families are asymptomatic and are detected only by careful study. In other kindreds, hyperparathyroidism occurs as part of the constellation known as the *multiple endocrine neoplasia (MEN) syndromes* or of the *hyperparathyroidism-jaw tumor syndrome.*

Neonatal severe hyperparathyroidism has been reported in approximately 50 infants. Symptoms develop shortly after birth and consist of anorexia, irritability, lethargy, constipation, and failure to thrive. Roentgenograms reveal subperiosteal bone resorption, osteoporosis, and pathologic fractures. Symptoms may be mild, resolving without treatment, or may have a rapidly fatal course if diagnosis and treatment are delayed. Histologically, the parathyroid glands show diffuse hyperplasia. Affected siblings have been observed in some kindreds, and parental consanguinity has been reported in several kindreds.

Most cases have occurred in kindreds with the clinical and biochemical features of *familial hypocalciuric hypercalcemia.* These infants may be homozygous or heterozygous for the mutation in the Ca^{2+}-sensing receptor gene, whereas most individuals with one copy of this mutation exhibit autosomally dominant familial hypocalciuric hypercalcemia.

MEN type I is an autosomal dominant disorder characterized by hyperplasia or neoplasia of the endocrine pancreas (which secretes gastrin, insulin, pancreatic polypeptide, or occasionally glucagon), the anterior pituitary (which usually secretes prolactin), and the parathyroid glands. In most kindreds, hyperparathyroidism is usually the presenting manifestation, with a prevalence approaching 100% by 50 yr of age but occurring only rarely in children younger than 18 yr of age. In the past, after an affected family was identified, it was necessary to perform repeated metabolic screening for many years to detect other affected family members. With appropriate DNA probes, it is now possible to detect carriers of the gene with 99% accuracy at birth, avoiding unnecessary biochemical screening programs.

The gene for MEN type I is on chromosome 11q13; it appears to function as a tumor suppressor gene and follows the two-hit hypothesis of tumor development. The first mutation (germinal) is inherited and is recessive to the dominant allele; this does not result in tumor formation. A second mutation (somatic) is required to eliminate the normal allele, which then leads to tumor formation.

Hyperparathyroidism-Jaw Tumor syndrome is an autosomal dominant disorder characterized by parathyroid adenomas and fibro-osseous jaw tumors. Affected patients may also have polycystic kidney disease, renal hamartomas, and Wilms tumor. Although the condition affects adults primarily, it has been diagnosed as early as age 10.

MEN type II may also be associated with hyperparathyroidism (see Chapter 579.2).

Transient neonatal hyperparathyroidism has occurred in a few infants born to mothers with hypoparathyroidism (idiopathic or surgical) or with pseudohypoparathyroidism. In each case, the maternal disorder had been undiagnosed or inadequately treated during pregnancy. The cause of the condition is chronic intrauterine exposure to hypocalcemia with resultant hyperplasia of the fetal parathyroid glands. In the newborn, manifestations involve the bones primarily, and healing occurs between 4 and 7 mo of age.

CLINICAL MANIFESTATIONS. At all ages, the clinical manifestations of hypercalcemia of any cause include muscular weakness, anorexia, nausea, vomiting, constipation, polydipsia, polyuria, loss of weight, and fever. When hypercalcemia is of long duration, calcium may be deposited in the renal parenchyma (nephrocalcinosis), with progressively diminished renal function. Renal calculi may occur and may produce renal colic and hematuria. Osseous changes may produce pain in the back or extremities, disturbances of gait, genu valgum, fractures, and tumors. Height may decrease from compression of vertebrae; the patient may become bedridden. Detection of completely asymptomatic patients is increasing with the advent of automated panel assays that include serum calcium determinations.

Abdominal pain is occasionally prominent and may be associated with acute pancreatitis. Parathyroid crisis may occur, manifested by serum calcium levels greater than 15 mg/dL and progressive oliguria, azotemia, stupor, and coma. In infants, failure to thrive, poor feeding, and hypotonia are common. Mental retardation, convulsions, and blindness may occur as sequelae of long-standing hypercalcemia.

LABORATORY FINDINGS. The serum calcium level is elevated; 39 of 45 children with adenomas had levels greater than 12 mg/dL. The hypercalcemia is more severe in infants with parathyroid hyperplasia; concentrations ranging from 15–20 mg/dL are common, and values as high as 30 mg/dL have been reported. Even when total serum calcium is borderline or only slightly elevated, ionized calcium levels are often increased. The serum phosphorus level is reduced to about 3 mg/dL or less, and the level of serum magnesium is low. The urine may have a low and fixed specific gravity, and serum levels of nonprotein nitrogen and uric acid may be elevated. In patients with adenomas who have skeletal involvement, serum phosphatase levels are elevated, but in infants with hyperplasia the levels of alkaline phosphatase may be normal even when there is extensive involvement of bone.

Serum levels of PTH measured by carboxy terminal antisera are elevated, especially in relation to the level of calcium. Results may vary markedly from one laboratory to another, depending on the antibody used. Calcitonin levels are normal. Acute hypercalcemia can stimulate calcitonin release, but with prolonged hypercalcemia, hypercalcitoninemia does not occur.

The most consistent and characteristic roentgenographic finding is resorption of subperiosteal bone, best seen along the margins of the phalanges of the hands. In the skull, there may be gross trabeculation or a granular appearance resulting from focal rarefaction; the lamina dura may be absent. In more advanced disease, there may be generalized rarefaction, cysts, tumors, fractures, and deformities. About 10% of patients have roentgenographic signs of rickets. Roentgenograms of the abdomen may reveal renal calculi or nephrocalcinosis.

DIFFERENTIAL DIAGNOSIS. Other causes of hypercalcemia may result in a similar clinical pattern and must be differentiated from hyperparathyroidism (Table 583–1). A low serum phosphorus level with hypercalcemia is characteristic of primary hyperparathyroidism; elevated levels of PTH are also diagnostic. With hypercalcemia of any cause except hyperparathyroidism and familial hypocalciuric hypercalcemia, PTH levels are suppressed. Pharmacologic doses of corticosteroids lower the serum calcium level level to normal in patients with hypercalcemia from other causes but generally do not affect the calcium level in patients with hyperparathyroidism.

TREATMENT. Surgical exploration is indicated in all instances. All glands should be carefully inspected; if an adenoma is discovered, it should be removed; very few instances of carcinoma are known in children. Most neonates with severe hypercalcemia require total parathyroidectomy; less severe hypercalcemia may remit spontaneously in others. A portion of a parathyroid gland may be autografted into the forearm; four infants treated in this fashion were able to maintain normocalcemia without supplementary treatment, but no long-term outcome has yet been reported. The patient should be carefully observed postoperatively for the development of hypocalcemia and tetany; intravenous administration of calcium gluconate may be required for a few days. The serum calcium level then gradually returns to normal, and under ordinary circumstances, a diet high in calcium and phosphorus must be maintained for only several months after operation.

TABLE 583–1 Etiologic Classification of Hypercalcemia

Parathyroid hormone (PTH) excess
- Primary hyperparathyroidism
  - Adenoma
    - Sporadic
    - Autosomal dominant
    - Hyperparathyroidism-jaw tumor syndrome
  - Hyperplasia or adenoma
    - Multiple endocrine neoplasia type I
      - Mutation in MEN1 gene (11q13)
    - Multiple endocrine neoplasia 2A and 2B
      - Mutation in RET proto-oncogene
    - Parathyroid hyperplasia of infancy
      - Inactivating mutation of Ca^{2+}-sensing receptor
      - Secondary to maternal hypoparathyroidism
  - Ectopic PTH production
    - Nonendocrine malignancies

Parathyroid hormone-related peptide (PTHrP) excess
- Nonendocrine malignancies
- Benign hypertrophy of breasts

Ca^{2+}-sensing receptor inactivating mutation
- Heterozygous-familial hypoacalciuric hypercalcemia
- Neonatal hyperparathyroidism

Activating mutation of PTH/PTHrP receptor
- Jansen-type metaphyseal chondrodysplasia

Inactivating mutations of PTH/PTHrP receptor

Blomstrand Chondrodysplasia

Vitamin D excess
- Iatrogenic
- Ectopic production
  - Sarcoidosis, tuberculosis, granulomatous lesions, subcutaneous fat necrosis
  - Excessively fortified milk

Unknown cause
- Williams syndrome (7q11.23 deletion)

Other
- Hypophosphatasia
  - Mutation of tissue nonspecific alkaline phosphatase gene
- Prolonged immobilization
- Thyrotoxicosis
- Hypervitaminosis A
- Leukemia

Arteriography and selective venous sampling with radioimmunoassay of PTH for preoperative localization and differentiation of a single adenoma from hyperplasia have been replaced by imaging methods. Computed tomography, real-time ultrasonography, and subtraction scintigraphy using ^{99m}Tc-pertechnetate and 201Tl have each proved effective in 50–90% of adults. These procedures are rarely required by the expert parathyroid surgeon but may be advisable before re-exploration in cases of persistent or recurrent hyperparathyroidism.

PROGNOSIS. The prognosis is good if the disease is recognized early and there is appropriate surgical treatment. When extensive osseous lesions are present, deformities may be permanent. A search for other affected family members is indicated.

OTHER CAUSES OF HYPERCALCEMIA

FAMILIAL HYPOCALCIURIC HYPERCALCEMIA (FAMILIAL BENIGN HYPERCALCEMIA). Patients with this disorder are usually asymptomatic, and the hypercalcemia comes to light by chance during routine investigation for other conditions. The parathyroid glands are normal, PTH levels are inappropriately normal, and subtotal parathyroidectomy does not correct the hypercalcemia. Serum levels of magnesium are high normal or mildly elevated. The rate of calcium to creatinine clearance is usually decreased despite hypercalcemia. The disorder is inherited in an autosomal dominant manner and is caused by a mutant gene on chromosome 3q2. Penetrance is near 100%, and affected individuals can be diagnosed early in childhood by serum and urinary calcium concentrations. Detection of other affected family members is important to avoid inappropriate parathyroid surgery. The basic defect in this condition results from inactivating mutations in the Ca^{2+}-sensing receptor gene. This G protein–coupled receptor senses the level of free Ca^{2+} in the blood and triggers the pathway to increase extracellular Ca^{2+} in the face of hypocalcemia. This receptor functions in the parathyroid and kidney to regulate calcium homeostasis; inactivating mutations lead to an increased set point with respect to serum Ca^{2+}, resulting in mild to moderate hypercalcemia in heterozygotes.

GRANULOMATOUS DISEASES. Hypercalcemia occurs in 30–50% of children with sarcoidosis and less often in patients with other granulomatous diseases such as tuberculosis. Levels of PTH are suppressed, and levels of $1,25[OH]_2D_3$ are elevated. The source of ectopic $1,25[OH]_2D_3$ is the activated macrophage, through stimulation by interferon-α from T lymphocytes, which are present in abundance in granulomatous lesions. Unlike renal tubular cells, the 1α-hydroxylase in macrophages is unresponsive to homeostatic regulation. Oral administration of prednisone (2 mg/kg/24 hr) lowers serum levels of $1,25[OH]_2D_3$ to normal and corrects the hypercalcemia.

HYPERCALCEMIA OF MALIGNANCY. Hypercalcemia frequently occurs in adults with a wide variety of solid tumors but is identified much less often in children. It has been reported in infants with malignant rhabdoid tumors of the kidney or congenital mesoblastic nephroma and in children with neuroblastoma, medulloblastoma, leukemia, Burkitt lymphoma, dysgerminoma, and rhabdomyosarcoma. Serum levels of PTH are rarely elevated. In most patients, the hypercalcemia associated with malignancy is caused by elevated levels of parathyroid hormone–related peptide (PTHrP) and not PTH. Rarely, tumors produce $1,25[OH]_2D_3$ or PTH ectopically.

MISCELLANEOUS CAUSES OF HYPERCALCEMIA. Hypercalcemia may occur in infants with subcutaneous *fat necrosis*. Levels of PTH are normal. In one infant, the level of $1,25[OH]_2D_3$ was elevated, and biopsy of the skin lesion revealed granulomatous infiltration, suggesting that the mechanism of the hypercalcemia was akin to that seen in patients with other granulomatous disease. In another infant, although $1,25[OH]_2D_3$ was normal, PTH was suppressed, suggesting the hypercalcemia was not PTH-related. Treatment with prednisone is effective.

Hypophosphatasia, especially the severe infantile form, is usually associated with mild to moderate hypercalcemia (Chapter 709). Serum levels of phosphorus are normal, and those of alkaline phosphatase are subnormal. The bones exhibit rachitic-like lesions on roentgenograms. Urinary levels of phosphoethanolamine, inorganic pyrophosphate, and pyridoxal 5′-phosphate are elevated; each is a natural substrate to a *tissue-nonspecific* (liver, bone, kidney) *alkaline phosphatase enzyme*. Missense mutations of the tissue-nonspecific alkaline phosphatase enzyme gene result in an inactive enzyme in this autosomal recessive disorder.

Idiopathic hypercalcemia of infancy is manifested by failure to thrive and hypercalcemia during the 1st yr of life followed by spontaneous remission. Serum levels of phosphorus and PTH are normal. The hypercalcemia results from increased absorption of calcium. Vitamin D may be involved in the pathogenesis. Both normal and elevated levels of $1,25[OH]_2D_3$ have been reported. An excessive rise in the level of $1,25[OH]_2D_3$ in response to PTH administration years after the hypercalcemic phase suggests that vitamin D has a role in the pathogenesis. A blunted calcitonin response to intravenous calcium has also been reported.

Ten per cent of patients with *Williams syndrome* also exhibit associated infantile hypercalcemia. The phenotype consists of feeding difficulties, slow growth, elfin facies, renovascular disorders, and a gregarious personality. The IQ score of 50 to 70 is curiously accompanied by enhanced quantity and quality of vocabulary, auditory memory, and social use of language. A submicroscopic deletion at chromosome 7q11.23, which includes deletion of one elastin allele, occurs in 90% of patients and seems to account for the vascular problems. Definitive diagnosis can be established by specific fluorescent in situ hybridization. The hypercalcemia and central nervous system symptoms may be caused by deletion of adjacent genes. Hypercalcemia has been successfully controlled with either prednisone or calcitonin.

Hypervitaminosis D resulting in hypercalcemia from drinking milk that has been incorrectly fortified with vitamin D has been reported. Serum levels of 25[OH]D are a better indicator of hypervitaminosis D than $1,25[OH]_2D_3$ because 25[OH]D has a longer half-life.

Prolonged immobilization may lead to hypercalcemia and occasionally to decreased renal function, hypertension, and encephalopathy. Children having hypophosphatemic rickets and undergoing surgery with subsequent long-term immobilization are at risk for hypercalcemia and should therefore have their vitamin D supplementation decreased or discontinued.

Jansen-type metaphyseal chondrodysplasia is a rare genetic disorder characterized by short-limbed dwarfism and severe but asymptomatic hypercalcemia (Chapter 707). Circulating levels of PTH and PTHrP are undetectable. These patients have an activating PTH–PTHrP receptor mutation that results in aberrant calcium homeostasis and abnormalities of the growth plate.

Aaltonen J, Bjorses P, Su Lee Y, et al: An autoimmune disease, APECED, caused by mutations in a novel gene featuring two PHD-type zinc-finger domains. Nat Genet 17:399, 1997.

Ahonen P, Myllarniemi S, Sipla I, Perheentupa J: Clinical variation of autoimmune polyendocrinopathy-candidiasis-ectodermal dystrophy (APECED) in a series of 68 patients. N Engl J Med 322:1829, 1990.

Allbery SM, Swischuk LE, John SD: Hypercalcemia associated with dysgerminoma: Case report and imaging findings. Pediatr Radiol 28:183, 1990.

Bassett JH, Forbes SA, Thakker RV, et al: Characterization of mutations in patients with multiple endocrine neoplasia type I. Am J Hum Genet 62:232, 1998.

Body JJ, Chanoine JP, Dumon JC, Delange F: Circulating calcitonin levels in healthy children and subjects with hypothyroidism from birth to adolescence. J Clin Endocrinol Metab 77:565, 1993.

Brown EM, Pollak M, Hebert SC, et al: Calcium-Ion-Sensing Cell-Surface Receptors (review). N Engl J Med 333:234, 1995.

Burgess JR, Shepherd JJ, Greenaway TM, et al: Spectrum of pituitary disease in multiple endocrine neoplasia type I (MEN 1): Clinical, biochemical, and radiological features of pituitary disease in a large MEN 1 kindred. J Clin Endocrinol Metab 81:2642, 1996.

Burtis WJ, Brady TG, Orloff JJ, et al: Immunochemical characterization of circulating parathyroid hormone–related protein in patients with hormonal hypercalcemia of cancer. N Engl J Med 322:1106, 1990.

Clapman DS: Why testicles are cool. Nature 371:109, 1994.

Chesney RW: Requirements and upper limits of vitamin D intake in the term neonate, infant, and older child. J Pediatr 116:159, 1990.

Cook JS, Stone MS, Hansen JR: Hypercalcemia in association with subcutaneous fat necrosis of the newborn: Studies of calcium-regulating hormones. Pediatrics 90:93, 1992.

Cooper L, Wertheimer J, Levey R, et al: Severe primary hyperparathyroidism in a neonate with two hypercalcemic parents: Management with parathyroidectomy and heterotopic autotransplantation. Pediatrics 78:263, 1986.

Damiani D, Agwar CH, Bueno VS, et al: Primary hyperparathyroidism in children: Patient report and review of literature. J Pediatr Endocrinol Metab 11:83, 1998.

DiGeorge AM: Congenital absence of the thymus and its immunologic consequences, concurrence with congenital hypoparathyroidism. In: Bergsma D, Good RA (eds): Birth Defects. Original Article Series, No. 1, Vol IV. New York, The National Foundation, 1968.

Ewart AK, Morris CA, Atkinson D, et al: Hemizygosity at the elastin locus in a developmental disorder, Williams syndrome. Nat Genet 5:11, 1993.

Fedde KN, Michell MP, Whyte MP, et al: Aberrant properities of alkaline phosphatase in patients with clinical expressivity in severe forms of hypophosphatasia. J Clin Endocrinol Metab 81:2587, 1996.

Gillis D, Hirsch HJ, Peylan-Ramu N, et al: Parathyroid adenoma after radiation in an 8-year old boy. J Pediatr 132:892, 1998.

Hobbs MR, Pole AR, Pidisirng GN, et al: Hyperparathyroidism-jaw tumor syndrome: The HRPT2 locus is within a 0.7-cM region on chromosome 1q. Am J Hum Genet 64:518, 1999.

Iiri T, Herzmark P, Nakimoto JM, et al: Rapid GDP release from Gs_{α} in patients with gain and loss of endocrine function. Nature 371:164, 1994.

Jacabus CH, Holick MF, Shao G, et al: Hypervitaminosis D associated with drinking milk. N Engl J Med 326:1173, 1992.

Jobert AS, Zhang P, Courineau A, et al: Absence of functional receptors for parathyroid hormone and parathyroid hormone-related peptide in Blomstrand Chondrodysplasia. J Clin Invest 102:34, 1998.

Kahn KT, Uma R, Farag TI, et al: Kenny-Caffey syndrome in six Bedouin sibships: Autosomal recessive inheritance is confirmed. Am J Med Genet 69:126, 1997.

Key LL, Thorne M, Pitzer B, et al: Management of neonatal hyperparathyroidism with parathyroidectomy and autotransplantation. J Pediatr 116:923, 1990.

Khosla S, Johansen KL, Ory SJ, et al: Parathyroid hormone–related peptide in lactation and in umbilical cord blood. Mayo Clin Proc 65:1408, 1990.

Kovacs CS, Kronenberg HM: Maternal-fetal calcium and bone metabolism during pregnancy, puerperium and lactation. Endocr Rev 18:832, 1997.

Learoyd DL, Twigg SM, Robinson BG, et al: The practical management of multiple endocrine neoplasia. Trends Endocrinol Metab 6:273, 1995.

Levitt M, Gessert C, Finberg L: Inorganic phosphate (laxative) poisoning resulting in tetany in an infant. J Pediatr 82:479, 1973.

Li Y, Song Y-H, Muir A, et al: Autoantibodies to the extracellular domain of the calcium-sensing receptor in patients with acquired hypoparathyroidism. J Clin Invest 97:910, 1996.

Marx SJ: Familial multiple endocrine neoplasia type 1. Mutation of a tumor suppressor gene. Trends Endocrinol Metab 76:82, 1989.

McKay C, Furman WL: Hypercalcemia complicating childhood malignancies. Cancer 72:256, 1993.

Meij IC, Saar K, vanden Heuvel LPS, et al: Hereditary isolated renal magnesium loss maps to chromosome 11q23. Am J Hum Genet 64:180, 1999.

Miric A, Vechio JD, Levine MA: Heterogeneous mutations in the gene encoding the α-subunit of the stimulatory G protein of adenylyl cyclase in Albright hereditary osteodystrophy. J Clin Endocrinol Metab 76:1560, 1993.

Morris CA, Demsey SA, Leonard CD, et al: Natural history of Williams syndrome: Physical characteristics. J Pediatr 113:318, 1988.

Nagamine K, Peterson P, Shimizu N, et al: Positional cloning of the APECED gene. Nat Genet 17:393, 1997.

Nakamoto JM, Sandstrom AT, Van Dop C, et al: Pseudohypoparathyroidism type Ia from maternal but not paternal transmission of a Gs_α gene mutation. Am J Med Genet 77:261, 1998.

Panvari R, Hershkovitz E, Kanis A, et al: Homozygosity and linkage-disequalibrium mapping of the syndrome of congenital hypoparathyroidism, growth and mental retardation, and dysmorphism to a 1-cM interval on chromosome 1q42-43. Am J Hum Genet 63:163, 1998.

Patten JL, Johns DR, Valle D, et al: Mutation in the gene encoding the stimulating G protein of adenylate cyclase in Albright's hereditary osteodystrophy. N Engl J Med 322:1412, 1990.

Pearce SH: Multiple endocrine neoplasia type I (MEN 1): Recent advances (commentary). Clin Endocrinol 47:513, 1997.

Pearce SH, Williamson C, Thaker RV, et al: A familial syndrome of hypocalcemia with hypercalciuria due to mutations in the calcium-sensing receptor. N Engl J Med 335:1115, 1996.

Pollak MR, Brown EM, WuChou YH, et al: Mutations in the human $Ca2^+$-sensing receptor gene cause familial hypocalciuric hypercalcemia and neonatal severe hyperthyroidism. Cell 75:1297, 1993.

Pollak MR, WuChou YH, Marx SJ, et al: Familial hypocalciuric hypercalcemia and neonatal severe hyperparathyroidism. Effects of mutant gene dosage on phenotype. J Clin Invest 93:1108, 1994.

Reichel H, Koeffler HP, Norman AW: The role of the vitamin D endocrine system in health and disease. N Engl J Med 320:980, 1989.

Sanjad SA, Sakati NA, Abu-Osba YK, et al: A new syndrome of congenital hypoparathyroidism, severe growth failure and dysmorphic features. Arch Dis Child 66:193, 1992.

Schipani E, Langman CB, Juppner H, et al: Constitutively activated receptors for parathyroid hormone and parathyroid hormone–related peptide in Jansen's metaphyseal chondrodysplasia. N Engl J Med 335:708, 1996.

Shalev H, Phillip M, Landau D, et al: Clinical presentation and outcome in primary familial hypomagnesaemia. Arch Dis Child 78:127, 1998.

Stewart AF, Broadus A: Parathyroid hormone–related proteins: Coming of age in the 1990's. J Clin Endocrinol Metab 71:1410, 1990.

Tean BT, Farnebo F, Larson C, et al: Familial isolated hyperparathyroidism maps to the hyperparathyroidism-jaw tumor locus in 1q21–q32 in a subset of families. J Clin Endocrinol Metab 83:2114, 1998.

Tengan CH, Kiyomoto BH, Moraes CT, et al: Mitochondrial encephalomyopathy and hypoparathyroidism associated with a duplication and a deletion of mitochondrial deoxyribonucleic acid. J Clin Endocrinol Metab 83:125, 1998.

Thomas BR, Bennett JD: Symptomatic hypocalcemia and hypoparathyroidism in two infants of mothers with hyperparathyroidism and familial benign hypercalcemia. J Perinatol 15:23, 1995.

Trump D, Dixon PH, Mumm S, et al: Localization of X-linked idiopathic hypoparathyroidism to a 1.5 Mb region on Xq26-q27. J Med Genet 35:905, 1998.

Tyni T, Rapola J, Pihko H: Hypoparathyroidism in a patient with long-chain 3-hydroxyacyl-coenzyme A dehydrogenase deficiency caused by the G1528C mutation. J Pediatr 131:766, 1997.

Walder RY, Shalev H, Sheffield VC, et al: Familial hypomagnesemia maps to chromosome 9q not to the X chromosome: Genetic linkage mapping and analysis of a balanced translocation breakpoint. Hum Mol Genet 6:1491, 1997.

Watanabe T, Bai M, Yasuda T, et al: Familial hypoparathyroidism: Identification of a novel gain of function mutation in transmembrane domain 5 of the calcium-sensing receptor. J Clin Endocrinol Metab 83:2497, 1998.

Weinstein LS, Shuhva Y: The role of genomic imprinting of G_s α in the pathogenesis of Albright hereditary osteodystrophy. Trends Endocrinol Metab 10:81, 1999.

Whyte MP: Hypophosphatasia and the role of alkaline phosphatase in skeletal mineralization. Endocr Rev 15:439, 1994.

Whyte MP, Weldon VV: Idiopathic hypoparathyroidism presenting with seizures during infancy: X-linked recessive inheritance in a large Missouri kindred. J Pediatr 99:608, 1981.

Winter WE, Silverstein JH, MacLaren NK, et al: Autosomal dominant hypoparathyroidism with variable, age-dependent severity. J Pediatr 103:387, 1983.

SECTION 4

Disorders of the Adrenal Glands

Lenore S. Levine ■ Angelo M. DiGeorge

CHAPTER 584

The Physiology of the Adrenal Gland

The adrenal gland is composed of two endocrine systems, the medullary and the cortical systems. The chromaffin cells of the adrenal medulla are derived from neuroectoderm, whereas the cells of the adrenal cortex are derived from mesoderm. Mesodermal cells also contribute to the development of the gonads and the liver. The adrenal glands and gonads have in common certain enzymes involved in steroid synthesis, and an inborn error in steroidogenesis in one tissue may also be present in the other.

ADRENAL CORTEX. The adrenal cortex consists of three zones: the zona glomerulosa, the outermost zone located immediately beneath the capsule; the zona fasciculata, the middle zone; and the zona reticularis, the innermost zone, lying next to the adrenal medulla. The zona fasciculata is the largest of the zones, constituting about three fourths of the cortex; the zona glomerulosa composes about 15% and the zona reticularis about 10%. Glomerulosa cells are small with a lower cytoplasmic:nuclear ratio, intermediate number of lipid inclusions, and smaller nuclei containing more condensed chromatin than the cells of the other two zones. The cells of the zona fasciculata are large with a high cytoplasmic:nuclear ratio and many lipid inclusions that give the cytoplasm a foamy, vacuolated appearance. The cells are arranged in radial cords. The cells of the zona reticularis are arranged in irregular anastamosing cords. The cytoplasmic:nuclear ratio is intermediate and the compact cytoplasm has relatively little lipid content.

The zona glomerulosa cells produce aldosterone, the most potent natural mineralocorticoid in humans. The zona fasciculata produces cortisol, the most potent natural glucocorticoid in humans, and the zona fasciculata and zona reticularis produce the adrenal androgens.

Adrenal Steroidogenesis. For the synthesis of these hormones a series of enzymatic steps is required (see Fig. 586–1). P450 scc (CYP11AI), found in the adrenal mitochondria, catalyzes the conversion of cholesterol to pregnenolone. This is the first rate-limiting step in steroid hormone synthesis and involves three reactions—20α-hydroxylation, 22-hydroxylation, and side chain cleavage. P450 scc is coded for by the CYP11AI gene located on the long arm of human chromosome 15. 3βHSD/isomerase (3βHSD II), a microsomal enzyme coded for by the gene HSD3B2 on the short arm of chromosome 1, converts pregnenolone to progesterone, and 17-OH pregnenolone to 17-OH progesterone.

P450c17 (CYP17), found in the endoplasmic reticulum, catalyzes the conversion of pregnenolone and progesterone to 17-OH pregnenolone and 17-OH progesterone (17-hydroxylation), respectively, as well as side chain cleavage at C17 (17,20-lyase activity) to form dehydroepiandrosterone (DHEA) and androstenedione. The CYP 17 gene is located on the long arm of chromosome 10. 21-Hydroxylation of progesterone and 17-hydroxyprogesterone to 11-deoxycorticosterone (DOC) and 11-deoxycortisol (S), respectively, is mediated by P450c21 (CYP21A2), located in the endoplasmic reticulum. This enzyme is encoded by the CYP21A2 gene, located within the HLA complex on the short arm of chromosome 6. P450c11 (CYP11B1) and P450c18 (CYP11B2) are two closely related enzymes found in the inner mitochondrial membrane. P450c11 catalyzes the conversion of 11-deoxycortisol to cortisol, and DOC to corticosterone (B), and is found abundantly in the zona fasciculata. P450c18 (CYP11B2), a far less abundant enzyme, is found only in the zona glomerulosa, where it has 11β-hydroxylase, 18-hydroxylase, and 18-methyl oxidase activities, and thus catalyzes all the steps necessary to convert DOC to aldosterone. P450c11 and P450c18 are encoded by two tandemly duplicated genes, CYP11B1 and CYP11B2, respectively, located on the long arm of chromosome 8.

Although adrenal steroid cells can synthesize cholesterol de novo from acetate, 80% of the cholesterol precursor for adrenal cortex hormone formation is provided by the circulating plasma lipoproteins. Specific cell surface receptors for low-density lipoprotein (LDL) bind the circulating LDL and internalize it by receptor-mediated endocytosis. It is then stored in vesicles or hydrolyzed to liberate free cholesterol to be used for steroid hormone synthesis.

Adrenocorticotropic hormone (ACTH) increases the number of LDL receptors on the cell surface, stimulates cholesterol esterase activity, and inhibits cholesterol ester synthetase, thus increasing the amount of free intracellular cholesterol. The transport of free cholesterol through the cytosol to the inner mitochondrial membrane, where P450 scc is located, appears to be affected by a number of proteins whose role is not clearly defined. StAR (steroidogenic acute regulatory protein), a 30-kd protein, is rapidly induced by cyclic adenosine monophosphate and functions to enhance cholesterol delivery to the inner mitochondrial membrane.

Hypothalamic-Pituitary-Adrenal Axis. Glucocorticoid secretion is regulated by ACTH produced in the pituitary. ACTH is released in secretory bursts of varying amplitude throughout the day and night. The normal diurnal rhythm of cortisol secretion is caused by the varying amplitudes of ACTH pulses. Pulses of ACTH and cortisol occur every 30 to 120 minutes, are highest at about the time of waking, are low in late afternoon and evening, and reach their lowest point an hour or two after sleep begins. ACTH acts by binding to its cell surface receptor on adrenal cortical cells, leading to adenylate cyclase activation and increased cyclic adenosine monophosphate concentration, by which most ACTH action is mediated. The acute effect of ACTH is stimulation of cholesterol release, transport of cholesterol into mitochondria, binding of cholesterol to P450 scc, and release of newly synthesized pregnenolone. The long-term effect of ACTH stimulation is to increase the uptake of LDL cholesterol and the formation of the steroidogenic enzymes. Corticotropin-releasing hormone (CRH), synthesized by neurons of the parvicellular division of the hypothalamic paraventricular nucleus, is the most important stimulator of ACTH secretion. Arginine vasopression (AVP) augments CRH action. Neural stimuli from the brain cause the release of CRH and AVP (see Chapter 566). AVP and CRH are secreted in the hypophyseal–portal circulation in a pulsatile manner. This pulsatile secretion appears to be responsible for the pulsatile (ultradian) release of ACTH. Although not definitively established, it has been suggested that the circadian rhythm of corticotropin release is induced by the circadian rhythmic hypothalamic secretion, regulated by the suprachiasmatic nucleus with input from other areas of the brain. Cortisol exerts a negative feedback effect on the synthesis and secretion of ACTH, CRH, and AVP. ACTH inhibits its own secretion, a feedback effect mediated at the level of the hypothalamus. Thus the secretion of cortisol is a result of the interaction of the hypothalamus, pituitary, and adrenal glands, and other neural stimuli.

Renin-Angiotensin-Aldosterone System. The major regulators of aldosterone secretion are the renin-angiotensin system and potassium. Renin produced by the juxtaglomerular apparatus of the kidney reacts with renin substrate, an α_2-globulin produced by the liver, to yield the inactive decapeptide angiotensin I. Angiotensin-converting enzyme in the lungs and other tissues rapidly cleaves angiotensin I to the biologically active octapeptide angiotensin II. Cleavage of angiotensin II produces the heptapeptide angiotensin III. Angiotensin II and III are potent stimulators of aldosterone secretion; angiotensin II is a more potent vasopressor agent. The angiotensins act on the adrenal through their cell surface receptors. Sodium deprivation, decreased blood volume, decreased arterial pressure, and decreased renal blood flow result in activation of the juxtaglomerular apparatus, increased renin secretion, and stimulation of aldosterone secretion. Potassium directly increases aldosterone secretion by the adrenal cortex. Both angiotensin and potassium act by intracellular signal transduction mechanisms to stimulate conversion of cholesterol to pregnenolone. ACTH normally plays a minor role in the regulation of aldosterone secretion.

ADRENAL STEROIDS

Glucocorticoids. Glucocorticoids have a 21-carbon structure and are produced by the zona fasciculata; they are also referred to as 17-hydroxycorticosteroids or simply as corticosteroids. Cortisol, also known as compound F or hydrocortisone, is the principal glucocorticoid produced in humans.

Glucocorticoids affect the metabolism of most tissues. They enter the cell by passive diffusion and attach to specific intracellular receptor proteins, which then bind to the cell nucleus to regulate RNA and protein synthesis. Steroid hormone receptors may be found in the cystolic and nuclear fractions of a tissue homogenate. The receptors for glucocorticoids (type II) and mineralocorticoids (type I) are similar. The type I receptor binds mineralocorticoids and glucocorticoids. It appears that the mineralocorticoid-responsive tissues (e.g., kidney) exclude the glucocorticoid from the type I receptor by converting cortisol to cortisone, catalyzed by the enzyme 11β-hydroxysteroid dehydrogenase. Specificity depends on prereceptor enzyme activity. In many tissues, glucocorticoids have a catabolic effect, resulting in increased degradation of protein; primarily affected are muscles, skin, and connective, adipose, and lymphoid tissues. Glucocorticoids are anabolic in the liver, where they stimulate a number of enzymes, increase protein and glycogen content, and enhance the liver's capacity for gluconeogenesis.

Patients with cortisol excess (e.g., Cushing syndrome) have increased glucose production, and those with deficiency of cortisol (Addison's disease) have decreased gluconeogenesis, with hypoglycemia. The effects of insulin and androgens are antagonistic to those of glucocorticoids. Glucocorticoids also have important effects on the immune and nervous systems.

The 17-hydroxycorticosteroids are excreted in urine; cortisol itself is also excreted in urine in amounts of less than 1% of the adrenal production. Levels of cortisol and of its precursors and metabolites can be measured by radioimmunoassay and by high-performance liquid chromatography in biologic fluids and tumor tissues.

Many synthetic analogs of cortisone and hydrocortisone and available. Prednisone and prednisolone are derivatives with an additional double bond in ring A. They are four times as potent in anti-inflammatory and carbohydrate activity as the natural steroids but have less effect on salt and water retention. Halogenated derivatives have different effects; 9α-fluorohydrocortisone has approximately 15 times more anti-inflammatory activity than does hydrocortisone but is more than 125 times as active in salt and water retention. Betamethasone and dexamethasone are approximately 25 times as potent as cortisol and have little effect on the retention of water and electrolytes. These analogs are usually used in pharmacologic doses for their anti-inflammatory or immunosuppressive properties.

Mineralocorticoids. Aldosterone, the most potent mineralocorticoid produced in humans, is the 18-aldehyde of corticosterone and is produced in the zona glomerulosa. The principal action of aldosterone is the maintenance of electrolyte equilibrium, which, in turn, contributes to the stabilization of blood volume and blood pressure. Aldosterone controls sodium reabsorption (and hence water reabsorption) in the distal tubule of the kidney.

Androgens. Androgens are produced by the zona fasciculata and zona reticularis. They are capable of increasing retention of nitrogen, potassium, phosphorus, and sulfate. They promote growth and have androgenic effects, which are most conspicuous when adrenal hyperplasia or adrenal tumors induce precocious growth and development of male secondary sex characteristics. The adrenal androgens seem to be partly responsible for the development of axillary and pubic hair.

Dehydroepiandrosterone sulfate (DHEAS) is the most abundant adrenal androgen in the circulation. It is derived from adrenal secretion or from peripheral sulfation of DHEA secreted by the adrenal gland. DHEAS levels are low during childhood but begin to rise before the other hormonal changes of puberty take place in a process called adrenarche (see Chapter 571). The zona reticularis is probably the major source of these adrenarcheal changes. Aside from a relationship of these hormones to the growth of axillary and pubic hair, their function remains unknown; they do not appear to initiate puberty. Levels are low in patients with Addison disease and in those with adrenal insufficiency secondary to ACTH deficiency. For many years, a separate adrenal cortical androgen-stimulating hormone has been proposed but has not been identified. Marked elevations of DHEAS occur in patients with virilizing adrenal cortical tumors, lesser elevations occur in patients with congenital adrenal hyperplasia, and modest elevations occur in children with isolated precocious adrenarche.

ADRENAL MEDULLA. The principal hormones of the adrenal medulla are the physiologically active catecholamines: dopamine, norepinephrine, and epinephrine. The sequence of their biosynthetic reactions is shown in Figure 590–1. Catecholamine synthesis also occurs in the brain, in sympathetic nerve endings, and in chromaffin tissue outside the adrenal medulla. Metabolites of catecholamines are excreted in the urine. The principal ones are 3-methoxy-4-hydroxy-mandelic acid (VMA), metanephrine, and normetanephrine. Measurement of metanephrines and catecholamines is used to detect functioning tumors of the adrenal medulla.

The proportions of epinephrine and norepinephrine in the adrenal gland vary with age. In early fetal stages, there is practically no epinephrine, and at birth norepinephrine is predominant. In adults, norepinephrine makes up only 10–30% of the pressor amines in the medulla. Both epinephrine and norepinephrine raise the mean arterial blood pressure, norepinephrine without changing the cardiac output. By increasing peripheral vascular resistance, norepinephrine increases systolic and diastolic blood pressures with only a slight reduction in the pulse rate. Epinephrine increases the pulse rate and, by decreasing the peripheral vascular resistance, decreases the diastolic pressure. The hyperglycemic and calorigenic effects of norepinephrine are much less pronounced than are those of epinephrine.

FETAL DEVELOPMENT. The primordium of the fetal adrenal gland can be recognized at 3–4 wk of gestation just cephalad to the developing mesonephros. At 5–6 wk, the gonadal ridge develops into the steroidogenic cells of the gonads and adrenal cortex; the adrenal and gonadal cells separate, the adrenal cells migrate retroperitoneally, and the gonadal cells migrate caudally. At 6–8 wk of gestation, the gland rapidly enlarges, the cells of the inner cortex differentiate to form the fetal zone, and the outer subcapsular rim remains as the definitive zone. The primordium of the adrenal cortex is invaded at this time by sympathetic neural elements that differentiate into the chromaffin cells capable of synthesizing and storing catecholamines. The methyl transferase, which converts norepinephrine to epinephrine, develops later. By the end of the 8th wk of gestation, the encapsulated adrenal gland is associated with the upper pole of the kidney. By 9–12 wk of gestation, the cells of the fetal zone are capable of active steroidogenesis. In the fetus of 2 mo, the adrenals are larger than the kidneys, but from the 4th mo, the kidneys grow rapidly, becoming twice as large as the adrenals by the end of the 6th mo. In the full-term infant, the adrenal gland is one-third the size of the kidney, and the combined weight of both glands is 7–9 g. At birth, the inner fetal cortex makes up about 80% of the gland and the outer "true" cortex, 20%. Within a few days the fetal cortex begins to involute, undergoing a 50% reduction by 1 mo of age. By 1 yr, the adrenal glands each weigh less than 1 g. Adrenal growth thereafter results in adult adrenal glands reaching a combined weight of 8 g. The zonae fasciculata and glomerulosa are fully differentiated by about 3 yr of age. The zona reticularis may not be fully differentiated until puberty.

Early fetal adrenal growth appears to be independent of ACTH, but, at least from midterm until term, ACTH is essential for adrenal growth and maturation. At which stage of fetal development feedback regulation of ACTH by cortisol is established has not been fully defined, but clinical experience suggests that normal pituitary-adrenal feedback relationships are operative in the first trimester.

Two transcription factors are critical for the development of the adrenal glands: steroidogenic factor-1 (SF-1) and DAX-1 (*d*osage-sensitive sex reversal, *a*drenal hypoplasia congenita, *X*-chromosome). Disruption of SF-1, encoded on chromosome 9q33, results in adrenal and gonadal agenesis, absence of pituitary gonadotopes, and an underdeveloped ventral medial hypothalamus. Mutations in the DAX-1 gene, encoded on Xp21, result in congenital adrenal hypoplasia and hypogonadotropic hypogonadism.

Fetoplacental Unit. LDL cholesterol synthesized by the fetal liver is the major substrate for steroid synthesis in the fetal adrenal gland. This gland has low 3β-HSD activity and high steroid sulfokinase activity. The placenta is low in 17-hydroxylase activity and high in steroid sulfatase activity. The major steroid products of the fetal adrenal gland are DHEA and DHEAS and, by 16α-hydroxylation in the liver, 16α-OH DHEAS. The placenta uses DHEA and DHEAS as substrates for estrone and estradiol and 16α-OH DHEAS as a substrate for estriol. Placental estrone and estradiol are derived equally from fetal and maternal precursors; estriol is almost exclusively produced from the fetal precursor. In addition to providing substrate for the placental synthesis of estrogens, the fetal adrenal gland also produces significant amounts of cortisol, much of which is converted to cortisone by the enzyme 11β-HSD. As term approaches, fetal cortisol concentration increases as a result of increased cortisol secretion and decreased conversion of cortisol to cortisone. Low levels of aldosterone are found in midgestation, but aldosterone secretory capacity appears to increase near term.

Bamberger CM, Schulte HM, Chrousos GP: Molecular determinants of glucocorticoid receptor function and tissue sensitivity to glucocorticoids. Endocr Rev 17:245, 1996.

Carlstedt-Duke J: Glucocorticoid receptors: Structure and function. Clin Cour 16:12, 1997.

Funder JW: Mineralocorticoids, glucocorticoids, receptors and response elements. Science 259:1132, 1993.

Gomez MT, Malazowski S, Winterer J, et al: Urinary free cortisol values in children and adolescents. J Pediatr 118:256, 1991.

Guiochon-Mantel A, Milgrom E: Cytoplasmic-nuclear trafficking of steroid hormone receptors. Trends Endocrinol Metab 4:322, 1993.

Harshfield GA, Alpert BS, Pullam DA: Renin-angiotensin aldosterone system in healthy subjects ten to eighteen years. J Pediatr 122:563, 1993.

Lin D, Sugawara T, Straun JF, et al: Role of steroidogenic acute regulatory protein in adrenal and gonadal steroidogenesis. Science 267:1828, 1995.

Linder BL, Esteban NV, Yergey AL, et al: Cortisol production rate in childhood and adolesence. J Pediatr 117:892, 1990.

Miller WL: Molecular biology of steroid hormone synthesis. Endocr Rev 9:295, 1988.

Stewart PM, Edwards CRW: Specificity of the mineralocorticoid receptor. Crucial role of 11β-hydroxysteroid dehydrogenase. Trends Endocrinol Metab 1:225, 1990.

CHAPTER 585
Adrenocortical Insufficiency

Deficient production of cortisol or aldosterone may result from a wide variety of congenital or acquired lesions of the hypothalamus, pituitary gland, or adrenal cortex (Table 585–1). Depending on the pathologic lesions, symptoms may be severe or mild, appear abruptly or insidiously, begin in infancy or later, and be permanent or temporary.

ETIOLOGY

Corticotropin Deficiency. Congenital hypoplasia or aplasia of the pituitary is almost always associated with secondary hypoplasia of the adrenals as well as with other hormonal deficiencies. These congenital defects are usually associated with abnormalities of the skull and brain such as anencephaly and holoprosencephaly. Such infants have a considerable residuum of pituitary function, and the hypoplasia of the pituitary is probably secondary to a hypothalamic deficiency of corticotropin-releasing hormone (CRH). The adrenals are characteristically small with normal architecture, a well-defined permanent zone, and a reduced fetal zone. The disorder is usually sporadic, although a few cases of autosomal recessive inheritance have occurred. Isolated deficiency of corticotropin (adrenocorticotropic hormone [ACTH]) has been reported, including in several sets of siblings. Idiopathic hypopituitarism and destructive lesions in the area of the pituitary, such as craniopharyngioma, are the most common causes of ACTH deficiency; the defect is in the hypothalamus in many patients. Isolated deficiency of CRH has been documented in an Arabic kindred as an autosomal recessive trait. In rare instances, autoimmune hypophysitis has been the cause of ACTH deficiency.

Adrenal Hypoplasia Congenita. The onset of hypoadrenalism usually begins in the neonatal period but may be delayed until 10 yr of age; marked intrafamilial variability of onset has been reported in several instances. Increasing pigmentation, salt-losing symptoms, and low levels of all adrenal steroids are the presenting manifestations. Histologic examination of the hypoplastic adrenal cortex reveals disorganization and cytomegaly, findings not present in the adrenals from ACTH-deficient patients. The disorder affects primarily boys and has been shown to be caused by a mutation of the DAX-1 gene, a new member of the nuclear hormone receptor family, located on Xp21. It has been known for more than 20 years that boys with adrenal hypoplasia congenita (AHC) do not undergo puberty owing to hypogonadotropic hypogonadism (HHG), but the reason for this association has been unclear. It is now known that both AHC and HHG are caused by the same

TABLE 585–1 Etiologic Classification of Adrenocortical Hypofunction

Corticotropin-releasing hormone deficiency
- Isolated deficiency
- Multiple deficiencies
  - Congenital defects (e.g., anencephaly, septo-optic dysplasia)
  - Destructive lesions (e.g., tumor)
  - Idiopathic (e.g., idiopathic hypopituitarism)

Corticotropin deficiency
- Isolated
- Autosomal recessive
- Multiple deficiencies
  - Pituitary hypoplasia or aplasia
  - Destructive lesions (e.g., craniopharyngioma)
  - Autoimmune hypophysitis

Primary adrenal hypoplasia or aplasia
- X-linked
  - With Duchenne muscular dystrophy and glycerol kinase deficiency (Xp21 deletion)
  - With hypogonadotropic hypogonadism (DAX-1 mutation)

Familial glucocorticoid deficiency
- Corticotropin-receptor mutations
- With alacrima, achalasia, and neurologic disorders (triple A syndrome)

Defects of steroid biosynthesis
- Lipoid adrenal hyperplasia (StAR mutation)
- 3β-Hydroxysteroid dehydrogenase deficiency
  - Classic
    - Salt loser
    - Non–salt loser
  - Mild or nonclassic
- 21-Hydroxylase (P450C21) deficiency
  - Classic
    - Salt loser
    - Non–salt loser
  - Nonclassic or mild
- Isolated aldosterone (P450C18) deficiency

Pseudohypoaldosteronism (aldosterone unresponsiveness)

Adrenoleukodystrophy (peroxisomal membrane protein defect)
- Isolated adrenal involvement
- With neurologic involvement

Acid lipase deficiency
- Wolman disease, fatal neonatal form

Destructive lesions of adrenal cortex
- Granulomatous lesions (e.g., tuberculosis)

Autoimmune adrenalitis (idiopathic Addison disease)
- Isolated
- Associated with hypoparathyroidism or mucocutaneous candidiasis (type I autoimmune polyglandular syndrome), or both
- Associated with autoimmune thyroid disease and insulin-dependent diabetes (type II autoimmune polyglandular syndrome)

Neonatal hemorrhage

Acute infection (Waterhouse-Friderichsen syndrome)

Mitochondrial disorders

Acquired immunodeficiency syndrome

Iatrogenic
- Abrupt cessation of exogenous corticosteroids or corticotropin
- Removal of functioning adrenal tumor
- Adrenalectomy for Cushing disease
- Drugs
  - Aminoglutethimide
  - Mitotane (o, p-DDD)
  - Metyrapone
  - Ketoconazole

Fetal adrenal suppression–maternal hypercortisolism
- Endogenous
- Therapeutic

mutated DAX-1 gene. Cryptorchidism, often noted in these boys, is probably an early manifestation of HHG.

AHC also occurs as part of a contiguous gene deletion syndrome together with Duchenne muscular dystrophy, glycerol kinase deficiency, or mental retardation, or a combination of these conditions. Prenatal diagnosis of AHC is possible.

Familial Glucocorticoid Deficiency. This form of chronic adrenal insufficiency is characterized by isolated deficiency of glucocorticoids, elevated levels of ACTH, and normal aldosterone production. The salt-losing manifestations present in most other forms of adrenal insufficiency do not occur; instead, patients present primarily with hypoglycemia, seizures, and increased pigmentation during the 1st decade of life. The disorder affects both sexes equally and is inherited in an autosomal recessive manner. Histologically, there is marked adrenocortical atrophy with relative sparing of the zona glomerulosa. A number of mutations in the gene for the ACTH receptor have been described in some (approximately 40%) but not all these patients.

Another syndrome of ACTH resistance occurs in association with achalasia of the gastric cardia and alacrima (triple A or Allgrove syndrome). These patients also have autonomic dysfunction, mental retardation, and other neurologic disorders that in some instances are progressive. This syndrome is also inherited in an autosomal recessive fashion, but thus far no mutations of the ACTH receptor have been detected.

Inborn Defects of Steroidogenesis. The most common causes of adrenocortical insufficiency in infancy are the salt-losing forms of congenital adrenal hyperplasia (see Chapter 586.1). Approximately 75% of infants with the 21-hydroxylase defect, all infants with lipoid adrenal hyperplasia, and most infants with a deficiency of 3β-hydroxysteroid dehydrogenase manifest salt-losing symptoms in the newborn period. In these defects, there is a deficiency in the synthesis of both cortisol and aldosterone, and there are elevated levels of steroids that are formed prior to the enzymatic defect.

Isolated Deficiency of Aldosterone. This is a rare autosomal recessive disorder in which conversion of corticosterone (B) to aldosterone is impaired. There are two forms of the disorder, corticosterone methyloxidase I (CMO I) deficiency, in which conversion of B to 18-hydroxycorticosterone (18OHB) is defective, and corticosterone methyloxidase II (CMO II) deficiency, in which there is impaired conversion of 18OHB to aldosterone. The disorders can be differentiated biochemically. In CMO I deficiency, the ratio of B to 18OHB is increased, and 18OHB is usually decreased. In CMO II deficiency, there is overproduction of 18OHB and a markedly increased 18OHB:aldosterone ratio. CMO I and CMO II deficiencies result from mutations in the aldosterone synthase gene (CYP11B2). Aldosterone synthase (P450c18) mediates the three final steps in the synthesis of aldosterone. A number of mutations in the CYP11B2 gene have been described.

Infants with aldosterone synthase deficiency may have severe electrolyte abnormalities with hyponatremia, hyperkalemia, and acidosis, with hyperreninemia and hypoaldosteronism in the newborn period. Alternatively, they may present later with failure to thrive and poor growth. Adults often are asymptomatic.

Treatment consists of administration of enough salt or 9α-fluorohydrocortisone (0.05–0.3 mg daily), or both, to return plasma renin levels to normal. With increasing age, the salt-losing manifestations improve, and it may appear that therapy can be discontinued; however, levels of plasma renin rise and growth decelerates, indicating chronic salt depletion. The biosynthetic defect persists and can be demonstrated in adults. This autosomal recessive defect is especially frequent in Iranian Jews. Carrier detection and prenatal diagnosis are possible.

Pseudohypoaldosteronism. This salt-losing syndrome also presents in the neonate; however, levels of aldosterone in plasma and urine are markedly elevated. Levels of plasma renin activity are also elevated, indicating hyperactivity of the renin-angiotensin system. The defect is target organ unresponsiveness to aldosterone. Administration of mineralocorticoids is ineffective; the condition is treated by supplementary dietary salt, which may be discontinued as the condition improves. The syndrome appears to be heterogeneous. In some patients, salt loss involves only the renal tubules, whereas in others the salivary and sweat glands may be involved, and occasionally the colonic mucosal cells may be affected. In the more than 70 reported patients, autosomal dominant and autosomal recessive forms have been identified. In the patients studied to date, the gene for the aldosterone receptor was normal, and linkage analysis studies appear to exclude mutations in the human mineralocorticoid receptor as the cause of the autosomal recessive form of the disorder. Mutations in the α subunit coded for on chromosome 12, and the β and δ subunits coded for on chromosome 16, of the epithelial sodium channel have been demonstrated in patients with autosomal recessive pseudohypoaldosteronism type 1.

Addison Disease. Destruction of the adrenal cortex during childhood is one of the more common causes of adrenal insufficiency. Tuberculosis, a common cause of adrenal destruction in the past, is much less prevalent. The most common cause is autoimmune destruction of the glands. The glands may be so small that they are not visible at autopsy, and only remnants of tissue are found in microscopic sections. Usually the medulla is not destroyed, and there is marked lymphocytic infiltration in the area of the former cortex. In advanced disease, all adrenal cortical function is lost, but early in the clinical course, isolated cortisol deficiency or isolated aldosterone deficiency may occur. Most patients have antiadrenal cytoplasmic antibodies in their plasma. Many affected patients have immunoglobulins that block the growth and steroidogenic effects of ACTH. Autoantibodies to 21-hydroxylase have been found in most patients with Addison's disease and have been demonstrated to inhibit 21-hydroxylase activity. How the various antibodies act in concert with cell-mediated processes to cause disease is under investigation.

Addison disease often occurs as a component of two syndromes, each consisting of a constellation of autoimmune disorders. *Type I autoimmune polyendocrinopathy* is also known as *autoimmune polyendocrinopathy-candidiasis-ectodermal dystrophy.* Chronic mucocutaneous candidiasis is most often the first manifestation, followed by hypoparathyroidism and then by Addison disease. Other closely associated autoimmune disorders include gonadal failure, alopecia, vitiligo, keratopathy, enamel hypoplasia, nail dystrophy, intestinal malabsorption, and chronic active hepatitis. Hypothyroidism and type I diabetes mellitus occur in fewer than 10% of affected patients. The disorder is inherited as an autosomal recessive disorder, and the gene has been assigned to chromosome 21q22.3. Some components of the syndrome continue to develop as late as the 5th decade. The presence of antiadrenal antibodies and steroidal cell antibodies in these patients usually indicates a high likelihood of Addison disease developing or, in females, ovarian failure. Autoantibodies to 21-OH, 17α-OH, and P450 scc enzymes have been reported in patients with type I autoimmune polyendocrinopathy.

Type II autoimmune polyendocrinopathy consists of Addison disease associated with autoimmune thyroid disease or insulin-dependent diabetes. Gonadal failure, vitiligo, alopecia, and chronic atrophic gastritis, with or without pernicious anemia, may occur. HLA-D3 and HLA-D4 predominate in these patients. The disorder is more common in females and most often occurs in many generations of the same family. Antiadrenal antibodies, steroid cell antibodies, and antibodies to 21-OH, 17α-OH, and P450 scc enzymes are also found in these patients.

Adrenoleukodystrophy. In this disorder, adrenocortical deficiency is associated with demyelination in the central nervous system (see Chapters 83.2 and 608.3). High levels of very long chain fatty acids are found in tissues and body fluids, resulting from impairment of their degradation in the peroxisomes. Neonatal adrenoleukodystrophy (ALD) is a rare autosomal recessive disorder. Infants present with neurologic deterioration and have or acquire evidence of adrenocortical dysfunction. Most patients have severe mental retardation and die before 5 yr of age.

The more frequent form of ALD is an X-linked disorder with various presentations. The most common clinical picture is of a degenerative neurologic disorder appearing in childhood or adolescence and progressing to severe dementia and deterioration of vision, hearing, speech, and gait, with death occurring within a few years. A milder form of X-linked ALD is adrenomyeloneuropathy that begins in later adolescence or early adulthood. Many patients have evidence of adrenal insufficiency at the time of neurologic presentation, but Addison disease may precede the neurologic symptoms by many years. X-linked ALD may present as isolated Addison disease. The therapeutic approaches of uncertain efficacy include diets restricted in very long chain fatty acids and bone marrow transplantation. The gene for ALD has been identified, and mutations and deletions of this gene have been described. The gene codes for a peroxisomal membrane protein whose function is unknown. More than 100 mutations in the gene have been identified in ALD. The variability of clinical presentation, even within families, is not understood and may be due to modifier genes or other unknown factors.

Hemorrhage Into Adrenal Glands. This may occur in the neonatal period as a consequence of difficult labor or asphyxia. The hemorrhage may be sufficiently extensive to result in death from exsanguination or hypoadrenalism. Scrotal hematoma may be the presenting sign. Often, the hemorrhage is asymptomatic initially and is identified by later calcification of the adrenal gland. On rare occasions, gradual impairment in function resulting from progressive fibrosis or cystic changes may culminate in adrenocortical insufficiency in infancy or childhood. Fetal adrenal hemorrhage has also been reported. Another cause of hemorrhage into the adrenal glands is the Waterhouse-Friderichsen syndrome, the characteristic state of shock resulting from meningococcemia (see Chapter 173). Adrenal hemorrhage may also occur as a result of child abuse.

Mitochondrial Disorders. Cases in which adrenal insufficiency may have been due to a mitochondrial disorder have been reported. In one case, there was a defect in oxidative phosphorylation characterized by chronic lactic acidosis, lipid storage myopathy, bilateral cataracts, and primary adrenal insufficiency. Mitochondrial deletions or duplications were ruled out and the molecular defect was not identified. In another case, a large-scale mitochondrial DNA deletion was identified in a girl with adrenal insufficiency, sensorineural hearing loss, short stature, and hypoparathyroidism. Future studies in patients with unexplained adrenal insufficiency may provide evidence of mitochondrial disorders.

Abrupt Cessation of Administration of Corticotropin or a Corticosteroid. This condition may result in adrenal insufficiency, manifesting glucocorticoid but not mineralocorticoid deficiency. Symptoms are most likely to occur if these substances have been given in large doses for a long time to patients who are subsequently subjected to stressful situations such as severe infections or surgical procedures.

Drugs. Ketoconazole, an antifungal drug, can cause adrenal insufficiency by inhibiting adrenal enzymes. Rifampicin and anticonvulsive drugs such as phenytoin and phenobarbital reduce the effectiveness and bioavailability of corticosteroid replacement therapy by inducing steroid-metabolizing enzymes in the liver. Mitotane (o,p′ DDD), used in the treatment of adrenal carcinoma, is suppressive and cytotoxic to the adrenal gland and may also alter extra-adrenal cortisol metabolism. Signs of adrenal insufficiency occur in a substantial percentage of patients treated with mitotane.

Acquired Immunodeficiency Syndrome. Frank adrenal insufficiency is rare in patients infected with the human immunodeficiency virus. However, a variety of subclinical abnormalities in the hypothalamic-pituitary-adrenal axis have been reported. In addition, drugs used in the treatment of acquired immunodeficiency syndrome may affect adrenal hormone homeostasis. Adrenal function should be evaluated in patients presenting with symptoms of adrenal insufficiency, such as hypoglycemia, hyponatremia, or hyperkalemia.

CLINICAL MANIFESTATIONS. The age at onset of symptoms and the clinical manifestations depend on the specific causative factor involved. In patients with adrenal hypoplasia, defects in steroidogenesis, or pseudohypoaldosteronism, symptoms and signs begin shortly after birth and are characteristic of salt loss. Failure to thrive, vomiting, lethargy, anorexia, and dehydration occur; circulatory collapse may be fatal.

In older children with Addison disease, the onset is usually more gradual and is characterized by muscular weakness, lassitude, anorexia, loss of weight, general wasting, and low blood pressure. Abdominal pain may simulate an acute abdominal process, and there may be an intense craving for salt. If the condition is not recognized and treated, adrenal crisis may supervene. The patient suddenly becomes cyanotic, the skin is cold, and the pulse is weak and rapid. The blood pressure falls, and respirations are rapid and labored. In the absence of immediate and intensive therapy, the course is rapidly fatal. In patients with inadequately treated chronic adrenal insufficiency, crises may be precipitated by infection, trauma, excessive fatigue, or drugs such as morphine, barbiturates, laxatives, thyroid hormone, or insulin.

Increased pigmentation of the skin should always alert the clinician to the possibility of adrenocortical insufficiency. This manifestation occurs in conditions in which there is a deficiency of cortisol as well as excessive secretion of ACTH, as in primary adrenal hypoplasia, familial glucocorticoid deficiency, adrenoleukodystrophy, and Addison disease. Pigmentation may be first apparent on the face and hands and is most intense around the genitals, umbilicus, axillae, nipples, and joints. Scars and freckles may be especially pigmented. Areas of depigmentation (vitiligo) may be interspersed with dark areas. The exposed areas of the skin are the most intensely affected, and failure of a suntan to disappear may be the first clue to the condition. In the buccal mucosa, the pigmentation is usually bluish brown.

The presenting manifestations may be those of hypoglycemia, particularly in the neonate with congenital adrenal hypoplasia. Patients with adrenocortical insufficiency are deficient in gluconeogenic substrates; the hypoglycemia may therefore be associated with ketosis and confused with ketotic hypoglycemia (see Chapter 88).

In young children with familial glucocorticoid deficiency, salt-losing manifestations do not occur, and the symptoms consist primarily of increased pigmentation and hypoglycemia. Symptoms may begin shortly after birth and almost always appear by 5 yr of age. Many affected children have received other treatment for seizures before the hypoglycemic cause was recognized.

Pigmentation does not occur in patients with a deficiency of ACTH. Hypoglycemia is the usual presenting manifestation. Hyperkalemia does not occur because of preserved aldosterone secretion, but hyponatremia may be present.

In conditions known to have a genetic basis, it is important to evaluate fully the adrenocortical function of siblings.

LABORATORY FINDINGS. When salt-losing manifestations are present, the levels of sodium and chloride in the serum are usually low and that of potassium elevated, with increased plasma renin activity. Urinary excretion of sodium and chloride is increased, urinary potassium is decreased, and there is acidosis. The nonprotein nitrogen level in plasma is elevated if dehydration is present. Hypoglycemia may be striking or may become manifested only after prolonged fasting. The blood eosinophils may be increased in number. When hemorrhage, adrenal cysts, or tuberculosis has been a causative factor, roentgenograms of the abdomen may reveal calcifications in the area of the adrenals. Ultrasonography, computed tomography, and magnetic resonance imaging may also be helpful. A small and narrow roentgenographic shadow of the heart reflects hypovolemia. Electrocardiographic changes reflect potassium levels.

The most definitive test is measurement of the plasma or serum levels of cortisol before and after administration of ACTH; resting levels are low, and no increase occurs after administration of ACTH. Occasionally, normal resting levels that do not increase after administration of ACTH indicate an absence of adrenocortical reserve. A low initial level followed by a significant response to ACTH may indicate adrenal insufficiency secondary to endogenous insufficiency of ACTH. Traditionally, the ACTH stimulation has been performed by giving 0.250 mg of ACTH 1–24 by rapid intravenous infusion. Recently a low-dose test (0.5–1 μg ACTH 1–24/1.73 m^2) has been proposed to be a more sensitive test of pituitary-adrenal reserve. Levels of ACTH are elevated in disorders of primary cortisol deficiency and are low when the adrenal insufficiency is secondary to a hypothalamic or pituitary disorder. Testing with CRH may be helpful in localizing the defect.

Measurement of plasma or serum levels of cortisol precursors is necessary in infants in whom congenital adrenal hyperplasia is suspected. Aldosterone levels are usually low in patients with salt-losing congenital adrenal hyperplasia, adrenal hypoplasia, or Addison disease. Measurement of aldosterone is necessary in infants suspected of having isolated defects of aldosterone synthesis (in whom it is low) and in those suspected of having pseudohypoaldosteronism (in whom it is usually elevated). In patients with familial glucocorticoid deficiency, aldosterone levels are normal and rise appropriately with salt deprivation. Levels of plasma renin activity (PRA) are elevated in patients with subtle or overt salt-wasting due to aldosterone deficiency or aldosterone resistance. The PRA:aldosterone ratio is increased in disorders of aldosterone synthesis even when aldosterone levels can be maintained in the normal range.

TREATMENT. Treatment for acute adrenal insufficiency or for adrenal crisis must be immediate and vigorous. If the cause of adrenal insufficiency has not been established, a blood sample should be obtained before therapy for determination of levels of ACTH, cortisol, aldosterone, PRA, 17α-hydroxyprogesterone, and adrenal androgens. Intravenous administration of 5% glucose in 0.9% saline solution should be given to correct the hypoglycemia and the sodium loss. Concomitantly, a water-soluble form of hydrocortisone, such as hydrocortisone hemisuccinate, should be given intravenously. High levels are achieved instantaneously, and large doses can be used safely. As much as 25 mg for infants and 75 mg for older children should be given intravenously at 6-hr intervals for the first 24 hr. These doses may be reduced during the next 24 hr if progress is satisfactory. Adequate fluid and sodium repletion is achieved by the intravenous saline administration, aided by the mineralocorticoid effect of high doses of hydrocortisone. After the first 48 hr, if oral intake is satisfactory, intravenous fluids may be discontinued and the corticosteroid given orally as cortisol in doses of 5–20 mg at 8-hr intervals. Further reduction can then be accomplished until maintenance levels and a stable clinical situation are achieved. Florinef (9α-fluorohydrocortisone), a mineralocorticoid, can be added orally at 0.05–0.3 mg daily.

After the acute manifestations are under control, most patients require chronic replacement therapy for their aldosterone and cortisol deficiencies. The cortisol may be given orally in daily doses of 5–10 mg/24 hr in two or three divided doses for infants and 10–20 mg/24 hr in two or three divided doses for children and adolescents. Fluorhydrocortisone is continued orally in doses of 0.05–0.3 mg daily. Measurements of plasma renin activity are useful in monitoring the adequacy of mineralocorticoid replacement. During situations of stress, such as periods of infection or operative procedures, the dose of hydrocortisone should be increased.

Overdosage with fluorhydrocortisone results in hypertension and may lead to cardiac enlargement and edema because of excessive retention of sodium chloride and water; excessive loss of potassium may produce weakness or paralysis.

Patients with primary ACTH deficiency or with familial glucocorticoid deficiency do not require a salt-retaining hormone because their ability to secrete aldosterone is intact. Patients with isolated defects in aldosterone synthesis do not require cortisol; a salt-retaining hormone may be required, but in milder forms the addition of salt to the diet is adequate to maintain homeostasis. In patients with pseudohypoaldosteronism, administration of salt-retaining hormones does not correct the urinary sodium loss; therapy must consist of supplementation with sodium chloride. In newborn infants with adrenal hemorrhage, vitamins K and C and transfusions with whole blood may be indicated.

Patients with apparent Addison disease must be differentiated from those with familial glucocorticoid deficiency and adrenoleukodystrophy (see Chapter 83.2); absence of salt-losing manifestations and presence of alacrima suggest familial glucocorticoid deficiency, and elevated levels of very long chain fatty acids are diagnostic of adrenoleukodystrophy. The presence of antiadrenal antibodies suggests an autoimmune pathogenesis; these patients must be closely observed for the development of other associated autoimmune disorders. Infants with congenital adrenal hypoplasia should undergo chromosomal analysis to search for a mutation or deletion of the Xp21 region; elevated levels of creatine phosphokinase indicate an association with Duchenne muscular dystrophy, and elevated levels of triglycerides suggest glycerol kinase deficiency. DNA probe analysis for the gene defect, glycerol kinase enzyme assay, and negative dystrophin staining of muscle tissue permit confirmation of the components of this complex.

Aaltonen J, Bjorses P, Sandkuijl L, et al: An autosomal locus causing autoimmune disease: Autoimmune polyglandular disease type I assigned to chromosome 21. Nat Genet 8:83, 1994.

Ahonen P, Myllarniemi S, Spila I, et al: Clinical variation of autoimmune polyendocrinopathy-candidiasis-ectodermal dystrophy (APECED) in a series of 68 patients. N Engl J Med 322:1824, 1990.

Arai K, Tsigos C, Suzuki Y, et al: No apparent mineralocorticoid receptor defect in a series of sporadic cases of pseudohypoalderosteronism. J Clin Endocrinol Metab 80:814, 1995.

Armanini D, Kuhnle U, Strasser T, et al: Aldosterone-receptor deficiency in pseudohypoaldosteronism. N Engl J Med 313:1178, 1985.

Aubourg P, Chaussain J-L: Adrenoleukodystrophy presenting as Addison's's disease in children and adults. Trends Endocrinol Metab 2:49, 1991.

Baker JR Jr: Autoimmune endocrine disease. JAMA 278:1931, 1997.

Balducci R, Municchi G, Toscano V, et al: Complex glycerol kinase deficiency: An unusual cause of salt-wasting in males. Clin Endocrinol 42:437, 1995.

Betterle C, Volpato M, Smith BR, et al: II. Adrenal cortex and steroid 21-hydroxylase autoantibodies in children with organ-specific autoimmune diseases: Markers of high progression to clinical Addison's disease. J Clin Endocrinol Metab 82:939, 1997.

Burris TP, Weiwen G, McCabe ERB: The gene responsible for adrenal hypoplasia congenita, DAX-1, encodes a nuclear hormone receptor that defines a new class within the superfamily. Recent Prog Horm Res 51:241, 1996.

Carey DE: Isolated ACTH deficiency in childhood: Lack of response to corticotropin-releasing hormone alone and in combination with arginine vasopressin. J Pediatr 107:925, 1985.

Chang SS, Grunder S, Hanukoglu A, et al: Mutations in subunits of the epithelial sodium channel cause salt wasting with hyperkalaemic acidosis, pseudohypoaldosteronism type 1. Nat Genet 12:248, 1996.

Chung E, Hanukoglu A, Rees M, et al: Exclusion of the locus for autosomal recessive pseudohypoaldosteronism type I from the mineralocorticoid receptor gene region on human chromosome 4q by linkage analysis. J Clin Endocrinol Metab 80:3341, 1995.

Clark AJL, Weber A: Molecular insights into inherited ACTH resistance syndromes. Trends Endocrinol Metab 5:209, 1994.

Corvol P, Funder J: The enigma of pseudohypoaldosteronism. J Clin Endocrinol Metab 79:25, 1994.
Dickstein G, Arad E, Shechner C: Low-dose ACTH stimulation test. Endocrinologist 7:285, 1997.
Dodd A, Rowland SA, Hawkes SLJ, et al: Mutations in the aadrenoleukodystrophy gene. Hum Mutat 9:500, 1997.
Freda PU, Papadopoulos AD, Wardlaw SL, et al: Spectrum of adrenal dysfunction in patients with acquired immunodeficiency syndrome. Trends Endocrinol Metab 8:173, 1997.
Grant DB, Dunger DB, Smith I, Hyland K: Familial glucocorticoid deficiency with achalasia of the cardia associated with mixed neuropathy, long-tract degeneration and mild dementia. Eur J Pediatr 151:85, 1992.
Hoffbauer LC, Heufelder AE: Endocrine implications of human immunodeficiency virus infection. Medicine 75:262, 1996.
Kletter GB, Gorski JL, Kelch RP: Congenital adrenal hypoplasia and isolated gonadotropin deficiency. Trends Endocrinol Metab 2:123, 1991.
Kuhnle U, Nielsen MD, Tietze U, et al: Pseudohypoaldosteronism in eight families: Different forms of inheritance are evidence for various genetic defects. J Clin Endocrinol Metab 70:638, 1990.
Kruse K, Sippell WG, Schnakenburg KV: Hypogonadism in congenital adrenal hypoplasia: Evidence for a hypothalamic origin. J Clin Endocrinol Metab 58:12, 1984.
Lee PDK, Patterson BD, Hintz RL, et al: Biochemical diagnosis and management of corticosterone methyloxidase type II deficiency. J Clin Endocrinol Metab 62:225, 1986.
Miele V, Galluzo M, Patti G, et al: Scrotal hematoma due to neonatal adrenal hemorrhage: The value of ultrasonography in avoiding unnecessary surgery. Pediatr Radiol 27:672, 1997.
Moser HW: Adrenoleukodystrophy: Phenotype, genetics, pathogenesis and therapy. Brain 120:1485, 1997.
Moser HW, Moser AE, Singh J, et al: Adrenoleukodystrophy: Survey of 303 cases: Biochemistry, diagnosis, and therapy. Ann Neurol 16:628, 1984.
Muscatelli F, Strom TM, Walker AP, et al: Mutations in the DAX-1 gene give risk to both X-linked adrenal hypoplasia congenita and hypogonadotropic hypogonadism. Nature 372:672, 1994.
Nicolino M, Ferlin T, Forest M, et al: Identification of a large-scale mitochondrial deoxyribonucleic acid deletion in endocrinopathies and deafness: Report of two unrelated cases with diabetes mellitus and adrenal insufficiency, respectively. J Clin Endocrinol Metab 82:3063, 1997.
Nimkin K, Teeger S, Wallach MT, et al: Adrenal hemorrhage in abused children: Imaging and postmortem findings. AJR 162:661, 1994.
North K, Korson MS, Krawiecki N, et al: Oxidative phosphorylation defect associates with primary adrenal insufficiency. J Pediatr 128:688, 1996.
Oelkers W: Adrenal insufficiency. N Engl J Med 335:1206, 1996.
Peter M, Fawaz L, Drop SLS, et al: Hereditary defect in biosynthesis of aldosterone: Aldosterone synthase deficiency 1964–1997. J Clin Endocrinol Metab 82:3525, 1997.
Peter M, Partsch C-J, Sippell WG: Multisteroid analysis in children with terminal aldosterone biosynthesis defects. J Clin Endocrinol Metab 80:1622, 1995.
Prader A, Zachmann M, Illig R: Luteinizing hormone deficiency in hereditary congenital adrenal hypoplasia. J Pediatr 86:421, 1975.
Rahman S, Ohlsson A, Fong KW, Glanc P: Fetal adrenal hemorrhage in a diamniotic, dichorionic twin: Case report and review of controversies in diagnosis and management. J Ultrasound Med 16:297, 1997.
Song Y-H, Connor EL, Muir A, et al: Autoantibody epitope mapping of the 21-hydroxylase antigen in autoimmune Addison's disease. J Clin Endocrinol Metab 78:1108, 1994.
Strautnieks SS, Thompson RJ, Gardiner RM, Chung E: A novel splice-site mutation in the δ subunit of the epithelial sodium channel gene in three pseudohypoaldosteronism type 1 families. Nat Genet 13:248, 1996.
Weintraub N, Sprecher E, Josefsberg Z, et al: Standard and low-dose short adrenocorticotropin test compared with insulin-induced hypoglycemia for assessment of the hypothalamic-pituitary-adrenal axis in children with idiopathic multiple pituitary hormone deficiencies. J Clin Endocrinol Metab 83:88, 1998.
White PC: Disorders of aldosterone biosynthesis and action. N Engl J Med 331:250, 1994.
Winqvist O, Söderbergh A, Kämpe O: The autoimmune basis of adrenocortical destruction in Addison's disease. Mol Med Today 2:282, 1996.
Yao-Hua S, Connor EL, Muir A, et al: Autoantibody epitope mapping of the 21-hydroxylase antigen in autoimmune Addison's disease. J Clin Endocrinol Metab 78:1108, 1994.

CHAPTER 586
Adrenal Disorders and Genital Abnormalities

Disorders of adrenal hormone synthesis with signs of adrenal hyper- or hypofunction, or both, and associated genital abnormalities occur in congenital adrenal hyperplasia and virilizing adrenal tumors (Table 586–1).

586.1 Congenital Adrenal Hyperplasia

PATHOGENESIS. Congenital adrenal hyperplasia (CAH) is a family of autosomal recessive disorders of adrenal steroidogenesis leading to a deficiency of cortisol. The deficiency of cortisol results in increased secretion of corticotropin, which, in turn, leads to adrenocortical hyperplasia and overproduction of intermediary metabolites. Severe and mild forms of these disorders, caused by variations in the severity of the genetic mutations, have been reported. Depending on the enzymatic step that is deficient, there may be signs, symptoms, and laboratory findings of mineralocorticoid deficiency or excess; incomplete virilization or premature androgenization of the affected male; and virilization or sexual infantilism in the affected female (Fig. 586–1, Table 586–2).

Deficiency of 21-hydroxylase accounts for 90% of affected patients. This P450 enzyme (P450c21) hydroxylates progesterone and 17-hydroxyprogesterone (17-OHP) to yield 11-deoxycorticosterone (DOC) and 11-deoxycortisol (see Fig. 586–1). There

TABLE 586–1 Etiologic Classification of Adrenocortical Hyperfunction

- Excess androgen
  - Congenital adrenal hyperplasia
    - 21-Hydroxylase (P450c21) deficiency
    - 11β-Hydroxylase (p450c11) deficiency
    - 3β-Hydroxysteroid dehydrogenase defect
  - Tumor
    - Carcinoma
    - Adenoma
- Excess cortisol (Cushing syndrome)
  - Bilateral adrenal hyperplasia
    - Hypersecretion of corticotropin (Cushing disease)
    - Ectopic secretion of corticotropin
    - Exogenous corticotropin
  - Adrenocortical nodular dysplasia
  - Pigmented nodular adrenocortical disease (Carney complex)
  - Tumor
    - Carcinoma
    - Adenoma
- Excess mineralocorticoid (hypertensive hypokalemic syndrome)
  - Primary hyperaldosteronism
    - Aldosterone-secreting adenoma
    - Bilateral micronodular adrenocortical hyperplasia
    - Glucocorticoid-suppressible aldosteronism
    - Tumor
      - Adenoma
      - Carcinoma
  - Desoxycorticosterone excess
    - Congenital adrenal hyperplasia
      - 11β-Hydroxylase (P450c11)
      - 17α-Hydroxylase (P450c17)
    - Tumor (carcinoma)
  - Apparent mineralocorticoid excess
    - 11β-Hydroxysteroid dehydrogenase deficiency
- Excess estrogen (adrenal feminization syndrome)
  - Carcinoma
  - Adenoma
- Mixed hypercorticism–tumor

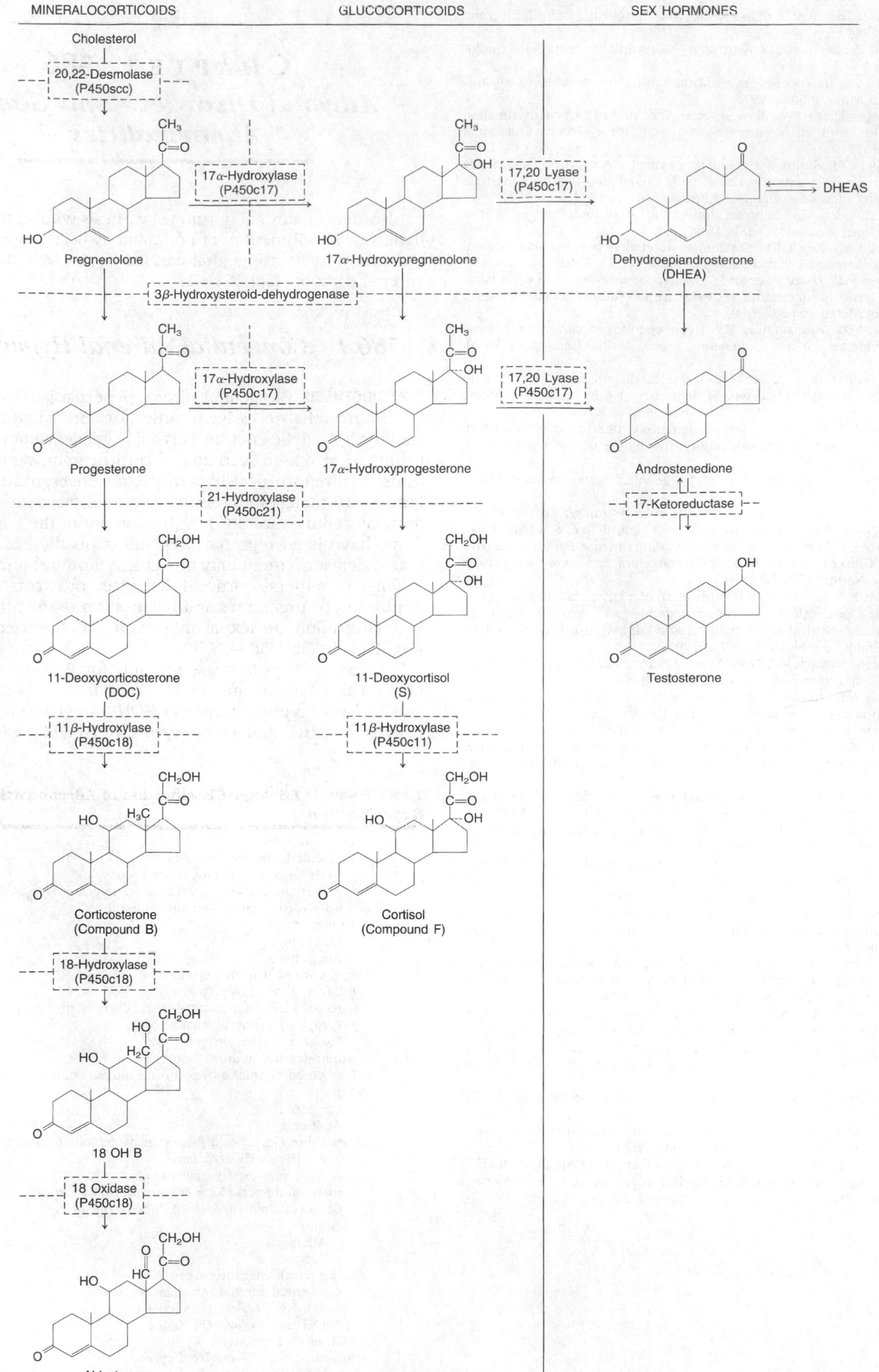

Figure 586–1 The synthesis of cortisol and aldosterone is shown to the left of the vertical line. To the right of the solid vertical line are the predominant adrenal androgens that lead to conversion to testosterone. Note that a single polypeptide, P450c17, catalyzes both 17-hydroxylase and 17,20-lyase activities. Likewise, polypeptide P450c18 mediates the last three steps in aldosterone synthesis.

TABLE 586–2 Diagnosis and Treatment of Congenital Adrenal Hyperplasia

Disorder	Signs and Symptoms	Laboratory Findings	Therapeutic Measures
Lipoid congenital adrenal hyperplasia	Salt-wasting crisis Male pseudohermaphroditism	Low levels of all steroid hormones, with decreased or absent response to ACTH Decreased or absent response to hCG in male pseudohermaphroditism ↑ ACTH ↑ PRA	Glucocorticoid and mineralocorticoid administration Sodium chloride supplementation Gonadectomy of male pseudohermaphrodite Sex hormone replacement consonent with sex of rearing
3β-HSD deficiency	Classic form: Salt-wasting crisis Male and female pseudohermaphroditism Precocious pubarche Disordered puberty	↑ ↑ Baseline and ACTH-stimulated Δ5 steroids (pregnenolone, 17-OH pregnenolone, DHEA, and their urinary metabolites) ↑ ACTH ↑ PRA Suppression of elevated adrenal steroids after glucocorticoid administration	Glucocorticoid and mineralocorticoid administration Sodium chloride supplementation Surgical correction of genitals and sex hormone replacement as necessary consonent with sex of rearing
3β-HSD deficiency	Nonclassic form: Precocious pubarche, disordered puberty, menstrual irregularity, hirsutism, acne, infertility	↑ Baseline and ACTH-stimulated Δ5 steroids (pregnenolone, 17-OH pregnenolone, DHEA, and their urinary metabolites) ↑ Δ5/Δ4 serum and urinary steroids Suppression of elevated adrenal steroids after glucocorticoid administration	Glucocorticoid administration
21-OH deficiency	Classic form: Salt-wasting crisis Female pseudohermaphroditism Postnatal virilization	↑ ↑ Baseline and ACTH-stimulated 17-OH progesterone and pregnanetriol ↑ ↑ Serum androgens and urinary metabolites ↑ ACTH ↑ PRA Suppression of elevated adrenal steroids after glucocorticoid administration	Glucocorticoid and mineralocorticoid replacement Sodium chloride supplementation Vaginoplasty and clitoral recession in female pseudohermaphroditism
21-OH deficiency	Nonclassic form: Precocious pubarche, disordered puberty, menstrual irregularity, hirsutism, acne, infertility	↑ Baseline and ACTH-stimulated 17-OH progesterone and pregnanetriol ↑ Serum androgens and urinary metabolites Suppression of elevated adrenal steroids after glucocorticoid administration	Glucorticoid administration
11β-Hydroxylase deficiency	Classic form: Female pseudohermaphroditism Postnatal virilization in males and females Hypertension	↑ ↑ Baseline and ACTH-stimulated compound S and DOC and their urinary metabolites ↑ ↑ Serum androgens and their urinary metabolites ↑ ACTH ↓ PRA Hypokalemia Suppression of elevated steroids after glucocorticoid administration	Glucocorticoid administration Vaginoplasty and clitoral recession in female pseudohermaphroditism
11β-Hydroxylase deficiency	Nonclassic form: Precocious pubarche, disordered puberty, menstrual irregularity, hirsutism, acne, infertility	↑ Baseline and ACTH-stimulated compound S and DOC and their urinary metabolites ↑ Serum androgens and their urinary metabolites Suppression of elevated steroids after glucocorticoid administration	Glucocorticoid administration
17α-OH/17,20-lyase deficiency	Male pseudohermaphroditism Sexual infantilism Hypertension	↑ ↑ DOC, 18-OH DOC, corticosterone, 18-hydroxycorticosterone Low 17-α-hydroxylated steroids and poor response to ACTH Poor response to hCG in male pseudohermaphroditism ↓ PRA ↑ ACTH Hypokalemia Suppression of elevated adrenal steroids after glucocorticoid administration	Glucocorticoid administration Surgical correction of genitals and sex hormone replacement in male pseudohermaphroditism consonant with sex of rearing Sex hormone replacement in female

ACTH = adrenocorticotropic hormone (corticotropin); hCG = human chorionic gonadotropin; PRA = plasma renin activity; DOC = deoxycorticosterone
(Adapted from Miller WL, Levine LS: Molecular and clinical advances in congenital adrenal hyperplasia. J Pediatr 111:1, 1987.)

are two steroid 21-hydroxylase genes (CYP21A and CYP21B), which alternate in tandem with two genes for the fourth component of complement (C4A and C4B) on the short arm of chromosome 6 between the HLA-B and HLA-DR loci. Several other genes are located in this cluster. The CYP21B gene is the active gene; the CYP21A gene is 98% homologous to the CYP21B gene but is a pseudogene. The majority of mutations causing 21-hydroxylase deficiency are recombinations between the active CYP21B gene and the adjacent CYP21A pseudogene, resulting in microconversions (which appear as point mutations) and accounting for approximately 75% of cases of 21-hydroxylase deficiency. Large gene conversions and gene deletions also occur. Most patients are compound heterozygotes having a different mutation on each allele. The severity of disease expression is determined by the activity of the less severely affected of the two alleles. The classic disorder occurs in salt-wasting and simple virilizing forms. The salt-wasting form is found in patients with gene deletions or gene conversions, or both. However, point mutations are also found in patients with salt-wasting forms. A milder nonclassic form also occurs, with a high frequency reported among Ashkenazi Jews.

Newborn screening programs, using capillary heel blood on filter paper disks, have been developed to detect 21-hydroxylase deficiency. Data on more than 7.5 million neonates screened indicate that the disorder occurs in 1/21,000 newborns in Japan, 1/10,000–16,000 newborns in Europe and North America, and 1/300 newborns in Yupik Eskimos of

Alaska. About 75% of affected infants have the salt-losing, virilizing form, and 25% have the simple virilizing form of the disorder. The nonclassic form is not reliably detected by newborn screening.

Deficiency of 11β-hydroxylase accounts for 5–8% of cases of adrenal hyperplasia. This P450c11 enzyme mediates the 11-hydroxylation of 11-deoxycortisol to cortisol. Deficiency of 11β-hydroxylase occurs relatively frequently in Israeli Jews of North African origin; in this ethnic group, a point mutation (Arg448 to His) has been found in the CYP11B1 gene encoded on chromosome 8q22. Other mutations have also been identified. This disorder presents in a classic, severe form and a nonclassic, milder form.

Hypertension is a distinctive clinical feature of the disorder but is absent in the first few years of life. Virilization occurs as in 21-hydroxylase deficiency. The serum characteristically contains large amounts of both 11-deoxycortisol and DOC. The elevated levels of DOC are thought to cause the hypertension and prevent symptoms of salt loss. Prenatal diagnosis is possible by measuring levels of 11-deoxycortisol in amniotic fluid or in maternal urine during pregnancy and by DNA probes in chorionic villus cells or amniocytes.

Deficiency of 3β-hydroxysteroid dehydrogenase (3β-HSD) occurs in fewer than 5% of patients with adrenal hyperplasia. This enzyme is required for conversion of Δ5 steroids (pregnenolone, 17-hydroxypregnenolone, dehydroepiandrosterone [DHEA]) to Δ4 steroids (progesterone, 17-hydroxyprogesterone, and androstenedione). Deficiency of the enzyme results in decreased synthesis of cortisol, aldosterone, and androstenedione but increased secretion of DHEA (see Fig. 586–1). The 3β-HSD enzyme expressed in the adrenal cortex and gonad is encoded by the HSD3B2 gene located on chromosome 1. A number of mutations in the HSD3B2 gene have been described in patients with 3β-HSD deficiency. Severe and milder forms of the disorder occur. In the classic form of the disease, there is often a salt-wasting crisis in the newborn; boys are incompletely virilized and have hypospadias, and girls are mildly virilized. Postnatally, continued excessive DHEA secretion results in early development of pubic or axillary hair, or both. In the nonclassic, milder form, salt wasting and ambiguity of the genitals do not occur, and affected individuals may present with precocious pubarche or with hirsutism, menstrual disorders, and infertility. Polycystic ovaries may be found on examination. The hallmark of this disorder is the marked elevation of the Δ5 steroids preceding the enzymatic block. Patients may also have elevated levels of 17-hydroxyprogesterone because of the extra-adrenal 3β-HSD activity that occurs in peripheral tissues; these patients may be mistaken for patients with 21-hydroxylase deficiency. The ratio of 17-hydroxyprogesterone:17-hydroxypregnenolone is markedly elevated, however, in 3β-HSD deficiency, in contrast to the decreased ratio in 21-hydroxylase deficiency. The demonstration of normal HSD3B2 in children and adults diagnosed as having mild nonclassic 3β-HSD deficiency by hormonal criteria has resulted in the recommendation that new hormonal criteria for the diagnosis of nonclassic 3β-HSD deficiency be established.

Lipoid adrenal hyperplasia is a rare disorder, reported in fewer than 100 patients, the majority of whom are Japanese. In this disorder there is marked accumulation of cholesterol and lipids in the adrenal cortex and gonads, leading to severe impairment of steroidogenesis as well as cortisol, aldosterone, and sex hormone deficiencies. As a consequence, genetic males are phenotypically female and females exhibit no genital abnormality. Salt-losing manifestations are usual, and many infants have died in early infancy. Because adrenal steroid levels are low in this form of adrenal hyperplasia, affected infants are apt to be confused with those with adrenal hypoplasia. Imaging studies of the adrenal gland demonstrating massive adrenal enlargement in the newborn would help establish the diagnosis of lipoid CAH. Mutational analysis of the P450 scc genes in patients with lipoid adrenal hyperplasia demonstrated normal P450 scc genes and cDNA sequences. Studies have now established that congenital lipoid adrenal hyperplasia is due to a mutation in the gene for steroidogenic acute regulatory protein (StAR), a mitochondrial protein that promotes the movement of cholesterol from the outer to the inner mitochondrial membrane. Lipoid adrenal hyperplasia is thus the only form of CAH that is not caused by a defective steroidogenic enzyme. The elucidation of the molecular abnormality has made possible the understanding of the clinical variability in this disorder—the varied age at onset of symptoms of aldosterone and cortisol deficiency, the severe impairment of testicular function, and the less severe impairment in ovarian function, with spontaneous puberty reported in 46,XX patients.

17-Hydroxylase deficiency has been described in more than 125 patients. A single polypeptide, P45017, catalyzes two distinct reactions: 17-hydroxylation of pregnenolone and progesterone, and the 17,20-lyase reaction mediating conversion of 17-hydroxypregnenolone and 17-hydroxyprogesterone to DHEA and Δ4-androstenedione, respectively, the C-19 steroid precursors of testosterone and estrogen (see Fig. 586–1). The enzyme is encoded on chromosome 10, and the gene is expressed in both the adrenal cortex and the gonads. The deficiency results in overproduction of DOC, leading to hypertension, hypokalemia, and suppression of renin and aldosterone. In addition, there is an inability to synthesize normal amounts of sex hormones. Affected males are incompletely virilized and present as phenotypic females or with sexual ambiguity (male pseudohermaphroditism). Affected females usually present with failure of sexual development at the expected time of puberty. Patients have been described with complete or partial combined 17-hydroxylase/17,20-lyase deficiencies or with deficiencies of only one of these activities. The gene has been cloned. Approximately 20 different genetic lesions have been reported. This defect must be considered in the differential diagnosis of male pseudohermaphroditism or of testicular feminization. 17-Hydroxylase deficiency in females must be considered in the differential diagnosis of primary hypogonadism (see Chapter 596).

CLINICAL MANIFESTATIONS. The clinical manifestations in CAH depend on which hormones are deficient and which are overproduced (see Table 586–2). Most patients with CAH have the defect in 21-hydroxylation. In newborn screening programs, about 75% of infants in whom this condition is detected are salt losers, whereas without screening only about 50% of clinically diagnosed infants are salt losers, presumably because of undiagnosed neonatal deaths.

Non-Salt–Losing Congenital Adrenal Hyperplasia. In the male with 21-hydroxylase deficiency, the main clinical manifestations are those of premature isosexual development. The infant usually appears normal at birth, but signs of sexual and somatic precocity may appear within the first 6 mo of life or develop more gradually, becoming evident at 4–5 yr of age or later. Enlargement of the penis, scrotum, and prostate; appearance of pubic hair; and development of acne and a deep voice are noted. Muscles are well developed, and bone age is advanced for chronological age. Although affected patients are tall in early childhood, premature closure of the epiphyses causes growth to stop relatively early, and adult stature is stunted (Fig. 586–2).

The testes are prepubertal in size so that they appear relatively small in contrast to the enlarged penis. Occasionally, ectopic adrenocortical cells in the testes of patients with adrenal hyperplasia become hyperplastic just as the adrenal glands do, producing enlargement of the testes (see Chapter 594). Mental development is usually normal, but the abnormal physical development may result in behavioral problems.

In the female, CAH due to 21-hydroxylase deficiency results

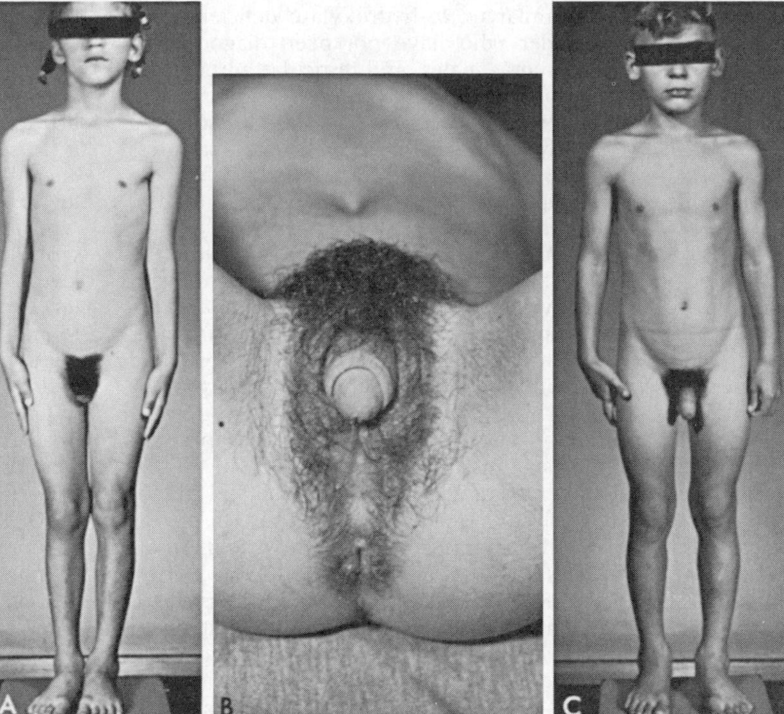

Figure 586–2 *A,* A 6-yr-old girl with congenital virilizing adrenal hyperplasia. The height age was 8.5 yr; the bone age was 13 yr; and urinary 17-ketosteroids were 50 mg/24 hr. *B,* Notice the clitoral enlargement and labial fusion. *C,* Five-yr-old brother of girl in *A* was not considered to be abnormal by the parents. The height age was 8 yr; the bone age was 12.5 yr; and the urinary 17-ketosteroids were 36 mg/24 hr.

in female pseudohermaphroditism (Fig. 586–3). Because the disorder of steroidogenesis begins early in fetal life, there is almost always evidence of some degree of masculinization at birth. It is manifested by enlargement of the clitoris and varying degrees of labial fusion. The vagina usually has a common opening with the urethra (urogenital sinus). The clitoris may be so enlarged that it resembles a penis, and, because the urethra opens below this organ, a mistaken diagnosis of hypospadias and cryptorchidism is sometimes made. Females with a complete male phenotype have been reported; there is complete labial fusion, a phallic urethra, and an external meatus at the tip of the penis. The severity of the virilization is in general greater in salt-losing CAH than in non–salt-losing CAH. The internal genital organs are those of a normal female.

After birth, the masculinization progresses. Pubic and axillary hair develop prematurely, acne appears, and the voice assumes a masculine quality. Affected girls are tall for their age, and ossification is advanced; they show good muscular development and, in general, have the body build of a boy (see Fig. 586–2). Although the internal genitals are female, breast development and menstruation do not occur unless the excessive production of androgens is suppressed by adequate treatment.

A number of virilized female pseudohermaphrodites whose condition was not diagnosed until later childhood or adult life have been erroneously reared as males. These patients have behaved in every way as males, including having sexual intercourse and satisfactory (albeit infertile) marriages.

With the *11β-hydroxylase defect,* salt-losing manifestations do not occur. Most patients are hypertensive, but several have been normotensive or have had intermittent hypertension only. Several prepubertal children with this defect presented with gynecomastia. Virilization occurs in all patients and is as severe or more severe than that occurring with the 21-

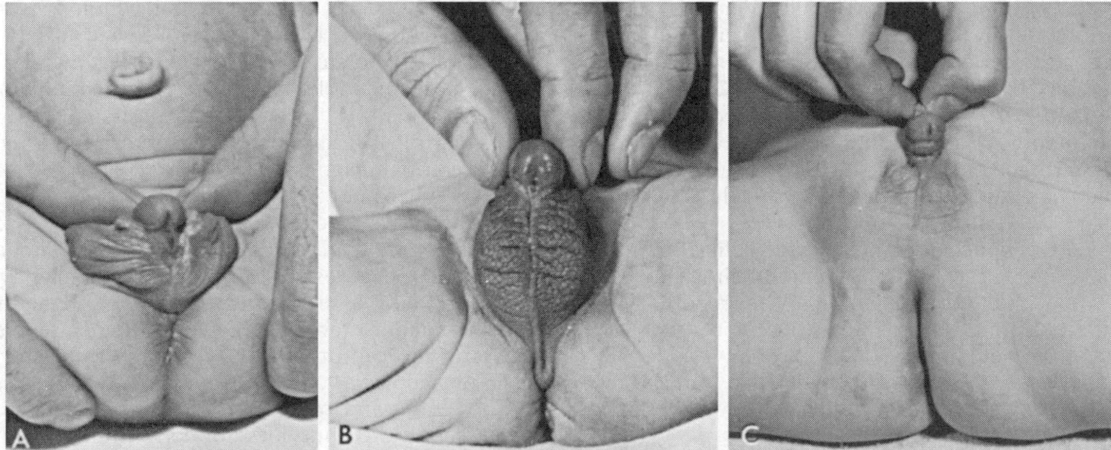

Figure 586–3 Three female pseudohemaphrodites with untreated congenital adrenal hyperplasia. All were erroneously assigned male sex at birth, and each had normal female sex-chromosome complement. Infants *A* and *B* were salt losers and were diagnosed in early infancy. Infant *C* was referred at 1 yr of age because of bilateral cryptorchidism. Notice the completely penile urethra; such complete degrees of masculinization in females with adrenal hyperplasia are rare; most of these infants are salt losers.

hydroxylase defect. Similar to 21-hydroxylase deficiency, females with this disorder who have not been diagnosed in infancy have been reared as males, and testicular adrenal rest tumors have been reported in affected males.

Salt wasting also does not occur in 17-hydroxylase/17,20 lyase deficiency, and hypertension and hypokalemia are present secondary to excessive DOC secretion. Males have varying degrees of sexual ambiguity and females have sexual infantilism as a result of the gonadal steroid deficiency.

Salt-Losing Congenital Adrenal Hyperplasia. In patients with the salt-losing variants, symptoms begin shortly after birth with failure to regain birthweight, progressive weight loss, and dehydration. Vomiting is prominent, with anorexia. Disturbances in cardiac rate and rhythm may occur, with cyanosis and dyspnea. Without treatment, collapse and death may occur within a few weeks.

In females, virilization of the external genitals in an infant with the these manifestations directs attention to the correct diagnosis. In the male, the genitals appear normal, and clinical manifestations are likely to be confused with those of pyloric stenosis, intestinal obstruction, heart disease, cow's milk intolerance, or other causes of failure to thrive.

Familial homogeneity of the defect is usually observed for the salt-losing and non–salt-losing forms. Under conditions of stress or sodium deprivation, salt losing may be provoked in compensated patients.

Patients with the 3β-HSD defect are usually salt losers but are less virilized. In females, virilization is usually mild, with slight to moderate clitoral enlargement. It may be mild enough to escape detection. In the male, varying degrees of hypospadias may occur, with or without bifid scrotum or cryptorchidism. During adolescence and adulthood, hirsutism, irregular menses, and polycystic ovarian disease occur in females. Males manifest variable degrees of hypogonadism, although appropriate male secondary sexual development may occur. A persistent defect of testicular 3β-HSD is demonstrated, however, by the high Δ5:Δ4 steroid ratio in testicular effluent. Patients with lipoid adrenal hyperplasia are salt losers, and their phenotype is female in both 46,XX and 46,XY individuals. 46,XY phenotypic females have testicular failure with hypergonadotropic hypogonadism. Females, however, may undergo feminization at puberty with menstrual bleeding; they too, however, progress to hypergonadotropic hypogonadism.

Nonclassic 21-Hydroxylase Deficiency. In this attenuated form, affected females have normal genitals at birth. Males and females may present with precocious pubarche and early development of pubic and axillary hair. Hirsutism, acne, menstrual disorders, and infertility may develop later in life. Some females and males are completely asymptomatic. The disorder results from a combination of a severe CYP21B deficiency gene (found in the classic form of the disease) and a mild CYP21B (nonclassic) deficiency gene, or a combination of two mild CYP21B deficiency genes. About 70% of alleles are associated with HLA-B14, DR1. A mutation in codon 281 occurs in all or nearly all patients who carry the HLA-B14, DR1 haplotype. Other mutations have been reported in patients with the nonclassic disorder.

Nonclassic 3β-HSD deficiency and 11-OH deficiency have also been reported with a clinical presentation similar to that of nonclassic 21-hydroxylase deficiency. The reported frequency of, and hormonal criteria for, these disorders vary widely and remain to be definitively established.

It is estimated that 0.1% of North American whites have nonclassic 21-hydroxylase deficiency, with the highest frequency occurring in Ashkenazi Jews.

LABORATORY FINDINGS (see Table 586–2). Patients with salt-losing disease may have low serum concentrations of sodium and chloride and elevated levels of potassium and blood urea nitrogen. Plasma levels of renin are elevated and serum aldosterone is inappropriately low for the renin level. In classic 21-hydroxylase deficiency, serum levels of 17-OHP are markedly elevated and are especially helpful in diagnosis, but they are normally high during the first 2–3 days of life and may range as high as levels found in affected patients; by the 3rd day, however, levels in normal infants fall, and those in affected infants rise to clearly diagnostic levels. Sick, unaffected infants and prematures may have elevated levels of 17-OHP. Blood levels of cortisol are usually low in patients with the salt-losing type of disease. They are often normal in those with the simple virilizing type but inappropriately low in relation to the ACTH level. A large part of the virilization is caused by increased levels of testosterone; the excess 17-OHP is partially diverted to androstenedione, which is converted to testosterone in the periphery (see Fig. 586–1). Levels of urinary 17-ketosteroids and pregnanetriol are elevated; 24-hr urine collections are difficult and often unnecessary, however, because radioimmunoassay permits serum or plasma measurement of levels of the steroids involved in all forms of CAH.

In the late-onset variant of CAH, basal circulating levels of 17-OHP are not as high as in the classic form and may even be normal. There is, however, a diagnostic rise in the level 60 min following an intravenous bolus of 0.25 mg of ACTH (1–24).

In patients with the 11-hydroxylase defect, plasma levels of DOC and 11-deoxycortisol (compound S) are elevated, and plasma renin activity and aldosterone are suppressed.

The 3β-HSD defect is characterized by markedly elevated Δ5 steroids such as 17-hydroxypregnenolone. 17-OHP levels are also elevated, however, and the condition may be confused with the 21-hydroxylase defect. It is necessary to determine the ratios of Δ5 to Δ4 steroids in plasma or urine for definitive diagnosis. Plasma renin activity is elevated in the salt-wasting form.

Adrenal and gonadal steroid hormone levels are low in lipoid adrenal hyperplasia, with a decreased or absent response to stimulation (ACTH, human chorionic gonadotropin). Plasma renin levels are increased.

Cortisol and sex steroids are low in 17-hydroxylase/17,20-lyase deficiency with a poor response to stimulation, whereas deoxycorticosterone and corticosterone levels are elevated. Plasma renin activity and aldosterone are suppressed.

Affected females with CAH have an XX karyotype; males have a normal XY chromosome constitution. Injection of contrast medium into the urogenital sinus of female pseudohermaphrodites usually demonstrates a vagina and uterus. Ultrasonography is also helpful in demonstrating the presence of a uterus in female pseudohermaphrodites and its absence in male pseudohermaphrodites.

DIAGNOSIS. CAH in an infant or child should always alert one to the diagnosis in later siblings. The salt-losing form of the disorder must be suspected in any infant who fails to thrive and, especially, in female infants with ambiguous external genitals. When virilization occurs postnatally in males or females, a virilizing adrenocortical tumor must be considered in the differential diagnosis.

An adrenal tumor may be palpable or suggested on pyelography by displacement of the adjacent kidney. Ultrasonography, computed tomography (CT), or magentic resonance imaging (MRI) may be necessary if hormonal studies have ruled out CAH. Urinary 17-ketosteroid excretion and plasma levels of dehydroepiandrosterone sulfate (DHEAS) are elevated with CAH and cortical tumors, but very high values favor the diagnosis of neoplasm. Administration of hydrocortisone quickly reduces these and other elevated steroid levels to normal in patients with CAH but does not do so in those with a virilizing tumor. By inhibiting secretion of corticotropin, corticosteroids reduce the excessive stimulation of the adrenals in patients with CAH, whereas adrenocortical tumors are not subject to pituitary regulation.

In males with CAH, the testes are small for the degree of

virilization, whereas in those with true precocious puberty or with Leydig cell tumors, the testes are enlarged for age. However, testicular enlargement may be present with adrenal rest tumors or when true precocious puberty occurs in CAH.

Females with this condition must be differentiated from those with other causes of ambiguous external genitalia. Only in this condition are adrenal cortical steroid levels elevated. Males with the 3β-HSD defect may be confused with female pseudohermaphrodites because they lack normal virilization of the external genitals. These male patients are 46,XY and also have elevated adrenal Δ5 steroids.

Detection of the heterozygous carrier of 21-hydroxylase deficiency has been performed by measuring the ratio of 17-OHP to 11-deoxycortisol or cortisol 60 min after an intravenous bolus injection of 0.25 mg of ACTH (1–24) and, in families with an affected individual, by HLA genotyping. Molecular DNA techniques should be used for genetic counseling when available, either alone or in combination with hormonal measurements and HLA genotyping.

Molecular techniques can now be used for genetic counseling for all forms of CAH.

Prenatal Diagnosis and Treatment. Prenatal diagnosis of 21-hydroxylase is possible in the 1st trimester by DNA analysis and HLA genotyping of chorionic villus cells. In the 2nd trimester, the diagnosis can be established by measuring 17-OHP and androstenedione in amniotic fluid as well as by HLA typing and DNA analysis of amniotic fluid cells. Prenatal treatment by maternal dexamethasone administration of more than 50 affected female infants has been reported. In approximately one fourth, the genitals were normal; in one half, there was mild virilization with clitoromegaly or partial labial fusion; and in one fourth, therapy was unsuccessful and the infants had marked genital virilization. Possible reasons for unsuccessful treatment are late onset of treatment, inadequate dosage, and variations in maternal and placental metabolism of the administered steroid. Recommendations for pregnancies at risk consist of administration of dexamethasone, a steroid that readily crosses the placenta, by the 5th wk of pregnancy in an amount of 20–25 μg/kg prepregnancy maternal weight in two or three divided doses. First-trimester chorionic villus biopsy is then performed to determine the sex and genotype of the fetus; therapy is continued only if the fetus is an affected female. There is insufficient information to determine whether or to what degree such a regimen will be effective or whether there are long-term risks to the treatment. Maternal side effects have included edema, excessive weight gain, hypertension, glucose intolerance, cushingoid facial features, and severe striae with permanent scarring. Prenatal diagnosis and treatment of 11β-hydroxylase deficiency and prenatal diagnosis of lipoid CAH have also been reported. DNA analysis of chorionic villus cells can be used for the prenatal diagnosis of all forms of CAH.

TREATMENT. Administration of glucocorticoids inhibits excessive production of androgens and prevents progressive virilization. A variety of glucocorticoids and dosage schedules have been used for this purpose. We recommend hydrocortisone (10–20 mg/m²/24 hr) administered orally in two or three divided doses. Infants usually require 2.5–5 mg two to three times daily and children 5–10 mg two to three times daily. Doses must be individualized by monitoring growth and hormonal levels. Patients with disturbances of electrolyte regulation (salt-losing disease) and elevated plasma renin activity require a mineralocorticoid and sodium supplementation in addition to the glucocorticoid. Maintenance therapy with 9α-fluorohydrocortisone (0.05–0.3 mg daily) and sodium chloride, 1–3 g, is usually sufficient to normalize plasma renin activity. Patients with non–salt-losing disease may also manifest elevated plasma renin activity and require a mineralocorticoid.

The protocol for monitoring these patients varies with personal preference. Measurements of urinary levels of 17-ketosteroids and pregnanetriol are no longer necessary. Serum levels of 17-OHP, androstenedione, testosterone, and renin, measured preferably at 8–9 A.M., prior to taking the morning medication, usually provide adequate indices of control. Careful monitoring for signs of cortisol or androgen excess, growth and weight gain, pubertal development, and osseous maturation are important.

The administration of hydrocortisone must be continued indefinitely in all patients with classic forms of CAH. Increased doses are indicated during periods of stress such as infection or surgery for patients with salt-losing and non–salt-losing CAH, including those with the 11-hydroxylase defect, because they all have defective adrenal reserve.

The enlarged clitoris of female infants usually requires surgical correction; a good age for this elective surgery is 6–12 mo. Recession of the clitoris should be performed rather than its removal; the clitoris is freed and repositioned beneath the pubis with preservation of the glans, corporal components, and all neural and vascular elements. Vaginoplasty and correction of the urogenital sinus is usually performed at the time of clitoral surgery. Later revision may be necessary. Parents should be reassured that complete sexual gratification, including orgasm, can be achieved. The menarche occurs at the appropriate age in most girls in whom good control has been achieved. However, it is not exceptional for adolescents past the age of 16 yr not to have begun menstruating; such delay is probably related to suboptimal control.

Children with non–salt-losing disease, particularly males, are frequently not diagnosed until 3–7 yr of age, at which time osseous maturation may be 5 yr or more in advance of chronologic age. Institution of treatment slows growth and osseous maturation to more nearly normal rates in some children; in others, especially if the bone age is 12 yr or more, spontaneous gonadotropin-dependent puberty may occur, therapy with hydrocortisone having suppressed production of adrenal androgens and permitted release of pituitary gonadotropins if the appropriate level of hypothalamic maturation is present. This form of superimposed true precocious puberty may now be effectively treated with a luteinizing hormone–releasing hormone analog.

Males with 21-hydroxylase deficiency, 11β-hydroxylase deficiency, or 3β-HSD deficiency who have had inadequate corticosteroid therapy, may acquire unilateral or bilateral adrenal rest testicular tumors, which may or may not regress with increased steroid dosage. Testicular MRI, ultrasonography, and color flow Doppler examination help define the character and extent of disease. Testis-sparing surgery for steroid-unresponsive tumors has been reported.

Prolonged, inadequate adrenal suppression may also result in adenomatous changes in the adrenal gland, and large adrenal tumors have been reported in untreated adults in the 6th decade of life. Several studies have documented an increased frequency of adrenal incidentalomas in individuals homozygous or heterozygous for 21-hydroxylase deficiency.

Those disorders (lipoid CAH, 17-OHP/17,20-lyase deficiency, 3β-HSD deficiency) associated with gonadal sex hormone deficiency require sex hormone replacement to induce and sustain puberty consonant with the sex of rearing.

Outcome and Controversies. Although glucocorticoid administration has been used for the treatment of CAH for almost 50 yr, the optimal mode of therapy remains elusive. Dosage regimens vary in regard to the glucocorticoid given, number of daily doses, timing of administration of medication, and whether higher doses are given in the morning or evening. Although successful treatment with achievement of normal height, puberty, sexual function, and fertility has been reported, short stature, disordered puberty, menstrual irregularity, infertility, inadequate vaginal reconstruction, and lack of sexual function are frequent. Cross-gender development and gender change from female to male have been reported. It is hoped that more precise methods of monitoring patients and improved surgical techniques will alleviate some of these problems. Because it is recognized that patients with Addison disease are more easily and successfully treated than are CAH patients, adrenalectomy of patients with salt-wasting 21-OH deficiency has been suggested as a possible mode of therapy. This would eliminate the difficult problem of achieving adequate suppression of adrenal androgens while avoiding the problems of glucocorticoid excess and would permit simply providing glucocorticoid and mineralocorticoid replacement therapy as in Addison disease. Adrenalectomy has now been reported in both 21-OH deficiency and 11β-OH deficiency. Long-term follow-up of a large number of patients is necessary to determine the safety and efficacy of this mode of therapy.

Preliminary results of a study using a combination of an antiandrogen (to block androgen effect), an aromatase inhibitor (to block conversion of androgen to estrogen), and a reduced hydrocortisone dose have also been reported. Again, long-term studies are required to determine whether this regimen will result in improvement in final outcome.

The practice of sex assignment of infants with intersex conditions based on expected sexual functioning and fertility in adulthood, with early surgical correction of the external genitals and, if necessary, castration, to conform with the sex assignment has been questioned. Both lay and medical opponents of this practice state that it ignores any prenatal biased gender role predisposition and precludes the patient from having any decision as to his or her own preferred sexual identity and what surgical correction of the genitals should be performed. They say treatment should be aimed primarily at educating patient, family, and others about the medical condition, its treatment, and how to deal with the intersex condition. Surgery should be delayed until the patient decides on what, if any, correction should be performed. Whether this would be a successful practice in our society requires long-term follow-up studies.

586.2 Virilizing Adrenocortical Tumors

Adrenocortical tumors are rare in childhood. They occur in all age groups but most commonly in children less than 10 yr of age. In 2–10% of cases, the tumors are bilateral. Symptoms of endocrine hyperfunction are present in more than 90% of children with adrenal tumors. Virilization is the most common presenting symptom. In males, this produces a clinical picture similar to that of simple virilizing CAH-accelerated growth velocity and muscle development, acne, penile enlargement, and the precocious development of pubic and axillary hair. In females, virilizing tumors of the adrenal gland cause masculinization of a previously normal female with clitoral enlargement, growth acceleration, acne, deepening of the voice, and premature pubic and axillary hair development.

CAH is almost always associated with genital abnormalities at birth. However, virilization in CAH may have its onset during childhood, and an adrenal adenoma is known to have caused intrauterine clitoral enlargement and mild labial fusion. Instances of an adrenal cortical carcinoma arising in the newborn period are known.

In addition to virilization, 20–40% of children with adrenal cortical tumors also have Cushing syndrome—hypertension, obesity, and moon facies. Although virilization may occur alone (50–80%), it is unusual to have Cushing syndrome (glucocorticoid excess) alone in children with adrenal tumors.

Tumors of the adrenal gland (with or without Cushing syndrome) may be associated with **hemihypertrophy**, usually occurring during the first few years of life. These tumors are also associated with the Beckwith-Wiedemann syndrome and other congenital defects, particularly genitourinary tract and central nervous system abnormalities and hamartomatous defects.

Germ line mutations in p53 have been found in patients with isolated adrenal carcinoma as well as in patients with familial clustering of unusual malignancies. Loss of heterozygosity of the 11p15 region and IGF-II gene overexpression have also been reported in sporadic adrenocortical carcinomas.

Urinary 17-ketosteroids and serum levels of DHEA, DHEAS, and androstenedione are usually elevated, often markedly in patients with virilizing adrenal tumors. Serum levels of testosterone are also usually increased as a result of peripheral conversion of androstenedione, but infants with predominantly testosterone-secreting adenomas are known. Many adrenocortical tumors have 11β-hydroxylase deficiency and secrete increased amounts of deoxycorticosterone; these patients are hypertensive, and the tumor is usually malignant. Ultrasonography, MRI, and CT are indicated and can detect masses as small as 1.5 cm. Preoperatively, the presence of metastatic disease should be determined by MRI or CT of the chest, abdomen, and pelvis. Carcinomas are three times more common than adenomas. Differentiation between benign and malignant tumors by histologic criteria often is not possible.

The *treatment* is surgical; a transperitoneal approach is usually recommended. Some of these neoplasms are highly malignant and metastasize widely, but cure with regression of the masculinizing features may follow removal of less malignant encapsulated tumors. Bilateral tumors occur in 2–10% of cases.

A neoplasm of one adrenal gland may produce atrophy of the other, because excessive production of cortisol by the tumor suppresses ACTH stimulation of the normal gland. Consequently, adrenal insufficiency may follow surgical removal of the tumor. This situation can be avoided by giving 10–25 mg of hydrocortisone every 6 hr, starting on the day of operation and continuing for 3–4 days postoperatively. Adequate quantities of water, sodium chloride, and glucose must also be provided. Incomplete resection, tumors weighing more than 100 g, tumors larger than 200 cm^3, age greater than 3.5 yr at diagnosis, symptoms for more than 6 mo, and a marked increase in urinary 17-ketosteroids and 17-hydroxysteroids have been associated with poor prognosis. Postoperatively, patients should be closely monitored biochemically, with frequent determinations of adrenal androgen levels, urinary steroids, and imaging studies. Recurrent symptoms or biochemical abnormalities should prompt a careful search for metastatic disease. Metastases primarily involve liver, lung, and regional lymph nodes. The majority of metastatic recurrences appear within 1 yr of tumor resection. Repeat surgical resection of metastatic lesions should be performed if possible and adjuvant therapy instituted. Radiotherapy has not been generally helpful. Antineoplastic agents, such as cisplatin and etoposide, ifosfamide and carboplatin, and 5-fluorouracil and leucovorin have had limited use in children and their success is not established. Therapy with o,p′-DDD—mitotane, an adrenolytic agent—may relieve the symptoms of hypercortisolism or virilization in recurrent disease but does not appear to improve survival. Other agents that interfere with adrenal steroid synthesis, such as ketoconazole, aminoglutethimide, and metyrapone, may also relieve symptoms of steroid excess but do not improve survival.

Bose HS, Sugawara T, Strauss III JF, et al: The pathophysiology and genetics of congenital lipoid adrenal hyperplasia. N Engl J Med 355:1870, 1996.

Burr IM, Sullivan J, Graham T, et al: A testosterone-secreting tumour of the adrenal producing virilization in a female infant. Lancet 2:643, 1973.

Clark RV, Albertson BD, Munabi A, et al: Steroidogenic enzyme activities, morphology, and receptor studies of a testicular adrenal rest in a patient with congenital adrenal hyperplasia. J Clin Endocrinol Metab 70:1408, 1990.

Diamond M: Prenatal predisposition and the clinical management of some pediatric conditions. J Sex Marital Ther 22:139, 1996.

Diamond M, Sigmundson HK: Sex reassignment at birth. Arch Pediatr Adolesc Med 151:298, 1997.

Eldar-Geva T, Hurwitz A, Vecsei P, et al: Secondary biosynthetic defects in women with late-onset congenital adrenal hyperplasia. N Engl J Med 323:855, 1990.

Fardella CE, Hum DW, Homoki J, Miller WL: Point mutation of Arg 440 to His in cytochrome P450c17 causes severe 17α-hydroxylase deficiency. J Clin Endocrinol Metab 79:160, 1994.
Forest MG: Prenatal diagnosis, treatment, and outcome in infants with congenital adrenal hyperplasia. Curr Opin Endocrinol Diabetes 4:209, 1997.
Fraumeni JF Jr, Miller RW: Adrenocortical neoplasms with hemihypertrophy, brain tumors, and other disorders. J Pediatr 70:129, 1967.
Geley S, Kapelari K, Jöhrer K, et al: CYP11B1 mutations causing congenital adrenal hyperplasia due to 11β-hydroxylase deficiency. J Clin Endocrinol Metab 81:2896, 1996.
Geller DH, Auchus RJ, Mendonca BB, Miller WL: The genetic and functional basis of isolated 17,20-lyase deficiency. Nat Genet 17:201, 1997.
Hendren WH, Atala A: Repair of the high vagina in girls with severely masculinized anatomy from the adrenogenital syndrome. J Pediatr Surg 30:91, 1995.
Holler W, Scholz S, Knon D, et al: Genetic differences between the salt-wasting simple virilizing and nonclassical types of congenital adrenal hyperplasia. J Clin Endocrinol Metab 60:757, 1985.
Karnak I, Senocak ME, Gogus S, et al: Testicular enlargement in patients with 11-hydroxylase deficiency. J Pediatr Surg 32:756, 1997.
Kuhnle U, Bullinger M: Outcome of congenital adrenal hyperplasia. Pediatr Surg Int 12:511, 1997.
Laue L, Merke DP, Jones JV, et al: A preliminary study of flutamide, testolactone, and reduced hydrocortisone dose in the treatment of congenital adrenal hyperplasia. J Clin Endocrinol Metab 81:3535, 1996.
Lee PDK, Winter RJ, Green OC: Virilizing adrenocortical tumors in childhood: Eight cases and a review of the literature. Pediatrics 76:437, 1985.
Levine LS, Pang S: Prenatal diagnosis and treatment of congenital adrenal hyperplasia. *In:* Milunsky A (ed): Genetic Disorders and the Fetus: Diagnosis, Prevention and Treatment. Baltimore, The Johns Hopkins University Press, 1998, pp 529–549.
Luton LP, Cerdas S, Billaud L, et al: Clinical features of adrenocortical carcinoma, prognostic factors, and the effect of mitotane therapy. N Engl J Med 322:1195, 1990.
Mason JI: The 3β-hydroxysteroid dehydrogenase gene family of enzymes. Trends Endocrinol Metab 6:199, 1993.
Mayer SK, Oligny LL, Deal C, et al: Childhood adrenocortical tumors: Case series and reevaluation of prognosis—a 24-year experience. J Pediatr Surg 32:911, 1997.
Mendonca BB, Lucon AM, Menezes CAV, et al: Clinical, hormonal and pathological findings in a comparative study of adrenocortical neoplasms in childhood and adulthood. J Urol 154:2004, 1995.
Meyer-Bahlburg HFL, Gruen RS, New MI, et al: Gender change from female to male in classical congenital adrenal hyperplasia. Horm Behav 30:319, 1996.
Michalkiewicz EL, Sandrini R, Bugg MF, et al: Clinical characteristics of small functioning adrenocortical tumors in children. Med Pediatr Oncol 28:175, 1997.
Miller WL: Gene conversions, deletions, and polymorphisms in congenital adrenal hyperplasia. Am J Hum Genet 42:4, 1988.
Miller WL: Genetics, diagnosis, and management of 21-hydroxylase deficiency. J Clin Endocrinol Metab 78:241, 1994.
Miller WL: Congenital lipoid adrenal hyperplasia: The human gene knockout for the steroidogenic acute regulatory protein. J Mol Endocrinol 19:227, 1997.
Nasir J, Royston C, Walton C, et al: 11β-hydroxylase deficiency: management of a difficult case by laparoscopic bilateral adrenalectomy. Clin Endocrinol 45:225, 1996.
Pang S: Genetics of 3β-hydroxysteroid dehydrogenase deficiency disorder. Growth Genet Horm 12:5, 1996.
Pang S, Shook MK: Current status of neonatal screening for congenital adrenal hyperplasia. Curr Opin Pediatr 9:419, 1997.
Pang S, Levine LS, Stoner E, et al: Nonsalt-losing congenital adrenal hyperplasia due to 3β-hydroxysteroid dehydrogenase deficiency with normal glomerulosa function. J Clin Endocrinol Metab 56:808, 1983.
Premawardhana LD, Hughes IA, Read GF, Scanlon MF: Longer term outcome in females with congenital adrenal hyperplasia (CAH): the Cardiff experience. Clin Endocrinol 46:327, 1997.
Reiner WG: Sex assignment in the neonate with intersex or inadequate genitalia. Arch Pediatr Adolesc Med 151:1044, 1997.
Rescoria FJ, Vane DW, Fitzgerald JF, et al: Vasoactive intestinal polypeptide-secreting ganglioneuromatosis affecting the entire colon and rectum. J Pediatr Surg 23:635, 1988.
Ribeiro RC, Neto RS, Schell MJ, et al: Adrenocortical carcinoma in children: A study of 40 cases. J Clin Oncol 8:67, 1990.
Sanchez R, Rheaume E, LaFlamme N, et al: Detection and functional characterization of the novel missense mutation Y254D in type II 3β-hydroxysteroid dehydrogenase (3βHSD) gene in a female patient with nonsalt-losing 3βHSD deficiency. J Clin Endocr Metab 78:561, 1994.
Sandrini R, Ribeiro RC, DeLacerda L: Childhood adrenocortical tumors. J Clin Endocrinol Metab 82:2027, 1997.
Soliman AT, AlLamki M, AlSalmi I, et al: Congenital adrenal hyperplasia complicated by central precocious puberty: Linear growth during infancy and treatment with gonadotropin-releasing hormone analog. Metabolism 46:513, 1997.
Speiser PW, Agdere L, Ueshiba H, et al: Aldosterone synthesis in salt-wasting congenital adrenal hyperplasia with complete absence of adrenal 21-hydroxylase. N Engl J Med 324:145, 1991.
Speiser PW, New MI, White PC: Molecular genetic analysis of nonclassic steroid 11-hydroxylase deficiency associated with HLA-B14,DR1. N Engl J Med 319:19, 1988.
Strachan T: Molecular pathology of congenital adrenal hyperplasia. Clin Endocrinol 32:373, 1990.
Therrell Jr BL, Berenbaum SA, Manter-Kapanke V, et al: Results of screening 1.9 million Texas newborns for 21-hydroxylase-deficient congenital adrenal hyperplasia. Pediatrics 101:538, 1998.
Urabe K, Kimura A, Harada F, et al: Gene conversions in steroid 21-hydroxylase genes. Am J Hum Genet 46:1178, 1990.
Van Wyk JJ, Gunther DF, Ritzen EM, et al: The use of adrenalectomy as a treatment for congenital adrenal hyperplasia. J Clin Endocrinol Metab 81:3180, 1996.
White PC, Tusie-Luna MJ, New MI, Speiser PW: Mutations in steroid 21-hydroxylase (CPY21). Hum Mutat 3:373, 1994.
White PC, Pascoe L: Disorders of steroid 11β-hydroxylase isozymes. Trends Endocrinol Metab 3:229, 1992.
Yanase T, Simpson ER, Waterman MR: 17α-hydroxylase/17.20-lyase deficiency: From clinical investigation to molecular definition. J Clin Endocrinol Metab 12:91, 1991.
Zachmann M: Prismatic cases: 17, 20-desmolase (17,20-lyase) deficiency. Clin Endocrinol Metab 81:457, 1996.

CHAPTER 587
Cushing Syndrome

Cushing syndrome, a characteristic pattern of obesity with associated hypertension, is the result of abnormally high blood levels of cortisol resulting from hyperfunction of the adrenal cortex. The syndrome may be corticotropin (adrenocorticotropic hormone [ACTH])–dependent or ACTH-independent.

ETIOLOGY. In infants, Cushing syndrome is most often caused by a *functioning adrenocortical tumor,* usually a malignant carcinoma but occasionally a benign adenoma. More than 50% of cortical tumors occur in children 3 yr of age or younger, and 85% occur in children 7 yr or younger. Patients with cortical tumors often exhibit a mixed form of hypercortisolism because of overproduction of other steroids such as androgens, estrogens, and aldosterone.

Primary pigmented nodular adrenocortical disease is a distinctive form of ACTH-independent Cushing syndrome, usually presenting before 20 yr of age. It may occur as an isolated event or as a familial disorder with or without other manifestations. The adrenal glands are small and have characteristic multiple, small (<4 mm in diameter), pigmented (black) nodules containing large cells with cytoplasm and lipofuscin; between the nodules, there is cortical atrophy. Although previous reports suggested that the condition is caused by circulating immunoglobulins directed toward the ACTH receptor, with ensuing stimulation of adrenal steroidogenesis, this has not been confirmed. This adrenal disorder occurs as a component of **Carney complex**, an autosomal dominant disorder consisting of centrofacial lentigines and blue nevi, cardiac and cutaneous myxomas, sexual precocity in boys with large cell calcifying Sertoli cell tumors, functioning pituitary tumors, thyroid tumors, and pigmented melanotic schwannomas. In a study of 11 families with Carney complex, the genetic defect was mapped to chromosome 2p16 by linkage analysis and appears to be associated with a gain of function mutation.

ACTH-independent Cushing syndrome with nodular hyperplasia and adenoma formation occurs in cases of *McCune-Albright syndrome,* with symptoms beginning in infancy or childhood. McCune-Albright syndrome is caused by a somatic mutation of $G_{s\alpha}$, resulting in inhibition of guanosine triphosphatase activity and constitutive activation of adenylate cyclase. When the mutation is present in adrenal tissue, cortisol and cell division are stimulated independently of ACTH. Other tissues in which activating mutations may occur are bone (producing fibrous dysplasia), gonads, thyroid, and pituitary. Clinical manifestations depend on which tissues are affected.

In children older than 7 yr of age with Cushing syndrome, *bilateral adrenal hyperplasia*, an ACTH-dependent form of Cushing syndrome, is usually found. Covert pituitary adenomas (microadenomas) occur in most patients with Cushing disease, and resection of these tumors results in correction of the hypercorticism. Immunostaining of the adenoma frequently produces positive results for ACTH. In some children, the pituitary tumors become overt after adrenalectomy *(Nelson syndrome)*; these consist principally of chromophobe cells and produce increased levels of β-lipotropin, β-endorphin, and ACTH. ACTH-secreting pituitary tumors in infants with Cushing syndrome are extremely rare.

Bilateral hyperplasia of the adrenals may also result from *ectopic production of ACTH*. Cushing syndrome in children has been associated with islet cell carcinoma of the pancreas, neuroblastoma or ganglioneuroblastoma, hemangiopericytoma, Wilms tumor, and thymic carcinoid. These cases are uncommon in children.

Prolonged exogenous administration of ACTH or hydrocortisone or its analogs results in a clinical pattern identical to the spontaneous disorder and is frequently referred to as *cushingoid syndrome*.

CLINICAL MANIFESTATIONS. Symptoms may begin in the neonatal period and have been recognized in at least 35 infants younger than 1 yr of age. Early in life, girls outnumber boys 3:1, and adrenocortical tumors (e.g., carcinoma, adenoma) are the usual causative lesions. The disorder appears to be more severe and the clinical findings more flagrant in infants than when the onset occurs in older children. The face is rounded, with prominent cheeks and a flushed appearance (moon facies). The chin is doubled, there is a buffalo hump, and generalized obesity is common. Signs of abnormal masculinization due to the androgen production of tumors occurs frequently; accordingly, there may be hypertrichosis on the face and trunk, pubic hair, acne, deepening of the voice, and enlargement of the clitoris in girls. Growth is impaired, with length falling below the 3rd percentile, except when significant virilization produces normal or even accelerated growth. Hypertension is common and may lead to heart failure. An increased susceptibility to infection may lead to fatal sepsis. Infants with Cushing syndrome, despite a robust appearance, are usually fragile. Occasionally, the condition is associated with hemihypertrophy or other congenital defects.

In older children, bilateral hyperplasia of the adrenals is the most common lesion, and the sex incidence is equal. In addition to obesity, short stature is a common presenting feature. Gradual onset of obesity and deceleration or cessation of growth may be the only early manifestations. Purplish striae on the hips, abdomen, and thighs are common. Pubertal development may be delayed, or amenorrhea may occur in girls past menarche. Weakness, headache, deterioration in schoolwork, and emotional lability may be prominent. Hypertension is usual. Renal stones have occurred in older children and in infants.

LABORATORY FINDINGS. Cortisol levels in blood are normally elevated at 8 A.M. and decrease to less than 50% by 8 P.M. except in children younger than 3 yr of age, in whom a diurnal rhythm is not always established. In patients with Cushing syndrome, this diurnal rhythm is lost, and cortisol levels at 8 P.M. are usually elevated. Urinary excretion of free cortisol is almost always increased; normal values are 20–90 μg/24 hr. Urinary excretion of 17-hydroxycorticosteroids is usually increased (>5 mg/m²/24 hr). In questionable cases, a single-dose dexamethasone suppression test may be helpful; a dose of 0.3 mg/m² given at 11 P.M. results in a plasma cortisol level of less than 5 μg/dL at 8 A.M. the next morning in normal children.

Additional laboratory findings in Cushing syndrome are polycythemia, lymphopenia, and eosinopenia. The glucose tolerance test result may point to diabetes despite elevated levels of insulin. Levels of serum electrolytes are usually normal, but potassium may be decreased.

After the diagnosis of Cushing syndrome has been established, it is necessary to determine whether it is ACTH-dependent or -independent. ACTH concentrations alone usually are not helpful in the differential diagnosis because of the large range of normal basal levels. Corticotropin-releasing hormone (CRH) testing and the two-step dexamethasone suppression test are useful. After an intravenous bolus of CRH (1 μg/kg), patients with ACTH-dependent Cushing syndrome have an exaggerated ACTH and cortisol response, but those with adrenal tumors show no increase in ACTH and cortisol. The two-step dexamethasone suppression test consists of administration of dexamethasone, 30 and 120 μg/kg/24 hr, divided into four doses and given for two consecutive days each. In children with ACTH-dependent Cushing syndrome, the larger dose, but not the smaller dose, suppresses urinary free cortisol or 17-hydroxycorticosteroids to less than 50% of baseline, and serum levels of cortisol decrease to less than 7 μg/dL. Occasional paradoxical results have been reported.

Osseous maturation is usually moderately retarded but may be normal; in virilized children, the bone age is likely to be advanced. Osteoporosis is common and is most evident in roentgenograms of the spine. A severe decrease in bone mineral density has been demonstrated by dual-energy x-ray absorptiometry (DEXA). Pathologic fractures may be detected. Levels of growth hormone, both secreted spontaneously and stimulated, are suppressed but return to normal when the hypercortisolism is corrected. Diminution of muscle mass and increased deposition of adipose tissue may be noticed in roentgenograms of the extremities. The thymic shadow is absent because excessive cortisol produces involution. Computed tomography detects virtually all adrenal tumors larger than 1.5 cm in diameter. Adrenal scintigraphy with radiocholesterol is rarely indicated except for those patients with pigmented micronodular adrenal hyperplasia, for whom it may be more accurate than computed tomography. Magnetic resonance imaging is the screening method of choice to detect ACTH-secreting pituitary adenomas; the addition of gadolinium contrast increases the sensitivity of detection. Bilateral inferior petrosal blood sampling to measure concentrations of ACTH before and after CRH administration may be required to localize the tumor when a pituitary adenoma is not visualized.

DIFFERENTIAL DIAGNOSIS. Cushing syndrome is frequently suspected in children with obesity, particularly when striae and hypertension are present. The differential diagnosis is complicated by the fact that elevated urinary concentrations of corticosteroids are frequently secondary to obesity itself. Children with simple obesity are usually tall, but those with Cushing syndrome are short or have a decelerating growth rate. The excretion of urinary corticosteroids is rapidly suppressed by oral administration of low doses of dexamethasone in uncomplicated obesity. Elevated levels of cortisol and ACTH without clinical evidence of Cushing syndrome occur in patients with generalized glucocorticoid resistance. Affected patients may be asymptomatic or exhibit hypertension, hypokalemia, and precocious pseudopuberty; these manifestations are caused by increased mineralocorticoid and adrenal androgens in response to elevated ACTH levels. Several mutations of the glucocorticoid receptor have been reported.

TREATMENT. If the lesion is a benign cortical adenoma, unilateral adrenalectomy is indicated. Such adenomas are occasionally bilateral; then the treatment of choice is subtotal adrenalectomy. In either instance, an excellent therapeutic result is achieved by removing the tumor. Adrenocortical carcinomas frequently metastasize, especially to the liver and lungs, and the prognosis may be unfavorable despite removal of the primary lesion. Rarely, the tumors are bilateral and require total adrenalectomy. It is often impossible to differentiate benign from malignant tumors by histologic appearance alone.

Trans-sphenoidal pituitary microsurgery is the treatment of choice in Cushing disease in children, and a number of reports on long-term outcome of surgery in children have been published. Duration of follow-up and remission rates have varied, but the overall success rate with follow-up of less than 10 yr is approximately 60–80%. Low postoperative serum or urinary cortisol concentrations appear to be predictive of long-term remission in the majority of, but not all, cases. Reoperation or pituitary irradiation is performed when relapse occurs.

Cyproheptadine, a centrally acting serotonin antagonist that blocks ACTH release, has been used to treat Cushing disease in adults; remissions are usually not sustained after discontinuation of therapy. This agent is rarely used in children. Inhibitors of adrenal steroidogensis (metyrapone, ketoconozole, aminoglutethimide) have been used preoperatively to normalize circulating cortisol levels and reduce perioperative morbidity and mortality.

Management of patients undergoing adrenalectomy requires adequate preoperative and postoperative replacement therapy with a corticosteroid. Tumors that produce corticosteroids usually lead to atrophy of the normal adrenal tissue, and replacement with cortisol may be required. Postoperative complications have included sepsis, pancreatitis, thrombosis, poor wound healing, and sudden collapse, particularly in infants with Cushing syndrome. Substantial catch-up growth, pubertal progress, and increased bone density occur, but bone density remains abnormal and adult height is often compromised.

Bitton RN, Cobbs R, Schneider BS: Development of Nelson syndrome in a patient with recurrent Cushing disease: Analysis of secretory behavior of the pituitary tumor. Am J Med 84:319, 1988.

Boston BA, Mandel S, LaFranchi S, Bliziotes M: Activating mutation in the stimulatory guanine nucleotide-binding protein in an infant with Cushing's syndrome and nodular adrenal hyperplasia. J Clin Endocrinol Metab 79:890, 1994.

Brönnegåard M, Carlstedt-Duke J: The genetic basis of glucocorticoid resistance. Trends Endocrinol Metab 6:160, 1995.

Devoe DJ, Miller WL, Conte FA, et al: Long-term outcome in children and adolescents after transsphenoidal surgery for Cushing's disease. J Clin Endocrinol Metab 82:3196, 1997.

Karl M, Lamberts SWJ, Detera-Wadleigh SD, et al: Familial glucocorticoid resistance caused by a splice site deletion in the human glucocorticoid receptor. J Clin Endocrinol Metab 76:683, 1993.

Kaye TB, Crapo L: The Cushing syndrome: An update on diagnostic tests. Am J Intern Med 112:424, 1990.

Leinung MC, Kane LA, Scheithauer BW, et al: Long-term follow-up of transsphenoidal surgery for the treatment of Cushing's disease in childhood. J Clin Endocrinol Metab 80:2475, 1995.

Levy SR, Cerdas S, Billard L, et al: Cushing's syndrome in infancy secondary to pituitary adenoma. Am J Dis Child 136:605, 1982.

Magiakou MA, Mastorakos G, Oldfield EH, et al: Cushing's syndrome in children and adolescents. N Engl J Med 331:629, 1994.

Malchoff CD, Javier EC, Malchoff DM, et al: Primary cortisol resistance presenting as isosexual precocity. J Clin Endocrinol Metab 70:503, 1990.

Malchoff CD, MacGillivray D, Malchoff DM: Adrenocorticotropic hormone–independent adrenal hyperplasia. Endocrinologist 6:79, 1996.

Mampalam TH, Tyrell JB, Wilson CB: Transphenoidal microsurgery for Cushing disease. Ann Intern Med 109:487, 1988.

McArthur RG, Bahn RC, Hayles AB: Primary adrenocortical nodular dysplasia as a cause of Cushing's syndrome in infants and children. Mayo Clin Proc 57:58, 1982.

Muguruza MTG, Chrousos GP: Periodic Cushing syndrome in a short boy: Usefulness of the ovine corticotropin-releasing hormone test. J Pediatr 115:270, 1990.

Ray DW: Molecular mechanisms of glucocorticoid resistance. J Endocrinol 149:1, 1996.

Stratakis CA, Carney JA, Lin J-P, et al.: Carney Complex, a familial multiple neoplasia and lentiginosis syndrome. J Clin Invest 97:699, 1996.

Styne DM, Isaac R, Miller WL, et al: Endocrine, histological and biochemical studies of adrenocorticotropin-producing islet cell carcinoma of the pancreas in childhood with characterization of pro-opiomelanocortin. J Clin Endocrinol Metab 57:723, 1983.

Styne DM, Grumbach MM, Kaplan SL, et al: Treatment of Cushing's disease in childhood and adolescents by transphenoidal microadenomectomy. N Engl J Med 310:889, 1984.

Weber A, Trainer PJ, Grossman AB, et al: Investigation, management and therapeutic outcome in 12 cases of childhood and adolescent Cushing's syndrome. Clin Endocrinol 43:19, 1995.

Wolffraat NM, Drexhage HA, Wiersinga WM, et al: Immunoglobulins of patients with Cushing's syndrome due to pigmented adrenocortical micronodular dysplasia stimulate in vitro steroidogenesis. J Clin Endocrin Metab 66:301, 1988.

CHAPTER 588
Excess Mineralocorticoid Secretion

The principal mineralocorticoid secreted by the adrenal gland is aldosterone. Increased secretion may result from a primary defect of the adrenal gland (primary hyperaldosteronism) or from factors that activate the renin-angiotensin system (secondary hyperaldosteronism). Patients with primary hyperaldosteronism usually have hypertension or hypokalemia, or both; those with secondary hyperaldosteronism do not.

Deoxycorticosterone is a precursor of aldosterone, with only about 1/30th the sodium-retaining potency of aldosterone (see Fig. 586–1). Overproduction of deoxycorticosterone occurs with two distinct defects of adrenal steroidogenesis. The first defect involves 11-hydroxylation, which also leads to androgen excess and presents clinically as the hypertensive form of congenital adrenal hyperplasia (see Chapter 586.1). The second defect involves 17-hydroxylation, producing hypogonadism in the female and pseudohermaphroditism in the male because the synthesis of androgens and estrogens, as well as that of cortisol, is impaired.

ETIOLOGY. Primary aldosteronism encompasses disorders characterized by excessive aldosterone secretion independent of the renin-angiotensin system. These disorders, rare in children, are characterized by hypertension, hypokalemia, and suppression of the renin-angiotensin system.

Aldosterone-secreting adenomas are unilateral and have been reported in children as young as 3.5 yr of age; they mainly affect girls.

Bilateral micronodular adrenocortical hyperplasia tends to occur in older children and is more frequent in males.

Primary aldosteronism due to *unilateral adrenal hyperplasia* has been reported infrequently in children.

Glucocorticoid-suppressible aldosteronism, also known as *glucocorticoid-remediable aldosteronism*, is an ACTH-dependent autosomal dominant form of hyperaldosteronism. The hyperaldosteronism is rapidly suppressed by glucocorticoid administration, with normalization of the biochemical abnormalities and, in young patients, the hypertension. In this disorder, there is marked overproduction of 18-hydroxycortisol and 18-oxocortisol, hybrid steroids having the characteristics of zona glomerulosa and zona fasciculata steroids. The regulation of aldosterone secretion by ACTH and the oversecretion of the hybrid steroids is caused by crossover events between the CYP11B1 gene (which encodes P450c11) and the CYP11B2 gene (which encodes aldosterone synthase or P450c18). A "hybrid" gene is produced, having the regulatory sequence of CYP11B1 and the coding sequences of the aldosterone synthase gene. This results in the ectopic expression of aldosterone synthase in the adrenal fasciculata. At-risk family members should be investigated for this easily treated cause of hypertension. The biochemical abnormality can be demonstrated in normotensive individuals. It has been suggested that blood pressure in affected patients is higher when the disorder is inherited from the mother than when it is inherited from the father.

CLINICAL MANIFESTATIONS. Some affected children have no symptoms, the diagnosis being established after incidental discovery of moderate hypertension. Others have severe hypertension (up to 240/150 mm Hg), with headache, dizziness, and visual disturbances. Chronic hypokalemia may lead to "clear cell nephrosis," polyuria, nocturia, enuresis, and polydipsia. Muscle weakness and discomfort, tetany, intermittent paralysis, fatigue, and growth failure affect these children.

LABORATORY FINDINGS. Hypertension, hypokalemia, and suppressed plasma renin activity are the hallmarks of hyperaldosteronism. The serum pH, carbon dioxide content, and sodium concentrations may be elevated and the serum chloride and magnesium levels decreased. Serum levels of calcium are normal, even in children who manifest tetany. The urine is neutral or alkaline, and kaliuresis is present. Plasma and urine levels of aldosterone are increased, and plasma levels of renin are persistently low. Aldosterone does not decrease with sodium chloride administration, and renin does not respond to salt and fluid restriction. In patients with glucocorticoid-suppressible aldosteronism, urinary and plasma levels of 18-oxocortisol and 18-hydroxycortisol are markedly increased.

DIFFERENTIAL DIAGNOSIS. After establishing the diagnosis of primary aldosteronism, it is necessary to determine the cause. All children should have a therapeutic trial with dexamethasone before invasive studies are performed. Daily administration of 0.25 mg every 6 hr results in marked suppression of aldosterone and disappearance of hypertension in those patients with the glucocorticoid-suppressible variant of hyperaldosteronism. If there is no response to dexamethasone, computed tomography may help detect an adrenal adenoma, but the tumors are often quite small. If computed tomographic scans are normal, adrenal vein catheterization is indicated. High concentrations of aldosterone are found in only one adrenal vein when an adenoma is present and in both when bilateral hyperplasia is the cause. Cortisol levels should be obtained simultaneously to compare adrenal vein aldosterone and cortisol ratios. If adrenal vein catheterization is not successful, exploratory laparotomy may be required to establish the diagnosis. Some investigators have recommended adrenal vein sampling in all cases, even when a mass is visualized, to document secretory activity of the mass in view of the now-recognized frequency of adrenal incidentalomas.

Hyperaldosteronism occurs in many other conditions in which it is a normal homeostatic response. In such *secondary hyperaldosteronism*, plasma renin activity is high or rises with a low-salt diet, whereas in primary hyperaldosteronism the renin-angiotensin system is suppressed. Increased aldosterone secretion occurs in edematous disorders with reduced effective volume, such as nephrotic syndrome, congestive cardiac failure, and cirrhosis of the liver. Increased secretion of aldosterone also occurs in conditions in which compromise of renal perfusion results in increased secretion of renin, such as in stenosis of the renal artery. Wilms tumor and juxtaglomerular cell tumors may also secrete renin and cause secondary hyperaldosteronism.

In *pseudohypoaldosteronism*, the increased levels of aldosterone are due to a target organ unresponsiveness to aldosterone, with ensuing activation of the renin-angiotensin system (see Chapter 585).

Bartter and *Gitelman syndromes* are also characterized by hypokalemic alkalosis, hypochloremia, and hyperaldosteronism, but hypertension is absent and renin secretion is increased (see Chapter 539). The characteristic presentation of Bartter syndrome is severe neonatal dehydration after a preterm delivery complicated by polyhydramnios. Hypercalciuria and nephrocalcinosis are an integral part of the disease. Mutations in the Na-K-2 Cl cotransporter (NKCC2) gene have been described as the cause of Bartter syndrome, which result in reduced sodium and chloride reabsorption in the thick ascending loop of Henle. Gitelman syndrome, in contrast, presents at an older age, predominantly with musculoskeletal signs and symptoms and with hypocalcemia and hypomagnesemia. This disorder appears to result from mutations in the gene coding for the Na-Cl cotransporter of the distal collecting tubule (TSC), mapped to chromosome 16.

Liddle syndrome is an autosomal dominant form of hypertension, usually accompanied by hypokalemia. Renin is suppressed. In contrast to disorders with hyperaldosteronism, however, aldosterone levels are low. Blood pressure and hypokalemia improve with sodium restriction and the potassium-sparing diuretic triamterene. Mutations in the β subunit of the renal epithelial sodium channel, coded for on chromosome 16, and in the δ subunit of the renal epithelial sodium channel, coded for on chromosome 12, have been demonstrated in patients with Liddle's syndrome.

11β-Hydroxysteroid dehydrogenase (11β-HSD) deficiency has been reported in approximately 20 children. Onset occurs in early childhood with failure to thrive, polyuria and polydipsia secondary to the effects of hypokalemia, and severe hypertension. Strokes have occurred in young children. Although clinically the disorder mimics that seen in patients with elevated aldosterone levels, renin and aldosterone levels are low (low-renin hypertension). The condition was thought to be caused by production of an undetected mineralocorticoid and was therefore named the *syndrome of apparent mineralocorticoid excess*. However, the disorder is caused by a deficiency of the enzyme that converts cortisol to cortisone. Plasma levels of cortisol are normal, but those of cortisone are low, and the ratio of the urinary tetrahydro products of cortisol to cortisone is characteristically elevated.

How this glucocorticoid defect can cause such profound mineralocorticoid effects has been elucidated. Type I mineralocorticoid receptors (kidney, parotid glands, colon) have equal affinity for aldosterone and cortisol. Under normal conditions, 11β-HSD acts as a paracrine protector for the mineralocorticoid receptor in the proximal tubules of the kidney; by converting cortisol to cortisone at this site, it can no longer bind to the receptor. In the absence of this enzyme and with failure of conversion of cortisol to cortisone, cortisol binds to the mineralocorticoid receptor and elicits effects similar to those of aldosterone. The disorder has been reported in siblings in several kindreds and is inherited in an autosomal recessive manner. Molecular genetic studies in 15 kindreds have demonstrated mutations in HSD11B2, the gene encoding the type II 11-βHSD enzyme, the kidney isozyme, in all patients. The well-known hypertensive effect of glycorrhetinic acid, a constituent of licorice, is now known to be caused by its inhibition of renal 11β-HSD.

TREATMENT. Glucocorticoid-suppressible hyperaldosteronism is managed by daily administration of glucocorticoid, often prednisone. The treatment of an aldosterone-producing adenoma is surgical removal. This has been performed primarily by laparotomy and adrenalectomy. However, successful enucleation of aldosterone-producing adenomas as well as laparoscopic adrenalectomy have been reported. Pharmacologic treatment of hyperaldosteronism due to bilateral adrenal hyperplasia with spironolactone often results in normalization of blood pressure and serum potassium levels.

If the side effects of spironolactone are unacceptable, amiloride may be used, and other antihypersive agents added as necessary. In patients whose condition cannot be controlled medically, unilateral adrenalectomy may be considered.

Treatment of secondary hyperaldosteronism is directed toward the specific causative disorder.

Abasiyanik A, Oran B, Kaymakci A, et al: Conn syndrome in a child, caused by adrenal adenoma. J Pediatr Surg 31:430, 1996.

Bryer-Ash M, Wilson DM, Tune BM, et al: Hypertension caused by an aldosterone-secreting adenoma. Occurrence in a 7-year-old child. Am J Dis Child 138:673, 1984.

Fallo F, Kuhnle U, Boscaro M, Sonino N: Abnormality of aldosterone and cortisol late pathways in glucocorticoid-remediable aldosteronism. J Clin Endocrinol Metab 79:772, 1994.

Findling JW, Raff H, Hansson JH, Lifton RP: Liddle's syndrome: Prospective

genetic screening and suppressed aldosterone secretion in an extended kindred. J Clin Endocrinol Metab 82:1071, 1997.
Gomez-Sanchez CE, Gill JR Jr, Ganguly A, et al: Glucocorticoid-suppressible aldosteronism: A disorder of the adrenal transitional zona. J Clin Endocrinol Metab 67:444, 1988.
Gordon RD: Primary aldosteronism. J Endocrinol Invest 18:495, 1995.
Lifton RP, Dluhy RG: The molecular basis of a hereditary form of hypertension, glucocorticoid-remediable aldosteronism. Trends Endocrinol Metab 4:57, 1993.
Simon DB, Lifton RP: The molecular basis of inherited hypokalemic alkalosis: Bartter's and Gitelman's syndromes. Am J Physiol 271:F961, 1997.
White PC: Inherited forms of mineralocorticoid hypertension. Hypertension 28:927, 1996.
White PC, Mune T, Agarwal AK: 11β-Hydroxysteroid dehydrogenase and the syndrome of apparent mineralocorticoid excess. Endocr Rev 18:135, 1997.
Young WF Jr: Primary aldosteronism: Update on diagnosis and treatment. Endocrinologist 7:213, 1997.

CHAPTER 589
Feminizing Adrenal Tumors

Adrenocortical tumors have been reported in approximately a dozen boys with excessive production of estrogens and heterosexual precocious puberty. The tumors may produce only estrogen, estrogen and androgen, or rarely estrogen and cortisol (Fig. 589–1). Gynecomastia was the initial manifestation, appearing from 6 mo–14 yr of age. Growth and development were otherwise normal, or concomitant virilization was sometimes evidenced by acne, deep voice, phallic enlargement, and advanced osseous maturation. The testes were not enlarged. Hypertension is common in affected adults but has not been observed in children. The levels of estrogens and often of androgens in plasma and urine are markedly elevated. Tumors may be carcinomas or benign adenomas and may appear calcified on roentgenograms. Gynecomastia regresses after removal of the tumor, and hormone values return to normal.

Estrogen-secreting adrenocortical tumors have been reported in at least 12 girls ranging in age from 6 mo–10 yr. The majority of the tumors were adenomas, some of which also elaborated androgens (with virilization) or mineralocorticoids (with hypertension). In addition to elevated plasma and urinary levels of estrogens, there were usually elevated levels of 17-ketosteroids in urine and of adrenal steroids (i.e., dehydroepiandrosterone and its sulfate) in plasma. Plasma gonadotropin levels are suppressed, and GnRH stimulation does not elicit a response. Computed tomography usually localizes the tumor.

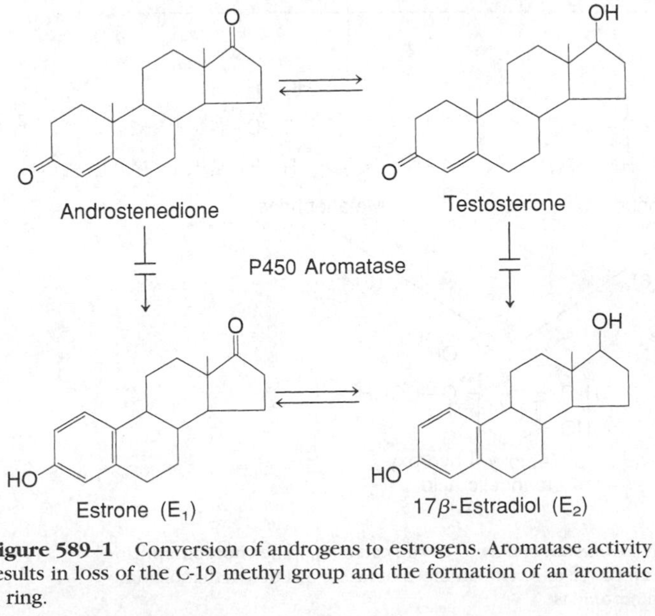

In a study of an adult male with a feminizing adrenocortical tumor, a high level of aromatase activity and expression of the CYP19 (P450arom) gene, absent in normal adrenal tissue, were found in tumor tissue. The tumor was thus able to aromatize androstenedione to estrone, and the peripheral conversion of estrone to estradiol resulted in the feminizing symptoms.

Androstenedione ⇌ Testosterone; P450 Aromatase; Estrone (E_1) ⇌ 17β-Estradiol (E_2)

Figure 589–1 Conversion of androgens to estrogens. Aromatase activity results in loss of the C-19 methyl group and the formation of an aromatic A ring.

Comite F, Schiebinger RJ, Alertson BD, et al: Isosexual precocious pseudopuberty secondary to a feminizing adrenal tumor. J Clin Endocrinol Metab 58:435, 1984.
Ghazi AAM, Mofid D, Rahimi F, et al: Oestrogen and cortisol producing adrenal tumour. Arch Dis Child 71:358, 1994.
Howard CP, Takahashi H, Hayles AB: Feminizing adrenal adenoma in a boy. Case report and literature review. Mayo Clin Proc 52:354, 1977.
LaFranchi SH, Hanna CE, Mandel SH: Feminizing adrenal adenoma secreting estrone presenting as prepubertal gynecomastia. J Pediatr Endocrinol 3:261, 1989.
Sultan C, Descomps B, Garandeau P, et al: Pubertal gynecomastia due to an estrogen-producing adrenal adenoma. J Pediatr 95:744, 1979.
Young J, Bulun SE, Agarwal V, et al: Aromatase expression in a feminizing adrenocortical tumor. J Clin Endocrinol Metab 81:3173, 1996.

CHAPTER 590
Pheochromocytoma

The pheochromocytoma, a catecholamine-secreting tumor, arises from the chromaffin cells. The most common site of origin is the adrenal medulla; however, tumors may develop anywhere along the abdominal sympathetic chain and are likely to be located near the aorta at the level of the inferior mesenteric artery or at its bifurcation. They also appear in the periadrenal area, the urinary bladder or ureteral walls, the thoracic cavity, and the cervical region. Ten per cent occur in children, in whom they present most frequently between 6 and 14 yr of age. Tumors vary from about 1–10 cm in diameter; they are found more often on the right side than on the left. In more than 20% of affected children, the adrenal tumors are bilateral, and in 30–40% of children, tumors are found in both the adrenal and extra-adrenal areas or only in an extra-adrenal area.

Pheochromocytoma may be inherited as an autosomal dominant trait. In affected families, the ages of patients at the time of diagnosis have varied from the 1st to 5th decades of life; more than half the patients have had multiple tumors.

Pheochromocytomas may also be associated with other syndromes such as neurofibromatosis and von Hippel-Lindau disease and as a component of multiple endocrine neoplasia (MEN) syndromes MEN IIA and MEN IIB. Germ-line mutations of the RET proto-oncogene on chromosome 10 (10q11.2) have been found in families with MEN IIA, and germ-line mutations in a tumor suppressor gene on chromosome 3 have been identified in von Hippel-Lindau syndrome. Pheochromocytoma is also associated with tuberous sclerosis, Sturge-Weber syndrome, and ataxia-telangiectasia.

CLINICAL MANIFESTATIONS. The clinical features of pheochromocytoma result from excessive secretion of epinephrine and norepinephrine. All patients have hypertension at some time. The hypertension in children is more often sustained rather than paroxysmal, as it is in adults. Paroxysms should particularly suggest pheochromocytoma as a diagnostic possibility. When there are paroxysms of hypertension, the attacks are usually infrequent at first but become more frequent and eventually give way to a continuous hypertensive state. Between attacks of hypertension, the patient may be free of symptoms. During attacks, the patient complains of headache, palpitations, abdominal pain, and dizziness; pallor, vomiting, and sweating also occur. Convulsions and other manifestations of hypertensive encephalopathy may occur. In severe cases, precordial pains radiate into the arms, and pulmonary edema and cardiac and hepatic enlargement may develop. The child has a good appetite but because of hypermetabolism does not gain weight, and severe cachexia may develop. Polyuria and polydipsia can be sufficiently severe to suggest diabetes insipidus. Growth failure may be striking. The blood pressure may range from 180–260 systolic and 120–210 diastolic, and the heart may be enlarged. Ophthalmoscopic examination may reveal papilledema, hemorrhages, exudate, and arterial constriction.

LABORATORY FINDINGS. The urine contains protein, a few casts, and occasionally glucose. Gross hematuria suggests that the tumor is in the bladder wall. Polycythemia is occasionally observed. The diagnosis is established by demonstration of elevated blood or urinary levels of catecholamines and their metabolites.

Pheochromocytomas produce norepinephrine and epinephrine; however, norepinephrine in plasma is derived from the adrenal gland and adrenergic nerve endings, but epinephrine is derived primarily from the adrenal gland. In contrast to adults, the predominant catecholamine in children is norepinephrine, and total urinary catecholamine excretion usually exceeds 300 μg/24 hr. Urinary excretion of vanillylmandelic acid (VMA, 3-methoxy-4-hydroxymandelic acid), the major metabolite of epinephrine and norepinephrine, and of metanephrine (Fig. 590–1) is also increased. Catecholamine levels can be measured by radioimmunoassay and high-performance

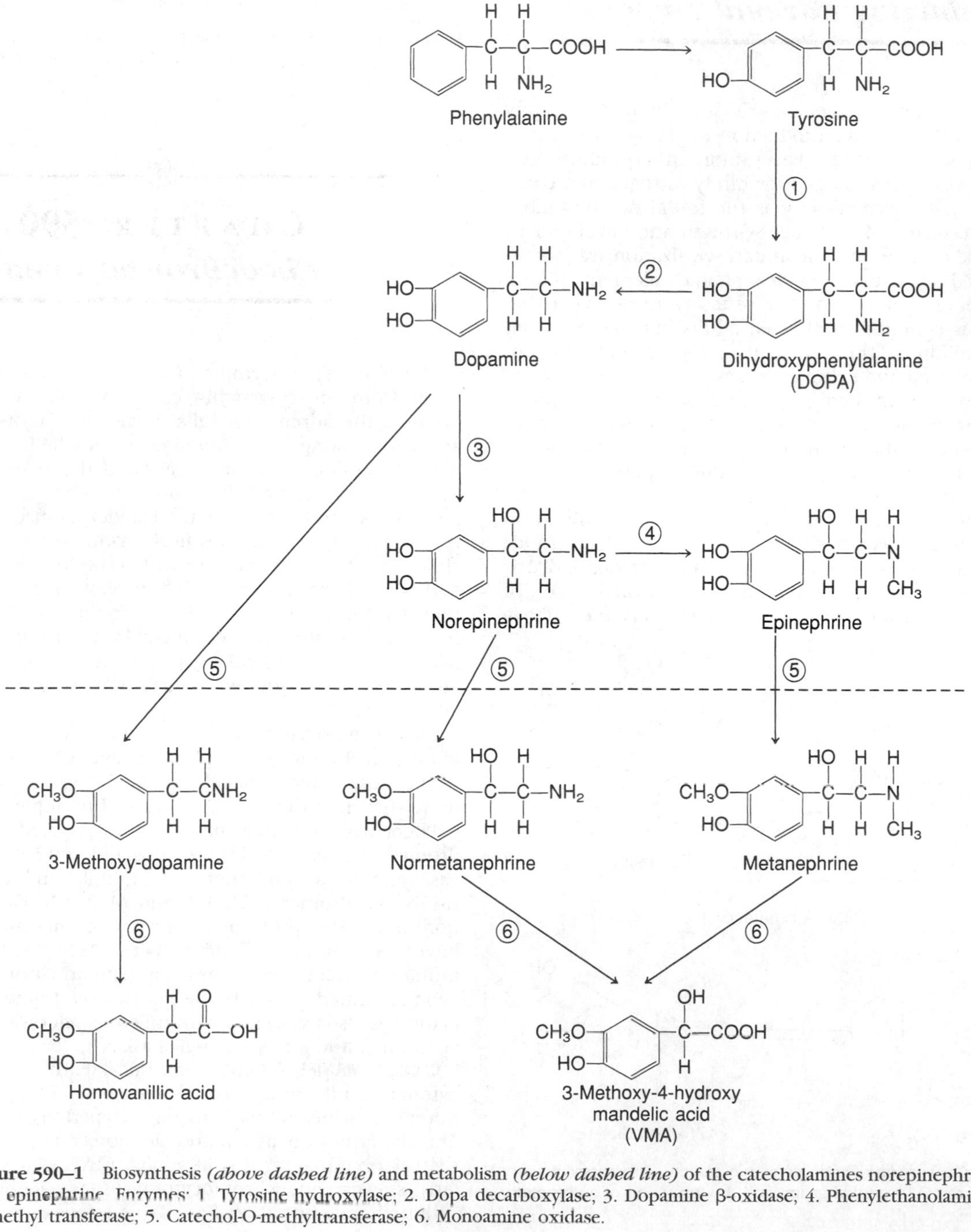

Figure 590–1 Biosynthesis *(above dashed line)* and metabolism *(below dashed line)* of the catecholamines norepinephrine and epinephrine. Enzymes: 1. Tyrosine hydroxylase; 2. Dopa decarboxylase; 3. Dopamine β-oxidase; 4. Phenylethanolamine-N-methyl transferase; 5. Catechol-O-methyltransferase; 6. Monoamine oxidase.

liquid chromatography methods. Excretion of catecholamine metabolites may be similar in children with neuroblastoma and pheochromocytoma, but levels are usually higher in those with pheochromocytoma, and neuroblastoma does not usually produce hypertension. Daily urinary excretion of these compounds by unaffected children increases with age; and vanilla-containing foods and fruits can produce falsely elevated levels of VMA. Certain drugs interfere with fluorometric determinations of catecholamines.

Most tumors in the area of the adrenal gland are readily localized by ultrasonography or by computed tomography or magnetic resonance imaging; their frequent bilateral occurrence must not be forgotten. Extra-adrenal tumors, anywhere from the neck to the bladder, may be difficult to detect. ^{131}I-metaiodobenzylguanidine is taken up by chromaffin tissue anywhere in the body and is useful for localizing small tumors. Venous catheterization with sampling of blood at different levels for catecholamine determinations is now only rarely necessary for localizing the tumor.

DIFFERENTIAL DIAGNOSIS. The various causes of hypertension in children, such as renal or renovascular disease; coarctation of the aorta; acrodynia; thallium intoxication; hyperthyroidism; Cushing syndrome; 11β-hydroxylase, 17β-hydroxylase, and 11β-hydroxysteroid dehydrogenase deficiency; primary aldosteronism; adrenal cortical tumors; and essential hypertension must be considered. A nonfunctioning kidney may result from compression of a ureter or of a renal artery by a pheochromocytoma. Paroxysmal hypertension may be associated with porphyria or familial dysautonomia. Urinary excretion of VMA is low in familial dysautonomia because of a defect in release rather than in synthesis of catecholamines. Cerebral disorders, diabetes insipidus, diabetes mellitus, and hyperthyroidism must also be considered in the differential diagnosis. Hypertension in patients with neurofibromatosis may be caused by renal vascular involvement and by concurrent pheochromocytoma.

Neuroblastoma, ganglioneuroblastoma, and ganglioneuroma frequently produce catecholamines. Secreting neurogenic tumors commonly produce hypertension, excessive sweating, flushing, pallor, rash, polyuria, and polydipsia. Chronic diarrhea may be associated with these tumors, particularly with ganglioneuroma, and at times may be sufficiently persistent to suggest the celiac syndrome.

TREATMENT. Removal of these tumors results in cure, but the operation is not without danger. Careful preoperative, intraoperative, and postoperative management is essential. Preoperative α- and β-adrenergic blockade is required. Because these tumors are often multiple in children, a thorough transabdominal exploration of all the usual sites offers the best chance of finding all of them. Appropriate choice of anesthesia and expansion of blood volume with appropriate fluids during surgery are critical to avoid a precipitous drop in blood pressure during operation or within 48 hr postoperatively. Manipulation and excision of these tumors result in marked increases in catecholamine secretion that cause rises in blood pressure and heart rate. Surveillance must continue postoperatively.

Although these tumors often appear malignant histologically, the only accurate indicators of malignancy are the presence of metastatic disease or local invasiveness that precluded complete resection, or both. Pediatric malignant pheochromocytoma is rare, occurring less frequently than in adults, and appears to occur more frequently in extra-adrenal, than adrenal, sites. Prolonged follow-up is indicated because functioning tumors at other sites may become manifested many years after the initial operation. Examination of relatives of affected patients may reveal other persons harboring unsuspected tumors. In one family with 10 affected individuals, the highest blood pressures and urinary concentrations of catecholamines were found in the children, but some of the affected adults were normotensive and had only moderately elevated urinary concentrations of catecholamines and VMA.

OTHER CATECHOLAMINE-SECRETING NEURAL TUMORS. See Chapters 345 and 504.

Bravo EL: Evolving concepts in the pathophysiology, diagnosis and treatment of pheochromocytoma. Endocr Rev 15:356, 1994.

Ein SH, Weitzman S, Thorner P, et al: Pediatric malignant pheochromocytoma. J Pediatr Surg 29:1197, 1994.

CHAPTER 591
Adrenal Calcification

591.1 Adrenal Masses

Calcification within the adrenal glands may occur in a wide variety of situations, some serious and others of no obvious consequence. Adrenal calcifications are often detected as incidental findings in roentgenographic studies of the abdomen in infants and children. The physician may elicit a history of anoxia or trauma at birth. Hemorrhage into the adrenal gland at or immediately after birth is probably the common factor that leads to subsequent calcification. Although it is advisable to assess the adrenocortical reserve of such patients, there is rarely any functional disorder.

Neuroblastomas, ganglioneuromas, cortical carcinomas, pheochromocytomas, and cysts of the adrenal gland may be responsible for calcifications, particularly if hemorrhage has occurred within the tumor. Calcification in such lesions is almost always unilateral.

In the past, tuberculosis was a common cause of calcification within the adrenals and of Addison disease. Calcifications may also develop in the adrenal glands of children who recover from the Waterhouse-Friderichsen syndrome; such patients are usually asymptomatic. Infants with *Wolman disease*, a rare lipid disorder due to deficiency of lysosomal acid lipase, have extensive bilateral calcifications of the adrenal glands. The disorder is lethal within the 1st yr of life, with infants dying from complications of massive storage of lipids in most tissues. Mutations in the gene encoding the human lysosomal acid lipase–cholesterol esterase have been identified in a patient with Wolman disease (see Chapter 83).

Anderson RA, Byrum RS, Coates PM, Sando GN: Mutations at the lysosomal acid cholesteryl ester hydrolase gene locus in Wolman disease. Proc Natl Acad Sci USA 91:2718, 1994.

Bilal MM, Brown JJ: MR imaging of renal and adrenal masses in children. Magn Reson Imaging Clin N Am 5:179, 1997.

Hill EE, Williams JA: Massive adrenal haemorrhage in the newborn. Arch Dis Child 34:178, 1959.

Jarvis JL, Seaman WB: Idiopathic adrenal calcification in infants and children. Am J Roentgenol 82:510, 1959.

Stevenson J, MacGregor AM, Connelly P: Calcification of the adrenal glands in young children: A report of three cases with a review of the literature. Arch Dis Child 36:316, 1961.

591.2 Adrenal Incidentaloma

As a result of the widespread use of computed tomography and magnetic resonance imaging, adrenal masses are being discovered with increasing frequency in patients undergoing abdominal imaging for reasons unrelated to the adrenal gland. Single adrenal masses have been reported in 1–4% of abdominal computed tomographic examinations. The unexpected discovery of such a mass presents the clinician with a dilemma in terms of diagnostic steps to undertake and treatment interventions to recommend. The differential diagnosis of adrenal incidentaloma includes benign lesions such as cysts, hemorrhagic cysts, hematomas, and myelolipomas. These lesions can usually be differentiated on computed tomography or magnetic resonance imaging. If a known benign lesion is excluded, additional evaluation is required to determine the nature of the lesion. Included in the differential diagnosis of lesions requiring additional evaluation are benign adenomas, functional or nonfunctional; pheochromocytomas; adrenocortical carcinoma; and metastasis from extra-adrenal primary carcinoma. Careful history, physical examination, and endocrine evaluation must be performed to seek evidence of autonomous cortisol, androgen, mineralocorticoid, or catecholamine secretion. If the adrenal mass is nonfunctional and larger than 6 cm, current recommendations are to proceed with surgical resection of the mass; if it is less than 3 cm, it is recommended that it be followed clinically with periodic reimaging. Masses between 3 and 6 cm are problematic and treatment must be individualized. Nuclear scan or fine-needle aspiration, or both, may be helpful in defining the mass.

Barzon L, Scaroni C, Sonino N, et al: Incidentally discovered adrenal tumors: Endocrine and scintigraphic correlates. J Clin Endocrinol Metab 83:55, 1998.
Bondanelli M, Campo M, Trasforino G, et al: Evaluation of hormonal function in a series of incidentally discovered adrenal masses. Metabolism 46:107, 1997.
Li BDL, Douglass HO: Management of the incidentally discovered adrenal mass or "incidentaloma." J La State Med Soc 149:291, 1997.

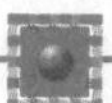

SECTION 5

Disorders of the Gonads

Robert Rapaport

CHAPTER 592
Development and Function of the Gonads

EMBRYONIC GONADAL DIFFERENTIATION. The undifferentiated, bipotential fetal gonad arises from a thickening of the urogenital ridge, close to the region that forms the kidney and adrenal cortex. At 6 wk of gestation, the gonad contains germ cells, stromal cells that will become Leydig cells in testes, or theca, interstitial or hilar cells in the ovary, and supporting cells that will develop into Sertoli cells in testes or granulosa cells in ovaries. In the absence of a testis-determining factor, thought to be the SRY (sex-determining region on the Y chromosome), the gonad develops into an ovary.

A 46,XX complement of chromosomes is necessary for the development of normal ovaries. Both the long and the short arms of X chromosomes bear genes for normal ovarian development. The DSS (dosage sensitive-sex reversal) locus associated with the DAX 1 gene responsible for X-linked congenital adrenal hypoplasia may contain a gene that controls ovarian differentiation. Autosomal genes also play a role in normal ovarian organogenesis and testicular development. Several conditions of gonadal dysgenesis are associated with chromosomal abnormalities. A deletion affecting the short arm of the X chromosome produces the typical somatic anomalies of Turner syndrome.

Development of the testis requires a Y chromosome, but the short arm of the Y chromosome is critical for sex determination; a testis-determining factor at this site has been identified, and the gene for it has been cloned and designated SRY. During male meiosis, the Y chromosome must segregate from the X chromosome so that both X and Y chromosomes do not occur in the same spermatozoa. The major portion of the Y chromosome is composed of Y-specific sequences that do not pair with the X chromosome. However, a minor portion of the Y chromosome shares sequences with the X chromosome, and pairing does occur in this region. The genes and sequences in this area recombine between the sex chromosomes behaving like autosomal genes. Therefore the term *pseudoautosomal* is used to describe the genetic behavior of these genes. The SRY gene is localized to the 35-kilobase portion proximal to this pairing and exchange (pseudoautosomal) region of the Y chromosome. It contains a high-mobility group nonhistone protein (HMG box), suggesting that SRY may be a transcriptional regulator of other, some as yet unidentified, genes involved in sex differentiation. These include SOX 9, an SRY-related gene, containing a shared motif homologous with the high-mobility group box 9 (HMG box 9) of SRY, located on chromosome 17 that results in sex reversal and campomelic dysplasia, steroidogenic factor 1 (SF-1) on chromosome 9q33, and the Wilms tumor genes (WTI) on chromosome 11p13 needed for early gonadal, adrenal, and renal development. When recombination events extend beyond the pseudoautosomal region, X- and Y-specific DNA may be transferred between the chromosomes. Such aberrant recombinations result in X chromosomes carrying SRY, resulting in XX males, or Y chromosomes that have lost SRY, resulting in XY females. SRY in some unknown way induces the indifferent genital ridge to develop into a testis.

FUNCTION OF THE TESTES. In the 1st trimester of pregnancy, levels of placental chorionic gonadotropin peak (8–12 wk) and stimulate the fetal Leydig cells to secrete testosterone, the main hormonal product of the testis. This period is critical for normal virilization of the XY fetus. Defects in this process lead to different forms of male pseudohermaphroditism (see Chapter 598.2). After virilization occurs, fetal levels of testosterone decrease but are maintained at low levels in the latter half of pregnancy by luteinizing hormone (LH) secreted by the fetal pituitary; this is required for continued penile growth.

Shortly after birth, a transient increase of gonadotropins, especially LH, occurs, leading to a sharp increase in serum levels of testosterone, which peak at about 1–3 mo of age (80–400 ng/dL). Thereafter, levels of gonadotropins subside, and by 6 mo of age, levels of testosterone decrease to the low prepubertal levels (10–20 ng/mL) that persist until the beginning of puberty. The significance of the neonatal testosterone surge is unknown. Neonates with testicular torsion and atrophy have very low levels of testosterone and markedly elevated levels of follicle-stimulating hormone (FSH) and LH. The development of nocturnal pulsatile secretion of LH marks the advent of puberty (see Chapter 571).

Within specific target cells, about 6–8% of testosterone is converted by 5-reductase to dihydrotestosterone, another potent androgen (see Fig. 598–1), and about 0.3% is acted on by aromatase to produce estradiol (see Fig. 589–1). Approximately half of circulating testosterone is bound to *sex hormone-binding globulin* (SHBG) and half to albumin; only 2% circulates in the free form. Plasma levels of SHBG are low at birth, rise rapidly during the 1st 10 days of life, and then remain stable until the onset of puberty. Thyroid hormone may play a role in this physiologic increase because neonates with athyreosis have very low levels of SHBG.

Müllerian-inhibiting substance (MIS), also called *antimüllerian hormone,* a 145-kd homodimeric glycoprotein hormone, is the earliest secreted product of the Sertoli cells of the fetal testis. Produced as a prohormone, its C-terminal fragment needs to be removed before it is active by way of a plasma membrane receptor. Its transcription in immature Sertoli cells is activated by the nuclear receptor SF-1 (steroidogenic factor 1). The gene for MIS has been cloned and mapped to chromosome 19. The gene for the MIS receptor (cloned and mapped to chromosome 12) is expressed in Sertoli cells and also in fetal müllerian duct and fetal and postnatal granulosa cells. During sexual differentiation, MIS causes involution of the embryologic precursors of the cervix, uterus, and fallopian tubes (müllerian ducts).

MIS is secreted in males by Sertoli cells both during fetal and postnatal life. In females, it is secreted by granulosa cells only postnatally. Hence, the serum concentration of MIS in males is highest at birth, whereas in females it is detected only at puberty. After puberty, both sexes have similar serum concentrations of MIS.

Inhibin is another glycoprotein hormone secreted by the Sertoli cells of the testes and granulosa and theca cells of the ovary. Inhibin A consists of an α subunit disulfide linked to the β A subunit, whereas inhibin B consists of the same α subunit linked to the β B subunit.

Activins are dimers of the B subunits—either homodimers (BA/BA, BB/BB) or heterodimers (BA/BB). Inhibins selectively inhibit, whereas activins stimulate pituitary FSH secretion. By means of immunoassays specific for inhibin A or B, it has been shown that inhibin A is absent in males and is present mostly in the luteal phase in women. Inhibin B is the principal form of inhibin in males and females during the follicular phase. Inhibin B may be used as a marker of Sertoli cell function in males. FSH stimulates inhibin B secretion in females and males, but only in males is there also evidence for a gonadotropin-independant way of its regulation.

Like inhibin and activin, follistatin (a single-chain glycosylated protein) is produced by gonads and other tissues such as the hypothalamus, kidney, adrenal gland, and placenta. Follistatin inhibits FSH secretion principally by binding activins, blocking activins' effects at the level of both ovary and pituitary.

An additional plethora of peptides are known to be involved as mediators of the development and function of the testis. They include neurohormones such as growth hormone–releasing hormone, gonadotropin-releasing hormone (GnRH), corticotropin-releasing hormone, oxytocin, arginine vasopressin, somatostatin, substance P, and neuropeptide Y; growth factors such as insulin-like growth factors (IGFs) and IGF-binding proteins, transforming growth factor β (TGF-β), fibroblast, platelet-derived, and nerve growth factors; vasoactive peptides; and immune-derived cytokines such as tumor necrosis factor and interleukins IL-1, IL-2, IL-4, and IL-6.

Considerable attention will continue to be focused on the complex endocrine and, especially, paracrine, autocrine, and intracrine effects of these regulatory peptides.

Clinical patterns of pubertal changes vary widely (see Chapters 14 and 571). In 95% of boys, enlargement of the genitals begins between 9.5 and 13.5 yr, reaching maturity from 13–17 yr. In a minority of normal boys, puberty begins after 15 yr of age. In some boys, pubertal development is completed in less than 2 yr, but in others, it may take longer than 4.5 yr. The adolescent growth spurt occurs later in boys than in girls at corresponding levels of sexual maturation; for example, the peak velocity of change in height is not attained in boys until the genitals are well developed, but in girls the growth rate is usually at its maximum when the nipple and areola have developed but before there is any other significant breast development.

The median age of sperm production *(spermarche)* is 14 yr. This event occurs in midpuberty as judged by pubic hair, testes size, evidence of growth spurt, and testosterone levels. Nighttime levels of FSH are in the adult male range at the time of spermarche; the first conscious ejaculation occurs at about the same time.

FUNCTION OF THE OVARIES. Without the presence of the SRY gene, the undifferentiated gonad can be identified histologically as an ovary by 10–11 wk of gestation. Oocytes are present from the 4th mo of gestation and reach a peak of 7 million by 5 mo of gestation. For normal maintenance, oocytes need granulosa cells to form primordial follicles. Normal X chromosomes are needed for the maintenance of the oocytes. In contrast to somatic cells, in which only one X chromosome is active, both are active in germ cells. At birth, the ovaries contain about 1 million active follicles, which decrease to 0.5 million by menarche. Thereafter, they decrease at a rate of 1000/mo, and at an even higher rate after the age of 35 yr.

The hormones of the fetal ovary are provided in most part by the fetoplacental unit. As in males, peak gonadotropin secretion occurs in fetal life and then again at 2–3 mo of life, with the lowest levels at about 6 yr of age. In both infancy and childhood, gonadotropin levels are higher in females than in males.

The most important estrogens produced by the ovary are estradiol-17 (E_2) and estrone (E_1); estriol is a metabolic product of these two, and all three estrogens may be found in the urine of mature females. Estrogens also arise from androgens in the adrenal gland and in the testis; the pathway for this conversion is shown in Figure 589–1. This conversion explains why in certain types of male pseudohermaphroditism, feminization occurs at puberty; in 17-ketosteroid reductase deficiency, for example, the enzymatic block results in markedly increased secretion of androstenedione, which is converted in the peripheral tissues to estradiol and estrone; these estrogens, in addition to those directly secreted by the testis, result in gynecomastia. The ovary also synthesizes progesterone, a progestational steroid; the adrenal cortex and testis synthesize progesterone as a precursor for other adrenal and testicular hormones.

As in the testis (see earlier), a host of other hormones with autocrine, paracrine, and intracrine effects have been identified in the ovary. They include inhibins, activins, relaxin, and growth factors IGF-I, TGF-α and β, and cytokines.

Plasma levels of estradiol increase slowly but steadily with advancing sexual maturation and correlate well with clinical evaluation of pubertal development, skeletal age, and rising levels of FSH. Levels of LH do not rise until secondary sexual characteristics are well developed. Estrogens, like androgens, inhibit secretion of both LH and FSH (negative feedback). In females, estrogens also provoke the surge of LH secretion that occurs in the midmenstrual cycle. The capacity for this positive feedback is another maturational milestone of puberty.

The average age at menarche in American girls is 12.5–13 yr, but the range of "normal" is wide, and 1–2% of "normal" girls have not menstruated by 16 yr of age. The age of onset of pubertal signs varies, with recent studies suggesting earlier ages then previously thought, especially in the United States

African American population (see Chapter 14). Menarche generally correlates closely with skeletal age (see Chapters 14 and 571). Maturation and closure of the epiphyses is at least partially estrogen-dependent, as demonstrated by a 28-yr-old, normally masculinized male with incomplete closure of the epiphyses who proved to have complete estrogen insensitivity because of an estrogen-receptor defect.

DIAGNOSTIC AIDS. Improved, sensitive, and specific assays for pituitary and gonadal hormones that can be measured in small amounts of blood have contributed to rapid advances in the understanding of normal and aberrant hypothalamic-pituitary-gonadal interactions. For example, in infant males measurements of LH, FSH, and testosterone can detect pituitary-testicular defects. Leydig cell integrity in childhood can be determined by the testosterone response following human chorionic gonadotropic administration such as 5,000 IU daily for 3 days. The integrity as well as the maturity of the hypothalamic-pituitary-gonadal axis in males and females can be assessed by the administration of GnRH or a GnRH analog.

Normal inhibin B levels have been documented in infant boys; inhibin B may be a marker for granulosa cell tumors. Estrogen-receptor assays may be clinically useful in the management of various ovarian cancers. MIS measurements are useful in the evaluation of children with nonpalpable gonads and intersex problems.

THERAPEUTIC AIDS. Phytoestrogens, a family of plant compounds such as soy and flax products, have been shown to have both estrogenic and antiestrogenic properties. Their potential health consequences, so far based largely on population studies, are being investigated. Naturally occurring estrogens administered orally are rapidly destroyed by gastrointestinal and liver enzymes; accordingly, they are usually given as conjugates or esters. The most widely used oral preparations are equine conjugated estrogens (e.g., Premarin) and ethinyl estradiol. Estrogen-containing skin patches for transdermal absorption are also used. With improvements in the understanding of estrogen and estrogen receptor interactions, a new class of compounds called selective estrogen-receptor modulators have been synthesized. For example, raloxifene, a nonsteroidal benzothiophene derivative acts as an estrogen agonist in bone and liver and as an estrogen antagonist in breast and uterus. Androgens such as testosterone are generally injected intramuscularly as long-acting esters (enanthate or cypionate, most commonly) because of their potency and steady response. Transdermal testosterone patches applied to the scrotal or nonscrotal areas have to date been used mostly in adults with hypogonadism because of the difficulty in titrating the doses needed during childhood and adolescence. Oral preparations, such as methyltestosterone or fluoxymesterone, do not produce as potent an androgenic response and may be hepatotoxic. Testosterone undecenoate, another oral preparation, is used in Europe but not in the United States. Sublingual (microspheres or pellets) and buccal (absorption via the buccal mucosa) preparations of testosterone are in development.

CHAPTER 593
Hypofunction of the Testes

Testicular hypofunction may be primary in the testis (primary hypogonadism) or secondary to deficiency of pituitary gonadotropic hormones (secondary hypogonadism). Patients with primary hypogonadism have elevated levels of gonadotropin (hypergonadotropic); those with secondary hypogonadism have low or absent levels (hypogonadotropic).

593.1 Hypergonadotropic Hypogonadism in the Male (Primary Hypogonadism)

Defects of androgen production involving the fetal testis and resulting in male pseudohermaphroditism are discussed in Chapter 598.1.

ETIOLOGY. Congenital anorchia occurs in 0.6% of boys with nonpalpable testes (1/20,000 males). These boys have normal external genitals, indicating that a noxious factor damaged the fetal testes of the genetic male fetus sometime after sexual differentiation had taken place (14th wk of fetal life). Hence, some refer to this condition as vanishing testes syndrome. The condition has been reported in monozygotic twins. Low levels of testosterone (<10 ng/dL) and markedly elevated levels of luteinizing hormone (LH) and follicle-stimulating hormone (FSH) are found in the early postnatal months; thereafter, levels of gonadotropins tend to decrease even in agonadal children, rising to castration levels as the pubertal years approach. Stimulation with human chorionic gonadotropin (hCG) fails to evoke an increase in the levels of testosterone. Serum levels of müllerian-inhibiting substance are undetectable or low.

A syndrome of rudimentary testes has been described in which the testes are exceedingly small; this appears to be inherited as an autosomal or X-linked recessive trait. The cause is unknown. Atrophy of the testes may follow damage to the vascular supply as a result of unskillful manipulation of the testes during surgical procedures for correction of cryptorchidism or as a result of bilateral torsion of the testes. Acute orchitis in pubertal or adult males with mumps may also damage the testes; usually, only the reproductive function of the testes is impaired. The routine immunization of all prepubertal males with mumps vaccine should prevent this complication.

Testicular damage is a frequent consequence of chemotherapy and radiotherapy for cancer. The frequency and extent of damage depend on the agent used, total dosage, duration of therapy, and post-therapy interval of observation. Another important variable is age at therapy; germ cells are less vulnerable in prepubertal than in pubertal and postpubertal boys. Chemotherapy is most damaging if more then one agent is used. The use of alkylating agents such as cyclophosphamide in prepubertal children does not impair pubertal development, even though there may be biopsy evidence of germ cell damage. Most chemotherapeutic agents produce azoospermia and infertility more commonly then Leydig cell damage. Interleukin-2 can depress Leydig cell function, whereas interferon-α does not seem to affect gonadal function.

Radiation damage is dose-dependent (see Chapter 718). Temporary azoospermia can be seen with doses greater then 0.3 Gy, with permanent azoospermia seen with doses greater then 8 Gy. Leydig cells are more resistent to radiation. Mild damage as determined by elevated LH levels can be seen with up to 6 Gy; doses greater then 30 Gy cause hypogonadism in most. Whenever possible, testes should be shielded from radiation. Testicular function should be carefully evaluated in adolescents after multimodal treatment for cancer in childhood. Replacement therapy with testosterone and counseling concerning fertility may be indicated.

The term *hypogonadism* has been widely used to describe aspects in children with a variety of multiple malformation syndromes. The term often refers simply to cryptorchidism, a small phallus, or a scrotal anomaly. In many of these syndromes little is known about the function of the testes; hyper- or hypogonadotropic hypogonadism has been proved in some instances.

In patients with Prader-Willi syndrome, both hypogonadotropic hypogonadism and hypergonadotropic hypogonadism, perhaps secondary to cryptorchidism and its treatment, have been reported. Small testes and azoospermia are seen in patients with the Sertoli cell–only syndrome (germ cell aplasia or Del Castillo syndrome).

Various degrees of hypogonadism also occur in a significant percentage of patients with chromosomal aberrations such as Klinefelter syndrome or XX males.

CLINICAL MANIFESTATIONS. Primary hypogonadism may be suspected at birth if the testes and penis are abnormally small. The condition often is not noticed until puberty when secondary sex characteristics fail to develop. Facial, pubic, and axillary hair is scant or absent; there is neither acne nor regression of scalp hair; and the voice remains high pitched. The penis and scrotum remain infantile and may be almost obscured by pubic fat; the testes are small or absent. Fat accumulates in the region of the hips and buttocks and sometimes in the breasts and on the abdomen. The epiphyses close late in life; therefore, extremities are long. The span is several inches longer than the height, and the distance from the symphysis pubis to the soles of the feet is much greater than that from the symphysis to the vertex. The proportions of the body are described as eunuchoid. (The upper to lower segment ratio is considerably less then 0.9.) Many individuals with milder degrees of hypogonadism may be detected only by appropriate studies of the pituitary-gonadal axis. Examination of the testes should be performed routinely by pediatricians; testicular volumes as determined by comparison with standard orchidometers should be recorded.

DIAGNOSIS. Levels of serum FSH and, to a lesser extent, of LH are elevated to greater than age-specific normal values. These elevated levels indicate that even in the prepubertal child there is an active hypothalamic-gonadal feedback relationship. After the age of 11 yr, FSH and LH levels rise significantly, reaching the castrate range. Measurements of random plasma testosterone levels in prepubertal boys are not helpful because they are ordinarily low in normal prepubertal children, rising during puberty to attain adult levels. During puberty, these levels correlate better with testicular size, stage of sexual maturity, and bone age than with chronological age. In patients with primary hypogonadism, testosterone levels remain low at all ages. There is an attenuated rise or no rise following administration of hCG, in contrast to normal males in whom hCG produces a significant rise in plasma testosterone at any stage of development. Measurements of serum müllerian-inhibiting substance and inhibin levels may give an indication of gonadal presence and function.

NOONAN SYNDROME

ETIOLOGY. The term *Noonan syndrome* has been applied to males and females who have certain phenotypic features that occur also in females with Turner syndrome. These boys and girls have normal karyotypes. Noonan syndrome occurs in 1/2,000 live births. The disorder is usually sporadic, but affected siblings of the same and of different genders have been reported. Total or partial expression is present in 20% of relatives. Reports of male-to-male transmission suggest an autosomal dominant gene with variable expressivity. The gene has been mapped to chromosome 12q.

CLINICAL MANIFESTATIONS. The most common abnormalities are short stature, webbing of the neck, pectus carinatum or pectus excavatum, cubitus valgus, right-sided congenital heart disease, and characteristic facies. Hypertelorism, epicanthus, and downward slanted palpebral fissures, ptosis, micrognathia, and ear abnormalities are common. Other abnormalities such as clinodactyly, hernias, and vertebral anomalies occur less frequently. Moderate mental retardation occurs in 25% of patients. High-frequency sensorineural hearing loss is common. The cardiac defect is most often pulmonary valvular stenosis, hypertrophic cardiomyopathy, or atrial septal defect. Hepatosplenomegaly; several hematologic diseases, including low clotting factors XI and XII; acute lymphoblastic leukemia; and chronic myelomonocytic leukemia have been described in patients with Noonan syndrome. Features of both Noonan syndrome and type 1 neurofibromatosis have been reported, but linkage has been excluded. It is now thought that Noonan-like features can be part of the phenotypic variation of the NF-I gene mutation, suggesting the possible existance of a Noonan syndrome locus also on chromosome 17q. A few patients with NF-I and features of Noonan syndrome were subsequently reported as having Turner syndrome. Males frequently have cryptorchidism and small testes; they may be hypogonadal or normal. Puberty is delayed 2 yr on average; adult height is achieved by the end of the 2nd decade and usually reaches the lowest limit of the normal population.

TREATMENT. Human growth hormone has resulted in improvement in growth velocity comparable to that seen in patients with Turner syndrome without adverse effects on cardiac ventricular wall thickness, at least in the short term. The ultimate safety and efficacy of this treatment in improving final height is yet to be determined.

KLINEFELTER SYNDROME (also see Chapters 78 and 570)

ETIOLOGY. Approximately 1/500 to 1/1,000 newborn males has a 47,XXY chromosome complement, representing the most common sex chromosomal aneuploidy in males. The incidence approximates 1% among the mentally retarded, clustering among patients with IQs greater than 50 and among children admitted to psychiatric hospitals or referred to psychiatric clinics. In infertile males, the incidence is 3%. The chromosomal aberration most often results from meiotic nondisjunction of an X chromosome during parental gametogenesis; the extra X chromosome is maternal in origin in 54% and paternal in origin in 46% of patients. Increased maternal age predisposes to meiotic nondisjunction and to this syndrome, but in most instances maternal age is not advanced.

The 47,XXY complement is the most common chromosomal pattern in persons with Klinefelter syndrome (80%); some have mosaic patterns: 46,XY/47,XXY, 46,XY/48,XXYY, 45,X/46,XY/47,XXY, or 46,XX/47,XXY. Rarely, occurrence of more than two X chromosomes may result in Klinefelter variants: 48,XXXY, 49,XXXYY, 49,XXXXY, 50,XXXXYY, 47,XXY/48,XXXY, 47,XXY/49,XXXXY, or 48,XXYY karyotype. Even with as many as four X chromosomes, the Y chromosome determines a male phenotype. In most patients with four or five X chromosomes, all the additional chromosomes come from the same parent and are not associated with increased parental age.

CLINICAL MANIFESTATIONS. The diagnosis is rarely made before puberty because of the paucity or subtleness of clinical manifestations in childhood. Because behavioral or psychiatric disorders may often be apparent long before defects in sexual development, the condition should be considered in all boys with mental retardation and in children with psychosocial, learning, or school adjustment problems. Affected children may be anxious, immature, excessively shy, or aggressive, and they may engage in antisocial acts. Fire-setting behavior has been observed in some of these children. In a prospective study, a group of children with 47,XXY karyotypes identified at birth exhibited relatively mild deviations from normal during the first 5 yr of life. None had major physical, intellectual, or emotional disabilities; some were inactive, with poorly organized motor function and mild delay in language acquisition. Problems often first become apparent after the child begins school. Full-scale IQ scores may be normal, with verbal IQ being somewhat decreased. Verbal cognitive defects and underachievement in reading, spelling, and mathematics are common. By late adolescence, most boys with Klinefelter syndrome have generalized learning disabilities and are four to five grade levels behind. Despite these difficulties, most complete high school.

The patients tend to be tall, slim, and underweight and to have relatively long legs, but body habitus can vary markedly. The testes tend to be small for age, but this sign may become apparent only after puberty, when normal testicular growth fails to occur. The phallus tends to be smaller than average, and cryptorchidism or hypospadias may occur in a few patients.

Pubertal development may be delayed. Some degree of androgen deficiency is usually detected, although some children may undergo almost normal virilization. About 80% of adults have gynecomastia; they have sparser facial hair, most shaving less often than daily. The most common testicular lesions are spermatogenic arrest and Sertoli cell predominance. The sperm have a high incidence of sex chromosomal aneuploidy. Azoospermia and infertility are usual, although rare instances of fertility are known. Testicular sperm extraction followed by intracytoplasmic sperm injection can result in the birth of healthy infants. Antisperm antibodies have been detected in one quarter of tested specimens.

The height of patients with Klinefelter syndrome tends to be increased. There is an increased incidence of pulmonary disease, varicose veins, and cancer of the breast. Among 93 unselected male breast cancer patients, 7.5% were found to have Klinefelter syndrome. Mediastinal germ cell tumors have been reported; some of these tumors produce hCG and cause precocious puberty in young boys. They may also be associated with leukemia, lymphoma, and other hematologic neoplasias. The highest cancer risk (relative risk 2.7) occurs in the 15–30 yr age group.

In adults with XY/XXY mosaicism, the features of Klinefelter syndrome are decreased in severity and frequency. Children with mosaicism have a better prognosis for virilization, fertility, and psychosocial adjustment.

Klinefelter Variants. When the number of X chromosomes exceeds two, the clinical manifestations, including mental retardation and impairment of virilization, are more severe. The XXYY variant is the most common variant (1/50,000 male births). In most, mental retardation occurs with IQ scores between 60 and 80, but 10% have IQs greater then 110. The XXYY male phenotype is not distinctively different from that of the XXY patient, except that XXYY adults tend to be taller than the average XXY patient. The 49,XXXXY variant is sufficiently distinctive to be detected in childhood. Its incidence is estimated to be 1/80,000 to 1/100,000 male births. The disorder arises from sequential nondisjunction in meiosis. Affected patients are severely retarded, have short necks, and typical coarse facies with wide-set eyes with a mild upward slant of the fissures, epicanthus, strabismus, a wide and flat upturned nose, a large open mouth, and large malformed ears. The testes are small and may be undescended, the scrotum is hypoplastic, and the penis is very small. Defects suggestive of Down syndrome (e.g., short incurved terminal 5th phalanges, single palmar creases, and hypotonia) and other skeletal abnormalities (including defects in the carrying angle of the elbows and restricted supination) are common. The most frequent radiographic abnormalities are radioulnar synostosis or dislocation, elongated radius, pseudoepiphyses, scoliosis or kyphosis, coxa valga, and retarded osseous age. Most patients with such extensive changes have a 49,XXXXY chromosome karyotype; several mosaic patterns have also been observed: 48,XXXY/49,XXXXY (Fig. 593–1); 48,XXXY/49,XXXXY/50,XXXXXY; and 48,XXXY/49,XXXXY/50,XXXXYY.

The 48 XXXY variant is relatively rare. The characteristic features are generally less severe then in those patients with 49,XXXXY and more severe than in 47,XXY patients. Mild mental retardation, delayed speech and motor development, and immature but passive and pleasant behavior are associated with this condition.

Very few patients have been described with 49,XYYY and 49,XXYYY karyotypes. Dysmorphic features and mental retardation are common to both.

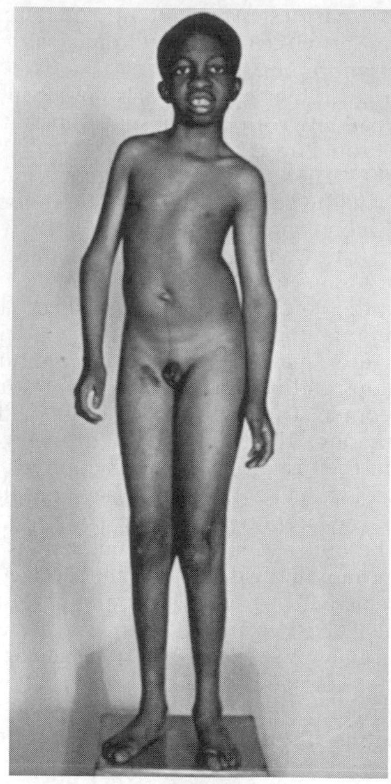

Figure 593–1 A 12-yr-old boy with 48,XXXY/49,XXXXY mosaicism who has prognathism, epicanthal folds, scoliosis, very small testes, severe mental retardation, clinodactyly, and radioulnar synostoses.

LABORATORY FINDINGS. Most males with this condition go through life undiagnosed. The chromosomes should be examined in all patients suspected of having Klinefelter syndrome, particularly those attending child guidance, psychiatric, and mental retardation clinics. Before 10 yr of age, boys with 47,XXY Klinefelter syndrome have normal basal plasma levels of FSH and LH. Responses to gonadotropin-stimulating hormone and to hCG are also normal. The testes show normal growth early in puberty, but by midpuberty testicular growth stops, gonadotropins become elevated, and testosterone levels are slightly low. Inhibin B levels are low in men with the syndrome. Elevated levels of estradiol, resulting in a high estradiol:testosterone ratio, account for the development of gynecomastia during puberty. Despite hypogonadism, most have normal bone mass.

Testicular biopsy before puberty may reveal only a deficiency or absence of germinal cells. After puberty, the seminiferous tubular membranes are hyalinized, and there is adenomatous clumping of Leydig cells. Sertoli cells predominate. Azoospermia is characteristic, and infertility is the rule.

TREATMENT. Replacement therapy with a long-acting testosterone preparation depends on the age of the patient. It should begin at 11–12 yr of age. The enanthate ester may be used in a starting dose of 25–50 mg injected intramuscularly every 3–4 wk, with 50-mg increments every 6–9 mo until a maintenance dose for adults (200–250 mg every 3–4 wk) is achieved. At that time, testosterone patches may be substituted for the injections. For older boys, larger initial doses and increments can achieve more rapid virilization. Testosterone treatment leads to an increase in prostate volume and prostate-specific antigen levels. Fertility can be accomplished by an intracytoplasmic sperm injection technique

XX MALES

This disorder is thought to occur in 1 of 20,000 newborn males. Affected individuals have a male phenotype, small testes, a small phallus, and no evidence of ovarian or müllerian duct tissue; they appear, therefore, to be distinct from the XX true hermaphrodite (see Chapter 598.3). This disorder resembles Klinefelter syndrome, but stature is greater in the latter. Undescended testes and hypospadias occur in a minority of patients. The histologic features of the testes are essentially the same as in Kleinfelter syndrome. Patients with the condition usually come to medical attention in adult life because of hypogonadism, gynecomastia, or infertility. Hypergonadotropic hypogonadism occurs secondary to testicular failure. A few cases have been diagnosed perinatally as a result of discrepancies between prenatal ultrasonography and karyotype findings.

In 80% of XX males with normal male external genitals, one of the X chromosomes carries the SRY gene. The exchange from the Y to the X chromosome occurs during paternal meiosis, when the short arms of the Y and X chromosomes pair. XX males inherit one maternal X chromosome and one paternal X chromosome containing the translocated male-determining gene. Such exchanges occur because of the proximity of the SRY gene to the pseudoautosomal region where recombination between X and Y chromosomes normally occurs in meiosis. Most XX males who are identified before puberty have hypospadias or micropenis; this group of patients usually lacks Y-specific sequences, suggesting other mechanisms for virilization (see Chapter 592).

45,X MALES (also see Chapter 592)

Of the few male patients recognized with a 45,X karyotype, Yp sequences have been translocated to an autosomal chromosome. In one instance, the terminal short arm of the Y chromosome was translocated onto an X chromosome.

XYY MALES

The 47,XYY male does not have hypogonadism; this condition is discussed here for easy comparison with the XXY and the XX male syndromes.

Approximately 1/1,000 newborn males has an XYY chromosome pattern. When this disorder was first discovered in adults, studies of XYY individuals in mental or penal institutions created a stereotype of affected individuals as having deviant behavior marked by physical aggressiveness and violence. The rate at which XYY males are found in mental or penal settings may be 20 times higher then the rate of the condition of birth. Adults with this karyotype may be relatively impulsive, antisocial, and likely to break the law, but they are not especially aggressive. Unselected 47,XYY boys detected in screening programs tend to exhibit attention deficits, impulsive behavior, inadequate interactions, and poor self-image. Patients with 48,XXYY and 48,XYYY karyotypes tend to have similar deviant behavior.

The XYY adult has few phenotypic manifestations. He tends to be tall and to have severe nodulocystic acne. In affected persons, genital abnormalities have been observed, but cryptic mosaicism, such as X/XYY, is a possibility in these instances. Prolonged PR intervals on electrocardiography and radioulnar synostosis occur more often than in the general population. Renal agenesis and cystic dysplasia of the kidney, as well as hematologic malignancies, have been reported. No clear-cut endocrine abnormalities have been found. This condition poses a serious dilemma for counseling of parents of infants or children discovered to have this sex chromosome complement. The risks for some developmental disability may not be trivial, but neither do they appear to be as dire as earlier thought. Still, the most common reason for a 47,XYY male to be karyotyped is developmental delay or behavioral problems, or both. Children with sex chromosome abnormalities are at an increased risk of learning disabilities, cognitive skill impairments, and difficulties in psychosocial adaptation. Stable, supportive, and compassionate family environments promote improved adaptation of these children and adolescents.

593.2 Hypogonadotropic Hypogonadism in the Male (Secondary Hypogonadism)

In hypogonadotropic hypogonadism, there is deficiency of FSH or LH, or both. The primary defect may lie in the anterior pituitary or in the hypothalamus as a deficiency of gonadotropin-releasing hormone (GnRH). The testes are normal but remain in the prepubertal state because stimulation by gonadotropins is lacking.

ETIOLOGY

Hypopituitarism. Most causes of hypopituitarism may be associated with deficiency of gonadotropins and hypogonadotropic hypogonadism (see Chapter 567). In patients with organic lesions in or near the pituitary, whether congenital or acquired, the gonadotropin deficiency is pituitary in origin. In most patients with "idiopathic" hypopituitarism, the defect is in the hypothalamus, caused by a deficiency of GnRH. Microphallus (<2.5 cm) in the newborn male with growth hormone deficiency suggests the likelihood of gonadotropin deficiency, and diagnostic confirmation is feasible; after 6 mo of age, gonadotropin deficiency can rarely be established with certainty until the teenage years.

Isolated Deficiency of Gonadotropin. Usually, this disorder involves the hypothalamus rather than the pituitary. It affects about 1/10,000 males and 1/50,000 females and encompasses a heterogeneous group of entities. GnRH deficiency may be complete or partial; it may occur sporadically or in families. *Kallmann syndrome*, one of the most frequent genetic forms of hypogonadotropic hypogonadism, is characterized by its association with anosmia or hypo-osmia. The X-linked disorder is caused by several mutations of the KAL gene at Xp22.3. The association reflects the failure of olfactory axons and GnRH-expressing neurons to migrate from their common origin in the olfactory placode to the brain. The KAL gene is also expressed in various parts of the brain. It appears that the KAL gene product functions in the guidance of neuronal migration.

Some kindreds contain anosmic individuals with or without hypogonadism; others contain hypogonadal individuals who are anosmic. Cleft lip and palate, hypotelorism, median facial clefts, sensorineural hearing loss, unilateral renal aplasia, neurologic deficits, and other findings occur in some affected patients. When Kallmann syndrome is caused by terminal or interstitial deletions of the Xp22.3 region, it may be associated with other contiguous gene syndromes such as steroid sulfatase deficiency, chondrodysplasia punctata, X-linked ichthyosis, or ocular albinism. Autosomal recessive and autosomal dominant forms of Kallmann syndrome have been reported.

As in patients with Kallmann syndrome, children with *X-linked congenital hypoplasia* have associated hypogonadotropic hypogonadism due to impaired GnRH secretion. In these patients, there is a mutation of the DAX-1 gene at Xp21.2–21.3, Conditions occasionally associated with these patients because of the contiguous gene syndrome include glycerol kinase deficiency, Duchenne muscular dystrophy, and ornithine transcarbamyltransferase deficiency (see Chapter 584).

Several genetic defects involving the hypothalmic-pituitary-gonadal axis have been identified. They involve the function of either hormones or their receptors. Depending on both the level and nature of the mutation, hypogonadism, precocious puberty, or sexual ambiguity may develop. A compound heterozygote mutation of the GnRH-receptor gene, located on the long arm of chromosome 4, has been identified as the cause of hypogonadotropic hypogonadism in a family. A mutation in the gene for the β subunit of LH at the level of the pituitary causes hypogonadotropic hypogonadism. At the level of the gonads, LH-receptor defects have led to Leydig cell hypoplasia and undervirilization in genetic males. A boy was reported with micropenis and normal testes that did not produce testosterone even after repeated courses of hCG. Vanishing Leydig cell syndrome was thought to be a possibility (by analogy with the vanishing testes syndrome): Normally functioning Leydig cells must have been present in the first trimester of pregnancy, but because of LH receptor defect, inadequate testosterone production in the 2nd and 3rd trimesters led to an underdeveloped penis at birth. A novel mutation of the β subunit of FSH also has been described as the cause of hypogonadism in an 18-yr-old man evaluated for delayed puberty (Table 593–1).

Other Disorders. Hypogonadotropic hypogonadism has been observed in a few patients with polyglandular autoimmune syndrome, in some with elevated melatonin levels, and in a variety of other syndromes such as Bardet-Biedl, Prader-Willi, multiple lentigines, and several syndromes of ataxia. The sites of most of these defects are unknown.

DIAGNOSIS. Levels of gonadotropins and gonadal steroids remain in the prepubertal range, and nocturnal pulsatile secretion of LH does not occur. The gonadotropin response to stimulation with GnRH or a more potent analog of GnRH is markedly blunted. These findings are also consistent with those observed in normal adolescents with the variant known as constitutional delayed puberty; it is difficult to distinguish between the two conditions. Many different tests, including stimulation tests with GnRH, thyrotropin-releasing hormone, metoclopramide, and domperidone, have yielded inconclusive results. The measurement of a single, 8 A.M. testosterone level may be a good indicator of impending puberty. A value of more then 0.7 nmol/L (20 mg/dL) was noted in boys, all of whom had an increase in testicular volume to greater than 4 mL by 15 mo and 77% by 12 mo. In contrast, of boys with testosterone levels lower then 0.7 nmol/L, only 25% entered puberty by 15 yr of age. The use of a GnRH analog or the GnRH test following 36 hr of "priming" of the hypothalamic-pituitary-gonadal axis with pulsatile GnRH administration may distinguish adolescents with hypogonadism from those with delayed puberty.

Gonadotropin deficiency is likely if the patient has evidence of another pituitary deficiency, such as a deficiency of growth hormone, particularly if it is associated with corticotropin (adrenocorticotropic hormone [ACTH]) deficiency. The presence of anosmia usually indicates permanent gonadotropin deficiency, but occasional instances of markedly delayed puberty (18–20 yr of age) have been observed in anosmic individuals. Although anosmia may be present in the family or in the patient from early childhood, its existence is rarely volunteered, and direct questioning is necessary in all patients with delayed puberty. Magnetic resonance imaging may detect anomalous olfactory lobes and sulci in some patients. Prolactinomas are increasingly recognized as a cause of delayed puberty and should be excluded by determination of serum levels of prolactin.

Probes are available to establish the diagnosis in heterozygotes and newborn infants with the X-linked form of Kallmann syndrome. During the first 3–4 mo of life, unaffected infants demonstrate the usual physiologic rise in gonadotropins and gonadal steroids, and the response to GnRH exceeds that seen in prepubertal children.

TREATMENT. Constitutional delayed puberty should be ruled out before a diagnosis of isolated deficiency of GnRH is established and treatment is initiated. Testicular volume of less than 4 mL by 14 yr of age occurs in about 3% of boys, but true hypogonadotropic hypogonadism is a rare condition. Even relatively moderate delays in sexual development and growth may result in significant psychologic distress and require attention. Initially, an explanation of the variations characteristic of puberty and reassurance suffice for the majority of boys. If by 15 yr of age there is no clinical evidence of puberty beginning, and the testosterone level is less than 50 ng/dL, a brief course of testosterone is indicated. Testosterone enanthate, 100 mg intramuscularly once monthly for 4–6 mo, usually results in an increase in the signs of secondary sexual characteristics and an increase in growth velocity; it may initiate puberty and may differentiate constitutional delay in puberty from isolated gonadotropin deficiency. The age of initiation of this treatment must be individualized.

Patients with established deficiency of gonadotropins should be treated with the same program of repository testosterone as that used for those with primary testicular deficiency (see Chapter 593.1). With this therapy, the testes will remain small. Treatment with hCG, given subcutaneously or intramuscularly in doses of 500–1,000 IU, three times weekly, stimulates growth of the testes and spermatogenesis. If, after 6–12 mo of therapy, sufficient growth of the testes has not occurred, human menopausal gonadotropin may be added in doses of 37.5–150 IU, three times weekly. It may require up to 2 yr of treatment to achieve adequate spermatogenesis in adults. Recombinantly produced gonadotropins are able to stimulate gonadal growth and function.

A more physiologic, but cumbersome, form of treatment consists of episodic administration (subcutaneously or intravenously) of GnRH. Long-term therapy has been provided with a programmable peristaltic infusion pump. Most patients require about 2 yr of treatment to maximize testicular growth and achieve spermatogenesis.

TABLE 593–1 Known Gene Defects Causing Hypogonadism

Defect	Clinical Condition	Affected Gender
Gonadotropin-Releasing Hormone		
KAL-1	Kallmann syndrome	Both
DAX-1	X-linked adrenal hypoplasia and hypogonadotropic hypogonadism	Male
Receptor	Familial hypogonadotropic hypogonadism	Both
Luteinizing Hormone		
β Subunit	Pubertal delay, Leydig cell hypoplasia, infertility	Male
Receptor	Male pseudohermaphroditism, Leydig cell hypoplasia, micropenis Amenorrhea	Both
Follicle-Stimulating Hormone		
β Subunit	Pubertal delay Amenorrhea	Both
Receptor	Ovarian failure Ovarian germ cell tumors	Female

Abramsky L, Chapple J: 47,XXY (Klinefelter syndrome) and 47,XYY: Estimated rates of and indication for postnatal diagnosis with implications for prenatal counselling. Prenat Diagn 17:363, 1997.
Anderson A, Toppari J, Haavisto A, et al: Longitudinal reproductive hormone profiles in infants: Peak of inhibin B levels in infant boys exceeds levels in adult men. J Clin Endocrinol Metab 83:675, 1998.
Bader-Meunier B, Tchernia G, Mielot F, et al: Occurrence of myeloproliferative disorder in patients with Noonan syndrome. J Pediatr 130:885, 1997.
Bahuau M, Houdayer C, Assouline B, et al: Novel recurrent nonsense mutation causing neurofibromatosis type 1 (NF1) in a family segregating both NF1 and Noonan syndrome. Am J Med Genet 75:254, 1998.
Bender BG, Harmon RJ, Linden MG, Robinson A: Psychosocial adaptation of 39 adolescents with sex chromosome abnormalities. Pediatrics 96:302, 1995.
Cotterill AM, McKenna WJ, Brady AF, et al: The short-term effects of growth hormone therapy on height velocity and cardiac ventricular wall thickness in children with Noonan syndrome. J Clin Endocrinol Metab 81:2291, 1996.
Crowne EC, Shalet SM: Management of constitutional delay in growth and puberty. Trends Endocrinol Metab 1:239, 1990.
DeRoux N, Young J, Misrahi M, et al: A family with hypogonadotropic hypogonadism and mutations in the gonadotropin-releasing hormone receptor. N Engl J Med 337:1597, 1997.
Dobs AS, Hoover DR, Chen MC, Allen R: Pharmacokinetic characteristics, efficacy, and safety of buccal testosterone in hypogonadal males: A pilot study. J Clin Endocrinol Metab 83:33, 1998.
Ehrmann DA, Rosenfield RL, Cuttler L, et al: A new test of combined pituitary testicular function using the gonadotropin-releasing hormone agonist nafarelin in the differentiation of gonadotropin deficiency from delayed puberty: Pilot studies. J Clin Endocrinol Metab 69:963, 1989.
Fauser BCJM, VanHeusden AM: Manipulation of human ovarian function: Physiological concepts and clinical consequences. Endocr Rev 18:71, 1997.
Foresta C, Galeazzi C, Bettella A, et al: High incidence of sperm sex chromosomes aneuploidies in two patients with Klinefelter's syndrome. J Clin Endocrinol Metab 83:203, 1998.
Fuleihan GEH: Tissue-specific estrogens—the promise for the future. N Engl J Med, 337:1686, 1997.
Gnessi J, Fabbri A, Spera G: Gonadal peptides as mediators of development and functional control of the testis: An integrated system with hormones and local environment. Endocr Rev 18:541, 1997.
Hayes FJ, Hall JE, Boepple PA, Crowley WF: Differential control of gonadotropin secretion in the human: Endocrine role of inhibin. J Clin Endocrinol Metab 826:1835, 1998.
Hultborn R, Hanson C, Kopf I, et al: Prevalence of Klinefleter's syndrome in male breast cancer patients. Anticancer Res 17:4293, 1997.
Kotlar TJ, Young RH, Albanese C, et al: A mutation in the follicle-stimulating hormone receptor occurs frequently in human ovarian sex cord tumors. J Clin Endocrinol Metab 82:1020, 1997.
Latronico AC, Anasti J, Arnhold IJ, et al: Brief report: Testicular and ovarian resistance to luteinizing hormone caused by inactivating mutations of the luteinizing hormone–receptor gene. N Engl J Med 334:507,1996.
Layman LC, Lee EJ, Peak DB, et al: Delayed puberty and hypogonadism caused by mutations in the follicle stimulating hormone β-subunit gene. N Engl J Med 337:607, 1997.
Lee MM, Donahoe PK, Silverman BL, et al: Measurements of serum mullerian inhibiting substance in the evaluation of children with nonpalpable gonads. N Engl J Med 336:1480, 1997.
MacLean HE, Warne GL, Zajac JD: Intersex disorders: Shedding light on male sexual differentiation beyond SRY. Clin Endocrinol 46:101, 1997.
Matthews CH, Borgato S, Beck-Peccoz, et al: Primary amenorrhoea and infertility due to a mutation in the β-subunit of follicle-stimulating hormone. Nat Genet 5:83, 1993.
Meyer J, Sudbeck P, Held M, et al: Mutational analysis of the SOX9 gene in campomelic dysplasia and autosomal sex reversal: Lack of genotype/phenotype correlations. Hum Mol Genet 6:9108, 1997.
Misrahi M, Meduri G, Pissard S, et al: Comparison of immunocytochemical and molecular features with the phenotype in a case of incomplete male pseudohermaphroditism associated with a mutation of the luteinizing hormone receptor. J Clin Endocrinol Metab 82:2159, 1997.
Muller J: Hypogonadism and endocrine metabolic disorders in Prader-Willi syndrome. Acta Paediatr Suppl 423:58, 1997.
Numabe H, Nagafuchi S, Nakahuri Y, et al: DNA analysis of XX and XX-hypospadiac males. Hum Genet 90:211, 1992.
Olsen NJ, Kovacs WJ: Gonadal steroids and immunity. Endocr Rev 17:369, 1996.
Palermo GD, Schlegel PN, Sills, ES: Births after intracytoplasmic injection of sperm obtained by testicular extraction from men with nonmosaic Klinefelter's syndrome. N Engl J Med 338:588, 1998.
Phillip M, Arbelle JE, Segev Y, Parvari R: Male hypogonadism due to a mutation in the gene for the β-subunit of follicle-stimulating hormone. N Engl J Med 338:1729, 1998.
Ranke MB, Heidemann P, Knupter C, et al: Noonan syndrome: Growth and clinical manifestations in 144 cases. Eur J Pediatr 148:220, 1988.
Revelli A, Massobrio M, Tesarik J: Nongenomic actions of steroid hormones in reproductive tissues. Endocr Rev 19:3, 1998.
Romano AA, Blethen SL, Dana K, Noto RA: Growth hormone treatment in Noonan syndrome: the National Cooperative Growth Study experience. J Pediatr 128:S18, 1996.
Rosenfeld RL: Diagnosis and management of delayed puberty. J Clin Endocrinol Metab 70:559, 1990.
Rovet J, Netley C, Keenan M, et al: The psychoeducational profile of boys with Klinefelter syndrome. J Learn Disabil 29:180, 1996.
Sengul A, Gul D, Sayli BS, et al: Antisperm antibody and Klinefelter syndrome: Does autoimmunity play a role in the pathogenesis? Urol Int 57:77, 1996.
Smals AGH, Hermus ARM, Boers GHJ, et al: Predictive value of luteinizing hormone releasing hormone (LHRH) bolus testing before and after 36-hour pulsatile LHRH administration in the differential diagnosis of constitutional delay of puberty and male hypogonadotropic hypogonadism. J Clin Endocrinol Metab 78:602, 1994.
Stavrou SS, Zhu YS, Cai LQ, et al: A novel mutation of the human luteinizing hormone receptor in 46XY and 46XX sisters. J Clin Endocrinol Metab 83:2091, 1998.
Than DM, Gardner CD, Haskell WL: Clinical Review 97, Potential health benefits of dietary phytoestrogens: A review of the clinical, epidemiological and mechanistic evidence. J Clin Endocrinol Metab 83:2223, 1998.
Toledo SPA, Brunner HG, Kraaij R, et al: An inactivating mutation of the luteinizing hormone receptor causes amenorrhea in a 46,XX female. J Clin Endocrinol Metab 81:3850, 1996.
VanDop C, Burstein S, Conte FA, et al: Isolated gonadotropin deficiency in boys: Clinical characteristics and growth. J Pediatr 111:684, 1987.
Wu FC, Brown DC, Butler GE, et al: Early morning plasma testosterone is an accurate predictor of imminent pubertal development in prepubertal boys. J Clin Endocrinol Metab 76:26, 1993.
Yeung SCJ, Chiu AC, Vassilopolor-Sellin R, Gagel RF: The endocrine effects of nonhormonal antineoplastic therapy. Endocr Rev 19:144, 1998.

CHAPTER 594

Pseudoprecocity Resulting from Tumors of the Testes

Leydig cell tumors of the testes are rare causes of precocious pseudopuberty and cause asymmetric enlargement of the testes. Leydig cells are sparse before puberty; tumors derived from them are more common in the adult. The reported cases in children include one member in each of two pairs of identical twins. These tumors are usually unilateral and benign. Reinke crystalloids are a characteristic microscopic feature but occur in fewer than 50% of Leydig cell tumors. A gsp mutation was described in one testicular Leydig cell tumor. In adult testes, testicular germ cell tumors, but not Sertoli cell tumors or Leydig cell tumors, exhibit biallelic expression of the human H19 gene.

The *clinical manifestations* are those of puberty in the male; onset occurs usually from 5–9 yr of age. Gynecomastia has been described. The tumor of the testis can usually be readily felt; the contralateral unaffected testis is normal in size for the age of the patient.

Plasma levels of testosterone are markedly elevated. Follicle-stimulating hormone and luteinizing hormone levels are suppressed, and there is no response to gonadotropin-releasing hormone. Ultrasonography may aid in the detection of small nonpalpable tumors.

Treatment consists of surgical removal of the affected testis. Progression of virilization ceases, and partial reversal of the signs of precocity may occur.

Testicular adrenal rests may develop into tumors that mimic Leydig cell tumors; in the absence of Reinke crystals, these two tumors cannot be differentiated histologically. Adrenal rest tumors are usually bilateral and occur in children with congenital adrenal hyperplasia, usually salt-losing patients, during adolescence or young adult life. The stimulus for the growth of the adrenal rests is inadequate corticosteroid suppressive therapy, and treatment with adequate doses almost always results in their regression. Definite evidence of the origin of these tumors has been achieved by demonstrating their 21-hydroxylase activity. The misdiagnosis of these tumors in patients with congenital adrenal hyperplasia has led to unnecessary orchidectomy.

Fragile X syndrome is the most frequent cause of hereditary mental retardation, with an incidence of 1/2,000 births. It is caused by the amplification of a polymorphic CGG repeat in the 5′ untranslated region of the FMRI gene at Xp17.3. Amplified beyond 200 units, the repeat CGG sequence leads to methylation of the promoter region of FMRI and to a lack of gene product (FMRP). A cardinal characteristic of the condition is testicular enlargement (macro-orchidism), reaching 40–50 mL after puberty. Although the condition has been recognized in a child as young as 5 mo of age, affected boys younger than 6 yr of age rarely have testicular enlargement; by 8–10 yr of age, most have testicular volumes greater than 3 mL. The testes are enlarged bilaterally, are not nodular, and are histologically normal. Results of hormonal studies are normal. Direct DNA analysis searching for CGG repeat sequences permits definitive diagnosis (see Chapter 76).

Sex cord tumors with annular tubules of the testes can cause breast development in young boys. These tumors usually are associated with Peutz-Jeghers syndrome; they occur bilaterally, are multifocal, and are detectible by ultrasonography. Excessive production of aromatase ($P450_{arom}$) causes feminization of these boys.

In boys with *unilateral cryptorchidism*, the contralateral testis is about 25% larger than normal for age. Testicular enlargement has also been noted in boys with Henoch-Schönlein purpura and lymphangiectasia. Epidermoid and dermoid cysts of the testes have been reported rarely.

Clark RV, Albertson BD, Monabi A, et al: Steroidogenic enzyme activities, morphology and receptor studies of a testicular rest in a patient with congenital adrenal hyperplasia. J Clin Endocrinol Metab 70:1408, 1990.
Coen P, Kulin H, Ballantine T, et al: An aromatase-producing sex-cord tumor resulting in prepubertal gynecomastia. N Engl J Med 324:317, 1991.
Combes-Moukousky ME, Kottler ML, Valensi P, et al: Gonadal and adrenal catheterization during adrenal suppression and gonadal stimulation in a patient with bilateral testicular tumors and congenital adrenal hyperplasia. J Clin Endocrinol Metab 79:1390, 1994.
Fragoso MCBV, Latronico AC, Carvalho FM, et al: Activating mutation of the stimulatory G protein (gsp) as a putative cause of ovarian and testicular human stromal Leydig cell tumors. J Clin Endocrinol Metab 83:2074, 1998.
Hoogeveen AT, Oostra BA: The fragile X syndrome. J Inherit Metab Dis 20:139, 1997.
Nisula BC, Loriaux DL, Sherins RJ, et al: Benign bilateral testicular enlargement. J Clin Endocrinol Metab 38:440, 1974.
Rosenberg T, Gilboa Y, Golik A, et al: Pseudoprecocious puberty in a young boy due to interstitial cell adenomas of the testis. Helv Paediatr Acta 39:79, 1984.

CHAPTER 595
Gynecomastia

Gynecomastia, or the occurrence of mammary tissue in the male, is a common condition. It is almost always a sign of estrogen-androgen imbalance, but its cause is often obscure. It occurs in most newborn males as a result of stimulation by maternal hormones; the effect disappears in a few weeks.

During early to midpuberty, approximately two thirds of boys develop various degrees of subareolar hyperplasia of the breasts. *Physiologic pubertal gynecomastia* may involve only one breast, and it is not unusual for both breasts to enlarge at disproportionate rates or at different times. Tenderness of the breast is common but transitory. Spontaneous regression may occur within a few months; it rarely persists longer than 2 yr. Mean concentrations of follicle-stimulating hormone, luteinizing hormone, prolactin, testosterone, estrone, and estradiol are the same as in boys without gynecomastia. When levels are correlated with stage of puberty, a decreased ratio of testosterone to estradiol is found in boys with gynecomastia. Cultured pubic skin fibroblasts from boys with gynecomastia show excessive aromatase activity. *Treatment* usually consists of reassuring the boy and his family of the physiologic and transient nature of the phenomenon. Surgical removal of the breast is rarely indicated; when enlargement is striking and persistent and causes serious emotional disturbance to the patient, removal may be justified. One technique involves endoscopically assisted transaxillary removal of glandular tissue.

Benign, self-limited, and usually transient gynecomastia has been reported in prepubertal children during the initiation of therapy with human growth hormone.

Occasionally, breast development may mimic female breast development (to Tanner stages 3–5) and fails to regress. *Familial gynecomastia* has occurred in several kindreds as an X-linked or autosomal dominant sex-limited trait. Levels of gonadotropins, testosterone, prolactin, and steroid-binding globulins are normal. Increased peripheral conversion of C19-steroids to estrogens (increased aromatization) has been found in familial and sporadic cases of gynecomastia and may explain some instances of this condition.

A report of the *syndrome of aromatase excess* in a father and his son and daughter suggests autosomal dominant inheritance. There was gynecomastia in the 9-yr-old boy and macromastia and isosexual precocity in his 7.5-yr-old sister. Excess aromatase activity was shown in skin fibroblasts and transformed lymphocytes in vitro. This was associated with $P450_{arom}$ polymorphism that suggested a sequence change in the $P450_{arom}$ promoter region.

In prepubertal children with gynecomastia, an *exogenous source of estrogens* must be sought. Accidental or therapeutic exposure to small amounts of exogenous estrogens by inhalation, percutaneous absorption, or ingestion may cause gynecomastia. Increased pigmentation of the nipple and areola should suggest this cause. Exposure to medications that decrease levels of androgens, especially free androgens, increase estradiol or displace androgens from breast androgen receptors may result in gynecomastia.

Several other pathologic conditions may cause gynecomastia. It has been observed in children with congenital virilizing adrenal hyperplasia (for example 11β-hydroxylase deficiency). It may be associated with Leydig cell tumors of the testis or with feminizing tumors of the adrenal gland. Several boys with the *Peutz-Jeghers syndrome* and gynecomastia had *sex-cord tumors with annular tubules* of the testes. The testes may not be enlarged; the tumor is usually multifocal and bilateral. Excessive aromatase production accounts for the gynecomastia. This condition occurs in patients with Klinefelter syndrome and with other types of testicular failure (hypergonadotropic states). It is a common finding in boys with certain types of male pseudohermaphroditism, particularly Reifenstein syndrome, the androgen insensitivity syndromes, and in patients with the 17-ketosteroid reductase defect. When gynecomastia is associated with galactorrhea, a prolactinoma should be considered. In a pubertal boy with fibrolamellar carcinoma of the liver, the associated gynecomastia and elevated estrogen level were attributed to increased aromatization of circulating androgens by the tumor. In an 8-yr-old boy with a calcifying Sertoli cell tumor, the gynecomastia was postulated to be the result of peripheral aromatization of androgens derived from Leydig cells newly differentiated from intestital cells stimulated by the tumor.

In adults, gynecomastia occurs with liver cirrhosis, with digitalis therapy for congestive heart failure, bronchogenic carcinoma, administration of various nonsteroidal therapeutic agents, and heavy marijuana smoking. Ketoconazole, an antifungal drug, causes gynecomastia by directly inhibiting testosterone synthesis.

August GP, Chandra R, Hung W: Prepubertal male gynecomastia. J Pediatr 80:259, 1972.
Braunstein GD: Gynecomastia. N Engl J Med 328:490, 1993.
Bulard J, Mowszowicz I, Schaison G: Increased aromatase in pubic skin fibro-

blasts from patients with isolated gynecomastia. J Clin Endocrinol Metab 64:618, 1987.
Hochberg Z, Even L, Zadik Z: Mineralocorticoids in the mechanism of gynecomastia in adrenal hyperplasia caused by 11β-hydroxylase deficiency. J Pediatr 118:258, 1991.
Lee PA: The relationship of concentrations of serum hormones to pubertal gynecomastia. J Pediatr 86:212, 1975.
Maclaren NK, Migeon CJ, Raiti S: Gynecomastia with congenital virilizing adrenal hyperplasia (11β-hydroxylase deficiency). J Pediatr 86:579, 1975.
Malozowski S, Stadel BV: Prepubertal gynecomastia during growth hormone therapy. J Pediatr 126:659, 1995.
Nydick M, Bustos J, Dale JH Jr, et al: Gynecomastia in adolescent boys. JAMA 178:449, 1961.
Ohyama T, Takada A, Fujikawa M, Hosokawa K: Endoscope-assisted transaxillary removal of glandular tissue in gynecomastia. Ann Plast Surg 40:62, 1998.
Stratakis CA, Vottero A, Brodies A, et al: The aromatase excess syndrome is associated with feminization of both sexes and autosomal dominant transmission of aberrant P450 aromatase gene transcription. J Clin Endocrinol Metab 83:1348, 1998.

CHAPTER 596
Hypofunction of the Ovaries

Hypofunction of the ovaries may be caused by congenital failure of development, postnatal destruction (primary or hypergonadotropic hypogonadism), or lack of stimulation by the pituitary (secondary or hypogonadotropic hypogonadism). Many chronic diseases may result in the latter type of hypofunction.

596.1 Hypergonadotropic Hypogonadism in the Female (Primary Hypogonadism)

Diagnosis of hypergonadotropic hypogonadism before puberty is difficult. Except in the case of Turner syndrome, most affected patients have no prepubertal clinical manifestations.

TURNER SYNDROME (also see Chapter 78)

In 1938, Turner described a syndrome consisting of sexual infantilism, webbed neck, and cubitus valgus in adult females. Ullrich in 1930 had described an 8-yr-old girl with short stature and many of the same phenotypic features. The term *Ullrich-Turner syndrome* is frequently used in Europe but rarely in the United States. The chromosomal nature of the condition was discovered in 1959.

PATHOGENESIS. Half the patients with Turner syndrome have a 45,X chromosomal complement. About 15% of patients are mosaics for 45,X and a normal cell line (45,X/46,XX). Other mosaics with isochromosomes, 45,X/46,X,i(Xq); with rings, 45,X/46,X,r(X); or fragments, 45,X/46fra, occur less often. The single X is of maternal origin in 70% of 45,X patients. The mechanism of chromosome loss is unknown, and the risk for the syndrome does not increase with maternal age. The genes involved in the Turner phenotype are X-linked genes that escape inactivation. A major locus involved in the control of linear growth has been mapped within the pseudoautosomal region of the X chromosome (PAR 1). SHOX, a homeobox-containing gene of 170 Kb of DNA within the PAR 1, is thought to be important for controlling growth in children with Turner syndrome and in patients having idiopathic short stature. Genes for the control of normal ovarian function are postulated to be on Xp and perhaps two "supergenes" on Xq.

Turner syndrome occurs in about 1/1,500–2,500 liveborn females. The frequency of the 45,X karyotype at conception is about 3.0%, but 99% of these are spontaneously aborted, accounting for 5–10% of all abortuses. Mosaicism (45,X/46,XX) occurs in a proportion higher than that seen with any other aneuploid state, but the mosaic Turner constitution is rare among the abortuses; these findings indicate preferential survival for mosaic forms.

The normal fetal ovary contains about 7 million oocytes, but these begin to disappear rapidly after the 5th mo of gestation. At birth, there are only 2 million (1 million active follicle); by menarche, there are 400,000–500,000; and at menopause, 10,000 remain. In the absence of one X chromosome, this process is accelerated, and nearly all oocytes are gone by 2 yr of age. In aborted 45,X fetuses, the number of primordial germ cells in the gonadal ridge appears to be normal, suggesting that the normal process is accelerated in patients with Turner syndrome. Eventually, the ovaries are described as "streaks" and consist only of connective tissue, but a few germ cells may persist.

CLINICAL MANIFESTATIONS. Many patients with Turner syndrome are recognizable at birth because of a characteristic edema of the dorsa of the hands and feet and loose skin folds at the nape of the neck. Low birthweight and decreased length are common. Clinical manifestations in childhood include webbing of the neck, a low posterior hairline, small mandible, prominent ears, epicanthal folds, high arched palate, a broad chest presenting the illusion of widely spaced nipples, cubitus valgus, and hyperconvex fingernails. The diagnosis is often first suspected at puberty when sexual maturation fails to occur.

Short stature, the cardinal finding in all girls with Turner syndrome, may be present with minimal other clinical manifestations. During the first 3–5 yr of life, the rate of growth may be normal, albeit in the lower percentiles; thereafter, it begins to decelerate and results in significant short stature. Sexual maturation fails to occur at the expected age. The mean adult height is 143–144 cm in the United States and most of northern Europe, but 140 cm in Argentina and 147 cm in Scandinavia (Fig. 596–1). The height is well correlated with the mid-parental height (average of the parents' heights). Specific growth curves have been developed for girls with Turner syndrome.

Associated defects are common. Complete cardiologic evaluation, including echocardiography, reveals isolated nonstenotic bicuspid aortic valves in about one third to one half of patients. In later life, bicuspid aortic valve disease can progress to dilatation of the aortic root. Less frequent defects include aortic coarctation (20%), aortic stenosis, mitral valve prolapse, and anomalous pulmonary venous drainage. In a study of 170/393 females with Turner syndrome in Denmark, 38% of patients with 45,X chromosomes had cardiovascular malformations compared with 11% of those with mosaic monosomy X; the most common were aortic valve abnormalites and aortic coarctation. Web neck in patients with or without recognized syndromes is associated with both flow and nonflow-related heart defects. Among patients with Turner syndrome, those with web neck have a much greater chance of having coarctation of the aorta then do those without web necks. Approximately one quarter to one third of patients have renal malformations on ultrasonographic examination (50% of those with 45,X karyotypes). The more serious defects include pelvic kidney, horseshoe kidney, double collecting system, complete absence of one kidney, and ureteropelvic junction obstruction. Idiopathic hypertension is also common. When the ovaries were examined by ultrasonography, older studies found a significant decrease in percentage of detectable ovaries from infancy to later childhood. A subsequent report found no such age-related differences in a cross sectional (N = 142) and longitudinal study (N = 38) conducted in Italy; 27–46% of patients had detectable ovaries at various ages; 76% of those with X mosaicism and 26% of those with 45,X karotypes had detectable ovaries.

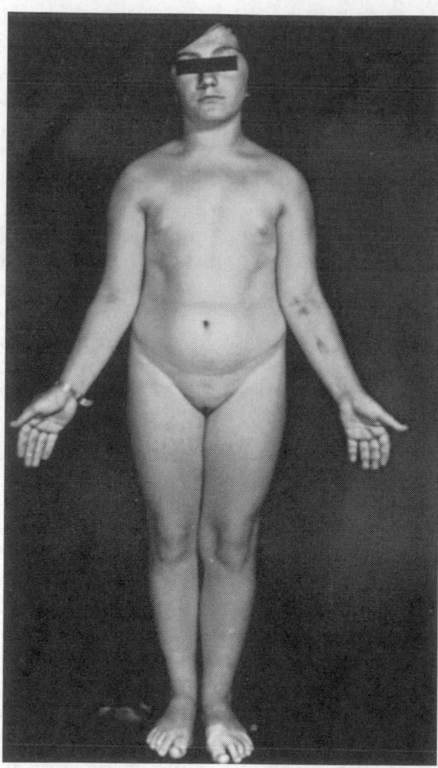

Figure 596–1 Turner syndrome in a 15-yr-old girl exhibiting failure of sexual maturation, short stature, cubitus valgus, and a goiter. There is no webbing of the neck. Karyotyping revealed 45, X/46, XX chromosome complement, and the urinary gonadotropin level was over 96 mouse units/24 hr; T4 was 2.2 μg/dL.

Sexual maturation usually fails to occur, but 10–20% of girls have spontaneous breast development, and a small percentage may have menstrual periods. More than 60 pregnancies have been reported for spontaneously menstruating patients with Turner syndrome. Premature menopause, increased risk of miscarriage, and offspring with increased risk of trisomy 21 have been reported in these women. A woman with a 45,X/46,X,r(X) karotype treated with hormone replacement therapy had three pregnancies resulting in a normal 46,XY male infant, a spontaneous abortion, and a healthy term female with Turner syndrome 45X/46Xr(X).

Antithyroid antibodies, thyroid peroxidase, or thyroglobulin antibodies occur in 30–50% of patients. The prevalence increases with advancing age. Ten to 20% have autoimmune thyroid disease, with or without the presence of a goiter. Age-dependent abnormalities in carbohydrate metabolism characterized by abnormal glucose tolerance and insulin resistance and, only rarely, frank type II diabetes occur in patients with Turner syndrome. Cholesterol levels are elevated in adolescence, regardless of body mass index or karyotype.

Inflammatory bowel disease, both Crohn disease and ulcerative colitis; gastrointestinal bleeding due to abnormal mesenteric vasculature; and delayed gastric emptying time have all been reported.

Sternal malformations can be detected by lateral chest radiography. An increased carrying angle at the elbow is usually not clinically significant. Scoliosis occurs in about 10% of adolescent girls. Reported eye findings include anterior segment dysgenesis and keratoconus. Pigmented nevi become more proeminent with age; melanocytic nevi are common. Essential hyperhidrosis, torus mandibularis, and alopecia areata occur rarely.

Recurrent bilateral otitis media develops in about 75% of patients. Sensorineural hearing deficits are common, and the frequency increases with age. Problems with gross and fine motor–sensory integration, failure to walk before 15 mo of age, and early language dysfunction often raise questions about developmental delay, but intelligence is normal in most patients. However, mental retardation does occur in patients with 45,X/46,X,r(X); the ring chromosome is unable to undergo inactivation and leads to two functional X chromosomes. In adults, deficits in perceptual spatial skills are more common than they are in the general population. Evidence suggests the existence of an imprinted X-linked locus that affects cognitive function. Patients with Turner syndrome with a 45,X karyotype whose X chromosome was of paternal origin were significantly better adjusted and had superior verbal and higher order executive function skills then did those whose X chromosome was of maternal origin.

The prevalence of mosaicism depends in large part on the techniques used for studying chromosomal patterns. The use of fluorescent in situ hybridization and reverse transcription–polymerase chain reaction (PCR) have increased the reported prevalence of mosaic patterns to as high as 60–74%.

Mosaicism involving the Y chromosome occurs in 5%: an additional half of 3% who do not have identified chromosomal fragments may contain Y material. Whether or not clinically virilized, these individuals have a high risk for the development of gonadoblastoma (15–25%). Therefore, prophylactic gonadectomy should be performed even in the absence of magnetic resonance imaging or computed tomographic evidence of tumors. The gonadoblastoma locus on the Y chromosome (GBY) maps close to the Y centromere. The presence of only the SRY (sex determining region on Y) locus is not sufficient to confer increased susceptibility for the development of gonadoblastoma. A careful study of 53 patients with Turner syndrome by nested PCR excluded low-level Y mosaicism in almost all cases. A second round of PCR detected SRY on the distal short arm of the Y chromosome in only two subjects. Therefore, routine PCR for Y chromosome detection for the purpose of assigning gonadoblastoma risk does not seem indicated.

In patients with 45,X/46,XX mosaicism, the abnormalities are attenuated and fewer; short stature is as frequent as it is in the 45,X patient and may be the only manifestation of the condition other than ovarian failure (see Fig. 596–1).

LABORATORY FINDINGS. Chromosomal analysis must be considered in all short girls. In a systematic search, using Southern blot analysis of leukocyte DNA, Turner syndrome was detected in 4.8% of girls referred to an endocrinology service because of short stature. Girls referred with already recognized Turner phenotypes were excluded from analysis. Patients with a marker chromosome in some or all cells should be tested for DNA sequences at or near the centromere of the Y chromosome.

Ultrasonography of the heart, kidneys, and ovaries is indicated after the diagnosis is established. The most common skeletal abnormalities are shortening of the 4th metatarsal and metacarpal bones, epiphyseal dysgenesis in the joints of the knees and elbows, Madelung deformity, scoliosis and, in older patients, inadequate osseous mineralization.

Plasma levels of gonadotropins, particularly follicle-stimulating hormone (FSH), are markedly elevated to greater than those of age-matched controls during infancy; at about 2–3 yr of age, a progressive decrease in levels occurs until they reach a nadir at 6–8 yr of age, and by 10–11 yr, they rise to adult castrate levels.

Thyroid antiperoxidase antibodies should be checked periodically and, if positive, levels of thyroxine and thyroid-stimulating hormone should be obtained. Extensive studies have failed to establish that growth hormone deficiency plays a primary role in the pathogenesis of the growth disorder. Defects in normal secretory patterns of growth hormone are seen in adolescents but not younger girls with Turner syndrome. In vitro, monocytes and lymphocytes show decreased sensitivity to insulin-like growth factor I.

The American Academy of Pediatrics has published a comprehensive guide to the health supervision of children with Turner syndrome.

TREATMENT. Treatment with recombinant human growth hormone increases height velocity and ultimate stature in most but not all children. Many girls achieve heights of greater than 150 cm with early initiation of treatment. By adjusting growth hormone doses according to growth velocity measures, 80% of 14 patients achieved final adult height better than 2 S.D. less than the mean for the general population (mean height 155 cm). Although some believe that growth hormone treatment should be initiated in early childhood, many wait until there is evidence of growth velocity attenuation on specific Turner syndrome growth curves before instituting therapy. The starting dose of growth hormone is 0.375 mg/kg/wk, higher than the initial dose in classically growth hormone–deficient children. Growth hormone therapy does not significantly aggravate carbohydrate tolerance in patients with Turner syndrome.

Replacement therapy with estrogens is indicated, but there is little consensus about the optimal age at which to initiate treatment. The psychologic preparedness of the patient to accept therapy must be taken into account. The improved growth achieved by girls treated with growth hormone permits initiation of estrogen replacement at 12–13 yr. However, even with growth hormone treatment, greater gains in height are achieved when estrogen replacement is delayed until 14–15 yr of age. Careful consideration should be given to the sometimes conflicting psychologic consequences of delaying estrogen therapy for the purpose of achieving better ultimate height. The availability of very low dose estrogen replacement therapy in the future may obviate the need to chose between appropriate pubertal replacement and optimizing height potential.

Premarin, a conjugated estrogen, 0.3–0.625 mg, or Estrace, 0.5 mg (micronized estradiol), given daily for 3–6 mo is usually effective in inducing puberty. The estrogen then is cycled (taken on days 1–23), and Provera, a progestin, is added (taken on days 10–23) in a dose of 5–10 mg daily. In the remainder of the calendar month, during which no treatment is given, withdrawal bleeding usually occurs.

Prenatal chromosome analysis for advanced maternal age has revealed a frequency of 45,X/46,XX that is 10 times higher than when diagnosed postnatally. Most of these patients have no clinical manifestations of Turner syndrome, and levels of gonadotropins are normal. Awareness of this mild phenotype is important in counseling patients.

Psychosocial support for these girls is an integral component of treatment. The Turner Syndrome Society, which has local chapters in the United States, and similar groups in Canada and other countries provide a valuable support system for these patients and their families in addition to that given by the health care team.

Successful pregnancies have been carried to term using ovum donation and in vitro fertilization.

In adult women with Turner syndrome, there seems to be a high prevalence of undiagnosed bone mineral density, lipid, and thyroid abnormalities. Glucose intolerance, diminished first-phase insulin response, elevated blood pressure, and lowered fat free mass are common. Glucose tolerance worsens, but fat free mass and blood pressure and general physical fitness improve with sex hormone replacement.

In an analysis of a cohort of 597 women with cytogenetically proven Turner syndrome in Danemak (Danish Cytogenetic Register), neoplasms were identified in 20 women. Only one case, a Wilms tumor, was diagnosed in childhood. Colon cancer was observed in five patients for a relative risk of 6.9. No case of dysgerminoma or gonadoblastoma was found even in the 20 women with Y chromosomes.

Careful and appropriate health maintenance should be continued for patients with Turner syndrome throughout their lifetimes.

XX GONADAL DYSGENESIS

Some phenotypically and genetically normal females have gonadal lesions identical to those in 45,X patients but without somatic features of Turner syndrome; their condition is termed *pure gonadal dysgenesis* or *pure ovarian dysgenesis*. Here we discuss only those with the XX chromosome constitution. XY gonadal dysgenesis, also termed *Swyer syndrome*, is discussed later in the section on male pseudohermaphroditism. These two conditions are distinct entities; XX and XY gonadal dysgenesis have not been reported in the same family.

The disorder is rarely recognized in children because the external genitals are normal, no other abnormalities are visible, and growth is normal. At pubertal age, sexual maturation fails to take place. Plasma gonadotropin levels are elevated. Delay of epiphyseal fusion results in a eunuchoid habitus. Pelvic ultrasonography reveals streak ovaries.

Affected siblings, parental consanguinity, and failure to uncover mosaicism all point to female-limited autosomal recessive inheritance. The disorder appears to be especially frequent in Finland (1/8,300 liveborn girls). In this population, a mutation in the FSH receptor gene (on chromosome 2p) was demonstrated as the cause of the condition. In some patients, XX gonadal dysgenesis has been associated with sensorineural deafness *(Perrault syndrome)*. A patient with this condition and concommital growth hormone deficiency and virilization has also been reported. There may be distinct genetic forms of this disorder. Tumors of the gonads have not been reported in these patients. Treatment consists of estrogen replacement therapy.

45,X/46,XY GONADAL DYSGENESIS

45,X/46,XY gonadal dysgenesis, also called *mixed gonadal dysgenesis*, has extreme variability, which may extend from a Turner-like syndrome to a male phenotype with a penile urethra; it is possible to delineate three major clinical phenotypes. Short stature is a major finding in all affected children.

Some patients have no evidence of virilization; they have a female phenotype and often have the somatic signs of Turner syndrome. The condition is discovered prepubertally when chromosomal studies are made in short girls, or later when chromosomal studies are made because of failure of sexual maturation. Fallopian tubes and the uterus are present. The gonads consist of intra-abdominal undifferentiated streaks; chromosome study of the streak often reveals an XY cell line. The streak gonad differs somewhat from that in girls with Turner syndrome; in addition to wavy connective tissue, there are often tubular or cordlike structures, occasional clumps of granulosa cells, and frequently mesonephric or hilar cells.

Some children have mild virilization manifested only by prepubertal clitorimegaly. Normal müllerian structures are present, but at puberty virilization occurs. These patients usually have an intra-abdominal testis, a contralateral streak gonad, and bilateral fallopian tubes.

Most children present with frank ambiguity of the genitals in infancy. A testis and vas deferens are found on one side in the labioscrotal fold, and a streak gonad is identified on the contralateral side. Despite the presence of a testis, fallopian tubes are often present bilaterally. An infantile or rudimentary uterus is almost always present.

Other genotypes and phenotypes have been described. About 25% of 200 analyzed patients have a dicentric Y chromosome (45,X/46,X,dic Y). In some patients, the Y chromosome may be represented by only a fragment (45,X/45,X

+fra); application of Y-specific probes can establish the origin of the fragment. It is not clear why the same genotype (45,X/46,XY) can result in such diverse phenotypes.

Children with a female phenotype present no problem in gender of rearing. Patients who are only slightly virilized are usually assigned a female gender of rearing before a diagnosis is established. Patients with ambiguity of the genitals are readily confused with various types of male pseudohermaphrodism. In most but not all instances, these children are best reared as females; the short stature, the ease of genital reconstruction, and the predisposition of the gonad to the development of malignancy favor this choice. In some patients followed to adulthood, the putative normal testis proves to be dysgenetic with eventual loss of Leydig and Sertoli cell function. (See also Chapter 593.) In an analysis of 22 Australian patients with mixed gonadal dysgenesis, no significant associations or correlations were found between internal and external phenotypes or endocrine function and gonadal morphologic features. The sex of rearing was determined by the appearance of the external genitals. In 11 patients, basal and human chorionic gonadotropin–stimulated testosterone levels were lower then in control subjects.

Gonadal tumors, usually gonadoblastomas, occur in about 25% of these children. A gonadoblastoma locus has been localized to a region near the centrome of the Y chromosome (GBY). These germ cell tumors are preceded by the changes of carcinoma in situ. Accordingly, both gonads should be removed in all patients reared as girls, and the undifferentiated gonad should be removed in the patients reared as males.

In the past, all patients came to clinical attention because of their abnormal phenotypes. However, 45,X/46,XY mosaicism is found in about 7% of fetuses with true chromosome mosaicism encountered prenatally. Of 76 infants with 45,X/46,XY mosaicism diagnosed prenatally, 72 had a normal male phenotype, 1 had a female phenotype, and only 3 males had hypospadias. Of 12 males whose gonads were examined, only 3 were abnormal. These data must be taken into account when counseling a family in which a 45,X/46,XY infant is discovered prenatally.

XXX, XXXX, AND XXXXX FEMALES

XXX FEMALES. The 47,XXX chromosomal constitution is the most frequent X chromosome abnormality in females, occurring in almost 1/1,000 liveborn females. In 68%, this condition is caused by maternal meiotic nondisjunction, but most 45,X and half of 47,XXY constitutions are caused by paternal sex chromosome errors. The phenotype is that of a normal female; affected infants and children are not recognized.

Sexual development and menarche are normal. Most pregnancies have resulted in normal infants. By 2 yr of age, delays in speech and language become evident, and lack of coordination, poor academic performance, and immature behavior are seen. These girls tend to be tall and gangly, manifest behavior disorders, and are placed in special education classes. There is marked variability within the syndrome, and a small proportion of affected girls are well coordinated, socially outgoing, and academically superior.

XXXX AND XXXXX FEMALES. The great majority of females with these rare karotypes have been mentally retarded. Commonly associated defects are epicanthal folds, hypertelorism, clinodactyly, transverse palmar creases, radioulnar synostosis, and congenital heart disease. Sexual maturation is often incomplete and may not occur at all. Nevertheless, three women with the tetra-X syndrome gave birth, but no pregnancies were reported in 49,XXXXX women. Most 48,XXXX women tend to be tall, with an average height of 169 cm, whereas short stature is a common feature of the 49,XXXXX phenotype.

NOONAN SYNDROME

Girls with Noonan syndrome show certain anomalies that also occur in girls with 45,X Turner syndrome, but they have normal 46,XX chromosomes. The most common abnormalities are the same as those described for males with Noonan syndrome (see Chapter 593.1). The phenotype differs from Turner syndrome in several respects. Mental retardation is often present, the cardiac defect is most often pulmonary valvular stenosis or an atrial septal defect rather than an aortic defect, normal sexual maturation usually occurs but is delayed 2 yr on average, and premature ovarian failure has been reported.

OTHER OVARIAN DEFECTS

An increasing number of other young women with no chromosomal abnormality are found to have streak gonads that may contain only occasional germ cells, if any. Gonadotropins are increased. *Cytotoxic drugs,* especially alkylating agents such as cyclophosphamide and busulfan, procarbazine, etoposide, and exposure of the ovaries to radiation for the treatment of malignancy are increasingly frequent causes of ovarian failure. A study of young women with Hodgkin disease found that combination chemotherapy and pelvic irradiation may be more deleterious than either therapy alone. Teenagers are more likely than older women to retain or recover ovarian function after irradiation or combined chemotherapy; normal pregnancies have occurred after such treatment. Current treatment regimens may result in some ovarian damage in most girls treated for cancer. The LD_{50} for the human oocyte has been estimated to be about 4 Gy; doses as low as 6 Gy have produced primary amenorrhea. Ovarian transposition before abdominal and pelvic irradiation in childhood can preserve ovarian function by decreasing the ovarian exposure to less then 4–7 Gy.

Autoimmune ovarian failure occurs in 60% of children older than 13 yr of age with *type I autoimmune polyendocrinopathy* (Addison disease, hypoparathyroidism, candidiasis). Affected girls may not develop sexually, or secondary amenorrhea may occur in young women. The ovaries may have lymphocytic infiltration or appear simply as streaks. Most affected patients have circulating steroid cell antibodies and autoantibodies to 21-hydroxylase.

The condition also occurs in young women as an isolated event or in association with other autoimmune disorders, leading to secondary amenorrhea *(premature ovarian failure).* It occurs in 0.9% of women younger than 40 years of age. Premature ovarian failure is a heterogeneous disorder with many causes: chromosomal, genetic, enzymatic, infectious, or iatrogenic. About 70% of sera from affected adult patients contain antibodies against the ovaries (steroid cell antibodies). Some adults treated with immunosuppressive doses of glucocorticoids resume menses and become pregnant; in one case, fertility returned spontaneously 7 yr after the onset of autoimmune ovarian failure. In 2–10%, "idiopathic" ovarian failure is associated with adrenal autoimmunity.

Galactosemia, particularly the classic form of the disease, usually results in ovarian damage, beginning during intrauterine life. Levels of FSH and luteinizing hormone (LH) are elevated early in life. Ovarian damage may be due to deficient uridine diphosphate–galactose (see Chapter 84.2). The Denys-Drash syndrome, due to a WT-1 mutation, can result in ovarian dysgenesis.

Ataxia-telangiectasia may be associated with ovarian hypoplasia and elevated gonadotropins; the cause is unknown. Gonadoblastomas and dysgerminomas have occurred in a few girls.

Hypergonadotrophic hypogonadism has been postulated to also occur because of the resistence of the ovary to both endogenous and exogenous gonadotropins (Savage syndrome). Antiovarian antibodies or FSH receptor abnormalities may cause this condition. Mutation of the FSH receptor gene has been reported as an autosomal recessive condition (see under XX Gonadal Dysgenesis). Two females with 46,XX chromosomes presenting in primary amenorrhea with elevated gonadotropin levels were found to have inactivating mutations of the LH receptor gene. This suggests that LH action is needed for normal follicular development and ovulation.

596.2 Hypogonadotropic Hypogonadism in the Female (Secondary Hypogonadism)

Hypofunction of the ovaries can result from failure to secrete normal levels of gonadotropins. The defect may lie in the anterior pituitary or, more commonly, in the hypothalamus.

ETIOLOGY

Hypopituitarism (also see Chapter 567). Congenital or acquired lesions in or near the pituitary almost always result in impaired secretion of gonadotropins and other pituitary hormones. In children with idiopathic hypopituitarism, the defect is usually found in the hypothalamus. In these patients, administration of gonadotropin-releasing hormone (GnRH) results in increased plasma levels of FSH and LH, establishing the integrity of the pituitary gland.

Isolated Deficiency of Gonadotropins. This heterogeneous group of disorders is sorted out with the help of the GnRH test. In most children, the pituitary is normal, the defect residing in the hypothalamus.

Several sporadic instances of anosmia with hypogonadotropic hypogonadism have been reported. Anosmic hypogonadal females have also been reported in kindreds with Kallmann syndrome, but hypogonadism more frequently affects the males in these families. Mutations in the gene for the β subunit of FSH and LH have been reported.

Some autosomal recessive disorders such as the Laurence-Moon-Biedl, multiple lentigines, and Carpenter syndromes appear in some instances to include gonadotropic hormone deficiency. Girls with Prader-Willi syndrome may have hypogonadotropic hypogonadism. Girls with severe thalassemia may have gonadotropin deficiency due to pituitary damage caused by chronic iron overload secondary to multiple transfusions. Anorexia nervosa (discussed elsewhere) frequently results in hypogonadotropic hypogonadism (see Chapter 112).

DIAGNOSIS. The diagnosis may be apparent in patients with other deficiencies of pituitary tropic hormones, but as in males, it is difficult to differentiate isolated hypogonadotropic hypogonadism from physiologic delay of puberty. Repeated measurements of FSH and LH, particularly during sleep, may reveal the rising levels that herald the onset of puberty. Stimulation testing with GnRH or one of its analogs may help establish the diagnosis.

POLYCYSTIC OVARIES (STEIN-LEVENTHAL SYNDROME)

The classic polycystic ovaries syndrome (PCOS) is characterized by obesity, hirsutism, and secondary amenorrhea, with bilaterally enlarged polycystic ovaries, but these manifestations may not all be present (also see Chapter 560). Onset usually occurs at puberty or shortly thereafter; menstrual irregularities and hirsutism are the most frequent complaints. In the reproductive years, the condition is the most common cause of anovulatory infertility. Several terms have gained acceptance in describing these patients: *functional ovarian hyperandrogenism* and, especially in adults, *chronic hyperandrogenic anovulation.* There seems to be a strong relationship between premature adrenarche and the subsequent development of PCOS. The enlarged ovaries can often be felt on combined rectal and abdominal palpation and are always demonstrable by ultrasonography (see Chapter 560).

The cause of the disorder in most patients is unsettled despite intensive investigation. PCOS is a heterogeneous condition that may be associated with several distinct entities, such as 21-hydroxylase deficiency, deficiency of 3-hydroxysteroid dehydrogenase, and deficiency of ovarian 17-ketoreductase, the enzyme that converts androstenedione to testosterone and estrone to estradiol. However, in most patients with PCOS, the elevated plasma level of free testosterone or androstenedione is not suppressed by dexamethasone, ruling out an adrenal cause of the disorder. In some patients, serum levels of total testosterone may not be elevated, but serum levels of free testosterone are, and sex hormone–binding globulins are markedly diminished. About 75% of patients have an increased ratio of LH to FSH levels, an increased amplitude and frequency of plasma LH levels, and an exaggerated response to GnRH. Inhibin B levels are high at baseline and lack normal pulsatile changes. Premenarcheal girls may have an early morning rise in LH rather than the characteristic nocturnal one. The perturbances of LH secretion are believed to bring about hyperplasia of theca cells, arrested follicular development, and impaired estradiol production. These effects lead to hyperandrogenemia and irregular cycles or amenorrhea. In children having congenital virilizing syndromes, the hypothalamic-pituitary axis appears to be programmed for hypersecretion of LH at puberty, leading to hyperandrogenism even when adrenal androgens are thought to be adequately suppressed.

There is an association between hyperandrogenism and insulin resistance. Especially in obese patients, PCOS may be associated with hyperinsulinism, insulin resistance, and acanthosis nigricans. Because of the high prevalence of PCOS, it needs to be counted among the most common conditions associated with glucose intolerance and type II diabetes. The insulin resistance seems to be related to excessive serine phosphorylation of the insulin receptor. The same process, serine phosphorylation, is important in regulating the activity of P450c17, a major enzyme involved in androgen biosynthesis. Therefore, some have postulated this defect as the single abnormality that may be responsible for both the insulin resistance and hyperandrogenism seen in PCOS.

For *diagnosis* of PCOS, measurements of serum LH, FSH, prolactin, free testosterone, and sex hormone–binding globulin as well as dehydroepiandrosterone-sulfate are helpful. Complex stimulation and inhibitory pharmacologic manipulation have been used to distinguish between adrenal and ovarian causes of hyperandrogenism. Basal and adrenocorticotropic hormone (1–24)–stimulated adrenal steroid levels may reveal subtle adrenal steroidogenic defects.

A deficiency of 17-ketoreductase is suggested when there are affected brothers or when the estrone:estradiol and androstenedione:testosterone ratios are increased. Women treated with valproate for epilepsy before 20 yr of age often have PCOS and elevated serum testosterone levels, but their levels of LH are normal.

The optimal method of *treatment* is still evolving. The mainstay of therapy is ovarian suppression with new-generation oral contraceptives containing nonandrogenic progestins such as desogetrel (Desogen). Spironolactone, in addition to oral contraceptives, has been the main pharmacologic agent available in the United States to diminish hirsutism. Further suppression can be achieved with testolactone, a compound with antiandrogen and weak progestin properties. Attention to the obesity is important because its correction often leads to correction of the insulin resistance. Oral agents to treat type II diabetes may be used in the future to improve insulin resistance in patients with PCOS. D-*Chiro*-inositol treatment of women with PCOS improves insulin action, thus enhancing ovarian function while decreasing serum androgen levels. This approach stimulates postreceptor insulin action. Naltrexone, an opioid antagonist, was recently found to decrease insulin secretion in hyperinsulinemic patients with PCOS. Electrolysis and laser therapy are the main nonpharmacologic treatment modalities for hirsutism.

Ahonen P, Myllärniemi S, Sipila I, et al: Clinical variation of autoimmune polyendocrinopathy-candidiasis-ectodermal dystrophy (APECED) in a series of 68 patients. N Engl J Med 322:1829, 1990.

Aittomaki K, Lucena JLD, Pakarinen P, et al: Mutation in the follicle-stimulating hormone receptor gene causes hereditary hypergonadotropic ovarian failure. Cell 82:959, 1995.

Ala-Fossi SL, Maenpaa J, Koivisto AR, et al: Prognostic significance of p53 expression in ovarian granulosa cell tumors. Gynecol Oncol 66:475, 1997.

Barnes RB, Rosenfield RL, Ehrmann DA, et al: Ovarian hyperandrogynism as a result of congenital virilizing disorders: Evidence for perinatal masculinization of neuroendocrine function in women. J Clin Endocrinol Metab 79:1328, 1994.

Berdahl LD, Wenstrom KD, Hanson JW: Web neck anomaly and its association with congenital heart disease. Am J Med Genet 56:304, 1995.

Binder G, Kock A, Wajs E, Ranke MB: Nested polymerase chain reaction study of 53 cases with Turner syndrome: Is cytogenetically undetected Y mosaicism common? J Clin Endocrinol Metab 80:3532, 1995.

Blumenthal AL, Allanson JE: Turner syndrome in a mother and daughter: r(X) and fertility. Clin Genet 52:187, 1997.

Carel JC, Mathivon L, Gendrel C, et al: Near normalization of final height with adapted doses of growth hormone in Turner syndrome. J Clin Endocrinol Metab 83:1462, 1998.

Chang HJ, Clark RD, Bachman H: The phenotype of 45,X/46,XY mosaicism: An analysis of 92 prenatally diagnosed cases. Am J Hum Genet 46:156, 1990.

Dunaif A: Insulin resistance and the polycystic ovary syndrome: Mechanism and implications for pathogenesis. Endocr Rev 18:774, 1997.

Garcia-Rudaz C, Martinez AS, Heinrick JJ, et al: Growth of Argentinian girls with Turner syndrome. Ann Hum Biol 22:533, 1995.

Gicquel C, Gaston V, Cabrol S, LeBouc Y: Assessment of Turner syndrome by molecular analysis of the X chromosome in growth-retarded girls. J Clin Endocrinol Metab 83:1472, 1998.

Gravholt CH, Juul S, Naeraa RW, Hansen J: Prenatal and postnatal prevalence of Turner syndrome: A registry study. Br Med J 312:16, 1996.

Gravholt CH, Naeraa RW, Nyhold B, et al: Glucose metabolism, lipid metabolism and cardiovascular risk factors in adult Turner syndrome. Diabetes Care 21:1062, 1998.

Guido M, Pavone V, Ciampelli M, et al: Involvement of ovarian steroids in the opioid-mediated reduction of insulin secretion in hyperinsulinemic patients with polycystic ovary syndrome. J Clin Endocrinol Metab 83:1742, 1998.

Hochberg Z, Aviram M, Rubin D, et al: Decreased sensitivity to insulin-like growth factor I in Turner syndrome: A study of monocytes and T lymphocytes. Eur J Clin Invest 27:543, 1997.

Hoek A, Schoemaker J, Dreshage HA: Premature ovarian failure and ovarian autoimmunity. Endocr Rev 18:107, 1997.

Iezzoni JC, Kap-Herr CV, Golden W, Gaffey MJ: Gonadoblastomas in 45,X/46XY mosaicism. Am J Clin Pathol 108:197203, 1997.

Lin AE, Lippe B, Rosenfeld RD: Further delineation of aortic dilation, dissection, and rupture in patients with Turner syndrome. Pediatrics 102: e12, 1998. www.Pediatrics.org/cgi/content/full/102/1/e/2.

Linssen WHJP, Bent MJV, Brunner HG, Poels PJE: Deafness, sensory neuropathy, and ovarian dysgenesis: A new syndrome or a broader spectrum of Perrault syndrome. Am J Med Genet 51:81, 1994.

Lo KWK, Lam SK, Cheung TH, et al: Gonadoblastoma in patient with Turner syndrome. J Obstet Gynecol Res 22:35, 1996.

Lockwood GM, Muttukrishna S, Groome NP, et al: Mid-follicular phase pulses of inhibin B are absent in polycystic ovarian syndrome and are initiated by successful laparoscopic ovarian diathermy: A possible mechanism regulating emergence of the dominant follicle. J Clin Endocrinol Metab 83:1730, 1998.

Matthews CH, Borgato S, Beck-Peccoz P, et al: Primary amenorrhea and infertility due to a mutation in the β-subunit of follicle-stimulating hormone. Nat Genet 5:83, 1993.

Mazzanti L, Cacciari E, Bergamaschi R, et al: Pelvic ultrasonography in patients with Turner syndrome: Age-related findings in different karyotypes. J Pediatr 131:135, 1997.

Migeon BR, Luo S, Jani M, Jeppesen P: The severe phenotype of females with tiny ring X chromosomes are associated with inability of these chromosomes to undergo X inactivation. Am J Med Genet 55:497, 1994.

Muller J, Shakkeback NE, Ritzen M, et al: Carcinoma in situ of the testis in children with 45,X/46,XY gonadal dysgenesis. J Pediatr 106:431, 1985.

Nester J, Jakubowicz D, Reamer P, et al: Ovulatory and metabolic effects of D-*Chiro*-inositol in polycystic ovary syndrome. N Engl J Med 340:1314, 1999.

Pasquino AM, Passeri F, Pucarelli I, et al: Spontaneous pubertal development in Turner syndrome. J Clin Endocrinol Metab 82:1810, 1997.

Plotnick L, Attie KM, Blethen SL, et al: Growth hormone treatment of girls with Turner syndrome: The National Cooperative Growth Study experience. Pediatrics 102:479, 1998.

Radetti G, Mazzanti K, Paganini C, et al: Frequency of clinical and laboratory features of thyroiditis in girls with Turner syndrome. Acta Paediatr 84:909, 1995.

Rao E, Weiss B, Fukami M, et al: Pseudoautosomal deletions encompassing a novel homeobox gene cause growth failure in idiopathic short stature and Turner syndrome. Nat Genet 16:54, 1997.

Rongen-Westerlaken C, Corel K, van den Broeck J, et al: Reference values for height, height velocity and weight in Turner syndrome. Acta Paediatr 86:937, 1997.

Rosenfeld RL, Pesovic N, Deveine N, et al: Optimizing estrogen replacement treatment on Turner syndrome. Pediatrics 102:486, 1998.

Schorry EK, Lovell AM, Milatovich A, Saal HM: Ullrich-Turner syndrome and neurofibromatosis-1. Am J Med Genet 66:423, 1996.

Seashore MR, Cho S, Desposito F, et al: Health supervision for children with Turner syndrome. Pediatrics 96:1166, 1995.

Sempe M, Hansson Bodallaz C, Limoni C: Growth curves in untreated Ullrich-Turner syndrome: French reference standards 1–22 years. Eur J Pediatr 155:862, 1996.

Skuse DH, James RS, Bishop DVM, et al: Evidence from Turner symdrome of an imprinted X-linked locus affecting cognitive function. Nature 387:705, 1997.

Sills I, Rapaport R, Skuza K, Horlick M: 46,XX pure gonadal dysgenesis with growth hormone deficiency and impaired 3β-hydroxysteroid dehydrogenase activity. Am J Med Genet 42:100, 1992.

Sybert VP: Cardiovascular malformations and complicaions in Turner syndrome. Pediatrics 101: E11, 1998. www.Pediatrics.org/cgi/content/full/101/1/e11.

Tanaka Y, Sasaki Y, Nishihira H, et al: Ovarian juvenile granulosa cell tumor associated with Maffucci's syndrome. Am J Clin Pathol 97:523, 1992.

Thibaud E, Ramirez M, Brauner R, et al: Preservation of ovarian function by ovarian transposition performed before pelvic irradiation during childhood. J Pediatr 121:880, 1992.

Yeh J, Rebar RW, Liu JH, et al: Pituitary function in isolated gonadotropin deficiency. Clin Endocrinol 31:375, 1989.

Young RH, Dickersin GR, Scully RE: Juvenile granulosa cell tumor of the ovary. A clinicopathologic analysis of 125 cases. Am J Surg Pathol 8:575, 1984.

Wilson R, Chu CE, Donaldson MDC, et al: An increased incidence of thyroid antibodies in patients with Turner syndrome and their first degree relatives. Autoimmunity 25:47, 1996.

Zinn AR, Page DC, Fisher EMC: Turner syndrome: The case of the missing X chromosome. Trends Genet 9:90, 1993.

CHAPTER 597

Pseudoprecocity Due to Lesions of the Ovary

Ovarian tumors are rare in pediatrics, and yet ovarian malignancies are the most common genital neoplasms in adolescence. More then 60% are germ cell tumors, most of which are dysgerminomas that can secrete tumor markers and hormones (see Chapter 509). Next most common are epithelial cell tumors (~20%), and nearly 10% are sex cord–stromal tumors (granulosa, Sertoli cell, and mesenchymal tumors). Multiple tumor markers can be seen in ovarian tumors, including α-fetoprotein, human chorionic gonadotropin (hCG), carcinoembryonic antigen, oncoproteins, p105, p53, K-ras mutations, cyclin D1, epidermal growth factor–related proteins and receptors, cathepsin B, and others.

Functioning lesions of the ovary consist of benign cysts or malignant tumors. The majority synthesize estrogens; a few synthesize androgens.

ESTROGENIC LESIONS OF THE OVARY. These lesions cause isosexual precocious sexual development but account for only a small percentage of all cases of precocity. Benign ovarian follicular cysts are the most common tumors associated with isosexual precocious puberty in girls; they may rarely be gonadotropin-dependent.

Juvenile Granulosa Cell Tumor. In childhood, the most common neoplasm of the ovary with estrogenic manifestations is the granulosa cell tumor, although it composes only about 10% of all ovarian tumors. These tumors have distinctive histologic features that differ from those encountered in older women (adult granulosa cell tumor). Follicles are often irregular, Call-Exner bodies are rare, and luteinization is frequent. The tumor may be solid or cystic, or both. They are usually benign. In a few instances, this tumor has been associated with multiple enchondromas *(Ollier disease)* and, in fewer still, with multiple subcutaneous hemangiomas *(Maffucci syndrome)*.

Clinical Manifestations and Diagnosis. The tumor has been observed in newborns and may manifest with sexual precocity at 2 yr of age or younger; about half of these tumors have occurred before 10 yr of age. The mean age at diagnosis is 7.5 yr. The tumors are almost always unilateral. The breasts become enlarged, rounded, and firm and the nipples prominent. The external genitals resemble those of a normal girl at puberty, and the uterus is enlarged. A white vaginal discharge is followed by irregular or cyclic menstruation. Ovulation, however, does not occur. The presenting manifestation may be abdominal pain or swelling. Pubic hair is usually absent unless there is mild virilization.

A mass is readily palpable in the lower portion of the abdomen in most children by the time sexual precocity is evident. The tumor may be small, however, and escape detection even on careful rectal and abdominal examination; such tumors are usually detectable by ultrasonography. Most such tumors are diagnosed at very early stages of malignancy (FIGO, International Federation of Gynecology and Obstetrics, stage I).

Plasma estradiol levels are markedly elevated. Plasma levels of gonadotropins are suppressed and do not respond to gonadotropin-releasing hormone stimulation. Levels of müllerian-inhibiting substance, inhibin, and α-fetoprotein may be elevated. Osseous development is moderately advanced.

Treatment and Prognosis. The tumor should be removed as soon as the diagnosis is established. Prognosis is excellent because fewer than 5% of these tumors in children are malignant. In adults with granulosa cell tumors, p53 expression is associated with unfavorable prognosis. Vaginal bleeding immediately after removal of the tumor is common. Signs of precocious puberty abate and may disappear within a few months after the operation. The secretion of estrogens returns to normal.

Sex cord tumor with annular tubules is a distinctive tumor, thought to arise from granulosa cells, that occurs primarily in patients with Peutz-Jeghers syndrome. These tumors are multifocal, bilateral, and usually, but not always, benign. The presence of calcifications aids ultrasonographic detection. Increased aromatase production by these tumors results in gonadotropin-independent precocious puberty. Inhibin A and B levels are elevated and decrease after tumor removal. In one study, 9 of 13 sex cord stromal tumors exhibited FSH-receptor mutations, suggesting a role for such mutation in the development of these tumors.

Chorioepithelioma has been reported only rarely. This very malignant tumor is thought to arise from a pre-existing teratoma. The usually unilateral tumor produces large amounts of hCG, which stimulates the contralateral ovary to secrete estrogens and progesterone. Elevated levels of hCG are diagnostic.

Follicular Cyst. Small ovarian cysts (<0.7 cm in diameter) are common in prepubertal children. At puberty and in girls with true isosexual precocious puberty, larger cysts (1–6 cm) are often seen; these are secondary to stimulation by gonadotropins. However, similar larger cysts occur occasionally in young girls with precocious puberty in the absence of LH and FSH. Because surgical removal or spontaneous involution of these cysts results in regression of pubertal changes, there is little doubt that they are its cause. The mechanism of production of these autonomously functioning cysts is unknown. Such cysts may form only once, or they may disappear and recur, resulting in waxing and waning of the signs of precocious puberty. They may be unilateral or bilateral. The sexual precocity that occurs in young girls with McCune-Albright syndrome is usually associated with autonomous follicular cysts caused by a somatic-activating mutation of the G protein occurring early in development (see Chapter 572.6). Gonadotropins are suppressed, and estradiol levels are often markedly elevated, but they may fluctuate widely and even return to normal. Gonadotropin-releasing hormone stimulation fails to evoke an increase in gonadotropins. Because gonadotropins are suppressed in these children, the mechanism of ovarian stimulation is unknown. Ultrasonography is the method of choice for the detection and monitoring of such cysts. A short period of observation to ascertain a lack of spontaneous resolution is advisable before cyst aspiration or cystectomy is considered. Cystic neoplasms must be considered in the differential diagnosis.

ANDROGENIC LESIONS OF THE OVARY. Virilizing ovarian tumors are rare at all ages but particularly so in prepubertal girls. The *arrhenoblastoma* has been reported as early as 14 days of age, but few cases have been reported in girls younger than 16 yr of age.

The *gonadoblastoma* occurs exclusively in dysgenetic gonads, particularly in phenotypic females who have a Y chromosome in their genotype (46,XY; 45,X/46,XY; 45,X/46,X fra). The tumor may be bilateral. Virilization occurs with some but not all tumors. The clinical features are the same as those seen in patients with virilizing adrenal tumors and include accelerated growth, acne, clitoral enlargement, and growth of sexual hair. A palpable, abdominal mass is found in only about 50% of patients. Plasma levels of testosterone and androstenedione are elevated, and those of gonadotropins are suppressed. Ultrasonography, computed tomography, and magnetic resonance imaging usually localize the lesion. The dysgenetic gonad of phenotypic females with a Y chromosome should be removed prophylactically. When a unilateral tumor is removed, the contralateral dysgenetic gonad should also be removed. In an immunohistochemical study of two gonadoblastomas expression of WT-1, p53, and MIS as well as inhibin were all demonstrated.

Virilizing manifestations occur occasionally in girls with *juvenile granulosa cell tumors*. Adrenal rests and hilus cell tumors rarely lead to virilization. Activating mutations of G protein genes have been described in ovarian (and testicular) tumors. GSP mutations, usually seen in gonadal tumors associated with McCune-Albright syndrome, were also noted in four of six Leydig cell tumors (three ovarian, one testicular). Two granulosa cell tumors and one thecoma of 10 ovarian tumors studied were found to have gip 2 mutations.

Calaminus G, Wessalowski R, Harms D, Gobel U: Juvenile granulosa cell tumors of the ovary in children and adolescents: Results from 33 patients registered in a prospective cooperative study. Gynecol Oncol 65:447, 1997.

Dewhurst J, Pryse-Davies J, Helm W, et al: Diagnosis and management of granulosa/theca cell tumors of childhood. Pediatr Adolesc Gynecol 3:131, 1985.

Fotiou SK: Ovarian malignancies in adolescence. Ann NY Acad Sci 816:338, 1997.

Hussong J, Crussi FG, Chou PM: Gonadoblastoma: Immunohistochemical localization of müllerian-inhibiting substance, inhibin, WT-1, and p53. Mod Pathol 10:1101, 1997.

Kotlar TJ, Young RH, Albanese, C, et al: A mutation in the follicle-stimulating hormone receptor occurs frequently in human ovarian sex cord tumors. J Clin Endocrinol Metab 82:1020, 1997.

Lazar EL, Stolar CJ: Evaluation and management of pediatric solid ovarian tumors. Semin Pediatr Surg 7:29, 1998.

Lyons, J, Landis CA, Harsh, G, et al: Two G protein oncogenes in human endocrine tumors. Science 249:655, 1990.

Silverman LA, Gitelman SE: Immunoreactive inhibin, müllerian inhibitory substance, and activin as biochemical markers for juvenile granulosa cell tumors. J Pediatr 129:918, 1996.

Yamashita K, Yamoto M, Shikone T, et al: Production of inhibin A and inhibin B in human ovarian sex cord stromal tumors. Am J Obstet Gynecol 177:1450, 1997.

Zalel Y, Piura B, Elchalal U, et al: Diagnosis and management of malignant germ cell ovarian tumors in young females. Int J Gynecol Obstet 55:1, 1996.

Chapter 598
Hermaphroditism (Intersexuality)

Hermaphroditism implies a discrepancy between the morphology of the gonads and that of the external genitals. Many chromosomal aberrations resulting in ambiguity of the external genitals were discussed earlier in this section. In this chapter, conditions of aberrant sexual differentiation that are imposed on the XX or XY genotype (female and male pseudohermaphrodites) are discussed (Table 598–1). An increasing number of such conditions are understood through advances in the knowledge about molecular biology of normal sexual differentiation. The category known as true hermaphroditism, with few exceptions, is still a poorly understood heterogeneous group of disorders.

SEXUAL DIFFERENTIATION (see also Chapter 592). In normal differentiation, the final form of all sexual structures is consistent with normal sex chromosomes (either XX or XY). A 46,XX complement of chromosomes is necessary for the development of normal ovaries. Development of the male phenotype is complex. Maleness requires a Y chromosome and, specifically, an intact SRY gene, which, in association with other genes such as SOX 9, SF-1, and WT-1, and an as yet unknown mechanism, directs the undifferentiated gonad to become a testis. As previously mentioned, aberrant recombinations may result in X chromosomes carrying SRY, resulting in XX males, or Y chromosomes that have lost SRY, resulting in XY females.

Müllerian-inhibiting substance (MIS), the first testicular hormone produced at 6–7 wk of gestation, causes the müllerian ducts to regress; in its absence, they persist. MIS activation in the testes may require the SF-1 gene for activation. By about 8 wk of gestation, the Leydig cells of the testis begin to produce testosterone. During this critical period of male differentiation, testosterone secretion is stimulated by placental human chorionic gonadotropin (hCG), which peaks at 8–12 wk. In the latter half of pregnancy, lower levels of testosterone are maintained by luteinizing hormone secreted by the fetal pituitary. Testosterone initiates virilization of the wolffian duct into the epididymis, vas deferns, and seminal vesicle. Development of the external genitals also requires dihydrotestosterone (DHT), an active metabolite of testosterone. DHT is necessary to fuse the genital folds to form the penis and scrotum. A functional androgen receptor, controlled by an X-linked gene, is required for testosterone and DHT to produce these virilizing changes.

In the XX fetus with normal long and short arms of the X, the bipotential gonad develops into an ovary by about the 10th–11th wk. This occurs only in the absence of SRY, testosterone, and MIS and may require a normal gene in the DSS locus. The female phenotype develops independently of the fetal gonads, but maleness is imposed on a basically female potential by the hormones of the fetal testis. Estrogen is unnecessary for normal prenatal sexual differentiation, as demonstrated by 46,XX patients with aromatase deficiency and by mice without estradiol receptors.

TABLE 598–1 Etiologic Classification of Hermaphroditism

- Female pseudohermaphroditism
  - Androgen exposure
    - Fetal source
      - 21-Hydroxylase (P450 c21) deficiency
      - 11β-Hydroxylase (P450 c11) deficiency
      - 3β-Hydroxysteroid dehydrogenase II (3β-HSD II) deficiency
      - Aromatase ($P450_{arom}$) deficiency
    - Maternal source
      - Virilizing ovarian tumor
      - Virilizing adrenal tumor
      - Androgenic drugs
  - Undetermined origin
    - Associated with genitourinary and gastrointestinal tract defects
- Male pseudohermaphroditism
  - Defects in testicular differentiation
    - Denys-Drash syndrome (mutation in WT1 gene)
    - WAGR syndrome (*W*ilms tumor, *a*niridia, *g*enitourinary malformation, *r*etardation)
      - Deletion of 11p13
    - Camptomelic syndrome (autosomal gene at 17q24.3–q25.1) and SOX 9 mutation
    - XY pure gonadal dysgenesis (Swyer syndrome)
      - Mutation in SRY gene
      - Unknown cause
    - XY gonadal agenesis
  - Deficiency of testicular hormones
    - Leydig cell aplasia
    - Mutation in LH receptor
    - Lipoid adrenal hyperplasia (P450 scc) deficiency; mutation in StAR (steroidogenic acute regulatory protein)
    - 3β-HSDII deficiency
    - 17-Hydroxylase/17, 20-lyase (P450 c17) deficiency
    - Persistent müllerian duct syndrome
      - Gene mutations, müllerian-inhibiting substance (MIS)
      - Receptor defects for MIS
  - Defect in androgen action
    - 5α-Reductase II mutations
    - Androgen receptor defects
      - Complete androgen insensitivity syndrome
      - Partial androgen insensitivity syndrome
      - (Reinfenstein and other syndromes)
      - Smith-Lemli-Opitz syndrome
        - Defect in conversion of 7-dehydrocholesterol to cholesterol
- True hermaphroditism
  - XX
  - XY
  - XX/XY chimeras

598.1 Female Pseudohermaphroditism

In the female pseudohermaphrodite, the genotype is XX and the gonads are ovaries, but the external genitals are virilized. Because there is no MIS (the gonads are ovaries not testes), the uterus, tubes, and ovaries develop. The varieties and causes of female pseudohermaphroditism are relatively few. Most instances result from exposure of the female fetus to excessive exogenous or endogenous androgens during intrauterine life. The changes consist principally of virilization of the external genitals (clitoral hypertrophy and labioscrotal fusion).

CONGENITAL ADRENAL HYPERPLASIA (see Chapter 586.1). This is the most common cause of female pseudohermaphroditism. Females with the 21-hydroxylase and 11-hydroxylase defects are the most highly virilized, although minimal virilization also occurs with the type II 3β-hydroxysteroid dehydrogenase defect. Salt losers tend to have greater degrees of virilization than do non–salt-losing patients. Masculinization may be so intense that a complete penile urethra results, and the condition may mimic a male with cryptorchidism (Chapter 586.1).

AROMATASE DEFICIENCY. In genotypic females, aromatase deficiency during fetal life leads to female pseudohermaphroditism and results in hypergonadotropic hypogonadism at puberty because of ovarian failure to synthesize estrogen (see Section 4 and Fig. 589–1).

Two 46,XX infants had enlargement of the clitoris and posterior labial fusion at birth. In one instance, maternal serum and urinary levels of estrogen were very low, and serum levels of androgens were high. Cord serum levels of estrogen were also extremely low, but those of androgen were elevated. The second patient also had virilization of unknown cause since birth, but the aromatase deficiency was not diagnosed until 14 yr of age, when she had further virilization and failed to go into puberty. At that time, she had elevated levels of gonadotropins and androgens but low estrogens, and ultrasonography revealed large ovarian cysts bilaterally. These two patients demonstrate the important role of aromatase in the conversion of androgens to estrogens. Additional female, and male, patients with aromatase deficiency due to mutations in the $P450_{arom}$ (CYP19) gene are known. Two siblings were described. The 28-yr-old XY proband was 177.6 cm tall (+2.5 SD) after having received hormonal replacement therapy; her 24-yr-old brother was 204 cm tall (+3.7 SD), and had a bone age of 14 yr. Low-dose estradiol replacement, carefully adjusted to maintain normal age-appropriate levels, may be indicated for affected females even prepubertally.

VIRILIZING MATERNAL TUMORS. Rarely, the female fetus has been virilized during fetal life by a maternal androgen-producing tumor. In a few cases, the lesion was a benign adrenal adenoma, but all others were ovarian tumors, particularly androblastomas, luteomas, and Krukenberg tumors. Maternal virilization may be manifested by enlargement of the clitoris, acne, deepening of the voice, decreased lactation, hirsutism, and elevated levels of androgens. In the infant, there is enlargement of the clitoris of varying degrees, often with labial fusion. Mothers of children with unexplained female pseudohermaphroditism should undergo measurements of their own levels of plasma testosterone, dehydroepiandrosterone sulfate, and androstenedione.

ADMINISTRATION OF ANDROGENIC DRUGS TO WOMEN DURING PREGNANCY. Testosterone and 17-methyltestosterone have been reported to cause female pseudohermaphroditism in some instances. The greatest number of cases, however, have resulted from the use of certain progestational compounds for the treatment of threatened abortion. In recent years, most of these progestins have been replaced by nonvirilizing ones.

Infants with female pseudohermaphroditism and caudal anomalies have been reported for whom no virilizing agent could be identified. In such instances, the disorder is usually associated with other congenital defects, particularly of the urinary and gastrointestinal tracts. Y-specific DNA sequences, including SRY, are absent. In one recent case, a scrotal raphe and elevated testosterone levels were found, but the cause remains unknown.

598.2 Male Pseudohermaphroditism

In the male pseudohermaphrodite, the genotype is XY, but the external genitals are incompletely virilized, ambiguous, or completely female. When gonads can be found, they are invariably testes; their development may range from rudimentary to normal. Because the process of normal virilization in the fetus is so complex, it is not surprising that there are many varieties of male hermaphroditism.

DEFECTS IN TESTICULAR DIFFERENTIATION

The first step in male differentiation is conversion of the indifferent gonad to a testis. In the XY fetus, if there is a deletion of the *short arm of the Y chromosome* or of the SRY gene, male differentiation does not occur. The phenotype is female; müllerian ducts are well developed because of the absence of MIS, but gonads consist of undifferentiated streaks. By contrast, even extreme deletions of the *long arm of the Y chromosome* (Yq-) have been found in normally developed males, most of whom are azoospermic and have short stature, indicating that the long arm of the Y chromosome normally has genes that prevent these manifestations. In other syndromes in which the testes fail to differentiate, Y chromosomes are morphologically normal.

DENYS-DRASH SYNDROME. The constellation of nephropathy with ambiguous genitals or Wilms tumor are the major characteristics of this syndrome. Most reported cases have been 46,XY. Müllerian ducts are often present, indicating a global deficiency of fetal testicular function. Patients with 46,XX karyotype have normal external genitals. The onset of proteinuria in infancy progresses to nephrotic syndrome and end-stage renal failure by 3 yr of age, with focal or diffuse mesangial sclerosis being the most consistent histopathologic finding. Wilms tumor usually develops in children younger than 2 yr of age and is frequently bilateral. Gonadoblastomas have been reported.

Several mutations of the Wilms tumor gene (WT1), located on chromosome 11p13, have been found. WT1 functions as a tumor-suppressor gene and transcriptional factor and is expressed in the genital ridge and fetal gonads. Nearly all reported mutations have been near or within the zinc finger coding region. In most patients, nephrotic syndrome rather then Wilms tumor is the most consistent finding. However, one report found a zinc finger domain mutation in the WT1 alleles of a patient without any genitourinary abnormalities, suggesting that some cases of sporadic Wilms tumor may carry the Denys-Drash WT1 mutation.

WAGR SYNDROME. This acronymic syndrome consists of *W*ilms tumor, *a*niridia, *g*enitourinary malformations, and *r*etardation. Only 46,XY males have genital abnormalities, ranging from cryptorchidism to severe deficiency of virilization. Gonadoblastomas have developed in the dysgenetic gonads. Wilms tumor usually occurs by 2 yr of age. These children have a deletion of one copy of chromosome 11p13, which may be visible on karyotype analysis. The deleted region encompasses the aniridia gene *(*PAX6) and the Wilms tumor suppressor gene (WT1), which is critical for testicular development.

CAMPTOMELIC SYNDROME (see Chapter 701). This form of short-limbed dysplasia is characterized by anterior bowing of the femur and tibia and by malformations of other organs. It is usually lethal in early infancy. About 75% of reported 46,XY patients exhibit sex reversal with a completely female phenotype; the external and internal genitals are female. Some 46,XY patients have ambiguous genitals. The gonads appear to be ovaries but histologically may contain elements of ovaries and testes.

The gene responsible for the condition is SOX 9 (*S*RY-related HMG-bo*x* gene) and is on 17q24–q25. This gene is structurally related to SRY and also directly regulates the type II collagen gene (COL 2A1) development. The same mutations may result in different gonadal phenotypes. Gonadoblastoma was reported in a patient with this condition. The inheritance is autosomal dominant.

XY PURE GONADAL DYSGENESIS (SWYER SYNDROME). The designation "pure" distinguishes this condition from forms of gonadal dysgenesis that are of chromosomal origin and associated with somatic anomalies. Affected patients have normal stature and a female phenotype, including vagina, uterus, and fallopian tubes, but at pubertal age, breast development and menarche fail to occur. None of the defects associated with 45,X children is present. Patients present at puberty with hypergonadotropic primary amenorrhea. Familial cases suggest an X-linked or a sex-limited dominant autosomal transmission. Most of the patients examined have had mutations of the SRY gene. None had a SOX 9 gene mutation. The gonads consist of almost totally undifferentiated streaks despite the presence of a cytogenetically normal Y chromosome. The primitive gonad cannot accomplish any testicular function, including suppression of müllerian ducts. There may be hilar cells in the gonad capable of producing some androgens; accordingly, some virilization, such as clitoral enlargement, may occur at the age of puberty. The streak gonads may undergo neoplastic changes, such as gonadoblastomas and dysgerminomas, and should be removed shortly after diagnosis, regardless of age.

Pure gonadal dysgenesis also occurs in XX individuals (see Chapter 596.1).

XY GONADAL AGENESIS SYNDROME (EMBRYONIC TESTICULAR REGRESSION SYNDROME). In this rare syndrome, the external genitals are slightly ambiguous but more nearly female. Hypoplasia of the labia, some degree of labioscrotal fusion, a small clitoris-like phallus, and a perineal urethral opening are present. No uterus, no gonadal tissue, and usually no vagina can be found. At the age of puberty, no sexual development occurs, and gonadotropin levels are elevated. Most children have been reared as females. In several patients with XY gonadal agenesis in whom no gonads could be found on exploration, significant rises in testosterone followed stimulation with hCG, indicating Leydig cell function somewhere. Siblings with the disorder are known.

In this condition, it is presumed that testicular tissue was active long enough during fetal life for MIS to inhibit development of müllerian ducts but not long enough for testosterone production to result in virilization. In one patient, no deletion of the Y chromosome was found using Y-specific DNA probes. Testicular degeneration seems to occur between the 8th and 12th fetal wk. Regression of the testis before the 8th wk of gestation results in Swyer syndrome; between the 14th and 20th wk of gestation, it results in the rudimentary testis syndrome; and after the 20th wk, it results in anorchia.

In *bilateral anorchia,* testes are absent, but the male phenotype is complete; it is presumed that tissue with fetal testicular function was active during the critical period of genital differentiation but that sometime later it was damaged. Bilateral anorchia in identical twins and unilateral anorchia in identical twins and in siblings suggest a genetic predisposition. Coexistence of anorchia and the gonadal agenesis syndrome in a sibship is evidence for a relationship between the disorders.

A retrospective review of urologic explorations revealed absent testes in 21% of 691 testes. Of those, 73% had blind-ending cord structures with the suggested site of the vanishing testes being the inguinal canal (59%), the abdomen (21%), superficial inguinal ring (18%), and scrotum (2%). It was suggested that the presence of cord structures on laparoscopy should prompt inguinal exploration because viable testicular tissue was found in four of these children. No hormonal data (hCG stimulation tests, MIS levels) were reported.

DEFECTS IN TESTICULAR HORMONES

Five genetic defects have been delineated in the enzymatic synthesis of testosterone by fetal testis, and a defect in Leydig cell differentiation has been described. These defects produce male pseudohermaphroditism through inadequate masculinization of the XY fetus (Fig. 598–1). Because levels of testosterone are normally low before puberty, an hCG stimulation test must be used in children to assess the ability of the testes to synthesize testosterone.

LEYDIG CELL APLASIA. Patients with aplasia or hypoplasia of the Leydig cells usually have female phenotypes, but there may be mild virilization. Testes, epididymis, and vas are present; the uterus and fallopian tubes are absent. There are no secondary sexual changes at puberty; pubic hair may be normal. Plasma levels of testosterone are low and do not respond to hCG; luteinizing hormone (LH) levels are elevated. The Leydig cells of the testes are absent or markedly deficient. The defect may involve a lack of receptors for LH. In children, hCG stimulation is necessary to differentiate the condition from the androgen insensitivity syndromes (AIS). There is male-limited autosomal recessive inheritance. The human LH receptor is a member of the G-protein–coupled superfamily of receptors that contain seven transmembrane domains. Several inactivating mutations of the LH receptor have been described in males with hypogonadism suspected of having Leydig cell hypoplasia or aplasia.

High serum LH and low follicle stimulating hormone were noted in one male with hypogonadism due to a mutation in the gene for the β subunit of follicle-stimulating hormone (See Table 593–1).

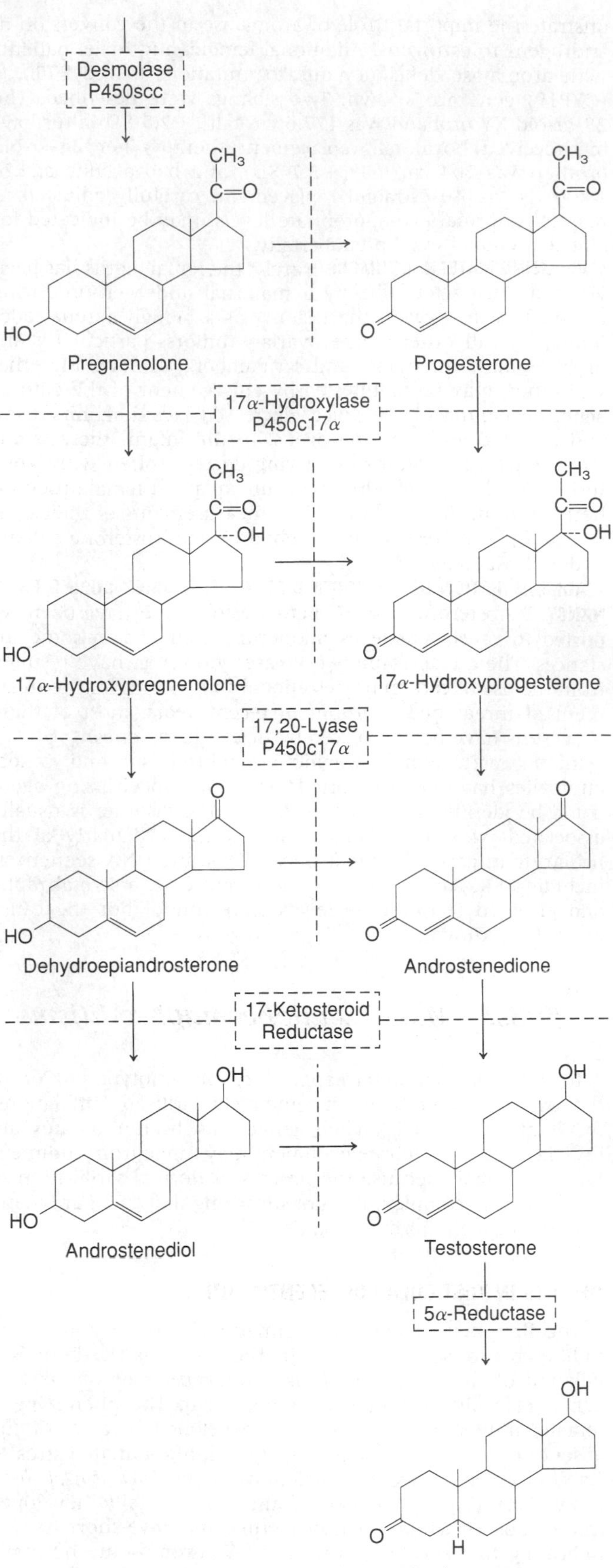

Figure 598–1 Biosynthesis of androgens. The dotted lines indicate enzymatic defects associated with male pseudohermaphroditism. The vertical dotted line indicates a defect in 3β-hydroxysteroid dehydrogenase. A single polypeptide, P450c17, catalyzes both 17α-hydroxylase and 17,20-lyase activities

LIPOID ADRENAL HYPERPLASIA (also see Chapter 586). The most severe form of congenital adrenal hyperplasia derives its name from the appearance of the enlarged adrenal glands resulting from accumulation of cholesterol and cholesterol esters. It was previously thought to be due to defective P450scc activity, the enzyme responsible for side-chain cleavage of a carbon unit from cholesterol to form pregnenolone. It has now been proved that it is due to diminished delivery of the substrate cholesterol to the inner mitochondrial membrane and to the P450scc system. That process is regulated by steroidogenic acute regulatory protein (StAR), mutations of which were documented in children with lipoid adrenal hyperplasia.

All serum steroid levels are low or undetectable, whereas corticotropin and plasma renin levels are elevated. The phenotype is female in genetic females and males; genetic males have no müllerian structures because the testes can produce normal MIS but no steroid. These children present with acute adrenal crisis and salt wasting in infancy. Most patients are 46,XY. In a few patients, ovarian steroidogenesis is present at puberty.

The regulatory role of StAR-independent steroidogenesis is illustrated by 46,XX 4-mo-old twins with lipoid adrenal hyperplasia. One died at 15 mo because of cardiac complications related to coarctation of the aorta. The adrenal glands had characteristic lipid deposits. The surviving twin had spontaneous puberty with feminization at 11.5 yr with menarche at 13.8 yr. When restudied at the age of 15 yr, a homozygous frameshift-inactivating mutation in her StAR gene was discovered. This and the fact that she survived as a baby until 4 mo of age without replacement therapy with detectable serum aldosterone levels supports the hypothesis that StAR-independent steroidogenesis was able to proceed until enough intracellular lipid accumulated to destroy steroidogenic activity. Partial defects in only partially virilized males and delayed onset of salt wasting have been described. Complete P450scc defects may be incompatible with life because only this enzyme can convert cholesterol to pregnenolone, which then becomes progesterone, a hormone essential for the maintenance of normal mammalian pregnancy. At 6–7 wk of gestation, when maternal corpus luteum progesterone synthesis stops, the placenta, which does not express StAR, produces progesterone by StAR-independent steroidogenesis using the P450scc enzyme system.

3β-HYDROXYSTEROID DEHYDROGENASE DEFICIENCY. Males with this form of congenital adrenal hyperplasia (see Chapter 586) have various degrees of hypospadias, with or without bifid scrotum and cryptorchidism and, rarely, a complete female phenotype. Affected infants usually acquire salt-losing manifestations shortly after birth. Incomplete defects, occasionally seen in boys with premature pubarche, as well as late-onset nonclassic forms have been reported. These children have point mutations of the gene for type II 3β-hydroxysteroid enzyme, resulting in impairment of steroidogenesis in the adrenals and gonads; the impairment may be unequal between adrenals and gonads. Normal pubertal changes in some boys could be explained by the normally present type I 3β-hydroxysteroid dehydrogenase present in many peripheral tissues. There is no correlation between degree of salt wasting and degree of phenotypic abnormality.

DEFICIENCY OF 17-HYDROXYLASE/17,20 LYASE. A single enzyme (P450c17) encoded by a single gene on chromosome 10q24.3 has both 17-hydroxylase and 17,20 lyase activities in adrenal and gonadal tissues (Chapter 586). Many different genetic lesions have been reported. Genetic males usually present with a complete female phenotype or, less often, with various degrees of undervirilization from labioscrotal fusion to perineal hypospadias and cryptorchidism. Pubertal development fails to occur in both genetic sexes.

In the classic disorder, there is decreased synthesis of cortisol by the adrenals and of sex steroids by the adrenals and gonads (see Fig. 598–1 and Fig. 586–1). Levels of deoxycorticosterone (DOC) and corticosterone are markedly increased and lead to the hypertension and hypokalemia characteristic of this form of male pseudohermaphroditism. Although levels of cortisol are low, the elevated corticotropin and corticosterone levels maintain a eucorticoid state. The renin-aldosterone axis is suppressed because of the strong mineralocorticoid effect of elevated DOC. Virilization does not occur at puberty; levels of testosterone are low and those of gonadotropins are increased. Because fetal production of MIS is normal, no müllerian duct remnants are present. In phenotypic XY females, gonadectomy and replacement therapy with hydrocortisone and sex steroids are indicated.

The defect follows autosomal recessive inheritance. Affected XX females are usually not detected until young adult life, when they fail to experience normal pubertal changes and are found to have hypertension and hypokalemia. This condition should be suspected in patients presenting with primary amenorrhea and hypertension whose chromosomal complement is either 46,XX or 46,XY.

DEFICIENCY OF 17-KETOSTEROID REDUCTASE. This enzyme, also called *17β-hydroxysteroid dehydrogenase (17β-HSD)*, is the last in the testosterone biosynthetic pathway; it is necessary to convert androstenedione to testosterone and also dehydroepiandrosterone to androstenediol and estrone to estradiol. Enzymatic defects in fetal testicular tissue give rise to males with complete or near-complete female phenotype in 46,XY males. Müllerian ducts are absent, and a shallow vagina is present. The diagnosis is based on the ratio of testosterone to androstenedione; in prepubertal children, prior stimulation with hCG is necessary.

The defect is inherited in an autosomal recessive fashion. At least four different types of 17β-HSD are recognized, each coded by a different gene or different chromosomes. One of the best studied forms, type III, is the enzyme defect that is especially common in a highly inbred Arab population in the Gaza strip. The gene for the disorder is at 9q22 and is expressed only in the testes, where it converts androstenedione to testosterone. Most patients are diagnosed at puberty because of the failure to menstruate and virilization. Testosterone levels at puberty may approach normal, presumably as a result of peripheral conversion of androstenedione to testosterone; at this time, some patients spontaneously adopt a male gender role.

Type I 17β-HSD, encoded by a gene on chromosome 17q21, converts estrone to estradiol and is found in placenta, ovary, testis, liver, prostate, adipose tissue, and endometrium. Type II, whose gene is on chromosome 16q24 has activities that are opposite to those of types I and III (convert testosterone to andostenedione and estrone to estradiol). Type IV is similar in action to type II. A late-onset form of 17-ketosteroid reductase deficiency presents as gynecomastia in young adult males.

PERSISTENT MÜLLERIAN DUCT SYNDROME. In this disorder, there is persistence of müllerian duct derivatives in otherwise completely virilized males. Cases have been reported in siblings and identical twins. Cryptorchidism is present in 80% of affected males, and during surgery for this or inguinal hernia, the condition is uncovered when a fallopian tube and uterus are found. The degree of müllerian development is variable and may be asymmetric. Testicular function is normal in most, but testicular degeneration has been reported. Some affected males acquire testicular tumors after puberty. In a study of 38 families, 16 families had defects in the MIS gene, located on the short arm of chromosome 19. They had low MIS levels. In 16 families with high MIS levels, the defect was in the MIS type II receptor gene, with 10/16 having identical 27 base pair deletions on exon 10 in at least one allele.

Treatment consists of removal of as many of the müllerian structures as possible without causing damage to the testis, epididymis, or vas deferens.

DEFECTS IN ANDROGEN ACTION

In the following group of disorders, fetal synthesis of testosterone is normal, and defective virilization results from inherited abnormalities in androgen action.

5α-REDUCTASE DEFICIENCY. Decreased production of dihydrotestosterone (DHT) in utero results in severe ambiguity of the external genitals of the affected male fetus. Biosynthesis and peripheral action of testosterone are normal.

The phenotype most commonly associated with this condition results in boys who have a small phallus, bifid scrotum, urogenital sinus with perineal hypospadias, and a blind vaginal pouch. Testes are in the inguinal canals or labioscrotal folds and are normal histologically. There are no müllerian structures. Wolffian structures—the vas deferens, epididymis, and seminal vesicles—are present. Most affected patients have been identified as females. At puberty, virilization occurs; the phallus enlarges, the testes descend and grow normally, and spermatogenesis occurs. There is no gynecomastia. Beard growth is scanty, acne is absent, the prostate is small, and recession of the temporal hairline fails to occur. These findings are consistent with studies in animals that show virilization of the wolffian duct to be caused by the action of testosterone itself, although masculinization of the urogenital sinus and external genitals depends on the action of DHT during the critical period of fetal masculinization. Growth of facial hair and of the prostate also appears to be DHT-dependent.

The adult height reached is close to that of the father and other male siblings. There is, however, significant phenotypic heterogeneity. This has lead to a classification of such patients into five types of steroid 5α-reductase deficiency (SRD) ranging from complete female (type 5), to partial female (type 4), ambiguous (type 3), predominantely male with micropenis (type 2), and completely male phenotype without apparent undervirilization (type 1).

Several different gene defects leading to steroid 5α-reductase deficiency have been identified in the 5α-reductase type 2 gene, located on the short arm of chromosome 2, in patients from throughout the world. Familial clusters have been reported from the Dominican Republic, Turkey, Papua New Guinea, Brazil, Mexico, and the Middle East. There is no correlation between severity of the genetic defect and phenotype.

The disorder is inherited as an autosomal recessive trait but is limited to males; normal homozygous females with normal fertility indicate that in females, DHT has no role in sexual differentiation or in ovarian function later in life. The clinical diagnosis should be made as early as possible in infancy; it should be distinguished from AIS. The biochemical diagnosis is based on finding normal serum testosterone levels, normal or low DHT levels with markedly increased basal and, especially, hCG-stimulated testosterone:DHT ratios (>17), and high ratios of urinary etiocholanolone to androsterone and 5β to 5α metabolities. Children with androgen insensitivity have normal hepatic 5α reduction and, thus, a normal ratio of tetrahydrocortisol to 5α-tetrahydrocortisol as opposed to those with SRD.

Most but, importantly, not all children reared as females in childhood have changed to male around the time of puberty. It appears that exposures to testosterone in utero, neonatally, and at puberty contribute to the formation of male gender identity. Much more needs to be learned about the influences of hormones such as androgens as well as the influences of cultural, social, psychologic, genetic, and other biologic factors in gender identity and behavior. Infants with this condition should be reared as boys whenever practical. Treatment of male infants with DHT results in phallic enlargement.

ANDROGEN INSENSITIVITY SYNDROMES. The AIS compose the most common forms of male pseudohermaphroditism, occurring with a presumed frequency of 1/20,000 genetic males. This group of heterogeneous X-linked disorders is due to several identified defects in the androgen receptor gene, located on Xq11–12.

Clinical Manifestations. The clinical spectrum of patients with AIS, all of whom have a 46,XY chromosomal complement, range from phenotypic females (in complete AIS) to males with various forms of ambiguous genitals and undervirilization (partial AIS, or clinical syndromes such as Reifenstein's syndrome) to phenotypically normal-appearing males with infertility. In addition to normal 46,XY chromosomes, the presence of testes and normal or elevated testosterone levels are common to all such children.

In complete AIS, an extreme form of failure of virilization, genetic males appear female at birth and are invariably reared accordingly. The external genitals are female. The vagina ends blindly in a pouch, and the uterus is absent. In about one third of patients, unilateral or bilateral fallopian tube remnants are found. The testes are usually intra-abdominal but may descend into the inguinal canal; they consist largely of seminiferous tubules. At puberty, there is normal development of breasts, and the habitus is female, but menstruation does not occur, and sexual hair is absent. Adult heights of these women are commensurate with those of normal males despite profound congenital deficiency of androgenic effects.

The testes of affected adult patients produce normal male levels of testosterone and DHT. Failure of normal male differentiation during fetal life reflects defective response to androgens at that time, but the absence of müllerian ducts indicates normal fetal testicular production of MIS. The absence of androgenic effects is caused by a striking resistance to the action of endogenous or exogenous testosterone at the cellular level.

Prepubertal children with this disorder are often detected when inguinal masses prove to be testes or when a testis is unexpectedly found during herniorrhaphy in a phenotypic female. About 1–2% of girls with an inguinal hernia prove to have this disorder. In infants, elevated gonadotropin levels should suggest the diagnosis. In adults, amenorrhea is the usual presenting symptom. In prepubertal children, the condition must be differentiated from other types of XY male pseudohermaphroditism in which there is complete feminization. These include XY gonadal dysgenesis (Swyer syndrome), true agonadism, Leydig cell aplasia including LH receptor defects, and 17-ketosteroid reductase deficiency; all of these conditions, unlike complete AIS, are characterized by low levels of testosterone as neonates and during adult life and by failure to respond to hCG during the prepubertal years. Although patients with complete AIS present with unambiguously female external genitals at birth, those with partial AIS have a wide variety of phenotypic presentations ranging from perineoscrotal hypospadias, bifid scrotum, and cryptorchidism to extreme undervirilization appearing as clitoromegaly and labial fusion. Some forms of partial AIS have been known as specific syndromes. Patients with *Reifenstein syndrome* have incomplete virilization characterized by hypogonadism, severe hypospadias, and gynecomastia. *Gilbert-Dreyfuss* and *Lubs* are additional syndromes now classified under the partial AIS category. In all such cases, abnormalities in the androgen receptor gene have been identified.

Diagnosis. The diagnosis of patients with partial AIS may be particularly difficult in infancy. In some, especially those sufficiently virilized in infancy, the diagnosis is not suspected until puberty when there is inadequate virilization with lack of facial hair or voice change and the appearance of gynecomastia. Azoospermia and infertility are common. Increasingly, androgen receptor defects are being recognized in adults who have a small phallus and testes and infertility.

Treatment and Prognosis. In patients with complete AIS whose sexual orientation is unambiguously female, the testes should be removed as soon as they are discovered. Laparoscopic removal of Y-bearing gonads has been performed in patients with AIS and in those with gonadal dysgenesis. In one third of patients, malignant tumors, usually seminomas, develop by 50 yr of age. Several teenaged girls have acquired seminomas. Replacement therapy with estrogens is indicated at the age of puberty.

Normal breasts develop in affected girls who have not had their testes removed by the age of puberty. In these individuals, production of estradiol results from aromatase activity. The absence of androgenic activity also contributes to the feminization of these women.

The psychosexual and surgical management of patients with partial AIS is extremely complex and depends in large part on the presenting phenotype. Osteopenia is now recognized as a feature of AIS.

Molecular analyses have suggested that phenotype may depend in part on somatic mosaicism of the androgen receptor gene. This was based on the case of a 46,XY patient who had a premature stop codon in exon 1 of the AR gene but who also had evidence of virilization (pubic hair and clitoral enlargement) explained by the discovery of the wild-type alleles on careful examination of the sequencing gel. The presence of mosaicism shifts the phenotype to a higher degree of virilization then expencted from the genotype of the mutant allele alone.

Genetic counseling is difficult in families with androgen receptor gene mutation. In addition to lack of genotype-phenotype correlations, a recent study documented a high rate (27%) of de novo mutations in families.

Sex hormone–binding globulin reduction following exogenous androgen administration (stanozolol) has been shown to correlate with the severity of the receptor defect and may become a useful clinical tool. Successful therapy with supplemental androgens has been reported in patients with partial AIS and various mutations of the androgen receptor in the DNA-binding domain and the ligand-binding domain.

UNDETERMINED CAUSES

Other XY male pseudohermaphrodites display great variability of the external and internal genitals and various degrees of phallic and müllerian development. Testes may be histologically normal or rudimentary, or there may only be one. Even the newer techniques may find no recognized cause of pseudohermaphroditism in a substantial number of children. Some ambiguity of genitals is associated with a wide variety of chromosomal aberrations, which must always be considered in the differential diagnosis, the most common being the 45,X/46,XY syndrome (see Chapter 596.1). It may be necessary to examine several tissues in order to establish mosaicism. Other complex genetic syndromes, many resulting from single gene mutations, are associated with varying degrees of ambiguity of the genitals, particularly in the male. These entities must be identified on the basis of the associated extragenital malformations.

Smith-Lemli-Opitz syndrome is an autosomal recessive disorder characterized by prenatal and postnatal growth retardation, microcephaly, ptosis, anteverted nares, broad alveolar ridges, syndactyly of the 2nd and 3rd toes, and severe mental retardation. Genotypic males usually have genital ambiguity and, occasionally, complete sex reversal with female genital ambiguity or complete sex reversal with female external genitals. Müllerian duct derivatives are usually absent. Affected 46,XX patients have normal genitals. Two types of Smith-Lemli-Opitz syndrome have been recognized: the classic form (type I) described earlier and the acrodysgenital syndrome, which is usually lethal within 1 yr and is associated with severe malformations, postaxial polydactyly, and extremely abnormal external genitals (type II). Pyloric stenosis is associated with Smith-Lemli-Opitz syndrome type I and Hirschprung disease with type II. Cleft palate, skeletal abnormalities, and one case of a lipoma of the pituitary gland have been seen in type II cases.

Low plasma cholesterol with elevated 7-dehydrocholesterol, its precursor, are found in both types. There is no correlation between plasma cholesterol levels and severity of disease. A translocation and deletion on chromosome 7q32–34 has been reported.

Male pseudohermaphroditism also has been described in siblings with the α-thalassenia–mental retardation syndrome.

598.3 True Hermaphroditism

In true hermaphroditism, both ovarian and testicular tissues are present, either in the same or in opposite gonads. Affected patients have ambiguous genitals, varying from normal female with only slight enlargement of the clitoris to almost normal male external genitals.

About 70% of all patients have a 46,XX karyotype; 97% of affected African blacks are 46,XX. Fewer than 10% of true hermaphrodites are 46,XY. About 20% have 46,XX/46,XY mosaicism. Half of these are derived from more than one zygote and are chimeras (chi 46,XX/46,XY). The presence of paternal and both maternal alleles for some blood groups are demonstrated. A true hermaphrodite chimera, 46 XX/46 XY, was reported as resulting from embryo amalgamation after in vitro fertilization. Each embryo was derived from an independent, separately fertilized ovum.

Examination of 46,XX true hermaphrodites with Y-specific probes has detected fewer than 10% with a portion of the Y chromosome including the SRY gene. True hermaphroditism is usually sporadic, but a number of siblings have been reported. The cause of most cases of true hermaphroditism is unknown.

The most frequently encountered gonad in true hermaphrodites is an ovotestis, which may be bilateral; if unilateral, the contralateral gonad is usually an ovary but may be a testis. The ovarian tissue is normal, but the testicular tissue is dysgenetic. The presence and function of testicular tissue can be determined by measuring basal and hCG-stimulated testosterone levels and MIS levels. Patients who are highly virilized, have good testicular function, and have no uterus are usually reared as males. If a uterus exists, virilization is mild, and testicular function minimal, assignment of female sex may be indicated. Selective removal of gonadal tissue inconsistent with sex of rearing is indicated.

Pregnancies with living offspring have been reported in 46,XX true hermaphrodites reared as females, but, to date, apparently only one male true hermaphrodite has fathered a child. About 5% of patients acquire gonadoblastomas, dysgerminomas, or seminomas.

DIAGNOSIS AND MANAGEMENT. In the neonate, ambiguity of the genitals requires emergency medical attention to decide on the sex of rearing as early in life as possible. The family of the infant needs to be informed of the child's condition as early, completely, compassionately, and honestly as possible. Caution must be used to avoid feelings of guilt, shame, and discomfort. Guidance needs to be provided to alleviate both short-term and long-term concerns and allow the child to grow up in a completely supportive and entirely unambiguous environment. The initial care is best provided by a team of professionals that include neonatologists and pediatric specialists, endocrinologists, radiologists, urologists, psychologists, and geneticists, all of whom remain focused foremost on the needs of the child. Management of the potential psychologic upheaval that these disorders can generate in the child or the family is of paramount importance and requires physicians and other health care professionals with sensitivity, training, and experience in this field. After the appropriate sex of rearing has been established, parents should be left with no ambiguity in their minds as to the gender of the child.

While awaiting the results of chromosomal analysis, pelvic ultrasonography or magnetic resonance imaging is indicated to determine the presence of a uterus and ovaries. Presence of a uterus and absence of palpable gonads usually suggests a virilized XX female. A search for the source of virilization should be undertaken; this includes studies of adrenal hormones to rule out varieties of congenital adrenal hyperplasia, and studies of androgens and estrogens occasionally may be necessary to rule out aromatase deficiency. Female pseudohermaphrodites should be reared as females even when highly virilized.

The absence of a uterus, with or without palpable gonads, almost always indicates male pseudohermaphroditism and an XY karyotype. Measurements of levels of gonadotropins, testosterone, MIS, and DHT are necessary to determine whether testicular production of androgen is normal. Male pseudohermaphrodites who are totally feminized may be reared as females. However, certain significantly feminized infants, such as those with 5α-reductase deficiency, should be reared as males because these children virilize normally at puberty. An infant with a comparable degree of feminization resulting from an androgen-receptor defect is best reared as a female. Infants with 45,X/46,XY whose phenotype varies from almost completely male to completely female are usually reared as females because they are generally short in stature and have a uterus; they require gonadectomy.

When receptor disorders are suspected in the XY male with a small phallus (micropenis), a course of three monthly intramuscular injections of testosterone enanthate (25–50 mg) may assist in the differential diagnosis as well as in treatment.

In some mammals, the female exposed to androgens prenatally or in early postnatal life exhibits aberrant sexual behavior in adult life. Most, but not all, girls who have undergone fetal masculinization from congenital adrenal hyperplasia or from maternal progestin therapy have no such problems in sexual identity, although during childhood they may appear to prefer male playmates and activities over female playmates and feminine play with dolls in mothering roles.

Advances in visualization procedures, hormonal assays, molecular methodology as well as surgical techniques should make for more rapid, accurate, and appropriate diagnosis and management of the infant and child with intersex. It has been thought that it is more feasible to reconstruct the external genitals to create a functional female, particularly when a vagina is present, than to create a functional male phallus. Hence, in the absence of reasonable prospects for a well-functioning male phallus, the intersex infants have in the past always been assigned a female gender. Considerable controversy currently exists regarding these decisions. A poorly functioning female external genital system may be no better then a poorly functioning male phallus. In addition, sexual functioning is to a large extent more dependent on other neurohormonal and behavioral factors then the physical appearance and functional ability of the genitals. This concept is given added support by a case report of a 46,XY subject whose penis was accidentally ablated and was subsequently reared as a female. At puberty this individual switched to male and continues to successfully live as such.

Similarly, controversy exists regarding the timing of the performance of invasive procedures, such as surgery. Whenever possible without endangering the physical or psychological health of the child, an expert multidisciplinary team should consider deferring elective surgical repairs and gonadectomies until the child can participate in the informed consent for the procedure.

The pediatrician and pediatric endocrinologist, along with the appropriate additional specialists, should provide ongoing compassionate, supportive care to the patient and the patient's family throughout childhood and adolescence. Support groups are available for patients and families with many of the conditions discussed.

Affara NA, Chalmers IJ, Ferguson-Smith MA: Analysis of the SRY gene in 22 sex-reversed XY females identifies four new point mutations in the conserved DNA binding domain. Hum Mol Genet 2:785, 1993.

Bell DM, Leung KK, Wheatley SC, et al: SOX9 directly regulates the type-II collagen gene. Nat Genet 16:174, 1997.

Bose HS, Pescovitz OH, Miller WL: Spontaneous feminization in a 46,XX female patient with congenital lipoid adrenal hyperplasia due to a homozygous frameshift mutation in the steroidogenic acute regulatory protein. J Clin Endocrinol Metab 82:1511, 1997.

Cameron FJ, Montalto J, Byrt, E, et al: Gonadal dysgenesis: Associations between clinical features and sex of rearing. Endocr J 44:95, 1997.

Canto P, Vilchis F, Chavez B, et al: Mutations of the 5α-reductase tyep 2 gene in eight Mexican patients from six different pedigrees with 5α-reductase-2 deficiency. Clin Endocrinol 46:155, 1997.

Castro-Magana M, Angulo M, Uy J: Male hypogonadism with gynecomastia caused by late-onset deficiency of testicular 17-ketosteroid reductase. N Engl J Med 328:1297, 1993.

Conte FA, Grumbach MM, Ito Y, et al: A syndrome of female pseudohermaphroditism, hypergonadotropic hypogonadism, and multicystic ovaries associated with missense mutations in the gene encoding aromatase ($P450_{arom}$). J Clin Endocrinol Metab 78:1287, 1994.

Cormier-Daire V, Wolf C, Munnich A, et al: Abnormal cholesterol biosynthesis in the Smith-Lemli-Opitz and the lethal acrodysgenital syndromes. Eur J Pediatr 155:656, 1996.

Damiani D, Fellous M, McElreavey K, et al: True hermaphroditism: Clinical aspects and molecular studies in 16 cases. Eur J Endocr 136:201, 1997.

Diamond M, Sigmundson K: Sex reassignment at birth. Arch Pediatr Adolesc Med 151:298, 1997.

Fardella CE, Hum DW, Homoki J, Miller WL: Point mutation of Arg 440 to His in cytochrome P450c17 causes severe 17β-hydroxylase deficiency. J Clin Endocrinol Metab 79:160, 1994.

Frade Costa EM, Bilharinho Mendonca B, Inacio M, et al: Management of ambiguous genitalia in pseudohermaphrodites: New perspectives on vaginal dilation. Fertil Steril 67:229, 1997.

Geissler WM, Davis DL, Wu L, et al: Male pseudohermaphroditism caused by mutation of testicular 17β-hydroxysteroid dehydrogenase 3. Nat Genet 7:34, 1994.

Ghahremani M, Chan CB, Bistritzer T, et al: A novel mutation H373Y in the Wilms tumor suppressor gene, WT1, associated with Denys-Drash syndrome. Hum Hered 46:336, 1996.

Hadjiathanasiou CG, Brauner R, Lortat-Jacob S, et al: True hermaphroditism: Genetic variants and clinical management. J Pediatr 125:738, 1994.

Hiort O, Sinnecker GHG, Holterbus PM, et al: Inherited and de novo androgen receptor gene mutations: Investigation of single-case families. J Pediatr 132:939, 1998.

Hochberg Z, Chayen R, Reiss N, et al: Clinical, biochemical and genetic findings in a large pedigree of male and female patients with 5α-reductase 2 deficiency. J Clin Endocrinol Metab 81:2821, 1996.

Holterhus PM, Bruggenwirth HT, Hiort O, et al: Mosaicism due to a somatic mutation of the androgen receptor gene determines phenotype in androgen insensitivity syndrome. J Clin Endocrinol Metab 82:3584 1997.

Imbeaud S, Belville C, Messika-Zeitoun L, et al: A 27 base-pair deletion of the anti-Müllerian type II receptor gene is the most common cause of the persistent müllerian duct syndrome. Hum Mol Genet 5:1269, 1996.

Kremer H, Karaaij R, Toledo SPA, et al: Male pseudohermaphroditism due to a homozygous missense mutation of the luteinizing hormone receptor gene. Nat Genet 9:160, 1995.

Krob G, Braun A, Kuhnle U: True hermaphroditism: Geographical distribution, clinical findings, chromosomes and gonadal histology. Eur J Pediatr 153:2, 1994.

Lefebvre V, Huang W, Harley VR, et al: SOX9 is a potent activator of the chondrocyte-specific enhancer of the pro alpha1 (II) collagen gene. Mol Cell Biol 17:2336, 1997.

McElreavey K, Rappaport R, Vilain E, et al: A minority of 46,XX true hermaphrodites are positive for the Y DNA sequence including SRY. Hum Genet 90:121, 1992.

McPherson EW, Clemens MM, Gibbons RJ, et al: X-linked α-thalassemia/mental retardation (ATR-X) syndrome: A new kindred with severe genital anomalies and mild hematologic expression. Am J Med Genet 55:302, 1995.

Mebarki F, Sanchez R, Rheaumes E, et al: Nonsalt-losing male pseudohermaphroditism due to the novel homozygous N100S mutation in the type II 3β-hydroxysteroid dehydrogenase gene. J Clin Endocrinol Metab 80:2127, 1995.

Mendonca BB, Inacio M, Costa EMF, et al: Male pseudohermaphroditism due to steroid 5α-reductase 2 deficiency. Medicine 75:64, 1996.

Merry C, Sweeney B, Puri P: The vanishing testis: Anatomical and histological findings. Eur Urol 31:65, 1997.

Miller WL: Why nobody has p450scc (20,22 desmoslase) deficiency. J Clin Endocrinol Metab 83:1299, 1998.

Monno S, Mizushima Y, Toyoda N, et al: A new variant of the cytochrome P450c17 (CYP17) gene mutation in three patients with 17 α-hydroxylase deficiency. Ann Hum Genet 61:275, 1997.

Morishima A, Grumbach MM, Simpson ER, et al: Aromatase deficiency in male

and female siblings caused by a novel mutation and the physiological role of estrogens. J Clin Endocrinol Metab 80:3689, 1995.
Mueller RF: The Denys-Drash syndrome. J Med Genet 31:471, 1994.
Mullis PE, Yoshimura N, Kuhlmann B, et al: Aromatase deficiency in a female who is compound heterozygote for two new point mutations in the $P450_{arom}$ gene: impact of estrogens on hypergonadotropic hypogonadism, multicystic ovaries, and bone densitometry in childhood. J Clin Endocrinol Metab 82:1739, 1997.
Quigley CA, French FS: Androgen insensitivity syndromes. Curr Ther Endocrinol Metab 5:342, 1994.
Reardon W, Gibbons RJ, Winter RM, Baraitser M: Male pseudohermaphroditism in sibs with the α-thalassemia/mental retardation (ATR-X) syndrome. Am J Med Genet 55:285, 1995.
Saenger P: New developments in congenital lipoid adrenal hyperplasia and steroidogenic acute regulatory protein. Pediatr Clin North Am 44:397, 1997.
Sinnecker GHG, Hiort O, Dibbelt L, et al: Phenotypic classification of male pseudohermaphroditism due to steroid 5α-reductase 2 deficiency. Am J Med Genet 63:223, 1996.
Sinnecker GHG, Hirot O, Nitsche EM: Functional assessment and clinical classification of androgen sensitivity in patients with mutations of the androgen receptor gene. Eur J Pediatr 156:7, 1997.
Smith EP, Boyd J, Frank GR, et al: Estrogen resistance caused by a mutation in the estrogen-receptor gene in a man. N Engl J Med 331:1056, 1994.
Wagner T, Wirth J, Meyer J, et al: Autosomal sex reversal and camptomelic dysplasia are caused by mutations in and around the SRY-related gene SOX9. Cell 79:1111, 1994.
Warne GL, Zajac JD, MacLean HE: Androgen insensitivity syndrome in the era of molecular genetics and the Internet: A point of view. J Pediatr Endocrinol Metab 11:3, 1998.
Weidemann W, Peters B, Romalo G, et al: Response to androgen treatment in a patient with partial androgen insensitivity and a mutation in the deoxyribonucleic acid-binding domain of the androgen receptor. J Clin Endocrinol Metab 83:1173, 1998.

SECTION 6

Diabetes Mellitus in Children

CHAPTER 599 *Diabetes Mellitus*

Mark A. Sperling

599.1 Introduction and Classification

Diabetes mellitus is a syndrome of metabolic disease characterized by hyperglycemia. It is caused by deficiency of insulin secretion or insulin action, or both, and results in abnormal metabolism of carbohydrate, protein, and fat. It is the most common endocrine-metabolic disorder of childhood and adolescence, with important consequences for physical and emotional development. Individuals affected by type I diabetes confront serious burdens that include an absolute daily requirement for exogenous insulin, the need to monitor their own metabolic control, and the need to pay constant attention to dietary intake. Morbidity and mortality stem from acute metabolic derangements and from long-term complications that affect small and large vessels and result in retinopathy, nephropathy, neuropathy, ischemic heart disease, and arterial obstruction with gangrene of the extremities. The acute clinical manifestations can be fully understood in the context of current knowledge about the secretion and action of insulin. Genetic and other etiologic considerations point to autoimmune mechanisms as factors in the genesis of type I diabetes, and there is a consensus that the long-term complications are related to metabolic disturbances. These considerations form the basis of therapeutic approaches to this disease.

Diabetes mellitus is not a single entity but rather a heterogeneous group of disorders in which there are distinct genetic patterns as well as other etiologic and pathophysiologic mechanisms that lead to impairment of glucose tolerance. A classification of diabetes and other categories of glucose intolerance is presented in Table 599–1. Three major forms of diabetes and several forms of carbohydrate intolerance are identified.

TYPE I DIABETES. This condition is characterized by severe insulinopenia and dependence on exogenous insulin to prevent ketosis and to preserve life; it was, therefore, formerly termed insulin-dependent diabetes mellitus (IDDM). The natural history of this disease indicates that there are preketotic, non–insulin-dependent phases both before and after the initial diagnosis. The onset occurs predominantly in childhood, but it may come at any age. Hence, such terms as *juvenile diabetes, ketosis-prone diabetes,* and *brittle diabetes* have been abandoned in favor of type I diabetes. Type I diabetes is characterized by pancreatic islet β-cell destruction mediated by immune mechanisms. This form is clearly distinct by virtue of its association with certain histocompatibility antigens (human leukocyte antigens [HLAs]); the presence of circulating antibodies to cytoplasmic and cell surface components of islet cells; antibodies to insulin in the absence of prior exposure to exogenous injection of insulin; antibodies to glutamic acid decarboxylase (GAD), the enzyme that converts glutamic acid to λ-aminobutyric acid (GABA), found abundantly in the innervation of pancreatic islets; antibodies to other islet components such as tyrosine phosphatase (IA-2, IA-2B); lymphocytic infiltration of islets early in the disease; and other autoimmune disease. In some patients with apparent type I diabetes, evidence of autoimmunity is lacking, so that the cause of the β-cell destruction remains unknown. This idiopathic category is distinct from identifiable causes of B-cell destruction that include drugs or chemicals, viruses, mitochondrial gene defects, pancreatectomy, and ionizing radiation to the abdomen. Of those who fit this category, the majority are of African or Asian origin. They may present with ketoacidosis but have extensive periods of remission with variable insulin deficiency, more akin to type II diabetes. Diabetes in children is commonly insulin-dependent and falls into the type I immune-mediated category.

TYPE II DIABETES. Persons in this subclass (formerly known as adult-onset diabetes, maturity-onset diabetes [MOD], or non–insulin-dependent diabetes mellitus [NIDDM]) are not insulin-dependent and only infrequently develop ketosis; however, some may need insulin for correction of symptomatic hyperglycemia, and ketosis may develop in some during severe infections or other stress. This category includes the most prevalent form of diabetes, which is characterized by insulin resistance with an associated and often progressive defect in insulin secretion. Many persons in this category are obese and inactive.

The serum concentration of insulin may be elevated early in the evolution of disease; it is generally less when compared with that in controls matched for weight, age, and stage of puberty by the time diabetes is clinically apparent. In the majority of instances, the onset of non–insulin-dependent diabetes mellitus occurs after age 40, but it may occur at any age. Its prevalence in childhood and adolescence is increasing dramatically in the United States, where it may account for as many as one third of newly diagnosed patients, especially in obese black American adolescents. In some individuals, it may represent slowly evolving type I diabetes mellitus. As an initial approach, weight reduction is indicated in those children who are obese.

Abnormal carbohydrate tolerance may also occur in children who have a strong family history of type II diabetes in a pattern suggestive of dominant inheritance; this pattern of diabetes has been termed maturity-onset diabetes of the young (MODY), and it may require treatment with insulin. In this type of diabetes, there is no association with HLAs, autoimmunity, or islet cell antibodies. Specific genetic disorders involving mutations in the gene encoding pancreatic β-cell and liver glucokinase and the nuclear transcription factors hepatocyte nuclear factor 4α and hepatic nuclear factor 1α are the cause of hyperglycemia in many affected families. MODY is described more fully further on. A defect in the gene regulating glucose transport into the pancreatic β cell, GLUT-2 transporter, may be responsible for other forms of non–insulin-dependent diabetes mellitus. The molecular genetic basis of type II diabetes now includes defects in glucokinase, hepatocyte nuclear factors 4α and 1α, GLUT-2 glucose transporter, glycogen synthase, insulin receptors, Rad (Ras associated with diabetes), and possibly apolipoprotein C-III.

TABLE 599–1 Etiologic Classifications of Diabetes Mellitus

Type I diabetes* (β-cell destruction, usually leading to absolute insulin deficiency)	Drug- or chemical-induced
Immune mediated	Vacor
Idiopathic	Pentamidine
Type II diabetes* (may range from predominantly insulin resistance with relative insulin deficiency to a predominantly secretory defect with insulin resistance)	Nicotinic acid
Other specific types	Glucocorticoids
Genetic defects of β-cell function	Thyroid hormone
Chromosome 12, HNF-1α (formerly MODY-3)	Diazoxide
Chromosome 7, glucokinase (formerly MODY-2)	β-Adrenergic agonists
Chromosome 20, HNF-4α (formerly MODY-1)	Thiazides
Mitochondrial DNA	Dilantin
Others	β-Interferon
Genetic defects in insulin action	Others—cyclosporine, tacrolimus
Type A insulin resistance	Infections
Leprechaunism	Congenital rubella
Rabson-Mendenhall syndrome	Cytomegalovirus
Lipoatrophic diabetes	Others—hemolytic uremic syndrome
Others	Uncommon forms of immune-mediated diabetes
Diseases of the exocrine pancreas	"Stiff-man" syndrome
Pancreatitis	Cytomegalovirus
Trauma, pancreatectomy	Others
Neoplasia	Other genetic syndromes sometimes associated with diabetes
Cystic fibrosis	Down syndrome
Hemochromatosis	Klinefelter syndrome
Fibrocalculous pancreatopathy	Turner syndrome
Pancreatic resection	Wolfram syndrome
Others	Friedreich ataxia
Endocrinopathies	Huntington chorea
Acromegaly	Lawrence-Moon-Beidel syndrome
Cushing's disease	Myotonic dystrophy
Glucagonoma	Porphyria
Pheochromocytoma	Prader-Willi syndrome
Hyperthyroidism	Others
Somatostatinoma	Gestational diabetes mellitus
Aldosteronoma	Neonatal diabetes mellitus
Others	Transient—without recurrence
	Transient—recurrence 7–20 yr later
	Permanent from onset

**Patients with any form of diabetes may require insulin treatment at some stage of the disease. Such use of insulin does not, of itself, classify the patient.*

TABLE 599–2 Diagnostic Criteria for Diabetes Mellitus

New Criteria	Criteria of the Recent Past
Symptoms* of diabetes plus a random plasma glucose ≥200 mg/dL (11.1 mmol/L)	Symptoms* of diabetes plus a random plasma glucose ≥200 mg/dL (11.1 mmol/L)
or	*or*
Fasting plasma glucose ≥126 mg/dL (7.0 mmol/L)	Fasting plasma glucose ≥140 mg/dL (7.8 mmol/L)
or	*or*
2-hr plasma glucose during the oral glucose tolerance test ≥200 mg/dL	2-hr plasma glucose plus one other glucose value during the oral glucose tolerance test ≥200 mg/dL

**Symptoms include polyuria, polydipsia, and unexplained weight loss with glucosuria and ketonuria.*

OTHER SPECIFIC TYPES OF SECONDARY DIABETES. This subclass contains a variety of types of diabetes, for some of which the etiologic relationship is known. Examples include diabetes secondary to exocrine pancreatic diseases, such as cystic fibrosis; endocrine diseases other than pancreatic diseases (e.g., Cushing syndrome); and ingestion of certain drugs or poisons (e.g., the rodenticide Vacor). Certain genetic syndromes, including those with abnormalities of the insulin receptor, also are included in this category. There are no associations with HLAs, autoimmunity, or islet cell antibodies among the entities in this subdivision.

Table 599–2 details the current criteria for the diagnosis of diabetes mellitus. It should be noted that a fasting blood glucose that exceeds 126 mg/dL (7.0 mM) is now the accepted criterion for diagnosing diabetes. Formerly, the criterion was a fasting blood glucose of greater than 140 mg/dL (7.8 mM).

IMPAIRED GLUCOSE TOLERANCE. The term *impaired glucose tolerance* (IGT) refers to a metabolic stage that is intermediate between normal glucose homeostasis and diabetes. A fasting glucose concentration of 109 mg/dL (6.1 mmol/L) has been chosen as the upper limit of "normal." Although this choice is somewhat arbitrary, it is near the level above which acute-phase insulin secretion is lost in response to intravenous administration of glucose and is associated with a progressively greater risk of the development of micro- and macrovascular complications.

Many individuals with IGT are euglycemic in their daily lives and may have normal or nearly normal glycated hemoglobin levels. Individuals with IGT often manifest hyperglycemia only when challenged with the oral glucose load used in the standardized oral glucose tolerance test.

In the absence of pregnancy, IGT is not a clinical entity but rather a risk factor for future diabetes and cardiovascular disease. This may be observed as an intermediate stage in any of the disease processes listed in Table 599–1. IGT is associated with the *insulin resistance syndrome* (also known as syndrome X or the metabolic syndrome), which consists of insulin resistance, compensatory hyperinsulinemia to maintain glucose homeostasis, obesity (especially abdominal or visceral obesity), dyslipidemia of the high-triglyceride or low-high-density lipoprotein type, or both, and hypertension. Insulin resistance is directly involved in the pathogenesis of type II diabetes. IGT appears as a risk factor for this type of diabetes at least in part because of its correlation with insulin resistance. The diagnostic criteria for IGT are presented in Table 599–3.

599.2 Type I Diabetes Mellitus (Immune-Mediated)

EPIDEMIOLOGY. In the United States, the prevalence of diabetes among school-age children is about 1.9/1,000. The frequency, however, is highly correlated with increasing age; the range is

TABLE 599–3 Diagnostic Criteria for Impaired Glucose Tolerance

New Criteria	Criteria of the Recent Past
Fasting plasma glucose <126 mg/dL (7.0 mmol/L)	Fasting plasma glucose <140 mg/dL (7.8 mmol/L)
plus	*plus*
2-hr plasma glucose during the OGTT <200 mg/dL (11.1 mmol/L) but ≥140 mg/dL	2-hr plasma glucose during the OGTT ≥140 mg/dL (7.8 mmol/L but <200 mg/dL) (11.1 mmol/L)
	plus
	0.5-hr or 1-hr or 1.5-hr plasma glucose during the OGTT ≥200 mg/dL

OGTT = oral glucose tolerance test.

Report of the Expert Committee on the Diagnosis and Classification of Diabetes Mellitus: Diabetes Care 20(Suppl 1):S5, 1999.

1 case/1,430 children at 5 yr of age to 1 in 360 children at 16 yr. In relation to racial or ethnic backgrounds, there is also a broad range of nearly 40 new cases/100,000 population/yr in Finland to about 1/100,000 in Japan (Fig. 599–1). Among black Americans, the occurrence of IDDM is between one third and two thirds of that seen in American whites. These observations have implications for genetic counseling (see later). The annual incidence in the United States is about 12–15 new cases/100,000 of the child population. Girls and boys are almost equally affected; there is no apparent correlation with socioeconomic status. Peaks of presentation occur in two age groups: at 5–7 yr of age and at the time of puberty. Nonetheless, a growing number of patients are presenting between 1 and 2 yr of age. The first peak corresponds to the time of increased exposure to infectious agents coincident with the beginning of school; the latter, to the pubertal growth spurt induced by gonadal steroids, increased pubertal growth hormone secretion (which antagonizes insulin action), and the emotional stresses accompanying puberty. These possible cause-and-effect relationships remain to be proved. The prevalence and incidence of IDDM in childhood in the United States and elsewhere may reflect the population's distribution of susceptibility genes encoded on the DQ β-chain of the HLA system.

Seasonal and long-term cyclic variations occur in the incidence of IDDM. Newly recognized cases appear with greater frequency in the autumn and winter months in the Northern and Southern Hemispheres. Seasonal variations are most apparent in the adolescent years. Attempts to link a pattern of long-term cyclicity with the incidence of mumps or other viral infections, when allowance was made for a 4-yr time lag, have not been successful. There is, however, a definite increased incidence of diabetes in children with congenital rubella. These associations with viral infections suggest a potential role for viruses as direct or indirect triggering mechanisms in the etiology of diabetes.

ETIOLOGY AND PATHOGENESIS. The basic cause of the initial clinical findings in this predominant form of diabetes in childhood is the sharply diminished secretion of insulin. At diagnosis, basal insulin concentrations in plasma may be normal, but insulin production in response to a variety of potent secretagogues is blunted and usually totally disappears over a period of months to years, rarely exceeding 5 yr. In certain individuals

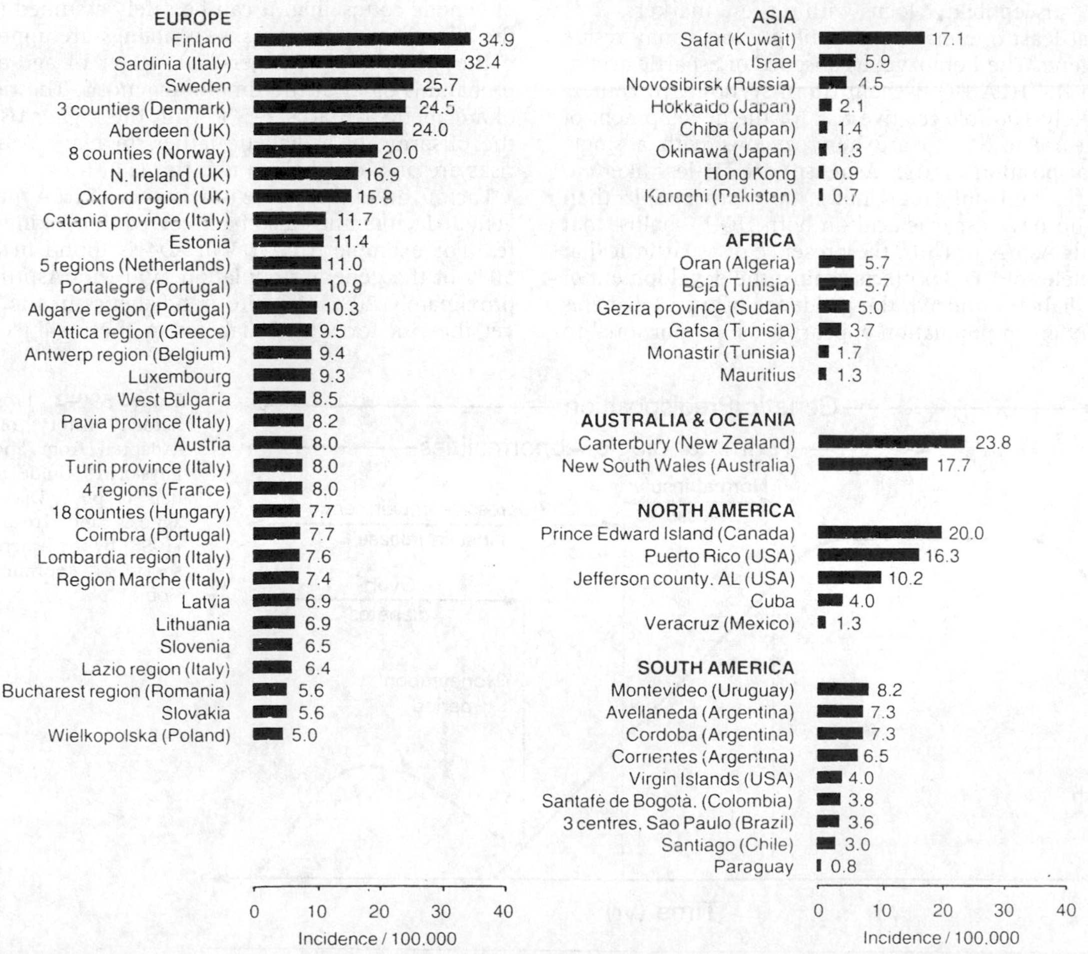

Figure 599–1 Incidence rates of type I diabetes mellitus by region and country. (From LaPorte RA, et al: The DiaMond Project. Pract Diabetes Int 12:93, 1995.)

considered at high risk for the development of type I diabetes, such as the nonaffected identical twin of a diabetic or siblings with various markers of immunity to β cells—for example, GAD65 antibody or insulin autoantibodies, a progressive decline in insulin-secreting capacity has been noted for months to years before the clinical appearance of symptomatic diabetes, which usually becomes manifested when insulin-secreting reserve is 20% or less of normal (Fig. 599–2).

The mechanisms that lead to failure of pancreatic β-cell function increasingly point to the likelihood of autoimmune destruction of pancreatic islets in predisposed individuals. Type I diabetes has long been known to have an increased prevalence among persons with disorders such as Addison disease, Hashimoto thyroiditis, and pernicious anemia, in which autoimmune mechanisms are known to be pathogenic. These conditions, as well as type I diabetes mellitus, are known to be associated with an increased frequency of certain HLAs, in particular HLA-B8, -DR3, -BW15, and -DR4. Located on chromosome 6, the HLA system is the major histocompatibility complex, consisting of a cluster of genes that code transplantation antigens and play a central role in immune responses (see Chapter 77).

Increased susceptibility to a number of diseases has been related to one or more of the identified HLA antigens. Inheritance of HLA-D3 or -D4 antigens appears to confer a two- to threefold increased risk for the development of type I diabetes. When both D3 and D4 are inherited, the relative risk for the development of diabetes is increased by 7- to 10-fold. Analysis of DNA polymorphisms after digestion by specific restriction endonucleases has revealed further heterogeneity in the HLA-D region among individuals with and without diabetes despite the possession in both DR3 or DR4 markers, suggesting a yet to be defined "susceptibility" locus within these markers.

In whites, at least one major susceptibility locus may reside in the $DQ\beta_1$ gene. The homozygous absence of aspartic acid at position 57 of the HLA DQ β-chain (nonAsp/nonAsp) confers an approximately 100-fold relative risk for the development of type I diabetes. Those who are heterozygous with a single aspartic acid at position 57 (nonAsp/Asp) are far less likely to acquire diabetes and only marginally more susceptible than individuals who have aspartic acid on both DQ β-chains, that is, homozygous Asp/Asp. Thus, the presence of aspartic acid at one or both alleles of DQ β protects against the development of autoimmune diabetes. Indeed, the incidence of type I diabetes mellitus in any given population appears to be proportional to the gene frequency of nonAsp alleles in that population. In addition, arginine at position 52 of the DQ β chain confers marked susceptibility to IDDM. Position 57 of the DQ β and position 52 of DQ β are at critical locations of the HLA molecule that permit or prevent antigen presentation to T-cell receptors and activate the autoimmune cascade. In addition to the genetic susceptibility loci related to the HLA system or chromosome 6, a minimum of 11 other loci on 9 different chromosomes has been associated with an increased risk of the development of diabetes. None provide as strong an association as HLA, which accounts for about one third of familial clustering. A region of variable number of tandem repeats in the region of the insulin gene on chromosome 11 may account for about 10% of the genetic risk.

These observations provide a rational framework for the long-recognized association of type I diabetes with genetic factors on the basis of the increased incidence in some families, the incomplete concordance rates in monozygotic twins, and ethnic and racial differences in prevalence. For example, type I diabetes among black Americans is associated with the same HLA genes as it is in American whites. From multiple family pedigrees and HLA typing data, it has been determined that if a sibling shares both HLA-D haplotypes with an index case, the risk for IDDM in that individual is 12–20%; for a sibling sharing one haplotype, the risk is 5–7%; and with no haplotypes in common, the risk is only 1–2%. HLA typing is not recommended for routine practice because of its expense. When measurement of spontaneous antibodies to insulin, islet cell antibodies including antibodies to GAD and IA-2, and assessment of insulin secretory reserve are considered together, it may be possible to predict, and hence delay or prevent, the clinical appearance of type I diabetes. In general, for purposes of genetic counseling, it can be safely assumed that in whites, the overall recurrence risks to siblings are approximately 6% if the proband is younger than 10 yr of age and 3% if the proband is older at the time of diagnosis. The risk to offspring of a diabetic parent is 2–5%, with the higher risk occurring in the offspring of a diabetic father. In black Americans, these risks are only one half to two thirds of those in whites.

Factors other than pure inheritance of HLA markers or other genetic factors must also be involved in evoking clinical diabetes. For example, HLA-D3 or -D4 is found in approximately 50% of the general population, and (nonAsp/nonAsp) in approximately 20% of white nondiabetics in the United States, yet the risk for type I diabetes in these subjects is only one

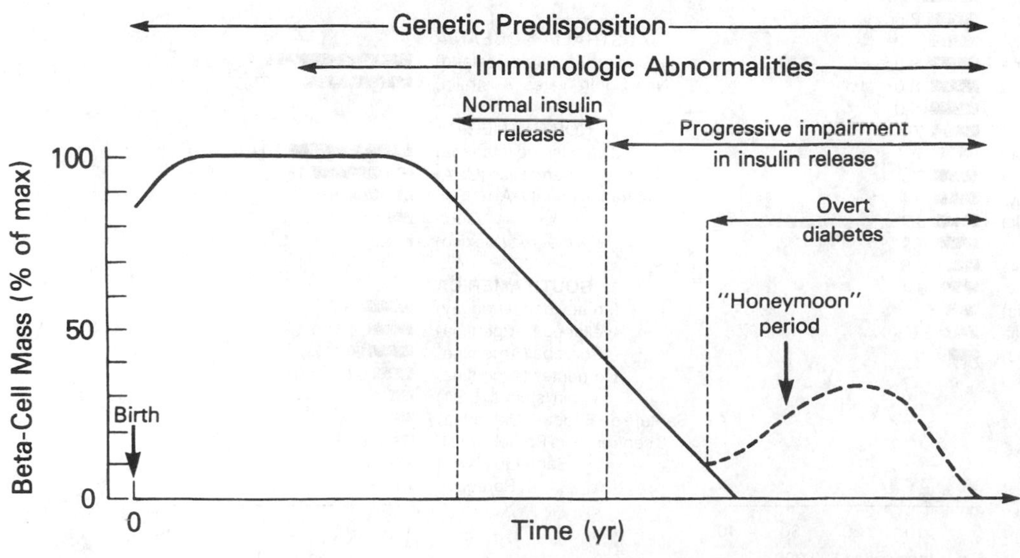

Timing of trigger in relation to immunologic abnormalities is unknown. Note that overt diabetes is not apparent until insulin secretory reserves are <10–20% of normal.

Figure 599–2 Proposed scheme of natural history of β-cell defect. (Adapted from Sperling MA [ed]: Physician's Guide to Insulin-Dependent [Type 1] Diabetes Mellitus: Diagnosis and Treatment. Copyright [1988] by the American Diabetes Association. Reprinted with permission.)

tenth of that in an HLA identical sibling of an index case possessing these markers. Even siblings sharing only one haplotype have a 6- to 10-fold greater risk of the development of type I diabetes compared with the normal population. In addition, about 10% of patients with type I diabetes do not possess either HLA-D3 or -D4, although most white diabetics lack at least one aspartic acid at position 57 of the DQ β chain. Most compelling is the fact that the concordance rate among identical twins of whom one has IDDM is only 30–50%, suggesting the participation of environmental triggering factors or other genetic factors such as the postnatal selection of certain autoreactive T-cell clones that bear receptors recognizing "self." This postnatal process occurs within the thymus and implies that identical twins are not identical with respect to the T-cell receptor repertoire they possess.

Triggering factors might include viral infections. In animals, a number of viruses can cause a diabetic syndrome, the appearance and severity of which depend on the genetic strain and immune competence of the species of animal tested. In humans, epidemics of mumps, rubella, and coxsackievirus infections have been associated with subsequent increases in the incidence of type I diabetes; the acute onset of diabetes mellitus, presumably induced by coxsackievirus B4, has been described. The viruses may act by directly destroying β cells, by persisting in pancreatic β cells as slow viral infections, or by triggering a widespread immune response to several endocrine tissues. The virus may induce initial β-cell damage that results in the presentation of previously masked or altered antigenic determinants. It is also possible that the virus shares some antigenic determinants with those present on or in β-cells, including GAD, so that antibodies formed in response to the virus may interact with these shared determinants of β-cells, resulting in their destruction, an example of molecular mimicry. Molecular mimicry is also invoked as a possible mechanism in bovine serum albumin–mediated islet antibodies because many patients with new-onset diabetes have IgG antibodies to bovine serum albumin, specifically a 17–amino acid peptide that also occurs on islet membranes. Another protein component of cow's milk, β-casein has also been implicated. Implicit in these findings is the possibility that early exposure to cow's milk may be a factor in triggering diabetes, thus explaining the reported lower incidence of diabetes among breast-fed infants. Antecedent stress and exposure to certain chemical toxins also have been implicated in the development of type I diabetes. Histologic examination of the pancreas from patients with type I diabetes who die of incidental causes has revealed lymphocytic infiltration around the islets of Langerhans. Later, the islets become progressively hyalinized and scarred, a process suggesting an ongoing inflammatory response, possibly autoimmune in nature.

Considerable evidence now supports an autoimmune basis for the development of type I diabetes. Some 80–90% of newly diagnosed patients with type I diabetes have islet-cell antibodies (ICAs) directed at cell surface or cytoplasmic determinants in their islet cells; the prevalence of these antibodies decreases with the duration of established disease. In contrast, after pancreatic transplantation, ICAs may reappear in patients whose sera had become negative for ICAs prior to transplantation. Taken together, these findings suggest that ICAs disappear as the antigens in the form of pancreatic islets are destroyed and reappear when fresh antigen (transplanted islets) is presented. Studies in identical twins and in family pedigrees demonstrate that the existence of ICAs may precede by months to years the appearance of symptomatic type I diabetes. In vitro, ICAs may impair insulin secretion in response to secretagogues and can be shown to be cytotoxic to islet cells, especially in the presence of complement or T cells from patients with type I diabetes. As many as 80% of patients may have antibodies to GAD, and some 30–40% may have spontaneous anti-insulin antibodies at initial diagnosis. In young children less than 5 yr at diagnosis, almost 100% have insulin autoantibodies that probably were present before clinical manifestations of diabetes. There is also some evidence of abnormal T-cell function with an alteration in the ratio of suppressor to killer T cells at the onset of the disease. Tissue damage of pancreatic β cells is mediated by the Th1 subset of T lymphocytes producing various cytokines, some of which invoke apoptosis of β cells via nitric oxide–induced expression of Fas. These findings suggest that type I diabetes, like other autoimmune diseases such as Hashimoto's thyroiditis, is a disease of "autoaggression," in which autoantibodies, in cooperation with complement, T cells, or other factors, induce destruction of the insulin-producing islet cells. Thus, the inheritance of certain genes intimately associated with the HLA system and other genes appears to confer a predisposition toward autoimmune disease, including diabetes, when triggered by an appropriate stimulus such as a virus. Although it is known that some patients with IDDM have none of the frequently associated HLAs, the evidence in favor of an immune basis of islet cell destruction was sufficiently compelling to have fostered several studies of different immunosuppressive agents in the treatment of newly diagnosed diabetics. These immunosuppressive agents must be considered experimental and should not be viewed as established or recommended therapy. Indeed, the toxic nature and side effects of some of the drugs used (such as cyclosporine), as well their overall poor effectiveness in maintaining a remission after the disease is clinically manifested, led to abandonment of these agents in children.

Figure 599–2 summarizes current concepts of the etiology of type I diabetes as an autoimmune disease, the tendency toward which is inherited through the HLA system and in which autoimmune destruction of β cells is triggered by an as yet unidentified agent. The slope of decline in insulin varies, and the point at which clinical features appear corresponds to an approximately 80% destruction of the insulin secretory reserve. This process may take months to years, usually in adolescent and older patients, and weeks in the very young patient. Higher titers of spontaneous autoinsulin antibodies and islet cell antibodies are characteristic of the more active islet cell destruction typically seen in the younger patient and may prove useful in predicting evolving diabetes.

PREDICTION AND PREVENTION. Although no currently available marker or test can accurately predict the development of type I diabetes mellitus, there is increased evidence that type I diabetes may be predictable. It has been proposed that the presence of high titers of islet cell, GAD, and insulin autoantibodies combined with a markedly diminished first-phase response to insulin after an intravenous pulse of glucose, corresponding to the 5th percentile or less for age, can be used to predict the onset of type I diabetes reliably. Although there is disagreement on this point, the data are sufficiently persuasive to have fostered national trials in Europe and the United States to predict and possibly prevent the clinical onset of type I diabetes through immune intervention strategies.

The United States Diabetes Prevention Trial I (DPT-I) sponsored by the National Institutes of Health, is based on promising pilot data that suggested preservation of insulin secretion and prevention of progression to diabetes mellitus in at-risk individuals treated with insulin. Daily subcutaneous insulin, coupled with intensive intravenous insulin every 9 months, prevented diabetes for at least 3 yr in five subjects considered to be at risk because of islet cell and insulin autoantibodies and diminished first-phase insulin response. Among seven similar at-risk subjects who chose not to be treated, six acquired IDDM within 3 yr.

The European Nicotinamide Diabetes Intervention Trial (ENDIT) is a multicenter trial that will screen approximately 22,000 first-degree relatives of patients with type I diabetes to identify 500 considered to be at high risk for developing this disease. These at-risk individuals will be treated with nicotin-

TABLE 599–4 Influence of Feeding (High Insulin) or of Fasting (Low Insulin) on Some Metabolic Processes in Liver, Muscle, and Adipose Tissue*

	High Plasma Insulin (Postprandial State)	Low Plasma Insulin (Fasted State)
Liver	Glucose uptake Glycogen synthesis Absence of gluconeogenesis Lipogenesis Absence of ketogenesis	Glucose production Glycogenolysis Gluconeogenesis Absence of lipogenesis Ketogenesis
Muscle	Glucose uptake Glucose oxidation Glycogen synthesis Protein synthesis	Absence of glucose uptake Fatty acid and ketone oxidation Glycogenolysis Proteolysis and amino acid release
Adipose tissue	Glucose uptake Lipid synthesis Triglyceride uptake	Absence of glucose uptake Lipolysis and fatty acid release Absence of triglyceride uptake

**Insulin is considered to be the major factor governing these metabolic processes. Diabetes mellitus may be viewed as a permanent low-insulin state that, untreated, results in exaggerated fasting.*

amide or a placebo in a double-blind fashion. The advantages purported to nicotinamide are that it is not known to be toxic or harmful in humans at the recommended doses. Its proposed protective effects in delaying diabetes are, based on small preliminary results, by mechanisms possibly involving enhancement of DNA repair in pancreatic β cells. These strategies are experimental and not appropriate for current clinical practice.

PATHOPHYSIOLOGY. The progressive destruction of β cells leads to a progressive deficiency of insulin, a major anabolic hormone. Normally, insulin secretion in response to feeding is exquisitely modulated by the interplay of neural, hormonal, and substrate-related mechanisms to permit controlled disposition of ingested foodstuff as energy for immediate or future use; mobilization of energy during the fasted state depends on low plasma levels of insulin. Thus, in normal metabolism there are regular swings between the postprandial, high-insulin anabolic state and the fasted, low-insulin catabolic state that affect liver, muscle, and adipose tissue (Table 599–4). Type I diabetes mellitus, as it evolves, becomes a permanent low-insulin catabolic state in which feeding does not reverse, but rather exaggerates, these catabolic processes. It is important to emphasize that liver is more sensitive than muscle or fat to a given concentration of insulin; that is, endogenous glucose production from the liver through glycogenolysis and gluconeogenesis can be restrained at insulin concentrations that do not fully augment glucose utilization by peripheral tissues.

Consequently, with progressive failure of insulin secretion, the initial manifestation is postprandial hyperglycemia; fasting hyperglycemia indicates excessive endogenous glucose production and is a late manifestation reflecting severe insulin deficiency.

Although insulin deficiency is the primary defect, several secondary changes that involve the stress hormones (epinephrine, cortisol, growth hormone, and glucagon) accelerate and exaggerate the rate and magnitude of metabolic decompensation. Increased plasma concentrations of these counterregulatory hormones magnify metabolic derangements by further impairing insulin secretion (epinephrine), by antagonizing its action (epinephrine, cortisol, growth hormone), and by promoting glycogenolysis, gluconeogenesis, lipolysis, and ketogenesis (glucagon, epinephrine, growth hormone, and cortisol) while decreasing glucose utilization and glucose clearance (epinephrine, growth hormone, cortisol).

With progressive insulin deficiency, excessive glucose production and impairment of its utilization result in hyperglycemia with glucosuria when the renal threshold of approximately 180 mg/dL is exceeded. The resultant osmotic diuresis produces polyuria, urinary losses of electrolytes, dehydration, and compensatory polydipsia. These evolving manifestations, especially dehydration, represent physiologic stress, resulting in hypersecretion of epinephrine, glucagon, cortisol, and growth hormone, which amplifies and perpetuates metabolic derangements and accelerates metabolic decompensation. The acute stress of trauma or infection may likewise accelerate metabolic decompensation to ketoacidosis in evolving or established diabetes. Hyperosmolality, commonly encountered as a result of progressive hyperglycemia, contributes to the symptoms, especially to cerebral obtundation in diabetic ketoacidosis (DKA). Serum osmolality has important implications in the therapy of DKA and can be estimated by the following formula:

$$\text{Serum osmolality in mOsm/kg} = [\text{Serum Na}^+\ (\text{mEq/L}) + \text{K}^+\ (\text{mEq/L}) \times 2] + \frac{\text{glucose mg/dL}}{18} + \frac{\text{BUN mg/dL}}{3}$$

The combination of insulin deficiency and elevated plasma values of the counterregulatory hormones also is responsible for accelerated lipolysis and impaired lipid synthesis, with resulting increased plasma concentrations of total lipids, cholesterol, triglycerides, and free fatty acids. The hormonal interplay of insulin deficiency and glucagon excess shunts the free fatty acids into ketone body formation; the rate of formation of these ketone bodies, principally β-hydroxybutyrate and acetoacetate, exceeds the capacity for peripheral utilization and renal excretion. Accumulation of these ketoacids results in metabolic acidosis and compensatory rapid deep breathing in an attempt to excrete excess CO_2 (Kussmaul respiration). Acetone, formed by nonenzymatic conversion of acetoacetate, is responsible for the characteristic fruity odor of the breath. Ketones are excreted in the urine in association with cations and thus further increase losses of water and electrolyte (Table 599–5). With progressive dehydration, acidosis, hyperosmolality, and diminished cerebral oxygen utilization, consciousness becomes impaired, and the patient ultimately becomes comatose. Thus, insulin deficiency produces a profound catabolic state—an exaggerated state of starvation in which all of the initial clinical features can be explained on the basis of known alterations in intermediary metabolism mediated by insulin deficiency in combination with counterregulatory hormone excess. Because the counterregulatory hormonal changes are secondary, the severity and duration of the symptoms reflect the extent of primary insulinopenia.

CLINICAL MANIFESTATIONS. The classic presentation of diabetes in children is a history of polyuria, polydipsia, polyphagia, and weight loss. The duration of these symptoms varies but is often less than 1 mo. A clue to the existence of polyuria may be the onset of enuresis in a previously toilet-trained child. An insidious onset characterized by lethargy, weakness, and weight loss is also common. The loss of weight despite an increased dietary intake is readily explicable by the following illustration: The average healthy 10-yr-old child has a daily caloric intake of

TABLE 599–5 Fluid and Electrolyte Maintenance Requirements and Estimated Losses in Diabetic Ketoacidosis

	Approximate Daily Maintenance Requirements*	Approximate Accumulated Losses†
Water	1500 mL/m²	100 mL/kg (range 60–100 mL/kg)
Sodium	45 mEq/m²	6 mEq/kg (range 5–13 mEq/kg)
Potassium	35 mEq/m²	5 mEq/kg (range 4–6 mEq/kg)
Chloride	30 mEq/m²	4 mEq/kg (range 3–9 mEq/kg)
Phosphate	10 mEq/m²	3 mEq/kg (range 2–5 mEq/kg)

**Maintenance is expressed in surface area to permit uniformity because fluid requirements change as weight increases. See also Chapter 53.*

†Losses are expressed per unit of body weight because the losses remain relatively constant in relation to total body weight.

2,000 calories or more, of which approximately 50% are derived from carbohydrate. With the development of diabetes, daily losses of water and glucose may be as much as 5 L and 250 g, respectively. This represents 1,000 calories lost in the urine or 50% of the average daily caloric intake. Therefore, despite the child's compensatory increased intake of food and water, the calories cannot be utilized, excessive caloric losses continue, and increasing catabolism and weight loss ensue. Weight loss and enuresis in a child should alert the clinician to the possible existence of diabetes mellitus.

Pyogenic skin infections and monilial vaginitis in adolescent females are occasionally present at the time of diagnosis of diabetes. They are rarely the sole clinical manifestations of diabetes in children, and a careful history invariably reveals the coexistence of polyuria and polydipsia.

Ketoacidosis is responsible for the initial presentation of many (approximately 25%) diabetic children. The early manifestations may be relatively mild and consist of vomiting, polyuria, and dehydration. In more prolonged and severe cases, Kussmaul's respiration is present, and there is an odor of acetone on the breath. Abdominal pain or rigidity may be present and may mimic appendicitis or pancreatitis. Cerebral obtundation and ultimately coma ensue. Laboratory findings include glucosuria, ketonuria, hyperglycemia, ketonemia, and metabolic acidosis. Leukocytosis is common, and nonspecific serum amylase may be elevated; serum lipase is usually not elevated. In those with abdominal pain, it should not be assumed that these findings are evidence of a surgical emergency before a period of appropriate fluid, electrolyte, and insulin therapy has been tried to correct dehydration and acidosis; the abdominal manifestations frequently disappear after several hours of such treatment. A precipitating event such as infection should be sought.

DIAGNOSIS. Children in whom the diagnosis of diabetes mellitus must be considered may, for practical purposes, be divided into three general categories: (1) those who have a history suggestive of diabetes, especially polyuria with polydipsia and failure to gain or a loss of weight in spite of a voracious appetite; (2) those who have a transient or persistent glucosuria; and (3) those who have clinical manifestations of metabolic acidosis with or without stupor or coma. In all instances, the diagnosis of diabetes mellitus is dependent on the demonstration of hyperglycemia in association with glucosuria with or without ketonuria. When classic symptoms of polyuria and polydipsia are associated with hyperglycemia and glucosuria, the glucose tolerance test is not needed to support the diagnosis.

Renal glucosuria may be an isolated congenital disorder or a manifestation of the Fanconi syndrome and other renal tubular disorders caused by severe heavy metal intoxication, ingestion of certain drugs (e.g., outdated tetracycline), or inborn errors of metabolism (cystinosis). When vomiting, diarrhea, inadequate intake of food, or a combination of these factors is a complicating feature in any of these conditions, starvation ketosis may ensue, simulating DKA. The absence of hyperglycemia eliminates the possibility of diabetes. It is also important to recognize that not all urinary sugar is glucose, and infrequently galactosemia, pentosuria, and the fructosurias will require consideration as diagnostic possibilities.

The discovery of glucosuria, with or without a mild degree of hyperglycemia, during a hospital admission for trauma or infection or even during the associated emotional upheaval may, but usually does not, herald the existence of diabetes; in most of these instances, the glucosuria remits during recovery. Because this circumstance may indicate a limited capacity for insulin secretion, which is unmasked by elevated plasma concentrations of stress hormones, these patients should be rechecked at a later date for the possibility of hyperglycemia or clinical features of diabetes mellitus, or both. In these circumstances, a glucose tolerance test may be useful to establish a diagnosis; glucose tolerance testing should be performed several weeks after recovery from the acute illness using a glucose loading dose adjusted for weight. Evidence indicates that the test is most likely to be abnormal in patients in whom islet cell antibodies or insulin autoantibodies are detected. Such testing is increasingly available; those with positive ICAs or insulin autoantibodies should be educated about the symptoms of diabetes mellitus.

Screening procedures, such as postprandial determinations of blood glucose or screening oral glucose tolerance tests, have yielded low detection rates in children, even among those considered at risk, such as siblings of diabetic children. Accordingly, such screening procedures are not recommended in children.

Diabetic Ketoacidosis. This disorder must be differentiated from acidosis or coma due to other causes, including hypoglycemia, uremia, gastroenteritis with metabolic acidosis, lactic acidosis, salicylate intoxication, sepsis, and intracranial lesions. DKA exists when there is hyperglycemia (glucose greater than 300 mg/dL), ketonemia (ketones strongly positive at a greater than 1:2 dilution of serum), acidosis (pH less <7.30 and bicarbonate <15 mEq/l), glucosuria, and ketonuria in addition to the clinical features described. Precipitating factors, even for the initial presentation, include stress such as trauma, infections, vomiting, and psychologic disturbances. Recurrent episodes of ketoacidosis in established diabetics often represent deliberate errors in recommended insulin dosage, unusual stress responses that indicate psychologic disturbances and, at times, pleas to be removed from the home environment perceived to be stressful or intolerable. DKA also should be distinguished from nonketotic hyperosmolar coma.

Nonketotic Hyperosmolar Coma. This syndrome is characterized by severe hyperglycemia (blood glucose greater than 600 mg/dL), absence of or only slight ketosis, nonketotic acidosis, severe dehydration, depressed sensorium or frank coma, and various neurologic signs that may include grand mal seizures, hyperthermia, hemiparesis, and positive Babinski signs. Respirations are usually shallow, but coexistent metabolic (lactic) acidosis may be manifested by Kussmaul breathing. Serum osmolarity is commonly 350 mOsm/kg or higher. This condition is uncommon in children; among adults, mortality rates have been as high as 40–70%, possibly in part because of delays in recognition and in institution of appropriate therapy. In children, there has been a high incidence of pre-existing neurologic damage. Profound hyperglycemia may develop over a period of days and, initially, the obligatory osmotic polyuria and dehydration may be partially compensated by increasing fluid intake. With progression of disease, thirst becomes impaired, possibly because of alteration of the hypothalamic thirst center by hyperosmolarity and possibly, in some instances, because of a pre-existing defect in the hypothalamic osmoregulating mechanism.

The low production of ketones is attributed mainly to the hyperosmolarity, which in vitro blunts the lipolytic effect of epinephrine and the antilipolytic effect of residual insulin; blunting of lipolysis by the therapeutic use of β-adrenergic blockers may contribute to the syndrome. Depression of consciousness is closely correlated with the degree of hyperosmolarity in this condition as well as in DKA; hemoconcentration may also predispose to cerebral arterial and venous thromboses.

Treatment of nonketotic hyperosmolar coma is directed at rapid repletion of the vascular volume deficit and very slow correction of the hyperosmolar state (see the discussion of the management of ketoacidosis further on). One-half isotonic saline (0.45% NaCl; some use normal saline) is administered at a rate estimated to replace 50% of the volume deficit in the first 12 hr, and the remainder is administered during the ensuing 24 hr. The rate of infusion and the saline concentration are titrated to result in a slow decline of serum osmolality.

When the blood glucose concentration approaches 300 mg/dL, the hydrating fluid should be changed to 5% dextrose in 0.2 normal (N) saline. Approximately 20 mEq/L of potassium chloride should be added to each of these fluids to prevent hypokalemia. Serum potassium and plasma glucose concentrations should be monitored at 2-hr intervals for the first 12 hr and at 4-hr intervals for the next 24 hr to permit appropriate adjustments of administered potassium and insulin.

Insulin can be given by continuous intravenous infusion beginning with the 2nd hr of fluid therapy. Because blood glucose may decrease dramatically with fluid therapy alone, the intravenous loading dose should be 0.05 U/kg of regular (fast-acting) insulin followed by 0.05 U/kg/hr of the same insulin, rather than 0.1 U/kg/hr as advocated for patients with DKA. Some do not use a loading dose. During the recovery period, therapy with insulin and diet and monitoring of the patient should be the same as that described for patients recovering from DKA (See Table 599–5 and related text).

TREATMENT. The management of IDDM may be divided into three phases depending on the initial presentation: that of ketoacidosis, the postacidotic or transition period for establishment of metabolic control, and the continuing phase of guidance of the diabetic child and his or her family. Each of these phases has separate goals, although in practice they merge into a continuum. For purposes of management, the transition period corresponds to patients presenting with polyuria, polydipsia, and weight loss but without biochemical decompensation to ketoacidosis.

Ketoacidosis. The immediate aims of therapy are expansion of intravascular volume; correction of deficits in fluid, electrolyte, and acid-base status; and initiation of insulin therapy to correct intermediary metabolism. Treatment should be instituted as soon as the clinical diagnosis is confirmed by the presence of hyperglycemia and ketonemia. Determinations of blood pH and electrolytes should also be obtained; an electrocardiogram may be useful to provide a rapid reference for the existence of hyperkalemia. If sepsis is suspected as a possible precipitating factor, blood culture should be performed and the urine examined for the presence of bacteria and leukocytes. A flow sheet to record chronologically the rate and composition of fluid input, urine output, amount of insulin administered, and the acid-base and electrolyte values of the blood is most useful. Catheterization of the bladder is not routinely recommended in children; bag collection or condom drainage permits an assessment of urinary output, but catheterization may be indicated in comatose patients.

Fluid and Electrolyte Therapy (Table 599–6). The expansion of reduced intravascular volume and correction of depleted fluid and electrolyte stores are most important in the treatment of DKA. It must be stressed, however, that exogenous insulin is essential to arrest further metabolic decompensation and to restore intermediary metabolism.

The amount of dehydration is commonly about 10%; initial fluid therapy can be based on this estimate, with subsequent adjustments related to clinical and laboratory data. The initial hydrating fluid should be isotonic saline (0.9%). Because of the hyperglycemia, hyperosmolarity is universal in DKA; thus, even 0.9% saline is hypotonic relative to the patient's serum osmolality. A gradual decline in osmolality is desirable because too rapid a decline has been implicated in the development of cerebral edema, one of the major complications of diabetic therapy in children. For the same reason, the rate of fluid replacement is adjusted to provide only 50–60% of the calculated deficit within the initial 12 hr; the remaining 40–50% is

TABLE 599–6 Fluid and Electrolyte Therapy for Diabetic Ketoacidosis

Recommendations for replacement of fluid losses and for maintenance of a 30-kg (surface area 1.0 m²) child with assumed 10% dehydration. Duration of treatment: 36 hours.

Replacement Fluids	Approximate Accumulated Losses with 10% Dehydration	Approximate Requirements for Maintenance (36 hr)	Approximate Totals for Replacement and Maintenance (36 hr)
Water (mL)	3,000	2,250	5,500
Sodium (mEq)	180	65	250
Potassium (mEq)	150	50	200
Chloride (mEq)	120	45	165
Phosphate (mEq)	90	15	100

Replacement Schedule (continuous intravenous infusion)

Approximate Duration	*Fluid (Composition)*	*Sodium (mEq)*	*Potassium (mEq)*	*Chloride (mEq)*	*Phosphate (mEq)*
Hour 1	500 mL of 0.9% NaCl (isotonic saline)	75	—	75	—
Hour 2	500 mL of 0.45% NaCl (0.5 isotonic saline) plus 20 mEq of KCl	35	20	55	—
Hour 3–12 (200 mL/hr for 10 hr)	2,000 ml of 0.45% NaCl with 30 mEq/L of potassium phosphate	150	60	150	40
Subtotal initial 12 hr	3,000 mL	260	80	280	40
Next 24 hr 100 mL/hr	5% glucose in 0.2% NaCl with 40 mEq/L of potassium phosphate	75	100	75	60
Total over 36 hours	5,400 mL	335	180	355	100

Note: All replacement values should be halved if dehydration is estimated to be 5%. Maintenance requirements remain the same.

Additional Guidelines

A diabetic flow sheet *with laboratory data appropriately recorded must be maintained in the patient's chart.*

Insulin therapy by continuous low-dose intravenous method: *Priming dose—bolus injection of 0.1 U/kg of regular insulin intravenously followed immediately by continuous intravenous infusion of 0.1 U/kg/hr of regular insulin beginning with 2nd hr.*

Directions for making insulin infusion: *Add 50 U of regular insulin to 500 mL of isotonic saline. Flush 50 mL through the tubing to saturate insulin-binding sites. For 30-kg patient, infuse at rate of 30 mL/hr. When the blood glucose concentration approaches 300 mg/dL, continue the insulin infusion at a reduced rate, or add glucose to the infusate until acidosis is resolved, then start insulin therapy by subcutaneous injections of 0.2–0.4 U/kg of insulin at intervals of 6 hr.*

Bicarbonate therapy: *For pH >7.20, no therapy necessary. For pH 7.10–7.20, 40 mEq/m² of bicarbonate over 2 hr; then re-evaluate. For pH <7.10, 80 mEq/m² of bicarbonate over 2 hr; then re-evaluate. New diabetics, <2 yr of age, with diabetic ketoacidosis and 10% dehydration, or any diabetic with pH <7.00, should be managed in an intensive care unit or equivalent setting.*

TABLE 599–7 Intermittent Insulin Regimen for Diabetic Ketoacidosis

Blood Glucose	Total Insulin Dose	Intravenous Dose	Intramuscular or Subcutaneous Dose	Frequency
>600 mg/dL	1 U/kg	0.5 U/kg	0.5 U/kg	Every 2–4 hr
300–600 mg/dL	0.5 U/kg	0.25 U/kg	0.25 U/kg	Every 2–4 hr

When blood glucose approaches 300 mg/dL, the intravenous infusion for fluid and electrolyte replacement should contain 5% glucose (see Table 599–6 for rate of administration). Continue subcutaneous injections of insulin at 0.2–0.4 U/kg every 6 hr and monitor blood glucose concentration at the same time. If blood glucose concentration rises, increase the next insulin dose by 50%; if glucose concentration falls, decrease the next insulin dose by 50%. Continue this insulin regimen for 24 hr after oral intake of fluid and food is established. See text for subsequent management.

administered during the next 24 hr. Also, administration of glucose (5% solution in 0.2 N saline) is initiated when blood glucose concentration approaches 300 mg/dL in order to limit the decline of serum osmolality and reduce the risk of the development of cerebral edema (Tables 599–6 and 599–7).

Administration of potassium should be started early. Total body potassium may be considerably depleted during acidosis, even when the serum potassium concentration is normal or elevated. Although potassium moves from intracellular to extracellular sites during acidosis, the reverse occurs during correction of acidosis, particularly when exogenous insulin and glucose are available in the circulation. This shift of potassium back to the intracellular compartment may result in life-threatening hypokalemia. Hence, after the initial fluid replacement of approximately 20 mL/kg of isotonic saline (0.9%) has been provided, potassium should be added to subsequent infusates if urinary output is adequate; the serum potassium concentration should then be monitored periodically. An electrocardiogram provides a rapid assessment of serum potassium concentration; T waves are peaked in hyperkalemia and are low and associated with U waves in hypokalemia (See Chapter 430.2). Because the total potassium deficit cannot be replaced within the initial 24 hr of treatment, potassium supplementation should be continued as long as fluids are administered intravenously (see Table 599–6).

It is almost inevitable that the patient will receive an excess of chloride, which may aggravate acidosis. The extent of acidosis, however, can be reduced by substitution of phosphate, which is also significantly depleted in DKA. Moreover, phosphate in conjunction with glycolysis is essential for the formation of 2,3-diphosphoglycerate (2,3-DPG), which governs the oxygen dissociation curve. During deficiency of 2,3-DPG, the oxygen dissociation curve is shifted to the left, that is, more oxygen is retained by hemoglobin and less is available to the tissues, a situation that predisposes to lactic acidosis. Acidosis per se tends to shift the oxygen dissociation curve toward the right (Bohr effect) and thus partially "compensates" for 2,3-DPG deficiency. As acidosis resulting from the accumulation of ketones is corrected by the provision of insulin, with or without administration of bicarbonate, the effects of 2,3-DPG deficiency may no longer be "compensated" and the release of oxygen to tissues may again be impaired. Exogenous phosphate, by contributing to the formation of 2,3-DPG, permits the oxygen dissociation curve to shift to the right and thus facilitates release of oxygen to tissues and aids in the correction of acidosis. Furthermore, resistance to insulin action is associated with hypophosphatemia. Hence, the administration of potassium phosphate is recommended as outlined in Table 599–6. Because excessive use of phosphate may result in hypocalcemia, serum calcium levels should be measured periodically. Symptomatic hypocalcemia should be corrected with calcium gluconate and potassium chloride, which should be temporarily substituted for potassium phosphate.

Alkali Therapy. With provision of fluids, electrolytes, glucose, and insulin, metabolic acidosis is usually corrected through the interruption of ketogenesis, the metabolism of ketones to bicarbonate, and the generation of bicarbonate by the distal renal tubule. Concerns over the therapeutic administration of bicarbonate center on four issues: (1) by shifting the oxygen dissociation curve to the left, alkalosis may diminish the release of oxygen to tissues and hence predispose to lactic acidosis; (2) alkalosis accelerates the entry of potassium into cells and hence may produce hypokalemia; (3) provision of bicarbonate according to the calculated base deficit overcorrects and may result in alkalosis; and, perhaps most important, (4) bicarbonate may lead to worsening of cerebral acidosis while the plasma pH is being restored to normal because HCO_3^- combines with H^+ and dissociates to CO_2 and H_2O. Whereas bicarbonate passes the blood-brain barrier slowly, CO_2 diffuses freely, thereby exacerbating cerebral acidosis and possibly cerebral depression. Conversely, severe acidosis, with a blood pH of 7.1 or less, diminishes respiratory minute volume, may produce hypotension by means of peripheral vasodilation, impairs myocardial function, and may be a factor in insulin resistance. For these reasons, administration of bicarbonate is recommended only when the pH is 7.2 or less (see Table 599–6). At pH 7.1–7.2, 40 mEq of HCO_3^-/m^2, and at less than pH 7.1, 80 mEq of HCO_3^-/m^2 should be infused over a period of 2 hr; acid-base status should then be re-evaluated prior to further alkali therapy. Many have a conservative approach to the use of alkali. Bicarbonate should not be given by bolus infusion because it may precipitate cardiac arrhythmias.

The major life-threatening complication in children treated for DKA is *cerebral edema.* Clinically, cerebral edema develops several hours after the institution of therapy, when clinical and biochemical indices may suggest improvement. The manifestations are those of raised intracranial pressure and include headache, alteration and deterioration in alertness and conscious state, "delirious outbursts," bradycardia, vomiting, diminished responsiveness to painful stimuli, and diminished reflexes. There may be a change in papillary responsiveness with unequal pupils or fixed dilated pupils. Polyuria, secondary to development of diabetes insipidus, may be erroneously attributed to osmotic diuresis secondary to hyperglycemia, although diabetes mellitus and diabetes insipidus coexist. Prompt recognition of the condition as it evolves, and prompt therapy with mannitol and hyperventilation, can be lifesaving. Increasingly, evidence points to the conclusion that subclinical cerebral edema occurs in many patients treated with fluids and insulin for DKA, and that in only a minority does it become clinically manifested as a medical emergency.

The evidence that patients treated for DKA acquire subclinical cerebral edema includes increasing cerebrospinal fluid pressure documented by continuous intrathecal monitoring during therapy of DKA in adults and evidence from sequential computed tomography of the head that ventricular size is narrower, compatible with brain swelling, during therapy than several days after recovery from DKA. Excessive use of fluids (with failure of the serum sodium to rise), excessive use of bicarbonate, compensatory responses to intracellular acidosis through the Na^+/H^+ exchanger, and large doses of insulin during treatment have all been implicated. The reason that a majority of patients have subclinical brain swelling, whereas only a minority (1–2%) manifest clinically apparent cerebral edema, may be related to the intracranial pressure-volume curve, which shows a steep exponential rise in intracranial pressure beyond a critical extent of cerebral volume.

For these reasons, it is prudent to anticipate clinical cerebral edema in all children treated for DKA by limiting the rate of fluid administration to 4.0 L/m^2/24 hr or less, avoiding the excessive use of bicarbonate as outlined earlier, and being alert to the clinical manifestations of raised intracranial pressure. Once raised intracranial pressure becomes clinically manifested, reduction of the rate of fluid administration, use of mannitol at 10–20 g/m^2 intravenously and repeated at 2- to 4-hr intervals, and hyperventilation are warranted. Preliminary retrospective evidence suggests that these measures, instituted promptly, are lifesaving and may avoid neurologic sequelae.

Insulin Therapy. The continuous low-dose intravenous infusion method, in which a priming dose of 0.1 U/kg of regular insulin is followed by a constant infusion of 0.1 U/kg/hr is outlined in Table 599–6. Some do not use a priming dose. This method is effective, simple, and physiologically sound and has gained wide acceptance as the preferred method of administering insulin during DKA. It provides a constant steady concentration of insulin in plasma that approximates the peak attained in normal individuals during an oral glucose tolerance test. Presumably, the same steady concentration is attained at the cellular level and permits a steady metabolic response without the fluctuations that must occur with intermittent injections of insulin. Concern that the insulin may adhere to glass and tubing has proved to be unfounded, and effective delivery of insulin can be provided without the use of albumin or gelatin added to the infusate. Moreover, insulin infusion can be provided by gravity drip without the use of a special pump, although such a pump is helpful. A separate infusion set for insulin connected to the infusion line used for fluid and electrolyte therapy is recommended so that adjustments in the dosage of each can be made independently. After the amount of insulin for the initial 6–8 hr has been calculated, this quantity is added to a 250- or 500-mL bottle of 0.9% saline (see Table 599–6 for specific instructions).

When the blood glucose concentration approaches 300 mg/dL, the ongoing potassium requirement is added to 5% glucose in 0.2 N saline, and the rate of insulin infusion may sometimes be reduced from 0.1 to 0.05 U/kg/hr providing that acidosis is being corrected. The rate of insulin infusion should, however, be periodically adjusted according to the patient's recovery from acidosis and the blood glucose response of each individual.

In treating DKA, it is commonly observed that blood glucose concentration corrects more quickly than the pH or plasma bicarbonate. Insulin must be provided by infusion or subcutaneous injection as long as acidosis persists, even if the glucose level is approaching 300 mg/dL. It may be necessary to add glucose to the infusate while continuing insulin infusion at a rate of 0.05 to 0.1 U/kg/hr until acidosis is corrected. If acidosis persists despite these measures, a cause such as gram-negative sepsis should be considered.

When acidosis has been corrected, the continuous infusion may be discontinued and insulin given immediately by subcutaneous injection at a dose of 0.2–0.4 U/kg every 6 to 8 hr while maintaining the glucose infusion until the child can fully tolerate food. Subcutaneous injections of regular insulin at doses of 0.2–0.4 U/kg every 6–8 hr before meals should be continued for a full 24-hr after the child is eating. The blood glucose level should be monitored before and 2 hr after each meal and the insulin dose adjusted to maintain the blood glucose concentration in the range of 80–180 mg/dL. The total dose of regular insulin used in this representative day serves as a guide for subsequent insulin treatment with a combination of intermediate and short-acting insulin as described later.

Insulin treatment during DKA can also be administered by repeated intramuscular or subcutaneous bolus injections; a portion of the dose is also usually injected intravenously. One such regimen based on body weight is outlined in Table 599–7; if plasma ketones are only moderately elevated, the recommended doses may be half of those listed. Administration of insulin as the fast-acting form is repeated every 2–4 hr, and blood glucose values and acid-base status are monitored as during the continuous intravenous insulin approach. When the blood glucose concentration has fallen to approximately 300 mg/dL, subsequent insulin therapy at a dose of 0.2–0.4 U/kg may be given subcutaneously every 6–8 hr while maintaining an infusion of 5% glucose in 0.2 N saline with potassium added (see Table 599–6) until acidosis is resolved and the child can tolerate solid foods. Sips of clear liquid, broth, or carbonated beverages may be given during this interval. Subcutaneous injections of regular insulin at doses of 0.2–0.4 U/kg every 6–8 hr before meals are continued for a full 24-hr after the child is eating, when the switch to combined intermediate and short-acting insulins can be made as described. Use of intermediate-acting insulin can usually begin within 36 hr after commencing therapy for ketoacidosis.

Ketonemia and ketonuria may persist despite clinical improvement. The nitroprusside reaction that is routinely used to measure "ketones" reacts with acetoacetate and weakly with acetone but not with β-hydroxybutyrate. The usual ratio of β-hydroxybutyrate to acetoacetate is approximately 3:1 but is commonly as much as 8:1 or more in patients with DKA. With correction of acidosis, β-hydroxybutyrate dissociates to acetoacetate, which is identified by the nitroprusside reaction. Hence, persistence of ketonuria for a day or more may not reliably reflect the clinical improvement and should not be interpreted as a poor therapeutic response.

Key steps in the management of DKA are summarized in Table 599–8.

Postacidotic Phase or Transition Period for Establishment of Metabolic Control. DKA is usually corrected within 36 to 48 hr by the foregoing therapeutic regimen. At this time, food and fluids are usually tolerated orally, and insulin can be given by subcutaneous injection. The child who presents with classic symptoms and documented hyperglycemia, in the absence of clinical dehydration and ketoacidosis, can be considered as requiring treatment at this transition stage. For such children, subcutaneous injections of fast-acting insulin are begun at doses of 0.1–0.25 U/kg every 6–8 hr before meals with simultaneous monitoring of blood glucose concentration and adjustment of the insulin dose for 1–2 days. The initial dose of insulin is lower because these children generally have lower blood glucose concentration and are more sensitive to insulin than are those presenting with DKA. One to 2 days of fast-acting insulin therapy are needed to estimate the total daily insulin requirement as a guide to subsequent use of combined intermediate- and short-acting forms.

The aims of therapy during the transitional period are to treat any recognized precipitating cause for DKA such as infection, stabilize the patient's metabolic control by adjusting the insulin dosage, institute an appropriate nutritional pattern for the child, and educate the parents and patient in the principles of diabetic management. These principles include techniques of insulin injection, as well as techniques for monitoring blood and urine glucose levels and urinary ketone spill, understanding nutritional requirements, recognizing hypoglycemia (insulin shock) and its management, and having the ability to make adjustments to insulin dosage during minor illnesses and for regularly planned exercise. This education is best carried out by the coordinated participation of physician, dietitian, and nurse educator who have special training in diabetes. For newly diagnosed patients, this phase commonly lasts 5–10 days; less time may be required for stabilization and re-education of previously diagnosed patients. Ongoing education and adjustment of insulin dosage are continued after discharge from the hospital through patient visits and inquiries by telephone; during this phase, gradual reductions in insulin dosage

TABLE 599–8 Steps in Management of Diabetic Ketoacidosis

1. *Confirm Diagnosis*
   Obtain
      Blood glucose
      Serum electrolytes
      Acid-base status—pH; HCO_3^-
   Consider
      Urine microscopy/culture
      Chest film
      Blood culture
      Throat culture
      Electrocardiography
   Consider intensive care–like setting if:
      pH <7.00
      Age <2 yr
      Unconscious
      Blood glucose >1000 mg/dL
2. *Begin intravenous fluids*
   20 mL/kg of 0.9% (normal)
   Saline (NaCl) over 1 hr
3. *Reassess the patient—what precipitated this episode?*
   Delayed diagnosis
   Noncompliance
   Infection
   Trauma
4. *Follow protocol*
   Guidelines in Table 599–6—Begin insulin 0.1 U/kg/hr with hour 2 of intravenous therapy as outlined in Table 599–6
5. Measure glucose every hour; electrolytes and acid-base every 2–4 hr for the first 24 hr
6. Continue treatment with insulin even if glucose approaches 300 mg/dL (17 mM) as long as acidosis persists. Consider adding 5–10% glucose in intravenous line or occasionally reducing insulin to 0.05 U/kg/hr.
7. If acidosis is not resolving (or improving) despite fluids and insulin of 0.1 U/kg/hr consider:
      Severe sepsis causing lactic acidosis or insulin degradation, or both
      Error in insulin dose
8. In children less than 10 yr (especially less than 5 yr) anticipate possible clincial cerebral edema after 4–6 hr of treatment. The following herald evolving edema:
      Headache
      Change in conscious level or response
      Unequal dialated pupils
      Delirium
      Incontinence
      Vomiting
      Bradycardia
9. *If cerebral edema is clinically apparent*
   Reduce intravenous solution rate
   Give mannitol 1 g/kg intravenously (10–20 g/m_2)
   Repeat in 2–4 hr.

are frequently required, and the patients should be so advised (see later section on residual β-cell function). The details and rationale for insulin and dietary therapy as well as other aspects of long-term management are provided in the following section on insulin regimens.

The immediate goals in the management of children with type I diabetes are to provide adequate nutrition and exogenous insulin in a manner that prevents polydipsia and polyuria, including nocturia; avoids ketoacidosis and severe hypoglycemia; and permits normal growth and development with an active life pattern. These goals are achievable by most patients and their parents if they come to understand the principles of the pathophysiology and management of this disease. Ongoing supervision by the physician is essential and should be provided in a manner that avoids undue anxiety and psychologic dependence on the part of the child or parents or a sense of guilt on the part of the parents.

Evidence is now compelling that the long-term complications of diabetes are related to the degree of day-to-day metabolic control. Therefore, one should aim for as nearly normal metabolism as possible. The achievement of completely normal metabolism, however, is not possible by the standard pattern of treatment that consists of two to three daily injections of insulin and attention to nutritional intake and exercise. In highly motivated individuals and their care providers, however, near-normal metabolism can now be achieved in one of two ways. The first consists of monitoring blood glucose values at home with appropriate adjustment of insulin dosage administered at least three to four times a day and close attention to nutritional intake, which can be effective. The second method is continuous subcutaneous insulin infusion by a pump worn externally, which can be programmed to provide a basal rate of delivery with meal-related increments. This is also an effective means for highly selected patients. For the majority of pediatric patients, however, these newer approaches are not acceptable or applicable, and routine management rests on three pillars: the provision of insulin and guidance with respect to its dosage, attention to nutritional intake, and exercise.

CONTINUING GUIDANCE

Insulin Regimens. The diurnal pattern of insulin concentration in the plasma of normal persons is characterized by a basal level on which secretory episodes that coincide with intake of food are superimposed. Each rise in plasma insulin concentration during feeding is synchronous with, and proportional to, the rise in blood glucose. Plasma insulin concentrations, however, do not reflect total insulin secretion. Because insulin is secreted into the portal circulation, its first target organ is the liver, the key organ governing the initial disposal of a glucose load (See Table 599–4). The liver extracts approximately 50% of the insulin presented to it from the portal circulation.

Currently available insulins and their duration of *action* are listed in Tables 599–9 and 599–10. They are classified as short-, intermediate-, and long-acting types; each is available in a concentration of 100 U/mL (U-100); higher concentrations are available for the unusual patient who has high resistance to insulin. Appropriate dilutions can be prepared for younger patients requiring low doses. Refinements in manufacture are now responsible for animal forms of insulin that have distinctly less contamination than formerly with other pancreatic hormones such as proinsulin, glucagon, pancreatic polypeptide, and somatostatin. Antibodies to these and other contaminants have been demonstrated in the sera of insulin-treated diabetics. It is unclear whether these new and more highly purified insulins facilitate metabolic control, but they probably do result in fewer local and systemic allergic reactions, including lipoatrophy and lipohypertrophy. Insulins extracted from beef and pork pancreas and marketed separately or as a mixture of the two forms of insulin are still available. Human insulin, synthesized in bacteria via recombinant DNA technology (synthetic) or by chemical modification of pork insulin (semisynthetic), is now routinely available for therapy. Human insulin may be less allergenic and less likely to induce antibody formation, but the limited data available do not indicate any significant advantages over highly purified pork insulin. Human insulin, synthetically produced by recombinant DNA techniques, is likely to become the predominantly available insulin. A synthetically modified human insulin, Lispro, has the property of extremely rapid onset of action within 15 min of injection, peak effect within 1–1.5 hr, and shortened duration with dissipation of effect within 3 hr. Therefore, it is useful in children because it can be injected at the time of feeding or even at its conclusion, allowing for better correlation of insulin dose to food intake.

Because exogenous insulins are injected subcutaneously rather than directly into the portal vein, their rate of absorption may be variable, and because the dose injected is determined empirically, it lacks the precision of endogenously secreted insulin. Therefore, a single injection of intermediate-acting insulin cannot duplicate the pattern of normal insulin secretion, and periods of excessive plasma insulin that may produce hypoglycemia or periods of inadequate insulin that permit hyperglycemia, or both, are virtually inevitable. Even with injections of regular fast-acting insulin prior to each meal, normalization of blood glucose values is not entirely achieved, although the degree of control is improved. Thus, the regimen of insulin administration selected for the diabetic child must represent a compromise designed to achieve as nearly normal an intermediary metabolism as possible to permit normal growth and development, avoid frequent hypoglycemic reactions, and minimize the untoward consequence of unrestrained hyperglycemia.

At the onset of diabetes, or after recovery from ketoacidosis, the total daily dose of insulin is about 0.5–1.0 U/kg. The actual total daily requirement of insulin is estimated from the representative 24-hr period when only regular insulin was administered before each meal during the transition phase after resolution of ketoacidosis, or during the initial management of less severely affected patients as outlined earlier. Long-acting insulins are not often used in children. In most instances, one of the intermediate insulins is employed, but because of its delayed action, a fast-acting (regular) insulin is usually combined with it. With the single daily dose combined regimen, approximately two thirds of the total dose is an intermediate-acting insulin (e.g., NPH, Lente) and the remainder is regular insulin; the injection is given 30 min before breakfast or with breakfast if Lispro is the regular (short-acting) insulin used. The two types of insulins should always be drawn into the syringe in the same sequence (regular first) so that the residual insulin in the "dead space" is always the same type; thus, greater stability of the patient can be assured once a therapeutic dose is established. Disposable syringes with fine needles, minimal dead space, and easy-to-read calibration for use with U-100 insulin are available. For small children, syringes calibrated to a maximum of 50 U are also available; in some European countries diluted insulins are marketed.

In order to avoid hypoglycemia, *the single daily dose regimen* combining intermediate- and short-acting insulin is initially calculated on the basis of two thirds of the total daily dose or approximately 0.5 U/kg. Step increases or decreases of 10–15% can then be made daily during the initial phase in educating patients and their families until the desired degree of control

TABLE 599–9 Common Types of Available Insulins

Product	Manufacturer	Form	Strength
Rapid-Acting (Onset 0.5–4 hr)			
Humulin R (regular)	Lilly	Human	U-100
Humulin BR (buffered regular) or external insulin pumps only)	Lilly	Human	U-100
Humalog*	Lilly	Human, modified	U-100
Novolin R (regular)	Novo Nordisk	Human	U-100
Novolin R PenFill (regular)	Novo Nordisk	Human	U-100
Velosulin Human (regular buffered)	Novo Nordisk	Human	U-100
Iletin II Regular	Lilly	Beef	U-100
Iletin II Regular	Lilly	Pork	U-100, U-500
Purified Pork R (regular)	Novo Nordisk	Pork	U-100
Velosulin (regular)	Novo Nordisk	Pork	U-100
Iletin I Regular	Lilly	Beef, pork	U-100
Regular	Novo Nordisk	Pork	U-100
Iletin I Semilente	Lilly	Beef, pork	U-100
Semilente	Novo Nordisk	Beef	U-100
Intermediate-Acting (Onset 2–4 hr)			
Humulin L (Lente)	Lilly	Human	U-100
Humulin N (NPH)	Lilly	Human	U-100
Insulatard Human NPH	Novo Nordisk	Human	U-100
Novolin L (Lente)	Novo Nordisk	Human	U-100
Novolin N (NPH)	Novo Nordisk	Human	U-100
Novolin N PenFill (NPH)	Novo Nordisk	Human	U-100
Iletin II Lente	Lilly	Beef	U-100
Iletin II NPH	Lilly	Beef	U-100
Iletin II Lente	Lilly	Pork	U-100
Iletin II NPH	Lilly	Pork	U-100
Insulatard NPH	Novo Nordisk	Pork	U-100
Purified Pork Lente	Novo Nordisk	Pork	U-100
Purified Pork N (NPH)	Novo Nordisk	Pork	U-100
Iletin I Lente	Lilly	Beef, pork	U-100
Iletin I NPH	Lilly	Beef, pork	U-100
Lente	Novo Nordisk	Beef	U-100
NPH	Novo Nordisk	Beef	U-100
Long-Acting (Onset 4 6 hr)			
Humulin U (Ultralente)	Lilly	Human	U-100
Iletin I (Ultralente)	Lilly	Beef, pork	U-100
Ultralente	Novo Nordisk	Beef	U-100
Mixtures			
Humulin 70/30 (70% NPH, 30% Regular)	Lilly	Human	U-100
Humulin 50/50 (50% NPH, 50% Regular)	Lilly	Human	U-100
Mixtard (70% NPH, 30% Regular)	Novo Nordisk	Pork	U-100
Mixtard Human 70/30 (70% NPH, 30% Regular)	Novo Nordisk	Human	U-100
Novolin 70/30 (70% NPH, 30% Regular)	Novo Nordisk	Human	U-100
Novolin 70/30 PenFill (70% NPH, 30% Regular)	Novo Nordisk	Human	U-100

**Humalog is the trade name of insulin Lispro, a synthetic human insulin analog that is rapid-acting and of short duration. It differs from human insulin in that the amino acids at positions 28 (proline) and 29 (lysine) of the insulin β-chain have been reversed, hence "Lispro." Although equivalent in potency to human insulin, the onset of Lispro's effect is more rapid but of shorter duration (see Table 599–10).*

TABLE 599–10 Insulins by Relative Comparative Action Curves

Insulin	Onset (hr)	Peak (hr)	Usually Effective Duration (hr)	Usual Maximal Duration (hr)
Animal				
Regular	0.5–2.0	3–4	4–6	6–8
NPH	4–6	8–14	16–20	20–24
Lente	4–6	8–14	16–20	20–24
Ultralente	8–14	10–16	24–36	24–36
Human				
Regular	0.5–1.0	2–3	3–6	4–6
Lispro	0.25–0.5	1–2	2–3	3–4
NPH	2–4	4–10	10–16	14–18
Lente	3–4	4–12	12–18	16–20
Ultralente	6–10	?	18–20	20–30

is achieved. The initial phase of recovery of metabolic equilibrium is characterized by a period of replenishment of body stores of glycogen, protein, and fat that were depleted during the evolution of diabetes. Thus, insulin requirements for the first few days may on occasion be found to be even greater than 1 U/kg/24 hr. Adjustments in the dose of insulin are made in relation to the pattern of blood glucose values monitored before each meal or the excretion of glucose, or both. If the predominant hyperglycemia or glucosuria occurs in late morning, the quick-acting form of insulin is increased by 10–15%. If the predominant hyperglycemia or glucosuria occurs in late afternoon or evening, the intermediate-acting insulin is increased by 10–15%. Should hypoglycemic reactions occur in midmorning to noon, the quick-acting form of insulin is reduced by 10–15%, and if hypoglycemia occurs in late afternoon or evening, the intermediate-acting insulin is decreased by 10–15%. In anticipation of increased exercise at home, the daily dose of insulin should be decreased by about 10% at the time of discharge from the initial hospitalization.

Although children can be managed with a single daily injection of insulin, *two daily injections* are now routinely recommended as standard (Fig. 599–3). When there is persistent nocturia associated with excessive fasting hyperglycemia and morning glucosuria in response to a single daily injection of insulin, dividing the total daily dose into two injections is clearly indicated. In this plan, two thirds of the daily total dose is given before breakfast and one third before the evening meal; each injection consists of intermediate- and short-acting insulins in proportions of 2:1–3:1. For example, assuming a total daily dose of 1 U/kg for a 30-kg child, 14 U of NPH or Lente combined with 6 U of regular or Lispro insulin would be given before breakfast, and 6 U of NPH or Lente with 4 U of regular or Lispro insulin before the evening meal. As with the single daily dose regimen, stepwise increases or decreases, each consisting of 10–15% should be made to minimize hypoglycemic reactions and undue hyperglycemia (see preceding paragraph for guidelines).

At least two daily injections of insulin are especially applicable for infants and children less than 5 yr of age, in whom intake of food and extent of activity are not always predictable, and for adolescents, especially during the pubertal growth spurt. At least two daily injections tend to result in smoother metabolic control with fewer hypoglycemic reactions and less uncontrolled hyperglycemia. This approach is also more effective when the evening meal is the major one (see under Nutritional Management). With an explanation of the rationale, acceptance of this twice-daily regimen by patients and parents is usually good and twice-daily insulin is now considered standard therapy. When compliance is erratic, as particularly occurs with adolescents, one injection is preferable to none. The physician should in all instances attempt to determine the regimen that will be in the best interests of the patient. For children who insist on only one daily injection of insulin, the daily dose is adjusted according to carefully kept records of blood or urinary glucose values until the best possible degree of metabolic control is achieved. In this way, confidence in the patient-family-physician relationship is maintained and a sense of guilt in patient or family is avoided. However, erratic administration of insulin and particularly inadvertent or deliberate omission of insulin is the most common cause of recurrent DKA.

In special circumstances, such as highly motivated older adolescents or with particularly committed, capable parents, *three or more daily injections* of insulin based on frequent blood glucose monitoring can be administered. This kind of intensive

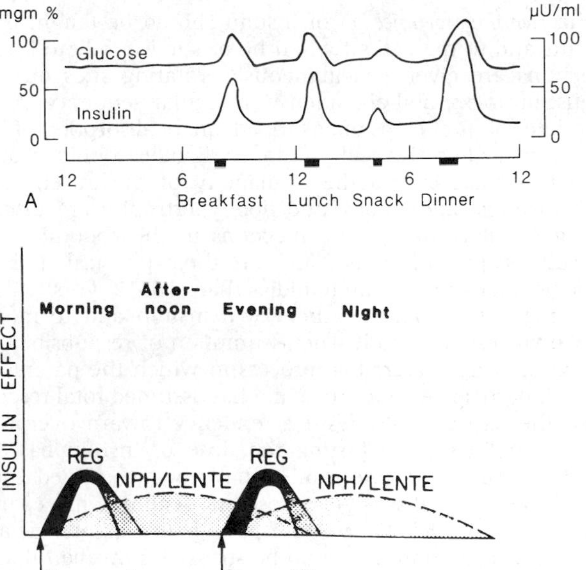

Figure 599–3 *A,* Schematic representation of the normal relationship of food intake, blood glucose, and serum insulin concentration. Note that glucose concentration is maintained between 80 and 120 mg/dL. Note also the precise release of insulin that has passed through the portal circulation synchronous with and proportional to the food-induced glycemic excursions. Compare and contrast these patterns with the time pattern of insulin action followed by subcutaneous injection. *B,* Standard combined split-dose insulin regimen in treatment of insulin-dependent diabetes in children. The combined regular (short-acting) and NPH or lente (intermediate-acting) injection in the morning before breakfast is approximately one half to two thirds of the total daily insulin dose with an ~2:1 ratio of intermediate to short acting. The remaining one third to one half of daily insulin is given before supper in the same proportion of 2:1 intermediate to short acting. Individual adjustments in the total dose and preparations used depend on blood glucose profiles. Compare and contrast with the normal relationship between meals and insulin in part A. (B from Schade DS, et al: Intensive Insulin Therapy. Belle Mead, NJ, Excerpta Medica, 1983.)

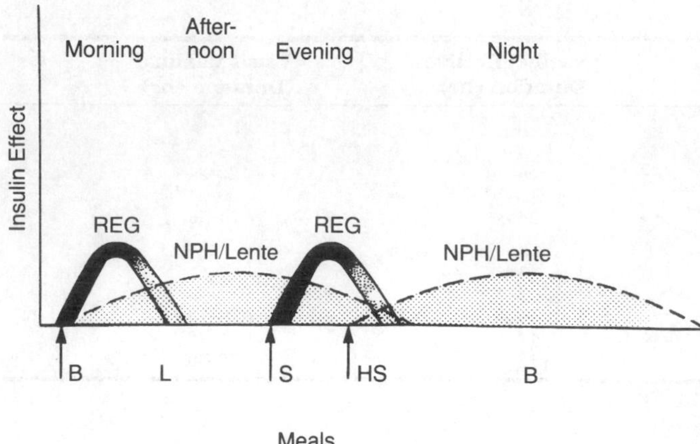

Figure 599–4 Three-dose insulin regimen intended to reduce the likelihood of the Somogyi or the dawn phenomenon. The morning dose comprises a combined short- and intermediate-acting insulin of about one half to two thirds of the total daily dose. The short-acting dose before supper covers the anticipated glycemic elevation with dinner. The intermediate-acting insulin is delayed until bedtime so that the peak effect is delayed. (From Schade DS, Santiago JV, Skyler JS, et al: Intensive Insulin Therapy. Princeton, NJ, Excerpta Medica, 1983.)

therapy improves glycemic control toward normal, diminishes the risk of microvascular complications, but is often associated with more severe and frequent hypoglycemic reactions (Fig. 599–4).

The *technique of injection* of insulin should be taught to the parents and to the patient when he or she is ready to learn it. Injections are given subcutaneously, rotating sites on arms, thighs, buttocks, and abdomen in a regular sequence. An appropriate rotation helps to ensure adequate absorption of insulin, prevent fibrosis, and minimize lipodystrophic changes. With this rotation and the availability of the purer, single-peak insulins, lipoatrophy and lipohypertrophy are unusual. Younger children may find injections in the abdominal wall difficult or painful. Depending on their physical and psychologic maturity, children older than 10–12 yr should be encouraged to administer their own insulin and to monitor their own responses to it. The assumption of responsibility for self-monitoring is a gradual process in which the parents and child all participate. Once the child has assumed total responsibility, the parents must resist a tendency toward overprotection. Guidelines for adjusting the dose of insulin based on blood or urinary glucose profiles have been outlined earlier, and those for adjusting the dose of insulin with exercise, illness, and "brittle" diabetes are provided in greater detail in the following section. It should be stressed, however, that the adolescent growth spurt is regularly associated with an increase in insulin requirements, which become lower when puberty is completed. These changes in insulin requirement are the consequence of parallel changes of increased growth hormone secretion during puberty, an event associated with increased endogenous insulin secretion in the nondiabetic individual.

Hypersensitivity to insulin is uncommon in children. Local skin reactions are characterized by erythema or urticaria, with burning, itching, and tenderness within hours or sooner after an injection. These reactions usually resolve spontaneously over a period of days but may require a change from mixed beef-pork to pure pork or human insulin or from NPH to Lente insulin because of allergy to protamine in the former; antihistamines may be used if necessary. Generalized reactions with severe urticaria or angioedema are extremely rare and may also resolve spontaneously, but a change in the type of insulin is usually indicated, for example, from a mixed beef-pork preparation to a pure pork or human preparation. Desensitization may also be necessary, as may a course of systemic corticosteroid therapy for 1–2 wk. Rarely, insulin resistance develops in response to a local tissue enzyme that destroys injected insulin. Some of these patients have benefited from the addition of a protease enzyme inhibitor to the insulin solution; others have required chronic intravenous infusion and are best managed in a hospital with a specialized diabetes unit.

After several months of insulin therapy, nearly all patients will have acquired *antibodies to insulin*. In the majority, these do not interfere with the metabolic response. They may, however, promote instability by creating a reservoir of insulin that may be released at unpredictable times. Rarely, children with antibodies acquire true resistance to insulin and require more than 2 U of insulin/kg/24 hr. A change to a preparation of pure pork, pure beef, or human insulin usually resolves this problem; in some instances, a period of corticosteroid therapy or a course of desensitization may be necessary. Antibodies causing allergy are usually of the IgE class; IgA and IgM antibodies may be responsible for resistance to insulin.

Nutritional Management. Because the word *diet* may connote restriction and denial and constitute a source of anxiety or rebellion, or both, on the part of parent or patient, its use should be avoided. Instructional discussion can be provided under terms such as "nutritional requirements" and "meal plans." Actually, there are no special nutritional requirements for the diabetic child other than those for optimal growth and development. However, because the capacity to secrete insulin in response to the intake of food is negligible in the diabetic child, and because the dose of insulin is predicated on caloric intake, regularity of the eating pattern for the determined insulin regimen becomes paramount. In outlining nutritional requirements for the child on the basis of age, sex, weight, and activity, food preferences, including any based on cultural and ethnic backgrounds, must be considered. General guidelines are usually applicable, but individualization for each child should be programmed.

Total recommended *caloric intake* is based on size or surface area and can be obtained from standard tables (Tables 599–11 and 599–12). The caloric mixture should comprise approximately 55% carbohydrate, 30% fat, and 15% protein. In general, approximately 70% of the carbohydrate content should be derived from complex carbohydrates such as starch, and intake of sucrose and highly refined sugars should be limited. Complex carbohydrates require prolonged digestion and absorption so that plasma glucose levels rise slowly, whereas glucose in refined sugars, including those in carbonated beverages, is rapidly absorbed and may cause wide swings in the metabolic pattern; carbonated beverages should therefore be

TABLE 599–11 Calorie Needs for Children and Young Adults

Age	Kcal Required/Kg Body Weight*
Children	
0–12 mo	120
1–10 yr	100–75
Young women	
11–15 yr	35
≥16 yr	30
Young men	
11–15 y r	80–50 (65)
16–20 yr	
Average activity	40
Very physically active	50
Sedentary	30

Numbers in parentheses are means.

**Gradual decline in calories per unit weight as age increases.*

From Nutrition Guide for Professionals: Diabetes Education and Meal Planning. Alexandria, VA, and Chicago, IL, The American Diabetes Association and The American Dietetic Association, 1988.

TABLE 599–12 Summary of Nutrition Guidelines for Children and/or Adolescents with Type 1 Diabetes Mellitus

Nutrition Care Plan

Promotes optimal compliance.
Incorporates goals of management: normal growth and development, control of blood glucose, maintenance of optimal nutritional status, and prevention of complications. Uses staged approach.

Nutrient Recommendations and Distribution

Nutrient	*(%) of Calories*	*Recommended Daily Intake*
Carbohydrate	Will vary	High fiber, especially soluble fiber; optimal amount unknown
Fiber	>20 g per day	
Protein	12–20	
Fat	<30	
Saturated	<10	
Polyunsaturated	6–8	
Monounsaturated	Remainder of fat allowance	
Cholesterol		300 mg
Sodium		Avoid excessive; limit to 3,000–4,000 mg if hypertensive

Additional Recommendations

Energy: If using measured diet, re-evaluate prescribed energy level at least every 3 mo.
Protein: High-protein intakes may contribute to diabetic nephropathy. Low intakes may reverse preclinical nephropathy. Therefore, 12–20% of energy is recommended; lower end of range is preferred. In guiding toward the end of the range, a staged approach is useful.
Alcohol: Safe use of moderate alcohol consumption should be taught as routine anticipatory guidance as early as junior high.
Snacks: Snacks vary according to individual needs (generally three snacks per day for children; midafternoon and bedtime snacks for junior high children or teens).
Alternative sweeteners: Use of a variety of sweeteners is suggested.
Educational techniques: No single technique is superior. Choice of educational method used should be based on patient needs, Knowledge of variety of techniques is important. Follow-up education and support are required.
Eating disorders: Best treatment is presention. Unexplained poor control or severe hypoglycemia may indicate a potential eating disorder.
Exercise: Education is vital to prevent delayed or immediate hypoglycemia and to prevent worsened hyperglycemia and ketosis.

From Connell JE, Thomas-Doberson D: Nutritional Management of children and adolescents with insulin-dependent diabetes mellitus: A review by the Diabetes Care and Education Dietetic Practice Group. J Am Diet Assoc 91:1556, 1991.

of the sugar-free variety. Because sucrose, as part of total carbohydrate, does not impair overall blood glucose control in type I diabetes, priority should be given to total calories and total carbohydrate consumed rather than its sourcc. In the United States, the ban on saccharin as an artificial sweetener has been removed pending further evidence of its toxic or teratogenic effect. Although in children there is concern about the potential cumulative effect, available data do not support an association of modcratc amounts with bladder cancer. Other non-nutritive sweeteners such as aspartame are used in a variety of products. Sorbitol and xylitol should not be used as artificial sweeteners; they are products of the polyol pathway and are implicated in some of the complications of diabetes.

Diets with *high fiber content* are useful in improving control of blood glucose in diabetic subjects. In addition, moderate amounts of sucrose consumed with fiber-rich foods such as whole meal bread may have no more glycemic effect than their low-fiber, sugar-free equivalents. The concept of biologic equivalence or of a "glycemic index" of foods is currently under investigation. When completed, these studies may provide a listing of foods with more predictable and desirable effects on blood glucose and serum lipid patterns for patients with diabetes.

The *intake of fat* is adjusted so that the polyunsaturated:saturated ratio is increased to about 1.2:1.0, in contrast to the estimated American average of 0.3:1.0. Dietary fats derived from animal sources are, therefore, reduced and replaced by polyunsaturated fats from vegetable sources. Substituting margarine for butter, vegetable oil for animal oils in cooking, and lean cuts of meat, poultry, and fish for fatty meats, such as bacon, is advisable. The intake of cholesterol is also reduced by these measures and by limiting the number of egg yolks consumed. These simple measures reduce serum low-density lipoprotein cholesterol, a predisposing factor to atherosclerotic disease. Less than 10% of calories should be derived from saturated fats, up to 10% from polyunsaturated fats, and the remaining fat-derived calories from monounsaturated fats. Table 599–12 summarizes current nutritional guidelines for children and adolescents with type I diabetes mellitus.

The total daily caloric intake may be divided to provide 20% at breakfast, 20% at lunch, and 30% at dinner, leaving 10% for each of the midmorning, midafternoon, and evening snacks, if they are desired. In older children, the midmorning snack may be omitted and its caloric equivalent added to lunch. Special brochures and pamphlets describing sample meal plans for children are usually available from regional diabetes associations; their use should be encouraged as part of the educational process. Meal plans are often based on groups of food exchanges; within each of the exchange lists of the foods that are principal sources of carbohydrates, proteins, and fats, there is a wide variety of foods that can be substituted or exchanged. For practical purposes there are few restrictions so that each child can select a diet based on personal taste or preferences with the help of the physician or dietitian, or both. Emphasis should be placed on regularity of food intake and on constancy of carbohydrate intake. Occasional excesses for birthdays and other parties are permissible and tolerated in order not to foster rebellion and stealth in obtaining desired food. Similarly, cakes and even candies are permissible on special occasions as long as the food exchange value and carbohydrate content are adjusted in the meal plan. Adjustments in meal planning must constantly be made to meet the needs as well as the desires of each child, although a consistent eating pattern with appropriate supplements for exercise, the pubertal growth spurt, and pregnancy in a diabetic adolescent are important for metabolic control. *There is also an increased frequency of eating disorders among young women with diabetes.* Thus, expectations and educational advice regarding nutrition must be dealt with in a sensitive careful manner, especially in adolescents.

Monitoring. Success in the daily management of the diabetic child can be measured to a considerable extent by the competence acquired by the family, and subsequently by the child, in assuming responsibility for daily "diabetic care." Their initial and ongoing instruction in conjunction with their supervised experience can lead to a sense of confidence in making intermittent adjustments in insulin dosage for dietary deviations, unusual physical activity, and even for some minor intercurrent illnesses as well as for otherwise unexplained repeated hypoglycemic reactions and excessive glucosuria. Within limits, such acceptance of responsibility should make them independent of the physician for their ordinary care. Independence is good provided that the physician maintains ongoing interested supervision and shared responsibility with the family and the child.

Self-monitoring is an essential component of managing diabetes and necessitates a regimen that includes measurements of blood and urinary glucose and, at times, ketones as well as the keeping of a standardized record of these results and the corresponding data of dietary deviations, unusual physical activity, hypoglycemic reactions, intercurrent illness, the daily dose of insulin, and other items of possible relevance. Many of these records may be patently unreliable for a number of reasons. There may be self-delusion, reliance on memory with charting just prior to the visit to the physician, attempts to please the physician and avoid rebuke, as well as reluctance to perform some aspects of the blood or urinary tests. Despite these problems, asking patients to keep records is justified. Initially, following diagnosis and institution of the treatment plan, the parent or patient is apt to be particularly attentive to a prescribed regimen. It is after some months of satisfactory experience that parents or patients tend to become less attentive to detail. When the physician apparently accepts the contrived report, the parent or child may come to find more and more reasons for noncompliance. When the physician mistrusts the report, he or she may think it justifiable to make evaluations of his or her own selection (see later). Should this data be counter to those in the parent's or child's report, the physician can then attempt to clarify the situation with them in a manner that does not undermine their mutual confidence. Such situations test the physician's skill in the management of patients with persistent but not confining illness.

Short-term (daily) blood glucose monitoring has been markedly enhanced by the availability of strips impregnated with glucose oxidase that permit blood glucose measurement from a drop of blood. The blood glucose concentration can be approximated directly by comparison to a color scale or accurately by a portable calibrated reflectance meter. Many meters now contain a memory "chip" enabling recall of each measurement, its average over a given interval, and the ability to display the pattern on a computer screen by means of appropriate adaptor links. Such information is a useful educational tool for verifying degree of control and modifying recommended regimens. A small spring-loaded device that automates capillary bloodletting in a relatively painless fashion is also commercially available. Parents and patients should be taught to use these devices and measure blood glucose three to four times daily—before breakfast, lunch, and supper, and before retiring at night. Initially, at diagnosis, the blood glucose measurement should also be performed at 3–4 A.M. to exclude inappropriate nocturnal hypoglycemia and avoid the Somogyi phenomenon (see later). Ideally, the blood glucose concentration should range from approximately 80 mg/dL in the fasting state to 140 mg/dL after meals. In practice, however, a range of 60–240 mg/dL is acceptable. Blood glucose measurements that are consistently at or outside these limits, in the absence of an identifiable cause such as exercise or dietary indiscretion, are an indication for a change in the insulin dose. For example, if the fasting blood glucose is high, the evening dose of intermediate-acting insulin is increased by 10–15%; if the noon glucose level exceeds set limits, the morning regular insulin is increased by 10–15%; if the presupper glucose is high, the morning intermediate-acting insulin is increased by 10–15%; and if the prebedtime glucose measurement is high, the evening dose of regular insulin is increased by 10–15%. Similarly, reductions in the insulin type and dose should be made if the corresponding blood glucose measurements are consistently below desirable limits.

Daily blood glucose measurements should be continued as long as they are acceptable to the patient. Practical considerations require a reduction in the frequency of blood glucose monitoring at home; few children tolerate capillary blood letting four times daily for prolonged periods. Consequently, after the initial stabilization period of several weeks, when the routine of insulin administration and meal plan is established, some suggest that home blood glucose monitoring be performed only 2–3 days per week, varying the days each week to allow a representative profile in time. Monitoring of urine glucose spill is performed on those days when blood glucose measurements are omitted. However, blood glucose measurement should be performed if there are symptoms suggestive of hypoglycemia or if urine glucose spill persists at 2% or greater. When more precise adjustments are deemed necessary, the physician may request a fractional 24-hr collection of urine. The urine should be collected in three fractions: 8 A.M.–2 P.M.; 2 P.M to 8 P.M.; and 8 P.M. to 8 A.M. Assessment of volume and semiquantitative or quantitative glucose values in each sample permits a rational basis for adjusting the respective doses of the rapid- and intermediate-acting insulins. In highly motivated adolescents and young adults who become sufficiently knowledgeable about managing their diabetes, self-monitoring of blood glucose levels before and 2 hr after meals, in conjunction with multiple daily injections of insulin, adjusted as necessary, can maintain near-normal glycemia for prolonged periods.

A reliable index of long-term glycemic control is provided by measurement of *glycosylated hemoglobin.* Glycohemoglobin (HbA_{1c}) represents the fraction of hemoglobin to which glucose has been nonenzymatically attached in the bloodstream. The formation of HbA_{1c} is a slow reaction that is dependent on the prevailing concentration of blood glucose; it continues irreversibly throughout the red blood cell's life span of approximately 120 days. The higher the blood glucose concentration and the longer the red blood cell's exposure to it, the higher will be the fraction of HbA_{1c}, which is expressed as a percentage of total hemoglobin. Because a blood sample at any given time contains a mixture of red blood cells of varying ages, exposed for varying times to varying blood glucose concentrations, an HbA_{1c} measurement reflects the average blood glucose concentration of the preceding 2–3 mo. When measured by standardized methods to remove labile forms, the fraction of HbA_{1c} is not influenced by an isolated episode of hyperglycemia. Consequently, as an index of long-term glycemic control, a measurement of HbA_{1c} is superior to measurements of glycosuria or a single blood glucose determination. It is recommended that HbA_{1c} measurements be obtained three to four times/year in order to obtain a profile of long-term glycemic control. The more consistently lower the HbA_{1c} level, and hence the better the metabolic control, the more likely it is that microvascular complications such as retinopathy and nephropathy will be less severe, delayed in appearance, or avoided. Depending on the method used for determination, HbA_{1c} values may be spuriously elevated in thalassemia (or other conditions with elevated hemoglobin F) and spuriously lower in sickle cell disease. Although values of HbA_{1c} may vary according to the method used for measurement, in normal individuals, the HbA_{1c} fraction is usually less than 7%; in diabetics, values of 6–9% represent good metabolic control, values of 9–12%, fair control, and values greater than 12%, poor control (Table 599–13).

Exercise. Exercise is an integral component of growth and development. No form of exercise, including competitive sports of any kind, should be forbidden to the diabetic child, who should not be made to feel different or restricted. Examples of athletes with diabetes who have excelled in national or international sports are not rare. A major complication of

TABLE 599–13 Levels of Treatment: Biochemical and Clinical Characteristics

Minimal
HbA_{1c} 11.0–13.0% and GHb 13.0–15.0%
Many SMBG values of ≥300 mg/dL
Almost constantly positive urine glucose tests
Intermittent spontaneous ketonuria
Average
HbA_{1c} 8.0–9.0% and GHb 10.0–11.0%
Premeal SMBG 160–200 mg/dL
Intermittent positive urine glucose
Rare ketonuria
Intensive
HbA_{1c} 6.0–7.0% and GHb 7.0–9.0%
Premeal SMBG 70–120 mg/dL; postmeal SMBG <180 mg/dL
Essentially no positive urine glucose or ketones

SMBG = self-monitored blood glucose; HbA_{1c} = glycohemoglobin; GHb = glycosylated hemoglobin.

exercise in diabetic patients is the presence of a hypoglycemic reaction during or within hours after exercise. If hypoglycemia does not occur with exercise, adjustments in diet or insulin are not necessary, and glucoregulation is likely to be improved through the increased utilization of glucose by muscles. The major contributing factor to hypoglycemia with exercise is an increased rate of absorption of insulin from its injection site. Higher insulin levels dampen hepatic glucose production so that it is inadequate to meet the increased glucose utilization of exercising muscle. Regular exercise also improves glucoregulation by increasing insulin receptors. In patients who are in poor metabolic control, vigorous exercise may precipitate ketoacidosis because of the exercise-induced increase in the counterregulatory hormones.

In anticipation of vigorous exercise, one additional carbohydrate exchange may be taken prior to exercise, and glucose in the form of orange juice, carbonated beverage, or candy should be available during and after exercise. With experience and trial and error, each patient, guided by the physician, should develop an appropriate regimen for regularly planned exercise that is frequently associated with hypoglycemia; in such instances, the total dose of insulin may be reduced by about 10–15% on the day of the scheduled exercise. Prolonged exercise, such as long-distance running may require reduction of as much as 50% or more of the usual insulin dose.

Levels of Treatment. The intensity of treatment required for patients with diabetes mellitus must reflect mutually desirable goals negotiated between the physician and the patient and the family. These goals may change depending on the age of the patient, stage of physical and emotional maturity, understanding, commitment, financial resources available to the family, and their health beliefs as well as those of the physician. Goals that are not mutually acceptable are doomed to failure. Minimal levels of treatment are preferable to recurrent hospitalization for DKA; intensive therapy carries a significant risk for recurrent hypoglycemia, although it may reduce the risk of microvascular complications. The biochemical and clinical characteristics of minimal, average, and intensive treatment are summarized in Table 599–13.

Residual β-Cell Function (Honeymoon Period). After the initial stabilization period, some 75% of newly diagnosed diabetic children require progressive reductions in the daily dose of insulin from approximately 1 U/kg to 0.5 U/kg or less. Recurrent hypoglycemia is the manifestation that prompts a reduction in the insulin dose. A minority of children can even maintain normoglycemia for a time without any administered insulin; this complete remission occurs in less than 5% of diabetics, but even in these patients glucose tolerance tests demonstrate abnormal carbohydrate metabolism. The duration of this "honeymoon" phase is variable; it commonly lasts several weeks or months but may last as long as 1–2 yr. Residual insulin secretion, measured as C-peptide, is present during this remission period and to some extent in virtually all diabetic children in the initial year of their disease; in approximately 20% there is some C-peptide response even after 5 yr. Stable, well-controlled patients have higher C-peptide secretion than do nonstable patients, and the required dose of insulin is inversely correlated to the basal or the stimulated C-peptide response.

It is not completely clear why this residual insulin secretion is inadequate to prevent the evolution of diabetes, including ketoacidosis, but the reasons presumably relate to stress-provoked secretion of catecholamines that inhibit still further the insulin secretory capacity of the pancreatic β cells. In any event, the clinical remission phase is limited; with isolated exceptions, IDDM inevitably recurs. Although opinion varies, insulin treatment should be maintained unless a daily dose of 0.1 U/kg still causes hypoglycemia, in which case insulin treatment should be discontinued and the patient periodically tested for the re-emergence of glycosuria. The physician may decide to discontinue insulin treatment completely if it appears to be in the patient's best interests during this period. The patient and family, however, should not be led to believe that the disease is "cured," and they should continue to examine the child's urine for glucose.

Hypoglycemic Reactions (Insulin Shock). Virtually all diabetic children experience a hypoglycemic reaction at some time during the course of their disease. Almost one third of patients with type I diabetes mellitus have experienced hypoglycemic coma; about 1 in 10 patients experience severe hypoglycemia once annually, and about 1 in 20 experience repeated bouts of hypoglycemia. Hypoglycemia occurs suddenly or over a span of minutes in contrast to DKA, which develops over hours or days. The symptoms and signs are due to an outpouring of catecholamines, including pallor, sweating, apprehension, trembling, and tachycardia, as well as to cerebral glucopenia, including hunger, drowsiness, mental confusion, seizures, and coma. Mood and personality changes plus some abnormal physical patterns may be characteristic for an individual and provide an early clue to the more pronounced reaction. These symptoms may occur with a sudden drop in blood glucose to levels that do not meet the criteria for hypoglycemia (less than 60 mg/dL) in healthy individuals. For the same degree of hypoglycemia, children secrete more catecholamines than adults; children secrete catecholamines at glucose levels higher than those in adults and not traditionally considered hypoglycemia, for example, 60–70 mg/dL. As blood glucose falls toward these concentrations, subtle impairment in cognitive abilities may occur. However, these subtle effects of mild hypoglycemia do not impair long-term intellectual development.

The occurrence of hypoglycemia in a diabetic child indicates too much insulin relative to food intake and energy expenditure. Common causes include the evolution of the "honeymoon" phase (see earlier) after the initial diagnosis, deliberate or accidental errors in insulin dosage, inadvertent or deliberate reduction in caloric intake (often as a means to lose weight or manifestations of anorexia nervosa), and strenuous and sustained physical activity in the absence of increased caloric intake.

Many patients with IDDM lose their ability to secrete glucagon in response to hypoglycemia after 5 yr or more of diabetes and then rely almost solely on epinephrine secretion. The mechanism for the impairment of glucagon secretion is not clear. Epinephrine deficiency also may develop in long-standing diabetes if autonomic neuropathy develops as part of the complications of diabetes. Recurrent hypoglycemic episodes in association with near-normal metabolic control appear to result in a compensatory increase of glucose uptake in the brain. This mechanism preserves cerebral metabolism, reduces counterregulatory hormone responses, and results in the syndrome of "unawareness of hypoglycemia." The risk to the patient of severe hypoglycemia is thereby heightened. Avoidance of hypoglycemia results in recovery from unawareness and the restoration of appropriate counterregulatory hormone responses.

Modest decrements in plasma glucose concentration may cause early impairment in cognitive function before the activation of counterregulatory mechanisms but in the absence of typical hypoglycemic symptoms. Therefore, clinicians managing children with diabetes need to be alert to the possibility that symptoms consistent with hypoglycemia can occur at blood concentrations not previously considered in the hypoglycemic range; the former definition of hypoglycemia as 40 mg/dL or less for normal children is not applicable to those having diabetes mellitus.

Cerebral Glucopenia with Hypoglycemic Encephalopathy. Physicians caring for patients with IDDM should be aware of a syndrome of cerebral glucopenia with hypoglycemic encephalopathy. In these patients, prolonged severe hypoglycemia that is not recognized or treated may result in seizures and coma that lasts for hours despite correction of the blood glucose concentration. Such patients are often combative and use profane language. Several hours of glucose therapy may be necessary for recovery in such patients.

The most important factors in the management of hypoglycemia are an understanding by the patient and family of the symptoms and signs of the reaction, especially of the patient's individual pattern, and the avoidance of known precipitating factors. For management of an acute episode, a carbohydrate-containing snack or drink such as orange juice or a sugar-containing carbonated beverage or candy (equivalent to 5–10 g of glucose) should be taken. Patients, parents, and teachers should also be instructed in the administration of glucagon; 0.5 mg given intramuscularly is particularly useful when the patient is losing consciousness or is vomiting. If exercise has been the precipitating factor, the patient should be instructed to take additional calories prior to exercise as a preventative measure. If hypoglycemic episodes persist subsequently under similar circumstances, a reduction in the morning and evening dose of insulin by 10–15% for that day is indicated. The avoidance of severe hypoglycemic episodes should be a major objective of treatment; they have been implicated in epileptic seizures, and there is an increased frequency of abnormal electroencephalographic changes in diabetics.

The Somogyi Phenomenon, the Dawn Phenomenon, and Brittle Diabetes. Hypoglycemic episodes, which may be mild and manifest as late nocturnal or early morning sweating, night terrors, and headaches alternating rapidly, (within 4–5 hr), with ketosis, hyperglycemia, ketonuria, and excessive glucosuria, should suggest the possibility of the *Somogyi phenomenon*. This syndrome has been suitably described as "hypoglycemia begetting hyperglycemia" and is believed to be due to an outpouring of counterregulatory hormones in response to insulin-induced hypoglycemia. The coexistence of this brittle form of diabetes with daily doses of more than 2 U/kg of insulin suggests the presence of this phenomenon and the need to reduce the dose of insulin. The term *brittle diabetes* implies that control of blood glucose fluctuates widely and rapidly despite frequent adjustments of the dose of insulin.

The Somogyi phenomenon must be distinguished from the "dawn phenomenon," in which elevations of blood glucose concentration occur between 5 and 9 A.M. without preceding hypoglycemia. The dawn phenomenon is a normal event; it even occurs in patients treated by continuous subcutaneous infusion of insulin unless the rate of insulin infusion is increased in the early morning hours. The dawn phenomenon reflects the waning effects of biologically available insulin probably as a consequence of increased clearance of insulin and nocturnal surges of growth hormone that antagonize insulin's metabolic effects; the normal early morning rise in cortisol is not responsible for this phenomenon. Together, the Somogyi and dawn phenomena are the most common causes of instability or "brittleness" in diabetic children. To distinguish between the dawn and Somogyi phenomena, blood glucose concentrations should be measured at 3, 4, and 7 A.M. If blood glucose concentrations are greater than 80 mg/dL in the first two samples and markedly higher in the last, the dawn phenomenon is likely; an increase in the evening dose of intermediate insulin of 10–15% may be helpful. It may also be helpful to delay the evening dose of intermediate-acting insulin by 2–3 hr so that its delayed peak effect coincides with the anticipated timing of the dawn phenomenon, and excessive increases of blood glucose are avoided or blunted (see Fig. 599–4). Conversely, if the 3 or 4 A.M. blood glucose measurement is 60 mg/dL or less followed by rebound hyperglycemia at 7 A.M., the Somogyi phenomenon is likely; a reduction of the evening intermediate-acting insulin of 10–15% or a delay in its injection until approximately 9 P.M., is indicated (see Fig. 599–4).

In other patients with brittle diabetes, better control is often achieved by instituting a change from two to three daily injections of insulin or by changing to pure pork or human insulin, which may circumvent problems with antibodies that bind insulin. In young children, especially toddlers, the use of Lispro insulin may be beneficial because it can be given even after meals so that the dose can be adjusted according to the actual food consumed. Its shorter duration of action makes Lispro highly useful as the evening insulin to avoid nocturnal hypoglycemia. Attention should also be directed to psychologic problems that may be the basis for deliberate errors in insulin or nutritional intake.

Psychologic Aspects. Diabetes in a child affects the lifestyle and interpersonal relationships of the entire family. Feelings of anxiety and guilt are common in parents. Similar feelings, coupled with denial and rejection, are equally common in children, particularly during the rebellious teenage years. No specific personality disorder or psychopathology is characteristic of diabetes; similar feelings are observed in families with other chronic disorders.

In children with diabetes, these feelings find expression in nonadherence to instructions regarding nutritional and insulin therapy and in noncompliance with self-monitoring. Deliberate overdosage with insulin, resulting in hypoglycemia, or omission of insulin, often in association with excesses in nutritional intake and resulting in ketoacidosis, may be pleas for psychologic help or manipulative attempts to escape an environment perceived as undesirable or intolerable; occasionally, they may be manifestations of suicidal intent. Frequent admissions to the hospital for ketoacidosis or hypoglycemia should arouse suspicion of an underlying emotional conflict. Overprotection on the part of parents is common and often is not in the best interest of the patient. Feelings of being different or of being alone, or both, are common and may be justified in view of the restrictive schedules imposed by testing of urine and blood, administration of insulin, and nutritional limitations. Furthermore, concern about the likelihood of complications developing and the decreased life span of patients with type I diabetes fosters anxiety. Unfortunately, misinformation abounds about the risks of the development of diabetes in siblings or offspring and of pregnancy in young diabetic women. Even appropriate information often causes further anxiety.

Many, but not all, of these problems can be averted through continued empathic counseling based on correct information and attempts to build attitudes of normality in the patient and a feeling of being a productive member of society. Recognizing the potential impact of these problems, peer discussion groups have been organized in many locales; feelings of isolation and frustration tend to be lessened by the sharing of common problems. Summer camps for diabetic children afford an excellent opportunity for learning and sharing under expert supervision. Education about the pathophysiology of diabetes, insulin dose, technique of administration, nutrition, exercise, and hypoglycemic reactions can be reinforced by medical and paramedical personnel. The presence of numerous peers with similar problems offers new insights to the diabetic child. Residential treatment for children and adolescents with difficult to manage type I diabetes is an option available only in some centers.

The physician managing a child or adolescent with diabetes should be aware of his or her pivotal role as counselor and advisor and should anticipate the common emotional problems of the patient. When emotional problems are clearly responsible for poor compliance with the medical regimen, referral for psychologic help is indicated. Such help is often available in pediatric centers where psychologists form part of the management team for diabetic children.

Management During Infections. Systemic and local infections are no more common in diabetic children than in nondiabetic ones. During intercurrent illnesses, either infectious or traumatic, diabetic children nearly always require additional insulin, especially during prolonged serious episodes that necessitate inactivity. In the latter situations, when hyperglycemia persists or glucosuria is excessive, a good working rule is to add 10–20% of the total daily dose as regular (short-acting) insulin prior to each meal. Subsequent increases or decreases should then be based on careful monitoring of blood and urinary glucose values.

Patients who are vomiting should nevertheless take some insulin; approximately 50% of the daily dose is a general rule, followed by careful monitoring of blood or urinary glucose and subsequent adjustments of the dose of insulin as indicated. If vomiting continues and the patient cannot tolerate clear liquids, admission is recommended to a facility where intravenous therapy with glucose, electrolytes, and insulin can be given.

Management During Surgery. The objectives of management are prevention of hypoglycemia during anesthesia, severe loss of fluids, and diabetic acidosis. The regimens described here are generally applicable, but vigilance and individual adjustments for each patient are necessary to achieve these goals.

When surgery is elective, the patient should be admitted to the hospital 24 hr prior to surgery; during this time the usual nutritional requirements and insulin dose are provided. Supplemental regular insulin may be given to achieve better control of blood glucose when the need is demonstrated. On the morning of surgery, an infusion of 5% glucose in 0.45% saline solution plus 20 mEq/L of potassium chloride is begun; initially 1 U of regular insulin is added to the infusate for each 4 g of administered glucose. The rate of infusion should provide maintenance fluid requirements plus estimated losses during surgery. The blood glucose concentration should be monitored at periodic intervals before, during, and after surgery; concentrations of approximately 120–150 mg/dL should be the goal; this can be achieved by varying the rate of infusion of the glucose and electrolyte mixture or the amount of insulin added. This regimen may be discontinued when the patient is awake and capable of taking food and fluid orally. Prior to reinstitution of the patient's usual diet, regular insulin may be administered at a dose of 0.25 U/kg at 6-hr intervals; appropriate adjustments in the dose are based on blood or urinary concentrations of glucose.

An equally effective plan that is particularly useful for *surgery of short duration* is as follows: On the morning of surgery half of the usual morning dose of insulin is administered subcutaneously, and intravenous infusion of the electrolyte and glucose solution described in the preceding paragraph, but minus the insulin, is initiated. After surgery, regular insulin in a dose of 0.25 U/kg is administered subcutaneously; subsequent doses at 6-hr intervals are adjusted on the basis of blood glucose concentrations until the patient is ready for his or her usual dietary pattern.

For *emergency surgery,* an intravenous infusion is initiated that provides 5–10% glucose in 0.45% saline solution, 20 mEq of potassium chloride/L, and 1 U of regular insulin for each 2–4 g of glucose. Blood glucose concentration should be maintained at approximately 120–150 mg/dL. When possible, rehydration and metabolic balance should precede the surgery. After surgery, the regimen described earlier can be instituted.

For *minor surgery* under local anesthesia, the usual insulin and dietary regimens can be maintained. If there should be extensive vomiting, the losses can usually be compensated with a glucose solution administered intravenously.

NEUROVASCULAR AND OTHER COMPLICATIONS: RELATION TO GLYCEMIC CONTROL. The increasingly prolonged survival of the diabetic child is associated with an increasing prevalence of complications that affect the microcirculation of the eye (retinopathy), kidney (nephropathy), and nerves (neuropathy) as well as the large vessels (atherosclerosis) and the lens (cataracts). Retinopathy is present in 45–60% of insulin-dependent diabetics after 20 yr of known disease and in 20% after 10 yr; lens opacities are present in at least 5% of those younger than 19 yr of age. Diabetic nephropathy is also common; it is present in about 40% after 25 yr of IDDM when the onset was in childhood; this complication may account for about 50% of deaths in long-term insulin-dependent diabetics.

Various biochemical pathways may be responsible for these complications. For example, the process of glycosylation of erythrocyte hemoglobin, which is directly proportional to the blood glucose concentration, also involves other serum and tissue proteins; it has been implicated in basement membrane thickening in the glomeruli. There is evidence that activation of the polyol pathway and disturbances in myoinositol metabolism are related to cataracts and neuropathy, respectively. In humans, typical lesions of diabetic nephropathy develop in normal kidneys within several years after they have been transplanted to diabetics with chronic renal failure. By contrast, the early histologic changes of diabetic nephropathy regress when kidneys of a diabetic are transplanted to a nondiabetic recipient with chronic renal failure. Therefore, it appears that the diabetic environment and not the genetic background predisposes to these renal changes. Genetic factors clearly play a role, however, because only 30–40% of patients affected by type I diabetes mellitus eventually experience end-stage renal disease, and only 50% experience proliferative retinopathy.

There is a relationship between the degree of metabolic control and the appearance, progression, and severity of retinopathy, nephropathy, and neuropathy. In the United States, a multicenter randomized trial compared the effects of intensive treatment versus standard therapy on microvascular complications. Subjects in the customary treatment group received no more than twice-daily insulin, tested blood glucose levels once daily, followed standard nutrition and exercise regimens, and maintained a HbA_{1c} level significantly higher than those in the intensively treated group who used multiple (three to four) daily injections of insulin or continuous subcutaneous insulin infusion via programmable pumps coupled with frequent self-monitoring of blood glucose levels to maintain blood glucose concentrations as near to normal as possible. Intensive therapy reduced the risk of the development of clinically significant retinopathy, including severe nonproliferative and proliferative retinopathy, by 35–75%. Intensive therapy similarly reduced the development and progression of diabetic nephropathy and the development of neuropathy. However, intensive therapy was associated with a two- to threefold increase in episodes of severe hypoglycemia as well as excessive weight gain. The relationship between development or progression of a microvascular complication was linearly related to the level of glycosylated hemoglobin, suggesting that there is not a set point of metabolic control above which complications develop exponentially or below which complications may be avoided. Similar results have been reported from European trials. Moreover, the importance of metabolic control for limiting the development of diabetic nephropathy extends to adolescents and to those who ultimately may require a renal transplant. In such patients, there is a causal relationship between the development of nephropathy in the kidney transplanted to the diabetic recipient and the degree of hyperglycemia. In those whose renal function begins to deteriorate as a result of diabetic nephropathy, the use of angiotensin-converting enzyme inhibitors protects against deterioration in renal function. These angiotensin-converting enzyme inhibitors are significantly more protective than is blood pressure control alone.

Because of this established relationship between the development of complications and metabolic control, physicians should encourage their patients to achieve the best possible metabolic control that is compatible with their psychologic, social, physical, and emotional well-being. Although the preadolescent may be naturally protected against the development of microvascular complications, the principles of metabolic control and their potential impact on future complications must be imparted from the outset.

Other complications in diabetic children include dwarfism associated with a glycogen-laden enlarged liver (Mauriac syndrome), osteopenia, and a **syndrome of limited joint mobility** associated with tight, waxy skin; growth impairment; and maturational delay. The Mauriac syndrome is related to underinsulinization; it is now rare because of the availability of the longer-acting insulins. The syndrome of limited joint mobility is frequently associated with the early development of diabetic microvascular complications, such as retinopathy and nephropathy, which may appear before 18 yr of age. None of these complications have been demonstrated in a nondiabetic identical twin, even after 20 yr of recognized diabetes in his or her insulin-dependent twin. As indicated, genetic predisposition to the development of diabetic vascular complications does, however, play a role.

PROGNOSIS. Type I diabetes mellitus is not a benign disease. In one study on the long-term outcome of 45 children less than 12 yr of age at the time of diagnosis, there were deaths within 10–25 yr of diagnosis: three deaths were directly attributable to diabetes, and two deaths were due to suicide; three patients attempted suicide unsuccessfully. Visual, renal, neuropathic, and other complications were relatively frequent. Furthermore, although diabetic children eventually attain a height within the normal adult range, puberty may be delayed, and the final height may be less than the genetic potential. From studies in identical twins, it is apparent that despite seemingly satisfactory control, the diabetic twin manifests delayed puberty and a substantial reduction in height when onset of disease occurs before puberty. These observations indicate that in the past, conventional criteria for judging control were inadequate and that adequate control of IDDM was almost never achieved by routine means.

The introduction of portable devices that can be programmed to provide continuous subcutaneous infusion of insulin with meal-related pulses is one approach to the resolution of these long-term problems. In selected individuals, nearly normal patterns of blood glucose and other indices of metabolic control, including HbA_{1c}, have been maintained for several years. This approach, however, should be reserved for highly motivated persons committed to rigorous self-monitoring of blood glucose, who are alert to the potential complications such as mechanical failure of the infusion device causing hyper- or hypoglycemia and infections at the site of needle implantation.

The changing pattern of metabolic control already is having a profound influence on reducing the incidence and severity of certain complications. For example, after 20 yr of diabetes, there is a decline in the incidence of nephropathy in type I diabetes in Sweden among children diagnosed in 1971–1975 compared with those diagnosed in the preceding decade. Also, in the majority of patients with microalbuminuria in whom it was possible to obtain good glycemic control, microalbuminuria disappeared. Thus, prognosis is related to metabolic control.

PANCREAS AND ISLET TRANSPLANTATION. In an attempt to cure IDDM, transplantation of a segment of the pancreas or of isolated islets has been increasingly performed in humans. These procedures are both technically demanding and associated with the risks and complications of rejection and its treatment by immunosuppression. Hence, segmental pancreas transplantation is generally performed in association with transplantation of a kidney for a patient with end-stage renal disease due to diabetic nephropathy in whom the immunosuppressive regimen is indicated for the renal transplant. Several thousand such transplants have been performed in adults worldwide during the past 25 yr. With experience and newer immunosuppressive agents, functional survival of the pancreatic graft may be achieved for up to several years, during which time patients may be in metabolic control with no or minimal exogenous insulin and reversal of some of the microvascular complications. However, because children and adolescents with diabetes mellitus are not likely to have end-stage renal disease from their diabetes, pancreas transplantation as a primary treatment in children cannot be recommended or its risk justified. Complications of immunosuppression include the development of malignancy.

Some of the new antirejection drugs, notably cyclosporine and FK-506 (tacrolimus), are themselves toxic to the islets of Langerhans, impairing insulin secretion and even causing diabetes. Attempts to transplant isolated islets have been equally challenging because of rejection. Research continues to improve techniques for the yield, viability, and reduction of immunogenicity of the islets of Langerhans for transplantation. Transplanting islets coated or microencapsulated with a film of protective chemicals that permit diffusion of insulin and nutrients, but prevent T-cell contact and hence avoid rejection, are being investigated.

599.3 Type II Diabetes

Type II diabetes is the most common form of diabetes in the population at large. Onset is usually after age 40 yr and is most prevalent among obese individuals who lack physical activity. Individuals with type II diabetes have resistance to insulin's effects in lowering glucose and variable degrees of relative insulin deficiency. Although obesity itself is associated with insulin resistance, diabetes does not develop until there is some degree of failure of insulin secretion. Thus, when measured, insulin secretion in response to glucose or other stimuli is always lower in persons with type II diabetes than in their controls matched for age, sex, weight, and equivalent glucose concentration. Autoimmune destruction of pancreatic β-cells does not occur, hence there are no circulating ICAs, insulin autoantibodies, or antibodies to GAD. Insulin deficiency is rarely absolute, so patients usually do not need insulin to survive, although glycemic control may be improved by exogenous insulin. Ketoacidosis, when it occurs, is associated with the stress of another illness such as severe infection and may resolve when the stressful illness resolves.

The disease may remain undiagnosed for months to years because hyperglycemia is so moderate that symptoms are not as dramatic as the polyuria and weight loss accompanying type I diabetes; in fact, weight gain may continue. However, the prolonged hyperglycemia may be accompanied, in time, by the development of micro- and macrovascular complications. Type II diabetes occurs more frequently in certain ethnic or racial groups, such as Pacific Islanders, Pima Indians, and black

Americans. It also occurs in individuals with hypertension and dyslipidemia. There is a strong genetic component, stronger than in type I diabetes; for example, concordance rates among identical twins are virtually 100% for type II and only 30–50% for type I. However, the genetic basis for type II diabetes is complex and incompletely defined, and no single identified defect predominates as does the HLA association with type I. Acanthosis nigricans may be a marker for insulin resistance, hyperinsulinemia, and eventually type II diabetes. Hirsutism, associated with the polycystic ovary syndrome, premature adrenarche, or mild mutations in steroidogenic enzymes, is frequently associated with insulin resistance in children and adolescents and may be a harbinger of the future development of type II diabetes mellitus (Chapter 596).

Type II diabetes mellitus is increasing dramatically among children, especially adolescents in the United States, accompanying the rise in obesity in the pediatric population. Formerly rare, the incidence of type II diabetes among children diagnosed with diabetes at one medical center rose from 4% before 1992 to 16% in 1994. In that report, among those aged 10–19 yr, type II diabetes mellitus accounted for one third of all newly diagnosed children with diabetes in 1994. Overall, the incidence of adolescent type II diabetes increased 10-fold from 0.7 to 7.2/100,000/yr in the reported Midwest metropolitan area. The mean age of presentation was 13.8 yr and most children were markedly obese. Both black and white American adolescents were affected, but twice as many black Americans were affected, and one quarter of these but none of the whites presented with DKA. Thus, presentation in DKA for obese adolescents, especially black Americans, does not imply future dependence on insulin. The increasing incidence of type II diabetes and its association with obesity in children and adolescents is a cause of concern.

A particular form of type II diabetes is *type A insulin resistance with acanthosis nigricans.* This syndrome is characterized by severe insulin resistance and acanthosis nigricans in the absence of obesity or lipoatrophy; affected females also have hyperandrogenism, possibly as a secondary manifestation of the hyperinsulinemia with stimulation of androgen synthesis by ovarian theca cells (Chapter 596). Glucose intolerance is variable and includes symptomatic diabetes. The hyperandrogenism presents with clinical and biochemical findings suggestive of polycystic ovary syndrome. Some patients, predominantly black females with obesity, acanthosis nigricans, and accelerated growth suggestive of gigantism, may represent insulin resistance due to obesity with downregulation of the insulin receptor. The gigantism may represent a "spill over" effect of insulin acting via the insulin growth factor 1 receptor, rather than the insulin receptor.

TREATMENT. Treatment for type II diabetes should target weight loss and increasing physical activity as an initial approach. These approaches, however, are frequently unsuccessful. Sulfonylurea compounds that stimulate endogenous insulin secretion and biguanides that diminish hepatic glucose production may be used in these children and adolescents. A class of pharmaceutical agents, the thiozolidinediones, enhance insulin action by decreasing hepatic glucose production and facilitating glucose disposal in muscle and fat. Because they act as insulin enhancers, they are used in conjunction with sulfonylureas, exogenous insulin, and metformin. These agents, the "glitazones," are not approved for use in children in the United States; undue liver toxicity has been reported with their use.

IMPAIRED GLUCOSE TOLERANCE. The term *impaired glucose tolerance* is suggested as a replacement for terms such as asymptomatic diabetes, chemical diabetes, subclinical diabetes, borderline diabetes, or latent diabetes in order to avoid the stigma associated with the term *diabetes mellitus,* which may influence the choice of vocation, eligibility for health or life insurance, and self-image. Furthermore, although impaired glucose tolerance represents a biochemical intermediate between normal glucose metabolism and that of diabetes, experience has shown that few children with impaired glucose tolerance go on to acquire diabetes; estimates range from 0–10%. There is disagreement about whether the degree of glucose intolerance is useful as a prognostic index of the likelihood of progression, but there is evidence that among the few instances of progression, the insulin response during glucose tolerance testing is severely impaired. Islet cell or insulin autoantibodies as well as the HLA-DR3 or -DR4 haplotype are commonly found in those who go on to diabetes. In the majority of children with impaired glucose tolerance, particularly the obese, insulin responses during oral glucose tolerance tests are higher than the mean for age-adjusted, but not weight-adjusted, controls; these individuals have some resistance to the effects of insulin rather than a total inability to secrete it.

In normal children, the glucose response during an oral glucose tolerance test is similar at all ages. In contrast, plasma insulin responses during the test increase progressively within the age span of about 3–15 yr and are significantly higher during puberty so that interpretation of these responses requires comparison with age- and puberty-adjusted responses.

The performance of the glucose tolerance test should be standardized according to currently accepted criteria. These include at least 3 days of a well-balanced diet containing approximately 50% of calories from carbohydrates, fasting from midnight until the time of the test in the morning, and a dose of glucose for the test of 1.75 g/kg but not more than 75 g. Plasma samples are obtained prior to ingestion of the glucose and at 1, 2, and 3 hr thereafter. The arbitrarily designated response to the test that identifies "impaired glucose tolerance" is a fasting plasma glucose value of less than 126 mg/dL and a value at 2 hr of more than 140 mg/dL but less than 200 mg/dL (see Table 599–3). Determination of serum insulin responses during the glucose tolerance test is not a prerequisite for reaching a diagnosis; the magnitude of the response, however, may have prognostic value.

In children with impaired glucose tolerance but without fasting hyperglycemia, repeated oral glucose tolerance tests are not recommended. Investigations in such children indicate that the degree of impaired glucose tolerance tends to remain stable or may actually improve over a period of years, except in patients with markedly subnormal insulin responses. Consequently, apart from reduction in weight for the obese child, no therapy is indicated. In particular, the use of oral hypoglycemic agents should be restricted to investigational studies. If fasting hyperglycemia or characteristic symptoms of diabetes develop, the affected children will have the characteristics of type II diabetes, previously known as NIDDM (see Table 599–1 and the related text of Chapter 599.1).

599.4 Other Specific Types of Diabetes

GENETIC DEFECTS OF β-CELL FUNCTION

Maturity-Onset Diabetes of Youth. This is a genetically and clinically heterogeneous subtype of diabetes mellitus characterized by early onset between the ages of 9 and 25 yr of age, autosomal dominant inheritance, and a primary defect in insulin secretion. Three maturity-onset diabetes of youth (MODY) genes have been identified. MODY 1 results from a mutation in the hepatocyte nuclear factor-4α gene located on the long arm of chromosome 20. MODY 2 is due to a mutation in the gene for glucokinase located on the short arm of chromosome 7. MODY 3 is due to a gene mutation for hepatic nuclear factor-1α located on the long arm of chromosome 12. Strict criteria for the diagnosis of MODY include diabetes in at least three generations with autosomal dominant transmission and diagnosis before age 25 yr in at least one affected subject.

Mutations in the glucokinase gene responsible for MODY 2 result in mild, chronic hyperglycemia due to mild reductions in pancreatic β-cell response to glucose. As a result, this is usually a relatively mild form of diabetes with mild fasting hyperglycemia and impaired glucose tolerance in the majority of patients, which can be treated with small doses of exogenously administered insulin. Patients affected with mutations in hepatic nuclear factor 4α or 1α show more severe abnormalities of carbohydrate metabolism varying from impaired glucose tolerance to severe diabetes and often progressing from a mild to a severe form over time. About one third of these patients will require insulin and are prone to the development of vascular complications. In general, patients with MODY 2 and defects in the glucokinase gene may demonstrate normal insulin responses to intravenous glucose when blood glucose concentrations are maintained at greater than 7 mM. A defective glucokinase has been likened to a defective glucose sensor in the pancreatic β-cell. By contrast, patients with MODY 1 and MODY 3 have more severe impairment of insulin secretion, and this defect cannot be overcome by priming with glucose infusion.

By definition, the absence of a family history suggestive of autosomal dominant inheritance makes a diagnosis of MODY virtually untenable. In such circumstances, the appearance of diabetes in a relatively young person would most likely represent evolving type I diabetes, and therefore evaluation for markers of autoimmunity are warranted. Milder, slowly evolving type I diabetes could be confused with type II diabetes.

Distinction among the present forms of MODY has clinical relevance in counseling because of the lesser likelihood of vascular complications in MODY 2 and, therefore, the need to treat appropriately with insulin, if necessary, in patients with MODY 1 and MODY 3. Molecular analysis for the currently known gene mutations on chromosomes 20, 7, and 12 are likely to become available for routine clinical use in the future to facilitate diagnosis and management. An additional form of MODY due to heterozygous mutation in a homeodomain transcription factor called insulin promoter factor-1 (IPF-1) has also been described.

Primary or secondary defects in *GLUT-2 type of glucose transporter,* an insulin-independent form, also may be associated with diabetes. GLUT-2 rapidly transports glucose into β-cells for subsequent phosphorylation by glucokinase, which eventually leads to insulin secretion. The phenomenon of glucose toxicity, in which there is a loss or reduction in the first-phase insulin response to a pulse of glucose, may be the result of secondary downregulation of GLUT-2 transporters.

MODY also may be a manifestation of a *polymorphism in the glycogen synthase gene.* This enzyme is crucially important for storage of glucose as glycogen in muscle. Patients with this defect are notable for marked resistance to insulin and hypertension as well as a strong family history of diabetes.

Mitochondrial Gene Defects. Point mutations in mitochondrial DNA are sometimes associated with diabetes mellitus and deafness. One mutation is identical to the mutation in MELAS (myopathy, encephalopathy, lactic acidosis, and strokelike syndrome), but this syndrome is not associated with diabetes so that the phenotypic expression of the same defect varies. Another form of IDDM, sometimes associated with mitochondrial mutations, is the Wolfram syndrome.

Wolfram syndrome is characterized by diabetes insipidus, diabetes mellitus, optic atrophy, and deafness—thus the acronym DIDMOAD. Wolfram syndrome is caused by mitochondrial dysfunction, possibly by a nuclear gene mapped to the short arm of chromosome 4. Some patients with diabetes appear to have severe insulinopenia, whereas others have significant insulin secretion as judged by C-peptide. In two patients who were tested, islet cell antibodies were not detected, whereas HLA typing revealed DR2, which is generally considered "protective" for diabetes. In some patients with diabetes and deafness, a mutation in mitochondrial tRNA has been detected; in others, this mutation is absent. In a survey in Britain, 45 patients were identified, for an overall prevalence of 1/770,000. The sequence of appearance of the stigmas was nonautoimmune IDDM in the 1st decade; central diabetes insipidus and sensorineural deafness in two thirds to three quarters of the patients in the 2nd decade; renal tract anomalies in about one half of the patients in the 3rd decade; and neurologic complications such as cerebellar ataxia and myoclonus in one half to two thirds of the patients in the 4th decade. Other features included primary gonadal atrophy in the majority of males and a progressive neurodegenerative course with neurorespiratory death at a median age of 30 yr. Absence of maternal diabetes or deafness and absence of the previously reported mitochondrial gene defect suggests autosomal recessive inheritance.

Diabetes Mellitus of the Newborn

Transient. Onset of persistent IDDM before the age of 6 mo is most unusual. The syndrome of transient diabetes mellitus in the newborn infant has its onset in the 1st wk of life and persists only several weeks to months before spontaneous resolution. It occurs most often in infants who are small for gestational age and is characterized by hyperglycemia and pronounced glycosuria, resulting in severe dehydration and at times metabolic acidosis but with only minimal or no ketonemia or ketonuria. Insulin responses to glucose or tolbutamide are low to absent; basal plasma insulin concentrations, however, are normal. After spontaneous recovery, the insulin responses to these same stimuli are brisk and normal, implying a functional delay in β-cell maturation with spontaneous resolution. Occurrence of the syndrome in consecutive siblings has been reported. There are also reports of patients with classic type I diabetes who formerly had transient diabetes of the newborn. It remains to be determined whether this association of transient diabetes in the newborn followed much later in life by classic IDDM is a chance occurrence or causally related. This syndrome should be distinguished from severe hyperglycemia that may occur in hypertonic dehydration; this condition usually occurs in infants beyond the newborn period, who respond promptly to rehydration with a minimal requirement for insulin (see Chapter 176).

Administration of insulin is mandatory during the active phase of diabetes mellitus in the newborn. One to 2 U/kg/24 hr of an intermediate-acting insulin in two divided doses usually results in dramatic improvement and accelerated growth and gain in weight. Attempts at gradually reducing the dose of insulin may be made as soon as recurrent hypoglycemia becomes manifested or after 2 mo of age.

Permanent. Diabetes mellitus in the newborn period may be permanent if associated with the rare syndrome of pancreatic agenesis. Long-term follow up of a cohort of patients with neonatal diabetes revealed that almost one half had permanent diabetes, one third had transient diabetes, and about one fourth had transient diabetes that recurred when they were 7–20 yr old. The majority of all these infants were small at birth. Instances of affected twins and families with more than one affected infant have been reported.

Abnormalities of the Insulin Gene. Diabetes of variable degrees may also result from *defects in the insulin gene* from faulty processing of proinsulin to insulin, an autosomal dominant defect, to various amino acid substitutions that impair the effectiveness of insulin at the receptor level. However, these defects are notable for the high concentration of insulin as measured by radioimmunoassay, whereas defects in glucokinase, MODY-1, MODY-3, and GLUT-2 are characterized by relative or absolute deficiency of insulin secretion for the prevailing glucose concentrations.

GENETIC DEFECTS OF INSULIN ACTION. Type A insulin resistance is discussed earlier in this chapter and in Chapters 599.1 and 599.2. Two other mutations in the insulin receptor gene with relevance for children are leprechaunism and Rabson-Mendenhall syndrome.

Leprechaunism. This is a syndrome characterized by intrauterine growth retardation, fasting hypoglycemia, and postprandial hyperglycemia in association with profound resistance to insulin, whose serum concentrations may be 100-fold that of comparable age-matched infants during an oral glucose tolerance test. Various defects of the insulin receptor have been described, thereby attesting to the important role of insulin and its receptor in fetal growth and possibly in morphogenesis. However, even probable complete absence of functional insulin receptors due to homozygous inheritance of a missense mutation in the insulin-receptor gene resulted in normal organogenesis and a live born infant who had a severe form of leprechaunism. Most of these patients die in the 1st yr of life.

Rabson-Mendenhall Syndrome. This entity is defined by clinical manifestations that appear to be intermediate between those of acanthosis nigricans with insulin resistance type A and leprechaunism. The features include extreme insulin resistance, acanthosis nigricans, abnormalities of the teeth and nails, and pineal hyperplasia. It is not clear whether this syndrome is entirely distinct from leprechaunism; however, patients with Rabson-Mendenhall tend to live beyond the 1st yr of life. Defects in the insulin-receptor gene have been described in this syndrome.

CYSTIC FIBROSIS. Because of improvements in the medical care of children with cystic fibrosis, many survive to the late teenage and early adult years. In addition to the primary insufficiency of pancreatic exocrine function, there is an increasing incidence of pancreatic endocrine dysfunction manifested as glucose intolerance that occasionally progresses to overt diabetes mellitus (see Chapter 416). When hyperglycemia develops, the accompanying metabolic derangements are usually mild and, if insulin therapy becomes necessary, relatively low doses usually suffice for adequate management. Ketoacidosis is uncommon but may occur with progressive deterioration of islet cell function. Treatment with insulin is as outlined for type I diabetes, but dietary management may be limited by the constraints of the primary disturbance.

AUTOIMMUNE DISEASES. Chronic lymphocytic thyroiditis (Hashimoto thyroiditis) is frequently associated with type I diabetes in children. As many as one in five insulin-dependent diabetics may have thyroid antibodies in their serum; the prevalence is 2–20 times greater than that observed in control populations. Only a small proportion of these diabetics, however, acquire clinical hypothyroidism; the interval between diagnosis of diabetes and thyroid disease averages about 5 yr. Periodic palpation of the thyroid gland is indicated in all diabetic children; if the gland feels firm or enlarged, or both, serum measurements of thyroid antibodies and thyroid-stimulating hormone (TSH) should be obtained. A TSH level of greater than 10 μU/mL indicates existing or incipient thyroid dysfunction that warrants replacement with thyroid hormone. Deceleration in the rate of growth may also be due to thyroid failure and is, in itself, a reason for securing serum measurements of thyroxine and TSH concentrations.

When diabetes and thyroid disease coexist, the possibility of *adrenal insufficiency* should also be considered. It may be heralded by decreasing insulin requirements, increasing pigmentation of the skin and buccal mucosa, salt craving, weakness, asthenia and postural hypotension, or even frank addisonian crisis as evidence of primary adrenal failure. This syndrome is most unusual in the 1st decade of life, but it may become apparent in the 2nd decade or later.

Circulating antibodies to gastric parietal cells and to intrinsic factor are two to three times more common in patients with type I diabetes than in control subjects. There are good correlations of antibodies to gastric parietal cells with atrophic gastritis and of antibodies to intrinsic factor with *malabsorption of vitamin* B_{12}. Although the possibility of megaloblastic anemia should be considered in children with type I diabetes, its occurrence is rare.

A *variant of the multiple endocrine deficiency syndrome* is characterized by type I diabetes—idiopathic intestinal mucosal atrophy with associated inflammation and severe malabsorption, IgA deficiency, and circulating antibodies to multiple endocrine organs including the thyroid, adrenal, pancreas, parathyroid, and gonads. In addition, nondiabetic family members have an increased frequency of vitiligo, Graves disease, and multiple sclerosis as well as low complement levels and antibodies to endocrine tissues.

ENDOCRINOPATHIES. The endocrinopathies listed in Table 599–1 are only rarely encountered as a cause of diabetes in childhood. They may accelerate the manifestations of diabetes in those with inherited or acquired defects in insulin secretion or action.

DRUGS. The immunosuppressive agents cyclosporin and tacrolimus are toxic to β cells, causing insulin-dependent diabetes in a significant proportion of patients treated with these agents. Their toxicity to pancreatic β cells was a contributing factor in limiting their usefulness to arrest ongoing autoimmune destruction of β cells. Streptozotocin and the rodenticide Vacor also are toxic to β cells, causing diabetes.

Genetic Syndromes Associated with Diabetes Mellitus. A number of rare genetic syndromes associated with IDDM or carbohydrate intolerance have been described (see Table 599–1). These syndromes represent a broad spectrum of diseases ranging from premature cellular aging, as in the Werner and Cockayne syndromes (see Chapter 716), to excessive obesity associated with hyperinsulinism, resistance to insulin action, and carbohydrate intolerance as in the Prader-Willi syndrome (see Chapter 77). Some of these syndromes are characterized by primary disturbances in the insulin receptor or in antibodies to the insulin receptor without any impairment in insulin secretion. Although rare, these syndromes provide unique models to understand the multiple causes of disturbed carbohydrate metabolism from defective insulin secretion or from defective insulin action at the cell receptor or postreceptor level.

Epidemiology, Etiology, Pathology, Classification, and Prevention

Alberti KGMM: Preventing insulin dependent diabetes mellitus. Br Med J 307:1435, 1993.

Atkinson MA, Ellis TM: Infants diets and insulin-dependent diabetes: Evaluating the "cows' milk hypothesis" and a role for anti-bovine serum albumin immunity. J Am Coll Nutr 16:334, 1997.

Atkinson MA, Maclaren NK: The pathogenesis of insulin-dependent diabetes mellitus. N Engl J Med 331:1428, 1994.

Bach JF: Insulin-dependent diabetes mellitus as an autoimmune disease. Endocr Rev 15:516, 1994.

Carel JC, Bougneres PF: Treatment of prediabetic patients with insulin: Experience and future. Horm Res 45(Suppl 1):44, 1996.

Ferner RE: Drug-induced diabetes. Baillieres Clin Endocrinol Metab 6:849, 1992.

Froguel P, Zouali H, Vionnet N, et al: Familial hyperglycemia due to mutations in glucokinase. N Engl J Med 328:697, 1993.

Gottlieb PA, Eisenbarth GS: Diagnosis and treatment of pre-insulin dependent diabetes. Annu Rev Med 49:391, 1998.

Green A, Gale EAM, Patterson CC: Incidence of childhood-onset insulin-dependent diabetes mellitus: The Eurodiab Ace study. Lancet 399:905, 1992.

Groop LC, Kankuri J, Schalin-Janti C, et al: Association between polymorphism of the glycogen synthase gene and non–insulin dependent diabetes mellitus. N Engl J Med 328:10, 1993.

Kahn BB: Type 2 diabetes: When insulin secretion fails to compensate for insulin resistance. Cell 92:593, 1998.

Karvonen M, Tuomilehto J, Libman I, LaPorte R: A review of the recent epidemiological data on the worldwide incidence of type 1 (insulin-dependent) diabetes mellitus. World Health Organization DIAMOND Project Group. Diabetologia 36:883, 1993.

Mandrup-Poulsen T: Diabetes. Br Med J 316:1221, 1998.

Report of the expert committee on the diagnosis and classification of diabetes mellitus. Diabetes Care 22(suppl 1):55, 1999.

Schatz DA, Maclaren NK: Cow's milk and insulin-dependent diabetes mellitus. JAMA 276:647, 1996.

Skyler JS, Marks JB: Immune intervention in type 1 diabetes mellitus. Diabetes Rev 1:15, 1993.

Solimena M, DeCamilli P: Coxsackieviruses and diabetes. Nat Med 1:25, 1995.

Sperling MA: Diabetes mellitus. *In:* Sperling MA (ed): Pediatric Endocrinology. Philadelphia, WB Saunders, 1996, pp 229–263.

Sperling MA: Aspects of the etiology, prediction, and prevention of insulin-dependent diabetes mellitus in childhood. Pediatr Clin North Am 44:269, 1997.

Tuomi T, Groop LC, Zimmet PZ, et al: Antibodies to glutamic acid decarboxylase reveal latent autoimmune diabetes mellitus in adults with a non–insulin-dependent onset of disease. Diabetes 42:359, 1993.

Weir GC: A defective β-cell glucose sensor as a cause of diabetes. N Engl J Med 328:729, 1993.

Yoon JW: The role of viruses and environmental factors in the induction of diabetes. Curr Top Microbiol Immunol 164:95, 1990.

Genetics

Cordell HJ, Todd JA: Multifactorial inheritance in type 1 diabetes. Trends Genet 11:499, 1995.

Davies JL, Kawaguchi Y, Bennett ST, et al: A genome-wide search for human type 1 diabetes susceptibility genes. Nature 371:130, 1994.

Faas S, Trucco M: The genes influencing the susceptibility to IDDM in humans. J Endocrinol Invest 17:477, 1994.

Ghosh S, Schork NJ: Genetic analysis of NIDDM. The study of quantitative traits. Diabetes 45:1, 1996.

Johns DR: Mitochondrial DNA and disease. N Engl J Med 333:638, 1995.

Leahy JL, Boyd AE II: Diabetes genes in non–insulin-dependent diabetes mellitus. N Engl J Med 328:56, 1993.

Owerbach D, Gabbay KH: The search for IDDM susceptibility genes: the next generation. Diabetes 45:544, 1996.

Pratley RE, Thompson DB, Prochazka M, et al: An autosomal genomic scan for loci linked to prediabetic phenotypes in Pima Indians. J Clin Invest 101:1757, 1998.

Stassi G, Maria RD, Trucco G, et al: Nitric oxide primes pancreatic beta cells for Fas-mediated destruction in insulin-dependent diabetes mellitus. J Exp Med 186:1193, 1997.

Stoffers DA, Stanojevic V, Habener JF: Insulin promotor factor-1 gene mutation linked to early-onset type 2 diabetes mellitus directs expression of a dominant negative isoprotein. J Clin Invest 102:232, 1998.

Velho G, Froguel P: Genetic, metabolic and clinical characteristics of maturity onset diabetes of the young. Eur J Endocrinol 138:233, 1998.

Zamani M, Cassiman JJ: Reevaluation of the importance of polymorphic HLA class II alleles and amino acids in the susceptibility of individuals of different populations to type 1 diabetes. Am J Med Genet 76:183, 1998.

Diabetic Ketoacidosis

Durr JA, Hoffman, WH, Sklar AH, et al: Correlates of brain edema in uncontrolled IDDM. Diabetes 41:627, 1992.

Finberg L: Fluid management of diabetic ketoacidosis. Pediatr Rev 17:46, 1996.

Foster DW, McGarry JD: The metabolic derangements and treatment of diabetic ketoacidosis. N Engl J Med 309:159, 1983.

Genuth SM: Diabetic ketoacidosis and hyperglycemic hyperosmolar coma. Curr Ther Endocrinol Metab 6:438, 1997.

Hale PM, Rezvani I, Braunstein AW, et al: Factors predicting cerebral edema in young children with diabetic ketoacidosis and new onset type 1 diabetes. Acta Paediatr 86:626, 1997.

Hammond P, Wallis S: Cerebral edema in diabetic ketoacidosis. Br Med J 305:203, 1992.

Krane EJ, Rockoff MA, Wallman JK, et al: Subclinical brain swelling in children during treatment of diabetic ketoacidosis. N Engl J Med 312:1147, 1985.

Rosenbloom AL: Intracerebral crisis during treatment of diabetic ketoacidosis. Diabetes Care 13:22, 1990.

Sperling MA: Diabetic ketoacidosis. Pediatr Clin North Am 31:591, 1984.

Tattersall RB: Brittle diabetes revisited: The Third Arnold Bloom Memorial Lecture. Diabet Med 14:99, 1997.

Management of Type I Diabetes in Children

Becker DJ, Sperling MA: Sucrose in the diet of children with insulin-dependent diabetes mellitus. J Pediatr 119:586, 1991.

Bohannon NJ: Effective use of insulin. A balancing act. Postgrad Med 95:52, 1994.

Bolli GB, Gerich JE: The "dawn phenomenon"—a common occurrence in both non-insulin and insulin-dependent diabetes mellitus. N Engl J Med 310:746, 1984.

Bolli GB, Gottesman IS, Campbell PJ, et al: Glucose counterregulation and waning of insulin in the Somogyi phenomenon (posthypoglycemic hyperglycemia). N Engl J Med 311:1214, 1984.

Geffken GR, Lewis C, Bennett S, et al: Residential treatment for youngsters with difficult-to-manage insulin dependent diabetes mellitus. J Pediatr Endocrinol Metab 10:517, 1997.

Goldstein DE: Understanding GHb assays: A guided tour for clinicians. Clin Diabetes 4:7, 1986.

Jacobson AM, Anderson BJ: Psychosocial problems in children. In: DeFronzo RA (ed): Current Management of Diabetes Mellitus. St. Louis, CV Mosby, 1998, pp 8–13.

Menon RK, Sperling MA: Childhood Diabetes. Med Clin North Am 72:1565, 1988.

Rami B, Schober E: Postprandial glycaemia after regular and Lispro insulin in children and adolescents with diabetes. Eur J Pediatr 156:838, 1997.

Rutledge KS, Chase HP, Klingensmith GJ, et al: Effectiveness of postprandial Humalog in toddlers with diabetes. Pediatrics 100:968, 1997.

Sperling MA: The scylla and charybdis of blood glucose control in children with diabetes mellitus. J Pediatr 130:339, 1997.

Zinman B: The physiologic replacement of insulin. N Engl J Med 321:363, 1989.

Long-Term Outcome of Childhood Diabetes: Relation of Control to Development of Complications

Bojestig M, Arnqvist HJ, Hermansson G, et al: Declining incidence of nephropathy in insulin-dependent diabetes mellitus. N Engl J Med 330:15, 1994.

Bojestig M, Arnqvist HJ, Karlberg BE, Ludvigsson J: Glycemic control and prognosis in type 1 diabetic patients with microalbuminuria. Diabetes Care 19:313, 1996.

Diabetes Control and Complications Trial: Are continuing studies of metabolic control and microvascular complications in insulin-dependent diabetes mellitus justified? N Engl J Med 318:246–250, 1988.

Leslie ND, Sperling MA: Relation of metabolic control to complications in diabetes mellitus. J Pediatr 108:491, 1986.

Lewis EJ, Hunsicker LG, Bain RP, et al: The effect of angiotensin-converting enzyme inhibition on diabetic nephropathy. N Engl J Med 329:1456, 1993.

Makita Z, Radoff S, Rayfield EJ, et al: Advanced-glycosylation end products in patients with diabetic nephropathy. N Engl J Med 325:936, 1991.

Nathan DM: Long-term complications of diabetes mellitus. N Engl J Med 328:1676, 1993.

Reichard P, Nilsson BY, Rosenqvist U: The effect of long-term intensified insulin treatment on the development of microvascular complications of diabetes mellitus. N Engl J Med 329:304, 1993.

Rosenbloom AL: Skeletal and joint manifestations of childhood diabetes. Pediatr Clin North Am 31:569, 1984.

Sandman DD, Shore AC, Tooke JE: Relation of skin capillary pressure in patients with insulin-dependent diabetes mellitus to complications and metabolic control. N Engl J Med 327:760, 1992.

The absence of a glycemic threshold for the development of long-term complications: The perspective of the Diabetes Control and Complications Trial. Diabetes 45:1289, 1996.

Wang PH: Tight glucose control and diabetic complications. Lancet 342:129, 1993.

Diseases and Syndromes Associated with Diabetes

Barrett TG, Bundey SE: Wolfram (DIAMOAD) syndrome. J Med Genet 34:838, 1997.

DeFronzo RA: Classification and diagnosis of diabetes mellitus. *In:* Ralph A. DeFronzo (ed): Current Management of Diabetes Mellitus. St. Louis, CV Mosby, 1998, pp 8–13.

Jones KL: Non-insulin dependent diabetes in children and adolescents: The therapeutic challenge. Clin Pediatr 37:103, 1998.

Krook A, Brueton L, O'Rahilly S: Homozygous nonsense mutation in the insulin receptor gene in an infant with leprechaunism. Lancet 342:277, 1993.

Low L, Chernausek SD, Sperling MA: Acromegaloid patients with type-A insulin resistance: Parallel defects in insulin and insulin-like growth factor-I receptors and biological responses in cultured fibroblasts. J Clin Endocrinol Metab 69:329, 1989.

Morrison EY, McKenzie K: The Mauriac syndrome. West Indian Med J 38:180, 1989.

Pinhas-Hamiel O, Dolan LM, Daniels SR: Increased incidence of non–insulin-dependent diabetes mellitus among adolescents. J Pediatr 128:608, 1996.

Pinhas-Hamiel O, Dolan LM, Zeitler PS: Diabetic ketoacidosis among obese African American adolescents with NIDDM. Diabetes Care 20:484, 1997.

Rotig A, Cormier V, Chatelain P, et al: Deletion of mitochondrial DNA in a case of early-onset diabetes mellitus, optic atrophy, and deafness. J Clin Invest 91:1095, 1993.

Sullivan MM, Denning CR: Diabetic microangiopathy in patients with cystic fibrosis. Pediatrics 84:642, 1989.

Taylor SI, Cama A, Accili D, et al: Mutations in the insulin receptor gene. Endocr Rev 13:566, 1992.

Watkins PB, Whitcomb RW: Hepatic dysfunction associated with troglitazone. N Engl J Med 338:916, 1998.

Winter WE, Maclaren NK, Riley WJ, et al: Congenital pancreatic hypoplasia: A syndrome of exocrine and endocrine pancreatic insufficiency. J Pediatr 109:465, 1986.

Winter WE, Maclaren NK, Riley WJ, et al: Maturity-onset diabetes of youth in black Americans. New Engl J Med 316:285, 1987.

Diabetes of the Newborn

Alcolado JC, Thomas AW: Maternally inherited diabetes mellitus: The role of mitochondrial DNA defects. Diabetic Med 12:102, 1995.

Blethen SL, White NH, Santiago JV, et al: Plasma somatomedins, endogenous insulin secretion, and growth in transient neonatal diabetes mellitus. J Clin Endocrinol Metab 52:144, 1981.

Geffner ME, Clare-Salzler M, Kaufman DL, et al: Permanent diabetes developing after transient neonatal diabetes. Lancet 341:1095, 1993.

Pagliara AS, Karl IE, Kipnis DB: Transient neonatal diabetes: Delayed maturation of the pancreatic beta cell. J Pediatr 82:97, 1973.

Schiff D, Colle E, Stern L: Metabolic and growth patterns in transient neonatal diabetes. N Engl J Med 287:119, 1972.

Shield JPH, Baum JD: Is transient neonatal diabetes a risk factor for diabetes in later life? Lancet 341:693, 1993.

von Muhlendahl KR, Herkenhoff H: Long-term course of neonatal diabetes. N Engl J Med 333:704, 1995.

Hypoglycemia and Diabetes

Amiel SA, Simonson DC, Sherwin RS: Exaggerated epinephrine responses to hypoglycemia in normal and insulin-dependent diabetic children. J Pediatr 110:832, 1987.

Amiel SA, Tamborlane WV, Simonson DC, et al: Defective glucose counterregulation after strict glycemic control of insulin-dependent diabetes mellitus. N Engl J Med 316:1376, 1987.

Bergada I, Suissa S, Dufresne J, et al: Severe hypoglycemia in IDDM children. Diabetes Care 12:239, 1989.

Bolli GB, Fanelli CG: Unawareness of hypoglycemia. N Engl J Med 333:1771, 1995.

DeFeo P, Gallai V, Mazzota G, et al: Modest decrements in plasma glucose concentration cause early impairment in cognitive function and later activation of glucose counterregulation in the absence of hypoglycemic symptoms in normal man. J Clin Invest 82:436, 1988.

Gerich JE: Lilly Lecture, 1988. Glucose counterregulation and its impact on diabetes mellitus. Diabetes 37:1608, 1988.

Jones TW, Borg WP, Borg MA, et al: Resistance to neuroglycopenia: An adaptive response during intensive insulin treatment of diabetes. J Clin Endocrinol Metab 82:1713, 1997.

Jones TW, Borg WP, Boulware SD, et al: Enhanced adrenomedullary response and increased susceptibility to neuroglycopenia: Mechanisms underlying the adverse effects of sugar ingestion in healthy children. J Pediatr 126:171, 1995.

Silverstein JH, Gordon G, Pollock BH, et al: Long-term glycemic control influences the onset of limited joint mobility in type I daibetes. J Pediatr 132:944, 1998.

Pancreas and Islet Transplantation

Alejandro R, Lehmann R, Ricordi C, et al: Long-term function (6 years) of islet allografts in type 1 diabetes. Diabetes 46:1983, 1997.

Brouhard BH, Rogers DG: Pancreatic and islet replacement therapy for insulin-dependent diabetes mellitus. Clin Pediatr 32:258, 1993.

Humar A, Gruessner RW, Sutherland DE: Living related donor pancreas and pancreas-kidney transplantation. Br Med Bull 53:879, 1997.

Larsen JL, Stratta RJ: Consequences of pancreas transplantation. J Invest Med 42:62, 1994.

Mitanchez D, Doiron B, Chen R, et al: Glucose-stimulated genes and prospects of gene therapy for type 1 diabetes. Endocr Rev 18:520, 1997.

Robertson RP, Kendall D, Teuscher A, et al: Long-term metabolic control with pancreatic transplantation. Transplant Proc 26:386, 1994.

Soon-Shiong P, Heintz RE, Merideth N, et al: Insulin independence in a type 1 diabetic patient after encapsulated islet transplantation. Lancet 343:950, 1994.

Sutherland DE: Present status of pancreas transplantation alone in non-uremic diabetic patients. Transplant Proc 26:379, 1994.

PART XXVI

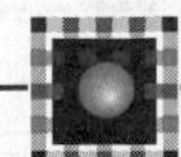

The Nervous System

Robert H. A. Haslam

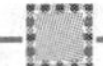

CHAPTER 600
Neurologic Evaluation

The neurologic evaluation seeks to assess the integrity of the central nervous system (CNS) by means of a thorough history and physical examination and thus to determine the location (and causes) of abnormal function.

HISTORY

The history is the most important component of the evaluation of a child with a neurologic problem. The history should carefully document in chronological order the onset of symptoms and a thorough description of their frequency, duration, and associated characteristics. Most children beyond the age of 3–4 yr are capable of contributing to their history, particularly about facts relating to the present illness. It is essential to obtain a comprehensive review of the function and interaction of all organ systems, because abnormalities of the CNS may initially present with clinical manifestations (e.g., vomiting, pain, constipation, or urinary tract disorders) implicating other systems. A detailed history might suggest that the child's vomiting is due to increased intracranial pressure (ICP), that the pain behind the eye may be caused by migraine headaches or multiple sclerosis, and that the constipation and urinary dribbling may be due to a spinal cord tumor.

It is important to start with a concise description of the chief complaint within its developmental context. For example, parents may be concerned that their child cannot talk. The seriousness of this problem depends on many factors, including the age of the patient, the normal range of language development for age, the parent/child interaction, function of the auditory system, and the intellectual level of the child. A comprehensive understanding of developmental milestones is essential in order to ascertain the relative importance of the parents' observations (see Chapters 9–16).

After the chief complaint and history of present illness are elicited, a review of the pregnancy, labor, and delivery is indicated, particularly if a congenital disorder is suspected (see Chapters 90–104). Was the mother exposed to a viral illness during the pregnancy, and what is the mother's rubella, HIV, and syphilis immune status? The history should also include information about the quantity of cigarette and alcohol consumption, toxin exposure, and drug use (legal and illicit) that are known to have adverse effects on fetal development. Decreased or absent fetal activity may be associated with the congenital myopathies and other neuromuscular disorders. Seizures in utero occasionally occur and suggest placental insufficiency or rare inborn errors of metabolism, such as pyridoxine dependence. Seizure activity in utero is difficult to evaluate, particularly in a primigravida. The fact that fetal seizures occurred during pregnancy is often realized retrospectively after the mother has had an opportunity to observe her infant's seizures. The mother's postpartum health may provide a clue to the cause of her infant's neurologic problem; for example, maternal fever, drug dependence, cervical or vaginal vesicles (e.g., herpes simplex), hemorrhage, petechiae, or the presence of an abnormal placenta.

The history of the birthweight, length, and head circumference is particularly important. It may be necessary to obtain the infant's hospital records to determine the head circumference, particularly if congenital microcephaly is a consideration, and the Apgar score, for suspected asphyxia. Several indicators of neurologic dysfunction during the newborn period can reliably be obtained from the history. The fact that a full-term infant was unable to breathe spontaneously and required ventilatory assistance may suggest a CNS abnormality. Poor, uncoordinated sucking or a full-term infant who requires an inordinate amount of time to feed suggests a neurologic disorder requiring careful evaluation. If such an infant requires gavage feeding, there is almost certainly a significant problem. All of the aforementioned abnormalities may be common to a premature infant, particularly a very low birthweight infant, and do not necessarily signify a poor neurologic outcome. Additional important information in the newborn period includes the presence of jaundice, its degree, and management. The physician should also attempt to assess the activity, sleep patterns, the nature of the cry, and the general well-being of the newborn infant from the history.

The most important component of a neurologic history is a child's developmental assessment (see Chapters 9–16). Careful evaluation of a child's developmental milestones usually determines the presence of a global delay in language and gross and fine motor or social skills or a delay in a particular subset of development. An abnormality in development from birth suggests an intrauterine or perinatal cause. Slowing of the rate of acquisition of skills later in infancy or childhood may imply an acquired abnormality of the nervous system. A loss of skills (regression) over time strongly suggests an underlying degenerative disease of the CNS. The ability of parents to precisely recall the timing of their children's developmental milestones is extremely variable. Some are very reliable and others are uncertain, particularly if the patient in question has a significant neurodevelopmental problem. Table 600–1 provides some guidelines with regard to the upper range of normal skills that are usually recalled by the parents and that, if not present, should alert the physician. It is often helpful to request photographs taken at an earlier age or to review the family's baby book, because milestones for a child may have been dutifully recorded. Parents (particularly mothers) are usually aware when their children have a developmental problem, and the physician should show appropriate concern.

Family history is extremely important in the neurologic evaluation of a child. Parents are sometimes unwilling to dis-

TABLE 600–1 Screening Scheme for Developmental Delay: Upper Range

Age (mo)	Gross Motor	Fine Motor	Social Skills	Language
3	Supports weight on forearms	Opens hands spontaneously	Smiles appropriately	Coos, laughs
6	Sits momentarily	Transfers objects	Shows likes and dislikes	Babbles
9	Pulls to stand	Pincer grasp	Plays pat-a-cake, peek-a-boo	Imitates sounds
12	Walks with one hand held	Releases an object on command	Comes when called	1–2 meaningful words
18	Walks upstairs with assistance	Feeds from a spoon	Mimics actions of others	At least 6 words
24	Runs	Builds a tower of six blocks	Plays with others	2–3 word sentences

cuss family members with debilitating neurologic disorders or may be unaware of them, particularly if they are institutionalized. However, most parents are extremely cooperative in securing medical information about family members, particularly if it may have relevance for their child. The history should document the ages and well-being of all close relatives and the presence of neurologic disease, including epilepsy, migraine, cerebrovascular accidents, developmental delay, and heredofamilial disorders. The sex and age at death of miscarriages or live-born siblings, including the results of postmortem examinations, should be obtained because this information may have a direct bearing on the patient's condition. It should also be determined whether the parents are related, because the incidence of metabolic and degenerative disorders affecting the CNS is increased significantly in children of consanguineous marriages.

Finally, an attempt should be made to learn about the patient as a person. The child's performance in school, both academically and socially, may shed light on the diagnosis, particularly if there has been an abrupt change. A description of the child's personality before and after the onset of symptoms may provide a clue to the cause of the disorder. Discussions with the day-care worker or kindergarten or school teacher may provide useful information that is not available from the parent.

NEUROLOGIC EXAMINATION

Neurologic examination of a child begins at the outset of the interview. Observation during interaction with the parents, while playing, or during the time when little attention is directed to the child can provide useful information (Chapters 6 and 17). It may be obvious that the child has characteristic facies, an unusual posture, or an abnormality of motor function manifested by a gait disturbance or hemiparesis. Furthermore, much can be learned from observing the child's behavior during the interview. A normally inquisitive child or toddler may play independently but soon wishes to become involved with the interview process. A child with an attention disorder may display inappropriate behaviors in the examining room, whereas a neurologically abnormal child may appear lethargic or disinterested or may show complete lack of awareness of the environment. The degree of interaction between the parent and the child should be noted. Because the neurologic examination of a newborn or premature infant requires a somewhat modified approach from that of an older child, the differences in the examination are highlighted for both age groups (see also Chapters 6 and 90).

The examination should be conducted in a setting that is nonthreatening and enjoyable for a child. The more it seems like a game, the greater will be the degree of cooperation. Children may be most comfortable on a parent's lap or interacting on the floor of the examination room. It is unwise to force a child to sit on the examining table or to demand that all clothes be removed at the beginning of the procedure. Cooperation is essential for a comprehensive neurologic examination; as a child's confidence increases, so too does the level of participation. Several methods may be used to assess *mental status, cognitive function,* and the level of *alertness,* depending on the age of the child. Simple puzzles may be useful. A child's ability to tell a story or to draw a picture is often a powerful method for assessing cognitive function or for determining the developmental level. The manner in which a child plays with toys or explores the function of a new object or game is an excellent indicator of intellectual curiosity. The level of alertness of a newborn infant depends on many factors, including the time of the last feeding, the room temperature, and the gestational age. Sequential assessment of the infant is valuable in determining changes in neurologic function. Prematures less than 28 wk of gestation do not consistently demonstrate periods of alertness, whereas gentle physical stimulation applied to a slightly older infant arouses the child from sleep and results in a brief period of alertness. Sleep and waking patterns are well developed at term.

The examiner must take advantage of the opportunities provided by the patient; if the circumstances permit, evaluation of muscle power and tone or cerebellar function might precede the cranial nerve examination. However, if a hearing assessment is considered to be important from the historical information, attention should be directed initially to that portion of the examination so that full cooperation can be achieved before the interest and curiosity of the child are lost.

THE HEAD. The *size* and *shape* of the head should be documented carefully. A tower-head, or oxycephalic skull, suggests premature closure of sutures and is associated with various forms of inherited craniosynostosis (see Chapter 601.12). A broad forehead may indicate hydrocephalus and a small head microcephaly. The observation of a square or a box-shaped skull should suggest chronic subdural hematomas because the long-standing presence of fluid in the subdural space causes enlargement of the middle fossa. Inspection of the scalp should include observation of the venous pattern, because increased ICP and thrombosis of the superior sagittal sinus can produce marked venous distention.

An infant has two *fontanels* at birth: a diamond-shaped open anterior fontanel that is situated in the midline at the junction of the coronal and sagittal sutures and a posterior fontanel placed between the intersection of the occipital and parietal bones that may be closed at birth or, at the most, admit the tip of a finger. The posterior fontanel is usually closed and nonpalpable after the first 6–8 wk of life; its persistence suggests underlying hydrocephalus or the possibility of congenital hypothyroidism. The anterior fontanel varies greatly in size, but the usual measurement approximates 2×2 cm. The average time of closure is 18 mo, but the fontanel may normally close as early as 9–12 mo. A very small or absent anterior fontanel at birth may indicate premature fusion of the sutures or microcephaly, whereas a very large fontanel could signify a variety of problems (see Table 90–1). *The fontanel is normally slightly depressed and pulsatile and is best evaluated when an infant is held upright and is asleep or feeding.* A bulging fontanel is a reliable indicator of increased ICP, but vigorous crying can cause a protuberant fontanel in a normal infant.

Palpation of a newborn's skull characteristically shows overriding of the cranial sutures for the first several days of life due to the pressures exerted on the skull during its descent through the pelvis. Marked over riding of the sutures beyond a few days is cause for alarm and suggests the possibility of an underlying abnormality of the brain. Palpation may uncover cranial defects or *craniotabes*, a peculiar softening of the parietal bone so that gentle pressure produces a sensation similar to indenting a Ping-Pong ball. Craniotabes is often associated with prematurity.

Auscultation of the skull is an important adjunct to a neurologic examination. *Cranial bruits* are most prominent over the anterior fontanel, temporal region, or the orbits and are best heard through the diaphragm of the stethoscope. Soft symmetric bruits may be discovered in normal children younger than 4 yr or in association with a febrile illness. Arteriovenous malformations of the middle cerebral artery or vein of Galen may produce a loud bruit. Murmurs arising from the heart or great vessels frequently are transmitted to the cranium. A child with severe anemia is often found to have a skull bruit that disappears when the anemia is corrected. Increased ICP resulting from hydrocephalus, tumor, subdural effusions, or purulent meningitis frequently produces significant intracranial bruits. *Demonstration of a loud or localized bruit is usually significant and warrants further investigation.*

Correct *measurement of the head circumference* is important. It should be performed on every patient, at every visit, and should be recorded on a suitable head growth chart. A nondistensible plastic measuring tape should be used. The tape is placed over the midforehead and is extended circumferentially to include the most prominent portion of the occiput so that the greatest volume of the cranium is measured. The head circumferences of the parents and siblings should also be recorded if the patient is found to have an abnormal skull. Errors in the accurate measurement of a newborn skull are frequent and result from scalp edema, over-riding of the sutures, intravenous fluid infiltration, and the presence of a cephalohematoma. The average rate of head growth in a healthy premature infant is 0.5 cm in the first 2 wk, 0.75 cm during the 3rd wk, and 1.0 cm in the 4th wk and thereafter until the 40th wk of development. The head circumference of a term infant at birth measures 34–35 cm, 44 cm by 6 mo, and 47 cm by 1 yr of age (see Chapters 9 and 10).

CRANIAL NERVES

Olfactory Nerve (1). Anosmia, loss of smell, is most commonly found in association with an upper respiratory tract infection in children and therefore is a transient abnormality. A fracture of the base of the skull and cribriform plate as well as a frontal lobe tumor also may produce anosmia. Occasionally, a child who recovers from purulent meningitis or who develops hydrocephalus has a diminished sense of smell. Rarely, anosmia is congenital. Although not a routine component of the examination, smell can be tested reliably as early as the 32nd wk of gestation. Care should be taken to use appropriate stimuli, such as coffee, peppermint, and other substances, that are familiar to the child; strongly aromatic substances should be avoided.

Optic Nerve (2). Examination of the optic disc and retina is an important component of the neurologic examination. To visualize a good portion of the retina, dilation of the pupil is necessary. One drop of a combination of 1% cyclopentolate hydrochloride, 2.5% phenylephrine hydrochloride, and 1% tropicamide repeated every 15 min three times effectively produces mydriasis. Mydriatics should not be used if a patient's pupil reaction is necessary to follow the level of consciousness or if a cataract is present. Examination of an infant's retina is enhanced by providing a nipple or soother and by placing the head on one side. The physician gently strokes the patient to maintain arousal, while examining the closest eye. An older child should be placed in the parent's lap and should be distracted by bright objects or toys that are presented during the ophthalmologic examination. The optic nerve is salmon-pink in a child but is gray-white in the newborn, particularly in a blond infant. This normal finding may cause confusion and may lead to the improper diagnosis of optic atrophy.

Papilledema rarely occurs in infancy because the skull sutures are capable of separating to accommodate the expanding brain. Papilledema in an older child may be recognized by the following changes in the optic nerve and surrounding retina (Fig. 600–1):

1. The optic nerve becomes hyperemic.
2. The small capillaries that normally cross the optic nerve are no longer visualized as they become constricted.
3. The larger veins become dilated, and the accompanying arterioles become constricted.
4. The border of the optic nerve becomes indistinct from the surrounding retina, particularly along the temporal edge.
5. Subhyaloid, flame-shaped hemorrhages appear in the retina surrounding the optic nerve.
6. In some cases, a macular star develops owing to retinal edema in the region of the macula. Visual acuity and color vision remain intact in acute papilledema as contrasted with optic neuritis, but the blind spot is increased in both.

Retinal hemorrhages occur in 30–40% of all full-term newborn infants. The hemorrhages are more common after vaginal delivery than after cesarean section and are not associated with birth injury or with neurologic complications. They disappear spontaneously by 1–2 wk of age.

Vision. (see also Part XXVIII). Normal 28-wk-old premature infants blink when a bright light is directed to the eyes, and by 32 wk infants maintain eye closure until the light source is removed. At 37 wk, normal prematures turn the head and the eyes to a soft light, and by term, visual fixation and the ability to follow a brilliant target are present. During a period of alertness, optokinetic nystagmus can be demonstrated in a newborn. Visual acuity in term infants approximates 20/150 and reaches the adult level of 20/20 by about 6 mo of age. Children who are too young to read the standard letters on the Snellen Eye Chart may learn the "E game" by pointing a finger in the direction that the "E" is oriented. Children as

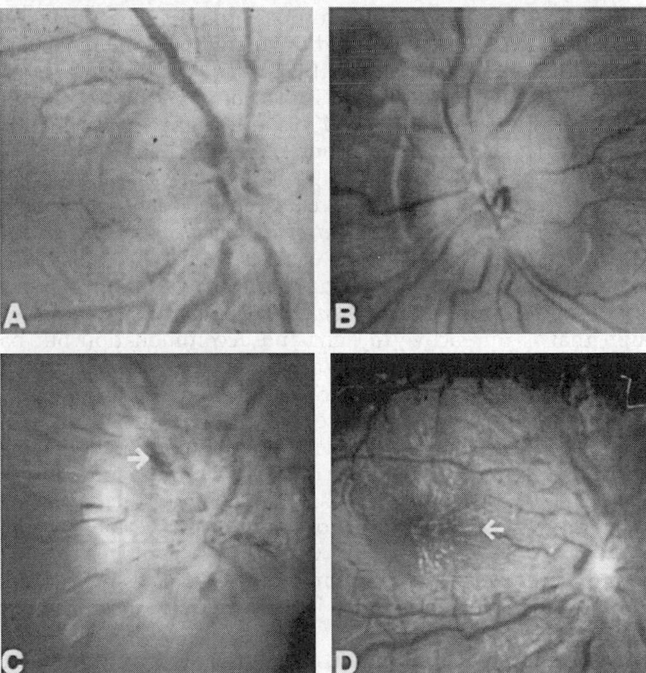

Figure 600–1 *A*, Mild papilledema. Blurred disc margins and venous congestion. *B*, Moderate papilledema. Disc edematous and raised. Vessels buried within substance of nerve tissue. *C*, Severe papilledema. Hemorrhages are evident within disc *(arrow)*, and there are microinfarcts (soft exudates) in the nerve fiber layer. *D*, Macular star *(arrow)* with edema residues distributed within the Henle layer of the macula. See also color section.

young as 2½ or 3 yr of age with normal vision will identify the objects on the Allen Chart at a distance of 15–20 ft. Peripheral vision may be tested in an infant by bringing an object from behind the patient into the peripheral field of vision that normally produces a visual recognition response. The examiner should be sure that the object rather than a sound produces the visual response.

The *pupil* is difficult to examine in premature infants owing to the poorly pigmented iris and the resistance to lid opening. The pupil reacts to light by the 29th–32nd wk of gestation. The equality of the pupils, their size, and reaction to light may be affected by drugs, a space-occupying brain lesion, metabolic disorders, and abnormalities of the midbrain and optic nerves, *Horner syndrome* is characterized by miosis, ptosis, enophthalmos, and ipsilateral anhidrosis of the face. It may be congenital or may result from a lesion involving the sympathetic nervous system in the brain stem, cervical spinal cord, or the sympathetic plexus in juxtaposition to the carotid artery. Localization of the lesion within the sympathetic nervous system is aided by the pupillary response to a series of topical drugs, including cocaine, epinephrine, hydroxyamphetamine, and phenylephrine. Visual fields are tested in an infant by advancing a brightly colored (red) object from behind the child's head through the peripheral field of vision and noting when the child first looks at the object. Suspension of the object by a string prevents the infant from focusing on the examiner's hand and arm.

Oculomotor (3), Trochlear (4), and Abducens Nerves (6). The eye is moved by the extraocular muscles that are innervated by the oculomotor, trochlear, and abducens nerves. The oculomotor nerve innervates the superior, inferior, and medial rectus as well as the inferior oblique and the levator palpebrae superioris muscles. Complete paralysis of the oculomotor nerve causes ptosis, dilation of the pupil, displacement of the eye outward and downward, and impairment of adduction and elevation. The trochlear nerve supplies the superior oblique muscle, and isolated paralysis causes the eye to deviate upward and outward, often with an associated head tilt. The abducens nerve innervates the lateral rectus muscle so that its paralysis causes medial deviation of the eye and the inability to abduct beyond the midline. In an older child, the *red glass test* is used to assess extraocular palsies. A red glass is placed over one eye, and the patient is requested to follow a white light in all fields of direction. The child sees only one red/white light in the direction of normal muscle function but notes a separation of the red and white images that is greatest in the plane of action of the affected muscle. *Internuclear ophthalmoplegia* results from a lesion in the brain stem and consists of paralysis of medial rectus function of the adducting eye and nystagmus confined to the abducting eye. *Internal ophthalmoplegia* refers to a dilated pupil that is unreactive to light and accommodation but has normal extraocular function, and *external ophthalmoplegia* is associated with ptosis and paralysis of all eye muscles with preservation of the pupillary response. *Nystagmus* is an involuntary rapid movement of the eye that may be horizontal, vertical, rotatory, pendular, or mixed. Jerk nystagmus is used to describe a fast and slow phase. As a general rule, horizontal nystagmus occurs with an abnormality of the peripheral labyrinth or with a lesion of the vestibular system in the brain stem or cerebellum and as a consequence of drugs, particularly phenytoin. Vertical nystagmus is indicative of brain stem dysfunction.

Complete ocular movement may be demonstrated as early as 25 wk of gestation using the *doll's eye maneuver.* This technique is used to examine horizontal and vertical eye movements in an infant or an uncooperative or comatose patient. If the head is suddenly turned to the right, the eyes look to the left in a symmetric fashion. Horizontal eye movements in the opposite direction may then be evaluated if the head is turned to the left. Vertical movements may be assessed in a similar fashion by rapid flexion and extension of the head. Normal infants and children follow a toy or interesting object in all directions. The rapid on-off occlusion ("blinking light") of a light source is a reliable test for visual following in uncooperative children. The examiner observes the completeness and flow of the eye movements and determines the presence or absence and the direction of nystagmus, diplopia, opsoclonus, ocular bobbing, or other abnormal eye positions. Premature infants tend to have slightly disconjugate eyes at rest, with one eye horizontally displaced from the other by 1 or 2 mm. Skew deviation of the eyes (vertical displacement) is always abnormal and requires investigation. Strabismus is discussed in Chapter 630.

Trigeminal Nerve (5). The sensory distribution of the face is divided into three areas: the ophthalmic area, the maxillary area, and the mandibular area. Each region may be tested by light touch and by pinprick, and may be compared with the opposite side. The corneal response is elicited by touching the cornea with a small pledget of cotton and by observing the eye closure response. Trigeminal nerve function in premature infants is best documented by facial grimacing from a pinprick (away from the eye) or by stimulating the nostril with a cotton tip. Motor function may be tested by examination of the masseters, pterygoid, and temporalis muscles during mastication as well as by evaluation of the jaw jerk.

Facial Nerve (7). Decreased voluntary movement of the lower face with flattening of the nasolabial angle on the ipsilateral side indicates an upper motor neuron or supranuclear corticospinal lesion. A lower motor neuron lesion tends to involve upper and lower facial muscles equally. Facial nerve paralysis may be congenital or secondary to trauma, infection, intracranial tumor, hypertension, toxins, or myasthenia gravis. Taste for the anterior two thirds of the tongue may be tested in a cooperative child by placing a solution of saline or glucose on one side of the extended tongue. Normal children can identify the substance with little difficulty.

Auditory Nerve (8). Screening for hearing loss is an important component of the neurologic examination, because a hearing deficit is not readily recognized by parents (see Chapter 643). Normal newborns pause briefly during sucking when a bell is presented, but after several stimuli the pauses will cease as habituation occurs. Neurologically abnormal infants will not habituate. Normal hearing infants, turn their head toward a bell, rattle, or crumpled paper and by 3 mo of age will look in the direction of the sound source. Normally intelligent, hearing-impaired toddlers are visually alert and respond appropriately to physical stimuli. Temper tantrums and abnormal speech are common symptoms in a hearing-impaired child. Audiometry or brain stem–evoked potential testing is mandatory for any child suspected of having a hearing loss (see Chapter 643). The risk factors that indicate a need for testing during the first few months of life include a family history of deafness, prematurity, severe asphyxia, use of ototoxic drugs in the newborn period, hyperbilirubinemia, congenital anomalies of the head or neck, bacterial meningitis, and congenital infections due to rubella, toxoplasmosis, herpes, and cytomegalovirus. Parental concern is often a reliable indicator of hearing impairment and warrants a formal hearing assessment.

Vestibular function may be evaluated by the *caloric test.* Approximately 5 mL of ice water is delivered by syringe into the external auditory canal with the patient's head elevated 30 degrees from the horizontal position. In obtunded or comatose patients with an intact brain stem, there is prompt deviation of the eyes to the side of the stimulus. A much smaller quantity of ice water (0.5 mL) is used in alert, awake subjects. In normal subjects, introduction of ice water produces nystagmus with the quick component in the opposite direction to the stimulated labyrinth. No response implies severe dysfunction of the brain stem and medial longitudinal fasciculus. If the otoscopic examination reveals a ruptured tympanic membrane, the test should not be performed in that ear.

Glossopharyngeal Nerve (9). This nerve supplies innervation to the stylopharyngeus muscle. An isolated lesion of the 9th cranial nerve is rare. The nerve is tested by observing the gag response to tactile stimulation of the posterior pharyngeal wall. Taste for the posterior one third of the tongue is provided by the sensory portion of the glossopharyngeal nerve.

Vagus Nerve (10). A unilateral injury of the vagus nerve produces weakness and asymmetry of the ipsilateral soft palate and a hoarse voice due to paralysis of a vocal cord. Bilateral lesions may produce respiratory distress as a result of vocal cord paralysis as well as nasal regurgitation of fluids, pooling of secretions, and an immobile, low-lying soft palate. Isolated lesions of the vagus nerve may occur postoperatively after a thoracotomy due to separation of the recurrent laryngeal nerve, and these lesions are not uncommon during the neonatal period in children with the type II Chiari malformation. If a lesion involving the vagus nerve is suspected, visualization of the vocal cords is necessary. To test for a cough in a neonate/infant, the examiner applies gentle pressure to the trachea at the suprasternal notch.

Accessory Nerve (11). Paralysis and atrophy of the sternomastoid and trapezius muscles result from lesions of the accessory nerve. The sternomastoid muscle has two origins, sternal and clavicular, and is tested by forceful rotation of the head and neck against the examiner's hand. Motor neuron disease, myotonic dystrophy, and myasthenia gravis are the most common conditions producing weakness and atrophy of these muscles.

Hypoglossal Nerve (12). The hypoglossal nerve innervates the tongue. Examination of the tongue includes an assessment of its motility, size, and shape and the presence of atrophy or fasciculations. Malfunction of the hypoglossal nucleus or nerve produces wasting, weakness, and fasciculations of the tongue. If the injury is bilateral, tongue protrusion is not possible and dysphagia may be present. Werdnig-Hoffmann disease (infantile spinal muscular atrophy—SMA type 1) and congenital anomalies in the region of the foramen magnum are the principal causes of hypoglossal nerve involvement.

MOTOR EXAMINATION. The motor examination includes an assessment of the integrity of the musculoskeletal system and a search for abnormal movements that may indicate a disorder of the peripheral nervous system or the CNS. The components of the motor examination include testing of strength (power), muscle bulk, tone, posture, locomotion and motility, deep tendon reflexes, and the presence of primitive reflexes, when applicable.

Strength. Testing of muscle strength is relatively straightforward in cooperative children. It may begin by requesting that the child squeeze the examiner's fingers, flex and extend the wrist and elbow, and adduct and abduct the shoulder against resistance. Shoulder girdle muscle strength may be evaluated in a newborn or infant by supporting the child by the axillae. Patients with weakness are unable to support body weight and slip through the examiner's hands. Distal power can be tested in an infant by evaluating the palmar grasp; a child with weakness will not adequately grasp or will show abnormalities in the manipulation of objects. A normal 3- to 4-yr-old child cooperates in testing extension or flexion of the muscles of the foot, knee, and hip. Examination of the pelvic girdle and proximal lower extremity muscles is also performed by observing the child climb steps or stand up from a prone position. Weakness in these muscles causes the child to use the hands to "climb up" the legs in order to assume an upright position, a maneuver called *Gowers sign* (Fig. 600–2). Infants with diminished power in the lower extremities tend to have decreased spontaneous activity in the legs and refuse to support body weight when suspended by the axillae. It is important not only

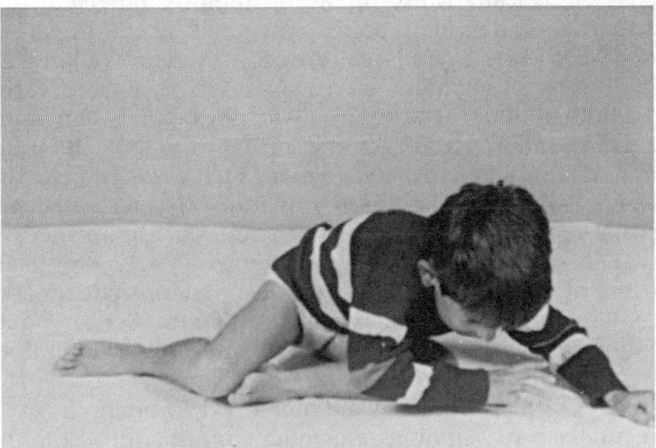

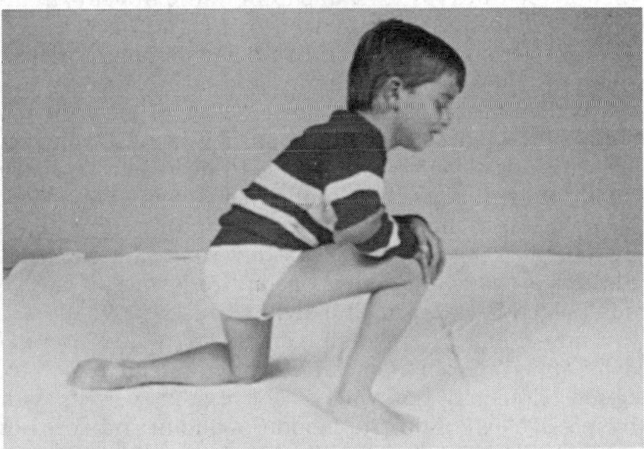

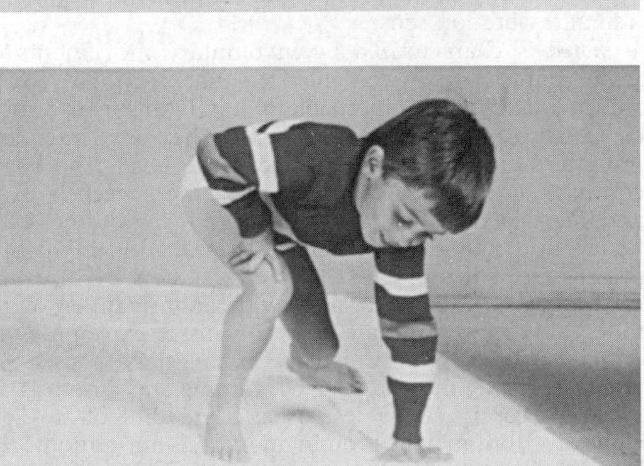

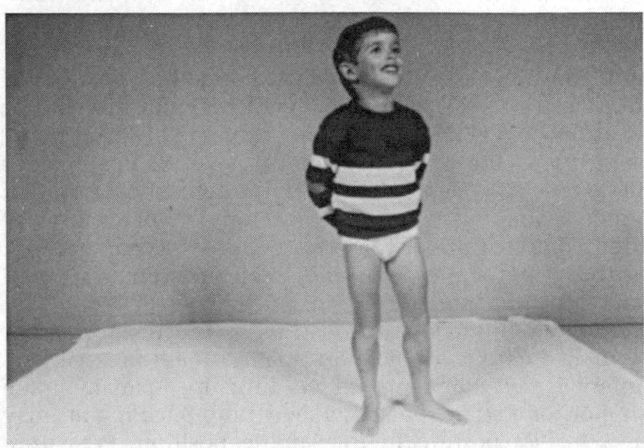

Figure 600–2 Gowers sign. A boy with hip girdle weakness due to Duchenne muscular dystrophy.

to assess individual muscle groups but also to carefully compare muscle power between the upper and lower extremities as well as the opposite extremities. Muscle power in a cooperative child is graded by a scale of 0–5 as follows: 0 = no contraction; 1 = flicker or trace of contraction; 2 = active movement, with gravity eliminated; 3 = active movement against gravity; 4 = active movement against gravity and resistance; and 5 = normal power. Examination of muscle power should include the muscles of respiration. Observation of the action of the intercostal muscles, diaphragmatic movement, and the use of accessory muscles of respiration should be documented. Finally, evaluation of power should include an assessment of muscle bulk and nutrition. Weakness may be associated with muscle atrophy and fasciculations. Because most infants have excess body fat, muscle fasciculations and atrophy are most commonly demonstrated in the denervated tongue in this age group.

Tone. Muscle tone is tested by assessing the degree of resistance when an individual joint is moved passively. Tone undergoes considerable change and assumes different forms depending on age. A premature or newborn infant is relatively hypotonic compared with a child. Tone in this age group is tested by various maneuvers (see Chapter 93 and Fig. 93–3). When the upper extremity of a normal term infant is pulled gently across the chest, the elbow normally does not quite reach the midsternum (*scarf sign*). The elbow of a hypotonic infant extends beyond the midline with ease. Measurement of the popliteal angle is a useful method to document tone in the legs of a newborn. The examiner flexes the child's lower extremity on the abdomen and extends the knee. Normal term infants allow extension of the knee to approximately 80 degrees. Abnormalities of tone consist of spasticity, rigidity, and hypotonia.

Spasticity is characterized by an initial resistance to passive movement, followed by a sudden release called the *clasp-knife* phenomenon. Spasticity is most apparent in the upper extremity flexors and lower extremity extensor muscles. It is associated with brisk tendon reflexes and an extensor plantar reflex, clonus, diminished active movements, and disuse atrophy. *Clonus* may be demonstrated in the lower extremity by sudden dorsiflexion of the foot with the knee partially flexed. Whereas sustained clonus is always abnormal, 5–10 beats in a newborn is a normal finding unless the clonus is asymmetric. Spasticity results from a lesion that involves upper motor neuron tracts and may be unilateral or bilateral. *Rigidity,* the result of a basal ganglia lesion, is characterized by constant resistance to passive movement of both extensor and flexor muscles. As the extremity is undergoing passive movement, a typical *cogwheel* (caused by superimposition of an extrapyramidal tremor on rigidity) sensation may be evident. The rigidity persists with repetitive passive extension and flexion of a joint and does not give way or release, such as with spasticity. Children with spastic lower extremities drag the legs while crawling (commando style) or walk on tiptoes. Patients with marked spasticity or rigidity develop a posture of *opisthotonos,* in which the head and the heels are bent backward and the body bowed forward (Fig. 600–3). *Decerebrate* rigidity is characterized by marked extension of the extremities resulting from dysfunction or injury to the brain stem at the level of the superior colliculi. *Hypotonia* refers to abnormally diminished tone and is the most common abnormality of tone in neurologically compromised premature or full-term neonates. Demonstration of hypotonia may reflect pathology of the cerebral hemispheres, cerebellum, spinal cord, anterior horn cell, peripheral nerve, myoneural junction, or muscle. An unusual position or posture in an infant is a reflection of abnormal tone. A hypotonic infant is *floppy* and may have difficulty in maintaining head support or a straight back while sitting. Such infants may assume a *frog-leg* posture in the supine position. Premature infants of 28 wk of gestation tend to extend all extremities at rest, but by 32 wk there is evidence of flexion, particularly in the lower extremities. A normal full-term infant's posture is characterized by flexion of all extremities.

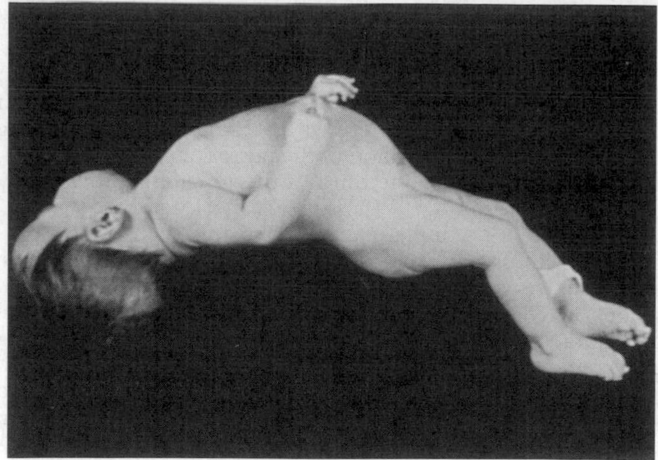

Figure 600–3 Opisthotonus in a brain-injured infant.

Motility and Locomotion. Premature infants of less than 32 wk of gestation display random, slow, writhing movements interspersed with rapid, myoclonic-like activity of the extremities. Beyond 32 wk, the motor activity is primarily flexor. Observation of crawling, walking, or running may uncover movement disorders, most of which are most likely to be apparent during motion and to disappear with rest or sleep. *Ataxia* refers to incoordination of movement or a disturbance of balance. It may be primarily truncal or may be limited to the extremities. Truncal ataxia is characterized by unsteadiness during sitting or standing and results primarily from involvement of the cerebellar vermis. Abnormalities of the cerebellar hemispheres characteristically cause intention tremor unaffected by visual attention. Ataxia may be demonstrated by the finger-to-nose and heel-to-shin tests, heel-to-toe or tandem walking, and, in infants by observation of reaching for or playing with toys. Additional abnormalities associated with cerebellar lesions include dysmetria (errors in measuring distances), rebound (inability to inhibit a muscular action, such as when the examiner suddenly releases the flexed arm and the patient inadvertently strikes the face), and disdiadochokinesia (diminished performance of rapid alternating movements). Hypotonia, dysarthria, nystagmus, and decreased deep tendon reflexes are common features of cerebellar abnormalities. Sensory ataxia is found with diseases of the spinal cord and peripheral nerves. In these disorders, the *Romberg sign* is positive (patient is unsteady with eyes closed but not open), and there are often related sensory findings including abnormalities in joint position and vibration sense.

Chorea is characterized by involuntary movements of the major joints, trunk, and the face that are rapid and jerky. Affected children are incapable of extending their arms without producing abnormal movements. They have a tendency to pronate the arms when held above the head. The hand grip contracts and relaxes *(milkmaid sign)*, the speech is explosive and inarticulate, the deep tendon reflexes of the knee are "hung up," and patients may have difficulty in maintaining protrusion of the tongue. *Athetosis* is a slow, writhing movement that is often associated with abnormalities of muscle tone. It is most prominent in the distal extremities and is enhanced by voluntary activity or emotional upset. Speech and swallowing may be affected. Chorea and athetosis are the result of basal ganglia lesions and are difficult to separate clinically. Both may be prominent in the same patient. *Dystonia* is an involuntary, slow, twisting movement that primarily involves the proximal muscles of the extremities, trunk, and neck.

Deep Tendon Reflexes and the Plantar Response. The deep tendon reflexes are readily elicited in most infants and children. In premature and term infants, the biceps, knee, and ankle jerks are the most reliable deep tendon reflexes. They are graded from 0 (absent) to 4 (markedly hyperactive), with 2 being normal. The ankle reflex is difficult to obtain by percussing the Achilles tendon in this age group. Gentle dorsiflexion of the foot and tapping the plantar surface with the reflex hammer usually elicits a response. The knee jerk in an infant may produce a crossed adductor response (tapping the patellar tendon in one leg causes contraction in the opposite extremity), which, if present, does not become abnormal until 6–7 mo of age. The deep tendon reflexes are absent or decreased in primary disorders of the muscle (myopathy), nerve (neuropathy), and myoneural junction and in abnormalities of the cerebellum. They are characteristically increased in upper motor neuron lesions. Asymmetry of deep tendon reflexes suggests a lateralizing lesion. The plantar response is obtained by stimulation of the external portion of the sole of the foot, beginning at the heel and extending to the base of the toes. Firm pressure from the examiner's thumb is a useful method for eliciting the response. The *Babinski reflex* is characterized by extension of the great toe and by fanning of the remaining toes. Too vigorous stimulation may produce withdrawal, which may be misinterpreted as a Babinski response. Most newborn infants show an initial flexion of the great toe on plantar stimulation. As with adults, asymmetry of the plantar response between extremities is a useful lateralizing sign in infants and children.

Primitive Reflexes. Primitive reflexes appear and disappear in sequence during specific periods of development (Table 600–2). Their absence or persistence beyond a given time frame signifies dysfunction of the CNS. Some primitive reflexes, such as the snout or *rooting reflex*, reappear during old age or with specific degenerative diseases involving the cerebral cortex. Although many primitive reflexes have been described, the Moro, grasp, tonic neck, and parachute reflexes are the most important. The *Moro reflex* is obtained by placing the infant in a semi-upright position. The head is momentarily allowed to fall backward, with immediate resupport by the examiner's hand. The child symmetrically abducts and extends the arms and flexes the thumbs, followed by flexion and adduction of the upper extremities. An asymmetric response may signify a fractured clavicle, brachial plexus injury, or a hemiparesis. Absence of the Moro reflex in a term newborn is ominous, suggesting significant dysfunction of the CNS. The *grasp* response is elicited by placing a finger or object in the open palm of each hand. Normal infants grasp the object, and with attempted removal, the grip is reinforced. The *tonic neck* reflex is produced by manually turning the head to one side while supine. Extension of the arm occurs on that side of the body corresponding to the direction of the face, while flexion develops in the contralateral extremities. An obligatory tonic neck response, by which the infant remains "locked" in the fencer's position, is always abnormal and implies a CNS disorder. The *parachute reflex* is demonstrated by suspending the child by the trunk and by suddenly producing forward flexion as if the child were to fall. The child spontaneously extends the upper extremities as a protective mechanism. The parachute reflex appears before the onset of walking.

TABLE 600–2 Timing of Selected Primitive Reflexes

Reflex	Onset	Fully Developed	Duration
Palmar grasp	28 wk	32 wk	2–3 mo
Rooting	32 wk	36 wk	Less prominent after 1 mo
Moro	28–32 wk	37 wk	5–6 mo
Tonic neck	35 wk	1 mo	6–7 mo
Parachute	7–8 mo	10–11 mo	Remains throughout life

SENSORY EXAMINATION. Sensory examination is difficult to perform in an infant or uncooperative child. Furthermore, the understanding child soon tires of the examination because it requires considerable attention to repetitious and uninteresting tasks. The more this part of the neurologic examination can be made to simulate a game, the greater is the likelihood that a child will cooperate. Fortunately, disorders involving the sensory system are less common in the pediatric population than among adults; thus, this component of the neurologic assessment is less important for infants and children than for adolescents and adults. While the infant is distracted by a parent or an interesting toy, the examiner touches the patient with a piece of cotton or a fragment of a torque depressor. Normal children indicate an awareness of the stimulus by pausing during play, withdrawing the extremity, crying, or looking at and touching the stimulated area. Unfortunately, a child quickly loses patience and soon begins to disregard the examiner. It is critical, therefore, that the area in question is tested efficiently and, if necessary, re-examined at an appropriate time.

Identification of a sensory level in association with a *spinal cord lesion* can be very difficult in an infant. Observation may suggest a difference in color, temperature, or perspiration, with the skin cooler and dry below the spinal cord level. Touching the skin lightly above the level evokes a response that is usually in the form of a squirming movement or physical withdrawal. The superficial abdominal reflexes may be absent. A child with a spinal cord lesion may have evidence of rectal sphincter incontinence that is manifested by a patulous anus, by the absence of contraction of the sphincter when the skin in the anal region is stimulated with a sharp object (anal wink), and by a lack of contraction of the anal sphincter during the rectal examination. In boys, the presence of the cremasteric reflex is also valuable. Children 4–5 yr of age are capable of detailed sensory testing, including joint position, vibration, temperature, stereognosis, two-point discrimination, double simultaneous extinction, light touch, and pain. The success of the sensory examination depends on the ingenuity and the patience of the examiner.

GAIT AND STATION. Observation of a child's gait is an important aspect of a neurologic examination. The *spastic gait* is characterized by stiffness and by stepping like a tin soldier. Spastic children may walk on tiptoes because of tightness or contractures of the Achilles tendons. *Hemiparesis* is associated with a decreased arm swing on the affected side and a lateral circular motion of the leg (*circumduction gait*). Extrapyramidal movements, such as dystonia or chorea, may become apparent while the child is walking or running. Cerebellar ataxia produces a broad-based unsteady gait, and if severe, the child requires support to prevent falling. Heel-to-toe or tandem walking is performed poorly in patients with abnormalities of the cerebellum. A *waddling gait* results from weakness of the proximal hip girdle. Affected children often develop a compensatory lordosis and have difficulty in climbing stairs. Weakness or hypotonia of the lower extremities may result in genu recurvatum and flat feet, which causes a clumsy, tentative gait. *Scoliosis* may cause an abnormal gait and can result from disorders of muscle and spinal cord.

GENERAL EXAMINATION

Physical examination of other organ systems is an essential component of a neurologic examination. For example, cutaneous lesions suggest a neurocutaneous syndrome (see Chapter 605); hepatosplenomegaly suggests inborn errors of metabolism, storage diseases, HIV, or malignancy; and dysmorphic features suggest various syndromes (see Chapter 104). Heart murmurs raise the possibility of rheumatic fever (chorea), tuberous sclerosis (cardiac rhabdomyoma), cerebral abscess or thrombosis (cyanotic heart disease), or cerebral vascular occlusion (endocarditis).

SOFT NEUROLOGIC SIGNS. These signs should be interpreted cautiously because they are present in normal children during various stages of neurodevelopment. A soft neurologic sign may be defined as a particular form of deviant performance on a motor or sensory test in the neurologic examination that is abnormal for a particular age. Testing for the presence of soft neurologic signs involves the observation of a series of timed motor tasks and a comparison of the quality and the precision of the patient's movement with normal controls of similar age and sex. The tests include repetitive and successive finger movements, hand pats, arm, pronation-supination movements, foot taps, hopping, and tandem walking. There is considerable variation in the expression of these signs, depending on age, sex, and maturation of the nervous system. For example, minimal choreoathetoid movements in the fingers of the extended arms are normal at 4 yr of age but disappear by 7 or 8 yr of age. Neurodevelopment of girls is more accelerated than that of boys for many motor tasks, including hopping, skipping, and fine balance maneuvers. Although intellectually normal children may demonstrate a soft neurologic sign, the finding of two or more persistent soft signs correlates significantly with neurologic dysfunction, including attention deficit disorder, learning disorders, and cerebral palsy. Because specific soft signs lack association with a particular disability and can occur in a normal child, it is unwise to label a child who shows several soft neurologic signs. It is more appropriate to monitor such a patient closely and to ensure that a developmental disability has been precluded.

SPECIAL DIAGNOSTIC PROCEDURES

LUMBAR PUNCTURE AND CEREBROSPINAL FLUID EXAMINATION. Examination of the cerebrospinal fluid (CSF) is essential in confirming the diagnosis of meningitis, encephalitis, and subarachnoid hemorrhage and is often helpful in evaluating demyelinating, degenerative, and collagen vascular diseases and the presence of tumor cells within the subarachnoid space. Preparation of a patient is important in order to successfully complete the procedure. An experienced assistant has a vital role in positioning, restraining, and comforting the patient. The skin is thoroughly prepared with a cleansing agent, and the patient is placed in the lateral recumbent position. The physician should be gowned and gloved; the patient should be draped. The neck and legs of the patient are flexed by an assistant to enlarge the intervertebral spaces. The ideal interspace for lumbar puncture (LP) is L3–L4 or L4–L5, which is determined by drawing an imaginary horizontal line from one anterior superior spine of the ilium to the other. The skin and underlying tissue are anesthetized with a local anesthetic or by placing on the skin 30 min before the procedure a patch that contains a eutectic mixture of local anesthetics including lidocaine and prilocaine (EMLA). A 22-gauge, 1- to 2-in, sharp, beveled spinal needle with a properly fitting stylet is introduced into the midsagittal plane directed slightly in the cephalic direction. The stylet is removed frequently as the needle is slowly advanced to determine whether CSF is present. A pop is felt as the needle penetrates the dura and enters the subarachnoid space. A manometer and a three-way stopcock may be attached to obtain an opening pressure. The opening pressure in the recumbent and relaxed position averages 100 mm of fluid; the range in the flexed lateral decubitus position is 60–180 mm of fluid. The most common cause of an elevated opening pressure is a crying, uncooperative, and struggling patient. The pressure is recorded most reliably with a child positioned comfortably with the head and the legs extended. Sick neonates may be placed in the upright position for a spinal tap, because decreased ventilation and perfusion abnormalities leading to respiratory arrest are more common in the recumbent position in this age group.

The *contraindications* for performing an LP include: (1) raised ICP owing to a suspected mass lesion of the brain or spinal cord, which may develop transtentorial herniation or herniation of the cerebellar tonsils after the procedure. Inspection of the eyegrounds for the presence of papilledema is mandatory before proceeding with an LP; (2) symptoms and signs of pending cerebral herniation in a child with probable meningitis. These include decerebrate or decorticate posture, a generalized tonic seizure, abnormalities of pupil size and reaction, with absence of the oculocephalic response and fixed oculomotor deviation of the eyes. Pending herniation is also associated with respiratory abnormalities, including hyperventilation, Cheyne-Stokes respiration, ataxic breathing, apnea, and respiratory arrest. These children must be treated immediately with appropriate intravenous antibiotics and transported to a critical care unit for stabilization and imaging studies before an LP is contemplated. LP is the primary diagnostic procedure in children with suspected bacterial meningitis in the absence of overwhelming sepsis or shock, or symptoms and signs of brain herniation. Because the clinical status of children with untreated bacterial meningitis may rapidly deteriorate, deferral of the LP and appropriate antibiotic therapy while awaiting the results of a CT could be the determining factor between recovery or severe complications and death; (3) *on rare occasions*, an LP is temporarily withheld from a critically ill, moribund patient because the procedure may produce cardiorespiratory arrest. In this situation, blood cultures are drawn; antibiotics and supportive care are administered; and when the patient is stabilized, an LP may be accomplished safely under more controlled circumstances; (4) a skin infection at the site of the LP. If examination of the CSF is urgent in such a patient, a ventricular or cisterna magna tap performed by a skilled physician is indicated; and (5) thrombocytopenia, with a platelet count less than 20×10^9/L, may cause uncontrolled bleeding in the subarachnoid or subdural space.

Normal CSF is the color of water. Cloudy CSF results from an elevated white blood cell (WBC) or red blood cell (RBC) count. Normal CSF contains up to 5/mm^3 WBCs, and a newborn may have as many as 15/mm^3. Polymorphonuclear (PMN) cells are always abnormal in a child, but 1–2/mm^3 may be present in a normal neonate. The presence of PMN cells raises suspicion of a pathologic process. An elevated PMN count suggests bacterial meningitis or the early phase of an aseptic meningitis (Chapter 174). CSF lymphocytosis indicates aseptic, tuberculous, or fungal meningitis; demyelinating diseases; brain or spinal cord tumor; immunologic disorders including collagen vascular diseases; and chemical irritation (e.g., postmyelogram, intrathecal methotrexate).

A Gram stain of the CSF is essential in the investigation of suspected bacterial meningitis; an acid-fast stain or India ink preparation is used if tuberculous or fungal meningitis is a possibility. The fluid is placed on appropriate culture media based on the clinical findings and on the CSF analysis.

Normal CSF contains no RBCs. The presence of RBCs indicates a traumatic tap or a subarachnoid hemorrhage. Bloody CSF should be centrifuged immediately. The supernatant of a bloody tap is clear, but it is xanthochromic in the presence of a subarachnoid hemorrhage. Progressive clearing of bloody CSF is noted during collection of the fluid in the case of a traumatic tap. The presence of crenated RBCs does not differentiate a traumatic tap from a subarachnoid hemorrhage. In addition to a subarachnoid hemorrhage, xanthochromia may result from hyperbilirubinemia, carotenemia, and a markedly elevated CSF protein.

The normal *CSF protein* ranges from 10–40 mg/dL in a child to as high as 120 mg/dL in a neonate. The CSF protein falls to the normal childhood range by 3 mo of age. The CSF protein may be elevated in many processes, including infectious, immunologic, vascular, and degenerative diseases as well as tumors of the brain and spinal cord. The CSF protein is increased after a bloody tap by approximately 1 mg/dL for every 1,000 mm³. Elevation of CSF immunoglobulin G (IgG), which normally represents approximately 10% of the total protein, is observed in subacute sclerosing panencephalitis, postinfectious encephalomyelitis, and in some cases of multiple sclerosis. If the diagnosis of multiple sclerosis is suspected, the CSF should be tested for the presence of oligoclonal bands.

The *CSF glucose* content is about 60% of the blood glucose in a healthy child. To prevent a spuriously elevated blood/CSF glucose ratio in a case of suspected meningitis, it is advisable to collect the blood glucose before the LP when the child is relatively calm. Hypoglycorrhachia is found in association with diffuse meningeal disease, particularly bacterial and tuberculous meningitis. In addition, widespread neoplastic involvement of the meninges, subarachnoid hemorrhage, fungal meningitis, and, on occasion, aseptic meningitis can produce a low CSF glucose level.

The CSF may also be examined for specific *antigens* (e.g., latex agglutination for suspected meningitis) and in investigation of a series of metabolic diseases (e.g., lactate, amino acids, endolase determination).

SUBDURAL TAP. This procedure may be indicated to establish the diagnosis of a subdural effusion or hematoma. A blunt, short-beveled No. 20 gauge needle and stylet are used for the procedure. The subdural space is approached at the lateral border of the anterior fontanel or along the upper margin of the coronal suture at least 2–3 cm from the midline to prevent injury to the underlying sagittal sinus. After adequate cleansing and preparation of the skull, including shaving of the hair from the operative site, the patient is placed in the supine position and is firmly held by an attendant. After a local anesthetic, the needle and stylet are slowly advanced through the skin and underlying tissue with a z-like movement until the dura is entered with a sudden popping sensation. Considerable care is taken to prevent advancement of the needle into the cerebral cortex, which in an infant is approximately 1.5 cm from the skin surface. A hemostat attached approximately 5–7 mm from the beveled end of the needle should provide an adequate safeguard. The subdural fluid, which may squirt out under pressure, is collected and sent for protein analysis, cell count, and culture. The color of the fluid may be xanthochromic, bright red, or oily brown (depending on the age of the subdural collections). Bilateral subdural taps may be indicated, because subdural collections are bilateral in most cases. The amount of fluid removed with each tap should be limited to a total of 15–20 mL from each side in order to prevent rebleeding from a sudden shift of the intracranial contents. At the termination of the procedure, a sterile dressing is applied, and the child is placed in a sitting position that tends to prevent leakage of fluid from the puncture site. (See Chapter 174 for a discussion of subdural fluid associated with meningitis.)

VENTRICULAR TAP. A ventricular tap is used for the removal of CSF in the management of life-threatening increased ICP associated with hydrocephalus, when conservative measures have failed. The procedure should not be undertaken by a pediatrician except when the patient's life is in jeopardy and a neurosurgeon is not available. For an infant, the procedure is similar to a subdural tap. A No. 20 gauge ventricular needle with a stylet is placed in the lateral border of the anterior fontanel and is directed toward the inner canthus of the ipsilateral eye. The needle is advanced slowly, and the stylet is removed frequently to determine the presence of CSF. The ventricle is usually encountered about 4 cm from the skin surface.

NEURORADIOLOGIC PROCEDURES. A *skull roentgenogram* is occasionally a useful diagnostic procedure. It may demonstrate fractures, intracranial calcification, craniosynostosis, congenital anomalies, or bony defects and evidence of increased ICP. Acute increased ICP is characterized by separation of the sutures, whereas erosion of the posterior clinoid processes, enlargement of the sella turcica, and an increase in convolutional markings indicate long-standing intracranial hypertension.

CT scanning is an important diagnostic procedure for emergencies and for less emergent disorders. CT scanning is a noninvasive procedure that uses conventional x-ray techniques. Sedation is usually required for infants and young children, because a lack of head movement is essential during the study. Pentobarbital, 4 mg/kg IM 30 min before the CT scan, with a supplementary dose of 2 mg/kg IM 1–1½ hr later if necessary, is usually effective. Chloral hydrate, 50–75 mg/kg PO 45 min before the procedure, is an alternate method of sedation. CT scanning is useful in demonstrating congenital malformations of the brain, including hydrocephalus and porencephalic cysts, subdural collections, cerebral atrophy, intracranial calcification, intracerebral hematoma, brain tumors and areas of cerebral edema, infarction, and demyelination (Table 600–3). Intravenous injection of radiographic contrast medium enhances areas of increased vascular permeability due to abnormalities of the blood-brain barrier and highlights abnormal collections of blood vessels in an arteriovenous malformation.

MRI is a noninvasive procedure and is especially well suited

TABLE 600–3 Preferred Imaging Procedures in Neurologic Diseases

Neurologic Disease	Imaging Procedure
Cerebral or cerebellar ischemic infarction	CT in the first 12–24 hr; MRI after 12–24 hr (diffusion-weighted and perfusion-weighted MRI augments the findings, especially in the first 24 hr, and even before 8 hr)
Cerebral or cerebellar hemorrhage	CT in the first 24 hr; MRI after 24 hr; MRI and endovascular angiography for suspected arteriovenous malformation
Transient ischemic attack	MRI to identify lacunar or other small lesions; ultrasound studies of the carotid arteries; magnetic resonance angiography
Arteriovenous malformation	CT for acute hemorrhage; MRI and endovascular angiography as early as possible
Cerebral aneurysm	CT for acute subarachnoid hemorrhage; CT angiography or endovascular angiography to identify the aneurysm; TCD to detect vasospasm
Brain tumor	MRI without and with injection of contrast material
Craniocerebral trauma	CT initially; MRI after initial assessment and treatment
Multiple sclerosis	MRI without and with injection of contrast material
Meningitis or encephalitis	CT without and with injection of contrast material initially; MRI after initial assessment and treatment
Cerebral or cerebellar abscess	CT without and with injection of contrast material for initial diagnosis or, if stable, MRI instead of CT; MRI without and with injection of contrast material subsequently
Granuloma	MRI without and with injection of contrast material
Dementia	MRI; PET; SPECT
Movement disorders	MRI; PET
Neonatal and development disorders	Ultrasound in unstable premature neonates; otherwise MRI
Epilepsy	MRI; PET; SPECT
Headache	CT in patients suspected of having structural disorders

PET = positron-emission tomography; SPECT = single-photon-emission computed tomography; TCD = transcranial Doppler ultrasonography.
From Gilman S: Imaging the brain. N Engl J Med 338:812, 1998.

for the study of neoplasms, cerebral edema, demyelination, degenerative diseases, and congenital anomalies, particularly of the posterior fossa and spinal cord (Table 600–3). MRI is capable of detecting small plaques in patients with multiple sclerosis and areas of localized gliosis in children with uncontrolled seizures. MRI is routinely used in the evaluation of children who are potential candidates for epilepsy surgery. Intracerebral calcifications are not detected by MRI. The contrast agent, gadolinium-DTPA, is useful during MRI, especially to highlight lesions associated with a disrupted blood-brain barrier. Functional MRI (fMRI) is a noninvasive technique for detecting and mapping with high resolution the hemodynamic changes produced by localized brain activity during specific cognitive and/or sensorimotor function. It is useful for presurgical localization of critical brain functions (and is very promising as a tool for investigating the development and plasticity of these functions).

Radionuclide brain scan uses a radioactive material such as ^{99}Tc, which concentrates in regions where the blood-brain barrier has been disrupted. It is useful in the investigation of herpes encephalitis and cerebral abscess. *Positron emission tomography* (PET) provides unique information on brain metabolism and perfusion by measuring blood flow, oxygen uptake, and glucose consumption. PET is an expensive technique that has been used primarily in adults, but its use for the study of epilepsy and metabolic and neurobehavioral disorders in the pediatric population holds considerable promise. *Single photon emission computerized tomography* (SPECT), using ^{99m}Tc hexamethyl propylenamine oxime (Tc 99m-HMPAO) is a sensitive and inexpensive technique to study regional cerebral blood flow. SPECT is particularly useful in investigating cerebral vascular disease in children (systemic lupus erythematosus), as well as herpes encephalitis, and for localization of focal epileptiform discharges and recurrent brain tumors. *Cerebral angiography* is reserved for the study of vascular disorders. The procedure requires a general anesthetic in most children. Cerebral angiography, using subtraction techniques, is particularly useful for the delineation of arteriovenous malformations, aneurysms, arterial occlusions, and venous thrombosis. In most cases, a four-vessel study (internal carotids and vertebral arteries) is accomplished. *MRA* (angiography) may reduce the need for contrast invasive angiography. *Cranial ultrasonography* for the detection of intracranial hemorrhage, hydrocephalus and intracranial tumors, is limited to infants with a patent fontanel. The procedure is used intraoperatively in older children for placing shunts, locating small tumors, and directing needle biopsies. *Myelography* was used in the past for demonstrating congenital anomalies, tumors, and vascular malformations of the spinal cord. MRI is superior in most cases to contrast myelography and is not associated with arachnoiditis, which occasionally complicates injection of contrast material into the subarachnoid space.

ELECTROENCEPHALOGRAPHY. An *electroencephalogram* (EEG) provides a continuous recording of electrical activity between reference electrodes placed on the scalp. Although the genesis of the electrical activity is not certain, it likely originates from postsynaptic potentials in the dendrites of cortical neurons. Even with amplification of the electrical activity, not all potentials are recorded owing to the buffering effect of the scalp, muscles, bone, vessels, and subarachnoid fluid. The EEG waves are classified according to their frequency as delta (1–3/sec), theta (4–7/sec), alpha (8–12/sec), and beta (13–20/sec). These waves are altered by many factors, including age, state of alertness, eye closure, drugs, and disease states. The maturational changes between the neonatal period and childhood are evident in Figure 600–4. High-voltage slow and sharp waves (K complexes) and sleep spindles (regular 12–14/sec waves) confined to the central regions occur during sleep in a normal EEG. Abnormalities of waveform include spikes and slow waves. Spikes are characteristically paroxysmal, sharp, and of high voltage followed by a slow wave. Spikes and slow waves are associated with epilepsy, but some normal patients may have this EEG finding. Focal spikes are often associated with irritative lesions, including cysts, slow-growing tumors, and glial scar tissue. Epileptiform activity may be enhanced by activation procedures, including hyperventilation, photic stimulation, and sleep deprivation. Slow waves may be focal, in which case a circumscribed lesion such as a hematoma, tumor, infarction, or a localized infectious process may be considered; generalized slow waves suggest a metabolic, inflammatory, or more widespread process.

EEG/polygraphic/video monitoring provides precise characterization of seizure types, which allows for specific medical or surgical management. In addition, the physician is more accurately able to differentiate epileptic seizures from paroxysmal events that mimic epilepsy, including pseudoseizures. EEG/polygraphic/video monitoring provides for measurement of seizure discharges and for study of the efficacy of various

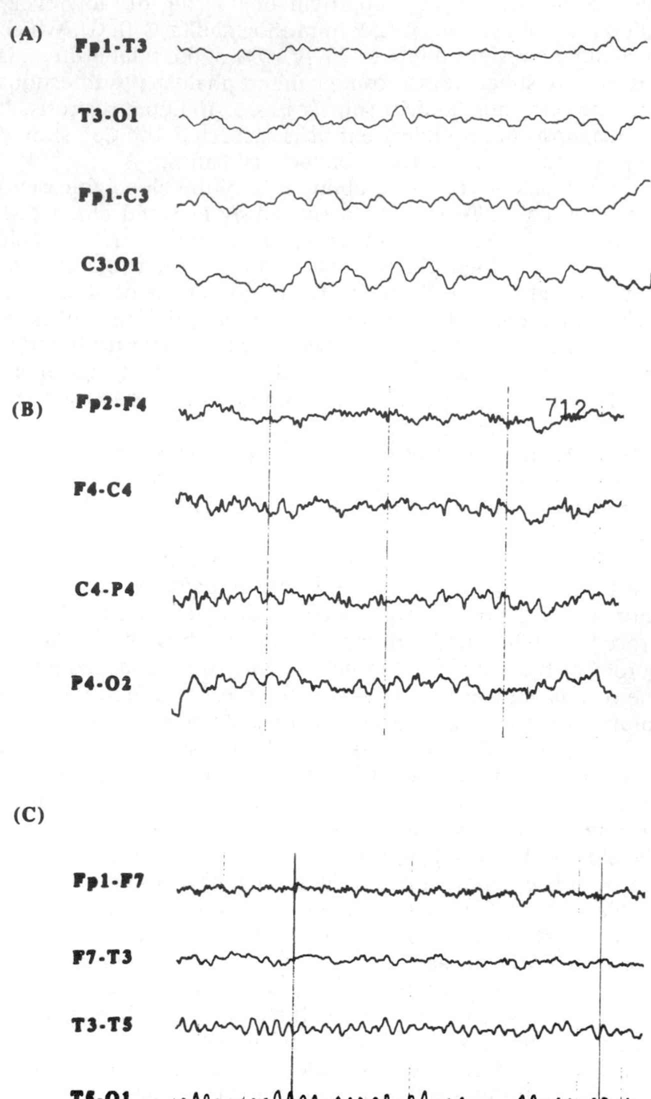

Figure 600–4 *A*, Normal waking record in a term infant. The background rhythm consists of low-amplitude 3- to 4-Hz activity. *B*, An 8-mo-old infant with occipital θ (5 Hz) and superimposed frontal β waves. *C*, Normal 9 yr old. Note the regular α rhythm in the occipital region.

therapeutic regimens. Finally, polygraphic/EEG with video monitoring simultaneously records physiologic and EEG changes; it is particularly useful in neonates in whom the characterization of seizures is difficult.

Magnetic source imaging (MSI) is an advanced neurophysiologic technique that combines magnetoencephalography (MEG) and MRI to measure the magnetic field generated by a series of neurons. MSI is particularly useful for the investigation of patients who may be candidates for epilepsy surgery.

EVOKED POTENTIALS. An evoked potential is an electrical response that follows stimulation of the CNS by a specific stimulus of the visual, auditory, or sensory system. Clinical application of evoked potentials in infants and children has increased dramatically during the past decade. Stimulation of the visual system by a flash or patterned stimulus, such as a black-and-white checkerboard, produces *visual evoked potentials* (VEPs), which are recorded over the occiput and averaged in a computer. Abnormal VEPs result from lesions involving the visual system from the retina to the visual cortex. Neurodegenerative diseases, such as Tay-Sachs, Krabbe, Pelizaeus-Merzbacher disease, and neuronal ceroid lipofuscinoses, show characteristic VEP abnormalities. Lesions of the optic nerve and chiasm also produce abnormalities in the VEP response. The VEP, using patterned stimuli, is useful particularly in assessing visual function in at-risk neonates. Flash VEPs are also very useful in predicting outcome in term infants after asphyxia. *Brain stem auditory evoked potentials* (BAEPs) may be used to objectively measure hearing acuity, particularly in a neonate or uncooperative child when routine hearing assessment techniques have failed. BAEPs are abnormal in many neurodegenerative diseases in children and are an important tool in evaluating patients with suspected tumors of the cerebellopontine angle. BAEPs are helpful in the assessment of brain stem function in comatose patients, because the waveforms are unaffected by drugs or by the level of consciousness. They are not accurate in predicting neurologic recovery and outcome. *Somatosensory evoked potentials* (SSEPs) are obtained by stimulating a peripheral nerve (peroneal, median) and by recording the electrical response over the cervical region and contralateral parietal somatosensory cortex. The SSEP determines the functional integrity of the dorsal column–medial-lemniscal system and is useful in monitoring spinal cord function during operative procedures, such as scoliosis, the repair of coarctation of the aorta, and myelomeningocele. SSEPs are abnormal in many neurodegenerative disorders in children and are the most accurate evoked potential in the assessment of neurologic outcome following a severe CNS insult.

Ellis R: Lumbar cerebrospinal fluid opening pressure measured in a flexed lateral decubitus position in children. Pediatrics 93:622, 1994.

Gilman S: Imaging the brain. Parts I and II. N Engl J Med 338:812, 889, 1998.

Gooding CA, Bras RC, Lallemand DP, et al: Nuclear magnetic resonance imaging of the brain in children. J Pediatr 104:509, 1984.

Haslam RHA: Role of computed tomography in the early management of bacterial meningitis. J Pediatr 119:157, 1991.

Mizrahi EM: Electroencephalographic/polygraphic/video monitoring in childhood epilepsy. J Pediatr 105:1, 1984.

Packer RJ, Zimmerman RA, Sutton LN, et al: Magnetic resonance imaging of spinal cord disease of childhood. Pediatrics 78:251, 1986.

Portnoy JM, Olson LC: Normal cerebrospinal fluid values in children: Another look. Pediatrics 75:484, 1985.

Taylor MJ: Evoked potentials in paediatrics. *In:* Halliday AM (ed): Evoked Potentials in Clinical Testing, 2nd ed. Edinburgh, Churchill Livingstone, 1993, p 489.

CHAPTER 601
Congenital Anomalies of the Central Nervous System

601.1 Neural Tube Defects

(Dysraphism)

Neural tube defects account for most congenital anomalies of the central nervous system (CNS) and result from failure of the neural tube to close spontaneously between the 3rd and 4th wk of in utero development. Although the precise cause of neural tube defects remains unknown, evidence suggests that many factors, including radiation, drugs, malnutrition, chemicals, and genetic determinants (mutations in folate-responsive or folate-dependent pathways), may adversely affect normal development of the CNS from the time of conception. In some cases, an abnormal maternal nutritional state or exposure to radiation before conception may increase the likelihood of a CNS congenital malformation. The major neural tube defects include spina bifida occulta, meningocele, myelomeningocele, encephalocele, anencephaly, dermal sinus, tethered cord, syringomyelia, diastematomyelia, and lipoma involving the conus medullaris.

The human nervous system originates from the primitive ectoderm that also develops into the epidermis. The ectoderm, endoderm, and mesoderm form the three primary germ layers that are developed by the 3rd wk. The endoderm, particularly the notochordal plate and the intraembryonic mesoderm, induces the overlying ectoderm to develop the neural plate during the 3rd wk of development (Fig. 601–1*A*). Failure of normal induction is responsible for most of the neural tube defects. Rapid growth of cells within the neural plate causes further invagination of the neural groove and differentiation of a conglomerate of cells, the neural crest, which migrate laterally on the surface of the neural tube (Fig. 601–1*B*). The notochordal plate becomes the centrally placed notochord, which acts as a foundation around which the vertebral column ultimately develops. With formation of the vertebral column, the notochord undergoes involution and becomes the nucleus pulposus of the intervertebral disks. The neural crest cells differentitate to form the peripheral nervous system, including the spinal and autonomic ganglia as well as the ganglia of cranial nerves V, VII, VIII, IX, and X. In addition, the neural crest forms the leptomeninges, as well as Schwann cells, which are responsible for myelinization of the peripheral nervous system. The dura is believed to arise from the paraxial mesoderm.

During the 3rd wk of embryonic development, invagination of the neural groove is completed and the neural tube is formed by separation from the overlying surface ectoderm (Fig. 601–1*C*). Initial closure of the neural tube is accomplished in the area corresponding to the future junction of the spinal cord and medulla and moves rapidly both caudally and rostrally. For a brief period, the neural tube is open at both ends, and the neural canal communicates freely with the amniotic cavity (Fig. 601–1*D*). Failure of closure of the neural tube allows excretion of fetal substances (e.g., α-fetoprotein [AFP], acetylcholinesterase) into the amniotic fluid, serving as biochemical markers for a neural tube defect. Prenatal screening of maternal serum for AFP during 16–18 wk gestation has proved to be an effective method for identifying pregnancies at risk for fetuses with neural tube defects in utero. Normally,

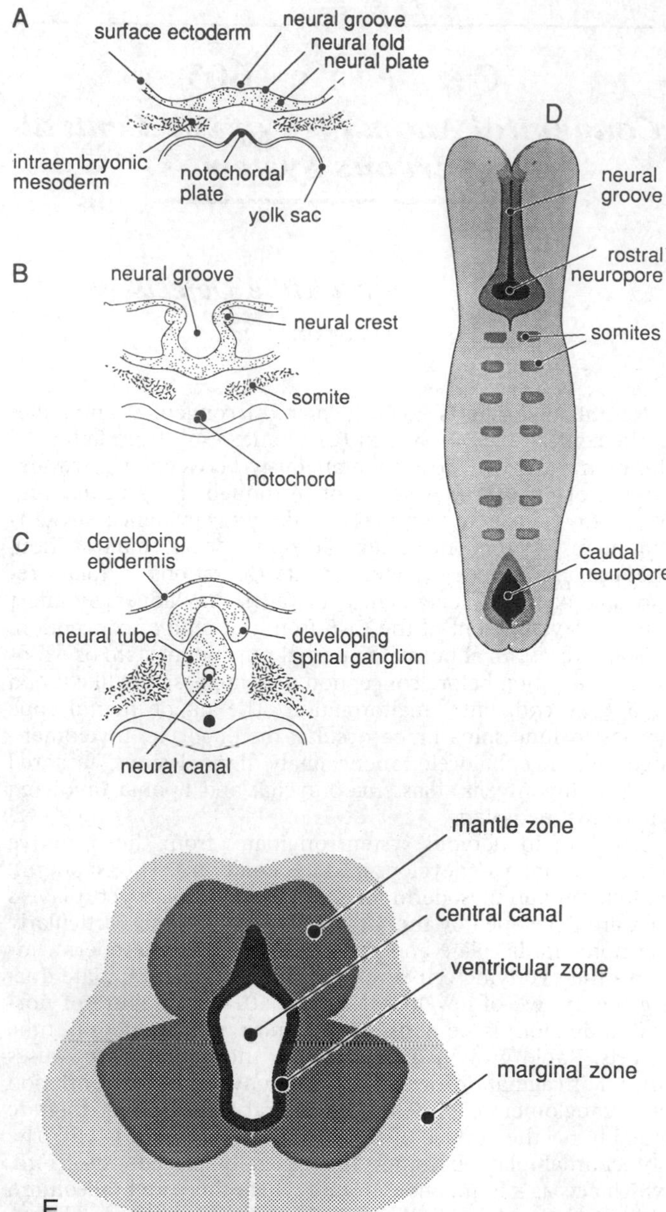

Figure 601–1 Diagrammatic illustration of the developing nervous system. *A,* Transverse sections of the neural plate during the 3rd week. *B,* Formation of the neural groove and the neural crest. *C,* The neural tube is developed. *D,* Longitudinal drawing showing the initial closure of the neural tube in the central region. *E,* Cross-sectional drawing of the embryonic neural tube (primitive spinal cord).

the rostral end of the neural tube closes on the 23rd day and the caudal neuropore closes by a process of secondary neurulation by the 27th day of development, before the time that many women realize they are pregnant.

601.2 Spina Bifida Occulta

This common anomaly consists of a midline defect of the vertebral bodies without protrusion of the spinal cord or meninges. Most individuals are asymptomatic and lack neurologic signs, and the condition is usually of no consequence. In some cases, patches of hair, a lipoma, discoloration of the skin, or a dermal sinus in the midline of the low back signifies an underlying spina bifida occulta. A spine roentgenogram shows a defect in closure of the posterior vertebral arches and laminae, typically involving L5 and S1. There is no abnormality of the meninges, spinal cord, or nerve roots. Spina bifida occulta is occasionally associated with more significant developmental abnormalities of the spinal cord, including syringomyelia, diastematomyelia, and a tethered cord. A *dermoid sinus* usually forms a small skin opening, which leads into a narrow duct, sometimes indicated by protruding hairs, a hairy patch, or a vascular nevus. Dermoid sinuses occur in the midline at the site of occurrence of meningoceles or encephaloceles, that is, the lumbosacral region or occiput. Dermoid sinus tracts may pass through the dura, acting as a conduit for the spread of infection. Recurrent meningitis of occult origin should prompt careful examination for a small sinus tract in the posterior midline region, including the back of the head.

601.3 Meningocele

A meningocele is formed when the meninges herniate through a defect in the posterior vertebral arches. The spinal cord is usually normal and assumes a normal position in the spinal canal, although there may be tethering, syringomyelia, or diastematomyelia. A fluctuant midline mass that may transilluminate occurs along the vertebral column, usually in the low back. Most meningoceles are well covered with skin and pose no threat to the patient. Careful neurologic examination is mandatory. Asymptomatic children with normal neurologic findings and full-thickness skin covering the meningocele may have surgery delayed. Before surgical correction of the defect, the patient must be thoroughly examined with the use of plain roentgenograms, ultrasonography, and MRI to determine the extent of neural tissue involvement, if any, and associated anomalies, including diastematomyelia, tethered spinal cord, and lipoma. Those patients with leaking cerebrospinal fluid (CSF) or a thin skin covering should undergo immediate surgical treatment to prevent meningitis. A CT scan of the head is recommended for children with a meningocele because of the association with hydrocephalus in some cases. An anterior meningocele projects into the pelvis through a defect in the sacrum. Symptoms of constipation and bladder dysfunction develop owing to the increasing size of the lesion. Female patients may have associated anomalies of the genital tract, including a rectovaginal fistula and vaginal septa. Plain roentgenograms demonstrate a defect in the sacrum, and CT scanning or MRI outlines the extent of the meningocele.

601.4 Myelomeningocele

Myelomeningocele represents the most severe form of dysraphism involving the vertebral column and occurs with an incidence of approximately 1/1,000 live births.

ETIOLOGY. The cause of myelomeningocele is unknown, but as with all neural tube closure defects, a genetic predisposition exists; the risk of recurrence after one affected child rises to 3–4% and increases to approximately 10% with two previous abnormal pregnancies. Nutritional and environmental factors unboubtedly have a role in the etiology of myelomeningocele. Studies have provided strong evidence that maternal periconceptional use of folic acid supplementation reduces the incidence of neural tube defects in pregnancies at risk by at least 50%. To be effective, folic acid supplementation should be initiated before conception and continued until at least 12 wk of gestation when neurulation is complete. The U.S. Public Health Service has recommended that all women who are of childbearing age and who are capable of becoming pregnant take 0.4 mg of folic acid daily and that women who have previously had a pregnancy resulting in a neural tube defect be treated with 4 mg of folic acid daily, beginning 1 mo before the time the pregnancy is planned. The modern diet provides about half the daily requirement of folic acid. In order to increase folic acid intake, fortification of flour, pasta, rice, and cornmeal with 0.15 mg folic acid per 100 g was mandated by the United States and Canada in 1998. Unfortunately, the added folic acid will be insufficient to meet the minimal requirements to prevent neural tube defects (4 mg daily). Therefore, informative educational programs remain essential for women planning a pregnancy. Certain drugs are also known to increase the risk of myelomeningocele. Valproic acid, an effective anticonvulsant, causes neural tube defects in approximately 1–2% of pregnancies if the drug is administered during pregnancy.

CLINICAL MANIFESTATIONS. The condition produces dysfuction of many organs and structures, including the skeleton, skin, and genitourinary tract, in addition to the peripheral nervous system and the CNS. A myelomeningocele may be located anywhere along the neuraxis, but the lumbosacral region accounts for at least 75% of the cases. The extent and degree of the neurologic deficit depend on the location of the myelomeningocele. A lesion in the low sacral region causes bowel and bladder incontinence associated with anesthesia in the perineal area but with no impairment of motor function. Newborns with a defect in the midlumbar region typically have a saclike cystic structure covered by a thin layer of partially epithelialized tissue (Fig. 601–2). Remnants of neural tissue are visible beneath the membrane, which may occasionally rupture and leak CSF. Examination of the infant shows a flaccid paralysis of the lower extremities, an absence of deep tendon reflexes, a lack of response to touch and pain, and a high incidence of postural abnormalities of the lower extremities (including clubfeet and subluxation of the hips). Constant urinary dribbling and a relaxed anal sphincter may be evident. Thus, a myelomeningocele in the midlumbar region tends to produce lower motor neuron signs due to abnormalities and disruption of the conus medullaris. Infants with myelomeningocele typically have an increasing neurologic deficit as the myelomeningocele extends higher into the thoracic region. However, patients with a myelomeningocele in the upper thoracic or the cervical region usually have a very minimal neurologic deficit and in most cases do not have hydrocephalus.

Hydrocephalus in association with a type II Chiari defect develops in at least 80% of patients with myelomeningocele. Generally, the lower the deformity in the neuraxis (e.g., sacrum), the less likely is the risk of hydrocephalus. Ventricular enlargement may be indolent and slow growing or may be rapid, causing a bulging anterior fontanel, dilated scalp veins, setting-sun appearance of the eyes, irritability, and vomiting associated with an increased head circumference. Not infrequently, infants with hydrocephalus and Chiari II malformation develop symptoms of hindbrain dysfunction, including difficulty feeding, choking, stridor, apnea, vocal cord paralysis, pooling of secretions, and spasticity of the upper extremities, which, if untreated, can lead to death. This *Chiari crisis* is due to downward herniation of the medulla and cerebellar tonsils through the foramen magnum.

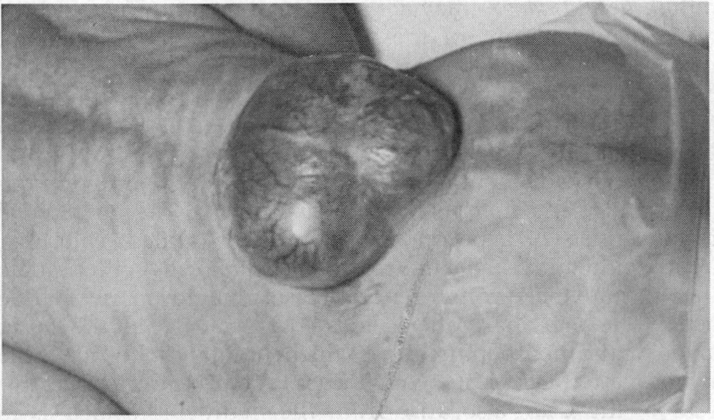

Figure 601–2 A lumbar myelomeningocele is covered by a thin layer of skin.

TREATMENT. Management and supervision of a child and family with a myelomeningocele require a *multidisciplinary team approach*, including surgeons, physicians, and therapists, with one individual (often a pediatrician) acting as the advocate and coordinator of the treatment program. The news that a newborn child has a devastating condition such as myelomeningocele causes parents to feel considerable grief and anger. They need time to learn about the handicap and the associated complications and to reflect on the various procedures and treatment plans. The parents must be given the facts by a knowledgeable individual in an unhurried and nonthreatening setting. If possible, discussions with other parents of children with neural tube defects are helpful in resolving important questions and issues.

Surgery can be delayed for several days (with the exception of a CSF leak) to allow the parents to begin to adjust to the shock and to prepare for the multiple procedures and inevitable problems that lie ahead. Evaluation of other congenital anomalies and renal function can also be initiated before surgery. Some centers have attempted to develop criteria for determining which infants will be treated aggressively and which will receive only supportive care. The most-quoted exclusion criteria, developed in the United Kingdom, consist of the following: marked paralysis of the legs; thoracolumbar or thoracolumbosacral lesions; kyphosis or scoliosis; associated birth injury; other congenital defects of the heart, brain, or gastrointestinal tract; and a grossly enlarged head. However, selective criteria have little prognostic value, and as a result, most pediatric centers aggressively treat the majority of infants with myelomeningocele. After repair of a myelomeningocele, most infants require a shunting procedure for hydrocephalus. If symptoms or signs of hindbrain dysfunction appear, early surgical decompression of the medulla and cervical cord is indicated. Clubfeet may require casting, and dislocated hips may require operative procedures.

Careful evaluation and reassessment of the *genitourinary system* are some of the most important components of the management. Teaching the parents, and ultimately the patient, to regularly catheterize a neurogenic bladder maintains a low residual volume that prevents urinary tract infections and reflux leading to pyelonephritis and hydronephrosis. Periodic urine cultures and assessment of renal function, including serum electrolytes and creatinine as well as renal scans, intravenous pyelograms, and ultrasonography, are obtained according to the progress of the patient and the results of the physical examination. This approach to urinary tract management has greatly reduced the need for surgical diversionary procedures and has significantly decreased the morbidity and mortality associated with progressive renal disease in these patients. Some children can become continent with surgical implantation of an artificial urinary sphincter at a later age. Although *incontinence of fecal matter* is common and is socially unacceptable during the school years, it does not pose the same risks as urinary incontinence. Many children can be bowel-trained with a regimen of timed enemas or suppositories that allows evacuation at a predetermined time once or twice a day. Also see Chapter 20.

Functional *ambulation* is the wish of each child and parent and may be possible, depending on the level of the lesion and on intact function of the iliopsoas muscles. Almost every child with a sacral or lumbosacral lesion obtains functional ambulation; approximately half of the children with higher defects will ambulate with the use of braces and canes.

PROGNOSIS. For a child who is born with a myelomeningocele and who is treated aggressively, the mortality rate is approximately 10–15%, and most deaths occur before age 4 yr. At least 70% of survivors have normal intelligence, but learning problems and seizure disorders are more common than in the general population. Previous episodes of meningitis or ventriculitis adversely affect the ultimate intelligence quotient. Because myelomeningocele is a chronic handicapping condition, periodic multidisciplinary follow-up is required for life.

601.5 Encephalocele

Two major forms of dysraphism affect the skull, resulting in protrusion of tissue through a bony midline defect, called *cranium bifidum*. A *cranial meningocele* consists of a CSF-filled meningeal sac only, and a *cranial encephalocele* contains the sac plus cerebral cortex, cerebellum, or portions of the brain stem. Microscopic examination of the neural tissue within an encephalocele often reveals abnormalities. The cranial defect occurs most commonly in the occipital region at or below the inion, but in certain parts of the world frontal or nasofrontal encephaloceles are more prominent. These abnormalities are one tenth as common as neural tube closure defects involving the spine. The etiology is presumed to be similar to that for anencephaly and myelomeningocele, because examples of each have been reported in the same family.

Infants with a cranial encephalocele are at increased risk for developing hydrocephalus due to aqueduct stenosis, Chiari malformation, or the Dandy-Walker syndrome. Examination may show a small sac with a pedunculated stalk or a large cystlike structure that may exceed the size of the cranium. The lesion may be completely covered with skin, but areas of denuded skin can occur and require urgent surgical management. Transillumination of the sac may indicate the presence of neural tissue. A plain roentgenogram of the skull and cervical spine is indicated to define the anatomy of the vertebra. Ultrasonography is most helpful in determining the contents of the sac, obviating the need for a CT scan in most cases. Children with a cranial meningocele generally have a good prognosis, whereas patients with an encephalocele are at risk for visual problems, microcephaly, mental retardation, and seizures. Generally, children with neural tissue within the sac and associated hydrocephalus have the poorest prognosis. *Meckel-Gruber syndrome* is a rare autosomal recessive condition that is characterized by an occipital encephalocele, cleft lip or palate, microcephaly, microphthalmia, abnormal genitalia, polycystic kidneys, and polydactyly. Encephaloceles may be diagnosed in utero by determination of AFP levels and ultrasound measurement of the biparietal diameter.

601.6 Anencephaly

An anencephalic infant presents a distinctive appearance with a large defect of the calvarium, meninges, and scalp associated with a rudimentary brain, which results from failure of closure of the rostral neuropore. The primitive brain consists of portions of connective tissue, vessels, and neuroglia. The cerebral hemispheres and cerebellum are usually absent, and only a residue of the brain stem can be identified. The pituitary gland is hypoplastic, and the spinal cord pyramidal tracts are missing owing to the absence of the cerebral cortex. Additional anomalies include folding of the ears, cleft palate, and congenital heart defects in 10–20% of cases. Most anencephalic infants die within several days of birth. The incidence of anencephaly approximates 1/1,000 live births, and the greatest frequency is in Ireland and Wales. The recurrence risk is approximately 4% and increases to 10% if a couple has had two previously affected pregnancies. Many factors have been implicated as the cause of anencephaly (in addition to a genetic basis), including low socioeconomic status, nutritional and vitamin deficiencies, and a large number of environmental and toxic factors. It is very likely that several noxious stimuli interact on a genetically susceptible host to produce anencephaly. Fortunately, the frequency of anencephaly has been decreasing during the past two decades. Approximately 50% of cases of anencephaly are associated with polyhydramnios. Couples who have had an anencephalic infant should have successive pregnancies monitored, including amniocentesis, determination of AFP levels, and ultrasound examination between the 14th and 16th wk of gestation.

Charney EB, Weller SC, Sutton LN, et al: Management of the newborn with myelomeningocele: Time for a decision-making process. Pediatrics 75:58, 1985.

Copp AJ, Brook FA, Estibeiro JP, et al: The embryonic development of mammalian neural tube defects. Prog Neurobiol 35:363, 1990.

Fernandes ET, Reinberg Y, Vernier R, et al: Neurogenic bladder dysfunction in children: Review of pathophysiology and current management. J Pediatr 124:1, 1994.

Haddow JE, Palomaki GE, Knight GJ, et al: Reducing the need for amniocentesis in women 35 years of age or older with serum markers for screening. N Engl J Med 330:1114, 1994.

Hannigan KF: Teaching intermittent self-catheterization to young children with myelodysplasia. Dev Med Child Neurol 21:365, 1979,

Lemire RJ, Beckwith JB, Warkany J: Anencephaly. New York, Raven Press, 1978.

Lorber J, Salfiedl S: Results of selective treatment of spina bifida cystica. Arch Dis Child 56:822, 1981.

McLone DG: Results of treatment of children born with a myelomeningocele. Clin Neurosurg 30:407, 1983.

McLone DG, Czyzewski D, Raimondi AJ, et al: Central nervous system infections as a limiting factor in the intelligence of children with myelomeningocele. Pediatrics 70:338, 1982.

MRC Vitamin Study Research Group: Prevention of neural tube defects: Results of the Medical Research Council Vitamin Study. Lancet 338:131, 1991.

Norman D, Brant-Zawadski M, Yeates A, et al: Magnetic resonance imaging of the spinal cord and canal: Potentials and limitations. AJNR 5:9, 1985.

Opitz JM, Howe JJ: The Meckel syndrome. Birth Defects 5:167, 1969.

Robert E, Guibaud P: Maternal valproic acid and congenital neural tube defects. Lancet 2:937, 1982.

601.7 Disorders of Neuronal Migration

Disorders of neuronal migration may result in minor abnormalities with little or no clinical consequence (e.g., small heterotopia of neurons) or devastating abnormalities of the CNS (e.g., mental retardation, lissencephaly, schizencephaly) (Fig. 601–3). One of the most important mechanisms in the control of neuronal migration is the radial glial fiber system that guides neurons to their proper site. Migrating neurons attach to the radial glial fiber and then disembark at predetermined sites to ultimately form the precisely designed six-layered cerebral cortex. The product of a mouse gene called *reelin* directs the new neuron to reach its final destination in the brain. Another mouse gene (*mdab1*) may act as a signaling pathway triggered by *reelin*. Mutations of these genes in mice produce major neuronal migration abnormalities. The severity and the extent of the disorder are related to numerous factors, including the timing of a particular insult and a host of environmental and genetic factors.

The embryonic neural tube consists of three zones: ventricular, mantle, and marginal (see Fig. 601–1*E*). The ependymal layer consists of a pluripotential, pseudostratified, columnar neuroepithelium. Specific neuroepithelial cells differentiate into primitive neurons or neuroblasts that form the mantle layer. The marginal zone is formed from cells in the outer layer of the neuroepithelium, which ultimately becomes the white matter. Glioblasts, which act as the primitive supportive cells of the CNS, also arise from the neuroepithelial cells in the ependymal zone. They migrate to the mantle and marginal zones and become future astrocytes and oligodendrocytes. It is

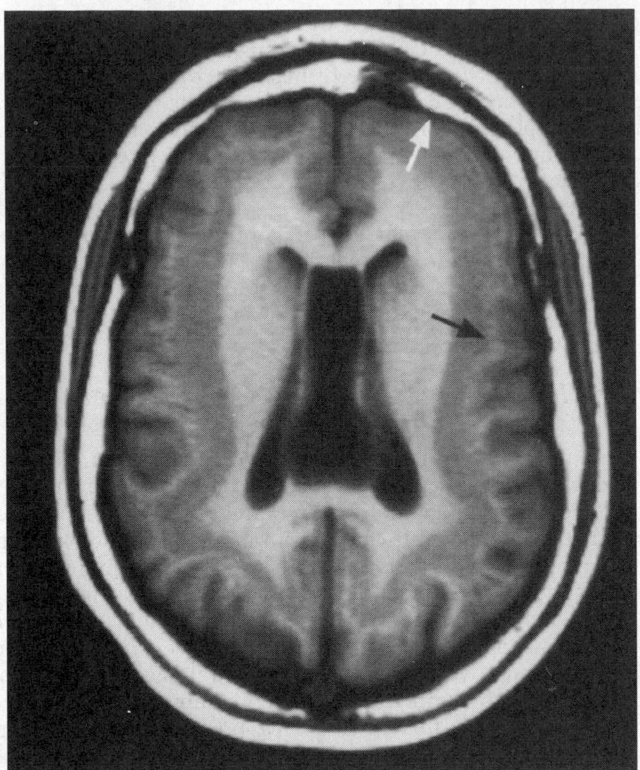

Figure 601–3 T1 weighted MRI scan demonstrating band heterotopia. A thin layer of white matter (*black arrow*) lies between the band of heterotopic gray matter and the cortical surface. Failure of cortical organization with lissencephaly is present in both frontal lobes (*white arrow*).

likely that microglia originate from mesenchymal cells at a later stage of fetal development when blood vessels begin to penetrate the developing nervous system.

LISSENCEPHALY

Lissencephaly or agyria is a rare disorder that is characterized by the absence of cerebral convolutions and a poorly formed sylvian fissure, giving the appearance of a 3–4 mo fetal brain. The condition is probably a result of faulty neuroblast migration during early embryonic life and is usually associated with enlarged lateral ventricles and heterotopias in the white matter. There is a four-layered cortex, rather than the usual six, with a thin rim of periventricular white matter and numerous gray heterotopia visible by microscopic examination. Clinically, these infants present with failure to thrive, microcephaly, marked developmental delay, and a severe seizure disorder. Ocular abnormalities are common, including hypoplasia of the optic nerve and microphthalmia. Lissencephaly can occur as an isolated finding; however, in about 15% of cases it is associated with the *Miller-Dieker syndrome* (MDS). These children have characteristic facies, including a prominent forehead, bitemporal hollowing, anteverted nostrils, a prominent upper lip, and micrognathia. About 90% of children with MDS have visible or submicroscopic chromosomal deletions of 17p13.3. The gene LIS-1 (lissencephaly 1) in 17p13.3 is deleted in patients with MDS. CT and MRI scans typically show a smooth brain with an absence of sulci (Fig. 601–4).

SCHIZENCEPHALY

Schizencephaly is the presence of unilateral or bilateral clefts within the cerebral hemispheres due to an abnormality of morphogenesis. The cleft may be fused or unfused and, if unilateral and large, may be confused with a porencephalic cyst. Not infrequently, the borders of the cleft are surrounded by abnormal brain, particularly microgyria. CT scan is diagnostic and clearly demonstrates the size and extent of the cleft. Many patients are severely mentally retarded, with seizures that are difficult to control, and microcephalic, with spastic quadriparesis when the clefts are bilateral.

PORENCEPHALY

Porencephaly is the presence of cysts or cavities within the brain that result from development defects or acquired lesions, including infarction of tissue. *True porencephalic* cysts are most frequently located in the region of the sylvian fissure and typically communicate with the subarachnoid space, the ventricular system, or both. They represent developmental abnormalities of cell migration and are often associated with other malformations of the brain, including microcephaly, abnormal patterns of adjacent gyri, and encephalocele. Affected infants tend to have many problems, including mental retardation, spastic quadriparesis, optic atrophy, and seizures. *Pseudoporencephalic cysts* characteristically develop during the perinatal or postnatal period and result from abnormalities (infarction, hemorrhage) of arterial or venous circulation. These cysts tend to be unilateral; they do not communicate with a fluid-filled cavity; and they are not asociated with abnormalities of cell migration or CNS malformations. Infants with pseudoporencephalic cysts present with hemiparesis and focal seizures during the 1st year of life.

HOLOPROSENCEPHALY

Holoprosencephaly, a developmental disorder of the brain, results from defective cleavage of the prosencephalon. The abnormality is classified into three groups, alobar, semilobar, and lobar, depending on the degree of the cleavage abnormality (Fig. 601–5). Facial anormalities including cyclopia, cebocephaly, and premaxillary agenesis are common, as the prechordal mesoderm that induces the prosencephalon is also responsible for induction of the median facial structures. The most severe form, alobar holoprosencephaly, is typically associ-

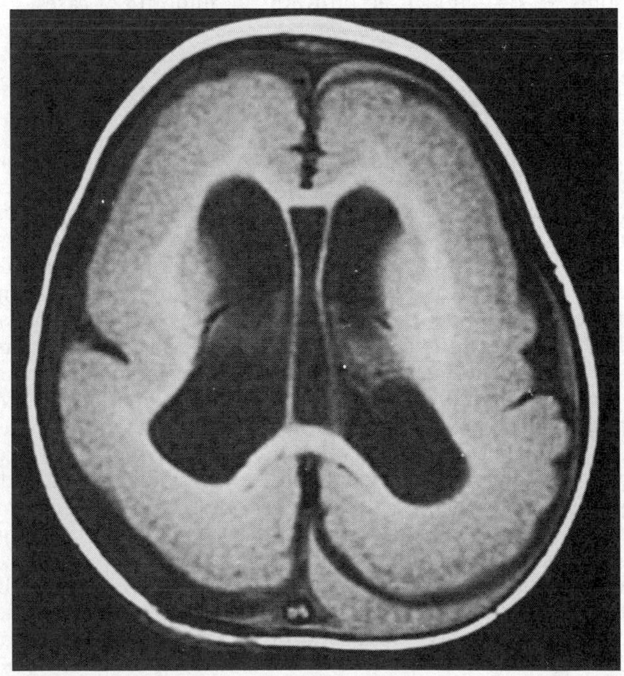

Figure 601–4 MRI of an infant with lissencephaly. Note the absence of cerebral sulci and the maldeveloped sylvian fissures associated with enlarged ventricles.

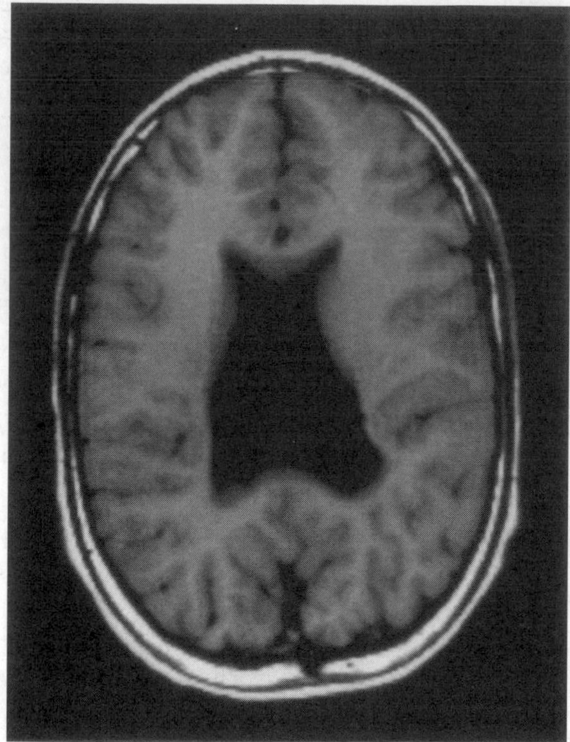

Figure 601–5 Lobar holoprosencephaly. T_1 weighted MRI scan demonstrates failure of separation of the hemispheres and a persistent fused ventricle.

ated with neuronal migration disorders. Alobar holoprosencephaly is characterized by a single ventricle, an absent falx, and fused basal ganglia. Affected infants usually die during infancy. The incidence of holoprosencephaly ranges from 1/5000 to 1/16,000. A prenatal diagnosis can be confirmed by ultrasound after the 10th wk of gestation. The cause of holoprosencephaly is unknown. Chromosomal abnormalities, including deletions of chromosomes 7q and 3p as well as trisomy 13, 18, and 21, account for the minority of cases.

601.8 Agenesis of the Corpus Callosum

Agenesis of the corpus callosum consists of a heterogeneous group of disorders that vary in expression from severe intellectual and neurologic abnormalities to the asymptomatic and normally intelligent individual. The corpus callosum develops from the commissural plate that lies in proximity to the anterior neuropore. An insult to the commissural plate during early embryogenesis causes agenesis of the corpus callosum. When agenesis of the corpus callosum is an isolated phenomenon, the patient may be normal, whereas individuals with neurologic symptoms, including mental retardation, microcephaly, hemiparesis, diplegia, and seizures, have associated brain anomalies due to cell migration defects, such as heterotopias, microgyria, and pachygyria (broad, wide gyri) in addition to the absence of the corpus callosum. The anatomic features are best depicted on a CT scan or by MRI and show widely separated frontal horns with an abnormally high position of the third ventricle between the lateral ventricles. The MRI precisely outlines the extent of the corpus callosum defect. Absence of the corpus callosum may be inherited as an X-linked recessive trait or as an autosomal dominant trait. The condition may be associated with specific chromosomal disorders, particularly 8-trisomy and 18-trisomy. *Aicardi syndrome* represents a complex disorder that affects many systems and is typically associated with agenesis of the corpus callosum. Patients are almost all female, suggesting a genetic abnormality of the X chromosome (it may be lethal in males during fetal life). Seizures become evident during the first few months and are typically resistant to anticonvulsants. An electroencephalogram (EEG) shows independent activity recorded from both hemispheres as a result of the absent corpus callosum. All patients are severely mentally retarded and may have abnormal vertebrae that may be fused or only partially developed (e.g.,hemivertebra). Abnormalities of the retina, including circumscribed pits or lacunae and coloboma of the optic disc, are the most characteristic findings of Aicardi syndrome.

601.9 Agenesis of the Cranial Nerves

Absence of the cranial nerves or the corresponding central nuclei has been described in several conditions and includes the optic nerve, congential ptosis, Marcus Gunn phenomenon (sucking jaw movements causing simultaneous eyelid blinking; this congenital synkinesis results from abnormal innervation of the trigeminal and oculomotor nerves), the trigeminal and auditory nerves, and cranial nerves IX, X, XI, and XII. *Möbius syndrome* is characterized by bilateral facial weakness, which is often associated with abducens nerve paralysis. Hypoplasia or agenesis of brain stem nuclei as well as absent or decreased numbers of muscle fibers has been reported. Affected infants present in the newborn period with facial weakness, causing feeding difficulties due to a poor suck. The immobile, dull facies may give the incorrect impression of mental retardation; the prognosis for normal development is excellent in most cases.

601.10 Microcephaly

Microcephaly is defined as a head circumference that measures more than three standard deviations below the mean for age and sex. This condition is relatively common, particularly among the mentally retarded population. Although there are many causes of microcephaly, abnormalities in neuronal migration during fetal development, including heterotopias of neuronal cells and cytoarchitectural derangements, are found in many brains. Microcephaly may be subdivided into two main groups: primary (genetic) microcephaly and secondary (nongenetic) microcephaly. A precise diagnosis is important for genetic counseling and for prediction for future pregnancies.

ETIOLOGY. Primary microcephaly refers to a group of conditions that usually have no other malformations and follow a mendelian pattern of inheritance or are associated with a specific genetic syndrome. Affected infants are usually identified at birth because of a small head circumference. The more common types include familial and autosomal dominant microcephaly and a series of chromosomal syndromes that are summarized in Table 601–1. Secondary microcephaly results from a large number of noxious agents that may affect a fetus in utero or an infant during periods of rapid brain growth, particularly the first 2 yr of life.

CLINICAL MANIFESTATIONS. A thorough family history should be taken, seeking additional cases of microcephaly or disorders affecting the nervous system. It is important to measure a patient's head circumference at birth. A very small head circumference implies a process that began early in embryonic or fetal development. An insult to the brain that occurs later in life, particularly beyond the age of 2 yr, is less likely to produce severe microcephaly. Serial head circumference measurements are more meaningful than a single determination, particularly when the abnormality is minimal. In addition, the head circumference of each parent and sibling should be recorded.

TABLE 601–1 Causes of Microcephaly

Causes	Characteristic Findings
Primary (Genetic)	
1. Familial (autosomal recessive)	• Incidence 1/40,000 births • Typical appearance with slanted forehead, prominent nose and ears; severely mentally retarded and prominent seizures; surface convolutional markings of the brain poorly differentiated and disorganized cytoarchitecture
2. Autosomal dominant	• Nondistinctive facies, up-slanting palpebral fissures, mild forehead slanting, and prominent ears • Normal linear growth, seizures readily controlled, and mild or borderline mental retardation
3. Syndromes	
Down (21-trisomy)	• Incidence 1/800 • Abnormal rounding of occipital and frontal lobes and a small cerebellum; narrow superior temporal gyrus, propensity for Alzheimer's neurofibrillary alterations, and ultrastructure abnormalities of cerebral cortex
Edward (18-trisomy)	• Incidence 1/6,500 • Low birthweight, microstomia, micrognathia, low-set malformed ears, prominent occiput, rocker-bottom feet, flexion deformities of fingers, congenital heart disease, increased gyri, heterotopias of neurons
Cri-du-chat (5 p-)	• Incidence 1/50,000 • Round facies, prominent epicanthic folds, low-set ears, hypertelorism, and characteristic cry • No specific neuropathology
Cornelia de Lange	• Prenatal and postnatal growth delay, synophrys, thin down-turning upper lip • Proximally placed thumb
Rubinstein-Taybi	• Beaked nose, downward slanting of palpebral fissures, epicanthic folds, short stature with broad thumbs and toes
Smith-Lemli-Opitz	• Ptosis, scaphocephaly, inner epicanthic folds, anteverted nostrils • Low birthweight, marked feeding problems
Secondary (Nongenetic)	
1. Radiation	• Microcephaly and mental retardation most severe if exposure before 15th wk of gestation
2. Congenital infections	
Cytomegalovirus	• Small for dates, petechial rash, hepatosplenomegaly, chorioretinitis, deafness, mental retardation, and seizures • Central nervous system calcification and microgyria
Rubella	• Growth retardation, purpura, thrombocytopenia, hepatosplenomegaly, congenital heart disease, chorioretinitis, cataracts, and deafness • Perivascular necrotic areas, polymicrogyria, heterotopias, subependymal cavitations
Toxoplasmosis	• Purpura, hepatosplenomegaly, jaundice, convulsions, hydrocephalus, chorioretinitis, and cerebral calcification
3. Drugs	
Fetal alcohol	• Growth retardation, ptosis, absent philtrum and hypoplastic upper lip, congenital heart disease, feeding problems, neuroglial heterotopia, and disorganization of neurons
Fetal hydantoin	• Growth delay, hypoplasia of distal phalanges, inner epicanthic folds, broad nasal ridge, and anteverted nostrils
4. Meningitis/encephalitis	• Cerebral infarcts, cystic cavitation, diffuse loss of neurons
5. Malnutrition	• Controversial cause of microcephaly
6. Metabolic	• Maternal diabetes mellitus and maternal hyperphenylalaninemia
7. Hyperthermia	• Significant fever during 1st 4–6 wk has been reported to cause microcephaly, seizures, and facial anomalies • Pathologic studies show neuronal heterotopias • Further studies showed no abnormalities with maternal fever
8. Hypoxic-ischemic encephalopathy	• Initially diffuse cerebral edema; late stages characterized by cerebral atrophy

Laboratory investigation of a microcephalic child is determined by the history and physical examination. If the cause of the microcephaly is unknown, the mother's serum phenylalanine level should be determined. High phenylalanine serum levels in an asymptomatic mother can produce marked brain damage in an otherwise normal nonphenylketonuric infant. A karyotype is obtained if a chromosomal syndrome is suspected or if the child has abnormal facies, short stature, and additional congenital anomalies. CT scanning or MRI may be useful in identifying structural abnormalities of the brain or intracerebral calcification. Additional studies include a fasting plasma and urine amino acid analysis; serum ammonium determination; *to*xoplasmosis, *r*ubella, *c*ytomegalovirus, and *h*erpes simplex (TORCH) titers of the mother and child; and a urine sample for the culture of cytomegalovirus.

TREATMENT. Once the cause of microcephaly has been established, the physician must provide accurate and supportive genetic and family counseling. Because many children with microcephaly are also mentally retarded, the physician must assist with placement in an appropriate program that will provide for maximum development of the child (Chapter 37.2).

Barth PG: Disorders of neuronal migration. Can J Neurol Sci 14:1, 1987.

Dobyns WB, Reiner O, Carrozzo R, et al: A human brain malformation associated with deletion of L1S1 gene located at chromosome 17p13. JAMA 270:2838, 1993.

Dobyns WB, Stratton RF, Greenberg F: Syndromes with lissencephaly. 1: Miller-Dieker and Norman-Roberts syndromes and isolated lissencephaly. Am J Med Genet 18:509, 1984.

Harwood-Nash DC: Congenital craniocerebral abnormalities and computed tomography. Semin Roentgenol 12:39, 1977.

Haslam RHA: Microcephaly. *In*: Vinken PJ, Bruyn G, Klawans HL (eds): Handbook of Clinical Neurology. Amsterdam, Elsevier Science Publishers, 1987, pp 267–284.

Miller GM, Stears JC, Guggenheim MA, et al: Schizencephaly: A clinical and CT study. Neurology 34:997, 1984.

Molina JA, Mateos F, Merino M, et al: Aicardi syndrome in two sisters. J Pediatr 115:282, 1989.

Nerdich JA, Nussbaum RL, Packer TCJ, et al: Heterogeneity of clinical severity and molecular lesions in Aicardi syndrome. J Padiatr 116:911, 1990.

Parrish ML, Roessmann U, Levinsohn MW: Agenesis of the corpus callosum: A study of the frequency of associated malformations. Ann Neurol 6:349,1979.

Reiner D, Carrozzo R, Shen Y, et al: Isolation of a Miller-Dieker lissencephaly gene containing G protein β-subunit-like repeats. Nature 364:717, 1993.

Sheldon M, Rice DS, D'Arcangelo G, et al: Scrambler and yotari disrupt the disabled gene and produce a reeler-like phenotype in mice. Nature 389:730, 1997.

Sudarshan A, Goldie WD: The spectrum of congenital facial diplegia (Moebius syndrome). Pediatr Neurol 1:180, 1985.

601.11 Hydrocephalus

Hydrocephalus is not a specific disease; rather, it represents a diverse group of conditions that result from impaired circulation and absorption of CSF or, in the rare circumstance, from increased production by a choroid plexus papilloma.

PHYSIOLOGY. The CSF is formed primarily in the ventricular system by the choroid plexus, which is situated in the lateral, third, and fourth ventricles. Although most CSF is produced in the lateral ventricles, approximately 25% originates from extrachoroidal sources, including the capillary endothelium within the brain parenchyma. There is active neurogenic control of CSF formation as the choroid plexus is innervated by adrenergic and cholinergic nerves. Stimulation of the adrenergic system diminishes CSF production, whereas excitation of the cholinergic nerves may double the normal CSF production rate. In a normal child, approximately 20 mL of CSF is produced per hour. The total volume of CSF approximates 50 mL in an infant and 150 mL in an adult. Most of the CSF is extraventricular. CSF is formed by the choroid plexus in several stages; through a series of intricate steps, a plasma ultrafiltrate is ultimately processed into a secretion, the CSF.

CSF flow results from the pressure gradient that exists between the ventricular system and venous channels. Intraventricular pressure may be as high as 180 mm H_2O in the normal state, whereas the pressure in the superior sagittal sinus is in the range of 90 mm H_2O. Normally, CSF flows from the lateral ventricles through the foramina of Monro into the third ventricle. It then traverses the narrow aqueduct of Sylvius, which is approximately 3 mm in length and 2 mm in diameter in a child, to enter the fourth ventricle. The CSF exits the fourth ventricle through the paired lateral foramina of Luschka and the midline foramen of Magendie into the cisterns at the base of the brain. Hydrocephalus resulting from obstruction within the ventricular system is called *obstructive* or *noncommunicating hydrocephalus*. The CSF circulates from the basal cisterns posteriorly through the cistern system and over the convexities of the cerebral hemispheres. CSF is absorbed primarily by the arachnoid villi through tight junctions of their endothelium by the pressure forces that were noted earlier. CSF is absorbed to a much lesser extent by the lymphatic channels directed to the paranasal sinuses, along nerve root sleeves, and by the choroid plexus itself. Hydrocephalus resulting from obliteration of the subarachnoid cisterns or malfuncion of the arachnoid villi is called *nonobstructive* or *communicating hydrocephalus*.

PATHOPHYSIOLOGY AND ETIOLOGY. Obstructive or noncommunicating hydrocephalus develops most commonly in children because of an abnormality of the aqueduct or a lesion in the fourth ventricle. *Aqueductal stenosis* results from an abnormally narrow aqueduct of Sylvius that is often associated with branching or forking. In a small percentage of cases, aqueductal stenosis is inherited as a sex-linked recessive trait. These patients occasionally have minor neural tube closure defects, including spina bifida occulta. Rarely, aqueductal stenosis is associated with neurofibromatosis. *Aqueductal gliosis* may also give rise to hydrocephalus. As a result of neonatal meningitis or a subarachnoid hemorrhage in a premature infant, the ependymal lining of the aqueduct is interrupted and a brisk glial response results in complete obstruction. Intrauterine viral infections may also produce aqueductal stenosis followed by hydrocephalus, and mumps meningoencephalitis has been reported as a cause in a child. A vein of Galen malformation can expand to become large and, because of its midline position, obstruct the flow of CSF. Lesions or malformations of the posterior fossa are prominent causes of hydrocephalus, including posterior fossa brain tumors. Chiari malformation, and the Dandy-Walker syndrome.

Nonobstructive or communicating hydrocephalus most commonly follows a subarachnoid hemorrhage, which is usually a result of intraventricular hemorrhage in a premature infant. Blood in the subarachnoid spaces may cause obliteration of the cisterns or arachnoid villi and obstruction of CSF flow. Pneumococcal and tuberculous meningitis have a propensity to produce a thick, tenacious exudate that obstructs the basal cisterns, and intrauterine infections may also destroy the CSF pathways. Finally, leukemic infiltrates may seed the subarachnoid space and produce communicating hydrocephalus.

CLINICAL MANIFESTATIONS. The clinical presentation of hydrocephalus is variable and depends on many factors, including the age at onset, the nature of the lesion causing obstruction, and the duration and rate of rise of the intracranial pressure, (ICP). In an infant, an accelerated rate of enlargement of the head is the most prominent sign. In addition, the anterior fontanel is wide open and bulging, and the scalp veins are dilated. The forehead is broad, and the eyes may deviate downward because of impingement of the dilated suprapineal recess on the tectum, producing the setting-sun eye sign. Long-tract signs including brisk tendon reflexes, spasticity, clonus (particularly in the lower extremities), and Babinski sign are common owing to stretching and disruption of the corticospinal fibers originating from the leg region of the motor cortex. In an older child, the cranial sutures are partially closed so that the signs of hydrocephalus may be more subtle. Irritability, lethargy, poor appetite, and vomiting are common to both age groups, and headache is a prominent symptom in older patients. A gradual change in personality and deterioration in academic productivity suggest a slowly progressive form of hydrocephlus. Serial measurments of the head circumference indicate an increased velocity of growth. Percussion of the skull may produce a "cracked-pot" or *Macewen sign,* indicating separation of the sutures. A foreshortened occiput suggests Chiari malformation, and a prominent occiput suggests the Dandy-Walker malformation. Papilledema, abducens nerve palsy, and pyramidal tract signs, which are most evident in the lower extremities, are apparent in most cases.

Chiari malformation consists of two major subgroups, Type I typically produces symptoms during adolescence or adult life and is usually not associated with hydrocephalus. Patients complain of recurrent headache, neck pain, urinary frequency, and progressive lower extremity spasticity. The deformity consists of displacement of the cerebellar tonsils into the cervical canal. Although the pathogenesis is unknown, the prevailing theory suggests that obstruction of the caudal portion of the fourth ventricle during fetal development is responsible. The type II Chiari malformation is characterized by progressive hydrocephalus and a myelomeningocele. This lesion represents an anomaly of the hindbrain, probably due to a failure of pontine flexure during embryogenesis, and results in elongation of the fourth ventricle and kinking of the brain stem, with displacement of the inferior vermis, pons, and medulla into the cervical canal (Fig. 601–6). Approximately 10% of type II malformations produce symptoms during infancy consisting of stridor, weak cry, and apnea, which may be relieved by shunting or by posterior fossa decompression. A more indolent

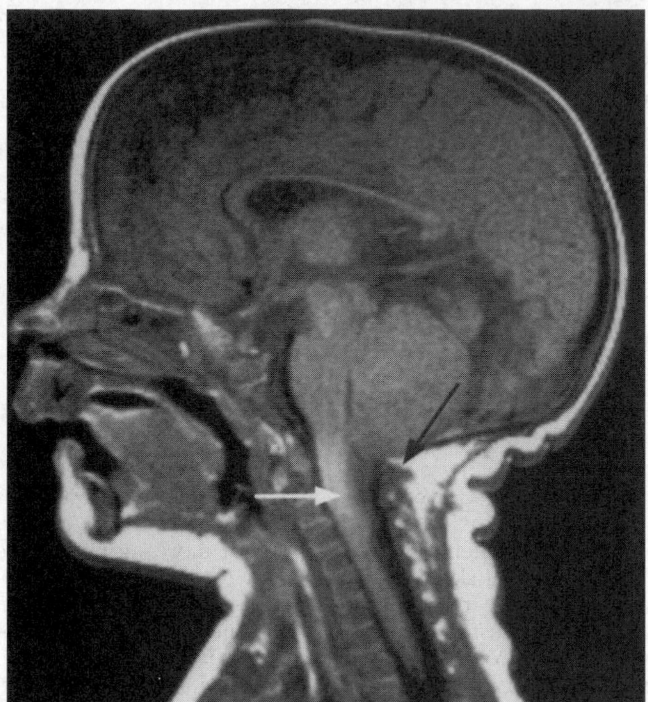

Figure 601–6 A midsagittal T1 weighted MRI of a patient with type II Chiari malformation. The cerebellar tonsils (*white arrow*) have descended below the foramen magnum (*black arrow*). Note the small slitlike 4th ventricle, which has been pulled into a vertical position.

form consists of abnormalities of gait, spasticity, and increasing incoordination during childhood. Plain skull radiographs show a small posterior fossa and a widened cervical canal. CT scanning with contrast and MRI display the cerebellar tonsils protruding downward into the cervical canal and the hindbrain abnormalities. The anomaly is treated by surgical decompression.

The *Dandy-Walker malformation* consists of a cystic expansion of the fourth ventricle in the posterior fossa, which results from a developmental failure of the roof of the 4th ventricle during embryogenesis (Fig. 601–7). Approxiamtely 90% of patients have hydrocephalus, and a significant number of children have associated anomalies, including agenesis of the posterior cerebellar vermis and corpus callosum. Infants present with a rapid increase in head size and a prominent occiput. Transillumination of the skull may be positive. Most children have evidence of long-tract signs, cerebellar ataxia, and delayed motor and cognitive milestones, probably owing to the associated structural anomalies. The Dandy-Walker malformation is managed by shunting the cystic cavity (and on occasion the ventricles as well) in the presence of hydrocephalus.

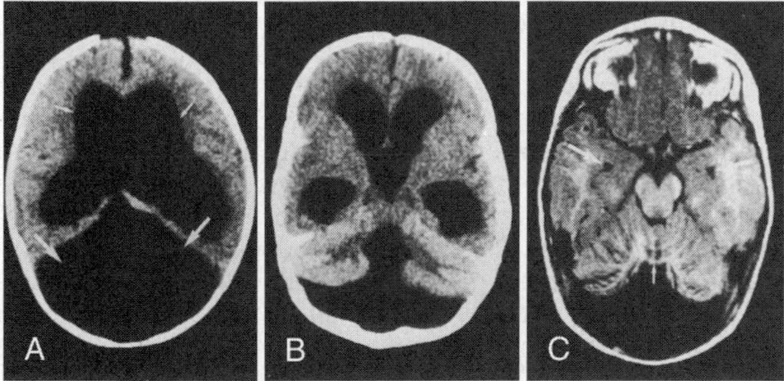

Figure 601–7 Dandy-Walker cyst. *A*, Axial CT scan (preoperative) showing large posterior fossa cyst (Dandy-Walker cyst; *large arrows*) and dilated lateral ventricles (*small arrows*), a complication secondary to CSF pathway obstruction at the 4th ventricular outlet. *B*, Same patient, with a lower axial CT scan showing splaying of the cerebellar hemispheres by the dilated 4th ventricle (Dandy-Walker cyst). The dilated ventricles proximal to the 4th ventricle again show CSF obstruction due to the Dandy-Walker cyst. *C*, MRI of the same patient showing decreased size of the Dandy-Walker cyst and temporal horns (*arrows*) following shunting. The incomplete vermis (*small arrow*) now becomes recognizable.

DIAGNOSIS AND DIFFERENTIAL DIAGNOSIS. Investigation of a child with hydrocephalus begins with the history. Familial cases suggest X-linked hydrocephalus secondary to aqueductal stenosis. A past history of prematurity with intracranial hemorrhage, meningitis, or mumps encephalitis is important to ascertain. Multiple café-au-lait spots and other clinical features of neurofibromatosis point to aqueductal stenosis as the cause of hydrocephalus. Examination includes careful inspection, palpation, and auscultation of the skull and spine. The occipitofrontal head circumference is recorded and compared with previous measurements. The size and configuration of the anterior fontanel are noted, and the back is inspected for abnormal midline skin lesions, including tufts of hair, lipoma, or angioma that might suggest spinal dysraphism. The presence of a prominent forehead or abnormalities in the shape of the occiput may suggest the pathogenesis of the hydrocephalus. A cranial bruit is audible in association with many cases of vein of Galen arteriovenous malformation. Transillumination of the skull is positive with massive dilatation of the ventricular system or in the Dandy-Walker syndrome. Inspection of the eyegrounds is mandatory because the finding of chorioretinitis suggests an intrauterine infection such as toxoplasmosis as a cause of the hydrocephalus. Papilledema is observed in older children but is rarely present in infants because the cranial sutures separate as a result of the increased pressure. Plain skull films typically show separation of the sutures, erosion of the posterior clinoids in an older child, and an increase in convolutional markings (beaten-silver appearance) with longstanding increased ICP. The CT scan and/or MRI along with ultrasonography in an infant are the most important studies to identify the specific cause of hydrocephalus.

The head may appear enlarged and be confused with hydrocephalus secondary to a thickened cranium resulting from chronic anemia, rickets, osteogenesis imperfecta, and epiphyseal dysplasia. Chronic subdural collections can produce bilateral parietal bone prominence. Various metabolic and degeneraive disorders of the CNS produce megalencephaly due to abnormal storage of substances within the brain parenchyma. These disorders include lysosomal diseases (e.g., Tay-Sachs, gangliosidosis, and the mucopolysaccharidoses), the aminoacidurias (e.g., maple syrup urine disease [MSUD]), and the leukodystrophies (e.g., metachromatic, Alexander disease, and Canavan disease). In addition, cerebral gigantism and neurofibromatosis are characterized by increased brain mass. Familial megalencephaly is inherited as an autosomal dominant trait and is characterized by delayed motor milestones and hypotonia but normal or near-normal intelligence. Measurement of the parent's head circumference is necessary to establish the diagnosis. *Hydranencephaly* may be confused with hydrocephalus. The cerebral hemispheres are absent or represented by membranous sacs with remnants of frontal, temporal, or occipital cortex dispersed over the membrane. The midbrain and brain stem are relatively intact (Fig. 601–8). The cause of hydranencephaly is unknown, but bilateral occlusion of the internal carotid arteries during early fetal development would explain most of the pathologic abnormalities. Affected infants may have a normal or enlarged head circumference at birth that grows at an excessive rate postnatally. Transillumination shows an absence of the cerebral hemispheres. The child is irritable, feeds poorly, develops seizures and spastic quadriparesis, and has little or no cognitive devel-

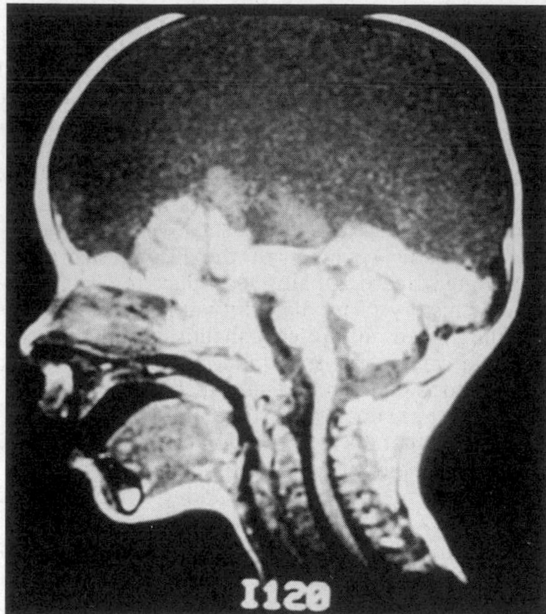

Figure 601–8 Hydranencephaly. MRI showing the brain stem and spinal cord with remnants of the cerebellum and the cerebral cortex. The remainder of the cranium is filled with CSF.

opment. A ventriculoperitoneal shunt prevents massive enlargement of the cranium.

TREATMENT. Therapy for hydrocephalus depends on the cause. Medical management, including the use of acetazolamide and furosemide, may provide temporary relief by reducing the rate of CSF production, but long-term results have been disappointing. Most cases of hydrocephalus require extracranial shunts, particularly a ventriculoperitoneal shunt (occasionally a ventriculostomy suffices). The major complication of shunts is bacterial infection, usually due to *Staphylococcus epidermidis* (Chapter 182). With meticulous preparation, the shunt infection rate can be reduced to less than 5%. The results of intrauterine surgical management of fetal hydrocephalus have been poor, possibly because of the high rate of associated cerebral malformations in addition to the hydrocephalus.

PROGNOSIS. This depends on the cause of the dilated ventricles and not on the size of the cortical mantle at the time of operative intervention. Hydrocephalic children are at increased risk for various developmental disabilities. The mean intelligence quotient is reduced compared with the general population, particularly for performance tasks as compared with verbal abilities. Most children have abnormalities in memory function. Visual problems are common, including strabismus, visuospatial abnormalities, visual field defects, and optic atrophy with decreased acuity secondary to increased ICP. The visual-evoked potential latencies are delayed and take some time to recover after correction of the hydrocephalus. Although most hydrocephalic children are pleasant and mild mannered, some children show aggressive and delinquent behavior. Accelerated pubertal development in patients with shunted hydrocephalus or meningomyelocele is relatively common, possibly because of increased gonadotropin secretion in response to increased ICP. It is imperative that hydrocephalic children receive long-term follow-up in a multidisciplinary setting.

Cochrane DD, Myles ST, Nimrod C, et al: Intrauterine hydrocephalus and ventriculomegaly: Associated abnormalities and fetal outcome. Can J Neurol Sci 12:51, 1985.

Cull C, Wyke MA: Memory function of children with spina bifida and shunted hydrocephalus. Dev Med Child Neurol 26:177, 1984.

De Myer W: Megalencephaly in children. Neurology 22:634, 1972.

Dennis M, Fitz CR, Netley CT, et al: The intelligence of hydrocephalic children. Arch Neurol 38:607, 1981.

Fernell E, Hagberg G, Hagberg B: Infantile hydrocephalus epidemiology: An indicator of enhanced survival. Arch Dis Child 70:123, 1994.

Fitzsimmons JS: Laryngeal stridor and respiratory obstruction in association with myelomeningocele. Dev Med Child Neurol 15:553, 1973.

Greene M, Benacerraf B, Crawford J: Hydranencephaly: US appearance during in utero evolution. Radiology 156:779, 1985.

Hirsch JF, Pierre-Kahn A, Renier D, et al: The Dandy-Walker malformation. J Neurosurg 61:515, 1984.

Hoffman HJ, Hendrick EB, Humphreys RP: Manifestations and management of Arnold-Chiari malformations in patients with myelomeningocele. Childs Brain 1:255, 1975.

Jackson JC, Blumhagen JD: Congenital hydrocephalus due to prenatal intracranial hemorrhage. Pediatrics 72:344, 1983.

Löppönen T, Saukkonen A-L, Serlo W, et al: Accelerated pubertal development in patients with shunted hydrocephalus. Arch Dis Child 74:490, 1996.

601.12 Craniosynostosis

Craniosynostosis is defined as premature closure of the cranial sutures and is classified as primary or secondary. *Primary craniosynostosis* refers to closure of one or more sutures due to abnormalities of skull development, whereas *secondary craniosynostosis* results from failure of brain growth and expansion and is not discussed further. The incidence of primary craniosynostosis approximates 1/2,000 births. The cause is unknown in the majority of children; however, genetic syndromes account for 10–20% of cases.

DEVELOPMENT AND ETIOLOGY. A review of skull development is helpful in understanding the genesis of craniosynostosis. During early development, the brain is enveloped by a film of mesenchyme. By the 2nd mo, osseous tissue is evident in that portion of the mesenchyme corresponding to the cranium, and cartilaginous tissue is formed at the base of the skull. The bones of the cranium are well developed by the 5th mo of gestation (frontal, parietal, temporal, and occipital) and are separated by sutures and fontanels. The brain grows rapidly during the first several years of life and is normally not impeded because of equivalent growth along the suture lines. The cause of craniosynostosis is unknown, but the prevailing hypothesis suggests that abnormal development of the base of the skull creates exaggerated forces on the dura that act to disrupt normal cranial suture development. Dysfunctional osteoblasts or osteoclasts are not responsible for craniosynostosis.

CLINICAL MANIFESTATIONS AND TREATMENT. Most cases of craniosynostosis are evident at birth and are characterized by a skull deformity that is a direct result of premature suture fusion. Palpation of the suture reveals a prominent bony ridge, and fusion of the suture may be confirmed by plain skull roentgenograms or bone scan in ambiguous cases.

Premature closure of the sagittal suture produces a long and narrow skull, or *scaphocephaly*, the most common form of craniosynostosis. Scaphocephaly is associated with a prominent occiput, a broad forehead, and a small or absent anterior fontanel. The condition is sporadic and more common in males and often causes difficulties during labor because of cephalopelvic disproportion. Scaphocephaly does not produce increased ICP or hydrocephalus, and results of neurologic examination of affected patients are normal.

Frontal plagiocephaly is the next most common form of craniosynostosis and is characterized by unilateral flattening of the forehead, elevation of the ipsilateral orbit and eyebrow, and a prominent ear on the corresponding side. The condition is more common in females and is the result of premature fusion of a coronal and sphenofrontal suture. Surgical intervention produces a cosmetically pleasing result.

Occipital plagiocephaly is most often a result of positioning during infancy and is more common in an immobile or handicapped child, but fusion or sclerosis of the lambdoid suture can cause unilateral occipital flattening and bulging of the ipsilateral frontal bone. *Trigonocephaly* is a rare form of cranio synostosis due to premature fusion of the metopic suture. These children have a keel-shaped forehead and hypotelorism and are at risk for associated developmental abnormalities of the forebrain. *Turricephaly* refers to a cone-shaped head due to premature fusion of the coronal and often sphenofrontal and frontoethmoidal sutures. The *kleeblattschädel deformity* is a peculiarly shaped skull that resembles a cloverleaf. Affected children have very prominent temporal bones, and the remainder of the cranium is constricted. Hydrocephalus is a common complication.

Premature fusion of only one suture rarely causes a neurologic deficit. In this situation, the sole indication for surgery is to enhance the child's cosmetic appearance, and the prognosis depends on the suture involved and on the degree of disfigurement. Neurologic complications, including hydrocephalus and increased ICP, are more likely to occur when two or more sutures are prematurely fused, in which case operative intervention is essential.

The most prevalent genetic disorders associated with craniosynostosis include Crouzon, Apert, Carpenter, Chotzen, and Pfeiffer syndromes. *Crouzon syndrome* is characterized by premature craniosynostosis and is inherited as an autosomal dominant trait. The shape of the head depends on the timing and order of suture fusion but most often is a compressed back-to-front diameter or brachycephaly due to bilateral closure of the coronal sutures. The orbits are underdeveloped, and ocular proptosis is prominent. Hypoplasia of the maxilla and orbital hypertelorism are typical facial features.

Apert syndrome has many features in common with Crouzon syndrome. However, Apert syndrome is usually a sporadic condition, although autosomal dominant inheritance may occur. It is associated with premature fusion of multiple sutures, including the coronal, sagittal, squamosal, and lambdoid sutures. The facies tend to be asymmetric, and the eyes are less proptotic than in Crouzon syndrome. Apert syndrome is characterized by syndactyly of the 2nd, 3rd, and 4th fingers, which may be joined to the thumb and the 5th finger. Similar abnormalities often occur in the feet. All patients have progressive calcification and fusion of the bones of the hands, feet, and cervical spine.

Carpenter syndrome is inherited as an autosomal recessive condition, and the many fusions of sutures tend to produce the kleeblattschädel skull deformity. Soft-tissue syndactyly of the hands and feet is always present, and mental retardation is common. Additional but less common abnormalities include congenital heart disease, corneal opacities, coxa valga, and genu valgum.

Chotzen syndrome is charaterized by asymmetric craniosynostosis and plagiocephaly. The condition is the most prevalent of the genetic syndromes and is inherited as an autosomal dominant trait. It is associated with facial asymmetry, ptosis of the eyelids, shortened fingers, and soft tissue syndactyly of the 2nd and 3rd fingers.

Pfeiffer syndrome is most often associated with turricephaly. The eyes are prominent and widely spaced, and the thumbs and great toes are short and broad. Partial soft tissue syndactyly may be evident. Most cases appear to be sporadic, but autosomal dominant inheritance has been reported.

Mutations of the fibroblast growth factor receptor (FGFR) gene family have been shown to be associated with phenotypically specific types of craniosynostosis. Mutations of the $FGFR_1$ gene located on chromosome 8 result in Pfeiffer syndrome; a similar mutation of the $FGFR_2$ gene causes Apert syndrome. Identical mutations of the $FGFR_2$ gene may result in both Pfeiffer and Crouzon phenotypes.

Each of the genetic syndromes poses a risk of additional anomalies, including hydrocephalus, increased ICP, papilledema, optic atrophy due to abnormalities of the optic foramina, respiratory problems secondary to a deviated nasal septum or choanal atresia, and disorders of speech and deafness. Craniectomy is mandatory for management of increased ICP, and a multidisciplinary craniofacial team is essential for the long-term follow-up of affected children. Craniosynostosis may be surgically corrected with good outcomes and relatively low morbidity and mortality, especially for nonsyndromic infants.

Cohen MM: Craniosynostosis update. Am J Med Genet 4(suppl):99, 1987.

Rutland P, Pulleyn LJ, Reardon W, et al: Identical mutations in the $FGFR_2$ gene cause both Pfeiffer and Crouzon syndrome phenotypes. Nature Genet 56:334, 1995.

Sloan GM, Wells KC, Raffel C, et al: Surgical treatment of craniosynostosis: Outcome analysis of 250 consecutive patients. Pediatrics 100:1, 1997.

CHAPTER 602
Seizures in Childhood

Seizures are a common neurologic disorder in the pediatric age group and occur in 3–5% of children. Epilepsy occurs in 0.5–1.0% of the population and begins in childhood in 60% of cases; 30,000 children and adolescents are diagnosed each year with epilepsy in the United States. Seizures do not constitute a diagnosis but are a symptom of an underlying central nervous system (CNS) disorder that requires a thorough investigation and management plan. In most children, a cause of the seizure cannot be determined, and a diagnosis of idiopathic epilepsy is made. Although the outcome for most uncomplicated seizures in children is good, 10–20% have persistent seizures refractory to drugs, and these pose a diagnostic and management challenge. The terms *seizure* and *convulsion* may be incorrectly used interchangeably with *epilepsy*. A *seizure* (convulsion) is defined as a paroxysmal involuntary disturbance of brain function that may be manifested as an impairment or loss of consciousness, abnormal motor activity, behavioral abnormalities, sensory disturbance, or autonomic dysfunction. Some seizures are characterized by abnormal movements without loss or impairment of consciousness. *Epilepsy* is defined as recurrent seizures unrelated to fever or to an acute cerebral insult.

EVALUATION. The *history* should attempt to define factors that may have promoted the convulsion and to provide a detailed description of the seizure and the child's postictal state. Some seizure types are inherited: autosomal dominant nocturnal frontal lobe epilepsy, familial benign neonatal convulsions, familial benign infantile convulsions, autosomal dominant febrile seizures, partial epilepsy with auditory symptoms, and autosomal dominant frontal lobe progressive epilepsy with mental retardation.

Children who have a propensity to develop epilepsy may experience the first convulsion in association with a viral illness or a low-grade fever. Seizures that occur during the early morning hours or with drowsiness, particularly during the initial phase of sleep, are common in childhood epilepsy. In retrospect, irritability, mood swings, headache, and subtle personality changes may precede a seizure by several days. Some parents can accurately predict the timing of the next seizure on the basis of changes in the child's disposition.

Most parents vividly recall their child's initial convulsion and can describe it in detail. The first step in an evaluation is to determine whether the seizure has a focal onset or is generalized. *Focal seizures* may be characterized by motor or sensory symptoms and include forceful turning of the head and eyes to one side, unilateral clonic movements beginning in the face or extremities, or a sensory disturbance such as paresthesias or pain localized to a specific area. Focal seizures in an adult usually indicate a localized lesion, but investigation of focal seizures during childhood may be nondiagnostic. Motor seizures may be focal or generalized and tonic-clonic, tonic, clonic, myoclonic, or atonic. *Tonic seizures* are characterized by increased tone or rigidity, and atonic seizures are characterized by flaccidity or by lack of movement during a convulsion. *Clonic seizures* consist of rhythmic muscle contraction and relaxation, and myoclonus is most accurately described as shocklike contraction of a muscle. The duration of the seizure and state of consciousness (retained or impaired) should be documented. The history should determine whether an aura preceded the convulsion and the behavior of the child immediately preceding the seizure. The most common aura experienced by children consists of epigastric discomfort or pain and a feeling or fear. The posture of the patient, presence and distribution of cyanosis, vocalizations, loss of sphincter control (particularly of the urinary bladder), and postictal state (including sleep and headache) should be noted.

Some parents can precisely act out or recreate a seizure. The physical portrayal by the parent or caregiver is often surprisingly similar to the actual convulsion and is much more accurate than the verbal description. Aside from the description of the seizure pattern, the frequency, time of day, precipitating factors, and alternation in the type of convulsive disorder are important. Although generalized tonic-clonic seizures are readily documented, the frequency of absence seizures is often underestimated by parents. A prolonged personality change or intellectual deterioration may suggest a degenerative disease of the CNS, whereas constitutional symptoms, including vomiting and failure to thrive, might indicate a primary metabolic disorder or a structural lesion. It is essential to obtain details of prior anticonvulsant medication and the child's response to the regimen and to determine whether drugs that may potentiate seizures, including chlorpromazine or methylphenidate, were prescribed.

Examination of a child with a seizure disorder should be geared toward the search for an organic cause. Blood pressure is recorded, and the child's head circumference, length, and weight are plotted on a growth chart and compared with previous measurements. The finding of unusual facial features or associated physical findings such as hepatosplenomegaly point to an underlying metabolic or storage disease as the cause of the neurologic disorder. A search for vitiliginous lesions of tuberous sclerosis using an ultraviolet light source, examination for adenoma sebaceum, shagreen patch, multiple café-au-lait spots, or a nevus flammeus, and the presence of retinal phakoma would indicate a neurocutaneous disorder as the cause of the seizure. Localizing neurologic signs such as a subtle hemiparesis with hyperreflexia, an equivocal Babinski, and a downward-drifting extended arm with eyes closed might suggest a contralateral hemispheric structural lesion, such as a slow-growing temporal lobe glioma, as the cause of the seizure disorder. Unilateral growth arrest of the thumbnail, hand, or extremity in a child with a focal seizure disorder suggests a chronic condition such as a porencephalic cyst, arteriovenous malformation, or cortical atrophy in the opposite hemisphere. The eyegrounds must be examined for the presence of papilledema, retinal hemorrhages, chorioretinitis, coloboma, and macular changes as well as retinal phakoma. Hyperventilation for a 3- or 4-min period produces an immediate seizure in virtually all children with absence epilepsy.

CLASSIFICATION OF SEIZURES

It is important to classify the type of seizure for several reasons. First, the seizure type may provide a clue to the cause of the seizure disorder. In addition, precise delineation of the seizure may allow a firm basis for making a prognosis and choosing the most appropriate treatment. A child with generalized tonic-clonic epilepsy is usually readily controlled with anticonvulsants, whereas a patient with multiple seizure types or partial seizures may fare less well. Infants with benign myoclonic epilepsy have a more favorable outlook than patients with infantile spasms. Similarly, a school-aged child who has benign partial epilepsy with centrotemporal spikes (rolandic epilepsy) has an excellent prognosis and is unlikely to require a prolonged course of anticonvulsants. Clinical classification of seizures may be difficult because the manifestations of different seizure types may be similar. For example, the clinical features of a child with absence seizures may be almost identical to those of another patient with complex partial epilepsy. An electroencephalogram (EEG) is a useful adjunct to the classification of epilepsy because of the variability of seizure expressivity in this age group. A classification combining the clinical description of the seizure with the EEG findings has improved the delineation of childhood epilepsy (Table 602–1).

TABLE 602–1 International Classification of Epileptic Seizures

Partial Seizures

- Simple partial (consciousness retained)
    - Motor
    - Sensory
    - Autonomic
    - Psychic
- Complex partial (consciousness impaired)
    - Simple partial, followed by impaired consciousness
    - Consciousness impaired at onset
- Partial seizures with secondary generalization

Generalized Seizures

- Absences
    - Typical
    - Atypical
- Generalized tonic-clonic
- Tonic
- Clonic
- Myoclonic
- Atonic
- Infantile spasms

Unclassified Seizures

Epilepsy in children has also been classified by syndrome. Using the age at onset of seizures, cognitive development and neurologic examination, description of seizure type and the EEG findings including the background rhythm, it has been possible to classify approximately 50% of childhood seizures into specific syndromes. The *syndromic* classification of seizures provides a distinct advantage over previous classifications by improving management with appropriate anticonvulsant medication, identifying potential candidates for epilepsy surgery, and providing patients and families with a reliable and accurate prognosis. Examples of epilepsy syndromes include infantile spasms (West syndrome), benign myoclonic epilepsy of infancy, the Lennox-Gastaut syndrome, febrile convulsions, Landau-Kleffner syndrome, benign childhood epilepsy with centrotemporal spikes (rolandic epilepsy), Rasmussens encephalitis, juvenile myoclonic epilepsy (Janz syndrome), and Lafora disease (progressive myoclonic epilepsy).

602.1 Partial Seizures

Partial seizures account for a large proportion of childhood seizures, up to 40% in some series. Partial seizures may be classified as *simple* or *complex*; consciousness is maintained with simple seizures and is impaired in patients with complex seizures.

SIMPLE PARTIAL SEIZURES (SPS). Motor activity is the most common symptom of SPS. The movements are characterized by asynchronous clonic or tonic movements, and they tend to involve the face, neck, and extremities. *Versive seizures* consisting of head turning and conjugate eye movements are particularly common in SPS. Automatisms do not occur with SPS, but some patients complain of aura (e.g., chest discomfort and headache), which may be the only manifestation of a seizure. Unfortunately, children have difficulty in describing aura and often refer to it as "feeling funny" or "something crawling inside me." The average seizure persists for 10–20 sec. *The distinguishing characteristic of SPS is that the patients remain conscious and may verbalize during the seizure. Furthermore, no postical phenomenon follows the event.* SPS may be confused with tics; however, *tics* are characterized by shoulder shrugging, eye blinking, and facial grimacing and primarily involve the face and shoulders (Chapter 21). Tics can be briefly suppressed, but partial seizures cannot be controlled. The EEG may show spikes or sharp waves unilaterally or bilaterally or a multifocal spike pattern in patients with SPS.

COMPLEX PARTIAL SEIZURES (CPS). A CPS may begin with a simple partial seizure with or without an aura, followed by impaired consciousness; conversely, the onset of the CPS may coincide with an altered state of consciousness. An *aura* consisting of vague, unpleasant feelings, epigastric discomfort, or fear is present in approximately one third of children with SPS and CPS. *The presence of an aura always indicates a focal onset of the seizure.* Because partial seizures are difficult to document in infants and children, the frequency of their association with CPS may be underestimated. Impaired consciousness in infants and children is difficult to appreciate. There may be a brief blank stare or a sudden cessation or pause in activity that is frequently overlooked by the parent. Furthermore, the child is unable to communicate or to describe the periods of impaired consciousness in most cases. Finally, the periods of altered consciousness may be brief and infrequent, and only an experienced observer or an EEG may be able to identify the abnormal event.

Automatisms are a common feature of CPS in infants and children, occurring in approximately 50–75% of cases; the older the child, the greater is the frequency of automatisms. Automatisms develop after the loss of consciousness and may persist into the postical phase, but they are not recalled by the child. The automatic behavior observed in infants is characterized by alimentary automatisms, including lip smacking, chewing, swallowing, and excessive salivation. These movements can represent normal infant behavior and are difficult to distinguish from the automatisms of CPS. Prolonged and repetitive alimentary automatisms associated with a blank stare or with a lack of responsiveness almost always indicate CPS in an infant. Automatic behavior in older children consists of semipurposeful, incoordinated, and unplanned gestural automatisms, including picking and pulling at clothing or the bed sheets, rubbing or caressing objects, and walking or running in a nondirective, repetitive, and often fearful fashion.

Spreading of the epileptiform discharge during CPS can result in secondary generalization with a tonic-clonic convulsion. During the spread of the ictal discharge throughout the hemisphere, contralateral versive turning of the head, dystonic posturing, and tonic or clonic movements of the extremities and face including eye blinking may be noted. The average duration of a CPS is 1–2 min, which is considerably longer than an SPS or an absence seizure.

CPS are associated with interictal EEG anterior temporal lobe sharp waves or focal spikes, and multifocal spikes are a frequent finding. Approximately 20% of infants and children with CPS have a normal routine interictal EEG. In these patients, a sleep-deprived EEG study, zygomatic leads during EEG, prolonged EEG recording, or a video-EEG study of the hospitalized patient weaned from anticonvulsants are techniques that can be used to increase the identification of spikes and sharp waves (Fig. 602–1*A*). In addition, some children with CPS have interictal sharp waves or spikes originating from the frontal, parietal, or occipital lobes. Radiographic studies including CT scanning and especially MRI are most likely to identify an abnormality in the temporal lobe of a child with CPS. These lesions include mesial temporal sclerosis, hamartoma, postencephalitic gliosis, subarachnoid cysts, infarction, arteriovenous malformations, and a slow-growing glioma.

BENIGN PARTIAL EPILEPSY WITH CENTROTEMPORAL SPIKES (BPEC). BPEC is a common type of partial epilepsy in childhood and has an excellent prognosis. The clinical features, EEG findings (rolandic foci), and lack of a neuropathologic lesion are characteristic and readily separate BPEC from CPS. BPEC occurs between the ages of 2 and 14 and has a peak age of onset of 9–10 yr. The disorder occurs in normal children with an unremarkable past history and normal neurologic examination. There is often a positive family history of epilepsy. The seizures are usually partial, and motor signs and somatosensory symptoms are often confined to the face. Oropharyngeal symptoms include tonic contractions and paresthesias of the tongue, unilateral numbness of the cheek (particularly along the gum), guttural noises, dysphagia, and excessive salivation. Unilateral tonic-clonic contractures of the lower face frequently accompany the oropharyngeal symptoms, as do clonic movements or paresthesias of the ipsilateral extremities. Consciousness may be intact or impaired, and the partial seizure may proceed to secondary generalization. Approximately 20% of children experience only one seizure, the majority have infrequent seizure, and about one quarter have repeated clusters of seizures. BPEC occurs during sleep in 75% of patients, whereas CPS tends to be observed during waking hours. The EEG pattern is diagnostic for BPEC and is characterized by a repetitive spike focus localized in the centrotemporal or rolandic area with normal background activity (Fig. 602–1*A*). Anticonvulsants are necessary for patients who have frequent seizures but should not be prescribed automatically after the initial convulsion. Carbamazepinie is the preferred drug, which is continued for at least 2 yr or until 14–16 yr of age, when spontaneous remission of BPEC usually occurs.

RASMUSSEN ENCEPHALITIS. This subacute inflammatory encephalitis is one cause of *epilepsia partialis continua.* A nonspecific febrile illness may have preceded the onset of focal seizures, which may be very frequent or continuous. The onset is usually before age 10 yr. Sequelae include hemiplegia, hemianopia, and aphasia. The EEG reveals diffuse paroxymal activity with a slow background. The disease is progressive and potentially lethal but more often becomes self-limited with significant neurologic deficits. The disease may be due to autoantibodies that bind to and stimulate the glutamate receptors. Studies have identified cytomegalovirus in several surgical specimens of patients with Rasmussen encephalitis.

602.2 Generalized Seizures

ABSENCE SEIZURES. Simple (typical) absence (petit mal) seizures are characterized by a sudden cessation of motor activity or speech with a blank facial expression and flickering of the eyelids. These seizures, which are uncommon before age 5 yr, are more prevalent in girls; they are never associated with an aura; they rarely persist longer than 30 sec; and they are not associated with a postictal state. These features tend to differentiate absence seizures from complex partial seizures. Children with absence seizures may experience countless seizures daily, whereas complex partial seizures are usually less frequent. Patients do not lose body tone, but their head may fall forward slightly. Immediately after the seizure, patients resume preseizure activity with no indication of postictal impairment. Automatic behavior frequently accompanies simple absence seizures. Hyperventilation for 3–4 min routinely produces an absence seizure. The EEG shows a typical 3/sec spike

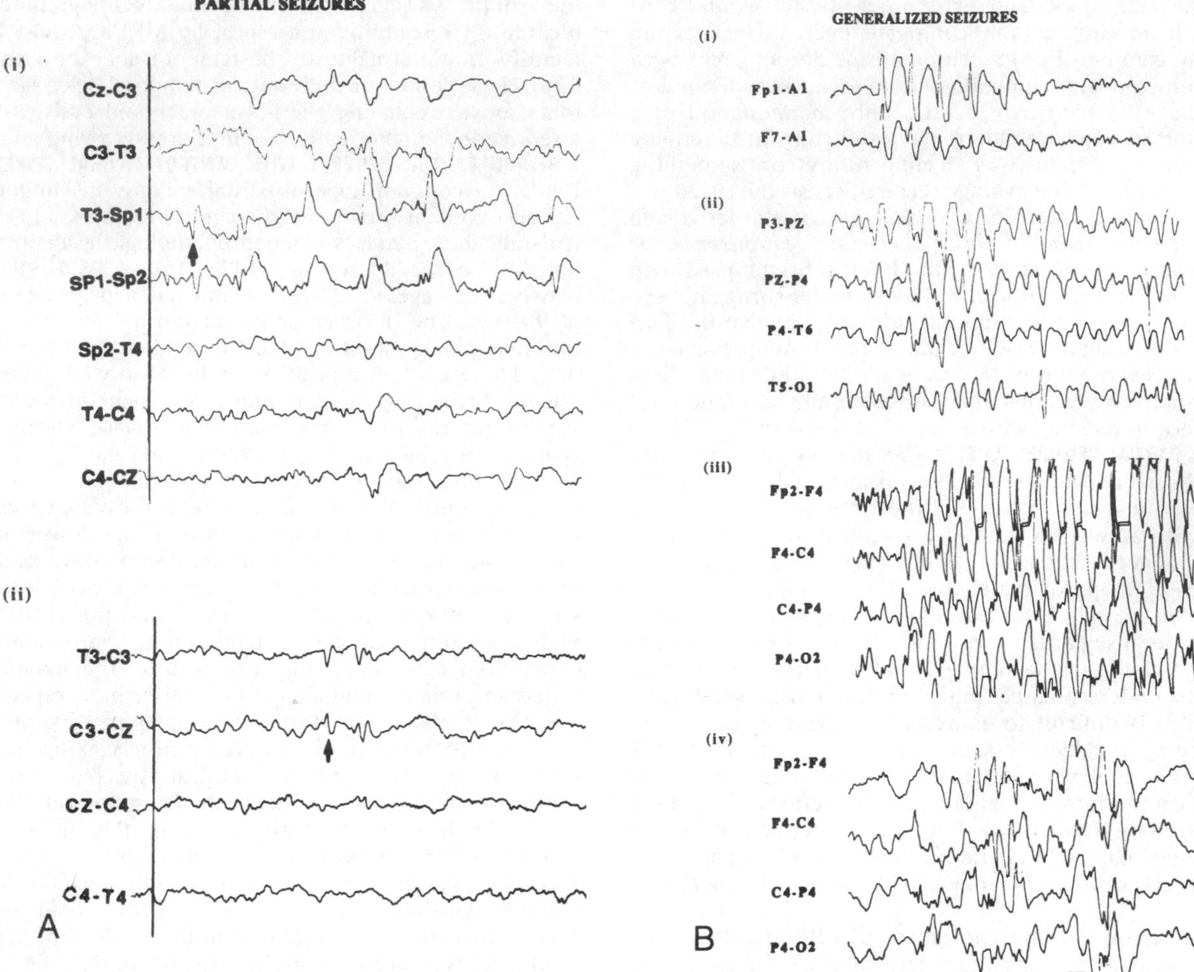

Figure 602–1 *A*, An EEG of partial seizures: (i) spike discharges from the left temporal lobe *(arrow)* in a patient with CPS, (ii) left parietal central spikes *(arrow)* characteristic of BPEC. *B*, Representative EEGs of generalized seizures: (i) 3/sec spike and wave discharge of absence seizures with normal background activity, (ii) complex myoclonic epilepsy (Lennox-Gastaut syndrome) with interictal slow spike waves, (iii) juvenile myoclonic epilepsy showing 6/sec spike and waves enhanced by photic stimulation, and (iv) hypsarrhythmia with an irregular high-voltage spike and wave activity.

and generalized wave discharge (Fig. 602–1*B*). Complex (atypical) absence seizures have associated motor components consisting of myoclonic movement of the face, fingers, or extremities and, on occasion, loss of body tone. These seizures produce atypical EEG spike and wave discharges at 2–2.5/sec.

GENERALIZED TONIC-CLONIC SEIZURES. These seizures are extremely common and may follow a partial seizure with a focal onset (second generalization) or occur de novo. They may be associated with an aura, suggesting a focal origin of the epileptiform discharge. It is important to inquire about the presence of an aura, because its presence and site of origin may indicate the area of pathology. Patients suddenly lose consciousness and in some cases emit a shrill, piercing cry. Their eyes roll back, their entire body musculature undergoes tonic contractions, and they rapidly become cyanotic in association with apnea. The clonic phase of the seizure is heralded by rhythmic clonic contractions alternating with relaxation of all muscle groups. The clonic phase slows toward the end of the seizure, which usually persists for a few minutes, and patients often sigh as the seizure comes to an abrupt stop. During the seizure, children may bite their tongue but rarely vomit. Loss of sphincter control, particularly the bladder, is common during a generalized tonic-clonic seizure.

Tight clothing and jewelry around the neck should be loosened, the patient should be placed on one side, and the neck and jaw should be gently hyperextended to enhance breathing. The mouth should not be opened forcibly by an object or by a finger because the patient's teeth may be dislodged and aspirated, or significant injury to the oropharyngeal cavity may result. Postictally, children initially are semicomatose and typically remain in a deep sleep from 30 min to 2 hr. If patients are examined during the seizure or immediately postictally, they may demonstrate truncal ataxia, hyperactive deep tendon reflexes, clonus, and a Babinski reflex. The postictal phase is often associated with vomiting and an intense bifrontal headache. *Idiopathic seizure* is a term applied when the cause of a generalized seizure cannot be ascertained. Many factors are known to precipitate generalized tonic-clonic seizures in children, including low-grade fever associated with infections, excessive fatigue or emotional stress, and various drugs including psychotropic medications, theophylline, and methylphenidate, particularly if the seizures are poorly controlled by anticonvulsant drugs.

MYOCLONIC EPILEPSIES OF CHILDHOOD. This disorder is characterized by repetitive seizures consisting of brief, often symmetric muscular contractions with loss of body tone and falling or slumping forward, which has a tendency to cause injuries to the face and the mouth. Myoclonic epilepsies include a heterogeneous group of conditions with multiple causes and variable outcomes. However, at least five distinct subgroupings can be identified; these represent the broad spectrum of myoclonic epilepsies in the pediatric population.

Benign Myoclonus of Infancy. Benign myoclonus begins during infancy and consists of clusters of myoclonic movements confined to the neck, trunk, and extremities. The myoclonic activity may be confused with infantile spasms; however, the EEG is normal in patients with benign myoclonus. The prognosis is good, with normal development and the cessation of myoclonus by 2 yr of age. An anticonvulsant is not indicated.

Typical Myoclonic Epilepsy of Early Childhood. Children who develop typical myoclonic epilepsy are near normal before the onset of seizures, with an unremarkable pregnancy, labor, and delivery and intact developmental milestones. The mean age of onset is approximately 2½ yr, but the range spreads from 6 mo to 4 yr. The frequency of myoclonic seizures varies; they may occur several times daily, or children may be seizure free for weeks. A few patients have febrile convulsions or generalized tonic-clonic afebrile seizures that precede the onset of myoclonic epilepsy. Approximately half of patients occasionally have tonic-clonic seizures in addition to the myoclonic epilepsy. The EEG shows fast spike wave complexes of ≥2.5 Hz and a normal background rhythm in most cases. At least one third of the children have a positive family history of epilepsy, which suggests a genetic etiology in some cases. The long-term outcome is relatively favorable. Mental retardation develops in the minority, and more than 50% are seizure free several years later. However, learning and language problems and emotional and behavioral disorders occur in a significant number of these children and require prolonged follow-up by a multidisciplinary team.

Complex Myoclonic Epilepsies. These consist of a heterogeneous group of disorders with a uniformly poor prognosis. Focal or generalized tonic-clonic seizures beginning during the 1st year of life typically antedate the onset of myoclonic epilepsy. The generalized seizure is often associated with an upper respiratory tract infection and a low-grade fever and frequently develops into status epilepticus. Approximately one third of these patients have evidence of delayed developmental milestones. A history of hypoxic-ischemic encephalopathy in the perinatal period and the finding of generalized upper motor neuron and extrapyramidal signs with microcephaly constitute a common pattern among these children. A family history of epilepsy is much less prominent in this group compared with typical myoclonic epilepsy. Some children display a combination of frequent myoclonic and tonic seizures, and when interictal slow spike waves are evident in the EEG, the seizure disorder is classified as the **Lennox-Gastaut syndrome.** This syndrome is characterized by the triad of intractable seizures of various types, a slow spike wave EEG during the awake state, and mental retardation. Patients with complex myoclonic epilepsy routinely have interictal slow spike waves and are refractory to anticonvulsants (Fig. 602–1*B*). The seizures are persistent, and the frequency of mental retardation and behavioral problems is approximately 75% of all patients. Treatment with valproic acid or the benzodiazepines may decrease the frequency or intensity of the seizures. The ketogenic diet should be considered for those patients whose seizures are refractory to anticonvulsants.

Juvenile Myoclonic Epilepsy (Janz Syndrome). Juvenile myoclonic epilepsy usually begins between the ages of 12 and 16 yr and accounts for approximately 5% of the epilepsies. A gene locus has been identified on chromosome 6p21. Patients note frequent myoclonic jerks on awakening, making hair combing and tooth brushing difficult. As the myoclonus tends to abate later in the morning, most patients do not seek medical advice at this stage and some deny the episodes. A few years later, early morning generalized tonic-clonic seizures develop in association with the myoclonus. The EEG shows a 4–6/sec irregular spike and wave pattern, which is enhanced by photic stimulation (Fig. 602–1*B*). The neurologic examination is normal, and the majority respond dramatically to valproate, which is required lifelong. Discontinuance of the drug causes a high rate of recurrence of seizures.

Progressive Myoclonic Epilepsies. This heterogeneous group of rare genetic disorders uniformly has a grave prognosis. These conditions include Lafora disease, myoclonic epilepsy with ragged-red fibers (MERRF) (see Chapter 607.2), sialiosis type 1 (see Chapter 608.4), ceroid lipofuscinosis (see Chapter 608.2), juvenile neuropathic Gaucher disease, and juvenile neuroaxonal dystrophy. *Lafora disease* presents in children between 10 and 18 yr with generalized tonic-clonic seizures. Ultimately, myoclonic jerks appear; these become more apparent and constant with progression of the disease. Mental deterioration is a characteristic feature and becomes evident within 1 yr of the onset of seizures. Neurologic abnormalities, particularly cerebellar and extrapyramidal signs, are prominent findings. The EEG shows polyspike-wave discharges, particularly in the occipital region, with progressive slowing and a disorganized background. The myoclonic jerks are difficult to control, but a combination of valproic acid and a benzodiazepine (e.g., clonazepam) is effective in controlling the generalized seizures. Lafora disease is an autosomal recessive disorder, and the diagnosis may be established by examination of a skin biopsy specimen for characteristic periodic acid–Schiff positive inclusions, which are most prominent in the eccrine sweat gland duct cells. The gene for Lafora disease is located on 6p24 and it encodes a protein, tyrosine phosphatase.

INFANTILE SPASMS. Infantile spasms usually begin between the ages of 4 and 8 mo and are characterized by brief symmetric contractions of the neck, trunk, and extremities. There are at least three types of infantile spasms: flexor, extensor, and mixed. *Flexor spasms* occur in clusters or volleys and consist of sudden flexion of the neck, arms, and legs onto the trunk, whereas *extensor spasms* produce extension of the trunk and extremities and are the least common form of infantile spasm. *Mixed infantile spasms,* consisting of flexion in some volleys and extension in others, is the most common type of infantile spasm. Clusters or volleys of seizures may persist for minutes, with brief intervals between each spasm. A cry may precede or follow an infantile spasm, accounting for the confusion with colic in a few cases. The spasms occur during sleep or arousal but have a tendency to develop while patients are drowsy or immediately on awakening. The EEG that is most commonly associated with infantile spasms is referred to as *hypsarrhythmia,* which consists of a chaotic pattern of high-voltage, bilaterally asynchronous, slow-wave activity (Fig. 602–1*B*), or a modified hypsarrhythmia pattern.

Infantile spasms are typically classified into two groups: *cryptogenic* and *symptomatic.* A child with cryptogenic infantile spasms has an uneventful pregnancy and birth history as well as normal developmental milestones before the onset of seizures. The neurologic examination and the CT and MRI scans of the head are normal, and there are no associated risk factors. Approxiamately 10–20% of infantile spasms are classified as cryptogenic, and the remainder are classified as symptomatic. Symptomatic infantile spasms are related directly to several prenatal, perinatal, and postnatal factors. Prenatal and perinatal factors include hypoxic-ischemic encephalopathy with periventricular leukomalacia, congenital infections, inborn errors of metabolism, neurocutaneous syndromes such as tuberous sclerosis, cytoarchitectural abnormalities including lissencephaly and schizencephaly, and prematurity. Postnatal conditions include CNS infections, head trauma (especially subdural hematoma and intraventricular hemorrhage), and hypoxic-ischemic encephalopathy. In the past, immunization, particularly with the pertussis antigen, had been implicated as a cause of infantile spasms. The fact that infantile spasms and immunizations often occur simultaneously around 6 mo of age has now been shown to be a coincidence of timing rather than a cause and effect. Infants with cryptogenic infantile spasms have a good prognosis, whereas those with the symptomatic type have an 80–90% risk of mental retardation. The underlying CNS disorder has the major role in the neurologic outcome. Several theories have been advanced with regard to the pathogenesis of infantile spasms, including dysfunction of the monoaminergic neurotransmitter system in the brain stem, derangement of neuronal structures in the brain stem, and an abnormality of the immune system. One hypothesis implicates corticotropin-releasing hormone (CRH), a putative neurotransmitter, metabolized in the inferior olive. CRH acts on the pituitary to enhance the release of adrenocorticotropic hormone (ACTH); ACTH and glucocorticoids suppress the metabolism and secretion of CRH by a feedback mechanism. It is proposed that specified stresses or injury to an infant during a critical period of neurodevelopment causes CRH overproduction, resulting in neuronal hyperexcitability and seizures. The number of CRH receptors reaches a maximum in an infant's brain followed by spontaneous reduction with age, perhaps accounting for the eventual resolution of infantile spasms, even without therapy. Exogenous ACTH and glucocorticoids suppress CRH synthesis, which may explain their effectiveness in treating infantile spasms. The therapy of infantile spasms follows in the treatment section.

LANDAU-KLEFFNER SYNDROME (LKS). This is a rare condition of unknown causes, more common in boys, with a mean onset of 5.5 yr. LKS is often confused with autism, as both conditions are associated with a loss of language function. LKS is characterized by loss of language skills in a previously normal child. At least 70% have an associated seizure disorder. Language regression may be sudden or the speech loss protracted. The aphasia may be primarily receptive or expressive, and auditory agnosia may be so severe that the child is oblivious to everyday sounds. Hearing is normal, but behavioral problems, including irritability and poor attention span, are particularly common. Formal testing often shows normal performance and visual-spatial skills despite poor language. The seizures are of several types, including focal or generalized tonic-clonic, atypical absence, partial complex, and occasionally myoclonic. High-amplitude spike and wave discharges predominate and tend to be bitemporal but can be multifocal or generalized. In the evolutionary stages of the condition, the EEG findings may be normal. The spike discharges are always more apparent during non-REM sleep; thus, a child suspected of LKS should have an EEG during sleep, particularly if the awake record is normal. If the sleep EEG is normal but a high index of suspicion for the diagnosis of LKS continues, the child should be referred to a tertiary pediatric epilepsy center for prolonged EEG recording and specific neuroimaging studies. CT and MRI studies typically yield normal results, and positron emission tomography (PET) scans have demonstrated either unilateral or bilateral hypometabolism or hypermetabolism. Microscopic examination of surgical specimens has shown minimal gliosis but no evidence of encephalitis.

Valproic acid is the anticonvulsant of choice; however, some children require a combination of valproic acid and clobazam to control their seizures. If the seizures and aphasia persist, a trial of steroids should be considered. One recommended schedule consists of oral prednisone, 2 mg/kg/24 hr for 1 mo, tapered to 1 mg/kg/24 hr for an additional month. With clinical improvement, the prednisone is reduced further to 0.5 mg/kg/24 hr for up to 6–12 mo. It is imperative to initiate speech therapy and maintain treatment for several years, as improvement in language function occurs over a prolonged period. Some centers advocate an operative procedure, subpial transection, when medical management fails. Methylphenidate should be considered for patients with severe hyperactivity and inattention. Seizures, if poorly controlled, may be potentiated by methylphenidate; however, anticonvulsants are usually protective. Intravenous immunoglobulin may be helpful in LKS. Some children experience a recurrence of aphasia and seizures after apparent recovery. Most children with LKS have a significant abnormality of speech function during adulthood. The onset of LKS at an early age (<2 yr) uniformly tends to be associated with a poor prognosis for recovery of speech.

602.3 Febrile Seizures

Febrile convulsions rarely develop into epilepsy, and they spontaneously remit without specific therapy. They are the most common seizure disorder during childhood, with a uniformly excellent prognosis. However, a febrile convulsion may signify a serious underlying acute infectious disease such as sepsis or bacterial meningitis, and thus each child must be carefully examined and appropriately investigated for the cause of the associated fever (Chapter 170). Febrile seizures are age dependent and are rare before 9 mo and after 5 yr of age. The peak age of onset is approximately 14–18 mo of age, and the incidence approaches 3–4% of young children. A strong family history of febrile convulsions in siblings and parents suggests a genetic predisposition. Linkage studies in several large families have mapped the febrile seizure gene to chromosomes 19p and 8q13–21. An autosomal dominant inheritance pattern is demonstrated in some families.

CLINICAL MANIFESTATIONS. The convulsion is associated with a rapidly rising temperature and usually develops when the core temperature reaches 39°C or greater. The seizure is typically generalized, tonic-clonic of a few seconds to 10-min duration, followed by a brief postictal period of drowsiness. Febrile seizures persisting longer than 15 min suggest an organic cause such as an infectious or toxic process and require thorough investigation. Because the seizure is no longer present by the time the child reaches the hospital, a physician's most important responsibility is to determine the cause of the fever and to rule out meningitis. *If any doubt exists about the possibility of meningitis, a lumbar puncture with examination of the cerebrospinal fluid (CSF) is indicated.* Viral infections of the upper respiratory tract, roseola, and acute otitis media are most frequently the causes of febrile convulsions.

An EEG is not warranted after a simple febrile seizure. An EEG is indicated for atypical febrile seizures or for a child at risk for developing epilepsy. Atypical febrile seizures include a seizure persisting for more than 15 min, repeated convulsions for several hours or days, and a focal seizure. Approximately 50% of children have recurrent febrile seizures, and a small minority have numerous recurrent seizures. The risk factors for development of epilepsy as a complication of febrile seizures include a positive family history of epilepsy, initial febrile seizure before 9 mo of age, a prolonged or atypical febrile seizure, delayed developmental milestones, and abnormal neurologic findings. The incidence of epilepsy is approximately 9% when several risk factors are present, compared with an incidence of 1% in children who have febrile convulsions and no risk factors.

TREATMENT. Routine treatment of a normal infant who has simple febrile convulsions includes a careful search for the cause of the fever, active measures to control the fever including the use of antipyretics, and reassurance of the parents. Short-term anticonvulsant prophylaxis is not indicated. Prolonged anticonvulsant prophylaxis for preventing recurrent febrile convulsions is controversial and no longer recommended. Antiepileptics such as phenytoin and carbamazepine have no effect on febrile seizures. Phenobarbital has been ineffective in preventing recurrent febrile seizures and may decrease cognitive function in treated children compared with untreated children. Sodium valproate is effective in the management of febrile seizures, but the potential risks of the drug do not justify its use in a disorder with an excellent prognosis irrespective of treatment. Oral diazepam is recommended as an effective and safe method of reducing the risk of recurrence of febrile seizures. At the onset of each febrile illness, diazepam, 0.3 mg/kg q8h PO (1 mg/kg/24 hr), is administered for the duration of the illness (usually 2–3 days). The side effects are usually minor, but symptoms of lethargy, irritability, and ataxia may be reduced by adjusting the dose.

MECHANISMS OF SEIZURES

Although the precise mechanisms of seizures are unknown, several physiologic factors appear to be responsible for the development of a seizure. To initiate a seizure, there must be a group of neurons that are capable of generating a significant burst discharge and a GABAergic inhibitory system. Seizure discharge transmission ultimately depends on excitatory glutamatergic synapses. Evidence suggests that excitatory amino acid neurotransmitters (glutamate, aspartate) may have a role in producing neuronal excitation by acting on specific cell receptors. It is known that seizures may arise from areas of neuronal death and that these regions of the brain may promote development of novel hyperexcitable synapses that can cause seizures. For example, lesions in the temporal lobe (including slow-growing gliomas, hamartomas, gliosis, and arteriovenous malformations) cause seizures, and when the abnormal tissue is removed surgically, the seizures are likely to cease. Further, convulsions may be produced in experimental animals by the phenomenon of *kindling*. In this model, repeated subconvulsive stimulation of the brain (e.g., amygdala) ultimately leads to a generalized convulsion. Kindling may be responsible for the development of epilepsy in humans after an injury to the brain. In humans, it has been proposed that recurrent seizure activity from an abnormal temporal lobe may produce seizures in the contralateral normal temporal lobe by transmission of the stimulus via the corpus collosum.

Seizures are more common in infants and in immature experimental animals. Certain seizures in the pediatric population are age specific (e.g., infantile spasms); this observation suggests that the underdeveloped brain is more susceptible to specific seizures than is the brain of an older child or adult. Genetic factors account for at least 20% of all cases of epilepsy. Using linkage analyses, the chromosomal location of several familial epilepsies has been identified, including benign neonatal convulsions (20q and 8q), juvenile myoclonic epilepsy (6p), and progressive myoclonic epilepsy (21q22.3). The genetic defect of benign familial neonatal convulsions has been characterized by the identification of submicroscopic deletion of chromosome 20q13.3. Study of the cDNAs spanning the deleted region identified one encoding a novel voltage-gated potassium channel, $KCNQ_2$. It is very likely that in the near future the molecular basis of additional epilepsies, such as benign rolandic epilepsy and absence seizures, will be identified. It is also known that the substantia nigra has an integral role in the development of generalized seizures. Electrographic seizure activity spreads within the substantia nigra, causing an increase in uptake of 2-deoxyglucose in adult animals, but there is little or no metabolic activity within the substantia nigra when immature animals have a convulsion. It has been proposed that the functional immaturity of the substantia nigra may have a role in the increased seizure susceptibility of the immature brain. Additionally, the γ-aminobutyric acid (GABA)-sensitive substantia nigra pars reticulata (SNR) neurons play a part in preventing seizures. It is likely that substantia nigra outflow tracts modulate and regulate seizure dissemination but are not responsible for the onset of seizures. Additional research will likely focus on the causes of neuronal hyperexcitability, additional inhibitory mechanisms, the search for nonsynaptic mechanisms of seizure propagation, and GABA receptor abnormalities.

DIAGNOSIS OF SEIZURES

The investigation of a seizure depends on many factors, including the age of the patient, the type and frequency of the seizure, and the presence or absence of neurologic findings and constitutional symptoms. The minimum work-up for the first afebrile seizure in an otherwise healthy child includes a fasting glucose, calcium, magnesium, and serum electrolyte levels and a routine EEG. Demonstration of paroxysmal discharges on the EEG during a clinical seizure is diagnostic of epilepsy, but seizures rarely occur in the EEG laboratory. A normal EEG does not preclude the diagnosis of epilepsy, because the interictal recording is normal in approximately 40% of patients. Activation procedures, including hyperventilation, eye closure, photic stimulation, and, when indicated, sleep deprivation and special electrode placement (e.g., zygomatic leads), substantially increase the positive yield. Seizure discharges are more likely to be recorded in infants and children than in adolescents or adults. Patients who are taking an anticonvulsant and who are scheduled for a routine EEG should not have the medication decreased or discontinued before the study, as status epilepticus could result.

Prolonged EEG monitoring with simultaneous closed-circuit video recording is reserved for complicated cases of protracted and unresponsive seizures. It provides an invaluable method for recording ictal seizure events that are rarely obtained during routine EEG studies. This technique is extremely helpful in the classification of seizures because it can accurately determine the location and frequency of seizure discharges while recording alterations in the level of consciousness and the presence of clinical signs. Patients with pseudoseizures can be readily distinguished from those with true epilepsy, and seizure type (e.g., complex partial vs generalized) can be more precisely identified. Determination of seizure type is critical in the investigation of a child who may be a candidate for epilepsy surgery.

The role of *CT scanning* or *MRI* in the investigation of seizures is controversial. The yield in routine use of these procedures in patients with a first afebrile seizure and normal results of neurological examination is negligible. In studies of children with chronic seizure disorder, the results are similar. Although approximately 30% of these children show a structural abnormality (e.g., focal cortical atrophy or dilated ventricles), only a small minority benefit from active intervention as a result of CT scanning. Thus, CT scanning or MRI should be reserved for patients in whom an intracranial lesion is suspected on the basis of the history or abnormal neurologic finding. Indications for an MRI include complex partial seizures, the presence of focal neurologic signs during or after the seizure, seizures of increasing frequency or severity, a changing seizure pattern, evidence of increased intracranial pressure or trauma, and a first seizure in all adolescents.

Examination of the CSF is indicated if the seizure is potentially related to an infectious process, subarachnoid hemorrhage, or a demyelinating disorder. Specific metabolic tests are outlined in the sections on neonatal seizures and status epilepticus.

602.4 Treatment of Epilepsy

The first step in the management of epilepsy is to ensure that the patient has a seizure disorder and not a condition that mimics epilepsy (see later). It is sometimes difficult to be certain about the cause of a paroxysmal event in a normal child. A negative result on a neurologic examination and EEG usually supports the approach of watchful waiting rather than administration of an anticonvulsant. The true cause of the paroxysmal disorder eventually becomes apparent. Although there is not uniform agreement, most would concur that antiepileptics should be withheld from a previously healthy child with the first afebrile convulsion if there is a negative family history, normal results of an examination and EEG, and a cooperative and compliant family. Approximately 70% of these children will not experience another convulsion. Approximately 75% of those patients with two or three unprovoked seizures have additional seizures. A recurrent seizure, particularly if it occurs in close proximity to the first seizure, is an indication to begin an anticonvulsant. Table 602–2 suggests an approach to a child with a suspected seizure disorder.

The second step involves choosing an anticonvulsant. The drug of choice depends on the classification of the seizure, determined by the history and EEG findings. The goal for every patient should be the use of only one drug with the fewest possible side effects for the control of seizures. The drug is increased slowly until seizure control is accomplished or until undesirable side effects develop. The child's serum anticonvulsant level should be monitored during this stage, and the dose should be altered accordingly. Table 602–3 summarizes the common antiepileptic drugs used in childhood epilepsy and highlights the recommended daily dose, therapeutic serum levels, and common side effects. A suggested loading dose is indicated for drugs that are useful for the treatment of status epilepticus. Physicians should be familiar with the pharmacokinetics of the anticonvulsant and its toxic actions and should monitor the child on a regular basis to gauge the seizure control while watching for unwanted side effects.

Routine serum monitoring of anticonvulsant levels is not recommended because the practice is not cost effective. There are several important indications for anticonvulsant drug monitoring: (1) at the onset of anticonvulsant therapy to confirm that the drug level is within the therapeutic range; (2) for noncompliant patients and families; (3) at the time of status epilepticus; (4) during accelerated growth spurts; (5) for patients on polytherapy, especially valproic acid, phenobarbital, and lamotrigine because of drug interactions; (6) for uncontrolled seizures or seizures that have changed in type; (7) for symptoms and signs of drug toxicity (e.g., toxicity due to a metabolite of carbamazepine, carbamazepine-10,11 epoxide); (8) for patients with hepatic or renal disease; and (9) for children with cognitive or physical disabilities, especially those taking phenytoin, in whom toxicity may be difficult to evaluate. Good clinical judgment is more reliable in achieving seizure control than over-reliance on therapeutic drug monitoring.

There is controversy about whether routine blood tests (complete blood count [CBC], liver function studies) are indicated during anticonvulsant therapy. Because most serious adverse anticonvulsant drug reactions develop during the initial 2–3 mo of therapy, monthly blood screening for the first 3 mo is recommended. Subsequently, routine blood tests are ordered only when clinically indicated.

Anticonvulsants that are introduced during childhood may

TABLE 602–2 An Approach to the Child with a Suspected Convulsive Disorder

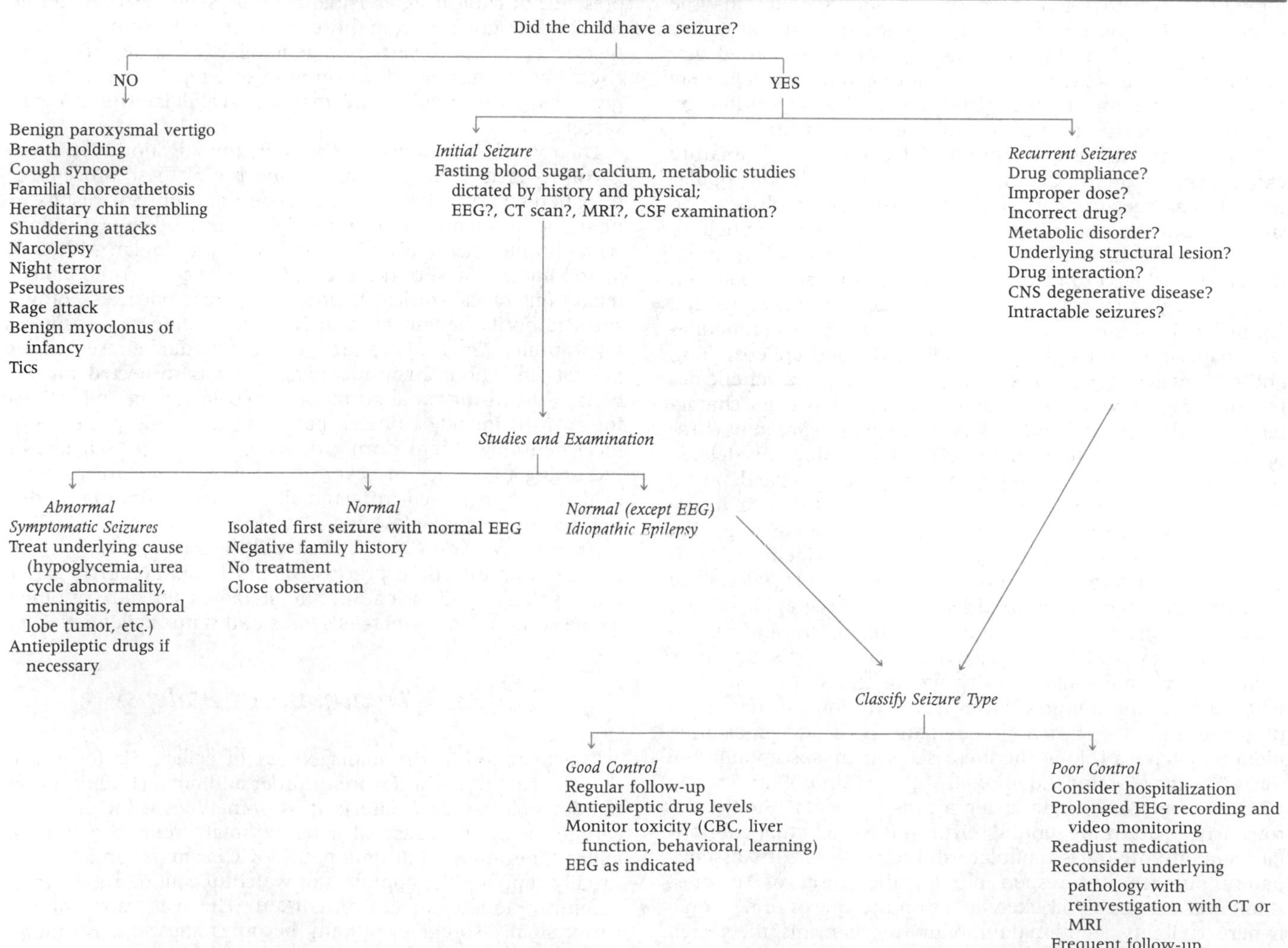

EEG = electroencephalogram; CBC = complete blood count; CNS = central nervous system.

TABLE 602–3 Common Anticonvulsant Drugs

Drug	Seizure Type	Oral Dose	Loading Dose (IV)	Therapeutic Serum Level (μg/mL)	Side Effects and Toxicity
Carbamazepine (Tegretol)	Generalized tonic-clonic Partial	Begin 10 mg/kg/24 hr Increase to 20–30 mg/kg/24 hr tid	—	8–12	Dizziness, drowsiness, diplopia, liver dysfunction, anemia, neutropenia, SIADH, blood dyscrasias rare, hepatotoxic effects
*Clobazam (Frisium)	Adjunctive therapy when seizures poorly controlled	0.25–1 mg/kg/24 hr bid or tid	—	—	Dizziness, fatigue, weight gain, ataxia and behavior problems
Clonazepam (Rivotril)	Absence Myoclonic Infantile spasms Partial Lennox-Gastaut Akinetic	Children <30 kg: Begin 0.05 mg/kg/24 hr Increase by 0.05 mg/kg/wk Maximum 0.2 mg/kg/24 hr bid or tid Children >30 kg: 1.5 mg/kg/24 hr tid, not to exceed 20 mg/24 hr	—	>0.013	Drowiness, irritability, agitation, behavioral abnormalities, depression, excessive salivation
Ethosuximide (Zarontin)	Absence May increase tonic-clonic seizures	Begin 20 mg/kg/24 hr Increase to maximum of 40 mg/kg/24 hr or 1.5 g/24 hr, whichever is less	—	40–100	Abdominal discomfort, skin rash, liver dysfunction, leukopenia
Gabapentin (Neurontin)	Adjuntive therapy when seizures poorly controlled	Children: 20–50 mg/kg/24 hr tid Adolescence: 900–3,600 mg/24 hr tid	—	Not necessary to monitor	Somnolence, dizziness, ataxia, headache, tremor, vomiting, nystagmus, fatigue and weight gain
Lamotrigine (Lamictal)	Adjunctive therapy when seizures poorly controlled Broad-spectrum anticonvulsant activity in various seizure types including: complex partial, absence, myoclonic, clonic, tonic-clonic, and Lennox-Gastaut	Individualized based on age and additional anticonvulsants (see Chapter 602.4)	—	—	Rash, dizziness, ataxia, somolence, diplopia, headache, nausea, vomiting
*Nitrazepam (Mogadon)	Absence Myoclonic Infantile spasms	Begin 0.2 mg/kg/21 hr Increase slowly to 1 mg/kg/24 hr tid	—	—	Similar to clonazepam, hallucinations
Paraldehyde	Generalized status epilepticus	Make a 5% solution by adding 1.75 mL of paraldehyde to D5W with total volume of 35 mL	150–200 mg/kg Maintenance, 20 mg/kg/hr	10–40	
Phenobarbital	Generalized tonic-clonic Partial Status epilepticus	3–5 mg/kg/24 hr bid	20 mg/kg 20–30 mg/kg in the neonate	15–40	Hyperactivity, irritability, short attention span, temper tantrums, altered sleep pattern, Stevens-Johnson syndrome, depression of cognitive function
Phenytoin (Dilantin)	Generalized tonic-clonic Partial Status epilepticus	3–9 mg/kg/24 hr bid	20 mg/kg	10–20	Hirsutism, gum hypertrophy, ataxia, skin rash, Stevens-Johnson sydrome, nystagmus, nausea, vomiting, drowsiness, coarsening facial features, blood dyscrasias
Primidone (Mysoline)	Generalized tonic-clonic Partial	Children <8 yr: 10–25 mg/kg/24 hr tid or qid Children >8 yr: usual maintenance dose, 750–1,500 mg/24 hr tid or qid	—	5–12	Aggressive behavior, personality changes, similar to phenobarbital
Topiramate (Topimax)	Adjunctive therapy for poorly controlled seizures Refractory complex partial seizures	1–9 mg/kg/24 hr bid	—	—	Fatigue, cognitive depression
Tiagabine (Gabitril)	Adjunctive therapy for complex partial seizures	Average dose, 6 mg tid	—	—	Asthenia, dizziness, poor attention span, nervousness, tremor
Valproic acid (Depakene, Epival)	Generalized tonic-clonic Absence Myoclonic Partial Akinetic	Begin 10 mg/kg/24 hr Increase by 5–10 mg/kg/wk Usual dose, 30–60 mg/kg/24 hr tid or qid	Intravenous preparation now available Studies in children under way	50–100	Nausea, vomiting, anorexia, amenorrhea, sedation, tremor, weight gain, alopecia, hepatotoxicity
*Vigabatrin (Sabril)	Infantile spasms Adjunctive therapy for poorly controlled seizures	Begin 30 mg/kg/24 hr once daily or bid Maintenance dose, 30–100 mg/kg/24 hr once daily or bid	—	—	Hyperactivity, agitation, excitement, somnolence, weight gain Note: Reports of visual field constriction, optic pallor or atrophy, and optic neuritis

**Not available in the United States.*
SIADH = syndrome of inappropriate secretion of antidiuretic hormone.

be required during adolescence and the childbearing years. Unfortunately, some anticonvulsants, including phenytoin, valproic acid, carbamazepine, and primidone, are associated with the occurrence of specific birth defects, including facial and limb anomalies and spinal dysraphism. Whether the teratogenic effect is secondary to the mother's epilepsy or the anticonvulsant medication is still debated. Meanwhile, the pediatrician should counsel the family about the possibile relationship and should avoid prescribing an anticonvulsant to a pregnant patient unless it is absolutely necessary.

If complete seizure control is accomplished by an anticonvulsant, a minimum of 2 seizure-free years is an adequate and safe period of treatment for a patient with no risk factors. Prominent risk factors include age greater than 12 yr at onset, neurologic dysfunction (motor handicap or mental retardation), a history of prior neonatal seizures, and numerous seizures before control is achieved. In a child with complete seizure control for a minimum of 2 yr and low risk factors, the chance of recurrence is approximately 20–25%, particularly during the first 6 mo after discontinuation of the anticonvulsant. Those children with the best prognosis following anticonvulsant withdrawal are those with benign epilepsy with rolandic spikes and those with idiopathic generalized seizures. CPS and juvenile myoclonic seizures are more likely to recur. When the decision is made to discontinue the drug, the weaning process should occur for 3–6 mo, because abrupt withdrawal may cause status epilepticus.

Possible sites of action, dose, and side effects of anticonvulsants are noted in Figure 602–2 and Table 602–3.

BENZODIAZEPINES. The benzodiazepines exert anticonvulsant activity by binding to a specific GABA site that enhances the opening frequency of the chloride channel without affecting open or burst duration (see Fig. 602–2). The drugs *diazepam* and *lorazepam* IV are used for initial management of status epilepticus (see Chapter 602.3). *Clonazepam* is useful for the management of the Lennox-Gastaut syndrome, myoclonic, akinetic, and absence seizures. The elimination half-life is 18–50 hr. Clonazepam may increase serum phenytoin concentrations when used together, and additional CNS depression may occur when combined with other CNS depressant drugs. Clonazepam is supplied in 0.5 mg and 2 mg tablets. *Nitrazepam* is useful for the management of myoclonic seizures. The elimination half-life is 18–57 hr. The drug may increase CNS depression when used with additional depressants. Nitrazepam is supplied in 5 and 10 mg tablets. *Clobazam* is indicated as adjunctive therapy for complex partial seizures. The half-life is 10–30 hr. Clobazam may increase the serum drug levels of carbamazepine, phenytoin, phenobarbital, and valproic acid when used concomitantly. Clobazam is supplied in 10 mg tablets.

CARBAMAZEPINE. This drug is effective for the management of generalized tonic-clonic and partial seizures. Carbamazepine acts similarly to phenytoin by decreasing the sustained repetitive firing of neurons by blocking sodium-dependent channels and by decreasing depolarization-dependent calcium uptake. Significant leukopenia (<1,000 neutrophils/mL^3) and hepatotoxicity may rarely develop, particularly during the initial 3–4 mo of therapy. Therefore, a CBC and differential and SGOT

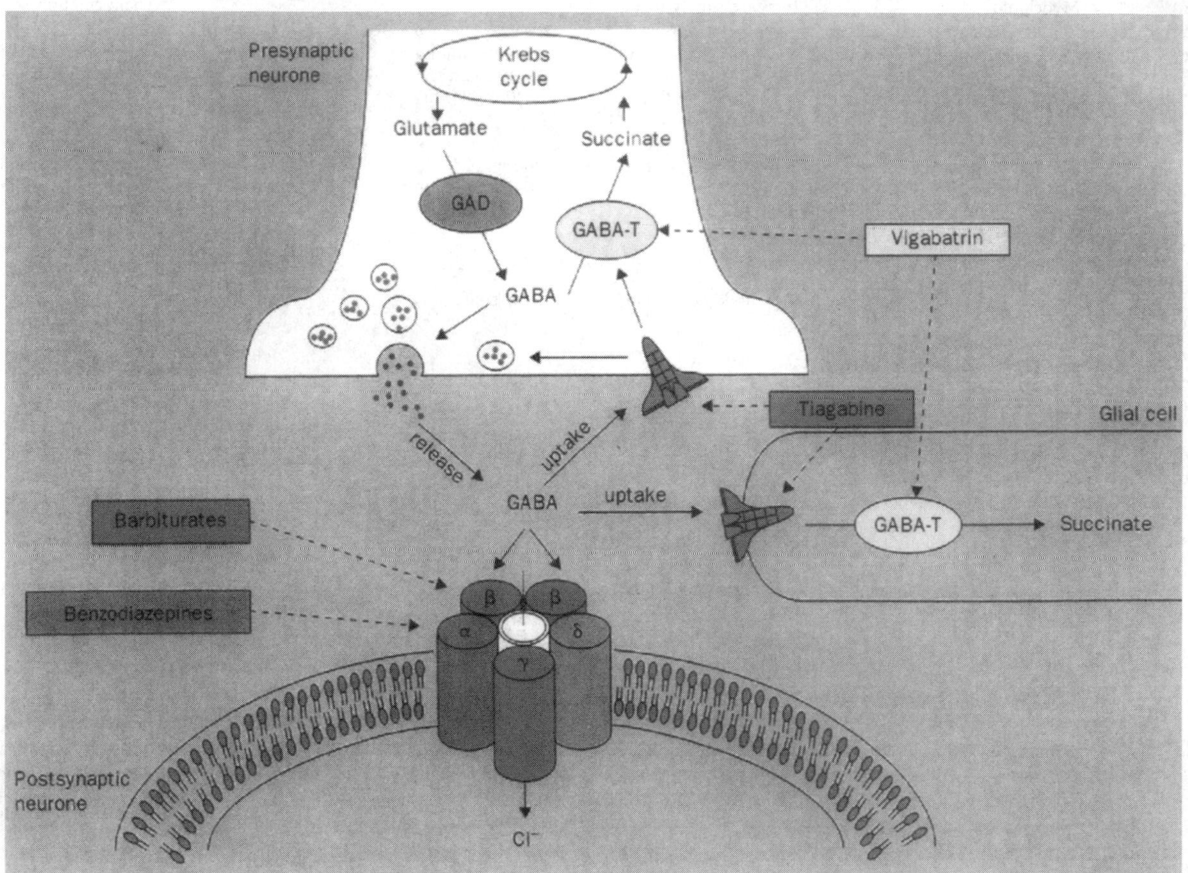

Figure 602–2 Pharmacologic effects of antiepileptic drugs at $GABA_A$ receptor. GABA = γ-aminobutyric acid. GAD = glutamic acid decarboxylase. GABA-T = GABA-transaminase. Barbiturates bind to β-subunit of $GABA_A$ receptor to potentiate action of endogenous agonist GABA and prolong opening time of chloride ion channel. Benzodiazepines bind to α-subunit of $GABA_A$ to potentiate action of GABA and increase frequency of opening of chloride ion channel. Vigabatrin irreversibly binds to GABA-transaminase to inhibit degradation of inhibitory neurotransmitter GABA. Tiagabine blocks uptake of synaptically released GABA into both presynaptic neurones and glial cells, allowing GABA to remain at site of action for longer periods. (From Leach JP, Brodie MJ: Tiagabine. Lancet 351:203, 1998.)

and SGPT levels should be obtained on a monthly basis during this period, although serious idiosyncratic drug reactions may develop despite normal liver function tests results and routine blood work. Subsequent laboratory testing is determined by the presence of adverse symptoms or signs. The parents should be informed of untoward drug effects and instructed to report them immediately to the physician. Erythromycin should be used cautiously with carbamazepine because the two drugs compete for metabolism by the liver. The plasma concentration of carbamazepine is lowered by phenytoin, phenobarbital, and valproic acid. Carbamazepine-10,11-epoxide, which is an active metabolite of carbamazepine, may produce toxicity despite therapeutic carbamazepine levels, particularly when valproic acid is added to the drug regimen. Carbamazepine is supplied in suspension 20 mg/mL, chewtabs 100 and 200 mg tablets, and in a controlled release (CR) form, 200 and 400 mg tablets. The half-life is 8–20 hr, and the drug should be given two or three times daily.

ETHOSUXIMIDE. Ethosuximide provides its anticonvulsant action by blocking calcium channels associated with thalamocortical circuitry. Ethosuximide is an effective drug for the management of typical absence epilepsy and has a half-life of 60 hr. When used with phenobarbital or primidone, ethosuximide may reduce the serum levels of those anticonvulsants. Ethosuximide is supplied in syrup, 50 mg/mL, and in 250 mg capsules.

GABAPENTIN. This anticonvulsant is used as an add-on drug for patients with refractory complex partial and secondarily generalized tonic-clonic seizures. The mechanism of action results from binding of the drug to neuronal membranes (glutamate synapses) and increased brain GABA turnover. The plasma half-life of gabapentin is 5–7 hr. The drug is rapidly absorbed from the gastrointestinal tract, does not bind to plasma proteins, and is not metabolized. Gabapentin has no significant drug interactions and is relatively free of dose-related CNS adverse effects. Gabapentin is recommended for children 12 yr and older. Gabapentin is supplied in 100 mg, 300 mg and 400 mg capsules.

LAMOTRIGINE. Lamotrigine is a phenyltriazine compound used as an add-on drug for the management of complex partial and generalized tonic-clonic seizures. Lamotrigine is effective as monotherapy for some children with the Lennox-Gastaut syndrome and generalized absence seizures. Pharmacologic studies suggest the drug acts at voltage-sensitive sodium channels to stabilize neuronal membranes and inhibit neuronal release, particularly glutamate. The plasma elimination half-life is 22–37 hr. In children, the recommended starting dose is 2 mg/kg/24 hr for 2 wk divided into two doses, followed by 5 mg/kg/24 hr for an additional 2 wk. The maintenance dose is 5–15 mg/kg/24 hr. If lamotrigine is added to valproate therapy, the starting dose of lamotrigine should be reduced to 0.5 mg/kg/24 hr because valproate inhibits the metabolism of lamotrigine. In this case, the maintenance dose of lamotrigine is 1–5 mg/kg/24 hr. The therapeutic serum levels have been reported as 1–4 mg/L or 3.9–15.6 μmol/L. Common side effects include nausea, headache, dizziness, blurred vision, diplopia, and ataxia. A maculopapular skin rash develops in about 3% of patients. The Stevens-Johnson syndrome, angioedema, or toxic epidermal necrolysis occasionally results, usually during the first month of therapy, especially in association with valproate. Because these skin disorders may be fatal, the anticonvulsants must be immediately discontinued. Lamotrigine is supplied in 25, 50, 100, and 200 mg tablets.

PHENOBARBITAL AND PRIMIDONE. These are relatively safe anticonvulsants that are particularly useful for generalized tonic-clonic seizures. Unfortunately, approximately 25% of children undergo severe behavioral changes on these drugs. Neurologically abnormal children are at greater risk. Furthermore, there is evidence that phenobarbital may adversely affect the cognitive performance of children treated on a long-term basis. Valproic acid interferes with the metabolism of phenobarbital causing elevated phenobarbital plasma levels and toxicity despite the usual daily doses. Phenobarbital acts on the GABA receptor to increase the chloride channel open duration (see Fig. 602–2). The plasma half-life is 48–150 hr. Phenobarbital is supplied in an elixir (4 mg/mL) and in 15, 30, 60, and 100 mg tablets and injectable, 30 and 120 mg/mL. Primidone is prepared in a suspension, 50 mg/mL, and in 125 and 250 mg tablets. The plasma half-life of primidone is 10–21 hr. Phenobarbital is prescribed twice daily, and primidone is prescribed three times a day. Routine blood work is not indicated for these anticonvulsants.

PHENYTOIN. Phenytoin acts by decreasing the sustained repetitive firing of single neurons by blocking sodium-dependent channels and by decreasing depolarization-dependent calcium uptake. Phenytoin is used for primary and secondary generalized tonic-clonic seizures, partial seizures, and status epilepticus. The plasma half-life is 7–42 hr. Phenytoin has many drug interactions that may increase or decrease other concomitantly used anticonvulsants (see Table 602–3). Phenytoin is supplied in a suspension, 6 mg/mL and 25 mg/mL; chewable tablets, 50 mg; capsules, 100 mg; and injectable, 100 mg/2 mL and 250 mg/5 mL.

TIAGABINE. Tiagabine inhibits seizure activity by blocking reuptake of the neuroinhibitory transmitter GABA into neuronal and glial cells (see Fig. 602–2). The drug is effective in the management of complex partial seizures as an add-on drug. Tiagabine is supplied in 4, 12, 16, and 20 mg tablets.

TOPIRAMATE. Topiramate produces anticonvulsant action by blocking voltage-dependent sodium channels. The drug is used as adjunctive therapy for refractory complex seizures with or without secondary generalization. The elimination half-life is 21 hr. Phenytoin, carbamazepine, and valproic acid may decrease the concentration of topiramate. Topiramate is dispensed in 25, 100, and 200 mg tablets.

VALPROIC ACID. Valproic acid is a broad-spectrum anticonvulsant. It acts by blocking voltage-dependent sodium channels and increases calcium-dependent potassium conductance. The elimination half-life is 6–16 hr. This drug is useful for the management of many seizure types, including generalized tonic-clonic, absence, atypical absence, and myoclonic seizures. It rarely induces behavioral changes but is associated with mild gastrointestinal disturbances, alopecia, tremor, and hyperphagia. Two rare but serious side effects of valproate are a Reye-like syndrome and irreversible hepatotoxicity. A small number of children develop progressive lethargy and coma with elevated serum ammonia and decreased levels of serum carnitine. Valproic acid may block the metabolism of carnitine, producing the altered state of consciousness in these patients. Discontinuation of valproic acid leads to recovery over several days. Another small group of patients, particularly children younger than 2 yr and having specific neurologic syndromes, who are treated with several anticonvulsants simultaneously, are at significant risk (1:800) for developing an idiosyncratic potentially fatal hepatotoxic syndrome, characterized by abdominal pain, anorexia, weight loss, and retching within a few weeks to months of beginning valproate therapy. These patients have normal results of liver function studies during the initial stages; thus, significant and persistent gastrointestinal symptoms are cause for alarm during the initial few months of valproate therapy. If reduction in the valproate dose does not provide immediate relief, the physician should discontinue the drug. To decrease the risk of fatal hepatotoxicity, a series of screening tests for an underlying metabolic disorder are indicated for a child younger than 2 yr and having a seizure disorder of unknown cause, before initiation of valproic acid therapy. The tests include determinations of serum ammonium, amino acids, blood gases, a lactate-pyruvate ratio, urinary organic acids, and free and total serum carnitine. The incidence of fatal valproic acid–induced hepatotoxicity has decreased dramatically in recent years owing to less use of the drug in epileptic children younger than 2 yr and the knowledge that monotherapy is much less likely to result in fatal liver disease. Valproic acid also may cause a decrease in serum-free carnitine levels by inhibition of plasmalemmal carnitine uptake. Some studies suggest that carnitine deficiency is a major cause of valproate hepatotoxicity and that supplementation with L-carnitine, 50–100 mg/kg/24 hr, may prevent this fatal complication. Until further data are available, it is recommended that L-carnitine supplementation be provided to those children at greatest risk for hepatotoxicity (see earlier). In older children on valproic acid therapy, L-carnitine supplementation should be administered if there are clinical symptoms suggestive of carnitine deficiency (weakness, lethargy, hypotonia) or if a significant decrease in the serum-free carnitine levels is measured on a periodic basis. Valproic acid is available in a syrup, 50 mg/mL; 250 and 500 mg capsules; and 125, 250, and 500 mg tablets.

Depakote sprinkle capsules (divalproex sodium, a stable coordination compound composed of sodium valproate and valproic acid) are useful for children who are unable to tolerate valproate suspension, tablets, or capsules. The contents of the Depakote capsule are sprinkled onto soft food that does not require chewing. Depakote sprinkle capsules are supplied in 125 mg capsules.

VIGABATRIN. Vigabatrin acts by binding to a specific GABA receptor, causing an increase in GABA levels and inhibition of neurotransmission (see Fig. 602–2). The drug is effective in the management of infantile spasms, particularly in children with tuberous sclerosis. Vigabatrin is also useful as adjunctive therapy for poorly controlled seizures. The plasma half-life is 5–8 hr. Vigabatrin may cause a reduction in plasma phenobarbital and phenytoin levels. The drug is supplied in 500 mg tablets and 500 mg sachets.

ACTH. This is the preferred drug for the management of infantile spasms, although the dose and duration of therapy are not uniform. Prednisone is equally effective. A common schedule includes ACTH, 20 units IM daily for 2 wk, and if no response occurs the dose is increased to 30 and then 40 units IM daily for an additional 4 wk. Unless seizure control is complete the ACTH is replaced with oral prednisone, 2 mg/kg/24 hr for 2 wk. If the seizures persist, prednisone is given for an additional 4 wk. The side effects of ACTH include hyperglycemia, hypertension, electrolyte abnormalities, gastrointestinal disturbances, infection, and transient brain shrinkage observed by CT scanning. ACTH and prednisone are equally effective for the treatment of cryptogenic and symptomatic seizures, and control can be expected in approximately 70% of patients. There is no relationship between the ease or degree of seizure control and ultimate neurologic and cognitive outcome. The response to medication is usually apparent within a few weeks of therapy, but one third of patients who respond suffer relapse when the ACTH or prednisone is discontinued.

KETOGENIC DIET. This treatment should be considered for the management of recalcitrant seizures, particularly for children with complex myoclonic epilepsy with associated tonic-clonic convulsions. The diet restricts the quantity of carbohydrate and protein, and most calories are provided as fat. Some children older than 2–3 yr will not tolerate this fatty, unpalatable diet. Because the diet demands precise weighing of foodstuffs and is time consuming to prepare, it is not tolerated by all families. Some children respond to a liberalized ketogenic diet that substitutes medium-chain triglycerides for the high-fat content of the former diet. Although the mechanism of action of the ketogenic diet is unknown, some evidence shows that it exerts an anticonvulsant effect secondary to elevated levels of β-hydroxybutyrate and acetoacetate resulting from the ketosis. The use of valproic acid is contraindicated in association with the ketogenic diet, because the risk of hepatotoxicity is enhanced.

SURGERY FOR EPILEPSY. Surgery should be considered for children with intractable seizures unresponsive to anticonvulsants. Until recently, surgery was reserved for adults with long-standing seizures with a focal onset. Studies have now shown that certain children, particularly those with focal seizures, are also candidates for surgery. Although the history and neurologic examination may suggest a focal onset of seizure activity, an EEG is critical in documenting the localization and extent of the epileptogenic discharges. Prolonged EEG recording with video monitoring, frequently necessary on more than one occasion, is essential for precise localization of the epileptogenic area. It is often helpful to decrease or discontinue the anticonvulsant in hospitalized patients to increase the probability of recording ictal and interictal epileptogenic activity. In those cases when the EEG with the use of sphenoidal electrodes does not adequately localize the focus, placement of subdural electrodes may provide invaluable information. Subdural electrodes are particularly useful in the investigation of epileptogenic foci in sites other than the temporal lobe. EEG studies are complemented by neuropsychologic testing, the Wada (intracarotid injection of amobarbital to establish the dominant hemisphere) test, single photon emission CT (SPECT) or positron emission tomography (PET) scanning, and neuroimaging procedures including CT scanning, MRI, and functional MRI (fMRI). Some centers use magnetic source imaging/magnetoelectroencephalograms (MSI/MEG), which localized seizure discharges more precisely than other techniques. The results of surgery in children with a well-defined focus of epileptogenic activity supported by an identical structural lesion on CT scanning or MRI are extremely favorable and are comparable to those in adults with similar pathology. Further refinement in electrophysiologic testing and neuroimaging will undoubtedly lead to even better surgical results in children with anticonvulsant-unresponsive epilepsy.

COUNSELING THE PARENTS. Most parents are initially frightened by the diagnosis of epilepsy and require support and accurate information. Physicians should anticipate questions, including inquiries about the duration of the seizure disorder, side effects of medication and convulsions, etiology, social and academic repercussions, and parental guilt. Parents usually wish to know if restrictions should be placed on the child and whether the teacher should be informed. Others inquire about the genetic implications, including the risks for future children. Parents should be encouraged to treat their child as normally as possible. For most children with epilepsy, restriction of physical activity is unnecessary except that they must be attended by a responsible adult while bathing and swimming. The mechanism of the seizure and what epilepsy means should be explained, and the purpose and side effects of the specific anticonvulsant should be reviewed. Parents who understand the fundamental action and purpose of anticonvulsants and the need for a specific drug regimen are generally very compliant. Counseling should include first-aid measures to be used if the seizure recurs. Fortunately, most parents and children readily adapt to the seizure disorder and to the requirement for long-term anticonvulsants. Most children with epilepsy are well controlled on medication, have normal intelligence, and can be expected to lead normal lives. These children require careful monitoring of their academic performance because learning disabilities are more common in children with epilepsy than in the general population. Cooperation and understanding among the parents, physician, teacher, and child enhance the outlook for patients with epilepsy.

Annegers JF, Hauser WA, Coan SP, et al: A population-based study of seizures after traumatic brain injuries. N Engl J Med 338:20, 1998.

Baram TZ: Pathophysiology of massive infantile spasms: Perspective on the putative role of the brain adrenal axis. Ann Neurol 33:231, 1993.

Baram TZ, Mitchell WG, Tournay A, et al: High-dose corticotropin (ACTH) versus prednisone for infantile spasms: A prospective, randomized, blinded study. Pediatrics 97:375, 1996.

Berg AT, Shinnar S, Darefsky AS, et al: Predictors of recurrent febrile seizures. Arch Pediatr Adolesc Med 151:371, 1997.

Berkovic SF, Andermann F, Carpenter S, et al: Progressive myoclonus epilepsies: Specific causes and diagnosis. N Engl J Med 315:296, 1986.
Cross JH, Jackson GD, Neville BGR, et al: Early detection of abnormalities in partial epilepsy using magnetic resonance. Arch Dis Child 69:104, 1993.
Delgado-Escueta AV, Enrile-Bacsal FE: Juvenile myoclonic epilepsy of Janz. Neurology 34:285, 1984.
Devinsky O: Cognitive and behavioral effects of antiepileptic drugs. Epilepsia 36(Suppl 2):S46, 1995.
Duchowny M, Harvey AS: Pediatric epilepsy syndromes: An update and critical review. Epilepsia 37(Suppl 1):S26, 1996.
Duchowny MS: Complex partial seizures of infancy. Arch Neurol 44:911, 1987.
Gross-Tsur V, Manor O, van der Meore J: Epilepsy and attention deficit hyperactivity disorder: Is methylphenidate safe and effective? J Pediatr 130:40, 1997.
Hauser WA, Rich SS, Lee JRJ, et al: Risk of recurrent seizures after two unprovoked seizures. N Engl J Med 338:429, 1998.
Holmes GL: Partial seizures in children. Pediatrics 77:725, 1986.
Lagae LG, Silberstein J, Gillis PL, et al: Successful use of intravenous immunoglobins in Landau-Kleffner syndrome. Pediatr Neurol 18:165, 1998.
Leach JP, Brodie MJ: Tiagabine. Lancet 351:203, 1998.
Maher J, McLachlan RS: Febrile convulsions in selected large families: A single-major-locus mode of inheritance? Dev Med Child Neurol 39:79, 1997.
Minassian BA, Lee JR, Henbrick JA, et al: Mutations in a gene encoding a novel protein tyrosine phosphate cause progressive myoclonus epilepsy. Nat Genet 20:171, 1998.
Neville BGR: Epilepsy in childhood. Br Med J 315:924, 1997.
Offringa M, Bossuyt PMM, Lubsen J, et al: Risk factors for seizure recurrence in children with febrile seizures. A pooled analysis of individual patient data from five studies. J Pediatr 124:574, 1994.
Sandramouli S, Robinson R, Tsaloumas M, et al: Retinal haemorrhages and convulsions. Arch Dis Child 76:449, 1997.
Singh NA, Charlier C, Stauffer D, et al: A novel potassium channel gene, $KCNQ_2$, is mutated in an inherited epilepsy of newborns. Nat Genet 18:25, 1998.
Verity CM: Do seizures damage the brain? The epidemiological evidence. Arch Dis Child 78:78, 1998.
Vining EPG, Freeman JM, Pillas DJ, et al: Why would you remove half a brain? The outcome of 58 children after hemispherectomy—the Johns Hopkins experience: 1968 to 1996. Pediatrics 100:163, 1997.
Wallace SJ: First tonic-clonic seizures in childhood. Lancet 349:1009, 1997.

602.5 Neonatal Seizures

Neonates are at particular risk for the development of seizures because metabolic, toxic, structural, and infectious diseases are more likely to be manifested during this time than at any other period of life. Neonatal seizures are dissimilar from those in a child or adult because generalized tonic-clonic convulsions tend not to occur during the 1st mo of life. The arborization of axons and dendritic processes as well as myelination is incomplete in the neonatal brain. A seizure discharge therefore cannot readily be propagated throughout the neonatal brain to produce a generalized seizure. At least five seizure types are recognizable in newborn infants.

CLINICAL MANIFESTATIONS AND CLASSIFICATION. *Focal seizures* consist of rhythmic twitching of muscle groups, particularly those of the extremities and face. These seizures are often associated with localized structural lesions as well as with infections and subarachnoid hemorrhage. *Multifocal clonic* convulsions are similar to focal clonic seizures but differ in that many muscle groups are involved, frequently several simultaneously. *Tonic seizures* are characterized by rigid posturing of the extremities and trunk and are sometimes associated with fixed deviation of the eyes. *Myoclonic seizures* are brief focal or generalized jerks of the extremities or body that tend to involve distal muscle groups. *Subtle seizures* consist of chewing motions, excessive salivation, and alterations in the respiratory rate including apnea, blinking, nystagmus, bicycling or pedaling movements, and changes in color.

Neonatal seizures may be difficult to recognize clinically, and some neonatal behaviors that were considered previously to be convulsions are not substantiated by the EEG recording. Nonetheless, several clinical features distinguish seizures from nonepileptic activity in neonates. Autonomic changes such as tachycardia and elevation of the blood pressure are common with seizures but do not occur with nonepileptic events. Nonepileptic movements are suppressed by gentle restraint, but true seizures are not. Nonepileptic phenomena are enhanced by sensory stimuli that have no influence on seizures. Correct classification of neonatal seizures is important for appropriate selection of anticonvulsant therapy. Studies using polygraphic EEG recording with video monitoring have greatly enhanced the characterization of neonatal seizures and their medical management.

EEG CLASSIFICATION OF NEONATAL SEIZURES

Clinical Seizure with a Consistent EEG Event. In this category, a clinical seizure occurs in relationship to seizure activity recorded on the EEG and includes focal clonic, focal tonic, and some myoclonic seizures. These seizures are clearly epileptic and are likely to respond to an anticonvulsant.

Clinical Seizures with Inconsistent EEG Events. Neonates may have a clinical seizure without a corresponding seizure discharge. This is observed with all generalized tonic seizures and subtle seizures and with some myoclonic seizures. These infants tend to be neurologically depressed or comatose as a result of hypoxic-ischemic encephalopathy. Seizures in this category are likely to be of nonepileptic origin and may not require or respond to antiepileptics.

Electrical Seizures with Absent Clinical Seizures. Electrical seizures associated with a markedly abnormal background EEG may develop in comatose infants who are not on anticonvulsants. Conversely, electrical seizures may persist in patients with focal tonic or clonic seizures without clinical signs after the introduction of an anticonvulsant.

ETIOLOGIC DIAGNOSIS. The most common cause of neonatal seizures, hypoxic-ischemic encephalopathy, is discussed in Chapter 95.7. Many additional disorders are likely to cause seizures, including metabolic, infectious, traumatic, structural, hemorrhagic, embolic, and maternal disturbances. Because seizures in neonates may indicate a serious, life-threatening, and potentially reversible disease, it is imperative that a timely and organized approach to the investigation of neonatal seizures be carried out.

Careful neurologic examination of the infant may uncover the cause of the seizure disorder. Examination of the retina may show the presence of chorioretinitis, suggesting a congenital infection in which case TORCH titers of mother and infant are indicated. The *Aicardi syndrome*, which occurs exclusively in infant girls, is associated with coloboma of the iris and retinal lacunae, refractory seizures, and absence of the corpus callosum. Inspection of the skin may show hypopigmented lesions characteristic of tuberous sclerosis or the typical crusted vesicular lesions of incontinentia pigmenti; both neurocutaneous syndromes are associated with generalized myoclonic seizures beginning early in life. An unusual body odor suggests an inborn error of metabolism.

Blood should be obtained for determinations of glucose, calcium, magnesium, electrolytes, and blood urea nitrogen (BUN). If hypoglycemia is a possibility, a serum Dextrostix testing is indicated so that treatment can be initiated immediately. See Chapter 103.2 for a discussion of the diagnosis and treatment of hypoglycemia. Hypocalcemia may occur in isolation or in association with hypomagnesemia. A lowered serum calcium level is often associated with birth trauma or a CNS insult in the perinatal period. Additional causes include maternal diabetes, prematurity, the DiGeorge syndrome, and high-phosphate feedings. See Chapters 55.9 and 102 for a full discussion. Hypomagnesemia (<1.5 mg/dL) is often associated with hypocalcemia and occurs particularly in infants of malnourished mothers. In this situation, the seizures are resistant to calcium therapy but respond to intramuscular magnesium, 0.2 mL/kg of a 50% solution of $MgSO_4$. See Chapter 102 for diagnosis and treatment of hypomagnesemia. Serum electrolyte measurement may indicate significant hyponatremia (serum sodium <135 mEq/L) or hypernatremia (serum sodium >150 mEq/L) as a cause of the seizure disorder.

A *lumbar puncture* is indicated in virtually all neonates with seizures, unless the cause is obviously related to a metabolic disorder such as hypoglycemia or hypocalcemia secondary to feeding of high concentrations of phosphate. These latter infants are normally alert interictally and usually respond promptly to appropriate therapy. The CSF findings may indicate a bacterial meningitis or aseptic encephalitis (see Chapters 105 and 106). Prompt diagnosis and appropriate therapy improve the outcome for these infants. Bloody CSF indicates a traumatic tap or a subarachnoid/intraventricular bleed. Immediate centrifugation of the specimen may assist in differentiation of the two disorders. A clear supernatant suggests a traumatic tap, and a xanthochromic color suggests a subarachnoid bleed. However, mildly jaundiced normal infants may have a yellowish discoloration of the CSF that makes inspection of the supernatant less reliable in the newborn period.

Many *inborn errors of metabolism* cause generalized convulsions in the newborn period. Because these conditions are often inherited in an autosomal recessive or X-linked recessive fashion, it is imperative that a careful family history be obtained to determine if siblings or close relatives developed seizures or expired at an early age. Serum ammonia determination is useful for screening for suspected urea cycle abnormalities, such as ornithine transcarbamylase, arginosuccinic lysate, and carbamylphosphate synthetase deficiencies. In addition to having generalized clonic seizures, these infants present during the first few days of life with increasing lethargy progressing to coma, anorexia and vomiting, and a bulging fontanel. If the blood gases show an anion gap and a metabolic acidosis with hyperammonemia, urine organic acids should be immediately determined to investigate the possibility of methylmalonic or propionic acidemia. Maple syrup urine disease (MSUD) should be suspected when a metabolic acidosis occurs in association with generalized clonic seizures, vomiting, and muscle rigidity during the 1st wk of life. The result of a rapid screening test using 2,4-dinitrophenylhydrazine that identifies ketoderivatives in the urine is positive in MSUD. Additional metabolic causes of neonatal seizures include nonketotic hyperglycemia, a lethal condition characterized by markedly elevated plasma and CSF glycine levels, persistent generalized seizures, and lethargy rapidly leading to coma; ketotic hyperglycinemia in which seizures are associated with vomiting, fluid and electrolyte disturbances, and a metabolic acidosis; and Leigh's disease suggested by elevated levels of serum and CSF lactate or an increased lactate/pyruvate ratio. Biotinidase deficiency should also be considered. A comprehensive description of the diagnosis and management of these metabolic diseases is discussed in Part X.

Unintentional *injection of a local anesthetic* into a fetus during labor can produce intense tonic seizures. These infants are often thought to have had a traumatic delivery because they are flaccid at birth, they have abnormal brain stem reflexes, and they show signs of respiratory depression that sometimes requires ventilation. Examination may show a needle puncture of the skin or a perforation or laceration of the scalp. An elevated serum anesthetic level confirms the diagnosis. The treatment consists of supportive measures and promotion of urine output by administering intravenous fluids with appropriate monitoring to prevent fluid overload.

Benign familial neonatal seizures, an autosomal dominant condition, begins on the 2nd–3rd day of life, with a seizure frequency of 10–20/day. Patients are normal between seizures, which stop in 1–6 mo. *Fifth-day fits* occur on day 5 of life (4–6 days) in normal-appearing neonates. The seizures are multifocal and are present for less than 24 hr. The prognosis is good.

Pyridoxine dependency, a rare disorder, must be considered when generalized clonic seizures begin shortly after birth with signs of fetal distress in utero. These seizures are particularly resistant to conventional anticonvulsants, such as phenobarbital or phenytoin. The history may suggest that similar seizures occurred in utero. Some cases of pyridoxine dependency are reported to begin later in infancy or in early childhood. This condition is inherited as an autosomal recessive. Although the precise biochemical defect is unknown, pyridoxine is essential for the synthesis of glutamic acid decarboxylase, which in turn is required for the synthesis of GABA. In affected infants, large amounts of pyridoxine are required to maintain adequate production of GABA. When pyridoxine-dependent seizures are suspected, 100 to 200 mg of pyridoxine should be administered intravenously during the EEG, which should be promptly completed once the diagnosis is considered. The seizures will abruptly cease, and the EEG will normalize during the next few hours. However, not all cases of pyridoxine dependency respond dramatically to the initial bolus of IV pyridoxine. Therefore, A 6-wk trial of oral pyridoxine (10–20 mg daily) is recommended for those infants in whom a high index of suspicion continues after a negative response to IV pyridoxine. In the future, measurement of CSF and plasma pyridoxal-5-phosphate may prove to be the more precise method of confirming the diagnosis of pyridoxine dependency. These children require lifelong supplementation of oral pyridoxine, 10 mg/day. Generally, the earlier the diagnosis and therapy with pyridoxine, the more favorable will be the outcome. Untreated children have persistent seizures and are uniformly severely mentally retarded (see also Chapter 44.6).

Drug withdrawal seizures can present in the newborn nursery but may take several weeks to develop because of prolonged excretion of the drug by the neonate. The incriminated drugs include barbiturates, benzodiazepines, heroin, and methadone. The infant may be jittery, irritable, and lethargic and may show myoclonus or frank clonic seizures. The mother may deny the use of drugs; a serum or urine analysis may identify the responsible agent (see Chapter 102).

Infants with focal seizures, suspected stroke or intracranial hemorrhage, and severe *cytoarchitectural abnormalities* of the brain including lissencephaly, schizencephaly, which clinically may appear normal or microcephalic, should undergo MRI or CT imaging. Indeed, many recommend imaging of all neonates with seizures unexplained by serum glucose, calcium, or electrolyte disorders. Infants with chromosome abnormalities and adrenoleukodystrophy are also at risk for seizures and should be evaluated with investigation of a karyotype and serum long-chain fatty acids, respectively.

TREATMENT. Anticonvulsants should be used in the treatment of infants with seizures secondary to hypoxic-ischemic encephalopathy or an acute intracranial bleed (Chapters 95.2 and 95.7). The dose and administration of phenobarbital, diazepam, and other medications for the treatment of neonatal seizures are discussed in Chapter 95.7. The greater use of EEG recording in infants with subtle seizures has identified a number of patients with abnormal movements unrelated to seizure discharges; anticonvulsants are not indicated for this group of neonates.

PROGNOSIS. This depends mainly on the primary cause of the disorder or the severity of the insult. In the case of hypoglycemic infants of a diabetic mother or hypocalcemia associated with excessive phosphate feedings, the prognosis is excellent. Conversely, a child with intractable seizures due to severe hypoxic-ischemic encephalopathy or a cytoarchitectural abnormality of the brain usually does not respond to anticonvulsants and is susceptible to status epilepticus and early death. The challange for the physician is to identify patients who will recover with prompt treatment and to avoid delays in diagnosis that could lead to severe, irreversible neurologic damage.

Donn S, Grasela T, Goldstein G: Safety of a higher loading dose of phenobarbital in the term newborn. Pediatrics 74:1061, 1985.

Gilman JT, Gal P, Duchowny MS, et al: Rapid sequential phenobarbital treatment of neonatal seizures. Pediatrics 83:674, 1989.

Gospe SM, Olin KL, Keen CL: Reduced GABA synthesis in pyridoxine-dependent seizures. Lancet 343:1133, 1994.

Herzlinger RA, Krandall SR, Vaughan HG: Neonatal seizures associated with narcotic withdrawal. J Pediatr 91:683, 1977.
Hillman L, Hillman R, Dodson WE: Diagnosis, treatment and follow-up of neonatal mepivacaine intoxication secondary to paracervical and pudendal blocks during labor. J Pediatr 95:472, 1979.
Hunt AD, Stokes J, McCrory WW, et al: Pyridoxine dependency: Report of a case of intractable convulsions in an infant controlled by pyridoxine. Pediatrics 13:140, 1964.
Kellaway P, Mizrahi EM: Neonatal seizures, *In:* Luders H, Lesser RP (eds): Epilepsy, Electroclinical Syndromes. New York, Springer-Verlag, 1987, pp 13–47.
Koren G, Warwicke B, Rajchgot R, et al: Intravenous paraldehyde for seizure control in newborn infants. Neurology 36:108, 1986.
Legido A, Clancy RR, Berman P: Neurologic outcome after electroencephalographically proven neonatal seizures. Pediatrics 88:583, 1991.
Mizrahi E, Kellaway P: Characterizations and classification of neonatal seizures. Neurology 37:1837, 1987.
Painter MJ, Pippenger C, Wasterlain C, et al: Phenobarbital and phenytoin in neonatal seizures: Metabolism and tissue distribution. Neurology 31:1107, 1981.
Sillanpää M, Jalava M, Kaleva O, et al: Long-term prognosis of seizures with onset in childhood. N Engl J Med 338:1715, 1998.
Volpe JJ: Neonatal seizures: Current concepts and revised classification. Pediatrics 84:422, 1989.

602.6 Status Epilepticus

Status epilepticus is defined as a continuous convulsion lasting longer than 30 min or the occurrence of serial convulsions between which there is no return of consciousness. Status epilepticus may be classified as generalized (tonic-clonic, absence) or partial (simple, complex, or with secondary generalization). Generalized tonic-clonic seizures predominate in cases of status epilepticus. Status epilepticus is a medical emergency that requires an organized and skillful approach in order to minimize the associated mortality and morbidity.

ETIOLOGY. There are three major subtypes of status epilepticus in children: prolonged *febrile seizures; idiopathic status epilepticus,* in which a seizure develops in the absence of an underlying CNS lesion or insult; and *symptomatic status epilepticus,* when the seizure occurs as a result of an underlying neurologic disorder or a metabolic abnormality. A febrile seizure lasting for more than 30 min, particularly in a child younger than 3 yr of age, is the most common cause of status epilepticus. The idiopathic group includes epileptic patients who have had sudden withdrawal of anticonvulsants (especially benzodiazepines and barbiturates) followed by status epilepticus. Epileptic children who are given anticonvulsants on an irregular basis or who are noncompliant are more likely to develop status epilepticus. Status epilepticus may also be the initial presentation of epilepsy. Sleep deprivation and an intercurrent infection tend to render epileptic patients more susceptible to status epilepticus. The mortality and morbidity among patients with prolonged febrile seizures and idiopathic status epilepticus are low. Status epilepticus owing to other causes has a much higher mortality, and the cause of death usually is directly attributable to the underlying abnormality. Unlike those with idiopathic status epilepticus, many of these children have not previously had a convulsion. Severe anoxic encephalopathy presents with seizures during the first few days of life, and the ultimate prognosis relates partly to the ease in controlling the seizures. A prolonged convulsion may be the initial manifestation of encephalitis, and epilepsy may be a long-term complication of meningitis. Infants with congenital malformations of the brain (e.g., lissencephaly or schizencephaly) may have recurrent episodes of status epilepticus that are frequently refractory to anticonvulsants. Inborn errors of metabolism may present with status epilepticus in newborns. Affected infants often have a progressive loss of consciousness associated with failure to thrive and excessive vomiting. Electrolyte abnormalities, hypocalcemia, hypoglycemia, drug intoxication, Reye syndrome, lead intoxication, extreme hyperpyrexia, and brain tumors, particularly in the frontal lobe, are additional causes of status epilepticus.

PATHOPHYSIOLOGY. The relationship between the neurologic outcome and the duration of status epilepticus is unknown in children and adults. Some evidence shows that the period of status epilepticus that produces neuronal injury in a child is less than that for an adult. In primates, pathologic changes can occur in the brain of ventilated animals after 60 min of constant seizure activity when metabolic homeostasis is maintained. Thus, cell death may result from excessively increased metabolic demands by continually discharging neurons. The most vulnerable areas of the brain include the hippocampus, amygdala, cerebellum, middle cortical area, and thalamus. Characteristic acute pathologic changes consist of venous congestion, small petechial hemorrhages, and edema. Ischemic cellular changes are the earliest histologic finging, followed by neuronophagia, microglial proliferation, cell loss, and increased numbers of reactive astrocytes. Prolonged seizures are associated with lactic acidosis, an alteration in the blood-brain barrier, and elevation of ICP and temperature. A series of complex, poorly understood hormonal and biochemical changes ensues. Circulating levels of prolactin, ACTH, cortisol, glucagon, growth hormone, insulin, epinephrine, and cyclic nucleotides are elevated during status epilepticus in the animal. Neuronal concentrations of calcium, arachidonic acid, and prostaglandins rise and may promote cell death. Initially, the animal may be hyperglycemic, but hypoglycemia ultimately occurs. Inevitably, dysfunction of the autonomic nervous system develops and may lead to hypotension and shock. These series of biochemical changes are not unique to status epilepticus because they may also follow severe mechanical and stress injuries. Constant tonic-clonic muscle activity during a seizure may produce myoglobinuria and acute tubular necrosis.

Several investigations have shown significant increases in cerebral blood flow and metabolic rate during status epilepticus. In animals, approximately 20 min of status epilepticus produces regional oxygen insufficiency, which promotes cell damage and necrosis. The studies have led to the concept of a critical period during status epilepticus when irreversible neuronal changes may develop. This *transitional period* varies between 20 and 60 min in animals during constant seizure activity. Treatment of children should be directed to supporting vital functions and to controlling the convulsions as expeditiously as possible, because the precise transitional period in humans is unknown.

TREATMENT. *Initial treatment* of patients begins with an assessment of the respiratory and cardiovascular systems. Children should be transferred to an intensive care unit if possible. The oral airway is secured and inspected for patency, and the pulse, temperature, respirations, and blood pressure are recorded. Excessive oral secretions are removed by gentle suction, and a properly fitting face mask attached to oxygen is applied. If patients do not respond to oxygen by mask or are difficult to ventilate by an Ambu bag, consideration should be given to intubation and assisted ventilation. A nasogastric tube is placed in position, and an IV catheter is immediately inserted. If hypoglycemia is confirmed by Dextrostix, a rapid infusion of 5 mL/kg of 10% dextrose is provided. Blood is obtained for a CBC and for determination of electrolytes (including calcium, phosphorus, and magnesium), glucose, creatinine, lactate, and anticonvulsant levels, if indicated. Blood and urine may be obtained for metabolic studies and toxicology, keeping in mind that some drugs potentiate or precipitate status epilepticus, (e.g., amphetamines, cocaine, phenothiazines, theophylline in toxic levels, and tricyclic antidepressants). Arterial blood gases should be determined, and it is wise to monitor oxygen saturation (SaO_2) with an oximeter. Examination of the CSF is imperative if meningitis or encephalitis is considered, unless there is a contraindication to the procedure. In this case, appropriate antibiotics should be administered, followed by imaging studies, before a lumbar puncture is attempted. If the seizures are refractory to the front-line anticonvulsants, or the patient is paralyzed and is on a respirator, continuous EEG monitoring is important to monitor the frequency of seizure discharges, their location, and the response to anticonvulsant therapy.

A physical and neurologic examination should be carried out concurrently to assess evidence of trauma; papilledema, a bulging anterior fontanel, or lateralizing neurologic signs suggesting increased ICP; manifestations of sepsis or meningitis; retinal hemorrhages that may indicate a subdural hematoma; Kussmaul breathing and dehydration suggestive of metabolic acidosis or irregular respirations signifying brain stem dysfunction; evidence of failure to thrive, a peculiar body odor, or abnormal hair pigmentation that suggests an inborn error of metabolism; and constriction or dilatation of pupils suggesting a toxin or drugs as the cause of the status epilepticus. A comprehensive examination should be undertaken once the seizures are under control. Further investigation of the patient including neuroradiologic studies depends on the physical and neurologic findings and on a precise history of the seizure type and frequency.

Drugs should always be delivered IV in the management of status epilepticus; the intramuscular (IM) route is unreliable because some drugs are bounded by muscle. One of the major problems in the management of status epilepticus is the inappropriate use of anticonvulsants. An unsuitably low drug dose is too often given, and with lack of response, another antiepileptic is introduced immediately. Care should be given with regard to how the anticonvulsant is delivered. Phenytoin forms a precipitate in glucose solutions and is rendered ineffective. Other drugs interact with plastic containers or are altered by sunlight (e.g., paraldehyde). It is essential to have resuscitation equipment at the bedside and the ability to intubate and ventilate the patient immediately if respiratory depression should supervene.

A benzodiazepine (diazepam, lorazepam, or midazolam) may be used initially, because these are effective for immediate control of prolonged tonic-clonic seizures in most children. Diazepam should be given IV directly into the vein (not the tubing) in a dose of 0.1–0.3 mg/kg at a rate no greater than 2 mg/min for a maximum of three doses. Respiratory depression and hypotension can occur, especially if administered with a barbiturate. Diazepam is effective in the management of tonic-clonic status, but the drug has a short half-life and seizures thus recur unless a longer acting anticonvulsant is administered simultaneously. Lorazepam is an equally effective short-term anticonvulsant, with a greater duration of action and decreased likelihood of producing hypotension and respiratory arrest. The recommended dose is 0.05–0.1 mg/kg administered slowly, IV. The dose of midazolam is 0.15–0.3 mg/kg IV. If an IV line cannot be established or the child is some distance from a medical center, rectal diazepam or lorazepam can be used safely. Diazepam diluted in 3 mL 0.9% NaCl is placed into the rectum by a syringe and a flexible tube at a dose of 0.3–0.5 mg/kg. The effective dose of rectal lorazepam is 0.05–0.1 mg/kg. Therapeutic serum levels occur within 5–10 min. Sublingual lorazepam may be used to treat children with serial seizures that tend to develop into status epilepticus while the children are at home. The dose of sublingual lorazepam is 0.05–0.1 mg/kg. The tablet is placed under the patient's tongue and dissolves in a few seconds.

After administration of diazepam or lorazepam, several options are available for further management. If the convulsive activity ceases after diazepam or lorazepam therapy or if the seizures persist, *phenytoin* is given immediately. The loading dose of phenytoin is 15 up to 30 mg/kg IV (given in 10 mg/kg increments) at the rate of 1 mg/kg/min. Phenytoin may be safely added to half-normal or normal saline but not to glucose solutions; the undiluted drug can cause pain, irritation, and phlebitis of the vein. An electrocardiogram tracing is recommended during the loading phase to identify arrhythmias and bradycardia, a rare complication in children. Systemic hypotension may also complicate IV phenytoin. If the seizures do not recur, a maintenance dose of 3–9 mg/kg divided into two equal doses daily is begun 12–24 hr later. Serum phenytoin levels should be monitored because the maintenance dose varies considerably with age. Phenytoin is not always effective in controlling tonic-clonic status epilepticus, in which case an alternative drug is necessary. In some centers, *phenobarbital* is initiated before phenytoin. It is given in a loading dose of 15–20 mg/kg or in neonates 20–30 mg/kg IV during 10–30 min. With control of the seizures, the maintenance dose is 3–5 mg/kg/24 hr divided into two equal doses.

If the status epilepticus is not controlled by the preceding strategy, the physician must make some important therapeutic decisions, because it is likely the *transitional period* has passed. The choices for further drug management include paraldehyde, a diazepam infusion, barbiturate coma, or general anesthesia. By this stage, the patient is usually sedated and may show signs of respiratory depression, necessitating elective intubation and assisted ventilation.

Constant IV infusion of either midazolam (0.20 mg/kg bolus, 1–5 μg/kg/min infusion) or propofol (1–2 mg/kg, 2–10 mg/kg/hr infusion) has been effective in managing seizures during status epilepticus unresponsive to other anticonvulsants. If seizures continue, serious consideration is given to induction of barbiturate coma. In an intensive care unit, the patient is placed on a ventilator and a continuous EEG monitor. The initial IV loading dose of thiopental is 2–4 mg/kg and is then titrated to achieve a burst suppression EEG pattern. Barbiturate coma is continued for at least 48 hr, followed by cessation of thiopental until the serum phenobarbital level falls to the therapeutic range. Barbiturate coma requires careful monitoring because hypotension due to myocardial depression often requires pressor therapy.

Paraldehyde is relatively safe for administration to children. A 5% solution of paraldehyde is prepared by adding 1.75 mL of paraldehyde (1 g/mL) to D5W to a total volume of 35 mL. The loading dose is 150–200 mg/kg IV slowly for 15–20 min, and then seizure control is maintained with an infusion of 20 mg/kg/hr in a 5% concentration in a glass bottle, because the drug is incompatible with plastic. The IV drip rate may be lowered as the seizures and EEG improve. The drug should be freshly opened, because outdated paraldehyde can deteriorate to acetylaldehyde and acetic acid.

General anesthesia is an alternative adjunct to the management of status epilepticus if conventional drug therapy is not effective or if barbiturate coma is not an option. Several agents have been used successfully, including halothane and isoflurane. General anesthesia probably acts by reversing cerebral anoxia and the concomitant metabolic abnormalities, allowing the previously administered anticonvulsants to exert their effect. The major disadvantage of general anesthesia is that it must be administered by well-trained personnel with anesthetic gas scavenging equipment for prolonged periods.

Valproic acid has been an effective anticonvulsant in the management of several types of seizures. Valproic acid is available as an injectable and may be given IV. Preliminary studies recommend a loading dose of IV valproic acid, 10–15 mg/kg. IV valproic acid may become a useful drug for status epilepticus.

The use of anticonvulsant therapy after status epilepticus is controversial. There is little question that a long-term antiepileptic should be maintained in children with a progressive neurologic disorder or with a history of recurrent seizures before the onset of status epilepticus. However, it is unlikely that a lengthy period of anticonvulsant treatment is necessary after an initial attack of idiopathic status epilepticus, particularly when a prolonged febrile seizure was the cause. Anticonvulsant therapy is maintained arbitrarily for 3 mo in this case and is discontinued if the child remains asymptomatic.

PROGNOSIS. The neurologic outcome after status epilepticus has improved significantly since the advent of modern pediatric intensive care units and the aggressive management of prolonged seizures. The mortality rate of status epilepticus is approximately 5% in most series. The greatest number of deaths occur in the symptomatic group, most of whom have a serious and life-threatening CNS disorder known before the onset of status epilepticus. In the absence of a progressive neurologic insult or metabolic disorder, the morbidity from status epilepticus is low. The fact that long-term sequelae such as hemiplegia, extrapyramidal syndromes, mental retardation, and epilepsy are more common in children younger than 1 yr following status epilepticus is related to the fact that this group is more likely to have a premorbid underlying CNS disorder than are older children.

Aicardi J, Chevrie JJ: Consequences of status epilepticus in infants and children. Adv Neurol 34:115, 1983.

Curless RG, Holzman BH, Ramsay RE: Paraldehyde therapy in childhood status epilepticus. Arch Neurol 40:447, 1983.

Dulac O, Aicardi J, Rey E, et al: Blood levels of diazepam after single rectal administration in infants and children. J Pediatr 93:1039, 1978.

Koul RL, Aithala GR, Chacko A, et al: Continuous midazolam infusion as treatment of status epilepticus. Arch Dis Child 76:445, 1997.

Kreisman NR, Rosenthal M, LaManna JC, et al: Cerebral oxygenation during recurrent seizures. Adv Neurol 34:231, 1983.

Lowenstein DH, Alldredge BK: Status epilepticus. N Engl J Med 338:970, 1998.

Maytal J, Shinnar S, Moshe SL, et al: Low morbidity and mortality of status epilepticus in children. Pediatrics 83:323, 1989.

Working Group on Status Epilepticus: Treatment of convulsive status epilepticus. JAMA 270:854, 1993.

Yager JY, Seshia SS: Sublingual lorazepam in childhood serial seizures. Am J Dis Child 142:931, 1988.

Young RSK, Ropper AH, Hawkers D, et al: Pentobarbital in refractory status epilepticus. Pediatr Pharmacol 3:63, 1983.

602.7 Rickets Associated with Anticonvulsant Therapy

Russel W. Chesney

A small group of children receiving chronic anticonvulsant therapy will present with calcium-deficient rickets, despite apparently adequate vitamin D intake. This condition is more common after the combination of phenobarbital and phenytoin, but it has been associated with almost all anticonvulsant drugs. Affected patients have reduced serum levels of 25(OH)D and may have normal levels of $1,25(OH)_2D$. Because these anticonvulsants induce hepatic cytochrome P-450 hydroxylation enzyme activities, 25(OH)D is readily converted to more polar, inactive metabolites, thus accounting for lower serum 25(OH)D concentrations. However, this condition is much more complex because many patients have a low intake of dairy products, which represent the major dietary source of calcium, and very poor exposure to sunlight. This condition is more common in institutionalized children. Thus, the relatively normal serum $1,25(OH)_2D$ values are actually subnormal in relation to the degree of hypocalcemia, hypophosphatemia, and secondary hyperparathyroidism.

In children receiving chronic anticonvulsant therapy, the serum values of calcium, phosphate, and alkaline phosphatase activity should be evaluated periodically. This form of rickets usually can be prevented by providing an extra 500–1,000 IU of vitamin D_2 each day and by ensuring that the dietary intake of calcium is adequate.

CHAPTER 603
Conditions That Mimic Seizures

Several conditions share common features with epilepsy. Because these disorders may be associated with altered levels of consciousness, tonic or clonic movements, or cyanosis, they are often confused with epilepsy. Affected children may be inappropriately placed on many anticonvulsants with no response and some risk; conditions that mimic epilepsy are refractory to antiepileptic drugs. The treatment of these children differs significantly from those with epilepsy.

BENIGN PAROXYSMAL VERTIGO

Benign paroxysmal vertigo (BPV) typically develops in toddlers and is relatively rare beyond 3 yr of age. The attacks develop suddenly and are associated with ataxia, causing the child to fall or refuse to walk or sit. Horizontal nystagmus may be evident during the duration of the attack. The child appears frightened and pale. Nausea and vomiting may be prominent. Consciousness and the ability to verbalize are not disturbed, lethargy or drowsiness do not follow completion of the episode. The attacks vary in duration (seconds to minutes), frequency (daily to monthly), and intensity. A rotational sensation (vertigo) is verbalized by older children with BPV. These children are susceptible to motion sickness and may develop migraine headaches several years later, suggesting a relationship between BPV and migraine. Neurologic evaluation characteristically yields negative results, except for the finding of abnormal vestibular function detected by ice water caloric testing. Patients with clusters of attacks usually respond to dimenhydrinate, 5 mg/kg/24 hr with a maximum of 300 mg/24 hr PO, IM, IV, or per rectum.

NIGHT TERRORS

Night terrors are common, particularly in boys between 5 and 7 yr of age (Chapter 22). They occur in 1–3% of children and are usually short-lived. A night terror has a sudden onset, usually between midnight and 2.00 A.M. during stage 3 or 4 of slow-wave sleep. The child screams and appears frightened, with dilated pupils, tachycardia, and hyperventilation. There is little or no verbalization; the child may thrash violently, cannot be consoled, and is unaware of parents or surroundings. Sleep follows in a few minutes, and there is total amnesia the following morning. Approximately one third of children with night terrors experience somnambulism. An underlying emotional disorder should be explored in children with persistent and prolonged night terrors. A short course of diazepam or imipramine may be considered for treatment of protracted night terrors while the family dynamics are under investigation.

BREATH-HOLDING SPELLS

A breath-holding spell can be a frightening experience for parents because the infant becomes lifeless and unresponsive owing to cerebral anoxia at the height of the attack. There are two major types of breath-holding spells: the more common cyanotic form and the pallid form. Also see Chapter 25.

CYANOTIC SPELLS. A cyanotic breath-holding spell is usually predictable and is always provoked by upsetting or scolding an infant. The episode is heralded by a brief, shrill cry followed by forced expiration and apnea. There is rapid onset of generalized cyanosis and a loss of consciousness that may be associated with repeated generalized clonic jerks, opisthotonos, and bradycardia. Results of an interictal electroencephalogram (EEG) are normal. A breath-holding spell can occur repeatedly within a few hours or it can recur sporadically, but it is always stereotyped. Breath-holding spells are rare before 6 mo of age; they peak at about 2 yr of age, and they abate by 5 yr of age. The management of breath-holding spells concentrates on the support and reassurance of the parents. Some parents feel that whatever the physician recommends, they must splash cold water on the face, turn the child upside down, or initiate mouth-to-mouth resuscitation and even cardiopulmonary resuscitation. A thorough examination followed by an explanation of the mechanism of breath-holding spells is reassuring for most parents. The counseling session should emphasize the need for both parents to be consistent and not reinforce the child's behavior after the child recovers from the spell. This may be accomplished by placing the child safely in bed and by refusing to cuddle, play, or hold the child for a given period of time until recovery is complete.

PALLID SPELLS. These spells are much less common than cyanotic breath-holding spells, but they share several characteristics. Pallid spells are typically initiated by a painful experience, such as falling and striking the head or a sudden startle. The child stops breathing, rapidly loses consciousness, becomes pale and hypotonic, and may have a tonic seizure. Bradycardia with periods of asystole of longer than 2 sec may be recorded. The interictal EEG is normal. Pallid spells can in some cases be induced spontaneously in the laboratory by ocular compression that produces the oculocardiac reflex by afferent stimulation of the trigeminal nerve and by efferent inhibition of the heart by way of the vagus nerve. This procedure should not be attempted by an inexperienced physician, and appropriate resuscitation equipment should be readily available. Most children respond to conservative measures as outlined for cyanotic spells, but a trial of an anticholinergic, oral atropine sulfate 0.01 mg/kg/24 hr in divided doses with a maximum daily dose of 0.4 mg, which increases the heart rate by blocking the vagus nerve, may be considered in refractory cases. Atropine should not be prescribed during very hot weather because an episode of hyperpyrexia may be initiated.

SYNCOPE

SIMPLE SYNCOPE. Syncope follows an alteration in brain metabolism, the consequence of decreased cerebral blood flow, usually secondary to systemic hypotension. Decreased blood flow causes loss of consciousness, and the concomitant ischemia influences the higher cortical centers to release their inhibiting influence on the reticular formation within the brain stem. Neuronal discharges from the reticular formation then produce brief tonic contractions of the muscles of the face, trunk, and extremities in approximately 50% of patients with syncope. During a syncopal episode, a child may have fixed upward deviation of the eyes that can be confused with epilepsy. Simple syncope results from vasovagal stimulation and is precipitated by pain, fear, excitement, and extended periods of standing still, particularly in a warm environment. The EEG shows transient slowing during the attack but no seizure discharges. Simple syncope is uncommon before 10–12 yr of age but is quite prevalent in adolescent females. Tilt-table testing is an effective method of producing symptoms, including hypotension, in the majority of children with unexplained syncope. Most patients with positive tilt-table test results have vasovagal syncope, which if recurrent responds favorably to oral β-adrenergic blocking agents. Syncope can usually be differentiated from a seizure because of its short duration, associated symptoms of nausea and perspiration, and complete orientation after the event.

COUGH SYNCOPE. This is most common in asthmatic children. It often occurs shortly after the onset of sleep, and the coughing paroxysm abruptly awakens the child. The patient's face becomes plethoric, and the child perspires, becomes agitated, and is frightened. Loss of consciousness is associated with generalized muscle flaccidity, vertical upward gaze, and clonic muscle contractions lasting for several seconds. Urinary incontinence is frequent. Recovery begins within seconds, and consciousness is usually restored a few minutes later. The child has no recollection of the attack except for the events surrounding the paroxysm of coughing. Coughing produces a marked increase in intrapleural pressure followed by a lowered venous return to the right side of the heart and an associated decrease in right ventricular output. Reduction of left ventricular filling follows, and a rapidly diminished cardiac output results in altered cerebral blood flow, cerebral hypoxia, and a loss of consciousness. The cornerstone of management for asthmatic children with cough syncope is an aggressive approach to the prevention of bronchoconstriction.

THE PROLONGED QT SYNDROME. The incidence of the prolonged QT syndrome is 1/10,000 to 1/15,000. The prolonged QT syndrome is characterized by sudden loss of consciousness during exercise or an emotional and stressful experience (see Chapter 442.4). Loss of consciousness in association with exercise or stress is rarely due to epilepsy, and in every case a cardiac cause must be considered. The onset of the condition is typically in late childhood or adolescence, although onset in infancy may mimic sudden infant death syndrome. During the period of syncope, various cardiac arrhythmias are evident, particularly ventricular fibrillation. The child may recover within minutes or die during the event. The electrocardiogram (ECG) may show prolongation of the QT interval, due to abnormal lengthening of the QT interval, especially during carefully monitored exercise. QT intervals corrected for heart rate of 0.46 msec or greater support the diagnosis. There are at least two varieties of the syndrome: those due to acquired heart disease (myocarditis, mitral valve prolapse, electrolyte abnormalities, drug induced) and two congenital forms. The QT syndrome may be inherited as an autosomal recessive trait (Jervell and Lange-Nielsen syndrome) that is associated with deafness or as autosomal dominant (Romano-Ward syndrome). Mutations in a cardiac potassium channel gene [KvLQT1], linked to chromosome 11p15.5, account for about 50% of the long-QT syndrome inherited as an autosomal dominant (type 1 or LQT1). LQT2 results from a mutation in a second potassium channel gene (HERG), which is linked to chromosome 7q35–36. Type 3 long QT syndrome is the result of a mutation to a cardiac sodium channel gene (SCN5A) linked to chromosome 3p21–24, and a fourth type of long QT syndrome has been linked to chromosome 4q25–27. The gene for type 4 LQT has not been determined. All family members of an affected patient should have a 12-lead ECG. Further testing may include carefully supervised exercise tests or Holter monitoring. β-Adrenergic-antagonist drugs are usually effective and may be lifesaving. Permanent implantable cardiac pacing or left cervicothoracic sympathectomy may also be considered if drug therapy is not effective. Parents should be taught cardiopulmonary resuscitation, because exercise restriction and drug therapy may be ineffective for some children.

PAROXYSMAL KINESIGENIC CHOREOATHETOSIS

This disorder is characterized by a sudden onset of unilateral or occasionally bilateral choreoathetosis or dystonic posturing of a leg or an arm and associated facial grimacing and dysarthria. The condition is precipitated by sudden movement, particularly on arising from a sitting position, or by excitement and stress. The attacks rarely persist for longer than a minute and are never associated with loss of consciousness. The age of onset is typically between 8 and 14 yr, but the condition may begin as early as 2 yr. The child may have several attacks daily, or they may be intermittent, occurring once or twice a month. Results of neurologic examination, EEG, and neuroimaging studies are normal, and neuropathologic studies in a few cases showed no abnormalities. Most reported cases are familial, suggestive of autosomal recessive inheritance. The attacks can be prevented by the use of anticonvulsants, particularly phenytoin. The attacks of paroxysmal kinesigenic choreoathetosis tend to diminish in frequency during adulthood, and the anticonvulsant can be successfully weaned at that time.

SHUDDERING ATTACKS

Shuddering attacks have their onset at 4–6 mo of age and may persist to 6–7 yr of age. They produce an interesting posture, with sudden flexion of the head and trunk and shuddering or shivering movements similar to what must occur if ice-cold water is poured down the back of an unsuspecting individual. These children may have 100 attacks/day followed by several symptom-free weeks. Shuddering attacks may be the childhood precursor of benign essential tremor, because examination of parents and relatives reveals a high incidence of that common condition.

BENIGN PAROXYSMAL TORTICOLLIS OF INFANCY

Infants with benign paroxysmal torticollis have recurrent attacks of head tilt associated with pallor, agitation, and vomiting with an onset between 2 and 8 mo of age. During the attack, the child resists passive head movement. There is no loss of consciousness, and spontaneous remission occurs by 2–3 yr of age. As with benign paroxysmal vertigo, abnormalities in vestibular function have been documented in these patients. Children with persistent torticollis should be investigated for abnormalities of the cervical vertebrae including dislocation or fracture, or a tumor located in the posterior fossa. Some infants with benign paroxysmal torticollis develop migraine headaches later in childhood.

HEREDITARY CHIN TREMBLING

Hereditary chin trembling may be confused with epilepsy owing to repeated episodes of rapid 3/sec chin trembling movements. These brief attacks are precipitated by stress, anger, and frustration and are inherited as an autosomal dominant trait. Findings on the neurologic examination and EEG are normal.

NARCOLEPSY AND CATAPLEXY

See also Chapters 20.5 and 383. Narcolepsy is a disorder that rarely begins before adolescence and is characterized by paroxysmal attacks of irrepressible daytime sleep, which is sometimes associated with transient loss of muscle tone (cataplexy). The incidence of narcolepsy is 1/2000. An EEG shows that the recurrent sleep attacks consist of rapid eye movement (REM) sleep. Patients with narcolepsy are easily aroused and become spontaneously alert, whereas a convulsion is followed by a deep sleep, postictal drowsiness, lethargy, and often a headache. Cataplexy is also occasionally confused with epilepsy. Patients with cataplexy experience sudden loss of muscle tone and fall to the floor because of laughter, stress, or frightening experiences. Cataplectic patients do not lose consciousness but lie without moving for a few minutes until normal body tone returns. Treatment consists of scheduled naps, amphetamines, methylphenidate, tricyclic antidepressants, and counseling with respect to occupational safety and driving. The stimulant and antidepressant drugs commonly produce side effects including anxiety, euphoria, hypersomnolence, and the development of tolerance. Modafinil acetamide, 200 mg PO daily, is superior to the stimulant drugs in the management of narcolepsy and has fewer adverse side effects.

RAGE ATTACKS OR EPISODIC DYSCONTROL SYNDROME

The *episodic dyscontrol syndrome*, a nonepileptic condition, can be confused with complex partial seizures. Patients develop sudden and recurrent attacks of violent physical behavior with minimal provocation. The attacks consist of kicking, scratching, biting, and shouting (including abusive and profane language). An affected child or adolescent cannot seem to control the behavior and may seem momentarily psychotic throughout the attack. The episode is followed by fatigue, amnesia, and sincere remorse. A routine EEG may show nonspecific abnormalities in patients with the rage syndrome. The EEG in such patients during the attack remains normal; this condition is thus distinguished from complex partial seizures, which always show an abnormal EEG during an attack.

MASTURBATION

Masturbation or self-stimulation behavior may occur in girls between the ages of 2 mo and 3 yr. These children have repetitive stereotyped episodes of tonic posturing associated with copulatory movements, but without manual stimulation of the genitalia. The child suddenly becomes flushed and perspires, may grunt and breathe irregularly, but has no loss of consciousness. The masturbatory activity has a sudden onset, usually persists for a few minutes (rarely hours), and tends to occur during periods of stress or boredom. The examination should include a search for evidence of sexual abuse or abnormalities of the perineum, but in most cases a cause is not found. Treatment consists of reassurance that the self-stimulatory activity will subside by 3 yr of age and that no specific therapy is required.

PSEUDOSEIZURES

The diagnosis of a pseudoseizure should be made only after a thorough history and physical examination and exclusion of "true" seizures by prolonged EEG recording when indicated. Pseudoseizures occur typically between 10 and 18 yr of age and are more frequent among girls. Pseudoseizures occur in many patients with a past history of epilepsy and in some with ongoing true seizures. A pseudoseizure may be quite realistic but frequently is bizarre, with unusual postures, verbalizations, and uncharacteristic tonic or clonic movements. There are several distinguishing features of a pseudoseizure, including lack of cyanosis, normal reaction of the pupil to light, no loss of sphincter control, normal plantar responses, and the absence of tongue biting or injury during the attack. Many patients moan or cry during a pseudoseizure, and some patients can be persuaded to have an attack on request by the physician. Patients with pseudoseizures are likely to have a neurotic personality documented by formal psychologic testing. It is not unusual to find a patient taking three or four anticonvulsants, which, of course, have no effect. The most reliable method of differentiating epilepsy from suspected pseudoseizures is to record an attack. The EEG shows an excess of muscle artifact during the pseudoseizure but a normal background rhythm devoid of seizure discharges. After a true epileptic seizure, there is a significant increase in serum prolactin, whereas there is no change from the baseline at the termination of a pseudoseizure.

Ackerman MJ, Clapham DE: Ion channels—basic science and clinical disease. N Engl J Med 336:1575, 1997.

Broughton RJ, Fleming JAE, George CFP, et al: Randomized double-blind placebo-controlled crossover trial of modafinil in the treatment of excessive daytime sleepiness in narcolepsy. Neurology 49:444, 1997.

Fleisher DR, Morrison A: Masturbation mimicking abdominal pain or seizures in young girls. J Pediatr 116:810, 1990.
Grossman BJ: Trembling of the chin—an inheritable dominant character. Pediatrics 19:453, 1957.
Haslam RHA, Freigang B: Cough syncope mimicking epilepsy in asthmatic children. Can J Neurol Sci 12:45, 1985.
Kertesz A: Paroxysmal kinesigenic choreoathetosis. An entity within the paroxysmal choreoathetosis syndrome. Description of 10 cases, including 1 autopsied. Neurology 17:680, 1967.
Koenigsberger MR, Chutorian AM, Gold AP, et al: Benign paroxysmal vertigo of childhood. Neurology 20:1108, 1970.
Lombroso CT, Lerman P: Breath-holding spells (cyanotic and pallid infantile syncope). Pediatrics 39:563, 1967.
Mount LA, Reback S: Familial paroxysmal choreoathetosis. Arch Neurol Psychiatry 44:841, 1940.
O'Marcaigh AS, MacLellan-Tobert SG, Porter CJ: Tilt-table testing and oral metoprolol therapy in young patients with unexplained syncope. Pediatrics 93:278, 1994.
Pritchard PB, Wannamaker BB, Sagel J, et al: Serum prolactin and cortisol levels in evaluation of pseudoepileptic seizures. Ann Neurol 18:87, 1985.
Ruckman RN: Cardiac causes of syncope. Pediatr Rev 9:101, 1987.
Schneider S, Rice DR: Neurologic manifestations of childhood hysteria. J Pediatr 94:153, 1979.
Snyder CH: Paroxysmal torticollis in infancy. Am J Dis Child 117:458, 1969.
Vanasse M, Bedard P, Andermann F: Shuddering attacks in children: An early clinical manifestation of essential tremor. Neurology 26:1027, 1976.
Zarcone V: Narcolepsy. N Engl J Med 288:1156, 1973.

CHAPTER 604
Headaches

Headache is a common problem in pediatrics. The effect that headaches have on a child's academic performance, memory, personality, and interpersonal relationships, as well as school attendance, depends on their etiology, frequency, and intensity. A headache may occasionally indicate a severe underlying disorder (e.g., a brain tumor), and thus careful evaluation of children with recurrent, severe, or unconventional headaches is mandatory. Infants and children respond to a headache in an unpredictable fashion. Most toddlers cannot communicate the characteristics of a headache, but rather they may become irritable and cranky, vomit, prefer a darkened room because of photophobia, or repeatedly rub their eyes and head. Children are poor historians when describing a headache and its associated symptoms. The most important causes of headache in children include migraine, increased intracranial pressure (ICP), and psychogenic factors or stress. Refractive errors, strabismus, sinusitis, and malocclusion of the teeth are much less common causes of significant headaches in children.

604.1 Migraine

Migraine is defined as a recurrent headache with symptom-free intervals and at least three of the following symptoms or associated findings: abdominal pain, nausea or vomiting, throbbing headache, unilateral location, associated aura (visual, sensory, motor), relief following sleep, and a positive family history. It is the most important and frequent type of headache in the pediatric population. Most migraine headaches are not severe and are readily managed by conservative measures without requiring medical attention. The youngest child reported to have developed migraine was 1 yr of age. The incidence of migraine among school-aged children between 7 and 15 yr of age was 4% in a comprehensive Swedish study. Girls are more likely to develop a migraine as adolescents, whereas boys are in the slight majority among children under 10 yr old with migraine headaches. More than half undergo spontaneous prolonged remission after the 10th birthday. As adults, 5–10% of men and 15–20% of women have migraines. The cause of migraine headaches is unknown, but an inherited predisposition to vasomotor instability appears to be an important underlying factor. Hormonal changes, food allergies, personality traits characterized by high achievement, stress, bright flashing lights, and excessive sound all have been implicated. Increased levels of circulating serotonin and substance P, a vasodilating polypeptide, may act directly on the extracranial and intracranial vessels.

CLINICAL MANIFESTATIONS AND CLASSIFICATION. Migraine may be classified into subgroups, including common and classic migraine, migraine variants, cluster headaches, and complicated migraine. Cluster headaches rarely occur in children.

Common Migraine (migraine without aura). This migraine is not associated with an aura and is the most prevalent type of migraine in children. The headache is throbbing or pounding and tends to be unilateral at onset or throughout its duration and located in the bifrontal or temporal regions. It may not be hemicranial in children and is less intense compared with the migraine in adults. The headache usually persists for 1–3 hr, although the pain may last for as long as 24 hr. The pain may inhibit daily activity, because physical activity aggravates the pain. A characteristic feature of childhood migraine is intense nausea and vomiting, which may be more bothersome than the headache. The vomiting may be associated with abdominal pain and fever; thus, conditions such as appendicitis and a systemic infection may be erroneously confused with the primary diagnosis. Additional symptoms include extreme paleness, photophobia, lightheadedness, phonophobia, osmophobia (aversion to odors), and paresthesias of the hands and feet. A family history, particularly on the maternal side, is present in approximately 90% of children with common migraine. Thus, considerable caution should be exercised when making the diagnosis of a common migraine in the absence of a positive family history.

Additional features of all migraines may include near synchrony with perimenstrual or periovulation timing, gradual appearance after sustained exercise, relief with sleep, stereotypical prodromes (hypersomnia, food craving, irritability, moods), precipitation by food or odors, and migraines after a letdown or high period of stress. Manifestations suggestive of a more serious condition include rapid onset of the first or worst headache of the patient's life, a change in the characteristics of the headaches, a progressive headache lasting for days, headache associated with Valsalva maneuver, chronic systemic signs (weight loss, fever), persistent focal neurologic manifestations, seizures, loss of consciousness, nuchal rigidity, cranial bruits, abnormal visual fields, or papilledema (see Table 604–1).

Classic Migraine (migraine with an aura). In this disorder, an aura precedes the onset of the headache. Visual auras are rarely present in young children with migraine, but when they occur they may take the form of blurred vision, scotoma (an area of depressed vision within the visual field), photopsia (flashes of light), fortification spectra (brilliant white zigzag lines), or irregular distortion of objects. Some patients also have vertigo and lightheadedness during this stage of the headache. Sensory symptoms include perioral paresthesias and numbness of the hands and feet. Distortions of body image may predominate as a prelude to a classic migraine headache. After the aura, a patient with classic migraine develops typical symptoms of a common migraine as described earlier.

Migraine Variants. These variants include cyclic vomiting, acute confusional states, and benign paroxysmal vertigo. The last condition is discussed in Chapter 603. *Cyclic vomiting* is characterized by recurrent, sometimes monthly bouts of severe vomiting that may be so intense that dehydration and electrolyte abnormalities occur, particularly in an infant. Systemic symptoms such as fever, abdominal pain, and diarrhea are initially absent, but they may become prominent in association with excessive fluid losses secondary to vomiting. The vomiting may be protracted and persist for several days. The child may appear pale and frightened but does not lose consciousness. After a period of deep sleep, the child awakens and resumes normal play and eating habits as if the vomiting had not occurred. Many children with cyclic vomiting have a positive family history of migraine, and as they grow older and become verbal, they describe a typical migraine headache that leaves little doubt about the diagnosis and the association of the cyclic vomiting with the condition. Cyclic vomiting is treated with rectally administered antiemetics such as dimenhydrinate or ondansetron and careful attention to fluid replacement if the vomiting is excessive. Additional causes of cyclic vomiting include intestinal obstruction (e.g., malrotation, intermittent volvulus, duodenal web, duplication cysts, superior mesenteric artery compression, and internal hernias), peptic ulcer, gastritis, giardiasis, chronic pancreatitis, and Crohn's disease. Abnormal gastrointestinal motility and pelviureteric junction obstruction also can cause cyclic vomiting. Metabolic causes include disorders of amino acid metabolism (i.e., heterozygote ornithine transcarbamylase deficiency), organic acidurias (e.g., propionic acidemia, methylmalonic acidemia), fatty acid oxidation defects (e.g., medium-chain acyl-CoA dehydrogenase deficiency), disorders of carbohydrate metabolism (e.g., hereditary fructose intolerance), acute intermittent porphyria, and structural central nervous system (CNS) lesions (e.g., posterior fossa brain tumors, subdural hematoma or effusions).

Acute confusional states may be a manifestation of migraine. Migraine may present in a bizarre fashion, particularly in children, characterized by confusion, hyperactivity, disorientation, unresponsiveness, memory disturbances, vomiting, and lethargy. The neurologic examination shows defects of the sensorium, delayed responses to stimuli including touch and pain, and occasionally plantar extensor responses. The differential diagnosis includes toxic (drugs of abuse, ingestions) encephalopathy (particularly in an adolescent), encephalitis, acute psychosis, postictal state, petit mal (absence) status epilepticus, head trauma, and sepsis. The episode of acute confusion may persist for several hours and characteristically clears spontaneously after sleep; patients have no recall of the confusional state. The diagnosis is usually made in retrospect as a patient or family recalls the onset of a severe headache or visual symptoms preceding the acute attack of confusion, and a family history of migraine is established. Acute confusional states as a component of migraine probably result from localized cerebral edema due to increased vascular permeability during the headache. The EEG shows regional areas of slowing (2–4 cps) during and shortly after the attack but routinely returns to normal within a few days.

Complicated Migraine. Complicated migraine refers to the development of neurologic signs during a headache that persist after termination of the headache. The presence of neurologic signs in association with a headache suggests the possibility of an underlying structural lesion and requires a thorough investigation. There are three subsets of complicated migraine.

Brain stem signs predominate in patients with *basilar migraine,* owing to vasoconstriction of the basilar and posterior cerebral arteries. The major symptoms include vertigo, tinnitus, diplopia, blurred vision, scotoma, ataxia, and an occipital headache. The pupils may be dilated, and ptosis may be evident. Alterations in consciousness followed by a generalized seizure may result. After the attack there is a complete resolution of the neurologic symptoms and signs. Most affected children have a strongly positive family history of migraine. Many develop classic migraine as adolescents or adults. Relatively minor head trauma may precipitate an episode of basilar migraine. The condition has been described in children of both sexes, with girls younger than 4 yr at particular risk.

Ophthalmoplegic migraine is relatively rare in children. These patients develop a third-nerve palsy ipsilateral to the headache during the attack, owing to altered blood supply to the oculomotor nerve. The major differential diagnosis is a congenital aneurysm compressing the oculomotor nerve. *Amaurosis fugax* (acute, reversible, monocular blindness) may also be a variant of complicated migraine.

Hemiplegic migraine is characterized by the onset of unilateral sensory or motor signs during an episode of migraine. Hemisyndromes are more common in children than in adults and may be characterized by numbness of the face, arm, and leg; unilateral weakness; and aphasia. More than one attack is uncommon in the pediatric age group. The neurologic signs may be transient or may persist for days. It is unusual for a child to develop a completed stroke after a single episode. Hemiplegic migraine in an older child or adolescent has a relatively good prognosis, and a positive family history of similar hemiplegic events is often elicited. Familial hemiplegic migraine (FHM) is an autosomal dominant disorder. FHM is characterized by hemiplegia during the headache and, in some kindreds, progressive cerebellar atrophy. Mutations of the CACNL1A4 gene located on chromosome 19p13.1 are found in the majority of patients with FHM. Additional mutations may be identified in the calcium channel gene CACNL1A4, which would establish the genetic basis of the more common types of migraine.

Some children with migraine develop the syndrome of *alternating hemiplegia,* which has its onset during infancy. Acute hemiplegia may be the initial manifestation of migraine and may recur, affecting one side and then the other. Frequent episodes of vasoconstriction associated with ischemia may result in irreversible cerebral injury leading to mental retardation and epilepsy in this subgroup of children.

DIAGNOSIS AND DIFFERENTIAL DIAGNOSIS. A thorough history and physical examination suffice to establish the diagnosis in most cases. Basilar migraine may be confused with several conditions, including congenital malformations of the skull and cervical vertebrae, posterior fossa tumors, toxins and drugs, and metabolic abnormalities including Leigh disease and pyruvate decarboxylase deficiency. In children with hemiplegic migraine, an arteriovenous malformation, MELAS (mitochondrial myopathy, encephalopathy, lactic acidosis, and stroke), cerebral tumor, Todd paralysis, clotting disorders, hemoglobinopathies such as sickle cell disease, and metabolic conditions including homocystinuria should be considered. A lipid profile should be obtained in children with migraine and a positive family history of premature myocardial infarction or cerebrovascular accident. Migraines may occur in patients with systemic lupus erythematosus and patients abusing cocaine. The organization of laboratory tests and radiologic studies depends on the constellation of symptoms and findings during the neurologic examination. A CT scan or MRI is indicated if the headache is associated with an unusual constellation of symptoms or signs (see earlier) or when increased ICP is suspected (Table 604–1).

TREATMENT. Migraine may be prevented or ameliorated by *avoiding certain initiating stimuli.* A few children can identify specific factors that uniformly result in a headache. The most common precipitators of migraine headaches are stress, fatigue, and anxiety. An affected child may be under undue stress because of difficulties at home or school, particularly when unrealistic pressures or demands are placed on the patient. Children who experience recurrent migraine headaches during the school year may have a learning disability or may have been placed in a too highly competitive classroom. Reassessment of the child's school placement and academic abilities may be the most important step in the management of the headache disorder. Some studies implicate certain foods as a cause of migraine, particularly nuts, chocolate, cola drinks, hot dogs, spicy meats, kippers, and Chinese food (monosodium glutamate). Elimination of the incriminating foodstuff is indi-

TABLE 604–1 Indications for Neuroimaging a Child with Headaches

Abnormal neurologic signs
Recent school failure, behavioral change, fall-off in linear growth rate
Headache awakens child during sleep; early morning headache, with increase in frequency and severity
Periodic headaches and seizures coincide, especially if seizure has a focal onset
Migraine and seizure occur in the same episode, and vascular symptoms precede the seizure (20–50% risk of tumor or arteriovenous malformation)
Cluster headaches in child; any child <5 or 6 yr whose principal complaint is a headache
Focal neurologic symptoms or signs developing during a headache (i.e., complicated migraine)
Focal neurologic symptoms or signs (except classic visual symptoms of migraine) develop during the aura, with fixed laterality; focal signs of the aura persisting or recurring in the headache phase
Visual graying out occurring at the peak of a headache instead of the aura
Brief cough headache in a child or adolescent

Modified from Barlow CF: Headaches and Migraine in Childhood. Philadelphia, JB Lippincott, 1984, p 205.

cated if the history suggests a relationship between the ingestion of a particular food and the onset of headache. Avoidance of bright flashing lights, sun exposure, excessive physical exertion, mild head trauma, loud noises, hunger, fatigue, motion sickness, and drugs (including alcohol and oral contraceptives) is indicated when the history suggests a direct relationship. It is important to note that the frequency and severity of migraine headaches are reduced significantly in at least 50% of pediatric patients who undergo a careful history and neurologic examination followed by reassurance from the physician.

Management of an acute attack of migraine should include the use of *analgesics* and *antiemetics*. Most migraine headaches in children can be treated by the judicious use of *acetaminophen* or *ibuprofen*, particularly if the headaches are mild, infrequent, and of short duration. Additional agents for more severe migraine include naproxen, ketorolac, codeine, butorphanol, and meperidine. The *ergotamine preparations* (ergotamine tartrate or dihydroergotamine) should be considered for older children and adolescents with severe, classic migraine headaches and are most efficacious during the early stages of the migraine attack. The usual dose is 1 mg, which may be administered orally, subcutaneously, or per rectum in the form of a suppository. A repeat dose may be given 30 min later. Ergotamine should not be prescribed for patients with hemiplegic episodes. The ergotamines are frequently ineffective in children because they must be used early in the evolution of the headache. Most children either are unaware of an aura or fail to communicate the onset of the headache to their parents. *Chlorpromazine* is a useful drug in the short term (5–6 days) to "break-up" migraine. The dose is 2 mg/kg/24 hr PO divided every 4–6 hr or 4 mg/kg/24 hr per rectum divided every 6–8 hr. Intravenous chlorpromazine, 0.5–1.0 mg/kg, is often effective in the management of acute migraine in an ambulatory setting. An antiemetic such as *dimenhydrinate*, 5 mg/kg/24 hr in four divided doses, is the mainstay of treatment when vomiting is the major symptom. The child usually prefers to rest in a quiet, darkened room and typically awakens, refreshed and headache free, several hours later after a deep sleep. *Sumatriptan*, a specific and selective 5-hydroxytryptamine receptor agonist, is effective in treating the acute phase of both classic and common migraine headaches in adults. The drug may be administered subcutaneously, nasally, or orally, and the adverse effects, including hot flushes, nausea and vomiting, fatigue, and drowsiness, are usually minor and transient. Hypertension and coronary vasospasm have been reported in adults. The drug is not licensed at present for patients younger than 18 yr. Studies in young children have shown that sumatriptan is much less effective than in adolescents and adults and that there is no difference between the drug and placebo.

The decision to use *continuous daily medication* is based on the severity and frequency of the headaches and on the impact of the migraine on the child's daily activities, including school attendance and performance as well as participation in recreation. The use of prophylactic drugs should be considered if a child experiences more than two to four severe episodes monthly or is unable to attend school regularly. Although few drugs have been subjected to well-designed clinical trials in children, propranolol, a β-adrenergic blocker, is the drug of choice in most centers. Additional β blockers include atenolol, metoprolol, and nadolol. Other drugs used for migraine prophylaxis include calcium channel blockers (flunarizine, verapamil), tricyclic antidepressants (amitriptyline, nortriptyline), nonsteroidal anti-inflammatory agents, and serotonin receptor antagonists (methylsergide—not used under age 10 yr and not for more than 3 mo, or pizotyline). If a drug is effective, it is usually maintained for 1 yr, particularly during the school term.

Behavior management is an effective method for the treatment of migraine in some children and adolescents. Biofeedback and self-hypnosis are replacing pharmacologic treatment in some centers because of the undesirable side effects of drugs and the concern that some may produce chemical dependency. Biofeedback can be mastered by most children over 8 yr of age and has been effective in many clinical trials. Several studies of migrainous children show a significant decrease in frequency and no change in intensity of headaches in those treated by self-hypnosis compared with those taking the placebo or propranolol. Many pediatric headache clinics employ social workers skilled in pain management. Children respond favorably to being taught imagery and may often learn to control the pain associated with migraine without the use of medication.

604.2 Organic Headaches

A headache may be the earliest symptom of increased ICP. The headache results from tension or traction of the cerebral blood vessels and dura and occurs initially in a sporadic fashion, primarily in the early hours in the morning or shortly after the patient arises. The headache is diffuse and generalized and is more prominent over the frontal and occipital reigons. Its onset may be insidious, and the pain is enhanced by any activity that raises the ICP (e.g., coughing, sneezing, or straining during a bowel movement). As the ICP increases, the child becomes lethargic and irritable, and the headache becomes constant. Early morning vomiting is often associated with increased ICP. Causes of organic headaches in children include brain tumors, particularly those located in the posterior fossa, hydrocephalus, meningitis and encephalitis, cerebral abscess, subdural hematoma, chronic lead poisoning, and pseudotumor cerebri. Additional causes of organic headaches in children that may not be associated with increased ICP include arteriovenous malformations, berry aneurysm, collagen vascular diseases affecting the CNS, hypertensive encephalopathy, acute subarachnoid hemorrhage, and stroke. The management of organic headaches depends on the cause. The initial step includes a thorough history and physical examination, including recording of the blood pressure and inspection of the eyegrounds. Ordering of laboratory tests and neuroradiologic procedures depends on the clues provided by the history and physical examination.

604.3 Tension or Stress Headaches

Stress or tension headaches are relatively uncommon in the pediatric age group, particularly before puberty, and are often difficult to differentiate from migraine headaches. The two are often associated in the same patient. Tension headaches infrequently appear in the morning hours but are most apparent during the school day, particularly coinciding with a test or similarly anxiety-provoking circumstance. Although these headaches can be continuous and persist for weeks, they tend to wax and wane and build in intensity during the day. The headache is described as hurting or aching but is rarely perceived as throbbing. Most tension headaches in children are distributed in the frontal region, but they may localize over the vertex or the occipital area. Unlike migraine or headaches associated with increased ICP, tension headaches are not, as a rule, associated with nausea and vomiting.

The *diagnosis* of tension headache is made by exclusion at the completion of the history and physical examination. Studies such as an EEG or a CT scan are rarely necessary. Management consists of a search for possible underlying emotional or stressful factors. Most children have considerable insight into the origin of tension headaches and, when given the opportunity, will share concerns and conflicts. A poor self-image, fear of school failure, and lack of self-confidence are common factors. A depressed child occasionally presents with severe headaches. These patients may also complain of sudden mood changes, weight loss, anorexia, disturbed sleep, fatigue, and withdrawal from social activities.

Treatment of tension headaches begins with reassurance and an explanation about how stress may cause a headache. Anxiety and stress may unconsciously produce constant isometric contraction of the temporalis, masseter, or trapezius muscles, which leads to the characteristic dull, aching headache. Steps should be introduced to remove obvious anxiety-provoking situations. Acetaminophen and other mild analgesics are often all that are required to treat a tension headache. Sedatives and antidepressants are rarely necessary. Children with severe tension headaches may benefit from a brief hospitalization, particularly if an underlying depressive illness is under consideration. In the hospital setting, the child's interaction with other patients, nursing and medical staff, and family is observed while a plan is formulated for counseling or psychiatric intervention. In most cases, the child's headaches are considerably relieved during the period of observation. As with migraine headaches, biofeedback and self-hypnosis exercises are effective in the treatment of some patients with tension headaches.

Borge AIH, Nordhagen R, Moe B, et al: Prevalence and persistence of stomach ache and headache among children. Follow-up of a cohort of Norwegian children from 4 to 10 years of age. Acta Paediatr 83:433, 1994.
Ferrari MD: Sumatriptan in the treatment of migraine. Neurology 43(Suppl 3):S43–S47, 1993.
Forsythe WI, Gillies D, Sills MA: Propranolol in the treatment of childhood migraine. Dev Med Child Neurol 26:737, 1984.
Gardner K, Barmada MM, Ptacek LJ, et al: A new locus for hemiplegic migraine maps to chromosome 1q31. Neurology 49:1231, 1997.
Gascon G, Barlow C: Juvenile migraine, presenting as an acute confusional state. Pediatrics 45:628, 1970.
Hämäläinen ML, Hoppu K, Santavuouri P: Sumatriptan for migraine attacks in children: A randomized placebo-controlled study. Neurology 48:1100, 1997.
Hämäläinen ML, Hoppu K, Valkeila E, et al: Ibuprofen and acetaminophen for the acute treatment of migraine in children: A double-blind, randomized, placebo controlled, crossover study. Neurology 48:103, 1997.
Igarashi M, May WN, Golden GS: Pharmacologic treatment of childhood migraine. J Pediatr 120:653, 1992.
Olness H, MacDonald JT, Uden DL: Comparison of self-hypnosis and propranolol in the treatment of juvenile classic migraine. Pediatrics 79:593, 1987.
Presnky AL, Sommer D: Diagnosis and treatment of migraine in children. Neurology 29:506, 1979.
Pryse-Phillips WEM, Dodick DW, Edmeads JG, et al: Guidelines for the diagnosis and management of migraine in clinical practice. Can Med Assoc J 156:1273, 1997.
Schwartz BS, Stewart WF, Simon D, et al: Epidemiology of tension-type headache. JAMA 279:381, 1998.
Verret S, Steel JC: Alternating hemiplegia of childhood: A report of eight patients with complicated migraine beginning in infancy. Pediatrics 47:675, 1971.

CHAPTER 605
Neurocutaneous Syndromes

The neurocutaneous syndromes include a heterogeneous group of disorders characterized by abnormalities of both the integument and central nervous system (CNS). Most disorders are familial and believed to arise from a defect in differentiation of the primitive ectoderm. Disorders classified as neurocutaneous syndromes include neurofibromatosis, tuberous sclerosis, Sturge-Weber disease, von Hippel–Lindau disease, ataxia telangiectasia (see Chapter 605), linear nevus syndrome, hypomelanosis of Ito (see Chapter 659), and incontinentia pigmenti (see Chapter 658).

605.1 Neurofibromatosis

Neurofibromatosis (NF) (von Recklinghausen disease) is a common autosomal dominant disorder. The condition is protean, because virtually every system and organ may be affected, and progressive in that distinctive features may be present at birth but the development of complications is delayed for decades. NF is the consequence of an abnormality of neural crest differentiation and migration during the early stages of embryogenesis (see also Chapter 658).

CLINICAL MANIFESTATIONS AND DIAGNOSIS. There are two distinct forms of NF. NF-1 is the most prevalent type, with an incidence of 1/4,000, and is diagnosed if any two of the following signs are present: (1) *Six or more café-au-lait macules over 5 mm is greatest diameter in prepubertal individuals and over 15 mm in greatest diameter in postpubertal individuals.* Café-au-lait spots are the hallmark of neurofibromatosis and are present in almost 100% of patients. They are present at birth but increase in size, number, and pigmentation, especially during the first few years of life. The spots are scattered over the body surface, with predilection for the trunk and extremities and sparing of the face. (2) *Axillary or inguinal freckling* consists of multiple hyperpigmented areas 2–3 mm in diameter. (3) *Two or more iris Lisch nodules.* Lisch nodules are hamartomas located within the iris and are best identified with a slit-lamp examination. They are present in more than 74% of patients with NF-1 but are not a component of NF-2. The prevalence of Lisch nodules increases with age, from only 5% of children less than 3 yr of age, to 42% among children 3–4 yr of age, and to 100% of adults 21 yr of age or older. (4) *Two or more neurofibromas or one plexiform neurofibroma.* Neurofibromas typically involve the skin, but they may be situated along peripheral nerves and blood vessels and within viscera including the gastrointestinal tract. These cutaneous lesions appear characteristically during adolescence or pregnancy, suggesting a hormonal influence. They are usually small, rubbery lesions with a slight purplish discoloration of the overlying skin. Plexiform neurofibromas are usually evident at birth and result from diffuse thickening of nerve trunks that are frequently located in the orbital or temporal region of the face. The skin overlying a plexiform neurofibroma may be hyperpigmented to a greater degree than a café-au-lait spot. Plexiform neurofibromas may produce overgrowth of an extremity and a deformity of the corresponding bone. (5) *A distinctive osseous lesion* such as sphenoid dysplasia (which may cause pulsating exophthalmos) or cortical thinning of long bones with or without pseudoarthrosis. Scoliosis is the most common orthopedic manifestation of NF-1, although it is not specific enough to be included as a diagnostic criterion. (6) *Optic gliomas* are present in approximately 15% of patients with NF-1. These relatively benign tumors consist of glial cells and a mucinous material. Most patients with optic gliomas are asymptomatic and have normal or near-normal vision, but approximately 20% have visual disturbances or evidence of precocious sexual development secondary to tumor invasion of the hypothalamus. Children rarely are aware of unilateral visual loss; thus, diagnosis may be delayed. Patients with a unilateral optic glioma typically display an afferent pupillary defect. To test for this, each eye is alternatively stimulated by a bright light source (swinging flashlight test). The affected pupil dilates rather than constricts, whereas light in the unaffected eye causes both pupils to constrict equally. Patients with NF-1 and a plexiform neuroma of the eyelid have a high association with an ipsilateral optic glioma. The MRI findings of an optic glioma include diffuse thickening, localized enlargement, or a distinct focal mass originating from the optic nerve or chiasm. (7) *A first-degree relative with NF-1 whose diagnosis was based on the aforementioned criteria*. The NF-1 gene on chromosome region 17q11.2 encodes all mRNA of 11–13 kb containing at least 59 exons and produces neurofibromin.

Children with NF-1 are susceptible to *neurologic complications*. MRI studies of selected children have shown abnormal signals in the globus pallidus, thalamus, and internal capsule. These probably represent low-grade glioma or hamartoma that is not detected by CT scanning (Fig. 605–1). These findings may account for the high incidence of learning disabilities, attention deficit disorders, and abnormalities of speech among affected children. Complex partial and generalized tonic-clonic seizures are a frequent complication. Hydrocephalus is a rare manifestation secondary to aqueductal stenosis, whereas macrocephaly with normal-sized ventricles is a common finding. The cerebral vessels may develop stenosis, aneurysms, or stenosis resulting in moyamoya disease (see Fig. 609–1). Neurologic sequelae include transient cerebrovascular ischemic attacks, hemiparesis, and cognitive defects. Not surprisingly, *psychologic disturbances* are prevalent owing to the seriousness and uncertainty of the disease. Precocious puberty may become evident in the presence or absence of lesions of the optic chiasm and hypothalamus. *Malignant neoplasms* are also a significant problem in patients with NF-1. A neurofibroma occasionally differentiates into a neurofibrosarcoma or malignant schwannoma. Patients with NF-1 are at risk for hypertension, which may result from renal vascular stenosis or a pheochromocytoma. The incidence of pheochromocytoma, rhabdomyosarcoma, leukemia, and Wilms' tumor is higher than in the general population. There is an unusual association involving myeloid leukemia, juvenile xanthogranuloma, and NF-1. However, tumors of the CNS (including optic gliomas, meningiomas of the brain and spinal cord, neurofibromas, astrocytomas, and neurilemmomas) account for significant morbidity and mortality because of their increased frequency in patients with NF-1.

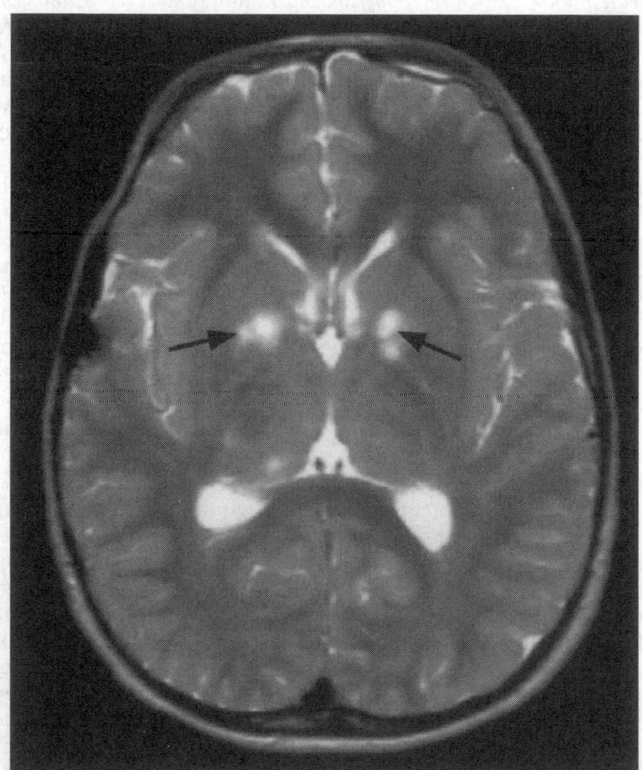

Figure 605–1 T2 weighted MRI of a patient with neurofibromatosis. Note the high-signal areas in the basal ganglia (*black arrows*), which represent hamartomas.

NF-2 accounts for 10% of all cases of NF, with an incidence of 1/50,000, and may be diagnosed when one of the following is present: (1) *bilateral eighth nerve masses* consistent with acoustic neuromas as demonstrated by CT scanning or MRI. (2) *A parent, sibling or child with NF-2* and either unilateral eighth nerve masses or any two of the following: neurofibroma, meningioma, glioma, schwannoma, or juvenile posterior subcapsular lenticular opacities. **Bilateral acoustic neuromas** are the most distinctive feature of NF-2. Symptoms of hearing loss, facial weakness, headache, or unsteadiness may appear during childhood, although signs of a cerebellopontine angle mass are more commonly present in the 2nd and 3rd decades of life. Although café-au-lait spots and skin neurofibromas are classic findings in NF-1, they are much less common in NF-2. Posterior subcapsular lens opacities are identified in approximately 50% of patients with NF-2. As with NF-1, CNS tumors, including schwann cell and glial tumors, and meningiomas are common in patients with NF-2. Linkage analysis has shown that the gene for NF-2 is located near the center of the long arm of chromosome 22q1.11.

TREATMENT. Because there is no specific treatment for NF, management includes genetic counseling and early detection of treatable conditions or complications. The National Institutes of Health consensus statement suggests that tests should be dictated by findings on clinical evaluation. Laboratory tests in asymptomatic patients are unlikely to be of value, particularly evoked potentials, an electroencephalogram (EEG), CT, or MRI. It is recommended that the child have a detailed history and physical examination by a pediatrician and a thorough annual ophthalmologic examination by a pediatric ophthalmologist. A parent with NF has a 50% chance of transmitting the disease with each pregnancy. The type of NF (NF-1 and NF-2) "breeds true" for successive generations. Because approximately half of all cases of NF result from fresh mutations, each parent should be carefully examined (including a search for Lisch's nodules) before counseling for the risk of affected future pregnancies. Standard DNA diagnostic analysis is not practical for the prenatal diagnosis of the NF-1 gene because of the large size of the gene and the significant number of mutations. However, prenatal diagnosis is feasible if the mutation causing the condition is known in the affected parent. The majority of NF-2 cases are the result of a mutation. Examination of fetal DNA for the characteristic single-strand conformational polymorphism of an altered DNA sequence provides accurate prenatal testing. In familial cases, when affected and unaffected family members are available, linkage can be established, making prenatal diagnosis available with a certain degree of accuracy.

605.2 Tuberous Sclerosis

Tuberous sclerosis (TS) is inherited as an autosomal dominant trait with an estimated frequency of 1/6000. The TS gene is located on chromosomes 9q34 (TSC_1) and 16p13 (TSC_2), but at least half of the cases are sporadic owing to new mutations. The 8.6 kb TSC_1 transcript encodes a protein of 130 kd called hamartin. The TSC_2 gene encodes the protein tuberin. TS is an extremely heterogeneous disease with a wide clinical spectrum varying from severe mental retardation and incapacitating seizures to normal intelligence and a lack of seizures, often within the same family. As a rule, the younger the patient presents with symptoms and signs of TS, the greater is the likelihood of mental retardation. The disease affects many organ systems other than the skin and brain, including the heart, kidney, eyes, lungs, and bone.

PATHOLOGY. The characteristic brain lesions consist of tubers. Tubers are located in the convolutions of the cerebral hemispheres and are typically present in the subependymal region, where they undergo calcification and project into the ventricular cavity, producing a candle-dripping appearance. Tubers in the region of the foramen of Monro may cause obstruction of cerebrospinal fluid (CSF) flow and hydrocephalus. The microscopic appearance of the tuber consists of decreased numbers of neurons and a proliferation of astrocytes and the presence of oddly shaped multinucleated giant neurons. MRI is useful for identification of the lesions. Generally, the greater the number of tubers, the more neurologically impaired is the patient.

CLINICAL MANIFESTATIONS. TS may present during infancy with infantile spasms and a hypsarrhythmic EEG pattern. Careful examination of the skin on the trunk and extremities shows the typical hypopigmented skin lesions that have been likened to an ash leaf in more than 90% of cases in this age group. Visualization of the hypopigmented lesions is enhanced by the use of a Wood's ultraviolet lamp (see Chapter 561). The CT scan typically shows calcified tubers in the periventriuclar area, but these may not be apparent until 3–4 yr of age (Fig. 605–2). The seizures may be difficult to control, and at a later age they may develop into myoclonic epilepsy. In Europe and Canada, infantile spasms associated with TS are treated with vigabatrin (rather than adrenocorticotropic hormone), with good results. Vigabatrin is not available in the United States. There is a high incidence of mental retardation in young patients with TS and infantile spasms.

During childhood, TS presents most often with a generalized seizure disorder and pathognomonic skin lesions. Sebaceous adenomas develop between 4 and 6 yr of age; they appear as tiny red nodules over the nose and cheeks and are sometimes confused with acne. Later, they enlarge, coalesce, and assume a fleshy appearance. A **shagreen patch** is also characteristic of TS and consists of a roughened, raised lesion with an orange-peel consistency located primarily in the lumbosacral region. Subungual or periungual fibromas arise from the stratum lucidum of the finger and toe in many patients with TS during adolescence. Retinal lesions consist of two types: mulberry tumors that arise from the nerve head or round, flat gray lesions (phakoma) in the region of the disc (Fig. 605–3). Brain tumors are much less common in TS compared with NF, but a tuber occasionally differentiates into a malignant astrocytoma. Approximately 50% of children with TS have rhabdomyomas of the heart, which may be detected in a fetus at risk by an echocardiogram. The rhabdomyomas may be numerous or located at the apex of the left ventricle, and although they can cause congestive heart failure and arrhythmias, they tend to slowly resolve spontaneously. The kidneys in most patients are involved by hamartomas or polycystic disease, resulting in hematuria, pain, and, in some cases, renal failure. Angiomyolipomas may produce generalized cystic or fibrous pulmonary changes in the lung and lead to spontaneous pneumothorax.

DIAGNOSIS. Diagnosis of TS relies on a high index of suspicion when assessing a child with infantile spasms. A careful search for the typical skin and retinal lesions should be completed in all patients with a seizure disorder. Head CT scan or MRI confirms the diagnosis in most cases.

TREATMENT. Management consists of seizure control and baseline studies, including renal ultrasonography, an echocardiogram, and a chest roentgenogram with follow-up as indicated. Symptoms and signs of increased intracranial pressure suggest obstruction of the foramen of Monro by a tuber or malignant transformation of a tuber, and warrant immediate investigation and surgical intervention.

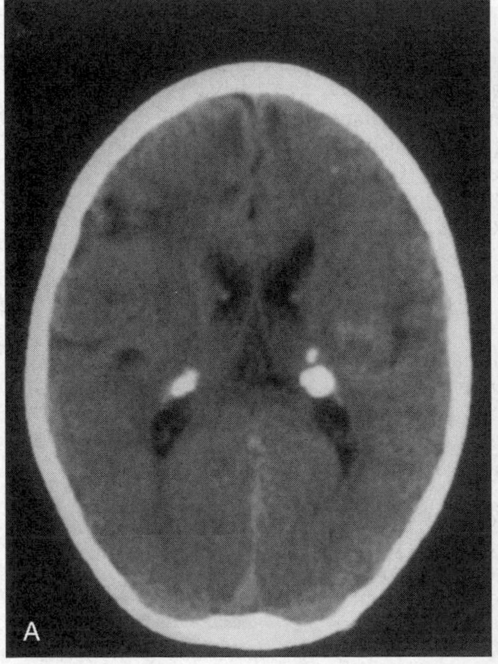

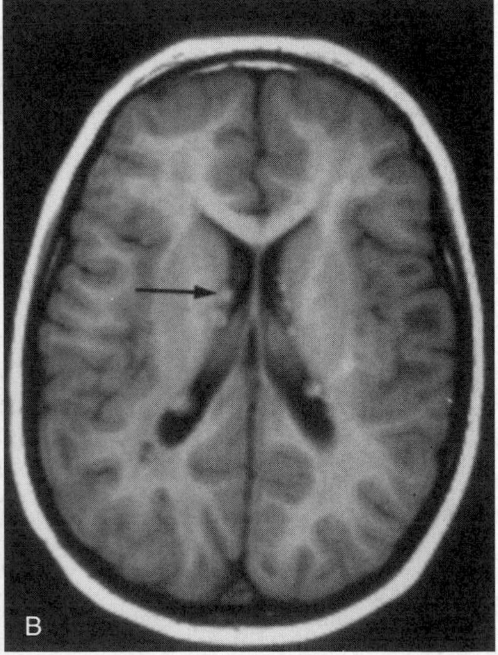

Figure 605–2 Tuberous sclerosis. *A*, CT scan with subependymal calcifications characteristic of tuberous sclerosis. *B*, The MRI demonstrates multiple subependymal nodules in the same patient (*black arrow*). Parenchymal tubers are also visible on both the CT and the MRI scan as low-density areas in the brain parenchyma.

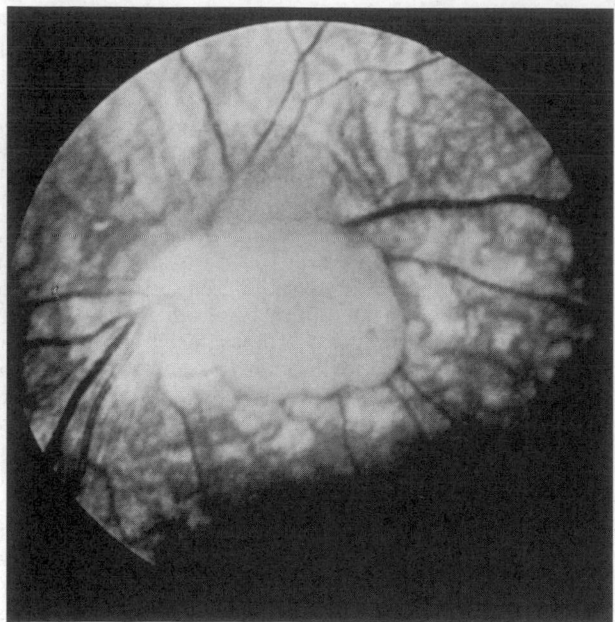

Figure 605–3 An astrocytoma of the retina (mulberry tumor) in a patient with tuberous sclerosis.

605.3 Sturge-Weber Disease

Sturge-Weber disease consists of a constellation of symptoms and signs including a facial nevus (port-wine stain), seizures, hemiparesis, intracranial calcifications, and, in many cases, mental retardation. It occurs sporadically, with a frequency of approximately 1/50,000.

ETIOLOGY. The condition is thought to result from anomalous development of the primordial vascular bed during the early stages of cerebral vascularization. At this stage, the blood supply to the brain, meninges, and face is undergoing reorganization, while the primitive ectoderm in the region differentiates into the skin of the upper face and the occipital lobe of the cerebrum. The overlying leptomeninges are richly vascularized, and the brain beneath becomes atrophic and calcified, particularly in the molecular layer of the cortex, in patients with Sturge-Weber disease.

CLINICAL MANIFESTATIONS. The facial nevus is present at birth and tends to be unilateral and always involves the upper face and eyelid. The nevus may also be evident over the lower face, trunk, and in the mucosa of the mouth and pharynx. Not all children with facial nevi have Sturge-Weber disease (Chapter 656). Buphthalmos and glaucoma of the ipsilateral eye are a common complication. Seizures develop in most patients during the 1st year of life. They are typically focal tonic-clonic and contralateral to the side of the facial nevus. The seizures tend to become refractory to anticonvulsants and are associated with a slowly progressive hemiparesis in many cases. Although neurodevelopment appears to be normal during the 1st year of life, mental retardation or severe learning disabilities are present in at least 50% during later childhood, probably the result of prolonged generalized seizures and increasing cerebral atrophy secondary to local hypoxia and use of numerous anticonvulsants.

DIAGNOSIS. The skull radiograph shows intracranial calcification in the occipitoparietal region in most patients. This characteristically assumes a serpentine or railroad-track appearance. The CT scan highlights the extent of the calcification that is usually associated with unilateral cortical atrophy and ipsilateral dilatation of the lateral ventricle (Fig. 605–4).

TREATMENT. Management of Sturge-Weber disease is multifaceted and somewhat controversial. Seizure frequency and the significant risk for mental retardation influence the treatment plan. For patients with well-controlled seizures and normal or near-normal development, management is straightforward and conservative. However, increasing evidence shows that a hemispherectomy or lobectomy may prevent the development of mental retardation, in patients with recalcitrant seizures, particularly if the surgery is accomplished during the 1st year of life. Because of the risk of glaucoma, regular measurements of intraocular pressure with a tenonometer is indicated. The facial nevus is often a target for ridicule by classmates, leading to psychologic trauma. Flashlamp-pulsed laser therapy holds considerable promise for clearing of the port-wine stain. Finally, because of the high frequency of developmental disabilities, special educational facilities are frequently required.

605.4 von Hippel–Lindau Disease

As with most of the neurocutaneous syndromes, von Hippel–Lindau disease affects many organs, including the cerebellum, spinal cord, medulla, retina, kidney, pancreas, and epididymis. von Hippel–Lindau disease is inherited as an autosomal dominant trait with variable penetrance and delayed expression. The gene for von Hippel–Lindau disease has been mapped to chromosome 3p25. The major neurologic features of the condition include cerebellar hemagioblastomas and retinal angiomata. Patients with cerebellar hemangioblastoma present in early adult life or beyond with symptoms and signs of increased intracranial pressure. A smaller number of patients have hemangioblastoma of the spinal cord, producing abnormalities of proprioception and disturbances of gait and bladder dysfunction. The CT scan typically shows a cystic cerebellar lesion with a vascular mural nodule. Total surgical removal of the tumor is curative. Approximately 25% of patients with cerebellar hemangioblastoma have retinal angiomas.

Retinal angiomas are characterized by small masses of thin-walled capillaries that are fed by large and tortuous arterioles and venules. They are usually located in the peripheral retina

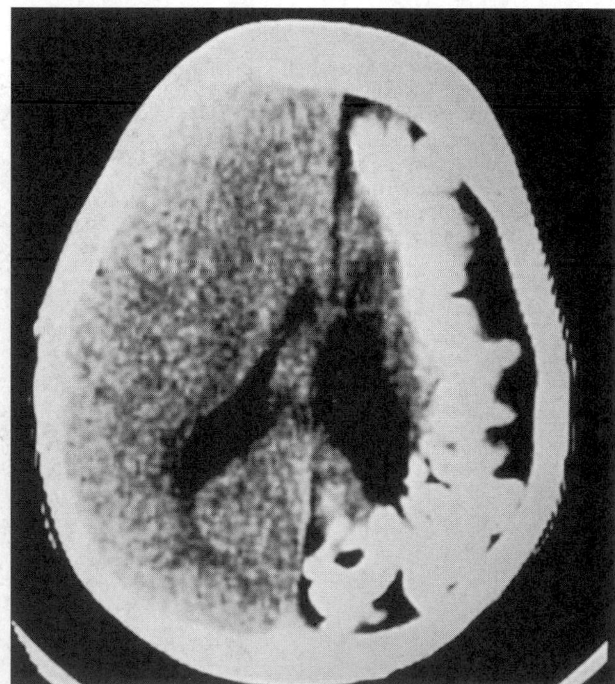

Figure 605–4 A CT scan of a patient with Sturge-Weber syndrome, showing unilateral calcification and atrophy of a cerebral hemisphere.

so that vision is unaffected. However, exudation in the region of the angiomas may lead to retinal detachment and visual loss. Retinal angiomas are treated with photocoagulation and cryocoagulation, with good results. Cystic lesions of the kidneys, pancreas, liver, and epididymis as well as pheochromocytoma are frequently associated with von Hippel–Lindau disease. Renal carcinoma is the most common cause of death. Regular follow-up and appropriate imaging studies are necessary to identify lesions that may be treated at an early stage.

605.5 Linear Nevus Syndrome

This sporadic condition is characterized by a facial nevus and neurodevelopmental abnormalities. The nevus is located on the forehead and nose and tends to be midline in its distribution. It may be quite faint during infancy but later becomes hyperkeratotic, with a yellow-brown appearance. More than half of the patients have a seizure disorder and are mentally retarded. The seizures may be generalized myoclonic or focal motor. Most patients have normal results of CT studies, although hemimegalencephaly with hamartomatous changes has been reported. Focal neurologic signs including hemiparesis and homonymous hemianopia are more common in this group.

605.6 PHACE Syndrome

Large facial hemangiomas may be associated with a Dandy-Walker malformation, vascular anomalies (coarctation of aorta, aplasia or hypoplastic carotid arteries, aneurysmal carotid dilation, aberrant left subclavian artery), glaucoma, cataracts, microphthalmia, optic nerve hypoplasia, and ventral defects (sternal clefts). There is a female predominance. Airway hemangiomas may produce obstruction. The syndrome denotes *p*osterior fossa malformations, *h*emangiomas, *a*rterial anomalies, *c*oarctation of the aorta and other cardiac defects, and *e*ye abnormalities. Interferon-α is of value in the management of the hemangiomas.

American Academy of Pediatrics Committee on Genetics: Health supervision for children with neurofibromatosis. Pediatrics 96:368, 1995.
Crossen MH, de Goede-Bolder A, van den Broek KM, et al: A prospective 10 year follow up study of patients with neurofibromatosis type 1. Arch Dis Child 78:408, 1998.
Frieden IJ, Reese V, Cohen D: The association of posterior fossa brain malformations, hemangiomas, arterial anomalies, coarctation of the aorta and cardiac defects, and eye abnormalities. Arch Dermatol 132:307, 1996.
Gutmann DH, Aylsworth A, Carey JC, et al: The diagnostic evaluation and multidisciplinary management of neurofibromatosis 1 and neurofibromatosis 2. JAMA 278:51, 1997.
Hoffman KJ, Harris EL, Bryan RN, et al: Neurofibromatosis type 1: The cognitive phenotype. J Pediatr 124:51, 1994.
Hurst RW, Newman SA, Cail WS: Multifocal intracranial MR abnormalities in neurofibromatosis. AJNR 9:293, 1988.
Jozwiak S, Pedich M, Rajszys P, et al: Incidence of hepatic hamartomas in tuberous sclerosis. Arch Dis Child 67:1363, 1992.
Jozwiak S, Kawalec W, Dluzewska J, et al: Cardiac tumors in tuberous sclerosis: Their incidence and course. Eur J Pediatr 153:155, 1994.
Latif F, Tory K, Gmarra J, et al: Identification of the von Hippel–Landau disease tumor suppressor gene. Science 260:1317, 1993.
Lazaro C, Gaona A, Ravella A, et al: Prenatal diagnosis of neurofibromatosis 1: From flanking RFLPS to intragene microsatellite markers. Prenat Diagn 15:129, 1995.
Lovejoy FH, Boyle LE: Linear nevus sebaceous syndrome: Report of two cases and a review of the literature. Pediatrics 52:382, 1973.
Maher ER, Kaelin WG Jr: von Hippel-Lindau disease. Medicine 76:381, 1997.
Martuza RL, Eldridge R: Neurofibromatosis 2 (bilateral acoustic neurofibromatosis). N Engl J Med 318:684, 1988.
O'Callaghan FJK, Shiell AW, Osborne JP, et al: Prevalence of tuberous sclerosis estimated by capture-recapture analysis. Lancet 351:1490, 1998.
Rizzo JF, Lessell S: Cerebrovascular abnormalities in neurofibromatosis type 1. Neurology 44:1000, 1994.
Roach ES, Williams MD, Laster MD: Magnetic resonance imaging in tuberous sclerosis. Arch Neurol 44:301, 1987.
Seizinger BR, Martuza RL, Gusella JF: Loss of genes on chromosome 22 in tumorigenesis of human acoustic neuroma. Nature 322:644, 1986.
Tan OT, Sherwood K, Gilchrest BA: Treatment of children with port-wine stains using the flashlamp-pulsed tunable dye laser. N Engl J Med 320:416, 1989.
van Slegtenhorst M, de Hoogt R, Hermans C, et al: Identification of the tuberous sclerosis gene TSC_1 on chromosome 9q34. Science 277:805, 1997.
Webb DW, Clarke A, Fryer A, et al: The cutaneous features of tuberous sclerosis: A population study. Br J Dermatol 135:1, 1996.

CHAPTER 606
Movement Disorders

Abnormalities of movement in children constitute a wide range of conditions with multiple causes. The type of movement disorder assists in localization of the pathologic process, whereas the onset, age, and degree of the abnormal motor activity and associated neurologic findings help to classify the disorder and organize the investigation. Movement disorders are rarely limited to one form such as ataxia; the examination usually demonstrates additional abnormal movements such as tremor or chorea.

606.1 Ataxias

Congenital anomalies of the posterior fossa, including the Dandy-Walker syndrome, Chiari malformation, and encephalocele, are prominently associated with ataxia because of their destruction or replacement of the cerebellum (Chapter 601). **Agenesis of the cerebellar vermis** presents in infancy with generalized hypotonia and decreased deep tendon reflexes. Delayed motor milestones and truncal ataxia are typical. A familial variety (Joubert disease) is inherited as an autosomal recessive trait. Affected children typically have abnormalities of respiration during infancy, characterized by alternating periods of hyperpnea and apnea. In addition to ataxia, mental retardation and abnormal eye movements have been described. MRI is the method of choice for investigating congenital abnormalities of the cerebellum, vermis, and related structures.

The major *infectious causes of ataxia* include cerebellar abscess, acute labyrinthitis, and acute cerebellar ataxia. **Acute cerebellar ataxia** occurs primarily in children 1–3 yr of age and is a diagnosis by exclusion. The condition often follows a viral illness, such as varicella, coxsackievirus, or echovirus infection, by 2–3 wk and is thought to represent an autoimmune response to the viral agent affecting the cerebellum (see Chapters 174, 243, and 246). The onset is sudden, and the truncal ataxia can be so severe that the child is unable to stand or sit. Vomiting may occur initially, but fever and nuchal rigidity are absent. Horizontal nystagmus is evident in approximately 50% of cases, and if the child is able to speak, dysarthria may be impressive. Examination of the cerebrospinal fluid (CSF) reveals typically normal results at the onset of ataxia; however, a slight pleocytosis of lymphocytes (10–30/mm^3) is not unusual. Later in the course, the CSF protein undergoes a moderate elevation. The ataxia begins to improve in a few weeks but may persist for as long as 2 mo. The prognosis for complete recovery is excellent; however, a small number have long-term sequelae, including behavioral and speech disorders as well as ataxia and incoordination. **Acute labyrinthitis** may be difficult to differentiate from acute cerebellar ataxia in a toddler. The condition is associated with middle-ear infections and intense vertigo, vomiting, and abnormalities in labyrinthine function, particularly ice water caloric testing.

Toxic causes of ataxia include alcohol, thallium (which is used occasionally in homes as a pesticide), and the anticonvulsants, particularly phenytoin when serum levels reach or exceed 30 μg/mL (120 μmol/L).

Brain tumors, including tumors of the cerebellum and frontal lobe as well as neuroblastoma, may present with ataxia. Frontal lobe tumors may cause ataxia owing to destruction of the association fibers connecting the frontal lobe with the cerebellum. Neuroblastoma may be associated with an encephalopathy characterized by progressive ataxia, myoclonic jerks, and opsoclonus (nonrhythmic horizontal and vertical oscillations of the eyes).

Several *metabolic disorders* are characterized by ataxia, including abetalipoproteinemia, arginosuccinic aciduria, and Hartnup disease. **Abetalipoproteinemia** (Bassen-Kornzweig disease) begins in childhood with steatorrhea and failure to thrive (see Chapter 83.3). A blood smear shows acanthocytosis and decreased serum levels of cholesterol and triglycerides, and the serum β-lipoproteins are absent. Neurologic signs become evident by late childhood and consist of ataxia, retinitis pigmentosa, peripheral neuritis, abnormalities in position and vibration sense, muscle weakness, and mental retardation. Vitamin E is undetectable in the serum of patients with neurologic symptoms.

Degenerative diseases of the central nervous system (CNS) represent an important group of ataxic disorders of childhood because of the genetic consequences and poor prognosis. **Ataxia-telangiectasia,** an autosomal recessive condition, is the most common of the degenerative ataxias and is heralded by ataxia beginning at about age 2 yr and progressing to loss of ambulation by adolescence (see Chapter 126.12). Ataxia telangiectasia is caused by mutations in the ATM gene located at 11q22–q23. Oculomotor apraxia, defined as having difficulty fixating smoothly on an object and therefore overshooting the target with lateral movement of the head followed by refixating the eyes, is a frequent finding, as is horizontal nystagmus. The telangiectasia becomes evident by midchildhood and is found on the bulbar conjunctiva, over the bridge of the nose, and on the ears and exposed surfaces of the extremities. Examination of the skin shows a loss of elasticity. Abnormalities of immunologic function that lead to frequent sinopulmonary infections include decreased serum and secretory IgA as well as diminished IgG_2, IgG_4 and IgE levels in more than 50% of patients. Children with ataxia-telangiectasia have a 50- to 100-fold greater chance of developing lymphoreticular tumors (lymphoma, leukemia, and Hodgkin disease) as well as brain tumors, compared with the normal population. Additional laboratory abnormalities include an increased incidence of chromosome breaks, particularly of chromosome 14, and elevated levels of α-fetoprotein. Death results from infection or tumor dissemination.

Friedreich ataxia is inherited as an autosomal recessive trait. The majority of patients are homozygous for a GAA repeat expansion in the noncoding region of the X25 gene, which is located on chromosome 9q13. The gene encodes a 210 amino acid, frataxin. The onset of ataxia is somewhat later than in ataxia-telangiectasia but usually occurs before age 10 yr. The ataxia is slowly progressive and involves the lower extremities to a greater degree than the upper extremities. The Romberg test result is positive; the deep tendon reflexes are absent (particularly the Achilles), and the plantar response is extensor. Patients develop a characteristic explosive, dysarthric speech, and nystagmus is present in most children. Although patients may appear apathetic, their intelligence is preserved. They may have significant weakness of the distal musculature of the hands and feet. Typically noted is a marked loss of vibration and position sense owing to degeneration of the posterior columns and indistinct sensory changes in the distal extremities. Friedreich ataxia is also characterized by skeletal abnormalities, including high-arched feet (pes cavus) and hammer toes as well as progressive kyphoscoliosis. Results of electrophysiologic studies including visual, auditory brain stem, and somatosensory evoked potentials are often abnormal. Hypertrophic cardiomyopathy with progression to intractable congestive heart failure is the cause of death for most patients. Several forms of *spinocerebellar ataxia* are similar to Friedreich's ataxia. **Roussy-Levy disease** has, in addition, atrophy of the muscles of the lower extemity with a similar pattern of wasting observed in Charcot-Marie-Tooth disease; **Ramsay Hunt syndrome** has an associated myoclonic epilepsy.

The **olivopontocerebellar atrophies** (OPCA) include at least five familial subtypes with dominant inheritance that usually have the onset of ataxia, cranial nerve palsies, and abnormal sensory findings in the 2nd or 3rd decade. However, some cases have been described in children, particularly of Finnish ancestry, with rapidly progressive ataxia, nystagmus, dysarthria, and seizures. Classifications of the hereditary ataxias are based on biochemical analysis; aspartic acid and glutamic acid contents in the inferior olive and the Purkinje cell layer of the cerebellum are significantly decreased.

Rare forms of progressive cerebellar ataxia have been described in association with **vitamin E deficiency.** Additional degenerative ataxias include **Pelizaeus-Merzbacher disease,** neuronal ceroid lipofuscinoses, and late onset GM_2 gangliosidosis (see Chapter 608).

606.2 Chorea

Sydenham chorea is the most common acquired chorea of childhood and is the sole neurologic manifestation of rheumatic fever (Chapter 184.1). The pathogenesis of Sydenham chorea is probably an autoimmune response of the CNS to group A streptococcal organisms. The majority of children with Sydenham chorea have antineuronal antibodies, which develop in response to group A β-hemolytic streptococcal infections. Antineuronal antibodies cross react with the cytoplasm of subthalamic and caudate nuclei neurons. Some pediatric patients with tics and obsessive-compulsive disorder (features also associated with Sydenham chorea) have antineuronal antibodies suggesting that Tourette syndrome and other childhood neuropsychiatric disorders in some cases may be secondary to an autoimmune process. The primary pathologic findings, possibly the result of the cellular response to antineuronal antibodies, consist of vasculitis of the cortical arterioles with round cell infiltration of the gray and white matter in the surrounding area. The cerebral cortex, caudate nucleus, and subthalamic nuclei are most prominently involved. Chorea is likely a result of functional overactivity of the dopaminergic system.

The three major features of Sydenham chorea include chorea, hypotonia, and emotional lability. The chorea is usually symmetric, although children may have the choreic movements limited to one side of the body. The movements, which are rapid and jerky, are prominent in the face, trunk, and distal extremities and dart from one muscle group to another; they are increased by stress, and disappear during sleep. The onset may be abrupt, but the chorea typically has a slowly progressive course. Hypotonia may be a prominent sign, and when combined with severe chorea, the child may be incapable of feeding, dressing, or walking. The speech is often involved and is sometimes unintelligible. Periods of uncontrollable crying and extreme mood swings are characteristic, perhaps in part as a result of the motor handicap and feelings of helplessness. Several typical signs are associated with Syden ham chorea, including the "milkmaid's grip" (relaxing and tightening hand shake), the "choreic hand" (spooning of the extended hand by flexion at the wrist and extension of the fingers), the "darting tongue" (the tongue cannot be protruded for longer than a few seconds), and the "pronator sign" (the arms and palms turn outward when held above the head). Sydenham chorea may persist for several months and as long as 1–2 yr. About 20% of children experience a recurrence of chorea within 2 yr of the intial episode. Cases with minimal signs are treated conservatively with avoidance of stress as much as possible. Incapacitating chorea is managed with a trial of diazepam followed by phenothiazines or haloperidol if the former is unsuccessful.

Although the phenothiazines and haloperidol are effective drugs in the treatment of Sydenham chorea, long-term use may be complicated by the development of another movement disorder, **tardive dyskinesia**. Tardive dyskinesa is characterized by stereotypical facial movements, particularly by lip smacking and protrusion and retraction of the tongue. The movement disorder may gradually disappear but in some patients persists after discontinuing the drug. Because patients with Sydenham chorea are at risk for the development of rheumatic carditis, particularly mitral stenosis, a regimen of daily penicillin prophylaxis should be instituted and maintained until adulthood. A much rarer cause of chorea during childhood, *paroxysmal kinesigenic choreoathetosis*, is discussed in Chapter 603.

Systemic lupus erythematosus (SLE) may present or be associated with neurologic symptoms and signs including seizures, organic brain syndromes (psychoses), aseptic meningitis, and various isolated neurologic signs including chorea. Chorea may be the presenting sign of SLE, particularly in children. Antiphospholipid antibodies are present in the serum in the majority of these patients. The presence of circulating antiphospholipid antibodies is associated with a high incidence of venous and arterial occlusions. Any child with chorea of unknown cause should be investigated for the possibility of antiphospholipid antibodies.

Huntington disease is a progressive degenerative disorder of the CNS of unknown cause. It affects about 1/10,000 individuals and is inherited as an autosomal dominant trait. Huntington disease is associated with an expanded sequence of CAG repeats in a gene on chromosome 4p16.3. The onset of symptoms of progressive chorea and presenile dementia occurs most typically between 35 and 55 yr of age. The disease is rare in the pediatric population; fewer than 1% of cases have the onset of symptoms before 10 yr of age. Rigidity and dystonia are the most common neurologic findings in children. Chorea tends to involve proximal muscles, and the abnormal movements are often incorporated into semipurposeful acts in an attempt to mask the abnormality. Mental deterioration and behavioral problems are prominent in children. Generalized tonic-clonic seizures are common and are typically resistant to anticonvulsants. Cerebellar signs are present in 50% and oculomotor apraxia occurs in approximately 20% of cases. The course of the disease is more rapid in children, with an average duration of 8 yr until death compared with 14 yr in adults. CT scanning, although nondiagnostic, shows the mean bifrontal to bicaudate ratio to be decreased, indicating atrophy of the caudate nucleus and putamen. MRI shows hyperdensity of the putamen in adults with the akinetic-rigid form. There is no specific therapy for Huntington disease, but once the diagnosis is confirmed, the pediatrician should provide genetic counseling to the family so that risks for additional cases in future generations are understood. Molecular biologic testing (CAG trinucleotide repeat) is available but is inappropriate for children under the age of consent. Presymptomatic adult patients who test positive respond similarly to patients with cancer when the diagnosis is confirmed.

Other causes of chorea include atypical seizures, drug intoxication (eg., phenytoin, amitriptyline, and fluphenazine), hormonally induced seizures (e.g., oral contraceptives, pregnancy/chorea gravidarum), Lyme disease, hypoparathyroidism, hyperthyroidism, and Wilson disease (see Chapter 357.2). Chorea also may occur after cardiac surgery and circulatory arrest, possibly relating to the steal phenomenon, duration of the cooling period, and acid-base disturbances.

606.3 Dystonias

Dystonia is a slow, intermittent twisting motion that produces exaggerated turning and posture of the extremities and trunk. The principal causes of dystonia include perinatal asphyxia (see Chapters 95.2 and 95.7), dystonia musculorum deformans, drugs, Wilson disease (hepatolenticular degeneration), and Hallervorden-Spatz disease.

Dystonia musculorum deformans (DMD) is a slowly progressive disorder that typically begins during childhood. The cause is unknown, but an abnormality of catecholamine metabolism within the CNS has been proposed. DMD is inherited as an autosomal dominant trait. One form occurs primarily in the Ashkenazi Jewish popultion, with an incidence of approximately 1/1,000. The disorder results from mutations in the DYT_1 gene located on chromosome 9q34. The initial manifestation of the disease during childhood is often unilateral posturing of the lower extremity, particuarly the foot, which assumes an extended and rotated position causing tiptoe walking. Because the dystonic movement is initially intermittent and is aggravated by stress, patients are often labeled as hysterical. Ultimately, all four extremities and the axial musculature are affected as well as the muscles of the face and tongue, and thus speech and swallowing become impaired. Patients with generalized dystonia, including those with involvement of the muscles of swallowing, may respond to large doses of trihexyphenidyl (Artane). The initial dose is 2 mg/24 hr, slowly increasing to 60–80 mg/24 hr or until untoward side effects (urinary retention, mental confusion, or blurred vision) occur. Additional drugs that have been effective include carbamazepine, levodopa, bromocriptine, and diazepam.

Dopa-responsive dystonia (DRD), a variant of childhood-onset idiopathic torsion dystonia, is more common in females and typically presents at a mean age of 6.5 yr with dystonic posturing of a lower extremity. The gene for dopa-sensitive dystonia is located on chromosome 148 and encodes for the enzyme GTP cyclohydrolase 1. DRD responds remarkably to small daily doses (50–250 mg) of levodopa given with an inhibitor of peripheral catabolism. The dystonia is diurnal, improving with sleep but becoming apparent and sometimes incapacitating during the daytime. Signs of Parkinson disease may ultimately become evident, including bradykinesia, tremors, and cogwheel rigidity. The disease is familial, with an autosomal dominant inheritance.

Segmental dystonia, including writer's cramp, blepharospasm and buccomandibular dystonia, is more common in adults and tends to be limited to a specific group of muscles. Adults with segmental dystonia, particularly blepharospasm, may respond to local injections of botulinum toxin, which holds promise for some children with generalized DMD. Cryothalamectomy with the placement of a lesion in the ventrolateral thalamus is reserved primarily for patients with extremity involvement.

Certain *drugs* are capable of producing an acute dystonic reaction in children. Therapeutic doses of phenytoin or carbamazepine may rarely cause progressive dystonia in children with epilepsy, particularly in those who have an underlying structural abnormality of the brain. Children may have an idiosyncratic reaction to the phenothiazines, characterized by acute dystonic posturing that is sometimes confused with encephalitis. Intravenous diphenhydramine, 1–2 mg/kg/dose, may rapidly reverse the drug-related dystonia.

Wilson disease is a rare (incidence of 1/40,000 to 1/100,000 live births) autosomal recessive inborn error of copper transport characterized by cirrhosis of the liver and degenerative changes in the CNS, particularly the basal ganglia (see Chapter 357.2). The gene (WND) for Wilson disease has been mapped to chromosome 13q14–21. It has been determined that there are multiple mutations in the Wilson disease gene, accounting for the variability in presentation of the condition. The precise cause is unknown, but the basic mechanism relates to decreased excretion of biliary copper, owing partly to a lysosomal defect of the liver cells. The initial symptoms and signs in children younger than 10 yr relate to acute or subacute hepatic failure, which is frequently misinterpreted as infectious hepatitis. The neurologic manifestations of Wilson disease rarely appear before age 10 yr, and the initial sign is often progressive dystonia. Tremors of the extremities develop, unilaterally at first, but they eventually become coarse, generalized, and incapacitating (the so-called wing-beating tremor). Signs of progressive basal ganglia destruction include drooling, a fixed smile owing to retraction of the upper lip, dysarthria, dysphonia, rigidity, contractures, dystonia, and choreoathetosis. The Kayser-Fleischer ring, which is best seen with the slit lamp, is pathognomonic and results from deposition of copper in Descemet membrane. In the untreated state, patients typically become bedridden and demented and die in coma within a few years from the onset of the disease. The MRI or CT scan shows ventricular dilatation in advanced cases with atrophy of the cerebrum and lesions in the thalamus and basal ganglia (Fig. 606–1). The treatment of Wilson disease is discussed in Chapter 357.2.

Hallervorden-Spatz disease is a rare degenerative disorder inherited as an autosomal recessive trait. Linkage analysis indicates that the gene is located on chromosome 20p13. The condition usually begins during childhood and is characterized by progressive dystonia, rigidity, and choreoathetosis. Spasticity, extensor plantar responses, dysarthria, and intellectual deterioration become evident during adolescence, and death usually occurs by early adulthood. MRI shows lesions of the globus pallidus, including low signal intensity in T2-weighted images (corresponds to iron pigments) and an anteromedial area of high signal intensity or "eye-of-the-tiger" sign (corresponding to areas of vacuolation). Neuropathologic examination indicates excessive accumulation of iron-containing pigments in the globus pallidus and substantia nigra.

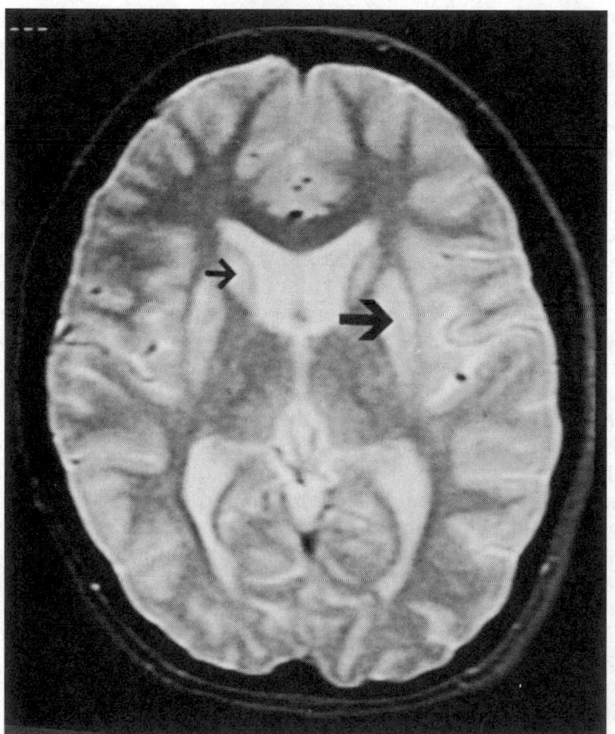

Figure 606–1 Wilson disease. MRI, T2 image showing increased density of the caudate *(small arrow)* and the putamen *(large arrow)*.

Athetosis is most commonly associated with perinatal brain insults and is occasionally the major movement disorder of *phenothiazine idiosyncrasy.* Choreoathetosis may occur after hypothermic bypass surgery for congenital heart disease. Rigidity is associated with progressive destructive or neurodegenerative conditions,including Krabbe disease.

Tremor is an involuntary movement characterized by rhythmic oscillations of a part of the body, which may be more prominent during rest or with movement. **Jitteriness,** defined as rhythmic tremors of equal amplitude around a fixed axis, is the most common involuntary movement of healthy full-term infants. Jitteriness is most apparent when an infant is crying or being examined (e.g., Moro response) and is abnormal when an infant is awake and alert and when the tremor persists beyond the second week of life. Organic causes of jitteriness include sepsis, intracranial hemorrhage, hypoxic encephalopathy, hypoglycemia, hypocalcemia, hypomagnesemia, prenatal exposure to maternal marijuana, and the narcotic abstinence syndrome. **Essential tremor** is a familial condition, inherited as an autosomal dominant trait. It may begin during childhood and usually is slowly progressive. The tremor has a frequency of 4–9 Hz, primarily affects the distal upper extremities, is typically postural, and commonly disappears with rest. If the tremor causes difficulty in writing or activities of daily living, a trial of propranolol hydrochloride or primidone usually provides a favorable response. **Primary writing tremor** occurs only during the action of writing and is characterized by a jerky tremor, often responsive to β blockers or anticholinergics. Drugs that can cause tremor include amphetamines, valproic acid, neuroleptics, tricyclic antidepressants, caffeine, and theophylline. Tremor may be the initial manifestation of a metabolic disorder, including hypoglycemia, thyrotoxicosis, neuroblastoma, and pheochromocytoma. Children recovering from a severe head injury may develop a proximal tremor that is enhanced by movement and responds to propranolol. Wilson disease often presents with a postural tremor associated with kinetic movement. These patients may also develop a wing-beating tremor of the shoulders when the upper arms are abducted and the elbows flexed. Hereditary dystonia-parkinsonism syndrome often displays a proximal tremor in addition to the characteristic dystonic movements.

606.4 Tics

Tics are spasmodic, involuntary, repetitive, stereotyped movements that are nonrhythmic, often exacerbated by stress, and may affect any muscle group. Tics can be classified into three subgroups: transient tics of childhood, chronic tics, and Gilles de la Tourette syndrome (TS). **Transient tic disorder** is the most common movement abnormality of childhood (see Chapter 21). The tics are more prevalent in boys, and the family history is often positive. They consist of eye blinking or facial movements and occasional throat-clearing noises. The disorder persists from weeks to less than a year and does not require drug therapy. **Chronic motor tic disorder** occurs in children and persists throughout adult life. The tics characteristically involve up to three muscle groups simultaneously and may occur throughout life. Evidence shows that the gene for TS may be expressed as simple transient tic of childhood and chronic motor tics, suggesting considerable overlap of these conditions.

Gilles de la Tourette syndrome is a lifelong condition, with a prevalence of approximately 1/2,000, that has an onset between 2 and 21 yr of age. TS is probably inherited in most cases as autosomal dominant, and the gene has been mapped to chromosome 18q22.1 (see Chapter 21). TS has four components, not all of which may be present in each patient: motor tics, vocal tics, obsessive-compulsive behavior, and attention deficit hyperactivity disorder (ADHD). These symptoms may wax and wane and are always enhanced by stress and anxiety. TS is a lifelong condition, and the ultimate prognosis can usually be determined by the severity of the symptons during adolescence. Motor tics are associated with numerous fluctuating movements of the face, eyelids, neck, and shoulders. Ultimately, the tics are accompanied by vocalizations (vocal tics), including throat clearing, sniffling, barking, coprolalia (obscene words), echolalia (repetition of words addressed to the patient), palilalia (repetition of one's own words), and echokinesis (imitation of movement of others). The vocalizations are uncontrollable and frequently jeopardize patients' social interaction with other children. Compulsive behavior, including touching, licking, repetitive thoughts, and motor actions, and a greater than 50% incidence of ADHD are common to TS.

Medication should be considered when the motor tics or vocalizations interfere significantly with a child's social and academic interactions, although behavior management and biofeedback programs have been successful for some patients. Several reports implicate stimulant medications (methylphenidate) as the cause of TS. Methylphenidate may unmask TS but not cause it.

All children who have ADHD and who are treated with stimulant medication should be monitored closely for the onset of tics. The decision to continue the stimulant medication should be determined by the severity of the ADHD and tic disorder. Haloperidol, a dopamine-blocking agent, is effective in the treatment of approximately 50% of children with TS. The initial dose is 0.25 mg/24 hr, and the drug is increased weekly by 0.25 mg to the usual dose range of 2–6 mg/24 hr, although some children can tolerate larger doses. Side effects include cognitive impairment, lethargy, fatigue, depression, restlessness, acute dystonic reactions, drug-induced parkinsonism, akathisia, and tardive dyskinesia syndromes, including tardive dystonia in children. Additional drugs that may prove useful include penfluridol, pimozide, and clonidine. Clonidine, an α_2-presynaptic noradrenergic agonist, is begun at a dose of 0.05 mg/24 hr and gradually increased to a maximum of 0.125–0.2 mg/24 hr. Several weeks of clonidine therapy may be needed to control the vocal and motor tics. The major side effects are lethargy, fatigue, and drowsiness. Approximately 50% of patients with TS experience obsessive-compulsive symptoms. The tricyclic antidepressant clomipramine is effective in approximately 60% of patients. Other useful antidepressant drugs include sertraline, fluoxetine, and fluvoxamine. Because TS is a chronic disorder associated with many social, behavioral, and learning problems, pediatricians can have an important role in the multidisciplinary management as an advocate for children.

Aron AM, Freeman JM, Carter S: The natural history of Sydenham's chorea. Am J Med 38:83, 1965.

Bebin EM, Bebin J, Currier RD, et al: Morphometric studies in dominant olivopontocerebellar atrophy: Comparison of cell losses with amino acid decreases. Arch Neurol 47:188, 1990.

Boder E, Sedgwick RP: Ataxia-telangiectasia: A familial syndrome of progressive cerebellar ataxia, oculocutaneous telangiectasia and frequent pulmonary infection. Pediatrics 21:526, 1958.

Bray PF: Coincidence of neuroblastoma and acute cerebellar encephalopathy. J Pediatr 75:983, 1969.

Campuzano V, Montermini L, Malto MD, et al: Friedreich's ataxia: Autosomal recessive disease caused by an intronic GAA triplet repeat expansion. Science 271:1423, 1996.

Cervera R, Asherson RA, Font J, et al: Chorea in the antiphospholipid syndrome. Medicine 76:203, 1997.

Chamberlain S, Farrall M, Shaw J, et al: Genetic recombination events which position the Friedreich ataxia locus proximal to the D9S15/D9S5 linkage group on chromosome 9q. Am J Hum Genet 52:99, 1993.

Eldridge R: The torsion dystonia: Literature review and genetic and clinical studies. Neurology 20:1, 1970.

Gatti RA: Candidates for the molecular defect in ataxia telangiectasia. Adv Neurol 61:127, 1993.

Golden GS: Tics and Tourette's: A continuum of symptoms? Ann Neurol 4:145, 1978.

Hansotia P, Cleeland CS, Chun RWM: Juvenile Huntington's chorea. Neurology 18:217, 1968.

Holinski-Feder E, Baldwin Jedele K, Hörtnagel K: Large intergenerational variation in age of onset in two young patients with Huntington's disease presenting as dyskinesia. Pediatrics 100:896, 1997.

Joubert M, Eisenring JJ, Robb JP, et al: Familial agenesis of the cerebellar vermis. Neurology 19:824, 1969.

Konigsmark BW, Weiner LP: The olivopontocerebellar atrophies: A review. Medicine 49:227, 1970.

Parker S, Zuckerman B, Bauchner H, et al: Jitteriness in full-term neonates: Prevalence and correlates. Pediatrics 85:17, 1990.

Swedo SE, Leonard HL, Miltleman BB, et al: Identification of children with pediatric autoimmune neuropsychiatric disorders associated with streptococcal infections by a marker associated with rheumatic fever. Am J Psychiatry 154:110, 1997; 155:264, 1998.

Suchowersky O: Gilles de la Tourette syndrome. Can J Neurol Sci 22:48, 1994.

Thomas GR, Forbes JR, Roberts EA, et al: The Wilson disease gene: spectrum of mutations and their consequences. Nat Genet 9:210, 1995.

Vakili S: Hallervorden-Spatz syndrome Arch Neurol 34:729, 1977.

Van Caillie-Bertrand M, Degenhart HJ, Visso HKA, et al: Oral zinc sulphate for Wilson's disease. Arch Dis Child 60:656, 1985.

Weiss S, Carter S: Course and prognosis of acute cerebellar ataxia in children. Neurology 9:711, 1959.

Wong PC, Barlow CF, Hickey PR, et al: Factors associated with choreoathetosis after cardiopulmonary bypass in children with congenital heart disease. Circulation 86 (Suppl II):118, 1992.

Chapter 607
Encephalopathies

Encephalopathy is a generalized disorder of cerebral function that may be acute or chronic, progressive or static. The etiology of the encephalopathies in children includes infectious, toxic (e.g., carbon monoxide, drugs, lead), metabolic, and ischemic causes. Hypoxic-ischemic encephalopathy is discussed in Chapter 95.7.

607.1 Cerebral Palsy

See also Chapters 37 and 93.2.

Cerebral palsy (CP) is a static encephalopathy that may be defined as a nonprogressive disorder of posture and movement, often associated with epilepsy and abnormalities of speech, vision, and intellect resulting from a defect or lesion of the developing brain. CP is a common disorder, with an estimated prevalence of 2/1,000 population. The condition was first described almost 150 yr ago by Little, an orthopedic surgeon. He suggested that the primary causes included birth trauma and asphyxia, as well as prematurity, and that improved obstetric care would significantly reduce the incidence of CP. During the past 2–3 decades, considerable advances have been made in obstetric and neonatal care, but unfortunately, there has been virtually no change in the incidence of CP.

EPIDEMIOLOGY AND ETIOLOGY. The Collaborative Perinatal Project, in which approximately 45,000 children were regularly monitored from pregnancy to the age of 7 yr, reported the prevalence of CP to be 4/1,000 live births. Birth asphyxia was an uncommon cause of CP; moreover, most high-risk pregnancies resulted in neurologically normal children. Although a cause of CP could not be identified in most cases, a substantial number of children with CP had congenital anomalies external to the central nervous system (CNS), and these may have placed them at increased risk for developing asphyxia during the perinatal period. An Australian study comparing children with spastic CP with a group of matched controls had similar findings. Fewer than 10% of children with CP had evidence of intrapartum asphyxia. Intrauterine exposure to maternal infection (e.g., chorioamnionitis, inflammation of placental membranes, umbilical cord inflammation, foul-smelling amniotic fluid, maternal sepsis, temperature greater than 38°C during labor, and urinary tract infection) is associated with a significant increase in the risk of CP in normal birthweight infants. The prevalence of CP has increased among low birthweight infants, particularly those weighing less than 1,000 g at birth, primarily because of intracerebral hemorrhage and periventricular leukomalacia. These studies suggest that future developments aimed at enhancing perinatal care will have minimal impact on the incidence of CP and that research might be directed more profitably to the field of developmental biology in order to understand the pathogenesis of CP.

CLINICAL MANIFESTATIONS. CP may be classified by a description of the motor handicap in terms of physiologic, topographic, and etiologic categories and functional capacity (Table 607–1). The physiologic classification identifies the major motor abnormality, whereas the topographic taxonomy indicates the involved extremities. CP is also commonly associated with a spectrum of developmental disabilities, including mental retardation, epilepsy, and visual, hearing, speech, cognitive, and behavioral abnormalities. The motor handicap may be the least of the child's problems.

Infants with *spastic hemiplegia* have decreased spontaneous movements on the affected side and show hand preference at a very early age. The arm is often more involved than the leg and difficulty in hand manipulation is obvious by 1 yr of age. Walking is usually delayed until 18–24 mo, and a circumductive gait is apparent. Examination of the extremities may show growth arrest, particularly in the hand and thumbnail, especially if the contralateral parietal lobe is abnormal, because extermity growth is influenced by this area of the brain. Spasticity is apparent in the affected extremities, particularly the ankle, causing an equinovarus deformity of the foot. An affected child often walks on tiptoes because of the increased tone, and the affected upper extremity assumes a dystonic posture when the child runs. Ankle clonus and a Babinski sign may be present, the deep tendon reflexes are increased, and weakness of the hand and foot dorsiflexors is evident. About one third of patients with spastic hemiplegia have a seizure disorder that usually develops during the first year or two, and approximately 25% have cognitive abnormalities including mental retardation. A CT scan or MRI may show an atrophic cerebral hemisphere with a dilated lateral ventricle contralateral to the side of the affected extremities. Intrauterine thromboembolism with focal cerebral infarction may be one cause; CT or MRI at birth in infants with focal seizures often demonstrates the area of infarction. Spastic hemiplegia is more common than spastic diplegia in low birthweight infants.

Spastic diplegia is bilateral spasticity of the legs. The first indication of spastic diplegia is often noted when an affected infant begins to crawl. The child uses the arms in a normal reciprocal fashion but tends to drag the legs behind more as a rudder (commando crawl) rather than using the normal four-limbed crawling movement. If the spasticity is severe, application of a diaper is difficult owing to excessive adduction of the hips. Examination of the child reveals spasticity in the legs with brisk reflexes, ankle clonus, and a bilateral Babinski sign. When the child is suspended by the axillae, a scissoring posture of the lower extremities is maintained. Walking is significantly delayed; the feet are held in a position of equinovarus; and the child walks on tiptoes. Severe spastic diplegia is characterized by disuse atrophy and impaired growth of the lower extremities and by disproportionate growth with normal development of the upper torso. The prognosis for normal intellectual development is excellent for these patients, and the likelihood of seizures is minimal. The most common neuropathologic finding is periventricular leukomalacia, particularly in the area where fibers innervating the legs course through the internal capsule.

Spastic quadriplegia is the most severe form of CP because of marked motor impairment of all extremities and the high association with mental retardation and seizures. Swallowing difficulties are common owing to supranuclear bulbar palsies, and they often lead to aspiration pneumonia. At autopsy, the central white matter is disrupted by areas of necrotic degeneration that may coalesce into cystic cavities. Neurologic examination shows increased tone and spasticity in all extremities, decreased spontaneous movements, brisk reflexes, and plantar extensor responses. Flexion contractures of the knees and elbows are often present by late childhood. Associated developmental disabilities, including speech and visual abnormalities, are particularly prevalent in this group of children. Children with spastic quadriparesis often have evidence of athetosis and may be classified as having mixed CP.

Athetoid CP is relatively rare, especially since the advent of aggressive management of hyperbilirubinemia and the prevention of kernicterus. Affected infants are characteristically hypotonic and have poor head control and marked head lag. Feeding may be difficult, and tongue thrust and drooling may be prominent. The athetoid movements may not become evident until 1 yr of age and tend to coincide with hypermyelination of the basal ganglia, a phenomenon called **status marmoratus.** Speech is typically affected owing to involvement of the oropharyngeal muscles. Sentences are slurred, and voice modulation is impaired. Generally, upper motor neuron signs are not present, seizures are uncommon, and intellect is preserved in most patients.

DIAGNOSIS. A thorough history and physical examination should preclude a progressive disorder of the CNS, including degenerative diseases, spinal cord tumor, or muscular dystrophy. Depending on the severity and the nature of the neurologic abnormalities, a baseline electroencephalogram (EEG) and CT

TABLE 607–1 Various Classification Systems for Cerebral Palsy

Physiologic	Topographic	Etiologic	Functional
Spastic	Monoplegia	Prenatal (e.g., infection, metabolic, anoxia, toxic, genetic, infarction)	Class I—no limitation of activity
Athetoid	Paraplegia		
Rigid	Hemiplegia		Class II—slight to moderate limitation
Ataxic	Triplegia		
Tremor	Quadriplegia	Perinatal (e.g., anoxia)	Class III—moderate to great limitation
Atonic	Diplegia		
Mixed	Double hemiplegia	Postnatal (e.g., toxins, trauma, infection)	Class IV—no useful physical activity
Unclassified			

Adapted from Minear WL: A classification of cerebral palsy. Pediatrics 18:841, 1956.

scan may be indicated to determine the location and extent of structural lesions or associated congenital malformations. Additional studies may include tests of hearing and visual function. As CP is usually associated with a wide spectrum of developmental disorders, a multidisciplinary approach is most helpful in the assessment and treatment of such children.

TREATMENT. A team of physicians from various specialties as well as the occupational and physical therapists, speech pathologist, social worker, educator, and developmental psychologist provide important contributions to the treatment of these children. Parents should be taught how to handle their child in daily activities such as feeding, carrying, dressing, bathing, and playing in ways that limit the effects of abnormal muscle tone. They also need to be instructed in the supervision of a series of exercises designed to prevent the development of contractures, especially a tight Achilles tendon. There is no proof that physical or occupational therapy prevents development of CP in infants at risk or that it corrects the neurologic deficit, but ample evidence shows that therapy optimizes the development of an abnormal child.

Children with spastic diplegia are treated initially with the assistance of adaptive equipment, such as walkers, poles, and standing frames. If a patient has marked spasticity of the lower extremities or evidence of hip dislocation, consideration should be given to performing surgical soft tissue procedures that reduce muscle spasm around the hip girdle, including an adductor tenotomy or psoas transfer and release. A rhizotomy procedure in which the roots of the spinal nerves are divided has produced considerable improvement in selected patients with severe spastic diplegia. A tight heel cord in a child with spastic hemiplegia may be treated surgically by tenotomy of the Achilles tendon. Quadriplegia is managed with motorized wheelchairs, special feeding devices, modified typewriters, and customized seating arrangements.

Communication skills may be enhanced by the use of Bliss symbols, talking typewriters, and specially adapted computers including artificial intelligence computers to augment motor and language function. Significant behavior problems may substantially interfere with the development of a child with CP; their early identification and management are important, and the assistance of a psychologist or psychiatrist may be necessary. Learning and attention deficit disorders and mental retardation are assessed and managed by a psychologist and educator. Strabismus, nystagmus, and optic atrophy are common in children with CP; thus, an ophthalmologist should be included in the initial assessment. Lower urinary tract dysfunction should receive prompt assessment and treatment. Several drugs have been used to treat spasticity, including dantrolene sodium, the benzodiazepines, and baclofen. These medications are generally ineffective but should be considered if severe spasticity is not controlled by other measures. Intrathecal baclofen has been used successfully in selected children with severe spasticity. This experimental therapy requires a team approach and constant follow-up for complications of the infusion pumping mechanism and infection. Botulinum toxin is undergoing study for the management of spasticity in specific muscle groups, and the preliminary findings show a positive response in those patients studied. Patients with incapacitating athetosis occasionally respond to levodopa, and children with dystonia may benefit from carbamazepine or trihexyphenidyl.

*607.2 Mitochondrial Encephalomyophathies**

Mitochondrial diseases are a complex family of disorders with many clinical manifestations that can be caused by mutations of nuclear DNA (nDNA) or mitochondrial DNA (mtDNA). They can affect various developmental stages, tissues, or systems, resulting in a diversity of clinical phenotypes that span all age groups. Biochemically, they can present with a tissue-specific or generalized monoenzymopathy, tissue-specific multienzymopathy, or generalized multienzymopathy. In the respiratory chain, oxidative phosphorylation is mediated by five intramitochondrial enzyme complexes (complexes I–V) that are responsible for producing the ATP required for normal cellular function. The maintenance and assembly of oxidative phosphorylation requires coordinated regulation of nuclear DNA and mitochondrial DNA genes. Human mtDNA is a small (16.5 kb) circular, double-stranded molecule that has been completely sequenced and encodes 13 structural proteins, all of which are subunits of the respiratory chain complexes, as well as 2 ribosomal RNAs and 22 tRNAs needed for translation. The nuclear DNA is responsible for synthesizing approximately 70 subunits, transporting them to the mitochondria via chaperone proteins, ensuring their passage across the inner mitochondrial membrane, and coordinating their correct processing and assembly.

MtDNA is unique from nDNA for the following reasons: (1) its genetic code differs from nDNA; (2) it is tightly packed with information because it contains no introns; (3) it is subject to spontaneous mutations at a higher rate than nDNA; (4) it has less efficient repair mechanisms; and (5) it is present in hundreds or thousands of copies per cell and is transmitted by maternal inheritance. MtDNA is contributed only by the oocyte in the formation of the zygote. If a mutation in mtDNA occurs in the ovum or zygote, it may be passed on randomly to subsequent generations of cells. Some receive few or no mutant genomes (normal or wild-type homoplasmy), others receive a mixed population of mutant and wild-type mtDNAs (heteroplasmy), and others receive primarily or exclusively mutant genomes (mutant homoplasmy). The important implications of maternal inheritance and heteroplasmy are as follows: (1) Inheritance of the disease is maternal, but both sexes are equally affected; (2) phenotypic expression of a mtDNA mutation depends on the relative proportions of mutant and wild type genomes, with a minimum critical number of mutant genomes being necessary for expression (threshold effect); (3) at cell division, the proportion may shift in daughter cells (mitotic segregation), leading to a corresponding phenotypic change; and (4) subsequent generations are affected at a higher rate than in autosomal dominant diseases. The critical number of mutant mtDNAs required for the threshold effect may vary, depending on the vulnerability of the tissue to impairments of oxidative metabolism as well as on the vulnerability of the same tissue over time that may increase with aging. Diseases of mitochondrial oxidative phosphorylation can be divided into three groups: (1) defects of nDNA, (2) defects of mtDNA, and (3) defects of communication between the nuclear and mitochondrial genome.

Using a broader classification system, mitochondrial diseases caused by defects of nDNA include defects of substrate transport (plasmalemmal carnitine transporter, carnitine palmitoyltransferase I and II, carnitine acylcarnitine translocase defects), defects of substrate oxidation (pyruvate dehydrogenase complex, pyruvate carboxylase, intramitochondrial fatty acid oxidation defects), defects of the Krebs cycle (α-ketoglutarate dehydrogenase, fumarase, aconitase defects), and defects of the respiratory chain (complexes I to V) including defects of oxidation/phosphorylation coupling (Luft syndrome) and defects of mitochondrial protein transport. These diseases follow mendelian inheritance. Diseases caused by defects of mtDNA can be divided into those due to point mutations that are maternally inherited (Leber hereditary optic neuropathy and MELAS, MERRF, and NARP syndromes—see later) and those due to deletions or duplications that tend to be sporadic (Kearns-Sayre and Pearson marrow/pancreas syndromes). Fi-

*Written with the collaboration of Dr. Ingrid Tein.

nally, diseases caused by defects of communication between the nuclear and mitochondrial genome follow mendelian inheritance and include multiple mtDNA deletions, which are autosomal dominant, and mtDNA depletion syndromes, which are generally autosomal recessive.

MITOCHONDRIAL ENCEPHALOMYOPATHY, LACTIC ACIDOSIS, AND STROKE-LIKE EPISODES (MELAS). Children with MELAS may be normal for the first several years, but they gradually display delayed motor and cognitive development and short stature. The clinical syndrome is characterized by (1) strokelike episodes most commonly in the posterior temporal, parietal, and occipital lobes (with CT or MRI evidence of focal brain abnormalities); (2) lactic acidosis, ragged red fibers (RRF), or both; and (3) at least two of the following: focal or generalized seizures, dementia, recurrent migraine headaches, and vomiting. In one series, onset was before age 15 in 62% of patients and hemianopia or cortical blindness was the most common manifestation. Cerebrospinal fluid protein is often increased. The MELAS 3243 mutation can also be associated with different combinations of exercise intolerance, myopathy, ophthalmoplegia, pigmentary retinopathy, hypertrophic or dilated cardiomyopathy, cardiac conduction defects, deafness, endocrinopathy (diabetes mellitus), and proximal renal tubular dysfunction. MELAS is a progressive disorder that has been reported in siblings. It is punctuated with episodes of stroke leading to dementia. Regional hypoperfusion can be detected by single-photon emission CT (SPECT) studies. Neuropathology may show cortical atrophy with infarct-like lesions in both cortical and subcortical structures, basal ganglia calcifications, and ventricular dilatation. Muscle biopsy specimens usually, but not always, show RRF. Mitochondrial accumulations and abnormalities have been shown in smooth muscle cells of intramuscular vessels and of brain arterioles and in the epithelial cells and blood vessels of the choroid plexus, producing a mitochondrial angiopathy. Muscle biochemistry has shown complex I deficiency in many cases; however, multiple defects have also been documented involving complexes I, III, and IV. Inheritance is maternal, and there is a highly specific, although not exclusive, point mutation at nt 3243 in the $tRNA^{Leu (UUR)}$ gene of mtDNA in approximately 80% of patients. An additional 7.5% have a point mutation at nt 3271 in the $tRNA^{Leu (UUR)}$ gene. A third mutation has been identified at nt 3252 in the $tRNA^{leu (UUR)}$ gene. Because the number of mutant genomes is lower in blood than in muscle, muscle is the preferable tissue for examination. The prognosis in patients with the full syndrome is poor. Therapeutic trials have included corticosteroids and coenzyme Q10. Lowering the serum lactate concentration with dichloroacetate has led to marked clinical improvement in some but not all cases.

MYOCLONUS EPILEPSY AND RAGGED-RED FIBERS (MERRF). This syndrome is characterized by progressive myoclonic epilepsy, mitochondrial myopathy, and cerebellar ataxia with dysarthria and nystagmus. Onset may be in childhood or in adult life, and the course may be slowly progressive or rapidly downhill. Other features include dementia, sensorineural hearing loss, optic atrophy, peripheral neuropathy, and spasticity. Because some patients have abnormalities of deep sensation and pes cavus, the condition may be confused with Friedreich ataxia. As with MELAS syndrome, a significant number of patients have a positive family history and short stature. This condition is maternally inherited. Pathologic findings include elevated serum lactate concentrations, RRF on muscle biopsy, and marked neuronal loss and gliosis affecting in particular the dentate nucleus and inferior olivary complex with some dropout of Purkinje's cells and neurons of the red nucleus. Pallor of the posterior columns of the spinal cord and degeneration of the gracile and cuneate nuclei are noted. Muscle biochemistry has shown variable defects of complex III, complexes II and IV, complexes I and IV, or complex IV alone. More than 80% of cases are caused by a heteroplasmic G to A point mutation at nt 8344 of the $tRNA^{Lys}$ gene of mtDNA. Additional patients have been reported with a T to C mutation at nt 8356 in the $tRNA^{Lys}$ gene. There is no specific therapy, although coenzyme Q10 appeared to be beneficial in a mother and daughter with the MERRF mutation.

LEBER HEREDITARY OPTIC NEUROPATHY (LHON). LHON is characterized by onset usually between the ages of 18 and 30 yr of acute or subacute visual loss due to severe bilateral optic atrophy, although children as young as 5 yr have been reported. There is a marked male predominance: At least 85% are young men. This suggests an X-linked factor that modulates the expression of the mitochondrial DNA point mutation. The classic ophthalmologic features include circumpapillary telangiectatic microangiopathy and pseudoedema of the optic disc. Variable features may include cerebellar ataxia, hyperreflexia, Babinski sign, psychiatric symptoms, peripheral neuropathy, or cardiac conduction abnormalities (pre-excitation syndrome). Some cases have been associated with widespread white matter lesions as seen with multiple sclerosis. Lactic acidosis and RRF tend to be conspicuously absent in LHON. More than eleven mtDNA point mutations have been described, including a usually homoplasmic G to A transition at nt 11,778 of the ND4 subunit gene of complex I, which leads to replacement of a highly conserved arginine residue by histidine at the 340th amino acid and which accounts for approximately 50–70% of cases in Europe and over 90% of cases in Japan. Certain LHON pedigrees with other point mutations are associated with complex neurologic disorders and may have features in common with MELAS syndrome and with infantile bilateral striatal necrosis.

ATPase SUBUNIT 6 MUTATION (NARP). This maternally inherited disorder presents with either Leigh syndrome or with developmental delay, retinitis pigmentosa, dementia, seizures, ataxia, proximal weakness, and sensory neuropathy (NARP syndrome). It is due to a point mutation at nt 8993 within the ATPase subunit 6 gene. The severity of the disease presentation appears to have close correlation with the percentage of mutant mtDNA in leukocytes

KEARNS-SAYRE SYNDROME (KSS). The criteria for KSS include a triad of (1) onset before age 20 yr, (2) progressive external ophthalmoplegia (PEO) with ptosis, and (3) pigmentary retinopathy. In addition, there must be at least one of the following: heart block, cerebellar syndrome, or cerebrospinal fluid protein greater than 100 mg/dL. Other nonspecific but common features include dementia, sensorineural hearing loss, and multiple endocrine abnormalities, including short stature, diabetes mellitus, and hypoparathyroidism. The prognosis is poor, despite placement of a pacemaker, and progressively downhill, with death by the third or fourth decade. Unusual clinical presentations can include renal tubular acidosis and Lowe syndrome. There are also a few overlap cases of children with KSS and strokelike episodes. Muscle biopsy shows RRF and variable cytochrome oxidase (COX)–negative fibers. Most patients have mtDNA deletions, and some have duplications. These may be new mutations accounting for the generally sporadic nature of KSS. A few pedigrees have shown autosomal dominant transmission.

Sporadic PEO with RRF is a clinically benign condition characterized by adolescent or young adult-onset ophthalmoplegia, ptosis, and proximal limb girdle weakness. It is slowly progressive and compatible with a relatively normal life. The muscle biopsy material demonstrates RRF and COX-negative fibers. Approximately 50% of patients with PEO have mtDNA deletions, and there is no family history.

LEIGH DISEASE (SUBACUTE NECROTIZING ENCEPHALOMYOPATHY). There are at least four known genetically determined causes of Leigh disease: pyruvate dehydrogenase complex deficiency, complex I deficiency, complex IV (COX) deficiency, and complex V (ATPase) deficiency. These defects may occur sporadically or be inherited by autosomal recessive transmission, as in the case of COX deficiency, by X-linked transmission as in the case of PDH $E_1\alpha$ deficiency, or by maternal transmission as in complex V (ATPase 6 nt 8993 mutation) deficiency. Most cases become apparent during infancy with feeding and swallowing problems, vomiting, and failure to thrive. Delayed motor and language milestones may be evident, and generalized seizures, weakness, hypotonia, ataxia, tremor, pyramidal signs, and nystagmus are prominent findings. Intermittent respirations with associated sighing or sobbing are characteristic and suggest brain stem dysfunction. Some patients have external ophthalmoplegia, ptosis, optic atrophy, and decreased visual acuity. Abnormal results on CT or MRI scan consist of bilaterally symmetric areas of low attenuation in the basal ganglia. Pathologic changes consist of focal symmetric areas of necrosis in the thalamus, basal ganglia, tegmental gray matter, periventricular and periaqueductal regions of the brain stem, and posterior columns of the spinal cord. Microscopically, these *spongiform* lesions show cystic cavitation with neuronal loss, demyelination, and vascular proliferation. Elevations in serum lactate levels are characteristic. The overall outlook is poor, but a few patients experience prolonged periods of remission.

REYE SYNDROME. This encephalopathy is associated with pathologic features characterized by fatty degeneration of the viscera (microvesicular steatosis) and mitochondrial abnormalities and biochemical features consistent with a disturbance of mitochondrial metabolism (see Chapter 360). Sporadic Reye syndrome can occur in the context of influenza B virus and salicylate ingestion, in the idiosyncratic valproic acid hepatotoxicity reaction in individuals who may have an underlying genetic predisposition, and in Jamaican vomiting sickness (due to the hypoglycin toxin).

Recurrent Reye-like syndrome is encountered in children with genetic defects of fatty acid oxidation, such as the plasmalemmal carnitine transporter, carnitine palmitoyltransferase I and II, carnitine acylcarnitine translocase, medium- and long-chain acyl-CoA dehydrogenase, multiple acyl CoA dehydrogenase, and long-chain L-3 hydroxyacyl-CoA dehydrogenase or trifunctional protein deficiencies. These disorders are manifested by recurrent hypoglycemic, hypoketotic encephalopathy, and are inherited in an autosomal recessive pattern. Other potential inborn errors of metabolism presenting with Reye syndrome include urea cycle defects (e.g., ornithine transcarbamylase, carbamylphosphate synthetase) and certain of the organic acidurias (e.g., glutaric aciduria type I), respiratory chain defects, and defects of carbohydrate metabolism (e.g., fructose intolerance).

607.3 Other Encephalopathies

ZELLWEGER SYNDROME (CEREBROHEPATORENAL SYNDROME [CHRS]). This rare, lethal disorder is inherited as an autosomal recessive trait. It represents the prototype of a group of peroxisomal disorders that have overlapping symptoms, signs, and biochemical abnormalities (see Chapter 83.2). Infants with Zellweger syndrome have dysmorphic facies consisting of frontal bossing and a large anterior fontanel. The occiput is flattened, and the external ears are abnormal. A high-arched palate, excessive skinfolds of the neck, severe hypotonia, and areflexia are usually evident. Examination of the eyes reveals searching nystagmoid movements, bilateral cataracts, and optic atrophy. Generalized seizures become evident early in life, associated with severe global developmental delay and a significant bilateral hearing loss. The cause of the severe neurologic abnormalities is related to an arrest of migrating neuroblasts during early development, resulting in cerebral pachygyria with neuronal heterotopia (see Chapter 601.7). Hepatomegaly is a prominent finding shortly after birth, often associated with a history of prolonged neonatal jaundice. Patients with Zellweger syndrome rarely survive beyond 1 yr of age.

ACQUIRED IMMUNODEFICIENCY SYNDROME (AIDS) ENCEPHALOPATHY. Encephalopathy is an unfortunate and common manifestation in infants and children with HIV infection (see Chapter 268). Neurologic signs in congenitally infected patients may appear during early infancy or may be delayed to as late as 5 yr of age. The encephalopathy may have an acute onset with a relentless progressive course, but in some cases the process is either static or is characterized by insidious deterioration. The primary features of AIDS encephalopathy include an arrest in brain growth, evidence of developmental delay, and the evolution of neurologic signs including weakness with pyramidal tract signs, ataxia, myoclonus, pseudobulbar palsy, and seizures.

LEAD ENCEPHALOPATHY. See Chapter 721.

BURN ENCEPHALOPATHY. An encephalopathy develops in approximately 5% of children with significant burns during the first several weeks of hospitalization (see also Chapter 70). There is no single cause of burn encephalopathy but rather a combination of factors that include anoxia (smoke inhalation, carbon monoxide poisoning, laryngospasm), electrolyte abnormalities, bacteremia and sepsis, cortical vein thrombosis, a concomitant head injury, cerebral edema, drug reactions, and emotional distress. Seizures are the most common clinical manifestation of burn encephalopathy, but altered states of consciousness, hallucinations, and coma may also occur. Management of burn encephalopathy is directed to a search for the underlying cause and treatment of hypoxemia, seizures, specific electrolyte abnormalities, or cerebral edema. The prognosis for complete neurologic recovery is generally excellent, particularly if seizures are the primary abnormality.

HYPERTENSIVE ENCEPHALOPATHY. Hypertensive encephalopathy is most commonly associated with renal disease in children, including acute glomerulonephritis, chronic pyelonephritis, and end-stage renal disease (see Chapters 451 and 543). In some cases, hypertensive encephalopthy is the initial manifestation of underlying renal disease. Marked systemic hypertension produces vascoconstriction of the cerebral vessels, which leads to vascular permeability, causing areas of focal cerebral edema and hemorrhage. The onset may be acute, with seizures and coma, or more indolent, with headache, drowsiness and lethargy, nausea and vomiting, blurred vision, transient cortical blindness, and hemiparesis. Examination of the eyegrounds may be nondiagnostic in children, but papilledema and retinal hemorrhages may occur. Treatment is directed at restoration of a normotensive state and control of seizures with appropriate anticonvulsants.

RADIATION ENCEPHALOPATHY. Although techniques for administering radiation therapy to the brain have improved considerably and the incidence of serious side effects has decreased significantly, radiation encephalopathy remains an important complication. *Acute radiation encephalopathy* is most likely to develop in young patients who have received large daily doses. Excessive radiation injures vessel endothelium, resulting in enhanced vascular permeability, cerebral edema, and numerous hemorrhages. The child may suddenly become irritable and lethargic, complain of headache, or present with focal neurologic signs and seizures. Patients occasionally develop hemiparesis due to an infarct secondary to vascular occlusion of the cerebral vessels. Steroids are often beneficial in reducing the cerebral edema and reversing the neurologic signs. *Late radiation encephalopathy* develops months to years after the completion of therapy. It is rare in children. The condition is characterized by headaches and slowly progressive focal neurologic signs, including hemiparesis and seizures. Although the cause of late radiation encephalopathy is unknown, a CT scan shows cerebral atrophy and low-density lesions. Some children with acute lymphatic leukemia treated with a combination of intrathecal methotrexate and cranial irradiation develop neurologic signs months or years later, consisting of increasing lethargy, loss of cognitive abilities, dementia, and focal neurologic signs and seizures (see Chapter 501). The CT scan shows calcifications in the white matter, and the postmortem examination demonstrates a necrotizing encephalopathy. This devastating complication of the treatment of leukemia has prompted re-evaluation of the use of cranial radiation in the treatment of these children.

Albright AL, Barron WB, Fasick MP, et al: Continuous intrathecal baclofen infusion for spasticity of cerebral origin. JAMA 270:2475, 1993.
Ciafaloni E, Ricci E, Shanske S, et al: MELAS: Clinical features, biochemistry and molecular genetics. Ann Neurol 31:391, 1992.
Fukuhara N, Tokiguchi S, Shirakawa K, et al: Myoclonus epilepsy associated with ragged-red fibres (mitochondrial abnormalities): Disease entity or a syndrome? J Neurol Sci 47:117, 1980.
Gaffney G, Flavell V, Johnson A, et al: Cerebral palsy and neonatal encephalopathy. Arch Dis Child 70:195, 1994.
Goto Y, Itami N, Kajii N, et al: Renal tubular involvement mimicking Barter syndrome in a patient with Kearns-Sayre syndrome. J Pediatr 116:904, 1990.
Goto Y, Nonaka I, Horai S: A mutation in the $tRNA^{Leu(UUR)}$ gene associated with the MELAS subgroup of mitochondrial encephalomyopathies. Nature 348:651, 1990.
Grether JK, Nelson KB: Maternal infection and cerebral palsy in infants of normal birth weight. JAMA 278:207, 1997.
Karpati G, Carpenter S, Larbrisseau A, et al: The Kearns-Shy syndrome: A multisystem disease with mitochondrial abnormality demonstrated in skeletal muscle and skin. J Neurol Sci 19:133, 1973.
Kobayashi M, Morishita H, Sugiyama N, et al: Two cases of NADH-coenzyme Q reductase deficiency: Relationship to MELAS syndrome. J Pediatr 110:223, 1987.
Koman LA, Mooney JF, Smith B, et al: Management of cerebral palsy with botulinum-A toxin: Preliminary investigation. J Pediatr Orthop 13:489, 1993.
Kuban RCR, Leviton A: Cerebral palsy. N Engl J Med 330:188, 1994.
Mohnot D, Snead OC, Benton JW: Burn encephalopathy in children. Ann Neurol 12:42, 1982.
Monnens L, Heymans H: Peroxisomal disorders: Clinical characterization. J Inherit Metab Dis 10(Suppl 1):23, 1987.
Moraes CT, DiMauro S, Zeviani M, et al: Mitochondrial DNA deletions in progressive external ophthalmoplegia and Kearns-Sayre syndrome. N Engl J Med 320:1293, 1989.
Park TS, Owen AH: Surgical management of spastic diplegia in cerebral palsy. N Engl J Med 326:745, 1992.
Pavlakis SG, Phillips PC, Di Mauro S, et al: Mitochondrial myopathy, encephalopathy, lactic acidosis, and strokelike episodes: A distinctive clinical syndrome. Ann Neurol 16:481, 1984.
Peacock WJ, Staudt LA: Selective posterior rhizotomy: Evolution of theory and practice. Pediatr Neurosurg 92:128, 1991.
Pharoah POD, Platt MJ, Cooke T: The changing epidemiology of cerebral palsy. Arch Dis Child 75:F169, 1996.
Robinson BH, Taylor J, Sherwood WG: The genetic heterogeneity of lactic acidosis: Occurrence of recognizable inborn errors of metabolism in a pediatric population with lactic acidosis. Pediatr Res 14:956, 1980.
Sheline GE: Irradiation injury of the human brain: A review of clinical experience. *In*: Gilbert HA, Kagan AR (eds): Radiation Damage to the Nervous System. New York, Raven Press, 1980.
Shoffner JM, Lott M, Lezza AMS, et al: Myoclonic epilepsy and ragged-red fiber disease (MERRF) is associated with a mitochondrial DNA $tRNA^{Lys}$ mutation. Cell 61:931, 1990.
Wallace DC, Singh G, Lott MT, et al: Mitochondrial DNA mutation associated with Leber's hereditary optic neuropathy. Science 242:1427, 1988.

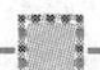

CHAPTER 608
Neurodegenerative Disorders of Childhood

Neurodegenerative disorders of childhood encompass a large number of heterogeneous diseases that result from specific genetic and biochemical defects, chronic viral infections, and toxic substances and a significant group of conditions of unknown cause. In the past, children with suspected neurodegenerative disorders were subjected to brain and rectal biopsies, but with the advent of modern neuroimaging techniques and specific biochemical molecular diagnostic tests, these invasive procedures are now rarely necessary. Nevertheless, the most important component of the investigation continues to be a thorough history and physical examination. The hallmark of a neurodegenerative disease is progressive deterioration of neurologic function with loss of speech, vision, hearing, or locomotion, often associated with seizures, feeding difficulties, and impairment of intellect. The age of onset, rate of progression, and principal neurologic findings determine whether the disease is primarily affecting the white or gray matter. Upper motor neuron signs are prominent early in the former, and convulsions, intellectual, and visual impairment in the latter. A precise history confirms regression of developmental milestones, and the neurologic examination localizes the process within the nervous system. Although the outcome is invariably fatal and current therapeutic attempts have been unsuccessful, it is important to make the correct diagnosis so that genetic counseling may be offered and prevention strategies can be implemented. For all conditions in which the specific enzyme defect is known, prevention by prenatal diagnosis (chorionic villus sampling or amniocentesis) is possible. Carrier detection is also often possible by enzyme assay. Table 608–1 summarizes the heredity, biochemical defects, and specific diagnostic abnormality in the inherited neurodegenerative disorders. Additional age of onset–related categorization is noted in Table 608–2.

The inherited neurodegenerative disorders include the sphingolipidoses, neuronal ceroid lipofuscinoses, adrenoleukodystrophy, and sialidosis. The sphingolipidoses are characterized by intracellular storage of a normal lipid component of the cell membrane owing to a defect in catabolism of the compound. The sphingolipidoses are subclassified into six categories: Niemann-Pick disease, Gaucher disease, GM_1 gangliosidosis, GM_2 gangliosidosis, Krabbe disease, and metachromatic leukodystrophy. Niemann-Pick disease and Gaucher disease are discussed in Chapter 83.4. The spinocerebellar degenerative diseases (Friedreich ataxia, ataxia-telangiectasia, olivopontocerebellar atrophy, and abetalipoproteinemia) and degenerative disorders of the basal ganglia (Huntington disease, dystonia musculorum deformans, Wilson disease, and Hallervorden-Spatz disease) are included in Chapter 606. Finally, a miscellaneous group of degenerative diseases is discussed in this section, including multiple sclerosis, Pelizaeus-Merzbacher disease, Alexander disease, Canavan spongy degeneration, kinky hair disease, Rett syndrome, and subacute sclerosing panencephalitis.

608.1 Sphingolipidoses

GANGLIOSIDOSES

See also Chapter 83.4.

Gangliosides are glycosphingolipids, normal constituents of the neuronal and synaptic membranes. The basic structure of GM_1 ganglioside consists of an oligosaccharide chain attached to a hydroxyl group of ceramide and sialic acid bound to galactose. The gangliosides are catabolized by sequential cleavage of the sugar molecules by specific exoglycosidases. Abnormalities in catabolism result in an accumulation of the ganglioside within the cell. Defects in ganglioside degradation can be classified into two groups, the GM_1 gangliosidoses and the GM_2 gangliosidoses.

GM_1 GANGLIOSIDOSES. The three subtypes of GM_1 gangliosidoses are classified according to age at presentation: infantile (type 1), juvenile (type 2), and adult (type 3). The condition is inherited as an autosomal recessive trait and results from a marked deficiency of acid β-galactosidase. This enzyme may be assayed in leukocytes and cultured fibroblasts. The acid β-galactosidase gene has been mapped to chromosome 3p14.2. Prenatal diagnosis is possible by measurement of acid β-galactosidase in cultured amniotic cells.

TABLE 608–1 Heredity and Biochemical Defects in the Neurodegenerative Disorders

Neurodegenerative Disorder	Mode of Inheritance	Biochemical Defect	Specimen for Analysis
Sphingolipidosis			
GM_1 gangliosidosis	AR	β-Galactosidase	Serum, leukocytes, skin fibroblasts
GM_2 gangliosidosis			
Tay-Sachs disease	AR	Hexosaminidase A	Serum, leukocytes, skin fibroblasts
Sandhoff disease	AR	Hexosaminidase A and B	Serum, leukocytes, skin fibroblasts
Krabbe disease	AR	Galactocerebrosidase	Leukocytes and skin fibroblasts
Metachromatic leukodystrophy	AR	Arylsulfatase A	Leukocytes and skin fibroblasts
Neuronal Ceroid Lipofuscinoses	AR	?	EM of skin biopsy
Adrenoleukodystrophy	XLR	VLCFA oxidation	Plasma, skin fibroblasts
Sialidosis	AR	Neuraminidase	Skin fibroblasts

AR = autosomal recessive; EM = electron microscopy; XLR = X-linked recessive; VLCFA = very long chain fatty acid.

Infantile GM_1 gangliosidosis presents at birth or during the neonatal period with anorexia, poor sucking, and inadequate weight gain. Development is globally retarded, and generalized seizures are prominent. The phenotype is striking and shares many characteristics with Hurler syndrome. The facial features are coarse, the forehead is prominent, the nasal bridge is depressed, the tongue is large (macroglossia), and the gums are hypertrophied. Hepatosplenomegaly is present early in the course owing to accumulation of foamy histiocytes, and kyphoscoliosis is evident owing to anterior beaking of the vertebral bodies. The neurologic examination is dominated by apathy, progressive blindness, deafness, spastic quadriplegia, and decerebrate rigidity. A cherry red spot in the macular region is visualized in approximately 50% of cases. The **cherry red spot** is characterized by an opaque ring (sphingolipid-laden retinal ganglion cells) encircling the normal red fovea (Fig. 608–1). Children rarely survive beyond age 2–3 yr, and death is due to aspiration pneumonia.

Juvenile GM_1 gangliosidosis has a delayed onset beginning about 1 yr of age. The initial symptoms consist of incoordination, weakness, ataxia, and regression of language. Thereafter, convulsions, spasticity, decerebrate rigidity, and blindness are

TABLE 608–2 Select "Intrinsic" Conditions Associated with Developmental Regression

Age at Onset (yr)	Condition	Comments
<2—with hepatomegaly (see Chapter 81)	Fructose intolerance	Vomiting, hypoglycemia, poor feeding, failure to thrive (when given fructose)
	Galactosemia	Lethargy, hypotonia, icterus, cataract, hypoglycemia (when given lactose)
	Glycogenosis (glycogen storage disease) types I–IV	Hypoglycemia, cardiomegaly (II)
	Mucopolysaccharidosis tpes I and II	Coarse facies, stiff joints
	Niemann-Pick disease, infantile type	Gray matter disease, failure to thrive
	Tay-Sachs disease	Seizures, cherry red macula, edema, coarse facies
	Zellweger (cerebrohepatorenal) syndrome	Hypotonia, high forehead, flat facies
	Gaucher disease type II	Extensor posturing, irritability
<2—without hepatomegaly	Krabbe disease	Irritability, extensor posturing, optic atrophy and blindness
	Rett syndrome	Girls with deceleration of head growth, loss of hand skills, hand wringing, impaired language skills, gait apraxia
	Maple syrup urine disease	Poor feeding, tremors, myoclonus, opisthotonos
	Phenylketonuria	Light pigmentation, eczema, seizures
	Menkes kinky hair disease	Hypertonia, irritability, seizures, abnormal hair
	Subacute necrotizing encephalopathy of Leigh	White matter disease
	Cerebro-oculofacioskeletal syndrome (of Pena and Shokeir)	Reduced white matter, failure to thrive
	Canavan disease	White matter disease
	Pelizaeus-Merzbacher disease	White matter disease
2-5	Niemann-Pick disease types III and IV	Hepatosplenomegaly, gait difficulty
	Wilson disease	Liver disease, Kayser-Fleischer ring, deterioration of cognition is late
	Gangliosidosis type II	Gray matter disease
	Ceroid lipofuscinosis	Gray matter disease
	Mitochondrial encephalopathies (e.g., myoclonic epilepsy, ragged-red fibers [MERRF])	Gray matter diseases
	Ataxia-telangiectasia	Basal ganglia disease
	Huntington's disease (chorea)	Basal ganglia disease
	Hallervorden-Spatz syndrome	Basal ganglia disease
	Metachromatic leukodystrophy	White matter disease
	Adrenoleukodystrophy	White matter disease, behavior problems, falling school performance, quadriparesis
	Subacute sclerosing panencephalitis	Diffuse encephalopathy, myoclonus, may occur years after measles
5–15	Adrenoleukodystrophy	See above for adrenoleukodystrophy
	Multiple sclerosis	White matter disease
	Neuronal ceroid lipofuscinosis, juvenile and adult (Spielmeyer-Vogt and Kuf disease)	Gray matter disease
	Schilder disease	White matter disease, focal neurologic symptoms
	Refsum disease	Peripheral neuropathy, ataxia, retinitis pigmentosa
	Sialidosis II, juvenile form	Cherry red macula, myoclonus, ataxia, coarse facies

From *Liptak G:* In: *Kliegman R (ed): Practical Strategies in Pediatric Diagnosis and Therapy. Philadelphia, WB Saunders, 1996, p 503.*

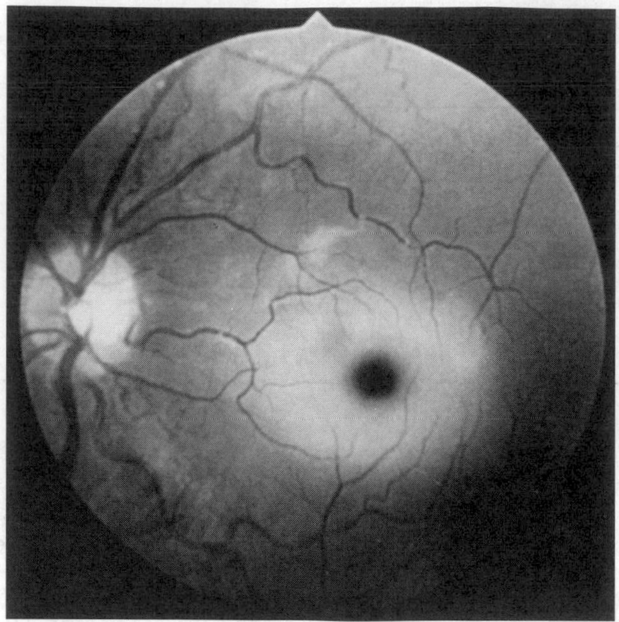

Figure 608–1 A cherry red spot in a patient with GM_1 gangliosidosis. Note the whitish ring of sphingolipid-laden ganglion cells surrounding the fovea.

the major findings. Unlike the infantile type, this type is not usually marked by coarse facial features and hepatosplenomegaly. Radiographic examination of the lumbar vertebrae may show minor beaking. Children rarely survive beyond 10 yr of age. *Adult GM_1 gangliosidosis* is a slowly progressive disease consisting of spasticity, ataxia, dysarthria, and a gradual loss of cognitive function.

GM_2 GANGLIOSIDOSES. The GM_2 gangliosidoses are a heterogeneous group of autosomal recessive inherited disorders that consist of several subtypes, including Tay-Sachs disease (TSD), Sandoff disease, juvenile GM_2 gangliosidosis, and adult GM_2 gangliosidosis. *TSD* is most prevalent in the Ashkenazi Jewish population and has a carrier rate of approximately 1/30. TSD is due to mutations in the HEXA gene located on chromosome 15q23–q24. Affected infants appear normal until approximately 6 mo of age, except for a marked startle reaction to noise that is evident soon after birth. Affected children then begin to lag in developmental milestones, and by 1 yr of age they lose the ability to stand, sit, and vocalize. Early hypotonia develops into progressive spasticity, and relentless deterioration follows, with convulsions, blindness, deafness, and cherry red spots in almost all patients (see Fig. 608–1). Macrocephaly becomes apparent by 1 yr of age and results from the 200- to 300-fold normal content of GM_2 ganglioside deposited within the brain. Few children live beyond 3–4 yr of age, and death is usually associated with aspiration or bronchopneumonia. A deficiency of the isoenzyme hexosaminidase A is found in tissues of patients with TSD. Mass screening for prenatal diagnosis of TSD is a reliable and cost-effective method of prevention because the condition occurs in a defined population (Ashkenazi Jews). An accurate and inexpensive carrier detection test is available (serum or leukocyte hexosaminidase A), and the disease can be reliably diagnosed by chorionic villus sampling during the 1st trimester of pregnancy in couples at risk (heterozygote parents).

Sandhoff disease is very similar to TSD in the mode of presentation, including progressive loss of motor and language milestones beginning at 6 mo of age. Seizures, cherry red spots, macrocephaly, and doll-like facies are present in most patients; however, children with Sandhoff disease may also have splenomegaly. The visual evoked potentials (VEPs) are normal early in the course of Sandhoff disease and TSD but become abnormal or absent as the disease progresses. The auditory brain stem responses (ABRs) show prolonged latencies. The diagnosis of Sandhoff disease is established by finding deficient levels of hexosaminidase A and B in serum and leukocytes. Children usually succumb by 3 yr or age. Sandhoff disease is due to mutations in the HEXB gene located on chromosome 5q13.

Juvenile GM_2 gangliosidosis develops in midchildhood, initially with clumsiness followed by ataxia. Signs of spasticity, athetosis, loss of language, and seizures gradually develop. Progressive visual loss is associated with optic atrophy, but cherry red spots rarely occur in juvenile GM_2 gangliosidosis. A deficiency of hexosaminidase is variable (total deficiency to near normal) in these patients. Death occurs around 15 yr of age. *Adult GM_2 gangliosidosis* is characterized by a myriad of neurologic signs, including slowly progressive gait ataxia, spasticity, dystonia, proximal muscle atrophy, and dysarthria. Generally, visual acuity and intellectual function are unimpaired. Hexosaminidase A or A and B activity is reduced significantly in the serum and leukocytes.

KRABBE DISEASE (GLOBOID CELL LEUKODYSTROPHY). Krabbe disease (KD) is a rare autosomal recessive neurodegenerative disorder characterized by severe myelin loss and the presence of globoid bodies in the white matter. The gene for KD(GALC) is located on chromosome 14q24.3–q32.1. The disease results from a marked deficiency of the lysosomal enzyme galactocerebroside β-galactosidase, which cleaves a galactose moiety from the ceramide portion of galactocerebroside. KD is a disorder of myelin destruction rather than abnormal myelin formation. Normally, myelination begins during the 3rd trimester, corresponding with a rapid rise of galactocerebroside β-galactosidase activity in the brain. In patients with KD, galactocerebroside cannot be metabolized during the normal turnover of myelin because of deficiency of galactocerebroside β-galactosidase. When galactocerebroside is injected into the brains of experimental animals, a globoid cell reaction ensues. It has been postulated that a similar phenomenon occurs in humans, nonmetabolized galactocerebroside stimulates the formation of globoid cells that reflect the destruction of oligodendroglial cells. Because oligodendroglial cells are responsible for the elaboration of myelin, their loss results in myelin breakdown, thus producing additional galactocerebroside and causing a vicious circle of myelin destruction.

The symptoms of KD become evident during the first few months of life and include excessive irritability and crying, unexplained episodes of hyperpyrexia, feeding problems, vomiting, and failure to thrive. During the initial stage of KD. children are often treated for colic or "milk allergy" with frequent formula changes. Generalized seizures may appear early in the course of the disease. Alterations in body tone with rigidity and opisthotonos and visual inattentiveness owing to optic atrophy become apparent as the disease progresses. During the later stages of the illness, blindness, deafness, absent deep tendon reflexes, and decerebrate rigidity constitute the major physical findings. A nonenhanced CT scan of the head may show symmetric increased densities in the caudate nuclei and thalami. Most patients expire by 2 yr of age.

Late-onset KD has been described beginning in childhood or during adolescence. Patients present with optic atrophy and cortical blindness, and their condition is often confused with the adrenoleukodystrophies. Slowly progressive gait disturbances, including spasticity and ataxia, are prominent. As with classic KD, globoid cells are abundant in the white matter, and leukocytes are deficient in galactocerebroside β-galactosidase. An examination of the cerebrospinal fluid (CSF) shows an elevated protein content, and the nerve conduction velocities are markedly delayed owing to segmental demyelination of the peripheral nerves. The VEPs decrease gradually in amplitude with no response in the late stages of the disease, and the ABRs are characterized by the presence of only waves I and II. CT scans and MRI studies highlight the marked decrease in white matter, especially of the cerebellum and centrum semiovale, with sparing of the subcortical u fibers. Prenatal diagnosis is possible by the assay of galactocerebroside β-galactosidase activity in chorionic villi or in cultured amniotic fluid cells.

METACHROMATIC LEUKODYSTROPHY (MLD). This disorder of myelin metabolism is inherited as an autosomal recessive trait and is characterized by a deficiency of arylsulfatase A activity. Several mutations in the gene encoding for arylsulfatase A have been identified. The gene is located on chromosome 22q13–13qter, and DNA diagnosis is possible. The absence or deficiency of arylsulfatase A leads to accumulation of cerebroside sulfate within the myelin sheath of the central nervous system (CNS) and peripheral nervous system owing to the inability to cleave sulfate from galactosyl-3-sulfate ceramide. The excessive cerebroside sulfate is thought to cause myelin breakdown and destruction of oligodendroglia. Prenatal diagnosis of MLD is made by assay of arylsulfatase A in chorionic villi or cultured amniotic fluid cells. Cresyl violet applied to tissue specimens produces metachromatic staining of the sulfatide granules, giving the disease its name. Six disorders are included in the MLD group of diseases, classified by the age at onset and enzyme deficiency. Three conditions are briefly discussed: the classic or late infantile, juvenile, and adult leukodystrophies.

Late infantile MLD begins with insidious onset of gait disturbances between 1 and 2 yr of age. The child initially appears awkward and frequently falls, but locomotion is gradually impaired significantly and support is required in order to walk. The extremities are hypotonic, and the deep tendon reflexes are absent or diminished. Within the next several months, the child can no longer stand, and deterioration in intellectual function becomes apparent. The speech is slurred and dysarthric, and the child appears dull and apathetic. Visual fixation is diminished, nystagmus is present, and examination of the retina shows optic atrophy. Within 1 yr from the onset of the disease, the child is unable to sit unsupported, and progressive decorticate postures develop. Feeding and swallowing are impaired owing to pseudobulbar palsies, and a feeding gastrostomy is required. Patients ultimately become stuporous and die of aspiration or bronchopneumonia by age 5–6 yr. Neurophysiologic evaluation shows progressive changes in the VEPs, ABRs, and somatosensory evoked potentials (SSEPs), and the nerve conduction velocities (NCVs) of the peripheral nerves are significantly reduced. CT and MRI images of the brain indicate diffuse symmetric attenuation of the cerebellar and cerebral white matter, and examination of the CSF shows an elevated protein content. Bone marrow transplantation is a promising experimental therapy for the management of late infantile MLD. Favorable outcomes have been reported only in patients treated very early in the course of the disease. The total number of patients treated is relatively small and the follow-up too short to draw conclusions about the efficacy of bone marrow transplantation.

Juvenile MLD has many features in common with late infantile MLD, but the onset of symptoms is delayed to 5–10 yr of age. Deterioration in school performance and alterations in personality may herald the onset of the disease. This is followed by incoordination of gait, urinary incontinence, and dysarthria. Muscle tone becomes increased, and ataxia, dystonia, or tremor may be present. During the terminal stages, generalized tonic-clonic convulsions are prominent and are difficult to control. Patients rarely live beyond midadolescence. *Adult MLD* occurs from the 2nd to 6th decade. Abnormalities in memory, psychiatric disturbances, and personality changes are prominent features. Slowly progressive neurologic signs, including spasticity, dystonia, optic atrophy, and generalized convulsions lead eventually to a bedridden state characterized by decorticate postures and unresponsiveness.

608.2 Neuronal Ceroid Lipofuscinoses

Neuronal ceroid lipofuscinoses constitutes the most common class of neurodegenerative diseases in children and consist of three disorders inherited as autosomal recessive traits. They are characterized by the storage of an autofluorescent substance within neurons and other tissues. *Infantile type* (*Haltia-Santavuori*) begins toward the end of the 1st year of life with myoclonic seizures, intellectual deterioration, and blindness. Optic atrophy and brownish discoloration of the macula are evident on examination of the retina, and cerebellar ataxia is prominent. The electroretinogram (ERG) typically shows small-amplitude or absent waveforms. Death occurs at approximately 10 yr or age. The gene defect causing the infantile form has been assigned to chromosome 1p32. *Late infantile* (*Jansky-Bielschowsky*) is the most common type of neuronal ceroid lipofuscinosis. The presenting manifestation is myoclonic seizures beginning between 2 and 4 yr of age in a previously normal child. Dementia and ataxia are combined with a progressive loss of visual acuity and microcephaly. Examination of the retina shows marked attenuation of vessels, peripheral black "bone spicule" pigmentary abnormalities, optic atrophy, and a subtle brown pigment in the macular region. The ERG is abnormal early in the course owing to deposition of the abnormal storage substance within the rod and cone area of the retina. VEPs are characteristic and consist of markedly enlarged responses followed by absent waveforms with progression of the disease. The autofluorescent material is deposited in neurons, fibroblasts, and secretory cells. Electron microscopic examination of the storage material in skin or conjunctival biopsy material typically shows curvilinear bodies or "fingerprint profiles." The gene for late infantile neuronal ceroid lipofuscinosis has not been localized.

Juvenile type (*Spielmeyer-Vogt*) is characterized by progressive visual loss and intellectual impairment beginning between 5 and 10 yr of age. The funduscopic changes are similar to those for the late infantile type. The ERG is also abnormal early in the course of the disease, but in the juvenile type the VEPs typically are characterized by small amplitude waves and, later, absence of waveforms as the disease progresses. Myoclonic seizures are not as prominent as in the late infantile type of neuronal ceroid lipofuscinosis, but dystonic posturing is marked during the late stages of the disease. Elevated urine dolichol levels are a nonspecific finding. Ultrastructural abnormalities of skin biopsy samples are present in most cases. The gene for the juvenile form of neuronal ceroid lipofuscinosis is located on chromosome 16p12.1.

608.3 Adrenoleukodystrophy

See Chapter 83.2.

The adrenoleukodystrophies consist of a group of CNS degenerative disorders that are often associated with adrenal cortical insufficiency, are inherited by X-linked recessive transmission, and are not responsive to any known treatments. *Classic adrenoleukodystrophy* (ALD) becomes symptomatic between 5 and 15 yr of age with evidence of academic deterioration, behavioral disturbances, and gait abnormalities. Generalized seizures are common in the early stages. Upper motor neuron signs include spastic quadriparesis and contractures, ataxia, and marked swallowing disturbances secondary to pseudobulbar palsy. These dominate the terminal stages of the illness. Hypoadrenalism is present in approximately 50% of cases, and adrenal insufficiency characterized by abnormal skin pigmentation (tanning without exposure to sun) may precede the onset of neurologic symptoms. CT scans and MRI studies of patients indicate periventricular demyelination beginning posteriorly; this advances progressively to the anterior regions of the cerebral white matter. ABRs, VEPs, and SSEPs may be normal initially but ultimately show prolonged latencies and abnormal waveforms. Death supervenes within 10 yr of the onset of the neurologic signs. The incidence of ALD approximates 1/20,000 boys. The gene for ALD consists of 10 exons spanning 20 kb of genomic DNA. The gene is located on Xq28.

Adrenomyeloneuropathy begins with a slowly progressive spastic paraparesis, urinary incontinence, and onset of impotence during the 3rd or 4th decade despite the fact that adrenal insufficiency may have been present since childhood. Cases of typical ALD have occurred in families in whom the propositus presented with adrenomyeloneuropathy. One of the most difficult problems in the management of X-linked ALD is the common observation that affected individuals in the same family may have quite different clinical courses. For example, in one family one affected boy had severe classical ALD culminating in death by age 10 yr, another affected male (e.g., a brother) had late-onset adrenomyeloneuropathy, and a third had no symptoms at all. Counseling families with presymptomatic males is extraordinarily difficult because there is no reliable method for predicting the clinical course.

Neonatal ALD is characterized by marked hypotonia, severe psychomotor retardation, and early onset of seizures. It is inherited as an autosomal recessive condition. Visual inattention is secondary to optic atrophy. Results of adrenal function tests are normal, but adrenal atrophy is evident post mortem. Correction of adrenal insufficiency is ineffective in halting neurologic deterioration.

608.4 Sialidosis

Sialidosis is inherited as an autosomal recessive trait and results from accumulation of a sialic acid–oligosaccharide complex secondary to a deficiency in the lysosomal enzyme neuraminidase. The lysosomal sialidase gene has been mapped to chromosome 6p21.3. Urinary excretion of sialic acid–containing oligosaccharides is increased significantly in affected patients. *Sialidosis type I,* the cherry red spot–myoclonus syndrome (CRSM), usually presents during the 2nd decade of life, when a patient complains of visual deterioration. Inspection of the retina shows a cherry red spot, but, unlike patients with TSD, visual acuity declines slowly in individuals with CRSM. Myoclonus of the extremities is gradually progressive and often debilitating and eventually renders patients nonambulatory. The myoclonus is triggered by voluntary movement, touch, and sound and is not controlled with anticonvulsants. Generalized convulsions responsive to antiepileptic drugs have been reported in most patients. *Sialidosis type II* may be subdivided into infantile and juvenile forms, depending on the age at presentation. In addition to cherry red spots and myoclonus, these patients have somatic involvement, including coarse facial features, corneal clouding (rarely), and dysostosis multiplex, producing anterior beaking of the lumbar vertebrae. Examination of lymphocytes shows vacuoles in the cytoplasm; biopsy of the liver demonstrates cytoplasmic vacuoles in Kupffer cells; and membrane-bound vacuoles are found in Schwann cell cytoplasm, all attesting to the multiorgan nature of sialidosis type II. No distinctive neuroimaging findings or abnormalities in electrophysiologic studies are noted in this group of disorders. Patients with sialidosis have been reported to live beyond the 5th decade.

Some cases of what appears to be sialidosis type II are the result of combined deficiencies of β-galactosidase and α-neuraminidase due to deficiency of a "protective protein" that prevents premature intracellular degradation of the two enzymes. Clinically, affected patients are indistinguishable from those with sialidosis type II, either the infantile or juvenile form, caused by isolated α-neuraminidase deficiency. The diagnosis may be missed if β-galactosidase testing is done and testing of α-neuraminidase activity in fibroblasts is not completed.

608.5 Miscellaneous Disorders

MULTIPLE SCLEROSIS

Multiple sclerosis (MS) is a chronic, remitting disorder characterized by multiple white lesions in the CNS separated by time and location. The condition is rare in the pediatric population, and onset before age 10 yr occurs in 0.2–2% of all cases. There is a greater incidence of MS in females in the pediatric age group compared with adults. The cause of MS is unknown, but interactive genetic, immunologic, and infectious factors are probably responsible. The most frequent presenting symptom is unilateral weakness or ataxia. Headache is an important early component of the disease and is often severe, prolonged, and generalized. Ill-defined paresthesias involving the lower extremities, distal portions of the hands and feet, and the face are common. Visual symptoms including diplopia, blurred vision, or sudden visual loss secondary to optic neuritis are also important early manifestations of MS. Vertigo, dysarthria, and sphincter disturbances are relatively uncommon. *Neuromyelitis optica* (*Devic disease*) is a variant of classic MS and consists of optic neuritis and transverse myelitis, which occur conjointly.

The pathology of MS consists of demyelination with the formation of plaques. No reliable laboratory test unequivocally confirms the diagnosis of MS, except for an autopsy. MRI is the neuroimaging technique of choice; small plaques of 3–4 mm can be identified, particularly those located in the brain stem and spinal cord (Fig. 608–2).

The treatment of MS is supportive, and particular attention is given to the management of a neurogenic bladder. No evidence shows that corticosteroids alter the long-term course of the disease, but they may expedite recovery after an acute attack. Studies indicate that interferon β-1b given subcutaneously every other day or interferon β-1a given intramuscularly every day on a weekly basis are effective in the treatment of MS by decreasing disease activity and disease burden, as shown by serial gadolinium-enhanced lesions in brain MRI scan in adults. The prognosis for childhood MS is similar to that in adults; recovery is often complete, and progression of the disease tends to be slow, with long periods of remission in most cases. Promising immunologic therapy, including the use of intravenous immunoglobulins, is currently being investigated.

PELIZAEUS-MERZBACHER DISEASE

This disease consists of a group of disorders that are characterized by nystagmus and abnormalities of myelin. The classic form is inherited as an X-linked recessive trait caused by abnormalities in the proteolipid protein (PLP) gene, which is essential for CNS myelin formation and oligodendrocyte differentiation. It is recognized by nystagmus and roving eye movements with head nodding during infancy. The gene is located on chromosome Xq22. Molecular diagnosis of Pelizaeus-Merzbacher disease is possible using mutation analysis. However, as with most X-linked diseases, the molecular diagnosis of Pelizaeus-Merzbacher disease is complex because exonic mutations are present in only 10–25% of patients with the disease. A child's developmental milestones are delayed, and ataxia, choreoathetosis, and spasticity ultimately develop. Optic atrophy and dysarthria are associated findings, and death occurs in the 2nd or 3rd decade. The major pathologic finding is a loss of myelin with intact axons, suggesting a defect in the

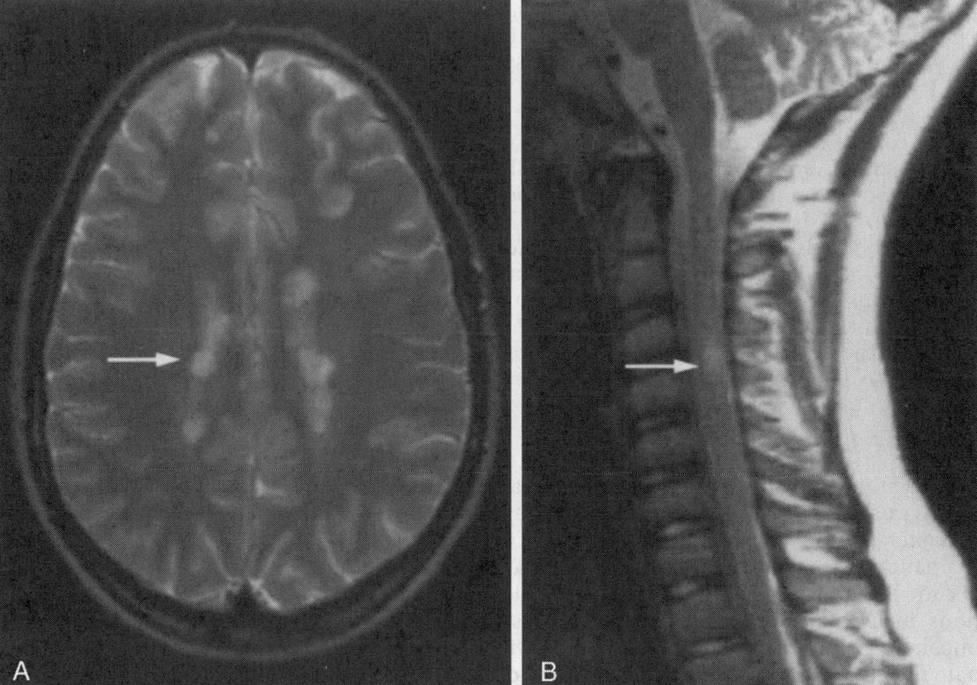

Figure 608–2 Multiple sclerosis. *A*, T2 weighted MRI of brain demonstrates multiple lesions located in the white matter characteristic of multiple sclerosis (*white arrow*). *B*, T1 weighted MRI of spine indicates a demyelinating plaque of multiple sclerosis in the midcervical region (*white arrow*).

function of oligodendroglia. Studies point to a genetic defect in the biosynthesis of proteolipid apoprotein, a protein that is concerned with the differentiation and maintenance of oligodendrocytes. An MRI scan shows a symmetric pattern of delayed myelination. Multimodal evoked potential studies demonstrate an interesting pattern early in the course, consisting of loss of waves III–V on the ABR. This finding is useful in the investigation of nystagmus in infant boys. VEPs show prolonged latencies, and SSEPs show absent cortical responses or delayed latencies.

ALEXANDER DISEASE

Alexander disease is a rare disorder that occurs sporadically and causes progressive macrocephaly during the 1st year of life. Pathologic examination of the brain discloses deposition of eosinophilic hyaline bodies in a perivascular distribution throughout the brain and beneath the pia mater. Degeneration of white matter is most prominent in the frontal lobes, and a CT scan during this stage shows corresponding attenuation of the cerebral white matter. Affected children develop progressive loss of intellect, spasticity, and unresponsive seizures causing death by 5 yr of age.

CANAVAN SPONGY DEGENERATION

See Chapter 82.13.

MENKES DISEASE

Menkes disease (kinky hair disease) is a progressive neurodegenerative condition inherited as a sex-linked recessive trait. The MNK gene is organized in 23 exons spanning approximately 150 kb. The gene has been mapped to Xq13.3. Symptoms begin during the first few months of life and include hypothermia, hypotonia, and generalized myoclonic seizures. The facies are distinctive, with chubby, rosy cheeks and kinky, colorless, friable hair. Microscopic examination of the hair shows several abnormalities, including trichorrhexis nodosa (fractures along the hair shaft) and pili torti (twisted hair). Feeding difficulties are prominent and lead to failure to thrive. Severe mental retardation and optic atrophy are constant features of the disease. Low serum copper and ceruloplasmin levels have been found consistently in patients with Menkes disease, and a defect in copper absorption and transport across the gut has been shown to be the cause of the condition. Neuropathologic changes include tortuous degeneration of the gray matter, and marked changes in the cerebellum with loss of the internal granule cell layer and necrosis of the Purkinje cells.

Death occurs by 3 yr of age in untreated patients. Copper-histidine therapy has been shown to be effective in preventing neurologic deterioration in some patients with Menkes disease, particularly if treatment is begun during the neonatal period or, preferably, with the fetus. Copper is essential during the early stages of CNS development, and its absence probably accounts for the neuropathologic changes. Copper-histidine is given subcutaneously in a dose of 50–150 μg elemental copper/kg/24 hr for the duration of the child's life. The serum copper and ceruloplasmin levels return to the normal range within 2–3 wk of commencing therapy. The *occipital horn syndrome*, a skeletal dysplasia caused by different mutations in the same gene as that involved in Menkes disease, is a relatively mild disease. The two diseases are often confused, because the biochemical abnormalities are identical. Resolution of the uncertainty about treatment of patients with Menkes disease will require careful genotype-phenotype correlation, along with further clinical trials of copper therapy.

RETT SYNDROME

Rett syndrome, a neurodegenerative disorder of unknown cause, occurs exclusively in girls and has a prevalance of approximately 1/15,000 to 1/22,000. There are no biologic markers for the disease, the diagnosis is established by the history and clinical findings. The etiology of Rett syndrome is presumed to be related to X-linked dominant inheritance, which is lethal to male fetuses. Development proceeds normally until 1 yr of age, when regression of language and motor milestones and acquired microcephaly become apparent. An ataxic gait or fine tremor of hand movements is an early neurologic finding. Most children develop peculiar sighing respirations with intermittent periods of apnea that may be associated with cyanosis. The hallmark of Rett syndrome is repetitive hand-wringing movements and a loss of purposeful and spontaneous use of the hands; these may not appear until 2–3 yr of age. Austistic behavior is a typical finding in all patients. Generalized tonic-clonic convulsions occur in the majority and are usually well controlled by anticonvulsants. Feeding disorders and poor weight gain are common. After the initial period of neurologic regression, the disease process appears to plateau, with persistence of the autistic behavior. Death occurs during adolescence or during the third decade. Cardiac arrhythmias may result in sudden, unexpected death. Postmortem studies show significantly reduced brain weight (60–80% of normal) with a decrease in the number of synapses, associated with a decrease in dendritic length and branching.

SUBACUTE SCLEROSING PANENCEPHALITIS

Subacute sclerosing panencephalitis is a rare, progressive slow-virus infection of the CNS caused by a measles-like virus (Chapter 240.1). The number of reported cases has decreased dramatically to 0.06 case/million population, paralleling the decline in reported measles cases. The initial clinical manifestations include personality changes, aggressive behavior, and impaired cognitive function. Myoclonic seizures soon dominate the clinical picture. Later, generalized tonic-clonic convulsions, hypertonia, and choreoathetosis become evident, followed by progressive bulbar palsy, hyperthermia, and decerebrate postures. Funduscopic examination early in the course of the disease reveals papilledema in approximately 20% of the cases. Optic atrophy, chorioretinitis, and macular pigmentation are observed in most patients. The *diagnosis* is established by the typical clinical course and one of the following: (1) measles antibody detected in the CSF, (2) a characteristic EEG consisting of bursts of high-voltage slow waves interspersed with a normal background in the early stages, and (3) typical histologic findings in the brain biopsy or postmortem specimen. *Treatment* with a series of antiviral agents has been attempted without success. Death occurs usually within 1–2 yr from the onset of symptoms.

Baram TZ, Goldman AM, Percy AK: Krabbe disease: Specific MRI and CT findings. Neurology 36:111, 1986.

Boustany RMN, Alroy J, Kolodny EH: Clinical classification of neuronal ceroid lipofuscinosis subtypes. Am J Med Genet 5(Suppl):47, 1988.

Chelly J, Tümer Z, Tonnesen T, et al: Isolation of a candidate gene for Menkes disease that encodes a potential heavy binding protein. Nature Genet 3:14, 1993.

De Meirleir LJ, Taylor MJ, Logan WJ: Multimodal evoked potential studies in leukodystrophies of children. Can J Neurol Sci 15:26, 1988.

Duquette P, Murray TJ, Pleines J, et al: Multiple sclerosis in childhood: Clinical profile in 125 patients. J Pediatr 111:359, 1987.

Dyken PR, Cunningham SC, Ward LC: Changing character of subacute sclerosing panencephalitis in the United States. Pediatr Neurol 5:339, 1989.

Farrell K, Chuang S, Becker LE: Computed tomography in Alexander's disease. Ann Neurol 15:605, 1984.

Fazekas F, Deisenhammer F, Strass-Fuchs S, et al: Randomised placebo-controlled trial of monthly intravenous immunoglobulin therapy in relapsing-remitting multiple sclerosis. Lancet 349:589, 1997.

Inoue K, Osaka H, Sugiyama N, et al: A duplicated PLP gene causing Pelizaeus-Merzbacher disease detected by comparative multiplex PCR. Am J Hum Genet 59:32, 1996.

Jarvela I, Vesa J, Santavuori P, et al: Molecular genetics of neuronal ceroid lipofuscinoses. Pediatr Res 32:645, 1992.

Johnson WG: The clinical spectrum of hexosaminidase deficiency disease. Neurology 31:1453, 1981.

Kelley RI, Datta NS, Dobyns WB, et al: Neonatal adrenoleukodystrophy: New cases, biochemical studies and differentiation from Zellweger and related peroxisomal polydystrophy syndromes. Am J Med Genet 23:869, 1986.

Kolodny EH: Metachromic leukodystrophy and multiple sulfatase deficiency. *In*: Rosenberg RN, Prusiner SB, DiMauro S, et al (eds): The Molecular and Genetic Basis of Neurological Disease. Stoneham, MA, Butterworth-Heinemann, 1993, p 497.

Kozinetz CA, Skender MI, MacNaughton N, et al: Epidemiology of Rett syndrome: A population-based registry. Pediatrics 91:445, 1993.

Krivit W, Shapiro EG, Peters C, et al: Hematopoietic stem-cell transplantation in globoid-cell leukodystrophy. N Engl J Med 338:1119, 1998.

Lowden JA, O'Brien JS: Sialidosis: A review of human neuraminidase deficiency. Am J Hum Genet 31:1, 1979.

McKhann GM: Metachromatic leukodystrophy: Clinical and enzymatic parameters. Neuropediatrics 15(Suppl):4, 1984.

Mobley WC, White CL, Tennekoon G, et al: Neonatal adrenoleukodystrosphy. Ann Neurol 12:204, 1982.

Moser HW, Moser AE, Singh I, et al: Adrenoleukodystrophy: Survey of 303 cases: Biochemistry, diagnosis, and therapy. Ann Neurol 16:628, 1984.

Mosser J, Douar A-M, Sarde C-D, et al: Putative X-linked adrenoleukodystrophy gene shares unexpected homology with ABC transporters. Nature 361:726, 1993.

Neufeld EF: Lysosomal storage diseases. Annu Rev Biochem 60:259, 1991.

Nishimoto J, Nanba E, Inui K, et al: GM_1-gangliosidosis (genetic β-galactosidase deficiency): Identification of four mutations in different clinical phenotypes among Japanese patients. Am J Hum Genet 49:566, 1991.

O'Brien JS: Beta-galactosidase deficiency, ganglioside sialidase deficiency. *In*: Scriver CR, Beaudet AL, Sly WS, Valle D (eds): The Metabolic Basis of Inherited Disease, 6th ed. New York, McGraw-Hill, 1989.

Percy AK: The inherited neurodegenerative disorders of childhood: Clinical assessment. J Child Neurol 2:82, 1987.

Percy AK: Second International Rett Syndrome Workshop and Symposium. J Child Neurol 8:97, 1993.

Pshezhetsky AV, Richard C, Michaud L, et al: Cloning, expression and chromosomal mapping of human lysosomal sialidase and characterization of mutations in sialidoses. Nat Genet 15:316, 1997.

Rapin I, Goldfischer S, Katzman R, et al: The cherry-red spot myoclonus syndrome. Ann Neurol 3:234, 1978.

Sarkar B, Lingertat-Walsh K, Clarke JTR: Copper-histidine therapy for Menkes disease. J Pediatr 123:828, 1993.

Strautnieks S, Rutland P, Winter RM, et al: Pelizaeus-Merzbacher disease: Detection of mutations Thr 181-Pro and Leu 223-Pro in the proteolipid protein gene, and prenatal diagnosis. Am J Hum Genet 51:871, 1992.

Tümer Z, Horn N: Menkes disease: Recent advances and new aspects. J Med Genet 34:265, 1997.

Wood AJJ: Management of multiple sclerosis. N Engl J Med 337:1604, 1997.

Zeman W, Dyken P: Neuronal ceroid-lipofuscinosis (Batten's disease): relationship to amaurotic family idiocy? Pediatrics 44:570, 1969.

Zoghbi HY: Molecular genetics and neurobiology of neurodegenerative and neurodevelopmental disorders. Pediatr Res 41:722, 1997.

CHAPTER 609
Acute Stroke Syndromes

Hemiplegia secondary to vascular disorders occurs in children with an incidence of 1–3/100,000 per year. The pediatric causes of stroke are distinctive compared to adult causes. Types of stroke include arterial and venous thrombosis, intracranial hemorrhage, arterial embolism, and various miscellaneous conditions. The cause of stroke in children is established in approximately 75% of cases (Table 609–1). Because the mode of presentation of acute stroke syndromes is not uniform, a brief description of the most prevalent forms of pediatric stroke follows.

609.1 Arterial Thrombosis/Embolism

Arterial thrombosis and embolism may involve major cerebral arteries (internal carotid or anterior, middle, and posterior cerebral artery occlusion) or smaller cerebral arteries. Certain thrombotic processes affect large vessels and others more commonly involve small arteries. *Thrombosis of the internal carotid artery* may result from blunt trauma to the posterior pharynx due to a fall on a pencil or popsicle stick in the child's mouth. The injury produces a tear in the intima of the vessel wall; this may lead to formation of a dissecting aneurysm. Cerebral symptoms result from shedding of emboli from the thrombus. The onset of symptoms may be delayed for up to 24 hr after the accident, with a stuttering but progressive flaccid hemiple-

TABLE 609–1 Causes of Stroke in Children

I. Cardiac Disease
- A. Congenital
  1. Aortic stenosis
  2. Mitral stenosis; mitral prolapse
  3. Ventricular septal defects
  4. Patent ductus arteriosus
  5. Cyanotic congenital heart disease involving right-to-left shunt
- B. Acquired
  1. Endocarditis (bacterial, SLE)
  2. Kawasaki disease
  3. Cardiomyopathy
  4. Atrial myxoma
  5. Arrhythmia
  6. Paradoxical emboli through patent foramen ovale
  7. Rheumatic fever
  8. Prosthetic heart valve

II. Hematologic Abnormalities
- A. Hemoglobinopathies
  1. Sickle cell (SS) disease
  2. Sickle (SC) disease
- B. Polycythemia
- C. Leukemia/lymphoma
- D. Thrombocytopenia
- E. Thrombocytosis
- F. Disorders of coagulation
  1. Protein C deficiency
  2. Protein S deficiency
  3. Factor V Leiden
  4. Antithrombin III deficiency
  5. Lupus anticoagulant
  6. Oral contraceptive pill use
  7. Pregnancy and the postpartum state
  8. Disseminated intravascular coagulation
  9. Paroxysmal nocturnal hemoglobinuria
  10. Inflammatory bowel disease (thrombosis)

III. Inflammatory Disorders
- A. Meningitis
  1. Viral
  2. Bacterial
  3. Tuberculosis
- B. Systemic infection
  1. Viremia
  2. Bacteremia
  3. Local head and neck infections
- C. Drug-induced inflammation
  1. Amphetamine
  2. Cocaine
- D. Autoimmune disease
  1. Systemic lupus erythematosus
  2. Juvenile rheumatoid arthritis
  3. Takayasu arteritis
  4. Mixed connective tissue disease
  5. Polyarteritis nodosum
  6. Primary CNS vasculitis
  7. Sarcoidosis
  8. Behçet's syndrome
  9. Wegener granulomatosis

IV. Metabolic Disease Associated with Stroke
- A. Homocystinuria
- B. Pseudoxanthoma elasticum
- C. Fabry disease
- D. Sulfite oxidase deficiency
- E. Mitochondrial disorders
  1. MELAS
  2. Leigh syndrome
- F. Ornithine transcarbamylase deficiency

V. Intracerebral Vascular Processes
- A. Ruptured aneurysm
- B. Arteriovenous malformation
- C. Fibromuscular dysplasia
- D. Moyamoya disease
- E. Migraine headache
- F. Postsubarachnoid hemorrhage vasospasm
- G. Hereditary hemorrhagic telangiectasia
- H. Sturge-Weber syndrome
- I. Carotid artery dissection
- J. Post varicella

VI. Trauma and Other External Causes
- A. Child abuse
- B. Head trauma/neck trauma
- C. Oral trauma
- D. Placental embolism
- E. ECMO therapy

ECMO = extracorporeal membrane oxygenation; MELAS = mitochondrial encephalomyopathy, lactic acidosis, and stroke; CNS = central nervous system.
From Riukin M: In: *Kliegman R (ed): Practical Strategies in Pediatric Diagnosis and Therapy. Philadelphia, WB Saunders, 1996.*

gia, lethargy, and aphasia if the dominant hemisphere is involved. Focal motor seizures are a common complication.

A retropharyngeal abscess may produce an identical clinical picture, but in this case the arterial thrombosis results from inflammation of the intima. A cerebral angiogram or MRI/magnetic resonance angiography (MRA) typically demonstrates occlusion of the internal carotid artery, and a CT/MRI scan shows a hypodense lesion outlining the area of infarction.

Embolization of cerebral vessels, although rare in children, may also produce acute hemiparesis. Cardiac abnormalities are the most common overall cause of thromboembolic stroke in children. Cardiac causes include arrhythmias (particularly atrial fibrillation), myxoma, paradoxical emboli through a patent foramen ovale, and bacterial endocarditis that results in a mycotic aneurysm. Air emboli may complicate surgery, and fat emboli occur with fracture of long bones. Septic emboli may seed the cerebral vessels and evolve into an area of cerebritis leading to a cerebral abscess.

Cyanotic congenital heart disease in children younger than 2 yr may cause thrombosis, particularly of the middle cerebral artery. These patients are particularly vulnerable when the oxygen saturation is significantly decreased together with a viral illness or dehydration. Cardiac procedures, including catheterization and complex cardiac surgery operations (e.g., Fontan), can result in arterial thrombosis from embolization of a clot. If a cardiac cause of arterial thrombosis is suspected, the child must have an echocardiogram as part of the investigation.

Occlusive vascular disorders, some of which are unique in children, are important causes of acute hemiplegia in the pediatric population. *Basal arterial occlusion with telangiectasia* or *moyamoya ("puff of smoke") disease* has a characteristic angiogram (Fig. 609–1). The condition is more common in girls and often presents with headache and bilateral upper motor neuron signs. It may also present with chorea. The prognosis for recovery is poor, with intermittent episodes of transient ischemic attacks coupled with progressive neurologic signs and severe disability. Surgical procedures designed to enhance cerebral flow (superficial temporal artery to middle cerebral artery shunt and laying the superficial temporal artery on the arachnoid membrane) have variable results. *Occlusion of distal arteries* is associated with diabetes mellitus, neurofibromatosis, sickle cell disease, postvaricella angiopathy, head and neck radiation, oral contraceptives, and illicit drug use (amphetamines, cocaine). Patients present with unilateral neurologic signs, and recovery is often complete owing to the small area of infarction. Patients with *thrombosis of small arteries,* including the perforating striate vessels, due to polyarteritis nodosa and homocystinuira, generally have a progressive debilitating course characterized by bilateral signs and high mortality.

609.2 Venous Thrombosis

Venous sinus thrombosis may be subdivided into septic and nonseptic causes. The symptoms and signs may evolve over days and in neonates are characterized by diffuse neurologic signs and seizures, whereas focal neurologic signs are more

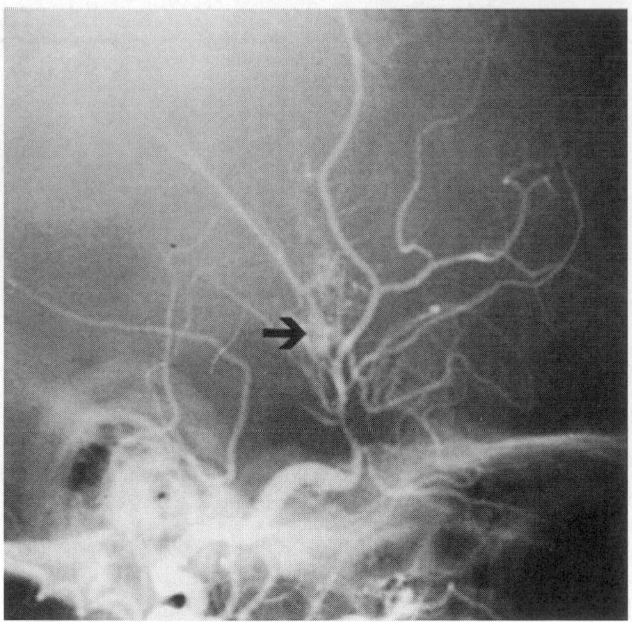

Figure 609–1 Cerebral angiogram showing idiopathic supraclinoid-internal carotid arteriopathy with classic moyamoya collaterals *(arrow)*.

prominent in children. Dilated scalp veins, a bulging anterior fontanel, and symptoms and signs of increased intracranial pressure may be present.

Septic causes of venous sinus thrombosis include encephalitis and bacterial meningitis. Hemiplegia is a relatively common complication of *bacterial meningitis* due to thrombosis of the superficial cortical and deep penetrating veins. Additional infectious causes of septic sinus thrombosis in children include *otitis media* and *mastoiditis* with involvement of the dural vessels, and retrograde orbital infections producing *cavernous sinus thrombosis*. *Aseptic causes* include *severe dehydration* in infancy, which may cause thrombosis of the superior sagittal sinus and the superficial cortical veins due to hyperviscosity and sludging of blood. Conditions resulting in hypercoagulopathy, cyanotic congenital heart diseases, and leukemic infiltrates of cerebral veins are additional causes of nonseptic acute hemiplegia of childhood. Deficiencies of inhibitors of coagulation, including protein C, protein S, antithrombosis III, heparin cofactor II, and dysfunctional plasminogen or fibrinogen are additional causes of venous sinus thrombosis.

609.3 Intracranial Hemorrhage

Intracranial hemorrhage may occur in the subarachnoid space, or the bleeding may be primarily located in the parenchyma of the brain. Subarachnoid bleeding is characterized by severe headache, nuchal rigidity, and progressive loss of consciousness, and intracerebral bleeding is characterized by focal neurologic signs and seizures. Intracranial hemorrhage is a common event in premature infants and is discussed in Section 95.2.

Arteriovenous malformations result from failure of normal capillary bed development between arteries and veins during embryogenesis. Arteriovenous malformations produce abnormal shunting of blood, causing an expansion of vessels and a space-occupying effect or rupture of a vein and intracerebral bleeding. Arteriovenous malformations are typically located in the cerebral hemisphere, but they may be situated in the cerebellum, brain stem, or spinal cord. Although the malformation may remain asymptomatic throughout life, rupture and bleeding can occur at any age. Children with arteriovenous malformations frequently have a history of seizures and migraine-like headaches. Typical migraine alternates from one side of the head to the other, whereas headaches associated with an arteriovenous malformation classically remain on the same side. Auscultation of the skull is positive for a high-pitched bruit in approximately 50% of cases. Rupture of an arteriovenous malformation causes a severe headache, vomiting, nuchal rigidity due to subarachnoid bleeding progressive hemiparesis, and a focal or generalized seizure. Cavernous angiomas may be familial and are of lower risk for spontaneous hemorrhage. An **arteriovenous malformation of the vein of Galen** during infancy can cause high-output congestive heart failure secondary to shunting of large volumes of blood or progressive hydrocephalus and increased intracranial pressure due to obstruction of the cerebrospinal fluid (CSF) pathways. Vein of Galen malformations are difficult to treat and are associated with a poor prognosis.

Cerebral aneurysms producing symptoms in children are relatively rare. In contrast to those in adults, aneurysms in children tend to be large and are located at the carotid bifurcation or on the anterior and posterior cerebral arteries rather than the circle of Willis. The aneurysmal dilatation results from a congenital weakness of the vessel, and in some cases a deficiency or type III collagen has been demonstrated. In children, there is an association between cerebral aneurysms and coarctation of the aorta and bilateral polycystic kidney disease. Although most ruptured aneurysms bleed into the subarachnoid space, causing an intense headache, nuchal rigidity, and coma, intracerebral hemorrhage and progressive hemiparesis also occur. Additional causes of intracerebral hematoma include hematologic disorders, particularly thrombocytopenic purpura and hemophilia. Finally, trauma can produce hemiparesis due to intracerebral bleeding or a subdural or epidural hematoma. A contrast CT scan or MRI with gadolinium and MRA is useful for identifying large arteriovenous malformations; however four-vessel cerebral angiography is the study of choice for investigating arteriovenous malformations and cerebral aneurysm.

609.4 Differential Diagnosis of Strokelike Events

Alternating hemiplegia of childhood is occasionally associated with migraine, but in most cases the cause is unknown. It develops in infants between 2 and 18 mo of age and is characterized by intermittent episodes of hemiplegia alternating from one side of the body to the other. Rarely, both sides are involved during an attack. Choreoathetois and dystonic movements are commonly observed in the hemiparetic extremity. Symptoms spontaneously regress with sleep but recur with awakening. The hemiplegia persists for minutes to weeks and then resolves spontaneously. The condition has a poor prognosis with progressive mental retardation and developmental disabilities. Results of neuroimaging and metabolic studies are negative. Several *metabolic diseases* are associated with strokelike episodes in children, including mitochondrial encephalomyolopathy (MELAS, see Chapter 607.2), ornithine transcarbamylase deficiency, pyruvate dehydrogenase deficiency, and homocystinuria. *Todd paralysis* may be confused initially with a stroke. The hemiparesis follows a focal seizure, but the weakness and neurologic signs disappear completely within 24 hr of the convulsion. Although the cause of Todd paralysis remains unknown, the hemiparesis probably results from an inhibitory phenomenon, possibly related to neurotransmitter dysfunction. Additional causes of hemiparesis include *cerebral tumor, encephalitis* (particularly herpes), *focal postviral encephalitis*, and *status epilepticus*. In some pediatric series of unexplained stroke, *lipid abnormalities*, including elevated triglycerides and low lev els of high-density lipoprotein cholesterol, have been found in approximately 20% of the cases. The family histories of these children reveal an increased incidence of premature coronary heart disease and early ischemic cerebrovascular diseases. Screening of at-risk families identifies children who may benefit from long-term dietary management.

INVESTIGATION OF STROKE. The most critical component of the investigation is a thorough history and physical examination, searching for an underlying disease process; evidence of trauma; an infectious, metabolic, or hematologic disorder; neurocutaneous syndrome; increased intracranial pressure; or hydrocephalus. Appropriate tests for infectious diseases, metabolic disorders, and hematologic disorders are based on the results of the history and physical examination. An EEG may be helpful in localizing the disease process but rarely establishes the diagnosis. A brain scan is extremely useful in cases of focal encephalitis, cerebritis, cerebral abscess, and infarction. A CT scan or MRI is mandatory in the investigation of children with acute hemiparesis. A cerebral angiogram is essential for those children in whom a CT scan or MRI is nondiagnostic. In these cases, a four-vessel cerebral angiogram should be planned. Electrocardiography and echocardiography may help to exclude intrinsic cardiac diseases or an arrhythmia as a cause of the stroke. Finally, the basic investigations for a child with an unexplained stroke syndrome should be organized to eliminate the following conditions: (1) vasculitis and connective tissue diseases (ESR, C3, C4, RF, ANA), (2) lipid disorders, (3) coagulation disorders, (4) hematologic disorders (sickle cell disease, thrombocytopenia), (5) metabolic disorders (homocystinuria, Fabry disease, MELAS), and (6) an infectious etiology (meningitis and encephalitis).

Treatment of Stroke. Several studies using low molecular weight heparin in children have shown the agent to be effective, safe, and well tolerated. The contraindications for the use of an antithrombotic agent include significant intracerebral hemorrhage and hypertension. The treatment for some causes of stroke are specific for the condition (e.g., repeated blood transfusions for sickle cell disease and stroke, immunosuppressant therapy for vasculitis, and surgical evacuation of a large blood clot). The rehabilitation requirements of children after a stroke are usually significant and include speech therapy, occupational and physical therapy, psychologic services, and special education. These treatment regimens are most effectively provided in a multidisciplinary setting.

Bourgeois M, Aicardi J, Goutières F: Alternating hemiplegia of childhood. J Pediatr 122:673, 1993.

Christodoulou J, Qureshi IA, McInnes RR, et al: Ornithine transcarbamylase deficiency presenting with strokelike episodes. J Pediatr 122:423, 1993.

David M, Andrew M: Venous thromboembolic complications in children. J Pediatr 123:337, 1993.

Fisher M, Bogousslavsky J: Further evolution toward effective therapy for acute ischemic stroke. JAMA 279:1298, 1998.

Ganesan V, Kirkham FJ: Mechanisms of ischaemic stroke after chickenpox. Arch Dis Child 76:522, 1997.

Kelly JJ, Mellinger JF, Sundt TM: Intracranial arteriovenous malformations in childhood. Ann Neurol 3:338, 1978.

Lees KR: Does neuroprotection improve stroke outcome? Lancet 351:1447, 1998.

Martin PJ, Enevoldson TP, Humphrey PRD: Causes of ischaemic stroke in the young. Postgrad Med J 73:855, 1997.

Pitner SE: Carotid thrombosis due to intraoral trauma. N Engl J Med 274:764, 1966.

Rivkin MJ, Volpe JJ: Strokes in children. Pediatr Rev 17:265, 1996.

Seeler RA, Royal JE, Powe L, et al: Moya-moya in children with sickle cell anemia and cerebrovascular occlusion. J Pediatr 93:808, 1978.

Thompson JR, Harwood-Nash DC, Fitz CR: Cerebral aneurysms in children. Am J Roentgenol 188:163, 1973.

Tomsick TA, Lukin RR, Chambers AA, et al: Neurofibromatosis and intracranial arterial occlusive disease. Neuroradiology 11:229, 1976.

Watanabe K, Negoro T, Maehara M, et al: Moyamoya disease presenting with chorea. Pediatr Neurol 6:40, 1990.

Wiznitzer M, Masaryk TJ: Cerebrovascular abnormalities in pediatric stroke: Assessment using parenchymal and angiographic magnetic resonance imaging. Ann Neurol 29:585, 1991.

CHAPTER 610
Brain Abscess

Brain abscesses can occur in children of any age but are most common between 4 and 8 yr. The causes of brain abscess include embolization due to congenital heart disease with right-to-left shunts (especially tetralogy of Fallot), meningitis, chronic otitis media and mastoiditis, sinusitis, soft tissue infection of the face or scalp, orbital cellulitis, dental infections, penetrating head injuries, immunodeficiency states, and infection of ventriculoperitoneal shunts. The pathogenesis is undetermined in 10–15% of cases. Cerebral abscesses are evenly distributed between the two hemispheres, and approximately 80% of cases are divided equally between the frontal, parietal, and temporal lobes. Brain abscesses in the occipital lobe, cerebellum, and brain stem account for about 20% of the cases. Most brain abscesses are single, but 30% are multiple and may involve more than one lobe. An abscess in the frontal lobe is often caused by extension from sinusitis or orbital cellulitis, whereas abscesses located in the temporal lobe or cerebellum are frequently associated with chronic otitis media and mastoiditis. Abscesses resulting from penetrating injuries tend to be singular and caused by *Staphylococcus aureus*, whereas those resulting from septic emboli, congenital heart disease, or meningitis often have several organisms.

ETIOLOGY. The responsible bacteria include *S. aureus*, streptococci (*viridans*, pneumococci, microaerophilic), anaerobic organisms (gram-positive cocci, *Bacteroides* spp, *Fusobacterium* spp, *Prevotella* spp, *Actinomyces* spp, and *Clostridium* spp), and gram-negative aerobic bacilli (enteric rods, *Proteus* spp, *Pseudomonas aeruginosa*, *Citrobacter diversus*, and *Haemophilus* spp). One organism is cultured from the majority of abscesses (70%), two from 20%, and three or more in 10% of cases. Abscesses associated with mucosal infections (sinusitis) frequently have anaerobic bacteria.

CLINICAL MANIFESTATIONS. The early stages of cerebritis and abscess formation are associated with nonspecific symptoms, including low-grade fever, headache, and lethargy. The significance of these symptoms is generally not recognized, and an oral antibiotic is often prescribed with resultant transient relief. As the inflammatory process proceeds, vomiting, severe headache, seizures, papilledema, focal neurologic signs (hemiparesis), and coma may develop. A cerebellar abscess is characterized by nystagmus, ipsilateral ataxia and dysmetria, vomiting, and headache. If the abscess ruptures into the ventricular cavity, overwhelming shock and death usually ensue.

DIAGNOSIS. The peripheral white blood cell count can be normal or elevated, and the blood culture is positive in only 10%. Examination of the cerebrospinal fluid (CSF) shows variable results; the white blood cells and protein may be minimally elevated or normal. The glucose level may be slightly low, and CSF cultures are rarely positive. Because examination of the CSF is seldom useful and a lumbar puncture may cause herniation of the cerebellar tonsils, the procedure should not be undertaken in a child suspected of having a brain abscess. The electroencephalogram (EEG) shows corresponding focal slowing, and the radionuclide brain scan indicates an area of enhancement due to disruption of the blood-brain barrier in greater than 80% of cases. CT and MRI are the most reliable methods of demonstrating cerebritis and abscess formation (Fig. 610–1). The CT findings of cerebritis are characterized by a parenchymal low-density lesion, and MRI T2-weighted images indicate increased signal intensity. An abscess cavity shows a ring-enhancing lesion by contrast CT, and the MRI

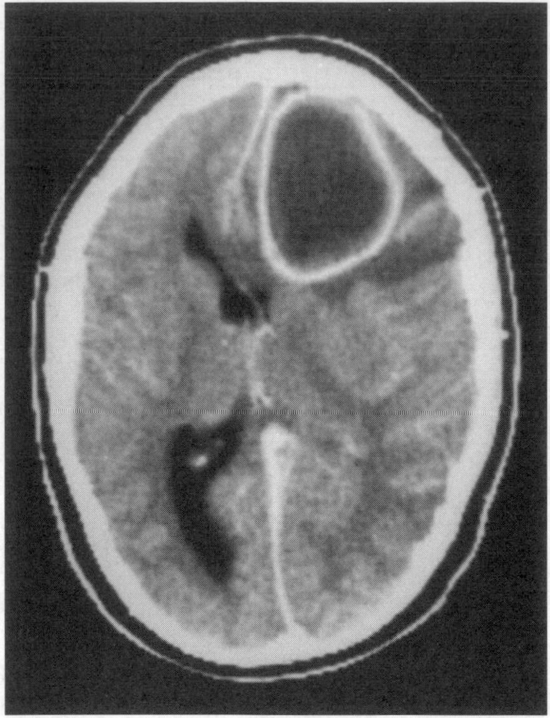

Figure 610–1 CT with contrast. Note the large wall-enhancing abscess in the left frontal lobe. The lesion is causing a shift of the brain to the right. The patient had no neurologic signs until just prior to the CT scan because the abscess is located in the frontal lobe, a "silent" area of the brain.

also demonstrates an abscess capsule with gadolinium administration.

TREATMENT. The initial management of a brain abscess includes prompt diagnosis and institution of an antibiotic regimen that is based on the probable pathogenesis and most likely organism. In cases in which the cause is unknown, the dual combination of a third-generation cephalosporin and metronidazole is commonly used. If there is a history of head trauma or neurosurgery, a combination of nafcillin or vancomycin with a third-generation cephalosporin and metronidazole is given. The choice of antibiotics should be altered when the culture and sensitivity results become available. An abscess resulting from a penetrating injury, head trauma, or sinusitis should be treated with a combination of nafcillin or vancomycin, cefotaxime or ceftriaxone, and metronidazole. Monotherapy with meropenem, which has good activity against gram-negative bacilli, anaerobes, staphylococci, and streptococci, including virtually all antibiotic-resistant pneumococci, is a reasonable alternative. In contrast, the initial treatment of a lesion resulting from cyanotic heart disease is penicillin and metronidazole. Abscesses secondary to an infected ventriculoperitoneal shunt may be initially treated with vancomycin and ceftazidime. When otitis media or mastoiditis is the likely cause, nafcillin or vancomycin in combination with ceftazidime and metronidazole is indicated. In those cases in which *Citrobacter* meningitis (often in neonates) leads to abscess formation, a third-generation cephalosporin is used, typically in combination with an aminoglycoside. In immunocompromised patients, broad antibiotic coverage is used, and amphotericin B therapy should be considered. Surgical management of brain abscesses has changed since the advent of CT. In the early stages of cerebritis or with multiple abscesses, antibiotics may be used alone. An encapsulated abscess, particularly if the lesion is causing a mass effect or increased intracranial pressure, should be treated by a combination of antibiotics and aspiration. Surgical excision of an abscess is rarely required, because the procedure may be associated with greater morbidity compared with aspiration of a cavity. Surgery is indicated if gas is present in the abscess, if it is multiloculated, if it is located in the posterior fossa, or if a fungus is identified. Associated infectious processes, such as mastoiditis, sinusitis, or a periorbital abscess, may require surgical drainage. The duration of antibiotic therapy depends on the organism and response to treatment but usually is 4–6 wk.

PROGNOSIS. Mortality due to brain abscesses has decreased significantly, to approximately 5–10% with the use of CT or MRI and prompt antibiotic and surgical management. Factors associated with high mortality at the time of admission include multiple abscesses, coma, and lack of CT facilities. Long-term sequelae occur in at least 50% of survivors and include hemiparesis, seizures, hydrocephalus, cranial nerve abnormalities, and behavior and learning problems.

Brook I: Aerobic and anaerobic bacteriology of intracranial abscesses. Pediatr Neurol 8:210, 1992.

Saez-Lloreus XJ, Umana NA, Odio CN, et al: Brain abscesses in infants and children. Pediatr Infect Dis J 8:449, 1989.

Sjolin J, Lilja A, Erikson N, et al: Treatment of brain abscess with cefotaxime and metronidazole: Prospective study on 15 consecutive patients. Clin Infect Dis 17:857, 1993.

Smith RR: Neuroradiology of intracranial infection. Pediatr Neurosurg 18:92, 1992.

CHAPTER 611
Brain Tumors in Children

(See also Chapters 498 and 508)

Brain tumors are second only to leukemia as the most prevalent malignancy in childhood, and they account for the most common solid tumors in this age group. Brain tumors can present at any age, but each tends to have a peak age incidence. Metastatic brain tumors are common in adults but relatively rare in children.

EPIDEMIOLOGY. Approximately two thirds of all intracranial tumors occurring in children between the ages of 2 and 12 yr are infratentorial (located in the posterior fossa). In adolescents and infants younger than 2 yr, tumors occur with equal frequencies in the posterior fossa and the supratentorial region.

PATHOLOGY AND PATHOGENESIS. The two major histologic types of brain tumors in children are glial cell tumors and those of primitive neuroectodermal cell origin. Glial cell tumors are the most common and consist of various cell types with variable prognoses, including the astrocytoma, ependymoma, and glioblastoma multiforme. Neuroectodermal tumors probably arise from a primitive, undifferentiated cell line and are prominent throughout the central nervous system (CNS), involving the cerebellum (medulloblastoma), cerebrum, spinal cord, and pineal gland (pineoblastoma) (see Chapter 499). Some tumors are unique because they originate from embryonic remnants, such as the craniopharyngioma, which arises from Rathke pouch; dermoid and epidermoid tumors originating from the invagination of epithelial cells during the closure of the neural tube; and the chordoma, which develops from traces of the embryonic notochord. The pathogenesis of brain tumors is complex because many factors influence their development. Conditions that result from abnormalities of neural crest development have a high association with tumors of the CNS. Both types of neurofibromatosis are associated with an increased incidence of specific brain tumors: optic glioma and low-grade astrocytoma in NF 1 and acoustic neuroma and meningioma in NF 2. Some patients who received radiation for scalp disorders during childhood develop cranial tumors years later, and second brain tumors occasionally develop after radiation for the treatment of a primary brain tumor or prophylactic radiation for acute lymphoblastic leukemia.

The evolution of brain tumors may involve sequential mutation or deletion of specific genes. For example, in gliomas, deletion of 17p is found at high frequency in all grades of the tumor, while in high-grade glioma an additional loss of 9p occurs. In the case of glioblastoma multiforme, the most malignant variant, an addition or loss of a portion of chromosome 10 occurs in many tumors. Other tumors are associated with nonrandom chromosome loss: the meningioma with a portion of chromosome 22 and medulloblastoma with a segment of 17p, not related to the p53 tumor suppressor gene. Various growth factors appear to have prominent roles in the development and progression of brain tumors. An aberrant receptor site for epidermal growth factor (EGFR) has been demonstrated in gliomas, while alteration of platelet-derived growth factor receptor and increased expression of its ligand, platelet-derived growth factor, have been shown in meningiomas. The precise roles and relationship of the molecular oncogene events remain to be clarified.

CLINICAL MANIFESTATIONS. Brain tumors present in many ways, depending on the location, type, and rate of growth of the tumor and the age of the child. Generally, there are two distinct patterns of presentation: symptoms and signs of increased intracranial pressure (ICP) and focal neurologic signs. Tumors located within the posterior fossa primarily produce symptoms and signs of increased ICP due to obstruction of CSF pathways and the development of hydrocephalus. Supratentorial tumors are more likely to be associated with focal abnormalities, including long-tract signs and seizures.

Alterations in personality are often the first symptoms of a brain tumor, irrespective of its location. The child, beginning weeks or months before the discovery of the tumor, may have become lethargic, irritable, hyperactive, or forgetful or may perform poorly academically. It is not certain whether the behavioral changes result from increased ICP, the site of the lesion, or both. After the tumor has been removed and amelioration of the increased ICP, significant reversal of the behavioral problems usually occurs.

Increased ICP is characterized by headache, vomiting, diplopia, and papilledema, and in infants, a bulging fontanel and increasing head size (macrocrania) develop. The *headache* initially tends to occur in the morning and is relieved with standing, as venous flow away from the head is enhanced in the upright position. The headache is described as dull, generalized, and steady and may be intermittent and worsened by coughing or sneezing or during defecation. The headache is typically associated with *vomiting*, which often relieves the headache. Tumors that occupy the fourth ventricle are often associated with pernicious vomiting. Children who present with vomiting as the initial symptom of a brain tumor are frequently subjected to a series of gastrointestinal investigations. A thorough history and neurologic examination would obviate those tests in many cases. *Diplopia* is a common symptom of posterior fossa tumors. Children do not usually complain of double vision, because they seem to readily suppress the image of the affected eye. Examination of the eye movements shows strabismus owing to involvement of the abducens, oculomotor nerve, or, rarely, the trochlear nerve. Some children with diplopia compensate by tilting the head in an attempt to align the two images. *Head tilting* and *nuchal rigidity* may also indicate herniation of the cerebellar tonsils. In this situation, a lumbar puncture may enhance the herniation and result in death. *Nystagmus* is a prominent sign associated with posterior fossa tumors. Unilateral cerebellar tumors cause horizontal nystagmus, which is exaggerated on looking to the side of the lesion. Tumors located in the posterior cerebellar vermis or fourth ventricle produce nystagmus in all directions of gaze. Brain stem tumors may result in horizontal, vertical, and rotatory nystagmus. *Papilledema* (Fig. 600–1) is the cardinal finding of increased ICP, but it is important to remember that in infants, separation of the cranial sutures and bulging of the anterior fontanel may decompress the contents of the skull. The head may continue to accelerate in size without associated symptoms and signs of increased ICP. In this case, papilledema may be conspicuous by its absence. A rapid rise or prolonged increase in ICP may result in coma with alterations in the vital signs. Bradycardia, an irregular pulse, and systemic hypertension occur associated with alterations in the respiratory pattern. Initially, hyperventilation is noted, which, without intervention, progresses to ataxic and irregular breathing followed by respiratory arrest.

Supratentorial tumors may also be associated with symptoms and signs of increased ICP. However, focal neurologic signs including hemiparesis and complex partial seizures predominate, particularly with a temporal lobe tumor. The greatest oversight in the examination of a child with headache and vomiting is failure to examine the retina and optic nerve. *Obscuration of vision* characterized by blurring is a serious symptom that indicates marked vasoconstriction of cerebral vessels and impending cerebellar herniation. *Visual loss*, manifesting as clumsiness or, in infants, developmental delay associated with roving eye movements or nystagmus, is a feature of optic tract gliomas or of impingement of pituitary or suprasellar masses on the optic chiasm.

Ataxia is often associated with posterior fossa tumors, although it is interesting that some large tumors cause absolutely no abnormality of movement. Tumors of the cerebellar vermis characteristically cause truncal ataxia that is enhanced with sitting or standing, and involvement of the anterior cerebellum results in marked gait disturbances that are typically broad based. Tumors of a cerebellar hemisphere produce ipsilateral extremity ataxia and dysdiadochokinesia. The following sections highlight the pathology, management, and prognosis of the major brain tumors in the pediatric age group.

INFRATENTORIAL TUMORS. The *cerebellar astrocytoma* is the most common posterior fossa tumor of childhood and has the best prognosis. These neoplasms tend to be cystic and have a mural nodule of solid tumor; however, they can be solid with little or no cystic cavitation. Those tumors with cystic cavities are filled with a thickened xanthochromic fluid. Cerebellar astrocytomas may be midline involving the vermis or confined to a hemisphere, and although usually of low grade, they are capable of invading the cerebellar peduncles (Fig. 611–1). The tumor causes hydrocephalus and symptoms and signs of increased ICP by obstructing the aqueduct of Sylvius or fourth ventricle. Histologically, the astrocytoma is characterized by protoplasmic and fibrillary astrocytes arranged in a radial fashion interspersed with Rosenthal's fibers. The treatment is surgical resection, and the 5-yr survival is greater than 90%. Radiation therapy is reserved for patients with high-grade astrocytomas or in whom postoperative tumor progression is evident by clinical and radiologic investigation.

The *medulloblastoma* is the next most common posterior fossa tumor in the pediatric age group and is the most prevalent brain tumor in children younger than 7 yr. Although the cell site of origin of the medulloblastoma is unknown, in some cases it originates from the roof of the fourth ventricle and grows rapidly to fill the fourth ventricle or invade the adjacent cerebellar hemisphere. This tumor may spread over the cerebral convexities or along the CSF pathways and is capable of metastasizing to extracranial sites. Microscopically, the tumor is vascular and cellular and is characterized by deeply staining nuclei with scant cytoplasm arranged in pseudorosettes. The prognosis and treatment depend on the size and dissemination of the tumor, and the age of the child. All children with a diagnosis of medulloblastoma require neuroimaging of the neuraxis, preferably by MRI or by CT myelography if MRI is

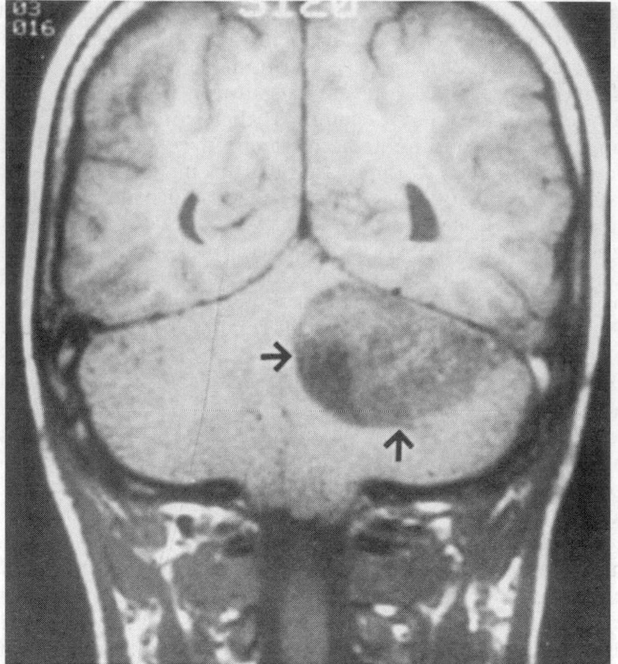

Figure 611–1 A coronal MRI scan of a large, primarily solid, cerebellar astrocytoma *(arrows)*.

not available. All patients are treated with surgical extirpation, followed by irradiation. Irradiation is directed to the entire neuraxis because of the propensity for medulloblastomas to seed to remote sites. The standard irradiation dose is 5,400 cGy to the posterior fossa and 3,600 cGy to the neuraxis. High risk patients with dissemination of the tumor are treated with surgery, radiation, and chemotherapy following diagnosis. Standard risk patients are routinely treated with surgery and radiation. Because many standard risk patients relapse following treatment, many centers treat all patients with a combination of chemotherapy and radiation. The 5 yr survival of these combined groups now approaches 80%–90% in many studies. Chemotherapy agents used for the treatment of medulloblastoma include vincristine, cyclophosphamide, cis-platinum, and etoposide. In very young patients (younger than 3 yr), most centers follow surgery with chemotherapy and withhold radiation therapy to a later age when the brain is more tolerant of the effects of radiation.

Brain stem gliomas are the third most frequent posterior fossa tumor in children. These tumors are of two types: those that produce diffuse infiltration in the pons, extending throughout the brain stem, which at postmortem examination are found to be anaplastic astrocytomas, and low-grade focal tumors (exophytic cervicomedullary or localized tectal lesions) in the midbrain and medulla (Fig. 611–2). The prognosis for the former is grave, whereas a focal brain stem tumor confined to the midbrain or the cervical medullary junction and the dorsally exophytic brain stem gliomas have excellent survival rates after surgery alone. The symptoms and signs result from invasion and destruction of cranial nerve nuclei and the pyramidal tracts. The most common cranial nerve symptoms include diplopia and facial weakness due to abducens and facial nerve involvement. Later, dysarthria, dysphagia, and dysphonia may result owing to infiltration of the cranial nuclei in the medulla. Pyramidal tract involvement is manifested by gait disturbances and the presence of generalized upper motor neuron signs. Changes in personality are particularly common with brain stem gliomas and include lethargy, irritability, and aggressive behavior.

Clinical manifestations of increased ICP including papilledema occur late (if at all) in the course, because the CSF pathways remain patent in most cases until the tumor has become massive.

The surgical treatment of brain stem gliomas is controversial. With newer radioimaging techniques, particularly MRI, the diagnosis is usually apparent and biopsy is unnecessary. If there is uncertainty after neuroimaging, a stereotactic biopsy is warranted. The primary treatment is irradiation, and although some brain stem gliomas are radiosensitive, the mean 5-yr survival is approximately 20%. Diffuse intrinsic pontine tumors have a 2-yr survival of only 10%. In view of the very poor prognosis and response to radiotherapy, the role of hyperfractionated radiation therapy (smaller, more frequent doses ultimately resulting in a higher total dose) was investigated, and this radiotherapy mode was found not to be beneficial. Chemotherapy has not proved efficacious for the management of brain stem gliomas. Low-grade focal tumors of the midbrain or medulla have an excellent prognosis after radical excision. Patients are observed, and radiotherapy is withheld unless the residual tumor shows evidence of regrowth.

Ependymomas account for approximately 10% of childhood posterior fossa tumors. These lesions arise from within the fourth ventricle and cause hydrocephalus and signs of increased ICP due to obstruction of the CSF pathways. Aside from vomiting, headache, and diplopia, nuchal rigidity and torticollis may result owing to herniation of the cerebellar tonsils. Ataxia and focal neurologic signs are usually absent; however, papilledema is a consistent finding in a symptomatic child. The histologic picture consists of rosettes of ependymal cells with cilia protruding into the central cavity. Treatment includes surgical removal and radiation therapy to the tumor region, with a 5-yr survival approximating 50%. If the tumor histology reveals an aggressive anaplastic ependymoma, radiation should be delivered to the entire craniospinal region, because these tumors readily disseminate and are associated with a much less favorable prognosis. Chemotherapy is ineffective.

Additional tumors that have a proclivity for the posterior fossa include several benign tumors, such as a choroid plexus papilloma of the fourth ventricle, dermoids, epidermoids, chordomas, and teratomas. Although generally nonmalignant, these lesions are capable of producing significant morbidity and death owing to their location, size, and possibility of obstructing the normal flow of CSF.

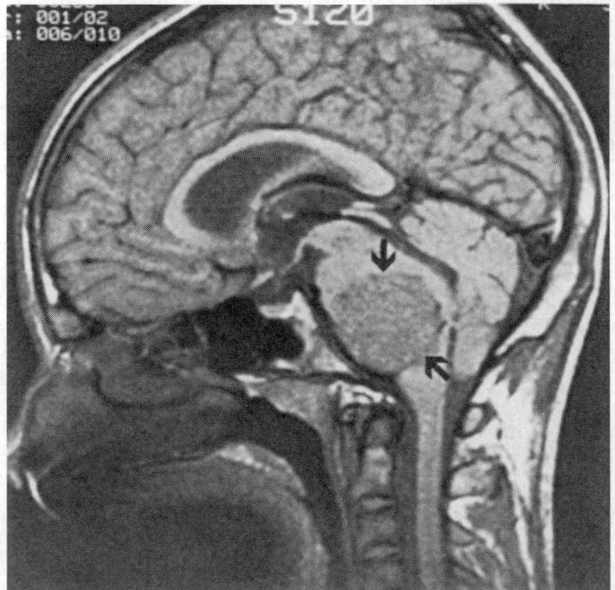

Figure 611–2 MRI scan of a solid brain stem glioma, an anaplastic astrocytoma *(arrows)*.

SUPRATENTORIAL TUMORS. *Craniopharyngioma* is one of the most common supratentorial tumors in children. The tumor may be confined to the sella turcica, or it can extend through the diaphragma sella and compress the optic nerve system, pons, or third ventricle, producing hydrocephalus. The tumor consists of a solid and cystic areas that have a tendency to calcify. Approximately 90% of craniopharyngiomas show calcification on the plain skull roentgenogram or CT scan. Many children with craniopharyngioma are referred to endocrine clinics because of short stature due to pituitary-hypothalamic involvement. Pressure or injury to the optic chiasm typically produces bitemporal visual field defects, although most children are unaware of peripheral visual loss until the time of testing. Papilledema and symptoms of increased ICP are evident when hydrocephalus is prominent. The treatment is a craniotomy using a subfrontal approach. With complete or near-total removal, 60% of patients experience no further recurrence. The role of radiation therapy is still debated, but most centers favor radiation to the sellar region postoperatively only in those cases in which tumor removal is incomplete and recurrence follows. Endocrine disorders, including diabetes insipidus, hypothyroidism, growth hormone, and adrenocortical deficiency, may develop postoperatively and warrant close follow-up. There is no effective chemotherapeutic agent.

Optic nerve gliomas present with decreased visual acuity and pallor of the discs. These tumors are primarily low-grade astrocytomas, and approximately 25% of patients have associated neurofibromatosis (see Chapter 605.1). Because the natural history of optic gliomas is variable, treatment is most often delayed until there is evidence of clinical or radiologic progression. Irradiation is effective in halting tumor growth and preserving vision but has major neurodevelopmental consequences in young infants. Chemotherapy is effective in arresting growth of the tumor in up to 70% of cases and should be the treatment of first choice. The glioma may invade the optic chiasm and hypothalamus, producing visual field defects or the **diencephalic syndrome**. Affected children are anorectic and emaciated and have little or no subcutaneous tissue but normal linear growth. Their behavior is not in keeping with the nutritional state, because they are often hyperalert and euphoric. Approximately 25% have a coarse horizontal nystagmus. Conversely, tumor invasion of the hypothalamus can result in an insatiable appetite, obesity, diabetes insipidus, and hypogonadism. Resection of the optic glioma confined to an optic nerve produces blindness in the affected eye but prevents recurrence or extension through the chiasm; it may be the preferred therapy if the eye is already blind from tumor invasion. Optic chiasm gliomas with hypothalamic involvement may be treated with chemotherapy (carboplatinum and vincristine) in children younger than 3 yr, and this may delay the requirement for radiation therapy. Radiotherapy in older patients with chiasmatic/hypothalamic gliomas results in an excellent prognosis, with 10-yr survival rates of almost 90%.

Astrocytoma and related glial tumors (ependymoma and oligodendrogliomas) have a less favorable prognosis when located in the cerebral hemisphere than when they are confined to the cerebellum. These patients may have a chronic history of complex partial epilepsy, particularly if the tumor is located within the temporal lobe. Neurologic examination frequently reveals subtle upper motor neuron signs or contralateral growth arrest of the extremities. Surgical excision of a low-grade astrocytoma results in at least an 80% 5-yr survival. High-grade astrocytomas have a much greater mortality, with only a 30% survival after surgery and radiation therapy. Chemotherapy may add marginally to survival rates.

A series of *tumors peculiar to children arise in the region of the pineal gland*, including varieties of germ cell tumors, pinealomas, pineoblastomas, and teratomas. These tumors are remarkably different in degrees of malignancy and invasion of surrounding structures. They may cause obstruction of the CSF pathways, resulting in macrocrania and hydrocephalus. Pressure by the tumor on the quadrigeminal plate produces **Parinaud syndrome,** consisting of paralysis of conjugate upward movement of the eyes and poorly reactive pupils. There is no uniform agreement about the management of pineal area tumors, because of the heterogeneity of the tumors and the variable response to radiotherapy. Most would concur that a tissue diagnosis is preferable before initiation of therapy. Modern surgical techniques, including the use of an operating microscope, have significantly decreased the morbidity and mortality and have allowed total resection of some tumors in the pineal region. Germ cell tumors, both germinoma and nongerminomas, are chemosensitive. The 5-yr survival for germinomas treated with chemotherapy (cis-platinum, bleomycin, and etoposide) with a reduced radiation dose and field approximates 90%. Results are not as favorable with nongerminoma tumors. A radiosensitive germinoma has a 5-yr survival greater than 75%. Some tumors (e.g., pinealomas) are resistant to radiation and are more likely to respond to chemotherapy (cis-platinum and etoposide), whereas others such as mature teratomas may be treated exclusively by surgery.

The *choroid plexus papilloma* produces slowly progressive hydrocephalus due to excessive production of CSF. The most common location is the lateral ventricle, followed by the third and fourth ventricles. These tumors arise from the choroid plexus epithelium and protrude into the ventricular cavity. The prognosis is excellent after surgical removal. Malignant choroid plexus carcinoma is extremely vascular and invasive. Cure requires complete resection, which may be facilitated by preoperative chemotherapy.

In *leukemia,* infiltrates may invade the leptomeninges, causing increased ICP due to infiltration of the pacchionian granulations, or may involve the brain parenchyma and, in combination with an acute hermorrhage, result in a mass lesion. Finally, cranial nerves, particularly the facial nerve, or peripheral nerves, such as the peroneal and sciatic nerves, may be invaded by leukemic infiltrates, resulting in weakness, pain, and sensory phenomena.

LABORATORY FINDINGS. MRI is the best technique for delineation of brain tumors in children. Aside from the lack of ionizing radiation, the MRI study provides a superior image of the posterior fossa structures compared with a CT scan. Furthermore, the fine detail in MRI has identified cerebral tumors that are not visible with CT scanning. In addition, MRI is more accurate in defining the extent of an infiltrating tumor. Metastases to the spinal cord can be identified by noninvasive MRI enhanced with the contrast agent gadolinium; contrast myelography is a complementary study for small metastatic lesions in that region. Children with tumors of the sella turcica should undergo a series of baseline endocrine studies, including measurements of growth hormone, thyroid-stimulating hormone, adrenocorticotrophic hormone (ACTH), luteinizing hormone, follicle-stimulating hormone, antidiuretic hormone, and prolactin, because these hormones may require replacement if they are deficient. Nongerminomatous germ cell tumors in the pineal gland are associated with elevated CSF human chorionic gonadotropin and α-fetoprotein levels. Monoclonal antibodies are proving helpful in differentiating medulloblastoma from CNS lymphoma antigens. CSF tumor cells may be examined at the time of surgery or as a component of routine follow-up. Positive CSF cytology immediately postoperatively is common, but the interpretation of the finding is not certain, because seeding and new growth may not occur.

PROGNOSIS. Neuropsychologic deficits, including changes in cognitive behavior, verbal performance, perceptual-motor function, and academic achievement, have been reported as frequent complications of cranial radiation therapy. Neurophysiologic abnormalities consisting of generalized slowing of the EEG and increased evoked potential latencies have also been noted. After irradiation, CT scanning and MRI have shown various lesions involving the cortex and myelin, including calcification, ventricular dilatation, white matter hypodensities, and cortical atrophy. Generally, the younger the patient, the greater is the disability. However, there is little correlation between the site of the pathology as identified by imaging studies and the cognitive disorder. Abnormalities in linear growth and radiation-induced hypothyroidism are common after radiation therapy, secondary to growth hormone dysfunction. Baseline endocrine studies should be carried out on all newly diagnosed patients before the initiation of therapy and careful monitoring of growth is essential in the follow-up of these children. Second malignancies are rare after treatment of a primary brain tumor in children. Prospective studies evaluating the age of the child and specific therapeutic regimens are required to better understand the consequences of cranial radiation therapy.

Newer therapeutic modalities, such as implantation of radiation seeds (brachytherapy) and the use of focal and focused radiation, add promise for the treatment of brain tumors in children. The role of autologous stem cell rescue to allow the use of higher concentrations of chemotherapeutic agents is under investigation. Molecular biologic studies are also likely to define the mechanisms of tumor behavior and provide a method for more effective therapy in the future.

Davis FG, Freels S, Grutsch J, et al: Survival rates in patients with primary malignant brain tumors stratified by patient age and tumor histological type: An analysis based on surveillance, epidemiology, and end results (SEER) data, 1973–1991. J Neurosurg 88:1, 1998.

Duffner PK, Horowitz ME, Krischer JP, et al: Postoperative chemotherapy and delayed radiation in children less than three years of age with malignant brain tumors. N Engl J Med 328:1725, 1993.

Edwards MSB, Hudgins RJ, Wilson CB, et al: Pineal region tumors in children. J Neurosurg 68:689, 1988.

Epstein F, McCleary EL: Intrinsic brain-stem tumors of childhood: Surgical indications. J Neurosurg 64:11, 1986.

Glaser AW, Buxton N, Walker D, et al: Corticosteroids in the management of central nervous system tumours. Arch Dis Child 76:76, 1997.

Horowitz ME, Mulhern RK, Kun LE, et al: Brain tumors in the very young child. Cancer 61:428, 1988.

Kadota RP, Allen JB, Hartman GA, et al: Brain tumors in children. J Pediatr 114:511, 1989.

Lashford LS, Walker DA: Improving care for central nervous system tumours: A mood for change. Arch Dis Child 76:88, 1997.

Listernick R, Charrow J, Greenwald M, et al: Natural history of optic pathway tumors in children with neurofibromatosis type 1: A longitudinal study. J Pediatr 125:63, 1994.

Marsh WR, Laws ER Jr: Intracranial ependymomas. Progr Exp Tumor Res 30:175, 1987.

Packer RJ, Batnitzky S, Cohen ME: Magnetic resonance imaging in the evaluation of intracranial tumors of childhood. Cancer 56:1767, 1985.

Packer RJ, Sutton LN, Goldwein JW, et al: Improved survival with the use of adjuvant chemotherapy in the treatment of medulloblastoma. J Neurosurg 74:433, 1991.

Shrieve DC, Wara WM, Edwards MSB, et al: Hyperfractionated radiation therapy for gliomas of the brainstem in children and in adults. Int J Radiat Oncol Biol Phys 24:599, 1992.

Shuper A, Horev G, Kornreich L, et al: Visual pathway glioma: An erratic tumor with therapeutic dilemmas. Arch Dis Child 76:259, 1997.

Strickler HD, Rosenberg PS, Devesa SS, et al: Contamination of poliovirus vaccines with simian virus 40 (1955–1963) and subsequent cancer rates. JAMA 279:292, 1998.

Sznajder L, Abrahams C, Parry DM, et al: Multiple schwannomas and meningiomas associated with irradiation in childhood. Arch Intern Med 156:1873, 1996.

Tores CF, Rebsamen S, Silber JH, et al: Surveillance scanning of children with medulloblastoma. N Engl J Med 330:892, 1994.

Weil MD, Lamborn K, Edwards MSB, et al: Influence of a child's sex on medulloblastoma outcome. JAMA 279:1474, 1998.

CHAPTER 612
Pseudotumor Cerebri

Pseudotumor cerebri is a clinical syndrome that mimics brain tumors and is characterized by increased intracranial pressure (ICP) with a normal cerebrospinal fluid (CSF) cell count and protein content and normal ventricular size, anatomy, and position.

ETIOLOGY. There are many explanations for the development of pseudotumor cerebri, including alterations in CSF absorption and production, cerebral edema, abnormalities in vasomotor control and cerebral blood flow, and venous obstruction. The causes of pseudotumor are numerous and include *metabolic disorders* (galactosemia, hypoparathyroidism, pseudohypoparathyroidism, hypophosphatasia, prolonged corticosteroid therapy, possibly growth hormone treatment, hypervitaminosis A, vitamin A deficiency, Addison's disease, obesity, menarche, oral contraceptives, and pregnancy), *infections* (roseola infantum, chronic otitis media and mastoiditis, Guillain-Barré syndrome), *drugs* (nalidixic acid, tetracycline, nitrofurantoin, isotretinoin), *hematologic disorders* (polycythemia, hemolytic and iron-deficiency anemia, Wiskott-Aldrich syndrome), and *obstruction of intracranial drainage by venous thrombosis* (lateral sinus or posterior sagittal sinus thrombosis, head injury, and obstruction of the superior vena cava).

CLINICAL MANIFESTATIONS. The most frequent symptom is headache, and although vomiting also occurs, it is rarely as persistent and pernicious as that associated with a posterior fossa tumor. Diplopia secondary to paralysis of the abducens nerve is a frequent complaint. Most patients are alert and lack constitutional symptoms. Examination of the infant characteristically reveals a bulging fontanel and a "cracked-pot sound" or Macewen sign (percussion of the skull produces a resonant sound) due to separation of the cranial sutures. Papilledema with an enlarged blind spot is the most consistent sign in a child beyond infancy. Early optic nerve edema may be noted with ultrasonography. An inferior nasal defect may be detected on formal tangent screen testing. The presence of focal neurologic signs indicates a process other than pseudotumor cerebri.

TREATMENT. The prime goal in management should be discovery and treatment of the underlying cause. Pseudotumor cerebri is mainly a self-limited condition, but optic atrophy and blindness are the most significant complications. Consideration should be given to treating sinus thrombosis with anticoagulation. For many patients, repeated follow-up and monitoring of the visual acuity are all that is required. Serial visual evoked potentials are useful if the visual acuity cannot be reliably documented. For others, the initial lumbar tap that follows a CT or MRI scan is diagnostic and therapeutic. The spinal needle produces a small rent in the dura that allows CSF to escape the subarachnoid space, thus reducing the ICP. Several additional lumbar taps and the removal of sufficient CSF to reduce the opening pressure by 50% occasionally lead to resolution of the process. Acetazolamide, 10–30 mg/kg/24 hr, and corticosteroids have been effective for some patients. Rarely, a lumboperitoneal shunt or subtemporal decompression is necessary if the aforementioned approaches are unsuccessful and optic nerve atrophy supervenes. Some centers are performing optic nerve sheath fenestration. Finally, any patient whose increased ICP proves to be refractory to treatment warrants consideration for repeat neuroradiologic studies. A slow-growing tumor or obstruction of a venous sinus may become evident at the time of reinvestigation.

Baker R, Baumann R, Buncic J: Idiopathic intracranial hypertension (pseudotumor cerebri) in pediatric patients. Pediatr Neurol 5:5, 1989.
Shuper A, Snir M, Barash D: Ultrasonography of the optic nerves: Clinical application in children with pseudotumor cerebri. J Pediatr 131:734, 1997.
Soler D, Cox T, Bullock P, et al: Diagnosis and management of benign intracranial hypertension. Arch Dis Child 78:89, 1998.

CHAPTER 613
Spinal Cord Disorders

613.1 Spinal Cord Tumors

In children, spinal cord tumors account for aproximately 20% of neuraxial tumors and are classified according to anatomic position (Fig. 613–1). *Intramedullary tumors* arise within the substance of the cord and grow slowly by infiltration, usually in the cervical region. The most common intramedullary tumor is a low-grade astrocytoma, followed by an ependymoma. *Extramedullary, intradural tumors* tend to be benign and arise from neural crest tissue. Tumors in this area include neurofibroma, ganglioneuroma, and meningioma. *Extramedullary, extradural tumors* characteristically are metastatic lesions, particularly neuroblastoma, sarcoma, and lymphoma.

CLINICAL MANIFESTATIONS. Most children with spinal cord tumors present with a combination of gait disturbance, scoliosis, and back pain, depending on the locale of the tumor. Intramedullary gliomas are slow growing. Progressive difficulties in locomotion and sphincter disturbances are the earliest symptoms. Glial tumors in the cervical cord produce lower motor neuron signs in the upper extremities and upper motor neuron signs in the legs. Denervation of the intercostal muscles decreases chest wall movement and results in a weak cough. Loss of pain, temperature, and light touch sensation is evident in the lower extremities, and a cord level can be documented by light touch and pain sensation or by somatosensory evoked potentials. With extramedullary tumors, the presenting symptom is often back pain. The child has difficulty in sleeping because of pain and maintains a tripod posture while attempting to assume the supine position. If the tumor is attached to a nerve root, segmental pain, paresthesia, and weakness are evident. Extramedullary, extradural tumors have a propensity to cause an acute block of the cerebrospinal fluid (CSF) pathways owing to rapid growth within a confined space. Such children present with a flaccid paraplegia, urinary retention, and a patulous anus. Some extramedullay tumors produce the **Brown-Séquard syndrome,** which consists of ipsilateral weakness, spasticity, and ataxia, with contralateral loss of pain and temperature sensation. Papilledema is observed in a few patients, usually in association with markedly elevated CSF protein levels that presumably interfere with normal CSF flow dynamics.

DIAGNOSIS. It is important to establish the diagnosis of a spinal cord tumor as early as possible, because surgical management is facilitated and irreversible damage to the cord may be prevented. In approximately 40% of the cases, routine roentgenograms show abnormalities including widening of the interpediculate distance, destruction or sclerosis of the adjacent vertebral bodies or pedicles, and widening of vertebral foramen on an oblique view in the case of a neurofibroma or ganglioneuroma. MRI is the most important diagnostic test to establish the diagnosis. Intramedullary tumors produce a fusiform swelling of the cord, often with a complete block of the CSF (Fig. 613–2). Neurofibromas tend to create a circular indentation of the cord, and extramedullary tumors show various degrees of blockage.

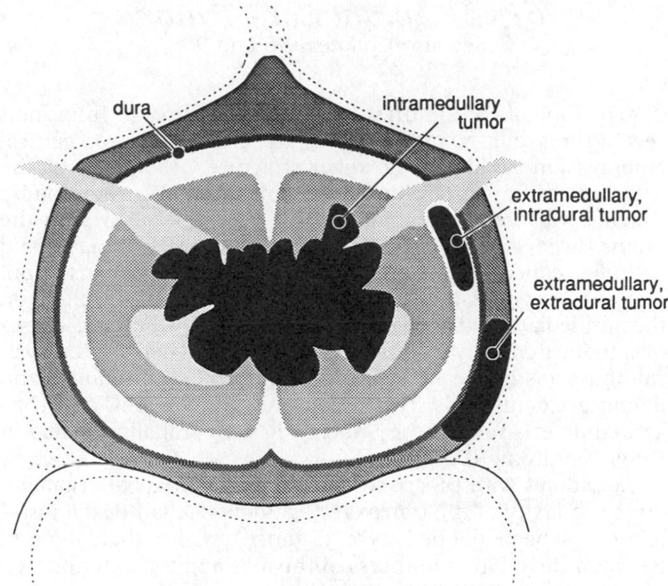

Figure 613–1 Diagram of the location of spinal cord tumors in children.

TREATMENT. With modern surgical techniques, many tumors can be totally and safely resected. Surgical removal of benign extramedullary tumors is associated with a good prognosis. For children with a primary neuroblastoma presenting with a sudden onset of paraplegia secondary to metastases in the extradural space, immediate radiation therapy may circumvent the need for a laminectomy.

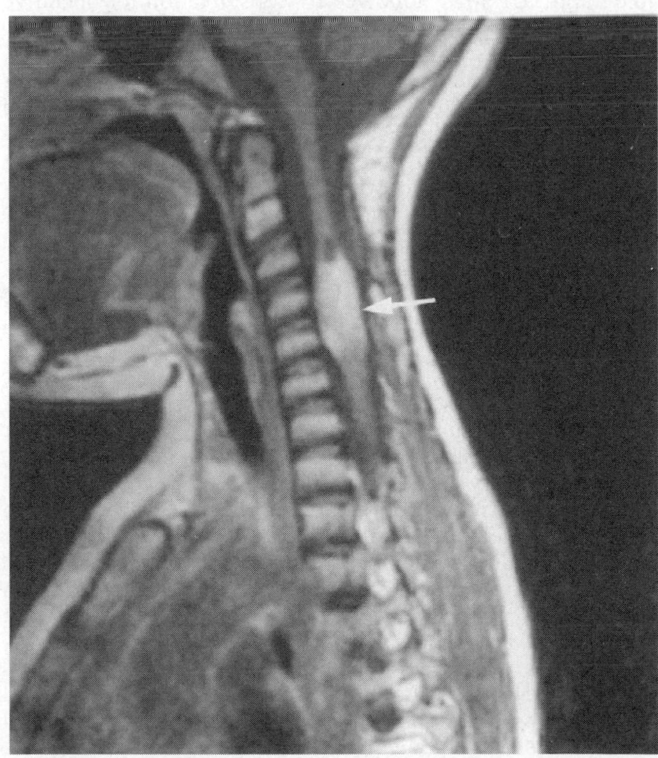

Figure 613–2 T1 weighted MRI of a spinal cord tumor (*white arrow*). The fusiform expansion of the cervical cord enhances following intravenous gadolinium injection.

613.2 Spinal Cord Trauma

See also Chapters 58 and 95.

Acute spinal cord injuries in children may result from indirect trauma due to hyperflexion, hyperextension, or vertical compression accidents; however, fracture dislocation of the vertebral column or epidural bleeding may also compromise spinal cord integrity secondary to a mass effect. As with the brain, the degree of injury to the spinal cord is variable and includes concussion, contusion, laceration, and transection. Recovery depends on the extent of the trauma as well as on the immediate and long-term management. Common causes of spinal cord injury include traumatic breech deliveries, physical abuse (as in the shaken baby syndrome), automobile and diving accidents, falls from playground equipment, and congenital defects such as the underlying vertebral abnormality in Down syndrome (DS).

Individuals with DS are susceptible to atlantoaxial instability owing to laxity of the transverse ligaments. Atlantoaxial instability has been defined as a distance greater than 4.5 mm between the odontoid process of the axis and the anterior arch of the atlas. Spinal cord compression (myelopathy) may be a consequence of atlantoaxial instability. There is not a consensus about the usefulness of radiograph screening in predicting spinal cord injury in children with DS. It is recommended that (1) lateral roentgenograms of the neck in the flexion position be obtained at 5–8 yr, 10–12 yr, and 18 yr in individuals with DS, because atlantoaxial instability can develop during periods of growth; (2) children with atlantoaxial instability be advised not to participate in risky sports, such as tumbling, diving, and football; (3) radiographs of the neck be obtained before operative procedures or therapeutic programs that involve active neck movement or manipulation; (4) parents and physicians be made aware of the symptoms and signs of cord compression (neck pain, urinary and fecal incontinence, head tilt, gait abnormalities, ataxia, hyperreflexia, weakness, spasticity, and quadriplegia); and (5) there be prompt investigation (neck radiographs, CT, MRI) followed by consideration for operative intervention in patients with signs of myelopathy.

A patient with *severe cord injury* presents with **spinal shock**, consisting of flaccidity, areflexia, and loss of sensation. This may persist for up to 4 wk and results from dysfunction of synaptic activity in the pathways caudal to the injury. Ultimately, reflex flexor movements develop, followed by extensor reflex activity associated with hyperactive deep tendon reflexes, spasticity, and an automatic bladder. *Fracture dislocations at the C5–C6 level* are the most common acute cause of spinal cord injuries and are characterized by a flaccid quadriparesis, loss of sphincter function, and a sensory level corresponding to the upper sternum. A transverse injury in the high cervical cord level (C1–C2) causes respiratory arrest and death in the absence of ventilatory support. Fractures in the low thoracic (T12–L1) region may produce the **conus medullaris syndrome,** which includes a loss of urinary and rectal sphincter control, flaccid weakness, and sensory disturbances of the legs. Spinal cord injury may occur in the absence of a vertebral fracture. A **central cord lesion** may result from contusion and hemorrhage and typically involves the upper extremities to a greater degree than the legs. There are lower motor neuron signs in the upper extremities and upper motor neuron signs in the legs, bladder dysfunction, and loss of sensation caudal to the lesion. Recovery may be considerable, particularly in the lower extremities.

Spinal cord injuries should be managed by stabilization and immobilization of the spine at the accident site using a cervical collar or sandbags. An adequate airway should be maintained, respiratory support should be provided, and shock should be treated with appropriate volume expanders. High-dose intravenous methylprednisolone (30 mg/kg bolus followed by 5.4 mg/kg/hr ×23 hr) should be started immediately even before transport. If steroids are started within 3–8 hr of the injury, they should be continued for 48 hr. After transportation, roentgenograms of the spine, including oblique views, should be obtained. Approximately 50% of children with severe cord injuries show no abnormality on the spine roentgenogram. Fracture dislocations are treated with traction, immobilization, and, if the injury is unstable, vertebral fusion. Laminectomy and inspection of the cord are reserved for patients with progression of neurologic signs and appearance on CT or MRI scan that suggests an epidural or intraspinal hemorrhage. Additional therapeutic measures include management of bladder and gastrointestinal disturbances, nutritional and skin care, and a rigorous multidisciplinary rehabilitation program.

613.3 Tethered Cord

During fetal development, the spinal cord occupies the entire length of the vertebral column, but owing to differential growth the conus medullaris in a child ultimately assumes a position at the level of L1. Normal regression of the distal embryonic spinal cord produces a slender, threadlike filum terminale that is attached to the coccyx. A tethered cord results when a thickened ropelike filum terminale persists and anchors the conus at or below the L2 level. Neurologic signs may develop as a result of abnormal tension on the spinal cord, compromising blood supply, particularly during flexion and extension movements. Diastematomyelia may coexist with a tethered cord. Inspection of the back shows a midline skin lesion in approximately 70% of cases, such as a lipoma, cutaneous hemangioma, tuft of hair, hyperpigmentation, or a dermal pit. The clinical presentation varies, and signs may be evident at birth or may be delayed until adulthood. Infants may have asymmetric growth in a foot or leg associated with talipes cavus deformities and muscle wasting due to prolonged denervation. Abnormalities in bladder function with overflow incontinence, progressive scoliosis, and diffuse pain in the lower extremities are more common findings in a child. Plain roentgenograms of the lumbosacral spine demonstrate spina bifida in most cases. CT scanning with a small amount of metrizamide or MRI precisely outlines the level of the conus medullaris and the filum terminale. Surgical transection of the thickened filum terminale tends to halt progression of neurologic signs and prevents the development of dysfunction in asymptomatic patients.

613.4 Diastematomyelia

Diastematomyelia is division of the spinal cord into two halves by projection of a fibrocartilaginuous or bony septum originating from the posterior vertebral body and extending posteriorly. It represents a disorder of neural tube fusion with the persistence of mesodermal tissue from the primitive neurenteric canal acting as the septum. The defect involves the lumbar vertebrae (L1–L3) in approximately 50% of cases and tends to be associated with abnormalities of the vertebral bodies, including fusion defects, hemivertebra, hypoplasia, kyphoscoliosis, spina bifida, and myelomeningocele. A midline abnormality of the skin, such as a cutaneous hemangioma, provides a clue to the possibility of an underlying abnormality. The neurologic signs are thought to result from flexion and extension movements of the cord, which produce traction and additional trauma by the impaling septum. The clinical presentation of diastematomyelia varies, and in some cases patients may remain asymptomatic. Most often, unilateral foot abnormalities, including talipes equinovarus, claw toes, atrophy of the gastrocnemius, and loss of pain and temperature sensation, are apparent in a preschool child. A more progressive course may ensue, characterized by bilateral weakness and muscle atrophy in the lower extremities, absent ankle jerks, urinary incontinence, and low back pain. Plain roentgenograms of the vertebrae may not detect the septum owing to lack of calcification; thus CT scanning or MRI is the study of choice. The treatment of symptomatic patients is excision of the bony spur or septum and lysis of the adjacent adhesions.

613.5 Syringomyelia

Syringomyelia is a cystic cavity within the spinal cord that may communicate with the CSF pathways or remain localized and noncommunicating. *Syringobulbia* exists when the cystic cavity extends into the medulla. Although the pathogenesis of communicating syringomyelia is unknown, the prevailing hypothesis suggests a constriction of the central canal at the level of the foramen magnum during embryogenesis. CSF may pass caudad through the narrowed canal, especially during periods of increased intracranial pressure (e.g., sneezing, coughing), and produce dilatation of the central canal. Because of the constriction, CSF is prevented from flowing in a cephalic direction. Communicating syringomyelia is frequently associated with the Chiari type I malformation, whereas the noncommunicating syrinx is associated with cord tumors, vascular accidents, trauma, and arachnoiditis. Because of its slow evolution, syringomyelia rarely produces symptoms during childhood.

Interruption of the anterior white commissure at the level of the cervical cord disrupts the lateral spinothalamic tracts, causing an asymmetric loss of pain and temperature sensation in the upper extremities, with preservation of light touch (dissociation of sensation). Progressive enlargement of the cavity impinges on the anterior horn cells and corticospinal tracts, resulting in muscle wasting of the hands, absent deep tendon reflexes in the upper extremities, and upper motor neuron signs in the lower extremities. A rapidly progressive scoliosis may be the initial manifestation of syringomyelia. Trophic ulcers associated with vasomotor disturbances of the hands and arms indicate the loss of appreciation of pain. CT scanning with intrathecal injection of metrizamide outlines an enlarged spinal cord in the region of the syrinx, and a delayed scan displays the contrast medium within the cavity. MRI is the study of choice (Fig. 613–3). The management is surgical and depends on the site and cause of the syringomyelia. Decompression of the foramen magnum and the upper cervical vertebrae is recommended when the syrinx is associated with a Chiari type I or II anomaly. Additional procedures include insertion of a tissue plug in the open end of the central canal, draining the cystic cavity into the subarachnoid space, and percutaneous aspiration of the syrinx, which may result in marked improvement in neurologic function for prolonged periods.

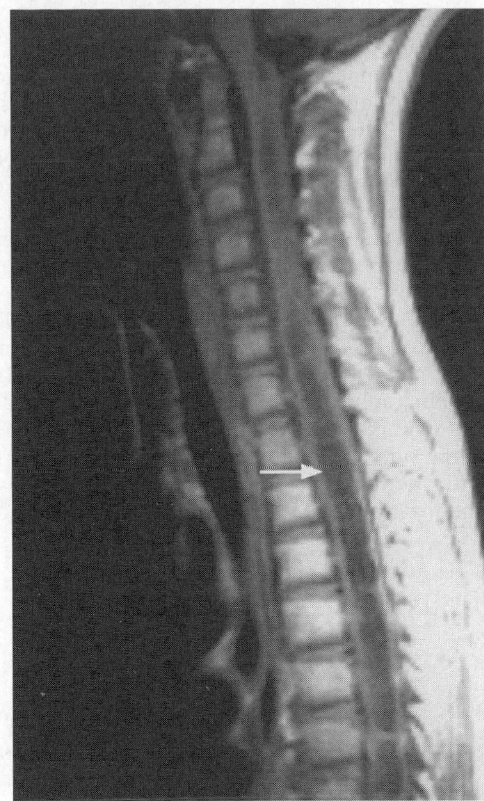

Figure 613–3 T1 weighted MRI of upper spinal cord showing an extensive syringomyelia (*white arrow*).

613.6 Transverse Myelitis

Transverse myelitis is characterized by abrupt onset of progressive weakness and sensory disturbances in the lower extremities. A history of a preceding viral infection accompanied by fever and malaise is documented in most cases. Several viruses have been implicated, including Epstein-Barr virus and herpes, influenza, rubella, mumps, and varicella viruses. At least three hypotheses have been proposed to explain the pathogenesis of transverse myelitis: cell-mediated autoimmune response, direct viral invasion of the spinal cord, and an autoimmune vasculitis. Pathologic examination of the cord shows marked softening and perivascular cuffing by lymphocytes, supporting an immunologic basis for the disorder.

Low back or abdominal pain and paresthesias of the legs are prominent symptoms in the early stages. The leg muscles are weak and flaccid, and a sensory level is present, usually in the midthoracic region. Pain, temperature, and light touch sensation are affected, but joint position and vibration sense may be preserved. Sphincter disturbances are common, in which case catheterization of the bladder is necessary. Fever and nuchal rigidity are present early in most cases. The neurologic deficit evolves for 2–3 days and then plateaus, with flaccidity gradually changing to spasticity and with the concomitant development of upper motor neuron signs in the lower extremities. Examination of the CSF shows moderate lymphocyte pleocytosis and a normal or slightly elevated protein level. CT scanning or MRI reveals mild fusiform swelling in the affected region. Spontaneous recovery occurs over a period of weeks or months and is complete in approximately 60% of cases. Residual deficits include bowel and bladder dysfunction and weakness in the lower extremities. Management is directed to bladder care and physiotherapy. No evidence shows that steroids influence the course or the outcome of transverse myelitis. The differential diagnosis includes meningitis, infectious polyneuropathy (Guillain-Barré syndrome), poliomyelitis, neuromyelitis optica (Devic disease), spinal cord neoplasm, epidural abscess, and a vascular malformation.

613.7 Arteriovenous Malformation

An arteriovenous malformation of the spinal cord consists of a collection of tortuous dilated veins that are usually located on the dorsal aspect of the thoracic cord. The malformation may cause neurologic symptoms by its mass effect on the cord or by the "steal" phenomenon, by which blood is shunted through the abnormal veins, bypassing the spinal cord, which produces transient and in some cases progressive loss of neurologic function. Patients occasionally present with acute paraparesis and a sensory deficit due to a subarachnoid bleed from the malformation. More commonly, gradual onset of gait abnormalities, low back pain, and bowel and bladder dysfunction is noted. The deep tendon reflexes are absent or reduced in the lower extremities, and the Babinski reflex is present. In approximately one third of cases, a midline cutaneous angioma overlies the arteriovenous malformation, and a spinal bruit may occasionally be auscultated. Roentgenograms of the spine may show erosion of the pedicles; however, contrast myelography and selective spinal angiography are required to delineate the blood supply and the extent of the malformation. The malformation is removed by surgical excision with the use of an operating microscope or is obliterated by embolization.

Bracken MB, Shepard MJ, Holford TR, et al: Administration of methylprednisolone for 24 or 48 hours or tirilazad mesylate for 48 hours in the treatment of acute spinal cord injury. JAMA 277:1597, 1997.
Cahan LD, Bentson JR: Considerations in the diagnosis and treatment of syringomyelia and Chiari malformation. J Neurosurg 57:24, 1982.
Committee on Sports Medicine & Fitness 1994–1995, American Academy of Pediatrics: Atlantoaxial instability in Down syndrome: Subject review. Pediatrics 96:151, 1995.
Cremers MJG, Bol E, deRoos F, et al: Risk of sports activities in children with Down's syndrome and atlantoaxial instability. Lancet 342:511, 1993.
DiJunno JF, Formal CS: Chronic spinal cord injury. N Engl J Med 330:550, 1994.
Haft H, Ransohoff J, Carter S: Spinal cord tumors in children. Pediatrics 23:1152, 1959.
Hendrick EB, Hoffman HJ, Humphreys RP: The tethered spinal cord. Clin Neurosurg 30:457, 1982.
Hilal S, Marton D, Pollack E: Diastematomyelia in children. Radiology 112:609, 1974.
McAtee-Smith J, Hebert AA, Rapini R, et al: Skin lesions of the spinal axis and spinal dysraphism. Arch Pediatr Adolesc Med 148:740, 1994.
Pueschel SM, Findley TW, Furia J, et al: Atlantoaxial instability in Down syndrome: Roentgenographic, neurologic and somatosensory evoked potential studies. J Pediatr 110:515, 1987.
Riche MC, Modenesi-Freitas J, Djindjian M, et al: Arteriovenous malformations (AVM) of the spinal cord in children: Review of 38 cases. Neuroradiology 22:171, 1982.

PART XXVII

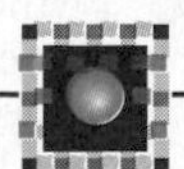

Neuromuscular Disorders

Harvey B. Sarnat

The term *neuromuscular disease* refers to disorders of the motor unit and excludes suprasegmental disorders, such as cerebral palsy, even though muscle tone, strength, function, and reflexes are influenced by cerebral disease. The *motor unit* consists of four components: (1) a motor neuron in the brain stem or ventral horn of the spinal cord; (2) its axon that, together with other axons, forms the peripheral nerve; (3) the neuromuscular junction; and (4) all muscle fibers innervated by a single motor neuron. The size of the motor unit varies among different muscles and with the precision of muscular function required. In large muscles, such as the glutei and quadriceps femoris, hundreds of muscle fibers are innervated by a single motor neuron; in small finely tuned muscles, such as the stapedius or the extraocular muscles, a 1:1 ratio may prevail. The motor unit is influenced by suprasegmental or upper motor neuron control that alters properties of muscle tone, precision of movement, reciprocal inhibition of antagonistic muscles during movement, and sequencing of muscle contractions to achieve smooth, coordinated movements. Suprasegmental impulses also augment or inhibit the monosynaptic stretch reflex.

Diseases of the motor unit are common in children. These neuromuscular diseases may or may not be genetically determined, congenital or acquired, acute or chronic, and progressive or static. Because specific therapy is available for many diseases and because of genetic and prognostic implications, precise diagnosis is important; laboratory confirmation is required for most diseases because of overlapping clinical manifestations.

Many chromosomal loci have been identified with specific neuromuscular diseases as a result of genetic linkage studies and the isolation and cloning of a few specific genes. In some cases, such as Duchenne muscular dystrophy, the genetic defect has been shown to be a deletion of nucleotide sequences and is associated with a defective protein product, *dystrophin;* in other cases, such as myotonic muscular dystrophy, the genetic defect is an expansion rather than a deletion in a codon (a set of three consecutive nucleotide repeats that encodes for a single amino acid), with many copies of a particular codon. Some diseases, such as nemaline rod myopathy and limb-girdle muscular dystrophy, present with autosomal dominant and autosomal recessive traits in different pedigrees; these different mendelian genotypes are different diseases despite many common phenotypic features and shared histopathologic findings in a muscle biopsy specimen. Among the several clinically defined mitochondrial myopathies, specific mtDNA deletions and tRNA point mutations are recognized. The inheritance patterns and chromosomal and mitochondrial loci of common neuromuscular diseases affecting infants and children are summarized in Table 615–1. ■

CHAPTER 614

Evaluation and Investigation

CLINICAL MANIFESTATIONS. Examination of the neuromuscular system includes an assessment of muscle bulk, tone, and strength. Tone and strength should not be confused: Passive tone is range of motion around a joint; active tone is physiologic resistance to movement. Head lag when an infant is pulled to a sitting position from supine is a sign of weakness, not of low tone. Hypotonia may be associated with normal strength or with weakness; enlarged muscles may be weak or strong; thin, wasted muscles may be weak or have unexpectedly normal strength. The distribution of these components is of diagnostic importance. In general, myopathies follow a proximal distribution of weakness and muscle wasting (with the notable exception of myotonic muscular dystrophy); neuropathies are generally distal in distribution (with the notable exception of juvenile spinal muscular atrophy). Involvement of the face, tongue, palate, and extraocular muscles provides an important distinction in the differential diagnosis. Tendon stretch reflexes are generally lost in neuropathies and in motor neuron diseases and are diminished but preserved in myopathies. A few specific clinical features are important in the diagnosis of some neuromuscular diseases. Fasciculations of muscle, which are often best seen in the tongue, are a sign of denervation. Sensory abnormalities indicate neuropathy. Fatigable weakness is characteristic of neuromuscular junctional disorders. Myotonia is specific for a few myopathies.

Some features do not distinguish myopathy from neuropathy. Muscle pain or myalgias are associated with acute disease of either myopathic or neurogenic origin. Both acute dermatomyositis and acute polyneuropathy (Guillain-Barré syndrome) are characterized by myalgias. Muscular dystrophies and spinal muscular atrophies are not associated with muscle pain. Myalgias also occur in several metabolic diseases of muscle and in ischemic myopathy. Contractures of muscles, whether present at birth or developing later in the course of an illness, occur in both myopathic and neurogenic diseases.

Infant boys who are weak in late fetal life and in the neonatal period often have undescended testicles. The testicles are actively pulled into the scrotum from the anterior abdominal wall by a pair of cords that consist of smooth and striated muscle called the *gubernaculum* (Fig. 614–1). The gubernaculum is weakened in many congenital neuromuscular diseases, including spinal muscular atrophy, myotonic muscular dystrophy, and many congenital myopathies.

The thorax of infants with congenital neuromuscular disease often has a funnel shape, and the ribs are thin and radiolucent owing to intercostal muscle weakness during intrauterine growth. This phenomenon is characteristically found in infantile spinal muscular atrophy but also occurs in myotubular myopathy, neonatal myotonic dystrophy, and other disorders. Because of the small muscle mass, birthweight may be low for gestational age.

Generalized hypotonia and motor developmental delay are the most common presenting manifestations of neuromuscular disease in infants and young children. These features may also be expressions of neurologic disease, endocrine and systemic

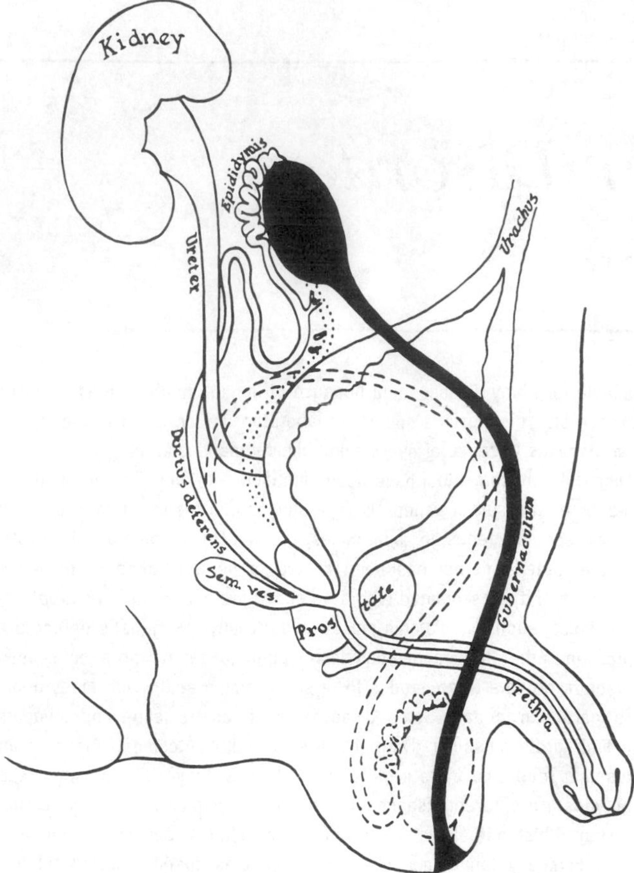

Figure 614–1 Undescended testes are common in male neonates with neuromuscular disease already symptomatic at birth, regardless of the etiology. The gubernaculum is a cylinder of striated muscle surrounding a core of smooth muscle that actively pulls the testicle into the scrotum in late gestation. Weakness of the gubernaculum in a generalized myopathy of fetal life prevents or delays the descent of the testis. Reproduced with permission from Sarnat HB, Sarnat MS: Disorders of muscle in the newborn. *In*: Moss AJ, Stern L (eds): Pediatrics Update, 4th ed. New York, Elsevier-North Holland, 1983.

metabolic diseases, and Down syndrome, or they may be nonspecific neuromuscular expressions of malnutrition or chronic systemic illness. A prenatal history of decreased fetal movements and intrauterine growth retardation are often found in patients who are symptomatic at birth.

LABORATORY FINDINGS

Serum Enzymes. Several lysosomal enzymes are released by damaged or degenerating muscle fibers and may be measured in serum. The most useful of these enzymes is the *creatine phosphokinase* (CK), which is found in only three organs and may be separated into corresponding isozymes: MM for skeletal muscle, MB for cardiac muscle, and BB for brain. Serum CK determination is by no means a universal screening test for neuromuscular disease because many diseases of the motor unit may not be associated with elevated enzymes. However, the CK level is characteristically elevated in certain diseases, such as Duchenne muscular dystrophy, and the magnitude of increase is characteristic for particular diseases.

Nerve Conduction Velocity (NCV). Motor and sensory nerve conduction may be measured electrophysiologically by using surface electrodes. Neuropathies of various types are detected by decreased conduction. The site of a traumatic nerve injury may also be localized. The nerve conduction at birth is about half of the mature value achieved by age 2 yr. Tables are available for normal values at various ages in infancy, including for preterm infants. Because the NCV study measures only the fastest conducting fibers in a nerve, 80% of the total nerve fibers must be involved before slowing in conduction is detected.

Electromyography (EMG). EMG is less useful in pediatrics than in adult medicine, in part because of technical difficulties in recording young children and in part because the best results require patients' cooperation for full relaxation and maximal voluntary contraction of a muscle. Most children are too frightened to provide such cooperation. EMG requires insertion of a needle into the belly of a muscle and recording the electric potentials in various states of contraction. Characteristic patterns distinguish denervation from myopathic involvement. The specific type of myopathy is not usually definitively diagnosed, but certain specialized myopathic conditions, such as myotonia, may be demonstrated. An EMG may falsely raise the serum CK level.

EMG combined with repetitive electrical stimulation of a motor nerve supplying a muscle to produce tetany is useful in demonstrating myasthenic decremental responses. Small muscles, such as the abductor digiti quinti of the hypothenar eminence, are used for such studies.

Muscle Biopsy. The muscle biopsy is the most important and specific diagnostic study of muscle. Not only are neurogenic and myopathic processes distinguished, but also the type of myopathy and specific enzymatic deficiencies may be determined. The vastus lateralis (quadriceps femoris) is the muscle that is most commonly sampled. The deltoid muscle should be avoided in most cases because it normally has a 60–80% predominance of type I fibers so that the distribution patterns of fiber types are difficult to recognize. Muscle biopsy is a simple outpatient procedure that may be performed under local anesthesia with or without femoral nerve block. Needle biopsies, advocated by some physicians, require an incision in the skin similar to open biopsy, and numerous samples must be taken to conduct an adequate examination of the tissue; needle biopsies are as traumatic as open biopsies and provide inferior specimens.

Histochemical studies of frozen sections of the muscle are obligatory in all pediatric muscle biopsies because many congenital and metabolic myopathies cannot be diagnosed from paraffin sections using conventional histologic stains. Immunohistochemistry is a useful supplement in some cases, such as for demonstrating dystrophin in suspected Duchenne muscular dystrophy or merosin in congenital muscular dystrophy. A portion of the biopsy specimen should be fixed for potential electron microscopy, but ultrastructure has additional diagnostic value only in selected cases. Muscle biopsy sample interpretation is complex and should be performed by an experienced pathologist.

Nerve Biopsy. The most commonly sampled nerve is the sural nerve, which is a pure sensory nerve that supplies a small area of skin on the lateral surface of the foot. Whole or fascicular biopsy specimens of this nerve may be taken. When the sural nerve is severed behind the lateral malleolus of the ankle, regeneration of the nerve occurs in more than 90% of cases so that permanent sensory loss is not experienced. The sural nerve is often involved in many neuropathies that are clinically predominantly motor.

Electron microscopy should be performed on most nerve biopsy specimens because the most important morphologic alterations cannot be appreciated at the resolution of a light microscope. Teased fiber preparations are sometimes useful in demonstrating segmental demyelination, axonal swellings, and other specific abnormalities, but this time-consuming procedure is not done routinely. Special stains may be applied to even ordinary frozen or paraffin sections of nerve biopsy material to demonstrate myelin, axoplasm, and metabolic products.

Electrocardiography (ECG). Cardiac evaluation is important if myopathy is suspected because of involvement of the heart in muscular dystrophies and in inflammatory and metabolic myopathies. ECG often detects early cardiomyopathy or conduction defects that are clinically asymptomatic. Serial pulmonary function tests should be performed in muscular dystrophies and in other chronic or progressive diseases of the motor unit.

CHAPTER 615

Developmental Disorders of Muscle

A heterogeneous group of congenital neuromuscular disorders is sometimes known as the *congenital myopathies,* but in some of these disorders the assumption that the pathogenesis is primarily myopathic is unjustified. Most congenital myopathies are nonprogressive conditions, but some patients show slow clinical deterioration accompanied by additional changes in their muscle biopsy material. Most of the diseases in the category of congenital myopathies are hereditary; others are sporadic. Although clinical features, including phenotype, may raise a strong suspicion of a congenital myopathy, the definitive diagnosis is determined by the histopathologic findings in the muscle biopsy sample. In a few conditions for which the defective gene has been identified, the diagnosis may be established by the specific molecular genetic probe on lymphocytes. The morphologic and histochemical abnormalities differ considerably from those of the muscular dystrophies, spinal muscular atrophies, and neuropathies. Many are reminiscent of the embryologic development of muscle, thus suggesting possible defects in the genetic regulation of muscle development.

MYOGENIC REGULATORY GENES AND GENETIC LOCI OF INHERITED DISEASES OF MUSCLE (Table 615–1). A family of four myogenic regulatory genes shares encoding transcription factors of "basic helix-loop-helix" (bHLH) proteins associated with common DNA nucleotide sequences. These proto-oncogenes direct the differentiation of striated muscle from any undifferentiated mesodermal cell; some are so strongly expressed that they convert partially differentiated mesenchymal cells, such as fibroblasts or chondroblasts, into myoblasts. The earliest bHLH gene to program the differentiation of myoblasts is myogenic factor 5 (*myf-5*). The second gene, *myogenin,* promotes fusion of myoblasts to form myotubes. *Herculin* (also known as *mrf-4* and *myf-6*) and *MyoD1* are the other two myogenic genes. In mice, *MyoD1* and *myf-5* may substitute their functions so that if either is deleted the muscle still develops normally, but the absence of both genes results in amyoplasia. Each of these four genes can activate the expression of at least one other and, under certain circumstances, can autoactivate as well. The expression of *myf-5* and of *herculin* is transient in early ontogenesis but returns later in fetal life and persists into adult life. The human locus of the *MyoD1* gene is on chromosome 11, very near to the domain associated with embryonal rhabdomyosarcoma. The genes encoding *myf-5* and *herculin* are on chromosome 12 and that for *myogenin* is on chromosome 1. The precise role of the myogenic genes in developmental myopathies is not yet defined.

TABLE 615–1 Inheritance Patterns and Chromosomal or Mitochondrial Loci of Neuromuscular Diseases Affecting the Pediatric Age Group

Disease	Transmission	Locus
Duchenne/Becker's muscular dystrophy	XR	Xp21.2
Emery-Dreifuss muscular dystrophy	XR	Xq28
Myotonic muscular dystrophy (Steinert)	AD	19q13
Facio-scapulo-humeral muscular dystrophy	AD	4q35
Limb-girdle muscular dystrophy	AD	5q
Limb-girdle muscular dystrophy	AR	15q
Congenital muscular dystrophy with merosin deficiency	AR	6q2
Congenital muscular dystrophy (Fukuyama)	AR	8q31–33
Myotubular myopathy	XR	Xq28
Myotubular myopathy	AR	Unknown
Nemaline rod myopathy	AD	1q21–q23
Nemaline rod myopathy	AR	2q21.2–q22
Congenital muscle fiber–type disproportion	AR	Unknown
Central core disease	AD	19q13.1
Myotonia congenita (Thomsen)	AD	7q35
Myotonia congenita (Becker)	AR	7q35
Paramyotonia congenita	AD	17q13.1–13.3
Hyperkalemic periodic paralysis	AD	17q13.1–13.3
Hypokalemic periodic paralysis	AD	1q31–q32
Glycogenosis II (Pompe; acid maltase deficiency)	AR	17q23
Glycogenosis V (McArdle; myophosphorylase deficiency)	AR	11q13
Glycogenosis VII (Tarui; phosphofructokinase deficiency)	AR	1cenq32
Glycogenosis IX (phosphoglycerkinase deficiency)	XR	Xq13
Glycogenosis X (phosphoglyceromutase deficiency)	AR	7p12–p13
Glycogenosis XI (lactate dehydrogenase deficiency)	AR	11p15.4
Muscle carnitine deficiency	AR	Unknown
Muscle carnitine palmityltransferase deficiency 2	AR	1p32
Spinal muscular atrophy (Werdnig-Hoffmann; Kugelberg-Welander)	AR	5q11–q13
Familial dysautonomia (Riley-Day)	AR	9q31–33
Hereditary motor-sensory neuropathy (Charcot-Marie-Tooth; Déjerine-Sottas)	AD	17p11.2
Hereditary motor-sensory neuropathy (axonal type)	AD	1p35–p36
Hereditary motor-sensory neuropathy (Charcot-Marie-Tooth-X)	XR	Xq13.1
Mitochondrial myopathy (Kearns-Sayre)	Maternal; sporadic	Single large mtDNA deletion
Mitochondrial myopathy (MERRF)	Maternal	tRNA point mutation at position 8344
Mitochondrial myopathy (MELAS)	Maternal	tRNA point mutation at positions 3243 and 3271

AD = autosomal dominant; AR = autosomal recessive; XR = X-linked recessive; MERRF = mitochondrial encephalomyopathy with ragged-red fibers; MELAS = mitochondrial encephalomyopathy with lactic acidosis and strokelike episodes; mtDNA = mitochondrial deoxyribonucleic acid; tRNA = transfer ribonucleic acid.

615.1 Myotubular Myopathy

The term *myotubular myopathy* implies a maturational arrest of fetal muscle during the myotubular stage of development at 8–15 wk of gestation. It is based on the morphologic appearance of myofibers: A row of central nuclei lie within a core of cytoplasm; contractile myofibrils form a cylinder around this core (Fig. 615–1). Many challenge this interpretation and use the more neutral term *centronuclear myopathy* when referring to this myopathy. But this term is too nonspecific because internal nuclei occur in many unrelated myopathies.

PATHOGENESIS. Although the pathogenesis has sometimes been suggested to be neurogenic, spinal motor neurons are normal in number and morphology. Peripheral nerves also usually have normal ultrastructure and conduction velocity. Persistently high fetal concentrations of vimentin and desmin are demonstrated in myofibers of infants with myotubular myopathy. These intermediate filament proteins serve as cytoskeletal elements in fetal myotubes, attaching nuclei and mitochondria to the sarcolemmal membranes to preserve their

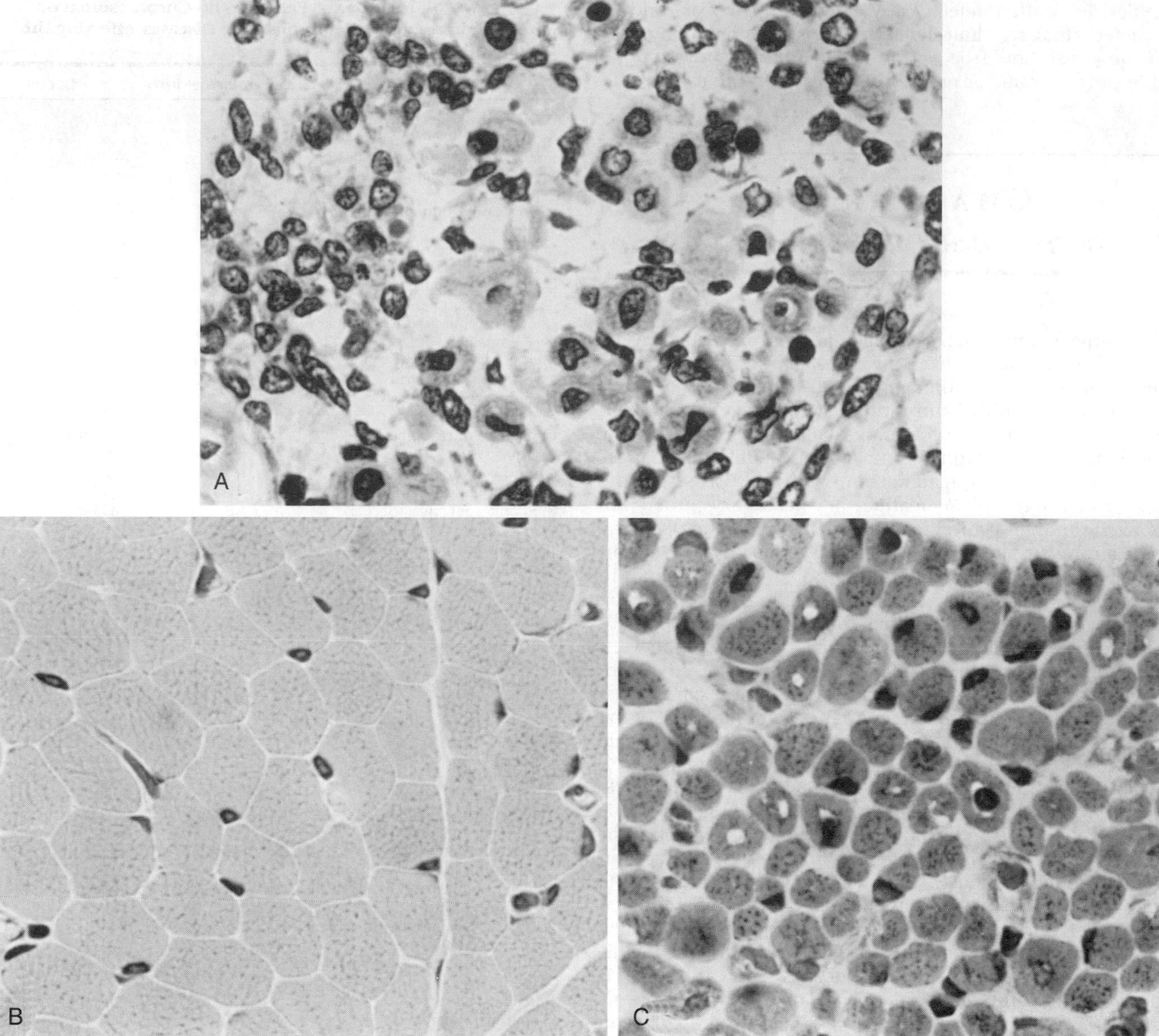

Figure 615–1 *A*, Cross-section of muscle from a 14-wk-old human fetus; *B*, normal full-term neonate; and *C*, term neonate with X-linked recessive myotubular myopathy. Myofibers have large central nuclei in the fetus and in myotubular myopathy, and nuclei are at the periphery of the muscle fiber in the term neonate as in the adult. (Hematoxylin & eosin, ×500.)

central positions. As intracellular organization changes with maturation, the nuclei move to the periphery and mitochondria are redistributed between myofibrils. At the same time, vimentin and desmin diminish. Vimentin disappears altogether by term, and desmin remains only in trace amounts. Persistent fetal vimentin and desmin in muscle fibers may be one mechanism of "maturational arrest."

CLINICAL MANIFESTATIONS. Decreased fetal movements are perceived in late gestation. Polyhydramnios is a common complication because of pharyngeal weakness of the fetus and inability to swallow amniotic fluid. At birth, affected infants have a thin muscle mass involving axial, limb-girdle, and distal muscles; severe generalized hypotonia; and diffuse weakness. Respiratory efforts may be ineffective, requiring ventilatory support. Gavage feeding may be required because of weakness of the muscles of sucking and deglutition. The testicles are often undescended. Facial muscles may be weak, but infants do not have the characteristic facies of myotonic dystrophy. Ophthalmoplegia is observed in a few cases. The palate may be high. The tongue is thin, but fasciculations are not seen. Tendon stretch reflexes are weak or absent. Myotubular myopathy is not associated with cardiomyopathy; mature cardiac muscle fibers normally have central nuclei. Congenital anomalies of the central nervous system or of other systems are not associated.

The original case described as "myotubular myopathy" in 1966 was in an adolescent boy with mild weakness. Many subsequent cases in older children and adults with centronuclear myopathy and variable weakness have been reported, but their relation to the severe neonatal disease is uncertain.

LABORATORY FINDINGS. Serum levels of creatine phosphokinase (CK) are normal. The electromyogram (EMG) does not show evidence of denervation, and results are usually normal or show minimal nonspecific myopathic features in early infancy. Nerve conduction velocity may be slow but is usually normal. The electrocardiogram (ECG) appears normal. Roentgenograms of the chest show no cardiomegaly; the ribs may be thin.

DIAGNOSIS. The muscle biopsy findings are diagnostic at birth, even in premature infants. More than 90% of muscle fibers are small and have centrally placed, large vesicular nuclei in a single row. Spaces between nuclei are filled with sarcoplasm containing mitochondria. Histochemical stains for oxidative enzymatic activity and glycogen reveal a central distribution as in fetal myotubes. The cylinder of myofibrils shows mature histochemical differentiation with adenosine triphosphatase (ATPase) stains. The connective tissue of muscle, spindles, blood vessels, intramuscular nerves, and motor end plates are mature. Ultrastructural features in neonatal myotubular myopathy, other than those that define the disease, are also mature. Vimentin and desmin show strong immunoreactivity in muscle fibers in myotubular myopathy and no demonstrable activity in normal term neonatal muscle. The molecular genetic marker in blood is available and is useful not only for confirming the diagnosis but also for early prenatal diagnosis.

GENETICS. X-linked recessive inheritance is the most common trait; most patients are boys. The mothers of affected infants are clinically asymptomatic, but their muscle biopsy specimen shows scattered small centronuclear fibers with increased vimentin and desmin. Autosomal dominant and autosomal recessive forms are also reported but are rarer.

Genetic linkage on the X chromosome has been localized to the Xq28 site, a locus different from the Xp21 gene of Duchenne and Becker muscular dystrophies. A deletion in the responsible MTM1 gene has been identified. It encodes a protein, myotubularin, with a putative tyrosine phosphatase domain. Although only a single gene is involved, five distinct point mutations of the MTM1 gene account for only 27% of cases; many different alleles may produce the same clinical disease.

PROGNOSIS. About 75% of severely affected neonates die within the first few weeks or months of life. Survivors do not experience a progressive course but have major physical handicaps, rarely walk, and remain severely hypotonic.

615.2 Congenital Muscle Fiber-Type Disproportion (CMFTD)

This condition occurs as an isolated "congenital myopathy" but also develops in association with various unrelated disorders that include nemaline rod disease, Krabbe disease (globoid cell leukodystrophy) early in the course before expression of the neuropathy, cerebellar hypoplasia and certain other brain malformations (see later), fetal alcohol syndrome, some glycogenoses, multiple sulfatase deficiency, Lowe syndrome, rigid spine syndrome, and some infantile cases of myotonic muscular dystrophy.

PATHOGENESIS. The association of CMFTD with cerebellar hypoplasia (see later) suggests that the pathogenesis may be an abnormal suprasegmental influence on the developing motor unit during the stage of histochemical differentiation of muscle between 20 and 28 wk of gestation. Muscle fiber types and growth are determined by innervation and are mutable even in adults. Although CMFTD does not actually correspond with any normal stage of development, it appears to be an embryologic disturbance of fiber type differentiation and growth.

CLINICAL MANIFESTATIONS. As an isolated condition not associated with other diseases, CMFTD is a nonprogressive disorder present at birth. Patients have generalized hypotonia and weakness, but the weakness is usually not severe and respiratory distress and dysphagia are rare. Mild congenital contractures are often present. Poor head control and developmental delay for gross motor skills are common in infancy. Walking is usually delayed until 18–24 mo but is eventually achieved. Because of the hypotonia, subluxation of the hips may occur. Muscle bulk is reduced. The muscle wasting and hypotonia are proportionately greater than the weakness, and the child may be stronger than expected during examination.

The facies of children with CMFTD often raise suspicion, especially if the child is referred for assessment of developmental delay and hypotonia. The head is dolichocephalic, and facial weakness is present. The palate is usually high arched. Thin muscles of the trunk and extremities give a thin, wasted appearance. Patients do not complain of myalgias. The clinical course is benign and nonprogressive. The facies and body habitus of many children with CMFTD may be indistinguishable from those of nemaline rod myopathy (see later), which also includes CMFTD as a component.

LABORATORY FINDINGS. Serum CK, ECG, EMG, and nerve conduction velocity results all are normal in simple CMFTD. If other diseases are associated, laboratory investigation of those conditions discloses the specific features.

DIAGNOSIS. CMFTD is diagnosed by a muscle biopsy sample that shows a disproportion in both size and relative ratios of histochemical fiber types: Type I fibers are uniformly small, and type II fibers are hypertrophic; type I fibers are more numerous than those of type II. Degeneration of myofibers and other primary myopathic features are absent. The biopsy result is diagnostic at birth.

GENETICS. Many cases of simple CMFTD are sporadic, although autosomal recessive inheritance is well documented in some families. CMFTD may also be associated with cerebellar hypoplasia.

TREATMENT. No drug therapy is available. Physiotherapy may be helpful for some patients in strengthening muscles that do not receive sufficient exercise in daily activities. Mild congenital contractures often respond well to gentle range of motion exercises and rarely require plaster casting or surgery.

615.3 Nemaline Rod Myopathy

Nemaline rods (derived from the Greek *nema*, meaning "thread") are rod-shaped inclusion-like abnormal structures within muscle fibers. They are difficult to demonstrate histologically with conventional hematoxylin-eosin stain but are easily seen with special stains. They are not foreign inclusion bodies but rather consist of excessive Z-band material with a similar ultrastructure (Fig. 615–2). Chemically, the rods are composed of actin, α-actinin, tropomyosin-3, and the protein nebulin. Nemaline rod formation may be an unusual reaction of muscle fibers to injury because these rod structures have rarely been found in other diseases. They are most abundant in the congenital myopathy known as nemaline rod disease. Most rods are within the myofibrils (cytoplasmic), but intra-

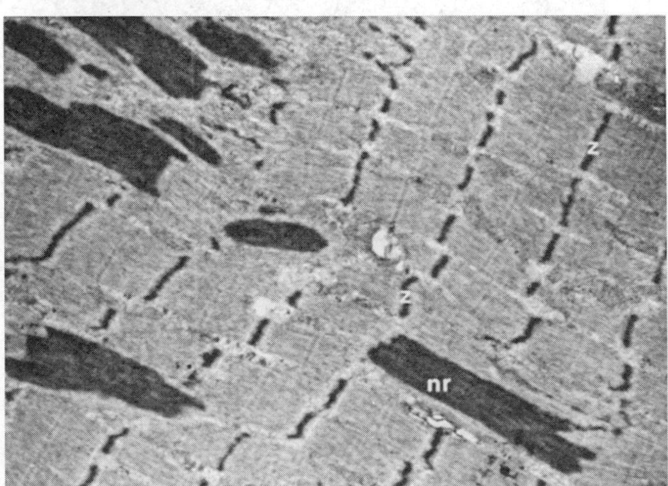

Figure 615–2 Electron micrograph of the muscle from a patient shown in Figure 615-4. Nemaline rods (nr) are seen within many myofibrils. They are identical in composition to the normal Z bands (z) (×6.000).

nuclear rods are occasionally demonstrated by electron microscopy; how they form in the nucleus is unknown.

CLINICAL MANIFESTATIONS. Severe infantile and juvenile forms of the disease are known. Patients resemble those with CMFTD, except that they are more severely affected. Generalized hypotonia, weakness including bulbar-innervated and respiratory muscles, and a very thin muscle mass are characteristic (Fig. 615–3). The head is dolichocephalic, and the palate high arched or even cleft. Muscles of the jaw may be too weak to hold it closed (Fig. 615–4). Infants may be severely weak at birth; some die in the neonatal period. Survivors are confined to an electric wheelchair and are usually unable to overcome gravity. Both proximal and distal muscles are involved. Gastrostomy may be needed for chronic dysphagia. In the juvenile form, patients are ambulatory and are able to perform most tasks of daily living. Weakness is not usually progressive, but some patients have more difficulty over time or enter a phase of progressive weakness. Cardiomyopathy is an uncommon complication.

LABORATORY FINDINGS. Serum CK level is normal. The muscle biopsy sample shows CMFTD or at least fiber type I predominance in addition to the nemaline rods. In some patients, uniform type I fibers are seen with few or no type II fibers. Focal myofibrillar degeneration and an increase in lysosomal enzymes have been found in a few severe cases associated with progressive symptoms. Intranuclear nemaline rods correlate with the most severe clinical manifestations.

GENETIC ASPECTS. Autosomal dominant and autosomal recessive forms of nemaline rod disease are well documented, and an X-linked dominant form in girls may occur. Autosomal dominant nemaline rod myopathy has been mapped to the 1q21–23 locus; the responsible gene, *TPM3*, programs tropomyosin-3, an important component of the Z band. The more common autosomal recessive form results from a defective gene at the 2q21.2–q22 locus that produces *nebulin*, a large molecule also needed for Z-band integrity.

615.4 Central Core Disease

This autosomal dominant disease, caused by an abnormal gene at the 19q13.1 locus, is characterized pathologically by central cores within muscle fibers in which only amorphous, granular cytoplasm is found with an absence of myofibrils and organelles. Histochemical stains show a lack of enzymatic activities of all types within these cores. Infantile hypotonia, proximal weakness, muscle wasting, and involvement of facial muscles and neck flexors are the typical features. The course is nonprogressive, and the weakness is not usually severely disabling. Congenital dislocated hips and skeletal deformities are common. Scoliosis occurs even without much axial weakness.

Central core disease is consistently associated with **malignant hyperthermia,** and all patients should have special precautions with pretreatment by dantrolene before an anesthetic agent is administered. The serum CK value is normal in central core disease except during crises of malignant hyperthermia. See Chapter 618.2.

Variants of central cores, called *minicores* and *multicores*, are described in some families, but **minicore myopathy** is probably a different genetic disease. Children with this disorder are hypotonic in early infancy and follow a benign course but often develop progressive kyphoscoliosis or a rigid spine in adolescence. Some children with Prader-Willi syndrome have focal loss of myofilaments resembling early central cores.

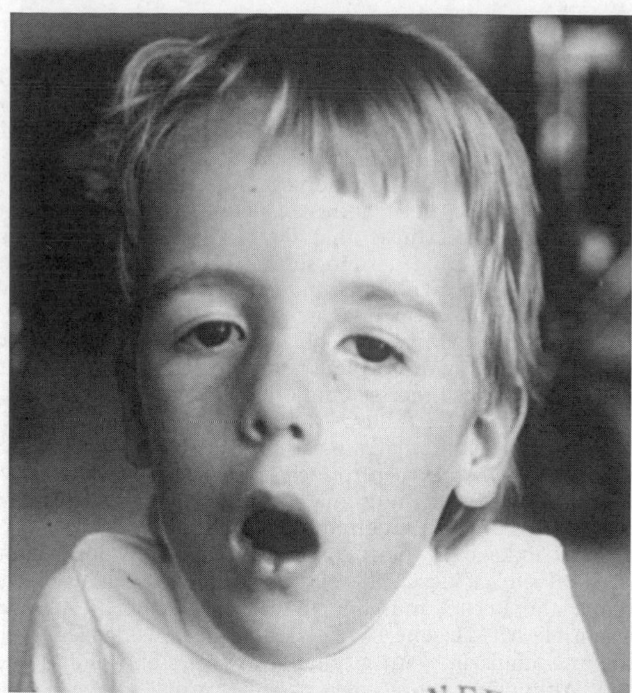

Figure 615–4 Infantile form of nemaline rod disease in a 6-yr-old boy. Facial weakness and generalized muscle wasting are severe. The head is dolichocephalic. The mouth is usually open because the masseters are too weak to lift the mandible against gravity for more than a few seconds.

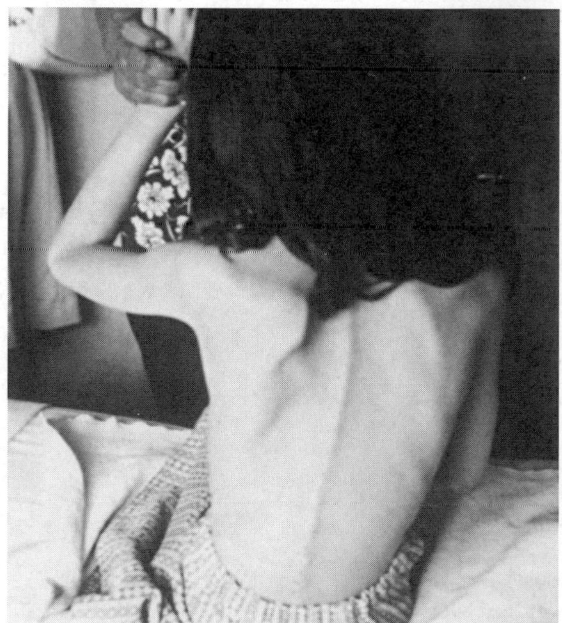

Figure 615–3 Back of a 13-yr-old girl with juvenile form of nemaline rod disease. The paraspinal muscles are very thin, and winging of the scapulae is evident. The muscle mass of the extremities is also greatly reduced both proximally and distally.

615.5 Brain Malformations and Muscle Development

Infants with *cerebellar hypoplasia* are hypotonic and developmentally delayed. Muscle biopsy is sometimes performed to exclude a congenital myopathy. Such biopsy material may show delayed maturation of muscle, fiber-type predominance, or CMFTD. Other malformations of the brain may also be associated with abnormal histochemical patterns, but supratentorial lesions are less likely than brain stem or cerebellar lesions to alter muscle development. Abnormal descending impulses along bulbospinal pathways probably alter discharge patterns of lower motor neurons that determine the histochemical differentiation of muscle. The corticospinal tract does not participate because it is not yet functional during this period of fetal life.

615.6 Amyoplasia

Congenital absence of individual muscles is common and is often asymmetric. A common aplasia is the *palmaris longus muscle* of the ventral forearm, which is absent in 30% of normal subjects and is fully compensated by other flexors of the wrist. Unilateral absence of a *sternocleidomastoid muscle* is one cause of congenital torticollis. Absence of one *pectoralis major muscle* is part of the **Poland anomalad**.

When innervation does not develop, such as in the lower limbs in severe cases of *myelomeningocele*, muscles may fail to develop. In *sacral agenesis*, the abnormal somites that fail to form bony vertebrae may also fail to form muscles from the same defective mesodermal plate, a disorder of induction resulting in segmental amyoplasia. Skeletal muscles of the extremities fail to differentiate from embryonic myomeres if the long bones do not form. Absence of one long bone, such as the radius, is associated with variable aplasia or hypoplasia of associated muscles, such as the *carpi flexor radialis*.

Generalized amyoplasia due to defective myogenic regulatory genes is documented in mice and is theoretical in humans but would result in spontaneous fetal loss. End-stage neurogenic atrophy of muscle is sometimes called *amyoplasia*, but this use is semantically incorrect.

615.7 Muscular Dysgenesis

(Proteus Syndrome Myopathy)

The *Proteus syndrome* is a disturbance of cellular growth involving ectodermal and mesodermal tissues. The cause is unknown, but it is not a mendelian trait. It presents as asymmetric overgrowth of the extremities, verrucous cutaneous lesions, angiomas of various types, thickening of bones, hemimegalencephaly, and excessive growth of muscles without weakness. Histologically, the muscle is a unique *muscular dysgenesis*. Abnormal zones are adjacent to zones of normal muscle formation and do not follow anatomic boundaries. The disorder may be due to abnormal paracrine growth factors. Historically the "elephant man," who was exploited for his grotesque features in late 19th century London and became a popular sensation, was long misdiagnosed as having neurofibromatosis but is now recognized to have had Proteus syndrome.

615.8 Benign Congenital Hypotonia

Benign congenital hypotonia is not a disease but is a descriptive term for infants or children with nonprogressive hypotonia of unknown origin. The hypotonia is not usually associated with weakness or developmental delay, although some children acquire gross motor skills more slowly than normal. Tendon stretch reflexes are normal or hypoactive. There are no cranial nerve abnormalities, and intelligence is normal.

The *diagnosis* is one of exclusion after results of laboratory studies including muscle biopsy and imaging of the brain with special attention to the cerebellum are normal. No known molecular genetic basis for this syndrome has been identified.

The *prognosis* is generally good; no specific therapy is required. Contractures do not develop. Hypotonia persists into adult life. The disorder is not always as "benign" as its name implies, because a common complication is recurrent dislocation of joints, especially the shoulders. Excessive motility of the spine may result in stretch injury, compression, or vascular compromise of nerve roots or of the spinal cord. These are particular hazards for patients who perform gymnastics or who become circus performers because of agility of joints without weakness or pain.

615.9 Arthrogryposis

(See Chapter 631)

Arthrogryposis multiplex congenita is not a disease but is a descriptive term that signifies numerous congenital contractures. The etiologies encompass both neurogenic and primary myopathic diseases, but most cases, and indeed the most severe cases, are not due to neuromuscular disease. Myopathies that have a high incidence of either minor congenital contractures or extensive arthrogryposis include myotonic muscular dystrophy, many congenital myopathies, and intrauterine viral myositis. Neurogenic diseases causing arthrogryposis include infantile spinal muscular atrophy and the Pena-Shokeir and Marden-Walker syndromes (see Chapter 631).

Barth PG, Dubowitz V: X-linked myotubular myopathy. A long-term follow-up study. Eur J Paediatr Neurol 1:49, 1998.

De Gouyon BM, Zhao W, Laporte J, et al: Characterization of mutations in the myotubularin gene in twenty-six patients with X-linked myotubular myopathy. Hum Mol Genet 6:1499, 1997.

Iannaccone ST: Myogenes and myotubes. J Child Neurol 7:180, 1992.

Martinez BA, Lake BD: Childhood nemaline myopathy: A review of clinical presentation in relation to prognosis. Dev Med Child Neurol 29:815, 1987.

Miller JB: Myoblasts, myosins, MyoDs, and the diversification of muscle fibers. Neuromuscul Disord 1:7, 1991.

Sarnat HB: Cerebral dysgeneses and their influence on fetal muscle development. Brain Dev 8:495, 1986.

Sarnat HB: New insights into the pathogenesis of congenital myopathies. J Child Neurol 9:193, 1994.

Sarnat HB: Ontogenesis of striated muscle. *In:* Polin RA, Fox WW (eds): Neonatal and Fetal Medicine: Physiology and Pathophysiology, 2nd ed. Philadelphia, WB Saunders, 1998.

Shimomura C, Nonaka I: Nemaline myopathy: Comparative muscle histochemistry in the severe neonatal, moderate congenital, and adult-onset forms. Pediatr Neurol 5:25, 1989.

Wallgren-Pattersson C, Clarke A, Samson F, et al: The myotubular myopathies: Differential diagnosis of the X-linked recessive, autosomal dominant and autosomal recessive forms and present state of DNA studies. J Med Genet 32:673, 1995.

CHAPTER 616
Muscular Dystrophies

The term *dystrophy* means abnormal growth, derived from the Greek *trophe*, meaning "nourishment." *Muscular dystrophy* implies much more than simply aberrant growth or nutrition of muscle fibers. A muscular dystrophy is distinguished from all other neuromuscular diseases by four obligatory criteria: (1) It is a primary myopathy; (2) it has a genetic basis; (3) the course is progressive; (4) degeneration and death of muscle fibers occur at some stage in the disease. This definition excludes neurogenic diseases such as spinal muscular atrophy, nonhereditary myopathies such as dermatomyositis, nonprogressive and non-necrotizing congenital myopathies such as congenital muscle fiber–type disproportion (CMFTD), and nonprogressive inherited metabolic myopathies. Some metabolic myopathies may fulfill the definition of a progressive muscular dystrophy but are not traditionally classified as dystrophies. An example is muscle carnitine deficiency. Conversely, all muscular dystrophies might eventually be reclassified as metabolic myopathies once the biochemical defects are better defined.

Muscular dystrophies are a group of unrelated diseases, each transmitted by a different genetic trait and each differing in its clinical course and expression. Some are severe diseases at birth or lead to early death; others follow very slow progressive courses over many decades, may be compatible with normal longevity, or may not even become symptomatic until late adult life. Some categories of dystrophies, such as limb-girdle muscular dystrophy, are not homogeneous diseases but rather syndromes encompassing several distinct myopathies. Relationships between the various muscular dystrophies are resolved by molecular genetics rather than by similarities or differences in clinical and histopathologic features.

616.1 Duchenne and Becker Muscular Dystrophies

Duchenne muscular dystrophy is the most common hereditary neuromuscular disease affecting all races and ethnic groups. Its incidence is 1:3,600 liveborn infant boys. This disease is inherited as an X-linked recessive trait. The abnormal gene is on the X chromosome at the Xp21 locus and is one of the largest genes identified. Becker muscular dystrophy is the same fundamental disease as Duchenne dystrophy, with a genetic defect at the same locus, but clinically follows a milder and more protracted course.

Duchenne recognized most of the characteristic clinical features in 1861: hypertrophy of the calves, progressive weakness, intellectual impairment, and proliferation of connective tissue in muscle.

CLINICAL MANIFESTATIONS. Infant boys are only rarely symptomatic at birth or in early infancy, although some are already mildly hypotonic. Early gross motor skills, such as rolling over, sitting, and standing, are usually achieved at the appropriate ages or may be mildly delayed. Poor head control in infancy may be the first sign of weakness. Distinctive facies are not a feature because facial muscle weakness is a late event. Walking is often accomplished at the normal age of about 12 mo, but hip girdle weakness may be seen in subtle form as early as the 2nd year. Toddlers may assume a lordotic posture when standing to compensate for gluteal weakness. An early **Gowers sign** is often evident by age 3 yr and is fully expressed by age 5 or 6 yr (see Fig. 600–2). A **Trendelenburg gait**, or hip waddle, appears at this time.

The length of time that a patient remains ambulatory varies greatly. Some patients are confined to a wheelchair by 7 yr of age; most patients continue to walk with increasing difficulty until age 10 yr without orthopedic intervention. With orthotic bracing, physiotherapy, and sometimes minor surgery (e.g., Achilles' tendon lengthening), most are able to walk until age 12 yr. Ambulation is important not only for postponing the psychologic depression that accompanies the loss of an aspect of personal independence but also because scoliosis usually does not become a major complication as long as a patient remains ambulatory, even for as little as 1 hr/day; scoliosis often becomes rapidly progressive after confinement to a wheelchair.

The relentless progression of weakness continues into the 2nd decade. The function of distal muscles is usually relatively well enough preserved, allowing the child to continue to use eating utensils, a pencil, and a computer keyboard. Respiratory muscle involvement is expressed as a weak and ineffective cough, frequent pulmonary infections, and decreasing respiratory reserve. Pharyngeal weakness may lead to episodes of aspiration, nasal regurgitation of liquids, and an airy or nasal voice quality. The function of the extraocular muscles remains well preserved. Incontinence due to anal and urethral sphincter weakness is an uncommon and very late event.

Contractures most often involve the ankles, knees, hips, and elbows. Scoliosis is common. The thoracic deformity further compromises pulmonary capacity and compresses the heart. Scoliosis may be uncomfortable or painful. Enlargement of the calves **(pseudohypertrophy)** and wasting of thigh muscles is a classic feature. The enlargement is due to hypertrophy of some muscle fibers, infiltration of muscle by fat, and proliferation of collagen. After the calves, the next most common site of muscular hypertrophy is the tongue, followed by muscles of the forearm. Fasciculations of the tongue do not occur.

Unless ankle contractures are severe, ankle jerks remain well preserved until terminal stages. The knee jerks may be present until about 6 yr of age but are less brisk than the ankle jerks and are eventually lost. In the upper extremities, the brachioradialis reflex is usually stronger than the biceps or triceps brachii reflexes.

Cardiomyopathy is a constant feature of this disease. The severity of cardiac involvement does not necessarily correlate with the degree of skeletal muscle weakness. Some patients die early of severe cardiomyopathy while still ambulatory; others in terminal stages of the disease have well-compensated cardiac function.

Intellectual impairment occurs in all patients, although only 20–30% have an intelligence quotient (IQ) less than 70. The majority have learning disabilities that still allow them to function in a regular classroom, particularly if remedial help is available. A few patients are profoundly mentally retarded, but there is no correlation with the severity of the myopathy. Epilepsy is slightly more common than in the general pediatric population.

The degenerative changes and fibrosis of muscle constitute a painless process. Myalgias and muscle spasms do not occur. Calcinosis of muscle is rare.

Death occurs usually at about 18 yr of age. The causes of death are respiratory failure in sleep, intractable heart failure, pneumonia, or occasionally aspiration and airway obstruction.

In *Becker muscular dystrophy,* boys remain ambulatory until late adolescence or early adult life. Calf pseudohypertrophy, cardiomyopathy, and elevated serum levels of creatine phosphokinase (CK) are similar to Duchenne dystrophy. Learning disabilities are less frequent. The onset of weakness is later in Becker than in Duchenne disease. Death often occurs in the mid to late 20s; fewer than half of patients are still alive by age 40 yr; these survivors are severely disabled.

LABORATORY FINDINGS. The serum CK level is consistently greatly elevated in Duchenne muscular dystrophy, even in presymptomatic stages, including at birth. The usual serum concentration is 15,000–35,000 IU/L (normal <160 IU/L). A normal serum CK level is incompatible with the diagnosis of Duchenne dystrophy, although in terminal stages of the disease the serum CK value may be considerably lower than it was a few years earlier because there is less muscle to degenerate. Other lysosomal enzymes present in muscle, such as aldolase and aspartate aminotransferase (AST), are also increased but are less specific.

Cardiac assessment by echocardiography, electrocardiogram (ECG), and chest roentgenogram is essential and should be repeated periodically. After the diagnosis is established, patients should be referred to a pediatric cardiologist for long-term cardiac care.

Electromyogram (EMG) shows characteristic myopathic features but is not specific for Duchenne muscular dystrophy. No evidence of denervation is found. Motor and sensory nerve conduction velocities are normal.

DIAGNOSIS. The *muscle biopsy material* is diagnostic and shows

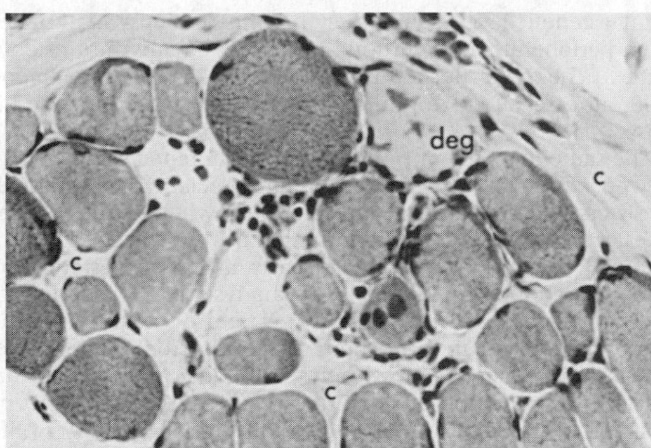

Figure 616–1 Muscle biopsy of a 4-yr-old boy with Duchenne muscular dystrophy. Both atrophic and hypertrophic muscle fibers are seen, and some fibers are degenerating (deg). Connective tissue (c) between muscle fibers is increased. (Hematoxylin & eosin, ×400).

characteristic changes (Figs. 616–1 and 616–2). Myopathic changes include endomysial connective tissue proliferation, scattered degenerating and regenerating myofibers, foci of mononuclear inflammatory cell infiltrates as a reaction to muscle fiber necrosis, mild architectural changes in still functional muscle fibers, and many dense fibers. These hypercontracted fibers probably result from segmental necrosis at another level, allowing calcium to enter the site of breakdown of the sarcolemmal membrane and trigger a contraction of the whole length of the muscle fiber.

The decision about whether muscle biopsy should be performed to establish the diagnosis sometimes presents problems. If there is a family history of the disease, particularly in the case of an involved brother whose diagnosis has been confirmed, a patient with typical clinical features of Duchenne muscular dystrophy and high concentrations of serum CK probably does not need to undergo biopsy. The result of the polymerase chain reaction (PCR) may also influence whether to perform a muscle biopsy (see next paragraph). A first case in a family, even if the clinical features are typical, should have the diagnosis confirmed to ensure that another myopathy is not masquerading as Duchenne dystrophy. The most common muscles sampled are the vastus lateralis (quadriceps femoris) and the gastrocnemius.

A specific *molecular genetic diagnosis* is possible by demonstrating deficient or defective dystrophin by immunohistochemical staining of sections of muscle biopsy tissue or by DNA analysis from peripheral blood. Confirmation of the diagnosis by one of these methods should be done in every case. If the blood PCR is diagnostic, muscle biopsy may be deferred, but if it is normal and clinical suspicion is high, the more specific dystrophin immunocytochemistry test performed on muscle biopsy sections detects the one third of cases that do not show a PCR abnormality.

GENETIC ETIOLOGY AND PATHOGENESIS. Despite the X-linked recessive inheritance in Duchenne muscular dystrophy, about 30% of patients are new mutations, and the mother is not a carrier. The female carrier state usually shows no muscle weakness or any clinical expression of the disease, but affected girls are occasionally encountered, usually having much milder weakness than boys. These symptomatic girls are explained by the Lyon hypothesis in which the normal X chromosome becomes inactivated, and the one with the gene deletion is active (see Chapter 78). The full clinical picture of Duchenne dystrophy has occurred in several girls with Turner's syndrome in whom the single X chromosome must have had the Xp21 gene deletion.

The asymptomatic carrier state is associated with elevated serum CK values in 80% of cases. The level of increase is usually in the magnitude of hundreds or a few thousand but does not have the extreme values noted in affected males. Prepubertal girls who are Duchenne carriers also have increased serum CK values, with highest levels at 8–12 yr of age. Approximately 20% of Duchenne carriers have normal serum

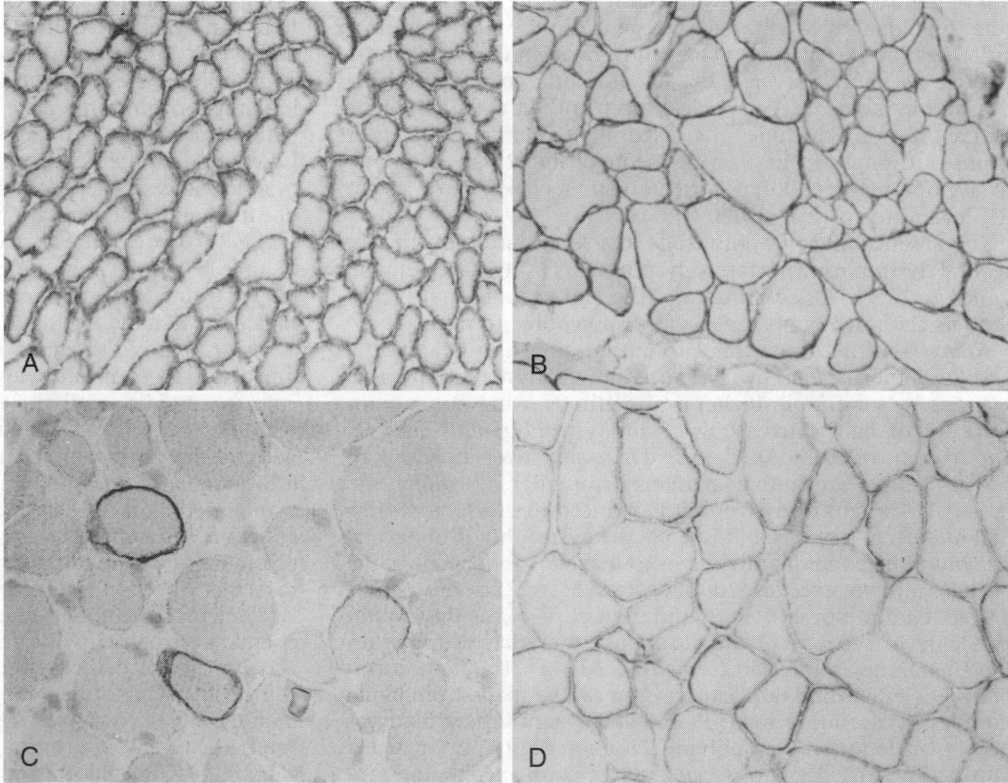

Figure 616–2 Dystrophin is demonstrated by immunohistochemical reactivity in the muscle biopsies of *(A)* a normal term male neonate; *(B)* a 10-year-old boy with limb-girdle muscular dystrophy; *(C)* a 6-year-old boy with Duchenne muscular dystrophy; and *(D)* a 10-year-old boy with Becker muscular dystrophy. In the normal condition and also in non-X-linked muscular dystrophies in which dystrophin is not affected, the sacrolemmal membrane of every fiber is strongly stained, including atrophic and hypertrophic fibers. In Duchenne dystrophy, most myofibers express no detectable dystrophin, but a few scattered fibers known as "revertant fibers" show near-normal immunoreactivity. In Becker muscular dystrophy, the abnormal dystrophin molecule is expressed as thin, pale staining of the sarcolemma in which reactivity varies not only between myofibers but also along the circumference of individual fibers (×250).

CK values. If the mother of an affected boy has normal CK levels, it is unlikely that her daughter can be identified as a carrier by measuring CK. Muscle biopsy of suspected female carriers may detect an additional 10% in whom serum CK is not elevated; a specific genetic diagnosis using PCR on peripheral blood is definitive.

Detection of the carrier state by serum CK or muscle biopsy will become obsolete because of discoveries in the molecular genetics of Duchenne muscular dystrophy. The Xp21 site of the Duchenne gene has more than 2,000 kilobases (kb), but Duchenne DNA encompasses only 14 kb; the entire gene sequence has been mapped.

A 427 kd cytoskeletal protein known as *dystrophin* is encoded by the gene at the Xp21.2 locus. This subsarcolemmal protein attaches to the sarcolemmal membrane overlying the A band and M band of the myofibrils and consists of four distinct regions or domains: the N-terminus contains 250 amino acids and is related to the N-actin binding site of α-actinin; the second domain is the largest, with 2,800 amino acids, and contains many repeats, giving it a characteristic rod shape; a third cysteine-rich domain is related to the C-terminus of α-actinin; and the final C-terminus domain of 400 amino acids is unique to dystrophin and to a dystrophin-related protein encoded by chromosome 6. Dystrophin is first detected in developing human fetal muscle at 11 wk gestation. Dystrophin mRNA normally is detected in cardiac and smooth muscle as well as in skeletal muscle and brain. All of these tissues show various degrees of clinical involvement.

The molecular defects in the dystrophinopathies are of various types: intragenic deletions, duplications, or point mutations of nucleotides. About 65% of patients have deletions, and only 7% exhibit duplications. The site or size of the intragenic abnormality does not always correlate well with the phenotypic severity; in both Duchenne and Becker forms, the mutations are mainly near the middle of the gene, involving deletions of exons 46–51. Phenotypic or clinical variations are explained by the alteration of the translational reading frame of mRNA, which results in unstable, truncated dystrophin molecules and severe, classic Duchenne dystrophy; mutations that preserve the reading frame still permit translation of coding sequences further downstream on the gene and produce a semifunctional dystrophin, expressed clinically as Becker muscular dystrophy. An even milder form of adult onset, formerly known as *quadriceps myopathy,* is also due to an abnormal dystrophin molecule. The clinical spectrum of the dystrophinopathies not only includes the classical Duchenne and Becker forms but ranges from a severe neonatal muscular dystrophy to asymptomatic children with persistent elevation of serum CK levels greater than 1,000 IU/L.

The absence of dystrophin leads to a secondary reduction in several dystrophin-associated glycoproteins in the sarcolemma, which results in loss of linkage to the extracellular matrix and renders the sarcolemma even more susceptible to necrosis.

Analysis of the dystrophin protein requires a muscle biopsy and is demonstrated by Western blot analysis or in tissue sections by immunohistochemical methods using either fluorescence or light microscopy of antidystrophin antisera (see Fig. 616–2). In classic Duchenne dystrophy, levels of less than 3% of normal are found; in Becker muscular dystrophy, the molecular weight of dystrophin is reduced to 20–90% of normal in 80% of patients, but in 15% the dystrophin is of normal size but reduced in quantity, and 5% have an abnormally large protein due to excessive duplications or repeats of codons. Selective immunoreactivity of different parts of the dystrophin molecule in sections of muscle biopsy material distinguishes the Duchenne and Becker forms (Fig. 616–3). The demonstration of deletions and duplications also can be made from blood samples by the more rapid PCR, which identifies as many as 98% of deletions by amplifying 18 exons but cannot detect duplications. The diagnosis can thus be confirmed at the molecular genetic level from either the muscle biopsy material or from peripheral blood, although as many as one third of boys with Duchenne or Becker dystrophy have a false normal blood PCR; all cases of dystrophinopathy are detected by muscle biopsy.

The same methods of DNA analysis from blood samples may be applied for carrier detection in female relatives at risk, such as sisters and cousins, and to determine whether the mother is a carrier or whether a new mutation occurred in the embryo. Prenatal diagnosis is possible as early as 12 wk gestation by sampling chorionic villi for DNA analysis by Southern blot or PCR and is confirmed in aborted fetuses with Duchenne dystrophy by immunohistochemistry for dystrophin in muscle.

TREATMENT. There is now neither a medical cure for this disease nor a method of slowing its progression. Much can be done to treat complications and to improve the quality of life of affected children. *Cardiac decompensation* often responds well to digoxin, at least in early stages. *Pulmonary infections* should be promptly treated. Patients should avoid contact with children who have obvious respiratory or other contagious illnesses. Immunizations for influenza virus and routine vaccinations are indicated.

Preservation of a good *nutritional state* is important. Duchenne muscular dystrophy is not a vitamin deficiency disease, and excessive doses of vitamins should be avoided. Adequate calcium intake is important to minimize osteoporosis in boys confined to a wheelchair, and fluoride supplements may also be given, particularly if the local drinking water is not fluoridated. Because sedentary children burn fewer calories than active children and because of depression as an additional factor, these children tend to eat excessively and gain weight. Obesity makes a patient with myopathy even less functional because part of the limited reserve muscle strength is dissipated in lifting the weight of excess subcutaneous adipose tissue. Dietary restrictions with supervision may be needed.

Physiotherapy delays but does not always prevent contractures. At times, contractures may actually be useful in functional rehabilitation. For example, if contractures prevent extension of the elbow beyond 90 degrees and the muscles of the upper limb no longer are strong enough to overcome gravity, the elbow contractures are functionally beneficial in fixing an otherwise flail arm and in allowing the patient to eat and write. Surgical correction of the elbow contracture may be technically feasible, but the result may be deleterious. Physiotherapy contributes little to muscle strengthening because patients usually are already using their entire reserve for daily function, and exercise cannot further strengthen involved muscles. Excessive exercise may actually accelerate the process of muscle fiber degeneration.

The discovery of the dystrophin molecule, the gene encoding it, and the specific mutations in Duchenne and Becker muscular dystrophies raises the theoretical potential of a cure by molecular genetic engineering. One experimental approach is *myoblast transfer therapy,* in which normal myoblasts from the muscle of a genetically close relative, usually the father, are cultured in vitro and then injected into dystrophic muscles with the expectation that they will form healthy myofibers with normal dystrophin to replace degenerating fibers. A major drawback is the requirement for immunosuppression to prevent rejection of the foreign cells. The results in cases without rejection phenomena have not been encouraging. Another possible but unproven approach is the introduction by intramuscular injection of a recombinant dystrophin gene.

Other investigational treatment of human patients with Duchenne dystrophy involves the use of *prednisone or other steroids.* Glucocorticoids decrease the rate of apoptosis or programmed cell death of myotubes during ontogenesis and theoretically may decelerate the myofiber necrosis in muscular dystrophy. Strength usually improves initially, but the long-term complications of chronic steroid therapy, including considerable

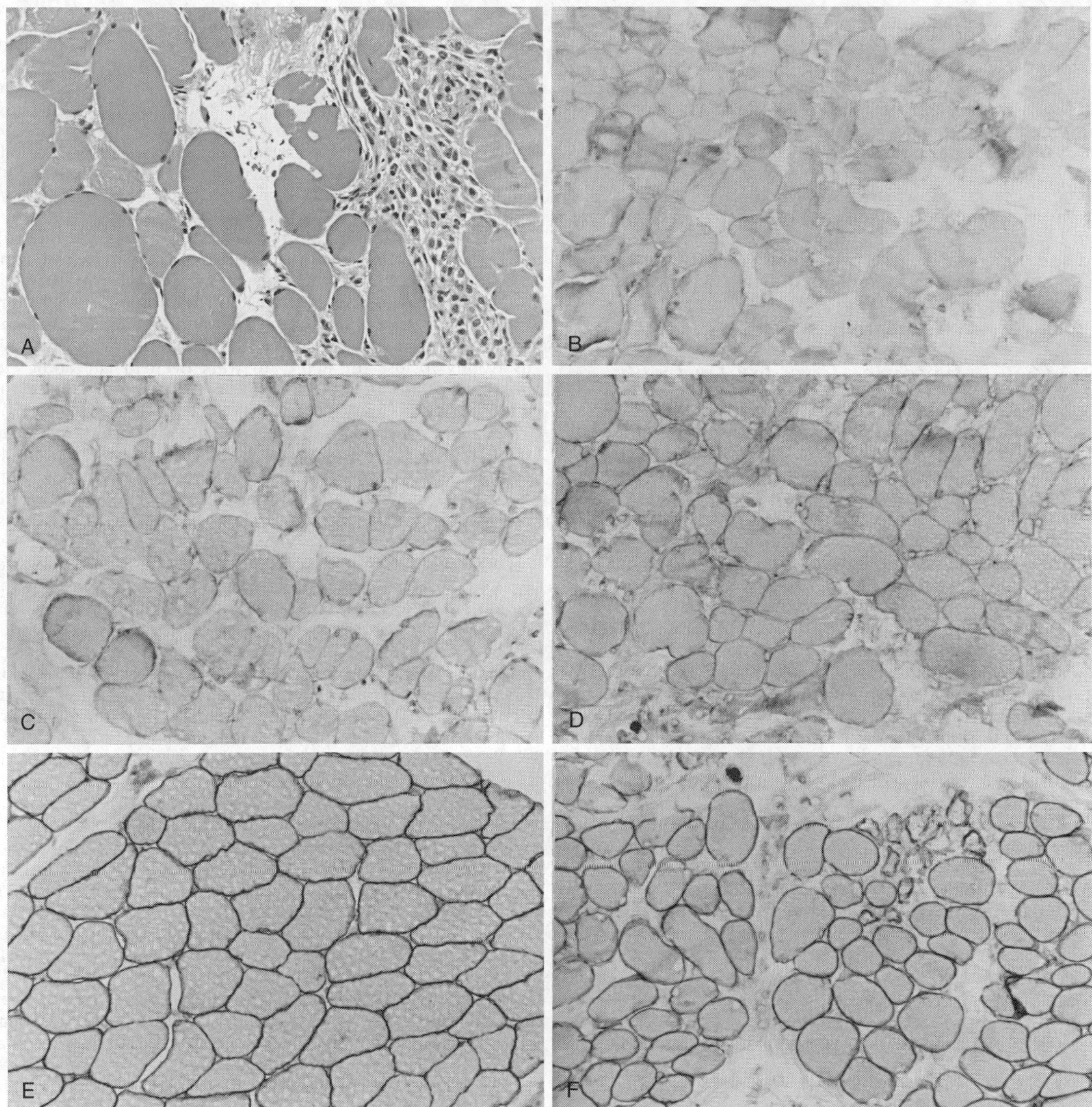

Figure 616–3 Quadriceps femoris muscle biopsy of a 4-yr-old boy with Becker muscular dystrophy. *A*, Myofibers vary greatly in size, with both atrophic and hypertrophic forms; at the right is a zone of degeneration and necrosis infiltrated by macrophages, similar to Duchenne muscular dystrophy. (Hematoxylin-eosin, X 250). Immunoreactivity using antibodies against the dystrophin molecule in the rod domain *(B)*, carboxyl-terminus *(C)*, and amino-terminus *(D)* all show deficient but not totally absent dystrophin expression; most fibers of all sizes retain some dystrophin in parts of the sarcolemma but not around the entire circumference in cross section. Alternatively, the prominence of dystrophin is less, appearing weak, when compared with the simultaneously incubated normal control from another child of similar age *(E)*. *F*, Merosin expression is normal in this Becker patient, in both large and small myofibers and is lacking only in frankly necrotic fibers. Compare with classic Duchenne muscular dystrophy illustrated in Figure 616–2 and with Figure 616–6.

weight gain and osteoporosis, may offset this advantage or even result in greater weakness than might have occurred in the natural course of the disease.

616.2 Emery-Dreifuss Muscular Dystrophy

Emery-Dreifuss muscular dystrophy, also known as *scapuloperoneal* or *scapulohumeral muscular dystrophy,* is a rare X-linked recessive dystrophy. The locus is on the long arm within the large Xq28 region that includes other mutations that cause myotubular myopathy, neonatal adrenoleukodystrophy and the Bloch-Sulzberger type of incontinentia pigmenti; it is far from the Duchenne muscular dystrophy gene on the short arm of the X chromosome.

Clinical manifestations begin in middle childhood, but many patients survive to late adult life because of the slow progression of its course. Hypertrophy of muscles does not occur.

Contractures of elbows and ankles develop early, and muscle becomes wasted in a scapulohumeroperoneal distribution. Facial weakness does not occur; this disease is thus distinguished clinically from autosomal dominant scapulohumeral and scapuloperoneal syndromes of neurogenic origin. Myotonia is absent. Intellectual function is normal. Cardiomyopathy is severe and is often the cause of death. The serum CK value is only mildly elevated, further distinguishing this disease from other X-linked recessive muscular dystrophies.

Nonspecific myofiber necrosis and endomysial fibrosis are seen in the muscle biopsy sample. Many centronuclear fibers and selective histochemical type I muscle fiber atrophy may cause confusion with myotonic dystrophy. Treatment should be supportive.

616.3 Myotonic Muscular Dystrophy

Myotonic dystrophy **(Steinert disease)** is the second most common muscular dystrophy in North America, Europe, and Australia, having an incidence of 1:30,000 general population. It is inherited as an autosomal dominant trait.

Myotonic dystrophy is an example of a genetic defect causing dysfunction in multiple organ systems. Not only is striated muscle severely affected, but smooth muscle of the alimentary tract and uterus is also involved; cardiac function is altered; and patients have multiple and variable endocrinopathies, immunologic deficiencies, cataracts, dysmorphic facies, intellectual impairment, and other neurologic abnormalities.

CLINICAL MANIFESTATIONS. In the usual clinical course, excluding the severe neonatal form, infants may appear almost normal at birth, or facial wasting and hypotonia may already be early expressions of the disease. The facial appearance is characteristic, consisting of an inverted V-shaped upper lip, thin cheeks, and scalloped, concave temporalis muscles (Fig. 616–4). The head may be narrow, and the palate is high and arched because the weak temporal and pterygoid muscles in late fetal life do not exert sufficient lateral forces on the developing head and face.

Weakness is mild in the 1st few years. Progressive wasting of distal muscles becomes increasingly evident, particularly involving intrinsic muscles of the hands. The thenar and hypothenar eminences are flattened, and the atrophic dorsal interossei leave deep grooves between the fingers. The dorsal forearm muscles and anterior compartment muscles of the lower legs also become wasted. The tongue is thin and atrophic. Wasting of the sternocleidomastoids gives the neck a long, thin, cylindric contour. Proximal muscles also eventually undergo atrophy, and scapular winging appears. Difficulty with climbing stairs and Gowers sign are progressive. Tendon stretch reflexes are usually preserved.

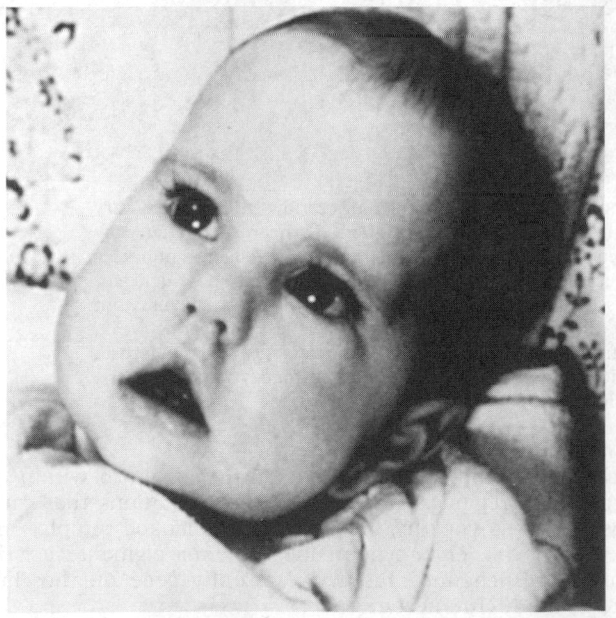

Figure 616–4 Facial weakness, inverted V-shaped upper lip, and loss of muscle mass in the temporal fossae are characteristic of myotonic muscular dystrophy, even in infancy, as seen in this 8-mo-old girl.

The distal distribution of muscle wasting in myotonic dystrophy is an exception to the general rule of myopathies having proximal and neuropathies distal distribution patterns. The muscular atrophy and weakness in myotonic dystrophy are slowly progressive throughout childhood and adolescence and continue into adulthood. It is rare for patients with myotonic dystrophy to lose the ability to walk even in late adult life, although splints or bracing may be required to stabilize the ankles.

Myotonia, a characteristic feature shared by few other myopathies, does not occur in infancy and is usually not clinically or even electromyographically evident until about age 5 yr. Exceptional patients develop it as early as age 3 yr. Myotonia is a very slow relaxation of muscle after contraction, regardless of whether that contraction was voluntary or was induced by a stretch reflex or electrical stimulation. During physical examination, myotonia may be demonstrated by asking the patient to make tight fists and then to quickly open the hands. It may be induced by striking the thenar eminence with a rubber percussion hammer, and it may be detected by watching the involuntary drawing of the thumb across the palm. Myotonia may also be demonstrated in the tongue by pressing the edge of a wooden tongue blade against its dorsal surface and by observing a deep furrow that disappears slowly.

The severity of myotonia does not necessarily parallel the degree of weakness, and the weakest muscles often have only minimal myotonia. Myotonia is not a painful muscle spasm. Myalgias do not occur in myotonic dystrophy.

The *speech* of patients with myotonic dystrophy is often articulated poorly and is slurred because of the involvement of the muscles of the face, tongue, and pharynx. Difficulties with swallowing sometimes occur. Aspiration pneumonia is a risk in severely involved children. Incomplete external ophthalmoplegia may sometimes result from extraocular muscle weakness.

Smooth muscle involvement of the *gastrointestinal tract* results in slow gastric emptying, poor peristalsis, and constipation. Some patients have encopresis associated with anal sphincter weakness. Women with myotonic dystrophy may have ineffective or abnormal uterine contractions during labor and delivery.

Cardiac involvement is usually manifested as heart block in the Purkinje conduction system and arrhythmias rather than as cardiomyopathy, unlike most other muscular dystrophies.

Endocrine abnormalities involve many glands and appear at any time during the course of the disease so that re-evaluation of endocrine status must be done annually in the 1st few years and every several years after that. **Hypothyroidism** is common; hyperthyroidism may occur rarely. Adrenocortical insufficiency may lead to an **addisonian crisis** even in infancy. **Diabetes mellitus** is common in patients with myotonic dystrophy; some children have a disorder of insulin release rather than defective insulin production. Onset of puberty may be precocious or, more often, delayed. Testicular atrophy and testosterone deficiency are common in adults and are responsible for a high incidence of male infertility. Ovarian atrophy is rare. Frontal baldness is also characteristic in males and often begins in adolescence.

Immunologic deficiencies are common in myotonic dystrophy. The plasma IgG is often low.

Cataracts occur frequently in myotonic dystrophy. They may be congenital, or they may begin at any time during childhood or adult life. Early cataracts are detected only by slit lamp examination; periodic examination by an ophthalmologist is recommended. Visual evoked potentials are often abnormal in children with myotonic dystrophy and are unrelated to cataracts. They are not usually accompanied by visual impairment.

About half of the patients with myotonic dystrophy are intellectually impaired, but severe mental retardation is unusual. The remainder are of average or occasionally above average intelligence. Epilepsy is not common.

A **severe neonatal form of myotonic dystrophy** appears in a minority of involved infants born to mothers with myotonic dystrophy. Clubfoot deformities alone or more extensive congenital contractures of many joints may involve all extremities and even the cervical spine. Generalized hypotonia and weakness are present at birth. Facial wasting is prominent. Some infants require gavage feeding or even ventilator support for respiratory muscle weakness or apnea. One or both leaves of the diaphragm may be nonfunctional. The abdomen becomes distended with gas in the stomach and intestine because of poor peristalsis due to smooth muscle weakness. The distention further compromises respiration. Inability to empty the rectum may compound the problem. About 75% of severely affected neonates die within the 1st yr.

LABORATORY FINDINGS. The classic myotonic EMG is not found in infancy but may appear in toddlers or during the early school years. The levels of serum CK and other serum enzymes from muscle may be normal or only mildly elevated in the hundreds (never the thousands).

An ECG should be performed annually in early childhood. Ultrasonic imaging of the abdomen may be indicated in affected infants to determine diaphragmatic function. Roentgenograms of the chest and abdomen and contrast studies of gastrointestinal motility may be needed.

Endocrine assessment should be undertaken to determine thyroid and adrenal cortical function and to verify carbohydrate metabolism (glucose tolerance test). Immunoglobulins should be examined, and if needed, more extensive immunologic studies should be performed.

DIAGNOSIS. The muscle biopsy specimen often shows many muscle fibers with central nuclei and selective atrophy of histochemical type I fibers, but degenerating fibers are usually few and widely scattered, and there is little or no fibrosis of muscle. Intrafusal fibers of muscle spindles are also abnormal. In young children with the common form of the disease, the biopsy material may even appear normal or may at least not show myofiber necroses, which is a striking contrast with Duchenne muscular dystrophy. In the severe neonatal form of myotonic dystrophy, the muscle biopsy sample reveals maturational arrest in various stages of development. It is likely that the sarcolemmal membrane of muscle fibers not only has abnormal properties of electrical polarization but is also incapable of responding to trophic influences of the motor neuron. Muscle biopsy is not usually required for diagnosis, which in typical cases can be based on the clinical manifestations. It is recommended in severe neonatal cases because the biopsy may be of prognostic as well as of diagnostic value. Molecular genetic diagnosis from a blood sample and prenatal diagnosis are possible.

GENETICS. The genetic defect in myotonic muscular dystrophy is on chromosome 19 at the 19q13 locus. It consists of an expansion of the gene rather than a deletion with numerous repeats of the cytosine-thymine-guanine (CTG) codon. Rarely, the disease is associated with no detectable repeats, perhaps a spontaneous correction of a previous expansion but a phenomenon still incompletely understood. Both clinical and genetic expressivity may vary between siblings or between an affected parent and child. In the severe neonatal form of the disease, the mother is the transmitting parent in 94% of cases, a fact not explained by increased male infertility alone. Genetic analysis reveals that such infants usually have many more repeats of the CTG codon, as many as 2,500, than do patients with the more classic form of the disease that have more than 50 repeats, typically 80–130, compared with the 35–40 repeats of normal alleles. Myotonic dystrophy often exhibits a pattern of *anticipation* in which each successive generation has a tendency to be more severely involved than the previous generation.

TREATMENT. There is no specific medical treatment, but the cardiac, endocrine, gastrointestinal, and ocular complications can often be treated. Physiotherapy and orthopedic treatment of contractures in the neonatal form of the disease may be beneficial.

Myotonia may be diminished, and function may be restored by drugs that raise the depolarization threshold of muscle membranes, such as mexiletine, phenytoin (PHT), carbamazepine (CBZ), procainamide, and quinidine sulfate. These drugs also have cardiotropic effects; thus, cardiac evaluation is important before prescribing them. PHT and CBZ are used in doses similar to their use as anticonvulsants (see Chapter 602.4); serum concentrations of 40–80 μmol/L for PHT and 35–50 μmol/L for CBZ should be maintained. If a patient's disability is due mainly to weakness rather than to myotonia, these drugs will be of no value.

OTHER MYOTONIC SYNDROMES

Most patients with myotonia have myotonic dystrophy. Myotonia is not specific for this disease and occurs in several rarer conditions.

Myotonic chondrodystrophy **(Schwartz-Jampel disease)** is a rare congenital disease characterized by generalized muscle hypertrophy and weakness. Dysmorphic phenotypical features and the roentgenographic appearance of long bones are reminiscent of Morquio disease (see Chapter 85), but abnormal mucopolysaccharides are not found. Dwarfism, joint abnormalities, and blepharophimosis are present. Several patients have been the products of consanguinity, suggesting autosomal recessive inheritance.

EMG reveals continuous electrical activity in muscle fibers closely resembling or identical to myotonia. Muscle biopsy reveals nonspecific myopathic features, which are minimal in some cases and pronounced in others. The sarcotubular system is dilated.

Myotonia congenita **(Thomsen disease)** is a channelopathy and is characterized by weakness and generalized muscular hypertrophy so that affected children resemble bodybuilders. Myotonia is prominent and may develop at age 2–3 yr, earlier than in myotonic dystrophy. The disease is clinically stable and is apparently not progressive for many years. Muscle biopsy specimens show minimal pathologic changes, and the EMG demonstrates myotonia. Various families are described as showing either autosomal dominant **(Thomsen disease)** or recessive (**Becker disease,** not to be confused with Becker/Duchenne muscular dystrophy) inheritance. Rarely, myotonic dystrophy and myotonia congenita coexist in the same family. Both the autosomal dominant and autosomal recessive forms of myotonia congenita have been mapped to the same 7q35 locus. This gene is important for the integrity of chloride channels of the sarcolemma.

Paramyotonia is a temperature-related myotonia that is aggravated by cold and alleviated by warm external temperatures. Patients have difficulty when swimming in cold water or if they are dressed inadequately in cold weather. Paramyotonia congenita is a defect in a gene at the 17q13.1–13.3 locus, the identical locus identified in hyperkalemic periodic paralysis. By contrast with myotonia congenita, paramyotonia is a disorder of the sodium channel. Myotonic dystrophy also is a sodium channelopathy.

In **sodium channelopathies**, exercise produces increasing myotonia, whereas in **chloride channelopathies,** exercise reduces the myotonia. This is easily tested during examination by asking patients to close the eyes forcefully and open them repeatedly; it becomes progressively more difficult in sodium channel disorders and progressively easier in chloride channel disorders.

616.4 Limb-Girdle Muscular Dystrophy

This term encompasses a group of progressive hereditary myopathies that mainly affect muscles of the hip and shoulder girdles. Distal muscles also eventually become atrophic and weak. Hypertrophy of the calves and ankle contractures develop in some forms (Fig. 616–5), causing potential confusion with Becker muscular dystrophy.

The initial symptoms and signs rarely appear before middle or late childhood or may be delayed until early adult life. Low back pain may be a presenting complaint because of the lordotic posture resulting from gluteal muscle weakness. Confinement to a wheelchair usually becomes obligatory at about 30 yr of age. The rate of progression varies from one pedigree to another but is uniform within a kindred. Although weakness of neck flexors and extensors is universal, facial, lingual, and other bulbar-innervated muscles are rarely involved. As weakness and muscle wasting progress, tendon stretch reflexes become diminished. Cardiac involvement is unusual. Intellectual function is generally normal. The clinical differential diagnosis of limb-girdle muscular dystrophy includes juvenile spinal muscular atrophy **(Kugelberg-Welander disease),** myasthenia gravis, and metabolic myopathies.

Most cases of limb-girdle muscular dystrophy are of autosomal recessive inheritance, but some families express an autosomal dominant trait. The latter often follows a benign course with little functional impairment.

The EMG and muscle biopsy show confirmatory evidence of muscular dystrophy, but none of the findings are specific enough to make the definitive diagnosis without additional clinical criteria. In some cases, adhalen, a dystrophin-related glycoprotein of the sarcolemma, is deficient; this specific defect may be demonstrated in the muscle biopsy material by immunocytochemistry. Increased serum CK level is usual, but the magnitude of elevation varies among families. The ECG is usually unaltered.

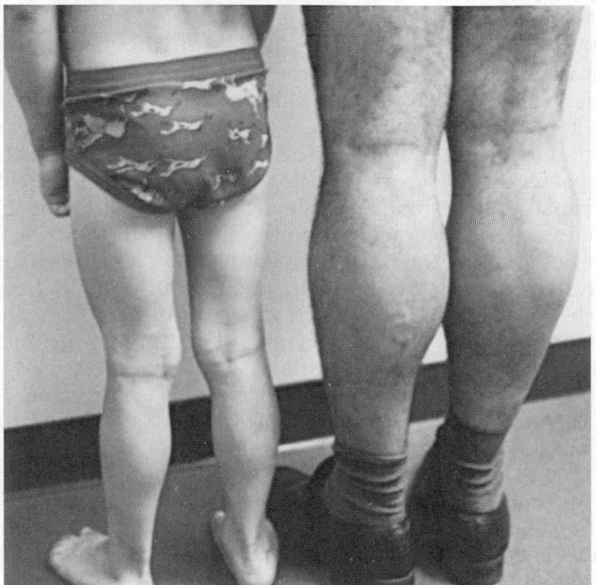

Figure 616–5 Posterior aspect of the legs of a father and his 6-yr-old son with a rare autosomal dominant muscular dystrophy. Hypertrophy of the calves resembles Duchenne muscular dystrophy, but the clinical course is benign and causes little disability throughout life.

Adhalen is *alpha-sarcoglycan*; other limb-girdle dystrophies due to deficiencies in *beta-*, *gamma-*, and *delta*-sarcoglycan also occur. Each of these may be diagnosed by immunochemistry of muscle biopsy tissue. There is more variation in both clinical course and myopathologic involvement in the sarcoglycanopathies than in the dystrophinopathies.

In the autosomal dominant form of limb-girdle muscular dystrophy, a genetic defect has been localized to the long arm of chromosome 5. In the autosomal recessive disease, it is on the long arm of chromosome 15. A mutated dystrophin-associated protein in the sarcoglycan complex (sarcoglycanopathy) is responsible for some cases of autosomal recessive limb-girdle muscular dystrophy.

616.5 Facioscapulohumeral Muscular Dystrophy

Facioscapulohumeral (FSH) muscular dystrophy, also known as **Landouzy-Déjèrine disease,** is probably not a single disease entity but a group of diseases with similar clinical manifestations. Autosomal dominance is the rule; the phenomenon of *genetic anticipation* is often found within several generations of a family, the succeeding more severely involved at an earlier age than the preceding. The genetic defect in autosomal dominant FSH muscular dystrophy is at the 4q35 locus.

CLINICAL MANIFESTATIONS. FSH dystrophy shows the earliest and most severe weakness in facial and shoulder girdle muscles. The facial weakness differs from that of myotonic dystrophy; rather than an inverted V-shaped upper lip, the mouth in FSH dystrophy is rounded and appears puckered because the upper and lower lips protrude. Inability to close the eyes completely in sleep is a common expression of upper facial weakness; some patients have extraocular muscle weakness, although ophthalmoplegia is rarely complete. FSH dystrophy has been reported in association with Möbius syndrome on rare occasions. Pharyngeal and tongue weakness may be absent and is never as severe as the facial involvement. Hearing loss and retinal vasculopathy are associated features, particularly in cases of FSH dystrophy with early childhood onset.

Scapular winging is prominent, often even in infants. Flattening or even concavity of the deltoid contour is seen, and the biceps and triceps brachii muscles are wasted and weak. Muscles of the hip girdles and thighs also eventually lose strength and undergo atrophy, and Gowers sign and a Trendelenburg gait appear. Contractures are rare. Finger and wrist weakness occasionally is the first symptom. Weakness of the anterior tibial and peroneal muscles may lead to footdrop; this complication usually occurs only in advanced cases with severe weakness. Lumbar lordosis and kyphoscoliosis are common complications of axial muscle involvement. Calf hypertrophy is not a feature.

FSH muscular dystrophy may also be a mild disease causing minimal disability. Clinical manifestations may not be expressed in childhood and are delayed into middle adult life. Unlike most other muscular dystrophies, asymmetry of weakness is common.

LABORATORY FINDINGS. Serum, levels of CK and other enzymes vary greatly, ranging from normal or near normal to elevations of several thousand. ECG should be performed, although the anticipated findings are usually normal. EMG reveals nonspecific myopathic muscle potentials.

DIAGNOSIS AND DIFFERENTIAL DIAGNOSIS. Muscle biopsy distinguishes more than one form of FSH, consistent with clinical evidence that several distinct diseases are embraced by the term *FSH dystrophy.* Muscle biopsy and EMG also distinguish the primary myopathy from a neurogenic disease with a similar distribution of muscular involvement. The general histopathologic findings in the muscle biopsy material are extensive proliferation of connective tissue between muscle fibers, extreme variation in fiber size with many hypertrophic as well as atrophic myofibers, and scattered degenerating and regenerating fibers. An *"inflammatory" type of FSH muscular dystrophy* is also distinguished, characterized by extensive lymphocytic infiltrates within muscle fascicles. Despite the resemblance of this form to inflammatory myopathies, such as polymyositis, there is no evidence of autoimmune disease, and steroids and immunosuppressive drugs do not alter the clinical course. A precise histopathologic diagnosis has important therapeutic implications. Mononuclear cell "inflammation" in a muscle biopsy sample of infants younger than 2 yr is usually FSH dystrophy.

TREATMENT. Physiotherapy is of no value in regaining strength or in retarding progressive weakness or muscle wasting. Footdrop and scoliosis may be treated by orthopedic measures. Cosmetic improvement of the facial muscles of expression may be achieved by reconstructive surgery, which grafts a fascia lata to the zygomatic muscle and to the zygomatic head of the *quadratus labiae superioris* muscle.

616.6 Congenital Muscular Dystrophy

The term *congenital* muscular dystrophy is misleading because all muscular dystrophies are genetically determined. It is used to encompass several distinct diseases with a common characteristic of severe involvement at birth but that ironically usually follow a benign clinical course. Autosomal recessive inheritance is the rule.

CLINICAL MANIFESTATIONS. Infants often have contractures or *arthrogryposis* at birth and are diffusely hypotonic. The muscle mass is thin in the trunk and extremities. Head control is poor. Facial muscles may be mildly involved, but ophthalmoplegia, pharyngeal weakness, and weak sucking are not common. A minority have severe dysphagia and require gavage or gastrostomy. Tendon stretch reflexes may be hypoactive or absent. Arthrogryposis is common in all forms of congenital muscular dystrophy (see Chapter 615.9).

One form of congenital muscular dystrophy, the **Fukuyama type,** is the 2nd most common muscular dystrophy in Japan (following Duchenne dystrophy); it has also been reported in children of Dutch, German, Scandinavian, and Turkish ethnic backgrounds. In the Fukuyama variety, severe cardiomyopathy and malformations of the brain usually accompany the skeletal muscle involvement. Signs and symptoms related to these organs are prominent: cardiomegaly and heart failure, mental retardation, seizures, microcephaly, and failure to thrive. The genetic defect in Fukuyama congenital muscular dystrophy has been identified at the 8q31–33 locus in Japanese patients.

Neurologic disease may accompany forms of congenital muscular dystrophy other than Fukuyama disease. Mental and neurologic status are the most variable features; an apparently normal brain and normal intelligence do not preclude the diagnosis if other manifestations indicate this myopathy. The cerebral malformations that occur are not consistently of one type and vary from severe dysplasias (holoprosencephaly, lissencephaly) to milder conditions (agenesis of the corpus callosum, focal heterotopia of the cerebral cortex and subcortical white matter, cerebellar hypoplasia). Congenital muscular dystrophy is a consistent association with cerebral dysgenesis in

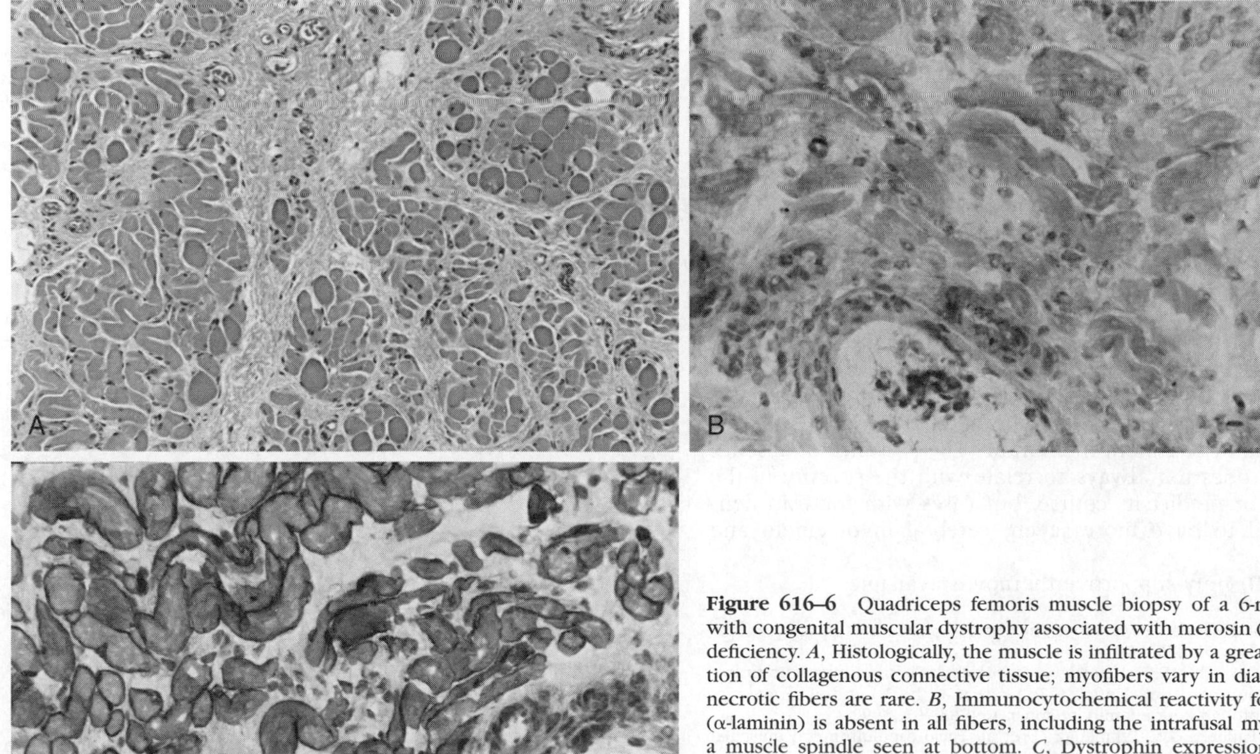

Figure 616–6 Quadriceps femoris muscle biopsy of a 6-mo-old girl with congenital muscular dystrophy associated with merosin (α-laminin) deficiency. *A*, Histologically, the muscle is infiltrated by a great proliferation of collagenous connective tissue; myofibers vary in diameter, but necrotic fibers are rare. *B*, Immunocytochemical reactivity for merosin (α-laminin) is absent in all fibers, including the intrafusal myofibers of a muscle spindle seen at bottom. *C*, Dystrophin expression (rod domain) is normal. Compare with Figures 616-2, 616-3, and 616-7.

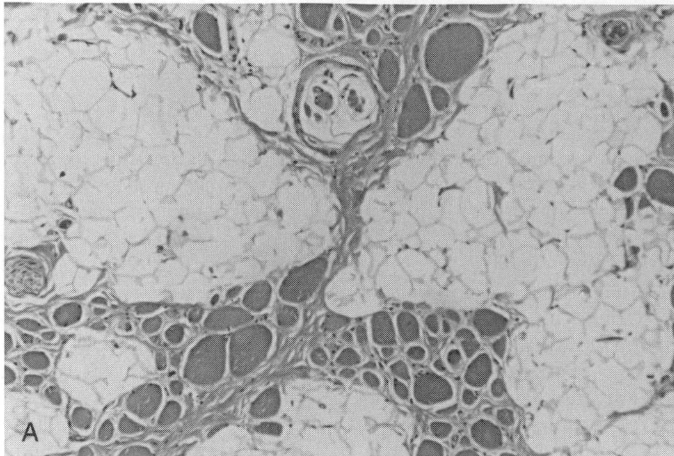

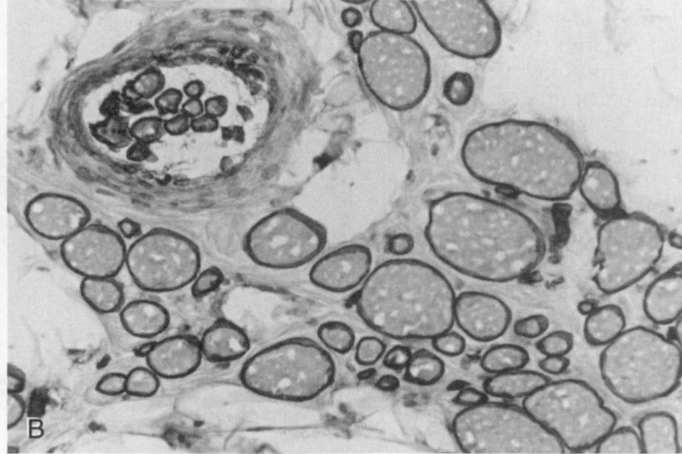

Figure 616–7 Quadriceps femoris muscle biopsy of a 2-yr-old girl with congenital muscular dystrophy. *A*, The fascicular architecture of the muscle is severely disrupted, and muscle is replaced by fat and connective tissue; remaining small groups of myofibers of variable size are seen, including a muscle spindle at top. *B*, Merosin expression is normal in both extrafusal fibers of all sizes and in intrafusal spindle fibers. The severity of the myopathy does not relate to the presence or absence of merosin in congenital muscular dystrophy. Compare with Figure 616–6.

the **Walker-Warburg syndrome** and in **muscle-eye-brain disease of Santavuori.** The neuropathologic findings are those of neuroblast migratory abnormalities in the cerebral cortex, cerebellum, and brain stem.

LABORATORY FINDINGS. Serum CK level is usually moderately elevated from several hundred to many thousand IU/L; only marginal increases are sometimes found. EMG shows nonspecific myopathic features. Investigation of all forms of congenital muscular dystrophy should include cardiac assessment and an imaging study of the brain. Muscle biopsy is essential for the diagnosis.

DIAGNOSIS. Muscle biopsy is diagnostic in the neonatal period or thereafter. An extensive proliferation of endomysial collagen envelops individual muscle fibers even at birth, also causing them to be rounded in cross-sectional contour by acting as a rigid sleeve, especially during contraction. The perimysial connective tissue and fat are also increased, and the fascicular organization of the muscle may be disrupted by the fibrosis. Tissue cultures of intramuscular fibroblasts exhibit increased collagen synthesis, but the structure of the collagen is normal. Muscle fibers vary in diameter, and many show central nuclei, myofibrillar splitting, and other cytoarchitectural alterations. Scattered degenerating and regenerating fibers are seen. No inflammation or abnormal inclusions are found. Immunocytochemical reactivity for merosin (α-laminin) at the sarcolemmal region is absent in about half the cases and normally expressed in the others (Figs. 616–6 and 616–7). Merosin is a protein that binds the sarcolemmal membrane of the myofiber to the basal lamina or basement membrane. The presence or absence of merosin does not always correlate with the severity of the myopathy or predict its course, but cases with merosin deficiency tend to have more severe cerebral involvement and myopathy.

TREATMENT. Only supportive therapy is available.

Angelini C, Fanin N, Freda MP, et al: The clinical spectrum of sarcoglycanopathies. Neurology 52:176, 1999.

Brook JD, McCurrach ME, Harley HG, et al: Molecular basis of myotonic dystrophy: Expansion of a trinucleotide (CTG) repeat at the 3N end of a transcript encoding a protein kinase family member. Cell 68:799, 1992.

Brouwer OF, Padberg GW, Wijmenga C, et al: Facioscapulohumeral muscular dystrophy in early childhood. Arch Neurol 51:387, 1994.

Dubowitz V: Prednisone in Duchenne dystrophy. Neuromuscul Disord 1:161, 1991.

Duggan DJ, Gorospe JR, Fanin N, et al: Mutations in the sarcoglycan genes in patients with myopathy. N Engl J Med 336:618, 1997.

Egger J, Kendall BE, Erdohazi M, et al: Involvement of the central nervous system in congenital muscular dystrophies. Dev Med Child Neurol 25:32, 1983.

Fukuyama Y, Osawa M, Saito K (eds): Congenital Muscular Dystrophies. New York, Elsevier, 1997.

Links TP, Smit AJ, Molenaar WM, et al: Familial hypokalemic periodic paralysis: clinical, diagnostic and therapeutic aspects. J Neurol Sci 122:33, 1994.

Miller G, Wessel HB: Diagnosis of dystrophinopathies: Review for the clinician. Pediatr Neurol 9:3, 1993.

Monsieurs KG, Van Broeckhoven C, Martin JJ, et al: Gly241Arg mutation indicating malignant hyperthermia susceptibility: Specific cause of chronically elevated serum creatine kinase activity. J Neurol Sci 154:62, 1998.

Moxley RT III: Myotonic disorders in childhood: Diagnosis and treatment. J Child Neurol 12:116, 1997.

Rose MR: Neurological channelopathies. Br Med J 316:1104, 1998.

Santavuori P, Valanne L, Autti T, et al: Muscle-eye-brain disease. Clinical features, visual evoked potentials and brain imaging in 20 patients. Eur J Paediatr Neurol 1:41, 1998.

Sarnat HB, O'Connor T, Byrne PA: Clinical effects of myotonic dystrophy on pregnancy and the neonate. Arch Neurol 33:459, 1976.

Sewry CA, Philpot J, Sorokin LM, et al: Diagnosis of merosin (laminin-2) deficient congenital muscular dystrophy by skin biopsy. Lancet 347:582, 1996.

Tokgozoglu LS, Ashizawa T, Pacifico A, et al: Cardiac involvement in a large kindred with myotonic dystrophy. JAMA 274:813, 1995.

Tsilfidis C, MacKenzie AE, Mettler G, et al: Correlation between CTG trinucleotide repeat length and frequency of severe congenital myotonic dystrophy. Nature Genet 1:192, 1992.

Voit T: Congenital muscular dystrophies: 1997 update. Brain Dev 20:65, 1998.

Wijmenga C, Frants RR, Hewitt JE, et al: Molecular genetics of facioscapulohumeral muscular dystrophy. Neuromuscul Disord 3:487, 1993.

CHAPTER 617
Endocrine Myopathies

THYROID MYOPATHIES. (See also Part XXV, Section 2.) Thyrotoxicosis causes proximal weakness and wasting accompanied by myopathic electromyogram (EMG) changes. Thyroxine binds to myofibrils and in excess impairs contractile function. Hyperthyroidism may also induce myasthenia gravis and hypokalemic periodic paralysis (see later).

Hypothyroidism, whether congenital or acquired, consistently produces hypotonia and a proximal distribution of weakness. Although muscle wasting is most characteristic, one form of cretinism, the **Kocher-Debré-Sémélaigne syndrome,** is characterized by generalized pseudohypertrophy of weak muscles. Infants may have a herculean appearance reminiscent of myotonia congenita. The serum creatine phosphokinase (CK) level is elevated in hypothyroid myopathy and returns to normal after thyroid replacement therapy. Muscle biopsy material reveals myopathic changes including myofiber necrosis and sometimes central cores.

Both the clinical and pathologic features of hyperthyroid myopathy and hypothyroid myopathy resolve after appropriate treatment of the thyroid disorder.

HYPERPARATHYROIDISM. (See also Chapter 583.) Most patients with primary hyperparathyroidism develop weakness, fatigability, and muscle wasting that are reversible after removal of the parathyroid adenoma.

STEROID-INDUCED MYOPATHY. Both natural **Cushing disease** and the iatrogenic **Cushing syndrome** due to exogenous corticosteroid administration may cause progressive proximal weakness, increased serum CK levels, and a myopathic EMG and muscle biopsy specimen (see Chapter 587). Myosin filaments may be selectively lost. Fluorinated steroids, such as dexamethasone, are the most likely to produce *steroid myopathy.* In patients with dermatomyositis or other myopathies treated with steroids, it is sometimes difficult to distinguish refractoriness of the disease from steroid-induced weakness, especially after long-term steroid administration. All patients who have been taking steroids for long periods develop a reversible type II myofiber atrophy; this is a *steroid effect* but is not steroid myopathy unless it progresses to become a necrotizing myopathy.

Hyperaldosteronism (Conn syndrome) is accompanied by episodic and reversible weakness similar to that of periodic paralysis (see Chapter 587). The proximal myopathy may become irreversible in chronic cases. Elevated CK levels and even myoglobinuria sometimes occur during acute attacks.

Gellerra C, Verderio E, Floridia G, et al: Assignment of the human carnitine palmitoyltransferase (CPT1) to chromosome 1p32. Genomics 24:195, 1994.
Hilton-Jones D, Squier M, Taylor D, et al: Metabolic Myopathies. Philadelphia, WB Saunders, 1995.
Lestienne P, Ponsot G: Kearns-Sayre syndrome with muscle mitochondrial DNA deletion. Lancet 1:885, 1988.
Mastaglia FL, Ojeda VJ, Sarnat HB, et al: Myopathies associated with hypothyroidism. Aust N Z J Med 18:799, 1988.
Tsujino S, Shanske S, DiMauro S, et al: Molecular genetic heterogeneity of myophosphorylase deficiency (McArdle's disease). N Engl J Med 329:241, 1993.

CHAPTER 618
Metabolic Myopathies

618.1 Potassium-Related Periodic Paralysis

Episodic weakness or paralysis known as *periodic paralysis* is associated with transient alterations in serum potassium levels, usually hypokalemia but occasionally hyperkalemia. The disorder is inherited as an autosomal dominant trait. It is precipitated in some patients by hyperaldosteronism or hyperthyroidism, by administration of amphotericin B, or by ingestion of licorice. The defective genes are at the 17q13.1–13.3 locus in *hyperkalemic periodic paralysis,* the same as in paramyotonia congenita, and at the 1q31–32 locus in *hypokalemic periodic paralysis.*

In childhood, periodic paralysis is often an episodic event; patients are unable to move after awakening and gradually recover muscle strength during the next few minutes or hours. Muscles that remain active in sleep, such as the diaphragm and cardiac muscle, are not affected. Patients are normal between attacks, but in adult life the attacks become more frequent, and the disorder causes progressive myopathy with permanent weakness even between attacks.

Alterations in serum potassium level occur only during acute episodes and are accompanied by T-wave changes in the electrocardiogram (ECG). The creatine phosphokinase (CK) level may be mildly elevated at those times. Muscle biopsy findings are often normal between attacks, but during an attack a vacuolar myopathy is demonstrated. The vacuoles are dilated sarcoplasmic reticulum and invaginations of the extracellular space into the cytoplasm, and they may be filled with glycogen. Hypoglycemia does not occur.

618.2 Malignant Hyperthermia

(See also Chapters 73 and 615.4)

This syndrome is usually inherited as an autosomal dominant trait. It occurs in all patients with central core disease but is not limited to that particular myopathy. The gene is at the 19q13.1 locus in both central core disease and malignant hyperthermia without this specific myopathy. One candidate gene is the ryanodine receptor, a tetrameric calcium release channel in the sarcoplasmic reticulum. It occurs rarely in Duchenne's and other muscular dystrophies, in various other myopathies, and in an isolated syndrome not associated with other muscle disease. Affected children sometimes have peculiar facies. All ages are affected, including premature infants whose mothers underwent general anesthesia for cesarean section.

Acute episodes are precipitated by exposure to general anesthetics and occasionally to local anesthetic drugs. Patients suddenly develop extreme fever, rigidity of muscles, and metabolic and respiratory acidosis; the serum CK level rises to as high as 35,000 IU/L. Myoglobinuria may result in tubular necrosis and acute renal failure.

The muscle biopsy during an episode of malignant hyperthermia or shortly afterward shows widely scattered necrosis of muscle fibers **(rhabdomyolysis).** Between attacks, the muscle biopsy findings are normal unless there is an underlying chronic myopathy.

It is important to recognize patients at risk for malignant hyperthermia because the *attacks may be prevented by administering dantrolene sodium before an anesthetic is given.* Identification of patients at risk, such as siblings of those who have experienced an episode, is done by the caffeine contracture test: A portion of fresh muscle biopsy tissue in a saline bath is attached to a strain gauge and exposed to caffeine and other drugs; an abnormal spasm is diagnostic. The gene defect of the ryanodine receptor is present in 50% of patients; gene testing is available only for this genetic group.

618.3 Glycogenoses

(See also Chapter 84)

Glycogenosis I **(von Gierke disease)** is not a true myopathy because the deficient liver enzyme, glucose-6-phosphatase, is not normally present in muscle. Nevertheless, children with this disease are hypotonic and mildly weak for uncertain reasons.

Glycogenosis II **(Pompe disease)** is an autosomal recessively inherited deficiency of the glycolytic lysosomal enzyme acid maltase. The defective gene is at locus 17q23. Two forms are described. The infantile form is a severe generalized myopathy and cardiomyopathy. Patients have cardiomegaly and hepatomegaly and are diffusely hypotonic and weak. The serum CK level is greatly elevated. Muscle biopsy reveals a vacuolar myopathy with abnormal lysosomal enzymatic activities such as acid and alkaline phosphatases (Fig. 618–1). Death in infancy or early childhood is usual.

The late childhood or adult form is a much milder myopathy without cardiac or hepatic enlargement. It may not become clinically expressed until later childhood or early adult life but may be symptomatic as myopathic weakness and hypotonia even in early infancy. The serum CK level is greatly elevated, and the muscle biopsy findings are diagnostic even in the presymptomatic stage.

The diagnosis of glycogenosis II is confirmed by quantitative assay of acid maltase activity in muscle or liver biopsy tissue. A rare KM variant of the milder form of acid maltase deficiency may show muscle acid maltase activity in the low normal range with only intermittent decreases to subnormal values, but the muscle biopsy findings are similar though milder.

Glycogenosis III **(Cori-Forbes disease)**, deficiency of debrancher enzyme (amylo-1,6-glucosidase), is the most common of the glycogenoses but also the least severe. Hypotonia, weakness, hepatomegaly, and fasting hypoglycemia in infancy are common, but these features often resolve spontaneously, and patients become asymptomatic in childhood and adult life. Others experience slowly progressive distal muscle wasting, hepatic cirrhosis, and heart failure. Minor myopathic findings including vacuolation of muscle fibers are found in the muscle biopsy specimen.

Glycogenosis IV **(Andersen disease)** is a deficiency of brancher enzyme, resulting in the formation of an abnormal glycogen molecule, amylopectin, in the liver, reticuloendothelial cells, and skeletal and cardiac muscle. Hypotonia, generalized weakness, muscle wasting, and contractures are the usual signs of myopathic involvement. Most patients die before age 4 yr because of hepatic or cardiac failure. A few children without neuromuscular manifestations have been described.

Glycogenosis V **(McArdle disease)** is due to muscle phosphorylase deficiency inherited as an autosomal recessive trait at locus 11q13. Exercise intolerance is the cardinal clinical feature. Physical exertion results in cramps, weakness, and myoglobinuria, but strength is normal between attacks. The serum CK level is elevated only during exercise. A characteristic clinical feature is lack of the normal rise in serum lactate level during ischemic exercise because of inability to convert pyruvate to lactate under anaerobic conditions in vivo. Myophosphorylase deficiency may be demonstrated histochemically and biochemically in the muscle biopsy tissue.

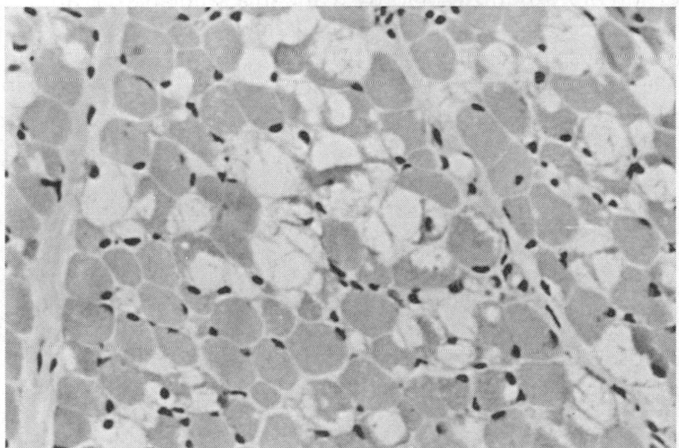

Figure 618–1 Muscle biopsy of a 2-yr-old boy with glycogenosis II (Pompe disease; acid maltase deficiency). More than half of the myofibers have large vacuoles replacing contractile myofibrils and cytoplasmic organelles. Special stains show glycogen storage and abnormally strong activity of lysosomal enzymes. (Hematoxylin & eosin, ×250.)

A rare *neonatal form of myophosphorylase deficiency* causes feeding difficulties in early infancy, may be severe enough to result in neonatal death, or may follow a course of slowly progressive weakness resembling a muscular dystrophy.

The long-term prognosis is good. Patients must learn to moderate their physical activities, but they do not develop severe chronic myopathic handicaps or cardiac involvement.

Glycogenosis VII **(Tarui disease)** is muscle phosphofructokinase deficiency. Although this disease is rarer than glycogenosis V, the symptoms of exercise intolerance, clinical course, and inability to convert pyruvate to lactate are identical. The distinction is made by biochemical study of the muscle biopsy specimen. It is transmitted as an autosomal recessive trait at the 1cenq32 locus.

618.4 Mitochondrial Myopathies

(See also Chapter 607.2)

Several diseases involving muscle, brain, and other organs are associated with structural and functional abnormalities of mitochondria, producing defects in aerobic cellular metabolism, the electron transport chain, and the Krebs cycle. The structural aberrations are best demonstrated by electron microscopy of the muscle biopsy sample, revealing abnormally shaped cristae and fusion of cristae to form paracrystalline structures. Histochemical study of sections of muscle biopsy material reveal abnormal clumping of oxidative enzymatic activity, sometimes increased neutral lipids because of impaired lipid metabolism, and ragged-red muscle fibers with accumulations of membranous material beneath the muscle fiber membrane, best demonstrated by special stains. These characteristic histochemical and ultrastructural changes in the muscle biopsy specimen are most consistently seen only with point mutation in mitochondrial tRNA; the large mtDNA deletions of 5 or 7.4 kb (the single mitochondrial chromosome has 16.5 kb) are associated with defects in mitochondrial respiratory oxidative enzyme complexes, but minimal or no morphologic or histochemical changes may be noted in the muscle biopsy specimen, even by electron microscopy; hence, the quantitative biochemical studies of the muscle tissue are needed to confirm the diagnosis.

Several distinct mitochondrial diseases that primarily affect striated muscle or muscle and brain are identified. The *Kearns-Sayre syndrome* is characterized by the triad of progressive external ophthalmoplegia, pigmentary degeneration of the retina, and onset before age 20 yr. Heart block, cerebellar deficits, and high cerebrospinal fluid protein content are often associated. Visual evoked potentials are abnormal. Patients usually do not experience weakness of the trunk or extremities or dysphagia. Most cases are sporadic.

Chronic progressive external ophthalmoplegia may be isolated or accompanied by limb muscle weakness, dysphagia, and dysarthria. A few patients described as having *ophthalmoplegia plus* have additional central nervous system (CNS) involvement. Autosomal dominant inheritance is found in some pedigrees, but most cases are sporadic.

Myoclonic epilepsy and *ragged-red fibers (MERRF)* and the *MELAS syndrome*, an acronym for mitochondrial myopathy, encephalopathy, lactic acidosis, and strokelike episodes, are other mitochondrial disorders affecting children. The latter is characterized by stunted growth, episodic vomiting, seizures, and recurrent cerebral insults causing hemiparesis, hemianopia or even cortical blindness, and dementia. The disease behaves as a degenerative disorder, and children die within a few years. Ragged-red fibers are characteristic of combined defects in oxidative respiratory complexes I and IV.

Other "degenerative" diseases of the CNS that also involve myopathy with mitochondrial abnormalities include *Leigh sub-*

acute necrotizing encephalopathy (see Chapter 84.4) and *cerebrohepatorenal (Zellweger) disease* (see Chapter 83.2). Another recognized mitochondrial myopathy is *cytochrome-c-oxidase deficiency. Oculopharyngeal muscular dystrophy* is also fundamentally a mitochondrial myopathy. Many other rare diseases with only a few case reports are suspected of being mitochondrial disorders.

Mitochondrial DNA is distinct from the DNA of the cell nucleus and is inherited exclusively from the mother; mitochondria are present in the cytoplasm of the ovum but not in the head of the sperm, the only part that enters the ovum at fertilization. The rate of mutation of mitochondrial DNA is 10 times higher than that of nuclear DNA. The mitochondrial respiratory enzyme complexes each have subunits encoded either in mtDNA or in nuclear DNA. For example, complex II (succinate dehydrogenase, a Krebs cycle enzyme) has 4 subunits, all encoded in nuclear DNA; complex III (ubiquinol or cytochrome-b-oxidase) has 9 subunits, only one of which is encoded in mtDNA and 8 of which are programmed by nuclear DNA; complex IV (cytochrome-c-oxidase) has 13 subunits, only 3 of which are encoded by mtDNA. For this reason, mitochondrial diseases of muscle may be transmitted as autosomal recessive traits rather than by strict maternal transmission even though all mitochondria are inherited from the mother.

In the Kearns-Sayre syndrome, a single large mtDNA deletion has been identified; in the MERRF and MELAS syndrome of mitochondrial myopathy, point mutations occur in tRNA (see Table 615–1).

There is no effective treatment of mitochondrial cytopathies, but various "cocktails" are often used empirically to try to overcome the metabolic deficits. These include oral carnitine supplements, riboflavin, coenzyme Q_{10}, ascorbic acid (vitamin C), vitamin E, and other antioxidants. Though some anecdotal reports are encouraging, no controlled studies that prove efficacy are published.

618.5 Lipid Myopathies

(See Chapter 83.4)

Considered as metabolic organs, skeletal muscles are the most important sites in the body for long-chain fatty acid metabolism because of their large mass and their rich density of mitochondria where fatty acids are metabolized. Hereditary disorders of lipid metabolism that cause progressive myopathy are an important, relatively common, and often treatable group of muscle diseases.

Muscle carnitine deficiency is an autosomal recessive disease involving deficient transport of dietary carnitine across the intestinal mucosa. Carnitine is acquired from dietary sources but is also synthesized in the liver and kidneys from lysine and methionine; it is the obligatory carrier of long- and medium-chain fatty acids into muscle mitochondria.

The clinical course may be one of sudden exacerbations of weakness or may resemble a progressive muscular dystrophy with generalized proximal myopathy and sometimes facial, pharyngeal, and cardiac involvement. Symptoms usually begin in late childhood or adolescence or may be delayed until adult life. Progression is slow but may end in death.

Serum CK level is mildly elevated. Muscle biopsy material shows vacuoles filled with lipid within muscle fibers in addition to nonspecific changes suggestive of a muscular dystrophy. Mitochondria may appear normal or abnormal. Carnitine measured in muscle biopsy tissue is reduced, but serum carnitine level is normal.

Treatment stops the progression of the disease and may even restore lost strength if the disease is not too advanced. It consists of special diets low in long-chain fatty acids. Steroids may enhance fatty acid transport. Specific therapy with L-carnitine taken by mouth in large doses overcomes the intestinal barrier in some patients. Some patients also improve when given supplementary riboflavin, and other patients seem to improve with propranolol.

Systemic carnitine deficiency is a disease of impaired renal and hepatic synthesis of carnitine rather than a primary myopathy. Patients with this autosomal recessive disease experience progressive proximal myopathy and show muscle biopsy changes similar to those of muscle carnitine deficiency; however, the onset of weakness is earlier and may be evident at birth. Endocardial fibroelastosis also may occur. Episodes of acute hepatic encephalopathy resembling Reye syndrome may occur. Hypoglycemia and metabolic acidosis complicate acute episodes.

The concentration of carnitine is reduced in serum as well as in muscle and liver. A similar clinical syndrome may be a complication of the renal Fanconi syndrome, because of excessive urinary loss of carnitine or during chronic hemodialysis.

Treatment with L-carnitine improves the maintenance of blood glucose and serum carnitine levels but does not reverse the ketosis or acidosis or improve exercise capacity.

Muscle carnitine palmityltransferase (CPT) deficiency presents as episodes of rhabdomyolysis, coma, and elevated serum CK level that may be indistinguishable from Reye syndrome. CPT transfers long-chain fatty acid–acyl-CoA residues to carnitine on the outer mitochondrial membrane for transport into the mitochondria. Exercise intolerance and myoglobinuria resemble glycogenoses V and VII (see earlier). Fasting hypoglycemia may also occur. Genetic transmission is autosomal recessive owing to a defect on chromosome 1 at the 1p32 locus.

618.6 Vitamin E Deficiency Myopathy

Deficiency of vitamin E in experimental animals produces a progressive myopathy closely resembling a muscular dystrophy. Myopathy and neuropathy are recognized in humans who lack adequate intake of this antioxidant. Patients with chronic malabsorption, those undergoing long-term dialysis, and premature infants who do not receive vitamin E supplements are particularly vulnerable. Treatment with high doses of vitamin E may reverse the deficiency.

CHAPTER 619 Disorders of Neuromuscular Transmission and of Motor Neurons

619.1 Myasthenia Gravis

Myasthenia gravis is a disease caused by an immune-mediated neuromuscular blockade. The release of acetylcholine (ACh) into the synaptic cleft by the axonal terminal is normal, but the postsynaptic muscle membrane or *motor end plate* is less responsive than normal. A decreased number of available ACh receptors is due to circulating receptor-binding antibodies in most cases of acquired myasthenia. The disease is generally nonhereditary and is an autoimmune disorder. A rare familial myasthenia gravis is probably an autosomal recessive trait and is not associated with plasma anti-ACh antibodies. Infants born to myasthenic mothers may have a transient neonatal myasthenic syndrome secondary to placentally transferred anti-ACh receptor antibodies, distinct from congenital myasthenia gravis.

CLINICAL MANIFESTATIONS. Ptosis and some degree of extraocular muscle weakness are the earliest and most constant signs in myasthenia gravis. Older children may complain of diplopia, and young children may hold open their eyes with their fingers or thumbs if the ptosis is severe enough to obstruct vision. The pupillary responses to light are preserved. Dysphagia and facial weakness are also common, and in early infancy feeding difficulties are often the cardinal sign of myasthenia. Poor head control due to weakness of the neck flexors is also prominent. Involvement may be limited to bulbar-innervated muscles, but the disease is systemic and weakness involves limb-girdle muscles and distal muscles of the hands in most cases. Fasciculations of muscle, myalgias, and sensory symptoms do not occur. Tendon stretch reflexes may be diminished but are rarely lost.

Rapid fatigue of muscles is a characteristic feature of myasthenia gravis that distinguishes it from most other neuromuscular diseases. Ptosis increases progressively as patients are asked to sustain an upward gaze for 30–90 sec. Holding the head up from the surface of the examining table while lying supine is very difficult, and gravity cannot be overcome for more than a few seconds. Repetitive opening and closing of the fists produces rapid fatigue of hand muscles, and patients cannot elevate their arms for more than 1–2 min because of fatigue of the deltoids. A carefully taken history also discloses that patients are more symptomatic late in the day or when tired. Dysphagia may interfere with eating, and the muscles of the jaw soon tire when an affected child chews.

If untreated, myasthenia gravis is usually progressive and may become life threatening because of respiratory muscle involvement and the risk of aspiration, particularly at times when the child is otherwise unwell with an upper respiratory infection. Familial myasthenia gravis usually is not progressive.

Infants born to myasthenic mothers may have respiratory insufficiency, inability to suck or swallow, and generalized hypotonia and weakness. They may show little spontaneous motor activity for several days to weeks. Some require ventilatory support and feeding by gavage during this period. After the abnormal antibodies disappear, the infants have normal strength and are not at increased risk for developing myasthenia gravis in later childhood. The syndrome of **transient neonatal myasthenia gravis** is to be distinguished from a rare and often hereditary **congenital myasthenia gravis** not related to maternal myasthenia that is nearly always a permanent disorder without spontaneous remission. An abnormality of the ACh receptor channels appearing as high conductance and excessively fast closure may be due to a point mutation in a subunit of the receptor affecting a single amino acid residue. Children with congenital myasthenia gravis do not experience myasthenic crises and rarely exhibit elevations of anti-ACh antibodies in plasma.

Myasthenia gravis is occasionally secondary to hypothyroidism, usually *Hashimoto thyroiditis*. Other collagen vascular diseases may also be associated. Thymomas, noted in some adults, rarely coexist with myasthenia gravis in children; nor do carcinomas of the lung occur, which produce a unique form of myasthenia in adults, the *Eaton-Lambert syndrome*.

LABORATORY FINDINGS AND DIAGNOSIS. Myasthenia gravis is one of the few neuromuscular diseases in which an *electromyogram* (EMG) is more specifically diagnostic than a muscle biopsy. A decremental response is seen in response to repetitive nerve stimulation; the muscle potentials diminish rapidly in amplitude until the muscle becomes refractory to further stimulation. Motor nerve conduction velocity remains normal. This unique EMG pattern is the electrophysiologic correlate of the fatigable weakness observed clinically and is reversed after a cholinesterase inhibitor is administered. A myasthenic decrement may be absent or difficult to demonstrate in muscles that are not involved clinically. This feature may be confusing in early cases or in patients showing only weakness of extraocular muscles.

Anti-ACh antibodies should be assayed in the plasma but are inconsistently demonstrated. About one third of adolescents show elevations, but anti-ACh receptor antibodies are only occasionally demonstrated in the plasma of prepubertal children. Other serologic tests of autoimmune disease, such as antinuclear antibodies and abnormal immune complexes, should also be sought. If these are positive, more extensive autoimmune disease involving vasculitis or tissues other than muscle is likely. A thyroid profile should always be examined. The serum creatine phosphokinase (CK) level is normal in myasthenia gravis.

The heart is not involved, and the electrocardiogram (ECG) findings remain normal. Roentgenograms of the chest often reveal an enlarged thymus, but the hypertrophy is not a *thymoma*. It may be further defined by tomography or by CT imaging of the anterior mediastinum.

The role of *muscle biopsy* in myasthenia gravis is limited. It is not required in most cases, but about 17% of patients show inflammatory changes sometimes called **lymphorrhages** that are interpreted by some physicians as a mixed myasthenia-polymyositis immune disorder. Muscle biopsy tissue in myasthenia gravis shows nonspecific type II muscle fiber atrophy, similar to that seen with disuse atrophy, steroid effects on muscle, polymyalgia rheumatica, and many other conditions. The ultrastructure of motor end plates shows simplification of the membrane folds.

A *clinical test for myasthenia gravis* is administration of a short-acting cholinesterase inhibitor, usually edrophonium chloride. A small test dose is given intravenously (IV) initially to ensure that the patient is not allergic; if tolerated, the full dose of 0.2 mg/kg (maximum dose 10 mg) is given IV a few minutes later. Children weighing less than 30 kg should be given only 1–2 mg total dose. Within a few seconds, the ptosis and ophthalmoplegia improve, and fatigability of other muscles is greatly decreased. The effects last only 1–2 min. Edrophonium should not be given to young infants because cardiac arrhythmias may result. An alternative with fewer cardiogenic side effects is intramuscular (IM) neostigmine. If the initial test dose of 0.04 mg/kg produces negative results, the infant may be retested 4 hr later with 0.08 mg/kg. A maximal effect occurs in 20–40 min. Because of muscarinic side effects, such as abdominal distention, diarrhea, and profuse tracheal secretions, 0.01 mg/kg of atropine may be given just before the neostigmine.

TREATMENT. Some patients with mild myasthenia gravis require no treatment. *Cholinesterase-inhibiting drugs* are the primary therapeutic agents. Neostigmine methylsulfate (0.04 mg/kg) may be given IM every 4–6 hr, but most patients tolerate oral neostigmine bromide, 0.4 mg/kg every 4–6 hr. If dysphagia is a major problem, the drug should be given about 30 min before meals to improve swallowing. Pyridostigmine is an alternative; the dose required is about four times greater than that of neostigmine, but it may be slightly longer acting. Overdoses of cholinesterase inhibitors produce cholinergic crises; atropine blocks the muscarinic effects but does not block the nicotinic effects that produce additional skeletal muscle weakness.

Because of the autoimmune basis of the disease, long-term *steroid treatment* with prednisone may be effective. *Thymectomy* should be considered and may provide a cure. Thymectomy is most effective in patients with high titers of anti-Ach-receptor antibodies in the plasma and who are symptomatic for less than 2 yr. Thymectomy is ineffective in congenital and familial forms of myasthenia gravis. Treatment of hypothyroidism usually abolishes an associated myasthenia without the use of cholinesterase inhibitors or steroids.

Plasmapheresis is effective treatment in some children, particularly those who do not respond to steroids, but plasma exchange therapy may provide only temporary remission. *Intravenous immunoglobulin* (IVIG) is sometimes beneficial and might be tried before plasmapheresis because it is less invasive. Both plasmapheresis and IVIG appear to be most effective in patients with high circulating levels of anti-ACh receptor antibodies.

Neonates with transient maternally transmitted myasthenia gravis require cholinesterase inhibitors for only a few days or occasionally for a few weeks, especially to allow feeding. No other treatment is usually necessary.

COMPLICATIONS. Children with myasthenia gravis do not tolerate neuromuscular blocking drugs, such as succinylcholine and pancuronium, and may be paralyzed for weeks after a single dose. An anesthesiologist should carefully review myasthenic patients who require a surgical anesthetic. Also, certain antibiotics may potentiate myasthenia and should be avoided; these include the aminoglycosides (gentamicin and others).

PROGNOSIS. This is difficult to predict. Some patients undergo spontaneous remission after a period of months or years; others have a permanent disease extending into adult life. Immunosuppression, thymectomy, and treatment of associated hypothyroidism may provide a cure.

OTHER CAUSES OF NEUROMUSCULAR BLOCKADE

Organophosphate chemicals, commonly used as insecticides, may cause a myasthenia-like syndrome in children exposed to these toxins (see Chapter 722).

Botulism results from ingestion of food containing the toxin of *Clostridium botulinum,* a gram-positive, spore-bearing, anaerobic bacillus (see Chapter 208). Honey is a frequent source of contamination. The incubation period is short, only a few hours, and symptoms begin with nausea, vomiting, and diarrhea. Cranial nerve involvement soon follows, with diplopia, dysphagia, weak suck, facial weakness, and absent gag reflex. Generalized hypotonia and weakness then develop and may progress to respiratory failure. Neuromuscular blockade is documented by EMG with repetitive nerve stimulation. Respiratory support may be required for days or weeks until the toxin is cleared from the body. No specific antitoxin is available. Guanidine, 35 mg/kg/24 hr, may be effective for extraocular and limb muscle weakness but not for respiratory muscle involvement.

Tick paralysis is a disorder of ACh release from axonal terminals due to a neurotoxin that blocks depolarization. It also affects large myelinated motor and sensory nerve fibers. This toxin is produced by the wood tick or dog tick, insects common in the Appalachian and Rocky Mountains of North America. The tick embeds its head into the skin, usually the scalp, and neurotoxin production is maximal about 5–6 days later. Motor symptoms include weakness, loss of coordination, and sometimes an ascending paralysis resembling Guillain-Barré syndrome. Tendon reflexes are lost. Sensory symptoms of tingling paresthesias may occur in the face and extremities. The diagnosis is confirmed by EMG and nerve conduction studies and by identifying the tick. The tick must be removed completely, and the buried head not left beneath the skin. Patients then recover completely within hours or days.

619.2 Spinal Muscular Atrophies

Spinal muscular atrophies (SMA) are degenerative diseases of motor neurons that begin in fetal life and continue to be progressive in infancy and childhood. The progressive denervation of muscle is compensated in part by reinnervation from an adjacent motor unit, but giant motor units are thus created with subsequent atrophy of muscle fibers when the reinnervating motor neuron eventually becomes involved. Upper motor neurons remain normal.

SMA is classified into a severe infantile form, also known as **Werdnig-Hoffmann disease** or SMA type 1; a late infantile and more slowly progressive form, SMA type 2; and a more chronic or juvenile form, also called **Kugelberg-Welander disease,** or SMA type 3. These distinctions are clinical and are based on age of onset, severity of weakness, and clinical course; muscle biopsy does not distinguish types 1 and 2, although type 3 shows a more adult than perinatal pattern of denervation-reinnervation. Some patients are transitional between types 1 and 2 or between types 2 and 3 in terms of clinical function. A variant of SMA, **Fazio-Londe disease,** is a progressive bulbar palsy resulting from motor neuron degeneration more in the brain stem than the spinal cord.

ETIOLOGY. The etiology of SMA is a pathologic continuation of a process of programmed cell death that is normal in embryonic life. A surplus of motor neuroblasts and other neurons is generated from primitive neuroectoderm, but only about half survive and mature to become neurons; the excess cells have a limited life cycle and degenerate. If the process that arrests physiologic cell death fails to intervene by a certain stage, neuronal death may continue in late fetal life and postnatally. The survivor motor neuron (SMN) gene arrests apoptosis (programmed cell death) of motor neuroblasts.

CLINICAL MANIFESTATIONS. The cardinal features of SMA type 1 are severe hypotonia; generalized weakness; thin muscle mass; absent tendon stretch reflexes; involvement of the tongue, face, and jaw muscles; and sparing of extraocular muscles and sphincters. Infants who are symptomatic at birth may have respiratory distress and are unable to feed. Congenital contractures, ranging from simple clubfoot to generalized arthrogryposis, occur in about 10% of severely involved neonates. Infants lie flaccid with little movement, unable to overcome gravity. They lack head control. More than two thirds die by 2 yr of age, and many early in infancy.

In type 2 SMA, affected infants are usually able to suck and swallow, and respiration is adequate in early infancy. They show progressive weakness, but many survive into the school years or beyond, though confined to an electric wheelchair and severely handicapped. Nasal speech and problems with deglutition develop later. Scoliosis becomes a major complication in many patients with long survival.

Kugelberg-Welander disease is the mildest SMA (type 3), and patients may appear normal in infancy. The progressive weakness is proximal in distribution, particularly involving shoulder girdle muscles. Patients are ambulatory. Symptoms of bulbar muscle weakness are rare. Longevity may extend well into middle adult life. Fasciculations are a specific clinical sign of denervation of muscle. In thin children, they may be seen in the deltoid, biceps brachii, and occasionally the quadriceps femoris, but the continuous involuntary wormlike movements may be masked by a thick pad of subcutaneous fat. Fasciculations are best observed in the tongue, where almost no subcutaneous connective tissue separates the muscular layer from the epithelium. If the intrinsic lingual muscles are contracted, such as in crying or when the tongue protrudes, fasciculations are more difficult to see than when the tongue is relaxed.

The outstretched fingers of children with SMA often show a characteristic tremor due to fasciculations and weakness. It should not be confused with a cerebellar tremor. Myalgias are not a feature of SMA.

The heart is not involved in SMA. Intelligence is normal, and children often appear brighter than their normal peers because the effort they cannot put into physical activities is redirected to intellectual development, and they are often exposed to adult speech more than to juvenile language because of the social repercussions of the disease.

LABORATORY FINDINGS. The serum CK level may be normal but more commonly is mildly elevated in the hundreds. A CK level of several thousand is occasionally demonstrated. Results of motor nerve conduction studies are normal, an important feature distinguishing SMA from peripheral neuropathy. The EMG shows fibrillation potentials and other signs of denervation of muscle.

DIAGNOSIS. Muscle biopsy tissue in SMA reveals a characteristic pattern of perinatal denervation that is unlike that of mature muscle. Groups of giant type I fibers are mixed with fascicles of severely atrophic fibers of both histochemical types (Fig. 619–1). In juvenile SMA, the pattern may be more similar to adult muscle that has undergone many cycles of denervation and reinnervation. Neurogenic changes in muscle also may be demonstrated by EMG, but the results are less definitive than by muscle biopsy in infancy.

Sural nerve biopsy sometimes shows mild sensory neuropathic changes, and sensory nerve conduction velocity may be slowed. At autopsy, mild degenerative changes are seen in sensory neurons of dorsal root ganglia and in somatosensory nuclei of the thalamus, but these alterations are not perceived clinically as sensory loss or paresthesias. The most pronounced neuropathologic lesions are the extensive neuronal degeneration and gliosis in the ventral horns of the spinal cord and brain stem motor nuclei, especially the hypoglossal nucleus.

GENETICS. Molecular genetic diagnosis by DNA probes in blood samples or in muscle biopsy or chorionic villi tissues are available not only for diagnosis of suspected cases but also for prenatal diagnosis. Most cases are inherited as an autosomal recessive trait. The incidence of SMA is 1/25,000, affecting all ethnic groups; it is the second most common neuromuscular disease, following Duchenne muscular dystrophy. The genetic locus for all three of the common forms of SMA is on chromosome 5, a deletion at the 5q11–q13 locus, indicating that they are variants of the same disease rather than different diseases. A few families with autosomal dominant inheritance are described, and a rare X-linked recessive form is reported. Carrier testing by dosage analysis is available.

TREATMENT. No medical treatment is able to delay the progression. Supportive therapy includes orthopedic care with particular attention to scoliosis and joint contractures, mild physiotherapy, and mechanical aids for assisting the child to eat and to be as functionally independent as possible. Most children learn to use a computer keyboard with great skill but cannot use a pencil easily.

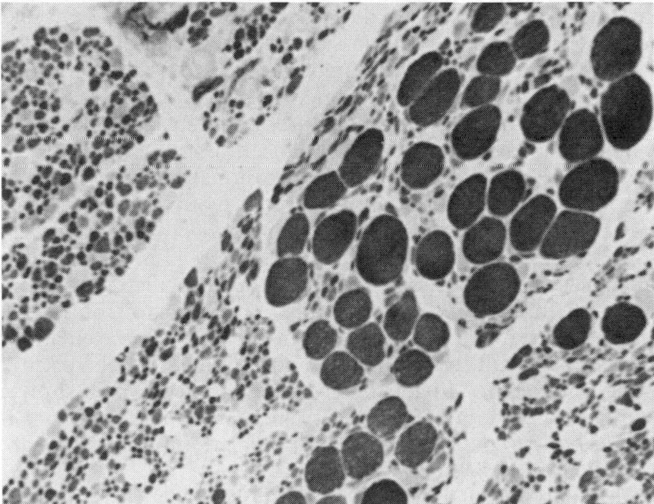

Figure 619–1 Muscle biopsy of neonate with infantile spinal muscular atrophy. Groups of giant type I (darkly stained) fibers are seen within muscle fascicles of severely atrophic fibers of both histochemical types. This is the characteristic pattern of perinatal denervation of muscle. Myofibrillar ATPase, preincubated at pH 4.6. (×400.)

619.3 Other Motor Neuron Diseases

Motor neuron diseases other than SMA are rare in children. *Poliomyelitis* used to be a major cause of chronic disability, but since the routine use of polio vaccine, this viral infection is now rare (see Chapter 243.1). *Other enteroviruses*, such as Coxsackie and ECHO viruses, or the live polio vaccine virus, may also cause an acute infection of motor neurons with symptoms and signs similar to poliomyelitis, although usually milder. Specific polymerase chain reaction tests and viral cultures of cerebrospinal fluid are diagnostic.

A *juvenile form of amyotrophic lateral sclerosis* is rare. Upper motor neuron loss as well as lower motor neuron loss is evident clinically, unlike SMA. The course is progressive and is ultimately fatal.

The *Pena-Shokeir* and *Marden-Walker syndromes* are progressive motor neuron degenerations associated with severe arthrogryposis and congenital anomalies of many organ systems. *Pontocerebellar hypoplasias* are progressive degenerative diseases of the central nervous system that begin in fetal life; one form also involves motor neuron degeneration resembling a spinal muscular atrophy, but the SMN gene or chromosome 5 is normal.

Motor neurons become involved in several metabolic diseases of the nervous system, such as gangliosidosis (Tay-Sachs disease), ceroid lipofuscinosis (Batten disease), and glycogenosis II (Pompe disease), but the signs of denervation may be minor or obscured by the more prominent involvement of other parts of the central nervous system or of muscle.

Disorders of Neuromuscular Transmission

Afifi AK, Bell WE: Tests for juvenile myasthenia gravis: Comparative diagnostic yield and prediction of outcome. J Child Neurol 8:403, 1993.

Anlar B, Özdirim E, Renda Y, et al: Myasthenia gravis in childhood. Acta Paediatr 85:838, 1996.

Engel AG, Uchitel OD, Walls TJ, et al: Newly recognized congenital myasthenic syndrome associated with high conductance and fast closure of the acetylcholine receptor channel. Ann Neurol 34:38, 1993.

Pickett J, Berg B, Chaplin E, et al: Syndrome of botulism in infancy: Clinical and electrophysiologic studies. N Engl J Med 295:770, 1976.

Spinal Muscular Atrophies

Devriendt K, Lammens M, Schollen E, et al: Clinical and molecular genetic features of congenital spinal muscular atrophy. Ann Neurol 40:731, 1996.

Hageman G, Willemse J, van Ketel BA, et al: The heterogeneity of the Pena-Shokeir syndrome. Neuropediatrics 18:45, 1987.

Roy N, Mahedevan N, McLean M, et al: The gene for neuronal apoptosis inhibitory protein is partially deleted in individuals with spinal muscular atrophy. Cell 80:167, 1995.

Sees JN Jr, Towfighi J, Robins DB, Ladda RL: Marden-Walker syndrome: Neuropathologic findings in two siblings. Pediatr Pathol 10:807, 1990.

Souchon F, Simard LR, Lebrun S, et al: Clinical and genetic study of chronic (types II and III) childhood onset spinal muscular atrophy. Neuromuscul Disord 6:419, 1996.

Talbot K: What's new in the molecular genetics of spinal muscular atrophy? Eur J Paediatr Neurol 5/6:149, 1997.

CHAPTER 620

Hereditary Motor-Sensory Neuropathies

The hereditary motor-sensory neuropathies (HMSN) are a group of progressive diseases of peripheral nerves. Motor components generally dominate the clinical picture, but sensory and autonomic involvement are expressed later.

620.1 Peroneal Muscular Atrophy

(Charcot-Marie-Tooth Disease; HMSN Type I)

This disease is the most common genetically determined neuropathy and has an overall prevalence of 3.8/100,000. It is transmitted as an autosomal dominant trait with 83% expressivity; the 17p11.2 locus is the site of the abnormal gene. The gene product is *peripheral myelin protein P22* (PMP). A much rarer X-linked HMSN type I results from a defect at the Xq13.1 locus, causing mutations in the gap junction protein *connexin-32.*

CLINICAL MANIFESTATIONS. Most patients are asymptomatic until late childhood or early adolescence, but young children sometimes show signs of gait disturbance as early as the 2nd yr. The peroneal and tibial nerves are the earliest and most severely affected. Child patients are often described as being clumsy, falling easily, or tripping over their own feet. The onset of symptoms may be delayed until after the 5th decade.

Muscles of the anterior compartment of the lower legs become wasted, and the legs have a characteristic storklike contour. The muscular atrophy is accompanied by progressive weakness of dorsiflexion of the ankle and eventual footdrop. The process is bilateral but may be slightly asymmetric. Pes cavus deformities may develop because of denervation of intrinsic foot muscles, further destabilizing the gait. Atrophy of muscles of the forearms and hands is usually not as severe as that of the lower extremities, but in advanced cases contractures of the wrists and fingers produce a claw hand. Proximal muscle weakness is a late manifestation and is usually mild. Axial muscles are not involved.

The disease is slowly progressive throughout life, but patients occasionally show accelerated deterioration of function over a few years. Most patients remain ambulatory and have normal longevity, although orthotic appliances are required to stabilize the ankles.

Sensory involvement mainly affects large myelinated nerve fibers that convey proprioceptive information and vibratory sense, but the threshold for pain and temperature may also increase. Some children complain of tingling or burning sensations of the feet, but pain is rare. Because the muscle mass is reduced, the nerves are more vulnerable to trauma or compression. Autonomic manifestations may be expressed as poor vasomotor control with blotching or pallor of the skin of the feet and inappropriately cold feet.

Nerves often become palpably enlarged. Tendon stretch reflexes are lost distally. Cranial nerves are not affected. Sphincter control remains well preserved. Autonomic neuropathy does not affect the heart, gastrointestinal tract, or bladder. Intelligence is normal.

Davidenkow syndrome is a variant of HMSN type I with a scapuloperoneal distribution.

LABORATORY FINDINGS AND DIAGNOSIS. Motor and sensory nerve conduction velocities are greatly reduced, sometimes as slow as 20% of normal conduction time. Electromyogram (EMG) and muscle biopsy are not usually required for diagnosis, but they show evidence of many cycles of denervation and reinnervation. Serum creatine phosphokinase (CK) level is normal. Cerebrospinal fluid (CSF) protein may be elevated, but no cells appear in the CSF.

Sural nerve biopsy is diagnostic. Large- and medium-sized myelinated fibers are reduced in number, collagen is increased, and characteristic *onion bulb formations* of proliferated Schwann cell cytoplasm surround axons. This pathologic finding is called *interstitial hypertrophic neuropathy.* Extensive segmental demyelination and remyelination also occur.

The definitive molecular genetic diagnosis may be made in blood.

TREATMENT. Stabilization of the ankles is a primary concern. In early stages, stiff boots that extend to midcalf often suffice, particularly when patients walk on uneven surfaces such as ice and snow or stones. As the dorsiflexors of the ankles weaken further, lightweight plastic splints may be custom made to extend beneath the foot and around the back of the ankle. They are worn inside the socks and are not visible, reducing self-consciousness. External short leg braces may be required when footdrop becomes complete. Surgical fusion of the ankle may be considered in some cases.

The leg should be protected from traumatic injury. In advanced cases, compression neuropathy during sleep may be prevented by placing soft pillows beneath or between the lower legs. Burning paresthesias of the feet are not common but are often abolished by phenytoin or carbamazepine. No medical treatment is available to arrest or slow the progression.

In new cases without a family history, both parents should be examined, and nerve conduction studies should be performed.

620.2 Peroneal Muscular Atrophy, Axonal Type

(HMSN Type II)

This disease is clinically similar to HMSN type I, but the rate of progression is slower and the disability is less. EMG shows denervation of muscle. Sural nerve biopsy reveals axonal degeneration rather than the demyelination and whorls of Schwann cell processes typical in type I. The locus is on chromosome 1 at 1p35–p36; this is a different disease than HMSN type I though both are transmitted as autosomal dominant traits.

620.3 Dejerine-Sottas Disease

(HMSN Type III)

This interstitial hypertrophic neuropathy of autosomal dominant transmission is similar to HMSN type I but is more severe. Symptoms develop in early infancy and are rapidly progressive. Pupillary abnormalities, such as lack of reaction to light or **Argyll-Robertson pupil,** are common. Kyphoscoliosis and pes cavus deformities complicate about 35% of cases. Nerves become palpably enlarged at an early age.

The onion-bulb formations seen in the sural nerve biopsy specimen are more pronounced. Hypomyelination also occurs.

The genetic locus of 17p11.2 is identical to that of HMSN type I or Charcot-Marie-Tooth disease. The clinical and pathologic differences may be phenotypic variants of the same disease, analogous to the situation in Duchenne and Becker muscular dystrophies. An autosomal recessive form of Dejerine-Sottas disease is also described but is incompletely documented.

620.4 Roussy-Lévy Syndrome

This syndrome is defined as a combination of HMSN type I and cerebellar deficit resembling Friedreich's ataxia, but it does not have cardiomyopathy.

620.5 Refsum Disease

(See Chapter 83.2)

This rare disease is due to an enzymatic block in β-oxidation of phytanic acid to pristanic acid. Phytanic acid is a branched-chain fatty acid that is derived mainly from dietary sources: spinach, nuts, and coffee. Phytanic acid is greatly elevated in plasma, CSF, and brain tissue. The CSF shows an albuminocytologic dissociation with a protein concentration of 100–600 mg/dL.

Clinical onset is usually between 4 and 7 yr of age, with intermittent motor and sensory neuropathy. Ataxia, progressive neurosensory hearing loss, retinitis pigmentosa and loss of night vision, ichthyosis, and liver dysfunction also develop in various degrees. Motor and sensory nerve conduction velocities are delayed. Treatment is by dietary management and periodic plasma exchange.

620.6 Fabry Disease

This rare X-linked recessive trait results in storage of *ceramide trihexose* because of deficiency of the enzyme *ceramide trihexosidase,* which cleaves the terminal galactose from ceramide trihexose (ceramide–glucose-galactose-galactose), resulting in tissue accumulation of this trihexose lipid in central nervous system (CNS) neurons, Schwann cells and perineurial cells, ganglion cells of the myenteric plexus, skin, kidneys, blood vessel endothelial and smooth muscle cells, heart, sweat glands, cornea, and bone marrow.

CLINICAL MANIFESTATIONS. The presentation is in late childhood or adolescence, with recurrent episodes of burning pain and parestheias of the feet and lower legs so severe that patients are unable to walk. These episodes are often precipitated by fever or by physical activity. Objective sensory and motor deficits are not demonstrated on neurologic examination, and reflexes are preserved. Characteristic skin lesions are seen in the perineal region, scrotum, buttocks, and periumbilical zone as flat or raised red-black telangiectasia known as ***angiokeratoma corporis diffusum***. Hypohydrosis may be present. Corneal opacities, cataracts, and necrosis of the femoral heads are inconstant features. The disease is progressive. Hypertension and renal failure are usually delayed until early adult life. Recurrent strokes result from vascular wall involvement. Death occurs in the 5th decade owing to cerebral infarction or renal failure.

LABORATORY FINDINGS. Motor and sensory nerve conduction velocities are normal to only mildly slow, showing preservation of large myelinated nerve fibers. CSF protein is normal. Proteinuria is present early in the course.

Pathologic features are usually first detected in skin or sural nerve biopsy specimens. Crystalline glycosphingolipids appear as *zebra bodies* in lysosomes of endothelial cells, in smooth myocytes of arterioles, and in Schwann cells, best demonstrated by electron microscopy. Nerves show a selective loss of small myelinated fibers and relative preservation of large and medium-sized axons, contrasting with most axonal neuropathies in which large myelinated fibers are most involved.

Assay for the deficient enzyme may be performed from skin fibroblasts, leukocytes, and other tissues. This test permits detection of the asymptomatic female carrier state and provides a reliable means of prenatal diagnosis.

620.7 Giant Axonal Neuropathy

This rare autosomal recessive disease with onset in early childhood is a progressive mixed peripheral neuropathy. Ataxia and nystagmus usually develop. Most affected children have been noted to have peculiar curly reddish hair. Focal axonal enlargements are seen in both the peripheral nervous system and the CNS, but the myelin sheath is intact. The disease is thought to be a disorder of neurofilament synthesis or organization.

620.8 Congenital Hypomyelinating Neuropathy

This disorder is a lack of normal myelination of motor and sensory peripheral nerves but not of CNS white matter. It is not a degeneration or loss of previously formed myelin, thus differentiating it from a leukodystrophy. Schwann cells are preserved, and axons are normal. Cases in siblings suggest autosomal recessive inheritance.

The condition is present from birth; hypotonia and developmental delay are the hallmark clinical findings. Many patients present clinically as having congenital insensitivity to pain. Cranial nerves are inconsistently involved, and respiratory distress and dysphagia are rare complications. Tendon reflexes are absent. Arthrogryposis is present at birth in at least half the cases. It is uncertain whether the condition is progressive; myelination of nerves proceeds at a slow rate and remains incomplete. Motor and sensory nerve conduction velocities are slow. The diagnosis is confirmed by sural nerve biopsy, which shows lack of myelination of large and small fibers and sometimes interstitial hypertrophic reactive changes. Muscle biopsy may show mild neurogenic atrophy but not the characteristic alterations of spinal muscular atrophy. No inflammation is demonstrated in muscle or nerve.

620.9 Tomaculous Neuropathy

This hereditary neuropathy is characterized by redundant overproduction of myelin around each axon in an irregular segmental fashion so that tomaculous (i.e., sausage-shaped) bulges occur in the individual myelinated nerve fibers. The nerves are particularly prone to pressure palsies, and patients present with recurrent mononeuropathies secondary to minor trauma. It is transmitted as an autosomal dominant trait, and the locus has been identified at 17p11.2. Sural nerve biopsy is diagnostic, but special "teased fiber" preparations should be made to demonstrate the myelin abnormalities most clearly. The genetic defect is a deletion of exons in the PMP 22 gene.

620.10 Leukodystrophies

Several hereditary degenerative diseases of white matter of the CNS also cause peripheral neuropathy. The most important are Krabbe disease (globoid cell leukodystrophy), metachromatic leukodystrophy, and adrenoleukodystrophy (see Chapter 83).

Balestrini MR, Cavaletti G, D'Angelo A, et al: Infantile hereditary neuropathy with hypomyelination. Neuropediatrics 22:65, 1991.
Boylan KB, Ferriero DM, Greco CM, et al: Congenital hypomyelination neuropathy with arthrogryposis multiplex congenita. Ann Neurol 31:337, 1992.
Chance PF, Alderson MK, Leppig KA, et al: DNA deletion associated with hereditary neuropathy with liability to pressure palsies. Cell 72:143, 1993.
Flanigan KM, Crawford TO, Griffin JW, et al: Localization of the giant axonal neuropathy gene to chromosome 16q24. Ann Neurol 43:143, 1998.
Ouvrier RA: Giant axonal neuropathy: A review. Brain Dev 11:207, 1989.
Roa BB, Garcia CA, Pentao L, et al: Evidence for a recessive PMP22 point mutation in Charcot-Marie-Tooth disease type 1A. Nat Genet 5:189, 1993.
Ronen GM, Lowry N, Wedge JH, et al: Hereditary motor-sensory neuropathy

type I presenting as scapuloperoneal atrophy (Davidenkow syndrome): Electrophysiological and pathological studies. Can J Neurol Sci 13:264, 1986.

CHAPTER 621
Toxic Neuropathies

Many *chemicals* (organophosphates), *toxins*, and *drugs* are capable of causing peripheral neuropathy. *Heavy metals* are well-known neurotoxins. Lead poisoning, especially if chronic, causes mainly a motor neuropathy selectively involving large nerves, such as the common peroneal, radial, or median nerves, a condition known as **mononeuritis multiplex** (see Chapter 721). Arsenic produces painful burning paresthesias and motor polyneuropathy.

Antimetabolic drugs, especially vincristine, cisplatin and taxol produce polyneuropathies as complications of chemotherapy for neoplasms.

Chronic uremia is associated with toxic neuropathy and myopathy. The neuropathy is due to excessive levels of circulating parathormone. Reduction in serum parathyroid hormone levels is accompanied by clinical improvement and a return to normal of nerve conduction velocity.

CHAPTER 622
Autonomic Neuropathies

622.1 Familial Dysautonomia

Familial dysautonomia **(Riley-Day syndrome)** is an autosomal recessive disorder that is common in Eastern European Jews, among whom the incidence is 1/10,000–20,000, and the carrier state is estimated to be 1%. It is rare in other ethnic groups. The defective gene is at the 9q31–q33 locus.

PATHOLOGY. This disease of the peripheral nervous system is characterized pathologically by a reduced number of small unmyelinated nerve fibers that carry pain, temperature, and taste sensations and that mediate autonomic functions. Large myelinated afferent nerve fibers that relay impulses from muscle spindles and Golgi tendon organs are also deficient. The degree of demonstrable anatomic change in peripheral and especially autonomic nerves is variable. Fungiform papillae of the tongue (taste buds) are absent or reduced in number.

CLINICAL MANIFESTATIONS. The disease is expressed in infancy by poor sucking and swallowing. Aspiration pneumonia may occur. Feeding difficulties remain a major symptom throughout childhood. Vomiting crises may occur. Excessive sweating and blotchy erythema of the skin are common, especially at mealtime or when the child is excited. Breath-holding spells followed by syncope are common in the first 5 yr. As affected children become older, insensitivity to pain becomes evident and traumatic injuries are frequent. Corneal ulcerations are common. Newly erupting teeth cause tongue ulcerations. Walking is delayed or clumsy or appears ataxic because of poor sensory feedback from muscle spindles. The ataxia is probably related more to deficient muscle spindle feedback and to vestibular nerve dysfunction than to cerebellar involvement. Tendon stretch reflexes are absent. Scoliosis is a serious complication in the majority of patients and usually is progressive. Normal overflow tearing with crying does not usually develop until 2–3 mo of age but fails to develop after that time or is severely reduced in children with familial dysautonomia.

About 40% of patients have generalized major motor seizures, some of which are associated with acute hypoxia during breath-holding, some with extreme fevers but most without an apparent precipitating event. Body temperature is poorly controlled; both hypothermia and extreme fevers occur. Intellectual function is usually impaired but is unrelated to epilepsy. Puberty is often delayed, especially in girls. Speech is often slurred or nasal.

After 3 yr of age, **autonomic crises** begin, usually with attacks of cyclic vomiting lasting 24–72 hr or even several days. Retching and vomiting occur every 15–20 min and are associated with hypertension, profuse sweating, blotching of the skin, apprehension, and irritability. Prominent gastric distention may occur, causing abdominal pain and even respiratory distress. Hematemesis may complicate pernicious vomiting.

Allgrove syndrome is a clinical variant, involving alacrima, achalasia, autonomic dysfunction with orthostatic hypotension and altered heart rate variability, and sensorimotor polyneuropathy, usually presenting in adolescence. Cholinergic dysfunction may be demonstrated.

LABORATORY FINDINGS. Electrocardiography discloses prolonged correcting QT intervals with lack of appropriate shortening with exercise, a reflection of the aberration in autonomic regulation of cardiac conduction. Chest roentgenograms show atelectasis and pulmonary changes resembling cystic fibrosis. Urinary vanillylmandelic acid (VMA) level is decreased, and homovanillic acid (HVA) is increased. Plasma level of dopamine β-hydroxylase (the enzyme that converts dopamine to epinephrine) is diminished. Sural nerve biopsy shows a decreased number of unmyelinated fibers. An electroencephalogram (EEG) is useful for evaluating seizures.

DIAGNOSIS. Slow intravenous infusion of norepinephrine produces an exaggerated pressor response. The hypotensive response to infusion of methacholine is increased. Intradermal injection of 1:1,000 histamine phosphate fails to produce a normal axon flare, and local pain is absent or diminished. Because the skin of a normal infant reacts more intensely to histamine, a 1:10,000 dilution should be used. Instillation of 2.5% methacholine into the conjunctival sac produces miosis in patients with familial dysautonomia and no detectable effect on a normal pupil; this is a nonspecific sign of parasympathetic denervation due to any cause, however. Methacholine is applied to only one eye in this test, with the other eye serving as a control; the pupils are compared at 5-min intervals for 20 min.

TREATMENT. Symptomatic treatment includes special attention to the respiratory and gastrointestinal systems, methylcellulose eye drops or topical ocular lubricants to replace tears and prevent corneal ulceration, orthopedic management of scoliosis and joint problems, and appropriate anticonvulsants for epilepsy. Chlorpromazine is an effective antiemetic and may be given as rectal suppositories during autonomic crises. It also reduces apprehension and lowers the blood pressure. Dehydration and electrolyte disturbances should be anticipated. Bethanechol may be an alternative drug for cyclic vomiting. It is also useful for enuresis, another common complication, and augments tear production. Protection from injuries is important because of the lack of pain as a protective mechanism. Scoliosis often requires surgical treatment.

Intravenous gamma globulin (IVIg) results in dramatic improvement in the hypotension and pupillary areflexia in some cases and may deserve a clinical trial in severely disabled children, but most patients would be expected to have little benefit.

PROGNOSIS. This is poor. Most patients die in childhood, usually of chronic pulmonary failure or aspiration.

622.2 Other Autonomic Neuropathies

MYENTERIC PLEXUS NEUROPATHIES. *Aganglionic megacolon* ***(Hirschsprung disease)*** is a failure of embryonic development of parasympathetic neurons in the submucosal and myenteric plexuses of segments of the colon and rectum. Nerves between the longitudinal and circular layers of smooth muscle of the gut wall are hypertrophic; ganglion cells are absent (see Chapter 332.3).

CONGENITAL INSENSITIVITY TO PAIN AND ANHIDROSIS. This hereditary disorder of uncertain genetic transmission affects boys much more frequently than girls and presents in early infancy. Patients have episodes of high fever related to warm environmental temperatures because they do not perspire. Frequent burns and traumatic injuries result from apparent lack of pain perception. Intelligence is normal. Nerve biopsy reveals an almost total absence of unmyelinated nerve fibers that convey impulses of pain, temperature, and autonomic functions. Some cases of hypomyelinating neuropathy present clinically as congenital insensitivity to pain (see Chapter 620.8).

REFLEX SYMPATHETIC DYSTROPHY. This disorder is a form of local causalgia, usually involving a hand or foot but not corresponding to the anatomic distribution of a peripheral nerve. A continuous burning pain and hyperesthesia are associated with vasomotor instability in the affected zone, resulting in increased skin temperature, erythema, and edema due to vasodilatation and hyperhydrosis. In the chronic state, atrophy of skin appendages, cool and clammy skin, and disuse atrophy of underlying muscle and bone occur. More than one extremity is occasionally involved. The pain is disabling and is exacerbated by the movement of an associated joint, although no objective signs of arthritis are seen; immobilization provides some relief. The most common preceding event is local trauma in the form of a contusion, laceration, sprain, or fracture that occurred days or weeks earlier.

Several theories of pathogenesis have been proposed to explain this phenomenon. The most widely accepted is reflexive overactivity of autonomic nerves in response to injury, and regional sympathetic blockade often affords temporary relief. Physiotherapy also is helpful. Some cases resolve spontaneously after weeks or months, but others continue to be symptomatic and require sympathectomy. A psychogenic component is suspected in some cases but is difficult to prove.

Axelrod FB, Gouge TH, Ginsburg HB, et al: Fundoplication and gastrostomy in familial dysautonomia. J Pediatr 118:388, 1991.

Axelrod FB, Nachtigal P, Dancis J: Familial dysautonomia: Diagnosis, pathogenesis and management. Adv Pediatr 21:75, 1974.

Blumenfeld A, Slaugenhaupt SA, Axelrod FB, et al: Localization of the gene for familial dysautonomia on chromosome 9 and definition of DNA markers for genetic diagnosis. Nat Genet 4:160, 1993.

Bonica JJ: Causalgia and other reflex sympathetic dystrophies. *In:* Bonica JJ (ed): The Management of Pain, 2nd ed. Philadelphia, Lea & Febiger, 1990, pp 220–243.

Chu ML, Berlin D, Axelrod FB: Allgrove syndrome: Documenting cholinergic dysfunction by autonomic testing. J Pediatr 129:156, 1996.

Heafield MTE, Gammage MD, Nightingale S, et al: Idiopathic dysautonomia treated with intravenous gammaglobulin. Lancet 347:28, 1996.

CHAPTER 623
Guillain-Barré Syndrome

Guillain-Barré syndrome is a postinfectious polyneuropathy that causes demyelination in mainly motor but sometimes also sensory nerves. This syndrome affects people of all ages and is not hereditary. The disorder closely resembles experimental allergic polyneuritis in animals.

CLINICAL MANIFESTATIONS. The paralysis usually follows a nonspecific viral infection by about 10 days. The original infection may have caused only gastrointestinal (especially *Campylobacter jejuni*) or respiratory tract (especially *Mycoplasma pneumoniae*) symptoms. Weakness begins usually in the lower extremities and progressively involves the trunk, the upper limbs, and finally the bulbar muscles, a pattern formerly known as **Landry ascending paralysis.** Proximal and distal muscles are involved relatively symmetrically, but asymmetry is found in 9% of patients. The onset is gradual and progresses over days or weeks. Particularly in cases with an abrupt onset, tenderness on palpation and pain in muscles is common in the initial stages. Affected children are irritable. Weakness may progress to inability or refusal to walk and later to flaccid tetraplegia. Paresthesias occur in some cases.

Bulbar involvement occurs in about half of cases. Respiratory insufficiency may result. Dysphagia and facial weakness are often impending signs of respiratory failure. They interfere with eating and increase the risk of aspiration. Extraocular muscle involvement is rare, but in an uncommon variant, oculomotor and other cranial neuropathies are severe early in the course. The **Miller-Fisher syndrome** consists of acute external ophthalmoplegia, ataxia, and areflexia. Papilledema is found in some cases, although visual impairment is not clinically evident. Urinary incontinence or retention of urine is a complication in about 20% of cases but is usually transient.

Tendon reflexes are lost, usually early in the course, but are sometimes preserved until later. This variability may cause confusion when attempting early diagnosis.

The clinical course is usually benign, and spontaneous recovery begins within 2–3 wk. Most patients regain full muscular strength, although some are left with residual weakness. The tendon reflexes are usually the last function to recover. Improvement usually follows a gradient inverse to the direction of involvement, with recovery of bulbar function first and lower extremity weakness resolving last. Bulbar and respiratory muscle involvement may lead to death if the syndrome is not recognized and treated.

The autonomic nervous system may also be involved in some cases. Lability of blood pressure and cardiac rate, postural hypotension, episodes of profound bradycardia, and occasional asystole occur. Cardiovascular monitoring is important. A few patients require insertion of a temporary venous cardiac pacemaker.

Chronic relapsing polyradiculoneuropathy and *chronic unremitting polyradiculoneuropathy* are chronic forms of Guillain-Barré syndrome that recur intermittently or do not improve for a period of months and years. About 7% of children with Guillain-Barré syndrome suffer relapse. Patients are usually severely weak and may have a flaccid tetraplegia with or without bulbar and respiratory muscle involvement.

Congenital Guillain-Barré syndrome is described rarely, presenting as generalized hypotonia, weakness, and areflexia in an affected neonate, fulfilling all electrophysiologic and cerebrospinal fluid (CSF) criteria, and in the absence of maternal neuromuscular disease. Treatment may not be required, and there is gradual improvement over the first few months and no evidence of residual disease by a year of age. In one case, the mother had ulcerative colitis treated with prednisone and mesalamine from the 7th month until delivery at term.

LABORATORY FINDINGS AND DIAGNOSIS. CSF studies are essential for diagnosis. The CSF protein is elevated to more than twice the upper limit of normal, glucose level is normal, and there is no pleocytosis. Fewer than ten white blood cells/mm^3 are found. The results of bacterial cultures are negative, and viral cultures rarely isolate specific viruses. The dissociation between high CSF protein and a lack of cellular response in a patient with an acute or subacute polyneuropathy is diagnostic of Guillain-Barré syndrome.

Motor nerve conduction velocities are greatly reduced, and sensory nerve conduction time is often slow. An electromyogram shows evidence of acute denervation of muscle. Serum creatine phosphokinase (CK) level may be mildly elevated or normal. Muscle biopsy is not usually required for diagnosis; specimens appear normal in early stages and show evidence of denervation atrophy in chronic stages. Sural nerve biopsy tissue shows segmental demyelination, focal inflammation, and wallerian degeneration but also is usually not required for diagnosis.

Serologic testing for *Campylobacter* infection helps establish the cause if results are positive but does not alter the course of treatment. Results of stool cultures are rarely positive because the infection is self-limited and only occurs for about 3 days, and the neuropathy follows the acute gastroenteritis.

TREATMENT. Patients in early stages of this *acute* disease should be admitted to the hospital for observation because the ascending paralysis may rapidly involve respiratory muscles during the next 24 hr. Patients with slow progression may simply be observed for stabilization and spontaneous remission without treatment. Rapidly progressive ascending paralysis is treated with intravenous immunoglobulin (IVIg), administered for 2, 3, or 5 days. Plasmapheresis, steroids, and/or immunosuppressive drugs are alternatives, if IVIg is ineffective. Supportive care, such as respiratory support, prevention of decubiti in children with flaccid tetraplegia, and treatment of secondary bacterial infections, is important.

Chronic relapsing polyradiculoneuropathy or unremitting chronic neuropathy is also treated with IVIg. Plasma exchange, sometimes requiring as many as ten exchanges daily, is an alternative. Remission in these cases may be sustained, but relapses may occur within days, weeks, or even after many months; relapses usually respond to another course of plasmapheresis. Steroid and immunosuppressive drugs are another alternative, but their effectiveness is less predictable. High-dose pulsed methylprednisolone given intravenously is successful in some cases. The prognosis in chronic forms of the Guillain-Barré syndrome is more guarded than in the acute form, and many patients are left with major residual handicaps.

Even if *Campylobacter jejuni* infection is documented by stool culture or serologic tests, treatment of the infection is not necessary because it is self-limited, and the use of antibiotics does not alter the course of the polyneuropathy.

Abd-Allah SA, Jansen PW, Ashwan S, et al: Intravenous immunoglobulin as therapy for pediatric Guillain-Barré syndrome. J Child Neurol 12:376, 1997.
Evans OB, Vedanarayanan V: Guillain-Barré syndrome. Pediatr Rev 18:10, 1997.
Farcas P, Avnunv A, Frisher S, et al: Efficacy of repeated intravenous immunoglobulin in severe unresponsive Guillain-Barré syndrome. Lancet 350:1747, 1997.
Jackson AH, Barquis GD, Shah BL: Congenital Guillain-Barré syndrome. J Child Neurol 11:407, 1996.
Massachusetts Medical Society: Tick paralysis—Washington, 1995. MMWR 45:325, 1996.
Plasma Exchange/Sandoglobulin Guillain-Barré Syndrome Trial Group: Randomised trial of plasma exchange, intravenous immunoglobulin, and combined treatments in Guillain-Barré syndrome. Lancet 349:225, 1997.
Rees JH: *Campylobacter jejuni* infection and Guillain-Barré syndrome. N Engl J Med 333:1374, 1995.
Shahar E, Shorer Z, Roifman CM, et al: Immune globulins are effective in severe pediatric Guillain-Barré syndrome. Pediatr Neurol 16:32, 1997.
Shuaib A, Becker WJ: Variants of Guillain-Barré syndrome: Miller-Fisher syndrome, facial diplegia and multiple cranial nerve palsies. Can J Neurol Sci 14:611, 1987.

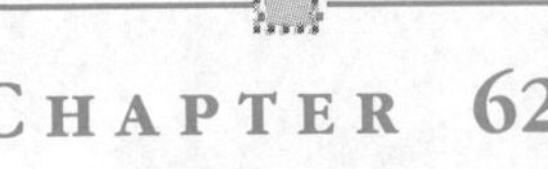

CHAPTER 624
Bell Palsy

Bell palsy is an acute unilateral facial nerve palsy that is not associated with other cranial neuropathies or brain stem dysfunction. It is a common disorder at all ages from infancy through adolescence and usually develops abruptly about 2 wk after a systemic viral infection. The preceding infection is due to the Epstein-Barr virus in about 20% of cases; Lyme disease (see Chapter 219), herpes simplex virus, and mumps virus are identified in many others. The disease is believed to be a postinfectious allergic or immune demyelinating facial neuritis rather than an active viral invasion of the nerve or of its motor neurons or origin. At times, it is associated with hypertension.

CLINICAL MANIFESTATIONS. The upper and lower portions of the face are paretic, and the corner of the mouth droops. Patients are unable to close the eye on the involved side and may develop an exposure keratitis at night. Taste on the anterior two thirds of the tongue is lost on the involved side in about half of cases; this finding helps to establish the anatomic limits of the lesion as being proximal or distal to the chorda tympani branch of the facial nerve. Numbness and paresthesias do not occur.

TREATMENT. Protection of the cornea with methylcellulose eye drops or an ocular lubricant is especially important at night. Steroids do not induce remission and are not recommended. Surgical decompression of the facial canal, theoretically to provide more space for the swollen facial nerve, has not proved to be of value.

PROGNOSIS. The prognosis is excellent. More than 85% of cases recover spontaneously with no residual facial weakness; another 10% have mild facial weakness as a sequela; only 5% are left with permanent severe facial weakness. In chronic cases that do not recover within a few weeks, electrophysiologic examination of the facial nerve helps to determine the degree of neuropathy and regeneration. In chronic cases, other causes of facial neuropathy should be considered, including facial nerve tumors such as schwannomas and neurofibromas, infiltration of the facial nerve by leukemic cells or by a rhabdomyosarcoma of the middle ear, brain stem infarcts or tumors, and traumatic injury of the facial nerve.

FACIAL PALSY AT BIRTH. This is usually a compression neuropathy from forceps application during delivery and recovers spontaneously in a few days or weeks in most cases. Congenital Bell's palsy should not be diagnosed. *Congenital absence of the depressor angularis oris muscle* causes facial asymmetry, especially when an affected infant cries. It is not a facial nerve lesion but is a cosmetic defect that does not interfere with feeding. Infants with **Möbius syndrome** may have bilateral or, less commonly, unilateral facial palsy; this syndrome is usually due to symmetrical calcified infarcts in the tegmentum of the pons and medulla oblongata during midgestation or late fetal life though rarely may be a developmental anomaly of the brain stem.

Davidoff F: Herpes simplex virus and Bell palsy. Ann Intern Med 124:63, 1996.
Shapiro ED, Gerber MA: Lyme disease and facial nerve palsy. Arch Pediatr Adolesc Med 151:1183, 1997.

PART XXVIII

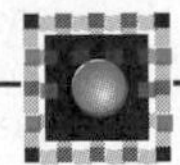

Disorders of the Eye

Scott E. Olitsky ■ Leonard B. Nelson

CHAPTER 625
Growth and Development

At birth, the eye of a normal full-term infant is approximately 65% of adult size. Postnatal growth is maximal during the 1st yr, proceeds at a rapid but decelerating rate until the 3rd yr, and continues at a slower rate thereafter until puberty, after which little change occurs. In general, the anterior structures of the eye are relatively large at birth but thereafter grow proportionately less than the posterior structures. This results in a progressive change in the shape of the globe; it becomes more spherical.

In an infant, the *sclera* is thin and translucent, with a bluish tinge. The *cornea* is relatively large in newborns (averaging 10 mm) and attains adult size (nearly 12 mm) by the age of 2 yr or earlier. Its curvature tends to flatten with age, with progressive change in the refractive properties of the eye. A normal cornea is perfectly clear. In infants born prematurely, the cornea may have a transient opalescent haze. The anterior chamber in a newborn appears shallow, and the angle structures, important in the maintenance of normal intraocular pressure, must undergo further differentiation after birth. The *iris*, typically light blue or gray at birth in white individuals, undergoes progressive change of color as the pigmentation of the stroma increases in the first 6 mo of life. The pupils of a newborn infant tend to be small and are often difficult to dilate. Remnants of the pupillary membrane (anterior vascular capsule) are often evident on ophthalmoscopic examination as cobweb-like lines crossing the pupillary aperture, especially in preterm infants.

The *lens* of a newborn infant is more spherical than that of an adult; its greater refractive power helps to compensate for the relative shortness of the young eye. The lens continues to grow throughout life; new fibers added to the periphery continually push older fibers toward the center of the lens. With age, the lens becomes progressively more dense and more resistant to change of shape during accommodation.

The *fundus* of a newborn's eye is less pigmented than that of an adult; the choroidal vascular pattern is highly visible, and the retinal pigmentary pattern often has a fine peppery or mottled appearance. In some darkly pigmented infants, the fundus has a gray or opalescent sheen. In a newborn, the macular landmarks, particularly the foveal light reflex, are less well defined and may not be readily apparent. The peripheral retina appears pale or grayish, and the peripheral retinal vasculature is immature, especially in premature infants. The optic nerve head color varies from pink to slightly pale, sometimes grayish. Within 4–6 mo, the appearance of the fundus approximates that of the mature eye.

Superficial retinal hemorrhages may be observed in many newborn infants. These are usually absorbed promptly and rarely leave any permanent effect. Conjunctival hemorrhages also may occur at birth and are resorbed spontaneously without consequence.

Remnants of the primitive hyaloid vascular system may also be seen as small tufts or wormlike structures projecting from the disc (Bergmeister's papilla) or as a fine strand traversing the vitreous; in some cases, only a small dot (Mittendorf's dot) remains on the posterior aspect of the lens capsule.

An infant's eye is somewhat hyperopic (farsighted). The general trend is for hyperopia to increase from birth until 7 yr. Thereafter, the level of hyperopia tends to decrease rapidly until age 14. Elimination of the hyperopic state may occur during this time. If the process continues, myopia (nearsightedness) develops. A slower continuation of the decrease in hyperopia, or increase in myopia, continues into the 3rd decade of life. The refractive state at any time in life depends on the net effect of many factors: the size of the eye, the state of the lens, and the curvature of the cornea.

Newborn infants tend to keep their eyes closed much of the time, but normal newborns can see, respond to changes in illumination, and fixate points of contrast. The *visual acuity* in newborns is estimated to be in the range of 20/400. One of the earliest responses to a formed visual stimulus is an infant's regard for the mother's face, evident especially during feeding. By 2 wk of age, an infant shows more sustained interest in large objects, and by 8–10 wk of age a normal infant can follow an object through an arc of 180 degrees. The acuity improves rapidly and may reach 20/30–20/20 by the age of 2–3 yr.

Many normal infants may have imperfect coordination of the *eye movements* and *alignment* during the early days and weeks, but proper coordination should be achieved by 3–6 mo, usually sooner. Persistent deviation of an eye in an infant requires evaluation.

Tears often are not present with crying until after 1–3 mo.

Archer SM, Sondhi N, Helveston EM: Strabismus in infancy. Ophthalmology 96:133, 1989.

Friendly DS: Development of vision in infants and young children. Pediatr Clin North Am 40:693, 1993.

Gordon RA, Donzis PB: Refractive development of the human eye. Arch Ophthalmol 103:785, 1985.

Khodadoust AA, Ziai M, Biggs SL: Optic disc in normal newborns. Am J Ophthalmol 66:502, 1968.

Krishnamohan VK, Wheeler MB, Testa MA, et al: Correlation of postnatal regression of the anterior vascular capsule of the lens to gestational age. J Pediatr Ophthalmol Strabismus 19:28, 1982.

Roarty JD, Keltner JL: Normal pupil size and anisocoria in newborn infants. Arch Ophthalmol 108:94, 1990.

Robb RM: Increase in retinal surface area during infancy and childhood. J Pediatr Ophthalmol Strabismus 19:16, 1982.

Spieres A, Isenberg SJ, Inkelis SH: Characteristics of the iris in 100 neonates. J Pediatr Ophthalmol Strabismus 26:28, 1989.

CHAPTER 626
Examination of the Eye

Examination of the eyes is a routine part of the periodic pediatric assessment beginning in the newborn period. The primary care physician is very important in detecting both obvious and insidious, asymptomatic eye diseases. Screening in schools and community programs can also be effective in detecting problems early. The American Academy of Ophthalmology recommends preschool vision screening as a means of reducing preventable visual loss (Table 626–1). This testing should be done by primary providers during well child visits. Children should be examined by an ophthalmologist whenever a significant ocular abnormality or vision defect is noted or suspected. Children who are at high risk for ophthalmologic problems, such as genetically inherited ocular conditions and various systemic disorders, should also be examined by an ophthalmologist.

Basic examination, whether done by a pediatrician or an ophthalmologist, must include evaluation of visual acuity and the visual fields, assessment of the pupils, ocular motility and alignment, a general external examination, and an ophthalmoscopic examination of the media and fundi. When indicated, biomicroscopy (slit-lamp examination), cycloplegic refraction, and tonometry are performed by an ophthalmologist. Special diagnostic procedures, such as ultrasonic examination, fluorescein angiography, electroretinography (ERG), or visual evoked response (VER) testing, are also indicated for specific conditions.

VISUAL ACUITY. Many tests of visual acuity exist. Which test is used depends on a child's age and ability to cooperate, as well as a clinician's preference and experience with each test. The most common visual acuity test in infants is an assessment of their ability to fixate and follow a target. If appropriate targets are used, this reflex can be demonstrated by about 6 wk of age. The test is performed by seating the child comfortably in the caretaker's lap. The object of visual interest, usually a bright-colored toy, is slowly moved to the right and to the left. The examiner observes whether the infant's eyes turn toward the object and follow its movements. The examiner can use a thumb to occlude one of the infant's eyes in order to test each eye separately. Although a sound-producing object might compromise the purity of the visual stimulus, in practice, toys that squeak or rattle heighten an infant's awareness and interest in the test.

TABLE 626–1 Vision Screening Schedule for Infants and Children

Age	Screening Test	Findings Requiring Referral
Newborn–3 mo	Red reflex test	Opacity of the cornea, cataract, retinal detachment or disorder
	Corneal light reflex test	Ocular misalignment (strabismus)
	External examination	Structural defect
6–12 mo	Red reflex test	As above
	Corneal light reflex test	As above
	Occlusion of each eye separately	Amblyopia if child resists occlusion unequally
	Fixation and following	Amblyopia if unable to do
3 yr	Red reflex test	As above
	Corneal light reflex test	As above
	Visual acuity test	Refractive error, amblyopia
	Stereoacuity	Refractive error, amblyopia
5 yr	Same as 3 yr	As above

From Catalano RA, Nelson LB: Pediatric Ophthalmology. A Text Atlas. Norwalk, CT, Appleton & Lange, 1994.

The human face is a better target than test objects. The examiner can exploit this by moving his or her face slowly in front of the infant's face. If the appropriate following movements are not elicited, the test should be repeated with the caretaker's face as the test stimulus. It should be remembered that even children with poor vision may follow a large object without apparent difficulty, especially if only one eye is affected.

An objective measurement of visual acuity is usually possible when children reach 2½–3 yr. Children this age are tested using a schematic picture or other illiterate eye chart. Each eye should be tested separately. It is essential to prevent peeking. The examiner should hold the occluder in place and observe the child throughout the test. The child should be reassured and encouraged throughout the test, because many children are intimidated by the procedure and fear a "bad grade" or punishment for errors.

The **E test,** in which a child points in the direction of the letter, is the most widely used visual acuity test for preschool children. Right-left presentations are more confusing than up-down presentations. With pretest practice, this test can be performed by most children 3–4 yr.

An adult-type **Snellen acuity chart** can be used at about 5 or 6 yr if the child knows letters. An acuity of 20/40 is generally accepted as normal for 3-yr-old children. At age 4 yr, 20/30 is typical. By age 5 or 6 yr, most children attain 20/20 vision.

Optokinetic nystagmus (the response to a sequence of moving targets; "railroad" nystagmus) can also be used to assess vision; this can be calibrated by targets of various sizes (stripes or dots) or by a rotating drum at specified distances. The VER, an electrophysiologic method of evaluating the response to light and special visual stimuli, such as calibrated stripes or a checkerboard pattern, can also be used to study visual function in selected cases. Preferential looking tests are also used for evaluating vision in infants and children who cannot respond to standard acuity tests. This is a behavioral technique based on the observation that, given a choice, an infant prefers to look at patterned rather than unpatterned stimuli. Preferential looking tests cannot be directly correlated to standard visual acuity data. Because these tests require the presence of a skilled examiner, their use is often limited to research protocols involving preverbal children.

VISUAL FIELD ASSESSMENT. Like visual acuity testing, visual field assessment must be geared to a child's age and abilities. Formal visual field examination (perimetry and scotometry) can often be accomplished in school-aged children. The examiner must often rely on confrontation techniques and finger counting in quadrants of the visual field. In many children, only testing by attraction can be accomplished; the examiner observes a child's response to familiar objects brought into each of the four quadrants of the visual field of each eye in turn. The child's bottle, a favorite toy, and lollipops are particularly effective attention-getting items. These gross methods can often detect diagnostically significant field changes such as the bitemporal hemianopia of a chiasmal lesion or the homonymous hemianopia of a cerebral lesion.

COLOR VISION TESTING. This can be accomplished whenever a child is able to name or trace the test symbols; these may either be numbers or X's, O's, triangles, or other symbols. Color vision testing is not frequently necessary in young children, but parents sometimes request it, particularly if their child seems to be slow in learning colors. Defective color vision is common in males but is rare in females. Achromatopsia, a total color vision defect with subnormal visual acuity, nystagmus, and photophobia, is encountered occasionally. A change in color discrimination can be a sign of optic nerve or retinal disease.

PUPILLARY EXAMINATION. This includes evaluation of both the direct and consensual reactions to light, the reaction on near gaze, and the response to reduced illumination, noting the size and symmetry of the pupils under all conditions. Special care must be taken to differentiate the reaction to light from the reaction to near gaze; a child's natural tendency is to look directly at the approaching light, inducing the near gaze reflex when one is attempting to test only the reaction to light; accordingly, every effort must be made to control fixation. The swinging flashlight test is especially useful for detecting unilateral or asymmetric prechiasmatic afferent defects in children (see Marcus Gunn pupil, Chapter 629).

OCULAR MOTILITY. This is tested by having a child follow an object into the various positions of gaze. Movements of each eye individually (ductions) and of the two eyes together (versions, conjugate movements, and convergence) are assessed. Alignment is judged by the symmetry of the corneal light reflexes and by the response to alternate occlusion of each eye (see cover tests for strabismus, Chapter 630).

BINOCULAR VISION. A determination of the degree of binocular vision is commonly performed by an ophthalmologist. The **Titmus test** is probably the most frequently used test; a series of three-dimensional images are shown to the child while he or she wears a set of Polaroid glasses. The level of difficulty with which these images can be detected correlates with the degree of binocular vision that is present. Other tests may also be used to detect the presence of abnormal binocular adaptations secondary to poor vision or strabismus.

EXTERNAL EXAMINATION. This begins with general inspection in good illumination, noting size, shape, and symmetry of the orbits, position and movement of the lids, and the position and symmetry of the globes. Viewing the eyes and lids from above aids in detecting orbital asymmetry, lid masses, proptosis (exophthalmos), and abnormal pulsations. Palpation is also important in detecting orbital and lid masses.

The lacrimal apparatus is assessed by looking for evidence of tear deficiency, overflow of tears (epiphora), and erythema and swelling in the region of the tear sac or gland. The sac is massaged to check for reflux when obstruction is suspected. The presence and position of the puncta are also checked.

The lids and conjunctiva are specifically examined for focal lesions, foreign bodies, and inflammatory signs; loss and maldirection of lashes should also be noted. When necessary, the lids can be everted in the following manner: (1) instruct the patient to look down; (2) grasp the lashes of the patient's upper lid between the thumb and index finger of one hand; (3) place a probe, a cotton-tipped applicator, or the thumb of the other hand at the upper margin of the tarsal plate; and (4) pulling the lid down and outward, evert it over the probe, using the instrument as a fulcrum. Foreign bodies commonly lodge in the concavity just above the lid margin and are exposed only by fully everting the lid.

The anterior segment of the eye is then evaluated with oblique focal illumination, noting luster and clarity of the cornea, depth and clarity of the anterior chamber, and features of the iris. Transillumination of the anterior segment aids in detecting opacities and in demonstrating atrophy or hypopigmentation of the iris; these latter signs are important when ocular albinism is suspected. When necessary, fluorescein dye can be used to aid in diagnosing abrasions, ulcerations, and foreign bodies.

BIOMICROSCOPY (SLIT-LAMP EXAMINATION). This provides a highly magnified view of the various structures of the eye and an optical section through the media of the eye—that is, the cornea, aqueous humor, lens, and vitreous. Lesions can be identified and localized according to their depth within the eye; the resolution is sufficient to detect individual inflammatory cells in the aqueous and vitreous. With the addition of special lenses and prisms, the angle of the anterior chamber and regions of the fundus also can be examined with a slit lamp. Biomicroscopy is often crucial in trauma and in examining for iritis. It is also helpful in diagnosing many metabolic diseases of childhood.

FUNDUS EXAMINATION (OPHTHALMOSCOPY). This is best done with the pupil dilated unless there are neurologic or other contraindications. Tropicamide (Mydriacyl), 0.5–1%, and phenylephrine (Neo-Synephrine), 2.5%, are recommended as mydriatics of short duration. These are safe for most children, but the possibility of adverse systemic effects must be recognized. For very small infants, more dilute preparations may be advisable. Beginning with posterior landmarks, the disc and the macula, the four quadrants are systematically examined by following each of the major vessel groups to the periphery. More of the fundus can be seen if a child is directed to look up, down, right, and left. Even with care, only a limited amount of the fundus can be seen with a direct or handheld ophthalmoscope. For examination of the far periphery, an indirect ophthalmoscope is used, and full dilation of the pupil is essential.

It should be noted that before the retina is examined, an ophthalmoscope is used to examine the clarity of the media. With a high plus lens (+8 or +10) in place, an ophthalmoscope can also be used for examination of external lesions and foreign bodies, because it provides magnification and good illumination.

REFRACTION. This determines the refractive state of the eye—that is, the degree of nearsightedness, farsightedness, or astigmatism. Retinoscopy provides an objective determination of the amount of correction needed and can be performed at any age. In young children, it is best done with cycloplegia. Subjective refinement of refraction involves asking patients for preferences in the strength and axis of corrective lenses; it can be accomplished in many school-aged children. Refraction and determination of visual acuity with appropriate corrective lenses in place are essential steps in deciding whether or not a patient has a visual defect or amblyopia. Photoscreening cameras have been developed to aid ancillary medical personnel in screening for abnormal refractive errors in preverbal children.

TONOMETRY. This measures intraocular pressure; it may be performed with a portable, stand-alone instrument or by the applanation method with the slit lamp. Alternative methods are pneumatic and electronic tonometry. When accurate measurement of the pressure is necessary in a child who cannot cooperate, it may be performed with sedation or general anesthesia. A gross estimate of pressure can be made by palpating the globe with the index fingers placed side by side on the upper lid above the tarsal plate.

American Academy of Ophthalmology Preferred Practice Patterns Committee, Pediatrics Ophthalmology Panel: Pediatric eye evaluations: Preferred practice pattern. Abstracts of Clinical Care Guidelines, April 7, 1998.

American Academy of Ophthalmology: Preferred Practice Pattern: Comprehensive Pediatric Eye Evaluation. San Francisco, American Academy of Ophthalmology, 1992.

American Academy of Pediatrics, Committee on Practice and Ambulatory Medicine, Section on Ophthalmology: Eye examination and vision screening in infants, children and young adults. Pediatrics 98:153, 1996.

Fulton A: Screening preschool children to detect visual and ocular disorders. Arch Ophthalmol 110:1553, 1992.

Isenberg SJ: Clinical application of the pupil examination in neonates. J Pediatr 118:650, 1991.

Reinecke RD: Screening 3-year olds for visual problems: Are we gaining or falling behind? Arch Ophthalmol 105:1497, 1987.

Simons K: Preschool vision screening: Rationale, methodology and outcome. Surv Ophthalmol 41:3, 1996.

Teller DY, McDonald MA, Preston KI, et al: Assessment of visual acuity in infants and children: The acuity card procedure. Dev Med Child Neurol 28:779, 1986.

Chapter 627
Abnormalities of Refraction and Accommodation

Emmetropia is the state in which parallel rays of light come to focus on the retina with the eye at rest (nonaccommodating). Such an ideal optical state is common, but the opposite condition, ametropia, often exists. Three principal types occur: hyperopia (farsightedness), myopia (nearsightedness), and astigmatism. The majority of children are physiologically hyperopic at birth, but a significant number, especially those born prematurely, are myopic, and they often have some degree of astigmatism. With growth, the refractive state tends to change and should be evaluated periodically.

Measurement of the refractive state of the eye (refraction) can be accomplished objectively and subjectively. The objective method involves focusing a beam of light from a retinoscope onto a patient's retina through lenses of various powers placed in front of the eye. This method is precise and can be carried out at any age, because it requires no response from a patient. In infants and children, it is best done after instillation of eye drops that produce *mydriasis* (dilatation of the pupil) and *cycloplegia* (relaxation of accommodation); those used most commonly are tropicamide (Mydriacyl), cyclopentolate (Cyclogyl), homatropine hydrobromide, and atropine sulfate. The subjective method involves placing various lenses in front of the eye and having the patient report which lenses provide the clearest image of the letters on the chart. This method depends on a patient's ability to discriminate and communicate, but it can be used for some children and can be helpful in determining the best refractive correction for children who are developmentally capable.

HYPEROPIA. If parallel rays of light come to focus posterior to the retina with the eye in a state of rest (nonaccommodating), hyperopia or farsightedness exists. This may result because the anteroposterior diameter of the eye is too short, because the refractive power of the cornea or lens is less than normal, or because the lens is dislocated posteriorly.

In hyperopia, accommodation is used to bring objects into focus for both far and near gaze. If the accommodative effort required is not too great, the child has clear vision and is comfortable with both distant and close work. In high degrees of hyperopia requiring greater accommodative effort, vision may be blurred, and the child may complain of eyestrain, headaches, or fatigue. Squinting, eye rubbing, lid inflammation, and lack of interest in reading are frequent manifestations. If the induced discomfort is great enough, a child does not make an effort to see well and may develop bilateral amblyopia (ametropic amblyopia). Esotropia may also be associated (convergent strabismus, accommodative esotropia, Chapter 630). Convex lenses (spectacles or contact lenses) of sufficient strength to provide clear vision and comfort are prescribed when indicated. Even children who have high degrees of hyperopia but who have good vision will happily wear glasses because they provide comfort by eliminating the excessive accommodation required to see well. Preverbal children should also be given glasses for high levels of hyperopia in order to prevent the development of esotropia or amblyopia.

MYOPIA. In myopia, parallel rays of light come to focus anterior to the retina. This may result because the anteroposterior diameter of the eye is too long, because the refractive power of the cornea or lens is greater than normal, or because the lens is dislocated forward. The principal symptom is blurred vision for distant objects. The far point of clear vision varies inversely with the degree of myopia; as the myopia increases, the far point of clear vision comes closer. With myopia of 1 diopter, for example, the far point of clear focus is 1 m from the eye; with myopia of 3 diopters, the far point of clear vision is only 1/3 m from the eye. Thus, myopic children tend to hold objects and reading matter close, prefer to be close to the blackboard, and may be uninterested in distant activities. Frowning and squinting are common, because the visual acuity is improved when the lid aperture is reduced; the effect is similar to that achieved by closing or "stopping down" the aperture of the diaphragm of a camera.

Myopia is infrequent in infants and preschool children. It is more common in preterm infants and in infants with a history of retinopathy of prematurity. A hereditary tendency to myopia is also observed, and children of myopic parents should be examined at an early age. The incidence of myopia increases during the school years, especially during the preteen and teen years. The degree of myopia also increases with age during the growing years.

Concave lenses (spectacles or contact lenses) of appropriate strength to provide clear vision and comfort are prescribed. Changes are usually needed periodically, sometimes in 1–2 yr, sometimes every few months. Excessive accommodation during near work has been considered by some to lead to progression of myopia. Based on this philosophy, some practitioners advocate the use of cycloplegic agents, bifocals, intentional undercorrection of myopic refractive errors, or mandatory removal of myopic glasses for near work in an effort to retard the progression of myopia. The value of such treatment has not been scientifically proved.

In most cases, myopia is not a result of pathologic alteration of the eye and is referred to as simple or physiologic myopia. Some children may have pathologic myopia, a rare condition caused by a pathologically abnormal axial length of the eye; this is usually associated with thinning of the sclera, choroid, and retina and often with some degree of uncorrectable visual impairment. Tears or breaks in the retina may occur as it becomes increasingly thin, leading to the development of retinal detachments. Myopia may also occur as a result of other ocular abnormalities, such as keratoconus, ectopia lentis, congenital stationary night blindness, and glaucoma and is also a major feature of *Stickler syndrome*.

ASTIGMATISM. In astigmatism, the refractive power of the various meridians of the eye differs. Most cases are caused by irregularity in the curvature of the cornea; some astigmatism results from changes in the lens. Mild degrees of astigmatism are very common and may produce no symptoms. With greater degrees there may be distortion of vision. In an effort to achieve a clearer image, a person with astigmatism uses accommodation or frowns or squints to obtain a pinhole effect. Symptoms include eyestrain, headache, and fatigue. Eye rubbing and lid hyperemia, indifference to schoolwork, and holding reading matter close are common manifestations in childhood. Cylindric or spherocylindric lenses are used to provide optical correction when indicated. Glasses may be needed constantly or only part time, depending on the degree of astigmatism and the severity of the attendant symptoms. In some cases, contact lenses are used.

Infants and children with corneal irregularity resulting from injury, periorbital and eyelid hemangiomas, and ptosis are at increased risk for astigmatism and attendant amblyopia.

ANISOMETROPIA. When the refractive state of one eye is significantly different from the refractive state of the other eye, anisometropia exists. If uncorrected, one eye may always be out of focus, leading to the development of amblyopia, or lazy eye. Early detection and correction are essential if normal visual development in both eyes is to be achieved.

ACCOMMODATION. During accommodation, the ciliary muscle contracts, the suspensory fibers of the lens relax, and the lens assumes a more rounded shape to bring rays of light into focus on the retina. The amplitude of accommodation is greatest during childhood and gradually diminishes with age. The physiologic decrease in accommodative ability that occurs with age is called *presbyopia*.

Disorders of accommodation in children are relatively rare. Premature presbyopia is occasionally encountered in youngsters. The most common cause of paralysis of accommodation in children is intentional or inadvertent use of cycloplegic substances, topically or systemically; included are all the anticholinergic drugs and poisons, as well as plants and plant substances having these effects. Neurogenic causes of accommodative paralysis include lesions affecting the oculomotor nerve (3rd cranial nerve) in any part of its course. Differential diagnosis includes tumors, degenerative diseases, vascular lesions, trauma, and infectious diseases. Systemic disorders that may cause impairment of accommodation include botulism, diphtheria, Wilson's disease, diabetes mellitus, and syphilis. Adie's tonic pupil may also lead to a deficiency of accommodation after some viral illnesses (see Chapter 629). Rarely, inability to accommodate is caused by a congenital defect of the ciliary muscle. An apparent defect in accommodation may be psychogenic in origin; it is common for a child to feign inability to read when it can be demonstrated that visual acuity and ability to focus are normal.

Brodstein RS, Brodstein DE, Olson RJ, et al: The treatment of myopia with atropine and bifocals: A long-term prospective study. Ophthalmology 91:1373, 1984.

Catalano RA, Nelson LB: Pediatric Ophthalmology: A Text Atlas. Norwalk, CT, Appleton & Lange, 1994.

Curtin BJ: The etiology of myopia. *In*: Curtin BJ (ed): The Myopias: Basic Science and Clinical Management. Philadelphia, Harper & Row, 1985, pp 113–124.

Fulton AB, Dobson V, Salem D, et al: Cycloplegic refractions in infants and young children. Am J Ophthalmol 90:239, 1980.

Gordon RA, Donzis PB: Refractive development of the human eye. Arch Ophthalmol 103:785, 1985.

Gordon RA, Donzis PB: Myopia associated with retinopathy of prematurity. Ophthalmology 93:1593, 1986.

Mantyjarvi MI: Changes in refraction in schoolchildren. Arch Ophthalmol 103:790, 1985.

Schoenleber DB, Crouch ER: Bilateral hypermetropic amblyopia. J Pediatr Ophthalmol Strabismus 24:75, 1987.

Slataper FJ. Age norms of refraction and vision. Arch Ophthalmol 43:466, 1950.

Spencer JB, Mets MB: Refractive abnormalities in childhood. Ophthalmol Clin North Am 2:265, 1990.

CHAPTER 628
Disorders of Vision

AMBLYOPIA. Amblyopia is the decrease in visual acuity, unilateral or bilateral, that occurs in visually immature children as a result of a lack of a clear image falling on the retina. The unformed retinal image may occur secondary to a deviated eye (strabismic amblyopia), an unequal need for vision correction between the eyes (anisometropic amblyopia), a high refractive error in both eyes (ametropic amblyopia), or a media opacity within the visual axis (deprivation amblyopia).

Under normal conditions, the development of visual acuity proceeds rapidly in infancy and early childhood. Anything that interferes with the formation of a clear retinal image during this early developmental period can produce amblyopia. Amblyopia may occur only during the critical period of development, before the cortex has become visually mature, within the first decade of life. The younger a child, the more susceptible he or she is to the development of amblyopia.

The *diagnosis* of amblyopia is confirmed when a complete ophthalmologic examination reveals reduced acuity that is unexplained by an organic abnormality. If the history and ophthalmologic examination do not support the diagnosis of amblyopia in a child with poor vision, consideration must be given to other causes (i.e., neurologic, psychologic). Amblyopia is usually asymptomatic and detected only by screening programs. Screening is easier in older children. However, just as amblyopia is less likely to occur in an older child, it is also more resistant to treatment at that age. Amblyopia is reversed more rapidly in younger children whose visual system is less mature, although screening is more difficult. The key to the successful treatment of amblyopia is early detection and prompt intervention.

Treatment generally first consists of removing any media opacity or prescribing appropriate glasses, if needed, so that a well-formed retinal image can be produced in each eye. The sound eye is then covered (occlusion therapy) or blurred with glasses or drops (penalization therapy) to stimulate proper visual development of the more severely affected eye. In many cases, best results are achieved with complete and constant occlusion throughout the waking hours by the use of adhesive eye patches; in some cases, part-time occlusion is sufficient or preferred. Occluders placed on spectacles allow peeking, and the adjustable headband type of cloth or plastic occluder is too easily removed by a child. In selected cases, an opaque contact lens or a contact lens of sufficiently high power to blur the vision in the better eye is used. Most children and their families tolerate occlusion therapy well. In some cases, a child resists therapy because of the severity of the vision defect, the cosmetic blemish of the patching, or related psychologic disturbances. The goals of treatment must be thoroughly understood and the treatment carefully supervised. Close monitoring of amblyopia therapy is essential, especially in the very young, to avoid deprivation amblyopia in the good eye. Many families need reassurance and support throughout the trying course of treatment.

DIPLOPIA. Diplopia, or double vision, is most frequently a result of malalignment of the visual axes—that is, displacement or deviation of the eye. It is common in heterophoria, in heterotropia of recent onset (particularly when caused by acquired nerve palsy), and in proptosis. Occluding one eye relieves the diplopia; affected children commonly squint, cover one eye with a hand, or assume abnormal head postures (a face turn or head tilt) to alleviate the bothersome sensation. These mannerisms, especially in preverbal children, are important clues to diplopia. The onset of diplopia in any child warrants prompt evaluation; it may signal the onset of a serious problem such as increased intracranial pressure, a brain tumor, an orbital mass, or myasthenia gravis.

Monocular diplopia results from dislocation of the lens or some defect in the media or macula.

SUPPRESSION. In the presence of strabismus, diplopia occurs secondary to two separate images falling on the retina. In a visually immature child, a process that may occur in the cortex eliminates the disability of seeing double. This active process is termed *suppression*, and it occurs only in children. Although suppression eliminates the annoying symptom of diplopia, it is the potential awareness of a second image that tends to keep our eyes properly aligned. Once suppression develops, it may allow an intermittent strabismus to become constant or strabismus to redevelop later in life even after successful treatment during childhood.

AMAUROSIS. Amaurosis is partial or total loss of vision; the term is usually reserved for profound impairment, blindness, or near blindness. When amaurosis exists from birth, primary consideration in differential diagnosis must be given to developmental malformations, damage consequent to gestational or perinatal infection, anoxia or hypoxia, perinatal trauma, and the genetically determined diseases that can affect the eye itself or the visual pathways (Table 628–1). In certain cases, the reason for amaurosis can be readily determined by objective

TABLE 628–1 Etiologies of Childhood Amaurosis (Blindness)

Congenital

Optic nerve hypoplasia or aplasia
Optic coloboma
Congenital hydrocephalus
Hydranencephaly
Porencephaly
Micrencephaly
Encephalocele, particularly occipital type
Morning glory disc
Aniridia
Anterior microphthalmia
Peter's anomaly
Persistent pupillary membrane
Glaucoma
Cataracts
Persistent hyperplastic primary vitreous

Phakomatoses

Tuberous sclerosis
Neurofibromatosis (special association with optic glioma)
Sturge-Weber syndrome
von Hippel–Lindau disease

Tumors

Retinoblastoma
Optic glioma
Perioptic meningioma
Craniopharyngioma
Cerebral glioma
Posterior and intraventricular tumors when complicated by hydrocephalus
Pseudotumor cerebri

Neurodegenerative Diseases

Cerebral storage disease
Gangliosidoses, particularly Tay-Sachs disease (infantile amaurotic familial idiocy), Sandhoff's variant, generalized gangliosidosis
Other lipidoses and ceroid lipofuscinoses, particularly the late-onset amaurotic familial idiocies such as those of Jansky-Bielschowsky and of Batten-Mayou-Spielmeyer-Vogt
Mucopolysaccharidoses, particularly Hurler's syndrome and Hunter's syndrome
Leukodystrophies (dysmyelination disorders), particularly metachromatic leukodystrophy and Canavan's disease
Demyelinating sclerosis (myelinoclastic diseases), especially Schilder's disease and Devic's neuromyelitis optica
Special types: Dawson's disease, Leigh's disease, the Bassen-Kornzweig syndrome, Refsum's disease
Retinal degenerations: retinitis pigmentosa and its variants, and Leber's congenital type
Optic atrophies: congenital autosomal recessive type, infantile and congenital autosomal dominant types, Leber's disease, and atrophies associated with hereditary ataxias—the types of Behr, of Marie, and of Sanger-Brown

Infectious Processes

Encephalitis, especially in the prenatal infection syndromes due to *Toxoplasma gondii*, cytomegalovirus, rubella virus, *Treponema pallidum*, herpes simplex
Meningitis; arachnoiditis
Chorioretinitis
Endophthalmitis
Keratitis

Hematologic Disorders

Leukemia with central nervous system involvement

Vascular and Circulatory Disorders

Collagen vascular diseases
Arteriovenous malformations—intracerebral hemorrhage, subarachnoid hemorrhage
Central retinal occlusion

Trauma

Contusion or avulsion of optic nerves, chiasm, globe, cornea
Cerebral contusion or laceration
Intracerebral, subarachnoid, or subdural hemorrhage

Drugs and Toxins

Other

Retinopathy of prematurity
Sclerocornea
Conversion reaction
Optic neuritis
Osteopetrosis

Modified from Kliegman R: Practical Strategies in Pediatric Diagnosis and Therapy. Philadelphia, WB Saunders, 1996.

ophthalmic examination; examples are severe microphthalmia, corneal opacification, dense cataracts, chorioretinal scars, macular defects, retinal dysplasia, and severe optic nerve hypoplasia. In some cases, an intrinsic retinal disease may not be apparent on initial ophthalmoscopic examination; an example is **Leber congenital retinal amaurosis**. In this retinal dystrophy, the fundus may appear normal or near normal for some time before ophthalmoscopically appreciable signs of retinal degeneration (e.g., pigmentary deposits, arteriolar attenuation, optic disc pallor) develop. In such cases, electroretinography is important in diagnosis, because the electroretinographic response in this condition is markedly reduced or absent. In many cases of amaurosis, the defect lies not in the eye or optic nerve but in the brain, requiring neurologic and neuroradiologic evaluation, including CT or MRI.

Amaurosis that develops in a child who once had useful vision has different implications (Table 628–1). In the absence of obvious ocular disease (e.g., cataract, chorioretinitis, retinoblastoma, retinitis pigmentosa), consideration must be given to many neurologic and systemic disorders that can affect the visual pathways. Amaurosis of rather rapid onset may indicate an encephalopathy (hypertension), infectious or parainfectious processes, vasculitis, migraine, leukemia, toxins, or trauma. It may be caused by acute demyelinating disease affecting the optic nerves, chiasm, or cerebrum. In some cases, precipitous loss of vision is a result of increased intracranial pressure, rapidly progressive hydrocephalus, or dysfunction of a shunt. More slowly progressive visual loss suggests tumor or neurodegenerative disease. Gliomas of the optic nerve and chiasm and craniopharyngiomas are primary diagnostic considerations in children who show progressive loss of vision.

Clinical manifestations of impairment of vision vary with the age and abilities of a child, the mode of onset, and the laterality and severity of the deficit. The first clue to amaurosis in an infant may be nystagmus or strabismus, the vision defect itself passing undetected for some time. Timidity, clumsiness, or behavioral change may be the initial clues in the very young. Deterioration in school progress and indifference to school activities are common signs in an older child. School-aged children often try to hide their disability and, in the case of very slowly progressive disorders, may not themselves realize the severity of the problem; some detect and promptly report small changes in their vision.

Any evidence of loss of vision requires prompt and thorough ophthalmic evaluation. Complete delineation of childhood amaurosis and its cause usually requires extensive investigation involving neurologic evaluation, electrophysiologic tests, neuroradiologic procedures, and sometimes metabolic and genetic studies. Furthermore, attendant special educational, social, and emotional needs must be met.

NYCTALOPIA. Nyctalopia, or night blindness, is vision that is defective in reduced illumination. It generally implies impairment in function of the rods, particularly in dark adaptation time and perceptual threshold. *Stationary congenital night blindness* may occur as an autosomal dominant, autosomal recessive, or X-linked recessive condition. It may be associated with myopia, nystagmus, and disc anomaly. *Progressive night blindness* usually indicates primary or secondary retinal, choroidal, or vitrioretinal degeneration (see Chapter 637); it occurs also in vitamin A deficiency or as a result of retinotoxic drugs such as quinine.

PSYCHOGENIC DISTURBANCES. Vision problems of psychogenic origin are common in school-aged children. Both conversion reactions and willful feigning are encountered. The usual manifestation is a report of reduced visual acuity in one or both eyes. Another common manifestation is constriction of the visual field. In some cases, the symptom is diplopia or polyopia. See Chapters 19 and 22.

Important clues to the diagnosis are inappropriate affect, excessive grimacing, inconsistency in performance, and suggestibility. Thorough ophthalmologic examination is essential to differentiate organic from functional visual disorders.

Affected children usually fare well with reassurance and positive suggestion. In some cases, psychiatric care is indicated. In all cases, the approach must be supportive and nonpunitive.

DYSLEXIA. Dyslexia is the inability to develop the capability to read at an expected level despite an otherwise normal intellect. The terms reading disability and dyslexia are often used interchangeably. Most dyslexic individuals also display poor writing ability. Dyslexia is a primary reading disorder and should be differentiated from secondary reading difficulties due to mental retardation, environmental or educational deprivation, and physical, or organic, diseases. Because there is no one standard test for dyslexia, the diagnosis is usually made by comparing reading ability with intelligence and standard reading expectations. Dyslexia is a language-based disorder and is not caused by any defect in the eye or visual acuity per se, nor is it attributable to a defect in ocular motility or binocular alignment. Although ophthalmologic evaluation of children with a reading problem is recommended to diagnose and correct any concurrent ocular problems such as a refractive error, amblyopia, or strabismus, treatment directed to the eyes themselves cannot be expected to correct developmental dyslexia (Chapter 29.3).

American Academy of Ophthalmology: Policy Statement: Learning Disabilities, Dyslexia, and Vision. San Francisco, American Academy of Ophthalmology, 1992.

Barnet AB, Manson JI, Wilmer E: Acute cerebral blindness in childhood. Six cases studied clinically and electrophysiologically. Neurology 30:1147, 1970.

Catalano RA, Simon JW, Krohel GB, et al: Functional visual loss in children. Ophthalmology 93:385, 1986.

Duffy FH, Burchfield JL, Snodgrass SR: The pharmacology of amblyopia. Ophthalmology 86:489, 1978.

Flynn JT: Amblyopia revisited. J Pediatr Ophthalmol Strabismus 28:171, 1991.

Francois J: Diagnosis of blindness in the infant. Ann Ophthalmol 2:533, 1970.

Hittner HM, Borda RP, Justice J Jr: X-linked recessive congential stationary night blindness, myopia, and tilted discs. J Pediatr Ophthalmol 18:15, 1981.

Jastrzebski GR, Hoyt CS, Marg E: Stimulus deprivation amblyopia in children: Sensitivity, plasticity, and elasticity (SPE). Arch Ophthalmol 102:1030, 1984.

Kushner BJ: Functional amblyopia associated with organic ocular lesions. Am J Ophthalmol 91:39, 1981.

Mellor DH, Fields AR: Dissociated visual development: Electrodiagnostic studies in infants who are "slow to see." Dev Med Child Neurol 22:327, 1980.

Olitsky SE, Nelson LB: Reading disorders in children. Ophthalmol Clin North Am 2:309, 1996.

Stager DR: Amblyopia and the pediatrician. Pediatr Ann 8:91, 1977.

Tongue AC: Low vision examination in children with visual impairment. J Pediatr Ophthalmol Strabismus 17:175, 1980.

Vellutino F: Dyslexia. Sci Am 25:20, 1987.

Von Noorden GK: Amblyopia: A multidisciplinary approach. Invest Ophthalmol Vis Sci 26:1704, 1985.

CHAPTER 629

Abnormalities of Pupil and Iris

ANIRIDIA. The term aniridia is a misnomer because iris tissue is usually present, although it is hypoplastic (Fig. 629–1). Two thirds of the cases are dominantly transmitted with a high degree of penetrance. The other one third of cases are sporadic and are considered to be new mutations. The condition is bilateral in 98% of all patients regardless of the means of transmission and is found in approximately 1/50,000 persons.

Aniridia is a panocular disorder and should not be thought of as an isolated iris defect. Macular and optic nerve hypoplasia are commonly present and lead to decreased vision and sensory nystagmus. The visual acuity is measured as 20/200 in most patients, although the vision may occasionally be better. Other ocular deformities are common and may involve the lens and cornea. The cornea may be small, and a cellular infiltrate (pannus) occasionally develops in the superficial layers of the peripheral cornea. Clinically this appears as a gray opacification. Lens abnormalities include cataract formation and partial or total lens dislocation. Glaucoma develops in as many as 75% of individuals with aniridia.

One fifth of sporadic aniridic patients may develop **Wilms tumor** (Chapter 505.1). Of particular interest is the association of aniridia, genitourinary anomalies, mental retardation, and a partial deletion of the short arm of chromosome 11. Among

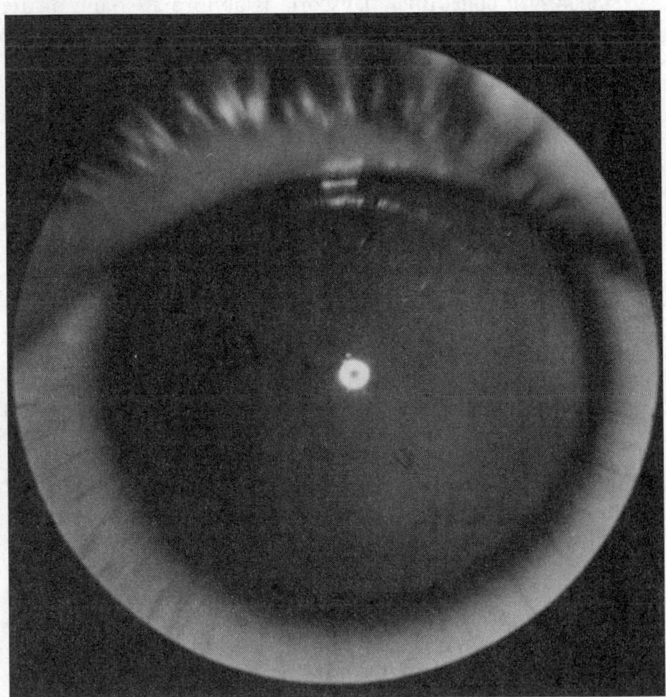

Figure 629–1 Aniridia. Minimal iris tissue. (From Nelson LB, Spaeth GL, Nowinski TS, et al: Aniridia: A review. Surv Ophthalmol 28:621, 1984.)

individuals thus affected, the appearance of Wilms tumor is more common. It is thought that only patients with sporadic aniridia are at risk for developing Wilms tumor, although Wilms tumor has occurred in a patient with familial aniridia. Wilms tumor usually presents before the 3rd yr. Therefore, these children should be screened using renal ultrasonography every 3–6 mo, until approximately age 5 yr.

The gene for aniridia had been localized to the 11p13 region. This gene may be involved in properly directing the interactions between the optic cup, surface ectoderm, and neural crest cells during early formation of the iris and other ocular structures.

COLOBOMA OF THE IRIS. This developmental defect may present as a defect in a sector of the iris, a hole in the substance of the iris, or a notch in the pupillary margin. Simple colobomas are frequently transmitted as an autosomal dominant trait and may occur alone or in association with other anomalies. A coloboma is formed when the embryonic fissure fails to close completely. Because of the anatomic location of the embryonic fissure, an iris coloboma is always located inferiorly, giving the iris a keyhole appearance. An iris coloboma may be the only externally visible part of an extensive malclosure of the embryonic fissure that also involves the fundus and optic nerve. Therefore, all children with an iris coloboma should undergo a full ophthalmologic examination.

MICROCORIA. Microcoria (congenital miosis) appears as a small pupil that does not react to light or accommodation and that dilates poorly, if at all, with medication. The condition may be unilateral or bilateral. In bilateral cases, the degree of miosis may be different in each eye. The eye may be otherwise normal or may demonstrate other abnormalities of the anterior segment. Congenital microcoria is usually transmitted as an autosomal dominant trait, although it may occur sporadically.

CONGENITAL MYDRIASIS. In this disorder, the pupils appear dilated, do not constrict significantly to light or near gaze, and respond minimally to miotic agents. The iris is otherwise normal, and affected children are usually healthy. Trauma, pharmacologic mydriasis, and neurologic disorders should be considered. Many apparent cases of congenital mydriasis show abnormalities of the central iris structures and may be considered a form of aniridia.

DYSCORIA AND CORECTOPIA. Dyscoria is abnormal shape of the pupil, and corectopia is abnormal pupillary position. They may occur together or independently as congenital or acquired anomalies.

Congenital corectopia is usually bilateral and symmetric and rarely occurs as an isolated anomaly; it is usually accompanied by dislocation of the lens (ectopia lentis et pupillae), and the lens and pupil are commonly dislocated in opposite directions. Ectopia lentis et pupillae is transmitted as an autosomal recessive disorder; consanguity is common.

When acquired, distortion and displacement of the pupil are frequently a result of trauma or intraocular inflammation. Prolapse of the iris after perforating injuries of the eye leads to peaking of the pupil in the direction of the perforation. Posterior synechiae (adhesions of the iris to the lens) are commonly seen when inflammation due to any cause occurs in the anterior segment.

ANISOCORIA. This is inequality of the pupils. The difference in size may be due to local or neurologic disorders. As a rule, if the inequality is more pronounced in the presence of bright focal illumination or on near gaze, there is a defect in pupillary constriction and the larger pupil is abnormal. If the anisocoria is worse in reduced illumination, a defect in dilation exists and the smaller pupil is abnormal. Neurologic causes of anisocoria (parasympathetic or sympathetic lesions) must be differentiated from local causes such as synechiae (adhesions), congenital iris defects (colobomas, aniridia), and pharmacologic effects. Simple central anisocoria may occur in otherwise healthy individuals.

DILATED FIXED PUPIL. Differential diagnosis of a dilated unreactive pupil includes internal ophthalmoplegia caused by a central or peripheral lesion, Hutchinson's pupil of transtentorial herniation, tonic pupil, pharmacologic blockade, and iridoplegia secondary to ocular trauma.

The most common cause of a dilated unreactive pupil is purposeful or accidental instillation of a cycloplegic agent, particularly atropine and related substances. Central lesions, such as a pinealoma, may cause internal ophthalmoplegia in children. Because the external surface of the oculomotor nerve carries the fibers responsible for pupillary constriction, compression of the nerve along its intracranial course may be associated with internal ophthalmoplegia, even before the development of ptosis or an ocular motility deficit. Although ophthalmoplegic migraine is a common cause of a 3rd nerve palsy with pupillary involvement in children, an intracranial aneurysm must also be considered in the differential diagnosis. The "blown pupil" of transtentorial herniation, occurring with increasing intracranial pressure, is generally unilateral, and patients usually are obviously ill. The pilocarpine test can help differentiate neurologic iridoplegia from pharmacologic blockade. In the case of neurologic iridoplegia, the dilated pupil constricts within minutes after instillation of 1 or 2 drops of 0.5–1% pilocarpine; if the pupil has been dilated with atropine, pilocarpine has no effect. Because pilocarpine is a long-acting drug, this test is not to be used in acute situations in which pupillary signs must be carefully monitored. Because of the consensual pupil response to light, it is important to realize that even complete uniocular blindness does not cause a unilaterally dilated pupil.

TONIC PUPIL. This is typically a large pupil that reacts poorly to light (the reaction may be very slow or essentially nil), reacts poorly and slowly to accommodation, and redilates in a slow, tonic manner. The features of tonic pupil are explained by cholinergic supersensitivity of the sphincter after peripheral (postganglionic) denervation and imperfect reinnervation. A distinctive feature of a tonic pupil is its sensitivity to dilute cholinergic agents. Instillation of 0.125% pilocarpine causes significant constriction of the involved pupil and has little or no effect on the unaffected side. The condition is usually unilateral.

Tonic pupil may develop after the acute stage of a partial or complete iridoplegia. It can be seen after trauma to the eye or orbit and may occur in association with toxic or infectious conditions. In those in the pediatric age group, tonic pupil is uncommon. Infectious processes (primarily viral syndromes) and trauma are the primary causes. Features of tonic pupil may also be seen in infants and children with familial dysautonomia (Riley-Day syndrome), although the significance of these findings has been questioned. Tonic pupil has also been reported in young children with Charcot-Marie-Tooth disease. The occurrence of tonic pupil in association with decreased deep tendon reflexes in young women is referred to as **Adie's syndrome**.

MARCUS GUNN PUPIL. This relative afferent pupillary defect indicates an asymmetric, prechiasmatic, afferent conduction defect. It is best demonstrated by the swinging flashlight test; this allows comparison of the direct and consensual pupillary responses in both eyes. With patients fixing on a distant target (to control accommodation), a bright focal light is directed alternately into each eye in turn. In the presence of an afferent lesion, both the direct response to light in the affected eye and the consensual response in the fellow eye are subnormal. Swinging the light to the better or normal eye causes both pupils to react (constrict) normally. Swinging the light back to the affected eye causes both pupils to redilate to some degree, reflecting the defective conduction. This is a very sensitive and useful test for detecting and confirming optic nerve and retinal disease. A subtle relative afferent defect may be found in some children with amblyopia.

HORNER SYNDROME. The principal signs of oculosympathetic paresis (Horner syndrome) are homolateral miosis, mild ptosis, and apparent enophthalmos with slight elevation of the lower lid. Patients may also have decreased facial sweating, increased amplitude of accommodation, and transient decrease in intraocular pressure. If paralysis of the ocular sympathetic fibers occurs before the age of 2 yr, heterochromia iridis with hypopigmentation of the iris may occur on the affected side.

Oculosympathetic paralysis may be caused by a lesion in the midbrain, brain stem, upper spinal cord, neck, middle fossa, or orbit. Congenital oculosympathetic paresis resulting from birth trauma, often as part of Klumpke brachial palsy, is common, although the ocular signs, particularly the anisocoria, may pass undetected for years. Horner syndrome is also seen in some children after thoracic surgery, as for congenital heart disease. Congenital Horner syndrome may occur in association with vertebral anomalies and with enterogenous cysts. In some infants and children, Horner's syndrome is the presenting sign of tumor in the mediastinal or cervical region, particularly neuroblastoma. Rare causes of Horner syndrome, such as vascular lesions, also occur in the pediatric age group. In some cases, no cause of Horner syndrome can be identified. Occasionally, the condition is familial.

When the cause of Horner syndrome is in question, investigative procedures should be implemented, including chest radiography, CT, MRI of the head and neck, and 24-hr urinary catecholamine assay. Examining old photographs and old records can sometimes be helpful in establishing the age of onset of Horner syndrome.

The *cocaine test* is useful in diagnosing oculosympathetic paralysis; a normal pupil dilates within 20–45 min after instillation of 1 or 2 drops of 4% cocaine, whereas the miotic pupil of an oculosympathetic paresis dilates poorly, if at all, with cocaine. In some cases there is denervation supersensitivity to dilute phenylephrine; 1 or 2 drops of a 1% solution dilates the affected but not the normal pupil. Furthermore, instillation of 1% hydroxyamphetamine hydrobromide dilates the pupil only if the postganglionic sympathetic neuron is intact.

PARADOXICAL PUPIL REACTION. Some children exhibit paradoxical constriction of the pupils to darkness. An initial brisk constriction of the pupils occurs when the light is turned off, followed by slow redilation of the pupils. The response to direct light stimulation and the near response are normal. The mechanism is not clear, but paradoxical constriction of the pupils in reduced light can be a sign of retinal or optic nerve abnormalities. The phenomenon has been observed in children with congenital stationary night blindness, albinism, retinitis pigmentosa, Leber congenital retinal amaurosis, and Best disease. It has also been observed in those with optic nerve anomalies, optic neuritis, optic atrophy, and possibly amblyopia.

PERSISTENT PUPILLARY MEMBRANE. Involution of the pupillary membrane and anterior vascular capsule of the lens is usually completed during the 5th–6th mo of fetal development. It is common to see some remnants of the pupillary membrane in newborns, particularly in premature infants. These membranes are nonpigmented strands of obliterated vessels that cross the pupil and may secondarily attach to the lens or cornea. The remnants tend to atrophy in time and usually present no problem. In some cases, however, significant remnants that remain obscure the pupil and interfere with vision. Rarely, there is patency of the vascular elements; hyphema may result from rupture of persistent vessels.

Intervention must be considered to minimize amblyopia in infants with extensive persistent pupillary membrane of sufficient degree to interfere with vision in the early months of life. In some cases, mydriatics and occlusion therapy may be effective, but in others surgery may be needed to provide an adequate pupillary aperture.

HETEROCHROMIA. In heterochromia, the two irides are of different color (heterochromia iridum), or a portion of an iris differs in color from the remainder (heterochromia iridis). Simple heterochromia may occur as an autosomal dominant characteristic. Congenital heterochromia is also a feature of **Waardenburg syndrome**, an autosomal dominant condition characterized principally by lateral displacement of the inner canthi and puncta, pigmentary disturbances (usually a median white forelock and patches of hypopigmentation of the skin), and defective hearing. Change in the color of the iris may occur as a result of trauma, hemorrhage, intraocular inflammation (iridocyclitis, uveitis), intraocular tumor (especially retinoblastoma), intraocular foreign body, glaucoma, iris atrophy, oculosympathetic palsy (Horner syndrome), or melanosis oculi.

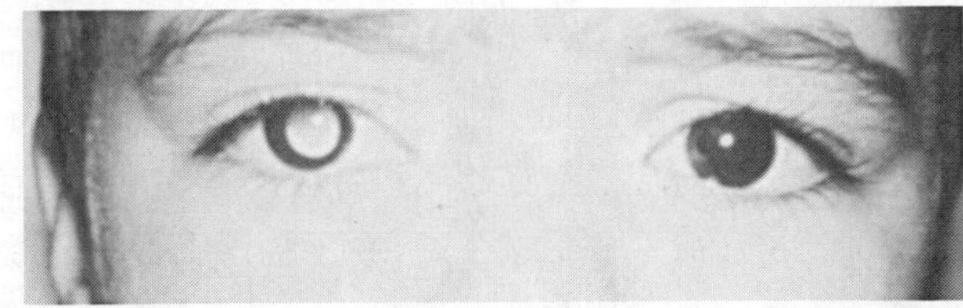

Figure 629–2 Leukocoria. White pupillary reflex in a child with retinoblastoma.

OTHER IRIS LESIONS. Discrete nodules of the iris, referred to as **Lisch nodules**, are commonly seen in patients with neurofibromatosis. Lisch nodules represent melanocytic hamartomas of the iris and vary from slightly elevated pigmented areas to distinct ball-like excrescences. Lisch nodules are found in 92–100% of individuals older than 5 yr and having neurofibromatosis. Slit-lamp identification of these nodules may help to fulfill the criteria required to confirm the diagnosis of neurofibromatosis.

In leukemia there may be infiltration of the iris, sometimes with hypopyon, an accumulation of white blood cells in the anterior chamber, which may herald relapse or involvement of the central nervous system.

The lesion of juvenile xanthogranuloma (nevoxanthoendothelioma) may occur in the eye as a yellowish fleshy mass or plaque of the iris. Spontaneous hyphema (blood in the anterior chamber), glaucoma, or a red eye with signs of uveitis may be associated. A search for the skin lesions of xanthogranuloma (see also Chapter 83.3) should be made in any infant or young child with spontaneous hyphema. In many cases, the ocular lesion responds to topical corticosteroid therapy.

LEUKOKORIA. This includes any white pupillary reflex, or so-called *cat's-eye reflex*. Primary diagnostic considerations in any child with leukokoria are cataract, persistent hyperplastic primary vitreous, cicatricial retinopathy of prematurity, retinal detachment and retinoschisis, larval granulomatosis, and retinoblastoma (Fig. 629–2). Also to be considered are endophthalmitis, organized vitreous hemorrhage, leukemic ophthalmopathy, exudative retinopathy (as in *Coat disease*), and a few rare conditions such as medulloepithelioma, massive retinal gliosis, the retinal pseudotumor of Norrie's disease, the so-called pseudoglioma of the *Bloch-Sulzberger syndrome*, retinal dysplasia, and the retinal lesions of the phakomatoses. A white reflex may also be seen with fundus coloboma, large atrophic chorioretinal scars, and ectopic medullation of retinal nerve fibers. Leukokoria is an indication for prompt and thorough evaluation.

The diagnosis can often be made by direct examination of the eye by ophthalmoscopy and biomicroscopy. Ultrasonographic and radiologic examinations are often helpful. In some cases, the final diagnosis rests with a pathologist.

Cross HE: Ectopia lentis et pupillae. Am J Ophthalmol 88:381, 1979.
Francois J: Differential diagnosis of leukokoria in children. Ann Ophthalmol 10:1375, 1978.

Frank JW, Kushner BJ, France TD: Paradoxic pupillary phenomenon: A review of patients with pupillary constriction to darkness. Arch Ophthalmol 106:1564, 1988.
Greenwald MJ, Folk ER: Afferent pupillary defects in amblyopia. J Pediatr Ophthalmol Strabismus 20:63, 1983.
Hersh JH, Douglas C, Houston J, et al: Familial iridoplegia. J Pediatr Ophthalmol Strabismus 24:49, 1982.
Ivanov I, Shuper A, Shohat M, et al: Aniridia: Recent achievements in paediatric practice. Eur J Pediatr 154:795, 1995.
Jaffe N, Cassady JR, Filler RM, et al: Heterochromia and Horner syndrome associated with cervical and mediastinal neuroblastoma. J Pediatr 87:75, 1975.
Krishnamohan VK, Wheeler MD, Testa MA, et al: Correlation of postnatal regression of the anterior vesicular capsule of the lens to gestational age. J Pediatr Ophthalmol Strabismus 19:28, 1982.
Lewis RA, Riccardi VM: Von Recklinghausen neurofibromatosis: Incidence of iris hamartomata. Ophthalmology 88:348, 1981.
Lowenfeld IE: "Simple, central" anisocoria: A common condition seldom recognized. Trans Am Acad Ophthalmol Otolaryngol 83:832, 1977.
Maloney WF, Younge BR, Moyer NJ: Evaluation of the causes and accuracy of pharmacologic localization in Horner's syndrome. Am J Ophthalmol 90:394, 1980.
Polomeno RC, Milot J: Congenital miosis. Can J Ophthalmol 14:43, 1979.
Schachat AP, Jabs DA, Graham ML, et al: Leukemic iris infiltration. J Pediatr Ophthalmol Strabismus 25:135, 1988.
Thompson HS: Segmental palsy of the iris sphincter in Adie's syndrome. Arch Ophthalmol 96:1615, 1978.
Thompson HS, Newsome DA, Loewenfeld IE: The fixed dilated pupil: Sudden iridoplegia or mydriatic drops? A simple diagnostic test. Arch Ophthalmol 86:21, 1971.
Woodruff G, Buncic JR, Morin JD: Horner syndrome in children. J Pediatr Ophthalmol Strabismus 25:40, 1988.

CHAPTER 630
Disorders of Eye Movement and Alignment

STRABISMUS

Strabismus, or misalignment of the eyes, is one of the most common eye problems encountered in children, affecting approximately 4% of children younger than 6 yr. This important ocular disorder can result in vision loss (amblyopia) in one eye and can have significant psychologic effects. Early detection and treatment of strabismus is essential to prevent permanent visual impairment. Of children with strabismus, 30–50% develop secondary visual loss (amblyopia). Restoration of proper alignment of the visual axis must occur at an early stage of visual development to allow these children a chance to develop normal binocular vision.

DEFINITIONS. The word *strabismus* means "to squint or to look obliquely." Many terms are used in discussing strabismus.

Orthophoria is the ideal condition of exact ocular balance. It implies that the oculomotor apparatus is in perfect equilibrium so that the eyes remain coordinated and aligned in all positions of gaze and at all distances. Even when fusion is interrupted, as by occlusion of one eye, truly orthophoric individuals maintain perfect alignment. Orthophoria is seldom encountered, because the majority of individuals have a small latent deviation (heterophoria).

Heterophoria is a latent tendency for the eyes to deviate. This latent deviation is normally controlled by fusional mechanisms that provide binocular vision or avoid diplopia (double vision). The eye deviates only under certain conditions, such as fatigue, illness, or stress, or during tests that interfere with maintenance of these normal fusional abilities (such as covering one eye). If the amount of heterophoria is large, it may give rise to bothersome symptoms, such as transient diplopia (double vision), headaches, or asthenopia (eyestrain). Some degree of heterophoria is found in normal individuals; it is usually asymptomatic.

Heterotropia is a misalignment of the eyes that is apparent. It occurs because of an inability of the fusional mechanism to control the deviation. Tropias can be alternating, involving both eyes, or unilateral. In an alternating tropia, there is no preference for fixation of either eye, and both eyes drift at an equal rate. Vision usually develops normally in both eyes because each eye is used in turn. A unilateral tropia is a more serious situation because only one eye is constantly maligned. The undeviated eye becomes the preferred eye, resulting in loss of vision or amblyopia of the deviated eye.

It is common in ocular misalignments to describe the type of deviation present because this indicates different causes and treatments of the strabismus. The prefixes *eso-*, *exo-*, *hyper-*, and *hypo-* are added to the terms *-phoria* and *-tropia* to delineate further the type of deviation. *Esophorias* and *esotropias* are inward or convergent deviations of the eyes, commonly known as *crossed eyes*. *Exophorias* and *exotropias* are divergent or outward-facing eye deviations, *walleyed* being the lay term. Hyperdeviations and hypodeviations designate upward or downward deviations of an eye. In cases of unilateral strabismus, the deviating eye is often part of the description of the misalignment (left esotropia).

DIAGNOSIS. Many techniques are used to assess ocular alignment and movement of the eyes to aid in diagnosing strabismic disorders. In a child with strabismus or any other ocular disorder, assessment of visual acuity is mandatory. Decreased vision in one eye requires evaluation for ocular deviation or other ocular abnormalities, which may be difficult to discern on a quick screening evaluation. Even strabismic deviations of only a few degrees in magnitude, too small to be evident by gross inspection, may lead to amblyopia and devastating vision loss.

Corneal light reflex tests are perhaps the most rapid and easily performed diagnostic tests for strabismus. They are particularly useful in children who are uncooperative and in those who have poor ocular fixation. To perform Hirschberg's corneal reflex test, the examiner projects a light source onto the cornea of both eyes simultaneously as a child looks directly at the light. Comparison should then be made of the placement of the corneal light reflex in each eye. In straight eyes, the light reflection appears symmetric and, because of the relationship between the cornea and the macula, slightly nasal to the center of each pupil. If strabismus is present, the reflected light is asymmetric and appears off center in one eye. Krimsky's method of the corneal reflex test uses prisms placed over one or both eyes to align the light reflections. The amount of prism needed to align the reflections is used to measure the degree of deviation of the eye.

Cover tests for strabismus require a child's attention and cooperation, good eye movement capability, and reasonably good vision in each eye. If any of these are lacking, the results of these tests may not be valid. These tests consist of the cover-uncover test and the alternate-cover test. In the cover-uncover test, a child looks at an object in the distance, preferably 6 m away. An eye chart is commonly used for fixation in children older than 3 yr. For younger children, a brightly colored or noise-making toy helps hold their attention for the test. As the child looks at the distant object, the examiner covers one eye and watches for movement of the uncovered eye. If no movement occurs, there is no apparent misalignment of that eye. After one eye is tested, the same procedure is repeated on the other eye. When performing the alternate-cover test, the examiner rapidly covers and uncovers each eye, shifting back and forth from one eye to another like a windshield wiper. If the child has any ocular deviation, the eye rapidly moves as the cover is shifted to the other eye. Both the cover-uncover test and the alternate-cover test should be performed at both distance and near fixation, with and without glasses. The cover-uncover test differentiates tropias, or manifest deviations, from latent deviations, called *phorias*.

CLINICAL MANIFESTATIONS AND TREATMENT. The etiologic classification of strabismus is complex, and the causative types must be distinguished; these are nonparalytic and paralytic types.

Nonparalytic Strabismus. Nonparalytic strabismus is the most common type. The individual extraocular muscles usually have no defect. The amount of deviation is constant, or relatively constant, in the various directions of gaze.

ESODEVIATIONS. Esodeviations are the most common type of ocular misalignment in children and represent well over 50% of all ocular deviations.

Pseudostrabismus (pseudoesotropia) is one of the most common reasons a pediatric ophthalmologist is asked to evaluate an infant. This condition is characterized by the false appearance of strabismus when the visual axes are aligned accurately. This appearance may be caused by a flat, broad nasal bridge; prominent epicanthal folds; or a narrow interpupillary distance. The observer may see less white sclera nasally than would be expected, and the impression is that the eye is turned in toward the nose, especially when the child gazes to either side. Parents frequently comment that when their child looks to the side, the eye almost disappears from view. Pseudoesotropia can be differentiated from a true misalignment of the eyes when the corneal light reflex is centered in both eyes and when the cover-uncover test shows no refixation movement. Once pseudoesotropia has been confirmed, parents can be reassured that the child will outgrow the appearance of esotropia. As the child grows, the bridge of the nose becomes more prominent and displaces the epicanthal folds, and the medial sclera becomes proportional to the amount visible on the lateral aspect. It should be emphasized that it is the appearance of crossing that the child will outgrow. Many parents of children with pseudoesotropia erroneously believe that their child has an actual esotropia that will resolve on its own. Because true esotropia can develop later in children with pseudoesotropia, parents and pediatricians should be cautioned that reassessment is required if the apparent deviation does not improve.

Congenital esotropia is a confusing term. Few children who are diagnosed with this disorder are actually born with an esotropia. Most reports in the literature have therefore considered infants with confirmed onset earlier than 6 mo as having the same condition, which some observers have redesignated infantile esotropia.

The characteristic angle of congenital esodeviations is large and constant. Owing to the large deviation, cross-fixation is frequently encountered. This is a condition in which the child looks to the right with the left eye and to the left with the right eye. With cross-fixation, each eye is reluctant to turn away from the nose (abduction); this condition simulates a 6th nerve palsy. Abduction can be demonstrated by the doll's head maneuver or by patching one eye for a short time. Children with congenital esotropia tend to have refractive errors similar to those of normal children of the same age. This contrasts with the characteristic high level of farsightedness associated with accommodative esotropia (see below). Amblyopia is common in children with congenital esotropia.

The primary goal of treatment in congenital esotropia is to eliminate or reduce the deviation as much as possible. Ideally, this results in normal sight in each eye, in straight-looking eyes, and in the development of binocular vision. Early treatment is more likely to lead to the development of binocular vision, which helps to maintain long-term ocular alignment. Once any associated amblyopia is treated, surgery is performed to align the eyes. Even with successful surgical alignment, it is common for vertical deviations to develop in children with a history of congenital esotropia. One form of vertical deviation results from overaction of the inferior oblique muscles. When this occurs, side gaze produces an upshoot of the eye closest to the nose. Dissociated vertical deviation also develops in children with infantile esotropia. In this type of deviation, one eye drifts up slowly with no movement of the other eye. Surgery may be necessary to treat either or both of these conditions.

It is important that parents realize that early successful surgical alignment is only the beginning of the treatment processes. Because many children may redevelop strabismus or amblyopia, they need to be monitored closely during the visually immature period of life.

Accommodative esotropia is defined as a "convergent deviation of the eyes associated with activation of the accommodative (focusing) reflex." It usually occurs in a child who is between 2 and 3 yr of age and who has a history of acquired intermittent or constant crossing. Amblyopia occurs in the majority of cases.

The mechanism of accommodative esotropia involves uncorrected hyperopia, accommodation, and accommodative convergence. The image entering a hyperopic (farsighted) eye is blurred. If the amount of hyperopia is not significant, the blurred image can be sharpened by accommodating (focusing of the lens of the eye). Accommodation is closely linked with convergence (eyes turning inward). If a child's hyperopic refractive error is large or if the amount of convergence that occurs in response to each unit of accommodative effort is great, esotropia may develop.

To treat accommodative esotropia, the full hyperopic (farsighted) correction is initially prescribed. These glasses eliminate a child's need to accommodate and therefore eliminate the esotropia (Fig. 630–1). Although many parents are initially concerned that their child will not want to wear glasses, the benefits of binocular vision and decreasing the focusing effort required to see clearly provide a strong stimulus to wear glasses, and they are generally accepted well. The full hyperopic correction sometimes straightens the eye position at distance fixation but leaves a residual deviation at near fixation; this may be observed or treated with bifocal lenses, antiaccommodative drops, or surgery.

It is important to warn parents of children with accommodative esotropia that the esodeviation may appear to increase without glasses after the initial correction is worn. Parents frequently state that before wearing glasses, their child had a small esodeviation, whereas after removal of the glasses the esodeviation is now quite large. Parents often blame the increased esodeviation on the glasses. This apparent increase is due to a child's using the appropriate amount of accommodative effort after the glasses have been worn. When these children remove their glasses, they continue to use an accommodative effort in order to bring objects into proper focus and increase the esodeviation.

Most children maintain straight eyes once initially treated. Because hyperopia generally decreases with age, many but not all patients outgrow the need to wear glasses to maintain alignment. In some patients, a residual esodeviation persists even when wearing their glasses. This condition commonly occurs when there is a delay between the onset of accommodative esotropia and treatment. In others, the esotropia may initially be eliminated with glasses but crossing redevelops and is not correctable with glasses. The crossing that is no longer correctable with glasses is the deteriorated or nonaccommodative portion. Surgery for this portion of the crossing is indicated to regain binocular vision.

EXODEVIATIONS. Exodeviations are the second most common type of misalignment. The divergent deviation may be intermittent or constant. *Intermittent exotropia* is the most common exodeviation in childhood. It is characterized by outward drifting of one eye, which usually occurs when a child is fixating at distance. The deviation is generally more frequent with fatigue or illness. Exposure to bright light may cause reflex closure of the exotropic eye. Because the eyes initially can be kept straight most of the time, visual acuity tends to be good in both eyes and binocular vision is initially normal.

The age of onset of intermittent exotropia varies but is often

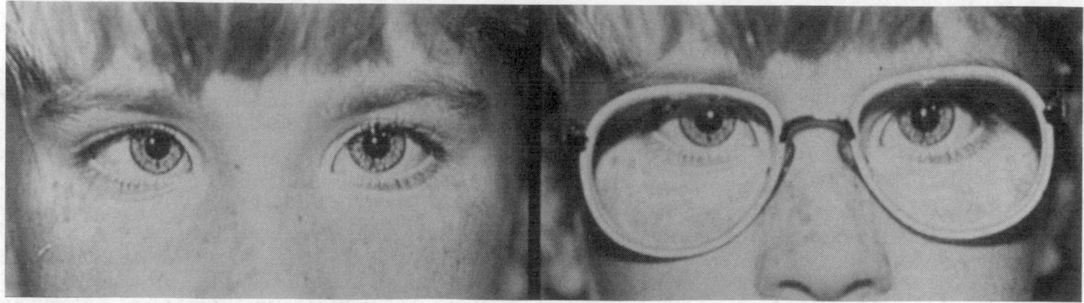

Figure 630–1 Accommodative esotropia; control of deviation with corrective lenses.

between age 6 mo and 4 yr. The decision to perform eye muscle surgery is based on the amount and frequency of the deviation. If the deviation is small and infrequent, it is reasonable just to observe the child. If the exotropia is large or increasing in frequency, surgery is indicated to maintain normal binocular vision.

Constant exotropia may rarely be congenital. Exotropia also may be associated with neurologic disease or abnormalities of the bony orbit, as in Crouzon's syndrome. Exotropia that occurs later life may represent a deterioration of an intermittent exotropia that was present in childhood. Surgery can restore binocular vision even in long-standing cases.

Paralytic Strabismus. When an eye muscle is paretic or palsied, a characteristic muscle imbalance occurs in which the deviation of the eye varies according to the direction of gaze. Recent onset of a paretic muscle can be suggested by the symptom of double vision that increases in one direction, the findings of an ocular deviation that increases in the field of action of the paretic muscle, and an increase in the deviation when the child fixates with the paretic eye. It is important to differentiate an extraocular muscle paresis or palsy from a comitant deviation because noncomitant forms of strabismus are often associated with trauma, systemic disorders, or neurologic abnormalities.

Third Nerve Palsy. In the pediatric population, 3rd nerve palsies are usually congenital. The congenital form is often associated with a developmental anomaly or birth trauma. Acquired 3rd nerve palsies in children can be an ominous sign and may indicate a neurologic abnormality such as an intracranial neoplasm or an aneurysm. Other less serious causes include an inflammatory or infectious lesion, head trauma, postviral syndromes, and migraines.

A 3rd nerve palsy, whether congenital or acquired, usually results in an exotropia. In this situation, the exotropia is associated with a hypotropia, or downward deviation of the affected eye, as well as complete or partial ptosis of the upper lid. This characteristic deviation results from the action of the remaining unopposed muscles, the lateral rectus muscle and the superior oblique muscle. If the internal branch of the 3rd nerve is involved, pupillary dilation may be noted as well. Eye movements are usually limited nasally, in elevation and in depression. In addition, clinical findings and treatment may be complicated in congenital and traumatic cases of 3rd nerve palsy owing to misdirection of regenerating nerve fibers, referred to as **aberrant regeneration**. This results in anomalous and paradoxical eyelid, eye and pupil movement such as elevation of the eyelid, constriction of the pupil, or depression of the globe on attempted medial gaze.

Fourth Nerve Palsy. These palsies can be congenital or acquired. Because the 4th nerve has a long intracranial course, it is susceptible to damage resulting from head trauma. In children, however, 4th nerve palsies are more frequently congenital than traumatic. A palsied 4th nerve results in weakness in the superior oblique muscle, which causes an upward deviation of the eye, a hypertropia. Because the antagonist muscle, the inferior oblique, is relatively unopposed, the affected eye demonstrates an upshoot when looking toward the nose. Children typically present with a head tilt to the shoulder opposite the affected eye, their chin down and their face turned away from the affected side. This position is assumed to minimize the deviation and the associated double vision. Because the abnormal head posture maintains the child's ocular alignment, amblyopia is uncommon. Because no abnormality exists in the neck muscles, attempts to correct the head tilt by exercises and neck muscle surgery are ineffective. Recognition of a superior oblique paresis can be difficult because deviation of the head and the eye may be minimal. Eye muscle surgery can be performed to improve the ocular alignment and eliminate the abnormal head posture.

Sixth Nerve Palsy. These palsies produce markedly crossed eyes with limited ability to move the afflicted eye laterally. Children frequently present with their head turned toward the palsied muscle, a position that helps preserve binocular vision. The esotropia is largest when the eye is moved toward the affected muscle.

Congenital 6th nerve palsies are rare. Decreased lateral gaze in infants is often associated with other disorders, such as congenital esotropia or Duane's retraction syndrome. In neonates, a transient 6th nerve paresis can occur; it usually clears spontaneously by 6 wk. It is believed that increased intracranial pressure associated with labor and delivery is the contributing factor. A benign 6th nerve palsy, which is painless and acquired, can be noted in infants and older children. This is frequently preceded by a febrile illness or upper respiratory tract infection and may be recurrent. Complete resolution of the palsy is usual.

Acquired 6th nerve palsies in childhood are often an ominous sign because the 6th nerve is susceptible to increased intracranial pressure associated with hydrocephalous and intracranial tumors. Other causes of 6th nerve defects in children include trauma, vascular malformations, meningitis, and Gradenigo's syndrome. In this latter syndrome, otitis media precipitates a mastoiditis with associated petrositis and edema of the dura. These events result in pinching the 6th nerve against the petrosphenoidal ligament as the nerve passes between the ligament and the dura on its intracranial course. The 6th nerve palsy resolves with antibiotic treatment.

Strabismus Syndromes. Special types of strabismus have unusual clinical features. Most of these disorders are caused by structural anomalies of the extraocular muscles or adjacent tissues.

Double Elevator Palsy. A monocular elevation deficit in both abduction and adduction is referred to as double elevator palsy. It may represent a paresis of both elevators, the superior rectus and inferior oblique muscles, or a possible restriction to elevation from a fibrotic inferior rectus muscle. When an affected child fixates with the nonparetic eye, the paretic eye is hypotropic and the ipsilateral upper eyelid may appear ptotic. Fixation with the paretic eye causes a hypertropia of the nonparetic eye and a disappearance of the ptosis.

Duane Syndrome. This congenital disorder of ocular motility is characterized by retraction of the globe on adduction. This is attributed to anomalous innervation, which results in cocontraction of the medial and lateral rectus muscles on attempted adduction of the affected eye. Within the spectrum of Duane's syndrome, patients may exhibit impairment of abduction, impairment of adduction, or upshoot or downshoot of the involved eye on adduction. They may have esotropia, exotropia, or relatively straight eyes. Many exhibit compensatory posturing for the defect in horizontal eye movement. Some develop amblyopia. Surgery to improve ocular motility and alignment or to reduce a noticeable face turn can be helpful in selected cases.

Duane's syndrome usually occurs sporadically. It is sometimes inherited as an autosomal dominant trait. It usually occurs as an isolated condition but may occur in association with various other ocular and systemic anomalies.

Möbius Syndrome. The distinctive features of Möbius syndrome are congenital facial paresis and abduction weakness. The facial palsy is commonly bilateral, frequently asymmetric, and often incomplete, tending to spare the lower face and platysma. Ectropion, epiphora, and exposure keratopathy may develop. The abduction defect may be unilateral or bilateral. Esotropia is common. The cause is unknown. Whether the primary defect is maldevelopment of cranial nerve nuclei, hypoplasia of the muscles, or a combination of central and peripheral factors is unclear. Gestational factors such as trauma, illness, and intake of various drugs, particularly thalidomide, have been implicated. Some familial cases have been reported. Associated developmental defects may include ptosis, palatal and lingual palsy, hearing loss, pectoral and lingual muscle defects, micrognathia, syndactyly, supernumerary digits, or the absence of hands, feet, fingers, or toes. Surgical correction of the esotropia is indicated in selected cases, and any attendant amblyopia should be treated.

Brown Syndrome. In this syndrome, elevation of the eye in the adducted position is restricted or absent. An associated downward deviation of the affected eye in adduction is common. A compensatory tilt of the head may occur. Various causes have been described. Some cases have been attributed to structural abnormalities such as a tight superior oblique tendon, congenital shortening or thickening of the superior oblique tendon sheath, or connective tissue trabeculae between the superior oblique tendon and the trochlea. No anatomic abnormality is sometimes found.

Acquired Brown syndrome may follow trauma to the orbit involving the region of the trochlea or sinus surgery. It may also occur with inflammatory processes, particularly sinusitis and juvenile rheumatoid arthritis.

Acquired inflammatory Brown syndrome may respond to treatment with steroids. Surgery may be helpful for children with true congenital Brown syndrome.

Parinaud Syndrome. This eponym designates a palsy of vertical gaze, isolated or associated with pupillary or nuclear oculomotor (cranial nerve III) paresis. It indicates a lesion affecting the mesencephalic tegmentum. The ophthalmic signs of midbrain disease include vertical gaze palsy, dissociation of the pupillary responses to light and to near focus, general pupillomotor paralysis, corectopia, dyscoria, accommodative disturbances, pathologic lid retraction, ptosis, extraocular muscle paresis, and convergence paralysis. Some cases have associated spasms of convergence, convergent retraction nystagmus, and vertical nystagmus, particularly on attempted vertical gaze. Combinations of these signs are referred to as the Koerber-Salus-Elschnig or sylvian aqueduct syndrome.

A principal cause of vertical gaze palsy and associated mesencephalic signs in children is tumor of the pineal gland or 3rd ventricle. Differential diagnosis includes trauma and demyelinating disease. In children with hydrocephalus, impairment of vertical gaze and pathologic lid retraction are referred to as the *setting-sun sign.* A transient supranuclear disorder of gaze is sometimes seen in healthy neonates.

CONGENITAL OCULAR MOTOR APRAXIA

This congenital disorder of conjugate gaze is characterized by a defect in voluntary horizontal gaze, compensatory jerking movement of the head, and retention of slow pursuit and reflexive eye movements. Additional features are absence of the fast (refixation) phase of optokinetic nystagmus and obligate contraversive deviation of the eyes on rotation of the body. Affected children typically are unable to look quickly to either side voluntarily in response to a command or in response to an eccentrically presented object but may be able to follow a slowly moving target to either side. To compensate for the defect in purposive lateral eye movements, children jerk their head to bring the eyes into the desired position and may also blink repetitively in an attempt to change fixation. The signs tend to become less conspicuous with age.

The pathogenesis of congenital ocular motor apraxia is unknown. It may be a result of delayed myelination of the ocular motor pathways. Structural abnormalities of the central nervous system have been found in a few patients, including agenesis of the corpus callosum and cerebellar vermis, porencephaly, hamartoma of the foramen of Monro, and macrocephaly. Many children with congenital ocular motor apraxia show delayed motor and cognitive development.

A disorder of eye movement resembling congenital ocular motor apraxia may occur in patients with certain metabolic

TABLE 630–1 Specific Patterns of Nystagmus

Pattern	Description	Associated Conditions
Latent nystagmus	Conjugate jerk nystagmus toward viewing eye	Congenital vision defects, occurs with occlusion of eye
Manifest latent nystagmus	Fast jerk to viewing eye	Strabismus, congenital idiopathic nystagmus
Periodic alternating	Cycles of horizontal or horizontal-rotary that change direction	Caused by both visual and neurologic conditions
Seesaw nystagmus	One eye rises and intorts as other eye falls and extorts	Usually associated with optic chiasm defects
Nystagmus retractorius	Eyes jerk back into orbit or toward each other	Caused by pressure on mesencephalic tegmentum (Parinaud syndrome)
Gaze-evoked nystagmus	Jerk nystagmus in direction of gaze	Caused by medications, brain stem lesion, or labyrinthine dysfunction
Gaze-paretic nystagmus	Eyes jerk back to maintain eccentric gaze	Cerebellar disease
Downbeat nystagmus	Fast phase beating downward	Posterior fossa disease, drugs
Upbeat nystagmus	Fast phase beating upward	Brain stem and cerebellar disease; some visual conditions
Vestibular nystagmus	Horizontal-torsional or horizontal jerks	Vestibular system dysfunction
Asymmetric or monocular nystagmus	Pendular vertical nystagmus	Disease of retina and visual pathways
Spasmus nutans	Fine, rapid, pendular nystagmus	Torticollis, head nodding; idiopathic or gliomas of visual pathways

From Kliegman R: Practical Strategies in Pediatric Diagnosis and Therapy. Philadelphia, WB Saunders, 1996.

TABLE 630–2 Specific Patterns of Non-Nystagmus Eye Movements

Pattern	Description	Associated Conditions
Opsoclonus	Multidirectional conjugate movements of varying rate and amplitude	Hydrocephalus, diseases of brain stem and cerebellum, neuroblastoma
Ocular dysmetria	Overshoot of eyes on rapid fixation	Cerebellar dysfunction
Ocular flutter	Horizontal oscillations with forward gaze and sometimes with blinking	Cerebellar disease, hydrocephalus, or central nervous system neoplasm
Ocular bobbing	Downward jerk from primary gaze, remain for a few seconds, then drift back	Pontine disease
Ocular myoclonus	Rhythmic to-and-fro pendular oscillations of the eyes, with synchronous nonocular muscle movement	Damage to red nucleus, inferior olivary nucleus, and ipsilateral dentate nucleus

From Kliegman R: Practical Strategies in Pediatric Diagnosis and Therapy. Philadelphia, WB Saunders, 1996.

neurodegenerative diseases (particularly Gaucher disease) or with ataxia-telangiectasia, or as a sign of brain tumor.

NYSTAGMUS

Nystagmus (rhythmic oscillations of one or both eyes) may be caused by an abnormality in any one of the three basic mechanisms that regulate position and movement of the eyes: the fixation, conjugate gaze, or vestibular mechanisms. In addition, physiologic nystagmus may be elicited by appropriate stimuli (Table 630–1).

Congenital pendular nystagmus is commonly associated with ocular and visual defects; it typically occurs with albinism, aniridia, achromatopsia, congenital cataracts, congenital macular lesions, congenital optic atrophy, and high refractive errors. In some instances, pendular nystagmus occurs as a dominant or X-linked characteristic without obvious ocular abnormalities. Rhythmic movements of the head may be associated.

Congenital jerky nystagmus is characterized by horizontal jerky oscillations with gaze preponderance; the nystagmus is coarser in one direction of gaze than in the other, with the jerk toward the direction of gaze. There is usually a point of reversal or a null point in which the nystagmus lessens and the vision improves; compensatory posturing, turning the head to bring the eyes into the position of least nystagmus, is characteristic. The cause of congenital jerky nystagmus is unknown; in some instances it is familial. Eye muscle surgery may be performed to eliminate head deviation by bringing the point of best vision into straight-ahead gaze.

Acquired nystagmus requires prompt and thorough evaluation. Worrisome pathologic types are the gaze-paretic or gaze-evoked oscillations of cerebellar, brain stem, or cerebral disease.

Nystagmus retractorius or *convergent nystagmus* is repetitive jerking of the eyes into the orbit or toward each other. It is usually seen with vertical gaze palsy as a feature of **Parinaud's** or **Koerber-Salus-Elschnig** (sylvian aqueduct) **syndrome**. The causal condition may be neoplastic, vascular, or inflammatory. In children, nystagmus retractorius suggests particularly the presence of pinealoma or hydrocephalus.

Spasmus nutans is a special type of acquired nystagmus in childhood (see also Chapter 606). In its complete form, it is characterized by the triad of pendular nystagmus, head nodding, and torticollis. The nystagmus is characteristically very fine, very rapid, horizontal, and pendular; it is often asymmetric, sometimes unilateral. Signs usually develop within the first year or two of life. Components of the triad may develop at various times. In many cases, the condition is benign and self-limited, usually lasting a few months, sometimes years. The cause of this classic type of spasmus nutans, which resolves spontaneously, is unknown. Many children exhibiting signs resembling those of spasmus nutans have underlying brain tumors, particularly hypothalamic and chiasmal optic gliomas. Appropriate neurologic and neuroradiologic evaluation and careful monitoring of infants and children with nystagmus are therefore recommended.

OTHER ABNORMAL EYE MOVEMENTS

To be differentiated from true nystagmus are certain special types of abnormal eye movements, particularly opsoclonus, ocular dysmetria, and flutter (Table 630–2).

OPSOCLONUS. Opsoclonus and ataxic conjugate movements are spontaneous, nonrhythmic, multidirectional, chaotic movements of the eyes. The eyes appear to be in agitation, with bursts of conjugate movement of varying amplitude in varying directions. Opsoclonus is most often associated with encephalitis. It may be the first sign of neuroblastoma.

OCULAR MOTOR DYSMETRIA. This is analogous to dysmetria of the limbs. Affected individuals show a lack of precision in performing movements of refixation, characterized by an overshoot (or undershoot) of the eyes with several corrective to-and-fro oscillations on looking from one point to another. Ocular motor dysmetria is a sign of cerebellar or cerebellar pathway disease.

FLUTTER-LIKE OSCILLATIONS. These intermittent to-and-fro horizontal oscillations of the eyes may occur spontaneously or on change of fixation. They are characteristic of cerebellar disease.

Anthony JH, Ouvrier RA, Wise G: Spasmus nutans: A mistaken identity. Arch Neurol 37:373, 1980.
Awner S, Catalano RA: Nystagmus. *In*: Nelson LB (ed): Harley's Pediatric Ophthalmology, 4th ed. Philadelphia, WB Saunders, 1998.
Birch EE, Stager DR, Everett ME: Random dot stereoacuity following surgical correction of infantile esotropia. J Pediatr Ophthalmol Strabismus 32:231, 1995.
Bixenman WW, von Noorden GK: Benign recurrent VI nerve palsy in childhood. J Pediatr Ophthalmol Strabismus 18:29, 1981.
Catalano RA, Nelson LB: Pediatric Opthalmology: A Text Atlas. Norwalk, CT, Appleton & Lange, 1994.
Cogan DG: Heredity of congenital ocular motor apraxia. Trans Am Acad Ophthalmol Otolaryngol 76:60, 1972.
DeRespinis PA, Caputo AR, Wagner RS, et al: Duane's retraction syndrome. Surv Ophthalmol 38:257, 1993.
Harley RD: Paralytic strabismus in children: Etiologic incidence and management of the third, fourth and sixth nerve palsies. Ophthalmology 87:24, 1980.
Hoyt CS, Mousel DK, Weber AA: Transient supranuclear disturbance of gaze in healthy neonates. Am J Ophthalmol 89:708, 1980.
Ing M: Early surgical alignment for congenital esotropia. Ophthalmology 90:132, 1983.
Kushner BJ: Ocular causes of abnormal head postures. Ophthalmology 86:2115, 1979.
Lavery MA, O'Neill JF, Chau FC, et al: Acquired nystagmus in early childhood: A presenting sign of intracranial tumor. Ophthalmology 91:425, 1984.
Metz HS: Double elevator palsy. Arch Ophthalmol 97:901, 1979.
Miller MT, Ray V, Owens P, et al: Möbius and Möbius-like syndromes (TTV-OFM, OMLH). J Pediatr Ophthalmol Strabismus 26:176, 1989.
Miller NR: Solitary oculomotor nerve palsy in children. Am J Ophthalmol 83:106, 1977.
Mohindra I, Zwann J, Held R, et al: Development of acuity and stereopsis in infants with esotropia. Ophthalmology 92:691, 1985.
Morre RT, Morin JD: Bilateral acquired inflammatory Brown's syndrome. J Pediatr Ophthalmol Strabismus 22:26, 1985.
Morris RJ, Scott WE, Dickey CF: Fusion after surgical alignment of longstanding strabismus in adults. Ophthalmology 100:135, 1993.
Nelson LB, Wagner RS, Simon JW, et al: Congenital esotropia. Surv Ophthalmol 31:363, 1987.
Norton EWD, Cogan DG: Spasmus nutans: A clinical study of twenty cases followed two years or more since onset. Arch Ophthalmol 52:442, 1954.
Olitsky SE, Nelson LB: Strabismus disorders. *In*: Nelson LB (ed): Harley's Pediatric Ophthalmology, 4th ed. Philadelphia, WB Saunders, 1998.

Raab EL: Etiologic factors in accommodative esodeviation. Trans Am Ophthalmol Soc 80:657, 1982.
Rappaport L, Urlon D, Strand K, et al: Concurrence of congenital oculomotor apraxia and other motor problems: An expanded syndrome. Dev Med Child Neurol 29:85, 1987.
Richard JM, Parks M: Intermittent exotropia: Surgical results in different age groups. Ophthalmology 90:1172, 1983.
Richards BW, Jones FR, Younge BR: Causes and prognosis in 4,278 cases of paralysis of the oculomotor, trochlear and abducens cranial nerves. Am J Ophthalmol 113:489, 1992.
Shetty T, Rosman NP: Opsoclonus in hydrocephalus. Arch Ophthalmol 88:585, 1972.
von Noorden GK, Murray E, Wong SY: Superior oblique paralysis: A review of 270 cases. Arch Ophthalmol 104:1771, 1986.
Wang FM, Wertenbaker C, Behrens MM, et al: Acquired Brown's syndrome in children with juvenile rheumatoid arthritis. Ophthalmology 91:23, 1984.
Wilson ME, Eustis HS, Parks MM: Brown's syndrome. Surv Ophthalmol 34:153, 1989.
Zaret CR, Behrens MM, Eggers HM: Congenital ocular motor apraxia and brain stem tumor. Arch Ophthalmol 98:328, 1980.

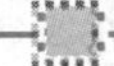

CHAPTER 631
Abnormalities of the Lids

PTOSIS. In *blepharoptosis,* the upper eyelid droops below its normal level. Congenital ptosis is usually a result of a localized dystrophy of the levator muscle in which the striated muscle fibers are replaced with fibrous tissue. The condition may be unilateral or bilateral and can be familial, transmitted as a dominant trait.

Parents often comment that the eye looks smaller because of the drooping eyelid. The lid crease is decreased or absent where the levator muscle would normally insert below the skin surface. Because the levator is replaced by fibrous tissue, the lid does not move downward fully in downgaze (lid lag). If the ptosis is severe, affected children often attempt to raise the lid by lifting their brow or adapting a chin-up head posture to maintain binocular vision. **Marcus Gunn jaw-winking ptosis** accounts for 5% of ptosis in children. In this syndrome, an abnormal synkinesis exists between the fifth and third cranial nerves; this causes the eyelid to elevate with movement of the jaw. The wink is produced by chewing or sucking and may be more noticeable than the ptosis itself.

Although ptosis in children is often an isolated finding, it may occur in association with other ocular or systemic disorders. Systemic disorders include myasthenia gravis, muscular dystrophy, and botulism. Ocular disorders include mechanical ptosis secondary to lid tumors, blepharophimosis syndrome, congenital fibrosis syndrome, combined levator/superior rectus maldevelopment, and congenital or acquired 3rd nerve palsy. A complete ophthalmic and systemic examination is therefore important in the evaluation of a child with ptosis.

Amblyopia may occur in children with ptosis. The amblyopia may be secondary to the lid's covering the visual axis (deprivation) or induced astigmatisim due to the weight of the lid on the globe (anisometropia). When amblyopia occurs, it should generally be treated before treating the ptosis.

Treatment of ptosis in a child is indicated for elimination of an abnormal head posture, improvement in the visual field, prevention of amblyopia, and restoration of a normal eyelid appearance. The timing of surgery depends on the degree of ptosis, its cosmetic and functional severity, the presence or absence of compensatory posturing, the wishes of the parents, and the discretion of the surgeon. Surgical treatment is determined by the amount of levator function that is present. A levator resection may be used in children with moderate to good function. In patients with poor or absent function, a frontalis suspension procedure may be necessary. This technique requires that a suspension material be placed between the frontalis muscle and the tarsus of the eyelid. It allows patients to use their brow and frontalis muscle more effectively to raise their eyelid. Amblyopia remains a concern even after surgical correction and should be monitored closely.

EPICANTHAL FOLDS. These vertical or oblique folds of skin extend on either side of the bridge of the nose from the brow or lid area, covering the inner canthal region. They are present to some degree in most young children and become less apparent with age. The folds may be sufficiently broad to cover the medial aspect of the eye, making the eyes appear crossed (pseudoesotropia). Epicanthal folds are a common feature of many syndromes, including chromosomal aberrations (trisomies) or disorders of single genes.

LAGOPHTHALMOS. This is a condition in which complete closure of the lids over the globe is difficult or impossible. It may be paralytic, because of a facial palsy involving the orbicularis muscle, or spastic, as in thyrotoxicosis. It may be structural when retraction or shortening of the lids results from scarring or atrophy consequent to injury (burns) or disease. Infants with collodion membrane may have temporary lagophthalmos caused by the restrictive effect of the membrane on the lids. Lagophthalmos may accompany proptosis or buphthalmos when the lids, although normal, cannot effectively cover the enlarged or protuberant eye. A degree of physiologic lagophthalmos may occur normally during sleep, but functional lagophthalmos in an unconscious or debilitated patient can be a problem.

In patients with lagophthalmos, exposure of the eye may lead to drying, infection, corneal ulceration, or perforation of the cornea; the result may be loss of vision, even loss of the eye. In lagophthalmos, protection of the eye by artificial tear preparations, ophthalmic ointment, or moisture chambers is essential. Gauze pads are to be avoided, because the gauze may abrade the cornea. In some cases, surgical closure of the lids (tarsorrhaphy) may be necessary for long-term protection of the eye.

LID RETRACTION. Pathologic retraction of the lid may be myogenic or neurogenic. Myogenic retraction of the upper lid occurs in thyrotoxicosis, in which it is associated with three classic signs: a staring appearance **(Dalrymple sign),** infrequent blinking **(Stellwag sign),** and lag of the upper lid on downward gaze **(von Graefe sign).**

Neurogenic retraction of the lids may occur in conditions affecting the anterior mesencephalon. Lid retraction is a feature of the syndrome of the sylvian aqueduct. In children, it is commonly a sign of hydrocephalus. It may occur with meningitis. Paradoxical retraction of the lid is seen in the Marcus Gunn jaw-winking syndrome. It may also be seen with attempted eye movement after recovery from a 3rd nerve palsy if aberrant regeneration of the oculomotor nerve fibers has occurred.

Simple staring and the physiologic or reflexive lid retraction ("eye popping"), in contrast to pathologic lid retractions, occur in infants in response to a sudden reduction in illumination or as a startle reaction.

ECTROPION, ENTROPION, AND EPIBLEPHARON. *Ectropion* is eversion of the lid margin; it may lead to overflow of tears (epiphora) and subsequent maceration of the skin of the lid, to inflammation of exposed conjunctiva, or to superficial exposure keratopathy. Common causes are scarring consequent to inflammation, burns, or trauma, or weakness of the orbicularis muscle as a result of facial palsy; these forms may be corrected surgically. Protection of the cornea is essential. Ectropion is also seen in certain children who have faulty development of the lateral canthal ligament; this may occur in Down syndrome.

Entropion is inversion of the lid margin, which may cause discomfort and corneal damage because of the inward turning of the lashes (trichiasis). A principal cause is scarring secondary to inflammation such as occurs in trachoma or as a sequela of Stevens-Johnson syndrome. There is also a rare congenital form. Surgical correction is effective in many cases.

Epiblepharon is commonly seen in childhood and may be confused with entropion. In epiblepharon, a roll of skin beneath the lower eyelid lashes causes the lashes to be directed vertically and to touch the cornea. Unlike entropion, the eyelid margin itself is not rotated toward the cornea. Epiblepharon usually resolves spontaneously. If corneal scarring begins to occur, surgical correction may be necessary.

BLEPHAROSPASM. This spastic or repetitive closure of the lids may be caused by irritative disease of the cornea, conjunctiva, or facial nerve; fatigue or uncorrected refractive error; or common tic. Thorough ophthalmic examination for pathologic causes, such as trichiasis, keratitis, conjunctivitis, or foreign body, is indicated. Local injection of botulinum toxin may give relief but frequently must be repeated.

BLEPHARITIS. This inflammation of the lid margins is characterized by erythema and crusting or scaling; the usual symptoms are irritation, burning, and itching. The condition is commonly bilateral and chronic or recurrent. The two main types are staphylococcal and seborrheic. In *staphylococcal blepharitis,* ulceration of the lid margin is common, the lashes tend to fall out, and conjunctivitis and superficial keratitis are often associated. In *seborrheic blepharitis,* the scales tend to be greasy, the lid margins are less red, and ulceration usually does not occur. The blepharitis is often of mixed type.

Thorough daily cleansing of the lid margins with a cloth or moistened cotton applicator to remove scales and crusts is important in the treatment of both forms. Staphylococcal blepharitis is treated with an antistaphylococcal antibiotic applied directly to the lid margins. When a child also has seborrhea, concurrent treatment of the scalp is important.

Pediculosis of the eyelashes may produce a clinical picture of blepharitis. The lice can be smothered with opthalmic-grade petrolatum ointment applied to the lid margin and lashes. Nits should be mechanically removed from the lashes.

HORDEOLUM. Infection of the glands of the lid may be acute or subacute; tender focal swelling and redness are noted. The usual agent is *Staphylococcus aureus.* When the meibomian glands are involved, the lesion is referred to as an *internal hordeolum;* the abscess tends to be large and may point through either the skin or the conjunctival surface. When the infection involves the glands of Zeis or Moll, the abscess tends to be smaller and more superficial and points at the lid margin; it is then referred to as an *external hordeolum* or *stye.*

Treatment is frequent warm compresses and, if necessary, surgical incision and drainage. In addition, topical antibiotic preparations are often used. Untreated, the infection may progress to cellulitis of the lid or orbit, requiring the use of systemic antibiotics.

CHALAZION. A chalazion is a granulomatous inflammation of a meibomian gland characterized by a firm, nontender nodule in the upper or lower lid. This lesion tends to be chronic and differs from internal hordeolum in the absence of acute inflammatory signs. Although many chalazia subside spontaneously, excision may be necessary if they become large enough to distort vision (by inducing astigmatism by exerting pressure on the globe) or to be a cosmetic blemish.

COLOBOMA OF THE EYELID. This cleftlike deformity may vary from a small indentation or notch of the free margin of the lid to a large defect involving almost the entire lid. If the gap is extensive, xerosis, ulceration, and corneal opacities may result from exposure. Early surgical correction of the lid defect is recommended. Other deformities frequently associated with lid colobomas include dermoid cysts or dermolipomas on the globe; they often occur in a position corresponding to the site of the lid defect. Lid colobomas may also be associated with extensive facial malformation, as in mandibulofacial dysostosis (Franceschetti's or Treacher Collins syndrome).

TUMORS OF THE LID. A number of lid tumors arise from surface structures (the epithelium and sebaceous glands). *Nevi* may appear in early childhood; most are junctional. Compound nevi tend to develop in the prepubertal years, dermal nevi at puberty. *Malignant epithelial tumors* (basal cell carcinoma, squamous cell carcinoma) are rare in children, but the basal cell nevus syndrome and the malignant lesions of xeroderma pigmentosum and of Rothmund-Thomson syndrome may develop in childhood.

Other lid tumors arise from deeper structures (the neural, vascular, and connective tissues). *Capillary hemangiomas* are especially common in children. Many tend to regress spontaneously, although they may show alarmingly rapid growth in infancy. In many cases, the best management of such hemangiomas is patient observation, allowing spontaneous regression to occur (see Chapter 656). In the case of a rapidly expanding lesion, which may cause amblyopia by obstructing the visual axis or inducing astigmatism, corticosteroid and interferon treatment should be considered. *Nevus flammeus* (port-wine stain), a noninvoluting hemangioma, occurs as an isolated lesion or in association with other signs of Sturge-Weber syndrome. Affected patients should be monitored for the development of glaucoma. *Lymphangiomas* of the lid appear as firm masses at or soon after birth and tend to enlarge slowly during the growing years. Associated conjunctival involvement, appearing as a clear, cystic, sinuous conjunctival mass, may provide a clue to the diagnosis. In some cases there is also orbital involvement. The treatment is surgical excision. *Plexiform neuromas* of the lids occur in children with neurofibromatosis, often with ptosis as the first sign. The lid may take on an S-shaped configuration. The lids may also be involved by other tumors, such as retinoblastoma, neuroblastoma, and rhabdomyosarcoma of the orbit; these conditions are discussed elsewhere.

Anderson RL, Baumgarten SA: Amblyopia in ptosis. Arch Ophthalmol 98:1068, 1980.

Crawford JS: Congenital eyelid anomalies in children. J Pediatr Ophthalmol Strabismus 21:140, 1984.

Crawford JS, Iliff CE, Stasier OG: Symposium on congenital ptosis. J Pediatr Ophthalmol Strabismus 19:245, 1982.

Johnson CC: Epicanthus and epiblepharon. Arch Ophthalmol 96:1030, 1978.

Masaki S: Congenital bilateral facial paralysis. Arch Otolaryngol 94:260, 1971.

McCully JP, Dougherty JM, Deneau DG: Classification of chronic blepharitis. Ophthalmology 89:1173, 1982.

Moainie R, Kopelowitz N, Rosenfeld W, et al: Congenital eversion of the eyelids: A report of two cases treated with conservative management. J Pediatr Ophthalmol Strabismus 19:326, 1982.

Pico G: Congenital ectropion and distichiasis. Etiologic and hereditary factors. A report of cases and review of the literature. Am J Ophthalmol 47:363, 1959.

Pratt SG, Beyer CK, Johnson CC: The Marcus Gunn phenomenon: A review of 71 cases. Ophthalmology 91:27, 1984.

Schaefer DP, Schaefer AJ: Blepharoptosis: Classification, evaluation and treatment in the pediatric age group. Ophthalmol Clin North Am 2:277, 1996.

Stigmar G, Crawford JS, Ward CM, et al: Ophthalmic sequelae of infantile hemangiomas of the eyelid and orbit. Am J Ophthalmol 85:806, 1978.

Zak TA: Congenital primary upper eyelid entropion. J Pediatr Ophthalmol Strabismus 21:69, 1984.

CHAPTER 632
Disorders of the Lacrimal System

THE TEAR FILM. The tear film, which bathes the eye, is actually a complex structure composed of three layers. The innermost mucin layer is secreted by the goblet and epithelial cells of the conjunctiva and the acinar cells of the lacrimal gland. It adds stability and provides an attachment for the tear film to the conjunctiva and cornea. The middle aqueous layer constitutes 98% of the tear film and is produced by the main lacrimal gland and accessory lacrimal glands. It contains various electrolytes and proteins as well as antibodies. The outermost lipid layer is produced largely from the sebaceous meibomian glands of the eyelid and retards evaporation of the tear film. Tears drain medially into the punctal openings of the lid margin and flow through the canaliculi into the lacrimal sac and then through the nasolacrimal duct into the nose.

DACRYOSTENOSIS AND DACRYOCYSTITIS. *Congenital nasolacrimal duct obstruction* (CNLDO), or dacryostenosis, is the most common disorder of the lacrimal system, occurring in up to 6% of newborn infants. It is usually caused by a failure of canalization of the epithelial cells that form the nasolacrimal duct as it enters the nose (valve of Hasner). Signs of CNLDO may be present at the time of birth, although the condition may not become evident until normal tear production develops. Signs of CNLDO include an excessive tear lake, overflow of tears onto the lid and cheek, and reflux of mucoid material that is produced in the lacrimal sac. Erythema or maceration of the skin may result from irritation and rubbing produced by dripping of tears and discharge. If the blockage is complete, these signs may be severe and continuous. If obstruction is only partial, the nasolacrimal duct may be capable of draining the basal tear film that is produced. However, under periods of increased tear production (exposure to cold, wind, sunlight) or increased closure of the distal end of the nasolacrimal duct (nasal mucosal edema), tear overflow may become evident or may increase.

Infants with CNLDO may develop acute infection and inflammation of the nasolacrimal sac (dacryocystitis), inflammation of the surrounding tissues (pericystitis), or rarely periobital cellulitis. With dacryocystitis, the sac area is swollen, red, and tender, and patients may have systemic signs of infection such as fever and irritability.

The primary treatment of uncomplicated nasolacrimal obstruction is a regimen of nasolacrimal massage, usually two to three times a day, accompanied by cleansing of the lids with warm water. Topical antibiotics are used for significant mucopurulent drainage. Most cases of CNLDO resolve spontaneously, 96% before 1 yr of age. For cases that do not resolve by 1 yr, the nasolacrimal duct may be probed, with a cure rate of approximately 90%. Most pediatric ophthalmologists repeat simple probing once or twice before proceeding to placement of tubes or more extensive reconstructive surgery (dacryocystorhinostomy).

Acute dacryocystitis or *cellulitis* requires prompt treatment with antibiotics. In such cases, some form of definitive surgical intervention is usually indicated.

A *mucocele* is an unusual presentation of a nonpatent nasolacrimal sac that is obstructed both proximally and distally. Mucoceles can be seen at birth or shortly after birth as a bluish subcutaneous mass just below the medial canthal tendon. Initial treatment should include warm compresses and gentle massage of the lacrimal sac. At the earliest sign of inflammation, probing should be performed.

It is important to remember that not all tearing in infants and children is caused by nasolacrimal obstruction. Tearing may also be a sign of glaucoma, intraocular inflammation, or external irritation, such as that from a corneal abrasion or foreign body.

DACRYOADENITIS. Dacryoadenitis, or inflammation of the lacrimal gland, is uncommon in childhood. It may occur with mumps (in which case it is usually acute and bilateral, subsiding in a few days or weeks) or with infectious mononucleosis. *Staphylococcus aureus* may produce a suppurative dacryoadenitis. Chronic dacryoadenitis is associated with certain systemic diseases, particularly sarcoidosis, tuberculosis, and syphilis. Some systemic diseases may produce enlargement of the lacrimal and salivary glands **(Mikulicz syndrome)**.

ALACRIMA AND "DRY EYE." Marked deficiency of tears may occur as an isolated unilateral or bilateral congenital defect or in association with other nervous system anomalies, such as aplasia of cranial nerve nuclei. It occurs congenitally in familial dysautonomia (Riley-Day syndrome) and in the anhidrotic type of ectodermal dysplasia; it may occur with glucocorticoid deficiency, sometimes in association with swallowing dysfunction. An acquired abnormality of any layer of the tear film may produce a dry eye. Commonly acquired disorders that may lead to a decreased or unstable tear film include Sjögren's syndrome, Stevens-Johnson syndrome, vitamin A deficiency, ocular pemphigoid, trachoma, chemical burns, irradiation, and meibomian gland dysfunction. Any tear deficiency can lead to corneal ulceration, scarring, or infection. Treatment includes correction of the underlying disorder when possible and frequent instillation of an artificial tear preparation. In some cases, occlusion of the lacrimal puncta is helpful. In severe cases, tarsorrhaphy may be necessary to protect the cornea.

Caccamise WC, Townes PL: Congenital absence of the lacrymal puncta associated with alacrima and aptyalism. Am J Ophthalmol 89:62, 1980.

El-Mansoury J, Calhoun JH, Nelson LB, et al: Results of late probing for congenital nasolacrimal duct obstruction. Ophthalmology 93:1052, 1986.

Geffner ME, Lippe BM, Kaplan SA, et al: Selective ACTH insensitivity, achalasia, and alacrima: A multisystem disorder presenting in childhood. Pediatr Res 17:532, 1983.

MacEwen CJ, Young JDH: Epiphora during the first year of life. Eye 5:596, 1991.

Manson AM, Cheng KP, Mumma JV, et al: Congenital dacryocele. Ophthalmology 98:1744, 1991.

Mondino BJ, Brown SI: Hereditary congenital alacrima. Arch Ophthalmol 94:1478, 1976.

Paul TO: Medical management of congenital nasolacrymal duct obstruction. J Pediatr Ophthalmol Strabismus 22:68, 1985.

Wagner RS: Lacrimal disorders. Ophthalmol Clin North Am 2:229, 1996.

Young JDH, MacEwen CJ: Managing congenital lacrimal obstruction in general practice. Br Med J 315:293, 1997.

CHAPTER 633
Disorders of the Conjunctiva

CONJUNCTIVITIS. The conjunctiva reacts to a wide range of bacterial and viral agents, allergens, irritants, toxins, and systemic diseases. Conjunctivitis is common in childhood and may be infectious or noninfectious (Table 633–1).

OPHTHALMIA NEONATORUM. Ophthalmia neonatorum, a form of conjunctivitis occurring in infants younger than 4 wk, is the most common eye disease of newborns. Its many different etiologic agents vary greatly in their virulence and outcome. For instance, silver nitrate instillation may result in a mild self-limited conjunctivitis, whereas *Neisseria gonorrhoeae* and *Pseudomonas* are capable of causing corneal perforation, blindness, and death. The risk of conjunctivitis in newborns depends

TABLE 633–1 The Red Eye

Condition	Etiology	Signs and Symptoms	Treatment
Bacterial conjunctivitis	*Haemophilus influenzae, Haemophilus aegyptius, Streptococcus pneumoniae* *Neisseria gonorrhoeae*	Mucopurulent unilateral or bilateral discharge, normal vision, photophobia Conjunctival injection and edema (chemosis); gritty sensation	Topical antibiotics, parenteral ceftriaxone for gonococcus, *H. influenzae*
Viral conjunctivitis	Adenovirus, ECHO virus, coxsackievirus	As above; may be hemorrhagic, unilateral	Self-limited
Neonatal conjunctivitis	*Chlamydia trachomatis,* gonococcus, chemical (silver nitrate), *Staphylococcus aureus*	Palpebral conjunctival follicle or papillae; as above	Ceftriaxone for gonococcus and erythromycin for *C. trachomatis*
Allergic conjunctivitis	Seasonal pollens or allergen exposure	Itching, incidence of bilateral chemosis (edema) greater than that of erythema, tarsal papillae	Antihistamines, steroids, cromolyn
Keratitis	Herpes simplex, adenovirus, *Streptococcus pneumoniae, Staphylococcus aureus, Pseudomonas, Acanthamoeba,* chemicals	Severe pain, corneal swelling, clouding, limbus erythema, hypopyon, cataracts; contact lens history with amebic infection	Specific antibiotics for bacterial/fungal infections; keratoplasty, acyclovir for herpes
Endophthalmitis	*S. aureus, S. pneumoniae, Candida albicans,* associated surgery or trauma	Acute onset, pain, loss of vision, swelling, chemosis, redness; hypopyon and vitreous haze	Antibiotics
Anterior uveitis (iridocyclitis)	JRA, Reiter's syndrome, sarcoidosis, Behçet's disease, Kawasaki's disease, inflammatory bowel disease	Unilateral/bilateral; erythema, ciliary flush, irregular pupil, iris adhesions; pain, photophobia, small pupil, poor vision	Topical steroids, plus therapy for primary disease
Posterior uveitis (choroiditis)	Toxoplasmosis, histoplasmosis, *Toxocara canis*	No signs of erythema, decreased vision	Specific therapy for pathogen
Episcleritis/scleritis	Idiopathic autoimmune disease (e.g., SLE, Henoch-Schönlein purpura)	Localized pain, intense erythema, unilateral; blood vessels bigger than in conjunctivitis; scleritis may cause globe perforation	Episcleritis is self-limiting; topical steroids for fast relief
Foreign body	Occupational exposure	Unilateral, red, gritty feeling; visible or microscopic size	Irrigation, removal; check for ulceration
Blepharitis	*S. aureus, Staphylococcus epidermidis,* seborrheic, blocked lacrimal duct; rarely molluscum contagiosum, *Phthirus pubis, Pediculus capitis*	Bilateral, irritation, itching, hyperemia, crusting, affecting lid margins	Topical antibiotics, warm compresses
Dacryocystitis	Obstructed lacrimal sac: *S. aureus, H. influenzae,* pneumococcus	Pain, tenderness, erythema and exudate in area of lacrimal sac (inferomedial to inner canthus); tearing (epiphora); possible orbital cellulitis	Systemic, topical antibiotics; surgical drainage
Dacryoadenitis	*S. aureus, Streptococcus,* CMV, measles, EBV, enteroviruses; trauma, sarcoidosis, leukemia	Pain, tenderness, edema, erythema over gland area (upper temporal lid); fever, leukocytosis	Systemic antibiotics; drainage of orbital abscesses
Orbital cellulitis (postseptal cellulitis)	Paranasal sinusitis: *H. influenzae, S. aureus, S. pneumoniae,* streptococci Trauma: *S. aureus* Fungi: *Aspergillus, Mucor* spp. if immunodeficient	Rhinorrhea, chemosis, vision loss, painful extraocular motion, proptosis, ophthalmoplegia, fever, lid edema, leukocytosis	Systemic antibiotics, drainage of orbital abscesses
Periorbital cellulitis (preseptal cellulitis)	Trauma: *S. aureus,* streptococci Bacteremia: pneumococcus, streptococci, *H. influenzae*	Cutaneous erythema, warmth, normal vision, minimal involvement of orbit; fever, leukocytosis, toxic appearance	Systemic antibiotics

From Behrman R, Kliegman R: Nelson's Essentials of Pediatrics, 3rd ed. Philadelphia, WB Saunders, 1998.
CMV = cytomegalovirus; EBV = Epstein-Barr virus; JRA = juvenile rheumatoid arthritis; SLE = systemic lupus erythematosus.

on frequencies of maternal infections, prophylactic measures, circumstances during labor and delivery, and postdelivery exposures to microorganisms.

Epidemiology. Conjunctivitis during the neonatal period is usually acquired during vaginal delivery and reflects the sexually transmitted diseases prevalent in the community. In 1880, 10% of European children developed gonococcal conjunctivitis at birth. Ophthalmia neonatorum was the leading cause of blindness during that period. The epidemiology of this condition changed dramatically in 1881, when Crede reported that 2% silver nitrate solution instilled in the eyes of newborns reduced the incidence of gonococcal ophthalmia from 10% to 0.3%.

During the 20th century, the incidence of gonococcal ophthalmia neonatorum decreased in industrialized countries secondary to widespread use of silver nitrate prophylaxis and prenatal screening and treatment of maternal gonorrhea. Gonococcal ophthalmia neonatorum has an incidence of 0.3/1,000 live births in the United States. In comparison, *Chlamydia trachomatis* is the most common organism causing ophthalmia neonatorum in the United States, with an incidence of 8.2/1,000 births.

Clinical Manifestations. The clinical manifestations of the various forms of ophthalmia neonatorum are not specific enough to allow an accurate diagnosis. Although the timing and character of the signs are somewhat typical for each cause of this condition, there is considerable overlap and physicians should not rely solely on clinical findings. Regardless of its cause, ophthalmia neonatorum is characterized by redness and chemosis (swelling) of the conjunctiva, edema of the eyelids, and discharge, which may be purulent.

Ophthalmia neonatorum is a potentially blinding condition. The infection may also have associated systemic manifestations that require treatment. Therefore, any newborn infant who develops signs of conjunctivitis needs a prompt and comprehensive evaluation to determine the agent causing the infection and the appropriate treatment.

The onset of inflammation caused by silver nitrate drops usually occurs within 6–12 hr after birth, with clearing by 24–48 hr. The usual incubation period for conjunctivitis due to *N. gonorrhoeae* is 2–5 days and for that due to *C. trachomatis* is 5–14 days. Gonococcal infection may be present at birth or delayed beyond 5 days of life owing to partial suppression by ocular prophylaxis. Gonococcal conjunctivitis may also begin in infancy after inoculation by the contaminated fingers of adults. The time of onset of disease with other bacteria is highly variable.

Gonococcal conjunctivitis begins with mild inflammation and a serosanguineous discharge. Within 24 hr, the discharge becomes thick and purulent, and tense edema of the eyelids with marked chemosis occurs. If proper treatment is delayed, the infection may spread to involve the deeper layers of the conjunctivae and the cornea. Complications include corneal ulceration and perforation, iridocyclitis, anterior synechiae, and rarely panophthalmitis. Conjunctivitis caused by *C. trachomatis* (inclusion blennorrhea) may vary from mild inflammation to severe swelling of the eyelids with copious purulent discharge. The process involves mainly the tarsal conjunctivae; the corneas are rarely affected. Conjunctivitis due to *Staphylococcus aureus* or other organisms is similar to that produced by *C. trachomatis.* Conjunctivitis due to *Pseudomonas aeruginosa* is uncommon, is acquired in the nursery, and is a potentially serious process. It is characterized by the appearance on day 5–18 of edema, erythema of the lids, purulent discharge, pannus formation, endophthalmitis, sepsis, shock, and death.

Diagnosis. Conjunctivitis appearing after 48 hr should be evaluated for a possibly infectious cause. Gram stain of the purulent discharge should be performed, and the material cultured. If a viral etiology is suspected, a swab should be submitted in tissue culture media for virus isolation. In chlamydial conjunctivitis, the diagnosis is made by examining Giemsa-stained epithelial cells scraped from the tarsal conjunctivae for the characteristic intracytoplasmic inclusions, by isolating the organisms from a conjunctival swab using special tissue culture techniques, by immunofluorescent staining of conjunctival scrapings for chlamydial inclusions, or by tests for chlamydial antigen. The differential diagnosis includes dacrocystitis, caused by congenital lacrimal duct obstruction with lacrimal sac distention (dacrocystocele).

Treatment. Treatment of infants in whom gonococcal ophthalmia is suspected and the Gram stain shows the characteristic intracellular gram-negative diplococci should be initiated immediately with ceftriaxone, 50 mg/kg/24 hr for one dose not to exceed 125 mg. In addition, the eye should be irrigated initially with saline every 10–30 min, gradually increasing to 2-hr intervals, until the purulent discharge has cleared. An alternative regimen includes the use of cefotaxime (100 mg/kg/24 hr given IV or IM every 12 hr for 7 days or 100 mg/kg as a single dose). Treatment is extended if sepsis or other extraocular sites are involved (meningitis, arthritis). Inclusion blennorrhea is treated with oral erythromycin (50 mg/kg/24 hr in four divided doses) for 2 wk. This cures conjunctivitis and may prevent subsequent chlamydial pneumonia. *Pseudomonas* neonatal conjunctivitis is treated with systemic antibiotics, including an aminoglycoside, plus local saline irrigation and gentamicin ophthalmic ointment. Staphylococcal conjunctivitis is treated with parenteral methicillin and local saline irrigation.

Prognosis and Prevention. Before the institution of topical ophthalmic prophylaxis at birth, gonococcal ophthalmia was a common cause of blindness or permanent eye damage. If properly applied, this form of prophylaxis is highly effective unless infection is present at birth. Drops of 0.5% erythromycin or 1% silver nitrate are instilled directly into the open eyes at birth using wax or plastic single-dose containers. Saline irrigation after silver nitrate application is unnecessary. Silver nitrate is ineffective against active infection. Povidone-iodine (2% solution) may also be an effective prophylactic agent.

Identification of maternal gonococcal infection and appropriate treatment has become a standard element of routine prenatal care. An infant born to a woman who has untreated gonococcal infection should receive a single dose of ceftriaxone, 50 mg/kg (maximum 125 mg) IV or IM, in addition to topical prophylaxis. The dose should be reduced for premature infants. Penicillin (50,000 units) should be used if the mother's gonococcal isolate is known to be penicillin sensitive.

Neither topical prophylaxis nor topical treatment prevents the afebrile pneumonia that occurs in 10–20% of infants exposed to *C. trachomatis.* Although chlamydial conjunctivitis is often a self-limiting disease, chlamydial pneumonia may have serious consequences. It is important that infants with chlamydial disease receive systemic treatment. Treatment of colonized pregnant women with erythromycin may prevent neonatal disease.

ACUTE PURULENT CONJUNCTIVITIS. This is characterized by more or less generalized conjunctival hyperemia, edema, mucopurulent exudate, and various degrees of ocular discomfort. It is usually a result of bacterial infection. The most frequent causes are nontypable *Haemophilus influenzae* (associated with ipsilateral otitis media), pneumococci, staphylococci, and streptococci. Conjunctival smear and culture are helpful in differentiating specific types. These common forms of acute purulent conjunctivitis usually respond well to warm compresses and frequent topical instillation of antibiotic drops. Brazilian purpuric fever due to *Haemophilis aegyptius* manifests as conjunctivitis and sepsis. *N. gonorrhoeae* and *Chlamydia* are relatively common causes of acute purulent conjunctivitis in children beyond the newborn period, especially in adolescents. These infections require specific testing and treatment.

VIRAL CONJUNCTIVITIS. This is generally characterized by a watery discharge. Follicular changes (small aggregates of lymphocytes) are often found in the palpebral conjunctiva. Conjunctivitis resulting from adenovirus infection is relatively common, sometimes with corneal involvement (see later). Outbreaks of conjunctivitis caused by enterovirus are also encountered; this type may be hemorrhagic. Conjunctivitides are commonly associated with such systemic viral infections as the childhood exanthems, particularly measles. These are self-limited.

EPIDEMIC KERATOCONJUNCTIVITIS. This is caused by adenovirus type 8 and is transmitted by direct contact. It initially presents as a sensation of a foreign body beneath the lids, with itching and burning. Edema and photophobia develop rapidly, and large oval follicles appear within the conjunctiva. Preauricular adenopathy and a pseudomembrane on the conjunctival surface occur frequently. Subepithelial corneal infiltrates may develop and may cause blurring of vision; these usually disappear but may permanently reduce visual acuity. Corneal complications are less common in children than in adults. Children may have associated upper respiratory tract infection and pharyngitis. No specific therapy is available. Emphasis must be placed on prevention of spread of the disease.

MEMBRANOUS AND PSEUDOMEMBRANOUS CONJUNCTIVITIS. These types can be encountered in a number of diseases. The classic membranous conjunctivitis is that of diphtheria, accompanied by a fibrin-rich exudate that forms on the conjunctival surface and permeates the epithelium; the membrane is removed with difficulty and leaves raw bleeding areas. In pseudomembranous conjunctivitis, the layer of fibrin-rich exudate is superficial and can often be stripped easily, leaving the surface smooth. This type occurs with many bacterial and viral infections, including staphylococcal, pneumococcal, streptococcal, or chlamydial conjunctivitis, and in epidemic keratoconjunctivitis. It is also found in vernal conjunctivitis and in Stevens-Johnson disease.

ALLERGIC CONJUNCTIVITIS. This is usually accompanied by intense itching, tearing, and conjunctival edema. It is commonly seasonal. Cold compresses and decongestant drops give symptomatic relief. Topical mast cell stabilizers or prostaglandin inhibitors may also help. In selected cases, topical corticosteroids are used under an ophthalmologist's supervision.

VERNAL CONJUNCTIVITIS. This usually begins in the prepubertal years and may recur for many years. Atopy appears to have a role in its origin, but the pathogenesis is uncertain. Extreme itching and tearing are the usual complaints. Large, flattened, cobblestone-like papillary lesions of the palpebral conjunctivae are characteristic. A stringy exudate and a milky conjunctival pseudomembrane are frequently present. Small elevated lesions of the bulbar conjunctiva adjacent to the limbus (limbal form) may be found. Smear of the conjunctival exudate reveals many eosinophils. Topical corticosteroid therapy and cold compresses afford some relief. Topical mast cell stabilizers or prostaglandin inhibitors are useful when long-term control is needed.

CHEMICAL CONJUNCTIVITIS. This can result when an irritating substance enters the conjunctival sac (as in the acute but benign conjunctivitis caused by silver nitrate in newborns). Other common offenders are household cleaning substances, sprays, smoke, smog, and industrial pollutants. Alkalis tend to linger in the conjunctival tissues and continue to inflict damage for hours or days. Acids precipitate the proteins in tissues and so produce their effect immediately. In either case, prompt, thorough, and copious irrigation is crucial. Extensive tissue damage, even loss of the eye, can result, especially if the offending agent is an alkali.

OTHER CONJUNCTIVAL DISORDERS. *Subconjunctival hemorrhage* is manifested by bright or dark red patches in the bulbar conjunctiva and may result from injury or inflammation. It commonly occurs spontaneously. It may occasionally result from severe sneezing or coughing. Rarely it may be a manifestation of a blood dyscrasia.

Pinguecula is a yellowish-white, slightly elevated mass on the bulbar conjunctiva, usually in the interpalpebral region. It represents elastic and hyaline degenerative changes of the conjunctiva. No treatment is required except for cosmetic reasons, in which case simple excision suffices.

Pterygium is a fleshy triangular conjunctival lesion that may encroach on the cornea. It typically occurs in the nasal interpalpebral region. The pathologic findings are similar to those of a pinguecula. The development of pterygia is related to exposure to ultraviolet light, and it therefore is more commonly found among people who live near the equator. Removal is suggested when the lesion encroaches far onto the cornea. Recurrence after removal is common.

Dermoid cyst and *dermolipoma* are benign lesions, clinically similar in appearance. They are smooth, elevated, round to oval lesions of various sizes. The color varies from yellowish white to fleshy pink. The most frequent site is the upper outer quadrant of the globe; they also commonly occur near or straddling the limbus. Dermolipoma is composed of adipose and connective tissue. Dermoid cysts may also contain glandular tissue, hair follicles, and hair shafts. Excision for cosmetic reasons is feasible. Dermolipomas are often connected to the extraocular muscles, making their complete removal impossible without sacrificing ocular motility.

Conjunctival nevus is a small, slightly elevated lesion that may vary in pigmentation from pale salmon to dark brown. It is usually benign, but careful observation for progressive growth or changes suggestive of malignancy is advised.

Symblepharon is a cicatricial adhesion between the conjunctiva of the lid and the globe; the lower lid is usually affected. It follows operation or injuries, especially burns due to lye, acids, or molten metals. It is a serious complication of Stevens-Johnson syndrome. It may interfere with motion of the eyeball and may cause diplopia. The adhesions should be separated and the raw surfaces kept from uniting during healing. Grafts of oral mucous membrane may be necessary.

Abelson MB, Schaefer K: Conjunctivitis of allergic origin: Immunologic mechanisms and current approaches to therapy. Surv Ophthalmol 38(Suppl):115, 1993.

Arstikaitis MJ: Ocular aftermath of Stevens-Johnson syndrome. Arch Ophthalmol 90:376, 1973.

Brook I: Anaerobic and aerobic bacterial flora of acute conjunctivitis in children. Arch Ophthalmol 98:833, 1980.

Catalano RA, Nelson LB: Conjunctivitis. *In*: Dershervitz RA (ed): Ambulatory Pediatric Care, 2nd ed. Philadelphia, JB Lippincott, 1992.

Clark SW, Culbertson WW, Forster RK: Clinical findings and results of treatment in an outbreak of acute hemorrhagic conjunctivitis in southern Florida. Am J Ophthalmol 99:45, 1983.

Fischer MC: Conjunctivitis in children. Pediatr Clin North Am 34:1447, 1987.

Hammerschlag MR, Cummings C, Roblin PM, et al: Efficacy of neonatal ocular prophylaxis for the prevention of chlamydial and gonococcal conjunctivitis. N Engl J Med 320:769, 1989.

Isenberg SJ, Apt L, Yoshimora R, et al: Bacterial flora of the conjunctiva at birth. J Pediatr Ophthalmol Strabismus 23:284, 1986.

Knopf HLS, Hierholzer JC: Clinical and immunologic responses in patients with viral keratoconjunctivitis. Am J Ophthalmol 80:661, 1975.

Matobu A: Ocular viral infections. Pediatr Infect Dis 3:358, 1984.

O'Hara MA: Ophthalmia neonatorum. Pediatr Clin North Am 40:715, 1993.

Schnall BM, Nelson LB: Ophthalmia neonatorum. Semin Ophthalmol 5:107, 1990.

Chapter 634
Abnormalities of the Cornea

MEGALOCORNEA. This is a nonprogressive symmetric condition characterized by an enlarged cornea (>12 mm in diameter) and an anterior segment in which there is no evidence of previous or concurrent ocular hypertension. High myopia is frequently present and may lead to reduced vision. A frequent complication is the development of lens opacities in adult life. All modes of inheritance have been described, although X-linked recessive is most common; therefore, this disorder most commonly afflicts males. Systemic abnormalities that may be associated with megalocornea include Marfan's syndrome, craniosynostosis, and Alport's syndrome. The cause of the enlargement of the cornea and the anterior segment is unknown, but possible explanations include a defect in the growth of the optic cup and an arrest of congenital glaucoma. The region on the X chromosome responsible for this disorder has been identified.

Pathologic corneal enlargement caused by glaucoma is to be differentiated from this anomaly. Any progressive increase in the size of the cornea, especially when accompanied by photophobia, lacrimation, or haziness of the cornea, requires prompt ophthalmologic evaluation.

MICROCORNEA. Microcornea, or *anterior microphthalmia,* is an abnormally small cornea in an otherwise relatively normal eye. It may be familial, transmission being dominant more often than recessive. More commonly, a small cornea is just one feature of an otherwise developmentally abnormal or microphthalmic eye; associated defects include colobomas, microphakia, congenital cataract, glaucoma, and aniridia.

KERATOCONUS. This is a disease of unclear pathogenesis characterized by progressive thinning and bulging of the central cornea, which becomes cone shaped. Although familial cases are known, most cases are sporadic. Eye rubbing and contact lens wear have been implicated as pathogenic, but the evidence to support this is equivocal. The incidence is increased in individuals with atopy, Down syndrome, Marfan's syndrome, and retinitis pigmentosa.

Most cases are bilateral, but involvement may be asymmetric. The disorder usually presents and progresses rapidly during adolescence; progression slows and stabilizes when patients reach full growth. Descemet's membrane may occasionally be stretched beyond its elastic breaking point, causing an acute rupture in the membrane with resultant sudden and marked corneal edema (acute hydrops) and decrease in vision. The corneal edema resolves as endothelial cells cover the defective area. Some degree of corneal scarring occurs, but the visual acuity is often better than before the initial incident. Signs of keratoconus include Munson's sign (bulging of the lower eyelid on looking downward) and the presence of a Fleischer ring (a deposit of iron in the epithelium at the base of the cone). Corneal transplantation is indicated if satisfactory visual acuity cannot be attained with the use of hard contact lenses.

NEONATAL CORNEAL OPACITIES. Loss of the normal transparency of the cornea in neonates may occur secondary to either intrinsic hereditary or extrinsic environmental causes (Table 634–1).

SCLEROCORNEA. In sclerocornea, the normal translucent cornea is replaced by sclera-like tissue. Instead of a clearly demarcated cornea, white, feathery, often ill-defined and vascularized tissue develops in the peripheral cornea, appearing to blend with and extend from the sclera. The central cornea is usually clearer, but total replacement of the cornea with sclera may occur. The curvature of the cornea is often flatter, similar to the sclera. Potentially coexisting abnormalities include a shallow anterior chamber, iris abnormalities, and microphthalmos. This condition is usually bilateral. In approximately 50% of cases, a dominant or recessive inheritance has been described. Sclerocornea has been reported in association with numerous systemic abnormalities including limb deformities, craniofacial defects, and genitourinary disorders. In generalized sclerocornea, early keratoplasty should be considered in an effort to provide vision.

PETERS ANOMALY. Peters anomaly is a central corneal opacity (leukoma) that is present at birth. It is often associated with iridocorneal adhesions that extend from the iris collarette to the border of the corneal opacity. Approximately one half of patients have other ocular abnormalities, which may include cataracts, glaucoma, and microcornea. As many as 80% of cases may be bilateral, and 60% are associated with systemic malformations that may affect any major organ system. Some investigators have divided Peters anomaly into two types: a mesodermal or neuroectodermal form (type I), which shows no associated lens changes, and a surface ectodermal form (type II), which does. Histologic findings include a focal absence of Descemet's membrane and corneal endothelium in the region of the opacity. Peters anomaly may be caused by incomplete migration and differentiation of the precursor cells of the central corneal endothelium and Descemet's membrane or a defective separation between the primitive lens and cornea during embryogenesis.

DERMOIDS. Epibulbar dermoids are choristomas. They are often present at birth and may increase in size with age. They occur most frequently in the lower temporal quadrant. They most commonly straddle the limbus and extend into the peripheral cornea. Rarely, they may be confined entirely to the cornea or conjunctiva. Epibulbar dermoids may cause visual disturbance by encroaching on the visual axis or by contributing to the development of astigmatism.

A dermoid usually appears as a well-circumscribed rounded or oval, gray or pinkish-yellow mass with a dry surface from which short hairs may protrude. It may affect only the superficial layers of the cornea, although full-thickness involvement is common. Associated ocular anomalies include eyelid and iris colobomas, microphthalmos, and retinal and choroidal defects. Thirty per cent of dermoids are associated with systemic abnormalities. Many of the associated anomalies involve developmental defects of the first branchial arch (vertebral anomalies, dystoses of the facial bones and dental anomalies, and Goldenhar syndrome). Epibulbar dermoids are found in 75% of cases of Goldenhar syndrome.

DENDRITIC KERATITIS. Infection of the cornea with the virus of herpes simplex produces a characteristic lesion of the corneal epithelium, referred to as a *dendrite*; it has a branching treelike pattern that can be demonstrated by fluorescein staining. The acute episode is accompanied by pain, photophobia, tearing, blepharospasm, and conjunctival infection. Specific treatment

TABLE 634–1 STUMPED: Differential Diagnosis of Neonatal Corneal Opacities

Diagnosis	Laterality	Opacity	Ocular Pressure	Other Ocular Abnormalities	Natural History	Inheritance
S—Sclerocornea	Unilateral or bilateral	Vascularized, blends with sclera, clearer centrally	Normal (or elevated)	Cornea plana	Nonprogressive	Sporadic
T—Tears in endothelium and Descemet's membrane						
Birth trauma	Unilateral	Diffuse edema	Normal	Possible hyphema, periorbital ecchymoses	Spontaneous improvement in 1 mo	Sporadic
Infantile glaucoma	Bilateral	Diffuse edema	Elevated	Megalocornea, photophobia and tearing, abnormal angle	Progressive unless treated	Autosomal recessive
U—Ulcers						
Herpes simplex keratitis	Unilateral	Diffuse with geographic epithelial defect	Normal	None	Progressive	Sporadic
Congenital rubella	Bilateral	Disciform or diffuse edema, no frank ulceration	Normal or elevated	Microphthalmos, cataract, pigment epithelial mottling	Stable, may clear	Sporadic
Neurotrophic—exposure	Unilateral or bilateral	Central ulcer	Normal	Lid anomalies, congenital sensory neuropathy	Progressive	Sporadic
M—Metabolic (rarely present at birth) (mucopolysaccharidoses IH, IS; mucolipidoses type IV)*	Bilateral	Diffuse haze, denser peripherally	Normal	Few	Progressive	Autosomal dominant
P—Posterior corneal defect	Unilateral or bilateral	Central, diffuse haze or vascularized leukoma	Normal or elevated	Anterior chamber cleavage syndrome	Stable, sometimes early clearing or vascularization	Sporadic, autosomal recessive
E—Endothelial dystrophy						
Congenital hereditary endothelial dystrophy	Bilateral	Diffuse corneal edema, marked corneal thickening	Normal	None	Stable	Autosomal dominant or recessive
Posterior polymorphous dystrophy	Bilateral	Diffuse haze, normal corneal thickness	Normal	Occasional peripheral anterior synechiae	Slowly progressive	Autosomal dominant
Congenital hereditary stromal dystrophy	Bilateral	Flaky, feathery stromal opacities; normal corneal thickness	Normal	None	Stable	Autosomal dominant
D—Dermoid	Unilateral or bilateral	White vascularized mass, hair, lipid arc	Normal	None	Stable	Sporadic

**Mucopolysaccharidosis IH (Hurler's syndrome); mucopolysaccharidosis IS (Scheie's syndrome).*
From Nelson LB, Calhoun JH, Harley RD: Pediatric Ophthalmology, 3rd ed. Philadelphia, WB Saunders, 1991, p 210.

may include mechanical debridement of the involved corneal epithelium to remove the source of infection and eliminate an antigenic stimulus to inflammation in the adjacent stroma. Medical treatment involves the use of 5-iodo-2′-deoxyuridine (IDU), topical vidarabine, or, most commonly, trifluridine. In addition, a cycloplegic agent is useful to relieve pain from spasm of the ciliary muscle. Overly aggressive topical antiviral treatment itself can be toxic to the cornea and should be avoided. Recurrent infection and deep stromal involvement can lead to corneal scarring and loss of vision.

Topical use of corticosteroids causes exacerbation of superficial herpetic disease of the eye; eye drops combining steroids and antibiotics are therefore to be avoided in treatment of red eye unless there are clear-cut indications for their use and close supervision during therapy.

Infants born to mothers infected with herpes simplex virus should be examined carefully for signs of ocular involvement. Intravenous acyclovir is required for treatment of ocular herpes in newborns.

CORNEAL ULCERS. The usual signs and symptoms are focal or diffuse corneal haze, hyperemia, lid edema, pain, photophobia, tearing, and blepharospasm. *Hypopyon* (pus in the anterior chamber) is common. Corneal ulcers require prompt treatment. They result most frequently from traumatic lesions that become secondarily infected. Many organisms are capable of infecting the cornea. One of the most troublesome is *Pseudomonas aeruginosa;* it can rapidly destroy stromal tissue and lead to corneal perforation. *Neisseria gonorrhoeae* also is particularly damaging to the cornea. Indolent ulcers may be caused by fungi, often in association with the use of contact lenses. In each case, scrapings of the cornea must be studied in an effort to identify the infectious agent and to determine the best therapy. Although aggressive local treatment is generally needed to save the eye, systemic treatment may be necessary in some cases as well. Perforation or scarring resulting from corneal ulceration is an important cause of blindness throughout the world and is estimated to be responsible for 10% of blindness in the United States.

Unexplained corneal ulcers in infants and young children should raise the question of a sensory defect, as in Riley-Day or Goldenhar-Gorlin syndrome, or of a metabolic disorder such as tyrosinemia.

PHLYCTENULES. These are small, yellowish, slightly elevated lesions usually located at the corneal limbus; they may encroach on the cornea and extend centrally. A small corneal ulcer is often found at the head of the advancing lesion, with a fascicle of blood vessels behind the head of the lesion. Although once thought to represent a sign of systemic tuberculin infection, phylctenular keratoconjunctivitis is now accepted as a morphologic expression of delayed hypersensitivity to diverse antigens. In children, it commonly occurs as a result of a hypersensitivity reaction of the conjunctiva or cornea to bacterial products. Treatment usually consists of eliminating the underlying disorder, usually staphylococcal blepharitis or meibomianitis, and suppressing the immune response with the use of topical corticosteroid therapy. A superficial stromal pannus and scarring sometimes remain after treatment.

INTERSTITIAL KERATITIS. This denotes inflammation of the corneal stroma. The most common cause is syphilis, interstitial keratitis being one of the characteristic late manifestations of congenital syphilis. The corneal changes in congenital syphilis occur in two phases. The acute phase presents between the ages of 5 and 10 yr, with an intense keratitis that may last for several months and causes a severe reduction in vision. The acute effects of syphilis are due in most part to the host immune response, such as mononuclear cell infiltrates, proliferative vascular changes, and occasionally granuloma formation. The deep inflammation produces pain, photophobia, tearing, circumcorneal injection, and corneal haze. The acute episode is followed by a chronic stage with significant regression in the corneal findings along with a parallel improvement in visual acuity. Although the corneal findings may regress with time, "ghost vessels," which represent the previous vascular changes, and patchy corneal scarring remain and serve as permanent stigmata of the disease.

Cogan's syndrome is a nonluetic interstitial keratitis associated with hearing loss and vestibular symptoms. Although its cause is unknown, a systemic vasculitis is suspected. Prompt treatment is required to avoid permanent hearing loss. Both the corneal changes and the auditory involvement may respond to the use of immunosuppressive agents.

Less frequently, interstitial keratitis is caused by other infectious diseases, such as tuberculosis or leprosy.

CORNEAL MANIFESTATIONS OF SYSTEMIC DISEASE. Several metabolic diseases produce distinctive corneal changes in childhood. Refractile polychromatic crystals are deposited throughout the cornea in cystinosis. Corneal deposits producing various degrees of corneal haze also occur in certain of the mucopolysaccharidoses, particularly MPS IH (Hurler), MPS IS (Scheie), MPS I H/S (Hurler-Scheie compound), MPS IV (Morquio), MPS VI (Maroteaux-Lamy), and sometimes MPS VII (Sly). Corneal deposits may develop in patients with GM_1 (generalized) gangliosidosis. In Fabry's disease, fine opacities radiating in a whorl or fanlike pattern occur, and corneal changes can be important in identifying the carrier state. A spraylike pattern of corneal opacities may also be seen in the Bloch-Sulzberger syndrome. In Wilson's disease, the distinctive corneal sign is the Kayser-Fleischer ring, a golden brown ring in the peripheral cornea resulting from changes in Descemet's membrane. Pigmented corneal rings may develop in neonates with cholestatic liver disease. Corneal changes may occur in autoimmune hypoparathyroidism, and band keratopathy in patients with hypercalcemia. Transient keratitis may occur with rubeola, sometimes with rubella.

Allen NB, Cox CC, Cobo M, et al: Use of immunosuppressive agents in the treatment of severe ocular and vascular manifestations of Cogan's syndrome. Am J Med 88:296, 1990.

Beauchamp GR, Gillette TE, Friendly DS: Phlyctenular keratoconjunctivitis. J Pediatr Ophthalmol Strabismus 18:22, 1981.

Deckard PS, Bergstrom TJ: Rubeola keratitis. Ophthalmology 88:810, 1981.

Dunn LL, Annable WL, Kliegman RM: Pigmented corneal rings in neonates with liver disease. J Pediatr 110:771, 1987.

Elliott JH, Feman SS, O'Day DM, et al: Hereditary sclerocornea. Arch Ophthalmol 103:676, 1985.

Goldberg MF, Payne JW, Brunt PW: Ophthalmologic studies of familial dysautonomia. Arch Ophthalmol 80:732, 1966.

Hutchison DS, Smith RE, Haughton PB: Congenital herpetic keratitis. Arch Ophthalmol 93:70, 1975.

Kraft SP, Judisch GF, Grayson DM: Megalocornea: A clinical and echographic study of an autosomal dominant pedigree. J Pediatr Ophthalmol Strabismus 21:190, 1984.

Laibson PR, Waring GO: Diseases of the cornea. *In*: Nelson LB, Calhoun JH, Harley RD (eds): Pediatric Ophthalmology, 3rd ed. Philadelphia, WB Saunders, 1991.

Mackey DA, Buttery RG, Wise GM, et al: Description of X-linked megalocornea with identification of the gene locus. Arch Ophthalmol 109:829, 1991.

Mohandessan MM, Romano PE: Neuroparalytic keratitis in Goldenhar-Gorlin syndrome. Am J Ophthalmol 85:111, 1978.

Schanzlin DJ, Goldberg DB, Brown SI: Transplantation of congenitally opaque corneas. Ophthalmology 87:1253, 1980.

Traboulsi EI, Maumenee IH: Peters' anomaly and associated congenital malformations. Arch Ophthalmol 110:1739, 1992.

Tso MOM, Fine BS, Thorpe HE: Kayser-Fleischer ring and associated cataract in Wilson's disease. Am J Ophthalmol 79:479, 1975.

Yang LLH, Lambert SR, Fernhoff PM, et al: Peters' anomaly: Associated congenital malformations and etiology. Invest Ophthalmol Vis Sci 36:S41, 1995.

CHAPTER 635
Abnormalities of the Lens

CATARACTS. A cataract is any opacity of the lens. Some are clinically unimportant, others significantly affect visual function, and many are associated with ocular or systemic disease.

Differential Diagnosis. The differential diagnosis of cataracts in infants and children includes a wide range of developmental disorders, infectious and inflammatory processes, metabolic diseases, and toxic and traumatic insults (Table 635–1). Cataracts may also develop secondary to intraocular processes, such as retinopathy of prematurity, persistent hyperplastic primary vitreous, retinal detachment, retinitis pigmentosa, and uveitis.

DEVELOPMENTAL VARIANTS. Early developmental processes may lead to various congenital lens opacities. Discrete dots or white plaquelike opacities of the lens capsule are common and sometimes involve the contiguous subcapsular region. Small opacities of the posterior capsule may be associated with persistent remnants of the primitive hyaloid vascular system (the common Mittendorf's dot), whereas those of the anterior capsule may be associated with persistent strands of the pupillary membrane or vascular sheath of the lens. Congenital cataracts of this type are usually stationary and rarely interfere with vision; in some, progression occurs.

PREMATURITY. A special type of lens change seen in some preterm newborns is the so-called cataract of prematurity. The appearance is of a cluster of tiny vacuoles in the distribution of the Y sutures of the lens. They can be visualized with an ophthalmoscope and are best seen with the pupil well dilated. The pathogenesis is unclear. In most cases, the opacities disappear spontaneously, often within a few weeks.

MENDELIAN INHERITANCE. Many cataracts unassociated with other diseases are hereditary. The most common mode of inheritance is autosomal dominant. Penetrance and expressivity vary. Autosomal recessive inheritance occurs less frequently; it is sometimes found in populations with high rates of consanguinity. X-linked inheritance of cataracts unassociated with disease is relatively rare, whereas cataracts occurring in association with X-linked disease are seen in Lowe's syndrome, Alport's syndrome, and Fabry's disease.

CONGENITAL INFECTION SYNDROME. Cataracts in infants and children frequently are a result of prenatal infection. Lens opacity may occur in any of the major congenital infection syndromes (e.g., toxoplasmosis, cytomegalovirus, syphilis, rubella, herpes simplex virus). Cataracts may also occur secondary to other perinatal infections, including measles, poliomyelitis, influenza, varicella-zoster, and vaccinia.

TABLE 635–1 Differential Diagnosis of Cataracts

Developmental Variants

Prematurity (Y suture vacuoles) with or without retinopathy of prematurity

Genetic Disorders

Simple Mendelian Inheritance

Autosomal dominant (most common)
Autosomal recessive
X-linked

Major Chromosomal Defects

Trisomy disorders (13, 18, 21)
Turner's syndrome (45 X)
Deletion syndromes (11p13, 18p, 18q)
Duplication syndromes (3q, 20p, 10q)

Multisystem Genetic Disorders

Alport's syndrome (hearing loss, renal disease)
Alström's disease (nerve deafness, diabetes mellitus)
Apert's syndrome (craniosynostosis, syndactyly)
Cockayne's syndrome (premature senility, skin photosensitivity)
Conradi's syndrome (chondrodysplasia punctata)
Crouzon's syndrome (dysostosis craniofacialis)
Hallermann-Streiff syndrome (microphthalmia, small pinched nose, skin atrophy, and hypotrichosis)
Hypohidrotic ectodermal dysplasia (anomalous dentition, hypohidrosis, hypotrichosis)
Ichthyosis (keratinizing disorder with thick, scaly skin)
Incontinentia pigmenti (dental anomalies, mental retardation, cutaneous lesions)
Lowe's syndrome (oculocerebrorenal syndrome: hypotonia, renal disease)
Marfan's syndrome
Meckel-Gruber syndrome (renal dysplasia, encephalocele)
Myotonic dystrophy
Nail-patella syndrome (renal dysfunction, dysplastic nails, hypoplastic patella)
Marinesco-Sjögren syndrome (cerebellar ataxia, hypotonia)
Nevoid basal cell carcinoma syndrome (autosomal dominant, basal cell carcinoma erupts in childhood)
Peters' anomaly (corneal opacifications with iris-corneal dysgenesis)
Reiger syndrome (iris dysplasia, myotonic dystrophy)
Rothmund-Thomson syndrome (poikiloderma: skin atrophy)
Rubinstein-Taybi syndrome (broad great toe, mental retardation)
Smith-Lemli-Opitz syndrome (toe syndactyly, hypospadias, mental retardation)
Sotos' syndrome (cerebral gigantism)
Spondyloepiphyseal dysplasia (dwarfism, short trunk)
Werner's syndrome (premature aging in 2nd decade of life)

Inborn Errors of Metabolism

Abetalipoproteinemia (absent chylomicrons, retinal degeneration)
Fabry disease (α-galactosidase A deficiency)
Galactokinase deficiency
Galactosemia (galactose-1-phosphate uridyltransferase deficiency)
Homocystinemia (subluxation of lens, mental retardation)
Mannosidosis (acid α-mannosidase deficiency)
Niemann-Pick (sphingomyelinase deficiency)
Refsum's syndrome (phytanic acid α-hydrolase deficiency)
Wilson's disease (accumulation of copper leads to cirrhosis and neurologic symptoms)

Endocrinopathies

Hypocalcemia (hypoparathyroidism)
Hypoglycemia
Diabetes mellitus

Congenital Infections

Toxoplasmosis
Cytomegalovirus infection
Syphilis
Rubella
Perinatal herpes simplex infection
Measles (rubeola)
Poliomyelitis
Influenza
Varicella-zoster

Ocular Anomalies

Microphthalmia
Coloboma
Aniridia
Mesodermal dysgenesis
Persistent pupillary membrane
Posterior lenticonus
Persistent hyperplastic primary vitreous
Primitive hyaloid vascular system

Miscellaneous Disorders

Atopic dermatitis
Drugs (corticosteroids)
Radiation
Trauma

Idiopathic

Metabolic Disorders. Cataracts are a prominent manifestation of many metabolic diseases, particularly certain disorders of carbohydrate, amino acid, calcium, and copper metabolism. A primary consideration in any infant with cataracts is the possibility of galactosemia (see Chapter 84.2). In classic infantile galactosemia, galactose-1-phosphate uridyl transferase deficiency, the cataract is typically of the zonular type, with haziness or opacification of one or more of the perinuclear layers of the lens; haziness or clouding of the nucleus also often occurs. In its early stages, the cataract generally has a distinctive oil droplet appearance and is best detected with the pupil fully dilated. Progression to complete opacification of the lens may occur within weeks. With early treatment (galactose-free diet), the lens changes may be reversible.

In galactokinase deficiency, cataracts are the sole clinical manifestation. The cataracts are usually zonular and may appear in the first months or years of life or later in childhood.

In children with juvenile-onset diabetes mellitus, lens changes are uncommon. Some develop snowflake-like white opacities and vacuoles of the lens. Others develop cataracts that may progress and mature rapidly, sometimes in a matter of hours or days, especially during adolescence. An antecedent event may be the sudden development of myopia caused by changes in the optical density of the lens.

Congenital lens opacities may be seen in children of diabetic and prediabetic mothers. Hypoglycemia in neonates can also be associated with early development of cataracts. Ketotic hypoglycemia is also associated with cataracts.

An association between cataracts and hypocalcemia is well established. Various lens opacities may be seen in patients with hypoparathyroidism.

The oculocerebral renal syndrome of Lowe is associated with cataracts in infants. Affected male children frequently have dense bilateral cataracts at birth, often in association with glaucoma and miotic pupils. Punctate lens opacities are frequently present in heterozygous females.

The distinctive sunflower cataract of Wilson disease is not commonly seen in children. Various lens opacities may be seen in children with certain of the sphingolipidoses, mucopolysaccharidoses, and mucolipidoses, particularly Niemann-Pick disease, mucosulfatidosis, Fabry disease, and aspartylglycosaminuria.

Chromosomal Defects. Lens opacities of various types may occur in association with chromosomal defects, including 13-, 18-, and 21-trisomy; Turner syndrome; and a number of deletion (11p13, 18p, 18q) and duplication syndromes (3q, 20p, 10q).

Drugs, Toxic Agents, and Trauma. Of the various drugs and toxic agents that may produce cataracts, corticosteroids are of major importance in the pediatric age group. Steroid-related cataracts characteristically are posterior subcapsular lens opacities. The incidence and severity vary. The relative significance of dose, mode of administration, duration of treatment, and individual susceptibility is controversial, and the pathogenesis of steroid-induced cataracts is unclear. The effect on vision depends on the extent and density of the opacity. In many cases, the acuity is only minimally or moderately impaired. Reversibility of steroid-induced cataracts may occur in some cases. All children being treated with long-term steroids should have periodic eye examinations.

Trauma to the eye is a major cause of cataracts in children. Opacification of the lens may result from contusion or penetrating injury. Cataracts are an important manifestation of child abuse. Other physical agents, such as radiation, can also damage the lens and produce cataracts.

Miscellaneous Disorders. The list of multisystem syndromes and diseases associated with lens opacities and other eye anomalies is extensive. The clinical features of some of the major disorders are presented in Table 635–2.

Treatment. The treatment of cataracts that significantly interfere with vision includes the following: (1) surgical removal of lens material to provide an optically clear visual axis; (2) correction of the resultant aphakic refractive error with spectacles, contact lenses, or, in appropriate cases, intraocular lens implantation; and (3) correction of any associated sensory deprivation amblyopia. Because spectacles may not be possible or are contraindicated in children after cataract removal, the use of contact lenses for visual rehabilitation is a medical necessity. They should not be thought of as a cosmetic option to glasses. Treatment of the amblyopia may be the most demanding and difficult step in the visual rehabilitation of infants or children with cataracts.

Prognosis. Prognosis depends on many factors, including the nature of the cataract, the underlying disease, age of onset, age of intervention, duration and severity of any attendant amblyopia, and presence of any associated ocular abnormalities (e.g., microphthalmia, retinal lesions, optic atrophy, glaucoma, nystagmus, strabismus). Persistent amblyopia is the most common cause of poor visual recovery after cataract surgery in children. Secondary conditions and complications may develop in children who have had cataract surgery, including inflammatory sequelae, secondary membranes, glaucoma, retinal detachment, and changes in the axial length of the eye. All these should be considered in planning treatment.

ECTOPIA LENTIS. Normally, the lens is suspended in place behind the iris diaphragm by the zonular fibers of the ciliary body. Abnormalities of the suspensory system resulting from a developmental defect, disease, or trauma may result in instability or displacement of the lens. Displacement of the lens is classified as luxation (dislocation—complete displacement of the lens) or as subluxation (partial displacement—shifting or tilting of the lens). Symptoms include blurring of vision, which is often the result of refractive changes such as myopia, astigmatism, or aphakic hyperopia. Some patients experience diplopia. An important sign of displacement is iridodenesis, a tremulousness of the iris caused by the loss of its usual support. Also, the anterior chamber may appear deeper than normal. Sometimes the equatorial region ("edge") of the displaced lens may be visible in the pupillary aperture. On ophthalmoscopy, this may appear as a black crescent. Also, the difference between the phakic and aphakic portions can be appreciated when focusing on the fundus.

Differential Diagnosis. A major cause of lens displacement is trauma. Displacement may occur as a result of ocular disease, such as uveitis, intraocular tumor, congenital glaucoma, high myopia, megalocornea, or aniridia, or in association with cataract. There are also heritable forms of ectopia lentis and those associated with systemic disease.

Displacement of the lens occurring as a heritable ocular condition unassociated with systemic abnormalities is referred to as *simple ectopia lentis*. Simple ectopia lentis is usually transmitted as an autosomal dominant condition. The lens is generally displaced upward and temporally. The ectopia may be present at birth or may appear later in life. Another form of heritable dislocation is *ectopia lentis et pupillae*. In this condition, both the lens and pupil are displaced, usually in opposite directions. This condition is generally bilateral, with one eye being almost a mirror image of the other. Ectopia lentis et pupillae is a recessive condition, although variable expression with some intermingling with simple ectopia lentis has been reported.

Systemic disorders associated with displacement of the lens include Marfan syndrome, homocystinuria, Weill-Marchesani syndrome, and sulfite oxidase deficiency. Ectopia lentis occurs in approximately 80% of patients with Marfan syndrome, and in about 50% of patients the ectopia is evident by the age of 5 yr. In most cases, the lens is displaced superiorly and temporally; it is almost always bilateral and relatively symmetric. In homocystinuria, the lens is usually displaced inferiorly and somewhat nasally. It occurs early in life and is often evident by 5 yr of age. In Weill-Marchesani syndrome the displacement

TABLE 635–2 Clinical Features and Ocular Changes in Developmental Pediatric Syndromes

CNS Anomalies

- Anencephaly (see Chapter 601.6)
  - Optic nerve aplasia or hypoplasia
- Holoprosencephaly (see Chapter 601.7)
  - Hypotelorism; in extreme form, cyclopia; in some cases, iris coloboma
- Cyclopia
  - A single eye of variable complexity, usually accompanied by a proboscis-like structure on the forehead; often associated with holoprosencephaly; sometimes fusion of both eyes with duplication of lenses, corneas, and other structures; rosette formation in the retina; optic nerve rudimentary or absent; orbit diamond shaped
- Arnold-Chiari malformation (see Chapter 601.11)
  - Nystagmus, usually vertical, often downbeat; ocular motor palsies with diplopia; sometimes skew deviation
- Dandy-Walker syndrome (see Chapter 601.11)
  - Ophthalmic manifestations of increased intracranial pressure
- Septo-optic dysplasia (deMorsier syndrome)
  - Malformation of anterior midline structures (agenesis of septum pellucidum, primitive optic ventricle, with hypoplasia of optic nerves, chiasm, and infundibulum); sometimes associated endocrine abnormalities; vision defects, strabismus, nystagmus; in some cases, other anomalies of eyes

Craniostenosis Syndromes (see Chapter 601.12)

- Apert syndrome (acrocephalosyndactyly)
  - Orbits shallow, eyes protuberant (proptosis) and widely spaced; antimongoloid slant of palpebral fissures; ocular motor abnormalities (strabismus, partial ophthalmoplegia, nystagmus); papilledema; optic atrophy; cataracts; sometimes dislocated lenses; occasionally iris and fundus colobomas
- Carpenter syndrome (acrocephalopolysyndactyly)
  - Orbits shallow; lateral displacement of medial canthi; epicanthus; antimongoloid slant of palpebral fissures; optic atrophy; microcornea and corneal opacities in some cases
- Crouzon syndrome (dysostosis craniofacialis)
  - Eyes protuberant (proptosis) and widely spaced; luxation of globe may occur; antimongoloid slant of palpebral fissures; strabismus; papilledema; optic atrophy; vision loss; cataracts in some patients
- Kleeblattschädel syndrome (cloverleaf skull)
  - Shallow orbits with proptosis; high risk of corneal ulceration

Miscellaneous Craniofacial Defects and Syndromes

- Frontonasal dysplasia (median cleft-face syndrome)
  - Hypertelorism (radiographic interorbital distance 2 SD above normal for age); in some cases, anophthalmia, microphthalmia, epibulbar dermoids, lid colobomas, congenital cataracts
- Opitz's syndrome
  - Hypertelorism, particularly associated with hypospadias; antimongoloid slant of palpebral fissures; epicanthus; strabismus
- Waardenburg's syndrome
  - Lateral displacement of medial canthi and inferior puncta; heterochromia iridis, total or partial; in some cases both irides completely blue (isochromia); fundus pigmentary changes in some cases
- Oculodentodigital dysplasia (Meyer-Schwickerath syndrome)
  - Hypotelorism, microphthalmos, microcornea, dental anomalies and enamel hypoplasia, camptodactyly, syndactyly, and other skeletal defects; persistent pupillary membrane; glaucoma
- Hallermann-Streiff syndrome (dyscephalia oculomandibulofacialis)
  - Microphthalmos, cataract, sparse eyebrows and lashes, blue sclerae, nystagmus
- Pierre Robin syndrome
  - Congenital glaucoma; retinal detachment; strabismus
- Treacher Collins syndrome (mandibulofacial dysostosis; Franceschetti-Klein syndrome)
  - Antimongoloid slant of palpebral fissures; underdevelopment of supraorbital ridges, colobomas of lower eyelids and in some cases of iris or choroid
- Goldenhar syndrome (oculoauriculovertebral dysplasia)
  - Antimongoloid slant of palpebral fissures; colobomata of eyelid, upper lid more commonly involved than lower; hypoplasia or coloboma of iris; hypertelorism; sometimes microphthalmos

Chromosomal Abnormalities

- 21-Trisomy (Down syndrome; see Chapter 78)
  - Mongoloid slant of palpebral fissures; epicanthus; dacryostenosis; blepharitis; Brushfield spots of iris; peripheral thinning of iris stroma; keratoconus and corneal hydrops; cataracts; high refractive errors; strabismus; nystagmus; increased vessels at disc
- 18-Trisomy (Edwards syndrome; see Chapter 78)
  - Ptosis; short palpebral fissures; epicanthus; hypoplastic supraorbital ridges; microphthalmia; corneal opacities; anisocoria; cataracts; fundus and disc colobomas; retinal hypopigmentation
- 13-Trisomy (Patau's syndrome; see Chapter 78)
  - Microphthalmos; anophthalmos; cyclopia in some cases; dysgenesis of anterior segment (iris hypoplasia, iris adhesions, chamber angle abnormalities); corneal opacities; congenital glaucoma; cataracts; persistent hyperplastic primary vitreous; retinal dysplasia; colobomas of iris, ciliary body, fundus; intraocular cartilage, optic nerve hypoplasia
- 9-Trisomy
  - Antimongoloid slant of palpebral fissures; deeply set eyes; corectopia; strabismus
- 8-Trisomy
  - Dysmorphic skull; strabismus
- Syndrome 45X (Turner, and mosaic variants; see Chapter 78)
  - Ptosis; epicanthus; blue sclerae; defective color vision; cataracts; strabismus; nystagmus
- 47,XXY; 48,XXXY; 49,XXXXY (Klinefelter) syndromes (see Chapter 593)
  - Hypertelorism; epicanthus; Brushfield spots of iris; myopia; strabismus
- Partial deletion short arm chromosome 4 (4p −) (see Chapter 78)
  - Ptosis; hypertelorism; epicanthus; colobomata
- Partial deletion short arm chromosome 5 (5p −) (cri-du-chat syndrome; see Chapter 67)
  - Antimongoloid slant of palpebral fissures; hypertelorism; epicanthus; strabismus
- Partial deletion short arm chromosome 9 (9p −) (see Chapter 78)
  - Mongoloid slant of palpebral fissures; epicanthus; arched brows
- Partial deletion long arm chromosome 13 (13q −)
  - Ptosis; epicanthus; hypertelorism; microphthalmos; colobomas; retinoblastoma
- Partial deletion long arm chromosome 18 (18q −) (see Chapter 78)
  - Horizontal palpebral fissures; epicanthus; deeply set eyes; optic disc pallor; tapetoretinal degeneration; nystagmus
- Partial deletion, long arm chromosome 21 (21q −)
  - Downward slanting palpebral fissures
- Partial deletion long arm chromosome 22 (22q −)
  - Ptosis; epicanthus
- Extrachromosomal material (cat-eye syndrome)
  - Antimongoloid slant of palpebral fissures; epicanthus; hypertelorism; microphthalmos; colobomas of iris, fundus, optic nerve; macular defects; pale discs; cataracts; strabismus; nystagmus

Disorders of Amino Acid Metabolism

- Albinism*
  - Defect in the formation of melanin; several forms:
    - (1) *Oculocutaneous albinism, tyrosinase negative;* generalized hypopigmentation; iris blue or gray; generalized hypopigmentation of eye; typical pink or orange reflex; fundus bright, with increased choroidal vascular pattern; macula/fovea poorly defined (hypoplastic); photophobia; nystagmus; subnormal vision; often high refractive error
    - (2) *Oculocutaneous albinism, tyrosinase positive;* pigmentation may increase with age; iris blue, yellow, or brownish; color increasing with age; photophobia; nystagmus; subnormal vision, which may improve with age
    - (3) *Amish* or *yellow* mutant; generalized albinism in which a yellowish pigment is produced instead of melanin, providing some skin and hair color
    - (4) *Hermansky-Pudlak syndrome;* tyrosine-negative albinism associated with a hemorrhagic diathesis; iris blue-gray to brown; photophobia; nystagmus; slight to moderate vision defect
    - (5) *Cross syndrome;* tyrosine positive; a syndrome of hypopigmentation, gingival fibromatosis, spasticity, athetoid movements, and microphthalmos; iris blue-gray, microphthalmos; cataracts; severe vision defect; nystagmus
    - (6) *Ocular albinsim;* pigment deficiency limited to the eye; generalized ocular hypopigmentation; macular hypoplasia; nystagmus (in blacks, fundus tessellated)
- Alkaptonuria (see Chapter 82.2)
  - Black discoloration of sclera, most noticeable at insertion of extraocular muscles
- Tyrosinemia (Richner-Hanhart syndrome; see Chapter 82.2)
  - Corneal ulceration, "herpetiform"
- Cystinosis (see Chapter 537.3)
  - Accumulation of refractile crystals in cornea (best seen with slit lamp, but corneal haze may be detected grossly); photophobia; pigmentary retinopathy; fundi generally hypopigmented, with fine to coarse spotty pigmentation, most marked peripherally; vision usually normal to nearly normal
- Homocystinemia, type I (see Chapter 82.3)
  - Ectopia lentis; cataract; secondary glaucoma; peripheral cystic degeneration of retina
- Sulfite oxidase deficiency (see Chapter 82.4)
  - Subluxation of lens; spherophakia; strabismus
- Hartnup's disease (see Chapter 82.5)
  - Photophobia; nystagmus; strabismus
- Maple syrup urine disease (see Chapter 82.6)
  - Strabismus, varying with condition of child

Table continued on following page

TABLE 635–2 Clinical Features and Ocular Changes in Developmental Pediatric Syndromes *Continued*

The Mucopolysaccharidoses (MPS)

Hurler's syndrome (MPS IH; α-L-iduronidase deficiency; see Chapter 85)
Hypertelorism, prominent eyes; puffy lids; heavy brows; deposition of MPS and attendant cellular changes throughout most regions of eye, particularly the conjunctiva, cornea, sclera, iris, ciliary body, retina, and optic nerve; characteristic corneal clouding, clinically evident early in life, and progressing to dense milky "ground-glass" haze, often with associated photophobia; progressive retinal degeneration with pigmentary dispersion and clumping, arteriolar attenuation and disc pallor, and reduced ERG; optic atrophy; vision loss, principally because of corneal, retinal, and optic nerve changes; hydrocephalus and cerebral changes; glaucoma in some cases

Scheie syndrome (MPS IS; α-L-iduronidase deficiency; see Chapter 85)
Progressive corneal clouding, diffuse but sometimes more dense peripherally than centrally; progressive retinal degeneration; visual symptoms, field loss, and night blindness often commencing in 2nd or 3rd decade; glaucoma in some cases

Hurler-Scheie Compound (MPS IH/S; α-L-iduronidase deficiency; see Chapter 85)
Corneal clouding, diffuse and progressive; glaucoma in some cases; vision loss because of corneal clouding or optic nerve effects of arachnoid cysts

Hunter syndrome (MPS II; iduronosulfate sulfatase deficiency)
Phenotypically similar to MPS IH; both mild and severe forms occur; progressive retinal degeneration with pigmentary changes, arteriolar attenuation, optic atrophy, vision, loss, reduced ERG; corneas macroscopically (clinically) clear, but microscopic corneal changes documented; papilledema secondary to hydrocephalus in some cases

Sanfilippo syndrome (MPS III; type A [heparin sulfate sulfatase deficiency], B [*N*-acetyl-α-D-glucosaminidase deficiency], and C [acetyl-Co A:α-glucosaminide *N*-acetyl transferase deficiency])
Retinal changes in some patients—arteriolar narrowing; reduced ERG; corneas clinically clear but some microscopic changes reported

Morquio's syndrome (MPS IV; galactosamine-6-sulfate sulfatase deficiency in classic form, β-galactosidase deficiency reported in variants; see Chapter 85)
Fine corneal clouding in many patients; slowly progressive; often not clinically apparent for several years

Maroteaux-Lamy syndrome (MPS VI; arylsulfatase-B deficiency; see Chapter 85)
Diffuse corneal clouding, usually evident within 1st few yr of life; tortuosity of retinal vessels in some patients; papilledema and 6th nerve paresis in some patients with hydrocephalus

Sly's syndrome (MPS VII; β-D-glucuronidase deficiency)
Some diversity of phenotype; corneas clear or cloudy; corneal haze of either fine or coarse type

Di Ferrenti syndrome (MPS VIII; *N*-acetylglucosamine-6-sulfate sulfatase deficiency)
Short stature; mild dysostosis multiplex; odontoid hypoplasia; hepatosplenomegaly; mental retardation; ophthalmologic abnormalities not yet described

The Sphingolipidoses

Generalized gangliosidosis (GM_1 gangliosidosis type 1; β-galactosidase deficiency; see Chapter 608.1)
Diffuse corneal clouding (MPS accumulation); macular cherry red spot of retinal ganglioside accumulation; retinal vascular tortuosity and retinal hemorrhages; optic atrophy; vision loss, nystagmus, strabismus

Juvenile GM_1 gangliosidosis (GM_1 gangliosidosis type 2; β-galactosidase deficiency; see Chapter 608.1)
Corneas clinically clear; histologic changes of retinal ganglioside storage without clinically obvious signs; optic atrophy and vision loss; nystagmus and strabismus

Tay-Sachs disease (GM_2 gangliosidosis type 1; hexosaminidase A deficiency; see Chapter 608.1)
Macular cherry red spot; optic atrophy (demyelination and degeneration of optic nerves, chiasm, and tracts); progressive loss of vision, caused by ocular and cerebral abnormalities; sequential deterioration of eye movements

Sandhoff variant (GM_2 gangliosidosis type 2; hexosaminidase A and B deficiency; see Chapter 608.1)
Macular cherry red spot; optic atrophy and progressive loss of vision; corneas clinically clear or slightly opalescent; histologic evidence of storage cytosomes in cornea

Juvenile GM_2 gangliosidosis (GM_2 gangliosidosis type 3; partial deficiency of hexosaminidase; see Chapter 608.1)
Retinal pigmentary degeneration; macular changes (cherry red spot type) in some cases; optic atrophy; blindness later in course of disease

Krabbe globoid cell leukodystrophy (galactosyl ceramide lipidosis; galactosylceramide β-galactosidase deficiency)
Cortical blindness and optic atrophy caused by degenerative changes in brain and visual pathways; nystagmus; strabismus

Gaucher's disease (glycosyl ceramide lipidosis; glucosyl ceramide β-glucosidase deficiency; see Chapter 83.4)
Paralytic strabismus caused by brain stem and cranial nerve involvement in neuronopathic forms; nystagmus; macular changes (grayness) in some cases; retinal hemorrhages secondary to anemia, thrombocytopenia; discrete white spots in or on retina reported in juvenile form; pingueculae (wedge-shaped conjunctival lesions) in chronic non-neuronopathic form; possibly corneal clouding

Niemann-Pick disease (sphingomyelin lipidoses; sphingomyelinase deficiency; see Chapter 83.4)
Grayish macular haze in classic infantile neuronopathic form (type A), and in subacute neurovisceral or juvenile form (type C); corneal clouding, lens opacities in some cases (type A); vertical gaze palsy in some patients

Fabry disease (glycosphingolipid lipidosis; α-galactosidase A deficiency; see Chapter 83.4)
Corneal dystrophy related to epithelial lipid deposits (radiating lines/whorls in affected males and in carrier females); aneurysmal dilatation and tortuosity of conjunctival and retinal vessels; renovascular signs of renal hypertension; papilledema; orbital and lid edema; cataracts (spokelike posterior cortical lens opacities—anterior lens opacities in some cases)

Farber disease (ceramide lipidosis; ceramidase deficiency; see Chapter 83.4)
Cherry red–like spot; grayish posterior pole; retinal pigmentary mottling; granulomas in and around eye

Ceroid Lipofuscinoses (see also Chapters 83.4 and 608.2)

Infantile (Finnish variant; unsaturated fatty acid lipidosis)
Microcephaly; marked atrophy of brain; loss of vision; granular inclusions; ataxia; myoclonus; profound dementia, decorticate state; onset 1–2 yr; death by 10 yr

Late infantile (Jansky-Bielschowsky)
Intellectual deterioration, seizures, ataxia; pigmentary retinal degeneration, in some cases, predominantly macular; ERG abnormal; optic atrophy; inclusions of curvilinear type; onset 2–4 yr; death by 10 yr

Juvenile (Batten-Mayou-Spielmeyer-Vogt)
Intellectual deterioration, seizures, ataxia, progressive loss of motor function; pigmentary retinal degeneration, resembling retinitis pigmentosa, with progressive loss of vision; in some cases predominantly macular degeneration; ERG abnormal; optic atrophy as a late manifestation; mixed inclusion bodies including curvilinear and fingerprint types, and lipofuscin in brain; onset 5–8 yr, sometimes later; death in teens or 20s

Late juvenile or adult (Kuf's)
Behavior disturbances and intellectual impairment; ataxia, spasticity, myoclonic seizures; vision and fundi usually normal; macular degeneration in some cases; mostly lipofuscin in brain; onset in childhood, adolescence, or eary adult life

Cherry red spot myoclonus syndrome
Macular cherry red spot; vision loss; intention myoclonus; variable inclusions in brain; light inclusions in hepatocytes and Kupffer's cells; onset in childhood; survival to adulthood

Leukodystrophies (see also Chapter 608.1)

Metachromatic leukodystrophy (arylsulfatase A deficiency)
Retinal degeneration resembling retinitis pigmentosa; in some cases, early macular involvement (macular grayness with accentuation of central red spot); optic atrophy; vision loss; strabismus and nystagmus

Pelizaeus-Merzbacher syndrome
"Eye rolling" (rhythmic eye movements) noted soon after birth, sometimes with rotary movements of the head; optic atrophy as a late manifestation

Canavan's disease
Vacuolation of ganglion cell layer of retina reportedly detectable with slit lamp; retinal pigmentary changes; optic atrophy; blindness early in course; ERG normal; VER reduced; strabismus, roving eye movements, and nystagmus

Demyelinating Scleroses (see Chapter 608.5)

Schilder disease (encephalitis periaxialis diffusa)
Involvement of visual pathways, producing retrobulbar neuritis, optic atrophy, central scotomas, chiasmal syndromes, homonymous field defects; disorders of cortical gaze functions; nystagmus

Multiple sclerosis
Optic neuritis (episodic loss of vision, typically a central scotoma, unilateral more often than bilateral, often with retrobulbar pain); other visual pathway lesions (various field defects); internuclear ophthalmoplegia; supranuclear gaze palsies; nystagmus; sheathing of peripheral retinal vessels in some cases

Neuromyelitis optica (Devick disease)
Optic neuritis (usually papillitis with visible disc edema), with resultant optic atrophy; other visual pathway lesions (various visual field defects); in some cases extraocular muscle palsies, conjugate gaze palsies, nystagmus, pupil abnormalities

TABLE 635–2 Clinical Features and Ocular Changes in Developmental Pediatric Syndromes *Continued*

Hamartomatoses and Phakomatoses

Tuberous sclerosis (Bourneville's disease; see Chapter 605.2)
Retinal phakomas (glial hamartomas, ranging from small flat or slightly elevated white or yellowish lesions to large elevated refractile yellowish multinodular or cystic masses often likened to an unripe mulberry); fibroangioma of the lids; in some, papilledema or optic atrophy, vision defects, pupil or ocular motor signs related to CNS changes (tumors, hydrocephalus); occasionally iris or pigmentary changes

Neurofibromatosis (von Recklinghausen syndrome; see Chapter 605.1)
Plexiform neuromas of eyelids, often producing ptosis; episcleral and conjunctival neurofibromas; prominent corneal nerves; Lisch's iris nodules; uveal hypercellularity; glaucoma (related to angle anomalies, uveal hypercellularity, neovascularization, or synechiae); hamartomas (phakomas) of disc and retina; fundus pigmentary changes likened to café-au-lait spots; optic gliomas and vision loss (presenting with proptosis, strabismus, nystagmus if intraorbital—with signs of increased intracranial pressure, hydrocephalus, or diencephalic syndrome when intracranial); orbital asymmetry; orbital wall defects; pulsatile exophthalmos, intraorbital neurofibromas, with proptosis

Angiomatosis of the retina and cerebellum (von Hippel–Lindau disease; see Chapter 605.4)
Retinal hemangioblastoma (reddish or yellowish globular mass with paired vessels coursing to and from the lesion, sometimes likened to a toy balloon in the fundus); may lead to hemorrhage, exudates, retinal detachment

Encephalofacial angiomatosis (Sturge-Weber syndrome; see Chapter 605.3)
Lid and conjunctival involvement of facial nevus flammeus; choroidal hemangioma; dilated and tortuous retinal vessels; glaucoma, congenital or later in infancy or childhood (related to possible angle anomalies, vascular lesion, or hypersecretion); visual field defects associated with CNS lesions; hemianopia in some cases)

Angiomatosis of mid-brain and retina (Wyburn-Mason syndrome)
Extensive vascular malformations involving principally the midbrain and eye; angiomatosis of the retina; vessels dilated and tortuous; angiomatosis affecting optic nerve and orbit

Neurocutaneous Syndromes

Ataxia-telangiectasia (Louis-Barr syndrome; see Chapter 606.1)
Telangiectasias of bulbar conjunctivae, usually by the age of 4–6 yr; apraxic disorder of conjugate eye movements; horizontal and vertical gaze performed in halting dyssynergic fashion; difficulty in maintaining eccentric gaze; sometimes convergence defect; nystagmus

Sjögren-Larsson syndrome (see Chapter 664)
Chorioretinal lesions; discrete defects in retinal pigment epithelium of unknown cause; circumscribed symmetric lesions of varying size in and about the macula in approximately 25% of cases

Incontinentia pigmenti (Bloch-Sulzberger syndrome; see Chapter 658)
Intraocular retrolental masses ("pseudogliomas") and membranes, apparently secondary to an underlying retinal vascular disorder characterized by aneurysmal dilatation, abnormal arteriovenous connections, and vasoproliferative changes; sometimes intraocular hemorrhage and inflammation; microphthalmos; corneal opacities; cataracts; optic atrophy

Linear nevus sebaceus of Jadassohn (see Chapter 658)
Coloboma of the eyelids, iris, and fundus; corectopia; epibulbar lipodermoids; orbital teratomas; proptosis; aberrant lacrimal gland; corneal vascularization; ocular motor palsies; nystagmus; defective vision

Xerodermic idiocy of de Sanctis and Cacchione (see Chapter 658)
Atrophy of eyelids; loss of cilia, ectropion, entropion, symblepharon, ankyloblepharon; drying and infection of conjunctiva; ulceration of cornea; iritis; photophobia

Klippel-Trenaunay-Weber syndrome (see Chapter 656)
Conjunctival telangiectasia; choroidal hemangioma; iris coloboma; heterochromia; glaucoma; strabismus

Special Neurobiothrophies

Subacute sclerosing panencephalitis (Dawson disease; Van Bogaert disease; see Chapter 240.1)
Focal retinitis (edema, hemorrhage, pigmentary changes), with chorioretinal scarring (usually macular or paramacular, usually bilateral)—may precede other neurologic manifestations; papilledema; optic atrophy; visual symptoms of retinal and optic nerve involvement; field defects of cerebral involvement; nystagmus; extraocular muscle palsies; ptosis

Subacute necrotizing encephalomyopathy (Leigh disease; see Chapter 607.2)
Abnormal eye movements (bizarre rolling eye movements, disconjugate eye movements, horizontal and vertical nystagmus, saccadic ocular movements); extraocular muscle palsies (sometimes complete external ophthalmoplegia); blepharoptosis; progressive optic atrophy and vision loss; sometimes retinal changes (diminished macular reflex); afferent and efferent pupil defects

Hepatolenticular degeneration (Wilson's disease; see Chapter 357.2)
Kayser-Fleischer ring of cornea (copper deposition in periphery of Descemet's membrane, particularly in deepest zone adjacent to endothelium, seen as granules of golden, greenish, grayish, or brown hue); Sonnenblumenkatarakt ("sunflower" cataract); occasionally ocular motor abnormalities (jerky oscillations of eyes, involuntary upward deviation of eyes, or paresis of upward gaze); accommodation sometimes affected; in some cases, optic neuritis secondary to penicillamine therapy

Trichopoliodystrophy (Menkes disease; kinky hair disease; see Chapter 607.3)
Decrease in retinal ganglion cells, thinning of retinal nerve fiber layer, and partial atrophy of optic nerve; progressive vision loss; abnormal ERG; microcysts of pigment epithelium of iris

Abetalipoproteinemia (acanthocytosis; Bassen-Kornzweig disease; see Chapter 83.3)
Pigmentary retinal degeneration with progressive impairment of visual function (pigment dispersion, arteriolar attenuation, disc pallor, impaired dark adaptation); cataracts, ptosis, and ocular motor abnormalities; in some cases, progressive exotropia, paresis of medial recti, and dissociated nystagmus on lateral gaze

Heredopathia atactica polyneuritiformis (Refsum syndrome; phytanic acid α-hydrolase deficiency; see Chapters 83.2 and 620.5)
Pigmentary retinal degeneration (pigmentary clumping, arteriolar attenuation, optic atrophy, progressive impairment of night vision and visual field); ERG abnormal; sometimes vitreous opacities, cataracts, cornea guttata, miosis; ophthalmoparesis; nystagmus

Familial dysautonomia (Riley-Day syndrome; see Chapter 622.1)
Depressed or absent corneal sensation, with corneal ulceration and scarring common; defective lacrimation; tortuosity of retinal vessels; tonic pupil in some cases; myopia and exotropia common

Congenital familial sensory neuropathy with anhidrosis (Pinsky-DiGeorge syndrome; see Chapter 622.2)
Defective corneal sensation, with defective lacrimation; corneal ulceration and scarring may result

Disorders of Connective Tissues, Bones, and Joints

Arachnodactyly (Marfan syndrome; see Chapter 705)
Ectopia lentis (lens dislocation, usually upward) and iridodonesis (tremulous iris); microphakia, spherophakia; cataract; myopia; glaucoma; retinal changes; degeneration, detachment

Cutis hyperelastica (Ehlers-Danlos syndrome; see Chapter 665)
Epicanthus; blue sclera; keratoconus; subluxation of lens; retinal detachment

Pseudoxanthoma elasticum (see Chapter 665)
Angioid streaks (breaks in Bruch's membrane appearing as dark lines in the fundus radiating from the disc); tendency to retinal hemorrhage

Osteogenesis imperfecta (see Chapter 704)
Blue sclera; prominent eyes; in some cases, megalocornea, keratoconus, corneal opacities

Polyostotic fibrous dysplasia (McCune-Albright syndrome; see Chapter 572.6)
Thickening of bones of orbit

Osteopetrosis (Albers-Schönberg disease; "marble bones"; see Chapter 702)
Vision loss and extraocular muscle palsies, caused by bony overgrowth of cranial foramina; in some cases, retinal degeneration, optic atrophy

Chondrodystrophia calcificans congenita (Conradi syndrome; see Chapter 664)
Cataract, optic atropy; hypertelorism

Spondyloepiphyseal dysplasia congenita (see Chapter 698)
Myopia; retinal detachment; cataract; buphthalmos

Spondyloepiphyseal dysplasia variants (see Chapter 698)
Punctate corneal dystrophy without impairment of vision

Hereditary onycho-osteodysplasia (nail-patella syndrome)
Dark "cloverleaf" pigmentation of iris; cataract; microphakia; microcornea; keratoconus; ptosis

Progressive arthro-ophthalmopathy (Stickler's syndrome)
Pain and stiffness of joints with bony enlargement; kyphosis, cleft palate; Pierre Robin anomaly; deafness; progressive myopia; retinal detachment; glaucoma

Dermatologic Disorders

Focal dermal hypoplasia (Goltz syndrome; see Chapter 654)
Nystagmus; strabismus; microphthalmos; coloboma

Hypohidrotic (anhidrotic) ectodermal dysplasia (see Chapter 654)
Deficiency of tears, leading to keratopathy, photophobia; stenosis of the lacrimal puncta; cataracts; lashes and brows sparse

Dyskeratosis congenita (see Chapter 654)
Bullous conjunctivitis, with minimal scarring of cornea; chronic blepharitis; loss of lashes and ectropion; keratinization of lacrimal puncta

Ichthyosis (see Chapter 664)
Conjunctivitis, ectropion, and corneal erosions in lamellar and sex-linked forms; cataracts in congenital and vulgaris forms

Table continued on following page

Basal cell nevus syndrome (see Chapter 676)
  Prominent supraorbital ridges; hypertelorism or dystopia canthorum; cataracts; coloboma; vision defects; strabismus
Juvenile xanthogranuloma (nevoxanthoendothelioma; see Chapter 676)
  Xanthogranuloma in ocular tissues, as infiltrates in orbit, iris, episclera, ciliary body; presenting signs may be proptosis, heterochromia, spontaneous hyphema, uveitis, glaucoma
Poikiloderma congenitale (Rothmund-Thomson syndrome; see Chapter 662)
  Sparse eyebrows and eyelashes; cataracts (onset 2–7 yr); corneal dystrophy
Bloom syndrome (see Chapter 662)
  Conjunctivitis; conjunctival telangiectasias; drusen at posterior pole of fundus

Syndromes of Multiple Developmental Abnormalities

Cornelia de Lange syndrome
  Microbrachycephaly, short neck, low hairline, anteverted nares, micrognathism, and low-set ears; physical and mental retardation; limb defects including micromelia-phocomelia, oligodactyly, polydactyly; cardiac and urogenital anomalies; synophrys (confluent eyebrows) and long, curly eyelashes; ptosis; epicanthus; microphthalmos with eccentric pupils; corneal opacities; optic atrophy; strabismus
Fraser syndrome
  Facial, genitourinary, skeletal anomalies (including lateral cleft of nostril, ear deformity, renal agenesis, hydronephrosis, hypospadias, cryptorchidism, syndactyly); cerebral defects, meningoencephalocele;cryptophthalmos (eye hidden, fused lids—absence of palpebral fissure), sometimes with symblepharon (adhesion of lid to globe); microphthalmos in some cases; flat supraorbital ridge
Rieger syndrome
  Various dental and limb anomalies; occasionally intellectual retardation, muscular dystrophy, and myotonic dystrophy; dysplasia of anterior segment of the eye; posterior embryotoxon (prominence and anterior displacement of Schwalbe's line), often with bands of iris tissue attached (Axenfeld syndrome); iris hypoplasia; glaucoma; cataracts; ectopia lentis; colobomas; micro- or megalocornea; strabismus; ptosis; optic atrophy
Peters syndrome
  Skeletal anomalies; developmental defects of the gastrointestinal tract and CNS; hydrocephalus and mental retardation; central defect of Descemet's membrane, with central corneal leukoma, shallow anterior chamber, peripheral anterior synechia; cataracts
Lenz syndrome
  Microcephaly, mental retardation; short stature, digital anomalies, and dental defects; colobomatous microphthalmos; blepharoptosis; nystagmus; strabismus
Meckel syndrome (Meckel-Gruber syndrome)
  Microcephaly, occipital encephalocele, or anencephaly; polycystic kidneys; polydactyly; congenital heart disease; genital abnormalities; microphthalmos, anophthalmos, cryptophthalmos; sclerocornea; partial aniridia; cataract; retinal dysplasia; optic nerve hypoplasia
Otopalatodigital syndrome (Rubinstein-Taybi syndrome)
Intellectual and growth retardation; abnormally broad thumbs and broad great toes; characteristic facies with hypoplasia of maxilla and mandible, beaked nose, posterior rotation of ears; hypertrichosis; cryptorchidism; cardiac and renal anomalies; hypertelorism, with epicanthus, ptosis, and antimongoloid slant of palpebral fissures; cataract, colobomas, strabismus
Seckel syndrome
  Growth retardation with small head circumference and characteristic face, narrow with beaklike nose ("bird head"); micrognathia and apparent prominence of maxilla; sometimes musculoskeletal and genitourinary anomalies; hypertelorism, with antimongoloid slant of palpebral fissures, prominent eyes; strabismus
Freeman-Sheldon syndrome
  Syndrome characterized by masklike face with small pursed mouth, "whistling face"; ulnar deviation of the hand and fingers; talipes equinovarus; deep-set eyes; epicanthus, blepharophimosis, ptosis; strabismus
Aicardi's syndrome
  Agenesis of the corpus callosum, with cortical heterotopia; seizures; mental retardation; costovertebral anomalies; multiple discrete chorioretinal defects of varying size; sometimes microphthalmos
Wildervanck syndrome
  Association of the Klippel-Feil malformation with congenital deafness and Duane syndrome; unilateral or bilateral (congenital defect in abduction with retraction of the globe or attempted adduction of the affected eye); epibulbar dermoid cysts
Falls-Kertesz syndrome
  Pterygium coli; later onset of lymphedema of lower extremities; distichiasis of all four lids; partial ectropion of lower lids
Kartagener syndrome (see Chapter 417)
  Pigmentary retinal disorder; cataracts

Miscellaneous Multisystem Disorders

Oculocerebrorenal syndrome (Lowe syndrome; see Chapter 537.4)
  Congenital cataracts in affected males; fine lens opacities in carrier females; glaucoma; rarely, microphthalmos
Cerebrohepatorenal syndrome (Zellweger syndrome) (congenital adrenoleukodystrophy)
  Profound hypotonia, growth retardation, and failure to thrive; hepatomegaly, jaundice, hypoprothrombinemia; renal cortical cysts; characteristic facies; flat profile; accumulation of iron in various organs; mild hypertelorism, flat supraorbital ridges, and epicanthal folds, cataracts; glaucoma (also, nonglaucomatous corneal haze); vitreous opacities; optic nerve hypoplasia; retinal pigmentary disorder (fundi generally hypopigmented with fine to coarse spotty pigmentation, most marked peripherally)
Laurence-Moon-Biedl syndrome (see Chapter 43)
  Pleomorphic pigmentary retinal degeneration (retinitis pigmentosa type, with prominent macular involvement in some cases), with progressive vision impairment
Prader-Willi syndrome
  Hypotonia, hypomentia, hypogonadism, and obesity, with tendency to diabetes mellitus; strabismus
Cockayne syndrome (see Chapter 662)
  Pigmentary retinal degeneration; optic atrophy, cataracts; photophobia
Werner syndrome
  Syndrome of premature aging; in the 2nd decade, with cessation of growth, graying of the hair, alopecia, scleroderma-like changes of the skin, atherosclerosis, and diabetes mellitus; hypogonadism, increased risk of neoplasia; cataracts, juvenile onset; pigmentary retinal degeneration ("retinitis pigmentosa"); macular degeneration; glaucoma
Asphyxiating thoracic dysplasia (Jeune's syndrome; see Chapter 424.2)
  Pigmentary retinal degeneration, with progressive vision impairment in some cases
Alstrom's disease
  Nerve deafness, diabetes mellitus, and obesity in childhood; pigmentary retinal degeneration; cataracts
Renal-retinal dystrophy
  Interstitial nephritis; progressive pigmentary retinal degeneration, with attenuation of arterioles, reduced ERG, optic atrophy, and loss of vision
Usher's syndrome
  Nerve deafness; pigmentary retinal degeneration ("retinitis pigmentosa"); cataracts
  Norrie's disease
A syndrome of retinal malformation, mental retardation, and deafness; congenital retinal pseudoglioma; persistent hyperplastic primary vitreous, with vision loss; degenerative changes with phthisis bulbi; corneal opacities; cataracts

Congenital Infection Syndromes

Congenital rubella (see Chapter 241)
  Ophthalmic sequelae, both teratogenic and inflammatory; bilateral or unilateral effects; persistence of virus in the eye for months or years; microphthalmia; cataract (usually a dense, pearly, nuclear opacity with relatively clearer cortical rim); iris hypoplasia, atrophy synechiae (pupils often difficult to dilate); congenital glaucoma; transient nonglaucomatous corneal clouding in a newborn; retinopathy (pigmentary mottling "salt and pepper," focal or generalized, without loss of function); acute maculopathy (submacular neovascularization) as a delayed complication later in childhood in some cases, with attendant vision impairment; optic atrophy; vision defects and ocular motor abnormalities (nystagmus, strabismus) related not only to ocular involvement but also to effects of encephalomyelitis
Congenital cytomegalovirus infection (see Chapter 248)
  Chorioretinitis (single or multifocal atrophic and pigmented fundus lesions, more often peripheral than macular—sometimes perivascular retinal exudates and hemorrhages); anterior uveitis, conjunctivitis, and corneal clouding; optic atrophy; optic nerve hypoplasia; coloboma; microphthalmos; vision defects with strabismus, nystagmus
Congenital toxoplasmosis (see Chapter 280)
  Retinochoroditis (retinitis, with secondary choroiditis; often with exudate into vitreous in early stages, resulting in single or multifocal atrophic and pigmented scars); often large macular lesions; satellite lesions and recurrent inflammation common in later years caused by persistence of organism in eye; vision loss, optic atrophy, retinal detachment, cataract, and glaucoma common; attendant oculomotor abnormalities (strabismus, nystagmus) attributed to ocular and/or CNS involvement; congenital anomalies of eye (e.g., microphthalmos)
Congenital syphilis (see Chapter 215)
Perivascular infiltration by *T. pallidum*, with inflammation in the cornea, uvea, retina, and optic nerve; persistence of the organism in the eye for years; interstitial keratitis, usually appearing after age 5 or 6 yr (iridocyclitis and intense photophobia in acute phase, vascularization and corneal opacification later, with decreased vision); retinopathy ("salt and pepper" pigmentary changes, frequently with arteriolar attenuation and disc pallor); retinal periphlebitis, sometimes with vascular occlusion; exudative uveitis in some cases; phthisis may result; disc edema; optic atrophy

**To be differentiated from these forms of albinism is the Chédiak-Higashi syndrome in which the defect is in the morphology of the melanosomes, not in the formation of melanin. Ocular signs include hypopigmentation of iris and fundus, photophobia, nystagmus, and papilledema with lymphocytic infiltration of the optic nerve.*
ERG = electroretinogram; VER = visual evoked response; CNS = central nervous system.

of the lens is often downward and forward, and the lens tends to be small and round.

Ectopia lentis is also associated occasionally with other conditions, including Ehler-Danlos, Sturge-Weber, Crouzon's, or Klippel-Feil syndrome; oxycephaly; and mandibulofacial dysostosis. A syndrome of dominantly inherited blepharoptosis, high myopia, and ectopia lentis has also been described.

Treatment and Prognosis. Displacement of the lens often results only in optical problems; in other cases, however, more serious complications may develop, such as glaucoma, uveitis, retinal detachment, or cataract. Management must be individualized according to the type of displacement, its etiology, and the presence of any complicating ocular or systemic conditions. For many patients, optical correction by spectacles or contact lenses can be provided. Manipulation of the iris diaphragm with mydriatic or miotic drops may sometimes help improve vision. In selected cases, the best treatment is surgical removal of the lens. In many children, treatment of any associated amblyopia must be instituted early. In addition, for children with ectopia lentis, safety precautions should be taken to prevent injury to the eye.

MICROSPHEROPHAKIA. The term *microspherophakia* refers to a small, round lens that may occur as an isolated anomaly (probably autosomal recessive) or in association with other ocular abnormalities, such as ectopia lentis, myopia, or retinal detachment (possibly autosomal dominant). Microspherophakia may also occur in association with various systemic disorders, including Marfan syndrome, Marchesani syndrome, Alport syndrome, mandibulofacial dysostosis, and Klinefelter's syndrome.

ANTERIOR LENTICONUS. Anterior lenticonus is a rare bilateral condition in which the anterior surface of the lens bulges centrally. It may be accompanied by lens opacities or other eye anomalies and is a prominent feature of Alport syndrome. The increased curvature of the central area may cause high myopia.

POSTERIOR LENTICONUS. Posterior lenticonus, which occurs more commonly than anterior lenticonus, is characterized by a circumscribed round or oval bulge of the posterior lens capsule and cortex, restricted to the 2 to 7 mm central (axial) region. In the early stages, by the red reflex test, this may look like an oil droplet. It occurs in infants and young children, and it tends to increase with age. Usually the lens material within and surrounding the capsular bulge eventually becomes opacified. Posterior lenticonus usually occurs as an isolated ocular anomaly. It is generally unilateral but may be bilateral. It is believed to be sporadic, although autosomal dominant heredity has been suggested in some cases. Infants or children with posterior lenticonus may require lens surgery for progressive cataract, optical correction, amblyopia treatment, and care of secondary conditions, such as strabismus.

Bateman JB, Spence MA, Marazita ML, et al: Genetic linkage analysis of autosomal dominant congenital cataracts. Am J Ophthalmol 101:218, 1986.
Buckley EG: Pediatric cataracts and lens anomalies. *In*: Nelson LB (ed): Harley's Pediatric Ophthalmology, 4th ed. Philadelphia, WB Saunders, 1998.
Casper DS, Simon JW, Nelson LB, et al: Familial simple ectopia lentis. A case study. J Pediatr Ophthalmol Strabismus 22:227, 1985.
Cheng KP, Hiles DA, Biglan AW, et al: Visual results after early surgical treatment of unilateral congenital cataracts. Ophthalmology 98:903, 1991.
Chrousos GA, Parks MM, O'Neill JF: Incidence of chronic glaucoma, retinal detachment and secondary membrane surgery in pediatric aphakic patients. Ophthalmology 91:1238, 1984.
Chugh KS, Sakhuja V, Agarwal A, et al: Hereditary nephritis (Alport's syndrome)—clinical profile and inheritance in 28 kindreds. Nephrol Dial Transplant 8:690, 1993.
Cotlier E: Congenital varicella cataract. Am J Ophthalmol 86:627, 1978.
Cross HE, Jensen AD: Ocular manifestations in the Marfan syndrome and homocystinuria. Am J Ophthalmol 75:405, 1973.
Cumming RG, Mitchell P, Leeder SR: Use of inhaled corticosteroids and the risk of cataracts. N Engl J Med 337:8, 1997.
Forman AR, Loreto JA, Tina LU: Reversibility of corticosteroid-associated cataracts in children with the nephrotic syndrome. Am J Ophthalmol 84:75, 1977.
Gelbart SS, Hoyt CS, Jastrebski G, et al: Long-term visual results in bilateral congenital cataracts. Am J Ophthalmol 93:615, 1982.
Gillum WN, Anderson RL: Dominantly inherited blepharoptosis, high myopia, and ectopia lentis. Arch Ophthalmol 100:282, 1982.
Goldberg MF: Clinical manifestations of ectopia lentis et pupillae in 16 patients. Ophthalmology 95:1080, 1988.
Hiles DA: Intraocular lens implantation in children with monocular cataracts, 1974–1983. Ophthalmology 91:1231, 1984.
Jaafar MS, Robb RM: Congenital anterior polar cataract: A review of 63 cases. Ophthalmology 91:249, 1984.
Khalil M, Saheb N: Posterior lenticonus. Ophthalmology 91:1429, 1984.
Kirkam TH: Mandibulofacial dysostosis with ectopia lentis. Am J Ophthalmol 70:947, 1979.
Levin AV, Edmonds SA, Nelson LB, et al: Extended-wear contact lenses for the treatment of pediatric aphakia. Ophthalmology 95:1107, 1988.
Nelson LB: Diagnosis and management of congenital and developmental cataracts. Semin Ophthalmol 5:154, 1990.
Nelson LB, Calhoun JH, Simon JW, et al: Progression of congenital anterior polar cataracts in childhood. Arch Ophthalmol 103:1842, 1985.
Nelson LB, Maumenee IH: Ectopia lentis. Surv Ophthalmol 27:143, 1982.
Olitsky SE, Nelson LB: Intraocular lens implantation in children. *In*: Wilson RP (ed): Year Book of Ophthalmology, St. Louis, CV Mosby 1997, p 227.
Parks MM: Visual results in aphakic children. Am J Ophthalmol 94:441, 1982.
Rasoby R, Ben Ezra D: Congenital and traumatic cataracts: The effect on ocular axial length. Arch Ophthalmol 106:1066, 1988.
Simon JW, Mehta N, Simmons ST, et al: Glaucoma after pediatric lensectomy/vitrectomy. Ophthalmology 98:670, 1991.
Wets B, Milot JA, Polomeno RC, et al: Cataracts and ketotic hypoglycemia. Ophthalmology 89:999, 1982.

CHAPTER 636
Disorders of the Uveal Tract

UVEITIS (IRITIS, CYCLITIS, CHORIORETINITIS). The uveal tract (the inner vascular coat of the eye, consisting of the iris, ciliary body, and choroid) is subject to inflammatory involvement in a number of systemic diseases, both infectious and noninfectious, and in response to exogenous factors, including trauma and toxic agents (Table 636–1). Inflammation may affect any one portion of the uveal tract preferentially or all parts together.

Iritis may occur alone or in conjunction with inflammation of the ciliary body as iridocyclitis or in association with pars planitis. Pain, photophobia, and lacrimation are the characteristic symptoms of acute anterior uveitis, but the inflammation may develop insidiously without disturbing symptoms. Signs of anterior uveitis include conjunctival hyperemia, particularly in the perilimbal region (ciliary flush) and cells and protein ("flare") in the aqueous humor (Fig. 636–1). Inflammatory deposits on the posterior surface of the cornea (keratic precipitates [KP]) and congestion of the iris may also be seen. More chronic cases may show degenerative changes of the cornea (band keratopathy), lenticular opacities (cataract), development of glaucoma, and impairment of vision. The cause of anterior uveitis is often obscure; primary considerations in children are rheumatoid disease, particularly pauciarticular rheumatoid arthritis, Kawasaki disease, Reiter syndrome, and sarcoidosis. Iritis may be secondary to corneal disease, such as herpetic keratitis or a bacterial or fungal corneal ulcer, or to a corneal abrasion or foreign body. Traumatic iritis and iridocyclitis are especially common in children.

Iridocyclitis that occurs in children with arthritis deserves special mention. Unlike most forms of anterior uveitis, it rarely creates pain, photophobia, or conjunctival hyperemia. Loss of vision may not be noticed until severe and irreversible damage has occurred. Because of the lack of symptoms and the high incidence of uveitis in these children, routine periodic screening is necessary.

Choroiditis, inflammation of the posterior portion of the uveal

TABLE 636–1 Uveitis in Childhood

Anterior Uveitis

Juvenile rheumatoid arthritis (pauciarticular)
Sarcoidosis
Trauma
Tuberculosis
Kawasaki disease
Ulcerative colitis
Reiter syndrome
Spirochetal (syphilis, leptospiral)
Heterochromic iridocyclitis (Fuchs')
Viral (herpes simplex, herpes zoster)
Ankylosing spondylitis
Stevens-Johnson syndrome
Idiopathic
Drugs

Posterior Uveitis (choroiditis—may involve retina)

Toxoplasmosis
Parasites (toxocariasis)
Sarcoidosis
Tuberculosis
Viral (rubella, herpes simplex, human immunodeficiency virus, cytomegalovirus)
Subacute sclerosing panencephalitis
Idiopathic

Anterior and/or Posterior Uveitis

Sympathetic ophthalmia (trauma to other eye)
Vogt-Koyanagi-Harada syndrome (uveo-otocutaneous syndrome: poliosis, vitiligo, deafness, tinnitus, uveitis, aseptic meningitis, retinitis)
Behçet's syndrome
Lyme disease

tract, invariably also involves the retina; when both are obviously affected, the condition is termed *chorioretinitis*. The causes of posterior uveitis are numerous; the more common are toxoplasmosis, histoplasmosis, cytomegalic inclusion disease, sarcoidosis, syphilis, tuberculosis, and toxocariasis (Fig. 636–2). Depending on the etiology, the inflammatory signs may be diffuse or focal. Vitreous reaction often occurs as well. With many types, the result is atrophic chorioretinal scarring demarcated by pigmentation, often with visual impairment. Secondary complications include retinal detachment, glaucoma, or phthisis.

Panophthalmitis is inflammation involving all parts of the eye. It is frequently suppurative, most often as a result of a perforating injury or of septicemia. It produces severe pain, marked congestion of the eye, inflammation of the adjacent orbital tissues and eyelids, and loss of vision. In many cases, the eye is lost despite intensive treatment of the infection and inflammation. Enucleation of the eye or evisceration of the orbit may be necessary.

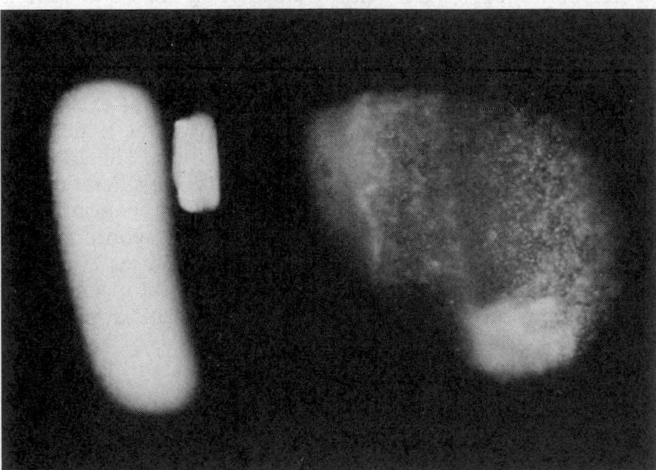

Figure 636–1 Cell and flare in the anterior chamber. The flare represents protein leakage. (Courtesy of Peter Buch, C.R.A.)

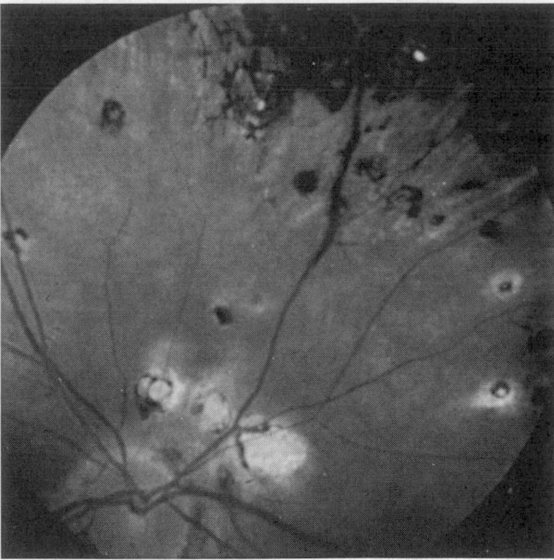

Figure 636–2 Focal atrophic and pigmented scars of chorioretinitis.

Sympathetic ophthalmia is a rare type of inflammatory response that affects both eyes after perforating injury of one eye. It may occur weeks, months, or even years after the injury. A hypersensitivity phenomenon is the most probable cause. Loss of vision in the uninjured (sympathizing) eye may result. Removal of the injured eye prevents the development of sympathetic ophthalmia but does not stop the progression of the disease once it has occurred. Therefore, early enucleation should be considered if there is no hope of visual recovery after a severe injury.

TREATMENT. The various forms of intraocular inflammation are treated according to their etiologic factors. When infection is proved or suspected, appropriate systemic antimicrobial therapy is used. In some cases, subconjunctival or intravitreal injection of antibiotics is indicated. Prevention or reduction of inflammatory sequelae is also important; in selected cases, topical or systemic corticosteroids are used. Systemic immunosuppressive agents may also be required. Cycloplegic agents, particularly atropine, are also used to reduce inflammation and to prevent adhesion of the iris to the lens, especially in anterior uveitis.

Albert DM, Diaz-Rohena R: A historical review of sympathetic ophthalmia and its epidemiology. Surv Ophthalmol 34:1, 1989.

Cochereau-Massin I, LeHoang P, Lautier-Frau M, et al: Efficacy and tolerance of intravitreal ganciclovir in cytomegalovirus retinitis in acquired immune deficiency syndrome. Ophthalmology 98:1348, 1991.

Contreras F, Pereda J: Congenital syphilis of the eye with lens involvement. Arch Ophthalmol 96:1052, 1978.

Giannini EH, Brewer EJ, Kuzmina N, et al: Methotrexate in resistant juvenile rheumatoid arthritis: Results of the U.S.A.–U.S.S.R. double-blind, placebo-controlled trial. N Engl J Med 326:1043, 1992.

Giles CL: Uveitis in children. *In:* Nelson LB (ed): Harley's Pediatric Ophthalmology, 4th ed. Philadelphia, WB Saunders, 1998.

Guidelines for ophthalmic examinations in children with juvenile rheumatoid arthritis: Section on rheumatology and section on ophthalmology. Pediatrics 92:295, 1993.

Hoover DL, Khan JA, Giangiacomo J: Pediatric ocular sarcoidosis. Surv Ophthalmol 30:215, 1986.

Kanski JJ: Juvenile arthritis and uveitis. Surv Ophthalmol 34:253, 1990.

Kimura SJ: Uveitis in children: Analysis of 274 cases. Trans Am Ophthalmol Soc 62:171, 1964.

Regillo CD, Shields CL, Shields JA, et al: Ocular tuberculosis. JAMA 266:1490, 1991.

Shields JA: Ocular toxocariasis: A review. Surv Ophthalmol 28:361, 1984.

Smith ME, Zimmerman LE, Harley RD: Ocular involvement in congenital cytomegalic inclusion disease. Arch Ophthalmol 76:696, 1966.

Stern GA, Romano PE: Congenital ocular toxoplasmosis: Possible occurrence in siblings. Arch Ophthalmol 96:615, 1978.
Wilkinson CP, Welch RB: Intraocular toxocara. Am J Ophthalmol 71:921, 1971.
Winterkorn JMS: Lyme disease: Neurologic and ophthalmologic manifestations. Surv Ophthalmol 35:191, 1990.

CHAPTER 637
Disorders of the Retina and Vitreous

RETINOPATHY OF PREMATURITY (ROP). This retinal vasculopathy occurs almost exclusively in preterm infants (see Chapter 93.2). It may be acute (early stages) or chronic (late stages). Clinical manifestations range from mild, usually transient changes of the peripheral retina to severe progressive vasoproliferation, scarring, and potentially blinding retinal detachment. ROP includes all stages of the disease and its sequelae. Retrolental fibroplasia (RLF), the previous name for this disease, described only the cicatricial stages.

Pathogenesis. Beginning at 16 wk of gestation, retinal angiogenesis normally proceeds from the optic disc to the periphery, reaching the outer rim of the retina (ora serrata) nasally at about 36 wk and extending temporally by approximately 40 wk. Injury to the process results in various pathologic and clinical changes. The first observation in the acute phase is cessation of vasculogenesis. Rather than a gradual transition from vascularized to avascular retina, there is an abrupt termination of the vessels, marked by a line in the retina. The line may then grow into a ridge composed of mesenchymal and endothelial cells. Cell division and differentiation may later resume, and vascularization of the retina may proceed. Alternatively, there may be progression to an abnormal proliferation of vessels out of the plane of the retina, into the vitreous, and over the surface of the retina. Cicatrization and traction on the retina may follow, leading to detachment.

The risk factors associated with ROP are not fully known, but prematurity and the associated retinal immaturity at birth represent the major factors. Hyperoxia is also a major factor, but other problems, such as respiratory distress, apnea, bradycardia, heart disease, infection, hypoxia, hypercarbia, acidosis, anemia, and the need for transfusion are thought by some to be contributory factors. Generally, the lower the birthweight and the sicker the infant, the greater is the risk for ROP.

The basic pathogenesis of ROP is still unknown. Exposure to the extrauterine environment including the necessarily high inspired oxygen concentrations produces cellular damage, perhaps mediated by free radicals. Later in the course of the disease, peripheral hypoxia develops and vascular endothelial growth factors are produced in the nonvascularized retina. These growth factors stimulate abnormal vasculogenesis, and neovascularization may occur. This may then lead to scarring and vision loss.

Classification. The currently used international classification of ROP describes the location, extent, and severity of the disease. To delineate location, the retina is divided into three concentric zones, centered on the optic disc. Zone I, the posterior or inner zone, extends twice the disc-macular distance, or 30 degrees in all directions from the optic disc. Zone II, the middle zone, extends from the outer edge of zone I to the ora serrata nasally and to the anatomic equator temporally. Zone III, the outer zone, is the residual crescent that extends from the outer border of zone II to the ora serrata temporally, this area of the retina being vascularized. The extent of involvement is described by the number of circumferential clock hours involved.

The phases and severity of the disease process are classified into five stages. Stage 1 is characterized by a demarcation line that separates vascularized from avascular retina (Fig. 637–1*A*). This line lies within the plane of the retina and appears relatively flat and white. Often noted is abnormal branching or arcading of the retinal vessels that lead into the line. Stage 2 is characterized by a ridge; the demarcation line has grown, acquiring height, width, and volume and extending up and out of the plane of the retina. It may change from white to pink. Vessels may leave the plane of the retina to enter the ridge. Stage 3 is characterized by the presence of a ridge and by the development of extraretinal fibrovascular tissue. Stage 4 is characterized by subtotal retinal detachment caused by traction from the proliferating tissue in the vitreous or on the retina. Stage 4 is subdivided into two phases: (1) subtotal retinal detachment not involving the macula and (2) subtotal retinal detachment involving the macula. Stage 5 is total retinal detachment.

When signs of posterior retinal vascular changes accompany the active stages of ROP, the term *plus disease* is used. Patients reaching the point of dilatation and tortuosity of the retinal vessels also frequently demonstrate the associated findings of engorgement of the iris, pupillary rigidity, and vitreous haze.

Clinical Manifestations and Prognosis. In more than 90% of at-risk infants, the course is one of spontaneous arrest and regression of the usually asymmetric disease process, with little or no

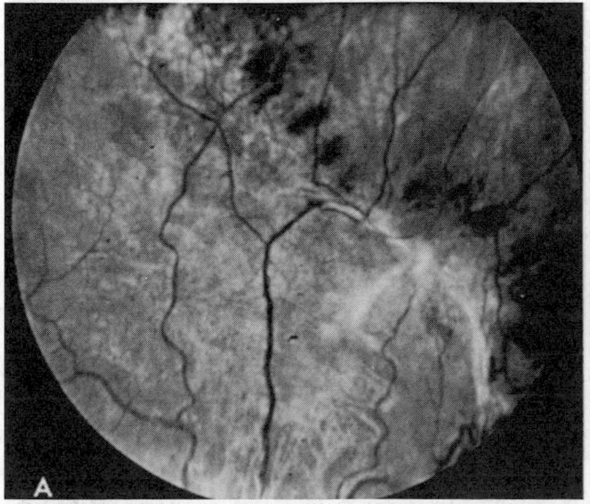

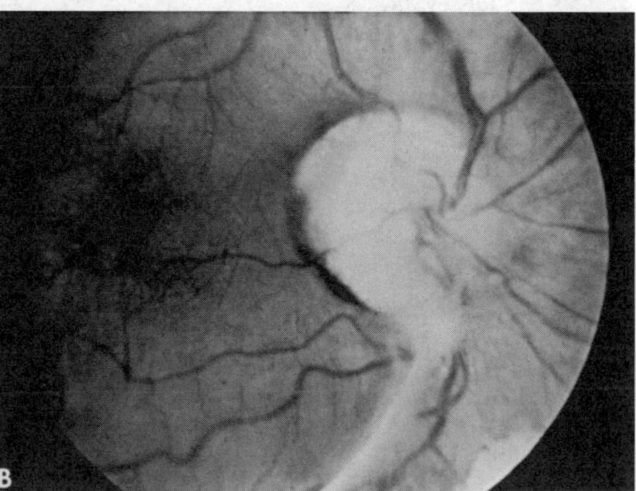

Figure 637–1 *A*, Developing retinopathy of prematurity in the temporal periphery. *B*, "Dragged disc" phenomenon in cicatricial retinopathy of prematurity.

residual effects or visual disability. Fewer than 10% of infants have progression toward severe disease, with significant extraretinal vasoproliferation, cicatrization, detachment of the retina, and impairment of vision.

Some children with arrested or regressed ROP are left with demarcation lines, undervascularization of the peripheral retina, or abnormal branching, tortuosity, or straightening of the retinal vessels. Some are left with retinal pigmentary changes, dragging of the retina (so-called dragged disc), ectopia of the macula, retinal folds, or retinal breaks (Fig. 637–1*B*). Others proceed to total retinal detachment, which commonly assumes a funnel-like configuration. The clinical picture is often that of a retrolental membrane, producing leukokoria (a white reflex in the pupil). Some patients develop cataract, glaucoma, and signs of inflammation. The end stage is often a painful blind eye or a degenerated phthisical eye. The spectrum of ROP also includes myopia, which is often progressive and of significant degree in infancy. The incidence of anisometropia, strabismus, amblyopia, and nystagmus may also be increased.

Diagnosis. Systematic ophthalmologic examination of infants at risk is recommended. Guidelines vary but generally include infants weighing less than 1,500 g at birth and those born before 28 wk gestational age. Infants born weighing over 1,500 g and having an unstable clinical course and thought to be at high risk should also be examined for ROP. The initial examination should be performed between 4 and 6 wk of chronological age or at 31–33 wk postconceptional age. ROP is diagnosed most often at 32–44 wk post conception. The examination can be stressful to fragile preterm infants, and the dilating drops can have untoward side effects; thus, discretion must be used in timing the eye examination, and infants must be carefully monitored during and after the examination. Follow-up is based on the initial findings and risk factors but is usually 2 wk or less.

Treatment. In selected cases, cryotherapy or laser photocoagulation of the avascular retina reduces the more severe complications of progressive ROP. Advances in vitreoretinal surgical techniques have led to limited success in reattaching the retina in infants with total retinal detachment (stage 5 ROP), but the visual results are often disappointing.

Prevention. Prevention of ROP ultimately depends on prevention of premature birth and its attendant problems. Despite advances in technology and the meticulous care given to high-risk infants in modern nurseries, ROP continues to occur. Oxygen alone is neither sufficient nor necessary to produce ROP, and no safe level of oxygen has yet been determined. Each infant must be treated with whatever is necessary to sustain life and neurologic function. Some investigators have suggested the use of supplemental vitamin E for its antioxidant properties in infants at risk for ROP. Its efficacy has not been proved; at certain dosage levels, it may produce untoward side effects (see Chapter 93.2).

PERSISTENT HYPERPLASTIC PRIMARY VITREOUS (PHPV). PHPV includes a spectrum of manifestations caused by the persistence of various portions of the fetal hyaloid vascular system and associated fibrovascular tissue.

During development of the eye, the hyaloid artery extends from the optic disc to the posterior aspect of the lens; it sends branches into the vitreous and ramifies to form the posterior portion of the vascular capsule of the lens. The posterior portion of the hyaloid system normally regresses by the 7th fetal mo and the anterior portion by the 8th fetal mo. Small remnants of the system, such as a tuft of tissue at the disc (Bergmeister's papilla) or a tag of tissue on the posterior capsule of the lens (Mittendorf's dot), are common findings in healthy persons. More extensive remnants and associated complications constitute PHPV. Two major forms are described, anterior PHPV and posterior PHPV. Variability is great, and mixed or intermediate forms occur.

The usual *clinical manifestation* of anterior PHPV is the presence of a vascularized plaque of tissue on the back surface of the lens in an eye that is microphthalmic or slightly smaller than normal. The condition is usually unilateral and may occur in infants with no other abnormalities and no history of prematurity. The fibrovascular tissue tends to undergo gradual contracture. The ciliary processes become elongated, and the anterior chamber may become shallow. The lens usually is smaller than normal and may be clear but often becomes cataractous and may swell or absorb fluid. Large or anomalous vessels of the iris may be present. The anterior chamber angle may have abnormalities. In time, the cornea may become cloudy.

Anterior PHPV is usually noted in the 1st wk or mo of life. The most frequent presenting signs are leukokoria (white pupillary reflex), strabismus, and nystagmus. The course is usually progressive and the outcome poor. Major complications are spontaneous intraocular hemorrhage, swelling of the lens caused by rupture of the posterior capsule, and glaucoma. The eye may eventually deteriorate.

Surgery is performed in an effort to prevent complications,

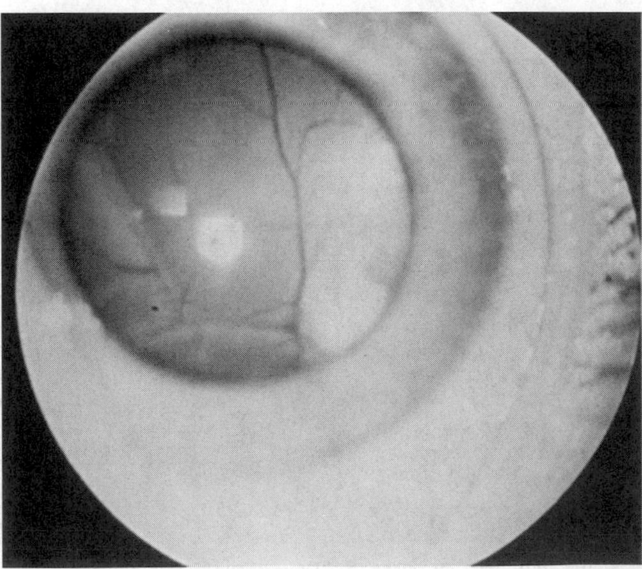

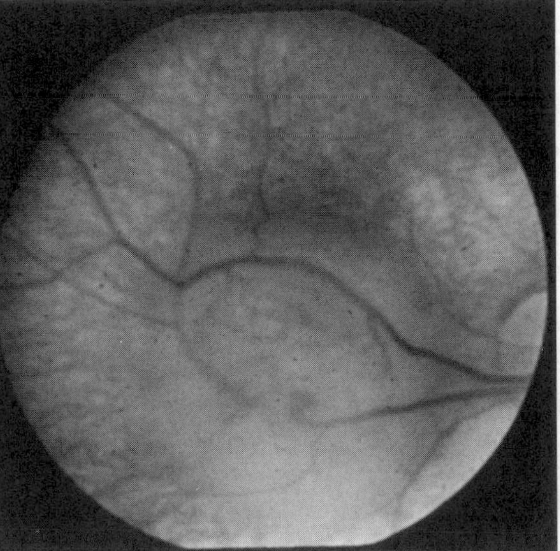

Figure 637–2 Retinoblastoma.

to preserve the eye and a reasonably good cosmetic appearance, and, in some cases, to salvage vision. Surgical *treatment* usually involves aspirating the lens and excising the abnormal tissue. If useful vision is to be attained, refractive correction and aggressive amblyopia therapy are required. In some cases, the affected eye is enucleated, because distinguishing between this white mass and retinoblastoma can be difficult. Ultrasonography and CT are valuable diagnostic aids.

The spectrum of posterior PHPV includes fibroglial veils around the disc and macula, vitreous membranes and stalks containing hyaloid artery remnants projecting from the disc, and meridional retinal folds. Traction detachment of the retina may occur. Vision may be impaired, but the eye is usually retained.

RETINOBLASTOMA (also see Chapter 508). Retinoblastoma (Fig. 637–2) is the most common primary malignant intraocular tumor of childhood. It occurs in approximately 1/18,000 infants; 250–300 new cases are diagnosed in the United States annually. Hereditary and nonhereditary patterns of transmission occur; there is no sex or race predilection. The hereditary form is usually bilateral and multifocal, whereas the nonhereditary form is generally unilateral and unifocal. Fifteen per cent of unilateral cases are hereditary. Bilateral cases often present earlier than unilateral cases. Unilateral tumors are often large by the time they are discovered. The average age at diagnosis is 15 mo for bilateral cases, compared with 25 mo for unilateral cases. It is unusual for a child to present with a retinoblastoma after 2 yr. Rarely, the tumor is discovered at birth, during adolescence, or even in adulthood.

The *clinical manifestations* of retinoblastoma vary, depending on the stage at which the tumor is detected. The initial sign in the majority of patients is a white pupillary reflex (leukokoria). Leukokoria results because of the reflection of light off the white tumor. The second most frequent initial sign of retinoblastoma is strabismus. Less frequent presenting signs include pseudohypopyon (tumor cells layered inferiorly in front of the iris), caused by tumor seeding in the anterior chamber of the eye; hyphema (blood layered in front of the iris), secondary to iris neovascularization; vitreous hemorrhage; or signs of orbital cellulitis. On examination, the tumor appears as a white mass, sometimes small and relatively flat, sometimes large and protuberant. It may appear nodular. Vitreous haze or tumor seeding may be evident.

The retinoblastoma gene is a recessive suppressor gene located on chromosome 13 at the 13q14 region. Because of the hereditary nature of retinoblastoma, family members of affected children should undergo a complete ophthalmologic examination and genetic counseling. Newborn siblings and children of affected patients should be referred to an ophthalmologist shortly after birth, when the peripheral retina can be evaluated without the need for an examination under anesthesia.

The *diagnosis* of a retinoblastoma is made by direct observation by an experienced ophthalmologist. Ancillary testing such as CT scanning or ultrasonography may help to confirm the diagnosis and demonstrate calcification within the mass. A definitive diagnosis occasionally cannot be made, and removal of the eye must be considered to avoid the possibility of lethal metastasis of the tumor. Because a biopsy can lead to spread of the tumor, histologic confirmation before enucleation is not possible in most cases. Therefore, removal of a blind eye in which the diagnosis of retinoblastoma is a consideration is appropriate.

Treatment varies, depending on the size and location of the tumor as well as whether it is unilateral or bilateral. Advanced tumors may be treated by enucleation. Other treatment modalities include the use of external beam irridation, radiation plaque therapy, laser or cryotherapy, and chemotherapy.

The *prognosis* for children with retinoblastoma depends on the size and extension of the tumor. When confined to the eye, most tumors can be cured. The prognosis for long-term survival is poor when the tumor has extended into the orbit or along the optic nerve.

RETINITIS PIGMENTOSA. This progressive retinal degeneration is characterized by pigmentary changes, arteriolar attenuation, usually some degree of optic atrophy, and progressive impairment of visual function. Dispersion and aggregation of the retinal pigment produce various ophthalmoscopically visible changes, ranging from granularity or mottling of the retinal pigment pattern to distinctive focal pigment aggregates with the configuration of bone spicules (Fig. 637–3). Other ocular findings include subcapsular cataract, glaucoma, and keratoconus.

Impairment of night vision or dark adaptation is often the first *clinical manifestation*. Progressive loss of peripheral vision, often in the form of an expanding ring scotoma or concentric contraction of the field, is usual. There may be loss of central vision. Retinal function, as measured by electroretinography (ERG), is characteristically reduced. Manifestations commonly begin in childhood. The disorder may be autosomal recessive, autosomal dominant, or sex linked.

A special form of retinitis pigmentosa is **Leber congenital retinal amaurosis**, in which the retinal changes tend to be pleomorphic, with various degrees of pigment disorder, anteriolar attenuation, and optic atrophy. The retina may appear normal during infancy. Vision impairment is usually evident soon after birth, and the ERG findings are abnormal early.

Clinically similar, secondary pigmentary retinal degenerations to be differentiated from retinitis pigmentosa occur in a wide variety of metabolic diseases, neurodegenerative processes, and multifaceted syndromes. Examples include the progressive retinal changes of the mucopolysaccharidoses (particularly the syndromes of Hurler, Hunter, Scheie, and Sanfilippo) and certain of the late-onset gangliosidoses (the syndromes of Batten-Mayou, Spielmeyer-Vogt, and Jansky-Bielschowsky), the progressive retinal degeneration that is associated with progressive external ophthalmoplegia (Kearns-Sayre syndrome), and the retinitis pigmentosa–like changes in the Laurence-Moon and Bardet-Biedl syndromes. The retinal manifestations of abetalipoproteinemia (Bassen-Kornzweig syndrome) and Refsum syndrome are similar to those found in retinitis pigmentosa. The diagnosis of these latter two disorders in a patient with presumed retinitis pigmentosa is important because treatment is possible. There is also an association of retinitis pigmentosa and congenital hearing loss, as in Usher's syndrome.

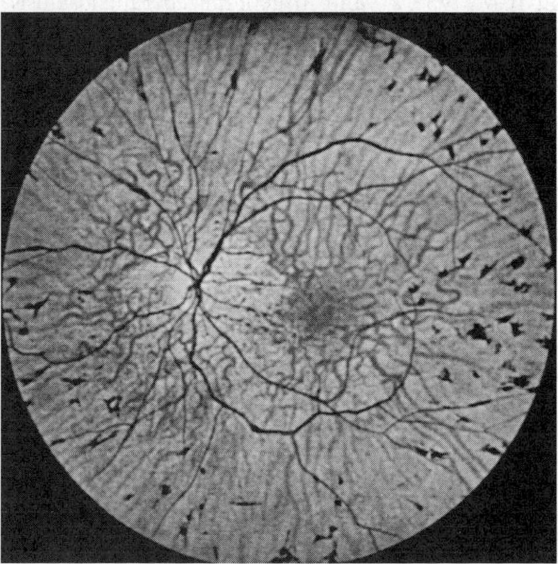

Figure 637–3 Retinitis pigmentosa.

STARGARDT DISEASE (FUNDUS FLAVIMACULATUS). This autosomal recessive retinal disorder is characterized by slowly progressive bilateral macular degeneration and vision impairment. It usually appears at 8–14 yr of age, and affected children are often initially misdiagnosed as having functional visual loss. The foveal reflex becomes obtunded or appears grayish, pigment spots develop in the macular area, and macular depigmentation and chorioretinal atrophy eventually occur. Macular hemorrhages also may develop. Some patients also have white or yellow spots beyond the macula or pigmentary changes in the periphery; the term *fundus flavimaculatus* is commonly used for this condition. It is now recognized that Stargardt disease and fundus flavimaculatus represent different parts on the spectrum of the same disease. Central visual acuity is reduced, often to 20/200, but total loss of vision does not occur. ERG findings vary. The condition is not associated with central nervous system (CNS) abnormalities and is to be differentiated from the macular changes of many progressive metabolic neurodegenerative diseases. The genetic mutation responsible for Stargardt's macular dystrophy has been identified.

BEST'S VITELLIFORM DEGENERATION. This macular dystrophy is characterized by a distinctive yellow or orange discoid subretinal lesion in the macula, resembling the intact yolk of a fried egg. Diagnosis is usually made between 3 and 15 yr of age, with a mean age of presentation of 6 yr. Vision is usually normal at this stage. The condition may be progressive; the yolklike lesion may eventually degenerate ("scramble") and result in pigmentation, chorioretinal atrophy, and vision impairment. The condition is usually bilateral. There is no association with systemic abnormalities. Inheritance is usually autosomal dominant. In vitelliform macular degeneration, the ERG response is normal. The electro-oculogram findings are abnormal in affected patients and carriers, and this test is useful in diagnosis and in genetic counseling.

CHERRY RED SPOT. Because of the special histologic features of the macula, certain pathologic processes affecting the retina produce an ophthalmoscopically visible sign referred to as a cherry red spot, a bright to dull red spot at the center of the macula surrounded and accentuated by a grayish-white or yellowish halo. The halo is a result of a loss of transparency of the retinal ganglion cell layer secondary to edema, lipid accumulation, or both. Because ganglion cells are not present in the fovea, the retina surrounding the fovea is opacified but the fovea transmits the normal underlying choroidal color (red), accounting for the presence of the cherry red spot. A cherry red spot typically occurs in certain sphingolipidoses, principally in Tay-Sachs disease (GM_2 type 1), in the Sandhoff variant (GM_2 type 2), and in generalized gangliosidosis (GM_1 type 1). Similar but less distinctive macular changes occur in some cases of metachromatic leukodystrophy (sulfatide lipidosis), in some forms of neuronopathic Niemann-Pick disease, and in certain mucolipidoses. The cherry red spot that characteristically occurs as a result of retinal ischemia secondary to vasospasm, ocular contusion, or occlusion of the central retinal artery must be differentiated from the cherry red spot of neurodegenerative disease.

PHAKOMAS. These are the herald lesions of the hamartomatous disorders. In Bourneville disease (tuberous sclerosis), the distinctive ocular lesion is a refractile, yellowish, multinodular cystic lesion arising from the disc or retina; the appearance of this typical lesion is often compared to that of an unripe mulberry (Fig. 637–4). Equally characteristic and more common in tuberous sclerosis are flatter, yellow to whitish retinal lesions, varying in size from minute dots to large lesions approaching the size of the disc. These lesions are benign astrocytic proliferations. Rarely, similar retinal phakomas occur in von Recklinghausen disease (neurofibromatosis). In von Hippel–Lindau disease (angiomatosis of the retina and cerebellum) the distinctive fundus lesion is a hemangioblastoma; this vascular lesion usually appears as a reddish globular mass with large paired arteries and veins passing to and from the lesion. In Sturge-Weber syndrome (encephalofacial angiomatosis), the fundus abnormality is a choroidal hemangioma; the hemangioma may impart a dark color to the affected area of the fundus, but the lesion is best seen with fluorescein angiography.

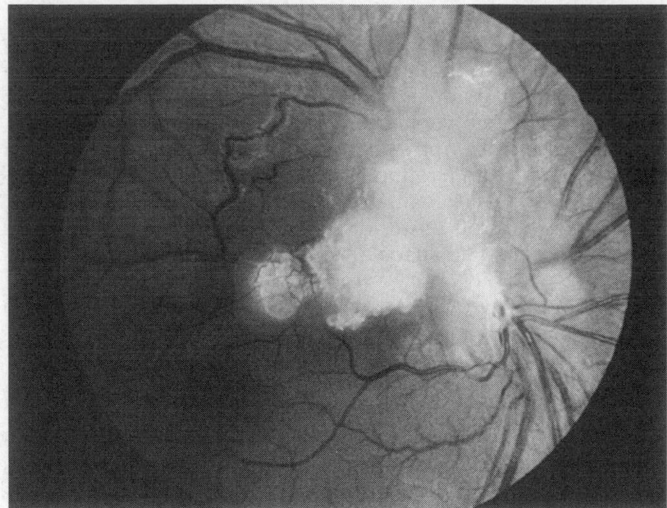

Figure 637–4 Retinal phakoma of tuberous sclerosis.

RETINOSCHISIS. *Congenital hereditary retinoschisis,* also referred to as *juvenile X-linked retinoschisis,* is a bilateral vitreoretinal dystrophy that appears early in life, often in infancy. It is characterized by splitting of the retina into inner and outer layers. The usual ophthalmoscopic finding in affected males is an elevation of the inner layer of the retina, most commonly in the inferotemporal quadrant of the fundus, often with round or oval holes visible in the inner layer. Schisis of the fovea is virtually pathognomonic and is found in almost 100% of patients. Ophthalmoscopically, this appears in early stages as small, fine striae in the internal limiting membrane. These striae radiate outward in a petaloid or spokewheel configuration. In some cases, frank retinal detachment or vitreous hemorrhage occurs.

Vision impairment varies from mild to severe; visual acuity may worsen with age, but good vision is often retained. Carrier females are asymptomatic, but linkage studies may be useful to help detect carriers.

RETINAL DETACHMENT. A retinal detachment is a separation of the outer layers of the retina from the underlying retinal pigment epithelium (RPE). During embryogenesis, the retina and RPE are initially separated. During ocular development, they join together and are held in apposition to each other by various physiologic mechanisms. Pathologic events leading to a retinal detachment return the retina-RPE to its former separated state. The detachment can occur as a congenital anomaly but more commonly arises secondary to other ocular abnormalities or trauma. Three types of detachment are described; each may occur in children. *Rhegmatogenous detachments* result from a break in the retina that allows fluid to enter the subretinal space. In children, these are usually a result of trauma (such as child abuse) but may occur secondary to myopia or ROP or after congenital cataract surgery. *Tractional retinal detachments* result when vitreoretinal membranes pull on the retina. They can occur in diabetes, sickle cell disease, and ROP. *Exudative retinal detachments* result when exudation exceeds absorption. This can be seen in Coats disease, retinoblastoma, and ocular inflammation.

The presenting sign of retinal detachment in an infant or child may be loss of vision, secondary strabismus or nystagmus, or leukokoria (white pupillary reflex). In addition to direct examination of the eye, special diagnostic studies such as ultrasonography and neuroimaging (CT, MRI) may be necessary to establish the cause of the detachment and the appropriate treatment. Prompt care is essential if vision is to be salvaged.

COATS' DISEASE. This exudative retinopathy of unknown cause is characterized by telangiectasis of retinal vessels with leakage of plasma to form intraretinal and subretinal exudates and by retinal hemorrhages and detachment. The condition is usually unilateral. It predominantly affects boys, usually appearing in the first decade. The condition is nonfamilial and for the most part occurs in otherwise healthy children. The most frequent presenting signs are blurring of vision, leukokoria, and strabismus. Rubeosis of the iris, glaucoma, and cataract may develop. Treatment with photocoagulation or cryotherapy may be helpful.

FAMILIAL EXUDATIVE VITREORETINOPATHY (FEV). This progressive retinovascular disorder is of unknown cause, but clinical and angiographic findings suggest an aberration of vascular development. Avascularity of the peripheral temporal retina is a significant finding in most cases, with abrupt cessation of the retinal capillary network in the region of the equator. The avascular zone often has a wedge- or V-shaped pattern in the temporal meridian. Glial proliferation or well-marked retinochoroidal atrophy may be found in the avascular zone. Excessive branching of retinal arteries and veins, dilatation of the capillaries, arteriovenous shunt formation, neovascularization, and leakage from retinal vessels of the farthest vascularized retina occur. Vitreoretinal adhesions are usually present at the peripheral margin of the vascularized retina. Traction, retinal dragging and temporal displacement of the macula, falciform retinal folds, and retinal detachment are common. Intraretinal or subretinal exudation, retinal hemorrhage, and recurrent vitreous hemorrhages may develop. Patients may also develop cataracts and glaucoma. Vision impairment of varying severity occurs. The condition is usually bilateral. FEV is usually an autosomal dominant condition with incomplete penetrance. Asymptomatic family members often display a zone of avascular peripheral retina.

The findings in FEV may resemble those of ROP in the cicatricial stages, but unlike ROP, the neovascularization of FEV seems to develop years after birth and most patients with FEV have no history of prematurity, oxygen therapy, prenatal or postnatal injury or infection, or developmental abnormalities. FEV is also to be differentiated from Coats' disease, angiomatosis of the retina, peripheral uveitis, and other disorders of the posterior segment.

HYPERTENSIVE RETINOPATHY. In the early stages of hypertension, no retinal changes may be observable. Generalized constriction and irregular narrowing of the arterioles are usually the first signs in the fundus. Other alterations include retinal edema, flame-shaped hemorrhages, cotton-wool spots (retinal nerve fiber layer infarcts) and papilledema (Fig. 637–5). These changes are reversible if the disease can be controlled in the early stages, but in long-standing hypertension, irreversible changes may occur. Thickening of the vessel wall may produce a silver- or copper-wire appearance. Hypertensive retinal changes in a child should alert the physician to renal disease, pheochromocytoma, collagen disease, and cardiovascular disorders, particularly coarctation of the aorta.

DIABETIC RETINOPATHY. The retinal changes of diabetes mellitus are classified as nonproliferative or proliferative. *Nonproliferative diabetic retinopathy* is characterized by retinal microaneurysms, venous dilatation, retinal hemorrhages, and exudates. The microaneurysms appear as tiny red dots. The hemorrhages may be of both the dot and blot type, representing deep intraretinal bleeding, and the splinter or flame-shaped type, involving the superficial nerve fiber layer. The exudates tend to be deep and to appear waxy. There may also be superficial nerve fiber infarcts called *cytoid bodies* or cotton-wool spots, as well as retinal edema. These signs may wax and wane. They are seen primarily in the posterior pole, around the disc and macula, well within the range of direct ophthalmoscopy. Involvement of the macula may lead to decreased vision.

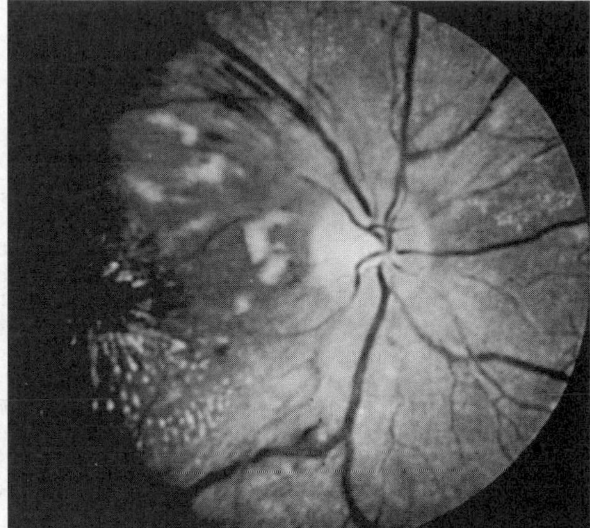

Figure 637–5 Hypertensive retinopathy.

Proliferative retinopathy, the more serious form, is characterized by neovascularization and proliferation of fibrovascular tissue on the retina, extending into the vitreous. Neovascularization may occur on the optic disc (NVD), elsewhere on the retina (NVE), or on the iris and in the anterior chamber angle (NVI, or rubeosis irides) (Fig. 637–6). Traction on these new vessels leads to hemorrhage and eventually scarring. The vision-threatening complications of proliferative diabetic retinopathy are retinal and vitreous hemorrhages, cicatrization, traction, and retinal detachment. Neovascularization of the iris may lead to secondary glaucoma if not treated promptly.

Diabetic retinopathy involves the alteration and nonperfusion of retinal capillaries, retinal ischemia, and neovascularization, but its pathogenesis is not yet completely understood, either in terms of location of the primary pathogenetic mechanism (retinal vessels vs surrounding neuronal or glial tissue) or the specific biochemical factors involved. The better the degree of long-term metabolic control, the lower is the risk of diabetic retinopathy.

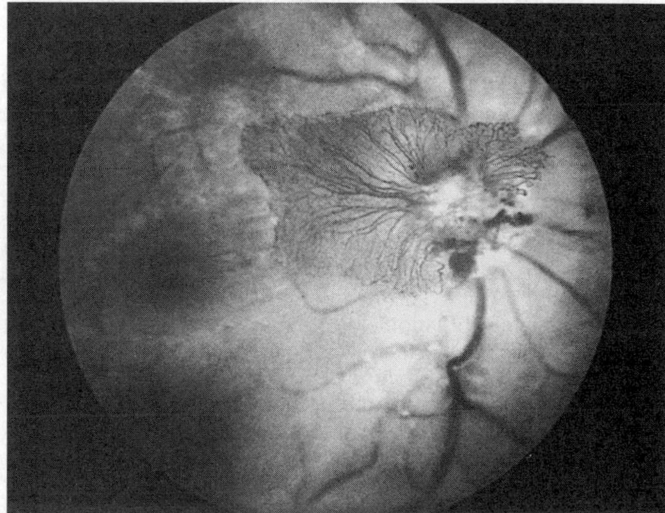

Figure 637–6 Proliferative diabetic retinopathy with neovascularization of the disc (NVD).

Clinically, the prevalence and course of retinopathy relate to a patient's age and to duration of disease. Detectable microvascular changes are rare in prepubertal children, with the prevalence of retinopathy increasing significantly after puberty, especially after the age of 15 yr. The incidence of retinopathy is low during the first 5 yr of disease and increases progressively thereafter, with the incidence of proliferative retinopathy becoming substantial after 10 yr and with increased risk of visual impairment after 15 yr or more. Periodic ophthalmologic evaluation is recommended for all patients with diabetes mellitus.

In addition to retinopathy, patients with juvenile-onset diabetes may develop optic neuropathy, characterized by swelling of the disc and blurring of vision. Patients with diabetes may also develop cataracts, even at an early age, sometimes with rapid progression.

Macular edema is the leading cause of visual loss in diabetic persons. Photocoagulation may be used to decrease the risk of continued vision loss in patients with macular edema. Proliferative retinopathy causes the most severe vision loss and can lead to total loss of vision and even loss of the eye.

Patients who have proliferative disease and who display certain high-risk characteristics should undergo panretinal photocoagulation (PRP) to preserve their central vision. Neovascularization of the iris is also treated with PRP to stop the development of neovascular glaucoma. Vitrectomy and other intraocular surgery may be necessary in patients with nonresolving vitreous hemorrhage or traction retinal detachment. The value of technologic advances, such as insulin infusion pumps and pancreatic transplants, in preventing ocular complications is under investigation (see Chapter 599).

SUBACUTE BACTERIAL ENDOCARDITIS. At some time during the course of the disease, retinopathy is present in approximately 40% of cases of subacute bacterial endocarditis. The lesions include hemorrhages, hemorrhages with white centers *(Roth's spots)*, papilledema, and, rarely, embolic occlusion of the central retinal artery.

BLOOD DISORDERS. In primary and secondary anemias, retinopathy in the form of hemorrhages and cotton-wool patches may occur. Vision can be affected if hemorrhage occurs in the macular area. The hemorrhages may be light and feathery or dense and preretinal. In polycythemia vera, the retinal veins are dark, dilated, and tortuous. Retinal hemorrhages, retinal edema, and papilledema may be observed. In leukemia, the veins are characteristically dilated, with sausage-shaped constrictions; hemorrhages, particularly white-centered hemorrhages and exudates, are common during the acute stage. In the sickling disorders, fundus changes include vascular tortuosity, arterial and venous occlusions, "salmon patches," refractile deposits, pigmented lesions, arteriolar-venous anastomoses, and neovascularization (with "sea-fan" formations), sometimes leading to vitreous hemorrhage and retinal detachment. Individuals with Hb SC and Hb S-β-thalassemia hemoglobinopathies are at a higher risk for the development of retinopathy than are those with SS disease. It is thought that the more anemic state of those patients with SS disease offers protection from vascular occlusions in the retina.

TRAUMA-RELATED RETINOPATHY. Retinal changes may occur in patients who suffer trauma to other parts of the body. The occurrence of retinal hemorrhages in infants who have been physically abused is well documented (see Chapter 35). Retinal, subretinal, subhyaloid, and vitreous hemorrhages have been described. Often there are no signs of direct trauma to the eye, periocular region, or head. Such cases may result from violent shaking of an infant, and permanent retinal damage may result. Retinal, subhyaloid, and vitreous hemorrhages are common in patients with traumatic and nontraumatic subarachnoid hemorrhage, an association referred to as *Terson's syndrome*.

In patients with head or chest trauma, a traumatic retinal angiopathy known as *Purtscher retinopathy* may occur. This is characterized by retinal hemorrhage, cotton-wool spots, possible disc swelling, and decreased vision. The pathogenesis is unclear, but there is evidence for arteriolar obstruction in this condition. A Purtscher-like fundus picture may also occur in several nontraumatic settings, such as acute pancreatitis, lupus erythematosus, and childbirth.

MEDULLATED NERVE FIBERS. Myelination of the optic nerve fibers normally terminates at the level of the disc, but in some individuals ectopic medullation extends to nerve fibers of the retina. The condition is most commonly seen adjacent to the disc, although more peripheral areas of the retina may be involved. The characteristic ophthalmoscopic picture is a focal white patch with a feathered edge or brush-stroke appearance. Because the macula is generally unaffected, the visual prognosis is good. A relative or absolute visual field defect corresponding to areas of ectopic medullation is usually the only associated ocular abnormality. Extensive unilateral involvement, however, has been associated with ipsilateral myopia, amblyopia, and strabismus. If unilateral high myopia and amblyopia are present, appropriate optical correction and occlusion therapy should be instituted. For unknown reasons, the disorder is more commonly encountered in patients with craniofacial dysostosis, oxycephaly, neurofibromatosis, and Down syndrome.

COLOBOMA OF THE FUNDUS. The term *coloboma* describes a defect such as a gap, notch, fissure, or hole. The typical fundus coloboma is a result of malclosure of the embryonic fissure, which leaves a gap in the retina, RPE, and choroid, thus baring the underlying sclera. The defect may be extensive, involving the ciliary body, iris, and even lens, or it may be localized to one or more portions of the fissure. The usual appearance is of a well-circumscribed, wedge-shaped white area extending inferonasally below the disc, sometimes involving or engulfing the disc. In some cases there is ectasia or cyst formation in the area of the defect. Less extensive colobomatous defects may appear as only single or multiple focal punched-out chorioretinal defects or anomalous pigmentation of the fundus in the line of the embryonic fissure. Colobomas may occur in one or both eyes. A visual field defect usually corresponds to the chorioretinal defect. Visual acuity may be impaired, particularly if the defect involves the disc or macula.

Fundus colobomas may occur in isolation as sporadic defects or as an inherited condition. Isolated colobomatous anomalies are commonly inherited in an autosomal dominant manner with highly variable penetrance and expressivity. Family members of affected patients should receive appropriate genetic counseling. Colobomas may also be associated with such abnormalities as microphthalmia, glioneuroma of the eye, cyclopia, or an encephaly. They occur in children with various chromosomal disorders, including 13-trisomy, 18-trisomy, triploidy, cat-eye syndrome, and 4p−. Ocular colobomata also occur in many multisystem disorders, including the CHARGE* association, Joubert, Aicardi, Meckel, Warburg, and Rubinstein-Taybi syndromes; linear sebaceous nevus; Goldenhar and Lenz microphthalmia syndromes; and Goltz focal dermal hypoplasia.

Aaby AA, Kushner BJ: Acquired and progressive myelinated nerve fibers. Arch Ophthalmol 103:542, 1985.

Abramson DH, Frank CM, Susman M, et al: Presenting signs of retinoblastoma. J Pediatr 132:505, 1998.

Barr CC, Glaser JS, Blankenship G: Acute disc swelling in juvenile diabetes: Clinical profile and natural history of 12 cases. Arch Ophthalmol 98:2185, 1980.

Bateman JB, Riedner E, Levin LS, et al: Heterogeneity of retinal degeneration and hearing impairment syndromes. Am J Ophthalmol 90:755, 1980.

Berson EL, Rosner B, Siminoff E: Risk factors for genetic typing and detection in retinitis pigmentosa. Am J Ophthalmol 89:763, 1980.

*C = coloboma; H = heart disease; A = atresia choanae; R = retarded growth and development and/or CNS anomalies; G = genetic anomalies and/or hypogonadism; E = ear anomalies and/or deafness.

Burns RP, Lourien EW, Cibis AB: Juvenile sex-linked retinoschisis: Clinical and genetic studies. Trans Am Acad Ophthalmol Otolaryngol 75:1011, 1971.
Chang M, McLean IW, Merritt JC: Coats' disease: A study of 62 histologically confirmed cases. J Pediatr Ophthalmol Strabismus 21:163, 1984.
Cryotherapy for Retinopathy of Prematurity Cooperative Group: Multicenter trial of cryotherapy for retinopathy of prematurity. Arch Ophthalmol 114:417, 1996.
Drack AV: Preventing blindness in premature infants. N Engl J Med 338:1620, 1998.
Duane TD, Osher RH, Green WR: White-centered hemorrhages: Their significance. Ophthalmology 87:66, 1980.
Eagle RC, Lucier AC, Bernardino VB Jr, et al: Retinal pigment epithelial abnormalities in fundus flavimaculatus. Ophthalmology 87:1189, 1980.
Early Treatment Diabetic Retinopathy Research Study Group: Photocoagulation for diabetic macular edema. Early treatment diabetic retinopathy study report 1. Arch Ophthalmol 103:1796, 1985.
Goldberg MF, Mafee M: Computed tomography for diagnosis of persistent hyperplastic primary vitreous (PHPV). Ophthalmology 90:442, 1983.
Hardwig P, Robertson DM: Von Hippel–Lindau disease: A familial, often lethal, multi-system phakomatosis. Ophthalmology 91:263, 1984.
Jackson RL, Ide CH, Guthrie RA, et al: Retinopathy in adolescents and young adults with onset of insulin-dependent diabetes in childhood. Ophthalmology 89:7, 1982.
Juan Verdaguer T: Juvenile retinal detachment. Am J Ophthalmol 93:145, 1982.
Knobloch WH, Layer JM: Clefting syndromes associated with retinal detachment. Am J Ophthalmol 73:517, 1972.
Kushner BJ, Sondheimer S: Medical treatment of glaucoma associated with cicatricial retinopathy of prematurity. Am J Ophthalmol 94:313, 1982.
Mann E, Kut LJ, Lee CB: Rheumatogenous retinal detachment in infancy. Arch Ophthalmol 95:1774, 1971.
Matthews JD, Weiter JJ, Kolodny EH: Macular halos associated with Niemann-Pick type B disease. Ophthalmology 93:933, 1986.
Miyakulo H, Hashimoto K, Miyakulo S: Retinal vascular pattern in familial exudative vitreoretinopathy. Ophthalmology 91:1524, 1984.
Mohler CW, Fine SL: Long-term evaluation of patients with Best's vitelliform dystrophy. Ophthalmology 88:688, 1981.
Noble KG, Carr RE: Leber's congenital amaurosis: A retrospective study of 33 cases and a histopathological study of one case. Arch Ophthalmol 96:818, 1978.
Noble KG, Carr RE: Stargardt's disease and fundus flavimaculatus. Arch Ophthalmol 97:1281, 1979.
Nyboer JH, Robertson DM, Gomez MR: Retinal lesions in tuberous sclerosis. Arch Ophthalmol 94:1277, 1976.
Pagon RA: Ocular coloboma. Surv Ophthalmol 25:223, 1981.
Pierce EA, Foley ED, Smith LE: Regulation of vascular endothelial growth factor by oxygen in a model of retinopathy of prematurity. Arch Ophthalmol 114:1219, 1996.
Quinn GE, Dobson V, Repka MX, et al: Development of myopia in infants with birthweights less than 1251 grams. Ophthalmology 99:329, 1992.
Reynolds JD: Retinopathy of prematurity. Ophthalmol Clin North Am 2:149, 1996.
Reynolds JD, Hardy RJ, Kennedy KA, et al: Lack of efficacy of light reduction in preventing retinopathy of prematurity. N Engl J Med 338:1572, 1998.
Ridgeway EW, Jaffe N, Walton DS: Leukemic ophthalmopathy in children. Cancer 38:1744, 1976.
Riley FC, Campbell RJ: Double phakomatosis. Arch Ophthalmol 97:518, 1979.
Rosenthal AR: Ocular manifestations of leukemia. Ophthalmology 90:899, 1983.
Salazar FG, Lamiell JM: Early identification of retinal angiomas in a large kindred with von Hippel–Lindau disease. Am J Ophthalmol 89:540, 1980.
Screening examination of premature infants for retinopathy of prematurity. A joint statement of the American Academy of Pediatrics, the American Association for Pediatric Ophthalmology and Strabismus and the American Academy of Ophthalmology. Pediatrics 100:273, 1997.
Shields CL, De Potter P, Himelstein BP, et al: Chemoreduction in the initial management of intraocular retinoblastoma. Arch Ophthalmol 114:1330, 1996.
Shields CL, Shields JA: Genetics of retinoblastoma. *In*: Tasman WS, Jaeger EA (eds): Duane's Foundation of Clinical Ophthalmology. Philadelphia, JB Lippincott, 1997.
Straatsma BR, Foos RY, Heckenlively JR, et al: Myelinated retinal nerve fibers. Am J Ophthalmol 91:25, 1981.
Walsh JB: Hypertensive retinopathy: Description, classification and prognosis. Ophthalmology 89:1127, 1982.
Wright K, Anderson ME, Walker E, et al: Should fewer premature infants be screened for retinopathy of prematurity in the managed care era? Pediatrics 102:31, 1998.

CHAPTER 638
Abnormalities of the Optic Nerve

OPTIC NERVE APLASIA. This rare congenital anomaly is typically unilateral. The optic nerve, retinal ganglion cells, and retinal blood vessels are absent. A vestigial dural sheath usually connects with the sclera in a normal position, but no neural tissue is present within this sheath. Optic nerve aplasia typically occurs sporadically in an otherwise healthy person. A wide variety of ocular abnormalities may occur, but colobomas are the most frequent associated finding.

OPTIC NERVE HYPOPLASIA. Hypoplasia of the optic nerve is a nonprogressive condition characterized by a subnormal number of optic nerve axons with normal mesodermal elements and glial supporting tissue. In typical cases, the nerve head is small and pale, with a pale or pigmented peripapillary halo or double ring sign.

This anomaly is associated with defects of vision and of visual fields of varying severity, ranging from blindness to normal or near-normal vision. It may be associated with systemic anomalies that most commonly involve the central nervous system (CNS). Protean CNS defects such as hydranencephaly or anencephaly or more focal lesions compatible with continued development of a patient may accompany optic nerve hypoplasia, but unilateral or bilateral optic nerve hypoplasia may be found without any concomitant defects.

Optic nerve hypoplasia is a principal feature of *septo-optic dysplasia of de Morsier*, a developmental disorder characterized by the association of anomalies of the midline structures of the brain with hypoplasia of the optic nerves, optic chiasm, and optic tracts; typically noted are agenesis of the septum pellucidum, partial or complete agenesis of the corpus callosum, and malformation of the fornix, with a large chiasmatic cistern. Patients may have hypothalamic abnormalities and endocrine defects, ranging from panhypopituitarism to isolated deficiency of growth hormone, hypothyroidism, or diabetes insipidus. Neonatal hypoglycemia and seizures are important presenting signs in affected infants.

Bilateral, subtle hypoplasia may be difficult to diagnose from the appearance of the disc alone because no comparison with a contralateral uninvolved eye is possible. However, it is important to establish the diagnosis because this eliminates confusion with optic atrophy or glaucoma and may explain the cause of decreased vision in a patient unresponsive to amblyopia therapy. Endocrine function should be watched closely in patients with optic nerve hypoplasia.

The etiology of optic nerve hypoplasia remains unclear. Early gestational injuries to midline CNS structures with secondary axonal injury or a disruption of normal neuronal guidance mechanisms that affect both optic nerve and cerebral neurons may account for these commonly associated disorders. Optic nerve hypoplasia may occur with somewhat increased frequency in infants of diabetic mothers and has been associated with maternal use of dilantin, quinine, LSD, and alcohol during pregnancy.

MORNING GLORY DISC ANOMALY. This term describes a congenital malformation of the optic nerve characterized by an enlarged, excavated, funnel-shaped disc with an elevated rim, resembling a morning glory flower. White glial tissue is present in the central part of the disc. The retinal vessels are abnormal and appear at the peripheral disc and course over the elevated pink rim in a radial fashion. Pigmentary mottling of the peripapillary region is usually seen. Most cases are unilateral. Females are affected twice as often as males. Visual acuity is usually severely reduced, and retinal detachment occurs in approximately one third of involved eyes. The association between basal encephaloceles and the morning glory disc anomaly has been well established.

TILTED DISC. In this congenital anomaly, the vertical axis of the optic disc is directed obliquely, so that the upper temporal portion of the nerve head is more prominent and anterior to the lower nasal portion of the disc. The retinal vessels emerge from the upper temporal portion of the disc rather than from the nasal side. Often noted is a peripapillary crescent or conus. Associated visual field defects and myopic astigmatism may be found. Clinical recognition of the tilted disc syndrome is important to avoid confusion of its disc and visual field signs with those of papilledema and intracranial tumor.

DRUSEN OF THE OPTIC NERVE. These globular, acellular bodies are thought to arise from axoplasmic derivatives of disintegrating nerve fibers. Drusen may be buried within the optic nerve, producing elevation of the optic nerve head (which can be confused with papilledema), or they may be partially or completely exposed, appearing as refractile bodies at the surface of the disc. Visual field defects and spontaneous peripapillary nerve fiber layer hemorrhages may occur in association with drusen. Drusen may occur as an autosomal dominant condition. They have also been observed in children with various neurologic disorders, including primary megalencephaly, seizures, learning disorders, mental retardation, schizophrenia, tuberous sclerosis, Down syndrome, and intracranial tumors.

PAPILLEDEMA. The term *papilledema* ("choked disc") is reserved to describe swelling of the nerve head secondary to increased intracranial pressure (ICP). *Clinical manifestations* of papilledema include edematous blurring of the disc margins, fullness or elevation of the nerve head, partial or complete obliteration of the disc cup, capillary congestion and hyperemia of the nerve head, generalized engorgement of the veins, loss of spontaneous venous pulsation, nerve fiber layer hemorrhages around the disc, and peripapillary exudates. In some cases, edema extending into the macula may produce a fan- or star-shaped figure. In addition, concentric peripapillary retinal wrinkling (Paton's lines) may be noted. Transient obscuration of vision may occur, lasting seconds and associated with postural changes. Vision, however, is usually normal in acute papilledema. Normally, when the ICP is relieved, the papilledema resolves and the disc returns to a normal or nearly normal appearance within 6–8 wk. Sustained chronic papilledema or long-standing unrelieved increased ICP may, however, lead to permanent nerve fiber damage, atrophic changes of the disc, macular scarring, and impairment of vision. In cases of impending or progressive vision loss caused by papilledema in patients with benign intracranial hypertension, decompression of the optic nerve by slitting the sheath may preserve vision.

The *pathophysiology* of papilledema is probably as follows: elevation of intracranial subarachnoid cerebrospinal fluid (CSF) pressure, elevation of CSF pressure in the sheath of the optic nerve, elevation of tissue pressure in the optic nerve, stasis of axoplasmic flow and swelling of the nerve fibers in the optic nerve head, and secondary vascular changes and the characteristic ophthalmoscopic signs of venous stasis. Associated neurophthalmic signs of increased ICP in infants and children include abducent palsy and attendant esotropia, lid retraction, paresis of upward gaze, tonic downward deviation of the eyes, and convergent nystagmus.

The common *causes* of papilledema in childhood are intracranial tumors and obstructive hydrocephalus, intracranial hemorrhage, the cerebral edema of trauma, meningoencephalitis and toxic encephalopathy, and certain metabolic diseases. Whatever the cause, the optic disc signs of increased ICP in early childhood may occasionally be modified by the distensibility of the young skull. In the absence of conditions associated with early closure of sutures and early obliteration of the fontanel (craniosynostosis, Crouzon and Apert syndromes), infants with increased ICP may not develop papilledema.

The *differential diagnosis* of papilledema includes structural changes of the disc ("pseudopapilledema," "pseudoneuritis," drusen, and medullated fibers), with which it may be confused, and the disc swelling of hypertension and diabetes mellitus. Unless retinal hemorrhage or edema involves the macular area, the preservation of good central vision and the absence of an afferent pupillary defect (Marcus Gunn pupil) help to differentiate acute papilledema from the edema of the optic nerve head found in acute optic neuritis.

Papilledema is a neurologic emergency. It can be accompanied by other signs of increased ICP, including headaches, nausea, and vomiting. Neuroimaging should be performed; if no intracranial masses are detected, a lumbar puncture in the lateral position and determination of CSF pressure should follow.

OPTIC NEURITIS. This is any inflammation, demyelinization, or degeneration of the optic nerve with attendant impairment of function. The process is usually acute, with rapidly progressive loss of vision. It may be unilateral or bilateral. Pain on movement of the globe or pain on palpation of the globe may precede or accompany the onset of visual symptoms.

When the retrobulbar portion of the nerve is affected without ophthalmoscopically visible signs of inflammation at the disc, the term *retrobulbar neuritis* is applied. When there is ophthalmoscopically visible evidence of inflammation of the nerve head, the term *papillitis* or *intraocular optic neuritis* is used. When there is involvement of both the retina and papilla, the term *optic neuroretinitis* is used.

In childhood, optic neuritis may occur as an isolated condition or as a manifestation of a neurologic or systemic disease. It may occur with bacterial meningitis or with viral infection (often accompanying encephalomyelitis following an exanthem). It may signify one of the many demyelinizing diseases of childhood. Although a significant percentage of adults who experience an episode of optic neuritis eventually develop other symptoms associated with multiple sclerosis, children with optic neuritis are seemingly at less risk. Bilateral optic neuritis in children may be associated with **neuromyelitis optica** (Devic disease). This syndrome is characterized by rapid and severe bilateral visual loss accompanied by transverse myelitis and paraplegia. Optic neuritis may also be secondary to an exogenous toxin or drug—for example, with lead poisoning or as a complication of long-term high-dose treatment with chloramphenicol or vincristine therapy. Extensive pediatric neurologic and ophthalmic investigation, including neuroradiologic and electrophysiologic studies, is usually required.

In most cases of acute optic neuritis, some improvement in vision begins within 1–4 wk after onset, and vision may improve to normal or near normal within weeks or months. The course varies with etiology. Although central vision may fully recover, it is common to find permanent defects in other areas of visual function (contrast sensitivity, color, brightness sense, and motion perception).

A *treatment* trial demonstrated that intravenous corticosteroids may help to speed the visual recovery in young adults but do not alter the long-term visual outcome. Therefore, their use has been reserved by some physicians for cases with severe vision loss or significant discomfort. Orally administered corticosteroids should not be used because they are associated with a significant increase in the recurrence rate of optic neuritis. It is unknown to what degree the results of the aforementioned trial may be extrapolated to optic neuritis in childhood.

LEBER OPTIC NEUROPATHY. This entity is characterized by sudden loss of central vision occurring in the 2nd and 3rd decades of life, primarily affecting young males. A characteristic peripapillary telangiectatic microangiopathy occurs not only in the presymptomatic phase of involved eyes but also in a high number of asymptomatic offspring in the female line. Disc hyperemia and edema mark the acute phase of visual loss. One eye is usually affected before the other. In time, progressive optic atrophy and vision loss usually ensue. The tortuous angiopathy becomes less obvious. Although visual function after the initial loss generally remains stable, a significant and sometimes complete recovery may occur in as many as one third of affected individuals. This recovery may take place years or decades after the initial episode of acute vision loss. The peripapillary angiopathy, the lack of short-term remission, and the degree of symmetry serve to distinguish most cases of Leber's disease from the optic neuritis of multiple sclerosis.

Leber optic neuropathy is maternally inherited and is caused by defective cytoplasmic mitochondrial DNA. Multiple point mutations in the mitochondrial DNA which lead to the development of the disorder have been found. Because of the mitochondrial nature of the disorder, skeletal and cardiac muscle disorders, including electrocardiographic abnormalities, may also be encountered in affected individuals.

OPTIC ATROPHY. This denotes degeneration of optic nerve axons, with attendant loss of function. The ophthalmoscopic signs of optic atrophy are pallor of the disc and loss of substance of the nerve head, sometimes with enlargement of the disc cup. The associated vision defect varies with the nature and site of the primary disease or lesion.

Optic atrophy is the common expression of a wide variety of congenital or acquired pathologic processes. The cause may be traumatic, inflammatory, degenerative, neoplastic, or vascular; intracranial tumors and hydrocephalus are principal causes of optic atrophy in children. In some cases, progressive optic atrophy is hereditary. Dominantly inherited infantile optic atrophy is a relatively mild heredodegenerative type that tends to progress through childhood and adolescence. Autosomal recessively inherited congenital optic atrophy is a rare condition that is evident at birth or develops at a very early age; the visual defect is usually profound. **Behr optic atrophy** is a hereditary type associated with hypertonia of the extremities, increased deep tendon reflexes, mild cerebellar ataxia, some degree of mental deficiency, and possibly external ophthalmoplegia. This disorder afflicts principally males from 3 to 11 yr of age. Some forms of heredodegenerative optic atrophy are associated with sensorineural hearing loss, as may occur in some children with juvenile-onset (insulin-dependent) diabetes mellitus. In the absence of an obvious cause, optic atrophy in an infant or child warrants extensive etiologic investigation.

OPTIC NERVE GLIOMA. Optic nerve glioma, more properly referred to as **juvenile pilocytic astrocytoma**, is the most frequent tumor of the optic nerve in childhood. This neuroglial tumor may develop in the intraorbital, intracanalicular, or intracranial portion of the nerve; the chiasm is often involved.

The tumor is a cytologic benign hamartoma that is generally stationary or only slowly progressive. The principal manifestations when the tumor occurs in the intraorbital portion of the nerve are unilateral loss of vision, proptosis, and deviation of the eye; optic atrophy or congestion of the optic nerve head may occur. Chiasmal involvement may be attended by defects of vision and visual fields (often bitemporal hemianopia), increased ICP, papilledema or optic atrophy, hypothalamic dysfunction, pituitary dysfunction, and sometimes nystagmus or strabismus. Juvenile pilocytic astrocytomas occur with increased frequency in patients with neurofibromatosis.

Treatment of optic pathway gliomas is controversial. The best management is usually periodic observation. Surgical removal may be appropriate when the tumor is confined to the intraorbital, intracanalicular, or prechiasmal portion of the nerve if a patient has unsightly proptosis with complete or nearly complete loss of vision of the affected eye. When the chiasm is involved, resection is not advocated and radiation and chemotherapy may be necessary.

TRAUMATIC OPTIC NEUROPATHIES. Injury to the optic nerve may result from both direct and indirect trauma. Direct trauma to the optic nerve is a result of a penetrating injury to the orbit with transection or contusion of the nerve. Blunt trauma to the orbit may also lead to severe visual loss if the traumatic force is transmitted to the optic canal and causes disruption of the blood supply to the intracanalicular portion of the nerve. Treatment may include high-dose corticosteroids or optic canal decompression.

Anderson RL, Panje WR, Gross CE: Optic nerve blindness following blunt forehead trauma. Ophthalmology 89:445, 1982.
Barr CC, Glaser JS, Blankenship G: Acute disc swelling in juvenile diabetes: Clinical profile and natural history of 12 cases. Arch Ophthalmol 98:2185, 1980.
Brown MD, Voljavec AS, Lott MT, et al: Leber's hereditary optic neuropathy: A model for mitochondrial neurodegenerative diseases. FASEB J 6:2791, 1992.
Costin G, Murgpree AL: Hypothalamic-pituitary function in children with optic nerve hypoplasia. Am J Dis Child 139:249, 1985.
Haik BG, Greenstein SH, Smith ME, et al: Retinal detachment in the morning glory anomaly. Ophthalmology 91:1638, 1984.
Hayreh SS: Optic disc edema in raised intracranial pressure. VI. Associated visual disturbances and their pathogenesis. Arch Ophthalmol 95:1566, 1977.
Hoover DL, Robb RM, Petersen RA: Optic disc drusen and primary megalencephaly in children. J Pediatr Ophthalmol Strabismus 26:81, 1989.
Hotchkiss ML, Green WR: Optic nerve aplasia and hypoplasia. J Pediatr Ophthalmol Strabismus 16:225, 1979.
Hoyt CS: Autosomal dominant optic atrophy: A spectrum of disability. Ophthalmology 87:245, 1980.
Kazarian EL, Gager WE: Optic neuritis complicating measles, mumps and rubella vaccination. Am J Ophthalmol 86:544, 1978.
Leys D, Petit H, Block AM, et al: Neuromyelitis optica (Devic's disease). Four cases. Rev Neurol (Paris) 143:722, 1987.
Listernick R, Louis DN, Packer RJ, et al: Optic pathway gliomas in children with neurofibromatosis 1: Consensus statement from the NF1 optic pathway glioma task force. Ann Neurol 41:143, 1997.
Margalith D, Jan JE, McCormick AQ, et al: Clinical spectrum of congenital optic nerve hypoplasia: Review of 51 patients. Dev Med Child Neurol 26:311, 1984.
Nikoskelainen E, Hoyt WF, Nummelin K: Ophthalmoscopic findings in patients with Leber's hereditary optic neuropathy. I. Fundus findings in asymptomatic family members. Arch Ophathalmol 100:1597, 1982.
Optic Neuritis Study Group: Visual function 5 years after optic neuritis. Experience of the optic neuritis treatment trial. Arch Ophthalmol 115:1545, 1997.
Repka MX, Miller NR: Optic atrophy in children. Am J Ophthalmol 106:191, 1988.
Rosenberg MA, Savino PJ, Glaser JS: A clinical analysis of pseudopapilledema. I: Population, laterality, acuity, refractive error, ophthalmoscopic characteristics, and coincident disease. Arch Ophthalmol 97:65, 1979.
Sergott RC, Savino PJ, Bosley TM: Modified optic nerve sheath decompression provides long-term visual improvement for pseudotumor cerebri. Arch Ophthalmol 106:1384, 1988.
Singh G, Lott MT, Wallace DC: A mitochondrial DNA mutation as a cause of Leber's hereditary optic neuropathy. N Engl J Med 320:1300, 1989.
Skarf B, Hoyt CS: Optic nerve hypoplasia in children: Association with anomalies of the endocrine and CNS. Arch Ophthalmol 102:62, 1984.
Traboulsi EI, O'Neill JE: The spectrum in the morphology of the so-called "morning glory disc anomaly." J Pediatr Ophthalmol Strabismus 25:93, 1988.
Weiss AH, Beck RW: Neuroretinitis in childhood. J Pediatr Ophthalmol Strabismus 26:198, 1989.

CHAPTER 639
Childhood Glaucoma

Glaucoma is a general term used to indicate damage to the optic nerve with visual field loss that is caused by or related to elevated pressure within the eye. It is classified according to the age of the affected individual at presentation and the association of other ocular or systemic conditions. Glaucoma that begins within the first 3 yr of life is called *infantile* (congenital); that which begins between the ages of 3 and 30 yr is called *juvenile*.

Primary glaucoma indicates that the cause is an isolated anomaly of the drainage apparatus of the eye (trabecular meshwork). More than 50% of infantile glaucoma is primary. In secondary glaucoma, other ocular or systemic abnormalities are associated, even if a similar developmental defect of the trabecular meshwork is also present. Primary infantile glaucoma occurs with an incidence of only 0.03%.

CLINICAL MANIFESTATIONS. The symptoms of infantile glaucoma include the classic triad of epiphora (tearing), photophobia (sensitivity to light), and blepharospasm (eyelid squeezing). Each can be attributed to corneal irritation. Only about 30% of affected infants demonstrate the classic symptom complex. Other signs include corneal edema, corneal and ocular enlargement, conjunctival injection, and visual impairment.

The sclera and cornea are more elastic in early childhood than later in life. An increase in intraocular pressure (IOP) therefore leads to an expansion of the globe, including the cornea, and the development of buphthalmos ("ox eye"). If the cornea continues to enlarge, breaks occur in the endothelial basement membrane (Descemet's membrane) and may lead to permanent corneal scarring. These breaks in Descemet's membrane (Haab's striae) are visible as horizontal edematous lines that cross or curve around the central cornea. They rarely occur beyond 3 yr of age or in corneas less than 12.0 mm in diameter. The cornea also becomes edematous and cloudy, with increased IOP. The corneal edema leads to tearing and photophobia. Glaucoma should be considered in a child suspected of having a nasolacrimal duct obstruction if any of these other signs or symptoms are present.

Children with unilateral glaucoma generally present early because the difference in the corneal size between the eyes can be noticed. When the disease is bilateral, parents may not recognize the increased corneal size. Many parents view the large eyes as attractive and do not seek help until other symptoms develop.

Cupping of the optic nerve head is detected by ocular examination. The optic nerve of an infant is easily distended by excessive pressure. Deep, central cupping readily occurs and may regress with normalization of pressure.

Some infants and children with early-onset glaucoma have more extensive maldevelopment of the anterior segment of the eye. The neurocrestopathies, once known as mesodermal dysgenesis, comprise a spectrum of conditions relating to abnormal embryologic development of the anterior segment. They are usually bilateral and may include abnormalities of the iris, cornea, and lens. Other ocular anomalies that may be associated with glaucoma in infants and children are aniridia, cataract, spherophakia, and ectopia lentis. Glaucoma may also develop secondary to persistent hyperplastic primary vitreous or retinopathy of prematurity.

Trauma, intraocular hemorrhage, ocular inflammatory disease, and intraocular tumor are also important causes of glaucoma in the pediatric population. Systemic disorders associated with glaucoma in infants and children are Sturge-Weber syndrome, von Recklinghausen disease, Lowe syndrome, Marfan syndrome, congenital rubella, a number of chromosomal syndromes, and juvenile xanthogranuloma.

DIAGNOSIS AND TREATMENT. The diagnosis of infantile glaucoma is made on recognition of the signs and symptoms. Although measurement of IOP may be helpful in monitoring treatment response, it is not a vital part of the diagnostic process. Once the diagnosis is established, treatment is started promptly. Unlike adult glaucoma, in which medication is often the first line of therapy, for infantile glaucoma the treatment is primarily surgical. Procedures used to treat glaucoma in children include surgery to establish a more normal anterior chamber angle (goniotomy and trabeculotomy), to create an exit site for aqueous fluid to exit the eye (trabeculectomy and seton surgery), or to reduce aqueous fluid production (cyclocryotherapy and photocyclocoagulation). Many children frequently require several operations to lower and maintain their IOP adequately, and long-term medical therapy may be necessary as well. Although vision may be reduced secondary to glaucomatous optic nerve damage or corneal scarring, amblyopia is the most common cause of loss of vision in these children.

Bardelli AM, Hadjistilianou T: Congenital glaucoma associated with other abnormalities in 150 cases. Glaucoma 9:10, 1987.

Barsoum-Homsy M, Chevrette L: Incidence and prognosis of childhood glaucoma: A study of 63 cases. Ophthalmology 93:1323, 1986.

Cibis GW, Tripathi RC, Tripathi BJ: Glaucoma in Sturge-Weber syndrome. Ophthalmology 91:1061, 1984.

Ginsberg J, Bove KE, Fogelson MH: Pathological features of the eye in the oculocerebrorenal (Lowe) syndrome. J Pediatr Ophthalmol Strabismus 18:16, 1981.

Kushner BJ, Sondheiner S: Medical treatment of glaucoma associated with cicatricial retinopathy of prematurity. Am J Ophthalmol 94:313, 1982.

McPherson SD Jr, Berry DP: Goniotomy vs external trabeculotomy for developmental glaucoma. Am J Ophthalmol 95:427, 1983.

Netland P, Walton D: Glaucoma drainage implants in pediatric patients. Ophthalmic Surg Lasers 24:723, 1993.

Quigley HA: Childhood glaucoma: Results with trabeculotomy and study of reversible cupping. Ophthalmology 89:219, 1982.

Rubin SE, Marcus CH: Glaucoma in childhood. Ophthalmol Clin North Am 2:215, 1996.

Seidman DJ, Nelson LB, Calhoun JH, et al: Signs and symptoms in the presentation of primary infantile glaucoma. Pediatrics 77:399, 1986.

Stern JH, Catalono RA: Current status of diagnostic and therapeutic measures in infantile glaucoma. Semin Ophthalmol 5:166, 1990.

CHAPTER 640
Orbital Abnormalities

HYPERTELORISM AND HYPOTELORISM. *Hypertelorism* is wide separation of the eyes or an increased interorbital distance, which may occur as a morphogenetic variant, a primary deformity, or a secondary phenomenon in association with developmental abnormalities, such as frontal meningocele or encephalocele or the persistence of a facial cleft. Often associated are strabismus, generally exotropia, and sometimes optic atrophy.

Hypotelorism refers to narrowness of the interorbital distance, which may occur as a morphogenetic variant alone or in association with other anomalies, such as epicanthus or holoprosencephaly or secondary to a cranial dystrophy, such as scaphocephaly.

EXOPHTHALMOS AND ENOPHTHALMOS. Protrusion of the eye is referred to as *exophthalmos* or *proptosis*. It may be caused by shallowness of the orbits, as in many craniofacial malformations, or by increased tissue mass within the orbit, as with neoplastic, vascular, and inflammatory disorders. Ocular complications include exposure keratopathy, ocular motor disturbances, and optic atrophy with loss of vision.

Posterior displacement or sinking of the eye back into the orbit is referred to as *enophthalmos*. This may occur with orbital fracture or with atrophy of orbital tissue.

ORBITAL CELLULITIS. This is a condition involving inflammation of the tissues of the orbit, with proptosis, limitation of movement of the eye, edema of the conjunctiva (chemosis), and inflammation and swelling of the eyelids. Patients often feel some discomfort, usually with general symptoms of toxicity, fever, and leukocytosis. Also see Chapter 193.

Orbital cellulitis may follow direct infection of the orbit from a wound, metastatic deposition of organisms during bacteremia, or more often direct extension or venous spread of infection from contiguous sites such as the lids, conjunctiva, globe, lacrimal gland, nasolacrimal sac, or commonly the paranasal sinuses. In some cases, primary or metastatic tumor in the orbit can produce the clinical picture of orbital cellulitis. The most common cause of orbital cellulitis in children is paranasal sinusitis. Frequent pathogenic organisms include nontypable *Haemophilus influenzae, Staphylococcus aureus,* group A β-hemolytic streptococci, *Streptococcus pneumoniae,* and anaerobic bacteria.

The orbital inflammatory *clinical manifestations* of paranasal sinusitis vary with the location and extent of involvement. Stage 1 is swelling of the lids—the edema of impaired venous drainage or the reactive inflammation of underlying periostitis; in this stage, the infection is still confined to the sinus. The 2nd stage is subperiosteal abscess, a collection of pus between the periosteum and the wall of the orbit, often with localized tenderness, displacement of the globe, and some limitation of eye movement. The 3rd stage is true orbital cellulitis, diffuse inflammation of the tissues within the orbit, with proptosis and impairment of ocular motility. The 4th stage is orbital abscess, resulting from localization of infection in the orbit or from extension of a subperiosteal abscess through the periosteum.

The potential for complications is great. Involvement of the optic nerve may result in loss of vision. Extension of infection from the orbit into the cranial cavity may lead to cavernous sinus thrombosis or meningitis or to epidural, subdural, or brain abscesses.

Orbital cellulitis must be recognized promptly and treated aggressively (Chapter 193). Hospitalization and systemic antibiotic therapy are usually indicated. In some cases, surgical intervention is necessary to drain infected sinuses or a subperiosteal or orbital abscess.

PERIORBITAL CELLULITIS. Inflammation of the lids and periorbital tissues without signs of true orbital involvement (such as proptosis or limitation of eye movement) is generally referred to as periorbital or preseptal cellulitis. This is common in young children and may be caused by trauma, by an infected wound, or by abscess of the lid or periorbital region (e.g., pyoderma, hordeolum, conjunctivitis, dacryocystitis, insect bite). It may be associated with respiratory infection or more often bacteremia, often with *H. influenzae* type b, streptococci, or pneumococci. What initially appears to be periorbital or preseptal cellulitis may be the first sign of sinusitis that may occasionally progress to true orbital cellulitis. Prompt antibiotic therapy and careful monitoring for signs of sepsis and local progression are essential. See Chapter 381.2.

ORBITAL INFLAMMATION. Inflammatory disease involving the orbit may be primary or secondary to systemic disease. Idiopathic orbital inflammation (orbital pseudotumor) represents a wide spectrum of clinical entities. Symptoms at the time of presentation may include pain, eyelid swelling, proptosis, and fever. The inflammation may involve a single extraocular muscle (myositis) or the entire orbit. Confusion with orbital cellulitis is common but can be differentiated by the lack of associated sinus disease, its appearance on CT scan, and lack of improvement with systemic antibiotics. Treatment includes the use of high-dose systemic corticosteroids. Immunotherapy or radiation treatment may be necessary for resistant or recurrent cases.

Thyroid-related ophthalmopathy (TRO) is believed to be secondary to an immune mechanism, leading to inflammation and deposition of mucopolysaccharides and collagen in the extraocular muscles and orbital fat. Involvement of the extraocular muscles may lead to a restrictive strabismus. Lid retraction and exophthalmos may cause corneal exposure and infection or perforation. Involvement of the posterior orbit can compress the optic nerve. Treatment of TRO may include the use of systemic corticosteroids, radiation of the orbit, eyelid surgery, strabismus surgery, or orbital decompression to eliminate symptoms and protect vision. The degree of orbital involvement is often independent of the status of the systemic disease.

Other systemic disorders that may cause inflammatory disease within the orbit include lymphoma, sarcoidosis, amyloidosis, polyarteritis nodosa, systemic lupus erythematosus, dermatomyositis, Wegener's granulomatosis, and juvenile xanthogranuloma.

TUMORS OF THE ORBIT. Various tumors occur in and about the orbit in childhood. Among benign tumors, the most common are vascular lesions (principally hemangiomas) and dermoids. Among malignant neoplasms, rhabdomyosarcoma, lymphosarcoma, and metastatic neuroblastoma are the most frequent. Optic gliomas and retinoblastomas that extend into the orbit also occur.

The effects of orbital tumors vary with their locations and growth patterns. The principal signs are proptosis, resistance to retroplacement of the eye, and impairment of eye movement. A palpable mass may be found. Other significant signs are ptosis, optic nerve head congestion, optic atrophy, and loss of vision. Bruit and visible pulsation of the globe are important clues to vascular lesions.

Evaluation of orbital tumors includes ultrasonography, MRI, and CT. Pseudotumor of the orbit also must be considered in children with signs of a mass lesion.

Barone SR, Aiuto LT: Periorbital and orbital cellulitis in the *Haemophilus influenzae* vaccine era. J Pediatr Ophthalmol Strabismus 34:293, 1997.

Haik BG, Jakobiec FA, Ellsworth RM, et al: Capillary hemangioma of the lids and orbit: An analysis of the clinical features and therapeutic results in 101 cases. Ophthalmology 86:760, 1979.

Hawkins DB, Clark RW: Orbital involvement in acute sinusitis: Lessons from 24 childhood patients. Clin Pediatr 16:464, 1977.

Mottow LS, Jakobiec FA: Idiopathic inflammatory orbital pseudotumor in childhood. Arch Ophthalmol 96:1410, 1978.

Pollard ZF, Calhoun J: Deep orbital dermoid with draining sinus. Am J Ophthalmol 79:310, 1975.

Shields JA: Diagnosis and Management of Orbital Tumors. Philadelphia, WB Saunders, 1989.

Shields JA, Bakewell B, Augsberger JJ, et al: Space-occupying orbital masses in children: A review of 250 consecutive biopsies. Ophthalmology 93:379, 1988.

Utresky SH, Kennerdell JS, Gupta JP: Graves' ophthalmopathy in childhood and adolescence. Arch Ophthalmol 98:1963, 1980.

Weiss A, Friendly D, Eglin K, et al: Bacterial periorbital cellulitis in childhood. Ophthalmology 90:195, 1983.

CHAPTER 641
Injuries to the Eye

About one third of all blindness in children results from trauma. Children and adolescents account for a disproportionate number of episodes of ocular trauma. Boys age 11–15 yr are the most vulnerable; their injuries outnumber those in girls by a ratio of about 4:1. The majority of injuries are related to sports, toy darts, other projectiles, sticks, stones, fireworks, and air-powered BB guns. The last cause particularly devastating ocular and orbital injuries. Much of the trauma is avoidable. See Chapter 57.

ECCHYMOSES AND SWELLING OF THE EYELIDS. These are common after blunt trauma. Hemorrhage into the lids and periorbital region ("black eye" or "shiner") is usually of no consequence and absorbs spontaneously, but it should prompt careful examination of the eye for deeper, more serious injury, such as a blowout fracture of the orbit, an intraocular hemorrhage, or rupture of the globe.

LACERATIONS OF THE EYELIDS. These require careful management. Horizontal laceration of the upper lid may involve the levator, the tarsal plate, or the orbital septum. Faulty repair can result in ptosis, distortion of the lid, or herniation of orbital fat. Lacerations involving the lid margins require meticulous surgical apposition to prevent notching, eversion, or inversion of the margin or misdirection of the lashes that might lead to epiphora (tear overflow), wetting defects of the cornea, and chronic irritation. Lacerations situated near the medial canthus may involve the punctum, canaliculi, or nasolacrimal duct and require microsurgical repair by an experienced ophthalmic surgeon. In all cases of lid laceration, examination of the globe for perforating injury is mandatory.

SUPERFICIAL ABRASIONS OF THE CORNEA. When the corneal epithelium is scratched, abraded, or denuded, it exposes the underlying epithelial basement layer and superficial corneal nerves. This is accompanied by pain, tearing, photophobia, and decreased vision. Corneal abrasions are detected by instilling fluorescein dye and inspecting the cornea using a blue-filtered light. A slit lamp is ideal for this examination, but a hand-held Wood's lamp is adequate for young children.

Treatment of a corneal abrasion is directed at promoting healing and relieving pain. Abrasions are treated with frequent applications of a topical antibiotic ointment until the epithelium is completely healed. The use of a semi-pressure patch does not improve healing time or decrease pain. Furthermore, an improperly applied patch may itself abrade the cornea. A topical cycloplegic agent (cyclopentolate hydrochloride 1%) can relieve the pain from ciliary spasm in patients with large abrasions. Topical anesthetics should not be given at home because they retard epithelial healing and inhibit the natural blinking reflex.

FOREIGN BODY ON OR IN THE CORNEA OR CONJUNCTIVA. This usually produces acute discomfort, lacrimation, and inflammation. Most foreign bodies can be detected by examination in good light with the aid of magnification; a direct ophthalmoscope set on a high plus lens (+10 or +12) is helpful. In many cases, slit-lamp examination is necessary, especially if the particle is deep or metallic. Some conjunctival foreign bodies tend to lodge under the upper eyelid, causing the sensation of corneal foreign body as they come into contact with the globe on eyelid movement; they may also produce vertically oriented linear corneal abrasions. Finding these abrasions should lead to a suspicion of such a foreign body, and eversion of the lid may be necessary (Chapter 626). If a foreign body is suspected but not found, further examination is indicated. If the history suggests injury with a high-velocity particle, roentgenographic examination of the eye may be needed to explore the possibility of intraocular foreign body.

Removal of a foreign body can be facilitated by instillation of a drop of topical anesthetic. Many foreign bodies can be removed by irrigating or by gently wiping them away with a moistened cotton-tipped applicator. Embedded foreign bodies should be treated by an ophthalmologist. Removal of corneal foreign bodies may leave epithelial defects, which are treated as corneal abrasions. Metallic foreign bodies may cause rust to form in the corneal tissues; examination by an ophthalmologist a day or two after removal of a foreign body is recommended, because a rust ring would require further treatment (curettage).

LACERATIONS AND PERFORATING WOUNDS OF THE CORNEA OR SCLERA. These require immediate referral to an ophthalmologist and prompt surgical repair if the eye and vision are to be saved. Important clues to perforating injury of the eye are collapse of the anterior chamber, distortion and displacement of the pupil, and protrusion of dark tissue (uvea) into the wound. Emergency treatment consists of protecting the injured eye from further damage by applying a sterile bandage and a rigid eye shield. If these medical supplies are not on hand, an adequate eye shield can be fashioned from a plastic or styrofoam cup or from a piece of cardboard bent into a box or cone shape. Manipulation should be kept to a minimum, and no medication should be instilled except under the direction of an ophthalmologist.

HYPHEMA. This is the presence of blood in the anterior chamber of the eye. It may occur with either a blunt or perforating injury. Hyphema appears as a bright or dark red fluid level between the cornea and iris or as a diffuse murkiness of the aqueous humor. Children with hyphema have pain and may be somnolent. The treatment of hyphema usually includes bed rest, with the head elevated 30–45 degrees to promote settling and resorption of the blood. Hospitalization and sedation may be necessary to ensure compliance in some children. In most cases, topical mydriatics, topical or oral corticosteroids, or oral aminocaproic acid are used to prevent rebleeding. Secondary bleeding typically occurs 3–5 days after the initial hemorrhage, increasing the risk of sequelae. The blood in the anterior chamber may produce elevation of intraocular pressure and blood staining of the cornea. These complications may affect vision. In such cases, surgical evacuation of the clot and irrigation of the anterior chamber may be necessary. Patients with sickle cell disease or trait are at higher risk for acute loss of vision and rebleeding and may require more aggressive intervention. Individuals with a history of traumatic hyphema have an increased incidence of glaucoma later in life.

CHEMICAL INJURIES. Chemical burns of the cornea and adnexal tissue are among the most urgent of ocular emergencies. Alkali burns are usually more destructive than acid burns because they react with fats to form soaps, which damage cell membranes, allowing further penetration of the alkali into the eye. Acids generally cause less severe, more localized tissue damage. The corneal epithelium offers moderate protection against weak acids, and little damage occurs unless the pH is 2.5 or less. Most stronger acids precipitate tissue proteins, creating a physical barrier against their further penetration.

Mild acid or alkali burns are characterized by conjunctival injection and swelling and mild corneal epithelial erosions. The corneal stroma may be mildly edematous, and the anterior chamber may have mild to moderate cell and flare. With strong acids, the cornea and conjunctiva rapidly become white and opaque. The corneal epithelium may slough, leaving a relatively clear stroma; this appearance may initially mask the severity of the burn. Severe alkali burns are characterized by corneal opacification.

Emergency treatment of a chemical burn begins with copious immediate irrigation with water or saline. Local debridement and removal of foreign particles should be performed while still irrigating. If the nature of the chemical injury is unknown, the use of pH test paper is helpful in determining whether the agent was basic or acidic. Irrigation should continue for at least 30 min or until 2 L of irrigant has been instilled in mild cases and for 2–4 hr or until 10 L of irrigant has been instilled in severe cases. At the end of irrigation, the pH should be within a normal range (7.3–7.7). The pH should be checked again approximately 30 min after irrigation to ensure that it has not changed.

FRACTURES. A *direct orbital floor fracture* is a floor fracture associated with an orbital rim fracture. An *indirect orbital floor fracture* is an isolated floor fracture and is more commonly known as a blowout fracture. Floor fractures are common when objects larger than the orbital opening, such as a ball, fist, or the dashboard of an automobile, strike the orbit, particularly the inferior lateral orbit.

The most obvious clinical sign of an orbital floor fracture is limitation of upward gaze. Additional signs include lower eyelid ecchymosis, nosebleed, orbital emphysema, and hypesthesia of the ipsilateral cheek and upper lip. The last results from disruption of the infraorbital nerve as it traverses the orbital floor.

The best imaging techniques to visualize orbital fractures are plain-film radiography and CT. The Waters view best demonstrates the orbital floor and maxillary sinus.

Treatment for children with acute orbital fractures includes antibiotic prophylaxis, nasal decongestants, and ice packs. If entrapment of the extraocular muscles (resulting in restriction of movement of the eye and diplopia) and herniation of orbital fat or of the eye itself (resulting in enophthalmos) occur, then surgical repair may be necessary.

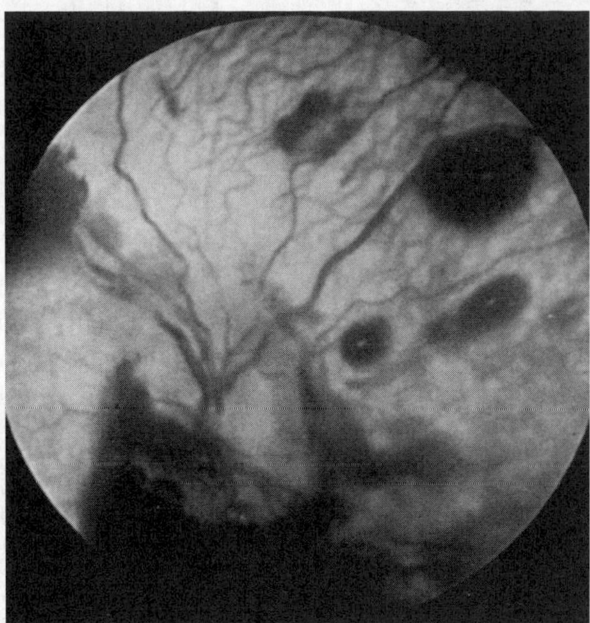

Figure 641–1 Retinal hemorrhages in the abused child with subdural hematoma.

PENETRATING WOUNDS OF THE ORBIT. These demand careful evaluation for possible damage to the eye, the optic nerve, or the brain. Examination should include investigation for retained foreign body. Orbital hemorrhage and infection are common with penetrating wounds of the orbit; such injuries must be treated as emergencies.

CHILD ABUSE. This is a major cause of injuries to the eye and orbital region. The manifestations are numerous and may have a prominent role in recognition of this syndrome. The possibility of nonaccidental trauma must be considered in any child with ecchymosis or laceration of the lids, hemorrhage in or about the eye, cataract or dislocated lens, retinal detachment, or fracture of the orbit (Fig. 641–1). Also see Chapter 35.

FIREWORKS-RELATED INJURIES. Injuries related to the use of fireworks can be the most devastating of all ocular trauma that occurs in children. At least one fifth of emergency room visits for fireworks-related injuries are for ocular trauma. In the United States, a majority of these injuries take place around Independence Day, and most occur despite adult supervision.

SPORTS-RELATED OCULAR INJURIES AND THEIR PREVENTION. Although sports injuries occur in all age groups, far more children and adolescents participate in high-risk sports than do adults. The greater number of participating children, their athletic immaturity, and the increased likelihood of their using inadequate or improper eye protection account for their disproportionate share of sports-related eye injuries. See Chapter 690.

The sports with the highest risk of eye injury are those in which no eye protection can be worn, including boxing, wrestling, and martial arts. High-risk sports include those that use a rapidly moving ball or puck, bat, stick, racquet, or arrow (baseball, hockey, lacrosse, racquet sports, and archery) or involve aggressive body contact (football and basketball). Related to both risk and frequency of participation, the highest percentage of eye injuries are in basketball and baseball.

Protective eyewear, designed for a specific activity, is available for most sports. For basketball, racquet sports, and other recreational activities that do not require a helmet or face mask, molded polycarbonate sports goggles that are secured to the head by an elastic strap are suggested. For hockey, football, lacrosse, and baseball (batter), specific helmets with polycarbonate face shields and guards are available. Children should also wear sports goggles under the helmets. For baseball, goggles and helmets should be worn for batting, catching, and base running; goggles alone are usually sufficient for other positions.

American Academy of Pediatrics Committee on Sports Medicine and Fitness, American Academy of Ophthalmology Committee on Eye Safety and Sports Ophthalmology: Protective eyewear for young athletes. Pediatrics 98:311, 1996.

Catalono RA: Eye injuries and prevention. Pediatr Clin North Am 40:827, 1993.

Deutsch TA, Weinreb RN, Goldberg MF: Indications for surgical management of hyphema in patients with sickle cell trait. Arch Ophthalmol 102:566, 1984.

Gottsch JD: Hyphema: Diagnosis and management. Retina 10(Suppl 1):S65, 1990.

Hofman RF, Paul TO, Pentelei-Molner J: The management of corneal birth trauma. J Pediatr Ophthalmol Strabismus 18:45, 1981.

Kaiser PK: A comparison of pressure patching versus no patching for corneal abrasions due to trauma or foreign body removal. Corneal Abrasion Patching Study Group. Ophthalmology 102:1936, 1995.

Lavrich JB, Goldberg DS, Nelson LB, et al. Visual outcome of severe eye injuries during the amblyopiagenic years. Binocular Vision 9:39, 1994.

Levin AV: Ocular manifestations of child abuse. Ophthalmol Clin North Am 3:249, 1990.

Nelson LB, Wilson TW, Jeffers JB: Eye injuries in childhood: Demography, etiology and prevention. Pediatrics 84:438, 1989.

Pfister RR: Chemical injuries of the eye. Ophthalmology 90:1246, 1983.

Serious eye injuries associated with fireworks—United States, 1990–1994. MMWR Morbid Mortal Wkly Rep 44:449, 1995.

Smith GA, Knapp JF, Barnett TM, et al: The rocket's red glare, the bombs bursting in air: Fireworks-related injuries to children. Pediatrics 98, 1 1996.

PART XXIX

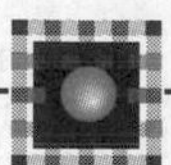

The Ear*

Margaret Kenna

Chapter 642
Clinical Manifestations

Eight prominent signs and symptoms are associated primarily with diseases of the ear and temporal bone. These are discussed in the paragraphs that follow.

OTALGIA. This is usually associated with inflammation of the external and middle ear, but it may also arise from involvement of the teeth, temporomandibular joint, or pharynx. In young infants, pulling or rubbing the ear or general irritability, especially when either is associated with fever, may be the only sign of ear pain. Nonetheless, pulling the ear is not diagnostic of ear pathology.

PURULENT OTORRHEA. This is a sign of otitis externa, otitis media with perforation of the tympanic membrane or drainage from the middle ear through a patent tympanostomy tube, or both. Bloody discharge may be associated with acute or chronic inflammation, trauma, neoplasm, foreign body, or blood dyscrasias. Clear drainage suggests either a perforation of the drum with a serous middle-ear effusion or a cerebrospinal fluid leak draining through a defect in the external auditory canal or from the middle ear through the tympanic membrane.

HEARING LOSS. This results from disease of either the external or middle ear (conductive hearing loss) or from pathology in the inner ear, retrocochlear structures, or central auditory pathways (sensorineural hearing loss). The most common cause of hearing loss in children is otitis media.

SWELLING. Swelling around the ear is most commonly a result of inflammation (external otitis, perichondritis, mastoiditis), trauma (hematoma), or, on rare occasions, neoplasm.

VERTIGO. This is not a common complaint in children; the child or parent may not volunteer information about balance unless asked directly. *Vertigo*, a specific type of dizziness, is defined as any hallucination, illusion, or sensation of motion; *dizziness* refers to any altered orientation in space and is less specific than vertigo. The most frequent cause of dizziness in young children is eustachian tube–middle-ear disease, but true vertigo may also be caused by labyrinthitis, perilymphatic fistula between the inner and middle ear due to a congenital inner ear defect, trauma, cholesteatoma in the mastoid or middle ear, vestibular neuronitis, benign paroxysmal positional vertigo, Ménière disease, or disease of the central nervous system. Older children may describe a feeling of spinning or turning, whereas younger children may express the dysequilibrium only by falling, stumbling, or clumsiness.

NYSTAGMUS. Unidirectional, horizontal, or jerk nystagmus, usually associated with vertigo, is vestibular in origin.

TINNITUS. Although infrequently described spontaneously by children, tinnitus is common, especially in patients with eustachian tube–middle-ear disease or with conductive or sensorineural hearing loss. Children often describe tinnitus if asked directly about it, including laterality and the quality of the sound.

FACIAL PARALYSIS. This is an infrequent but frightening condition for both children and parents. When resulting from disease within the temporal bone in children, it most commonly occurs as a complication of acute or chronic otitis media or cholesteatoma. It may also be due to Bell palsy, the Ramsay Hunt syndrome (herpes zoster oticus), Lyme disease, fracture, neoplasm, or infection of the temporal bone. Congenital facial paralysis may be due to birth trauma or congenital abnormality of the 7th nerve or may be associated with other cranial nerve abnormalities and craniofacial anomalies.

PHYSICAL EXAMINATION. Adequately examining the entire child, paying special attention to the head and neck, can reveal a condition that may predispose to or be associated with ear disease. The facial appearance and the character of speech may be important clues to an abnormality of the ear or hearing. Many of the craniofacial anomalies, such as cleft palate, mandibulofacial dysostosis (Treacher Collins syndrome) and 21-trisomy (Down syndrome), are associated with disorders of the ear. Mouth breathing and hyponasality may indicate intranasal or postnasal obstruction; hypernasality is a sign of velopharyngeal insufficiency. Examining the oropharyngeal cavity may uncover an overt cleft palate or a submucous cleft, both of which predispose to otitis media with effusion. A bifid uvula may also be associated with middle-ear disease. Further examination may reveal posterior nasal or pharyngeal inflammation and discharge. Nasal polyposis, severe deviation of the nasal septum, or a nasopharyngeal tumor may be associated with otitis media.

The *position* of the patient for examination of the ear, nose, and throat depends on the patient's age, ability to cooperate, clinical setting, and preference of the examiner. The child can be examined on an examination table or in the parent's lap. The presence of a parent or assistant is usually necessary to help restrain the baby, because, undue movement may prevent adequate evaluation (Fig. 642–1). Some clinicians prefer to place an infant prone on the table, whereas others prefer the patient to be supine. Use of the examining table may also be desirable for older infants who are uncooperative or when a procedure, such as microscopic evaluation or tympanocentesis, is performed. Infants and young children who are not struggling too actively can be evaluated adequately while sitting on the parent's lap. When necessary, a child may be restrained firmly on a adult's lap if the parent folds the child's wrists and arms over the child's own abdomen with one hand and holds the child's head against the parent's chest with the other hand. If necessary, the child's legs can be held between the parent's knees and thighs. Some infants can be examined by placing their head on the parent's knee. Cooperative children sitting in a chair or on the edge of an examination table can usually be evaluated successfully. The examiner should hold the otoscope with the hand or finger placed firmly against the child's head or face, so that the otoscope moves with the head rather than causes trauma or pain to the ear canal if the child moves suddenly. Pulling up and out on the pinna usually straightens the ear canal enough to allow exposure of the tympanic mem-

*Modified from sections in the 15th edition by James Arnold.

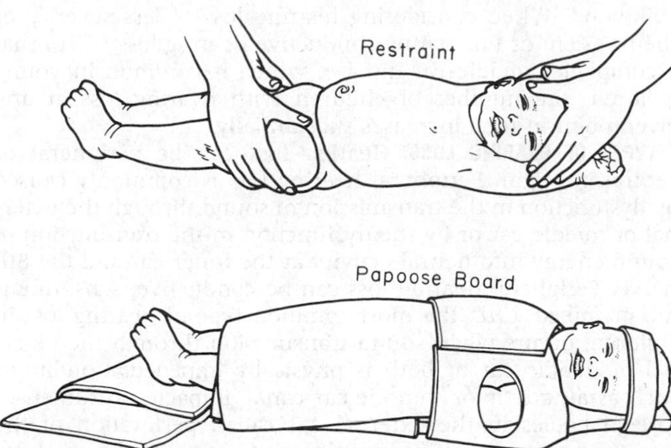

Figure 642–1 Methods of restraining an infant for examination and for procedures such as tympanocentesis or myringotomy. (From Bluestone CD, Klein JO: Otitis Media in Infants and Children, 2nd ed. Philadelphia, WB Saunders, 1995, p 91.)

brane. In young infants, the tragus must be moved forward and out of the way.

Examining the ear itself is the most critical assessment. The auricle and external auditory meatus should be examined first, because the presence or absence of signs of infection in these areas may aid later in the differential diagnosis or evaluation of complications of otitis media. For instance, eczematoid external otitis may result from acute otitis media with discharge, or inflammation of the posterior auricular area may indicate a periosteitis or subperiosteal abscess extending from the mastoid air cells. The presence of preauricular pits or skin tags should also be noted, because affected children have a slightly higher incidence of sensorineural hearing loss.

Before adequate visualization of the external canal and tympanic membrane is possible, obstructing cerumen must often be removed from the canal. **Removal of cerumen** can usually be accomplished by using an otoscope with a surgical head and a wire loop or a blunt cerumen curette or by irrigating the ear canal *gently* with warm water (irrigate only in the presence of an intact eardrum!). Instillation of hydrogen peroxide (3% solution), Domeboro solution, or alcohol in the ear canal for 2–3 min softens cerumen and may facilitate removal with subsequent irrigation. Use of some commercial preparations (trolamine polypeptide oleate–condensate [Cerumenex] or carbamide peroxide [Debrox]) may cause dermatitis of the external canal and is not routinely recommended; if used, it should always be under a physician's supervision. The absence of cerumen associated with inflammation of the ear canal often indicates external otitis. Abnormalities of the external auditory canal include stenosis, edema, otorrhea, and the presence of foreign bodies or abnormal-appearing debris (not just normal-looking cerumen). Whitish flaky debris in the ear canal may indicate the presence of a cholesteatoma, whereas thick whitish "clumpy" debris suggests external otitis. The external canal of newborns is filled with vernix caseosa, which is soft and pale yellow and should disappear shortly after birth.

The tympanic membrane and its mobility are properly assessed by using a pneumatic otoscope. The normal tympanic membrane is in the neutral position; a drum that is bulging is a condition that may be caused by increased (positive) middle-ear air pressure, by an effusion within the middle ear, or by both; visualization of the malleus handle and short process is obscured by a bulging drum. Retraction of the tympanic membrane usually indicates negative middle-ear pressure, but it may also result from previous middle-ear or tympanic membrane disease and subsequent fixation of the ossicles, ossicular ligaments, or tympanic membrane. When retraction is present, the short process of the malleus is prominent and the long process is foreshortened.

The normal tympanic membrane has a ground-glass or waxed paper appearance; a blue or yellow appearance usually indicates a middle-ear effusion. A red tympanic membrane alone may not indicate pathology, because the blood vessels of the drum head may be engorged as a result of crying, sneezing, or blowing the nose. A normal tympanic membrane is also translucent, allowing the observer to look through it to visualize the middle-ear landmarks—incudostapedial joint, promontory, round window niche, and frequently the chorda tympani nerve. If a middle-ear effusion is present medial to a translucent drum, an air-fluid level or bubbles of air mixed with the fluid may be visible. Inability to visualize the middle-ear structures indicates opacification of the drum, usually caused by thickening of the tympanic membrane, a middle-ear effusion, or both. Assessment of the light reflex is generally not helpful, as a middle ear full of fluid reflects the light at least as well as a normal middle-ear space without fluid.

Normal and abnormal middle-ear pressures are reflected in the pattern of **tympanic membrane mobility** when positive and then negative pressures are applied to the external canal using a pneumatic otoscope; a rubber ring around the tip of the distal end of the ear speculum may help to obtain a better seal in the external auditory canal. Normal middle-ear pressure is reflected by the neutral position of the tympanic membrane as well as by its brisk response to both positive and negative pressures.

The eardrum may be retracted, usually because negative middle-ear pressure is present. The normally compliant membrane is maximally retracted by even moderate negative middle-ear pressure and hence cannot visibly be deflected inward further with applied positive pressure in the ear canal. Negative pressure produced by releasing the rubber bulb of the pneumatic otoscope, however, causes a return of the eardrum toward the neutral position if a negative pressure equivalent to that in the middle ear can be created by releasing the rubber bulb; retracted tympanic membranes may occur in both the presence and absence of middle-ear fluid, and if the middle-ear fluid is mixed with air, the tympanic membrane may still have some mobility. When the middle-ear pressure is even more negative, there may be only slight outward mobility of the tympanic membrane because of the limited negative pressure that can be applied through most otoscopes. When assessing the mobility of the tympanic membrane in which negative middle-ear pressure is present, return of the tympanic membrane to the resting retracted position after the application of negative external canal pressure should not be confused with movement to applied positive pressure. This "rebound" of the eardrum after applied negative pressure may lead the examiner to conclude erroneously that the tympanic membrane is mobile to both positive and negative pressures and that, therefore, the middle-ear pressure is normal. If the eardrum is severely retracted with extremely high negative middle-ear pressure or in the presence of a middle-ear effusion or both, the examiner should not be able to produce significant outward movement with pneumatic otoscopy.

The tympanic membrane that exhibits fullness (bulging) moves to applied positive pressure but not to applied negative pressure if the pressure within the middle ear is positive and air, with or without an effusion, is present. A full tympanic membrane and positive middle-ear pressure without a middle-ear effusion are frequently found in neonates and in young infants who are crying during the otoscopic examination; in older infants and children, the same situation may be encountered when the nose is obstructed. However, in the initial stage of acute otitis media, the tympanic membrane may be full, with the characteristic findings of pneumatic otoscopy described before, because air is usually present within the middle ear. When the middle-ear–mastoid air cell system is filled with

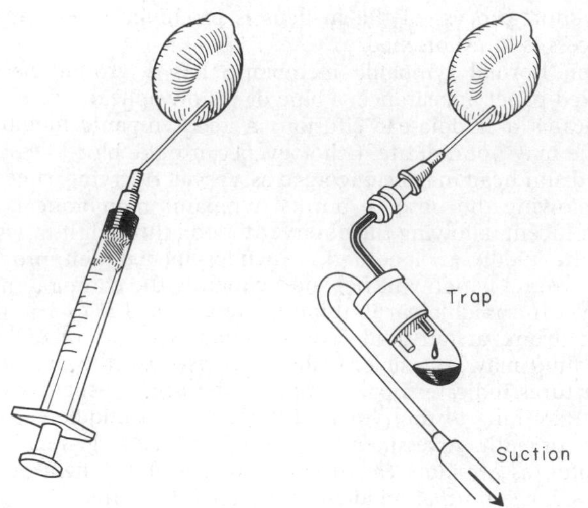

Figure 642–2 Tympanocentesis can be performed with a needle attached to a tuberculin syringe *(left)* or by using an Alden-Senturia collection trap (Storz Instrument Co, St. Louis). (From Bluestone CD, Klein JO: Otitis Media in Infants and Children, 2nd ed. Philadelphia, WB Saunders, 1995, p 127.)

an effusion and little or no air is present, the mobility of the bulging tympanic membrane is severely decreased or absent in response to both applied positive and negative pressures.

Aspiration of the middle ear is the definitive method of verifying the presence and type of a middle-ear effusion. Diagnostic tympanocentesis is performed by inserting, through the inferior portion of the tympanic membrane, an 18-gauge spinal needle attached to a syringe or a collection trap (Fig. 642–2). Alcohol cleansing and culturing of the ear canal should precede tympanocentesis and culture of the middle-ear aspirate. External ear canal culture helps to determine whether organisms cultured from the middle ear are contaminants from the external canal or true pathogens from the middle ear.

Further diagnostic studies of the ear and hearing include audiometric evaluation, impedance audiometry (tympanometry), acoustic reflectometry, and specialized eustachian tube function studies. Diagnostic imaging studies, including CT and MRI, often provide further information about anatomic abnormalities and the extent of inflammatory processes or neoplasms. Specialized assessment of labyrinthine function should be considered in the evaluation of a child with a suspected vestibular disorder (Chapter 647).

CHAPTER 643
Hearing Loss

INCIDENCE AND PREVALENCE. Although estimates vary because of differences in criteria for defining hearing impairment, the age group surveyed, and the testing methods used, from 1–2 newborns / 1,000 live births have moderate (30–50 dB), severe (50–70 dB) or profound (70 dB or greater) bilateral sensorineural hearing loss (SNHL), including 0.5–1 / 1,000 with bilateral SNHL exceeding 75 dB. An additional 1–2 / 1,000 may have milder or unilateral impairments; by age 19 yr, the prevalence doubles. Unilateral SNHL of 45 dB or greater occurs in 3/1,000 U.S. school children; hearing loss of 26 dB or greater occurs in 13/1,000. Onset of hearing loss can occur at any time in childhood. When considering hearing loss of less severity or the transient or fluctuating conductive hearing loss (CHL) that accompanies middle-ear disease, which is common in young children, the number of children with hearing loss at any given point in time increases substantially.

TYPES OF HEARING LOSS. Hearing loss can be peripheral or central in origin. Peripheral hearing loss is commonly caused by dysfunction in the transmission of sound through the external or middle ear or by the dysfunction in the transduction of sound energy into neural activity at the inner ear and the 8th nerve. Peripheral hearing loss can be conductive, sensorineural, or mixed. *CHL*, the most common type of hearing loss in children, occurs when sound transmission through the external or middle ear or both is physically impeded. Conditions such as an atretic or stenotic ear canal, impacted cerumen or foreign bodies in the external ear canal, perforation of the tympanic membrane, interruption or fixation of the ossicular chain, otitis media with effusion, otosclerosis, and cholesteatoma can cause conductive hearing loss. Damage to or maldevelopment of structures in the inner ear, such as destruction of hair cells because of noise, disease, or ototoxic agents, cochlear malformation, perilymphatic fistula of the round or oval window membrane, and lesions of the acoustic division of the 8th nerve cause *SNHL*. A combined CHL and SNHL is considered a *mixed hearing loss*.

Auditory deficits originating along the central auditory nervous system pathways from the proximal 8th nerve to the cerebral cortex are generally considered central (also called retrocochlear) hearing losses. Tumors or demyelinating disease of the 8th nerve and cerebellopontine angle can cause hearing deficits but spare the outer, middle, and inner ear. These causes of hearing loss are rare in children. Other forms of central auditory deficits, known as central auditory processing disorders, include those that make it difficult even for children with normal hearing to listen selectively in the presence of noise, to combine information from the two ears properly, to process speech when it is slightly degraded, and to integrate auditory information that is delivered faster than at a slow rate. These deficits are often manifested as poor attention or academic achievement or as behavior problems in school. Strategies for coping with such disorders are available, and identification and documentation of the central auditory processing disorder is often valuable because parents and teachers are made aware of a valid reason for the child's poor attention or behavior and adjustments can be made.

ETIOLOGY. The etiology of a hearing impairment depends on whether the hearing loss is conductive or sensorineural. CHL may be congenital or acquired. Anomalies of the pinna, external ear canal, tympanic membrane, and ossicles are the most common causes of the CHL. Less commonly, congenital cholesteatoma or (very rarely) other masses in the middle ear may present as CHL. The majority of CHL is acquired; otitis media in its various forms is the most common cause. Tympanic membrane perforation (trauma, tympansotomy tubes, otitis media), ossicular discontinuity (infection, cholesteatoma, trauma), tympanosclerosis, acquired cholesteatoma, or masses in the ear canal or middle ear (Langerhans' cell histiocytosis, salivary gland tumors, glomus tumors, rhabdomyosarcoma) may also present as CHL. Uncommon diseases affecting the middle ear and temporal bone that may present with CHL include otosclerosis, osteopetrosis, fibrous dysplasia, and osteogenesis imperfecta.

SNHL may be congenital or acquired. Causes of SNHL include genetic, infectious, autoimmune, anatomic, traumatic, ototoxic, and idiopathic factors. The most common infectious cause of congenital SNHL is cytomegalovirus (CMV), with which 1/100 newborns in the United States are infected. Of these, 6,000–8,000 infants will have clinical manifestations, including approximately 75% with SNHL. Congenital CMV warrants special attention because it is associated with hearing loss in its symptomatic and asymptomatic forms; the hearing loss may be progressive. Some children with congenital CMV have suddenly lost residual hearing at age 4–5 yr. Other less common congenital infectious causes of SNHL include toxoplasmosis and syphilis. Congenital CMV, toxoplasmosis, and syphilis all may also present with delayed onset of SNHL months to years after birth. Rubella, once the most common viral cause of congenital SNHL, is now very uncommon because of effective vaccination programs. Prenatal infection with herpes is rare, and hearing loss as the only manifestation is very unusual.

Other postnatal infectious causes of SNHL include bacterial meningitis. Group B streptococcal sepsis is encountered in newborns, and *Streptococcus pneumoniae* is the most common cause of bacterial meningitis that results in SNHL after the neonatal period. *Haemophilus influenzae*, once the most common cause of meningitis resulting in SNHL, is now rare owing to the Hib vaccine.

Uncommon infectious causes of SNHL include bacterial meningitis, Lyme disease, parvovirus B19, and varicella. Mumps, rubella, and rubeola, all once common causes of SNHL in children, are rare owing to vaccination programs.

Genetic causes of SNHL are probably responsible for as many as 50% of SNHL cases. These disorders may be associated with other abnormalities, may be part of a named syndrome, or may exist in isolation. SNHL often occurs with abnormalities of the ear and eye and with disorders of the metabolic, musculoskeletal, integumentary, renal, and nervous systems. Autosomal dominant hearing losses account for about 10% of all cases of childhood SNHL. Waardenburg (types I and II) and branchio-otorenal syndromes represent two of the most common autosomal dominant syndromic types of SNHL. Autosomal recessive genetic SNHL, both syndromic and nonsyndromic, accounts for about 38% of all childhood cases of SNHL. Usher syndrome (types I, II, and III), Pendred syndrome, and the Jervell and Lange-Nielsen syndrome (a form of the long Q-T syndrome) are three of the most common-syndromic recessive types of SNHL. Whereas children with an easily identified syndrome or with anomalies of the outer ear may be identified as being at risk for hearing loss and monitored adequately, nonsyndromic children present greater difficulty. Mutations of the connexin-26 gene have been identified in autosomal recessive and autosomal dominant and in sporadic nonsyndromic patients with SNHL. Sex-linked disorders associated with SNHL, thought to account for 1–2% of SNHL, include Norrie syndrome, the otopalatal digital syndrome, and Alport syndrome. Chromosomal abnormalities such as 13–15-trisomy, 18-trisomy, and 21-trisomy can also be accompanied by hearing impairment. Patients with Turner syndrome have monosomy for all or part of one X chromosome and may have CHL, SNHL, or mixed hearing loss. The hearing loss may be progressive. Mitochondrial genetic abnormalities may also result in SNHL.

Agenesis or malformation of cochlear structures, including Scheibe, Mondini, Alexander, and Michel anomalies, and enlarged vestibular aqueducts and semicircular canal anomalies may be genetic. These anomalies probably occur before the 8th wk of gestation and result from arrest in normal development, aberrant development, or both. Many of these anomalies have also been described in association with other congenital conditions such as intrauterine infections (CMV, rubella). These abnormalities are quite common; in as many as 20% of children with SNHL, obvious or subtle temporal bone abnormalities are seen on high-resolution CT scanning or MRI.

CHL can also be genetic. Conditions, diseases, or syndromes that include craniofacial abnormalities are often associated with conductive hearing loss and possibly with SNHL. Pierre Robin, Treacher Collins, Klippel-Feil, and Crouzon and branchio-otorenal syndromes and osteogenesis imperfecta are often associated with hearing loss. Congenital anomalies causing CHL include malformations of the middle-ear structures and atresia of the external auditory canal.

Many genetically determined causes of hearing impairment, including both syndromic and nonsyndromic, do not express themselves until some time after birth. Alport, Alstrom, and Down syndromes, von Recklinghausen's disease, and Hunter-Hurler syndrome are genetic diseases that may have SNHL as a late manifestation.

SNHL may also occur secondary to exposure to toxins, chemicals, and antimicrobials. Early in pregnancy, the embryo is vulnerable to the effects of toxic substances. Ototoxic drugs, including aminoglycosides, loop diuretics and chemotherapeutic agents (cisplatin) may also cause SNHL. Congenital SNHL may occur secondary to exposure to these drugs as well as to thalidomide and retinoids. Certain chemicals, such as quinine, lead, and arsenic, may cause hearing loss both prenatally and postnatally.

Trauma, including temporal bone fractures, inner ear concussion, head trauma, iatrogenic trauma (surgery, extracorporeal membrane oxygenation [ECMO]), radiation, and noise may also cause SNHL. Other very uncommon causes of SNHL in children include immune disease (systemic or limited to the inner ear), metabolic abnormalities, and neoplasms of the temporal bone.

Table 643–1 lists some factors that place a newborn at risk

TABLE 643–1 Indicators Associated With Sensorineural and/or Conductive Hearing Loss

For use with neonates (birth through age 28 days) when universal screening is not available
Family history of hereditary childhood sensorineural hearing loss
In utero infection, such as cytomegalovirus, rubella, syphilis, herpes simplex, or toxoplasmosis
Craniofacial anomalies, including those with morphologic abnormalities of the pinna and ear canal
Birth weight less than 1500 g (3.3 lb)
Hyperbilirubinemia at a serum level requiring exchange transfusion
Ototoxic medications, including but not limited to the aminoglycosides, used in multiple courses or in combination with loop diuretics
Bacterial meningitis
Apgar scores of 0 to 4 at 1 min or 0 to 6 at 5 min
Mechanical ventilation lasting 5 days or longer
Stigmata or other findings associated with a syndrome known to include a sensorineural and/or conductive hearing loss

For use with infants (age 29 days through 2 yr) when certain health conditions develop that require rescreening
Parent/caregiver concern regarding hearing, speech, language, and/or developmental delay
Bacterial meningitis and other infections associated with sensorineural hearing loss
Head trauma associated with loss of consciousness or skull fracture
Stigmata or other findings associated with a syndrome known to include a sensorineural and/or conductive hearing loss
Ototoxic medications, including but not limited to chemotherapeutic agents or aminoglycosides used in multiple courses or in combination with loop diuretics
Recurrent or persistent otitis media with effusion for at least 3 mo

For use with infants (age 29 days through 3 yr) who require periodic monitoring of hearing
(Some newborns and infants may pass initial hearing screening but require periodic monitoring of hearing to detect delayed-onset sensorineural and/or conductive hearing loss. Infants with these indicators require hearing evaluation at least every 6 mo until age 3 yr, and at appropriate intervals thereafter.)
Indicators associated with delayed-onset sensorineural hearing loss include:
Family history of hereditary childhood hearing loss
In utero infection, such as cytomegalovirus, rubella, syphilis, herpes simplex, or toxoplasmosis
Neurofibromatosis type II and neurodegenerative disorders
Indicators associated with conductive hearing loss include:
Recurrent or persistent otitis media with effusion
Anatomic deformities and other disorders that effect eustachian tube function
Neurodegenerative disorders

Adapted from American Academy of Pediatrics, Joint Committee on Infant Hearing: Joint Committee on Infant Hearing 1994 Position Statement. Pediatrics 95:152, 1995.

for hearing impairment. These factors account for about 50% of cases of moderate to profound SNHL in neonates.

EFFECTS OF HEARING IMPAIRMENT. These depend on the nature and degree of the hearing loss and on the individual characteristics of the child. Hearing loss may be unilateral or bilateral, conductive, sensorineural, or mixed; mild, moderate, severe, or profound; of sudden or gradual onset; stable, progressive, or fluctuating; and selective in the region of the acoustic spectrum affected (or it can affect most of the audible spectrum). Factors such as intelligence, medical or physical condition (including accompanying syndromes), family support, age at onset, age at time of identification, and promptness of intervention also affect the impact of hearing loss on a child.

Most hearing-impaired children have some usable hearing. Only 6% of those in the hearing-impaired population have bilateral profound hearing loss. Hearing loss very early in life can affect the development of speech and language, social and emotional development, behavior, attention, and academic achievement. Some cases of hearing impairment are misdiagnosed because affected children have sufficient hearing to respond to environmental sounds, can learn some language, and have some speech but, when challenged in the classroom, cannot perform to full potential.

Even mild or unilateral hearing loss may have a detrimental effect on the development of a young child and on school performance. Children with such hearing impairments have greater difficulty when listening conditions are unfavorable (background noise and poor acoustics), as may occur in a classroom. The fact that schools are auditory-verbal environments is unappreciated by those who minimize the impact of hearing impairment on learning. Hearing loss should be considered in any child with speech and language difficulties, below-par performance, poor behavior, or inattention in school (Table 643–2).

Children with moderate, severe, or profound hearing impairment and those with other handicapping conditions are often educated in classes or schools for children with special needs. The auditory management and choices about modes of communication and education for children with hearing handicaps must be individualized because these children are not a homogeneous group. A team approach to individual case management is essential because each child and family unit represents unique needs and abilities.

HEARING SCREENING. Because hearing impairment can have a major impact on the development of a child and because the earlier the impairment is identified the better is the prognosis, early identification through screening programs is widely and strongly advocated. Data from the Colorado newborn screening program suggest that if hearing-impaired infants are identified and treated by age 6 mo, they (with the exception of children with bilaterally profound impairment) should develop the same level of language as their age-matched peers who are not hearing impaired. This is compelling support for the establishment of mandated newborn hearing screening programs for all children. The American Academy of Pediatrics endorses the goal of universal detection of hearing loss in infants before 3 mo of age, with appropriate intervention no later than 6 mo of age.

Until mandated screening programs are established, many hospitals will continue to use other criteria to screen for hearing loss. Some use the high-risk criteria (see Table 643–1) to decide which infants to screen, some screen all infants who require intensive care, and some do both. The problem with using high-risk criteria to screen is that 50% of the cases of hearing impairment will be missed because the infants are hearing impaired but do not meet any of the high-risk criteria, or they develop hearing loss after the neonatal period. Past screening methods include observing behavioral responses to uncalibrated noisemakers, using automated systems such as the Crib-o-gram or the auditory response cradle (in which movement of the infant in response to sound is recorded by motion sensors), and evoked potentials and otoacoustic emissions (OAE) testing. Sixteen states now have mandated newborn hearing screening programs for all newborns whether high risk or not; other states should follow. The currently recommended hearing screening techniques are either auditory brainstem evoked responses (ABR) or OAE. The ABR test, an auditory evoked electrophysiologic response that

TABLE 643–2 Hearing Handicap as a Function of Average Hearing Threshold Level of the Better Ear

Average Threshold Level (dB) at 500–2,000 Hz (ANSI)	Description	Common Causes	What Can Be Heard Without Amplification	Degree of Handicap (if Not Treated in 1st yr of Life)	Probable Needs
0–15	Normal range	Conductive hearing loss	All speech sounds	None	None
16–25	Slight hearing loss	Otitis media, TM perforation, tympanosclerosis; eustachian tube dysfunction; some SNHL	Vowel sounds heard clearly, may miss unvoiced consonant sounds	Mild auditory dysfunction in laguage learning. Difficulty in perceiving some speech sounds	Consideration of need for hearing aid; speech reading; Auditory training Speech therapy Preferential seating Appropriate surgery
25–30	Mild	Otitis media, TM perforation, tympanosclerosis, severe eustachian dysfunction, SNHL	Hears only some of speech sounds, the louder voiced sounds	Auditory learning dysfunction Mild language retardation Mild speech problems Inattention	Hearing aid Lip reading Auditory training Speech therapy Appropriate surgery
30–50	Moderate hearing loss	Chronic otitis, ear canal/middle ear anomaly, SNHL	Misses most speech sounds at normal conversational level	Speech problems Language retardation Learning dysfunction Inattention	All of the above, plus consideration of special classroom situation
50–70	Severe hearing loss	SNHL or mixed loss due to a combination of middle-ear disease and sensorineural involvement	Hears no speech sound of normal conversations	Severe speech problems Language retardation Learning dysfunction Inattention	All of the above; probable assignment to special classes
70+	Profound hearing loss	SNHL or mixed	Hears no speech or other sounds	Severe speech problems Language retardation Learning dysfunction Inattention	All of the above; probable assignment to special classes or schools

ANSI = American National Standards Institute; TM = tympanic membrane; SNHL = sensorineural hearing loss

Modified from Northern JL, Downs MP: Hearing in Children, 4th ed. Baltimore, Williams & Wilkins, 1991.

correlates highly with hearing, has been used successfully and cost effectively to screen newborns and to identify further the degree and type of hearing loss. OAE tests, used successfully in many newborn screening programs, are inexpensive and provide a sensitive indication of the presence of hearing loss. Results are relatively easy to interpret. OAEs are absent if hearing is worse than 30–40 dB, no matter what the cause, and thus ABR must be used to evaluate these children further.

Many children become hearing impaired after the neonatal period and therefore are not identified by newborn screening programs. It is often not until children are in preschool or kindergarten that hearing screening takes place. Consequently, primary care physicians and pediatricians should be alert to the signs and symptoms of childhood hearing impairment, so that those with hearing impairment who are not screened formally can be identified as early as possible.

Identification of Hearing Impairment. The impact of hearing impairment is greatest on an infant who has yet to develop language; therefore, identification, diagnosis, description, and treatment should begin as soon as possible. In general, infants with a prenatal or perinatal history that puts them at risk (see Table 643–1) or those who have failed a formal hearing screening should be closely monitored by a clinical audiologist experienced in the evaluation and treatment of hearing-impaired children until a reliable assessment of auditory function has been obtained. The primary physician is important in encouraging families to cooperate with the follow-up plan. Infants who are born at risk but who have not been screened as neonates (often because of transfer from one hospital to another) should have a hearing screening by a pediatric audiologist by age 3 mo.

Hearing-impaired infants who are born at risk or screened for hearing loss in a neonatal hearing screening program account for only a portion of those in the pediatric hearing-impaired population. Those who are congenitally deaf because of autosomal recessive inheritance or subclinical congenital infection are often not identified until the 2nd or 3rd yr of life. Usually, the more severe the hearing loss, the earlier is the age at identification, but identification occurs later than the age necessary for an optimal outcome. Children with normal hearing have developed an extensive language by age 3 yr. Parental concern about hearing and any delayed development of speech and language should alert the practitioner; parental concern usually precedes formal identification and diagnosis of hearing impairment by 6 mo–1 yr. Primary care physicians are uniquely able to respond to the concerns of parents and to monitor the development of speech and language. Table 643–3 presents guidelines for screening language development in young children, and Table 643–4 provides guidelines for identifying children with abnormal auditory behavior. Failure to fulfill these criteria should be reason for referral for an audiologic evaluation.

Clinical Audiologic Evaluation. Even the youngest infants can be evaluated for auditory function. When hearing impairment is suspected in a young child, reliable and valid estimates of auditory function can be obtained. Successful treatment strategies for hearing-impaired children rely on prompt identification and ongoing assessment to define the dimensions of auditory function. Cooperation among the pediatrician and those specializing in such areas as audiology, speech and language pathology, education, and child development is necessary to optimize auditory-verbal development. Therapy for hearing-impaired children includes considering (and often fitting) an amplification device; monitoring hearing and auditory skills, counseling parents and families, advising teachers, and dealing with public agencies.

TABLE 643–3 Criteria for Referral for Audiologic Assessment

Age (mo)	Referral Guidelines for Children with "Speech" Delay
12	No differentiated babbling or vocal imitation
18	No use of single words
24	Single-word vocabulary of ≤10 words
30	Fewer than 100 words; no evidence of two-word combinations; unintelligible
36	Fewer than 200 words; no use of telegraphic sentences, clarity <50%
48	Fewer than 600 words; no use of simple sentences; clarity ≤80%

From Matkin ND: Early recognition and referral of hearing-impaired children. Pediatr Rev 6:151, 1984. Reproduced by permission of Pediatrics.

TABLE 643–4 Guidelines for Referral of Children Suspected of Having Hearing Loss

Age (mo)	Normal Development
0–4	Should startle to loud sounds, quiet to mother's voice, momentarily cease activity when sound is presented at a conversational level
5–6	Should correctly localize to sound presented in a horizontal plane, begin to imitate sounds in own speech repertoire or at least reciprocally vocalize with an adult
7–12	Should correctly localize to sound presented in any plane Should respond to name, even when spoken quietly
13–15	Should point toward an unexpected sound or to familiar objects or persons when asked
16–18	Should follow simple directions without gestural or other visual cues; can be trained to reach toward an interesting toy at midline when a sound is presented
19–24	Should point to body parts when asked; by 21–24 mo, can be trained to perform play audiometry

From Matkin ND. Early recognition and referral of hearing-impaired children. Pediatr Rev 6:151, 1984. Reproduced by permission of Pediatrics.

Audiometry. The technique of the audiologic evaluation varies as a function of the age or developmental level of the child, the reason for the evaluation, and the child's otologic condition or history. An audiogram provides the fundamental description of hearing sensitivity (Fig. 643–1). Hearing thresholds are assessed as a function of frequency using pure tones (sine waves) at octave intervals from 250–8,000 Hz. Earphones are typically used, and hearing is assessed independently for each ear. Air-conducted signals are presented through earphones (or loudspeakers) and are used to provide information about the sensitivity of the auditory system. These same test sounds can be delivered to the ear through an oscillator that is placed on the head, usually on the mastoid. Such signals are considered bone-conducted signals because the bones of the skull are vibrated and sound energy is transmitted directly to the inner ear, essentially bypassing the outer and middle ears. In a normal ear, the air and bone conduction thresholds are the same; they are also the same in those with SNHL. In those with CHL, the air and bone conduction thresholds differ. This is called the air-bone gap; it indicates the amount of hearing loss attributable to dysfunction in the outer and/or middle ear. With mixed hearing loss, both the bone and air conduction thresholds are abnormal and there is an air-bone gap.

Speech Recognition Threshold. Another measure useful in describing auditory function is the speech recognition threshold (SRT), which is the lowest intensity level at which a score of approximately 50% correct is obtained on a task of recognizing spondee words. Spondee words are two-syllable words or phrases that have equal stress on each syllable (baseball, hotdog, pancake). Listeners must be familiar with all the words for a valid test result to be obtained. The SRT should correspond to the average of pure-tone thresholds at 500, 1,000, and 2,000 Hz, the pure-tone average (PTA). The SRT is relevant because much of the rationale for assessing hearing in children involves determining the adequacy for development and use of speech and language. It also serves to check the validity of the evaluation because children with nonorganic hearing loss (malingerers) often have a large discrepancy between the PTA and SRT. Audiometric configuration can also affect the SRT-

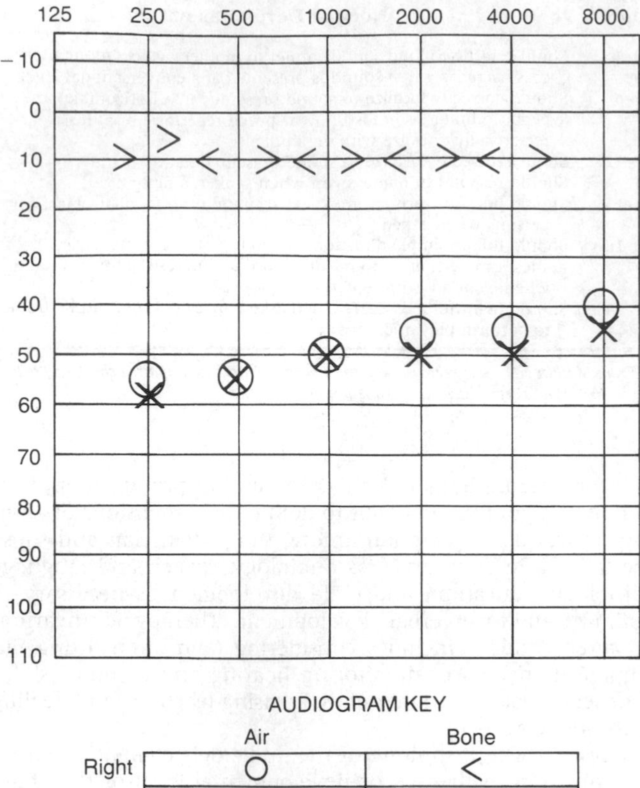

Figure 643–1 Audiogram demonstrating a bilateral conductive hearing loss.

PTA relationship and should be considered before assessing the possibility of malingering.

The basic battery of hearing tests concludes with an assessment of a child's ability to understand monosyllabic words when presented at a comfortable listening level. Performance on such word intelligibility tests assists in the differential diagnosis of hearing impairment and provides a measure of how well a child performs when speech is presented at loudness levels similar to those encountered in the environment.

Play Audiometry. For children at or above the developmental level of a 5- or 6-yr-old, conventional test methods can be used. For children 2-1/2–5 yr old, play audiometry can be used. Responses in play audiometry are usually conditioned motor activities associated with a game, such as dropping blocks in a bucket, placing rings on a peg, stringing beads, or completing a puzzle. The technique can be used to obtain a reliable audiogram for a preschool child. For those who will not or cannot repeat words clearly for the SRT and word intelligibility tasks, pictures can be used with a pointing response.

Visual Reinforcement Audiometry. For those between the ages of about 5–6 mo and 2-1/2 yr, visual reinforcement audiometry (VRA) is commonly used. The technique incorporates a head-turning response with activation of an animated (mechanical) toy reinforcer. If infants are properly conditioned, VRA can provide reliable estimates of hearing sensitivity for tones and speech sounds. In most applications of VRA, sounds are presented by loudspeakers in a sound field, so no ear-specific information is obtained. Assessment of an infant is often designed to rule out hearing loss that would affect the development of speech and language. Normal sound field response levels of infants indicate sufficient hearing for this purpose despite the possibility of different hearing levels in the two ears.

Behavioral Observation Audiometry. For those younger than 5 mo, behavioral hearing assessment is limited to unconditioned, reflexive responses to complex (not frequency-specific) test sounds, such as noise, speech, or music presented using calibrated signals from a loudspeaker or uncalibrated noisemakers. Response levels can vary widely within and among infants and usually do not represent a reliable estimate of sensitivity. Behavioral observation audiometry (BOA) is a screening device.

Assessment of a child with suspected hearing loss is not complete until pure-tone hearing thresholds and SRTs have been obtained in each ear (until a reliable audiogram has been obtained). Estimates of hearing responsivity obtained using BOA or VRA in a sound field (loudspeakers) cannot be used satisfactorily to describe hearing in both ears.

Acoustic Immittance Testing. This is a standard part of the clinical audiologic test battery and includes tympanometry. Acoustic immittance testing is a useful objective assessment technique that provides information about the status of the middle ear. It is helpful in the diagnosis and management of otitis media with effusion, one of the leading causes of mild to moderate hearing loss in young children. Tympanometry may also be performed by physicians.

TYMPANOMETRY. This technique provides a graph of the ability of the middle ear to transmit sound energy (admittance, or compliance) or impede sound energy (impedance) as a function of air pressure in the external ear canal. Because most immittance test instruments measure acoustic admittance, the term *admittance* is used here. The principles apply to whatever units of measure are used.

A probe is inserted into the entrance of the external ear canal so that an airtight seal is obtained. The probe varies air pressure, presents a tone, and measures sound pressure level in the ear canal through the probe assembly. The sound pressure measured in the ear canal relative to the known intensity of the probe signal is used to estimate the acoustic admittance of the ear canal and middle-ear system. Admittance can be expressed in a unit called a millimho (mmho) or as a volume of air (mL) with equivalent acoustic admittance. The test is performed so that an estimate of the volume of air enclosed between the probe tip and tympanic membrane can be made. The acoustic admittance of this volume of air is deducted from the overall admittance measure to obtain a measure of the admittance of the middle-ear system alone. Estimating ear canal volume also has some diagnostic benefit because an abnormally large value is consistent with the presence of an opening in the tympanic membrane (perforation or tube).

With elimination of the admittance of the air mass in the external auditory canal, it is assumed that the remaining admittance measure accurately reflects the admittance of the entire middle-ear system. Its value is largely controlled by the dynamics of the tympanic membrane. Abnormalities of the tympanic membrane can dictate the shape of tympanograms and thus obscure abnormalities that lie beyond the tympanic membrane. In addition, the frequency of the probe tone, the speed and direction of the air pressure change, and the air pressure at which the tympanogram is initiated all are factors that can influence the outcome of tympanometric assessment.

When air pressure in the ear canal is equal to that in the middle ear, the middle-ear system is functioning optimally. Therefore, the ear canal pressure at which there is the greatest flow of energy (admittance) should be a reasonable estimate of the air pressure in the middle-ear space. This pressure is determined by finding the admittance maximum (peak) on the tympanogram and obtaining its value on the *x*-axis. The value on the *y*-axis at the tympanogram peak is an estimate of peak admittance. This peak measure is sometimes referred to

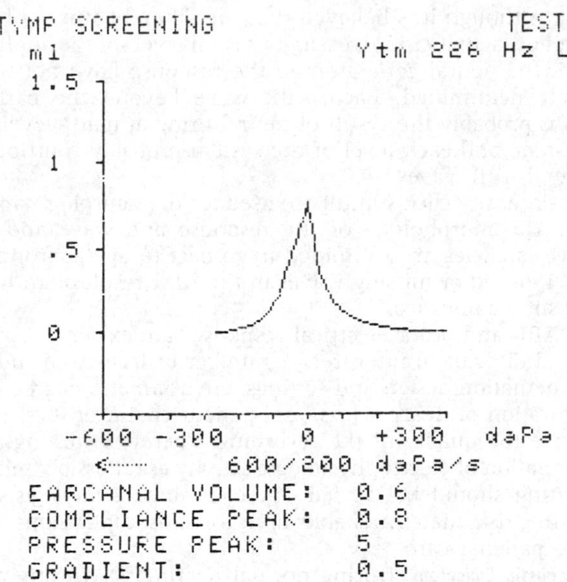

Figure 643–2 Admittance tympanogram of a normal ear of a 7-yr-old child. Ear canal volume, compliance peak (i.e., peak admittance in mL using the y-axis scale), and tympanometric peak pressure and gradient are all within normal limits. For this instrument, the gradient can range from 0 to 1.0, and the sharpest peaks get the highest values.

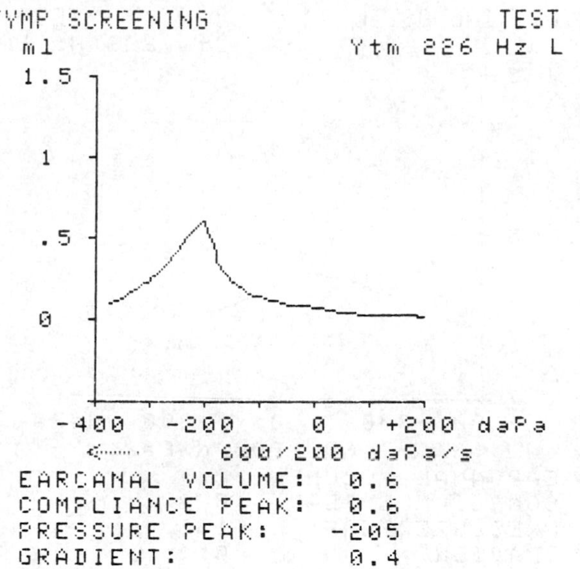

Figure 643–3 Admittance tympanogram of the same ear as that shown in Figure 643–2, only 2 wk earlier. On this occasion, tympanometric peak pressure is abnormal. Whereas the other variables are in the normal range, peak admittance and gradient are both slightly reduced relative to the values shown in Figure 643–2.

as static acoustic admittance, even though it is estimated from a dynamic measure (Fig. 643–2). Table 643–5 presents the norms for peak admittance based on admittance tympanometry for normal adults and children.

Acoustic Reflex Test. This is also part of the immittance test battery. With a properly functioning middle-ear system, admittance at the tympanic membrane changes on activation of the stapedius and tensor tympani muscles. In healthy ears, the stapedial reflex occurs after exposure to loud sounds. Admittance instruments are designed to present reflex activating signals (pure tones of various frequencies or noise), either to the same or the contralateral ear, while monitoring admittance. Very small admittance changes that are time locked to presentations of the signal are considered to be a result of middle-ear muscle reflexes. Absence of admittance changes can occur when the hearing loss is sufficient to prevent the signal from reaching the loudness level necessary to elicit the reflex or when a middle-ear condition affects the ability to monitor a small admittance change. Reflexes cannot usually be measured in those with CHL because of the examiner's inability to measure any change in admittance in an ear with an abnormal transfer system. As a result, the acoustic reflex test is useful in the differential diagnosis of hearing impairment. The acoustic reflex also has applications to the assessment of SNHL and the integrity of the neurologic components of the reflex arc, including cranial nerves VII and VIII.

TABLE 643–5 Norms for Peak (Static) Admittance (in mL) Using a 226-Hz Probe Tone for Children and Adults

		Speed of Air Pressure Sweep	
		*≤50 da/Pa/sec**	*200 da/Pa/sec†*
Children (3–5 yr)	Lower limit	0.30	0.36
	Median	0.55	0.61
	Upper limit	0.90	1.06
Adults	Lower limit	0.56	0.27
	Median	0.85	0.72
	Upper limit	1.36	1.38

**Ear canal volume measurement based on admittance at lowest tail of tympanogram.*
†Ear canal measurement based on admittance at lowest tail of tympanogram for children and at +200 da/Pa for adults.

Adapted from Margolis RH, Shanks JE: Tympanometry: Basic Principles of Clinical Application. In: *Rintelman WS (ed): Hearing Assessment, 2nd ed. Austin, TX, PRO-ED, 1991, pp 179–245.*

Tympanometry in Otitis Media with Effusion. Children with otitis media often have high negative tympanometric peak pressure (Fig. 643–3) or reduced peak admittance values. However, in regard to the diagnosis of middle-ear effusion, the tympanometric measure that has the greatest sensitivity and specificity is the tympanogram shape rather than its peak pressure (poor predictive value) or peak admittance (fair predictive value). This shape is sometimes referred to as the tympanometric gradient or tympanometric width; it measures the degree of roundness or "peakedness" of the tympanogram. The more rounded the peak (or, ultimately, an absent peak), the higher is the probability that an effusion is present (Fig. 643–4). Some instruments compute gradient automatically but others do not. Various ways to compute this gradient can be used; thus, until the measure becomes standardized, the individual characteristics of the instrument used must be known and applied accordingly.

Auditory Brain Stem Response. The ABR test is used for neonatal newborn hearing screening, to confirm hearing loss in young children, to obtain ear-specific information in young children, and to test children who cannot, for whatever reason, cooperate with behavioral test methods. It is also important in the diagnosis of auditory dysfunction and of disorders of the auditory nervous system. The ABR test is a far-field recording of minute electrical discharges from numerous neurons. The stimulus, therefore, must be able to cause simultaneous discharge of the large numbers of neurons involved. Stimuli with very rapid onset, such as clicks or tone bursts, must be used. Unfortunately, the rapid onset required to create a measurable ABR also causes energy to be spread in the frequency domain, reducing the frequency-specificity of the response.

The ABR result is not affected by sedation or general anesthesia. Infants and children from about 6 mo–4 yr of age are routinely sedated to avoid problems related to the electrical interference caused by muscle activity during testing. Also, ABR testing can be performed in the operating room when a child is anesthetized for another procedure.

The ABR is recorded as five to seven waves. Waves I, III,

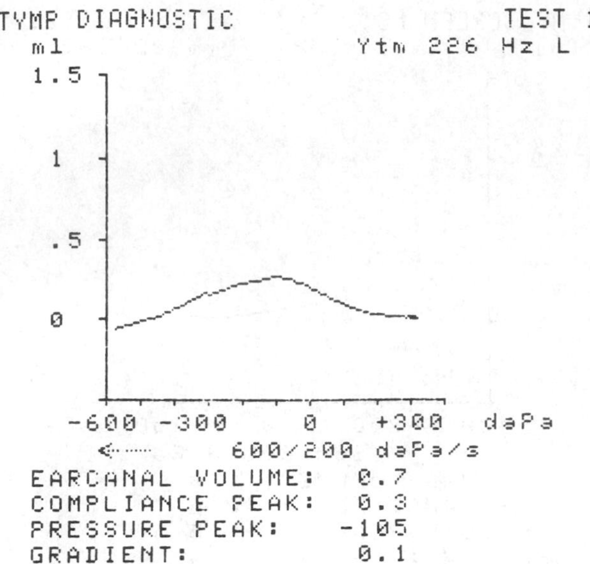

Figure 643–4 Admittance tympanogram of the left ear of a 4-yr-old child with middle-ear effusion. Note that the peak admittance and gradient are both very low, whereas the tympanometric peak pressure is grossly within normal limits.

and V can be obtained consistently in all age groups. Waves II and IV appear less consistently, between and within subjects. The latency of each wave (time of occurrence of the wave peak after stimulus onset) increases, and the amplitude decreases with reductions in stimulus intensity or loudness. Developmental change occurs in the latency of the various waves; latency decreases with increasing age, with the earliest waves reaching mature latency values earlier in life than the later waves.

The ABR test commonly has two major uses in a pediatric setting: (1) It is used as an audiometric test, providing information about the ability of the peripheral auditory system to transmit information to the auditory nerve and beyond, and (2) it is used in the differential diagnosis or monitoring of central nervous system pathology. For the audiometric approach, a search is conducted for the minimum stimulus intensity that yields an observable ABR. Plotting latency versus intensity for various waves also aids in the differential diagnosis of hearing impairment. A major advantage of auditory assessment using the ABR test is that ear-specific threshold estimates can be obtained on infants or otherwise difficult-to-test patients. ABR thresholds using click stimuli are correlated best with behavioral hearing thresholds in the higher frequencies (1,000–4,000 Hz). Measurement of the responsivity of the peripheral auditory system to low-frequency stimuli requires different stimuli (tone bursts or filtered clicks) or the use of masking, neither of which isolates the low-frequency region of the cochlea in all cases. ABR responses for low frequencies should be interpreted by those knowledgeable and experienced in ABR testing.

The ABR test does not assess "hearing." It reflects auditory neuronal electric responses that can be correlated to behavioral hearing thresholds, but a normal ABR result only suggests that the auditory system, up to the level of the midbrain, is responsive to the stimulus used. Conversely, a failure to elicit an ABR indicates an impairment of the system's synchronous response but does not necessarily mean that there is no "hearing." The behavioral response to sound is sometimes normal when no ABR can be elicited (neurologic demyelinating disease). The ABR test may be used to infer whether and at what level of the auditory system an impairment exists. Hearing losses that are sudden, progressive, or unilateral are indications for ABR testing. Although it is believed that the different waves of the ABR reflect activity in increasingly rostral levels of the auditory system, the neural generators of the response have not been precisely determined. Each ABR wave beyond the earliest waves is probably the result of neural firing at many levels of the system, and each level of the system probably contributes to several ABR waves.

High-intensity click stimuli are used for the neurologic application. The morphology of the response and wave and interwave latencies are examined in respect to age-appropriate forms. Delayed or missing waves in the ABR result often have diagnostic significance.

The ABR and other electrical responses are extremely complex and difficult to interpret. A number of factors, including instrumentation design and settings, environment, degree and configuration of hearing loss, and patient characteristics, may influence the quality of the recording. Therefore, testing and interpretation of electrophysiologic activity as it possibly relates to hearing should be carried out by trained audiologists to avoid the risk that unreliable or erroneous conclusions will affect a patient's care.

Otoacoustic Emissions. During normal hearing, OAEs originate from the hair cells in the cochlea and are detected by sensitive amplifying processes. They travel from the cochlea through the middle ear to the external auditory canal, where they can be detected using miniature microphones. Transient evoked OAEs (TEOAEs) may be used to check the integrity of the cochlea. In the neonatal period, detection of OAEs can be accomplished during natural sleep, and TEOAEs can be used as screening tests in infants and children for hearing at the 30 dB level of hearing loss. They are less time consuming and elaborate than ABR and are more sensitive than behavioral tests in young children. TEOAEs are reduced or absent owing to various dysfunctions in the inner ear. They are absent in patients with more than 30 dB of hearing loss and thus cannot be used to determine hearing threshold; rather, they provide a screen for whether hearing is present (30–40 dB or greater) or absent. Diseases such as otitis media or congenitally abnormal middle ear structures reduce the transfer of TEOAEs and may incorrectly indicate a cochlear hearing disorder. If a hearing loss is suspected by the absence of OAE, ABR testing should be used for confirmation and identification of the type, degree, and laterality of hearing loss.

Acoustic reflectometry uses a hand-held instrument that is placed next to the opening of a child's ear canal and delivers an 80-dB sound that varies in frequency from 2,000–4,500 Hz in a 100-msec period. The instrument measures the total level of reflected and transmitted sound. Some investigators and physicians have found this useful to help gauge the presence or absence of middle-ear fluid. It does not, however, provide any information about hearing; if the presence of chronic fluid is suggested by this instrument, audiometric evaluation should be obtained.

TREATMENT. Once a hearing loss is identified, a full developmental and speech and language evaluation is needed. Parental counseling as well as involvement in all stages of the evaluation and eventual treatment or rehabilitation is mandatory. A conductive hearing loss can often be corrected through treatment of a middle-ear effusion or surgical correction of the abnormal sound-conducting mechanism. Children with SNHL should be evaluated for possible hearing aid use. Audiologists with special experience and training in working with children are required. Hearing aids may be fitted for children as young as 2 mo. Compelling evidence from the hearing screening program in Colorado shows that identification and amplification before age 6 mo makes a very significant difference in the speech and language abilities of affected children, compared with those cases identified and amplified after the age of 6 mo. In these children, repeat audiologic testing is needed to reliably identify the degree of hearing loss and to fine-tune the use of hearing aids. The best educational approach to children with significant hearing loss is a subject of ongoing controversy. Because we live in a predominantly speaking world, some have advocated only an auditory and oral approach to hearing therapy. Because affected children often are slow to develop communication skills, a total communication approach has also been advocated; this blends the use of sign language, lip reading, hearing aids, and speaking as appropriate for each individual child. The appropriate program for each child depends on the patient, family, and resources available.

The use of a surgically placed cochlear implant in children with severe to profound hearing loss and little or no help from conventional hearing aids improves the development of communication skills. This is currently approved for use in the United States in children age 2 yr and older. Some members of the hearing-impaired community object to its use in children who have no decision in the matter and who may develop excellent communication abilities using more conventional therapeutic strategies.

CHAPTER 644
Congenital Malformations

The external and middle ears, derived from the 1st and 2nd branchial arches and grooves, grow throughout puberty, but the inner ear, which develops from the otocyst, reaches adult size and shape by mid-fetal development. The ossicles are derived from the 1st and 2nd arches (malleus and incus), and the stapes arises from the 2nd arch and the otic capsule. The ossicles achieve adult size and shape by the 15th wk of gestation for the malleus and incus and 18th wk for the stapes. Although the pinna, ear canal, and tympanic membrane continue to grow after birth, congenital abnormalities of these structures develop during the 1st half of gestation. Malformed external and middle ears may be associated with serious renal anomalies, mandibulofacial dysostosis, hemifacial microsomia, and other craniofacial malformations. In any of the congenital abnormalities of the temporal bone and soft tissue structures of the ear, abnormalities of the facial nerve may be present. Deformed external and middle ears may also be associated with malformations of the inner ear and both conductive and sensorineural hearing loss. Any child born with even a minor abnormality of the pinna, external auditory canal, or eardrum should have a complete audiometric evaluation in the neonatal period.

PINNA MALFORMATIONS. Severe malformations of the external ear are rare, but minor deformities are common. Isolated abnormalities of the external ear occur in approximately 1% of children. A *pit*-like depression just in front of the helix and above the tragus may represent a cyst or an epidermis-lined fistulous tract; these are common, with an incidence of approximately 8/1,000 children. These do not require surgical removal unless there is recurrent infection. Accessory *skin tags,* with an incidence of 1–2/1,000, may be on narrow pedicles and can be removed by simple ligation: if the pedicle is broad based or contains cartilage, the defect should be corrected surgically. An unusually prominent or *"lop" ear* results from lack of bending of the cartilage that creates the antihelix. It may be improved cosmetically in the neonatal period by applying a firm framework (sometimes soldering wire is used) attached by Steri-Strips to the pinna and worn continuously for weeks to months. Otoplasty can be considered in children age 5 yr or older; by this time, the pinna has reached about 80% of its adult size. *Microtia* includes fairly subtle abnormalities of the size, shape, and location of the pinna (and frequently the ear canal) as well as abnormalities with only a few nubbins of cartilage and skin or no pinna and ear canal at all (anotia). Microtic ears are often more anterior and inferior in placement than normal auricles; the facial nerve function and location may frequently be abnormal. Surgery to correct microtia is considered for both cosmetic and functional reasons; children who have some pinna can wear regular glasses, a hearing aid, and earrings and feel more normal in appearance. If the microtia is severe, some patients may opt for creation and attachment of a prosthetic ear, which cosmetically closely resembles a real ear. Surgery to correct severe microtia may involve a multistage procedure including ribgrafts and local soft tissue flaps.

CONGENITAL EXTERNAL AUDITORY CANAL STENOSIS. Stenosis or atresia of the ear canal often occurs in association with malformation of the auricle and middle ear; minor stenoses may occur in isolation. In some genetic syndromes, such as trisomy 21, ear canals are narrow. Audiometric evaluation should be undertaken as soon as possible. Further diagnosis and surgical planning is often aided by CT, sometimes supplemented by MRI, of the temporal bone. Milder cases of ear canal stenosis usually do not require surgical enlargement unless the patient develops significant recurrent/chronic external otitis or severe cerumen impactions that affect hearing. Reconstructive ear canal and middle-ear surgery for atresia is generally considered for patients older than 5 yr with bilateral deformities resulting in a significant conductive hearing loss. Reconstruction is undertaken to improve hearing to a point where the child may not need a hearing aid, or at least to provide an ear canal and pinna so that the child can derive improved benefit from an air conduction hearing aid. Most children with significant hearing loss secondary to bilateral atresia wear bone conduction hearing aids for the first several years of life (because they do not have ear canals) but often do not want to continue to do so as they get older. The development of bone-anchored hearing aids may provide an option for some of these children when they are older. CT evidence of an adequate middle-ear cleft and mastoid is required to consider the surgery; the position of the facial nerve, which is frequently in an abnormal location in these children, also needs to be considered.

CONGENITAL MIDDLE-EAR MALFORMATIONS. Children may have congenital abnormalities of the middle ear as an isolated defect or in association with other abnormalities of the temporal bone, especially the ear canal and pinna, or as part of a syndrome. Affected children usually have conductive hearing losses but may have mixed conductive and sensorineural hearing losses. The most common abnormalities involve the ossicles, with the incus being the most commonly affected. Other uncommon abnormalities of the middle ear include persistent stapedial artery, high-riding jugular bulb, a dehiscent facial nerve, and abnormalities of the shape and volume of the aerated portion of the middle ear and mastoid; all present problems for a surgeon. Depending on the type of abnormality and the presence of other anomalies, surgery may be possible to improve the hearing of some children with middle-ear abnormalities causing hearing loss.

CONGENITAL INNER EAR MALFORMATIONS. Congenital inner ear malformations are uncommon; they are identified as a result of improvements in imaging modalities, especially CT and MRI. As many as 20% of children with sensorineural hearing loss may have anatomic abnormalities identified on CT or MRI. Congenital perilymphatic fistula (PLF) of the oval or round window membrane may present as a rapid-onset, fluctuating, or progressive sensorineural hearing loss with or without vertigo and is often associated with congenital inner ear abnormalities. PLFs may need to be repaired to prevent possible spread of infection from the middle ear to the labyrinth, stabilize hearing loss, and improve vertigo.

Congenital malformations of the inner ear are usually associated with sensorineural hearing loss of various degrees from mild to profound. These malformations may occur as isolated anomalies or in association with other syndromes, genetic abnormalities, or structural abnormalities of the head and neck.

CONGENITAL CHOLESTEATOMA. Congenital cholesteatomas occur 80% of the time in the anterior-superior portion of the middle ear, although they can present in other locations. The middle ear and mastoid are well aerated, and an affected child frequently has no prior history of otitis media or other middle ear disease. A common theory is that these represent a congenital rest of epithelial tissue (the epidermoid formation) that persists beyond 33 wk of gestation, when it would ordinarily disappear. Other theories include squamous metaplasia of the middle ear, entrance of squamous epithelium through a nonintact eardrum into the middle ear, ectodermal implants between the 1st and 2nd brachial arch remnants, and residual amniotic fluid squamous debris. Congenital cholesteatomas usually appear as a white, cystlike structure medial to or within an intact tympanic membrane. Cholesteatoma, either congenital or acquired, should be suspected when deep retraction pockets, keratin debris, chronic drainage, aural granulation tissue, or a mass behind or involving the tympanic membrane is present. As a result, erosion of the ossicles of the middle ear, pressure on the facial nerve, erosion into the inner ear, or exposure of the dura may occur. Besides acting as a benign tumor, the keratinaceous debris of a cholesteatoma is a perfect culture medium and may become a focus of infection for severe chronic otitis media. Cholesteatoma should be removed surgically.

Chapter 645
Diseases of the External Ear

EXTERNAL OTITIS (OTITIS EXTERNA)

In an infant, the outer two thirds of the ear canal is cartilaginous and the inner third is bony, whereas in an older child and adult only the outer third is cartilaginous. In the bony portion the epithelium is thinner than in the cartilaginous portion, there is no subcutaneous tissue, and epithelium is tightly applied to the underlying periosteum; hair follicles, sebaceous glands, and apocrine glands arc scarce or absent. The skin in the cartilaginous area has well-developed dermis and subcutaneous tissue and contains hair follicles, sebaceous glands, and apocrine glands. The highly viscid secretions of the sebaceous glands and the watery, pigmented secretions of the apocrine glands in the outer portion of the canal combine with exfoliated surface cells of the skin to form a protective, waxy, water-repellent coating (cerumen). The normal flora of the external canal consists mainly of aerobic bacteria and includes coagulase-negative staphylococci, *Corynebacterium* (diphtheroids), *Micrococcus* spp., and occasionally *Staphylococcus aureus*, viridans streptococci, and *Pseudomonas aeruginosa*. Excessive wetness (swimming, bathing, or increased environmental humidity), dryness (dry ear canal skin and lack of cerumen), and the presence of other skin pathology (previous infection, eczema or other forms of dermatitis) and trauma (digital or foreign body) make the skin of the canal vulnerable to infection by the normal flora or virulent exogenous bacteria.

ETIOLOGY. External otitis (also called "swimmer's ear," although it occurs without swimming) is most commonly caused by *P. aeruginosa*, but *S. aureus*, *Enterobacter aerogenes*, *Proteus mirabilis*, *Klebsiella pneumoniae*, streptococci, coagulase-negative staphylococci, diphtheroids, and fungi such as *Candida* and *Aspergillus* may also be isolated. External otitis results from the loss of protective cerumen and chronic irritation and maceration from excessive moisture in the canal. Inflammation of the ear canal due to herpesvirus, varicella-zoster, other skin exanthems, and severe eczema may also cause or predispose to external otitis.

CLINICAL MANIFESTATIONS. The predominant symptom is ear pain, often severe, accentuated by manipulation of the pinna and especially by pressure on the tragus. The severity of the pain and tenderness may be disproportionate to the degree of inflammation, because the skin of the external ear canal is closely adherent to the underlying perichondrium and periosteum. Itching is a frequent precursor of pain and is usually characteristic of chronic inflammation of the canal or resolving acute otitis externa. Conductive hearing loss may result from edema of the skin and tympanic membrane, serous or purulent secretions, or the progressive meatal skin thickening associated with long-standing external otitis.

Edema of the ear canal, erythema, and thick, clumpy otorrhea are prominent signs of the acute disease. The cerumen is usually white and soft in consistency, as opposed to its usual yellow, gold, or brown color and firmer consistency. The canal frequently is so tender and swollen that the entire ear canal and tympanic membrane cannot be adequately visualized, and complete otoscopic examination may be delayed until the acute swelling subsides. If the tympanic membrane can be visualized, it may appear either normal or opaque; the mobility of the membrane may be normal or, if thickened, reduced in response to positive and negative pressure.

Other physical findings may include palpable and tender lymph nodes in the periauricular and, especially, preauricular areas. Rarely, facial paralysis, other cranial nerve abnormalities, vertigo, or sensorineural hearing loss is present. If so, *necrotizing (malignant) external otitis* is probable. This invasive infection of the temporal bone and skull base requires immediate culture, intravenous antibiotics, and imaging studies to evaluate the extent of the disease. Surgical intervention to obtain cultures or debride devitalized tissue may be necessary. *P. aeruginosa* is the most common causative organism of necrotizing otitis externa. Fortunately, necrotizing external otitis is rare in children and occurs most commonly in immunocompromised or severely malnourished children.

DIAGNOSIS. Diffuse external otitis may be confused with furunculosis, otitis media, and mastoiditis. Furuncles occur in the hair-bearing part of the ear canal, usually at the junction of the lateral aspect of the canal and the concha. It usually causes a localized swelling of the canal limited to one quadrant, whereas external otitis is associated with concentric swelling and involves the whole ear canal. In otitis media, the eardrum may be perforated, severely retracted, or bulging and immobile; hearing is usually impaired. If the middle ear is draining through a perforated eardrum membrane or tympanostomy tube, secondary infection of the ear canal, with associated pain and swelling, may occur; if the membrane is not visible owing to drainage or ear canal swelling, it may be very difficult to distinguish acute otitis media with drainage from an acute otitis externa. Pain on manipulation of the auricle and significant lymphadenitis are not common features of acute middle-ear disease. In some patients with external otitis, the periauricular edema is so extensive that the auricle is pushed forward, creating a condition that may be confused with acute mastoiditis and a subperiosteal abscess; in mastoiditis, the postauricular fold is obliterated, whereas in external otitis the fold is usually better preserved. When the edema over the mastoid process is due to mastoiditis, a history of otitis media and hearing loss is usual; tenderness is noted over the mastoid antrum or tip and not on movement of the auricle, as in external otitis. Sagging of the posterior external canal wall may also occur with acute mastoiditis.

TREATMENT. Topical otic preparations containing neomycin (active against gram-positive organisms and some gram-negative organisms, notably *Proteus* spp.) with either colistin or polymyxin (active against gram-negative bacilli, notably *Pseudomonas* spp.) and corticosteroids are effective in treating most forms of acute diffuse external otitis. Newer preparations of ear drops contain fewer potentially ototoxic antibiotics. If canal edema is marked, a wick should be inserted into the outer third of the ear canal and the topical drops applied to the wick several times a day for 24–48 hr; the wick can be removed after these applications and the otic medication instilled three to four times per day. After 2 or 3 days of this treatment, the edema of the ear canal is usually markedly improved and the medial portion of the ear canal and tympanic membrane better seen. Acetic acid preparations (2%), with or without corticosteroids, or half-strength Burow's solution (aluminum acetate, 1:20) are probably equally effective. When the pain is severe, oral analgesics (ibuprofen, codeine) and dry heat may be necessary.

As the inflammatory process subsides, cleaning the canal with cotton-tipped applicators or, more effectively, irrigating with 2% acetic acid to remove the debris enhances the effectiveness of the topical medications. In subacute and chronic infections, periodic cleansing of the canal is essential. In severe, acute, diffuse external otitis associated with fever and lymphadenitis from which bacteria have been cultured, oral and, on occasion, parenteral antibiotics are indicated; the choice of drug depends on the antibiotic susceptibility of the organism cultured from the ear canal. A fungal infection (otomycosis) of the external auditory canal may be treated by applying clotrimazole, nystatin, or other antifungal agents. Agents used in the treatment of fungal otitis external include *m*-cresyl acetate 25%, gentian violet 2%, and thimerosal 1:1,000.

PREVENTION. Preventing external otitis may be necessary for individuals susceptible to recurrences, especially children who swim. The most effective prophylaxis is instillation of dilute alcohol or acetic acid (2%) immediately after swimming or bathing. During an acute episode of otitis externa, patients should not swim and the ears should be protected from water during bathing.

OTHER DISEASES OF THE EXTERNAL EAR

FURUNCULOSIS. This is caused by *S. aureus* and affects only the hair-containing outer third of the ear canal. Mild forms are treated with oral antibiotics active against *S. aureus*; if an abscess develops, incision and drainage may be necessary.

ACUTE CELLULITIS. Acute cellulitis of the auricle and external auditory canal is usually caused by Group A *Streptococcus* and occasionally by *S. aureus*. The skin is red, hot, and indurated, without a sharply defined border. Fever may be present with little or no exudate in the canal. Parenteral administration of penicillin G or a penicillinase-resistant penicillin is the therapy of choice.

PERICHONDRITIS/CHONDRITIS. Perichondritis is an infection involving the skin and perichondrium of the auricular cartilage; extension of infection to the cartilage is termed chondritis. The ear canal, especially the lateral aspect, may also be involved. Early perichondritis may be difficult to differentiate from cellulitis (earlier) because both are characterized by skin that is red, edematous, and tender. The main cause of perichondritis/chondritis and cellulitis is trauma (accidental or iatrogenic, laceration or contusion), including ear piercing (especially through the cartilage). The most commonly isolated organism in perichondritis/chondritis is *P. aeruginosa*, although other gram-negative and occasionally gram-positive organisms may be found. Treatment involves systemic, often parenteral, antibiotics; surgery to drain an abscess or remove nonviable skin or cartilage may also be needed. Removal of all ear jewelry is mandatory in the presence of infection.

DERMATOSES. Various dermatoses (seborrheic, contact, infectious eczematoid, or neurodermatoid) are common causes of inflammation of the external canal and can be precursors of acute diffuse external otitis caused by scratching and the introduction of infecting organisms.

Seborrheic dermatitis is characterized by greasy scales that flake and crumble as they are detached from the epidermis; associated changes in the scalp, forehead, cheeks, brow, postauricular areas, and concha are usual.

Contact dermatitis may be caused by topical otic medications such as neomycin, polymyxin, and colistin, which may produce erythema, vesiculation, edema, and weeping. Poison ivy, oak, and sumac may also produce contact dermatitis. Earrings are another source of contact dermatitis.

Infectious eczematoid dermatitis is caused by a purulent infection of the external canal, middle ear, or mastoid; the purulent drainage infects the skin of the canal, auricle, or both. The lesion is weeping, erythematous, or crusted.

Atopic dermatitis occurs in children with a familial or personal history of allergy; the auricle, particularly the postauricular fold, becomes thickened, scaly, and excoriated.

Neurodermatitis is recognized by the intense itching and erythematous, thickened epidermis localized to the concha and orifice of the meatus.

Treatment of these dermatoses depends on the type but should include application of the aural medication described for external otitis, elimination of the source of infection or contact when identified, and management of any underlying dermatologic problem. In addition to topical antibiotics (or antifungals), topical steroids are helpful if contact dermatitis, atopic dermatitis, or eczematoid dermatitis is suspected.

HERPES SIMPLEX. This may appear as vesicles on the auricle and lips. The lesions eventually become encrusted and dry and may be confused with impetigo. Topical application of a 10% solution of carbamide peroxide in anhydrous glycerol is symptomatically helpful. The *Ramsay Hunt* syndrome (herpes zoster oticus) may present with herpes vesicles in the ear canal and on the pinna and with facial paralysis. Other cranial nerves may be affected as well, especially the 8th nerve. The current recommended treatment of herpes zoster oticus includes systemic antiviral agents, such as acyclovir, and corticosteroids. As many as 50% of patients with Ramsay Hunt syndrome do not have complete recovery of their facial nerve function.

BULLOUS MYRINGITIS. This is commonly associated with an acute upper respiratory tract infection. The ear is very painful and hemorrhagic or serous blisters or bullas form on the tympanic membrane. The disease is difficult to differentiate from acute otitis media, because early in the course of acute otitis the membrane may appear to have bullas. The organisms involved are probably the same as those causing acute otitis media, including both bacteria and viruses. Treatment consists of antibiotic therapy of the type generally used for acute otitis media. Incision of the bullas, although not necessary, promptly relieves the pain.

EXOSTOSES AND OSTEOMAS. Exostoses represent benign hyperplasia of the perichondrium and underlying bone of the external ear canal and are frequently found in people who swim often in cold water. Exostoses are broad based, often multiple and bilateral. Osteomas are benign bony growths in the ear canal; their cause is uncertain. They are usually solitary and attached by a narrow pedicle to the tympanosquamous or tympanomastoid suture line. Both are more common in males; exostoses are more common than osteomas. Treatment is usually not required, although large masses may cause cerumen impaction and ear canal obstruction. If this occurs, surgical intervention is warranted.

CHAPTER 646
Otitis Media and Its Complications

After respiratory tract infections, inflammation of the middle ear, otitis media (OM), is the most prevalent disease of childhood. An estimated 25 million yearly visits to pediatricians are related to OM; it is the most common diagnosis for children in the United States and the second most common in medicine overall. In the past 2 decades, the number of visits to pediatricians for OM has increased dramatically, from 9.9 million visits in 1975 to 24.5 million in 1990. This probably reflects a combination of factors including a true change in disease pattern, more children in child care, increased awareness by health care providers, improved technical capabilities including improved illumination with halogen lights and pneumatic bulbs in otoscopes, and the use of sensitive tests such as tympanometry and acoustic reflectometry. Unfortunately, the exact incidence of OM in a given population may be hard to determine because it is significantly both overdiagnosed and underdiagnosed. Correct diagnosis and treatment of OM are important because it is so prevalent and because significant life-threatening complications may occasionally occur. More commonly, acute inflammation of the middle ear is followed by persistent middle-ear effusion for a variable period. The latter can cause significant conductive hearing loss, which may adversely affect speech and language development.

DEFINITION. OM is inflammation of the middle ear, without reference to pathogenesis or etiology. The other areas of the temporal bone that are contiguous with the middle ear, including the mastoid, petrous apex, and perilabyrinthine air cells, may also be involved. OM can be further divided into acute OM (AOM) without effusion, AOM with effusion, OM with effusion (OME), chronic suppurative OM with or without cholesteatoma, and atelectasis of the tympanic membrane/middle ear/mastoid. AOM is usually suppurative or purulent, but serous effusions may also have an acute onset. The many other descriptions of OME include serous, secretory, mucoid, nonsuppurative, and "glue ear." Because it is often difficult to judge the type of effusion through an intact tympanic membrane, OME is a useful, all-inclusive term. Chronic suppurative OM implies a nonintact tympanic membrane (perforation or tympanostomy tube present) with 6 wk or more of middle-ear drainage.

EPIDEMIOLOGY. Nearly two thirds of children have at least one episode of AOM by 3 yr of age; 50% of children have two or more episodes. Infants and young children are at highest risk for OM, with the peak between 6 and 13 mo of age. In one study, 2% of children had experienced at least one episode of AOM by 2 mo, 34% by 12 mo, and 59% by 24 mo. For asymptomatic OME, 10% have had at least one episode by 2 mo, and 78% by 12 mo. After a single episode of AOM, about 40% of children have OME that persists for 4 wk, and 10% have an effusion that is still present at 3 mo. The incidence of the disease tends to decrease as a function of age, with a marked decrease after age 6 yr. The incidence is higher in boys, children in large daycare settings, those exposed to secondhand smoke, non–breast-fed infants, and those with HIV or biologic siblings or parents with a significant history of OM. OM is most common during the winter months because many episodes are associated with an upper respiratory tract infection (URI). Children who live in developing areas or in crowded conditions have statistically more middle-ear disease than other children, as do Native Americans and Alaskan and Canadian Inuits. Children with cleft palate and other craniofacial anomalies are at increased risk for OM.

PATHOPHYSIOLOGY. The high incidence of acute and recurrent OM in children probably reflects a combination of factors, with eustachian tube dysfunction being a common underlying factor and the child's susceptibility to recurrent URI being of importance. The eustachian tubes open into the anterior middle-ear space and connect that structure with the nasopharynx. They are lined by respiratory epithelium and surrounded for a short distance near the middle ear by bone; for most of their length, they are surrounded by cartilage. A child's eustachian tubes are different from an adult's in that they are more horizontal and their nasopharyngeal opening, the torus tubarius, is likely to have numerous lymphoid follicles surrounding it. Also in a child, adenoids may fill the nasopharynx, mechanically blocking the nose and eustachian tube orifice or acting as a source of infection that may contribute to edema and dysfunction of the eustachian tube. The eustachian tubes are normally closed at rest and open with swallowing by action of the tensor veli palatini, which extends from the skull base and inserts laterally into the soft palate. The eustachian tubes protect the middle ear from nasopharyngeal secretions, provide drainage into the nasopharynx of secretions produced within the middle ear, and permit equilibration of air pressure with atmospheric pressure in the middle ear. Mechanical or functional obstruction of the eustachian tubes can result in negative middle-ear pressure and eustachian tube dysfunction. Intrinsic mechanical obstruction can result from edema due to infection, allergy, or other causes, and extrinsic obstruction from obstructive adenoids or nasopharyngeal tumors. Persistent collapse of the eustachian tubes during swallowing can result in functional obstruction related to decreased tubal stiffness, an inefficient active opening mechanism, or both. Functional obstruction is common in infants and younger children because the amount and stiffness of the cartilage support of the tubes are less than in older children and adults. Because the eustachian tubes are intimately involved with muscles attached to the soft palate and because it is part of the skull base, patients with anomalies in these areas, such as cleft palate, have a much higher incidence of eustachian tube dysfunction and chronic OME.

Eustachian tube obstruction results in negative middle-ear pressure and, if persistent, in a transudative middle-ear effusion. Drainage of the effusion is inhibited by impaired mucociliary transport and by sustained negative pressure. When the eustachian tubes are not totally obstructed mechanically, contamination of the middle ear space from nasopharyngeal secretions may occur by reflux (especially when the tympanic membrane has a perforation or when a tympanostomy tube is present), by aspiration (from high negative middle-ear pressure), or by insufflation during crying, nose blowing, sneezing, and swallowing when the nose is obstructed. Rapid alterations in ambient pressure or barotrauma during deep-water diving or flying can also result in acute middle-ear effusion that may be hemorrhagic. Infants and young children have a shorter eustachian tube than older children and adults, which makes them more susceptible to reflux of nasopharyngeal secretions into the middle-ear space and to the development of AOM.

Young children suffer an increased frequency of viral URI. These infections probably lead to edema of the eustachian tube mucosa, causing increased eustachian tube dysfunction. Reactive enlargement of lymphoid tissue, such as the adenoids or tissue at the eustachian tube orifice, may also mechanically block tube function and provide a site of inflammation. The presence of viral infection has been shown to increase bacterial adhesion in nasopharyngeal tissue.

The number of children in child-care centers in the United States has significantly increased in the past 2 decades; children in these centers are more prone to URI. This may account in part for the parallel increase in middle-ear problems during this time. Elevated levels of cotinine, a metabolite of nicotine, also correlate with an increased incidence of both OME and

AOM in children, indicating that passive exposure to cigarette smoke increases ear problems, probably by acting as an irritant to respiratory epithelium and having an adverse effect on ciliary motion and mucociliary clearance. Children with well-documented allergies appear to have approximately the same incidence of recurrent ear problems as those without allergies. However, on an individual basis, allergic factors probably play a part in some children's recurrent ear infections.

Young children have an immature, developing immune system, which is another factor leading to a high incidence of otitis in this age group. The incidence of humoral immune problems affecting respiratory epithelium does appear to be increased in children who have not responded to prophylactic antibiotics or ventilation tube placement and who have had recurrent infections involving the sinonasal or the lower respiratory tract.

ETIOLOGY. The most commonly identified pathogens associated with OM are *Streptococcus pneumoniae* (30–50%), non–typable *Haemophilus influenzae* (20–30%), and *Moraxella catarrhalis* (1–5%). Additionally, other bacteria, including *S. aureus* and gram-negative enteric organisms such as *Escherichia coli, Klebsiella* spp., and *Pseudomonas aeruginosa,* are infrequently isolated in a small percentage of patients. In neonates and young infants, *S. pneumoniae* and *H. influenzae* are still the most common pathogens; *S. aureus*, group B *Streptococcus*, gram-negative enteric pathogens, and other organisms associated with local and systemic infection, especially in former high-risk neonates, are identified as much as 20% of the time.

Infants and children in intensive care settings, especially if the stay is prolonged and they are immunocompromised, may have unusual organisms isolated from middle-ear fluid. Nasotracheal intubation is a risk for sinusitis and OM. Other uncommon organisms that have been isolated from middle-ear fluid include *Mycoplasma pneumoniae, Chlamydia trachomatis,* and *Mycobacterium tuberculosis. Alloiococcus otitidis* has been isolated under very careful culture conditions from chronic middle-ear fluid; other unusual organisms may be reported as isolated cases.

Although anaerobic organisms have been consistently identified in middle-ear cultures, the consensus is that their role is a minor one. *Peptostreptococcus, Fusobacterium* spp, and *Bacteroides* spp. are the most commonly isolated. In chronic suppurative OM, however, anaerobes are often found, sometimes in more abundance than aerobic organisms. The management of these organisms, even when isolated in large numbers, remains unclear.

An increasing number of β-lactamase-producing bacteria have been identified in the middle ear, including approximately 35% of *H. influenzae*, nearly 80% of *M. catarrhalis*, and many *S. aureus* and anaerobes. Approximately 4% of β-lactamase-negative *H. influenzae* isolates are ampicillin resistant. Reduced susceptibility of *S. pneumoniae* to penicillin has increased dramatically over the past decade to 20–25% (5–7% highly resistant), with reduced susceptibility to third-generation cephalosporins in 10% of isolates (4% highly resistant); the reduced antibiotic susceptibilities of *S. pneumoniae* occur independently. The exact percentages for all resistant organisms varies somewhat with the geographic area and population studied. The mechanisms for the different types of resistance vary; thus, numerous strategies in terms of antimicrobial use are needed. Factors promoting the development of bacterial resistance include repeated and prolonged exposure to antimicrobials, including prophylaxis, incomplete courses of antimicrobials, and unwarranted, inappropriate administration.

Viruses may be causative or copathogenic organisms, along with bacteria; viruses that have been directly isolated from middle ear fluid include respiratory syncytial virus (RSV), rhinovirus, influenzavirus, adenovirus, enteroviruses, and parainfluenza viruses. In a small number of cases, cytomegalovirus (CMV) and herpes simplex virus have also been isolated. OM is a complication of viral exanthems, such as measles and Epstein-Barr virus.

646.1 Acute Otitis Media

CLINICAL MANIFESTATIONS. Children with an URI often develop the symptoms of AOM: otalgia, fever, hearing loss, and generalized malaise. Other symptoms may include otorrhea, irritability, and lethargy, followed less often by anorexia, nausea, vomiting, diarrhea, and headache. Fever occurs in approximately 30–50% of patients; temperatures exceeding 40°C are uncommon and suggest bacteremia or another complication. In infants, the symptoms may be less localizing, and fever, irritability, diarrhea, vomiting, or malaise may be quite prominent. Older children may complain of tinnitus, vertigo, and hearing loss; smaller children may not be able to complain about these specific symptoms but may appear to be off balance. Any child with a fever without a focus should be evaluated for a middle-ear infection (Chapter 172).

DIAGNOSIS. The diagnosis of AOM is based on clinical symptoms combined with visualization of the tympanic membrane. Examination with a pneumatic otoscope reveals a hyperemic, opaque, bulging tympanic membrane with poor mobility; purulent otorrhea with tympanic membrane perforation may be present (Fig. 646–1). The usual middle ear landmarks frequently are obscured. Uncommonly, bullas appear on the lateral aspect of the tympanic membrane; children with bullas on the tympanic membrane often have severe ear pain. In children who have small ear canals or large amounts of cerumen or who are very uncooperative, seeing the eardrum may be difficult. Cerumen should be gently cleaned using a fine wire loop through the open or operating head of an otoscope. If there is a question of tympanic membrane perforation, irrigation of the ear canal should not be performed. If the membrane cannot be seen because of cerumen, edema, or drainage, an otolaryngology consultation should be considered before starting therapy.

If a child is in extreme pain or culture of the middle-ear fluid is desired, tympanocentesis with aspiration of the middle-ear fluid should be considered. Tympanocentesis should also be considered in seriously ill children or those who appear toxic; children who clinically continue to be symptomatic despite antibiotic therapy; patients already receiving antibiotic agents with onset of AOM; patients who develop suppurative intratemporal or intracranial complications of OM; newborn or immunologically deficient patients with OM, in whom unusual organisms may cause infection.

DIFFERENTIAL DIAGNOSIS. A red tympanic membrane is often associated with an infectious process of the tympanic mem-

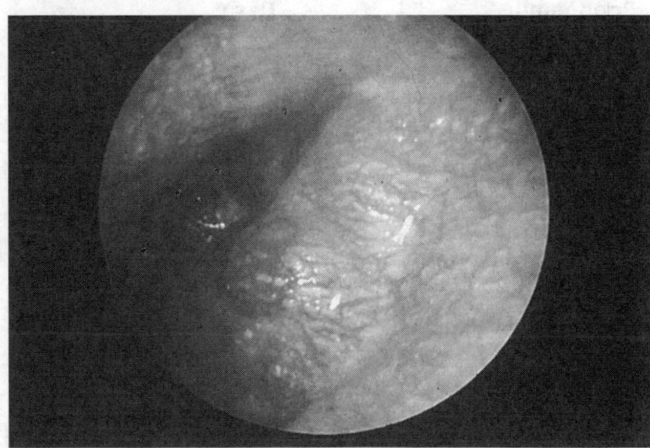

Figure 646–1 Acute left otitis media. See also color section.

brane and middle ear; a normal membrane can become red in a crying child, just as the cheeks can turn red. If pneumatic otoscopy is performed properly, an immobile eardrum usually denotes significant negative middle-ear pressure or fluid. A retracted tympanic membrane moves better with negative pressure. Structural abnormalities of the membrane should also be identified. Focal thickening of the membrane associated with chronic infections and prior ventilation tube placement is called *tympanosclerosis*. This is a hyaline degeneration of the middle fibrous layer of the tympanic membrane that may be calcified. If there has been a prior perforation or ventilation tube placement, the tympanic membrane may heal without this normal middle fibrous layer. The resulting thinned portion of the membrane is prone to retraction when negative middle-ear pressure is present. The most superior portion of the tympanic membrane is called the pars flaccida. In this location, the collagen bundles are less organized, and the eardrum is more prone to retraction. Deep retraction pockets may lead to squamous epithelium within the middle ear and mastoid cavities, causing a *cholesteatoma* that may grow by the enzymatic activity of the skin tissues and by accumulation of squamous debris within the cholesteatoma. Rarely, middle-ear masses, such as a glomus tympanicum, may be able to be seen through or abutting an intact eardrum; this situation may confuse the observer. Similarly, foreign bodies of the ear canal may be mistaken for a thickened, discolored tympanic membrane.

TREATMENT. Empirical treatment is based on knowledge of the most common bacterial organisms found in AOM (Table 646–1). There is no single oral antimicrobial agent that eradicates all AOM pathogens. Amoxicillin is the initial antibiotic of choice, because it is usually effective against the most commonly encountered bacteria, has the best pharmacodynamic profile against multiple-drug resistant *S. pneumoniae* of any of the available oral agents, has a long record of safety, and is inexpensive. Patients with AOM may be treated with high-dose amoxicillin (80–90 mg/kg/24 hr in three divided doses), which is well tolerated. Treatment is continued for 10 days. Patients assessed to be at low risk for resistant *S. pneumoniae* may be treated with the traditional dose of amoxicillin (40–45 mg/kg/24 hr in three divided doses). Risk factors to consider for resistant *S. pneumoniae* include recent antimicrobial exposure, young age (<2 yr), and childcare attendance. Tympanocentesis to identify the infecting organism should be considered for patients who are immunocompromised or who have persistent symptoms despite multiple courses of different antibiotics.

Treatment failure can be defined by lack of clinical improvement, such as persistent ear pain or fever, and by objective findings, such as tympanic membrane bulging or otorrhea, after 3 days of therapy. Nonspecific signs such as persistent middle ear effusion or coryza, which may indicate persistent viral infection, should not be interpreted as signs of treatment failure. Few comparative studies are available to guide therapy for treatment failures. There are compelling data for effectiveness of treatment of AOM with cefuroxime axetil (30 mg/kg/24 hr in two divided doses) orally; amoxicillin-clavulanate (80–90 mg/kg/24 hr of amoxicillin; 6.4 mg/kg/24 hr of clavulanate [requires newer formulation]) orally; or ceftriaxone (50 mg/kg) as a single intramuscular injection daily for 3 days. These alternatives should be used for patients who fail to respond to amoxicillin, for presence of resistant organisms determined by tympanocentesis, or coexisting illness requiring a second-line medication. However, many of the other drugs approved by the Food and Drug Administration lack evidence of efficacy against drug-resistant *S. pneumoniae*. There are promising but insufficient data at this time to recommend cefpodoxime and cefprozil, but many of the traditional second-line drugs should now be considered ineffective for AOM, including trimethoprim-sulfamethoxazole and erythromycin-sulfisoxazole. The clinical effectiveness of the newer macrolides, clarithromycin and azithromycin, in the era of multiple drug–resistant *S. pneumoniae* remains to be established. Some of these drugs, however, may be used for selected cases based on susceptibility testing of middle ear fluid isolates obtained by tympanocentesis.

Supportive therapy, including analgesics, antipyretics, and local heat, is usually helpful. An oral decongestant (pseudoephedrine hydrochloride) may relieve some nasal congestion, and antihistamines may help patients with known or suspected nasal allergy. Antihistamines, decongestants, and corticosteroids are not effective in the actual treatment of AOM, however.

If a patient's clinical manifestations of acute infection increase during the first 24 hr despite antimicrobial therapy, a suppurative complication of OM should be suspected. The child should be re-examined, and tympanocentesis and middle ear culture performed. Similarly, if a patient continues to have appreciable pain, fever, or both after 24–48 hr, tympanocentesis with culture of the middle-ear fluid should be considered as both a diagnostic and therapeutic procedure. If a diagnostic aspiration is not performed, antimicrobials effective against resistant organisms prevalent in the community should be administered.

Because it is well established that middle-ear fluid often persists after an episode of AOM, follow-up for a single episode

TABLE 646–1 Treatment Recommendations for Acute Otitis Media in Children

Antibiotics in Prior Month	Day 0	Clinically Defined Treatment Failure on Day 3	Clinically Defined Treatment Failure on Days 10 to 28
No	High-dose amoxicillin (80–90 mg/kg/24 hr) *or* Traditioinal dose amoxicillin (40–45 mg/kg/24 hr)	High-dose amoxicillin-clavulanate (80–90 mg/kg/24 hr of amoxicillin, 6.4 mg/kg/24 hr of clavulanate)[1] Cefuroxime axetil (30 mg/kg/24 hr) *or* Ceftriaxone (50 mg/kg intramuscularly as a single injection)	Same as day 3
Yes	High-dose amoxicillin (80–90 mg/kg/24 hr) High-dose amoxicillin-clavulanate (80–90 mg/kg/24 hr of amoxicillin, 6.4 mg/kg/24 hr of clavulanate)[1] *or* Cefuroxime axetil (30 mg/kg/24 hr)	Ceftriaxone (50 mg/kg intramuscularly as a single injection, daily for 3 days)[2] Clindamycin (40 mg/kg/24 hr)[3] *or* Tympanocentesis	High-dose amoxicillin-clavulanate (80–90 mg/kg/24 hr of amoxicillin, 6.4 mg/kg/24 hr of clavulanate) Cefuroxime axetil Ceftriaxone (50 mg/kg intramuscularly) *or* Tympanocentesis

[1]*Requires newer formulation, or combination with amoxicillin.*
[2]*Ceftriaxone has documented efficacy in AOM treatment failures if three daily doses are given.*
[3]*Clindamycin is not effective against* Haemophilus influenzae *or* Moraxella catarrhalis.
Adapted from Dowell SF, Butler JC, Giebink GS, et al: Acute otitis media: Management and surveillance in an era of pneumococcal resistance—a report from the Drug-resistant Streptococcus pneumoniae *Therapeutic Working Group. Pediatr Infect Dis J 18:4, 1999.*

of AOM can occur several weeks after the initial diagnosis if the child is otherwise clinically well. At the time of follow-up, the tympanic membrane should no longer be red and bulging and the middle-ear fluid may have started to resolve. Statistically, in patients who have had a single episode of AOM middle-ear fluid may still remain in up to 40% of patients at 1 mo, 20% at 2 mo, and 10% at 3 mo. Periodic follow-up is indicated for patients with persistent middle-ear fluid or patients who have had recurrent episodes of OM. If the middle-ear fluid is persistent, patients should be treated as described in Chapter 646.2.

Some physicians believe that AOM is overtreated. Their concerns are based on the fact that (1) AOM will resolve without medical intervention in 60–80% of cases (usually due to *H. influenzae, M. catarrhalis*); (2) AOM is frequently misdiagnosed (a red eardrum in a crying child is mistaken for an actual infection) and therefore likely to be treated inappropriately; (3) the antimicrobials prescribed may not be the most appropriate ones (using a macrolide for a first episode of AOM versus amoxicillin); and (4) the full course of the prescribed antimicrobial is not taken, making resistance more likely in the long term for that organism. However, before the use of antimicrobials, significant morbidity and death were commonly associated with AOM. Therefore, the current recommendation to treat symptomatic AOM with antimicrobials should be followed, keeping in mind that correct diagnosis and appropriate use of antimicrobials is important. Prevention may be possible with the use of xylitol-containing gum, lozenges, or syrup and in the future by the conjugated pneumococcal vaccine.

646.2 Persistent Middle-Ear Effusion

If middle-ear effusion persists after the initial therapy for AOM, one or more of the following options have often been suggested for use during the next, subacute phase. However, none of these have been demonstrated to be more effective than observation in randomized controlled trials: (1) a course of an antimicrobial different from the initial agent (the new antimicrobial agent may be effective against an organism resistant to the previous one); (2) a topical or systemic nasal decongestant, antihistamine, or combination of these drugs; (3) systemic corticosteroids; and (4) eustachian tube–middle-ear inflation. Although individual children may have a short-term response with one of these methods, there is no proven statistical difference in terms of long-term resolution of middle-ear fluid or recurrence rates of AOM between methods. It is therefore reasonable to observe children who have asymptomatic (except for hearing loss) middle-ear effusion still present after an acute episode of OM, examining the patient 2 mo after the initial visit, at which time most patients are effusion free. Treatment with another antimicrobial, which is effective against resistant bacteria, may be indicated if a child has any signs or symptoms of persistent infection, such as otalgia, or if such organisms have been isolated from subacute effusions in the community.

If at 3 mo the middle-ear fluid is still present, either as a result of AOM or middle-ear effusion that occurred secondary to a URI, further therapy should be considered. If a child with persistent middle-ear fluid continues to be clinically symptomatic with pain, fever, imbalance, disturbed sleep, or very significant hearing loss, more aggressive management is indicated (see section on OME Chapter 646.4).

646.3 Recurrent Acute Otitis Media

Some children suffer recurrent episodes of AOM with almost every URI, have moderate symptoms, respond well to therapy, and have fewer episodes with advancing age. Others have end-to-end otitis, severe symptoms, or persistent middle-ear effusion with superimposed episodes of AOM. Children with occasional AOM that completely clears between episodes may be treated as previously outlined, but if the episodes are frequent and close together (three to four episodes in 6 mo or six episodes in a year), especially if they are very symptomatic, further evaluation and management are warranted. Prophylactic antibiotics may be used effectively for children with recurrent AOM that clears between episodes (amoxicillin 20 mg/kg/24 hr, or sulfisoxazole 50 mg/kg/24 hr, orally once daily at bedtime for 6 mo in the winter and spring). However, with the emergence of many resistant bacterial organisms, the routine use of prophylactic antimicrobials for many months has come into question. Prophylaxis for recurrent AOM might be considered for short periods, such as vacations, holidays, and the few months from spring until the summer. However, in otherwise normal children with intact immune systems, long periods of prophylaxis may not be appropriate and other possible interventions should be considered. If a child is in a large daycare setting, change to a smaller setting or home care should be considered. If there is cigarette smoking in the home, this should be stopped. If the child goes to bed with a bottle, anecdotal evidence shows that stopping this practice reduces the episodes of AOM. Some evidence also suggests that gastroesophageal reflux (GER) may play a part in some children with recurrent AOM, and treatment of the GER may help in the management of AOM. Xylitol may also be effective in gum, lozenges, or syrup but requires further study.

Children with significant recurrent AOM should have a baseline immune evaluation; children with IgG subclass deficiencies and poor responses to polysaccharide vaccines may be more likely to have significant OM. Giving these children, especially those older than 2 yr, the pneumococcal vaccine may help. Finally, although it has been hard to link allergy and otitis in large numbers of children, there does appear to be a relationship in some children; allergy evaluation and appropriate treatment may be warranted.

Myringotomy and ventilating tubes are also effective and should be considered for children failing to respond to medical management. Preventive efficacy of antimicrobial chemoprophylaxis or myringotomy with tympanostomy tube insertion has been demonstrated in clinical trials. Adenoidectomy has not been proved to be of significant benefit in children with recurrent AOM, although it can be considered in children with severe OM when additional modalities of management are being sought.

646.4 Otitis Media with Effusion

OME is a middle-ear effusion lacking the clinical manifestations of acute infection, such as otalgia and fever. It is often a result of AOM and in this situation generally clears by 3 mo in 90% of children. The duration (not the severity) of the effusion can be divided into acute (<3 wk), subacute (3 wk–3 mo), and chronic (>3 mo). The effusions may be serous (thin), mucoid (thick), purulent, or a combination (Fig. 646–2).

CLINICAL MANIFESTATIONS. Children with truly asymptomatic OME should have, by definition, no symptoms of AOM. However, these children often seem inattentive, complain of hearing loss, or have hearing loss documented by audiometric evaluation. They may appear to be off balance or dizzy and sometimes complain of otalgia or tinnitus. Children who are otherwise asymptomatic in the daytime may be restless sleepers at night.

PHYSICAL EXAMINATION. The tympanic membrane is often retracted and moves poorly or not at all with pneumatic otos-

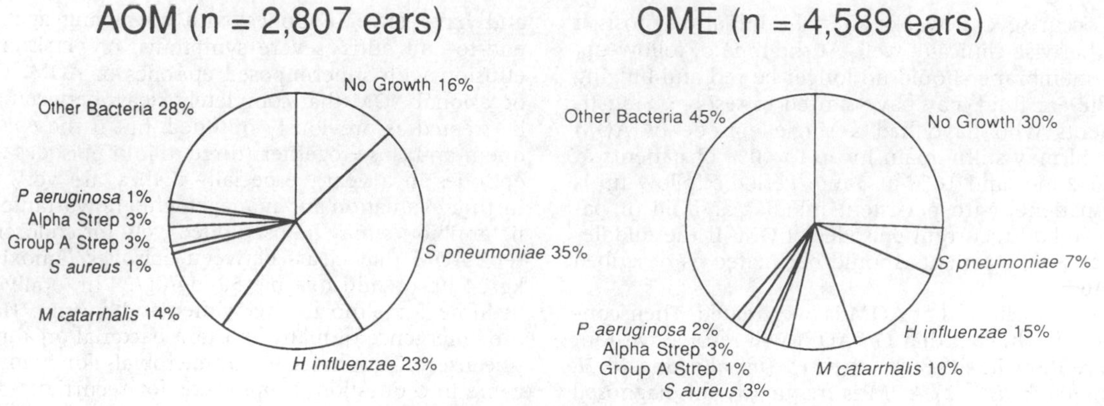

AOM (n = 2,807 ears)

No Growth 16%
Other Bacteria 28%
P aeruginosa 1%
Alpha Strep 3%
Group A Strep 3%
S aureus 1%
M catarrhalis 14%
H influenzae 23%
S pneumoniae 35%

OME (n = 4,589 ears)

Other Bacteria 45%
No Growth 30%
S pneumoniae 7%
H influenzae 15%
P aeruginosa 2%
Alpha Strep 3%
Group A Strep 1%
S aureus 3%
M catarrhalis 10%

Figure 646–2 Comparison of distribution of isolates in 2807 effusions from patients with acute otitis media and 4,589 effusions from patients with otitis media with effusion at the Pittsburgh Otitis Media Research Center between 1980 and 1989. *AOM*, acute otitis media; *OME*, otitis media with effusion. (Total percentages are greater than 100% because of multiple organisms.) (From Bluestone CD, Klein JO: Otitis Media in Infants and Children, 2nd ed. Philadelphia, WB Saunders, 1995.)

copy. If a significant amount of middle-ear fluid is found, the middle-ear landmarks may be obscured; if the tympanic membrane is very retracted, the malleus may be very prominent, and the incudostapedial joint may be seen as the eardrum drapes tightly over it. The tympanic membrane is usually opaque but may also be translucent, with an air-fluid level or air bubbles seen behind it. The middle-ear fluid may be whitish, yellow, or almost bluish. It may occasionally appear to be hemorrhagic if there has been recent acute infection (Fig. 646–3). Occasionally, even when there is little effusion, the tympanic membrane is retracted and its mobility impaired, usually because of negative middle-ear air pressure. There is usually no associated erythema unless the child is crying vigorously and the tympanic membrane has turned pink, in which case differentiation from AOM may be difficult.

AUDIOMETRIC FINDINGS. Conductive hearing loss of various degrees is usually present. Tympanometry may show significant negative pressure or a flat tracing.

TREATMENT. If the fluid has persisted for 3 mo or less and the child is not significantly symptomatic, treatment other than watchful waiting may not be indicated, as the fluid often resolves. However, if the fluid has persisted longer than 3 mo, is bilateral, and is associated with hearing loss, treatment should be considered. If a child has an underlying sensorineural hearing loss or is significantly symptomatic, treatment should be considered sooner than 3 mo. Although the significance of any associated conductive hearing loss continues to be vigorously debated, some evidence shows that such a loss

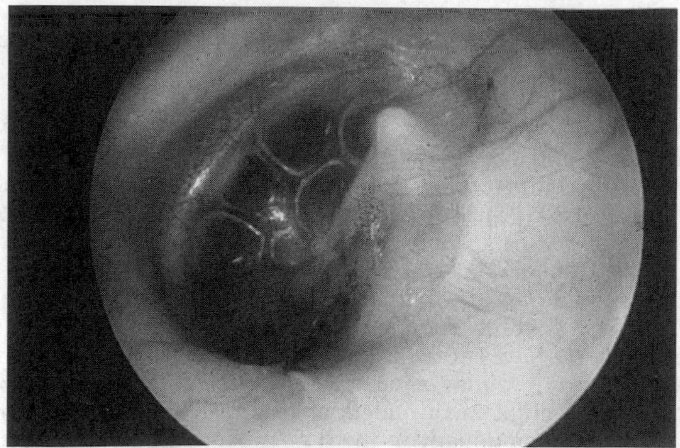

Figure 646–3 Otitis media with effusion of left ear. Retracted ear drum, prominent short process of malleus, and air bubbles seen anteriorly through the tympanic membrane. See also color section.

may impair cognitive and language development in some children and may hamper social and educational skills owing to impaired communication. Because of these concerns, many clinicians believe treatment is indicated under certain conditions. For example, treatment may be indicated for a child with bilateral chronic middle-ear effusions and a marked hearing loss. Treatment may not be needed as soon for a child having a unilateral, asymptomatic OME and only a mild hearing loss and without serious secondary changes in the tympanic membrane. In addition to conductive or sensorineural hearing loss, other conditions to be considered in deciding whether to treat and which therapy to use include (1) occurrence of OME in young infants who are unable to communicate their symptoms; (2) vertigo; (3) otalgia; (4) alterations of the tympanic membrane such as severe atelectasis, especially a deep retraction pocket in the posterosuperior quadrant, the pars flaccida, or both; (5) middle-ear changes such as adhesive otitis media or ossicular involvement; (6) persistence of the effusion for 3 mo or longer; and (7) frequently recurrent episodes over many months, resulting in an increasing percentage of time with middle-ear effusion.

One of the most popular treatments for OME previously was an orally administered combination of a decongestant and antihistamine. However, in many studies, this has been shown to be ineffective in infants and children with acute, subacute, and chronic OME. The efficacy of topical intranasal and systemic corticosteroid therapy is unproven, although several studies pose arguments for both sides. The risks of systemic corticosteroid therapy generally outweigh many of the possible benefits. The method of Politzer or using the Valsalva maneuver to open the eustachian tubes has generally proved ineffective in long-term management of OME.

Either observation or a trial of antibiotics and control of environmental risk factors are indicated treatment options for children with acute or subacute effusions (Fig. 646–4). Antibiotics should especially be considered for symptomatic effusions. Because bacteria similar to those found in AOM have been isolated from a significant proportion of middle-ear aspirates in children with OME, the antibiotic chosen and duration of treatment should be the same as that recommended for AOM (see Fig. 646–2). In clinical trials, both amoxicillin and amoxicillin-clavulanate have been shown to be somewhat more effective than placebo. Repeated courses of antimicrobials for asymptomatic OME are not indicated.

If the effusion persists for 3 mo or longer or if there have been frequent recurrences of episodes of AOM in addition to the underlying OME, patients require further evaluation for hearing loss, respiratory allergy, adenoid tissue obstructing the nose and nasopharynx or acting as a reservoir of infectious

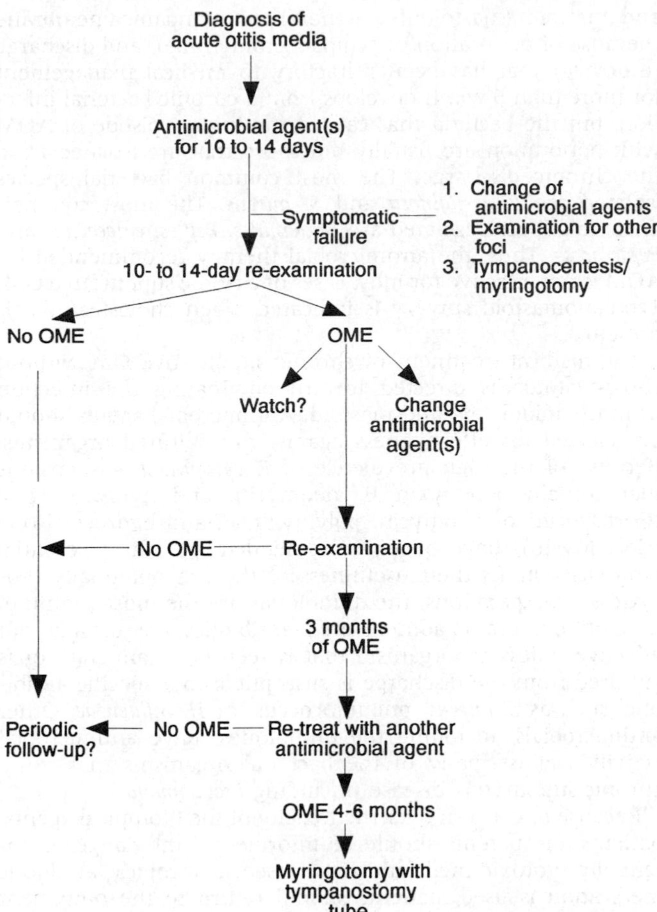

Figure 646–4 Recommended management plan for children with acute otitis media. Otitis media with effusion (OME). (Modified from Bluestone CD, Klein JO: Otitis Media in Infants and Children, 2nd ed. Philadelphia, WB Saunders, 1995.)

organisms, an immunologic disorder, or anatomic abnormalities such as submucous cleft palate or a tumor of the nasopharynx. If a child has significant hearing loss, myringotomy with insertion of tympanostomy tubes is an additional option after a trial of antibiotics (Fig. 646–4). The rationale for this procedure is to improve middle-ear ventilation.

Myringotomy and insertion of ventilation tubes may also be helpful in patients with atelectasis of the tympanic membrane or when pain, hearing loss, vertigo, or tinnitus is present in association with OME. Ventilation tubes may prevent permanent structural damage and cholesteatoma if a deep retraction pocket develops in the posterosuperior quadrant or in the attic (pars flaccida) portion of the tympanic membrane. Myringotomy with aspiration of the middle-ear effusion but without tube placement may be appropriate in those children in whom the procedure can be performed without the aid of a general anesthetic, especially if the myringotomy is being performed for severe otalgia and to obtain culture of the middle-ear fluid. The need for a repeat myringotomy may suggest that the placement of a ventilating tube be considered.

Adenoidectomy for chronic OME may benefit some children. Because the effectiveness of adenoidectomy for chronic OME is not significantly related to adenoid size, the selection of children who might benefit from adenoidectomy should be related to the potential benefits weighed against the costs and potential risks. For children who have recurrent or chronic OME and who had one or more myringotomy and tympanostomy tube operations in the past, adenoidectomy may be a reasonable option. The presence of upper airway obstruction, recurrent acute or chronic adenoiditis, or sinusitis is an additional indication in the consideration of adenoidectomy for children who have chronic OME.

646.5 Atelectasis of the Tympanic Membrane–Middle Ear and High Negative Pressure

Atelectasis of the tympanic membrane may be acute or chronic, generalized or localized, mild or severe. The tympanic membrane may be retracted or collapsed. High negative middle-ear pressure may be present or absent. When middle-ear effusion is also present, the clinical picture is the same as with acute or chronic OME. The membrane may appear draped over the ossicles, allowing the observer to see the short process of the malleus and the incudo-stapedial joint. An effusion may be evident by the presence of an air-fluid level or bubbles behind a severely retracted tympanic membrane.

Atelectasis is not usually associated with clinical symptoms and is diagnosed on otoscopy or suspected when the audiogram result is abnormal. A child may have a severely retracted translucent tympanic membrane with evidence of high negative pressure by pneumatic otoscopy (immobile to applied positive pressure and decreased or absent mobility to applied negative pressure) or a high negative middle-ear pressure tracing on the tympanogram. The otoscopist can look through the tympanic membrane and see if an effusion is present. Some children with such findings on otoscopic (and tympanometric) examination may not have any complaint, whereas others may have a feeling of fullness in the ear, otalgia, tinnitus, hearing loss, and even vertigo. The condition may be self-limited, and in some it may be physiologic because of temporary eustachian tube obstruction. In others, especially those with symptoms, the condition is pathologic and should be managed in a manner similar to that used when an effusion is present. Worsening or deepening of a retraction pocket or increasing conductive hearing loss is an indication for intervention in the severely atelectatic tympanic membrane.

The evaluation of children with atelectasis caused by high negative pressure is similar to that described for those with chronic OME. Management is also similar and ranges from watchful waiting to tympanostomy tube insertion, depending on the duration, frequency, and severity of the problem. If a chronic retraction pocket has developed, tympanoplasty may be necessary to correct the defect because a cholesteatoma can develop at the retraction pocket site.

646.6 Complications and Sequelae

Since the advent of antimicrobial therapy, the intracranial suppurative complications of otitis media are uncommon, although they still occasionally are encountered, especially in situations where the children do not have adequate access to regular medical care. However, intratemporal complications, those occurring within the middle ear, mastoid, and adjacent structures of the temporal bone, are common.

HEARING LOSS. This is the most common complication and morbid outcome of OM that may be caused by one or more of the intratemporal complications. Most frequently noted is a fluctuating or persistent conductive hearing loss associated with acute or chronic middle-ear effusions or, in the absence of an effusion, with high negative pressure within the middle ear. The audiogram usually reveals a mild to moderate conductive loss. Infrequently, there may be a sensorineural component, usually at the higher frequencies and usually in long-standing chronic middle-ear disease. The conductive hearing loss is usually reversible with resolution of the effusion, but permanent conductive hearing loss can result from irreversible changes secondary to recurrent acute or chronic inflammation (adhesive otitis, tympanosclerosis, ossicular discontinuity). Rarely, very significant sensorineural loss may occur, usually as a result of suppurative labyrinthitis.

Persistent or episodic conductive hearing loss in children may impair their cognitive, language, and emotional development, but the degree and duration of the hearing loss required to produce such deficits are unknown. Many studies suggest that children do suffer such long-term effects when OM occurs early in life. The scientific evidence, however, remains incomplete. Some experts are skeptical about the available data and have concluded that no causal link can be established between early, recurrent middle-ear effusion and language delay or learning problems. Several studies, however, have shown an association between early OM and later deficits. Prolonged duration of middle-ear effusions, which is associated with significant loss of hearing, may be detrimental to a child's ability to develop speech and language optimally when the OM occurs early in life.

PERFORATION. Perforation of the tympanic membrane frequently occurs when the central portion of the eardrum spontaneously ruptures during an episode of AOM. A large number of temporary perforations are created by surgical treatment of OM with tympanostomy tubes. Approximately 1/200 children develops a long-term perforation as a result of the placement of tympanostomy tubes.

OTORRHEA. More than 1 million tympanostomy tubes are inserted annually for the treatment of recurrent AOM and OME, and approximately 50–65% of patients develop otorrhea at least once while the tubes are in place and patent. The organisms, most frequently cultured from acute discharge through a tympanostomy tube, are the same as those cultured from acute middle-ear effusions when tympanocentesis was performed (*S. pneumoniae, H. influenzae*, and *M. catarrhalis*). Group A *Streptococcus*, when present and untreated, has been associated with acute, spontaneous perforation of the tympanic membrane.

Antimicrobial therapy for patients with acute perforation of the membrane is the same as that for AOM when a perforation is not present. When chronic aural discharge is present, culturing the drainage is desirable. The antimicrobial regimen can then be adjusted according to the results of the Gram stain, culture, and antibiotic susceptibility testing. Patients may also benefit from otic drops instilled into the external canal because the topical medication may treat or prevent an external canal infection and hasten the resolution of the middle-ear infection. In addition, ototopical drops may prevent bacteria in the external canal (*Staphylococcus* and *Pseudomonas*) from entering the middle ear and causing a chronic infection. Healing of the tympanic membrane frequently follows cessation of the suppurative process in the middle ear, but the perforated tympanic membrane may remain open after an episode of AOM. When the perforation is present with no signs of healing and there are no signs of OM for several months, the perforation is considered to be chronic and possibly permanent. Many infants and young children may benefit from the open tympanic membrane (acting perhaps as a "tympansotomy tube"), but for patients older than 5 yr, the perforation should be evaluated for repair (tympanoplasty) to restore the eustachian tube–middle-ear air cushion.

If otorrhea persists despite adequate antimicrobial therapy or if the drainage seems to be coming from an apparent posterosuperior or attic (pars flaccida) defect, a cholesteatoma should be suspected. Aural polyps, which appear as red, friable masses, may protrude through one of these defects, possibly indicating the presence of a cholesteatoma.

CHRONIC SUPPURATIVE OTITIS MEDIA WITH MASTOIDITIS. This stage of ear disease is marked by chronic infection of the middle ear and mastoid (mastoiditis), a nonintact tympanic membrane (because of perforation or tympanostomy tube), and discharge (otorrhea) that has been refractory to medical management for more than 6 wk. It develops from a chronic bacterial infection, but the bacteria that caused the initial episode of AOM with perforation are usually not those that are isolated from the chronic discharge. The most common bacterial species isolated are *P. aeruginosa* and *S. aureus*. The most common anaerobic species isolated are *Bacteroides, Peptostreptococcus*, and *Peptococcus*. Thus, the antimicrobial therapy recommended for AOM is not effective for most cases of chronic suppurative OM. Tympanomastoid surgery is indicated when cholesteatoma is present.

The medical treatment of chronic suppurative OM without cholesteatoma is directed toward eliminating the infection from the middle ear and mastoid. Antimicrobial agents should be selected for effectiveness against the cultured organisms. Because of the high prevalence of *P. aeruginosa*, suspensions that contain polymyxin B, neomycin, and hydrocortisone (Cortisporin) or neomycin, polymyxin E, and hydrocortisone (Coly-Mycin), have been recommended, but their potential ototoxicity limits their usefulness of the less potentially ototoxic otic preparations, the quinolones are the most common. In children, orally administered antibiotics are usually not effective unless an organism that is seen on Gram stain or is cultured from the discharge is susceptible to a specific antibiotic, such as *S. aureus*, pneumococcus, or *H. influenzae*. Other antimicrobials, including the quinolones, have antimicrobial activity against many of the bacterial organisms that cause chronic suppurative disease (including *Pseudomonas*).

Because of concern over the toxicity of the ototopical agents, patients and parents should be informed of the danger if potentially ototoxic medications are used. If a topical antibiotic medication is used, patients should return to the outpatient facility daily so that the discharge can be thoroughly aspirated. The discharge rapidly improves with this type of treatment, usually within 1–2 wk.

As an alternative, it is recommended that children be given a parenteral antipseudomonal (or other appropriate drug). The middle ear is aspirated daily through the existing tube or perforation. In most children, the middle ear is free of discharge and the signs of OM greatly improve or disappear within 7–10 days.

When the discharge fails to respond to intensive medical therapy, surgery on the middle ear and mastoid is indicated. In a study of 36 pediatric patients with chronic suppurative OM, in which all received parenteral antimicrobial therapy and daily aural cleansing, 89% had their initial infection resolved with medical therapy alone and 11% required tympanomastoidectomy.

If the infection is eliminated using these methods, prevention of recurrence is usually achieved by the following: (1) prophylactic antimicrobial therapy, (2) removal of the tympanostomy tube, or (3) surgical repair of the tympanic membrane defect. The appropriate choice depends on the age of the patient and the function of the eustachian tube.

ACQUIRED CHOLESTEATOMA. Long-standing middle-ear and mastoid disease, including deep retraction pockets, may lead to formation of a cholesteatoma. This saclike structure within the middle ear is lined by keratinized, stratified, squamous epithelium and contains desquamated epithelium or keratin. White, shiny, greasy debris accompanied by a foul-smelling discharge may be observed. Tympanomastoid surgery is the only effective therapy for cholesteatoma; if it is delayed, the disease can invade and destroy other structures of the temporal bone and can spread to the intracranial cavity.

MASTOIDITIS. Mastoiditis is classified into acute and chronic forms. Acute mastoiditis is further subdivided into pathologic stages, which are the basis for management. In almost every child with AOM, the mastoid air cells are also inflamed; thus, acute mastoiditis is a natural extension and part of the pathologic process of an acute middle-ear infection. No specific signs or symptoms of the mastoid infection are present in this most common stage of acute mastoiditis. The hearing loss, otalgia, and fever are primarily a result of the acute infection within the middle ear. CT scans of the mastoid area are usually interpreted as "cloudy mastoids," which is indicative of the general inflammation. No mastoid osteitis is evident on the CT scan. The process is usually reversible because the middle-ear-mastoid effusion resolves, either as a natural process or as a result of treatment of the acute infection. If resolution of the infection does not occur at this stage, one or more of the following conditions may develop: (1) acute mastoiditis with periosteitis, (2) acute mastoid osteitis (with or without a subperiosteal abscess), or (3) chronic mastoiditis.

Acute Mastoiditis with Periosteitis. This occurs when the infection within the mastoid air cells spreads to the periosteum covering the mastoid process, causing periosteitis. The condition should not be confused with the presence of a subperiosteal abscess because management of the latter condition requires incision and drainage of the abscess and possibly complete simple (cortical) mastoidectomy; the former, however, usually responds to immediate but less aggressive surgical intervention, including myringotomy with or without ventilation tube placement and parenteral antimicrobials.

Prompt improvement of the periosteal involvement should occur within 24–48 hr after the tympanic membrane has been opened for drainage and appropriate antimicrobial therapy has begun. Clinically, the ear should no longer be protruding forward, and the posterior auricular sulcus should not be red and should be better defined than at the time of initial presentation. Surgical drainage of the mastoid (complete simple mastoidectomy) should be performed if the symptoms of the acute infection, such as fever and otalgia, persist, if the postauricular involvement does not improve, or if a subperiosteal abscess develops.

Failure to institute immediate treatment at this stage may result in the development of acute mastoid osteitis with or without a subperiosteal abscess or, more dangerous to a child, a suppurative intratemporal or intracranial complication such as lateral sinus thrombosis, extradural abscess, or meningitis.

Acute Mastoid Osteitis (Acute Coalescent Mastoiditis, Acute Surgical Mastoiditis). This occurs when an infection within the mastoid progresses, causing destruction of the bony trabeculae that separate the mastoid cells and coalescence of the cells. Essentially, a mastoid empyema is present. The primary clinical manifestations include swelling, redness, and tenderness to the touch over the mastoid bone. The pinna is displaced outward and downward, and swelling or sagging of the posterosuperior canal wall may also be noted. A purulent discharge may issue through a perforation in the tympanic membrane. Ear drainage may be persistent, and the ear canal filled with pus and debris. Alternatively, a nipple-like protrusion may be seen at the site of a small tympanic membrane perforation. A fluctuant subperiosteal abscess or even a drainage fistula from the mastoid to the postauricular area may be present. Patients may be toxic and febrile, with systemic signs of acute illness. In the subacute disease, fever may be prolonged and low grade, with occasional temperature spikes.

The diagnosis should be suspected on the basis of clinical signs. CT scans of the temporal bone may reveal one or more of the following: (1) haziness, distortion, or destruction of the mastoid outline; (2) fuzziness of the shadows of cellular walls as a result of demineralization, atrophy, or ischemia of the bony septa; (3) a decrease in the density and cloudiness of the areas of pneumatization because of inflammatory swelling of the air cells; and (4) in long-standing cases, a chronic osteoblastic inflammatory reaction that may obliterate the cellular structure. Small abscess cavities in sclerotic bone may be confused with pneumatic cells. CT scans are also helpful in ruling out the coexistence of other suppurative intratemporal or intracranial complications of OM.

Antimicrobial agents are the mainstay of treatment of acute disease. If the case is otherwise uncomplicated (no prior infection), *S. pneumoniae* or *H. influenzae* is probably responsible. For coalescent mastoiditis, a complete, simple ("cortical") mastoidectomy should also be performed, especially when the mastoid empyema has extended outside the mastoid bone. Appropriate systemic antimicrobial therapy should also be given. The procedure should be considered an emergency, but the timing of the operation must depend on a child's status, failure to control infection during the acute stage of mastoid osteitis may lead to a chronic infection within the mastoid bone or to a suppurative complication.

Chronic Mastoiditis. Chronic mastoiditis is invariably associated with chronic suppurative OM. The mastoid may be poorly pneumatized or sclerotic. The chronic infection should be controlled by medical treatment, but when extensive granulation tissue and osteitis are present in the mastoid, mastoidectomy is usually necessary to eliminate the chronic mastoid osteitis, especially if a cholesteatoma is present.

PETROSITIS. This may result from acute or chronic infections of the pneumatized apical and perilabyrinthine cells of the temporal bone. The triad of OM, paralysis of the external rectus muscle, and pain in the ipsilateral orbit or retro-orbital area with headache constitutes petrous apicitis (Gradenigo's syndrome).

ADHESIVE OTITIS. This is a result of healing after chronic inflammation of the middle ear. The mucous membrane is thickened by proliferation of fibrous tissue, which frequently impairs the movement of the ossicles and tympanic membrane and may result in significant conductive hearing loss.

TYMPANOSCLEROSIS. This is a complication of chronic middle-ear inflammation characterized by whitish plaques involving the middle layer of the tympanic membrane and nodular deposits in the submucosal layers of the middle ear. There is hyalinization with deposition of calcium and phosphate crystals, and conductive hearing loss may result from the ossicles' embedding in the deposits.

OSSICULAR DISCONTINUITY. This is a result of rarefying osteitis secondary to chronic middle-ear inflammation. The long process of the incus is commonly involved, but the crural arch of the stapes, the body of the incus, or the manubrium of the malleus may also be eroded. The conductive hearing loss that frequently results can often be corrected surgically.

FACIAL PARALYSIS. This may occur during an episode of AOM or during chronic middle-ear, often suppurative, disease. Because the facial nerve is congenitally dehiscent in its middle ear course as much as 50% of the time, it is not surprising that facial nerve dysfunction may occur secondary to infection; remarkably, this is uncommon. When it occurs as an isolated complication of AOM, a myringotomy with culture of the middle ear contents should be performed and parenteral antibiotics administered. The paralysis usually improves rapidly without further surgery (facial nerve decompression). Mastoidectomy is not indicated unless mastoid osteitis is present. However, urgent surgical intervention is indicated when facial paralysis develops in a child who has chronic suppurative OM with or without cholesteatoma.

SUPPURATIVE LABYRINTHITIS. This may result from direct invasion of bacteria through the round or oval windows during an episode of AOM. When chronic OM is present, the infection may penetrate the windows or enter through a fistula of the bony horizontal semicircular canal. Patients may have vertigo, nystagmus, tinnitus, hearing loss, nausea, and vomiting. Treatment consists of intensive parenteral antibiotic therapy, myringotomy, and possibly tube insertion. Mastoidectomy with labyrinthectomy may prevent spread to the intracranial cavity.

CHOLESTEROL GRANULOMA. Cholesterol granuloma is a sequela of chronic OME. It has been described as "idiopathic hemotympanum" because the tympanic membrane appears to be dark blue. The treatment of choice is middle-ear and mastoid surgery.

NECK ABSCESS. Neck muscles such as the sternocleidomastoid and posterior belly of the digastric attach to the mastoid tip, and occasionally, a mastoid infection breaks through deep to these muscles and presents as an abscess in the neck called a *Bezold abscess*. In all cases of cervical infection, it is important to visualize the tympanic membrane and to consider the possible role of OM and mastoiditis.

INFECTIOUS ECZEMATOID DERMATITIS. This may be associated with an infection of the external auditory canal (see Chapter 645) or may be secondary to a discharge from the middle ear and mastoid. Management should be directed toward resolving the middle ear-mastoid infection.

INTRACRANIAL SUPPURATIVE COMPLICATIONS. These include meningitis, otitis hydrocephalus, lateral sinus thrombosis, intracranial abscess, and epidural and subdural abscess. The incidence of suppurative intracranial complications of OM has declined greatly because of the use of antimicrobial agents. They occur most often in association with chronic suppurative OM and mastoiditis, with or without cholesteatoma. The middle ear and mastoid air cells are adjacent to important structures, including the dura of the posterior and middle cranial fossa, the sigmoid venous sinus of the brain, and the inner ear. Suppuration in the middle ear, mastoid, or both may spread to these structures through progressive thrombophlebitis, bony erosion, or direct extension, resulting in meningitis, extradural abscess, subdural empyema, focal encephalitis, brain abscess, lateral (sigmoid) sinus thrombosis, and otic hydrocephalus. The numerous complications frequently depend on the route of infection.

Any child who has acute or chronic OM and who develops one or more of the following signs or symptoms, especially while receiving medical treatment, should be suspected of having a suppurative intracranial complication: persistent headache, lethargy, malaise, irritability, change in personality, severe otalgia, persistent or recurrent fever, nausea, and vomiting. High fever is rarely present in children with chronic suppurative OM; when present, it should suggest an impending intracranial complication. The following are definitive clinical manifestations requiring an intensive search for an intracranial complication: meningismus, focal seizures, ataxia, blurred vision, papilledema, diplopia, hemiplegia, aphasia, dysdiadochokinesia, intention tremor, dysmetria, and hemianopia. Conversely, children with intracranial infection, such as meningitis or a brain abscess, should have middle-ear-mastoid disease ruled out as the origin of, or concomitant with, the central nervous system (CNS) disease.

Diagnosis of intracranial complications is greatly improved by the use of CT. MRI also provides excellent definition of intracranial suppuration and its consequences (edema, herniation, thrombosis, hydrocephalus), but it does not provide the bony detail needed to evaluate the mastoid.

MENINGITIS. Meningitis may occur because of (1) direct invasion, in which a suppurative focus in the middle ear or mastoid spreads through the dura and extends to the pia-arachnoid, causing generalized meningitis; (2) suppuration in an adjacent area, such as a subdural abscess, brain abscess, or lateral sinus thrombophlebitis, which causes the meninges to become inflamed, and (3) hematogenous spread with concurrent infection, in which OM arises by contiguous spread from an infectious focus in the upper respiratory tract, and meningitis results from invasion of the blood from the upper respiratory focus. The latter is the most common route.

EXTRADURAL ABSCESS. Extradural (epidural) abscess usually results from the destruction of bone adjacent to the dura by cholesteatoma, infection, or both. This occurs when granulation tissue and purulent material collect between the lateral aspect of the dura and adjacent temporal bone. Dural granulation tissue within a bony defect is more common than an actual accumulation of pus. When an abscess is present, a dural sinus thrombosis, or less commonly a subdural or brain abscess, may also be present. If extensive bony destruction has occurred because of acute mastoid osteitis (acute coalescent mastoiditis), an extradural abscess may develop in the area of the sigmoid dural sinus with sigmoid sinus thrombosis.

Clinical manifestations may include severe earache, low-grade fever, and headache in the temporal region with deep, local, throbbing pain. There may be no signs or symptoms. An asymptomatic extradural abscess may occasionally be found in patients undergoing elective mastoidectomy for cholesteatoma. When otorrhea occurs, it is characteristically profuse, creamy, and pulsatile. Compression of the ipsilateral jugular vein may increase the rate of discharge and the degree of pulsation. Patients usually have no accompanying fever (but malaise and anorexia may be observed) and no neurologic signs; the intracranial pressure (ICP) is normal, and it is difficult to detect any displacement of the brain. The cerebrospinal fluid (CSF) cell count and pressure are normal unless meningitis is also present. CT scanning may reveal a large extradural abscess.

The *treatment* of extradural abscess consists of surgical drainage. A mastoidectomy is performed, enough bone is removed so that the dura of the middle and posterior fossas may be inspected directly, the extradural abscess is identified and removed (and sometimes a drain is also inserted), and the otologic procedure that can provide optimal exteriorization of the diseased area is completed by removing all the granulation tissue until normal dura is found.

SUBDURAL EMPYEMA. A subdural empyema is a collection of purulent material within the potential space between the dura externally and arachnoid membrane internally. It may develop as a direct extension of infection or, more rarely, by thrombophlebitis through venous channels. It is a rare complication of OM and mastoiditis.

Children with subdural empyema are extremely toxic and febrile. They usually have the signs and symptoms of a locally expanding intracranial mass. Severe headache in the temporoparietal area is usually present. CNS findings may include seizures, hemiplegia, dysmetria, belligerent behavior, somnolence, stupor, deviation of the eyes, dysphagia, sensory deficits, meningismus, and a positive Kernig sign. Hemiplegia and jacksonian epilepsy in a child with suppurative disease of the middle ear and mastoid usually indicate a subdural empyema. CT scanning is often diagnostic. The peripheral white blood cell count is high, and there is a predominance of polymorphonuclear leukocytes. The CSF glucose concentration is normal, and no microorganisms are seen on smear or culture of the CSF. If a patient has signs of increased ICP, lumbar puncture is contraindicated.

Treatment of subdural empyema includes intensive intravenous antimicrobial therapy, anticonvulsants, and neurosurgical drainage of the empyema through bur holes or craniectomy. Corticosteroids are occasionally needed to diminish severe edema. Mastoid surgery to locate and drain the source of infection may be performed concurrently with the neurosurgical intervention or occasionally may be delayed until after neurosurgical intervention has yielded some improvement in neurologic status. The condition has a significant mortality rate, and more than 50% of children who recover have some residual neurologic deficit.

FOCAL OTITIC ENCEPHALITIS. Edematous and inflamed focal areas of brain may occur as a complication of acute or chronic OM or of the other suppurative complications of these disorders. The signs and symptoms of this focal otic encephalitis may be similar to those of a brain abscess or subdural empyema, except that the suppuration within the brain is absent. Ataxia, nystagmus, vomiting, and giddiness suggest a possible focus within the cerebellum, whereas drowsiness, disorientation, restlessness, seizures, and coma suggest a cerebral focus. Headache may be present. CT or needle aspiration may be necessary to preclude an abscess. If an abscess is not present, the focal encephalitis should be treated by administering high-dose intravenous antimicrobial agents and by carrying out an appropriate otologic surgical procedure to remove the source of infection as soon as possible. Failure to control the source of the infection within the temporal bone, as well as the focal encephalitis, may result in the development of a brain abscess. Anticonvulsive medication is given when a patient has cerebral involvement.

OTOGENIC BRAIN ABSCESS (also see Chapter 610). Otogenic abscess of the brain may result directly from acute or chronic middle-ear and mastoid infection (with or without cholesteatoma) or may follow the development of an adjacent infection, such as lateral sinus thrombophlebitis, petrositis, or meningitis. The dura overlying the infected mastoid is invaded along vascular pathways or by adherence of the dura to underlying infected bone. Chronic OM or mastoiditis (with or without cholesteatoma) may lead to erosion of the tegmen tympani by pressure necrosis and perforation of the bone, with resultant inflammation of the dura and invasion by pathogenic organisms. An extradural abscess occurs, with subsequent infiltration of the dura, and spreads to the subdural space. A localized subdural abscess or leptomeningitis ensues. Invasion of brain tissue follows. The abscess is located closest to the primary source of infection. Thus, temporal lobe abscesses follow invasion through the tegmen tympani or petrous bone. Cerebellar abscesses occur when the infectious focus is the posterior surface of the petrous bone or thrombophlebitis of the lateral sinus. The former occurs more frequently than the latter, and numerous abscesses are common.

Signs and symptoms of invasion of the CNS usually occur about 1 mo after an episode of AOM or an acute exacerbation of chronic OM. Most children are febrile, although systemic signs, including fever and chills, vary and may be absent. Signs of a generalized CNS infection include severe headache, vomiting, drowsiness, seizures, irritability, personality change, altered levels of consciousness, anorexia and weight loss, and meningismus. Temporal lobe abscesses are associated with seizures in some children, may be associated with visual field deficits (optic radiation involvement), or may be silent. Cerebellar abscesses cause vertigo, nystagmus, ataxia, dysmetria, and symptoms of hydrocephalus. Patients may have persistent purulent ear drainage, suggesting the primary site of infection. See Chapter 610 for treatment.

LATERAL SINUS THROMBOSIS. Lateral and sigmoid sinus thrombosis or thrombophlebitis arises from inflammation in the adjacent mastoid. The superior and petrosal dural sinuses are also intimately associated with the temporal bone but are rarely affected. The mastoid infection in contact with the sinus walls produces inflammation of the adventitia followed by penetration of the venous wall. Formation of a thrombus occurs after the infection has spread to the intima. The mural thrombus may become infected and propagate, occluding the lumen. Embolization of septic thrombi or extension of infection into the tributary vessels may cause further disease. This complication is still common in children and can be caused by both acute and chronic OM and mastoiditis.

The clinical signs of lateral sinus thrombosis include (1) general fever, headache, and malaise (with the formation of the infectious mural thrombus, patients may have spiking fever and chills); (2) CNS—headache, papilledema, signs of increased ICP, altered states of consciousness, and seizures; (3) metastatic disease caused by infected thrombi and septic infarcts—pneumonia, septic infarcts, empyema, bone and joint infection, and, less commonly, thyroiditis, endocarditis, ophthalmitis, and abscess of the kidney; (4) spread to skin and soft tissues—cellulitis or abscess; and (5) signs of intracranial complications, including meningitis, cavernous sinus thrombosis, and brain abscess.

CT and MRI are invaluable in making the diagnosis, and their use must precede a lumbar puncture. Variations in CSF pressure can occur; thus, demonstration by the Queckenstedt test is contraindicated because of the risk of herniation. In some cases, leakage of red blood cells and subsequent xanthochromia may occur.

Treatment includes the use of antimicrobial agents and surgery. Administration of anticoagulant medication is controversial because of the risks of releasing septic emboli or causing uncontrollable hemorrhage in the mastoid. The sinus should be uncovered, and any perisinus abscesses drained. The lateral sinus should be opened, and the thrombus removed if there is septic thrombophlebitis.

OTITIC HYDROCEPHALUS. This syndrome consists of increased ICP without other abnormalities of the CSF, complicating acute or chronic OM. The pathogenesis is unknown, but because the ventricles are not dilated, the term *benign intracranial hypertension* may also be appropriate. The disease is frequently associated with lateral sinus thrombosis. Symptoms include a headache that is often intractable, blurring of vision, nausea, vomiting, and diplopia. Signs include a draining ear, abducens paralysis of one or both lateral rectus muscles, and papilledema.

CT should be performed before lumbar puncture to prevent brain herniation. The CSF pressure sometimes exceeds 300 mm H_2O, and the ventricles are of normal or small size. Although usually benign, otitic hydrocephalus may evolve to loss of vision secondary to optic atrophy (see Chapter 612).

Treatment includes the use of antimicrobial agents, mastoidectomy, normalization of ICP by medications (acetazolamide, furosemide), repeated lumbar punctures, or a lumboperitoneal shunt. An aggressive approach is warranted because of the possibility of optic atrophy.

CHAPTER 647
The Inner Ear and Diseases of the Bony Labyrinth

The function and anatomy of the inner ear may be affected by infectious organisms, including viruses, bacteria, and protozoa. Genetic abnormalities may also be responsible for abnormal anatomy and function. Other acquired diseases of the labyrinthine capsule include otosclerosis, osteopetrosis, Langerhans' cell histiocytosis, fibrous dysplasia, and other types of bony dysplasia. All of these can cause hearing loss, both conductive and sensorineural, as well as vestibular dysfunction.

VIRUSES. Viral causes of sensorineural hearing loss (SNHL) include congenital rubella and congenital cytomegalovirus (CMV), as well as mumps, postnatal rubella, and rubeola (measles). Fifth disease, caused by parvovirus B19, is an infrequent cause of SNHL. Many other viruses are occasionally associated with SNHL. The most common cause of congenital viral sensorineural hearing loss currently is CMV. An estimated 1% of all liveborn infants in the United States are infected with CMV; between 6,000 and 8,000 have clinical manifestations. Of the 6,000–8,000, approximately 75% have hearing loss. In addition, 10–15% of the "asymptomatic" children with congenital CMV have SNHL. In as many as 50%, hearing loss, which is usually bilateral though often asymmetric, progresses and worsens over weeks to years. Stabilization or improvement in the hearing loss may be possible by using ganciclovir in very young infants with congenital CMV (Chapter 248).

Before the introduction of an effective vaccine, rubella was responsible for as many as 60% of the newly identified cases of childhood SNHL. Fortunately, vaccination in most developed countries has reduced the rate of rubella by more than 97%, although rubella may still occur in children from countries where the vaccine has not completely eliminated the disease. Similarly, measles and mumps, though now uncommon causes of SNHL in the United States because of successful vaccination programs, may still result in SNHL in children who get these diseases.

Herpes simplex encephalitis may also be associated with SNHL; the hearing loss is more common in those children with congenital herpesvirus infection. Acyclovir and other antiviral agents may help the hearing loss and other central nervous system manifestations.

TOXOPLASMOSIS. *Toxoplasma gondii* is a protozoan that may cause congenital SNHL. Estimates are that about 3,000 children are born in the United States yearly with congenital toxoplasmosis, with about 5–10% showing severe clinical signs and symptoms at birth. Symptoms may also occur throughout a child's life, causing chorioretinitis. Approximately 25% of untreated patients have SNHL. If infection is documented during the fetal period, medical therapy may be able to prevent some of the clinical manifestations, including SNHL (Chapter 280).

BACTERIAL MENINGITIS. Since the introduction of the Hib vaccine, *Streptococcus pneumoniae* and *Neisseria meningitidis* have become the leading causes of bacterial meningitis in children. Hearing loss occurs more commonly with *S. pneumoniae*, with an estimated incidence of 15–20%. Approximately 60% of those hearing losses are bilateral, though often asymmetric. If the hearing loss is present at the time of presentation with meningitis, and especially if it is severe to profound, the likelihood of significant improvement is small. However, if the hearing loss develops after admission for treatment and is not severe, stabilization or improvement is possible. Late progression of SNHL has also been noted in some children years after meningitis. In the United States and may other developed countries, bacterial meningitis is one of the major causes of profound deafness leading to cochlear implantation in children.

All studies since 1988 have shown favorable trends in the course and outcome of adjunctive dexamethasone for hearing loss and other neurologic deficits associated with bacterial meningitis (Chapter 174.1), although the effectiveness, especially for *S. pneumoniae* and *N. meningitidis* meningitis, has not reached statistical significance in all individual trials because of the few number of cases in some studies. A recent meta-analysis of 11 studies conducted from 1988 to 1996 showed a beneficial effect of dexamethasone to reduce severe hearing loss associated with *H. influenzae* type b meningitis regardless of the timing of administration of dexamethasone (before or with antibiotics vs. later) or of the antibiotic used. For pneumococcal meningitis, the meta-analysis showed a benefit of dexamethasone only when given early and only for protection against severe hearing loss. There were still too few cases even by meta-analysis of hearing loss with meningococcal meningitis to assess the benefit of dexamethasone.

SYPHILIS. Congenital syphilis may cause SNHL in 3–38% of children; the exact incidence is difficult to ascertain, because the hearing loss may not occur until adolescence or even adulthood. When the condition is identified, treatment with antibiotics and steroids may improve the hearing loss.

OTHER DISEASES OF THE INNER EAR. *Labyrinthitis* may be a complication of direct spread of acute or chronic otitis media and mastoiditis but may also complicate bacterial meningitis as a result of organisms entering the labyrinth through the internal auditory meatus, endolymphatic duct, perilymphatic duct, vascular channels, or hematogenous spread. Clinical manifestations of labyrinthitis may include vertigo, disequilibrium, deep-seated ear pain, nausea, vomiting, nystagmus, and SNHL. Acute suppurative labyrinthitis, characterized by abrupt, severe onset of these symptoms, requires intensive antimicrobial therapy. If it is secondary to otitis media, it may require otologic surgery to remove cholesteatoma or drain the middle ear and mastoid, in addition to antibiotics. Acute serous labyrinthitis, with milder symptoms of vertigo and hearing loss, may occur secondary to middle-ear infection as well. Fortunately, it usually responds well to antibiotics and steroids, with improvement in both the vertigo and hearing loss. Chronic labyrinthitis, most commonly associated with cholesteatoma, presents with SNHL and vestibular dysfunction that develops over time; surgery is required to remove the cholesteatoma. Chronic labyrinthitis may also uncommonly occur secondary to long-standing otitis media, with the slow development of SNHL, usually starting in the higher frequencies, and possibly with vestibular dysfunction. Additionally, and more commonly, children with chronic middle-ear fluid are often unsteady or off balance, a situation that immediately improves when the fluid resolves.

Otosclerosis, an autosomal dominant disease that affects only the temporal bones, causes abnormal bone growth that can cause fixation of the stapes in the oval window, resulting in progressive hearing loss. The hearing loss is usually conductive at first, but SNHL may develop. Females and whites are affected most commonly. The onset of otosclerosis generally occurs in teenagers or young adults. Corrective surgery to replace the stapes with a mobile prosthesis is often successful.

Osteogenesis imperfecta (OI) is a systemic disease that may involve both the middle and inner ears. Many different genetic types of OI, with varying clinical presentations, have been described. Hearing loss occurs in about 20% of young children and as many as 90% of adults. The hearing loss is most commonly conductive owing to abnormalities of the ossicles, but SNHL may occur if other areas of the otic capsule become affected. If the hearing loss is severe enough, a hearing aid may be a preferable alternative to surgical correction of the fixed stapes, because stapedectomy in children with OI can be technically very difficult and the disease and the hearing loss may be progressive (Chapter 704).

Osteopetrosis, a very uncommon skeletal dysplasia, may involve the temporal bone, including the middle ear and ossicles, resulting in a moderate to severe, generally conductive hearing loss. Recurrent facial nerve paralysis may also occur owing to excess bone deposition; each time it occurs, less facial function may return (Chapter 704).

CHAPTER 648

Traumatic Injuries of the Ear and Temporal Bone

AURICLE AND EXTERNAL AUDITORY CANAL. *Hematoma*, an accumulation of blood between the perichondrium and the cartilage, may follow trauma to the pinna. Immediate needle aspiration or, when the hematoma is extensive or recurrent, incision and drainage and a pressure dressing are necessary to prevent perichondritis, which can result in a cauliflower ear deformity.

Frostbite of the auricle should be managed by rapidly rewarming the exposed pinna with warm irrigation or warm compresses.

Foreign bodies in the external canal are common in childhood. These can often be removed without general anesthesia if the child is informed about the procedure (if old enough to understand it) and is properly restrained; if an adequate headlight, surgical head otoscope, or otomicroscope is used for visualizing the object; and if appropriate instruments, such as alligator forceps, wire loops or a blunt cerumen curette, or suction are used, depending on the shape of the object. Gentle irrigation of the ear canal with body temperature water or saline may also result in removal of very small objects (this should be attempted only if the examiner is certain that the tympanic membrane is intact). Conversely, attempted removal of an object when a child is struggling and when visualization and tools are inadequate often results in a terrified child with a swollen and bleeding ear canal that mandates a trip to the operating room for removal of the object. General anesthesia and an otomicroscope are necessary for removal of more difficult foreign bodies, especially those that are large, round, or deeply embedded in the canal just lateral to the tympanic membrane or those objects that have resulted in a marked amount of swelling of the ear canal skin, making visualization of the object difficult. After a foreign body is removed from the external canal, the tympanic membrane should be carefully inspected for possible traumatic perforation or for a pre-existing middle-ear effusion. If a foreign body has resulted in acute inflammation of the canal, treatment as described for acute diffuse external otitis should be instituted. Insects in the canal may be pretreated with lidocaine or mineral oil; they either exit spontaneously or with continued lavage.

TYMPANIC MEMBRANE AND MIDDLE EAR. Traumatic perforation of the tympanic membrane usually occurs as a result of a sudden external compression (a slap) or penetration by a foreign object (a stick or cotton-tipped applicator). The perforation may be linear or stellate and is most frequently in the anterior portion of the pars tensa when it is caused by compression; it may be in any quadrant of the tympanic membrane when caused by a foreign object. Systemic antibiotics and topical otic medications are not required unless suppurative otorrhea is present. Spontaneous healing usually occurs. If the membrane does not heal within several months, surgery to repair the tympanic membrane should be considered. As long as the perforation is present, otorrhea may occur at any time during periods of upper respiratory tract infection because the middle-ear air cushion is lost, permitting reflux of nasopharyngeal secretions into the middle-ear cavity. Water entering the middle ear from the ear canal, which can occur during swimming (or, less commonly, bathing), may also result in otorrhea. Perforations resulting from penetrating foreign bodies are less likely to heal than those caused by compression. Implantation of epithelium from a traumatic perforation can also result in a cholesteatoma. Audiometric examination usually reveals a conductive hearing loss as well, with larger air-bone gaps generally occurring secondary to larger perforations. Immediate surgical exploration is indicated if the injury is accompanied by one or more of the following: vertigo, nystagmus, severe tinnitus, moderate to severe hearing loss, or cerebrospinal fluid (CSF) otorrhea. At the time of exploration, it is necessary to inspect the ossicles, especially the stapes, as they may have been dislocated or fractured; sharp objects may have penetrated the oval or round windows. If the stapes has been subluxed or dislocated into the oval window or if either the oval or round window has been penetrated, SNHL results.

Perilymphatic fistula (PLF) may occur after sudden barotrauma or an increase in CSF pressure. This condition is more common than generally appreciated and should always be suspected in a child who develops a sudden or fluctuating SNHL, vertigo, or both after physical exertion, deep water diving, flying in an airplane, playing a wind instrument, significant head trauma, or any activity that suddenly increases the pressures within the middle ear or the labyrinth. The leak characteristically is at the oval or the round window; PLF's probably occur if the oval or round windows are congenitally abnormal or if there is pre-existing anatomic abnormality of the cochlea or semicircular canals. PLFs occasionally close spontaneously, but immediate surgical repair of the fistula is usually needed to control the vertigo and to stop any progression of the SNHL. Even appropriate surgery does not usually restore the SNHL that has already occurred.

TEMPORAL BONE FRACTURES. Children are particularly prone to basilar skull fractures, which usually involve the temporal bone. Seventy to 80% of temporal bone fractures are longitudinal and are commonly manifested by bleeding from a laceration of the external canal or tympanic membrane; hemotympanum (blood accumulating behind an intact eardrum); conductive hearing loss resulting from laceration of the tympanic membrane, hemotympanum, or ossicular injury; delayed onset of facial paralysis (which usually improves spontaneously); and temporary CSF otorrhea or rhinorrhea (from CSF running down the eustachian tube). Transverse fractures of the temporal bone have a graver prognosis than longitudinal fractures and are often associated with immediate facial paralysis. Facial paralysis may improve if caused by edema, but surgical decompression of the nerve is often recommended if there is no evidence of clinical recovery and facial nerve studies are unfavorable. If the facial nerve has been transected, surgical decompression and anastomosis offer the possibility of at least some functional recovery. Transverse fractures are also associated with severe SNHL, vertigo, nystagmus, tinnitus, nausea, and vomiting associated with loss of cochlear and vestibular function; hemotympanum; rarely, external canal bleeding; and CSF otorrhea, either in the external auditory canal or behind the tympanic membrane, which may exit the nose via the eustachian tube.

If temporal bone fracture is suspected or seen on radiographs, gentle examination of the pinna and ear canal is indicated; lacerations or avulsion of soft tissue is common with temporal bone fractures. *Battle sign,* ecchymosis over the mastoid, may also be seen. Vigorous removal of external auditory canal blood clots, tympanocentesis, or application of otic preparations are not indicated, because inadvertent removal of clots may also further dislodge the ossicles or reopen CSF leaks. Some have advocated prophylactic parenteral administration of antibiotics when CSF otorrhea or rhinorrhea is present, but this is controversial. If a patient is afebrile and the drainage is not cloudy, watchful waiting without antibiotics is indicated. Surgical intervention is reserved for children who require repair of the perforated tympanic membrane (that fails to heal spontaneously), who have suffered dislocation of the ossicular chain, or who need decompression of the facial nerve. SNHL can also follow a blow to the head without an obvious fracture of the temporal bone (labyrinthine concussion).

ACOUSTIC TRAUMA. This results from exposure to high-intensity sound (fireworks, gunfire, rock music, heavy machinery) and is initially manifested by a temporary decrease in hearing threshold, most commonly at 4,000 Hz on an audiometric examination, and tinnitus. If the sound exceeds 85 dB but less than 140 dB, the loss is usually temporary (after a rock concert), but both the hearing loss and the tinnitus may become permanent with chronic noise exposure, with the frequencies from 3,000–6,000 Hz most often involved. Sudden, extremely loud (>140 dB), short-duration noises with loud peak components (gunfire, bombs) may cause permanent hearing loss after a single exposure. Avoiding chronic exposure to loud noise and trying to protect the ears from sudden loud sounds are preventive measures. Hearing loss due to chronic noise exposure should be entirely preventable.

CHAPTER 649
Tumors of the Ear and Temporal Bone

Benign tumors of the external canal include *osteomas* and *monostotic* and *polyostotic fibrous dysplasia*. Osteomas present as bony masses in the canal and require removal only if hearing is impaired or external otitis results; osteomas may be confused clinically with exostoses.

Eosinophilic granuloma, which may occur in isolation or as part of the systemic Langerhans' cell histiocytosis, should be suspected in patients with otalgia, otorrhea, hearing loss, abnormal tissue within the middle ear or ear canal, and roentgenographic findings of a sharply delineated destructive lesion of the temporal bone. Definitive diagnosis is made by biopsy. Treatment depends on the site of the lesion and whether it is "eosinophilic granuloma," a unifocal or multifocal lesion of the bone that has a more benign course. Depending on the site, it may be treated by surgical excision, curettage, or local radiation (Chapter 515). If the lesion is part of a systemic presentation of Langerhans' cell histiocytosis, chemotherapy in addition to local therapy (surgery with or without radiation) is indicated. Long-term follow-up is indicated whether the temporal bone lesion is a single isolated one or part of a multisystem disease.

Symptoms and signs of *rhabdomyosarcoma* originating in the middle ear or ear canal include a mass or polyp in the middle ear or ear canal, bleeding from the ear, otorrhea, otalgia, facial paralysis, and hearing loss. Other cranial nerves may be involved as well. Diagnosis is based on biopsy, but the extent of disease is determined by both CT and MRI of the temporal bone, skull base, and brain. Classification is generally according to the stage as outlined in the current International Rhabdomyosarcoma Study group system. Management usually involves a combination of chemotherapy, radiation, and surgery (Chapter 506.1).

Non-Hodgkin lymphoma and leukemia may also present in the temporal bone, although as presentation of the initial lesion in these diseases it is rare. Although primary neoplasms of the middle ear are very uncommon in children, they include adenoid cystic carcinoma, adenocarcinoma, and squamous cell carcinoma. Benign tumors of the temporal bone include glomus tumors. The initial signs and symptoms of the more common nasopharyngeal neoplasms (angiofibroma, rhabdomyosarcoma, epidermoid carcinoma) may be associated with insidious onset of chronic otitis media with effusion (often unilateral); a high index of suspicion is needed for diagnosing these tumors accurately.

Adair-Bischoff CE, Sauve RS. Environmental tobacco smoke and middle ear disease in preschool-age children. Arch Pediatr Adolesc Med 152:127, 1998.

American Academy of Otolaryngology—Head and Neck Surgery Subcommittee on Cochlear Implants. Status of cochlear implantation in children. J Pediatr 118:1, 1991.

American Academy of Pediatrics, The Otitis Media Guideline Panel: Managing otitis media with effusion in young children. Pediatrics 94:766, 1994.

American Academy of Pediatrics; Joint Committee on Infant Hearing. 1994 Position Statement. Pediatrics 95:152, 1995.

American Academy of Pediatrics, Task Force on Newborn and Infant Hearing: Newborn and infant hearing loss: Detection and intervention. Pediatrics 103:527, 1999.

Barnett ED, Klein JO, Hawkins KA, et al: Comparison of spectral gradient acoustic reflectometry and other diagnostic techniques for detection of middle ear effusion in children with middle ear disease. Pediatr Infect Dis J 17:556, 1998.

Barsky-Firkser L, Sun S: Universal newborn hearing screenings: A three-year experience. Pediatrics 99:1, 1997.

Berman S, Roark R, Luckey D: Theoretical cost effectiveness of management options for children with persistent middle ear effusions. Pediatrics 93:353, 1994.

Bluestone CD, Klein JO: Otitis Media in Infants and Children, 2nd ed. Philadelphia, WB Saunders, 1995.

Bluestone CD, Klein JO: Intracranial suppurative complications of otitis media and mastoiditis. *In:* Bluestone CD, Stool SE, Kenna MA (eds): Pediatric Otolaryngology, 3rd ed. Philadelphia, WB Saunders, 1996, pp 636–648.

Bluestone CD, Klein JO: Intratemporal complications and sequelae of otitis media. *In:* Bluestone CD, Stool SE, Kenna MA (eds): Pediatric Otolaryngology, 3rd ed. Philadelphia, WB Saunders, 1996, pp 583–635.

Bluestone CD, Klein JO: Otitis media, atelectasis, and eustachian tube dysfunction. *In*: Bluestone CD, Stool SE, Kenna MA (eds): Pediatric Otolaryngology, 3rd ed. Philadelphia, WB Saunders, 1996, pp 388–582.

Bluestone CD: Otitis media and congenital perilymphatic fistula as a cause of sensorineural hearing loss in children. Pediatr Infect Dis J 7:S141, 1988.

Breiman RF, Butler JO, Tenover FC, et al: Emergence of drug-resistant pneumococcal infections in the United States. JAMA 271:1831, 1994.

Clinical Practice Guideline No. 12: Otitis Media with Effusion in Young Children. Publication No. 94-0622, Rockville, MD, U.S. Dept of HHS, Public Health Services. Agency for Health Care Policy and Research, 1994.

Cohen R, Levy C, Boucherat M, et al: A multicenter, randomized, double-blind trial of 5 versus 10 days of antibiotic therapy for acute otitis media in young children. J Pediatr 133:634, 1998.

Cox LC: Otoacoustic emissions as a screening tool for sensorineural hearing loss. J Pediatr 130:685, 1997.

Dowell SF, Butler JC, Giebink GS, et al: Acute otitis media: Management and surveillance in an era of pneumococcal resistance—a report from the Drug-resistant *Streptococcus pneumoniae* Therapeutic Working Group. Pediatr Infect Dis J 18:1, 1999.

Eilers RE, Oller DK: Infant vocalizations and early diagnosis of severe hearing impairment. J Pediatr 124:199, 1994.

Gates GA, Avery CA, Prihoda TJ, et al: Effectiveness of adenoidectomy and tympanostomy tubes in the treatment of chronic otitis media with effusion. N Engl J Med 317:1444, 1987.

Hayden GF, Schwartz RH: Characteristics of earache among children with acute otitis media. Am J Dis Child 139:721, 1985.

Herbert RL, King GE, Bent JP: Tympanostomy tubes and water exposure. Arch Otolaryngol Head Neck Surg 124:1118, 1998.

Hough JVD, Stuart WD: Middle ear injuries in skull trauma. Laryngoscope 78:899, 1968.

Isaacson G, Rosenfeld RM: Care of the child with tympanostomy tubes: A visual guide for the pediatrician. Pediatrics 93:924, 1994.

Kaleida PH, Casselbrant ML, Rockette HE, et al: Amoxicillin or myringotomy or both for acute otitis media: Results of a randomized clinical trial. Pediatrics 87:466, 1991.

Konigsmark BW, Gorlin RJ: Genetic and Metabolic Deafness. Philadelphia, WB Saunders, 1976.

Kozyrskyi AL, Hildes-Ripstein GE, Longstaffe SEA, et al: Treatment of acute otitis media with a shortened course of antibiotics. JAMA 279:1736, 1998.

Lench N, Houseman M, Newton V, et al: Connexin-26 mutations in sporadic nonsyndromal sensorineural deafness. Lancet 351:415, 1998.

Lim DJ, Bluestone CD, Casselbrant ML (eds): Recent advances in otitis media—report of the sixth research conference. Ann Otol Rhinol Laryngol 107 (Suppl 174):9, 1998.

Mandel EM, Rockette HE, Bluestone CD, et al: Efficacy of amoxicillin with and without decongestant-antihistamine for otitis media with effusion in children. N Engl J Med 316:432, 1987.

Mandel EM, Rockette HE, Bluestone CD, et al: Myringotomy with and without tympanostomy tubes for chronic otitis media with effusion. Arch Otolaryngol Head Neck Surg 115:1217, 1989.

Maniglia AJ, Goodwin WJ, Arnold JE, et al: Intracranial abscesses secondary to nasal, sinus and orbital infections in adults and children. Arch Otolaryngol Head Neck Surg 115:1424, 1989.

Mason JA, Herrmann KR'. Universal infant hearing screening by automated auditory brainstem response measurement. Pediatrics 101:221, 1998.

McIntyre PB, Berkey CS, King SM, et al: Dexamethasone as adjunctive therapy in bacterial meningitis. A meta-analysis of randomized clinical trials since 1988. JAMA 278:925, 1997.

Mehl AL, Thomson V: Newborn hearing screening: The great omission. Pediatrics 101(1):E4, 1998.

Morell R J, Kim H J, Hood L J, et al: Mutations in the connexin 26 gene (GJB2) among Ashkenazi jews with nonsyndromic recessive deafness. N Engl J Med 339:1500, 1998.

Niskar AS, Kieszak SM, Holmes A, et al: Prevalence of hearing loss among children 6 to 19 years of age. JAMA 279:1071, 1998.

Nozza RJ: The assessment of hearing and middle ear function in children. *In:* Bluestone CD, Stool SE, Kenna MA (eds): Pediatric Otolaryngology, 3rd ed. Philadelphia, WB Saunders, 1996, pp 165–206.

Orlin MN, Effgen SK, Handler SD: Effect of otitis media with effusion on gross motor ability in preschool-aged children: Preliminary findings. Pediatrics 99:334, 1997.

Paradise JL: Short-course antimicrobial treatment for acute otitis media. Not best for young children. JAMA 278:1640, 1997.

Paradise JL, Rockette HE, Colburn DK, et al: Otitis media in 2253 Pittsburgh-area infants: Prevalence and risk factors during the first two years of life. Pediatrics 99:318, 1997.

Pitkäranta A, Virolainen A, Jero J, et al: Detection of rhinovirus, respiratory syncytial virus, and coronavirus infections in acute otitis media by reverse transcriptase polymerase chain reactions. Pediatrics 102:291, 1998.
Post JC, Preston RA, Aul JJ, et al: Molecular analysis of bacterial pathogens in otitis media with effusion. JAMA 273:1598, 1995.
Reichler MR, Allphin A, Breiman R, et al: The spread of multiply-resistant *Streptococcus pneumoniae* at a day care center in Ohio. J Infect Dis 166:1346, 1992.
Rosenfeld RM, Vertress JE, Carr J, et al: Clinical efficacy of antimicrobial drugs for acute otitis media: Meta-analysis of 5400 children from thirty-three randomized trials. J Pediatr 124:355, 1994.
Samuel J, Fernandes CMC, Steinberg JL: Intracranial otogenic complications: A persisting problem. Laryngoscope 96:272, 1986.
Shurin PA, Rehmus JM, Johnson CE, et al: Bacterial polysaccharide immune globulin for prophylaxis of acute otitis media in high-risk children. J Pediatr 123:801, 1993.
Teele DW, Klein JO, Rosner BA: Otitis media with effusion during the first three years of life and development of speech and language. Pediatrics 74:282, 1984.
Uhari M, Kontiokari T, Niemelä M: A novel use of xylitol sugar in preventing acute otitis media. Pediatrics 102:879, 1998.
Wright PF: Xylitol sugar and acute otitis media. Pediatrics 102:971, 1998.
Yoshinaga-Itano C, Sedey AL, Coulter DK, et al: Language of early- and later-identified children with hearing loss. Pediatrics 102:1161, 1998.
Zorowka PG: Otoacoustic emissions: A new method to diagnose hearing impairment in children. Eur J Pediatr 152:626, 1993.

PART XXX

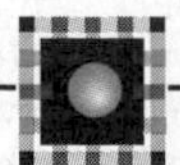

The Skin

Gary L. Darmstadt

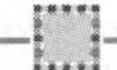

CHAPTER 650
*Morphology of the Skin**

EPIDERMIS. The mature epidermis is a stratified epithelial tissue composed predominantly of *keratinocytes*. The lowest keratinocyte layer, the basal cell layer, is constantly renewing the epidermis by mitotic division of the basal cells. Keratinocyte stem cells originate from hair follicles. Individual keratinocytes mature through a process of epidermal differentiation that results in the barrier portion of the epidermis, the stratum corneum. When composed of mature, differentiated keratinocytes, the stratum corneum is 10–50 μm thick. Damage to the stratum corneum increases skin permeability and may increase the potential for skin or systemic infection or systemic toxicity to topically applied medications or chemicals.

The continuous renewal of the surface keratinocytes of the epidermis normally proceeds in an orderly fashion as the cells of the basal cell layer move upward to the stratum corneum. The total life span from mitotic division of the basal cell until loss from the stratum corneum is approximately 28 days. In hyperproliferative diseases such as psoriasis, the movement of the cells is more rapid. The newly arrived keratinocytes in the stratum corneum are not fully differentiated and form a defective barrier. Keratinocytes are joined together by attachment plaques, the desmosomes. Cytoplasmic tonofibrils project to the desmosome and aid in cell attachment. Autoantibodies to various desmosomal adhesion molecules cause acantholysis (detachment of joined keratinocytes with bullae formation).

In addition to keratinocytes, the epidermis contains three additional cell types. The *melanocytes* are pigment-forming cells, which are responsible for skin color. Melanocytes produce melanosomes containing melanin. Epidermal melanocytes are derived from the neural crest and migrate to the skin during embryonic life. They reside in the interfollicular epidermis and in the hair follicles and increase in number in the epidermis by mitosis or migration of additional cells into the epidermis. *Merkel cells* are nerve-associated epidermal cells that may be important in the sensation of touch and in skin development. *Langerhans cells* are dendritic cells of the mononuclear phagocyte system. They contain a specific organelle, the Birbeck granule. These cells are derived from bone marrow and participate in immune reactions in the skin, playing an active part in antigen presentation and processing.

DERMIS. The dermis forms a tough, pliable, fibrous supporting structure between the epidermis and the subcutaneous fat. It consists of collagen and elastic and reticulin fibers embedded in an amorphous ground substance; it contains blood vessels, lymphatics, neural structures, eccrine and apocrine sweat glands, hair follicles, sebaceous glands, and smooth muscle. Morphologically, the dermis can be divided into two layers: the superficial papillary layer that interdigitates with the rete ridges of the epidermis and the deeper reticular layer that lies beneath the papillary dermis. The papillary layer is less dense and more cellular, whereas the reticular layer appears more compact because of the coarse network of interlaced collagen and elastic fibers.

The junction of the epidermis and dermis is the *basement membrane zone*. This complex structure is a result of contributions from both epidermal and mesenchymal cells. The dermoepidermal junction extends from the basal cell plasma membrane to the uppermost region of the dermis. Ultrastructurally, the basement membrane appears as a trilaminar structure, consisting of a *lamina lucida* immediately adjacent to the basal cell plasma membrane, a central *lamina densa*, and the *subbasal lamina* on the dermal side of the lamina densa. Several structures within this zone act to anchor the epidermis to the dermis. The plasma membrane of basal cells contains electron-dense plates known as hemidesmosomes; tonofilaments course within basal cells to insert at these sites. Anchoring filaments originate in the plasma membrane, primarily near the hemidesmosomes, and insert into the lamina densa. Anchoring fibrils, composed predominantly of type VII collagen, extend from the lamina densa into the uppermost dermis where they insert into anchoring plaques. The composition of the basement membrane as well as its role in skin disease, particularly the vesiculobullous disorders, is the subject of intensive investigation. Molecular defects in basement membrane components have been shown to underlie several of the blistering diseases (see Chapter 660).

The predominant dermal cell is a spindle-shaped *fibroblast* that is responsible for the synthesis of collagen, elastic fibers, and mucopolysaccharides. Phagocytic histiocytes, mast cells, and motile leukocytes are also present. The gelatinous ground substance serves as a supporting medium for the fibrillar and cellular components and as a storage place for a substantial portion of body water. Nutrients are supplied to both epidermis and dermis by the dermal blood vessels.

SUBCUTANEOUS TISSUE. Panniculus, or subcutaneous tissue, consists of fat cells and fibrous septa that divide it into lobules and anchor it to the underlying fascia and periosteum. Blood vessels and nerves are also present in this layer, which serves as a storage depot for lipid, an insulator to conserve body heat, and a protective cushion against trauma.

APPENDAGEAL STRUCTURES. These structures are derived from aggregates of epidermal cells that become specialized during early embryonic development. Small buds (primary epithelial germs) appear during the 3rd fetal mo and give rise to hair follicles, sebaceous and apocrine glands, and the attachment bulges for the arrector pili muscles. Eccrine sweat glands are derived from separate epidermal downgrowths that arise during the 2nd fetal mo and are completely formed by the 5th mo. Formation of nails is initiated during the 3rd intrauterine mo.

HAIR FOLLICLES. The hair follicle is the most prominent structure in the pilary complex, which includes the sebaceous

*Modified from N. Esterly, 14th edition, and G. Darmstadt and A. Lane, 15th edition.

gland, the arrector pili muscle, and, in areas such as the axillae, an apocrine gland. Hair follicles are distributed throughout the skin, except in the palms, soles, lips, and glans penis; if destroyed, they cannot regenerate. Individual follicles extend from the surface of the epidermis to the deep dermis, where the matrix cells with the dermal papilla form a bulbous hair root. The growing hair consists of a bulb and a matrix from which the keratinized hair shaft is generated; the shaft consists of an inner medulla, a cortex, and an outer cuticular layer.

Human hair growth is cyclical, with alternate periods of growth (anagen) and rest (telogen). The length of the anagen phase varies from months to years. At birth, all hairs are in the anagen phase. Subsequent generative activity lacks synchrony, so that an overall random pattern of growth and shedding prevails. Scalp hair usually grows about 1 cm/mo.

The types of hair are fetal lanugo, terminal, and vellus. *Lanugo* hair is thin and short; this hair is shed before term and is replaced by vellus hair by 36–40 wk of gestation. *Terminal hair* is long and coarse and is found on the scalp, beard, eyebrows, eyelashes, and axillary and pubic areas. *Vellus hair* is short, soft, and frequently unpigmented and is distributed over the rest of the body. During puberty, androgenic hormone stimulation causes pubic, axillary, and beard hair to change from vellus hair to terminal hair.

SEBACEOUS GLANDS. These glands occur in all areas except the palms of the hands and soles and dorsa of the feet, but they are most numerous on the face, upper chest, and back. Their ducts open into the hair follicles except on the lips, prepuce, and labia minora, where they emerge directly onto the mucosal surface. These holocrine glands are saccular structures that are often branched and lobulated and consist of a proliferative basal layer of small flat cells peripheral to the central mass of lipidized cells. The latter cells disintegrate as they move toward the duct and form the lipid secretion known as sebum, which consists of cellular debris, triglycerides, phospholipids, and cholesterol esters. Sebaceous glands depend on hormonal stimulation and are activated by androgens at puberty. Fetal sebaceous glands are stimulated by maternal androgens, and their lipid secretion, together with desquamated stratum corneum cells, constitutes the vernix caseosa.

APOCRINE GLANDS. The apocrine glands are located in the axillae, areolae, perianal and genital areas, and the periumbilical region. These large, coiled, tubular structures continuously secrete an odorless milky fluid that is discharged in response to adrenergic stimuli, usually a result of emotional stress. Bacterial decomposition of apocrine sweat accounts for the unpleasant odor associated with perspiration. Apocrine glands remain dormant until puberty, when they enlarge and secretion begins in response to androgenic activity. The secretory coil of the gland consists of a single layer of cells enclosed by a layer of contractile myoepithelial cells. The duct is lined with a double layer of cuboidal cells and opens into the pilosebaceous complex. Although apocrine glands do not function in thermoregulation, they are involved in certain disease processes.

ECCRINE SWEAT GLANDS. These glands are distributed over the entire body surface, including the palms and soles, where they are most abundant. Those on the hairy skin respond to thermal stimuli and serve to regulate body temperature by delivering water to the skin surface for evaporation; in contrast, sweat glands on the palms and soles respond mainly to psychophysiologic stimuli.

Each eccrine gland consists of a secretory coil located in the reticular dermis or subcutaneous fat and a secretory duct that opens onto the skin surface. Sweat pores can be identified on the epidermal ridges of the palm and fingers with a magnifying lens but are not readily visualized elsewhere. Two types of cells compose the single-layered secretory coil: small dark cells and large clear cells; these rest on a layer of contractile myoepithelial cells and a basement membrane. The glands are supplied by sympathetic nerve fibers, but the pharmacologic mediator of sweating is acetylcholine rather than epinephrine. Sweat consists of water, sodium, potassium, calcium, chloride, phosphorus, lactate, and small quantities of iron, glucose, and protein. The composition varies with the rate of sweating but is always hypotonic in normal children.

NAILS. Nails are specialized protective epidermal structures that form convex, translucent, tight-fitting plates on the distal dorsal surfaces of the fingers and toes. The nail plate, which is derived from a metabolically active matrix of multiplying cells situated beneath the posterior nail fold, grows forward at a rate of approximately 1 cm every 3 mo. The nail plate is bounded by the lateral and posterior nail folds; a thin eponychium (the cuticle) protrudes from the posterior fold over a crescent-shaped white area called the lunula. The pink color reflects the underlying vascular bed.

Goldsmith LA: Physiology, Biochemistry, and Molecular Biology of the Skin, 2nd ed. New York, Oxford University Press, 1991.

CHAPTER 651
Evaluation of the Patient

HISTORY AND PHYSICAL EXAMINATION. Although many skin disorders are easily recognized by simple inspection, a painstaking history and physical examination are often necessary for accurate assessment. In all cases, the entire body surface, mucous membranes, conjunctiva, hair, and nails should be examined thoroughly under adequate illumination. The color, turgor, texture, temperature, and moisture of the skin and the growth, texture, caliber, and luster of the hair and nails should be noted. Skin lesions should be palpated, inspected, and classified on the bases of morphology, size, color, texture, firmness, configuration, location, and distribution. One must also decide whether the changes are those of the primary lesion itself or whether the clinical pattern has been altered by a secondary factor such as infection, trauma, or therapy.

Primary lesions are classified as macules, papules, patches, plaques, nodules, tumors, vesicles, bullae, pustules, wheals, and cysts. A *macule* represents an alteration in skin color but cannot be felt. When the lesion is larger than 1 cm, the term *patch* is used. *Papules* are palpable solid lesions smaller than 0.5–1 cm, whereas *nodules* are larger in diameter. *Tumors* are usually larger than nodules and vary considerably in mobility and consistency. *Vesicles* are raised, fluid-filled lesions less than 0.5 cm in diameter; when larger, they are called *bullae*. *Pustules* contain purulent material. *Wheals* are flat-topped, palpable lesions of variable size and configuration that represent dermal collections of edema fluid. *Cysts* are circumscribed, thick-walled lesions that are located deep in the skin; they are covered by a normal epidermis and contain fluid or semisolid material. Aggregations of papules and pustules are referred to as *plaques*.

Primary lesions may change into secondary lesions, or secondary lesions may develop over time where no primary lesion existed. Primary lesions are usually more helpful for diagnostic purposes than secondary lesions. Secondary lesions include scales, ulcers, erosions, excoriations, fissures, crusts, and scars. *Scales* consist of compressed layers of stratum corneum cells that are retained on the skin surface. *Erosions* involve focal loss of the epidermis, and they heal without scarring. *Ulcers* extend into the dermis and tend to heal with scarring. Ulcerated lesions inflicted by scratching are often linear or angular in configuration and are called *excoriations*. *Fissures* are caused by splitting or cracking; they usually occur in diseased skin. *Crusts* consist of matted, retained accumulations of blood, serum, pus, and epithelial debris on the surface of a weeping lesion. *Scars* are end-stage lesions that can be thin, depressed and atrophic, raised and hypertrophic, or flat and pliable; they are composed of fibrous connective tissue. *Lichenification* is a thickening of skin with accentuation of normal skin lines that is caused by chronic irritation (rubbing, scratching) or inflammation.

If the diagnosis is not clear after a thorough examination, one or more diagnostic procedures may be indicated. Besides those discussed here, others are identified in appropriate subsections (e.g., scrapings of scabies lesions and smears, cultures of vesicles and pustules for detection of virus or bacteria).

BIOPSY OF SKIN. Biopsy of skin is required for diagnosis in children only occasionally. *Punch biopsy* is a simple, relatively painless procedure and usually provides adequate tissue for examination if the appropriate lesion is sampled. The selection of a fresh, well-developed primary lesion is extremely important to obtain an accurate diagnosis. The site of the biopsy should have relatively low risk for damage to underlying dermal structures. The skin is anesthetized by application of Emla cream and/or intradermal injection of 1 or 2% lidocaine (Xylocaine), with or without epinephrine, with a 27- or 30-gauge needle after cleansing of the site. A punch, 3 or 4 mm in diameter, is pressed firmly against the skin and rotated until it sinks to the proper depth. All three layers (epidermis, dermis, subcutis) should be contained in the plug. The plug should be lifted gently with forceps or extracted with a needle and separated from the underlying tissue with an iris scissors. Bleeding abates with firm pressure and with suturing. The biopsy specimen should be placed in 10% formaldehyde solution (Formalin) for appropriate processing.

WOOD'S LAMP. The Wood's lamp transmits ultraviolet light mainly in a wavelength of 365 nm. The examination, which is performed in a darkened room, is useful in detecting hypopigmented macules and certain superficial fungal infections of the scalp. Blue-green fluorescence is detectable at the base of each infected hair shaft in ectothrix and in some endothrix infections. Scales and crusts may appear pale yellow, but this is not evidence of a fungal infection. Dermatophyte lesions of the skin (tinea corporis) do not fluoresce; macules of tinea versicolor, however, have a golden fluorescence under a Wood's lamp. *Erythrasma*, an intertriginous infection due to *Corynebacterium minutissimum*, may fluoresce pink-orange, whereas *Pseudomonas aeruginosa* is yellow-green under a Wood's lamp. Discrete areas of altered pigment can often be visualized more clearly by using a Wood's lamp, particularly if the pigmentary change is epidermal. Hyperpigmented lesions appear darker, and hypopigmented lesions lighter than the surrounding skin.

POTASSIUM HYDROXIDE (KOH) PREPARATION. This provides a rapid and reliable method for detecting fungal elements of both yeasts and dermatophytes. Scaly lesions should be scraped at the active border for optimal recovery of mycelia and spores. Vesicles should be unroofed, and the blister top should be clipped and placed on a slide for examination. In tinea capitis, infected hairs must be plucked from the follicle; scales from the scalp do not usually contain mycelia. A few drops of 20% KOH are added to the specimen, which is then gently heated over an alcohol lamp until it begins to bubble; alternatively, ample time (approximately 10–20 min) can be allowed for dissolution of the keratin. Alternatively, dimethyl sulfoxide (DMSO) can be included in the KOH solution. The preparation is examined under low-intensity light for fungal elements.

TZANCK SMEAR. This is useful in the diagnosis of some viral infections (herpes simplex, varicella, herpes zoster, eczema herpeticum) and for the detection of acantholytic cells in pemphigus. An intact, fresh blister should be ruptured and drained of fluid. The base of the blister is then scraped with a dull-edged instrument, taking care to avoid drawing a significant amount of blood; the material is smeared on a clear glass slide and air dried. Staining with Giemsa stain is preferable, but Wright stain is acceptable. Balloon cells and multinucleated giant cells are diagnostic of herpesvirus infection; acantholytic epidermal cells are characteristic of pemphigus.

The *direct fluorescent assay* is more sensitive and specific. The keratinocytes are scraped from the base of the blister as described earlier. The laboratory stains the slide with labeled antibodies specific for varicella zoster virus or herpes simplex virus. Observation of the slide with a fluorescence microscope documents the presence of the specific virus within the cells.

IMMUNOFLUORESCENCE STUDIES. Immunofluorescence studies of skin can be used to detect tissue-fixed antibodies to skin components and complement; characteristic staining patterns are specific for certain skin disorders. Serum can be used for identi-

TABLE 651–1 Immunofluorescent Findings in Immune-Mediated Cutaneous Diseases

Disease	Involved Skin	Uninvolved Skin	Direct IF	Indirect IF	Other Antibodies
Dermatitis herpetiformis	Negative	Positive	Granular IgA ± C in papillary dermis	None	IgA antireticulum in 20–70%. Antigliadin antibodies with celiac disease
Bullous pemphigoid	Positive	Positive	Linear IgG and C band in BMZ, occasionally IgM, IgA, IgE	IgG to BMZ in 70%	None
Pemphigus (all variants)	Positive	Positive	IgG in intercellular spaces of epidermis between keratinocytes	IgG to intercellular space	None
Pemphigus foliaceus	Positive	Positive	IgG to desmosomal glycoprotein, desmoglein$_1$	Same as direct IF	None
Herpes gestationis	Positive	Positive	C3 at BMZ, occasionally IgG	IgG anti-BMZ	None
Linear IgA bullous dermatosis (chronic bullous dermatosis of childhood)	Positive	Positive	Linear IgA at BMZ, occasionally C	Low titer, rare IgA, anti-BMZ	None
Discoid lupus erythematosus	Positive	Negative	Linear IgG, IgM, IgA, and C3 at BMZ (lupus band)	None	ANA negative
Systemic lupus erythematosus	Positive	Variable; exposed to sun, 30–50%; nonexposed, 10–30%	Linear IgG, IgM, C3 at BMZ (lupus band)	None	ANA Anti-Ro (SSA) Anti-RNP Anti-DNA Anti-Sm
Henoch-Schönlein purpura	Positive	Negative	IgA around vessel walls	None	IgA rheumatoid factor, occasionally

C = complement; IF = immunofluorescent findings; Ig = immunoglobulin; ANA = antinuclear antibody; BMZ = basement membrane zone at the dermoepidermal junction.

fying circulating antibodies. Skin biopsy specimens for direct immunofluorescence preparations should be obtained from involved sites except in those diseases for which paralesional skin or uninvolved skin is required (Table 651–1). A punch biopsy sample is obtained, and the tissue is placed in a special transport medium or immediately frozen in liquid nitrogen for transport or storage. Thin cryostat sections of the specimen are incubated with fluorescein-conjugated antibodies to the specific antigens.

Serum of patients can be examined by indirect immunofluorescence techniques using sections of normal human skin, guinea pig lip, or monkey esophagus as substrate. The substrate is incubated with fresh or thawed frozen serum and then with fluorescein-conjugated antihuman globulin. If the serum contains antibody to epithelial components, its specific staining pattern can be seen on fluorescence microscopy. By serial dilution, the titer of circulating antibody can be estimated.

Gately LE, Nesbitt LT: Update on immunofluorescent testing in bullous diseases and lupus erythematosus. Dermatol Clin 12:133, 1994.

CHAPTER 652
Principles of Therapy

Competent skin care requires a specific diagnosis, knowledge of the natural course of the disease, and appreciation of primary vs secondary lesions. If the diagnosis is uncertain, it is better to err on the side of less rather than more aggressive treatment. Even when the diagnosis is clear, an acute dermatitis may require gentle and bland therapy initially.

In the use of topical medication, consideration of vehicle is as important as the specific therapeutic agent. Acute weeping lesions respond best to wet compresses, followed by lotions or creams. For dry, thickened, scaly skin or when treating a contact-allergic reaction possibly due to a component of a topical medication, an ointment base is preferable. Gels and solutions are most useful for the scalp and other hairy areas. The site of involvement is of considerable importance because the most desirable vehicle may not be cosmetically or functionally appropriate, such as an ointment on the face or hands. A patient's preference should also play a part in the choice of vehicle because compliance is poor if a medication is not acceptable to a patient.

Most *lotions* are mixtures of water and oil that can be poured. After the water evaporates, the small amount of remaining oil covers the skin. Some *shake lotions* are a suspension of water and insoluble powder; as the water evaporates, cooling the skin, a thin film of powder covers the skin. *Creams* are emulsions of oil and water that are viscous and do not pour (more oil than in lotions). *Ointments* have oils and a small amount of water or no water at all; they feel greasy, lubricate dry skin, trap water, and may be occlusive. Ointments without water usually require no preservatives because microorganisms require water to survive.

Therapy should be kept as simple as possible, and specific written instructions about the frequency and duration of application should be provided. Physicians should become familiar with one or two preparations in each category and should learn to use them appropriately. Prescribing nonspecific proprietary medications that may contain sensitizing agents should be avoided. Certain preparations such as topical antihistamines and sensitizing anesthetics are never indicated.

WET DRESSINGS. These dressings decrease pruritus, burning, and stinging sensations; they are indicated for acutely inflamed moist or oozing dermatitis. Although various astringent and antiseptic substances may be added to the solution, tap water compresses are just as effective.

Open Wet Dressings. These dressings cool and dry the skin by evaporation and cleanse by removing crusts and exudate that cause further irritation if permitted to remain. The solution should be cool or tepid and consist of tap water, isotonic saline, or aluminum acetate (Burow's solution) in a 1:20 or 1:40 dilution. Potassium permanganate is messy and offers no advantage. Boric acid can be toxic if absorbed and should *never* be used for compresses. Dressings of multiple layers of Kerlix, gauze, or soft cotton material should be saturated with the solution and remoistened as often as necessary. Compresses should be applied for 10–20 min at least every 4 hr and should be continued usually for 24–48 hr.

Closed Wet Dressings. These dressings are indicated for abscesses. The solution should be warm, and the dressings should be covered with plastic to prevent evaporation. Closed wet dressings, if prolonged, cause maceration because they prevent evaporation and heat loss.

BATH OILS, COLLOIDS, SOAPS. *Bath oil* has little benefit in the treatment of children. It offers little moisturizing effect while increasing the risk of injury during a bath. Bath oil may lubricate the surface of the bathtub, causing an adult or child to fall when stepping into the tub. Tar bath solutions (Balnetar, Zetar) can be prescribed and may be helpful for psoriasis and atopic dermatitis. *Colloids* such as starch powder or colloidal oatmeal (Aveeno) are soothing and antipruritic for some patients when added to the bath water. Oilated Aveeno contains mineral oil and lanolin derivatives for lubrication if the skin is dry. These can also lubricate the bathtub surface. Ordinary toilet *soaps* may be irritating and drying if patients have dry skin or dermatitis. Examples of soaps that are usually not harmful to skin are Dove, Lowila, Aveeno, Neutrogena, Basis, Alpha Keri, and Oilatum. When skin is acutely inflamed, avoidance of soap is advised. Some patients find that lipid-free cleansers containing cetyl alcohol (Cetaphil) are soothing.

LUBRICANTS. Lubricants, such as lotions, creams, and ointments, can be used as emollients for dry skin and as vehicles for topical agents such as corticosteroids and keratolytics. In general, ointments are the most effective emollients. Numerous commercial preparations are available in addition to standard products such as petrolatum, cold cream, stearin-lanolin cream, and hydrophilic ointment. Some patients do not tolerate ointments, and some may be sensitized to a component of the lubricant; some preservatives of creams (most commonly parabens) are sensitizers. Useful lubricating lotions include Lubriderm, Nutraderm, and Nivea. Creams include Eucerin, Neutrogena, Nutraderm, Purpose, Vanicream, and Complex 15. Aquaphor is a cosmetically acceptable alternative to petrolatum. These preparations can be applied several times a day if necessary. Maximal effect is achieved when they are applied *immediately* to damp skin after a bath or shower. Sarna lotion contains menthol and camphor in an emollient vehicle for control of pruritus and dryness.

SHAMPOOS. Special shampoos containing sulfur, salicylic acid, antiseptics, and selenium sulfide (Selsun, Exsel) are useful for conditions in which there is scaling of the scalp. Most shampoos also contain surfactants and detergents. Shampoos with sulfur or salicylic acid include Ionil, Sebulex, Fostex, and Vanseb. Those with only antiseptic agents include DHS-Zinc, Danex, and Head and Shoulders. Tar-containing shampoos such as T-Gel, Ionil-T, Sebutone, and Polytar are useful for psoriasis and severe seborrheic dermatitis. In general, they can be used as frequently as necessary to control scaling, but use should be limited to avoid irritation. Patients should be instructed to leave the lathered shampoo in contact with the scalp for 5–10 min.

SHAKE LOTIONS. These lotions are useful antipruritic agents;

they consist of a suspension of powder in a liquid vehicle. A water-dispersible oil may be added for lubrication. Calamine lotion is acceptable but tends to cake on the skin. A prototype lotion is zinc oxide 20 g, talc 20 g, glycerin 20 g, Alpha Keri 5 g, and water to make 120 g. These preparations can be used effectively in combination with wet dressings for exudative dermatitis. Cooling occurs as the lotion evaporates and moisture is absorbed by the powder deposited on the skin.

POWDERS. Powders are hygroscopic and serve as absorptive agents in areas of excessive moisture. When dry, powders decrease friction between two surfaces. They are most useful in the intertriginous areas and between the toes, where maceration and abrasion may result from friction on movement. Coarse powders may cake; therefore, they should be of fine particle size and inert unless medication has been incorporated in the formulation. Zeasorb is a bland, finely milled, general purpose powder that can be applied to any area of the body.

PASTES. These contain a fine powder in an ointment vehicle and are not often prescribed in current dermatologic therapy; in certain situations, however, they can be used effectively to protect vulnerable or damaged skin. For example, a stiff zinc oxide paste is bland and inert and can be applied to the diaper area to prevent further irritation due to diaper dermatitis. Zinc paste should be applied in a thick layer completely obscuring the skin and is removed more easily with mineral oil than with soap and water.

KERATOLYTIC AGENTS. *Urea-containing agents* are hydrophilic; they hydrate the stratum corneum and make the skin more pliable. In addition, because urea dissolves hydrogen bonds and epidermal keratin, it is effective in treating scaling disorders. Concentrations of 10–25% are available in several commercial lotions and creams (Carmol 20, Carmol 10, Nutraplus, Aquacare HP), which can be applied once or twice daily as tolerated. *Salicylic acid* is an effective keratolytic agent and can be incorporated into various vehicles in concentrations up to 6% to be applied two to three times daily. Salicylic acid preparations should not be used in treating small infants or on large surface areas or denuded skin; percutaneous absorption may result in salicylism. The *α-hydroxy acids*, particularly *lactic acid* and *glycolic acid*, are available in commercial preparations (Lacticare, LacHydrin, Aqua Glycolic) or can be incorporated in an ointment vehicle such as petrolatum or Aquaphor in concentrations up to 5%. Eucerin Plus Creme contains both urea and lactic acid. The α-hydroxy acid preparations are useful for the treatment of keratinizing disorders and may be applied once or twice daily. Some patients complain of burning; in this case, the frequency of application should be decreased.

TAR COMPOUNDS. Tars are obtained from bituminous coal, shales, petrolatum (coal tars), and wood. They are antipruritic and astringent and appear to promote normal keratinization. They may be useful for chronic eczema and psoriasis, and their efficacy may be increased if the affected area is exposed to ultraviolet (UV) light after the tar has been removed. *Tars should not be used in acute inflammatory lesions.* Tars are often messy and unacceptable because they may stain and they have an odor. Tars may be incorporated into shampoos, bath oils, lotions, and ointments. A useful preparation for pediatric patients is liquor carbonis detergens (LCD) 2–5% in a cream or ointment vehicle. Tar gels (Psorigel, Estargel, Aquatar) and tar in a light body oil (T-Derm) are relatively pleasant cosmetic preparations that cause minimal staining of skin and fabrics. Tars can also be incorporated into a vehicle with a topical corticosteroid. The frequency of application varies from one to three times daily, according to tolerance. Many children refuse to use tar preparations because of their odor and staining characteristics.

ANTIFUNGAL AGENTS. These agents are now available as powders, lotions, creams, and ointments for the treatment of dermatophyte and yeast infections. Nystatin, naftifine (Naftin), and amphotericin B are specific for *Candida* and are ineffective in other fungal disorders. Tolnaftate is effective against dermatophytes but not effective for yeast. The spectrum for ciclopirox olamine includes the dermatophytes, *Malassezia furfur*, and *Candida albicans*. The azoles—miconazole, clotrimazole, econazole, oxiconazole, and ketoconazole (Nizoral)—have a similar broad spectrum. Terbinafine has greater activity against dermatophytes but poorer activity against yeasts than the azoles. The topical antifungal agents should be applied one to two times a day for most fungal infections. All have low sensitizing potential; however, additives such as preservatives and stabilizers in the vehicles may cause allergic contact dermatitis. Whitfield's ointment (6% benzoic acid and 3% salicylic acid) is a potent keratolytic agent that has also been used for the treatment of dermatophyte infections. Irritant reactions are common.

TOPICAL ANTIBIOTICS. Topical antibiotics have been used to treat local cutaneous infections for many years, although their efficacy, with the exception of mupirocin (Bactroban), has been questioned. Ointments are the preferred vehicle, and combinations with other topical agents, such as corticosteroids, are in general inadvisable. Whenever possible, the etiologic agent should be identified and treated specifically. Antibiotics in wide use as systemic preparations should be avoided because of the risk of sensitization. The sensitizing potential of certain other antibiotics (e.g., neomycin, nitrofurazone [Furacin]) should be kept in mind. Mupirocin is the most effective topical agent currently available and has been documented to be as effective as oral erythromycin in treatment of impetigo. Polysporin and bacitracin are not as effective as mupirocin or oral antibiotics.

TOPICAL CORTICOSTEROIDS. Topical corticosteroids are potent anti-inflammatory agents and effective antipruritic agents. Successful therapeutic results have been achieved in a wide variety of skin conditions. In general, corticosteroids fall into two classes: nonfluorinated preparations, such as hydrocortisone (Hytone), desonide (Tridesilon, Des Owen), hydrocortisone butyrate (Locoid), and mometasone furoate (Elocon); and fluorinated compounds including triamcinolone (Kenalog; Aristocort), flurandrenolide (Cordran), fluocinolone (Synalar), betamethasone (Valisone, Benisone, Flurobate), and amcinonide (Cyclocort). The nonfluorinated steroids are usually of lesser potency and may cause fewer local and systemic side effects, whereas fluorinated steroids are potentially more harmful, particularly with long-term use. Other fluorinated compounds, for example, fluorocinonide (Lidex), halcinonide (Halog), betamethasone dipropionate (Diprolene), and clobetasol propionate (Temovate), are extremely potent and should be prescribed with care. Some of these compounds are formulated in several strengths based on their clinical efficacy and vasoconstrictive ability. Physicians using topical steroids should become familiar with several preparations and with the potency of the preparations used.

Virtually all corticosteroids can be obtained in various vehicles, including creams, ointments, solutions, gels, and aerosols. Absorption is enhanced by an ointment or gel vehicle, but the vehicle should be selected on the basis of the type of disorder and the site of involvement. Frequency of application should be determined by the potency of the preparation and the severity of the eruption. In general, applying a *thin film* two times daily suffices. Adverse local effects include cutaneous atrophy, striae, telangiectasia, hypopigmentation, and increased hair growth.

In selected circumstances, corticosteroids may be administered by intralesional injection (acne cysts, keloids, psoriatic plaques, alopecia areata, persistent insect bite reactions). This method of administration should be used only by physicians who are experienced with this technique of dermatologic therapy.

SUNSCREENS. Sunscreens are of two general types: those that reflect all wavelengths of UV and visible spectrums, such as zinc oxide and titanium dioxide; and a heterogeneous group of chemicals that selectively absorb energy of various wavelengths within the UV spectrum. Some sunscreens permit tanning without burning; others prevent both. In addition to the spectrum of light that is blocked, other factors to be considered include cosmetic acceptance, sensitizing potential, retention on skin while swimming or sweating, required frequency of application, and cost. Effective opaque total barrier agents are zinc oxide ointment, Covermark, Dermablend, and RVPaque. Para-aminobenzoic acid (PABA)–ethanol (Pabanol, PreSun) and cinnamate-benzophenone combinations (Maxafil, Solbar, Uval) effectively prevent transmission of solar UVB and at least some UVA wavelengths. PABA esters (Eclipse, Pabafilm, Sundown) afford partial protection. Lip protectants that absorb in the UVB range (Sunstick, Blistik, PreSun) are also available for patients with photo-induced lip disorders such as recurrent herpesvirus infections. Sunscreens are designated by sun protection factor (SPF). The SPF is defined as the amount of time to develop a mild sunburn with the sunscreen compared with the amount of time without the sunscreen. A minimum SPF factor of 15 is required for most fair-skinned individuals to prevent sunburn. The higher the SPF, the better the protection is against UVB rays. Examples of sunscreens offering maximal protection are Supershade, Photoplex, and Total Eclipse. The efficacy of these agents depends on careful attention to instructions for use. PABA-containing sunscreens should be applied at least 30 min before sun exposure to permit penetration of the epidermis. Most patients with photosensitivity eruptions require protection by agents that absorb UVB wavelengths; patients with porphyria, phototoxic eruptions, and some types of solar urticaria require agents with a broader spectrum of prevention (see Chapter 662).

Sunscreens do not give complete protection against all harmful UV light. Sun avoidance is also important during the times when the sun is most intense, such as during midday. Clothing and hats also offer additional sun protection.

McGregor J, Young A: Sunscreens, suntans and skin cancer. Br Med J 312:1621, 1996.
Morelli JG, Weston WL: Soaps and shampoos in pediatric practice. Pediatrics 80:634, 1987.
Nilsson EJ, Henning CG, Magnusson J: Topical corticosteroids and *Staphylococcus aureus* in atopic dermatitis. J Am Acad Dermatol 27:29, 1992.
Yohn JJ, Weston WL: Topical glucocorticosteroids. Curr Probl Dermatol 2:33, 1990.

CHAPTER 653
Diseases of the Neonate

Minor evanescent lesions of newborn infants, particularly when florid, may cause undue concern. Most of the entities described in this chapter are relatively common, benign, and transient; they do not require therapy.

SEBACEOUS HYPERPLASIA. Minute, profuse, yellow-white papules are frequently found on the forehead, nose, upper lip, and cheeks of a term infant; they represent hyperplastic sebaceous glands. These tiny papules diminish gradually in size and disappear entirely within the first few weeks of life.

MILIA. Milia are superficial epidermal inclusion cysts that contain laminated keratinized material. The lesion is a firm papule, 1–2 mm in diameter, and pearly, opalescent white. Milia may occur at any age but in neonates are most frequently scattered over the face and gingivae and on the midline of the palate, where they are called *Epstein pearls*. Milia exfoliate spontaneously in most infants and may be ignored; those that appear in scars or sites of trauma in older children may be gently unroofed and the contents extracted with a fine-gauge needle.

SUCKING BLISTERS. Solitary or scattered superficial bullae on the upper limbs of infants at birth are presumed to be induced by vigorous sucking on the affected part in utero. Common sites are the radial aspect of the forearm, thumb, and index finger. These bullae resolve rapidly without sequelae and should be distinguished from sucking pads (calluses), which are found on the lips in the first few months and are due to combined intracellular edema and hyperkeratosis. The diagnosis can be confirmed by observing the neonate suck the affected area.

CUTIS MARMORATA. When a newborn infant is exposed to low environmental temperatures, an evanescent, lacy, reticulated red and/or blue cutaneous vascular pattern appears over most of the body surface. This vascular change represents an accentuated physiologic vasomotor response that disappears with increasing age, although it is sometimes discernible even in older children. Persistent and pronounced cutis marmorata occurs in Menkes disease, familial dysautonomia, and Cornelia de Lange, Down, and trisomy 18 syndromes. Cutis marmorata telangiectatica congenita is clinically similar, but the lesions are more intense, may be segmental, are persistent, and may be associated with loss of dermal tissue, epidermal atrophy, and ulceration. The condition improves in the first year of life, however, with half showing decreased vascular markings. The congenital form is associated with microcephaly, micrognathia, cleft palate, dystrophic teeth, glaucoma, short stature, and skull asymmetry.

HARLEQUIN COLOR CHANGE. This rare but dramatic vascular event occurs in the immediate newborn period and is most common in infants of low birthweight. It probably reflects an imbalance in the autonomic vascular regulatory mechanism. When the infant is placed on his or her side, the body is bisected longitudinally into a pale upper half and a deep red dependent half. The color change lasts only for a few minutes and occasionally affects only a portion of the trunk or face. The pattern may be reversed by changing the infant's position. Muscular activity causes generalized flushing and obliterates the color differential. Repeated episodes may occur but do not indicate permanent autonomic imbalance.

SALMON PATCH (NEVUS SIMPLEX). Salmon patches are small, pale pink, ill-defined, vascular macules that occur most commonly on the glabella, eyelids, upper lip, and nuchal area of 30–40% of normal newborn infants. These lesions, which represent localized vascular ectasia, persist for several months and may become more visible during crying or changes in environmental temperature. Most lesions on the face eventually fade and disappear completely, but those on the posterior neck and occipital areas often persist. The facial lesions should not be confused with a port-wine stain, which is a permanent lesion. The salmon patch is usually symmetric, with lesions on both eyelids or both sides of midline. Port-wine stains are often larger and unilateral, and they usually end along the midline (see Chapter 656).

MONGOLIAN SPOTS. These blue or slate-gray macular lesions have variably defined margins; they occur most commonly in the presacral area but may be found over the posterior thighs, legs, back, and shoulders. They may be solitary or numerous and often involve large areas. More than 80% of black, Asian, and East Indian infants have these lesions, whereas the incidence in white infants is less than 10%. The peculiar hue of these macules is due to the dermal location of melanin-containing melanocytes that are presumed to have been arrested in their migration from neural crest to epidermis. Mongolian spots usually fade during the first few years of life but occasionally persist. Malignant degeneration does not occur. Widespread numerous lesions, particularly those in unusual sites, are unlikely to disappear. The characteristic appearance and

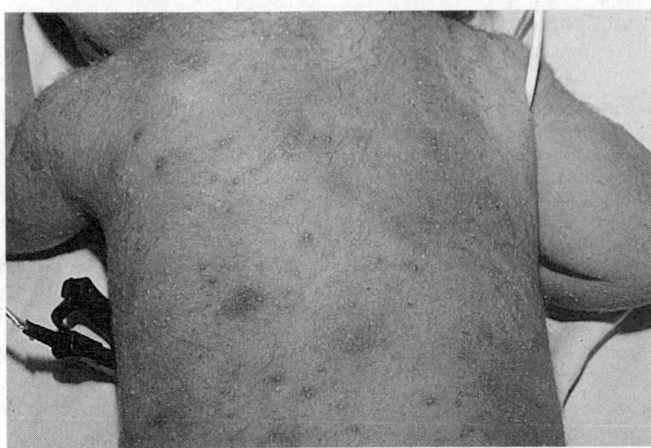

Figure 653–1 Erythema toxicum on the trunk of a newborn infant. See also color section.

congenital onset distinguish these spots from the bruises of child abuse.

ERYTHEMA TOXICUM. This benign, self-limited, evanescent eruption occurs in approximately 50% of full-term infants; preterm infants are affected less commonly. The lesions are firm, yellow-white, 1–2 mm papules or pustules with a surrounding erythematous flare (Fig. 653–1). At times, splotchy erythema is the only manifestation. Lesions may be sparse or numerous and clustered in several sites or widely dispersed over much of the body surface. Palms and soles are usually spared. Peak incidence occurs on the 2nd day of life, but new lesions may erupt during the 1st few days as the rash waxes and wanes. Onset may occasionally be delayed for a few days to weeks in premature infants. The pustules form below the stratum corneum or deeper in the epidermis and represent collections of eosinophils that also accumulate around the upper portion of the pilosebaceous follicle. The eosinophils can be demonstrated in Wright-stained smears of the intralesional contents. Cultures are sterile.

The cause of erythema toxicum is unknown. The lesions can mimic pyoderma, candidosis, herpes simplex, transient neonatal pustular melanosis, and miliaria but can be differentiated by the characteristic infiltrate of eosinophils and the absence of organisms on a stained smear. The course is brief, and no therapy is required. Incontinentia pigmenti and eosinophilic pustular folliculitis also have eosinophilic infiltration but can be distinguished by their distribution, histologic type, and chronicity.

TRANSIENT NEONATAL PUSTULAR MELANOSIS. Pustular melanosis, which is more common in black than in white infants, is a transient, benign, self-limited dermatosis of unknown cause that is characterized by three types of lesions: (1) evanescent superficial pustules; (2) ruptured pustules with a collarette of fine scale, at times with a central hyperpigmented macule; and (3) hyperpigmented macules (Fig. 653–2). Lesions are present at birth, and one or all types of lesions may be found in a profuse or sparse distribution. Pustules represent the early phase of the disorder, and macules, the late phase. The pustular phase rarely lasts more than 2–3 days; hyperpigmented macules may persist for as long as 3 mo. Sites of predilection are the anterior neck, forehead, and lower back, although the scalp, trunk, limbs, palms, and soles may be affected.

Biopsy tissue during the active phase shows an intracorneal or subcorneal pustule filled with polymorphonuclear leukocytes, debris, and an occasional eosinophil. The macules are characterized only by increased melanization of epidermal cells. Cultures and smears can be used to distinguish these pustules from those of erythema toxicum and pyoderma because they do not contain bacteria or dense aggregates of eosinophils. No therapy is required.

INFANTILE ACROPUSTULOSIS. Infantile acropustulosis generally has its onset at 2–10 mo of age; lesions are occasionally noted at birth. Black males have a predisposition for this eruption, but infants of both sexes and all races may be affected. The cause is unknown.

The lesions are initially discrete erythematous papules that become vesiculopustular within 24 hr and subsequently crust before healing. They are intensely pruritic, and a fresh out-

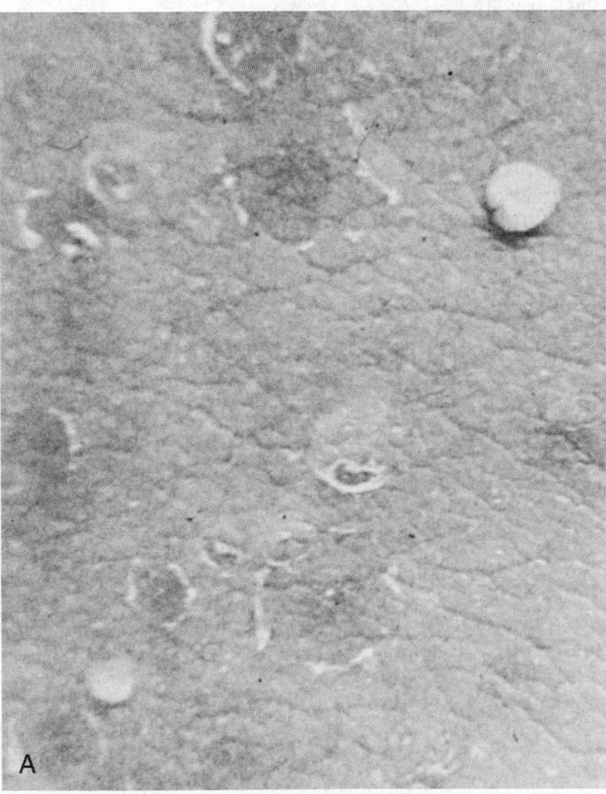

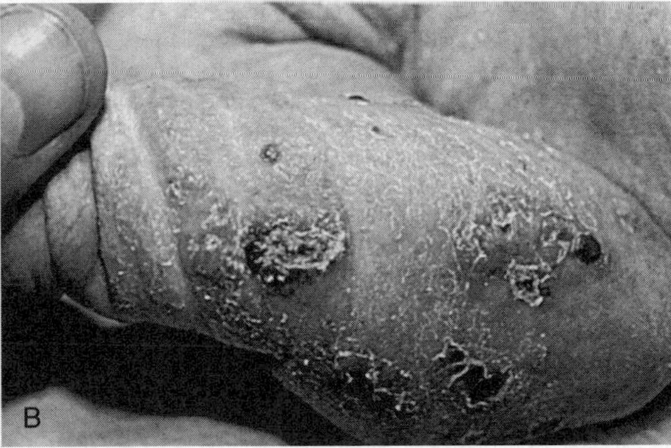

Figure 653–2 *A* and *B,* Transient neonatal pustular melanosis showing pustules, rings of scales, and hyperpigmented macules.

break is usually accompanied by fretfulness and irritability. Preferred sites are the palms of the hands and soles and sides of the feet, where the lesions may develop in profusion. A less dense eruption may be found on the dorsum of the hands and feet, ankles, and wrists. Pustules occasionally may occur elsewhere on the body. Each episode lasts 7–14 days, during which time pustules continue to appear in crops. After a 2–4 wk remission, a new outbreak follows. This cyclic pattern continues for about 2 yr; permanent resolution is often preceded by longer intervals of remission between periods of activity. Infants with acropustulosis are otherwise well.

Wright-stained smears of intralesional contents show abundant neutrophils or, occasionally, a predominance of eosinophils. Histologically, well-circumscribed, subcorneal, neutrophilic pustules, with or without eosinophils, are noted.

The *differential diagnosis* in neonates includes transient neonatal pustular melanosis, erythema toxicum, milia, cutaneous candidosis, and staphylococcal pustulosis. In older infants and toddlers, additional diagnostic considerations include scabies; dyshidrotic eczema; pustular psoriasis; subcorneal pustular dermatosis; and hand-foot-and-mouth disease. A therapeutic trial of a scabicide is warranted in equivocal cases.

Therapy is directed at minimizing discomfort for infants. Topical corticosteroid preparations or oral antihistamines decrease the severity of the pruritus and an infant's irritability. Dapsone 2 mg/kg/24 hr PO bid has been effective but has potentially serious side effects—notably, hemolytic anemia and methemoglobinuria—and should be used with caution.

EOSINOPHILIC PUSTULAR FOLLICULITIS. This is described as recurrent crops of pruritic, coalescing, follicular papulopustules on the face, trunk, and extremities. Fifty per cent of patients have peripheral eosinophilia exceeding 5%, and about one third (32%) have leukocytosis (>10,000/mm^3).

Infants with eosinophilic pustular folliculitis (EPF) make up less than 10% of all cases reported. The clinical and histologic appearance of this disorder in infants closely resembles that in immunocompetent adults, with minor exceptions. In infants, the lesions are most prominent on the scalp, although they also occur on the trunk and extremities and occasionally are found on the palms and soles. Also, the classic annular and polycyclic appearance with centrifugal enlargement is not seen in infants. Histopathologically, adults have an eosinophilic infiltrate that invades sebaceous glands and the outer root sheath of hair follicles, often leading to spongiosis in the outer root sheath. The eosinophilic infiltrate in most infants, however, is perifollicular, without spongiosis in the outer root sheath. Because of the slightly different clinical findings and course of EPF in immunocompetent adults compared with infants or patients with acquired immunodeficiency syndrome, it has been proposed that EPF should be subclassified into classic human immunodeficiency virus–related and infantile forms. The differential diagnosis includes erythema toxicum neonatorum, infantile acropustulosis, localized pustular psoriasis, pustular folliculitis, and transient neonatal pustular melanosis.

The pathogenesis of EPF is linked epidemiologically to sebaceous gland activity because lesions appear most commonly in association with hair follicles in areas of the body with a high density of sebaceous glands. Most theories on the pathogenesis of EPF invoke immunologic mechanisms in the initiation of lesions. Proposed etiologic factors in EPF include a cyclooxygenase–generated metabolite with chemotactic properties; an exaggerated response to skin saprophytes or dermatophytes, leading to eosinophilic infiltration and destruction of the follicle; or autoantibodies directed against the intercellular substance of the lower epidermis or the cytoplasm of basal cells of the epidermis and the outer sheath of hair follicles.

Response of EPF to therapy has been variable, and no one specific treatment is the therapy of choice. In general, antimicrobials and medicated shampoos have been ineffective; mid-potency topical corticosteroids have been modestly effective in the treatment of scalp lesions in infants.

Alper JC, Holmes LB: The incidence and significance of birthmarks in a cohort of 4,641 newborns. Pediatr Dermatol 1:58, 1983.

Alper J, Holmes LB, Mihm MC: Birthmarks with serious medical significance: Nevocellular nevi, sebaceous nevi, and multiple café au lait spots. J Pediatr 95:696, 1979.

Darmstadt GL, Tunnessen WW, Sweren RJ: Eosinophilic pustular folliculitis. Pediatrics 89:1095, 1992.

Jacobs AH, Walton RG: The incidence of birthmarks in the neonate. Pediatrics 58:281, 1976.

Jennings JL, Burrows WM: Infantile acropustulosis. J Am Acad Dermatol 9:733, 1983.

Karlsson J, Telang G, Tunnessen W: Cutis marmorata telangiectatica congenita. Arch Pediatr Adolesc Med 151:950, 1997.

Chapter 654
Cutaneous Defects

SKIN DIMPLES. Cutaneous depressions over bony prominences and in the sacral area, at times associated with pits and creases, may occur in normal children and in association with dysmorphologic syndromes. It has been postulated that skin dimples develop in utero as a result of interposition of tissue between a sharp bony point and the uterine wall, which leads to decreased subcutaneous tissue formation. A rare benign autosomal dominant anomaly presents with dimples near the acromion bilaterally in association with deletion of the long arm of chromosome 18. Dimples tend to occur over the patella in congenital rubella, over the lateral aspects of the knees and elbows in prune-belly syndrome, on the pretibial surface in camptomelic dwarfs, and in the shape of an H on the chin in whistling-face syndrome. Sacral dimples occur as part of multiple syndromes, including Bloom syndrome, Smith-Lemli-Opitz syndrome, 4p deletion syndrome, spina bifida occulta, and diastomyelia.

REDUNDANT SKIN. Loose folds of skin must be differentiated from a congenital defect of elastic tissue or collagen such as cutis laxa, Ehlers-Danlos syndrome, or pseudoxanthoma elasticum. Redundant skin over the posterior part of the neck is common in the Turner, Noonan, Down, and Klippel-Feil syndromes; more generalized folds of skin occur in infants with trisomy 18 and short-limbed dwarfism.

AMNIOTIC CONSTRICTION BANDS. Partial or complete constriction bands that produce defects in extremities and digits are found in 1/10,000–1/45,000 otherwise normal infants. Constrictive tissue bands are caused by primary amniotic rupture, with subsequent entanglement of fetal parts, particularly limbs, in shriveled fibrotic amniotic strands. This event is probably sporadic, with negligible risk of recurrence. Formation of constrictive tissue bands is associated with abdominal trauma, amniocentesis, and hereditary defects of collagen such as Ehlers-Danlos syndrome or osteogenesis imperfecta. Constriction bands on the limbs may be removed by plastic surgical procedures.

Adhesive bands involve the craniofacial area and are associated with severe defects such as encephalocele and facial clefts. Adhesive bands result from broad fusion between disrupted fetal parts and an intact amniotic membrane. The craniofacial defects do not appear to be caused by constrictive amniotic bands but result from a vascular disruption sequence with or without cephaloamniotic adhesion.

The *limb–body wall complex* (LBWC) involves vascular disruption early in development, affecting several embryonic structures; it includes at least two of the following three characteristics: exencephaly or encephalocele with facial clefts, thoraco- and/or abdominoschisis, and limb defects. Amniotic rupture may be the cause of embryonic vascular disruption, leading to the LBWC; the LBWC, however, has been reported in the absence of amniotic rupture.

PREAURICULAR SINUSES AND PITS. Pits and sinus tracts anterior to the pinna may be a result of imperfect fusion of the tubercles of the first and second branchial arches. These anomalies may be unilateral or bilateral, may be familial, are more common in females and blacks, and at times are associated with other anomalies of the ears and face. Preauricular pits are present in branchio-otorenal dysplasia, an autosomal dominant disorder that consists of external ear malformations, branchial fistulas, hearing loss, and renal anomalies. When the tracts become chronically infected, retention cysts may form and drain intermittently; such lesions may require excision.

ACCESSORY TRAGI. An accessory tragus typically appears as a single pedunculated, flesh-colored papule in the preauricular region anterior to the tragus. Less commonly, accessory tragi are multiple, unilateral or bilateral, and may be located in the preauricular area, on the cheek along the line of the mandible, or on the lateral aspect of the neck anterior to the sternocleidomastoid muscle. In contrast to the rest of the pinna, which develops from the second branchial arch, the tragus and accessory tragi derive from the first branchial arch. Accessory tragi may occur as isolated defects or in chromosomal first branchial arch syndromes that include anomalies of the ears and face such as cleft lip, cleft palate, and mandibular hypoplasia. Accessory tragus is consistently found in *oculoauriculovertebral syndrome (Goldenhar syndrome).* Surgical excision is appropriate.

BRANCHIAL CLEFT AND THYROGLOSSAL CYSTS AND SINUSES. Cysts and sinuses in the neck may be formed along the course of the first, second, third, or fourth branchial clefts as a result of improper closure during embryonic life. Second branchial cleft cysts are the most common. The lesions may be unilateral or bilateral (2–3%) and may open onto the cutaneous surface or drain into the pharynx. Secondary infection is an indication for systemic antibiotic therapy. These anomalies may be inherited as autosomal dominant traits.

Thyroglossal cysts and fistulas are similar defects located in or near the midline of the neck; they may extend to the base of the tongue. A pathognomonic sign is vertical motion of the mass with swallowing and tongue protrusion. Cysts in the tongue base may be differentiated from an undescended lingual thyroid by radionuclide scanning. Unlike branchial cysts, a thyroglossal duct cyst often appears after an upper respiratory infection.

SUPERNUMERARY NIPPLES. Solitary or multiple accessory nipples may occur in a unilateral or bilateral distribution along a line from the anterior axillary fold to the inguinal area. They are more common in black (3.5%) than white (0.6%) children. Accessory nipples may or may not have an areola and may be mistaken for congenital nevi. They may be excised for cosmetic reasons. Rarely, they undergo malignant change. Renal or urinary tract anomalies may occur in children with this finding.

APLASIA CUTIS CONGENITA (CONGENITAL ABSENCE OF SKIN). Developmental absence of skin is usually noted on the scalp as multiple or solitary (70%), noninflammatory, well-demarcated, oval or circular 1–2 cm ulcers. The appearance of lesions varies, depending on when they occurred during intrauterine development. Those that form early in gestation may heal before delivery and appear as an atrophic, fibrotic scar with associated alopecia, whereas more recent defects may present as an ulceration. Most occur at the vertex just lateral to the midline, but similar defects may also occur on the face, trunk, and limbs, where they are often symmetric. The depth of the ulcer varies. Only the epidermis and upper dermis may be involved, resulting in minimal scarring or hair loss, or the defect may extend to the deep dermis, subcutaneous tissue, and, rarely, to the periosteum, skull, and dura.

No unifying theory can account for all lesions of aplasia cutis congenita. *Diagnosis* is made on the basis of physical findings indicative of in utero disruption of skin development. Lesions are sometimes mistakenly attributed to scalp electrodes or obstetric trauma. Rather, they appear to be due to various factors, including genetic factors, teratogens, compromised vasculature to the skin, and trauma.

Although most individuals with aplasia cutis congenita have no other abnormalities, these lesions may be associated with isolated physical anomalies or with a number of malformation syndromes. Scalp lesions may be seen in association with distal limb reduction anomalies, generally with autosomal dominant inheritance, or sporadically in association with epidermal and organoid nevi. Aplasia cutis congenita may also be found in association with an overt or underlying embryologic malformation, such as meningomyelocele, gastroschisis, omphalocele, or spinal dysraphism. Aplasia cutis congenita in association with fetus papyraceus is apparently due to ischemic or thrombotic events in the placenta and fetus. Blistering or skin fragility and/or absence or deformity of nails in association with aplasia cutis congenita is a well-recognized presentation of epidermolysis bullosa. Maternal ingestion of the teratogen methimazole or intrauterine herpes simplex virus or varicella-zoster virus infection may also be associated with lesions of aplasia cutis congenita. Finally, aplasia cutis congenita may also occur in the setting of a malformation syndrome such as several of the ectodermal dysplasias, trisomy 13 or 14, deletion of the short arm of chromosome 4, Johanson-Blizzard syndrome, focal facial dermal dysplasia, or focal dermal hypoplasia. Cutis aplasia may be confused with traumatic skin injury from monitoring devices and spontaneous atrophic patches (anetoderma) of prematurity.

Major *complications* are hemorrhage, secondary local infection, and meningitis. If the defect is small, recovery is uneventful, with gradual epithelialization and formation of a hairless atrophic scar over a period of several weeks (Fig. 654–1). Small bony defects usually close spontaneously during the 1st yr of life. Large or numerous scalp defects may require excision and primary closure, if feasible; rotation of a flap to fill the defect; or the use of tissue expanders. Truncal and limb defects, despite large size, usually epithelialize and form atrophic scars, which can later be revised, if necessary.

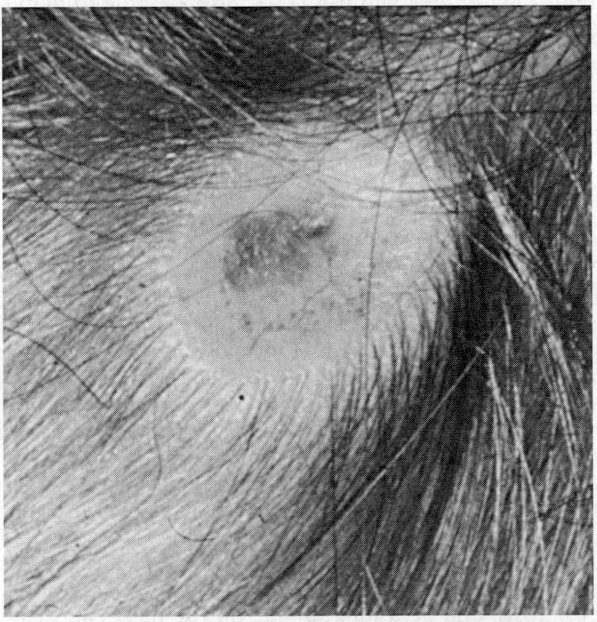

Figure 654–1 Healing solitary lesion of aplasia cutis congenita.

FOCAL FACIAL ECTODERMAL DYSPLASIA (BITEMPORAL APLASIA CUTIS CONGENITA, ECTODERMAL DYSPLASIA OF THE FACE). This rare disorder is characterized by congenital atrophic scarlike lesions on the temples. Sweating is absent over the defects, the lateral one third of the eyebrows is sparse, and linear vertical wrinkles are present on the forehead. Autosomal dominant and autosomal recessive inheritance have been documented; both subgroups of patients lack associated facial anomalies. A subgroup, identified as *Setler syndrome,* is marked by full lips, coarse facies, and rugae around the lips and chin. Growth and development are generally normal.

FOCAL DERMAL HYPOPLASIA (GOLTZ SYNDROME). This rare congenital mesoectodermal and ectodermal disorder is characterized by dysplasia of connective tissue in the skin and skeleton. It presents with numerous soft tan papillomas. Other cutaneous findings include linear atrophic lesions; reticulated hypopigmentation and hyperpigmentation; telangiectasias; congenital absence of skin; angiofibromas presenting as verrucous excrescences; and papillomas of the lips, tongue, circumoral region, vulva, and anus and the inguinal, axillary, and periumbilical areas. Partial alopecia, sweating disorders, and dystrophic nails are additional less common ectodermal anomalies. The most frequent skeletal defects include syndactyly, clinodactyly, polydactyly, and scoliosis. Osteopathia striata are fine parallel vertical stripes noted on radiographs in the metaphyses of long bones; these are highly characteristic of focal dermal hypoplasia but not pathognomonic. Many ocular abnormalities, the most common of which are colobomas, strabismus, nystagmus, and microphthalmia, are also characteristic. Small stature, dental defects, soft tissue anomalies, and peculiar dermatoglyphic patterns are also common. Mental deficiency occurs occasionally.

This familial disorder occurs principally in girls. It has been postulated that an X-linked dominant gene, lethal in hemizygous males, may account for the sex distribution. The linear pattern of skin and bone lesions may be due to random X-inactivation in females. Cases of father-daughter transmission, evidence for an autosomal locus 9q32-qter, and the unusually high (10%) proportion of males with the disorder, however, argue against X-linked dominance with lethality in males. Affected males may have an early half chromatid mutation or autosomal dominant inheritance affecting the germ line.

The primary defect has been hypothesized by some to be a deficiency of collagen caused by a fibroblastic defect. Others suggest that the cutaneous defects represent heterotopic proliferations of fatty nevi within the dermis, resulting from dysplasia, not hypoplasia, followed by herniation of subcutaneous fat.

This disorder is often confused with incontinentia pigmenti because of the sex predilection for females, the linear distribution of skin lesions, and the initial inflammatory phase, which are features of both disorders. The cutaneous lesions may also superficially resemble epidermal nevi. *Treatment* should be directed at amelioration of specific anomalies; genetic counseling is advisable.

DYSKERATOSIS CONGENITA (ZINSSER-ENGMAN-COLE SYNDROME). This rare familial syndrome consists classically of the triad of reticulated hyperpigmentation of the skin, dystrophic nails, and mucous membrane leukoplakia. It usually affects males and is inherited most often in an X-linked recessive fashion, although autosomal recessive or dominant inheritance has been reported. Onset occurs during childhood, most commonly as nail dystrophy, at age 5–13 yr. The nails become atrophic and ridged longitudinally, and there is considerable loss of the nail plate. Skin changes usually appear 2–3 yr after onset of nail changes and consist of reticulated gray-brown pigmentation, atrophy, and telangiectasia, especially on the neck, face, and chest. Hyperhidrosis and hyperkeratosis of the palms and soles, acrocyanosis, and occasional bullae on the hands and feet are also characteristic. Blepharitis, ectropion, and excessive tearing as a result of atresia of the lacrimal ducts are occasional manifestations. Vesiculobullous lesions may occur on the oral mucous membranes and result in ulceration, formation of epithelial tags, atrophic changes of the tongue, and oral leukokeratosis. Oral leukokeratosis generally presents after the 3rd decade of life and may give rise to squamous cell carcinoma. Similar changes have been noted in the urethral and anal mucosae. The scalp hair, eyebrows, and lashes may become sparse. Hypoplastic anemia, at times of the Fanconi variety, may present at age 10 yr or older in up to 50% of patients. Impaired cell-mediated immunity and other T-cell abnormalities have also been noted. The primary causes of death are infections, including *Pneumocystis carinii,* and carcinoma. In one large series, 12% of patients had tumors, most commonly oral and anal squamous cell carcinoma, pancreatic adenocarcinoma, or Hodgkin's disease. The *differential diagnosis* includes the ectodermal dysplasias, pachyonychia congenita, poikilodermas, epidermolysis bullosa, keratoderma of the palms and soles, and lichen sclerosus et atrophicus. The abnormalities noted in skin biopsy specimens are those of poikiloderma.

Treatment includes biopsy of leukoplakic sites to identify malignancies. Etretinate may cause regression of leukoplakia, and orally administered β-carotene has some utility for treatment of leukoplakia and as a preventive agent for oral cancer. Aplastic anemia may be treated by administration of androgens or granulocyte-macrophage colony–stimulating factor or bone marrow transplantation.

CUTIS VERTICIS GYRATA. This bizarre alteration of the scalp, which is more common in males, may be present from birth or may develop during adolescence. The scalp is characterized by convoluted elevated folds, 1–2 cm in thickness, usually in the fronto-occipital axis. Unlike the lax skin of other disorders, the convolutions cannot generally be flattened by traction. Primary cutis gyrata is often associated with mental retardation, ocular defects, abnormal size and shape of the head, seizures, and spasticity. Secondary cutis gyrata may be due to chronic inflammatory diseases; tumors; nevi; acromegaly; and pachydermoperiostosis, a syndrome characterized by hypertrophy of the skin and bones.

Drachtman RA, Alter BP: Dyskeratosis congenita: Clinical and genetic heterogeneity. Am J Pediatr Hematol Oncol 14:297, 1992.

Drolet B, Prendiville J, Golden J, et al: Membranous aplasia cutis with hair collars. Arch Dermatol 131:1427, 1995.

Frieden IJ: Aplasia cutis congenita: A clinical review and proposal for classification. J Am Acad Dermatol 14:646, 1986.

Howell JB, Freeman RG: Cutaneous defects of focal dermal hypoplasia: An ectomesodermal dysplasia syndrome. J Cutan Pathol 16:237, 1989.

Kowalski DC, Fenske NA: The focal facial dermal dysplasias: Report of a kindred and proposed new classification. J Am Acad Dermatol 27:575, 1992.

Moerman P, Fryns JP, Vandenberghe K, et al: Constrictive amniotic bands, amniotic adhesions, and limb-body wall complex: Discrete disruption sequences with pathogenetic overlap. Am J Med Genet 42:470, 1992.

Prizant T, Lucky A, Frieden I, et al: Spontaneous atrophic patches in extremely premature infants. Arch Dermatol 132:671, 1996.

Sebben JE: The accessory tragus—No ordinary skin tag. J Dermatol Surg Oncol 15:304, 1989.

CHAPTER 655
Ectodermal Dysplasias

Ectodermal dysplasia is a heterogeneous group of disorders characterized by a constellation of findings involving defects of two or more of the following: the teeth, skin, and appendageal structures, including hair, nails, and eccrine and sebaceous glands. Disturbances in tissue derived from embryologic layers other than ectoderm are common.

HYPOHIDROTIC (ANHIDROTIC) ECTODERMAL DYSPLASIA. This syndrome is manifested as a triad of defects: partial or complete absence of sweat glands, anomalous dentition, and hypotrichosis. It is usually inherited as an X-linked recessive trait, with full expression only in males; however, an autosomal recessive mode of inheritance may be operative in some families.

Heterozygotic females may have no or variable *clinical manifestations*, including dental defects, sparse hair, and reduced sweating; because of random X-inactivation, they are mosaics of functionally normal and abnormal cells. Affected children, unable to sweat, may experience episodes of high fever in warm environments and may be mistakenly considered to have fever of unknown origin. This is particularly the case in infancy, when the facial changes are not easily appreciated. The typical facies is characterized by frontal bossing; malar hypoplasia; a flattened nasal bridge; recessed columella; thick, everted lips; wrinkled, hyperpigmented periorbital skin; and prominent, low-set ears (Fig. 655–1). The skin over the entire body is dry, finely wrinkled, and hypopigmented, often with a prominent venous pattern. Extensive peeling of the skin is a clinical clue to diagnosis in the newborn period. The paucity of sebaceous glands may account for the dry skin. The hair is sparse, unruly, and lightly pigmented, and eyebrows and lashes are sparse or absent. Anodontia or hypodontia with widely spaced, conical teeth is a consistent feature (see Fig. 655–1). Less commonly, stenotic lacrimal puncta, corneal opacity, cataracts, hypoplastic or absent mammary glands, and conductive hearing loss have been observed. The incidence of atopic diseases in these children is relatively high. Poor development of mucous glands in the respiratory and gastrointestinal tract may result in increased susceptibility to respiratory infection, purulent rhinitis, dysphonia, dysphagia, and diarrhea. Sexual development is usually normal. Approximately 30% of affected boys die during the first 2 yr of life of hyperpyrexia or respiratory infection.

The sweating deficit is a reflection of hypoplasia or absence of eccrine glands; this may be *diagnosed* by skin biopsy. The palmar skin is an appropriate site for biopsy. Reduction or absence of sweating can be documented by pilocarpine iontophoresis or by topical application of *o*-phthalaldehyde to the palmar skin. Sweat pores are not visible in the palmar ridges of affected children and are decreased in number in carrier females. Applying a 2% solution of iodine in alcohol to the back, followed by applying a suspension of cornstarch in castor oil, also allows highlighting of sweat glands by the appearance of a black dot; this test may be useful for detecting female carriers. Linkage analysis has been used for prenatal and early neonatal diagnosis.

Treatment of these children includes protecting them from exposure to high ambient temperatures. Early dental evaluation is necessary so that prostheses can be provided for cosmetic reasons and for adequate nutrition. The use of artificial tears prevents damage to the cornea in patients with defective lacrimation. Alopecia may necessitate the wearing of a wig to improve appearance.

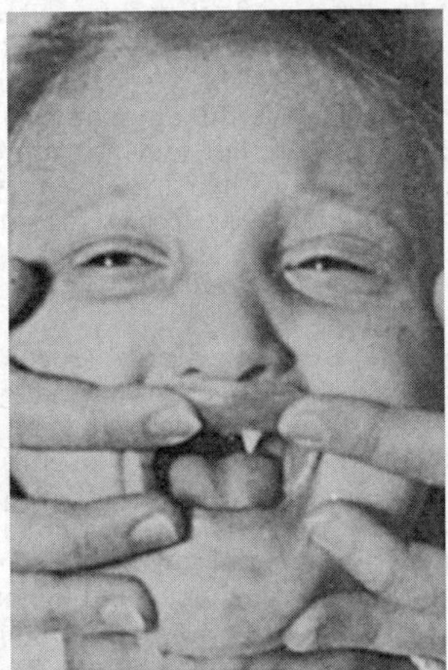

Figure 655–1 Hypohidrotic ectodermal dysplasia is characterized by pointed ears, wispy hair, periorbital hyperpigmentation, midfacial hypoplasia, and pegged teeth.

HIDROTIC ECTODERMAL DYSPLASIA (CLOUSTON SYNDROME). Dystrophic, hypoplastic, or absent nails; sparse hair; and hyperkeratosis of the palms and soles are the salient features of this autosomal dominant disorder. The dentition is usually normal, although small teeth and numerous caries are occasionally found. Conjunctivitis and blepharitis are common. Sweating is always normal. Absence of eyebrows and lashes and hyperpigmentation over the knees, elbows, and knuckles have been noted in some affected individuals.

EEC SYNDROME. Ectrodactyly (split hand and foot), ectodermal dysplasia, cleft lip and palate, and tear duct abnormalities constitute the EEC syndrome, which is probably inherited as an autosomal dominant trait of low penetrance and variable expressivity. The ectodermal dysplasia consists of dry, poorly pigmented skin; light-colored, wispy, sparse scalp hair and eyebrows; and absence of lashes. Decreased numbers of hair follicles and sebaceous glands have been demonstrated by biopsy. Nails may be dystrophic. Clinical expression of the EEC syndrome is variable; any one of these signs may be absent, except the ectodermal signs. Associated defects include anomalies of the hands and feet, nail hypoplasia, granulomatous perlèche frequently complicated by candidosis, defective dentition, deafness, ocular abnormalities (blepharophimosis, strabismus), and abnormalities of the urinary tract. Sweating usually is normal.

Clarke A, Burn J: Sweat testing to identify female carriers of X linked hypohidrotic ectodermal dysplasia. J Med Genet 28:330, 1991.

Clarke A, Phillips DIM, Brown R, et al: Clinical aspects of X-linked hypohidrotic ectodermal dysplasia. Arch Dis Child 62:989, 1987.

Freire-Maia N, Pinheiro M: Ectodermal dysplasias. Some recollections and a classification. *In*: Salinas CF, Opitz JM, Paul NW (eds): Recent Advances in Ectodermal Dysplasias, Vol 24. New York, Alan R. Liss, 1988, p 3.

Rodini ESO, Richieri-Costa A: EEC syndrome: Report on 20 new patients, clinical and genetic considerations. Am J Med Genet 37:42, 1990.

Zonana J: Hypohidrotic (anhidrotic) ectodermal dysplasia: Molecular genetic research and its clinical application. Semin Dermatol 12:241, 1993.

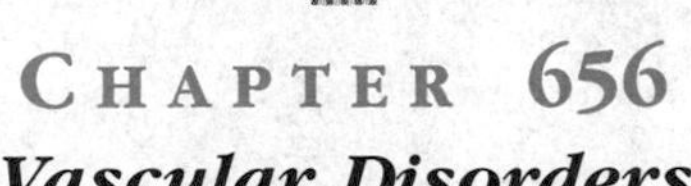

CHAPTER 656
Vascular Disorders

Developmental vascular anomalies may occur as isolated defects or as part of a syndrome. They can be separated into two major categories: hemangiomas and vascular malformations. Hemangiomas are proliferative hamartomas of vascular endothelium that are present at birth or, more commonly, become apparent in the first few (e.g., 3–5) weeks of life, predictably enlarge, and then spontaneously involute. Hemangiomas are the most common tumor of infancy, occurring in 1–2% of newborns and 10% of white infants in the first year of life. With rare exceptions, they occur sporadically and without a genetic basis. Malformations are present at birth and are derived from capillaries, veins, arteries, or lymphatics or any combination thereof. Malformations do not regress but usually enlarge over time.

PORT-WINE STAIN (NEVUS FLAMMEUS, PORT-WINE NEVUS). Port-wine stains are always present at birth. These vascular malformations consist of mature dilated dermal capillaries and represent a permanent developmental defect. The lesions are macular, sharply circumscribed, pink to purple, and tremendously varied in size (Fig. 656–1). The head and neck region is the most common site of predilection, and most lesions are unilateral. The mucous membranes can be involved. As a child matures into adulthood, the port-wine stain may become darker in color and pebbly in consistency, and it may occasionally develop elevated areas that bleed spontaneously.

True port-wine stains should be distinguished from the most common vascular malformation, the salmon patch of neonates, which is, in contrast, a relatively transient lesion (see Chapter 653). Stretching the skin horizontally or placing firm pressure on a glass slide over the involved skin decreases the red color of both lesions and is not diagnostic. When a port-wine stain is localized to the trigeminal area of the face, specifically around the eyelids, the diagnosis of *Sturge-Weber syndrome* (glaucoma, leptomeningeal venous angioma, seizures, hemiparesis contralateral to the facial lesion, intracranial calcification) must be considered (see Chapter 605.3). Early screening for glaucoma is important to prevent additional damage to the eye. Port-wine stains also occur as a component of *Klippel-Trenaunay-Weber syndrome* and with moderate frequency in other syndromes, including the *Cobb* (spinal arteriovenous malformation, port-wine stain), *Proteus, Beckwith-Wiedemann,* and *Bonnet-Bechaume-Blanc* syndromes. In the absence of associated anomalies, morbidity from these lesions may include a poor self-image, hypertrophy of underlying structures, and traumatic bleeding.

The most effective treatment for port-wine stains is the flashlamp-pumped–pulsed dye laser. This therapy is targeted at the lesion and avoids thermal injury to the surrounding normal tissue. After such treatment, the texture and pigmentation of the skin are generally normal without scarring. Therapy can begin in infancy when the surface area of involvement is smaller, although the response appears to be similar regardless of age when treated. Other therapies include masking with cosmetics (Covermark, Dermablend), cryosurgery, excision, grafting, and tattooing.

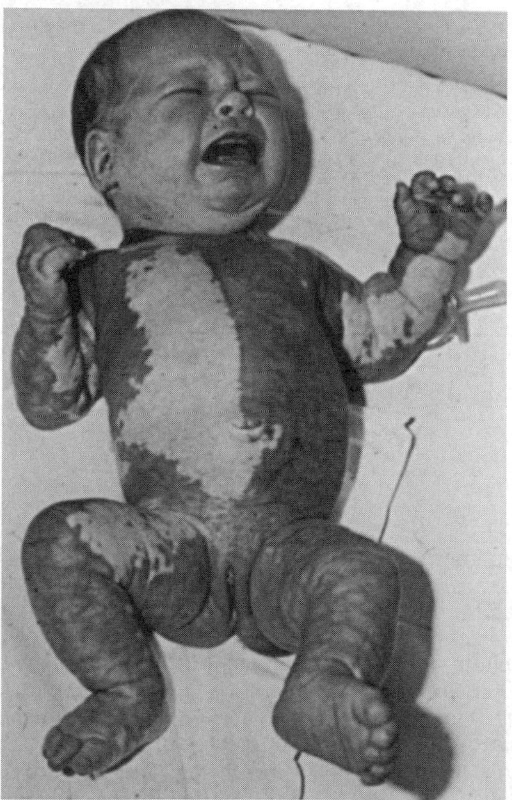

Figure 656–1 Widespread nevus flammeus in an infant with Klippel-Trenaunay-Weber syndrome.

HEMANGIOMA. Superficial hemangiomas are bright red, protuberant, compressible, sharply demarcated lesions that may occur on any area of the body. Although sometimes present at birth, they more often appear within the first 2 mo, heralded by an erythematous or blue mark or an area of pallor, which subsequently develops a fine telangiectatic pattern before the phase of expansion. The presenting sign may occasionally be an ulceration of the perineum or lip. Girls are affected more often than boys. Favored sites are the face, scalp, back, and anterior chest; lesions may be solitary or multiple. Most superficial hemangiomas undergo a phase of rapid expansion, followed by a stationary period, and finally by spontaneous involution. Regression may be anticipated when the lesion develops blanched or pale gray areas that indicate fibrosis. The course of a particular lesion is unpredictable, but approximately 60% of these lesions involute completely by the age of 5 yr, with 90–95% by the age of 9 yr. Spontaneous involution cannot be correlated with size or site of involvement, but lip lesions seem to persist most often. Complications include ulceration, secondary infection, and, rarely, hemorrhage. The location of a lesion may interfere with a vital function (eyelid with vision, urethra with urination). Hemangiomas in a "beard" distribution may be associated with upper airway or subglottic involvement. Respiratory symptoms should suggest a tracheobronchial lesion.

In the usual patient who has no serious complications or extensive overgrowth that results in tissue destruction and severe disfigurement, *treatment* consists of expectant observation. Because almost all lesions resolve spontaneously, therapy is rarely indicated and may, in fact, cause further harm. Parents require repeated reassurance and support. After spontaneous resolution, approximately 10% of patients are left with small cosmetic defects, such as puckering or discoloration of skin. These defects can be eliminated or minimized by judicious plastic repair if desired. In the rare case in which intervention is required, early therapy by the flashlamp-pumped–pulsed dye laser may be beneficial in decreasing growth of the hemangioma and in inducing more rapid resolution of an ulcerated hemangioma. Excision may be advisable in lesions that have remained large for several years; the extent of scarring anticipated should influence the final decision. Radiation can be hazardous and should be considered only in life-threatening situations, such as the Kasabach-Merritt syndrome (see later). Elastic bandages may reduce the amount of tissue distortion resulting from rapid growth, but they are appropriate only in selected patients with large hemangiomas. Systemic or intralesional administration of corticosteroids and interferon-α (IFN-α) may be indicated for infants at risk for serious sequelae from exceptionally large or rapidly growing hemangiomas in vital areas (see later).

Hemangiomas that are more deeply situated appear more diffuse and ill-defined than superficial hemangiomas. The lesions are cystic, firm, or compressible, and the overlying skin may appear normal in color or have a bluish hue. Mixed hemangiomas have both superficial and deep components. Deep hemangiomas progress from a growth phase to a stationary phase to a period of involution. These lesions are as likely to regress as superficial hemangiomas, and the outcome cannot be predicted from size or site of involvement. A course of expectant observation should be followed in most cases. If involvement of underlying structures is suspected, appropriate radiologic studies should be performed for elucidation. Rarely, these lesions impinge on vital structures, interfere with functions such as vision or feeding (Fig. 656–2), cause grotesque disfigurement because of rapid growth, or are associated with life-threatening complications such as thrombocytopenia and hemorrhage (see Kasabach-Merritt syndrome).

If *treatment* becomes necessary, a course of prednisone (2–5 mg/kg/24 hr) is effective in some infants. Termination of growth and sometimes regression may be evident after approximately 4 wk of therapy. When a response is obtained, the dose should be decreased gradually. Alternate-day corticosteroid therapy has also been administered with success. Intralesional corticosteroid injection with the patient anesthetized can also induce rapid involution of a localized hemangioma. IFN-α therapy may also be effective. Spastic diplegia is a rare complication of interferon therapy.

Syndromes associated with hemangiomas include Klippel-Trenaunay-Weber, Maffuci, Gorham (cutaneous hemangiomas with massive osteolysis), and Bannayan-Riley-Ruvalcaba (macrocephaly lipomas, hemangiomas—autosomal dominant inheritance).

KASABACH-MERRITT SYNDROME. This syndrome is a combination of a rapidly enlarging vascular anomaly, thrombocytopenia, microangiopathic hemolytic anemia, and an acute or chronic consumption coagulopathy. The vascular lesion has been presumed to be a hemangioma but alternatively may be a tufted angioma or a kaposiform hemangioendothelioma with lymphatic-like vessels. The *clinical manifestations* are usually evident during early infancy, but the onset occasionally is later. The vascular lesion is usually cutaneous and is only rarely located in viscera. The associated platelet defect may lead to precipitous hemorrhage accompanied by ecchymoses, petechiae, and a rapid increase in size of the vascular lesion. Severe anemia as a result of hemorrhage or microangiopathic hemolysis may ensue. The platelet count is depressed, but the bone marrow contains increased numbers of normal or immature megakaryocytes. The thrombocytopenia has been attributed to sequestration or increased destruction of platelets within the hemangioma. Hypofibrinogenemia and decreased levels of consumable clotting factors are relatively common (see Chapter 488).

Treatment includes management of thrombocytopenia, anemia, and consumptive coagulopathy by administering platelets and by transfusion of red blood cells and fresh frozen plasma. Heparinization is controversial but has benefited some patients when combined with transfusions. Arteriovenous shunts in large lesions may produce high-output heart failure requiring digitalization (see Chapter 488). Treatment of these lesions includes systemic steroids, embolization, radiation therapy, aminocaproic acid (inhibits fibrinolysis), cyclophosphamide, pentoxifylline, or recombinant IFN-α, which may inhibit proliferation of endothelial and smooth muscle cells. The mortality rate is 20–30%.

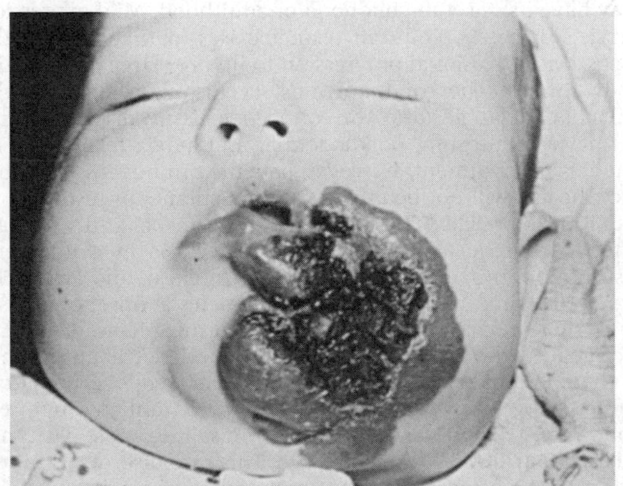

Figure 656–2 Large hemangioma with central crusted ulcer.

DISSEMINATED HEMANGIOMATOSIS. This is a serious condition in which numerous hemangiomas are widely distributed. The skin usually has many small red or purple papular hemangiomas, but infrequently they may be sparse or absent. The internal hemangiomas may involve any of the viscera; the liver, gastrointestinal tract, central nervous system, and lungs are the most common sites. Although involvement falls along a continuum, three entities have been described: (1) benign neonatal hemangiomatosis, with widespread cutaneous hemangiomas in the absence of apparent visceral involvement; (2) disseminated neonatal hemangiomatosis, with myriad small (2 mm–2 cm) papular hemangiomas on the skin and generally also in internal organs; and (3) hemangiomatosis of the liver. In cases of benign neonatal hemangiomatosis, spontaneous regression of the lesions without complications is probable. Multiple hemangiomas may also occur in several rare syndromes, such as macrocephaly combined with pseudopapilledema or with lipomas. Ultrasound and computed tomographic (CT) scanning are indicated to determine the extent of visceral or neural involvement. The disorder is often fatal because of high-output cardiac failure, visceral hemorrhage, obstruction of the respiratory tract, or compression of central neural tissue. In some cases, systemic corticosteroid therapy alone or in combination with IFN-α, surgery, or irradiation has been lifesaving.

BLUE RUBBER BLEB NEVUS. This syndrome consists of numerous vascular malformations of the skin, mucous membranes, and gastrointestinal tract. Typical lesions are blue-purple and rubbery in consistency; they vary in size from a few millimeters to a few centimeters in diameter. They are sometimes painful or tender. The nodules occasionally are present at birth but usually appear in childhood. New lesions may continue to develop throughout life. Large disfiguring and irregular blue marks may also occur. The lesions, which can rarely be located in the liver, spleen, and central nervous system in addition to the skin and gastrointestinal tract, do not involute spontaneously. Recurrent gastrointestinal hemorrhage may lead to severe anemia. Palliation can be achieved by excision of involved bowel. Cutaneous angiomas have been successfully removed by laser therapy.

PYOGENIC GRANULOMA (LOBULAR CAPILLARY HEMANGIOMA, TELANGIECTATIC GRANULOMA). A pyogenic granuloma is a small red, glistening, sessile or pedunculated papule that often has a discernible epithelial collarette (Fig. 656–3). The surface may be weeping and crusted or completely epithelialized. Pyogenic granulomas initially grow rapidly, may ulcerate, and bleed easily when traumatized because they consist of exuberant granulation tissue. They are relatively common in children, particularly on the face, arms, and hands. Those located on a finger or hand may appear as a subcutaneous nodule. Lesions that develop on the oral mucosa during pregnancy are called *granuloma gravidarum*. Pyogenic granulomas generally arise at sites of injury, but a history of trauma often cannot be elicited. Clinically, they resemble and are often indistinguishable from small hemangiomas. Microscopically, an early lesion resembles an early capillary hemangioma. Collarette formation at the base of the tumor and edema of the stroma may allow differentiation from a capillary hemangioma.

Pyogenic granulomas are benign but a nuisance because they bleed easily with trauma and may recur if incompletely removed. Numerous satellite papules have developed after incomplete removal of pyogenic granulomas from the back, particularly in the interscapular region. Small lesions may regress after cauterization with silver nitrate; larger lesions require excision and electrodesiccation of the base of the granuloma. They also have been treated successfully with the flashlamp-pumped–pulsed dye laser.

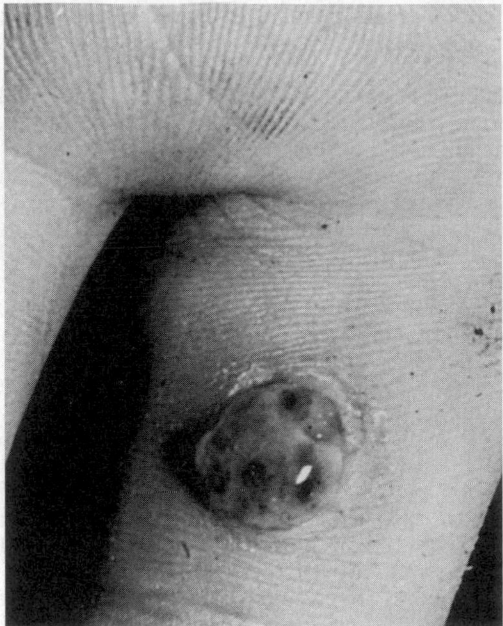

Figure 656–3 Pyogenic granuloma with a moist surface and epithelial collarette at the base.

MAFFUCCI SYNDROME. The association of numerous vascular and, occasionally, lymphatic malformations with nodular enchondromas in the metaphyseal or diaphyseal portion of long bones is known as Maffucci syndrome. Vascular lesions typically are soft, compressible, asymptomatic blue to purple subcutaneous masses that grow in proportion to a child's growth and stabilize by adult life. Mucous membranes or viscera also may be involved. Onset occurs during childhood. Bone lesions may produce limb deformities and pathologic fractures. Malignant transformation of enchondromas (chondrosarcoma, angiosarcoma) or primary malignancies (ovarian, fibrosarcoma, glioma, pancreatic) may be a complication (Chapters 512 and 514).

KLIPPEL-TRENAUNAY-WEBER SYNDROME. A cutaneous vascular malformation in combination with bony and soft tissue hypertrophy and venous varicosities constitutes the triad of defects of this nonheritable disorder. The anomaly is present at birth and usually involves a lower limb but may involve more than one and portions of the trunk or face (see Fig. 656–1). Enlargement of the soft tissues may be gradual and may involve the entire extremity, a portion of it, or selected digits. The vascular lesion most often is a nevus flammeus, generally localized to the hypertrophied area. Venous blebs and/or vesicular lymphatic lesions may be present on their surface. Thick-walled venous varicosities typically become apparent ipsilateral to the vascular malformation after the child begins to ambulate. The deep venous system may be absent, hypoplastic, or obstructed, resulting in lymphedema. Arteriovenous fistulas can develop, and bruits may be audible in the affected part. This disorder can be confused with Maffucci syndrome or, if the surface vascular lesion is minimal, with Milroy disease. Pain, limb swelling, and cellulitis may occur. Thrombophlebitis, dislocations of joints, gangrene of the affected extremity, congestive heart failure, hematuria secondary to angiomatous involvement of the urinary tract, rectal bleeding from lesions of the gastrointestinal tract, pulmonary lesions, and malformations of the lymphatic vessels are infrequent complications. Arteriograms, venograms, and CT or MRI scans may delineate the extent of the anomaly, but surgical correction or palliation is often difficult. The indications for radiologic studies of viscera and bones are best determined by clinical evaluation. Supportive care includes compression bandages for varicosities; surgical treatment may help carefully selected patients. Leg-length differences should be treated with orthotic devices to prevent the development of spinal deformities. Corrective bone surgery may eventually be needed to treat significant leg-length discrepancy.

HEREDITARY HEMORRHAGIC TELANGIECTASIA (OSLER-WEBER-RENDU DISEASE). This disorder is inherited as an autosomal dominant trait. One involved gene encodes endoglin, a membrane glycoprotein on endothelial cells that binds transforming growth factor-β. Affected children may experience recurrent epistaxis before detection of the characteristic skin and mucous membrane lesions. The mucocutaneous lesions, which usually develop at puberty, are 1–4 mm, sharply demarcated red to purple macules, papules, or spider-like projections, each composed of a tightly woven mat of tortuous telangiectatic vessels. The nasal mucosa, lips, and tongue are usually involved; less commonly, cutaneous lesions occur on the face, ears, palms, and nail beds. Vascular ectasias may also arise in the conjunctivae, larynx, pharynx, gastrointestinal tract, bladder, vagina, bronchi, brain, and liver.

Massive hemorrhage is the most serious complication and may result in severe anemia. Bleeding may occur from the nose, mouth, gastrointestinal tract, genitourinary tract, and lungs; epistaxis often is the only complaint, however, occurring in 80% of patients. Approximately 15–20% of patients with arteriovenous malformations in the lungs present with stroke due to embolic abscesses. Persons with hereditary hemorrhagic telangiectasia have normal levels of clotting factors and an intact clotting mechanism. In the absence of serious complications, life span is normal. Local lesions may be ablated temporarily with chemical cautery or electrocoagulation. More drastic surgical measures may be required for lesions in critical sites such as the lung or gastrointestinal tract. Anemia should be treated with iron.

SPIDER ANGIOMAS. A vascular spider (nevus araneus) consists of a central feeder artery with many dilated radiating vessels and a surrounding erythematous flush, varying from a few millimeters to several centimeters in diameter. Pressure over the central vessel causes blanching; pulsations visible in larger nevi are evidence for the arterial source of the lesion. Spider angiomas are associated with conditions in which there are increased levels of circulating estrogens, such as cirrhosis and pregnancy, but they also occur in up to 15% of normal preschool-aged children and 45% of school-aged ones. Sites of predilection in children are the dorsum of the hand, forearm, face, and ears. Angiomas can be obliterated by application of liquid nitrogen, electrocoagulation, or pulsed dye laser; they may also regress spontaneously.

GENERALIZED ESSENTIAL TELANGIECTASIA. A rare and presumably nevoid anomaly of unknown cause, essential telangiectasia may have its onset in childhood or adulthood. Mild expression consists of patchy retiform telangiectases, particularly on the limbs, with occasional progression to involve large areas of the body surface. The condition must be distinguished from the secondary telangiectasias of connective tissue diseases, xeroderma pigmentosum, poikiloderma, and ataxia-telangiectasia. There is no treatment; however, patients can be reassured that their health will not be affected by the cutaneous disorder.

UNILATERAL NEVOID TELANGIECTASIA. This unusual entity is characterized by the appearance of telangiectasia in a unilateral distribution, primarily on the face, neck, chest, and arms. The acquired form occurs particularly in females at onset of menses or during pregnancy. The congenital form predominantly affects males who lack endocrine abnormalities. The appearance of these lesions usually coincides with elevated levels of circulating estrogens, whatever the cause. When initiated by pregnancy, the telangiectasia may fade or disappear post partum.

HEREDITARY BENIGN TELANGIECTASIA. This rare disorder is inherited as an autosomal dominant trait and develops during childhood. The face, upper trunk, and arms are the areas of predilection. The condition is progressive but remains limited to the skin.

CUTIS MARMORATA TELANGIECTATICA CONGENITA (CONGENITAL GENERALIZED PHLEBECTASIA). This benign vascular anomaly represents dilatation of superficial capillaries and veins and is apparent at birth. Involved areas of skin have a reticulated red or purple hue that resembles physiologic cutis marmorata but is more pronounced and relatively unvarying (Fig. 656–4). The lesions may be restricted to a single limb and a portion of the trunk or may be more widespread. Port-wine stain may also be associated. The lesions become more pronounced during changes in environmental temperature, physical activity, or crying. In some cases, the underlying subcutaneous tissue is underdeveloped, and ulceration may occur within the reticulated bands. Rarely, defective growth of bone and other congenital abnormalities may be present. No specific therapy is indicated; the expected course is one of gradual improvement, with partial or complete resolution by adolescence.

ATAXIA-TELANGIECTASIA (see Chapter 126.12). This disorder *(Louis-Bar syndrome)* is transmitted as an autosomal recessive trait. The characteristic telangiectasias develop at about 3 yr of age, first on the bulbar conjunctivae and later on the nasal bridge, malar areas, external ears, hard palate, upper anterior chest, and antecubital and popliteal fossae. Additional cutaneous stigmata include café-au-lait spots, premature graying of the hair, and sclerodermatous changes.

ANGIOKERATOMAS. Several forms of angiokeratomas have been described, but some do not occur during childhood or adolescence. Angiokeratomas, characterized by ectasia of superficial dermal vessels and hyperkeratosis of the overlying epidermis, look like flat hemangiomas with a verrucous, irregular surface. *Angiokeratoma of Mibelli,* probably transmitted in an autosomal dominant pattern, is characterized by 1–8 mm red, purple, or black scaly, verrucous, occasionally crusted papules and nodules that appear on the dorsum of the fingers and toes and on the knees and the elbows. Less commonly, palms, soles, and ears may be affected. In many patients, onset has followed frostbite or chilblains. These nodules bleed freely after injury and may involute in response to trauma. *Angiokeratoma circumscriptum* is a rare solitary lesion that presents as a plaque of blue-red papules or nodules with a verrucous surface. These usually develop during infancy and early childhood, and they increase in size at adolescence. The lower limb is the site of predilection. They may be effectively eradicated by cryotherapy, fulguration, excision, or laser ablation.

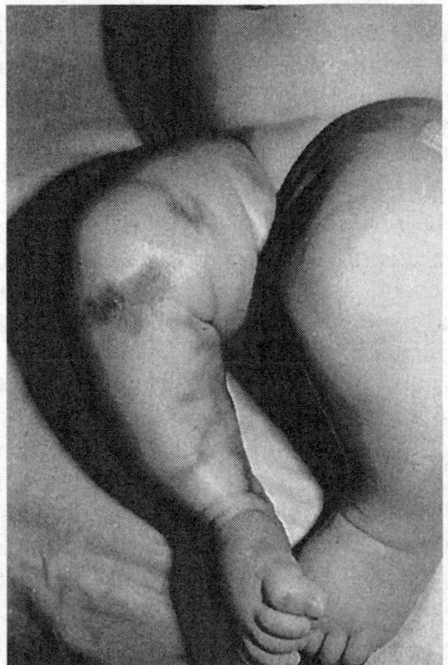

Figure 656–4 Marbled pattern of cutis marmorata telangiectatica congenita on the right leg. See also color section.

ANGIOKERATOMA CORPORIS DIFFUSUM (FABRY DISEASE) (see Chapter 83). This inborn error of glycolipid metabolism is an X-linked recessive disorder that is fully penetrant in males and is of variable penetrance in carrier females. Angiokeratomas have their onset before puberty and occur in profusion over the genitalia, hips, buttocks, and thighs and in the umbilical and inguinal regions. They consist of 0.1–3 mm red to blue-black papules that may have a hyperkeratotic surface. Telangiectasias are seen in the mucosa and conjunctiva. On light microscopy, these angiokeratomas appear as blood-filled, dilated, endothelium-lined vascular spaces. Granular lipid deposits are demonstrable in dermal macrophages, fibrocytes, and endothelial cells.

Additional *clinical manifestations* include recurrent episodes of fever and agonizing pain, cyanosis and flushing of the acral limb areas, paresthesias of the hands and feet, corneal opacities detectable by slit-lamp examination, and hypohidrosis. Renal and cardiac involvement are the usual causes of death. The biochemical defect is a deficiency of the lysosomal enzyme α-galactosidase, with accumulation of ceramide trihexoside in tissues, particularly vascular endothelium, and excretion in urine. There is no specific therapy. Similar cutaneous lesions have also been described in another lysosomal enzyme disorder, α-L-fucosidase deficiency, and in sialidosis, a storage disease with neuraminidase deficiency.

NEVUS ANEMICUS. Although present at birth, nevus anemicus may not be detectable until early childhood. The nevus consists of solitary or numerous sharply delineated pale macules that are most often on the trunk but may also occur on the neck or limbs. These nevi may simulate plaques of vitiligo, leukoderma, or nevoid pigmentary defects, but they can be readily distinguished by their response to firm stroking. Stroking evokes an erythematous line and flare in normal surrounding skin, but the skin of a nevus anemicus does not redden. Although the cutaneous vasculature appears normal histologically, the blood vessels within the nevus do not respond to injection of vasodilators. It has been postulated that the persistent pallor may represent a sustained localized adrenergic vasoconstriction.

LYMPHANGIOMAS (see Chapter 514).

Barlow CF, Priebe CJ, Mulliken JB, et al: Spastic diplegia as a complication of interferon alfa-2a treatment of hemangiomas of infancy. J Pediatr 132:527, 1998.

Boon LM, Enjolras O, Mulliken JB, et al: Congenital hemangioma: Evidence of accelerated involution. J Pediatr 128:329, 1996.

Enjolras O, Wassef M, Mazoyer E, et al: Infants with Kasabach-Merritt syndrome do not have "true" hemangiomas. J Pediatr 130:631, 1997.

Esterly NB: Cutaneous hemangiomas, vascular stains and malformations and associated syndromes. Curr Probl Dermatol 7:65, 1995.

Ezekowitz RAB, Mulliken JB, Folkman J: Interferon-alfa-2a therapy for life-threatening hemangiomas of infancy. N Engl J Med 326:1456, 1992.

Guttmacher AE, Marchuk DA, White RI: Hereditary hemorrhagic telangiectasia. N Engl J Med 333:918, 1995.

Klein JA, Barr RJ: Bannayan-Zonana syndrome associated with lymphangiomyomatous lesions. Pediatr Dermatol 7:48, 1990.

Lacour M, Syed S, Linward J, et al: Role of the pulsed dye laser in the management of ulcerated capillary haemangiomas. Arch Dis Child 74:161, 1996.

Orlow SJ, Isakoff MS, Blei F: Increased risk of symptomatic hemangiomas of the airway in association with cutaneous hemangiomas in a "beard" distribution. J Pediatr 131:643, 1997.

Picascia DD, Easterly NB: Cutis marmorata telangiectatica congenita: A report of 22 cases. J Am Acad Dermatol 20:1098, 1989.

Sadan N, Wolach B: Treatment of hemangiomas of infants with high doses of prednisone. J Pediatr 128:141, 1996.

Tallman B, Tan OT, Morelli JG, et al: Location of port-wine stains and the likelihood of ophthalmic and/or central nervous system complications. Pediatrics 87:323, 1991.

Tay YK, Weston WL, Morelli JG: Treatment of pyogenic granuloma in children with the flashlamp-pumped pulsed dye laser. Pediatrics 99:368, 1997.

Van der Horst CMAM, Koster PHL, De Borgie CAJM, et al: Effect of the timing of treatment of port-wine stains with the flash-lamp-pumped pulsed dye laser. N Engl J Med 338:1028, 1998.

CHAPTER 657
Cutaneous Nevi

Nevus skin lesions are characterized histopathologically by collections of well-differentiated cell types normally found in the skin. Vascular nevi are described in Chapter 656. Melanocytic nevi are subdivided into two broad categories: those that appear after birth, or acquired nevi, and those that are present at birth, the congenital nevi.

ACQUIRED MELANOCYTIC NEVUS. Melanocytic nevi are a benign cluster of melanocytic nevus cells that arise as a result of proliferation of melanocytes at the epidermal-dermal junction. Nevus cells may have the same origin as melanocytes and are probably identical to them. An alternative, less popular theory is that nevus cells are of dual origin, with superficially located cells arising from melanocytes *(melanocytic nevus)* and cells in the deeper layers arising from Schwann cells *(neuroid nevus)*.

Epidemiology. The number of acquired melanocytic nevi increases gradually during childhood, sharply at adolescence, and more slowly in early adulthood. It reaches a plateau in number during the third or fourth decade and then slowly decreases thereafter. The mean number of melanocytic nevi in an adult is 25–35. The greater the number of nevi present, the greater is the risk for development of melanoma. Sun exposure during childhood, particularly intermittent, intense exposure of an individual with light skin and a propensity to burn and freckle rather than tan, is an important determinant of the number of melanocytic nevi that develop. Increased numbers of nevi are also associated with immunosuppression and administration of chemotherapy.

Clinical Manifestations. Nevocellular nevi have a well-defined life history and are classified as junctional, compound, or dermal in accordance with the location of the nevus cells in the skin. In childhood, more than 90% of nevi are junctional; melanocyte proliferation occurs at the junction of the epidermis and dermis to form nests of cells. *Junctional nevi* appear anywhere on the body in various shades of brown; they are relatively small, discrete, flat, and variable in shape. The melanized nevus cells are cuboidal or epithelioid in configuration and occur in nests on the epidermal side of the basement membrane. Although some nevi, particularly those on the palms, soles, and genitalia, remain junctional throughout life, most become compound as melanocytes migrate into the papillary dermis to form nests at both the epidermal-dermal junction and within the dermis. If the junctional melanocytes stop proliferating, nests of melanocytes remain only within the dermis, forming an intradermal nevus. With maturation, *compound* and *intradermal nevi* may become raised, dome shaped, verrucous, or pedunculated. Slightly elevated lesions are usually compound. Distinctly elevated lesions are usually intradermal. With age, the dermal melanocytic nests regress and the nevi gradually disappear.

Prognosis and Treatment. Acquired pigmented nevi are benign, but a very small percentage undergo malignant transformation. Suspicious changes such as rapid increase in size; development of satellite lesions; variegation of color, particularly with shades of red, brown, gray, black, and blue; pigmentary incontinence; notching or irregularity of the borders; and changes in texture such as scaling, erosion, ulceration, and induration; or regional lymphadenopathy are indications for excision and histopathologic evaluation. Most of these changes are due to irritation, infection, or maturation; darkening and gradual increase in size and elevation normally occur during adolescence and should not be cause for concern. Consideration should be given to the presence of risk factors for development of melanoma and the parents' wishes about removal of the nevus. If doubt remains about the benign nature of a nevus, excision is a safe and simple outpatient procedure that may be justified to allay anxiety.

ATYPICAL MELANOCYTIC NEVUS. Atypical nevocellular nevi occur both in an autosomal dominant familial melanoma-prone setting (familial mole-melanoma syndrome, dysplastic nevus syndrome, BK mole syndrome) and as a sporadic event. Only 2% of all pediatric melanomas occur in individuals with this familial syndrome, and 10% of those with the syndrome have a melanoma develop before age 20 yr. Malignant melanoma has been reported in children with the dysplastic nevus syndrome as early as age 10 yr. Risk for development of melanoma is essentially 100% in individuals with dysplastic nevus syndrome and two family members who have had melanomas. The term *atypical mole syndrome* has been proposed to describe lesions in those individuals without an autosomal dominant familial history of melanoma but with more than 50 nevi, some of which are atypical. The lifetime risk of melanoma associated with dysplastic nevi in this context is estimated to be 5–10%.

Atypical nevi tend to be large (5–15 mm) and round to oval. They have irregular margins, variegated color, and elevation of a portion of the lesion. These nevi are most common on the posterior trunk, suggesting that intermittent, intense sun exposure has a role in their genesis. They may also occur, however, in sun-protected areas such as the breasts, buttocks, and scalp. Atypical nevi do not usually develop until puberty, although scalp lesions may be present earlier. Histopathologically, atypical nevi demonstrate disordered proliferation of atypical intraepidermal melanocytes, lymphocytic infiltration, fibroplasia, and angiogenesis. It may be helpful to obtain histopathologic documentation of dysplastic change by biopsy to identify these individuals. It is prudent to excise borderline atypical nevi in immunocompromised children or in those treated with x-irradiation or chemotherapeutic agents. Although chemotherapy has been associated with the development of a greater number of melanocytic nevi, it has not been directly linked to increased risk for development of melanoma. The threshold for removal of clinically atypical nevi is also lower at sites that are difficult to observe, such as the scalp. Children with atypical nevi should have a complete skin examination every 6–12 mo. Parents must be counseled about the importance of sun protection and avoidance and instructed to look for early signs of melanoma on a regular basis, approximately every 3–4 mo.

CONGENITAL MELANOCYTIC NEVUS. Congenital melanocytic nevi are present in approximately 1% of newborn infants. These nevi have been categorized by size: giant congenital nevi are more than 20 cm in diameter (adult size), small congenital nevi are less than 2 cm in diameter, and intermediate nevi are in between in size. Histopathologically, congenital nevi are characterized by the presence of nevus cells in the lower reticular dermis; between collagen bundles; surrounding cutaneous appendages, nerves, and vessels in the lower dermis; and occasionally extending to the subcuticular fat. Identification is often uncertain, however, because they may have the histologic features of ordinary junctional, compound, or intradermal nevi. Some nevi that were not present at birth display histopathologic features of congenital nevi. Furthermore, congenital nevi may be difficult to distinguish clinically from other types of pigmented lesions, adding to the difficulty that parents may have in identifying nevi that were present at birth. The clinical differential diagnosis includes mongolian spots, café-au-lait spots, smooth muscle hamartoma, and dermal melanocytosis (nevi of Ota and Ito).

Sites of predilection of *small congenital nevi* are the lower trunk, upper back, shoulders, chest, and proximal limbs. The lesions may be flat, elevated, verrucous, or nodular and may be various shades of brown, blue, or black. Given the difficulty in identifying small congenital nevi with certainty, data regarding their malignant potential are controversial. Based on historical criteria, it is estimated that approximately 15% of melanomas arise within small congenital nevi. With histopathologic criteria, a congenital nevus has been found in association with approximately 3–8% of melanomas. Removal of all small congenital nevi is not warranted, particularly in view of the fact that development of melanoma in a small congenital nevus is an exceedingly rare event before puberty. A number of factors must be weighed in the decision about whether or not to remove a nevus, including its location and ability to be monitored clinically, the potential for scarring, the presence of other risk factors for melanoma, and the presence of atypical clinical features.

Giant congenital pigmented nevi (<1/20,000 births) occur most commonly on the posterior trunk but may also appear on the head or the extremities. These nevi are of special significance because of their association with leptomeningeal melanocytosis and their predisposition for development of malignant melanoma. Leptomeningeal involvement occurs most often when the nevus is located on the head or midline on the trunk, particularly when associated with "satellite" melanocytic nevi. Nevus cells within the leptomeninges and brain parenchyma may cause increased intracranial pressure, hydrocephalus, seizures, retardation, and motor deficits and may result in melanoma. Malignancy can be identified by careful cytologic examination of the cerebrospinal fluid for melanin-containing cells. Asymptomatic leptomeningeal melanosis was noted on MRI scans of approximately one third of individuals with a giant congenital nevus. The overall incidence of malignant melanoma arising in a giant congenital nevus is estimated to be approximately 5–10%, and approximately 3% of all melanomas arise within a giant congenital nevus. Approximately half of all melanomas that arise within a giant congenital nevus do so by age 5 yr. The mortality rate is approximately 45%. Management of giant congenital nevi remains controversial and should involve the parents, pediatrician, dermatologist, and plastic surgeon. If the nevus lies over the head or spine, an MRI scan may allow detection of neural melanosis; its presence makes gross removal of a nevus from the skin a futile effort. In the absence of neural melanosis, early excision and repair aided by tissue expanders or grafting may reduce the burden of nevus cells and thus the potential for development of melanoma, but at the cost of many potentially disfiguring surgeries. Even then, nevus cells deep within subcutaneous tissues may evade excision. Random biopsies of the nevus are not helpful, but biopsy of newly expanding nodules is indicated. Follow-up is recommended every 6 mo for 5 yr and every 12 mo thereafter. Serial photographs of the nevus may aid in detecting changes.

MELANOMA. Malignant melanoma accounts for 1–3% of all pediatric malignancies and is the most common cancer in young adults age 25–29 yr. Melanoma develops primarily in white individuals, on the head and trunk in males and on the extremities in females. Risk factors for development of melanoma include the presence of the familial atypical mole-melanoma syndrome or xeroderma pigmentosum; increased number of melanocytic nevi, either acquired nevi, giant congenital nevus, or atypical nevi; fair complexion; excessive sun exposure, especially intense sunlight intermittently; a personal or family (i.e., 1st-degree relative) history of a previous melanoma; and immunosuppression. Fewer than 5% of childhood melanomas develop within giant congenital nevi or in those with the familial atypical mole-melanoma syndrome. Approximately 40–50% of the time, melanoma develops at a site where there was no apparent nevus. The mortality rate from melanoma is related primarily to tumor thickness and the level of invasion into the skin. The overall mortality rate reaches approximately 40%, regardless of whether it arises in a child or adult. Given the lack of effective therapy for melanoma, prevention and early detection are the most effective measures. Avoidance of intense midday sun exposure between 10 A.M. and 3 P.M.; use of protective clothing such as a hat, long sleeves, and pants; and use of sunscreen should be emphasized. Early detection includes frequent clinical and photographic examinations for patients at risk (dysplastic nevus syndrome) and prompt response to rapid changes in nevi (size, shape, color, inflammation, bleeding or crusting, and sensation).

HALO NEVUS (LEUKODERMA ACQUISITUM CENTRIFUGUM). Halo nevi occur primarily in children and young adults, most commonly on the back (Fig. 657–1). Development of the halo may coincide with puberty or pregnancy. Several pigmented nevi frequently develop a halo simultaneously. Subsequent disappearance of the central nevus over several months is the usual outcome, and the depigmented area may or may not become repigmented. Excision and histopathologic examination of the lesion is indicated only when the nature of the central lesion is in question. An acquired melanocytic nevus occasionally develops a peripheral zone of depigmentation over a period of days to weeks. Histopathologically, there is a dense inflammatory infiltrate of lymphocytes and histiocytes in addition to the nevus cells. The pale halo reflects disappearance of the melanocytes. This phenomenon is associated with congenital nevi, blue nevi, Spitz nevi, dysplastic nevi, neurofibromas, and primary and secondary malignant melanoma and occasionally with poliosis, Vogt-Koyanagi-Harada syndrome, and pernicious anemia. Patients with vitiligo have an increased incidence of halo nevi. Individuals with halo nevi have circulating antibodies against the cytoplasm of malignant melanoma cells, and their lymphocytes display enhanced killing of melanoma cells in culture.

SPITZ NEVUS (SPINDLE AND EPITHELIOID CELL NEVUS). Spitz nevus presents most commonly during the first 2 decades of life as a pink to red, smooth, dome-shaped, firm, hairless papule on the face, shoulder, or upper limb. Most are less than 1 cm in diameter, but they can achieve a size of 3 cm. Rarely, they occur as numerous grouped lesions. Visually similar lesions include pyogenic granuloma, hemangioma, nevocellular nevus, juvenile xanthogranuloma, and basal cell carcinoma, but histologically these entities are distinguishable. Spitz nevus may be difficult to distinguish histopathologically from malignant melanoma because nuclear atypia is a common feature, particularly after local recurrence of the nevus. Local recurrence after excision may occur up to 5% of the time. If a nevus arouses clinical suspicion that it may be a melanoma,

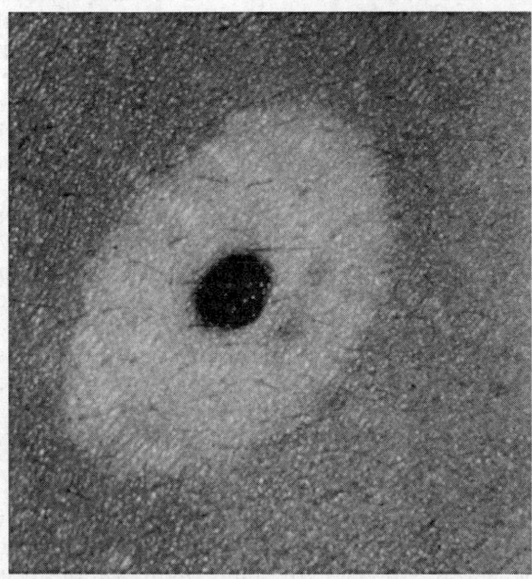

Figure 657–1 Well-developed halo nevus.

an excisional biopsy of the entire lesion is recommended. If the margins of excision of a Spitz nevus are positive, re-excision of the site is prudent to avoid difficulties in histopathologic interpretation of the lesion in the future.

ZOSTERIFORM LENTIGINOUS NEVUS (AGMINATED LENTIGENES). This nevus is a unilateral, linear, bandlike collection of numerous 2–10 mm brown or black macules on the face, trunk, or limbs. The nevus may be present at birth or may develop during childhood. Seen histopathologically are increased numbers of melanocytes in elongated rete ridges of the epidermis.

NEVUS SPILUS (SPECKLED LENTIGINOUS NEVUS). This nevus is a flat brown patch within which are darker, flat or raised brown melanocytic elements. These nevi vary considerably in size and can occur anywhere on the body. Nevus spilus is rare at birth and is commonly acquired during late infancy or early childhood. Dark elements within the nevus are usually present initially and tend to increase in number gradually over time. The darker macules represent nevus cells in a junctional or dermal location; the patch has increased numbers of melanocytes in a lentiginous epidermal pattern. The malignant potential of these nevi is uncertain; nevus spilus is found more commonly in individuals with melanoma compared with matched controls. The nevi need not be excised, unless atypical features or recent clinical changes are noted.

NEVUS OF OTA. Nevus of Ota is more common in females and in Asian and black patients. This nevus consists of a permanent patch composed of blue, black, and brown, partially confluent macules. The intensity of pigmentation may vary from day to day, and enlargement and darkening may occur with time. Some areas of the nevus occasionally are raised. The macular nevi resemble mongolian spots in color and occur unilaterally in the areas supplied by the 1st and 2nd divisions of the trigeminal nerve. Nevus of Ota differs from a mongolian spot, not only by its distribution but also by having a speckled rather than a uniform appearance. It also has a greater concentration of elongated, dendritic dermal melanocytes located in the upper rather than the lower portion of the dermis. Nevus of Ota is sometimes present at birth; in other cases, it may arise during the 1st or 2nd decade of life. Patchy involvement of the conjunctiva, hard palate, pharynx, nasal mucosa, buccal mucosa, or tympanic membrane occurs in some patients. Malignant change is exceedingly rare. Laser therapy may effectively decrease the pigmentation.

Nevus of Ito is localized to the supraclavicular, scapular, and deltoid regions. This nevus tends to be more diffuse in its distribution and less mottled than the nevus of Ota. The only available treatment is masking with cosmetics or laser therapy.

BLUE NEVI. The *common blue nevus* is a solitary, asymptomatic, smooth, dome-shaped, blue to blue-gray papule less than 10 mm in diameter on the dorsal aspect of the hands and feet. Rarely, common blue nevi form large plaques. Blue nevus is nearly always acquired, often during childhood and more commonly in females. Microscopically, it is characterized by groups of intensely pigmented spindle-shaped melanocytes in the dermis. This nevus is benign.

The *cellular blue nevus* is typically 1–3 cm in diameter and occurs most frequently on the buttocks and in the sacrococcygeal area. In addition to collections of deeply pigmented dermal dendritic melanocytes, cellular islands composed of large spindle-shaped cells are noted in the dermis and may extend into the subcutaneous fat. The cellular blue nevus has a low but definite incidence of malignant transformation; therefore, excision is the treatment of choice. A *combined nevus* is the association of a blue nevus with an overlying melanocytic nevus.

The blue-gray that is characteristic of these nevi is an optical effect caused by dermal melanin. Longer wavelengths of visible light penetrate to the deep dermis and are absorbed there by melanin; shorter-wavelength blue light cannot penetrate deeply but instead is reflected back to the observer.

ACHROMIC NEVUS (NEVUS DEPIGMENTOSUS). These nevi are usually present at birth; they are localized macular hypopigmented patches or streaks, often with bizarre, irregular borders. They can resemble hypomelanosis of Ito clinically, except that they are more localized and often unilateral. Small lesions may also resemble the white leaf macules of tuberous sclerosis. They appear to represent a focal defect in transfer of melanosomes to keratinocytes.

EPIDERMAL NEVI. These may be visible at birth or may develop within the first months or years of life. They affect both sexes equally and usually occur sporadically. Epidermal nevi are hamartomatous lesions characterized by hyperplasia of the epidermis and/or adnexal structures in a focal area of the skin. Proliferation of nevocellular nevus cells is not present in these lesions.

Epidermal nevi are classified into a number of variants, depending on the morphology and extent of the nevus and the epidermal structure that is predominant. An epidermal nevus may appear initially as a discolored, slightly scaly patch that, with maturation, becomes more linear, thickened, verrucous, and hyperpigmented. *Systematized* refers to a diffuse or extensive distribution of lesions, and *ichthyosis hystrix* indicates that the distribution is extensive and bilateral. Morphologic types include pigmented papillomas, often in a linear distribution; unilateral hyperkeratotic streaks involving a limb and perhaps a portion of the trunk; velvety hyperpigmented plaques; and whorled or marbled hyperkeratotic lesions in localized plaques (Fig. 657–2) or over extensive areas of the body along Blaschko lines. An inflammatory linear verrucous variant is markedly pruritic and tends to become erythematous, scaling, and crusted.

The histologic pattern evolves as the lesion matures, but epidermal hyperplasia of some degree is apparent in all stages of development. One or another dermal appendage may predominate in a particular lesion. These nevi must be distinguished from lichen striatus, lymphangioma circumscriptum, shagreen patch of tuberous sclerosis, congenital hairy nevi, linear porokeratosis, linear lichen planus, linear psoriasis, the verrucous stage of incontinentia pigmenti, and nevus sebaceus (Jadassohn). Keratolytic agents such as retinoic acid or salicylic acid may be moderately effective in reducing scaling and controlling pruritus, but definitive *treatment* requires full-thickness excision; recurrence is usual if more superficial removal is attempted. Alternatively, the nevus may be left intact. Rarely, basal cell carcinoma or squamous cell carcinoma has developed in a verrucous epidermal nevus that shows sudden growth, nodularity, or erosions.

Epidermal nevi are occasionally associated with other abnormalities of the skin and soft tissues, eyes, and nervous, cardio-

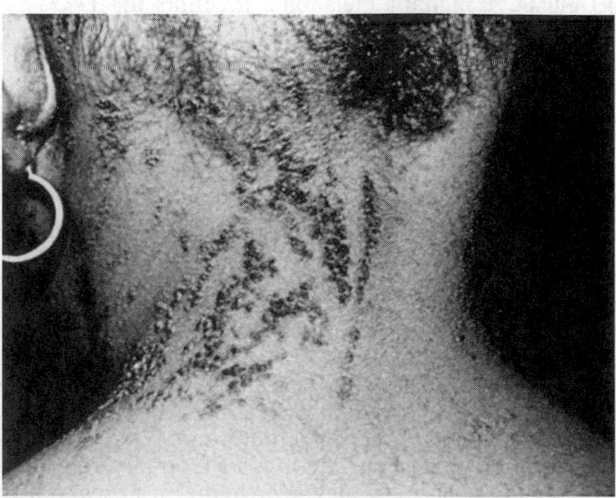

Figure 657–2 Verrucous streaky epidermal nevus on the neck.

vascular, musculoskeletal, and urogenital systems. In these instances, referred to as *epidermal nevus syndrome,* a mosaic phenotype is expressed. This syndrome, however, is not a distinct clinical entity. The well established syndromes that involve a type of epidermal nevus and distinct birth defects include the sebaceous nevus, Proteus, and CHILD (congenital hemidysplasia with ichthyosiform erythroderma and limb defects) syndromes.

Nevus Sebaceus (Jadassohn). This is a relatively small, sharply demarcated, oval or linear, yellow-orange, elevated plaque that is usually devoid of hair and occurs on the head and neck of infants. It may occur occasionally on the trunk. Although the lesion is characterized histopathologically by an abundance of sebaceous glands, all elements of the skin are represented. It is frequently flat and inconspicuous in early childhood. With maturity, usually during adolescence, the lesions become verrucous and studded with large rubbery nodules. The changing clinical appearance reflects the histologic pattern, which is characterized by a variable degree of hyperkeratosis, hyperplasia of the epidermis, malformed hair follicles, and often a profusion of sebaceous glands and the presence of ectopic apocrine glands. It is believed that these nevi form from pleuripotential primary epithelial germ cells, which can dedifferentiate into various epithelial tumors. Consequently, during adulthood, these nevi are frequently complicated by secondary malignancies and benign adnexal tumors, most commonly basal cell carcinoma or syringocystadenoma papilliferum. Diagnosis can be established by biopsy; the treatment of choice is total excision before adolescence. Sebaceous nevi associated with central nervous system, skeletal, and ocular defects represent a variant of the epidermal nevus syndrome.

Becker Nevus (Becker Melanosis). This form of epidermal nevus develops predominantly in males, during childhood or adolescence, initially as a hyperpigmented patch. The lesion commonly develops hypertrichosis, limited to the area of hyperpigmentation, and evolves into a unilateral, slightly thickened, irregular, hyperpigmented plaque. The most common sites are the upper torso and upper arm. Histopathologically, the nevus shows an increased number of basal melanocytes and variable epidermal hyperplasia. Becker melanosis is commonly associated with a smooth muscle hamartoma, which may appear as slight perifollicular papular elevations or slight induration. Stroking such a lesion may induce smooth muscle contraction and make the hairs stand up. Androgen sensitivity may have a role in the development of Becker melanosis. The nevus is benign, has no risk for malignant change, and is very rarely associated with other anomalies.

NEVUS COMEDONICUS. This is an uncommon organoid nevus of epithelial origin that consists of linear plaques of plugged follicles that simulate comedones; they may be present at birth or may appear during childhood. The horny plugs represent keratinous debris within dilated, malformed pilosebaceous follicles. The lesions are most often unilateral and may develop at any site. Rarely, they are associated with other congenital malformations, including skeletal defects, cerebral anomalies, and cataracts. Although these lesions are often asymptomatic, some individuals experience recurrent inflammation, resulting in cyst formation, fistulas, and scarring. There is no effective treatment except full-thickness excision; palliation of larger lesions may be achieved by regular applications of a retinoic acid preparation.

CONNECTIVE TISSUE NEVUS. This is a hamartoma of collagen, elastin, and/or glycosaminoglycans of the dermal extracellular matrix. It may occur as a solitary defect or as a manifestation of an associated disorder. These nevi may occur at any site but are most common on the back, buttocks, arms, and thighs. They are skin-colored, ivory, or yellow plaques, 2–15 cm in diameter, composed of many tiny papules or grouped nodules that are frequently difficult to appreciate visually because of the subtle color changes. The plaques have a rubbery or cobblestone consistency on palpation. Biopsy findings are variable and include increased amounts and/or degeneration or fragmentation of dermal collagen, elastic tissue, or ground substance. Similar lesions occurring with tuberous sclerosis are called shagreen patches; however, shagreen patches consist only of excessive amounts of collagen. The association of many small papular connective tissue nevi with osteopoikilosis is called *dermatofibrosis lenticularis disseminata* (Buschke-Ollendorf syndrome).

SMOOTH MUSCLE HAMARTOMA. This hamartoma is a developmental anomaly resulting from hyperplasia of the smooth muscle (arrector pili) associated with hair follicles. It is usually evident at birth or shortly thereafter as a flesh-colored or lightly pigmented plaque with overlying hypertrichosis on the trunk or limbs. Transient elevation or a rippling movement of the lesion, caused by contraction of the muscle bundles, can sometimes be elicited by stroking the surface. Smooth muscle hamartoma can be mistaken for congenital pigmented nevus, but the distinction is important because it has no risk for malignant melanoma and need not be removed.

Ackerman AB, Milde P: Naming acquired melanocytic nevi. Common and dysplastic, normal and atypical, or Unna, Miescher, Spitz, and Clark? Am J Dermatopathol 14:447, 1992.

Berg P, Lindelöf B: Differences in malignant melanoma between children and adolescents. Arch Dermatol 133:295, 1997.

Casso EM, Grin-Jorgensen CM, Grant-Kels JM: Spitz nevi. J Am Acad Dermatol 27:901, 1992.

Ceballos PI, Ruiz-Maldonado R, Mihm MC: Melanoma in children. N Engl J Med 332:656, 1995.

De David M, Orlow SJ, Provost N, et al: Neurocutaneous melanosis: Clinical features of large congenital melanocytic nevi in patients with manifest central nervous system melanosis. J Am Acad Dermatol 35:529, 1996.

Frieden IJ, Williams ML, Barkovich AJ: Giant congenital melanocytic nevi: Brain magnetic resonance findings in neurologically asymptomatic children. J Am Acad Dermatol 31:423, 1994.

Gallagher RP, McClean DI, Yang CP, et al: Anatomic distribution of acquired melanocytic nevi in white children. Arch Dermatol 125:466, 1990.

Gallagher RP, McClean DI, Yang CP, et al: Suntan, sunburn, and pigmentation factors and the frequency of acquired melanocytic nevi in children. Arch Dermatol 126:770, 1990.

Green MH, Clark WH, Tucker MA, et al: Acquired precursors of cutaneous malignant melanoma. (The familial dysplastic nevus syndrome.) N Engl J Med 312:91, 1985.

Jacobs AH, Walton RG: The incidence of birthmarks in the neonate. Pediatrics 58:281, 1976.

Kaplan EN: The risk of malignancy in large congenital nevi. Plast Reconstr Surg 53:421, 1974.

Marghoob AA, Orlow SJ, Kopf AW: Syndromes associated with melanocytic nevi. J Am Acad Dermatol 29:373, 1993.

Rhodes AR: Congenital nevi: Should these be excised? JAMA 262:1696, 1989.

Rothman KE, Esterly N: Dysplastic nevi in children. Pediatr Dermatol 7:218, 1990.

Ruiz-Maldonado R, Orozco-Covarrubias ML: Malignant melanoma in children. Arch Dermatol 133:363, 1997.

Shpall S, Frieden I, Chesney M, et al: Risk of malignant transformation of congenital melanocytic nevi in blacks. Pediatr Dermatol 11:204, 1994.

Tucker M, Halpern A, Holly E, et al: Clinically recognized dysplastic nevi. JAMA 277:1439, 1997.

Williams ML, Pennella R: Melanoma, melanocytic nevi, and other melanoma risk factors in children. J Pediatr 124:833, 1994.

Williams ML, Sagebiel RS, Vasconez LO: Special symposium. The management of congenital nevocytic nevi. Pediatr Dermatol 2:143, 1984.

CHAPTER 658
Hyperpigmented Lesions

DISORDERS OF PIGMENT. Increased skin color may be generalized or localized and may result from various defects in melanocyte formation, differentiation, migration, or distribution or in the production or distribution of melanin. Some of these aberrations are a manifestation of systemic disease (hyperpigmentation of Addison disease); others represent generalized or focal developmental defects (piebaldism); and still others may be nonspecific and the result of cutaneous inflammation (postinflammatory hyperpigmentation).

EPHELIDES, OR FRECKLES. These are light or dark brown macules usually less than 3 mm in diameter, with a poorly defined margin, that occur in sun-exposed areas, such as the face, upper back, arms, and hands. They are induced by exposure to sun, particularly during the summer, and may fade or disappear during the winter. They are more common in fair-haired individuals, appear first during the preschool years, and are determined by an autosomal dominant gene. Histologically, they are marked by increased melanin pigment in epidermal basal cells, which have more numerous and larger dendritic processes than the melanocytes of the surrounding paler skin. The lack of melanocytic proliferation or elongation of epidermal rete ridges distinguishes them from lentigines. Freckles have been identified as a risk factor for melanoma independent of melanocytic nevi.

LENTIGINES. Lentigines, often mistaken for freckles or junctional nevi, are small (<3 cm), round, dark brown macules that can appear anywhere on the body. They are unrelated to sun exposure and remain permanently. Histologically, they have elongated, club-shaped, epidermal rete ridges with increased numbers of melanocytes and dense epidermal deposits of melanin. No nests of melanocytes are found. The lesions are benign and, when few, may be viewed as a normal occurrence.

Lentigines may increase in number and darken excessively in Addison disease and during pregnancy. *Lentiginosis profusa* involves innumerable small, pigmented macules that are present at birth or appear during childhood. There are no associated abnormalities, and mucous membranes are spared. *LAMB syndrome* consists of lentigines of the face and vulva, atrial myxoma, mucocutaneous myxomas, and blue nevi. The *multiple lentigines (LEOPARD) syndrome* is an autosomal dominant entity consisting of a generalized, symmetric distribution of lentigines in association with electrocardiogram abnormalities, ocular hypertelorism, pulmonary stenosis, abnormal genitals (cryptorchidism, hypogonadism, hypospadias), growth retardation, and sensorineural deafness. Other features include hypertrophic obstructive cardiomyopathy and pectus excavatum or carinatum.

The *Peutz-Jeghers syndrome* is characterized by melanotic macules on the lips and mucous membranes and by gastrointestinal (GI) polyposis. It is inherited as an autosomal dominant trait. Onset is noted during infancy and early childhood when pigmented macules appear on the lips and buccal mucosa. The macules are usually a few millimeters in size but may be as large as 1–2 cm. Macules also appear occasionally on the palate, gums, tongue, and vaginal mucosa. Cutaneous lesions may develop on the nose, hands, and feet; around the mouth, eyes, and umbilicus; and as longitudinal bands or diffuse hyperpigmentation of the nails. Pigmented macules often fade from the lips and skin during puberty and adulthood but generally do not disappear from mucosal surfaces. Buccal mucosal macules are the most constant feature of the disorder; in some families, however, occasional members may be affected only with the pigmentary changes. Indistinguishable pigmentary changes beginning in adult life also occur sporadically in individuals without intestinal involvement.

Polyposis usually involves the jejunum and ileum but may also occur in the stomach, duodenum, colon, and rectum. Episodic abdominal pain, diarrhea, melena, and intussusception are frequent complications. Patients have a significantly increased risk of GI tract and non–GI tract tumors at a young age. GI cancer has been reported in approximately 2–3% of patients; the lifetime relative risk of GI malignancy is 13. The relative risk of non–GI tract malignancies is 9, including ovarian, cervical, and testicular tumors. Peutz-Jeghers syndrome must be differentiated from other syndromes associated with multiple lentigines *(Laugier-Hunziker syndrome)*, from ordinary freckling, from *Gardner syndrome*, and from *Cronkhite-Canada syndrome*, a disorder characterized by GI polyposis; alopecia; onychodystrophy; and diffuse pigmentation of the palms, volar aspects of the fingers, and dorsal hands. Treatment of Peutz-Jeghers melanotic macules has been successful, in some cases, with carbon dioxide, ruby, or argon lasers.

CAFÉ-AU-LAIT SPOTS. These are uniformly hyperpigmented, sharply demarcated macular lesions, the hues of which vary with the normal degree of pigmentation of the individual: They are tan or light brown in white individuals and may be dark brown in black children. Café-au-lait spots vary tremendously in size and may be large, covering a significant portion of the trunk or limb. Generally, the borders are smooth, but some have an exceedingly irregular border. The lesions are characterized by increased numbers of melanocytes and melanin in the epidermis but lack the clubbed rete ridges that typify lentigines. One to three café-au-lait spots are common in normal children; approximately 10% of normal children have café-au-lait macules. They may be present at birth or develop during childhood.

Large, often asymmetric café-au-lait spots with irregular borders are characteristic of patients with *McCune-Albright syndrome* (see Chapter 572.6). This disorder includes polyostotic fibrous dysplasia of bone, leading to pathologic fractures; precocious puberty; and numerous hyperfunctional endocrinopathies. The macular hyperpigmentation may be present at birth or develop late in childhood. Cutaneous pigmentation typically is most extensive on the side showing the most severe bone involvement. The full syndrome with precocious puberty occurs only in girls. A mutation in the gene for the α subunit of G_s, resulting in stimulation of cyclic adenosine monophosphate formation, occurs in these patients.

Neurofibromatosis Type 1 (von Recklinghausen disease). The café-au-lait spot is the most familiar cutaneous hallmark of this autosomal dominant neurocutaneous syndrome (see Chapter 605.1). These lesions also occur with certain other disorders, including other types of neurofibromatosis (Table 658–1). Included in the criteria for this diagnosis is the presence of five or more café-au-lait spots more than 5 mm in diameter in prepubertal patients or six or more café-au-lait spots more than 15 mm in diameter in postpubertal children. Multiple café-au-lait macules commonly produce a freckled appearance of non–sun-exposed areas such as the axillae (Crowe sign), the inguinal and inframammary regions, and under the chin.

INCONTINENTIA PIGMENTI (BLOCH-SULZBERGER DISEASE). This rare, heritable, multisystem ectodermal disorder features dermatologic, dental, and ocular abnormalities. The phenotype is produced by functional mosaicism caused by random X-inactivation of an X-linked dominant gene that is lethal in males. The paucity of affected males, the occurrence of female-to-female transmission, and an increased frequency of spontaneous abortions in carrier females supports this supposition. The gene is linked to the Xq28 region.

Clinical Manifestations. This disease has four phases, not all of which may occur in a given patient. The *first phase* is evident at birth or during the first few weeks of life and consists of erythematous linear streaks and plaques of vesicles that are most pronounced on the limbs and circumferentially on the trunk. The lesions may be confused with those of herpes

TABLE 658–1 Disorders with Café-au-Lait Spots

Neurofibromatosis	Basal cell nevus syndrome
McCune-Albright syndrome	Gaucher disease
Russell-Silver syndrome	Chédiak-Higashi syndrome
Ataxia telangiectasia	Hunter syndrome
Fanconi anemia	Maffucci syndrome
Tuberous sclerosis	Multiple mucosal neuroma syndrome
Bloom syndrome	Watson syndrome

simplex, bullous impetigo, or mastocytosis, but the linear configuration is unique. Histopathologically, epidermal edema and eosinophil-filled intraepidermal vesicles are present. Eosinophils also infiltrate the adjacent epidermis and dermis. Blood eosinophilia up to 65% also is common. The first stage generally resolves by 4 mo of age, but mild, short-lived recurrences of blisters may develop during febrile illnesses of childhood. In the *second phase*, as blisters on the distal limbs resolve, they become dry and hyperkeratotic, forming verrucous plaques. The verrucous plaques rarely affect the trunk or face and generally involute within 6 mo. Epidermal hyperplasia, hyperkeratosis, and papillomatosis are characteristic. The *third* or *pigmentary stage* is the hallmark of incontinentia pigmenti. It generally develops over weeks to months and may overlap the earlier phases, be evident at birth, or, more commonly, begin to appear within the first few weeks of life. Hyperpigmentation more often is apparent on the trunk than the limbs and is distributed in macular whorls, reticulated patches, flecks, and linear streaks that follow Blaschko lines. The axillae and groin are invariably affected. The sites of involvement are not necessarily those of the preceding vesicular and warty lesions. The pigmented lesions, once present, persist throughout childhood (Fig. 658–1). They generally begin to fade by early adolescence, however, and often have disappeared by age 16 yr. Occasionally, the pigmentation remains permanently, particularly in the groin. The lesion, histopathologically, shows vacuolar degeneration of the epidermal basal cells and melanin in melanophages of the upper dermis as a result of incontinence of pigment. In the *fourth stage*, hypopigmented, hairless, anhidrotic patches or streaks occur as a late manifestation of incontinentia pigmenti; they may develop, however, before the hyperpigmentation of stage three has resolved. The lesions develop mainly on the flexor aspect of the lower legs and less often on the arms and trunk.

Although skin lesions may constitute the only manifestation, approximately 80% of affected children have other defects. Alopecia, which may be scarring and patchy or diffuse, is most common on the vertex and occurs in up to 40% of patients. Hair may be lusterless, wiry, and coarse. Dental anomalies, which are present in up to 80% of patients and are persistent throughout life, consist of late dentition, hypodontia, conical teeth, and impaction. Central nervous system manifestations, including motor and cognitive developmental retardation, seizures, microcephaly, spasticity, and paralysis, are found in up to one third of affected children. Ocular anomalies, such as neovascularization, microphthalmos, strabismus, optic nerve atrophy, cataracts, and retrolenticular masses, occur in more than 30% of children. Nonetheless, more than 90% of patients have normal vision. The ocular and central nervous system lesions may be secondary to an occlusive vasculopathy. Less common abnormalities include dystrophy of nails (ridging, pitting) and skeletal defects.

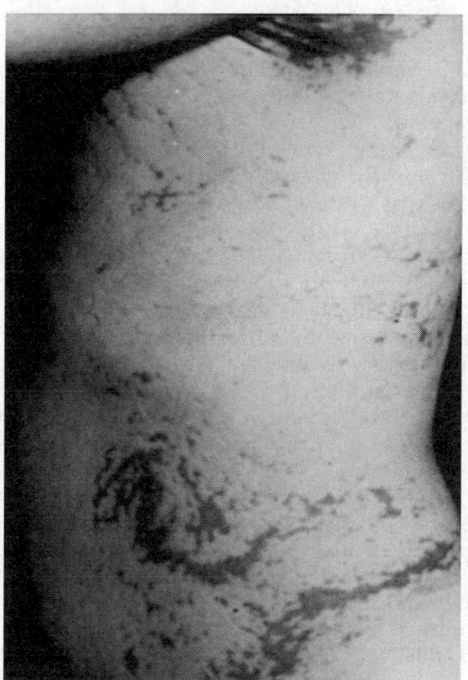

Figure 658–1 Whorled macular hyperpigmentation of incontinentia pigmenti.

Diagnosis of incontinentia pigmenti is made on clinical grounds, although major and minor criteria have been established to aid in diagnosis. Wood's lamp examination may be useful in older children and adolescents to highlight pigmentary abnormalities.

Treatment. The choice of investigative studies and the plan of management depend on the occurrence of particular noncutaneous abnormalities because the skin lesions are benign. The high incidence of associated major anomalies warrants genetic counseling.

POSTINFLAMMATORY PIGMENTARY CHANGES. Either hyperpigmentation or hypopigmentation can occur as a result of cutaneous inflammation. Alteration in pigmentation usually follows a severe inflammatory reaction but may result from mild dermatitis. Dark-skinned children are more likely to show these changes than fair-skinned ones. Although altered pigmentation may persist for weeks to months, patients can be reassured that these lesions are usually temporary. These changes must be distinguished from nevoid lesions and diseases manifested by pigmentary alterations such as vitiligo.

Bolognia JL, Orlow SJ, Glick SA: Lines of Blaschko. J Acad Dermatol 31:157, 1994.

Gutman D, Aylsworth A, Carey J, et al: The diagnostic evaluation and multidisciplinary management of neurofibromatosis1 and neurofibromatosis 2. JAMA 278:51, 1997.

Hizawa K, Iida M, Matsumoto T, et al: Neoplastic transformation arising in Peutz-Jeghers polyposis. Dis Colon Rectum 36:953, 1993.

Landy SJ, Donnai D: Incontinentia pigmenti (Bloch-Sulzberger syndrome). J Med Genet 30:53, 1993.

Lee A, Goldberg M, Gillard J, et al: Intracranial assessment of incontinentia pigmenti using magnetic resonance imaging, angiography, and spectroscopic imaging. Arch Pediatr Adolesc Med 149:573, 1995.

Spigelman AD, Murday V, Phillips RKS: Cancer and the Peutz-Jeghers syndrome. Gut 30:1588, 1989.

CHAPTER 659
Hypopigmented Lesions

ALBINISM. Several types of congenital oculocutaneous albinism consist of partial or complete failure of melanin production in the skin, hair, and eyes despite the presence of normal number, structure, and distribution of melanocytes. The various forms of albinism, including nine autosomal recessive and one rare autosomal dominant variants, may be distinguished by clinical manifestations, morphology of the melanosomes, and the hair bulb incubation test, in which hair bulbs are plucked and incubated with tyrosine to determine whether tyrosinase is present. Tyrosinase is the copper-containing enzyme that catalyzes at least three steps in melanin biosynthesis (see Chapter 82.2). Tyrosinase-positive variants, which are characterized by darkening of the hair bulb on incubation with tyrosine, are most common.

Ocular albinism, which involves only the eyes, presents in

X-linked and autosomal dominant forms, and one autosomal recessive form. Two of these types are associated with deafness. Female carriers of the X-linked types may show irregular retinal pigmentation.

Tyrosinase-negative or type 1 oculocutaneous albinism is characterized by greatly reduced or absent tyrosinase activity. Type 1A albinism, the most severe form, is characterized by a lack of visible pigment in hair, skin, and eyes. This is manifested as photophobia, nystagmus, defective visual acuity, white hair, and white skin. The irises are blue-gray in oblique light and prominent pink in reflected light. Type 1B or yellow mutant albinism presents at birth with white hair, pink skin, and gray eyes. This type is particularly prevalent in Amish communities. Progressively, however, the hair becomes yellow-red, the skin tans lightly on exposure to the sun, and the irises may accumulate some brown pigment, with a resultant improvement in visual acuity. Photophobia and nystagmus are present but are mild. Numerous different allelic mutations in the tyrosinase gene account for types 1A and 1B albinism. In whites, no single mutant tyrosinase allele accounts for a significant fraction of the total, and this fact complicates molecular approaches to carrier detection and prenatal diagnosis.

The phenotype of *tyrosinase-positive or type 2 albinism* ranges from nearly normal to closely resembling type 1 albinism. Little or no melanin is present at birth, but pigment, particularly red-yellow pigment, may accumulate rapidly during childhood to produce straw-colored or light brown skin in whites. Progressive improvement in visual acuity and nystagmus occurs with aging. Blacks may have yellow-brown skin, dark-brown freckles in sun-exposed areas, and brown coloration of the irises. The defect in type 2 albinism has been mapped to chromosome 15 (the P gene) and may involve a tyrosine-specific transport protein. Deletions in this region also result in the Prader-Willi and Angelman syndromes, which include hypopigmentation.

The *Hermansky-Pudlak syndrome* is tyrosinase-positive albinism, with variable pigmentation, in association with a platelet storage pool deficiency and a hemorrhagic diathesis. Additional features include accumulation of a ceroid-like pigment in cells of the reticuloendothelial system, pulmonary fibrosis, and granulomatous colitis.

The *Cross-McKusick-Breen syndrome* consists of tyrosinase-positive albinism with ocular abnormalities, retardation, spasticity, and athetosis. Some patients have darkly pigmented hairs distributed among hair without color in the eyebrows and eyelashes.

Because of the absence of normal protection by adequate amounts of epidermal melanin, persons with albinism are predisposed to develop actinic keratoses and cutaneous carcinoma secondary to skin damage by ultraviolet light. Protective clothing and a broad-spectrum sunscreen preparation (see Chapter 652) should be worn during exposure to sunlight.

PARTIAL ALBINISM (PIEBALDISM). This congenital autosomal dominant disorder is characterized by sharply demarcated amelanotic patches that occur most frequently on the forehead, anterior scalp (producing a white forelock), ventral trunk, elbows, and knees. Islands of normal pigmentation may be present within the amelanotic areas. The plaques are a result of a permanent localized absence of melanocytes and melanosomes or reduced numbers of abnormally large melanocytes. Piebaldism results from mutations in the *KIT* proto-oncogene, which encodes the cellular transmembrane tyrosinase kinase for mast/stem cell growth factor. The pattern of depigmentation is thought to stem from defective melanocyte proliferation or migration from the neural crest during development. Piebaldism must be differentiated from vitiligo, which may be progressive and is not usually congenital; nevus depigmentosus; and Waardenburg syndrome.

WAARDENBURG SYNDROME. This congenital syndrome is characterized by lateral displacement of the medial canthi with dystopia canthorum (99%), broad nasal root (80%), heterochromic irises (25%), congenital deafness (20%), a white forelock (17%), and cutaneous hypopigmentation. A few patients have skin changes identical to piebaldism. Premature graying may develop in the 3rd decade. Waardenburg syndrome is inherited as an autosomal dominant trait with variable penetrance. It is due to defective migration and differentiation of neural crest cells.

CHÉDIAK-HIGASHI SYNDROME (see Chapter 130.3).

TUBEROUS SCLEROSIS (see Chapter 605.2). This disorder is a multisystemic disorder affecting primarily tissues derived from ectoderm but also involving organs of mesodermal and endodermal origin, particularly the eyes, kidneys, and heart. The classic clinical triad is skin lesions in association with epilepsy and mental retardation.

Etiology and Epidemiology. This is an autosomal dominant condition with variable expression. Mutations have been mapped to chromosome 9q34.3 (TSC1) and 16p13.3 (TSC2). The TSC2 product is tubern, which has sequence homology with a GTPase-activating protein and may have a role in regulating cellular growth by acting as a growth suppressor gene. TSC1 also is postulated to act as a growth suppressor. Approximately half of cases are due to new mutations. The most reliable early cutaneous sign is the white- or ash-leaf macule, which presents at birth or in early infancy, often years before other signs of the disease. Ash-leaf macules also appear in 2–3/1,000 normal newborns. They are sharply demarcated, pale, 0.5–3 cm lesions that often assume the shape of a mountain ash leaflet.

Clinical Manifestations. Single or multiple ash-leaf lesions are most often found on the trunk (Fig. 659–1*A*) but also occur on the face and limbs. Small, confetti-like hypopigmented macules are also present in some instances, reflecting inadequate melanization of the melanosomes in melanocytes. *Adenoma sebaceum* is the most commonly recognized cutaneous marker of tuberous sclerosis; the lesions appear on the face during middle to late childhood or adolescence in approximately 80% of patients. These red-brown or flesh-colored, smooth, glistening, telangiectatic 1–10 mm papules may extend from the nasolabial folds to the cheeks and chin (Fig. 659–1*B*). The presence of telangiectasias and the lack of comedones and pustules help to distinguish this eruption from acne vulgaris. *Adenoma sebaceum* is a misnomer because these growths are angiofibromas rather than tumors of the sebaceous glands. Similar fibromatous nodules may be scattered on the forehead, trunk, and limbs. Large, skin-colored, irregularly thickened plaques with an orange peel or cobblestone texture *(shagreen patch)* may occur in the lumbosacral area. At puberty, firm, flesh-colored *periungual fibromas* (Fig. 659–1*C*) emerge on the nail folds of some children; gingival fibromas may also occur, unassociated with the administration of anticonvulsant medications. Café-au-lait spots occur with increased frequency but are not as numerous as in neurofibromatosis. Mental deficiency occurs in 60–70%, nearly all of whom have epilepsy. Epilepsy is also present in approximately 70% of those patients without mental retardation. Epilepsy begins in infancy or early childhood and is often progressively more severe. Cardiac rhabdomyomas are present in approximately one half of infants but regress in most cases; mechanical obstruction is a potential complication. Rarely, the presenting sign of tuberous sclerosis is hematuria, caused by a renal angiomyolipoma, which occurs exclusively in this condition. Seventy-five per cent of patients with tuberous sclerosis die before the age of 25 yr, most commonly as a complication of epilepsy, of intercurrent infection, or occasionally of cardiac failure or pulmonary fibrosis.

HYPOMELANOSIS OF ITO (INCONTINENTIA PIGMENTI ACHROMIANS). This congenital skin disorder affects children of both sexes and is frequently associated with defects in several organ systems. There is no evidence for genetic transmission; chromosomal

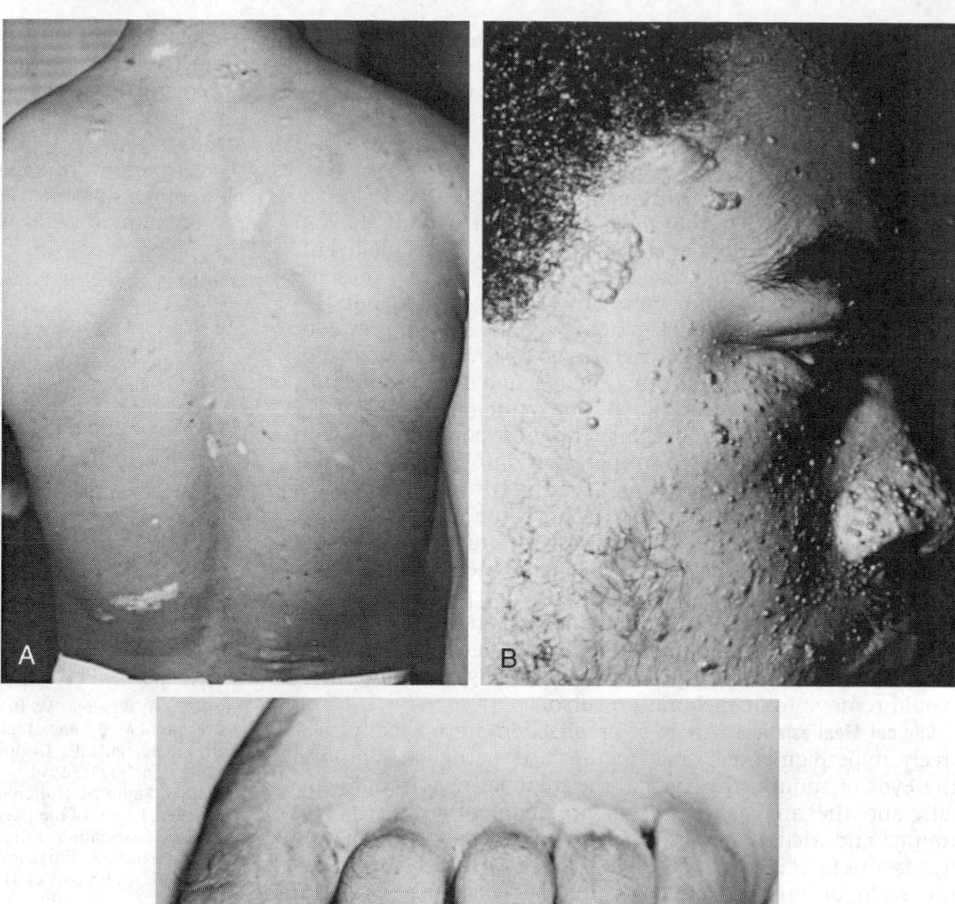

Figure 659–1 Tuberous sclerosis. *A,* Multiple white-leaf macules, small papular fibromas, and shagreen patch on lower back. *B,* Angiofibromas and angiofibromatous plaques on the temple. *C,* Periungual fibromas.

mosaicism and chromosomal translocations have been reported. Hypomelanosis of Ito currently is a descriptive rather than definitive diagnosis.

The skin lesions of hypomelanosis of Ito are generally present at birth but may be acquired within the first 2 yr of life. The lesions are similar to a negative image of that present in incontinentia pigmenti, consisting of bizarre, patterned, hypopigmented macules arranged over the body surface in sharply demarcated whorls, streaks, and patches that follow the lines of Blaschko (Fig. 659–2). The palms, soles, and mucous membranes are spared. The hypopigmentation remains unchanged throughout childhood but fades during adulthood. The degree of depigmentation varies from hypopigmented to achromic. Neither inflammatory nor vesicular lesions precede the development of the pigmentary changes as in incontinentia pigmenti. Histopathologic changes in the hypopigmented areas include fewer and smaller melanocytes and a decreased number of melanin granules in the basal cell layer than normal. Inflammatory cells and pigment incontinence are lacking.

The most commonly associated abnormalities involve the nervous system, including mental retardation (70%), seizures (40%), microcephaly (25%), and muscular hypotonia (15%). The musculoskeletal system is the second most frequently involved system, affected by scoliosis and thoracic and limb deformities. Minor ophthalmologic defects (strabismus, nystagmus) are present in 25% of patients, and 10% have cardiac defects. The differential diagnosis includes systematized nevus depigmentosus, which is a stable leukoderma not associated with systemic manifestations. Differentiation from incontinentia pigmenti, particularly the hypopigmented fourth stage,

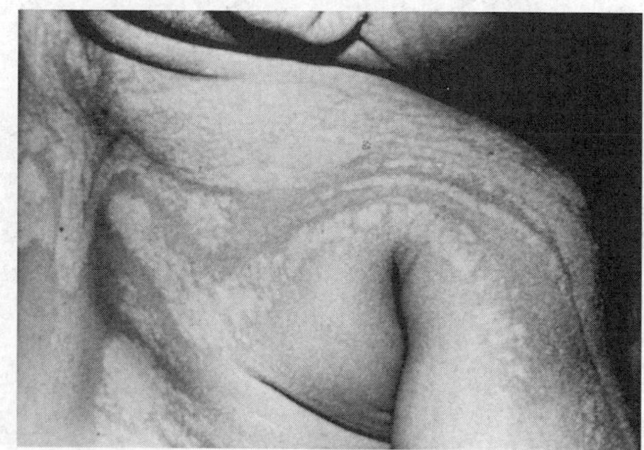

Figure 659–2 Marbled hypopigmented streaks of hypomelanosis of Ito (incontinentia pigmenti achromians).

is critical for genetic counseling because incontinentia pigmenti, unlike hypomelanosis of Ito, is inherited.

VITILIGO. Approximately half of cases of this acquired pigmentary defect present before age 20 yr. The lesions are sharply circumscribed, depigmented macules that vary in size and shape.

Epidemiology and Etiology. Although no clear-cut pattern of genetic transmission is established, 30–40% of patients have a positive family history. Associated abnormalities include uveitis and premature graying of hair. *Vogt-Koyanagi syndrome* presents with vitiligo, uveitis, and premature graying of hair but also involves the central nervous system. Vitiligo is more prevalent in patients with thyroid disease (hypo- or hyperthyroidism), adrenal insufficiency, pernicious anemia, and diabetes mellitus. The cause of vitiligo is unknown, but trauma appears to have a role in induction of the lesions. The most popular theory on the pathogenesis of vitiligo proposes an autoimmune mechanism, based on the finding that organ-specific autoantibodies to thyroid, gastroparietal, and adrenal tissue are found more frequently in the serum of patients with vitiligo than in the general population. Alternatively, a neurogenic theory purports that a compound that is released at peripheral nerve endings in the skin may inhibit melanogenesis, and a self-destruct theory suggests that melanocytes destroy themselves as a result of a defective protective mechanism that normally would remove toxic melanin precursors.

Clinical Manifestations. Areas of predilection are normally relatively hyperpigmented, such as the face, particularly around the eyes or mouth, the axillae, the inguinal region and genitals, and the areolas. Sites that are frequently subjected to trauma and friction are also likely to be affected, including the hands and feet, elbows, knees, and ankles (Fig. 659–3). When the scalp or brow is affected, the hair may lose pigment. The distribution of involvement is generally symmetric but occasionally is unilateral or dermatomal.

The course of vitiligo varies; some lesions may remit spontaneously while others are developing, but relentlessly progressive depigmentation may occur. Spontaneous repigmentation occurs in 10–20% of patients, most commonly in lesions that are in a sun-exposed distribution. Histopathologically, melanocytes are absent from involved sites and repopulate the epidermis from the hair follicle epithelium when repigmentation occurs. Although the diagnosis is usually made clinically, the disappearance of melanocytes can be confirmed by DOPA stains or electron microscopy of specimens obtained from depigmented skin.

Treatment. This usually involves administration of oral or topical psoralen compounds in conjunction with exposure to sunlight or an ultraviolet light source. Repigmentation may be partial or complete, but many months of therapy may be required. High-potency topical steroids are sometimes effective in repigmenting small areas of vitiligo or early lesions in areas not amenable to phototherapy (lips). Small lesions may be camouflaged by application of a specially prepared makeup (Covermark, Dermablend). Because of the absence of melanin, vitiliginous skin burns readily on sun exposure and should be protected at all times with an appropriate sunscreen.

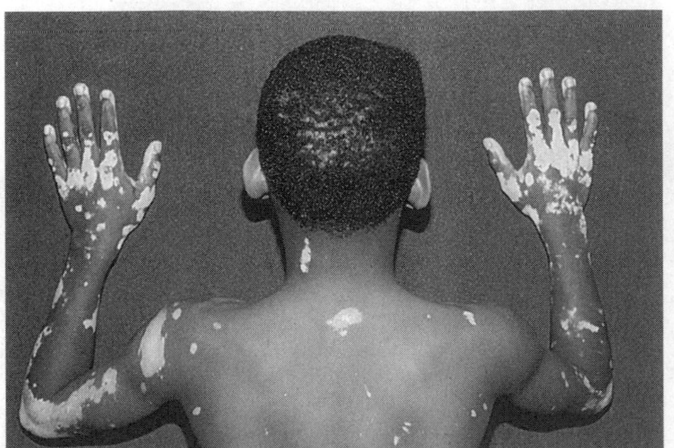

Figure 659–3 Multiple, sharply demarcated, symmetric, depigmented areas of vitiligo.

Bologna J, Pawelek JM: Biology of hypopigmentation. J Am Acad Dermatol 19:217, 1988.

Cui J, Arita Y, Bystryn JC: Cytolytic antibodies to melanocytes in vitiligo. J Invest Dermatol 100:812, 1993.

da-Silva EO: Waardenburg I syndrome: A clinical and genetic study of two large Brazilian kindreds, and literature review. Am J Med Genet 40:65, 1991.

Glover M, Brett EM, Atherton DJ: Hypomelanosis of Ito: Spectrum of the disease. J Pediatr 115:75, 1989.

Grimes PE: Vitiligo: An overview of therapeutic approaches. Dermatol Clin 11:325, 1993.

Janniger CK: Childhood vitiligo. Cutis 51:25, 1993.

Janniger CK, Schwartz RA: Tuberous sclerosis: Recent advances for the clinician. Cutis 51:167, 1993.

Kuster W, Happle R: Neurocutaneous disorders in children. Curr Opin Pediatr 5:436, 1993.

Mosher DB, Fitzpatrick TB: Piebaldism. Arch Dermatol 124:364, 1988.

Naughton GK, Reggiardo D, Bystryn J-C: Correlation between vitiligo antibodies and extent of depigmentation in vitiligo. J Am Acad Dermatol 15:978, 1986.

Nordlund JJ, Halder RM, Grimes P: Management of vitiligo. Dermatol Clin 11:27, 1993.

Northrup H, Wheless JW, Bertin TK, et al: Variability of expression in tuberous sclerosis. J Med Genet 30:41, 1993.

Pinto FJ, Bolognia JL: Disorders of hypopigmentation in children. Pediatr Clin North Am 38:991, 1991.

Roach ES, Smith M, Huttenlocher P, et al: Diagnostic criteria: Tuberous sclerosis complex. Report of the Diagnostic Criteria Committee of the National Tuberous Sclerosis Association. J Child Neurol 7:221, 1992.

Ruiz-Maldonado R, Toussaint S, Tamayo L, et al: Hypomelanosis of Ito: Diagnostic criteria and report of 41 cases. Pediatr Dermatol 9:1, 1992.

Schwartz MF Jr, Esterly NB, Fretzin DF, et al: Hypomelanosis of Ito (incontinentia pigmenti achromians): A neurocutaneous syndrome. J Pediatr 90:236, 1977.

Spritz RA: Molecular genetics of oculocutaneous albinism. Semin Dermatol 12:167, 1993.

Thibaut H, Parizel PM, Van Goethem J, et al: Tuberous sclerosis: CT and MRI characteristics. Eur J Radiol 16:176, 1993.

Vanderhooft S, Francis J, Pagon R: Prevalence of hypopigmented macules in a healthy population. J Pediatr 129:355, 1996.

Winship I, Young K, Martell P, et al: Piebaldism: An autonomous autosomal dominant entity. Clin Genet 39:330, 1991.

CHAPTER 660
Vesiculobullous Disorders

Many diseases are characterized by vesiculobullous lesions; they vary considerably in cause, age of occurrence, and pattern. Some of them (varicella) are discussed in other chapters; some are described in other chapters of this part because the vesiculobullous lesions represent only a transient stage of the disease (incontinentia pigmenti) or are seen only on occasion (mastocytosis). The morphology of the blister often provides a visual clue to the location of the lesion within the skin. Blisters localized to the epidermal layers are thin walled, relatively flaccid, and easily ruptured. Subepidermal blisters are tense, thick walled, and more durable. Biopsies of blisters can be diagnostic because the level of cleavage within the skin and associated findings such as the nature of the inflammatory infiltrate are characteristic for a particular disorder. Other diagnostic procedures such as immunofluorescence and electron microscopy can often help to distinguish vesiculobullous disorders that have nearly identical histopathologic findings (Table 660–1).

TABLE 660–1 Sites of Blister Formation and Diagnostic Studies for the Vesiculobullous Disorders

Disorder	Blister Cleavage Site	Cutaneous Diagnostic Studies
Acrodermatitis enteropathica	IE	—
Bullous impetigo	GL	Smear, culture
Bullous pemphigoid	SE (junctional)	Direct and indirect immunofluorescence studies
Candidosis	SC	KOH preparation, culture
Chronic bullous dermatosis of childhood	SE	Direct immunofluorescence studies
Dermatitis herpetiformis	SE	Direct immunofluorescence studies
Dermatophytosis	IE	KOH preparation, culture
Dyshidrotic eczema	IE	—
EB simplex	IE	Electron microscopy; immunofluorescence mapping
Hands and feet	IE	Electron microscopy: immunofluorescence mapping
Junctional EB (letalis)	SE (junctional)	Electron microscopy; immunofluorescence mapping
Recessive dystrophic EB	SE	Electron microscopy; immunofluorescence mapping
Dominant dystrophic EB	SE	Electron microscopy; immunofluorescence mapping
Epidermolytic hyperkeratosis	IE	—
Erythema multiforme	SE	—
Erythema toxicum	SC, IE	Smear for eosinophils
Incontinentia pigmenti	IE	Smear for eosinophils
Insect bites	IE	—
Mastocytosis	SE	Smear for mast cells
Miliaria crystallina	IC	—
Pachyonychia congenita	IC	—
Pemphigus foliaceus	GL	Direct and indirect immunofluorescence studies Tzanck smear
Pemphigus vulgaris	SB	Direct and indirect immunofluorescence studies Tzanck smear
Pseudomonas infection	IE, SE	Smear, culture
Scabies	IE	Scraping
Staphylococcal scalded skin syndrome	GL	Frozen section biopsy
Syphilis	SE	Dark-field preparation
Toxic epidermal necrolysis (Lyell)	SE	Frozen section biopsy
Transient neonatal pustular melanosis	SC, IE	Smear for cells
Viral blisters	IE	Tzanck smear for herpesvirus infections

GL = granular layer; IC = intracorneal; IE = intraepidermal; SB = suprabasal; SC = subcorneal; SE = subepidermal; EB = epidermolysis bullosa; KOH = potassium hydroxide.

ERYTHEMA MULTIFORME. Erythema multiforme (EM) has numerous morphologic manifestations on the skin, varying from erythematous macules, papules, vesicles, bullae, or urticaria-appearing plaques to patches of confluent erythema. The eruption appears most commonly in patients between the ages of 10 and 30 yr and usually is asymptomatic, although a burning sensation or pruritus may be present. The *diagnosis* of EM is established by finding the classic lesion: doughnut-shaped, target-like (iris, or bull's eye) papules with an erythematous outer border, an inner pale ring, and a dusky purple to necrotic center.

EM is characterized by an abrupt, symmetric cutaneous eruption, most commonly on the extensor upper extremities; lesions are relatively sparse on the face, trunk, and legs. The eruption often appears initially as red macules or urticarial plaques that expand centrifugally to form lesions up to 2 cm in diameter with a dusky to necrotic center. Lesions of a particular episode typically appear within 72 hr and remain fixed in place. Oral lesions may occur, but other mucosal surfaces are spared. Approximately 25% of cases of EM appear to be confined to the oral mucosa, with a predilection for the vermilion border of the lips and the buccal mucosa, generally sparing the gingivae. Prodromal symptoms generally are absent. Lesions typically resolve without sequelae in about 2 wk, and progression to Stevens-Johnson syndrome does not occur.

Although EM may present initially with urticarial lesions, unlike urticaria, a given lesion of EM does not fade within 24 hr. Serum sickness–like reaction (SSLR) to cefaclor also has been described as presenting with EM-like lesions. Although the lesions may develop a dusky to purple center, in most cases the eruption of cefaclor-induced SSLR is pruritic, transient, and migratory and is probably urticarial rather than true EM.

The *differential diagnosis* of EM also includes bullous pemphigoid, pemphigus, linear IgA dermatosis, graft versus host disease, bullous drug eruption, urticaria, viral infections such as herpes simplex, Reiter disease, Kawasaki disease, Behçet's disease, allergic vasculitis, erythema annulare centrifugum, and periarteritis nodosa. EM that primarily involves the oral mucosa may be confused with a handful of other conditions, including bullous pemphigoid, pemphigus vulgaris, vesiculobullous or erosive lichen planus, Behçet's syndrome, recurrent aphthous stomatitis, and primary herpetic gingivostomatitis.

Among the numerous factors implicated in the *etiology* of EM, infection with herpes simplex virus (HSV) is the most common. HSV labialis and, less commonly, HSV genitalis have been implicated in 60% of episodes of EM and are believed to trigger nearly all episodes of recurrent EM, frequently in association with sun exposure, despite the presence of robust HSV-specific immunity. HSV antigens and DNA are present in skin lesions of EM but are absent in nonlesional skin. Presence of the human leukocyte antigens B62, B35, and DR53 is associated with an increased risk of HSV-induced EM, particularly the recurrent form. Most patients experience a single self-limited episode of EM. Lesions of HSV-induced recurrent EM typically develop 10–14 days after onset of recurrent HSV eruptions, have a similar appearance from episode to episode, but may vary in frequency and duration in a given patient. Not all episodes of recurrent HSV evolve into EM in susceptible patients.

The *pathogenesis* of EM is unclear, but it may be a host-specific cell-mediated immune response to an antigenic stimulus, resulting in damage to keratinocytes. Cytokines released by activated mononuclear cells and keratinocytes may contribute to epidermal cell death and constitutional symptoms.

Microscopic findings of EM, as with the gross appearance of the cutaneous eruption, are variable but are significant *diagnostically.* Early lesions typically show slight intercellular edema, rare dyskeratotic keratinocytes, and basal vacuolation in the epidermis and a perivascular lymphohistiocytic infiltrate with edema in the upper dermis. More mature lesions show an accentuation of these characteristics and the development of lymphocytic exocytosis and an intense, perivascular and interstitial mononuclear infiltrate, lacking in significant numbers of eosinophils or neutrophils, in the upper third of the dermis. The entire epidermis becomes necrotic in severe cases.

Treatment of EM is supportive. Topical emollients and systemic antihistamines and nonsteroidal anti-inflammatory agents do not alter the course of the disease but may provide symptomatic relief. No controlled, prospective studies support the use of corticosteroids in the management of EM. Rather, glucocorticoid therapy may be permissive of HSV replication and make EM episodes more frequent or continuous. Prophylactic oral acyclovir given for 6 mo may be effective in controlling recurrent episodes of HSV-associated EM. On discontinuation of acyclovir, both HSV and EM may recur, although episodes may be less frequent and more mild.

STEVENS-JOHNSON SYNDROME. Cutaneous lesions in Stevens-Johnson syndrome generally consist initially of erythematous macules that rapidly and variably develop central necrosis to form vesicles, bullae, and areas of denudation on the face, trunk, and extremities. The skin lesions typically are more widespread than in EM and are accompanied by involvement of two or more mucosal surfaces, namely the eyes, oral cavity, upper airway or esophagus, gastrointestinal tract, or anogenital mucosa. A burning sensation, edema, and erythema of the lips and buccal mucosa are often the presenting signs, followed by development of bullae, ulceration, and hemorrhagic crusting. Lesions may be preceded by a flulike upper respiratory illness. Pain from mucosal ulceration is often severe, but skin tenderness is minimal to absent, in contrast to toxic epidermal necrolysis. Corneal ulceration, anterior uveitis, panophthalmitis, bronchitis, pneumonitis, myocarditis, hepatitis, enterocolitis, polyarthritis, hematuria, and acute tubular necrosis leading to renal failure may occur. Disseminated cutaneous bullae and erosions may result in significant blood loss, increased insensible fluid loss, and a high risk of bacterial superinfection and sepsis. New lesions occur in crops, and complete healing may take 4–6 wk; ocular scarring and visual impairment and strictures of the esophagus, bronchi, vagina, urethra, or anus may remain. Nonspecific laboratory abnormalities in Stevens-Johnson syndrome include leukocytosis, elevated erythrocyte sedimentation rate and liver transaminase levels, and decreased serum albumin values. Toxic epidermal necrolysis is the most severe disorder in the clinical spectrum of the disease, involving considerable constitutional toxicity and extensive necrolysis of the mucous membranes and more than 30% of the body surface area.

Mycoplasma pneumoniae is the most convincingly demonstrated infectious cause of Stevens-Johnson syndrome; the organism also has been detected in lesional skin. Drugs, particularly sulfonamides, nonsteroidal anti-inflammatory agents (butazones, pyrazolones, ibuprofen, piroxicam, and salicylates), and anticonvulsants (phenytoin), are the agents most commonly precipitating Stevens-Johnson syndrome and toxic epidermal necrolysis (Table 660–2).

Treatment. Management of Stevens-Johnson syndrome is supportive and symptomatic. Ophthalmologic consultation is mandatory because ocular sequelae such as corneal scarring can lead to vision loss. Oral lesions should be managed with mouthwashes and glycerin swabs. Vaginal lesions should be observed closely and treated to prevent vaginal stricture or fusion. Topical anesthetics (diphenhydramine, dyclonine, and viscous lidocaine) may provide relief from pain, particularly when applied before eating. Denuded skin lesions can be cleansed with saline or Burow solution compresses. Antibiotic therapy is appropriate for secondary bacterial infection. Treatment may require admission to an intensive care unit; intravenous fluids; nutritional support; sheepskin or air-fluid bedding; daily saline or Burow solution compresses; paraffin gauze or hydrogel dressing of denuded areas; saline compresses on the eyelids, lips, or nose; analgesics; and urinary catheterization (when needed). A daily examination for infection and ocular lesions, which constitute the major cause of long-term morbidity, is essential. Systemic antibiotics are indicated for urinary or cutaneous infections and for suspected bacteremia because infection is the leading cause of death. Prophylactic systemic antibiotics, however, are not necessary. Although corticosteroids are sometimes advocated in early, severe cases of Stevens-Johnson syndrome, no prospective double-blind studies evaluating their efficacy have been reported. Most authorities discourage their use because of reports of increased morbidity and mortality (sepsis) with their administration.

TABLE 660–2 Potential Causes of Erythema Multiforme, Stevens-Johnson Syndrome, and Toxic Epidermal Necrolysis

Infectious Agents	Anticonvulsants
Herpes simplex 1, 2*	Phenytoin
Mycoplasma pneumoniae	Phenobarbital
Mycobacterium tuberculosis	Carbamazepine
Group A streptococci	Lamotrigine
Hepatitis B	Valproic acid
Epstein-Barr virus	**Other**
Francisella tularensis	Radiation therapy
Yersinia	Captopril
Enteroviruses	Etoposide
Histoplasma	Nonsteroidal anti-inflammatory agents
Coccidioides	Aspirin
Neoplasia	Sunlight
Leukemia	Pregnancy
Lymphoma	Allopurinol
Antibiotics	
Penicillin	
Sulfonamides	
Isoniazid	
Tetracyclines	
Cephalosporins	
Quinolones	

**Recurrent erythema multiforme.*
Drug reactions occur 1–3 wk after exposure.

TOXIC EPIDERMAL NECROLYSIS (LYELL SYNDROME)

Epidemiology and Etiology. The pathogenesis of toxic epidermal necrolysis is not proved but appears to involve a hypersensitivity phenomenon that results in damage primarily to the basal cell layer of the epidermis. This condition is triggered by many of the same factors that are responsible for Stevens-Johnson syndrome, principally drugs such as the sulfonamides, amoxicillin, phenobarbital, hydantoin, butazones, and allopurinol. Toxic epidermal necrolysis is defined by (1) widespread blister formation and morbilliform or confluent erythema, associated with skin tenderness; (2) absence of target lesions; (3) sudden onset and generalization within 24–48 hr; and (4) histologic findings of full-thickness epidermal necrosis and a minimal to absent dermal infiltrate. These criteria categorize toxic epidermal necrolysis as a separate entity from EM; some authorities, however, contend that toxic epidermal necrolysis represents the most severe form of the spectrum of EM. This condition is exceedingly rare in infants younger than 6 mo; only three such cases have been documented.

Clinical Manifestations. The prodrome consists of fever, malaise, localized skin tenderness, and diffuse erythema. Inflammation of the eyelids, conjunctivae, mouth, and genitals may precede skin lesions. Flaccid bullae may develop, although this is not a prominent feature. Characteristically, full-thickness epidermis is lost in large sheets. *Nikolsky sign* (denudation of the skin with gentle tangential pressure) is present but only in the areas of erythema. Conjunctivitis and oral lesions are usually not as severe as in Stevens-Johnson syndrome. Healing takes place over 14 or more days. Scarring, particularly of the eyes, may result in corneal opacity. The course may be relentlessly progressive, complicated by severe dehydration, electrolyte imbalance, shock, and secondary localized infection and septicemia. Loss of nails and hair may also occur. The differential diagnosis includes staphylococcal scalded skin syndrome, in which the blister cleavage plane is intraepidermal; graft versus host disease; chemical burns; drug eruptions; and pemphigus.

Anticonvulsant hypersensitivity syndrome is a multisystem reaction that appears approximately 4 wk to 3 mo after starting phenytoin, carbamazepine, phenobarbitone, or primidone. The mucocutaneous eruption may be identical to EM, Stevens-Johnson syndrome, or toxic epidermal necrolysis, but the reaction typically also includes lymphadenopathy, as well as fever, hepatitis, eosinophilia, and leukocytosis.

Treatment. Appreciation of the specific etiologic factor is crucial; particularly when the disorder is drug induced, its administration must be discontinued. Management is similar to that for severe burns and may be best accomplished in a burn unit. It may include strict reverse isolation, meticulous fluid and electrolyte therapy, use of an air-fluid bed, and daily cultures. Systemic antibiotic therapy is indicated when secondary infection is evident or suspected. Skin care consists of cleansing with isotonic saline or Burow solution and applications of mupirocin ointment. Biologic or hydrogel dressings alleviate pain and reduce fluid loss. Narcotics are often required for pain relief. Mouth and eye care may be necessary, such as for EM major. Early high-dose systemic corticosteroids are not of proven benefit.

EPIDERMOLYSIS BULLOSA. Diseases categorized under this general term are a heterogeneous group of congenital, hereditary blistering disorders. They differ in severity and prognosis, clinical and histologic features, and inheritance patterns (Table 660–3) but are all characterized by induction of blisters by trauma and exacerbation of blistering in warm weather. The disorders can be categorized under three major headings: epidermolysis bullosa simplex, junctional epidermolysis bullosa, and dystrophic epidermolysis bullosa.

Epidermolysis Bullosa Simplex. This is a nonscarring, autosomal dominant disorder. The defect in all types of epidermolysis bullosa simplex is in the central α-helical coil of keratin 5 or 14, which makes up intermediate filaments of the basal keratinocytes. Keratin 5 and 14 genes are located on chromosomes 17q and 12q, respectively. The intraepidermal bullae result from cytolysis of the basal cells.

Blisters are usually present at birth or during the neonatal period. Sites of predilection are the hands, feet, elbows, knees, legs, and scalp. Intraoral lesions are minimal, nails rarely become dystrophic and usually regrow even when they are shed, and dentition is normal. Bullae heal with minimal to no scar or milia formation. Secondary infection is the primary complication. The propensity to blister decreases with age, and the long-term prognosis is good. Blisters should be drained by puncturing, but the blister top should be left intact to protect the underlying skin. Erosions may be covered with mupirocin if there is evidence of infection and with a semipermeable dressing. Genetic counseling should be offered to families of affected children.

Localized *epidermolysis bullosa simplex of hands and feet* (Weber-Cockayne type) often presents when a child begins to walk; onset may be delayed, however, until puberty or early adulthood when heavy shoes are worn or the feet are subjected to increased trauma. Bullae are usually restricted to the hands and feet; rarely, they occur elsewhere such as the dorsal aspect of the arms and the shins. The disorder ranges from mildly incapacitating to crippling at times of severe exacerbations. *Generalized epidermolysis bullosa simplex* (Koebner type) is characterized at birth or during early infancy by blisters on the occiput, back, and legs and in childhood by blisters on the hands, feet, and other friction points. The *herpetiformis (Dowling-Meara) variant of epidermolysis bullosa simplex* is characterized by grouped blisters. During infancy, blistering may be severe and extensive, may involve mucous membranes, and may result in shedding of nails, formation of milia, and mild pigmentary changes, without scarring. After the first few months of life, warm temperatures do not appear to exacerbate blistering. Hyperkeratosis and hyperhidrosis of the palms and soles may develop, but generally, the condition improves with age.

Junctional Epidermolysis Bullosa. *Epidermolysis bullosa letalis* (Herlitz type) is an autosomal recessive condition that is life threatening; serious morbidity and disfigurement can be predicted from the complications. An afflicted infant is usually blistered at birth or develops lesions during the neonatal period, particularly on the perioral area, scalp, legs, diaper area, and thorax. In contrast to other variants of epidermolysis bullosa, the hands and feet tend to be relatively spared, with the exception of the distal digits and the nail plates; these are dystrophic or permanently lost. Mucous membrane involvement may be severe, and ulceration of the respiratory, gastrointestinal, and genitourinary epithelium has been documented in many affected children, although less frequently than in severe, recessive dystrophic epidermolysis bullosa. Healing is delayed, and vegetating granulomas, particularly in the generalized (Herlitz) variant, may persist for a long time. Large, moist, erosive plaques may provide a portal of entry for bacteria, and septicemia is a frequent cause of death. Mild atrophy may be seen in areas of recurrent blistering. Defective dentition with early loss of teeth as a result of rampant caries is characteristic. Growth retardation and recalcitrant anemia are almost invariable. In addition to infection, cachexia and circulatory failure are common causes of death. Most patients die within the first 3 yr of life.

A subepidermal blister is found on light microscopic examination, and electron microscopy demonstrates a cleavage plane in the lamina lucida, between the plasma membranes of the

TABLE 660–3 Characteristics of Epidermolysis Bullosa

Type	Predominant Inheritance	Level of Blister Formation	Features
Simplex (epidermolytic)	Autosomal dominant	Superficial; basal cell layer; above hemidesmosomes	Usually congenital onset; hands and feet involved; minimal mucosal lesions; no scarring; defects in keratins 5 or 14 of basal keratinocytes
Junctional (letalis)	Autosomal recessive	Lamina lucida, between bullous pemphigoid antigen and laminin; absent or rare hemidesmosomes	Congenital; localized or progressive; heals with scarring; pyloric atresia; mucosal lesions; dysplastic teeth; loss of nails; defects in basement membrane–associated proteins, e.g., laminin 5, bullous pemphigoid antigen 2, α6β4 integrin
Recessive dystrophic (dermolytic)	Autosomal recessive	Deep in dermis below the lamina densa; excessive production of abnormal dermal collagenase; absent anchoring fibrils	Congenital; mitten scarring of the hands and feet; marked deformities; mucosal lesions produce esophageal stricture or gastrointestinal perforation; varied clinical course; risk for aggressive squamous cell cancer of the skin, tongue, esophagus; defects in type VII collagen
Dominant dystrophic (dermolytic)	Autosomal dominant	Deep in dermis below the lamina densa, below type IV collagen layer; sparse anchoring fibrils	Congenital; hyperkeratotic lesions; variable severity; risk for squamous cell cancer; defects in type VII collagen

basal cells and the basal lamina. Absent or greatly reduced anchoring filaments are seen on electron micrographs, along with diminished or absent laminin 5. Junctional epidermolysis bullosa is due to mutations in proteins in the basement membrane zone involved in keratinocyte–lamina densa adherence, particularly laminin 5, a glycoprotein associated with anchoring filaments beneath the hemidesmosomes. Defects have also been described in other hemidesmosomal components, such as bullous pemphigoid antigen 2 and α6β4 integrin. Absence of laminin in amniocytes has been shown to be a prenatal marker for the Herlitz type of junctional epidermolysis bullosa.

Generalized atrophic benign epidermolysis bullosa, a milder autosomal recessive variant, presents with blistering at birth, is also nonscarring, and is characterized by identical histologic changes as the Herlitz type. It may be impossible to distinguish from the Herlitz variety for up to 2–3 yr. Pattern baldness with significant scalp atrophy is a prominent feature. The course is compatible with normal growth and life span.

Treatment for junctional epidermolysis bullosa is supportive, including genetic counseling for the family. The diet should provide adequate calories and supplemental iron. Infections should be treated promptly with antibiotics. Transfusions of packed red blood cells may be required if the patient does not respond to a combination of iron and erythropoietin therapy.

Dystrophic Epidermolysis Bullosa. *Dominant dystrophic epidermolysis bullosa* occurs sporadically in some cases, although an autosomal dominant mode of transmission has been documented in many families. Blisters may be present at birth and are often limited to the hands, feet, and sacrum. The lesions heal promptly, with the formation of soft, wrinkled scars; milia; and alterations in pigmentation. The general health is unimpaired; in many cases, the blistering process is rather mild, causing little restriction of activity and unimpaired growth and development. Mucous membrane involvement tends to be minimal, but nail loss is common.

The *Cockayne-Touraine variant* of dominant dystrophic epidermolysis bullosa presents during infancy or early childhood with blisters predominantly on the extremities, although widespread blistering may occur. The *albopapuloid Pasini form* presents during adolescence with blistering that may be widespread but occurs predominantly on the hands, feet, elbows, and knees and with flesh-colored papules called albopapuloid lesions on the trunk. Transient bullous dermolysis of the newborn affects a rare subset of patients with self-limited dystrophic disease; inheritance in most cases is autosomal dominant. Blistering at birth tends to be generalized but ceases within the first 1–2 yr. Resolution of clinical blistering and the immunohistochemically altered distribution of type VII collagen occur coincidentally. The blister is subepidermal in all variants, with separation beneath the basement membrane. On electron microscopy, anchoring fibrils, a major component of which is type VII collagen, are abnormal and decreased in number over the entire skin in the Pasini type but only in areas of blister predilection in the Cockayne-Touraine variant. The type VII collagen gene, located on the short arm of chromosome 3, is the major candidate gene for dystrophic epidermolysis bullosa.

Recessive dystrophic epidermolysis bullosa is probably the most incapacitating form of epidermolysis bullosa, although the clinical spectrum is wide. Some patients have blisters, scarring, and milia formation primarily on the hands, feet, elbows, and knees. Others at birth have extensive erosions and blister formation that seriously impede their care and feeding. Mucous membrane lesions are common and may cause severe nutritional deprivation, even in older children, whose growth may be retarded. During childhood, esophageal erosions and strictures, scarring of the buccal mucosa, flexion contractures of joints secondary to scarring of the integument, development of cutaneous carcinomas, and the development of digital fusion (Fig. 660–1) may significantly limit the quality of life.

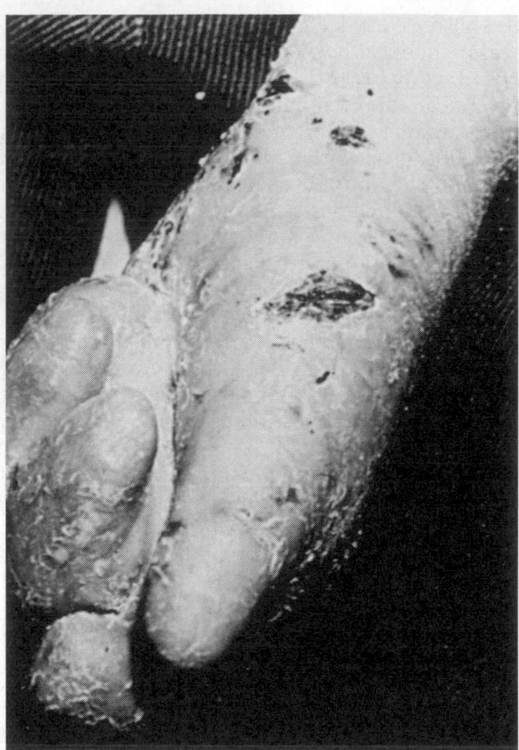

Figure 660–1 Mitten-hand deformity of recessive dystrophic epidermolysis bullosa.

The subepidermal bullae are located beneath the basement membrane, where anchoring fibrils are absent.

Although the skin becomes less sensitive to trauma with aging, the progressive and permanent deformities complicate management, and the overall prognosis is poor. Foods that traumatize the buccal or esophageal mucosa should be avoided. If esophageal scarring develops, a semiliquid diet and esophageal dilatations may be required. Alternatively, stricture excision or colonic interposition may be needed to relieve esophageal obstruction. In infants, severe oropharyngeal involvement may necessitate the use of special feeding devices such as a button gastrostomy tube. Continuous iron therapy for anemia; intermittent antibiotic therapy for secondary infections, which are a common cause of death; and periodic plastic procedures for release of digits may reduce morbidity.

PEMPHIGUS. Pemphigus occurs during childhood as pemphigus vulgaris or pemphigus foliaceus.

Pemphigus Vulgaris. This usually first appears as painful oral ulcers, which may be the only evidence of the disease for weeks or months. Subsequently, large, flaccid bullae emerge on nonerythematous skin, most commonly on the face, trunk, pressure points, groin, and axillae. Nikolsky sign is present. The lesions rupture and enlarge peripherally, producing painful raw, denuded areas that have little tendency to heal. When healing occurs, it is without scarring, but hyperpigmentation is common. Malodorous verrucous and granulomatous lesions may develop at sites of ruptured bullae, particularly in the skinfolds; as this becomes more pronounced, the condition may be more properly referred to as pemphigus vegetans.

Biopsy is best performed of a fresh small blister, which reveals a suprabasal (intraepidermal) blister containing loose, acantholytic epidermal cells that have lost their intercellular bridges and thus their contact with one another. IgG antibody to epidermal intercellular substance produces a characteristic pattern on direct immunofluorescence preparations of both involved and uninvolved skin of essentially all patients (see Table 651–1). Serum IgG antibody titers to the epidermal intercellular substance correlate with the clinical course of many patients; thus, serial determinations may have predictive value. Pemphigus antibodies are pathogenic. The antigen recognized by pemphigus vulgaris antibodies is a 130-kd glycoprotein known as desmoglein III that is complexed with plakoglobin, a plaque protein of desmosomes. The desmogleins are a subfamily of the cadherin cell adhesion molecules.

Neonatal pemphigus vulgaris develops in utero as a result of placental transfer of maternal antibodies from women who have active pemphigus vulgaris, although it may occur when the mother is in remission. High antepartum maternal titers of pemphigus vulgaris antibodies and increased maternal disease activity correlate with a poor fetal outcome, including demise.

The *differential diagnosis* includes EM, bullous pemphigoid, Stevens-Johnson syndrome, and toxic epidermal necrolysis. Because the course may rapidly lead to debility, malnutrition, and death, prompt diagnosis is essential. The disease is best treated initially with high-dose systemic corticosteroid therapy. Azathioprine, cyclophosphamide, methotrexate, and gold therapy all have been useful in maintenance regimens.

Pemphigus Foliaceus. This is extremely rare. It is characterized by intraepidermal blistering; the site of cleavage, however, is high in the epidermis rather than suprabasal as in pemphigus vulgaris. The superficial blisters rupture quickly, leaving erosions surrounded by erythema that heal with crusting and scaling. Nikolsky sign is present. Focal lesions are usually localized to the scalp, face, neck, and upper trunk. Mucous membrane lesions are minimal or absent. Pruritus, pain, and a burning sensation are frequent complaints. When generalized, the eruption may resemble exfoliative dermatitis or any of the chronic blistering disorders, but localized erythematous plaques simulate seborrheic dermatitis, psoriasis, impetigo, eczema, or lupus erythematosus. The clinical course varies but is generally more benign than that of pemphigus vulgaris. *Fogo selvagem*, which is edemic in certain areas of Brazil, is identical clinically, histopathologically, and immunologically to pemphigus foliaceus.

An intraepidermal acantholytic bulla high in the epidermis is diagnostic; it is imperative, however, to select an early lesion for biopsy. Tissue-bound and circulating intercellular epidermal antibodies bind to a 50-kd portion of the 160-kd desmosomal glycoprotein, desmoglein I (see Table 651–1). Long-term remission is usual after suppression of the disease by systemic corticosteroid therapy. Dapsone or a topical corticosteroid preparation is occasionally sufficient.

BULLOUS PEMPHIGOID. Bullous pemphigoid rarely occurs in children but must be considered in the differential diagnosis of any chronic blistering disorder.

Clinical Manifestations. The blisters typically arise in crops on a normal, erythematous, eczematous, or urticarial base. Bullae appear predominantly on the flexural aspects of the extremities, in the axillae, and on the groin and central abdomen. Infants have involvement of the palms, soles, and face more frequently than older children. Individual lesions vary greatly in size, are tense, and are filled with serous fluid that may become hemorrhagic or turbid. Oral lesions occur less frequently (50%) and are less severe than in pemphigus vulgaris but are found more commonly in children than in adults with bullous pemphigoid. Pruritus, a burning sensation, and subcutaneous edema may accompany the eruption, but constitutional symptoms are not prominent.

Diagnosis and Differential Diagnoses. Biopsy material should be taken from an early bulla arising on an erythematous base. A subepidermal bulla and a dermal inflammatory infiltrate, predominantly of eosinophils, can be identified histopathologically. In sections of a blister or perilesional skin, a band of immunoglobulin (usually IgG) and C3 can be demonstrated in the basement membrane zone by direct immunofluorescence (see Table 651–1). Indirect immunofluorescence studies of serum have positive results in approximately 70% of cases for IgG antibodies to the basement membrane zone; the titers, however, do not correlate well with the clinical course. The differential diagnosis includes bullous erythema multiforme, pemphigus, linear IgA dermatosis, bullous drug eruption, dermatitis herpetiformis, herpes simplex infection, and bullous impetigo, which can be differentiated by histologic examination, immunofluorescence studies, and cultures. The large, tense bullae of bullous pemphigoid can generally be distinguished from the smaller, flaccid bullae of pemphigus vulgaris. The major targets for bullous pemphigoid autoantibodies are proteins of 230 and 180 kd. The 230-kd protein is part of the hemidesmosome, whereas the 180-kd antigen localizes to both the hemidesmosome and the upper lamina lucida and is a transmembrane collagenous protein.

Treatment. Bullous pemphigoid can be successfully suppressed with systemic corticosteroid therapy alone or in combination with azathioprine, sulfapyridine, or dapsone. Ultimately, the condition usually remits permanently.

DERMATITIS HERPETIFORMIS. This is seen most commonly in children 2–7 yr of age. It is characterized by symmetric, grouped, small, tense, erythematous, stinging, intensely pruritic papules and vesicles. The eruption is pleomorphic, including erythematous, urticarial, papular, vesicular, and bullous lesions. Sites of predilection are the knees, elbows, shoulders, buttocks, and scalp; mucous membranes are usually spared. Hemorrhagic lesions may develop on the palms and soles. When pruritus is severe, excoriations may be the only visible sign.

Etiology. This is unknown; however, an association with gluten-sensitive enteropathy is found in 75–90% of patients. Aggressive gluten challenge generally unmasks the condition in the remainder of patients with dermatitis herpetiformis (see Chapter 340.8). Subepidermal blisters composed predominantly of neutrophils are found in dermal papillae on skin biopsy, and IgA and C3 can be detected in the dermal papillary tips of normal and perilesional skin in the sublamina densa region of the dermoepidermal junction by immunofluorescence studies. The frequent finding of immune complexes and autoimmune antibodies in serum and the association with histocompatibility antigen HLA-B8 in approximately 85% of patients suggest an immune mechanism. An antibody to smooth muscle endomysium is found in 70% of patients with dermatitis herpetiformis–associated gluten-sensitive enteropathy. Antibody titers correlate with the severity of intestinal disease; they decline rapidly on institution of a gluten-free diet. Enteric infection with adenovirus type 12 or 40 may increase the risk of developing gluten-sensitive enteropathy and dermatitis herpetiformis in genetically susceptible individuals.

Treatment. Dermatitis herpetiformis may mimic other chronic blistering diseases and may also resemble scabies, papular urticaria, insect bites, contact dermatitis, and papular eczema. The most effective treatment is oral administration of sulfapyridine or dapsone. These drugs provide immediate relief from the intense pruritus but must be used with caution because of possible serious side effects. Local antipruritic measures may also be useful. Jejunal biopsy is indicated to diagnose gluten-sensitive enteropathy because cutaneous manifestations may precede malabsorption. Enteropathy responds to a gluten-free diet more rapidly than skin lesions.

LINEAR IgA DERMATOSIS (CHRONIC BULLOUS DERMATOSIS OF CHILDHOOD). This rare dermatosis is most common in the 1st decade of life, with a peak incidence during the preschool years. The eruption consists of many large, tense bullae filled with clear or hemorrhagic fluid that develop on a normal or erythematous, urticarial base. Areas of predilection are the genitals and buttocks, the perioral region, and the scalp. Sausage-shaped bullae may be arranged in an annular or rosette-like fashion around a central crust (Fig. 660–2). Erythematous plaques with gyrate margins bordered by intact bullae may develop over larger areas. Pruritus may be absent or very intense, and systemic

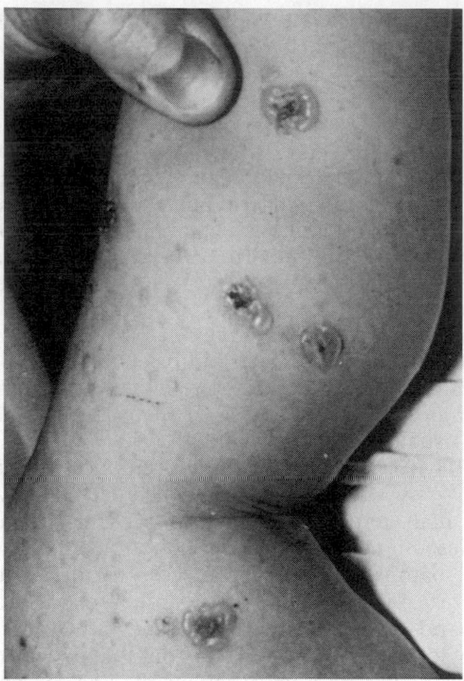

Figure 660–2 Rosette-like blisters around a central crust typical of linear IgA dermatosis (chronic bullous dermatosis of childhood).

signs or symptoms are absent. Gluten-sensitive enteropathy is not present, but there is a strong association with HLA-B8.

Etiology. The cause of the eruption is unknown. Histologic examination shows a subepidermal bulla infiltrated with a mixture of inflammatory cells. Neutrophilic abscesses may be noted in the dermal papillary tips, indistinguishable from those of dermatitis herpetiformis. The infiltrate may also be largely eosinophilic, resembling bullous pemphigoid. Therefore, direct immunofluorescence studies are required for a definitive *diagnosis;* lesional or perilesional skin demonstrates linear deposition of IgA and sometimes C3 at the dermoepidermal junction (see Table 651–1). Results of indirect immunofluorescence studies are sometimes positive for circulating antibodies. Immunoelectron microscopy has localized the immunoreactants to the sublamina densa, although a combined sublamina densa and lamina lucida pattern has also been seen. The linear IgA bullous dermatosis antigen has a molecular mass of 120 kd. The eruption can be distinguished by histopathologic and immunofluorescence studies from pemphigus, bullous pemphigoid, dermatitis herpetiformis, and EM. Gram stain and culture preclude the diagnosis of bullous impetigo, with which dermatitis herpetiformis is often confused on initial presentation. The lack of bullous formation in response to trauma differentiates epidermolysis bullosa.

Treatment. Many patients respond favorably to oral sulfapyridine or dapsone. During therapy with sulfapyridine, attention should be paid to maintaining urinary output and alkalization to avoid crystal formation within the renal parenchyma. Hematologic and biochemical studies must be obtained at regular intervals during treatment with either drug to avoid serious side effects. Children who do not respond to either of these drugs may benefit from oral therapy with a corticosteroid or a combination of these drugs. The usual course is 2–4 yr, although some children have persistent or recurrent disease; there are no long-term sequelae.

Assier H, Bastuji-Garin S, Revuz J, et al: Erythema multiforme with mucous membrane involvement and Stevens-Johnson syndrome are clinically different disorders with distinct causes. Arch Dermatol 131:539, 1995.

Bauer EA, Briggaman RA: Hereditary epidermolysis bullosa. *In*: Fitzpatrick TB, Eisen AZ, Wolff K, et al (eds): Dermatology in General Medicine, 4th ed. New York, McGraw-Hill, 1993, p 654.

Becker DS: Toxic epidermal necrolysis. Lancet 351:1417, 1998.

Castillo G: Chronic bullous disease of childhood: Linear IgA dermatosis of childhood. Dermatol Clin 1:231, 1983.

Christiano AM, Uitto J: Molecular complexity of the cutaneous basement membrane zone. Exp Dermatol 5:1, 1996.

Côté B, Wechsler J, Bastuji-Garin S, et al: Clinicopathologic correlation in erythema multiforme and Stevens-Johnson syndrome. Arch Dermatol 131:1268, 1995.

DEBRA Workshop Participants: Pathogenesis, clinical features, and management of nondermatologic complications of epidermolysis bullosa. Arch Dermatol 124:705, 1988.

Fine JD: Epidermolysis bullosa: Clinical aspects, pathology, and recent advances in research. Int J Dermatol 25:143, 1986.

Fine JD: Management of acquired bullous skin diseases. N Engl J Med 333:1475, 1995.

Fridge JL, Vichinsky EP: Correction of the anemia of epidermolysis bullosa with intravenous iron and erythropoietin. J Pediatr 132:871, 1998.

Goodyear HM, Abrahamson EL, Harper JI: Childhood pemphigus foliaceus. Clin Exp Dermatol 16:229, 1991.

Kakourou T, Klontza D, Soteropoubu F, et al: Corticosteroid treatment of erythema multiforme major (Stevens-Johnson syndrome) in children. Eur J Pediatr 156:90, 1997.

Nemeth AJ, Klein AD, Gould EW, et al: Childhood bullous pemphigoid: Clinical and immunologic features, treatment, and prognosis. Arch Dermatol 127:378, 1991.

Patterson R, Miller M, Kaplan M, et al: Effectiveness of early therapy with corticosteroids in Stevens-Johnson syndrome: Experience with 41 cases and a hypothesis regarding pathogenesis. Ann Allergy 73:27, 1994.

Rabinowitz LG, Esterly NB: Inflammatory bullous diseases in children. Dermatol Clin 11:565, 1993.

Roujeau JC, Kelly JP, Naldi L, et al: Medication use and the risk of Stevens-Johnson syndrome or toxic epidermal necrolysis. N Engl J Med 333:1600, 1995.

Roujeau JC, Stern RS: Severe adverse cutaneous reactions to drugs. N Engl J Med 331:1272, 1994.

Sahn EE: Vesiculopustular lesions of neonates and infants. Curr Opin Pediatr 6:442, 1994.

Tay YK, Huff C, Weston WL: *Mycoplasma pneumoniae* infection is associated with Stevens-Johnson syndrome, not erythema multiforme (von Hebra). J Am Acad Dermatol 35:757, 1996.

Weston WL: What is erythema multiforme? Pediatr Ann 25:106, 1996.

Weston WL, Morelli JG: Herpes simplex virus-associated erythema multiforme in prepubertal children. Arch Pediatr Adolesc Med 151:1014, 1997.

CHAPTER 661
Eczema

Eczema is a generic designation for a particular type of reaction pattern in the skin, which includes exudation, lichenification, and pruritus. Acute eczematous lesions are characterized by erythema, weeping, oozing, and the formation of microvesicles within the epidermis. Chronic lesions are generally thickened, dry, and scaly, with coarse skin markings (lichenification) and altered pigmentation. Many types of eczema occur in children; the most common is atopic dermatitis (see Chapter 146), although seborrheic dermatitis, allergic and irritant contact dermatitis, nummular eczema, and dyshidrosis also are relatively common in childhood. Various dermatoses that have pruritus as a common feature may become eczematized owing to scratching. Atopic skin is sensitive to many factors that increase pruritus, such as soap, wool, cool air, and food allergens.

Once the diagnosis of eczema has been established, it is important to classify the eruption more specifically for proper management. Pertinent historical data often provide the clue. In some instances, the subsequent course and character of the eruption permit classification. Histologic changes are relatively nonspecific, but all types of eczematous dermatitis are characterized by intraepidermal edema known as spongiosis.

CONTACT DERMATITIS. This form of eczema can be subdivided into irritant dermatitis, resulting from nonspecific injury to the skin, and allergic contact dermatitis, in which the mechanism is a delayed hypersensitivity reaction. Irritant dermatitis is more frequent in children, particularly during the early years of life.

Irritant contact dermatitis can result from prolonged or repetitive contact with various substances that include saliva, citrus juices, bubble bath, detergents, abrasive materials, strong soaps, and proprietary medications. Saliva is probably one of the most common offenders; it may cause dermatitis on the face and in the neck folds of a drooling infant or a retarded child. Older children who habitually lick their lips, frequently without awareness, because of dryness may develop a striking, sharply demarcated perioral rash (Fig. 661–1*A*). Among the exogenous irritants, citrus juices, proprietary medications, and bubble bath preparations are relatively common; bubble bath dermatitis can be a cause of severe pruritus. Excessive accumulation of sweat and moisture as a result of wearing occlusive shoes may also be responsible for irritant dermatitis.

Clinically, irritant contact dermatitis may be indistinguishable from atopic dermatitis or allergic contact dermatitis. A detailed history and consideration of the sites of involvement, the age of the child, and contactants usually provide clues to the etiologic agent. The propensity to develop irritant dermatitis varies considerably among children; some may respond to minimal injury, making it difficult to identify the offending agent by history. In general, irritant contact dermatitis clears after removal of the stimulus and after temporary treatment with a topical corticosteroid preparation. Education of patients and parents about the causes of contact dermatitis is crucial to successful therapy.

Diaper dermatitis can be regarded as the prototype of irritant contact dermatitis. As a reaction to overhydration of the skin, friction, maceration, and prolonged contact with urine and feces, retained diaper soaps, and topical preparations, the skin of the diaper area may become erythematous and scaly, often with papulovesicular or bullous lesions, fissures, and erosions. The eruption can be patchy or confluent, but the genitocrural folds are often spared. Chronic hypertrophic, flat-topped papules and infiltrative nodules may simulate syphilitic lesions. Secondary infection with bacteria and yeasts is common; discomfort may be marked because of intense inflammation. Such conditions as allergic contact dermatitis, seborrheic dermatitis, candidosis, atopic dermatitis, and rare disorders such as histiocytosis X and acrodermatitis enteropathica should be considered when the eruption is persistent or recalcitrant to simple therapeutic measures.

Diaper dermatitis often responds to simple measures; however, some infants seem predisposed to diaper dermatitis, and management may be difficult. The damaging effects of overhydration of the skin and prolonged contact with feces and ammoniac urine can be obviated by frequent changing of diapers and meticulous washing of the genitals. Disposable diapers containing a superabsorbent material may help to maintain a relatively dry environment. Frequent topical applications of a bland protective barrier agent (petrolatum or zinc oxide paste) after thorough gentle cleansing may suffice to prevent dermatitis. When the aforementioned measures are not sufficient to promote healing, a light application of 0.5–1% topical hydrocortisone ointment after each diaper change for a limited time is often effective. Secondary complications can result from prolonged use of corticosteroids, especially fluorinated compounds. Before initiating such therapy, the possibility of candidal infection should considered. Candidal infection can be identified by red-pink tender skin that has numerous 1–2-mm pustules and papules at the periphery of the dermatitis. Treatment with a topical anticandidal agent may be helpful.

Juvenile plantar dermatosis is a common form of irritant contact dermatitis occurring mainly in prepubertal children. The dermatitis characteristically involves the weight-bearing surfaces, is painful rather than pruritic, and causes a glazed appearance of the plantar skin. Fissuring may become extensive, producing considerable discomfort. The dermatitis results from alternating excessive hydration and rapid moisture loss, which causes chapping of the skin and cracking of the stratum corneum. Affected children often have hyperhidrosis, wear occlusive synthetic footwear, and subject their feet to rapid drying without moisturization. Immediate application of a thick emollient when socks and shoes are removed or immediately after swimming usually prevents this condition.

Allergic contact dermatitis is a T-cell–mediated hypersensitivity reaction that is provoked by application of an antigen to the

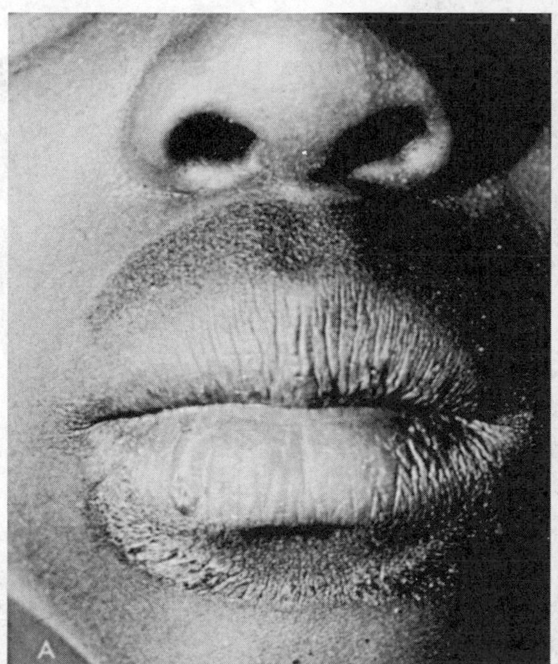

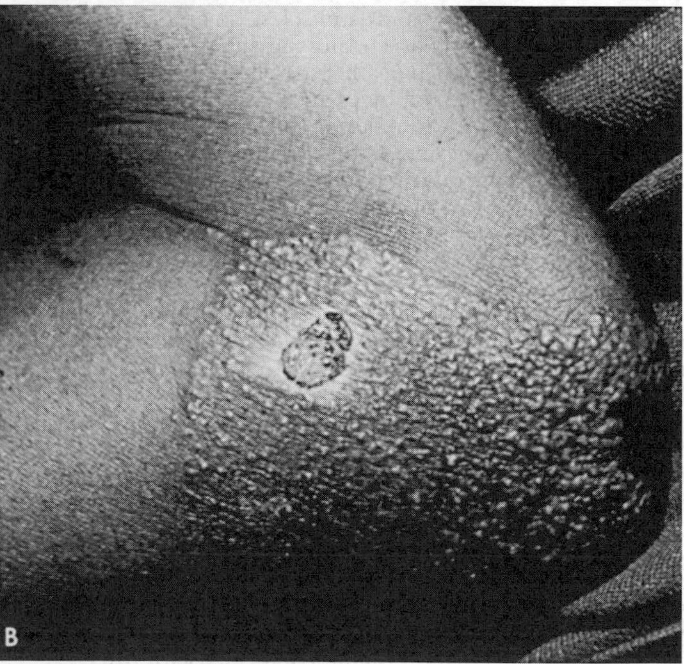

Figure 661–1 *A,* Perioral irritant contact dermatitis from lip licking. *B,* Allergic contact dermatitis to Merthiolate spray. Note the sharp angular border of vesicular eruption.

skin surface. The antigen penetrates the skin, where it is conjugated with a cutaneous protein, and the hapten-protein complex is transported to the regional lymph nodes by antigen-presenting Langerhans cells. A primary immunologic response occurs locally in the nodes and becomes generalized, presumably because of dissemination of sensitized T cells. Sensitization requires several days and, when followed by a fresh antigenic challenge, is manifested as allergic contact dermatitis. Generalized distribution may also occur if enough antigen finds its way into the circulation. Once sensitization has occurred, each new antigenic challenge may provoke an inflammatory reaction within 8–12 hr; sensitization to a particular antigen usually persists for many years.

Acute allergic contact dermatitis is an erythematous, intensely pruritic, eczematous dermatitis, which, if severe, may be edematous and vesiculobullous. The chronic condition has the features of long-standing eczema: lichenification, scaling, fissuring, and pigmentary change. The distribution of the eruption often provides a clue to the diagnosis. Volatile sensitizers usually affect exposed areas, such as the face and arms. Jewelry, topical agents, shoes, clothing, and plants cause dermatitis at points of contact.

Rhus dermatitis (poison ivy, poison sumac, poison oak) is often vesiculobullous and may be distinguished by linear streaks of vesicles where the plant leaves have brushed against the skin. Contrary to popular opinion, fluid from ruptured cutaneous vesicles does not spread the eruption; however, antigen retained on the skin, under the fingernails, and on clothing initiates new plaques of dermatitis if not removed by washing with soap and water. Antigen may also be carried by animals on their fur. The saplike allergen (oleoresin) is present on live and dead leaves, and sensitization to one plant produces cross reactions with the others.

Nickel dermatitis usually develops from contact with jewelry or metal closures on clothing and is seen most frequently on the earlobes, such as when nickel-containing posts rather than nonmetallic materials or stainless steel are used to keep a pierced tract open. Some children are exquisitely sensitive to nickel, with even the trace amounts found in gold jewelry provoking eruptions.

Shoe dermatitis typically affects the dorsum of the feet and toes, sparing the interdigital spaces; it is usually symmetric. Other forms of allergic contact dermatitis, in contrast to irritant dermatitis, rarely involve the palms and soles. Common allergens are the antioxidants and accelerators in shoe rubber and the chromium salts in tanned leather or shoe dyes. These substances are often leached out by excessive sweating.

Wearing apparel contains a number of sensitizers, including dyes, mordants, fabric finishes, fibers, resins, and cleaning solutions. Dye may be poorly fixed to clothing and leached out with sweating, as are the partially cured formaldehyde resins. The elastic in garments is also a frequent cause of clothing dermatitis.

Topical medications and cosmetics may be unsuspected as allergens, particularly if the medication is being used for a preexisting dermatitis. The most common offenders are neomycin, thimerosal (Merthiolate) (Fig. 661–1*B*), topical antihistamines (Caladryl), anesthetics (dibucaine [Nupercainal] and cyclomethycaine [Surfacaine]), preservatives (parabens), and ethylenediamine, a stabilizer present in many medications. All types of cosmetics can cause facial dermatitis; involvement of the eyelids is characteristic for nail polish sensitivity.

Contact dermatitis can be confused with other types of eczema, dermatophytoses, and vesiculobullous diseases. Patch testing may clarify the etiology. The essential principle in *treatment* is elimination of contact with the allergen. Acute dermatitis responds to cool compresses and topical application of a corticosteroid ointment. An antihistamine may be useful when taken orally. Massive acute bullous reactions or reactions that cause swelling around the eyes or genitals such as those of poison ivy may require treatment with a 2-wk tapering course of oral corticosteroids. If secondary infection has occurred, appropriate systemic antibiotic therapy should be given. Desensitization therapy is rarely indicated.

NUMMULAR ECZEMA. This disorder is unrelated to other types of eczema and is characterized by more or less coin-shaped eczematous plaques. Common sites are the extensor surfaces of the extremities (Fig. 661–2), buttocks, and shoulders. The plaques are relatively discrete, boggy, vesicular, severely pruritic, and exudative; when chronic, they often become thickened and lichenified. The cause is unknown. Most frequently, these lesions are mistaken for tinea corporis, but plaques of nummular eczema are distinguished by the lack of a raised, sharply circumscribed border, the lack of fungal organisms on a potassium hydroxide (KOH) preparation, and frequent weeping or bleeding when scraped. Secondary infection is common. Control of pruritus is usually achieved with a fluorinated corticosteroid preparation. Sedation with an antihistamine may be helpful, particularly at night. Antibiotics are indicated for secondary infection.

PITYRIASIS ALBA. This occurs mainly in children; the lesions are hypopigmented, round or oval, macular or slightly elevated patches with fine adherent scale (Fig. 661–3). They may be mildly erythematous and relatively well defined but lack a sharply marginated border. Lesions occur on the face, neck, upper trunk, and proximal portions of the arms. Itching is minimal or absent. The cause is unknown, but the eruption appears to be exacerbated by dryness and is often regarded as a mild form of eczema. Pityriasis alba is frequently misdiagnosed as tinea versicolor or corporis, each of which can be readily precluded by performing a KOH examination of surface scale. The lesions wax and wane but eventually disappear. Application of a lubricant may ameliorate the condition; if pruritus is troublesome, a topical 1% hydrocortisone preparation applied three to four times daily may be more effective. Normal pigmentation returns in weeks to months.

LICHEN SIMPLEX CHRONICUS. This lesion is characterized by a chronic pruritic, eczematous, circumscribed, solitary plaque that is usually lichenified and hyperpigmented. The most com-

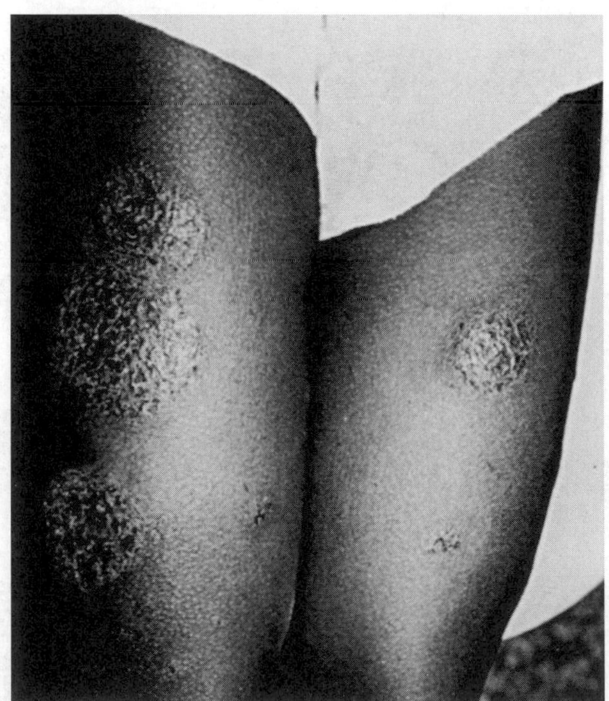

Figure 661–2 Multiple hyperpigmented scaly plaques of nummular eczema.

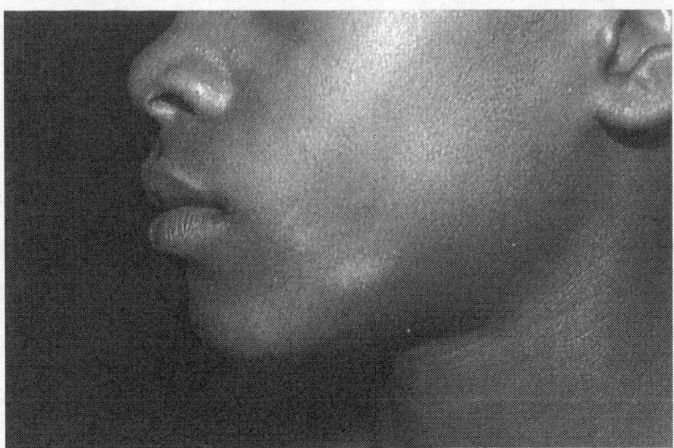

Figure 661–3 Patchy hypopigmented lesions with diffuse borders characteristic of pityriasis alba. See also color section.

mon sites are the posterior aspect of the neck, the dorsum of the feet, the wrists, and ankles. Trauma from rubbing and scratching accounts for persistence of the plaque, although the initiating event may be a transient lesion, such as an insect bite. Pruritus must be controlled to permit healing. A topical fluorinated corticosteroid preparation is often helpful, but constant irritation of the skin must be avoided. A covering to prevent scratching may be necessary.

DYSHIDROTIC ECZEMA (DYSHIDROSIS, POMPHOLYX). This is a recurrent, sometimes seasonal, blistering disorder of the hands and feet; it occurs in all age groups but is uncommon in infancy. The pathogenesis is not known; no genetic factor has been identified, although an increased incidence of atopy has been recorded in patients and their relatives. The disease is characterized by recurrent crops of intensely pruritic small vesicles on the hands and feet. Sites of predilection are the palms, soles, and lateral aspects of the fingers and toes. Primary lesions are noninflammatory and filled with clear fluid, which, unlike sweat, has a physiologic pH and contains protein. Larger vesicobullae may occur, and maceration and secondary infection are frequent because of scratching (Fig. 661–4). The chronic phase is characterized by thickened, fissured plaques that may cause considerable discomfort. Hyperhidrosis is common in many patients, but the association may be fortuitous. The diagnosis is made clinically. The disorder may be confused with allergic contact dermatitis, which usually affects the dorsal rather than the volar surfaces, and with dermatophytosis, which can be distinguished by a KOH preparation of the roof of a vesicle and by appropriate cultures.

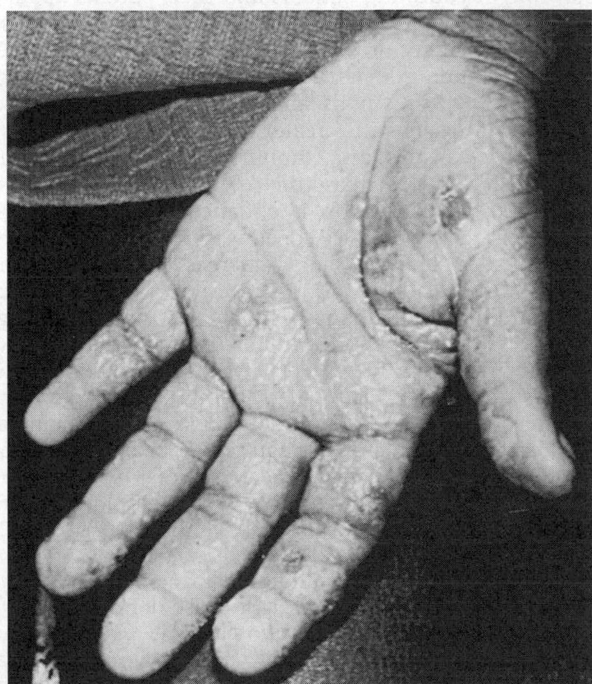

Figure 661–4 Vesicular palmar lesions of dyshidrotic eczema that have become secondarily infected.

Dyshidrotic eczema responds to wet dressings, followed by a topical corticosteroid preparation during the acute phase. Control of the chronic stage is difficult; lubricants containing mild keratolytic agents in conjunction with a potent topical fluorinated corticosteroid preparation may be indicated. Secondary bacterial infection should be treated systemically with an appropriate antibiotic. Patients should be told to expect recurrence and should protect their hands and feet from the damaging effects of excessive sweating, chemicals, harsh soaps, and adverse weather.

SEBORRHEIC DERMATITIS. This chronic inflammatory disease is most common in the pediatric age group, during infancy and adolescence, paralleling the distribution, size, and activity of the sebaceous glands. The cause is unknown, as is the role of the sebaceous glands in this disease. A generalized eruption with features of seborrheic dermatitis is extremely common in HIV-infected children and adolescents.

Clinical Manifestations. The disorder may begin within the 1st mo of life and may be most troublesome during the 1st yr. Diffuse or focal scaling and crusting of the scalp, sometimes called *cradle cap*, may be the initial and at times the only manifestation. A greasy, scaly, erythematous papular dermatitis, which is usually nonpruritic, may involve the face, neck, retroauricular areas, axillae, and diaper area. The dermatitis may be patchy and focal or may spread to involve almost the entire body (Fig. 661–5). Postinflammatory pigmentary changes are common, particularly in black infants. When the scaling becomes pronounced, the condition may resemble psoriasis and, at times, can be distinguished only with difficulty. The possibility of coexistent atopic dermatitis must be considered when there is an acute weeping dermatitis with pruritus. An intractable seborrhea-like dermatitis with chronic diarrhea and failure to thrive *(Leiner disease)* may reflect dysfunction of the immune system. A chronic seborrhea-like pattern, which responds poorly to treatment, may also result from cutaneous histiocytic infiltrates in infants with Langerhans cell histiocytosis X. Seborrheic dermatitis is a common cutaneous manifestation of AIDS among young adults and is characterized by thick, greasy scales on the scalp and large hyperkeratotic erythematous plaques on the face, chest, and genitals.

During adolescence, seborrheic dermatitis is more localized and may be confined to the scalp and intertriginous areas.

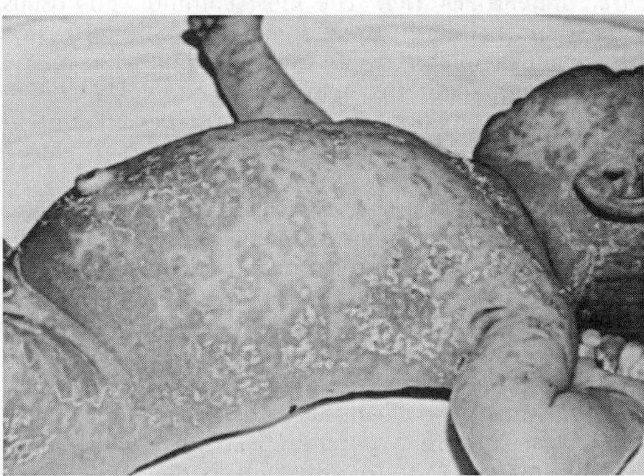

Figure 661–5 Widespread seborrheic dermatitis in an infant.

Also noted may be marginal blepharitis and involvement of the external auditory canal. Scalp changes may vary from diffuse, brawny scaling to focal areas of thick, oily, yellow crusts with underlying erythema. Loss of hair is not uncommon, and pruritus may be absent to marked. When the dermatitis is severe, erythema and scaling may occur at the frontal hairline, at the medial aspects of the eyebrows, and in the nasolabial and retroauricular folds. Red, scaly plaques may appear in the axillae, inguinal region, gluteal cleft, and umbilicus. On the extremities, seborrheic plaques may be more eczematous and less erythematous and demarcated.

Etiology. Seborrheic dermatitis is a condition that is reactivated in some patients by stressful situations, poor hygiene, and excessive perspiration. *Malassezia furfur* has also been implicated as a causative agent, although its role in the etiology of infantile seborrheic dermatitis is unclear. The *differential diagnosis* includes psoriasis, atopic dermatitis, dermatophytosis, and candidosis. Secondary bacterial infections and superimposed candidosis are not uncommon.

Treatment. Scalp lesions should be controlled with an antiseborrheic shampoo (selenium sulfide, sulfur, salicylic acid, zinc pyrithion, tar), used daily if necessary. Inflamed lesions usually respond promptly to topical corticosteroid therapy given two to four times daily. Topical antifungal agents effective against *Malassezia* have also been advocated as therapy. Wet compresses should be applied to the moist or fissured lesions before application of the steroid ointment. Many patients require continued use of an antiseborrheic shampoo for control. Response to therapy is usually rapid unless there are complicating factors or the diagnosis is in error.

Fergusson DM, Horwood J, Shannon FT: Early solid feeding and recurrent childhood eczema: A 10-year longitudinal study. Pediatrics 86:541, 1990.
Podmore P, Burrows D, Eady DJ, et al: seborrheic eczema—a disease entity or a clinical variant of atopic eczema? Br J Dermatol 115:341, 1986.
Rothe M, Grant-Kels J: Diagnostic criteria for atopic dermatitis. Lancet 348:769, 1996.
Ruzicka T, Bieber T, Schöpf E, et al: A short term trial of tacrolimus ointment for atopic dermatitis. N Engl J Med 337:816, 1997.
Tollesson A, Frithz A, Stenlund K: *Malassezia furfur* in infantile seborrheic dermatitis. Pediatr Dermatol 14:423, 1997.

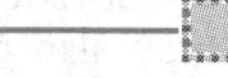

CHAPTER 662
Photosensitivity

Photosensitivity denotes a qualitatively or quantitatively abnormal cutaneous reaction to sunlight or artificial light.

ACUTE SUNBURN REACTION. The most common photosensitive reaction seen in children is acute sunburn. Sunburn is caused mainly by ultraviolet (UV) B radiation (290–320-nm wavelength). Sunlight contains many times more UVA (320–400 nm) than UVB radiation, but UVA must be encountered in much larger quantities than UVB radiation to produce sunburn.

Pathophysiology and Clinical Manifestations. Transmitted radiation below 300 nm is largely absorbed in the epidermis, whereas that above 300 nm is mostly transmitted to the dermis after variable epidermal melanin absorption. Children vary in susceptibility to UV radiation, depending on their skin type (amount of pigment) (Table 662–1). Immediate pigment darkening is due to UVA radiation–induced photo-oxidative darkening of existing melanin and its transfer from melanocytes to keratinocytes. This effect generally lasts for a few hours, and, like a UVA-induced tanning salon tan, is not photoprotective. UVB-induced effects appear 6–12 hr after initial exposure and reach a peak in 24 hr. Effects include redness, tenderness, edema, and blistering. The vasodilatation seen in UVB-induced erythema is mediated by prostaglandins E_2 and F_2. Delayed melanogenesis as a result of UVB radiation begins in 2–3 days and lasts several days to a few weeks. Manufacture of new melanin in melanocytes, transfer of melanin from melanocytes to keratinocytes, increase in size and arborization of melanocytes, and activation of quiescent melanocytes produces delayed melanogenesis. This effect reduces skin sensitivity to development of erythema by approximately two- to threefold. Additional effects and possible complications of sun exposure include increased thickness of the stratum corneum, recurrence or exacerbation of herpes simplex labialis, lupus erythematosus, and many other conditions (Table 662–2).

TABLE 662–1 Sun-Reactive Skin Types

Type	Demographics	Sunburn, Tanning History
I	Red hair, freckles, Celtic origin	Always burns easily, no tanning
II	Fair skin, fair-haired, blue-eyed, white	Usually burns, minimal tanning
III	Darker skinned white	Sometimes burns, gradual light brown tan
IV	Mediterranean background	Minimal to no burning, always tans
V	Middle eastern white, Mexican	Rarely burns, tans profusely dark brown
VI	Blacks	Never burns, pigmented black

Treatment. Acute severe sunburn should be managed with cool compresses; topical corticosteroids may diminish inflammation and pain, and oral prostaglandin inhibitors such as ibuprofen and indomethacin may decrease erythema and pain. Proprietary preparations containing topical anesthetics are relatively ineffective and potentially hazardous because of their propensity to cause contact dermatitis. A bland emollient is effective in the desquamative phase.

Prognosis and Prevention of Sequelae. The long-term sequelae of chronic and intense sun exposure are not often seen in children, but most individuals receive more than 50% of their lifetime UV dose by age 20 yr. Therefore, pediatricians have a pivotal role in educating patients and their parents about the harmful effects, potential malignancy risks, and irreversible skin damage that result from unduly prolonged exposure to the sun and tanning lights. Premature aging, senile elastosis, actinic keratoses, squamous and basal cell carcinomas, and melanomas all occur with greater frequency in sun-damaged skin. In particular, blistering sunburns in childhood and adolescence significantly increase the risk for development of *malignant melanoma*. Protection is enhanced by a wide variety of sunscreen agents. Physical opaque sunscreens (zinc oxide, titanium dioxide) block UV light, whereas chemical sunscreens (*p*-aminobenzoic acid [PABA], PABA esters, salicylates, benzophenones, dibenzoylmethanes, cinnamates) absorb damaging radiation. The benzophenones and dibenzoylmethanes provide protection in both the UVA and UVB ranges. Children with skin types I to III (see Table 662–1) require sunscreens with a sun protection factor (SPF) of at least 15. SPF is defined as the minimal dose of sunlight required to produce cutaneous erythema after applying a sunscreen, divided by the dose required with no use of sunscreen. Protective clothing (hats) and avoidance of sun exposure between 10:00 a.m. and 2:00 p.m. are additional prudent practices.

PHOTOSENSITIVE REACTIONS. Photosensitizers in combination with a particular wavelength of light cause dermatitis that can be classified as a phototoxic or a photoallergic reaction. Contact of the skin with the photosensitizer may occur externally, internally by enteral or parenteral administration, or by host synthesis of photosensitizers in response to an administered drug.

TABLE 662–2 Cutaneous Reactions to Sunlight

Sunburn

Photoallergic Drug Eruptions

Systemic drugs include tetracyclines (declomycin), psoralens, chlorthiazides, sulfonamides, barbiturates, griseofulvin, thiazides, quinidine, phenothiazines
Topical agents include coal tar derivatives, psoralens, halogenated salicylanilides (soaps), perfume oils (e.g., oil of bergamot), sunscreens (e.g., PABA, cinnamates, benzophenones)

Phototoxic Drug Eruptions

High doses of agents causing photoallergic eruptions; nalidixic acid, 5-fluorouracil, psoralens, furosemide, nonsteroidal anti-inflammatory agents (naproxen, piroxicam), sulfonamides, tetracyclines, phenothiazines, furocoumarins (e.g., lime, lemon, carrot, celery, dill, parsnip, parsley)

Genetic Disorder with Photosensitivity

Xeroderma pigmentosum
Bloom syndrome
Cockayne syndrome
Rothmund-Thomson syndrome

Inborn Errors of Metabolism

Porphyrias
Hartnup disease
Pellagra

Infectious Diseases Associated with Photosensitivity

Recurrent herpes simplex infection
Lymphogranuloma venereum
Viral exanthems (accentuated photodistribution; e.g., varicella)

Skin Disease Exacerbated or Precipitated by Light

Lichen planus
Darier disease
Lupus erythematosus
Dermatomyositis
Scleroderma
Solar urticaria
Polymorphous light eruptions (?)
Hydroa aestivale and vacciniforme (?)
Granuloma annulare
Psoriasis
Erythema multiforme
Sarcoid
Atopic dermatitis
Hailey-Hailey disease
Pemphigus
Acne rosacea
Bullous pemphigoid

Deficient Protection Due to Lack of Pigment

Vitiligo
Oculocutaneous albinism
Partial albinism
Phenylketonuria
Chédiak-Higashi syndrome
Piebaldism

Photoallergic reactions occur in only a small percentage of persons exposed to photosensitizers and light and require a time interval for sensitization to take place. Thereafter, dermatitis appears within approximately 24 hr of re-exposure to the photosensitizer and light. Photoallergic dermatitis is a T-cell–mediated delayed hypersensitivity reaction in which the drug, acting as a hapten, may combine with a skin protein to form the antigenic substance. Photoallergic reactions vary in morphology and may occur on partially covered and on light-exposed skin. Some of the important classes of drugs and chemicals responsible for photosensitivity reactions are listed in Table 662–2.

Phototoxic reactions occur in all individuals who accumulate adequate amounts of a photosensitizing drug or chemical within the skin. Prior sensitization is not required. Dermatitis develops within hours after exposure to radiation in the range of 285–450 nm. The eruption is confined to light-exposed areas and often resembles an exaggerated sunburn, but it may be urticarial or bullous. It results in postinflammatory hyperpigmentation. All the drugs that cause photoallergic reactions may also cause a phototoxic dermatitis if given in sufficiently high doses. Several additional drugs and contactants cause phototoxic reactions, notably the plant-derived furocoumarins (see Table 662–2). Differentiation from contact dermatitis as a result of poison ivy or oak may be difficult, but itching is prominent in contact dermatitis. In phytophotodermatitis, burning is prominent and is confined to sun-exposed areas, sparing the upper eyelids, beneath the nose and chin, and the retroauricular areas.

Although photodermatitis caused by drugs or chemicals may be diagnosed by photopatch testing, facilities for this diagnostic procedure are not widely available. A high index of suspicion combined with an appreciation of the distribution pattern of the eruption and a history of application or ingestion of a known photosensitizing agent is all that is required to make a diagnosis. Discontinuation of the offending medication or avoidance of sun exposure, oral administration of an antihistamine, and application of a topical corticosteroid to alleviate pruritus are appropriate therapeutic measures. Severe reactions may necessitate systemic corticosteroid therapy for a brief time.

PORPHYRIAS (see Chapter 87). Porphyrias are acquired or inborn abnormalities of specific enzymes in the heme biosynthetic pathway; they are diverse in their clinical manifestations. Two in particular occur in children and have photosensitivity as a consistent feature. Signs and symptoms may be negligible during the winter, when sun exposure is minimal.

Congenital erythropoietic porphyria (Günther disease) is a rare autosomal recessive disorder caused by a deficiency of uroporphyrinogen III cosynthase. This condition presents within the first few months of life with exquisite sensitivity to light, which may induce repeated severe bullous eruptions that result in mutilating scars. Hyperpigmentation, hyperkeratosis, vesiculation, and fragility of skin develop in light-exposed areas. Hirsutism in areas of mild involvement, scarring alopecia in severely affected areas, pink to red urine, brown teeth, hemolytic anemia, splenomegaly, and increased amounts of uroporphyrin I in urine, plasma, and erythrocytes and of coproporphyrin I in feces are additional characteristic manifestations. Urine from affected patients fluoresces reddish pink under a Wood light.

Erythropoietic protoporphyria is inherited as an autosomal dominant trait. It is due to decreased activity of ferrochelatase, which converts protoporphyrin to heme. Photosensitivity becomes apparent in early childhood and is manifested by pain, tingling, and a burning sensation within approximately 30 min of sun exposure, followed by erythema, edema, urticaria, and, rarely, vesicles on light-exposed areas. Nail changes consist of opacification of the nail plate, onycholysis, pain, and tenderness. Mild systemic symptoms of malaise, chills, and fever may accompany the acute skin reaction. Recurrent sun exposure produces a chronic eczematous dermatitis with thickened, lichenified skin, especially over the finger joints, and persistent violaceous erythema, ulcers, and pitted or linear, crusted atrophic scars on the face and rims of the ears. Pigmentation, hypertrichosis, skin fragility, and mutilation are uncommon. Liver disease is generally mild. Symptoms often improve spontaneously after age 10–11 yr.

The wavelengths of light mainly responsible for eliciting cutaneous reactions in porphyria are in the region of 400 nm. Window glass, which transmits wavelengths greater than 320 nm, is not protective, and artificial lights of a certain wavelength may be pathogenic. Patients must avoid direct sunlight, wear protective clothing, and use a sunscreen agent that effectively blocks wavelengths in the region of 400 nm. Administration of β-carotene (Solatene) quenches the fluorescence of the porphyrin molecule by yellowing the skin; its effectiveness in reducing photosensitivity in patients with protoporphyria has onset within 1–3 mo and is variable.

COLLOID MILIUM. This is a rare, asymptomatic disorder that occurs on the face (nose, upper lip, upper cheeks) and may extend to the dorsum of the hands and the neck as a profuse eruption of ivory to yellow, firm, tiny, grouped papules. Lesions appear before puberty on otherwise normal skin, unlike the adult variant that develops on sun-damaged skin. Onset may follow an acute sunburn or chronic sun exposure. Most cases reach maximal severity within approximately 3 yr and remain unchanged thereafter, although the condition may remit spontaneously after puberty. Histopathologic changes include well-circumscribed accumulations of fissured eosinophilic material, primarily in the upper dermis in contact with the epidermis. Basal cells, which are transformed into these colloid bodies, appear to be abnormally susceptible to degeneration after actinic exposure.

HYDROA VACCINIFORME. This vesicobullous disorder is more common in boys than in girls, begins in early childhood, but may remit at puberty. The peak incidence is in the spring and summer. Erythematous, pruritic macules develop symmetrically within hours of sun exposure over the ears, nose, lips, cheeks, and dorsal surfaces of the hands and forearms. Lesions progress to stinging tender papules and hemorrhagic vesicles and bullas. Severe lesions of hydroa vacciniforme resemble the vesicles of chickenpox; they become umbilicated, ulcerated, and crusted and heal with pitted scars and telangiectasias. Fever and malaise are noted occasionally during the acute phase. Histopathologically, lesions show intraepidermal multilocular vesicles, leading to focal epidermal and dermal necrosis. Noted early is a dermal perivascular mononuclear cell infiltrate that later surrounds areas of necrosis. This eruption should be distinguished from erythropoietic protoporphyria, which rarely shows vesicles. Pathogenesis of hydroa vacciniforme is unknown, but typical lesions have been reproduced with repeated doses of UVA light. A topical corticosteroid may be useful for the inflammatory phase of the eruption. Prophylactic broad-spectrum sunscreens may also be helpful, as may low-dose courses of UVB or psoralen with UVA (PUVA) therapy. β-Carotene and antimalarial agents are sometimes beneficial.

ACTINIC PRURIGO. This is a chronic familial photodermatitis that is inherited as an autosomal dominant trait among the Native Americans of North and South America. The first episode generally occurs in early childhood several hours to 2 days after intense sun exposure. Most patients are female and are sensitive to UVA radiation. Lesions are intensely pruritic, erythematous papules on the face, lower lip, distal extremities, and, in severe cases, buttocks. Facial lesions may heal with minute pitted or linear scarring. Lesions often become chronic, without periods of total clearing, merging into eczematous plaques that lichenify and may become secondarily infected. Associated features that distinguish this disorder from other photoeruptions and atopic dermatitis include cheilitis, conjunctivitis, and traumatic alopecia of the outer half of the eyebrows. Actinic prurigo is a chronic condition that generally persists into adult life, although it may improve spontaneously in the late teenage years. Broad-spectrum sunscreens such as butyl methoxydibenzoylmethane may be helpful in preventing the eruption, but antimalarials and β-carotene afford little to no protection. Topical corticosteroids palliate the pruritus and inflammation; thalidomide also may be effective.

SOLAR URTICARIA. This is a rare disorder induced by UV or visible irradiation. Primary solar urticaria is probably mediated by allergic type 1 hypersensitivity to a cutaneous or circulating irradiation-induced allergen, leading to mast cell degranulation and histamine release. This reaction occurs within 5–10 min of sun exposure, fades within 1–2 hr, and is characterized by widespread severe wheal formation, which may lead to faintness, headache, nausea, syncope, or bronchospasm. H_1-blocking antihistamines may be useful to prevent or abate the eruption. Secondary solar urticaria is due to photosensitization to exogenous chemicals or systemic drugs and may rarely be a presenting sign of erythropoietic protoporphyria. Treatment consists of avoidance of the photosensitizing wavelength of light and/or the drug.

POLYMORPHOUS LIGHT ERUPTION. Polymorphous light eruption develops most commonly in females younger than 30 yr. The first eruption typically appears after prolonged sun exposure during the spring or summer. Onset of the eruption is delayed by hours to days after sun exposure and lasts for hours to sometimes weeks. Areas of involvement tend to be symmetric and are characteristic for a given patient, including some but not all of the exposed or lightly covered skin on the face, neck, upper chest, and distal extremities. Lesions have various morphologies but most commonly are pruritic, 2–5-mm grouped erythematous papules or papulovesicles or edematous plaques that are more than 5 cm in diameter. Most cases involve sensitivity to UVA radiation, although some are UVB induced. Therapeutic approaches include sun avoidance, broad-spectrum sunscreens, topical or systemic corticosteroids, β-carotene, nicotinamide, antimalarials, or prophylactic UVB or PUVA phototherapy.

COCKAYNE SYNDROME. Onset of this autosomal recessive disorder is characterized by the appearance, at approximately 1 yr of age, of facial erythema in a butterfly distribution after sun exposure, followed by loss of adipose tissue and development of thin, atrophic, hyperpigmented skin, particularly over the face. Associated features include dwarfism; mental retardation; large, protuberant ears; long limbs; disproportionately large hands and feet, which are sometimes cool and cyanotic; pinched nose; carious teeth; unsteady gait with tremor; limitation of joint mobility; progressive deafness; cataracts; retinal degeneration; optic atrophy; decreased sweating and tearing; and premature graying of the hair. Diffuse extensive demyelination of the peripheral and central nervous systems ensues, and patients generally die of atheromatous vascular disease before the 3rd decade. Photosensitivity is due to deficient rates of repair of UV-induced damage, specifically within actively transcribing regions of DNA. The syndrome is distinguished from progeria (see Chapter 716) by photosensitivity and the ocular abnormalities.

XERODERMA PIGMENTOSUM. This is a rare autosomal recessive disorder that results from a defect in nucleotide excision repair. Ten complementation groups have been recognized, based on each group's separate defect in the ability to repair damaged DNA. The wavelength of light that induces the DNA damage ranges from 280–340 nm. Skin changes are first noted during infancy or early childhood in sun-exposed areas such as the face, neck, hands, and arms; lesions may occur, however, at other sites, including the scalp. The skin lesions consist of erythema, scaling, bullas, crusting, ephelides, telangiectasia, keratoses, basal and squamous cell carcinomas, and malignant melanomas. Ocular manifestations include photophobia, lacrimation, blepharitis, symblepharon, keratitis, corneal opacities, tumors of the lids, and possible eventual blindness. Neurologic abnormalities such as mental deterioration and sensorineural deafness may develop in approximately 20% of patients. Some patients with xeroderma pigmentosum have the clinical phenotype of Cockayne syndrome, suggesting that these two disorders may represent an overlapping spectrum of excision-repair defects. The association of xeroderma pigmentosum with microcephaly, mental retardation, dwarfism, and hypogonadism is known as *De Sanctis-Cacchione syndrome*.

This disease is a serious mutilating disorder, and the life span is often brief. Affected families should have genetic counseling. The disorder is detectable in cells cultured from amniotic fluid. Affected children should be totally protected from sun exposure; protective clothing, eyeglasses, and opaque broad-spectrum sunscreens should be used even for mildly affected children. Light from unshielded fluorescent bulbs and sunlight passing through glass windows are also harmful. Early detection and removal of malignancies is mandatory. Grafting of skin from non–light-exposed areas may be helpful, as is the use of topical antimitotic agents such as 5-fluorouracil.

ROTHMUND-THOMSON SYNDROME. This syndrome is also known as *poikiloderma congenitale* because of the striking skin changes; it is inherited as an autosomal recessive trait, although a preponderance of affected females has been reported. Skin changes are noted as early as 3 mo of age. Plaques of erythema and edema appear on the cheeks, forehead, ears, neck, dorsal portions of the hands, extensor surfaces of the arms, and buttocks and are replaced gradually by reticulated, atrophic, hyperpigmented, telangiectatic plaques. Light sensitivity is present in many cases, and exposure to the sun may provoke formation of bullae. Areas of involvement, however, are not strictly photodistributed. Short stature; frontal bossing; saddle nose; prognathism; small hands and feet; sparse eyebrows, eyelashes, pubic and axillary hair; sparse, fine, prematurely gray hair or alopecia; dystrophic nails; defective dentition; bony defects; and hypogenitalism are common. Cataracts commonly become apparent at 2–7 yr of age. Most patients have normal mental development and life expectancy. Keratoses and later squamous cell carcinomas may develop on exposed skin. In addition, the incidence of noncutaneous malignancies, particularly osteosarcoma, is higher than in the general population.

HARTNUP DISEASE (see Chapter 82.5). This is a rare inborn error of metabolism with autosomal recessive inheritance. Neutral amino acids, including tryptophan, are not transported across the brush border epithelium of the intestine and kidneys, resulting in deficiency of synthesis of nicotinamide and causing a photoinduced pellagra-like syndrome. The urine contains increased amounts of monoamine monocarboxylic amino acids. Cutaneous signs, which precede neurologic manifestations, initially develop during the early months of life when an eczematous, occasionally vesicobullous eruption is noted on the face and extremities in a glove-and-stocking photodistribution. Hyperpigmentation and hyperkeratosis may supervene and are intensified by further exposure to sunlight. Episodic flares may be precipitated by febrile illness, sun exposure, emotional stress, and poor nutrition. In most cases, mental development is normal, but some patients display emotional instability and episodic cerebellar ataxia. Neurologic symptoms are fully reversible. Administration of nicotinamide and protection from sunlight result in improvement of both cutaneous and neurologic manifestations. Neomycin may also be beneficial in abating neurologic symptoms by reducing the intestinal bacterial flora and minimizing formation of indole and indican.

BLOOM SYNDROME. The defect in Bloom syndrome is inherited in an autosomal recessive manner on chromosome 15, perhaps owing to absence of a DNA helicase. Erythema and telangiectasia develop during infancy in a butterfly distribution on the face after exposure to sunlight. A bullous eruption on the lips and telangiectatic erythema on the hands and forearms may develop. Café-au-lait spots, ichthyosis, acanthosis nigricans, and hypertrichosis are less constant cutaneous manifestations. Pre- and postnatal short stature and a distinctive facies consisting of a prominent nose and ears and a small, narrow face are generally found. Defective dentition, pilonidal cysts, sacral dimples, syndactyly, polydactyly, clinodactyly of the fifth fingers, shortened lower extremities, and clubfeet are additional inconstant features. Intellect is normal. Patients frequently have low levels of IgA, IgM, and IgG and are susceptible to infections. They are sensitive to UV radiation, and their rate of chromosomal breaks and sister chromatid exchanges is markedly increased. Affected children have an unusual tendency to develop lymphoreticular malignancies.

Council on Scientific Affairs: Harmful effects of ultraviolet radiation. JAMA 262:380, 1989.

Garzon MC, DeLeo VA: Photosensitivity in the pediatric patient. Curr Opin Pediatr 9:377, 1997.

Gonzales E, Gonzales S: Drug photosensitivity, idiopathic photodermatoses, and sunscreens. J Am Acad Dermatol 35:871, 1996.

Gould JW, Mercurio MG, Elmets CA: Cutaneous photosensitivity disease induced by exogenous agents. J Am Acad Dermatol 33:551, 1995.

Holzle E, Plewig G, von Kries R, et al: Polymorphous light eruption. J Invest Dermatol 88:32s, 1987.

Jung EG: The red face: Photogenodermatoses. Clin Dermatol 11:275, 1993.

Kraemer KW, Slor H: Xeroderma pigmentosum. Clin Dermatol 3:33, 1985.

Lane PR, Hogan DJ, Martel MJ, et al: Actinic prurigo: Clinical features and prognosis. J Am Acad Dermatol 26:683, 1992.

Poh-Fitzpatrick MB, Ramsay CA, Frain-Bell W, et al: Photodermatoses in infants and children. Pediatr Dermatol 5:189, 1988.

Soter NA: Acute effects of ultraviolet radiation on the skin. Semin Dermatol 9:11, 1990.

Vennos EM, Collins M, James WD: Rothmund-Thomson syndrome: Review of the world literature. J Am Acad Dermatol 27:750, 1992.

CHAPTER 663
Diseases of the Epidermis

PSORIASIS. This common, chronic skin disorder is first evident in approximately one third of affected individuals within the first 2 decades of life. When the onset occurs during childhood, about 50% have a positive family history of the disease, and girls are more frequently affected. The mode of transmission is unknown; a multifactorial type of inheritance has been proposed. There is an association with histocompatibility antigens (HLA)-BW17, -B13, -B16, -BW37, and -CW6. These HLA types are not associated with the pustular form of the disease. The pathogenesis is also unknown; epidermal turnover time, however, is distinctly accelerated compared with that of normal epidermis.

Clinical Manifestations. The lesions consist of erythematous papules that coalesce to form plaques with sharply demarcated, irregular borders. If they are unaltered by treatment, a thick silvery or yellow-white scale (resembling mica) develops; removal of it may result in pinpoint bleeding (Auspitz sign). The *Koebner*, or isomorphic, *response*, in which new lesions appear at sites of trauma, is a valuable diagnostic feature. Lesions may occur anywhere, but preferred sites are the scalp, knees (Fig. 663–1*A*), elbows, umbilicus, superior intergluteal fold, and genitals. Scalp lesions may be confused with seborrheic dermatitis, atopic dermatitis, or tinea capitis. Small raindrop-like lesions on the face are moderately common. Nail involvement, a valuable diagnostic sign, is characterized by pitting of the nail plate (Fig. 663–1*B*), detachment of the plate (onycholysis), yellowish-brown subungual discoloration, and accumulation of subungual debris.

Age is an important factor in determining the clinical pattern. Psoriasis is rare in neonates but may be severe and recalcitrant and pose a diagnostic problem. The initial lesions may involve the diaper area and mimic seborrheic dermatitis, eczematous diaper dermatitis, perianal streptococcal disease, or candidosis. Biopsy or prolonged observation may be required for definitive diagnosis. Other rare forms include psoriatic erythroderma, localized or generalized pustular psoriasis, and linear psoriasis. Hospitalization may be required for severe forms of the disease. *Guttate psoriasis*, a variant that occurs predominantly in children, is characterized by an explosive eruption of profuse, small, oval or round lesions that morphologically are identical to the larger plaques of psoriasis (Fig. 663–1*C*). Sites of predilection are the trunk, face, and proximal portions of the limbs. The onset frequently follows a recent streptococcal respiratory infection; a culture of the throat and serologic titers should be obtained. Guttate psoriasis has also been observed after perianal streptococcal infection, viral infections, sunburn, and withdrawal of systemic corticosteroid ther-

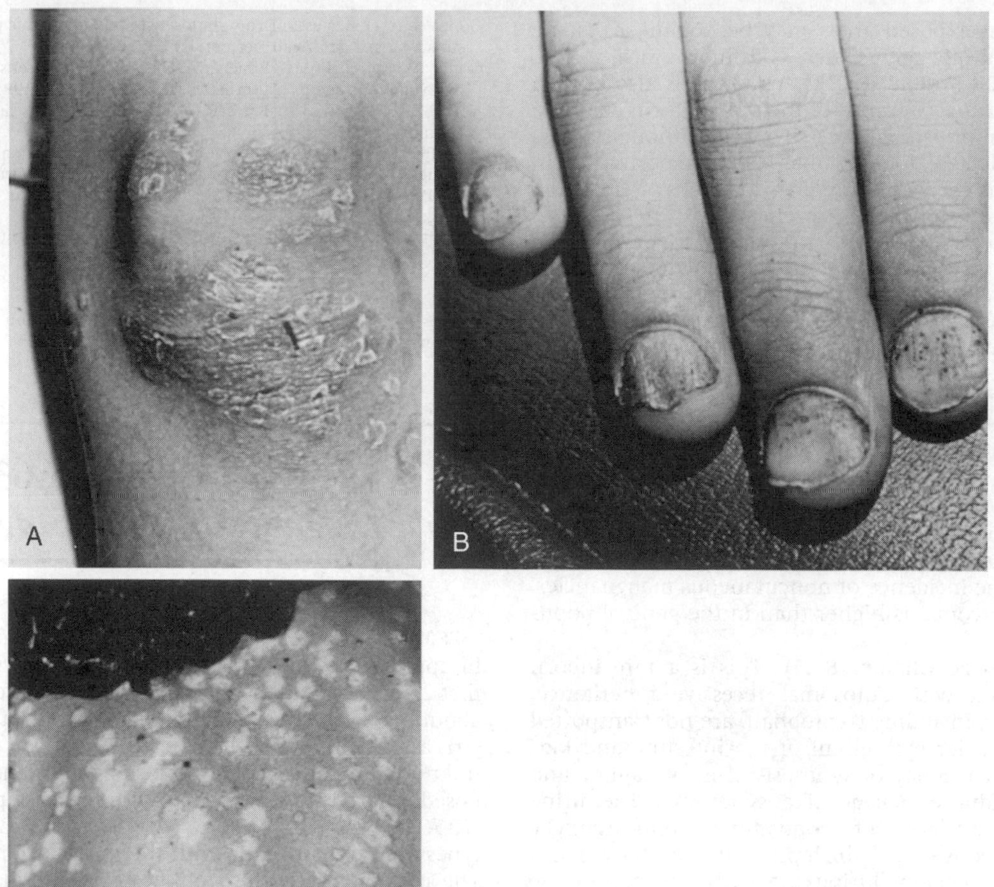

Figure 663–1 *A*, Chronic psoriatic plaques on the knee. *B*, Psoriatic nail changes of pitting and dystrophy. *C*, Guttate psoriasis in widespread distribution over the trunk.

apy. Psoriatic skin lesions may be induced, in a genetically susceptible host, by CD4+ T cells that were initially activated by streptococcal pyrogenic exotoxins acting as superantigens. The source of the streptococcal antigens can be the throat or the skin. Some of the superantigen-activated T cells recognize streptococcal M protein in the skin and appear to have cross reactivity with an abnormal keratin that has homology with streptococcal M protein. The autoreactive T cells may be responsible for the formation and maintenance of psoriatic skin lesions. The lesions may be confused with viral exanthems and guttate parapsoriasis (see later).

Diagnosis. This is based on the clinical manifestations. The differential diagnosis includes Reiter syndrome, which, in contrast to psoriasis, involves mucous membranes, and pityriasis rubra pilaris. When in doubt, histopathologic examination of an untreated lesion reveals characteristic changes of psoriasis.

Treatment. The therapeutic approach varies with the age of the child, type of psoriasis, sites of involvement, and extent of the disease. Therapy is mainly palliative and should not be overly aggressive. Physical and chemical trauma to the skin should be avoided as much as possible (see the Koebner response, earlier).

Tar preparations may be used in the form of an emulsion added to the daily bath, gel preparations, or ointments such as crude coal tar (1–5%) and liquor carbonis detergens (5–15%) in an emollient base alone or in conjunction with ultraviolet (UV) B light or natural sunlight. Sunlight occasionally has an adverse rather than a beneficial effect, and the use of tar preparations may have to be decreased during the summer to avoid phototoxic reactions. Salicylic acid ointment (1–3%) may provide an alternative for removal of scale, but extensive application may result in toxicity, particularly in small children. Topical corticosteroid preparations are effective during the first several weeks of therapy for an individual lesion, and then their effectiveness tends to decrease. Topical corticosteroids must be used with caution. Fluorinated compounds produce cutaneous atrophy if applied excessively or if occluded with polyethylene film for prolonged periods, and adrenal suppression may occur if systemic absorption is excessive. The preparation that is least potent but effective should be applied one to two times daily. The topical vitamin D analog calcipotriene may also be effective for limited lesions. It appears to have much less impact on calcium metabolism (e.g., 100-fold less) than calcitriol. Calcipotriene can burn and sting, which limits its usefulness in children. In addition, several weeks of therapy are necessary before benefit is seen. For scalp lesions, applications of a phenol and saline solution (Baker P & S) followed by a tar shampoo are effective in the removal of scales. A corticosteroid in a solution, lotion, or gel base may be applied when the scaling is diminished. Rarely, the more severe forms of psoriasis may require systemic therapy.

The use of psoralens and UV light (PUVA) is effective in severe psoriasis in adults, but the safety of PUVA has not been established for children. Methotrexate, oral retinoids (in combination with PUVA), and cyclosporine are used for the rare severe and generalized forms of psoriasis. The retinoid etretinate is useful in severe disorders, has a half-life of approximately 120 days, and may have serious side effects; dermatologic consultation is essential when its use is being considered. Acitretin may hold more promise for pediatric patients, because the half-life of this synthetic retinoid is 2–4 days. Psoriasis in infants and acute guttate psoriasis may flare with vigorous treatment and should be managed conservatively. Nail lesions are usually recalcitrant to therapy.

Prognosis. This is best for children with limited disease. Psoriasis is characterized by remissions and exacerbations; if present during adolescence, it is a lifelong disease. Arthritis may be an extracutaneous complication.

PITYRIASIS LICHENOIDES. This has historically encompassed pityriasis lichenoides et varioliformis acuta (PLEVA, Mucha-Habermann disease), which tends to develop acutely, and pityriasis lichenoides chronica (PLC), which follows a chronic course. The designation of pityriasis lichenoides as acute or chronic may more properly refer to morphologic appearance of the lesions, which is often hemorrhagic or necrotic in PLEVA, than to the duration of the disease. In a series of 89 pediatric cases, no correlation was found between the type of lesion at the onset of the eruption and the duration of the disease. Many patients have both acute and chronic lesions simultaneously, and transition of lesions from one form into another occurs occasionally. There is a correlation between the distribution of lesions and the duration of disease: (1) Disease characterized by diffusely distributed lesions may resolve relatively quickly (mean disease duration 11 mo); (2) centrally distributed lesions on the trunk, neck, and/or proximal extremities are intermediate in duration; and (3) disease located peripherally or acrally usually persists the longest (mean 31 mo). Pityriasis lichenoides most commonly presents in the 2nd and 3rd decades; approximately one third of cases present before age 20 yr.

Clinical Manifestations. PLC presents with generalized, multiple, asymptomatic 3–5-mm brown-red papules that are covered by a grayish mica-like scale. A useful clinical sign is the easy detachment of the adherent scale, revealing a shining surface. Lesions may be asymptomatic or may cause minimal pruritus and occasionally become infiltrated, vesicular, hemorrhagic, and crusted. Individual papules become flat and brownish over 2–6 wk, ultimately leaving a hyperpigmented or hypopigmented macule. Scarring is unusual. Lesions are most common on the trunk and extremities and generally spare the face, palmoplantar surfaces, scalp, and mucous membranes. The eruption persists for months to years and is characterized by polymorphous lesions in various stages of evolution. PLC histologically shows a parakeratotic, thickened corneal layer; epidermal spongiosis; a superficial perivascular infiltrate of macrophages and predominantly CD8+ lymphocytes, which may extend into the epidermis; and small numbers of extravasated erythrocytes in the papillary dermis.

PLEVA presents with an abrupt eruption of numerous papules that have a vesiculopustular and then a purpuric center, are covered by a dark adherent crust, and are surrounded by an erythematous halo. Constitutional symptoms of fever, malaise, headache, and arthralgias may be present for 2–3 days after the initial outbreak. Lesions are distributed diffusely on the trunk and extremities, as in PLC. Individual lesions heal within a few weeks, sometimes leaving a varioliform scar, and successive crops of papules produce the characteristic polymorphous appearance of the eruption. The condition is generally self-limited from several weeks to months. The histopathologic changes of PLEVA reflect its more severe nature compared with PLC. Intercellular and intracellular edema in the epidermis may lead to degeneration of keratinocytes. A dense perivascular mononuclear cell infiltrate that extends upward into the epidermis and downward into the reticular dermis, endothelial cell swelling, and extravasation of erythrocytes into the epidermis and dermis are additional characteristic features. Severe changes of vasculitis are exceptional. Differential diagnosis includes guttate psoriasis, pityriasis rosea, drug eruptions, secondary syphilis, viral exanthems, and lichen planus. The chronicity of pityriasis lichenoides helps to preclude pityriasis rosea, viral exanthems, and some drug eruptions. A skin biopsy helps to preclude other differential diagnoses.

A rare form of PLEVA has been described as presenting with fever and ulceronecrotic plaques up to 1 cm in diameter; those are most common on the anterior trunk and flexors of the proximal upper extremities. Arthritis and superinfection of cutaneous lesions with *Staphylococcus aureus* may also develop. The ulceronecrotic lesions appear within papules of PLEVA and heal with hypopigmented scarring in a few weeks. Leukocytoclastic vasculitis is occasionally seen histopathologically. The eruption may resemble erythema multiforme, but it generally spares the mucous membranes.

Etiology. The cause of pityriasis lichenoides in unknown, but sporadic outbreaks have led to an unsuccessful search for an infectious agent, despite the fact that human-to-human transmission has not been documented. Nevertheless, a popular hypothesis is that pityriasis lichenoides is a hypersensitivity reaction to an infectious organism. Cell-mediated mechanisms appear to be important in the pathogenesis because most infiltrating cells are cytotoxic-suppressor cells. Clonal gene rearrangement studies of the T-cell receptor and immunohistologic studies have led to the suggestion that PLEVA may be a T-cell lymphoproliferative process. The condition in two children with PLEVA was reported to evolve into cutaneous T-cell lymphoma. It has been postulated that the relatively greater proportion of cytotoxic-suppressor cells than helper-inducer T cells in lesions of PLEVA compared with those of lymphomatoid papulosis or T-cell lymphoma reflects the more effective host response in PLEVA.

Treatment. In general, pityriasis lichenoides should be considered a benign condition that does not alter the health of the child. A lubricant to remove excessive scaling may be all that is necessary if the patient is asymptomatic. The most appropriate treatment includes erythromycin (30–50 mg/kg/24 hr for 2 mo) in combination with natural sunlight. If this regimen is effective, erythromycin should then be tapered slowly over several months. The rare febrile ulceronecrotic form may be controlled effectively by systemic corticosteroids. Additional modalities that have been effective in some adult patients but are rarely appropriate for children include PUVA, tetracycline, dapsone, and methotrexate.

KERATOSIS PILARIS. This moderately common papular eruption may vary in extent from sparse lesions over the extensor aspects of the limbs to involvement of most of the body surface; typical areas of involvement include the upper extensor arms and the thighs, cheeks, and buttocks. The lesions may resemble gooseflesh; they are noninflammatory, scaly, follicular papules that do not coalesce. Irritation of the follicular plugs occasionally causes folliculitis. Because the lesions are associated with and accentuated by dry skin, they are often more prominent during the winter. They are more frequent in patients with atopic dermatitis and are most common during childhood and early adulthood, tending to subside during the 3rd decade of life. Mild or localized eruptions respond to lubrication with a bland emollient; more pronounced or widespread lesions require regular applications of a 10–25% urea cream, an α-hydroxy acid preparation such as lactic acid in an emollient or in combination with a corticosteroid, or topical retinoic acid. Therapy may improve the condition but does not cure it.

LICHEN SPINULOSUS. This uncommon disorder occurs principally in children and more frequently in boys. The cause is unknown. The lesions consist of sharply circumscribed irregular plaques of spiny, keratinous projections that protrude from the orifices of the pilosebaceous canals (Fig. 663–2). Plaques may occur anywhere on the body and are often distributed symmetrically on the trunk, elbows, knees, and extensor surfaces of the limbs. Although sometimes erythematous, the lesions are usually skin colored. They are readily palpable and represent keratotic follicular plugs. Lichen spinulosus is easily differentiated from keratosis pilaris because the latter lesions are never grouped to form plaques. More commonly, it is confused with papular eczema.

Treatment is usually unnecessary. For patients who regard the eruption as a cosmetic defect, keratolytic agents such as salicylic acid ointment (3–7%), urea-containing lubricants (10–25%), and retinoic acid preparations are often effective in flattening the projections. The plaques usually disappear spontaneously after several months or years.

PITYRIASIS ROSEA. This benign, common eruption occurs most frequently in children and young adults. Although a prodrome of fever, malaise, arthralgia, and pharyngitis may precede the eruption, children rarely complain of such symptoms. The cause of pityriasis rosea is unknown; a viral agent is suspected.

Clinical Manifestations. A *herald patch*, a solitary, round or oval lesion that may occur anywhere on the body and is often but not always identifiable by its large size, usually precedes the generalized eruption. Herald patches vary from 1–10 cm in diameter; they are annular in configuration and have a raised border with fine, adherent scales. Approximately 5–10 days after the appearance of the herald patch, a widespread, symmetric eruption becomes evident involving mainly the trunk and proximal limbs (Fig. 663–3). When the disease is extensive, the face, scalp, and distal limbs may be involved, or, in the inverse form of pityriasis rosea, only those sites may be affected. Lesions may appear in crops for several days. Typical lesions are oval or round, less than 1 cm in diameter, slightly raised, and pink to brown. The developed lesion is covered by a fine scale that gives the skin a crinkly appearance; some lesions clear centrally, producing a collarette of scale that is attached only at the periphery. Papular, vesicular, urticarial, hemorrhagic, and large annular lesions are unusual variants. The long axis of each lesion is usually aligned with the cutaneous cleavage lines, a feature that creates the so-called Christmas tree pattern on the back. Actually, conformation to skin lines is often more discernible in the anterior and posterior axillary folds and supraclavicular areas. Duration of the eruption varies from 2–12 wk. The lesions may be asymptomatic or mildly to severely pruritic.

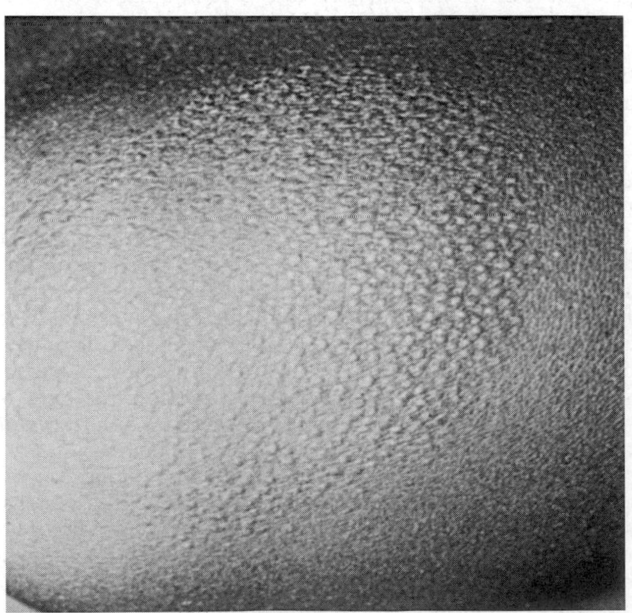

Figure 663–2 Sharply circumscribed plaque of follicular papules characteristic of lichen spinulosus.

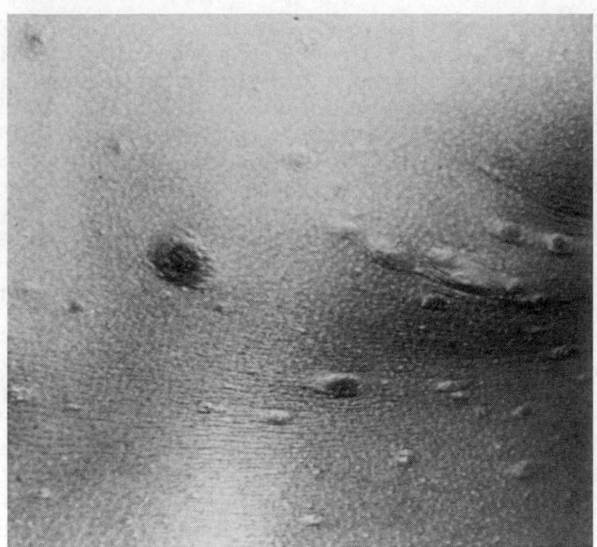

Figure 663–3 Ovoid, maculopapular lesions of pityriasis rosea. Note the distribution along the skin lines and the herald patch on the chest.

Diagnosis. This is clinical. The herald patch may be mistaken for tinea corporis, a pitfall that can be avoided if testing with a potassium hydroxide preparation is carried out. The generalized eruption resembles a number of other diseases; of these, secondary syphilis is the most important. Drug eruptions, viral exanthems, guttate psoriasis, PLC, and eczema can also be confused with pityriasis rosea.

Treatment. Therapy is unnecessary for asymptomatic patients. If scaling is prominent, a bland emollient may suffice. Pruritus may be suppressed by a lubricating lotion containing menthol and camphor or by an oral antihistamine for sedation, particularly at night, when itching may be troublesome. Occasionally, a nonfluorinated topical corticosteroid preparation may be necessary to alleviate pruritus. After the eruption has resolved, postinflammatory hypopigmentation or hyperpigmentation may be pronounced, particularly in black patients; these changes disappear during subsequent weeks to months.

PITYRIASIS RUBRA PILARIS. This rare chronic dermatosis often has an insidious onset with diffuse scaling and erythema of the scalp, which is indistinguishable from seborrheic dermatitis, and with thick hyperkeratosis of the palms and soles. The characteristic primary lesion is a firm, dome-shaped, tiny, acuminate papule, which is pink to red and has a central keratotic plug pierced by a vellus hair. Masses of these papules coalesce to form large, erythematous, sharply demarcated orangish plaques, within which islands of normal skin can be distinguished, creating a bizarre effect. Typical papules on the dorsum of the proximal phalanges are readily palpated. Gray plaques or papules resembling lichen planus may be found in the oral cavity. Dystrophic changes in the nails may occur and mimic those of psoriasis. In advanced stages, marked hyperkeratosis of the scalp and face may cause alopecia and ectropion. Differential diagnosis includes ichthyosis, seborrheic dermatitis, keratoderma of the palms and soles, and psoriasis.

Etiology. The cause is unknown. A genetic form with autosomal dominant transmission may account for some cases in childhood, but most appear to be sporadic. Attempts to link the disease with a defect in vitamin A metabolism have not been definitive. Skin biopsy may help to differentiate this condition from psoriasis and seborrheic dermatitis, which it resembles most closely.

Treatment. The numerous therapeutic regimens recommended are difficult to evaluate because the disease has a capricious course with exacerbations and remissions. Oral and topical retinoids and vitamin A have been used most frequently. When vitamin A or synthetic retinoids are administered orally, the child should be observed carefully for signs of toxicity (see Psoriasis, Treatment). In childhood, the *prognosis* for eventual resolution is relatively good.

DARIER DISEASE (KERATOSIS FOLLICULARIS). This rare genetic disorder is inherited as an autosomal dominant trait. Onset occurs usually during late childhood. Typical lesions are small, firm, skin-colored papules that are not always follicular in location. The lesions eventually acquire yellow, malodorous crusts; coalesce to form large, gray-brown, vegetative plaques; and usually involve the face, neck, shoulders, chest, back, and limb flexures in a symmetric distribution. Papules, fissures, crusts, and ulcers may appear on the mucous membranes of the lips, tongue, buccal mucosa, pharynx, larynx, and vulva. Hyperkeratosis of the palms and soles and nail dystrophy with subungual hyperkeratosis are variable features. Severe pruritus, secondary infection, offensive odor, and aggravation of the dermatosis on exposure to sunlight may occur. Darier disease is most likely to be confused with seborrheic dermatitis or juvenile flat warts. Histologic changes are diagnostic: Hyperkeratosis, intraepidermal separation with formation of suprabasal clefts, and dyskeratotic epidermal cells are characteristic features.

Treatment is nonspecific. Some patients have responded to topical vitamin A or retinoic acid, with or without occlusive dressings. Severe disease may be controlled with oral synthetic retinoids. Secondary infection may require local cleansing and systemically administered antibiotics. Affected individuals usually suffer more during the summer.

LICHEN NITIDUS. This chronic, benign, papular eruption is characterized by minute (1–2 mm), flat-topped, shiny, firm papules of uniform size; these are most often skin colored but may be pink or red. In black individuals, they are usually hypopigmented. Sites of predilection are the genitals, abdomen, chest, forearms, wrists, and inner aspects of the thighs. The lesions may be sparse or numerous and form large plaques; careful examination usually discloses linear papules in a line of scratch (Koebner phenomenon), a valuable clue to the diagnosis because it occurs in only a few diseases (Fig. 663–4). Lichen nitidus occurs in all age groups. The cause is unknown. Patients are usually asymptomatic and constitutionally well. The lesions may be confused with those of lichen planus and rarely coexist with them.

Widespread keratosis pilaris can also be confused with lichen nitidus, but the follicular localization of the papules and the absence of Koebner phenomenon in the former distinguish them. Verruca plana (flat warts), if small and uniform in size, may occasionally resemble lichen nitidus. Although the diagnosis can be made clinically, a biopsy is occasionally indicated. Histopathologically, the lichen nitidus papule consists of sharply circumscribed nests of lymphocytes and histiocytes in the upper dermis enclosed by clawlike epidermal rete ridges. The course of lichen nitidus spans months to years, but the lesions eventually involute completely. There is no effective therapy.

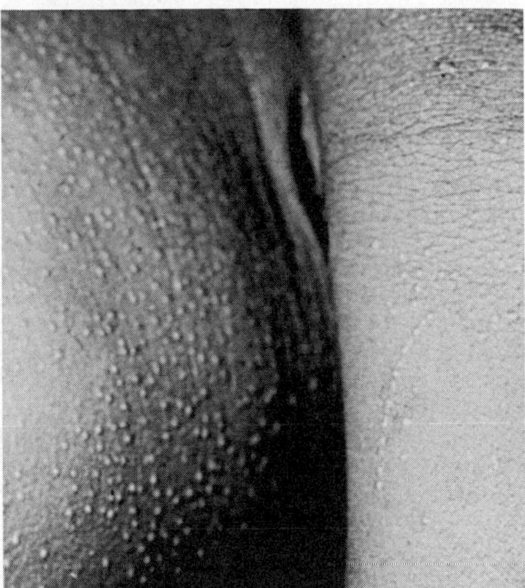

Figure 663–4 Tiny flat-topped papules of lichen nitidus on the arm and trunk. Note the Koebner response on the arm (papules in a line of scratch).

LICHEN STRIATUS. This benign, self-limited eruption consists of a continuous or discontinuous linear band of papules in a zosteriform distribution. The primary lesion is a flat-topped, red to violaceous papule covered with fine scale. Aggregates of these papules form multiple bands or plaques (Fig. 663–5). In black patients, the lesions may be hypopigmented. The cause and explanation for the linear distribution are unknown. The eruption evolves over a period of days or weeks in an otherwise healthy child, remains stationary for weeks to months, and finally remits without sequelae. Symptoms are usually absent; some children complain of itching. Nail dystrophy may occur when the eruption involves the posterior nail fold and matrix.

Lichen striatus is occasionally confused with other disorders. The initial plaque may resemble papular eczema or lichen nitidus until the linear configuration becomes apparent. Linear lichen planus and linear psoriasis are usually associated with

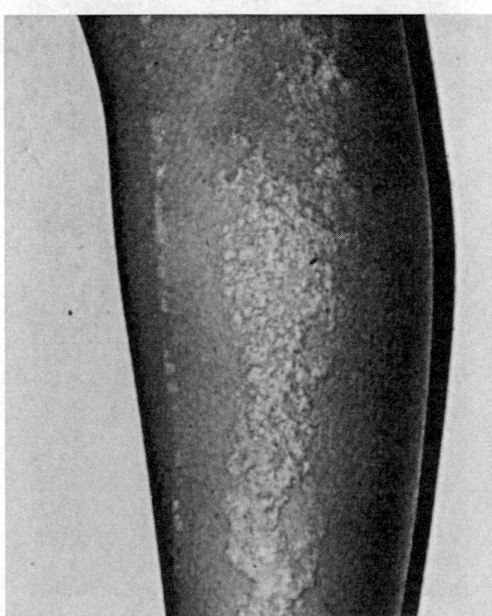

Figure 663–5 Multiple linear plaques and streaks of lichen striatus.

typical individual lesions elsewhere on the body. Linear epidermal nevi are permanent lesions that often become more hyperkeratotic and hyperpigmented than those of lichen striatus. A lubricating lotion containing menthol and camphor or a mild corticosteroid preparation provides sufficient relief when pruritus is a problem.

LICHEN PLANUS. This is a rare disorder in young children and uncommon in older ones. The primary lesion is a violaceous, sharply demarcated, polygonal papule with fine lines or thin white scales on the surface; papules may coalesce to form large plaques. The papules are intensely pruritic, and additional ones are often induced by scratching (Koebner phenomenon) so that lines of them are often detected (Fig. 663–6). Sites of predilection are the flexor surfaces of the wrists, forearms, and inner aspects of the thighs. Characteristic lesions of mucous membranes consist of pinhead-sized white papules that coalesce to form reticulated and lacy patterns on the oral mucosa and sometimes on the lips and tongue.

Acute eruptive lichen planus is probably the most common form in children. The lesions erupt in an explosive fashion, much like a viral exanthem, and spread to involve most of the body surface. Hypertrophic, linear, bullous, atrophic, annular, follicular, erosive, and ulcerative forms of lichen planus may also occur. Nail involvement may develop in the chronic forms but is rarely evident in children (see Chapter 669). The disorder may persist for months to years, but the acute eruptive form is most likely to involute permanently. Intense hyperpigmentation frequently persists for a long time after the resolution of lesions. The histopathologic findings of lichen planus are specific, and a biopsy is indicated if the diagnosis is unclear.

Treatment is directed at alleviation of the intense pruritus and amelioration of the skin lesions. Oral antihistamines and/or tranquilizers are often helpful. The skin lesions respond best to regular applications of a topical corticosteroid preparation. Rarely, systemic corticosteroid therapy is necessary to gain control of widespread, intractable lesions.

POROKERATOSIS. This rare, chronic, progressive disease is inherited as an autosomal dominant trait. Several forms have been delineated: solitary plaques, linear porokeratosis, hyperkeratotic lesions of the palms and soles, disseminated eruptive lesions, and superficial actinic porokeratosis. The last form, probably induced by excessive sun exposure, occurs more commonly in women. Other types of porokeratosis are more common in males and begin during childhood. Sites of predilection are the limbs, face, neck, and genitals. The primary lesion is a small, keratotic papule that enlarges peripherally so that the center becomes depressed, with the edge forming an elevated wall or collar. The configuration of the plaque may be round, oval, or gyrate; its elevated border is split by a thin groove from which minute cornified projections protrude. The enclosed central area is yellow, gray, or tan and sclerotic, smooth, and dry, whereas the hyperkeratotic border is a darker gray, brown, or black.

The differential diagnosis includes warts, epidermal nevi, lichen planus, granuloma annulare, and elastosis perforans serpiginosa. A skin biopsy discloses the characteristic cornoid lamella (plug of stratum corneum cells with retained nuclei), which is responsible for the invariable linear ridge of the lesion. The disease is slowly progressive but relatively asymptomatic. Lesions are sometimes responsive to applications of liquid nitrogen or occasionally may be surgically excised. Topical agents such as retinoic acid and 5-fluorouracil may be effective in some patients.

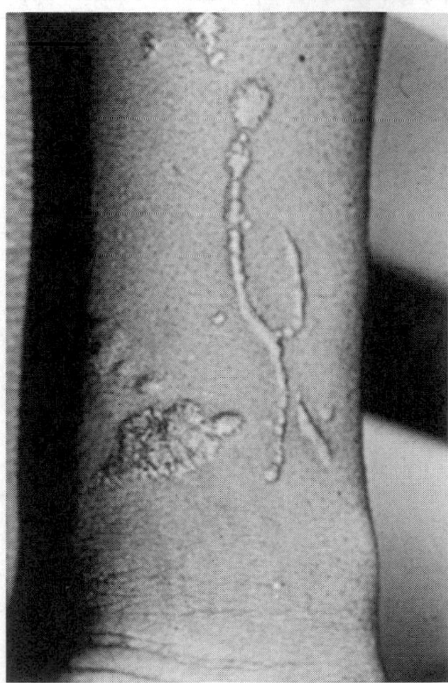

Figure 663–6 Violaceous polygonal papules of lichen planus. Note the striking Koebner response.

PAPULAR ACRODERMATITIS OF CHILDHOOD (GIANOTTI-CROSTI SYNDROME). This distinctive eruption is occasionally associated with malaise and low-grade fever but few other constitutional symptoms. The incidence peaks in early childhood. Occurrences are usually sporadic, but epidemics have been recorded. The skin lesion is a monomorphous, usually nonpruritic, dusky or coppery red, flat-topped, firm papule ranging in size from 1–5 mm. The papules appear in crops and may become profuse but remain discrete, forming a symmetric eruption on the face, buttocks, and limbs, including the palms and soles. The papules often have the appearance of vesicles; when opened, however, no fluid is obtained. The papules sometimes become hemorrhagic. Lines of papules (Koebner phenomenon) may be noted on the extremities. The trunk is relatively spared, as are the scalp and mucous membranes. Generalized lymphadenopathy and hepatomegaly (in those with hepatitis B viremia) constitute the only other abnormal physical findings. The eruption resolves spontaneously in about 15–60 days. Lymphadenopathy and hepatomegaly, if present, may persist for several months. This eruption in Italy was initially associated with primary liver infection by hepatitis B virus and surface antigenemia. Elevation of serum transaminase and alkaline phosphatase values without concomitant hyperbilirubinemia was usual. Skin biopsy was characterized by a perivascular mononuclear cell infiltrate and capillary endothelial swelling.

Generally, the disease is benign and is not associated with hepatitis in the United States. This eruption has been seen in children infected with Epstein-Barr virus, coxsackievirus A16, parainfluenza virus, and other viral infections. Papular acrodermatitis can be confused with lichen planus, erythema multiforme, histiocytosis X, and Henoch-Schönlein purpura.

ACANTHOSIS NIGRICANS. This is characterized by hyperpigmented, velvety, hyperkeratotic plaques that are most often localized to the neck, axillae, inframammary areas, groin, inner thighs, and anogenital region. The histologic changes are those of papillomatosis and hyperkeratosis rather than acanthosis or excessive pigment formation. Acanthosis nigricans has classically been associated with obesity; drugs such as nicotinic acid; endocrinopathies, including diabetes mellitus, Addison disease, Cushing syndrome, acromegaly, hypo- and hyperthyroidism, Stein-Leventhal syndrome, and hyperandrogenic or hypogonadal syndromes; many different syndromes such as Bloom, Crouzon, or Rud syndromes, Wilson disease, lipoatrophic diabetes, partial lipodystrophy, and leprechaunism; and malignancies, usually in adults with an abdominal adenocarcinoma. It may occasionally be familial, with autosomal dominant inheritance. Acanthosis nigricans is found in 7% of children and is nearly always associated with obesity; this form is termed pseudoacanthosis nigricans.

The skin lesions appear to be a manifestation of insulin resistance. The clinical severity and histopathologic features of acanthosis nigricans correlate positively with the degree of hyperinsulinism. It has been hypothesized that insulin resistance, with compensatory hyperinsulinism, leads to insulin binding to and activation of insulin-like growth factor receptors, promoting epidermal growth. In the malignant form, tumor-secreted growth factors and hyperinsulinemia could be pathogenic.

This skin disorder is extremely difficult to treat but may be improved by palliation of the underlying disorder, weight loss in the case of pseudoacanthosis nigricans, reduction in insulin resistance, and topical or oral retinoids.

Caputo R, Gelmetti C, Ermacora E, et al: Gianotti-Crosti syndrome: A retrospective analysis of 308 cases. J Am Acad Dermatol 26:207, 1992.

Farber EM, Muller RH, Jacobs AH, et al: Infantile psoriasis: A follow-up study. Pediatr Dermatol 3:237, 1986.

Forston JS, Schroeter AL, Esterly NB: Cutaneous T-cell lymphoma (parapsoriasis en plaque). An association with pityriasis lichenoides et varioliformis acuta in young children. Arch Dermatol 126:1449, 1990.

Gelmetti C, Rigoni C, Alessi E, et al: Pityriasis lichenoides in children: A long term follow-up of eighty-nine cases. J Am Acad Dermatol 23:473, 1990.

Luberti AA, Rabinowitz LG, Verrereli KO: Severe febrile Mucha-Habermann's disease in children: Case report and review of the literature. Pediatr Dermatol 8:51, 1991.

Rogers M: Pityriasis lichenoides and lymphomatoid papulosis. Semin Dermatol 11:73, 1992.

Stern R: Psoriasis. Lancet 350:349, 1997.

Taieb A, Youbi E, Grosshans E, et al: Lichen striatus: A Blaschko linear acquired inflammatory skin eruption. J Am Acad Dermatol 25:637, 1991.

Truhan AP, Herbert AA, Esterly NB: Pityriasis lichenoides in children: Therapeutic response to erythromycin. J Am Acad Dermatol 15:66, 1986.

CHAPTER 664
Disorders of Keratinization

DISORDERS OF CORNIFICATION. Disorders of cornification, also known as the ichthyoses, are a primary group of inherited conditions characterized clinically by patterns of scaling and histopathologically by hyperkeratosis. They are usually distinguishable on the basis of inheritance patterns, clinical features, associated defects, and histopathologic changes. Because some of these conditions cause disfigurement and considerable psychosocial stress, early diagnosis is helpful to predict probable course and prognosis and to provide supportive management for patients and families.

HARLEQUIN FETUS. This rare keratinizing disorder probably represents several genotypes with similar clinical manifestations. At birth, markedly thickened, ridged, and cracked skin forms horny plates over the entire body, disfiguring the facial features and constricting the digits. Severe ectropion and chemosis obscure the orbits, the nose and ears are flattened, and the lips are everted and gaping. Nails and hair may be absent. Joint mobility is restricted, and the hands and feet appear fixed and ischemic. Affected neonates have respiratory difficulty, suck poorly, and are subject to severe cutaneous infection. Most die within the 1st days to weeks of life, but patients occasionally survive beyond infancy and have severe ichthyosis and variable neurologic impairment. Ectropion and eclabium resolve, and the cracked, horny plated skin is replaced by large, thin scales with surrounding erythema.

Inheritance is autosomal recessive. Common morphologic abnormalities include hyperkeratosis, accumulation of lipid droplets within corneocytes, and absence of normal lamellar granules. One type has an altered catalytic subunit of 2A protein phosphorylase, which is encoded on chromosome 11. The basic defect of all types is suggested to be an abnormality of lamellar granules, which have an important role in desquamation.

Initial treatment includes high fluid intake to avoid dehydration from transepidermal water loss and use of a humidified heated incubator, emulsifying ointments, careful attention to hygiene, and oral retinoids such as etretinate. Survivors after retinoid therapy have shown severe congenital ichthyosiform erythroderma. Prenatal diagnosis has been accomplished by fetoscopy, fetal skin biopsy, and microscopic examination of cells from amniotic fluid taken at the 17th and 21st wk of gestation.

COLLODION BABY. These infants are covered at birth by a thick, taut membrane resembling oiled parchment or collodion, which is subsequently shed. The condition is usually a manifestation of congenital ichthyosiform erythroderma or lamellar ichthyosis; like a harlequin fetus, a collodion baby appears to be one phenotype for several genotypes. Infrequently, an affected infant has normal skin after the membrane is shed. Affected neonates have ectropion, flattening of the ears and nose, and fixation of the lips in an O-shaped configuration (Fig. 664–1). Hair may be absent or may perforate the horny covering. The membrane cracks with initial respiratory efforts and, shortly after birth, begins to desquamate in large sheets. Complete shedding may take several weeks, and a new membrane may occasionally form in localized areas.

Neonatal morbidity and deaths may be due to cutaneous infection, aspiration pneumonia (squamous material), hypothermia, or hypernatremic dehydration from excessive transcutaneous fluid losses as a result of increased skin permeability. The outcome is uncertain, and accurate prognosis is impossible with respect to the subsequent development of ichthyosis. Treatment with a high-humidity environment and application of nonocclusive lubricants may facilitate shedding of the membrane.

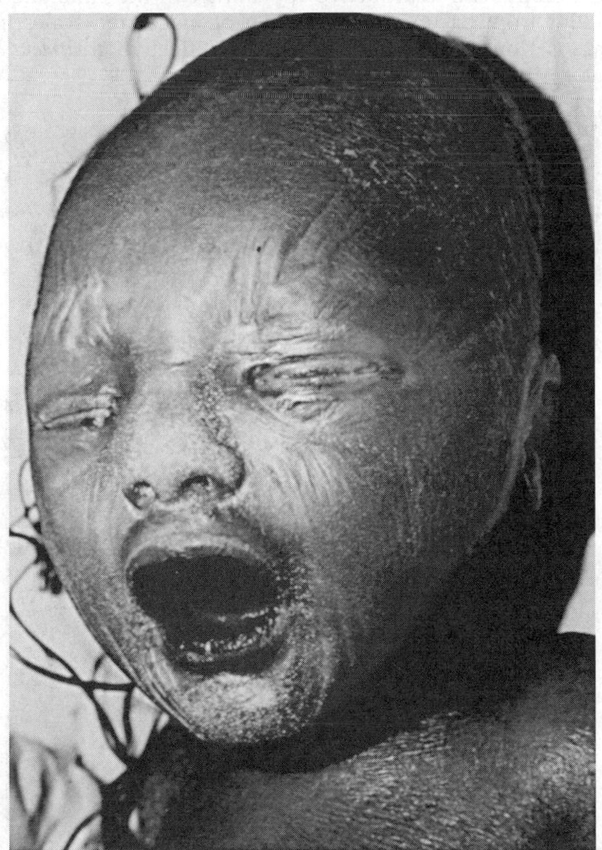

Figure 664–1 Typical facial appearance of a collodion baby.

LAMELLAR ICHTHYOSIS AND CONGENITAL ICHTHYOSIFORM ERYTHRODERMA (NONBULLOUS CONGENITAL ICHTHYOSIFORM ERYTHRODERMA). There are two major forms of autosomal recessively inherited ichthyosis. Both forms are present soon or shortly after birth and are the most common forms of ichthyosis to present as collodion babies, although most infants present with erythroderma and scaling.

After shedding of the collodion membrane, if present, *lamellar ichthyosis* evolves into large, quadilateral dark scales that are free at the edges and adherent at the center. Scaling is often pronounced and involves the entire body surface, including flexural surfaces. The face is often markedly involved, including ectropion and crumpled, small ears. The palms and soles are generally hyperkeratotic (Fig. 664–2). The hair may be sparse and fine, but the teeth and mucosal surfaces are normal. In contrast to congenital ichthyosiform erythroderma, there is little erythema. Neither form includes blistering.

In *congenital ichthyosiform erythroderma,* erythroderma tends to be persistent, and scales, although they are generalized, are finer and whiter than in lamellar ichthyosis. Erythema decreases in later life and may disappear in middle age, whereas scaling persists and may even worsen with age. Hyperkeratosis is particularly noticeable around the knees, elbows, and ankles. Palms and soles are uniformly hyperkeratotic. Some patients have sparse hair; cicatricial alopecia and nail dystrophy are found occasionally.

On histopathologic examination, lamellar ichthyosis is characterized by a markedly thickened stratum corneum and mild irregular epidermal thickening. Congenital ichthyosiform erythroderma has more epidermal thickening with parakeratosis but less hyperkeratosis and hypergranulosis than in lamellar ichthyosis. In congenital ichthyosiform erythroderma, there is a marked increase in the rate of epidermal cell production, considerably greater than the slightly increased rate observed in patients with lamellar ichthyosis.

Pruritus may be severe and responds minimally to antipruritic therapy. The unattractive appearance of the child and the malodor from bacterial colonization of macerated scales may create serious psychologic problems. Effective *treatment* includes prolonged baths with bath oil to remove excessive scales. Restriction of bathing, on the erroneous premise that accentuation of dryness will occur, only promotes malodor and accumulation of keratinous debris and contributes to pruritus and discomfort. A high-humidity environment in winter and air conditioning in summer reduce discomfort. Generous and frequent applications of emollients and keratolytic agents such as lactic or glycolic acid (5%), urea (10–25%), and retinoic acid (0.1% cream) may lessen the scaling to some extent, although these agents produce stinging if applied to fissured skin. Oral retinoids have a beneficial effect in these conditions but do not alter the underlying defect and, therefore, must be administered indefinitely. The long-term risks of these compounds (e.g., teratogenic effects and toxicity to bone) limit their usefulness. Ectropion requires ophthalmologic care and, at times, plastic procedures. Genetic counseling should be provided.

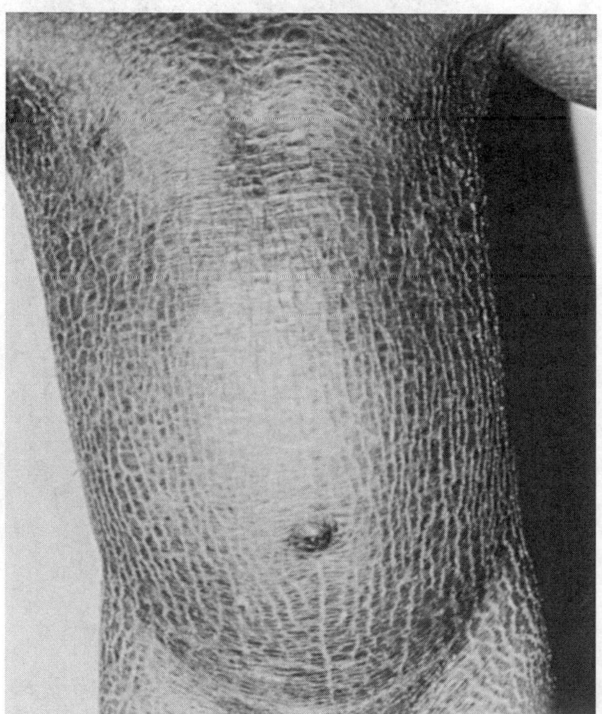

Figure 664–2 Generalized scaling of lamellar ichthyosis. Note the involvement of the axillary areas.

ICHTHYOSIS VULGARIS. This autosomal dominant ichthyosis is the most common of the disorders of keratinization, with an incidence of approximately 1/300 live births. Onset generally occurs sometime after birth during the 1st yr of life and, in most cases, is trivial, consisting only of slight roughening of the skin surface. In rare cases, infants have presented as collodian babies. Scaling is most prominent on the extensor aspects of the extremities, particularly the legs and back. Flexural surfaces are spared, and the abdomen, neck, and face are relatively uninvolved. Keratosis pilaris, particularly on the upper arms and thighs, accentuated markings and hyperkeratosis on the palms and soles, and atopy are relatively common. Scaling is most pronounced during the winter months and may abate completely during warm weather. The condition may improve and even disappear with age. There is no accompanying disorder of hair, teeth, mucosal surfaces, or other organ systems.

The histopathologic changes differ from those of other types of ichthyosis in that the hyperkeratosis is associated with a decreased or absent granular layer. Abnormally small and crumbly keratohyalin granules are found in epidermal cells on electron microscopy. The rate of epidermal proliferation is normal; rather, the hyperkeratosis is due to defective desquamation. Profilaggrin, which has a role in desmosome dissolution, is deficient.

Scaling may be diminished by use of bath oil and daily applications of an emollient or a lubricant containing urea, salicylic acid, or an α-hydroxy acid, such as lactic acid.

X-LINKED ICHTHYOSIS. X-linked ichthyosis is largely limited to males, although female carriers may display some clinical manifestations of the disorder. Skin peeling may be present at birth but typically abates until 3–6 mo of life. Scaling is most pronounced on the sides of the neck, lower face, preauricular areas, anterior trunk, and the limbs, particularly the legs. The elbow and knee flexures are generally spared but may be mildly involved. The palms and soles may be slightly thickened but are also usually spared. The condition gradually worsens in severity and extent. Keratosis pilaris is not present, and there is no increased incidence of atopy. Deep corneal opacities that do not interfere with vision develop during late childhood or adolescence and are a useful marker for the disease because they may also be present in carrier females. Cryptorchidism occurs in approximately 25% of affected males, although this may reflect an association with Kallmann syndrome, which also involves deletion on the short arm of the X chromosome. Testicular carcinoma occurs in some patients. Histologic changes include hyperkeratosis of the stratum corneum, a well-developed granular layer, and a hyperplastic epidermis.

As in ichthyosis vulgaris, the rate of epidermal proliferation is normal, and the hyperkeratosis is due to retention of corneocytes and delayed dissolution of the desmosomal disks. X-linked ichthyosis, however, involves a deficiency of steroid sulfatase, which hydrolyzes cholesterol sulfate and other sulfated steroids to cholesterol; cholesterol sulfate accumulates in the stratum corneum and plasma and may cause hyperkeratosis by inhibiting desmosomal proteolysis. Elevated cholesterol sulfate levels can be demonstrated in the serum, erythrocyte membranes, and epidermal cells and scales of affected males. Reduced enzyme activity can be detected in fibroblasts, keratinocytes, and leukocytes and, prenatally, in amniocytes or chorionic villus cells. In affected families, an affected male can be detected by restriction enzyme analysis of cultured chorionic villus cell DNA or amniocytes or by in situ hybridization, which identifies steroid sulfatase gene deletions prenatally in chorionic villus cells. A placental steroid sulfatase deficiency in carrier mothers results in low urinary and serum estriol values, prolonged labor, and insensitivity of the uterus to oxytocin and prostaglandins. The gene for steroid sulfatase is located on the short arm of the X chromosome (Xp22.3). Correction of steroid sulfatase deficiency is accomplished by gene transfer into tissue-cultured keratinocytes.

Hydration by bathing with bath oil and daily application of emollients and a urea-containing lubricant are usually effective *treatments*. Glycolic or lactic acid (5%) in an emollient base and propylene glycol 40–60% in water with occlusion overnight are alternative forms of therapy.

EPIDERMOLYTIC HYPERKERATOSIS (BULLOUS CONGENITAL ICHTHYOSIFORM ERYTHRODERMA). Epidermolytic hyperkeratosis is inherited as an autosomal dominant trait, although many cases are sporadic. The *clinical manifestations* are characterized by the onset at birth of generalized erythroderma and severe hyperkeratosis. The scales are small, hard, and verrucous; distinctive, parallel hyperkeratotic ridges develop over the joint flexures, including the axillary, popliteal, and antecubital fossas, and on the neck and hips. Erythema becomes less prominent after infancy; however, the hyperkeratosis persists throughout adult life. Recurrent blistering may be widespread in neonates and may cause diagnostic confusion with other blistering disorders. Blistering becomes accentuated at sites of trauma such as the knees, elbows, and lower limbs but is not problematic after age 7–8 yr. The palms and soles may be thickened, but the hair, nails, mucosa, and sweat glands are normal. Secondary bacterial infection is common and requires appropriate antibiotic therapy. Severely affected patients may have crumpled ears and ectropion.

The histopathologic pattern is *diagnostic* and consists of hyperkeratosis, a markedly thickened granular layer with an increased number of keratohyalin granules, clear spaces around nuclei, and indistinct cellular boundaries of cells in the upper epidermis. On electron microscopic examination, keratin intermediate filaments are clumped, and many desmosomes are attached to only one keratinocyte instead of connecting neighboring keratinocytes. Epidermolytic hyperkeratosis has been shown to be due to defects in either keratin 1 or 10 encoded in chromosome 12p, where the type II keratin genes are clustered. These keratins are required to form the keratin intermediate filaments in cells of the suprabasilar layers of the epidermis. Localized forms of the disease may resemble epidermal nevi (ichthyosis hystrix) or keratoderma of the palms and soles but share the distinctive histopathologic changes of epidermolytic hyperkeratosis. Prenatal diagnosis for affected families is now possible by examination of DNA extracts from chorionic villus cells or amniocytes, provided that the specific mutation in the affected parent is known.

Treatment is difficult. Morbidity is increased in the neonatal period as a result of prematurity, sepsis, and fluid and electrolyte imbalance. Bacterial colonization of macerated scales produces a distinctive malodor that can be controlled somewhat by use of an antibacterial cleanser. Intermittent oral antibiotics generally are necessary. Keratolytic agents are often poorly tolerated. Oral retinoids (e.g., etretinate, acitretin, isotretinoin) may produce significant improvement, even at relatively low doses. Genetic counseling should be provided.

ICHTHYOSIS LINEARIS CIRCUMFLEXA. This rare autosomal recessive disorder presents at birth or in the first few months of life with generalized erythema and scaling. The trunk and limbs have diffuse erythema and superimposed migratory, polycyclic, and serpiginous hyperkeratotic lesions, some with a distinctive double-edged margin of scale. Lichenification or hyperkeratosis tends to persist in the antecubital and popliteal fossas. The face and scalp may remain erythematous and scaling. Many hair shaft deformities, most notably trichorrhexis invaginata, have been described in more than half of patients. This type of ichthyosis is characteristic of patients with Netherton syndrome (see later). Nonspecific psoriasiform changes are found on histopathologic examination.

ERYTHROKERATODERMA VARIABILIS. This autosomal dominant disorder with genetic linkage to the Rh blood group usually presents in the early months of life, progresses in childhood, and stabilizes in adolescence. It is characterized by sharply demarcated hyperkeratotic plaques with geographic borders that develop in areas of normal skin or within discrete erythematous patches. Patches of erythema change shape or size within minutes to hours or days or migrate, and they may gradually became hyperkeratotic and fixed. The distribution is generalized but sparse; sites of predilection are the face, buttocks, axillae, and extensor surfaces of the limbs. The palms and soles may be thickened, but hair, teeth, and nails are normal. Histopathologic changes include hyperkeratosis, papillomatosis, and irregular hyperplasia of the epidermis.

Symmetric progressive erythrokeratoderma is an autosomal dominant disorder that presents in childhood with large, fixed, geographic and symmetric fine, scaling, hyperkeratotic, erythematous plaques primarily on the extremities, buttocks, face, ankles, and wrists. Palmoplantar keratoderma is also present. The primary feature distinguishing this from erythrokeratoderma variabilis is the lack of variable erythema, as seen in the latter condition. These two conditions may be manifestations of the same disorder.

ICHTHYOSIFORM DERMATOSES. Several syndromes that include ichthyosis as a constant feature have been established as rare but distinct entities.

Sjögren-Larsson Syndrome. This autosomal recessive inborn error of metabolism consists of ichthyosis of the lamellar or congenital ichthyosiform erythroderma types, mental retardation, and spasticity. The ichthyosis is generalized but is accentuated on the flexures and the lower abdomen and consists of erythroderma, fine scaling, larger platelike scales, and dark hyperkeratosis. A degenerative defect of retinal pigment epithelium has been detected in 20–30% of affected individuals. Glistening dots in the foveal area are a cardinal ophthalmologic sign. Motor and speech developmental delays are usually noted before 1 yr of age, and spastic diplegia or tetraplegia, epilepsy, and mental retardation generally become evident within the first 3 yr of life. Some patients may walk with the aid of braces, but most are confined to a wheelchair. The primary defect is an abnormality of fatty alcohol oxidation as a result of a deficiency of fatty aldehyde dehydrogenase, a component of the fatty alcohol–nicotinamide adenine dinucleotide oxidoreductase enzyme complex. This deficiency can be demonstrated in cultured skin fibroblasts of affected patients and carriers and, prenatally, in cultured chorionic villus cells and amniocytes from affected fetuses.

Netherton Syndrome. This autosomal recessive disorder is characterized by ichthyosis (usually ichthyosis linearis circumflexa but, occasionally, the lamellar or congenital ichthyosiform erythroderma types), trichorrhexis invaginata, and other hair shaft anomalies such as pili torti or trichorrhexis nodosa, and atopic diathesis (see Chapter 668). The ichthyosis is present in the first 10 days of life and may be especially marked around the eyes, mouth, and perineal area. The erythroderma often is intensified after infection. Infants may suffer from failure to thrive, recurrent bacterial and candidal infections, elevated serum IgE levels, and marked hypernatremic dehydration. Scalp hair is sparse and short and fractures easily; eyebrows, eyelashes, and body hair are also abnormal. The most frequent allergic manifestations are urticaria, angioedema, atopic dermatitis, and asthma. Some patients are mentally retarded. The characteristic hair abnormality is seen on electron microscopy as invagination of the distal end of the hair shaft into the proximal end.

Refsum Syndrome (see Chapter 83.2). This multisystem disorder is inherited as an autosomal recessive trait and becomes symptomatic during the 2nd or 3rd decade of life. The ichthyosis may be generalized, is relatively mild, and resembles ichthyosis vulgaris. The ichthyosis may also be localized to the palms and soles. Chronic polyneuritis with progressive paralysis and ataxia, atypical retinitis pigmentosa, anosmia, deafness, bony abnormalities, and electrocardiographic changes are the most characteristic features. This condition is diagnosed by lipid analysis of the blood or skin, which shows elevated phytanic acid levels. Dietary avoidance of phytanic acid–containing green vegetables and dairy products produces clinical improvement.

Chondrodysplasia Punctata (see Chapter 83.2). This includes several genetically heterogeneous disorders marked by ichthyosis and bone changes, principally *Conradi-Hunermann syndrome*, an X-linked dominant form affecting females only, and *rhizomelic dwarfism*, transmitted as an autosomal recessive trait. Nearly all with the X-linked dominant form and approximately 25% of patients with the recessive type have cutaneous lesions, ranging from severe, generalized erythema and scaling to mild hyperkeratosis. Rhizomelic chondrodysplasia punctata is associated with cataracts, hypertelorism, optic nerve atrophy, disproportionate shortening of the proximal extremities, psychomotor retardation, failure to thrive, and spasticity; most patients die during infancy. Numerous dysfunctional peroxisomal enzymes are found in patients with rhizomelic chondrodysplasia. Patients with the X-linked dominant form have asymmetric, variable shortening of the limbs and a distinctive ichthyosiform eruption at birth. Thick, yellow, tightly adherent keratinized plaques are distributed in a whorled pattern over the entire body, which may be intensely erythematous. The histologic changes include hyperkeratosis that penetrates to the depths of the hair follicles. The eruption typically resolves during infancy and may be superseded by a follicular atrophoderma and patchy alopecia.

Additional features in all variants include cataracts and abnormal facies with saddle nose and frontal bossing. The pathognomonic defect, termed chondrodysplasia punctata, is stippled epiphyses in the cartilaginous skeleton. This defect, which is seen in various settings and inherited disorders, often in association with peroxisomal deficiency, disappears by approximately age 3–4 yr.

Recessive X-linked chondrodysplasia punctata is due to a contiguous gene deletion affecting the recessive X-linked ichthyosis locus. These patients are deficient in steroid sulfatase activity, and their scaling resembles that in X-linked ichthyosis; peroxisomal function is normal.

Rud Syndrome. This consists of mental retardation, epilepsy, ichthyosis (type uncertain), and sexual infantilism. Associated defects of the skeleton, eyes, dentition, and hearing have also been reported.

A number of other rare syndromes with ichthyosis as a consistent feature include the following: ichthyosis with keratitis and deafness (KID syndrome); ichthyosis with defective hair having a banded pattern under polarized light and a low sulfur content (trichothiodystrophy), hypogonadism, and mental and growth retardation (Tay syndrome); multiple sulfatase deficiency; neutral lipid storage disease with ichthyosis (Chanarin-Dorfman syndrome); and CHILD syndrome (congenital hemidysplasia with ichthyosiform erythroderma and limb defects).

KERATODERMA OF PALMS AND SOLES (KERATOSIS PALMARIS ET PLANTARIS). Excessive hyperkeratosis of the palms and soles may occur as a manifestation of a focal or generalized congenital hereditary skin disorder or may result from such chronic skin diseases as psoriasis, eczema, pityriasis rubra pilaris, lupus erythematosus, or Reiter disease. The names of individual disorders have been based on descriptive titles, modes of inheritance, histopathologic findings, and biochemical defects.

Diffuse Hyperkeratosis of Palms and Soles (Unna-Thost Syndrome, Tylosis). This autosomal dominant disorder presents in the first few months of life with erythema that gradually progresses to sharply demarcated hyperkeratotic scaling plaques over the palms and soles. The margins of the plaques often remain red; plaques may extend along the lateral aspects of the hands and feet and onto the volar wrists and the heels. Hyperhidrosis is usually present, but hair, teeth, and nails are usually normal. Dermatophyte infections are common and difficult to treat. Mutations in the gene for keratin 1 on chromosome 12 appear to underlie the disorder. Striate and punctate forms of palmar and plantar hyperkeratosis represent distinct entities.

Epidermolytic Hyperkeratosis. This type of hyperkeratosis, which is localized to the palms and soles, is an autosomal dominant defect involving mutations in the gene for keratin 9 with clinical findings identical to those of the Unna-Thost type. There is no hyperhidrosis, however, and affected areas may blister. Histopathologic changes are characteristic.

Mal de Meleda (Keratoderma Palmoplantaris Transgrediens). This rare, progressive autosomal recessive condition is characterized by erythema and thick scales on the palms, fingers, soles, and flexor aspects of the wrists, knees, and elbows. Hyperhidrosis, nail thickening or koilonychia, and eczema may also occur.

Mutilating Keratoderma (Vohwinkel Syndrome). This is a progressive autosomal dominant disease with honeycombed hyperkeratosis of palms and soles, sparing the arches; starfish-like and linear keratoses on the dorsum of the hands, fingers, feet, and knees; and ainhum-like constriction of the digits that sometimes leads to autoamputation. This disorder may be associated with alopecia and hearing loss. Mutations of the gene for loricrin, a major protein of the cornified cell envelope, have been identified.

Papillon-Lefèvre Syndrome. This autosomal recessive erythematous hyperkeratosis of the palms and soles sometimes extends to the dorsal hands and feet, elbows, and knees later in childhood. This syndrome is characterized by periodontal inflammation, leading to loss of teeth by age 4–5 yr if untreated; a tendency to frequent pyogenic skin infections; nail dystrophy, including transverse nail grooves; hyperhidrosis; and ectopic calcification of the dura.

Keratoderma of palms and soles also occurs as a feature of some forms of ichthyosis and ectodermal dysplasia. *Richner-Hanhart syndrome* is an autosomal recessive palmoplantar keratoderma with corneal ulcers, progressive mental impairment, and a deficiency of tyrosine aminotransferase, which leads to tyrosinemia. *Pachyonychia congenita* is transmitted as an autosomal dominant trait with variable expressivity. The classic type I form *(Jadassohn-Lewandowski syndrome)* is due to mutations in the gene for keratin 16. Major features of the syndrome are onychogryphosis; palmoplantar keratoderma; follicular hyperkeratosis, especially of the elbows and knees; and oral leukokeratosis. The nail dystrophy is the most striking feature and may be present at birth or develop early in life. The nails are thickened and tubular, projecting upward at the free edge to form a conical roof over a mass of subungual keratotic debris. Repeated paronychial inflammation may result in shedding of the nails. The feature seen most consistently among patients with this condition is keratoderma of the palms and soles. Additional associated features include hyperhidrosis of the palms and soles, and bullae and erosions on the palms and soles. Some patients have shown a selective cell-mediated defect in recognition and processing of *Candida*. Surgical removal of the nails and excision of the nail matrix have been helpful in some patients.

Patients with palmoplantar hyperhidrosis may have macerated plaques that become secondarily infected and malodorous. Morbidity is lessened if the hyperkeratosis can be controlled by *treatment*; however, only mild palliation is achieved with applications of lubricants, keratolytic agents (urea, salicylic acid, lactic acid), and oral retinoids including etretinate, isotretinoin, and acitretin. Soaking in saline solution followed by debridement is a mainstay of treatment.

Bale SJ, Doyle SZ: The genetics of ichthyosis: A primer for epidemiologists. J Invest Dermatol 102:495, 1994.
DiGiovanna JJ, Bale SJ: Epidermolytic hyperkeratosis: Applied molecular genetics. J Invest Dermatol 102:390, 1994.
Huber M, Rettler I, Bernasconi K, et al; Mutations of keratinocyte transglutaminase in lamellar ichthyosis. Science 267:525, 1995.
Kousseff BG: Collodion baby, sign of Tay syndrome. Pediatrics 87:571, 1991.
Lavrijsen AP, Oestmann E, Hermans J, et al: Barrier function parameters in various keratinization disorders: Transepidermal water loss and vascular response to hexyl nicotinate. Br J Dermatol 129:547, 1993.
Paller AS: Laboratory tests for ichthyosis. Dermatol Clin 12:99, 1994.
Proksch E, Holleran WM, Menon GK, et al: Barrier function regulates epidermal lipid and DNA synthesis. Br J Dermatol 128:473, 1993.
Rabinowitz LG, Esterly NB: Atopic dermatitis and ichthyosis vulgaris. Pediatr Rev 15:220, 1994.
Rand RE, Baden HP: The ichthyoses—a review. J Am Acad Dermatol 8:285, 1983.
Rizzo WB: Sjögren-Larsson syndrome. Semin Dermatol 12:210, 1993.
Rizzo WB, Dammaum AL, Craft DA, et al: Sjögren-Larsson syndrome: Inherited defect in the fatty alcohol cycle. J Pediatr 115:228, 1989.
Williams ML: Ichthyosis: Mechanisms of disease. Pediatr Dermatol 9:365, 1992.
Williams ML, Elias PM: From basket weave to barrier. Unifying concepts for the pathogenesis of the diseases of cornification. Arch Dermatol 129:626, 1993.

CHAPTER 665
Diseases of the Dermis

KELOID. A keloid is a sharply demarcated, benign, dense growth of connective tissue that forms in the dermis after trauma. The lesions are firm, raised, pink, and rubbery; they may be tender or pruritic. Sites of predilection are the face, earlobes, neck, shoulders, upper trunk, sternum, and lower legs. Keloids are usually induced by trauma and commonly follow ear piercing, burns, scalds, and surgical procedures. Certain individuals, especially blacks, seem predisposed to keloid formation. In some cases, a familial tendency (recessive or dominant inheritance) or the presence of foreign material in the wound appears to have a pathogenic role. Keloids are a rare feature of Ehlers-Danlos syndrome, Rubinstein-Taybi syndrome, and pachydermoperiostosis. In both keloids and hypertophic scars, new collagen forms over a much longer period than in wounds that heal normally. Histopathologically, a keloid consists of whorled and interlaced hyalinized collagen fibers.

Keloids should be differentiated from hypertrophic scars, which remain confined to the site of injury and gradually involute over time. Young keloids may diminish in size if injected intralesionally at 4-wk intervals with triamcinolone suspension (10 mg/mL). At times, a more concentrated suspension is required. Large or old keloids may require surgical excision followed by intralesional injections of corticosteroid. The risk of recurrence at the same site argues against surgical excision alone. Placement of topical silicon gel sheeting over the keloid for several hours per day for several weeks may help some patients.

STRIAE CUTIS DISTENSAE. These thinned, depressed, erythematous bands of atrophic skin eventually become silvery, opalescent, and smooth. They occur most frequently in areas that have been subject to distention, such as the lower back, buttocks, thighs, breasts, abdomen, and shoulders. The most frequent causes are rapid growth, pregnancy, obesity, Cushing disease, or prolonged corticosteroid therapy. Adolescent striae tend to become less conspicuous with time. Histopathologically, striae distensae resemble scars.

CORTICOSTEROID-INDUCED ATROPHY. Both topical and systemic corticosteroid treatment can result in cutaneous atrophy. This is particularly common when a potent topical corticosteroid is applied under occlusion or to the intertriginous areas for a prolonged period. Affected skin is thin, fragile, smooth, and semitransparent, with telangiectasias and loss of normal skin markings. Histopathologically, one sees thinning of the stratum corneum and malpighii. Spaces between dermal collagen and elastic fibers are small, producing a more compact but thin dermis. The mechanism involves inhibition of synthesis of collagen type I, noncollagenous proteins, and total protein content of the skin; progressive reduction of dermal proteoglycans and glycosaminoglycans; and possibly prolonged vasoconstriction-induced ischemia. Retinoids applied topically restore these steroid-induced biochemical changes in the dermal connective tissue of the hairless mouse, without abrogating the beneficial anti-inflammatory effects.

GRANULOMA ANNULARE. This common dermatosis occurs predominantly in children and young adults. Typical lesions begin as erythematous, firm, smooth papules; they gradually enlarge to form annular plaques with a papular border and a normal, slightly atrophic or discolored central area (Fig. 665–1) up to several centimeters in size. Lesions may occur anywhere on the body, but mucous membranes are spared. Favored sites include the dorsum of the hands and feet. *Annular lesions* are often mistaken for tinea corporis because of the elevated advancing border; they differ in that they are not scaly. *Papular lesions*, another variant, may simulate rheumatoid nodules, particularly when grouped on the fingers and elbows. The disseminated papular form, which is provoked by light in some cases, is rare in children. *Subcutaneous granuloma annulare* is especially common in children; it tends to develop on the scalp and limbs, particularly in the pretibial area. These lesions are firm, usually nontender, skin-colored nodules. *Perforating granuloma annulare* is characterized by the development of a yellowish center in some of the superficial papular lesions as a result of transepidermal elimination of altered collagen.

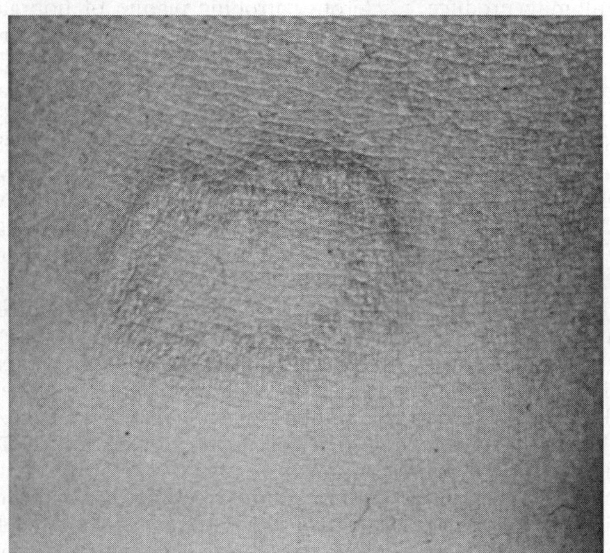

Figure 665–1 Annular lesion with a raised papular border and depressed center, characteristic of granuloma annulare.

A biopsy is occasionally required for diagnosis. The lesions consist of a granuloma with a central area of necrotic collagen; mucin deposition; and a peripheral palisading infiltrate of lymphocytes, histiocytes, and foreign body giant cells. The pattern resembles that of necrobiosis lipoidica and rheumatoid nodule (see Chapter 165), but subtle histologic differences usually permit differentiation. The cause of granuloma annulare is unknown. Affected children are usually healthy. Some cases of granuloma annulare, particularly the generalized form, may be associated with diabetes mellitus. The eruption persists for months to years, but spontaneous resolution without residual change is usual; 75% of lesions clear within 2 yr. Application of a potent topical corticosteroid preparation or intralesional injections of corticosteroid may hasten involution, but nonintervention is acceptable.

NECROBIOSIS LIPOIDICA. This rare disorder presents as erythematous papules that evolve into irregularly shaped, sharply demarcated, yellow, sclerotic plaques with central telangiectasia and a violaceous border. Scaling, crusting, and ulceration are frequent. Lesions develop most commonly on the shins. Slow extension of a given lesion over the years is usual, but long periods of quiescence or complete healing with scarring may occur.

Histopathologically, poorly defined areas of necrobiotic collagen are seen throughout, but primarily low in the dermis, associated with mucin deposition. Surrounding the necrobiotic, disordered areas of collagen is a palisading lymphohistiocytic granulomatous infiltrate. Some lesions are more characteristically granulomatous, with limited necrobiosis of collagen. Necrobiosis lipoidica must be differentiated clinically from xanthomas, morphea, granuloma annulare, and pretibial myxedema. Fifty to 75% of patients have diabetes mellitus; necrobiosis lipoidica occurs in 0.3% of all diabetic patients. The lesions persist despite good control of the diabetes but may improve minimally after applications of high-potency topical steroids or local injection of a corticosteroid.

LICHEN SCLEROSUS ET ATROPHICUS. This presents initially with ivory-colored, shiny, indurated papules, often with a violaceous halo. The surface shows prominent dilated pilosebaceous or sweat duct orifices that often contain yellow or brown horny plugs. The papules coalesce to form irregular plaques of variable size, which may develop hemorrhagic bullae in their margins. In the latter stages, atrophy results in a depressed plaque with a wrinkled surface. This disorder occurs more commonly in girls than in boys. Sites of predilection in girls are the vulvar, perianal, and perineal skin. Extensive involvement may produce a sclerotic, atrophic plaque of hourglass configuration; shrinkage of the labia and stenosis of the introitus may result. Vaginal discharge precedes vulvar lesions in approximately 20% of patients. In boys, the prepuce and glans penis are often involved, usually in association with phimosis; most boys with the disorder were not circumcised early in life. Sites elsewhere on the body that are most commonly involved include the upper trunk, the neck, the axillae, the flexor surfaces of wrists, and the areas around the umbilicus and the eyes. Pruritus may be severe.

In children, this disorder is most frequently confused with focal scleroderma (morphea) (see Chapter 161), with which it may coexist. In the genital area, it may be mistakenly attributed to sexual abuse. Biopsy is diagnostic, revealing hyperkeratosis with follicular plugging, hydropic degeneration of basal cells, a bandlike dermal lymphocytic infiltrate, homogenized collagen, and thinned elastic fibers in the upper dermis. The lesions may involute spontaneously, usually before or at the time of menarche; involution is more likely to occur in those in whom the disorder developed at a younger age. Leukoplakia and squamous cell carcinoma may rarely develop. Potent topical corticosteroids may provide relief from pruritus and produce clearing of lesions, including those in the genital area. Topical progesterone 1% and testosterone 2% preparations have also been used for genital lesions.

SCLEREDEMA (SCLEREDEMA ADULTORUM, SCLEREDEMA OF BUSCHKE). Approximately 30% of cases of scleredema develop before the age of 10 yr. Onset is sudden, with brawny edema of the face and neck that spreads rapidly to involve the thorax and arms in a sweater distribution; the abdomen and legs are usually spared. The face acquires a waxy, masklike appearance; the involved areas feel indurated and woody, are nonpitting, and are not sharply demarcated from normal skin. The overlying skin is normal in color and is not atrophic. Systemic involvement, which is uncommon, is marked by thickening of the tongue; dysarthria; dysphagia; restriction of eye and joint movements; and pleural, pericardial, and peritoneal effusions. Electrocardiographic changes may also be observed.

In 65–90% of cases, the disease follows an infection such as tonsillitis, pharyngitis, influenza, scarlet fever, measles, mumps, impetigo, or cellulitis after an interval of days or weeks; most cases follow a streptococcal infection. Onset may be heralded by a prodrome of fever, arthralgia, myalgia, and malaise. Onset in diabetic patients may occur insidiously. Laboratory data are not helpful. Some cases, however, are associated with immunoglobulin (Ig)G or IgA paraproteinemia. Skin biopsy demonstrates an increase in dermal thickness as a result of swelling and homogenization of the collagen bundles, which are separated by large interfibrous spaces. Increased amounts of mucopolysaccharides in the dermis can be identified by special stains.

The active phase of the disease persists for 2–8 wk; spontaneous and complete resolution usually occurs in 6 mo–2 yr. Recurrent attacks are unusual. The disorder must be differentiated from scleroderma, morphea, myxedema, trichinosis, dermatomyositis, sclerema neonatorum, and subcutaneous fat necrosis. There is no specific therapy.

LIPOID PROTEINOSIS (URBACH-WIETHE DISEASE, HYALINOSIS CUTIS ET MUCOSAE). This autosomal recessive disorder consists of infiltration of hyaline material into the skin, oral cavity, larynx, and internal organs. It may be noted initially in early infancy as hoarseness. Skin lesions appear during childhood and consist of yellowish papules and nodules that may coalesce to form plaques on the face, forearms, neck, genitals, dorsum of the fingers, and scalp, where they result in patchy alopecia. Similar deposits are found on the lips, undersurface of the tongue, fauces, uvula, epiglottis, and vocal cords. The tongue becomes enlarged and feels firm on palpation; patients may be unable to protrude their tongue. Translucent nodules along the margins of the eyelids, causing thickening of the eyelids, are the most characteristic clinical manifestation. Pocklike atrophic scars may develop on the face. Hypertrophic, hyperkeratotic nodules occur at sites of friction such as the elbows and knees; the palms may be diffusely thickened. The disease progresses until early adult life, but the prognosis is good. Involvement of the larynx can lead to respiratory compromise, particularly in infancy, necessitating tracheostomy. Associated anomalies include dental abnormalities, epilepsy, and recurrent parotitis as a result of infiltrates in the Stensen duct; virtually any organ can be involved. There is no specific treatment.

The distinctive histologic pattern includes dilatation of dermal blood vessels and infiltration of homogeneous eosinophilic extracellular hyaline material along capillary walls and around sweat glands. Hyaline material in homogeneous bundles, diffusely arranged in the upper dermis, produces a thickened dermis. The infiltrates appear to contain both lipid and mucopolysaccharide substances. Symmetric ossification lateral to the sella turcica in the medial temporal region, identifiable roentgenographically, is pathognomonic but is not always present. The biochemical defect is unknown but may represent a lysosomal storage disorder caused by single or numerous enzyme defects. Alterations in the distribution of collagens I, III, IV, and V have also been described.

MACULAR ATROPHY (ANETODERMA). Anetoderma is characterized by circumscribed areas of slack skin associated with loss of dermal substance. This disorder may have no associated underlying disease (primary macular atrophy) or may develop after an inflammatory skin condition (secondary macular atrophy) such as syphilis, lupus erythematosus, acne, varicella, leprosy, urticaria pigmentosa, or *Staphylococcus epidermidis* folliculitis. Lesions vary from 0.5–1 cm in diameter and, if inflammatory, may initially be erythematous. They subsequently become thin, wrinkled, and blue-white or hypopigmented. The lesions often protrude as small outpouchings that, on palpation, may be readily indented into the subcutaneous tissue because of the dermal atrophy. Sites of predilection include the trunk, thighs, upper arms, and less commonly the neck and face. Lesions remain unchanged for life; new lesions often continue to develop for years. There is no effective therapy, although some authorities have reported benefit from penicillin or pentoxifylline.

All types of macular atrophy show focal loss of elastic tissue on histopathologic examination, a change that is not recognizable unless special stains are used. The elastolysis may be due to release of elastase from inflammatory cells, such as macrophages, in contact with elastic fibers. Lesions of anetoderma occasionally resemble morphea, lichen sclerosus et atrophicus, focal dermal hypoplasia, atrophic scars, or end-stage lesions of chronic bullous dermatoses.

CUTIS LAXA (DERMATOMEGALY, GENERALIZED ELASTOLYSIS). Cutis laxa is a congenital autosomal recessive or autosomal dominant disorder. Affected newborn infants may appear prematurely aged. When onset appears to occur during childhood or adulthood, the disorder is termed *acquired cutis laxa*. Cutis laxa has developed after a febrile illness, inflammatory skin diseases such as lupus erythematosus or erythema multiforme, amyloidosis, urticaria, angioedema, and hypersensitivity reactions to penicillin, and in infants born to women who were taking penicillamine.

Clinical Manifestations. There may be widespread folds of lax skin, or changes may be mild and limited in extent, resembling anetoderma. Patients with severe cutis laxa have characteristic facial features, including an aged appearance with sagging jowls (bloodhound appearance), a hooked nose with everted nostrils, a short columella, a long upper lip, and everted lower eyelids. The skin is also lax elsewhere on the body and may resemble an ill-fitting suit (Fig. 665–2). Hyperelasticity and hypermobility of the joints are not present as they are in the Ehlers-Danlos syndrome. Many infants have a hoarse cry, probably as a result of laxity of the vocal cords. Tensile strength of the skin is normal. Histologically, elastic tissue is reduced throughout the dermis, with fragmentation, distention, and clumping of the elastic fibers.

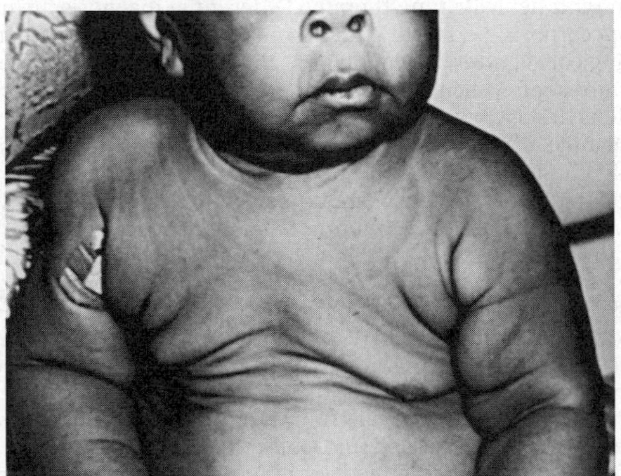

Figure 665–2 Pendulous folds of skin of an infant with cutis laxa. Note the long upper lip and upturned nose.

The dominant form of cutis laxa may develop at any age and is generally benign and mainly of cosmetic significance. When it presents in infancy, it may be associated with intrauterine growth retardation, ligamentous laxity, and delayed closure of fontanels. Affected males may be impotent and have infantile genitals and scanty body hair. Pulmonary emphysema and mild cardiovascular manifestations may also occur. In contrast, those with the more common recessive form of the disease are susceptible to severe complications, such as multiple hernias, rectal prolapse, diaphragmatic atony, diverticula of the gastrointestinal and genitourinary tracts, cor pulmonale, emphysema, pneumothoraces, peripheral pulmonary artery stenosis, and aortic dilatation. Characteristic facial features include downward slanting palpebral fissures; a broad, flat nose; and large ears. Skeletal anomalies, dental caries, growth retardation, and developmental delay also occur. Such patients often have a shortened life span.

The *pathogenesis* of cutis laxa is not well known. Abnormalities that have been described include excessive enzymatic destruction of elastin, decreased elastase inhibitor levels, and decreased elastin messenger RNA levels in fibroblasts.

EHLERS-DANLOS SYNDROME. This is a group of genetically heterogeneous connective tissue disorders. Affected children appear normal at birth, but skin hyperelasticity, fragility of the skin and blood vessels, and joint hypermobility develop. The essential defect is a quantitative deficiency of collagen. Ehlers-Danlos syndrome has been classified into 10 clinical forms.

I. Gravis Type. This autosomal dominant disorder is characterized by premature birth caused by rupture of membranes, skin hyperelasticity and fragility, easy bruising, generalized and severe joint hypermobility, scoliosis, and mitral valve prolapse. Insignificant lacerations may form gaping wounds that leave broad, atrophic, papyraceous scars. Additional cutaneous manifestations include molluscoid pseudotumors over pressure points from accumulations of connective tissue. Life expectancy is not reduced.

II. Mitis Type. This autosomal dominant form is characterized by mild skin and joint manifestations, the latter limited to hands and feet. The incidence of premature birth is not increased.

III. Benign, Hypermobile Type. This disorder has autosomal dominant inheritance and is manifested as generalized severe joint hypermobility and minimal skin manifestations. Osteoarthritis may develop prematurely.

IV. Ecchymotic (Sack) Type. This form may have autosomal dominant or autosomal recessive inheritance and shows the most pronounced dermal thinning of all; consequently, the underlying venous network is prominent. The skin has minimal hyperextensibility, and the joints are not hypermobile, except perhaps during childhood. Premature birth; extensive ecchymoses from trauma; a high incidence of keloids; rupture of the bowel, especially the colon; uterine rupture during pregnancy; rupture of the great vessels; dissecting aortic aneurysm; and stroke all contribute to the increased morbidity and shortened life span. Patients should be advised to avoid becoming pregnant, avoid activities such as trumpet playing that raise intracranial pressure as a result of a Valsalva maneuver, and minimize trauma to the skin. Defects that have been identified in affected patients include multiple deletions, exon skipping, or point mutations in the *COL3A1* gene of collagen III.

V. X-Linked Type. This is characterized by minimal joint hypermobility and skin hyperelasticity and moderate bruising, skin fragility, and scarring. The life span is normal. Lysyl oxidase was deficient in one family with this disorder.

VI. Autosomal Recessive Ocular Type. These patients have joint hyperextensibility, hypotonia, kyphoscoliosis, fragile cornea, keratoconus, skin hyperelasticity, and fragile bones. There is a mutation affecting a collagen structural protein. Patients lack lysyl hydroxylase, a crucial enzyme in collagen biosynthesis that catalyzes the formation of hydroxylysine, which cross-links collagen. Prenatal diagnosis is available by measuring lysyl hydroxylase activity in amniocytes. The diagnosis can also be confirmed by detecting decreased lysyl hydroxylase activity in cultured dermal fibroblasts. This form may respond to oral ascorbic acid.

VII. Arthrochalasis Multiplex Congenita. The A type is an autosomal recessive disorder characterized by short stature, marked joint hyperextensibility and dislocation, and moderate hyperelasticity and bruisability of skin. The defect is a failure of cleavage of the N-terminus propeptide of type I procollagen chains by procollagen N-proteinase caused by a mutation in the *COL1A1* gene that results in loss of the procollagen N-proteinase cleavage site. The B type, possibly autosomal dominant, is characterized by skin hyperelasticity and marked joint hypermobility. Mutations in the *COL1A2* gene cause loss of the N-proteinase cleavage site in the pro-α_2 (I) collagen chain. The type C disorder, known as dermatosparaxis, includes premature rupture of membranes; delayed closure of fontanels; skin fragility and laxity; easy bruisability; growth retardation; short limbs; umbilical hernia; and characteristic facies with micrognathia, jowls, and prominent, puffy eyelids. This disorder is due to a lack of N-proteinase activity.

VIII. Periodontitis Type. This autosomal dominant disorder is characterized by mild skin hyperelasticity, small joint hypermobility, bruisability, moderate cutaneous fragility, abnormal scarring, and severe periodontitis, leading to premature loss of teeth and alveolar bone. The proportion of type III collagen is reduced.

IX. X-Linked Recessive Skeletal Type. This form is characterized by occipital exostoses; widening and bowing of long bones at tendinous and ligamentous insertion sites; short, broad clavicles; mild skin hyperelasticity; bladder diverticula with spontaneous rupture; inguinal hernias; and chronic diarrhea. Defective copper transport results in low serum copper and ceruloplasm levels and diminished lysyl oxidase activity, an important copper-dependent enzyme required for collagen cross-linking. Menkes disease and X-linked cutis laxa also have altered copper metabolism and defective collagen fibril formation; these may be examples of type IX Ehlers-Danlos syndrome.

X. Dysfibronectinemic Type. This autosomal recessive disorder is characterized by fibronectin-correctable failure of platelet aggregation, easy bruisability, joint hypermobility, and skin hyperextensibility.

Differential Diagnosis. Ehlers-Danlos syndrome has been confused with cutis laxa, but the features of the two disorders differ considerably. The skin of patients with cutis laxa hangs in redundant folds, whereas the skin in Ehlers-Danlos syndrome is hyperextensible and snaps back into place when stretched. Because of the marked skin fragility in Ehlers-Danlos syndrome, minor trauma results in ecchymoses, bleeding, and poor healing with atrophic cigarette-paper scars, which are most prominent on the forehead and lower legs, and over pressure points. Surgical procedures are fraught with risk; dehiscence of wounds is common.

PSEUDOXANTHOMA ELASTICUM. This disorder of elastic tissue primarily affects the dermis, retina, and cardiovascular system.

Clinical Manifestations. Onset of skin manifestations often occurs during childhood, but the changes produced by early lesions are subtle and may not be recognized. The characteristic pebbly "plucked chicken skin" cutaneous lesions are asymptomatic, 1–2-mm yellow papules that are arranged in a linear or reticulated pattern or in confluent plaques. Preferred sites are the flexural neck, axillary and inguinal folds, umbilicus, thighs, and antecubital and popliteal fossas. As the lesions become more pronounced, the skin acquires a velvety texture and droops in lax, inelastic folds. The face is usually spared. Mucous membrane lesions may involve the lips, buccal cavity, rectum, and vagina. Involvement of the connective tissue of the media and intima of blood vessels, Bruch membrane of the eye, and endocardium or pericardium may result in visual disturbances; angioid streaks in Bruch membrane; intermittent claudication; cerebral and coronary occlusion; hypertension; and hemorrhage from the gastrointestinal tract, uterus, or mucosal surfaces. Affected women have an increased risk of miscarriage in the first trimester. Arterial involvement generally presents in adulthood, but claudication and angina have occurred in early childhood. There is no effective *treatment*, although laser therapy may help to prevent retinal hemorrhage.

Pathology and Pathogenesis. Histopathologic examination shows fragmented, swollen, and clumped elastic fibers in the middle and lower third of the dermis. The fibers stain positively for calcium. Collagen in the vicinity of the altered elastic fibers is reduced in amount and is split into small fibers. Aberrant calcification of the elastic fibers of the internal elastic lamina of arteries leads to narrowing of vessel lumina. It is hypothesized that an abnormal glycosaminoglycan is secreted by fibroblasts and deposited on the surface of elastic fibers, leading to fragmentation and calcification of the coated fibers. Candidate genes for pseudoxanthoma elasticum include the genes encoding elastin; the fibrillins, which form a microfibrillar coating around elastin; and lysyl oxidase, which catalyzes formation of the desmosines, the covalent interchain cross links that stabilize elastin polypeptides into their fibrillar structure. There are two autosomal dominant and two autosomal recessive forms of the disease. However, all affected patients tend to merge into a single classic phenotype involving the skin, eyes, and cardiovascular system, with considerable variability in expression of the disorder, particularly in the vascular and ophthalmologic complications.

ELASTOSIS PERFORANS SERPIGINOSA. This is an unusual skin disorder in which 1–3-mm, skin-colored, keratotic, firm papules tend to cluster in arcuate and annular patterns on the posterolateral neck and limbs and, occasionally, on the face and trunk. Onset usually occurs during childhood or adolescence. Histopathologically, a papule consists of a circumscribed area of epidermal hyperplasia that communicates with the underlying dermis by a narrow channel. Elastotic material is extruded from the channel. There is a great increase in the amount and size of elastic fibers in the upper dermis, particularly in the dermal papillae. The primary abnormality is probably in the dermal elastin, which provokes a cellular response that ultimately leads to extrusion of the abnormal elastic tissue. Approximately one third of cases occur in association with osteogenesis imperfecta, Marfan syndrome, pseudoxanthoma elasticum, Ehlers-Danlos syndrome, Rothmund-Thomson syndrome, and Down syndrome. It has also occurred in association with penicillamine therapy. Differential diagnosis includes tinea corporis, perforating granuloma annulare, reactive perforating collagenosis, lichen planus, creeping eruption, and porokeratosis of Mibelli. Treatment is ineffective; however, the lesions are asymptomatic and disappear spontaneously.

REACTIVE PERFORATING COLLAGENOSIS. This usually presents in early childhood with small papules on the dorsal areas of the hands and forearms, elbows, knees, and sometimes face and trunk. The condition is often familial and may be inherited in an autosomal recessive pattern. Over a period of several weeks, the papules increase in size to 5–10 mm, become umbilicated, and develop a keratotic plug in the center. Individual lesions resolve spontaneously in 2–4 mo, leaving a hypopigmented macule or scar. Lesions may recur in crops; may undergo a linear Koebner reaction; and may form in response to cold temperatures or superficial trauma such as abrasions, insect bites, and acne lesions. Histopathologically, collagen in the papillary dermis is engulfed within a cup-shaped perforation in the epidermis. The central crater contains pyknotic inflammatory cells and keratinous debris. The process appears to represent transepidermal elimination of altered collagen. Topical retinoic acid may reduce the number of lesions.

XANTHOMAS. See Chapter 83.3.

FABRY DISEASE. See Chapter 83.4.

MUCOPOLYSACCHARIDOSES. See Chapter 85. In several of these disorders, thick, inelastic, rough skin, particularly on the extremities, and generalized hirsutism are characteristic but nonspecific features. Telangiectasias on the face, forearms, trunk, and legs have been observed in Scheie and Morquio syndromes. In some patients with Hunter syndrome, distinctive ivory-colored, firm papulonodules with a corrugated surface texture are grouped into symmetric plaques on the upper trunk, arms, and thighs. Onset of these unusual lesions occurs during the 1st decade of life, and spontaneous disappearance has been noted.

MASTOCYTOSIS. Mastocytosis encompasses a spectrum of disorders that range from solitary cutaneous nodules to diffuse infiltration of skin associated with involvement of other organs. All the disorders are characterized by aggregates of mast cells in the dermis. Mast cell growth factor, which can be secreted by keratinocytes, stimulates the proliferation of mast cells and increases the production of melanin by melanocytes. Mastocytosis may be due to altered cutaneous metabolism of mast cell growth factor and, thus, may represent a hyperplastic rather than a neoplastic disorder.

Clinical Manifestations. Affected children can have intense pruritus. Systemic signs of histamine release, such as hypotension, syncope, headache, episodic flushing, tachycardia, wheezing, colic, and diarrhea, occur most frequently in the more severe types of mastocytosis. The local and systemic manifestations of the disease are due, at least partially, to release of histamine and heparin from mast cell granules; although heparin is present in significant amounts in mast cells, coagulation disturbances occur only rarely. The vasodilator prostaglandin D_2 or its metabolite appears to exacerbate the flushing response.

Mastocytomas are solitary lesions 1–5 cm in diameter. Lesions may be present at birth or arise during early infancy at any site; the wrist, neck, and trunk are sites of predilection. The lesions may present as recurrent, evanescent wheals or bullae; in time, however, an infiltrated, rubbery, pink, yellow, or tan plaque develops at the site of whealing or blistering (Fig. 665–3*A*). The surface acquires a pebbly, orange peel–like texture, and hyperpigmentation may become prominent. Stroking or trauma to the nodule may result in urtication (Darier sign) as a result of local histamine release; rarely, systemic signs of histamine release become apparent. The differential diagnosis includes recurrent bullous impetigo, nevi, and juvenile xanthogranuloma. Mastocytomas usually involute spontaneously during early childhood; troublesome lesions can be excised and do not recur. Only rarely do multiple cutaneous lesions develop.

Urticaria pigmentosa is the most common form of mastocytosis and occurs primarily in infants and children. Lesions may be present at birth but more often erupt in crops during the first several months to 2 yr of age. In some cases, early bullous or urticarial lesions fade, only to recur at the same

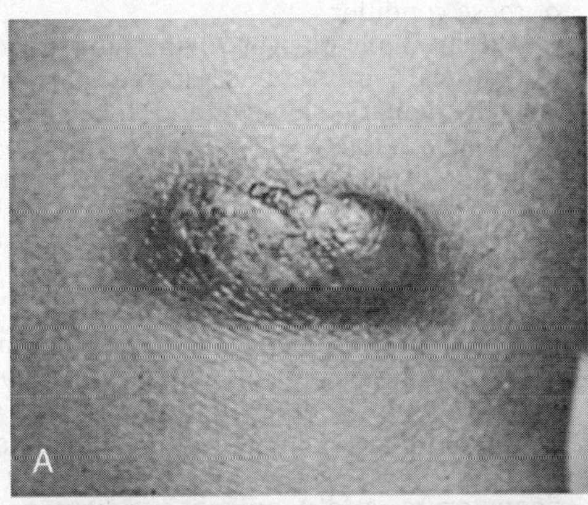

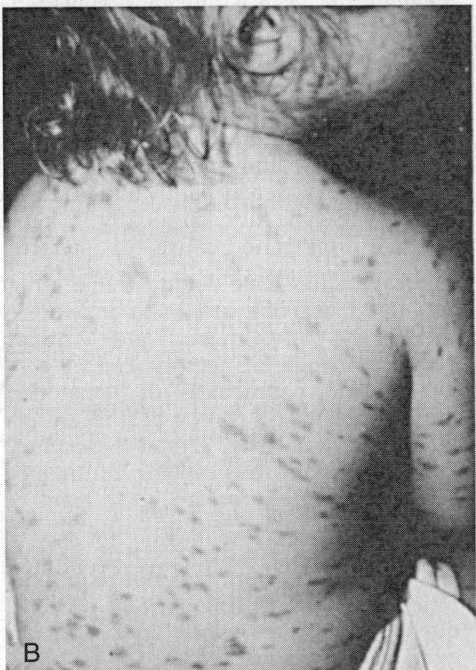

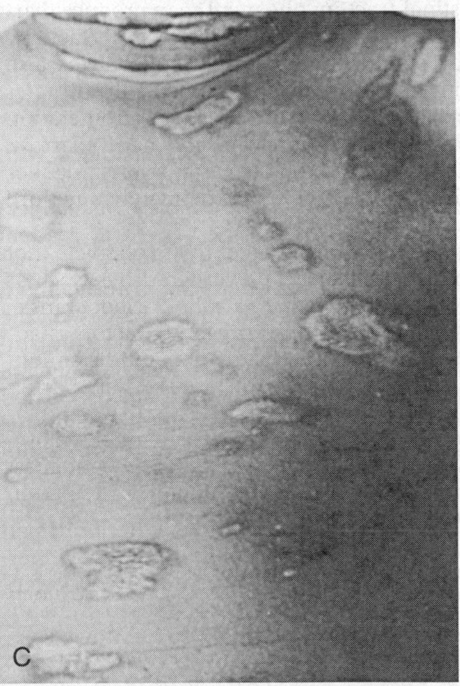

Figure 665–3 *A,* Solitary mastocytoma that is partially blistered. *B,* Hyperpigmented papular lesions of urticaria pigmentosa, some of which exhibit a surrounding flare. *C,* Infiltrated plaques of urticaria pigmentosa.

site, ultimately becoming fixed and hyperpigmented; in others, the initial lesions are hyperpigmented. Vesiculation usually abates by 2 yr of age. Individual lesions range in size from a few millimeters to several centimeters and may be macular, papular, or nodular; they range in color from yellow-tan to chocolate brown and often have ill-defined borders (Fig. 665–3*B*). Larger nodular lesions, like mastocytomas, may have a characteristic orange peel texture (Fig. 665–3*C*). Lesions of urticaria pigmentosa may be sparse or numerous and are often symmetrically distributed. Palms, soles, and face are sometimes spared, as are the mucous membranes. The rapid appearance of erythema and whealing in response to vigorous stroking of a lesion can usually be elicited; dermographism of intervening normal skin is also common. Urticaria pigmentosa can be confused with drug eruptions, postinflammatory pigmentary change, juvenile xanthogranuloma, pigmented nevi, ephelides, xanthomas, chronic urticaria, insect bites, and bullous impetigo.

Prognosis. This is good; spontaneous involution occurs in about 50% of patients by puberty; another 25% have partial resolution by adulthood. The incidence of systemic manifestations is very low.

Diffuse Cutaneous Mastocytosis. This variant is characterized by diffuse involvement of the skin rather than discrete hyperpigmented lesions. Affected patients are usually normal at birth and develop features of the disorder after the first few months of life. Rarely, the condition may present with intense generalized pruritus in the absence of visible skin changes. The skin usually appears thickened and pink to yellow and may have a doughy feel and a texture resembling an orange peel. Surface changes are accentuated in flexural areas. Recurrent bullae, intractable pruritus, and flushing attacks are common, as is systemic involvement.

Telangiectasia macularis eruptiva perstans is another variant that consists of telangiectatic hyperpigmented macules that are usually localized to the trunk. These lesions do not urticate when stroked. This form of the disease is seen in adolescents and adults primarily.

Systemic Mastocytosis. This disorder is marked by an abnormal increase in the number of mast cells in other than cutaneous tissues. It occurs in approximately 5–10% of patients with mastocytosis and is more common in adults than in children. Bone lesions may be silent but are detectable radiologically as osteoporotic or osteosclerotic areas, principally in the axial skeleton. Gastrointestinal tract involvement may produce diarrhea and steatorrhea. Mucosal infiltrates may be detectable by barium studies or by small bowel biopsy. Peptic ulcers also occur. Hepatosplenomegaly as a result of mast cell infiltrates and fibrosis has been described, as has mast cell proliferation in lymph nodes, kidneys, periadrenal fat, and bone marrow. Abnormalities in the peripheral blood, such as anemia, leukocytosis, and eosinophilia, are noted in approximately one third of patients.

Treatment. Flushing can be precipitated by excessively hot baths, vigorous rubbing of the skin, and certain drugs, such as codeine, aspirin, morphine, atropine, alcohol, tubocurarine, and polymyxin B. Avoidance of these triggering factors is advisable. For patients who are symptomatic, oral antihistamines may be palliative. H_1 receptor antagonists are the initial drugs of choice for systemic signs of histamine release. If H_1 antagonists are unsuccessful, H_2 receptor antagonists may be helpful in controlling pruritus or gastric hypersecretion. Oral mast cell–stabilizing agents, such as cromolyn sodium or ketotifen, may also be effective.

Golitz LE, Weston WL, Lane AT: Bullous mastocytosis: Diffuse cutaneous mastocytosis with extensive blisters mimicking scalded skin syndrome or erythema multiforme: Pediatr Dermatol 1:288, 1984.
Golkar L, Bernhard J: Mastocytosis. Lancet 349:1379, 1997.
Hacker SM, Ramos-Caro FA, Beers BB, et al: Juvenile pseudoxanthoma elasticum: Recognition and management. Pediatr Dermatol 10:19, 1993.
Helm KF, Gibson LE, Muller SA: Lichen sclerosus et atrophicus in children and young adults. Pediatr Dermatol 8:97, 1991.
Lebwohl M, Neldner K, Pope M, et al: Classification of pseudoxanthoma elasticum: Report of a consensus conference. J Am Acad Dermatol 30:103, 1994.
Lucky AW, Prose NS, Bove K, et al: Papular umbilicated granuloma annulare. A report of four pediatric cases. Arch Dermatol 128:1375, 1992.
Mulbauer JE: Granuloma annulare. J Am Acad Dermatol 3:217, 1980.
Murray JC: Keloids and hypertrophic scars. Clin Dermatol 12:27, 1994.
Tilstra DJ, Byers PH: Molecular basis of hereditary disorders of connective tissue. Annu Rev Med 45:149, 1994.
Yeowell HN, Pinnell SR: The Ehlers-Danlos syndromes. Semin Dermatol 12:229, 1993.

CHAPTER 666
Diseases of Subcutaneous Tissue

Diseases involving the subcutis are usually characterized by necrosis and/or inflammation; they may occur either as a primary event or as a secondary response to various stimuli or disease processes. Unfortunately, these disorders cannot all be distinguished by their histopathologic changes, which may merely reflect the stage of the lesion at the time of biopsy. The principal diagnostic criteria are the appearance and distribution of the lesions, associated symptoms, results of laboratory studies, and the natural history and exogenous provocative factors of these conditions.

CORTICOSTEROID-INDUCED ATROPHY. Injection of a corticosteroid intradermally can produce deep atrophy accompanied by surface pigmentary changes and telangiectasia. These changes occur approximately 2 wk after injection and may last for months. The deltoid area is most susceptible to this complication (see Chapter 665).

PANNICULITIS. Inflammation of fibrofatty subcutaneous tissue may primarily involve the fat lobule or, alternatively, the fibrous septum that compartmentalizes the fatty lobules. Lobular panniculitis that spares the subcutaneous vasculature includes poststeroid panniculitis, lupus erythematosus profundus, relapsing nodular nonsuppurative panniculitis *(Weber-Christian syndrome)*, pancreatic panniculitis, α_1-antitrypsin deficiency, subcutaneous fat necrosis of the newborn, sclerema neonatorum, cold panniculitis, subcutaneous sarcoidosis, and factitial panniculitis. Lobar panniculitis with vasculitis occurs in erythema induratum and occasionally as a feature of Crohn disease (see Chapter 337.2). Inflammation predominantly within the septum, sparing the vasculature, may be seen in erythema nodosum, necrobiosis lipoidica, scleroderma (see Chapter 161), and subcutaneous granuloma annulare (see Chapter 665). Septal panniculitis that includes inflammation of the vessels is found primarily in leukocytoclastic vasculitis and polyarteritis nodosa (see Chapter 167.3).

Poststeroid panniculitis has been observed in children who received high-dose corticosteroids orally for relatively short periods, usually for rheumatic fever. Within 1–2 wk after discontinuation of the drug, multiple subcutaneous nodules may appear on the cheeks, trunk, and arms. Nodules range in size from 0.5–4 cm, are erythematous or skin colored, and may be pruritic. The mechanism of the inflammatory reaction in the fat is unknown. Treatment is unnecessary because the lesions remit spontaneously over a period of months without scarring.

Lupus erythematosus profundus (lupus erythematosus panniculitis) presents with one to several firm, well-defined plaques or nodules 1 to several centimeters in diameter, most commonly on the face, buttocks, or proximal extremities. This condition may occur in patients with systemic or discoid lupus erythematosus and may precede or follow the development of other cutaneous lesions. The overlying skin is usually normal but may be erythematous, atrophic, poikilodermatous, or hyperkeratotic. Lesions may be painful and may ulcerate. On healing, a shallow depression generally remains; rarely, soft pink areas of anetoderma may result. The histopathologic changes are distinctive and may allow one to make the diagnosis in the absence of other cutaneous lesions of lupus erythematosus. The lupus band and antinuclear antibody test results are usually positive. Nodules tend to be persistent but may respond to antimalarials, oral or intralesional corticosteroids, or, in debilitating cases, immunosuppressive agents such as azathioprine or cyclophosphamide. Avoidance of sun exposure and trauma is also important.

α_1-Antitrypsin deficiency may present with cellulitis-like areas or red, tender nodules on the trunk or proximal extremities. (see Chapter 357.6). Nodules tend to ulcerate spontaneously and discharge an oily yellow fluid. Trauma is an inciting factor in some patients. Affected individuals have severe homozygous deficiency or rarely a partial deficiency of the protease inhibitor α_1-antitrypsin, which inhibits trypsin activity and the activity of elastase, serine proteases, collagenase, factor VIII, and kallikrein. Accordingly, panniculitis may be associated with panacinar emphysema, noninfectious hepatitis, cirrhosis, persistent cutaneous vasculitis, cold-contact urticaria, or acquired angioedema. Diagnosis can be substantiated by a decreased level of serum α_1-antitrypsin activity, although, because the protein behaves as an acute-phase reactant, the level may be elevated spuriously during an acute attack of pancreatitis. Some patients respond to dapsone or infusion of random-donor–derived α_1-protease inhibitor concentrate.

Pancreatic panniculitis presents most commonly on the pretibial regions, thighs, or buttocks as tender, erythematous nodules that may be fluctuant and occasionally discharge a yellowish oily substance. It presents most often in alcoholic males but may also occur in patients with pancreatitis as a result of cholelithiasis or abdominal trauma, with rupture of a pancreatic pseudocyst, with pancreatic ductal adenocarcinoma, or with pancreatic acinar cell carcinoma. Associated features may include arthropathy and synovitis, particularly in the ankles; eosinophilia; polyserositis; and painful osteolytic bone lesions with medullary necrosis. Microscopic changes consist of multiple foci of fat necrosis that contain ghost cells with thick, shadowy walls and no nuclei. A polymorphous inflammatory infiltrate surrounds the areas of fat necrosis. Pathogenesis of the panniculitis appears to be multifactorial, involving liberation of the lipolytic enzymes lipase, trypsin, and amylase into the circulation, causing adipocyte membrane damage and intracellular lipolysis. There is no correlation, however, between the occurrence of pancreatitis and the serum concentration of pancreatic enzymes.

Subcutaneous fat necrosis is an inflammatory disorder of adipose tissue that occurs primarily in the first 4 wk of life in full-term or post-term infants. Affected infants may have a history of perinatal asphyxia or a difficult labor and delivery. Typical lesions are asymptomatic, rubbery to firm, erythematous to violaceous plaques or nodules on the cheeks, buttocks, back, thighs, or upper arms (Fig. 666–1). Lesions may be focal or extensive and are generally asymptomatic, although they may be tender during the acute phase. Histopathologic changes are diagnostic and consist of necrosis of fat; a granulomatous cellular infiltrate composed of lymphocytes, histiocytes, multinucleated giant cells, and fibroblasts; and radially arranged clefts of crystalline triglyceride within fat cells and multinucleated giant cells. Calcium deposits are commonly found in areas of fat necrosis. Subcutaneous fat necrosis in infants may be due to ischemic injury under various circumstances such as maternal preeclampsia, birth trauma, asphyxia, and prolonged hypothermia; in many affected infants, however, no provocative factors are identified. Susceptibility has been attributed to differences in composition between the subcutaneous tissue of young infants and that of older infants, children, and adults.

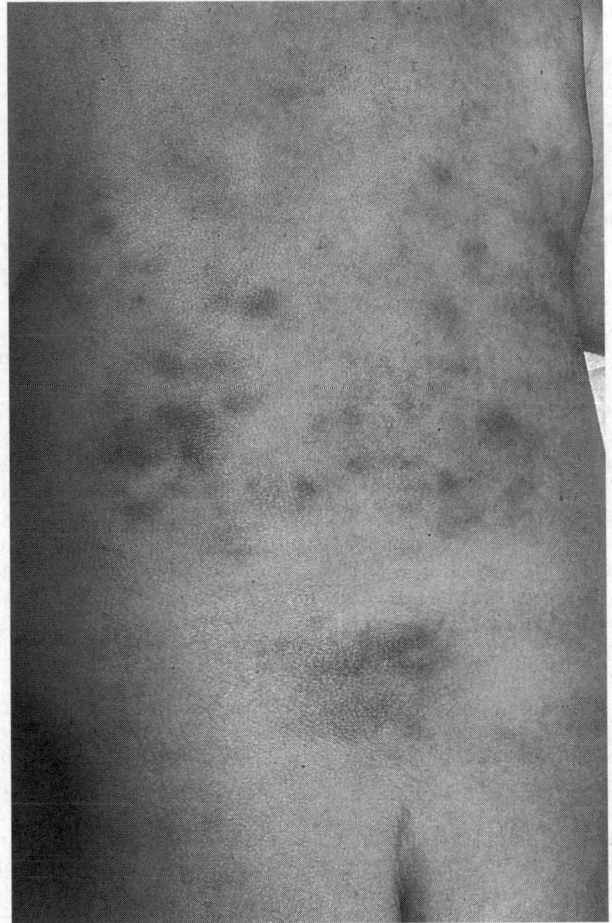

Figure 666–1 Red-purple nodular infiltration of skin of back caused by subcutaneous fat necrosis. See also color section.

Neonatal fat solidifies at a relatively high temperature because of its relatively greater concentration of high-melting-point saturated fatty acids such as palmitic and stearic acids.

Uncomplicated lesions involute spontaneously within weeks to months, usually without scarring or atrophy. Calcium deposition may occasionally occur within areas of fat necrosis, and this may sometimes result in rupture and drainage of liquid material. A rare but potentially life-threatening complication is *hypercalcemia*. This presents at 1–6 mo of age with lethargy, poor feeding, vomiting, failure to thrive, irritability, seizures, shortening of the QT interval, or renal failure. The origin of the hypercalcemia is unknown but is postulated to involve excess bone resorption through elevated levels of prostaglandin E or increased intestinal calcium uptake by unregulated extrarenal production of 1,25-dihydroxyvitamin D by macrophages in the granulomatous infiltrate. Subcutaneous fat necrosis can be confused with sclerema neonatorum, panniculitis, cellulitis, or hematoma. Because the lesions are self-limited, therapy is not required for uncomplicated cases. Needle aspiration of fluctuant lesions may prevent rupture and subsequent scarring. Treatment of hypercalcemia is aimed at enhancing renal calcium excretion by hydration and furosemide administration and at limiting dietary calcium and vitamin D intake. Reduction of intestinal calcium absorption and alteration of vitamin D metabolism may be accomplished by administration of corticosteroids.

Sclerema neonatorum is an uncommon disorder of adipose tissue that presents abruptly in preterm, gravely ill infants as diffuse, yellowish-white woody induration of the skin. Affected skin becomes stony in consistency, cold, and nonpitting.

The face assumes a masklike expression, and joint mobility may be compromised because of inflexibility of the skin. Histopathologic changes in sclerema neonatorum consist of an increase in the size of fat cells and an increase in the width of the fibrous connective tissue septa. In contrast to subcutaneous fat necrosis, with which it is most apt to be confused, fat necrosis, inflammation, giant cells, and calcium crystals are generally absent. Sclerema neonatorum almost always is associated with serious illness, such as sepsis, congenital heart disease, multiple congenital anomalies, or hypothermia. The appearance of sclerema in a sick infant should be regarded as an ominous prognostic sign. The outcome depends on the response of the underlying disorder to treatment.

Cold panniculitis may result in localized lesions in infants after prolonged cold exposure, especially on the cheeks, or after prolonged application of a cold object such as an ice cube, ice bag, or Popsicle to any area of the skin. Erythematous to bluish, indurated, ill-defined plaques or nodules arise within hours to a couple days of exposure, persist for 2–3 wk, and heal without residua. Recurrence of the lesions is common, however, thus emphasizing the importance of parental education in treating these patients. Histopathologic examination reveals an infiltrate of lymphoid and histiocytic cells around blood vessels at the dermal-subdermal junction; by the 3rd day, some of the fat cells in the subcutis may have ruptured and coalesced into cystic structures. Cold panniculitis may be confused with facial cellulitis caused by *Haemophilus influenzae* type b. Unlike the situation with buccal cellulitis, however, the area may be cold to the touch, and the patient is afebrile. Chilblains (pernio), a condition of acute or chronic cold injury, is characterized by localized symmetric erythematous to purplish edematous plaques and nodules in areas exposed to cold, typically acral areas (distal hands and feet, ears, face) (Chapter 71). Lesions develop 12–24 hr after cold exposure and may be associated with itching, burning, or pain. Blister formation and ulceration are rare. Vasospasm of arterioles due to cold exposure with resultant hypoxemia and localized perivascular mononuclear inflammation appears to be responsible for the disease. Frostbite due to extreme cold exposure is painful and histopathologically involves the epidermis, dermis, and subcutaneous fat. The pathogenic mechanism of cold panniculitis may be similar to that of subcutaneous fat necrosis, involving an increased propensity of fat to solidify in infants compared with that in older children and adults as a result of the higher percentage of saturated fatty acids in the subcutaneous fat of infants.

Factitial panniculitis results from subcutaneous injection by self or proxy of a foreign substance, the most common types of which include organic materials such as milk or feces; drugs such as the opiates or pentazocine; oily materials such as mineral oil or paraffin; and the synthetic polymer povidone. Indurated plaques, ulcers, or nodules that liquefy and drain may be noted clinically. The histopathologic picture is variable, depending on the injected substance, but may include the presence of birefringent crystals, oil cysts surrounded by fibrosis and inflammation, and an acute inflammatory reaction with fat necrosis. Vessels are characteristically spared.

LIPODYSTROPHY. Several rare conditions are associated with loss of fatty tissue in a partial or generalized distribution.

Partial lipodystrophy occurs more commonly in females than in males and generally begins during the 1st decade of life. There is gradual symmetric loss of subcutaneous tissue. Although the sites of loss are heterogeneous, loss of fat may occur primarily on the trunk and extremities, sparing the face; on the extremities, sparing both the face and trunk; or on the extremities and buttocks. The most common variant involves loss of fat from the face and the upper half of the body, resulting in a cadaverous facies and marked disproportion between the upper and lower halves of the body (Weir-Mitchell type). In some cases, there is a concurrent hypertrophy of the subcutaneous fat of the lower part of the body (Laignel-Lavastine and Viard types); others have hemilipodystrophy involving one half of the face or body. Loss of adipose tissue is not preceded by an inflammatory phase, and histopathologic examination reveals only absence of subcutaneous fat. Some patients have had hypocomplementemia (i.e., low C3) and associated renal disease, particularly progressive membranous mesangiocapillary glomerulonephritis, disordered glucose metabolism, or abnormal serum lipid profiles. The cause of the disorder is not understood, and there is no effective treatment, although dietary restrictions of fats and carbohydrates may be prudent. *Generalized lipodystrophy* may be congenital (Berardinelli-Seip syndrome) or acquired (Seip-Lawrence syndrome).

Congenital generalized lipodystrophy is a progressive multisystem disorder inherited as an autosomal recessive trait. The earliest manifestation is generalized loss of subcutaneous and visceral fat; it may be evident at birth or may occur during infancy. Associated cutaneous changes include prominent superficial veins, hirsutism, abundant curly scalp hair, and acanthosis nigricans. Patients have an anabolic syndrome with a voracious appetite; accelerated skeletal growth, resulting in tall stature; skeletal sclerosis; enlarged joints, especially of the hands and feet; accelerated muscle growth, resulting in a protuberant abdomen; and hypertrophic cardiomyopathy. Precocious enlargement of the genitals and mental deficiency and hemiplegia are seen commonly. Insulin resistance is present from birth. Hyperlipidemia, hyperinsulinism, and insulin-resistant nonketotic diabetes mellitus develop gradually and are reflected by increasing hepatomegaly caused by fatty infiltration and cirrhosis. Serum levels of growth hormone may be normal, but its secretion in response to stimuli may be disturbed. Hypothalamic releasing factors that are not ordinarily found in plasma have been identified in affected patients and suggest a lack of hypothalamic regulation. The underlying problem may be an insulin receptor or postreceptor defect. The acquired form is preceded by an undefined illness or an infection. Pathogenesis appears to involve autoimmune destruction of adipose tissue that results secondarily in an anabolic syndrome with insulin-resistant diabetes. When fat loss becomes generalized, the disease resembles the congenital form, although the anabolic features tend to be less striking. Pimozide, a selective dopamine blocker, or fenfluramine, a serotonergic agonist, may be helpful to some patients. Control of the diabetes with insulin is difficult to achieve, does not affect the course of the lipodystrophy, and is considered contraindicated by some authorities. Dietary fat regulation of energy consumption is the most important and efficacious intervention.

Localized lipoatrophy is an idiopathic condition that presents as annular atrophy at the ankles, a bandlike semicircular depression 2–4 cm in diameter on the thighs or, rarely, on the abdomen and upper groin as a centrifugally spreading, bluish, depressed plaque with an erythematous margin. It occurs predominantly in Japanese children.

Insulin lipoatrophy usually occurs approximately 6 mo–2 yr after initiation of relatively high doses of insulin. A dimple or well-circumscribed depression at the site of injection is typically seen, although loss of fat may extend beyond the site of injection, leading to an extensive, depressed plaque. Biopsy reveals a marked decrease or absence of subcutaneous tissue, without inflammation or fibrosis. In some patients, hypertrophy occurs clinically. In these cases, the mid-dermal collagen is replaced by hypertrophic fat cells on histopathologic sections. The mechanism of insulin lipoatrophy may be cross reaction of insulin antibodies with fat cells, as the incidence of this condition has decreased since the implementation of widespread use of highly purified insulins. Lesions may also be prevented by frequent alteration of injection sites.

Aronson IK, Zeitz HJ, Variakojis D: Panniculitis in childhood. Pediatr Dermatol 5:216, 1988.

Koransky JS, Esterly NB: Lupus panniculitis (profundus). J Pediatr 98:241, 1981.
Seip M, Trygstad O: Generalized lipodystrophy, congenital and acquired (lipoatrophy). Acta Paediatr 413 (Suppl):26, 1996.
Senior B, Gellis SS: The syndromes of total lipodystrophy and of partial lipodystrophy. Pediatrics 33:593, 1964.
Silverman RA, Newman AJ, LeVine MJ: Post-steroid panniculitis; a case report. Pediatr Dermatol 5:92, 1988.

CHAPTER 667
Disorders of the Sweat Glands

Eccrine glands are found over nearly the entire skin surface and provide the primary means, through evaporation of the water in sweat, for cooling the body. These glands have no anatomic relationship to hair follicles and secrete a relatively large amount of odorless aqueous sweat. In contrast, apocrine glands are limited in distribution to the axillas, anogenital skin, mammary glands, ceruminous glands of the ear, Moll glands in the eyelid, and selected areas of the face and scalp. The apocrine gland duct enters the pilosebaceous follicle at the level of the infundibulum and secretes a small amount of a complex, viscous fluid that, on alteration by microorganisms, produces a distinctive body odor. Some disorders of these two sweat glands are similar pathogenetically, whereas others are unique to a given gland.

ANHIDROSIS. *Neuropathic anhidrosis* results from a disturbance in the neural pathway from the control center in the brain to the peripheral efferent nerve fibers that activate sweating. Disorders in this category, which are characterized by generalized anhidrosis, include tumors of the hypothalamus and damage to the floor of the third ventricle. Pontine or medullary lesions may produce anhidrosis of the ipsilateral face or neck and ipsilateral or contralateral anhidrosis of the rest of the body. Peripheral or segmental neuropathies, caused by leprosy, amyloidosis, diabetes mellitus, alcoholic neuritis, or syringomyelia, may be associated with anhidrosis of the innervated skin. Various autonomic disorders are also associated with altered eccrine sweat gland function.

At the *level of the sweat gland*, drugs such as the anticholinergics atropine and scopolamine may paralyze the sweat glands. Acute intoxication with barbiturates or diazepam has produced necrosis of sweat glands, resulting in anhidrosis with or without erythema and bullae. Eccrine glands are largely absent throughout the skin or are present in a localized area among patients with anhidrotic ectodermal dysplasia and localized congenital absence of sweat glands, respectively. Infiltrative or destructive disorders that may produce atrophy of sweat glands by pressure or scarring include scleroderma, acrodermatitis chronica atrophicans, radiodermatitis, burns, Sjögren's disease, multiple myeloma, and lymphoma. Obstruction of sweat glands may occur in miliaria and in a number of inflammatory and hyperkeratotic disorders such as the ichthyoses, psoriasis, lichen planus, pemphigus, porokeratosis, atopic dermatitis, and seborrheic dermatitis. Occlusion of the sweat pore may also occur with the topical agents aluminum and zirconium salts, formaldehyde, or glutaraldehyde.

Diverse *disorders that are associated with anhidrosis by unknown mechanisms* include dehydration; toxic overdose with lead, arsenic, thallium, fluorine, or morphine; uremia; cirrhosis; endocrine disorders such as Addison disease, diabetes mellitus, diabetes insipidus, or hyperthyroidism; and inherited conditions such as Fabry disease, Franceschetti-Jadassohn syndrome, which combines features of incontinentia pigmenti and anhidrotic ectodermal dysplasia, and familial anhidrosis with neurolabyrinthitis.

Whereas anhidrosis may be complete, in many cases, what appears clinically to be anhidrosis is actually *hypohidrosis* caused by anhidrosis of many but not all eccrine glands. Compensatory, localized *hyperhidrosis* of the remaining functional sweat glands may occur, particularly in diabetes mellitus and miliaria. The primary complication of anhidrosis is hyperthermia, seen primarily in anhidrotic ectodermal dysplasia or in otherwise normal preterm or full-term *neonates* who have immature eccrine glands.

HYPERHIDROSIS. The numerous disorders that may be associated with increased production of eccrine sweat may also be classified into those with neural mechanisms involving an abnormality in the pathway from the neural regulatory centers to the sweat gland and those that are non-neurally mediated by direct effects on the sweat glands (Table 667–1). Excessive sweating of the palms and soles in response to emotional stimuli (volar hyperhidrosis) may respond to 10% glutaraldehyde soaks, 20% aluminum chloride in anhydrous ethanol applied under occlusion for several hours, iontophoretic therapy with anticholinergics, or in severe, refractory cases, cervicothoracic or lumbar sympathectomy. Axillary hyperhidrosis does not respond to topical glutaraldehyde or salts of aluminum, zirconium, or zinc. Aluminum chloride (Drysol) applied to the axillae at bedtime under occlusion, aided, if necessary, by oral administration of an anticholinergic agent such as glycopyrrolate, may produce a prompt and significant reduction in sweating. Cervicothoracic sympathectomy or selective surgical removal of the most highly sudoriferous eccrine glands in the axillae may be effective in refractory cases.

MILIARIA. This results from retention of sweat in occluded eccrine sweat ducts as a result of a keratinous plug in the sweat duct. Retrograde pressure may result in rupture of the duct and leakage of sweat into the epidermis and/or the dermis. The eruption is most often induced by hot, humid

TABLE 667–1 Causes of Hyperhidrosis

Cortical	***Vasomotor***
Emotional	Cold injury
Familial dysautonomia	Raynaud phenomenon
Congenital ichthyosiform erythroderma	Rheumatoid arthritis
Epidermolysis bullosa	***Neurologic***
Nail-patella syndrome	Abscess
Jadassohn-Lewandowsky syndrome	Familial dysautonomia
Pachyonychia congenita	Postencephalitic
Palmoplantar keratoderma	Tumor
Hypothalamic	***Miscellaneous***
Drugs	Chédiak-Higashi syndrome
Antipyretics	Compensatory
Emetics	Phenylketonuria
Insulin	Pheochromocytoma
Meperidine	Vitiligo
Exercise	**Medullary**
Infection	Physiologic gustatory sweating
Defervescence	Encephalitis
Chronic illness	Granulosis rubra nasi
Metabolic	Syringomyelia
Debility	Thoracic sympathetic trunk injury
Diabetes mellitus	**Spinal**
Hyperpituitarism	Cord transection
Hyperthyroidism	Syringomyelia
Hypoglycemia	**Changes in Blood Flow**
Obesity	Maffucci syndrome
Porphyria	Arteriovenous fistula
Pregnancy	Klippel-Trenaunay syndrome
Rickets	Glomus tumor
Infantile scurvy	Blue rubber bleb nevus syndrome
Cardiovascular	
Heart failure	
Shock	

weather, but it may also be caused by high fever. Infants who are dressed too warmly may develop this eruption indoors even during the winter.

In *miliaria crystallina,* asymptomatic, noninflammatory, pinpoint clear vesicles may suddenly erupt in profusion over large areas of the body surface, leaving brawny desquamation on healing (Fig. 667–1). The clarity of the fluid, superficiality of the vesicles, and absence of inflammation permit differentiation from other blistering disorders. This type of miliaria occurs most frequently in newborn infants because of the relative immaturity and delayed patency of the sweat duct and the tendency for infants to be nursed in relatively warm, humid conditions. It may also occur in older patients with hyperpyrexia. Histopathologically, an intracorneal or subcorneal vesicle is seen in communication with the sweat duct.

Miliaria rubra is a less superficial eruption characterized by erythematous, minute papulovesicles that may impart a prickling sensation. The lesions are usually localized to sites of occlusion or to flexural areas, such as the neck, groin, and axillae, where friction may have a role in their pathogenesis. Involved skin may become macerated and eroded. This lesion may be confused with or superimposed on other diaper area eruptions, including candidosis and folliculitis; lesions of miliaria rubra, however, are extrafollicular. Histopathologically, one sees focal areas of spongiosis and spongiotic vesicle formation in close proximity to sweat ducts that generally contain a keratinous plug. The keratinous plug does not form, however, until the later stages of the disease and therefore does not appear to be the primary cause of sweat duct obstruction. The initial obstruction is postulated to be due to swelling of the ductal epidermal cells, perhaps from imbibition of water. Miliaria rubra is generally reversible. Supplemental vitamin C may help to restore normal sweating in refractory cases. Prophylactic use of antibacterial agents may prevent development of miliaria rubra. Repeated attacks of miliaria rubra may lead to *miliaria profunda,* which is due to rupture of the sweat duct deeper in the skin at the level of the dermoepidermal junction. Severe, extensive miliaria rubra or miliaria profunda may result in disturbance of heat regulation. Lesions of miliaria rubra may become infected, particularly in malnourished or debilitated infants, leading to development of periporitis staphylogenes, which involves extension of the process from the sweat duct into the sweat gland.

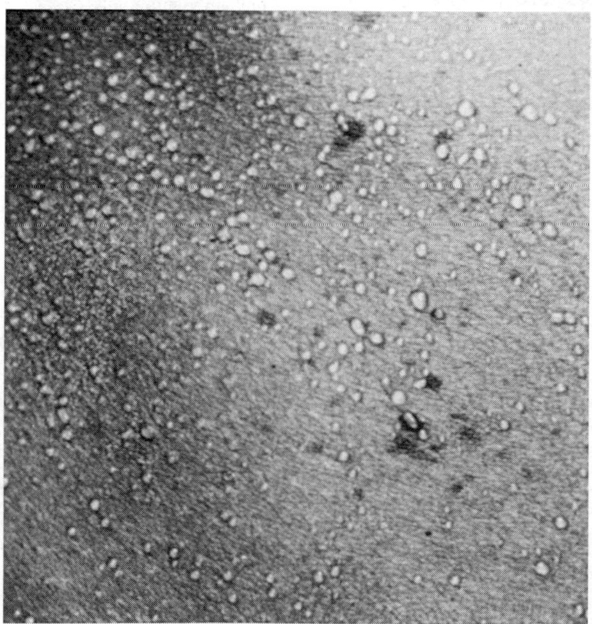

Figure 667–1 Superficial clear vesicles of miliaria crystallina in a patient with hyperpyrexia and lymphoma.

All forms of miliaria respond dramatically to cooling the patient by regulation of environmental temperatures and by removal of excessive clothing; administration of antipyretics is also beneficial to patients with fever. Topical agents are usually ineffective and may exacerbate the eruption.

BROMHIDROSIS. The excessive odor that characterizes bromhidrosis may result from alteration of either apocrine or eccrine sweat. Apocrine bromhidrosis develops after puberty as a result of the formation of short-chain fatty acids and ammonia by the action of anaerobic diphtheroids on axillary apocrine sweat. Treatments that may be helpful include cleansing with germicidal soaps; topical application of aluminum, zirconium, or zinc salts or gentamicin cream, all of which have antibacterial action; and axillary shaving. Eccrine bromhidrosis is caused by microbiologic degradation of stratum corneum that has become softened by excessive eccrine sweat. The soles of the feet and the intertriginous areas are the primary affected sites. Hyperhidrosis, warm weather, obesity, intertrigo, and diabetes mellitus are predisposing factors. In addition to local measures, oral anticholinergic drugs such as propantheline (Pro-Banthine) may decrease eccrine sweating but do not alter apocrine gland secretion. Topical aluminum chloride preparations such as Drysol are particularly useful for plantar eccrine bromhidrosis.

HIDRADENITIS SUPPURATIVA. This is a chronic, inflammatory, suppurative disorder of the apocrine glands in the axillae, the anogenital area, and occasionally the scalp, posterior aspect of the ears, female breasts, and periumbilical area. Onset of clinical manifestations, sometimes preceded by pruritus or discomfort, usually occurs during puberty or early adulthood. Solitary or multiple painful erythematous nodules, deep abscesses, and contracted scars are sharply confined to areas of skin containing apocrine glands. When the disease is severe and chronic, sinus tracts, ulcers, and thick, linear fibrotic bands develop. Hidradenitis suppurativa tends to persist for many years, punctuated by relapses and partial remissions. Complications include cellulitis, ulceration, and burrowing abscesses that may perforate adjacent structures, forming fistulas to the urethra, bladder, rectum, or peritoneum. Episodic inflammatory arthritis develops in some patients. A minority of patients have the follicular occlusion triad, which includes acne and perifolliculitis capitis. Early lesions are often mistaken for infected epidermal cysts, furuncles, scrofuloderma, actinomycosis, cat-scratch disease, granuloma inguinale, or lymphogranuloma venereum. Sharp localization to areas of the body that bear apocrine glands, however, should suggest hidradenitis. When involvement is limited to the anogenital region, the condition may be difficult to distinguish from Crohn disease and may coexist with it.

Histopathologically, early lesions are characterized by a keratinous plug in the apocrine duct or hair follicle orifice and by cystic distention of the follicle. The process generally but not necessarily extends into the apocrine gland. Later changes include inflammation within and around apocrine glands and the presence of groups of cocci within apocrine glands and in the adjacent dermis. Skin appendages may become obliterated by scarring. The disease is probably initiated by plugging of apocrine gland ducts with keratinous debris. Bacterial infection, particularly with *Staphylococcus aureus, Streptococcus milleri, Escherichia coli,* and possibly anaerobic streptococci, appears to be important in the progressive dilatation below the obstruction, leading to rupture of the duct, inflammation, sinus tract formation, and destructive scarring. Pathogenesis of hidradenitis suppurativa is controversial, but it appears to be an androgen-dependent condition.

Patients should be counseled to avoid tight-fitting clothes, because occlusion may exacerbate the condition. *Treatment* with topical antibiotic agents such as chlorhexidine, erythromycin, or clindamycin or with topical retinoids may be effective in early, indolent disease. Systemic antibiotics, chosen on the basis of bacterial culture (usually staphylococcal and streptococcal pathogens) and sensitivity tests, should be administered in the acute phase. Empirical therapy may be initiated with tetracycline, doxycycline, or minocycline if the patient is 8 yr or older; clindamycin and cephalosporins also are effective. Some patients require long-term treatment with tetracycline or erythromycin. Intralesional triamcinolone acetonide (5–10 mg/mL) is often helpful in early disease. The addition of prednisone, 40–60 mg/day for 7–10 days, tapering gradually as inflammation subsides, to the regimen of patients who respond poorly to antibiotics may decrease fibrosis and scarring. Oral contraceptive agents, which contain a high estrogen-to-progesterone ratio and low androgenicity of the progesterone, or oral retinoids may be helpful in some patients. Warm compresses encourage spontaneous rupture of abscesses; those that are "pointing" should be incised and drained. Ultimately, surgical measures may be required for control or cure.

FOX-FORDYCE DISEASE. This disease is most common in females and presents during puberty or the 3rd decade of life with pruritus in the axillae and, occasionally, in the anogenital region and around the breasts. Pruritus is exacerbated by emotional stress and stimuli that induce apocrine sweating. Skin-colored to slightly hyperpigmented dome-shaped follicular papules develop in the pruritic areas. Histopathologically, one sees keratinous plugging of the distal apocrine duct, rupture of the intraepidermal portion of the apocrine duct, paraductal microvesicle formation, and paraductal acanthosis. The condition generally remits during pregnancy, particularly in the third trimester. Oral contraceptive pills and topical corticosteroids or retinoic acid may help some patients.

Barth JH, Kealey T: Androgen metabolism by isolated human axillary apocrine glands in hidradenitis suppurativa. Br J Dermatol 125:304, 1991.

Holzle E, Kligman AM: The pathogenesis of miliaria rubra. Br J Dermatol 99:117, 1978.

Jackman PJH: Body odor—the role of skin bacteria. Semin Dermatol 1:143, 1982.

Sato K, Kang WH, Saga K, et al: Biology of sweat glands and their disorders. J Am Acad Dermatol 20:537, 1989.

CHAPTER 668
Disorders of Hair

Disorders of hair in infants and children may be due to intrinsic disturbances of hair growth, underlying biochemical or metabolic defects, inflammatory dermatoses, or structural anomalies of the hair shaft. Excessive and abnormal hair growth is referred to as hypertrichosis or hirsutism. Hypertrichosis is excessive hair growth at inappropriate locations; hirsutism is an androgen-dependent male pattern of hair growth in women. Hypotrichosis is deficient hair growth, and hair loss, partial or complete, is called alopecia. Alopecia may be classified as nonscarring or scarring; the latter type is rare in children and, if present, is most often due to prolonged or untreated inflammatory conditions such as pyoderma or tinea capitis.

HYPERTRICHOSIS

Hypertrichosis is rare in children and may be localized or generalized and permanent or transient. Hypertrichosis has many causes, some of which are listed in Table 668–1.

TABLE 668–1 Causes of and Conditions Associated with Hypertrichosis

Intrinsic Factors

Racial and familial forms such as hairy ears, hairy elbows, intraphalangeal hair, or generalized hirsutism

Extrinsic Factors

Local trauma
Malnutrition
Anorexia nervosa
Long-standing inflammatory dermatoses
Drugs
  Diazoxide, phenytoin, corticosteroids, Cortisporin, cyclosporine, androgens, anabolic agents, hexachlorobenzene, minoxidil, psoralens, penicillamine, streptomycin

Hamartomas or Nevi

Congenital pigmented nevocytic nevus, nevus pilosus, Becker nevus, congenital smooth muscle hamartoma, fawn-tail nevus associated with diastematomyelia

Endocrine Disorders

Virilizing ovarian tumors, Cushing syndrome, acromegaly, hyperthyroidism, hypothyroidism, congenital adrenal hyperplasia, adrenal tumors, gonadal dysgenesis, male pseudohermaphroditism, nonendocrine hormone–secreting tumors, polycystic ovary syndrome

Congenital and Genetic Disorders

Hypertrichosis lanuginosa, mucopolysaccharidosis, leprechaunism, congenital generalized lipodystrophy, de Lange syndrome, trisomy 18, Rubinstein-Taybi syndrome, Bloom syndrome, congenital hemihypertrophy, gingival fibromatosis with hypertrichosis, Winchester syndrome, lipoatrophic diabetes (Lawrence-Seip syndrome), fetal hydantoin syndrome, fetal alcohol syndrome, congenital erythropoietic or variegate porphyria (sun-exposed areas), porphyria cutanea tarda (sun-exposed areas), Cowden syndrome, Seckel syndrome, Gorlin syndrome, partial trisomy 3 q, Ambra syndrome

HYPOTRICHOSIS AND ALOPECIA

Some of the disorders associated with hypotrichosis and alopecia are listed in Table 668–2. True alopecia is rarely congenital; it is more often related to an inflammatory dermatosis, mechanical factors, drug ingestion, infection, endocrinopathy, nutritional disturbance, or disturbance of the hair cycle. Any

TABLE 688–2 Disorders Associated with Alopecia and Hypotrichosis

Congenital total alopecia: isolated autosomal recessive abnormality, progeria, hidrotic ectodermal dysplasia, Moynahan syndrome, atrichia with keratin cysts, Baraitser syndrome
Congenital localized alopecia: aplasia cutis, alopecia triangularis, epidermal nevus, hair follicle hamartoma, facial hemiatrophy (Romberg syndrome), male pattern baldness
Hereditary hypotrichosis: hypotrichosis with keratosis pilaris, Marie-Unna syndrome, phenylketonuria, arginosuccinic aciduria, hyperlysinemia, homocystinuria, orotic aciduria, Cockayne syndrome, Rothmund-Thomson syndrome, dyskeratosis congenita, Seckel syndrome, cartilage-hair hypoplasia, Conradi syndrome, pachyonychia congenita, Hallermann-Streiff syndrome, Treacher Collins syndrome, oculodentodigital, orofaciodigital, incontinentia pigmenti, focal dermal hypoplasia, keratosis follicularis, epidermolysis bullosa, ectodermal dysplasias, ichthyoses, loose anagen hair
Diffuse alopecia of endocrine origin: hypopituitarism, hypothyroidism, hypoparathyroidism, hyperthyroidism, diabetes mellitus
Alopecia of nutritional origin: marasmus, kwashiorkor, iron deficiency, zinc deficiency (acrodermatitis enteropathica), gluten-sensitive enteropathy, essential fatty acid deficiency, biotinidase deficiency
Disturbances of the hair cycle: telogen effluvium
Toxic alopecia: anagen effluvium
Autoimmune alopecia: alopecia areata
Traumatic alopecia: traction alopecia, trichotillomania
Cicatricial alopecia: lupus erythematosus, lichen planus pilaris, pseudopelade, scleroderma, dermatomyositis, infection (kerion, favus, tuberculosis, syphilis, folliculitis, leishmaniasis, herpes zoster, varicella), acne keloidalis, follicular mucinosis, cicatricial pemphigoid, lichen sclerosus et atrophicus, sarcoidosis
Hair shaft abnormalities: monilethrix, pili annulati, pili torti, trichorrhexis invaginata, trichorrhexis nodosa, woolly hair syndrome, Menkes disease, trichothiodystrophy, trichodento-osseous syndrome, trichorhinophalangeal syndrome, uncombable hair syndrome (spun glass hair, pili trianguli et canaliculi)

inflammatory condition of the scalp, such as atopic dermatitis or seborrheic dermatitis, if severe enough, may result in partial alopecia; hair growth returns to normal if the underlying condition is treated successfully, unless the hair follicle has been permanently damaged.

TELOGEN EFFLUVIUM. Telogen effluvium presents with sudden loss of large amounts of hair, often with brushing, combing, and washing of hair. Diffuse loss of scalp hair occurs from premature conversion of growing, or anagen, hairs, which normally constitute 80–90% of hairs, to resting, or telogen, hairs. Hair loss is noted 6 wk to 3 mo after the precipitating cause, which may include childbirth; a febrile episode; surgery; acute blood loss, including blood donation; sudden severe weight loss; discontinuation of high-dose corticosteroids or oral contraceptives; and psychiatric stress. Telogen effluvium also accounts for the loss of hair by infants during the first few months of life; friction from bedsheets, particularly in infants with pruritic, atopic skin, may exacerbate the problem. There is no inflammatory reaction; the hair follicles remain intact, and telogen bulbs can be demonstrated microscopically on shed hairs. Because more than 50% of the scalp hair is rarely involved, alopecia is usually not severe. Parents should be reassured that normal hair growth will return within approximately 6 mo.

TOXIC ALOPECIA (Anagen Effluvium). Anagen effluvium is an acute, severe, diffuse inhibition of growth of anagen follicles, resulting in loss of greater than 80–90% of scalp hair. Hairs become dystrophic, and the hair shaft breaks at the narrowed segment. Loss is diffuse, rapid (1–3 wk after treatment), and temporary, as regrowth occurs after the offending agent is discontinued. Causes of anagen effluvium include radiation; cancer chemotherapeutic agents such as antimetabolites, alkylating agents, and mitotic inhibitors; thallium; thiouracil; heparin; the coumarins; boric acid; and hypervitaminosis A.

TRACTION ALOPECIA (Marginal or Traumatic Alopecia). Traction alopecia is due to trauma to hair follicles by tight braids or ponytails, headbands, rubber bands, curlers, and rollers (Fig. 668–1*A*). Broken hairs and inflammatory follicular papules in circumscribed patches at the scalp margins are characteristic and may be subtended by regional lymphadenopathy. Children and parents must be encouraged to avoid devices that cause trauma to the hair and, if necessary, to alter the hair style. Otherwise, scarring of hair follicles may occur.

TRICHOTILLOMANIA. Compulsive pulling, twisting, and breaking of hair produces irregular areas of incomplete hair loss, most often on the crown and in the occipital and parietal areas of the scalp (Fig. 668–1*B*). Occasionally, eyebrows, eyelashes, and body hair are traumatized. Some plaques of alopecia may have a linear outline. The hairs remaining within the areas of loss are of various lengths and are typically blunt tipped because of breakage. The scalp appears normal, although chronic folliculitis may also occur. Trichophagy, resulting in trichobezoars, may complicate this disorder. The lifetime occurrence is 3% in girls and 1% in boys.

The *diagnosis* of trichotillomania is often difficult and may require biopsy confirmation. The *Diagnostic and Statistical Manual of Mental Disorders* diagnostic criteria include visible hair loss attributable to pulling; mounting tension preceding hair pulling; gratification or release of tension after hair pulling; and absence of hair pulling attributable to hallucinations, delusions, or an inflammatory skin condition. Histologic changes include coexistent normal and damaged follicles, perifollicular hemorrhage, atrophy of some follicles, and catagen transformation of hair. In late stages, perifollicular fibrosis may occur. Long-term repeated trauma may result in irreversible damage and permanent alopecia. Tinea capitis and alopecia areata must be considered in the differential diagnosis.

Trichotillomania is closely related to, and may be an expression of, obsessive-compulsive disorder in some children; in others, it is a benign habit disorder. *Treatment* of concurrent thumb sucking may be effective in the latter children. When trichotillomania occurs secondary to obsessive-compulsive disorder, clomipramine, fluoxetine, or trazodone may be helpful, particularly when combined with behavioral interventions.

ALOPECIA AREATA. Alopecia areata is characterized by rapid and complete loss of hair in round or oval patches on the scalp (Fig. 668–1*C*) and on other body sites. In *alopecia totalis,* all the scalp hair is lost; *alopecia universalis* involves all body and scalp hair. The lifetime incidence of alopecia areata is 1% of the population; approximately 60% of patients are younger than 20 yr of age.

Clinical Manifestations. Peripheral spread and confluence of plaques of alopecia areata often result in bizarre patterns. At the margin of active patches, the hairs can often be extracted with gentle traction and, on examination, demonstrate an attenuated or catagen bulb at the termination of a tapered, poorly pigmented shaft (i.e., exclamation hair). The skin within the plaques of hair loss appears normal. A perifollicular infiltrate of inflammatory round cells is found in biopsy specimens from active areas. In the chronic stages, the number of telogen hairs is increased, the diameter of hair fibers is reduced, and trichodystrophies such as trichorrhexis nodosa and trichomalacia may be found. Alopecia areata is associated with atopy; nail changes such as pits, ridges, opacification, serration of the free nail edge, dystrophy, and a red lunula; cataracts or lens opacification; and autoimmune diseases such as Hashimoto thyroiditis, Addison disease, pernicious anemia, ulcerative colitis, myasthenia gravis, collagen vascular diseases, and vitiligo. An increased incidence of alopecia areata has been reported in patients with Down syndrome (5–10%).

Etiology. The cause of alopecia areata is unknown. Emotional factors and stress have been suggested as triggering factors, but supportive evidence is tenuous. About 10–20% of patients have a family history of alopecia areata; the estimated risk for first-degree relatives is 6%. Inheritance is thought to be autosomal dominant with variable penetrance. The infrequent but striking association with autoimmune diseases has suggested an autoimmune pathogenesis. Some patients have serum antibodies to thyroglobulin, parietal cells, and adrenal gland, and autoantibodies to hair follicle antigens has been demonstrated.

Differential Diagnosis and Prognosis. Tinea capitis, seborrheic dermatitis, trichotillomania, traumatic alopecia, and lupus erythematosus should be considered. The course is unpredictable, but spontaneous resolution within 6–12 mo is usual, particularly when relatively small, stable patches of alopecia are present. Recurrences, however, are common. In general, onset at a young age, extensive or prolonged hair loss, numerous episodes, and associated atrophy are poor prognostic signs. Alopecia universalis, totalis, and *ophiasis,* a type of alopecia areata in which hair loss is circumferential, are also less likely to resolve.

Treatment. This is difficult to evaluate because the course is erratic and unpredictable. The use of high-potency topical fluorinated corticosteroids with occlusion at night is effective in some patients. Intradermal injections of steroid may also stimulate hair growth locally, but this mode of treatment is impractical in young children or in those with extensive hair loss. Systemic corticosteroid therapy has, on occasion, been associated with good results; however, the permanence of cure is questionable, and the side effects are a serious deterrent. Additional therapies that are sometimes effective include short-contact anthralin, topical minoxidil, and contact sensitization with squaric acid dibutylester or diphencyprone. Psoralen and ultraviolet A phototherapy may also be effective but has limited applicability in children. In general, parents and patients can be reassured that spontaneous remission usually occurs. New hair growth may initially be of finer caliber and lighter color, but replacement by normal terminal hair can be expected.

STRUCTURAL DEFECTS OF HAIR. Structural defects of the hair shaft

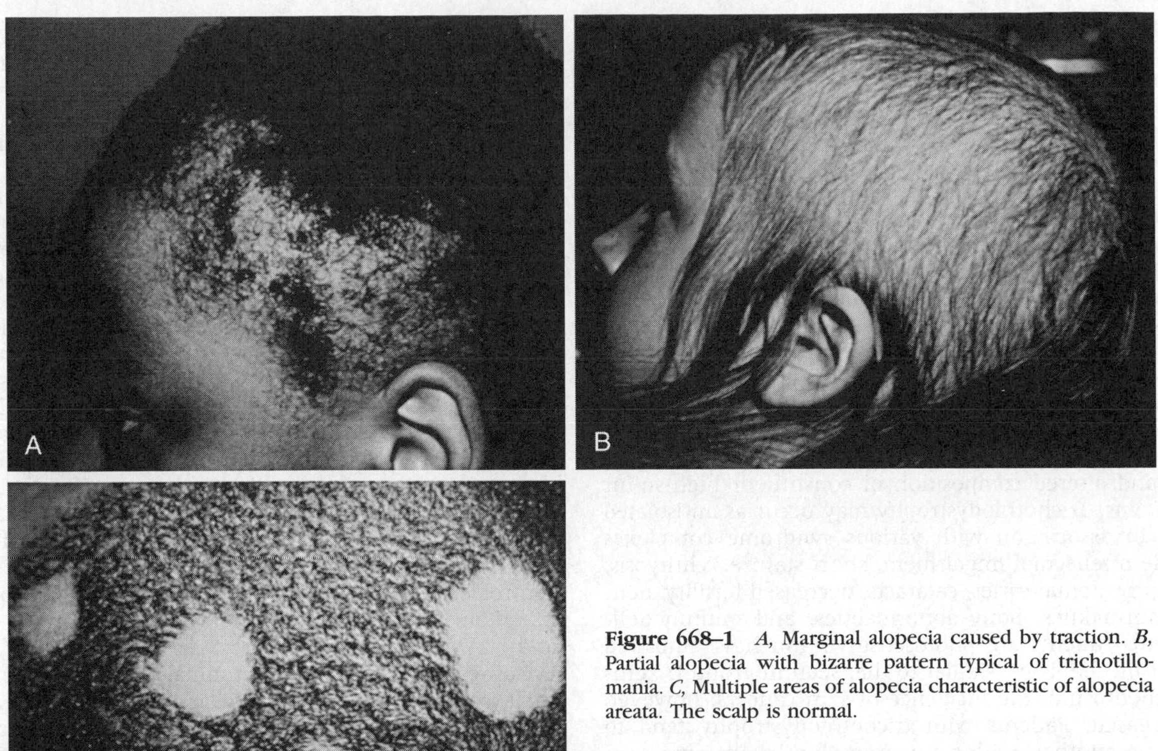

Figure 668–1 *A,* Marginal alopecia caused by traction. *B,* Partial alopecia with bizarre pattern typical of trichotillomania. *C,* Multiple areas of alopecia characteristic of alopecia areata. The scalp is normal.

may be congenital, reflect known biochemical aberrations, or relate to damaging grooming practices. All the defects can be demonstrated by microscopic examination of affected hairs, particularly by scanning and transmission electron microscopy.

TRICHORRHEXIS NODOSA. This is the most common of all hair shaft abnormalities. The hair is dry, brittle, and lusterless, with irregularly spaced grayish-white nodes on the hair shaft. Microscopically, the nodes have the appearance of two interlocking brushes. The defect results from a fracture of the hair shaft at the nodal points caused by disruption of the cells in the hair cortex. Trichorrhexis nodosa has been noted as an isolated congenital defect in some families, has been observed in some infants with Menkes syndrome or argininosuccinic aciduria, and may occur in Netherton syndrome or in association with ectodermal dysplasia and other hair shaft abnormalities such as pili annulati.

Acquired Trichorrhexis Nodosa. This, the most common cause of hair breakage, occurs in two forms. *Proximal defects* are found most frequently in black children, whose complaint is not of alopecia but of failure of their hair to grow. The hair is short, and longitudinal splits, knots, and whitish nodules can be demonstrated in hair mounts. Easy breakage is demonstrated by gentle traction on the hair shafts. A history of other affected family members may be obtained. The problem is thought to be caused by a combination of genetic predisposition and the cumulative mechanical trauma of rough combing and brushing, hair-straightening procedures, and "permanents." Patients must be cautioned to avoid damaging grooming techniques. A soft natural-bristle brush and a wide-toothed comb should be used. The condition is self-limited, with resolution in 2–4 yr if patients avoid damaging practices. *Distal trichorrhexis nodosa* is seen more frequently in white and Asian children. The distal portion of the hair shaft is thinned, ragged, and faded; white specks, sometimes mistaken for nits, may be noted along the shaft. Hair mounts reveal the paintbrush defect and the sites of excessive fragility and breakage. Localized areas of the moustache or beard may also be affected. Avoidance of traumatic grooming, regular trimming of affected ends, and the use of cream rinses to lessen tangling ameliorate this condition.

PILI TORTI. This is the second most common hair shaft abnormality. At age 3 mo–2 yr, patients present with spangled, brittle, coarse hair of different lengths over the entire scalp or with circumscribed alopecia. There is a structural defect in which the hair shaft is grooved and flattened at irregular intervals and is twisted on its axis to various degrees. Minor twists that occur in normal hair should not be misconstrued as pili torti. Curvature of the hair follicle apparently leads to the flattening and rotation of the hair shaft. Most cases of classic, isolated pili torti of early onset have autosomal dominant inheritance. Autosomal recessive forms have been described, however, and many cases are sporadic. Keratosis pilaris, nail dystrophy, and corneal opacity develop in some patients. Syndromes in which the hair shaft abnormalities of pili torti are seen in association with other cutaneous and systemic abnormalities include Menkes kinky hair, Bazex syndrome, Björnstad syndrome (pili torti with deafness), Crandall and Rapp-Hodgkin ectodermal dysplasia syndrome and trichothiodystrophy. It has also occurred in children treated with retinoids.

MONILETHRIX. This rare defect of the hair shaft is inherited as an autosomal dominant trait with variable age of onset, severity, and course. The hair appears dry, lusterless, and brittle, and it fractures spontaneously or with mild trauma. Eyebrows, lashes, body and pubic hair, and scalp hair may be affected. Monilethrix may be present at birth, but the hair is usually normal at birth and is replaced over the first few months of life by abnormal hairs; the condition sometimes is first apparent in childhood. Follicular papules may appear on the nape of the neck and the occiput and, occasionally, over the entire scalp. Short, fragile beaded hairs that emerge from the horny follicular plugs give a distinctive appearance. Keratosis pilaris and koilonychia of fingernails and toenails may also be present.

Microscopically, a distinctive, regular beading pattern of the hair shaft is evident, characterized by elliptic nodes that are separated by narrower internodes. Not all hairs have nodes, and both normal and beaded hairs may break. Patients should be advised to handle the hair gently to minimize breakage. Treatment is generally ineffective, although topical minoxidil and oral etretinate have helped some patients. Spontaneous improvement may occur at puberty, during pregnancy, and with use of oral contraceptive pills.

TRICHOTHIODYSTROPHY. Hair in trichothiodystrophy is sparse, short, brittle, and uneven; the scalp hair, eyebrows, or eyelashes may be affected. Microscopically, the hair is flattened, folded, and variable in diameter; has longitudinal grooving; and has nodal swellings that resemble those of trichorrhexis nodosa. Under a polarizing microscope, distinctive alternating dark and light bands are seen. The abnormal hair has a cystine content that is less than 50% of normal because of a major reduction and altered composition of constituent high-sulfur matrix proteins. Trichothiodystrophy may occur as an isolated finding or in association with various syndrome complexes that include intellectual impairment, short stature, ichthyosis, nail dystrophy, dental caries, cataracts, decreased fertility, neurologic abnormalities, bony abnormalities, and immunodeficiency. Some patients are photosensitive and have impaired DNA repair mechanisms, similar to that seen in group D xeroderma pigmentosum; the incidence of skin cancers, however, is not increased. Patients with trichothiodystrophy tend to resemble one another, with a receding chin, protruding ears, raspy voice, and sociable, outgoing personality. *Trichoschisis*, a fracture perpendicular to the hair shaft, is characteristic of the many syndromes that are associated with trichothiodystrophy. Perpendicular breakage of the hair shaft has also been described in association with other hair abnormalities, particularly monilethrix.

TRICHORRHEXIS INVAGINATA (Bamboo Hair). Short, sparse, fragile hair without apparent growth is characteristic of this condition, which is found primarily in association with Netherton syndrome (see Chapter 664). It has also been reported in other ichthyosiform dermatoses. The distal portion of the hair is invaginated into the cuplike proximal portion, forming a fragile nodal swelling. The abnormality is thought to result from a transient defect in keratinization of the inner root sheath and/or a partial defect in the conversion of sulfhydryl groups to disulfide bonds in the cortex. The abnormality may be identified in body and scalp hair and seems to abate as the child matures.

MENKES KINKY HAIR SYNDROME (Trichopoliodystrophy). Males with this sex-linked recessive trait are born to an unaffected mother after a normal pregnancy. Neonatal problems include hypothermia, hypotonia, poor feeding, seizures, and failure to thrive. Hair is normal to sparse at birth but is replaced by short, fine, brittle, light-colored hair that may have features of trichorrhexis nodosa, pili torti, or monilethrix. The skin is hypopigmented and thin cheeks typically appear plump, and the nasal bridge is depressed. Heterozygotes may have loss of skin pigmentation. Progressive psychomotor retardation is noted in early infancy. The disorder has been localized by linkage analysis to chromosome Xq13.3 and is due to a maldistribution of copper in the body. Copper uptake across the brush border of the small intestine is increased, but copper transport from these cells into the plasma is defective, resulting in low total body copper stores. Variable treatment success has been achieved with subcutaneous or intramuscular injection of copper salts.

PILI ANNULATI. Pili annulati is characterized by alternate light and dark bands of the hair shaft. When one is viewing the hair under the light microscope, the region that appeared bright in reflected light instead appears dark in the transmitted light as a result of focal aggregates of abnormal air-filled cavities within the hair shaft. The hair is not fragile. The defect may be autosomal dominant or sporadic. *Pseudopili annulati* is a variant of normal blond hair; an optical effect caused by the refraction and reflection of light from the partially twisted and flattened shaft creates the impression of banding.

WOOLLY HAIR DISEASE. This disorder presents at birth with peculiarly tight, curly, abnormal hair in a nonblack person. It becomes worse in childhood and ameliorates in adulthood. An autosomal dominant form, evident at birth or in infancy, consists of excessively curly, fragile hair. An autosomal recessive type includes scalp hair that is brittle, has a bleached appearance, and is markedly reduced in diameter; body hair is short and pale. Woolly hair nevus, a sporadic form, involves only a circumscribed portion of the scalp hair. The affected hair is fine, tightly curled, and light colored, and it grows poorly. It may be associated with a pigmented or epidermal nevus in another site of the body or with ocular defects. Microscopically, affected hairs are oval and show twisting 180 degrees on their axis.

UNCOMBABLE HAIR SYNDROME (Spun Glass Hair). The hair of patients with this syndrome appears disorderly, is often silvery blond, and may break because of repeated, futile efforts to control it. The condition is probably autosomal dominant in inheritance, is usually first noticed in the first 3 yr of life, and may spontaneously improve in childhood. Eyebrows and eyelashes are normal. A longitudinal depression along the hair shaft is a constant feature, and most hair follicles and shafts are triangular (pili trianguli et canaliculi). The shape of the hair varies along its length, however, preventing the hairs from lying flat.

Baumeister F, Schwarz H, Stengel-Rutkowski S: Childhood hypertrichosis: Diagnosis and management. Arch Dis Child 72:457, 1995.
Birnbaum PS, Baden HP: Heritable disorders of hair. Dermatol Clin 5:137, 1987.
Dawber R: Self-induced hair loss. Semin Dermatol 4:53, 1985.
Headington JT: Telogen effluvium. New concepts and review. Arch Dermatol 129:356, 1993.
Price VH: Trichothiodystrophy: update. Pediatr Dermatol 9:369, 1992.
Rittmaster R: Hirsutism. Lancet 349:191, 1997.
Thiers BH, Bergfeld WF, Fiedler-Weiss VC, et al: Alopecia areata symposium. Pediatr Dermatol 4:136, 1987.
Tobin DJ, Orentreich N, Fenton DA, et al: Antibodies to hair follicles in alopecia areata. J Invest Dermatol 102:721, 1994.
Verbov J: Hair loss in children. Arch Dis Child 68:702, 1993.

CHAPTER 669
Disorders of the Nails

Nail abnormalities in children may be manifestations of generalized skin disease, skin disease localized to the periungual region, systemic disease, drugs, trauma, or localized bacterial and fungal infections. Nail anomalies are also common in certain congenital disorders (Table 669–1).

Anonychia is absence of the nail plate, usually a result of a congenital disorder or trauma. It may be an isolated finding or

TABLE 669–1 Congenital Disease with Nail Defects

Large nails: Pachyonychia congenita, Rubinstein-Taybi syndrome, hemihypertrophy

Small or absent nails: Ectodermal dysplasias, nail-patella, dyskeratosis congenita, focal dermal hypoplasia, cartilage-hair hypoplasia, Ellis–van Creveld, Larsen, epidermolysis bullosa, incontinentia pigmenti, Rothmund-Thomson, Turner, popliteal web, trisomy 13, trisomy 18, Apert, Gorlin-Pindborg, long arm 21 deletion, otopalatodigital, fetal alcohol, fetal hydantoin, elfin facies, anonychia, acrodermatitis enteropathica

Other: Congenital malalignment of the great toenails, familial dystrophic shedding of the nails may be associated with malformations of the digits. *Koilonychia* is flattening and concavity of the nail plate with loss of normal contour, producing a spoon-shaped nail. Koilonychia occurs as an autosomal dominant trait or in association with hypochromic anemia, Plummer-Vinson syndrome, and hemochromatosis. The nail plate is relatively thin during the first 1–2 yr of life and consequently may be spoon shaped in otherwise normal children.

Leukonychia is a white opacity of the nail plate that may involve the entire plate or may be punctate or striate. The nail plate itself remains smooth and undamaged. Leukonychia can be traumatic or associated with infections such as leprosy and tuberculosis, dermatoses such as lichen planus and Darier disease, malignancies such as Hodgkin disease, anemia, and arsenic poisoning (Mees lines). Leukonychia of all nail surfaces is an uncommon hereditary autosomal dominant trait that may be associated with congenital epidermal cysts, renal calculi, and deafness. Paired parallel white bands that do not change position with growth of the nail and thus reflect a change in the nail bed are associated with hypoalbuminemia and are called Muehrcke lines. When the proximal portion of the nail is white and the distal 20–50% of the nail is red, pink, or brown, the condition is called half-and-half nails or Lindsay nails; this is seen most commonly in patients with renal disease but may occur as a normal variant. White nails of cirrhosis, or Terry nails, are characterized by a white ground-glass appearance of the entire or the proximal end of the nail and a normal pink distal 1–2 mm of the nail; this is associated with hypoalbuminemia.

Onycholysis indicates separation of the nail plate from the distal nail bed. Common causes are trauma, chronic exposure to moisture, hyperhidrosis, cosmetics, psoriasis, fungal infection (distal onycholysis), atopic or contact dermatitis, porphyria, drugs (bleomycin, vincristine, retinoid agents, indomethacin, thorazine), and drug-induced phototoxicity from tetracyclines or chloramphenicol. *Beau lines* are transverse grooves in the nail plate that represent a temporary disruption of formation of the nail plate. The line(s) first appear a few weeks after the event that caused the disruption in nail growth. A single transverse ridge appears at the proximal nail fold in most 4–6-wk-old infants and works its way distally as the nail grows; this line may reflect metabolic changes after delivery. At other ages, Beau lines are usually indicative of periodic trauma or episodic shutdown of the nail matrix secondary to a systemic disease such as measles, mumps, pneumonia, or zinc deficiency.

Nail changes may be particularly associated with various other diseases. Nail changes of *psoriasis* most characteristically include pitting, onycholysis, yellow-brown discoloration, and thickening. Nail changes in *lichen planus* include violaceous papules in the proximal nail fold and nail bed, leukonychia, longitudinal ridging, thinning of the entire nail plate, and *pterygium* formation, which is abnormal adherence of the cuticle to the nail plate or, if the plate is destroyed focally, to the nail bed. *Reiter disease* may include painless erythematous induration of the base of the nail fold; subungual parakeratotic scaling; and thickening, opacification, or ridging of the nail plate. *Dermatitis* that involves the nail folds may produce dystrophy, roughening, and coarse pitting of the nails. Nail changes are more common in atopic dermatitis than in other forms of dermatitis that affect the hands. *Darier disease* is characterized by red or white streaks that extend longitudinally and cross the lunula. Where the streak meets the distal end of the nail, a V-shaped notch may be present. Total leukonychia may also occur. Transverse rows of fine pits are characteristic of *alopecia areata*. In severe cases, the entire nail surface may be rough. Patients with *acrodermatitis enteropathica* may have tranverse grooves (Beau lines) and nail dystrophy as a result of periungual dermatitis.

Twenty-nail dystrophy is characterized by longitudinal ridging, pitting fragility, thinning, distal notching, and opalescent discoloration of all the nails. Patients have no associated skin or systemic diseases and no other ectodermal defects. Its occasional association with alopecia areata has led some authorities to suggest that 20-nail dystrophy may reflect an abnormal immunologic response to the nail matrix, whereas histopathologic studies have suggested that it may be a manifestation of lichen planus or spongiotic (eczematous) inflammation of the nail matrix. It also can be a feature of vitiligo or psoriasis. The disorder must be differentiated from fungal infections, psoriasis, nail changes of alopecia areata, and nail dystrophy secondary to eczema. Eczema and fungal infections rarely produce changes of all the nails simultaneously. The disorder is self-limited and eventually remits by adulthood.

Black pigmentation of an entire nail plate or linear bands of pigmentation (melanonychia striata) are common in black (90%) and Asian (10–20%) individuals but are unusual in whites (<1%). Most often, the pigment is melanin, which is produced by melanocytes of a junctional nevus in the nail matrix and nail bed and is of no consequence. Extension or alteration in the pigment should be evaluated by biopsy because of the possibility of malignant change. Bluish-black to greenish nails may be caused by *Pseudomonas* infection, particularly in association with onycholysis or chronic paronychia. The coloration is due to subungual debris and pyocyanin pigment from the bacterial organisms.

Splinter hemorrhages most often result from minor trauma but may also be associated with subacute bacterial endocarditis, vasculitis, severe rheumatoid arthritis, peptic ulcer disease, hypertension, chronic glomerulonephritis, cirrhosis, scurvy, trichinosis, malignant neoplasms, and psoriasis.

Clubbing of the nails (hippocratic nails) is characterized by swelling of the distal digit, an increase in the angle between the nail plate and the proximal nail fold (Lovibond angle) to greater than 180 degrees, and a spongy feeling when one pushes down and away from the interphalangeal joint because of an increase in fibrovascular tissue between the matrix and the phalanx. The pathogenesis is not known, but altered prostaglandin metabolism has been described. Nail clubbing is seen in association with diseases of numerous organ systems, including pulmonary, cardiovascular, gastrointestinal, and hepatic systems, and in healthy individuals as an idiopathic finding.

Habit tic deformity consists of a depression down the center of the nail with numerous horizontal ridges extending across the nail from it. One or both thumbs are usually involved as a result of chronic rubbing and picking at the nail with an adjacent finger.

Fungal infection of the nails has been classified into four types. *White superficial onychomycosis* presents with diffuse or speckled white discoloration of the surface of the toenails. It is caused primarily by *Trichophyton mentagrophytes*, which invades the nail plate. The organism may be scraped off the nail plate with a blade, but treatment is best accomplished by the addition of a topical azole antifungal agent. *Distal subungual onychomycosis* presents with foci of onycholysis under the distal nail plate or along the lateral nail groove, followed by development of hyperkeratosis and yellow-brown discoloration. The process extends proximally, resulting in nail plate thickening, crumbling, and separation from the nail bed. *T. rubrum* and occasionally *T. mentagrophytes* are most common on toenails; fingernail disease is almost exclusively due to *T. rubrum*, which may be associated with superficial scaling of the plantar surface of the feet and often of one hand. These dermatophytes are found most readily at the most proximal area of the nail bed or adjacent ventral portion of the nail plates that are involved. Topical therapies alone are ineffective in most cases, but nail evulsion in combination with topical antifungal agents may be effective. Because of their long half-life in the nail, terbinafine or itraconazole may be effective when given as pulse therapy

(1 wk of each mo for 3–4 mo). Either agent is superior to griseofulvin or ketoconazole. The risks, most concerning of which is hepatic toxicity, and costs of oral therapy must be weighed carefully against the benefits of treatment for a condition that generally causes only cosmetic problems.

Proximal white subungual onychomycosis occurs when the organism, generally *T. rubrum*, enters the nail through the proximal nail fold, producing yellow-white portions of the undersurface of the nail plate. The surface of the nail is unaffected. This occurs almost exclusively in immunocompromised patients and is a well-recognized manifestation of AIDS.

Candidal onychomycosis involves the entire nail plate in patients with chronic mucocutaneous candidiasis. It is also commonly seen in patients with AIDS. The organism, generally *Candida albicans*, enters distally or along the lateral nail folds, rapidly involves the entire thickness of the nail plate, and produces thickening, crumbling, and deformity of the plate. Topical azole antifungal agents may be sufficient for treatment of candidal onychomycosis in an immunocompetent host, but oral antifungal agents are necessary for treatment of those with immune deficiencies.

Paronychial inflammation may be acute or chronic and generally involves one or two nail folds on the fingers. Acute paronychia presents with erythema, warmth, edema, and tenderness of the proximal nail fold, most commonly as a result of pathogenic staphylococci or streptococci. Warm soaks and oral antibiotics such as clindamycin or amoxicillin plus clavulanic acid are generally effective; incision and drainage may be necessary in some cases. Development of chronic paronychia is favored by prolonged immersion in water, such as occurs in finger or thumb sucking; exposure to irritating solutions; nail fold trauma; or diseases including Raynaud's phenomenon, collagen vascular diseases, or diabetes. Swelling of the proximal nail fold is followed by separation of the nail fold from the underlying nail plate and suppuration. Foreign material, embedded in the dermis of the nail fold, becomes a nidus for inflammation and infection with *Candida* species and mixed bacterial flora. A combination of attention to predisposing factors; meticulous drying of the hands, including use of 4% thymol solution; and long-term antifungal, antibacterial, and topical anti-inflammatory agents may be required for successful treatment of chronic paronychia. The primary chancre of syphilis also may present on the finger as a relatively nontender paronychia.

Ingrown nails occur when the lateral edge of the nail, including spicules that have separated from the nail plate, penetrates the soft tissue of the lateral nail fold. Erythema, edema, and pain, most often involving the lateral great toes, are noted acutely; recurrent episodes may lead to formation of granulation tissue. Predisposing factors include compression of the side of the toe from poorly fitting shoes, particularly if the great toes are abnormally long and the lateral nail folds are prominent, and improper cutting of the nail in a curvilinear manner rather than straight across. Management includes proper fitting of shoes; allowing the nail to grow out beyond the free edge before cutting it straight across; warm water soaks; oral antibiotics if cellulitis affects the lateral nail fold; and, in severe, recurrent cases, application of silver nitrate to granulation tissue, nail avulsion, or excision of the lateral aspect of the nail followed by matricectomy.

Tumors in the paronychial area include pyogenic granulomas, mucous cysts, subungual exostoses, and junctional nevi. Periungual fibromas that appear during late childhood should suggest a diagnosis of tuberous sclerosis.

Nail-patella syndrome is an autosomal dominant disorder in which the nails are 30–50% their normal size and often have triangular or pyramidal lunulas. The thumbnails are always involved, although in some cases only the ulnar half of the nail may be affected or may be missing. The nails from the index finger to the little finger are progressively less damaged. The patella is also smaller than usual, and this anomaly may lead to knee instability. Bony spines arising from the posterior aspect of the iliac bones, overextension of joints, skin laxity, hyperhidrosis, and renal anomalies may also be present.

Pachyonychia congenita (see Chapter 664).

Yellow nail syndrome presents with thickened, excessively curved, slow-growing yellow nails without lunulas. All nails are affected in most cases. Associated systemic disease includes bronchiectasis, recurrent bronchitis, chylothorax, and focal edema of the limbs and face. Deficient lymphatic drainage, due to hypoplastic lymphatic vessels, is believed to lead to the manifestations of this syndrome.

Barth JH, Dawber RPR: Diseases of the nails in children. Pediatr Dermatol 12:275, 1987.
DeCoste SD, Imber MJ, Baden HP: Yellow nail syndrome. J Am Acad Dermatol 22:608, 1990.
Hazelrigg DE, Duncan C, Jarrett M: Twenty-nail dystrophy of childhood. Arch Dermatol 113:73, 1977.
Juhlin L, Baran R. *In*: Baran R, Dawber RPR (eds): Diseases of the Nails and Their Management. Oxford, Blackwell Scientific Publications, 1984, p 303.
Peluso AM, Tosti A, Piraccini BM, et al: Lichen planus limited to the nails in childhood: Case report and literature review. Pediatr Dermatol 10:36, 1993.
Stone OJ, Mullins JF: Chronic paronychia in childhood. Clin Pediatr 7:104, 1968.
Turano AF: Beau's lines in infancy. Pediatrics 41:996, 1968.

CHAPTER 670
Disorders of the Mucous Membranes

The mucous membranes may be involved in developmental disorders, infections, acute and chronic skin diseases, genodermatoses, and benign and malignant tumors. Some of the more common and distinctive diseases specific to mucous membranes are presented in this chapter.

CHEILITIS. Inflammation of the lips (cheilitis) and angles of the mouth (angular cheilitis or perlèche) are most commonly due to dryness, chapping, and lip licking; excessive salivation and drooling, particularly in children with neurologic deficits, may also cause chronic irritation. Lesions of oral thrush may occasionally extend to the angles of the mouth. Protection can be provided by frequent applications of a bland ointment such as petrolatum. Candidosis should be treated with an appropriate antifungal agent, and contact dermatitis of the perioral skin should be treated with a mild topical corticosteroid preparation and an emollient.

FORDYCE SPOTS. These are asymptomatic, minute, yellow-white papules on the vermilion border of the lips and buccal mucosa. These ectopic sebaceous glands may be found in otherwise normal individuals and require no therapy.

MUCOCELE. Mucous retention cysts are painless, bluish, fluctuant, tense, 2–10-mm papules on the lips, tongue, palate, or buccal mucosa. Traumatic severance of the duct of a minor salivary gland leads to submucosal retention of mucous secretion. Those on the floor of the mouth are known as *ranulas* when the submaxillary or sublingual salivary ducts are involved. Fluctuations in size are usual, and the lesions may disappear temporarily after traumatic rupture. Recurrence is prevented by excising the mucocele.

APHTHOUS STOMATITIS (CANKER SORES). Solitary or multiple painful ulcerations occur on the labial, buccal, or lingual mucosa and on the sublingual, palatal, or gingival mucosa. Lesions may present initially as erythematous, indurated papules that erode rapidly to form sharply circumscribed, necrotic ulcers with a gray fibrinous exudate and an erythematous halo. Minor aphthous ulcers are 2–10 mm in diameter and heal spontaneously in 7–10 days. Major aphthous ulcers are greater than

10 mm in diameter and take 10–30 days to heal. A third type of aphthous ulceration is herpetiform in appearance, presenting with a few to numerous grouped 1–2-mm lesions that tend to coalesce into plaques that heal over 7–10 days. Approximately one third of patients with recurrent aphthous stomatitis have a family history of the disorder.

The *etiology* of aphthous stomatitis is probably multifactorial; the condition probably represents an oral manifestation of a number of conditions. Altered local regulation of the cell-mediated immune system, after activation and accumulation of cytotoxic T cells, may contribute to the localized mucosal breakdown. Predisposing factors include trauma, emotional stress, low serum iron or ferritin levels, deficiency of vitamin B_{12} or folate, malabsorption in association with celiac or Crohn disease, menstruation accompanied by a fall in progestogens during the luteal phase, food hypersensitivity, and allergic or toxic drug reactions. It is a common misconception that aphthous stomatitis is a manifestation of herpes simplex virus infection. Recurrent herpes infections remain localized to the lips and rarely cross the mucocutaneous junction; involvement of the oral mucosa occurs only in primary infections.

Treatment of aphthous stomatitis is palliative. Use of 0.2% aqueous chlorhexidine gluconate mouthwash helps to maintain oral hygiene. Relief of pain, particularly before eating, may be achieved by use of a topical anesthetic such as viscous lidocaine (Xylocaine) or an oral rinse with a solution of elixir of diphenhydramine, viscous lidocaine, and 0.5% dyclonine hydrochloride. A topical corticosteroid in a mucosal adhering agent (0.1% triamcinolone in Orabase) may help to reduce inflammation, and topical tetracycline mouthwash may also hasten healing. In severe, debilitating cases, systemic therapy with corticosteroids, colchicine, or dapsone may be helpful.

COWDEN SYNDROME (MULTIPLE HAMARTOMA SYNDROME). This is an autosomal dominant condition that usually presents during the 2nd or 3rd decade with smooth, pink or whitish papules on the palatal, gingival, buccal, and labial mucosae. These benign fibromas may coalesce into a cobblestone appearance. Numerous flesh-colored papules also develop on the face, particularly around the mouth, nose, and ears; these papules most commonly are trichilemmomas, a benign neoplasm of the hair follicle. Associated findings may include acral keratotic papules, thyroid goiter, gastrointestinal polyps, fibrocystic breast nodules, and carcinoma of the breast or thyroid.

EPSTEIN PEARLS (GINGIVAL CYSTS OF THE NEWBORN). These are white keratin-containing cysts on the palatal or alveolar mucosa of approximately 80% of neonates. They cause no symptoms and are generally shed within a few weeks.

GEOGRAPHIC TONGUE (BENIGN MIGRATORY GLOSSITIS). This consists of single or multiple sharply demarcated, irregular, smooth red plaques on the dorsum of the tongue caused by transient atrophy of the filiform papillae and the surface epithelium, often with elevated gray margins composed of intervening filiform papillae that are increased in thickness. Symptoms of mild burning or irritation may occasionally be bothersome. Onset is rapid, and the pattern may change over hours to days. Geographic tongue is associated with scrotal tongue in nearly 50% of patients. Some patients have atopy; some feel that the condition is exacerbated by stress or by hot or spicy foods; and some have anemia, diabetes mellitus, Reiter disease, seborrheic dermatitis, or pustular psoriasis. Geographic tongue may be an oral manifestation of pustular psoriasis, with which it shares histologic features. No therapy other than reassurance is necessary.

SCROTAL (FISSURED) TONGUE. Approximately 1% of infants and 2.5% of children have many folds with deep grooves on the dorsal tongue surface. These impart a pebbled or wrinkled appearance. Some cases are congenital, caused by incomplete fusion of the two halves of the tongue; others develop in association with infection, trauma, malnutrition, or low vitamin A levels. Many patients with fissured tongue also have geographic tongue. Food particles and debris may become trapped in the fissures, resulting in irritation, inflammation, and halitosis. Careful cleansing with a mouth rinse and soft-bristled toothbrush is recommended.

BLACK HAIRY TONGUE. This is a dark coating on the dorsum of the tongue caused by hyperplasia and elongation of the filiform papillae; overgrowth of chromogenic bacteria and fungi and entrapped pigmented residues that adsorb to microbial plaque and desquamating keratin may contribute to the dark coloration. Changes often begin posteriorly and extend anteriorly on the dorsum of the tongue. The condition is most common in adults but may also present during adolescence. Poor oral hygiene and bacterial overgrowth, treatment with systemic antibiotics such as tetracycline (which promotes the growth of *Candida* species), and smoking are predisposing factors. Improved oral hygiene and brushing with a soft-bristled toothbrush may be all that are necessary for treatment. The filiform hyperplasia may also be decreased with topical keratolytic agents such as trichloroacetic acid, urea, or podophyllin.

ORAL HAIRY LEUKOPLAKIA. This occurs in approximately 25% of patients with AIDS but is rare in the pediatric population. It presents as a mostly asymptomatic white thickening and accentuation of the normal vertical folds of the lateral margins of the tongue. The mucosa is white and irregularly thickened but remains soft. Spread may occur occasionally to the ventral tongue surface, the floor of the mouth, the tonsillar pillars, and the pharynx. The condition appears to be due to Epstein-Barr virus, which is present in the upper layer of the affected epithelium. The plaques have no malignant potential. The disorder occurs predominantly in HIV-infected patients but may also be found in individuals who are immunosuppressed for other reasons, such as organ transplantation or leukemia and chemotherapy. The condition is generally asymptomatic and does not require therapy. Resolution of the plaques may be hastened, however, by use of antiviral agents such as acyclovir or local application of 0.1% vitamin A acid twice daily.

VINCENT GINGIVITIS (ACUTE NECROTIZING ULCERATIVE GINGIVITIS, FUSOSPIROCHETAL GINGIVITIS, TRENCH MOUTH). This disorder presents with punched-out ulceration, necrosis, and bleeding of interdental papillae. A grayish-white pseudomembrane may cover the ulcerations. Lesions may spread to involve the buccal mucosa, lips, tongue, tonsils, and pharynx and may be associated with dental pain, a bad taste, low-grade fever, and lymphadenopathy. It presents most commonly during the 2nd or 3rd decade, particularly in the context of poor dental hygiene, scurvy, or pellagra. A synergistic association between fusospirochetal organisms *(Fusobacterium nucleatum)* and *Borrelia vincenti* has been proposed to contribute to the pathogenesis.

Noma is a severe form of fusospirillary gangrenous stomatitis that presents primarily in malnourished children 2–5 yr of age who have had a preceding illness such as measles, scarlet fever, tuberculosis, malignancy, or immunodeficiency. It presents as a painful red, indurated papule on the alveolar margin, followed by ulceration and mutilating gangrenous destruction of tissue in the oronasal region. The process may also involve the scalp, neck, shoulders, perineum, and vulva. *Noma neonatorum* presents in the 1st mo of life with gangrenous lesions of the lips, nose, mouth, and anal regions. Affected infants are usually small for gestational age, malnourished, premature, and frequently ill, particularly with *Pseudomonas aeruginosa* sepsis. Care consists of nutritional support, conservative débridement of necrotic soft tissues, empirical broad-spectrum antibiotics such as penicillin and metronidazole, and in the case of noma neonatorum, antipseudomonal antibiotics.

Herbert AA, Berg JH: Oral mucous membrane diseases of childhood: I. Mucositis and xerostomia. II. Recurrent aphthous stomatitis. III. Herpetic stomatitis. Semin Dermatol 11:80, 1992.

Itin PH, Bircher AJ, Litzisdorf Y, et al: Oral hairy leukoplakia in a child: Confirmation of the clinical diagnosis by ultrastructural examination of exfoliative cytologic specimens. Dermatology 189:167, 1994.

Prose NS: Mucocutaneous disease in pediatric human immunodeficiency virus infection. Pediatr Clin North Am 38:977, 1991.

Sigal MJ, Mock D: Symptomatic benign migratory glossitis: Report of two cases and literature review. Pediatr Dent 14:392, 1992.

CHAPTER 671
Cutaneous Bacterial Infections

Skin complaints or findings are noted in 20–30% of children who attend general pediatric clinics. Bacterial skin infection is the single most common diagnosis among those with skin problems, accounting for 17% of all clinic visits. The most common bacterial skin infection of children is impetigo, which makes up approximately 10% of all skin problems.

IMPETIGO (see Chapters 182 and 184)

CLINICAL MANIFESTATIONS

Nonbullous Impetigo. There are two classic forms of impetigo: nonbullous and bullous. Nonbullous impetigo accounts for more than 70% of cases. Lesions typically begin on skin of the face or extremities that has been traumatized. The most common lesions that precede nonbullous impetigo include insect bites, abrasions, lacerations, chickenpox, scabies, pediculosis, and burns. A tiny vesicle or pustule forms initially (Fig. 671–1*A*) and rapidly develops into a honey-colored crusted plaque that is generally less than 2 cm in diameter (Fig. 671–1*B*). The infection may be spread to other parts of the body by the fingers, clothing, and towels. Lesions are associated with little to no pain or surrounding erythema, and constitutional symptoms are generally absent. Pruritus occurs occasionally, regional adenopathy is found in up to 90% of cases, and leukocytosis is present in approximately 50% of patients. Without treatment, most cases resolve spontaneously without scarring within approximately 2 wk. The differential diagnosis of nonbullous impetigo includes viral (herpes simplex, varicella-zoster), fungal (tinea corporis, kerion), and parasitic infections (scabies, pediculosis capitis), all of which may become impetiginized.

Staphylococcus aureus is the predominant organism of nonbullous impetigo in the United States; group A β-hemolytic streptococci (GABHS) are implicated in the development of some lesions. Staphylococci generally spread from the nose to normal skin and then infect the skin. In contrast, the skin becomes colonized with GABHS an average of 10 days before development of impetigo. GABHS then colonize the nasopharynx an average of 2–3 wk after the appearance of lesions of impetigo. The skin serves as the source for acquisition of GABHS in the respiratory tract and the probable primary source for spread of impetigo. Lesions of nonbullous impetigo that grow staphylococci in culture cannot be distinguished clinically from those that grow pure cultures of GABHS. Whereas *S. aureus* can be cultured from lesions of impetigo in children of all ages, GABHS is most commonly cultured from children of preschool age and is unusual before 2 yr of age, except in highly endemic areas. The staphylococcal types that cause nonbullous impetigo are variable but are not generally from phage group 2, the group that is associated with scalded skin and toxic shock syndromes. Several serotypes of GABHS, termed "impetigo strains," are found most frequently in lesions of nonbullous impetigo and are different from those that cause pharyngitis.

Bullous Impetigo. This is mainly an infection of infants and young children. Bullous impetigo is always caused by coagulase-positive *S. aureus;* approximately 80% are from phage group 2, among which 60% are type 71, and most of the remainder are types 3A, 3B, 3C, and 55. Flaccid, transparent bullae develop most commonly on skin of the face, buttocks, trunk, perineum, and extremities; neonatal bullous impetigo can begin in the diaper area. Rupture of bullae occurs easily, leaving a narrow rim of scale at the edge of a shallow, moist erosion. Surrounding erythema and regional adenopathy are generally absent. Unlike those of nonbullous impetigo, lesions of bullous impetigo are a manifestation of localized staphylococcal scalded skin syndrome and develop on intact skin.

DIAGNOSIS. Cultures of fluid from an intact blister or moist plaque should yield the causative agent; when the patient appears ill, blood cultures should also be obtained. On histopathologic examination, lesions of bullous impetigo show vesicle formation in the subcorneal or granular region, neutrophils and occasionally acantholytic cells within the blister, spongiosis, edema of the papillary dermis, and a mixed infiltrate of lymphocytes and neutrophils around blood vessels of the superficial plexus. Unless staphylococci can be cultured from the bullas or, less commonly, can be seen on Gram stain, it may be impossible to differentiate bullous impetigo from pemphigus foliaceous or subcorneal pustular dermatosis histopathologically. Nonbullous impetigo has histopathologic findings similar to those of the bullous variant, except that blister formation is slight.

The *differential diagnosis* of bullous impetigo in neonates includes epidermolysis bullosa, bullous mastocytosis, herpetic infection, and early scalded skin syndrome. In older children, allergic contact dermatitis, burns, erythema multiforme, chronic bullous dermatosis of childhood, pemphigus, and bullous pemphigoid must be considered, particularly if the lesions do not respond to therapy.

COMPLICATIONS. Potential but rare complications of either

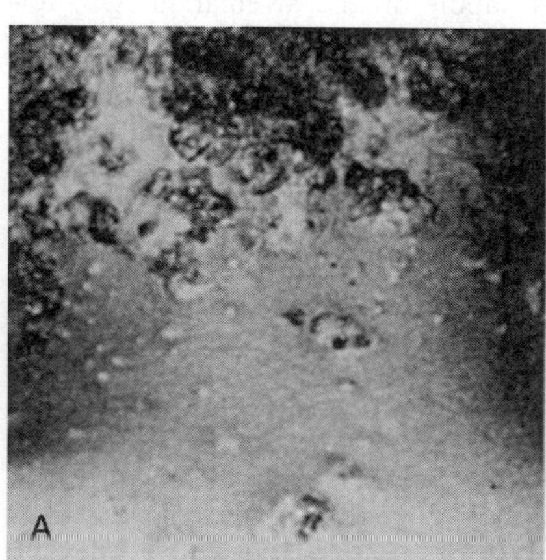

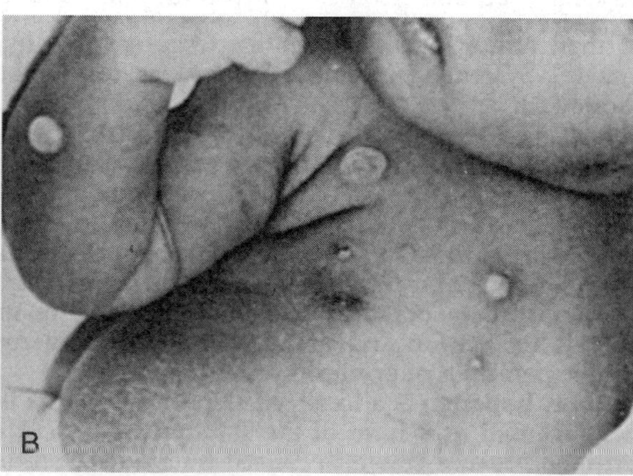

Figure 671–1 *A,* Multiple crusted and oozing lesions of streptococcal impetigo. *B,* Multiple tense and flaccid blisters of bullous impetigo on the trunk and arm of an infant.

nonbullous or bullous impetigo include osteomyelitis, septic arthritis, pneumonia, and septicemia; positive blood culture results are rare. Cellulitis has been reported in approximately 10% of patients with nonbullous impetigo but rarely follows the bullous form. Lymphangitis, suppurative lymphadenitis, guttate psoriasis, and scarlet fever occasionally follow streptococcal disease. There is no correlation between number of lesions and clinical involvement of the lymphatics or development of cellulitis in association with streptococcal impetigo.

Infection with nephritogenic strains of GABHS may result in acute poststreptococcal glomerulonephritis (Chapter 519.1). The clinical character of impetigo lesions that lead to poststreptococcal glomerulonephritis and those that do not differ. The most commonly affected age group is school-aged children 3–7 yr old. The latent period from onset of impetigo to development of poststreptococcal glomerulonephritis averages 18–21 days, which is longer than the 10-day latency period after pharyngitis. Poststreptococcal glomerulonephritis occurs epidemically after either pharyngeal or skin infection. Impetigo-associated epidemics have been caused by M groups 2, 49, 53, 55, 56, 57, and 60. Strains of GABHS that are associated with endemic impetigo in the United States have little or no nephritogenic potential. Acute rheumatic fever does not occur as a result of impetigo.

TREATMENT. Topical or systemic antibiotic treatment is superior to placebo or cleansing with 3% hexachlorophene soap. Furthermore, cleansing with 3% hexachlorophene soap adds little to no benefit over systemic antibiotics alone. Mupirocin is an ointment that is bactericidal by reversible inhibition of bacterial isoleucyl-transfer RNA synthetase. Applied topically three times daily for 7–10 days, it is equal to or greater in effectiveness, with fewer side effects, than oral erythromycin ethylsuccinate, 30–50 mg/kg/24 hr for 7–10 days. Rare instances of bacterial resistance to mupirocin have been reported, but most patients were treated irregularly or prophylactically for more than 2 wk.

Systemic therapy with a β-lactamase–resistant oral antibiotic should be prescribed for patients with widespread involvement; when lesions are near the mouth, where topical medication may be licked off; or in cases of evidence of deep involvement, including cellulitis, furunculosis, abscess formation, or suppurative lymphadenitis. In areas without a high prevalence of *S. aureus* resistance to erythromycin, erythromycin ethylsuccinate (40 mg/kg/24 hr divided three to four times daily for 7 days) or erythromycin estolate (30 mg/kg/24 hr divided three to four times daily) is the preferred oral therapy. If erythromycin resistance is widespread in the community, alternative oral antibiotics that have been shown to be effective in children for treatment of impetigo include dicloxacillin; amoxicillin plus clavulanic acid, clindamycin, and a cephalosporin such as cephalexin, cefaclor, cefadroxil, cefprozil, or cefpodoxime. The choice among these various agents may be guided primarily by issues of cost, local availability, and compliance. The macrolides clarithromycin or azithromycin may be advantageous primarily in instances of intolerance to erythromycin but will not provide cure rates superior to those of erythromycin. No evidence suggests that a 10-day course of therapy is superior to a 7-day one. If a satisfactory clinical response is not achieved within 7 days, however, a culture should be taken by swabbing beneath the lifted edge of a crusted lesion. If a resistant organism is detected, an appropriate antibiotic should be given for an additional 7 days.

SUBCUTANEOUS TISSUE INFECTIONS

The principal determination to be made about soft tissue infection is whether it is non-necrotizing or necrotizing; the former responds to antibiotic therapy alone, whereas the latter requires prompt surgical removal of all devitalized tissue in addition to antimicrobial therapy. Necrotizing soft tissue infections are potentially life-threatening conditions that are characterized by rapidly advancing local tissue destruction and systemic toxicity. Tissue necrosis distinguishes them from cellulitis; in cellulitis, an inflammatory infectious process involves subcutaneous tissue but does not destroy it. Necrotizing soft tissue infections characteristically present with a paucity of early cutaneous signs relative to the rapidity and degree of destruction of the subcutaneous tissues.

CELLULITIS. Cellulitis is characterized by infection and inflammation of loose connective tissue, with limited involvement of the dermis and relative sparing of the epidermis. A break in the skin due to previous trauma, surgery, or an underlying skin lesion predisposes to cellulitis. Cellulitis is also more common in individuals with lymphatic stasis, diabetes mellitus, or immunosuppression.

Etiology. *Streptococcus pyogenes* and *S. aureus* are the most common etiologic agents. Occasionally, *Streptococcus pneumoniae*, group G or C streptococci, and in neonates, group B streptococci or rarely *Escherichia coli* are the causal organism. In patients who are immunocompromised or have diabetes mellitus, a number of other bacterial or fungal agents may be involved, notably *Pseudomonas aeruginosa; Aeromonas hydrophila* and occasionally other Enterobacteriaceae; *Legionella* spp; the Mucorales, particularly *Rhizopus* spp, *Mucor* spp, and *Absidia* spp; and *Cryptococcus neoformans*. Children with relapsed nephrotic syndrome may develop cellulitis due to *E. coli*. In children age 3 mo to 3–5 yr, *Haemophilus influenzae* type b has been an important cause of facial cellulitis, but its incidence has declined significantly since institution of immunization against this organism.

Clinical Manifestations. Cellulitis presents clinically as an area of edema, warmth, erythema, and tenderness. The lateral margins tend to be indistinct because the process is deep in the skin, primarily involving the subcutaneous tissues in addition to the dermis. Application of pressure may produce pitting. Although distinction cannot be made with certainty in any particular patient, cellulitis due to *S. aureus* tends to be more localized and may suppurate, whereas infections due to *S. pyogenes* tend to spread more rapidly and may be associated with lymphangitis. Regional adenopathy and constitutional signs and symptoms of fever, chills, and malaise are common. Complications of cellulitis include subcutaneous abscess, osteomyelitis, septic arthritis, thrombophlebitis, bacteremia, and necrotizing fasciitis. Lymphangitis or glomerulonephritis also can follow infection with *S. pyogenes*.

Diagnosis. Aspirates from the site of inflammation, skin biopsy, and blood cultures allow identification of the causal organism in approximately 25% of cases of cellulitis. Yield of the causative organism is approximately one third when the site of origin of the cellulitis is apparent, such as an abrasion or ulcer. An aspirate taken from the point of maximum inflammation yields the causal organism more often than does a leading-edge aspirate. Lack of success in isolating an organism stems primarily from the low number of organisms present within the lesion.

Treatment. Empirical therapy for cellulitis should be directed by the history of the illness, the location and character of the cellulitis, and the age and immune status of the patient. Cellulitis in a neonate should prompt a full sepsis work-up, followed by initiation of empirical therapy intravenously with a β-lactamase–stable antistaphylococcal antibiotic such as methicillin and an aminoglycoside such as gentamicin or a cephalosporin such as cefotaxime. Treatment of cellulitis in an infant or child younger than about 5 yr should provide coverage for *S. pyogenes* and *S. aureus* as well as *H. influenzae* type b and *S. pneumoniae*. The evaluation should include a blood culture, and if the infant is younger than 1 year, if signs of systemic toxicity are present, or if an adequate examination cannot be carried out, a lumbar puncture should also be performed. In most cases of cellulitis on an extremity, regardless of age, *S.*

aureus and *S. pyogenes* are the cause and bacteremia is unlikely. Nevertheless, blood cultures should be obtained if sepsis is suspected. If fever, lymphadenopathy, and other constitutional signs are absent (e.g., white blood cell count < 15,000), treatment of cellulitis on an extremity may be initiated orally on an outpatient basis with a penicillinase-resistant penicillin such as dicloxacillin or cloxacillin or a first-generation cephalosporin such as cephalexin. If improvement is not noted or the disease progresses significantly within the first 24–48 hr of therapy, parenteral therapy is necessary. If fever, lymphadenopathy, or constitutional signs are present, therapy should be initiated parenterally. Oxacillin or nafcillin is effective in most cases, although if systemic toxicity is significant, consideration should be given to the addition of penicillin or clindamycin. Once the erythema, warmth, edema, and fever have decreased significantly, a 10-day course of treatment may be completed on an outpatient basis. Immobilization and elevation of an affected limb, particularly early in the course of therapy, may help to reduce swelling and pain.

NECROTIZING FASCIITIS. Necrotizing fasciitis is a subcutaneous tissue infection that involves the deep layer of superficial fascia but largely spares adjacent epidermis, deep fascia, and muscle.

Etiology. Relatively few organisms possess sufficient virulence to cause necrotizing fasciitis when acting alone. The most fulminant infections, associated with toxic shock syndrome and a high case-fatality rate, are caused by *S. pyogenes* (also see Chapter 184). Streptococcal necrotizing fasciitis in the absence of toxic shock syndrome may occur and is seldom fatal but may be associated with substantial morbidity. Necrotizing fasciitis can occasionally be caused by *S. aureus, Clostridium perfringens, Clostridium septicum, P. aeruginosa, Vibrio* spp, particularly *V. vulnificus,* and fungi of the order Mucorales, particularly *Rhizopus* spp, *Mucor* spp, and *Absidia* spp. Necrotizing fasciitis has also been reported on rare occasions to result from non–group A streptococci such as group B, C, F, or G streptococci, *S. pneumoniae*, or *H. influenzae* type b. Necrotizing fasciitis may be a polymicrobial infection. In most of these cases, a mixture of anaerobic bacteria and aerobic or facultative bacteria appear to act together to cause tissue necrosis. The most common aerobic or facultative bacteria are several species of hemolytic or nonhemolytic non–group A streptococci, *S. aureus, E. coli, Enterobacter* spp and various other Enterobacteriaceae, and *Pseudomonas* spp. The anaerobes present are similar to those found in subcutaneous abscesses: *Bacteroides* spp, *Peptostreptococcus* spp, *Peptococcus* spp, *Prevotella* spp, *Porphyromonas* spp, *Clostridium* spp, and *Fusobacterium* spp. Infections due to any one organism or combination of organisms cannot be distinguished clinically from one another, although development of crepitance signals the presence of *Clostridium* spp or gram-negative bacilli such as *E. coli, Klebsiella, Proteus* and *Aeromonas*.

Epidemiology. Necrotizing fasciitis may occur anywhere on the body; the most common locations, however, are the extremities, abdomen, and perineal region. Common predisposing conditions in neonates are omphalitis and balanitis after circumcision. The incidence of necrotizing fasciitis is highest in hosts with systemic or local tissue immunocompromise, such as those with diabetes mellitus, neoplasia, or peripheral vascular disease, and those recently having undergone surgery, those who abuse intravenous drugs, or those on immunosuppressive treatment, particularly with corticosteroids. The infection also can occur in healthy individuals after minor puncture wounds, abrasions, or lacerations; blunt trauma; surgical procedures, particularly of the abdomen, gastrointestinal or genitourinary tracts, or the perineum; or hypodermic needle injection. Since the mid-1980s, there has been a resurgence of fulminant necrotizing soft tissue infections due to *S. pyogenes,* which may occur in previously healthy individuals with little or no apparent compromise of immunologic or skin integrity. Necrotizing fasciitis due to *S. pyogenes* may occur after superinfection of varicella lesions. These children have tended to display onset, recrudescence, or persistence of high fever and signs of toxicity after the 3rd to 4th day of varicella.

Clinical Manifestations. Necrotizing fasciitis begins with acute onset of local swelling, erythema, tenderness, and heat. Fever is usually present, and pain, tenderness, and constitutional signs are out of proportion to cutaneous signs, especially with involvement of fascia and muscle. Lymphangitis and lymphadenitis are usually absent. The infection advances along the superficial fascial plane, and initially there are few cutaneous signs to herald the serious nature and extent of subcutaneous tissue necrosis that is occurring. Skin changes may appear over 24–48 hr as nutrient vessels are thrombosed and cutaneous ischemia develops. Early clinical findings include ill-defined cutaneous erythema and edema, which extend beyond the area of erythema. Additional signs include formation of bullae filled initially with straw-colored and later bluish to hemorrhagic fluid, and darkening of affected tissues from red to purple to blue. Skin anesthesia and finally frank tissue gangrene and slough develop owing to the ischemia and necrosis. Vesiculation or bulla formation, ecchymoses, crepitus, anesthesia, and necrosis are ominous and indicative of advanced disease. Children with varicella lesions initially may show no cutaneous signs of superinfection with invasive *S. pyogenes* such as erythema or swelling. Significant systemic toxicity may accompany necrotizing fasciitis, including shock, organ failure, and death. Advance of the infection in this setting can be rapid, progressing to death within hours. In general, patients with involvement of the superficial or deep fascia and muscle tend to be more acutely and systemically ill and have more rapidly advancing disease than those with infection confined solely to subcutaneous tissues above the fascia.

Diagnosis. Definitive diagnosis is made by surgical exploration, which should be undertaken as soon as the diagnosis is suspected. Necrotic fascia and subcutaneous tissue are gray and offer little resistance to blunt probing. Although MRI may aid in delineating the extent and tissue planes of involvement, this procedure should not delay surgical intervention. Frozen section incisional biopsy taken early in the course of the infection can aid management by decreasing the time to diagnosis and helping to establish margins of involvement. Gram stain of tissue can be particularly useful if chains of gram-positive cocci, indicative of infection with *S. pyogenes,* are seen.

Treatment. Early supportive care, surgical debridement, and parenteral antibiotic administration are mandatory. All devitalized tissue should be removed to freely bleeding edges, and repeat exploration is generally indicated within 24–36 hr to confirm that no necrotic tissue remains. This may need to be repeated on several occasions until devitalized tissue has ceased to form. Daily, meticulous wound care is also paramount.

Antibiotic therapy should be initiated parenterally as soon as possible with broad-spectrum agents against all potential pathogens. Most experts recommend initial empirical therapy with penicillin, ampicillin, or nafcillin; clindamycin; and an aminoglycoside for coverage against *S. pyogenes* and the broad spectrum of potential anaerobic and gram-negative pathogens.

Prognosis. The combined case fatality rate among children and adults with necrotizing fasciitis and toxic shock–like syndrome due to *S. pyogenes* has been approximately 60%. Death is less common in children, however, and in cases not complicated by toxic shock–like syndrome.

Bisno AL, Stevens DL: Streptococcal infections of skin and soft tissues. N Engl J Med 334:240, 1996.

Darmstadt GL, Marcy SM: Skin and soft tissue infection. *In*: Long SS, Prober CG, Pickering LK (eds): Principles and Practice of Pediatric Infectious Disease. New York, Churchill Livingstone, 1996.

Brogan TV, Nizet V, Waldhausen JHT, et al: Group A streptococcal necrotizing fasciitis complicating varicella: A series of ten patients. Pediatr Infect Dis J 14:588, 1995.

Peterson CL, Vugia DJ, Meyers HB, et al: Risk factors for invasive group A streptococcal infections in children with varicella: Case-control study. Pediatr Infect Dis J 15:151, 1996.

Stevens DL: Invasive group A streptococcal infections: The past, present and future. Pediatr Infect Dis J 13:561, 1994.

STAPHYLOCOCCAL SCALDED SKIN SYNDROME

(Ritter Disease)

CLINICAL MANIFESTATIONS. Staphylococcal scalded skin syndrome occurs predominantly in infants and children under 5 yr of age and includes a range of disease from localized bullous impetigo to generalized cutaneous involvement with systemic illness. Onset of the rash may be preceded by malaise, fever, irritability, and exquisite tenderness of the skin. Scarlatiniform erythema develops diffusely and is accentuated in flexural and periorificial areas. The conjunctivas are inflamed and occasionally become purulent. The brightly erythematous skin may rapidly acquire a wrinkled appearance, and in severe cases sterile, flaccid blisters and erosions develop diffusely. Circumoral erythema is characteristically prominent, as is radial crusting and fissuring around the eyes, mouth, and nose. At this stage, areas of epidermis may separate in response to gentle shear force (Nikolsky sign). As large sheets of epidermis peel away, moist, glistening, denuded areas become apparent, initially in the flexures and subsequently over much of the body surface (Fig. 671–2). This may lead to secondary cutaneous infection, sepsis, and fluid and electrolyte disturbances. The desquamative phase begins after 2–5 days of cutaneous erythema; healing occurs without scarring in 10–14 days. Patients may have pharyngitis, conjunctivitis, and superficial erosions of the lips, but intraoral mucosal surfaces are spared. Although some patients appear ill, many are reasonably comfortable except for the marked skin tenderness.

A presumed abortive form of the disease presents with diffuse, scarlatiniform, tender erythroderma, which is accentuated in the flexural areas but does not progress to blister formation. In these patients, Nikolsky sign may be absent. Although the exanthem is similar to that of streptococcal scarlet fever, strawberry tongue and palatal petechiae are absent. Staphylococcal scalded skin syndrome may be mistaken for a number of other blistering and exfoliating disorders, including bullous impetigo, epidermolysis bullosa, epidermolytic hyperkeratosis, pemphigus, drug eruption, erythema multiforme, and drug-induced toxic epidermal necrolysis. Toxic epidermal necrolysis can often be distinguished by a history of drug ingestion, the presence of Nikolsky sign only at sites of erythema, absence of perioral crusting, full-thickness epidermal necrosis, and a blister cleavage plane in the lowermost epidermis.

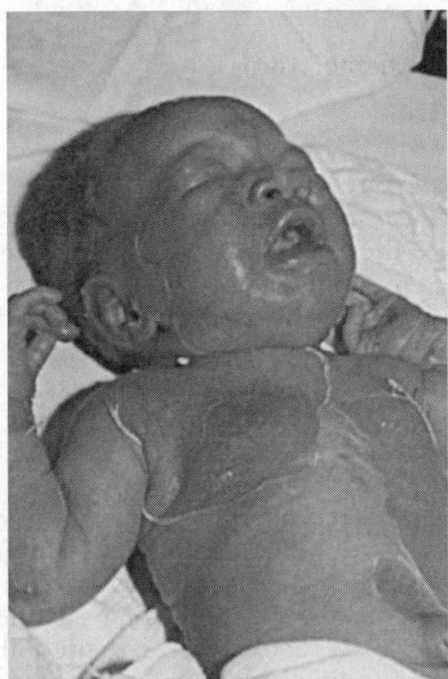

Figure 671–2 Infant with staphylococcal scalded skin syndrome. See also color section.

ETIOLOGY AND PATHOGENESIS. Staphylococcal scalded skin syndrome is caused predominantly by phage group 2 staphylococci, particularly strains 71 and 55, which are present at localized sites of infection. Foci of infection include the nasopharynx and, less commonly, the umbilicus, urinary tract, a superficial abrasion, conjunctivae, and blood. The clinical manifestations of staphylococcal scalded skin syndrome are mediated by hematogenous spread, in the absence of specific antitoxin antibody of staphylococcal epidermolytic or exfoliative toxins A or B. The toxins have reproduced the disease in both animal models and human volunteers. Decreased renal clearance of the toxins may account for the fact that the disease is most common in infants and young children. Epidermolytic toxin A is heat stable and is encoded by bacterial chromosomal genes; epidermolytic toxin B is heat labile and is encoded on a 37.5-kb plasmid. Histopathologically, the site of blister cleavage is subcorneal through the granular layer. The epidermolytic toxins appear to produce the granular layer split by binding to desmoglein I within desmosomes. Evidence suggests that the toxins are members of the trypsin-like serine protease family and may exert their action through proteolysis.

DIAGNOSIS. Intact bullae are consistently sterile, unlike those of bullous impetigo, but cultures should be obtained from all suspected sites of localized infection and from the blood to identify the source for elaboration of the epidermolytic toxins. The subcorneal, granular layer split can be identified on skin biopsy; absence of an inflammatory infiltrate is characteristic. In cases that demand a rapid diagnosis, the exfoliated corneal layer can be seen on a frozen biopsy specimen of the desquamating epidermis. Scattered acantholytic cells, which are evident in the cleftlike bullae, can also be seen in a Tzanck preparation.

TREATMENT. Systemic therapy, either orally, in cases of localized involvement, or parenterally, with a semisynthetic penicillinase-resistant penicillin, should be prescribed because the staphylococci are usually penicillin resistant. The skin should be gently moistened and cleansed with Burow solution, Dakin solution, or isotonic saline. Application of an emollient provides lubrication and decreases discomfort. Topical antibiotics are unnecessary. Recovery is usually rapid, but complications such as excessive fluid loss, electrolyte imbalance, faulty temperature regulation, pneumonia, septicemia, and cellulitis may cause increased morbidity.

ECTHYMA (see Chapters 184 and 203)

This resembles nonbullous impetigo in onset and appearance but gradually evolves into a deeper, more chronic infection. The initial lesion is a vesicle or vesiculopustule with an erythematous base that erodes through the epidermis into the dermis to form an ulcer with elevated margins. The ulcer becomes obscured by a dry, heaped-up, tightly adherent crust that contributes to the persistence of the infection and scar formation. Lesions may be spread by autoinoculation, may be as large as 4 cm, and occur most frequently on the legs. Predisposing factors include pruritic lesions, such as insect bites, scabies, or pediculosis, which are subject to frequent scratching; poor hygiene; and malnutrition. Complications include lymphangitis, cellulitis, and rarely poststreptococcal glomerulonephritis. The causative agent is usually GABHS; *S. aureus* is also cultured from most lesions but is probably a secondary pathogen. Crusts should be softened with warm compresses and removed with an antibacterial soap. Systemic antibiotic therapy, as for impetigo, is indicated; almost all lesions are responsive to treatment with penicillin.

Ecthyma gangrenosa is a necrotic ulcer covered with a gray-black eschar. It is usually a sign of *P. aeruginosa* sepsis and usually occurs in immunosuppressed patients. Ecthyma gangrenosum occurs in up to 6% of patients with systemic *P. aeruginosa* infection but can also occur as a primary cutaneous infection by inoculation. The lesion begins as a red or purpuric macule that vesiculates and then ulcerates; there is a surrounding rim of pink to violaceous skin. The punched-out ulcer develops raised edges with a dense, black, depressed, crusted center. Lesions may be single or multiple; patients with bacteremia commonly have lesions in apocrine areas. Clinically similar lesions may also develop as a result of infection with other agents such as *S. aureus, A. hydrophila, Enterobacter* species, *Proteus* species, *Pseudomonas cepacia, Serratia marcescens, Aspergillus* species, Mucorales, *E. coli,* and *Candida* species. Histopathologic examination reveals bacterial invasion of the adventitia and media of dermal veins but not arteries; the intima and lumina are spared. Blood cultures and skin biopsy for culture should be obtained, and empirical broad-spectrum, systemic therapy that includes coverage for *Pseudomonas* should be initiated as soon as possible.

BLASTOMYCOSIS-LIKE PYODERMA

(Pyoderma Vegetans)

This is an exuberant cutaneous reaction to bacterial infection, primarily in children who are malnourished and immunosuppressed. The organisms isolated most commonly from lesions are *S. aureus* and GABHS, but several other organisms have been associated with these lesions, including *P. aeruginosa, Proteus mirabilis,* diphtheroids, *Bacillus* species and *C. perfringens.* Hyperplastic, crusted plaques on the extremities are characteristic, sometimes forming from the coalescence of many pinpoint, purulent, crusted abscesses. Ulceration and sinus tract formation may develop, and additional lesions may appear at sites distant from the site of inoculation. Regional lymphadenopathy is common, but fever is not. Histopathologic examination reveals pseudoepitheliomatous hyperplasia and abscesses composed of neutrophils and/or eosinophils; giant cells are usually lacking. The differential diagnosis includes deep fungal infection, particularly blastomycosis and tuberculous and atypical mycobacterial infection. Underlying immunodeficiency should be ruled out, and the selection of antibiotics should be guided by susceptibility testing because the response to antibiotics is often poor.

BLISTERING DISTAL DACTYLITIS

This is a superficial blistering infection of the volar fat pad on the distal portion of the finger or thumb. More than one finger may be involved, as may the volar surfaces of the proximal phalanges, palms, and toes. Blisters are filled with a watery purulent fluid that contains polymorphonuclear leukocytes and chains of gram-positive cocci. Patients usually have no preceding history of trauma, and systemic symptoms are generally absent. Poststreptococcal glomerulonephritis has not occurred after blistering distal dactylitis. The infection is caused most commonly by GABHS but has also occurred as a result of infection with group B β-hemolytic streptococci and *S. aureus.* If left untreated, blisters may continue to enlarge and extend to the paronychial area. The infection responds to incision and drainage and a 10-day course of systemic penicillin or erythromycin therapy.

PERIANAL DERMATITIS

This presents most commonly in boys (70% of cases) between the ages of 6 mo and 10 yr as perianal dermatitis (90% of cases) and pruritus (80% of cases). The incidence of perianal dermatitis is not known precisely but ranges from 1/2,000 to 1/218 patient visits. The rash is superficial, erythematous, well marginated, nonindurated, and confluent from the anus outward. Acutely (<6-wk duration), the rash tends to be bright red, moist, and tender to touch. At this stage, a white pseudomembrane may be present. As the rash becomes more chronic, the perianal eruption may consist of painful fissures, a dried mucoid discharge, and little erythema or of psoriasiform plaques with yellow peripheral crust. In girls, the perianal rash may be associated with vulvovaginitis; the penis may be involved in boys. Approximately 50% of patients have rectal pain, most commonly described as burning inside the anus during defecation, and 33% have blood-streaked stools. Fecal retention is a frequent behavioral response to the infection. Patients have presented with guttate psoriasis. Although local induration or edema may occur, constitutional symptoms of fever, headache, and malaise are absent, suggesting that subcutaneous involvement, as in cellulitis, is absent. Familial spread of perianal dermatitis is common, particularly when family members bathe together or use the same water.

The *differential diagnosis* of perianal dermatitis includes psoriasis, seborrheic dermatitis, candidosis, pinworm infestation, sexual abuse, and inflammatory bowel disease. Differentiation from these other conditions can be accomplished by culturing a moderate to heavy growth of GABHS on 5% sheep blood agar. Perianal dermatitis may also be caused by *S. aureus.* Children with asymptomatic perianal colonization have light growth of GABHS on blood agar. Direct antigen studies for GABHS are also very sensitive (89%), but results may be falsely negative early in the course of the disease. Acute and convalescent sera for antistreptolysin O or anti-DNase B are not helpful in making the diagnosis. The index case and family members should be cultured initially, and follow-up cultures to document bacteriologic cure after a course of treatment are also recommended.

Treatment with a single 10-day course of oral penicillin produces resolution of the dermatitis and symptoms in most patients; however, recurrence rates of 40–50% have been reported, emphasizing the need for close follow-up, including repeat culture. Erythromycin estolate and ethylsuccinate are excellent alternative treatments for those who are allergic to penicillin, who have not responded to a course of penicillin, or who are infected with *S. aureus.* Clindamycin has also been used successfully to treat recurrent perianal dermatitis. Mupirocin has been used in conjunction with oral antibiotics to treat recurrences but has not been evaluated as a single-drug therapy.

ERYSIPELAS (see Chapter 184)

FOLLICULITIS

This superficial infection of the hair follicle is most often caused by *S. aureus* (Bockhart impetigo); coagulase-negative staphylococci are the cause occasionally. The lesions are typically small, discrete, dome-shaped pustules with an erythematous base, located at the ostium of the pilosebaceous canals. Hair growth is unimpaired, and the lesions heal without scarring. Favored sites include the scalp, buttocks, and extremities. Poor hygiene, maceration, and drainage from wounds and abscesses can be provocative factors. Folliculitis can also occur as a result of tar therapy or occlusive wraps; the moist environment encourages bacterial proliferation. In HIV-infected patients, *S. aureus* may produce confluent erythematous patches with satellite pustules in intertriginous areas and violaceous plaques composed of superficial follicular pustules in the scalp, axillas, or groin. *Candida* may cause satellite follicular papules and pustules surrounding erythematous patches of intertrigo, and *Malassezia furfur* produces pruritic 2–3-mm erythematous, perifollicular papules and pustules on the back, chest, and extremities, particularly in patients with diabetes mellitus or on corticosteroids or antibiotics. Diagnosis is made by examining potassium hydroxide–treated scrapings from lesions. Detection of *Malassezia* may require a skin biopsy, demonstrating clusters of yeast and short, branching hyphae ("spaghetti and meatballs") in widened follicular ostia mixed with keratinous debris. *Malassezia* may be cultured on Sabouraud's dextrose agar supplemented with gentamicin, vancomycin, and olive oil.

The causative organism of folliculitis can be identified by Gram stain and culture of purulent material from the follicular orifice. *Treatment* for folliculitis includes topical antibiotic cleansers such as chlorhexidine or hexachlorophene. Topical antibiotic therapy is usually all that is required for mild cases, but more severe cases may require use of penicillinase-resistant systemic antibiotics such as dicloxacillin or cephalexin. In chronic recurrent folliculitis, daily application of a benzoyl peroxide lotion or gel may facilitate resolution.

Folliculitis caused by Gram-negative organisms occurs primarily in patients with acne vulgaris treated long term with broad-spectrum systemic antibiotics. A superficial pustular form, caused by *Klebsiella, Enterobacter, E. coli*, or *P. aeruginosa*, occurs around the nose and spreads to the cheeks and chin. A deeper, nodular form of folliculitis on the face and trunk is caused by *Proteus*. Culture of infected follicles is necessary to establish the diagnosis. Treatment consists of incision and drainage of the deeper, larger cysts; topical neomycin or bacitracin; or selection of an oral antibiotic based on the sensitivity profile of the pathogenic organism. For severe, recalcitrant cases, 13-*cis*-retinoic acid, 1 mg/kg/24 hr, is helpful but should be administered only by experienced physicians because of side effects.

Sycosis barbae is a deeper, more severe recurrent inflammatory form of folliculitis caused by *S. aureus* that involves the entire depth of the follicle. Erythematous follicular papules and pustules develop on the chin, upper lip, and angle of the jaw, primarily in young black males. Papules may coalesce into plaques, and healing may occur with scarring. Affected individuals frequently are found to be *S. aureus* carriers. Treatment with warm saline compresses and topical antibiotics such as mupirocin generally clears the infection. More extensive, recalcitrant cases may require therapy with β-lactamase–resistant systemic antibiotics and elimination of *S. aureus* from sites of carriage.

Hot tub folliculitis is attributable to *P. aeruginosa*, predominantly serotype O-11. The lesions are pruritic papules and pustules or deeply erythematous to violaceous nodules that develop 8–48 hr after exposure and are most dense in areas covered by a bathing suit. Patients occasionally develop fever, malaise, and lymphadenopathy. The organism is readily cultured from pus. The eruption usually resolves spontaneously within 1–2 wk, often leaving postinflammatory hyperpigmentation, but topical agents with antipseudomonal activity, such as potassium permanganate and gentamicin cream, are sometimes necessary. Consideration should be given to use of systemic antibiotics (e.g., ciprofloxacin) in adolescent patients with constitutional symptoms. Immunocompromised children are susceptible to complications of *Pseudomonas* folliculitis (e.g., cellulitis) and should avoid hot tubs.

FURUNCLES AND CARBUNCLES

These follicular lesions may originate from a preceding folliculitis or may arise initially as a deep-seated, tender, erythematous, perifollicular nodule. Although lesions are initially indurated, central necrosis and suppuration follow, leading to rupture and discharge of a central core of necrotic tissue and destruction of the follicle. Healing occurs with scar formation. Sites of predilection are the hair-bearing areas on the face, neck, axillae, buttocks, and groin. Pain may be intense if the lesion is situated in an area where the skin is relatively fixed, such as in the external auditory canal or over the nasal cartilages. Patients with furuncles usually have no constitutional symptoms; however, bacteremia may occasionally ensue. Rarely, lesions on the upper lip or cheek may lead to cavernous sinus thrombosis. Infection of a group of contiguous follicles, with multiple drainage points, accompanied by inflammatory changes in surrounding connective tissue is a carbuncle. Carbuncles may be accompanied by fever, leukocytosis, and bacteremia.

ETIOLOGY. The causative agent is almost always *S. aureus*, which penetrates abraded perifollicular skin. Conditions predisposing to furuncle formation include obesity, hyperhidrosis, maceration, friction, and pre-existing dermatitis. Furunculosis is also more common in individuals with low serum iron levels, diabetes, malnutrition, HIV infection, or other immunodeficiency states. Recurrent furunculosis is frequently associated with carriage of *S. aureus* in the nares, axillas, or perineum or close contact with someone such as a family member who is a carrier. Other bacteria or fungi may occasionally cause furuncles or carbuncles; therefore, Gram stain and culture of the pus are indicated.

TREATMENT. This should include regular bathing with antimicrobial soaps and wearing of loose-fitting clothing, which minimize predisposing factors for furuncle formation. Frequent application of a hot, moist compress may facilitate drainage of lesions. Large lesions may be drained by a small incision. Carbuncles and large or numerous furuncles should be treated with systemic penicillinase-resistant antibiotics such as cloxacillin orally or oxacillin parenterally. Penicillin-allergic patients can be treated with a cephalosporin, clindamycin, or erythromycin. Treatment of recurrent cases has been successful by colonization of the individual with a less virulent strain of *S. aureus* such as 502A. The carriage state may be eliminated temporarily by application of mupirocin ointment for 5 days to the anterior nares. Attention to personal hygiene, use of an antibacterial soap, low-dose oral antistaphylococcal penicillin or clindamycin, and frequent handwashing may also be beneficial.

PITTED KERATOLYSIS

Pitted keratolysis occurs most frequently in humid tropical and subtropical climates, particularly in individuals whose feet are moist for prolonged periods, for example, as a result of hyperhidrosis, prolonged wearing of boots, or immersion in water. The lesions consist of 1–7-mm irregularly shaped superficial erosions of the horny layer on the soles, particularly at weight-bearing sites. Brownish discoloration of involved areas may be apparent. The condition is nearly always asymptomatic but frequently is malodorous. A rare, painful variant is manifested as thinned, erythematous to violaceous plaques in addition to the typical pitted lesions. The most likely etiologic agent is a species of *Corynebacterium*. Actinomycetes, dermatophili, and micrococci have also been isolated from lesions. Avoidance of moisture and maceration produces slow, spontaneous resolution of the infection. Therapeutic regimens that have been effective include topical application of 2% buffered glutaraldehyde, 20% formaldehyde solution (formalin) in Aquaphor, erythromycin, clindamycin, and the imidazoles.

ERYTHRASMA

This is a benign chronic superficial infection caused by *Corynebacterium minutissimum*. Predisposing factors include heat, humidity, obesity, skin maceration, and poor hygiene. Approximately 20% of healthy individuals have involvement of the toe webs. Other frequently affected sites are moist intertriginous areas such as the groin and axillas; the inframammary and perianal regions are involved occasionally. Sharply demarcated, irregularly bordered, brownish-red, slightly scaly patches are characteristic of the disease. Mild pruritus is the only constant symptom. *C. minutissimum* is a complex of related organisms that produce porphyrins that fluoresce brilliant coral-red under ultraviolet light. The diagnosis is readily made, and erythrasma is differentiated from dermatophyte infection and from tinea versicolor by Wood's lamp examination. Bathing within 20 hr of Wood's lamp examination, however, may remove the water-soluble porphyrins. Staining of skin scrapings with methylene blue or Gram stain reveals the pleomorphic, filamentous coccobacillary forms.

Most cases represent colonization, are asymptomatic, and require no therapy. Effective *treatment* can be achieved with topical erythromycin, clindamycin, miconazole, or Whitfield ointment or a 10–14-day course of oral erythromycin. Recurrence may be inhibited by frequent use of an antibacterial soap or an astringent such as 10–20% aluminum chloride in anhydrous ethyl alcohol.

ERYSIPELOID

This rare cutaneous infection is caused by inoculation of *Erysipelothrix rhusiopathiae* from contaminated animals, birds, fish, or their products. The localized cutaneous form is most common, characterized by well-demarcated diamond-shaped erythematous to violaceous patches at sites of inoculation. Local symptoms are generally not severe, constitutional symptoms are rare, and the lesions resolve spontaneously after weeks but can recur at the same site or develop elsewhere weeks to months later. The diffuse cutaneous form presents with lesions at several areas of the body in addition to the site of inoculation; it is also self-limited. The systemic form, caused by hematogenous spread, is accompanied by constitutional symptoms and may include endocarditis, septic arthritis, cerebral infarct and abscess, meningitis, and pulmonary effusion. Diagnosis is confirmed by skin biopsy, which reveals the gram-positive organisms, and culture. The treatment of choice is parenteral erythromycin or penicillin.

TUBERCULOSIS OF THE SKIN (see Chapters 212 and 214)

Cutaneous tuberculosis infection occurs worldwide, particularly in association with HIV infection, malnutrition, and poor hygiene. Primary cutaneous tuberculosis is rare in the United States but occurs with the greatest frequency in infants and children; the overall incidence of cutaneous tuberculosis among those with all forms of tuberculosis in the United States is approximately 1–2%. All forms of cutaneous disease are caused by *Mycobacterium tuberculosis*, by *Mycobacterium bovis*, and occasionally by the bacillus Calmette-Guérin (BCG), an attenuated form of *M. bovis*; the manifestations caused by a given organism are indistinguishable from one another. After invasion of the skin, mycobacteria either multiply intracellularly within macrophages, leading to progressive disease, or are controlled by the host immune reaction.

A primary lesion, a *tuberculous chancre*, results when *M. tuberculosis* or *M. bovis* gains access to the skin or mucous membranes through trauma. Sites of predilection are the face, lower extremities, and genitals. The initial lesion develops 2–4 wk after introduction of the organism into the damaged tissue. A red-brown papule gradually enlarges to form a shallow, firm, sharply demarcated ulcer; satellite abscesses may be present. Some lesions acquire a crust resembling impetigo, and others become heaped up and verrucous at the margins. The primary lesion occurs in one third of cases as a painless ulcer on the conjunctiva, gingiva, or palate and occasionally as a painless acute paronychia. Painless regional adenopathy appears approximately 3–8 wk after inoculation and may be accompanied by lymphangitis, lymphadenitis, or perforation of the skin surface, forming scrofuloderma. Erythema nodosum develops in approximately 10% of cases. Untreated lesions heal with scarring within approximately 12 mo but may reactivate, may form lupus vulgaris, or rarely may progress to the acute miliary form.

M. tuberculosis or *M. bovis* can be cultured from the skin lesion and local lymph nodes, but acid-fast staining of histologic sections, particularly of a well-controlled infection, often does not reveal the organism. Clinically, the differential diagnosis is broad, including a syphilitic chancre; deep fungal or atypical mycobacterial infection; leprosy; tularemia; cat scratch disease; sporotrichosis; nocardiosis; leishmaniasis; reaction to foreign substances such as zirconium, beryllium, silk or nylon sutures, talc, or starch; papular acne rosacea; and lupus miliaris disseminatum faciei. Spontaneous healing with scarring coincides with acquisition of immunity, at which time the skin lesions and infected nodes may become calcified. Antituberculous therapy is indicated (see Chapter 212).

Direct cutaneous inoculation of the tubercle bacillus into a previously infected individual with a moderate to high degree of immunity initially produces a small papule with surrounding inflammation. *Tuberculosis verrucosa cutis* (warty tuberculosis) forms when the papule becomes hyperkeratotic and warty, and several adjacent papules coalesce or a single papule expands peripherally to form a brownish-red to violaceous, exudative, crusted verrucous plaque. Irregular extension of the margins of the plaque produces a serpiginous border. Children have the lesion most commonly on the lower extremities after trauma and contact with infected material such as sputum or soil. Regional lymph nodes are involved only rarely. Spontaneous healing with atrophic scarring takes place slowly, over months to years; healing is also gradual with antituberculous therapy.

Lupus vulgaris is a rare, chronic, progressive form of cutaneous tuberculosis that develops in individuals with a moderate to high degree of tuberculin sensitivity induced by previous infection. The incidence is greater in cool, moist climates, particularly in females. Lupus vulgaris develops as a result of direct extension from underlying joints or lymph nodes; through lymphatic or hematogenous spread; or rarely, by cutaneous inoculation with BCG vaccine. It most commonly follows cervical adenitis or pulmonary tuberculosis. Approximately 33% of cases are preceded by scrofuloderma, and 90% of cases present on the head and neck, most commonly on the nose or cheek; involvement of the trunk is uncommon. A typical solitary lesion consists of a brownish-red, soft papule that has an apple-jelly color when examined by diascopy. Expansion of the papule peripherally, or occasionally the coalescence of several papules, forms an irregular lesion of variable size and form. One or several lesions may develop, including nodules or plaques that are flat and serpiginous, hypertrophic and verrucous, or edematous in appearance. Spontaneous healing occurs centrally, and lesions characteristically reappear within the area of atrophy. Chronicity is characteristic, and persistence and progression of plaques over many years is common. Lymphadenitis is present in 40% of those with lupus vulgaris, and 10–20% have infection of the lungs, bones, or joints. Vegetative masses and ulceration involving the nasal, buccal, or conjunctival mucosa; the palate; the gingiva; or the oropharynx may cause extensive deformities. Squamous cell carcinoma, with a relatively high metastatic potential, may develop, usually after several years of the disease. After a temporary impairment in immunity, particularly after measles infection (i.e., *lupus exanthematicus*), multiple lesions may form at distant sites as a result of hematogenous spread from a latent focus of infection. The histopathologic changes are those of a tuberculoid granuloma without caseation; and organisms are extremely difficult to demonstrate. The differential diagnosis includes sarcoidosis, leprosy, atypical mycobacterial infection, blastomycosis, chromoblastomycosis, actinomycosis, leishmaniasis, tertiary syphilis, leprosy, hypertrophic lichen planus, psoriasis, lupus erythematosus, lymphocytoma, and Bower disease. Small lesions can be excised; antituberculous drug therapy usually halts further spread and induces involution.

Scrofuloderma results from enlargement, cold abscess formation, and breakdown of a lymph node, most frequently in a cervical chain, with extension to the overlying skin. Linear or serpiginous ulcers and dissecting fistulas and subcutaneous tracts studded with soft nodules may develop. Spontaneous healing may take years, eventuating in cordlike keloid scars; lupus vulgaris may also develop. Scrofuloderma of a cervical lymph node often originates in the larynx and was linked in the past to ingestion of milk containing *M. bovis*. Lesions may also originate from an underlying infected joint, tendon, bone, or epididymis. The differential diagnosis includes syphilitic gumma, deep fungal infections, actinomycosis, and hidradenitis suppurativa. The course is indolent, and constitutional symptoms are typically absent. Antituberculous therapy is usually effective.

Orificial tuberculosis presents on the mucous membranes and periorificial skin after autoinoculation of mycobacteria from sites of progressive infection; it is a sign of advanced internal disease and carries a poor prognosis. Lesions appear as yellowish or red, painful nodules that form punched-out ulcers with inflammation and edema of the surrounding mucosa. Treatment consists of identification of the source of infection and initiation of antituberculous therapy.

Miliary tuberculosis (hematogenous primary tuberculosis) rarely presents cutaneously, most commonly in infants and in individuals who are immunosuppressed after chemotherapy or infection with measles or HIV. The eruption consists of crops of symmetrically distributed, minute, erythematous to purpuric macules, papules, or vesicles. The lesions may ulcerate, drain, crust, and form sinus tracts or may form subcutaneous gummas, especially in malnourished children with impaired immunity. Constitutional signs and symptoms are common, and a leukemoid reaction or aplastic anemia may develop. Tubercle bacilli are readily identified in an active lesion. A fulminant course should be anticipated, and aggressive antituberculous therapy is indicated.

Single or multiple *metastatic tuberculous abscesses* (tuberculous gummas) may develop on the extremities and trunk by hematogenous spread from a primary focus of infection during a period of decreased immunity, particularly in malnourished and immunosuppressed children. The fluctuant, nontender, erythematous subcutaneous nodules may ulcerate and form fistulas.

Vaccination with BCG characteristically produces a papule approximately 2 wk after vaccination. The papule expands in size, typically ulcerates within 2–4 mo, and heals slowly with scarring. In approximately 1–2 per million vaccinations, a complication caused specifically by the BCG organism occurs, including regional lymphadenitis, lupus vulgaris, scrofuloderma, and subcutaneous abscess formation.

Tuberculids are skin reactions that exhibit tuberculoid features histologically but do not contain detectable mycobacteria. The lesions appear in a host who usually has moderate to strong tuberculin reactivity, has a history of previous tuberculosis of other organs, and usually but not always shows a therapeutic response to antituberculous therapy. The cause of tuberculids is poorly understood. Most patients are in good health with no clear focus of disease at the time of the eruption. The most commonly observed tuberculid is the *papulonecrotic tuberculid*. Recurrent crops of symmetrically distributed, asymptomatic, firm, sterile, dusky-red papules appear on the extensor aspects of the limbs, the dorsum of the hands and feet, and the buttocks. The papules may undergo central ulceration and eventually heal, leaving sharply delineated, circular, depressed scars. The duration of the eruption is variable, but it usually disappears promptly after treatment of the primary infection. *Lichen scrofulosorum*, another form of tuberculid, is characterized by asymptomatic, grouped, pinhead-sized, often follicular pink or red papules that form discoid plaques, mainly on the trunk. Healing occurs without scarring.

Atypical mycobacterial infection may cause cutaneous lesions in children. *Mycobacterium marinum* is found in salt and freshwater and diseased fish; in the United States, it is most commonly acquired from tropical fish tanks and swimming pools. Traumatic abrasion of the skin serves as a portal of entry for the organism. Approximately 3 wk after inoculation, a single reddish papule develops and enlarges slowly to form a violaceous nodule or occasionally a warty plaque. The lesion occasionally breaks down to form a crusted ulcer or a suppurating abscess. Sporotrichoid erythematous nodules along lymphatics may also suppurate and drain. Lesions are most common on the elbows, knees, and feet of swimmers and the hands and fingers in aquarium-acquired infection. Systemic signs and symptoms are absent; regional lymph nodes occasionally become slightly enlarged but do not break down. Rarely, the infection becomes disseminated, particularly in an immunosuppressed host. A biopsy specimen of a fully developed lesion demonstrates a granulomatous infiltrate with tuberculoid architecture; intracellular organisms can usually be identified within the histiocytes with appropriate stains. The most effective antituberculous regimens include tetracycline, minocycline, and rifampin plus ethambutol. Application of heat to the affected site may be a useful adjunctive therapy. Spontaneous healing with scarring can be expected within several months to 2 yr (see Chapter 214).

Mycobacterium kansasii primarily causes pulmonary disease; skin disease is rare, often occurring in an immunocompromised host. Most commonly, sporotrichoid nodules develop after inoculation of traumatized skin. Lesions may develop into ulcerated, crusted, or verrucous plaques. The organism is relatively sensitive to antituberculous medications, which should be chosen on the basis of susceptibility testing.

M. scrofulaceum causes cervical lymphadenitis (scrofuloderma) in young children, typically in the submandibular region. Nodes enlarge over several weeks, ulcerate, and drain. The local reaction is nontender and circumscribed, constitutional symptoms are absent, and there generally is no evidence of lung or other organ involvement. Other atypical mycobacteria may cause a similar presentation, including *M. avium* complex, *M. kansasii*, and *M. fortuitum*. Treatment is accomplished by excision and antituberculous drugs (see Chapter 214).

Mycobacterium ulcerans causes a painless subcutaneous nodule after inoculation of abraded skin. Most infections occur in children in tropical rain forests. The nodule usually ulcerates, develops undermined edges, and may spread over large areas, most commonly on an extremity. Local necrosis of subcutaneous fat, producing a septal panniculitis, is characteristic. Ulcers persist for months to years before healing spontaneously with scarring and sometimes with lymphedema. Constitutional symptoms and lymphadenopathy are absent. Diagnosis is made by culturing the organism at 32–33°C. Treatment of choice is early excision of the lesion. Local heat therapy and oral chemotherapy may benefit some patients.

M. avium complex, composed of more than 20 subtypes, most commonly causes chronic pulmonary infection. Cervical lymphadenitis and osteomyelitis occur occasionally, and papules or purulent leg ulcers occur rarely by primary inoculation. Skin lesions may be an early sign of disseminated infection; the lesions may take various forms, including erythematous papules, pustules, nodules, abscesses, ulcers, panniculitis, and sporotrichoid spread along lymphatics. For treatment, see Chapter 214.

M. fortuitum complex is composed of two organisms: *M. fortuitum* and *M. chelonei*. These organisms cause disease in an immunocompetent host principally by primary cutaneous inoculation after traumatic injury, injection, or surgery. A nodule, abscess, or cellulitis develops 4–6 wk after inoculation. In an immunocompromised host, numerous subcutaneous nodules may form, break down, and drain. Treatment is based on identification and susceptibility testing of the organism.

Amren DP, Anderson AS, Wannamaker LW: Perianal cellulitis associated with group A streptococci. Am J Dis Child 112:546, 1966.
Barnett BO, Frieden IJ: Streptococcal skin diseases in children. Semin Dermatol 11:3, 1992.
Beyt BE Jr, Ortbals DW, Santa Cruz DJ: Cutaneous mycobacteriosis: Analysis of 34 cases with a new classification of the disease. Medicine (Baltimore) 60:95, 1980.
Cochran RJ, Rosen T, Landers T: Topical treatment for erythrasma. Int J Dermatol 20:562, 1981.
Darmstadt GL: Oral antibiotic therapy for uncomplicated bacterial skin infections in children. Pediatr Infect Dis J 16:227, 1997.
Darmstadt GL: Staphylococcal and streptococcal skin infections. *In*: Harahap M (ed): Diagnosis and Treatment of Skin Infections. Oxford, Blackwell Science, 1997, pp 7–115.
Darmstadt GL, Lane AT: Impetigo: An overview. Pediatr Dermatol 11:293, 1994.
Derrick CW, Reilly KM, Stallworth P, et al: Erythromycin in the treatment of streptococcal infections. Pediatr Infect Dis 5:172, 1986.
Dillon HC Jr, Reeves MSA: Streptococcal immune responses in nephritis after skin infection. Am J Med 56:333, 1974.
Doebbeling BN, Breneman DL, Neu HC, et al: Elimination of *Staphylococcus aureus* nasal carriage in health care workers: Analysis of six clinical trials with calcium mupirocin ointment. Clin Infect Dis 17:466, 1993.
Eady EA, Cove JH: Topical antibiotic therapy: Current status and future prospects. Drugs Exp Clin Res 16:423, 1990.
Elias PM, Levy W: Bullous impetigo. Occurrence of localized scalded skin syndrome in an adult. Arch Dermatol 112:856, 1976.
Ferrieri P, Dajani AS, Wannamaker LW, et al: Natural history of impetigo I. Site sequence of acquisition and familial patterns of spread of cutaneous streptococci. J Clin Invest 51:2851, 1972.
Gart GS, Forstall GJ, Tomecki KJ: Mycobacterial skin disease: Approaches to therapy. Semin Dermatol 12:352, 1993.
Hayden GF: Skin diseases encountered in a pediatric clinic. Am J Dis Child 139:36, 1985.
Hedstrom SA: Treatment and prevention of recurrent staphylococcal furunculosis: Clinical and bacteriologic follow up. Scand J Infect Dis 17:55, 1985.
Katz AR, Morens DM: Severe streptococcal infections in historical perspective. Clin Infect Dis 14:298, 1992.
Leyden JJ: Review of mupirocin ointment in the treatment of impetigo. Clin Pediatr 31:549, 1992.
McCray MK, Esterly NB: Cutaneous eruptions in congenital tuberculosis. Arch Dermatol 117:460, 1981.
Melish ME, Glasgow LA: Staphylococcal scalded skin syndrome: The expanded clinical syndrome. J Pediatr 78:958, 1971.
Rice TD, Duggan AK, DeAngelis C: Cost-effectiveness of erythromycin versus mupirocin for the treatment of impetigo in children. Pediatrics 89:210, 1992.
Tunnessen WW Jr: A survey of skin disorders seen in pediatric general and dermatology clinics. Pediatr Dermatol 1:219, 1984.
Tunnessen WW Jr: Practical aspects of bacterial skin infections in children. Pediatr Dermatol 2:255, 1985.

CHAPTER 672
Cutaneous Fungal Infections

TINEA VERSICOLOR

This common, innocuous, chronic fungal infection of the stratum corneum is caused by the dimorphic yeast *Malassezia furfur*. The synonyms *Pityrosporum ovale* and *P. orbiculare* were used previously to identify the causal organism.

ETIOLOGY. *M. furfur* is part of the indigenous flora, predominantly in the yeast form, and is found particularly in areas of skin that are rich in sebum production. Proliferation of filamentous forms occurs in the disease state. Predisposing factors include a warm, humid environment, excessive sweating, occlusion, high plasma cortisol levels, immunosuppression, malnourishment, and genetically determined susceptibility. The disease is most prevalent in adolescents and young adults.

CLINICAL MANIFESTATIONS. The lesions vary widely in color: In whites, they typically are reddish brown, whereas in blacks they may be either hypopigmented or hyperpigmented. The characteristic macules are covered with a fine scale; they often begin in a perifollicular location, enlarge, and merge to form confluent patches, most commonly on the neck, upper chest, back, and upper arms (Fig. 672–1*A*). Facial lesions are not unusual in adolescents, and lesions occasionally appear on the forearms, dorsum of the hands, and pubis. There may be little or no pruritus. Involved areas do not tan after sun exposure. A papulopustular perifollicular variant of the disorder may occur on the back, chest, and sometimes the extremities.

DIAGNOSIS. Examination with a Wood's lamp discloses a yellowish-gold fluorescence. A potassium hydroxide (KOH) preparation of scrapings is diagnostic, demonstrating groups of thick-walled spores and myriad short, thick, angular hyphae, resembling spaghetti and meatballs (Fig. 672–1*B*). Skin biopsy, including culture and special stains for fungi (e.g., periodic acid–Schiff), are often necessary to make the diagnosis in cases of primarily follicular involvement; organisms and keratinous debris can be seen within dilated follicular ostia.

Tinea versicolor must be distinguished from dermatophyte infections, seborrheic dermatitis, pityriasis alba, and secondary syphilis. Nonscaling pigmentary disorders, such as postinflammatory pigmentary change, may be mimicked if a patient has removed the scales by scrubbing. Disseminated candidiasis must be differentiated from *M. furfur* folliculitis.

TREATMENT. Many therapeutic agents can be used to treat this disease successfully; however, the causative agent, a normal human saprophyte, is not eradicated from the skin, and the disorder recurs in predisposed individuals. Appropriate topical therapy may include one of the following: a selenium sulfide suspension applied for 5–10 min each day for 2 wk; 25% sodium hyposulfite or thiosulfate lotion applied twice daily for 2–4 wk; lotions, ointments, or creams containing 3–6% salicylic acid twice daily for 2–4 wk; or miconazole, clotrimazole, ketoconazole, or terbinafine cream twice daily for 2–4 wk. Recurrent episodes continue to respond promptly to these agents. Oral therapy may be more convenient and may be achieved successfully with ketoconazole or fluconazole, 400 mg, repeated in 1 wk, or itraconazole, 200 mg/24 hr for 5–7 days.

DERMATOPHYTOSES

Dermatophytoses are caused by a group of closely related filamentous fungi with a propensity for invading the stratum corneum, hair, and nails. The three principal genera responsible for infections are *Trichophyton*, *Microsporum*, and *Epidermophyton*.

ETIOLOGY. *Trichophyton* species cause lesions of all keratinized tissue, including skin, nails, and hair; *T. rubrum* is the most common dermatophyte pathogen overall. *Microsporum* species principally invade the hair, and the *Epidermophyton* species invade the intertriginous skin. Dermatophyte infections are designated by the word *tinea* followed by the Latin word for the anatomic site of involvement. The dermatophytes are also classified according to source and natural habitat. Fungi acquired from the soil are called *geophilic*; they infect humans sporadically, inciting an inflammatory reaction. Dermatophytes that are acquired from animals are *zoophilic*; transmission may be through direct contact or indirectly by infected animal hair or clothing. Infected animals frequently are asymptomatic. Dermatophytes acquired from humans are referred to as *anthropophilic*; these infestations range from chronic low-grade to acute inflammatory disease. *Epidermophyton* infections are transmitted only by humans, but various species of *Trichophyton* and *Microsporum* can be acquired from both human and nonhuman sources.

EPIDEMIOLOGY. Host defense has an important influence on the severity of the infection. Disease tends to be more severe

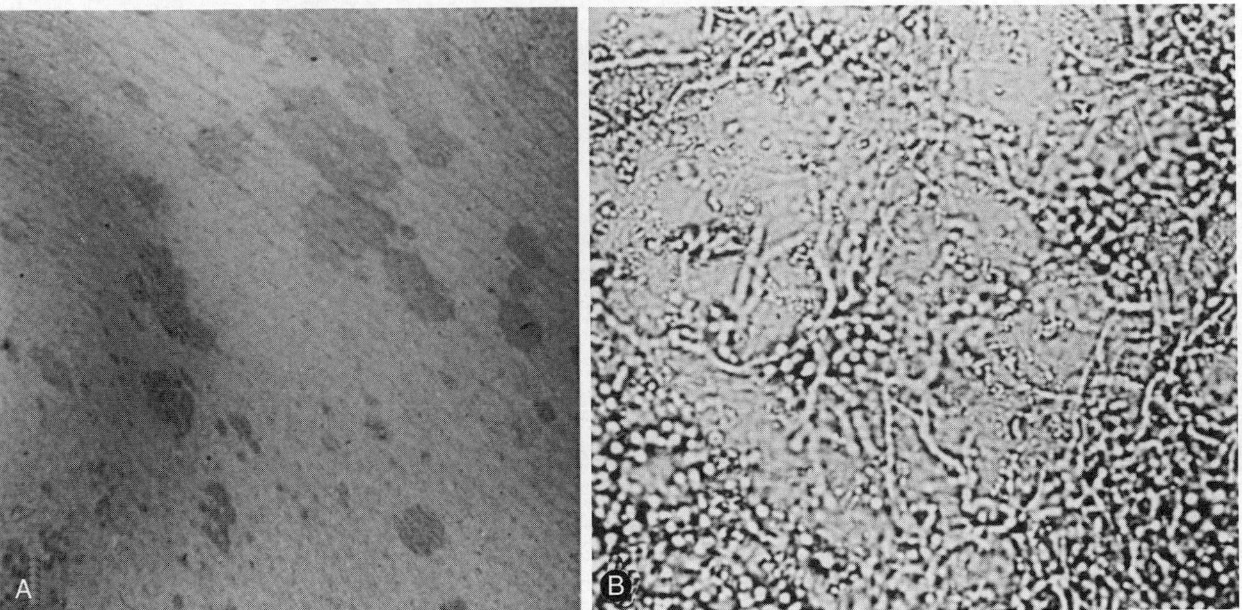

Figure 672–1 *A*, Hyperpigmented, sharply demarcated macules of varying sizes on the upper trunk characteristic of tinea versicolor. *B*, KOH preparation of *Malassezia furfur* demonstrating short, thick hyphae and clusters of spores.

in individuals with diabetes mellitus, lymphoid malignancies, immunosuppression, and states with high plasma cortisol levels, such as Cushing syndrome. Some dermatophytes, most notably the zoophilic species, tend to elicit more severe, suppurative inflammation in humans. Some degree of resistance to reinfection is acquired by most infected persons and may be associated with a delayed hypersensitivity response. No relationship has been demonstrated, however, between antibody levels and resistance to infection. The frequency and severity of infection are also affected by the geographic locale, the genetic susceptibility of the host, and the virulence of the strain of dermatophyte. Additional local factors that predispose to infection include trauma to the skin, hydration of the skin with maceration, occlusion, and elevated temperature.

Occasionally, a secondary skin eruption referred to as a *dermatophytid* or *"id" reaction* appears in sensitized individuals and has been attributed to circulating fungal antigens derived from the primary infection. The eruption occurs most frequently on the fingers, hands, and arms and is characterized by grouped papules and vesicles and, occasionally, by sterile pustules. Symmetric urticarial lesions and a more generalized maculopapular eruption also can occur. Id reactions are most often associated with tinea pedis but also occur with tinea capitis; in the latter case, a generalized papulovesicular follicular eruption may occur.

DIAGNOSIS. The important diagnostic procedures for the various dermatophyte diseases include examination of infected hairs with a Wood's lamp, microscopic examination of KOH preparations of infected material, and identification of the etiologic agent by culture. Hairs infected with common *Microsporum* species fluoresce a bright blue-green; most *Trichophyton*-infected hairs do not fluoresce.

CLINICAL MANIFESTATIONS. *Tinea capitis* is a dermatophyte infection of the scalp most often caused by *Trichophyton tonsurans,* occasionally by *Microsporum canis,* and much less commonly by other *Microsporum* and *Trichophyton* species. It is particularly common in black and Hispanic children age 4–14 yr. In *Microsporum* and some *Trichophyton* infections, the spores are distributed in a sheathlike fashion around the hair shaft (ectothrix infection), whereas *T. tonsurans* produces an infection within the hair shaft (endothrix). Endothrix infections may continue past the anagen phase of hair growth into telogen and are more chronic than infections with ectothrix organisms that persist only during the anagen phase. *T. tonsurans* is an anthropophilic species acquired most often by contact with infected hairs and epithelial cells that are on such surfaces as theater seats, hats, and combs. Dermatophyte spores may also be airborne within the immediate environment, and high carriage rates have been demonstrated in noninfected schoolmates and household members. *M. canis* is a zoophilic species that is acquired from cats and dogs.

The *clinical presentation* of tinea capitis varies with the infecting organism. The pattern produced by *Microsporum audouinii,* the most common cause of tinea capitis in the 1940s and 1950s, is characterized initially by a small papule at the base of a hair follicle. The infection spreads peripherally, forming an erythematous and scaly circular plaque *(ringworm)* within which the infected hairs become brittle and broken. Numerous confluent patches of alopecia develop, and patients may complain of severe pruritus. *M. audouinii* infection is no longer common in the United States. Endothrix infections such as those caused by *T. tonsurans* create a pattern known as "black-dot ringworm," characterized initially by many small circular patches of alopecia in which hairs are broken off close to the hair follicle. Another clinical variant presents with diffuse scaling with minimal hair loss secondary to traction; it strongly resembles seborrheic dermatitis, psoriasis, or atopic dermatitis. *T. tonsurans* may also produce a chronic and more diffuse alopecia (Fig. 672–2*A*). A severe inflammatory response produces elevated, boggy granulomatous masses *(kerions),* which are often studded with pustules (Fig. 672–2*B*). Fever, pain, and regional adenopathy are common, and permanent scarring and alopecia may result. The zoophilic organism *M. canis* or the geophilic organism *Microsporum gypseum* also may cause kerion formation. *Favus,* a chronic form of tinea capitis that is rare in the United States, is caused by the fungus *Trichophyton schoenleinii.* Favus starts as yellowish-red papules at the opening of hair follicles. The papules expand and coalesce to form cup-shaped, yellowish, crusted patches that fluoresce dull green under a Wood's lamp.

Tinea capitis can be confused with seborrheic dermatitis, psoriasis, alopecia areata, trichotillomania, and certain dystrophic hair disorders. When inflammation is pronounced, as in kerion, primary or secondary bacterial infection must also be considered. In adolescents, the patchy, moth-eaten type of alopecia associated with secondary syphilis may resemble tinea

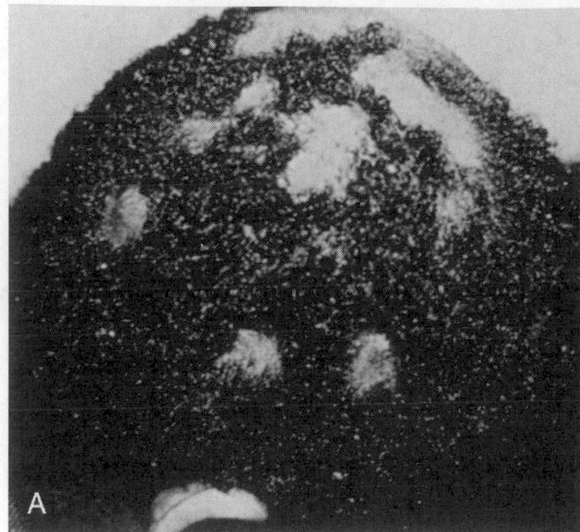

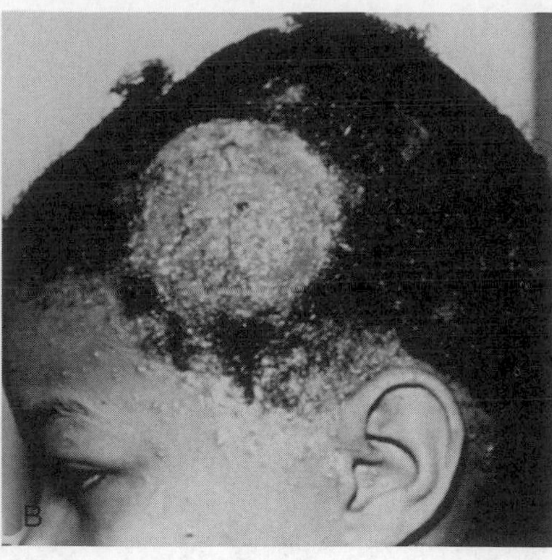

Figure 672–2 *A*, Patchy alopecia associated with tinea capitis. *B*, Elevated, boggy granuloma with multiple pustules (kerion) caused by inflammatory tinea capitis.

capitis. After prolonged tinea capitis has produced scarring, discoid lupus erythematosus and lichen planopilaris must also be considered in the differential diagnosis.

Microscopic examination of a KOH preparation of infected hair from the active border of a lesion discloses tiny spores surrounding the hair shaft in *Microsporum* infections and chains of spores within the hair shaft in *T. tonsurans* infections. Fungal elements usually are not seen in scales. A specific etiologic *diagnosis* of tinea capitis may be obtained by planting broken off infected hairs on Sabouraud's medium with reagents to inhibit growth of other organisms; such identification may require 2 wk or more.

Oral administration of griseofulvin microcrystalline (15 mg/kg/24 hr) is the recommended *treatment* for all forms of tinea capitis; it may be necessary for 8–12 wk and should be terminated only after fungal culture results are negative. Adverse reactions to griseofulvin are rare but include nausea, vomiting, headache, blood dyscrasias, phototoxicity, and hepatotoxicity. Oral itraconazole is useful in instances of griseofulvin resistance, intolerance, or allergy. Itraconazole is given for 4–6 wk at a dosage of 3–5 mg/kg/24 hr with food, typically 100 mg on alternate days in children weighing 10–20 kg, or 100 mg daily for children weighing 20–30 kg. Capsules are preferable to the syrup, which may cause diarrhea. Terbinafine also appears to be effective at a dosage of 3–6 mg/kg/24 hr for 4–6 wk or possibly in pulse therapy, although it has limited activity against *M. canis*. Neither itraconazole nor terbinafine is approved by the Food and Drug Administration for treatment of dermatophyte infections in the pediatric population. Topical therapy alone is ineffective; it may be an important adjunct because it may decrease the shedding of spores. For this purpose, vigorous shampooing with a 2.5% selenium sulfide or zinc pyrithione preparation is helpful. It is not necessary to shave the scalp.

Tinea corporis, infection of the glabrous skin, excluding the palms, soles, and groin, can be caused by most of the dermatophyte species, although *T. rubrum* and *T. mentagrophytes* are the most prevalent etiologic organisms. In children, infections with *M. canis* are also frequent. Tinea corporis can be acquired by direct contact with infected persons or by contact with infected scales or hairs deposited on environmental surfaces. *M. canis* infections are usually acquired from infected pets. Not infrequently, a single dermatophyte lesion is responsible for dissemination.

The most typical *clinical lesion* begins as a dry, mildly erythematous, elevated, scaly papule or plaque that spreads centrifugally as it clears centrally to form the characteristic annular lesion responsible for the designation ringworm (Fig. 672–3). At times, plaques with advancing borders may spread over large areas. Grouped pustules are another variant. Most lesions clear spontaneously within several months, but some may become chronic. Central clearing does not always occur, and differences in host response may result in wide variability in the clinical appearance, for example, granulomatous lesions called *Majocchi granuloma* due to penetration of organisms along the hair follicle to the level of the dermis, producing a fungal folliculitis and perifolliculitis, and the kerion-like lesions referred to as *tinea profunda*.

Many skin lesions, both infectious and noninfectious, must be differentiated from the lesions of tinea corporis. Those most frequently confused are granuloma annulare, nummular eczema, pityriasis rosea, psoriasis, seborrheic dermatitis, erythema chronicum migrans, and tinea versicolor. Microscopic examination of KOH wet mount preparations and cultures should always be obtained when fungal infection is considered. Tinea corporis usually does not fluoresce with a Wood's lamp.

Tinea corporis usually responds to *treatment* with one of the topical antifungal agents (e.g., miconazole, clotrimazole, econazole, ketoconazole, terbinafine, naftifine) twice daily for 2–4 wk. In unusually severe or extensive disease, a course of therapy with oral griseofulvin microcrystalline may be re-

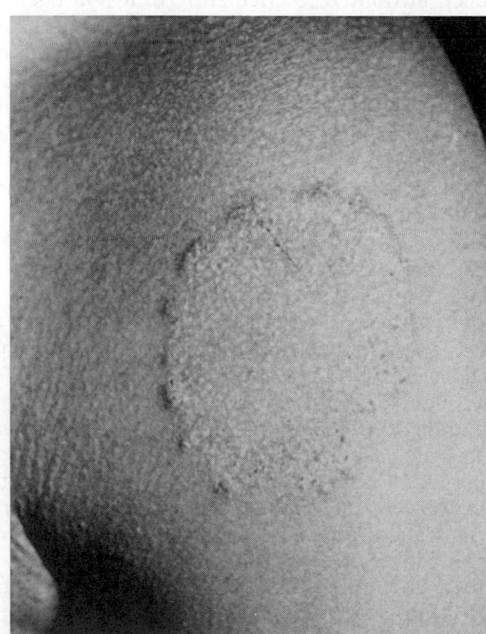

Figure 672–3 Circinate lesion of tinea corporis on the shoulder. Note the active papular border, scaling, and relative clearing centrally.

quired for several weeks. Itraconazole has produced excellent results in many cases with a 1–2-wk course of oral therapy.

Tinea cruris, infection of the groin, occurs most often in adolescent males and is usually caused by the anthropophilic species, *Epidermophyton floccosum* or *Trichophyton rubrum,* but occasionally by the zoophilic species *T. mentagrophytes.*

The initial *clinical lesion* is a small, raised, scaly, erythematous patch on the inner aspect of the thigh; this spreads peripherally, often developing numerous tiny vesicles at the advancing margin. It eventually forms bilateral, irregular, sharply bordered patches with hyperpigmented, scaly centers. In some cases, particularly in infections with *T. mentagrophytes,* the inflammatory reaction is more intense and the infection may spread beyond the crural region. The penis is usually not involved in the infection, an important distinction from candidosis. Pruritus may be severe initially but abates as the inflammatory reaction subsides. Bacterial superinfection may alter the clinical appearance, and erythrasma or candidosis may coexist. Tinea cruris is more prevalent in obese persons and in those who perspire excessively and wear tight-fitting clothing.

The *diagnosis* is confirmed by culture and by demonstrating septate hyphae on a KOH preparation of epidermal scrapings. Tinea cruris must be differentiated from intertrigo, allergic contact dermatitis, candidosis, and erythrasma. Bacterial superinfection must be precluded when there is a severe inflammatory reaction.

Patients should be advised to wear loose cotton underwear. Topical *treatment* with an imidazole is recommended for severe infection, especially because these agents are effective in mixed candidal-dermatophytic infections. Pure dermatophytic infection may also be treated with tolnaftate.

Tinea pedis (athlete's foot), infection of the toe webs and soles of the feet, is uncommon in young children but occurs with some frequency in preadolescent and adolescent males. The usual etiologic agents are *T. rubrum, T. mentagrophytes,* and *E. floccosum.*

Most commonly, the lateral toe webs (third to fourth and fourth to fifth interdigital spaces) and the subdigital crevice are fissured, with maceration and peeling of the surrounding skin. Severe tenderness, itching, and a persistent foul odor are characteristic. These lesions may become chronic. This type of infection may involve overgrowth by bacterial flora, including *Micrococcus sedantarius, Brevibacterium epidermidis,* and gram-negative organisms. Less commonly, a chronic diffuse hyperkeratosis of the sole of the foot occurs with only mild erythema. In many cases, two feet and one hand are involved. This type of infection is more refractory to treatment and tends to recur. An inflammatory vesicular type of reaction may occur with *T. mentagrophytes* infection; this type is most common in young children. These lesions involve any area of the foot, including the dorsal surface, and are usually circumscribed. The initial papules progress to vesicles and bullas that may become pustular (Fig. 672–4). A number of factors, such as occlusive footwear and warm, humid weather, predispose to infection. Tinea pedis may be transmitted in shower facilities and swimming pool areas.

Tinea pedis must be differentiated from simple maceration and peeling of the interdigital spaces, which is common in children. Infection with *Candida albicans* and various bacterial organisms (erythrasma) may cause confusion or may coexist with primary tinea pedis. Contact dermatitis, dyshidrotic eczema, atopic dermatitis, and juvenile plantar dermatitis also simulate tinea pedis. Fungal mycelia can be seen on microscopic examination of a KOH preparation or by culture; the fourth toe web provides a high yield of infected scales; a blister top can also be used.

Treatment for mild infections includes simple measures such as avoidance of occlusive footwear, careful drying between the toes after bathing, and the use of an absorbent antifungal powder such as zinc undecylenate. Topical therapy with an azole, such as clotrimazole, miconazole, ketoconazole, or econazole is curative in most cases; each of these agents is also effective against candidal infection. Tolnaftate can be used in uncomplicated dermatophyte infections. Several weeks of therapy may be necessary, and low-grade, chronic infections, particularly those caused by *T. rubrum,* may be refractory. In such patients, oral griseofulvin therapy may effect a cure, but recurrences are common.

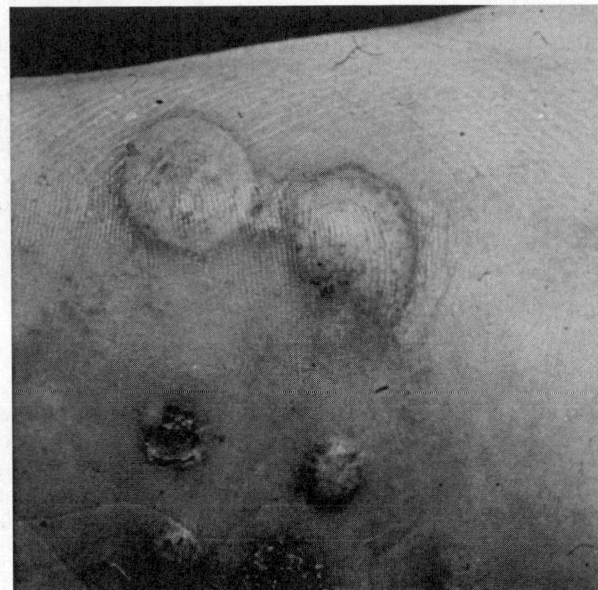

Figure 672–4 Multiple inflammatory bullae of tinea pedis.

Tinea unguium is a dermatophyte infection of the nail plate; it occurs most often in patients with tinea pedis, but it may occur as a primary infection. It can be caused by a number of dermatophytes, of which *T. rubrum* and *T. mentagrophytes* are the most common.

The most superficial form of tinea unguium (i.e., white superficial onychomycosis) is due to *T. mentagrophytes;* it is manifested by irregular single or numerous white patches on the surface of the nail unassociated with paronychial inflammation or deep infection. *T. rubrum* generally causes a more invasive, subungual infection that is initiated at the lateral distal margins of the nail and is often preceded by mild paronychia. The middle and ventral layers of the nail plate, and perhaps the naid bed, are the sites of infection. The nail initially develops a yellowish discoloration and slowly becomes thickened, brittle, and loosened from the nail bed. In advanced infection, the nail may turn dark brown to black and may crack or break off.

Tinea unguium must be differentiated from various dystrophic nail disorders. Changes due to trauma, psoriasis, lichen planus, and eczema all can be confused with tinea unguium. Nails infected with *C. albicans* have several distinguishing features, most prominently pronounced paronychial swelling. Thin shavings taken from the infected nail, preferably from the deeper areas, should be examined microscopically with KOH and cultured. Repeated attempts may be required to demonstrate the fungus.

The long half-life of itraconazole in the nail has led to promising trials of intermittent short courses of therapy (e.g., double the normal dose for 1 wk of each month for 3–4 mo). Oral terbinafine also shows promise for the treatment of onychomycosis. Griseofulvin and application of topical fungistatic agents to the nail bed often are ineffective and are not recommended.

Tinea nigra palmaris is a rare but distinctive superficial fungal infection that occurs principally in children and adolescents. It is caused by the dimorphic fungus *Exophiala werneckii*, which imparts a gray-black color to the affected palm. The characteristic lesion is a well-defined hyperpigmented macule; scaling and erythema are rare, and the lesions are asymptomatic. Tinea nigra is often mistaken for a junctional nevus, melanoma, or staining of the skin by contactants. Treatment with Whitfield's ointment, undecylenic acid ointment, miconazole, or tincture of iodine is most successful.

CANDIDAL INFECTIONS

(Candidosis, Candidiasis, and Moniliasis) (see Chapter 230)

The dimorphic yeasts of the genus *Candida* are ubiquitous in the environment, but *C. albicans* is the one that usually causes candidosis in children. This yeast is not part of the indigenous skin flora, but it is a frequent transient on skin and may colonize the human alimentary tract and the vagina as a saprophytic organism. Certain environmental conditions, notably elevated temperature and humidity, are associated with an increased frequency of isolation of *C. albicans* from the skin. Many bacterial species inhibit the growth of *C. albicans*, and alteration of normal flora by the use of antibiotics may promote overgrowth of the yeast.

ORAL CANDIDOSIS (THRUSH). See Chapter 230.

VAGINAL CANDIDOSIS (see Chapters 230 and 557). *C. albicans* is an inhabitant of the vagina in 5–10% of women, and vaginal candidosis is not uncommon in adolescent girls. A number of factors can predispose to this infection, including antibiotic therapy, corticosteroid therapy, diabetes mellitus, pregnancy, and the use of oral contraceptives. The infection is manifested by cheesy white plaques on an erythematous vaginal mucosa and by a thick white-yellow discharge. The disease may be relatively mild or may produce pronounced inflammation and scaling of the external genitals and surrounding skin with progression to vesiculation and ulceration. Patients often complain of severe itching and burning in the vaginal area. Before treatment is initiated, the diagnosis should be confirmed by microscopic examination and/or culture. The infection may be eradicated by insertion of nystatin or imidazole vaginal tablets, suppositories, creams, or foam. If these products are ineffective, the addition of oral nystatin tablets, 1–2 tablets tid for 14 days, may eliminate or decrease the candidal population in the gastrointestinal tract.

CONGENITAL CUTANEOUS CANDIDOSIS. See Chapter 230.

CANDIDAL DIAPER DERMATITIS. This is a ubiquitous problem in infants and, although relatively benign, is often frustrating because of its tendency to recur. Predisposed infants usually carry *C. albicans* in their intestinal tract, and the warm, moist, occluded skin of the diaper area provides an optimal environment for its growth. A seborrheic, atopic, or primary irritant contact dermatitis usually provides a portal of entry for the yeast.

The primary *clinical manifestation* consists of an intensely erythematous, confluent plaque with a scalloped border and a sharply demarcated edge. It is formed by the confluence of numerous papules and vesiculopustules; satellite pustules, those that stud the contiguous skin, are a hallmark of localized candidal infections. The perianal skin, inguinal folds, perineum, and lower abdomen are usually involved (Fig. 672–5). In males, the entire scrotum and penis may be involved with an erosive balanitis of the perimeatal skin; in females, the lesions may be found on the vaginal mucosa and labia. In some infants, the process is generalized, with erythematous lesions distant from the diaper area; in some cases, the generalized process may represent a fungal id (hypersensitivity) reaction.

The *differential diagnosis* includes other eruptions of the diaper area that may coexist with candidal infection. For this reason, it is important to establish a diagnosis by a KOH preparation or culture.

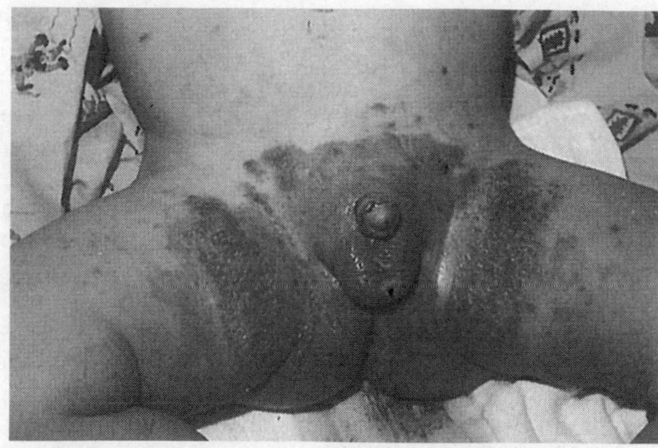

Figure 672–5 Erythematous confluent plaque with satellite pustules caused by candidal infection. See also color section.

Treatment consists of applications of an anticandidal agent (nystatin, miconazole, clotrimazole, ketoconazole) with each diaper change or four times daily. Ointments are better tolerated than creams; lotions and creams may cause a burning sensation when applied to irritated skin, and powder may cake and cause erosion due to friction during movement. The combination of a corticosteroid and an antifungal agent is justified if inflammation is severe but may confuse the situation if the diagnosis is not firmly established. Corticosteroid should not be continued for more than a few days. Protection of the diaper area by an application of thick zinc oxide paste overlying the anticandidal preparation may be helpful; the paste is more easily removed with mineral oil than with soap and water. *Fungal id reactions* gradually abate with successful treatment of the diaper dermatitis or may be treated with a mild corticosteroid preparation. When recurrences of diaper candidosis are frequent, it may be helpful to prescribe a course of oral anticandidal therapy to decrease the yeast population in the gastrointestinal tract. Some infants seem to be receptive hosts for *C. albicans* and may reacquire the organism from a colonized adult.

INTERTRIGINOUS CANDIDOSIS. This occurs most often in the axillas and groin, under the breasts, under pendulous abdominal fat folds, in the umbilicus, and in the gluteal cleft. Typical lesions are large, confluent areas of moist, denuded, erythematous skin with an irregular, macerated, scaly border. Satellite lesions are characteristic and consist of small vesicles or pustules on an erythematous base. With time, intertriginous candidal lesions may become lichenified, dry, scaly plaques. The lesions develop on skin subjected to irritation and maceration. Candidal superinfection is more likely to occur under conditions that lead to excessive perspiration, especially in obese children and in those with underlying disorders, such as diabetes mellitus. A similar condition, *interdigital candidosis*, commonly occurs in individuals whose hands are constantly immersed in water; fissures occur between the fingers and have red, denuded centers, with an overhanging white epithelial fringe. Similar lesions between the toes may be secondary to occlusive footwear. Treatment is the same as for other candidal infections.

PERIANAL CANDIDOSIS. Perianal dermatitis develops at sites of skin irritation as a result of occlusion, constant moisture, poor hygiene, anal fissures, and pruritus due to pinworm infestation. It may become superinfected with *C. albicans*, especially in children who are receiving oral antibiotic or corticosteroid medication. The involved skin becomes erythematous, macerated, and excoriated, and the lesions are identical to those of candidal intertrigo or candidal diaper rash. Application of a topical antifungal agent in conjunction with improved hygiene is usually effective. Underlying disorders such as pinworm infection must also be treated (see Chapter 284).

CANDIDAL PARONYCHIA AND ONYCHIA. See Chapter 669.

CANDIDAL GRANULOMA. This is a rare response to an invasive candidal infection of skin. The lesions appear as crusted, verrucous plaques and hornlike projections on the scalp, face, and distal limbs. Affected patients may have single or numerous defects in immune mechanisms and are often refractory to topical therapy. A systemic anticandidal agent may be required for palliation or eradication of the infection.

Abdel-Rahman SM, Powell DA, Nahata MC: Efficacy of itraconazole in children with *Trichophyton tonsurans* tinea capitis. J Am Acad Dermatol 38:443, 1998.
Allen H, Honig P, Leyden J, et al: Selenium sulfide: Adjunctive therapy for tinea capitis. Pediatrics 69:81, 1982.
Baley J, Silverman R: Systemic candidiasis: Cutaneous manifestations in low birth weight infants. Pediatrics 82:211, 1988.
DeCastro P, Jorizzo JL: Cutaneous aspects of candidosis. Semin Dermatol 4:165, 1985.
DeVroey C: Epidemiology of ringworm (dermatophytosis). Semin Dermatol 4:185, 1985.
Elewski B: Tinea capitis: Itraconazole in *Trichophyton tonsurans* infection. J Am Acad Dermatol 31:65, 1994.
Faergemann J: Pityrosporum infections. J Am Acad Dermatol 31:S18, 1994.
Frieden IJ, Howard R: Tinea capitis: Epidemiology, diagnosis, treatment, and control. J Am Acad Dermatol 31:S42, 1994.
Greer D: Treatment of symptom-free carriers in the management of tinea capitis. Lancet 348:350, 1996.
Gupta AK, Adam P: Terbinafine pulse therapy is effective in tinea capitis. Pediatr Dermatol 15:56, 1998.
Hubbard TW, de Triquet JM: Brush-culture method for diagnosing tinea capitis. Pediatrics 90:416, 1992.
Jacobs AH, O'Connell BM: Tinea in tiny tots. Am J Dis Child 140:1034, 1986.
Odom R: Pathophysiology of dermatophyte infections. J Am Acad Dermatol 5:S2, 1993.
Philpot CM, Shuttleworth D: Dermatophyte onychomycosis in children. Clin Exp Dermatol 14:203, 1989.
Rezabek GH, Friedman AD: Superficial fungal infections of the skin. Diagnosis and current treatment recommendations. Drugs 43:674, 1992.
Rosenthal JR: Pediatric fungal infections from head to toe: What's new? Curr Opin Pediatr 6:435, 1994.
Suarez S, Fallon-Friedlander S: Antifungal therapy in children: An update. Pediatr Ann 27:177, 1998.
Zienicke HC, Korting HC, Lukacs K, et al: Dermatophytosis in children and adolescents: Epidemiological, clinical, and microbiological aspects changing with age. J Dermatol 18:438, 1991.

CHAPTER 673
Cutaneous Viral Infections

WART
(Verruca)

Human papillomaviruses (HPV) cause a spectrum of disease from warts to squamous cell carcinoma of the skin and mucous membranes, including the larynx (see Chapter 257). The incidence of all types of warts is highest in children and adolescents. HPV is spread by direct contact and autoinoculation, but transmission by fomites can occur. The clinical manifestations of infection develop 1 mo or longer after inoculation and depend on the HPV type, of which more than 70 are recognized; the size of the inoculum; the immune status of the host; and the anatomic site.

CLINICAL MANIFESTATIONS. Cutaneous warts develop in 5–10% of children. *Common warts (verruca vulgaris),* caused most commonly by HPV types 2 and 4, occur most frequently on the fingers, dorsum of the hands, paronychial areas, face, knees, and elbows. They are well-circumscribed papules with a roughened, keratotic, irregular surface. When the surface is pared away, many black dots representing thrombosed dermal capillary loops are often visible. Periungual warts are often painful and may spread beneath the nail plate, separating it from the nail bed. *Plantar warts,* although similar to the common wart, are caused by HPV type 1 and are usually flush with the surface of the sole because of the constant pressure from weight bearing; they may be painful. Similar lesions (palmar) can also occur on the palms. They are sharply demarcated, often with a ring of thick callus. The surface keratotic material must sometimes be removed before the boundaries of the wart can be appreciated. Several contiguous warts (HPV type 4) may fuse to form a large plaque, the so-called *mosaic wart. Flat warts (verruca plana),* caused by HPV types 2, 3, and 10, are slightly elevated, minimally hyperkeratotic papules that usually remain less than 3 mm in diameter and vary in color from pink to brown. They may occur in profusion on the face, arms, dorsum of the hands, and knees. The distribution of several lesions along a line of cutaneous trauma is a helpful diagnostic feature. Lesions may be disseminated in the beard area by shaving and from the hairline onto the scalp by combing the hair. *Epidermodysplasia verruciformis,* caused primarily by HPV types 5 and 8, presents with many diffuse verrucous papules. Approximately 25% of cases are familial, occurring by autosomal recessive or X-linked inheritance, and 3–10% of patients have HPV-associated squamous cell carcinoma on sun-exposed skin.

Genital HPV infection occurs in nearly 40% of sexually active adolescents, most commonly as a result of infection with HPV types 6 and 11. *Condylomata acuminata (mucous membrane warts)* are moist, fleshy, papillomatous lesions that occur on the perianal mucosa (Fig. 673–1), labia, vaginal introitus, and perineal raphe and on the shaft, corona, and glans penis. Occasionally they obstruct the urethral meatus or the vaginal introitus. Because they are located in intertriginous areas, they may become moist and friable. When untreated, condylomata proliferate and become confluent, at times forming large cauliflower-like masses. Lesions can also occur on the lips, gingivae, tongue, and conjunctivae. Genital warts in children may occur after inoculation during birth through an infected birth canal; as a consequence of sexual abuse; or from incidental spread from cutaneous warts. A significant proportion of genital warts in children contain HPV types that are usually isolated from cutaneous warts. HPV infection of the cervix is a major risk factor for development of carcinoma, particularly if the infection is due to HPV types 16, 18, 31–33, 35, 39, 42, or 51–54. *Laryngeal (respiratory) papillomas* contain the same HPV types as in anogenital papillomas. Transmission is believed to occur from mothers with genital HPV infection to neonates who aspirate infectious virus during birth.

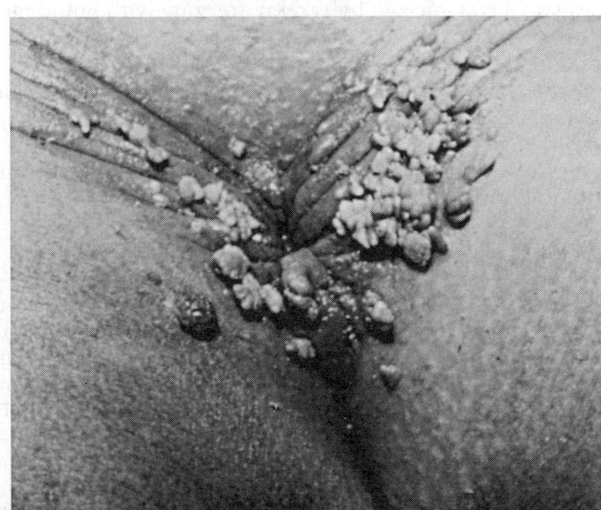

Figure 673–1 Condylomata acuminata in the perianal area of a toddler.

PATHOLOGY. The various types of warts differ in minor ways but share the basic changes of hyperplasia of the epidermal cells and vacuolation of the spinous keratinocytes, which may contain basophilic intranuclear inclusions (viral particles). Warts are confined to the epidermis and, contrary to the common misconception, do not have "roots." Parakeratosis, papillomatosis, and eosinophilic cytoplasmic inclusions, thought to represent altered keratohyalin, are additional variable histologic changes. Individuals with impaired cell-mediated immunity are particularly susceptible to HPV infection. Antibodies occur in response to infection but appear to have little protective effect.

DIFFERENTIAL DIAGNOSIS. Common warts are most often confused with molluscum contagiosum. Plantar and palmar warts may be difficult to distinguish from punctate keratoses, corns, and calluses. In contrast to calluses, warts obliterate normal skin markings. Juvenile flat warts mimic lichen planus, lichen nitidus, angiofibromas, syringomas, milia, and acne. Condylomata acuminata may resemble condylomata lata of secondary syphilis.

TREATMENT. Various therapeutic measures are effective in the treatment of warts. More than 50% of warts disappear spontaneously within 2 yr, but failure to treat incurs the risk of spread to other sites. Warts are epidermal lesions and do not produce scarring unless they are managed surgically or treated in an overly aggressive fashion. Hyperkeratotic lesions (common, plantar, and palmar warts) are more responsive to therapy if the excess keratotic debris is gently pared with a scalpel until thrombosed capillaries are apparent; further paring induces bleeding. Treatment is most successful when done regularly and frequently (e.g., every 2 wk).

Common warts can be destroyed by applications of liquid nitrogen or cantharidin or by light electrodesiccation and curettage. Daily applications of 10–17% lactic acid and 10–17% salicylic acid in flexible collodion is a slow but painless method of removal that is effective in some patients. Recalcitrant warts may respond to 5% 5-*fluorouracil ointment* rubbed into lesions daily. Care must be taken to avoid contact with adjacent normal skin, which may cause undue irritation, erosion, or postinflammatory hyperpigmentation. Plantar and palmar warts may be treated with salicylic and lactic acids in collodion or 40% salicylic acid or urea plasters. After prolonged soaking in lukewarm water, keratotic debris can be removed by an emery board or pumice stone. Occlusive taping for several days may also be effective. Condylomata respond best to weekly applications of 25% podophyllin in tincture of benzoin; the medication should be left on the warts for 4–6 hr and then removed by bathing. Condylomata localized to keratinized sites (e.g., buttocks) may not respond to podophyllin. Resistant lesions can usually be eradicated by weekly freezing with liquid nitrogen or by treatment with a carbon dioxide laser. Although intralesional injection of 1 million units of interferon-α or -β three times weekly for 3–4 wk appears to be effective against condylomata, this is not recommended because of a low incidence of effectiveness, high toxicity rate, and high cost. With all types of therapy, care should be taken to protect the surrounding normal skin from irritation.

MOLLUSCUM CONTAGIOSUM

The poxvirus that causes molluscum contagiosum is a large double-stranded DNA virus that replicates in the cytoplasm of host epithelial cells. The three types cannot be differentiated on the basis of clinical appearance, location of lesions, or a patient's age or sex. Type 1 virus causes most infections. The disease is acquired by direct contact with an infected person or from fomites and is spread by autoinoculation. School-aged children who are otherwise well and individuals who are immunosuppressed are affected most commonly. The incubation period is estimated to be 2 wk or longer.

CLINICAL MANIFESTATIONS. Discrete, pearly, skin-colored, dome-shaped, smooth papules vary in size from 1–5 mm. They typically have a central umbilication from which a plug of cheesy material can be expressed (Fig. 673–2). The papules may occur anywhere on the body, but the face, eyelids, neck, axillas, and thighs are sites of predilection. They may be found in clusters on the genitals or in the groin of adolescents and may be associated with other venereal diseases in sexually active individuals. Lesions commonly involve the genital area in children but in most cases are not acquired by sexual transmission; a search should be undertaken, however, for other signs of sexual abuse. Lesions on the eyelid margin can produce unilateral conjunctivitis; rarely, lesions may appear on the conjunctiva or cornea. Mild surrounding erythema or an eczematous dermatitis may accompany the papules. Lesions on patients with AIDS tend to be large and numerous, particularly on the face; exuberant lesions may also be found in children with leukemia and other immunodeficiencies. Children with atopic dermatitis are susceptible to widespread involvement in areas of dermatitis.

DIFFERENTIAL DIAGNOSIS. This includes trichoepithelioma, basal cell carcinoma, ectopic sebaceous glands, syringoma, hidrocystoma, keratoacanthoma, and warty dyskeratoma. In individuals with AIDS, cryptococcosis may be indistinguishable clinically from molluscum contagiosum; rarely, coccidioidomycosis, histoplasmosis, or *Penicillium marneffei* infection masquerades with molluscum-like lesions in an immunocompromised host.

PATHOLOGY AND DIAGNOSIS. The epidermis is hyperplastic and hypertrophied, extending into the underlying dermis and projecting above the skin surface. The molluscum papule consists of a lobulated adhesive mass of virus-infected epidermal cells. Eosinophilic viral inclusion bodies (Henderson-Patterson or molluscum bodies) become more prominent as the cells move upward from the basal layer to the stratum corneum. The central plug of material, which is composed of virus-laden cells, may be shelled out from a lesion (see Treatment) and examined under the microscope with 10% potassium hydroxide or Wright or Giemsa stain. The rounded, cup-shaped mass of homogeneous cells, often with identifiable lobules, is diagnostic. Specific antibody against molluscum contagiosum virus is detectable in most infected individuals but is of uncertain immunologic significance. Cell-mediated immunity is thought to be important in host defense.

TREATMENT. Molluscum contagiosum is a self-limited disease;

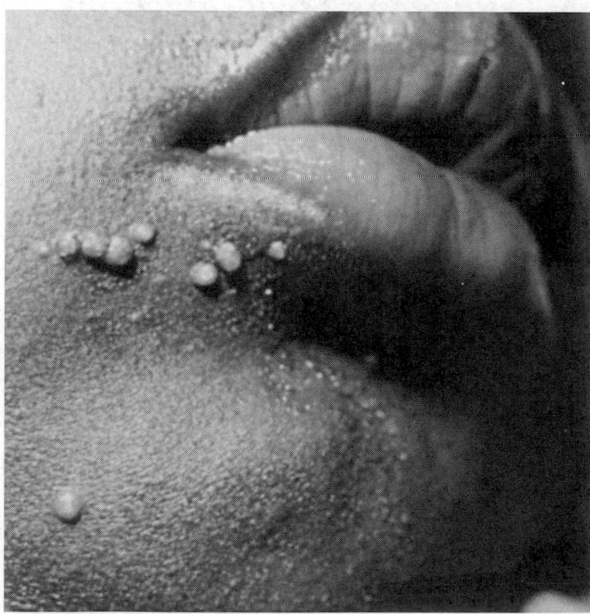

Figure 673–2 Grouped papules of molluscum contagiosum on the face.

the average attack lasts 6–9 mo. However, lesions can persist for years, can spread to distant sites, and may be transmitted to others. Affected patients should be advised to avoid shared baths and towels until the infection is clear. Infection may spread rapidly and produce hundreds of lesions in children with atopic dermatitis or immunodeficiency. A brief 6–9-sec application of liquid nitrogen is very effective and, in most instances, is the treatment of choice. The papules can also be destroyed by expressing the plug with a needle, a sharp curette, or a comedo extractor. Cantharidin 0.9% may be applied to each lesion without occlusion and frequently causes enough inflammation to facilitate spontaneous extrusion of the plug. Treatment of a few lesions is occasionally followed by resolution of the others. Sometimes, however, treatment with cantharidin results in formation of a rosette of new lesions encircling the site of treatment. Molluscum is an epidermal disease and should not be overtreated so that scarring results. A lesion-free period of 4 mo can be regarded as a cure.

Beutner KR: Cutaneous viral infections. Pediatr Ann 22:247, 1993.
Epstein WL: Molluscum contagiosum. Semin Dermatol 11:184, 1992.
Majewski S, Jablonska S: Human papillomavirus–associated tumors of the skin and mucosa. J Am Acad Dermatol 36:659, 1997.
Pauly CR, Artis WM, Jones HE: Atopic dermatitis, impaired cellular immunity, and molluscum contagiosum. Arch Dermatol 114:391, 1978.
Porter CD, Blake NW, Cream JJ, et al: Molluscum contagiosum virus. Mol Cell Biol Hum Dis Ser 1:233, 1992.
Rock B, Naghashfar Z, Barnett N, et al: Genital tract papillomavirus infections in children. Arch Dermatol 122:1129, 1986.
Schachner L, Hankin DE: Assessing child abuse in childhood condyloma acuminatum. J Am Acad Dermatol 12:157, 1985.

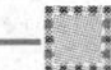

CHAPTER 674
Arthropod Bites and Infestations

ARTHROPOD BITES

Arthropod bites are a common affliction of children and occasionally pose a problem in diagnosis. A patient may be unaware of the source of the lesions or deny being bitten, making interpretation of the eruption difficult. In these cases, knowledge of the habits, life cycle, and clinical signs of the more common arthropod pests of humans may help lead to a correct diagnosis. The principal classes of arthropods that cause skin injury to humans are listed in Table 674–1. Some of the important dermatoses caused by arthropod bites and infestations are covered in this chapter; others are discussed in chapters addressing infectious organisms (see Part XVI).

CLINICAL MANIFESTATIONS. The type of reaction that occurs after an arthropod bite depends on the species of insect and the age group and reactivity of the human host. Arthropods may cause injury to a host by various mechanisms, including mechanical trauma, such as the lacerating bite of a tsetse fly; invasion of host tissues, as in myiasis; contact dermatitis, as seen with repeated exposure to cockroach antigens; granulomatous reaction to retained mouth parts; transmission of systemic disease; injection of irritant cytotoxic or pharmacologically active substances, such as hyaluronidase, proteases, peptidases, and phospholipases in sting venom; and induction of anaphylaxis. Most reactions to arthropod bites, however, depend on antibody formation to antigenic substances in saliva or venom. The type of reaction is determined primarily by the degree of previous exposure to the same or a related species of arthropod. When someone is bitten for the first time, no reaction develops. An immediate petechial reaction is occasionally seen, however, in newborn babies after a mosquito bite. After repeated bites, sensitivity develops, producing a pruritic papule approximately 24 hr after the bite; this is the most common reaction seen in young children. With prolonged, repeated exposure, a wheal develops within minutes after a bite, followed 24 hr later by papule formation; this combination of reactions is seen commonly in older children. By adolescence or adulthood, only a wheal may form, unaccompanied by the delayed papular reaction. Thus, adults may be unaffected in the same household as affected children. Ultimately, as a person becomes insensitive to the bite, no reaction occurs at all. This stage of nonreactivity is maintained only as long as the individual continues to be bitten regularly. Individuals in whom papular urticaria develops are in the transitional phase between development of primarily a delayed papular reaction and development of an immediate urticarial reaction.

Arthropod bites may occur as solitary, numerous, or profuse lesions, depending on the feeding habits of the perpetrator. For example, fleas tend to sample their host several times within a small localized area, whereas mosquitoes tend to attack a host at more randomly scattered sites. *Delayed hypersensitivity reactions* to insect bites, the predominant lesions in the young and uninitiated, are characterized by firm, persistent papules that may become hyperpigmented and are often excoriated and crusted. Pruritus may be mild or severe, transient or persistent. A central punctum is usually visible but may disappear as the lesion ages or is scratched. The *immediate hypersensitivity reaction* is characterized by an erythematous, evanescent wheal. If edema is marked, the wheal may be surmounted by a tiny vesicle. Certain beetles produce bullous lesions through the action of cantharidin, and hemorrhagic nodules and ulcers may be caused by various insects, including beetles and spiders. Bites on the lower extremities are more likely to be severe or persistent or become bullous than those located elsewhere. Complications of arthropod bites include development of impetigo, folliculitis, cellulitis, lymphangitis, and severe anaphylactic hypersensitivity reactions, particularly after the bite of certain Hymenoptera. The histopathologic changes are variable, depending on the arthropod, the age of the lesion, and the reactivity of the host. Acute urticarial lesions tend to show central vesiculation in which eosinophils are numerous. Papules most commonly show dermal edema and a mixed, superficial and deep perivascular inflammatory infiltrate, often including a number of eosinophils. At times, however, the dermal cellular infiltrate is so dense that a lymphoma is suspected. Retained mouth parts may stimulate a foreign body type of granulomatous reaction.

Papular urticaria occurs principally in the 1st decade of life, during the warmer months of the year. The most common culprits are species of fleas, mites, bedbugs, gnats, mosquitoes, chiggers, and animal lice. Individuals with papular urticaria have predominantly transitional lesions in various stages of evolution between delayed-onset papules and immediate-onset wheals. The most characteristic lesion is an edematous red-brown papule; an individual lesion frequently starts as a wheal that in turn is replaced by a papule. A given bite may incite an id reaction at distant sites of quiescent bites in the form of erythematous macules, papules, or urticarial plaques. The

TABLE 674–1 Arthropods That Cause Human Skin Disease

- Class Arachnida (four pairs of legs): mites, spiders, ticks
- Class Chilopoda: centipedes
- Class Diplopoda: millipedes
- Class Insecta (three pairs of legs):
  - Order Diptera: mosquitoes, flies
  - Order Siphonaptera: fleas
  - Order Hymenoptera: ants, bees, wasps
  - Order Anoplura: lice
  - Order Hemiptera: bedbugs, kissing bugs
  - Order Coleoptera: beetles
  - Order Lepidoptera: butterflies, moths

disorder is characterized by a temporary arrest at a transitional phase; after a season or two, however, the reaction progresses from a transitional to a primarily immediate hypersensitivity urticarial reaction.

One of the most commonly encountered arthropod bites is that due to human, cat, or dog *fleas* (family Pulicidae). Eggs, which are generally laid in dusty areas and cracks between floorboards, give rise to larvae that then form cocoons. The cocoon stage can persist for up to 1 yr, and the animal emerges in response to vibrations from footsteps, accounting for the assaults that frequently befall the new owners of a recently reopened dwelling. Adult dog fleas can live without a blood meal for approximately 60 days. Attacks from fleas are more likely to occur when the fleas do not have access to their usual host; for example, cat or dog fleas are more voracious and problematic when one visits an area frequented by the pet than when the pet is encountered directly. Flea bites tend to be grouped in lines or irregular clusters. Fleas are often not seen on the body of a pet; diagnosis of flea bites, however, is aided by examination of debris from the animal's bedding material. The debris is collected by shaking the bedding into a plastic bag and examining the contents for fleas or their eggs, larvae, or feces.

TREATMENT. This is directed at alleviation of pruritus by oral antihistamines, cool compresses, and soothing lotions such as calamine, to which 0.25% menthol and 0.5% phenol can be added. Topical corticosteroid creams are rarely effective, and topical antihistamines are potent sensitizers and have no role in the treatment of insect bite reactions. A short course of systemic steroids may be helpful if many severe reactions occur, particularly around the eyes. Insect repellents containing diethyltoluamide (DEET) may afford moderate protection against mosquitoes, fleas, flies, chiggers, and ticks but are relatively ineffective against wasps, bees, and hornets. DEET must be applied to exposed skin and clothing to be effective. The most effective protection against mosquitoes, the human body louse, and other blood-feeding arthropods is use of DEET and permethrin-impregnated clothing; these measures are not effective, however, against the phlebotomine sandfly, which transmits leishmaniasis. Advocates of treatment with B-complex vitamins or thiamine hydrochloride maintain that these agents impart an offensive odor to sweat, warding off mosquitoes; this claim has not been substantiated by clinical trials.

An effort should be made to identify and eradicate the etiologic agent. Pets should be carefully inspected; crawl spaces, eaves, and other sites of the house or outbuildings frequented by animals and birds should be decontaminated; and baseboard crevices, mattresses, rugs, furniture, and animal sleeping quarters should be decontaminated. Agents that are effective for ridding the home of fleas include lindane, pyrethroids, and organic thiocyanates. Flea-infested pets may be treated with powders containing rotenone, pyrethroids, malathion, or methoxychlor.

INFESTATIONS

SCABIES. Scabies is caused by burrowing and release of toxic or antigenic substances by the female mite *Sarcoptes scabiei* var. *hominis*. The most important factor that determines spread of scabies is the extent and duration of physical contact with an affected individual; the children and sexual partner of an affected individual are most at risk. Scabies is transmitted only rarely by fomites because the isolated mite dies within 2–3 days.

Clinical Manifestations. In an immunocompetent host, scabies is frequently heralded by intense pruritus, particularly at night. The first sign of the infestation often consists of 1–2-mm red papules, some of which are excoriated, crusted, or scaling. Threadlike burrows are the classic lesion of scabies but may not be seen in infants. In infants, bullae and pustules are relatively common; the eruption may also include wheals, papules, vesicles, and a superimposed eczematous dermatitis; and the palms, soles (Fig. 674–1*B*), face, and scalp are often affected. In older children and adolescents, the clinical pattern is similar to that in adults, in whom preferred sites are the interdigital spaces, wrist flexors, anterior axillary folds, ankles, buttocks, umbilicus and belt line, groin, genitals in men, and areolas in women (Fig. 674–1*A*); the head, neck, palms and soles are generally spared. Red-brown nodules, most often located in covered areas such as the axillas, groin, and genitals, predominate in the less common variant called nodular scabies. Untreated, scabies may lead to eczematous dermatitis, impetigo, ecthyma, folliculitis, furunculosis, cellulitis, lymphangitis, and id reaction. Children have been reported to develop glomerulonephritis as a result of streptococcal impetiginization of scabies lesions. In some tropical areas, scabies is the predominant underlying cause of pyoderma. A latent period of approximately 1 mo follows an initial infestation; thus, itching may be absent and lesions may be relatively inapparent in contacts who are asymptomatic carriers. On reinfestation, however, reactions to mite antigens are noted within hours.

Etiology and Pathogenesis. An adult female mite measures approximately 0.4 mm in length, has four sets of legs, and has a hemispheric body marked by transverse corrugations, brown spines, and bristles on the dorsal surface. A male mite is approximately half her size and is similar in configuration. After impregnation on the skin surface, a gravid female exudes a keratolytic substance and burrows into the stratum corneum, often forming a shallow well within 30 min. She gradually extends this tract by 0.5–5 mm/24 hr along the boundary with the stratum granulosum. She deposits one to three oval eggs and numerous brown fecal pellets (scybala) daily. When egg laying is completed, in 4–5 wk, she dies within the burrow. The eggs hatch in 3–5 days, releasing larvae that move to the skin surface to molt into nymphs. Maturity is achieved in about 2–3 wk. Mating occurs, and the gravid female invades the skin to complete the life cycle.

Diagnosis. This can often be made clinically but is confirmed by microscopic identification of mites (Fig. 674–1*C*), ova, and scybala in epithelial debris. Scrapings are most often positive when obtained from burrows, eczematous lesions, or fresh papules. A reliable method is application of a drop of mineral oil on the selected lesion, scraping of it with a No. 15 blade, and transfer of the oil and scrapings to a glass slide.

The *differential diagnosis* depends on the types of lesions present. Burrows are virtually pathognomonic for human scabies. Papulovesicular lesions are confused with papular urticaria, canine scabies, chickenpox, viral exanthems, drug eruptions, dermatitis herpetiformis, and folliculitis. Eczematous lesions may mimic atopic dermatitis and seborrheic dermatitis, and the less common bullous disorders of childhood may be suspected in infants with predominantly bullous lesions. Nodular scabies is frequently misdiagnosed as urticaria pigmentosa and histiocytosis X. The histopathologic appearance of nodular scabies, consisting of a deep, dense, perivascular infiltrate of lymphocytes, histiocytes, plasma cells, and atypical mononuclear cells, may mimic malignant lymphoid neoplasms.

Treatment. Application of permethrin 5% cream (Elimite) or 1% lindane cream or lotion to the entire body from the neck down, with particular attention to intensely involved areas, is standard therapy. Scabies is frequently found above the neck in infants, however, also necessitating treatment of the scalp. The medication is left on the skin for 8–12 hr; if necessary, it may be reapplied in 1 wk for another 8–12-hr period. Because lindane is potentially neurotoxic, the vulnerability of small infants to percutaneous absorption dictates caution in prescribing it for them. Signs of lindane toxicity include nausea, vomiting, weakness, tremors, irritability, disorientation, seizures, and respiratory compromise. Systemic absorption and toxicity of lindane can be minimized by not applying the medication

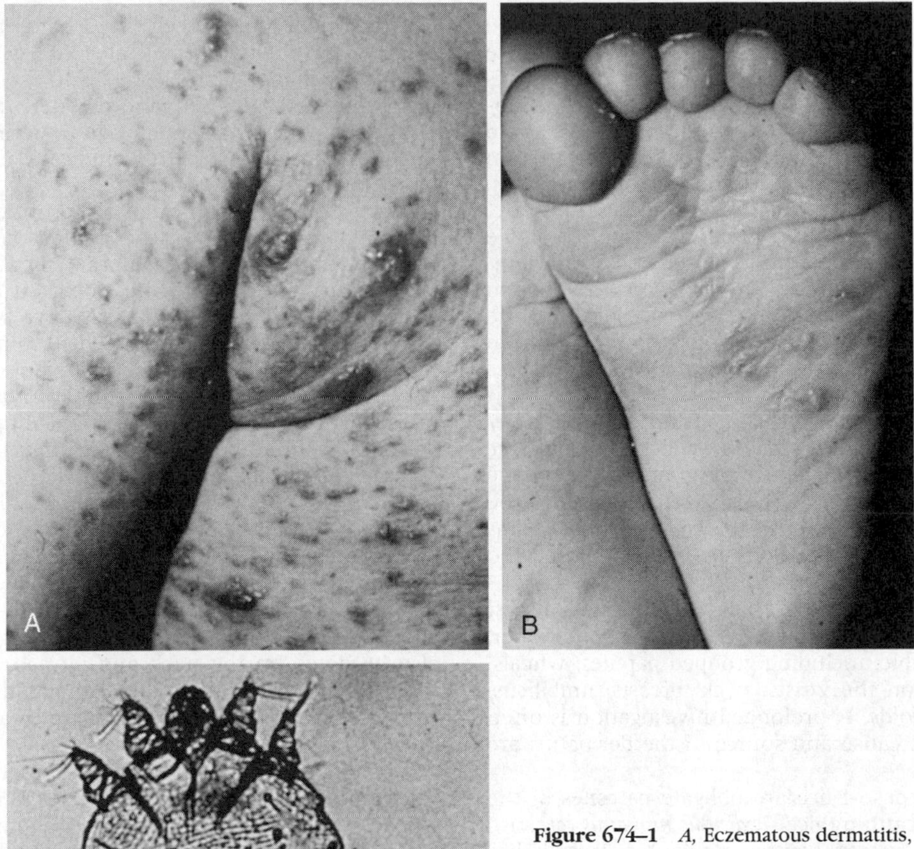

Figure 674–1 *A*, Eczematous dermatitis, papules, and nodules of human scabies. *B*, Vesiculopustular lesions of scabies on the soles of an infant. *C*, Human scabies mite obtained from scraping.

to warm, moist skin; not repeating an application within 7 days; and not using the medication on children who are underweight or malnourished or have extensive areas of inflamed, denuded, or secondarily infected skin. Permethrin 5% cream is a slightly more effective scabicide than lindane but is more expensive. It is poorly absorbed, rapidly metabolized by tissue esterases, and therefore of very low toxicity. For infants younger than 2 mo, alternative therapy includes 6% sulfur in petrolatum applied for three consecutive 24-hr periods. Topical sulfur ointment is messy, is malodorous, stains clothing, and commonly causes irritant dermatitis. No controlled studies of its efficacy and safety have been published in recent years. Permethrin 5% cream is a better alternative for infants. Crotamiton cream or lotion is not recommended because of lack of efficacy and toxicity data.

Transmission of mites is unlikely more than 24 hr after treatment. Pruritus, which is due to hypersensitivity to mite antigens, may persist for a number of days and may be alleviated by a topical corticosteroid preparation. If pruritus persists for more than 2 wk after treatment, the patient should be reexamined for mites. Nodules are extremely resistant to treatment and may take several months to resolve. The entire family should be treated, as should caretakers of the infested child. Clothing, bed linens, and towels should be thoroughly laundered.

Norwegian Scabies. This variant of human scabies is highly contagious and occurs mainly in individuals who are mentally and physically debilitated, particularly those who are institutionalized and those with Down syndrome; in patients with poor cutaneous sensation, such as those with leprosy or syringomyelia; in patients who have severe systemic illness such as leukemia or diabetes; and in immunosuppressed patients such as those with HIV infection. Affected individuals are infested by myriad mites that inhabit the crusts and exfoliating scales of the skin and scalp. The nails may become thickened and dystrophic; the subungual debris is densely populated by mites. The infestation is often accompanied by generalized lymphadenopathy and eosinophilia. On microscopic examination, one sees massive orthokeratosis and parakeratosis with numerous interspersed mites, psoriasiform epidermal hyperplasia, foci of spongiosis, and neutrophilic abscesses. Norwegian scabies is thought to represent a deficient host immune response to the organism. Management is difficult, requiring scrupulous isolation measures, removal of the thick scales, and repeated but careful applications of antiscabetic preparations. Ivermectin has been used successfully as single-dose therapy in refractory cases, particularly HIV-infected patients, although it is not approved by the Food and Drug Administration for treatment of scabies nor for any application in children younger than 5 yr.

Canine Scabies. This is caused by *S. scabiei* var. *canis*, the dog mite that is associated with mange. The eruption in humans, which is most frequently acquired by cuddling an infested puppy, consists of tiny papules, vesicles, wheals, and excoriated eczematous plaques. Burrows are not present because the mite infrequently inhabits human stratum corneum. The rash is pruritic and has a predilection for the arms, chest, and abdomen, the usual sites of contact with dogs. Onset is sudden and usually follows exposure by 1–10 days, possibly resulting from development of a hypersensitivity reaction to mite antigens. Recovery of mites or ova from scrapings of human skin is rare. The disease is self-limited because humans are not a suitable host; bathing and changing clothes are generally sufficient. Removal or treatment of the infested animal, however, is also necessary. Symptomatic therapy for itching is helpful. In rare cases in which mites are demonstrated in scrapings from an affected child, they can be eradicated by the same measures applicable to human scabies.

Other mites that occasionally bite humans include the *chigger* or harvest mite *(Eutrombicula alfreddugesi)*, which prefers to live on grass, shrubs, vines, and stems of grain. Larvae have hooked mouthparts, which allow the chigger to attach to the skin, but not to burrow, to obtain a blood meal, most commonly on the lower legs. *Avian mites* may affect those who come into close contact with chickens. Humans may occasionally be assaulted by avian mites that have infested a nest outside a window, an attic, heating vents, or an air conditioner. The dermatitis is variable, including grouped papules, wheals, and vesicular lesions on the wrists, neck, breasts, umbilicus, and anterior axillary folds. A prolonged investigation is often undertaken before the cause and source of the dermatitis are discovered.

PEDICULOSIS. Three types of lice are obligate parasites of the human host: body or clothing lice *(Pediculus humanus corporis)*, head lice *(Pediculus humanus capitis)*, and pubic or crab lice *(Phthirus pubis)*. Only the body louse serves as a vector of human disease (typhus, trench fever, relapsing fever). Body and head lice have similar physical characteristics; they are about 2–4 mm in length. Pubic lice are only 1–2 mm in length and are greater in width than length, giving them a crablike appearance. Female lice live for approximately 1 mo and deposit 3–10 eggs daily on the human host; body lice, however, generally lay eggs in or near the seams of clothing. The ova or nits are glued to hairs or fibers of clothing but not directly on the body. Ova hatch in 1–2 wk and require another week to mature; once the eggs hatch, the nits remain attached to the hair as empty sacs of chitin. Freshly hatched larvae die unless a meal is obtained within approximately 24 hr and every few days thereafter. Both nymphs and adult lice feed on human blood, injecting their salivary juices into the host and depositing their fecal matter on the skin. Symptoms of infestation do not appear immediately but develop as an individual becomes sensitized. *The hallmark of all types of pediculosis is pruritus.*

Pediculosis corporis is rare in children except under conditions of poor hygiene, especially in colder climates when the opportunity to change clothes on a regular basis is lacking. The parasite is transmitted mainly on contaminated clothing or bedding. The primary lesion is an intensely pruritic small red macule or papule with a central hemorrhagic punctum located on the shoulders, trunk, or buttocks. Additional lesions include excoriations, wheals, and eczematous, secondarily infected plaques. Massive infestation may be associated with constitutional symptoms of fever, malaise, and headache. Chronic infestation may lead to "vagabond's skin," which is manifested as lichenified, scaling, hyperpigmented plaques, most commonly on the trunk. Lice are found on the skin only transiently when they are feeding; at other times, they inhabit the seams of clothing. Nits are attached firmly to fibers in the cloth and may remain viable for up to 1 mo. Nits hatch when they encounter warmth from the host's body when the clothes are worn again. Therapy consists of improved hygiene and hot-water laundering of all infested clothing and bedding; a uniform temperature of 65°C, wet or dry, for 15–30 min kills all eggs and lice. Alternatively, eggs hatch and nymphs starve if clothing is stored for 2 wk at 75–85°F. For people who are unable to change clothes, the clothes may be dusted while inside out with 10% lindane powder; the effect lasts for approximately 1 mo. Lindane lotion or permethrin cream applied for 8–12 hr can be used to eradicate any eggs and lice that happen to be on body hair.

Pediculosis capitis is an intensely pruritic infestation of lice in the scalp hair. Head-to-head contact is the most important mode of transmission. In summer months in many areas of the United States and in the tropics at all times of the year, shared combs, brushes, or towels have a more important role in louse transmission. Translucent 0.5-mm eggs are laid near the proximal portion of the hair shaft and become adherent to one side of the hair shaft. A nit cannot be moved along or knocked off the hair shaft with the fingers. Secondary pyoderma, after trauma due to scratching, may result in matting together of the hair and cervical and occipital lymphadenopathy. Hair loss does not result from pediculosis but may accompany the secondary pyoderma. Head lice are a major cause of numerous pyodermas of the scalp, particularly in tropical environments. Lice are not always visible, but nits are detectable on the hairs, most commonly in the occipital region and above the ears, rarely on beard or pubic hair. Dermatitis may also be noted on the neck and pinnae. An id reaction, consisting of eythematous patches and plaques, may develop, particularly on the trunk. For unknown reasons, head lice infrequently infest blacks.

Brushing and combing of the hair regularly helps to reduce the number of lice and eggs and helps to minimize the severity of the infestion. The *treatment* of choice is permethrin 1% cream rinse (Nix) applied for 10 min with a repeat application in 7–10 days. Alternative treatments include natural pyrethrin shampoos (RID; A-200 pyrinate liquid, shampoo, or gel; R & C shampoo; Barc; Paratrol; Paranit; Triple X) and 1% lindane shampoo (Kwell) for 10 min with a repeat application in 7–10 days. All household members should be treated at the same time. Nits can be removed with a fine-toothed comb after a 1:1 vinegar:water rinse or, if tenacious, after application of a creme rinse containing 8% formic acid, which dissolves the chitin attaching the nits to the hair shafts. Clothing and bed linens should be laundered in very hot water or dry-cleaned; brushes and combs should be discarded or coated with a pediculicide for 15 min and then thoroughly cleaned in boiling water.

Pediculosis pubis is transmitted by skin-to-skin or sexual contact with an infested individual; the chance of acquiring the lice by one sexual exposure is approximately 95%. The infestation is usually encountered in adolescents, although small children may occasionally acquire pubic lice on the eyelashes. Patients experience moderate to severe pruritus and may develop a secondary pyoderma from scratching. Excoriations tend to be shallower and the incidence of secondary infection is lower than in pediculosis corporis. Maculae ceruleae are steel-gray spots, usually less than 1 cm in diameter, which may appear in the pubic area and on the chest, abdomen, and thighs. Oval translucent nits, which are firmly attached to the hair shafts, may be visible to the naked eye or may be readily identified by a hand lens or by microscopic examination (Fig. 674–2). Grittiness, as a result of adherent nits, may sometimes be detected when the fingers are run through infested hair. Adult lice are difficult to detect because of their lower level of activity and smaller, translucent body compared with head or body lice. Because pubic lice may occasionally wander or be transferred to other sites on fomites, terminal hair on the trunk, thighs, axillary region, beard area, and eyelashes should be examined for nits. The coexistence of other venereal diseases should be considered.

Treatment by a 10-min application of a pyrethrin preparation is usually effective. Retreatment may be required in 7–10

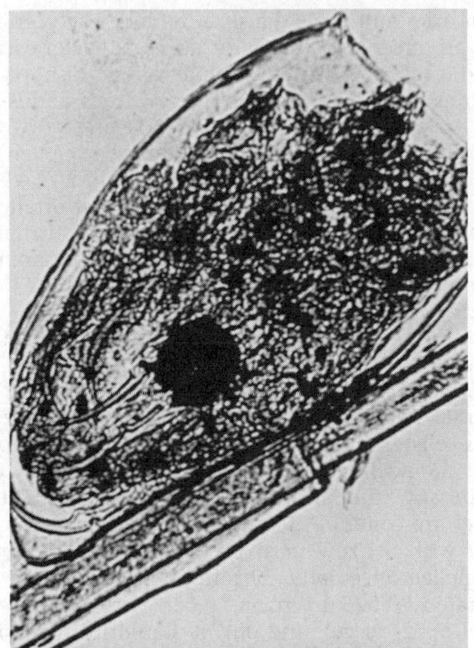

Figure 674–2 Intact nit on a human hair.

days. The shampoo form of lindane, which requires a 10-min application time, is an alternative choice, but lindane cream and lotion are no longer recommended for treatment of pubic lice. Infestation of eyelashes is eradicated by petrolatum applied three to five times/24 hr for 8–10 days. A less safe but effective alternative is 0.25% physostigmine ophthalmic ointment applied twice daily for 3 days. Clothing, towels, and bed linens may be contaminated with nit-bearing hairs and should be thoroughly laundered or dry-cleaned.

SEABATHER'S ERUPTION. Seabather's eruption is a severely pruritic dermatosis of inflammatory papules that develops within approximately 12 hr of bathing in salt water, primarily on body sites that were covered by a bathing suit. The eruption has been described primarily in waters of Florida and the Caribbean. Lesions, which may include pustules, vesicles, and urticarial plaques, are more numerous in those individuals who keep their bathing suit on for an extended period after leaving the water. The eruption may be accompanied by systemic symptoms of fatigue, malaise, fever, chills, nausea, and headache; approximately 40% of children younger than 16 yr had fever in one large series. Duration of the pruritus and skin eruption is 1–2 wk. Histopathologically, lesions consist of a superficial and deep perivascular and interstitial infiltrate of lymphocytes, eosinophils, and neutrophils. The eruption appears to be due to an allergic hypersensitivity reaction to venom from larvae of the thimble jellyfish *(Linuche unguiculata)*. Treatment is largely symptomatic; potent topical corticosteroids have been shown to provide relief to some patients.

Gurevitch AW: Scabies and lice. Pediatr Clin North Am 32:987, 1985.
Honig PJ: Arthropod bites, stings, and infestations: Their prevention and treatment. Pediatr Dermatol 3:189, 1986.
Ibarra J, Hall D: Head lice in school children. Arch Dis Child 75:471, 1996.
Meinking TL, Taplin D, Hermida JL, et al: The treatment of scabies with ivermectin. N Engl J Med 333:26, 1995.
Peterson C, Eichenfield L: Scabies. Pediatr Ann 25:97, 1996.
Taplin D, Meinking TL, Castillero PM, et al: Permethrin 1% cream rinse (Nix) for treatment of *Pediculus humanus* var *capitis* infestation. Pediatr Dermatol 3:344, 1986.
Taplin D, Meinking TL, Porcelain SL, et al: Permethrin 5% dermal cream: A new treatment for scabies. J Am Acad Dermatol 15:995, 1986.

CHAPTER 675
Acne

ACNE VULGARIS

Acne, particularly the comedonal form, occurs in approximately 80% of adolescents.

PATHOGENESIS. Lesions of acne vulgaris develop in sebaceous follicles, which consist of a large, multilobular sebaceous gland that drains its products into the follicular canal. The initial lesion of acne is a *comedo*, which is a dilated epithelium-lined follicular sac filled with lamellated keratinous material, lipid, and bacteria. An open comedo, known as a blackhead, has a patulous pilosebaceous orifice that permits visualization of the plug. An open comedo less commonly becomes inflammatory than a closed comedo or whitehead, which has only a pinpoint opening. An inflammatory papule or nodule develops from a comedo that has ruptured and extruded its follicular contents into the subadjacent dermis, inducing a neutrophilic inflammatory response. If the inflammatory reaction is close to the surface, a papule or pustule develops; if the inflammatory infiltrate develops deeper in the dermis, a nodule forms. Suppuration and an occasional giant cell reaction to the keratin and hair are the cause of nodulocystic lesions; these are not true cysts but liquefied masses of inflammatory debris.

The primary pathogenetic alterations in acne are (1) abnormal keratinization of the follicular epithelium, resulting in impaction of keratinized cells within the follicular lumen; (2) increased sebaceous gland production of sebum; (3) proliferation of *Propionibacterium acnes* within the follicle; and (4) inflammation. At puberty, the sebaceous gland enlarges and sebum production increases in response to the increased activities of androgens of primarily adrenal origin. Comedonal acne, particularly of the central face, is frequently the first sign of pubertal maturation. The prevalence and severity of acne correlate with pubertal development and amount of sebum production. Initiation of acne in prepubertal children age 7–10 yr has been shown to correlate significantly with the amount of wax esters in skin surface lipids and the concentration of serum dehydroepiandrosterone sulfate (DHEA-S), which is an androgenic steroid secreted primarily by the adrenal glands. DHEA-S levels are not elevated, however, in the serum of many individuals with acne. DHEA-S may act locally, however, to stimulate sebum production by the sebaceous glands after being metabolized in hair follicle dermal papillae and sebaceous glands by 5α-reductase to more potent androgens such as 5α-dihydrotestosterone. Other sex steroid hormones such as testosterone and estradiol may also have a role in enhancing sebum production. A significant number of women with acne (25–50%), particularly those with relatively mild papulopustular acne, note that their acne flares approximately 1 wk before menstruation. The pathogenesis of this phenomenon is unknown.

Freshly formed sebum consists of a mixture of triglycerides, wax esters, squalene, and sterol esters. Normal follicular bacteria produce lipases that hydrolyze sebum triglycerides to free fatty acids; those of medium chain length (C8–C14) may be provocative factors in initiating an inflammatory reaction. Sebum also provides a favorable substrate for proliferation of bacteria. Sebaceous follicles are colonized by organisms of three types: an anaerobic diphtheroid, *P. acnes*; coagulase-negative *Staphylococcus epidermidis*; and a dimorphic yeast, *Pityrosporum ovale*. Each of these organisms possesses lipolytic enzymes; however, *P. acnes* appears to be largely responsible for the formation of free fatty acids. It is probable that bacterial proteases, hyaluronidases, and hydrolytic enzymes produce biologically active extracellular materials that increase the permeability of the follicular epithelium. Chemotactic factors released by the intrafollicular bacteria attract neutrophils and monocytes. Lysosomal enzymes from the neutrophils, released in the process of phagocytizing the bacteria, further disrupt the integrity of the follicular wall and intensify the inflammatory reaction.

CLINICAL MANIFESTATIONS. Acne vulgaris is characterized by four basic types of lesions: open and closed comedones, papules, pustules, and nodulocystic lesions. One or more types of lesions may predominate; in its mildest form, which is often seen early in adolescence, lesions are limited to comedones on the central area of the face. Lesions may also involve the chest, upper back, and deltoid areas. A predominance of lesions on the forehead, particularly closed comedones, is often attributable to prolonged use of greasy hair preparations (pomade acne). Marked involvement on the trunk is most often seen in males. Lesions often heal with temporary postinflammatory erythema and hyperpigmentation; pitted, atrophic, or hypertrophic scars may be interspersed, depending on the severity, depth, and chronicity of the process. Diagnosis of acne is rarely difficult, although flat warts, folliculitis, and other types of acne may be confused with acne vulgaris.

TREATMENT. No evidence shows that early treatment, with the exception of isotretinoin, alters the course of acne. Acne can be controlled and severe scarring prevented, however, by judicious maintenance therapy that is continued until the disease process has abated spontaneously. Therapy must be individualized and aimed at preventing microcomedo formation through reduction of follicular hyperkeratosis, sebum production, the *P. acnes* population in follicular orifices, and free fatty acid production. Initial control takes at least 4–8 wk. It is also important to address the potentially severe emotional impact of acne on adolescents.

Diet. Little evidence shows that ingestion of particular foods can trigger acne flares. When a patient is convinced that certain dietary items exacerbate acne, it is prudent to omit those foods; however, it is unnecessary to impose unwarranted dietary restrictions.

Climate. Climate appears to influence acne in that improvement frequently occurs during summer and flares are more common during winter. Remission during summer may relate, in part, to the relative absence of stress. Emotional tension and fatigue seem to exacerbate acne in many individuals; the mechanism is unclear but has been proposed to relate to an increased adrenocortical response.

Cleansing. Cleansing with soap and water removes surface lipid and renders the skin less oily in appearance, but no evidence shows that surface lipid has a role in generating acne lesions. Only superficial drying and peeling are achieved by cleansing, and almost any mild soap or astringent is adequate. Repetitive cleansing can be harmful because it irritates and chaps the skin. Cleansing agents that contain abrasives and keratolytic agents, such as sulfur, resorcinol, and salicylic acid, may temporarily remove sebum from the skin surface. They exert a mild drying and peeling effect and suppress lesions to a limited degree. They do not, however, prevent microcomedones from forming. No evidence shows that preparations containing alcohol or hexachlorophene decrease acne because surface bacteria are not involved in the pathogenesis. Greasy cosmetic and hair preparations must be discontinued because they exacerbate pre-existing acne and cause further plugging of follicular pores. Manipulation and squeezing of facial lesions only ruptures intact lesions and provokes a localized inflammatory reaction.

Topical Therapy. The most effective topical preparations, particularly for comedones and papulopustular acne, include the benzoyl peroxide gels, retinoic acid, adapalene, and topical antibiotics. *Benzoyl peroxide* is an organic peroxide and oxidizing agent that dries and peels the skin, inhibits triglyceride hydrolysis and production of free fatty acids, is bacteriostatic for *P. acnes*, and causes follicular desquamation, disimpacting the follicle. Preparations are available in concentrations of 2.5%, 5%, and 10% prescription gels and 5% and 10% over-the-counter lotions. Benzoyl peroxide should be applied as a thin film, initially every other day, advancing over 2–3 wk to once-daily use as tolerated; the incidence of irritant or allergic contact dermatitis is 1%. Water-based gels are less irritating than alcohol-based ones, particularly for patients with atopic dermatitis or otherwise sensitive skin. Over-the-counter lotions are less effective than prescription gels.

Tretinoin (Retin-A), a derivative of retinoic acid, is the single most effective agent for treatment of comedonal acne. It affects keratinization in the sebaceous follicle by increasing turnover of epidermal cells and by decreasing the cohesiveness of the squamous cells; it thus aids in elimination of keratinous plugs. Erythema and peeling may be expected, particularly on initiation of therapy, and pustular flares from rupture of microcomedones are common. Flares may be minimized by starting treatment with benzoyl peroxide 2–3 wk before tretinoin. It may be applied once daily, 30 min after washing, in the form best tolerated (0.025% cream, 0.05% cream, 0.1% cream, 0.01% gel, 0.025% gel, and 0.05% liquid in increasing order of potency). Typically, 0.025% cream is prescribed initially; the strength of the formulation is increased sequentially until adequate control, without undue irritation, is achieved. Optimal results are not seen for 3–6 mo. Increased sensitivity to sunlight may occur, necessitating use of a sunscreen.

Adapalene (Differin gel), a derivative of naphthoic acid, is comedolytic and anti-inflammatory. A 0.1% gel may be more effective than 0.025% tretinoin gel and may have fever side effects.

Topical antibiotics for use in patients with acne include clindamycin and erythromycin; they may be applied once or twice daily. Although not as effective as orally administered antibiotics or benzoyl peroxide, they serve as a useful therapeutic adjunct by inhibiting growth of *P. acnes*. The effectiveness of a topical antibiotic is enhanced by concurrent use of benzoyl peroxide or tretinoin. Use of topical erythromycin or clindamycin has occasionally resulted in the emergence of resistant bacteria. *Azelaic acid* (Azelex cream) has antimicrobial and keratolytic properties. A 20% cream is as effective as 0.05% tretinoin cream.

All topical preparations must be used for 4–8 wk before their effectiveness can be assessed. They may be used alone but frequently are more effective when used together. A popular and effective combination is use of benzoyl peroxide gel in the morning and tretinoin at night.

Systemic Therapy. *Antibiotics*, especially tetracycline and its derivatives, are indicated for treatment of patients who cannot tolerate or have not responded to topical medications, who have moderate to severe inflammatory papulopustular and nodulocystic acne, and who have a propensity for scarring. The tetracyclines act by inhibiting bacterial lipases, causing a reduction in the concentration of free fatty acids; suppressing the normal follicular flora, mainly *P. acnes*; and inhibiting neutrophil chemotaxis and follicular inflammation. Tetracycline, minocycline, and doxycycline have been shown to suppress granuloma formation, perhaps by inhibition of protein kinase C, an important membrane signal transducer. For most adolescent patients, therapy may be initiated with tetracycline, 1 g/24 hr, divided twice daily, for at least 6 wk, followed by a gradual decrease to the minimal effective dose. The drugs are best administered in combination with topical benzoyl peroxide or tretinoin but not topical antibiotics. Tetracycline absorption is inhibited by food, milk, iron supplements, aluminum hydroxide gel, and calcium-magnesium salts. It should be taken on an empty stomach 1 hr before or 2 hr after meals. Side effects of tetracycline include vaginal candidosis, particularly in those who take tetracycline concurrently with oral contraceptives; gastrointestinal irritation; phototoxic reactions, including onycholysis and brown discoloration of nails; esophageal ulceration; inhibition of fetal skeletal growth; and staining of growing teeth, precluding its use during pregnancy and in those younger than 9 yr. Oral antibiotics may decrease the effectiveness of oral contraceptive pills. Alternatives to tetracycline include erythromycin, minocycline, doxycycline, clindamycin, and occasionally trimethoprim-sulfamethoxazole. A possible complication of prolonged systemic antibiotic use is proliferation of gram-negative organisms, particularly *Enterobacter, Klebsiella, Escherichia coli*, or *Pseudomonas aeruginosa*, producing severe, refractory folliculitis.

Women who have acne and hormonal abnormalities, who are unresponsive to antibiotic therapy, or who are not candidates for isotretinoin therapy should be considered for a trial of *hormonal therapy*. An effective combination is an antiandrogen such as cyproterone acetate or spironolactone, given on days 5–15 of the menstrual cycle, and ethinyl estradiol, a synthetic estrogen used in oral contraceptives that is a potent inhibitor of sebum production, given on days 5–26. Topically applied antiandrogens without systemic side effects are currently under investigation.

Isotretinoin (13-*cis*-retinoic acid, Accutane) is indicated for moderate to severe nodulocystic acne that has not responded to conventional therapy or has recurred quickly after several successful courses of conventional therapy; for severe, scarring acne such as acne conglobata and acne fulminans; and for acne that is associated with severe psychologic disturbance. The recommended dosage is approximately 0.5–1.0 mg/kg/24 hr; younger male patients and those with primarily truncal lesions tend to require doses at the upper end of this range. Four months of therapy is required for most patients; a standard course in the United States lasts 16–20 wk. At the end of one course of isotretinoin, approximately 30% are cured, 35% need conventional topical and/or oral medications to maintain adequate control, and 25% have relapses and need an additional course of isotretinoin. Dosages below 0.5 mg/kg/24 hr, or a cumulative dose of less than 120 mg/kg, are associated with a significantly higher rate of treatment failure and relapse. If the disease process is not in remission 2 mo after the first course of isotretinoin, a second course should be considered. Isotretinoin reduces sebum excretion by 80% within 1 mo, converts sebaceous units to epithelial buds, decreases the population of *P. acnes*, decreases ductal cornification, and inhibits neutrophil chemotaxis and thus decreases the inflammatory response. Isotretinoin therapy does not alter gonadal or adrenal functions but induces a significant local decrease in 5α-dihydrotestosterone formation in the skin.

Isotretinoin use has many side effects. It is teratogenic and is contraindicated in pregnancy; pregnancy should be avoided for 1 mo after discontinuation of therapy. Two or three forms of birth control are required, as are monthly pregnancy tests. Most patients experience cheilitis, xerosis, periodic epistaxis, and blepharoconjunctivitis. Increased serum triglyceride and cholesterol levels are also common; it is important to rule out pre-existent liver disease and hyperlipidemia before initiating therapy and to check the triglyceride response 4 wk after commencing therapy. Less common but significant side effects include arthralgias, myalgias, depression, temporary thinning of the hair, paronychia, increased susceptibility to sunburn, formation of pyogenic granulomas, and colonization of the skin with *Staphylococcus aureus*, leading to impetigo, secondarily infected dermatitis, and scalp folliculitis. Rarely, hyperostotic lesions of the spine develop after more than one course of isotretinoin. Concomitant use of tetracycline and isotretinoin is contraindicated because either drug, but particularly when used together, can cause benign intracranial hypertension.

Surgical Therapy. Intralesional injection of low-dose (3 mg/mL) midpotency glucocorticoids (e.g., triamcinolone) with a 30-gauge needle on a tuberculin syringe may hasten the healing of individual, painful nodulocystic lesions. Dermabrasion to minimize scarring should be considered only after the active process is quiescent.

DRUG-INDUCED ACNE

Pubertal and postpubertal patients who are receiving systemic corticosteroid therapy or potent topical steroids are predisposed to steroid-induced acne. This monomorphous folliculitis occurs primarily on the face, neck, chest (Fig. 675–1*A*), shoulders, upper back, arms, and, rarely, the scalp. Onset follows the initiation of steroid therapy by about 2 wk. The lesions are small erythematous papules or pustules that may erupt in profusion and are all in the same stage of development. Comedones may occur subsequently, but nodulocystic lesions and scarring are rare. Pruritus is occasional. The steroid appears to induce focal degeneration of the follicular epithelium, which incites a localized neutrophilic inflammatory response. Although steroid acne is relatively refractory if the medication is continued, the eruption may respond to use of tretinoin and a benzoyl peroxide gel. A prepubertal child with severe acne should be examined for endocrine disorders such as congenital adrenal hyperplasia. Studies of adrenal function are indicated in appropriate patients (see Chapter 585).

Other drugs that can induce acneiform lesions in susceptible individuals include isoniazid, phenytoin, phenobarbital, trimethadione, lithium carbonate, androgens (anabolic steroids), and vitamin B_{12}.

HALOGEN ACNE

Administration of medications containing iodides or bromides or, rarely, ingestion of massive amounts of vitamin-mineral preparations or iodine-containing "health foods" such as kelp may induce halogen acne. The lesions are often very inflammatory. Discontinuation of the provocative agent and appropriate topical preparations usually achieve reasonable therapeutic results.

CHLORACNE

Chloracne is due to external contact with, inhalation of, or ingestion of halogenated aromatic hydrocarbons, including polyhalogenated biphenyls, polyhalogenated naphthalenes (e.g., Halowax, which may be a component of wood preservatives and sealing compounds), and dioxins. Lesions are primarily comedonal; inflammatory lesions are infrequent but may include papules, pustules, nodules, and cysts. Healing occurs with atrophic or hypertrophic scarring. The face, postauricular regions, neck, axillas, genitals, and chest are involved most commonly. The nose is often spared. In cases of severe exposure, associated findings may include hepatitis, production of porphyrins, bulla formation on sun-exposed skin, hyperpigmentation, hypertrichosis, and palmar and plantar hyperhidrosis. Topical or oral retinoids may be effective; benzoyl peroxide and antibiotics are generally ineffective.

NEONATAL ACNE

Approximately 20% of normal neonates develop at least a few comedones within the 1st mo of life. Closed comedones predominate on the cheeks and forehead (see Fig. 675–1*B*); open comedones and papulopustules occur occasionally. The cause of neonatal acne is unknown but has been attributed to placental transfer of maternal androgens, hyperactive neonatal adrenal glands, and a hypersensitive neonatal end-organ response to androgenic hormones. Placental transfer of maternally ingested lithium and hydantoin may also cause acne in the neonate. The hypertrophic sebaceous glands involute

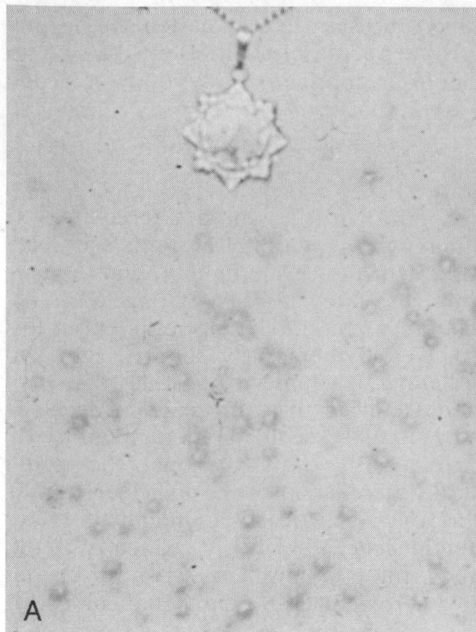

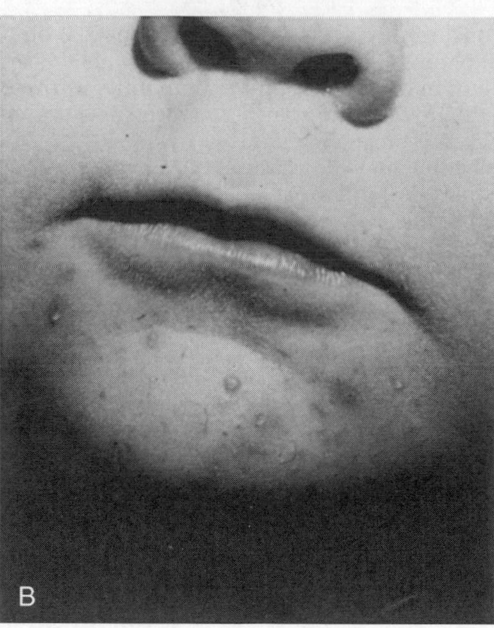

Figure 675–1 *A*, Monomorphous papular eruption of steroid acne. *B*, Acne in a male infant.

spontaneously over a few months, as does the acne. If desired, the lesions can be treated effectively with topical tretinoin and/or benzoyl peroxide.

INFANTILE ACNE

Infantile acne usually presents at 3–6 mo of life, more commonly in boys than girls. Acne lesions are more numerous, pleomorphic, severe, and persistent than in neonatal acne. Open and closed comedones predominate on the face; papules and pustules occur frequently, but only occasionally do nodulocystic lesions develop. Pitted scarring is rare. The course may be relatively brief, or the lesions may persist for many months, although the eruption generally resolves by age 3 yr. Use of topical benzoyl peroxide gel and tretinoin usually clears the eruption within a few weeks; oral erythromycin is necessary occasionally. A history of severe acne in one or both parents is often elicited, and the child is at risk for development of severe acne in adolescence. A child with refractory acne warrants a search for an abnormal source of androgens such as a virilizing tumor or congenital adrenal hyperplasia.

TROPICAL ACNE

A severe form of acne occurs in tropical climates and is believed to be due to the intense heat and humidity; hydration of the pilosebaceous duct pore may accentuate blockage of the duct. Affected individuals tend to have an antecedent history of adolescent acne that is quiescent at the time of the eruption. Lesions occur mainly on the entire back, chest, buttocks, and thighs, with a predominance of suppurating papules and nodules. Secondary infection with *S. aureus* may be a complication. The eruption is refractory to acne therapy if the environmental factors are not eliminated.

ACNE CONGLOBATA

Acne conglobata is a chronic progressive inflammatory disease that occurs mainly in men, more commonly in whites than in blacks, but it may begin during adolescence. Patients usually but not always have a history of pre-existing acne vulgaris. The principal lesion is the nodule, although one often finds a mixture of comedones with multiple pores, papules, pustules, nodules, cysts, abscesses, and subcutaneous dissection with formation of multichanneled sinus tracts. Severe scarring is characteristic. The face is relatively spared, but in addition to the back and chest, the buttocks, abdomen, arms, and thighs may be involved. Constitutional symptoms and anemia may accompany the inflammatory process. Coagulase-positive staphylococci and β-hemolytic streptococci are frequently cultured from lesions but do not appear to be involved primarily in the pathogenesis. Acne conglobata occasionally occurs in association with hidradenitis suppurativa and dissecting cellulitis of the scalp (as the follicular occlusion triad) and may be complicated by erosive arthritis and ankylosing spondyloarthritis. Endocrinologic studies are not revealing. Routine acne therapy is generally ineffective. Systemic therapy with a corticosteroid or sulfone may be required to suppress the intense inflammatory activity. Isotretinoin is the most effective form of therapy for some patients but may produce a flare after its initiation. Consequently, corticosteroids are often started before isotretinoin.

ACNE FULMINANS

(Acute Febrile Ulcerative Acne)

Acne fulminans is characterized by abrupt onset of extensive inflammatory, tender ulcerative acneiform lesions on the back and chest of male teenagers. The distinctive feature is the tendency for large nodules to form exudative, necrotic, ulcerated, crusted plaques. Lesions often spare the face and heal with scarring. A preceding history of mild papulopustular or nodular acne is noted in most patients. Constitutional symptoms and signs are common, including fever, debilitation, arthralgias, myalgias, weight loss, and leukocytosis. Blood cultures are sterile. Lesions of erythema nodosum sometimes develop on the shins. Osteolytic bone lesions may develop in the clavicle, sternum, and epiphyseal growth plates; affected bones appear normal or have slight sclerosis or thickening on healing. Salicylates may be helpful for the myalgias, arthralgias, and fever. Corticosteroids (1.0 mg/kg of prednisone) are started first; then approximately 1 wk later, isotretinoin (0.5 mg/kg) is added and continued for as long as inflammatory lesions persist, generally 3–4 mo. Dapsone may be effective if isotretinoin cannot be used. The corticosteroids are tapered over approximately 6 wk. Antibiotics are not indicated unless there is evidence of secondary infection. Compared with acne conglobata, acne fulminans presents in younger patients, is more explosive in onset, more commonly has associated constitutional symptoms and ulcerated crusted lesions, and less commonly has multiheaded comedones or involves the face.

Brown S, Shalita A: Acne vulgaris. Lancet 351:1871, 1998.
Hurwitz S: Acne vulgaris: Pathogenesis and management. Pediatr Rev 15:47, 1994.
Karvonen SL: Acne fulminans: Report of clinical findings and treatment of twenty-four patients. J Am Acad Dermatol 28:572, 1993.
Layton AM, Knaggs H, Taylor J, et al: Isotretinoin for acne vulgaris—10 years later: A safe and successful treatment. Br J Dermatol 129:292, 1993.
Leyden JJ: Therapy for acne vulgaris. N Engl J Med 336:1156, 1997.
Lucky AW, Biro FM, Simbartl LA, et al: Predictions of severity of acne vulgaris in young adolescent girls: Results of a five-year longitudinal study. J Pediatr 130:30, 1997.
Stainforth JM, Layton AM, Taylor JP, et al: Isotretinoin for the treatment of acne vulgaris: Which factors may predict the need for more than one course? Br J Dermatol 129:297, 1993.

CHAPTER 676
Tumors of the Skin

See also Chapter 513.

EPIDERMAL INCLUSION CYST (EPIDERMOID CYST). These are sharply circumscribed, dome-shaped, firm, freely movable, skin-colored nodules, often with a central dimple or punctum that is a plugged, dilated pore of a pilosebaceous follicle. Epidermoid cysts form most frequently on the face, neck, chest, or upper back and may periodically become inflamed and infected secondarily, particularly in association with acne vulgaris. The cyst wall may also rupture and induce an inflammatory reaction in the dermis. The wall of the cyst is derived from the follicular infundibulum; a mass of layered keratinized material that may have a cheesy consistency fills the cavity. Epidermoid cysts may arise from occlusion of pilosebaceous follicles, from implantation of epidermal cells into the dermis as a result of an injury that penetrates the epidermis, and from rests of epidermal cells. Multiple epidermoid cysts may be present in *Gardner syndrome* and the *nevoid basal cell carcinoma syndrome*. Excision of the cysts with removal of the entire sac and its contents is indicated, particularly if the cyst becomes recurrently infected. A fluctuant, infected cyst should first be incised, drained, and packed, and the patient should receive an antibiotic effective against *Staphylococcus aureus*. After the inflammation subsides, the cyst should be removed.

MILIUM. This is a pearly-white or yellowish, firm, 1–2-mm subepidermal keratin cyst. Milia in newborns is discussed in Chapter 653. Secondary milia occur in association with subepidermal blistering diseases, chronic corticosteroid-induced atrophy, 5-fluorouracil therapy, or after dermabrasion. They are retention cysts caused by hyperproliferation of injured epithelium and are indistinguishable histopathologically from primary milia; those that develop after blistering usually arise from the eccrine sweat duct, but they may develop from the hair follicle, sebaceous duct, or epidermis. A milium body differs from an epidermoid cyst only in its small size.

PILAR CYST (TRICHILEMMAL CYST). This is clinically indistinguishable from an epidermoid cyst. It presents as a smooth, firm, mobile nodule, predominantly on the scalp. These cysts occasionally develop on the face, neck, or trunk. The cyst may become inflamed and may occasionally suppurate and ulcerate. The cyst wall is composed of epithelial cells with indistinct intercellular bridges. The peripheral cell layer of the wall shows a palisade arrangement, which is not seen in an epidermoid cyst. No granular layer is present, the cyst cavity contains homogeneous eosinophilic keratinous material, and foci of calcification are seen in 25% of cases. The propensity to develop pilar cysts is inherited in an autosomal dominant manner; more than one cyst generally develops. Numerous pilar and epidermoid cysts, desmoid tumors, fibromas, lipomas, or osteomas may be associated with colonic polyposis or adenocarcinoma in Gardner syndrome. Pilar cysts shell out easily from the dermis.

PILOMATRICOMA. This is a benign tumor that presents as a 3–30-mm, firm, solitary, deep dermal or subcutaneous tumor on the head, neck, or upper extremities. The overlying epidermis is usually normal; the tumor may occasionally be located more superficially, however, tinting the overlying skin blue-red. Pilomatricomas may enlarge rapidly as a result of inflammation or hemorrhage and occasionally perforate the epidermis. Patients with both pilomatricoma and myotonic dystrophy are more likely to have several tumors and to have familial occurrence; in general, however, pilomatricomas are not hereditary. Histopathologically, irregularly shaped islands of epithelial cells are embedded in a cellular stroma. Calcium deposits are found in 75% of tumors.

TRICHOEPITHELIOMA. This is a smooth, round, firm, skin-colored 2–8-mm papule that is derived from immature hair follicles. Trichoepitheliomas generally occur singly on the face during childhood or early adulthood. Multiple trichoepitheliomas *(epithelioma adenoides cysticum)* are inherited autosomal dominantly, appear in childhood or at puberty, and gradually increase in number on the nasofacial folds, nose, forehead, and upper lip and occasionally on the scalp, neck, and upper trunk. Microscopically, these benign tumors are characterized by horn cysts composed of a fully keratinized center surrounded by basophilic cells in an adenoid network. Surgical excision is the therapy.

ERUPTIVE VELLUS HAIR CYSTS. These are asymptomatic, follicular, skin-colored, soft 1–3-mm papules on the chest. They may become crusted or umbilicated. Abnormal vellus hair follicles become occluded at the level of the infundibulum, resulting in retention of hairs within an epithelium-lined cystic dilatation of the proximal part of the follicle. Most cases are chronic, but spontaneous regression has been reported.

STEATOCYSTOMA MULTIPLEX. This condition usually presents in adolescence or early adulthood with numerous soft to firm cystic nodules that are adherent to the underlying skin and are a few millimeters to 3 cm in diameter. When punctured, the cysts may drain oily or cheesy material. Sites of predilection include the sternal region, axillas, arms, and scrotal skin. The multiply folded cyst wall is lined on the luminal side with a thick, homogeneous, eosinophilic horny layer and lacks a granular layer. Flattened sebaceous gland lobules are often visible in the cyst wall, and lanugo hairs may be present in the cystic cavity.

SYRINGOMA. These benign tumors are soft, small, skin-colored or yellowish-brown papules that develop on the face, particularly in the periorbital regions. Other sites of predilection include the axillas and umbilical and pubic areas. They often develop during puberty and are more frequent in females. Eruptive syringomas (eruptive hidradenoma) develop in crops over the anterior trunk during childhood or adolescence. A syringoma is derived from an intraepidermal sweat gland duct. They are of cosmetic significance only. Sparse lesions may be excised, but they are often too numerous to remove.

INFANTILE DIGITAL FIBROMA. This is a firm, smooth, erythematous or skin-colored nodule on the dorsal or lateral surfaces of the distal phalanges of the fingers and toes. More than 80% of tumors present in infancy; they may be present at birth. Lesions may be solitary or multiple and may present as "kissing" tumors on opposing digits. Generally, they are asymptomatic, but flexion deformity of the digits may occur. Clinically, the lesions resemble a fibroma, leiomyoma, angiofibroma, acquired digital fibrokeratoma, accessory digit, or mucous cyst. The diagnosis is confirmed by finding numerous spindle-shaped fibroblasts that contain small, dense, round eosinophilic cytoplasmic inclusion bodies composed of collections of actin microfilaments. A viral cause has been postulated. Local recurrence after simple excision of this tumor has been reported in 75% of patients. Because the tumor does not metastasize and may regress spontaneously within 2–3 yr, a course of expectant observation is advised. If functional impairment or flexion deformity of the digit becomes apparent, prompt full excision of the tumor is indicated.

DERMATOFIBROMA (HISTIOCYTOMA). These benign dermal tumors may be pedunculated, nodular, or flat and are usually well circumscribed and firm but occasionally feel soft on palpation. The overlying skin is usually hyperpigmented, may be shiny or keratotic, and dimples when the tumor is pinched. Dermatofibromas range in size from 0.5–10 mm, arise most frequently on the limbs, and are usually asymptomatic but may occasionally be pruritic. They are composed of fibroblasts, young and mature collagen, capillaries, and histiocytes in varying proportions, forming a nodule in the dermis that has poorly defined edges. The cause of these tumors is unknown, but trauma such as an insect bite or folliculitis appears to induce reactive fibroplasia. The differential diagnosis includes epidermal inclusion cyst, juvenile xanthogranuloma, hypertrophic scar, and neurofibroma. Dermatofibromas may be excised or left intact according to a patient's preference; they usually persist indefinitely but occasionally involute spontaneously.

JUVENILE XANTHOGRANULOMA. These are firm, dome-shaped, yellow, pink, or orange papules or nodules that vary in size from a few millimeters to approximately 4 cm in diameter. They usually present at birth or within the first several months of life; occasionally, they first appear in late childhood and, rarely, in adulthood. They are 10 times more common in white than in black individuals. Sites of predilection are the scalp, face, and upper trunk, where they may erupt in profusion or remain as solitary lesions. Nodular lesions may appear on the oral mucosa. Mature lesions are characterized histopathologically by a dermal infiltrate of lipid-laden histiocytes, admixed inflammatory cells, and Touton giant cells. The lesions may clinically resemble papulonodular urticaria pigmentosa, dermatofibromas, or xanthomas of hyperlipoproteinemia but can be distinguished from these entities histopathologically.

Affected infants are nearly always otherwise normal, and blood lipid values are not elevated. Café-au-lait macules are found on 20% of patients with juvenile xanthogranuloma. Xanthogranulomatous infiltrates occur occasionally in ocular tissues. This may result in glaucoma, hyphema, uveitis, heterochromia iridis, iritis, or sudden proptosis. There appears to be an association among juvenile xanthogranuloma, neurofibromatosis, and childhood leukemia, most frequently juvenile chronic myelogenous leukemia. There is no need to remove these benign lesions because most of them regress spontaneously during the first few years. Residual pigmentation and atrophy, but not scarring, may result.

LIPOMA. These benign collections of fatty tissue appear on the trunk, neck, and proximal portions of the limbs. They are soft, compressible, lobulated, subcutaneous masses that are movable against the overlying skin. Multiple lesions may occur occasionally, as in Gardner syndrome. Atrophy, calcification, liquefaction, or xanthomatous change may sometimes complicate their course. A lipoma is composed of normal fat cells and surrounded by a thin connective tissue capsule. They represent a cosmetic defect and may be surgically excised. Multiple lipomas, identical to those that occur singly, are inherited in an autosomal dominant fashion and often appear by the 3rd decade in patients with *familial multiple lipomatosis*. Lipomas may appear intra-abdominally, intramuscularly, and subcutaneously. *Congenital lipomatosis* presents during the first few months of life as large subcutaneous fatty masses on the chest, with extension into skeletal muscle. Congenital lipomatosis can also be a manifestation of Proteus syndrome. *Angiolipomas* usually present as numerous painful subcutaneous nodules on the arms and trunk.

BASAL CELL EPITHELIOMA (BASAL CELL CARCINOMA). Basal cell carcinoma is rare in children in the absence of a predisposing condition, such as nevoid basal cell carcinoma syndrome, xeroderma pigmentosum, nevus sebaceus of Jadassohn, arsenic intake, or exposure to irradiation. The lesions are pink, pearly, telangiectatic, smooth papules that enlarge slowly and may bleed or ulcerate. Sites of predilection are the face, scalp, and upper back. The differential diagnosis includes pyogenic granuloma, nevocellular nevus, epidermal inclusion cyst, closed comedo, dermatofibroma, and adnexal tumor. Depending on the site of occurrence and associated disease of the host, electrodesiccation and curettage or simple excision is usually curative. When the tumor is recurrent, larger than 2 cm in diameter, located on problematic anatomic areas such as the midface or ears, or is an aggressive histopathologic type, Mohs microscopically controlled surgery may be the most appropriate treatment.

NEVOID BASAL CELL CARCINOMA SYNDROME (BASAL CELL NEVUS SYNDROME, GORLIN SYNDROME). This autosomal dominant syndrome maps to a gene on chromosome 9q22.3. This tumor suppressor gene is part of the hedgehog signaling pathway and is important in determining embryonic patterning and cell fate in a number of structures in the developing embryo. Mutations in human patched gene produce dysregulation of several genes involved in organogenesis and carcinogenesis. Consequently, the syndrome includes a wide spectrum of defects involving the skin, eyes, central nervous and endocrine systems, and bones. The predominant features are early-onset basal cell carcinomas and mandibular cysts. Approximately 20% of those in whom a basal cell carcinoma develops before age 19 yr have this syndrome. Basal cell carcinomas appear between puberty and age 35 yr, erupting in crops of tumors that vary in size, color, and number and may be difficult to distinguish from other types of skin lesions. Sites of predilection are the periorbital skin, nose, malar areas, and upper lip, but the lesions can develop on the trunk and limbs and are not restricted to sun-exposed areas. Ulceration, bleeding, crusting, and local invasion can occur. Small milia, epidermal cysts, pigmented lesions, hirsutism, and palmar and plantar pits are additional cutaneous findings.

The facies of patients with this syndrome are characterized by temporoparietal bossing, prominent supraorbital ridges, a broad nasal root, ocular hypertelorism or dystopia canthorum, and prognathism. Keratinized cysts (odontogenic keratocysts) in the maxilla and mandible occur in most patients. They range in size from a few millimeters to several centimeters, may result in maldevelopment of the teeth, and cause pain, swelling of the jaw, facial deformity, bone erosion, pathologic fractures, and suppurating sinus tracts. Osseous defects such as anomalous rib development, spina bifida, kyphoscoliosis, and brachymetacarpalism occur in two thirds of patients, and ocular abnormalities including cataracts, glaucoma, coloboma, strabismus, and blindness occur in approximately one fourth. Some males have hypogonadism, with absent or undescended testes. Kidney malformations have also been reported. Neurologic manifestations include calcification of the falx, seizures, mental retardation, partial agenesis of the corpus callosum, hydrocephalus, and nerve deafness. The incidence of medulloblastoma, ameloblastoma of the oval cavity, fibrosarcoma of the jaw, teratoma, cystadenoma, cardiac fibroma, and ovarian fibroma is increased.

Treatment of these patients requires participation of various specialists according to individual clinical problems. Basal cell carcinomas should not be treated with irradiation. Most of the basal cell carcinomas have a clinically benign course, and it is often impossible to remove them all; those with an aggressive growth pattern and those on the central areas of the face, however, should be removed promptly. Oral retinoids have been shown to be helpful in preventing the development of new tumors in some patients. Genetic counseling is also indicated.

MUCOSAL NEUROMA SYNDROME (SIPPEL SYNDROME). Mucosal neuroma syndrome is inherited as an autosomal dominant trait and is easily recognized by characteristic physical features. An asthenic or marfanoid habitus is accompanied by scoliosis, pectus excavatum, pes cavus, and muscular hypotonia. Patients have thick, patulous lips and soft tissue prognathism simulating acromegaly. Multiple mucosal neuromas or neurofibromas appear as pink, pedunculated or sessile nodules on the anterior third of the tongue, at the commissures of the lips, and on the buccal mucosa and palpebral conjunctiva. Various ophthalmologic defects and intestinal ganglioneuromatosis with recurrent diarrhea are additional common findings. There is a high incidence of medullary thyroid carcinoma associated with high calcitonin levels, pheochromocytoma, and hyperparathyroidism. Periodic screening tests for the associated malignant tumors are mandatory.

Cerio R, Jones EW: Histiocytoma cutis: A tumour of dermal dendrocytes (dermal dendrocytoma). Br J Dermatol 120:197, 1989.
Coskey RJ, Dalrey KW: Recurring digital fibrous tumor of childhood: Review of the literature. J Pediatr Orthop 6:612, 1986.
Kimonis UE, Goldstein AM, Pastakia B, et al: Clinical manifestations in 105 persons with nevoid basal cell carcinoma syndrome. Am J Med Genet 69:299, 1997.
Milstone EG, Helwig EB: Basal carcinoma in children. Arch Dermatol 108:523, 1973.
Oro AE, Higgins KM, Ku Z, et al: Basal cell carcinomas in mice expressing sonic hedgehog. Science 276:817, 1997.
Roper SR, Spraker MK: Cutaneous histiocytosis syndromes. Pediatr Dermatol 3:19, 1985.
Rotte JJ, de Vaan GA, Koopman RJ: Juvenile xanthogranuloma and acute leukemia: A case report. Med Pediatr Oncol 23:57, 1994.
Taaffe, Wyatt EH, Bury HPR, et al: Pilomatricoma (Malherbe): A clinical and histopathologic survey of 78 cases. Int J Dermatol 27:477, 1988.
Wicking C, Bale AE: Molecular basis of the nevoid basal cell carcinoma syndrome. Curr Opin Pediatr 9:630, 1997.

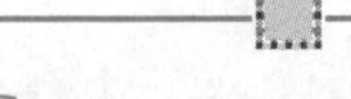

CHAPTER 677
Nutritional Dermatoses

ACRODERMATITIS ENTEROPATHICA. This is a rare autosomal recessive disorder caused by an inability to absorb sufficient zinc from the diet. Initial signs and symptoms usually occur during the first few months of life, often after weaning from breast to cow's milk. The cutaneous eruption consists of vesiculobullous, eczematous, dry, scaly, or psoriasiform skin lesions symmetrically distributed in the perioral, acral, and perineal areas and on the cheeks, knees, and elbows (Fig. 677–1). The hair often has a peculiar reddish tint, and alopecia of some degree is characteristic. Ocular manifestations include photophobia, conjunctivitis, blepharitis, and corneal dystrophy, detectable by slit-lamp examination. Associated manifestations include chronic diarrhea, stomatitis, glossitis, paronychia, nail dystrophy, growth retardation, irritability, delayed wound healing, intercurrent bacterial infections, and superinfection with *Candida albicans*. Lymphocyte function and free radical scavenging are impaired. Without treatment, the course is chronic and intermittent but often relentlessly progressive. When the disease is less severe, only growth retardation and delayed development may be apparent.

The *diagnosis* is established by the constellation of clinical findings and detection of a low plasma zinc concentration. Histopathologic changes in the skin are nonspecific and include parakeratosis and pallor of the upper epidermis. The variety of

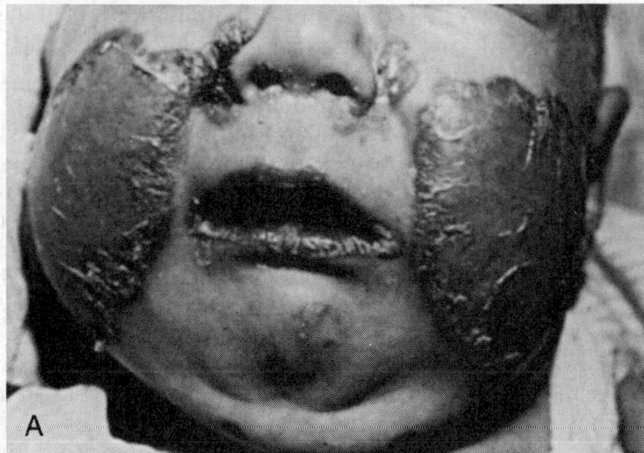

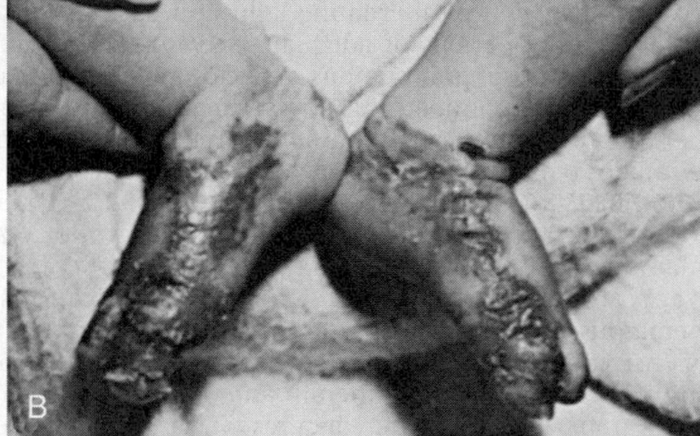

Figure 677–1 *A*, Psoriasiform facial lesions of zinc deficiency dermatitis. *B*, Similar lesions on the feet with secondary nail dystrophy.

manifestations of the syndrome may be due to the fact that zinc has a role in numerous metabolic pathways, including those of copper, protein, essential fatty acids, and prostaglandins, and zinc is incorporated into many zinc metalloenzymes.

Oral therapy with zinc compounds is the *treatment* of choice. Optimal doses range from 50 mg of zinc sulfate, acetate, or gluconate daily for infants up to 150 mg/24 hr for children; plasma zinc levels should be monitored, however, to individualize the dosage. Zinc therapy rapidly abolishes the manifestations of the disease. A syndrome resembling acrodermatitis enteropathica has been observed in patients with secondary zinc deficiency caused by long-term total parenteral nutrition without supplemental zinc or by chronic malabsorption syndromes. A rash similar to that of acrodermatitis enteropathica has also been reported in infants fed breast milk that is low in zinc and in those with maple syrup urine disease, organic aciduria, methylmalonic acidemia, biotinidase deficiency, essential fatty acid deficiency, severe protein malnutrition (e.g., kwashiorkor), and cystic fibrosis.

ESSENTIAL FATTY ACID DEFICIENCY. This causes a generalized, scaly dermatitis composed of thickened, erythematous, desquamating plaques. The eruption has been induced experimentally in animals fed a fat-free diet and has been observed in patients with chronic severe malabsorption such as in short-gut syndrome and in those sustained on a fat-free diet or fat-free parenteral alimentation. Linoleic (18:2 n-6) and arachidonic (20:4 n-6) acids are deficient, and an abnormal metabolite, 5,8,11-eicosatrienoic acid (20:3 n-9), is present in the plasma. Additional manifestations of essential fatty acid deficiency include alopecia, thrombocytopenia, and failure to thrive. The horny layer of the skin is cracked microscopically, the barrier function of the skin is disturbed, and transepidermal water loss is increased. Topical application of linoleic acid, which is present in sunflower seed and safflower oils, may ameliorate the clinical and biochemical skin manifestations. Appropriate nutrition should be provided.

KWASHIORKOR. Severe protein and essential amino acid deprivation in association with adequate caloric intake can lead to kwashiorkor, particularly at the time of weaning to a diet that consists primarily of corn, rice, or beans (see Chapter 42.2). Cutaneous erythema develops first and, in mild cases in white children, progresses to fine desquamation along natural skin lines and on the shins, outer thighs, and back. In dark-skinned children, characteristic early findings include circumoral pallor, cutaneous depigmentation, and development of purple patches. As the disease advances, well-marginated, slightly raised, purplish, waxy plaques appear, particularly in the diaper area and at sites of pressure such as the elbows, knees, and ankles and on the trunk. In severe cases, erosions and linear fissures develop. Sun-exposed skin is relatively spared, as are the feet and dorsal aspects of the hands. Nails are thin and soft, and hair is sparse, thin, and depigmented, sometimes displaying a flag sign of alternating light and dark bands that reflect alternating periods of adequate and inadequate nutrition. The cutaneous manifestations may closely resemble those of acrodermatitis enteropathica. The serum zinc level is often deficient, and in some cases, skin lesions of kwashiorkor heal more rapidly when zinc is applied topically.

CYSTIC FIBROSIS (see Chapter 416). Five to 10% of patients with cystic fibrosis develop protein-calorie malnutrition. Rash in infants with cystic fibrosis and malnutrition is rare but may appear by age 6 mo. The initial eruption consists of erythematous, scaling papules and progresses within 1–3 mo to extensive desquamating plaques. The rash is accentuated around the mouth and perineum and on the extremities (lower > upper). Alopecia may be present, but mucous membranes and nails are uninvolved.

PELLAGRA (see Chapter 44.5). This presents with edema, erythema, and burning of sun-exposed skin on the face, neck, and dorsal aspects of the hands, forearms, and feet. Lesions of pellagra may also be provoked by burns, pressure, friction, and inflammation. The eruption on the face frequently follows a butterfly distribution, and the dermatitis encircling the neck has been termed "Casal's necklace." Blisters and scales develop, and the skin increasingly becomes dry, rough, thickened, cracked, and hyperpigmented. Skin infections may be unusually severe. Pellagra develops in those with insufficient dietary intake or absorption of niacin and/or tryptophan. Administration of isoniazid, 6-mercaptopurine, or 5-fluorouracil may also produce pellagra. Nicotinamide supplementation and sun avoidance are the mainstays of therapy.

SCURVY (VITAMIN C OR ASCORBIC ACID DEFICIENCY) (see Chapter 44.9). This presents initially with follicular hyperkeratosis and coiling of hair on the upper arms, back, buttocks, and lower extremities. Perifollicular erythema and hemorrhage, particularly on the legs, advancing to involve large areas of hemorrhage; swollen, erythematous gums; stomatitis; and subperiosteal hematomas are also seen. The best method for confirmation of a clinical diagnosis of scurvy is a trial of vitamin C supplementation.

VITAMIN A DEFICIENCY (see Chapter 44.1). This deficiency presents initially with impairment of visual adaptation to the dark. Cutaneous changes include xerosis and hyperkeratosis and hyperplasia of the epidermis, particularly the lining of hair follicles and sebaceous glands. In severe cases, desquamation may be prominent.

Darmstadt GL, Schmidt CP, Wechsler DS, et al: Dermatitis as a presenting sign of cystic fibrosis. Arch Dermatol 128:1358, 1992.

Hansen AE, Wiese HF, Boelsche AN, et al: Role of linoleic acid in infant nutrition. Pediatrics 31:171, 1963.

Hansen RC, Lemen R, Revsin B: Cystic fibrosis manifesting with acrodermatitis enteropathica-like eruption. Arch Dermatol 119:51, 1983.

Hendricks WM: Pellagra and pellagra-like dermatoses: Etiology, differential diagnosis, dermatopathology, and treatment. Semin Dermatol 10:282, 1991.

Krieger I, Evans GW: Acrodermatitis enteropathica without hypozincemia: Therapeutic effect of a pancreatic enzyme preparation due to a zinc-binding ligand. J Pediatr 96:32, 1980.

Neldner KH, Hambidge KM: Zinc deficiency of acrodermatitis enteropathica. N Engl J Med 292:879, 1975.

PART XXXI

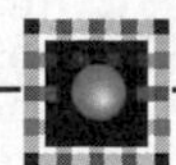

Bone and Joint Disorders

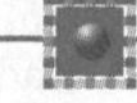

SECTION 1

Orthopedic Problems

George H. Thompson ▪ Peter V. Scoles

CHAPTER 678
Growth and Development

Musculoskeletal disorders in children and adolescents are common. Many of these disorders can be managed safely and effectively by the pediatrician provided that an accurate diagnosis is established. The differential diagnosis of pediatric musculoskeletal disorders involves all diagnostic categories: congenital, developmental, acquired, infectious, neuromuscular, neoplastic, and psychogenic.

Before beginning an evaluation of a child with an orthopedic problem, one must have a basic understanding of the effects of in utero positioning, the mechanism in which normal musculoskeletal growth occurs, and the relationships among skeletal growth, neurologic maturation, and normal developmental milestones.

IN UTERO POSITIONING. In the newborn, the imprint of the in utero position may be evident and confused with an abnormality. In utero positioning produces temporary joint and muscle contractures and affects the torsional alignment of the long bones, especially the lower extremities. Normal full-term newborns have 20–30 degree hip and knee flexion contractures. These resolve by 4–6 mo of age. The newborn hip externally rotates in extension 80–90 degrees and has limited internal rotation to 0–10 degrees. The lower leg frequently has inward rotation (internal tibial torsion), and the feet are supinated from their medial borders being wrapped against the posterolateral aspect of the opposite thigh. The top leg in the in utero position may show more changes than the bottom leg. The face may also be distorted, whereas the spine and upper extremities are less affected by the in utero position. The effects of in utero positioning, therefore, are physiologic in origin but may produce parental concerns. The child may be 3–4 yr old before the effects of the in utero position completely resolve.

GROWTH AND DEVELOPMENT. Each of the individual components of the skeletal system grow by different mechanisms. The long bones of the extremities (humerus, radius-ulna, femur, and tibia-fibula) have growth plates or physes at each end. Each contributes a varying proportion to the longitudinal growth of the individual bone as well as the extremity through a process termed *endochondral ossification.* The ends of each long bone are composed of the epiphyses. These are covered by articular cartilage and form the associated joints. Initially, the epiphyses are almost entirely cartilaginous and become progressively more ossified during growth. The articular cartilage also has growth potential, which contributes to the growth of the epiphysis. The perichondrial ring, which surrounds the physes, as well as the perichondrium around the epiphyses and periosteum, which surrounds the metaphysis and diaphyseal regions of the bone, contributes to apositional or circumferential growth.

Bones without physes, such as the pelvis, scapulae, carpals, and tarsals, grow by apositional bone growth from their surrounding perichondrium and periosteum. Other bones, such as the metacarpals, metatarsals, phalanges, and spine, grow by a combination of both apositional and endochondral ossification.

Trauma, infections, nutritional deficiencies (rickets), regional soft tissue processes, inborn errors of metabolism (mucopolysaccharidosis, mucolipidosis, Gaucher's disease, and disorders of cartilage), and other metabolic processes may affect each of these growth processes, producing a distinct alteration in the particular growth function.

DEVELOPMENTAL MILESTONES. Neurologic maturation, marked by the passage of motor milestones at regular intervals, is important for normal musculoskeletal development. The milestones for locomotion include independent sitting at 6 mo of age, crawling at 9 mo, walking without assistance at 12–15 mo, and running at 18 mo (see Chapter 11). There is a distinct relationship between skeletal form and gross motor function. Any process that produces a neurologic abnormality may cause a secondary delay in developmental milestones and an alteration of normal skeletal growth.

CHAPTER 679
Evaluation of the Child

The key to an accurate diagnosis is a careful history, a thorough physical examination, appropriate radiographic imaging, and occasionally laboratory testing. A glossary of common orthopedic terminology is provided in Table 679–1.

HISTORY. The history of the complaint is often the most important part of the evaluation. This is usually obtained from the parents or guardian, but the child, if old enough and cooperative, can also give useful information. The chief complaint is established first. This may include pain, deformity, joint stiffness, gait disturbance (limp, toe walking, in-toeing, out-toeing), swelling, or generalized muscle weakness. One must ascertain location and duration of symptoms; antecedent factors such as fever, trauma, radiation of pain, and neurologic symptoms; factors aggravating or alleviating the symptoms; and previous evaluations or treatment.

TABLE 679–1 Glossary of Orthopedic Terminology

Term	Definition
Abduction	Movement away from the midline
Adduction	Movement toward and possibly across the midline
Anteversion	Increased angulation of the femoral head and neck with respect to the knee in the frontal plane
Apophysis	Bone growth center that is not a growth plate or physis and that has a strong muscle insertion (e.g., greater trochanter of femur)
Arthroplasty	Surgical reconstruction of a joint
Arthrotomy	Surgical incision into a joint
Calcaneus	Dorsiflexion of hindfoot
Cavovarus	High longitudinal or medial arch of foot with plantar-flexed supinated forefoot and hindfoot varus
Cavus	High longitudinal arch of the foot (usually plantar-flexed forefoot)
Dislocation	Complete loss of contact between two joint surfaces
Equinus	Plantar flexion of the forefoot, hindfoot, or entire foot
Extension	Means to straighten; is the reverse of flexion
External or lateral rotation	Outward rotation away from the midline
Flexion	Means to bend
Internal or medial rotation	Inward rotation, toward the midline
Subluxation	Incomplete loss of contact between two joint surfaces
Valgum	Angulation of a bone or joint in which the apex is toward the midline; genu valgum results in knock-knee because the angulation of the knee is toward the midline
Varum	Angulation of a bone or joint away from the midline; genu varum results in bowleg because the angulation is away from the midline

In children with chronic symptoms, the past medical history is also important. The prenatal or pregnancy history should be obtained (see Chapters 90, 91, and 92). This includes maternal diseases or illnesses, vaginal bleeding, oligohydramnios, ingestion of toxic substances or medications, and trauma. The birth history should determine the length of pregnancy; duration of labor; type of difficulty, if any, with delivery; birth presentation; birthweight; and the Apgar score (see Chapters 93, 94, and 95). The condition of the child during the neonatal period is important (see Chapter 94). In older infants and young children, the presence and delay of developmental milestones for posture, locomotion, dexterity, social activities, and speech are important.

The family history may give clues to possible genetic disorders such as congenital syndromes, muscular dystrophy, skeletal dysplasias, and other disorders affecting the musculoskeletal system. It is important to inquire about specific problems, similar or not, on both the paternal and maternal sides.

PHYSICAL EXAMINATION. The physical examination of a child with a musculoskeletal disorder must be thorough. It includes the careful evaluation of the musculoskeletal and neurologic systems as well as an appropriate general physical examination. Many common musculoskeletal disorders can be diagnosed by the history and physical examination alone. The examination of the musculoskeletal system includes four parts: observation, palpation, assessment of joint range of motion, and gait assessment in ambulatory children.

Observation. The first part of the musculoskeletal examination begins with inspection of the body. This must be accomplished by observing the child undressed. If the child can stand, posture, truncal alignment, and symmetry of the extremities can be evaluated. The skin is assessed for cutaneous lesions. The presence of café au lait spots may be indicative of neurofibromatosis, whereas a maculopapular rash may indicate juvenile rheumatoid arthritis. Infants or young children may be examined on their parent's lap so that they feel more secure and are more likely to be cooperative.

Palpation. The involved joint, area of the extremity, or trunk that is of concern should be palpated for tenderness, masses, soft tissue swelling, and increased warmth. Abnormal joints should also be palpated for effusion, synovial thickening, increased warmth, and areas of tenderness.

Joint Range of Motion. The range of motion of the involved joint or joints should be assessed and recorded. If the opposite joint is normal, this range should also be recorded for comparison purposes. It must be remembered that the range of motion of joints changes from infancy through childhood and into adolescence.

Gait Assessment. Gait disturbances are one of the most common parental concerns in children. It is, therefore, important to have a thorough understanding of the development of normal gait. Human gait is dynamic, complex, and repetitive. The gait cycle is the time between right heel strike followed by left toe-off, left heel strike, and right toe-off and ends with right heel strike. The five events describe one gait cycle and include two phases: stance and swing. The stance phase is the period of time during which one of the two feet is on the ground. The swing phase is the portion of the gait cycle during which a limb is being advanced forward without ground contact.

Neurologic maturation is necessary for the development of gait and the normal progression of developmental milestones. The normal 1-yr-old child has a wide-based stance and rapid cadence with short steps. The elbows are flexed and reciprocal arm motion is not present. Foot strike occurs without initial heel strike. A 2-yr-old child shows increased velocity and step length and diminished cadence compared with a 1-yr-old. Most of the adult gait patterns are present in children by 3 yr of age, with changes of velocity, stride, and cadence continuing to 7 yr. The gait characteristics of a 7-yr-old child are similar to those of an adult.

Common gait disturbances include limp, torsional variations (in-toeing and out-toeing), and toe walking. In evaluating gait disturbance, it is important to observe the child walking and running. The child must be sufficiently undressed to allow visualization of the lower extremities and trunk during ambulation.

LIMPING. Limping is categorized into either painful (antalgic) or nonpainful (Trendelenburg gait) on the basis of the length of the stance phase. In a painful gait, the stance phase is shortened as the child decreases the time spent on the painful extremity. In a nonpainful gait, which is indicative of underlying proximal muscle weakness or hip instability, the stance phase is equal between the involved and uninvolved sides, but the child will lean or shift the center of gravity over the involved extremity for balance. If the disorder is bilateral, it produces a waddling gait. The differential diagnosis of limping is extensive. The vast majority of causes involve the lower extremity, but it must be remembered that spinal disorders, especially spinal cord or peripheral nerve disorders, can also produce limping and difficulty walking. Antalgic gaits are predominantly a result of trauma, infection, neoplasia, and rheumatologic disorders. Trendelenburg gaits are generally due to congenital, developmental, or muscular disorders. Thus, antalgic gaits are acute processes, whereas Trendelenburg gaits are chronic. The differential diagnosis of limping is presented in Table 679–2 and causes of limping according to age are seen in Table 679–3.

TORSIONAL VARIATIONS. Torsional variations—in-toeing and out-toeing—are the most common gait disturbances that cause parents to seek advice from their pediatrician (see Chapters 680 and 681). Many do not require treatment because they are physiologic in origin and improve and resolve with normal growth and development. They produce significant anxiety and require the pediatrician to have a clear understanding of the cause and natural history to reassure the family. The common causes of in-toeing and out-toeing are presented in Table 679–4. The presence of in-toeing and out-toeing does not imply an abnormality of the foot but rather only the direction in which the foot is pointing during ambulation. The causes for torsional variations can occur from proximal (hip) to distal (foot) in the involved extremity. Some causes, such as clubfoot, are obvious, whereas others can be subtle.

Toe Walking. Toe walking or equinus gait is a less common cause of gait disturbance. It can be a normal finding in children up to 3 yr of age. Persistent toe walking thereafter or acquired toe walking at a later age is considered abnormal and requires careful evaluation. The common causes of unilateral and bilateral toe walking are listed in Table 679–5. The differential diagnosis for persistent or acquired toe walking include (1) neuromuscular disorders, such as cerebral palsy, Duchenne muscular dystrophy, or spinal cord abnormalities (tethered cord); (2) congenital tendo-Achilles contracture; (3) leg length discrepancy; and (4) habit.

Neurologic Evaluation. After the musculoskeletal examination, a careful neurologic evaluation must be performed. This should include muscle strength testing, sensory assessment, and evaluation of deep tendon and pathologic reflexes, such as the Babinski reflex. The pertinent negative and positive findings should be recorded for future reference. Part of the neurologic evaluation should also include assessment of the spine. This includes the presence of deformity, such as scoliosis or kyphosis, as well as spinal mobility. The child's ability to forward flex and reverse the normal lumbar lordosis is a sign of normal mobility. Areas of tenderness and muscle spasm are determined by palpation.

RADIOGRAPHIC ASSESSMENT. Radiography is the principal method for the evaluation of the pediatric musculoskeletal system. This can include routine radiographs as well as special procedures such as technetium bone scans, computed tomography, magnetic resonance imaging (MRI), and ultrasonography.

TABLE 679–2 Differential Diagnosis of Limping

Antalgic	Trendelenburg
Congenital	**Developmental**
Tarsal coalition	DDH
Acquired	Leg length discrepancy
LCPD	**Neuromuscular**
SCFE	Cerebral palsy
Trauma	Poliomyetitis
Sprains, strains, contusions	
Fractures	
Occult	
Toddler's fracture	
Neoplasia	
Benign	
Unicameral bone cyst	
Osteoid osteoma	
Malignant	
Osteogenic sarcoma	
Ewing's sarcoma	
Leukemia	
Spinal cord tumors	
Infectious	
Septic arthritis	
Osteomyelitis	
Acute	
Subacute	
Diskitis	
Rheumatologic	
Hip monoarticular synovitis	

LCPD = Legg-Calvé-Perthes disease; SCFE = slipped capital femoral epiphysis; DDH = developmental dysplasia of the hip.

From Thompson GH: Gait disturbances. In: *Kliegman RM, Nieder ML, Super DM (eds): Practical Strategies of Pediatric Diagnosis and Therapy. Philadelphia, WB Saunders, 1996, pp 757–778.*

TABLE 679–3 Common Causes of Limping According to Age

Age	Antalgic	Trendelenburg	Leg Length Discrepancy
Toddler (1–3 yr)	Infection	Hip dislocation (DDH)	⊖
	Septic arthritis	Neuromuscular disease	
	Hip	Cerebral palsy	
	Knee	Poliomyetitis	
	Osteomyelitis		
	Diskitis		
	Occult trauma		
	Toddler's fracture		
	Neoplasia		
Childhood (4–10 yr)	Infection	Hip dislocation (DDH)	⊕
	Septic arthritis	Neuromuscular disease	
	Hip	Cerebral palsy	
	Knee	Poliomyetitis	
	Osteomyelitis		
	Diskitis		
	Transient synovitis, hip		
	LCPD		
	Tarsal coalition		
	Rheumatologic disorder		
	JRA		
	Trauma		
	Neoplasia		
Adolescence (11+ yr)	SCFE		⊕
	Rheumatologic disorder		
	JRA		
	Trauma		
	Tarsal coalition		
	Neoplasia		

LCPD = Legg-Calvé-Perthes disease; JRA = juvenile rheumatoid arthritis; SCFE = slipped capital femoral epiphysis; DDH = developmental dysplasia of the hip; ⊖ = absent; ⊕ = present.

From Thompson GH: Gait disturbances. In: *Kliegman RM, Nieder ML, Super DM (eds): Practical Strategies of Pediatric Diagnosis and Therapy. Philadelphia, WB Saunders, 1996, pp 757–778.*

Routine Radiography. This is the first step in the evaluation of most pediatric musculoskeletal disorders. Routine radiographs consist of anteroposterior and lateral views of the involved joint, bone, or area. Comparison views of the opposite side, if uninvolved, may be helpful in difficult situations but are usually not necessary. The type of radiographs for each anatomic area are discussed in the sections on specific disorders.

Technetium Bone Scans. These are particularly useful in looking for occult lesions when routine radiographs are normal. Common indications for bone scans include (1) early septic arthritis or osteomyelitis; (2) tumors, such as osteoid osteomas; (3) metastatic lesions; (4) occult fractures, such as child abuse or a toddler fracture of the tibia; and (5) inflammatory disorders.

Computed Tomography. Coronal and axial cross-section studies with computed tomography can be beneficial in evaluating complex disorders of the spine, pelvis, and feet. It allows visualization of the bone anatomy and the relationship of bones to contiguous structures, which routine radiographs do not.

Magnetic Resonance Imaging. This avoids ionizing radiation and is presumed not to produce biologically harmful effects. It produces excellent anatomic images of the musculoskeletal system, including the spinal cord and brain. It is especially

TABLE 679–4 Common Causes of In-Toeing and Out-Toeing

In-Toeing	Out-Toeing
Internal femoral torsion	External femoral torsion
Internal tibial torsion	External tibial torsion
Metatarsus adductus	Calcaneovalgus feet
Talipes equinovarus (clubfoot)	Hypermobile pes planus

From Thompson GH: Pediatric orthopedics (spine, hips, lower extremities, and feet). In: *Marcus RE (ed): Orthopedics. Los Angeles, Practice Management Information Corporation, 1991, pp 209–300.*

TABLE 679–5 Common Causes of Toe Walking (Equinus Gait)

Unilateral	Bilateral
Neuromuscular disorder	Neuromuscular disorder
Cerebral palsy (hemiplegia)	Cerebral palsy (diplegia)
Leg length discrepancy	Duchenne muscular dystrophy
Hip dislocation (DDH)	Congenital tendo-Achilles contracture
	Habitual

DDH = Developmental dysplasia of the hip.
From Thompson GH: Gait disturbances. In: Kliegman RM, Nieder ML, Super DM (eds): Practical Strategies of Pediatric Diagnosis and Therapy. Philadelphia, WB Saunders, 1996, pp 757–778.

useful for soft tissue lesions, allowing distinction among different muscles or muscle groups. Cartilage structures can be visualized, and different forms can be distinguished (articular cartilage of the knee can be distinguished from the fibrocartilage of the meniscus). MRI is helpful in visualizing joints that are unossified, which may occur in the shoulders, elbows, and hips of young infants. MRI distinguishes physiologic changes that occur in the bone marrow with respect to age and disease such as avascular necrosis. In children, MRI can be useful in the evaluation of (1) avascular necrosis of bone, especially the capital femoral epiphysis or femoral head; (2) bone and soft tissue neoplasms; (3) intra-articular abnormalities of the knee joint; and (4) assessment of intraspinal pathologic conditions.

Ultrasonography. Ultrasonography has no ionizing radiation, no contrast material to be administered, no biologically harmful effects, and can be repeated as often as necessary. The equipment is portable but relatively expensive. Scans can be obtained in any plane. The disadvantages of ultrasonography include the following: (1) bone is not penetrated, (2) static images are difficult to interpret, and (3) the results are heavily operator-dependent. The major indications for ultrasonography are (1) fetal studies of the extremities and spine, (2) developmental dysplasia of the hip, (3) joint effusions, (4) occult neonatal spinal dysraphism; (5) foreign bodies in soft tissues, and (6) popliteal cysts of the knee.

LABORATORY STUDIES. Occasionally, hematologic tests are necessary in the evaluation of the pediatric musculoskeletal system. These may include a complete blood count, erythrocyte sedimentation rate, and C-reactive protein for infectious disorders, such as septic arthritis or osteomyelitis. Rheumatoid factor, antinuclear antibodies, and human leukocyte antigen B27 screens are necessary for children with suspected rheumatologic disorders. Creatine phosphokinase, aldolase, serum glutamic-oxaloacetic transaminase, and dystrophin testing are indicated in children with suspected disorders of striated muscle such as Duchenne or Becker muscular dystrophy.

TALKING WITH PARENTS. Talking effectively with parents of children with musculoskeletal problems is critically important and challenging. Many problems are normal or physiologic variations that resolve with growth and development and require only observation. This is particularly true in torsional variations of the lower extremities, which can produce significant anxiety in the family. Establishing a strong rapport with the family is an important component in the patient-family-physician relationship. Active treatment is indicated when the disorder has the potential to produce disability and also when the treatment is effective in altering the natural history. In many instances, the treatment may not significantly improve the child's condition initially, but by altering the natural history, problems in adult life, such as degenerative osteoarthritis, will be avoided.

Several steps are helpful in establishing a working relationship with parents. The diagnosis should be accurate and accompanied by a clear explanation of the cause and natural history of the disorder. Treatment options, including observation, should be discussed along with the expected results, both short- and long-term. If observation is recommended, a follow-up evaluation should be performed to document resolution and give the family additional reassurance.

Finally, not all physiologic conditions resolve. A small percentage of these disorders may persist into adolescence. These may require treatment if problems are to be avoided in adult life. The longer a problem persists, the greater is the chance that the problem will not resolve and may require treatment.

Dabney KW, Lipton G: Evaluation of limp in children. Curr Opin Pediatr 73:88, 1995.

Forero N, Okamura LA, Larson MA: Normal ranges of hip motion in neonates. J Pediatr Orthop 9:391, 1989.

Hall TR, Kangarloo H: Magnetic resonance imaging of the musculoskeletal system in children. Clin Orthop 244:119, 1989.

Harcke HT, Grissom LE, Finkelstein MS: Evaluation of the musculoskeletal system with sonography. AJR 150:1253, 1988.

Harcke HT, Kumar SJ: Current concepts review: The role of ultrasound in the diagnosis and management of congenital dislocation and dysplasia of the hip. J Bone Joint Surg 73A:622, 1991.

Jones ET: Use of computed axial tomography in pediatric orthopaedics. J Pediatr Orthop 1:329, 1981.

Myers MR, Thompson GH: Imaging the child with a limp. Pediatr Clin North Am 44:637, 1997.

Shulman LH, Sala DA, Chu ML, et al: Developmental implications of idiopathic toe walking. J Pediatr 130:541, 1997.

Sutherland DH, Olsten R, Cooper L, et al: The development of gait. J Bone Joint Surg 62A:336, 1980.

Tachdjian MO: Clinical Pediatric Orthopaedics. The Art of Diagnosis and Principles of Management. East Norwalk, CT, Appleton & Lange, 1997.

Thompson GH: Gait disturbances. *In*: Kliegman RM, Nieder ML, Super DM (eds): Practical Strategies in Pediatric Diagnosis and Therapy. Philadelphia, WB Saunders, 1996, pp 757–778.

Thompson GH, Cooperman DR: Neonatal orthopaedics. *In*: Fonaroff AA, Martin RJ (eds): Neonatal-Perinatal Medicine, 6th ed. St. Louis, Mosby-Year Book, 1997, pp 1709–1742.

Todd FN, Lamoreaux LW, Skinner SR, et al: Variations in the gait of normal children. A graph applicable to the documentation of abnormalities. J Bone Joint Surg 71A:196, 1989.

CHAPTER 680
The Foot and Toes

The foot and toes are important in stance and locomotion. Abnormalities affecting the foot can produce pain and abnormal shoe wear and can adversely affect function. The foot articulates with the lower end of the tibia. The ankle joint is a box joint, which allows foot dorsiflexion and plantar flexion with essentially no rotation. The talus articulates with the distal end of the tibia. Support is achieved through the medial malleolus of the tibia and the lateral malleolus of the distal fibula. The foot is divided into three regions: hindfoot, midfoot, and forefoot. The toes are a portion of the forefoot.

The hindfoot is composed of the talus and calcaneus. The latter forms the heel. The joint between these two bones is the talocalcaneal or subtalar joint. This joint has a gliding and rotatory motion, which allows inversion and eversion of the hindfoot. This is important for walking on uneven ground.

The midfoot is composed of the navicular, cuboid, and the three cuneiform bones. The midfoot and hindfoot articulate through the transverse tarsal joint (calcaneocuboid and talonavicular joints). This joint is important for midfoot rotation and for walking on uneven ground. Deformity or malalignment of subtalar, talonavicular, or calcaneocuboid joints can have a significant effect on the alignment and function of the foot and produces abnormal stress on the ankle joint.

The forefoot is composed of the metatarsals and toes. The 1st metatarsal is unique because it has a single physeal plate that is located proximally. The lateral four metatarsals have a single physis located distally. The great toe is composed of proximal and distal phalanges and a single interphalangeal joint. The lateral four toes have proximal, middle, and distal phalanges that articulate through a proximal interphalangeal joint and a distal interphalangeal joint. All phalanges have their physeal plates located proximally. Normal function of the foot and toes requires a coordinated action between the extrinsic muscles of the calf and intrinsic muscles of the foot.

FOOT DISORDERS

680.1 Metatarsus Adductus

Congenital metatarsus adductus, a common problem among infants and young children, is also known as metatarsus varus if the forefoot is supinated as well as adducted. It occurs equally in males and females and is bilateral in approximately 50% of patients. There are hereditary tendencies; it tends to be more common in 1st-born than in later children as a result of the increased molding effect from the primigravida uterus and abdominal wall. There is an association with hip dysplasia; approximately 10% of children with metatarsus adductus may have acetabular dysplasia. Careful examination of the hips is necessary in any child with metatarsus adductus. Pelvic radiographs are obtained in suggestive cases.

CLINICAL MANIFESTATIONS. The forefoot is adducted and occasionally supinated. The hindfoot and midfoot are normal. The lateral border of the foot is convex, and the base of the 5th metatarsal appears prominent (Fig. 680–1). The medial border of the foot is concave. There is usually an increased interval between the 1st and 2nd toes, with the great toe being held in a greater varus position. Ankle dorsiflexion and plantar flexion are normal. Forefoot mobility can vary from flexible to rigid. This is assessed by stabilizing the hindfoot and midfoot in a neutral position with one hand and applying pressure over the 1st metatarsal head with the other. In the walking child with an uncorrected metatarsus adductus deformity, an in-toe gait and abnormal shoe wear may occur.

RADIOGRAPHIC EVALUATION. Radiographs of the foot are not routinely necessary in metatarsus adductus because they do not demonstrate forefoot mobility. Anteroposterior (AP) and lateral weight-bearing or simulated weight-bearing radiographs are indicated when there is rigidity or failure of spontaneous improvement with growth. The AP radiographs demonstrate adduction of the metatarsals at the tarsometatarsal articulation and an increased intermetatarsal angle between the 1st and 2nd metatarsals. The lateral four metatarsals appear to have increased closeness and occasionally overlap at their base. The hindfoot and midfoot are normal.

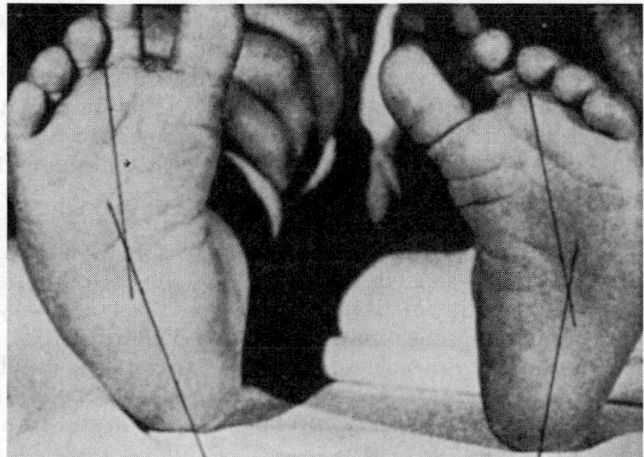

Figure 680–1 Metatarsus adductus. A line bisecting the hindfoot should pass through the second toe or between the second and third toes.

TREATMENT. The treatment of metatarsus adductus is predominantly nonoperative. There are limited indications for surgery.

Nonoperative. Most children with metatarsus adductus deformities respond to conservative treatment. The feet may be classified into three groups depending on forefoot flexibility. Type I feet are flexible and actively and passively overcorrect into mild abduction. Voluntary correction can be elicited by stimulating the peroneal musculature by stroking the lateral border of the foot. These feet usually require no treatment. Type II feet correct to the neutral position both passively and actively. These feet may benefit from an orthosis or corrective shoes such as straight or reverse last shoes. These are worn full-time (22 hr/day), and the condition is re-evaluated in 4–6 wk. If improvement occurs, treatment can be continued. If there is no improvement, serial plaster casts are necessary. Type III feet are rigid and do not correct to neutral. These feet are treated with serial casts. The best results are obtained when casting is initiated before 8 mo of age. Once correction has been achieved, orthoses or corrective shoes may be used for an additional 1–2 mo to maintain correction. Mild hallux varus, the "searching toe," may persist for several years after conservative correction and may be of concern to the parents. However, it eventually disappears with growth and the wearing of shoes.

Operative. Significant residual metatarsus adductus in children 4 yr of age and older may require surgical intervention. Children 4–6 yr of age usually require only a soft tissue release. Serial casting is performed postoperatively until forefoot correction has been obtained. This usually requires 2–3 mo. Children 6 yr of age or older require base of the metatarsal osteotomies or other osseous procedures to achieve satisfactory correction. The sequelae of mild residual metatarsus adductus are minimal.

680.2 Calcaneovalgus Feet

The calcaneovalgus foot is a relatively common finding in the newborn and is secondary to in utero positioning. This condition is manifested by a hyperdorsiflexed foot with forefoot abduction and increased heel valgus. It is usually associated with external tibial torsion. It is often unilateral but occasionally may be bilateral. In utero, the plantar surface of the foot was against the wall of the uterus, forcing it into a hyperdorsiflexed, abducted, and externally rotated position. The position also produces the external tibial torsion. When these two conditions are combined with the normal newborn increased external rotation of the hip (tight posterior capsule), it results in a lower extremity that appears excessively externally rotated.

CLINICAL MANIFESTATIONS. The infant typically presents with an out-toe position of the involved extremity. The dorsum of the foot can easily be brought into contact with the anterior aspect of the lower leg; the forefoot is abducted, and the heel is in valgus. This should not be confused with the neonatal maturity classification of Dubowitz (see Chapter 93). External tibial torsion (20–50 degrees) is a common associated finding. Ankle motion shows normal or almost normal plantar flexion.

Three conditions must be distinguished from the calcaneovalgus foot: (1) congenital vertical talus, (2) posteromedial bow of the tibia, and (3) neuromuscular abnormalities with paralysis of the gastrocnemius muscle. The differentiation can usually be made during the physical examination.

RADIOGRAPHIC EVALUATION. AP and lateral simulated weight-bearing radiographs of the feet may be necessary to differentiate between the calcaneovalgus foot and a congenital vertical talus. In a calcaneovalgus foot, the radiographs are normal or there may be increased hindfoot valgus and forefoot abduction. If a posteromedial bow of the tibia is suspected, AP and lateral radiographs of the tibia and fibula are necessary.

TREATMENT. The typical calcaneovalgus foot requires no treatment. The hyperdorsiflexion of the foot resolves during the 1st 6 mo of life. The external tibial torsion, however, persists and follows the same natural history as internal tibial torsion. Spontaneous improvement does not occur until the child begins to pull to stand and walk independently. It takes approximately 6–12 mo thereafter for complete correction to occur. The majority of infants with calcaneovalgus feet and external tibial torsion have normally aligned feet and lower extremities by 2 yr of age.

680.3 Talipes Equinovarus (Clubfoot)

A clubfoot is a common foot deformity that involves not only the foot but also the entire lower leg. It can be classified into three groups: (1) congenital, (2) teratologic, and (3) positional. The congenital clubfoot is usually an isolated abnormality, whereas the teratologic form is associated with a neuromuscular disorder, such as myelodysplasia, arthrogryposis multiplex congenita, or a syndrome complex. The congenital form has also been called *idiopathic* or *neurogenic* on the basis of possible causes. The positional clubfoot is a normal foot that has been held in a deformed position in utero.

The *cause* of clubfoot is unknown. There are inheritance factors, and these are currently considered multifactorial with a major influence from a single autosomal dominant gene. Biopsy studies of the extrinsic muscles of the calf have indicated a probable neuromuscular cause. There are fiber type disproportions and increased neuromuscular junctions within these muscles. These findings are in contrast to previous etiologic theories in which deformity of the talus was believed to be the primary abnormality. Although the talus is certainly deformed with medial deviation of the head and neck, this is considered to be a secondary deformity.

CLINICAL MANIFESTATIONS. The congenital form of clubfoot, which constitutes approximately 75% of all cases, is characterized by (1) the absence of other congenital abnormalities, (2) variable rigidity of the foot, (3) mild calf atrophy, and (4) mild hypoplasia of the tibia, fibula, and bones of the foot. It occurs more commonly in males (2:1) and is bilateral in 50% of cases. The probability for a random occurrence is approximately 1 in 1,000 births; within involved families, the probability is approximately 3% for subsequent siblings and 20–30% for offspring of involved parents.

Examination of the infant clubfoot demonstrates hindfoot equinus, hindfoot and midfoot varus, forefoot adduction, and variable rigidity. All these findings are secondary to the medial dislocation of the talonavicular joint. In the older child, the calf and foot atrophy are more obvious than in the infant, regardless of how well corrected or functional the foot. These findings are due to the causative aspects of clubfoot, not the method of treatment.

RADIOGRAPHIC EVALUATION. AP and lateral standing or simulated weight-bearing radiographs are used in the assessment of clubfeet. Non–weight-bearing radiographs are not helpful. Multiple different radiographic measurements can be made. The navicular bone, which is the primary site of deformity, does not ossify until 3 yr in the female and 4 yr in the male. This necessitates line measurements to determine the position of the unossified navicular bone and the overall alignment of the foot.

TREATMENT

Nonoperative. Conservative treatment is initiated in all infants, although a significant proportion of children later require surgery. Nonoperative treatment includes taping, the use of malleable splints, and serial plaster casts. Taping and malleable splints are particularly useful in premature infants until they attain an appropriate size for casting. Serial plaster casts are the major method of nonoperative treatment. Before the cast is applied, the foot is gently manipulated toward the corrected position. The cast is then applied and changed at 1–2 wk intervals. Complete correction, both clinically and radiographically, should be achieved by 3 mo of age. If this is accomplished, holding casts are then used for an additional 3–6 mo followed by orthoses or corrective shoes until the child is walking well. Failure to achieve clinical and radiographic correction by 3 mo of age is an indication for surgical treatment. Further attempts at conservative management may result in articular damage and a midfoot breech (rocker-bottom deformity).

Operative. The current method of surgical treatment is a complete soft tissue release. This is usually performed between 6 and 12 mo of age. Satisfactory long-term results can be expected in 80–90% of cases. Unsatisfactory results that require additional treatment are usually secondary to extrinsic muscle imbalance rather than incomplete correction. The use of tendon transfers and bone procedures, including arthrodeses (fusions), are primarily for salvage of recurrent clubfoot or incompletely corrected feet. Centralization of the tibialis anterior tendon has been particularly beneficial in young children with a dynamic pes varus, the most common residual abnormality. Triple arthrodeses are indicated in painful, deformed feet in adolescence.

680.4 Congenital Vertical Talus

Congenital vertical talus is an uncommon foot deformity with causes similar to those of talipes equinovarus. It must be distinguished from a calcaneovalgus foot, which is much more common. Typically, a congenital vertical talus is a rigid rocker-bottom deformity. The majority of these infants have an underlying disorder such as teratologic malformation (myelodysplasia and arthrogryposis multiplex congenita) or a syndrome such as trisomy 18.

CLINICAL MANIFESTATIONS. The characteristic of a congenital vertical talus is a rocker-bottom foot. There is hindfoot equinovalgus, a convex plantar surface, forefoot abduction and dorsiflexion, and rigidity. A careful physical examination must be performed on all children to look for an underlying disorder or syndrome.

RADIOGRAPHIC EVALUATION. Radiographic evaluation of a congenital vertical talus consists of an AP and lateral weight-bearing or simulated weight-bearing radiograph of the feet as well as a maximal plantar-flexed lateral view. This typically reveals the vertically oriented talus, the dorsal displacement and abduction of the midfoot on the hindfoot, hindfoot valgus, and mobility.

TREATMENT. As in clubfeet, nonoperative treatment is the initial method of treatment of congenital vertical talus, although most cases later require surgical correction.

Nonoperative. Serial casting after manipulation of the feet is performed beginning at birth. The forefoot is manipulated into equinus in an attempt to reduce the navicular onto the head of the talus. However, the success rate with nonoperative treatment is exceedingly low.

Operative. The operative management of congenital vertical talus is predominantly through a complete soft tissue release performed as a one-stage or two-stage procedure. Occasionally, in severe deformities, a naviculectomy may be necessary to realign the midfoot and hindfoot adequately. Fortunately, this is rarely necessary. In older children with persistent hindfoot valgus and pronation, a subtalar arthrodesis or a triple arthrodesis may be necessary to realign the foot and provide stability.

The goals of treatment of congenital vertical talus are pessimistic and include a plantigrade, pain-free foot that is able to wear shoes. Orthotic management is frequently necessary for a prolonged period postoperatively, if not for life, because of associated muscle weakness resulting from an underlying disorder.

680.5 Hypermobile Pes Planus (Flexible Flatfeet)

Hypermobile flatfeet or pronated feet are common sources of concern of parents. In general, these children are asymptomatic and have no functional limitations. Flatfeet are common in neonates and toddlers because of an associated laxity in the bone-ligament complexes of the feet and fat in the area of the medial longitudinal arch. These children usually demonstrate significant improvement by 6 yr of age. In the older child, flexible flatfeet are usually secondary to generalized ligamentous laxity, an autosomal dominant condition.

CLINICAL MANIFESTATIONS. In the non–weight-bearing position in the older child with a flexible flatfoot, the normal medial longitudinal arch is present, but in the weight-bearing position, the foot becomes pronated with varying degrees of pes planus and heel valgus. Instead of weight-bearing over the lateral column of the foot, weight is shifted medially, producing pronation. Subtalar motion is normal or slightly increased. Loss of subtalar motion indicates a rigid flatfoot. Common causes of rigid flatfeet include a tendo-Achilles contracture, tarsal coalitions, neuromuscular abnormalities (cerebral palsy), and familial trait.

RADIOGRAPHIC EVALUATION. Routine radiographs of asymptomatic flexible flatfeet are usually not indicated. AP and lateral weight-bearing radiographs are obtained if there is rigidity or symptoms. On the AP radiograph, there is excessive heel valgus. The lateral view shows distortion of the normal straight line relationship between the long axis of the talus and the 1st metatarsal with either a sag of the talonavicular or naviculocuneiform joint, resulting in flattening of the normal medial longitudinal arch.

TREATMENT. The treatment of flexible flatfeet is conservative. Affected children do not have symptoms predictably. Therefore, modified shoes and orthoses do not significantly alter the clinical or radiographic appearance of the feet. It should be emphasized that the diagnosis of flexible flatfeet is usually not possible until after 6 yr of age. Treatment is indicated for abnormal shoe wear or symptoms not attributable to other causes. Feet that are symptomatic with vigorous physical activities usually respond readily to the use of a commercially available medial longitudinal arch support. Custom-made supports are much more expensive and, in most cases, not any more effective.

680.6 Tarsal Coalition

Tarsal coalition, also known as peroneal spastic flatfoot, is a relatively common foot disorder characterized by a painful, rigid flatfoot deformity and peroneal (lateral calf) muscle spasm but without true spasticity. It represents a congenital fusion or failure of segmentation between two or more tarsal bones. However, any condition that alters the normal gliding and rotatory motion of the subtalar joint may produce the clinical appearance of a tarsal coalition. Thus, congenital malformations, arthritis or inflammatory disorders, infection, neoplasms, and trauma can be possible causes.

The most common tarsal coalitions occur at the medial talocalcaneal (subtalar) facet and between the calcaneus and navicular (calcaneonavicular) tarsal bones. Coalitions can be fibrous, cartilaginous, or osseous. Tarsal coalition occurs in approximately 1% of the general population; it appears to be inherited as a unifactorial autosomal dominant trait with nearly full penetrance. Approximately 60% of calcaneonavicular and 50% of the medial facet talocalcaneal coalitions are bilateral.

CLINICAL MANIFESTATIONS. The onset of symptoms usually occurs during the 2nd decade of life. Although mild limitation of subtalar motion and the flatfoot may have been present since early childhood, the onset of symptoms varies with the age at which the fibrous or cartilaginous bar begins to ossify and further decrease motion. The talonavicular coalition ossifies between 3 and 5 yr of age, the calcaneonavicular coalition between 8 and 12 yr, and the medial facet talocalcaneal coalition between 12 and 16 yr. The pain is typically felt laterally in the hindfoot and radiates proximally along the lateral malleolus and distal fibula (peroneal muscle spasm). Symptoms are frequently aggravated by sports or walking on uneven ground. Clinically, the foot is flat or pronated both in the weight-bearing and the non–weight-bearing positions. Subtalar and transverse tarsal joint motion is diminished or absent, and attempts at motion may produce pain.

RADIOGRAPHIC EVALUATION. The diagnosis of a tarsal coalition is confirmed radiographically. AP and lateral weight-bearing radiographs and an oblique radiograph of the foot should be obtained. Beaking of the anterior aspect of the talus on the lateral view is suspicious for a tarsal coalition. The oblique view demonstrates a calcaneonavicular coalition. Axial views through the hindfoot can be useful in the diagnosis of the medial facet talocalcaneal coalition. However, computed tomography is the procedure of choice in the evaluation of coalitions, especially those involving the subtalar joint.

TREATMENT. The treatment of symptomatic tarsal coalitions varies according to the type of coalition, age of the patient, extent of the coalition, presence or absence of degenerative osteoarthritis, and degree of disability. The treatment may be nonoperative or operative. Nonoperative treatment may consist of cast immobilization, shoe inserts, or orthotics. Operative management consists of excision of the coalition and interposition of muscle (calcaneonavicular) and fat or split flexor hallucis longus tendon (medial facet talocalcaneal) to prevent hematoma formation and reossification of the coalition (Fig. 680–2). Resections are effective in relieving pain, improving subtalar motion, and allowing resumption of normal activities. However, if degenerative osteoarthritis is present, a triple arthrodesis may be necessary.

680.7 Cavus Feet

Cavus feet represent an exaggeration in the medial longitudinal arch associated with hindfoot varus and occasionally adduction of the forefoot. When the latter occurs, the deformity is called a *cavovarus deformity.* This type of deformity appears most commonly during the middle childhood years. Both idiopathic and neuromuscular types(hereditary motor-sensory neuropathies)may be seen. In either case, a cavovarus foot is usually a progressive deformity, leading to considerable compromise of foot function. These deformities tend to be rigid. The most important aspect of the evaluation of a patient with a cavovarus foot is to establish an accurate diagnosis. Possible causes include spinal cord disease and peripheral neuropathies, such as Charcot-Marie-Tooth disease.

TREATMENT. Aggressive treatment is usually necessary for moderate to severe cavus feet. This usually involves reconstructive surgery. Special shoes and shoe modifications are not helpful from a therapeutic standpoint but sometimes may be warranted to provide relief from abnormal pressure during weight-bearing. Surgical correction by soft tissue balancing and occasionally by osseous procedures is usually necessary.

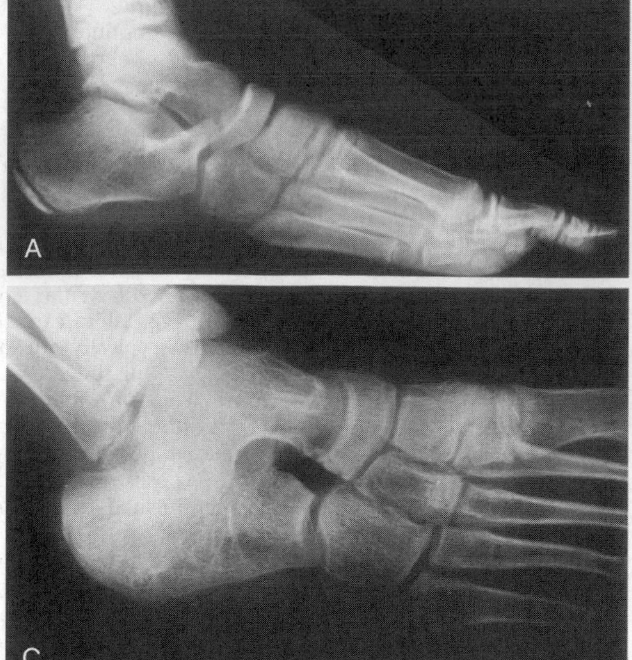

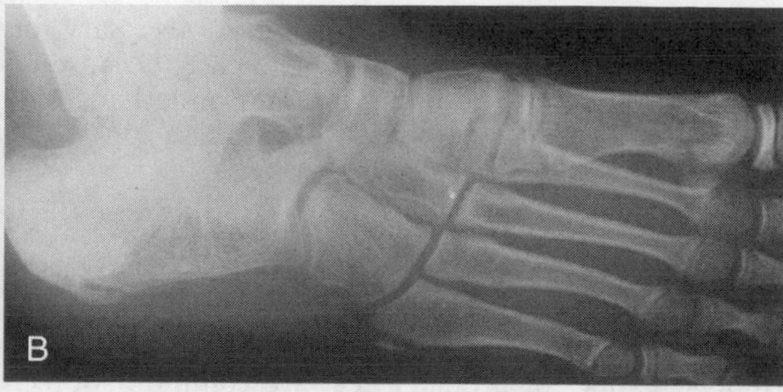

Figure 680–2 *A.* Standing lateral radiograph of the foot of a 12-yr-old girl with limited, painful subtalar joint motion. There is an extension of the anterior process of the calcaneus toward the navicular. This has been termed the "anteater's nose" and is indicative of calcaneonavicular coalition. *B.* The oblique radiograph demonstrates the calcaneonavicular coalition. The small, unossified area in the center of the coalition is actually cartilaginous and will ultimately form a complete osseous bridge. *C.* Oblique radiograph after excision of the coalition and interposition of the extensor digitorum brevis muscle to prevent reformation. This procedure restores subtalar joint motion and relieves discomfort.

680.8 Osteochondroses

Osteochondroses are pathologic processes that involve infarction, revascularization, resorption, and replacement of the affected bone. These are commonly termed *idiopathic avascular necrosis.* Both the tarsal navicular (*Köhler's disease*) and the head or epiphysis of the 2nd metatarsal (*Freiberg's disease*) may sustain avascular necrosis. These conditions are relatively uncommon and both produce pain, especially with activities. Symptomatic treatment is based on the severity of the child's complaint. Occasionally, a short leg cast and a non–weight-bearing stance with crutches may be helpful in relieving symptoms.

As the older child enters the period of pubescent growth spurt, the fibrocartilaginous insertion of major muscle groups to bone is vulnerable to microfracture, resulting in inflammatory and healing responses. The usual site of microfractures in the foot is the attachment of the tendo-Achilles (heel cord) to the posterior aspect of the calcaneus. This produces another osteochondrosis: *Sever's disease,* which is a common cause of heel pain. Symptoms wax and wane depending on the level of activity, and until skeletal maturity is achieved, the usual residual manifestation, if any, is bony enlargement at the tendon insertion site secondary to overgrowth during the healing response. Treatment is again symptomatic and includes the use of an anti-inflammatory agent and heel cord stretching.

680.9 Puncture Wounds of the Foot

For most puncture wound injuries, extensively cleansing the wound, ensuring prophylaxis for tetanus, and administering a broad-spectrum oral antibiotic are all that is needed. When infection occurs despite these measures, *Pseudomonas aeruginosa* and *Staphylococcus aureus* are the usual offending organisms. In *Pseudomonas* osteomyelitis, the puncture usually injured the bone or joint. This is most common when the puncture wound is through the sole of a sneaker. The heat and perspiration and the material within the sneakers tend to promote the growth of this organism. Treatment of established infections includes wound debridement to remove necrotic tissue. Broad-spectrum antibiotics are administered, including methicillin and gentamicin, pending the outcome of the cultures. Subsequent antibiotic treatment is based on the results of these tests. After surgery, further microbial therapy is continued for 10–14 days.

680.10 Toe Deformities

ADOLESCENT BUNIONS

Adolescent bunions, a common pediatric foot deformity, are more common in girls (3:1); there is frequently a positive family history. There are both intrinsic and extrinsic factors associated with this deformity. The intrinsic factors include metatarsus primus varus, oblique 1st metatarsal–medial cuneiform articulation, short 1st metatarsal, and pes planus. Extrinsic factors include abnormal shoe wear (narrow toe box with an elevated heel) and a subtle underlying neurologic disorder, such as mild cerebral palsy.

CLINICAL MANIFESTATIONS. An adolescent presenting with bunions requires careful evaluation. It must be determined whether it is the symptoms or the deformity, or both, that are of concern to the patient and the family. If pain is present, it must be ascertained whether it is due to activities and whether it produces functional limitation. It is also important to know what type of shoes are being worn when symptoms are present. When evaluating the foot, weight-bearing alignment, walking alignment, mobility of the 1st metatarsophalangeal joint, presence or absence of callous formation, and preferred shoe style must be determined.

RADIOGRAPHIC EVALUATION. AP and lateral weight-bearing radiographs of the feet are necessary in the assessment of adolescent bunions. This allows measurement of the (1) intermetatarsal angle, (2) hallux valgus angle, (3) alignment of the 1st metatarsal–medial cuneiform joint, and (4) pes planus. The normal intermetatarsal angle between the long axes of the 1st and 2nd metatarsals is 10 degrees or less, and the normal hallux valgus angle is 25 degrees or less. A short 1st metatarsal can be diagnosed from these radiographs.

TREATMENT

Nonoperative. Conservative management of adolescent bunions consists primarily of shoe modifications. It is important that footwear accommodate the width of the forefoot. Adolescents should be discouraged from wearing narrow-toed shoes with elevated heels. In the presence of a pes planus, an orthotic to restore the medial longitudinal arch may be beneficial.

Operative. The indications for surgical correction include an intermetatarsal angle between 12 and 18 degrees and failure of nonoperative management. The major indication for surgical treatment is symptoms, not cosmesis. Surgery rarely restores the foot to a completely normal appearance but is effective in narrowing the width of the forefoot, correcting the hallux valgus, improving weight-bearing alignment, and relieving symptoms. Surgery typically consists of a combination of a soft tissue and bone procedure. The osseous procedures are numerous and can be performed on the 1st metatarsal or medial cuneiform, or both.

CURLY TOES

The most common lesser toe deformity of childhood is curly toes. These represent a flexion deformity at the proximal interphalangeal joint with lateral rotation and varus alignment of the toe (Fig. 680–3). The 4th and 5th toes are the most commonly involved. Occasionally, the 2nd and 3rd toes are involved. The disorder is usually familial, bilateral, symmetric, and asymptomatic. The condition is secondary to short, tight flexor digitorum longus and flexor digitorum brevis tendons. The tightness in these tendons can be demonstrated by dorsiflexing the foot, which will increase the curling of the toes. Plantar flexion usually results in improvement. Radiographic evaluation of curly toe deformities is not necessary.

TREATMENT. In infants and young children, curly toe deformities should be observed because 25–50% resolve spontaneously. Taping or splinting is ineffective. At 3–4 yr of age, an open tenotomy of the toe flexor tendons can be performed. In older children and adolescents, a proximal interphalangeal joint fusion may be necessary.

OVERLAPPING FIFTH TOE

An overlapping 5th toe is a relatively common condition in which the 5th toe is adducted and overrides the 4th toe. It results in abnormal shoe wear and pain in approximately 50% of patients.

Examination of the 5th toe shows an extensor digitorum longus contracture. There is also a dorsal metatarsophalangeal joint contracture. The 5th toe is adducted, extended, and laterally rotated. It may be possible to realign the toe passively but the corrected position cannot be maintained. Radiographs are not necessary in the evaluation of an overlapping fifth toe.

TREATMENT. Nonoperative treatment is ineffective; it can be corrected surgically. The most common procedure consists of a racket-shaped incision around the base of the toe. The extensor digitorum longus tendon is released along with the dorsal joint contracture. This allows the toe to be placed into its normal position.

POLYDACTYLY

Polydactyly is a relatively common deformity. It usually involves the 5th toe. It occurs in approximately 2 in 1,000 births. Approximately 30% of patients have a positive family history. It is important to assess for syndromes and other organ anomalies as well as other digit deformities such as polydactyly of the hand and syndactyly of adjacent toes. Duplication of the great toe is also possible. There may be associated metatarsal abnormalities.

AP and lateral weight-bearing radiographs of both feet are obtained in the management of children with polydactyly. This demonstrates whether the duplication is articulated or rudimentary and whether there are metatarsal abnormalities.

TREATMENT. Rudimentary-type digits can be ligated at birth and allowed to autoamputate. Those that are articulated require excision at approximately 1 yr of age. The guidelines in polydactyly are to save the digit with best axial alignment, resect the projecting symptomatic toe, repair the capsule, balance the soft tissues, and shave any metatarsal prominences.

SYNDACTYLY

Syndactyly is a relatively common lesser toe condition. Cases of syndactyly are usually asymptomatic, and there may be a positive familial history. They can be classified into *zygosyndactyly* and *polysyndactyly.* In zygosyndactyly, there is complete or incomplete webbing. This usually occurs between the 2nd and 3rd toes. In polysyndactyly, there may be a duplication of the 5th toe, with a syndactyly between the 4th and 5th toes. Synostosis of the lateral metatarsals is common.

TREATMENT. Zygosyndactyly does not require treatment, but polysyndactyly may because of the associated anomalies.

HAMMER TOE

A hammer toe is similar to a curly toe except there is no malrotation of the involved toe. There is a flexion deformity at the proximal interphalangeal joint, and the metatarsophalangeal joint is extended. The metatarsal head may appear depressed. It is usually symmetric and bilateral, with the 2nd toe most commonly involved. The major problems with this deformity are painful calluses over the proximal phalangeal joint.

TREATMENT. Passive stretching and taping may be helpful in infants and young children. However, the majority require surgical correction of the contracted flexor digitorum longus and flexor digitorum brevis tendons. Occasionally, tendon transfers are required.

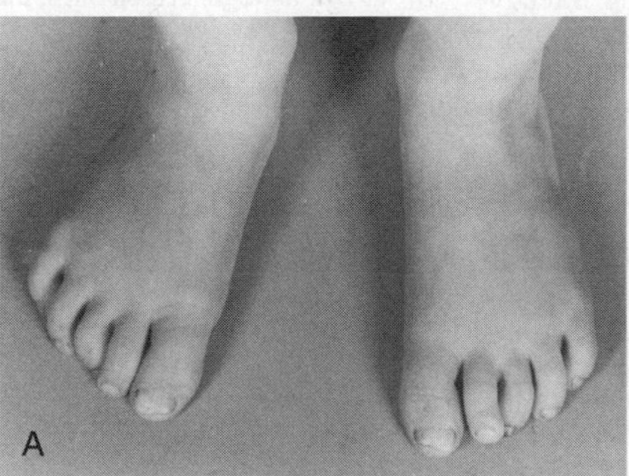

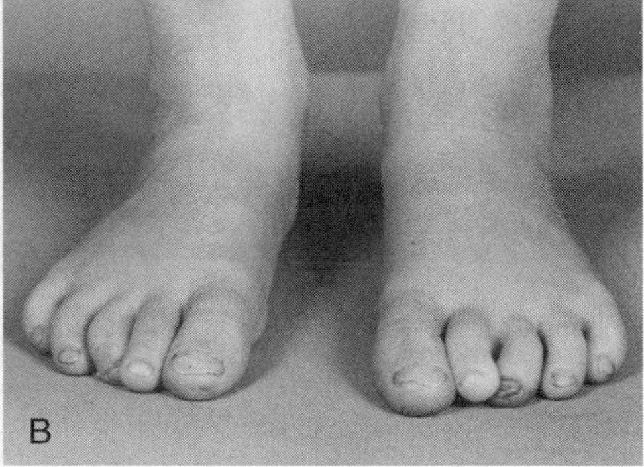

Figure 680–3 *A.* Bilateral curly toe deformities in a 4-yr-old. There is flexion and varus rotation of the lateral three toes. *B.* The frontal view better demonstrates the curling of the toes, especially the third toes.

MALLET TOE

Mallet toe is a flexion deformity at the distal interphalangeal joint. It may become symptomatic in adolescents as a result of a dorsal callosity or perhaps from nail bed irritation.

TREATMENT. Nonoperative treatment is usually ineffective. Correction is usually obtained by the release of the flexor digitorum longus tendon. Occasionally, in the adolescent, a distal interphalangeal joint fusion may be necessary.

CLAW TOE

Claw toes represent an extension contracture with dorsal subluxation of the metatarsophalangeal joint in association with flexion deformities of both the proximal and distal interphalangeal joints. They can occur idiopathically, but the majority are associated with a pes cavus deformity and are secondary to an underlying neurologic disorder, such as Charcot-Marie-Tooth disease. These deformities are complex and require careful assessment to determine the underlying cause.

TREATMENT. Claw toes are treated surgically, usually with soft tissue rebalancing and, occasionally, fusions of the proximal interphalangeal joint.

ANNULAR BANDS

Annular bands or constriction rings are relatively common congenital disorders that involve the toes and fingers. They may consist of simple constriction rings or rings with deformity of the distal part of the toe with swelling and lymphedema. Occasionally, the rings may be deep enough to have produced an amputation. Sometimes there will be an associated syndactyly with the adjacent toe. Annular bands of the lower extremity are frequently associated with clubfeet.

TREATMENT. The treatment of annular or constriction bands is predominantly observation. If there are deep rings with swelling and lymphedema, surgery may be necessary to relieve the congestion.

SUBUNGUAL EXOSTOSES

Subungual exostosis is an uncommon problem that primarily involves the great toe. It may simulate an ingrown toenail. On physical examination, there is a palpable mass beneath the toenail. The toe may appear irritated and similar to an infection; however, palpation reveals a mass rather than granulation tissue. Radiographs of the toe demonstrate exostosis of the distal phalanx.

TREATMENT. Subungual exostoses are managed by partial excision of the nail bed and removal of the underlying exostosis.

INGROWN TOENAIL

Ingrown toenails are relatively common in infants and young children and later in adolescents. These typically involve the medial and lateral borders of the great toe.

TREATMENT. Conservative treatment is usually effective. This consists of appropriate shoe modification, warm soaks, antibiotics, elevation of the nail edge, and proper nail-cutting techniques. If this fails, surgery with wedge section of the involved border, including the nail matrix, is usually effective.

680.11 *Painful Foot*

The causes of a painful foot can usually be determined from history and physical examination. The common causes are listed in Table 680–1. The specific treatment depends on the diagnosis and occasionally on the age of the child or adolescent.

TABLE 680–1 Differential Diagnosis of Foot Pain by Age

0–6 Yr	6–12 Yr	12–20 Yr
Poor-fitting shoes	Poor-fitting shoes	Poor-fitting shoes
Foreign body	Sever's disease	Stress fracture
Fracture	Enthesopathy (JRA)	Foreign body
Osteomyelitis	Foreign body	Ingrown toenail
Leukemia	Accessory navicular	Metatarsalgia
Puncture wound	Tarsal coalition	Plantar fasciitis
Drawing of blood	Ewing's sarcoma	Osteochondroses (avascular necrosis)
Dactylitis	Hypermobile flatfoot	Freiberg
JRA	Trauma (sprains, fractures)	Köhler
	Puncture wound	Achilles tendinitis
		Trauma (sprains)
		Plantar warts
		Tarsal coalition

JRA = juvenile rheumatoid arthritis.

680.12 *Shoes*

Clothing is worn for comfort, to enhance appearance, and for protection. Shoes should be selected on the same basis. Shoes are not corrective, and the foot does not need support for normal activities. The foot requires mobility to function normally. It has been demonstrated that populations that are predominantly barefoot have better feet than those that wear shoes. The best shoes for children are those that simulate the bare foot. They should be flexible, flat, and nonconstricting and made of material that breathes. Shoes do not have to be expensive.

Because overuse foot symptoms are common, especially in the athletic adolescent, shock-absorbing shoes are a good choice. The thick-cushioned sole absorbs some of the shock of impact and thereby decreases discomfort.

Shoe modifications are sometimes appropriate for a specific problem. A lift may be prescribed if the limb is short, and a shoe insert may be helpful for the stiff and deformed foot or to distribute the weight load more evenly over the sole.

Metatarsus Adductus

Crawford AH, Gabriel KR: Foot and ankle problems. Orthop Clin North Am 18:649, 1987.

Farsetti P, Weinstein SL, Ponseti IV: The long-term functional and radiographic outcomes of untreated and non-operatively treated metatarsus adductus. J Bone Joint Surg 76A:257, 1994.

Calcaneovalgus Foot

Gibson DA: Torsional variations in the lower limbs of children. Appl Ther 8:236, 1966.

Congenital Talipes Equinovarus (Clubfoot)

Cowell HR, Wein BK: Current concepts review: Genetic aspects of clubfoot. J Bone Joint Surg 62A:1381, 1980.

Handelsman J, Badalamente MA: Neuromuscular studies in clubfoot. J Pediatr Orthop 1:23, 1981.

Herzenberg JE, Carroll NC, Christofersen MR, et al: Clubfoot analysis with three-dimensional computer modeling. J Pediatr Orthop 8:257, 1988.

Howard CB, Benson MKD: Clubfoot: Its pathological anatomy. J Pediatr Orthop 13:654, 1993.

Ponseti IV: Current concepts review: Treatment of congenital club foot. J Bone Joint Surg 74A:448, 1992.

Thompson GH, Simons GW III: Congenital talipes equinovarus (clubfeet) and metatarsus adductus. *In:* Drennan JC (ed): The Child's Foot and Ankle. New York, Raven Press, 1992, pp 97–133.

Congenital Vertical Talus

Drennan JC: Instructional Course Lecture. Congenital vertical talus. J Bone Joint Surg 77A:1916, 1995.

Hypermobile Flatfoot

Bordelon FL: Hypermobile flatfoot in children: Comprehension, evaluation, and treatment. Clin Orthop 181:7, 1983.

Mosca VS: Instructional Course Lecture. Flexible flatfoot and skewfoot. J Bone Joint Surg 77A:1937, 1995.

Staheli LT, Chew DE, Corbet M: The longitudinal arch: A survey of 882 feet in normal children and adults. J Bone Joint Surg 69A:426, 1987.
Wenger DR, Mauldin D, Speck G, et al: Corrective shoes and inserts as treatment for a flexible flatfoot in infants and children. J Bone Joint Surg 71A:800, 1989.

Tarsal Coalition
Blakemore LC, Cooperman DR, Thompson GH: The rigid flatfoot: Tarsal coalitions. Foot Ankle Clin 1998, in press.
Gonzalez PK, Kumar SJ: Calcaneonavicular coalition treated by resection and interposition of the extensor digitorum brevis muscle. J Bone Joint Surg 72A:71, 1990.
Herzenberg JE, Goldner JL, Martinez S, et al: Computerized tomography of talocalcaneal tarsal coalitions: A clinical and anatomic study. Foot Ankle 6:273, 1986.
Kulik SA Jr, Clanton TO: Tarsal coalition. Foot Ankle Int 17:286, 1996.
Kumar SJ, Guille JT, Couto JC: Osseous and non-osseous coalition of the middle facet of the talocalcaneal joint. J Bone Joint Surg 74A:529, 1992.
Leonard MA: The inheritance of tarsal coalition and its relationship to spastic flat foot. J Bone Joint Surg 56B:520, 1974.
Thompson GH, Cooperman DR: Peroneal spastic flatfoot. *In:* Gould JS (ed): Operative Foot Surgery. Philadelphia, WB Saunders 1993, pp 858–877.

Puncture Wounds of the Foot
Laughlin TJ, Armstrong DJ, Caporusso J, Lavery LA: Soft-tissue and bone infections from puncture wounds in children. West J Med 166:126, 1997.

Adolescent Bunions
Coughlin MJ: Roger A. Mann Award. Juvenile hallux valgus: Etiology and treatment. Foot Ankle Int 16:682, 1995.
Thompson GH: Instructional Course Lecture. Bunions and toe deformities in adolescents and children. J Bone Joint Surg 77A:1924, 1995.

Curly Toes
Hamer AJ, Stanley D, Smith TW: Surgery for curly toe deformity: A double-blind, randomized, prospective trial. J Bone Joint Surg 75B:662, 1993.
Ross ERS, Menelaus MB: Open flexor tenotomy for hammer and curly toes in children. J Bone Joint Surg 66B:770, 1984.

Overlapping Fifth Toe
Black GB, Grogan DP, Bobechko WP: Butler arthroplasty for correction of the adducted fifth toe: A retrospective study of 36 operations between 1968 and 1982. J Pediatr Orthop 5:439, 1985.
DeBoeck H: Butler's operation for congenital overriding of the fifth toe: Retrospective 1–7 year study of 23 cases. Acta Orthop Scand 64:343, 1993.

Polydactyly
Crawford AH, Gabriel KR: Foot and ankle problems. Orthop Clin North Am 18:649, 1987.
Mubarak SJ, O'Brien TJ, Davids JR: Metatarsal epiphyseal bracket: Treatment by central physiolysis. J Pediatr Orthop 13:5, 1993.
Nogami H: Polydactyly and polysyndactyly of the fifth toe. Clin Orthop 204:216, 1986.
Phelps DA, Grogan DP: Polydactyly of the foot. J Pediatr Orthop 5:446, 1985.
Venn-Watson EA: Problems in polydactyly of the foot. Orthop Clin North Am 7:909, 1976.

Syndactyly
Meehan PL: Other conditions of the foot. *In:* Morrissy RT (ed): Lovell and Winter's Pediatric Orthopaedics. Philadelphia, JB Lippincott, 1990, pp 991–1021.

Hammer Toe
Newman RJ, Fitton JM: An evaluation of operative procedures in the treatment of hammer toe. Acta Orthop Scand 50:709, 1979.
Ross ERS, Menelaus MB: Open flexor tenotomy for hammer toes and curly toes in childhood. J Bone Joint Surg 66B:770, 1984.

Mallet Toe
Tachdjian MO: Pediatric Orthopedics. Philadelphia, WB Saunders, 1992, pp 2670–2671.

Claw Toes
Coughlin MJ, Mann RA: Lesser toe deformities. *In:* Mann RA (ed): Surgery of the Foot. St. Louis, CV Mosby, 1986, pp 132–148.
Myerson MS, Shereff MJ: The pathological anatomy of claw and hammer toes. J Bone Joint Surg 71A:45, 1989.

Annular Bands
Allington NJ, Kumar SJ, Guille JT: Clubfeet associated with congenital constriction bands of the ipsilateral lower extremity. J Pediatr Orthop 15:599, 1995.
Greene WB: One-stage release of congenital circumferential constriction bands. J Bone Joint Surg 75A:650, 1993.
Tada K, Yanenobu K, Swanson A: Congenital constriction band syndrome. J Pediatr Orthop 4:726, 1984.

Subungual Exostoses
Multhopp-Stephens H, Walling AK: Subungual (Dupuytren's) exostosis. J Pediatr Orthop 15:582, 1995.

Ingrown Toenails
Zuber TJ, Pfenninger JL: Management of ingrown toenails. Am Fam Physician 52:181, 1995.

Shoes
Staheli LT: Footwear for children. Am Acad Orthop Surg Instructional Course Lecture 43:193, 1994.

CHAPTER 681
Torsional and Angular Deformities

681.1 Normal Developmental Alignment

The most common torsion and angular changes of the lower extremity are related to normal in utero positioning or acquired disorders.

In the typical in utero position, the hips are flexed, abducted, and externally rotated; the knees are flexed and the lower legs are internally rotated; and the feet are in slight equinus, supinated, and in contact with the posterolateral aspect of the opposite thigh. The combination of external rotation of the hip and internal rotation of the lower leg produces a bowed appearance of the lower extremities when the child begins to ambulate. This is not true bowing but rather a torsional combination. *Physiologic genu varum* or bowlegs resolves with 6–12 mo of independent ambulation.

Physiologic genu valgum or knock-knees is seen between 3 and 4 yr of age. This is true genu valgum and not the result of a torsional combination. This, too, resolves with growth, with the normal adult knee alignment obtained between 5 and 8 yr of age. The mean tibiofemoral angle at birth is 15 degrees of varus (Fig. 681–1). This decreases to approximately 10 degrees by 1 yr of age. Neutral alignment occurs between 18 and 20 mo of age. The maximal valgus of 12 degrees occurs at 3–4 yr of age. The values are similar for boys and girls. By

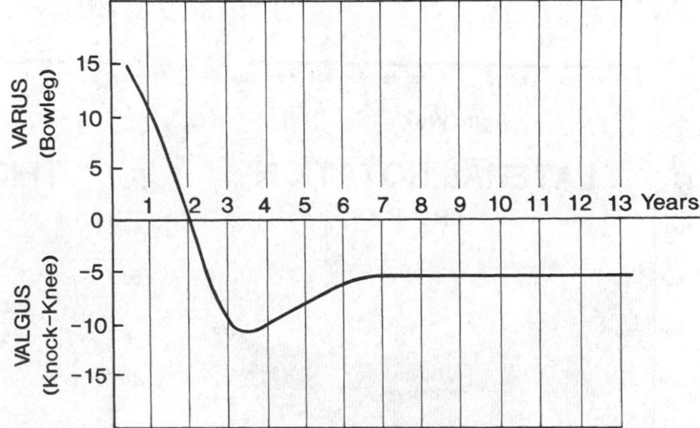

Figure 681–1 Graph demonstrating the normal development of the tibiofemoral or knee angle during growth. (Adapted from Salenius P, Vankka E: The development of the tibiofemoral angle in children. J Bone Joint Surg 57A:259, 1975.)

7 yr, the valgus alignment corrects to that of a normal adult (8 degrees in women; 7 degrees in men). Overall, 95% of developmental physiologic genu varum and genu valgum cases resolve with growth. This is also true for children with more pronounced physiologic varus or valgus, although some may not be completely corrected until adolescence.

TORSIONAL PROFILE

The torsional profile is beneficial in diagnosing and monitoring children with torsional variations (Fig. 681–2). The profile includes (1) foot progression angle, (2) hip rotation in extension, (3) thigh-foot angle, and (4) shape of the foot.

Foot Progression Angle

The foot progression angle represents the long axis of the foot with respect to the direction in which the child is walking (Fig. 681–3). Inward rotation is given a negative value and outward rotation a positive value. A normal foot progression angle in children and adolescence is 10 degree (range, −3 to 20 degrees). The foot progression angle serves only to define whether there is an in-toeing or out-toeing gait. The latter is considered abnormal when this angle exceeds 20 degrees.

Hip Rotation

Hip rotation in extension is assessed with the child prone, the thighs together, and the knees flexed 90 degrees (Fig. 681–4). In this position, the hip is in neutral alignment. As the lower leg is rotated outward, this produces internal rotation of the hip, whereas inward rotation produces external rotation. This is due to the anatomic shape of the proximal femur. The femoral neck normally has a 135-degree angle with the femoral shaft and 15 degrees of anterior rotation between femoral neck axis and the transcondylar axis of the distal femur. This angulation is known as femoral anteversion. By 1 yr of age there is approximately 45 degrees of internal and external rotation. Hip rotation should be symmetric. Asymmetric rotation may be indicative of a hip disorder, and radiographs of the pelvis are necessary.

Thigh-Foot Angle

With the child in the prone position for assessment of hip rotation, the long axis of the foot in the simulated weight-bearing position can be compared with the long axis of the thigh (Fig. 681–5). Inward rotation is given a negative value and outward rotation a positive value. Inward rotation is indic-

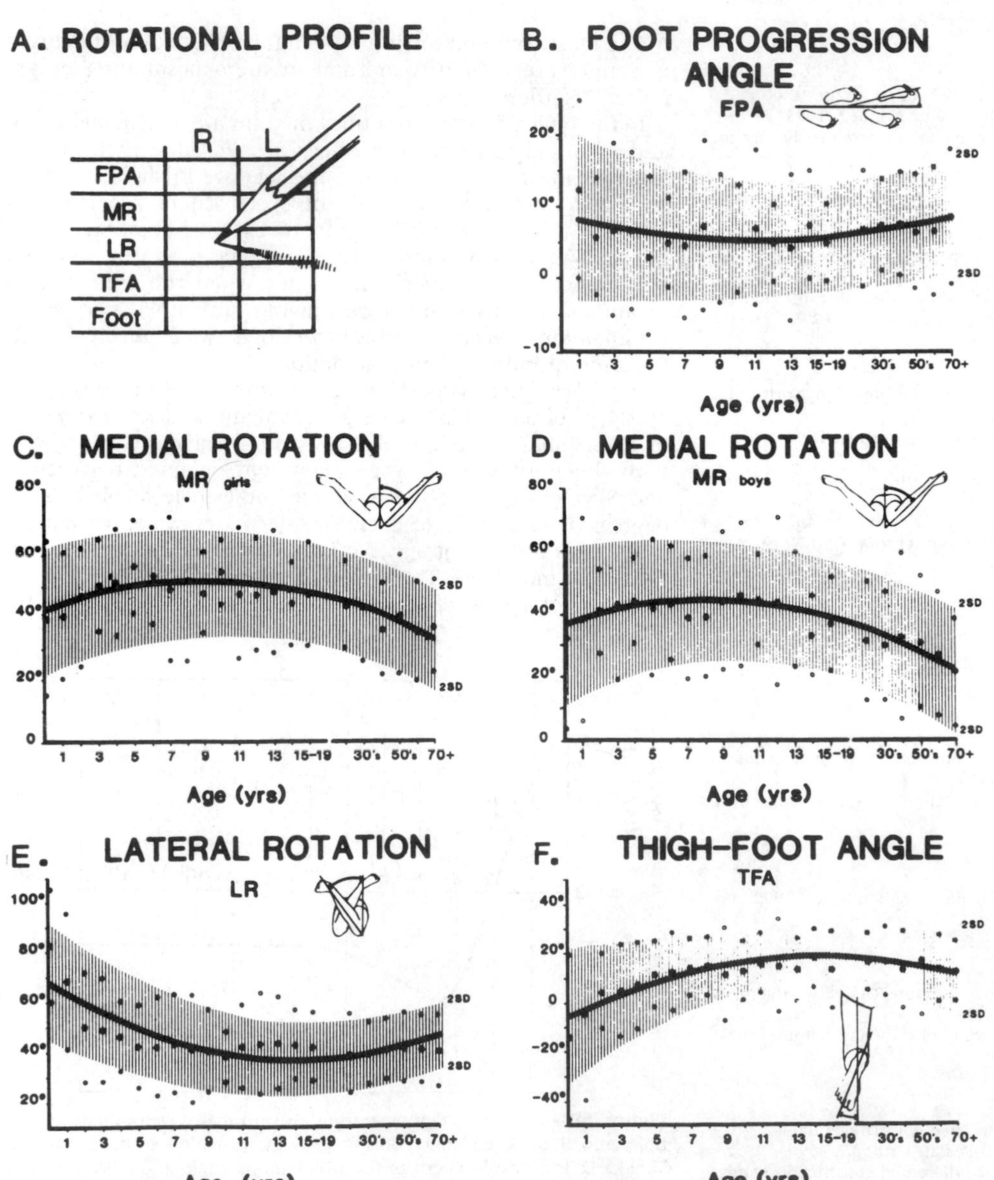

Figure 681–2 Range of normal values by age and sex with respect to the alignment of the lower extremity. *A,* Torsional profile. *B,* Foot progression angle (FPA) to determine the degree of in-toeing and out-toeing during ambulation. *C* and *D,* Medial (MR) or internal rotation of the hips in girls (*D*) and boys (*C*). *E,* Lateral (LR) or external rotation of the hips. *F,* Thigh-foot angle (TFA) to determine the degree of tibial torsion. Internal or medial tibial torsion is present if the angle is more than 20-30 degrees. (From Staheli LT: Torsional deformities. Pediatr Clin North Am 33:1373, 1986.)

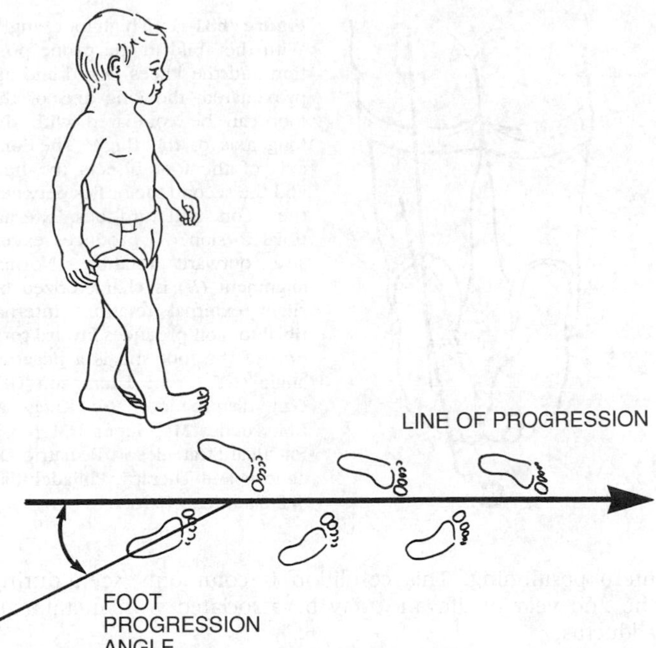

Figure 681–3 Foot progression angle. The long axis of the foot is compared with the direction in which the child is walking. If the long axis foot is directed outwardly, the angle is positive. If the foot is directed inwardly, the angle is negative and is indicative of in-toeing. (From Thompson GH: Gait disturbances. *In:* Kliegman RM, Nieder ML. Super DM [eds]: Practical Strategies in Pediatric Diagnosis and Therapy, Philadelphia, WB Saunders, 1996.)

ative of internal tibial torsion, whereas outward rotation represents external tibial torsion. Infants have a mean angle of −5 degrees (range, −35 to 40 degrees) as a consequence of normal in utero position. In middle childhood through adult life, the mean thigh-foot angle is 10 degrees (range, −5 to 30° degrees).

Foot Shape

With the child still in the prone position, the shape of the foot is easily assessed (Fig. 681–6). This position is helpful in the assessment of metatarsus adductus or a calcaneovalgus foot. The mobility of the ankle and subtalar region can also be evaluated with the child in this position.

TORSIONAL DEFORMITIES

The common causes of in-toeing and out-toeing are presented in Table 679–4.

In-Toe Gait

681.2 Internal Femoral Torsion

Internal femoral torsion is the most common cause of in-toeing in children 2 yr of age or older. It occurs more commonly in girls than boys (2:1). The majority of children with this condition have generalized ligamentous laxity. The cause of femoral torsion is controversial. Some believe that it is congenital and a result of persistent infantile femoral anteversion, whereas others believe it is acquired secondary to abnormal sitting habits.

CLINICAL MANIFESTATIONS. Clinical features of internal femoral torsion demonstrate that the entire lower leg is inwardly rotated during gait. Characteristically, there will be 80–90 degrees of internal rotation of the hip in the prone position (torsional profile). External rotation, as a consequence, is limited to 0 to 10 degrees (Fig. 681–7). There will be features of generalized ligamentous laxity, including elbow and finger hyperextension, thumb hyperabduction, knee recurvatum, and hypermobile pes planus. Affected children commonly sit in the "television" or "W" style position. It is believed that this position allows the lower leg to act as a lever, thereby producing torsional changes in the "biologically plastic" femora. This condition is also called femoral anteversion, implying an abnormality of the proximal femur. However, the torsion actually occurs throughout the femoral shaft and results in a change in the normal alignment between the hip and the knee.

RADIOGRAPHIC EVALUATION. Radiographic evaluation of internal femoral torsion is not routinely necessary, although a variety of radiographic techniques to measure femoral torsion have been described. Computed tomography and ultrasonography can assess the relationship between the proximal and distal femur. These studies are rarely indicated because the clinical measurements are equally accurate.

TREATMENT. The treatment of internal femoral torsion is predominantly by observation. Correction of abnormal sitting habits usually allows the torsion to resolve with normal growth and development. However, it takes 1–3 yr for complete correction to occur, depending on the age of the child when the sitting habits are corrected. The correction of sitting

Figure 681–4 Hip rotation in extension. This is measured with the child in the prone position and the knee flexed 90 degrees. The lower leg is vertically oriented. This is considered the neutral position. On outward rotation (*A*), the leg produces internal hip rotation, and on inward rotation (*B*), the leg produces external hip rotation. (From Thompson GH: Gait disturbances. *In:* Kliegman RM, Nieder ML, Super DM [eds]: Practical Strategies in Pediatric Diagnosis and Therapy. Philadelphia, WB Saunders, 1996.)

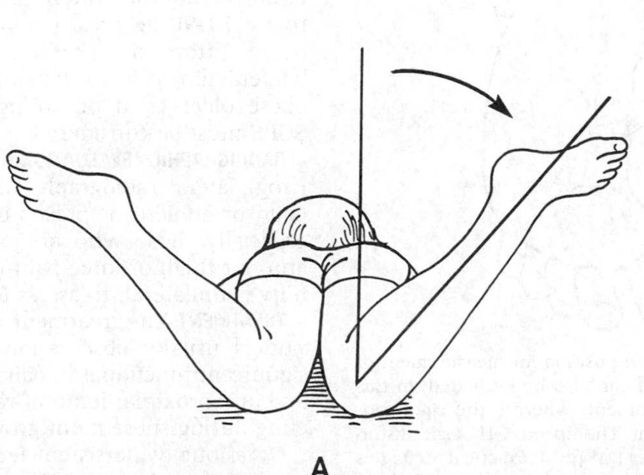

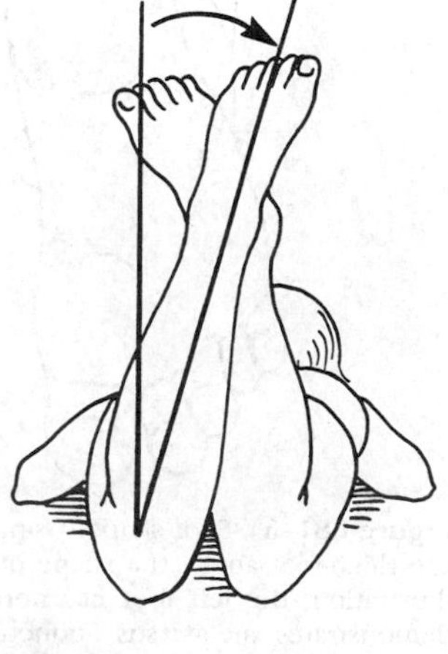

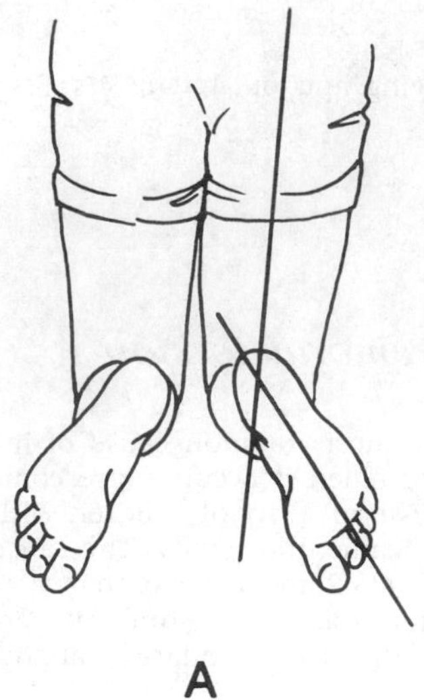

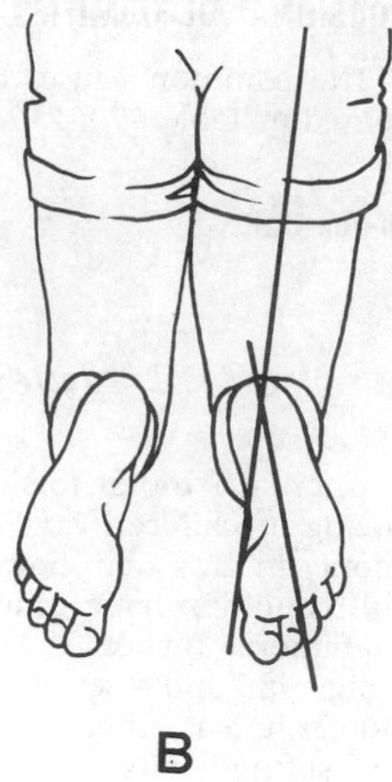

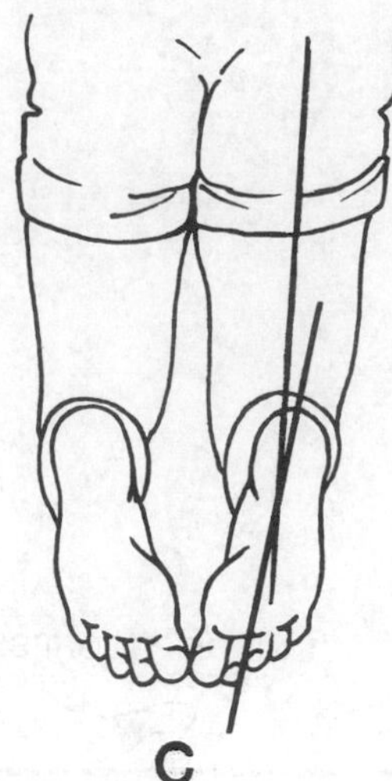

Figure 681–5 Thigh-foot angle. With the child in the prone position and the knees flexed and approximated, the long axis of the foot can be compared with the long axis of the thigh. The long axis of the foot bisects the heel and the second toe or lies between the second and third toes. External tibial torsion (*A*) produces excessive outward rotation. Normal alignment (*B*) is characterized by slight external rotation. Internal tibial torsion produces inward rotation of the foot and is a negative angle (*C*). (From Thompson GH: Gait disturbances. *In:* Kliegman RM, Nieder ML, Super DM [eds]: Practical Strategies in Pediatric Diagnosis and Therapy, Philadelphia, WB Saunders, 1996.)

habits can be difficult in preschool-age children and usually does not occur until they reach school age. The use of nighttime orthoses or daytime twister cables are of no value and may produce a compensatory external tibial torsion. The combination of internal femoral and compensatory external tibial torsion produces a pathologic genu valgum deformity. This can result in patellofemoral malalignment with patella subluxation or dislocation and pain.

Children 10 yr of age or older may not have enough remaining musculoskeletal growth for spontaneous correction to occur, and surgical intervention may be necessary. The procedures advocated include proximal femoral varus derotation osteotomy and simple derotation osteotomy of either the proximal or the distal femur. Sufficient derotation is performed to allow equal internal and external hip rotation postoperatively.

681.3 Internal Tibial Torsion

Internal tibial torsion is the most common cause of in-toeing in children younger than 2 yr and is secondary to normal in utero positioning. This condition is commonly seen during the 2nd year of life and may be associated with metatarsus adductus.

CLINICAL MANIFESTATIONS. The degree of tibial torsion can be measured by the prone thigh-foot angle (torsional profile).

RADIOGRAPHIC EVALUATION. Radiographic assessment is of no value in this predominantly clinical disorder.

TREATMENT. Treatment of internal tibial torsion is also by observation. This is a physiologic condition, and spontaneous resolution with normal growth and development can be anticipated. Significant improvement usually does not occur until the child begins to pull to stand and walk independently. Thereafter, it takes 6–12 mo and occasionally longer for complete correction to occur. Night splints are of no value and should be avoided. Persistent internal tibial torsion in an older child or adolescent may require surgical derotation; however, this rarely occurs.

Figure 681–6 Foot shape. Using the same position for measurement of the thigh-foot angle, the shape of the foot can also be evaluated. In this illustration, the left foot has normal alignment, whereas the right foot demonstrates metatarsus adductus. (From Thompson GH: Gait disturbances. *In:* Kliegman RM, Nieder ML, Super DM [eds]: Practical Strategies in Pediatric Diagnosis and Therapy. Philadelphia, WB Saunders. 1996.)

Out-Toe Gait

681.4 External Femoral Torsion

External femoral torsion, also known as femoral retroversion, is an uncommon disorder unless associated with a slipped capital femoral epiphysis (SCFE).

CLINICAL MANIFESTATIONS. The clinical examination of external femoral torsion shows excessive hip external rotation and limitation of internal rotation. Typically, the hip will externally rotate 70–90 degrees, whereas internal rotation is only 0–20 degrees (torsional profile). When idiopathic, it is usually a bilateral disorder. If the deformity is unilateral, especially in an obese older child or young adolescent, the presence of an SCFE must be considered.

RADIOGRAPHIC EVALUATION. Anteroposterior and Lauenstein (frog) lateral radiographs of the pelvis are necessary in any child or adolescent presenting with external femoral torsion, especially those who are obese or who have nontraumatic anterior thigh or knee pain (referred pain) or when the deformity is unilateral, to assess for a possible SCFE.

TREATMENT. The treatment of idiopathic external femoral torsion is usually observation because it ordinarily causes no significant functional impairment. A SCFE is treated surgically, and any proximal femoral retroversion improves with remodeling during subsequent growth.

Occasionally, persistent femoral retroversion after SCFE can produce functional impairment such as a severe out-toe gait

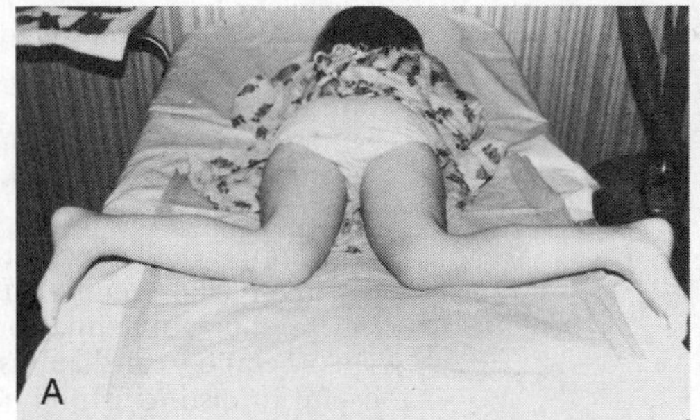
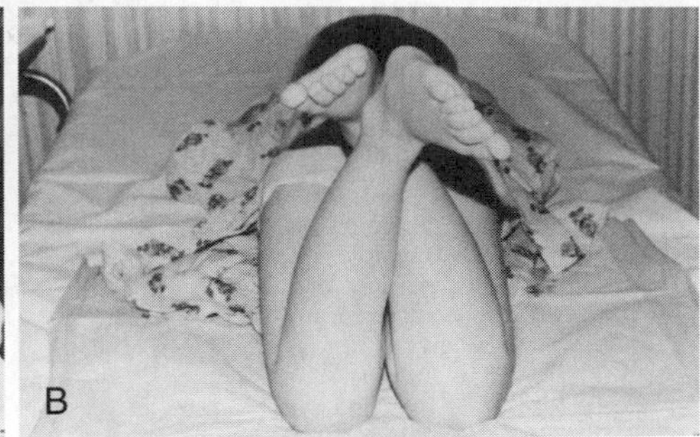

Figure 681–7 *A,* A 5-yr-old girl with bilateral internal femoral torsion. She has approximately 80 degrees of internal rotation bilaterally. *B,* External rotation is limited to approximately 15 degrees for a total arc of hip rotation of 90–95 degrees. (From Thompson GH: Gait disturbances. *In:* Kliegman RM. Nieder ML. Super DM [eds]: Practical Strategies in Pediatric Diagnosis and Therapy. Philadelphia, WB Saunders. 1996.)

and difficulty opposing one's knees in the sitting position. The latter can be disabling to adolescent females. Should this occur, a derotation osteotomy is beneficial.

681.5 External Tibial Torsion

External tibial torsion is a relatively common disorder and is frequently associated with a calcaneovalgus foot. It is secondary to a normal variation in in utero positioning.

CLINICAL MANIFESTATIONS. External tibial torsion is indicated by an abnormally positive thigh-foot angle (torsional profile), typically 30–50 degrees. There is a calcaneovalgus foot (Fig. 681–8).

RADIOGRAPHIC EVALUATION. Radiographic assessment for external tibial torsion is not necessary because there is no demonstrable radiographic abnormality.

TREATMENT. The treatment of external tibial torsion is observation. This condition follows the same clinical course as that of internal tibial torsion. Significant improvement does not occur during the 1st year of life. However, with the onset of independent ambulation, spontaneous improvement begins to occur and is typically complete by 2–3 yr of age.

ANGULAR DEFORMITIES

681.6 Genu Varum (Bowlegs)

The classification of genu varum is presented in Table 681–1. Physiologic genu varum and tibia vara (Blount's disease) are the most common disorders.

Physiologic Genu Varum

Physiologic bowlegs is a common torsional combination that is secondary to normal in utero positioning (Fig. 681–9). The tight posterior hip capsule results in an external rotation contracture. When it is combined with internal tibial torsion, it gives the clinical appearance of a bowleg deformity. Because it is physiologic, spontaneous resolution with normal growth and development can be anticipated. Significant improvement does occur during the 1st year of life. By 2 yr of age, the majority of children have straight or neutrally aligned lower extremities.

Tibia Vara

Idiopathic tibia vara, or Blount's disease, is an uncommon disorder characterized by abnormal growth of the medial aspect of the proximal tibial epiphysis, resulting in progressive varus angulation below the knee. Tibia vara can occur in any age group in a growing child and is classified as infantile (1–3 yr), juvenile (4–10 yr), and adolescent (11 yr or older). The juvenile and adolescent forms are commonly combined as late-onset tibia vara. All three groups share common characteristics, whereas the radiographic changes in the late-onset groups are less pronounced than those in the infantile form. Although the exact cause of tibia vara remains unknown, it appears to be secondary to growth suppression from increased compressive forces across the medial aspect of the knee.

CLINICAL MANIFESTATIONS. The infantile form of tibia vara is the most common; its characteristics include female and black predominance, marked obesity, approximately 80% bilateral involvement, a prominent medial metaphyseal beak, internal

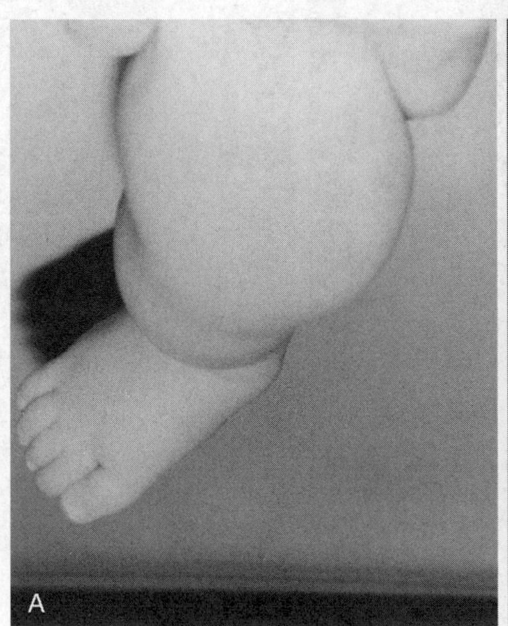
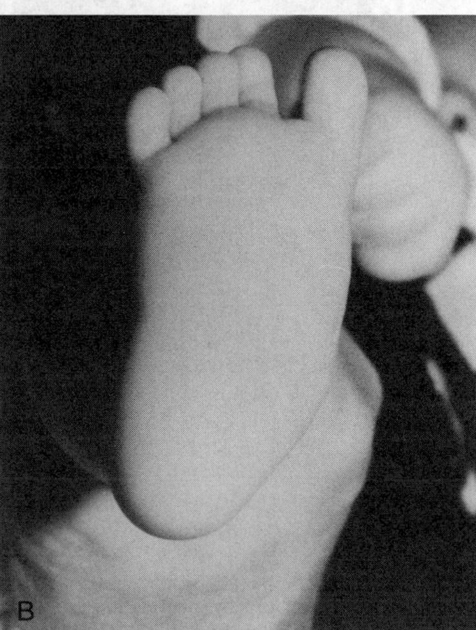

Figure 681–8 *A,* A 6-mo-old girl with an excessive external tibial torsion. This reverse, or anterior, thigh-foot angle shows approximately 50 degrees of external tibial torsion. *B,* The same infant demonstrates a calcaneovalgus foot with forefoot abduction and increased hindfoot valgus. There is also hyperdorsiflexibility of the foot in the ankle mortise. (From Thompson GH: Gait disturbances. *In:* Kliegman RM, Nieder ML, Super DM [eds]: Practical Strategies in Pediatric Diagnosis and Therapy. Philadelphia, WB Saunders. 1996.)

TABLE 681–1 Classification of Genu Varum (Bowlegs)

Physiologic

Asymmetric Growth

- Tibia vara (Blount's disease)
  - Infantile
  - Juvenile
  - Adolescent
- Focal fibrocartilaginous
- Physeal Injury
  - Trauma
  - Infection
  - Tumor

Metabolic Disorders

- Vitamin D deficiency (nutritional rickets)
- Vitamin D–resistant rickets
- Hypophosphatasia

Skeletal Dysplasia

- Metaphyseal dysplasia
- Achondroplasia
- Enchondromatosis

Modified from Thompson GH: Angular deformities of the lower extremities. In *Chapman MW (ed): Operative Orthopedics, 2nd ed. Philadelphia, JB Lippincott, 1993, pp 3131–3164.*

tibial torsion, and leg length discrepancy. The characteristics of the juvenile and adolescent forms (late-onset) include male and black predominance, marked obesity, normal or greater than normal height, approximately 50% bilateral involvement, slowly progressive genu varum deformity, pain rather than deformity as the primary initial complaint, no palpable proximal medial metaphyseal beak, minimal internal tibial torsion, mild medial collateral ligament laxity, and mild lower extremity length discrepancy. The differences among the three groups appear to be primarily due to age at onset, the amount of growth remaining, and the magnitude of the medial compression forces. The infantile group has the potential for the greatest deformity, and the adolescent group has the least.

RADIOGRAPHIC EVALUATION. Children with tibia vara are usually assessed radiographically with an anteroposterior standing radiograph of both lower extremities and a lateral radiograph of the involved extremity. Positioning the child in weight-bearing stance allows maximal presentation of the clinical deformity. The metaphyseal-diaphyseal angle can be measured and is useful in distinguishing between physiologic genu varum and early tibia vara. The latter is difficult to diagnose radiographically before 2 yr of age. Fragmentation with a protuberant step deformity and beaking of the proximal medial tibial metaphysis are the major features of the infantile group. The changes in the proximal medial tibial metaphysis are less conspicuous in the late-onset forms, which are characterized by wedging of the medial portion of the epiphysis, a mild posteromedial articular depression, a serpiginous cephalad curved physis, and mild or no fragmentation or beaking of the proximal medial metaphysis (Fig. 681–10).

Occasionally, arthrography, magnetic resonance imaging, or computed tomography may be necessary to assess the meniscus, the articular surface of the proximal tibia, or the integrity of the proximal tibial physis. These are usually reserved for the more severe deformities.

TREATMENT. The management of tibia vara may be both nonoperative and operative in the infantile form. Late-onset tibia vara is managed operatively.

Nonoperative. Orthotic management can be considered for children with infantile tibia vara who are 3 yr of age or younger with mild deformities. In approximately 50% of children meeting these criteria, the deformity may be adequately corrected. A knee-ankle-foot orthosis should be used with a single medial

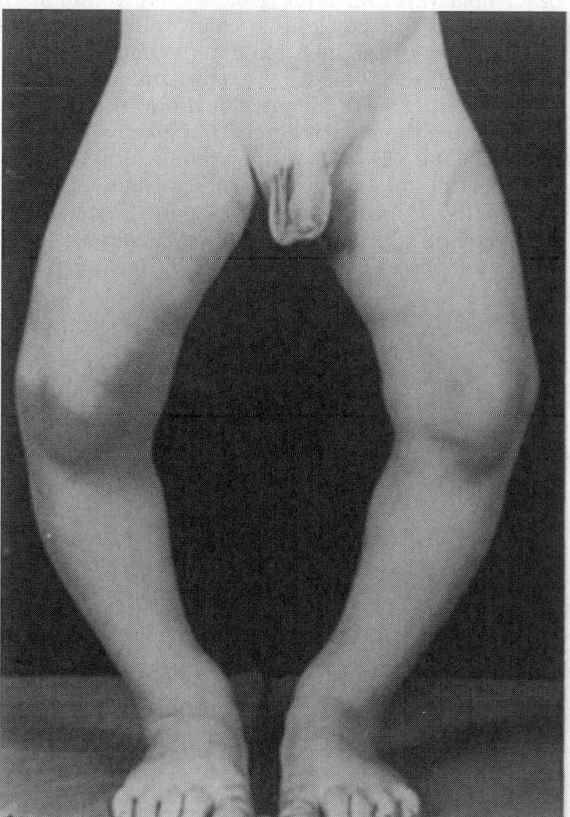

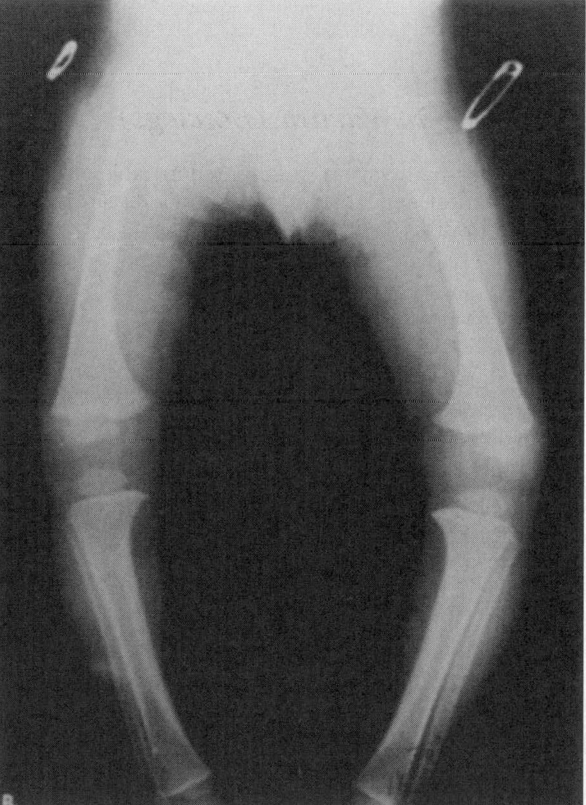

Figure 681–9 Infant with bilateral genu varum at 18 mo of age. This resolved spontaneously before 7 yr of age. *A,* Clinical photograph. *B,* Standing anteroposterior radiograph of the lower extremities. (From Tachdjian MO: Pediatric Orthopedics, 2nd ed. Philadelphia, WB Saunders, 1990.)

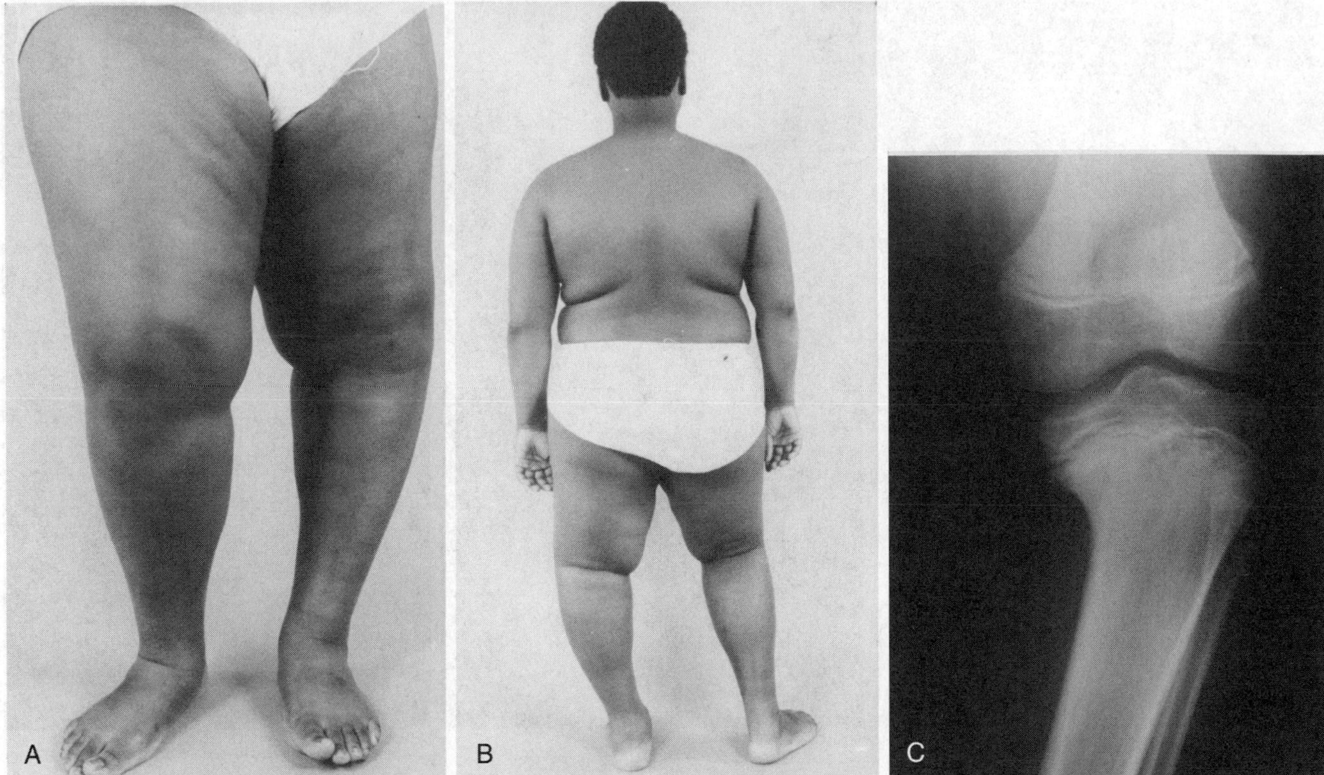

Figure 681–10 *A,* A 13-yr-old boy with late-onset, or adolescent, tibia vara. There is marked obesity and mild genu varum deformity of the left knee. *B,* Posterior view of the same child. *C,* Standing anteroposterior radiograph of the left knee demonstrating the tibia vara deformity but with less obvious changes than in the infantile form. The medial aspect of the proximal tibial epiphysis is narrow and the growth plate is irregular. The typical metaphyseal "beaking" is not present.

upright, without a knee hinge. Pads and straps should be placed over the distal femur and proximal tibia to apply a valgus force. The orthosis should be worn 22–23 hr each day. A maximal trial of 1 yr of orthotic management is currently recommended. If complete correction is not obtained after 1 yr or if progression occurs during this time, a corrective osteotomy is indicated.

Operative. The indications for surgical treatment of infantile tibia vara include age of 4 yr or more, failure of orthotic management, and more severe deformities. Proximal tibial valgus osteotomy and associated fibular diaphyseal osteotomy are usually the procedures of choice (Fig. 681–11). In late-onset tibia vara, correction is also necessary to restore the mechanical axis of the knee. The same surgical options as presented for older children with infantile tibia vara are applicable in these age groups. A proximal tibial valgus osteotomy and diaphyseal fibular osteotomy are the most common procedures.

681.7 Genu Valgum (Knock-Knees)

The classification of genu valgum is presented in Table 681–2. Fortunately, the pathologic causes, with the exception of post-traumatic disorders, are uncommon. As the spontaneous correction of physiologic bowlegs continues, there is typically an overcorrection, of variable degree, into mild genu valgum, or knock-knees. This physiologic angular variation, or genu valgum, is commonly seen between 3 and 5 yr of age. It is a true angular deformity that resolves spontaneously, with normal knee alignment being attained between 5 and 8 yr. Rarely is a knock-knee orthosis indicated. Surgery may be required in adolescence for a persistent deformity. Options include medial physeal stapling, medial hemiepiphysiodesis, and corrective osteotomy.

681.8 Congenital Angular Deformities of the Tibia and Fibula

The differential diagnosis of congenital angular deformities of the lower leg (Table 681–3) include posteromedial angulation, which is a benign process, and anterolateral angulation, which is a pathologic process.

CONGENITAL POSTEROMEDIAL TIBIAL ANGULATION (BOWING). This is an uncommon angular deformity that involves the distal one third of the tibia and fibula. There is a posteromedial bowing

TABLE 681–2 Classification of Genu Valgum (Knock-Knees)

Physiologic
Asymmetric Growth
Tibia valga
Physeal injury
Trauma following fracture of the proximal tibial metaphysis
Infection
Tumor
Metabolic Disorders
Renal osteodystrophy
Skeletal Dysplasia
Kniest's syndrome
Congenital Abnormalities
Congenital dislocation of the patella
Neuromuscular Disorders
Cerebral palsy
Myelodysplasia

From Thompson GH: Angular deformities of the lower extremities. In *Chapman MW (ed): Operative Orthopedics, 2nd ed. Philadelphia, JB Lippincott, 1993, pp 3131–3164.*

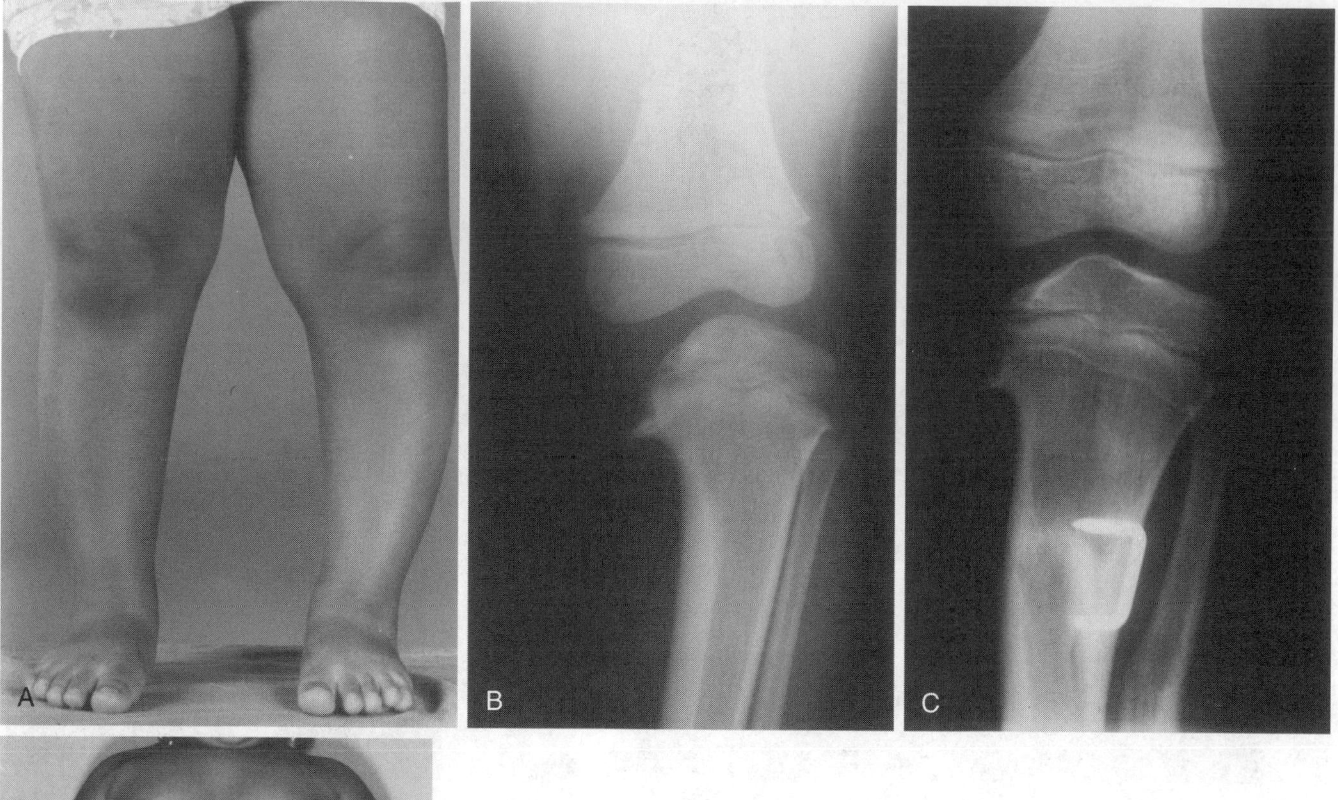

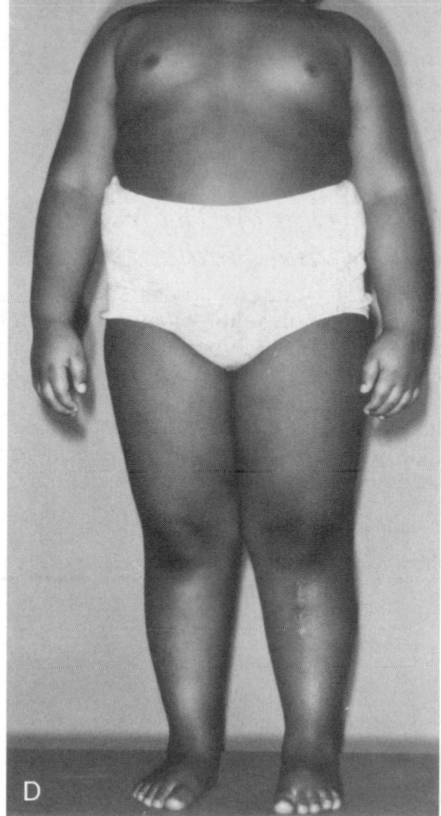

Figure 681–11 *A,* A 4-yr-old girl with infantile tibia vara. She is obese and has a moderate left genu varum deformity. *B,* Anteroposterior radiograph of the left knee demonstrating the genu varum deformity. There is narrowing and irregularity of the medial aspect of the proximal tibial epiphysis and beaking of the medial metaphysis. *C,* Repeat radiograph 2 yr after proximal tibial and diaphyseal fibular corrective osteotomy. The osteotomy is healed, and relatively normal growth is occurring in the proximal tibial epiphysis. *D,* Postoperative clinical photograph demonstrating symmetric alignment of the lower extremities.

in association with a calcaneovalgus foot. The clinical appearance can be dramatic. The diagnosis is confirmed radiographically and shows the posteromedial angulation without other osseous abnormalities. A significant portion of the calcaneovalgus foot is due to the position of the distal tibia and ankle.

The *cause* of the congenital posteromedial bowing is unknown. The natural history is characterized by spontaneous resolution by 3–5 yr of age. However, there is residual shortening in the tibia and fibula. The fibula is usually slightly shorter than the tibia. The mean growth inhibition is 12–13% (range, 5–27%). The mean leg length discrepancy at maturity is 4 cm (3–7 cm).

The *treatment* of congenital posteromedial bowing of the tibia and fibula is observation. All components of the deformity with the exception of leg length inequality resolve with growth and development. The child should have periodic radiographic leg length measurements to determine the degree of discrepancy and to predict the maximal discrepancy at maturity. This

TABLE 681–3 Differential Diagnosis of Congenital Angular Deformities of the Tibia and Fibula

Posteromedial Angulation

Anterolateral Angulation

Congenital pseudoarthrosis of the tibia
Congenital longitudinal deficiency of the tibia (paraxial tibial hemimelia)
Congenital longitudinal deficiency of the fibula (paraxial fibular hemimelia)

Modified from Thompson GH: Angular deformities of the lower extremities. In Chapman MW (ed): Operative Orthopedics, 2nd ed. Philadelphia, JB Lippincott, 1993, pp 3131–3164.

also allows information regarding the appropriate age for surgical intervention. Operative intervention for a defect other than leg length discrepancy is rarely indicated. A corrective osteotomy may be necessary in patients with severe deformity that is not improving with growth and development. Patients with discrepancies greater than 5 cm may be candidates for tibial lengthening.

CONGENITAL ANTEROLATERAL TIBIAL ANGULATION (BOWING). This type of bowing is associated with an underlying pathologic disorder (see Table 681–3). The diagnosis is made radiographically. *Congenital fibular hemimelia* represents a congenital absence of the fibula and usually the lateral portion of the foot, especially the fourth and fifth rays. *Congenital tibial hemimelia* represents a congenital absence of the tibia, either partial or total. Surgical reconstruction of these deformities is difficult, and most defects require amputation to achieve satisfactory function. *Congenital pseudoarthrosis* of the tibia is usually associated with neurofibromatosis. It represents a defect in the tibia that predisposes to pathologic fractures, which heal poorly. A variety of surgical techniques, including intramedullary rodding, electrical stimulation, and vascularized fibular transplants, have been used with varying success in this complex problem.

Torsional Malalignment

Internal and External Tibial and Femoral Torsion

Ruwe PA, Gage JR, Ozonoff MB, et al: Clinical determination of femoral anteversion: A comparison of established techniques. J Bone Joint Surg 74A:820, 1992.

Staheli LT: Instructional Course Lecture: Rotational problems in children. J Bone Joint Surg 75A:939, 1993.

Staheli LT, Corbett M, Wyss C, et al: Lower extremity rotational problems in children: Normal values to guide management. J Bone Joint Surg 67A:39, 1985.

Svenvingsen S, Terjesen T, Auflein M, et al: Hip rotation and in-toeing gait: A study of normal subjects from four years until adult age. Clin Orthop 251:177, 1990.

Thompson GH: Gait disturbances. *In*: Kliegman RM, Neider ML, Super DM (eds): Practical Strategies in Pediatric Diagnosis and Therapy. Philadelphia, WB Saunders, 1996, pp 757–778.

Angular Deformities

Physiologic Genu Varum and Genu Valgum

Cahuzac JPh, Vardon D, Sales de Gauzy J: Development of the clinical tibiofemoral angle in normal adolescents. A study of 427 normal subjects from 10 to 16 years of age. J Bone Joint Surg 77B:729, 1995.

Feldman MD, Schoenecker PL: Use of metaphyseal-diaphyseal angle in the evaluation of bowed legs. J Bone Joint Surg 75A:1602, 1993.

Greene WB: Genu varum and genu valgum in children: Differential diagnoses and guidelines for evaluation. Compr Ther 22:22, 1996.

Heath CH, Staheli LT: Normal limits of knee angle in white children-genu varum and genu valgum. J Pediatr Orthop 13:259, 1993.

Kling TF Jr: Angular deformities of the lower limbs in children. Orthop Clin North Am 18:513, 1987.

Mielke CH, Stevens PM: Hemiepiphyseal stapling for knee deformities in children younger than 10 years. A preliminary report. J Pediatr Orthop 16:423, 1996.

Salenius P, Vankka E: The development of the tibio-femoral angle in children. J Bone Joint Surg 57A:259, 1975.

Thompson GH: Angular deformities of the lower extremities in children. *In:* Chapman MW (ed): Operative Orthopedics, 2nd ed. Philadelphia, JB Lippincott, 1993, pp 3131–3164.

Vankka E, Salenius P: Spontaneous correction of severe tibiofemoral deformity in growing children. Acta Orthop Scand 53:567, 1982.

Tibia Vara

Doyle BS, Volk G, Smith CI: Infantile Blount's disease. Long-term follow-up of surgically treated patients at skeletal maturity. J Pediatr Orthop 16:469, 1996.

Feldman MD, Schoenecker PL: Use of metaphyseal-diaphyseal angle in the evaluation of bowed-legs. J Bone Joint Surg 75A:1602, 1993.

Greene WB: Instructional course lecture: Infantile tibia vara. J Bone Joint Surg 75A:130, 1993.

Henderson RC, Kemp GJ, Greene WB: Adolescent tibia vara: Alternatives for operative treatment. J Bone Joint Surg 74A:342, 1992.

Henderson RC, Kemp GJ, Hayes PRL: Prevalence of late-onset tibia vara. J Pediatr Orthop 13:255, 1993.

Johnston CE II: Infantile tibia vara. Clin Orthop 255:13, 1990.

Langenskiold A: Tibia vara: A critical review. Clin Orthop 264:195, 1989.

Loder RT, Johnston CE II: Infantile tibia vara. J Pediatr Orthop 7:639, 1987.

Schoenecker PL, Meade WC, Pierron RL, et al: Blount's disease: A retrospective review and recommendations for treatment. J Pediatr Orthop 5:181, 1985.

Thompson GH, Carter JR: Late-onset tibia vara (Blount's disease): Current concepts. Clin Orthop 255:24, 1990.

Zionts LE, Shean CJ: Brace treatment of early infantile tibia vara. J Pediatr Orthop 18:102, 1998.

Congenital Posteromedial Tibial Bowing

Hofmann A, Wenger DR: Posteromedial bowing of the tibia: Progression of discrepancy in leg lengths. J Bone Joint Surg 63A:384, 1981.

Pappas AM: Congenital posteromedial bowing of the tibia and fibula. J Pediatr Orthop 4:525, 1984.

CHAPTER 682
Leg Length Discrepancy

Leg length discrepancies are common in childhood, and many factors must be evaluated before management decisions can be made.

ETIOLOGY. The causes of leg length discrepancy are extensive; the common causes are presented in Table 682–1.

CLINICAL MANIFESTATIONS AND DIAGNOSIS. Signs and symptoms associated with leg length discrepancy, other than limping, are usually related to the underlying cause. Approximately 65% of the growth of the entire lower extremity comes from the distal femoral (37%) and proximal tibial (28%) physes. Thus, growth disturbances around the knee can have the most adverse effect on leg length. Determination of the *skeletal, or bone, age* allows for a relatively accurate assessment of remaining growth. The *Gruelich and Pyle Atlas* (1950) remains the standard by which bone age is determined from an anteroposterior radiograph of the left hand and wrist. It is possible to estimate the *ultimate discrepancy at maturity* using growth remaining ta-

TABLE 682–1 Common Causes of Leg Length Discrepancies

Congenital	**Infectious**
Proximal femoral focal deficiency	Pyogenic osteomyelitis with physeal damage
Coxa vara	**Trauma**
Hemiatrophy-hemihypertrophy (anisomelia)	Physeal injury with premature closure
Development dysplasia of the hip	Overgrowth
Developmental	Malunion (shortening)
Legg-Calvé-Perthes disease	**Tumor**
Neuromuscular	Physeal destruction
Polio	Radiation-induced physeal injury
Cerebral palsy (hemiplegia)	Overgrowth

Modified from Thompson GH: Gait disturbances. In: Kliegman RM, Nieder ML, Super DM (eds): Practical Strategies of Pediatric Diagnosis and Therapy. Philadelphia, WB Saunders, 1996, pp 757–778.

bles such as the Moseley straight-line graph (Fig. 682–1) and the Green-Anderson table. The former, the most commonly used today, uses scanographic and bone age data to determine the ultimate discrepancy. It can also be used to follow the response of treatment. The clinical methods available are less accurate than the radiographic techniques, but they are useful. The most common clinical measurement is leveling the pelvis. Blocks of various thickness may be placed beneath the foot on the involved side until the iliac crests are level. The thickness indicates the amount of discrepancy.

Adult sitting height is approximately 52% of total height in the male and 53% in the female. Thus, two times the predicted length of the normal leg at maturity gives a close approximation of the *anticipated adult height.* This height plays an important role in determining equalization. Lengthening procedures are more applicable in predicted short adults, whereas shortening procedures are generally used for predicted normal height or taller individuals. In either case, acceptable body proportions must be maintained.

Children with *neuromuscular disorders* such as spastic hemiplegia benefit from 1–2 cm of shortening on the involved side to improve the swing phase of gait and increased toe clearance. Only extremities that are neurologically normal should be considered for equalization of leg lengths.

Angular deformities and coexistent joint abnormalities are important considerations in children with leg length discrepancies. This is especially true when lengthening procedures are being considered. A child with a dysplastic acetabulum may subsequently experience a hip dislocation if femoral lengthening is attempted. Thus, any significant angular deformities or joint abnormalities should be corrected either before or simultaneously with leg length equalization.

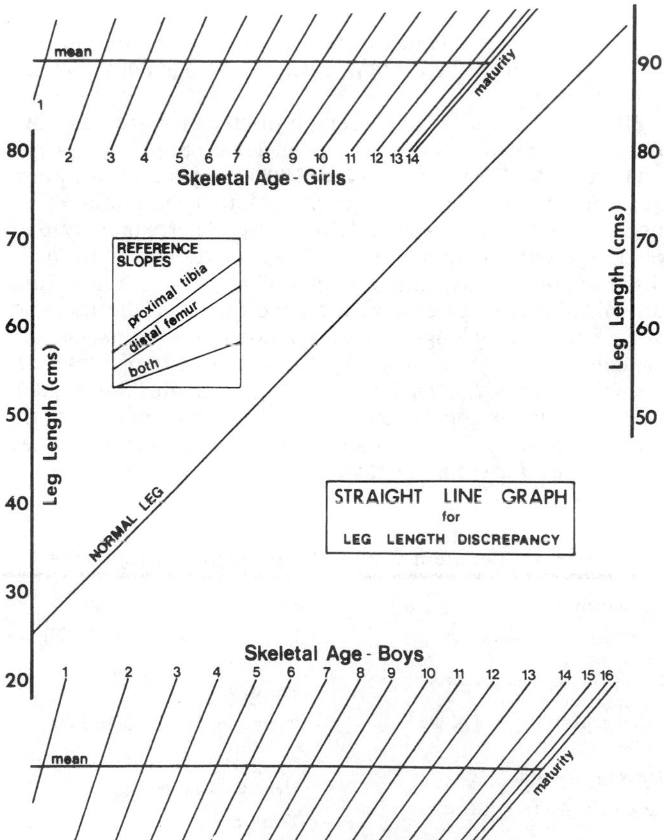

Figure 682–1 The Moseley straight-line graph for the assessment of leg length inequalities. This allows simultaneous correlation of the normal leg, short leg, and bone age of the child. It will accurately predict lengths of each extremity at skeletal maturity. The reference slopes are used as a guide in determining when appropriate treatment should be performed.

RADIOGRAPHIC EVALUATION. Radiographic evaluations are the most accurate methods of assessing leg lengths. Four different types of radiographic techniques are available. The *teleoroentgenogram* is a single exposure of both lower extremities. Its primary indication is for young children, usually younger than 5 yr. There is a small amount of magnification error present, but it has the advantage of demonstrating any associated angular deformity. The *orthoroentgenogram* consists of three separate, slightly overlapping exposures of the hips, knees, and ankles on a long cassette. Bone length is measured directly on the radiograph. There is less magnification, and it is relatively accurate and demonstrates angular deformities. The *scanogram* is a simple, accurate method of assessment. It consists of three narrow exposures of the hips, knees, and ankles on a standard cassette with a radiographic ruler laying next to the extremity. Thus, minimal magnification is present, and accurate measurements can be made. However, angular deformities cannot be fully visualized and, if present, can lead to errors in measurement. *Computed tomography* is the most accurate technique and also shows angular deformity.

TREATMENT. The psychologic status of the child as well as that of the parents is an important consideration in treatment selection. Some equalization techniques are simple and safe, whereas others, especially lengthening procedures, are complex with high complication rates that require strict cooperation by the child and parents. Discrepancies of greater than 2 cm at skeletal maturity usually require treatment because these often cause the patient to limp. Equalization can be achieved by nonsurgical and surgical methods. In general, the goals are to maintain an appropriate adult height (5 ft 6 inches in males, 5 ft in females) and adequate body proportions. Shortening procedures are preferred, and lengthening procedures should be used cautiously.

Orthotics and Prosthetics. Orthotic devices are generally indicated for discrepancies between 2 and 3 cm in skeletally mature individuals. A heel lift is frequently all that is necessary to provide the patient with a normal gait. Because of normal pelvic rotation during the gait cycle, complete equalization is not necessary. The smallest lift that will allow the patient to walk without a limp is all that is necessary. Prostheses are necessary for severe discrepancies or uncorrectable deformities.

Extremity Shortening Procedures. Three procedures are used to shorten the longer extremity. *Epiphysiodesis* is indicated in children who have 5 cm or less predicted discrepancy at maturity, have adequate remaining growth for satisfactory correction, and have a predicted relatively normal, corrected adult height. It requires accurate timing to achieve equalization of the leg lengths at maturity. The disadvantages of epiphysiodesis include shortened stature, surgery on the unaffected extremity, thc possibility of an angular growth deformity, and the irreversibility of the procedure itself. Percutaneous epiphysiodesis under fluoroscopic control is the most popular technique. This is an outpatient procedure that is effective and has a low complication rate. *Epiphyseal stapling* is performed to slow the rate of physeal growth. Three staples inserted extraperiosteally on each side of the physis are required to retard growth adequately. Once equalization has been achieved, the staples are removed, allowing normal growth to resume. Stapling on one side of the physis can be used to correct angular deformities around the knee. *Bone resection* is indicated for ultimate discrepancies of 5–6 cm in adults or adolescents who have inadequate remaining growth to undergo an epiphysiodesis. The femur can be shortened up to 6 cm and the tibia-fibula up to 3 cm before irreversible muscle weakness occurs.

Extremity Lengthening Procedures. The advantages of lengthening are equalization of significant leg length discrepancies, maintenance of ultimate adult height, preservation of normal body proportions, surgery on the affected limb, correction of existing angular deformities, and elimination of orthoses. The disadvantages are that it is technically difficult to perform and has a significant complication rate. Common complications include pin tract infection, wound infection, hypertension, hip and knee subluxation, ankle equinus, loss of correction, delayed union, metal failure, and fatigue fractures after metal removal. *Transiliac or pelvic lengthening osteotomies* can provide a gain of up to 3 cm in length. These procedures are generally reserved for individuals with mild discrepancies who have ipsilateral shortening with acetabular dysplasia, an asymmetric pelvis, or possibly decompensated scoliosis. The callotasis technique allows progressive *lengthening of the femur or tibia*. An osteotomy is performed after application of an external fixator lengthening system. There is no initial lengthening. After 7–10 days, lengthening is begun at 1.0 mm/day (0.25 mm every 6 hr). This allows elongation of the forming callus. Significant lengthening of the bone can be achieved with this technique. Once the desired length has been achieved, the callus is allowed to consolidate. The lengthening device is removed after consolidation. The entire process requires approximately 1 mo per centimeter lengthened. The advantages of this procedure over previous lengthening techniques is that it requires only one procedure, allows greater lengthening, and has a lower complication rate. Occasionally, *a combination of a transiliac, femoral, or tibial diaphyseal lengthening and possibly leg-shortening procedures* such as epiphysiodesis is necessary to equalize leg lengths. The combination of femoral diaphyseal lengthening and contralateral epiphysiodeses is useful for discrepancies of 8–10 cm when a single lengthening is insufficient for complete correction.

Aaron A, Weinstein D, Thickman D, et al: Comparison of orthoroentgenography and computed tomography in the measurement of limb-length discrepancy. J Bone Joint Surg 74A:897, 1992.

Anderson M, Green WT, Messner M: Growth and predictions of growth in the lower extremities. J Bone Joint Surg 45A:1, 1963.

Ballock RT, Weisner GL, Myers MT, Thompson GH: Current concepts. Hemihypertrophy: Concepts and controversies. J Bone Joint Surg 79A:1731, 1997.

Barry K, McManus F, O'Brien T: Leg lengthening by the transiliac method. J Bone Joint Surg 74B:275, 1992.

Gruelich WW, Pyle SI: Radiographic Atlas of Skeletal Development of the Hand and Wrist. 2nd ed. Stanford, CA, Stanford University Press, 1959.

Horton GA, Olney BW: Epiphysiodesis of the lower extremity: Results of the percutaneous technique. J Pediatr Orthop 16:180, 1996.

Moseley CF: A straight line graph for leg-length discrepancies. J Bone Joint Surg 59A:174, 1977.

Moseley CF: Leg length discrepancy. Orthop Clin North Am 18:529, 1987.

Paley D: Current techniques of limb lengthening. J Pediatr Orthop 8:73, 1988.

Shapiro F: Developmental patterns in lower extremity length discrepancies. J Bone Joint Surg 64A:639, 1982.

Velazquez RJ, Bell DF, Armstrong PF, et al: Complications of use of the Ilizarov technique in the correction of limb deformities in children. J Bone Joint Surg 75A:1148, 1993.

CHAPTER 683
The Knee

The knee is a unique joint because the tibiofemoral articulation is constrained only by soft tissues rather than by geometric fit. The distal femur is cam-shaped, allowing it to have a gliding, hinged motion. The major constraints of the knee are the medial and lateral collateral ligaments, the anterior and posterior cruciate ligaments, and the medial and lateral menisci. Weight is transmitted through both the articular cartilage and the menisci. A second important area of the knee is the patellofemoral joint. It is the common site of problems especially in adolescence.

Pain around the knee is one of the most common presenting complaints in older children and adolescents. This may be insidious in onset or the result of trauma. *Accumulation of fluid* (effusion) in the knee is indicative of an abnormal intra-articular process. Fluid accumulating after injury is usually blood (hemarthrosis) and is indicative of a potentially serious injury to one or more of the ligaments or menisci or an occult fracture. Recurrent effusions may indicate a chronic internal derangement such as a meniscal tear. Unexplained accumulation of fluid may occur with arthritis (septic, viral, postinfectious, juvenile rheumatoid arthritis, systemic lupus erythematosus), hemorrhage secondary to hemophilia, and overactivity. Occasionally, this fluid requires aspiration to relieve discomfort and to help establish the diagnosis. The presence of fat globules in the blood aspirated from a hemarthrosis may be indicative of an occult fracture. The presence of purulent material indicates septic arthritis or osteomyelitis.

PEDIATRIC KNEE DISORDERS

Overuse syndromes, ligament injuries, and meniscal tears may occur in children and adolescents and are discussed in the chapter on sports medicine (see Chapters 691.6 and 696).

683.1 Discoid Lateral Meniscus

CLINICAL MANIFESTATIONS AND DIAGNOSIS. Each meniscus is semilunar or "C"-shaped, but occasionally the lateral meniscus persists as a solid disk of cartilage and is referred to as a discoid lateral meniscus. The normal meniscus is attached around its periphery and glides anteriorly and posteriorly with knee motion, but a discoid meniscus is less mobile and may be torn. Occasionally, there is no peripheral attachment around the posterolateral aspect of the meniscus, which may allow it to become displaced anteriorly with knee flexion, producing a loud click or clunk. A tear or anterior displacement is most likely to occur in late childhood or early adolescence (11–15 yr). Physical examination may show a mild effusion and a positive McMurray test in which the displacement of the meniscus is both palpable and audible. Anteroposterior radiography of the knee may show only widening of the lateral aspect of the knee joint. Magnetic resonance imaging (MRI) or arthrography are required for definitive diagnosis.

TREATMENT. The treatment of discoid menisci is to excise tears and reshape the meniscus arthroscopically. Meniscal instability can occasionally be repaired or reconstructed concomitantly. Complete excision may be necessary if other procedures are unsuccessful.

683.2 Popliteal Cyst

Popliteal cyst (Baker cyst) is commonly seen during the middle childhood years. There is distention of the gastrocnemius and semimembranous bursa along the posterior aspect of the knee by synovial fluid from a tendon sheath or the knee joint. They are not associated with intra-articular pathologic conditions. Knee radiographs are normal. The diagnosis may be confirmed by ultrasonography or aspiration. *Treatment* is by observation, especially in children 10 yr of age and younger, because resolution over several years usually occurs. The only indications for surgical excision are the presence of symptoms or progressive enlargement.

683.3 Osteochondritis Dissecans

Osteochondritis dissecans commonly involves the knee and occurs when an area of bone adjacent to the articular cartilage becomes avascular and ultimately separates from the underlying bone. The exact cause is unknown, but trauma from the adjacent tibial spines is commonly implicated. The lateral portion of the medial femoral condyle is the most common site.

CLINICAL MANIFESTATIONS AND DIAGNOSIS. The child or adolescent typically presents with a vague knee pain. Occasionally, a mild effusion may be present. With the knee fully flexed, it is possible to palpate the involved area directly on the articular cartilage of the medial femoral condyle. This is usually tender.

Anteroposterior, lateral, and tunnel radiographs of the knee are necessary to establish the diagnosis and to follow the disease process. In younger children, the overlying articular cartilage usually remains intact. As revascularization occurs, the bone heals spontaneously. With increasing age, the risk increases for articular cartilage fracture and separation of the bony fragment, producing a loose body. MRI is helpful in determining the integrity of the articular cartilage.

TREATMENT. In children 11 yr of age and younger, the treatment is primarily by observation. Periodic radiographs and occasionally MRI scans may be necessary to assess the degree of healing. In adolescents 13 yr of age and older, especially those with a suspected loose body, arthroscopic surgical intervention may be necessary. This may consist of (1) excision of the loose body, (2) replacement and internal fixation, or (3) drilling of an intact lesion to promote revascularization and healing.

683.4 Osgood-Schlatter Disease

The patellar tendon inserts into the tibia tubercle, which is an extension of the proximal tibial epiphysis. This area is vulnerable to microfracture during late childhood or adolescence, especially in athletes, producing Osgood-Schlatter disease. It is most common in males. The natural history is usually benign. Physical examination demonstrates swelling, tenderness, and increased prominence of the tibia tubercle. Radiographs are usually necessary to rule out other lesions. Rest, restriction of activities and, occasionally, a knee immobilizer may be necessary, combined with an isometric exercise program. Anti-inflammatory medications usually are not beneficial. Complete resolution of symptoms through physiologic healing (physeal closure) of the tibia tubercle usually requires 12–24 mo.

PATELLOFEMORAL DISORDERS

The patellofemoral joint depends on balance among the restraining ligaments, muscle forces, and the articular anatomy of the patellofemoral groove. The patella has a "V"-shaped bottom that guides it through the matching groove (trochlea) in the distal femur. The force of the muscles pulling through the quadriceps mechanism and the patellar tendon does not act in a straight line because the patellar tendon inclines in a slightly lateral direction with respect to the line of the quadriceps. This lateral movement, coupled with the movement of the restraining ligaments, tends to move the patella in a lateral direction. The vastus medialis muscle is necessary to counteract the laterally acting forces. An abnormality of any one or a group of these factors may make the patellofemoral joint function abnormally. The usual clinical manifestation is knee pain that is aggravated by vigorous activities.

683.5 Idiopathic Adolescent Anterior Knee Pain Syndrome

The idiopathic adolescent anterior knee pain syndrome is a common patellofemoral disorder that was previously known as *chondromalacia patellae.* The term was used to describe a deranged patellar articular surface. There is now evidence to indicate that the articular surface is normal. The cause of the knee pain, which commonly occurs in early adolescence, is unknown.

CLINICAL MANIFESTATIONS AND DIAGNOSIS. The anterior peripatellar knee pain is poorly localized. Symptoms are usually produced by vigorous physical activities such as running. Typically, there is no history of injury. The child does not complain of locking, giving way, or recurrent effusion. Gait, range of motion, alignment of the lower extremity, knee stability, patellar tracking, and areas of focal tenderness should be evaluated. The presence of patellofemoral crepitation is common in normal individuals and does not indicate underlying knee disease. Routine radiographs, including anteroposterior, lateral, and tunnel views, are not particularly helpful in evaluating the cause of adolescent anterior knee pain. They may eliminate other sources of pain.

TREATMENT. The treatment is predominantly conservative and may include flexibility exercises, strengthening exercises (isometric quadriceps), contrast therapies (ice and heat), orthoses, and medications (nonsteroidal anti-inflammatory drugs). About 70–90% success can be anticipated. Rarely will arthroscopic evaluation of the knee and patellofemoral joint be necessary.

683.6 Patellar Subluxation and Dislocation

Patellar maltracking is usually due to a congenital deficiency or malalignment within the patellofemoral joint. This can consist of a high-riding patella (patella alta), genu valgum, hypoplasia of the lateral femoral condyle, ligamentous laxity, and malignant malalignment with internal femoral and external tibial torsion. Traumatic patellar subluxation and dislocation can occur as a result of a direct blow to the patella along its medial aspect, but this is uncommon.

CLINICAL MANIFESTATIONS AND DIAGNOSIS. Examination of a child with a maltracking patella that is predisposed to dislocation usually shows terminal subluxation of the patella when the knee is brought into full extension. There may be tenderness to palpation over the inferior surface of the lateral facet of the patella. Attempting to displace the patella laterally yields a subjective feeling of subluxation, resulting in the patient grabbing the examiner's hand. This has been termed the *apprehension sign.* The torsional profile should be performed for possible rotational abnormalities of the femur or tibia, or both. After an acute dislocation, there may be a hemarthrosis from capsular tearing or an osteochondral fracture.

Radiographs are necessary in the evaluation of patellar subluxation or after an acute dislocation. They should include anteroposterior, lateral, and skyline tangential views of the patella to assess for an osteochondral fracture from the lateral femoral condyle or the patella.

TREATMENT. The majority of children presenting with acute patellar dislocation can be treated nonoperatively. This normally consists of immobilization with the knee in extension for approximately 6 wk. The patient is started on isometric, straight leg-raising exercises as soon as possible. Once the immobilization is discontinued, the isometric exercise program should be continued until the knee is fully rehabilitated. Using this method, approximately 75% of patients do not have recurrent dislocations.

If patellar subluxation is due to dynamic muscle imbalance, a specific muscle rehabilitation program, such as strengthening the vastus medialis, may be successful.

In children and adolescents with recurrent dislocations or failure of conservative management for patellar subluxation, operative stabilization may be necessary. Depending on the disease, this may consist of an arthroscopic lateral release and, occasionally, a soft tissue reconstruction. The latter can be performed either proximally or distally depending on the age of the patient and the nature of the disease. Derotational osteotomies of the distal femur or proximal tibia, or both, are indicated if there is torsional malalignment.

Cash JD, Hughston JC: Treatment of acute patellar dislocation. Am J Sports Med 16:244, 1988.
Davids JR: Pediatric knee. Clinical assessment and common disorders. Pediatr Clin North Am 43:1067, 1996.
Dickhaut SC, Delee JC: The discoid lateral meniscus syndrome. J Bone Joint Surg 64A:1068, 1982.
Dinham JM: Popliteal cysts in children: The case against surgery. J Bone Joint Surg 57B:69, 1975.
Krause BPL, Williams JPR, Caterall A: The natural history of Osgood-Schlatter's disease. J Pediatr Orthop 10:65, 1990.
Nietosvaara Y, Aalto K, Kallio PE: Acute patella dislocation in children: Incidence and associated osteochondral fractures. J Pediatr Orthop 14:513, 1994.
Sandow MJ, Goodfellow JW: The natural history of anterior knee pain in adolescents. J Bone Joint Surg 67B:36, 1985.
Stanitski CL: Instructional course lecture: Anterior knee pain syndromes in the adolescent. J Bone Joint Surg 75A:1407, 1993.
Vahasarja V, Kinnunen P, Lanning P, Serlo W: Operative realignment of patellar malalignment in children. J Pediatr Orthop 15:281, 1995.

CHAPTER 684
The Hip

The hip is a ball-and-socket (femoral head and acetabulum, respectively) joint that allows for geometric motion, including flexion, extension, abduction, adduction, and internal and external rotation. The bulk of the femoral head is composed of the capital femoral epiphysis (CFE). The femoral head and acetabulum have a trophic relationship and are interdependent for normal growth and development. When this relationship is interrupted, abnormal hip development follows. Muscle balance and activity related to appropriate gross motor function are essential to the normal development of the hip.

The blood supply to the CFE is unique. The retinacular vessels lie on the surface of the femoral neck but are intracapsular. They enter the epiphysis from the periphery. This makes the blood supply vulnerable to damage from septic arthritis, trauma, and other vascular insults. If the blood supply is lost, avascular necrosis or osteonecrosis may occur. This can result in deformity, either acutely or as a consequence to abnormal growth and development, and predisposes to abnormal hip function and degenerative osteoarthritis as an adult.

684.1 Developmental Dysplasia of the Hip

Developmental dysplasia of the hip (DDH) usually occurs in the neonatal period. The hips at birth are rarely dislocated but rather "dislocatable." Dislocations tend to occur after delivery and, thus, are postnatal in origin, although the exact time when dislocations occur is controversial. Because they are not truly congenital in origin, the term *developmental dysplasia of the hip* is now used. DDH is classified into two major groups: typical, in a neurologically normal infant, and teratologic, in which there is an underlying neuromuscular disorder, such as myelodysplasia, arthrogryposis multiplex congenita, or a syndrome complex. Teratologic dislocations occur in utero and are therefore congenital. This discussion concentrates on typical DDH, which is the most common form.

ETIOLOGY. The cause of DDH is multifactorial, having physiologic, mechanical, and postural factors.

The positive family history (20%) and the generalized ligamentous laxity are related factors. The majority of children with DDH have generalized ligamentous laxity, which can predispose to hip instability. Maternal estrogens and other hormones associated with pelvic relaxation result in further, although temporary, relaxation of the newborn hip joint. There is a 9:1 female predominance.

Approximately 60% of children with typical DDH are first borns, and 30–50% were in the breech position. The frank breech position with the hips flexed and the knees extended is the position of highest risk. The breech position results in extreme hip flexion and limitation of hip motion. Increased hip flexion results in stretching of the already lax capsule and ligamentum teres. It also produces posterior uncoverage of the femoral head. Decreased hip motion leads to a lack of normal development of the cartilaginous acetabulum. There is also an association of congenital muscular torticollis (14–20%) and metatarsus adductus (1–10%) with DDH. The presence of either condition requires a careful examination of the hips.

Postnatal factors are also important determinants. Maintaining the hips in the position of adduction and extension may lead to dislocation. This puts the unstable hip under pressure because of the normal hip flexion and abduction contractures. An unstable femoral head, as a consequence, can be displaced from the acetabulum over several days or weeks.

PATHOANATOMY. Because hips are not dislocated at birth, the components of the hip joint, excluding the hip capsule and ligamentum teres, are relatively normal. There may be some variations in the shape of the cartilaginous acetabulum, especially if the child was in a breech position in utero. If a dislocation is allowed to occur, acetabular dysplasia and maldirection, excessive femoral anteversion (torsion), and hip muscle contractures develop.

CLINICAL MANIFESTATIONS. The Barlow test is the most important maneuver in examining the newborn hip. This provocative test to dislocate an unstable hip is performed by stabilizing the pelvis with one hand and then flexing and adducting the opposite hip and applying a posterior force (Fig. 684–1). If the hip is dislocatable, it is usually readily felt. After release of the posterior force, the hip usually relocates spontaneously. It has been estimated that only 1 in 100 newborn infants have clinically unstable hips (subluxation or dislocation), whereas only 1 in 800–1,000 of these infants eventually experience a true dislocation. The Ortolani test is a maneuver to reduce a recently dislocated hip. It is most likely to be positive in infants who are 1–2 mo of age because adequate time must have passed for the true dislocation to have occurred. In performing this test, the thigh is flexed and abducted, and the femoral head is lifted anteriorly into the acetabulum (see Fig. 684–1). If reduction is possible, the relocation will be felt as a "clunk," not an audible "click." After 2 mo of age, manual reduction of a dislocated hip is usually not possible because of the development of soft tissue contractures.

Limitation of hip abduction is indicative of soft tissue contractures and may indicate DDH. Conversely, hip abduction contractures may indicate dysplasia of the contralateral hip. An asymmetric number of thigh skinfolds and apparent shortening of an extremity and uneven knee levels when the supine infant's feet are placed together on the examining table with the hips and knees flexed (Galeazzi sign) indicate DDH with proximal displacement of the femoral head. Absent normal knee flexion contracture also occurs.

A common concern is the presence of *hip clicks* in infants. Hip clicks per se are not usually pathologic and are secondary to (1) breaking the surface tension across the hip joint, (2)

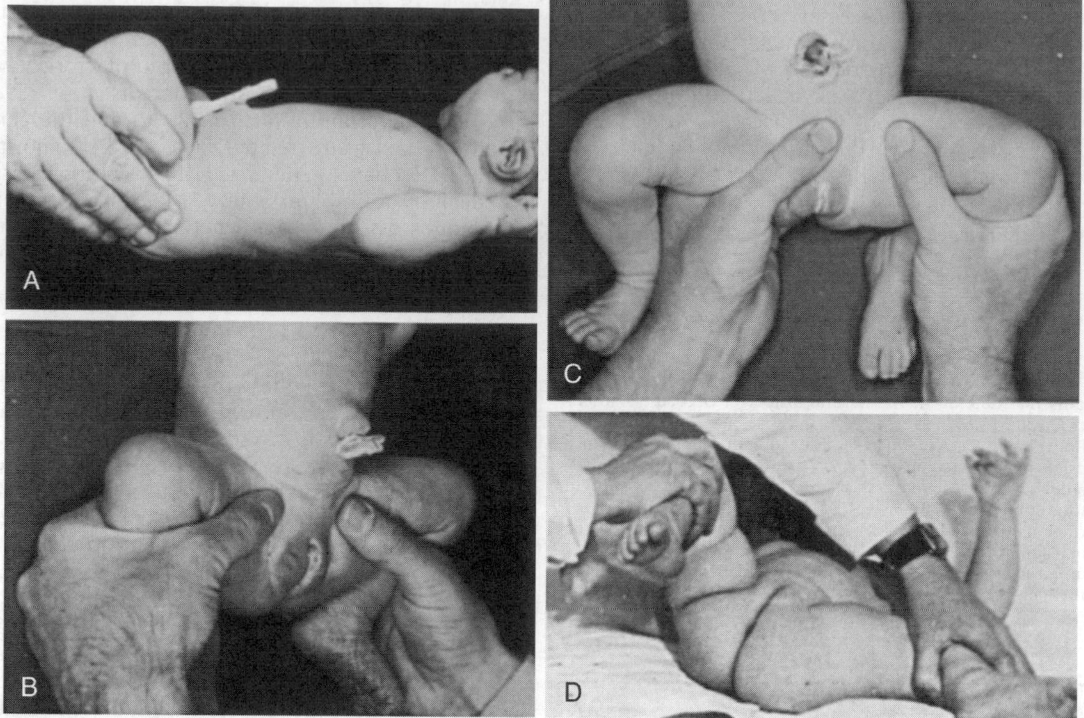

Figure 684–1 Newborn hip examination. *A*, The infant is laid on her back with the hips and knees flexed, and the examiner places the middle finger of each hand over each greater trochanter. *B*, The thumb of each hand is applied to the inner side of the thigh opposite the lesser trochanter. *C*, In a difficult infant, the pelvis may be steadied between a thumb over the pubis and fingers under the sacrum while the hip is tested (Barlow and Ortolani test) with the other hand. *D*, Limitation of hip abduction is also an early sign of developmental dislocation of the hip. Note the restriction in abduction of the right hip.

snapping of gluteal tendons, (3) patellofemoral motion, or (4) femorotibial (knee) rotation.

In older or walking children, complaints of limping, waddling, increased lumbar lordosis, toe walking, and leg length discrepancy may indicate an unrecognized DDH.

RADIOGRAPHIC EVALUATION. Hip stability as well as acetabular development may be assessed accurately in neonates and young infants by dynamic ultrasonography. Radiographic evaluation in older infants and children includes anteroposterior and Lauenstein (frog) lateral radiographs of the pelvis. The ossific nucleus of the femoral head does not appear until 3–7 mo of age, and it may be further delayed in DDH. Line measurements are usually made to determine the relationship of the femoral head to the acetabulum (acetabular index, quadrant assessment, Shenton's line, and the center edge angle of Wiberg) (Fig. 684–2). Arthrography, computed tomography, and magnetic resonance imaging scans may be beneficial in difficult cases, especially those involving older infants and children.

TREATMENT. The treatment of DDH should be individualized and depends on the patient's age and whether the hip is subluxated or dislocated.

Birth. When an unstable hip is recognized at birth, maintenance of the hip in the position of flexion and abduction ("human" position) for 1–2 mo is usually sufficient. This position maintains reduction of the femoral head and allows for tightening of the ligamentous structures as well as stimulation of normal growth and development. Methods that can be used to maintain the hip in this position include the Pavlik harness, Frejka splint, and a variety of abduction orthoses. Double and triple diapers, although controversial, are commonly used in newborns with dislocatable hips for 2–3 wk because the splints and harnesses usually do not initially fit satisfactorily. Treatment is continued until there is clinical stability of the hip, and ultrasonographic or radiographic measurements are normal.

Age 1–6 Months. During this age, a true dislocation may develop. As a consequence, treatment is directed toward reduction of the femoral head into the acetabulum. The Pavlik harness is the treatment of choice in this age group. The harness attempts to place the hips in the human position by flexing them more than 90 degrees (preferably 100–110 degrees) and maintaining relatively full, but gentle abduction (50–70 degrees). This redirects the femoral head toward the acetabulum. Usually, spontaneous relocation of the femoral head occurs within 3–4 wk. The Pavlik harness is approximately 95% successful in dysplastic or subluxated hips and 80% successful in true dislocations. If reduction is achieved, use of the harness is continued until radiographic parameters have returned to normal. If a spontaneous reduction does not occur, a surgical closed reduction is indicated. This consists of (1) preliminary skin traction for 1–3 wk to bring the femoral head opposite the acetabulum, (2) percutaneous adductor tenotomy, (3) closed reduction, (4) arthrography to assess the concentricity of the reduction, and (5) application of a hip spica cast in the "human" position. Treatment is continued until the radiographic parameters are within normal limits.

Age 6–18 Months. In the older infant, surgical closed reduction is the major method of treatment. If at the time of reduction there is significant instability, an open reduction may be indicated. This can be through a medial or anterior approach.

Age of 18 Months–8 Years. After 18 mo of age, the progressive deformities are so severe that open reduction followed by pelvic (innominate) osteotomy or femoral osteotomy, or both, are necessary to realign the hip. A femoral shortening derotation osteotomy is performed concomitantly if the reduction is tight, if there is excessive femoral anteversion, or if the child is 3 or 4 yr of age or older. Postoperatively, a hip spica cast is worn for 6–8 wk to allow healing. Thereafter, the child may be permitted to return to full activities gradually. Implanted metal is removed shortly after healing to prevent incorporation into the growing bone. Eighteen months of age is not an arbitrary age for these procedures. It has been demonstrated

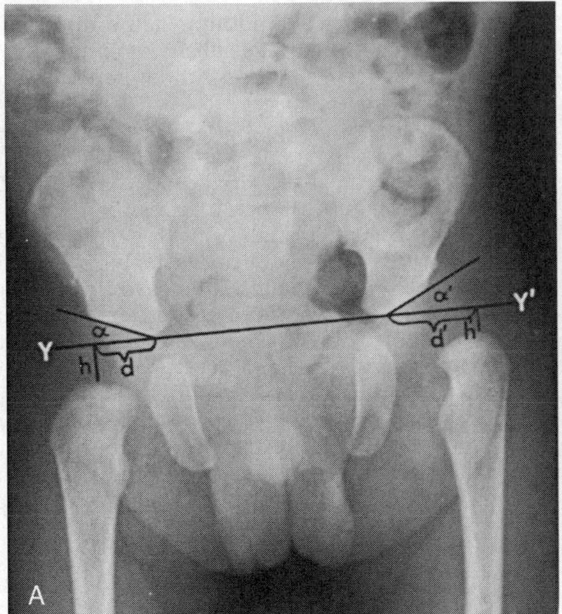

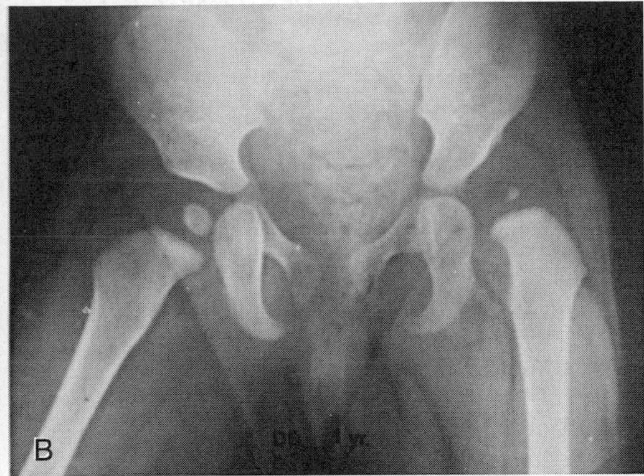

Figure 684–2 Pelvic radiographs demonstrating development dysplasia of the left hip. *A,* The Hilgenreiner method for identification of dysplasia of the hip before ossification of the capital femoral epiphysis; *a'* is greater than *a,* indicating greater obliquity of the acetabular roof. *d'* is greater than *d,* indicating lateral displacement of the femur. *b* is greater than *b',* indicating cephalad displacement of the femur. These relationships indicate dysplasia of the patient's left hip. *B,* Developmental dislocation of the left hip. The bony roof of the left acetabulum is quite oblique, and there is the beginning of a false acetabulum above its most lateral aspect. The left femur is displaced laterally and superiorly. The ossification center of the left capital femoral epiphysis is smaller than that of the right.

that approximately 25% of children who have a closed reduction performed between 9 and 12 mo of age, 50% who have one between 12 and 18 mo, and 75% who have one between 18 and 36 mo have residual acetabular dysplasia requiring a pelvic or femoral osteotomy at a later date.

COMPLICATIONS. The most important and severe complication of DDH is avascular necrosis of the CFE. This is an iatrogenic complication: reduction of the femoral head under pressure produces cartilaginous compression, and this can result in occlusion of the intra-articular, extraosseous epiphyseal vessels and produce CFE infarction, either partial or total. Revascularization follows, but abnormal growth and development may occur, especially if the physis is severely damaged. The hip is vulnerable to this complication before the development of the ossific nucleus (4–6 mo). The management outlined previously is designed to minimize this complication; with appropriate use of these treatments, the incidence of avascular necrosis is approximately 5–15%. Other potential complications in DDH include redislocation, residual subluxation, acetabular dysplasia, and postoperative complications, such as wound infections.

SEPTIC ARTHRITIS AND OSTEOMYELITIS

See Chapter 178 for a full discussion of septic arthritis and osteomyelitis. Diagnosis of septic arthritis and osteomyelitis is made by hip aspiration (arthrocentesis). This can be technically difficult and must always be performed under fluoroscopic control. If no fluid is obtained from the hip joint, an arthrogram should be obtained, documenting that the hip joint has been entered.

684.2 *Transient Monoarticular Synovitis*

Transient synovitis of the hip is one of the more common causes of limping in a normal child. It is characterized by acute onset of pain, limp, and mild restriction of motion, especially abduction and internal rotation. Septic arthritis and osteomyelitis of the hip must be excluded before this diagnosis can be confirmed. The cause remains uncertain, but possibilities include (1) active or recent systemic viral syndrome, (2) trauma, and (3) allergic hypersensitivity. Biopsy specimens from the hip joint have demonstrated synovial hypertrophy secondary to nonspecific inflammatory reaction.

CLINICAL MANIFESTATIONS. Transient monoarticular synovitis can occur in all age groups, but the mean age of onset is 6 yr; it occurs predominantly in the 3–8 yr age group. Approximately 70% of affected children have had a nonspecific upper respiratory tract infection 7–14 days before the onset of symptoms. There is usually an acute onset of symptoms with pain felt in the groin, anterior thigh, or knee; nontraumatic anterior thigh or knee pain may be referred from the hip. These children are usually ambulatory, and the hip is not held flexed, abducted, and laterally rotated unless a significant effusion is present. However, they walk with a painful, limping gait. They are usually afebrile or have a low-grade fever (temperature less than 38°C).

Laboratory values are usually normal, but occasionally a slight elevation in the erythrocyte sedimentation rate is seen. Arthrocentesis produces normal results, although a joint effusion of 1–3 mL is common.

RADIOGRAPHIC EVALUATION. Anteroposterior and Lauenstein (frog) lateral radiographs of the pelvis should be obtained and are usually normal. Ultrasonography of the hip may demonstrate a hip joint effusion. Technetium bone scan or magnetic resonance imaging may be of value in ruling out the presence of other lesions, such as infection or early Legg-Calvé-Perthes disease (LCPD). Transient monoarticular synovitis is a diagnosis of exclusion.

TREATMENT. Treatment for monoarticular synovitis of the hip is conservative. Bed rest and non–weight-bearing until the pain resolves, followed by limited activities thereafter are the treatments of choice. Most children are maintained on bed rest for less than 1 wk. They are then maintained on limited activities for 1–2 additional wk. This sometimes is difficult because children want to return to normal activities when their symptoms resolve. However, if the child is allowed to return to normal activities too early, exacerbation of symptoms may occur.

684.3 Legg-Calvé-Perthes Disease

LCPD is idiopathic osteonecrosis or avascular necrosis of the CFE, and the associated complications thereof, occurring in an immature, growing child. This osteochondrosis is caused by an interruption of the CFE blood supply. Its cause is unknown, but an association among protein C and protein S deficiency, thrombophilia, and hypofibrinolysis has been observed. It is primarily a disorder affecting males (4–5:1) and is bilateral in approximately 20% of children. Children with LCPD often have delayed bone age, disproportionate growth, and mild short stature.

CLINICAL MANIFESTATIONS. The clinical onset of LCPD occurs between the ages of 2 and 12 yr (mean, 7 yr). Most children present with mild or intermittent pain in the anterior thigh and a limp. The classic presentation has been described as a "painless limp." The pertinent early physical findings include antalgic gait; muscle spasm with mild restriction of motion, especially abduction and internal rotation; proximal thigh atrophy; and mild shortness of stature.

RADIOGRAPHIC EVALUATION: DIAGNOSIS AND PROGNOSIS. Anteroposterior and Lauenstein (frog) lateral radiographs of the pelvis should be obtained to establish the diagnosis (Fig. 684–3). The radiographic characteristics can be divided into five distinct stages representing a continuum of the disease process: (1) cessation of CFE growth, (2) subchondral fracture, (3) resorption (fragmentation), (4) reossification, and (5) healed or residual stage.

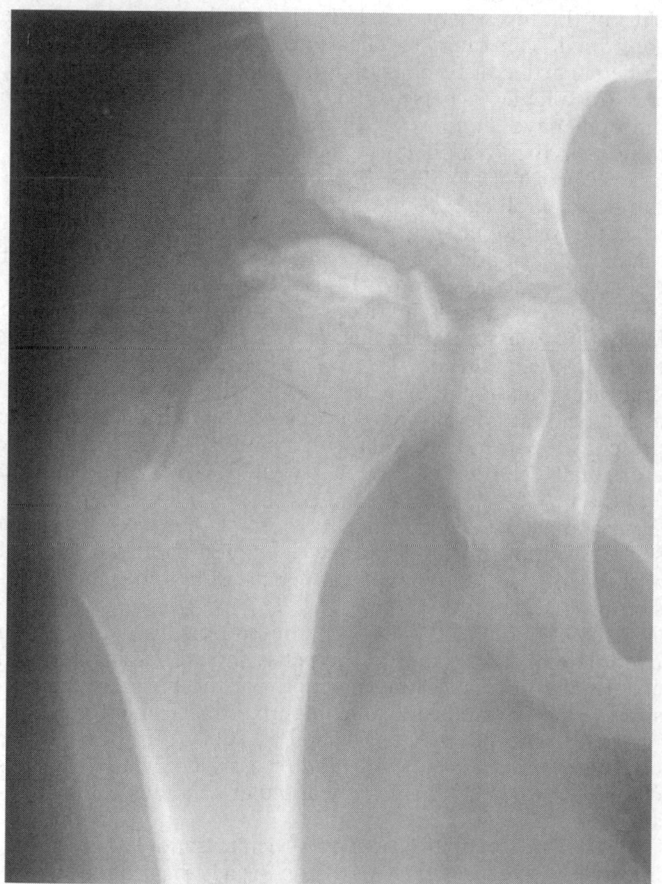

Figure 684–3 Anteroposterior radiograph of the right hip of an 8-yr-old male with LCPD. There is a collapsed yet dense CFE with early fragmentation. The small medial triangle of the CFE is uninvolved in the disease process.

There are three radiographic classification systems of the extent of CFE involvement. Catterall developed a four-group classification on the basis of the appearance of the CFE at maximal resorption. Although this classification has been helpful in the retrospective analysis of results, it has limited prognostic value because it is difficult to apply in the earliest phases of the disease process. Salter-Thompson used two groups and Herring and colleagues, three groups, depending on involvement or extent of involvement of the lateral portion of the CFE. When intact, this area acts as a supporting column or pillar that shields the involved portion of the CFE from compression, which can produce collapse, deformity, and possible extrusion. Involvement results in a poorer prognosis.

The short-term prognosis relates to the femoral head deformity at the completion of the healing stage. Adverse risk factors include older age at clinical onset, extensive CFE involvement, femoral head containment, reduced range of hip motion, and premature CFE closure. The long-term prognosis relates to the potential for osteoarthritis of the hip in adulthood. Older children with significant residual femoral head deformity are at risk for degenerative arthritis; the incidence is essentially 100% in children who are 10 yr of age or older at onset and who have residual femoral head deformity. This compares with a negligible risk in children who are 5 yr of age and younger at onset and 38% when onset occurs between 6 and 9 yr of age.

Two radiographic techniques evaluate the sphericity of the femoral head at the completion of the disease process, which correlates with the risk for degenerative osteoarthritis as an adult. In the Mose circle criteria, a transparent template with concentric circles is placed over the anteroposterior and Lauenstein lateral radiographs. If the variation of sphericity of the femoral head in the two views is 0–2 mm, the result is good; 2–3 mm, fair; and 3 mm or more, poor. Stulberg and colleagues' five-group classification is based on the shape of the femoral head and congruency with the acetabulum: class I, a spherical femoral head that is equal in size to the opposite uninvolved hip; class II, a spherical femoral head with coxa magna; class III, an oval femoral head with a congruent acetabulum; class IV, a flat femoral head with abnormalities of the femoral neck and acetabulum; and class V, a flat femoral head with a normal acetabulum. Classes I and II are spherical congruent hips, class III a nonspherical congruent hip, and classes IV and V incongruent hips.

TREATMENT. LCPD is a local, self-healing disorder. Prevention of femoral head deformity and secondary osteoarthritis are the only justifications for treatment. The treatment goals are (1) elimination of hip irritability; (2) restoration and maintenance of a good range of hip motion; (3) prevention of CFE collapse, extrusion, or subluxation; and (4) attainment of a spherical femoral head at healing. Current treatment methods use the concept of containment (i.e., the femoral head is contained within the acetabulum so that the latter acts as a mold for the reossifying CFE). This may be accomplished by nonsurgical and surgical techniques.

Observation. Expectant observation is appropriate for all children younger than 6 yr at clinical onset regardless of the extent of CFE involvement. These children must be monitored closely, both clinically and radiographically.

Intermittent Symptomatic Treatment. Temporary or periodic treatment with bed rest or abduction stretching exercises to maintain mobility can be used in conjunction with observation. Recurrent episodes of hip irritability with a temporary decrease in motion commonly occur during the phases of subchondral fracture and fragmentation, and the child may benefit from symptomatic treatment.

Definitive Early Treatment. Nonsurgical or surgical containment of the femoral head in the course of the disease is indicated when (1) the age at clinical onset is 6 yr or older (possibly 5 yr in girls), (2) the lateral portion of the CFE is involved, or (3) there is a loss of containment, as manifested by extrusion of the femoral head on anteroposterior radiograph.

Nonsurgical Containment. Abduction casts (Petrie) or orthoses can be used to contain the femoral head within the acetabulum. Containment is continued only until there is early radiographic subchondral reossification. Because this usually occurs 12–18 mo after clinical onset, nonsurgical containment methods can be limited to 18 mo or less with no adverse effect on the outcome. The Atlanta Scottish Rite Hospital orthosis is the most widely used because it allows reciprocal motion and ambulation without crutches or external support. The success of nonsurgical containment has been challenged on the grounds that it does not alter the natural history of untreated LCPD.

Surgical Containment. A pelvic or femoral osteotomy can be used to contain the femoral head. The results of surgical containment appear to be better than those of nonsurgical containment; approximately 85% of patients have Stulberg class I, II, or III.

Late Surgical Management for Deformity. If significant femoral head deformity prevents reduction of the femoral head into the acetabulum, an alternative method must be considered. Several surgical procedures at least partially correct the various existing deformities, thereby alleviating the associated symptoms.

684.4 Slipped Capital Femoral Epiphysis

Slipped capital femoral epiphysis (SCFE) is the most common adolescent hip disorder. Its cause is unknown, but an endocrine basis has been suggested because SCFE is frequently accompanied by abnormalities of growth. Sex hormones, growth hormone, and other hormones alter the rate of growth in the CFE and the rate of skeletal growth. SCFE occurs in adolescents who are either obese and have delayed skeletal maturation or are tall and thin and have had a recent growth spurt. In obese adolescents, a low level of sex hormones has been postulated, whereas in tall, thin individuals, an overabundance of growth hormone is implicated. SCFE can also occur as a complication of an underlying endocrine disorder such as hypothyroidism, pituitary disorders, pseudohypoparathyroidism, and others. When a SCFE occurs before puberty (10 yr of age or younger), an endocrine disorder (hypothyroidism, growth hormone deficiency) should be suspected.

RADIOGRAPHIC EVALUATION. Anteroposterior and Lauenstein (frog) lateral radiographs of the pelvis are used for assessment of SCFE (Fig. 684–4). Both hips must be evaluated and compared. The earliest sign of SCFE is widening of the physis without slippage, a preslip condition. As slippage occurs, the CFE remains in the acetabulum and the femoral neck rotates predominantly anteriorly (although occasionally superiorly), resulting in a varus, retroverted femoral head and neck. The degree of slippage between the CFE and the femoral neck can be classified as mild (0–33%), moderate (34–50%), and severe (greater than 50%) by radiographic measurement techniques.

DIAGNOSTIC CLASSIFICATION. SCFE is classified into four distinct clinical groups.

Preslip. The physis is wide, but slippage has not occurred. There may be mild discomfort, but the physical examination is usually normal. Preslips are frequently seen in the opposite hip of an adolescent with a previous SCFE.

Acute Slipped Capital Femoral Epiphysis. In acute SCFE, there are no or only mild antecedent symptoms such as pain or limp of less than 3 wk duration. Slippage occurs suddenly, usually without trauma, and the pain is so severe that the child is usually unable to stand or bear weight even with external support on the involved extremity. An acute SCFE is unstable.

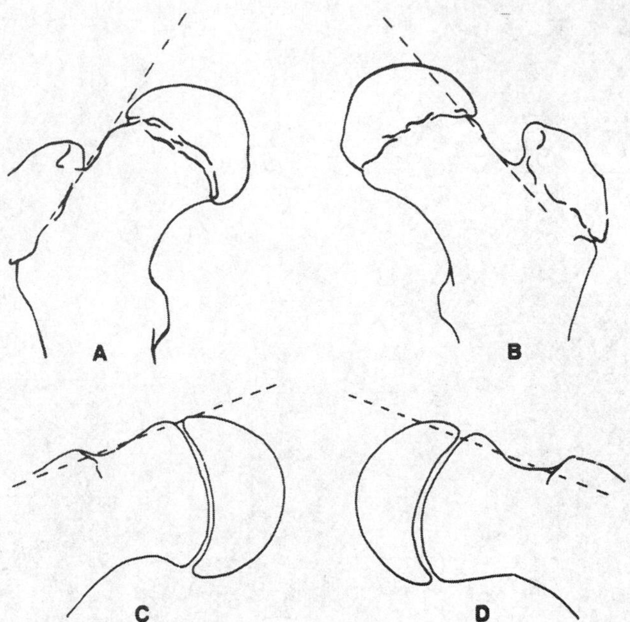

Figure 684–4 Slipped capital femoral epiphysis, anteroposterior view. A line superimposed on the superior femoral neck normally intersects part of the head (*B* and *D* are normal). With a slipped epiphysis, the line does not intersect the femoral head (*A* and *C*). Occasionally, the frog-leg view (*C* and *D*) is needed to demonstrate the slip. (From Chung S: Diseases of the developing hip joint. Pediatr Clin North Am 33:1457, 1986.)

Acute-on-Chronic Slipped Capital Femoral Epiphysis. In the acute-on-chronic SCFE, the CFE slips acutely on an existing chronic slip. These adolescents have had previous symptoms (pain, limp, out-toe gait) for several months or longer. This, too, is unstable and so painful that the child is unable to stand or bear weight on the involved side.

Chronic Slipped Capital Femoral Epiphysis. This is the most common type. There is usually a history of symptoms for several months. The symptoms typically worsen as the slip progresses. However, because there is continuity between the femoral neck and CFE, the symptoms are not severe, and the child is able to walk with a mildly antalgic, externally rotated gait. A chronic SCFE is stable (Fig. 684–5).

CLINICAL MANIFESTATIONS. The physical findings in SCFE depend on the degree of slippage and the classification. In the acute or acute-on-chronic unstable SCFE, the physical examination is limited as a result of severe pain with any attempted hip motion. In a chronic, stable SCFE, the patient has an antalgic gait, and the affected extremity is externally rotated. Hip range of motion demonstrates a lack of internal rotation and increased external rotation. Also, as the hip is flexed, it becomes progressively externally rotated. Limitation of flexion and abduction may also be present if there is a severe varus deformity of the proximal femur. Twenty percent of patients complain of knee pain only, although they have decreased hip rotation on physical examination. Adolescents, especially those who are obese, with nontraumatic anterior thigh or knee pain (referred pain) should be carefully evaluated for a SCFE.

TREATMENT. The goals of treatment for SCFE are to prevent further slippage and minimize complications. This is accomplished by performing an epiphysiodesis (closure) of the CFE. In situ pinning with one or two cannulated screws is the most popular technique. The screws can be inserted percutaneously under fluoroscopic control. Screw removal after CFE closure is controversial.

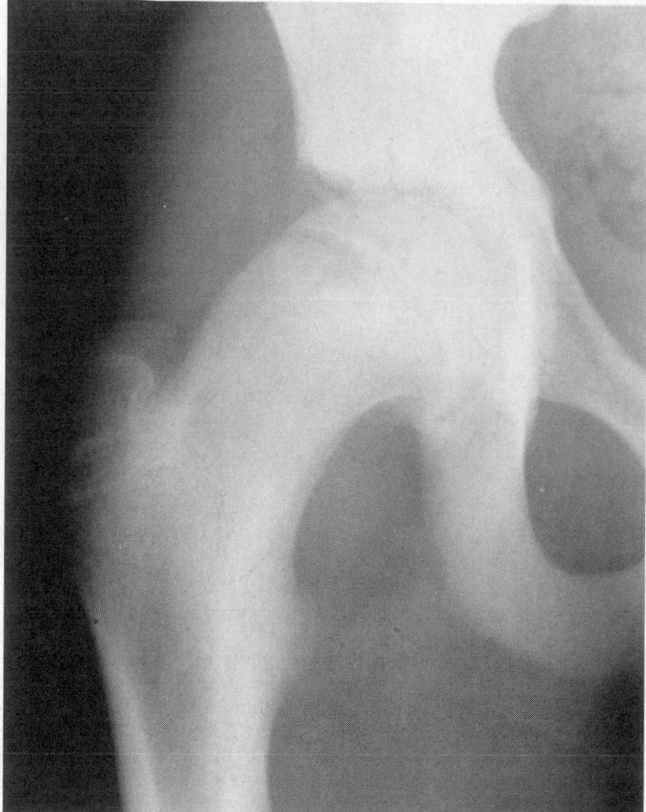

Figure 684–5 Anteroposterior radiograph of the right hip of a 13-yr-old male with a moderately severe chronic (stable) SCFE. Observe the physeal widening and the distorted relationship between the CFE and femoral neck.

COMPLICATIONS. The two serious complications in SCFE are osteonecrosis and chondrolysis. Osteonecrosis or avascular necrosis occurs as a result of injury to the retinacular vessels. This can be due to forced manipulation of an acute or unstable SCFE, compression from intracapsular hematoma, or direct injury during surgery. Partial forms of osteonecrosis may also occur after internal fixation as a result of disruption of the intraepiphyseal blood vessels. Chondrolysis is a degeneration of the articular cartilage of the hip. Its cause is unclear, but it (1) is associated with more severe slips, (2) occurs more frequently among blacks and females, and (3) is associated with pins or screws protruding out of the femoral head.

Developmental Dysplasia of the Hip

Allan DB, Gray RH, Scott TD, et al: The relationship between ligamentous clicks arising from the newborn hip and congenital dislocation. J Bone Joint Surg 67B:491, 1985.

Aronsson DD, Goldberg MJ, Kling TF Jr, et al: Developmental dysplasia of the hip. Pediatrics 94:201, 1994.

Baronciani D, Atti G, Andiloro F, et al: Electronic article. Screening for developmental dysplasia of the hip: From theory to practice. Pediatrics 99:85, 1997.

Gabuzda GM, Renshaw TS: Current concept review: Reduction of congenital dislocation of the hip. J Bone Joint Surg 74A:624, 1992.

Hansson G, Jacobsen S: Ultrasonography screening for developmental dysplasia of the hip. Acta Pediatr Scand 86:913, 1997.

Harcke HT, Kumar SJ: Current concepts review: The role of ultrasound in the diagnosis and management of congenital dislocation and dysplasia of the hip. J Bone Joint Surg 73A:622, 1991.

Hensinger RD: Congenital dislocation of the hip: Treatment in infancy to walking age. Orthop Clin North Am 18:597, 1987.

Hinderaker T, Daltveit AK, Irgens LM, et al: The impact of intra-uterine factors on neonatal hip instability. An analysis of 1,059,479 children in Norway. Acta Orthop Scand 65:239, 1994.

Hummer CD, MacEwen GD: The coexistence of torticollis and congenital dislocation of the hip. J Bone Joint Surg 54A:1255, 1972.

Keret D, MacEwen GD: Growth disturbance of the proximal part of the femur after treatment for congenital dislocation of the hip. J Bone Joint Surg 73A:410, 1991.

Malvitz TA, Weinstein SL: Closed reduction for congenital dysplasia of the hip. Functional and radiographic results after an average of thirty years. J Bone Joint Surg 76A:1777, 1994.

Schoenecker PL, Dollard PA, Sheridan JJ: Closed reduction of developmental dislocation of the hip in children older than 18 months. J Pediatr Orthop 15:763, 1995.

Viere RG, Birch JG, Herring JA, et al: Use of the Pavlik harness in congenital dislocation of the hip: An analysis of failures of treatment. J Bone Joint Surg 72A:238, 1990.

Viktor B, Bialik GM, Blazer S, et al: Developmental dysplasia of the hip: A new approach to incidence. Pediatrics 103:93, 1999.

Transient Monoarticular Synovitis

Hart JJ: Transient synovitis of the hip in children. Am Fam Physician 54:1587, 1996.

Hauseisen DC, Weiner DS, Weiner SD: The characterization of "transient synovitis of the hip" in children. J Pediatr Orthop 6:11, 1986.

Landin LA, Danielsson LG, Wattsgard C: Transient synovitis of the hip—its incidence, epidemiology and relation to Perthes disease. J Bone Joint Surg 69B:238, 1987.

Legg-Calvé-Perthes Disease

Bos CFA, Bloem JL, Bloem RM: Sequential magnetic resonance imaging in Perthes disease. J Bone Joint Surg 73B:219, 1991.

Catterall A: The natural history of Perthes disease. J Bone Joint Surg 53B:37, 1971.

Glueck CJ, Brandt G, Gruppo R, et al: Resistance to activated protein C and Legg-Perthes disease. Clin Orthop 338:139, 1997.

Herring JA, Neustadt JB, Williams JJ, et al: The lateral pillar classification of Legg-Calvé-Perthes disease. J Pediatr Orthop 12:143, 1992.

Herring JA: The treatment of Legg-Calvé-Perthes disease. A critical review of the literature. J Bone Joint Surg 76A:448, 1994.

Inoue A, Freeman MAR, Vernon-Roberts B, et al: The pathogenesis of Perthes disease. J Bone Joint Surg 58B:453, 1976.

McAndrews MP, Weinstein SL: A long-term follow-up of Legg-Calvé-Perthes disease. J Bone Joint Surg 66A:860, 1984.

Meehan PL, Angel D, Nelson JM: The Scottish Rite abduction orthosis for the treatment of Legg-Perthes disease. J Bone Joint Surg 74A:2, 1992.

Pinto MR, Peterson HA, Berquist TH: Magnetic resonance imaging in early diagnosis of Legg-Calvé-Perthes disease. J Pediatr Orthop 9:19, 1989.

Stulberg SD, Cooperman DR, Wallensten R: The natural history of Legg-Calvé-Perthes disease. J Bone Joint Surg 63A:1095, 1981.

Thompson GH, Salter RG: Legg-Calvé-Perthes disease: Current concepts and controversies. Orthop Clin North Am 18:617, 1987.

Slipped Capital Femoral Epiphysis

Aronson DD, Carlson WE: Slipped capital femoral epiphysis: A prospective study of fixation with a single screw. J Bone Joint Surg 74A:810, 1992.

Aronsson DD, Loder RT: Treatment of the unstable (acute) slipped capital femoral epiphysis. Clin Orthop 322:99, 1996.

Busch MT, Morrissey RT: Slipped capital femoral epiphysis. Orthop Clin North Am 18:637, 1987.

Carney BT, Weinstein SL, Noble J: Long-term follow-up of slipped capital femoral epiphysis. J Bone Joint Surg 73A:677, 1991.

Cooperman DR, Charles LM, Pathria M, et al: Post-mortem description of slipped capital femoral epiphysis. J Bone Joint Surg 74B:595, 1992.

Loder RT, Richards BS, Shapiro PS, et al: Acute slipped capital femoral epiphysis: The importance of physeal stability. J Bone Joint Surg 75A:1134, 1993.

Loder RT, Wittenberg B, DeSilva G: Slipped capital femoral epiphysis associated with endocrine disorders. J Pediatr Orthop 15:349, 1995.

Lubicky JP: Chondrolysis and avascular necrosis: Complications of slipped capital femoral epiphysis. J Pediatr Orthop 5B:162, 1996.

Mann DC, Weddington J, Richton S: Hormonal studies in patients with slipped capital femoral epiphysis without evidence of endocrinopathy. J Pediatr Orthop 8:543, 1988.

Siegel DB, Kasser JR, Sponseller P, et al: Slipped capital femoral epiphysis: A quantitative analysis of motion, gait, and femoral remodeling after in situ fixation. J Bone Joint Surg 73A:659, 1991.

CHAPTER 685
The Spine

Abnormalities in the vertebral column are a common nontraumatic pediatric musculoskeletal problem. They may be present at birth or may develop during childhood or adolescence. Some disorders worsen with growth and may lead to

TABLE 685–1 Classification of Spinal Deformities

Scoliosis
- ***Idiopathic***
  - Infantile
  - Juvenile
  - Adolescent
- ***Congenital***
  - Failure of formation
    - Wedge vertebrae
    - Hemivertebrae
  - Failure of segmentation
    - Unilateral bar
    - Bilateral bar
  - Mixed
- ***Neuromuscular***
  - Neuropathic diseases
    - Upper motor neuron
      - Cerebral palsy
      - Spinocerebellar degeneration (Friedreich's ataxia, Charcot-Marie-Tooth disease)
      - Syringomyelia
      - Spinal cord tumor
      - Spinal cord trauma
    - Lower motor neuron
      - Poliomyelitis
      - Spinal muscular atrophy
  - Myopathic diseases
    - Duchenne muscular dystrophy
    - Arthrogryposis
    - Other muscular dystrophies
- ***Syndromes***
  - Neurofibromatosis
  - Marfan's syndrome
- ***Compensatory***
  - Leg-length discrepancy

Kyphosis
- ***Postural Round-Back***
- ***Scheuermann's disease***
- ***Congenital Kyphosis***

Adapted from the Terminology Committee, Scoliosis Research Society: A glossary of scoliosis terms. Spine 1:57, 1976.

an unacceptable appearance, alterations in pulmonary function, and early degenerative osteoarthritis of the spine. A simplified classification of the common spinal abnormalities is presented in Table 685–1.

In the anteroposterior (frontal) plane, the vertebral bodies of the normal spine are stacked squarely one on the other with little or no deviation from vertical alignment. The vertebral end plates are parallel and the intervertebral disks are symmetric in height. In the sagittal plane, the spine has normal curvatures that provide balance and stability. The cervical and lumbar spine displays anterior convexity, termed *lordosis;* the thoracic spine and sacrum display posterior convexity and are *kyphotic.*

SCOLIOSIS

Alterations in normal spinal alignment that occur in the frontal plane are termed *scoliosis.* The majority of scoliotic deformities are idiopathic. Others can be congenital, associated with a neuromuscular disorder or syndrome, compensatory from a leg length discrepancy, or due to an intraspinal abnormality.

685.1 Idiopathic Scoliosis

ETIOLOGY AND EPIDEMIOLOGY. Idiopathic scoliosis is the most common form of scoliosis. It occurs in healthy, neurologically normal children, but its exact cause is unknown. The incidence is only slightly greater in girls than in boys, but scoliosis is more likely to progress and require treatment in girls than in boys. There appears to be a genetic component, but the disorder is not transmitted in a pure mendelian fashion. The daughters of affected mothers are more likely than other children to have scoliosis, but identical twins are not uniformly affected. The magnitude of curvature in an affected individual is not related to the magnitude of curvature in relatives. Involved children also tend to show subtle changes in proprioception and vibratory sensation, suggesting that abnormalities of spinal cord posterior column function may have a causative role.

Idiopathic scoliosis can be divided into three groups on the basis of age at onset: infantile (birth–3 yr); juvenile (4–10 yr); and adolescent (11 yr and older). Adolescent idiopathic scoliosis is much more common than juvenile-onset scoliosis; infantile idiopathic scoliosis is extraordinarily rare.

CLINICAL MANIFESTATIONS. A thorough history and physical examination is the first step in the evaluation of patients with suspected idiopathic scoliosis. Asymmetry of the posterior chest wall on forward bending (the Adams test) is the most striking and consistent abnormality in patients with scoliosis (Fig. 685–1). Rotation of the vertebral bodies within a curve toward the side of convexity of curvature displaces the attached ribs and overlying paraspinal musculature posteriorly

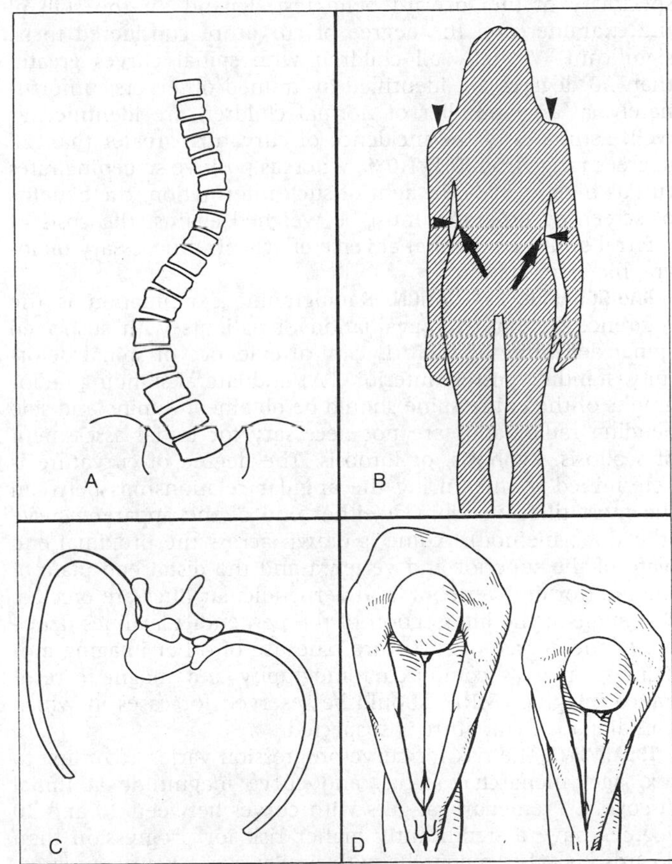

Figure 685–1 Structural changes in idiopathic scoliosis. *A,* As curvature increases, alterations in body configuration develop in both the primary and compensatory curve regions. *B,* Asymmetry of shoulder height, waistline, and the elbow-to-flank distance are common findings. *C,* Vertebral rotation and associated posterior displacement of the ribs on the convex side of the curve are responsible for the characteristic deformity of the chest wall in scoliosis patients. *D,* In the school screening examination for scoliosis, the patient bends forward at the waist. Rib asymmetry of even a small degree is obvious. (From Scoles PV: Spinal deformity in childhood and adolescence. *In:* Behrman RE, Vaughn VC III [eds]: Nelson Textbook of Pediatrics, Update 5. Philadelphia, WB Saunders, 1989.)

on the convex side of the curve and creates a depression on the concave side. Associated findings include asymmetry in shoulder height, apparent leg length discrepancy, flank asymmetry, and asymmetry of the anterior chest wall.

When the trunk is viewed from the side with the patient in the forward flexed position, the degree of *kyphosis* and *lordosis* can be evaluated. The upper region of the thoracic spine normally has a smooth, rounded curve that extends down to the midthoracic region. Flexible roundback that corrects easily when a child stands upright is common in adolescents. Sharp, abrupt, or accentuated forward angulation in the thoracic or thoracolumbar region is indicative of a kyphotic deformity. In the erect position, the lower lumbar spine is normally concave (lordotic). The magnitude of lordosis varies with age and among individuals of the same age. Children normally have less cervical lordosis and more lumbar lordosis than do adults or adolescents.

A careful neurologic evaluation is essential, especially in patients with apparent juvenile-onset scoliosis, atypical curve patterns, or back pain. The presence of café au lait spots, sacral dimpling, midline hairy patches, shoe size asymmetry, foot deformity, or a history of back pain or urinary incontinence suggest a nonidiopathic cause for the deformity.

School screening programs for early detection of scoliosis are common in North America. The forward bend test is the method employed; inclinometers to estimate the height of rib asymmetry are used in some centers. The sensitivity and specificity of the forward bend test depend on the skill of the examiner and the degree of curvature considered to be significant. Virtually all children with spinal curves greater than 20 degrees are identified by trained observers; unfortunately, a large number of normal children are identified as well. Estimates of the incidence of curvature greater than 20 degrees range from 0.1–1.0%, whereas positive screening rates run as high as 30%. In light of such information, the benefits of screening programs must be weighed against the costs of referral and the potential adverse effects of unnecessary radiographic examination.

RADIOGRAPHIC EVALUATION. Radiographic examination is the reference standard for evaluation of patients with suspected spinal deformity. If there is clinical evidence of spinal deformity, standing posteroanterior (PA) and lateral standing radiographs of the entire spine should be obtained. Supine and side bending radiographs are not necessary for initial assessment of scoliosis, kyphosis, or lordosis. The degree of curvature is determined by measuring the angular relationships between the most tilted vertebra at either end of the apparent curve (the Cobb method). A line is drawn across the proximal end plate of the superior end vertebra and the distal end plate of the inferior end vertebra, and perpendicular lines are erected. The angle at the intersection of the perpendicular lines determines the degree of curvature. The use of other imaging modalities, such as computed tomography and magnetic resonance imaging (MRI), should be reserved for cases in which nonidiopathic curvature is suspected.

TREATMENT. The risk for curve progression varies according to sex, age, menarchal status, and curve magnitude at initial discovery. Premenarchal girls with curves between 20 and 30 degrees have a significantly higher risk for progression than do girls 2 yr after menarche with similar curves; curve progression is likely in the first group, and uncommon in the second. Boys with curvature of the same magnitude appear to have similar risks of progression when judged by other maturation standards. Curves less than 30 degrees rarely progress after skeletal maturation is complete; curves greater than 45 or 50 degrees often continue to progress during adult life.

The rationale for treatment of patients with idiopathic scoliosis is based on the assumption that patients with progressive scoliosis will acquire unacceptable deformities, premature degenerative joint disease, and progressive cardiorespiratory compromise, and that treatment can positively affect these outcomes. Although there is conflicting data on the long-term fate of untreated scoliosis patients, it appears reasonable to assume that patients with high-magnitude deformities will both look and feel different than their age- and sex-matched peers.

The generally accepted methods of treatment of progressive idiopathic adolescent scoliosis are bracing and surgical correction. There is no evidence that exercise programs alter the outcome of scoliosis; transcutaneous electrical stimulation has been shown to have no effect. Most orthopedic surgeons recommend a trial of brace treatment for immature patients with curves less than 40 degrees. Although the efficacy of brace treatment has been questioned, current studies suggest a small decrease in the likelihoood of progression for patients treated with bracing when compared with age-, sex-, and curve-matched peers followed by observation alone. Bracing does not correct curvature; although improvement in Cobb angles is often noted during the active period of brace treatment, there are no studies that demonstrate consistent long-term maintenance of correction. A variety of spinal orthoses are employed; retrospective studies suggest little difference in outcome by brace type.

Surgical treatment is usually considered for patients with idiopathic curves greater than 45 degrees. Surgical treatment usually combines correction of deformity with permanently implanted internal fixation rods and posterior fusion of the involved vertebrae (Fig. 685–2). Occasionally, anterior spinal fusion and instrumentation may be indicated, especially in thoracolumbar and lumbar curves.

685.2 Congenital Scoliosis

Abnormalities of vertebral development during the first trimester of pregnancy often result in structural deformities of the spine that are evident at birth or become obvious in early childhood. Congenital scoliosis can be classified as (1) partial or complete failure of vertebral formation (wedge vertebrae or hemivertebrae), (2) partial or complete failure of segmentation (unsegmented bars), or (3) mixed. They may occur as an isolated deformity or in combination with other organ system malformations that are differentiating at the same time as the spine.

Congenital genitourinary malformations occur in 20% of children with congenital scoliosis. Unilateral renal agenesis is the most common abnormality. Duplication of ureters, horseshoe kidney, and genital anomalies also occur. Approximately 2% of children with associated genitourinary abnormalities have a silent, obstructive uropathy. Renal ultrasonography should be performed in all children with congenital scoliosis to assess for possible genitourinary problems. Other procedures, such as intravenous pyelography or MRI, may be necessary if the ultrasonogram is abnormal. Congenital heart disease occurs in 10–15% of children with congenital scoliosis.

A high percentage of patients with congenital scoliosis have associated defects of the spinal cord. *Spinal dysraphism* is the general term applied to such lesions; MRI studies suggest that they are present in as many as 40% of patients with congenital scoliosis. Spina bifida occulta is the most common and benign defect; myelomeningocele is the most severe. Other lesions include intradural and extradural lipomas, cysts and teratomas, and spinal cord tethers. In addition to spine asymmetry, physical examination in these patients often shows hairy patches, skin dimples, hemangiomas, and abnormalities of the feet and lower extremities. Asymmetric foot size, cavus feet, and calf atrophy strongly suggest the presence of spinal dysraphism in patients with congenital scoliosis. MRI is the procedure of choice for evaluating possible spinal dysraphism.

The risk for progression of spinal deformity in a child with congenital scoliosis depends on the growth potential of the

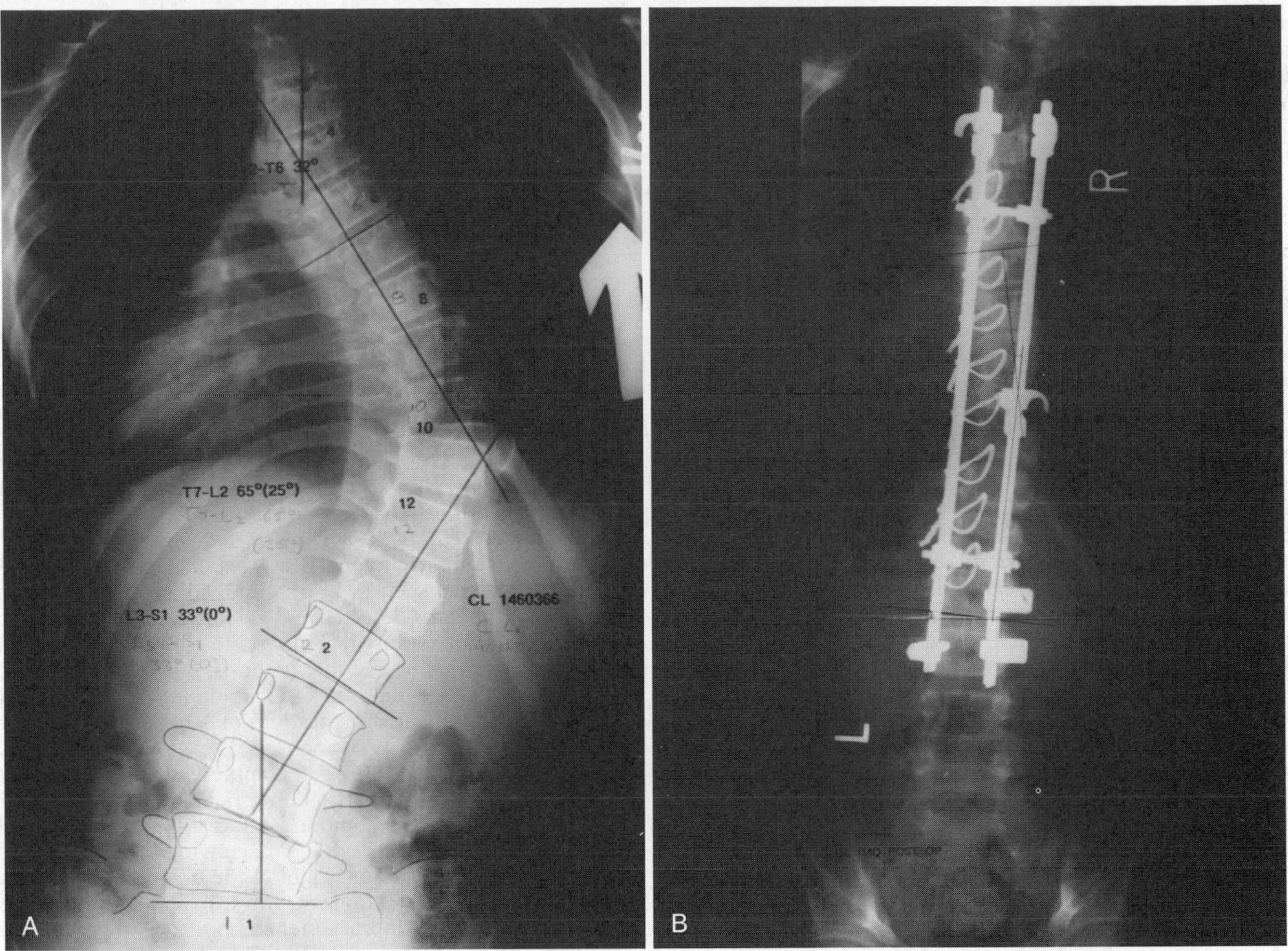

Figure 685–2 *A*, Preoperative standing posteroanterior radiograph of a 13-year-old girl with a severe right thoracic section. Note the Cobb measurement technique. The numbers in parentheses indicate the degree of correction of the deformity on side-bending radiographs. *B*, Postoperative radiograph demonstrating a selective right thoracolumbar fusion and instrumentation from T-3 to L-2. Note the spontaneous improvement in the compensatory left lumbar curve after correction of the structural right thoracolumbar curve.

malformed vertebra. Defects, such as block vertebra, have little growth potential and usually do not cause significant spinal deformity. Hemivertebrae may or may not cause significant deformity depending on location and their potential for growth. Unilateral unsegmented bars almost always produce progressive deformities. Approximately 25% of patients with congenital scoliosis do not demonstrate curve progression and do not require treatment. Most patients demonstrate some progression, and many require treatment. Patients are most at risk during periods of rapid growth before 2 and after 10 yr of age.

Early diagnosis and prompt treatment of progressive curves is essential. Orthotic treatment is of limited value because of the structural nature of congenital curvature. Often a combined anterior and posterior spinal fusion across the area of the deformity is required to halt progression and counteract the strong forces of growth. Anterior and posterior convex epiphysiodeses have been used to produce partial correction with growth. Hemivertebrae excision can also be considered. It is a serious mistake to defer treatment of progressive spinal curvatures while awaiting further spinal growth.

685.3 Neuromuscular Scoliosis, Syndromes, and Compensatory Scoliosis

Scolioisis is a common complication of many neuromuscular disorders of childhood. Muscle imbalance, soft tissue contracture, and progressive weakness predispose patients with disorders such as cerebral palsy, muscular dystrophies, and spinal muscular atrophy to scoliosis. In patients with myelodysplasia, structural malformations of the vertebral column complicate the problem. In general, the magnitude of the deformity depends on the severity of involvement, the pattern of weakness, and the progressive nature of the underlying disease process. Ambulatory patients with minimal involvement and cerebral palsy are much less likely to have significant spinal deformity than nonambulatory patients with profound involvement.

Progression of deformity in patients with neuromuscular scoliosis has serious consequences. Sitting and standing balance are altered, adversely affecting ambulation in marginal walkers and complicating seating support in nonambulators. Patients who must use their arms for trunk support lose a significant degree of independence. Severe curves decrease pulmonary reserve, compounding pre-existent respiratory problems.

Neuromuscular scoliosis can be treated safely and effectively in most instances, but the success of treatment depends on early recognition. Because scoliosis in most patients with neuromuscular disease progresses relentlessly once curvature begins, there is little reason to delay treatment once the deformity is identified. The forward bending test can be used for screening; the test may be performed in the sitting position for patients who cannot stand. Any asymmetry is an indication for radiographic evaluation. This should include PA and lateral standing radiographs of the entire spine. If the child or adolescent cannot stand, a sitting or supine (anteroposterior) radiograph is necessary.

The goal of treatment of neuromuscular scoliosis is to restore spinal alignment, stabilize respiratory function, and prevent progressive loss of independence. Nonambulatory patients are usually most comfortable, are more independent, and have better respiratory function when they are able to sit erect without external support. Unfortunately, options for treatment in neuromuscular scoliosis are limited. Orthotic management or bracing is usually not effective as definitive treatment in neuromuscular scoliosis. In young children, brace treatment may slow the rate of curve progression, allowing further spinal growth and delaying surgical intervention. For most patients with progressive deformity, surgery is necessary when treatment is indicated. Current instrumentation systems provide effective correction and eliminate the need for external support in the postoperative period. Most patients may be out of bed immediately after surgery.

SYNDROMES. Children with certain syndromes are also at increased risk for spinal deformities. Common syndromes include neurofibromatosis and Marfan syndrome. These children require periodic evaluation and prompt referral for orthopedic evaluation at the first sign of a spinal deformity.

COMPENSATORY SCOLIOSIS. Leg length inequality is a common cause of false-positive screening examinations (see Chapter 682). Discrepancies as small as 0.5 cm may produce asymmetry. The pelvis in such patients tilts toward the short side, producing a postural curve in the opposite direction. Because children with leg length inequality may also have idiopathic or congenital scoliosis, careful evaluation is necessary. Any child with a lower extremity inequality should be referred for orthopedic evaluation.

685.4 Kyphosis (Round-Back)

The normal thoracic spine has a convex alignment in the sagittal plane, termed *kyphosis*. The normal radiographic range of kyphosis is approximately 20 to 40 degrees; individuals with increased kyphotic alignment have the clinical sign of round-back. Round-back may be flexible or structural; structural round-back may be idiopathic or congenital in origin. Idiopathic round-back is sometimes referred to as Scheuermann disease.

Flexible Kyphosis

Round-back is a common concern of many parents of adolescents. They often are perceived by parents and teachers to sit and stand in a slouched position, and round-back is a common cause of referral from spine screening programs. Adolescents with postural round-back can correct the round-back appearance voluntarily in both the standing and prone positions. The overall angle of kyphosis my be increased on the standing lateral radiograph, but no vertebral abnormalities are present. A supine hyperextension lateral radiograph shows complete correction. It is commonly thought that such a posture leads to permanent deformity. Fortunately, there is no evidence that flexible round-back posture has adverse physical effects. A thoracic hyperextension exercise program may assist in strengthening the extensor muscles of the spine, but the patient has the ultimate responsibility for his or her posture. Orthotic treatment is not indicated for patients with flexible round-back.

Structural Kyphosis

Scheuermann's Disease (Idiopathic Kyphosis)

The term *Scheuermann's kyphosis* is used for nonflexible (structural) kyphosis that develops during adolescence in previously normal children. Mild increases in structural kyphosis are equally common in girls and boys; the condition may worsen slightly more often in boys than in girls. The absolute incidence of the disorder is unknown because small degrees of structural kyphosis are neither clinically obvious nor significant. Cadaver studies indicate that the vertebral changes associated with structural round-back occur in 7 or 8% of the population. The cause is unclear, but histologic specimens obtained at the time of surgical correction of severe deformity suggest that a disordered pattern of endochondral ossification similar to that found in slipped capital femoral epiphysis and tibia vara may be responsible. This may be the result of increased pressure on the anterior vertebral growth plates in some individuals with severe flexible round-back, but the relationship has not been clearly established.

CLINICAL MANIFESTATIONS. Patients with Scheuermann kyphosis present with thoracic kyphosis of greater degree and sharper contour than that seen in normal individuals. Unlike flexible round-back patients, affected individuals cannot actively correct the deformity. Many patients complain of occasional mild aching pain in the area of the kyphosis, but it is rarely severe or limiting. Careful neurologic examination is essential, but fortunately neurologic complications of Scheuermann's kyphosis are rare.

RADIOGRAPHIC EVALUATION. Radiographic assessment for kyphosis includes PA and lateral standing radiographs of the entire spine (Fig. 685–3). In addition to increased kyphotic angle, radiographic findings include (1) narrowing of disk space, (2) loss of the normal anterior height of the involved vertebra and elongation of the vertebral centrum, (3) wedging of 5 degrees or more in three or more vertebrae, and (4) irregularities of the end plates, sometimes called *Schmorl's nodes*.

TREATMENT. Treatment is dependent on the age of the patient, the degree of deformity, and the presence or absence of pain in the apical region. Scheuermann kyphosis appears to be primarily a cosmetic problem. There is little evidence that patients with kyphotic curves less than 70 or 80 degrees experience late progression, disabling pain, or neurologic compromise. Kyphotic deformities greater than 90 degrees are more likely to be aesthetically unacceptable, symptomatic, and progressive. There are few absolute guidelines for treatment, and decisions must be individualized. Mature patients with little or no pain and acceptable cosmetic alignment need no treatment. Immature patients with mild deformity may benefit from a hyperextension exercise program, whereas those with kyphotic deformities greater than 60 degrees require bracing if treatment is considered appropriate. Thoracic kyphosis usually requires a Milwaukee brace; in patients with thoracolumbar kyphosis, an underarm hyperextension orthosis can be used. Surgical treatment of Scheuermann disease is usually reserved for patients with severe and painful deformity who have completed growth. This usually involves a combination of anterior spinal release and fusion and posterior spinal fusion and instrumentation.

Congenital Kyphosis

Congenital kyphosis, or kyphotic deformity, is the result of vertebral malformations that occur during the first trimester. The most common abnormalities are congenital failure of formation of all or part of the vertebral centrum and failure of anterior segmentation of the spine (anterior unsegmented bar). Severe deformities are usually recognized at birth and rapidly progress thereafter. The less obvious deformities may not become obvious until later in childhood. Progressive congenital kyphosis is a serious problem; paraplegia may develop

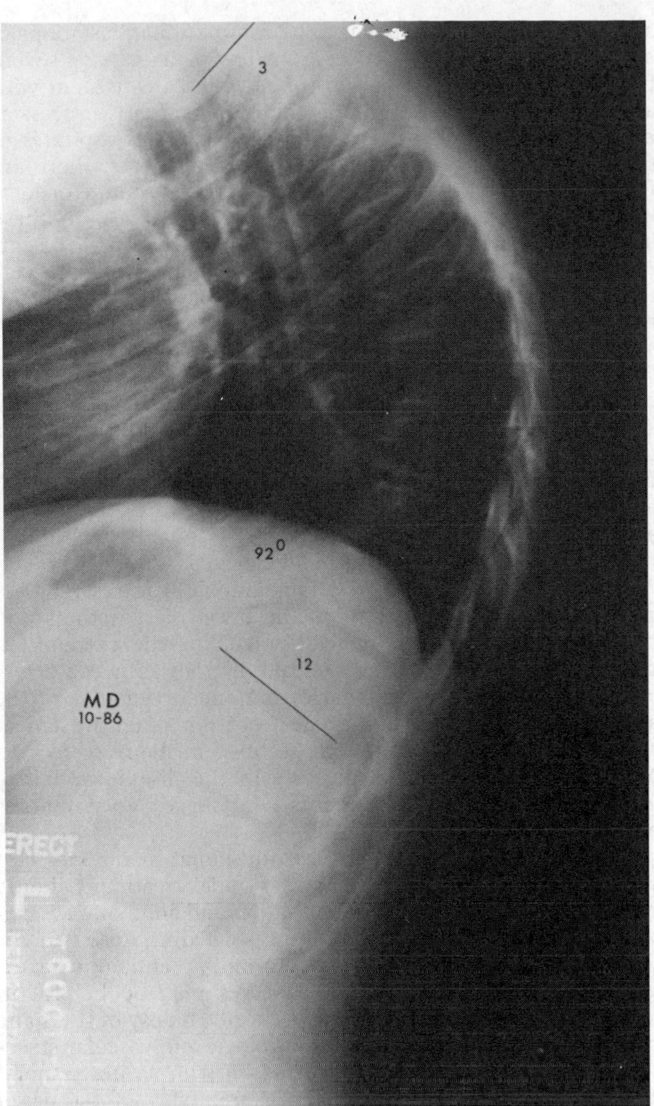

Figure 685–3 Standing lateral radiograph of a 14-year-old boy with severe Scheuermann kyphosis. This measures 92 degrees between T-3 and T-12. Note the wedging of the vertebrae at T-6, T-7, T-8, and T-9. The normal thoracic kyphosis is 40 degrees or less.

as a result of compression of the spinal cord against the apex of the deformity. Patients with congenital kyphosis should be referred for specialty evaluation as soon as the deformity is recognized. Brace treatment is not effective. Surgical intervention is often necessary, and the results of surgery are best if performed before significant deformity has developed.

685.5 Back Pain in Children

Back pain in children is unusual and should be viewed with concern. In contrast to adults, in whom back pain is frequently mechanical or psychologic in origin, back pain in children is frequently due to organic causes, especially in preadolescent children. Back pain lasting more than a few days requires careful investigation. It has been reported that approximately 85% of children with back pain lasting more than 2 mo have a specific diagnosable lesion: 33% post-traumatic (occult fracture, spondylolysis); 33% developmental (kyphosis, scoliosis); and 18% infection or tumor. Only in the remaining 15% is the diagnosis nonspecific.

CLINICAL MANIFESTATIONS. When confronted with a child with back pain, a careful history and physical evaluation are mandatory. The history includes the onset and duration of symptoms; antecedent factors; general health; family history; location, character, and radiation of pain; and neurologic symptoms, such as muscle weakness, sensory changes, and bowel or bladder dysfunction. Physical examination includes a complete musculoskeletal and neurologic evaluation. Spinal alignment, mobility, muscle spasm, and areas of tenderness are evaluated and recorded. The danger signs in childhood back pain include (1) persistent or increasing pain; (2) systemic symptoms, such as fever, malaise, or weight loss; (3) neurologic symptoms or findings; (4) bowel or bladder dysfunction; (5) young age, especially less than 4 yr (suspect tumor); and (6) painful left thoracic spine curvatures.

RADIOGRAPHIC AND LABORATORY EVALUATION. Plain radiographs are the first diagnostic procedure to use in the evaluation of pediatric back pain, usually PA and lateral standing radiographs of the spine with right and left oblique views of the involved area. However, MRI or bone scans may be necessary depending on the location of the pain and the differential diagnoses. Laboratory studies, such as a complete blood count with differential, erythrocyte sedimentation rate (ESR), and tests for the juvenile forms of arthritis (juvenile rheumatoid arthritis and ankylosing spondylitis) may be necessary in certain cases (see Chapter 156). Cerebrospinal fluid should be evaluated if myelography is performed.

DIFFERENTIAL DIAGNOSIS. The differential diagnosis in pediatric back pain is extensive and is presented in Table 685–2.

685.6 Spondylolysis and Spondylolisthesis

Spondylolysis is the term used to refer to a defect in the pars interarticularis, the posterior plate of bone that connects the

TABLE 685–2 Differential Diagnosis of Back Pain

Inflammatory Diseases

Diskitis (common before 6 yr)
Vertebral osteomyelitis (pyogenic, tuberculous)
Spinal epidural abscess
Pyelonephritis
Pancreatitis

Rheumatologic Diseases

Pauciarticular juvenile rheumatoid arthritis
Reiter's syndrome
Ankylosing spondylitis
Psoriatic arthritis

Developmental Diseases

Spondylolysis (common in adolescents)
Spondylolisthesis (common in adolescents)
Scheuermann's syndrome (common in adolescents)
Scoliosis (especially left thoracic)

Mechanical Trauma and Abnormalities

Hip-pelvic anomalies
Herniated disk
Overuse syndromes (common with athletic training and in gymnasts and dancers)
Vertebral stress fractures
Upper cervical spine instability

Neoplastic Diseases

Primary vertebral tumors (e.g., osteogenic sarcoma)
Metastatic tumor (e.g., neuroblastoma)
Primary spinal tumor (e.g., neuroblastoma, lipoma)
Malignancy of bone marrow (e.g., acute lymphocytic leukemia, lymphoma)
Benign tumors (e.g., eosinophilic granuloma, osteoid osteoma)

Other

After lumbar puncture
Conversion reaction
Juvenile osteoporosis

superior and inferior articular facets of a vertebral body. The abnormality most commonly occurs in the L5 vertebra and is sometimes associated with forward slip of the affected vertebra relative to the body of the first sacral vertebra termed *spondylolisthesis*. Spondylolysis may be congenital or acquired. Cadaver studies indicate that 5–7% of the general population has pars interarticularis defects; asymptomatic spina bifida occulta at L5 or S1 often accompanies the lesion. Most individuals with congenital spondylolysis have little or no pain and do not acquire spondylolisthesis. In such a patient, the abnormality is usually noted an incidental finding on radiographs made for other reasons. A small percentage of patients with spondylolysis acquire the lesion as a result of repetitive flexion exercises from activities such as gymnastics or diving. The lesion in such patients resembles a stress fracture and is more likely to be symptomatic. Spondylolisthesis, when present, is usually graded by the degree of slippage of one vertebra on the other: grade 1, less than 25%; grade 2, 25–50%; grade 3, 50–75%; grade 4, 75–100%; and grade 5, complete displacement.

CLINICAL MANIFESTATIONS. Symptomatic patients with spondylolysis usually present with low back pain and hamstring muscle spasm. Radicular symptoms are not common. Urinary retention or incontinence are uncommon, but when present imply serious compromise of the sacral nerve roots. Physical examination shows limitation of lumbar flexibility and tight hamstring muscles. When spondylolisthesis accompanies spondylolysis, lumbar lordosis is often reduced rather than accentuated, and sacral kyphosis is often present. The buttocks appear flattened and prominent, and the anterior abdominal wall is prominent. A palpable "step-off" at the lumbosacral area may be noted in patients with high-grade spondylolisthesis. The forward bend test for scoliosis should be performed because patients with spondylolysis may also have scoliosis. Careful neurologic examination is essential.

RADIOLOGIC EVALUATION. Initial radiographic examination in patients with suspected disorders of the lumbosacral region should include anteroposterior, lateral, and oblique radiographs of the lumbosacral spine. Large cassette films of the spine should be obtained if there is a suspicion of scoliosis. When there is a history of urinary dysfunction or physical signs of nerve root compromise, MRI of the thoracolumbar spine should be performed.

TREATMENT. Treatment of spondylolysis depends on the presence of symptoms. Progressive slippage has been reported in children and adolescents with asymptomatic spondylolysis, and such patients should be re-examined at 6-mo intervals. Repeat radiographs are probably not necessary in the absence of symptoms or physical signs of progression. When indicated, a single standing lateral film of the lumbosacral junction provides information for routine follow-up. Patients with painful spondylolysis, especially when a stress fracture is suspected, may benefit from a period of immobilization in a body jacket or underarm orthosis. If this does not relieve pain, surgical intervention may be required to repair the defect or stabilize the affected vertebrae.

Progressive spondylolisthesis causes deformity and disability. Since surgical reduction of severe slip is difficult and carries significant risks, progressive slips are best treated before a severe deformity develops. In general, painful spondylolisthesis, or asymptomatic spondylolisthesis with greater than 25% slip should be treated by an in situ posterior spinal fusion regardless of the age of the patient.

685.7 Disk Space Infection

Intervertebral diskitis is the term used for the association of back pain, progressive loss of intervertebral disk height, and erosion of adjacent vertebral end plates. The clinical findings and radiographic signs appear to be common manifestations of a number of underlying processes. A few patients have severe back pain, high fever, and signs of bacteremia consistent with acute osteomyelitis. In others, the inflammatory process is much less severe, even though blood cultures or aspirates of the involved area yield bacteria. In some patients, there are few symptoms and signs and no evidence of systemic or local infection despite progressive radiographic changes. In these instances, the lesion may be of traumatic or rheumatic origin.

CLINICAL MANIFESTATIONS. Symptoms in patients with intervertebral diskitis vary with age, and a high index of suspicion is required to establish the diagnosis. Very young children may simply be fussy and refuse to eat. Toddlers may cease walking. Older children and adolescents complain of back, abdominal, or pelvic pain. The physical findings in a child with a disk space infection are usually characteristic. The child maintains the spine in a straight, stiff, or splinted position and refuses to flex the lumbar spine. The normal lumbar lordosis is reversed, and there may be paravertebral muscle spasm. Fever is variable, and the systemic white blood cell count may be only mildly elevated. The ESR is usually elevated.

RADIOGRAPHIC EVALUATION. The radiographic features vary according to the interval between the onset of symptoms and the diagnosis. As in osteomyelitis involving the extremities, radiographic signs lag behind clinical symptoms. The characteristic findings of disk space (narrowing and irregularity of the adjacent vertebral body end plates) are not often present at the time of initial presentation. Technetium bone scans and MRI scans become abnormal early in the disease and may establish the diagnosis in patients with suggestive symptoms and signs.

TREATMENT. In patients with constitutional symptoms and signs suggestive of a bacterial cause, initial treatment should include a combination of immobilization and antibiotics. *Staphylococcus aureus* is the usual organism isolated in those patients with a clear bacterial cause, and appropriate antibiotic coverage should be initiated. Blood cultures may be helpful in identifying the organism. Aspiration needle biopsy of the spine carries some risks of damage to neurologic and vascular structures and is usualy reserved for children who do not respond to initial treatment with antibiotics. A minimum of 4–6 wk of antibiotic therapy should be used for patients with positive cultures, high white blood cell counts, or persistent elevation of the ESR. The appropriateness of antibiotics is less certain in patients with minimal symptoms, few signs, and normal laboratory studies. Immobilization alone may suffice in such cases. Surgical drainage is usually reserved for patients who do not respond to initial therapy or who have MRI evidence of abscess formation in the paravertebral area.

685.8 Intervertebral Disk Herniation

Intervertebral disk rupture is rare in children and uncommon in adolescents. In the United States, less than 1% of patients undergoing discectomy are younger than 16 yr. The frequency of symptomatic intervertebral disk herniation is more common in Asiatic populations than in whites, perhaps because of the smaller size of the spinal canal.

CLINICAL MANIFESTATIONS. Symptoms of intervertebral disk herniation in adolescents are similar to those in adults. The majority of affected patients report back pain; most have sciatic pain. About 30% complain of decreased sensation or paresthesia in the lower extremities. On physical examination, lumbar muscle spasm, scoliosis, and a decreased range of lumbar motion are common findings. A positive straight leg-raising test is present in most patients. Abnormal reflex patterns and lower extremity weakness are much less likely to be present in young patients than in adults. A history of trauma is occasionally present, and patients tend to be taller and slightly heavier than their peers. A positive family history of intervertebral disk disease is frequently present.

RADIOGRAPHIC EVALUATION. Radiographs often show loss of lumbar lordosis and lumbar scoliosis. Loss of intervertebral disk height is rarely noted on plain films. MRI is currently the study of choice for localization of the lesion.

TREATMENT. Most symptoms respond to bed rest followed by gradual resumption of activities. When sciatic pain, loss of reflexes, or weakness persist, surgical excision of the intervertebral disk is indicated. Fusion is not necessary unless there is accompanying evidence of spinal instability. Good results can be expected about 75% of the time. The incidence of recurrent symptoms requiring repeat surgery is about 25%.

685.9 Tumors

Back pain may be the presenting complaint in children who have a tumor involving the vertebral column or the spinal cord. Other associated symptoms may include weakness of the lower extremities, scoliosis, and loss of sphincter control. Both benign and malignant tumors may occur; most are benign (see Chapter 514). Common benign tumors include osteoid osteomas, osteoblastoma, solitary bone cysts, and eosinophilic granuloma. Malignant tumors may be osseous (osteogenic or Ewing's sarcoma), neurogenic (neuroblastoma), or metastatic in origin. Since the onset of symptoms usually precedes radiographic abnormality, radioisotope bone scans or MRI is necessary for localization and diagnosis. The treatment of tumors of the spinal column is complex and may involve a combination of surgery, radiotherapy, and chemotherapy. Side effects are common when combination therapy is required, and growth disturbances can be expected.

Idiopathic Scoliosis

Ceballas T, Ferrer-Torrelles M, Castillo F, et al: Prognosis in infantile idiopathic scoliosis. J Bone Joint Surg 62A:863, 1980.

Figueiredo UM, James JIP: Juvenile idiopathic scoliosis. J Bone Joint Surg 61B:36, 1979.

Lonstein JE, Carlson JM: The prediction of curve progression in untreated idiopathic scoliosis during growth. J Bone Joint Surg 66A:1061, 1984.

Lonstein, JE, Winter RB: The Milwaukee brace for the treatment of adolescent idiopathic scoliosis. J Bone Joint Surg 76A:1207, 1994.

Nachemson AL, Peterson LE: Effectiveness of treatment with a brace for girls who have adolescent idiopathic scoliosis. A prospective controlled study based on data from the brace study of the Scoliosis Research Society. J Bone Joint Surg 77A:815, 1995.

Noonan KJ, Weinstein SL, Jacobson WC, Dolan LA: Use of the Milwaukee brace for progressive idiopathic scoliosis. J Bone Joint Surg 78A:557, 1996.

Rowe DE, Bernstein SM, Riddick MF, et al: A meta-analysis of the efficiency of non-operative treatments for idiopathic scoliosis. J Bone Joint Surg 79A:664, 1997.

Schwend RM, Hennrikus W, Hall JE, Emans JB: Childhood scoliosis: Clinical indications for magnetic resonance imaging. J Bone Joint Surg 77A:46, 1995.

U.S. Preventive Services Task Force: Screening for adolescent idiopathic scoliosis. Policy Statement and Review. JAMA 269:2664, 1993.

Congenital Scoliosis

Callahan BC, Georgopoulos G, Eilert RE: Hemivertebral excision for congenital scoliosis. J Pediatr Orthop 17:96, 1997.

McMaster MJ: Occult intraspinal anomalies and congenital scoliosis. J Bone Joint Surg 66A:588, 1984.

McMaster MJ, Ohtsuka K: The natural history of congenital scoliosis: A study of 251 patients. J Bone Joint Surg 68B:588, 1986.

Thompson AG, Marks DS, Sayampanathan SR, Piggott H: Long-term results of combined anterior and posterior convex epiphysiodesis for congenital scoliosis due to hemivertebrae. Spine 20:1380, 1995.

Winter RB, Haven JJ, Moe JH, et al: Diastematomyelia and congenital spine deformities. J Bone Joint Surg 56A:27, 1974.

Winter RB, Moe JH, Eilers VE: Congenital scoliosis—a study of 234 patients treated and untreated. J Bone Joint Surg 50A:1, 1968.

Neuromuscular Scoliosis

Ferguson RI, Allen BL Jr: Consideration in the treatment of cerebral palsy patients with spinal deformities. Orthop Clin North Am 19:419, 1988.

Galasko GSB, Delaney C, Morris P: Spinal stabilization in Duchenne muscular dystrophy. J Bone Joint Surg 74B:210, 1992.

Piggott H: The natural history of scoliosis in myelodysplasia. J Bone Joint Surg 62B:54, 1980.

Smith AD, Koreska J, Moseley CF: Progression of scoliosis in Duchenne muscular dystrophy. J Bone Joint Surg 71A:1066, 1989.

Kyphosis—Scheuermann's and Congenital

Lowe TG: Current concepts review: Scheuermann disease. J Bone Joint Surg 72A:940, 1990.

Sachs B, Bradford D, Winter R, et al: Scheuermann's kyphosis: Follow-up of Milwaukee brace treatment. J Bone Joint Surg 69A:50, 1987.

Winter RB, Moe JH, Wang JF: Congenital kyphosis: Its natural history and treatment as observed in a study of 130 patients. J Bone Joint Surg 55A:223, 1973.

Spondylolysis and Spondylolisthesis

Bell DF, Ehrlich MG, Zaleski D: Brace treatment for symptomatic spondylolisthesis. Clin Orthop 236:192, 1988.

Dubousset J: Treatment of spondylolysis and spondylolisthesis in children and adolescents. Clin Orthop 33:77, 1997.

Hensinger RN: Current concepts review: Spondylolysis and spondylolisthesis in children and adolescents. J Bone Joint Surg 71A:1098, 1989.

Pizzutillo PD, Hummer CD III: Nonoperative treatment of painful adolescent spondylolysis or spondylolisthesis. J Pediatr Orthop 9:538, 1989.

Saraste H: Long-term clinical and radiographical follow-up of spondylolysis and spondylolisthesis. J Pediatr Orthop 7:631, 1987.

Seitsalo S, Osterman K, Hyvarinen H, et al: Severe spondylolisthesis in children and adolescents. J Bone Joint Surg 72B:259, 1990.

Disk Space Infection

Crawford AH, Kucharzyk DW, Ruda R, et al: Diskitis in children. Clin Orthop 266:70, 1991.

Scoles PV, Quinn TP: Intervertebral discitis in children and adolescents. Clin Orthop 162:31, 1982.

Szaly E, Green N, Heller R: Magnetic resonance imaging in the diagnosis of childhood discitis. J Pediatr Orthop 7:164, 1987.

Back Pain

Conrad EM III, Olszewski AD, Berger M, et al: Pediatric spine tumors with spinal cord compromise. J Pediatr Orthop 12:454, 1992.

Delamarter RB, Sachs BL, Thompson GH, et al: Primary neoplasms of the thoracic and lumbar spine: An analysis of 29 conservative cases. Clin Orthop 256:87, 1990.

King HA: Evaluating the child with back pain. Pediatr Clin North Am 33:1489, 1986.

Thompson GH: Instructional Course Lecture. Back pain in children. J Bone Joint Surg 75A:928, 1993.

Thompson GH: Back pain. *In*: Snyder RK (ed): Essentials of Musculoskeletal Care. The American Academy of Orthopaedic Surgeons. Rosemont, IL, 1997, pp 559–561.

CHAPTER 686
The Neck

Nonosseous and osseous abnormalities of the neck are relatively common in children. These are predominantly soft tissue, congenital, and neurologic in origin.

686.1 Torticollis

Torticollis (*torqueo L.*, to twist + *collum L.*, neck) is the term applied to the clinical finding of a twisted neck. In most instances, the head is tipped toward one side and the chin rotated toward the other. Torticollis is a sign, not a disease, and may be the result of a wide range of underlying pathophysiologic processes. Torticollis that is present at birth may be the result of developmental or traumatic lesions of the sternomastoid muscle or of congenital abnormalities of the cervical spine. Torticollis in later childhood may be the result of trauma, inflammatory processes, spinal syrinx, or central nervous system neoplasia. The differential diagnosis of torticollis is extensive and is presented in Table 686–1.

Muscular torticollis is the most common variety and is presumed to result from injury to the sternocleidomastoid muscle during delivery. Large infants who have had difficult vertex deliveries are at special risk. In affected infants, normal rotation of the neck during delivery may produce bleeding within the substance of the sternocleidomastoid muscle and a localized increase in pressure within the muscular compartment contained by the sternocleidomastoid fascia. Increased pressure produces focal ischemia; secondary fibrosis and contracture within the muscle result in the clinical finding of torticollis.

Swelling within the sternocleidomastoid muscle may be palpable in neonates with muscular torticollis; swelling diminishes shortly after birth, and the lesion may not be present in older infants. Contracture of the muscle results in the typical head tilt and rotation. In patients with a suggestive history and appropriate physical findings, a program of gentle passive stretching exercises started within the first month of life often results in resolution. The parents should be instructed to rotate the chin gently toward the side of head tilt while simultaneously bringing the head to the upright position. As range of motion improves, the chin can be rotated past neutral, and the head tilted toward the opposite side. Significant correction usually occurs within the first few months of life in patients with muscular torticollis. When deformity persists, the patient should be referred for orthopedic evaluation. Soft collars are not effective in treatment, and rigid devices produce secondary mandibular deformity. Surgical release of the sternomastoid muscle is occasionally required in such patients and should be performed before the development of secondary facial asymmetry (plagiocephaly).

Congenital malformations of the cervical spine may also produce torticollis. Malformation or congenital cervical scoliosis result in deformity of the neck that will not respond to stretching exercise programs. Infants with torticollis, in whom there is no history of possible birth trauma and no evidence of a mass within the sternocleidomastoid muscle, should have anteroposterior and lateral cervical spine radiographs before a program of manipulation is recommended. At best, such infants respond minimally to stretching exercises; at worst, passive manipulation may injure the cervical spinal cord.

Torticollis arising later in childhood in previously normal children requires careful evaluation. Although the most common causes are minor cervical muscle trauma or inflammation of the cervical muscles secondary to upper respiratory illness, torticollis may be a manifestation of more serious abnormalities of the brain or spinal cord. Untreated torticollis in older children may result in loss of the normal rotational motion of the upper cervical spine or rotational subluxation of the upper cervical segments. The evaluation and treatment of suspected rotational fixation and subluxation in children is complex and should be performed by experienced specialists.

TABLE 686–1 Differential Diagnosis of Torticollis (Wryneck)

Congenital	Neurologic
Muscular torticollis	Visual disturbances (nystagmus, superior oblique paresis)
Positional deformation	Dystonic drug reactions (phenothiazines, haloperidol, metoclopramide)
Hemivertebra (cervical spine)	Cervical cord tumor
Unilateral atlanto-occipital fusion	Posterior fossa brain tumor
Klippel-Feil syndrome	Syringomyelia
Unilateral absence of sternocleidomastoid	Wilson's disease
Pterygium colli	Dystonia musculorum deformans
Trauma	Spasmus nutans
Muscular injury (cervical muscles)	**Other**
Atlanto-occipital subluxation	Acute cervical disk calcification
Atlantoaxial subluxation	Sandifer syndrome (gastroesophageal reflux, hiatal hernia)
C2–3 subluxation	Benign paroxysmal torticollis
Rotary subluxation	Bone tumors (eosinophilic granuloma)
Fractures	Soft tissue tumor
Inflammation	Hysteria
Cervical lymphadenitis	
Retropharyngeal abscess	
Cervical vertebral osteomyelitis	
Rheumatoid arthritis	
Spontaneous (hyperemia, edema) subluxation with adjacent head and neck infection (rotary subluxation syndrome)	
Upper lobe pneumonia	

686.2 Klippel-Feil Syndrome

The clinical triad of short neck, low hairline, and restriction of neck motion in a patient with multiple coalitions of the cervical vertebrae defines this syndrome. There is an association of the Klippel-Feil triad with congenital abnormalities of the genitourinary tract, auditory system, spinal cord, and cardiovascular system, as well as with other abnormalities of the musculoskeletal system. **Sprengel anomaly** (congenital elevation of the scapula) is a common associated finding, and affected patients have a higher than expected incidence of scoliosis.

Affected children characteristically have low hairlines and short, sometimes webbed, necks. Decreased active and passive motion of the cervical spine is usually present, although the extent of restriction depends on the severity of the vertebral defects and may be difficult to detect in minimally affected patients. Torticollis may be present. Initial evaluation should include anteroposterior, lateral, and oblique views of the cervical spine. Flexion-extension lateral views, odontoid view, and computed tomography may be necessary if instability is suspected. Magnetic resonance imaging is recommended for patients with neurologic deficits.

Thirty to 40% of patients with Klippel-Feil abnormality have structural abnormalities of the urinary tract. Double collecting systems, renal aplasia, horseshoe kidney, and recurrent pyelonephritis are common. Patient may die of uremia. The extent of the cervical abnormality correlates poorly with the severity of the underlying genitourinary abnormality, and thorough evaluation of the genitourinary tract is indicated in all patients.

686.3 Atlantoaxial Instability

Instability of the upper cervical spine in children is uncommon but potentially devastating. In the normal upper cervical spine, flexion and extension take place at the occiput–first cervical vertebra (C1) articulation, and rotation occurs at the C1–2 joint. Neither joint is intrinsically stable, and both depend on the integrity of the ligaments and joint capsules that surround the joints to constrain motion. Developmental, traumatic, inflammatory, or metabolic lesions that affect the stability of the occiput-C1 or C1–2 joint have serious implications. Progresssive myelopathy may develop in patients with chronic instability; acute impingement and death are possible in patients with severe instability.

HYPOPLASIA AND ABSENCE OF THE ODONTOID PROCESS. Rudimentary formation (os odontoideum) or absence of the odontoid process is well documented in disorders such as Morquio's syndrome but has been also been reported in children with no demonstrable genetic or metabolic disorders. Absence of the odontoid may therefore be traumatic or congenital and is associated with varying degrees of upper cervical spine instability. In such patients, the proximal pole of the odontoid is absent, and the base of the odontoid is rounded off below the arch of the first cervical vertebra thereby resulting in C1–2 instability.

Symptoms vary depending on the degree of C1–2 instability. Preliminary evaluation should include controlled flexion and extension lateral radiographs of the cervical spine. Magnetic resonance imaging of the cervical spine performed in the neutral, flexed, and extended positions provides precise information on the size of the cervical canal, the position of the spinal cord within the canal, and the presence of spinal cord impingement. If available, anteroposterior and lateral tomography is also an excellent technique to identify small proximal ossicles. Transverse computed tomography and sagittal reconstruction provide detailed information regarding the craniovertebral junction.

In normal asymptomatic patients without radiographic evidence of instability, restriction of contact sports and close observation is appropriate. In patients with Morquio's syndrome, cervical stabilization should be considered even when such patients are asymptomatic and have little instability. In patients with cervical instability or abnormal neurologic findings, stabilization of the cervical spine is essential.

DOWN SYNDROME. The association of trisomy 21 (Down syndrome) with instability of the upper cervical spine is well known; estimates of the incidence of instability range from 10–25%. Reported abnormalities include occipito-atlantal instability, atlanto-axial instability, occipitalization of the atlas, and os odontoideum. The number of patients with *symptoms* related to C1–2 instability or other anomalies of the cervical spine is much lower. A minority of Down patients with cervical instablity have neurologic symptoms (see Chapter 78).

Patients with Down syndrome and upper cervical instability who have abnormal neurologic signs have highly variable manifestations. Obvious abnormalities such as incontinence, gait disturbances, and seizures may be the presenting symptoms in some patients, whereas others may be noted to have intermittent balance problems or decreased exercise tolerance. The incidence of instability increases with age. Unfortunately, significant neurologic injury, including quadraparesis or death, has been reported in previously asymptomatic patients.

The Orthopedic Section of the American Academy of Pediatrics has recommended screening of patients with Down syndrome with neurologic examination and lateral radiographs in the neutral, flexed, and extended positions. Patients with no neurologic abnormalities but with radiographic evidence of instability require further evaluation; at the least, they should be restricted from contact sports and followed periodically.

Patients with myelopathy and those with marked instability without myelopathy are candidates for cervical spine fusion. Decision-making is complicated by the lack of knowledge of the long-term outcome of patients with myelopathy treated nonoperatively and by the variability of outcome in patients treated surgically. Unfortunately, the results of surgical treatment of instability in Down syndrome are less predictable than that of instability in other conditions. Failure of fusion and graft resorption may occur, and the incidence of complications is high. It is not likely that pre-existent myelopathic changes will improve. Based on these findings, it has been recommended that patients with instability and no neurologic abnormality be treated nonoperatively. When operative intervention is necessary, all parties must be aware of the high potential for serious complications.

The occurrence of sudden death in previously normal patients with Down syndrome and the documented development of instability with increasing age raise the issue of whether all patients with Down syndrome should be restricted from potentially dangerous activities. Given the incomplete state of knowledge at this time, this judgment appears best made on a case by case basis.

Torticollis

Canale ST, Griffin DW, Hubbard CN: Congenital muscular torticollis: Long-term follow-up. J Bone Joint Surg 64A:810, 1982.

Davids J, Wenger D, Mubarak S: Congenital muscular torticollis: Sequela of intrauterine or perinatal compartment syndrome. J Pediatr Orthop 13:141, 1993.

Gupta AK, Roy DR, Conlon ES, Crawford AH: Torticollis secondary to posterior fossa tumors. J Pediatr Orthop 16:505, 1996.

Phillips W, Hensinger R: The management of rotary atlanto-axial subluxation in children. J Bone Joint Surg 71A:664, 1989.

Klippel-Feil Syndrome

Hensinger R, Lang J, MacEwen G: Klippel-Feil syndrome: A constellation of associated anomalies. J Bone Joint Surg 56A:246, 1974.

Pizzutillo PD, Woods M, Nicholson L, MacEwen GD: Risk factors in Klippel-Feil syndrome. Spine 19:2110, 1994.

Atlantoaxial Instability

Burke SW, French HG, Roberts JM, et al: Chronic atlanto-axial instability in Down syndrome. J Bone Joint Surg 67A:1356, 1985.

Doyle JS, Lauerman WC, Wood KB, Krause DR: Complications and long-term outcome of upper cervical spine arthrodesis in patients with Down syndrome. Spine 21:1223, 1996.

Fielding JW, Hensinger RN, Hawkins RJ: Os odontoideum. J Bone Joint Surg 62A:376, 1980.

Georgopoulos G, Pizzutillo PD, Lee MS: Occipito-atlantal instability in children: A report of five cases and review of the literature. J Bone Joint Surg 69A:429, 1987.

Hensinger RN: Congenital anomalies of the cervical spine. Clin Orthop 264:16, 1991.

Pueschal SM: Should children with Down syndrome be screened for atlantoaxial instability? Arch Pediatr Adolesc Med 152:123, 1998.

Pueschal SM, Scola FH, Tapper TB, Pezzulo JC: Skeletal anomalies of the upper cervical spine in children with Down syndrome. J Pediatr Orthop 10:607, 1990.

Sawark JF: Mucopolysaccharidoses, mucolipidoses, and homocystinuria, *In*: Weinstein, SL (ed): The Pediatric Spine. New York, Raven Press, 1994, pp 959–974.

CHAPTER 687
The Upper Limb

Upper limb disorders, with the exception of fractures, are less common in children and adolescents than are those involving the other areas of the musculoskeletal system.

SHOULDER

The shoulder joint is composed of the relatively small glenoid fossa of the scapula, which articulates with a proportionally larger hemispherical humeral head. The stability of the shoulder joint is provided by muscular and tendinous (rotator cuff) attachments. The shoulder has a relatively large range of motion because of this small articular surface and large muscle mass. Shoulder motion is a combination of glenohumeral and scapulothoracic motion.

687.1 Sprengel's Deformity

Failure of the scapula to descend to its normal location is termed *Sprengel's deformity.* The scapula is located at an abnormally high position with respect to the child's neck and thorax. This uncommon abnormality occurs with varying degrees of severity. Webbing of the skin between the neck and scapula and a low posterior hairline may be associated findings. In the severe form, a bone (omovertebral) may connect the scapula with the cervical spine and prevent scapulothoracic movement. There may also be associated muscle anomalies that further limit strength and stability of the shoulder girdle. In severe cases, the scapula is very high, producing a significant cosmetic deformity with markedly limited shoulder range of motion, particularly forward flexion and abduction. In the mild form, the scapula rides slightly high with less than normal motion. A Klippel-Feil anomaly (congenital fusion of one or more of the cervical spine vertebra) may also occur with Sprengel's deformity.

TREATMENT. The best outcome in severe Sprengel's deformity is achieved by surgically repositioning or, occasionally, partially resecting the scapula. An osteotomy of the clavicle is frequently necessary to bring the scapula to a more normal position. This improves the cosmetic appearance and increases shoulder motion, especially abduction.

687.2 Shoulder Dislocation

Traumatic dislocation of the shoulder is uncommon in childhood but increases in frequency during adolescence. Anterior dislocation is the most common type. It usually occurs when the shoulder is forced into abduction and external rotation. In young children, a Salter-Harris type II epiphyseal fracture is more likely to occur. Once a traumatic dislocation has occurred, there is damage to the anterior capsule and the associated musculature that may predispose to recurrent dislocation. The younger individuals are at the time of the initial dislocation, the more likely they are to experience recurrent dislocations.

TREATMENT. Closed reduction and immobilization in a shoulder immobilizer for 3–6 wk followed by rehabilitation is recommended for the first dislocation. However, some favor early reconstruction rather than instituting conservative treatment because of the risk of recurrent dislocations.

ELBOW

The elbow joint is composed of three bones: the distal humerus, the proximal radius, and the ulna. There are three articulations: the radiohumeral, the ulnohumeral, and the proximal radioulnar. There are anterior and posterior indentations on the distal surface of the humerus: the anterior coronoid and the posterior olecranon fossa. These accept the coronoid and olecranon processes of the proximal ulna. It allows the elbow to flex 150 degrees and extend to neutral. The proximal radius is a relatively flat, circular structure that allows pronation and supination of the forearm to occur with approximately 90 degrees of motion at each. Abnormalities involving the elbow typically produce pain and loss of motion.

687.3 Nursemaid's Elbow

The radial head is not as bulbous in infants and young children as it is in older children. During early childhood, the annular ligament that passes around the neck of the proximal radius just below the radial head provides stability between the radius and ulna. When longitudinal traction is applied to the upper extremity with the elbow in extension, the annular ligament can slide over the radial head and become partially entrapped in the radiohumeral joint (Fig. 687–1). This is known as nursemaid's elbow or subluxation of the radial head. It represents a soft tissue interposition in the elbow joint. The subluxation of the annular ligament is initiated by either a jerk on the arm when the child falls while the hand is being held by a parent or when the child is forcibly lifted by the hand. It may also occur if the child falls and holds onto an object for support but allows longitudinal traction to be applied across the elbow. The hand typically is held in a pronated position, and the child may refuse to use the hand and may cry when the elbow is moved.

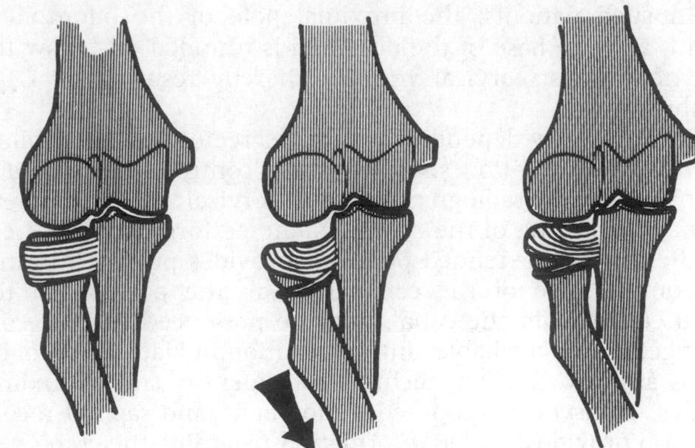

Figure 687–1 The pathology of nursemaid's, or pulled, elbow. The annular ligament is partially torn when the arm is pulled. The radial head moves distally, and when traction is discontinued, the ligament is carried into the joint. (From Rang M: Children's Fractures, 2nd ed. Philadelphia, JB Lippincott, 1983, p 193.)

TREATMENT. Rotating the hand and forearm to a supinated position with pressure over the radial head usually reduces the annular ligament and restores full, normal use of the extremity. With reduction of the annular ligament, there is a palpable "click" felt along the lateral aspect of the elbow. Radiographs are not usually necessary to make the diagnosis. When a child is sent for radiographic evaluation before the annular ligament is reduced, this click may inadvertently occur during positioning.

The parents should be educated about the mechanism of injury and encouraged to avoid lifting or holding the child up by the hands or forearm. Once a subluxation has occurred, there is a propensity for recurrent episodes. Usually, there is sufficient development of the radial head to prevent subluxation of the annular ligament by 4 yr of age.

687.4 Panner's Disease

Panner's disease is an osteochondrosis that involves the ossific nucleus of the capitellum, the lateral aspect of the distal humeral epiphysis. This disorder is most common in adolescence and occurs predominantly in those engaged in sport activities that involve throwing. Adolescents complain of pain and may have crepitation and loss of motion, particularly pronation and supination.

The diagnosis can usually be made from anteroposterior and lateral radiographs of the elbow. Occasionally, oblique radiographs may be beneficial. Additional radiographic studies, such as magnetic resonance imaging, may be helpful in identifying the extent of the lesion and determining whether the overlying articular cartilage is intact or disrupted.

TREATMENT. The treatment is usually conservative with restriction of activities. If the overlying articular cartilage is disrupted and joint fluid flows beneath the lesion, it may ultimately become a loose body. A loose osteocartilaginous fragment may be excised through an arthrotomy or arthroscopy. Occasionally, it is possible to repair the lesion by drilling it to allow for ingrowth of new blood vessels or by internal fixation with absorbable pins, which may allow the lesions to heal.

WRIST

The wrist is the articulation between the hand and the distal radius and ulna. The proximal row of carpal bones (scaphoid, lunate, and hamate) composes the articular surface of the hand. Anatomically, the distal radius has a 25-degree ulnar tilt and 12-degree volar angulation. The distal ulna is relatively flat, with the exception of the ulnar styloid, and has a small, triangle-shaped meniscus between its articulation with the hamate. There are three articulations: radiocarpal, ulnocarpal, and radioulnar. The wrist is not a common site for pediatric musculoskeletal disorders, with the exceptions of fractures involving the distal radius and ulna.

687.5 Ganglion

A synovial fluid-filled cyst around the wrist, a ganglion, is common in childhood. The usual site is the dorsum of the wrist near the radiocarpal joint; a common second site is over the volar radial aspect of the wrist. The disease is a defect in one of the joint capsules, which allows herniation of the synovium through the defect. If the synovium is ruptured, the fluid may be pumped into the soft tissues through the action of wrist motion; the fluid is subsequently walled off by reactive fibrous tissue.

TREATMENT. In children, ganglia are benign and tend to disappear over time. If a ganglion is sufficiently large, causes pain, or interferes with normal tendon functioning, aspiration of the cyst is sometimes helpful. Surgical excision of the cyst accompanied by removal of the tract that extends into the joint is curative.

687.6 Radial Clubhand

Absence of the radius, either total or partial, results in radial deviation of the hand and abnormal function. The ulna is usually hypoplastic as well as bowed, contributing to the shortness and deformity of the forearm and hand. This is an uncommon disorder but may be associated with a variety of other syndromes such as the VATER (vertebral defects, anal atresia, tracheoesophageal fistula with esophageal atresia, and radial and renal anomalies) or the Holt-Oram syndrome. Any child with a radial clubhand requires a careful evaluation for other disorders. The diagnosis is usually evident on physical examination, but radiographs show whether the radius is completely absent or whether there is a proximal remnant. Congenital absence of the thumb is a common accompaniment.

TREATMENT. The treatment of radial clubhand in infancy begins with serial casting or splinting in an attempt to center the carpus on the end of the ulna. Usually, a surgical procedure is ultimately necessary to centralize the hand adequately, provide stability, and place it into a position to maximize function. If the thumb is absent, a pollicization of the index finger can be performed to improve hand function.

HAND AND FINGERS

The hand and fingers are composed of the carpal and metacarpal bones proximally and the phalanges distally. The thumb has two phalanges (proximal and distal), whereas the fingers have three phalanges (proximal, middle, and distal). Thus, the thumb has an interphalangeal joint, and the fingers have proximal and distal interphalangeal joints. The thumb and fingers articulate with the metacarpals at the metacarpophalangeal joints. The hand has a delicate balance among the intrinsic muscle system, a powerful extrinsic muscle system, fine sensory innervation, and specialized skin to allow it to be a highly mobile, sensitive, delicate yet powerful appendage. Thumb and finger disorders, other than trauma, are relatively uncommon. When present, they tend to be due to congenital rather than developmental abnormalities.

TABLE 687–1 Syndromes Associated with Polydactyly

Carpenter's syndrome	Trisomy 13
Ellis–van Creveld syndrome	Orofaciodigital syndrome
Meckel-Gruber syndrome	Rubinstein-Taybi syndrome
Polysyndactyly	

TABLE 687–2 Syndromes Associated with Syndactyly

Apert's syndrome	Trisomy 21
Carpenter's syndrome	Fetal hydantoin syndrome
de Lange's syndrome	Laurence-Moon-Biedl syndrome
Holt-Oram syndrome	Fanconi's panctyopenia
Orofaciodigital syndrome	Trisomy 13
Polysyndactyly	Trisomy 18

687.7 Polydactyly

Extra digits, or polydactyly, occur as both simple and complex deformities. Skin tags and digit remnants are typically seen near the metacarpophalangeal joint of the small finger or the thumb. They do not have palpable bone in the base or possess voluntary motion and may simply be ligated or excised in the newborn period. Complex varieties require formal amputation, which is usually performed at approximately 1 yr of age. Syndromes in which polydactyly commonly occurs are listed in Table 687–1.

687.8 Syndactyly

Syndactyly also occurs in both simple and complex patterns. There should be concern about sharing of common important structures between the digits, such as the neurovascular bundle. There is also a tethering effect on the growth of the affected digits. Referral for delineation of specific disease and development of treatment strategies is indicated when the condition is recognized. Syndromes associated with syndactyly are presented in Table 687–2.

687.9 Congenital Trigger Thumb and Finger

A thickening in the tendon of the flexor hallucis longus (thumb) or the flexor digitorum longus (fingers) just below the first pulley of the digit may result in a triggering phenomenon. This thickening most likely is acquired rather than congenital. Each finger has a series of pulleys that prevent the tendons from bowstringing when flexed. This nodule may slide through the first pulley with a snapping, popping, or triggering sensation; this may or may not be painful. As the nodule enlarges because of the stimulation from triggering, it may ultimately be unable to pass beneath the pulley, resulting in a fixed flexion deformity of the interphalangeal joint of the thumb or the proximal interphalangeal joing and distal interphalangeal joints of the fingers. The nodule is typically palpable in the palm just proximal to the skin crease of the metacarpophalangeal joint. This is a clinical diagnosis and radiographs are not helpful.

TREATMENT. The treatment of a congenital trigger thumb or finger is a release of the first pulley. The normal excursion of the tendon does not allow the nodule to reach the next pulley. The release of the pulley does not cause bowstringing of the tendon.

Bora FW: The Pediatric Upper Extremity: Diagnosis and Management. Philadelphia, WB Saunders, 1986.
Satku K, Ganesh B: Ganglia in children. J Pediatr Orthop 5:13, 1985.
Steenwerckx A, DeSmet L, Fabry G: Congenital trigger digit. J Hand Surg 21A:909, 1996.
Wagner KT, Lyne ED: Adolescent traumatic dislocations of the shoulder with an open epiphysis. J Pediatr Orthop 3:61, 1983.

CHAPTER 688
Arthrogryposis

Arthrogryposis multiplex congenita refers to a symptom complex characterized by multiple joint contractures present at birth. The involved muscles are replaced partially or completely by fat and fibrous tissue. This is not a single disease because there are approximately 150 different syndromes occurring with multiple congenital contractures that are categorized as arthrogryposis. Although most children who have this nonprogressive disorder survive, some die in infancy as a result of involvement of respiratory muscles. One major form (amyoplasia) of arthrogryposis multiplex congenita refers to the classic syndrome in which there is involvement of the upper and lower extremities. Amyoplasia accounts for approximately 40% of children who have multiple congenital contractures.

688.1 Amyoplasia

The cause of amyoplasia is unknown, but children with this disorder have a decreased number of anterior horn cells in the spinal cord, suggesting a neuropathic cause. Other studies have shown that the disorder may be myopathic in origin. In the latter instance, diminution of in utero movement may be the final common pathway leading to contractures. Every child presenting with multiple joint contractures should have a complete musculoskeletal evaluation and genetics consultation.

CLINICAL MANIFESTATIONS. The distribution of involvement of multiple joint contractures is variable. The classic presentation involves the upper and lower extremities. The lower extremities are typically more involved than the upper extremities. Involvement of all four extremities is quadrimelic involvement. It is also possible that only the lower extremities or upper extremities (bimelic) may be involved. It is unusual to see only one extremity or a portion of one extremity (monomelic) involved.

The clinical features may include (1) adduction, internal rotation contractures of the shoulders; (2) fixed flexion or extension contractures of the elbow; (3) rigid volar flexion–ulnar deviation or dorsiflexion–radial deviation contractures of the wrists; (4) thumb and palm deformity; (5) rigid interphalangeal joints of the thumb and fingers; (6) flexion, abduction, external rotation hip contractures with dislocation of one or both hips; (7) fixed extension or flexion contractures of the knees; and (8) severe rigid bilateral clubfeet or congenital vertical tali.

RADIOGRAPHIC AND LABORATORY EVALUATION. Radiographs should be obtained of the involved joints in all children presenting with multiple joint contractures. Screening radiographs of the spine and pelvis are almost always necessary for evaluation of possible spinal deformity and underlying hip dysplasia. Routine laboratory studies are usually not helpful in evaluating amyoplasia. If an underlying syndrome is suspected, such as congenital muscular dystrophy, creatine phosphokinase determinations and chromosomal studies may be helpful.

TREATMENT. Correction of orthopedic deformities may be beneficial in maximizing walking or other functions. Each child must be treated individually with respect to potential rehabilitation and the possible treatment.

Physical Therapy. Physical therapy with passive range of motion exercises can be beneficial in improving the range of motion in involved joints. However, it rarely completely corrects the existing contractures. Splinting (daytime or nighttime, or both) of the extremities may also improve joint range of motion. This is particularly useful in the hands and wrists. Postoperative splinting is important in maintaining alignment and preventing recurrence.

Serial Casting. Serial casting can be helpful in further correcting soft tissue contractures after physical therapy has reached its maximal benefit. Serial casting is particularly useful in knee flexion contractures and in clubfeet. Casts are changed at weekly intervals, followed by a gentle manipulation of the involved area.

Orthoses. Orthotics can be beneficial in providing joint stability as well as maintaining alignment after satisfactory correction of contractures. The type of orthosis depends on the individual child's particular needs. It may be include an ankle-foot orthosis if there is only ankle and foot involvement, a knee-ankle-foot orthosis if there is concomitant knee involvement, and a hip-knee-ankle-foot orthosis if there is involvement of all the joints of the lower extremities. Should scoliosis develop, a spinal orthosis such as a thoracolumbar spinal orthosis may be tried; it may slow the rate of progression and delay surgical intervention.

Fracture Management. Perinatal fractures commonly occur in children with arthrogryposis. These should be suspected if there is localized deformity, soft tissue swelling, erythema, or irritability. Rigid joints and hypotonia contribute to the increased incidence of fractures. These typically involve the shafts as well as the epiphyseal regions and should be managed with appropriate immobilization until adequate healing has occurred. It is important that radiographs be obtained in all children suspected of having a fracture before any physical therapy is initiated.

Surgery. Surgery is usually necessary to achieve maximal correction of soft tissue contractures and joint deformities, reduce and stabilize dislocated hips, and correct foot deformities, and for partial correction and stabilization of spinal deformities.

UPPER EXTREMITIES. Surgical treatment of upper extremity deformities depends on the type and degree of contracture as well as the motor capabilities and functional needs of the patient. A child's compensatory or adaptive functioning of the upper extremities can be remarkable, and it is essential not to diminish function for cosmesis inadvertently. In bilateral involvement, it is preferable to have one extremity in extension and the other in flexion, but have them still be able to meet in the midline. This enhances function. Internal rotation contractures of the shoulder can be treated by soft tissue releases and proximal humeral derotation osteotomies at a level proximal to the deltoid insertion. Extension contractures of the elbow may benefit from posterior capsulotomy and triceps tenotomy or lengthening to allow restoration of passive or active flexion. Active flexion can be partially restored with a transfer of the pectoralis muscle and its neurovascular bundle. Wrist deformities may be managed by tendon transfers, proximal row carpectomy, or shortening dorsal wedge radial osteotomies.

LOWER EXTREMITIES. Most infants with clubfoot or vertical tali do not completely respond to passive stretching or serial casting. Complete soft tissue releases are usually required. Occasionally in a clubfoot, excision of the talus or talar decancellation may also be required to achieve a plantigrade foot.

Knee flexion contractures that are unresponsive to serial casting may benefit by a lengthening of the hamstring in association with a posterior knee capsulotomy. If this fails to correct the deformity to within 15–20 degrees of neutral, an extension osteotomy of the distal femur may be required. The value of walking with the knee extended is extremely beneficial. A recurrent flexion deformity may occur after an extension osteotomy if it is performed before adolescence. Knee extension contractures may also require treatment, especially if the child or adolescent is a nonambulator and cannot sit comfortably because of the extended position. Lengthening of the quadriceps mechanism may be beneficial.

Hip contractures may be improved by soft tissue releases. Occasionally, extension derotation osteotomies of the proximal femur may be helpful in completing the correction of the flexion, abduction, or external rotation contractures. Controversy exists as to whether bilateral dislocations of the hip should be reduced. If there is a unilateral dislocation, treatment is usually necessary to prevent leg length discrepancy, pelvic obliquity, and possible scoliosis. Open reduction is accompanied by soft tissue releases, shortening derotation varus osteotomies of the proximal femurs, and pelvic osteotomies.

SCOLIOSIS. Scoliosis is common in children with amyoplasia. The age at onset and patterns of deformity are variable. Orthotic management is usually effective only in slowing the rate of progression. In the majority of children, progression occurs slowly, and they ultimately require surgical intervention. Because of the associated soft tissue contractures, it is important that these curves not be allowed to become too severe because only partial correction will be obtained. Most children can be satisfactorily managed by a posterior spinal fusion and some type of segmental spinal instrumentation.

Axt MW, Niethard FU, Doderlein L, Weber M: Principles of treatment of the upper extremity in arthrogryposis multiplex congenita type I. J Pediatr Orthop 6B:179, 1997.

Banker BQ: Arthrogryposis multiplex congenita. *In*: Engel AG, Banker BQ (eds): Myology: Basic and Clinical. New York, McGraw-Hill, 1986, pp 2109–2150.

Daher YH, Lonstein JE, Winter RB, et al: Spinal deformities in patients with arthrogryposis: A review of 16 patients. Spine 10:609, 1985.

Diamond LS, Alegado R: Perinatal fractures in arthrogryposis multiplex congenita. J Pediatr Orthop 1:189, 1981.

Goldberg MJ: Syndromes of orthopaedic importance. *In*: Morrissy RT (ed): Lovell and Winter's Pediatric Orthopaedics, 4th ed. Philadelphia, Lippincott-Raven, 1996, pp 255–360.

Hall JG: Arthrogryposis multiplex congenita: Etiology, genetics, classification, diagnostic approach, and general aspects. J Pediatr Orthop 6B:159, 1997.

Murray C, Fixsen JA: Management of knee deformity in classical arthrogryposis multiplex congenita (amyoplasia congenita). J Pediatr Orthop 6B:186, 1997.

Sarwark JF, MacEwen GD, Scott CI Jr: Current concepts review: Amyoplasia (a common form of arthrogryposis). J Bone Joint Surg 72A:465, 1990.

Sells JM, Jaffe KM, Hall JG: Amyoplasia, the most common type of arthrogryposis: The potential for good outcome. Pediatrics 97:225, 1996.

Shapiro F, Specht L: Current concepts review: The diagnosis and orthopaedic treatment of childhood spinal muscular atrophy, peripheral neuropathy, Friedreich ataxia and arthrogryposis. J Bone Joint Surg 75A:1699, 1993.

Sodergard J, Hakamies-Blomqvist L, Saino K, et al: Arthrogryposis multiplex congenita: Perinatal and electromyographic findings, disability, and psychosocial outcome. J Pediatr Orthop 6B:167, 1997.

Staheli LT, Chew DE, Elliott JS, et al: Management of hip dislocations in children with arthrogryposis. J Pediatr Orthop 7:681, 1987.

Thompson GH: Arthrogryposis multiplex congenita. *In:* Staheli LT (ed): Pediatric Orthopaedic Secrets. Philadelphia, Hanley and Belfus, 1998, pp 371–375.

CHAPTER 689
Common Fractures

Fractures in children account for approximately 10–15% of all childhood injuries. The skeletal system of children is anatomically, biomechanically, and physiologically different from that in adults. This results in different fracture patterns, including epiphyseal fractures, problems of diagnosis, and management techniques.

The anatomic differences in the pediatric skeletal system include the presence of preosseous cartilage, physes, and a thicker, stronger, more osteogenic periosteum that produces callus more rapidly and in greater amounts. Biomechanically, the pediatric skeletal system can absorb more energy before deformation and fracture than can adult bone. This has been attributed to lower mineral content and the greater porosity of young bone. The increased porosity is due to larger, more abundant haversian canals. This results in a lower modulus of elasticity and lower bending strength. As maturation occurs, the porosity decreases and the cortical bone becomes thicker and stronger.

Ligaments frequently insert into epiphyses. As a consequence, traumatic forces applied to an extremity may be transmitted to the physes. The strength of the physes is enhanced by interdigitating mamillary bodies and the perichondrial ring. However, biomechanically the physes are not as strong as the ligaments or metaphyseal bone. The physis is most resistant to traction and least resistant to torsional forces. Thus, the majority of injuries to the physes are secondary to rotational and angular forces.

The thick periosteum of a child's bones is a major determinant in whether a fracture becomes displaced. The thick periosteum may also act as an impediment to closed reduction because of the hinging phenomenon, or it may help stabilize a fracture after reduction.

FRACTURE REMODELING. Remodeling occurs by a combination of periosteal resorption and new bone formation. Thus, anatomic alignment in certain pediatric fractures is not always necessary. The major factors affecting fracture remodeling include the child's age, proximity of the fracture to a joint, and relationship of a residual deformity to the plane of the joint axis of motion. The amount of remaining growth provides the basis for remodeling: The younger the child, the greater is the remodeling potential. Fractures adjacent to a physis undergo the greatest amount of remodeling provided that the deformity is in the plane of axis of motion for that joint. Fracture remodeling will be less effective in displaced intra-articular fractures, diaphyseal fractures, malrotation, and deformity not in the plane of joint axis of motion.

OVERGROWTH. Overgrowth, especially in long bones such as the femur, is due to physeal stimulation from the hyperemia associated with fracture healing. Femoral fractures in children younger than 10 yr frequently overgrow 1–3 cm. This is the reason for bayonet apposition of bone to compensate for the overgrowth that occurs over the next 1–2 yr. After 10 yr of age, overgrowth is less of a problem and anatomic alignment is recommended.

PROGRESSIVE DEFORMITY. Injuries to the physes can result in complete or partial closure. As a consequence, angular deformity or shortening, or both, can occur. The magnitude depends on the physis involved and the amount of growth remaining.

RAPID HEALING. Fractures in children heal faster than do those in adults. This is due to children's growth potential and thicker, more metabolically active periosteum. As children approach adolescence and maturity, the rate of healing slows and becomes similar to that of an adult's.

689.1 Pediatric Fracture Patterns

Pediatric fracture patterns result, in part, from the anatomic, biomechanical, and physiologic characteristics of a child's skeletal system. The majority of pediatric fractures can be managed by closed methods.

COMPLETE. Complete fractures are the most common type and occur when both sides of the bone are fractured. These fractures may be classified as spiral, transverse, oblique, or comminuted, depending on the direction of the fracture lines. Comminuted fractures are unusual in children.

BUCKLE OR TORUS FRACTURE. Compression of bone produces a buckle or torus fracture. These fractures typically occur in the metaphyseal areas in young children, especially in the distal radius. They are inherently stable and heal in 2–3 wk with simple immobilization.

GREENSTICK. When a bone is angulated beyond the limits of plastic deformation, a greenstick fracture may occur. This represents bone failure on the tension side and a plastic or bend deformity on the compression side. The energy was insufficient to result in a complete fracture.

PLASTIC DEFORMATION OR BEND FRACTURES. Traumatic bowing or bend deformities are due to plastic deformation of bone. The bone was angulated beyond its limit of plastic deformation, but the energy was insufficient to produce a fracture. Thus, no fracture line is visible radiographically. It is most commonly seen in the ulna and occasionally the fibula.

EPIPHYSEAL FRACTURES. Salter and Harris classified epiphyseal injuries into five groups: type I, separation through the physis, usually through the zones of hypertrophic and degenerating cartilage cell columns; type II, a fracture through a portion of the physis but extending through the metaphyses; type III, a fracture through a portion of the physis extending through the epiphysis and into the joint; type IV, a fracture across the metaphysis, physis, and epiphysis; and type V, a crush injury to the physis (Fig. 689–1). This classification allows generalized prognostic information regarding the risk for premature physeal closure and the indications for treatment. Type III and type IV epiphyseal fractures require anatomic alignment because of displacement of both the physis and the articular surface. Type V fractures are usually recognized in retrospect as a consequence of premature physeal closure. Type I and type II fractures usually can be managed by closed reduction techniques and do not require perfect alignment. A major exception is type II fractures of the distal femur. Fractures in this location have a poor prognosis unless almost anatomic alignment is obtained by either closed or open methods.

689.2 Clavicular Fractures

Fractures involving the junction of the middle and lateral aspects of the clavicle are common. These can be the result of birth injuries in newborns but are more typically the result of a fall on the outstretched arm or a direct blow to the clavicle. They are rarely associated with a neurovascular injury. Diagnosis is easily made by physical and radiographic evaluation. Anteroposterior radiograph of the clavicle and, occasionally, a cephalic view demonstrate the fracture. Typically, the fracture fragments are displaced and overlap 1–2 cm.

TREATMENT. The treatment of most clavicle fractures consists of an application of a figure-of-eight clavicle strap. This will extend the shoulders and minimize the amount of overlap of the fracture fragments. Rarely is anatomic alignment achieved, but this is not necessary. The fractures heal rapidly, usually in 3–6 wk. Commonly, a palpable mass of callus may be visible in thin children. This remodels satisfactorily in 6–12 mo.

689.3 Proximal Humerus Fractures

Salter-Harris type II fractures of the proximal humerus occur commonly in children and are due to a backward fall on the involved extremity with the elbow extended. Neurovascular injuries rarely occur. Diagnosis is made from anteroposterior and lateral radiographs of the shoulder or humerus.

TREATMENT. The treatment of these fractures is usually simple immobilization. Occasionally, a closed reduction may be necessary. A significant amount of deformity can be accepted because of the remodeling potential of this region; 80% of the growth of the humerus occurs from the proximal humeral epiphysis. A sling and swath and, occasionally, a coaptation splint may be necessary to provide satisfactory immobilization and comfort. In severely displaced fractures, closed reduction with immobilization may be necessary.

689.4 Distal Radius and Ulna Fractures

Torus, or buckle, fractures of the distal radial metaphysis are among the most common fractures of childhood. They are usually the result of a simple fall on the hand with the wrist in dorsiflexion. This is an impacted fracture, and there is minimal soft tissue swelling or hemorrhage. It is common for a child to present 1–2 days later because the initial injury was felt to be only a sprain or contusion. The clinical characteristics are nonspecific, usually with mild tenderness to palpation directly over the fracture. Diagnosis is confirmed by anteroposterior and lateral radiographs of the wrist.

TREATMENT. Treatment of torus fractures of the distal radius and ulna is by a short-arm cast. Fractures are typically healed in 3–4 wk.

689.5 Phalangeal Fractures

Phalangeal fractures in children are usually the result of a direct blow to the finger. They are typically trapped in doors or struck by another object. If the distal phalanx is involved,

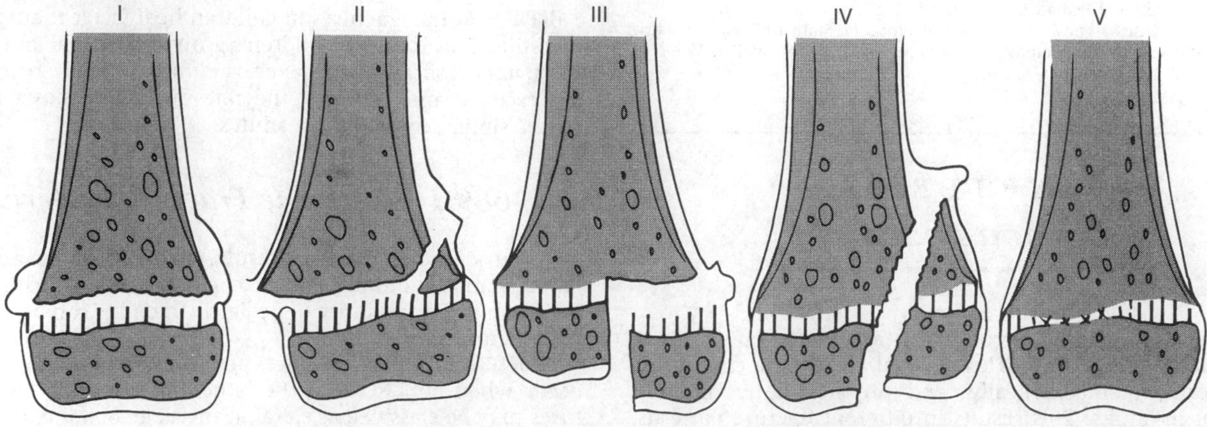

Figure 689–1 The types of growth plate injury as classified by Salter and Harris. (From Salter RB, Harris WR: Injuries involving the epiphyseal plate. J Bone Joint Surg 45A:587, 1963.)

there may be a subungual hematoma, which can be painful. This requires drainage. If the nail bed is avulsed or partially detached in association with a fracture, this is an open fracture and should be treated aggressively with irrigation, tetanus prophylaxis, and appropriate antibiotics. Occasionally, physeal involvement, especially Salter-Harris type II epiphyseal fracture, may occur. Anteroposterior and lateral radiographs of the digit confirm the fracture.

TREATMENT. The treatment of phalangeal fractures is usually by splint immobilization. Rarely is a closed reduction necessary. However, if there is angulation or malrotation, this procedure may necessary.

689.6 Toddler Fracture

Toddler fractures represent a spiral fracture of the distal one third of the tibia. They are usually the result of simple falls while running or playing. They may also occur when stepping on an object on the floor. These fractures occur in children between 2–4 yr and, occasionally, up to 6 yr of age. Clinical features include pain, refusal to walk, minimal soft tissue swelling, a slight increase in warmth to palpation over the fracture, and pain with palpation. These fractures may not be visible radiographically on anteroposterior and lateral radiographs of the tibia. Occasionally, oblique radiographs may reveal the fractures. The fracture can be detected by a technetium bone scan, but this is rarely necessary.

TREATMENT. Application of a long-leg cast in suspected cases relieves symptoms. Within 1–2 wk there is radiographic evidence of subperiosteal new bone formation. These fractures are usually healed within 3–4 wk.

689.7 Lateral Malleolar Fractures

A Salter-Harris type I separation of the distal fibular epiphysis is common in childhood. These fractures usually appear as ankle sprains. However, it must be remembered that ligaments are stronger than bone and that the epiphysis is more likely to separate than a ligament is to tear. Children present with soft tissue swelling and pain over the lateral malleolus. Careful palpation reveals that the bone is the site of greatest tenderness rather than the area over one of the three lateral ligaments. Anteroposterior, lateral, and mortise radiographs of the ankle are typically normal. The diagnosis can be confirmed by stress radiographs, but this is rarely necessary.

TREATMENT. Distal fibular epiphyseal separations require immobilization in a short-leg cast for 4–6 wk. Treatment is the same as that for a severe ankle sprain. This is why stress radiographs are rarely necessary. Follow-up radiographs show subperiosteal new bone formation in the metaphyseal region of the distal fibula.

689.8 Metatarsal Fractures

Fractures of the metatarsal shaft are usually the result of direct trauma to the dorsum of the foot. Children present with a history of injury followed by soft tissue swelling and, sometimes, ecchymosis. There is tenderness to palpation directly over the fracture. Diagnosis is obtained by anteroposterior and lateral radiographs of the foot.

Fractures of the tuberosity of the fifth metatarsal are also common. This has been termed dancer's fracture. It is an apophyseal avulsion fracture at the insertion peroneus brevis tendon. It typically occurs with the foot in an inverted position and the peroneal muscles contracting to realign the foot. The swelling, ecchymosis, and tenderness are limited to the tuberosity of the fifth metatarsal. Contraction of the peroneal musculature also increases discomfort. The diagnosis is confirmed radiographically.

TREATMENT. Metatarsal fractures are treated by a short-leg cast for 4–6 wk. Weight-bearing is allowed as tolerated. The one exception is the fifth metatarsal diaphyseal shaft fracture. This has an increased incidence of nonunion and should be treated by non–weight-bearing until there is radiographic evidence of early union.

689.9 Toe Phalangeal Fractures

Fractures of the lesser toes are common and are usually secondary to direct blows. They commonly occur when the child is barefoot. The toes are swollen, ecchymotic, and tender. There may be a mild deformity. Diagnosis is made radiographically.

TREATMENT. The lesser toes usually do not require closed reduction unless significantly displaced. If necessary, reduction can usually be accomplished with longitudinal traction on the toe. Casting is not usually necessary. "Buddy" taping of the fractured toe to an adjacent stable toe usually provides satisfactory alignment and relief of symptoms. Crutches may be beneficial for several days until the soft tissue swelling and discomfort decreases.

689.10 Operative Treatment

Certain pediatric fractures have better prognoses if the fractures are reduced, by either open or closed techniques, and then internally or externally stabilized (Table 689–1). Approximately 4–5% of pediatric fractures require surgery. The common indications for operative stabilization in children and adolescents with open physes include (1) displaced epiphyseal fractures, (2) displaced intra-articular fractures, (3) unstable fractures, (4) fractures in the multiply injured child, and (5) open fractures.

The principles of surgical management of pediatric fractures are distinctly different from those of mature adolescents and adults. Multiple closed reductions of an epiphyseal fracture are contraindicated because they may cause repetitive damage to

TABLE 689–1 Common Indications for Operative Stabilization

Indication	Location
Displaced epiphyseal fractures (usually Salter-Harris types III and IV)	Lateral condyle Radial head Phalanx Distal femur Proximal tibia Distal tibia
Displaced intra-articular fractures	Radial neck Olecranon Femoral neck Patella
Unstable fractures	Distal humerus (supracondylar) Radius-ulna diaphysis Phalanx Spine
Multiply injured child (especially with associated head and neurologic injury)	Femoral diaphysis Tibial diaphysis Pelvis Spine
Open fractures	Upper and lower extremities Severe soft tissue injury

Adapted from Thompson GH, Wilber JH, Marcus RE: Internal fixation of fractures in children and adolescents: A comparative analysis. Clin Orthop 188:10–20, 1984.

the germinal cells of the physis. Anatomic alignment at surgery is mandatory, especially for displaced intra-articular and epiphyseal fractures. When internal fixation is used, it should be simple (e.g., use of Kirschner wires, which can be removed as soon as the fracture is healed). Rigid fixation to allow immobilization of the extremity usually is not the goal; rather, stability sufficient to maintain anatomic alignment with supplemental immobilization, usually a plaster cast, is. Last, external fixators, when used, are removed as soon as possible and cast immobilization is substituted. The latter is indicated when soft tissue problems have been corrected or when the fracture is stable, or both.

SURGICAL TECHNIQUES. Three basic surgical techniques are used in the management of pediatric fractures. Open reduction and internal fixation may be required for displaced epiphyseal fractures, especially Salter-Harris types III and IV fractures, intra-articular fractures, and unstable fractures, such as those involving the forearm diaphysis, spine, and ipsilateral fractures of the femur and tibia (floating knee). Other indications include neurovascular injuries requiring repair and, occasionally, open fractures of the femur and tibia. Closed reduction and internal fixation is indicated for specific displaced epiphyseal, intra-articular, and unstable metaphyseal and diaphyseal fractures. Common indications include supracondylar fractures of the distal humerus, phalangeal, and femoral neck fractures. Anatomic alignment must be attained by a closed reduction before this method can be used. Failure to obtain anatomic alignment is an indication for an open reduction.

The indications for external fixation in pediatric fractures include (1) severe grade II and grade III open fractures; (2) fractures associated with severe burn; (3) fractures with bone or extensive soft tissue loss that may require reconstructive procedures, such as free vascularized grafts, skin grafts, or other procedures; (4) fractures requiring distractions such as those with significant bone loss; (5) unstable pelvic fractures; (6) fractures in children with associated head injuries and spasticity; and (7) fractures associated with vascular or nerve repairs or reconstruction. The advantages of external fixation include rigid mobilization of the fractures, separation of the management of the fractured limb and associated wounds, and patient mobilization for treatment of other injuries and transportation for diagnostic and therapeutic procedures. The majority of complications with external fixation are pin tract infections and refracture after pin removal.

Cramer KG, Limbird TJ, Green NE: Open fractures of the diaphysis of the lower extremity in children. J Bone Joint Surg 74A:218, 1992.

Green NE, Swiontkowski MF (eds): Skeletal Trauma in Children, Vol 3, 2nd ed. Philadelphia, WB Saunders, 1997.

Gustilo RB, Merkow RL, Templeman D: Current concepts review: The management of open fractures. J Bone Joint Surg 72A:299, 1990.

Loder RT: Pediatric polytrauma: Orthopaedic care in hospital course. J Orthop Trauma 1:48, 1987.

Mabrey JD, Fitch RD: Plastic deformation in pediatric fractures: Mechanism and treatment. J Pediatr Orthop 9:310, 1989.

Rockwood CA Jr, Wilkens KE, King RE: *In:* Fractures in Children, 3rd ed. Philadelphia, JB Lippincott, 1990.

Salter RB, Harris WR: Injuries involving the epiphyseal plate. J Bone Joint Surg 45A:587, 1963.

Scoles PV: Pediatric Orthopaedics in Clinic Practice, 2nd ed. Chicago, Year Book, 1988.

Staheli LT: Fundamentals of Pediatric Orthopedics. New York, Raven Press, 1992.

Tenenbien M, Reed MH, Block GB: The toddler's fracture revisited. Am J Emerg Med 8:208, 1990.

Thompson GH: Nailing children's fractures. Perspect Orthop Surg 2:40, 1991.

Tolo VT: External fixation in multiply injured children. Orthop Clin North Am 21:393, 1990.

Wilber JH, Thompson GH: The multiply injured child. *In:* Green NE, Swiontowski MF (eds): Skeletal Trauma in Children, 2nd ed. Philadelphia, WB Saunders, 1997, pp 71–102.

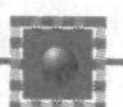

SECTION 2

Sports Medicine

Albert Hergenroeder ■ Joseph N. Chorley

Sports participation fosters physical fitness and overall health, provides opportunities for psychosocial development (teamwork, peer relations), improves decision-making abilities, and promotes self-confidence. Sports activity also provides children with an enjoyable experience as well as an opportunity to learn some skills that can be continued throughout life. Play is sometimes referred to as the "occupation" of a child. The role of physicians is to provide health services, counseling, instruction, and rehabilitation. Physicians need to avoid unnecessary restriction of a child's play and sports activities while trying to prevent injury. Activity should be restricted when the need is definite for an appropriate limited period and tailored to the young athlete's specific requirements. Alternatives are often appropriate. For example, swimming is often a good substitute for contact sports. The most stressful activities are those that involve competition or body contact, and these should be supervised by adults. It is prudent to advise parents that children and youth should be allowed normal activity when parents impose restrictions that are too stringent and confining. Alternately, parents and coaches should be advised against pressuring and demanding inappropriate activity for the sake of competition and their own gratification (see Overuse Injuries). ■

CHAPTER 690

Epidemiology and Prevention

Approximately 30 million children and adolescents participate in organized sports in the United States. Approximately 3 million injuries occur annually if injury is defined as time lost from the sport. More injuries occur in unorganized compared with organized sports. Within the same sport, injury rates for males equal those of females, with the exception of anterior cruciate ligament injuries, which are higher in females in the same sports. The majority of injuries are sprains and strains. Deaths in sports are rare, with the majority of nontraumatic deaths caused by cardiac diseases (see Chapter 442.6); the majority of traumatic deaths are caused by head and neck injuries. In the period 1982–1992, there were three times more nontraumatic than traumatic deaths.

Sports injuries in young children are predominantly due to

TABLE 690–1 Preparticipation Sports Examination

Component of the Physical Examination	Condition to be Detected
Vital signs	Hypertension, cardiac disease, brady/tachycardia
Height and weight	Obesity, eating disorders
Vision and pupil size	Legal blindness, absent eye, anisocoria
Lymph node	Infectious diseases, malignancy
Cardiac (performed standing and supine)	Heart murmur, prior surgery, rhythm
Pulmonary	Recurrent and exercise-induced bronchospasm, chronic lung disease
Abdominal	Organomegaly, abdominal mass
Skin	Contagious diseases (impetigo, herpes, staphylococcal, streptococcal)
Genitourinary	Varicocele, undescended testes, tumor
Musculoskeletal	Acute and chronic injuries, physical anomalies (scoliosis)

sprains, strains, fractures, contusions, and overuse syndromes. Ligamentous injuries, especially about the knee, are not common in children because the physes are weaker than the ligament and they usually break before a ligament tears. Thus, Salter-Harris type I injury should be considered when there is apparent injury about a joint and the initial radiographic findings are normal (Chapter 689). In adolescence, however, sports-related injuries become more similar to those of adults. Contusions, sprains, and fractures still occur, but ligament injuries about the knee increase in frequency as well as severity.

SPORTS INJURY PREVENTION

Sports injury prevention includes many strategies. Catastrophic injury rates have been reduced by enforcing rules that penalize dangerous play (e.g., spear tackling in football). Injury rates have also been reduced by removing environmental hazards, such as trampolines in gymnastics and stationary (vs breakaway) bases in softball, and modifying heat injury rates in soccer tournaments by adding water breaks and reducing the playing time. Mouth guards can reduce dental injuries, yet they are not worn routinely by athletes in any sport except football. A common reason for reinjury is lack of rehabilitation of old injuries; appropriate rehabilitation reduces injury rates. A common setting for detecting unrehabilitated injuries is the preparticipation sports examination (PSE).

PREPARTICIPATION SPORTS EXAMINATION. The PSE is an integral step in preparing for an athletic activity. Because as many as 75% of adolescents substitute the PSE for their annual health maintenance visit, the PSE should be a comprehensive annual health visit with emphasis on preventive health and adolescent primary care (see Chapters 14 and 108). The sports medicine–specific purposes include detecting medical conditions that delay or disqualify athletic participation owing to a risk of injury or death; detecting previously undiagnosed medical conditions; detecting medical conditions that need further evaluation or rehabilitation before participation; providing guidance for sports participation for patients with medical conditions; and meeting legal and insurance obligations. The PSE identifies possible problems in 1–8% of athletes but excludes fewer than 1% from participation.

State requirements for the frequency of a full PSE differ, ranging from before each athletic season, to annually, to on entry to a new school level (junior high, senior high, college). At least a focused interim evaluation should be carried out annually or sooner if a child or adolescent has had a medical problem since the last PSE. The PSE is optimally performed 6 wk before the start of practice so that rehabilitation of old injuries and evaluation of potential health problems can be completed to minimize absence from practices or games.

History and Physical Examination. The essential components of the PSE are the history and focused medical and musculoskeletal screening examinations. Identified problems require more investigation (Table 690–1). In the absence of symptoms, no screening laboratory tests are required.

TABLE 690–2 Medical Conditions and Sports Participation

Condition	May Participate?
Atlantoaxial instability (instability of the joint between cervical vertebrae 1 and 2) *Explanation:* Athlete needs evaluation to assess risk of spinal cord injury during sports participation.	Qualified yes
Bleeding disorder *Explanation:* Athlete needs evaluation.	Qualified yes
Cardiovascular diseases	
Carditis (inflammation of the heart) *Explanation:* Carditis may result in sudden death with exertion.	No
Hypertension (high blood pressure) *Explanation:* Those with significant essential (unexplained) hypertension should avoid weightlifting and powerlifting, bodybuilding, and strength training. Those with secondary hypertension (hypertension caused by a previously identified disease) or severe essential hypertension need evaluation.	Qualified yes
Congenital heart disease (structural heart defects present at birth) *Explanation:* Those with mild forms may participate fully; those with moderate or severe forms or who have undergone surgery need evaluation.	Qualified yes
Dysrhythmia (irregular heart rhythm) *Explanation:* Athlete needs evaluation because some types require therapy or make certain sports dangerous, or both.	Qualified yes
Mitral valve prolapse (abnormal heart valve) *Explanation:* Those with symptoms (chest pain, symptoms of possible dysrhythmia) or evidence of mitral regurgitation (leaking) on physical examination need evaluation. All others may participate fully.	Qualified yes
Heart murmur *Explanation:* If the murmur is innocent (does not indicate heart disease), full participation is permitted. Otherwise the athlete needs evaluation (see "Congenital heart disease" and "Mitral valve prolapse," above).	Qualified yes
Cerebral palsy *Explanation:* Athlete needs evaluation.	Qualified yes
Diabetes mellitus *Explanation:* All sports can be played with proper attention to diet, hydration, and insulin therapy. Particular attention is needed for activities that last 30 min or more.	Yes
Diarrhea *Explanation:* Unless disease is mild, no participation is permitted, because diarrhea may increase the risk of dehydration and heat illness. See "Fever," below.	Qualified no
Eating disorders Anorexia nervosa Bulimia nervosa *Explanation:* These patients need both medical and psychiatric assessment before participation.	Qualified yes

Table continued on following page

TABLE 690–2 Medical Conditions and Sports Participation *Continued*

Condition	May Participate?
Eyes	
Functionally one-eyed athlete Loss of an eye Detached retina Previous eye surgery or serious eye injury	Qualified yes
Explanation: A functionally one-eyed athlete has a best corrected visual acuity of <20/40 in the worse eye. These athletes would suffer significant disability if the better eye was seriously injured, as would those with loss of an eye. Some athletes who have previously undergone eye surgery or had a serious eye injury may have an increased risk of injury because of weakened eye tissue. Availability of eye guards approved by the American Society for Testing Materials (ASTM) and other protective equipment may allow participation in most sports, but this must be judged on an individual basis.	
Fever	No
Explanation: Fever can increase cardiopulmonary effort, reduce maximum exercise capacity, make heat illness more likely, and increase orthostatic hypotension during exercise. Fever may rarely accompany myocarditis or other infections that may make exercise dangerous.	
Heat illness, history of	Qualified yes
Explanation: Because of the increased likelihood of recurrence, the athlete needs individual assessment to determine the presence of predisposing conditions and to arrange a prevention strategy.	
HIV infection	Yes
Explanation: Because of the apparent minimal risk to others, all sports that the state of health allows may be played. In all athletes, skin lesions should be properly covered, and athletic personnel should use universal precautions when handling blood or body fluids with visible blood.	
Kidney: absence of one	Qualified yes
Explanation: Athlete needs individual assessment for collision/contact and limited contact sports.	
Liver: enlarged	Qualified yes
Explanation: If the liver is acutely enlarged, participation should be avoided because of risk of rupture. If the liver is chronically enlarged, individual assessment is needed before collision/contact or limited contact sports are played.	
Malignancy	Qualified yes
Explanation: Athlete needs individual assessment.	
Musculoskeletal disorders	Qualified yes
Explanation: Athlete needs individual assessment.	
Neurologic	
History of serious head or spine trauma, severe or repeated concussions, or craniotomy.	Qualified yes
Explanation: Athlete needs individual assessment for collision/contact or limited contact sports and for noncontact sports if there are deficits in judgment or cognition. Research supports a conservative approach to mangement of concussion.	
Convulsive disorder, well controlled	Yes
Explanation: Risk of convulsion during participation is minimal	
Convulsive disorder, poorly controlled	Qualified yes
Explanation: Athlete needs individual assessment for collision/contact or limited contact sports. Avoid the following noncontact sports: archery, riflery, swimming, weightlifting or powerlifting, strength training, or sports involving heights. In these sports, occurrence of a convulsion may be a risk to self or others.	
Obesity	Qualified yes
Explanation: Because of the risk of heat illness, obese persons need careful acclimatization and hydration.	
Organ transplant recipient	Qualified yes
Explanation: Athlete needs individual assessment.	
Ovary: absence of one	Yes
Explanation: Risk of severe injury to the remaining ovary is minimal.	
Respiratory	
Pulmonary compromise including cystic fibrosis	Qualified yes
Explanation: Athlete needs individual assessment, but generally all sports may be played if oxygenation remains satisfactory during a graded exercise test. Patients with cystic fibrosis need acclimatization and good hydration to reduce the risk of heat illness.	
Asthma	Yes
Explanation: With proper medication and education, only athletes with the most severe asthma have to modify their participation.	
Acute upper respiratory infection	Qualified yes
Explanation: Upper respiratory obstruction may affect pulmonary function. Athlete needs individual assessment for all but mild disease. See "Fever," above.	
Sickle cell disease	Qualified yes
Explanation: Athlete needs individual assessment. In general, if status of the illness permits, all but high-exertion, collision/contact sport may be played. Overheating, dehydration, and chilling must be avoided.	
Sickle cell trait	Yes
Explanation: It is unlikely that individuals with sickle cell trait (AS) have an increased risk of sudden death or other medical problems during athletic participation except under the most extreme conditions of heat, humidity, and possibly increased altitude. These individuals, like all athletes, should be carefully conditioned, acclimatized, and hydrated to reduce any possible risk.	
Skin: boils, herpes simplex, impetigo, scabies, molluscum contagiosum	Qualified yes
Explanation: While the patient is contagious, participation in gymnastics with mats, martial arts, wrestling, or other collision/contact or limited contact sports is not allowed. Herpes simplex virus probably is not transmitted via mats.	
Spleen, enlarged	Qualified yes
Explanation: Patients with acutely enlarged spleens should avoid all sports because of risk of rupture. Those with chronically enlarged spleens need individual assessment before playing collision/contact or limited contact sports.	
Testicle: absent or undescended	Yes
Explanation: Certain sports may require a protective cup.	

This table is designed to be understood by medical and nonmedical personnel. In the "Explanation" section, "needs evaluation" means that a physician with appropriate knowledge and experience should assess the safety of a given sport for an athlete with the listed medical condition. Unless otherwise noted, this is because the variability of the severity of the disease or of the risk of injury among specific sports, or both.

HIV = human immunodeficiency virus; AS = sickle cell trait.

Modified from Committee on Sports Medicine and Fitness, American Academy of Pediatrics: Medical conditions affecting sports participation. Pediatrics 4:757–758, 1994.

TABLE 690–3 Classification of Sports by Contact

Contact/ Collision	Limited Contact	Noncontact
Basketball	Baseball	Archery
Boxing*	Bicycling	Badminton
Diving	Cheerleading	Bodybuilding
Field hockey	Canoeing/kayaking (white water)	Bowling
Football	Fencing	Canoeing/kayaking (flat water)
Flag	Field	Crew/rowing
Tackle	High jump	Curling
Ice hockey	Pole vault	Dancing
Lacrosse	Floor hockey	Field
Martial arts	Gymnastics	Discus
Rodeo	Handball	Javelin
Rugby	Horseback riding	Shot put
Ski jumping	Racquetball	Golf
Soccer	Skating	Orienteering
Team handball	Ice	Powerlifting
Water polo	Inline	Race walking
Wrestling	Roller	Riflery
	Skiing	Rope jumping
	Cross-country	Running
	Downhill	Sailing
	Water	Scuba diving
	Softball	Strength training
	Squash	Swimming
	Ultimate Frisbee	Table tennis
	Volleyball	Tennis
	Windsurfing/surfing	Track
		Weightlifting

*Participation not recommended.

From Committee on Sports Medicine and Fitness, American Academy of Pediatrics: Medical conditions affecting sports participation. Am Acad Pediatr 94:757, 1994.

Seventy-five per cent of significant findings can be obtained by taking a history; a standardized questionnaire given to the parent and athlete is important. The questionnaire includes questions about previous medical, surgical, cardiac, pulmonary, neurologic, dermatologic, visual, psychologic, musculoskeletal, and menstrual problems, as well as about heat illness, medications, allergies, immunizations, and diet. The most common problems identified during a PSE are unrehabilitated injuries. An investigation of previous injuries including diagnostic tests, treatment, and present functional status is indicated. The most common musculoskeletal injuries identified are of the knee and ankle.

Orthopedic examination should proceed in a stepwise fashion for all joints and extremities. Specific testing for particular sports should be performed, such as ankle and knee examinations in twisting, rapid turning, and jumping sports; back examination for gymnasts and divers; and shoulder examination in overhead sports such as baseball and tennis. Particular attention is paid to limitations of joint range of motion in all directions and differences in extremity symmetry while at rest and during active contraction as well as signs of scoliosis (Chapter 685) and leg length differences (Chapter 682).

Psychologic assessment should determine attitudes and behaviors that would suggest the risk for burnout and overuse injuries. Burnout may be prevented by keeping sports fun, by having a proper perspective about winning and losing, and by taking time out from practice and competition. Pain is often reduced by rest, rehabilitation, and avoiding premature return to participation.

Sudden death during sports may result from cardiac disease such as hypertrophic or other cardiomyopathies, coronary artery disease (single or anomalous vessels, atherosclerosis), congenital heart disease (aortic stenosis), and ruptured aorta in Marfan's syndrome (see Chapter 705). In many cases the underlying heart disease is not suspected, and sudden death is the first sign of heart disease (Chapter 442.6). A chest roentgenogram, electrocardiogram, and echocardiogram are not recommended for screening but are indicated if there is concern about heart disease on the basis of history and physical examination.

Disqualification and limitations for sports participation among various medical conditions are noted in Table 690–2. Classification of sports activities is further delineated in Table 690–3. Students have a legal right to participate in a sport despite a disqualifying condition. Physicians must, nonetheless, provide complete information about the risks associated with participation in sports.

CHAPTER 691
Management of Musculoskeletal Injury

MECHANISM OF INJURY

Acute Injuries. The majority of musculoskeletal injuries are sprains, strains, and contusions; the mechanism may not be obvious. If the history of the injury is clear, such as a direct blow to the quadriceps muscle, the diagnosis is evident. The athlete may not remember what happened, so an important next question is, "What did you do immediately after the injury?" In general, the degree of disability immediately after the injury correlates with the severity. For instance, an athlete who suffers an acute knee injury and cannot bear weight to walk off the tennis court is more likely to have a serious injury than someone who can continue playing.

Overuse Injuries. Overuse injuries are caused by repetitive microtrauma that exceeds the body's rate of repair. This occurs in muscles, tendons, bone, bursas, cartilage, and nerves. Overuse injuries occur in all sports but more frequently in sports emphasizing repetitive motion (swimming, running, tennis, gymnastics). Parents' and coaches' excessively high expectations may add to the risk of an overuse injury in a young, eager-to-please athlete. Other factors include extrinsic (training errors, poor equipment or workout surface) and intrinsic biomechanical factors. Training error is the most frequently identified factor. At the beginning of the workout program, athletes may violate the "10% rule": Do not increase the duration or intensity of workouts more than 10% per week. Intrinsic factors include abnormal biomechanics (leg length discrepancy, pes planus, pes cavus, tarsal coalition, valgus heel, external tibial torsion, femoral anteversion), muscle imbalance, inflexibility, and medical conditions (deconditioning, nutritional deficits, amenorrhea, obesity). Runners should be asked about their shoes, orthotics or braces, running surface, pace, weekly mileage or time spent running per week, duration of the current regimen, and previous injuries and rehabilitation. When causative factors are identified, they can be eliminated or modified so that after rehabilitation the athlete does not return to the same regimen and suffer reinjury.

For athletes engaged in excessive training that causes an overuse injury, curtailing all sports is not always feasible. A rehabilitation program designed to return athletes to their sport as soon as possible while minimizing exposure to reinjury is indicated. Early identification of an overuse injury requires less alteration of the workout regimen.

The *inflammatory response after injury* is manifested as pain, spasm, edema, and, if unabated, scarring. Pain and spasm cause decreased use of the affected area. Although reduced use may protect the area, continued nonuse causes atrophy and decreased flexibility, strength, endurance, and proprioception. Stiff, weak structures with poor proprioception do not function normally and are vulnerable to reinjury. The goals of treatment are to control pain and spasm in order to rehabilitate flexibility, strength, and proprioceptive deficits (Table 691–1).

INITIAL EVALUATION OF THE INJURED EXTREMITY. Initially, the examiner should determine the quality of the peripheral pulses and capillary refill rate as well as the gross motor and sensory function to assess neurovascular injury. The first priorities are to maintain vascular and skeletal stability.

Criteria for immediate attention and rapid orthopedic consultation include vascular compromise (blood flow may be obstructed by a dislocated structure, so a skilled physician should reduce any obstructing dislocated joint); nerve compromise (peripheral nerve damage can be repaired after vascular and skeletal stability have been achieved); and open fracture (an open fracture should not be reduced immediately because of the risk of further contamination). The exposed wound should be covered with sterile saline-soaked gauze, and the injured limb should be padded and splinted. Pressure should be applied to any site of bleeding. Additional criteria include deep laceration over a joint, unreducible dislocation, grade III (complete) tear of a muscle-tendon unit, and displaced, significantly angulated fractures (depends on the bone involved, the degree of displacement and angulation, neurovascular status of the extremity). After the neurovascular assessment, the management of acute musculoskeletal trauma should follow the RICE (rest, ice, compression, elevation) guidelines.

THE TRANSITION FROM IMMEDIATE MANAGEMENT TO RETURN TO PLAY. Rehabilitation of a musculoskeletal injury should begin on the day of the injury.

Phase 1: Limit further injury, control swelling and pain, and minimize strength and flexibility losses. This requires the use of an appropriate device such as crutches or a sling, ice, compression, elevation, and analgesia. Crutches, air stirrups for ankle sprains, slings for arm injuries, and 4 to 8 in elastic wraps (for compression) are a reasonable inventory of office supplies. Ice in a plastic bag is placed directly on the skin for 20 min continuously, three to four times per day until the swelling resolves. Compression limits further bleeding and swelling but should not be so tight that it limits perfusion. Elevation of the extremity promotes venous return and limits swelling. Nonsteroidal anti-inflammatory medication or acetaminophen is indicated for analgesia.

TABLE 691–1 Staging of Overuse Injuries

	Grading Symptoms	Treatment
I	Pain only after activity Does not interfere with performance or intensity Generalized tenderness Disappears before next session	Modification of activity, consider cross-training, home rehabilitation program
II	Minimal pain with activity Does not interfere with performance More localized tenderness	Modification of activity, cross training, consider NSAIDs, home rehabilitation program
III	Pain interferes with activity and performance Definite area of tenderness Usually disappears between sessions	Significant modification of activity, strongly encourage cross-training, NSAIDs, home rehabilitation program, and outpatient physical therapy
IV	Pain with activities of daily living Pain does not disappear between sessions Marked interference with performance and training intensity	Discontinue activity temporarily, cross-training only, NSAIDs, home rehabilitation program and intensive outpatient physical therapy
V	Pain interferes with activities of daily living Signs of tissue injury (e.g., edema) Chronic or recurrent symptoms	Prolonged discontinuation of activity, cross-training only, NSAIDs, home rehabilitation program, and intensive outpatient physical therapy

NSAIDs = nonsteroidal anti-inflammatory drugs.

Pain-free isometric strengthening and range of motion should be initiated as soon as possible. Pain inhibits full muscle contraction; deconditioning results if the pain and resultant nonuse persist for days to weeks, thus delaying recovery. Education about the nature of the injury and the specifics of rehabilitation exercises including handouts with written instructions and drawings demonstrating the exercises are helpful.

Phase 2: Improve strength and range of motion (i.e., flexibility) while allowing the injured structures to heal. Protective devices are removed when the patient's strength and flexibility improve and activities of daily living are pain free. Flexibility can then be improved by a program of specific stretches, held for 15–20 sec for three to five repetitions, once or twice daily. A physical therapist or athletic trainer is invaluable in this treatment. Protective devices may need to be used for months during sports participation. Swimming, water jogging, and stationary cycling are good aerobic exercises that can allow the injured extremity to be rested or used pain free while maintaining cardiovascular fitness.

Phase 3: Achieve near normal strength and flexibility of the injured structures and further improve or maintain cardiovascular fitness. Strength and endurance are improved under controlled conditions using elastic bands and eventually free weights or exercise equipment. Proprioceptive training allows the athlete to redevelop a kinesthetic sense, which is critical to joint function and stability.

Phase 4: Return to exercise or competition without restriction. When the athlete has reached nearly normal flexibility, strength, proprioception, and endurance, he or she can start sports-specific exercises. The athlete will make the transition from the rehabilitation program to functional rehabilitation appropriate for the sport. Substituting sports participation for rehabilitation is inappropriate; rather, there should be progressive stepwise functional return to a full activity/play program. For instance, a basketball player recovering from an ankle injury might begin a walk-run-sprint-cut-program before returning to competition. At any point in this progression if pain is experienced, the athlete needs to stop, ice, take 1 to 2 days without running, continue to do ankle exercises, and then resume running at a lower intensity and progress accordingly.

Relative Rest and Return-to-Play Guidelines. Relative rest means that the athlete can do whatever he or she wants as long as the injured structures do not hurt during or within 24 hr of the activity. Going beyond relative rest delays recovery.

DIFFERENTIAL DIAGNOSES OF MUSCULOSKELETAL PAIN. The presenting complaint of musculoskeletal pain can be due to traumatic, rheumatologic, infectious, hematologic, and oncologic processes. Symptoms such as fatigue, weight loss, rash, multiple joint complaints, fever, chronic or recent illness, and persistence of pain suggest diagnoses other than sports-related trauma. Incongruity between the patient's history and physical examination findings should lead to further evaluation. A normal review of systems with a consistent history of the physical findings suggests a sports-related etiology.

691.1 Growth Plate Injuries

Twenty per cent of pediatric sports injuries seen in the emergency room are fractures. Twenty-five per cent of those fractures involve an epiphysis (Chapter 689). Growth in long bones occurs in three areas: the epiphyseal or growth plate, the articular surface (the cartilaginous covering of the bones), and the apophysis (the growth cartilage where major tendons attach to the bone). The growth plate can be acutely injured at the epiphysis (Salter-Harris fractures), the articular surface (osteochondritis dissecans), or the apophysis (avulsion fractures). Boys suffer about twice as many epiphyseal fractures as girls; the peak incidence of fracture is during peak height velocity (girls, 12 ± 2.5 yr; boys, 14 ± 2 yr).

The most common *epiphyseal injuries* are to the distal radius, followed by phalangeal and distal tibial fractures. Physeal injuries at the knee (distal femur and proximal tibia) are rare. Growth disturbance following a growth plate injury is a function of location, the part of the epiphysis fractured, and the vascular communication between the epiphysis and metaphysis. These factors influence the probability of physeal bar formation resulting in growth arrest at that growth plate. The areas making the largest contribution to longitudinal growth in the upper extremities are the proximal humerus and distal radius/ulna; in the lower extremities, they are the distal femur and the proximal tibia/fibula. Injuries to these areas are more likely to cause growth disturbance compared with epiphyseal injuries at the other end of these long bones. The part of the epiphysis fractured is described by the Salter-Harris classification system (see Fig. 689–1).

Osteochondritis dissecans (OCD) is avascular necrosis of the bone underlying the articular cartilage. The articular cartilage may flatten, soften, or break off. Some OCD lesions are asymptomatic (diagnosed on "routine" radiographs), whereas others are manifested as edema, pain, decreased range of motion, and mechanical symptoms (locking, popping, crepitus). Seventy-five per cent of OCD lesions are located on the medial side of the femoral notch on a non–weight-bearing surface and therefore may have minimal symptoms. Other joints where OCD lesions are identified are the ankle (talus) and elbow, usually involving the medial humeral epiphysis, capitellum, or radial head. OCD classically affects athletes in their second decade. The severity of the lesion is graded as follows: I—compression of the bone, cartilage intact; II—partial separation; III—loose fragment but still in place; and IV—loose fragment detached. Most grade I and II lesions heal spontaneously with protection of the injured joint from loading and torquing actions. If the lesion loosens, internal fixation or debridement may be required. The key to preventing complications is early diagnosis and treatment including non–weight-bearing or atraumatic activity until healing has occurred. Patients with OCD should be referred to an orthopedic surgeon.

Avulsion fractures occur when a forceful muscle contraction dislodges the apophysis from the bone. They occur most frequently around the hip, elbow, and ankle. Chronically increased traction at the muscle-apophysis attachment can lead to repetitive microtrauma, inflammation, and pain at the apophysis. The most common areas affected are the knee (*Osgood-Schlatter* and *Sindig-Larsen-Johannsen disease*), the ankle **(Sever disease),** and the medial epicondyle **(Little League elbow).** Traction apophysitis of the knee and ankle can be potentially treated in a primary care setting, following the principles discussed under rehabilitation. The main goal of treatment is to minimize the intensity and frequency of pain and disability. Exercises that increase the strength, flexibility, and endurance of the muscles attached at the apophysis, using the relative rest principle, are appropriate. Symptoms can last for 12–24 mo if untreated. As growth slows, symptoms abate. Traction apophysitis of the elbow should be referred to a pediatric orthopedic surgeon.

691.2 Shoulder Injuries

An acute shoulder injury characterized by radiating symptoms down the arm should suggest a coexisting neck injury. Neck pain and tenderness or limitation of cervical range of motion requires that the cervical spine be immobilized and that the athlete be transferred for imaging and further evaluation.

ACROMIOCLAVICULAR (AC) SEPARATION. This injury most commonly occurs when an athlete falls or collides with another player or object and the point of contact is the distal clavicle. Patients have discrete tenderness at the AC joint and may have an apparent step-off between the distal clavicle and the acromion. If a humeral fracture is present, point tenderness is noted over the fracture. If a patient has crepitance, the arm should be immobilized in a sling and the patient transferred to the emergency room. AC separations in skeletally immature patients should be immobilized in a sling, and patients should be sent for radiographs. Older athletes may not require radiography to evaluate a mild separation. Fractures require consultation with orthopedic surgeons. Assuming the radiographic results are negative, icing and pain-free range of motion exercises should be started. As the pain-free range improves, strengthening of the rotator cuff, deltoid, and trapezius muscles can start. When the AC joint is nontender and patients have sufficient strength to be functionally protected from a collision or fall and performs the maneuvers required for the sport, they can return to their sport. Surgery is not indicated for the majority of AC separations. Approximately 5% of AC separations are complicated by distal clavicular osteolysis, manifested as persistent pain for months and evidence of osteolysis radiographically. Distal claviclectomy is associated with alleviation of symptoms and full functional recovery.

ANTERIOR DISLOCATION. The common mechanisms of injury are falling onto an outstretched hand with a straight arm or making contact with another player with the shoulder abducted to 90 degrees and forcefully rotated externally. An example of the latter is football players' tackling another player only with their arms. Patients complain of pain and a shifting feeling. Patients with an anterior dislocation have a hollow region inferior to the acromion and a bulge in the anterior portion of the shoulder caused by anterior displacement of the humeral head. This differentiates it from a brachial plexus injury, but anterior dislocation can be complicated by injury to the brachial plexus. Abnormal sensation of the lateral deltoid region (axillary nerve) and the extensor surface of the proximal forearm (musculocutaneous nerve) and the ability to contract the middle deltoid (resisted abduction) and biceps isometrically should be noted. An attempt to reduce the anterior dislocation is indicated, assuming no crepitance is present. Once the dislocation is reduced and radiographs (anterior-posterior and West Point views) show a normal position, rehabilitation begins with isometric internal rotator strengthening. This can progress to elastic band exercises. The rotator cuff muscles are dynamic stabilizers of the shoulder anteriorly, and prevention of future anterior dislocations requires that their strength be restored. For 3 wk, no abduction beyond 10 degrees or external rotation beyond 90 degrees is allowed to permit anterior capsule healing. After 3 wk, as the internal rotator muscles strengthen, progressive strengthening of the rotator cuff muscles begins at greater degrees of abduction and external rotation. Patients can return to play when their strength, flexibility, and proprioception are equal to that of the uninvolved side so that they can protect the shoulder and perform the sports-specific activities pain free.

Patients with chronic shoulder pain may have symptoms due to repetitive stress, with some degree of *glenohumeral instability* causing inflammation in rotator cuff muscles and surrounding structures. Patients may have limitation of pain-free range of motion, a positive impingement sign, and reproduction of pain with resisted rotator cuff muscle testing. Rehabilitation consists of relative rest, including no throwing or whatever the causative activity is, icing, pain-free range of motion exercises, strengthening the rotator cuff muscles, and nonsteroidal anti-inflammatory medication. Strengthening the rotator cuff muscles is critical because they are the dynamic stabilizers of the glenohumeral joint. As patients become pain free and range of motion and strength approach that of the uninvolved shoulder, they can begin functional rehabilitation such as gently throwing a ball or swinging a racquet. If a patient continues to have pain despite these measures, other diagnosis should be considered. Weeks to months may often be required for an athlete to become pain-free.

Proximal humeral stress fracture (epiphysiolysis) is a rare cause of proximal shoulder pain and is suspected when shoulder pain does not respond to routine measures. Gradual onset of deep shoulder pain occurs in a young (open epiphyseal plates) athlete involved in repetitive overhead motion, such as in baseball, tennis, or swimming, but with no history of trauma. Tenderness is noted over the proximal humerus; the diagnosis is confirmed by detecting a widened epiphyseal plate on plain radiographs or increased uptake on nuclear scan.

691.3 Elbow Injuries

ACUTE INJURIES. The most common elbow dislocation is a posterior dislocation. The mechanism of injury is falling backward onto the outstretched arm with the elbow extended. Dislocation potentially compromises the brachial artery; rich collateral circulation makes distal arterial insufficiency unlikely. Intact radial and ulnar pulses are the best indicators of vascular integrity of the distal upper extremity. An obvious deformity is noted, with the olecranon process displaced prominently behind the distal humerus. Reduction is performed by gently applying longitudinal traction to the forearm with gentle upward pressure on the distal humerus. If reduction is not possible, the arm should be padded and placed in a sling and the patient transferred to the emergency room. Elbow injuries can compromise the radial, median, and ulnar nerves.

Supracondylar humeral fractures can result from the same mechanism of injury as elbow dislocations and can be complicated by coexisting injury to the brachial artery and to a lesser extent the median, radial, and ulnar nerves. A compartment syndrome may develop.

CHRONIC INJURIES. Overuse injuries occur primarily in throwing sports and sports that require repetitive wrist flexion or extension or demand weight bearing on hands (gymnastics). "Little League elbow" is a broad term for several different elbow problems.

Overuse, poor technique, unrehabilitated injuries, and poor overall conditioning can lead to injury at the elbow and shoulder. In throwing overhand, medial stretching and lateral compressive forces are placed on the elbow. Repetitive stress is also placed on the flexor and extensor muscle groups' insertions located on the medial and lateral epicondyles, respectively.

Medial elbow pain is a common complaint of young throwers. The stage of bone maturation assists in formulation of the diagnosis. In preadolescents, who still have maturing secondary ossification centers, *traction apophysitis of the medial epicondyle* is likely. Patients have tenderness along the medial epicondyle; this is exacerbated by valgus stress or resisted wrist flexion. Treatment includes no throwing for 4–6 wk, pain-free strengthening, and stretching of the flexor/pronator group followed by 1–2 wk of a progressive functional throwing program with accelerated rehabilitation. In adolescents, who have secondary ossification centers and whose epiphyseal plates have not fused, *avulsion fracture of the medial epicondyle* must be considered. In young adults, with fused epiphyses, the vulnerable structure is the *ulnar collateral ligament* (UCL). UCL tears are managed conservatively but may require surgery if the joint is unstable. Finally, *medial epicondylitis* is caused by overuse of the flexor-pronator muscle groups at their origin, the medial epicondyle, and occurs in sports requiring repetitive wrist flexion. Tenderness is felt over the medial epicondyle exacerbated by passive wrist extension or resisted wrist flexion. Treatment includes relative rest, analgesics, warm and cold modalities, stretching and strengthening wrist flexors, and counterforce bracing.

Lateral elbow compression during the throwing motion can cause problems at the radiocapitellar joint. *Panner's disease* is osteochondrosis of the capitellum that presents between age 7–12 yr. *OCD* of the capitellum presents at age 13–16 yr. Although patients with both conditions present with insidious onset of lateral elbow pain exacerbated by throwing, patients with OCD have mechanical symptoms (popping and locking) and, more frequently, decreased range of motion. Patients with Panner's disease have no mechanical symptoms and often have normal range of motion. The prognosis of Panner's disease is excellent, and treatment consists of relative rest (no throwing), brief immobilization, and repeat radiographics in 6–12 wk to assess bone remodeling.

Lateral epicondylitis, or "tennis elbow," is caused by repetitive contraction of the extensor muscles at their origin on the lateral epicondyle. Tenderness is elicited over the lateral epicondyle, and pain is felt with passive wrist flexion and resisted wrist extension. Treatment includes relative rest. This may require a wrist splint worn during daily activity and at night. Treatment also includes analgesic medication, warm and cold modalities, stretching and strengthening wrist extensors, and counterforce bracing. Functional rehabilitation, such as returning to playing tennis, should be gradual and progressive.

Other less common problems that cause elbow pain are *ulnar neuropathy, triceps tendinitis* and *olecranon apophysitis*, and *loose bodies*.

691.4 Back Injuries

Spondylolysis, a common cause of pain in athletes, is a stress fracture of the pars interarticularis (Chapter 685.6). It can occur at any vertebral level but is most likely in the lower lumbar area. Besides direct trauma that causes an acute fracture, the mechanism of injury is either a congenital defect, which is exacerbated by lumbar extension loading, or a stress fracture due to repetitive extension loading. Ballet, weightlifting, gymnastics, and football are examples of sports in which repetitive extension loading of the lumbar spine occurs. Patients present with pain without a single precipitating event. The diagnosis is often delayed. The pain is reproduced with lumbar extension while standing. The diagnosis is confirmed by finding a pars defect on an oblique lumbar spine radiograph. The defect is not easily seen on anterior-posterior and lateral views. The diagnosis is established by single photon emission CT or nuclear scan, the former being more sensitive.

Facet syndrome has similar history and physical examination findings as spondylolysis. It is caused by an instability in the facet joint, posterior to the pars interarticularis and at the interface of the inferior and superior articulating processes. Facet syndrome can be established by identifying facet abnormalities on CT or by exclusion, requiring a nondiagnostic radiograph and nuclear scan to rule out spondylolysis. *Spondylolythesis* results from anterior displacement of the vertebral body. This is a known complication of untreated spondylolysis and is diagnosed by a lateral lumbar radiograph.

Spondylolysis, spondylolythesis, and facet syndrome are injuries posterior to vertebral bodies. Treatment for posterior element injuries is conservative, directed at reducing the extension loading activity, often for 6–12 mo. Exercises attempt to increase the strength of the abdominal musculature and the flexibility of the lumbar extensor, hamstring, and quadriceps muscles. Extension loading exercises include jogging, overhead weightlifting, landing from the vault in gymnastics, and ballet. Walking and cycling are appropriate exercises during rehabilitation. Bracing to reduce lordosis is advocated by some. Surgery is rarely required for spondylolythesis.

Sciatica may be due to lumbar disk herniation and piriformis syndrome. **Lumbar disk herniation** presents with back pain radiating to the buttocks or down the leg (often below the knee) (Chapter 685.8). Physical examination findings include positive results of a straight leg raise test, sciatica that worsens when the patient bends forward (i.e., lumbar flexion), and possibly reduced strength, sensation, or deep tendon reflexes in the leg. MRI has a 30% false-positive rate in diagnosing disk protrusion in adults; MRI confirms the clinical diagnosis. Assuming the herniation is not large, the pain is not intractable, and the neurologic deficit improves with therapy, the treatment of choice is analgesia, anti-inflammatory medication, and physical therapy. Bed rest or surgery is rarely necessary.

The **piriformis syndrome** is manifested as sciatica because the sciatic nerve passes through the piriformis muscle in 25% of individuals, and in the remainder, it courses along the piriformis muscle. If the piriformis muscle is injured, the sciatic nerve can be secondarily involved, and sciatica ensues. Patients may have some reproduction of sciatica with the straight leg raise maneuver, but the pain is provoked with maneuvers that stretch or resist the piriformis muscle. The piriformis muscle is an external rotator of the hip. The "figure-of-four" test is done by externally rotating the ipsilateral hip by placing the foot on the contralateral quadriceps with the patient in the supine position and then bending the contralateral knee, causing stretch of the piriformis muscle. Pain would support the diagnosis of piriformis strain.

Sacroiliitis presents with lumbar pain that is usually chronic and without a history of trauma. Patients have a positive result of a **Patrick's test,** which includes external rotation of the ipsilateral hip by placing the foot on the contralateral quadriceps with the patient in the supine position, placing one hand on the contralateral anterior superior iliac spine, and then passively flexing the ipsilateral hip. A radiograph of the sacroiliac joints is indicated, and if results are positive, exploration for a rheumatologic disease (ankylosing spondylitis, juvenile rheumatoid arthritis, ulcerative colitis) is warranted. Treatment is with relative rest, nonsteroidal anti-inflammatory drugs, and physical therapy.

Less likely causes of sciatica are polyneuropathies and mass lesions that impinge on the sciatic nerve. Nerve conduction studies should be considered in these cases to establish a diagnosis. Other causes of lower back pain include infection (osteomyelitis, diskitis) and neoplasia (Chapter 685.5). These should be considered in patients with fever, other constitutional signs, or lack of response to initial therapy.

691.5 Hip and Pelvis Injuries

Hip and pelvis injuries represent a small percentage of sports injuries, but they are potentially severe and require prompt diagnosis. Hip pathology can present with knee pain and normal findings on knee examination.

Slipped capital femoral epiphysis (SCFE) usually presents in the 11–15 yr age range during the time of rapid linear bone growth (Chapter 684.4). There is a higher incidence in males (4:1), in African-Americans, and in the obese. Twenty-five per cent are bilateral but may not present synchronously. Pain and limitation of range of motion (especially internal hip rotation) are hallmarks. Radiographic examination shows the epiphysis displaced off the femur, which is described radiographically as "ice cream falling off the cone." If the condition is detected early, the epiphysis may show only slight widening. A bone scan or MRI may be required to diagnose an early or "preslip" SCFE. Non–weight bearing and urgent orthopedic referral are necessary.

Avulsion fractures occur in adolescents playing sports requiring sudden, explosive bursts of speed. Large muscles contract and create force greater than the strength of the attachment of the muscle to the apophysis. The most common sites of avulsion fractures (and the muscles that attach there) are the iliac crest (abdominal muscles), anterior superior iliac spine (sartorius), anterior inferior iliac spine (rectus femoris), lesser femoral trochanter (iliopsoas), and ischial tuberosity (hamstrings). Bilateral radiographs are required. When these fractures are nondisplaced or minimally displaced, healing occurs with conservative management in 4–12 wk. Surgery is reserved for displaced, large fracture fragments or failure of conservative management. Reinjury can occur with premature return to competition. Contact to the bone around the hip and pelvis causes exquisitely tender subperiosteal hematomas called **hip pointers.** Symptomatic care includes rest, ice, analgesia, and protection from reinjury.

A *stress fracture* may present with vague hip pain. If radiographs do not demonstrate a periosteal reaction consistent with a stress fracture, a bone scan or MRI may be required. Orthopedic consultation is necessary in femoral neck stress fractures because of their predisposition to nonunion. **Osteitis pubis** is an inflammation at the pubic symphysis that may be caused by excessive side-to-side rocking of the pelvis (hockey, roller-blading). Radiographic evidence (irregularity, sclerosis, widening of the pubic symphysis with osteolysis) may not be present until symptoms are present for 6–8 wk; bone scan and MRI are more sensitive to early changes. Relative rest for 6–12 wk may be required. *Legg-Calvé-Perthes disease* (avascular necrosis of the femoral head) also presents with insidious onset of limp and hip pain (Chapter 684.3). Classically, it presents in childhood. Treatment allows remodeling of the femoral head by containing it within the acetabulum. Containment may necessitate the use of a brace or surgery.

691.6 Knee Injuries

Knee complaints are the most common musculoskeletal complaint of adolescents. Acute knee injuries that cause immediate disability are likely to be due to fracture, patellar dislocation, internal derangement, or OCD. *Internal derangement* is a nonspecific term and includes injury to the cruciate and collateral ligaments or menisci (cartilage) (Chapter 683). The mechanism of injury is usually a weight-bearing event. After injury, if a player cannot bear weight within a few minutes, a fracture or internal derangement is more likely. If a player is able to bear weight and return to play after the injury, internal derangement is unlikely to have occurred.

Anterior cruciate ligament sprains occur from being hit directly, landing off balance from a jump, or quickly changing direction while running. *Posterior cruciate ligament sprains* occur from a direct blow to the region of the tibial tuberosity. *Medial collateral ligament sprains* result from a valgus blow (directed inward) to the outside of the knee. *Lateral collateral ligament sprains* are unusual as isolated injuries. *Meniscal tears* occur by the same mechanisms as the anterior cruciate ligament sprains.

Patellar dislocations occur most often as a noncontact injury when the quadriceps muscles forcefully contract to extend the knee while the lower leg is externally rotated. The patella is usually dislocated laterally, and this motion tears the medial patellar stabilizers, causing a rapidly enlarging medial hematoma. If a patient continually subluxates the patella or has hypermobile joints, little bleeding may ensue.

PHYSICAL EXAMINATION. The physician should inspect for hemarthrosis and obvious deformities; if these are present, the physician should assess neurovascular status and transfer the patient for emergency care. Assuming no gross deformities are present and neurovascular integrity is intact, initial maneuvers include full passive extension and gentle valgus stress to the knee while the knee is in extension. The patient's ability to contract the vastus medialis obliques should be noted. Point tenderness is consistent with fracture or injury to the underlying structure; a medial meniscal tear is manifested as tenderness along the medial joint line. Presence of swelling in the first 24 hr is diagnostic of internal derangement. Limitation in either passive flexion or extension while rotating the tibia (the McMurray or modified McMurray tests) implies a meniscal injury. Ligament injury is manifested as pain or laxity with the appropriate maneuver. Gross laxity with passive maneuvers implies fracture. Patients with patellar dislocation have pain and apprehension when the examiner gently tries to push the patella laterally (the "apprehension sign"). If the patella is dislocated, reduction is indicated.

INITIAL TREATMENT OF ACUTE KNEE INJURIES. If a patient cannot bear weight pain free or has clinical signs of instability, the knee should be immobilized, crutches given, and plain radiographs obtained. Straight-leg immobilizers offer no structural support. If any brace is used, a hinged brace is indicated. A brace with a lateral buttress is indicated for patients with acute patellar dislocation. Performing isometric quadriceps contractions pain free is necessary to maintain quadriceps strength and requires physical therapy. An elastic wrap or tubular stockinette can be applied for compression and the knee elevated throughout the day. Rehabilitation is indicated.

TREATMENT OF CHRONIC INJURIES. *Patellofemoral pain syndrome* (PFPS) is the most common cause of chronic anterior knee pain. It is worse going up stairs, after sitting for prolonged periods, or after squatting or running. The knee is usually stable. The mechanism of PFPS includes a relatively weak vastus medialis muscle with hamstring and quadriceps muscle inflexibility. The most common mechanism is overuse. The diagnosis is confirmed with peripatellar tenderness. Treatment was outlined earlier (see Chapter 691).

Osgood-Schlatter disease is a traction apophysitis that is a variant of PFPS, with the injury occurring at the insertion of the patellar tendon on the tibial tuberosity. Osgood-Schlatter disease is treated like patellofemoral syndrome, with the addition of a protective Osgood-Schlatter pad, which protects the tibial tubercle from direct trauma. Patients should miss little if any time from sports. *Iliotibial band tendinitis* is the most common cause of chronic lateral knee pain. Generally it is not associated with swelling and instability. Tenderness should be elicited along the iliotibial band as it courses over the lateral femoral condyle or at its insertion at Gerdy's tubercle, along the lateral tibial plateau; tightness of the iliotibial band is also noted. Treatment principles follow those for patellofemoral syndrome, except the emphasis is on improving strength, flexibility, and endurance of the iliotibial band.

691.7 Shin Splints and Stress Fractures of the Lower Leg

Shin splints, presenting with pain along the medial tibia, is an overuse injury of the lower leg. The pain initially appears toward the end of exercise, and if exercise continues without rehabilitation, the pain worsens, occurs earlier in the exercise period, and lasts longer after exercise. Tenderness is elicited over a 5–15-cm area of the posterior tibialis muscle body (just medial to the medial tibia) but not over the bone. This is to be distinguished from a *tibial stress fracture,* in which the tenderness is more discrete (2–5 cm) over the tibia. The tenderness is worse with a stress fracture.

The diagnosis can be made by history and physical examination. Findings on plain radiographs of the tibia are normal with shin splints and in tibial stress fractures within the first few weeks of the injury. Afterward, the radiograph may demonstrate periosteal reaction if a stress fracture is present. A bone scan is the most sensitive test to diagnose stress fractures; it demonstrates a single site of discrete tracer uptake. Increased uptake may be noted in the presence of shin splints but in a fusiform pattern. If results of the bone scan are normal, the diagnosis is likely to be shin splints.

The treatment of shin splints and tibial stress fractures is similar, involving relative rest accomplished by the use of appropriate running shoes. Fitness can be maintained with swimming, cycling, and water jogging. After 7–10 days, patients can start on the walk-run program. If pain worsens, 2–3 pain-free days are required before resuming the walk-jog program. Ice should be used daily. Orthotics to control pronation may be useful in patients who pronate. Stretching and strengthening the ankle dorsiflexors, plantar flexors, and everters can be useful. Analgesic medication can be used for shin splints but not routinely for stress fractures. Seven to 10 pain-free days are recommended before exercise walking is commenced; analgesics may mask the pain.

Stress fractures can occur in any bone in the lower extremity and are most common in the tibia and metatarsals. Stress fractures of the tarsal navicular, talus, proximal anterior third of the tibia, and femoral neck require consultation with an orthopedic surgeon.

691.8 Ankle Injuries

Ankle injuries are the most common acute athletic injury. Eighty-five per cent of ankle injuries are sprains, and 85% of those are inversion (foot planted with the lateral fibula moving toward the ground) injuries, 5% are eversion (foot planted with the medial malleolus moving toward the ground) injuries, and 10% are combined.

EXAMINATION AND INJURY GRADING SCALE. In obvious cases of fracture or dislocation, evaluating neurovascular status with as little movement as possible is the priority (Table 691–2). If no deformity is obvious, the next step is inspection for edema, ecchymosis, and anatomic variants. Key sites to palpate are the entire length of the fibula; the medial and lateral malleoli; the base of the fifth metatarsal; the anterior, medial, and lateral joint lines; the navicular and the Achilles' tendon complex. Assessment of active range of motion (patient alone) in dorsiflexion, plantar flexion, inversion, and eversion and resisted range of motion are indicated. Passive movement in a pain free range is seldom useful in the acute injury. The peroneal muscles are the most often injured and best assessed in the plantar flexed foot with resisted eversion.

Provocative testing of the ankle attempts to evaluate the integrity of the ligaments. In a patient with a markedly swollen, painful ankle, provocative testing is not helpful because of muscle spasm and involuntary guarding. The anterior

TABLE 691–2 Scheme for Grading Ankle Injuries

Severity	Signs and Symptoms	Disability
Grade I (mild)	Minimal swelling (clear definition of Achilles' tendon), small area of tenderness, little or no hemorrhage, minimal decreased range of motion	Little or no limp with walking, minimal difficulty hopping (7–10 days rest with optimal rehabilitation)
Grade II (moderate)	Moderate swelling (margin of Achilles' tendon less defined), more generalized tenderness, some hemorrhage, decreased range of motion	Obvious limping with walking, unable to run, unable to hop, unable to do toe raise (2–4 wk rest with optimal rehabilitation)
Grade III (severe)	Diffuse swelling (no clear margins of Achilles' tendon), widespread tenderness, hemorrhage evident, pronounced decreased range of motion	Unable to bear weight, involuntary guarding with examination (5–10 wk rest with optimal rehabilitation)

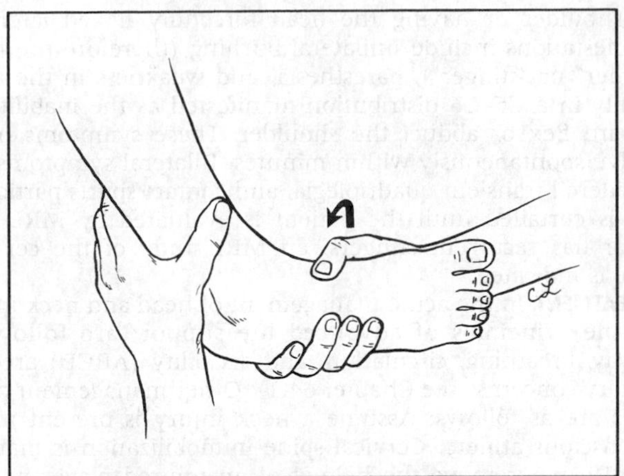

Figure 691–1 Inversion stress tilt test for ankle instability. (From Hergenroeder AC: Diagnosis and treatment of ankle sprains: A review. Am J Dis Child 144:809, 1990.)

drawer test assesses for anterior translation of the talus and competence of the anterior talofibular ligament (ATFL). The inversion stress test examines the competence of the ATFL and calcanoeofibular ligament (Fig. 691–1). In the acute setting, the integrity of the tibiofibular ligaments and syndesmosis is examined by the syndesmosis squeeze test as well as the peroneal subluxation test. If results of either of these tests are abnormal, orthopedic consultation should be sought.

Radiographs. Anterior/posterior, lateral, and mortise views of the ankle are obtained when patients have pain in the area of the malleoli, are unable to bear weight, or have bone pain over the posterior distal tibia or fibula (Ottawa rule). A foot series should be obtained when patients have pain in the area of the midfoot, are unable to bear weight, or have bone pain over the navicular or fifth metatarsal. It is important to differentiate an avulsion fracture of the proximal fifth metatarsal from the Jones fracture of the more distal portion of the proximal fifth metatarsal. The former is treated as an ankle sprain; the latter fracture has an increased risk of nonunion and requires orthopedic consultation. The *talar dome fractures* are manifested as an ankle sprain that does not improve. Radiographs on initial presentation may have subtle abnormalities. Inability to evert the ankle actively and pain over the peroneal retinaculum may indicate a *peroneal rupture or dislocation.*

REHABILITATION. This should begin the day of injury; for those with pain with movement, range of motion, isometric strengthening can be started. Important deficits to correct include loss of dorsiflexion, peroneal muscle weakness, and decreased proprioception. Until these deficits are restored, the ankle is vulnerable to reinjury. While standing on the uninjured side only, the athlete is instructed to hop five times as high as possible ("the five hop test"). If the athlete is able to hop as high on the injured side without pain, he or she can return to sports.

Recurrent ankle injuries are more likely in patients who have not undergone complete rehabilitation. Ankle sprains are less likely in players wearing high-top shoes. Taping the ankle with adhesive tape provides no functional support. If functional support is needed, an ankle brace such as an air stirrup or canvas brace is indicated. Ankle sprains with residual functional instability after 9–12 mo of adequate rehabilitation may require surgery.

691.9 Foot Injuries

Sever disease (calcaneal apophysitis) occurs at the insertion of the Achilles' tendon on the calcaneus. It is more common in boys (2:1); bilateral involvement occurs in 30%. Presentation is between age 8–13 yr. The chief complaint is activity-related heel pain. Tenderness is elicited at the insertion of the Achilles' tendon into the calcaneus, and heel cords are tight. Treatment includes relative rest, ice massage, stretching and strengthening of the Achilles' tendon, heel lifts (e.g., heel cups), and correcting abnormal foot morphology with orthotics or arch supports. With optimal management, symptoms improve in 4–8 wk. If there is no improvement, consideration should be given to less common causes of foot pain including plantar fasciitis, tarsal coalitions, Achilles' tendinitis, stress fractures, and OCD.

CHAPTER 692 *Head and Neck Injuries*

Head and neck injuries account for 90% of traumatic deaths and are the primary cause of permanent disability resulting from sports. The incidence of catastrophic neck injuries associated with quadriplegia is less than 1/100,000; between 1982 and 1992, 179 disabling injuries occurred. The incidence of sports-related catastrophic head and neck injuries has decreased secondary to improved equipment standards for helmets and enforcing rules to prohibit the use of the head as the point of initial contact when tackling.

HEAD INJURY. The most common head injury is the *concussion,* which is characterized by immediate and transient alteration of consciousness, disturbance of vision and equilibrium, and other similar symptoms as a result of mechanical force (also see Chapter 64.7). At least 250,000 sports-related minor head injuries occur annually. The cumulative effect of chronic concussions can cause permanent injury. Management of sports-related concussions is noted in Table 692 1.

An *epidural hematoma* is a rapidly accumulating hematoma between the dura and the cranium. Eighty-five per cent are associated with a skull fracture, and the most serious lacerate the middle meningeal artery. Most victims suffer loss of consciousness followed by a lucid, awake interval often associated with a severe headache. If untreated, this abruptly evolves to deterioration and death within 15–30 min. A *subdural hematoma* occurs when an artery or bridging vein is torn between the dura and the brain parenchyma. It is the most frequent, identifiable focal brain injury in sports and the most common cause of death in sports-related head injuries because it is also associated with cerebral contusion and edema. Patients may lose consciousness at the time of injury but recover in the acute setting. A *cerebral contusion,* bruising of the brain parenchyma, can present with focal symptoms at the site of injury (coup) or on the area opposite to the injury (contracoup). Cerebral contusions are associated with skull fractures (see Chapter 64.7).

NECK INJURIES. *Fracture with or without dislocation* is considered when a player has any head or neck injury or loss of consciousness but more specifically when the athlete has midline cervical pain, painful range of motion, tenderness over the cervical spine, or bilateral neurologic signs or symptoms following neck trauma. Patients should be immobilized and should have a full radiographic evaluation with anterior-posterior, lateral, oblique, and open-mouth views. If results are normal, patients should have flexion and extension views to evaluate for ligamentous instability. If patients have bilateral symptoms but normal findings on radiographs, a lesion impinging on the spinal cord, cord hematoma or edema, or

TABLE 692–1 Concussion Guidelines and Recommendations

Acute head injuries are usually divided into two categories:
1. Diffuse brain injuries—concussion and diffuse axonal injuries.
2. Focal brain injuries—all fractures and intracranial injuries.

It is not necessary to have loss of consciousness to have a concussion.* Several severity grading scales for concussion exist; one that is commonly used is the following:

Colorado Medical Society Guidelines

Grade	*Confusion*	*Amnesia*	*Loss of Consciousness*
I	+	–	–
II	+	+	–
III	+	+	+

Return-to-Play Criteria

Return-to-play criteria are based on prevention of the *second impact syndrome.* This syndrome is characterized by a loss of autoregulation of cerebral blood flow, manifest as a rapid increased intracranial pressure following a second head injury before full recovery from the initial head injury has occurred. Return to contact sports is based on the grade of the injury.

Recommendations for Return to Contact Sports Following a Concussion†

Grade	*Minimum Time to Return*	*Time Asymptomatic‡*
I	20 min	when examined
II	1 wk	1 wk
III	1 mo	1 wk

Recommendations for Return to Contact Sports Following Repeated Concussions

Grade	*Minimum Time to Return*	*Time Asymptomatic‡*
I (2nd time)	2 wk	1 wk
II (2nd time)	1 mo	1 wk
I (× 3), II (× 2), III (× 2)	Season over	1 wk

**In animal studies, there is evidence that there are microscopic changes in the brain after a concussion. These may not be evident in imaging studies, so the clinician must rely on history and neuropsychologic examination to follow a patient's progress. In college football players who experienced their first concussion, the neuropsychologic testing normalized in 5 days and symptoms of headache and memory resolved in 10 days.*

The chronic effects of repetitive boxing injuries include cortical atrophy and a cavum septum pellucidum (identified radiographically). Whether this occurs in other sports in which head injuries are common (football, ice hockey, wrestling) or in which the head is used as part of the game (soccer) is debatable. However, there appears to be no danger in the young soccer player occasionally heading the ball.

†Contact sports means any situation in which contact is possible, including practice.

‡A symptomatic athlete should not return to contact sports regardless of the initial diagnosis. Athletes with focal brain injuries are excluded from contact sports indefinitely. Patients with a neck injury can return to contact sports when they have full, pain-free range of motion, strength and sensation, and normal lordosis of the cervical spine.

stenotic cervical canal is possible, and a noncontrast MRI of the cervical spine is indicated.

Transient quadriplegia (<36 hr) is manifested as sensory changes that may be associated with motor paresis involving both arms, both legs, or all four extremities. Functional spinal narrowing due to congenital spinal stenosis, fused vertebrae, or a structural lesion that narrows the canal such as disk herniation is possible. These diagnoses are made by MRI. Players who have had a neck injury and functional spinal stenosis are at increased risk of permanent disability if they play contact sports. They must be excluded from contact sports.

Patients with a neck injury can return to contact sports when they have full, pain-free range of motion, strength and sensation, and normal lordosis of their cervical spine.

BRACHIAL PLEXUS INJURIES. The brachial plexus includes nerves originating from C5–T1 and emerging from the spinal column in the deep triangle of the neck. The upper trunk (C5–C6) can be contused or stretched during football when tackling with the shoulder or having the head forcefully flexed laterally. Manifestations include unilateral burning (therefore the term "burner" or "stinger"), paresthesia, and weakness in the arm, usually in a C5–C6 distribution manifested as the inability to forward flex or abduct the shoulder. These symptoms often resolve spontaneously within minutes. Bilateral symptoms are considered transient quadriplegia, and contact sports participation is curtailed until the patient is evaluated by MRI. If a player has recurrent stingers, an MRI study of the cervical spine is indicated.

TREATMENT. In the acute management of head and neck injuries, the principles of advanced life support are followed. Airway, breathing, circulation, and disability (ABCD) are the primary concerns (see Chapter 64.1). Other management principles are as follows: Assume a neck injury is present in an unconscious athlete. Cervical spine immobilization is mandatory. Do not remove the helmet of an injured player with a suspected neck injury. If access to a compromised airway is required, remove the face mask. Do not use ammonia smelling salts. The noxious stimulant causes involuntary withdrawal, which may cause secondary injury to an unstable cervical spine. Perform serial neurologic examinations. If the athlete is lucid, look for the signs indicative of a neck injury before the athlete is permitted to move. These include neck pain, painful range of motion, or bilateral neurologic signs.

Athletes with a head injury require transfer for evaluation and observation if they have a suspected skull fracture, deteriorating mental status or worsening headache, focal neurologic deficits or seizure, loss of consciousness for more than 5 min, confusion lasting longer than 30 min, persistent emesis, more than one concussion in a practice/game, or inadequate postinjury supervision.

CHAPTER 693
Heat Injuries

After heart disease, the second most common cause of nontraumatic death is heat illness. Seventy-five per cent of the energy produced by muscular contraction is heat, whereas 25% is converted into muscle work. Without proper heat dissipation mechanisms, intense exercise would elevate core body temperature by 1°C every 5 min and would approach heat stroke within 15–20 min of intense exercise. Heat illness is a continuum of clinical signs and symptoms that can be mild (heat stress) to fatal (heatstroke).

The body dissipates heat by radiation (60% heat transfer to the air), evaporation (20–25%), and convection (15%). With repeated exposure to heat for 8–12 days, the body acclimatizes. Children's ability to tolerate heat stress is not as effective as adults'.

Heat cramps, the most common heat injury, usually affect the calf and hamstring muscles. They respond to oral rehydration with electrolyte solution and with gentle stretching. *Heat syncope* is fainting after prolonged exercise attributed to poor vasomotor tone and depleted intravascular volume, and it responds to fluids, cooling, and supine positioning. *Heat edema* is mild edema of the hands and feet during initial exposure to heat; it resolves with acclimatization. *Heat tetany* is carpopedal tingling or spasms caused by heat-related hyperventilation. It responds to moving to a cooler environment and decreasing respiratory rate (or rebreathing by breathing into a bag).

Moderate heat injury is characterized by body temperature from 99–104°F. *Heat exhaustion* is manifested as headache, nausea, vomiting, dizziness, orthostasis, weakness, piloerection, and possibly syncope. The latter complaint should also suggest head trauma and cardiac conditions. Patients with moderate heat injury do not have serious central nervous system (CNS) dysfunction. Treatment includes moving to a cool environment, cooling the body with fans, removing excess clothing, and placing ice over the groin and axilla. If a patient is not able to tolerate oral rehydration, intravenous fluids are indicated. Patients should be monitored, including rectal temperature, for signs of heat stroke.

Severe heat injury is characterized by body temperature greater than 104°F and altered mental status. *Heat stroke* is a medical emergency; the mortality rate is 50%. Sports-related heatstroke is characterized by profuse sweating and is related to intense exertion, whereas "classic" heatstroke with dry, hot skin is of slower onset (days) in elderly or chronically ill persons exposed to summer heat waves. The physical response of a dehydrated athlete is to attempt to maintain the blood pressure by vasoconstriction, which makes it difficult to transfer heat peripherally. Treatment starts by addressing the airway, breathing, and circulation (ABC) and proceeds to aggressive cooling using ice water baths, cooling fans, and removal of excess clothing. Intravenous fluids at a rate of 800 mL/m^2 in the first hour with dextrose/saline solution improve intravascular volume and the body's ability to dissipate heat. In a previously healthy individual, the risk of pulmonary and cerebral edema is minimal compared with the risk of uncorrected hypovolemia.

Heat-related illness can be prevented. Preparticipation sports physical evaluation should include screening questions to identify predisposing risk factors such as obesity, lack of physical conditioning or acclimatization, prior heat injury, drugs/medications (amphetamines, LSD, alcohol, thyroid hormone, antihistamines, anticholinergics, haloperidol, phenothiazines, diuretics, laxatives, monoamine oxidase inhibitors, tricyclic antidepressants), or medical illnesses (febrile illness, diabetes mellitus and insipidus, diarrhea, CNS disorder, cystic fibrosis, malnutrition and eating disorders, dermatologic disorders with sweat gland dysfunction). Dehydration is common to all heat illness. Mild dehydration (2%) can decrease athletic performance and decrease normal thermoregulation. Thirst is not an adequate indicator of hydration status because it is initiated at 2–3% hydration. Athletes are advised to drink 8–12 oz of fluid before exercise and every 20 min during exercise. Free access to cold water, which is more efficiently absorbed than warm water, is effective and should be advocated to coaches. Scheduled breaks every 20–30 min with helmets off to get out of the heat can decrease the cumulative amount of heat exposure. Practices and competition should be scheduled in the early morning or late afternoon to avoid the hottest part of the day. Guidelines have been published about modification of activity related to the wet bulb temperature. Proper clothing such as shorts and T-shirts without helmets can improve heat dissipation. Proper supervision by an individual who can recognize and treat early heat illness can prevent progression to more severe injury. Prepractice and postpractice weight can be helpful in determining the amount of fluid needed to be replaced (16 oz or ½ L/lb weight loss).

Water is adequate for exercise lasting less than 1 hr. Fluids with electrolyte and carbohydrate should be reserved for exercise lasting for more than 1 hr. Most commercially available sports drinks have 6–8% carbohydrate; experimenting with different drinks or diluting standard sports drinks can decrease the side effects nausea, bloating, and abdominal pain. Salt pills should not be used because of their risk of causing hypernatremia and delayed gastric emptying.

CHAPTER 694
Female Athletes, Menstrual Problems, and the Risk for Osteopenia

Special concerns are related to overtraining in young women and its effect on reproductive function and bone mineral status (Chapters 116 and 121).

The majority of bone mass is acquired by the end of the 2nd decade. Sixty to 70% of adult bone mass is genetically determined, and the remaining is influenced by three controllable factors: exercise, calcium intake, and sex steroids, primarily estrogen. In general, exercise promotes bone mineralization in the majority of young women and is to be encouraged. However, in females with eating disorders and those who exercise to the point of excessive weight loss with amenorrhea or oligomenorrhea, exercise can be detrimental to bone mineral acquisition, resulting in *osteopenia*.

Menstrual dysfunction can occur in women participating in any sport. Athletes with amenorrhea have reduced bone mineral density, are at risk for stress fractures compared with their eumenorrheic athletic peers, and are at increased long-term risk for osteoporosis. Patients with athletic amenorrhea/oligomenorrhea do not have a history suggestive of other causes of amenorrhea. Young athletes with hypothalamic amenorrhea/oligomenorrhea and without an eating disorder appear fit, have an estimated ideal body weight greater than 85%, may have training bradycardia (resting pulse in the 50–60 beats range), and have no signs of other pathology. Patients with anorexia nervosa weigh less than 85% of estimated ideal body weight and may have evidence of starvation manifested as bradycardia, hypothermia, and orthostatic hypotension. The presence of normal genitourinary anatomy and normal breast development precludes other causes of amenorrhea.

The *treatment* of amenorrhea in athletes should include correction of any primary cause for the amenorrhea/oligomenorrhea. In young women who have hypothalamic amenorrhea for more than 6 mo and in whom counseling does not result in a behavioral change or who do not become eumenorrheic, treatment with oral contraceptive pills should be considered to improve bone mineral deposition. Measuring bone mineral can help with the treatment decision if osteopenia is identified. If amenorrhea persists beyond 12 mo regardless of the bone mineral density value, treatment with oral contraceptive pills may be recommended. See Chapter 116.

Adequate calcium intake is important. The current recommended daily allowance for calcium is 1,200 mg. Most adolescent females consume much less. An increase of calcium intake to 1,500 mg/day is suggested. Increased calcium intake alone in adolescent females with anorexia nervosa may not improve bone density because of increased calcium excretion and decreased absorption.

CHAPTER 695
Ergogenic Aids

Also see Chapter 113.9.

Ergogenic aids are any substance used for performance enhancement and include anabolic steroids, red blood cell transfusions, and creatine. With the exception of anabolic steroids, the efficacy of most aids has not been established despite anecdotal reports.

Male and female high school students have reported lifetime prevalence use of anabolic steroids of 4.2% and 2.7%, respectively. Pediatricians should discourage their use. Anabolic steroids at therapeutic doses increase strength and lean muscle mass when combined with increased caloric intake and exercise, compared with increased intake and exercise alone. Some athletes "stack" multiple formulations at many times the therapeutic dose for presumed enhanced efficacy. Short-term side effects of anabolic steroid use include liver toxicity (cholestatic jaundice, peliosis, hepatitis), endocrine abnormalities (gynecomastia, prostatic hypertrophy, hirsutism, impotence, decreased sperm count, testicular atrophy), hematologic changes (hypercoagulability, increased low-density lipoprotein and decreased high-density lipoprotein cholesterol), musculoskeletal problems (premature epiphyseal closure, muscle and tendon rupture), and possibly psychiatric disorders. Anabolic steroid use should be suspected in an athlete with a rapid increase in lean mass and strength that is beyond that expected in normal development. Physical findings include gynecomastia, acne, and marked striae.

Other supplements used by athletes are amino acids, growth hormone, insulin, erythropoietin, β blockers, DHEA, creatine, amphetamines, and cocaine, none of which is effective or recommended for young athletes. Creatine may increase lean body mass.

CHAPTER 696
Specific Sports and Associated Injuries*

GYMNASTICS. Competitive female gymnasts often begin the sport at 6 yr of age, achieve high-level competition at 16 yr of age, and retire at 18–20 yr of age. A similar activity pattern occurs in males at 9, 22, and 24–26 yr of age. In addition to mechanical or traumatic injuries, female gymnasts have delayed menarche and can have eating disorders.

Common problems include traumatic and overuse injuries, such as ankle sprain and wrist and spine injuries. The incidence of injury increases with the level of skill and is greatest in the floor exercise. Wrist pain may be due to chronic upper extremity weight bearing with distal radial physeal trauma. Ligamentous laxity may predispose to elbow or shoulder dislocation and ankle sprains. Spine problems include acute traumatic or overuse injuries such as pars interarticularis injury, resulting in spondylolysis and spondylolisthesis (Chapters 685.6 and 691.4). Therapy includes rest, immobilization, nonsteroidal anti-inflammatory drugs (NSAIDs), and, if pain persists, MRI or arthroscopic examination to rule out intra-articular tears, loose bodies, or ligamentous instability. Prevention includes wrist strengthening, flexibility exercises, and an ulnar variance brace.

SWIMMING. Shoulder injury is the most common overuse injury of competitive swimmers. *Swimmer shoulder* is rotator cuff tendinitis of the supraspinatus or biceps and is manifested as shoulder pain and tenderness of the supraspinatus tendon. The onset may be insidious. Supraspinatus tendinitis produces pain with active abduction between 60 and 100 degrees, whereas biceps tendinitis is demonstrated by resisting flexion of a straight supinated arm. Treatment includes ice, modification of stroke technique, rest, stretching, muscle strengthening, physiotherapy, and NSAIDs. Prevention includes avoiding overwork, proper technique, and strengthening and stretching exercises.

BASEBALL. Throwing injuries of the elbow and shoulder (especially among pitchers) are the most common baseball injuries. See Chapters 687.4 and 691.3.

BALLET. This very demanding activity is associated with delayed menarche and eating disorders in female dancers. Foot problems include metatarsal stress fractures, subungual hematomas, callus, sesamoiditis, bunion formation, proximal phalangeal epiphysitis, and accessory navicular pain syndrome. Ankle problems include inversion sprains, anterior and posterior impingement syndromes, and osteochondritis dissecans (OCD) of the talus. Leg problems include shin splints, tibial or fibular stress fracture, and compartment syndromes (see Running). Knee problems include Osgood-Schlatter disease, excessive recurvatum owing to lax ligaments (pseudo-genu varum), OCD, and patellar malalignment (subluxation dislocation) owing to lax ligaments. Hip problems include the medial snapping hip syndrome caused by the iliopsoas tendon's riding over the anterior hip capsule, tendinitis (piriformis, iliopsoas, rectus femoris), and subclinical slipped capital femoral epiphysis, usually affecting male dancers. Spine problems include Scheuermann's disease in males, idiopathic scoliosis in females, and purposeful excessive lumbar lordosis.

WRESTLING. Wrestlers have great fluctuations in weight to meet weight-matched competition standards. Such fluctuations are associated with fasting, dehydration, and then bingeing.

Wrestling holds may produce injury due to various torques or forces applied to the extremities and spine; wrestling throws with subsequent falls may produce concussions, neck strain, or spinal cord injury. "Stingers" and "burners" are neurogenic pain syndromes caused by traumatic stretching or pinching of the brachial plexus and shoulder injuries (see Football). Severe electric-like pain starts with impact and radiates from the shoulders to the fingertips. Numbness, weakness (predominantly of the abductor deltoid muscles), and tenderness over the paraspinous and trapezius muscles last a few seconds to 5 min. Treatment includes ice, NSAIDs, strengthening exercises, and, if severe, oral steroids, and cervical collar for 24–48 hr.

Shoulder subluxation is common but does not usually present with only pain and weakness. Patients are usually aware of their shoulder's slipping in and out (Chapters 687.2 and 691.2). Hand injuries are usually not severe and include recurrent metacarpophalangeal and proximal interphalangeal sprains. Treatment of hand injuries includes splinting and taping.

Knee injuries are common and potentially serious and include prepatellar bursitis, medial and lateral sprains, and medial and lateral meniscus tears. (See Chapters 683 and 691.6). Prepatellar bursitis is the most common knee problem. It is caused by a traumatic forceful impact to the mat or chronic trauma. Swelling occurs over the knee, and patients have no limitation of motion except full flexion. Treatment includes

*This chapter is modified from L.T. Staheli, 14th ed, and G.H. Thompson, 15th ed. A.C. Hergenroeder and J.N. Chorley made helpful suggestions for this addition, but the editors bear primary responsibility.

protective neoprene knee sleeves, NSAIDs, steroid application, aspiration of effusions, and bursectomy after the third recurrence.

Dermatologic problems include herpes simplex (herpes gladiatorum), impetigo, staphylococcal furunculosis or folliculitis, superficial fungal infections, and contact dermatitis.

FOOTBALL. Football injuries are common, in part owing to the popularity of the sport. Fortunately, most injuries are minor because the incidence of serious injuries has been reduced by prohibition of clipping blocks and "spearing" or head-butting tackling, improvement of techniques, equipment (pads; shoes with wider, more, and shorter cleats; helmet), preseason conditioning (strength and flexibility training), ankle taping, proper rehabilitation of injuries, and playing on grass rather than artificial surfaces.

Head and neck football injuries include concussion, neck sprain, brachial plexus trauma, and shoulder injuries ("stinger," "burner," see Wrestling) and often are unreported because athletes expect these problems. "Burners" represent a brachial plexus neurapraxia, possibly owing to lateral neck bending, manifesting without neck pain but with painful arm dysesthesia and deltoid muscle weakness. They are usually transient, with immediate recovery. Cervical collars (neck rolls) may reduce the risks of this injury, although this has not been proven.

Lumbar spine injury manifested as low back pain may represent spondylolysis. Shoulder trauma includes instability, rotator cuff, and tendinitis injury to the proximal humerus, shaft, and clavicular articulation. Rest, immobilization, and NSAIDs may be effective therapies for mild shoulder injuries. Repeated shoulder subluxation requires strengthening exercises, bracing, and possible surgical stabilization in the off season.

Contusions to the arm and thigh muscles are common, may produce large hematomas, and are at risk for the development of myositis ossificans.

Knee injuries are common reasons why a player seeks medical attention and include anterior cruciate (ACL), posterior cruciate (PCL), and collateral ligament tears. See Chapter 691.6. PCL injuries are usually isolated and respond to rehabilitation. Medial collateral ligament sprains are common, cause temporary disability, and may be rehabilitated with a brace.

Ankle sprains are frequent problems among football players and the risk of reinjury may be reduced by ankle taping or by reusable straps and supports. Turf toe, an injury to the first metatarsophalangeal joint (usually of the great toe), is caused by forceful dorsiflexion while playing on artificial turf in soft, lightweight, flexible shoes. Treatment of turf toe includes ice, NSAIDs, compression, and rest. Corticosteroid injections are not beneficial. Turf toe can be a season ending injury.

HOCKEY. Hockey is a collision sport associated with injuries caused by the puck and the stick, producing contusions, lacerations, or concussions, or by the players' bodies, the ice, and the boards, producing fractures, sprains, or concussions. The risk for injury is reduced by proper equipment (helmets with face masks) and rules regarding dangerous body contact (checking from behind, high sticking).

Specific hockey injuries include ankle sprains (dorsiflexion, eversion, and external rotation in contrast to the usual sprain of inversion in other sports), hip adductor strain, and various shoulder injuries from body contact. The latter include acromioclavicular sprain, dislocation, and clavicular fractures.

BASKETBALL AND VOLLEYBALL. Common physical activities of these two sports include shooting, jumping, pivoting, running, and sudden stopping, which increase the risks for ankle, knee, and finger injury. The latter may necessitate finger and hand guards.

Knee overuse injuries include patellar tendinitis ("jumper knee"), traction apophysitis (Osgood-Schlatter disease), physeal fractures of the distal femur and proximal tibia, fracture of the patella, and ligament sprains (medial collateral with or without anterior cruciate ligaments).

Ankle sprain is the most common injury and is usually caused by inversion with plantar flexion, placing the lateral ligaments at high tension. An avulsion fracture of the base of the fifth metatarsal at the insertion of the peroneus brevis tendon is another sequela of inversion ankle injuries. Achilles tendinitis is an overuse injury that may be exacerbated by rubbing of the tendon over high-top shoes. Foot pain may be due to retrocalcaneal bursitis, posterior tibial tendinitis, accessory tarsal navicular, calcaneal periostitis, plantar fasciitis, stress fracture of the tarsal navicular, Jones' stress fracture of the fifth metatarsal, sesamoiditis, blisters, subungual hematoma, and paronychia.

RUNNING. Running problems are due to an overuse (chronic repetitive motion) injury exacerbated by muscle imbalance, a minor skeletal deformity, or poor flexibility or overload trauma from repeated, poorly absorbed foot impact that ranges from three to eight times the athlete's body weight. Most problems ensue as the runner increases the distance or intensity of training. Minor variations (e.g., malalignment) in anatomy, which do not cause problems at rest, may predispose to injury at specific sites (patellofemoral stress, overpronation). Muscle fatigue, environmental temperature, and running surface (grass vs unyielding concrete) also contribute to injuries. Prevention of injuries is possible by using good-quality running shoes that match to an athlete's foot type, stretching, muscle-strengthening exercises, cross-training (bicycling, swimming), and rest.

Stress fractures may occur on the femoral neck, inferior pubic rami, subtrochanteric area, proximal femoral shaft, proximal tibia, fibula, navicular, metatarsal, sesamoid, and calcaneal apophysitis.

Muscle strains frequently affect the hamstrings, followed by the quadriceps, hip adductors, soleus, and gastrocnemius muscles. Tendinitis involving the tendon and its sheath is common in the Achilles' tendon, followed by the posterior tibial, peroneal, iliopsoas, and proximal hamstring tendons. Achilles tendinitis develops chronically; initially may get better during a run; is characterized by tenderness and crepitance if acute and nodularity if chronic; and must be distinguished from a retrocalcaneal bursitis. Treatment includes temporary abstinence from running (begin cross-training), a ½-in heel lift, heel cord stretching, and NSAIDs. Steroid injection is not indicated.

Anterior knee pain is usually due to patellofemoral stress syndrome (runners' knee), which results from excessive dynamic, usually lateral motion of the patellar tendon in relationship to the femoral intracondylar groove. Chondromalacia patellae may develop. Treatment includes stretching of the quadriceps and hamstring muscles, quadriceps-strengthening exercises, ice, and relative rest. Foot orthotics may be indicated if there is no improvement with the aforementioned treatment. Posterior knee pain is caused by gastrocnemius strain, whereas posteromedial pain is due to proximal tibial stress fractures or semimembranosus tendinitis, and lateral knee pain may be due to iliotibial band syndrome and popliteus tendinitis. Iliotibial band syndrome may be a combination of a bursitis and tendinitis owing to mechanical friction of the band (an extension of the tensor fasciae latae) over the lateral femoral epicondyle.

Shin splints is a descriptive term for pain over the anterior tibia and should be distinguished from tibial stress fractures and chronic compartment syndromes. (Chapter 691.7). Shin splints usually occur in new runners with overpronation. Treatment includes running on soft surfaces, shoe orthotics, NSAIDs, and relative rest (or cross-training).

Compartment syndromes involving the anterior, lateral, deep posterior, or superficial posterior may be induced by running, and they produce local pain confined to the muscle (not to the bone). During exercise, muscles gradually expand and if entrapped in unyielding fascia eventually develop increased intracompartment pressure. Pain usually prevents further training, thus limiting the risk of permanent nerve damage.

Plantar fasciitis is an inflammation of the supporting structure of the longitudinal arch owing to repetitive cyclic loading with foot strike. Pain increases with the first step out of bed in the morning and with running and is located on the medial aspect of the heel. Treatment is similar to that for shin splints.

SOCCER. Injuries in soccer include abrasions, contusions, muscle strains, and ligament sprains (ankle, knee) owing partly to body-to-body contact, falls, running, and kicking. Concussions are common in soccer.

Hip problems include the "hip pointer" (iliac crest contusion), iliac crest apophysitis, and chronic groin pain (muscle strain, hernia, osteitis pubis). Femoral neck stress fractures, slipped femoral capital epiphysis, and avulsion fractures of the pelvis or femur may also cause hip pain.

Knee problems include injuries to the medial collateral ligament, anterior collateral ligament, and menisci. Additional problems are similar to those in the section on running.

TENNIS. Common areas of injury in tennis include muscles and tendons of the elbow, shoulder, back, and abdomen. The risk for injury is increased by personal physical deficiencies (muscle imbalance, malalignment), prior injury, and poor technique. Acute injuries include ankle sprains, abdominal or leg muscle strains, and knee problems (patellofemoral syndrome, menisci); overuse injuries include tendinitis (shoulder, elbow, patellar, Achilles, plantar fascia) and apophysitis (elbow, knee, or calcis).

Shoulder tendinitis is caused by rotator cuff and biceps tendon inflammation. Subluxation of the glenohumeral joint may also be present.

Lateral tennis elbow tendinitis produces pain on backhand shots and tenderness over the extensor brevis origin. Medial elbow tendinitis is associated with pain at the medial epicondyle with wrist flexion and forearm pronation. Medial epicondylar apophysitis is noted in young tennis players and may be associated with ulnar nerve dysfunction if there is an avulsion fracture. Olecranon apophysitis is similar to Osgood-Schlatter disease and is marked by pain at the olecranon with elbow extension.

Wrist problems include an enlarged dorsal ganglion cyst, radiocarpal joint capsular (impingement) synovitis, and degenerative attrition (tears) of the triangular fibrocartilage.

Basic treatment includes rest, NSAIDs, ice, compression (acute phase), rehabilitation, learning proper mechanics, proper grip size, protective counterforce bracing (elbow, wrist), strengthening exercises, and gradual return to tennis. Surgery is rarely needed but is indicated for rotator cuff tendinitis (subluxation), patellofemoral or meniscal injury, and capitellar osteochondritis that has not responded to conservative measures.

SKIING. Injuries are related to falls (contusion, lacerations) and ski-specific mechanisms. Overall injuries have declined, partly because of better equipment (boots, bindings, poles) and slope conditions.

Thumb injuries resulting from falls with the thumb in abduction and hyperextension produce a sprain of the ulnar collateral ligament (skier's thumb). Complete tears with a 45-degree joint opening require surgical intervention, whereas smaller degrees may be treated with a thumb spica cast for 4 wk. A Salter-Harris type III fracture may also be present, and if the epiphyseal fracture is displaced, it requires open reduction and internal fixation.

Lower extremity injuries include ankle sprains (less common with good boots), fractures (often spiral) of the tibia ("boot top") and ankle, and ACL sprains with or without tibial eminence fracture. Hemarthrosis is present in severe ACL sprain. Some ACL sprains can be managed without surgery. However, for those that cannot, treatment of ACL sprains includes bracing, intra-articular reconstruction, and closed or open anatomic reduction of a tibial eminence fracture fragment.

American Academy of Pediatrics Committee on Sports Medicine and Fitness and American Academy of Ophthalmology Committee on Eye Safety and Sports Ophthalmology: Protective eyewear for young athletes. Pediatrics 98:311, 1996.

Cavanaugh RM Jr, Miller ML, Henneberger PK: The preparticipation athletic examination of adolescents: A missed opportunity? Curr Probl Pediatr 27:109, 1997.

Centers for Disease Control: Sports-related recurrent brain injuries—United States. JAMA 277:1190, 1997.

Chande VT: Decision rules for roentgenography of children with acute ankle injuries. Arch Pediatr Adolesc Med 149:255, 1995.

Committee on Sports Medicine and Fitness: Medical conditions affecting sports participation. Pediatrics 94:757, 1994.

Committee on Sports Medicine and Fitness: Cardiac dysrhythmias and sports. Pediatrics 95:786, 1995.

Committee on Sports Medicine and Fitness: Athletic participation by children and adolescents who have systemic hypertension. Pediatrics 99:637, 1997.

Decoster LC, Vailas JC, Lindsay RH, et al: Prevalence and features of joint hypermobility among adolescent athletes. Arch Pediatr Adolesc Med 151:989, 1997.

Dorsen PJ: Should athletes with one eye, kidney or testicle play contact sports? Phys Sportsmed 14:130, 1986.

Genuardi FJ, King WD: Inappropriate discharge instructions for youth athletes hospitalized for concussion. Pediatrics 95:216, 1995.

Maron BJ, Shirani J, Poliac LC, et al: Sudden death in young competitive athletes. JAMA 276:199, 1996.

Micheli LJ: Overuse injuries in children's sports: The growth factor. Orthop Clin North Am 14:337, 1983.

Micheli LJ, Wood R: Back pain in young athletes. Arch Pediatr Adolesc Med 149:15, 1995.

Pearson HA: Sickle cell trait and competitive athletics: Is there a risk? Pediatrics 83:613, 1989.

Stanitski CL, DeLee JC, Drez D Jr: Pediatric and Adolescent Sports Medicine, Vol 3. Philadelphia, WB Saunders, 1994.

Stiell IG, Wells GA, Hoag RH, et al: Implementation of the Ottawa knee rule for the use of radiography in acute knee injuries. JAMA 278:2075, 1997.

Sullivan JA: Ligament injuries of the knee in children. Clin Orthop 225:44, 1990.

Tofler IR, Stryer BK, Micheli LJ, et al: Physical and emotional problems of elite female gymnasts. N Engl J Med 335:281, 1996.

Warren WL, Bailes JE: On the field evaluation of athletic head injuries. Clin Sports Med 17:13, 1998.

Williams M, Branch J: Creatine supplementation and exercise performance: an update. J Am Coll Nutr 17:216, 1998.

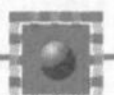

SECTION 3

The Skeletal Dysplasias

William A. Horton ■ Jacqueline T. Hecht

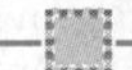

CHAPTER 697

General Considerations

The terms *skeletal dysplasias, bone dysplasias,* and *osteochondrodysplasias* refer to a genetically and clinically heterogeneous group of disorders of skeletal development and growth. Their prevalence is estimated to be about 1 in 4,000 births. They can be divided into the osteodysplasias typified by osteogenesis imperfecta (see Chapter 704) and the chondrodysplasias. The latter result from mutations of genes that are essential for skeletal development and growth. The clinical picture is dominated by skeletal abnormalities. The manifestations may be restricted to the skeleton, but in most cases, nonskeletal tissues are also involved. The disorders may be lethal in utero or mild with features that go undetected.

The chondrodysplasias are distinguished from other forms of short stature by a disproportionality of skeletal manifestations. They have been separated into individuals with predominantly short limbs and those with predominantly short trunks. Efforts to define the extent of clinical heterogeneity resulted in the delineation of more than 100 distinct entities. As the genetic mutations responsible for the chondrodysplasias were identified, it became apparent that many of these disorders result from mutations of a relatively small group of genes, the "chondrodysplasia genes."

An International Working Group on Bone Dysplasias named and classified these disorders based on genetic cause if known or on similarities of clinical and radiographic manifestations, which often imply a common pathogenesis and a common genetic basis, if the cause is unknown (Table 697–1). The classification differs substantially from previous ones, which were based mainly on radiographic grounds. Disorders previously thought to be different were grouped together, (e.g., pseudoachondroplasia, multiple epiphyseal dysplasia). By genetic definition, these are "allelic" disorders. In other instances, disorders believed to be related ended up in the different chondrodysplasia groups, (e.g., achondrogenesis types Ia and II) because the mutant genes differ.

The better defined chondrodysplasia groups, such as the achondroplasia and type II collagenopathy groups, contain graded series of disorders that range from very severe to very mild. This may be true for other groups as more mutations are found, and the full spectrum of clinical phenotypes associated

TABLE 697–1 Human Chondrodysplasias

Gene Locus	Chromosome Location	Protein	Protein Function	Clinical Phenotype	On-Line Mendelian Inheritance in Man	Inheritance	Mechanism
COL2A1	12q13.1-q13.3	Type II collagen α_1-Chain	Cartilage matrix protein	Achondrogenesis II	200610	AD*	Dominant negative
				Hypochondrogenesis	12014002	AD*	Dominant negative
				SED congenita	183900	AD	Dominant negative
				Kniest dysplasia	156550	AD	Dominant negative
				Late-onset SED		AD	Dominant negative
				Stickler dysplasia	108300	AD	Haploinsufficiency
COL11A1	1p21	Type XI collagen α_1-Chain	Cartilage matrix protein	Stickler-like dysplasia	184840	AD	Dominant negative
COL11A2	6p21.3	Type XI collagen α_2-Chain	Cartilage matrix protein	Stickler-like dysplasia	215150	AR	Loss of function
COL9A2	1p32.2-p33	Type IX collagen α_2-Chain	Cartilage matrix protein	Multiple epiphyseal dysplasia	600969	AD	Dominant negative
COMP	19p12-p13.1	Cartilage oligmeric matrix protein	Cartilage matrix protein	Pseudoachondroplasia	177170	AD	Dominant negative
				Multiple epiphyseal dysplasia	600969	AD	Dominant negative
COL10A1	6q21–q22.3	Type X collagen α_1-Chain	Hypertrophic cartilage matrix protein	Schmid metaphyseal chondrodysplasia	156500	AD	Haploinsufficiency
FGFR3	4p16.3	FGF receptor 3	Tyrosine kinase receptor for FGFs	Thanatophoric dysplasia I	187600	AD*	Gain of function
				Thanatophoric dysplasia II	187610	AD*	Gain of function
				Achondroplasia	100800	AD	Gain of function
				Hypochondroplasia	146000	AD	Gain of function
PTHrPR	3p21-p22	PTHrP receptor	G protein–coupled receptor for PTH and PTHrP	Jansen metaphyseal chondrodysplasia	156400	AD	Gain of function
DTDST	5q32-q33	DTD sulfate transporter	Transmembrane sulfate transporter	Achondrogenesis 1B	600972	AR*	Loss of function
				Atelosteogenesis II	256050	AR*	Loss of function
				Diastrophic dysplasia	222600	AR*	Loss of function
SOX9	17q24.3-q25.1	SRY box 9	Transcription factor	Camptomelic dysplasia	114290	AD	Haploinsufficiency
CBFA1	6p21	Core-binding factor α subunit	Transcription factor	Cleidocranial dysplasia	119600	AD	Haploinsufficiency
LMX1B	9q34.1		Transcription factor	Nail patella dysplasia	161200	AD	Haploinsufficiency
CTSK	1q21	Cathepsin K	Enzyme	Pycnodysostosis	265800	AR	Loss of function

AD = autosomal dominant; SED = spondyloepiphyseal dysplasia; AR = autosomal recessive; FGFs = fibroblast growth factors; DTD = diastrophic dysplasia.

TABLE 697–2 Major Problems Associated with Skeletal Dysplasias

Problem	Example
Lethality*	Thanatophoric dysplasia
Associated anomalies†	Ellis–van Creveld syndrome
Short stature	Spondyloepiphyseal dysplasia congenita
Cervical spine dislocations	Larsen syndrome
Severe limb bowing	Metaphyseal dysplasia type Schmid
Spine curvatures	Metatrophic dysplasia
Club feet	Diastrophic dysplasia
Fractures	Osteogenesis imperfecta
Pneumonias, aspirations	Camptomelic dysplasia
Hydrocephalus	Achondroplasia
Joint problems (hips, knees)	Most skeletal dysplasias
Hearing loss	Common (greatest with cleft palate)
Myopia/cataracts	Stickler syndrome
Immune deficiency‡	Cartilage-hair hypoplasia
Sudden infant death syndrome	Achondroplasia (rare)
Poor body image	Variable, but common to all
Sex reversal	Camptomelic dysplasia

*Mostly due to severely reduced size of thorax.
†See Table 673–3.
‡At least four additional disorders, all involving the metaphyses, can have immunodeficiency.

with mutations of a given gene are defined. These observations have changed the way these disorders are viewed. Previously, they were considered distinct entities with unique clinical, radiographic, and genetic features. The emerging view is that they are clinical phenotypes distributed along spectra of phenotypic abnormality associated with mutations of particular genes. For mutations of some genes such as *COL2A1*, the distribution is fairly continuous with clinical phenotypes merging into one another across a broad range. There is much less clinical overlap for mutations of some other genes, such as *FGFR3*, in which the distribution is discontinuous. Since most clinicians and most reference materials refer to the disorders as distinct entities, this vernacular continues to be used.

Although a few chondrodysplasias can be easily diagnosed, most require the analysis of information from the history, physical examination, skeletal radiographs, family history, and laboratory testing. The process involves recognizing complex patterns that are characteristic of the different disorders (Table 697–2). Comprehensive descriptions of disorders and references are on two Internet sites: On-Line Mendelian Inheritance in Man (OMIM) and the International Skeletal Dysplasia Web Site. OMIM numbers are given for disorders discussed in this and related chapters.

CLINICAL MANIFESTATIONS

Growth Related. The hallmark of the chondrodysplasias is disproportionate short stature. Although this refers to a disproportion between the limbs and the trunk, most disorders exhibit some shortening of both, and subtle degrees of disproportion may be difficult to appreciate, especially in premature, obese, or edematous infants. Disproportionate shortening of the limbs should be suspected if the upper limbs do not reach the midpelvis in infancy or the upper thigh after infancy. Disproportionate shortening of the trunk is indicated by a short neck, small chest, and protuberant abdomen. Skeletal disproportion is usually accompanied by short stature (i.e., length and height below the 3rd percentile), but these measurements are occasionally within the low-normal range early in the course of certain conditions.

In addition to limb-trunk disproportion, there may also be disproportionate shortening of different segments of the limbs; the particular pattern may provide clues for specific diagnoses. For example, shortening is greatest in the proximal segments (upper arms and legs) in achondroplasia; this is termed *rhizomelic* shortening. Disproportionate shortening of the middle segments (forearms and lower legs) is called *mesomelic* shortening; *acromelic* shortening involves the hands and feet.

With some exceptions, there is a strong correlation between the age of onset and the clinical severity. Many of the so-called lethal neonatal chondrodysplasias are evident by the time routine fetal ultrasound examinations are performed at the end of the 1st trimester of gestation. Gestational standards exist for long bone lengths; discrepancies are often detected between biparietal diameter of the skull and long bone lengths. Many disorders become apparent around the time of birth; others manifest during the 1st yr of life. A number of disorders present in early childhood and a few in late childhood or later.

Non-Growth Related. Although growth deficiency is a dominant feature, most patients also have problems unrelated to growth. Skeletal deformities, such as abnormal joint mobility, protuberances at and around joints, angular deformities, and so on, are common and usually symmetric. Skeletal abnormalities may adversely affect nonskeletal tissues. Impaired growth at the base of the skull and of vertebral pedicles reduces the size of the spinal canal in achondroplasia and may contribute to spinal cord compression. Short ribs reduce thoracic volume, which may compromise breathing in short trunk chondrodysplasias. Cleft palate is common to many disorders, presumably reflecting defective palatal growth.

Manifestations may be unrelated to the skeleton; they reflect expression of mutant genes in nonskeletal tissues. Examples include retinal detachment in spondyloepiphyseal dysplasia congenita, sex reversal in camptomelic dysplasia, congenital heart malformations in Ellis–van Creveld syndrome, immune deficiency in cartilage-hair hypoplasia, and renal dysfunction in asphyxiating thoracic dystrophy. These nonskeletal problems provide valuable clues to specific diagnoses and must be managed clinically (Table 697–3).

Family and Reproductive History. A careful family history may identify relatives with the condition; a mendelian inheritance pattern may be elicited. Because the presentation may vary substantially in some disorders, features that might be related to the disorder should be identified. Special attention should be given to mild degrees of short stature, disproportion, deformities, and other manifestations such as precocious osteoarthritis because they may be overlooked by the family. Physical examination of relatives may be useful as may the review of

TABLE 697–3 Associated Anomalies in Skeletal Dysplasias

Anomaly	Example
Heart defects	Ellis–van Creveld syndrome
Polydactyly	Short rib polydactyly, Majewski type
Cleft palate	Diastrophic dysplasia
Ear cysts	Diastrophic dysplasia
Hydrocephalus	Achondroplasia
Encephalocele	Dyssegmental dysplasia
Hemivertebrae	Dyssegmental dysplasia
Micrognathia	Camptomelic dysplasia
Nail dysplasia	Ellis–van Creveld syndrome
Conical teeth, oliogodontia	Ellis–van Creveld syndrome
Multiple oral frenulae	Ellis–van Creveld syndrome
Dentinogenesis imperfecta	Osteogenesis imperfecta
Pretibial skin dimples	Camptomelic dysplasia
Cataracts, retinal detachment	Stickler syndrome
Intestinal atresia	Saldino-Noonan
Renal cysts	Saldino-Noonan
Campodactyly	Diastrophic dysplasia
Craniosynostosis	Thanatophoric dysplasia
Ichthyosis	Chondrodystrophica punctata
Hitchhiker thumb	Diastrophic dysplasia
Facial hemangioma	Many severe dwarfing conditions
Sparse scalp hair	Cartilage-hair hypoplasia
Hypertelorism	Robinow syndrome
Hypoplastic nasal bridge	Acrodysostosis
Clavicular agenesis	Cleidocranial dysplasia
Genital hypoplasia	Robinow syndrome
Tail	Metatropic dysplasia
Omphalocele	Beemer-Langer
Blue sclera	Osteogenesis imperfecta

photographs, roentgenograms, and medical records of family members.

A reproductive history may reveal previous stillbirths, fetal losses, and other abnormal pregnancy outcomes resulting from a skeletal dysplasia. Pregnancy complications, such as polyhydramnios or reduced fetal movement, are common in bone dysplasias, especially neonatal lethal variants.

Even though most of the skeletal dysplasias are genetic, it is common to have no family history of the disorder. New mutations are common for autosomal dominant disorders, especially lethal disorders in the perinatal period (thanatophoric dysplasia, osteogenesis imperfecta). The majority of achondroplasia cases result from new mutations. Germ cell mosaicism, in which a parent has clones of mutant germ cells, has been observed in osteogenesis imperfecta and in other dominant disorders. A negative family history is common in recessive disorders.

Radiographic Features. Radiographic evaluation for a chondrodysplasia should include plain films of the entire skeleton. Efforts should be made to identify which bones and which parts of bones (epiphyses, metaphyses, diaphyses) are most affected. If possible, films taken at different ages should be examined because the radiographic changes evolve with time. Films taken before puberty are generally more informative because pubertal closure of the epiphyses obliterates many of the signs needed for a radiographic diagnosis.

DIAGNOSIS

If an infant or child is short with disproportionate features, a diagnosis is established by matching the observed clinical picture—defined primarily from clinical, family, and gestational histories; physical examination; and radiographic evaluation—with clinical phenotypes of well-documented disorders. Pediatricians should be able to gather most of this information and, in consultation with a radiologist, diagnose the common chondrodysplasias. There are a number of reference texts and online data bases that provide information about the disorders and comprehensive lists of current references. For less common disorders and for infants and children whose phenotypes do not closely match well-established clinical phenotypes, consultation with experts in the bone dysplasia field is warranted.

Laboratory testing has not been useful in diagnosing chondrodysplasias. An exception is osteogenesis imperfecta, in which analysis of collagen synthesis by skin fibroblasts has helped establish a diagnosis. Osteogenesis imperfecta is not a chondrodysplasia, but it is frequently in the differential diagnosis, especially for newborns with severe skeletal deformities (see Chapter 704).

Molecular genetic testing for chondrodysplasias may be useful, especially for disorders in which recurrent mutations occur (typical achondroplasia has the same *FGFR3* mutation). Mutation testing for achondroplasia is available; however, the diagnosis can usually be made clinically. The greatest utility for testing may be for prenatal diagnosis for couples in whom both parents have typical (heterozygous) achondroplasia. They are at a 25% risk for the much more severe homozygous achondroplasia, which can be detected by mutation analysis. Another example is in disorders due to mutations of *DTDST.* These disorders are inherited in an autosomal recessive manner, and a limited number of mutant alleles have been found. If the mutations are identified in the patient, they should be detectable in the parents and potentially used for prenatal diagnosis. Nonetheless, most chondrodysplasia mutations tend to be dispersed throughout host genes. This phenomenon makes their detection more difficult and currently reduces the usefulness of such testing for diagnostic purposes.

Many of the chondrodysplasias have distinct histologic changes of the skeletal growth plate. Sometimes such tissues obtained at biopsy or discarded from a surgical procedure are helpful diagnostically. It is uncommon to make a diagnosis histologically if it was not already suspected on clinical grounds. An exception is for the lethal neonatal chondrodysplasias, in which an aborted fetus is macerated, thus making a clinical and radiographic assessment difficult.

MOLECULAR GENETICS. A number of chondrodysplasia genes have been identified (see Table 697–1). They encode several categories of proteins, including cartilage matrix proteins, transmembrane receptors, ion transporters, and transcription factors. The number of identified gene loci is much smaller than anticipated from the number of recognized clinical phenotypes. The vast majority of patients have disorders that map to fewer than 10 loci; mutations at two loci (*COL2A1* and *FGFR3*) account for more than half of all cases. There may be a limited number of genes whose function is critical to skeletal development, especially linear bone growth; mutations in these genes give rise to a wide range of chondrodysplasia clinical phenotypes.

Mutations at the *COL2A1* and *FGFR3* loci illustrate different genetic characteristics. *COL2A1* mutations are distributed throughout the gene with few instances of recurrence in unrelated persons. In contrast, *FGFR3* mutations are restricted to a few locations within the gene, and occurrence of new mutations at these sites in unrelated individuals is the rule. There is a strong correlation between clinical phenotype and mutation site for *FGFR3,* but not *COL2A1,* mutations.

PATHOPHYSIOLOGY. Chondrodysplasia mutations act through different mechanisms. Most mutations involving cartilage matrix proteins cause disease when only one of the two copies (alleles) of the relevant gene is mutated. These mutations usually act through a *dominant negative mechanism* in which the protein products of the mutant allele interfere with the assembly and function of multimeric molecules that contain the protein products of both the normal and mutant alleles. For example, the type II collagen molecule is a triple helix composed of three collagen chains, which are the products of the type II collagen gene, *COL2A1.* When chains from both normal and mutant alleles are combined to form triple helices, most molecules contain at least one mutant chain. It is not known how many mutant chains are required to produce a dysfunctional molecule but, depending on the mutation, it theoretically could be as few as one.

Mutations involving type X collagen differ from the model just described. They map to the region of the chain that is responsible for chain recognition; the chains must recognize each other before they can assemble into collagen molecules. Mutations are thought to disrupt this process. As a result, none of the mutant chains is incorporated into molecules. This

TABLE 697–4 Lethal Neonatal Dwarfism

Usually Fatal*

Achondrogenesis (different types)
Thanatophoric dysplasia
Short rib polydactyly, Majewski type
Short rib polydactyly, Saldino-Noonan type
Homozygous achondroplasia
Osteopetrosis (congenital form)
Camptomelic dysplasia
Dyssegmental dysplasia, Silverman-Handmaker type
Osteogenesis imperfecta, type II
Hypophosphatasia (congenital form)
Chondrodysplasia punctata (rhizomelic form)

Often Fatal

Asphyxiating thoracic dystrophy (Jeune syndrome)

Occasionally Fatal

Ellis–van Creveld syndrome
Diastrophic dysplasia
Metatropic dwarfism
Kniest dysplasia

**A few prolonged survivors have been reported in most of these disorders.*

TABLE 697–5 Usually Nonlethal Dwarfing Conditions Recognizable at Birth or Within First Few Months of Life

Most Common
Achondroplasia
Osteogenesis imperfecta (types I, III, IV)
Spondyloepiphyseal dysplasia congenita
Diastrophic dysplasia
Ellis–van Creveld syndrome
Less Common
Chondrodysplasia punctata (some forms)
Kniest dysplasia (not severe congenital forms)
Metatrophic dysplasia
Langer mesomelic dysplasia

mechanism is termed *loss of function* because the products of the mutant allele are functionally absent. Mutations involving ion transport genes also act through a loss of function of the transporters. Alternatively, mutations of transmembrane receptors studied to date appear to act through a gain of function; the mutant receptors initiate signals in a constitutive manner independent of their normal ligands.

Regardless of genetic mechanism, the mutations ultimately disrupt endochondral ossification, the biologic process responsible for the development and linear growth of the skeleton. Indeed, a wide range of morphologic abnormalities of the skeletal growth plate, the anatomic structure in which endochondral ossification occurs, have been described in the chondrodysplasias.

DIAGNOSIS AND TREATMENT. The first step is to establish the correct diagnosis. This allows one to predict a prognosis and to anticipate the medical and surgical problems associated with a particular disorder. Establishing a diagnosis helps to distinguish between lethal disorders and nonlethal disorders in a premature or newborn infant (Tables 697–4 and 697–5). A poor prognosis for long-term survival may argue against initiating extreme lifesaving measures for thanatophoric dysplasia or achondrogenesis types Ib or II, whereas such measures may be indicated for infants with spondyloepiphyseal dysplasia congenita or diastrophic dysplasia, which carry a good prognosis if the infant survives the newborn period.

Since there is no definitive therapy to normalize bone growth in any of the disorders, management is directed at preventing and correcting skeletal deformities, treating nonskeletal complications, genetic counseling, and helping patients and families learn to cope. Each disorder has its own unique set of problems, and consequently management must be tailored to each disorder. Medical information for a few disorders can be found at the Dwarfism Web Site.

There are a number of problems common to many chondrodysplasias for which general recommendations can be made. For instance, children with most chondrodysplasias should avoid contact sports and other activities that cause injury or stress to joints. Good dietary habits should be established in childhood to prevent or minimize obesity in adulthood. Dental care should be started early to minimize crowding and malalignment of teeth. Children and relatives should be given the opportunity to participate in support groups, such as the Little People of America and Human Growth Foundation.

Two controversial approaches have been used to increase bone length. Surgical limb lengthening has been employed for a few disorders. Its greatest success has been in achondroplasia in which nonskeletal tissues tend to be redundant and easily stretched. The procedure is usually performed during adolescence. Injections of human growth hormone in pharmacologic doses comparable to those used to treat Turner's syndrome have also been tried in several disorders; the results have been equivocal.

Apajasalo M, Sintonen H, Rautonen J, Kaitila I: Health-related quality of life patients with genetic skeletal dysplasias. Eur J Pediatr 157:114, 1998.
Hall JG, Froster-Iskenius UG, Allanson JE: Handbook of Normal Physical Measurements. Oxford, Oxford University Press, 1989.
Horton WA: Molecular genetics of the human chondrodysplasias—1995. Eur J Hum Genet 3:357, 1995.
Lachman RS: Neurologic abnormalities in the skeletal dysplasias: A clinical and radiological perspective. Am J Med Genet 69:33, 1997.
Rimoin DL, Lachman RS: Chondrodysplasias. *In:* Rimoin DL, Connor JM, Pyeritz RE (eds): Emery and Rimoin's Principles and Practice of Medical Genetics, 3rd ed. New York, Churchill Livingstone, 1996, p 2779.
Spranger J, Maroteaux P: The lethal osteochondrodysplasias. Adv Hum Genet 19:1, 1995.
Spranger JW, Langer LOJ, Wiedemann H-R: Bone Dysplasias, An Atlas of Constitutional Disorders of Skeletal Development. Philadelphia, WB Saunders, 1974.
Taybi H, Lachman RS: Radiology of Syndromes, Metabolic Disorders, and Skeletal Dysplasias, 4th ed. New York, Mosby, 1996.

Online Resources

Medical Information on Dwarfism Web Site—http://www-bfs.ucsd.edu/dwarfism/medical.htm
On-Line Mendelian Inheritance in Man (OMIM)—http://www3.nebi.nlm.nih.gov/omim

CHAPTER 698
Disorders Involving Cartilage Matrix Proteins

Some bone and joint disorders result from functional disturbances of cartilage matrix proteins. They fall into four groups corresponding to the defective proteins: three collagens and the noncollagenous protein COMP (cartilage oligomeric matrix protein). The clinical phenotypes differ between and within the groups, especially the spondyloepiphyseal dysplasia (SED) group. In some groups, there is substantial variation in clinical severity.

SPONDYLOEPIPHYSEAL DYSPLASIAS

The term *spondyloepiphyseal dysplasia* refers to a heterogeneous group of disorders characterized by shortening of the trunk and to a lesser extent the limbs. Severity ranges from achondrogenesis type II to the slightly less severe, hypochondrogenesis (these two types are lethal in the perinatal period) to SED congenita and its variants including **Kniest dysplasia** (which are apparent at birth and are usually nonlethal), to late-onset SED (which may not be detected until adolescence or later). The radiographic hallmarks are abnormal development of the vertebral bodies and of epiphyses, the extent of which corresponds to the clinical severity. All the SEDs result from heterozygous mutations of *COL2A1*; they are autosomal dominant disorders. The mutations are dispersed through the gene; there is a poor correlation between the mutation's location and the resultant clinical phenotype.

LETHAL SPONDYLOEPIPHYSEAL DYSPLASIAS. Achondrogenesis type II (On-Line Mendelian Inheritance of Man [OMIM] 200610) is characterized by severe shortening of the neck and trunk and especially the limbs, and a large, soft head. Fetal hydrops and prematurity are common; infants are stillborn or die shortly after birth. Hypochondrogenesis (OMIM 12014002) refers to a clinical phenotype intermediate between achondrogenesis type II and SED congenita. It is typically lethal in the newborn period.

The severity of radiographic changes correlate with the clinical severity (Fig. 698–1). Both conditions produce short, broad tubular bones with cupped metaphyses. The pelvic bones are hypoplastic, and the cranial bones are not well mineralized. The vertebral bodies are poorly ossified in the entire spine in

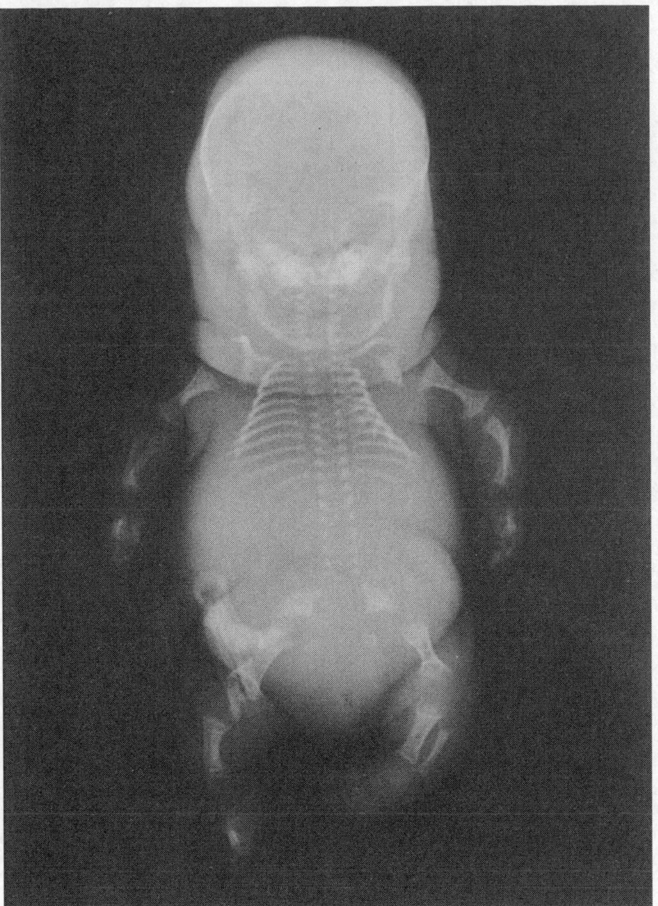

Figure 698–1 Stillborn with achondrogenesis type II. Note poor ossification of calvaria, vertebral bodies and sacrum, hypoplasia of pelvic bones, and short tubular bones with cupped metaphyses.

achondrogenesis type II and in the cervical and sacral spine in hypochondrogenesis. The pedicles are ossified in both.

SPONDYLOEPIPHYSEAL DYSPLASIA CONGENITA. The phenotype of this group, SED congenita (OMIM 183900), is apparent at birth. The head and face are usually normal, but a cleft palate is common. The neck is short and the chest is barrel-shaped (Fig. 698–2). Kyphosis and exaggeration of the normal lumbar lordosis are common. The proximal segments of the limbs are shorter than the hands and feet, which often appear normal. Some infants have clubfoot or exhibit hypotonia.

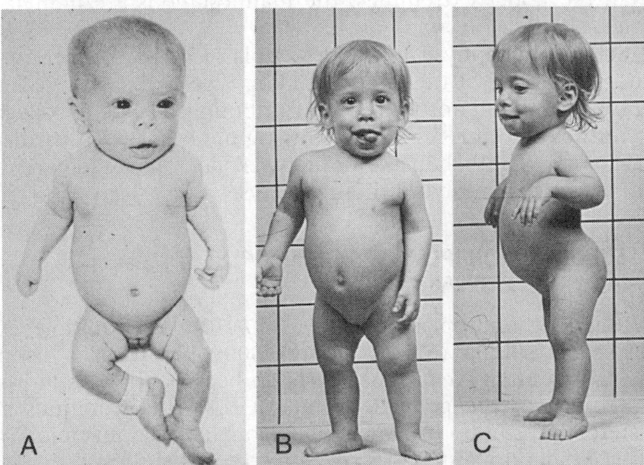

Figure 698–2 SED congenita is shown in infancy and early childhood. Note the short extremities, relatively normal hands, flat facies, and exaggerated lordosis.

Skeletal radiographs of the newborn reveal short tubular bones, delayed ossification of vertebral bodies, and proximal limb bone epiphyses (Fig. 698–3). Hypoplasia of the odontoid process; a short, square pelvis with a poorly ossified symphysis pubis; and mild irregularity of metaphyses are apparent.

Infants usually have normal developmental milestones; a waddling gait typically appears in early childhood. Childhood complications include respiratory compromise from spinal deformities and spinal cord compression due to cervicomedullary instability. The disproportionateness and shortening become progressively worse with age, and adult heights range from 95 to 128 cm. Myopia is typical; adults are predisposed to retinal detachment. Precocious osteoarthritis occurs in adulthood and requires surgical joint replacement.

KNIEST DYSPLASIA. The Kniest dysplasia variant of SED (OMIM 156550) presents at birth with a short trunk and limbs associated with a flat face, prominent eyes, enlarged joints, cleft palate, and clubfoot. Radiographs show vertebral defects and short tubular bones with epiphyseal irregularities and metaphyseal enlargement that gives rise to a dumbbell appearance.

Motor development is often delayed because of the joint deformities, although intelligence is normal. Hearing loss and myopia commonly develop during childhood, and retinal detachment may occur as a late complication. Joint enlargement progresses during childhood and becomes painful; it is accompanied by flexion contractures and muscle atrophy, which may be incapacitating by adolescence.

LATE-ONSET SPONDYLOEPIPHYSEAL DYSPLASIA. This term refers to a mild to very mild clinical phenotype characterized by slightly

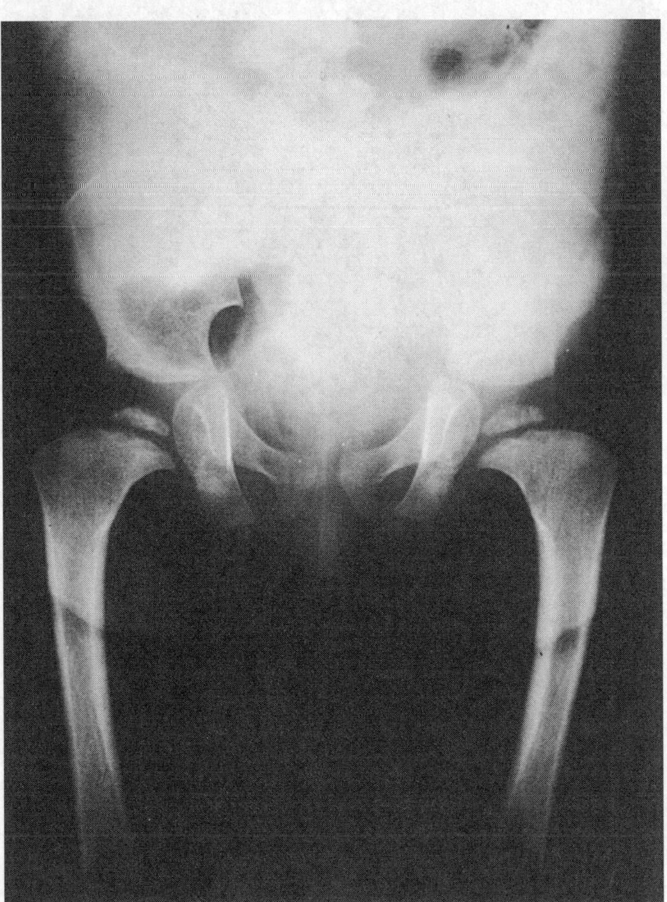

Figure 698–3 Radiograph of SED congenita pelvis demonstrating squared pelvis, hypoplastic capital femoral epiphyses, and femoral necks that are wide and short.

short stature associated with mild epiphyseal and vertebral abnormalities on roentgenograms. It is typically detected during childhood or adolescence but may go unrecognized until adulthood when precocious osteoarthritis appears. This designation is nosologically distinct from SED tarda, which is clinically similar but genetically maps to the X chromosome.

STICKLER DYSPLASIA (HEREDITARY OSTEOARTHROPHTHALMOPATHY)

Short stature is not a feature of Stickler dysplasia (OMIM 184840). It resembles SED because of its joint and eye manifestations. Mutations of genes encoding type XI collagen, which functionally interacts with type II collagen, have been identified in Stickler-like disorders (OMIM 184840, OMIM 215150). Stickler dysplasia is often identified in the newborn because of cleft palate and micrognathia (Pierre Robin anomaly). Infants typically have severe myopia and additional ophthalmologic complications, including choroidoretinal and vitreous degeneration; retinal detachment is common during childhood (Fig. 698–4). Sensorineural hearing loss may arise during adolescence, which is when symptoms of osteoarthritis may begin. Special attention must be given to the eye complications even in childhood.

SCHMID METAPHYSEAL DYSPLASIA

Schmid metaphyseal dysplasia (OMIM 156500) is one of several chondrodysplasias in which metaphyseal abnormalities dominate the radiographic features. It typically presents in early childhood with mild short stature, bowing of the legs, and a waddling gait (Fig. 698–5). Enlargement of joints, such as the wrist, may be found. Radiographs show flaring and irregular mineralization of the metaphyses of tubular bones of the proximal limbs (Fig. 698–6). Coxa vara is usually present and may require surgical correction. Short stature becomes more evident with age and affects the lower extremities more than the upper extremities; the manifestations are limited to the skeleton.

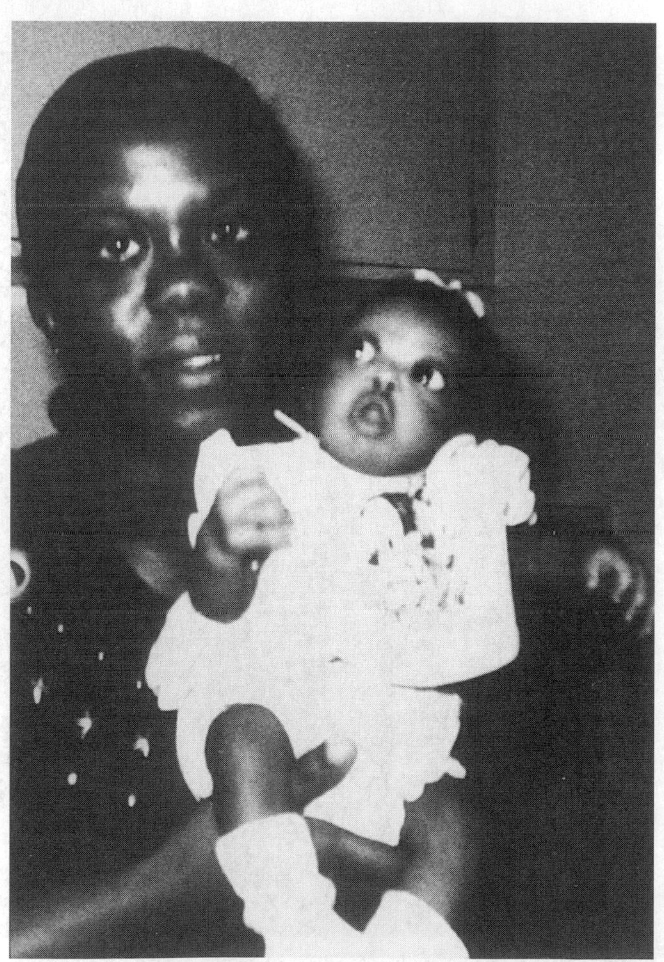

Figure 698–4 Stickler syndrome in mother and child. The facies are flat and the eyes are prominent.

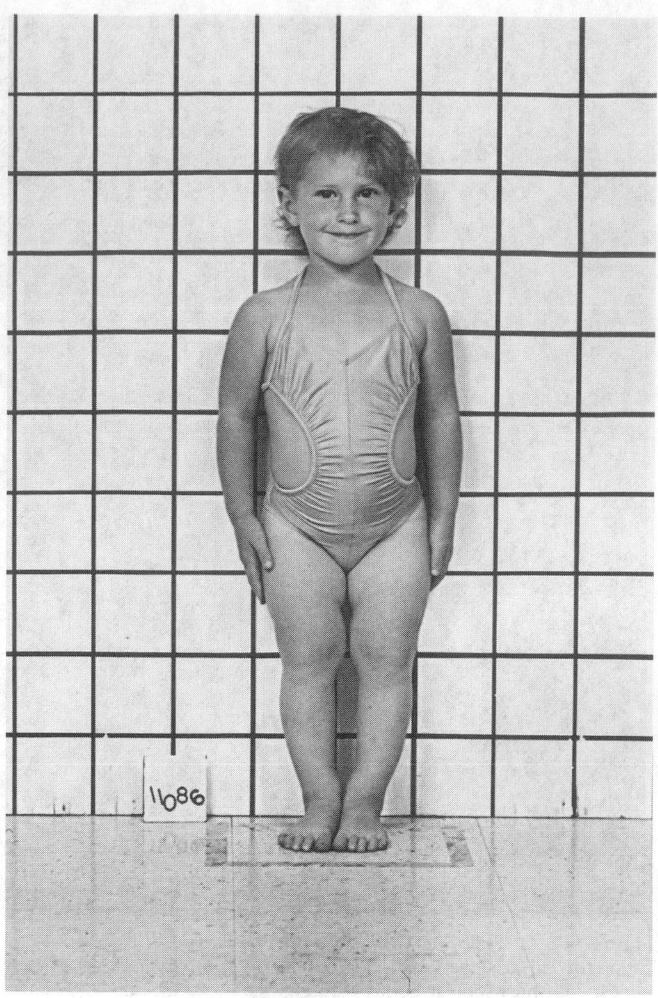

Figure 698–5 Female patient with metaphyseal dysplasia, type Schmid. The facies are normal and stature is mildly reduced. Mild tibia vara is present.

Schmid metaphyseal chondrodysplasia is duc to heterozygous mutations of the gene encoding type X collagen; it is an autosomal dominant trait. The distribution of type X collagen is restricted to the region of growing bone in which cartilage is converted into bone. This may explain why radiographic changes are confined to the metaphyses.

PSEUDOACHONDROPLASIA AND MULTIPLE EPIPHYSEAL DYSPLASIA

Pseudoachondroplasia (OMIM 177170) and multiple epiphyseal dysplasia (MED) (OMIM 600969) are two distinct phenotypes that are grouped together because they result from mutations of the gene encoding COMP. The mutations are heterozygous in both; they are autosomal dominant traits. The clinical phenotypes are restricted to skeletal tissues.

Newborns with pseudoachondroplasia are average in size and appearance. Gait abnormalities and short stature mainly affect the limbs and become apparent in late infancy. The short

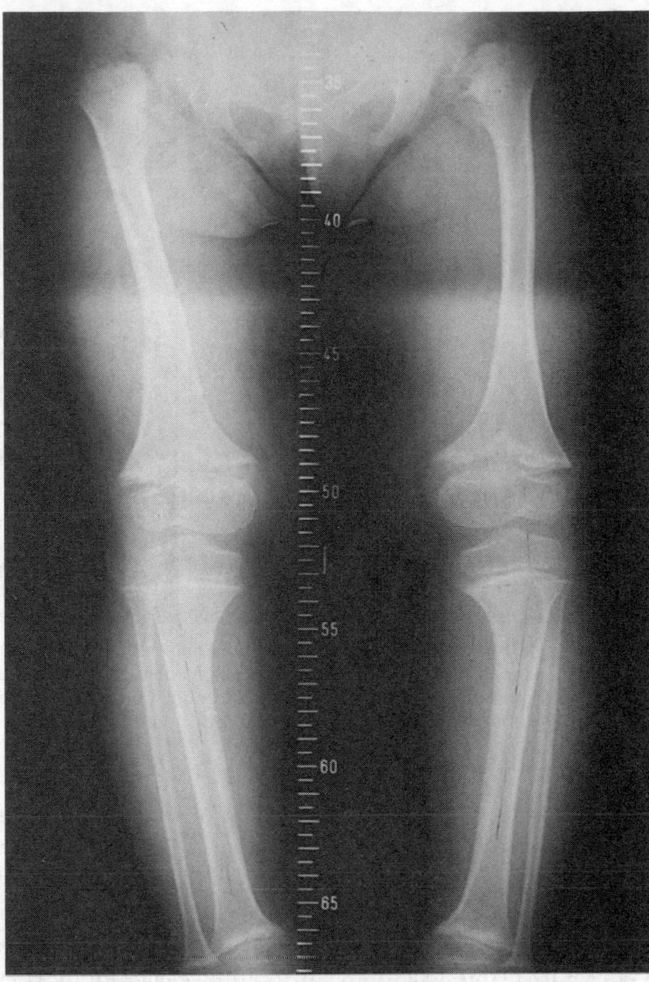

Figure 698–6 Radiographs of lower extremities in Schmid metaphyseal dysplasia showing short tubular bones and metaphyseal flaring and irregularities, abnormal capital femoral epiphyses, and femoral necks. The epiphyses are normal. Coxa vara is present.

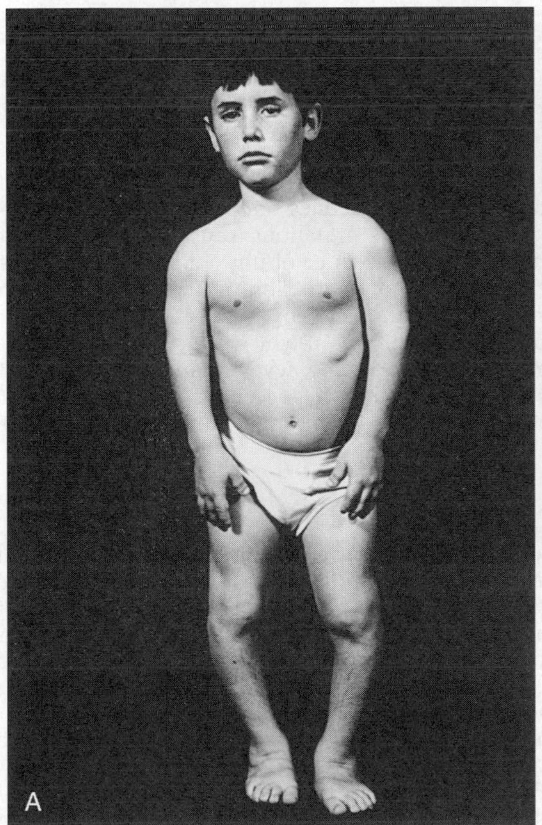

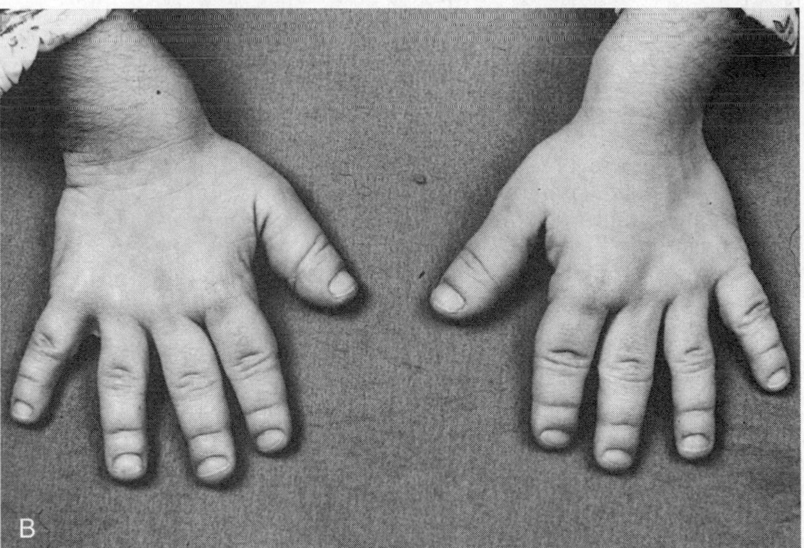

Figure 698–7 *A,* Pseudoachondroplasia in an adolescent male. The facies and head circumference are normal. There is shortening of all extremities and bowing of the lower extremities. *B,* Photograph of hands, demonstrating short stubby fingers.

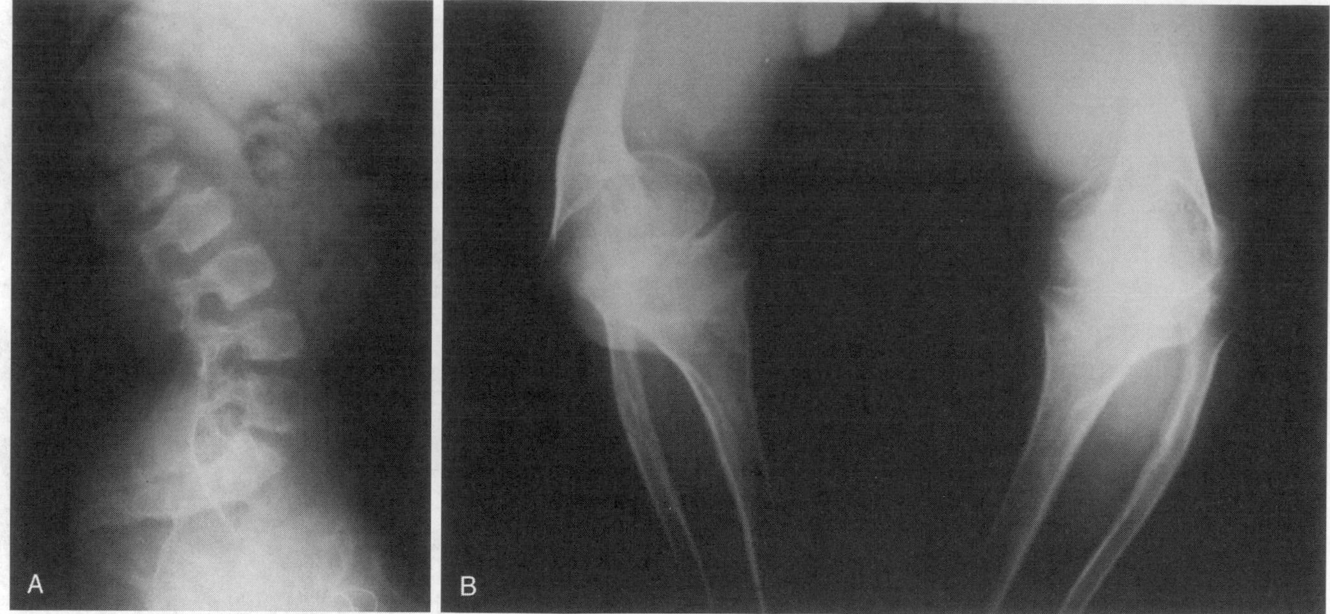

Figure 698–8 *A*, Lateral thoracolumbar spine radiograph of patient with pseudoachondroplasia showing central protrusion (tonguing) of the anterior aspect of upper lumbar and lower thoracic vertebrae. Note reduced heights (platyspondyly) and secondary lordosis. *B*, Lower extremity radiograph of patient with pseudoachondroplasia showing large metaphyses, poorly formed epiphyses, and marked bowing of the long bones.

stature becomes marked as the child grows and is associated with generalized joint laxity (Fig. 698–7). The hands are short, broad, and deviated in an ulnar direction; the forearms are bowed. Developmental milestones and intelligence are usually normal. Lumbar lordosis and deformities of the knee develop during childhood; the latter frequently requires surgical correction. Pain is common in weight-bearing joints during childhood and adolescence, leading to osteoarthritis late in the second decade of life. Adults range in height from 105 to 128 cm.

Skeletal roentgenograms show distinctive abnormalities of vertebral bodies and of both epiphyses and metaphyses of tubular bones (Fig. 698–8).

The MED phenotype has skeletal abnormalities that predominantly affect the epiphyses as noted on roentgenograms. Two classic forms are a severe Fairbank type, and a mild Ribbing type. Because of overlap in clinical features and because COMP mutations are found in both types, they may be considered clinical variants.

The more severe clinical phenotype has its onset during childhood, with mild short-limbed short stature, pain in weight-bearing joints, and a waddling gait. Radiographs show delayed and irregular ossification of epiphyses. More mildly affected individuals may not be recognized until adolescence or adulthood. Radiographic changes may be limited to the capital femoral epiphyses. In the latter case, mild MED must be distinguished from bilateral Legg-Perthes disease. Precocious osteoarthritis of hips and knees is the major complication in adults with MED. Adult heights range from 136 to 151 cm.

There are families with clinical and radiographic manifestations of MED that are not due to mutations of COMP. Some are linked to the gene encoding one of the type IX collagen chains. It has been suggested that COMP and type IX collagen interact functionally in cartilage matrix, thus explaining why mutations of different genes produce similar pictures.

Briggs MD, Mortier GR, Cole WG, et al: Diverse mutations in the gene for cartilage oligomeric matrix protein in a pseudoachondroplasia–multiple epiphyseal dysplasia disease spectrum. Am J Hum Genet 62:311, 1998.

McKeand J, Rotta J, Hecht JT: Natural history study of pseudoachondroplasia. Am J Med Genet 63:406, 1996.

Vikkula M, Metsaranta M, Ala-Kokko L: Type II collagen mutations in rare and common cartilage diseases. Ann Med 26:107, 1994.

Winterpacht A, Hilbert M, Schwarze U, et al: Kniest and Stickler dysplasia phenotypes caused by collagen type II gene (COL2A1) defect. Nat Genet 3:323, 1993.

CHAPTER 699

Disorders Involving Transmembrane Receptors

Disorders involving transmembrane receptors result from heterozygous mutations of genes encoding these receptors—*FGFR3* and *PTHrPR*. The mutations cause the receptors to become activated in the absence of physiologic ligands, which accentuates normal receptor function of negatively regulating bone growth. The mutations act by gain of negative function. In the *FGFR3* mutation group, in which the clinical phenotypes range from severe to mild, the severity appears to correlate with the extent to which the receptor is activated. Both *PTHrPR* and especially *FGFR3* mutations tend to recur in unrelated individuals.

ACHONDROPLASIA GROUP

The achondroplasia group represents a substantial percentage of patients with chondrodysplasias and contains thanatophoric dysplasia, the most common lethal chondrodysplasia with an incidence of 1 in 35,000 births; achondroplasia, the most common nonlethal chondrodysplasia with an incidence of 1 in 15,000 to 1 in 40,000 births, and hypochondroplasia. All three have mutations in a small number of locations in the *FGFR3* gene. There is a strong correlation between the mutation site and the clinical phenotype.

THANATOPHORIC DYSPLASIA. Thanatophoric dysplasia (TD) (On-Line Mendelian Inheritance of Man [OMIM] 187600, OMIM

187610) presents before or at birth. In the former situation, ultrasonographic examination in midgestation or later reveals a large head and very short limbs; the pregnancy is often accompanied by polyhydramnios and premature delivery. Very short limbs, short neck, long narrow thorax, and large head with midfacial hypoplasia dominate the clinical phenotype at birth (Fig. 699–1). The cloverleaf skull deformity known as **Kleeblattschädel** is sometimes found. Newborns have severe respiratory distress because of their small thorax. Although this distress can be treated by intense respiratory care, the long-term prognosis is poor.

Skeletal roentgenograms distinguish two slightly different forms called TD I and TD II. In the more common TD I, roentgenograms show large calvariae with a small cranial base, marked thinning and flattening of vertebral bodies visualized best on lateral view, very short ribs, severe hypoplasia of pelvic bones, and very short and bowed tubular bones with flared metaphyses (Fig. 699–2). The femurs are curved and shaped like a telephone receiver. TD II differs mainly in that there are longer and straighter femurs.

The TD II clinical phenotype is associated with mutations that map to codon 650 of *FGFR3,* causing the substitution of a glutamic acid for the lysine. This activates the tyrosine kinase activity of a receptor that transmits signals to intracellular pathways. Mutations of the TD I phenotype map mainly to two regions in the extracellular domain of the receptor, where they substitute cysteine residues for other amino acids. Free cysteine residues are thought to form disulfide bonds promoting dimerization of receptor molecules, leading to activation and signal transmission.

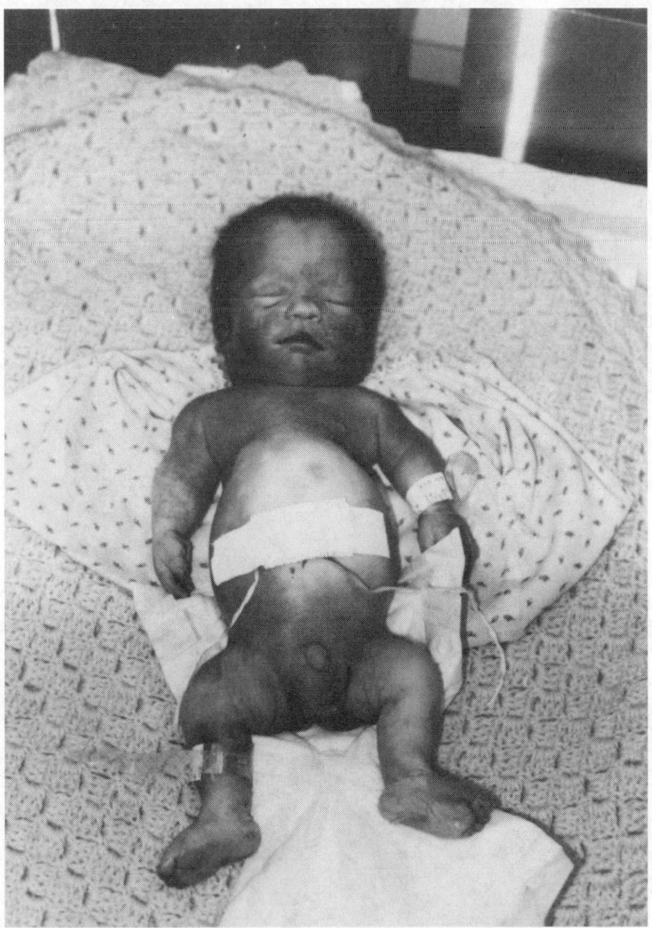

Figure 699–1 Stillborn infant with thanatophoric dysplasia. Limbs are very short, with upper limbs extending only two thirds of the way down the abdomen. The chest is narrow, exaggerating the protuberance of the abdomen. The head is relatively large.

TD I and TD II represent new mutations to normal parents. The recurrence risk is low. Because the mutated codons in TD are mutable for unknown reasons and because of the theoretical risk for germ cell mosaicism, parents are offered prenatal diagnosis for subsequent pregnancies.

ACHONDROPLASIA. Achondroplasia (OMIM 100800) is the prototype chondrodysplasia. It typically presents at birth with short limbs, a long narrow trunk, and a large head with midfacial hypoplasia and prominent forehead (Fig. 699–3). The limb shortening is greatest in the proximal segments, and the fingers often display a trident configuration. Most joints are hyperextensible, but extension is restricted at the elbow. A thoracolumbar gibbus is often found. Usually, birth length is slightly less than normal but occasionally plots within the low-normal range.

Diagnosis. Skeletal radiographs confirm the diagnosis (Fig. 699–4). The calvarial bones are large, whereas the cranial base and facial bones are small. The vertebral pedicles are short throughout the spine as noted on a lateral roentgenogram. The interpedicular distance, which normally increases from the first to the fifth lumbar vertebrae, decreases in achondroplasia. The iliac bones are short and round, and the acetabular roofs are flat. The tubular bones are short with mildly irregular and flared metaphyses. The fibula is disproportionately long compared with the tibia.

Clinical Manifestations. Infants usually exhibit delayed motor milestones, frequently not walking alone until 18–24 mo. This is due to hypotonia and mechanical difficulty balancing the large head on a normal-sized trunk and short extremities. Intelligence is normal unless central nervous system complications develop. As the child begins to walk, the gibbus usually gives way to an exaggerated lumbar lordosis.

Infants and children with achondroplasia progressively fall below normal standards for length and height. They can be plotted against standards established for achondroplasia. Adult heights typically range between 118 and 145 cm for males and between 112 and 136 cm for females. Surgical limb lengthening and human growth hormone treatment have been used to increase height; both are controversial.

There are several potential neurologic complications. Virtually all infants and children with achondroplasia have large heads, although only a fraction have true hydrocephalus. Head circumference should be carefully monitored using standards developed for achondroplasia, as should neurologic function in general. The spinal canal is stenotic, and spinal cord compression may occur at the foramen magnum and in the lumbar spine. The former most often presents in infants and small children; it may be associated with hypotonia, failure to thrive, quadriparesis, central and obstructive apnea, and sudden death. Surgical correction may be required for severe stenosis. Lumbar spinal stenosis usually does not present until early adulthood. Symptoms include paresthesias, numbness, and claudication in the legs. Loss of bladder and bowel control may be late complications.

Bowing of the legs is common and may need to be corrected surgically. Other common problems include dental crowding, articulation difficulties, obesity, and frequent episodes of otitis media, which may contribute to hearing loss.

Genetics. All patients with typical achondroplasia have mutations at *FGFR3* codon 380. The mutation maps to the transmembrane domain of the receptor and is thought to stabilize receptor dimers that enhance receptor signals, the consequences of which inhibit linear bone growth. Achondroplasia behaves as an autosomal dominant trait; most cases arise from a new mutation to normal parents.

Because of the high frequency of achondroplasia among dwarfing conditions, it is relatively common for adults with achondroplasia to marry. Such couples have a 50% risk of transmitting their condition, heterozygous achondroplasia, to each offspring, as well as a 25% risk for homozygous achon-

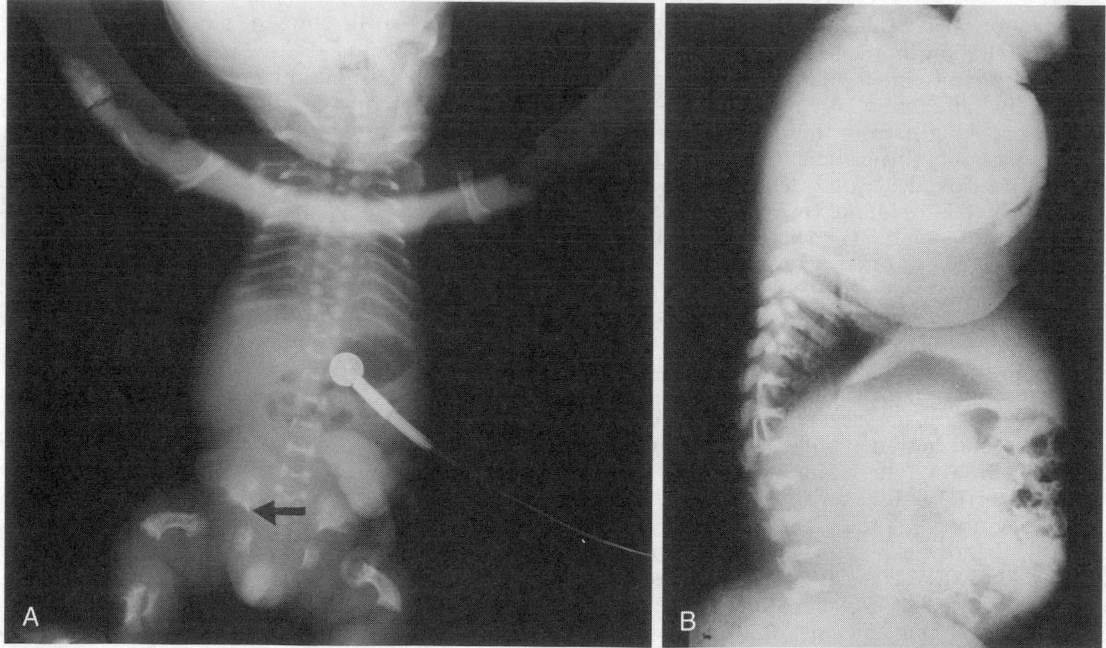

Figure 699–2 *A,* Neonatal radiograph of a child with thanatophoric dysplasia. Note medial acetabular spurs *(black arrow),* hypoplastic iliac bones, bowed femora with rounded protrusion of proximal femurs, hypoplastic thorax, and wafer-thin vertebral bodies. *B,* Lateral radiograph of the thoracolumbar spine in thanatophoric dysplasia, showing marked vertebral flattening and short ribs. Ossification defect of the central portion of the vertebral bodies is present.

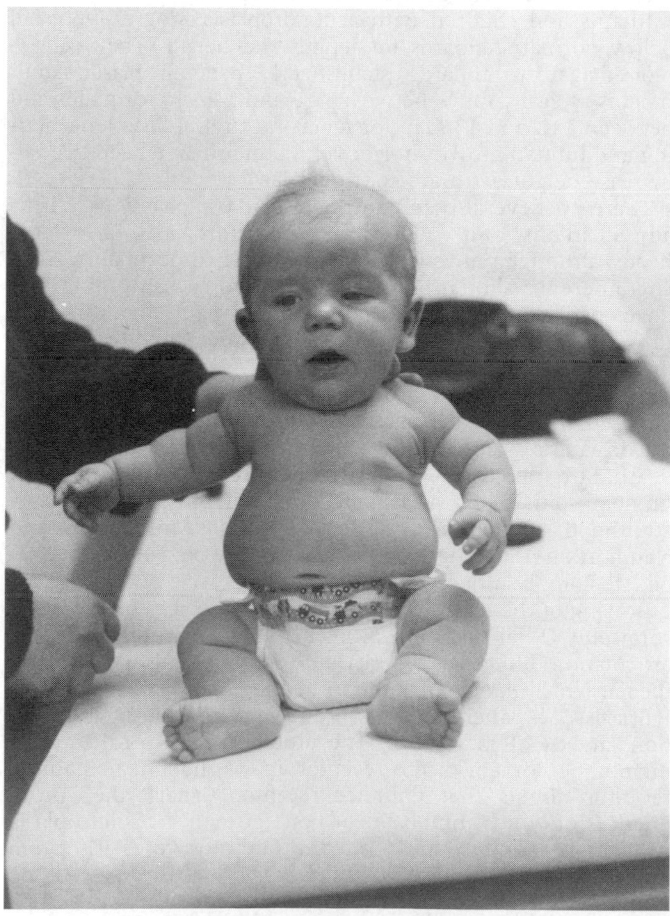

Figure 699–3 Infant with achondroplasia. The cranium is large and the forehead prominent. The nasal bridge is moderately flat, and the chest is small compared with the abdomen. Note medial arm and forearm creases, which reflect bowing at the sharpest concavity of the limbs.

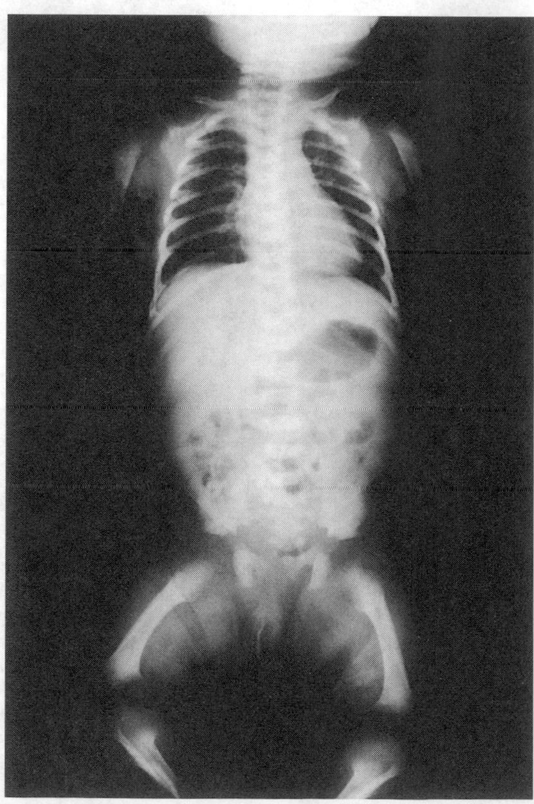

Figure 699–4 Radiograph of infant with achondroplasia, demonstrating interpedicular narrowing of the first through fifth lumbar vertebrae, short round iliac bones, and flat acetabular roofs. The tubular bones are short and show mild irregularities of the metaphyses.

droplasia. The latter condition exhibits intermediate severity between thanatophoric dysplasia and heterozygous achondroplasia and is usually lethal in the newborn period.

HYPOCHONDROPLASIA. Hypochondroplasia (OMIM 146000) resembles achondroplasia but is milder. Usually, it is not apparent until childhood, when mild short stature affecting the limbs becomes evident. Children have a stocky build and slight frontal bossing of the head. Radiographic changes are mild and consistent with the mild achondroplastic phenotype. Complications are rare; some patients are never diagnosed. Adult heights range from 116 to 146 cm. An *FGFR3* mutation at codon 540 has been found in many patients with hypochondroplasia.

JANSEN METAPHYSEAL DYSPLASIA

Jansen metaphyseal chondrodysplasia (OMIM 156400) is a rare, dominantly inherited chondrodysplasia characterized by severe shortening of limbs associated with an unusual facial appearance. Sometimes it is accompanied by clubfoot and hypercalcemia. At birth, a diagnosis can be made from these clinical findings and radiographs that show short tubular bones with characteristic metaphyseal abnormalities that include flaring, irregular mineralization, fragmentation, and widening of the physeal space. The epiphyses are normal.

The joints become enlarged and limited in mobility with age. Flexion contractures develop at the knees and hips, producing a bent-over posture. Intelligence is normal, although there may be hearing loss.

Jansen metaphyseal chondrodysplasia is the only disorder due to mutations of *PTHrPR.* This G protein–coupled transmembrane receptor serves as a receptor for both *PTH* and *PTHrP.* Signaling through this receptor serves as a brake on the terminal differentiation of cartilage cells at a critical step in bone growth. Since the mutations activate the receptor, they enhance the braking effect and thereby slow bone growth.

American Academy of Pediatrics Committee on Genetics: Health supervision for children with achondroplasia. Pediatrics 95:443, 1995.

Horton WA: Fibroblast growth factor receptor 3 and the human chondrodysplasias. Curr Opin Pediatr 9:437, 1997.

Mogayzel PJ Jr, Carroll JL, Loughlin GM, et al: Sleep-disordered breathing in children with achondroplasia. J Pediatr 132:667, 1998.

Pauli RM, Horton VK, Glinski LP, et al: Prospective assessment of risks for cervicomedullary-junction compression in infants with achondroplasia. Am J Hum Genet 56:732, 1995.

Rousseau F, Bonaventure J, Legeai-Mallet L, et al: Clinical and genetic heterogeneity of hypochondroplasia. J Med Genet 33:749, 1996.

Schipani E, Langman CB, Parfitt AM, et al: Constitutively activated receptors for parathyroid hormone and parathyroid hormone–related peptide in Jansen's metaphyseal chondrodysplasia. N Engl J Med 335:708, 1996.

Tavormina P, Shiang R, Thompson L, et al: Thanatophoric dysplasia (types I and II) caused by distinct mutations in fibroblast growth factor receptor 3. Nat Genet 9:321, 1995.

CHAPTER 700
Disorders Involving Ion Transporter

In order of decreasing severity, the disorders involving ion transporter include achondrogenesis type 1B, atelosteogenesis type II, and diastrophic dysplasia. They result from the functional loss of the sulfate ion transporter called *diastrophic dysplasia sulfate transporter* (DTDST). This protein transports sulfate ions into cells and is important for cartilage cells that add sulfate moieties to newly synthesized proteoglycans destined for cartilage extracellular matrix. Matrix proteoglycans are responsible for many of the properties of cartilage that allow it to serve as a template for skeletal development. The clinical manifestations result from defective sulfation of cartilage proteoglycans.

A number of mutant alleles have been found for the *DTDST* gene; they variably disturb transporter function. None is sufficient to cause disease alone; hence, the disorders are recessive traits requiring the presence of two mutant alleles. The phenotype is determined by the combination of mutant alleles; some alleles are in more than one disorder.

DIASTROPHIC DYSPLASIA (ON-LINE MENDELIAN INHERITANCE OF MAN [OMIM] 22600). This well-characterized disorder is recognized at birth by the presence of very short extremities, clubfoot, and short hands with proximal displacement of the thumb producing a hitchhiker appearance (Fig. 700–1). The hands are usually deviated in an ulnar direction. Bony fusion of the metacarpophalangeal joints (symphalangism) is common, as is restricted movement of many joints, including hips, knees, and elbows. The external ears frequently become inflamed soon after birth. The inflammation resolves spontaneously but leaves the ears fibrotic and contracted ("cauliflower" ear deformity). Many newborns have a cleft palate.

Roentgenograms reveal short and broad tubular bones with flared metaphyses and flat, irregular epiphyses (Fig. 700–2).

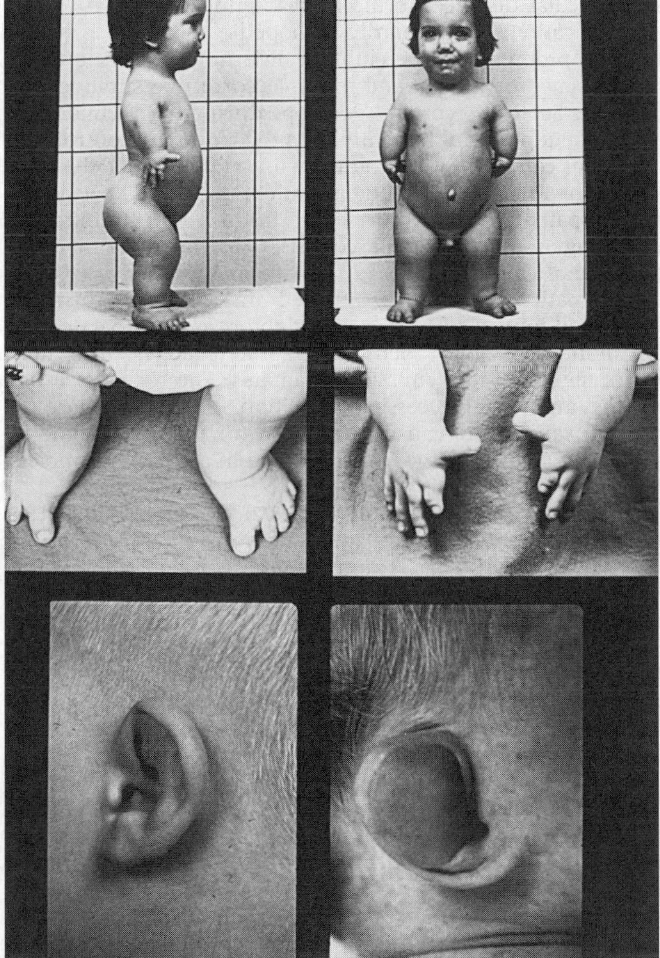

Figure 700–1 Child with diastrophic dysplasia. The extremities are dramatically shortened *(above).* Clubfoot is commonly observed *(middle-left).* The fingers are short, especially the index finger; the thumb characteristically is proximally placed and has a hitchhiker appearance *(middle-right).* The upper helix of the ears becomes swollen 3–4 wk postnatally *(lower left),* and this inflammation spontaneously resolves, leaving a cauliflower deformity of the pinnae *(lower right).*

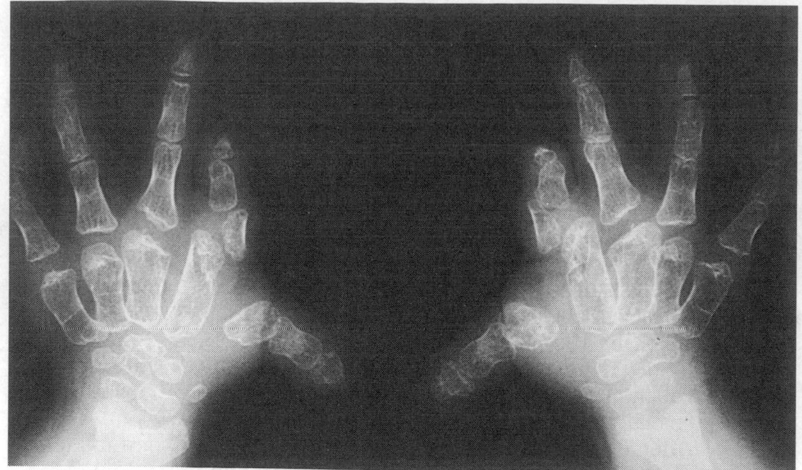

Figure 700–2 Radiograph of hands in diastrophic dysplasia. The metacarpals and phalanges are irregular and short. The first metacarpal is ovoid.

The capital femoral epiphyses are hypoplastic and the femoral heads broad. The ulnas and fibulas are disproportionately short. Carpal centers may be developmentally advanced; the first metacarpal is typically ovoid, and the metatarsals are twisted medially. There may be vertebral abnormalities, including clefts of cervical vertebral lamina and narrowing of the interpedicular distances in the lumbar spine.

Complications are primarily orthopedic and tend to be severe and progressive. The clubfoot deformity in the newborn resists usual treatments, and multiple corrective surgeries are common. Scoliosis typically develops during early childhood. It often requires multiple surgical procedures to control and sometimes compromises respiratory function in older children. Despite the orthopedic problems, patients typically have a normal life span and reach adult heights in the 105–130 cm range, depending on the severity of scoliosis. Growth curves are available for diastrophic dysplasia.

Some patients are mildly affected and exhibit slight short stature and joint contractures, no clubfoot or cleft palate, and correspondingly mild roentgenographic changes. The mild phenotype tends to recur within families. The recurrence risk for this autosomal recessive condition is 25%. Ultrasonographic examination can be employed for prenatal diagnosis, but if *DTDST* mutations can be identified in the parents, molecular genetic diagnosis is possible.

ACHONDROGENESIS TYPE 1B (OMIM 600972) AND ATELOSTEOGENESIS TYPE II (OMIM 256050). Both of the conditions are rare recessive lethal chondrodysplasias. The most serious is achondrogenesis type 1B, which demonstrates a severe lack of skeletal development usually detected in utero or after a miscarriage. The limbs are extremely short and the head is soft. Skeletal radiographs show poor to missing ossification of skull bones, vertebral bodies, fibulas, and ankle bones. The pelvis is hypoplastic, and the ribs are short. The femurs are short and exhibit a trapezoid shape with irregular metaphyses.

Infants with *atelosteogenesis type II* are stillborn or die soon after birth; prematurity is common. They exhibit very short limbs, especially the proximal segments. Clubfoot and dislocations of the elbows and knees may be detected. Hypoplasia of vertebral bodies, especially in the cervical and lumbar spine, is found on roentgenograms. The femurs and humeri are hypoplastic and display a club-shaped appearance. The distal limb bones, including the ulna and fibula, are poorly ossified.

Both disorders carry a 25% recurrence risk and are potentially detectable in utero by mutation analysis if the mutant alleles are present in the parents. Prenatal diagnosis should be possible with fetal ultrasonography.

Hall BD: Diastrophic dysplasia: Extreme variability within a sibship. Am J Med Genet 63:28, 1996.
Makitie O, Kaitila I: Growth in diastrophic dysplasia. J Pediatr 130:641, 1997.
Newbury-Ecob R: Atelosteogenesis type 2. J Med Genet 35:49, 1998.

CHAPTER 701
Disorders Involving Transcription Factors

There are three disorders involving transcription factors that result in bone dysplasias. One, camptomelic dysplasia, is historically considered a chondrodysplasia. The other two, cleidocranial dysplasia and nail-patella syndrome, have been regarded as dysostoses, or abnormalities of single bones. The mutant genes encode three transcription factors: *SOX9*, *CBFA1* and *LMX1B*, respectively, and are members of much larger gene families. For instance, *SOX9* is a member of the *SOX* family of genes related to the *SRY* (sex-determining region of the Y chromosome) gene; *CBFA1* belongs to the *runt* family of tran-

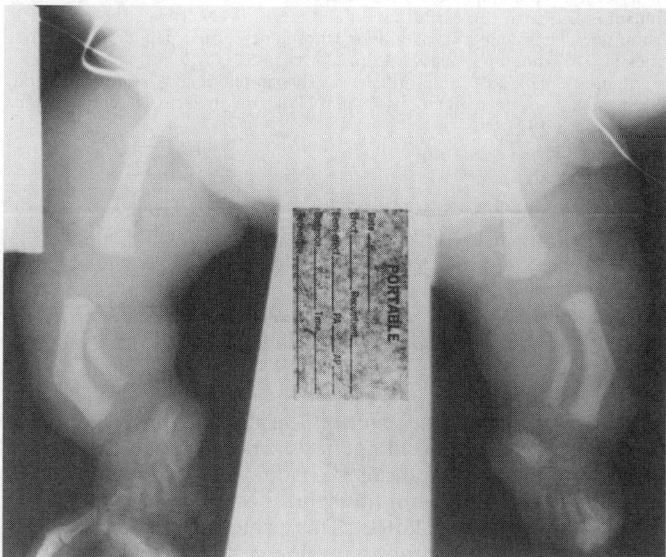

Figure 701–1 Radiograph of lower extremities of a child with camptomelic dysplasia. Note bowed femurs, which are not particularly wide as compared with the thick bowed tibiae and fibulae.

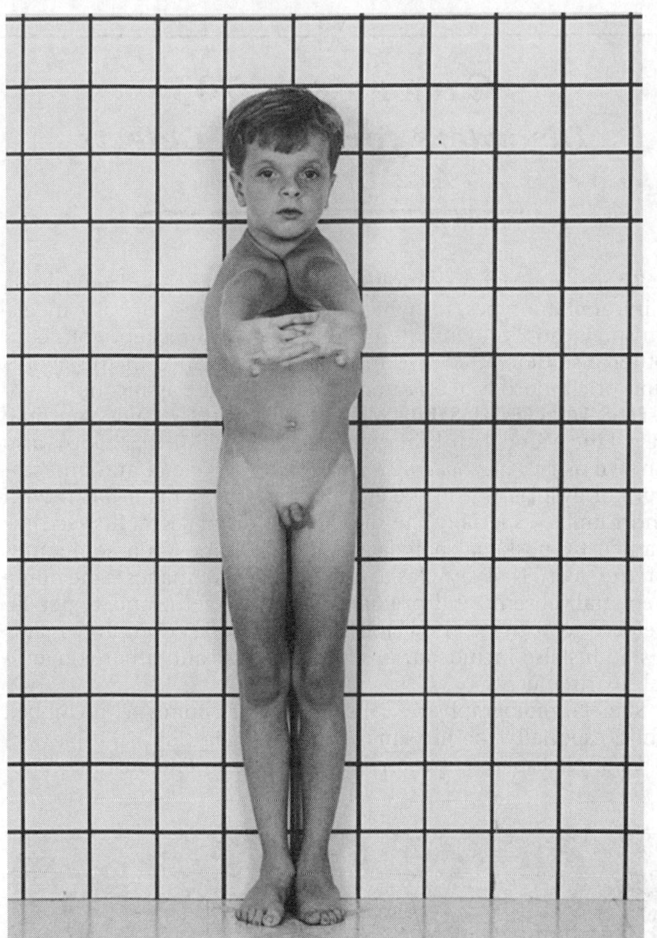

Figure 701–2 Cleidocranial dysplasia demonstrating approximation of the shoulder girdle in the midline. Prominent high foreheads and hypertelorism can be seen.

scription factor genes, and *LMX1B* is one of the *LIM* homeodomain gene family. All three disorders are due to haploinsufficiency of the respective gene products; the disorders are dominant traits.

CAMPTOMELIC DYSPLASIA. Apparent in newborn infants, camptomelic dysplasia (OMIM 114290) is characterized by bowing of long bones, especially in the lower legs, short bones, respiratory distress, and other anomalies that include defects of the cervical spine, central nervous system, heart, and kidneys. Several cases of sex reversal of XY males have been reported. Radiographs confirm the bowing and often show hypoplasia of the scapulas and pelvic bones (Fig. 701–1). Affected infants usually die from respiratory distress in the neonatal period.

CLEIDOCRANIAL DYSPLASIA. Cleidocranial dysplasia (OMIM 114290) is recognized in infants because of drooping shoulders, open fontanelles, prominent forehead, mild short stature, and dental abnormalities (Fig. 701–2). Radiographs reveal hypoplastic or absent clavicles, delayed ossification of the cranial bones with multiple ossification centers (wormian bones), and delayed ossification of pelvic bones. The course is usually uncomplicated except for dislocations, especially of the shoulders, and dental anomalies that require therapy.

NAIL-PATELLA SYNDROME. Dysplasia of the nails, absence or hypoplasia of the patella, abnormalities of the elbow, and spurs or "horns" extending from the iliac bones characterize the nail-patella syndrome (OMIM 119600), which is also called *osteo-onchodysostosis*. Some patients have nephritis that resembles chronic glomerulonephritis. There is a wide spectrum of severity; some patients present in early childhood, whereas others are asymptomatic as adults.

Dryer SD, Zhou G, Baldini A, et al: Mutations in MLX1B cause abnormal skeletal patterning and renal dysplasia in nail patella syndrome. Nat Genet 19:47, 1998.

Meyer J, Sudbeck P, Held M, et al: Mutational analysis of the SOX9 gene in camptomelic dysplasia and autosomal sex reversal: Lack of genotype/phenotype correlations. Hum Mol Genet 6:91, 1997.

Mundlos S, Otto F, Mundlos C, et al: Mutations involving the transcription factor CBFA1 cause cleidocranial dysplasia. Cell 89:773, 1997.

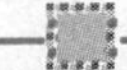

Chapter 702

Disorders Involving Defective Bone Resorption

Many bone dysplasias display increased bone density; most are rare. Osteopetrosis, which has many subtypes, and pyknodysostosis, and probably others in this category of bone dysplasias, result from defective bone resorption.

OSTEOPETROSIS. Two main forms of osteopetrosis have been delineated: a severe, autosomal recessive form (On-Line Mendelian Inheritance [OMIM] 259700) and a mild, autosomal dominant form [OMIM 166600]. The recessive and dominant forms of osteopetrosis have been genetically mapped to chromosomes 11q12-q13 and 1p21, respectively. The severe form is usually detected in infancy or earlier because of macrocephaly, hepatosplenomegaly, deafness, blindness, and severe anemia. Roentgenograms reveal diffuse bone sclerosis. Later films show a bone within a bone, which is characteristic. With time, infants typically fail to thrive and show psychomotor delay and worsening of cranial neuropathies and anemia. Dental problems, osteomyelitis of the mandible, and pathologic fractures are common. The most severely affected patients die during infancy; less severely affected individuals rarely survive beyond the 2nd decade. Those who survive beyond infancy usually have learning disorders but may have normal intelligence despite hearing and visual loss.

Clinical Manifestations. Most of the manifestations are due to failure to remodel growing bones. This leads to narrowing of cranial nerve foramina and encroachment on marrow spaces, which results in secondary complications, such as optic and facial nerve dysfunction, and anemia accompanied by compensatory extramedullary hematopoiesis in the liver and spleen.

The autosomal dominant form of osteopetrosis (Albers-Schönberg disease, osteopetrosis tarda, or marble bone disease) usually presents during childhood or adolescence with fractures and mild anemia and, less frequently, with cranial nerve dysfunction, dental abnormalities, or osteomyelitis of the mandible. Skeletal roentgenograms reveal a generalized increase in bone density and clubbing of metaphyses (Fig. 702–1). Alternating bands of lucent and dense bands produce a sandwich appearance to vertebral bodies. The radiographic changes are sometimes incidental findings in otherwise asymptomatic adolescents and adults. Treatment is symptomatic for the potential complications.

Treatment. The basic defect is thought to involve osteoclast differentiation because bone marrow transplantation with reconstitution of osteoclasts from donor cells has been successful in some patients. Calcitriol and interferon gamma have been used with some benefit in some patients. Symptomatic care, such as dental care, transfusions for anemia, and antibiotic treatment of infections, is important for patients who survive infancy.

PYKNODYSOSTOSIS. An autosomal recessive bone dysplasia, pyknodysostosis (OMIM 265800) presents in early childhood with short limbs, characteristic facies, an open anterior fontanelle, a large skull with frontal and occipital bossing, and

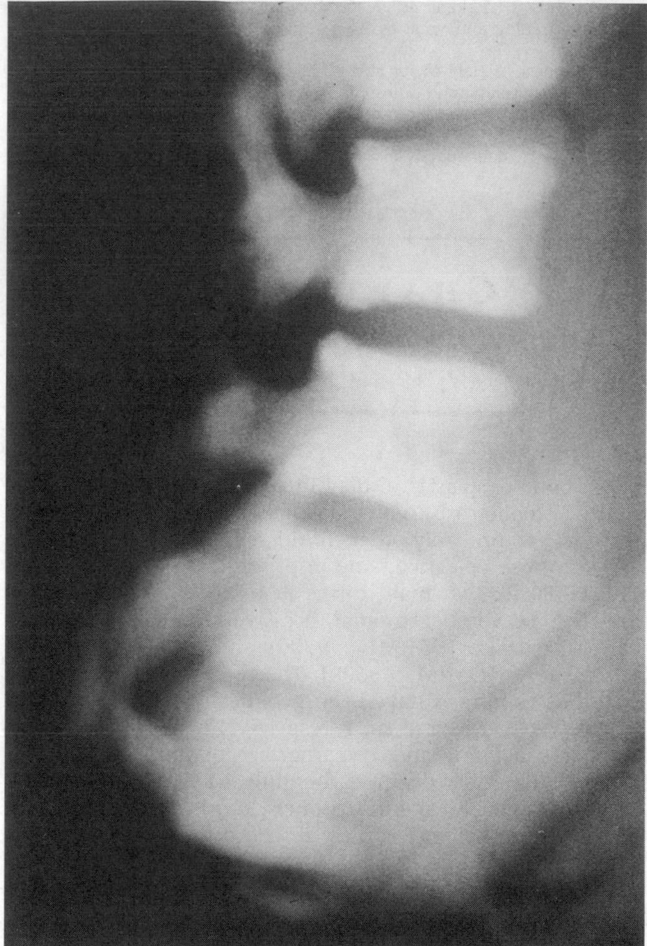

Figure 702–1 Lateral radiograph showing bone-in-bone appearance that is characteristic of osteopetrosis.

dental abnormalities. The hands and feet are short and broad, and the nails may be dysplastic. The sclerae may be blue. Minimal trauma often leads to fractures. Treatment is symptomatic and focused mainly on the management of dental problems and fractures. The prognosis is generally good, and patients typically reach heights of 130–150 cm.

Skeletal roentgenograms show a generalized increase in bone density. In contrast to many disorders in this group, the metaphyses are normal. Other changes include wide sutures and wormian bones in the skull, a small mandible, and hypoplasia of the distal phalanges.

Several mutations have been found in the gene encoding cathepsin K, a cysteine protease that is highly expressed in osteoclasts. The mutations predict loss of enzyme function, suggesting that there is an inability of osteoclasts to degrade bone matrix and remodel bones.

Charles JM, Key LL: Developmental spectrum of children with congenital osteopetrosis. J Pediatr 132:371, 1998.

Gelb BD, Shi GP, Chapman HA, et al: Pycnodysostosis, a lysosomal disease caused by cathepsin K deficiency. Science 273:1236, 1996.

Gerritsen EJ, Vossen JM, Fasth A, et al: Bone marrow transplantation for autosomal recessive osteopetrosis. A report from the Working Party on Inborn Errors of the European Bone Marrow Transplantation Group. J Pediatr 125:896, 1994.

Key LL Jr, Rodriguiz RM, Willi SM, et al: Long-term treatment of osteopetrosis with recombinant human interferon gamma. N Engl J Med 332:1594, 1995.

CHAPTER 703
Disorders for Which Defects Are Unknown

There are many chondrodysplasias, or chondrodysplasia clinical phenotypes, for which the genetic cause or basic mechanism is not known. Many illustrate features not found in other disorders and have historical significance in the evolution of chondrodysplasia nomenclature and classification.

ELLIS–VAN CREVELD SYNDROME. The Ellis–van Crevald syndrome (On-Line Mendelian Inheritance of Man [OMIM] 22550), also known as *chondroectodermal dysplasia,* is a skeletal and an ectodermal dysplasia. The skeletal dysplasia presents at birth with short limbs, especially the middle and distal segments, accompanied by postaxial polydactyly of the hands and sometimes of the feet. Nail dysplasia and dental anomalies—including neonatal, absent, and premature loss of teeth, and upper lip defects—constitute the ectodermal dysplasia. Common manifestations also include atrial septum defects and other congenital heart defects.

Skeletal radiographs reveal short tubular bones with clubbed ends, especially the proximal tibia and ulna (Fig. 703–1). Carpal bones display extra ossification centers and fusion; cone-

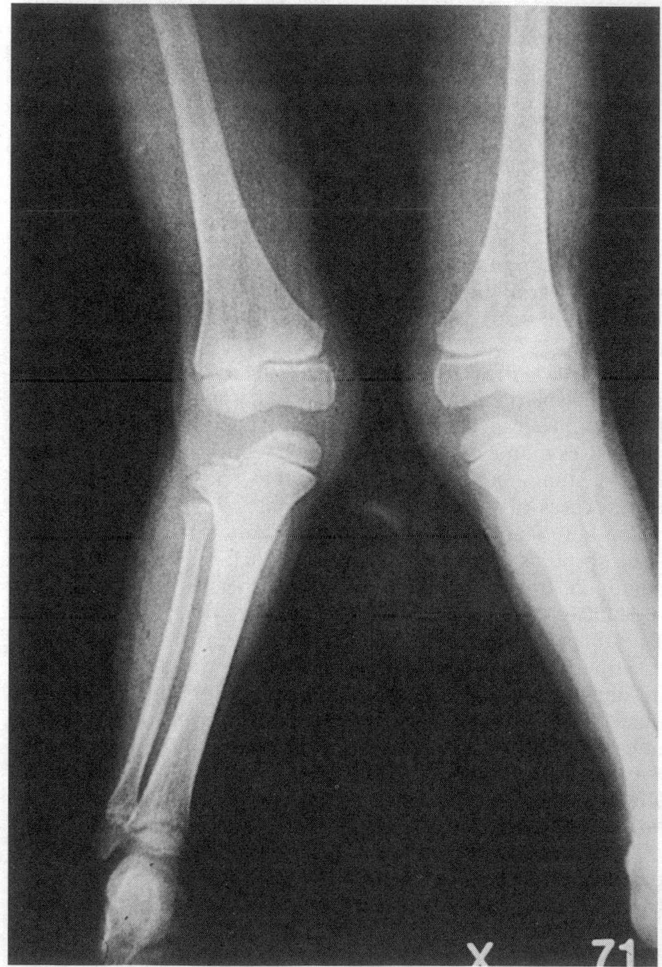

Figure 703–1 Radiograph of lower extremities in Ellis–van Creveld syndrome. Tubular bones are short and proximal fibula is short. Ossification is retarded in lateral tibia epiphyses, causing a knock-knee deformity.

shaped epiphyses are evident in the hands. A bony spur is often noted above the medial aspect of the acetabulum.

Ellis–van Creveld syndrome is an autosomal recessive trait that occurs most often in the Amish. Linkage studies have placed the responsible gene locus on chromosome 4p, although no candidate genes have been identified. About 30% of patients die of cardiac or respiratory problems during infancy. Life span is otherwise normal; adult heights range from 109–152 cm.

ASPHYXIATING THORACIC DYSTROPHY. Asphyxiating thoracic dystrophy (OMIM 208500), or Jeune syndrome, is an autosomal recessive chondrodysplasia that resembles Ellis–van Creveld syndrome. Newborn infants present with a long, narrow thorax and respiratory insufficiency associated with pulmonary hypoplasia. Neonates often die. Other neonatal manifestations include slightly short limbs and postaxial polydactyly.

Skeletal radiographs show very short ribs with anterior expansion. Tubular limb bones are short with bulbous ends; cone-shaped epiphyses occur in hand bones. The iliac bones are short and square with a spur above the medial aspect of the acetabulum.

If infants survive the neonatal period, respiratory function usually improves as the rib cage grows. Progressive renal dysfunction frequently develops during childhood. Intestinal malabsorption and hepatic dysfunction have also been reported.

SHORT-RIB POLYDACTYLY SYNDROMES. Four types of short-rib polydactyly syndrome (types I–IV) (OMIM 263530, 263520, 263510, 269860) have been described. All are lethal in the newborn period. Neonates present with respiratory distress, an extremely small thorax, very short extremities, polydactyly, and a variety of nonskeletal defects. Roentgenograms demonstrate very short ribs and tubular bones with changes characteristic for each type. All four types are autosomal recessive traits.

CARTILAGE-HAIR HYPOPLASIA. Cartilage-hair hypoplasia (OMIM 250250) is also known as metaphyseal chondrodysplasia—McKusick type. It is recognized during the 2nd year because of growth deficiency affecting the limbs, accompanied by flaring of the lower rib cage, a prominent sternum, and bowing of the legs. The hands and feet are short and the fingers are very short with extreme ligamentous laxity. The hair is thin, sparse, and light colored, and nails are hypoplastic. The skin is hypopigmented.

Radiographs show short tubular bones with flared, irregularly mineralized and cupped metaphyses (Fig. 703–2). The knees are more affected than are the hips, and the fibula is disproportionately longer than the tibia. The metacarpals and phalanges are short and broad. Spinal radiographs reveal mild platyspondyly.

Nonskeletal manifestations associated with cartilage-hair hypoplasia include immune deficiency (T-cell abnormalities, neutropenia, leukopenia, and susceptibility to chickenpox; children also may have complications from smallpox and polio vaccinations), malabsorption, celiac disease, and Hirschsprung disease. Adults are at risk for malignancy, especially skin tumors and lymphoma. Adults reach heights of 107–157 cm.

Cartilage-hair hypoplasia shows autosomal recessive inheritance. Although rare, its highest prevalence is in the Amish and Finnish populations. It has been genetically mapped to chromosome 9p13.

METATROPHIC DYSPLASIA. There are at least two forms of metatrophic dysplasia (OMIM 156530, 250600), an autosomal dominant and autosomal recessive form. Regardless of type, newborn infants present with a long narrow trunk and short extremities. A tail-like appendage sometimes extends from the base of the spine. Odontoid hypoplasia is common and may be associated with cervical instability. Kyphoscoliosis appears in late infancy and progresses through childhood, often becoming severe enough to compromise cardiopulmonary function. The joints are large and become progressively restricted in mobility, except in the hands. Contractures often develop in the hips and knees during childhood. Although severely affected infants may die at a young age from respiratory failure, patients usually survive, although they may become disabled as adults from the progressive musculoskeletal deformities. Adult heights range from 110–120 cm.

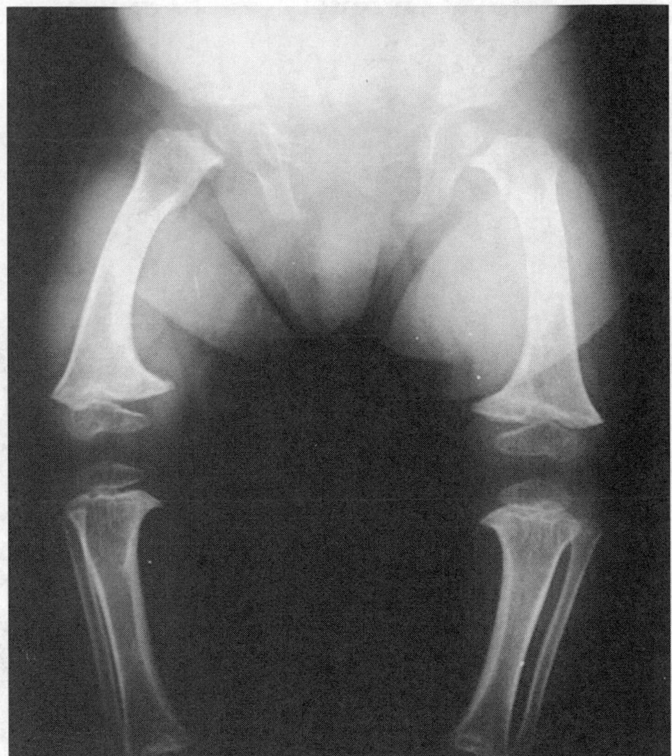

Figure 703–2 Radiograph of lower extremities in cartilage hair hypoplasia. The tubular bones are short and the metaphyses are flared and irregular. The fibula is disproportionately long compared with the tibia. The femoral necks are short.

Skeletal radiographs show characteristic changes dominated by severe platyspondyly and short tubular bones with expanded and deformed metaphyses that exhibit a dumbbell appearance (Fig. 703–3). The pelvic bones are hypoplastic and exhibit a halberd appearance because of a small sacrosciatic notch and a notch above the lateral margin of the acetabulum.

SPONDYLOMETAPHYSEAL DYSPLASIA—KOZLOWSKI TYPE. The Kozlowski type of spondylometaphyseal dysplasia (OMIM 184252) presents in early childhood with mild short stature involving mostly the trunk and a waddling gait. The hands and feet may be short and stubby. Radiographs show flattening of vertebral bodies. The metaphyses of tubular bones are widened and

TABLE 703–1 Juvenile Osteochondroses

Eponym	Affected Region	Age at Presentation
Legg-Calvé-Perthes disease	Capital femoral epiphysis	3–12 yr
Osgood-Schlatter disease	Tibial tubercle	10–16 yr
Sever disease	Os calcaneus	6–10 yr
Freiberg disease	Head of second metatarsal	10–14 yr
Scheuermann disease	Vertebral bodies	Adolescence
Blount disease	Medial aspect of proximal tibial epiphysis	Infancy or adolescence
Osteochondritis dissecans	Subchondral regions of knee, hip, elbow, and ankle	

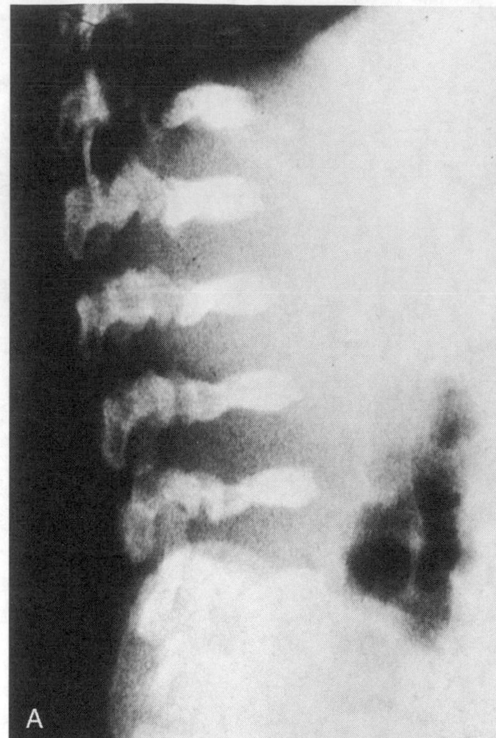

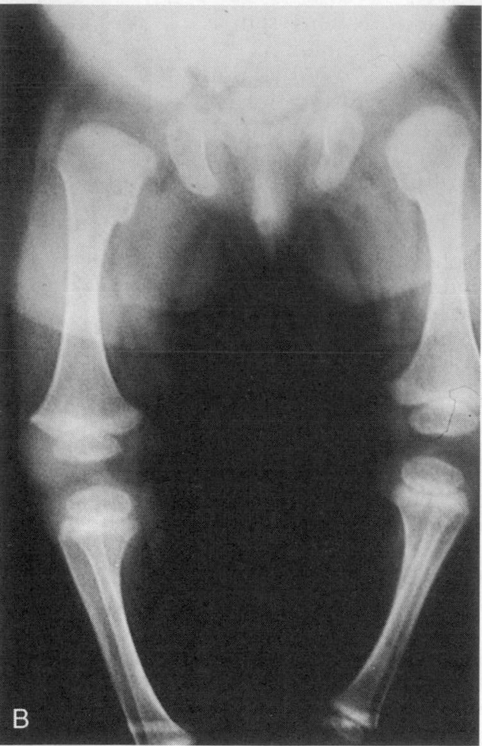

Figure 703–3 *A,* Radiograph of the lateral thoracolumbar spine in metatropic dysplasia showing severe platyspondyly. *B,* Radiograph of lower extremities in metatropic dysplasia showing short tubular bones with widened metaphyses. The femurs have a dumbbell appearance.

irregularly mineralized, especially at the proximal femur. The pelvic bones manifest mild hypoplasia.

Scoliosis may develop during adolescence. The disorder is otherwise uncomplicated, and manifestations are limited to the skeleton. Adults reach heights of 130–150 cm. The Kozlowski type of spondylometaphyseal dysplasia is an autosomal dominant trait.

JUVENILE OSTEOCHONDROSES. The juvenile osteochondroses are a heterogeneous group of disorders in which regional disturbances in bone growth cause noninflammatory arthropathies. They are summarized in Table 703–1. Some have localized pain and tenderness (Freiberg disease, Osgood-Schlatter disease, osteochondritis dissecans), whereas others present with painless limitation of joint movement (Legg-Calvé-Perthes disease, Scheuermann disease). Bone growth may be disrupted, leading to deformities. The diagnosis is usually confirmed radiographically, and treatment is symptomatic. The pathogenesis of these disorders is believed to involve ischemic necrosis of primary and secondary ossification centers. Although familial forms have been reported, these disorders usually occur sporadically.

Beck M, Roubicek M, Rogers JG, et al: Heterogeneity of metatropic dysplasia. Eur J Pediatr 140:231, 1983.

da Silva EO, Janovitz D, de Albuquerque SC: Ellis–van Creveld syndrome: Report of 15 cases in an inbred kindred. J Med Genet 17:349, 1980.

Makitie O, Sulisalo T, de la Chapelle A, et al: Cartilage-hair hypoplasia. J Med Genet 32:39, 1995.

Sharrard WJW: Abnormalities of the epiphyses and limb inequality. *In:* Sharrard WJW (ed): Paediatric Orthopaedics and Fracture, 3rd ed. Oxford, Blackwell Scientific Publications, 1993, p 719.

CHAPTER 704
Osteogenesis Imperfecta

Joan C. Marini

Osteoporosis, a feature of both inherited and acquired disorders, classically demonstrates fragility of the skeletal system and a susceptibility to long bone fractures or vertebral compressions from mild or inconsequential trauma. Osteogenesis imperfecta (OI) (brittle bone disease), the most common genetic cause of osteoporosis, is a generalized disorder of connective tissue caused by defects in type I collagen. The spectrum of OI is extremely broad, ranging from a form that is lethal in the perinatal period to a mild form in which the diagnosis may be equivocal in an adult.

ETIOLOGY. All types of osteogenesis imperfecta are caused by structural or quantitative defects in type I collagen, the primary component of the extracellular matrix of bone and skin. In about 10% of clinically indistinguishable cases, no biochemical defect of collagen protein can be demonstrated. It is not clear whether these cases represent limitations in biochemical detection or genetic heterogeneity of the disorder.

EPIDEMIOLOGY. OI is an autosomal dominant disorder that occurs in all racial and ethnic groups. The incidence of OI that is detectable in infancy is about 1 in 20,000. There is a similar incidence of the mild form, type I OI.

PATHOLOGY. The collagen structural mutations cause OI bone to be globally abnormal. The bone matrix contains abnormal type I collagen fibrils and relatively increased levels of types III and V collagen. In addition, several noncollagenous proteins of bone matrix are found in reduced amount. The hydroxyapatite crystals deposited on this matrix are poorly aligned with the long axis of fibrils.

PATHOGENESIS. Type I collagen is a heterotrimer, composed of two $\alpha 1(\text{I})$-chains and one $\alpha 2(\text{I})$-chain. The chains are synthesized as procollagen molecules with short globular extensions on both ends of the central helical domain. The helical domain is composed of uninterrupted repeats of the sequence Gly-X-Y, where gly is glycine, X is often proline, and Y is often hydroxyproline. The presence of glycine at every third residue is crucial to helix formation because its small side chain can be accommodated in the spatial constraints of the interior of the helical trimer. The chains are assembled into helices using crucial alignment sites in the carboxyl-terminal extension. Helix formation then proceeds linearly in a carboxyl to amino direction. Concomitant with helix assembly and formation, the chains are glycosylated at lysine residues.

The collagen structural defects are of two types: 85% are point mutations causing substitutions of glycine residues by other amino acids, 12% are single exon splicing defects. The clinically mild type I OI has a quantitative defect with mutations that cause one $\alpha1$(I) allele to be functionally null. These patients make a reduced amount of normal collagen.

The relationship between genotype and phenotype remains elusive for the structural mutations. Lethal and nonlethal mutations occur with about equal frequency on both chains. For $\alpha2$(I) mutations, lethal and nonlethal mutations occur in alternating regions along the chain. For mutations on the $\alpha1$(I)-chain, no model adequately predicts phenotype.

Osteogenesis imperfecta is an autosomal dominant disorder. A minority of OI cases with apparent recessive inheritance are due to parental mosaicism and are also dominant.

CLINICAL MANIFESTATIONS. OI has the triad of fragile bones, blue sclerae, and early deafness. OI was once divided into "congenita," the forms detectable at birth, and "tarda," the forms detectable later in childhood; this did not account for the variability of OI. The current classification divides OI into four types based on clinical and radiographic criteria.

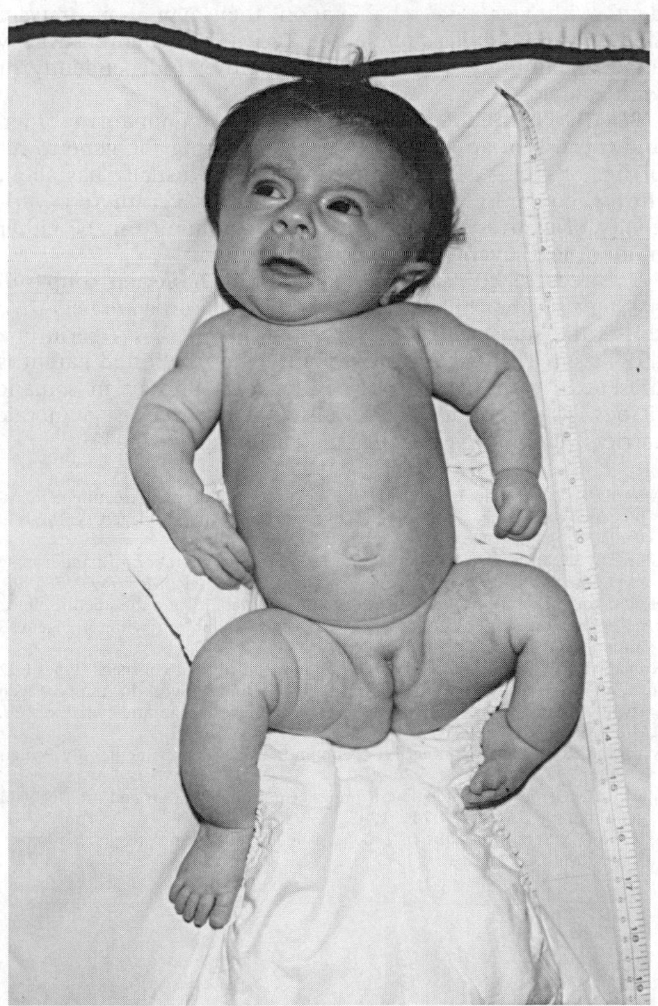

Figure 704–1 Infant with type III OI displays shortened bowed extremities, thoracic deformity, and relative macrocephaly.

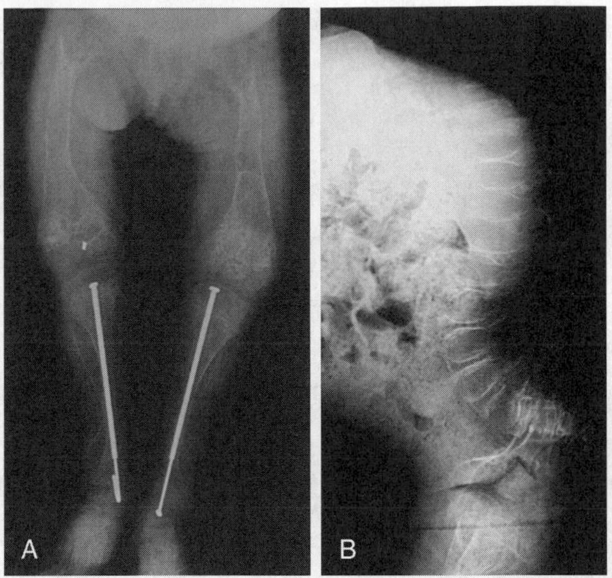

Figure 704–2 Typical features of type III OI radiographs in 6-yr-old child. *A,* Lower long bones are osteoporotic, with metaphyseal flaring, "popcorn" formation at growth plates, and placement of intramedullary rods. *B,* Vertebral bodies are compressed and osteoporotic.

Type I Osteogenesis Imperfecta (Mild). This form is sufficiently mild that it is often found in large pedigrees. Many type I families have blue sclerae, recurrent fractures in childhood, and presenile hearing loss (30–60%). Both types I and IV are divided into A and B subtypes, depending on the absence (A) or presence (B) of dentinogenesis imperfecta. Other possible connective tissue abnormalities include easy bruising, joint laxity, and slight short stature compared with family members. Fractures result from mild to moderate trauma and decrease after puberty.

Osteogenesis Imperfecta Type II (Perinatal Lethal). These infants may be stillborn or die in the 1st yr of life. Birthweight and length are small for gestational age. There is extreme fragility of the skeleton and other connective tissues. There are multiple intrauterine fractures of long bones, which have a crumpled appearance on roentgenograms. There is striking micromelia and bowing of extremities; the legs are held abducted at right angles to the body in the "frog-leg position." Multiple rib fractures create a beaded appearance and the small thorax contributes to respiratory insufficiency. The skull is large for body size with enlarged anterior and posterior fontanelles. Sclerae are dark blue-gray.

Osteogenesis Imperfecta Type III (Progressive Deforming). This is the severest nonlethal form of OI and results in significant physical disability. Birthweight and length are often low normal. There are usually in utero fractures. There is relative macrocephaly and triangular facies (Fig. 704–1). Postnatally, fractures occur from inconsequential trauma and heal with deformity. Disorganization of the bone matrix results in a "popcorn" appearance at the metaphyses (Fig. 704–2). The rib cage has flaring at the base, and pectal deformity is frequent. Virtually all type III patients have scoliosis and vertebral compression. Growth falls below the curve by the first year; all type III patients have extreme short stature. Scleral hue ranges from white to blue.

Osteogenesis Imperfecta Type IV (Moderately Severe). Patients with type IV OI may present at birth with in utero fractures or bowing of lower long bones. They may also present with

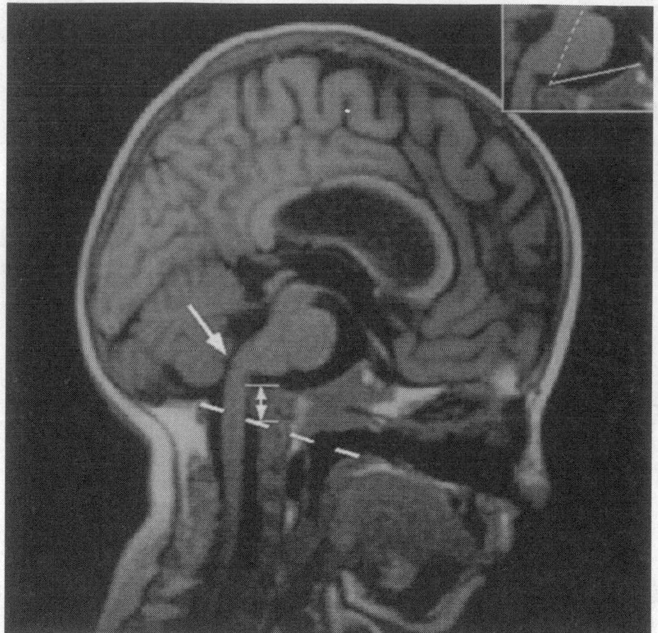

Figure 704–3 Typical features of basilar invagination shown in the sagittal MRI of an asymptomatic child with type III OI. There is invagination of the odontoid above Chamberlain's line causing compression and kinking at the pontomedullary junction *(arrow)*.

recurrent fractures after ambulation. Most children have moderate bowing even with infrequent fractures. Type IV children require orthopedic and rehabilitation intervention, but they are usually able to attain community ambulation skills. Fracture rates decrease after puberty. Radiographically, they are osteoporotic and have metaphyseal flaring and vertebral compressions. Type IV patients have moderate short stature. Scleral hue may be blue or white.

LABORATORY FINDINGS. The diagnosis is confirmed by collagen biochemical studies using fibroblasts cultured from a skin punch biopsy. Most collagen structural mutations cause a delay in helix formation, which results in overmodification of chains and the presence of broad or delayed bands on protein electrophoresis. In type I OI, the reduced amount of type I collagen results in an increase in the type III:type I collagen ratio detected by protein electrophoresis. Molecular techniques can identify the particular collagen mutation. This allows family members to be diagnosed using leukocyte DNA.

Severe OI can be detected prenatally by level II ultrasonography as early as 16 wk of gestation. OI and thanatophoric dysplasia may be confused. Fetal ultrasonography may not detect type IV OI and rarely detects type I OI. For recurrent cases, chorionic villus biopsy can be used for biochemical or molecular studies. Amniocytes produce false-positive biochemical studies but can be used for molecular studies in appropriate cases.

In the neonatal period, the normal to elevated alkaline phosphatase levels present in OI distinguish it from hypophosphatasia.

COMPLICATIONS. The morbidity and mortality of OI are cardiopulmonary. Recurrent pneumonias and transient cardiac failure occur in childhood and cor pulmonale is seen in adults.

Neurologic complications include basilar invagination, brain stem compression, hydrocephalus, and syringohydromyelia. Most types III and IV children have basilar invagination, but brain stem compression is infrequent. Basilar invagination is best detected with spiral computed tomography of the craniocervical junction (Fig. 704–3).

TREATMENT. There is no curative treatment for OI. For severe nonlethal OI, active physical rehabilitation in the early years allows children to attain a higher functional level than does orthopedic management alone. Type I and some type IV children are spontaneous ambulators. Type III and severe type IV children benefit from long leg plastic braces, gait aids, and a program of swimming and conditioning. Severely affected individuals require a wheelchair for community mobility but can acquire transfer and self-care skills.

Orthopedic management of OI is aimed at fracture management and correction of deformity to enable function. Fractures should be promptly splinted or cast; OI fractures heal well, and cast removal should be aimed at minimizing immobilization osteoporosis. Correction of long bone deformity requires an osteotomy procedure and placement of an intramedullary rod.

Treatments with calcium or fluoride supplements or calcitonin do not improve OI. Growth hormone improves bone histologic characteristics in growth-responsive children (usually types I and IV). Intravenous bisphosphonate treatment given each month may improve bone density and decrease bone turnover and new fractures. Bone marrow (mesenchymal cell) transplantation is an experimental approach to OI. OI teens may require psychologic support with body image issues.

PROGNOSIS. OI is a chronic condition that limits both life span and functional level. Infants with type II OI usually die within months to a year of life. An occasional child with radiographic type II and extreme growth deficiency may survive to the teen years. Type III OI individuals have a reduced life span with clusters of mortality from pulmonary causes in early childhood, the teen years, and the 40s. Types IV and I OI are compatible with a full life span.

Individuals with type III OI are usually wheelchair-dependent. With aggressive rehabilitation, they may attain transfer skills and household ambulation. Type IV OI children usually attain community ambulation skills either independently or with gait aids.

GENETIC COUNSELING. OI is an autosomal dominant disorder, and the risk of an affected individual passing the gene to his or her offspring is 50%. An affected child usually has about the same severity of OI as the parent; however, there is variability of expression, and the child's condition can be either more or less severe than that of the parent.

The recurrence risk to an apparently unaffected couple of having a second child with OI is empirically noted to be 5–7%; this is the statistical chance that one parent has a germ line mosaicism. The collagen mutation in the unaffected parent is present in some germ cells and may be present in somatic tissues. If genetic testing reveals that a parent is a mosaic carrier, the risk of recurrence may be as high as 50%.

Antoniazzi F, Bertoldo F, Mottes M, et al: Growth hormone treatment in osteogenesis imperfecta with quantitative defect of type I collagen synthesis. J Pediatr 129:432, 1996.

Glorieux FH, Bishop NJ, Plotkin H, et al: Cyclic administration of pamidronate in children with severe osteogenesis imperfecta. N Engl J Med 339:947, 1998.

Howitz E, Prockop D, Fitzpatrick L, et al: Transplantability and therapeutic effects of bone marrow-derived mesenchymal cells in children with osteogenesis imperfecta. Nat Med 5:309, 1999.

Kuivaniemi H, Tromp G, Prockop DJ: Mutations in fibrillar collagens (types I, II, III, and XI), fibril-associated collagen (type IX), and network-forming collagen (type X) cause a spectrum of diseases of bone, cartilage and blood vessels. Hum Mutat 9:300, 1997.

Marini JC: Osteogenesis imperfecta: Comprehensive management. Adv Pediatr 35:391, 1988.

Marini JC, Gerber NL: Osteogenesis imperfecta: Rehabilitation and prospects for gene therapy. JAMA 277:746, 1997.

Sillence DO, Senn A, Danks DM: Genetic heterogeneity in osteogenesis imperfecta. J Med Genet 16:101, 1979.

CHAPTER 705
Marfan Syndrome

Luther K. Robinson

Marfan syndrome is an autosomal dominantly inherited disorder with nearly complete penetrance but variable expressivity. The incidence of this disorder is about 1/10,000 births; nearly 30% of affected newborns represent sporadically occurring new mutations. Diagnosis of Marfan syndrome is based on clinical findings, some of which are age and maturation dependent.

PATHOGENESIS. Pathogenesis is related to abnormal biosynthesis of fibrillin 1, a 350-kd glycoprotein that is the major constituent of microfibrils that provide the scaffolding network of elastin and have an anchoring function in nonelastic tissue such as the suspensory ligament of the eye. The fibrillin locus lies within the long arm of chromosome 15 (15q21). To date, more than 100 mutations distributed throughout the fibrillin gene *(FBN1)* have been described, each appearing to be unique to a given affected family. The relatively even distribution of mutations throughout *FBN1* likely contributes to the phenotypic variability of the disorder.

CLINICAL MANIFESTATIONS. The diagnosis is made on the overall pattern of malformation (typically skeletal, cardiovascular, and ocular); many manifestations are age or maturation dependent. Tall stature may be present at birth and persist postnatally. Diminished subcutaneous tissue may suggest failure to thrive, but aggressive nutritional intervention (e.g., hyperalimentation) seldom is indicated. Hypotonia and ligamentous laxity may suggest developmental delays, but cognitive performance is usually normal.

Neonatal (infantile, congenital) Marfan syndrome is more severe than cases observed in older children and may have clinical similarity to congenital contractural arachnodactyly (CCA), presenting with hypotonia, arachnodactyly, joint laxity and dislocations, and flexion contractures. The face is long, and the skin is lax, with diminished recoil. The ears may appear large and pliant. Ocular examination may disclose megalocornea, iridodonesis, or frank lens dislocation. Cardiac examination often reveals mitral valve prolapse (MVP) with regurgitation or aortic root dilatation.

Older individuals display tall stature and a long, thin face with intermaxillary narrowness and dental crowding (Fig. 705–1). Ocular abnormalities reflect the connective tissue defect and include blue scleras, myopia, and suspensory ligament laxity with iridodonesis. Slit-lamp examination as early as infancy may disclose lens dislocation that may be congenital. Iridodonesis is a helpful clinical sign, but suspected cases of Marfan syndrome should have opthalmologic examinations, even in the absence of gross ocular abnormality.

Examination of the musculoskeletal system discloses dolichostenomelia (long, thin limbs), and the arm span substantially exceeds height. The lower segment (distance from pubis to heel) is increased in comparison with the upper segment (height minus lower segment) and contributes to a diminished upper segment/lower segment ratio (U_S/L_S). Hand findings are nonspecific and include long, thin fingers (arachnodactyly) that are hyperextensible. The thumb may be adducted across the narrow palm (Sternberg sign), and the thumb may appreciably overlap the fifth finger when encircling the wrist (wrist sign).

Long, gracile ribs may contribute to various sternal anomalies including pectus excavatum ("funnel chest") or pectus carinatum ("pigeon breast"). The risk of scoliosis among affected older children and adolescents is increased. The connective tissue defect contributes to increased distensibility of lung parenchyma and the dura, increasing the risks of spontaneous pneumothorax and dural ectasia, respectively.

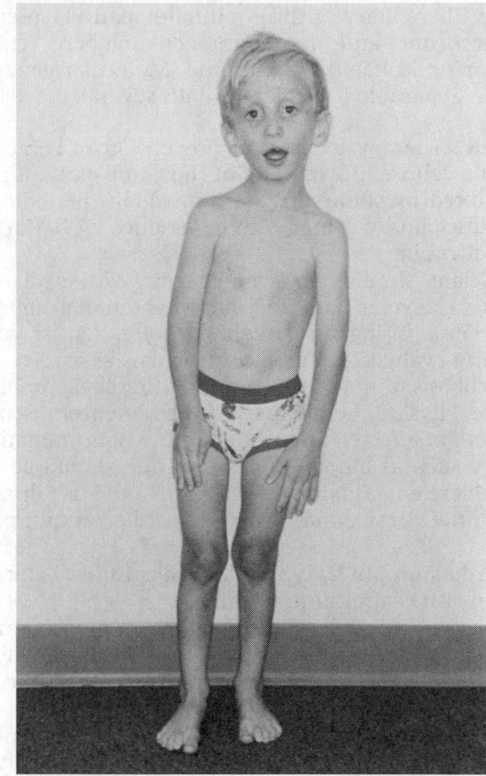

Figure 705–1 Marfan syndrome. Note the elongated facies, droopy lids, apparent dolichostenomelia, and mild scoliosis.

Progressive cardiovascular defects contribute to the substantial morbidity of Marfan syndrome. Echocardiography has permitted early detection of patients at risk of cardiovascular complications. As in adults, aortic root dilatation, whether or not accompanied by auscultatory evidence of aortic disease, occurs in 80–100% of cases and may be congenital. Frank aortic regurgitation is less common in children, in contrast to adults, perhaps because the amount and duration of distention required to cause aortic dysfunction is not manifested until later life. MVP occurs as frequently as aortic dilatation and tends to be progressive, in contrast to the more static lesion of idiopathic MVP. Progressive MVP is the most common cause of morbidity in children with Marfan syndrome and may be manifested as arrhythmias, heart failure, thromboemboli, or endocarditis.

DIAGNOSIS. Diagnosis of Marfan syndrome is based on clinical criteria. In general, diagnosis of a sporadic case, or new mutation, requires that the major manifestations of the disorder be present. In cases with an unequivocally affected first-degree relative, milder manifestations with at least one major manifestation are supportive of the diagnosis. Tall stature with an abnormally low U_S/L_S is the most consistent presenting feature. Echocardiography should show at least aortic root dilatation for age. Other abnormalities such as MVP, mitral regurgitation, or aortic regurgitation are supportive findings. A slit-lamp examination is indicated in all suspected cases.

Laboratory evaluation should document a negative urinary cyanide nitroprusside test result or specific amino acid studies to exclude cystathionine synthase deficiency (homocystinuria). Other conditions that should be excluded include idiopathic MVP, familial dissecting aortic dissection (cystic medial necrosis/annuloaortic ectasia, Erdheim disease), CCA, Stickler syndrome (hereditary arthro-ophthalmopathy), pseudoxanthoma elasticum, and the Shprintzen-Goldberg (craniosynostosis-marfanoid habitus) syndrome. Molecular genetic studies may be applicable to pedigrees with several affected family members.

TREATMENT. Therapy focuses on prevention of complications and genetic counseling. In view of the complexity of management required by some affected individuals, periodic referral to a interdisciplinary center with experience with Marfan syndrome is advisable.

Pediatricians should work in concert with pediatric subspecialists to develop and coordinate a rational approach to expectant monitoring and treatment of potential complications. Yearly evaluations for such problems as cardiac valvular disease, scoliosis, dislocations, or ophthalmologic problems are imperative. Physical therapy may improve neuromuscular tone and strength of affected infants. Moderate nontraumatic physical activity such as bicycling or swimming should be encouraged as tolerated. Maximal exertion should be discouraged because of the stresses that increased cardiac output places on the aorta.

Endocarditis prophylaxis should be instituted before dental or other invasive surgical procedures.

β-Adrenergic blockade with agents such as propranolol or atenolol may slow the progression of aortic dilatation and lessen the risk of catastrophic cardiovascular events. Acute aortic dissection may be managed by composite graft.

Optimal treatment of pregnant adolescents has not been established. The risk that cardiovascular abnormalities will worsen is of concern. Although substantial data are lacking, pregnant patients with minor cardiac manifestations and mild aortic root dilatation may tolerate pregnancy well and experience good maternal and fetal outcomes. Patients with aortic dilatation should be monitored echocardiographically at regular intervals. Although the β-adrenergic agents are not considered to be teratogenic, the prenatally exposed fetus of a woman with Marfan syndrome should be monitored in the newborn period for such drug-induced problems as hypotension, bradycardia, hypothermia, or hypoglycemia.

PROGNOSIS. Longevity in Marfan syndrome is diminished in comparison with population norms, primarily because of the increased risk of cardiovascular complications. Progressive dilatation of the aorta and aortic root may lead to aneurysm formation and dissection. These and other medical concerns pose not only medical but also psychologic stresses for affected children and their parents, especially during adolescence. Awareness of these issues and referral for support services may facilitate a positive perspective toward this condition.

GENETIC COUNSELING. The heritable nature of Marfan syndrome makes genetic counseling mandatory. About 15–30% of affected individuals are the first case in their families. Fathers in these sporadic cases have been, on average, 7–10 yr older than fathers in the general population. This paternal age effect suggests that these cases represent new dominant mutations with minimal recurrence risks to the future offspring of the normal parents. Each child of an affected individual has a 50% risk of inheriting the number 15 chromosome containing the mutant allele and thus being affected. Recurrence risk counseling is best managed by professionals with expertise in the issues surrounding the chronic nature of this condition.

American Academy of Pediatrics Committee on Genetics: Health supervision for children with Marfan syndrome. Pediatrics 98:978, 1996.

DePaepe A, Devereux RB, Dietz HC, et al: Revised criteria for the Marfan syndrome. Am J Med Genet 62:417, 1996.

Franke U, Furthmayer H: Marfan syndrome and other disorders of fibrillin. N Engl J Med 330:1384, 1994.

Lipscomb K, Clayton-Smith J, Harris R: Evolving phenotype of Marfan syndrome. Arch Dis Child 76:41, 1997.

Pereira L, Levran O, Ramirez F, et al: A molecular approach to stratification of cardiovascular risk in families with Marfan syndrome. N Engl J Med 331:148, 1994.

Rossiter JP, Morales AJ, Repke JT, et al: A prospective longitudinal evaluation of pregnancy in the Marfan syndrome. Am J Obstet Gynecol 173:1599, 1995.

Shores J, Berger KR, Murphy EA, et al: Progression of aortic dilatation and the benefit of long-term β-adrenergic-blockade in Marfan syndrome. N Engl J Med 330:1355, 1994.

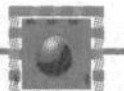

SECTION 4

Metabolic Bone Disease

Russell W. Chesney

CHAPTER 706

Bone Structure, Growth, and Hormonal Regulation

Also see Chapters 44.10, 44.11, 49, and 580.

Bone is a dynamic organ capable of rapid turnover, weight bearing, and withstanding the stresses of various physical activities. It is constantly being formed (modeling) and re-formed (remodeling). It is the major body reservoir for calcium, phosphorus, and magnesium. Disorders that affect this organ and the process of mineralization are designated metabolic bone diseases.

Because bone growth and turnover rates are high during childhood, many clinical features of metabolic bone diseases are more prominent in children than in adults. Advances in our knowledge of bone metabolism, the process of mineralization, interactions of the vitamin D–parathyroid hormone (PTH)–endocrine axis, and metabolism of vitamin D to active compounds have led to improved treatment of metabolic bone diseases.

The human skeleton consists of a protein matrix, largely composed of a collagen-containing protein, osteoid, on which is deposited a crystalline mineral phase. Although collagen-containing osteoid accounts for 90% of bone protein, other proteins are present, including osteocalcin, which contains γ-carboxyglutamic acid. Synthesis of osteocalcin is vitamin K and vitamin D dependent, and in high bone turnover states, serum osteocalcin values are often elevated.

The microfibrillar matrix of osteoid permits deposition of highly organized calcium phosphate crystals, including hydroxyapatite [C_{10} $(PO_4)_6 \cdot 6H_2O$] and octacalcium phosphate [Ca_8 $(H_2PO_4)_6 \cdot 5H_2O$], plus less organized amorphous calcium phosphate, calcium carbonate, sodium, magnesium, and citrate. Hydroxyapatite is deep within bone matrix, whereas amorphous calcium phosphate coats the surface of newly formed or remodeled bone.

Bone growth occurs in children by the process of calcification of the cartilage cells present at the ends of bone. In accord with the prevailing extracellular fluid (ECF) calcium and phosphate concentrations, mineral is deposited in those chondrocytes or cartilage cells set to undergo mineralization. The main function of the vitamin D–PTH–endocrine axis is to maintain the ECF calcium and phosphate concentrations at appropriate levels to permit mineralization.

Other hormones also appear to regulate the growth and mineralization of cartilage, including growth hormone acting through insulin-like growth factors, thyroid hormones, insulin, and androgens, and estrogens during the pubertal growth spurt. By contrast, supraphysiologic concentrations of glucocorticoids impair cartilage function and bone growth and augment bone resorption.

Rates of bone formation are coordinated with alterations in mineral metabolism at both the intestine and kidneys. Inadequate dietary intake or intestinal absorption of calcium causes a fall in serum levels of calcium and its ionized fraction. This serves as the signal for PTH synthesis and secretion, resulting in greater bone resorption to raise serum calcium level, enhanced distal tubular reabsorption of calcium, and higher rates of synthesis by the kidneys of 1,25-dihydroxy vitamin D (1,25[OH]$_2$D, or calcitriol), the most active metabolite of vitamin D (Fig. 706–1). Calcium homeostasis thus is controlled at the intestine, because the availability of 1,25(OH)$_2$D ultimately determines the fraction of ingested calcium that is absorbed.

By contrast, phosphate homeostasis is regulated by the kidneys, because intestinal phosphate absorption is nearly complete and renal excretion determines the serum level. Excessive intestinal phosphate absorption causes a fall in serum levels of ionized calcium and a rise in PTH secretion, resulting in phosphaturia, thus lowering serum phosphate level and permitting calcium level to rise. Hypophosphatemia blocks PTH secretion and promotes renal 1,25(OH)$_2$D synthesis. This latter compound also promotes greater intestinal phosphate absorption.

An understanding of the metabolism of vitamin D is necessary to appreciate metabolic bone disease and rickets (see Fig. 706–1). The skin contains 7-dehydrocholesterol, which is converted to vitamin D$_3$ by ultraviolet radiation; other inactive vitamin D sterols are also produced (see Chapter 44.10). Vitamin D$_3$ is then transported in the bloodstream to the liver by a vitamin D binding protein (DBP); DBP binds all forms of vitamin D. The plasma concentration of free or nonbound vitamin D is much lower than the level of DBP-bound vitamin D metabolities.

Vitamin D also can enter the metabolic pathway by ingestion of dietary vitamin D$_2$ (ergocalciferol) or vitamin D$_3$ (cholecalciferol), both of which are absorbed from the intestine because of the action of bile salts. After absorption, ingested vitamin D is transported by chylomicrons to the liver, where, along with skin-derived vitamin D$_3$, it is converted to 25-hydroxyvitamin D(25[OH]D) by the action of a hepatic microsomal enzyme requiring oxygen, NADPH, and magnesium to hydroxylate vitamin D at the 25th carbon atom. The 25(OH)D is next transported by DBP to the kidneys, where it undergoes further metabolism. 25(OH)D is the main circulating vitamin D metabolite in humans at a concentration of 20–80 ng/mL (Table 706–1). Because its synthesis is weakly regulated by feedback, its plasma level rises in summer and falls in winter. High vitamin D intake raises the plasma level of 25(OH)D to many times above normal, but the parent vitamin D itself is absorbed by adipose tissue.

In the kidneys, 25(OH)D undergoes further hydroxylation, depending on the prevailing serum concentration of calcium, phosphate, and PTH. If calcium or phosphate level is reduced or PTH level is elevated, the enzyme 25(OH)D-1-hydroxylase is activated and 1,25(OH)$_2$D is formed. This metabolite circulates at a level that is only 0.1% of the level of 25(OH)D (see Table 706–1) and acts on the intestine to increase the active transport of calcium and stimulate phosphate absorption. Because 1α-hydroxylase is a mitochondrial enzyme that is tightly feedback regulated, the synthesis of 1,25(OH)$_2$D declines after serum calcium or phosphate values return to normal. Excessive 1,25(OH)$_2$D is converted to an inactive metabolite. In the presence of normal or elevated serum calcium or phosphate

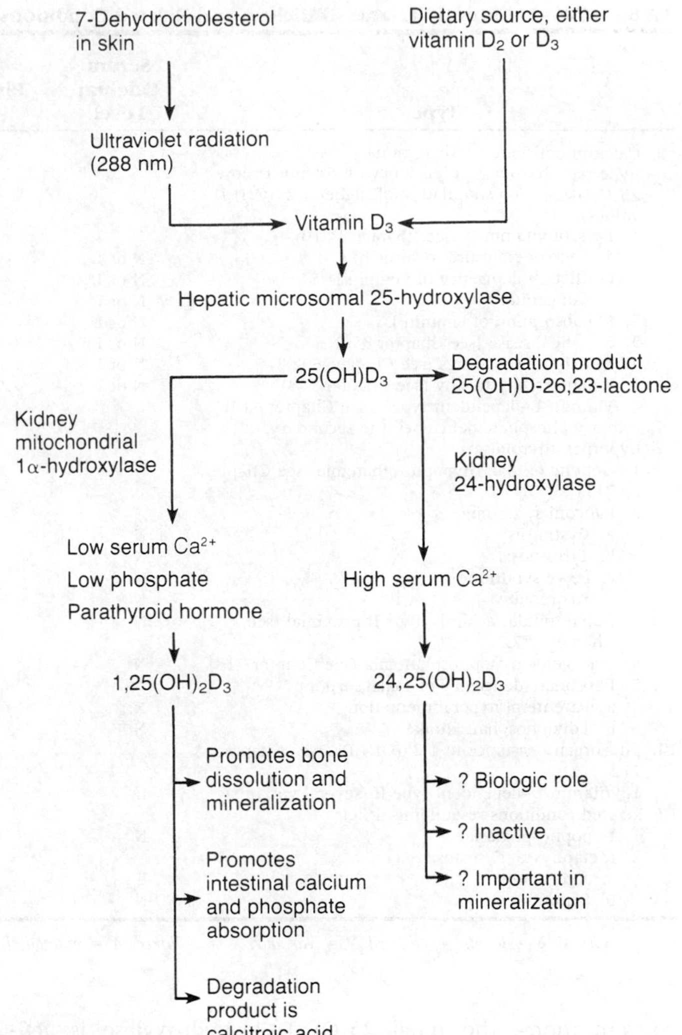

Figure 706–1 The metabolic pathway of vitamin D, indicating its conversion to the hormone 1,25(OH)$_2$D$_3$ and to 24,25(OH)$_2$D$_3$. Vitamin D$_2$ (ergosterol) of plant origin appears to undergo similar metabolic steps.

TABLE 706–1 Vitamin D Metabolic Values in Plasma of Normal Healthy Subjects

Metabolite	Plasma Value
Vitamin D$_2$	1–2 ng/mL
Vitamin D$_3$	1–2 ng/mL
25(OH)D$_2$	4–10 ng/mL
25(OH)D$_3$	12–40 ng/mL
Total 25(OH)D	15–50 ng/mL
24,25(OH)$_2$D	1–4 ng/mL
1,25(OH)$_2$D	
Infancy	70–100 pg/mL
Childhood	30–50 pg/mL
Adolescence	40–80 pg/mL
Adulthood	20–35 pg/mL

TABLE 706–2 Clinical Variants of Rickets and Related Conditions

Type	Serum Calcium Level	Serum Phosphorus Level	Alkaline Phosphatase Activity	Urine Concentration of Amino Acids	Genetics
I. Calcium deficiency with secondary hyperparathyroidism (deficiency of vitamin D; low 25(OH)D and no stimulation of higher $1,25(OH)_2D$ values)					
1. Lack of vitamin D (see Chapter 44.10)					
a. Lack of exposure to sunlight	N or L	L	E	E	
b. Dietary deficiency of vitamin D	N or L	L	E	E	
c. Congenital	N or L	L	E	E	
2. Malabsorption of vitamin D	N or L	L	E	E	
3. Hepatic disease (see Chapter 356)	N or L	L	E	E	
4. Anticonvulsive drugs (see Chapter 602.7)	N or L	L	E	E	
5. Renal osteodystrophy (see Chapter 543)	N or L	E	E	V	
6. Vitamin D–dependent type I (see Chapter 712)	L	N or L	E	E	AR
II. Primary phosphate deficiency (no secondary hyperparathyroidism)					
1. Genetic primary hypophosphatemia (see Chapter 711)	N	L	E	N	XD
2. Fanconi syndrome					
a. Cystinosis	N	L	E	E	AR
b. Tyrosinosis	N	L	E	E	AR
c. Lowe syndrome	N	L	E	E	XR
d. Acquired	N	L	E	E	
3. Renal tubular acidosis, type II proximal (see Chapter 537.5)	N	L	E	N	
4. Oncogenic hypophosphatemia (see Chapter 713)	N	L	E	N	
5. Phosphate deficiency or malabsorption					
a. Parenteral hyperalimentation	N	L	E	N	
b. Low phosphate intake	N	L	E	N	
III. End-organ resistance to $1,25(OH)_2D_3$, (see Chapter 712)					
1. Vitamin D–dependent type II (several variants)	L	L or N	E	E	AR
IV. Related conditions resembling rickets					
1. Hypophosphatasia	N	N	L	Phosphoethanolamine elevated	AR
2. Metaphyseal dysostosis					
a. Jansen type	E	N	E	N	AD
b. Schmid type	N	N	N	N	AD

N = normal; L = low; E = elevated; V = variable; X = X-linked; A = autosomal; D = dominant; R = recessive.

concentrations, the renal 25(OH)D-24-hydroxylase is activated, producing 24,25-dihydroxyvitamin D ($24,25[OH]_2D$), which is a pathway for the removal of excess vitamin D, because the serum levels of $24,25(OH)_2D$ (1–5 ng/mL) become higher after ingestion of large amounts of vitamin D. Although hypervitaminosis D and production of inactive metabolites can occur after oral dosing (see Chapter 44.12), extensive skin exposure to sunlight does not usually produce toxic levels of $25(OH)D_3$, suggesting natural regulation of the production of this metabolite in cutaneous tissue.

Serum $1,25(OH)_2D$ levels are higher in children than in adults, are not as subject to seasonal variability, and peak in the 1st yr of life and again during the adolescent growth spurt. These values must be interpreted in light of the prevailing serum calcium, phosphate, and PTH values and with regard to the entire vitamin D metabolite profile.

Mineral deficiency prevents the normal process of bone mineral deposition. If mineral deficiency occurs at the growth plate, growth slows and bone age is retarded—a condition called rickets. Poor mineralization of trabecular bone resulting in a greater proportion of unmineralized osteoid is the condition of osteomalacia. Rickets is found only in growing children before fusion of the epiphyses, whereas osteomalacia is present at all ages. All patients with rickets have osteomalacia, but not all patients with osteomalacia have rickets. These conditions should not be confused with osteoporosis, a condition of equal loss of bone volume and mineral, caused in childhood by glucocorticoid administration, found in Turner and Klinefelter syndromes, or as an idiopathic condition.

Rickets may be classified as calcium-deficient or phosphate-deficient rickets. Because both calcium and phosphate ions constitute bone mineral, the insufficiency of either type in the ECF that bathes the mineralizing surface of bone results in rickets and osteomalacia. The two types of rickets are distinguishable by their clinical manifestations (Table 706–2).

CHAPTER 707

Primary Chondrodystrophy

(Metaphyseal Dysplasia)

In this condition, bowing of the legs, short stature, and a waddling gait appear in the absence of abnormalities of serum levels of calcium and phosphate, alkaline phosphatase activity, or vitamin D metabolites. *Metaphyseal chondrodysplasia (Jansen type)* is typified by cupped and ragged metaphyses, which develop mottled calcification at the distal ends of bone over time. Hypercalcemia, with serum values of 13–15 mg/dL, may occur. The spine may also be deformed by the irregular growth of vertebrae. *Schmid type* of metaphyseal chondrodysplasia is less severe, although the roentgenographic appearance of the knees and extreme bowing of the lower limbs resemble signs seen in patients with familial hypophosphatemia. It is associated with defects in collagen type X. The hip abnormalities are more debilitating. Patients with both types of metaphyseal chondrodysplasia have lifelong short stature.

Metaphyseal dysotosis, or *Pyle disease,* results from defects in endochondral bone formation and metaphyseal modeling. The long ends of bones are splayed, resulting in an Erlenmeyer flask defect. Short stature is not present, and serum chemical levels are normal. Leonine features develop if the facial bones are involved.

No effective forms of treatment are available for the chondrodystrophies or dysostosis.

CHAPTER 708
Idiopathic Hypercalcemia

Excessive quantities of vitamin D used to enrich food for infants in post–World War II England have been associated with hypercalcemia. Although many infants were exposed to high levels of vitamin D, only a few developed hypercalcemia, failure to thrive, nephrolithiasis, and decline in renal function. These infants had roentgenographic evidence of osteosclerosis and dense bones at the metaphyses. This disorder disappeared with reduction in the vitamin D content of milk but has been reported sporadically when errors in vitamin D formulation of milk have occurred. It may also be observed when growing premature infants are not appropriately weaned from specialized preterm formula enriched with calcium and vitamin D. Subsequently, at least three separate forms of hypercalcemia of unknown origin have been described.

Williams syndrome, or the elfin facies syndrome, consists of a constellation of manifestations of which hypercalcemia is an infrequent finding. The characteristic facial features include a small mandible, prominent maxilla, and upturned nose. The upper lip has a Cupid's bow curve. Small peglike teeth with numerous caries are common. Feeding problems and failure to thrive during the 1st yr of life are usual. Mild mental retardation and an unusual "cocktail party patter" personality are typical. The types of cardiac lesions found separately or together include supravalvular aortic stenosis, peripheral pulmonary stenosis, hypoplasia of the aorta, coronary artery stenosis, and atrial or ventricular septal defects. Sudden death may be secondary to arrhythmias or coronary artery disease. In hypercalcemic patients, nephrocalcinosis and sclerotic long bones are sometimes evident.

Williams syndrome is sporadic, and some children have hypervitaminosis D without evidence of increased maternal or infantile vitamin D intake. In most cases, the circulating values for vitamin D metabolites are normal. Patients with this disorder slowly excrete an infused calcium load and have evidence of increased production of 25(OH)D from vitamin D. Impaired calcitonin secretion to an infused calcium load has also been reported. Treatment is directed at cardiac, social, and educational problems.

Children may also have mild idiopathic hypercalcemia, which is usually transient. Phenotypic features of Williams syndrome are not found. These patients have hypercalciuria and sometimes nephrocalcinosis, possibly resembling the English infants who received excessive vitamin D after World War II. However, no evidence for abnormalities in vitamin D metabolism has been found.

Familial hypocalciuric hypercalcemia is an autosomal dominant condition in which affected children have asymptomatic hypercalcemia without hypercalciuria. Pancreatitis may occur in some families, and in a few kindreds, neonates may present with life-threatening parathyroid hyperplasia. Instead of serum calcium levels of 12–15 mg/dL, typically found in the parent, these infants have levels exceeding 18 mg/dL. All of these children have had mild parathyroid hyperplasia despite hypercalcemia, suggesting that the parathyroid gland does not respond appropriately to the signal of hypercalcemia. The gene for the calcium-sensing receptor in parathyroid, kidney, and other tissues is abnormal in families with familial benign hypocalciuric hypercalcemia. This gene is located on chromosome 3 in 90% of families, and the gene defect impairs the responsiveness of the calcium receptor to ionized calcium. Vitamin D metabolism is normal. Only the infants with serious hyperparathyroidism require an emergency parathyroidectomy. Although serum magnesium level is elevated, it is not a serious concern.

CHAPTER 709
Hypophosphatasia

Hypophosphatasia is an autosomal recessive disorder that roentgenographically resembles rickets and is defined by low serum alkaline phosphatase activity. Hypophosphatasia is now recognized to be an inborn error of metabolism in which activity of the tissue-nonspecific (liver/bone/kidney) alkaline phosphatase is deficient. Single point mutations of the gene for alkaline phosphatase prevent the expression of the activity of this enzyme in vitro and indicate the necessity of this enzyme for normal skeletal mineralization. Missense mutations of the gene for the tissue nonspecific isoenzyme have been found, but other patients may have a regulatory defect involving this enzyme. Activity of the intestinal and placental enzyme is normal.

There is considerable heterogeneity in the severity of the disease. Some cases appear at birth, and diagnosis has even been made in utero by roentgenographic examination of a fetus. The disease may appear in a lethal neonatal or perinatal form (*congenital lethal hypophosphatasia*), a severe infantile form, or a milder form occurring in childhood or late adolescence (*hypophosphatasia tarda*). The lethal form is characterized by a moth-eaten appearance at the ends of the long bones, by severe deficiency of ossification throughout the skeleton, and by marked shortening of the long bones. Patients with the mild disease may present with bowing of the legs and variable statural shortening. Because calcium accumulation by mature chondrocytes does not occur, patients may appear to have rickets, and in the neonatal and infantile form they may have hypercalcemia.

Unusual clinical manifestations include wormian bones in the calvarium, poor calcification of the frontal, parietal, and occipital bones, and premature loss of deciduous or permanent teeth owing to hypoplasia of dental cementum. Because of the hypercalcemia in the infantile form, nephrocalcinosis is also found. In the childhood form, bone pain, frequent fractures, and milder skeletal deformities are evident, as well as premature tooth loss. The metaphyseal defect consists of irregular ossification, punched-out areas, and metaphyseal cupping.

In hypophosphatasia, large quantities of phosphoethanolamine are found in the urine because this compound cannot be degraded in the absence of adequate alkaline phosphatase activity. Plasma inorganic pyrophosphate and pyridoxal-5-phosphate are also elevated for the same reason. Although no satisfactory therapy has been found, infusion of plasma rich in alkaline phosphatase activity has been helpful in healing bone in short-term studies. The clinical course of this condition often improves spontaneously as an affected child matures, although early death due to renal failure or flail chest leading to pneumonia may also occur in the severe infantile form of the disorder. Rare patients presenting identical clinical and roentgenographic patterns have normal serum alkaline phosphatase activities. Their disease has been labeled *pseudohypophosphatasia* and may represent the presence of a mutant alkaline phosphatase isozyme that reacts to artificial substrates in an alkaline environment (i.e., in a test tube) but not in vivo with natural substrates.

CHAPTER 710
Hyperphosphatasia

Excessive elevation of the bone isozyme of alkaline phosphatase in serum and significant growth failure characterize hyperphosphatasia. Osteoid proliferation in the subperiosteal portion of bone results in separation of the periosteum from the bone cortex. Bowing and thickening of the diaphyses are common along with osteopenia. The disease usually has its onset by 2–3 yr of age, when painful deformity developing in the extremities leads to abnormal gait and sometimes fractures. Other common findings include pectus carinatum, kyphoscoliosis, and rib fraying. The skull is large, and the cranium is thickened (widened diploë) and may be deformed. Roentgenographically, the bony texture is variable; dense areas (showing a teased cotton-wool appearance) are interspersed with radiolucent areas and general demineralization. Long bones appear cylindric, lose metaphyseal modeling, and contain pseudocysts showing a dense, bony halo.

In this autosomal recessive disorder, serum levels of both calcium and phosphate are normal, whereas urinary leucine amino acid peptidase activity and serum acid phosphatase levels are increased. This disorder is often called *juvenile Paget disease* because as in adult-onset Paget disease, calcitonin may reduce the rapid bone turnover found in this disorder; in children, the disorder is more generalized and symmetric. This disorder is distinct from Paget disease because histology of bone reveals a lack of normal cortical bone remodeling and an absence of the classic mosaic pattern of lamellar bone found in that adult condition. Hence, the term *juvenile Paget disease* is inappropriate.

Transient hyperphosphatasia occurs between 2 mo and 2 yr of age, has no associated manifestations other than some mild gastrointestinal symptoms, and is usually detected during routine (screening) laboratory evaluation for some unrelated complaint. Both liver and bone isoenzyme fractions are elevated; there are no other manifestations of hepatic or bone dysfunction. The cause is unknown. Resolution usually occurs within 4–6 mo.

Familial hyperphosphatemia, an autosomal dominant trait, is another benign condition that is distinguished from the transient infantile form by persistent and asymptomatic elevations of serum alkaline phosphatase levels.

Bird LM, Billman GF, Lacro RV, et al: Sudden death in Williams syndrome: Report of ten cases. J Pediatr 129:296, 1996.

Brown EM, Bai M, Pollack M: Familial benign hypocalciuric hypercalcemia in metabolic bone diseases and clinically related disorders. *In:* Avioli LV, Krane SM (eds): Metabolic Bone Disease and Clinically Related Disorders, 3rd ed. San Diego, Academic Press, 1998, pp 479–500.

Chesney RW, DeLuca HF, Gertner JM, et al: Circulating levels of vitamin D metabolites in children with the Williams syndrome. N Engl J Med 313:888, 1985.

Culler FL, Jones KL, Deftos LJ: Impaired calcitonin secretion in patients with Williams syndrome. J Pediatr 107:720, 1985.

Hughes MR, Malloy PJ, O'Malley BW, et al: Genetic defects of the 1,25 dihydroxyvitamin D_3 receptor. J Recept Res 11:699, 1991.

Warman ML, Abbott M, Apra SS, et al: A type X collagen mutation causes Schmid metaphyseal chondrodysplasia. Nat Genet 5:79, 1993.

CHAPTER 711
Familial Hypophosphatemia

(Vitamin D–Resistant Rickets, X-Linked Hypophosphatemia)

The most commonly encountered non-nutritional form of rickets is familial hypophosphatemia. The usual mode of inheritance is X-linked dominant; some mothers of affected children exhibit clinical evidence of disease such as bowing or short stature, whereas others show only fasting hypophosphatemia. Autosomal recessive and sporadic forms have also been reported.

PATHOGENESIS. Pathogenic mechanisms involve defects in the proximal tubular reabsorption of phosphate and in the conversion of 25(OH)D to $1,25(OH)_2D$. The latter defect is evidenced by low-normal serum $1,25(OH)_2D$ levels despite hypophosphatemia and by the finding that further phosphate depletion of subjects with familial hypophosphatemia does not stimulate $1,25(OH)_2D$ synthesis as it does in normal subjects. Both a renal tubular reabsorption defect and reduced $1,25(OH)_2D$ synthesis are found in an animal model of this disease. In addition, oral phosphate supplementation alone cannot completely heal bone disease; the correction of osteomalacia requires $1,25(OH)_2D$ therapy. The activity of the Na^+-dependent phosphate transporter in the renal proximal tubule is reduced, resulting in excessive urinary phosphate excretion; this transporter protein is encoded on chromosome 5. Because the disorder has an X-linked inheritance pattern, the abnormal gene must represent a "nuisance" for a protein regulating phosphate reabsorption. The gene for this disorder is confined to Xp22.31–p21.3 on the X chromosome.

CLINICAL MANIFESTATIONS. Children with familial hypophosphatemia present with bowing of the lower extremities related to weight bearing at the age of walking. Tetany is not present, and the profound myopathy, rachitic rosary, and Harrison groove (pectus deformity) characteristic of calcium-deficient rickets are not evident (see Chapter 44.10). These children develop a waddling gait, smooth (rather than angular) bowing of the lower extremities, coxa vara, genu varum, genu valgum, and short stature. The adult height of untreated patients is 130–165 cm.

Pulp deformities and a lesion called **intraglobular dentin** are characteristic tooth abnormalities, although enamel defects are found only occasionally. By contrast, calcium-deficient rickets usually results in enamel defects. Periapical infections are found in both forms of rickets. Therapy of metabolic bone disease does not correct the defect in intraglobular dentin in this condition.

Roentgenographic findings include metaphyseal widening and fraying and coarse-appearing trabecular bone. Cupping of the metaphysis occurs at the proximal and distal tibia and at the distal femur, radius, and ulna.

LABORATORY FINDINGS. Patients have a normal or slightly reduced serum calcium level (9–9.4 mg/dL; 2.24–2.34 mM), a moderately reduced serum phosphate level (1.5–3 mg/dL; 0.48–0.96 mM), elevated alkaline phosphatase activity, and no evidence of secondary hyperparathyroidism. Urinary phosphate excretion is large, despite hypophosphatemia, indicating a defect in renal tubular phosphate reabsorption (Chapter 537.5). This disorder is typical of pure phosphate-deficient rickets, because aminoaciduria, glucosuria, bicarbonaturia, and kaliuria are never found. In potential obligate heterozygotes, who later develop disease, serum phosphate levels may remain normal for the first several months of life. The first laboratory abnormality is often a rise in serum alkaline phosphatase activity. The serum phosphate level probably remains normal for several months, because the glomerular filtration rate is quite low in neonates. Parathyroid hyperplasia with elevated serum parathyroid hormone (PTH) values is occasionally found, usually in sporadic cases.

TREATMENT. Oral phosphate supplements coupled with a vitamin D analog to offset the secondary hyperparathyroidism that may accompany an oral phosphate load is the preferred treatment. Oral phosphate is usually given every 4 hr at least five times a day, because urinary excretion is constant and patients quickly become hypophosphatemic. Young children should receive 0.5–1 g/24 hr, whereas older children require 1–4 g/24 hr. Phosphate can be given as Joulie solution (dibasic sodium phosphate, 136 g/L, and phosphoric acid, 58.8 g/L), which contains 30.4 mg of phosphate/mL. Thus, a 5 mL dose given every 4 hr five times daily provides 760 mg of phosphate. A capsule form of phosphate (Neutra-Phos) provides 250 mg of phosphorus per capsule. Patient compliance is readily assessed because almost all of this dose is excreted in a 24-hr urine collection. The main side effect of oral phosphate therapy is diarrhea, which often improves spontaneously.

Providing a vitamin D analog is important for complete bone healing and prevention of secondary hyperparathyroidism. Classically, vitamin D_2 was used at 2,000 IU/kg/24 hr, but more recently, dihydrotachysterol at a dosage of 0.02 mg/kg/24 hr or $1,25(OH)_2D$ at 50–65 ng/kg/24 hr has been effectively used.

Familial hypophosphatemia was previously treated with 50,000–200,000 IU/24 hr (1.25–10 mg) of vitamin D_2 but this caused hypervitaminosis D with nephrocalcinosis, hypercalcemia, and permanent renal damage (Chapter 44.12).

The term *vitamin D–resistant rickets* was used in the past to describe rickets in which patients failed to respond to a dose of vitamin D that would cure vitamin D deficiency. If appropriate doses of vitamin D or any of its metabolites fail to heal rickets, and if serum phosphate is not reduced, metaphyseal dysplasia should be considered (see Chapter 707).

With early diagnosis and good compliance, the bowing deformities can be minimized, and an adult height above 170 cm may be achievable. However, the influence of therapy on final height is controversial, because most patients remain short while in some studies good growth patterns are evident. Corrective osteotomies should always be deferred until rickets appears healed roentgenographically and until the serum alkaline phosphatase level is in the normal range. Surgery before bone healing may be followed by redevelopment of deformity and bowing. In some patients, aggressive medical management may obviate the need for surgical intervention. Patients undergoing osteotomy should stop taking all vitamin D preparations before surgery and should not start them again until they are again ambulating to avoid immobilization hypercalcemia. Because $1,25(OH)_2D$ has such a short half-life, it can be stopped just before surgery, whereas vitamin D_2 should be discontinued at least 1 mo before surgery. An additional advantage of $1,25(OH)_2D$ therapy is that it augments intestinal phosphate absorption and may improve phosphate balance. However, $1,25(OH)_2D$ should not be used without concomitant oral phosphate.

Certain patients have hypophosphatemia and hyperphosphaturia but no roentgenographic evidence of rickets. This condition, inherited as an autosomal dominant disorder, has been called *hypophosphatemic bone disease.* The serum concentrations of $1,25(OH)_2D$ are normal, and the renal tubular phosphate excretion defect is not as marked as in familial hypophosphatemic rickets. Short stature is not as prominent. Oral phosphate and $1,25(OH)_2D$ have been used to treat this disorder.

CHAPTER 712
Vitamin D–Dependent Rickets

(Pseudovitamin D Deficiency, Hypocalcemic Vitamin D–Resistant Rickets)

Vitamin D-dependent rickets appears at age 3–6 mo in children who have been receiving dosages of vitamin D (400–600 IU/24 hr) that ordinarily prevent rickets (Chapter 44.10). Serum calcium and phosphate levels are low, and alkaline phosphatase activity is elevated. This condition is a calcium-deficient form of rickets because patients have secondary hyperparathyroidism, aminoaciduria, glucosuria, renal tubular bicarbonate wasting, and renal tubular acidosis. These children also develop dental enamel hypoplasia. Although the rickets and biochemical features of this autosomal recessive disorder can be treated with a massive dose of vitamin D_2 (200,000–1 million IU/24 hr), the use of relatively low-dose $1,25(OH)_2D$ at 1–2 μg/24 hr heals this disorder. The current hypothesis to account for these findings is that the enzyme activity of 25(OH)D-1 α-hydroxylase is deficient or greatly reduced. As evidence of this hypothesis, the serum levels of $1,25(OH)_2D$ are low, despite hypocalcemia, hypophosphatemia, and elevated parathyroid hormone levels.

Some cases of vitamin D–dependent rickets fail to reverse after treatment either with high-dose vitamin D_2 or $1,25(OH)_2D$ at 1–2 μg/24 hr. Hypocalcemia, hypophosphatemia, aminoaciduria, and rickets persist in the presence of extremely high circulating levels of $1,25(OH)_2D$, usually above 180 pg/mL. Patients with hereditary $1,25(OH)_2D_3$-resistant rickets have (1) reduced or absent $1,25(OH)_2D_3$ binding to the human vitamin D nuclear receptor; (2) decreased affinity of this receptor for DNA so that transcription cannot occur; or (3) defective nuclear translocation or retention. An abnormal gene product is produced by the vitamin D receptor gene in these patients. A single amino acid substitution in an important DNA-binding site in the receptor may cause this disorder, thus preventing the binding of $1,25(OH)_2D$ and its receptor to the nucleus. Misuse and truncation mutations of the DNA binding or the steroid ($1,25[OH]_2D_3$) binding portions of the vitamin D receptor have been found. This form of the disease, which is particularly prevalent among children of 1st-cousin marriages, is termed *vitamin D dependence, type II,* or *hereditary resistance to $1,25(OH)_2D$.* Some patients have short stature and alopecia totalis. Rickets can sometimes be reversed by administration of 15–30 μg/24 hr of $1,25(OH)_2D$, but missing hair does not regrow.

CHAPTER 713
Oncogenous Rickets

(Primary Hypophosphatemic Rickets Associated with Tumor)

Rickets associated with a tumor of mesenchymal origin that resolves on removal of the tumor has been described in more than 90 cases. These tumors, which cause a phosphate-deficient form of rickets, are mostly benign, may become apparent only years after the development of rickets, and may be located in sites difficult to detect, such as the small bones of the hands and feet, the abdominal sheath, the nasal antrum, and the pharynx. This syndrome is also associated with the epidermal nevus syndrome, neurofibromatosis (von Recklinghausen disease), and linear nevus syndrome.

In addition to hypophosphatemia and hyperphosphaturia, glycinemia and glycinuria are sometimes found in this form of rickets. Evidence suggests that these tumors elaborate PEX, the phosphate-regulating gene product, which causes phosphaturia and impairs the conversion of 25(OH)D to $1,25(OH)_2D$. Serum 25(OH)D levels are normal, and serum $1,25(OH)_2D$ levels are low but rapidly rise to normal after tumor excision. Hypophosphatemia in this syndrome may be caused by ectopic production by tumor cells of a heat-labile factor with a molecular mass of 8–25 kD, which inhibits renal tubular reabsorption of phosphate. Surgery also cures the bone pain and myopathy, which, if untreated, may confine the child to a wheelchair. Children with acquired or late-appearing hypophosphatemic rickets should undergo bone roentgenographic examination or bone scan to search for tumors. If a tumor cannot be removed or is metastatic, treatment with $1,25(OH)_2D$ and oral phosphate is often beneficial.

PART XXXII

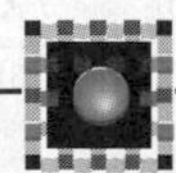

Unclassified Diseases

CHAPTER 714
Sudden Infant Death Syndrome

Carl E. Hunt

Sudden infant death syndrome (SIDS) is defined as the sudden death of an infant that is unexpected by history and unexplained by a thorough postmortem examination that includes a complete autopsy, investigation of the scene of death, and review of the medical history. An autopsy is essential in all sudden and unexpected infant deaths because the history and scene investigation do not preclude all known causes of sudden infant death (e.g., congenital cardiac or brain abnormalities and fatal child abuse) (Fig. 714–1).

SIDS has been recognized since biblical times. It is the most common cause of infant mortality in the United States after congenital anomalies and disorders relating to short gestation/low birthweight. SIDS is the most common cause of postneonatal infant mortality in developed countries, accounting for 35–55% of infant deaths between 1 mo and 1 yr of age (postneonatal infant mortality) and about 20% of all deaths in infants discharged from a neonatal intensive care unit (NICU). About 3,000 infants in the United States in 1996 died of SIDS, a rate of 0.74/1,000 live births. In full-term infants, SIDS is rare before 1 mo of age, the peak incidence is 2–4 mo, and 95% of all cases have occurred by 6 mo of age.

PATHOLOGY. The autopsy findings in SIDS victims are very subtle and yield only supportive, rather than conclusive, findings to explain SIDS. Mild pulmonary edema and diffuse intrathoracic petechiae are observed. Autopsy studies demonstrate structural evidence (tissue markers) of chronic asphyxia in nearly two thirds of SIDS victims. Infants discharged from a NICU and especially infants with a prior clinical diagnosis of bronchopulmonary dysplasia may have residual pulmonary abnormalities at autopsy, but a diagnosis of SIDS can nevertheless be established whenever the findings are not sufficient to explain a sudden and unexpected death.

Brain stem abnormalities in SIDS victims include focal astrogliosis, persistent dendritic spines, and hypomyelination. The primary areas of persisting brain stem dendritic spines are in the magnocellular nucleus of the reticular formation and dorsal and solitary nuclei of the vagal nerve. Significant increases in the number of reactive astrocytes in the medulla also have been observed in SIDS victims; these increases are not confined to areas related to respiratory neuroregulation. Substance P, a neuropeptide transmitter found in selected sensory neurons of the central nervous system, is present in increased amounts in the pons of SIDS victims. Quantitative three-dimensional anatomic studies indicate that a small subset of SIDS victims

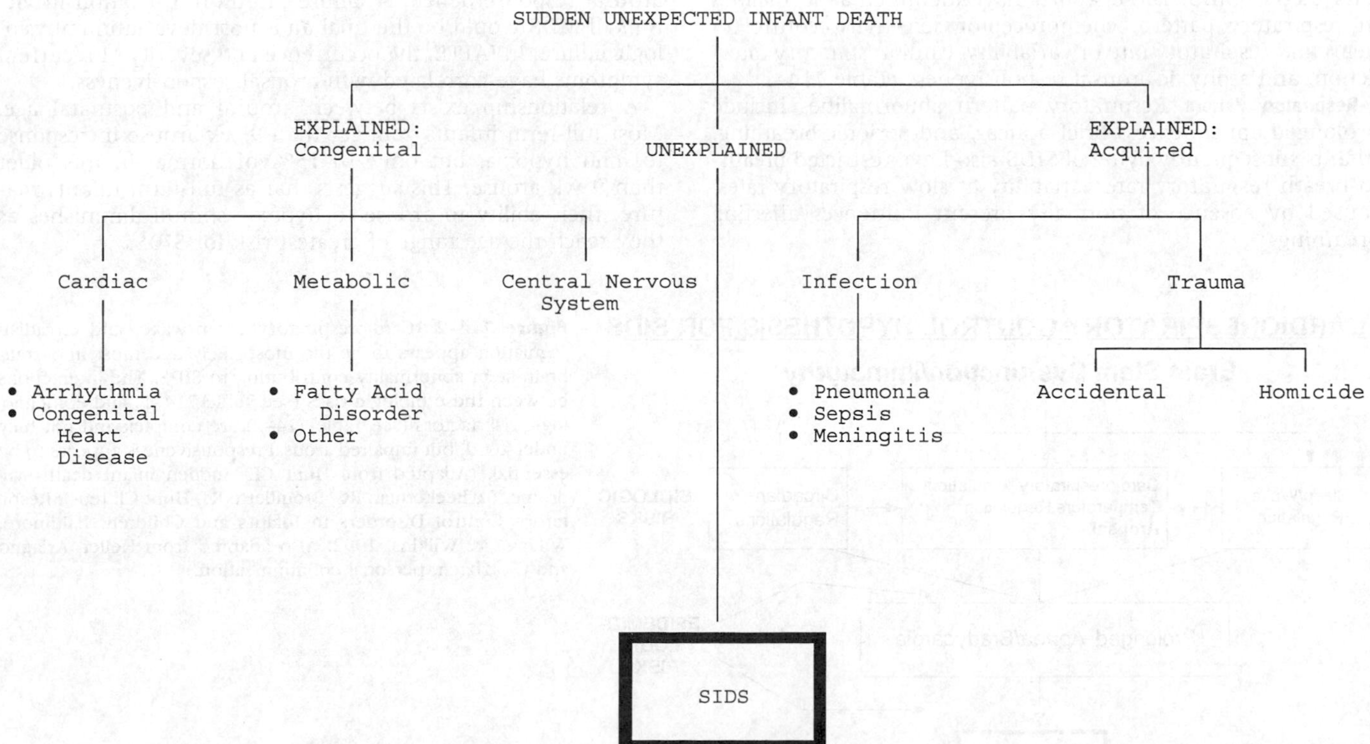

Figure 714–1 Differential diagnosis of sudden, unexpected death during infancy. An autopsy is necessary in order to exclude important but clinically undiagnosed congenital and acquired abnormalities. (Adapted from Hunt CE: Apnea and SIDS. Kliegman RM, Nieder ML, Super DM [eds]: *In:* Practical Strategies in Pediatric Diagnosis and Therapy. Philadelphia, WB Saunders, 1996.)

have hypoplasia of the arcuate nucleus; this region is a site of cardiorespiratory control in the ventral medulla and is integrated with other regions that regulate arousal and autonomic and chemosensory function. Neurotransmitter studies have also identified receptor abnormalities in the arcuate nucleus; significant decreases in binding to kainate receptors and muscarinic cholinergic receptors have been observed in some SIDS victims; and there is a positive correlation between decreased density of muscarinic cholinergic and kainate receptors. The neurotransmitter deficit in the arcuate nucleus in SIDS victims thus involves more than one receptor type relevant to carbon dioxide and blood pressure. Finally, tyrosine hydroxylase immunoreactivity in two brain stem areas, vagal nuclei and area reticularis superficialis ventrolateralis, suggests that adrenaline and noradrenaline neurons are altered in SIDS victims.

Other postmortem observations also suggest pre-existing, low-grade, chronic asphyxia. SIDS infants as a group have both prenatal and postnatal growth retardation and elevated blood cortisol levels. Elevated levels of hypoxanthine in vitreous humor have been reported in SIDS victims, suggesting a relatively long period of tissue hypoxia preceding the death. Because adenosine, a precursor of hypoxanthine, is a respiratory inhibitor, these observations thus indicate a potentially important interaction between asphyxia and hypoventilation; in response to asphyxia due to any cause, the secondary acceleration of adenosine monophosphate (AMP) catabolism and adenosine accumulation stimulate and then perpetuate hypoventilation, and hence, a vicious cycle may occur.

PATHOPHYSIOLOGY. The most compelling hypothesis to explain SIDS is a brain stem abnormality in cardiorespiratory control, including arousal responsiveness, and perhaps other autonomic controls such as blood pressure and sleep-wake regulation (Fig. 714–2). The postmortem data are consistent with this hypothesis. The clinical data to support this hypothesis were initially inferred from assessments of patients with idiopathic apparent life-threatening events (IALTE) or other infants at increased epidemiologic risk for SIDS (preterm infants, subsequent siblings of a previous SIDS victim), a few of whom later died of SIDS. These studies have identified abnormalities in respiratory pattern, chemoreceptor sensitivity, control of heart and respiratory rate or variability, cardiorespiratory interaction, and asphyxic arousal responsiveness (Table 714–1).

Respiratory Pattern. Respiratory pattern abnormalities include prolonged apnea, excess brief apneas, and periodic breathing. Infants subsequently dying of SIDS also have restricted breath-to-breath respiratory rate variability at slow respiratory rates, caused by absence of normally present influences affecting breathing.

TABLE 714–1 Biologic Risk Factors

Biologic markers or risk factors associated with SIDS. Interaction(s) with one or more epidemiologic risk factors (Table 714–2) are probably important, but such interactions are complex and not well understood:

Family history of SIDS
Idiopathic apparent life-threatening event (IALTE)
Prematurity
Deficient brain stem function:
- Arousal/gasping
- Ventilatory responsiveness
- Respiratory pattern
- Cardiac control
- Temperature regulation
- Other autonomic deficit(s), e.g., vagal tone, blood pressure

Hypothetical: Metabolic
- Infectious/inflammatory
- Immune

Chemoreceptor Sensitivity. Some infants at increased risk for SIDS have diminished ventilatory responsiveness to hypercarbia or hypoxia. However, chemoreceptor sensitivity studies have generally not been performed in preterm infants. Assessments of cardiorespiratory responses are too costly and time consuming for routine clinical use, and the extent of individual overlap between normal and at-risk infants precludes accurate identification of those infants who will later die of SIDS.

Arousal Responses. Absent arousal responsiveness renders infants incapable of responding effectively to sleep-related asphyxia, regardless of its cause. Infants at increased epidemiologic risk for SIDS (IALTE, preterm infants, and subsequent siblings of SIDS victims) and who have diminished ventilatory responsiveness to hypercarbia or hypoxia usually have a concomitant abnormality in hypercarbic or hypoxic arousal responsiveness. A deficit in arousal responsiveness may be a necessary prerequisite for SIDS to occur but may be insufficient to cause SIDS in the absence of other biologic or environmental risk factors. Victims of SIDS may also have deficient autoresuscitation (gasping) as a complement to the asphyxic arousal response deficit. A failure of autoresuscitation in victims of SIDS would be the final and most devastating physiologic failure. In IALTE, the occurrence and severity of recurrent symptoms have correlated with arousal responsiveness.

A relationship exists between arousal and postnatal age. Most full-term infants younger than 9 wk arouse in response to mild hypoxia, but only 10–15% of normal infants older than 9 wk arouse. This suggests that as full-term infants mature, their ability to arouse to hypoxic stimuli diminishes as they reach the age range of greatest risk for SIDS.

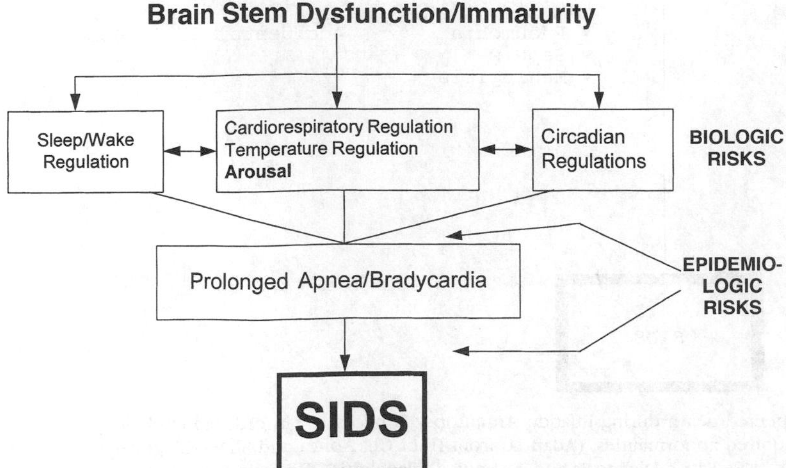

Figure 714–2 Cardiorespiratory, sleep/wake, and circadian regulation appears to be the most likely and most important brain stem abnormality contributing to SIDS. The interactions between these biologic risks (see Table 714-1) and epidemiologic risk factors (see Table 714-2) are complex and not fully understood, but impaired arousal responsiveness appears to be essential. (Adapted from Hunt CE: Sudden infant death syndrome. *In:* Beckerman RC, Brouillette RT, Hunt CE [eds]: Respiratory Control Disorders in Infants and Children. Baltimore, Williams & Wilkins, 1992. Also adapted from Heller, Ariagno and Glotzbach, personal communication.)

Current methods for assessing arousal responsiveness in infants are cumbersome and time consuming. Further, the overlap in individual values for healthy term controls and for infants at increased epidemiologic risk for SIDS prevents prospective identification of infants destined to die of SIDS.

Temperature Regulation. Increased body or environmental temperature is associated with SIDS. There are complex interactions between temperature regulation and cardiorespiratory control. The increased sleep-related sweating that does occur in some patients with IALTE may be caused by alveolar hypoventilation and secondary asphyxia, by autonomic dysfunction as part of a more generalized deficiency in brain stem function, or by overheating.

Cardiac Control. The ability to shorten Q-T interval as heart rate increases is impaired in some SIDS victims, suggesting that such infants may be predisposed to ventricular arrhythmias. Infants later dying of SIDS have higher heart rates in all sleep-waking states and diminished heart rate variability during wakefulness. Infants with SIDS also have significantly lower heart rate variation at a given respiratory frequency across all sleep-waking cycles than do normal infants. Even in early infancy, therefore, future SIDS victims differ in the extent to which cardiac and respiratory activity are coupled.

Part of the decreased heart rate variability and increased heart rate observed in infants who later die of SIDS may be related to decreased vagal tone. This could be related to vagal neuropathy, to brain stem damage in areas responsible for parasympathetic control of the heart, or to other factors. Furthermore, because the greatest reduction in all types of heart rate variability occurs while an infant is awake, these reductions may be related to the reduced mobility retrospectively reported in SIDS victims and observed in infants at increased risk for SIDS.

Home cardiorespiratory monitors with memory capability have recorded some terminal events in SIDS victims. In most instances, there has been sudden and rapid progression of severe bradycardia, too soon to be explained by progressive desaturation from prolonged central apnea. These observations are consistent with an abnormality in autonomic control of heart rate variability or with hypoxemia secondary to obstructive apnea as the precipitating mechanism for the severe bradycardia.

EPIDEMIOLOGY. No epidemiologic differences have been of sufficient sensitivity and specificity to permit prospective identification of SIDS victims. It is not possible to determine the relative importance of each individual risk factor or to measure the effect of combinations of risk factors (Table 714–2). Some of these factors are likely surrogates for more fundamental risk factors, and some are probably duplicative.

An increased SIDS risk is associated with numerous obstetric factors, suggesting that the in utero environment of future SIDS victims is suboptimal. Maternal smoking during pregnancy significantly increases the risk for SIDS; infants of smoking mothers also appear to die at a younger age. The risk of death is progressively greater as daily cigarette exposure increases and as the degree of maternal anemia worsens. Maternal smoking may potentiate hyperplasia of pulmonary neuroendocrine cells, and dysfunction of these cells may contribute to the pathophysiology of SIDS. Both animal and clinical studies indicate decreased ventilatory and arousal responsiveness to hypoxia secondary to fetal exposure to nicotine. The age-specific attenuation of hypoxic defenses following nicotine exposure focuses attention on brain catecholamine metabolism as a potential target for adverse fetal and neonatal influences.

Relative growth failure is evident postnatally and prenatally. The numbers of postneonatal regular care visits and of immunizations are significantly fewer in SIDS victims than in normal infants, suggesting that postneonatal care is also suboptimal. SIDS is associated with illnesses in the last two weeks of life and an increased frequency of doctor's office visits in the preceding week, especially for gastrointestinal illness or a droopy or listless appearance. Future SIDS victims have also been observed to have repeated fatigue during feedings and profuse sweating during sleep. The fatigue is unexplained except insofar as it may be secondary to an intercurrent acute illness. The sweating may be explained by intercurrent febrile illness or by thermal stress related to prone sleep position or overbundling but could also be indicative of an autonomic deficit.

Clinical Risk Groups (Table 714–3). Infants with an IALTE are at increased risk for SIDS. There is no consensus about the magnitude of this risk, but history of an IALTE has been reported in about 5% of SIDS victims. The risk of SIDS appears to be increased in infants with two or more IALTE, but no definitive incidence rates are available. There are no data about the extent, if any, to which home monitoring or any other intervention might decrease the risk of SIDS in infants with IALTE. Although most estimates indicate that at least 90–95%

TABLE 714–2 Epidemiologic Factors Associated with Increased Risk For SIDS

Uncertainty persists about which factors are causal, independent risks for SIDS. The extent and importance of interactions with biologic risk factors (Table 714–1) are not fully understood. From a practical perspective, only a few risk factors are modifiable.

Maternal and Antenatal Risk Factors

- Intrauterine hypoxia
- Fetal growth retardation
- Urinary tract infection
- Smoking
- Anemia
- Drug exposure (e.g., cocaine, heroin)
- Nutritional deficiency
- Less prenatal care
- Low socioeconomic status
- Decreased age, education
- Increased placental weight
- Increased parity
- Shorter interpregnancy interval

Infant Risk Factors

- Age (peak 2–4 mo)
- Asphyxia
- Bottle feeding
- Growth failure
- Male gender
- No pacifier (dummy)
- Prone (and side) sleep position
- Recent (febrile) illness
- Smoking exposure (fetal and postnatal)
- Soft sleeping surface, soft bedding
- Thermal stress

Other Risk Factors

- Colder season and climate; noncentral heating
- Race/ethnicity (e.g., African or Native American, Gypsy, Maori, Hawaiian, Filipino)

TABLE 714–3 General Incidence of SIDS in Infant Groups at Increased Epidemiologic Risk for SIDS*

Risk Group	Incidence of SIDS
Idiopathic apparent life-threatening event	Risk increased 3–5 times
Siblings	Risk increased at least 4–5 times
Preterm infants:	
1,500–2,499 g birthweight	Relative risk (RR) 2.64†
1,000–1,499 g birthweight	RR 3.68†
Racial:	
African-Americans	RR 1.7–2.0‡
Native Americans	RR 2.1‡
Intrauterine drug exposure	Risk increased 3–5 times

**The incidence of SIDS in the United States in 1996 was 0.74 deaths/1,000 live births.*
†RR 1.0 for full-term infants.
‡RR 1.0 for whites.

of all sudden, unexpected, and unexplained infant deaths are caused by SIDS, subsequent confessions or covert video recordings have confirmed that life-threatening or fatal child abuse can also be the cause of sudden and unexpected infant death. Filicide needs to be considered whenever the history, autopsy, or scene investigation yields suspicious findings.

Both recurrence risks for SIDS and for infant mortality from other causes are increased in subsequent siblings and to the same extent, 20.8 deaths/1,000 infants at risk. Among all second sibling deaths in families, the relative risk of dying of the same cause is 9.1 and of a dissimilar cause is 1.6. Epidemiologic studies of subsequent siblings indicate a wide range in the observed relative risk for repeat SIDS, 3.7–16.7. A familial metabolic disorder should be considered in families with more than one unexplained infant death, especially when the history is atypical for SIDS.

Numerous studies have identified low birthweight as a risk factor for SIDS. There is an inverse relationship between risk for SIDS and birthweight/gestational age. Below 1,000 g birthweight, however, the risk for SIDS has been observed to be less than in preterm infants weighing more than 1,000 g at birth, likely reflecting increasing reluctance to diagnose SIDS as the cause of death as the frequency and severity of (unrelated) autopsy abnormalities progressively increase. SIDS, however, should still be the correct diagnosis whenever the death was sudden, unexpected, and unexplained by the abnormalities found at autopsy. The epidemiologic characterists of preterm infants dying of SIDS are not substantially different from those observed in full-term infants, but the postnatal age of preterm infants dying of SIDS is about 5–7 wk older and the postconceptional age is 4–6 wks younger than for full-term infants. Early reports suggested a relationship between bronchopulmonary dysplasia (BPD) and risk for SIDS, but a prospective controlled study reported comparable incidences of IALTE in BPD and matched preterm infants and no deaths from SIDS among the 78 infants with BPD and 78 control preterm infants.

Infants with prenatal drug exposure to methadone, heroin, or cocaine also appear to have an increased risk of SIDS. There are no data to indicate to what extent, if any, the presence of additional risk factors for SIDS, such as prematurity, is contributory.

All studies of SIDS incidence show significantly higher rates in black infants than in white infants in the United States, independent of any other factors such as low birthweight, young maternal age, or high parity. Native Americans have a birthweight-specific SIDS rate that is at least as high as in black infants. SIDS rates in other racial groups in the United States are comparable or better than in white infants, but assimilation into the United States culture may be associated with increased rates to levels comparable to those observed in black Americans and Native Americans. Some ethnic groups in other countries also have increased SIDS rates, including Gypsy, Maori, Hawaiian, and Filipino infants.

Sleeping Position. A national back-to-sleep campaign was initiated in the United States in mid-1994 to advocate side or back sleeping during early infancy. The stimulus for this campaign was the aggregate experience from other countries of decrease of 50% or more in rates of SIDS after dramatic declines in prevalence of the prone sleep position to 10% or less. Prone prevalence rates in the United States progressively decreased from a high of 70–80% before 1992 and about 55% just before the campaign to the 18–30% range in 1996–1997 (1 and 3 mo of age, respectively). This significant decrease in prone prevalence was associated with a decrease in SIDS rates of about 35%, compared with an average annual decrease before 1992 of only about 2%. Annual SIDS rates thus decreased from 1.33/1,000 live births in 1989–1991 to 1.22/1,000 in 1993 and most recently to 0.74/1,000 (provisional) in 1996.

The initial back-to-sleep campaign recommendations considered side sleeping to be nearly equivalent to the supine position in reducing the risk of SIDS. More recently, however, epidemiologic data have identified both prone and side sleeping as risk factors for SIDS, with odds ratios (OR) of 13.9 and 3.5, respectively. The current back-to-sleep recommendations thus call for supine position for sleeping in all infants without medical contraindications (e.g., micrognathia or obstructive sleep apnea).

Preterm infants were initially excluded from all back-to-sleep campaigns. This exclusion was based on accumulated data at younger postnatal ages indicating that ventilation was optimal when sleeping prone, especially in the presence of lung disease. Epidemiologic studies, however, have now confirmed that preterm infants are also at greater risk for SIDS when sleeping prone or side; the OR for birthweights less than 2,500 g were 83 and 36.6 for prone and side, respectively. The current recommendation, therefore, is that supine should be the recommended sleeping position for all preterm infants and that supine sleeping should begin in the hospital before discharge from the NICU. Prone prevalence in the United States in 1997 among preterm infants less than 1,700 g birthweight remained significantly higher than in full-term infants, 30% and 18%, respectively.

The mechanism for the epidemiologic association between decreased prone/side prevalence and decreased risk for SIDS has not been established. However, there may be an interaction between prone/side sleep position and impaired cardiorespiratory control, especially impaired ventilatory and arousal responsiveness. Face-down or nearly face-down sleeping does occasionally occur in prone-sleeping infants and can result in episodes of airway obstruction and asphyxia in healthy full-term infants. These healthy infants all aroused before the face-down or face-nearly-down position became life-threatening, but infants with insufficient arousal responsiveness to asphyxia would be at risk for fatal asphyxia. Sleeping on a very soft surface would further increase the risk of life-threatening asphyxia in the face-down or nearly-down sleeping position. Some investigators attribute the risk of prone sleeping to thermal stress, hypothesizing that (face-down) prone sleeping causes a clinically significant degree of thermal stress. Any thermal stress could further compromise infants with deficient cardiorespiratory control. There thus may be links between epidemiologic risk factors such as soft bedding, prone sleep position, and thermal stress and biologic risk factors such as cardiorespiratory control deficits (e.g., arousal and temperature/metabolic control deficits).

As prone prevalence has decreased, prenatal and postnatal exposure to tobacco smoke has emerged as an important risk factor for SIDS. Elimination just of prenatal smoking exposure could theoretically reduce the risk of SIDS an additional 30%. The effect of prenatal smoking on SIDS rates does not appear to be mediated through an effect on birthweight. Bed sharing also has been a significant risk factor for SIDS in some studies and has been linked to mothers who smoke. Soft bedding, covers over the head, and sleeping under a comforter (duvet) have also emerged as more significant risk factors as prone prevalence has decreased.

PROSPECTIVE IDENTIFICATION. A major objective of SIDS research is to develop a screening test capable of accurately identifying those infants destined to die of SIDS. To be valid and practical, such a test must have a negligible false-negative rate and an acceptable false-positive rate. The pneumogram and polysomnogram (PSG) screening studies performed prospectively have focused primarily on respiratory pattern or cardiac abnormalities, and none has demonstrated sufficient sensitivity and specificity to be clinically useful as a screening test.

The extent to which incomplete maturation in cardiorespiratory control contributes to risk for IALTE or for SIDS remains unresolved. It is not known whether having a cardiorespiratory pattern value outside the 95th percentile has any clinical significance, nor is it known whether infants with a prior history of apnea of prematurity are at greater risk for SIDS than gestational age–matched infants without such a history. Even though 18.5% of SIDS victims are premature and the risk of SIDS progressively increases as birthweight decreases, those preterm infants destined to die of SIDS cannot be accurately identified prospectively.

New technologies using event recordings now permit home memory monitoring that can include respiratory pattern, heart rate, electrocardiography, and oxygenation. Thus, it is possible now to obtain ongoing home assessments of cardiorespiratory pattern. It is still not possible, however, to identify any specific cardiorespiratory pattern associated with increased risk for an IALTE or for SIDS.

INTERVENTION. The apnea hypothesis led to the hope that home electronic surveillance would reduce the risk for SIDS. Even though respiratory pattern abnormalities may not be a critical component of the cardiorespiratory control abnormalities that contribute to the risk for SIDS, home monitoring could still be effective if bradycardia or desaturation representative of life-threatening conditions were occurring sufficiently early to be amenable to intervention.

A major problem related to determining the efficacy of home monitoring has been uncertainty about the extent of monitor use or compliance. Anecdotal postmortem interviews with parents of SIDS victims dying with a monitor in the home have suggested that 50% or more of such families were not using the home monitor at the time death occurred. Fewer than 10% of monitor alarms are related to physiologic events; initial parental difficulties with movement, a loose lead, or other nonsignificant alarms may easily lead to parental frustration and noncompliance. Using memory monitors to identify and minimize problems with frequent false alarms in a timely manner should improve family compliance with recommended monitor use. Using memory monitors to document compliance and to identify cardiorespiratory patterns associated with true events, studies can now be performed to evaluate whether home electronic surveillance is effective in preventing life-threatening events and SIDS.

Both caffeine and theophylline have been used in apnea of prematurity and IALTE. Both of these methylxanthines improve respiratory pattern and reduce the frequency and severity of clinical symptoms. Caffeine has been observed to decrease the auditory arousal threshold in young adults, but there are no systematic evaluations of methylxanthines in infants with deficient arousal responsiveness or in infants identified as at increased epidemiologic risk for SIDS.

General

Hunt CE. Sudden infant death syndrome. *In:* Beckerman RC, Brouillette RT, Hunt CE (eds): Respiratory Control Disorders in Infants and Children. Baltimore, Williams & Wilkins. 1992, pp 90–211.

Pathology

Cutz E, Perrin DG, Hackman R, et al: Maternal smoking and pulmonary neuroendocrine cells in sudden infant death syndrome. Pediatrics 98:668, 1996.

Obonai T, Yasuhara M, Nakamura T, et al: Catecholamine neuron alteration in the brainstem of sudden infant death syndrome victims. Pediatrics 101:285, 1998.

Panigrahy A, Filiano JJ, Sleeper LA, et al: Decreased kainate receptor binding in the arcuate nucleus of the sudden infant death syndrome. J Neuropathol Exp Neurol 56:1253, 1997.

Pathophysiology

Hunt CE: Prone sleeping in healthy infants and victims of sudden infant death syndrome. J Pediatr 128:594, 1996.

Lewis KW, Bosque EM: Deficient hypoxia awakening response in infants of smoking mothers. J Pediatr 127:691, 1995.

Meny RG, Carroll JL, Carbone MT, et al: Cardiorespiratory recordings from infants dying suddenly and unexpectedly at home. Pediatrics 93:44, 1994.

Milerad J, Walsh WF: Nicotine attenuates the ventilatory response to hypoxia in the developing lamb. Pediatr Res 37:652, 1995.

Schechtman VL, Lee M, Wilson AJ, et al: Dynamics of respiratory patterning in normal infants and infants who subsequently died of the sudden infant death syndrome. Pediatr Res 40:571, 1996.

Southall DP, Plunkett MCB, Banks MW, et al: Covert video records of life-threatening child abuse: Lessons for child protection. Pediatrics 100:735, 1997.

Waters KA, Gonzales AJC, Morielli A, et al: Face-straight-down and face-near-straight-down positions in healthy, prone-sleeping infants. J Pediatr 128:616, 1996.

Epidemiology

Blair PS, Fleming PJ, Bensley D, et al: Smoking and the sudden infant death syndrome: Results from 1993–5 case-control study for confidential inquiry into stillbirths and deaths in infancy. Br Med J 313:195, 1996.

Fleming PJ, Blair PS, Bacon C, et al: Environment of infants during sleep and risk of the sudden infant death syndrome: Results of 1993–5 case-control study for confidential inquiry into stillbirths and deaths in infancy. Br Med J 313:191, 1996.

Guyer B, Martin JA, MacDorman MF, et al: Annual summary of vital statistics—1996. Pediatrics 100:905, 1997.

Lesko SM, Corwin MJ, Vezina RM, et al: Sleep position in infancy: A report from the Infant Care Practices Study. JAMA 280:336, 1998.

MacDorman MF, Cnattingius S, Hoffman HJ, et al: Sudden infant death syndrome and smoking in the United States and Sweden. Am J Epidemiol 146:249, 1997.

Malloy MH, Hoffman HJ: Prematurity, sudden infant death syndrome, and age of death. Pediatrics 96:464, 1995.

Mitchell EA, Tuohy PG, Brunt JM, et al: Risk factors for sudden infant death syndrome following the prevention campaign in New Zealand: A prospective study. Pediatrics 100:835, 1997.

Oyen N, Markestad T, Skjaerven R, et al: Combined effects of sleeping position and prenatal risk factors in sudden infant death syndrome: The Nordic epidemiological SIDS study. Pediatrics 100:613, 1997.

Oyen N, Skjaerven R, Irgens LM: Population-based recurrence risk of sudden infant death syndrome compared with other infant and fetal deaths. Am J Epidermiol 144:300, 1996.

Sawczenko A, Fleming PH: Thermal stress, sleeping position, and the sudden infant death syndrome. Sleep 19:S267, 1996.

Schwartz PJ, Stramba-Badrale M, Segantini A, et al: Prolongation of the QT interval and the sudden infant death syndrome. N Engl J Med 338:1709, 1998.

Taylor JA, Krieger JW, Reay DT, et al: Prone sleep position and SIDS in King County, Washington. J Pediatr 128:626, 1996.

Willinger M, Hoffman HJ, Wu KT, et al: Factors associated with the transitions to non-prone sleep position in the United States. JAMA 280:329, 1998.

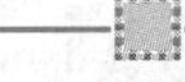

CHAPTER 715
Sarcoidosis

Margaret W. Leigh

Sarcoidosis, a chronic multisystem granulomatous disease of unknown cause, occurs most frequently in young adults but can occur during childhood. The initial clinical presentation is extremely variable, depending on the organ systems involved, but in most pediatric cases includes weight loss, cough, fatigue, bone and joint pain, and anemia. Definitive diagnosis requires demonstration of the characteristic noncaseating granulomatous lesions in an appropriate biopsy specimen. The granulomas in sarcoidosis resemble those caused by microbial agents (e.g., mycobacteria and fungi) or by hypersensitivity to organic agents. These similarities have led to speculation that microbes or organic dusts may be inciting agents. However, despite extensive studies, the etiology remains obscure.

Sarcoidosis has a worldwide distribution involving all ethnic groups; however, in the southeastern United States, sarcoidosis occurs more frequently in black Americans than in whites. Familial clustering of this disease has been observed and suggests a genetic predisposition; however, the mode of inheritance is unclear.

PATHOLOGY. The granulomatous lesions of sarcoidosis may occur in almost any organ of the body. Typically, the granulomas are not necrotic and contain epithelioid cells, macrophages, and giant cells in the center surrounded by a mixture of monocytes, lymphocytes, and fibroblasts. Activated lymphocytes and macrophages within the granulomas release various mediators, such as interleukin-1, interleukin-2, interferon, and other cytokines, that are thought to promote and maintain granulomatous lesions. During active disease, lymphocytes in and around the granulomas are predominantly helper T (CD4) lymphocytes. These lesions usually heal with complete preservation of the parenchyma; however, in approximately 20% of the lesions, fibroblasts proliferate at the periphery of the granuloma and may produce fibrotic scar tissue. Macrophages within sarcoidosis granulomas produce and secrete 1,25-$(OH)_2$-D_3, the active form of vitamin D typically produced in the kidneys. Excess vitamin D results in hypercalcemia and hypercalciuria in patients with sarcoidosis.

CLINICAL MANIFESTATIONS. In adults and children, the lung is the most frequently affected organ; pulmonary involvement is variable in its extent and characteristics. Parenchymal infiltrates, miliary nodules, and hilar and paratracheal lymphadenopathy (Fig. 715–1) occur. Pulmonary function tests primarily show restrictive changes. Peripheral lymphadenopathy, eye changes consisting of uveitis or iritis, skin lesions, and hepatic involvement occur frequently. Very young children (<4 yr old) have a distinct form of sarcoidosis consisting of a maculopapular erythematous rash, uveitis, and arthritis but minimal to no pulmonary changes. The arthritis, which can be confused with rheumatoid arthritis, produces large, painless, boggy synovial effusions of the tendon sheaths; there is little limitation of motion.

DIAGNOSIS. There are no specific diagnostic tests. An elevated erythrocyte sedimentation rate, hyperproteinemia, hypercalcemia, hypercalciuria, eosinophilia, and an elevated angiotensin-converting enzyme level are common. The Kveim test, consisting of intradermal injection of material from a sarcoid lesion and observation for the formation of a granuloma several weeks later, is used infrequently for diagnosis because of difficulty in obtaining a standardized test material and reports of varying sensitivity and specificity of the test. Biopsy of tissue from affected areas is the most valuable diagnostic measure. Significant eye disease and renal damage from hypercalciuria can occur without symptoms; therefore, all patients with sarcoidosis should be evaluated at the initial presentation and monitored at regular intervals for evidence of ocular disease and hypercalciuria.

Because of its protean manifestations, the *differential diagnosis* of sarcoidosis is extremely broad; it includes tuberculosis, the various pulmonary mycoses, lymphoma, Crohn disease, and inflammatory ocular lesions such as phlyctenular conjunctivitis.

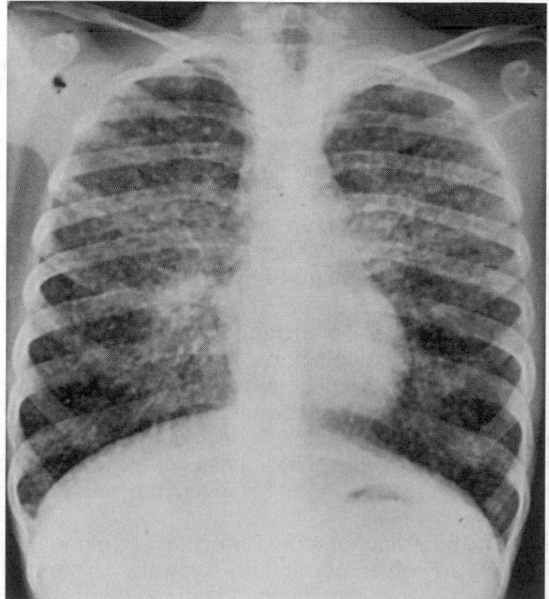

Figure 715–1 Sarcoidosis in a white 10-yr-old girl. There are widely disseminated peribronchial infiltrations, multiple small nodular densities, hyperaeration of the lungs, and hilar adenopathy.

TREATMENT. Treatment is symptomatic and supportive. Adrenal corticosteroids may suppress the acute manifestations, especially the inflammatory ocular lesions, progressive pulmonary disease, and hypercalcemia/hypercalciuria. Pulmonary function tests are useful in following the progress of lung involvement, and angiotensin-converting enzyme levels have been shown to correlate with disease activity.

The prognosis and natural history of sarcoidosis in children are uncertain. Spontaneous recovery may occur after a prolonged illness of several months to several years, or the condition may be very chronic, involving progressive lung disease. Eye involvement may lead to blindness.

Fink CW, Cimaz R: Early onset sarcoidosis: Not a benign disease. J Rheumatol 24:174, 1997.

Newman LS, Rose CS, Maier LA: Sarcoidosis. N Engl J Med 336:1224, 1997.

Pattishall EN, Kendig EL Jr: Sarcoidosis in children. Pediatr Pulmonol 22:195, 1996.

Sharma OP: Vitamin D, calcium, and sarcoidosis. Chest 109:535, 1996.

CHAPTER 716
Progeria

W. Ted Brown

Progeria is of considerable interest because of its striking features, which resemble accelerated aging. First reported in 1886 by Hutchinson and Gilford in England, it is also referred to as the Hutchinson-Gilford syndrome and has now been reported more than 100 times. This rare syndrome has a reported incidence of approximately 1/8 million. As a result of severe failure to thrive, affected children do not become sexually mature and reproduce. Hence, parent-to-child transmission has not been observed. Although two sets of identical twins have been noted, no examples of recurrence of classic progeria among siblings have been documented. Paternal age is significantly increased, but there is no increase in consanguinity, features associated with dominant mutations, and autosomal recessive inheritance, respectively. Therefore, each child with progeria most likely represents a new sporadic dominant mutation. The molecular basis of such mutations is unknown.

CLINICAL MANIFESTATIONS. Children with progeria usually appear normal in early infancy, but manifestations such as midfacial cyanosis, "sculpted nose," and "sclerodema" may suggest the existence of the syndrome at birth. Profound growth failure occurs during the 1st yr of life. The characteristic facies, alopecia, loss of subcutaneous fat, abnormal posture, stiffness of joints, and bone and skin changes usually become apparent during the 2nd yr of life (Fig. 716–1). Motor and mental development are normal. The clinical manifestations almost always present include short stature; weight distinctly low for height; diminished subcutaneous fat; head disproportionately large for face; micrognathia; prominent scalp veins; generalized alopecia; prominent eyes; delayed and abnormal dentition; pyriform thorax; short, dystrophic clavicles; "horse-riding" stance; wide-based shuffling gait; coxa valga, thin limbs, and prominent, stiff joints; and failure to complete sexual maturation.

Features frequently present are skin that is thin, taut, dry, wrinkled, and brown spotted in various areas; sclerodermatous

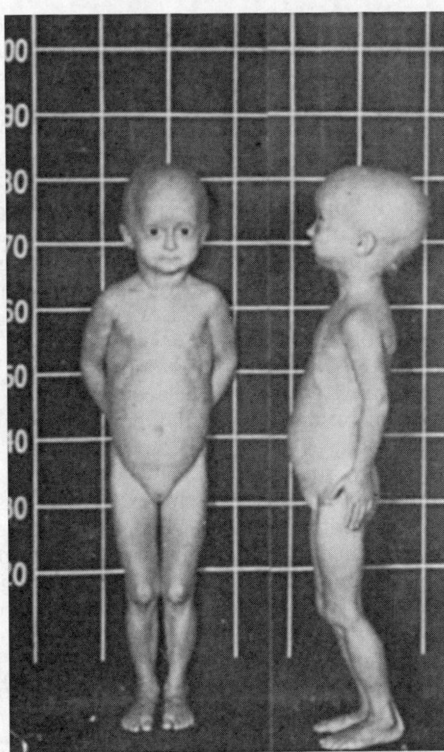

Figure 716–1 A 4.5-yr-old girl with height age of 1.75 yr and bone age of 4 yr. (From Wilkins L: Diagnosis and Treatment of Endocrine Disorders in Childhood and Adolescence, 3rd ed. Charles C Thomas, Springfield, IL, 1965.)

skin over the lower abdomen, proximal thighs, and buttocks; prominent superficial veins; loss of eyebrows and eyelashes; persistently patent anterior fontanel; sculpted, beaked nasal tip; faint nasolabial cyanosis; thin lips; protruding ears; absence of ear lobules; thin, high-pitched voice; dystrophic nails; and progressive radiolucency of the terminal phalanges and distal clavicles (acro-osteolysis). A *differential diagnosis* includes neonatal progeroid syndrome, Cockayne syndrome, Hallermann-Streif syndrome, and mandibular-acral dysplasia.

LABORATORY FINDINGS. Variable degrees of insulin resistance, occasionally insulin-dependent diabetes mellitus, abnormalities of collagen, increased metabolic rate, and inconsistent abnormalities of serum cholesterol and other lipids are found, but there are no demonstrable abnormalities of thyroid, parathyroid, pituitary, or adrenal function. Twenty-four-hour growth hormone levels are normal, but reduced levels of insulin-like growth factor I have been noted. Dramatically increased levels of hyaluronic acid occur in the urine of such patients. Variable decrease of DNA repair has also been observed.

PROGNOSIS. Children with progeria usually have severe atherosclerosis, and death occurs as a result of complications of cardiac or cerebrovascular disease generally between 5 and 20 yr, with a median life span of approximately 13 yr. Cataracts and tumors have infrequently been noted, but many changes associated with normal aging in adults such as presbycusis, presbyopia, arcus senilis, osteoarthritis, senile personality changes, or Alzheimer's disease are not found.

TREATMENT. No specific treatment for this condition exists. There is a progeria family support group. A Progeria Registry exists to help with diagnosis and to define more clearly the incidence and molecular basis of the disorder.

Abdenur JE, Brown WT, Friedman S, et al: Response to nutritional and growth hormone treatment in progeria. Metabolism 46:851, 1997.

Brown WT: Progeria: A human-disease model of accelerated aging. Am J Clin Nutr 55:122S, 1992.

DeBusk FL: The Hutchinson-Gilford progeria syndrome. J Pediatr 80:697, 1972.

CHAPTER 717

Chronic Fatigue Syndrome

Hal B. Jenson

Numerous terms (e.g., chronic mononucleosis, chronic Epstein-Barr virus [EBV] infection, and immune dysfunction syndrome) have been applied to the syndrome of easy fatigability associated with mild to debilitating somatic symptoms. This syndrome was formally defined by the Centers for Disease Control and Prevention (CDC) in 1988 as chronic fatigue syndrome because it is fatigue or profound tiredness that is the principal and invariable physical symptom. Chronic fatigue syndrome is neither a new disease nor the result of enhanced appreciation of previously unrecognized clinical illness. It is an illness that is the subjective experience of symptoms that encompass various clinical conditions of organic, psychologic, and mixed causes. No evidence shows that this is a single disease with characteristic physiologic or pathologic abnormalities or that it is caused by an identifiable etiologic agent, although the differential diagnosis includes many infectious and noninfectious diseases. Current understanding of this condition is derived largely from studies in adults and, to a lesser extent, in adolescents; little information is available about the existence of chronic fatigue syndrome in young children.

EPIDEMIOLOGY. Chronic fatigue is a common presenting symptom of adolescents and adults. Approximately 20% of adults in primary care clinics or in surveys complain of chronic fatigue; the incidence in children is unknown. Prevalence rates vary significantly, but chronic fatigue syndrome is encountered in all patient populations. The fatigue can be disabling. Most patients diagnosed with chronic fatigue syndrome are white, 25–45 yr of age, well educated, high achievers, and in above-average income brackets. These epidemiologic observations may be artifactual because assertive individuals may be less likely to accept being told by their physician that there is nothing physically wrong and are more likely to insist on referral to medical specialists. Women constitute 75% of patients. The minimum prevalence in the United States is estimated to be 4–10 cases/100,000 adults ≥18 yr of age. Most cases of chronic fatigue syndrome are sporadic and are not associated with secondary cases. No evidence shows that chronic fatigue syndrome can be transmitted from person to person, in utero to a fetus, or via donated blood.

PATHOGENESIS. The cause of chronic fatigue syndrome is unknown, and the hypothesis that infection with a known or new virus is the primary cause of the symptoms of chronic fatigue syndrome is unsubstantiated. However, most patients with chronic fatigue syndrome correlate the onset with a history of a virus-like illness such as infectious mononucleosis (EBV), influenza, varicella, or rubella or with nonspecific symptoms of sore throat, fever, myalgia, or diarrhea. In many cases, the clinical symptoms of depression, such as fatigue, lack of energy and interest, and inability to concentrate merge with or are intensified by the weakness often found during convalescence from a systemic infectious disease, resulting in disabling fatigue. Persistent fatigue after an otherwise uncomplicated primary infection is well recognized with many acute infections, especially EBV and influenza virus. Symptoms of fatigue and exhaustion may last for months to a few years and may be accompanied by signs of depression. Several studies of convalescence after acute systemic infection support the view that symptomatic recovery is critically dependent on the emotional state and attitude of the individual. Individuals with a propensity to succumb to illness are more likely to respond to acute infection with fatigue and depression-like symptoms than are individuals who do not have such vulnerability.

Several diverse and sometimes conflicting in vitro immunologic abnormalities (e.g., hypo- or hypergammaglobulinemia, immunoglobulin subclass deficiencies, elevated levels of circulating immune complexes, mild increased helper/suppressor lymphocyte ratios, natural killer cell dysfunction, monocyte dysfunction) have been reported in patients with chronic fatigue syndrome. A history of food, inhalant, or drug allergy is reported by approximately 67% of patients. No characteristic profile of immune dysfunction has been identified, and the magnitude of the immune abnormalities described is small and does not correlate with the severity of clinical symptoms.

CLINICAL MANIFESTATIONS. The symptoms of chronic fatigue syndrome are protean, with a spectrum of gradation from subtle to debilitating. Although the perception of fatigue is subjective and undoubtedly varies from individual to individual, fatigue as a symptom should not be dismissed as a minor ailment. The syndrome is characterized by numerous somatic complaints of at least 6 mo to several years' duration associated with significant impairment (below 50% of normal) of the work or school schedule, activities of daily living, exercise tolerance, and interpersonal relationships. Fatigue is generally manifested as lassitude, profound tiredness, weakness, intolerance to exertion with easy fatigability, significant sleeping during the day, and general malaise. Nocturnal sleeping is not usually changed and does not differ from that in unaffected individuals. Myalgias and low-grade fever in 50–95% of cases characteristically accompany fatigue. Headache and sore throat are common. A multitude of other physical symptoms (e.g., chest palpitations, visual blurring, nausea, dizziness, arthralgias, paresthesias, dry eyes and mouth, diarrhea, cough, night sweats, tender lymphadenopathy, rash) have been reported in 30–60% of cases. Emphasis on one particular physical symptom other than the constitutional symptoms of malaise and fatigability is somewhat uncommon and should prompt further investigation. Weight loss is uncommon in chronic fatigue syndrome. Symptoms of cognitive dysfunction are common and include confusion, difficulty in concentrating, impaired thinking, and forgetfulness. Adult patients often judge these as among the most debilitating symptoms.

Most patients diagnosed with chronic fatigue syndrome relate an abrupt onset to their symptoms, often as part of an initial virus-like illness characterized by low-grade fever accompanied by sore throat and cough. Less frequently, the initial symptoms indicate gastrointestinal tract involvement with nausea and diarrhea. Myalgia is a common symptom.

Symptoms in children appear to be similar to those in adolescents and adults. School absenteeism is a major problem. In a small retrospective study of 23 patients with a median age of 14 yr and a median duration of symptoms of 6 mo, 67% missed 2 wk or more of school and 33% required a home tutor.

Abnormal physical examination findings are conspicuously absent and provide reassurance to both the patient and the physician. Orthostatic intolerance with abnormal heart rate and blood pressure responses to tilt-table testing have been reported in adolescents diagnosed with chronic fatigue syndrome.

DIAGNOSIS. There are no pathognomonic signs or diagnostic tests for chronic fatigue syndrome; the diagnosis is a clinically defined condition based on inclusionary and exclusionary criteria (Fig. 717–1). Chronic fatigue syndrome is a diagnostic subset of chronic fatigue, a broader category defined as unexplained fatigue of 6 mo or longer, which in turn is a subset of prolonged fatigue, which is defined as fatigue lasting 1 mo or more.

Chronic fatigue syndrome is difficult to diagnose in children, who have trouble describing their symptoms and articulating their concerns. As with any chronic illness in childhood, careful attention must be directed to the family dynamics to identify and resolve family problems or psychopathology that may be contributing to a child's perceptions of his or her symptoms. The diagnosis of chronic fatigue syndrome in a child should be entertained with a great deal of caution. Applying the label of chronic fatigue syndrome may delay the diagnosis of a treatable medical illness, avoid the detection of psychologic problems or family dysfunction, and perpetuate inappropriate illness behaviors that may have a profound effect on the child's psychosocial development. Most patients, including children, with chronic fatigue syndrome attribute their symptoms to physical rather than psychologic causes.

The diagnosis of chronic fatigue syndrome can be made only after alternative medical and psychiatric causes of fatigue, many of which are treatable, have been excluded. These include any medical condition that may explain the presence of chronic fatigue, such as untreated hypothyroidism, sleep apnea, and narcolepsy, an adverse effect of medication, or severe obesity as defined by a body mass index [body mass index = weight in kg/ (height in meters)^2] of 45 or greater. A previously diagnosed medical condition whose resolution has not been documented and that may explain chronic fatigue should be clarified, such as unresolved cases of hepatitis B or C virus infection. The diagnosis of chronic fatigue syndrome should not be made in persons with prior diagnoses of a major depressive disorder with psychotic or melancholic features; bipolar affective disorders; schizophrenia of any subtype; delusional disorders of any subtype; dementias of any subtype; anorexia nervosa; bulimia nervosa; or alcohol or other substance abuse within 2 yr before the onset of the chronic fatigue or at any time afterward.

Fibromyalgia (fibrositis) is a relatively common rheumatic syndrome characterized by symptoms of chronic fatigue syndrome but with widespread musculoskeletal pain in addition to numerous specific tender point sites (see Chapter 168). Fibromyalgia may represent a subset of patients with chronic fatigue syndrome characterized by heightened musculoskeletal symptoms.

Although evaluation of each patient should be individualized, the initial laboratory evaluation should be limited to screening laboratory tests to provide reassurance of the lack of significant organic dysfunction (see Fig. 717–1). Further tests should be directed primarily toward excluding treatable diseases that may be suggested by the symptoms or physical findings that are present. Diagnostic evaluation of chronic fatigue should include psychologic evaluation for depression or anxiety disorders, which should precede exhaustive searches for organic causes.

TREATMENT. Development of definitive treatment for chronic fatigue syndrome awaits delineation of the causes of the symptoms. No specific therapeutic agents are recommended. No data suggest relief of symptoms or cure of chronic fatigue syndrome by dietary or vitamin supplements. Low-dose hydrocortisone is associated with some improvement in symptoms, but the associated adrenal suppression argues against its use. Therapy should be directed toward emotional support for patients and their families, relief of symptoms, and minimizing unnecessary and misleading diagnostic and therapeutic tests. This may include a combination of restoration of a normal sleep pattern, rehabilitation strategies including exercise for fatigue, and optimism. Psychologic or psychiatric intervention may be a principal component of supportive treatment.

Patients with severe limitation of activity should be started on a schedule of graded remobilization, determined by individual tolerance and, if warranted, physical therapy leading to a regular regimen of moderate exercise. Complete bed rest and lack of exercise only perpetuate immobility and lead to deconditioning; rapid remobilization, for whatever reason, usually exacerbates symptoms and should be avoided. Return to school should also be initiated gradually but systematically to

Clinical Evaluation and Classification of Chronic Fatigue

I. Clinically evaluate cases of chronic fatigue by:
  A. History and physical examination
  B. Mental status examination (abnormalities require appropriate psychiatric, psychologic, or neurologic examination)
  C. Tests (abnormal results that strongly suggest an exclusionary condition must be resolved)
    1. Screening lab tests: complete blood count, erythrocyte sedimentation rate, alanine aminotransferase, total protein, albumin, globulin, alkaline phosphatase, calcium, phosphorus, glucose, blood urea nitrogen, electrolytes, creatinine, thyroid stimulating hormone, and urinalysis
    2. Additional tests as clinically indicated to exclude other diagnosis

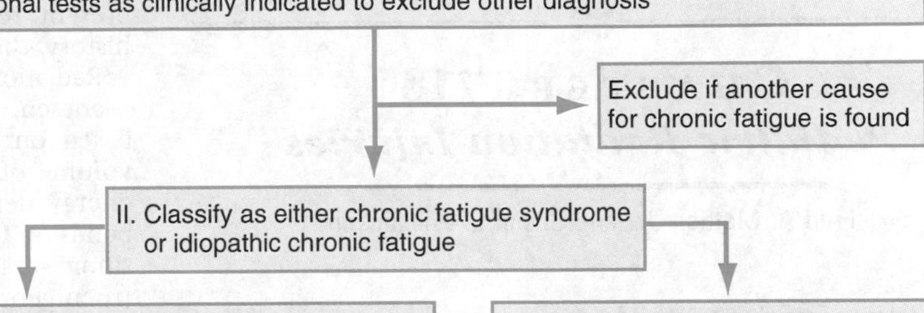
Exclude if another cause for chronic fatigue is found
II. Classify as either chronic fatigue syndrome or idiopathic chronic fatigue

A. Classify as chronic fatigue syndrome if both of the following criteria are met:
  a. Unexplained persistent or relapsing fatigue of new or definite onset that is not due to ongoing exertion, is not relieved by rest, and results in a substantial reduction in previous levels of activity.
  b. Four or more of the following symptoms are concurrently present for 6 months or longer:
    1) impaired memory or concentration (severe enough to reduce levels of occupational, social, or personal activities)
    2) sore throat
    3) tender cervical or axillary lymph nodes
    4) muscle pain
    5) multijoint pain (without joint swelling or redness)
    6) new headaches
    7) unrefreshing sleep
    8) postexertion malaise (lasting more than 24 hr)

B. Classify as idiopathic chronic fatigue if fatigue severity or symptom criteria for chronic fatigue syndrome are not met.

Figure 717–1 The clinical evaluation and classification of unexplained chronic fatigue. The case definition for chronic fatigue syndrome was proposed by the Centers for Disease Control and Prevention in 1988 (Holmes GP, Kaplan JE, Gantz NM, et al: Chronic fatigue syndrome: A working case definition. Ann Intern Med 108:387, 1998) and refined and simplified by an international working group in 1994 (Fukuda K, Straus SE, Hickie I, et al: The chronic fatigue syndrome: A comprehensive approach to its definition and study. Ann Intern Med 121:955, 1994).

resume normal attendance. Home tutoring may be an interim alternative. Patients and their families should clearly understand that no evidence shows that activity harms patients with chronic fatigue syndrome. Continued empathy and support by the treating physician are important in maintaining a physician-patient relationship conducive to identification and resolution of both organic and psychologic illness. Periodic medical re-evaluation approximately every 3 mo is warranted for early detection of other identifiable causes of chronic fatigue, especially with development of new symptoms.

PROGNOSIS. Chronic fatigue syndrome can persist for years with significant morbidity but no mortality. Patients have no long-term risks or increased rates of cancer, autoimmune disease, multiple sclerosis, opportunistic infections, or other complications.

The clinical course of chronic fatigue syndrome is highly variable. Patients should be instructed that their symptoms will likely wax and wane. Most adult patients never fully return to their preillness level of activity, but about 20% of patients return to their previous state of health for periods of at least 1 yr without any specific medical intervention. Some of these patients, however, subsequently have relapses. Approximately 60% of patients—adults, adolescents, and children—report gradual but marked improvement in symptoms over a period of 2–3 yr without specific therapy, although some patients appear to have no improvement or occasionally deteriorate. Patients who deal with stress by somatization and who deny the modulating role of psychosocial factors have a less favorable prognosis. The eventual clinical course is unpredictable, and many adult patients remain functionally impaired for years. Children and adolescents with chronic fatigue appear to have a more optimistic outcome, typically with an undulating course of gradual but substantial improvement, or complete resolution, 1–4 yr after diagnosis.

Carter BD, Edwards JF, Kronenberger WG, et al: Case control study of chronic fatigue in pediatric patients. Pediatrics 95:179, 1995.
Carter BD, Kronenberger WG, Edwards JF, et al: Psychological symptoms in chronic fatigue and juvenile rheumatoid arthritis. Pediatrics 103:975, 1999.
Fukuda K, Straus SE, Hickie I, et al: The chronic fatigue syndrome: A comprehensive approach to its definition and study. Ann Intern Med 121:953, 1994.
Gold D, Bowden R, Sixbey J, et al: Chronic fatigue. A prospective clinical and virologic study. JAMA 264:48, 1990.
Krilov LR, Fisher M, Friedman SB, et al: Course and outcome of chronic fatigue in children and adolescents. Pediatric 102:360, 1998.
Kruesi MJP, Dale J, Straus SE: Psychiatric diagnoses in patients who have chronic fatigue syndrome. J Clin Psychiatry 50:53, 1989.
Marshall GS: Report of a workshop of the epidemiology, natural history, and pathogenesis of chronic fatigue syndrome in adolescents. J Pediatr 134:395, 1999.
McKenzie R, O'Fallon A, Dale J, et al: Low-dose hydrocortisone for treatment of chronic fatigue syndrome. A randomized controlled trial. JAMA 280:1061, 1998.
Plioplys AV: Chronic fatigue syndrome should not be diagnosed in children. Pediatrics 100:270, 1997.
Smith MS, Mitchell J, Corey L, et al: Chronic fatigue in adolescents. Pediatrics 88:195, 1991.
Stewart JM, Gewitz MH, Wildon A, et al: Orthostatic intolerance in adolescent chronic fatigue syndrome. Pediatrics 103:116, 1999.
Wilson A, Hickie I, Lloyd A, et al: Longitudinal study of outcome of chronic fatigue syndrome. Br Med J 308:756, 1994.

PART XXXIII

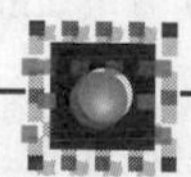

Environmental Health Hazards

CHAPTER 718
Pediatric Radiation Injuries

Fred A. Mettler, Jr., and Susan L. Williamson

Radiation injuries to children can usually be divided into four categories. External exposure from finding and handling lost highly radioactive metallic sources used in industrial radiography is one category. These exposures usually result in severe skin burns or in bone marrow depression. A second type of accident involves internal incorporation of radioactive substances. This can also cause bone marrow depression. The third type of exposure results from radiotherapy for childhood malignancies. These treatments have a normally accepted complication rate, but accidental overexposure can also result from miscalculations or machine malfunctions. Finally, potential neoplasms can occur years or decades after radiation exposure. Examples of these include a high rate of breast cancers in children treated for Hodgkin's disease and thyroid cancer in children exposed to radioiodine around Chernobyl.

Radiation accidents involving children per se are rare. Between 1946 and 1997, about 150 fatalities worldwide could be attributed to radiation accidents, and only several of these occurred in children. The rarity of radiation injuries makes their recognition difficult. The public perception about radiation also makes management difficult because patients, their families, and medical staff all are usually grossly misinformed about the effects of radiation exposure.

When radiation accident occurs, the pediatrician needs to be aware not only of the basic principles and management of the early phases of radiation injury but also of the later or delayed manifestations of radiation illness. In some accidents, children have presented with lethargy, nausea and vomiting, leukopenia, thrombocytopenia, or skin burns as manifestations of prolonged exposure to a highly radioactive source whose presence was not appreciated. Recognition of radiation exposure as the cause of these symptoms is necessary for the exposure to be terminated.

BASIC PRINCIPLES. Ionizing radiation may be either electromagnetic or particulate in nature. Ionizing electromagnetic radiation includes x-rays and gamma rays. These have no mass and are emitted either from a radiation-producing device (such as an x-ray machine or linear accelerator) or from radioactive materials. Gamma rays and x-rays easily penetrate body tissues, depending on their energy. They can deposit their potentially harmful energy deep in the body. Particulate radiations include alpha particles and beta particles. Alpha particles present a hazard only when they are inhaled, ingested, or deposited in an open wound because they have extremely poor penetration capability and are unable to penetrate the outer layer of skin or even a sheet of paper. Beta particles may penetrate as much as a few centimeters of tissue.

Although ionizing radiation is not appreciated by the human senses, it is easily detected, localized, and quantified through the use of various devices. If the radiation source is no longer present, recognition of radiation injury is made on the basis of history, the observed effects, and their temporal course.

Radiation was historically measured in three different units—roentgen, rad, and rem. The roentgen is a unit of exposure based on the number of ion pairs that are produced in a volume of air. The rad (roentgen absorbed dose) is based on energy deposited per gram of tissue. The absorbed dose depends on the type of radiation and the size, shape, and composition of the object absorbing the radiation. Finally, a rem (roentgen equivalent in man) takes into account the biologic effects of various kinds of radiation. For x-rays and gamma rays, a rad and a rem are essentially equivalent. Most literature now uses international units. These include the Gray (Gy), which is equal to 100 rads, and the Sievert (Sv), which is equal to 100 rem. Radioactivity was historically expressed in units of Curies (Ci). The international unit is the Becquerel (Bq), and 1 Curie equals 37 gigabecquerels (GBq). The following text uses the historical units followed by the international units in parentheses.

PATHOPHYSIOLOGY. Radiation injury involves energy deposited in a cell with subsequent formation of free radicals from water. Most of the free radicals that are formed recombine quickly because they are very reactive chemically, but they may occasionally interact with other nearby macromolecules.

At high radiation doses, parenchymal cells may die. The clinical effect may be insignificant if the cell is not critical to the survival of the individual. However, if a large number of cells are killed or they are essential, clinical symptoms become apparent. Not all cells in the body are equally radiosensitive. In general, rapidly dividing cells (such as the intestinal mucosa and bone marrow) are the most sensitive to cell killing by radiation, whereas cells that are slowly dividing or are nondividing (such as neurons) are quite resistant. Endothelial cells, arterioles, and capillaries have moderate radiosensitivity, and damage to these can reduce blood supply and result in effects months or several years after exposure.

At radiation doses less than 100 rads (1.0 Gy), most cell types survive, although they may be subject to transformation due to faulty repair of DNA breaks and there is the possibility of subsequent malignancy. Radiation-induced neoplasms (both benign and malignant) may occur after radiation exposure. Most leukemias (except chronic lymphocytic leukemia) can be induced by radiation. They usually appear from 2–15 yr after exposure. Tumors of solid organs can also occur, although the tissues have varying sensitivity. The thyroid, female breast, and lung are among the most sensitive. Most solid tumors appear 10–50 yr after exposure. Thyroid and bone cancer may appear as early as 5 yr. Over a wide dose range, the risk of a radiation-induced tumor for many tissues is directly proportional to the radiation dose. However, for a given dose, children appear to be at a two- to threefold greater risk of subsequent tumors than adults.

Although radiation principally affects DNA, and although genetic effects of radiation have been observed in animals, hereditary effects of radiation exposure have not been observed in large epidemiologic studies over several generations (i.e., the Hiroshima/Nagasaki survivors).

WHOLE BODY IRRADIATION

CLINICAL MANIFESTATIONS. Table 718–1 presents dose effect relationships for acute whole body penetrating irradiation. A

TABLE 718–1 Dose Effect Relationships After Acute Whole Body Radiation from Gamma or X-rays

Whole Body Absorbed Dose, Rads (Gy)	Findings
5 (0.05)	Asymptomatic
15 (0.15)	Asymptomtic (but chromosome aberrations may be present in cultured peripheral lymphocytes)
50 (0.5)	Asymptomatic (minor depression of white blood cells and platelets in a few persons)
100 (1.0)	Nausea and vomiting in approximately 10% of patients within 2 days of exposure
200 (2.0)	Nausea and vomiting in most persons exposed, with clear hematologic depression
400 (4.0)	Nausea, vomiting, and diarrhea within 48 hr. 50% mortality without medical treatment
600 (6.0)	100% mortality within 30 days due to bone marrow failure without medical treatment
5,000 (50.0)	Cardiovascular collapse and central nervous system damage, with death in 24–72 hr

large single exposure of penetrating radiation can result in *acute radiation syndrome*. The signs and symptoms of this syndrome result from damage to major organ systems that have different levels of radiation sensitivity, modulated by the rate at which the radiation exposure occurred. For example, 100 rads (1.0 Gy) delivered in a minute would be symptomatic but 1 rad (0.01 Gy)/day for 100 days would not.

The *hematopoietic syndrome* occurs from acute whole body doses of approximately 200–1,000 rad (2.0–10.0 Gy). A prodromal phase consists of nausea and vomiting within the first 12 hr, with symptoms usually lasting up to 48 hr. There follows a latent period of 2–3 wk during which patients may feel quite well. Although patients are asymptomatic, bone marrow impairment has occurred. The most obvious laboratory finding is lymphocyte depression (Table 718–2). Maximal bone marrow depression occurs approximately 30 days after exposure, when hemorrhage and infection can be major problems. If the bone marrow is not completely eradicated, a recovery phase then ensues. This radiation effect is similar to what occurs when whole body radiation therapy (given as 1,200 rads [12 Gy] in two treatments) is used to obliterate the bone marrow in leukemic children before bone marrow transplantation.

The *gastrointestinal (GI) syndrome* occurs from acute whole body doses of approximately 1,000–3,000 rad (10.0–30.0 Gy). Prompt onset of nausea, vomiting, and diarrhea follows. There is a latent period of approximately 1 wk and then recurrence of GI symptoms, sepsis, electrolyte imbalance, and ultimately death.

At dose levels over 3,000 rad (>30 Gy), the *cardiovascular/central nervous system (CNS) syndrome* predominates. Nausea, vomiting, prostration, hypotension, ataxia, and convulsions are almost immediate. Death usually occurs promptly.

TREATMENT. For the hematopoietic and GI syndromes, treatment is supportive involving transfusions, fluids, antibiotics, and antiviral agents. The cardiovascular/CNS syndrome is fatal within 1–14 days.

TABLE 718–2 Expected Outcome Based on Absolute Lymphocyte Count After Acute Penetrating Whole Body Irradiation

Minimal Lymphocyte Count Within First 48 Hr After Exposure	Prognosis
1,000–3,000 normal range	No significant injury
1,000–1,500	Significant but probably nonlethal injury, good prognosis
500–1,000	Severe injury, fair prognosis
100–500	Very severe injury, poor prognosis
Under 100	Lethal without compatible bone marrow donor

TABLE 718–3 Skin Changes After Single Acute Exposures

Absorbed Dose in Rads (Gy)	Findings
300 (3.0)	Threshold for erythema (100 keV diagnostic x-ray)
600 (6.0)	Threshold for erythema (10 MeV therapeutic x-ray)
1,500 (15.0)	Moist desquamation
2,000 (20.0)	Skin ulceration with slow healing
3,000+ (>30.0)	Gangrenous changes

LOCALIZED IRRADIATION

CLINICAL MANIFESTATIONS. Because localized exposure involves a small amount of tissue, systemic manifestations are less severe, and patients may survive even if local absorbed doses are very high. The hand is the most common site for accidental localized irradiation injuries, usually as a result of picking up or playing with lost radiation sources. The second most common site is the thigh and buttocks, predominately from placing unsuspected highly radioactive radiography sources in the pockets. Most industrial radiography sources are easily capable of causing skin erythema or radiation burns from only a few minutes of direct contact.

There are several major differences between thermal burns and radiation burns. The effects of a thermal burn are present almost immediately, and patients invariably know what it was that burned them. If patients present with burnlike symptoms but no known cause, radiation should be suspected as the cause. Table 718–3 lists the findings expected after localized skin doses.

The penetrability of the radiation is an important factor in the outcome of local radiation injury. In cases of low-energy β-irradiation, recovery and skin grafting are possibilities, even after high absorbed skin doses. Gamma and x-rays, on the other hand, penetrate substantially and cause progressive obliterative endarteritis that may result in necrosis and gangrene. Very few initial symptoms occur in the first 12 hr unless the dose has been extremely high. Under these circumstances, patients may complain of hypersensitivity and tingling.

Erythema is similar to that seen with a first-degree burn. If erythema is seen within the first 48 hr, ulceration will probably occur. The erythema may come in waves. That is, it will be present, disappear, and return days or 1–3 wk later. Transepidermal injury is similar to a second-degree thermal burn. Blister formation may occur at 1–2 wk with doses in the range of 10,000 rads (100 Gy) and at 3 wk at dose levels of 3,000–5,000 rads (30–50 Gy).

Some tissues that may receive localized radiation exposure are relatively radiosensitive. These include the lens of the eye and the gonads. Cataract formation may occur with single gamma ray exposures in the range of 200–500 rad (2.0–5.0 Gy). Such cataracts usually take between 2 mo to several years to develop. Gonadal exposure has occurred in several accidental situations. Oligospermia may take up to 2 mo to develop. Transient infertility may result from doses as low as 15 rads (0.15 Gy), and permanent sterility in men at dose levels between 300 and 600 rad (3.0–6.0 Gy). Both cataracts and infertility are common after whole body radiotherapy used to treat leukemia.

TREATMENT. Skin therapy is directed at prevention of infections. Treatment of localized injuries usually involves plastic surgery and grafting; if the radiation exposure was not very penetrating. The nature of the surgery depends on the dose at various depths in tissue and the location of the lesion. The full expression of radiation injury often is not apparent for 1–2 yr owing to slow arteriolar narrowing that can cause delayed necrosis. After relatively penetrating radiation, amputation may be necessary owing to obliterative changes in small vessels.

INTERNAL CONTAMINATION

EPIDEMIOLOGY. Accidents involving internal contamination are rare and generally are a result of misadministration in hospital settings or voluntary ingestion of unsuspected contaminated radioactive materials. Other relevant examples of potential internal contamination of children include that caused by breast-feeding mothers who have diagnostic nuclear medicine scans and radiation exposure of children when a parent or sibling receives a therapeutic dose of ^{131}I. Generally, patients given large activities (>30 mCi [1.1 GBq]) of radioiodine are hospitalized and isolated. When such patients are allowed to go home, they may still be excreting a moderate amount of activity through their urine (and to a lesser extent though saliva and sweat) for 1–2 wk, and it is best to have children use a separate bathroom and have their food prepared by somebody else, if possible, during this period. External exposure received by children as a result of radiation emanating directly from such a patient is not a problem.

CLINICAL MANIFESTATIONS. The hazards from internal contamination depend on the nature of the radionuclide (particularly in terms of its solubility in water, half-life, and radioactive emission), as well as the nature of the chemical compound. The signs and symptoms are similar to those described under whole body and local irradiation, depending on the dose and circumstances of ingestion.

TREATMENT. Internal contamination presents the physician with a dilemma. The most effective treatment requires knowledge of both the radionuclide and the chemical form, yet unless treatment is instituted very quickly, it rarely is effective. The general classes of treatment for internal contamination include removal, dilution, blocking, and chelation. Removal treatment involves cleaning a contaminated wound and performing stomach lavage or administration of cathartics in the case of ingestion. Administration of alginate-containing antacids (such as Gaviscon) also usually helps in removal by decreasing absorption in the GI tract. An example of blocking therapy is the administration of potassium iodine or other stable iodine-containing compounds in patients with known internal contamination with radioactive iodine. The stable iodine effectively blocks the thyroid, although the effectiveness decreases rapidly as time increases after the contamination occurred. Another example of blocking therapy is the use of Prussian blue in cases of internal contamination by cesium. Dilution therapy is used in cases of tritium (radioactive hydrogen as water) contamination. Forcing fluids promotes excretion. Finally, cases of internal contamination with transuranic elements (such as americium and plutonium) may require chelation therapy with calcium diethylene triaminepentaacetic acid (DTPA).

EXTERNAL CONTAMINATION

The presence of external radioactive contamination on a patient's skin is not an immediate medical emergency. Management involves removing and controlling the spread of radioactive materials. If a patient has suspected surface contamination and no physical injuries, decontamination can be performed relatively easily. If there is substantial physical trauma or other life-threatening injuries that are combined with external contamination, only after the patient has been stabilized physiologically should surface decontamination proceed. In many accident situations, essential medical care is inappropriately delayed by hospital emergency staff owing to fear of radiation or spread of contamination in the hospital.

Treatment of a patient who is externally contaminated and has other life-threatening injuries requires advance planning. The basic principles involved are as follows: (1) Bring the patient to a room where the traffic can be controlled. (2) While wearing protective clothing (universal precautions), remove the patient's clothing and treat nonradiation life-threatening injuries first. (3) Call the hospital Radiation Safety Officer. Only after the patient is medically stable, wash potentially contaminated areas with washcloths, lukewarm water, and regular soap. (4) Get a complete blood count, ask about nausea and vomiting, and consider possible therapy for internal contamination.

RADIATION THERAPY COMPLICATIONS AND ACCIDENTS

Radiation therapy uses high doses to kill malignant cells. Unfortunately, the sensitivity of normal cells is quite close to that of malignant cells, and to achieve significant cure rates, radiation oncologists also must accept a given percentage of serious complications, 5–10%. This leaves little room for error either in calculations of dose or in the actual mechanical functioning of the machine. Radiation therapy treatment protocols are reasonably standardized. Most radiotherapy regimens use about 5,000 rads (50 Gy) given in about 25 fractions over 5 wk. A radiotherapy treatment scheme that either uses doses much more than 10% higher than this or uses this dose with significantly fewer fractions poses a very high incidence of severe and potentially catastrophic complications.

The exact complications depend on the location of the treatment field. In children, because of the location of many childhood tumors, the CNS is commonly in the treatment field and suffers complications. Standard radiotherapy of the brain in children results in cortical atrophy in more than half of patients who received 2,000–6,000 rads (20–60 Gy); 26% have white matter changes (leukoencephalopathy), and 8% have calcifications (Fig. 718–1). The younger the age of the child at irradiation, the worse is the atrophy. Some patients also develop mineralizing microangiopathy (Fig. 718–2). Clinical findings after routine radiotherapy may include poor school performance and dysfunction of the pituitary and hypothalamus. As a result of overexposure, adverse effects may be severe and include lethargy, ataxia, spasticity, and progressive demen-

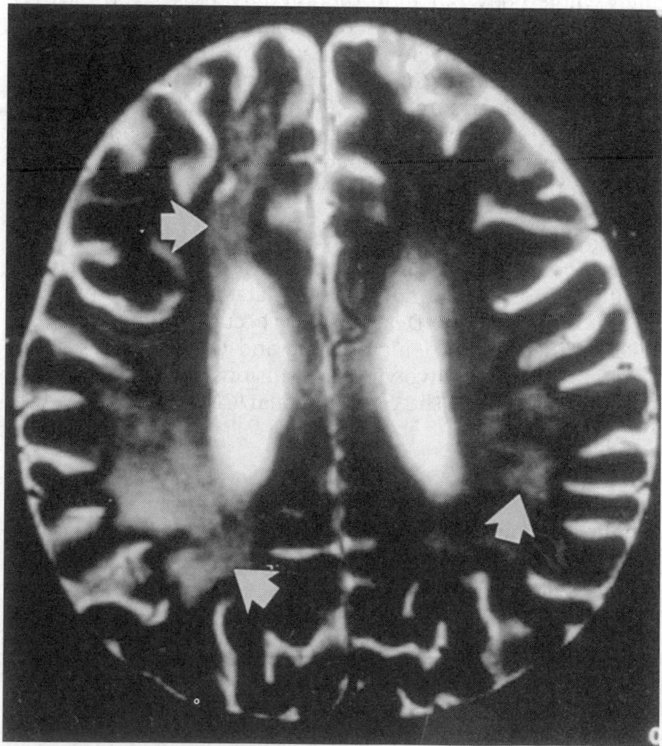

Figure 718–1 White matter changes after radiotherapy. A T2 weighted MRI scan of a child after radiotherapy demonstrates white matter changes *(arrows).*

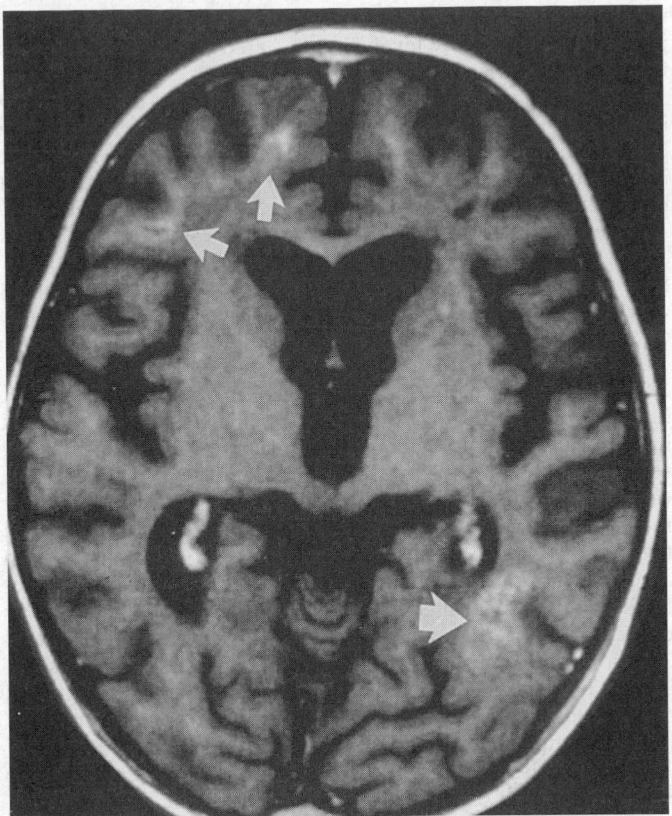

Figure 718–2 Generalized brain changes after radiotherapy. A T1 weighted MRI scan of a child shows both central and cortical atrophy as well as high signal areas *(arrows)* due to mineralizing microangiopathy.

tia. Radiation-induced changes of the brain are potentiated by methotrexate administered before, during, or after radiotherapy

Cerebral necrosis is a serious and irreversible complication of radiation-induced vascular disease. It is usually diagnosed 1–5 yr after irradiation but can occur up to a decade later. Radiation-induced necrosis occurs with a moderate probability when radiotherapy schemes exceed 4,000 rads (40 Gy) in 10 fractions, 5,000 rads (50Gy) in 20 fractions, 6,000 rads (60 Gy) in 30 fractions, or when individual fractions exceed 300 rads (3 Gy). The probability of necrosis is very high when treatment schemes exceed 5,000 rads (50 Gy) in 15 fractions, 6,000 rads (60 Gy) in 20 fractions, or 7,000 rads (70 Gy) in 30 fractions. Brain necrosis may be manifested by headache, increased intracranial pressure, seizures, sensory deficits, and psychotic changes.

Spinal cord irradiation may result in radiation myelitis, which may be either transient or permanent. Acute transient myelitis often appears 2–4 mo after irradiation. Patients with myelitis usually present with Lhermitte's sign, a sensation of little electrical shocks in the arms and legs occurring with neck flexion or other movements that stretch the spinal cord. Reversal of transient myelopathy usually occurs between 8–40 wk and does not necessarily progress to late delayed necrosis.

Delayed myelopathy occurs after a mean latent period of 20 mo, but it can occur earlier if the total dose or dose per fraction is high. This is usually manifested by discontinuous deterioriation and is irreversible. In the cervical and thoracic region, sensory dissociation develops, followed by spastic paresis and then flaccid paresis. In the lumbar cord, flaccid paresis is dominant. The mortality for high thoracic and cervical lesions reaches 70%, with death due to pneumonia and urinary tract infections. A 25–50% incidence of thoracic myelopathy occurs when treatment schemes exceed 6,000 rads (60 Gy) at 200 rads (2 Gy) per fraction, 4,000 rads (40 Gy) at 300 rads (3 Gy) per fraction, or 3,500 rads (35 Gy) at 400 rads (4 Gy) per fraction.

Radiotherapy also causes other effects specific to children. The effect on growth is most pronounced when children are younger than 6 yr and during their adolescent growth spurt. Scoliosis and hypoplasia of bones may occur if fractionated treatment schemes exceed 4,000 rads (40 Gy). Fractionated doses in excess of 2,500 rads (25 Gy) can result in slipped capital femoral epiphyses. An increase in the incidence of benign osteochondromas has also been reported after radiotherapy in children. Chest wall irradiation of girls with 1,500–2,000 rads (15–20 Gy) over 1 wk impairs breast development, and fractionated doses of 3,000–4,000 rads (30–40 Gy) cause fibrosis and atrophy of breast tissue. Virtually any tissues in a radiotherapy field may show disturbances in growth.

RADIATION CARCINOGENESIS

Radiation carcinogenesis is a potential late expression of radiation injury, and children are more sensitive to induction of tumors than adults. Breast cancer data from Hiroshima and Nagasaki indicate that per 100 rem (1.0 Sv), the relative risk in children is about 3.5 compared with 1.5 or so for women irradiated at 40 yr of age. Epidemiologic studies of children irradiated as infants for presumed thymic hyperplasia, of children treated with radiation for ringworm (tinea capitus) and for acne, and of children treated for hemangiomas and other disorders confirm that radiation can increase the risk of leukemia and cancer of the breast, thyroid, brain, skin, and other sites. The most recent example is the appearance of over 800 cases of thyroid cancer in children around Chernobyl. This has mostly occurred in children who were 0–2 yr of age at the time of the accident. There has been no increase in childhood leukemia or malformations in the Chernobyl children.

The incidence of second tumors is also increased in children who have received radiotherapy for childhood tumors, particularly neuroblastoma, retinoblastoma, and Hodgkin disease. A significant increase in soft tissue sarcomas has been noted in children treated for retinoblastoma, and genetic susceptibility has been implicated as well as radiation. In other large studies of children treated for childhood cancer, no increase in leukemia was observed, but there were increases in thyroid and breast cancer as well as bone sarcoma.

American Academy of Pediatrics: Risk of ionizing radiation exposure to children: A subject review. Pediatrics 101:717, 1998.

Barrett I: Slipped capital femoral epiphysis following radiotherapy. J Pediatr Orthop 5:263, 1985.

Furst C, Lundell M, Ahlback S, et al: Breast hypoplasia following irradiation of the female breast in infancy and early childhood. Acta Oncol 28:519, 1989.

Goldwein J, Meadows J: Influence of radiation on growth in pediatric patients. Clin Plast Surg 20:455, 1993.

Gutin PH, Leibel SA, Sheline GE: Radiation Injury to the Nervous System. New York, Raven Press, 1991.

Kasatkinan EP, Shilin DE, Rosenbloom AL, et al: Effects of low level radiation from Chermobyl accident in a population with iodine deficiency. Eur J Pediatr 156:916, 1997.

Mettler FA, Kelsey CA, Ricks R (eds): Medical Management of Radiation Accidents. Boca Raton, FL, CRC Press, 1991.

Mettler FA, Upton AC: Medical Effects of Ionizing Radiation, 2nd ed. Philadelphia, WB Saunders, 1995.

One Decade after Chernobyl, Summing up the Consequences of the Accident. Proceedings of an International Conference, Vienna, 8–12, April 1996, International Atomic Energy Agency, 1996.

Robertson W, Butler M, D'Angio G, et al: Leg length discrepancy following irradiation for childhood tumors. J Pediatr Orthop 11:284, 1991.

Scherer E, Streffer C, Trott KR (eds): Radiopathology of Organs and Tissues. New York, Springer-Verlag, 1991.

Schiebel-Jost P, Pfeil J, Niethard F, et al: Spinal growth after irradiation for Wilms tumor. Int Orthop 15:387, 1991.

Shore R: Issues and epidemiological evidence regarding radiation induced thyroid cancer. Radiat Res 131:98, 1992.

Sources and Effects of Ionizing Radiation, Report to the General Assembly 1993 and 1994, United Nations Committee on the Effects of Atomic Radiation, Vienna, 1993, 1994.

Tokunaga M, Land C, Tukapka S, et al: Incidence of female breast cancer in atomic bomb survivors, 1950–1985. Radiat Res 138:209, 1994.
Tucker MA, D'Angio G, Boice JD Jr, et al: Bone sarcomas linked to radiotherapy and chemotherapy in children. N Engl J Med 317:588, 1987.
Tucker MA, Meadows AT, Morris-Jones P, et al: Therapeutic radiation at young age linked to secondary thyroid cancer. Proc Am Soc Clin Oncol 5:827, 1986.
Wong FL, Boice JD Jr, Abramson DH, et al: Cancer incidence after retinoblastoma: Radiation dose and sarcoma risk. JAMA 278:1262, 1997.

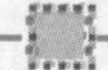

CHAPTER 719 Chemical Pollutants

Philip J. Landrigan and Ruth A. Etzel

Children today are at risk of exposure to more than 70,000 synthetic chemicals, most of which have been developed since World War II. Many are dispersed in the environment. Fewer than half have been tested for their potential hazards to children's health.

Children are uniquely vulnerable to chemical pollutants for several reasons:

1. They have proportionally greater exposures to many environmental pollutants than adults. Because they drink more water, eat more food, and breathe more air per kilogram of body weight, children are more heavily exposed to pollutants in water, food, and air. Children's hand-to-mouth behavior and their play close to the ground further magnify their exposures.
2. Children's metabolic pathways, especially in the first months after birth, are immature. In some instances, children are better able than adults to cope with environmental toxicants because they are unable to metabolize them to their active form. More commonly, however, children are less well able to detoxify and excrete chemical pollutants.
3. Infants and children are growing and developing, and their developmental processes are easily disrupted. The disability resulting from exposures to chemicals during periods of early vulnerability can be severe (Table 719–1).
4. Because children have many future years of life, they have time to develop multistage chronic diseases that may be triggered by early exposures.

CHEMICAL POLLUTANTS OF MAJOR CONCERN

AIR POLLUTANTS. Outdoor air pollutants of greatest concern are photochemical oxidants (especially ozone), oxides of nitrogen (NO_x), fine particulates, sulfur oxides, and carbon monoxide. These pollutants result principally from the combustion of fossil fuels. Automotive emissions are the major current source of air pollution worldwide.

Elevated levels of air pollutants, especially elevations of ozone and NO_x, are associated with respiratory problems in children, including decreased pulmonary expiratory flow, wheezing, and exacerbations of asthma. Fine particulate air pollution, even at low levels, is associated with slight increases in cardiopulmonary mortality.

Indoor air can also be an important source of respiratory irritation, because many children spend 80–90% of their time indoors. Indoor air pollution has become especially important in the United States since the energy crises of the 1970s, which led to the construction of tighter, more energy-efficient homes. Allergens in indoor air can contribute to respiratory problems and include cockroach, mite, mold, cat, and dog allergens. Some indoor molds produce extremely potent chemical toxins called mycotoxins. Environmental tobacco smoke is a major contributor to exacerbations of childhood asthma.

TABLE 719–1 Examples of the Vulnerability of Infants and Children to Chemical Pollutants

Diethylstilbestrol and adenocarcinoma of the vagina
Thalidomide and phocomelia
Mycotoxins and pulmonary hemorrhage
Fetal alcohol syndrome
Neurobehavioral toxicity of low-dose exposure to lead
Increased risk of cancer after intrauterine exposure to nitrosamine, vinyl chloride, or ionizing radiation
Developmental neurotoxicity of organophosphate insecticides

LEAD. Also see Chapter 721. Lead exposure occurs worldwide. Exposure is especially common in countries that still permit leaded gasoline. In the United States, pediatric blood lead levels have declined by more than 90% in the past 20 yr, principally as a result of removal of lead from gasoline. Nevertheless, the Centers for Disease Control and Prevention estimates that more than 900,000 children 1–6 yr of age still have blood lead levels of 10 μg/dL and above. Prevalence is especially high among poor minority children in inner cities. Lead-based paint is the major current source of exposure. Blood lead levels exceeding 10 μg/dL are associated with deficits in intellectual function, shortening of attention span, and increased risk of asocial behavior. The extent of injury is directly proportional to lead dose. Lead readily crosses the placenta, and antenatal exposures appear especially hazardous.

MERCURY. Also see Chapter 720. Children may be exposed to either inorganic or organic mercury. Inorganic mercury produces dermatitis, gingivitis, stomatitis, tremor, and acrodynia. Organic or methyl mercury is fat soluble, readily penetrates the central nervous system (CNS), and produces a neurotoxic syndrome. Exposure to organic mercury occurs principally through consumption of fish that have accumulated mercury deposited in lakes and oceans as atmospheric fallout from combustion of coal, which contains small quantities of mercury.

ASBESTOS. Between 1947 and 1973, asbestos was sprayed as insulation on classroom walls and ceilings in about 10,000 schools in the United States. Subsequent deterioration of this asbestos has released microscopic asbestos fibers into the air and thus posed a risk to children. Asbestos is a human carcinogen, and the two principal cancers caused by asbestos are lung cancer and mesothelioma. Federal law in the United States requires that all schools be inspected for asbestos and the results made public. Removal is required only when asbestos is visibly deteriorating or is within the reach of children. In most cases, placement of barriers (dry walls or drop ceilings) provides appropriate protection.

ENVIRONMENTAL TOBACCO SMOKE. Smoking during pregnancy poses a hazard to the fetus (Chapter 92). Infants born to women who smoke are, on the average, 10% smaller than infants born to nonsmoking women. Infants of parents who smoke have a higher risk of sudden infant death syndrome.

Passive smoking is also a hazard to children. Forty-three per cent of children younger than 12 yr in the United States live in a home with at least one smoker. Children exposed to environmental tobacco smoke have more lower respiratory illness, more middle-ear effusions, and more viral respiratory illnesses than unexposed children.

PESTICIDES. Pesticides are a diverse group of chemicals used to control insects, weeds, fungi, and rodents. Approximately 600 pesticides are registered with the U.S. Environmental Protection Agency.

Diet is a major route of children's exposure to pesticides. Children may also be exposed in homes or schools, on lawns, and in gardens. They may be exposed to pesticide drift from areas that have been sprayed. Children employed in agriculture or living in migrant farm camps may be exposed to many pesticides.

Pesticides can cause a range of chronic toxic effects: polyneuropathy and CNS dysfunction (organophosphates), hormonal disruption and reproductive impairment (DDT, kepone, dibromochloropropane), cancer (aldrin, dieldrin, chlorphenoxy herbicides [2, 4, 5-T]), and pulmonary fibrosis (paraquat). Pesticide exposures to children can be reduced by minimizing applications to lawns and gardens, by adapting techniques of integrated pest management, and by reducing pesticide applications to food crops.

Children can be acutely overexposed to pesticides (Chapter 722). The organophosphates and carbamates, both of which cause neurotoxicity through inhibition of acetylcholinesterase, cause the largest number of acute poisoning cases. Symptoms include meiosis (though not in all cases), excess salivation, abdominal cramping, vomiting, diarrhea, and muscle fasciculation. In severe cases, loss of consciousness, cardiac arrhythmias, and death by respiratory arrest occur. See Chapter 722 for treatment.

PCBs, DDT, DIOXINS, AND OTHER CHLORINATED HYDROCARBONS. Chlorinated hydrocarbons are used as insecticides (DDT), plastics (polyvinyl chloride [PVC]), electrical insulators (polychlorinated biphenyls, [PCBs]) and solvents (trichloroethylene). Highly toxic dioxins and furans can be formed during synthesis of chlorinated herbicides or as by-products of plastic combustion. All of these materials are widely dispersed in the environment. DDT and PCBs are highly persistent.

The embryo, fetus, and young child are at particularly high risk of injury from PCBs, DDT, and dioxins. All these compounds are lipid soluble. They readily cross the placenta, and they accumulate in breast milk. Intrauterine exposure to PCBs has been linked to persistent neurobehavioral dysfunction in children.

Fish from contaminated waters are a major source of children's exposure to PCBs. Children can be exposed *in utero* or through breast milk. To protect children and pregnant women in the United States against PCBs in fish, government agencies have issued fish consumption advisories for certain lakes and rivers. Combustion of medical wastes containing PVC is the principal current source of environmental dioxin.

ENVIRONMENTAL CARCINOGENS. Children may be exposed to carcinogenic pollutants in utero or after birth. The discovery that cancer of the vagina occurs in women after intrauterine exposure to diethylstilbestrol was the first recognition of transplacental carcinogenesis. Children are more likely than adults to develop leukemia and other malignancies after low-dose exposure to ionizing radiation in utero or early infancy (Chapter 718).

The U.S. National Cancer Institute (NCI) reports that incidence rates of leukemia and cerebral glioma, the two most common forms of childhood malignancy, have been increasing for the past 3 decades, despite greatly improved therapy and declining death rates. The cumulative increase in incidence of glioma is now about 40%. To some extent, these increases may reflect better diagnosis. Research is under way to determine whether intrauterine or postnatal exposures to chemical pollutants in the environment have also contributed to the reported increasing incidence of childhood cancer.

ROUTES OF EXPOSURE

TRANSPLACENTAL. Heavy metals and fat-soluble compounds such as PCBs and DDT readily cross the placenta. They may produce serious and irreversible toxic effects on the developing nervous, endocrine, and reproductive organs even at very low levels.

WATER. About 200 chemicals have been found in small amounts in various water supplies. Lead is especially common. In some older neighborhoods, lead in water derives from lead pipes. More commonly, it is dissolved (leached) from solder by soft, acidic water. Highest levels of lead occur in water that has been standing in pipes overnight; therefore, it is wise to run water for 2–3 min each morning before making up infant formula.

AIR. Vehicular emissions are the major source of urban air pollution. Diesel exhaust is a human carcinogen. In rural areas, wood smoke can contribute to air pollution. Children living in the vicinity of smelters and chemical production plants can be exposed to toxic industrial emissions such as lead, benzene, and 1,3-butadiene.

FOOD. Many chemicals are intentionally added to food to improve appearance, taste, texture, or preservation. Many such chemicals have been poorly tested for potential toxicity. Residues of many pesticides are found in both raw and processed foods.

WORK CLOTHES. Illnesses in children are at times traceable to contaminated dust from parents' work clothes; toxicity from lead, beryllium, dioxin, organophosphate pesticides, and asbestos has occurred. Prevention is achieved by providing facilities at work for changing and showering.

SCHOOLS. Children may be exposed in schools, kindergartens, and nurseries to lead paint, molds, asbestos, environmental tobacco smoke, pesticides, and hazardous arts and crafts materials. Substantial opportunities for prevention exist in the school environment, and pediatricians are often consulted for advice.

CHILD LABOR. Four to 5 million children and adolescents in the United States work for pay, and child labor is widespread around the world. Working children are at high risk of physical trauma and injury. Also, they may be exposed to a wide range of toxic chemicals including pesticides in agriculture and lawn work, asbestos in construction and building demolition, and benzene in pumping gasoline.

THE PHYSICIAN'S ROLE

Pediatricians should always be alert to the possibility that disease in a child has been caused by a chemical pollutant. In considering the origins of noninfectious disease, they should ask about the home environment, parental occupation, unusual exposures, and neighborhood factories. Especially when several unusual cases of disease or constellations of findings occur together, an environmental cause is possible. Any adolescent with a traumatic injury may have been injured at work.

The history is the single most important instrument for obtaining information on environmental exposures. Information about current and past exposures should routinely be sought through a few brief screening questions. Changes in patterns of exposure or new exposures may be especially important. If suspicious information is elicited, more detailed follow-up should be pursued. Accurate diagnosis of an environmental cause of disease can lead to better care of sick children and prevention of disease in other children.

American Academy of Pediatrics, Committee on Environmental Health: Ambient air pollution: Respiratory hazards to children. Pediatrics 91:1210, 1993.

American Academy of Pediatrics, Committee on Environmental Health: Environmental tobacco smoke: A hazard to children. Pediatrics 99:639, 1997.

American Academy of Pediatrics, Committee on Environmental Health: Toxic effects of indoor molds. Pediatrics 101:712, 1998.

American Academy of Pediatrics, Committee on Environmental Health: Risk of ionizing radiation exposure to children: A subject review. Pediatrics 101:717, 1998.

Bellinger D, Leviton A, Waternaux C, et al: Longitudinal analyses of prenatal and postnatal exposure and early cognitive development. N Engl J Med 315:1037, 1987.

Centers for Disease Control and Prevention: Asthma mortality and hospitalization among children and young adults—United States, 1980–1993. MMWR 45:350, 1996.

Environmental Defense Fund: Toxic Ignorance: The Continuing Absence of Basic Health Testing for Top-Selling Toxic Chemicals in the United States. Washington, DC, Environmental Defense Fund, 1997.

Etzel RA, Balk SJ (eds): Handbook of Environmental Health for Children. Elk Grove Village, IL, American Academy of Pediatrics (in press).
Etzel RA, Pattishall EN, Haley NJ, et al: Passive smoking and middle ear effusion among children in day care. Pediatrics 90:228, 1992.
Jacobson JL, Jacobson SW: Intellectual impairment in children exposed to polychlorinated biphenyls in utero. N Engl J Med 335:783, 1996.
Kenney LB, Miller BA, Gloeckler RL, et al: Increased incidence of cancer in infants in the U.S.: 1980–1990. Cancer 82:1396, 1998.
Longnecker MP, Rogan WJ, Lucier G: The human health effects of DDT (dichlorodiphenyltrichloroethane) and PCBs (polychlorinated biphenyls) and an overview of organochlorines in public health. Annu Rev Public Health 18:211, 1997.
National Academy of Sciences: Pesticides in the Diets of Infants and Children. Washington, DC, National Academy Press, 1993.
National Academy of Sciences: Toxicity Testing: Needs and Priorities. Washington, DC, National Academy Press, 1984.
Paulozzi L, Erickson JD, Jackson RJ: Hypospadias trends in two American surveillance systems. Pediatrics 100:831, 1997.
Pirkle JL, Flegal KM, Bernert JT, et al: Exposure of the US population to environmental tobacco smoke: the Third National Health and Nutrition Examination Survey, 1988–1991. JAMA 275:1233, 1996.
Rosenstreich DL, Eggleston P, Kattan M, et al: The role of cockroach allergy and exposure to cockroach in causing morbidity among inner-city children with asthma. N Engl J Med 336:1356, 1997.

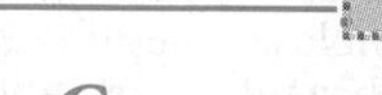

CHAPTER 720
Heavy Metal Intoxication

Collin S. Goto

Metals are electropositive elements characterized by properties such as luster, malleability, and the ability to conduct electricity. Severe illness may result when humans are exposed to the group known as the heavy metals. These substances have an immense range of industrial applications, and the majority of human poisonings result from occupational and household exposures or consumption of contaminated food, water, or medicinal preparations.

Heavy metal intoxication tends to result in diverse multiorgan toxicity through widespread disruption of vital cellular functions. After ingestion, gastrointestinal (GI), renal, hematologic, and nervous system toxicity are common. Inhalation of fumes and vapors may cause a severe pneumonitis, and skin exposure may result in various cutaneous abnormalities. The protean manifestations of heavy metal intoxication can easily be misdiagnosed unless a meticulous history of environmental exposure is obtained.

More than 50% of heavy metal exposures reported to poison control centers occur in the pediatric population (age <19 yr). Among the most common causes of heavy metal intoxication, arsenic and mercury are discussed in this section. Lead poisoning is discussed in Chapter 721.

ARSENIC

EPIDEMIOLOGY. Arsenic exists in the following forms: elemental arsenic, arsine gas, inorganic arsenic salts, and organic arsenic compounds. Children may be poisoned after exposure to inorganic arsenic found in pesticides, herbicides, dyes, homeopathic medicines, and certain folk remedies from China, India, and Southeast Asia. Soil deposits may contaminate artesian well water. Occupational exposure may occur in industries such as glass manufacturing, pottery, electronic components, semiconductors, mining, smelting, and refining. Organic arsenic compounds may be found in seafood, pesticides, and some veterinary pharmaceuticals. In contrast to mercury, the organic forms of arsenic found in seafood are nontoxic.

PHARMACOKINETICS. Elemental arsenic is insoluble in water and bodily fluids and therefore is insignificantly absorbed and nontoxic. Inhaled arsine gas is rapidly absorbed through the lungs. The inorganic arsenic salts are well absorbed through the GI tract and lungs. The organic arsenic compounds are well absorbed through the GI tract.

After acute exposure, arsenic is rapidly distributed to all tissues. Inorganic arsenic is methylated and eliminated predominantly by the kidneys, with about 95% excreted in the urine and 5% excreted in the bile. The majority of the arsenic is eliminated in the first few days, with the remainder slowly excreted over a period of several weeks.

PATHOPHYSIOLOGY. After exposure to arsine gas, absorbed arsine enters red blood cells (RBC) and is oxidized to arsenic dihydride and elemental arsenic. Complexing of these derivatives with RBC sulfhydryl groups results in cell membrane instability and massive hemolysis. The inorganic arsenic salts poison enzymatic processes vital to cellular metabolism. Trivalent arsenic binds to sulfhydryl groups, resulting in decreased production of adenosine triphosphate via the inhibition of enzyme systems such as the pyruvate dehydrogenase and alpha-ketoglutarate complexes. Pentavalent arsenic may be biotransformed to trivalent arsenic or substituted for phosphate in the glycolytic pathway, resulting in uncoupling of oxidative phosphorylation.

CLINICAL MANIFESTATIONS. Arsine gas is colorless, odorless, and nonirritating and is the most toxic form of arsenic. Inhalation causes no immediate symptoms. After a latent period of 2–24 hr, massive hemolysis occurs along with malaise, headache, weakness, dyspnea, nausea, vomiting, abdominal pain, hepatomegaly, pallor, jaundice, hemoglobinuria, and renal failure.

GI toxicity begins within minutes to hours of an acute ingestion of the inorganic arsenic salts, manifested by nausea, vomiting, abdominal pain, and diarrhea. Hemorrhagic gastroenteritis with extensive fluid loss and third spacing may result in hypovolemic shock. Cardiovascular toxicity includes QT interval prolongation, polymorphous ventricular tachycardia, congestive cardiomyopathy, pulmonary edema, and cardiogenic shock. Acute neurologic toxicity includes delirium, seizures, cerebral edema, encephalopathy, and coma. A delayed sensorimotor peripheral neuropathy may appear days to weeks after acute exposure, secondary to axonal degeneration. Early effects include painful dysesthesias, followed by diminished vibratory pain, touch, and temperature sensation, decreased deep tendon reflexes, and in the most severe cases, an ascending paralysis with respiratory failure mimicking Guillain-Barré syndrome. Other effects include fever, hepatitis, rhabdomyolysis, renal failure, hemolytic anemia, pancytopenia, and alopecia. Transverse white striae in the nails, known as Mees lines, become apparent 1–2 mo after exposure in only a small percentage of patients.

Chronic intoxication may present with fatigue, malaise, headache, chronic encephalopathy, peripheral sensorimotor neuropathy, leukopenia, anemia, chronic cough, gastroenteritis, and peripheral edema. Dermatologic manifestations, such as hypopigmentation, hyperpigmentation, and hyperkeratoses, take years to develop.

LABORATORY FINDINGS. The diagnosis of arsenic intoxication is based on characteristic clinical findings, a history of exposure, and elevated urinary arsenic levels, which confirm the exposure. A spot urine arsenic level should be determined for symptomatic patients before chelation, although the result may be negative acutely. Concentrations greater than 50 μg/L in a 24-hr urine collection are consistent with arsenic intoxication. It is important to remember that ingestion of seafood containing nontoxic arsenobetaine and arsenocholine can cause elevated urinary arsenic levels. Blood arsenic levels are rarely helpful owing to their high variability. Elevated arsenic levels in the hair or nails must be interpreted cautiously because of the possibility of external contamination. Abdominal radiographs may demonstrate ingested arsenic, which is radiopaque.

Later in the course of illness, a complete blood count may show anemia, thrombocytopenia, and leukocytosis followed by leukopenia, karyorrhexis, and basophilic stippling of RBCs. The serum levels of creatinine, bilirubin, and transaminases may be elevated; urinalysis may show proteinuria, pyuria, and hematuria; and examination of the cerebrospinal fluid may show elevated protein levels.

MERCURY

EPIDEMIOLOGY. Mercury exists in three states: elemental mercury, inorganic mercury salts, and organic mercury. Elemental mercury is present in thermometers, sphygmomanometers, barometers, batteries, and some latex paints produced before 1991. Workers in industries producing these products may expose their children to the toxin when mercury is brought home on contaminated clothing. Vacuuming of carpet contaminated with mercury and breaking of mercury fluorescent light bulbs may result in elemental mercury vapor exposure. Elemental mercury has also been used in folk remedies by Asian and Mexican populations for chronic stomach pain and by Latin Americans and Caribbean natives in occult practices. Dental amalgams containing elemental mercury release trace amounts of mercury vapor that do not pose a credible risk to health.

Inorganic mercury salts are found in pesticides, disinfectants, antiseptics, pigments, dry batteries, and explosives and as preservatives in some medicinal preparations.

Organic mercury in the diet, especially fish containing methyl mercury, is a major source of mercury exposure to the general population. Industries that may produce mercury-containing effluents include chlorine and caustic soda productions, mining and metallurgy, electroplating, chemical and textile manufacturing, paper and pharmaceutical manufacturing, and leather tanning. Mercury compounds in the environment are methylated to methyl mercury by soil and water microorganisms. Methyl mercury in the water rapidly accumulates in fish and other aquatic organisms, which are in turn consumed by humans.

PHARMACOKINETICS. Inhaled elemental mercury vapor is 80% absorbed by the lungs and rapidly distributed to the central nervous system (CNS) because of its high lipid solubility. The elemental mercury is oxidized by catalase to the mercuric ion, which is the reactive form causing cellular toxicity. Elemental mercury liquid is poorly absorbed from the GI tract, with less than 0.01% being absorbed. The half-life of elemental mercury in the tissues is about 60 days, with most of the excretion being in the urine.

Inorganic mercury salts are about 10% absorbed from the GI tract and cross the blood-brain barrier to a lesser extent than elemental mercury. Mercuric salts are more soluble than mercurous salts and therefore produce greater toxicity. Elimination occurs primarily in the urine, with a half-life of about 40 days.

Methyl mercury is the most avidly absorbed of the organic mercury compounds, with about 90% absorbed from the GI tract. Its lipophilic, short-chain alkyl structure enables methyl mercury to distribute rapidly across the blood-brain barrier and placenta. Methyl mercury is about 90% excreted in the bile, with the remainder being excreted in the urine. The half-life is 70 days.

PATHOPHYSIOLOGY. After absorption, mercury is distributed to all tissues, particularly the CNS and kidneys. Mercury reacts with sulfhydryl, phosphoryl, carboxyl, and amide groups, resulting in disruption of enzymes, transport mechanisms, membranes, and structural proteins. Widespread cellular dysfunction or necrosis results in the multiorgan toxicity characteristic of mercury poisoning.

CLINICAL MANIFESTATIONS. Five syndromes describe the clinical presentation of mercury poisoning: (1) acute inhalation of elemental mercury vapor, (2) acute ingestion of inorganic mercury salts, (3) chronic inorganic mercury intoxication, (4) acrodynia, and (5) methyl mercury intoxication.

Acute inhalation of elemental mercury vapor results in rapid onset of cough, dyspnea, chest pain, fever, chills, headaches, visual disturbances, and GI complaints. Depending on the severity of the exposure, the illness may be self-limited or may progress to necrotizing bronchiolitis, interstitial pneumonitis, pulmonary edema, and death due to respiratory failure. Younger children are more susceptible to pulmonary toxicity. Survivors may develop restrictive lung disease.

Acute ingestion of inorganic mercury salts can present in a few hours with corrosive gastroenteritis manifested by oropharyngeal burns, nausea, hematemesis, severe abdominal pain, hematochezia, cardiovascular collapse, acute tubular necrosis, and death.

Chronic inorganic mercury intoxication produces the classic triad of tremor, neuropsychiatric disturbances, and gingivostomatitis. The syndrome may result from chronic exposure to elemental mercury, inorganic mercury salts, or certain organic mercury compounds, all of which may be metabolized to mercuric ions. The tremor starts as a fine intention tremor of the fingers that is abolished during sleep, but it may later involve the face and progress to choreoathetosis and spasmodic ballismus. Mixed sensorimotor neuropathy and visual disturbances may also be present. The neuropsychiatric disturbances include emotional lability, delirium, headaches, memory loss, insomnia, anorexia, and fatigue. Renal dysfunction ranges from asymptomatic proteinuria to nephrotic syndrome.

Acrodynia, or pink disease, is a rare idiosyncratic hypersensitivity reaction to mercury that occurs predominantly in children. The symptom complex includes generalized pain, paresthesias, and an acral rash that may spread to involve the face. It is typically pink, papular, and pruritic and may progress to desquamation and ulceration. Morbilliform, vesicular, and hemorrhagic variants have been described. Other important features include anorexia, apathy, and hypotonia, especially of the pectoral and pelvic girdles. Irritability, tremors, diaphoresis, insomnia, hypertension, and tachycardia may be present. The outcome is good after removal of the source of mercury exposure.

Methyl mercury intoxication is also referred to as *Minamata disease* after the widespread mercury poisoning that occurred at Minamata Bay in Japan after the ingestion of contaminated fish. Methyl mercury poisoning presents with delayed neurotoxicity after a latent period of weeks to months, characterized by ataxia; dysarthria; paresthesias; tremors; movement disorders; impairment of vision, hearing, smell, and taste; memory loss; progressive dementia; and death. Infants exposed in utero are the most severely affected, with low birthweight, microcephaly, profound developmental delay, cerebral palsy, deafness, blindness, and seizures.

LABORATORY FINDINGS. The diagnosis of mercury intoxication is based on characteristic clinical findings, a history of exposure, and elevated blood or urine mercury levels, which confirm the exposure. Levels less than 2 μg/L in the blood and 10 μg/L in a 24-hr urine collection are considered normal. Although blood mercury levels may reflect acute exposure, they decrease as mercury redistributes into the tissues. Urine mercury levels are most useful for identifying chronic exposures, except in the case of methyl mercury, because methyl mercury undergoes minimal urinary excretion. Hair analysis for mercury is not reliable because hair reflects exogenous as well as endogenous mercury exposure. Abdominal radiographs may demonstrate ingested mercury.

Urinary markers of early nephrotoxicity include microalbuminuria, retinol binding protein, β_2-microglobulin, and N-acetyl-β-D-glucosaminidase. Early neurotoxicity may be detected with neuropsychiatric testing and nerve conduction studies, whereas severe CNS toxicity is apparent on CT or MRI.

TREATMENT

The principles of management for arsenic and mercury intoxication include prompt removal from the source of poisoning, aggressive stabilization and supportive care, decontamination, and chelation therapy. Once the diagnosis is suspected, the local poison control facility should be contacted and care coordinated with physicians who are familiar with the management of heavy metal poisoning.

Supportive care for patients exposed to arsine gas requires close monitoring for signs of hemolysis, including evaluation of the peripheral blood smear and urinalysis. Transfusion of packed RBCs may be necessary, as well as administration of intravenous fluids, sodium bicarbonate, and mannitol to prevent renal failure secondary to the deposition of hemoglobin in the kidneys. After inhalation of elemental mercury vapor, patients require careful monitoring of respiratory status, which may include pulse oximetry, arterial blood gas analysis, and chest radiography. Supportive care includes administration of supplemental oxygen and, in severe cases, intubation and mechanical ventilation. Acute ingestion of inorganic arsenic and mercury salts results in hemorrhagic gastroenteritis, cardiovascular collapse, and multiorgan dysfunction. Fluid resuscitation, pressor agents, and transfusion of blood products may be required for management of cardiovascular instability. Severe respiratory distress, coma with loss of airway reflexes, intractable seizures, and respiratory paralysis are indications for intubation and mechanical ventilation. Renal function must be carefully monitored for signs of renal failure and the need for hemodialysis.

GI decontamination after ingestion of the inorganic arsenic and mercury salts has not been well studied. Because of the corrosive effects of these compounds, emesis is not recommended, and endoscopy may be considered before gastric lavage. Although arsenic and mercury are not well adsorbed to activated charcoal, its use is generally advocated, especially if co-ingestants are suspected. Whole bowel irrigation is used to remove any radiopaque material remaining in the GI tract.

Chelation for acute arsenic and mercury poisoning is most effective when given as soon as possible after the exposure. Chelation should be continued until 24-hr urinary arsenic or mercury levels return to normal (<50 μg/L for arsenic and <10 μg/L for mercury), the patient is symptom free, or the remaining toxic effects are believed to be irreversible. The efficacy of chelation in chronic exposures is reduced because heavy metal in the tissue compartment is relatively unexchangeable and some degree of irreversible toxicity has already occurred.

Dimercaprol, also known as 2,3-dimercaptopropanol or British antilewisite (BAL), is the chelator of choice if a patient cannot tolerate oral therapy. This is often the case in critically ill patients and after ingestion of the corrosive inorganic arsenic and mercury salts. BAL is available suspended in peanut oil in 3-mL ampules at a concentration of 100 mg/mL for deep intramuscular (IM) injection. The recommended regimen is 3–5 mg/kg IM every 4 hr for the first 2 days, 2.5–3 mg/kg IM every 6 hr for the next 2 days, then 2.5–3 mg/kg every 12 hr for 1 wk. The BAL–heavy metal complex is excreted in the urine and bile. A period of 5 days between courses of chelation is recommended. Adverse effects of BAL include pain at the injection site, hypertension, tachycardia, diaphoresis, nausea, vomiting, abdominal pain, a burning sensation in the oropharynx, and a feeling of constriction in the chest. BAL may cause hemolysis in glucose-6-phosphate dehydrogenase (G6PD)–deficient individuals. It is important to note that BAL is contraindicated for chelation of methyl mercury because BAL redistributes methyl mercury to the brain from other tissue sites, resulting in increased neurotoxicity.

Oral agents are used in addition to BAL or when prolonged chelation is indicated and patients are able to tolerate oral therapy. Succimer, also known as 2,3-dimercaptosuccinic acid (DMSA), is an orally administered water-soluble derivative of BAL. DMSA is available in 100 mg capsules, and the recommended regimen is 10 mg/kg every 8 hr for the first 5 days, followed by 10 mg/kg every 12 hr for the next 2 wk. The DMSA–heavy metal complex is excreted in the urine and bile. A period of 2 wk between courses of chelation is recommended. Mild adverse effects include nausea, vomiting, diarrhea, loss of appetite, and transient elevations in liver enzyme levels. It may also cause hemolysis in G6PD-deficient patients.

D-penicillamine, or PCN, is another orally administered chelator used for arsenic and mercury intoxication. It is available in 125 and 250 mg capsules, and the recommended regimen is 25 mg/kg every 6 hr up to 250 mg/dose, for up to 1–2 wk. The PCN–heavy metal complex is excreted in the urine. Adverse effects include hypersensitivity rashes, leukopenia, thrombocytopenia, hemolytic anemia, agranulocytosis, hepatitis, pancreatitis, nausea, vomiting, and anorexia.

Davidson PW, Myers GJ, Cox C, et al: Effects of prenatal and postnatal methylmercury exposure from fish consumption on neurodevelopment. JAMA 280:701, 1998.

Ford MD: Heavy metals. *In:* Tintinalli JE, Ruiz E, Krome RL (eds): Emergency Medicine: A Comprehensive Study Guide, 4th ed. New York, McGraw-Hill, 1996, pp 833–841.

Kew J, Morris C, Aihie A, et al: Arsenic and mercury intoxication due to Indian ethnic remedies. Br Med J 306:506, 1993.

Kingston RL, Hall S, Sioris L: Clinical observations and medical outcome in 149 cases of arsenate ant killer ingestion. Clin Toxicol 31:581, 1993.

McLauchlan GA: Acute mercury poisoning. Anaesthesia 56:110, 1991.

Moromisato DY, Anas NG, Goodman G: Mercury inhalation poisoning and acute lung injury in a child. Chest 105:613, 1994.

Park MJ, Currier M: Arsenic exposures in Mississippi: A review of cases. South Med J 84:461, 1991.

Powell PP: Minamata disease: A story of mercury's malevolence. South Med J 84:1352, 1991.

Schwartz JG, Snider TE, Montiel MM: Toxicity of a family from vacuumed mercury. Am J Emerg Med 10:258, 1992.

Sue YJ: Mercury. *In:* Goldfrank LR, Flomenbaum NE, Lewin NA, et al (eds): Goldfrank's Toxicologic Emergencies, 5th ed. Norwalk, Appleton & Lange, 1994, pp 1051–1062.

Taueg C, Sanfilippo DJ, Rowens B, et al: Acute and chronic mercury poisoning from residential exposure to elemental mercury—Michigan, 1989–1990. Clin Toxicol 30:63, 1992.

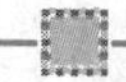

CHAPTER 721
Lead Poisoning

Sergio Piomelli

EPIDEMIOLOGY. Lead, a nonessential metal, is not a natural constituent of the human body; when present, it represents contamination of the internal milieu. An average blood lead level near 0 was found in an "unacculturated" population, the Yanomamo Indians, living at the remote source of the Orinoco River. In a study of children and adults living near the Himalayas, the average blood lead level was found to be 3 μg/dL; this very low level could be explained by the combustion of heating materials in huts without chimneys.

In the United States, the presence of lead in the environment has been pervasive, primarily because of vehicular emissions and lead paint in old deteriorated housing. In the 1970s, lead poisoning was a common and devastating illness, particularly for inner-city children. Lead encephalopathy was common, and thousands of children suffered marked brain damage.

The situation has profoundly changed, primarily because of the progressive elimination of lead in gasoline. According to the National Health and Nutritional Examination Survey, the average blood lead level of the entire United States population decreased from 12.2 μg/dL in 1980 to 3.2 μg/dL in 1991. In 1991, the prevalence of children age 1–5 yr with blood lead levels of 15 μg/dL or greater was 9%. The prevalence of children with blood lead levels of 20 μg/dL or greater (the level at which the Centers for Disease Control and Prevention [CDC] recommends medical intervention) was 1.1%. These figures refer to the entire nation; substantial differences in the percentages among various socioeconomic groups persist. However, blood lead levels decreased further by 1994; in the author's urban pediatric clinic, the average blood lead level declined from 5.2 μg/dL in 1991 to 3.2 μg/dL in 1994. The estimates of the prevalence of blood lead levels of 10 μg/dL or greater in children age 1–5 yr range from 2–9% in various areas. The percentage of children with blood lead level of 15 μg/dL or greater is now much lower than these values. The percentage of children with blood lead level of 20 μg/dL or greater is less than 1% throughout the United States and much lower in most areas. Lead levels vary greatly within the United States and within each city. The prevalence of blood lead levels of 20 μg/dL or greater is higher in children living in pre–World War II dilapidated housing; it is almost nonexistent among those living in recent housing.

The decline in the average blood lead level has been accompanied by a decrease in the frequency and severity of clinical lead intoxication. Lead encephalopathy has almost disappeared; most children tested by the current screening programs have blood lead levels well below 10 μg/dL. These remarkable results reflect primarily the effect of the reduction of vehicular lead emissions mandated by the Clean Air Act and demonstrate the effectiveness and importance of prevention. Nonetheless, many children, mostly those from poor urban areas, have an excessive body burden of lead and suffer unnecessary neuropsychologic damage. For these children and other children in many countries, lead poisoning continues to be a public health problem.

The major source of lead for children in the United States is the lead-containing paint present in most dwellings built before World War II; this is most dangerous when the paint is deteriorating. Lead-containing dust is taken up by small children through respiration and their normal hand-to-mouth activities. When lead-laden homes are renovated, lead dust is a particularly serious risk; children should always be removed from the premises during such renovations. Although airborne and dust-laden lead are continuous sources of low-level exposure, other nonpaint lead sources may at times provide an intense exposure, leading to rapid accumulation of a very toxic level of lead and provoking severe and acute lead poisoning. Acidic fruit juices stored in poorly glazed ceramic vessels, lead dust carried home by lead industry workers, fumes from burning batteries, some Asian cosmetics, and some Mexican folk medicines all have resulted in sporadic cases of lead poisoning in children. Sniffing of leaded gasoline by teenagers and older children is another cause of lead poisoning.

PATHOPHYSIOLOGY. The high toxicity of lead results from its avidity for the sulfhydryl (SH) group of proteins. Lead irreversibly binds to the SH group of a protein and thus impairs its function. Certain metabolic effects of lead can be detected even at minimal levels of exposure. The enzyme δ-aminolevulinic acid dehydratase, which catalyzes the formation of the porphobilinogen ring, a key step of the heme synthetic pathway, is progressively inhibited by lead in an exponential manner, without any threshold. Its inactivation can be reversed in vitro by removal of the lead with SH reagents. The loss of activity of the δ-aminolevulinic acid dehydratase is a continuously progressing phenomenon. However, at very low levels of lead exposure, the impact of partial inactivation of this enzyme is probably negligible, because the potential enzyme activity is largely in excess of the activity needed for heme synthesis. At higher levels of exposure, on the other hand, nearly complete inactivation of the enzyme results in serious clinical consequences; it leads to accumulation of δ-aminolevulinic acid, which is neurotoxic.

Another enzyme in the heme synthesis pathway that is severely damaged by lead is ferrochelatase, which catalyzes the final step of heme synthesis, the insertion of iron into the protoporphyrin IX ring. The result of an ineffective ferrochelatase is an accumulation of protoporphyrin in the erythrocytes. This, because of its fluorescence, is easily detected. This property permits a rapid and accurate measurement of the erythrocyte porphyrins (EP). EP is a useful adjunct in detecting childhood lead poisoning because it reflects the biochemical effects of lead; it also detects iron deficiency, a frequent and aggravating companion of lead poisoning.

Accumulation of protoporphyrin also sheds light on the pathogenesis of certain symptoms of lead poisoning. For instance, a defect in the heme-containing cytochrome P450 underlies the failure of the alcohol dehydrogenase system in workers of the lead industry that results in very prolonged hangovers (Monday morning colic). Organotypic neural tissue cultures exposed to lead demyelinate and accumulate fluorescent porphyrins; these effects can be prevented by the addition of heme to the system. Thus, the abnormalities of heme synthesis induced by lead underlie and parallel the neurologic abnormalities.

CLINICAL MANIFESTATIONS. There is no direct correlation between blood lead level and clinical manifestations. In practice, the probability of severe symptoms increases as the exposure to lead and blood lead levels rise. However, children with blood lead levels greater than 100 μg/dL may occasionally appear clinically well, and children with blood lead levels 30–35 μg/dL may be clearly symptomatic.

The most serious manifestation of lead poisoning is acute encephalopathy. This may appear without a prodrome or may be preceded by behavioral changes or lead colic, characterized by occasional vomiting, intermittent abdominal pain, and constipation. Encephalopathy includes persistent vomiting, ataxia, seizures, papilledema, impaired consciousness, and coma. If it is necessary for the diagnosis, a spinal tap may be carefully performed: This usually reveals mild pleocytosis, modest hyperproteinemia, and increased pressure. Peripheral neuropathy, which is common in adults, is rare in children, except for those with sickle cell disease. The symptoms of childhood lead poisoning in the absence of clear signs of encephalopathy are usually nonspecific and vague. Abdominal colic, behavioral abnormalities, attention disorders, hyperactivity, or severe unexplained retardation should lead one to suspect clinical lead poisoning.

Lead encephalopathy rarely occurs at blood lead levels below 100 μg/dL. However, children with elevated blood lead levels, even well below that level, may present with a constellation of neurologic symptoms. These are usually more obvious at higher blood level (hyperactivity, anorexia, decreased play activity). At lower levels, the neurologic abnormalities become progressively less evident; however, these cannot be discounted. Neurobehavioral abnormalities, demonstrated at low levels of lead exposure by epidemiologic studies, include lower intelligence and poor school performance. Needleman demonstrated significant neurobehavioral abnormalities when comparing two groups of children, one with high and the other with low lead in their deciduous teeth dentin. Peak blood lead levels in the affected children were approximately 35 μg/dL. The validity of this study was confirmed by the National Research Council. Similar neurobehavioral abnormalities have been shown at even lower levels of lead exposure. The effect of lead on children's intelligence has been established by several studies. An increase of blood lead from 10–20 μg/dL results in an average decrease in IQ of 1–2 points. Some consider this to be a trivial effect but current techniques for detecting neurobehavioral abnormalities are much less sensitive than those used to detect biochemical abnormalities. Subtle abnormalities are detectable only on large cohorts with sophisticated statistics. These may have little or physiologic relevance to the future intellectual capacity of individual children. Similar to this is the case of the demonstrable but physiologically irrelevant partial inactivation of the δ-aminolevulinic acid dehydratase by lead.

DIAGNOSIS. Of critical importance in the diagnosis is an accurate environmental history, particularly of exposure to lead-containing paint. History of pica, when present, is strongly suggestive; however, pica is not a prerequisite for lead poisoning. Children with a normal rate of hand-to-mouth activity ingest substantial amounts of lead from household dust when deteriorating lead-containing paint is present. Large radiopaque flakes of paint, when present on abdominal radiologic examination, are a clear indicator of pica. However, lead poisoning results mostly from ingestion of dust: The large flakes of paint themselves pass essentially unchanged through the intestine into the stool.

Environmental investigation should involve not only a child's own home but also other locations where the child spends considerable time, such as the grandmother's or baby sitter's residence. It is also important to consider the other nonpaint sources of exposure (see earlier). When the diagnosis of lead poisoning is established, technicians from the local Department of Health should be immediately dispatched to examine the involved homes.

Unless the symptoms of lead poisoning are obviously severe and evident, in most cases, the diagnosis needs to be established by blood lead testing. Lead poisoning is often diagnosed through a screening program in children who are apparently asymptomatic. Lead levels should preferably be measured on a venous blood sample. However, pragmatic considerations often make this difficult, particularly when the number of children to be tested is very large. In these situations, lead can be measured from blood samples obtained by finger puncture. If the finger puncture technique is impeccably executed by experienced technicians, the percentage of contaminated samples can be kept at less than 10%. The result of an elevated blood lead level obtained by finger puncture, however, should never be used as the only criterion to initiate therapy in an asymptomatic child: Therapy should be delayed until the result of a confirmatory venous blood lead level is available. If a child has symptoms of lead poisoning and a venous blood lead level cannot be rapidly obtained, supportive evidence should be used, such as measuring EP, an abdominal film to search for evidence of lead exposure, and radiography of the long bones to look for lead lines. (The latter finding is unspecific and may be present in other chronic illnesses.) None of these tests is, per se, diagnostic of lead poisoning, but each can, in critical situations, provide useful supportive information.

Measurements of blood lead levels are difficult and cumbersome. Such tests are rarely available in hospital laboratories. Most large cities and state laboratories provide blood lead analysis. Even in the best laboratories, however, the accuracy is only ± 2 μg/dL, and often it is only ± 4 μg/dL. Such a margin of error is acceptable when the blood lead level is high (≥30 μg/dL). When the blood lead level is low (≤15 μg/dL), however, the uncertainty creates difficulties in classification. Blood lead levels between 10 and 14 μg/dL should be confirmed before classifying a child on a single measurement as having "lead poisoning" according to the 1991 CDC definition.

Elevation of the EP level is an indication of alterations of the process of heme synthesis. It reflects either iron deficiency or lead poisoning. The EP level is most markedly elevated when both iron deficiency and lead poisoning coexist, a frequent occurrence, particularly in children from low socioeconomic levels in urban areas. Measurements of EP were used extensively to screen children in the 1970s when the frequency of elevated blood lead levels was very high. The EP level was then a very useful test for detecting the most severe cases of lead poisoning, because results are 100% positive when the blood lead level is 55 μg/dL or greater. However, at lower blood lead levels, the frequency of positive results declines; at a blood lead level of 32 μg/dL, only 50% of the children tested have positive results, and just a few children test positive when the blood lead level is 20 μg/dL or less. Because the current screening programs are directed at detecting lower blood lead levels, EP levels cannot be used anymore as primary screening tools. This test remains useful to diagnose iron deficiency, to assess the biochemical damage of lead, and to provide supportive evidence in symptomatic children when measurements of blood lead levels are not promptly available. EP measurements are also useful in follow-up of the effectiveness of long-term therapy. The EP level promptly rises within 24–48 hr of exposure, but because it is incorporated into the hemoglobin molecule itself, it persists for the entire red blood cell life span of 120 days. Thus, for children in treatment, a slow but progressive decline of the EP level reflects the elimination of lead from the body better than does the decline of blood lead level, which can be rapid but ephemeral after therapy.

DEFINITION AND CLASSIFICATION OF LEAD POISONING. The natural blood lead level is 0 μg/dL. Thus, any exposure to lead results in some biochemical damage that becomes continuously progressive with increasing levels. Thus, in a very precise sense, we all have *lead poisoning.* In practice, however, it is necessary to choose a threshold blood lead value below which the adverse effects of lead are "trivial" (i.e., physiologically irrelevant). The choice is always somewhat arbitrary, and this leads to further controversy.

In 1991, the CDC's expert panel designated all children with blood lead level of 10 μg/dL or more as having *"lead poisoning."* This unqualified definition gives equal importance to a blood lead level of 12 μg/dL as to one of 75 μg/dL or more. In the most recent revision of the CDC document, children with blood lead levels of 10–19 μg/dL are still defined as having lead poisoning. The wisdom of such rigid classification has been criticized by many, including representatives of the American Academy of Pediatrics.

The proposed CDC classification based on blood lead level (Table 721–1) is useful for providing approximate management guidelines and for helping large programs establish priorities. However, no rigid classification can replace sound clinical judgment in treating an individual child. Age, presence of iron deficiency, living conditions, and parental understanding should also be taken into consideration.

TREATMENT

Removing the Source of Lead Exposure. The most important aspect of therapy is to remove the child from the source of exposure to lead. In most cases, this is the only necessary action; only

TABLE 721–1 Centers for Disease Control and Prevention 1991 Classification and Recommendations

Blood Lead Level (μ/dL)		Action Recommended
0–9		No immediate concern
≥10		"Lead poisoning"
10–14	Environmental survey	If found in too many children, survey the community
15–19	Environmental survey	Education about lead exposure
20–24	Remove from lead source	Bring to medical attention
25–54	Remove from lead source	EDTA test: if positive, 25–44 EDTA; 45–54 EDTA or DMSA
55–69	Remove from lead source	Treat with EDTA or DMSA
≥70 or symptomatic	Emergency hospitalization	Treat with BAL and EDTA

Always return the child to a clean house.

EDTA = edetate calcium-disodium; DMSA = succimer; BAL = dimercaprol.

in more severe cases is treatment indicated. Removal from the source, however, must be complete. In the case of poor urban children, there often is more than one source; in addition to the child's own home, the grandmother's or the baby sitter's home may be equally contaminated. It is essential that children be removed from their own homes to a safer one that has been appropriately inspected by Health Department technicians. Similarly, while the child's home is being repaired, the child should stay out of it day and night. Repairs should be followed by cleaning with a high-efficiency particle accumulator (HEPA) vacuum cleaner, and the areas should be scrubbed with high-phosphate detergent two or three times, followed by HEPA vacuum cleaning again, before the child is allowed to return. Treatment of more severe cases requires chelation therapy.

Symptomatic Children and Children with Blood Lead Levels of More Than 70 μg/dL. In symptomatic children, regardless of blood lead level, the treatment is always given in a hospital. Children with blood lead levels of 70 μg/dL or more, even if asymptomatic, should always be considered as posing a medical emergency and should immediately be hospitalized for treatment. Treatment should consist of dimercaprol (BAL, 75 mg/m^2 every 4 hr; total daily dose of 450 mg/m^2), followed by edetate calcium-disodium (EDTA) (1,500 mg/m^2/24 hr by continuous infusion). It is important to start with BAL and to initiate the EDTA only 3–4 hr later. EDTA also binds zinc and renders even more complete the paralysis of the δ-aminolevulinic acid dehydratase (a zinc-dependent enzyme); this, in turn, results in a burst of neurotoxic δ-aminolevulinic acid in the blood, which may induce convulsions. Treatment should be continued for 5 days; the BAL may be suspended as soon as the blood lead level falls below 60 μg/dL. Repeated courses of treatment may be necessary for these children until their blood lead level returns to a safe range (≤ 20 μg/dL).

Management of the Encephalopathy. Treatment of these critically ill patients consists of controlling convulsions (if present), establishing urine flow, and administering the same chelation therapy as described earlier. Careful control of fluids is necessary to avoid aggravating the increased intracranial pressure (ICP). Intravenous EDTA, at the dosage recommended earlier, can be safely fitted into a controlled fluid administration. See Chapter 64.7 for management of increased ICP.

Asymptomatic Children with Blood Lead Levels of 45–69 μg/dL. Asymptomatic children with blood lead levels of 45–69 μg/dL almost always should be treated. The treatment may consist of EDTA alone (1,000 mg/m^2/24 hr intravenously, in a 24-hr infusion or in a short 20–30-min infusion) for 5 consecutive days. EDTA is best given intravenously. When the intravenous route is not possible, EDTA may be given intramuscularly; however, by this route it is extremely painful, and the pain is only partially alleviated if the drug is mixed with procaine. EDTA can be administered again, if necessary, after a 2-day interval.

An alternative therapy consists of Succimer (DMSA [Chemet]). DMSA can be given orally, has minimal side effects, and appears to be an excellent chelator. However, outpatient DMSA should never be used unless there is *absolute certainty* that the child's environment is perfectly clean. DMSA is administered for 5 days at a dose of 350 mg/m^2 every 8 hr for 5 consecutive days, followed by 2 wk more of therapy at reduced frequency (350 mg/m^2 every 12 hr) for a total of 19 days. Additional courses may be given, if needed, after a 2-wk interval. Repeated courses of treatment may be necessary to bring the blood lead into a safe range (≤ 20 μg/dL).

Asymptomatic Children with Blood Lead Levels of 20–45 μg/dL. When the blood lead level is in this range, it is preferable to perform an EDTA-provocative chelation test to ascertain the usefulness of treatment. This test consists of administration of EDTA (500 mg/m^2), preferably intravenously, in 5% dextrose, over 30 min, followed by urine collection of 8 hr duration. The urinary excretion of lead is measured, and the results are expressed as the following ratio:

$$\frac{\text{Lead excreted } (\mu g)}{\text{EDTA given (mg)}}$$

A ratio greater than 0.7 is considered an abnormal (positive) provocative test result. This suggests that treatment will be effective and is indicated. If the results of the EDTA provocative chelation test suggest treatment, only EDTA is administered, because at these blood lead levels, the use of DMSA is not approved by the Food and Drug Administration. EDTA should be given at a dose of 1,000 mg/m^2/24 hr, preferably on an outpatient basis.

Asymptomatic Children with Blood Lead Levels of 10–19 μg/dL. At these levels, no treatment or medical intervention is necessary; only general education is recommended. As a result of the CDC classification, physicians are requested to inform parents that their child with a blood lead level of 11 μg/dL has lead poisoning, although in most cases, a repeat analysis would yield a value of ≤9 μg/dL. Thus, it is recommended, when dealing with such borderline values, to repeat the blood lead level immediately (not wait 3 mo, as the CDC recommends) and to use caution and sensitivity to avoid unnecessary parental panic. Recommendations of household cleaning and attention to potential exposure should be offered to these and all other parents.

PREVENTION AND SCREENING. Today, the major source of lead in the United States remains old house paint. Lead poisoning will not completely disappear until the current housing stock is completely repaired and made lead free. This would represent a substantial cost, but it is the responsibility of a civilized society. In *Strategic Plan for Elimination of Childhood Lead Poisoning,* the CDC indicated the need and the cost effectiveness of eliminating lead from the homes where children live. However, in 1991, the CDC chose to emphasize universal screening by blood lead measurement, whether or not children live in a contaminated community. Screening should occur at 10–14 mo of age and again at approximately 2 yr of age. This approach has been criticized in the pediatric community, arguing for a targeted approach of screening all poor children. The recent HANES report reveals that dangerous lead levels (≥20 μg/dL) are currently still present in approximately 90,000 children in the United States. These significantly high levels are almost exclusively found in inner-city poor children. About 66% of children 1–5 yr old on Medicaid have elevated blood lead levels. Screening would be better directed to poor communities and children enrolled in Medicaid.

Annest JL, Pirkle JL, Maguk D, et al: Chronological trend in blood lead level between 1976 and 1980. N Engl J Med 308:1373, 1983.

Centers for Disease Control and Prevention: Preventing Lead Poisoning in Young Children. US Department of Health and Human Services, Public Health Service, 1991. Strategic Plan for Elimination of Childhood Lead Poisoning. US Department of Health and Human Services, Public Health Service, 1991. Screening Young Children for Lead Poisoning: Guidance for State and Local Public Health Officials. US Department of Health and Human Services, Public Health Service, 1997.

Harvey B: New lead screening guidelines from the Centers for Disease Control and Prevention: How will they affect pediatricians? Pediatrics 100:384, 1997.

Juberg DR, Kleiman CF, Kwon SC: Position paper of the American council on science and health: Lead and human health. J Expo Anal Environ Epidemiol 8:17, 1998.

Needleman HL, Gunnoe C, Leviton A, et al: Deficits in psychologic and classroom performance of children with elevated dentine lead levels. N Engl J Med 300:689, 1979.

Nordin J, Rolnick S, Ehlinger E, et al: Lead levels in high-risk and low-risk young children in the Minneapolis–St. Paul metropolitan area. J Fam Pract 45:515, 1997.

Patterson CC: Contaminated and natural lead environment of man. Arch Environ Health 11:344, 1985.

Piomelli S: Childhood lead poisoning in the '90s. Pediatrics 93:508, 1994.

Piomelli S, Rosen JF, Chisolm JJ, et al: Management of childhood lead poisoning. J Pediatr 105:523, 1984.

Pirkle JL, Brody DJ, Gunter EW, et al: The decline in blood lead levels in

the United States. The National Health and Nutritional Examination Surveys (NHANES). JAMA 272:294, 1994.
Pocock S, Smith M, Baghurst P: Environmental lead and children's intelligence: A systematic review of the epidemiologic evidence. Br Med J 309:1189, 1994.
Robertson WO: U.S. lead testing policies in question. [Letter.] Clin Pediatr 37:62, 1998.
Schwartz J: Low-level lead exposure and children's I.Q.: A meta-analysis and search for a threshold. Environ Res 56:42, 1994.
U.S. General Accounting Office: Medicaid: Elevated blood lead levels in children. GAO/HEHS-98-78.

CHAPTER 722
Poisonings: Drugs, Chemicals, and Plants

George C. Rodgers, Jr., and Nancy J. Matyunas

722.1 Epidemiology and Approach to Management

Of the more than 2 million human poisoning exposures reported annually to the Toxic Exposure Surveillance System (TESS) of the American Association of Poison Control Centers (AAPCC), more than 50% occurred in children 5 yr of age or younger. Almost all of these exposures are accidental and reflect the propensity for children in this age group to put virtually everything in their mouths. Also see Chapter 57.

More than 90% of toxic exposures in children occur in the home, and most involve only a single substance. Ingestion is the most common route of poisoning exposure (75% of cases), with the dermal, ophthalmic, and inhalation routes each occurring in about 6% of cases. Sixty per cent of cases involve nondrug products, most commonly cosmetics and personal care products, cleaning substances, plants, foreign bodies, and hydrocarbons. Pharmaceutical preparations comprise the remainder, with analgesics, cough and cold products, antimicrobial agents, and vitamins the most common categories. More than 75% of poisoning exposures can be managed at home without direct medical intervention, because either the product involved is not inherently very toxic or the quantity of the material involved is not sufficient to produce toxic effects. Table 722–1 is a partial list of nontoxic products commonly encountered by children. Death due to accidental poisoning in young children is not common owing to increased product safety measures (e.g., child-resistant packaging), increased poison prevention education, and improvements in medical management.

Poison prevention education should be an integral part of all well child visits, even before a child is mobile. Counseling parents and other caregivers about potential poisoning risks, how to "poison-proof" a child's environment, and what to do if a poisoning occurs diminishes the likelihood of serious morbidity or mortality from an exposure. See Chapter 5.

Poisoning exposures in children 6–12 yr of age are much less common (4% of exposures). Toxic exposures in adolescents are primarily intentional (suicide or abuse) or occupational. Pediatricians should be aware of the signs of drug abuse or suicidal ideation in this population and should aggressively intervene.

MANAGEMENT PLAN FOR POISONING AND OVERDOSE

HISTORY. Obtaining an accurate problem-oriented history is of paramount importance if a poisoning has occurred or is suspected. The following information should be obtained during the initial assessment:

Description of Toxins. Product names (brand, generic, or chemical) and ingredients, along with their concentrations, may be obtained from labels. Because many brand names that sound alike have very different ingredients, it is important to be precise. If the ingredient information is not readily available on the product, consultation with a Poison Control Center can usually provide this information rapidly.

Magnitude of Exposure. Determine how much of the substance has been ingested. This can be accomplished by counting the number of tablets or measuring the volume of liquid remaining. Because the toxicity of most agents is dose related, knowing the age and weight of the victim aids in assessment. For inhalation, ocular, or dermal exposures, the concentration of the offending agent and the length of contact time with the material should be determined.

Progression of Symptoms. Knowing the nature and progression of symptoms is helpful for assessing the need for immediate life support, the prognosis, and the type of intervention that may need to be performed. Several characteristic toxic syndromes (Table 722–2) are described, and evaluation of signs and symptoms may assist in identifying the offending agent.

Time of Exposure. For some products, toxic manifestations may be delayed for hours or days. Knowing the time lapse between exposure and the time until either medical evaluation or the onset of symptoms may influence therapeutic intervention.

Medical History. Underlying diseases may make a victim more susceptible to the effects of a toxin. Concurrent drug therapy may also influence the prognosis, because drugs may interact with the toxin. Pregnancy is a common precipitating factor in adolescent suicide attempts and may influence the treatment plan.

Demographic Information. This is particularly important to know if a parent or caregiver telephones the physician's office with a poisoning situation. Obtain the caller's telephone number and street address to allow for follow-up or to dispatch emergency personnel in the event phone contact is broken.

INITIAL MEDICAL CARE. If the patient is treated at home, follow-

TABLE 722–1 Common Nontoxic Products

Abrasives	Ink (black, blue—nonpermanent)
Antacids	Iodophil disinfectants (unless allergic)
Antibiotics	Laxatives
Ballpoint pen inks	Lipstick
Bathtub floating toys	Lubricating oils (unless aspirated)
Bath oil (castor oil and perfume)	Magazines
Body conditioners	Magic markers
Bubble bath soaps (detergents)	Makeup
Calamine lotion	Matches
Candles (beeswax or paraffin)	Mineral oil (unless aspirated)
Caps (toy pistols, potassium chlorate)	Newspaper (chronic ingestion may result in lead poisoning)
Chalk (calcium carbonate)	Paint—indoor latex
Children's toy cosmetics	Pencil lead (graphite, coloring)
Clay (modeling)	Petroleum jelly (Vaseline)
Contraceptive agents	Play-Doh
Corticosteroids	Polaroid picture coating fluid
Cosmetics	Porous—tip ink marking pens
Crayons (marked A.P. or C.P., gel)	Putty
Dehumidifying packets (silica or charcoal)	Rubber cement
Deodorants—underarm	Sachets
Fabric softeners	Shampoo
Fertilizers (if no insecticide or herbicides added)	Shaving creams and lotions
Fishbowl additives	Soap and soap products
Glues and pastes	Spackles
Golf ball (core may cause mechanical injury)	Suntan preparations
Grease	Sweetening agents (saccharin, aspartame)
Hand lotions and creams	Toothpaste (with and without fluoride)
Hydrogen peroxide (medicinal 3%)	Warfarin rodenticides (<0.5%)
Incense	Watercolor paints
Indelible markers	Zinc oxide

TABLE 722–2 Toxic Syndromes

Syndrome	Symptoms	Causes
Anticholinergic	Exocrine gland hyposecretion, thirst, flushed skin, mydriasis, hyperthermia, urinary retention, delirium, hallucinations, tachycardia, respiratory insufficiency	Belladonna alkaloids, jimsonweed, some mushrooms, antihistamines, tricyclic antidepressants, scopolamine
Cholinergic (muscarinic and nicotinic)	Exocrine gland hypersecretion, urination, nausea, vomiting, diarrhea, muscle fasciculations, miosis, weakness or paralysis, bronchospasm, tachycardia or bradycardia, convulsions, coma	Organophosphate and carbamate insecticides, some mushrooms, tobacco, black widow spider bites (severe)
Extrapyramidal	Tremor, rigidity, opisthotonos, torticollis, dysphonia, oculogyric crisis	Phenothiazines, haloperidol, metoclopramide
Hypermetabolic	Fever, tachycardia, hyperpnea, restlessness, convulsions, metabolic acidosis	Salicylates, some phenols, triethyltin, chlorophenoxy herbicides
Narcotic	Central nervous system depression, hypothermia, hypotension, hypoventilation, miosis	All narcotics, propoxyphene, heroin
Sympathomimetic	Excitation, psychosis, seizures, hypertension, tachypnea, hyperthermia, mydriasis	Amphetamines, phencyclidine, cocaine, crack cocaine, phenylpropanolamine, methylphenidate, theophylline, caffeine
Withdrawal	Abdominal cramps, diarrhea, lacrimation, sweating, "goose flesh," yawning, tachycardia, restlessness, hallucinations	Cessation of alcohol, barbiturates, benzodiazepines, narcotics

up assessment calls must be made approximately 0.5, 1, and 4 hr after exposure. Consultation with a Poison Control Center for assistance in monitoring such patients should be considered. Poison Control Centers are staffed by nurses, pharmacists, and physicians specially trained to respond to and monitor poisoning exposures. Any change in a patient's condition may alter the decision to treat at home. If a patient requires hospital treatment, the probability of the development of life-threatening symptoms dictates the mode of transportation used. After a decision to transport a patient is made, emergency department personnel should be notified so they can properly prepare. All product containers thought likely to be related to the exposure should be gathered up and taken with a patient. If a patient has vomited, the emesis should be saved and taken with the patient.

Once a patient has arrived in the appropriate medical care setting, initial attention should focus on life support, with primary emphasis on cardiorespiratory care. Shock, dysrhythmias, and seizures should be treated as for any other critically ill patient (see Chapter 64). There are few poisons for which there is an antidote. A list of antidotes is provided in Table 722–3.

PREVENTING ABSORPTION. Most toxins are rapidly absorbed from the gastrointestinal (GI) tract or the lungs. Many may also be well absorbed on dermal contact. Prompt action to remove the toxin from contact with the absorptive surface is crucial and may make the difference between no toxicity and major toxicity.

Dermal and ocular decontamination can be accomplished by flushing the affected area with tepid water. A minimum of 10 min is recommended for ocular exposures, although some chemicals, particularly alkaline corrosives, may require longer periods of flushing. For dermal exposures, mild soap and water can be used.

For inhaled toxins, decontamination is generally accomplished by removing the patient to fresh air or, if necessary, administering oxygen. In addition to supportive care, a few specific antidotes are used for some specific inhaled toxins. These are listed in Table 722–3.

Several procedures are used to prevent absorption of toxin from the stomach and GI tract, and each has limitations and risks. The decision to use one particular method over another should be based on whether the technique chosen is likely to be of sufficient value to merit the risk of the procedure. Timing is one limitation because many toxins are rapidly absorbed from the stomach. A decontamination procedure instituted after the drug is absorbed poses a risk to the patient with no potential for benefit. In general, most liquid drug products are essentially absorbed within 30 min of ingestion, and most solid dosage forms within 1–2 hr. Decontamination beyond this time is unlikely to be of value.

Emesis. The only emetic routinely used is **syrup of ipecac,** which contains two emetic alkaloids that work both in the central nervous system (CNS) and locally in the GI tract to produce vomiting. The onset of emesis is usually 20–30 min after dosing, with vomiting occurring in about 90–95% of patients. Several episodes of vomiting usually occur over a period of 1–2 hr. The recommended dose is 10 mL for infants 6–12 mo of age, 15 mL for children age 1–12 yr, and 30 mL for older children and adults. Ipecac should not be used in infants younger than 6 mo. Ipecac administration is followed by at least 8 ounces of water or other clear fluid. At best, emesis with syrup of ipecac removes about one-third of the stomach contents. Because of the delay in onset of emesis and poor yield, it should not be used as a general treatment for ingestions. The use of ipecac syrup has declined dramatically in the past 2 decades.

Gastric Lavage. This technique involves placing a tube into the stomach to aspirate contents, followed by flushing with aliquots of fluid, usually normal saline. Although gastric lavage has been widely used for many years, objective data do not document its efficacy, particularly in children, in whom only relatively small bore tubes can be used. The procedure is time consuming and, even under the best of circumstances, removes only a fraction of gastric contents. It should only be used in older children and only in select situations.

Activated Charcoal. The use of activated charcoal to prevent absorption of toxins has increased dramatically in the past 2 decades as data demonstrating its efficacy have accumulated. Activated charcoal is specially prepared to have a very large adsorptive surface area. Many but not all toxins are absorbed onto its surface, preventing absorption from the intestine. Some toxins, including heavy metals, lithium, hydrocarbons, and low molecular weight alcohols, are not significantly bound to charcoal; thus, activated charcoal should not be used to treat poisoning by these agents. In vitro, activated charcoal adsorbs about 1 g of toxin for each 10 g of charcoal; however, this relationship is generally not useful for clinical situations because the exact ingested dose is seldom known. The usual dose is 10–30 g for a child and 30–100 g for an adolescent or adult. Activated charcoal is commercially available mixed as a slurry in water or sorbitol, a cathartic. Flavoring may be added to improve palatability. In some serious poisonings, when life-threatening symptoms are present, repeated doses of activated charcoal may be useful to adsorb either toxin not bound by the first dose, or toxin may be recirculated through the gut. Under these circumstances, a cathartic should be used only with the first dose in order to prevent major fluid loss and dehydration. About 25% of patients receiving activated charcoal experience one episode of vomiting. Aspiration of activated charcoal into the lungs occasionally occurs. No evidence shows that aspiration of activated charcoal under such circum-

TABLE 722–3 Common Antidotes for Poisoning

Antidote	Use	Dose	Route	Adverse Effects/Warnings
N-Acetylcysteine (NAC, Mucomyst)	Acetaminophen; carbon tetrachloride and chloroform (experimental)	140/mg/kg loading, followed by 70 mg/kg every 4 hr for 17 doses	PO	Nausea, vomiting IV form not available in USA
Atropine	Organophosphate and carbamate pesticides; bradycardia due to atrioventricular conduction defects	0.05 mg/kg repeated every 5–10 min as needed. Dilute in 1–2 mL of NS for ET instillation.	IV/ET	Tachycardia, dry mouth, blurred vision, and urinary retention
BAL in oil (dimercoprol)	Arsenic, mercury, other metals	3–5 mg/kg every 4 hr, usually for 5–10 days	Deep IM	Local injection site pain and sterile abscess, nausea, vomiting, fever, salivation, nephrotoxicity
Benztropine (Cogentin)	Acute dystonic reactions	0.02 mg/kg (1 mg max)	IV/PO	Sedation, blurred vision, dry mouth, and tachycardia
Cyanide antidote kit	Cyanide Hydrogen sulfide (nitrites only)	Amyl nitrite: 1 crushable ampule Sodium nitrite: 0.33 mL/kg of 3% solution if hemoglobin level not known, otherwise based on tables with product Sodium thiosulfate: 1.6 mL (400 mg)/kg of 25% solution, may be repeated every 30–60 min to a maximum of 50 mL	Inhalation IV IV	Methemoglobinemia Methemoglobinemia
Deferoxamine (Desferal)	Iron	Infusion of 15 mg/kg/hr (max 6 g/24 hr) IM: 90 mg/kg/dose every 8 hr (max of 6 g/24 hr)	IV (preferred) IM	Hypotension (minimized by avoiding rapid infusion rates)
Digoxin-specific Fab antibodies (Digibind)	Digitalis glycosides (synthetic or natural)	One vial binds 0.6 mg of digitalis glycoside, ingested dose may be estimated from serum level (see table with product)	IV	Allergic reactions (rare), return of condition being treated with digitalis glycoside
Diphenhydramine (Benadryl)	Extrapyramidal symptoms, acute dystonic reactions, allergic reactions	5 mg/kg divide every 8 hr; 300 mg/24 hr max	IV/PO	Sedation or paradoxical agitation, ataxia
Dimercaptosuccinic acid (succimer, DMSA, Chemet)	Lead and probably mercury, arsenic, and perhaps other metals	10 mg/kg every 8 hr for 5 days, then 10 mg/kg every 12 hr for 14 days	PO	Nausea and vomiting; repeated courses may be needed
EDTA, calcium (calcium disodium, Versenate)	Lead, managanese, nickel, zinc, and perhaps chromium	1–1.5 g/m^2/24 hr in divided doses every 12 hr for 5 days	IM	Nausea, vomiting, fever, hypertension, arthralgias, allergic reactions, local inflammation, and nephrotoxicity (maintain adequate hydration)
Ethanol (ethyl alcohol)	Methanol, ethylene glycol	750 mg/kg loading dose followed by 80–150 mg/kg/hr infusion of 5% or 10% ethanol	IV/PO	Nausea, vomiting, sedation
Flumazenil (Romazicon)	Benzodiazepines	0.2 mg over 30 sec; if inadequate response, 0.3 mg over 30 sec; if inadequate response, 0.5 mg over 30 sec. No specific dose for children.	IV	Nausea, vomiting, facial flushing, agitation, headache, dizziness, seizures. Do not use for unknown or antidepressant ingestions *Note:* May not reverse respiratory depression
Fomepizole (4-methylpyrazole, Antizole)	Ethylene glycol; perhaps methanol	15 mg/kg load; 10 mg/kg every 12 hr for 4 doses; 15 mg/kg every 12 hr until level <20 mg/dL No specific dose for children.	IV	Infuse slowly over 30 min; increase doses to every 4 hr if dialysis is concurrent
Glucagon	β-blockers, calcium channel blockers, hypoglycemic agents	0.15 mg/kg bolus followed by infusion of 0.05–0.1 mg/kg/hr	IV	Hyperglycemia, nausea, and vomiting
Methylene blue	Methemoglobinemia	0.1–0.2 mL/kg of 1% solution, slow infusion, may be repeated every 30–60 min	IV	Nausea, vomiting, headache, dizziness
Naloxone (Narcan)	Narcotics Clonidine (inconsistent response)	0.01 mg/kg; if no effect, give 0.1 mg/kg; may be repeated as needed; may give continuous infusion	IV	Acute withdrawal symptoms if given to addicted patients
Physostigmine (Antilirium)	Anticholinergic agents	0.02 mg/kg; slow push	IV	Bradycardia, asystole, seizures, bronchospasm, vomiting, headache *Note:* Do not use with cyclic antidepressants
Pralidoxime (2-PAM, Protopam)	Organophosphate insecticides	25–50 mg/kg over 5–10 min (max 200 mg/min); can be repeated every 10–12 hr as needed	IV	Nausea, dizziness, headache, tachycardia, muscle rigidity, and bronchospasm (rapid administration)
Pyridoxine (vitamin B_6)	Isoniazid, *Gyromitra* mushrooms Ethylene glycol (investigational)	Isoniazid; dose = dose of isoniazid Mushrooms: 25 mg/kg Ethylene glycol: 50 mg/kg	IV	Uncommon

PO = oral; IV = intravenous; ET = endotracheal; IM = intramuscular; NS = normal saline.

stances is more serious than aspiration of gastric contents alone. If charcoal is given through a gastric tube, placement of the tube should be carefully confirmed before activated charcoal is given because instillation of charcoal directly into the lungs has disastrous effects.

Cathartics. Cathartics are commonly used in conjunction with activated charcoal to hasten the clearance of the charcoal-toxin complex, although no evidence shows that this is of value. Commonly used cathartics are sorbitol (maximum dose 1g/kg), magnesium sulfate (maximum dose 250 mg/kg), and magnesium citrate (maximum dose 250 mL/kg). Cathartics should be used with care in young children because of the risk of dehydration and electrolyte imbalance.

Whole Bowel Irrigation. Whole bowel irrigation involves instilling large volumes of a colonic lavage solution (Colyte, GoLYTELY) into the stomach to cleanse the entire GI tract. This technique has been successfully used to remove slowly absorbed products such as iron or sustained-release preparations. The procedure can be combined with the use of activated charcoal, if appropriate. Although very helpful in some situations, it should be used with caution in young children because of the possibility of fluid and electrolyte imbalance.

ENHANCING ELIMINATION. In practice, enhancing excretion is useful for only a minority of toxins. Dialytic techniques are not useful for drugs that are either highly protein bound or have a large volume of distribution. These techniques are also invasive and associated with risk. Certain procedures can be used for very specific agents.

Diuresis. For most toxins, renal clearance is not proportionate to urine volume; hence, producing diuresis alone does not increase elimination. Increasing the pH of the urine with intravenously administered bicarbonate increases the elimination of weak acids, such as salicylates and phenobarbital. Alternately, acidifying the urine to increase the elimination of weak bases such as amphetamine and phencyclidine is not clinically useful. This technique is termed *ion trapping*.

Dialysis. Hemodialysis and peritoneal dialysis have been used successfully to treat poisonings by select agents. Although hemodialysis is generally more efficient at removing toxins, peritoneal dialysis is often easier to perform in young children and may be sufficient. Few drugs or toxins are removed by dialysis in amounts sufficient to justify the risks and difficulty of dialysis. Examples of toxins for which dialysis may be useful in some cases include methanol, ethylene glycol, and large symptomatic ingestions of salicylate or theophylline.

Hemoperfusion. Hemoperfusion is a dialytic technique in which blood is passed through a column of activated charcoal or resin. It has been used successfully to treat large ingestions of salicylate, theophylline, and a few other selected agents. It is rarely used in small children because of the risks associated with its use.

LABORATORY EVALUATION. For some intoxications (e.g., salicylates, acetaminophen, iron, methanol, ethylene glycol), specific laboratory measurement is integral to the treatment plan. In other situations, specific measurement may assist in establishing a diagnosis but is not likely to change treatment. Examples include opioid toxicity, in which definitive treatment is unrelated to levels, or cyanide, in which treatment must be started rapidly and would be significantly delayed if the physician were to wait for laboratory confirmation. Comprehensive "drug screens" vary widely in their ability to detect toxins and generally add little information, particularly if the agent is known and a patient's symptoms are consistent with that agent. If a drug screen is obtained, it is important to know the specific drugs that are identified by the test. The best way to use the laboratory is to discuss the case with a Poison Control Center, medical toxicologist, or laboratory technologist and to provide appropriate samples and clinical data so that the most appropriate tests can be performed and properly interpreted.

American Academy of Clinical Toxicology and European Association of Poisons Centres and Clinical Toxicologists: Position Statement: Ipecac syrup. J Toxicol Clin Toxicol 35:699, 1997.

American Academy of Clinical Toxicology and European Association of Poisons Centres and Clinical Toxicologists: Position statement: Gastric lavage. J Toxicol Clin Toxicol 35:711, 1997.

American Academy of Clinical Toxicology and European Association of Poisons Centres and Clinical Toxicologists: Position statement: Single-dose activated charcoal. J Toxicol Clin Toxicol 35:721, 1997.

American Academy of Clinical Toxicology and European Association of Poisons Centres and Clinical Toxicologists: Position statement: Cathartics. J Toxicol Clin Toxicol 35:743, 1997.

American Academy of Clinical Toxicology and European Association of Poisons Centres and Clinical Toxicologists: Position statement: Whole bowel irrigation. J Toxicol Clin Toxicol 35:753, 1997.

Haddad LM, Shannon MW, Winchester, JF (eds): Clinical Mangement of Poisoning and Drug Overdose, 3rd ed. Philadelphia, WB Saunders, 1998.

Litovitz TL, Smilkstein M, Felberg L, et al: 1996 Annual Report of the American Association of Poison Control Centers Toxic Exposure Surveillance System. Am J Emerg Med 11:494, 1993; 15:447, 1997.

Rodgers GC, Matyunas NJ (eds): Handbook of Common Poisoning in Children, 3rd ed. Chicago, American Academy of Pediatrics, 1994.

722.2 *Acetaminophen*

Acetaminophen is the most widely used analgesic and antipyretic, in part because of the finding of a relationship between Reye syndrome and salicylates. Consequently, acetaminophen is commonly available in the home, where it can be accidentally ingested by young children or taken in an intentional overdose by adolescents.

PATHOPHYSIOLOGY. Acetaminophen toxicity results from the formation of a highly reactive intermediate metabolite, *N*-acetyl-*p*-benzoquinoneimine (NAPQI). When therapeutic doses are administered, only a small amount (4%) of a dose is metabolized by hepatic cytochrome P450 enzymes to NAPQI, which is immediately conjugated with glutathione to form a harmless mercapturic acid conjugate. When hepatic stores of glutathione are depleted to less than 70% of normal, the NAPQI metabolite combines with hepatic macromolecules to produce hepatic cellular damage. The acute toxic dose of acetaminophen is generally considered to be more than 150 mg/kg in children younger than 12 yr. A single ingestion of more than 7.5 g is considered a minimum toxic dose in adolescents and adults. In adults, renal damage and failure are associated with long-term ingestion. Repeated doses of acetaminophen at doses exceeding those recommended may lead to hepatic injury or failure in some children. It is unclear what doses may be associated with this problem or whether a subgroup of children may be at particular risk. Parents should be advised to follow closely the manufacturer's dosing guidelines.

CLINICAL AND LABORATORY MANIFESTATIONS. If untreated, patients who have acutely overdosed pass through four stages of toxicity (Table 722–4). Because symptoms early after ingestion are nonspecific, without a history of ingestion or high index of suspicion, pediatricians may not diagnose the ingestion. If a

TABLE 722–4 Stages in the Clinical Course of Acetaminophen Toxicity

Stage	Time Following Ingestion	Characteristics
I	½–24 hr	Anorexia, nausea, vomiting, malaise, pallor, diaphoresis
II	24–48 hr	Resolution of above; right upper quadrant abdominal pain and tenderness; elevated bilirubin, prothrombin time, hepatic enzymes; oliguria
III	72–96 hr	Peak liver function abnormalities; anorexia, nausea, vomiting, malaise may reappear
IV	4 days–2 wk	Resolution of hepatic dysfunction or complete liver failure

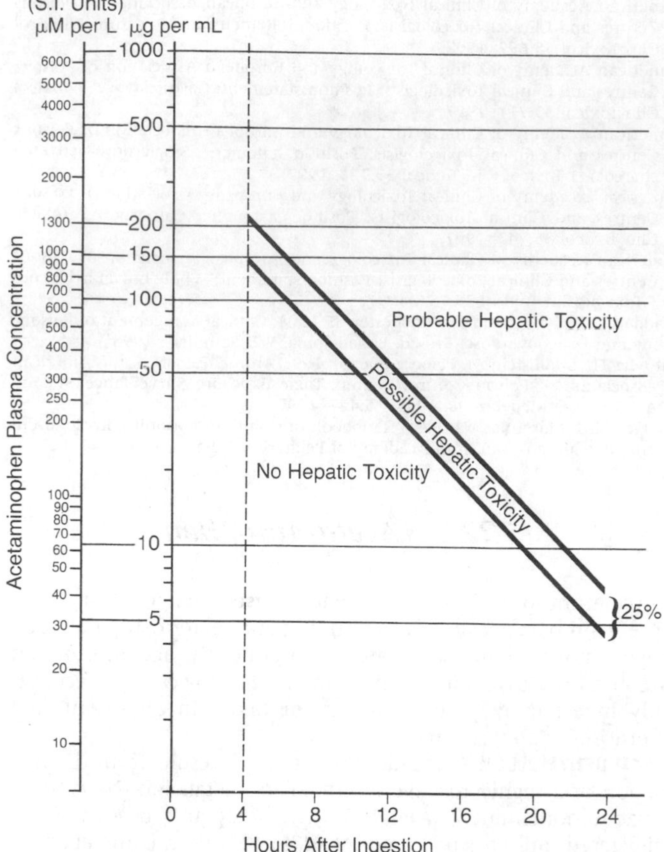

Figure 722–1 Rumack-Matthew nomogram for acetaminophen poisoning. Semilogarithmic plot of plasma acetaminophen levels versus time. *Cautions for the use of this chart*: (1) The time coordinates refer to time after *ingestion.* (2) Serum levels drawn before 4 hr may not represent peak levels. (3) The graph should be used only in relation to a single acute ingestion. (4) The lower *solid line* 25% below the standard nomogram is included to allow for possible errors in acetaminophen plasma assays and estimated time from ingestion of an overdose. (From Rumack BH, Hess AJ [eds]: Poisindex. Denver, 1995. Adapted from Rumack BH, Matthew H: Acetaminophen poisoning and toxicity. Pediatrics 55:871, 1975.)

history of acetaminophen ingestion is reported, a plasma level should be measured 4 hr or more after ingestion. Measurement earlier than 4 hr after ingestion cannot be used to determine the severity of an overdose because complete absorption may not yet have occurred. The level should be plotted on the Rumack-Matthews nomogram (Fig. 722–1) to determine whether antidotal treatment is indicated. Concomitant ethanol ingestion may produce hepatoxicity at lower than usual acetaminophen levels. Aspartate, alanine transaminase, and bilirubin levels, and prothrombin time should be followed daily in all patients with acetaminophen levels falling in the toxic range on the nomogram.

TREATMENT. In large acute overdose, when the need for antidotal treatment is anticipated and when treatment can be started within 1 to 2 hr of the ingestion, the use of activated charcoal should be considered. The antidote for acetaminophen poisoning is *N*-acetylcysteine (NAC or Mucomyst; see Table 722–3 for dosing). NAC serves as an available precursor for glutathione synthesis, thus replenishing glutathione stores and preventing the reaction of NAPQI with hepatocytes. NAC therapy should be initiated as soon as possible after the ingestion but may have value even if started 24–36 hr after the ingestion in severe cases. NAC is unpalatable and irritating to the GI tract and should be diluted to a 5% solution with soda or fruit juice to minimize vomiting. It may be given directly into the stomach or upper intestine by tube. An intravenous preparation is used in many countries and should soon be available in the United States. Intravenous NAC is equally effective as oral NAC but is given over a shorter period.

PROGNOSIS. Children younger than 6 yr are unlikely to develop significant toxicity after ingestion of even relatively large doses of acetaminophen. Nevertheless, at this time, children with a significant ingestion should have their plasma acetaminophen level measured and receive treatment with NAC if the level falls within the toxic range on the nomogram. Adolescents have a higher incidence (23.2%) of toxic plasma levels after ingestion than do children. Even if a serious case of hepatotoxicity develops, the mortality rate is less than 0.5%. Patients who recover have no sequelae when observed 3–12 mo after the acute toxicity. Severely affected patients may require liver transplantation (Chapter 367).

Brandwene EL, Williams SR, Tunget-Johnson C, et al: Refining the level for anticipated hepatotoxicity in acetaminophen poisoning. J Emerg Med 14:691, 1996.
Bond GR, Krenzelok EP, Normann SA, et al: Acetaminophen ingestion in childhood—cost and relative risk of alternative referral strategies. J Toxicol Clin Toxicol 32:513, 1994.
Cetaruk EW, Dart RC, Hurlbut KM, et al: Tylenol Extended Relief overdose. Ann Emerg Med 30:104, 1997.
Heubi JE, Barbacci MB, Zimmerman HJ: Therapeutic misadventures with acetaminophen: Hepatotoxicity after multiple doses in children. J Pediatr 132:22, 1998.
Luria JW, Ruddy R, Stephan M: Acute hepatic failure related to chronic acetaminophen intoxication. Pediatr Emerg Care 12:291, 1996.
Perry HE, Shannon MW: Efficacy of oral versus intravenous N-acetylcysteine in acetaminophen overdose: Result of an open-label, clinical trial. J Pediatr 132:149, 1998.
Rivers-Penera T, Gugig R, Davis J, et al: Outcome of acetaminophen overdose in pediatric patients and factors contributing to hepatotoxicity. J Pediatr 130:300, 1997.
Rumack BH, Peterson RG: Acetaminophen overdose: Incidence, diagnosis and management in 416 patients. Pediatrics 62:898, 1978.
Rumore MM, Blaiklock RG: Influence of age-dependent pharmacokinetics and metabolism of acetaminophen hepatotoxicity. J Pharm Sci 81:203, 1992.

722.3 Ibuprofen

Ibuprofen is involved in a growing number of accidental and intentional overdoses because of wider distribution and increased use as an antipyretic. Serious effects after overdose of ibuprofen are rare, occurring in fewer than 0.5% of cases reported to the AAPCC TESS database.

PATHOPHYSIOLOGY. Prostaglandins are involved in a wide variety of physiologic processes. Ibuprofen inhibits prostaglandin synthesis, and this disruption produces side effects reported with therapeutic use such as GI irritation, reduced renal blood flow, and platelet dysfunction. The toxic mechanism of ibuprofen in acute overdose has not been well described. In children, ingested doses less than 100 mg/kg do not cause toxicity, whereas doses greater than 400 mg/kg are capable of producing more serious effects, including seizures and coma.

CLINICAL AND LABORATORY MANIFESTATIONS. Symptoms usually develop within 4 hr of ingestion, and serious symptoms resolve within 24 hr. Common effects include nausea, vomiting, epigastric pain, drowsiness, lethargy, and ataxia. Anion gap metabolic acidosis, coma, transient apnea, renal failure, hypotension, and seizures are rare. Other reported effects include nystagmus, diplopia, headache, tinnitus, and transient deafness.

Symptoms may correlate with ibuprofen blood levels. A nomogram plotting blood levels vs time after ingestion has been developed in order to predict toxicity, but it requires further validation. In addition, testing of ibuprofen blood levels is not readily available, limiting the usefulness of the nomogram. Renal function studies and acid-base balance should be monitored after ingestion of large doses.

TREATMENT. Good supportive care is essential, and there is no antidotal therapy. Emesis is of little benefit, but activated charcoal can be administered. Extracorporeal removal methods have not been adequately evaluated and are not recommended.

Hall AH, Smolinske SC, Conrad FL, et al: Ibuprofen overdose: 126 cases. Ann Emerg Med 15:1308, 1986.
Hall AH, Smolinske SC, Kulig KW, et al: Ibuprofen overdose: A prospective study. West J Med 148:653, 1988.
Jenkinson ML, Fitzpatrick R, Streete PJ, et al: The relationship between plasma ibuprofen concentrations and toxicity in acute ibuprofen. Hum Toxicol 7:319, 1988.
McElwee NE, Veltri JC, Bradford DC, et al: A prospective, population-based study of acute ibuprofen overdose: Complications are rare and routine serum levels not warranted. Ann Emerg Med 19:657, 1990.
Perry SJ, Streete PJ, Volans GN: Ibuprofen overdose: The first two years of over-the-counter sales. Hum Toxicol 6:173, 1987.

722.4 *Antidepressants*

The cyclic antidepressants (CA) and the selective serotonin reuptake inhibitors (SSRIs) represent the two major classes of antidepressants of toxicologic significance. They are listed in Table 722–5.

CYCLIC ANTIDEPRESSANTS

PATHOPHYSIOLOGY. These agents block the neuronal reuptake of norepinephrine, 5-hydroxytryptamine, serotonin, and dopamine, in both the central and peripheral nervous systems. With therapeutic use, they also produce various degrees of sedation, α-blocking, and anticholinergic effects. Direct myocardial depressant effects (quinidine-like) result from inhibition of fast sodium channels, leading to the development of cardiac dysrhythmias. The toxic dose of these agents ranges from 5–20 mg/kg.

CLINICAL AND LABORATORY MANIFESTATIONS. The primary organ systems affected are the CNS and cardiovascular systems. Symptoms can occur as early as 30 min after ingestion, with serious symptoms usually developing within 6 hr of ingestion. The pattern of toxic effects that develop in children is slightly different from that described for adolescents and adults. CNS effects (drowsiness, seizures) occur more frequently in children than do cardiovascular effects. Drowsiness, lethargy, or coma has been reported in as many as one third of pediatric cases. Coma, when it occurs, has a mean duration of 6.4 hr but may last longer than 24 hr. Seizures develop in about 15% of cases and can occur without warning, but are usually brief and resolve without treatment. Adolescents with comparable blood CA levels suffer more significant toxicity than younger children.

TABLE 722–5 Antidepressant Agents

Generic Name	Common Trade Name
Cyclic Antidepressants	
Amitriptyline	Elavil, Endep
Amoxapine	Ascendin
Clomipramine	Anafranil
Doxepin	Sinequan
Desipramine	Tofranil
Imipramine	Norpramin
Maprotiline	Ludiomil
Mirtazapine	Remeron
Nortriptyline	Pamelor, Aventyl
Protriptyline	Vivactil
Venlafaxine	Effexor
Selective Serotonin Reuptake Inhibitors (SSRIs)	
Fluoxetine	Prozac
Fluvoxamine	Luvox
Nefazodone	Serzone
Paroxetine	Paxil
Sertraline	Zoloft

Tachycardia is common, likely secondary to the anticholinergic actions of CA, but does not usually compromise blood pressure. Hypertension may be noted early after ingestion but rarely requires treatment. Hypotension is also rare but is a poor prognostic sign. Cardiac findings include slowing of myocardial conduction, multifocal premature ventricular contractions, and ventricular tachycardia, flutter, and fibrillation. In addition to widening of the QRS complex, QT prolongation occurs with T-wave flattening or inversion, ST segment depression, right bundle branch block, and complete heart block.

Hypoventilation with respiratory arrest may occur without warning. Other reported effects include hyperthermia, choreiform movements, agitation, and twitching. An anticholinergic syndrome including mydriasis, disorientation, hallucinations, urinary retention, and diminished bowel sounds may be present but is not common.

The electrocardiogram (ECG) should be closely monitored for QRS widening and QT and QTc prolongation. QRS duration and axis deviation and the level of consciousness have been used as predictors of potential toxicity. ECG changes may not be useful predictors of toxicity in younger children because of normal variation. Blood levels of CA are not helpful in assessing or predicting the severity of the exposure but may aid in establishing a diagnosis.

TREATMENT. After general life support measures are instituted, including endotracheal intubation if indicated, efforts should be made to prevent absorption. Emesis is contraindicated because of the danger of aspiration from vomiting after onset of CNS depression. Activated charcoal should be administered. Repeated doses of activated charcoal to remove drug being reexcreted into the GI tract may be useful but only if bowel sounds are present.

Sodium bicarbonate in doses sufficient to achieve a serum pH of 7.45–7.55 should be administered to treat and prevent dysrhythmias. This is superior to artificial hyperventilation. Lidocaine is used if dysrhythmias develop despite serum alkalization or if dysrhythmias already exist. Quinidine and procainamide should not be used because they further depress cardiac conduction. Phenytoin (or fosphenytoin), once regarded as a key drug, is reserved for dysrhythmias that do not respond to sodium bicarbonate and lidocaine therapy.

Seizures, if they require treatment, usually respond to benzodiazepine therapy. Hypotension may respond to standard fluid therapy, although norepinephrine may be required. Severe, unresponsive hypotension is a poor prognostic sign. Hypertension usually is transient and does not require treatment.

Physostigmine, once promoted as an "antidote" for CA toxicity, is an exceptionally dangerous agent that can cause seizures and dysrhythmias and should not be used. Because of the large volumes of distribution and high degree of plasma protein binding of CAs, extracorporeal removal is not of value.

Asymptomatic children should be observed and the ECG monitored for at least 6 hr. If any manifestations (such as a QRS interval > 0.10 msec, conduction defects, altered mental status, hypotension, or hypoventilation) develop, continue monitoring in an intensive care unit for 24 hr. Only completely asymptomatic children should be discharged after 6 hr of observation.

SELECTIVE SEROTONIN REUPTAKE INHIBITORS

These drugs inhibit reuptake of serotonin in the CNS and have little or no effect on norepinephrine. They have minimal, if any, anticholinergic or α-blocking effects.

CLINICAL MANIFESTATIONS. Toxic effects are mild, with a usual onset of symptoms within 3 hr. Symptoms resolve within 24 hr in treated patients. Most cases in children remain asymptomatic (90% in one series). Primary organ systems affected are the CNS and GI tract. Drowsiness or hyperactivity and agitation are the most commonly reported effects. Tremor may also occur. Nausea, vomiting, and abdominal pain occur in fewer than 5% of children. Cardiovascular effects are rare, usually reported in adults who have co-ingested other agents. Adolescents have an increased incidence of symptoms, although they are still relatively minor. The toxic dose of these agents is not well defined.

Serotonin syndrome has been reported after accidental overdose of SSRIs. This is an idiosyncratic reaction that includes confusion and disorientation, agitation, coma, hyperthermia, myoclonus, hyperreflexia, tremor, and muscle rigidity. Therapy is supportive, but awareness and recognition of the syndrome is important to prevent complications caused by inappropriate interventions.

TREATMENT. Ipecac-induced emesis has been used without complication. Activated charcoal may be the more appropriate choice, however, considering the potential for CNS depression. There is no specific therapy other than general supportive care.

Borys DJ, Setzer SC, Ling LJ, et al: Acute fluoxetine overdose: A report of 234 cases. Am J Emerg Med 10:115, 1992.

James LP, Kearns GL: Cyclic antidepressant toxicity in children and adolescents. J Clin Pharmacol 35:343, 1995.

Klein-Schwartz W, Anderson B: Analysis of sertraline-only overdoses. Am J Emerg Med 14:456, 1996.

Mills KC: Serotonin syndrome: A clinical update. Med Toxicol 13:763, 1997.

Newton EH, Shih RD, Hoffman RS: Cyclic antidepressant overdose: A review of current management strategies. Am J Emerg Med 12:376, 1994.

722.5 *Salicylates*

The incidence of salicylate ingestion has declined, particularly in young children, as the use of alternative antipyretics has increased. Toxicity related to salicylates must still be considered in therapeutic situations as well as in cases of overdose. Methyl salicylate is the active ingredient in oil of wintergreen, a commonly used rubefacient.

PATHOPHYSIOLOGY. Salicylates directly or indirectly affect most organ systems in the body by uncoupling oxidative phosphorylation, inhibiting Krebs' cycle enzymes, and inhibiting amino acid synthesis. Various complex metabolic abnormalities result. Salicylates are gastric irritants, and nausea and vomiting usually occur early after overdose. Salicylates also decrease platelet adhesiveness. The acute toxic dose of salicylates is generally considered to be greater than 150 mg/kg.

CLINICAL AND LABORATORY MANIFESTATIONS

Phase 1. Salicylates directly stimulate the respiratory center, leading to hyperventilation and hyperpnea. An increased respiratory rate results in respiratory alkalosis and a compensatory alkaluria. Both potassium and sodium bicarbonate are excreted in the urine. This phase may last for as long as 12 hr after ingestion in an adolescent but may be inapparent in a young infant.

Phase 2. Hypokalemia is initially limited to renal tissue and is not reflected either in serum potassium level or the ECG. When sufficient potassium has been lost from the kidneys, an exchange of potassium for hydrogen ion occurs, and the urine becomes relatively acidic. This "paradoxical aciduria" occurs in the presence of a continued respiratory alkalosis. As this phase progresses, systemic hypokalemia develops. This phase may begin within hours after ingestion in a young child and may last as long as 12 to 24 hr in an adolescent.

Phase 3. Dehydration, hypokalemia, and progressive metabolic acidosis secondary to the accumulation of lactic acid and other metabolic acids eventually develop. All seriously poisoned patients are more than 5–10% dehydrated. Hyperpnea is the end response to acidosis rather than to primary respiratory center drive. The plasma salicylate level may be even higher than in earlier phases because of the inability to

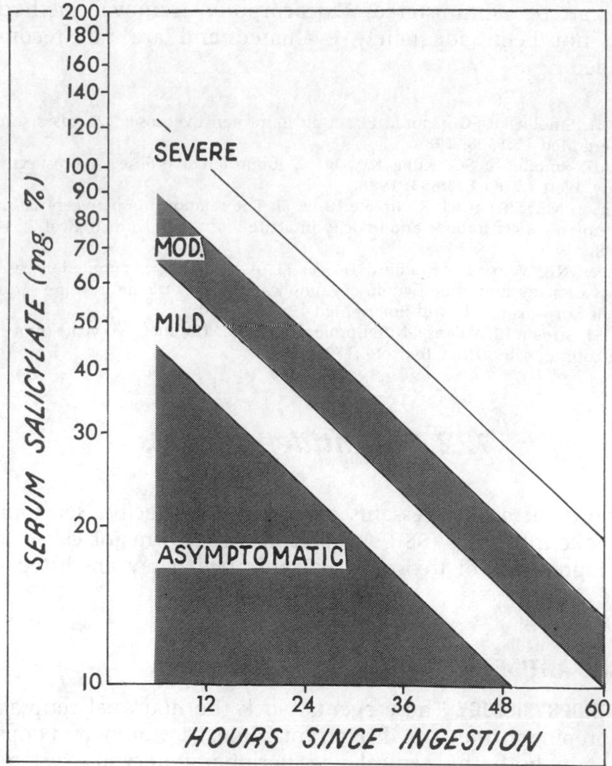

Figure 722–2 Nomogram relating serum salicylate concentration and expected severity of intoxication at varying intervals following the ingestion of a single dose of salicylate. (From Done AK: Salicylate intoxication: Significance of measurements of salicylate in blood in cases of acute ingestion. Pediatrics 26:800, 1960.)

excrete salicylate in an acid urine. This phase may begin 4–6 hr after ingestion in a young infant or 24 hr or more after ingestion in an adolescent. Patients with chronic salicylate poisoning usually present with metabolic acidosis.

Pulmonary edema or hemorrhage may develop in more severe cases. Hyperglycemia or hypoglycemia, particularly in infants, has also been observed. Death can result from pulmonary edema and respiratory failure, cerebral edema, hemorrhage, severe electrolyte imbalance, or cardiovascular collapse.

After a single acute ingestion, a plasma salicylate level should be measured no sooner than 6 hr after ingestion and plotted on the Done nomogram (Fig. 722–2) to gauge the severity of the ingestion. Levels obtained before a 6-hr time lapse may not reflect peak levels. The nomogram is used only to assess acute single ingestions. Patients with chronic salicylate toxicity may have a level within the therapeutic range (10–20 mg/dL). The level is low in relation to the severity of their illness, reflecting higher tissue concentrations of salicylate.

In overdose, salicylate pharmacokinetics are nonlinear; however, plotting plasma salicylate concentrations vs time on a semi-log scale helps evaluate the success of therapy and is recommended for all seriously poisoned patients. If the apparent half-life is greater than 10–15 hr, treatment may not be effective.

Urine pH and volume should be measured hourly in all seriously poisoned children. Plasma pH, glucose, potassium, and other electrolytes should be monitored at regular intervals. Prothrombin time should also be measured in all severely poisoned patients. Hepatotoxicity from salicylate in severe or chronic cases is demonstrated by results of liver function tests, bilirubin levels, and prothrombin abnormalities.

TREATMENT. Initial treatment should include gastric decontamination if a patient is seen soon after the ingestion. Salicylate tablets occasionally form into bezoars, which may be suspected if salicylate levels are rising or persistently elevated. Bezoars may be visualized with radiography using contrast.

In symptomatic patients, initial therapy includes rehydration and correction of electrolyte abnormalities (Chapter 55). Large quantities of potassium and bicarbonate may be needed if symptoms have been present for some time after an acute ingestion or in the case of chronic salicylate poisoning, because body stores of theses electrolytes may be severely depleted.

In overdose, urinary excretion of salicylate becomes an important route of elimination. Because salicylate is a weak acid (pKa ≈ 3.0), its urinary clearance is affected by urine pH. As metabolic acidosis produces a more acidic urine, a higher percentage of salicylate remains in the un-ionized form, which is reabsorbed from the glomerular filtrate. Urinary salicylate elimination can be increased using ion trapping, increasing urine pH to convert a greater percentage of salicylate to the ionized form, which is then excreted in the urine. Each 1-unit rise in urine pH increases urinary salicylate clearance fourfold. Urine pH should be raised to at least 7–7.5; this is accomplished using intravenous bicarbonate. It is important to remember that it may be impossible to alkalize the urine without adequately replenishing tissue stores of potassium. Acetazolamride (Diamox) and tris (hydroxymethyl) aminomethane (THAM) should not be used to achieve urine alkalization.

In severe cases of salicylate intoxication, (usually chronic ingestions or acute ingestions with serum levels >100 mg/dL), dialysis may be required both to remove salicylate and to correct electrolyte abnormalities. Hemodialysis is preferred over either peritoneal dialysis or charcoal hemoperfusion.

Brenner BE, Simon RR: Management of salicylate intoxication. Drugs 24:335, 1982.

Done AK: Salicylate intoxication: Significance of measurements of salicylates in blood in cases of acute ingestion. Pediatrics 26:800, 1960.

Krause DS, Wolf BA, Shaw LM: Acute aspirin overdose: Mechanisms of toxicity. Ther Drug Monit 14:441, 1992.

Leatherman JW, Schmitz PG: Fever, hyperdynamic schock, and multiple-system organ failure. A pseudo-sepsis syndrome associated with chronic salicylate intoxication. Chest 100:1391, 1991.

Snodgrass W, Rumack BH, Peterson RG: Salicylate toxicity following therapeutic doses in young children. J Toxicol Clin Toxicol 18:247, 1981.

722.6 *Iron*

Iron poisoning is the most common cause of childhood death due to poisoning. Iron-containing products are common in many homes and often resemble candy. The potential severity is based on the amount of elemental iron ingested. The amount of elemental iron ingested must be calculated on the basis of the number of tablets ingested and the percentage of elemental iron in the salt. Ferrous sulfate contains 20%, ferrous gluconate 12%, and ferrous fumarate 33% elemental iron. Multiple vitamin products containing iron list on the label the amount of iron per tablet as elemental iron.

PATHOPHYSIOLOGY. Iron is corrosive to the GI mucosa, resulting in localized GI effects. It also accumulates in the mitochondria and tissues to produce systemic effects. Iron causes venodilation and increased capillary permeability leading to hypotension. Reduced peripheral perfusion and mitochondrial damage result in lactic and citric acid accumulation, causing metabolic acidosis. Hepatic necrosis develops after serious poisoning, resulting in elevated liver function tests and coagulopathies. Drowsiness and coma develop as a result of hemodynamic instability or possibly a direct toxic effect of iron in the CNS. Although death has been reported after ingestion of as few as 10 ferrous sulfate tablets (a total of 650 mg elemental iron), more than 60 mg/kg of elemental iron is generally considered a toxic dose.

CLINICAL AND LABORATORY MANIFESTATIONS. Iron poisoning has historically been described as occurring in four phases; however, there is considerable overlap. Nausea, vomiting, diarrhea, and abdominal pain are the hallmark of iron poisoning and usually develop within 30 min–6 hr after ingestion. Hematemesis and bloody diarrhea may develop in more serious poisonings. The GI signs may subside over 6–12 hr; however, careful observation is warranted because systemic toxicity due to cellular damage may ensue, particularly in patients with severe GI signs, early hypotension, or drowsiness.

Gastric scarring and pyloric stenosis can develop 2–4 wk after a large ingestion or in instances when the iron tablets remain in prolonged contact with the GI mucosa. Stenosis may be symptomatic and occasionally requires surgical intervention.

Serum iron levels should be assessed after acute iron poisoning to assist with the clinical diagnosis. Iron levels should be obtained about 4 hr after ingestion. Serum iron levels less than 500 μg/dL, measured 4–8 hr after ingestion, correlate with a low risk of significant toxicity. Higher levels do not correlate well with clinical symptoms. Comparing serum iron levels with total iron-binding capacity is not a reliable indicator of potential toxicity. Other laboratory studies used to monitor patients include blood gases and pH, serum glucose, liver function tests, and coagulation studies.

Because iron is radiopaque, an abdominal roentgenogram may aid in the diagnosis of iron ingestion. Repeat roentgenograms may help with assessment of the efficiency of gastric decontamination methods. A negative result does not rule out iron ingestion because only undissolved tablets can be seen. Children's multiple vitamins are usually not visualized on roentgenogram because of the low concentration of iron and the rapid dissolution of the tablets.

TREATMENT. Good supportive and symptomatic care is essential in cases of iron poisoning. Ipecac-induced emesis can be used to remove tablets from the stomach; however, it may mask the GI symptoms caused by iron. Gastric lavage is not recommended because of its inefficiency in children, particularly because of the large size of many iron tablets. Activated charcoal does not adsorb iron and should not be used. Whole bowel irrigation may be of benefit to flush tablets from the intestine. If tablets adhere to the gastric mucosa, removal by endoscopic or surgical intervention (gastrotomy) or aggressive whole bowel irrigation has been attempted with mixed success.

Oral bicarbonate (2%), dilute phosphosoda (1:4), and magnesium hydroxide (milk of magnesia) react with iron to form less soluble, poorly absorbed iron salts, but they are inherently toxic and of questionable clinical benefit. Complexation of iron in the GI tract using oral deferoxamine is expensive, may increase iron absorption, and is generally not recommended.

Deferoxamine is a specific chelator of iron and is the "antidote" for moderate to severe iron intoxication (see Table 722–3). Indications for deferoxamine include a serum iron level greater than 500 μg/dL regardless of symptoms; serum iron level greater than 350 μg/dL along with moderate to severe symptoms; and moderate to severe symptoms regardless of the serum iron level. It should be administered as an intravenous infusion. The infusion should be continued until a patient is symptom free. The deferoxamine-iron complex may color the urine reddish (vin rosé), although this is an unreliable indicator of iron excretion.

Klein-Schwatrz W, Oderda GM, Gorman RL, et al: Assessment of management guidelines: Acute iron ingestion. Clin Pediatr 29:316, 1990.

Mills KC, Curry SC: Acute iron poisoning. Emerg Med Clin North Am 12:397, 1994.

Schauben JL, Augenstein WL, Cox J, et al: Iron poisoning: Report of three cases and a review of therapeutic intervention. J Emerg Med 8:309, 1990.

Tenenbein M: Whole bowel irrigation in iron poisoning. J Pediatr 111:145, 1987.

Yatscoff RW, Wayne EA, Tenenbein M: An objective criterion for the cessation of deferoxamine therapy in the acutely iron poisoned patient. J Toxicol Clin Toxicol 29:1, 1991.

722.7 Caustics

PATHOPHYSIOLOGY. Caustics include both acids and alkalies as well as a few common oxidizing agents such as bleach. Acids coagulate proteins, causing tissue necrosis. Alkalies digest and dissolve proteins, producing liquefaction necrosis with the risk of perforation, if the injury is located in the intestinal tract. The severity of the chemical burn produced depends on the pH and the concentration of the agent and the length of contact time. Agents with a pH below 2 or above 12 are more likely to produce significant injury.

CLINICAL MANIFESTATIONS. Ingestion of caustic materials may produce oral burns seen as reddened areas or whitish plaques. Symptoms include pain, drooling, vomiting, or difficulty or refusal to swallow. Circumferential burns of the esophagus are prone to cause strictures on healing, which may require repeated dilation or surgical correction. Strong acids may sometimes produce scarring around the pylorus, leading to delayed onset of gastric obstruction.

TREATMENT. Initial treatment of caustic exposure includes thorough removal of the product from the skin or eye by flushing with water. Ingested agents should be rinsed from the oral cavity. Emesis and lavage are contraindicated except under extraordinarily rare circumstances. Activated charcoal should not be used. Patients should be evaluated for evidence of esophageal burns, and if symptoms occur, oral fluids or solids should be withheld. The absence of visible oral injury does not preclude significant esophageal lesions. Endoscopy should be performed in symptomatic patients or those in whom injury is highly suspect on the basis of history. The use of corticosteroids and esophageal stents is controversial. Prophylactic antibiotics do not affect outcomes.

Berkovits RNP, Bos CE, Wijburg FA, et al: Caustic injury of the oesophagus. Sixteen years experience, and introduction of a new model oesophageal stent. J Laryngol Otol 110:1041, 1996.
Christensen HBT: Prediction of complications following unintentional caustic ingestion in children. Is endoscopy always necessary? Acta Paediatr 84:1177, 1995.
Gaudreault P, Parent M, McGuigan MA: Predictability of esophageal injury from signs and symptoms: A study of 378 children. Pediatrics 71:761, 1983.
Harley EH, Collins MD: Liquid household bleach ingestion in children: A retrospective review. Laryngoscope 107:122, 1997.
Penner GE: Acid ingestion: Toxicology and treatment. Ann Emerg Med 9:374, 1980.
Rothstein FC: Caustic injuries to the esophagus in children. Pediatr Toxicol 33:665, 1986.
Spitz L, Lakhoo K: Caustic ingestion. Arch Dis Child 68:157, 1993.

722.8 Methanol and Ethylene Glycol

Methanol is commonly found in windshield washer fluids, fuel additives, liquid fuel canisters, and industrial solvents. Ethylene glycol is commonly found in automobile radiator fluids. These solvents are well absorbed via inhalation or after skin contact; however, accidental ingestion is the most common route of exposure in children. The pathophysiology, clinical effects, and treatment of these two chemicals are similar. Although each parent compound is capable of producing mild toxicity, it is the metabolites of each product that are responsible for the serious clinical effects that can follow exposure.

METHANOL

PATHOPHYSIOLOGY. Methanol is metabolized in the liver by alcohol dehydrogenase to formaldehyde, which is further metabolized to formic acid by aldehyde dehydrogenase. Formic acid is metabolized via folate-dependent pathways to carbon dioxide and water. Toxicity is caused by formic acid, which inhibits mitochondrial respiration. The development of serious toxic effects is delayed as formic acid is generated and accumulates in blood and tissues.

CLINICAL AND LABORATORY MANIFESTATIONS. Drowsiness, mild inebriation, and gastric irritation, including nausea and vomiting, develop early after ingestion. The onset of serious effects, including profound metabolic acidosis and visual disturbances, are delayed up to 24 hr. Visual disturbances include blurred or cloudy vision, constricted visual fields, decreased acuity, and the "feeling of being in a snowstorm." Small children may not be able to describe these visual changes. Pupils may be dilated and unreactive to light, and retinal edema and optic disc hyperemia may be noted. Visual disturbances are usually reversible, but in significant poisonings, blindness has occasionally been permanent. An anion-gap metabolic acidosis develops; thus, serum electrolytes, pH, and acid-base balance should be monitored.

Children are usually discovered with an open container of product soon after an exposure, and determining if a significant exposure has occurred is usually a problem. Methanol blood measurements are usually available and can rule out an exposure; however, levels do not correlate with toxicity. Formic acid levels may correlate more closely with toxicity; however, the test is not routinely available. If tests of methanol level are not available, estimation of an osmolar gap has been recommended as a surrogate. Serum osmolarity is measured by the freezing point depression method and compared with a calculated serum osmolarity. The osmolar gap can be used to estimate the serum methanol level using the following formula:

$$\text{Osmolar gap} \times 3.2 = \text{estimated methanol level in mg/dL}$$

TREATMENT. Because methanol is rapidly absorbed, gastric decontamination is usually not of value. Methanol does not bind to activated charcoal. Metabolic acidosis is treated with intravenous sodium bicarbonate at doses of 1–2 mEq/kg.

Ethanol is considered the antidote for methanol poisoning (see Table 722–3). It is preferentially metabolized over methanol by alcohol dehydrogenase, which prevents the formation of formic acid. Unchanged methanol is excreted via the lungs and kidneys. Indications for ethanol therapy are a serum methanol level greater than 20 mg/dL, a symptomatic patient, or the ingestion of more than 0.4 mL/kg of 100% methanol. Assistance with ethanol dosing may be obtained through consultation with a medical toxicologist or Poison Control Center. Fomepizole (4-methylpyrazole, Antizole), a potent competitive inhibitor of alcohol dehydrogenase, is not currently approved for use in methanol poisoning in the United States.

Hemodialysis effectively removes methanol and formic acid and also is useful for correcting severe metabolic acidosis. The indications for hemodialysis are refractory metabolic acidosis, visual disturbances, or methanol blood levels greater than 50 mg/dL. Ethanol is also removed by dialysis, and doses thus must be increased during dialysis.

ETHYLENE GLYCOL

PATHOPHYSIOLOGY. Ethylene glycol is metabolized by alcohol dehydrogenase in the liver to glycoaldehyde, which is further converted to glycolic acid by aldehyde dehydrogenase. Glycolic acid is metabolized to glyoxylic acid and oxalic acid, which cause toxicity. The development of serious toxic effects is delayed while these acids are generated and accumulate in blood and tissues. Oxalic acid combines with serum and tissue calcium, causing hypocalcemia and the formation of calcium oxalate crystals.

CLINICAL AND LABORATORY MANIFESTATIONS. Ethylene glycol toxicity is described as occurring in three stages; however, there is considerable overlap in the stages. Early symptoms occur 1–12 hr after ingestion and include gastric irritation, with nausea and vomiting, and CNS effects, with drowsiness and inebriation. Metabolic acidosis begins to develop. From 12–24 hr after ingestion, cardiac dysrhythmias, muscle pain, and tetany due to hypocalcemia develop. Later in the clinical course, cardiac failure, seizures, cerebral edema, and renal failure occur. Renal failure is due to the deposition of calcium oxalate crystals in renal tubules.

Tests of ethylene glycol blood levels are not readily available, and results do not correlate well with toxicity. Glycolic acid and glyoxylic acid levels may correlate more closely with toxicity, but levels are not routinely available. Sodium fluorescene is an additive in many commercial antifreeze products. It is renally excreted and can be visualized in urine when illuminated with a Wood's lamp up to 6 hr after ingestion. This simple test may be used to verify ethylene glycol ingestion in children. Ethylene glycol levels can be estimated from an osmolar gap. The serum osmolarity is measured by the freezing point depression method and is compared with a calculated serum osmolarity. The osmolar gap can be used to estimate the serum ethylene glycol level using the following formula:

$$\text{Osmolar gap} \times 6.2 = \text{estimated ethylene glycol level in mg/dL.}$$

Calcium oxalate crystals are commonly found on urine microscopy but may not be evident early after exposure. Electrolytes, including calcium, should be monitored, as well as results of renal function studies and the ECG.

TREATMENT. Because ethylene glycol is rapidly absorbed, gastric decontamination is usually not of value. Activated charcoal does not bind ethylene glycol. Metabolic acidosis is treated with intravenous sodium bicarbonate at doses of 1–2 mEq/kg.

Ethanol is the antidote for ethylene glycol poisoning because it is preferentially metabolized over ethylene glycol by alcohol dehydrogenase, thus preventing formation of toxic metabolites (see Table 722–3). Unchanged ethylene glycol is then excreted via the lungs and kidneys. Indications for ethanol therapy are a serum ethylene glycol level greater than 25 mg/dL, a symptomatic patient, or ingestion of more than 0.4 mL/kg of 100% ethylene glycol. Assistance with ethanol dosing may be obtained through consultation with a medical toxicologist or Poison Center. Fomepizole (Table 722–3) is a potent competitive inhibitor of alcohol dehydrogenase that has been approved for use in ethylene glycol toxicity. It works like ethanol to inhibit ethylene glycol metabolism. Ease of dosing and lack of side effects are major advantages of fomepizole over ethanol. The high cost is a disadvantage. There is very limited experience with this agent in children. It should be reserved only for patients with known potentially toxic exposures when ethanol therapy is not an option.

Hemodialysis effectively removes ethylene glycol and its acid metabolites. It is also useful for correcting severe metabolic acidosis. The indications for hemodialysis are refractory metabolic acidosis, renal failure, or ethylene glycol blood levels exceeding 50 mg/dL. Ethanol is also removed by dialysis; thus, doses must be increased during dialysis. Fomepizole is also removed during dialysis, and dosage adjustment is necessary.

Church AS, Witting MD: Laboratory testing in ethanol, methanol, ethylene glycol and isopropanol toxicities. J Emerg Med 15:687, 1997.
Davis DP, Bramwell KJ, Hamilton RS, et al: Ethylene glycol poisoning: Case report of a record-high level and a review. J Emerg Med 15:653, 1997.
Glaser DS: Utility of the serum osmol gap in the diagnosis of methanol or ethylene glycol ingestion. Ann Emerg Med 27:343, 1996.
Jacobsen D, McMartin KE: Antidotes for methanol and ethylene glycol poisoning. J Toxicol Clin Toxicol 35:127, 1997.

722.9 Hydrocarbons

Hydrocarbons represent a wide array of chemical substances contained in thousands of commercial products. Many factors are involved in determining whether a particular exposure will produce systemic or local toxicity or both.

PATHOPHYSIOLOGY. The most important toxic effect of hydrocarbons is aspiration pneumonitis (also see Chapter 393.2). Aspiration usually occurs at the time of ingestion, when coughing and gagging are common, but can result from vomiting that commonly occurs after ingestion. The propensity of a hydrocarbon product to cause aspiration pneumonitis relates to its viscosity. Compounds with low viscosity such as mineral spirits, naphtha, kerosene, gasoline, and lamp oil spread rapidly across surfaces and cover large areas of the lungs when aspirated. Only small quantities (<1 mL) need be aspirated to produce significant injury. Pneumonitis does not result from dermal absorption of hydrocarbons or from ingestion in the absence of aspiration.

Hydrocarbons can be absorbed from ingestion, inhalation, or through the skin. Most hydrocarbons have anesthetic properties and can cause transient CNS depression. Several chlorinated solvents, most notably carbon tetrachloride, can produce hepatic toxicity. A few hydrocarbons have also been associated with renal toxicity. Benzene is known to cause cancer in humans after long-term exposure. The malignancy most commonly associated with benzene is acute myelogenous leukemia. Methylene chloride, found in some paint strippers, is metabolized to carbon monoxide (CO). Nitrobenzene, aniline, and related compounds produce methemoglobinemia. The diagnosis of methemoglobinemia (≥20%) is suggested if a drop of blood applied to filter paper remains brown as it dries. Methemoglobinemia is treated with the antidote methylene blue (see Table 722–3).

A number of volatile hydrocarbons, including toluene, propellants, refrigerants, and volatile nitrites, are commonly used as abuse agents by inhalation. Most of these substances can cause myocardial sensitization with the risk of dysrhythmias and sudden death. Chronic abuse of these agents can lead to cerebral atrophy and other serious complications.

All volatile hydrocarbons are lipid solvents and can cause defatting of the skin, producing local irritation or, with prolonged exposure, chemical burns.

CLINICAL AND LABORATORY MANIFESTATIONS. Transient, mild CNS depression is common after hydrocarbon ingestion. Aspiration pneumonitis is characterized by coughing, which usually is the first clinical finding. Chest roentgenograms may be unremarkable for as long as 8–12 hr after aspiration. Respiratory symptoms may remain mild or may rapidly progress to respiratory failure. Fever occurs later and may persist for as long as 10 days after ingestion. Accompanying leukocytosis may be misleading, because in most cases of aspiration pneumonitis, no bacteria are present in the lungs. Chest roentgenograms may remain abnormal long after a patient is clinically normal. Much later (2–3 wk after exposure), pneumatoceles may appear on the chest roentgenogram. See Chapter 393.2.

Older children, adolescents, and adults may be involved in chronic solvent abuse. Symptoms of CNS depression, congestive heart failure, headache, vertigo, ataxia, euphoria, and renal and hepatic damage may be seen acutely.

TREATMENT. Emesis, once thought to be useful, is contraindicated. Instillation of vegetable oils or mineral oil into the stomach in an attempt to prevent absorption is also contraindicated. In hydrocarbon-induced pneumonitis, corticosteroids should be avoided, because they do not provide any benefit and may be harmful. Likewise, antibiotics should not be given prophylactically. Fever and leukocytosis usually result from the pyrogenic effect of the agent; bacterial pneumonia occurs in only a very small percentage of cases. Respiratory failure has been successfully treated with both standard ventilation and with extracorporeal membrane oxygenation.

Anas N, Nanasonthi V, Ginsburg CM: Criteria for hospitalizing children who have ingested products containing hydrocarbons. JAMA 246:840, 1981.

Carder JR, Fuerst RS: Myocardial infarction after toluene inhalation. Pediatr Emerg Care 13:117, 1997.
Edminster SC, Bayer MJ: Recreational gasoline sniffing: Acute gasoline intoxication and latent organolead poisoning. J Emerg Med 3:365, 1985.
Flanagan RJ, Ruprah M, Meredith TJ, et al: An introduction to the clinical toxicology of volatile substances. Drug Safety 5:359, 1990.
Gurwitz D, Kattan M, Levison H, et al: Pulmonary function abnormalities in asymptomatic children after hydrocarbon pneumonitis. Pediatrics 62:789, 1978.
Meredith TJ, Ruprah M, Liddle A, et al: Diagnosis and treatment of acute poisoning with volatile substances. Hum Toxicol 8:277, 1989.

722.10 Toxic Gases

Although many industrial and naturally occurring gases pose a health risk by inhalation, only two, carbon monoxide (CO) and hydrogen cyanide, are considered in detail here. CO is a colorless, odorless gas produced during the combustion of any carbon-containing fuel. Hydrogen cyanide, as well as cyanide salts, is used in many industrial processes. Hydrogen cyanide is also produced during combustion of many plastics and fabrics and is released during metabolism of some chemicals, including the solvent acetonitrile.

Chlorine, chloramine, and hydrogen chloride are severe lung irritants and may cause a chemical pneumonitis. Nitrogen, propane, and methane are examples of simple asphyxiants.

CARBON MONOXIDE

PATHOPHYSIOLOGY. Toxicity develops through at least three mechanisms. First, CO binds to hemoglobin, displacing oxygen. Its affinity for hemoglobin is about 250 times that of oxygen. Second, CO impairs the ability of hemoglobin to release oxygen to tissues. Finally, CO also binds to cytochrome oxidase in tissues, impeding the use of oxygen. Although the relative contributions of these mechanisms to the overall toxicity of carbon monoxide are unclear, the net result is tissue hypoxia.

CLINICAL AND LABORATORY MANIFESTATIONS. Symptoms of CO poisoning are generally proportionate to the concentration of carboxyhemoglobin in the blood. Early symptoms are nonspecific and include headache, malaise, and nausea, which are often confused with the flu. At higher exposure levels, headaches become severe and dizziness, visual changes, and weakness may be present. Children may experience syncopal episodes as a first symptom. At high levels, coma, seizures, respiratory instability, and death may occur.

TREATMENT. Treatment of CO poisoning, in addition to general supportive care, requires administration of high concentrations of oxygen, which shortens the half-life of CO in the blood and tissues. Severely poisoned children benefit from hyperbaric oxygen therapy. After a significant exposure, some patients may experience delayed-onset neurotoxicity, which may be permanent. Aggressive early treatment of patients with significant symptoms may diminish the risk of neurologic sequelae.

HYDROGEN CYANIDE

PATHOPHYSIOLOGY. Cyanide exerts its toxicity by interfering with oxygen use in the cytochrome oxidase system, resulting in cellular hypoxia.

CLINICAL AND LABORATORY MANIFESTATIONS. Clinical symptoms occur rapidly after significant exposures and include headache, agitation and confusion, loss of consciousness, convulsions, and cardiac dysrhythmias. Death may occur. Severe metabolic acidosis occurs rapidly. Cyanide levels can be measured in the blood, but tests are not readily available and levels do not correlate well with symptoms. Severe metabolic acidosis in a patient with suspected cyanide exposure (e.g., fire victims) should be assumed to be cyanide poisoning.

TREATMENT. The cornerstone of treatment is rapid administration of high concentrations of oxygen, together with the use of the Cyanide Antidote Kit. This kit includes nitrites (amyl nitrite and sodium nitrite) used to produce methemoglobin, which effectively binds cyanide, and sodium thiosulfate, which hastens the metabolism of this cyanide-nitrite complex to regenerate hemoglobin and produce the less toxic thiocyanate. Hydroxocobalamin (vitamin B_{12a}), which reacts with cyanide to produce cyanocobalamin (vitamin B_{12}), is an alternative antidote but is not available in the United States.

Barillo DJ, Goode R, Esch V: Cyanide poisoning in victims of fire: Analysis of 364 cases and review of the literature. J Burn Care Rehabil 15:46, 1994.
Hardy KR, Thom SR: Pathophysiology and treatment of carbon monoxide poisoning. J Toxicol Clin Toxicol 32:613, 1994.
Geller RJ, Ekins BR, Iknoian RC: Cyanide toxicity from acetonitrile-containing false nail remover. Am J Emerg Med 9:268, 1991.
Meredith TJ, Ruprah M, Liddle A, et al: Diagnosis and treatment of acute poisoning with volatile substances. Hum Toxicol 8:277, 1989.
Salkowki AA, Penney DG: Cyanide poisoning in animals and humans: A review. Vet Hum Toxicol 36:455, 1994.

722.11 Plants

Exposure to plants, both inside the home and outside in backyards and fields, is one of the most common causes of accidental poisoning in children. Fortunately, ingestion of most plant parts (leaves, seeds, flowers) results in mild, self-limiting effects, and the treatment is symptomatic and supportive. Table 722–6 contains a list of plants considered to be nontoxic. This means that the inherent toxicity of the product is so low that the ingestion of small to moderate quantities of plant material is unlikely to produce toxic symptoms. Table 722–7 contains information describing the toxic effects following exposure to some common plants found in and around the home and yard.

The potential toxicity of a particular plant is highly variable, depending on the part of the plant involved (flowers are generally less toxic than the root or seed), the time of year, the growing conditions of the plant, and the route of exposure. Assessment of the potential severity following a plant exposure is also complicated by the difficulty in properly identifying the plant. Many plants are known by several common names, and the common name of the same plant may vary between communities. Poison Control Centers have access to individuals able to assist in the proper identification of plants. They also keep current on the common poisonous plants in their service area and the seasons in which they are more abundant; thus, consultation with a Poison Control Center is recommended if a potentially toxic plant is involved in the exposure. The literature describing plant exposure is often extrapolated from animal data or based on isolated case reports and thus is limited.

Gastrointestinal decontamination for potentially toxic ingestions includes the use of activated charcoal. Antidotes are

TABLE 722–6 Nontoxic Plants

African violet	Dracaena	Palm
Aluminum plant	Fern species (not asparagus fern)	Peperomia
Aralia, false	Fig	Petunia
Aster	Gardenia	Poke berries
Barberry	Geranium	Poinsettia
Begonia species	Hen and chicks	Pyracantha
Boston fern	Honeysuckle	Rose
Carnation	Impatiens	Rubber plant
Chinese evergreen	Jade plant	Schefflera
Christmas cactus	Kalanchoe	Snake plant
Coleus	Magnolia	Spider plant
Corn plant	Marigold	Violet
Dandelion	Mother-in-law's tongue	Wandering Jew
Daylily	Nasturtium	Yucca
Dogwood	Norfolk Island pine	

TABLE 722–7 Common Poisonous Plants

Common Plant Name	Toxic Constituent	Symptoms or Special Treatment
Black nightshade Climbing nightshade Deadly nightshade Horse nettle Jimsonweed Potato/tomato (foliage & sprouts)	Anticholinergic alkaloids such as atropine and solanine	Anticholinergic syndrome; gastroenteritis
Asparagus fern Caladium Dumbcane Elephant ear Jack-in-the-pulpit Peace lily Philodendron Pothos Rhubarb (leaves) Skunk cabbage	Calcium oxalate crystals	Irritation and edema of mucous membranes, edema, gastroenteritis; large ingestions may cause hypocalcemia
Christmas pepper Hot pepper	Capsicum	Irritation and burning sensation of skin and mucous membranes
Foxglove Lily-of-the-valley Oleander	Cardiac glycosides	Irritation of mucous membranes, cardiac toxicity; severe intoxication may require dioxin-specific FAB fragments
Water hemlock	Cicutoxin	Grand mal seizures
Fall crocus	Colchicine	Gastroenteritis, cardiotoxicity
Poison hemlock	Conine	Salivation, nausea, vomiting, diarrhea, seizures, coma, respiratory paralysis
Cherry, apple, peach, apricot, chokecherry (seeds, pits, leaves)	Hydrocyanic acid-containing glycosides	Very large amounts may cause dyspnea, seizures, coma
Morning glory (seeds)	Lysergic acid monoethylamide	Gastroenteritis, hallucinations
Amaryllis Daffodil Narcissus (bulb)	Lycorine	Vomiting, diarrhea
Tobacco Cardinal flower	Nicotine	Salivation, gastroenteritis
May apple	Podophylloresin	Vomiting, diarrhea, drowsiness, peripheral neuropathy
Pokeweed (leaves, root)	Podophyllotoxin-like resins	Vomiting, sweating, colic, drowsiness
Castor bean (chewed seeds)	Ricin	Burning sensation of mouth, throat; gastroenteritis, hepatotoxicity, seizures
Yew	Taxine	Vomiting, abdominal pain, respiratory depression
Euphorbia Spurges	Unknown acrid principle	Mucous membrane irritation
Mistletoe (berries)	Viscotoxin, phoratoxin, lectins	Gastroenteritis, cardiovascular collapse

not commonly used for plant exposures, and treatment is supportive and symptomatic.

Lampe KF, McConn MA: AMA Handbook of Poisonous and Injurious Plants. Chicago, American Medical Association, 1985.
Turner NJ, Szczawinski AF: Common Poisonous Plants and Mushrooms of North America. Portland, OR, Timber Press, 1991.

CHAPTER 723 Nonbacterial Food Poisoning

Stephen C. Aronoff

723.1 Mushroom Poisoning

Consumption of wild mushrooms, a favorite pastime in Europe, is increasingly popular in the United States, with concomitant increases in fatal cases of mushroom poisoning.

Four clinical syndromes and seven classes of toxins are associated with wild mushroom poisoning. The clinical syndromes are divided according to the predominant system involved and the rapidity of onset of symptoms. The toxins produced by wild mushrooms are categorized as follows: cyclopeptides, monomethylhydrazine, muscarine, coprine, ibotenic acid, psilocybin, and unknown.

GASTROINTESTINAL—DELAYED ONSET

Amanita Poisoning. Poisonings by species of *Amanita* and *Galerina* account for 95% of the fatalities due to mushroom intoxication, although the mortality rate for this group is 5–10%. Most species produce two classes of cyclopeptide toxins: (1) phalloidins, which are heptapeptides believed to be responsible for the early symptoms of *Amanita* poisoning; and (2) amanitotoxin, which is an octapeptide that inhibits RNA polymerase and subsequent production of messenger RNA. Cells with high turnover rates, such as those in the gastrointestinal (GI) mucosa, kidneys, and liver, are the most severely affected.

Histopathologically, Amanita poisoning causes cellular necrosis, which may occur throughout the GI tract, the most heavily exposed site. Acute yellow atrophy of the liver and necrosis of the proximal renal tubules are found in lethal cases.

The *clinical course* produced by poisoning with *Amanita* or *Galerina* species is biphasic, after an initial 6–12-hr latent period. Six to 24 hr after ingestion, nausea, vomiting, and severe abdominal pain ensue. Profuse watery diarrhea follows shortly thereafter and may last for 12–24 hr. During this time, as much as 9 L of fluid may be lost. Twenty-four to 48 hr after poisoning, jaundice, hypertransaminasemia (peaking at 72–96 hr), renal failure, and coma occur. Death occurs 4–7 days after the ingestion. A prothrombin time less than 10% of control is a poor prognostic factor.

Treatment of *Amanita* poisoning is both supportive and specific. Fluid loss from severe diarrhea during the early course of the illness is profound, requiring aggressive therapy for correction of this loss. In the late phase of the disease, management of renal and hepatic failure is also necessary.

Specific therapy for *Amanita* poisoning is designed to remove the toxin rapidly and to block binding at its target site. Oral activated charcoal and lactulose combined with fluid and electrolyte replacement are recommended as part of the initial treatment of children with *Amanita* poisoning. Forced diuresis should be avoided because this increases renal exposure.

Although cytochrome C protects mice from lethal doses of amanitotoxin, clinical trials with this agent have failed to demonstrate benefit. Intravenous penicillin G (250 mg/kg/24 hr) administered as a continuous infusion combined with silibinin, the water-soluble form of the flavolignone silymarin (in an intravenous dosage of 20–50 mg/kg/24 hr), acts synergistically to inhibit binding of both toxins and to interrupt enterohepatic recirculation of amanitotoxin. Hemodialysis and hemoperfusion are also recommended as part of the initial treatment for intoxicated children. Orthotopic liver transplantation is recommended for children in whom severe hepatic failure develops (Chapter 367).

Monomethylhydrazine Intoxication. Species of *Gyromitra* contain monomethylhydrazine (CH_3NHNH_2), which inhibits central nervous system (CNS) enzymatic production of γ-aminobutyric acid (GABA). Monomethylhydrazine also oxidizes iron in hemoglobin, resulting in methemoglobinemia. Children with *Gyromitra* poisoning develop vomiting, diarrhea, hematochezia, and abdominal pain within 6–24 hr of ingestion of the toxin. Symptoms of CNS depression and seizures develop later in the clinical course. Hemolysis and methemoglobinemia are potential life-threatening complications of monomethylhydrazine poisoning. Severe methemoglobinemia may require dialysis.

Hypovolemia due to GI fluid losses and seizures requires supportive intervention. Pyridoxal phosphate, the coenzyme that catalyzes the production of GABA, can reverse the effects of monomethylhydrazine when administered in high doses. Pyridoxine hydrochloride (25 mg/kg) is administered intravenously at a frequency dependent on clinical improvement. Parenteral administration of methylene blue is indicated if the methemoglobin concentration exceeds 30%. Blood transfusions may be required for significant hemolysis.

AUTONOMIC NERVOUS SYSTEM—RAPID ONSET

Muscarine Poisoning. Mushrooms of the genera *Inocybe* and, to a lesser degree, *Clitocybe* contain muscarine or muscarine-related compounds. These quaternary ammonium derivatives bind to postsynaptic receptors, producing an exaggerated cholinergic response.

The *clinical syndrome* is characterized by the following hypercholinergic response: The onset of symptoms is rapid (30 min–2 hr after consumption) and consists of diaphoresis, excessive lacrimation, salivation, miosis, urinary and fecal incontinence, and vomiting. Respiratory distress caused by bronchospasm and increased bronchopulmonary secretions is the most serious complication. The symptoms subside spontaneously within 6–24 hr.

Atropine sulfate, the *specific antidote,* is administered intravenously (0.1 mg/kg). This is repeated until the pulmonary symptoms resolve or the patient becomes overtly tachycardic.

Coprine Ingestion. *Coprinus atramentarius* and *Clitocybe clavipes* contain coprine. Like disulfiram (Antabuse), coprine inhibits the metabolism of acetaldehyde after ethanol ingestion. The clinical symptoms result from accumulation of acetaldehyde.

Coprine intoxication becomes apparent after ethanol ingestion and may occur up to 5 days after consuming the mushroom. Hyperemia of the face and trunk, tingling of the hands, metallic taste, tachycardia, and vomiting occur acutely. Hypotension may result from intense peripheral vasodilation.

The syndrome is typically self-limited and lasts only several hours. No specific antidote is available. If hypotension is severe, vascular re-expansion with isotonic parenteral solutions may be required. Small oral doses of propranolol have also been suggested.

CENTRAL NERVOUS SYSTEM—RAPID ONSET

Ibotenic Acid and Muscimol Intoxication. Although *Amanita muscaria* and *Amanita pantherina* may contain muscarine (see earlier), the toxins responsible for the CNS symptoms following ingestion of these mushrooms are muscimol and ibotenic acid. Muscimol, a hallucinogen, and ibotenic acid, an insecticide, have anticholinergic effects. One half to 3 hr after ingestion, CNS symptoms appear; obtundation, alternating lethargy and agitation, and, occasionally, seizures ensue. Nausea and vomiting are uncommon. If large amounts of muscarine are contained in the mushroom, symptoms of cholinergic crisis may also occur.

Specific therapy must be carefully selected. If an exaggerated cholinergic response is observed, atropine should be administered. Because ingestions of *A. muscaria* are frequently associated with anticholinergic findings, the acetylcholinesterase inhibitor physostigmine is used to reverse the delirium and coma. Seizures can be controlled with diazepam. Early treatment with ipecac (if the patient is conscious) and close observation are all that is required in most cases.

Indole Intoxication. Mushrooms belonging to the genus *Psilocybe* ("magic mushrooms") contain psilocybin and psilocin, two psychotropic compounds. Within 30 min after ingestion, patients experience euphoria and hallucinations, often accompanied by tachycardia and mydriasis. Fever and seizures have also been observed in children with psilocybin poisoning. These symptoms are short lived, usually lasting 6 hr after consumption of the mushroom. Severely agitated patients may respond to diazepam.

GASTROINTESTINAL—RAPID ONSET. Many mushrooms from various genera produce local GI symptoms. The causative toxins are diverse and largely unknown. Within 1 hr of ingestion, patients develop acute abdominal pain, nausea, vomiting, and diarrhea. Symptoms may last from hours to days, depending on the species of mushroom.

Treatment is mainly supportive. Children with large fluid losses may require parenteral fluid therapy. It is imperative to differentiate ingestion of mushrooms of this class from ingestions of Amanita and Galerina species containing cyclopeptide toxins.

723.2 Solanine Poisoning

Solanine is a mixture of several related toxins found in "greened" and sprouted potatoes. Potatoes exposed to light and allowed to sprout produce a number of alkaloid glycosides containing the cholesterol derivative solanidine. Two of these glycosides, α-solanine and α-chaconine, are found in highest concentration in the peels of greened potatoes and in the sprouts. The solanine alkaloids bind to serum cholinesterase, suggesting a possible pathophysiologic mechanism.

Clinical manifestations of solanine intoxication occur within 7–19 hr after ingestion. The most common symptoms are vomiting and diarrhea; in more severe instances of poisoning, fever, generalized abdominal pain, coma, and hypovolemic shock occur.

Treatment of solanine poisoning is largely supportive. In the most severe cases, symptoms resolve within 11 days. Atropine treatment has not been evaluated.

723.3 Seafood Poisoning

CIGUATERA FISH POISONING. Major outbreaks of ciguatera fish poisoning have been reported in Florida, Hawaii, and the Virgin Islands; however, with modern methods of transportation, the illness now occurs worldwide. Grouper is the most frequently identified source of the toxin, followed by snapper, kingfish, amberjack, dolphin, and barracuda. Poisoning has also been associated with farm-raised salmon.

The source of this poisoning is the dinoflagellate *Gambierdiscus toxicus*, a microscopic organism found in the food chain along coral reefs, which contains high concentrations of ciguatoxin and maitotoxin. After the organism is ingested by small fish, the toxin is absorbed and concentrated in fish flesh and muscle. Larger fish consume the smaller fish, and again the toxin is absorbed from the GI tract and concentrated in the musculature.

Ciguatoxin-1, a lipid with a molecular weight of approximately 1,100, increases the sodium permeability of excitable membranes. This action is inhibited by calcium and tetrodotoxin.

The onset of *clinical manifestations* after ingestion of fish containing ciguatoxin is rapid, usually occurring within 2–30 hr. The illness is often biphasic. The earliest symptoms are diarrhea, vomiting, and abdominal pain; the second phase includes myalgias and circumoral or extremity dysesthesias. The dysesthesia is characterized by reversal of hot and cold sensation. Tachycardia, bradycardia, and hypotension occur infrequently.

Treatment of ciguatera fish poisoning is supportive. Gastric lavage is recommended to remove any remaining toxin. Intravenous fluids may be required for severe diarrhea, and parenteral administration of calcium can be used to treat hypotension. In a few patients with coma or prolonged symptoms, mannitol has successfully reversed the neurologic manifestations of intoxication. However, further studies are needed before a recommendation for mannitol therapy can be made. Most cases are self-limited; symptoms may last up to 3 wk.

SCOMBROID (PSEUDOALLERGIC) FISH POISONING. Epidemics have been associated with ingestion of members of the Scombresocidae or Scombridae families, notably albacore, mackerel, tuna, bonita, and kingfish. Nonscombroid fish and marine mammals, such as mahi-mahi (dolphin) and bluefish, have also been linked to outbreaks of poisoning.

Scombrotoxin, either histamine or the product of the action of the toxin on fish flesh, is responsible for the clinical syndrome. Histidine is found in high concentrations in the flesh of scombroid fish; the action of bacterial decarboxylases during putrification converts the histidine to histamine. Fish containing more than 20 mg of histamine per 100 g of flesh are toxic. In patients receiving isoniazid, a potent histaminase blocker, ingestion of fish flesh containing lower concentration of histamine may be toxic.

The onset of *clinical manifestations* is acute and occurs within 10 min–2 hr after ingestion. The most common symptoms include diarrhea, flushing, diaphoresis, urticaria, nausea, and headache. Abdominal pain, tachycardia, oral burning, dizziness, respiratory distress, and facial swelling also occur. The illness is usually self-limited, terminating within 8–10 hr.

Treatment is mainly supportive. Gastric lavage decreases continued absorption of histamine. With severe diarrhea, fluid replacement may be necessary. Antihistamines have been variably successful. Four patients with severe toxicity treated with cimetidine (a histamine blocker) responded rapidly. Because data are limited, cimetidine or ranitidine should be reserved for severe cases.

PARALYTIC SHELLFISH POISONING. Filter-feeding mollusks, such as the black mussel and sea scallop, may become contaminated during dinoflagellate blooms or "red tides." The dinoflagellate *Ptychodiscus brevis* is often responsible for these red tides and contains several potent neurotoxins. Saxitoxin is the most important of the neurotoxins responsible for paralytic shellfish poisoning. This toxin prevents nerve conduction by inhibiting the sodium-potassium pump. Although six other toxins have been isolated from contaminated scallops, these toxins may be bioconverted to less toxic structures.

The onset of *clinical manifestations* of paralytic shellfish poisoning occurs rapidly, 30 min–2 hr after ingestion. Abdominal pain and nausea are common. Paresthesias are common and occur circumorally, in a stocking-glove distribution, or both. Perioral numbness or tingling, diplopia, ataxia, dysarthria, and the sensation of floating occur less commonly. Hot-cold reversal in temperature sensation is not unusual. In severe cases, respiratory failure due to diaphragmatic paralysis may result.

No antidote for paralytic shellfish poisoning is known. Supportive care, including mechanical ventilation, may be needed. Although the symptoms are usually self-limited and short lived, weakness and malaise may persist for weeks after ingestion.

Mushroom Poisoning

Benjamin DR: Mushroom poisoning in infants and children: The *Amanita pantherina/muscaria* group. Clin Toxicol 30:13, 1992.

Editorial: Mushroom poisoning. Lancet 2:351, 1980.

Hanrahan JP, Gordon MA: Mushroom poisoning: Case reports and a review of therapy. JAMA 251:1057, 1984.

Klein AS, Hart J, Brems JJ, et al: *Amanita* poisoning: Treatment and the role of liver transplantation. Am J Med 86:187, 1989.

Litten W: The most poisonous mushrooms. Sci Am 232:90, 1975.

McCormick DJ, Avbel AJ, Biggons RB: Nonlethal mushroom poisoning. Ann Intern Med 90:332, 1979.

McDonald A: Mushrooms and madness: Hallucinogenic mushrooms and some psychopharmacological implications. Can J Psychiatry 25:586, 1980.

Mitchell DH: *Amanita* mushroom poisoning. Annu Rev Med 31:51, 1980.

Sabeel AI, Kurkus J, Lindholm T: Intensive hemodialysis and hemoperfusion treatment of *Amanita* mushroom poisoning. Mycopathologia 131:107, 1995.

Solanine Poisoning

Editorial: Potato poisoning. Lancet 2:681, 1979.

McMillan M, Thompson JC: An outbreak of suspected solanine poisoning in school boys: Examination of criteria of solanine poisoning. Q J Med 48:227, 1979.

Ciguatera Fish Poisoning

DiNubile MJ, Hokama Y: The ciguatera poisoning syndrome from farm-raised salmon. Ann Intern Med 122:113, 1995.

Lawrence DN, Enriquez MB, Lumish RM, et al: Ciguatera fish poisoning in Miami. JAMA 244:254, 1980.

Morris JG, Lewin P, Hargrett NT, et al: Clinical features of ciguatera fish poisoning. Arch Intern Med 142:1090, 1982.

Palafox NA, Jain LG, Pinano AZ, et al: Successful treatment of ciguatera fish poisoning with intravenous mannitol. JAMA 259:2740, 1988.

Withers NW: Ciguatera fish poisoning. Annu Rev Med 33:97, 1982.

Scombroid Fish Poisoning

Blakesley ML: Scombroid poisoning: Prompt resolution of symptoms with cimetidine. Ann Emerg Med 12:104, 1983.

Gilbert RJ, Hobbs G, Murray CK, et al: Scombrotoxic fish poisoning: Features of the first 50 incidents to be reported in Britain (1976–9). Br Med J 281:71, 1980.

Hughes JM, Potter ME: Scombroid fish poisoning: From pathogenesis to prevention. N Engl J Med 324:766, 1991.

Morrow JD, Margolies GR, Rowland J, et al: Evidence that histamine is the causative toxin of scombroid fish poisoning. N Engl J Med 324:716, 1991.

Paralytic Shellfish Poisoning

Gessner BD, Middaugh JP: Paralytic shellfish poisoning in Alaska: A 20-year retrospective analysis. Am J Epidemiol 141:766, 1995.

Hughes JM, Merson MH: Fish and shellfish poisoning. N Engl J Med 295:1117, 1976.

Morris PD, Campbell DS, Taylor TJ, et al: Clinical and epidemiological features of neurotoxic shellfish poisoning in North Carolina. Am J Public Health 81:471, 1991.

Popkiss MEE, Horstman DA, Harpur D: Paralytic shellfish poisoning: A report of 17 cases in Cape Town. S Afr Med J 55:1017, 1979.

Shimizu Y, Yoshioka M: Transformation of paralytic shellfish toxins as demonstrated in scallop homogenates. Science 212:547, 1981.

Chapter 724
Envenomations

Steve Holve

The vast majority of bites and stings by spiders, snakes, and other venomous animals cause little more than local pain and never require medical attention. However, pediatricians should be prepared to identify and treat those few individuals who present with severe envenomation. Children, unfortunately, are at greater risk for severe reactions because of their smaller volume for venom distribution.

Symptoms of envenomation may be either IgE mediated, such as anaphylaxis in response to Hymenoptera stings, or venom mediated, as with the bites of poisonous spiders or snakes or the sting of scorpions. Immediate hypersensitivity reactions are treated emergently as indicated in Chapter 148, on anaphylaxis. In moderate and severe envenomation, species-specific antivenin has been shown to ameliorate symptoms and prevent death, but the use of antivenin carries significant risks. Appropriate assessment of the risk:benefit ratio in the use of antivenin is therefore the most important skill a physician can possess in treating envenomation.

ANTIVENINS. Animal venoms are species-specific mixtures of polypeptides, proteolytic enzymes, glycoproteins, and vasoactive substances. In theory, for every venom, an antivenin can potentially be produced. In the United States, only three antivenins approved by the Food and Drug Administration (FDA) are commercially available: antivenin polyvalent for pit viper (Crotalidae) bites; antivenin for coral snake *(Micrurus fulvius)* bites; and antivenin for black widow spider *(Latrodectus mactans)* bites. Other antivenins to more unusual species of snakes or scorpions are often available through local zoologic societies or the nearest Poison Control Center.

All antivenins are animal-derived (usually from horse serum) immunoglobulin that work by direct binding and neutralization of the proteins in venom. The animal origin of these products exposes patients to large amounts of foreign proteins that may cause both immediate and delayed hypersensitivity reactions.

Immediate hypersensitivity reactions (Chapter 148), especially, may be life threatening, and the incidence after administration of equine antivenin may be as high as 5–10%. Given the risk of anaphylaxis, antivenin should be given only in a setting in which full resuscitative measures including oxygen, endotracheal intubation, and epinephrine are available. Patients should be asked about medication allergies and previous exposure to antivenins. Skin testing using 0.02 mL of a 1:10 dilution of antivenin should be performed before intravenous infusion of antivenin. This testing should be performed only if antivenin is to be given, because fatal anaphylactic reactions have been reported with skin testing alone. A negative skin test response is reassuring, but the false-negative rate is as great as 20%. Conversely, a positive skin test result does not preclude the use of antivenin, because the false-positive rate is as high as 50%, but it does alert a clinician to the higher probability of a severe allergic reaction. In such instances, pretreatment with intravenous administration of diphenhydramine 1 mg/kg and methylprednisolone 1–2 mg/kg is required. Some toxicologists recommend pretreatment for all patients receiving antivenin.

If signs of immediate hypersensitivity develop during administration of antivenin, the infusion should be stopped until the patient is stabilized. If the severity of envenomation warrants continued infusion of antivenin, it may be resumed at a slower rate or simultaneously with administration of epinephrine. In such instances, consultation with the nearest toxicologist at a Poison Control Center is advisable.

Delayed hypersensitivity or *serum sickness* (Chapter 149) develops in up to 50% of patients who receive antivenin. Serum sickness results from deposition of antigen-antibody complexes on endothelial surfaces. It usually develops 5–21 days after exposure and may last for weeks. It is most commonly manifested as urticaria, pruritus, arthralgia, and malaise but rarely may present with immune complex glomerulonephritis, neuritis, or myocarditis. Intradermal skin tests have not been shown to predict the risk of serum sickness accurately. Prophylactic use of antihistamines and steroids has been postulated but not proved to reduce the risk of serum sickness but is definitely of benefit if symptoms develop.

It is hoped that in the near future, more purified antivenins of equine origin, antibody fragments, or antivenins from avian or ovine sources will become available, making the risk of allergic reactions significantly less.

SNAKEBITE. Of the more than 3,000 known species of snakes, only 200 are poisonous to humans. Ninety per cent of poisonous snakes are members of one of three families: the Hydrophidae, or poisonous sea snakes; the Elapidae, which includes the cobras, mambas, and coral snakes; and the Viperidae, or true vipers.

In the United States, 95% of poisonous snakebites are by the Crotalidae, or pit vipers, which are a subfamily of the true vipers. Pit vipers may be identified by their triangular heads, elliptical eyes, and the identifiable pit between the eyes and nose (Fig. 724–1). Members of the pit viper family in this country include the rattlesnakes, cottonmouths, and copperheads.

The other native poisonous snakes in this country are the coral snakes, which are found in Texas and the Southeast and are members of the Elapidae family. Coral snakes are small and have a small, rounded head and brightly colored bands of black and red separated by more narrow yellow bands. The rhyme "red on yellow, kill a fellow; red on black, venom lack" serves to differentiate the coral snake from the similar appearing but nonpoisonous scarlet king snake.

Epidemiology. Approximately 45,000 snakebites are reported in the United States each year, but only 8,000 of these bites are inflicted by venomous snakes. The large majority of snakebites

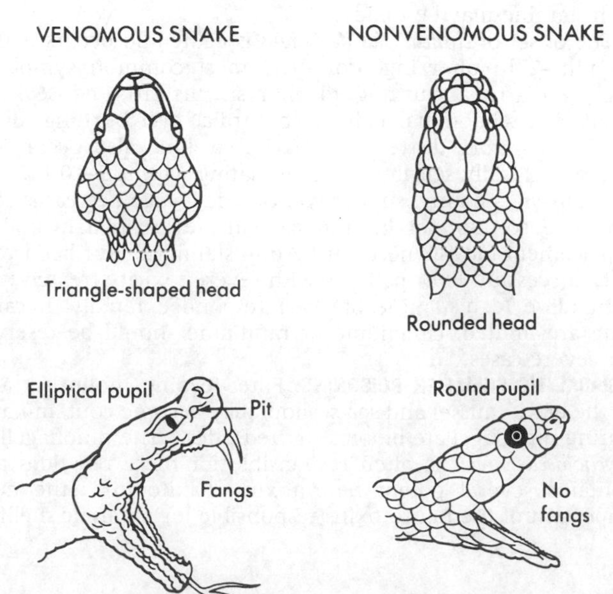

Figure 724–1 Identification of venomous snakes. (Modified from Rosen P, et al [eds]: Emergency Medicine, 3rd ed. St. Louis, CV Mosby, 1992.)

are in males younger than 30 yr and involve alcohol intoxication and a history of the victim's foolishly trying to capture or play with the snake. Despite these many bites, only 12–15 deaths are recorded each year. Unfortunately, children, because of their smaller body mass for venom distribution, are far more likely to have a serious systemic reaction to envenomation and account for more than half of the fatalities.

Pathogenesis. Snake venom is a mixture of polypeptides, proteolytic enzymes, and toxins, which are species specific. Venom from the Elapidae and the Hydrophidae is primarily neurotoxic and has a curare-like effect by blocking neurotransmission at the neuromuscular junction. Death due to envenomation results from respiratory depression. Crotalidae venom is cytolytic, causing tissue necrosis, vascular leak, and coagulopathies. Death due to pit viper bites results from hemorrhagic shock, adult respiratory distress syndrome, or renal failure.

Clinical Manifestations. Pit viper bites usually occur on the extremities; pain and swelling occur at the site within minutes. As the venom moves proximally, edema and ecchymosis advance and, in severe cases, bulla formation and tissue necrosis ensue. Systemic symptoms include nausea, vomiting, diaphoresis, weakness, tingling around the face, and muscle fasciculations. Rarely, patients may present in shock with generalized edema or cardiac arrhythmias. Complex clotting abnormalities often occur.

Bites of most Elapidae, including the coral snakes, are minimally painful because the venom has no cytotoxin. However, lack of immediate symptoms should not be mistaken for the absence of serious envenomation. The venom of the coral snake is primarily neurotoxic, and symptoms can rapidly progress in a few hours from mild drowsiness to cranial nerve palsies, weakness, and death due to respiratory failure.

Treatment. The first task is to determine if the bite was by a poisonous snake and if envenomation occurred. If the snake has been killed, it should be brought to the emergency department (ED) for identification. More than 80% of snakebites in the United States are by nonpoisonous snakes; these bites cause minimal pain and no swelling and require only local wound care.

If the bite is by a venomous snake, immediate care is directed toward decreasing lymphatic flow to limit the spread of venom into the circulation. Immobilization of the extremity, pressure at the site of envenomation, and a proximal tourniquet accomplish this goal. The tourniquet should be loose enough to insert a finger and allow arterial blood flow, because ischemia only exacerbates local tissue damage. Similarly, applying ice to the bite site or using excision and suction is believed to cause more tissue damage than benefit and should be avoided.

On arrival at the ED, the patient should have a large-bore intravenous line inserted and blood for baseline laboratory studies should be obtained. Initial blood tests should include type and cross match because a progressive coagulopathy may make later typing impossible. Other needed tests include complete blood and platelet counts; prothrombin and partial thromboplastin times; fibrinogen and fibrin degradation products; and blood urea nitrogen, creatinine, and creatine phosphokinase levels. These studies need to be repeated at intervals, depending on the severity of envenomation. Baseline vital signs and measurement of the circumference of the bitten extremity are obtained, and demarcation of ecchymosis and swelling marked on the limb so progression can be monitored. The wound can be cleaned and tetanus toxoid given if appropriate.

The decision to use antivenin depends on the severity and progression of symptoms. In general, rattlesnake envenomation requires antivenin and copperhead bites do not, with cottonmouth bites falling between these extremes. The severity of envenomation is commonly graded on a four-point scale (Table 724–1). Most pit viper envenomations cause symptoms

TABLE 724–1 Classification of Envenomation Severity

Grade 0	No envenomation
Grade 1	Minimal envenomation (local swelling and pain without progression)
Grade 2	Moderate envenomation (swelling, pain, or ecchymosis progressing beyond the site of injury; mild systemic or laboratory manifestations)
Grade 3	Severe envenomation (marked local response, severe systemic findings, and significant alteration in laboratory findings)

within 2 hr and almost always within 6 hr; if symptoms are not present, the bite may be presumed to have been "dry" and a grade 0 envenomation. A grade 1 envenomation with only localized swelling requires nothing more than pain control and careful observation. Unfortunately, children, because of their smaller size, are far more likely to have severe envenomation, and more than 75% of children have a grade 2 or 3 envenomation, which requires antivenin.

Antivenin is most effective if delivered within 4 hr of the bite and is of little value if administration is delayed beyond 12 hr. As discussed earlier, antivenin poses a small but significant risk of an immediate hypersensitivity reaction. Antivenin (Crotalidae) polyvalent is administered in increments of 5 vials and repeated as needed to neutralize circulating venom, as measured by normalization of clotting parameters and a halt in the progression of swelling of the affected limb. Children often require more antivenin than a similarly envenomated adult because of their small volume-to-venom ratio. The rapidity of administration and volume of antivenin are best decided in consultation with a toxicologist at the nearest Poison Control Center.

Any person who has been bitten by a coral snake should be administered 3 to 5 vials of antivenin (*M. fulvius*) prophylactically. After being bitten by a coral snake, victims may be asymptomatic for hours before suffering paralysis and respiratory failure. Antivenin is effective only if given before symptoms develop and is ineffective in reversing them once they have occurred.

Prognosis. Despite the potential for mortality and severe morbidity with poisonous snakebites, both can be minimized by early and judicious use of appropriate antivenin. Even extremities with marked tissue necrosis will return to full functioning with the resolution of swelling, and only rarely is delayed skin grafting required.

ARACHNID ENVENOMATION. The arachnids contain the largest number of known venomous species. More than 20,000 venomous spiders have been identified, but most are of no danger to humans because they lack either potent venom or fangs capable of penetrating the human skin. In the United States, the only significant morbidity is caused by spiders in two genera, *L. mactans* (the black widow spider) and *Loxosceles* (the fiddleback or brown recluse spider).

Latrodectism. The black widow is found throughout the United States, though more commonly in the South. The black widow is glossy black and has bright red or orange markings on the ventral surface of the abdomen, although only the species *L. mactans* has the classic hourglass markings. Females have a body length of 1.5 cm and a leg span of 4–5 cm. Males of the species are approximately half the size of females and pose no threat to humans because their fangs are too short to penetrate the skin. The black widow is commonly found in protected places such as under rocks, in woodpiles, and in outhouses or stables.

PATHOGENESIS. The venom of the black widow contains a potent neurotoxin, α-latrotoxin, which binds to presynaptic neuronal membranes, causing dramatic release of acetylcholine and norepinephrine at the neuromuscular junction. The outpouring of these neurotransmitters results in excessive muscle depolarization and autonomic hyperactivity.

Clinical Manifestations. The bite causes both local and systemic effects. A pinprick sensation is usually felt at the bite, which develops into a pale area of 2–3 mm with a red border. Within an hour, dull, crampy pain is felt around the site and gradually extends throughout the body. In the past, it was claimed that upper extremity bites present with chest tightness and grunting respirations whereas lower extremity bites present with abdominal pain and boardlike rigidity, but either may occur regardless of bite location. In addition to the severe muscle cramping, most children have nausea, vomiting, and diaphoresis, along with agitation and hypertension. In extremely rare instances, symptoms may progress to respiratory arrest and death.

Because of presentation with a painful, boardlike abdomen, the black widow spider bite can mimic acute appendicitis or peritonitis. A key point in the differential diagnosis is that most patients with black widow bites are hypertensive and agitated and tend to move about, seeking a comfortable position, whereas patients with a surgical abdomen are often hypotensive and try to lie still and avoid movement. Many past reports of deaths due to black widow bites were related to patients' mistakenly taken to surgery for a presumed acute abdomen. Therefore, obtaining an accurate history and making the correct diagnosis are the most important steps in managing black widow spider bites.

Treatment. Muscle cramping and agitation are the main causes of discomfort and can usually be well controlled with intravenous opiates for pain and benzodiazepines for muscle relaxation. Calcium infusions and dantrolene were previously used for muscle cramping, but neither is efficacious and they are no longer recommended.

Use of antivenin versus symptomatic treatment in black widow bites is determined by the knowledge that without treatment all symptoms will resolve in 24–48 hr but that symptoms can be excruciating. Conservative measures should be tried first before using antivenin if satisfactory pain control is not achieved. A decision tree for treatment is shown in Figure 724–2.

If antivenin is used, an intradermal test dose should be given and all precautions as listed in the earlier antivenin section should be followed. The risk of anaphylaxis is less than that associated with snake antivenin and is less than 1%. One vial of antivenin is usually sufficient, and symptoms of envenomation subside rapidly within 1–3 hr. As with other antivenin products, serum sickness may develop in 5–21 days.

Loxoscelism. Although the bite of a number of spiders can result in mild tissue reactions, only species of the genus *Loxosceles* can cause significant skin necrosis. Members of this genus are commonly known as the "fiddleback spider" because of the brown violin-shaped marking on the thorax or as the "brown recluse spider" because of their predilection for living in dark, undisturbed places such as woodpiles, closets, and basements.

Epidemiology. All species are dull colored and have a small body measuring 1 cm and legs extending up to 5 cm. The species with the most potent bite, *Loxosceles reclusa*, is found most commonly in the river country of mid-America but is also found in the South. Other less potent *Loxosceles* species are found throughout the United States, though their numbers decrease with more northern latitudes.

Clinical Manifestations. The venom of the brown recluse contains hyaluronidase, or spreading factor, and sphingomyelinase D, a protein that lyses cell walls. The bite is often unnoticed or felt only as a pinprick. It typically occurs when a spider is unknowingly trapped against the skin while the victim is putting on clothes; thus, the bite is often on the upper arm, lateral thorax, inner thigh, or rarely on the hands or face. Within 2 hr, a painful, sinking blue macule with a halo of inflammation occurs at the bite site, followed by systemic symptoms that include fever, chills, nausea, and vomiting. In a minority of cases but more commonly in small children, hemolysis can occur. The hemolysis is presumed secondary to toxin action because Coombs test results are negative and the coagulation system is not activated as measured by platelet counts, fibrin split products, and prothrombin time. In extremely rare instances, massive hemolysis can occur and may lead to disseminated intravascular coagulopathy or renal failure.

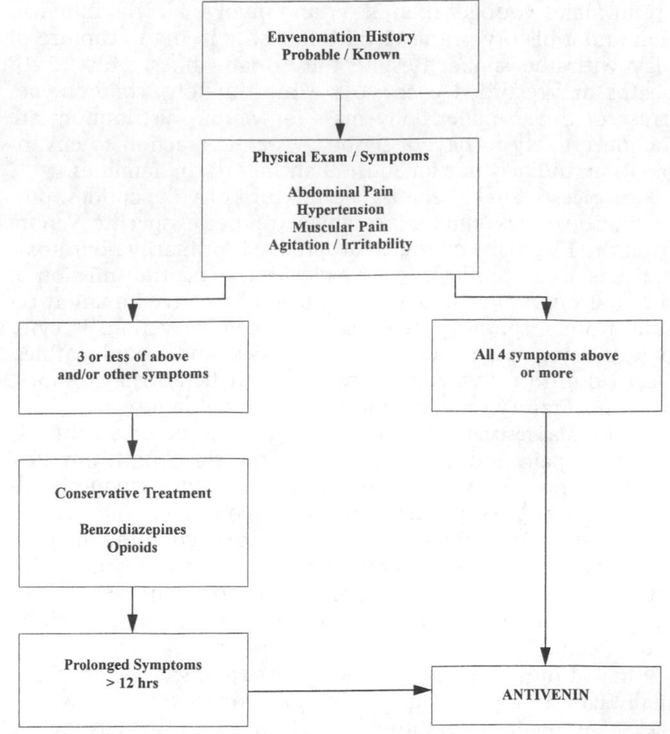

Figure 724–2 Decision process for treating pediatric black widow spider envenomation. (Courtesy of Robin Werstman, Loma Linda Children's Hospital, Loma Linda, CA.)

In addition to systemic symptoms of the bite, a hemorrhagic blister forms within 1–2 days. As the blister sloughs, it leaves the characteristic necrotic ulcer of brown recluse spider bites. Most ulcers remain 1–2 cm but can enlarge up to 15 cm in diameter and involve the full thickness of the skin and some underlying tissue.

Treatment and Prognosis. The outcome in brown recluse spider bites is excellent, and most bites resolve with supportive care alone. Patients with systemic symptoms or significant hemolysis should be admitted to the hospital for pain control and monitoring. Hydration and maintenance of urine output are essential if there is significant hemoglobinuria. Treatment of the ulcerative skin lesions is also supportive, with local wound care. Pain usually subsides in a few days although complete skin healing requires weeks. Hyperbaric oxygen to promote wound healing, dapsone for leukocyte inhibition, and cyproheptadine, a platelet aggregation inhibitor, all have been recommended to prevent enlargement of skin ulcers, but none has proven beneficial. In rare instances, large necrotic ulcers require delayed skin grafting.

SCORPION BITES. More than 1,000 species of scorpions are found worldwide; all of them are capable of delivering venom through a stinger located at the end of a six-segment tail. Of medical importance are the small number of species that belong to the family Butidae, which produce venom that is neurotoxic to humans. Among the most toxic species are those of the *Buthus (Leiurus)* in India and the Middle East, *Tityus* in Brazil and Trinidad, and *Centruroides* in Mexico and the desert Southwest of the United States. The majority of stings, even by toxic species, cause only a painful local reaction. However, given their small size, infants and young children who are stung are at risk for severe autonomic dysfunction, multisystem organ failure, and even death.

Pathogenesis. Scorpion venoms vary by species, but all have hyaluronidase, serotonin, histamine releasers, and neurotoxins, of which the neurotoxins are the most important component. These neurotoxins can bind to the presynaptic membranes, causing release of acetylcholine and stimulation of both the sympathetic and parasympathetic nervous systems.

Clinical Manifestations. The only medically significant scorpion species in the United States is *Centruroides elixicada,* which is found in the Southwest. Most stings cause an immediate local reaction that can vary from mild burning to severe pain. Severe envenomation causes autonomic dysfunction and generalized intoxication within a few hours of the sting. Symptoms include agitation, irritability, salivation, blurred vision, and tremulousness with signs of hypertension, tachycardia, tachypnea, and nystagmus. Rarely, in small children or infants, respiratory failure, convulsions, or coma may occur. In these cases, if a history of a sting is not elicited, a diagnosis of encephalitis may be entertained and the correct diagnosis of scorpion envenomation obscured by the fact that children with severe *Centruroides* envenomation may have mild cerebrospinal fluid pleocytosis.

Envenomation by other scorpion species may have specific features. Stings by *Tityus* species in South America are a major cause of pancreatitis, and envenomation by *Buthus* can cause severe hypertension, direct toxic myocarditis, and life-threatening myocardial ischemia.

Treatment. Localized pain can be treated with application of ice and analgesics; pain usually markedly diminishes within 24 hr. For *C. elixicada,* severe envenomation with intoxication or autonomic instability requires hospital admission for sedation and observation. Symptoms usually resolve within 24–48 hr. If cardiopulmonary compromise occurs, consideration should be given to administering antivenin. *Centruroides*-specific antivenin is not FDA approved but is available by contacting the Arizona Poison Control Center at (520)626–6016. It is prepared from goat serum and poses the same small risk of immediate anaphylaxis and later serum sickness as other antivenins produced from horse serum. The use of antivenin, if warranted, leads to complete resolution of symptoms within 1–2 hr. Antivenin for other scorpion species is available in countries where those species are found or through zoologic societies.

HYMENOPTERA STINGS. The insect order of Hymenoptera includes the ants, bees, and wasps, which are characterized by the presence of a stinger at the end of the abdomen through which venom is injected. They are found throughout the United States and worldwide.

Hymenoptera venom, a mixture of proteins and vasoactive substances, is not very potent; most stings cause only local reactions that can be treated with application of cold compresses and analgesics. However, 1–4% of the population is sensitized to hymenoptera venom and is at risk for immediate hypersensitivity reactions. Each year, 50–150 people in the United States die of anaphylaxis due to hymenoptera stings.

Any Hymenoptera envenomation that presents with urticaria, angioedema, wheezing, or hypotension should be treated aggressively for an immediate hypersensitivity reaction with intravenous fluids, oxygen, and epinephrine (see Chapter 148). In the past, any child who sustained a Hymenoptera sting and who had a systemic reaction and a positive result of a skin prick test with Hymenoptera venom was advised to have desensitization with venom-specific immunotherapy. Reports suggest that the clinical course of most children with venom sensitivity is much less severe than previously thought. Fewer than 20% of children with systemic reactions from an initial sting will have systemic reactions with subsequent stings. Measuring IgE or results of skin prick tests with Hymenoptera venom is also not predictive of future systemic reactions.

Children with large local reactions should receive corticosteroids and antihistamines. Children who have systemic reactions including wheezing do not require venom immunotherapy but should carry an emergency kit with epinephrine. Children who have had a life-threatening immediate hypersensitivity reaction should carry an epinephrine kit with them at all times and should undergo immunotherapy. More than 95% of these patients have lifelong protection after 3 yr of immunotherapy.

MARINE ENVENOMATION

Stingrays. Though found only in tropical and subtropical waters, stingrays cause more human envenomations than any other marine vertebrate. The stinging spines on their whiplike tails are retroserrated, and therefore they commonly cause a jagged laceration along with envenomation.

Minor punctures may resemble cellulitis, whereas more severe envenomations may cause marked tissue destruction and necrosis. Regardless of the appearance of the lesion, stingray envenomation is intensely painful for 24–28 hr. Systemic manifestations include nausea and vomiting and more rarely paralysis, hypotension, bradycardia, and seizures.

Treatment begins with thorough cleaning of the wound and tetanus prophylaxis. Because stingray toxins are heat labile, immersion in hot water denatures the protein elements of the venom and decreases pain. Additional analgesia should be provided as needed. Superinfection with aerobic and anaerobic organisms, including *Vibrio* spp, is common, and antibiotic prophylaxis should be considered.

Scorpionfish. Members of the family Scorpaenidae include the zebrafish, scorpionfish, and stonefish; all have venomous spines that become erect on stimulation. Envenomation by the Scorpaenidae causes immediate pain that may last for hours or days. Victims may suffer intense local tissue destruction in which superinfections are common. Systemic manifestations include vomiting, abdominal pain, headache, delirium, seizures, and cardiorespiratory failure. Therapy is similar to that for stingray envenomations. Envenomations with severe systemic symptoms benefit from antivenin administration.

Coelenterate Envenomations. Members of the phylum Cnidaria are common to the oceans of the world. Cnidarian species all share a common anatomic feature: miniscule capsules (cnidae) that contain a highly folded tubule that everts on contact, thereby injecting the venom.

Envenomation causes an immediate stinging sensation that may be associated with paresthesias, pruritus, and local edema. In more severe envenomations, systemic signs may include nausea and vomiting, myalgias, headache, and, more rarely, seizures, coma, and cardiorespiratory collapse. Most lethal envenomations have been attributed to the Pacific box jellyfish, *Chironex fleckeri,* which is indigenous to the waters off Australia, and the Atlantic Portuguese man-of-war, *Physalia physalis.*

Treatment of these envenomations begins in the ocean; the wounds should be rinsed in seawater because fresh water may lyse venom-producing cells (nematocysts), leading to further envenomation. Irrigation of the sting site with vinegar, rubbing alcohol, or baking soda is beneficial because it inhibits nematocyst discharge. Visible tentacle fragments should be removed with forceps, and microscopic fragments may be removed by gently shaving the affected area. Antihistamines and corticosteroids are indicated for swelling and urticaria.

Seabather's Eruption. Seabather's eruption is an intensely pruritic vesicular or maculopapular eruption that primarily affects the skin surfaces covered by swimwear. It is caused by exposure to the larvae of two species of the phylum Cnidaria: the sea anemone, *Edwardsiella lineata,* which is found off the coast of the northeastern United States; and the thimble jellyfish, *Linuche unguiculata,* which is the principal cause of seabather's eruption in Florida and the Caribbean.

Epidemics of seabather's eruption occur during summer months in which there are large quantities of larvae in the water. An intensely pruritic rash begins within 4–24 hr of exposure and may persist for days or weeks. Associated symptoms may include fever, chills, headache, malaise, conjunctivitis, and urethritis. Antihistamines are the mainstay of treatment, although corticosteroids, either applied topically or given systemically, may be beneficial in severe cases.

Antivenins

Weisman RS, Sandbeck S, Thompson V: Snake and spider antivenin. J Fla Med Assoc 83:192, 1996.

Snakebites

Davidson T, Schafer S: Rattlesnake bites: Guidelines for aggressive treatment. Postgrad Med 96:107, 1994.

Gaar G: Assessment and management of coral and other exotic snake envenomations. J Fla Med Assoc 83:178, 1996.

LoPoo JB, Bealer JF, Mantor PC, et al: Treating the snake bitten child in North America: A study of pit viper bites. J Pediatr Surg 33:1593, 1998.

Simon TL, Grace TG: Envenomation coagulopathy in wounds from pit vipers. N Engl J Med 305:443, 1981.

Arachnid and Insect Envenomations

Anderson PC: Spider bites in the United States. Dermatol Clin 15:307, 1997.

Bierman CW: Venom immunotherapy: Who should receive it? J Pediatr 126:257, 1995.

Hauk P, Friedl K, Kaufmehl K, et al: Subsequent insect stings in children with hypersensitivity to Hymenoptera. J Pediatr 126:185, 1995.

Montemarano AD, Gupta RK, Burge JR: Insect repellents and efficacy of sunscreens. Lancet 349:1670, 1997.

Sofer S, Shahak E, Gueron M: Scorpion envenomation and antivenom therapy. J Pediatr 124:973, 1994.

Visscher PK, Vetter RS, Comazine S: Removing bee stings. Lancet 348:301, 1996.

Woestman R, Perkin R, Van Stralen D: The black widow: Is she deadly to children? Pediatr Emerg Care 12:360, 1996.

Marine Envenomations

Auerbach PS: Marine envenomations. N Engl J Med 325:486, 1991.

PART XXXIV

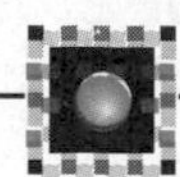

Laboratory Medicine, Drug Therapy, and Reference Tables

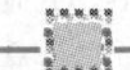

CHAPTER 725
Laboratory Testing in Infants and Children

John F. Nicholson and Michael A. Pesce

For a number of reasons (genetic heterogeneity, biologic and environmental variability, and inhomogeneity of subclinical health status), normal values for many laboratory tests do not show a gaussian bell-shaped curve of distribution. As a result, the population mean and standard deviation (SD) are frequently less useful than the range of normal values, generally given as the 95% normal range—that is, the range of values obtained in testing a normal population minus the lowest 2.5% and the highest 2.5%. As shown in Table 725–1, serum sodium in children, which is tightly controlled physiologically, has a distribution that is essentially gaussian; the mean value ± 2 SD gives a range very close to that actually observed in 95% of children. On the other hand, serum creatine kinase, which is subject to diverse influences and is not actively controlled, does not show a gaussian distribution, as evidenced by the lack of agreement between the range actually observed and that predicted by the mean value ± 2 SD.

A refinement of referencing that is used with increasing frequency is reporting the value obtained together with the percentile of normal values into which the value obtained falls. This method is useful when one is testing for risk factors such as in determination of serum cholesterol.

A further modification that is necessary for many tests performed in infants and children is calculating the age-related adjustment of the normal range. Both age adjustment and the use of percentiles are illustrated in the normal values for serum cholesterol in Table 726–6.

A final modification needed for reporting normal ranges is referencing to the Tanner stage of sexual maturation, which is most useful in assessing pituitary and gonadal function.

ACCURACY AND PRECISION OF LABORATORY TESTS. Technical accuracy is an important consideration in interpreting the results of a laboratory test. Because of improvements in methods of analysis and elimination of analytic interferences, the accuracy of most tests is limited primarily by their precision. Accuracy is a measure of the nearness of the test result to the actual value, whereas precision is a measure of the reproducibility of a result. No test can be more accurate than it is precise. Analysis of precision by repetitive measurements of a single sample gives rise to a gaussian distribution with a mean and SD. The estimate of precision is the coefficient of variation (CV):

$$CV = \frac{SD}{Mean} \times 100$$

The CV is not likely to be constant over the full range of values obtained in clinical testing, but it is about 5% in the normal range. The CV is generally not reported but is always known by the laboratory. It is particularly important in assessing the significance of changes in laboratory results. For example, a common situation is the need to assess hepatotoxicity incurred as a result of administration of a therapeutic drug and reflected in the serum alanine aminotransferase (ALT) value. If serum ALT increases from 25 U/L to 40 U/L, is the change significant? The CV for ALT is 7%. Using the value obtained plus or minus 2 × CV to express the extremes of imprecision, it can be seen that a value of 25 U/L is unlikely to reflect an actual concentration of greater than 29 U/L, and a value of 40 U/L is unlikely to reflect an actual concentration of less than 34 U/L. Therefore, the change in the value as obtained by testing is likely to reflect a real change in circulating ALT levels, and continued monitoring of ALT is indicated even though both values for ALT are within normal limits. "Likely" in this case is only a probability. Inherent biologic variability is such that the results of two successive tests may suggest a trend that will disappear on further testing.

The precision of a test may also be indicated by providing confidence limits for a given result. Ordinarily, 95% confidence limits are used, indicating that it is 95% certain that the value obtained lies between the two limits reported. Confidence limits are calculated using the mean and SD of replicate determinations:

$$95\% \text{ Confidence limits} = \text{Mean} \pm t \times SD$$

where t is a constant derived from the number of replications. In most cases t = 2.

SENSITIVITY, ACCURACY, AND TESTING PURPOSE. There are some circumstances in which sensitivity and accuracy of an analysis are reduced or increased as functions of clinical purpose. For example, ion exchange chromatography of plasma amino acids for the diagnosis of inborn errors of metabolism is usually performed at a sensitivity that allows measurement of all the amino acids with a single set of standards. The range of values is roughly 20–800 μmol/L, and accuracy is poor at values of 20 μmol/L or less. The detection of homocysteine in this type

TABLE 725–1 Gaussian and Nongaussian Laboratory Values in 458 Normal School Children Aged 7–14 Yr

	Serum Sodium (mM/L)	Serum Creatine Kinase (U/L)
Mean	141	68
SD*	1.7	34
Mean ± 2 SD	138–144	0–136
Actual 95% range	137–144	24–162

*SD = standard deviation.

of analysis suggests an inborn error of methionine metabolism. Adjusting the analysis to achieve greater sensitivity, one can accurately measure homocysteine in normal plasma (3–12 μmol/L). This more sensitive test is used in the assessment of cobalamin status and in the analysis of risk factors for atherosclerotic cardiovascular disease.

PREDICTIVE VALUE OF LABORATORY TESTS. Predictive value (PV) theory deals with the usefulness of tests as defined by their sensitivity (ability to detect a disease) and specificity (ability to define absence of a disease).

$$\text{Sensitivity} = \frac{\text{Number positive by test}}{\text{Total number positive}} \times 100$$

$$\text{Specificity} = \frac{\text{Number negative by test}}{\text{Total number without disease}} \times 100$$

$$\text{PV of a positive test} = \frac{\text{True positive results}}{\text{Total positive results}} \times 100$$

$$\text{PV of a negative test result} = \frac{\text{True negative results}}{\text{Total negative results}} \times 100$$

The problems addressed by PV theory are false-negative and false-positive test results. Both are major considerations in interpreting screening tests in general and neonatal screening tests specifically.

Testing for human immunodeficiency virus (HIV) seroreactivity serves to illustrate some of these considerations. If it is assumed that approximately 1,000,000 of 265,000,000 residents of the United States are infected with HIV (prevalence = 0.38%) and that 90% of those infected show appropriate antibodies, we can consider the usefulness of a simple test with 99% sensitivity and 99.5% specificity. If the total population of the United States were screened, it would be possible to identify most of those infected with HIV.

$$1{,}000{,}000 \times 0.9 \times 0.99 = 891{,}000\ (89.1\%)$$

There will be 109,000 false-negative test results. Even with a 99.5% specificity, the number of false-positive test results would be larger than the number of true-positive results.

$$264{,}000{,}000 \times 0.005 = 1{,}320{,}000$$

There will be 262,680,000 true-negative results.

$$\text{PV of positive test result} = \frac{891{,}000}{891{,}000 + 1{,}320{,}000} \times 100 = 40\%$$

$$\text{PV of negative test result} = \frac{262{,}680{,}000}{262{,}680{,}000 + 109{,}000} \times 100 = 99.96\%$$

Given the high cost associated with follow-up of false-positive test results, the anguish produced by a false-positive result, and the lack of curative therapy, it is easy to see why universal screening for HIV seropositivity received a low priority immediately after the introduction of testing for HIV infection.

By contrast, we can consider the screening of 100,000 individuals from groups at increased risk for HIV in whom the overall prevalence of disease is 10%, all other considerations being unchanged.

$$\text{True positive results} = 0.9 \times 0.99 \times 10{,}000 = 8{,}910$$

$$\text{False-positive results} = 0.005 \times 90{,}000 = 450$$

$$\text{False-negative results} = 10{,}000 - 8{,}910 = 1{,}090$$

$$\text{PV of positive test result} = \frac{8{,}910}{8{,}910 + 450} \times 100 = 95\%$$

$$\text{PV of negative test result} = \frac{89{,}500}{89{,}550 + 1{,}090} \times 100 = 99\%$$

These two hypothetical testing strategies illustrate that the diagnostic efficiency of testing heavily depends on the prevalence of the disease being tested for, even if the test is a superior one like the test for HIV antibodies. Because the treatment of pregnant women infected with HIV is effective in preventing vertical transmission of the infection, screening has now been expanded to all pregnant women. Effectiveness of current therapy to prevent neonatal infection has encouraged both patients and physicians to test more frequently, even when the neonatal risk of infection in untreated pregnancies is 30%.

NEONATAL SCREENING TESTS. Almost all the diseases detected in neonatal screening programs have a very low prevalence, and the tests are, for the most part, quantitative rather than qualitative. In general, the strategy is to use the initial screening test to separate a highly suspect group of patients from normal infants (i.e., to increase the prevalence) and then to follow this suspect group aggressively. This strategy is illustrated by a scheme used in screening newborns for congenital hypothyroidism, the prevalence of which is 25/100,000 liveborn infants. The initial test performed is for thyroxine in whole blood, and infants with the lowest 10% of test results are considered suspect. If all infants with hypothyroidism were in the suspect group, the prevalence of disease in this group would be 250/100,000 infants. The original samples obtained from the suspect group are retested for thyroxine and are tested for thyroid-stimulating hormone. This second round of testing results in an even more highly suspect group composed of 0.1% of the infants screened and having a prevalence of hypothyroidism of 25,000/100,000 subjects. This final group is aggressively pursued for further testing and treatment. Even with a 1,000-fold increase in prevalence, 75% of the population aggressively tested is euthyroid. The justifications advanced for the program are that treatment is easy and effective and that the alternative if undetected and untreated—long-term custodial care—is both unsatisfactory and expensive.

Current studies of neonatal screening for cystic fibrosis (CF) are driven by the hope that early treatment will dramatically alter the course of the disease. Initial screening for elevated blood levels of immunoreactive trypsinogen (IRT) serves to identify a population of newborns at high risk (1 in 5) for the disease. The difficulty of obtaining sweat tests in neonates and the severe psychic stress created by suggesting that an infant may have CF both require a refinement of screening tactics. If DNA analysis for some of the many mutations causing CF is performed on specimens with high IRT, the risk of disease in the group subjected to the sweat test can be increased to roughly 1 in 2. Refinement by measuring lactase in meconium (increased in CF) for infants with high IRT increases the sensitivity of the overall procedure by identifying affected individuals whose CF genes are either rare or unknown. This second refinement increases the false-positive rate by 0.5 unaffected neonates per affected neonate.

Because parent-infant bonding can be impaired when unaffected neonates are called back for further tests in screening programs, it is essential that screening programs address the psychologic needs of the families of those screened.

TESTING IN DIFFERENTIAL DIAGNOSIS. The use of laboratory tests in differential diagnosis satisfy PV theory because a correct differential diagnosis should result in a relatively high prevalence of the disease under consideration. An example of testing in differential diagnosis is the measurement of urinary vanillylmandelic acid (VMA) for diagnosis of neuroblastoma. A simple spot test for VMA is not useful in general screening programs because of the low prevalence of neuroblastoma (3/100,000) and the low sensitivity of the test (69%). Even though the specificity of urinary VMA is 99.6%, testing of 100,000 children would produce two true-positive test results, 400 false-positive results, and 1 false-negative result. The PV of a positive result in this setting is 0.5%, and the PV of a negative result is 99.99%, not much different from the assumption that neuroblastoma is not present at all. Testing for urinary VMA in a 3-yr-old child with an abdominal mass, however, gives a useful result because the prevalence of neuroblastoma is at least 50% in 3-yr-old children with abdominal masses. If 100 such children are tested and the prevalence of neuroblastoma in the group is assumed to be 50%, satisfactory PVs are obtained.

PV of positive test result =

$$\frac{0.69 \times 50}{(0.69 \times 50) + (0.004 \times 50)} \times 100 = 99\%$$

PV of negative test result =

$$\frac{0.996 \times 50}{(0.996 \times 50) + (0.31 \times 50)} \times 100 = 76\%$$

Here a test with a low sensitivity is powerful in differential diagnosis because the PV of a positive result is almost 100% in the setting of high prevalence.

PROBLEMS IN LABORATORY TESTING FOR DIFFERENTIAL DIAGNOSIS: SEROLOGIC TESTS FOR LYME DISEASE. Lyme disease, the consequence of tick-borne infection by *Borrelia burgdorferi,* has various manifestations in both early and late stages of infection (see Chapter 219). One manifestation (erythema chronicum migrans) occurs early, although not in all patients, and is pathognomonic. Direct demonstration of the organism is difficult, and serologic test results for Lyme disease are not reliably positive in young patients presenting early with erythema chronicum migrans. These results become positive after some weeks of infection and remain positive for years. In an older population being evaluated for late-stage Lyme disease, some individuals will have recovered from either clinical or subclinical Lyme disease and some will have active Lyme disease, with both groups having true-positive serologic test results. Of those individuals without Lyme disease, some will have true-negative serologic test results but a significant percentage will have antibodies to other organisms that cross-react with *B. burgdorferi* antigens.

This set of circumstances gives rise to a number of problems. First, the protean nature of Lyme disease makes it difficult to ensure a high prevalence of disease in subjects to be tested. Second, the most appropriate antibodies to be detected are imperfectly defined, leading to a wide variety of entry tests with varying rates of false positivity and false negativity. Third, the natural history of the antibody response to infection and the difficulty of demonstrating the causative organism directly combine to make the laboratory diagnosis of early Lyme disease difficult. Fourth, in the diagnosis of late-stage Lyme disease in older subjects, the laboratory diagnosis is plagued by misleading positive (either false-positive or true-positive but not clinically relevant) results of the entry test, typically an enzyme-linked immunosorbent assay, that uses whole *B. burgdorferi* organisms. A review of 788 patients referred to a specialty clinic with the diagnosis of Lyme disease revealed that diagnosis was correct in 180 patients, 156 patients had true seropositivity without active Lyme disease, and 452 had never had Lyme disease, even though 45% of them were seropositive by at least one test before referral.

Use of a more specific (and more costly) Western blot technique that allows definition of the actual bacterial antigens to which antibodies are directed offers good diagnostic value. The most promising test is amplification of bacterial DNA from body fluids (urine, synovial fluid, cerebrospinal fluid) by polymerase chain reaction. The test is specific, offers good sensitivity for active disease, and can demonstrate irradication of infection.

RISK FACTORS AND PREDICTIVE VALUE. When a given laboratory value within the spectrum of the reference range is considered a risk factor, it is generally true that, in the absence of clinical manifestations, the value has no predictive worth as an indicator of disease and has little worth in predicting the likelihood of future disease in any individual case.

American Academy of Pediatrics and American Thyroid Association: Newborn screening for congenital hypothyroidism. Pediatrics 180:745, 1987.

Castellani C, Bonizzato A, Cabrini G, et al: Newborn screening strategy for cystic fibrosis: A field study in area with high allelic heterogeneity. Acta Paediatr 86:497, 1997.

Clayton EW: Issues in state newborn screening programs. Pediatrics 90:641, 1992.

Galen RS, Gambino SR: Beyond Normality. New York, Academic Press, 1975.

Priem S, Rittig MG, Kamradt T, et al: An optimized PCR leads to rapid and highly sensitive detection of Borrelia burgdorferi in patients with Lyme borreliosis. J Clin Microbiol 35:685, 1997.

Steere AC, Taylor E, McHugh GL, et al: The overdiagnosis of Lyme disease. JAMA 269:1812, 1993.

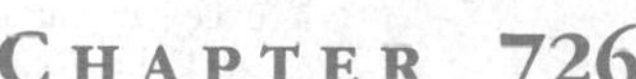

CHAPTER 726
Reference Ranges for Laboratory Tests and Procedures

John F. Nicholson and Michael A. Pesce

In the following tables, reference ranges apply to infants, children, and adolescents when possible. For many analyses, however, separate reference ranges for children and adolescents are not well delineated. When interpreting a test result, the reference range supplied by the laboratory performing the test should always be used. Refer to Figures 726–1 and 726–2 for estimations related to dosages.

In preparing the reference range listings, a number of abbreviations, symbols, and codes were used (Table 726–1).

TABLE 726–1 Prefixes Denoting Decimal Factors

Prefix	Symbol	Factor
Mega	M	10^6
Kilo	k	10^3
Hecto	h	10^2
Deka	da	10^1
Deci	d	10^{-1}
Centi	c	10^{-2}
Milli	m	10^{-3}
Micro	μ	10^{-6}
Nano	n	10^{-9}
Pico	p	10^{-12}
Femto	f	10^{-15}

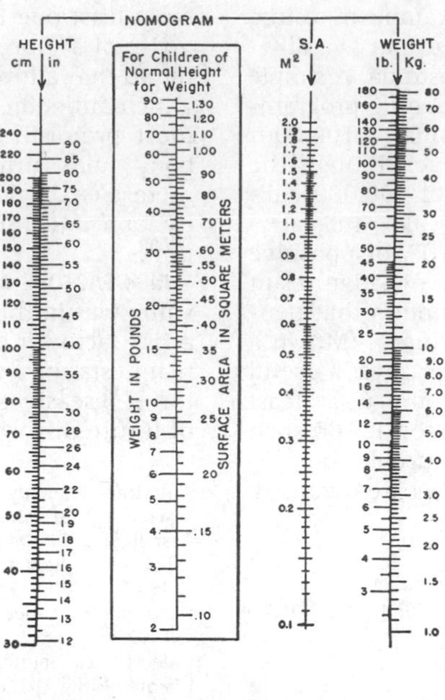

Alternative (Mosteller's formula):

$$\text{Surface area (m}^2\text{)} = \sqrt{\frac{\text{Height (cm)} \times \text{Weight (kg)}}{3600}}$$

Figure 726–1 Nomogram for estimation of surface area. The surface area is indicated where a straight line that connects the height and weight levels intersects the surface area column; or if the patient is roughly of average size, from the weight alone *(enclosed area)*. (Nomogram modified from data of E. Boyd by CD West.) (See also Briars G, Bailey B: Surface area estimation: pocket calculator v nomogram. Arch Dis Child 70:246, 1994.)

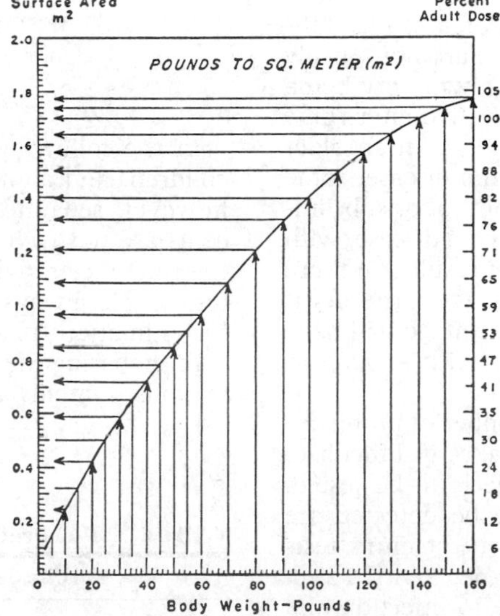

Figure 726–2 Relationship between body weight in pounds, body surface area, and adult dosage. The surface area values correspond with those set forth by Crawford and associates (1950). Note that the 100% adult dose is for a patient weighing about 140 lb and having a surface area of about 1.7 m². (From Talbot NB, et al: Metabolic Homeostasis—A Syllabus for Those Concerned with the Care of Patients. Cambridge, Harvard University Press, 1959.)

TABLE 726–2 Abbreviations

Ab	Absorbance
AU	Arbitrary unit
cap	Capillary
CH_{50}	Dilution required to lyse 50% of indicator red blood cell; indicates complement activity
CKBB	Brain isoenzyme creatine kinase
CKMB	Heart isoenzyme of creatine kinase
Cr	Creatinine
CSF	Cerebrospinal fluid
D	Day, days
F	Female
g	Gram
hr	Hour, hours
Hb	Hemoglobin
HbCO	Carboxyhemoglobin
hpf	High-power field
IU	International Unit of hormone activity
L	Liter
M	Male
mEq/L	Milliequivalents per liter
min	Minute, minutes
mm^3	Cubic millimeter; microliter (μL)
mmHg	Millimeters of mercury
mo	Month, months
mol	Mole
mOsm	Milliosmole
MW	Relative molecular weight
nm	Nanometer (wavelength)
Pa	Pascal
pc	Postprandial
RBC	Red blood cell(s); erythrocyte(s)
RT	Room temperature
s	Second, seconds
SD	Standard deviation
U	International Unit of enzyme activity
V	Volume
WBC	White blood cell(s)
WHO	World Health Organization
wk	Week, weeks
yr	Year, years

TABLE 726–3 Symbols

>	Greater than
≥	Greater than or equal to
<	Less than
≤	Less than or equal to
±	Plus/minus
≅	Approximately equal to

TABLE 726–4 Abbreviations for Specimens

S	Serum
P	Plasma
(H)	Heparin
(LiH)	Lithium heparin
(E)	Ethylenediaminetetraacetic acid (EDTA)
(C)	Citrate
(O)	Oxalate
W	Whole blood
U	Urine
F	Feces
CSF	Cerebrospinal fluid
AF	Amniotic fluid
(NaC)	Sodium citrate
(NH_4H)	Ammonium heparinate

TABLE 726–5 Key to Comments

30°, 37°	Temperature of enzymatic analysis (Celsius)
a	Values obtained are significantly method-dependent
b	Values in older males higher than those in older females
	Colorimetry
c	Values in older females higher than those in older males
d	Atomic absorption
e	Borate affinity chromatography
f	Cation-exchange chromatography
g	Ektachem, proprietary analytic system of Johnson & Johnson Clinical Diagnostics, Inc.
i	Electrophoresis
j	Enzymatic assay
k	Enzyme-amplified immunoassay
l	Fluorometric method
m	Fluorescence-activated cell sorting (FACS)
n	Fluorescence polarization
o	Gas chromatography
p	High-performance liquid chromatography (HPLC)
q	Indirect fluorescent antibody (IFA) assay
r	Ion-selective electrode
s	Nephelometry
t	Optical density
u	Radial immunodiffusion (RID)
v	Radioimmunoassay (RIA)

TABLE 726–6 Reference Ranges

Organization of Reference Values

I. ANALYSES OF BLOOD

A. Formed Elements, Indices, and Coagulation Factors

Analyte or Procedure	Specimen	Reference Values (USA)		Conversion Factor	Reference Values (SI)	Comments
Activated partial thromboplastin time (APTT)	P(C)	25–35 s Infants <90 s		×1	25–35 s Infants <90 s	
Clotting time Lee-White, 37°C	W	Glass tubes 5–8 min (5–15 min at RT) Silicone tubes about 30 min prolonged			Glass tubes 5–8 min (5–15 min at RT) Silicone tubes about 30 min prolonged	
Coagulation factor assays						
Factor I, see *Fibrinogen*						
Factor II	P(C)	0.5–1.5 U/mL or 60–150% of normal		×1	0.5–1.5 kU/L 60–150 AU	
Factor IV, see *Calcium*						
Factor V		0.5–2.0 U/mL or 60–150% of normal		×1	0.5–2.0 kU/L 60–150 AU	
Factor VII		65–135% of normal		×1	65–135 AU	
Factor VIII		60–145% of normal		×1	60–145 AU	
Factor VIII antigen		50–200% of normal		×1	50–200 AU	
Factor IX		60–140% of normal		×1	60–140 AU	
Factor X		60–130% of normal		×1	60–130 AU	
Factor XI		65–135% of normal		×1	65–135 AU	
Factor XII		65–150% of normal		×1	65–150 AU	
Factor XII (fibrin stabilizing factor, FSF)	W(C,O)	Minimal hemostatic level 0.02–0.05 U/mL 1–2% of normal		 ×1,000 ×1	 20–50 U/L or 1–2 AU	
Fibrin degradation products (D-dimer)	P(C)	Adults 68–494 μg/L Mean 207		×1	68–494 μg/L Mean 207	(Pittet et al)
Fibrinogen	(NaC)	Newborn: 125–300 mg/dL Adult: 200–400		×0.01	1.25–3.00 g/L 2.00–4.00	
Erythrocytes: Erythrocyte count (RBC count)	W(E)		millions of cells/mm³(μL)		$\times 10^{12}$ cells/L	
		Cord blood	3.9–5.5		3.9–5.5	
		1–3 d (cap)	4.0–6.6	×1	4.0–6.6	
		1 wk	3.9–6.3		3.9–6.3	
		2 wk	3.6–6.2		3.6–6.2	
		1 mo	3.0–5.4		3.0–5.4	
		2 mo	2.7–4.9		2.7–4.9	
		3–6 mo	3.1–4.5		3.1–4.5	
		0.5–2 yr	3.7–5.3		3.7–5.3	
		2–6 yr	3.9–5.3		3.9–5.3	
		6–12 yr	4.0–5.2		4.0–5.2	
		12–18 yr, M	4.5–5.3		4.5–5.3	
		F	4.1–5.1		4.1–5.1	

Test	Specimen		Conventional units	Factor	SI units	
		18–49 yr, M	4.5–5.9		4.5–5.9	
		F	4.0–5.2		4.0–5.2	
Hematocrit (HCT, Hct) Calculated from MCV and RBC count (electronic displacement or laser)	W(E)		% of packed red cells (V red cells/V whole blood cells ×100)		Volume fraction (V red cells/V whole blood)	
		1 d (cap)	48–69%	×0.01	0.48–0.69	
		2 d	48–75%		0.48–0.75	
		3 d	44–72%		0.44–0.72	
		2 mo	28–42%		0.28–0.42	
		6–12 yr	35–45%		0.35–0.45	
		12–18 yr, M	37–49%		0.37–0.49	
		F	36–46%		0.36–0.46	
		18–49 yr, M	41–53%		0.41–0.53	
		F	36–46%		0.36–0.46	
Hemoglobin (Hb)	W(E)		g/dL		mmol/L	
		1–3 d (cap)	14.5–22.5	×0.155	2.25–3.49	MW Hb = 64,500
		2 mo	9.0–14.0		1.40–2.17	
		6–12 yr	11.5–15.5		1.78–2.40	
		12–18 yr, M	13.0–16.0		2.02–2.48	
		F	12.0–16.0		1.86–2.48	
		18–49 yr, M	13.5–17.5		2.09–2.27	
		F	12.0–16.0		1.86–2.48	
	P(H)	see *Blood, chemical elements*				
Erythrocyte indices (RBC indices): Mean corpuscular hemoglobin (MCH)			pg/cell		fmol/cell	
		Birth	31–37	×0.0155	0.48–0.57	
		1–3 d (cap)	31–37		0.48–0.57	
		1 wk–1 mo	28–40		0.43–0.62	
		2 mo	26–34		0.40–0.53	
		3–6 mo	25–35		0.39–0.54	
		0.5–2 yr	23–31		0.36–0.48	
		2–6 yr	24–30		0.37–0.47	
		6–12 yr	25–33		0.39–0.51	
		12–18 yr	25–35		0.39–0.54	
	W(E)	18–49 yr	26–34		0.40–0.53	
Mean corpuscular hemoglobin concentration (MCHC)	W(E)		% Hb/cell or g Hb/dL RBC		mmol Hb/L RBC	
		Birth	30–36	×0.155	4.65–5.58	
		1–3 d (cap)	29–37		4.50–5.74	
		1–2 wk	28–38		4.34–5.89	
		1–2 mo	29–37		4.50–5.74	
		3 mo–2 yr	30–36		4.65–5.58	
		2–18 yr	31–37		4.81–5.74	
		>18 yr	31–37		4.81–5.74	
Mean corpuscular volume (MCV)	W(E)		μm^3		fL	
		1–3 d (cap)	95–121	×1	95–121	
		0.5–2 yr	70–86		70–86	
		6–12 yr	77–95		77–95	
		12–18 yr, M	78–98		78–98	
		F	78–102		78–102	
		18–49 yr, M	80–100		80–100	
		F	80–100		80–100	
Erythrocyte sedimentation rate (ESR) Westergren, modified			mm/hr	×1	mm/hr	
		Child	0–10		0–10	
		Adult M, <50	0–15		0–15	
	W(E)	F, <50	0–20		0–20	

Table continued on following page

TABLE 726–6 Reference Ranges *Continued*

Analyte or Procedure	Specimen	Reference Values (USA)		Conversion Factor	Reference Values (SI)	Comments
Wintrobe		Child	0–13		0–13	
		Adult M,	0–9		0–9	
		F,	0–20		0–20	
ZETA			41–54%		41–54 AU	
Leukocyte count (WBC)	W(E)	×1,000 cells/mm³ (μL)			×10⁹ cells/L	
		Birth	9.0–30.0	×10⁶	9.0–30.0	
		24 hr	9.4–34.0		9.4–34.0	
		1 mo	5.0–19.5		5.0–19.5	
		1–3 yr	6.0–17.5		6.0–17.5	
		4–7 yr	5.5–15.5		5.5–15.5	
		8–13 yr	4.5–13.5		4.5–13.5	
		Adult	4.5–11.0		4.5–11.0	
Leukocyte differential	W(E)		%		Number Fraction	
Myelocytes			0	×0.01	0	
Neutrophils—"bands"			3–5		0.03–0.05	
Neutrophils—"segs"			54–62		0.54–0.62	
Lymphocytes			25–33		0.25–0.33	
Monocytes			3–7		0.03–0.07	
Eosinophils			1–3		0.01–0.03	
Basophils			0–0.75		0–0.0075	
			Cells/mm³ (μL)		×10⁶ cells/L	
Myelocytes			0	×1	0	
Neutrophils—"bands"			150–400		150–400	
Neutrophils—"segs"			3,000–5,800		3,000–5,800	
Lymphocytes			1,500–3,000		1,500–3,000	
Monocytes			285–500		285–500	
Eosinophils			50–250		50–250	
Basophils			15–50		15–50	

Lymphocyte Subsets W(E)	Age: 2–3 mo	4–8 mo	12–23 mo	24–59 mo	in (Denny et al)
Median lymphocytes, total	5.68 × 10⁹/L	5.99 × 10⁹/L	5.16 × 10⁹/L	4.06 × 10⁹/L	
5th–95th centiles	2.92–8.84	3.61–8.84	2.18–8.27	2.40–5.81	
Median CD3 lymphocytes	4.03 × 10⁹/L	4.27 × 10⁹/L	3.33 × 10⁹/L	3.04 × 10⁹/L	
5th–9th centiles	2.07–6.54	2.28–6.45	1.46–5.44	1.61–4.23	
Median CD4 lymphocytes	2.83 × 10⁹/L	2.95 × 10⁹/L	2.07 × 10⁹/L	1.80 × 10⁹/L	
5th–95th centiles	1.46–5.11	1.69–4.60	1.02–3.60	0.90–2.86	
Median CD8 lymphocytes	1.41 × 10⁹/L	1.45 × 10⁹/L	1.32 × 10⁹/L	1.18 × 10⁹/L	
5th–95th centiles	0.65–2.45	0.72–2.49	0.57–2.23	0.63–1.91	
Median % lymphocytes	66	64	59	50	
5th–95th centiles	55–78	45–79	44–72	38–64	
Median % CD3 lymphocytes	72	71	66	72	
5th–95th centiles	60–87	57–84	53–81	62–80	
Median % CD4 lymphocytes	52	49	43	42	
5th–95th centiles	41–64	36–61	31–54	35–51	
Median % CD8 lymphocytes	25	24	25	30	
5th–95th centiles	16–35	16–34	16–38	22–38	

Analyte or Procedure	Specimen	%NaCl (g/dL)	% Hemolysis	Conversion Factor	NaCl (g/L)	Hemolyzed fraction
Osmotic fragility test (RBC Fragility) pH 7.4, 20°C	W(H)	0.30	97–100	×0.01 (hemolyzed fraction)	3.0	0.97–1.00
		0.35	90–99		3.5	0.90–0.99
		0.40	50–95		4.0	0.50–0.95
		0.45	5–45		4.5	0.05–0.45
		0.50	0–6		5.0	0.00–0.06
		0.55	0		5.5	0.00

Analyte or Procedure	Specimen	Reference Values (USA)		Conversion Factor	Reference Values (SI)		Comments
Osmotic fragility test (sterile incubation) at 37°C		%NaCl (g/dL)	% Hemolysis		NaCl (g/L)	Hemolyzed fraction	
		0.20	95–100	×0.01 (hemolyzed fraction)	2.0	0.95–1.00	
		0.30	85–100		3.0	0.85–1.00	
		0.35	75–100		3.5	0.75–1.00	
		0.40	65–100		4.0	0.65–1.00	
		0.45	55–95		4.5	0.55–0.95	
		0.50	40–85		5.0	0.40–0.85	
		0.55	15–70		5.5	0.15–0.70	
		0.60	0–40		6.0	0.00–0.40	
		0.65	0–10		6.5	0.00–0.10	
		0.70	0–5		7.0	0.00–0.05	
		0.85	0		8.5	0.00	
Partial thromboplastin time (PTT)	W(NaC)						
Nonactivated		60–85 s (platelin)			60–85 s		
Activated, see *Activated partial thromboplastin time*							
Platelet count (Thrombocyte count)	W(E)	$\times 10^3$/mm³ (μL)			$\times 10^9$/L		Buck
		Newborn 84–478 (after 1 wk, same as adult)		$\times 10^6$	84–478		
		Adult 150–400			150–400		
Prothrombin time (PT)							
One-stage (Quick)	W(NaC)	In general, 11–15 s (varies with type of thromboplastin)		× 1	11–15 s		
		Newborn prolonged by 2–3 s			Newborn prolonged by 2–3 s		
		International Normalized Ratio (INR) used only for patients receiving Coumarin			International Normalized Ratio (INR) used only for patients receiving Coumarin		
		Clinical Problem	Target INR		Clinical Problem	Target INR	
		Deep venous thrombosis	2.0–3.0		Deep venous thrombosis	2.0–3.0	
		Prosthetic heart valve	2.5–3.0		Prosthetic heart valve	2.5–3.0	
Two-stage modified (Ware and Seegers)	W(NaC)	18–22 s			18–22 s		
RBC count, see *Erythrocyte count*							
RBC fragility, see *Osmotic fragility*							
Red cell volume	W(H)	M 20–36 mL/kg F 19–31		×0.001	M 0.020–0.036 L/kg F 0.019–0.031		
Reticulocyte count	W(E,H,O)	Adults 0.5–1.5% of erythrocytes or 25,000–75,000/mm³ (μL)		×0.01 $\times 10^6$	0.005–0.015 (number fraction) or 25,000–75,000 $\times 10^6$/L		
			%		Number fraction		
	W(capillary)	1 day	0.4–6.0	×0.01	0.004–0.060		
		7 day	<0.1–1.3		<0.001–0.013		
		1–4 wk	<1.0–1.2		<0.001–0.012		
		5–6 wk	<0.1–2.4		<0.001–0.024		
		7–8 wk	0.1–2.9		0.001–0.029		
		9–10 wk	<0.1–2.6		<0.001–0.026		
		11–12 wk	0.1–1.3		0.001–0.013		
Sedimentation rate, see *Erythrocyte sedimentation rate*							
Sickle cell tests							
Sodium metabisulfite	W(E,H,O)	Negative					
Dithionite test	W(E,H,O)	Negative					

Table continued on following page

TABLE 726–6 Reference Ranges *Continued*

Analyte or Procedure	Specimen	Reference Values (USA)	Conversion Factor	Reference Values (SI)	Comments
Sucrose hemolysis and sugar-water tests for paroxysmal noctural hemoglobinuria (PNH)	W(C,O)	≤5% lysis 6–10% lysis questionable	×0.01	Lysed fraction ≤0.05 Lysed fraction 0.06–0.10 questionable	
Thrombin time	W(NaC)	Control time ± 2 s when control is 9–13 s		Control time ± 2 s when control is 9–13 s	
Thromboplastin time, activated, see *Activated partial thromboplastin time (APTT)*					
Tourniquet test		<5–10 petechiae in 2.5 cm circle on forearm (halfway between systolic and diastolic pressure for 5 min); 0–8 petechiae in 6 cm circle (50 mm Hg for 15 min); 10–20 petechiae in 5 cm circle (80 mm Hg)		<5–10 petechiae in 2.5 cm circle on forearm (halfway between systolic and diastolic pressure for 5 min); 0–8 petechiae in 6 cm circle (50 mm Hg for 15 min); 10–20 petechiae in 5 cm circle (80 mm Hg)	
WBC, see *Leukocyte*					
B. Chemical Elements					
Acetone					
Semiquantitative	S,P(O)	Negative (<3 mg/dL)		Negative (<0.5 mmol/L)	
Quantitative		0.3–2.0 mg/dL	×0.1722	0.05–0.34 mmol/L	
Adrenocorticotropic hormone (ACTH)	P(H)	pg/mL		ng/L	
		Cord: 130–160	×1	130–160	
		1–7 day postnatal 100–140		100–140	
		Adults			
		0800 hr 25–100		25–100	
		1800 hr <50		<50	
Alanine aminotransferase (ALT, SGPT)	S	0–5 day 6–50 U/L 1–19 yr 5–45	×1	6–50 U/L 5–45	37° bh (Lockitch, et al, 1988a)
Albumin	P	Premature 1 day 1.8–3.0 g/dL Full term <6 day 2.5–3.4 <5 yr 3.9–5.0 5–19 yr 4.0–5.3	×10	18–30 g/L 25–34 39–50 40–53	g (Meites)
Aldolase	S	10–24 mo 3.4–11.8 U/L 25 mo–16 yr 1.2–8.8	×1	3.4–11.8 U/L 1.2–8.8	j (Visnapu et al)
Aldosterone	S,P(E,E)	Supine			(Endocrine Sciences) *Ad lib* sodium intake
		Premature Infants			
		26–28 wk 5–635 ng/dL	×0.0277	0.14–17.6 nmol/L	
		31–35 wk 19–141		0.53–3.9	
		Full-Term Infants			
		3 day 7–184 ng/dL		0.19–5.1 nmol/L	
		1 wk 5–175		0.14–4.8	
		1–12 mo 5–90		0.14–2.5	
		Children Supine			
		1–2 yr 7–54 ng/dL		0.19–1.5 nmol/L	
		2–10 yr 3–35		0.1–0.97	
		10–15 yr 2–22		0.1–0.6	

Test	Specimen	Reference Range (Conventional)			Conversion Factor	Reference Range (International)		Source
		Adults		Supine				
				3–16 ng/dL		0.1–0.4 nmol/L		
		Children		Upright				
		2–10 years		5–80 ng/dL		0.14–2.2 nmol/L		
		10–15 years		4–48		0.11–1.3		
		Adults		Upright				
				7–30 ng/dL		0.19–0.83 nmol/L		
Alkaline phosphatase, serum, see *Phosphatase, alkaline*								
Amino acids, plasma	P(H)	0–30 day	>1 mo–16 yr	>16 yr				f (Nichols Institute Reference Laboratories)
Phosphoserine		0–30	0–12	3–7 μmol/L				
Taurine		74–216	22–192	27–168				
Aspartic acid		0–17	5–59	0–24				
Hydroxyproline		20–70	0–40	0–40				
Threonine		114–335	73–160	79–193				
Serine		94–243	90–226	73–167				
Asparagine		20–58	28–246	14–104				
Glutamic acid		0–50	0–210	0–88				
Glutamine		538–958	52–669	415–964				
Proline		107–177	67–238	102–336				
Glycine		224–514	89–360	120–554				
Alanine		236–410	142–484	210–661				
Citrulline		8–28	1–55	12–55				
2-Aminobutyric acid		6–29	0–42	3–38				
	P(H)	0–30 day	>1 mo–16 yr	>16 yr				
Valine		80–246	110–271	141–317 μmol/L				
Cysteine		70–167	0–106	16–167				
Methionine		9–41	0–90	6–40				
Isoleucine		27–53	34–85	36–98				
Leucine		46–109	55–165	75–175				
Tyrosine		42–99	29–86	21–87				
Phenylalanine		42–110	22–98	37–88				
Homocystine		0–0	0–0	0–0				
Tryptophan		17–71	24–79	20–95				
Omithine		49–151	15–143	30–106				
Lysine		114–269	68–266	83–238				
1-Methylhistidine		0–27	0–27	0–27				
Histidine		49–114	52–124	31–107				
3-Methylhistidine		0–10	0–6	0–4				
Arginine		22–88	5–187	36–145				
Aminolevulinic acid (ALA)	S	15–23 μg/dL (lower in child)			×0.076	1.1–1.8 μmol/L		
Ammonia	W	<30 day		21–95 μmol/L	×1	<30 day	21–95 μmol/L	(Diaz et al)
		1–12 mo		18–74		1–12 mo	18–74	
		1–14 yr		17–68		1–14 yr	17–68	
		>14 yr		19–71		>14 yr	19–71	
Amylase	S,P	1–19 yr		30–100 U/L	×1	30–100 U/L		(Lockitch et al, 1988a)
				% Pancreatic		Pancreatic Fraction		(Gillard et al)
Isoenzymes	S,P(H)	Cord—8 mo		0–34%	×0.01	0–0.34		
		9 mo–4 yr		5–56%		0.05–0.56		
		5–19 yr		23–59%		0.23–0.59		

Table continued on next page

TABLE 726–6 Reference Ranges *Continued*

Analyte or Procedure	Specimen	Reference Values (USA)	Conversion Factor	Reference Values (SI)	Comments
Androstenedione	S	Tanner / Age / Male			(Endocrine Sciences)
		1 / <9.8 yr / 8–50 ng/dL	×0.3479	0.28–1.74 nmol/L	
		2 / 9.8–14.5 / 31–65		1.08–2.26	
		3 / 10.7–15.4 / 50–100		1.74–3.48	
		4 / 11.8–16.2 / 48–140		1.67–4.87	
		5 / 12.8–17.3 / 65–210		2.26–7.30	
		Adult / 75–205		2.61–7.13	
	S	Tanner / Age / Female			
		1 / <9.2 yr / 8–50 ng/dL	×0.3479	0.28–1.74 nmol/L	
		2 / 9.2–13.7 / 42–100		1.46–3.48	
		3 / 10.0–14.4 / 80–190		2.78–6.61	
		4 / 10.7–15.6 / 77–225		2.68–7.83	
		5 / 11.8–18.6 / 80–240		2.78–8.35	
		Adult / Follicular / 85–275		2.96–9.57	
		Luteal / 85–275		2.96–9.57	
Anion gap (Sodium − (chloride + bicarbonate))	P(H)	7–16 mEq/L	×1	7–16 mEq/L	
Anti-deoxyribonuclease B titer (anti-DNase B titer)	S	Age / Upper limit of normal	×1	Age / Upper limit of normal	(Kaplan et al)
		4–6 yr / 240–480 U		4–6 yr / 240–480 U	
		7–12 yr / 480–800 U		7–12 yr / 480–800 U	
Antidiuretic hormone (hADH, vasopressin)	P(E)	Plasma Osmolarity mOsm/kg / Plasma ADH pg/mL		Plasma ADH ng/L	
		270–280 / <1.5	×1	<1.5	
		280–285 / <2.5		<2.5	
		285–290 / 1–5		1–5	
		290–295 / 2–7		2–7	
		295–300 / 4–12		4–12	
Anti-streptolysin-O titer (ASO titer)	S	Age / Upper limit of normal		Age / Upper limit of normal	(Kaplan et al)
		2–5 yr / 120–160 Todd units		2–5 yr / 120–160 Todd units	
		6–9 yr / 240 Todd units		6–9 yr / 240 Todd units	
		10–12 yr / 320 Todd units		10–12 yr / 320 Todd units	
α-1-Antitrypsin	S	0–5 day / 143–440 mg/dL	×0.01	1.43–4.40 g/L	(Lockitch et al, 1988b)
		1–9 yr / 147–245		1.47–2.45	
		9–19 yr / 152–317		1.52–3.17	
Apolipoproteins					(Baroni et al)
A-1	S	2–12 mo / 133 ± 27 mg/dL	×0.01	1.33 ± 0.27 g/L	
		2–10 yr / 143 ± 18		1.43 ± 0.18	
B	S	2–12 mo / 73 ± 16 mg/dL	×0.01	0.73 ± 0.16 g/L	
		2–10 yr / 78 ± 17		0.78 ± 0.17	
CII	S	2–12 mo / 47.0 ± 16 mg/L	×1	47.0 ± 16 mg/L	
		2–10 yr / 41.0 ± 16		41.0 ± 16	
CIII	S	2–12 mo / 76.0 ± 29 mg/L	×1	76.0 ± 29 mg/L	
		2–10 yr / 69.0 ± 22		69.0 ± 22	
E	S	2–12 mo / 41.0 ± 9 mg/L	×1	41.0 ± 9 mg/L	
		2–10 yr / 39.0 ± 10		39.0 ± 10	
Lipoprotein(a)	S	2–12 mo / 42.0 ± 36 mg/L	×1	42.0 ± 36 mg/L	
		2–10 yr / 64.0 ± 57		64.0 ± 57	
Ascorbic acid, see *Vitamin C*					

Test	Specimen	Group	Conventional	Conventional	Factor	SI	SI	Notes
Aspartate aminotransferase (AST, SGOT)	S	0–5 day	35–140 U/L		×1	35–140 U/L		37° b
		1–9 yr	15–55			15–55		(Lockitch et al, 1988b)
		10–19 yr	5–45			5–45		
Base excess	W(H)		mmol/L		×1	mmol/L		
		Newborn	(−10)–(−2)			(−10)–(−2)		
		Infant	(−7)–(−1)			(−7)–(−1)		
		Child	(−4)–(+2)			(−4)–(+2)		
		Thereafter	(−3)–(+3)			(−3)–(+3)		
Bicarbonate	S,P	Arterial	21–28 mmol/L		×1	21–28 mmol/L		
		Venous	22–29			22–29		
Bile acids, total	S, fasting	0.3–2.3 µg/mL			×1	0.3–2.3 mg/L		
	S, 2 hr pc	1.8–3.2 µg/mL				1.8–3.2 mg/L		
	F	120–225 mg/24 hr			×1	120–225 mg/L		
Bilirubin	S,P		Premature mg/dL	Full-term mg/dL		Premature µmol/L	Full-term µmol/L	
Total	S	Cord blood	<2.0	<2.0	×17.10	<34	<34	
		0–1 day	<8.0	<6.0		<137	<103	
		1–2 day	<12.0	<8.0		<205	<137	
		2–5 day	<16.0	<12.0		<274	<205	
		>5 day	<20.0	<10		<340	<171	
Bilirubin conjugated	S	0–0.2 mg/dL			×17.10	0–3.4 µmol/L		
Bleeding time (BBT)								
Ivy		Normal 2–7 min			×1	2–7 min		
		Borderline 7–11 min				7–11 min		
Simplate (G-D)		2.75–8 min				2.75–8 min		
Blood volume	W(H)	M 52–83 mL/kg			×0.001	M 0.052–0.083 L/kg		
		F 50–75 mL/kg				F 0.050–0.075 L/kg		
Brucellosis, agglutinins	S	≤1:8			×1	≤1:8		
C-peptide of insulin	S	Children 8:00 AM fasting	0.4–2.2 ng/mL		×1	0.4–2.2 µg/L		(Endocrine Sciences)
C-reactive protein	S	Cord blood	52–1,330 ng/mL		×1	52–1,330 µg/L		k (Unten and Hokama)
		2–12 yr	67–1,800			67–1,800		
Calcitonin	S,P(H,E)	Male	Female		×0.28	Male	Female	(Nichols Institute Reference Laboratories)
		3–26 pg/mL	2–17 pg/mL			0.8–7.2 pmol/L	0.6–4.7 pmol/L	
		Higher in newborn infants						
Calcium, ionized (Ca)	S,P(H),W(H)		mg/dL			mmol/L		
		Cord blood	5.0–6.0		×0.25	1.25–1.50		
		Newborn, 3–24 hr	4.3–5.1			1.07–1.27		
		24–48 hr	4.0–4.7			1.00–1.17		
		Thereafter	4.8–4.92			1.12–1.23		
		or	2.24–2.46 mEq/L		×0.5	1.12–1.23		
Calcium, total	S		mg/dL			mmol/L		
		Cord blood	9.0–11.5		×0.25	2.25–2.88		
		Newborn, 3–24 hr	9.0–10.6			2.3–2.65		
		24–48	7.0–12.0			1.75–3.0		
		4–7 d	9.0–10.9			2.25–2.73		
		Child	8.8–10.8			2.2–2.70		
		Thereafter	8.4–10.2			2.1–2.55		

Table continued on following page

TABLE 726–6 Reference Ranges *Continued*

Analyte or Procedure	Specimen	Reference Values (USA)	Conversion Factor	Reference Values (SI)	Comments
Carbon dioxide, partial pressure (P_{CO_2})	W(H)	mmHg		kPa	
		Newborn 27–40	×0.1333	3.6–5.3	
		Infant 27–41		3.6–5.5	
		Thereafter, M 35–48		4.7–6.4	
		F 32–45		4.3–6.0	
Carbon dioxide, total (t_{CO_2})	S,P(H)	mmol/L		mmol/L	
		Cord 14–22	× 1	14–22	
		Premature 14–27		14–27	
		Newborn 13–22		13–22	
		Infant 20–28		20–28	
		Child 20–28		20–28	
		Thereafter 23–30		23–30	
Carbon monoxide (carboxyhemoglobin)	W(E)	Nonsmokers <2% HbCO	×0.01	HbCO fraction <0.02	
		Smokers <10%		<0.10	
		Lethal >50%		>0.5	
Carnitine	P	Age / Total (μmol/L) / Free (μmol/L)		Age / Total (μmol/L) / Free (μmol/L)	(Schmidt-Sommerfeld, et al)
		1 day 36.4 ± 10.8 20.1 ± 6.7	×1	1 day 36.4 ± 10.8 20.1 ± 6.7	
		2–7 day 25.2 ± 4.1 14.9 ± 3.0		2–7 day 25.2 ± 4.1 14.9 ± 3.0	
		8–28 day 36.7 ± 10.5 27.6 ± 9.7		8–28 day 36.7 ± 10.5 27.6 ± 9.7	
		29 day–1 yr 47.6 ± 7.7 35.5 ± 6.5		29 day–1 yr 47.6 ± 7.7 35.5 ± 6.5	
		1–6 yr 54.4 ± 9.9 41.7 ± 7.9		1–6 yr 54.4 ± 9.9 41.7 ± 7.9	
		6–10 yr 56.2 ± 11.4 41.4 ± 10.0		6–10 yr 56.2 ± 11.4 41.4 ± 10.0	
		10–17 yr 53.4 ± 9.5 39.4 ± 8.7		10–17 yr 53.4 ± 9.5 39.4 ± 8.7	
		22–60 yr 54.0 ± 12.6 39.1 ± 8.6		22–60 yr 54.0 ± 12.6 39.1 ± 8.6	
β-Carotene	S	μg/dL		μmol/L	
		Infant 20–70	×0.0186	0.37–1.30	
		Child 40–130		0.74–2.42	
		Thereafter 60–200		1.12–3.72	
Catecholamines, fractionated	P(E)	Norepinephrine pg/mL			
		Supine 100–400	×5.911	591–2,364 pmol/L	
		Standing 300–900		1,773–5,320	
		Epinephrine pg/mL			
		Supine <70	×5.458	<382 pmol/L	
		Standing <100		<546	
		Dopamine (no postural change) <30 pg/mL	×6.528	<196 pmol/L (no postural change)	
Ceruloplasmin	S	0–5 day 5–26 mg/dL	×10	50–260 mg/L	cs (Lockitch et al, 1988b)
		1–19 yr 20–46 mg/dL		200–460 mg/L	
Chloride	S,P(H)	Cord blood 96–104 mmol/L	×1	96–104 mmol/L	
		Newborn 97–110		97–110	
		Thereafter 98–106		98–106	

Test	Specimen	Reference Range (Conventional)		Factor	Reference Range (SI)	
Cholesterol, total	S	1–3 yr	45–182 mg/dl	×0.0259	1.15–4.70 mmol/L	j (Lockitch et al, 1988a)
		4–6 yr	109–189		2.80–4.80	
	S	Male Percentiles Age 5 75 95 6–9 yr 126 172 191 mg/dL 10–14 yr 130 179 204 15–19 yr 114 167 198 Female Percentiles Age 5 75 95 6–9 yr 122 173 209 mg/dL 10–14 yr 124 174 217 15–19 yr 125 175 212		×0.0259	Male Percentiles Age 5 75 95 6–9 yr 3.26 4.45 4.94 mmol/L 10–14 yr 3.36 4.63 5.28 15–19 yr 2.95 4.32 5.12 Female Percentiles 5 75 95 6–9 yr 3.16 4.47 5.41 mmol/L 10–14 yr 3.21 4.50 5.61 15–19 yr 3.23 4.53 5.48	(Mayo Laboratories)
Chorionic gonadotropin	S,P(E)	Child and male undetectable				(Abbott)
β-Subunit (β-hCG)		F, post-conception	mIU/mL	×1	IU/l	
		1–2 wk	9–130		9–130	
		2–3 wk	75–2,600		75–2,600	
		3–4 wk	850–20,800		850–20,800	
		4–5 wk	4,000–100,200		4,000–100,200	
		5–10 wk	11,500–289,000		11,500–289,000	
		10–14 wk	18,300–137,000		18,300–137,000	
Complement components						
Total hemolytic complement activity (CH_{50})	P(E)	75–160 U/mL		×1	75–160 IU/L	
Total complement decay rate (functional)	P(E)	~10–20% Deficiency >50%		×0.01	~0.10–0.20 (fraction of decay rate) 0.50 (fraction of decay rate)	
Classic pathway components						
C1q	S		mg/dL		mg/L	
		Cord blood	1.0–14.9	×10	10–149	
		1 mo	2.2–6.2		22–62	
		6 mo	1.2–7.6		12–76	
		Adult	5.1–7.9		51–79	
C1r	S	2.5–3.8 mg/dL		×10	25–38	
C1s (C1 esterase)	S	2.5–3.8 mg/dL		×10	25–38	
C2	S		mg/dL		mg/L	
		Cord blood	1.6–2.8	×10	16–28	
		1 mo	1.9–3.9		19–39	
		6 mo	2.4–3.6		24–36	
		Adult	1.6–4.0		16–40	
C3	S		mg/dL	×10	mg/L	s (Meites)
		Cord blood	57–116		570–1,160	
		1–3 mo	53–131		530–1,310	
		3 mo–1 yr	62–180		620–1,800	
		1 yr–10 yr	77–195f		770–1,950	
		Adult	83–177		830–1,770	
C4	S		mg/dL	×10	mg/L	s (Meites)
		Cord blood	7–23		70–230	
		1–3 mo	7–27		70–270	
		3 mo–10 yr	7–40		70–400	
		Adult	15–45		150–450	

Table continued on following page

TABLE 726–6 Reference Ranges *Continued*

Analyte or Procedure	Specimen	Reference Values (USA)		Conversion Factor	Reference Values (SI)	Comments
C5	S		mg/dL		mg/L	
		Cord blood	3.4–6.2	×10	34–62	
		1 mo	2.3–6.3		23–63	
		6 mo	2.4–6.4		24–64	
		Adult	3.8–9.0		38–90	
C6	S		mg/dL		mg/L	
		Cord blood	1.0–4.2	×10	10–42	
		1 mo	2.2–5.2		22–52	
		6 mo	3.7–7.1		37–71	
		Adult	4.0–7.2		40–72	
C7	S	4.9–7.0 mg/dL		×10	49–70 mg/L	
C8	S	4.3–6.3 mg/dL		×10	43–63 mg/L	
C9	S	4.7–6.9 mg/dL		×10	47–69 mg/L	
Alternative pathway components						
C4 binding protein	S	18.0–32.0 mg/dL		×10	180–320 mg/L	
Factor B(C3 proactivator)						
RID	P(E)		mg/dL		mg/L	
		Cord blood	7.8–15.8	×10	78–158	
		1 mo	6.2–28.6		62–286	
		6 mo	16.9–29.3		169–293	
		Adult	14.7–33.5		147–335	
Nephelometry	S	Newborn	14–33 mg/dL	×10	140–330 mg/L	
		Adult	20–45		200–450	
Properdin	S		mg/dL		mg/L	
		Cord blood	1.3–1.7	×10	13–17	
		1 mo	0.6–2.2		6–22	
		6 mo	1.3–2.5		13–25	
		Adult	2.0–3.6		20–36	
Regulatory protein b1H-globulin (C3b inactivator accelerator)	S		mg/dL		mg/L	
		Cord blood	26–42	×10	260–420	
		1 mo	24–56		240–560	
		6 mo	33–61		330–610	
		Adult	40–72		400–720	
C1 inhibitor (esterase inhibitor)	P(E)	17.4–24.0 mg/dL		×10	174–240 mg/L	u
Complement decay rate (functional)	S	<20% decay		×0.01	<0.20 (fractional decay)	
		Deficiency >50% decay			>0.50 (fractional decay)	
C3b inactivator (KAF)	S		mg/dL		mg/L	
		Cord blood	1.8–2.6	×10	18–26	
		1 mo	1.5–3.9		15–39	
		6 mo	2.3–4.3		23–43	
		Adult	2.6–5.4		26–54	
S protein	S	41.8–60.0 mg/dL		×10	418–600 mg/L	

Test	Specimen	Group	Conventional units	Factor	SI units	Notes
Copper	S	0–5 d	9–46 μg/dL	×0.157	1.4–7.2 μmol/L	cd (Lockitch, et al., 1988c)
		1–9 yr	80–150		12.6–23.6	
		10–14 yr	80–121		12.6–19.0	
		15–19 yr	64–160		11.3–25.2	
Corticobinding globulin (CBG), see *Transcortin*						
Cortisol	S,P(H)		μg/dL		nmol/L	
		Newborn	1–24	×27.59	28–662	
		Adults, 0800 hr	5–23		138–635	
		1600 hr	3–15		82–413	
		2000 hr	≤50% of 0800 h	×0.01	Fraction of 0800 hr ≤0.50	
Creatine kinase	S	Cord blood	70–380 U/L	×1	70–380 U/L	30° b (Jedeikin et al)
		5–8 hr	214–1,175		214–1,175	
		24–33 hr	130–1,200		130–1,200	
		72–100 hr	87–725		87–725	
		Adult	5–130		5–130	
Creatine kinase isoenzymes	S		% MB / %BB			
		Cord blood	0.3–3.1 / 0.3–10.5			
		5–8 hr	1.7–7.9 / 3.6–13.4			
		24–33 hr	1.8–5.0 / 2.3–8.6			
		72–100 hr	1.4–5.4 / 5.1–13.3			
		Adult	0–2% / 0			
Creatinine						
Jaffe, kinetic, or enzymatic	S,P		mg/dL		μmol/L	
		Cord blood	0.6–1.2	×88.4	53–106	
		Newborn	0.3–1.0		27–88	
		Infant	0.2–0.4		18–35	
		Child	0.3–0.7		27–62	
		Adolescent	0.5–1.0		44–88	
		Adult M	0.6–1.2		53–106	
		F	0.5–1.1		44–97	
Jaffe, manual	S,P		0.8–1.5 mg/dL	×88.4	70–133 μmol/L	
Creatinine clearance (endogenous)	S,P, and U	Newborn	40–65 mL/min/1.73 m²			
		<40 yr, M	97–137			
		F	88–128			
			Decreases ~6.5 mL/min/decade			
Cyclic AMP	P(E)	Male	ng/mL 5.6–10.9	×3.04	Male nmol/L 17–33	
		Female	3.6–8.9		Female 11–27	
Dehydroepiandrosterone	S	Tanner / Age	Male			(Endocrine Sciences)
		1 / <9.8 yr	31–345 ng/dL	×0.0347	1.07–11.96 nmol/l	
		2 / 9.8–14.5	110–495		3.81–17.16	
		3 / 10.7–15.4	170–585		5.89–20.28	
		4 / 11.8–16.2	160–640		5.55–22.19	
		5 / 12.8–17.3	250–900		8.67–31.21	
		Adult	160–800		5.55–27.74	
			Female			
		1 / <9.2 yr	31–345 ng/dL		1.07–11.96 nmol/L	
		2 / 9.2–13.7	150–570		5.20–19.76	
		3 / 10.0–14.4	200–600		6.93–20.80	
		4 / 10.7–15.6	200–780		6.93–24.27	
		5 / 11.8–18.6	215–850		7.45–29.47	
		Adult Follicular	160–800		5.55–27.74	
		Luteal	160–800		5.55–27.74	

Table continued on following page

TABLE 726–6 Reference Ranges *Continued*

Analyte or Procedure	Specimen	Reference Values (USA)			Conversion Factor	Reference Values (SI)	Comments
Dehydroepiandrosterone sulfate (DHEA-Sulfate) (DHEA-S)		Tanner	Age	Male			(Endocrine Sciences)
		1	<9.8 y	13–83 µg/dL	×0.026	0.34–2.16 µmol/L	
		2	9.8–14.5	42–109		1.09–2.83	
		3	10.7–15.4	48–200		1.25–5.2	
		4	11.8–16.2	102–385		2.65–10.01	
		5	12.8–17.3	120–370		3.12–9.62	
			Adult	180–450		4.68–11.70	
		Tanner	Age	Female			
		1	<9.2 yr	19–114 µg/dL		0.49–2.96 µmol/L	
		2	9.2–13.7	34–129		0.88–3.35	
		3	10.0–14.4	32–326		0.83–8.48	
		4	10.7–15.6	58–260		1.51–6.76	
		5	11.8–18.6	44–248		1.14–6.45	
			Adult	60–255		1.56–6.63	
Deoxycorticosterone	S	Cord blood		111–372 ng/dL	×0.03026	3.4–11.3 nmol/L	(Endocrine Sciences)
		Newborn		Very High		Very High	
		1–12 months		7–49 ng/dL		0.2–1.5 nmol/L	
		Prepubertal (2–10 yr)		2–34 ng/dL		0.1–1 nmol/L	
		Pubertal and Adult		2–19 ng/dL		0.1–0.6 nmol/L	
11-Desoxycortisol Specific compound S	S	Cord Blood		295–554 ng/dL	×0.02886	8.51–16.00	(Endocrine Sciences)
		Full-term 3 d		13–147		0.38–4.24	
		Full-term 1–12 mo		<10–156		<0.29–4.50	
		Prepub. Child. (8:00 AM)		20–155		0.58–4.47	
		Pubertal and Adult (8:00 AM)		12–158		0.35–4.56	
Dihydrotestosterone (DHT)	S	Tanner	Age	Male			(Endocrine Sciences)
		1	<9.8	<3 ng/dL	×0.03443	<0.10 nmol/L	
		2	9.8–14.5	3–17		0.10–0.59	
		3	10.7–15.4	8–33		0.28–1.14	
		4	11.8–16.2	22–52		0.76–1.79	
		5	12.8–17.3	24–65		0.83–2.24	
			Adult	30–85		1.03–2.93	
	S	Tanner	Age	Female	×0.03443		
		1	<9.2 yr	<3 ng/dL		<0.10 nmol/L	
		2	9.2–13.7	5–12		0.17–0.41	
		3	10.0–14.4	7–19		0.24–0.65	
		4	10.7–15.6	4–13		0.14–0.45	
		5	11.8–18.6	3–18		0.10–0.62	
		Adult	Follicular	4–22		0.14–0.76	
			Luteal	4–22		0.14–0.76	
Disaccharide absorption test	S	Change in glucose from fasting value				Change in glucose from fasting value	
		Normal		>30 mg/dL	×0.055	Normal >1.67 mmol/L	
		Inconclusive		20–30		Inconclusive 1.11–1.67	
		Abnormal		<20		Abnormal <1.11	
Electrophoresis, hemoglobin, see *Hemoglobin electrophoresis*							

Test	Specimen	Conventional units	Factor	SI units	Comments
Epinephrine, see *Catecholamines, fractionated*					
Erythropoietin					
RIA	S	<5–20 mU/mL	×1	<5–20 U/L	
Hemagglutination		25–125		25–125	
Bioassay		5–18		5–18	
Estradiol	S	Tanner / Age / Male	×36.71		(Endocrine Sciences)
		1 <9.8 yr 0.5–1.1 ng/dL		18–40 pmol/L	
		2 9.8–14.5 0.5–1.6		18–59	
		3 10.7–15.4 0.5–2.5		18–92	
		4 11.8–16.2 1.0–3.6		37–132	
		5 12.8–17.3 1.0–3.6		37–132	
		Adult 0.8–3.5		29–128	
		Female			
		1 <9.2 yr 0.5–2.0 ng/dL		18–73 pmol/l	
		2 9.2–13.7 1.0–2.4		37–88	
		3 10.0–14.4 0.7–6.0		26–220	
		4 10.7–15.6 2.1–8.5		77–312	
		5 11.8–13.6 3.4–17		125–624	
		Adult Follicular 3–10		110–367	
		Luteal 7–30		257–1,100	
Estriol (E_3), free	S	Weeks of Gestation / μg/L		nmol/L	
		25 3.5–10.0	×3.47	12.1–34.7	
		28 4.0–12.5		13.9–43.4	
		30 4.5–14.0		15.6–48.6	
		32 5.0–16.0		17.4–55.5	
		34 5.5–18.5		19.1–64.2	
		36 7.0–25.0		24.3–86.8	
		37 8.0–28.0		27.8–97.2	
		38 9.0–32.0		31.2–111.0	
		39 10.0–34.0		34.7–118.0	
		40–41 10.5–25.0		36.4–86.8	
Estriol (E_3), total	S	Pregnancy (wk) / ng/mL		nmol/L	
		24–28 30–170	×3.467	104–590	
		28–32 40–220		140–760	
		32–36 60–280		208–970	
		36–40 80–350		280–1210	
		Adult. M and nonpregnant F <2		<7	
Estrogens, total	S	pg/mL		ng/L	
		Child <30	×1	<30	
		M 40–115		40–115	
		F, cycle—days			
		1–10 d 61–394		61–394	
		11–20 d 122–437		122–437	
		21–30 d 156–350		156–350	
		Prepubertal ≤40		≤40	

Table continued on following page

TABLE 726–6 Reference Ranges *Continued*

Analyte or Procedure	Specimen	Reference Values (USA)	Conversion Factor	Reference Values (SI)	Comments
Free fatty acids	S	Premature	×1	0.15–0.71 mmol/L	(Meites)
		10–55 d 0.15–0.71 mmol/L			
	W	1–12 mo 0.5–1.6 mmol/L	×1	0.5–1.6 mmol/L	(Bonnefont et al)
		1–7 y 0.6–1.5		0.6–1.5	
		7–15 y 0.2–1.1		0.2–1.1	
Ferritin	S	ng/mL		μg/L	
		Newborn 25–200	×1	25–200	
		1 mo 200–600		200–600	
		2–5 mo 50–200		50–200	
		6 mo–15 yr 7–140		7–140	
		Adult, M 15–200		15–200	
		F 12–150		12–150	
α-Fetoprotein (AFP)	S	Pregnancy Wk / Median ng/mL		Median μg/L	em
		15 34	×1	34	
		16 38		38	
		17 44		44	
		18 49		49	
		19 56.5		56.5	
		20 66		66	
Folate	S	Newborn 7.0–32 ng/mL	×2.265	15.9–72.4 nmol/L	
		Thereafter 1.8–9		4.1–20.4	
	W(E)	150–450 ng/mL RBCs		340–1020 nmol/L cells	
Follicle stimulating hormone (FSH)	S	Tanner / Age / Male			(Endocrine Sciences)
		1 <9.8 yr 0.26–3.0 mIU/mL	×1	0.26–3.0 U/L	
		2 9.8–14.5 1.8–3.2		1.8–3.2	
		3 10.7–15.4 1.2–5.8		1.2–5.8	
		4 11.8–16.2 2.0–9.2		2.0–9.2	
		5 12.8–17.3 2.6–11.0		2.6–11.0	
		Adult 2.0–9.2		2.0–9.2	
		Tanner / Age / Female			
		1 <9.2 yr 1.0–4.2 mIU/mL		1.0–4.2 U/L	
		2 9.2–13.7 1.0–10.8		1.0–10.8	
		3 10.0–14.4 1.5–12.8		1.5–12.8	
		4 10.7–15.6 1.5–11.7		1.5–11.7	
		5 11.8–18.6 1.0–9.2		1.0–9.2	
		Adult Follicular 1.8–11.2		1.8–11.2 mIU/mL	
		Midcycle 6–35		6–35	
		Luteal 1.8–11.2		1.8–11.2	
		Postmenopause 30–120		30–120	
Fructosamine	S	0–3 yr 1.56–2.27 mmol/L	×1	1.56–2.27 mmol/L	q (De Schepper et al)
		3–6 yr 1.73–2.34		1.73–2.34	
		6–9 yr 1.82–2.56		1.82–2.56	
		9–15 yr 2.02–2.63		2.02–2.63	

Test	Specimen	Reference range (conventional)		Factor	Reference range (SI)		Notes
Galactose	S	Newborn	0–20 mg/dL	×0.0555	0–1.11 mmol/L		
	P	5 mo–17 yr	0.0–0.5 mg/dL		0.0–0.03 mmol/L		j (Pesce and Boudorian, 1982a)
Galactose-1-PO_4	W(H)	5 mo–17 yr	0–44 µg/g Hb	×0.0038	0–0.17 µmoL/g Hb		l (Pesce and Boudorian, 1982b)
Galactose-1-PO_4 uridylyltransferase	W(H)	18–26 U/g Hb		×1	18–26 U/g Hb		(Pesce and Boudorian, 1977c)
Gastrin	S	Newborn	20–300 pg/mL	×1	20–300 ng/L		a (Endocrine Sciences)
		Children	<10–125		<10–125		
Glucagon	P(E)	Children and adults (fasting)	50–150 pg/mL	×1	50–150 ng/L		(Endocrine Sciences)
Glucose	S		mg/dL		mmol/L		
		Cord blood	45–96	×0.0555	2.5–5.3		
		Premature	20–60		1.1–3.3		
		Neonate	30–60		1.7–3.3		
		Newborn					
		1 day	40–60		2.2–3.3		
		>1 day	50–90		2.8–5.0		
		Child	60–100		3.3–5.5		
		Adult	70–105		3.9–5.8		
	W(H)	Adult	65–95		3.6–5.3		
Glucose, 2 hr post	S	<120 mg/dL		×0.0555	<6.7 mmol/L		
Glucose tolerance test (GTT) Oral dose, adult: 75 g Child: 1.75 g/kg of ideal weight up to maximum of 75 g	S	mg/dL: Normal	Diabetic	×0.0555	mmol/L: Normal	Diabetic	(American Diabetes Association)
		Fasting 70–105	≥126		3.9–5.8	≥7.0	
		60 min 120–170	≥200		6.7–9.4	≥11	
		90 min 100–140	≥200		5.6–7.8	≥11	
		120 min 70–120	≥200		3.9–6.7	≥11	
Glucose-6-phosphate dehydrogenase (G6PD) in erythrocytes Bishop, modified	W(E,H,C)	Adult			Adult		
		3.4–8.0 U/g Hb		×0.0645	0.22–0.52 mU/mol Hb		
		98.6–232 U/10^{12} RBC		$\times 10^{-3}$	0.10–0.23 nU/10^6 RBC		
		1.16–2.72 U/mL RBC		×1	1.16–2.72 kU/L RBC		
		Newborn: 50% higher			Newborn 50% higher		
Gammaglutamyltranspeptidase (GGT, GGTP)	S	Cord blood	37–193 U/L	×1	37–193 U/L		37°b (Knight and Haymond)
		0–1 mo	13–147		13–147		
		1–2 mo	12–123		12–123		
		2–4 mo	8–90		8–90		
		4 mo–10 yr	5–32		5–32		
		10–15 yr	5–24		5–24		

Table continued on following page

TABLE 726–6 Reference Ranges *Continued*

Analyte or Procedure	Specimen	Reference Values (USA)	Conversion Factor	Reference Values (SI)	Comments
Growth hormone (hGH) somatotropin	S,P(E,H)	Newborn 1 day 5–53 ng/mL 1 wk 5–27 1–12 mo 2–10	×1	5–53 μg/L 5–27 2–10	(Endocrine Sciences)
	Fasting, at rest	Child <0.7–6 ng/mL Adults <0.7–6		<0.7–6 μg/L <0.7–6	
Ham's test, see *Acidified serum test*					
Haptoglobin	S	0–1 mo <5.8–196 mg/dL 1 mo–19 yr 22–164	×0.01	<0.058–1.960 g/L 0.220–1.640	(Davis et al)
Hemoglobin total	W P(H)	see *Blood, formed elements . . .* <10 mg/dL <3 mg/dL with butterfly setup and 18-gauge needle	×0.155	<1.55 μmol/L <0.47 μmol/L with butterfly setup and 18-gauge needle	
HDL Cholesterol	S	1–13 yr 35–84 mg/dL 14–19 yr 35–65	×0.0259	0.9–2.15 mmol/L 0.90–1.65	ac (Meites)
Glycohemoglobin hemoglobin A_{1c}	W(H)	% of total Hb 1–5 yr 2.1–7.7 5–16 yr 3.0–6.2	×0.01	Fraction of total Hb 0.021–0.077 0.030–0.062	f (Meites)
Total glycohemoglobin	W(E)	4–16 yr 6.0–10.0%		0.060–0.100	e (Meites)
Hemoglobin A	W(E,C,H)	>95%	×0.01	Fraction of Hb: >0.95	
Hemoglobin A_2 (HbA_2)	W(E,O)	Adult: 1.5–3.5% (2 SD) Lower in infants <1 yr		Mass fraction 0.015–0.035 (2SD)	
Hemoglobin (Hb) electrophoresis	W(H,E,C)	HbA >95% HbA2 1.5–3.5% HbF <2%	×0.01	Mass fraction HbA >0.95 HbA2 0.015–0.035 HbF <0.02	
Hemoglobin F	W(E)				
Alkali denaturation		%HbF 1 day 63–92 5 day 65–88 3 wk 55–85 6–9 wk 31–75 3–4 mo <2–59 6 mo <2–9 Adult <2	×0.01	Mass fraction 0.62–0.92 0.65–0.88 0.55–0.85 0.31–0.75 <0.02–0.59 <0.02–0.09 <0.02	
Hemoglobin H (HbH) Isopropanol precipitation	W(H,E,C)	No precipitation at 40 min		No precipitation at 40 min	
Homocysteine	P	2 mo–18 yr 3.3–11.3 μmol/L	×1	3.3–11.3 μmol/L	(Vilaseca et al)

Test	Specimen	Reference range (conventional)	Factor	Reference range (SI)	Source
17-Hydroxyprogesterone (17-OHP)	S	Premature infants			(Endocrine Sciences)
		26–28 wks, day 4: 124–841 ng/dL	×0.03029	3.76–25.5 nmol/L	
		31–35 wks, day 4: 26–568		0.79–17.2	
		Full-term infants			
		3 day 7–77 ng/dL		0.2–2.33 nmol/L	
		1–12 mo			
		Male			
		Peak values of 40–200 ng/dL between 30 and 60 days.		Peak values of 1.21 to 6.1 nmol/L between 30 and 60 days	
		Female 13–106 ng/dL		0.39–3.21 nmol/L	
		Prepubertal children			
		3–90 ng/dL		0.09–2.73 nmol/L	
		Tanner / Age / Male			
		1 / <9.8 yr / 3–90 ng/dL		0.09–2.73 nmol/L	
		2 / 9.8–14.5 / 5–115		0.15–3.48	
		3 / 10.7–15.4 / 10–138		0.30–4.18	
		4 / 11.8–16.2 / 29–180		0.88–5.45	
		5 / 12.8–17.3 / 24–175		0.73–5.30	
		Adult / 27–199		0.82–6.03	
		Tanner / Age / Female			
		1 / <9.2 yr / 3–82 ng/dL		0.09–2.48 nmol/L	
		2 / 9.2–13.7 / 11–98		0.33–2.97	
		3 / 10.0–14.4 / 11–155		0.33–4.69	
		4 / 10.7–15.6 / 18–230		0.55–6.97	
		5 / 11.8–18.6 / 20–265		0.61–8.03	
		Adult / Follicular / 15–70		0.45–2.12	
		Luteal / 35–290		1.06–8.78	
β-Hydroxybutyrate		1–12 mo 0.1–1.0 mmol/L	×1	0.1–1.0 mmol/L	(Bonnefont et al)
		1–7 yr <0.1–0.9		<0.1–0.9	
		7–15 yr <0.1–0.3		<0.1–0.3	
Hypoxanthine	W	age			(Jung et al)
		12–36 hr 2.7–11.2 μmol/L	×1	2.7–11.2 μmol/L	
		3 day 1.3–7.9		1.3–7.9	
		5 day 0.6–5.7		0.6–5.7	
Immunoglobulin A (IgA)	S	Cord blood 1.4–3.6 mg/dL	×10	14–36 mg/L	s (Meites)
		1–3 mo 1.3–53		13–530	
		4–6 mo 4.4–84		44–840	
		7 mo–1 yr 11–106		110–1060	
		2–5 yr 14–159		140–1590	
		6–10 yr 33–236		330–2360	
		Adult 70–312		700–3120	
Immunoglobulin D (IgD)	S	Newborn: none detected		None detected	
		Thereafter: 0–8 mg/dL	×10	0–80 mg/L	
Immunoglobulin E (IgE)	S	M 0–230 IU/mL	×1	0–230 kIU/L	
		F 0–170		0–170	

Table continued on following page

TABLE 726–6 Reference Ranges *Continued*

Analyte or Procedure	Specimen	Reference Values (USA)		Conversion Factor	Reference Values (SI)	Comments
Immunoglobulin G (IgG)	S	Cord blood	636–1606 mg/dL	×0.01	6.36–16.06 g/L	s (Meites)
		1 mo	251–906		2.51–9.06	
		2–4 mo	176–601		1.76–6.01	
		5–12 mo	172–1069		1.72–10.69	
		1–5 yr	345–1236		3.45–12.36	
		6–10 yr	608–1572		6.08–15.72	
		Adult	639–1349		6.39–13.49	
IgG Subclasses	S	(mg/dL)		×10	(mg/L)	(Mayo Medical Laboratories)

Age	IgG1 (mg/dL)	IgG2 (mg/dL)	IgG3 (mg/dL)	IgG4 (mg/dL)	IgG1 (mg/L)	IgG2 (mg/L)	IgG3 (mg/L)	IgG4 (mg/L)
Cord	435–1084	143–453	27–146	1–47	4350–10840	1430–4530	70–1460	10–470
1–7 day	381–937	117–382	21–115	1–44	3810–9370	1170–3820	10–1150	10–440
8–14 day	327–790	92–310	16–85	1–40	3270–7900	920–3100	160–850	10–400
3–4 wk	218–496	40–167	4–23	1–33	2180–4960	400–1670	40–230	10–330
2 mo	194–480	35–164	4–36	1–30	1940–4800	350–1640	40–360	10–300
3 mo	167–447	28–157	4–52	1–24	1670–4470	280–1570	40–520	10–240
4 mo	143–394	23–147	4–65	1–14	1430–3940	230–1470	40–650	10–140
5 mo	158–392	24–132	6–68	1–13	1580–3920	240–1320	60–680	10–130
6 mo	175–390	24–115	8–72	1–11	1750–3900	240–1150	80–720	10–110
7 mo	190–388	25–100	10–75	1–10	1900–3880	250–1000	100–750	10–100
8 mo	200–417	26–123	10–76	1–16	2000–4170	260–1230	100–760	10–160
9 mo	211–450	26–149	10–77	1–22	2110–4500	260–1490	100–770	10–220
10–12 mo	241–543	28–221	10–80	1–39	2410–5430	280–2210	100–800	10–390
13–20 mo	281–692	30–343	10–88	1–68	2810–6920	300–3430	100–880	10–680
21 mo–36 mo	310–729	46–387	10–96	1–77	3100–7290	460–3870	100–960	10–770
3 yr	348–773	72–441	10–105	1–87	3480–7730	720–4410	100–1050	10–870
4 yr	370–804	88–455	11–108	1–97	3700–8040	880–4550	110–1080	10–970
5 yr	375–835	94–468	12–111	1–106	3750–8350	940–4680	120–1110	10–1060
6 yr	380–866	100–481	14–115	1–115	3800–8660	1000–4810	140–1150	10–1150
7 yr	385–896	105–494	16–118	1–124	3850–8960	1050–4940	160–1180	10–1240
8 yr	390–927	111–507	18–122	1–133	3900–9270	1110–5070	180–1220	10–1330
9 yr	395–958	117–520	19–125	1–142	3950–9580	1170–5200	190–1250	10–1420
10 yr	400–989	123–534	21–129	1–151	4000–9890	1230–5340	210–1290	10–1510
11 yr	405–1,020	128–547	23–132	1–160	4050–10200	1280–5470	230–1320	10–1600
12 yr	410–1,051	134–560	25–136	1–169	4100–10510	1340–5600	250–1360	10–1690
13 yr	415–1,081	140–573	27–139	1–178	4150–10810	1400–5730	270–1390	10–1780
14 yr	419–1,102	145–582	28–141	1–184	4190–11020	1450–5820	280–1410	10–1840
≥15 yr	423–1,112	149–586	29–142	1–187	4230–11120	1490–5860	290–1420	10–1870

Analyte or Procedure	Specimen	Reference Values (USA)		Conversion Factor	Reference Values (SI)	Comments
Immunoglobulin M (IgM)	S	Cord blood	6.3–25 mg/dL	×10	63–250 mg/L	s (Meites)
		1–4 mo	17–105		170–1050	
		5–9 mo	33–126		330–1260	
		10–1 y	41–173		410–1730	
		2–8 yr	43–207		430–2070	
		9–10 yr	52–242		520–2420	
		Adult	56–352		560–3520	
Insulin (12 hr fasting)	S,	Newborn	3–20 uU/mL	×1.0	3–20 mU/L	
		Thereafter	7–24		7–24	
Insulin with oral glucose tolerance test	S	Min	uU/mL		mU/L	
		0	7–24	×1	7–24	
		30	25–231		25–231	

Test	Specimen	Group	Conventional units	Factor	SI units	Reference
		60	18–276		16–166	
		120	16–166		4–38	
		180	4–38		18–276	
Insulin-like growth factor I IGFI/Somatomedin C	S	Age	Male			
		1–2 yr	31–160 ng/mL	×0.1307	4.05–21.96 nmol/L	(Endocrine Sciences)
		3–4	45–230		5.88–30.07	
		5–6	51–288		6.67–37.65	
		7–8	158–385		20.66–50.33	
		9–10	136–308		17.78–40.27	
		11–12	180–440		23.53–57.52	
		13–14	220–616		28.76–80.53	
		15–16	200–836		26.15–109.30	
		17–18	286–627		37.39–81.97	
		19–20	339–418		44.32–54.65	
		21–25	202–433		26.4–56.61	
	S	Puberty—Male				
		Tanner stage	Mean ± SD		Mean ± SD	
		1	215 ± 71 ng/mL		28.11 ± 9.28 nmol/L	
		2	320 ± 137		41.84 ± 17.91	
		3	475 ± 176		62.10 ± 23.01	
		4	500 ± 135		65.37 ± 17.65	
		5	490 ± 120		64.06 ± 15.69	
		Age	Female			
		1–2 yr	11–206 ng/mL		1.43–26.93 nmol/L	
		3–4	75–320		9.81–41.84	
		5–6	70–288		9.15–37.65	
		7–8	125–396		16.34–51.77	
		9–10	123–330		16.08–43.14	
		11–12	191–462		24.97–60.40	
		13–14	286–660		37.39–87.33	
		15–16	242–660		31.64–87.33	
		17–18	240–506		31.38–66.15	
		19–20	242–550		31.64–71.90	
		21–25	231–453		30.19–59.21	
		Puberty—Female				
		Tanner stage	Mean ± SD		Mean ± SD	
		1	255 ± 83 ng/mL		33.34 ± 10.85 nmol/L	
		2	410 ± 84		53.60 ± 10.98	
		3	492 ± 180		64.32 ± 23.53	
		4	505 ± 155		66.02 ± 20.26	
		Adult				
		(26–85 yr)	135–449 ng/mL			
		Prepubertal	334–642 ng/mL	×0.1333	44.53–85.60 nmol/L	(Endocrine Sciences)
		Pubertal	245–737		32.67–98.27	
		Adults	288–736		38.40–98.13	
Interleukin 6	P	Adults	<12.5 pg/mL	×1	<12.5 ng/L	(Krafte-Jacobs et al)
		Children	7 ± 1		7 ± 1	
Iron	S	All ages	22–184 μg/dL	×0.1791	4–33 μmol/L	(Lockitch et al, 1988c)
Iron-binding capacity, total (TIBC)	S	Infant	100–400 μg/dL	×0.179	17.90–71.60 μmol/L	
		Thereafter	250–400		44.75–71.60	

Table continued on following page

TABLE 726–6 Reference Ranges *Continued*

Analyte or Procedure	Specimen	Reference Values (USA)	Conversion Factor	Reference Values (SI)	Comments
Ketone bodies, qualitative	S	Negative	×1	Negative	(Bonnefont et al)
Ketone bodies, quantitative	W	1–12 mo 0.1–1.5 mmol/L 1–7 yr 0.15–2.0 7–15 yr <0.1–0.5		0.1–1.5 mmol/L 0.15–2.0 < 0.1–0.5	Sum of acetone, β-hydroxybutyrate and acetoacetate
LDL-Cholesterol (LDLC)	S,P(E)	mg/dL: M / F		mmol/l: M / F	
		Cord blood 10–50 / 10–50	×0.0259	0.26–1.30 / 0.26–1.30	
		1–9 yr 60–140 / 60–150		1.55–3.63 / 1.55–3.89	
		10–19 yr 50–170 / 50–170		1.30–4.40 / 1.30–4.40	
		20–29 yr 60–175 / 60–160		1.55–4.53 / 1.55–4.14	
		30–39 yr 80–190 / 70–170		2.07–4.92 / 1.81–4.40	
		40–49 yr 90–205 / 80–190		2.33–5.31 / 2.07–4.92	
		Recommended (desirable) range for adults <130 mg/dL		1.68–4.53	
L+-Lactate	W	1–12 mo 1.1–2.3 mmol/L 1–7 yr 0.8–1.5 7–15 yr 0.6–0.9	×1	1.1–2.3 mmol/L 0.8–1.5 0.6–0.9	(Bonnefont et al)
D-Lactate	P(H)	6 mo–3 yr 0.0–0.3 mmol/L	×1	0.0–0.3 mmol/L	j (Rosenthal and Pesce)
Lactate dehydrogenase	S	<1 yr 170–580 U/L 1–9 yr 150–500 10–19 yr 120–330	×1	170–580 U/L 150–500 120–330	37° a (Meites)
Isoenzymes	S	% of Total Activity: 1–6 yr / 7–19 yr LD1 20–38 / 20–35 LD2 27–38 / 31–38 LD3 16–26 / 19–28 LD4 5–16 / 7–13 LD5 3–13 / 5–12			
Lead	W(H)	μg/dL Child <10 Adult <40 Toxic ≥100	×0.0483	μmol/L <0.48 <1.93 ≥4.83	
Lipase	P,S	1–18 yr 3–32 U/L	×1	3–32 U/L	(Soldin et al, 1995)
Lipoprotein electrophoresis	S	Distinct β band; negligible chylomicron and pre–β-bands			
Long-acting thyroid stimulating hormone (LATS)	S	Undetectable		Undetectable	
Luteinizing hormone (LH)	S	Tanner / Age / Male			(Endocrine Sciences)
		1 / <9.8 yr / 0.02–0.3 mIU/mL	×1	0.02–0.3 U/L	
		2 / 9.8–14.5 / 0.2–4.9		0.2–4.9	
		3 / 10.7–15.4 / 0.2–5.0		0.2–5.0	Referred to WHO 2nd International Standard
		4–5 / 11.8–17.3 / 0.4–7.0		0.4–7.0	
		Adult / / 1.5–9		1.5–9	

Test	Specimen	Reference Range (Conventional)	Conversion Factor	Reference Range (SI)	Comments
		Tanner / Age / Female 1 / <9.2 yr / 0.02–0.18 mIU/mL 2 / 9.2–13.7 / 0.02–4.7 3 / 10.0–14.4 / 0.10–12.0 4–5 / 10.7–15.6 / 0.4–11.7 Adult / Follicular / 29 Midcycle / 18–49 Luteal / 2–11		0.02–0.18 U/L 0.02–4.7 0.10–12.0 0.4–11.7 2–9 18–49 2–11	
Magnesium	P(H)	0–6 day 1.2–2.6 mg/dL 7 d–2 yr 1.6–2.6 2–14 yr 1.5–2.3	×0.411	0.48–1.05 mmol/L 0.65–1.05 0.60–0.95	h (Meites)
Methemoglobin (MetHb)	W(E,H,C)	0.06–0.24 g/dL or 0.78 ± 0.37% of total Hb	×155 ×0.01	9.3–37.2 μmol/L 0.0078 ± 0.0037 (mass fraction)	
Methylmalonic acid	S	4–14 y 0.03–0.26 μmol/L	×1	0.03–0.26 μmol/L	(Straczek et al)
Microsomal antibodies, thyroid, see *Thyroid microsomal antibodies*					
Myoglobin	S	6–85 ng/mL	×1	6–85 μg/L	
Osmolality	S	Child, adult 275–295 mOsmol/kg H_2O			
Oxygen, partial pressure (Po_2)	W(H),arterial	mmHg Birth 8–24 5–10 min 33–75 30 min 31–85 >1 hr 55–80 1 day 54–95 Thereafter 83–108 (decreases with age)	×0.133	kPa 1.1–3.2 4.4–10.0 4.1–11.3 7.3–10.6 7.2–12.6 11–14.4	
Oxygen saturation	W(H),arterial	% Saturation Newborn 85–90% Thereafter 95–99%	×0.01	Fraction saturated 0.85–0.90 0.95–0.99	
Po_2, see *Oxygen, partial pressure*					
Po_2 at half saturation ($Po_2(0.5)$ or P_{50})	W(H),arterial	25–29 mm Hg	×0.133	3.3–3.9 kPa	
Parathyroid hormone (PTH) Intact (IRMA)	S	Cord blood ≤3.0 pg/mL 2 yr—Adult 9–65	×0.1053	≤0.32 pmol/L 0.95–6.8	(Nichols Institute Reference Laboratories)
pH	W(H),arterial	pH Premature (48 hr) 7.35–7.50 Birth, full term 7.11–7.36 5–10 min 7.09–7.30 30 min 7.21–7.38 >1 hr 7.26–7.49 1 d 7.29–7.45 Thereafter 7.35–7.45 Must be corrected for body temperature		H^+ concentration 31–44 nmol/L 43–77 50–81 41–61 32–54 35–51 35–44	
Phenylalanine	S	Premature 2.0–7.5 mg/dL Newborn 1.2–3.4 Thereafter 0.8–1.8	×60.54	120–450 μmol/L 70–210 50–110	

Table continued on following page

TABLE 726–6 Reference Ranges *Continued*

Analyte or Procedure	Specimen	Reference Values (USA)	Conversion Factor	Reference Values (SI)	Comments
Phosphatase, acid prostatic (RIA)	S	<3.0 ng/mL	×1	<3.0 µg/l	
Roy Brower, and Hayden 37°C		0.11–0.60 U/L	×1	0.11–0.60 U/L	
Phosphatase, alkaline	S	1–9 yr 145–420 U/L 10–11 yr 130–560 Male / Female 12–13 y 200–495 105–420 14–15 y 130–525 70–230 16–19 y 65–260 50–130	×1	1–9 yr 145–420 U/L 10–11 yr 130–560 Male / Female 12–13 y 200–495 105–420 14–15 y 130–525 70–230 16–19 y 65–260 50–130	37°C ah (Lockitch et al, 1988a)
Phospolipids, total	S,P(E)	mg/dL Newborn 75–170 Infant 100–275 Child 180–295 Adult 125–275	×0.01	g/L 0.75–1.70 1.00–2.75 1.80–2.95 1.25–2.75	
Phosphorus, inorganic	S,P(H)	0–5 d 4.8–8.2 mg/dL 1–3 yr 3.8–6.5 4–11 yr 3.7–5.6 12–15 yr 2.9–5.4 16–19 yr 2.7–4.7	×0.3229	1.55–2.65 mmol/L 1.25–2.10 1.20–1.80 0.95–1.75 0.90–1.50	h (Meites)
Plasma volume	P(H)	M 25–43 mL/kg F 28–45	×0.001	M 0.025–0.043 L/kg F 0.028–0.045	
Potassium	S	<2 mo 3.0–7.0 mmol/L 2–12 mo 3.5–6.0 >12 mo 3.5–5.0	×1	3.0–7.0 mmol/L 3.5–6.0 3.5–5.0	r (Meites) Increased by hemolysis; serum values systematically higher than plasma values
	P(H)	3.5–4.5 mmol/L		3.5–4.5 mmol/L	
Prealbumin (transthyretin)	P	2–6 mo 142–330 mg/L 6–12 mo 120–274 1–3 y 108–259	×1	142–330 mg/L 120–274 108–259	s (Sherry et al.)
Progesterone	S	Tanner / Age / Male 1 <9.8 yr <10–33 ng/dL 2 9.8–14.5 <10–33 3 10.7–15.4 <10–48 4 11.8–16.2 10–108 5 12.8–17.3 21–82 Adult 13–97	×0.03180	<0.32–1.05 nmol/L <0.32–1.05 <0.32–1.53 0.32–3.43 0.67–2.61 0.41–3.08	(Endocrine Sciences)
		Tanner / Age / Female 1 <9.2 yr <10–33 ng/dL 2 9.2–13.7 10–55 3 10.0–14.4 10–450 4 10.7–15.6 10–1300 5 11.8–18.6 10–950 Adult Follicular 15–70 Luteal 200–2500		<0.32–1.05 nmol/L <0.32–1.75 0.32–14.31 0.32–41.34 0.32–30.21 0.48–2.23 6.36–79.50	

Test	Specimen	Reference range (conventional)		Factor	Reference range (SI)		Source
Prolactin	S	Male	Female		Male	Female	(Endocrine Sciences)
		3–18	3–24 ng/mL	×0.0426	0.13–0.77	0.13–1.02 nmol/L	
		Higher in newborn infants			Higher in newborn infants		
Protein, total	S		g/dL		g/L		(Meites)
		Premature	4.3–7.6	×10	43–76		
		Newborn	4.6–7.4		46–74		
		1–7 yr	6.1–7.9	×10	61–79		
		8–12 yr	6.4–8.1		64–81		
		13–19 yr	6.6–8.2		66–82		
Protein electrophoresis	S		g/dL		g/L		
		Albumin					
		Premature	3.0–4.2	×10	30–42		
		Newborn	3.6–5.4		36–54		
		Infant	4.0–5.0		40–50		
		Thereafter	3.5–5.0		35–50		
		α1-Globulin					
		Premature	0.1–0.5		1–5		
		Newborn	0.1–0.3		1–3		
		Infant	0.2–0.4		2–4		
		Thereafter	0.2–0.3		2–3		
		α2-Globulin					
		Premature	0.3–0.7		3–7		
		Newborn	0.3–0.5		3–5		
		Infant	0.5–0.8		5–8		
		Thereafter	0.4–1.0		4–10		
		β-Globulin					
		Premature	0.3–1.2		3–12		
		Newborn	0.2–0.6		2–6		
		Infant	0.5–0.8		5–8		
		Thereafter	0.5–1.1		5–11		
		γ-Globulin					
		Premature	0.3–1.4		3–4		
		Newborn	0.2–1.0		2–10		
		Infant	0.3–1.2		3–12		
		Thereafter	0.7–1.2		7–12		
		Higher in blacks			Higher in blacks		
Pyruvate	W	7–17 yr	0.076 ± 0.026 mmol/l	×1	0.076 ± 0.026 mmol/L		(Pianosi et al.)
Renin (renin activity, plasma; PRA)	P(E)		ng/mL/hr		μg/L/hr		
		0–3 yr	<16.6	×1	<16.6		
		3–6 yr	<6.7		<6.7		
		6–9 yr	<4.4		<4.4		
		9–12 yr	<5.9		<5.9		
		12–15 yr	<4.2		<4.2		
		15–18 yr	<4.3		<4.3		
		Normal sodium diet					
		Supine	0.2–2.5		0.2–2.5		
		Upright	0.3–4.3		0.3–4.3		
		Low sodium diet					
		Upright	2.9–24		2.9–24		
Retinol-binding protein (RBP)	S	0–5 day	0.8–4.5 mg/dL	×10	8–45 mg/L		s (Lockitch, et al, 1988b)
		1–9 yr	1.0–7.8		10–78		
		10–13 yr	1.3–9.9		13–99		
		14–19 yr	3.0–9.2		30–92		

Table continued on following page

TABLE 726–6 Reference Ranges *Continued*

Analyte or Procedure	Specimen	Reference Values (USA)	Conversion Factor	Reference Values (SI)	Comments
Reverse triiodothyronine (rT3)	S	ng/dL		nmol/L	
		1–5 yr 15–71	×0.0154	0.23–1.1	
		5–10 yr 17–7		0.26–1.2	
		10–15 yr 19–88		0.29–1.36	
		Adults 30–80		0.46–1.23	
Selenium	S	0–5 day 5.7–9.4 μg/dL	×0.127	0.72–1.20 μmol/L	d (Lockitch et al, 1988c)
		1–9 yr 9.6–16.1		1.22–2.05	
		10–19 yr 10.3–18.5		1.31–2.35	
Sodium	S,P(LiH,NH_4H)	mmol/L		nmol/L	
		Newborn 134–146	×1	134–146	
		Infant 139–146		139–146	
		Child 138–145		138–146	
		Thereafter 136–146		136–146	
Somatomedin C, see *Insulin-like growth factor I*					
T3, see *Triiodothyronine*					
T4, see *Thyroxine*					
Testosterone	S	Tanner / Age / Male			(Endocrine Sciences)
		1 / <9.8 y / <3–10 ng/dL	×0.03467	<0.1–0.35 nmol/L	
		2 / 9.8–14.5 / 18–150		0.62–5.20	
		3 / 10.7–15.4 / 100–320		3.47–11.10	
		4 / 11.8–16.2 / 220–620		7.63–21.50	
		5 / 12.8–17.3 / 350–970		12.14–3363	
		Adult / 350–1030		12.14–35.71	
		Tanner / Age / Female			
		1 / <9.2 yr / <3–10 ng/dL		<0.1–0.35 nmol/L	
		2 / 9.2–13.7 / 7–28		0.24–0.97	
		3 / 10.0–14.4 / 15–35		0.52–1.21	
		4 / 10.7–15.6 / 13–32		0.45–1.11	
		5 / 11.8—18.6 / 20–38		0.69–1.32	
		Adult / 10–55		0.35–1.91	
Testosterone, free	S	Male / pg/mL / % Free		Male / pmol/L / Fraction Free	(Endocrine Sciences)
		Cord / 5–22 / 2.0–4.4	×3.4673	17–76 / 0.02–0.044	
		1–15 day / 1.5–31 / 0.9–1.7		5.2–107 / 0.009–0.017	
		1–3 mo / 3.3–18 / 0.4–0.8		11.4–62 / 0.004–0.008	
		3–5 mo / 0.7–14 / 0.4–1.1		2.4–49 / 0.004–0.011	
		5–7 mo / 0.4–4.8 / 0.4–1.0		1.4–16.6 / 0.0004–0.011	
		1–10 yr / 0.15–0.6 / 0.4–0.9		0.5–2.1 / 0.004–0.009	
		Pubertal / not defined		not defined	
		Adult / 52–280 / 1.5–3.2		180–971 / 0.015–0.032	
		Female / pg/mL / % Free		Female / pmol/l / Fraction Free	
		Cord / 4–16 / 2.0–3.9		13.9–55 / 0.02–0.039	
		1–15 day / 0.5–2.5 / 0.8–1.5		1.7–8.7 / 0.008–0.015	
		1–3 mo / 0.1–1.3 / 0.4–1.1		0.3–4.5 / 0.004–0.011	
		3–5 mo / 0.3–1.1 / 0.5–1.0		1.1–3.8 / 0.005–0.01	
		5–7 mo / 0.2–0.6 / 0.5–0.8		0.7–2.1 / 0.005–0.008	
		1–10 yr / 0.15–0.6 / 0.4–0.9		0.5–2.1 / 0.004–0.009	

Test	Specimen	Conventional units	Factor	SI units	Source
		Pubertal not defined Adult 1.1–6.3 0.8–1.4		not defined 3.8–21.8 0.008–0.014	
Thiamine (vitamin B1)	S	0–2.0 μg/dL	×37.68	0.0–75.4 nmol/L	
Thyroglobulin	S	Cord blood 14.7–101.1 ng/mL Birth–35 mo 10.6–92.0 3–11 yr 5.6–41.9 12–17 yr 2.7–21.9	×1	14.7–101.1 μg/L 10.6–92.0 5.6–41.9 2.7–21.9	(Nichols Institute Reference Laboratories)
Thyroid microsomal antibodies	S	Nondetectable (hemagglutination) or <1:10		Nondetectable (hemagglutination) or <1:10	q
Thyroid thyroglobulin	S				
Tanned RBC agglutination test		Children ≤ 1:4 dilution Thereafter ≤ 1:10		≤ 1:4 dilution ≤ 1:10	
Thyroid stimulating hormone	S	Premature (28–36 wk) 1st wk of life 0.7–27.0 mIU/L Term infants Birth–4 d 1.0–38.9 2–20 wk 1.7–9.1 5 mo–20 yr 0.7–6.4	×1	0.7–27.0 mIU/L 1.0–28.9 1.7–9.1 0.7–6.4	(Nichols Institute Reference Laboratories)
Thyroid uptake of radioactive iodine	Activity over thyroid gland	2 hr <6% 6 hr 3–20% 24 hr 8–30%	×0.01	2 hr <0.06 6 hr 0.03–0.20 24 hr 0.08–0.30	
Thyroid uptake of ^{99m}Tc04	Activity over thyroid gland	After 24 hr 0.4–3.0%	×0.01	Fractional uptake 0.004–0.03	
Thyrotropin releasing hormone (hTRH)	P	5–60 pg/mL	×2.759	14–165 pmol/L	
Thyroxine binding globulin (TBG)	S	mg/dL Cord blood 1.4–94 1–4 wk 1.0–9.0 1–12 mo 2.0–7.6 1–5 yr 2.9–5.4 5–10 yr 2.5–5.0 10–15 yr 2.1–4.6 Adult 1.5–3.4	×10	mg/L 14–94 10–90 20–76 29–54 25–50 21–46 15–34	
Thyroxine, total	S	Full-Term Infants 1–3 d 8.2–19.9 μg/dL 1 wk 6.0–15.9 1–12 mo 6.1–14.9 Prepubertal Children 1–3 yr 6.8–13.5 μg/dL 3–10 yr 5.5–12.8 Pubertal Children and Adults 4.2–13.0 μg/dL	×12.9	Full-Term Infants 1–3 d 106–256 nmol/L 1 wk 77–205 1–12 mo 79–192 Prepubertal Children 1–3 yr 88–174 nmol/L 3–10 yr 71–165 Pubertal Children and Adults 54–167 nmol/L	(Endocrine Sciences)

Table continued on following page

TABLE 726–6 Reference Ranges *Continued*

Analyte or Procedure	Specimen	Reference Values (USA)	Conversion Factor	Reference Values (SI)	Comments
Thyroxine, free	S	Newborn Infants 3 d 2.0–4.9 ng/dL Infants 0.9–2.6 ng/dL Prepubertal Children 0.8–2.2 ng/dL Pubertal Children and Adults 0.8–2.3 ng/dL	×12.9	Full-Term Infants 3 d 26–631 pmol/L Infants 12–33 pmol/L Prepubertal Children 10–28 pmol/L Pubertal Children and Adults 10–30 pmol/L	(Endocrine Sciences)
Thyroxine, total	W	Newborn screen (filter paper) 6.2–22 μg/dL	×12.9	80–283 nmol/L	
Transcortin	S	M 1.5–2.0 mg/dL F, Follicular 1.7–2.0 Luteal 1.6–2.1 Postmenopausal 1.7–2.5 Pregnancy, 21–28 wk 4.7–5.4 33–40 wk 5.5–7.0	×10	15–20 mg/L 17–20 16–21 17–25 47–54 55–70	
Transferrin (siderophilin)	S	95–385 mg/dL	×0.01	0.95–3.85 g/L	(Davis et al)
Triglycerides	S, after ≥12 hr fast	mg/dL: M / F Cord blood 10–98 / 10–98 0–5 yr 30–86 / 32–99 6–11 yr 31–108 / 35–114 12–15 yr 36–138 / 41–138 16–19 yr 40–163 / 40–128 20–29 yr 44–185 / 40–128 Recommended (desirable) levels	×0.01	g/L: M / F 0.10–.98 / 0.10–0.98 0.30–0.86 / 0.32–0.99 0.31–1.08 / 0.35–1.14 0.36–1.38 / 0.41–1.38 0.40–1.63 / 0.40–1.28 0.44–1.85 / 0.40–1.28	
Recommended (desirable)		For adults Male 40–160 mg/dL Females 35–135		For adults Males 0.40–1.60 g/l Females 0.35–1.35	
Triidothyronine, free	S	pg/dL Cord blood 20–240 1–3 d 200–610 6 wk 240–560 Adult (20–50 yr) 230–660	×0.01536	pmol/L 0.3–3.7 3.1–9.4 3.7–8.6 3.5–10.0	
Triiodothyronine resin uptake test (T3RU)	S	Newborn 26–36% Thereafter 26–35%	×0.01	Fractional uptake 0.26–0.36 0.26–0.35	
Triiodothyronine, total	S	ng/dL Cord blood 30–70 Newborn 75–260 1–5 yr 100–260 5–10 yr 90–240 10–15 yr 80–210 Thereafter 115–190	×0.0154	nmol/L 0.46–1.08 1.16–4.00 1.54–4.00 1.39–3.70 1.23–3.23 1.77–2.93	

Troponin	S	Children	0.03–0.14 ng/mL >0.15 (cardiac event)	×0.1	0.13–0.14 μg/L	
Tyrosine	S	 Premature Newborn Adult	mg/dL 7.0–24.0 1.6–3.7 0.8–1.3	×0.0552	mmol/L 0.39–1.32 0.088–0.20 0.044–0.07	
Urea nitrogen	S,P	 Cord blood Premature (1 wk) Newborn Infant/child Thereafter	mg/dL 21–40 3–25 3–12 5–18 7–18	×0.357	mmol urea/L 7.5–14.3 1.1–9 1.1–4.3 1.8–6,4 2.5–6.4	
Uric acid	S	1–5 yr 6–11 yr M 12–19 yr F 12–19 yr	1.7–5.8 mg/dL 2.2–6.6 3.0–7.7 2.7–5.7	×59.48	100–350 μmol/L 130–390 180–460 160–340	j (Meites)
Vitamin A (retinol)	S	1–6 yr 7–12 yr 13–19 yr	20–43 μg/dL 25–48 26–72	×0.0349	0.70–1.5 μmol/L 0.9–1.7 0.9–2.5	p (Lockitch, et al, 1988c)
Vitamin B, see *Thiamine*						
Vitamin B_2, see *Riboflavin*						
Vitamin B_6	P(E)	3.6–18 ng/mL		×4.046	14.6–72.8 nmol/L	
Vitamin B_{12}	S	Newborn Thereafter	175–800 pg/mL 140–700	×0.738	129–590 pmol/L 103–157	
Vitamin C	P(O,H,E)	0.6–2.0 mg/dL		×56.78	34–113 μmol/L	
Vitamin D, 25-hydroxy	S	1–30 day 31 d–1 yr	1.9–33.4 ng/mL 7.4–53.3	×1	1.9–33.4 μg/L 7.4–53.3	(Soldin et al, 1997)
Vitamin D3, 1,25-dihydroxy (calcitriol)	S	25–45 pg/mL		×2.4	60–108 nmol/L	
Vitamin E (tocopherol)	S	1–6 yr 7–19 yr	3.0–9.0 mg/L 4.4–10.4	×2.32	7–21 μmol/L 10–24	p (Lockitch, et al, 1988c)
Xylose absorption test 0.5 g/kg in H_2O, 25 g maximum	S	 Child, 1 hr Adult, 2 hr	mg/dL >20 >25	×0.0667	mmol/L >1.33 >1.67	
Zinc	S	1–19 yr	64–118 μg/dL	×0.1530	9.8–18.1 μmol/L	d (Lockitch et al, 1988c)

C. Analyses of Blood for Drugs of All Classes

		Peak		Trough			SI Peak		SI Trough		
Antibiotics:	***Specimen***	**Therapeutic**	**Toxic**	**Therapeutic**	**Toxic**	***Conversion Factor***	**Therapeutic**	**Toxic**	**Therapeutic**	**Toxic**	***Comment***
Amikacin	S	20–25 μg/mL	>30	1–4 μg/mL	>8	×1.708	34–43 μmol/L	>51	1.7–6.8	>14	kn (Taylor and Caviness)
Chloramphenicol	S	10–20 μg/mL	>25			×3.095	31–62 μmol/L	>77			k (Taylor and Caviness)
Gentamicin	S	6–10 μg/mL	>12	0.5–2.0	>2.0	×2.064	12–21 μmol/L	>25	1.0–4.1	>4.1	kn (Taylor and Caviness)
Netilmicin	S	6–10 μg/mL	>12	0.5–2.0	>2	×2.103	13–21 μmol/L	>25	1.1–4.2	>4.2	kn (Taylor and Caviness)
Tobramycin	S	6–10 μg/mL	>12	0.5–2.0	>2	×2.139	13–21 μmol/L	>26	1.1–4.3	>4.3	kn (Taylor and Caviness)
Vancomycin	S	30–40 μg/mL	>60	5–10	>20	×0.303	9.1–12.1 μmol/L	>18.2	1.5–3.0	>6.1	kn (Syva)

Table continued on following page

TABLE 726–6 Reference Ranges *Continued*

Other Drugs	Specimen	Reference Values	Conversion Factor	Reference Values (SI)	Comments
Acetaminophen	S,P(H,E)	Therapeutic 10–30 μg/mL Toxic >200	×6.62	66–200 μmol/L >1,300	n
Amphetamine	S,P(H,E)	Therapeutic 20–30 ng/mL Toxic >200	×7.396	150–220 nmol/L >1,500	
Amitriptyline (includes nortriptyline)	S	Therapeutic 100–250 ng/mL	×1	100–250 μg/L	(Syva)
Nortriptyline (only)		Therapeutic 50–150 ng/mL	×1	50–150 μg/L	
Caffeine	S,P	Therapeutic for neonatal apnea 5–20 μg/mL	×5.150	26–103 μmol/L	k (Syva)
Carbamazepine	S,P(H,E) at trough	Therapeutic 4–10 μg/mL Toxic >12	×4.233	17–42 μmol/L >51	kn
Chloral hydrate	S	As trichloroethanol Therapeutic 2–12 μg/mL Toxic >20	×6.694	13–80 μmol/L >134	
Diazepam	S,P(H,E) at trough	Therapeutic 100–1000 ng/mL Toxic >5000	×3.512	350–3500 nmol/L >17,500	
Digitoxin	S,P(H,E) 6 hr post	Therapeutic 20–35 ng/mL Toxic >45	×1.307	26–46 nmol/L >59	n
Digoxin	S,P(E,E) 12 hr post	ng/mL Therapeutic CHF 0.8–1.5 Arrhythmias 1.5–2.0 Toxic Child >2.5 Adult >3.0	× 1.281	nmol/L 1–1.9 1.9–2.6 >3.2 >3.8	kn
Diphenylhydantoin, see *Phenytoin*					
Doxepin (includes desmethyldoxepine)	S,P	Therapeutic 110–250 ng/mL	× 1	110–250 μg/L	(Syva)
Ethanol	W(O),S	Toxic 50–100 mg/dL Depression of CNS >100	× 0.2171	11–22 mmol/L >22	
Ethosuximide	S,P(H,E) at trough	Therapeutic 40–100 μg/mL Toxic >150	× 7.084	280–700 μmol/L >1,060	kn
Imipramine (includes desipramine)	S	Therapeutic 150–250 ng/mL	× 1	150–250 μg/L	k (Syva)
Lithium	S,P(not LiH)	12 hr after dose Therapeutic 0.6–1.2 mmol/L Toxic >2 mmol/L	× 1	0.6–1.2 mmol/L >2 mmol/L	
Lysergic acid diethylamide	P,(E) U	After hallucinogenic dose 0.005–0.009 μg/mL 0.001–0.050 μg/mL	× 3089	After hallucinogenic dose 15.5–27.8 nmol/L 3.1–155 nmol/L	

Methotrexate	S,P	After high-dose therapy Toxic >5 µmol/L at 24 hr Toxic >1 µmol/L at 48 hr	× 1	After high-dose therapy Toxic >5 µmol/l at 24 hr Toxic >1 µmol/l at 48 hr	kn
Paraldehyde	S,P(H,E)	Sedative 10–100 µg/mL Anticonvulsant 100–200 Toxic >200 Lethal >500	× 7.567	75–75 µmol/L >750–1,500 >1,500 >3,750	(Koren et al)
Phenacetin	P(E)	Therapeutic 1–20 µg/mL Toxic 50–250	× 5.580	5.6–110 µmol/L 280–1,400	
Phenobarbital	S,P(H,E) at trough	µg/mL Therapeutic 15–40 Toxic Slowness, ataxia, nystagmus 35–80 Coma with reflexes 65–117 Coma without reflexes >100	× 4.306	µmol/L 65–170 150–345 280–504 >430	kn
Phensuximide (both parent and *N*-desmethyl metabolite)	S,P(H,E)	Therapeutic 40–60 µg/mL	× 5.71	228–343 µmol/L	
Phenytoin	S,P(H,E)	Therapeutic 10–20 µg/mL	× 3.964	40–80 µmol/L	
Primidone	S,P(H,E) at trough	Therapeutic 5–12 µg/mL Toxic >15 Toxic (neonatal) >20	× 4.582	23–55 µmol/L >69 >92	(Taylor and Caviness)
Procainamide	S,P(H,E)	Therapeutic 4–10 µg/mL Toxic >10–12 µg/mL (Also consider concentration of metabolite *N*-acetylprocainamide [NAPA].)	× 4.25	17–42 µmol/L >42–51 µmol/L	
Propranolol	S,P(H,E) at trough	Therapeutic 50–100 ng/mL	× 3.856	190–380 nmol/L	
Quinidine	S,P(H,E)	Therapeutic 2–5 µg/mL Toxic >6	× 3.083	6.2–15.5 µmol/L >18.5	
Salicylate	S,P(H,E) at trough	Therapeutic 15–30 mg/dL Toxic >30	× 0.0724	1.1–2.2 mmol/L >18.5	
Theophylline	S,P(H,E)	µg/mL Therapeutic Bronchodilator 10–20 Neonatal apnea 5–10 Toxic >20	× 5.550	µmol/L 56–110 28–56 >110	kn
Valproic acid	S,P(H,E) at trough	Therapeutic 50–100 µg/mL Toxic >100	× 6.934	350–700 µmol/L >700	

II. ANALYSES OF URINE

A. Formed Elements

Sediment casts	U	Hyaline occasional (0–1) casts/hpf RBC not seen WBC not seen Tubular epithelial not seen Transitional and squamous epithelial not seen		Hyaline occasional (0–1) casts/hpf RBC not seen WBC not seen Tubular epithelial not seen Transitional and squamous epithelial not seen	

Table continued on following page

TABLE 726–6 Reference Ranges *Continued*

Other Drugs	Specimen	Reference Values		Conversion Factor	Reference Values (SI)		Comments
Cells		RBC 0–2/hpf WBC Males 0–3/hpf Females and children 0–5/hpf Epithelial few; more frequent in newborn Bacterial: unspun: no organism per oil immersion field Spun: <20 organisms/hpf			RBC 0–2/hpf WBC Males 0–3/hpf Females and children 0–5/hpf Epithelial few; more frequent in newborn Bacterial: unspun: no organisms per oil immersion field Spun: <20 organisms/hpf		
Specific gravity	U U, 24 hr	Adult 1.002–1.030 After 12 hr fluid restriction >1.025 1.015–1.025			Adult 1.002–1.030 After 12 hr fluid restriction >1.025		
Urine volume	U, 24 hr		mL/24 hr		L/24 hr		
		Newborn	50–300	× 0.001	0.050–0.300		
		Infant	350–550		0.350–0.550		
		Child	500–1000		0.500–1.000		
		Adolescent	700–1400		0.700–1.400		
		Thereafter, M	800–1800		0.800–1.800		
		F	600–1600		0.600–1.600		
		(varies with intake and other factors)					
B. Chemical Elements							
Acetone, semiquantiative	U	Negative			Negative		
Albumin	U	4–16 yr 3.35–18.3 mg/24 hr/1.73 m²					(Meites)
Aldosterone	U	Newborn:					
		1–3 days:	20–140 μg/g Cr	× 0.3139	6.28–43.94 nmol/mmol Cr		
			0.5–5 μg/24 hr	× 2.775	1.39–13.88 nmol/day		
		Prepubertal:					
		4–10 years	4–22 μg/g Cr	×0.3139	1.26–6.91 nmol/mmol Cr		
			1–8 μg/24 hr	× 2.775	2.78–22.20 nmol/day		
		Adults:	1.5–20 μg/g Cr	× 0.3139	0.47–6.28 nmol/mmol Cr		
			3–19 μg/24 hr	× 2.775	8.32–52.72 nmol/day		
Amino acids, urine	U	0–30 day	>1 mo		0–30 day	>1 mo	f (Nichols Institute Reference Laboratories)
		μmol/g Creatinine			mmol/mol Creatinine		
Phosphoserine		0–53	0–35	× 0.1131	0–6.0	0–4.0	
Taurine		1521–6922	0–1450		172–783	0–164	
Phosphoethanolamine		0–23	23–203		0–2.6	2.6–23	
Aspartic acid		78–172	0–82		8.8–19.5	0–9.3	
Hydroxyproline		210–2413	0–210		23.7–273	0–23.7	
Threonine		99–509	27–265		11.2–57.6	3.1–30	
Serine		80–1096	86–566		9.1–124	9.7–64	
Asparagine		0–438	0–107		0–49.5	0–12.1	
Glutamic acid		34–363	0–80		3.8–41.1	0–9	
Glutamine		256–1096	168–849		29–124	9.7–64	
Sarcosine		93–850	93–850		10.5–96.1	10.5–96.1	
Proline		74–537	0–57		8.4–60.7	0–6.4	
Glycine		1423–7143	0–2953		161–808	0–334	
Alanine		403–715	68–534		45.6–80.9	7.7–60.4	
Citrulline		9–212	8–106		1.0–24	0.9–12	
2-Aminobutyric acid		354–1061	44–221		40–120	5–25	
4-Aminoisobutyric acid		0–2643	0–2643				
Valine		18–314	7–50		2.0–35.5	0.8–5.6	
Cysteine		226–812	5–177		25.8–91.9	0.6–20	
Methionine		15–71	6–111		1.7–8	0.7–12.5	

Test	Specimen	Conventional		Factor	SI	
Homocitrulline		0–266	0–266		0–30.1	0–30.1
Crystathionine		27–111	3–23		3.1–12.5	0.3–2.6
Isoleucine		43–179	0–65		4.9–20.2	0–7.3
Leucine		17–72	15–57		1.9–8.1	1.7–6.5
Tyrosine		27–97	19–145		3–11	2.2–16.4
Phenylalanine		39–156	17–102		4.4–17.7	1.9–11.5
β-Alanine		0–1202	0–1202		0–136	0–136
3-Aminoisobutyric acid		0–111	0–111		0–12.5	0–12.5
		0–299	0–299			
Homocystine		0–0	0–0		0–0	0–0
Argininosuccinic acid		0–9	0–7		0–1.0	0–0.8
Ethanolamine		840–3492	57–308		95–395	6.5–34.8
Tryptophan		0–106	0–106		0–12	0–12
Hydroxylysine		0–106	0–106		0–12	0–12
Ornithine		34–156	1–44		3.9–17.7	0.1–5.0
Lysine		74–1282	0–548		8.4–145	0–62
1-Methylhistidine		72–425	0–691		8.1–48.1	0–78.2
Histidine		148–721	0–1353		16.7–81.6	0–153
3-Methylhistidine		115–401	19–413		13–45.4	2.1–46.7
Anserine		0–561	0–561		0–63.5	0–63.5
Carnosine		0–127	0–127		0–14.4	0–14.4
Arginine		50–73	8–32		5.6–8.3	0.9–3.6
Aminolevulinic acid (ALA)	U	1.3–7.0 mg/24 hr		× 7.626	9.9–53.4 μmol/24 hr	
Ammonia	U	500–1,200 mgN/24 hr		0.0714	36–86 mmol/24 hr	
Bilirubin	U	Negative			Negative	
Calcium, total	U	Ca in Diet	mg/24 hr		mmol/24 hr	
		Ca free	5–40	× 0.025	0.13–1.0	
		Low to average	50–150		1.25–3.8	
		Average (20 mmol/24 hr)	100–300		2.5–7.5	
Catecholamines, fractionated	U	Norepinephrine	μg/24 hr	× 5.911	nmol/24 hr	
		0–1 yr	0–10		0–59	
		1–2 yr	0–17		0–100	
		2–4 yr	4–29		24–171	
		4–7 yr	8–45		47–266	
		7–10 yr	13–65		77–384	
		Thereafter	15–80		87–473	
	U	Epinephrine	μg/24 hr		nmol/24 hr	
		0–1 yr	0–2.5	× 5.458	0–13.6	
		1–2 yr	0–3.5		0–19.1	
		2–4 yr	0–6.0		0–32.7	
		4–7 yr	0.2–10		1.1–55	
		7–10 yr	0.5–14		2.7–76	
		Thereafter	0.5–20		2.7–109	
		Dopamine	μg/24 hr		nmol/24 hr	
		0–1 yr	0–85	× 6.528	0–555	
		1–2 yr	10–140		65–914	
		2–4 yr	40–260		261–1697	
		Thereafter	65–400		424–2611	
Catecholamines, total, free	U		μg/24 hr		μg/ 24 hr	
		0–1 yr	10–15	× 1	10–15	
		1–5 yr	15–40		15–40	
		6–15 yr	20–80		20–80	
		Thereafter	30–100		30–100	

Table continued on following page

TABLE 726–6 Reference Ranges *Continued*

Other Drugs	Specimen	Reference Values	Conversion Factor	Reference Values (SI)	Comments
Chloride	U	Infant 2–10 mmol/24 hr Child 15–40 Thereafter 110–250 (varies greatly with chloride intake)	× 1	2–10 mmol/24 hr 15–40 110–250	
Copper	U	5–18 yr 0.36–7.56 mg/mol creatinine	× 15.7	6–119 μmol/mol creatinine	cd (Lockitch et al, 1988c)
Coproporphyrin	U	34–234 μg/24 hr	× 1.5	51–351 nmol/24 hr	
Cortisol free	U	μg/24 hr Child 2–27 Adolescent 5–55 Adult 10–100	× 2.759	nmol/day 5.5–74 14–152 27–276	
Creatinine	U	Premature 8.1–15.0 mg/kg/24 hr Full term 10.4–19.7 1.5–7 yr 10–15 7–15 yr 5.2–41	× 8.84	72–133 μmol/kg/24 hr 92–174 88–133 46–362	ah (Meites)
Cyclic AMP	U	<3.3 mg/24 hr or <1.64 mg/g creatinine	× 3.040	<10 μmol/24 hr <600 μmoles cAMP/mol creatinine	
Estradiol, urinary	U	Adult male 0–6 μg/24 hr Adult female Follicular 0–3 μg/24 hr Ovulatory peak 4–14 Luteal 4–10	× 3.671	Adult male 0–22 nmol/day Adult female Follicular 0–11 nmol/day Ovulatory peak 15–51 Luteal 15–37	
Estriol (E3), total	U	mg/24 hr Pregnancy (wk) 30 6–18 35 9–28 40 13–42 Decrease of >40% of previous value suggests fetus at risk	× 3.467	μmol/24 hr 21–62 31–97 45–146 Fraction of previous value of <0.60 suggests fetus at risk	
Estrogens, total	U, 24 hr	μg/24 hr Child <10 Adult male 5–25 Adult female Preovulation 5–25 Ovulation 28–100 Luteal peak 22–80 Pregnancy <45,000 Postmenopausal <10	× 1	μg/24 hr <10 5–25 5–25 28–100 22–80 <45,000 <10	
Ferric chloride test	U	Negative		Negative	
Galactose	U	Newborn ≤60 mg/dL Thereafter <14 mg/24 hr	× 0.0555 × 0.00555	≤3.33 mmol/L <0.08 mmol/24 hr	
Glucose Quantitative, enzymatic Qualitative	 U U	 <0.5 g/24 hr Negative	 × 5.55	 <2.8 mmol/ 24 hr Negative	
Hemoglobin (Hb)	U	Negative		Negative	

Test	Specimen		Reference range (conventional)	Conversion factor	Reference range (SI)	Notes
Homovanillic acid	U, 24 hr	0–1 yr	<32.2 mg/g Cr	×0.62	<20 mmol/mol Cr	p (Meites)
		2–4 yr	<22		<14	
		5–19 yr	<14		<8	
5-Hydroxyindoleacetic acid (5-HIAA)	U	3–8 yr				(Nichols Institute Reference Laboratories)
		0.4–5.6 mg/24 hr		× 8.8	3.5–49.3 μmol/24 hr	
		1.2–16.2 mg/g Cr		× 0.5917	0.71–9.6 mmol/mol Cr	
		9 yr and older				
		0.9–7 mg/24 hr		× 8.8	7.9–61.9 μmol/24 hr	
		1.3–8.7 mg/g Cr		× 0.5917	0.78–5.15 mmol/mol Cr	
Hydroxyproline, free and bound	U	3 day	33–112 μmol/24 hr	× 1	33–112 μmol/24 hr	q (Meites)
		10 day	148–225		148–225	
		20 day	229–310		229–310	
17-Hydroxycorticosteroids (17-OHCS)	U		mg/24 hr		μmol/24 hr	(Conversion based on hydrocortisone, MW 362)
		0–1 yr	0.5–1.0	× 2.76	1.4–2.8	
		Child	1.0–5.6		2.8–15.5	
		Adult, M	3.0–10.0		8.2–27.6	
		F	2.0–8.0		5.5–22	
		or 3–7 mg/g Cr		× 0.312	or 0.9–2.5 mmol/mol Cr	
17-Ketogenic steroids (17-KGS)	U		mg/24 hr		μmol/24 hr	(Conversion based on dehydroepiandrosterone, MW = 288)
		0–1 yr	<1.0	× 3.467	<3.5	
		1–10 yr	<5		<17	
		11–14 yr	<12		<42	
		Thereafter, M	5–23		17–80	
		F	3–15		10–52	
Ketone bodies, qualitative	U	Negative			Negative	
17-Ketosteroid (17-KS), total	U		mg/24 hr		μmol/24 hr	Zimmerman reaction (conversion based on dehydroepiandrosterone, MW = 288)
		14d–2 yr	<1	× 3.467	<3.5	
		2–6 yr	<2		<7	
		6–10 yr	1–4		3.5–14	
		10–12 yr	1–6		3.5–21	
		12–14 yr	3–10		10–35	
		14–16 yr	5–12		17–42	
		Thereafter,				
		M 18–30 yr	9–22		31–76	
		M >30 yr	8–20		28–70	
		F	6–15		21–52	
Lead	U, 24 hr	<80 μg/L		× 0.00483	<0.39 μmol/L	
Magnesium	U, 24 hr	1–6 mo				
		(breast milk)	0.04–1.55 mmol/L	× 1	0.04–1.55 mmol/L	
		(formula)	0.04–1.40		0.04–1.40	
Metanephrines, total	U, 24 hr	<1 yr	<15.9 μmol/g Cr	× 0.1131	<1.80 mmol/mol Cr	(Meites)
		1–2 yr	<14.8		<1.67	
		3–4 yr	<12.8		<1.45	
		5–8 yr	<11.7		<1.32	
		9–13 yr	<10.5		<1.19	
Methylmalonic acid	U	6–12 wk	0–57 mg/g Cr	× 0.9579	0–55 mmol/mol Cr	o (Meites)
Mucopolysaccharides	U	<2 yr	<50 μg/g Cr	× 0.1131	<5.7 mg/mmol Cr	(Meites)
		2–4 yr	<25		<2.8	
		4–15 yr	<20		<2.3	
Myoglobin	U	Negative			Negative	

Table continued on following page

TABLE 726–6 Reference Ranges *Continued*

Other Drugs	Specimen	Reference Values	Conversion Factor	Reference Values (SI)	Comments
Niacin (nicotinic acid)	U	0.3–1.5 mg/24 hr	× 8.113	2.43–12.17 μmol/24 hr	
Occult blood	U	Negative		Negative	
Organic acids	U	Adult			(Hoffman et al)
Lactic		115–407 μmol/g Cr	× 0.1132	13–46 mmol/mol Cr	
2-Hydroxyisobutyric		not detected		not detected	
Glycolic		159–486		18–55	
3-Hydroxybutyric		not detected–18		not detected–2.0	
3-Hydroxyisobutyric		36–168		4.1–19	
2-Hydroxyisovaleric		not detected		not detected	
3-Hydroxyisovaleric		61–221		6.9–25	
Methylmalonic		not detected		not detected	
4-Hydroxybutyric		2.7–51		0.3–5.8	
Ethylmalonic		3.57–37		0.4–4.2	
Succinic		4.4–141		0.5–16	
Fumaric		1.8–7		0.2–0.8	
Glutaric		5.3–23		0.6–2.6	
3-Methylglutaric		not detected		not detected	
Adipic		7–309		0.8–35	
Pyruvic		23–70		2.6–7.9	
Pyroglutamic		8–557		0.9–63	
2-Oxoisovaleric		not detected		not detected	
Acetoacetic		not detected		not detected	
Mevalonic		0.5–1.9		0.06–0.22	
2-Hydroxyglutaric		7–460		0.8–52	
3-Hydroxy-3-methyl-glutaric		not detected–88		not detected–10	
p-Hydroxyphenylacetic		31–195		3.5–22	
2-Oxoisocaproic		not detected		not detected	
Suberic		not detected–26		not detected–2.9	
Orotic		not detected		not detected	
cis-Aconitic		24–389		2.7–44	
Homovanillic		8–49		0.9–5.5	
Azeleic		11–137		1.3–5.5	
Isocitric		318–743		36–84	
Citric		619–1998		70–226	
Sebacic		not detected		not detected	
4-Hydroxyphenyllactic		1.8–23		0.2–2.6	
2-Oxoglutaric		35–654		4–74	
5-Hydroxyindoleacetic		not detected–64		not detected–72	
Succinylacetone		not detected		not detected	
Orotic acid	U	0–20.1 mg/g Cr	× 0.7247	0–14.6 mmol/mol Cr	ag (Meites)
Osmolality	U	50–1400 mOsmol/kg H_2O, depending on fluid intake. After 12 hr fluid restriction >850 mOsmol/kg H_2O		50–1400 mOsmol/kg H_2O, depending on fluid intake. After 12 hr fluid restriction >850 mOsmol/kg H_2O	
	U, 24 hr	300–900 mOsmol/kg H_2O		300–900 mOsmol/kg H_2O	
pH and Acidity	U	pH		H^+ concentration	
		Newborn/neonate 5–7		0.1–10 μmol/L	
		Thereafter 4.5–8 (average 6)		0.01–32 μmol/L (average 1.0 μmol/L)	
Phenylalanine	U	10 days–2 wk 1–2 mg/24 hr	× 6.054	6–12 μmol/24 hr	
		3–12 yr 4–18		24–110	
		Thereafter trace–17		trace–103	

Test	Specimen	Conventional units	Factor	SI units	Notes
Phenylpyruvic acid, qualitative	U	Negative by $FeCl_3$ test		Negative by $FeCl_3$ test	
Porphobilinogen (PBG) Quantitative Qualitative	 U U	 0–2.0 mg/24 hr Negative	 × 4.42	 0–8.8 μmol/24 hr Negative	
Potassium	U, 24 hr	2.5–125 mmol/L varies with diet		2.5–125 mmol/L varies with diet	
Pregnanetriol	U	mg/24 hr 2 wk–2 yr 0.02–0.2 2–5 yr <0.5 5–15 yr <1.5 >15 yr <2.0	 × 2.972	μmol/ 24 hr 0.06–0.6 <1.5 <4.5 <5.9	
Protein, total	U, 24 hr	1–14 mg/dL 50–80 mg/24 hr (at rest) <250 mg/24 hr after intense exercise	× 10 × 1	10–140 mg/L 50–80 mg/24 hr <250 mg/24 hr after intense exercise	
Electrophoresis		Average % Total Protein Albumin 37.9 α1-Globulin 27.3 α2-Globulin 19.5 β-globulin 8.8 γ-Globulin 3.3	 × 0.01	Fraction of Total 0.379 0.273 0.195 0.088 0.033	
Riboflavin (vitamin B_2)	U	μg/g Cr 1–3 yr 500–900 4–6 yr 300–600 7–9 yr 270–500 10–15 yr 200–400 Adult 80–269	 × 0.3	μmol/mol Cr 150–270 90–180 81–150 60–1200 24–81	
Sodium	U, 24 hr	40–220 (diet-dependent)		40–220	
Thiamine (Vitamin B_1)	U, acidified with HCl	μg/g Cr 1–3 yr 176–200 4–6 yr 121–400 7–9 yr 181–350 10–12 yr 181–300 13–15 yr 151–250 Thereafter 66–129	 × 0.426	μmol/mol Cr 75–85 52–170 77–149 77–128 64–107 28–55	
Vanillymandelic acid (VMA)	U	0–1 yr <18.8 mg/g Cr 2–4 yr <11 5–19 yr <8	× 0.5709	<11 mmol/mol Cr <6 <5	p (Meites)
Xylose absorption test 0.5 g/kg to 25 g maximum	U, 5 hr	Child 16–33% of ingested dose Adult g/5 hr 5 g dose >1.2 25 g dose >4.0	× 0.01 × 6.66	Fraction ingested dose 0.16–0.33 mmol/5 hr >8.00 >26.64	
Zinc	U	5–18 yr 10.1–95.9 mg/mol Cr	× 0.0153	0.15–1.47 mmol/mol Cr	d (Lockitch, et al, 1988c)

Table continued on following page

TABLE 726–6 Reference Ranges *Continued*

Other Drugs	Specimen	Reference Values	Conversion Factor	Reference Values (SI)	Comments
III. ANALYSES OF FECES					
A. Chemical Elements					
α-1-Antitrypsin	F	<1 yr (breast milk) <4.4 mg/g solid (formula) <2.9 6 mo–44 yr <1.7 mg/g solid (cow's milk, regular diet)			u (Meites)
Bile acids, total	F	120–225 mg/24 hr	× 1	120–225 mg/24 hr	
Calcium, total	F	Avg. 0.64 g/24 hr	× 25	16 mmol/24 hr	
Coproporphyrin	F, 24 hr	<30 μg/g dry weight 400–1,200 μg/24 hr	× 1.5	<45 nmol/g dry weight 600–1,800 nmol/dry	
Fat, fecal	F, 72 hr collection	g/24 hr Infant, breast-fed <1 0–6 yr <2 Adult <7 Adult (fat-free diet) <4 Coefficient of fat absorption (%) Infant, breast-fed >93 Infant, formula-fed >83 >1 yr ≥95	 × 1 × 0.01	g/24 hr <1 <2 <7 <4 Absorbed fraction >0.93 >0.83 ≥0.95	
Occult blood	F	Negative (<2 mL blood/24 hr in ~100–200 g stool)		Negative	
pH and Acidity	F	pH 7.0–7.5		H^+ concentration 31–100 nmol/L	
IV. ANALYSES OF CEREBROSPINAL FLUID					
A. Formed Elements					
Cell Count	CSF	cells/mm³ (μL) Premature 0–25 mononuclear 0–10 polymorphonuclear 0–1000 RBC Newborn 0–20 mononuclear 0–10 polymorphonuclear 0–800 RBC Neonate 0–5 mononuclear 0–10 polymorphonuclear 0–50 RBC Thereafter 0–5 mononuclear (numbers of cells in very young infants are greater than those in older individuals' CSF, without substantial implication for growth and development in most instances)	$\times 10^6$	$\times 10^6$ cells/L 0–25 0–10 0–1000 0–20 0–10 0–800 0–5 0–10 0–50 0–5	

Leukocyte differential count	CSF		%		Fraction	
		Lymphocytes	62 ± 34	× 0.01	0.62 ± 0.34	
		Monocytes	36 ± 20		0.36 ± 0.20	
		Neutrophils	2 ± −5		0.02 ± 0.05	
		Histiocytes	0-rare		0-rare	
		Ependymal cells*	0-rare		0-rare	
		Eosinophils	0-rare		0-rare	
		*Includes pia-arachnoid mesothelial cells.				
Cerebrospinal fluid pressure	CSF		70–180 mm water		70–180 mm water	
Cerebrospinal fluid volume	CSF	Child	60–100 mL	× 0.001	0.06–0.10 L	
		Adult	100–160		0.1–0.16	
B. Chemical Elements						
Amino acids in CSF	CSF					f (Dickinson and Hamilton)
Taurine			6.3 ± 1.8 μmol/L	× 1	6.3 ± 1.8 μmol/L	
Aspartic acid			0.9 ± 0.5		0.9 ± 0.5	
Threonine			25 ± 10		25 ± 10	
Serine + asparagine			38 ± 23		38 ± 23	
Glutamine			509 ± 144		509 ± 144	
Proline			0.6		0.6	
Glutamic acid			7.0 ± 4.9		7.0 ± 4.9	
Glycine			6.6 ± 1.8		6.6 ± 1.8	
Alanine			23 ± 9.4		23 ± 9.4	
Valine			14 ± 5.5		14 ± 5.5	
Half cystine			0.2		0.2	
Methionine			2.6 ± 1.6		2.6 ± 1.6	
Isoleucine			4.4 ± 1.3		4.4 ± 1.3	
Leucine			11 ± 3.6		11 ± 3.6	
Tyrosine			9.1 ± 5.0		9.1 ± 5.0	
Phenylalanine			9.2 ± 5.8		9.2 ± 5.8	
Ornithine			5.7 ± 1.8		5.7 ± 1.8	
Lysine			19 ± 6.6		19 ± 6.6	
Histidine			13 ± 4.4		13 ± 4.4	
Arginine			20 ± 5.8		20 ± 5.8	
Calcium, total	CSF		2.1–2.7 mEq/L or	× 0.50	1.05–1.35 mmol/L	
			4.2–5.4 mg/dL	× 0.25	1.05–1.35	
Chloride	CSF		118–132 mmol/L	× 1	118–132 mmol/L	
Glucose	CSF	Adult	40–70 mg/dL	× 0.0555	2.2–3.9 mmol/L	
Hypoxanthine	CSF	0–1 mo	1.8–5.5 μmol/L	× 1	1.8–5.5 μmol/L	(Jung et al)
Total protein column	CSF, Lumbar		8–32 mg/dL	× 10	80–320 mg/L	
Turbidimetry	CSF, Lumbar		mg/dL		mg/L	
		Premature	40–300		400–3,000	
		Newborn	45–120		450–1,200	
		Child	10–20		100–200	
		Adolescent	15–20		150–200	
		Thereafter	15–45		150–450	

Table continued on following page

TABLE 726–6 Reference Ranges *Continued*

Other Drugs	Specimen	Reference Values	Conversion Factor	Reference Values (SI)	Comments
Electrophoresis	CSF	% of Total		Fraction of Total	
		Prealbumin 2–7	× 0.01	0.02–0.07	
		Albumin 56–76		0.56–0.76	
		α1-Globulin 2–7		0.02–0.07	
		α2-Globulin 4–12		0.04–0.12	
		β-Globulin 8–18		0.08–0.18	
		γ-Globulin 3–12		0.03–0.12	
V. ANALYSES OF OTHER BODY FLUIDS					
A. Chemical Analyses					
1. Amnionic Fluid					
Amniotic fluid analysis Ab450nm	AF	28 wk 0–0.048 A 40 wk 0–0.02 A	× 1	0–0.048 A 0–0.02 A	t
Bilirubin	AF	28 wk <0.075 mg/dL (or Ab450 <0.048) 40 wk <0.025 mg/dL (or Ab450 <0.02)	× 17.10	<1.3 μmol/L (or Ab450 <0.048) <0.43 μmol/L (or Ab450 <0.02)	
Creatinine	AF	After 37 wk gestation >2.0 mg/dL	× 88.4	After 37 wk gestation >180 μmol/L	
Estriol (E3), free	AF	Wk — ng/mL (95% range)		nmol/L (95% range)	
		16–20 — 1.0–3.2	× 3.47	3.5–11.1	
		20–24 — 2.1–7.8		7.3–27.1	
		24–28 — 2.1–7.8		7.3–27.1	
		28–32 — 4.0–13.6		13.9–47.2	
		32–36 — 3.6–15.5		12.5–53.8	
		36–38 — 4.6–18.0		16.0–62.5	
		38–40 — 5.4–19.8		18.7–68.7	

Test	Specimen	Conventional Reference Interval		Factor	SI Reference Interval	Comments
α-Fetoprotein (AFP)	AF	Wk 15 16 17 18 19 20	Amniotic Fluid (Mean ISD) μg/mL 13.5 ± 3.42 11.7 ± 3.38 10.3 ± 3.03 9.5 ± 3.22 7.1 ± 2.86 5.7 ± 2.45			
Lecithin/sphingomyelin (L/S) ratio	AF	2.0–5.0 indicates probable fetal lung maturity (>3.0 in infants or diabetic mothers)			2.0–5.0 indicates probable fetal lung maturity (>3.0 in infants of diabetic mothers)	
Lecithin phosphorus	AF	>0.10 mg/dL indicates probable adequate fetal lung maturity		× 0.3229	>0.032 mmol/L indicates probable adequate fetal lung maturity	
2. Sweat						
Chloride	Sweat	Normal Indeterminate Cystic fibrosis	<40 mmol/L 45–60 >60	× 1	<40 mmol/L 40–60 >60	(Gibson et al)
Sodium	Sweat	Normal Indeterminate Cystic fibrosis	<40 mmol/L 40–60 >60	× 1	<40 mmol/L 40–60 >60	(Gibson et al)

Abbott Laboratories, Diagnostic Division, Abbott Park, IL, 1996.

American Diabetes Association: Report of the Expert Committee on the Diagnosis and Classification of Diabetes Mellitus. Diabetes Care 20:1183, 1997.

Baroni S, Scribano D, Valentini P, et al: Serum apolipoproteins A1, B, CII, CIII, E, and lipoprotein (a) in children. Clin Biochem 29:603, 1996.

Bonnefont JP, Specola NB, Vassault A, et al: The fasting test in children: Application to the diagnosis of pathological hypo- and hyperketotic states. Eur J Pediatr 150:80, 1990.

Buck ML: Anticoagulation with warfarin in infants and children. Ann Pharmacother 30:1316, 1996.

Davis ML, Austin C, Messner BL, et al: IFCC-standardized pediatric reference intervals for 10 serum proteins using the Beckman Array 360 System. Clin Biochem 29:489, 1996.

Diaz J, Tornel PL, Martinez P: Reference intervals for blood ammonia in healthy subjects, determined by microdiffusion. Clin Chem 41:1048, 1995.

De Schepper J, Derde MP, Goubert P, Gorus F: Reference values for fructosamine concentrations in children's sera: Influence of protein concentration, age and sex. Clin Chem 34:2444–2447, 1988.

Denny T, Yogev R, Gelman R, et al: Lymphocyte subsets in healthy children during the first five years of life. JAMA 267:1484, 1992.

Dickinson JC, Hamilton PB: The free amino acids of human spinal fluid determined by ion exchange chromatography. J Neurochem 13:1179, 1966.

Endocrine Sciences, Tarzana, CA.

Gibson LE, di Sant'Agnese PA, Schwachman H: Procedure for the quantitative iontophoretic sweat test for cystic fibrosis. Rockville, MD, Cystic Fibrosis Foundation, 1985, pp 1–4.

Gillard BK, Simbala JA, Goodglick L: Reference intervals for amylase isoenzymes in serum and plasma of infants and children. Clin Chem 29:1119, 1983.

Hoffman G, Aramaki S, Blum-Hoffman E, et al: Quantitative analysis for organic acids in biological samples: Batch isolation followed by gas chromatographic-mass spectrometric analysis. Clin Chem 35:587, 1989.

Instructions for Authors: Systeme International (SI) conversion factors for selected laboratory components. JAMA 281:19, 1999.

Jedeikin R, Makela SK, Shennan AT, et al: Creatine kinase isoenzymes in serum from cord blood and the blood of healthy full-term infants during the first three postnatal days. Clin Chem 28:317, 1982.

Jung D, Lun L, Zinsmeyer J, et al: The concentration of hypoxanthine and lactate in the blood of healthy and hypoxic newborns. J Perinat Med 13:43, 1985.

Kaplan EL, Rothermel CD, Johnson DR: Antistreptolysin O and anti-deoxyribonuclease B titers: Normal values for children ages 2 to 12 in the United States. Pediatrics 101:86, 1998.

Knight JA, Haymond RE: γ-Glutamyltransferase and alkaline phosphatase activities compared in serum of normal children and children with liver disease. Clin Chem 27:48, 1981.

Koren G, Butt W, Rajchgot P, et al: Intravenous paraldehyde for seizure control in neonates. Neurology 36:108, 1986.

Krafte-Jacobs B, Bock GH: Circulating erythropoietin and interleukin-6 concentrations increase in critically ill children with sepsis and septic shock. Crit Care Med 24:1455, 1996.

Lockitch G, Halstead AC, Albersheim S, et al: Age and sex specific pediatric reference intervals for biochemistry analytes as measured on the Ektachem-700 analyzer. Clin Chem 34:1622, 1988a.

Lockitch G, Halstead AC, Quigley G, MacCallum C: Age and sex specific pediatric reference intervals: Study design and methods illustrated by measurement of serum proteins with the Behring LN nephelometer. Clin Chem 34:1618, 1988b.

Lockitch G, Halstead AC, Wadsworth L, et al: Age and sex specific pediatric reference intervals and correlations for zinc, copper, selenium, iron, vitamins A and E, and related proteins. Clin Chem 34:1625, 1988c.

Mayo Medical Laboratories, Rochester, MN.

Meites S (ed): Pediatric Clinical Chemistry, Reference (Normal) Values. American Association for Clinical Chemistry, 3rd ed. Washington, DC, 1989.

Nichols Institute Reference Laboratories, San Juan Capistrano, CA.

Pesce MA, Boudorian S: Clinical significance of plasma galactose and erythrocyte galactose-1-phosphate measurements in transferase-deficient galactosemia and in individuals with below-normal transferase activity. Clin Chem 28:301, 1982a.

Pesce MA, Bodourian S, Nicholson JF: A new microfluorometric method for the measurement of galactose-1-phosphate in erythrocytes. Clin Chem Acta 118:177, 1982b.

Pesce MA, Bodourian S, Harris RC, Nicholson JF: Enzymatic micromethod for measuring galactose-1-phosphate uridylyltransferase in erythrocytes. Clin Chem 23:1711, 1977c.

Pianosi P, Seargeant L, Haworth JC: Blood lactate and pyruvate concentrations, and their ratio during exercise in healthy children: Developmental perspective. Eur J Appl Physiol 71:518, 1995.

Pittet JL, de Moerloose P, Reber G, et al: VIDAS D-dimer: Fast quantitative ELISA for measuring D-dimer in plasma. Clin Chem 42:410, 1996.

Rosenthal P, Pesce MA: Long-term monitoring of D-lactic acidosis in a child. J Pediatr Gastroenterol Nutr 4:674, 1985.

Schmidt-Sommerfeld E, Werner D, Penn D: Carnitine plasma concentrations in 353 metabolically healthy children. Eur J Pediatr 147:356, 1988.

Sherry B, Jack RM, Weber A, Smith AL: Reference interval for prealbumin for children two to 36 months old. Clin Chem 34:1878, 1988.

Soldin SJ, Bailey J, Beatey J, et al: Pediatric reference ranges for lipase. Clin Chem 41:593, 1995.

Soldin SJ, Hicks JM, Bailey J, et al: Pediatric reference ranges for 25 hydroxy vitamin D during the summer and winter. Clin Chem 43:S200, 1997.

Straczcek J, Felden F, Dousset B, et al: Quantification of methymalonic acid in serum measured by capillary gas chromatography-mass spectrometry as tert.-butyldimethylsilyl derivatives. J Chromatogr 620:1, 1993.

Syva Company, TDM Serum Sample Guide, 1986, Palo Alto, CA.

Taylor WJ, Caviness MHD (eds): A Textbook for the Clinical Application of Therapeutic Drug Monitoring. Irving, TX, Abbott Laboratories, Diagnostic Division, 1986.

Unten SK, Hokama Y: Enzyme immunoassay for C-reactive protein analysis. J Clin Lab Anal 1:205, 1987.

Vilaseca MA, Moyano D, Ferrer I, et al: Total homocysteine in pediatric patients. Clin Chem 43:690, 1997.

Visnapu LA, Karlson LK, Dubinsky EJ, et al: Pediatric reference ranges for serum aldolase. Am J Clin Pathol 91:476, 1989.

TABLE 726–7 Composition of Commonly Used Oral and Parenteral Solutions (Raymond Adelman and Michael Solhaug) (see related conversion Tables 726–8 to 726–10)

Fluid	CHO g/dL	Prot*	Calories per L	Na mEq/L	K mEq/L	Cl mEq/L	HCO_3† mEq/L	Ca mEq/L	P‡ mEq/L	Mg mEq/L	Osm§ mOsm/kg H_2O
Oral											
Apple juice¶	11.9	0.1	480		0.4	26		3	4.5		700
Coca-Cola¶	10.9		435	4.3	0.1		13.4				656
Ginger ale¶	9.0		360	3.5	0.1		3.6				565
Grape juice¶	16.6	0.2	672	0.4	30		32				1027
Grapefruit juice¶ (canned, sugar added)	17.8	0.6	736	0.2	35			6.5			591
Milk	4.9	3.5	670	22	36	28	30	60	54		260*
Orange juice¶	10.4	0.7	444	0.2	49		50				654
Pepsi-Cola	12.0		480	6.5	0.8		7.3				—
Pineapple juice (canned)¶	13.5	0.4	556	0.2	38			7.5	9		783
Prune juice¶	19	0.4	776	0.9	60			7	20		—
Root beer¶				3.5	3.9						588
Seven-Up¶	8.0		320	7.5	0.2			0.3			564
Tomato juice (canned, salted)¶	4.3		172	100	59	150	10	3	18		592
Gatorade	5.9		250	21	2.5	17			6.8		377
Hydra-lyte	2.5		100	84	10	59	15	<1	<1		300
Lytren	7.0		280	30	25	25	36	4	5	4	267**
Pedialyte	5.0		200	30	20	30	28	4		4	387
Rehydrate	2.5	0	100	75	25	65	30	0	0	0	305
Resol Solution	2.0	0	83	50	20	50	34	4	5	4	269
Ricelyte Oral Sol. (rice syrup solids)	3.0	0	140	50	25	45	34	0	0	0	200
Parenteral											
CHO†† in H_2O	5–10		200–400								266–532
Isotonic saline	0–5		0–200	154		154					292–558
1/2 isotonic saline	2.5–5		100–200	77		77					280–415
3% (M/2) saline				513		513					969
5% saline				855		855					1616
M/6 sodium lactate				167			167				
5% sodium bicarbonate				595			595				
Lactated Ringer's solution	0–5–10		0–20 0–40 0	130	4	109	28	3			261–531–801
Modified Butler 1 (a)	5		200	25	20	22	23		3	3	360
Modified Butler 2 (b)	5–10		200–400	56	25	49	26		12	5	423–719**
Talbot (c)	5		200	40	35	40	20		15		409
Human plasma protein fraction (d)		5		130	2	50	50				
Blood‡‡		3		95	4	50	40		2	1–2	
Dextran 10% (low mol. wt.) (e)	5		200								
Dextran 10% in saline (f)				154		154					
Dextran 6% (high mol. wt) (g)	5–10		200–400								
Dextran 6% in saline (h)				154		154					
Mannitol 20%§§											

Available Additives

Glucose 50%	0.5 g/mL
Sodium chloride	2.5 and 5 mEq/mL
Sodium acetate	2 and 4 mEq/mL
Sodium lactate	5 mEq/mL
Sodium bicarbonate	0.5 (4.2%) mEq/mL and 0.9 (7.5%) mEq/mL, 1 mEq/mL (8.4%)
Potassium acetate	2 and 4 mEq/mL
Potassium chloride	2 and 3 mEq/mL
Potassium phosphate	4.4 mEq/mL of potassium and 3 mM/ml phospate
Calcium gluconate 10%	9.3 mg (0.465 mEq/mL) elemental calcium
Calcium chloride 10%	27.3 mg (1.4 mEq/mL) elemental calcium
Ammonium chloride	5 mEq/mL
Magnesium sulfate	0.8 mEq/mL, 1 mEq/mL, and 4 mEq/mL available as the 10%, 12.5%, and 50% solutions

Table continued on following page

TABLE 726–7 Composition of Commonly Used Oral and Parenteral Solutions (Raymond Adelman and Michael Solhaug) (see related conversion Tables 726–8 to 726–10) *Continued*

Selected Commercial Preparations in the United States

(possible slight variations in composition from values in table)

(A, Abbott; B, Baxter; C, Cutter; M, McGaw; P, Pharmacia)

(a)	Ionosol MB in D5W (A); Isolyte P with 5% Dextrose (M)
(b)	Ionosol B in D5W (A); Electrolyte #2 with 10% Invert Sugar (C,M); 10% Travert in electrolyte #2 (B)
(c)	Ionosol T in D5W (A); Isolyte M (M)
(d)	Plasmatein (A); Plasmanate (C)
(e) (f)	LMD 10% (A); Dextran 40 (C,M); Rheomacrodex (P); Gentran 40 (B)
(g) (h)	Dextran 70 (A); Macrodex (P); Gentran 75 in 10% Travert (B)

**Protein or amino acid equivalent.*
†Actual or potential bicarbonate, such as acetate, lactate, citrate.
‡Calculated according to valence of 1.8.
§Osmolality except for values shown (**), which are osmolarity (in mOsm/L).
¶Composition varies slightly, depending on source.
***See § above.*
††Glucose (dextrose, fructose, or invert sugar).
‡‡Red cell contents not included in calculations.
§§Also available: mannitol 5%, 10%, 15%, and 20%.
(Sources: Pennington JAT (ed): Bowes & Church's Food Values of Portions Commonly Used. 17th ed. Philadelphia, Lippincott Williams & Wilkins, 1997; Olin BR (ed): Facts and Comparisons. Philadelphia, JB Lippincott, 1993; Murray BN, Peterson LJ: Unpublished observations. Additional Values in Wendland BE, Arbus GS: Oral fluid therapy: Sodium and potassium content and osmolality of some commercial soups, juices and beverages. Can Med Assoc J 121:564, 1979.)

TABLE 726–8 Method for Conversion of Milligrams to Milliequivalents per Liter (or to Millimoles per Liter)

mg = milligrams mL = milliliter

g = grams 1 mL = 1.000027 cc

dL = deciliter = 100 mL

$$\text{mEq/L (milliequivalents per liter)} = \frac{\text{mg/L}}{\text{equivalent weight}}$$

$$\text{Equivalent weight} = \frac{\text{atomic weight}}{\text{valence of element}}$$

For example: A sample of blood serum contains 10 mg of Ca in 1 dL (100 mL)

The valence of Ca is 2, and the atomic weight is 40. The equivalent weight of Ca is therefore 40 ÷ 2, or 20. The milliequivalents of Ca per liter are 10 (mg/dL) × 10 (dL/L) ÷ 20, or 5 milliequivalents per liter.

$$\text{mM/L (millimoles per liter)} = \frac{\text{mg/L}}{\text{molecular weight}}$$

Vol. % (volume per cent) = mM/L × 2.24 for a gas whose properties approach that of an ideal gas, such as oxygen or nitrogen. For carbon dioxide, the factor is 2.226.

TABLE 726–9 Factors for Conversion of Concentration Expressed in Milliequivalents per Liter to Milligrams per Deciliter (100 mL), and Vice Versa, for Common Ions That Occur in Physiologic Solutions

Element or Radical	mEq/L to mg/dL		mg/dL to mEq/L	
Sodium	1	2.30	1	0.4348
Potassium	1	3.91	1	0.2558
Calcium	1	2.005	1	0.4988
Magnesium	1	1.215	1	0.8230
Chloride	1	3.55	1	0.2817
Bicarbonate (HCO_3^-)	1	6.1	1	0.1639
Phosphorus valence 1	1	3.10	1	0.3226
Phosphorus valence 1.8	1	1.72	1	0.5814
Sulfur valence 2	1	1.60	1	0.625

Example: *to convert milliequivalents of magnesium per liter to milligrams per deciliter (100 mL), multiply by the factor 1.215; to convert milligrams of potassium per deciliter (100 mL) to milliequivalents per liter, multiply by the factor 0.2558.*

TABLE 726–10 Milliequivalents and Milligrams of Cations and Anions Present in a Millimole of Salts Commonly Used in Physiologic Solutions

Salt	mg/mmol Salt	Cation	mEq/mmol Salt	mg/mmol Salt	Anion	mEq/mmol Salt	mg/mmol Salt
Sodium chloride (NaCl)	58.5	Na^+	1	23.0	Cl^-	1	35.5
Potassium chloride (KCl)	74.6	K^+	1	39.1	Cl^-	1	35.5
Sodium bicarbonate ($NaHCO_3$)	84.0	Na^+	1	23.0	HCO_3^-	1	61.0
Sodium lactate ($CH_3CHOHCOONa$)	112.0	Na^+	1	23.0	$CH_3CHOHCOO^-$	1	89.0
Potassium phosphate monobasic (K_2HPO_4)	174.2	K^+	2	78.2	HPO_4^{2-}	2	96.0
Potassium phosphate dibasic (KH_2PO_4)	136.1	K^+	1	39.1	$H_2PO_4^-$	1	97.0
Calcium chloride, anhydrous ($CaCl_2$)	111.0	Ca^{2+}	2	40.0	Cl_2^{2-}	2	71.0
Calcium chloride dihydrate ($CaCl_2 \cdot 2H_2O$)	147.0	Ca^{2+}	2	40.0	Cl_2^{2-}	2	71.0
Magnesium chloride, anhydrous ($MgCl_2$)	95.2	Mg^{2+}	2	24.3	Cl_2^{2-}	2	71.0
Magnesium chloride hexahydrate ($MgCl_2 \cdot 6H_2O$)	203.3	Mg^{2+}	2	24.3	Cl_2^{2-}	2	71.0
Ammonium chloride (NH_4Cl)	53.5	NH_4^+	1	18.0	Cl^-	1	35.5

TABLE 726–11 Food Composition for Short Method of Dietary Analysis (Lewis A. Barness and John S. Curran)*

Food and Approximate Measure	Weight *g*	Food Energy *kcal*	Protein *g*	Fat *g*	Carbo-hydrate *g*	Calcium *mg*	Iron *mg*	Vitamin A *IU*	Thiamine *mg*	Ribo-flavin *mg*	Niacin *mg*	Ascorbic Acid *mg*
Milk, Cheese, Cream; Related Products												
Cheese: blue, cheddar (1 cu in, 17 g), cheddar process (1 oz), Swiss (1 oz)	30	105	6	9	1	165	0.2	345	0.01	0.12	Trace	0
cottage (from skim) creamed (½ c)	115	120	16	5	3	105	0.4	190	0.04	0.28	0.1	0
Cream: half-and-half (cream and milk) (2 tbsp)	30	40	1	4	2	30	Trace	145	0.01	0.04	Trace	Trace
For light whipping add 1 pat butter												
Milk: whole (3.5% fat) (1 c)	245	160	9	9	12	285	0.1	350	0.08	0.42	0.1	2
fluid, nonfat (skim) and buttermilk (from skim)	245	90	9	Trace	13	300	Trace	—	0.10	0.44	0.2	2
milk beverage (1 c): cocoa, chocolate drink made with skim milk. For malted milk add 4 tbsp half-and-half (270 g)	245	210	8	8	26	280	0.6	300	0.09	0.43	0.3	Trace
milk desserts, custard (1 c) 248 g, ice cream (8 fl oz) 142 g		290	8	17	29	210	0.4	785	0.07	0.34	0.1	1
cornstarch pudding (248 g), ice milk (1 c) 187 g		280	9	10	40	290	0.1	390	0.08	0.41	0.3	2
White sauce, med (½ c)	130	215	5	16	12	150	0.2	610	0.06	0.22	0.3	Trace
Egg: 1 Large	50	80	6	6	Trace	25	1.2	590	0.06	0.15	Trace	0
Meat, Poultry, Fish, Shellfish, Related Products												
Beef, lamb, veal: lean and fat, cooked, inc. corned beef (3 oz) (all cuts)	85	245	22	16	0	10	2.9	25	0.06	0.19	4.2	0
lean only, cooked; dried beef (2+ oz) (all cuts)	65	140	20	5	0	10	2.4	10	0.05	0.16	3.4	0
Beef, relatively fat, such as steak and rib, cooked (3 oz)	85	350	18	30	0	10	2.4	60	0.05	0.14	3.5	0
Liver: beef, fried (2 oz)	55	130	15	6	3	5	5.0	30,280	0.15	2.37	9.4	15
Pork, lean and fat, cooked (3 oz) (all cuts)	85	325	20	24	0	10	2.6	0	0.62	0.20	4.2	0
lean only, cooked (2+ oz) (all cuts)	60	150	18	8	0	5	2.2	0	0.57	0.19	3.2	0
ham, light cure, lean and fat, roasted (3 oz)	85	245	18	19	0	10	2.2	0	0.40	0.16	3.1	0
Luncheon meats: bologna (2 sl), pork sausage, cooked (2 oz), frankfurter (1), bacon, broiled or fried crisp (3 sl)		185	9	16	—	5	1.3	—	0.21	0.12	1.7	0
Poultry												
chicken: flesh only, broiled (3 oz)	85	115	20	3	0	10	1.4	80	0.05	0.16	7.4	0
fried (2+ oz)	75	170	24	6	1	10	1.6	85	0.05	0.23	8.3	0
turkey, light and dark, roasted (3 oz)	85	160	27	5	0	—	1.5	—	0.03	0.15	6.5	0
Fish and shellfish												
salmon (3 oz) (canned)	85	130	17	5	0	165	0.7	60	0.03	0.16	6.8	0
fish sticks, breaded, cooked (3–4)	75	130	13	7	5	10	0.3	—	0.03	0.05	1.2	0
mackerel, halibut, cooked	85	175	19	10	0	10	0.8	313	0.08	0.15	6.8	0
bluefish, haddock, herring, perch, shad, cooked (tuna canned in oil, 20 g)	85	160	19	8	2	20	1.0	60	0.06	0.11	4.4	0
clams, canned; crab meat, canned; lobster; oyster, raw; scallop; shrimp, canned	85	75	14	1	2	65	2.5	65	0.10	0.08	1.5	0
Mature Dry Beans and Peas, Nuts, Peanuts, Related Products												
Beans: white with pork and tomato, canned (1 c)	260	320	16	7	50	140	4.7	340	0.20	0.08	1.5	5
red (128 g), lima (96 g), cowpeas (125 g), cooked (½ c)		125	8	—	25	35	2.5	5	0.13	0.06	0.7	—
Nuts: almonds (12), cashews (8), peanuts (1 tbsp), peanut butter (1 tbsp), pecans (12), English walnuts (2 tbsp), coconut (¼ c)	15	95	3	8	4	15	0.5	5	0.05	0.9	—	
Vegetables and Vegetable Products												
Asparagus, cooked, cut spears (⅔ c)	115	25	3	Trace	4	25	0.7	1,055	0.19	0.20	1.6	30
Beans: green (½ c) cooked 60 g; canned 120 g		15	1	Trace	3	30	0.4	340	0.04	0.06	0.3	8
Lima, immature, cooked (½ c)	80	90	6	1	16	40	2.0	225	0.14	0.08	1.0	14
Broccoli spears, cooked (⅔ c)	100	25	3	Trace	4	90	0.8	2,500	0.09	0.20	0.8	90
Brussels sprouts, cooked (⅔ c)	85	30	3	Trace	5	30	1.0	450	0.07	0.12	0.7	75
Cabbage (110 g); cauliflower, cooked (80 g); and sauerkraut, canned (150 mg) (reduce ascorbic acid value by one third for kraut) (⅔ c)		20	1	Trace	4	35	0.5	80	0.05	0.05	0.3	37
Carrots, cooked (⅔ c)	95	30	1	Trace	7	30	0.6	10,145	0.05	0.05	0.5	6
Corn, 1 ear, cooked (140 g); canned (130 g) (½ c)		75	2	Trace	18	5	0.4	315	0.06	0.06	1.1	6
Leafy greens: collards (125 g), dandelions (120 g), kale (75 g), mustard (95 g), spinach (120 g), turnip (100 g cooked, 150 g canned) (⅔ c cooked and canned) (reduce ascorbic acid one half for canned)		30	3	Trace	5	175	1.8	8,570	0.11	0.18	0.8	45
Peas, green (½ c)	80	60	4	1	10	20	1.4	430	0.22	0.09	1.8	16

Table continued on following page

TABLE 726–11 Food Composition for Short Method of Dietary Analysis (Lewis A. Barness and John S. Curran)* *Continued*

Food and Approximate Measure	Weight *g*	Food Energy *kcal*	Protein *g*	Fat *g*	Carbo-hydrate *g*	Calcium *mg*	Iron *mg*	Vitamin A *IU*	Thiamine *mg*	Ribo-flavin *mg*	Niacin *mg*	Ascorbic Acid *mg*
Vegetables and Vegetable Products *Continued*												
Potatoes, baked, boiled (100 g), 10 pc.		85	3	Trace	30	10	0.7	Trace	0.08	0.04	1.5	16
French fried (55 g) (for fried, add 1 tbsp cooking oil)												
Pumpkin, canned (½ c)	115	40	1	1	9	30	0.5	7,295	0.03	0.06	0.6	6
Squash, winter, canned (½ c)	100	65	2	1	16	30	0.8	4,305	0.05	0.14	0.7	14
Sweet potato, canned (½ c)	110	120	2	—	27	25	0.8	8,500	0.05	0.05	0.7	15
Tomato, 1 raw, ⅔ c canned, ⅔ c juice	150	35	2	Trace	7	14	0.8	1,350	0.10	0.06	1.0	29
Tomato catsup (2 tbsp)	35	30	1	Trace	8	10	0.2	480	0.04	0.02	0.6	6
Other, cooked (beets, mushrooms, onions, turnips) (½ c)	95	25	1	—	5	20	0.5	15	0.02	0.10	0.7	7
Other, commonly served raw, cabbage (½ c, 50 g), celery (3 sm stalks, 40 g), cucumber (¼ med, 50 g), green pepper (½, 30 g), radishes (5, 40 g)		10	Trace	Trace	2	15	0.3	100	0.03	0.03	0.2	20
carrots, raw (½ carrot)	25	10	Trace	Trace	2	10	0.2	2,750	0.02	0.02	0.2	2
lettuce leaves (2 lg)	50	10	1	Trace	2	34	0.7	950	0.03	0.04	0.2	9
Fruits and Fruit Products												
Cantaloupe (½ med)	385	60	1	Trace	14	25	0.8	6,540	0.08	0.06	1.2	63
Citrus and strawberries: orange (1), grapefruit (½), juice (½ c), strawberries (½ c), lemon (1), tangerine (1)		50	1	—	13	25	0.4	165	0.08	0.03	0.3	55
Yellow, fresh: apricots (3), peach (2 med); canned fruit and juice (½ c) or dried, cooked, unsweetened: apricot, peaches (½ c)		85	—	—	22	10	1.1	1,005	0.01	0.05	1.0	5
Other, dried: dates, pitted (4), figs (2), raisins (¼ c)	40	120	1	—	31	35	1.4	20	0.04	0.04	0.5	—
Other, fresh apple (1), banana (1), figs (3), pear (1)		80	—	—	21	15	0.5	140	0.04	0.03	0.2	6
Grain Products												
Enriched and whole grain: bread (1 sl, 23 g), biscuit (½), cooked cereals (½ c), prepared cereals (1 oz), Graham crackers (2 lg), macaroni, noodles, spaghetti (½ c, cooked), pancake (1, 27 g), roll (½), waffle (½, 38 g)		65	2	1	16	20	0.6	10	0.09	0.05	0.7	—
Unenriched bread (1 sl, 23 g), cooked cereal (½ c), macaroni, noodles, spaghetti (½ c), popcorn (½ c), pretzel sticks, small (15), roll (½)		65	2	1	16	10	0.3	5	0.02	0.02	0.3	—
Desserts												
Cake, plain (1 pc), doughnut (1). For iced cake or doughnut add value for sugar (1 tbsp). For chocolate cake add chocolate (30 g)	45	145	2	5	24	30	0.4	65	0.02	0.05	0.2	—
Cookies, plain (1)	25	120	1	5	18	10	0.2	20	0.01	0.01	0.1	—
Pie crust, single crust (1/7 shell)	20	95	1	6	8	3	0.3	0	0.04	0.03	0.3	—
Flour, white, enriched (1 tbsp)	7	25	1	Trace	5	1	0.2	0	0.03	0.02	0.2	0
Fats and Oils												
Butter, margarine (1 pat, ½ tbsp)	7	50	Trace	6	Trace	1	0	230	—	—	—	—
Fats and oils, cooking (1 tbsp), French dressing (2 tbsp)	14	125	0	14	0	0	0	0	0	0	0	0
Salad dressings, mayonnaise type (1 tbsp)	15	80	Trace	9	1	2	0.1	45	Trace	Trace	Trace	0
Sugars, Sweets												
Candy, plain (½ oz), jam and jelly (1 tbsp), syrup (1 tbsp), gelatin dessert, plain (½ c), beverages, carbonated (1 c)		60	0	0	14	3	0.1	Trace	Trace	Trace	Trace	Trace
Chocolate fudge (1 oz), chocolate syrup (3 tbsp)		125	1	2	30	15	0.6	10	Trace	0.02	0.1	Trace
Molasses (1 tbsp), caramel (½ oz)		40	Trace	Trace	8	20	0.3	Trace	Trace	Trace	Trace	Trace
Sugar (1 tbsp)	12	45	0	0	12	0	Trace	0	0	0	0	0
Miscellaneous												
Chocolate, bitter (1 oz)	30	145	3	15	8	20	1.9	20	0.01	0.07	0.4	0
Sherbet (½ c)	96	130	1	1	30	15	Trace	55	0.01	0.03	Trace	2
Soups												
Bean, pea (green) (1 c)		150	7	4	22	50	1.6	495	0.09	0.06	1.0	4
Noodle, beef, chicken (1 c)		65	4	2	7	10	0.7	50	0.03	0.04	0.9	Trace
Clam chowder, minestrone, tomato, vegetable (1 c)		90	3	2	14	25	0.9	1,880	0.05	0.04	1.1	3

**See related conversion Tables 726–8 to 726–10.*

(From Wilson ED, Fisher KH, Fuqua ME: Principles of Nutrition, 2nd ed. New York, John Wiley & Sons, 1965, pp 528–533.)

TABLE 726–12 Nutritive Value of Baby Foods (Per Serving)*

Food	Serving g	Energy kcal	Protein g	Fat g	Carbo-hydrate g	Sodium mg	Calcium mg	Iron mg	Vitamin A IU	Thiamine mg	Ribo-flavin mg	Niacin mg	Ascorbic Acid mg
Cereals													
Barley	2.4	9	0.3	0.1	1.8	1	19	1.1		0.07	0.07	0.9	0
High protein	2.4	9	0.9	0.1	1.1	1	17	1.8		0.06	0.07	0.8	0
Mixed	2.4	9	0.3	0.1	1.8	1	18	1.5		0.06	0.07	0.8	0
Oatmeal	2.4	10	0.3	0.2	1.7	1	18	1.8		0.07	0.06	0.9	0
Rice	2.4	9	0.2	0.1	1.9	1	20	1.8		0.06	0.05	0.8	0
Dinners, Jar													
Beef and egg noodle	213	122	5.4	4.0	15.7	37	18	0.9	1,400	0.06	0.08	1.2	3
Chicken and noodles, jr.	213	109	4.1	3.0	16.1	36	36	0.8	1,900	0.06	0.07	1.1	3
Macaroni and ham, jr.	213	127	6.8	2.9	18.0	101	159	0.8	1,100	0.12	0.21	1.7	5
Turkey and rice, jr.	213	104	3.8	2.9	15.3	33	50	0.6	2,200	0.02	0.06	0.6	3
Spaghetti, tomato, beef, jr.	213	135	5.4	2.7	21.6	42	39	1.1	1,500	0.14	0.15	2.3	5
Fruits													
Applesauce, jr.	213	79	0.1	0.0	21.9	5	10	0.4	20	0.03	0.06	0.1	81
Applesauce, apricots, jr.	220	104	0.5	0.5	27.3	6	13	0.6	745	0.03	0.07	0.3	39
Bananas, tapioca, jr.	220	147	0.8	0.4	39.1	21	17	0.7	100	0.03	0.04	0.5	57
Peaches	220	157	1.3	0.4	41.6	10	11	0.6	400	0.03	0.07	1.4	42
Pears	213	93	0.6	0.2	24.7	4	18	0.5	70	0.03	0.06	0.4	47
Meats, Poultry													
Beef	99	105	14.3	4.9	0	65	8	1.6	100	0.01	0.16	3.3	2
Chicken	99	148	14.6	9.5	0	50	54	1.0	200	0.01	0.16	3.4	2
Ham	99	123	14.9	6.6	0	66	5	1.0	30	0.14	0.19	2.8	2
Lamb	99	111	15.0	5.2	2.5	73	7	1.6	30	0.02	0.20	3.2	2
Turkey	99	128	15.2	7.0	0	72	28	1.3	600	0.02	0.25	3.4	2
Egg Yolks	94	191	9.4	16.3	0.9	37	72	2.6	1,200	0.07	0.25	1.45	1
Vegetables													
Beans	206	51	2.5	0.3	11.8	3	133	2.2	900	0.04	0.21	0.7	17
Beets	128	43	1.7	0.1	9.8	106	18	0.4	40	0.01	0.06	0.2	4
Carrots	213	67	1.7	0.4	15.4	104	49	0.8	25,000	0.05	0.09	1.1	12
Mixed	213	88	3.1	0.8	17.4	77	24	0.9	9,000	0.06	0.07	1.4	5
Peas	213	113	7.0	1.1	19.0	15	34	1.9	700	0.15	0.13	2.0	9
Squash	213	51	1.8	0.4	12.0	3	50	0.7	4,000	0.02	0.14	0.8	17
Sweet potatoes	220	113	2.4	0.3	30.7	49	35	0.8	15,000	0.06	0.08	0.8	21

**See related conversion Tables 726–6 to 726–8.*
(Data from Pennington JAT (ed): Bowes and Church's Food Values of Portions Commonly Used, 15th ed. New York, Harper & Row, 1989.)

TABLE 726–13 Equivalent Temperature Readings (Celsius and Fahrenheit)*

C	F	C	F	C	F	C	F
0	32.0	37.2	99	39.2	102.6	41.2	106.2
20	68.0	37.4	99.3	39.4	102.9	41.4	106.5
30	86.0	37.6	99.7	39.6	103.3	41.6	106.9
31	87.8	37.8	100.1	39.8	103.7	41.8	107.2
32	89.6	38.0	100.4	40.0	104	42	107.6
33	91.4	38.2	100.8	40.2	104.4	43	109.4
34	93.2	38.4	101.2	40.4	104.7	44	111.2
35	95.0	38.6	101.5	40.6	105.1	100	212
36	96.8	38.8	101.8	40.8	105.4		
37	98.6	39.0	102.2	41.0	105.8		

**To convert Celsius (centigrade) readings to Fahrenheit, multiply by 1.8 and add 32. To convert Fahrenheit readings to Celsius, subtract 32 and divide by 1.8.*

CHAPTER 727

Principles of Drug Therapy

Michael D. Reed and Peter Gal

Clinical pharmacology is concerned with the integration of a drug's pharmacokinetic and pharmacodynamic profile to optimize drug therapy. *Pharmacokinetics* is the quantitative evaluation of each component of a compound's disposition—that is, the processes of absorption, distribution, metabolism, and excretion. The ability to estimate a drug's pharmacokinetic parameters accurately permits the determination of the dose and dose interval to achieve a defined target concentration, desired pharmacologic effect, or both. A drug concentration in a specific body fluid is, in theory, a reflection of the drug concentration in tissue, reflecting its concentration at its site of action, the receptor. A drug's concentration in blood (or other body fluid), however, is not necessarily equal to the drug's concentration in tissue or at its receptor site. It is important to appreciate the challenges involved in determining drug concentrations in body fluids, including physical access of that body fluid, available volume that can be safely removed, and the sensitivity and specificity of available laboratory methodology.

Pharmacodynamics involves the correlation of pharmacologic response to a measured drug concentration in blood (or other body fluid) that reflects the drug concentration at the receptor

TABLE 727–1 Physiologic Factors That Influence the Oral Absorption of Medications

Parameter	Neonate	Infant	Child
Gastric acid secretion	Reduced	Normal	Normal
Gastric emptying time	Decreased	Increased	Increased
Intestinal motility	Reduced	Normal	Normal
Biliary function	Reduced	Normal	Normal
Microbial flora	Acquiring	Adult pattern	Adult pattern

site. The pharmacologic or toxicologic effects of most drugs are a result of their interaction with micro- and macro-molecular components of cells. Rational prescribing of drugs depends on a fundamental understanding of a drug's pharmacokinetic and pharmacodynamic profile. Understanding the effect of age is essential to understanding pediatric drug therapy, because age is one of the most important variables that influences the processes responsible for a drug's disposition and action in children.

INFLUENCE OF AGE ON DRUG THERAPY. Drugs administered extravascularly must cross many physiologic membranes before entering the systemic circulation and being distributed to their site of action.

Gastrointestinal Absorption. Although certain xenobiotics and nutrients are absorbed by active transport or facilitated diffusion, most drugs are absorbed from the gastrointestinal tract by passive diffusion. A number of important patient variables can affect the rate and extent of a drug's gastrointestinal absorption, including pH-dependent diffusion; the presence, absence, and type of gastric contents; gastric emptying time; and gastrointestinal motility. These physiologic processes reflect a clear but highly variable dependence on a patient's age (Table 727–1). Despite the clear maturational changes observed in the functional capacity of these processes and their importance to intestinal drug absorption, the overall bioavailability of most orally administered medications in neonates and young infants is adequate. Whenever possible, the oral route for drug administration is preferred.

Alternative Routes of Drug Absorption. Another common means of extravascular drug administration in infants and children, other than the oral route, is the intramuscular route. Drugs administered intramuscularly should be water-soluble at physiologic pH to prevent precipitation and the resultant decreased, delayed, or erratic absorption from the injection site. Lipid solubility of a drug favors diffusion into the capillaries. Blood flow to and from the injection site should be adequate to ensure absorption into the systemic circulation. This physiologic requirement may be compromised in seriously ill infants and children with poor peripheral perfusion resulting from low cardiac output and respiratory disease.

The skin is another important but often overlooked organ for the absorption of various therapeutic agents and environmental chemicals. This is exemplified by the toxic effects noted in newborn infants exposed to hexachlorophene, aniline-containing disinfectant solutions, and hydrocortisone. The percutaneous absorption of a compound is directly related to the degree of skin hydration and inversely related to the thickness of the stratum corneum. The full-term newborn's integument is a more effective functional barrier than the skin of a premature infant. More importantly, however, the ratio of the newborn's skin surface area to body weight is approximately three times greater than that of an adult. Therefore, the amount of drug absorbed into the systemic circulation (bioavailability) for an identical percutaneous dose of a drug is approximately three times greater in an infant than in an adult. These characteristics of skin make topical creams and patch formulation of drugs important means of drug delivery in infants with adequate perfusion.

The effects of maturational changes on the bioavailability of a drug are unpredictable. A prolonged gastric emptying time and irregular intestinal peristaltic activity can lead to erratic rates of drug absorption, reducing the amount of drug absorbed, blunting or delaying the peak serum concentration, or both. Reducing the rate or amount of total drug absorbed into the body (or both) can be therapeutically important, leading to inadequate dosing, whereas blunting or delaying a drug's peak serum concentration may be of only minor clinical significance. The extent to which maturational changes influence gastrointestinal drug absorption also depends on the specific drug formulation administered. Solid dosage forms (tablets, capsules) must dissolve into solution before the drug can cross cell membranes. Most drugs administered to infants and young children are available in a liquid formulation, some as a suspension. In general, the rate of absorption is faster after administration of a liquid dosing formulation (liquid $>$ suspension) as compared with solid formulations (capsule $\geq$ tablet $>$ sustained/delayed-release tablet).

Drug Distribution. Understanding a drug's distribution characteristics in the body is important when selecting the dose. Although a drug's distribution volume (apparent volume of distribution, V_d) does not denote any real physiologic volume, an estimate of this pharmacokinetic parameter provides insight into the total amount of drug present in the body relative to its concentration in blood and thus the tissue distribution. Knowledge of a drug's V_d is important when selecting an initial loading dose or designing an optimal drug dosage regimen to attain a pre-selected target concentration. The value of the V_d for a number of drugs differs markedly among newborns (premature vs. full-term), infants, and children as compared with adults. These differences are a result of many important age-dependent variables, including the composition and size of body water compartments, protein binding characteristics, and hemodynamic factors, including cardiac output, regional blood flow, and membrane permeability. The absolute amounts and distribution of body water and fat depend on a child's age and are well characterized. Changes in body water compartment sizes and water distribution account for the differences observed in the V_d in infants and children.

The extent to which a drug is bound to circulating plasma proteins directly influences the distribution characteristics of the drug. Only the free, unbound drug can be distributed from the vascular space into other body fluids and tissues, where it binds to its receptor and stimulates a response. Drug binding to plasma proteins depends on a number of age-related variables, including the absolute amount of proteins available, their respective number of available binding sites, the affinity constant of the drug for the protein, the influence of pathophysiologic conditions, and the presence of endogenous substances, which may compete for protein binding (protein displacement interactions). These and other clinically important variables can affect drug protein binding relative to age. The extent to which a drug is bound to protein markedly influences its V_d and body clearance (Cl) as well as intensity of pharmacologic effects.

Albumin, α_1–acid glycoprotein, and lipoproteins are the most important circulating proteins responsible for drug binding in plasma. The absolute concentration of these proteins is influenced by age, nutrition, and disease. Basic drugs bind mainly to albumin, α_1–acid glycoprotein, and lipoprotein, whereas acidic and neutral compounds bind primarily to albumin. Serum albumin and total protein concentrations are decreased during infancy, approaching adult values by the age of 10–12 mo. A similar pattern of maturation is observed with α_1–acid glycoprotein; concentrations appear to be approximately three times lower in neonatal plasma compared with those in maternal plasma, achieving values comparable to those of adults by 12 mo of age.

In addition to drugs, several endogenous substances presenting in human plasma may bind to plasma proteins and compete for available drug-binding sites. During the neonatal period, free fatty acids, bilirubin, and 2-hydroxybenzoylglycine compete for albumin binding sites and influence the resultant balance between free and bound drug concentrations. Clinically significant protein binding displacement reactions occur only when a drug is more than 80–90% protein-bound, the drug's Cl is limited, and its apparent V_d is small, usually less than 0.15 L/kg. It is prudent to assess a drug's potential for displacement of bilirubin from protein-binding sites prior to its administration to premature and newborn infants.

Drug Metabolism. The moment a drug molecule is present within the body, the process of its removal begins. The overall rate of drug removal is described by the pharmacokinetic parameter clearance (Cl), or body Cl. A drug's body Cl is the summation of all clearance mechanisms involved in removing that compound from the body (see later, Clearance). The primary organ for drug metabolism is the liver, although the kidney, intestine, lung, adrenals, blood (phosphatases, esterases), and skin can also biotransform certain compounds. For most drugs (lipophilic weak acids or weak bases), biotransformation to more polar, water-soluble compounds facilitates their elimination from the body through the bile, kidney, or lung. Although the biotransformation of most drugs results in pharmacologically weaker or inactive compounds, parent compounds may be transformed into active metabolites or intermediates (theophylline to caffeine, carbamazepine to 10, 11-carbamazepine epoxide). Conversely, pharmacologically inactive parent compounds or prodrugs may be converted to an active moiety (chloramphenicol succinate to active chloramphenicol base, cefuroxime axetil to active cefuroxime) prior to subsequent biotransformation and body elimination.

Drug metabolism within the hepatocyte involves two primary enzymatic processes: phase I, or nonsynthetic, and phase II, or synthetic reactions. Phase I reactions include oxidation, reduction, hydrolysis, and hydroxylation reactions, whereas phase II reactions primarily involve conjugation with glycine, glucuronide, or sulfate. Most drug-metabolizing enzymes are located in the smooth endoplasmic reticulum of cells. Of these mixed-function oxidase systems, the cytochrome (CYP) P450 system has been studied in greatest detail. The CYP450 enzyme system is a supergene family with more than 13 primary enzymes and a number of isozymes of specific gene families. The specific subfamilies, or isozymes, most responsible for human drug metabolism involve CYP450 1A2, 2D6, 2C19, and 3A3/4. At birth, the concentration of drug-oxidizing enzymes in fetal liver (corrected for liver weight) is similar to that in adult liver. The activity of these oxidizing enzyme systems is reduced, however, which is reflected by a prolonged body elimination for drugs that depend on oxidation pathways in newborns (phenytoin, diazepam). Postnatally, the hepatic cytochrome P450 mono-oxygenase system appears to mature rapidly; metabolic activity similar to or in excess of the adult value is achieved by approximately 6 mo of age. An understanding of the substrates for specific isozymes and the effects certain drugs may have on isozyme activity (e.g., induction, inhibition) allows the clinician to predict the possibility of clinically important metabolic-based drug-drug interactions. Substrates, inducers, and inhibitors of specific isozymes important in human drug metabolism are outlined in Table 727–2.

The activity of certain hydrolytic enzymes, including blood esterases, is also reduced during the neonatal period. Blood esterases are important for the metabolic clearance of cocaine, and the reduced activity of these plasma esterases in the newborn may account for the delayed metabolism of cocaine in neonates.

Because elimination of metabolites is reduced in preterm and full-term infants, accumulation of active metabolites not considered clinically relevant in older infants, children, and adults may occur in infants. Such is the case with the N-methylation of theophylline to caffeine. This pathway becomes more important in neonates because theophylline is less readily metabolized, making it more available for N-methylation. Caffeine itself is normally metabolized prior to elimination, but in preterm infants with immature liver enzymes, the

TABLE 727–2 Important Cytochrome P450 Isozymes in Human Drug Metabolism: Isozyme Substrate, Inhibitors, and Inducers

Isoenzyme	Polymorphism	Substrate	Inhibitors	Inducers
1A2	Possible	Acetaminophen, caffeine, clomipramine, clozapine, imipramine, phenacetin, propranolol, tacrine, theophylline	Fluvoxamine, quinolones (e.g., ciprofloxacin)	Cruciferous vegetables, omeprazole, aromatic hydrocarbons, smoking
2C9	Yes	Diclofenac, ibuprofen, phenytoin, tolbutamide, S-warfarin	Fluconazole, isoniazid, itraconazole(?), ketoconazole(?), sulfaphenazole	Rifampin
2C19	Yes	Amitriptyline, citalopram, diazepam, imipramine, mephobarbital, olmeprazole, propranolol	Fluconazole, fluvoxamine, fluoxetine, omeprazole	Rifampin
2D6	Yes	Amitriptyline, citalopram, clomipramine, codeine, desipramine, dextromethorphan, doxepin, encainide, flecainide, fluoxetine, haloperidol, imipramine, loratadine, metoprolol, nortriptyline, paroxetine, perphenazine, propafenone, propranolol, risperidone, thioridazine, timolol, tramadol	Cimetidine, fluoxetine, norfluoxetine, nefazodone (plus metabolites), paroxetine, perphenazine, propoxyphene, quinidine, sertraline, thioridazine	
2E1	No	Acetaminophen, alcohol, chlorzoxazone, dapsone	Disulfiram, isoniazid	Ethanol, isoniazid
3A3/3A4	Possible	Alfentanil, alprazolam, amiodarone, amitriptyline, astemizole, carbamazepine, cisapride, cyclosporin, dapsone, diazepam, diltiazem, disopyramide, erythromycin, ethinylestradiol, imipramine, indinavir, lidocaine, loratadine, lovastatin, midazolam, nifedipine, nefazodone, progesterone, quinidine, ritonavir, saquinovir, tacrolimus (FK-506), terfenadine, testosterone, triazolam, verapamil	Cimetidine, citalopram, diltiazem, ethynylestradiol, fluconazole, fluvoxamine, fluoxetine, indinavir, norfluoxetine, itraconazole, ketoconazole, macrolides (clarithromycin, erythromycin), metronidazole, nefazodone, naringenin, ritanavir	Carbamazepine, dexamethasone, phenobarbital, phenytoin, rifampin

compound is mainly eliminated by the kidneys. This renal elimination is slow because of the immaturity of renal function in young infants, resulting in marked caffeine accumulation and potential toxicity.

Understanding the sequence of maturation of processes of drug metabolism is important when developing dosage recommendations for drugs that undergo extensive hepatic metabolism. An example of the consequences of failing to appreciate these processes is the tragedy that occurred after the administration of usual doses of chloramphenicol (75–100 mg/kg/24 hr) to premature and newborn infants (fatal gray-baby syndrome) and the resultant beneficial use of this compound in the same patient population when the dose was appropriately adjusted (15–50 mg/kg/24 hr) to compensate for the decreased hepatic ability for glucuronidation. Chloramphenicol glucuronide is the primary metabolite of chloramphenicol, which is then excreted through the kidneys.

The ultimate ability of children to metabolize drugs may be genetically modulated. Pharmacogenetic predisposition to slow drug metabolism along certain enzymatic pathways can provide important clues to patients at risk for drug toxicity.

Drug Excretion. The amount of drug that is filtered by the glomerulus per unit of time depends on the functional ability of the glomerulus, on the integrity of renal blood flow, and on the extent of drug-protein binding. The amount of drug filtered is inversely related to the degree of protein binding. Only the free drug is filtered by the glomerulus and excreted. Although highly variable, renal blood flow averages 12 mL/min at birth, approaching the adult value by approximately 5–12 mo of age. The glomerular filtration rate is approximately 2–4 mL/min in full-term infants, increases to approximately 8–20 mL/min by 2–3 days of life, and approaches the adult value by approximately 3–5 mo of age. Before 34 wk of gestation, glomerular filtration is markedly reduced and increases slowly.

PHARMACOKINETICS

Basic Concepts. Pharmacokinetics is the mathematical expression of the time course of drug movement in the body. It is clinically useful only when integrated with the drug's pharmacodynamic characteristics. Because the pharmacologic effects of most drugs are reversible, the time of onset, intensity, and duration of effect of a drug are proportional to the amount of drug in the body at any point in time. Pharmacokinetic-based methods can be used to predict drug concentration at any time after a dose is administered and can facilitate calculation of a drug dose to achieve a desired concentration. The recognition that a drug's pharmacologic effects, toxicologic effects, or both correlate best with its concentration in a biologic fluid (blood) rather than the absolute dose administered is the foundation of applied clinical pharmacokinetics.

The biodisposition of most drugs used clinically is best described using the principles of linear or first-order pharmacokinetics—that is, the serum concentration or, more appropriately, the amount of drug in the body is directly proportional to the dose administered. For example, if the dose of a drug that follows linear pharmacokinetics is doubled, its resultant concentration in blood (at steady state) also doubles. This characteristic of proportionality, combined with appropriate patient monitoring, is often used clinically to make adjustments in drug dosing (see later, Individualization of Drug Dose). In contrast, some drugs, such as phenytoin, salicylate, and alcohol, exhibit saturation kinetics; their elimination pathways become "saturated" and the resultant drug concentration in the blood changes disproportionately to the dose administered. Under usual clinical conditions, these drugs exhibit linear (first-order) elimination characteristics at low doses (low serum concentrations) but, as the amount of drug in the body increases with increasing dose, their elimination pathways become saturated. Such drugs are often called drugs that follow the principles of zero-order, or Michaelis-Menten, kinetics. The classic principles of elimination half-life (t1/2) and Cl do not apply to drugs that exhibit zero-order kinetics.

Drug Absorption and Bioavailability. To be effective, a drug must be absorbed from its site of administration into the systemic circulation, from where it is distributed to its site of action and eliminated from the body. Bioavailability is a measure of the amount of drug absorbed into the systemic circulation over a finite period. With few exceptions (prodrugs), a drug administered intravenously is 100% bioavailable. A drug's bioavailability is most often described as a fraction of the amount absorbed following extravascular drug administration relative to intravenous (IV) drug administration. Bioavailability is calculated as the ratio of the area under the drug concentration time curve (AUC) determined after extravascular drug administration to the drug AUC obtained after IV administration (i.e., AUC oral/AUC IV).

A drug's absorption profile is a composite that depends on both the bioavailability (amount) and the rate of absorption into the systemic circulation. A drug's rate and extent of absorption are influenced by a number of physicochemical and patient-related factors. For example, the presence of food in the stomach and duodenum can decrease the rate but generally does not affect the overall extent of absorption of many orally administered drugs. The clinical relevance of this interaction depends on whether the drug's efficacy is related to its peak serum concentration (decreased rate would blunt the peak concentration) or the total amount of drug in the body. Appreciating a drug's rate of absorption can be important in anticipating the onset of toxicologic symptoms in cases of drug overdose. In contrast, a disease or a drug interaction that results in a decrease in drug bioavailability would be expected to influence a patient's response to therapy. The concurrent administration of phenytoin and enteral tube feedings can markedly decrease phenytoin bioavailability. Such drug-food interactions may be easily overlooked as a cause of therapeutic failure.

Volume of Distribution. The V_d is the hypothetical volume of fluid in which a drug is distributed; it is a proportionality constant that relates the amount of drug in the body to its serum concentration. The apparent V_d is expressed by the equation $V_d = D/C_p$, where C_p is the peak concentration of drug following administration of the dose D. The V_d may be used to calculate the initial or loading dose (LD) of a drug needed to achieve a desired serum concentration (C_p). If a desired C_p is selected and an age-appropriate "average" V_d is known or obtained from the literature, a dose necessary to obtain that concentration can be easily calculated:

$$LD = C_p \text{ (mg/L)} \times V_d \text{ (L/Kg)} \times \text{patient's body weight (kg)}$$

Furthermore, it is apparent from this relationship that drug elimination from the body, or drug clearance, does not influence the initial or loading dose of a drug. For example, although a drug may be eliminated from the body only through the kidneys, the initial dose is the same for patients with normal renal function as for those with compromised or no renal function. The first dose of drug achieves an equilibrium concentration between body fluids and tissues.

Elimination Half-Life. A drug's elimination half-life (t1/2) is the time required for any given concentration in blood (or other biologic fluid) to decrease to half of the initial value—that is, the time required for half the amount of drug present in the fluid to be cleared. The t1/2 can be determined as t1/2 = 0.693/Kd, where Kd is equal to the slope of the terminal portion of the natural log of the linear serum concentration versus time curve. The t1/2 depends on both the drug's Cl and V_d. A more useful formula for t1/2, which reflects these important relationships, is $t1/2 = (0.693)(V_d)/Cl$. Thus, a change in t1/2 does not necessarily reflect a change in body Cl of a drug. This dependence of t1/2 on V_d is exemplified by the influence of extracorporeal membrane oxygenation (ECMO) on drug disposition. For most drugs, ECMO-induced changes are due to an increase in drug V_d rather than any change in drug Cl. Nevertheless, despite this important distinction, the t1/2 is often used clinically to adjust dosing intervals, primarily because it can easily be calculated in the clinic or at the patient's bedside. A drug's t1/2 can also be used to determine the time necessary to achieve the steady-state concentration—that is, the point at which the amount of drug administered (dose) is equivalent to the amount of drug cleared from the body. After three half-lives, 87.5% of a drug's steady-state concentration is achieved; after four half-lives, it is 93.8%; and after five half-lives, it is 100%. When integrated with a target concentration strategy, a drug's t1/2 is often used to determine a drug's dosage interval.

Clearance. Clearance (Cl) is the pharmacokinetic parameter that estimates the theoretical volume from which a drug is removed per unit of time. A drug's body clearance reflects the amount of drug removed or eliminated from the body per unit of time, whereas renal Cl reflects the amount of drug cleared by the kidneys per unit of time. Total body Cl is the summation of all Cl mechanisms for a given drug (Cl renal, Cl hepatic, Cl lung). The body Cl can be calculated as $Cl = (0.693)(V_d)/t1/2$ with the preferred mathematical method of drug dose/AUC where the dose is corrected for bioavailability. Knowledge of a drug's Cl is fundamental when determining the need for a drug and how often its dose must be repeated to maintain a given serum concentration. It is the most important pharmacokinetic parameter for determining the steady-state drug concentration for a given dose rate. Changes in organ function responsible for the removal of a drug from the body are reflected as a change in the drug Cl. A drug's body Cl is influenced by the integrity of blood flow and by the functional ability of the organs involved in removing the drug from the body.

INDIVIDUALIZATION OF DRUG DOSE. The clinical response to an average or usual recommended dose of drug can vary considerably, even when the dose is administered relative to a patient's body weight, surface area, and stage of maturation. This variation is a result of interindividual differences in drug pharmacokinetics and pharmacodynamics and a number of biologic variables, including genetic differences in metabolism and concurrent pathophysiology. Individual variability with respect to drug efficacy and possibly toxicity frequently necessitates the adjustment of dosage regimens for specific patients, especially when prescribing drugs with a low therapeutic index. For some drugs the dose may be adjusted according to the patient's immediate and readily quantifiable clinical response. For other drugs, dosage adjustment may be guided more appropriately by combining clinical response with measuring the concentration of drug in plasma or serum. Such an approach to therapy is often called a *target concentration strategy,* where a drug's pharmacologic or toxicologic response can be directly related to a specific serum concentration range.

Reported therapeutic concentration ranges for drugs are usually determined from studies of only a limited number of patients, mostly adults, and these therapeutic ranges represent an average (mean) value, and therefore only 49% of the population is encompassed within the two standard deviations that surround this mean value. Thus, the clinical monitoring of serum drug concentrations serves only as a guide to pharmacologic intervention and dose adjustment. Serum drug concentration values must be interpreted individually for each patient. For example, one patient may have a complete clinical response when the serum concentration of drug X is within the "low" portion of the therapeutic range or window. Conversely, the next patient, with the same disease of similar severity requiring the same drug X, may require a serum drug concentration above or below the reported therapeutic concentration range to achieve the same degree of positive therapeutic response. Toxicity, however, may limit how much above the therapeutic range the serum drug concentration may safely be raised. Therefore, therapeutic ranges for serum drug concentrations serve only as guidelines for therapy. Drug efficacy must be assessed by clinical response.

Serum drug concentration-time values or profiles may also be compared with previously determined patient-specific values or literature reports to assess patient compliance with a prescribed drug regimen. More commonly, the determination of a drug concentration in biologic fluid helps to achieve an optimal therapeutic regimen while reducing the likelihood of drug toxicity. Finally, the determination of a drug concentration in a biologic fluid provides a means to assess the influences, if any, of disease process or drug interaction on a drug's disposition profile.

Therapeutic drug monitoring is not appropriate, necessary, or practical for all drugs. Drugs with well-defined and easily recognizable and monitored pharmacodynamic effects do not warrant routine monitoring (diuresis with diuretics, lowering of blood pressure by an antihypertensive). For therapeutic drug monitoring to be of clinical value, a clear concentration-response or -toxicity relationship should be identifiable. Patient age and the extent or severity of disease can influence the relationships among drug concentration, efficacy, and toxicity. Unfortunately, a clear relationship between a specific serum drug concentration and effect is available for only a limited number of drugs in contrast with the large number of drugs with "recommended" therapeutic ranges.

A number of variables should be considered when designing strategies to monitor therapy using a serum drug concentration. When measuring a drug's concentration in blood, the pharmacokinetic characteristics of that drug must be recalled so that blood samples can be obtained at appropriate times in relation to administration of the drug. This permits proper interpretation of drug concentrations and therapeutic effects and helps avoid serious therapeutic errors. Peak drug concentrations in blood usually do not refer to the highest concentration achieved in blood with that drug but usually to the post-distribution peak drug concentration. Thus, a lag time often exists between the time of drug administration and the time that is recommended to obtain the "peak" blood sample. Also, most clinical determinations of drug concentrations in biologic fluids routinely measure (report) the total drug concentration in that fluid (free drug concentration plus concentration of drug bound to protein equals total drug concentration). This approach assumes a constant ratio of free to bound drug at various concentrations and under differing pathophysiologic conditions, which may not always be true; thus, caution must be exercised in its extrapolation. For example, clinically important imbalances between free and total drug concentrations have been observed with the drug phenytoin in critically ill trauma patients and in patients with severe renal disease. As a result, many laboratories are now beginning to report both free *and* total serum concentrations of drugs or have these results available on request. Despite these differences, it is generally unusual for an imbalance in this ratio to be clinically significant, except for those drugs whose protein binding, under normal circumstances, is greater than 90%.

Chronopharmacology is the effect of biologic rhythms on drug disposition and response. Many drugs are influenced pharmacokinetically and pharmacodynamically by this phenomenon. It is important to be aware of these situations and to time doses and blood sample collections appropriately.

ADDITIONAL CONSIDERATIONS

Method of Drug Administration. It is often assumed that drugs administered intravenously are administered rapidly and completely. Neither is always true. The length of time necessary to infuse the total dose of an intravenously administered drug depends on a number of factors, including the flow rate of the primary IV fluid, the dead space of the system into which the drug is injected, and the total volume in which the drug is diluted. Because most standard IV fluid delivery systems, including their tubing, are designed for adult use, they contain a large volume/unit of length. This introduces a relatively large dead space factor, which causes substantial infusion delays when operated at the slow flow rates necessary for infants and children.

Several steps can be taken to minimize problems with IV drug administration to small infants and children. These include the following: standardization and documentation of the total administration time; documentation of the volume and content of the solution used to "flush" an IV dose; standardization of specific infusion techniques (infusion duration, volumes) for drugs with a narrow therapeutic index; standardization of dilution and infusion volumes for drugs given by intermittent IV injection; avoidance of attaching lines for drug infusion to a central hub with other solutions infused concurrently at widely disparate rates; preferential use of large-gauge cannula; maintenance of the recommended solution at a specified height above the infusion site for use with a gravity-based controller; and the use of low-volume tubing and the most distal sites for access of the drug into an existing IV line.

Drug-Drug Interactions. When two or more drugs are administered to the same patient, the pharmacokinetic and pharmacodynamic properties of each agent may be modified by their combined interaction. Drugs may interact by a number of different mechanisms; these may be classified on the basis of pharmaceutics, pharmacokinetics, pharmacodynamics, or a combination thereof. These interactions may result in unpredictable clinical effects or toxicologic responses. Pharmaceutic interactions include those resulting in drug inactivation when compounds are mixed together physically prior to patient administration as in syringes, infusion tubing, or parenteral fluid preparations.

Pharmacokinetic interactions can occur when the disposition characteristics of one compound (absorption, distribution, metabolism, excretion, or a combination thereof) are influenced by those of another. This type of interaction may involve one or more aspects of a drug's pharmacokinetic profile. One drug may reduce the rate but not the overall extent of absorption, or a compound may displace a drug from its protein binding sites while concomitantly retarding its elimination from the body. Metabolic-based drug-drug interactions can occur whenever two compounds compete for the same metabolic site as described earlier and outlined in Table 727–2.

Drugs may interact pharmacodynamically and compete for the same receptor or physiologic system, thus altering a patient's response to drug therapy. The number of known, clinically important drug interactions, combined with the ever-increasing number of available pharmacologic agents, emphasizes the need to critically assess the possibility or presence of drug-drug interactions in any patient receiving multiple drugs.

Drugs in Human Milk. Almost all drugs administered to lactating women are secreted to some extent into their milk and may be ingested by the nursing infant. In general, drug use should be as minimal as possible during lactation; a few drugs have been reported to affect the nursing infant adversely (see Chapter 90). Obviously, it is not possible or desirable for lactating women to stop taking needed medications. If a question exists about the amount of drug a breast-feeding infant may be receiving or about possible drug effects on the infant, a sample of the mother's milk can be analyzed. Furthermore, up-to-date and specific information regarding breast milk distribution of medications and, most importantly, the amount a nursing infant would actually receive (absorb) can be obtained by consulting a clinical pharmacy/pharmacology service.

Prescribing Medications. Factors such as taste, smell, color, consistancy, dosing frequency, and cost affect the degree to which patients comply with their therapeutic drug regimen. Prescribing generically equivalent medications can sometimes reduce the cost of a drug. Such prescribing should be done only when it is clearly known that the generic brand affords equivalent bioavailability, bioeffectiveness, and patient acceptability. Unfortunately, complete bioequivalence data are not available for all drugs and, when in doubt, the prescribing physician should consult with the pharmacist.

A prescription issued by the prescribing physician should always direct the dispensing of just enough drug to treat the patient, leaving only a small amount of drug left over after the prescribed course of therapy has been completed. This small residual leaves some drug available for doses accidentally spilled or lost. Parents should be instructed to discard all remaining doses of a prescribed medication after the completed course of therapy to protect against accidental poisoning or improper self-medication at a later date. Patient medication instructions on the prescription should state the specific number of doses the patient should receive each day and the total duration of therapy (number of days of therapy). The number of times the prescribing physician allows the prescription to be refilled should be noted on the prescription label; if no refills are to be permitted, this should also be specified on the written prescription.

Compliance with the Prescribed Regimen. Little is know about the many factors that determine the degree of compliance with a physician's instructions, but it is clear that many patients frequently do not take medication consistently or in the manner intended or prescribed. Moreover, patients frequently take home remedies or medications not recommended or prescribed by their physician. A child's compliance with a prescribed therapeutic regimen is usually only as good as that of the parents. Compliance can often be maximized by carefully educating the family about the nature of the child's illness, the action of the medications prescribed, and the importance of following the instructions precisely. Often, if the instructions are written down clearly and in detail for the family and if the regimen results in minimal interference with the daily living schedule (particularly parental sleeping habits), compliance with the therapeutic regimen is improved. Collaboration between prescribing physician and dispensing pharmacist can often identify compliance problems and improve compliance through patient education.

Berlin CM Jr: Advances in pediatric pharmacology and toxicology. Adv Pediatr 44:545, 1997.
Choonara I, Gill A, Nunn A: Drug toxicity and surveillance in children. Br J Clin Pharmacol 42:407, 1996.
Gilman JT, Gal P: Pharmacokinetic and pharmacodynamic data collection in children and neonates: A quiet frontier. Clin Pharmacokinet 23:1, 1992.
Kearns GL, Reed MD: Clinical pharmacokinetics in infants and children: A reappraisal. Clin Pharmacokinet 17(Suppl 1):29, 1989.
Leeder JS, Kearns GL: Pharmacogenetics in pediatrics: Implications for practice. Pediatr Clin North Am 44:41, 1997.
May DG: Genetic differences in drug disposition. J Clin Pharmacol 34:881, 1994.
Tange SM, Grey VL, Senecal PE: Therapeutic drug monitoring in pediatrics: A need for improvement. J Clin Pharmacol 34:200, 1994.
TenEick AP, Nakamura H, Reed MD: Drug-drug interactions in pediatric psychopharmacology. Pediatr Clin North Am 45:1233, 1998.
Wilson JT, Kearns GL, Murphy D, Yaffe SJ: Paediatric labelling requirements: Implications for pharmacokinetic studies. Clin Pharmacokinet 26:308, 1994.

Chapter 728 Medications

Peter Gal and Michael D. Reed

TABLE 728–1 General Medications

Drug (Trade Names, Formulations)	Indications (Mechanism of Action) and Dosing	Comments (Cautions, Adverse Events, Monitoring)
Acetaminophen Analgesic, non-narcotic; antipyretic. Tempra; Tylenol; multiple generic and brand-name products. Caplet: 160 mg, 325 mg, 500 mg. Capsule: 325 mg, 500 mg. Drops: 100 mg/mL (15 mL); 120 mg/2.5 mL (35 mL). Granules, premeasured packs: 30 mg (32 s). Suppositories: 120 mg, 325 mg. Combination products with acetaminophen include cough and cold preparations and with codeine.	**Mild to moderate pain** (inhibits prostaglandin synthesis in CNS and peripheral pain impulse generation). **Fever** (inhibits hypothalamic heat regulation center). *Infants and children <12 yr:* 10–15 mg/kg/dose q4–6h *Children >12 yr and adults:* 325–650 mg q4–6h or 1,000 mg 3–4 times daily. Maximum 5 doses/24 hr (children) or 4 g/day (adults) administered PO or PR.	*Cautions:* Overdose can cause fatal hepatic necrosis. Treat acute overdoses with acetylcysteine. Chronic concurrent use with enzyme inhibitors, especially alcohol, can lead to hepatic necrosis. Avoid aspartame-containing products in patients with phenylketonuria (e.g., chewable tablets).
Acetazolamide Diuretic, carbonic anhydrase inhibitor. Dazamide; Diamox. Capsule, sustained release: 500 mg. Injection: 500 mg/5 mL. Tablet: 125 mg, 250 mg.	**Hydrocephalus due to communicating intraventricular hemorrhage** (carbonic anhydrase inhibition decreases CSF production). *Neonates:* 25 mg/kg q day to start and increase to bid, tid, and qid over 4–7 days. **Glaucoma** (carbonic anhydrase inhibition decreases formation of aqueous humor). *Children:* 8–30 mg/kg/day PO divided q6–8h or 20–40 mg/kg/day IV divided q6h. **Epilepsy, as adjunct to other drugs in refractory seizures** (undertain mechanism) *Children and adults:* 8–30 mg/kg/day in 1–4 divided doses (maximum 1 g/day). **Edema** (diuretic) *Children:* 5 mg/kg qd IV or PO. *Adults:* 250–375 mg q day IV or PO.	*Caution:* Used in combination with furosemide for hydrocephalus. Reduce dose and extend dosing interval if renal function is compromised. Avoid if patient has sulfa allergy. IM very painful because of alkaline pH of drug *Adverse events:* Metabolic acidosis, hypochloremia, hypokalemia, nausea, anorexia, drowsiness, fatigue, muscle weakness, renal calculi.
Acetylcysteine Antidote, acetaminophen; mucolytic agent. Mucomyst; Mucosil; Mucosol. Solution, as sodium: 10% [100 mg/mL] (4 mL, 10 mL, 30 mL); 20% [200 mg/mL] (4 mL, 10 mL, 30 mL, 100 mL).	**Mucolytic** (free sulfhydryl group opens up disulfide bonds in mucoproteins, lowering viscosity). Dose is based on 10% solution or diluted 20% solution (1:1) for inhalation. *Infants:* 2–4 mL tid–qid. *Children:* 6–10 mL tid–qid. *Adolescents:* 10 mL tid–qid. **Acute Acetaminophen Overdose** (provides alternative metabolic pathway for conjugation of toxic metabolites, restoring normal glutathione levels). *Children and adults:* 140 mg/kg loading dose, followed by 70 mg/kg q4h for 17 doses. Repeat dose if emesis occurs within 1 hr of administration.	*Cautions:* Give a bronchodilator 10–15 min before nebulized mucomyst to avoid bronchospasm. Follow treatment with chest percussion and suction to manage increased secretions. Dilute nebulized doses with saline or sterile water and oral solutions with soft drinks or orange juice. Prepare inhaled as 1:1 and PO as 1:3 solutions. *Adverse events:* Stomatitis nausea, vomiting, urticaria. *Monitoring:* Check acetaminophen concentration no earlier than 4 hr post overdose. Give complete acetylcysteine course regardless of acetaminophen concentrations.
Adenosine Antiarrhythmic agent, miscellaneous. Adenocard. Injection, preservative free: 3 mg/mL (2 mL).	**Paroxysmal supraventricular tachycardia (PSVT) treatment** (slows conduction time through the A-V node). *Neonates and children:* 0.05 mg/kg IV push, then increase bolus doses by 0.05 mg/kg every 2 min until a clinical response occurs or a maximum dose of either 0.25 mg/kg or 12 mg is achieved. *Adults:* 6 mg IV push, if no response in 2 min, give 12 mg IV push. May repeat 12 mg IV bolus if needed.	*Cautions:* Use a peripheral IV site. May cause bronchoconstriction in asthmatics. Methylxanthines (e.g., theophylline or caffeine) antagonize adenosine effects so higher adenosine doses are needed. Contraindicated in 2nd or 3rd degree A-V block or sick sinus syndrome. *Adverse events:* heart block, flushing, chest palpitations, bradycardia, hypotension, dyspnea, headache, dizziness, nausea. *Monitoring:* Continuous ECG, blood pressure, respirations.
Albumin Human Blood product derivative; plasma volume expander. Albuminar; Albumisol; Albutein; Buminate; Plasbumin. Injection: 5% [50 mg/mL] (50 mL, 250 mL, 500 mL, 1000 mL); 25% [250 mg/mL] (10 mL, 20 mL, 50 mL, 100 mL).	**Plasma volume expansion and treatment of hypovolemia** (increase intravascular oncotic pressure and mobilize fluid from interstitium to intravascular space). *Neonates:* 0.5–1 g/kg/dose (max 1 g/kg/day). *Infants and children:* 0.5–1 g/kg/dose (max 6 g/kg/day). *Adults:* 25 g/dose (max 250 g/day).	*Cautions:* 25% albumin may increase risk of IVH in preterm infants so 5% is preferred in these cases. Infusion should be over at least 2 hr in neonates. Infusion may be over 30–60 min for hypovolemia. *Adverse events:* Precipitation of heart failure, pulmonary edema, hypertension, tachycardia due to volume overload. Immune reactions (e.g., fever, chills, rash). Increased mortality in critically ill patients. *Monitoring:* Vital signs.

Table continued on following page

TABLE 728–1 General Medications *Continued*

Drug (Trade Names, Formulations)	Indications (Mechanism of Action) and Dosing	Comments (Cautions, Adverse Events, Monitoring)
Albuterol Adrenergic agonist agent; beta-2-adrenergic agonist agent; bronchodilator; sympathomimetic. Proventil; Ventolin; Volmax. Aerosol, oral: 90 μg/spray [200 inhalations] (17 g). Capsule, microfine, for inhalation, as sulfate (Rotacaps): 200 μg. Solution, inhalation, as sulfate: 0.083% [0.83 mg/mL] (3 mL); 0.5% [5 mg/mL] (20 mL). Syrup, as sulfate (strawberry flavor): 2 mg/5 mL (480 mL). Tablet, as sulfate: 2 mg, 4 mg. Tablet, extended release: 4 mg.	**Bronchodilator** (beta-2-agonist). **Inhalation Dose:** *Neonates, infants, children, and adults:* **Metered Dose Inhaler:** 1–2 puffs as prn, or 5-min prior to exercise or tid–qid. **Rotohaler:** 1–2 capsules prn, or q4–6h, or prior to exercise. **Nebulizer solution:** *Neonates:* 0.1–0.5 mg/kg/dose prn or q2–6h. *Children:* 1.25–2.5 mg prn or q4–6h. *Adults:* 1.25–5 mg prn or q4–6h. **Oral:** *Neonates:* 0.1–0.3 mg/kg/dose q6–8h. *Children < 6 yr:* 0.1–0.2 mg/kg/dose tid. *Children 6–12 yr:* 2 mg/dose tid–qid *Children >12 yr:* 2–4 mg tid–qid.	*Cautions:* Increased use or lack of effect may indicate loss of asthma control requiring medical attention. Better to use as prn or prior to exercise. *Adverse events:* Hyperglycemia, hypokalemia, tachycardia, palpitations, nervousness, CNS stimulation, insomnia, tremor. *Monitoring:* Evaluate clinical response and pulmonary function, e.g., peak flow meter (patient should achieve >80% of personal best peak expiratory flow rate after use). *Comments:* May mix albuterol nebulizer solution with cromolyn or ipratropium nebulizer solutions. Give MDI doses with an extender device.
Alfentanil Hydrochloride Analgesic, narcotic; general anesthetic. Alfenta Injection. Injection, preservative free: 500 μg/mL (2 mL, 5 mL, 10 mL, 20 mL).	**Analgesia, anesthesia** (narcotic analgesic). *Neonates, Infants, and Children <12 yr:* 5–15 μg/kg IV injected over 3–5 min or 0.5–3 μg/kg/min continuous infusion (limited experience and doses poorly established). *Adults:* IV continuous infusion 0.5–1.5 μg/kg/min.	*Cautions:* Bolus doses of 9–15 μg/kg caused chest wall rigidity in 9 of 20 newborns, compromising respiration in four patients. Use a skeletal muscle relaxant concurrently. Avoid in patients with increased intracranial pressure or severe respiratory depression. *Adverse events:* Bradycardia, hypotension, increased intracranial pressure, ADH release. *Comment:* Dose based on lean weight for obese patients.
Alglucerase Enzyme, glucocerebrosidase. Ceredase Injection. Injection: 10 units/mL (5 mL); 80 units/mL (5 mL).	**Enzyme replacement therapy for type I Gaucher disease** (replaces the missing enzyme beta-glucosidase needed to break down and thus avoid accumulation of glucosyl ceramide laden macrophages in bone liver and spleen). 20–60 units/kg IV infused over 1–2 hr. Typically repeated every 2 wk but varies from q2days to q4wk depending on response.	*Adverse events:* Fever, chills, abdominal discomfort, nausea, vomiting, local IV site. *Monitoring:* Resolution of anemia, thrombocytopenia, bleeding tendencies, and hepatosplenomegaly (within 6 mo). Improved bone mineralization (usually noted at 80–104 wk of therapy).
Allopurinol Antigout agent; uric acid–lowering agent. Lopurin; Zyloprim. Tablet: 100 mg, 300 mg.	**Prevent attacks of gouty arthritis and nephropathy.** **Prevent cancer chemotherapy-induced hyperuricemia** (inhibits xanthine oxidase thus preventing conversion of hypoxanthine to uric acid). *Children ≤ 10 yr:* 10 mg/kg/day in 2–3 divided doses. *Children >10 yr and Adults:* 200–600 mg/day in 2–3 divided doses. **Gout, chemotherapy-induced hyperuricemia** 600–800 mg/day in 2–3 divided doses starting 1–2 days prior to chemotherapy and continue for 3 days. Renal impairment: CrCl 10–50: reduce dose to 50%, CrCl <10: reduce dose to 30% of suggested.	*Cautions:* Discontinue at first sign of skin rash. *Adverse events:* Skin rashes including erythema multiforme, renal impairment, hepatitis, peripheral neuropathy, vasculitis. *Monitoring:* Uric acid levels decrease in 1–2 days with maximum effect seen in 1–3 wk.
Alprazolam Antianxiety agent. Benzodiazepine. Xanax. Tablet: 0.25 mg, 0.5 mg, 1 mg, 2 mg.	**Treatment of anxiety or panic attacks** (not certain but may be mediated through GABA). *Children:* 0.005–0.02 mg/kg/dose tid. *Adults:* 0.25–0.5 mg bid–tid, maximum 4 mg/day (anxiety) and 10 mg/day (panic).	*Cautions:* Abrupt discontinuation results in withdrawal reactions including seizures. Safety not established in children <18 yr. Pregnancy risk factor D. *Adverse events:* Drowsiness, confusion, sedation.
Alprostadil Prostoglandin. Prostin VR Pediatric Injection. Injection: 500 μg/mL (1 mL).	**Maintain patency of the ductus arteriosus in cyanotic heart lesions.** Direct vasodilation of ductus smooth muscle *Neonates and infants:* 0.05–0.1 μg/kg/min as continuous IV infusion, may gradually increase to maximum of 0.4 μg/kg/min or wean as low as 0.005 μg/kg/min depending on response.	*Adverse events:* Apnea, bradycardia, hypotension, tachycardia, flushing, seizure-like activity, cortical hyperostosis (with >6 mo use), diarrhea, gastric-outlet obstruction (if ≥ 5 days use). *Monitoring:* Therapeutic response includes increase in systemic blood pressure, improved oxygen saturation or Po_2, and less acidosis on blood pH. Discontinue immediately if severe apnea or bradycardia.
Aluminum Acetate Topical skin product. Acid Mantle; Bluboro; Boropak; Domeboro; PediBoro. Powder, to make topical solution: 1 packet/pint of water = 1:40 solution. Solution, otic: Aluminum acetate 1:10 with acetic acid 2% (60 mL). Tablet: 1 tablet/pint = 1:40 dilution.	**Astringent wet dressing for relief of inflammatory conditions of the skin; prophylaxis of swimmer's ear** *Children and adults:* Otic: instill 4–6 drops every 2–3 hr initially then every 4–6 hr until itching or burning resolves. Topical: soak the affected area in the solution for 15–30 min 2–4 times daily.	*Adverse events:* Local irritation.

TABLE 728–1 General Medications *(Continued)*

Drug (Trade Names, Formulations)	Indications (Mechanism of Action) and Dosing	Comments (Cautions, Adverse Events, Monitoring)
Aminocaproic Acid Hemostatic agent. Amicar. Injection: 250 mg/mL (20 mL, 96 mL, 100 mL). Syrup (raspberry flavor): 250 mg/mL (480 mL). Tablet: 500 mg.	**Treatment of excessive bleeding resulting from systemic hyperfibrinolysis (inhibits activation of plasminogen)** *Children:* Oral, IV load 100–200 mg/kg, maintenance 100 mg/kg every 6 hr or 33.3 mg/kg/hr continuous infusion. Traumatic hyphema: 100 mg/kg every 4 hr (max 30 g/day). *Adults:* load 5 g over 1 hr, then 1–1.25 g/hr until bleeding stops (max 30 g/day).	*Cautions:* Avoid in disseminated intravascular coagulation and hematuria of the upper urinary tract. Contains benzyl alcohol, so avoid in neonates <1500 g. *Adverse events:* Hypotension, bradycardia, arrythmias, dizziness, headache, nasal congestion. *Monitoring:* D-dimer or fibrin split products, activated clotting time (target 180–200 sec), serum potassium (especially if renal function decreased).
Aminophylline (Theophylline equivalent listed in brackets.) Bronchodilator; respiratory stimulant; theophylline derivative. Aminophyllin; Phyllocontin; Somophyllin; Truphylline. Injection, IV (Aminophyllin): 25 mg/mL [19.7 mg/mL] (10 mL, 20 mL). Liquid, oral: 105 mg/5 mL [90 mg/5 mL] (240 mL). Suppository, rectal (Truphylline): 250 mg [197.5 mg], 500 mg [395 mg]. Tablet (Aminophyllin): 100 mg [79 mg], 200 mg [158 mg]. Tablet, controlled release [12 hours] (Phyllocontin): 225 mg [178 mg]. Tablet, enteric coated: 100 mg [79 mg], 200 mg [158 mg]. See *Theophylline* for oral dosing.	**Apnea of prematurity, ventilator weaning in neonates, bronchodilator, weak pulmonary anti-inflammatory effects.** Increase contractility and decrease fatiguability of diaphragm and respiratory muscles, weak bronchodilator, CNS stimulation, decrease airway responsiveness to stimuli. Exact mechanisms for these effects remain controversial. *Neonates* (for apnea of prematurity, ventilator weaning, or bronchospasm): Loading dose: 6 mg/kg IV or PO. Maintenance dose: 2.5–3 mg/kg/dose q12h IV or PO. **Asthma chronic therapy (see *Theophylline*).** Use in acute therapy is of questionable value. If used as continuous IV infusion: *Children:* 6 wk–6 mo: 0.5 mg/kg/hr. 6 mo–1 yr: 0.7 mg/kg/hr. 1–9 yr: 1 mg/kg/hr. 9–12 yr: 0.9 mg/kg/hr. 12 yr–adult: 0.7 mg/kg/hr.	*Cautions:* May cause or worsen arrhythmias, seizures, or gastroesophageal reflux. Theophylline clearance is modified by numerous disease states and drugs requiring dosing adjustments guided by serum theophylline concentrations. Clearance is reduced by viral illnesses, fever >102°F for >24 hr, cor pulmonale, and drugs that inhibit P450 enzymes (cimetidine, verapamil, macrolides, quinolones); reduce dose by 50%. *Adverse events:* Feeding intolerance in neonates or GI discomfort in children and adults, nausea, vomiting, CNS irritability, agitation, tachycardia, and tachyarrhythmias. *Monitoring:* Theophylline blood levels correlate with clinical effects and toxicity. Target levels are somewhat controversial. *Neonates:* 6–15 mg/L (65% of neonates will not have apnea eliminated until levels exceed 10 mg/L if continuous electronic monitoring is performed. Levels above 10 mg/L are needed for ventilator weaning. Levels of 5–15 mg/L are sufficient for bronchodilation). *Children:* Theophylline alone is ineffective for acute asthma. For chronic asthma, theophylline levels of 5–15 mg/L are effective, but levels should exceed 10 mg/L for prevention of exercise-induced bronchospasm.
Amiodarone Hydrochloride Antiarrhythmic agent, class III. Cordarone. Tablet: 200 mg. Injection: 50 mg/mL (3 mL); Cordarone contains benzyl alcohol and polysorbate (Tween) 80. Injection, benzyl alcohol-free and polysorbate-free: 15 mg/mL (10 mL); Amio Aqueous contains an aqueous acetate buffer; available via orphan drug status or compassionate use from the manufacturer Academic Pharmaceuticals, Inc. (847) 735-1170.	**Management of resistant, life-threatening ventricular arrhythmias or PSVT unresponsive to less toxic agents** (class III antiarrhythmic agent, prolongs action potential and refractory period in myocardial tissue) **Oral Dose:** *Infants and children:* <1 yr: 600–800 mg/2.73 m^2/day in two divided doses. >1 yr: 10–15 mg/kg/day in two divided doses. *Adults:* 800 mg/day in two divided doses. Cut all doses in half, i.e., one dose per day after 1–4 wk of treatment or arrhythmias are controlled. **IV dose:** *Infants and children:* load 5 mg/kg over 1 h, then continuous infusion of 5–15 μg/kg/min. *Adults:* 150 mg over 10 min, then 0.5 mg/min.	*Cautions:* Use benzyl alcohol-free product in neonates. Minimize risk of torsade de pointes by correcting low potassium and magnesium. Inhibits cytochrome P450 enzymes, so many drugs that are metabolized will have markedly increased levels and effects including theophylline, phenytoin, warfarin, other antiarrhythmics, methotrexate, and cyclosporine. *Adverse events:* Proarrhythmia (may be brady- or tachy-arrhythmias or heart block); fatigue, malaise, nightmares, behavioral changes; hypothyroidism, hyperglycemia, elevated triglycerides, skin color changes (slate blue), photosensitivity, skin rash, liver toxicity (may be fatal or just increased liver enzymes), pulmonary toxicity (potentially fatal) includes pulmonary fibrosis, interstitial pneumonitis, hypersensitivity pneumonitis (present as cough, fever, dyspnea, chest x-ray changes), photophobia, thrombocytopenia. *Monitoring:* Pulmonary, liver, and thyroid function tests; chest x-ray, ECG, eye exam, and clinical signs and symptoms of toxicity. Amiodarone concentration: 2–4 μmol/L.
Amitriptyline Hydrochloride Antidepressant, tricyclic; antimigraine agent. Elavi; Emitrip; Endep. Injection: 10 mg/mL (10 mL) Tablet: 10 mg, 25 mg, 50 mg, 75 mg, 100 mg, 150 mg.	**Depression (increases CNS concentrations of serotonin and norepinephrine by inhibiting reuptake).** *Children:* 1–1.5 mg/kg/24 hr divided tid. *Adolescent:* 30–100 mg at bedtime or divided bid. (max 200 mg/day). *Adults:* 30–100 mg qd (max 300 mg/day). **Analgesic for neuropathic or chronic pain or migraine prophylaxis.** *Children:* 0.1 mg/kg at bedtime and advance over 2–3 wk to effect. Max 2 mg/kg at bedtime. *Adolescents:* 25 mg divided bid and increase dose to effect or maximum dose 200 mg/day. *Adults:* start 25 mg at bedtime and increase to effect or maximum dose 300 mg/day.	*Cautions:* Cardiac conduction abnormalities may occur, monitor ECG. Do not discontinue abruptly as withdrawal syndrome may occur. *Adverse events:* Dry mouth, constipation, weight gain, postural hypotension, drowsiness, confusion, headache, visual disturbance. *Monitoring:* Amitriptyline concentrations: therapeutic 100–250 ng/mL; nortriptyline concentrations: therapeutic 50–150 ng/mL.

Table continued on following page

TABLE 728–1 General Medications *Continued*

Drug (Trade Names, Formulations)	Indications (Mechanism of Action) and Dosing	Comments (Cautions, Adverse Events, Monitoring)
Ammonium Chloride Metabolic alkalosis, treatment agent: urinary acidifying agent. Generic. Injection: 26.75% [5 mEq/mL] (20 mL). Tablet: 500 mg. Tablet enteric coated: 500 mg.	**Systemic or urinary acidification (dissociation of ammonium and chloride then replacement of bicarbonate ions by chloride ions).** *Children:* 75 mg/kg/24 h IV divided q6h (max daily dose: 6 g). *Adults:* 1.5 g/dose IV q6h.	*Adverse events:* Hyperchloremia, hyperammonemia, hyperkalemia.
Amrinone Lactate Adrenergic agonist agent. Inocor. Injection: 5 mg/mL (20 mL).	**Treatment of low cardiac output states (increase cellular levels of cyclic AMP).** *Neonates:* 0.75 mg/kg IV bolus over 2–3 min then 3–5 μg/kg/min continuous infusion IV. *Infants and children:* 0.75 mg/kg IV bolus over 2–3 min then 5–10 μg/kg/min continuous infusion. *Adults:* 0.75 mg/kg IV bolus over 2–3 min then 5–10 μg/kg/min.	*Cautions:* Increased cardiac output may cause excess diuresis if diuretic doses are not adjusted. May repeat bolus doses if clinical response is inadequate. *Adverse effects:* Hypotension, arrhythmias, thrombocytopenia.
Antihemophilic Factor, Human Antihemophilic agent; blood product derivative. Alphanate; Hemofil M; Humate-P; Koate-HP; Koate-HS; Monoclate-P; Profilate OSD. Injection (approximate factor VIII activity per vial): 200 units, 250 units, 500 units, 750 units, 1,000 units, 1,250 units, 1,500 units; exact potency labeled on each vial.	**Factor VIII deficiency in hemophilia (provides factor VIII).** *All patients:* Units required = weight (kg) × 0.5 × desired increase factor VIII (% of normal).	*Adverse events:* Tachycardia, allergy, blood-borne viral infections. *Monitoring:* Plasma antihemophilic factor levels
Antipyrine and Benzocaine Otic agent, analgesic; otic agent, cerumenolytic. Allergan Ear Drops; Aurafair; Auralgan; Aurodex; Auroto; Oto; Otocalm Ear Solution, otic: antipyrine 5.4% and benzocaine 1.4% (10 mL, 15 mL).	**Temporary relief of ear pain and inflammation (topical anesthetic and antiinflammatory).** *All patients:* Fill ear canal, then moisten cotton pledget and place into meatus. May repeat every 1–2 hr until pain relief. Limit use to about 3 days.	*Adverse events:* Stinging, methemoglobinemia.
Antithrombin III. **Thrombate III.**	**Antithrombin III deficiency due to DIC or shock and surgery complications. Treatment of thrombosis in ATIII deficiency.** *All patients:* Dose (IU) = (120 − patient ATIII) × wt (kg).	*Monitoring:* Check ATIII levels, maintain between 80% and 120%.
Antivenin (Crotalidae) Polyvalent. Antivenom. Generic. Injection: Lyophilized serum, diluent (10 mL); one vacuum vial to yield 10 mL of antivenom.	**Antivenom for snake bite from North and South American Crotalids, i.e., rattlesnake, copperhead, cottonmouth, tropical moccasins, fer-de-lance, bushmaster.** Dosing based on severity of bite—mild: 5 vials, moderate: 10 vials, severe: > 15 vials.	*Cautions:* Sensitivity reactions, including anaphylaxis (treat with epinephrine and antihistamine and brief holding of dose).
Arginine Hydrochloride Diagnostic agent, growth hormone function; metabolic alkalosis, treatment agent. R-Gene. Injection: 10% [0.475 mEq chloride/mL] (500 mL).	**Pituitary function test (stimulates pituitary release of growth hormone and prolactin).** *Children:* 500 mg/kg over 30 min. *Adults:* 300 mL over 30 min.	*Adverse events:* Flushing, headache, hyperglycemia, hyperkalemia, metabolic acidosis. *Monitoring:* Plasma growth hormone concentrations.
Ascorbic Acid Nutritional supplement; urinary acidifying agent; vitamin, water soluble. Ascorbicap; C-Crystals; Cecon; Cetane; Cevalin; Ce-Vi-Sol; Dull-C; Flavorcee; Vita-C. Capsule, timed release: 500 mg. Crystals: 4 g/teaspoonful (1,000 g). Injection: 250 mg/mL (2 mL, 30 mL), 500 mg/mL (1 mL, 2 mL, 50 mL). Lozenge: 60 mg. Powder: 4 g/teaspoonful (1,000 g). Solution, oral: 35 mg/0.6 mL (50 mL), 100 mg/mL (50 mL). Syrup: 500 mg/5 mL (5 mL, 10 mL, 120 mL, 480 mL). Tablet: 25 mg, 50 mg, 100 mg, 250 mg, 500 mg, 1,000 mg. Tablet, chewable: 100 mg, 250 mg, 500 mg, 1,000 mg. Tablet, timed release: 500 mg, 1,000 mg, 1,500 mg.	**Scurvy.** *Children:* 100–300 mg/day. *Adults:* 100–250 mg bid. **Urinary acidification.** *Children:* 500 mg every 6 hr. *Adults:* 4–12 g/day in 3–4 divided doses.	*Adverse events:* GI upset, renal stones.
Asparaginase Antineoplastic agent, miscellaneous. Elspar. Injection: 10,000 units/vial.	**Cancer chemotherapy (inhibits protein synthesis to deprive cancer cells of asparagine)** *Children and adults:* Doses may vary depending on specific protocol being used; 6,000 units/m² IM, 3 times/wk for 3 wk as part of combination therapy. High-dose IM therapy: 25,000 units/m²/dose q wk × 9 doses. IV therapy: 1,000 units/kg/day for 10 days; or 200 units/kg/day × 28 days.	*Cautions:* Stop drug if any signs of renal failure or pancreatitis occur. Be prepared to treat anaphylaxis at each dose. *Adverse events:* Myelosuppression (WBC and platelets; is mild and rare) onset 7 days, nadir 14 days, recovery 21 days. Hepatotoxicity, pancreatitis, GI upset, azotemia, hyperglycemia, coagulopathy.

TABLE 728–1 General Medications *Continued*

Drug (Trade Names, Formulations)	Indications (Mechanism of Action) and Dosing	Comments (Cautions, Adverse Events, Monitoring)
Aspirin Analgesic, non-narcotic; anti-inflammatory agent; antiplatelet agent; antipyretic; nonsteroidal anti-inflammatory agent (NSAID), oral; salicylate. Anacin; A.S.A.; Ascriptin; Aspergum; Bayer Aspirin; Bufferin; Easprin; Ecotrin; Empirin; Gensan; Halfrin; Measurin ZORprin. Suppository, rectal: 60 mg, 120 mg, 125 mg, 130 mg, 195 mg, 200 mg, 300 mg, 325 mg, 600 mg, 650 mg, 1,200 mg. Tablet: 325 mg, 500 mg, 650 mg. Tablet, buffered: 325 mg with aluminum hydroxide 75 mg and magnesium hydroxide 75 mg, 325 mg with aluminum hydroxide 150 mg and magnesium hydroxide 150 mg, 500 mg with aluminum hydroxide 33 mg and magnesium hydroxide 150 mg. Chewable: 75 mg, 81 mg. Chewing gum: 227 mg. Controlled release: 800 mg. Enteric coated (delayed release): 80 mg, 165 mg, 325 mg, 500 mg, 650 mg, 975 mg. Timed release: 650 mg. Tablet, with caffeine: 400 mg and caffeine 32 mg; 500 mg and caffeine 32 mg.	**Pain, inflammation, fever (prostaglandin synthesis inhibition).** *Children:* 10–15 mg/kg/dose q4–6h. *Adults:* 650–1,000 mg/dose q4–6h (max 4 g/day). **Kawasaki disease (acute phase)** *Children:* 80–100 mg/kg/day divided every 6 hr. **Rheumatic fever** 60–100 mg/kg/day divided every 6 hr.	*Cautions:* Contraindicated in children <16 yr with chickenpox or flu-like symptoms due to risk of Reye syndrome. Discontinue if hearing loss or tinnitis occurs. *Adverse events:* Bleeding from gums or GI tract, gastric ulcers, bronchospasm in asthmatics, hearing loss, and tinnitis. *Monitoring:* Check serum concentration 2 hr after a dose for Kawasaki disease (target 150–300 μg/ml) or rheumatic fever (target: 250–400 μg/ml).
Astemizole Antihistamine. Hismanal. Tablet: 10 mg.	**Allergy and rhinitis (competative H1-receptor blocker)** *Children:* *<6 yr:* 0.2 mg/kg once daily. *6–12 yr:* 5 mg once daily. *>12 yr and adult:* 10–30 mg/day.	*Cautions:* Syncopal episodes may be a marker of arrhythmias including Q-T interval prolongation leading to fatal arrythmias. Discontinue if ECG shows Q-T prolongation, syncopal episode, or drugs that impair hepatic metabolism (e.g., erythromycin, ketoconazole) are added.
Atenolol Antianginal agent; Antihypertensive; beta-adrenergic blocker. Tenormin. Injection: 0.5 mg/mL (10 mL). Tablet: 25 mg, 50 mg, 100 mg.	**Hypertension, arrhythmias (competative beta 1-blocker).** *Children:* 0.8–1.5 mg/kg/day (max 2 mg/kg/day). *Adults:* 25–200 mg/day oral, 5 mg IV over 5 min.	*Cautions:* Avoid abrupt discontinuation, taper over 1–2 wk. *Adverse events:* Bradycardia, lethargy, headache, constipation, wheezing, dyspnea.
Atorvastatin Calcium Lipitor. Tablet: 10, 20, 40 mg.	**Hypercholesterolemia, including homozygous familial hypercholesterolemia (inhibit HMG-CoA reductase).** *Children >6 yr:* 10 80 mg/day. *Adults:* 10 80 mg/day.	*Adverse events:* Dyspepsia, flatulence, pancreatitis, hepatitis, myalgia, arthralgia. *Monitoring:* Plasma lipid profile.
Atracurium Besylate Neuromuscular blocker agent, nondepolarizing; skeletal muscle relaxant, paralytic. Tacrium. Injection: 10 mg/mL (5 mL, 10 mL).	**Neuromuscular blocker for muscle paralysis (binds to cholinergic receptor sites to block neural transmission).** *Children:* *<2 yr:* 0.3–0.4 mg/kg as needed. *>2 yr to Adult:* 0.4–0.5 mg/kg then 1 mg/kg 20 to 45 min after each initial block to maintain effect. Continuous IV infusion: 0.4–0.8 mg/kg/hr.	*Cautions:* Make sure airway and respiratory support are secure before use. Contains benzyl alcohol; neonatal use should be limited. Does not have sedative or analgesic properties, so adjunct sedative/analgesic should be used. *Monitoring:* Muscle twitch response to peripheral nerve stimulator.
Atropine Sulfate Anticholinergic agent; anticholinergic agent, ophthalmic; antidote, organophosphate poisoning; antispasmodic agent, gastrointestinal; bronchodilator; ophthalmic agent, mydriatic. Atropair Ophthalmic; Atropine-Care Ophthalmic; Atropisol Ophthalmic; Isopto Atropine Ophthalmic; I-Tropine Ophthalmic; Ocu-Tropin. Ophthalmic injection: 0.05 mg/mL (5 mL); 0.1 mg/mL (5 mL, 10 mL); 0.3 mg/mL (1 mL, 30 mL); 0.4 mg/mL (1 mL, 20 mL, 30 mL); 0.5 mg/mL (1 mL, 5 mL, 30 mL); 0.8 mg/mL (0.5 mL, 1 mL); 1 mg/mL (1 mL, 10 mL). Ointment, ophthalmic: 0.5% (3.5 g); 1% (3.5 g). Solution, ophthalmic: 0.5% (1 mL, 5 mL); 1% (1 mL, 2 mL, 5 mL, 15 mL); 2% (1 mL, 2 mL). Tablet: 0.4 mg. Tablet, soluble: 0.4 mg, 0.6 mg.	**Preoperative medication to inhibit secretions and salivation (blocks action of acetylcholine and antagonizes histamine and serotonin).** *Neonates and children:* <5 kg: 0.2 mg/kg 30 min preop then every 4–6 hr. >5 kg: 0.1–0.2 mg/kg/dose (max 0.4 mg/dose). *Adults:* 0.4–0.6 mg IV or SC 30 min preoperatively. **Treatment of sinus bradycardia** *Neonates and children:* 0.02 mg/kg (min dose 0.1 mg); IV or intratracheal (max 0.5 mg); may repeat 5 min later, one time. *Adults:* 0.5–1 mg every 5 min (max total dose 2 mg). **Antidote to organophosphate poisoning** 0.02–0.05 mg/kg every 10–20 min until atropine effect (tachycardia, mydriasis, fever), then every 1–4 hr for at least 24 hr.	*Cautions:* Avoid in narrow angle glaucoma, GI obstruction, thyrotoxicosis, tachycardia. *Adverse events:* Tachycardia, palpitations, delirium, ataxia, dry hot skin, tremor, impaired vision.

Table continued on following page

TABLE 728–1 General Medications *Continued*

Drug (Trade Names, Formulations)	Indications (Mechanism of Action) and Dosing	Comments (Cautions, Adverse Events, Monitoring)
Attapulgite Antidiarrheal. Children's Kaopectate; Diasorb; Donnagel; Kaopectate Advanced Formula; Kaopectate Maximum Strength Caplets; K-Pec; Parepectolin; Rheaban. Caplet: 750 mg. Liquid: 600 mg activated attapulgite/15 mL (180 mL, 240 mL, 360 mL, 480 mL); 750 mg activated attapulgite/15 mL (120 mL). Suspension: 600 mg/15 mL. Tablet, chewable: 300 mg, 600 mg, 750 mg.	**Uncomplicated diarrhea (Absorbent action).** *Children:* *3–6 yr:* 300–750 mg/dose (max 7 doses). *6–12 yr:* 600–1,500 mg/dose (max 7 doses). *>12 yr and adult:* 1,200–3,000 mg/dose (max 7 doses).	*Caution:* Do not use for diarrhea due to dysentary, enterocolitis, or toxigenic bacteria.
Auranofin Gold compound. Ridaura. Capsule: 3 mg [gold 29%].	**Treatment of active stage of rheumatoid or proriatic arthritis (immunomodulating effect).** *Children:* Initial dose: 0.1 mg/kg/day; usual maintenance dose: 0.15 mg/kg/day in 1–2 doses (max 0.2 mg/kg/day). *Adults:* 6 mg/day in 1–2 doses (max 9 mg/day in 1–3 doses).	*Adverse events:* Itching, skin rash, stomatitis, conjunctivitis, proteinuria, alopecia, glossitis, leukopenia, thrombocytopenia, hematuria, anemia, agranulocytosis, eosinophilia, peripheral neuropathy, interstitial penumonitis, angioedema, hepatotoxicity. *Monitoring:* Discontinue if WBC <4,000/mm³ or granulocytes <1,500/mm³ or platelets <100,000/mm³.
Aurothioglucose Gold compound. Solganal. Suspension, sterile: 50 mg/mL [gold 50%] (10 mL).	**Treatment of active rheumatoid or psoriatic arthritis (immunomodulator).** *Children:* 0.25 mg/kg/dose wk 1, increase 0.25 mg/kg/dose every wk to maintenance dose 0.75–1.0 mg/kg/dose weekly (max 25 mg/dose, total 20 doses). *Adults:* 10 mg wk 1, then 25 mg wk 2 and 3, then 50 mg/wk until cumulative dose 1 g given.	*Cautions:* Administer by deep IM injection. *Adverse events:* Same as for auranofin.
Azatadine Maleate Antihistamine. Optimine. Tablet: 1 mg.	**Treatment of allergy, allergic rhinitis and urticaria (antihistamine, anticholinergic).** *Children <12 yr:* not recommended. *Children >12 yr and adults:* 1–2 mg twice daily.	*Adverse events:* Sedation, dry mouth, thickened bronchial secretions.
Azathioprine Immunosuppressant agent. Imuran. Injection, as sodium: 100 mg (10 mL). Tablet: 50 mg.	**Prevent transplant rejection.** *Children and adults:* initial 2–5 mg/kg/day IV or PO, maintenance 1–3 mg/kg/day. **Treatment of autoimmune diseases, e.g., lupus, arthritis, nephrotic syndrome. (Inhibit synthesis of DNA, RNA, and proteins. Antagonize purine metabolism.)** *Adults:* 1 mg/kg/day × 6–8 wk.	*Cautions:* Chronic use causes increased risk of lymphoma and skin cancer. May cause irreversible bone marrow suppression. Reduce dose to 25% of normal if concurrent allopurinol used. *Adverse events:* Fever, chills, nausea, vomiting, diarrhea, thrombocytopenia, leukopenia, hepatotoxicity, skin rash.
Baclofen Skeletal muscle relaxant, nonparalytic. Lioresal. Injection, intrathecal: 0.5 mg/mL (20 ml); 2 mg/mL (5 mL). Tablet: 10 mg, 20 mg.	**Spasticity associated with MS or spinal cord lesions. Trigeminal neuralgia (inhibits transmission of monosynaptic and polysynaptic relfexes at the spinal cord level).** *Children:* 2–7 yr: 10–15 mg/day divided q8h and titrate up every 3 days (max 40 mg/day orally). *Adults:* 5 mg q8h and gradually increase by 5 mg every 3 days (max 80 mg/day orally). Intrathecal (adults only).	*Caution:* Avoid abrupt discontinuation, slowly titrate to discontinue. *Adverse events:* Drowsiness, vertigo, psychiatric reactions, ataxia, hypotonia.
Beclomethason Adrenal corticosteroid; anti-inflammatory agent; corticosteroid, inhalent (Oral); corticosteroid, nasal; glucocorticoid. Beclovent Oral Inhaler, Beconase AQ Nasal Inhaler, Beconase Nasal Inhaler, Vancenase AQ Inhaler, Vanceril Oral Inhaler. Inhalation: Nasal (Beconase, Vancenase): 42 μg/inhalation [200 metered doses] (16.8 g). Oral (Beclovent, Vanceril): 42 μg/inhalation [200 metered doses] (16.8 g). Spray, aqueous, nasal (Beconase AQ, Vancenase AQ): 42 μg/inhalation [200 metered doses] (25 g).	**Asthma (oral inhalation), rhinitis (nasal aerosol). (anti-inflammatory, immune modulator).** *Adults and children (inhaler):* 1–2 inhalations 2–4 times daily (maximum dose children: 10 puffs, adults: 20 puffs daily). *Adults and children (nasal spray):* 1 spray in each nostril 2–4 times daily.	*Adverse events:* Candida in mouth, burning and irritation of nasal mucosa, cough, hoarseness, headache. *Monitoring:* Inhaled corticosteroids should be administered via an extender device for better lung delivery and less local toxicity.

TABLE 728–1 General Medications *Continued*

Drug (Trade Names, Formulations)	Indications (Mechanism of Action) and Dosing	Comments (Cautions, Adverse Events, Monitoring)
Benzocaine Local anesthetic, oral; local anesthetic, topical. Americaine; Anbesol Maximum Strength; Babee Teething Lotion: BiCOZENE; chiggertox; Dermoplast; Foille Plus; Hurricaine; Orabase-B; OrabaseGel; Orabase-O, Orajel Brace-Aid Oral Anesthetic; Orajel Maximum Strength; Orajel Mouth-Aid; Rhulicaine; Solarcaine; Unguentine. Topical: Aerosol: 5% (97.5 mL, 105 mL) 20% (20 g, 60 g, 120 g). Cream: 5% (30 g, 454 g); 6% (28.4 g). Gel 15% (7 g). Liquid: with benzyl benzoate and soft soap (30 mL). Lotion: 8% (90 mL). Ointment: 5% (3.5 g, 30 g).	**Temporary relief of pain associated with minor skin injuries (local anesthetic).** *Children and adults:* apply to affected area as needed.	*Adverse events:* Local irritation or sensitization.
Benzonatate Topical anesthetic. Tessalon Perles.	**Relief of nonproductive cough (topical anesthetic action).** *Children <10 yr:* not indicated *Children >10 yr and adults:* 100 mg 3 times daily or q4h to maximum of 600 mg/day.	*Adverse events:* Sedation, numbness, dizziness, headache.
Benzoyl Peroxide Acne products, topical skin product. Benzoxyl; Benzac W; Clear by Design; Clearsil; Dermoxyl; Desquam-X; Loroxide; Oxy-5; PanOxyl; PanOxyl-AQ; Persa-Gel; pHisoAc-BP; Vanoxide. Cleansing bar: 5% (120 g); 10% (120 g). Cleansing lotion: 5% (120 mL, 150 mL, 240 mL); 10% (120 mL, 150 mL). Cream: 5% (30 g); 10% (30 g, 45 g). Facial mask: 5%. Gel: 2.5% (45 g, 60 g, 90 g); 5% (45 g, 60 g, 90 g, 120 g); 10% (45 g, 60 g, 90 g, 120 g). Lotion: 5% (30 mL, 42.5 mL, 60 mL); 5.5% (25 mL); 10% (30 mL, 42.5 mL, 60 mL). Stick 10%.	**Acne treatment (keratolytic and comedolytic effects and kill anaerobic bacteria).** *Children and adults:* Apply sparingly 1–3 times daily for 15 min. May increase strength and duration of exposure as tolerated.	*Adverse events:* Contact dermatitis, local irritation, stinging, or erythema.
Benztropine Mesylate Anticholinergic agent: antidote, drug-induced dystonic reactions; anti-Parkinson's agent. Cogentin. Injection: 1 mg/mL (2 mL). Tablet: 0.5 mg, 1 mg, 2 mg.	**Parkinsonism, drug-induced extrapyramidal reaction (block striatal cholinergic receptors).** *Children >3 yr:* 0.02–0.05 mg/kg/dose 1–2 times daily. *Adults:* 1–4 mg/day 1–2 times daily.	*Adverse events:* Tachycardia, drowsiness, nervousness, hallucinations, dry mouth, blurred vision, mydriasis.
Benzylpenicilloyl-polylysine Diagnostic agent, penicillin allergy skin test. Pre-Pen. Injection: 0.25 mL.	**Adjunct to assessing the risk of penicillin hypersensitivity (elicits type 1 urticarial reactions by IgE mediated reaction).** *Children and adults:* Scratch technique uses a 20-gauge needle to make a 3–5 mm scratch on dermis, apply a small drop of solution to scratch and rub it in gently with applicator. Intradermal injection of 0.1–0.2 ml of Pre-Pen and 0.9% saline in 2 sites at least 1 in apart.	*Monitoring:* Scratch test is positive if a pale wheal of 5–15 mm or more occurs within 10 minutes. Intradermal test is positive in 5–15 min. Discontinue antihistamines before performing tests (hydroxyzine and diphenhydramine for at least 4 days, astemizole for 6–8 wk).
Beractant Lung surfactant. Survanta. Suspension: 200 mg (8 mL).	**Prophylaxis and treatment of respiratory distress syndrome in premature infants (replace deficiency of endogenous surfactant).** *Neonates:* 4 mL/kg via endotracheal tube. May repeat every 6 hr up to a total of 4 doses. Rotate baby to right, then left and administer 1/2 dose on each side over 2–3 sec.	*Adverse events:* Bradycardia, hypotension, oxygen desaturation, pulmonary air leaks, airway obstruction, pulmonary hemorrhage, hypocarbia. *Monitoring:* Heart rate, oxygen saturation, and frequent atrerial blood gases. Adjust ventilator to minimize episodes of hyperoxia and hypocarbia.
Betamethasone Adrenal corticosteroid; anti-inflammatory agent; corticosteroid, systematic; corticosteroid, topical; glucocorticoid. Alphatrex Topical; Betalene Topical; Betatrex Topical; BetaVal Topical; Celestone Oral, Celestone Phosphate Injection; Celestone Soluspan; Cel-U-Jec Injection; Diprolene AF Topical; Diprolene Topical; Diprosine Topical; Maxivate Topical; Psorion Topical; Selestoject Injection; Teledar Topical; Uticort Topical; Valisone Topical. Base (Celestone): Syrup: 0.6 mg/5 mL. Tablet: 0.6 mg.	**Systemic use to stimulate fetal lung maturation in preterm labor. Topical use to treat inflammatory dermatoses.** *Children and adults:* Topical application of thin film to affected area 2–4 times daily. *Pregnant female:* 12 mg IM q24h for 2 doses.	*Adverse events:* Maternal pulmonary edema and hypertension, headache.

Table continued on following page

TABLE 728–1 General Medications *Continued*

Drug (Trade Names, Formulations)	Indications (Mechanism of Action) and Dosing	Comments (Cautions, Adverse Events, Monitoring)
Betamethasone *Continued* Benzoate (Uticort): Cream, emollient base: 0.025% (60 g). Gel, topical: 0.025% (15 g, 60 g). Lotion: 0.025% (60 mL). Dipropionate (Alphatrex, Diprosine, Maxivate, Teladar): Aerosol, topical: 0.1% (85 g). Cream: 0.05% (15 g, 45 g). Lotion: 0.05% (20 mL, 30 mL, 60 mL). Ointment, topical: 0.05% (15 g, 45 g). Diproprionate (Psorion): Cream: 0.05% (15 g, 45 g). Dipropionate, augmented (Diprolene, Diprolene AF): Cream, emollient base: 0.05% (15 g, 45 g). Gel, topical: 0.05% (15 g, 45 g). Lotion: 0.05% (30 mL, 60 mL). Ointment, topical: 0.05% (15 g, 45 g). Valerate (Betatrex, Beta-Val, Valisone): Cream: 0.01% (15 g, 60 g); 0.1% (15 g, 45 g, 110 g, 430 g). Lotion: 0.1% (20 mL, 60 mL). Ointment, topical: 0.1% (15 g, 45 g). Powder for compounding: 5 g, 10 g. Sodium phosphate (Celestone Phosphate, Selestoject): Injection: Equivalent to 3 g/mL (5 mL). Sodium phosphate and acetate (Celestone Soluspan): Injection, suspension: 6 mg/mL [3 mg betamethesone and betamethasone sodium phosphate and 3 mg betamethasone acetate per mL] (5 mL).		
Bethanechol Cholinergic agent. Duvoid; Myotonachol, Urecholine. Injection: 5 mg/mL (1 mL). Tablet: 5 mg, 10 mg, 25 mg, 50 mg.	**Treatment of nonobstructive urinary retention or gastroesophageal reflux (stimulate cholinergic receptors in smooth muscle in urinary and gastrointestinal tracts).** *Children:* 0.3–0.6 mg/kg/day divided into 3–4 doses. *Adults:* 10–50 mg 2–4 times/day.	*Adverse events:* Hypotension, abdominal cramps, diarrhea, vomiting, salivation, urinary frequency, bronchial constriction, sweating.
Biotin Biotinidase deficiency; treatment agent; vitamin, water soluble. Biotin Forte; Biotin Forte Extra Strength; Bio-Tn; d-Biotin. Tablet: 300 μg, 400 μg, 600 μg, 800 μg, 2.5 mg, 3 mg, 5 mg, 10 mg.	**Treatment of primary biotinidase deficiency or nutritional biotin deficiency, component of vitamin B complex (required for various metabolic functions).** *Children and adults:* Biotin deficiency: 5–20 mg once/day. Biotinidase deficiency: 5–10 mg once daily.	
Bisacodyl Laxative, stimulant. Bisacodyl Uniserts; Bisco-Lax; Carter's Little Pills; ClysodrastV; Dulcagen; Dulcolax; Fleet Laxative. Enema: 10 mg/30 mL. Powder: 1.5 mg with tannic acid 2.5 g per packet (25 s, 50 s). Suppository, rectal: 5 mg, 10 mg. Tablet, enteric coated: 5 mg.	**Treatment of constipation (direct smooth muscle irritation to stimulate gastrointestinal peristalsis).** *Children:* *<2 yr:* 5 mg rectal suppository. *>2 yr:* 10 mg rectal suppository. *>6 yr:* 5–10 mg oral at bedtime or before breakfast. *Adults:* 5–30 mg oral dose, 10 mg rectal suppository.	*Adverse events:* Fluid and electrolyte imbalance, abdominal cramps.
Bismuth Subsalicylate Antidiarrheal, gastrointestinal agent, gastric or duodenal ulcer treatment. Bismatrol; Pepto-Bismol. Liquid: 262 mg/15 mL (120 mL, 240 mL, 360 mL, 480 mL); 524 mg/15 mL (120 mL, 240 mL, 360 mL). Tablet, chewable: 262 mg.	**Treatment of diarrhea or gastrointestinal ulcer (adsorbs extra water and toxins in large intestine and kills bacterial pathogens).** *Child or adult:* Up to 8 doses/24 hr. *3–6 yr:* 1/3 tablet or 5 mL. *6–9 yr:* 2/3 tablet or 10 mL. *9–12 yr:* 1 tablet or 15 mL. *Adult:* 2 tablets or 30 mL.	*Cautions:* Avoid in patients with influenza or chickenpox because of salicylate content. *Adverse events:* Discoloration of tongue, grayish-black stools.
Bleomycin Antineoplastic agent, antibiotic type. Blenoxane. Powder for injection: 15 units.	**Palliative treatment for several cancers and sclerosing agent for malignant effusions (inhibit synthesis of DNA).** *Children and adults:* 10–20 units/m^2/dose IV, IM, SC (0.25–0.5 units/kg) 1–2 times per wk in combination regimens.	*Cautions:* Reduce dose in renal dysfunction. *Adverse events:* Interstitial pneumonitis, pulmonary fibrosis, nonproductive cough, phlebitis, leukopenia, thrombocytopenia, stomatitis, vomiting, alopecia, hyperkeratosis of hand and nails, desquamation, Raynaud phenomenon; avoid oxygen use.

TABLE 728–1 General Medications *Continued*

Drug (Trade Names, Formulations)	Indications (Mechanism of Action) and Dosing	Comments (Cautions, Adverse Events, Monitoring)
Bretylium Antiarrhythmic agent, class III. Bretylol. Injection: 50 mg/mL (10 mL, 20 mL); 100 mg/mL. INjection, premixed in D_5W: 1 mg/mL (500 mL); 2 mg/mL (250 mL); 4 mg/mL (250 mL, 500 mL).	**Treatment of serious or life-threatening arrhythmias (inhibits release of NE at postganglionic nerve endings).** *Children:* 2–5 mg/kg IV or IM, may repeat every 10–20 min to maximum 30 mg/kg. *Adults:* initial dose 5 mg/kg, then 10 mg/kg every 15–30 min to maximum 35 mg/kg. Note: Cardioversion/defibrillation must be attempted before and after each dose of bretylium.	*Adverse events:* Hypotension, increased PVCs, bradycardia, nasal congestion, sweating, hiccups. *Monitoring:* ECG, blood pressure.
Brompheniramine Antihistamine. Bromarest, Bromphen Elixir, Chlorphed, Cophene-B Injection, Dehist Injection, Dimetane Oral, NasahistB Injection, ND-Stat Injection, Oraminic II Injection, Sinusol-B Injection, Veltane Tablet. Elixir: 2 mg/5 mL with alcohol 3% (120 mL, 480 mL, 4,000 mL). Injection: 10 mg/mL (10 mL). Tablet: 4 mg, 8 mg, 12 mg. Tablet, sustained release: 8 mg, 12 mg.	**Treatment of allergic symptoms, e.g., rhinitis and urticaria (competes with histamine for H1-receptor sites).** *Children:* *<6 yr:* 0.125 mg/kg/dose every 6 hr (max 8 mg/day) oral. *6–12 yr:* 2–4 mg/dose every 6–8 hr (max 16 mg/day) oral. *Adults:* 4–8 mg/dose every 4–6 hr (max 24 mg/day) oral. IV, IM, SC route: *<12 yr:* 0.5 mg/kg/day divided every 6 hr. *>12 yr:* 10 mg/dose (max 40 mg/day).	*Adverse events:* Sedation, dry mouth.
Budesonide Adrenal corticosteroid; anti-inflammatory agent; corticosteroid, nasal, glucocorticoid. Rhinocort. Aerosol: 50 μg released per actuation to deliver ~32 μg to patient via nasal adapter [200 metered doses] (7 g). Pulmicort turbuhaler. Inhalation powder 200 μg/inhalation.	**Treatment of chronic rhinitis or asthma (suppress iflammation).** *Children >6 and adults:* Rhinocort nasal spray 2 puffs in each nostril twice daily or 4 puffs in each nostril once daily. *Children >6 yr:* Pulmicort Turbihaler 1–2 inhalations bid. *Adults:* 1–4 inhalations bid.	*Adverse events:* Oral thrush, dysphonia (minimize by rinsing mouth after dose).
Bumetanide Antihypertensive; diuretic, loop. Bumex Injection: 0.25 mg/mL (2 mL, 4 mL, 10 mL). Tablet: 0.5 mg, 1 mg, 2 mg.	**Management of edema or fluid overload states (prevent sodium and chloride reabsorption at the ascending loop of Henle and proximal tubule).** Oral, IV, IM *Neonates:* 0.01–0.05 mg/kg/dose every 24 to 48 hr. *Infants and children:* 0.015–0.1 mg/kg/dose every 6–24 hr (max 10 mg/day). *Adults:* 0.5–2 mg/dose (max 10 mg/day).	*Adverse events:* Electrolyte depletion, dehydration.
Bupivacaine Local anesthetic, injectable. Marcaine, Sensorcaine, Sensorcaine-MPF Bupivacaine. Injection: Preservative free: 0.25% [2.5 mg/mL]; 0.5% [5 mg/mL]; 0.75% [7.5 mg/mL]. With preservative: 0.25% [2.5 mg/mL]; 0.5% [5 mg/mL]. Bupivacaine and epinephrine [2:2,000,000] injection: Preservative free: 0.25% [2.5 mg/mL]; 0.5% [5 mg/mL]; 0.75% [7.5 mg/mL]. With preservative: 0.25% [2.5 mg/mL]; 0.5% [5 mg/mL]. Bupivacaine in dextrose [8.25% injection (spinal): Preservative free: 0.75% [7.5 mg/mL].	**Local anesthetic (block initiation and conduction of nerve impulses by decreasing permeability of neuron to sodium ions).** CAUDAL BLOCK *Children:* 1–3.7 mg/kg. *Adults:* 15–30 ml of 0.25% or 0.5%. EPIDURAL BLOCK *Children:* 1.25 mg/kg/dose. *Adults:* 10–20 ml of 0.25% or 0.5%. PERIPHERAL NERVE BLOCK 5 ml dose of 0.25% (12.5 mg) or 0.5% (25 mg); max 400 mg/day. SYMPATHETIC NERVE BLOCK 20–50 ml of 0.25% (no epinephrine).	*Cautions:* Excess doses may result in seizures, bradyarrhythmias, metabolic acidosis, apnea, and methemoglobinemia.
Bupropion Antidepressant. Wellbutrin. Tablet: 75 mg, 100 mg.	**Depression, attention deficit disorder, smoking cessation (block serotonin activity and norepinephrine reuptake).** *Children:* anecdotal experience had benefits at 75–100 mg 2–3 times/day. *Adults:* Begin 100 mg twice daily and may gradually increase to max of 450 mg/day.	*Adverse events:* Agitation, insomnia, headache, psychosis, confusion, anxiety, seizures, akathesia, fever, chills, dry mouth, constipation, nausea, vomiting.
Busulfan Antineoplastic agent, alkylating agent. Myleran. Tablet: 2 mg.	**Treatment of chronic myelogenous leukemia or as part of marrow ablation conditioning prior to bone marrow transplant (interferes with DNA alkylation).** *Children:* (for CML remission) 0.06–0.12 mg/kg once daily, titrate dose to keep leukocyte count >40,000/mm³; (for BMT conditioning) 1 mg/kg/dose every 6 hr for 16 doses. *Adults:* (for CML remission) 0.06 mg/kg/day.	*Adverse events:* Severe pancytopenia, leukopenia, thrombocytopenia, and bone marrow suppression (onset 7–10 days, nadir 14–21 days, recovery 28 days). *Monitoring:* CBC with differential and platelet count (discontinue if WBC <20,000/mm³). Hemoglobin, liver function tests.

Table continued on following page

TABLE 728–1 General Medications *Continued*

Drug (Trade Names, Formulations)	Indications (Mechanism of Action) and Dosing	Comments (Cautions, Adverse Events, Monitoring)
Caffeine, Citrated Central nervous system stimulant, nonamphetamine; respiratory stimulant Tablet: 65 mg [anhydrous caffeine 32.5 mg], caffeine citrate, caffeine benzoate.	**Treatment of apnea of prematurity (stimulate central inspiratory drive and sensitivity to carbon dioxide).** *Neonates:* oral (citrate or benzoate), IV (benzoate). Dose as caffeine base: loading dose 10 mg/kg. Maintenance dose: 5–10 mg/kg/day as 1 or 2 doses/day.	*Cautions:* Sodium benzoate displaces bilirubin from binding and should be avoided in neonates with elevated indirect bilirubin. *Adverse events:* Tachycardia, agitation, irritability, gastric irritation. *Monitoring:* Caffeine concentrations: therapeutic >10 μg/mL; toxic >50 μg/mL.
Calcifediol 25-hydroxycholecalciferol; 25-hydroxyvitamin D3; vit D–analog. Calderol. Capsule: 20 μg, 50 μg	**Treatment of metabolic bone disease associated with chronic renal failure (regulates serum calcium homeostasis as a vitamin D–analog).** *Infants:* 5–7 μg/kg/day. *Children and adults:* 20–100 μg/kg daily or every other day titrated to obtain normal serum calcium and phosphate levels.	*Cautions:* Avoid in hypercalcemia, hypervitaminosis D, malabsorption states. Ensure adequate calcium intake during use. *Adverse events:* Hypercalcemia, GI intolerance.
Calcitriol Vitamin D analog; 1,25 dihydroxycholecalciferol, vitamin, fat soluble. Calcijex, Rocaltrol. Capsule: 0.25 μg, 0.5 μg. Injection: 1 μg/mL (1 mL); 2 μg/mL (1 mL).	**Treatment of hypocalcemia and metabolic bone disease, reduce elevated parathyroid hormone levels, decrease severity of psoriatic lesions in psoriatic vulgaris (regulate serum calcium homeostasis and increase calcium absorption).** *Premature infants* (hypocalcemia): 0.05 μg/kg/day IV or 1 μg/day orally. *Children:* 0.01–0.08 μg/kg/day. *Adults:* 0.25–1 μg/day.	*Adverse events:* Hypercalcemia, vit D toxicity.
CALCIUM SALTS (oral and IV) Calcium Carbonate Elemental calcium listed in brackets. Antacid; calcium salt; electrolyte supplement, oral. Alka-Mints, Cal-Plus, Mylanta, Os-Cal, Tums. Capsule: 1,500 mg [600 mg]. Liquid: 1,000 mg/5 mL (360 mL). Lozenge: 600 mg [240 mg]. Powder: 6.5 g/packet [2.6]. Suspension, oral: 1,250 mg/5 mL [500 mg]. Tablet: 650 mg [260 mg], 1,500 mg [600 mg]. Tablet, chewable. **Calcium Chloride** Calcium salt, electrolyte supplement, parenteral. Cal Plus. Elemental calcium listed in brackets. Injection: 10% = 100 mg/mL [27.2 mg/mL] (10 mL) (1.4 mEq calcium/mL). **Calcium Glubionate** Calcium Salt; Electrolyte Supplement, Oral. Neo-Calglucon. Syrup: 1.8 g/5 mL [115 mg/5 mL] (480 mL) (1.2 mEq calcium/mL).	**Hypocalcemic tetany, cardiac distrubances of hyperkalemia (moderate nerve and muscle performance).** HYPOCALCEMIC TETANY *Neonates:* 2.4 mEq/kg/day in divided doses (if due to citrated blood transfusion give 0.45 mEq per 100 mL transfused blood). *Infants and children:* 10 mg/kg over 5–10 min (may repeat in 6–8 hr) followed by infusion with max dose of 200 mg/kg/day. *Adults:* 4.5–16 mEq repeated until response. CARDIAC ARREST *Infants and children:* 20 mg/kg IV and may repeat in 10 min. *Adults:* 2–4 mg/kg repeated every 10 min as needed. **Prevention of calcium depletion, relief of acid indigestion (source of calcium and neutralizes acid).** *Children:* *<6 mo:* 400 mg/day. *6–12 mo:* 600 mg/day. *1–5 yr:* 800 mg/day. *6–10 yr:* 800–1,200 mg/day. *>10 yr and adult:* 1,000–1,500 mg/day.	*Caution:* Make sure of IV access site to avoid severe IV burns; bradycardia. *Adverse events:* Constipation, hypercalcemia, milk-alkali syndrome. *Monitoring:* Continuous ECG; serum calcium, potassium, and magnesium levels. (Calcium Content of Salts: see table below)
Capsaicin Analgesic, topical; topical Skin Product. R-Gel, Zostrix-HP Topical, Zostrix Topical. Cream: 0.025% (45 g, 90 g); 0.075% (30 g, 60 g). Gel: 0.025% (15 mL, 30 mL).	**Topical treatment of pain associated with postherpetic neuralgia, rheumatoid arthritis, osteoarthritis, diabetic neuropathy, and postsurgical pain (induces release of substance P depleting peripheral nerves and preventing reaccumulation).** *Children >2 yr and adults:* apply to affected area at least 3–4 times daily.	*Adverse events:* Local itching, stinging, burning, and erythema.
Captopril Angiotensin-converting enzyme (ACE) inhibitors; antihypertensive. Capoten. Tablet: 12.5 mg, 25 mg, 50 mg, 100 mg.	**Management of hypertension and treatment of heart failure (ACE inhibitor).** *Premature newborns:* 0.01 mg/kg every 8–12 hr. *Neonates:* initial 0.05–0.1 mg/kg/dose every 8–24 hr and titrate upward to response (max dose 0.5 mg/kg/dose every 6–24 hr). *Infants:* initial 0.15–0.3 mg/kg/dose; and titrate upward (max 6 mg/kg/day in 1–4 divided doses). *Children:* initial 0.3–0.5 mg/kg/dose and titrate upward (max 6 mg/kg/day divided into 2–4 doses). *Older children:* initial 6.25–12.5 mg/kg/dose every 12–24 hr then titrate (max 6 mg/kg/day in 2–4 doses). *Adolescents and adults:* initial 12.5–25 mg/dose and titrate (max 450 mg/day).	*Cautions:* Use with caution in renal artery stenosis or patients with volume depletion. *Adverse events:* Cough, angioedema, oliguria, hyperkalemia.

Calcium Content of Salts:

Salt	mg of Calcium/ g salt (Elemental)	mEq Ca^{2+}/ g salt
Ca carbonate	400 mg	20 mEq
Ca chloride	270 mg	13.5 mEq
Ca glubionate	64 mg	3.2 mEq
Ca gluceptate	82 mg	4.1 mEq
Ca gluconate	90 mg	4.5 mEq
Ca lactate	130 mg	6.5 mEq
Ca phosphate	390 mg	19.3 mEq

TABLE 728–1 General Medications *Continued*

Drug (Trade Names, Formulations)	Indications (Mechanism of Action) and Dosing	Comments (Cautions, Adverse Events, Monitoring)
Carbamazepine Anticonvulsant, miscellaneous. Epitol, Tegretol. Suspension, oral (citrus-vanilla flavor): 100 mg/5 mL (450 mL). Tablet: 200 mg. Tablet, chewable: 100 mg. Tegretol XR: 100 mg, 200 mg, 400 mg (sustained-release product).	**Treatment of generalized tonic-clonic and partial seizures, pain relief in trigeminal neuralgia and diabetic neuropathy, bipolar disorders (limit influx of sodium ions across cell membranes or other unknown mechanisms).** *Children:* *<6 yr:* initial 5 mg/kg/day in 2–4 divided doses; may increase every 5–7 days by 5 mg/kg based on effect or toxicity and serum concentration. *6–12 yr:* initial 10 mg/kg/day in 2–4 divided doses; increase by 100 mg or 5 mg/kg/day at weekly intervals until therapeutic levels are achieved (usual dose 800–1,200 mg/day). *Adults:* initial 200 mg twice daily; increase by 200 mg at weekly intervals until therapeutic levels are achieved (usual dose 1.6 to 2.4 g/day in 3–4 divided doses).	*Caution:* Avoid in patients with bone marrow depression; may cross-react in patients with tricyclic antidepressant hypersensitivity. *Adverse events:* Sedation, dizziness, fatigue, ataxia, confusion, nausea, vomiting, blurred vision, nystagmus, bone marrow depression, leukopenia, neutropenia, thrombocytopenia, pancytopenia, aplastic anemia, hepatitis, hypersensitivity reactions. *Monitoring:* Serum concentrations correlate with clinical response (6–12 μg/mL), and neurologic and visual toxicity (>8 μg/mL but particularly >12 μg/mL). Drug dosing requirements will increase over first 4 wk because of hepatic enzyme induction by carbamazepine. Monitor serum concentrations to increase doses appropriately.
Carbamide Peroxide Otic agent, cerumenolytic. Auro Ear Drops, Gly-Oxide Oral, Proxigel Oral, Murine Ear Drops. Gel, oral: 11% (36 g). Solution, oral: 10% in glycerin (15 mL, 22.5 mL, 30 mL, 60 mL). Otic 6.5% in glycerin (15 mL, 30 mL).	**Relief of minor inflammation of oral mucosa including gums and lips, and removal of ear wax (release of hydrogen peroxide which inhibits bacteria and softens ear wax)** *Children and adults:* Gel: gently massage on affected area 4 times daily. Oral solution: apply several drops to affected area 4 times daily for up to 7 days (expectorate 2–3 min after each use). Otic solution: tilt head sideways and instill 5–10 drops twice daily for up to 4 days. Keep drops in ear canal for several minutes by tilting head and placing cotton in ear.	*Adverse events:* Local irritation.
Carbinoxamine and Pseudoephedrine Antihistamine/decongestant conbination. Carbiset Tablet; Carbodec Syrup; Rondec Drops. Drops: carbinoxamine maleate 2 mg and pseudocphedrine hydrochloride 25 mg/mL (30 mL with dropper). Syrup: carbinoxamine maleate 4 mg and pseudoephedrine hydrochloride 60 mg/5 mL (120 mL, 480 mL). Tablet: Film-coated: carbinoxamine maleate 4 mg and pseudoephedrine hydrochloride 60 mg. Sustained release: carbinoxamine maleate 8 mg and pseudoephedrine hydrochloride 120 mg.	**Temporary relief of nasal congestion, runny nose, sneezing, and allergy symptoms (antihistamine as H1-blocker, and decongestant as alpha- and beta-receptor stimulant).** *Children:* dose 4 times daily: *1–3 mo:* 1/4 dropper (0.25 mL). *3–6 mo:* 1/2 dropper (0.5 mL). *6–9 mo:* 3/4 dropper (0.75 mL). *9–18 mo:* 1 dropper (1.0 mL). *18 mo–6 yr:* 2.5 mL syrup. *6–12 yr:* 5 mL syrup or 1 tablet. *Children >12 yr and adults:* 1 tablet 4 times daily, or 1 sustained-release tablet twice/day.	*Cautions:* Avoid in narrow angle glaucoma, coronary argery disease, GI or GU obstruction, or MAO inhibitor therapy. *Adverse events:* Hypertension, tachycardia, drowsiness, sedation, thickening of bronchial secretions.
Carboplatin Antineoplastic agent, alkylating agent. Paraplatin Powder for injection, lyophilized: 50 mg, 150 mg, 450 mg.	**Treatment of multiple tumors including pediatric brain tumor and neuroblastoma (platination of DNA interferes with DNA function).** *Children:* Solid tumor: 300–600 mg/m² IV once every 4 wk. Brain tumor: 175 mg/m² IV once wk for 4 wk (2 wk recovery period between courses). *Adult:* 360 mg/m² IV once every 4 wk.	*Adverse events:* Neutropenia, leukopenia, thrombocytopenia, peripheral neuropathy, ototoxicity, abnormal liver and renal function, alopecia, nausea, vomiting. *Monitoring:* Neutrophil and platelet count affect dose selection as follows: platelets <50,000/mm³ or neutrophils <500/mm³: give 75% of recommended dose (nadir 14–21 days post dose).
Carmustine Antineoplastic agent, alkylating agent (nitrosourea). BiCNU Powder for injection: 100 mg/vial packaged with 3 mL of absolute alcohol for use as a sterile diluent.	**Treatment of cancers including brain tumor, Hodgkin disease and non-Hodgkin lymphoma, and multiple myeloma (inhibits key enzymatic reactions involved in DNA synthesis).** *Children:* 200–250 mg/m² IV every 4–6 wk as a single dose. *Adults:* 150–200 mg/m² IV every 6 wk as a single dose.	*Adverse events:* Nausea, vomiting, myelosuppression (nadir 4–6 wk post dose), alopecia, stomatitis, anorexia, diarrhea, dizziness, ataxia, pulmonary fibrosis, hepatic and renal dysfunction, retinitis, optic neuritis.
Carnitine Dietary supplement. Carnitor, Vitacarn. Capsule: 250 mg. Injection: 1 g/5 mL (5 mL). Liquid (cherry flavor): 100 mg/mL (10 mL). Tablet: 330 mg.	**Treatment of carnitine deficiency and improve utilization of IV fat emulsions by premature infants (facilitates long-chain fatty acid entry into the mitochondria and required in energy metabolism).** *Premature infants:* 8–16 mg/kg/day IV infusion. *Children:* 50–100 mg/kg/day in 2–3 divided doses orally, 50 mg/kg/dose every 4–6 hr IV (max dose 300 mg/kg/day). *Adults:* 0.33–1 g/dose 2–3 times daily orally, 50 mg/kg/dose every 4–6 hr (max 300 mg/kg/day).	*Adverse events:* Nausea, vomiting, abdominal cramps, body odor.

Table continued on following page

TABLE 728–1 General Medications *Continued*

Drug (Trade Names, Formulations)	Indications (Mechanism of Action) and Dosing	Comments (Cautions, Adverse Events, Monitoring)
Cascara Sagrada Laxative, stimulant. Liquid, aromatic fluid extract: 5 mL, 120 mL. Tablet: 325 mg.	**Temporary relief of constipation (direct chemical irritation of GI mucosa).** *Infants:* 1.25 mL once daily. *Children 2–11 yr:* 2.5 mL once daily. *>12 yr and adults:* 5 mL once daily.	*Cautions:* Fecal impaction, GI obstruction, GI bleeding. Onset of effect 6–10 hr, so give at bedtime. *Adverse events:* GI cramps, urine discolored red or brown.
Castor Oil Laxative, Stimulant. Alphamul, Emulsoil, Fleet, Purge. Emulsion, oral; Liquid, oral: 100% (60 mL, 120 mL, 480 mL).	**Bowel or rectal evacuation for surgery (stimulates peristalsis).** *Infants <2 yr:* 1–5 mL single dose. *Children 2–11 yr:* 5–15 mL. *>12 yrs and adult:* 15–60 mL	*Adverse events:* Electrolyte disturbances, abdominal cramps.
Charcoal Adsorbent, antidote. Actidose-Aqua, Actidose with Sorbitol, Charcocaps.	**Emergency treatment of poisoning by certain drugs and chemicals; gastrointestinal dialysis to promote elimination of certain drugs and toxins; treat diarrhea (adsorb toxic substance; interfere with enterohepatic recycling of certain drugs.** *Children and adults:* 1–2 g/kg or 5–10 times the weight of the ingested poison (limit sorbitol to 1–2 times daily); may repeat doses every 2–6 hr.	*Adverse events:* Constipation, black stools.
Chloral hydrate Hypnotic; sedative. Noctec; capsules: 250, 500 mg. Syrup: 250, 500 mg/5 ml. Suppository: 324 mg, 500 mg, 648 mg.	**Short-term sedative/hypnotic (mechanism unknown).** *Neonates:* 25 mg/kg/dose. *Infants and children:* 25–100 mg/kg/dose. *Adult:* 250–1,000 mg/dose. Doses may be repeated every 6–8 hr. Lower-end doses cause sedation, higher-end doses cause hypnosis.	*Cautions:* Repeat doses in neonates may cause accumulation of active metabolite trochloroethanol (TCE), which can cause hepatic toxicity and bilirubin displacement.
Chlorambucil Antineoplastic alkylating agent. Leukeran 2 mg tablet.	**Management of various cancers including Hodgkin and non-Hodgkin lymphoma, and CLL; and nephrotic syndrome (alkylation interferes with DNA replication and RNA transcription).** *Children and adults:* 0.1–0.2 mg/kg/day for 3–6 wk. Longer treatment doses are adjusted based on blood counts.	*Adverse events:* Bone marrow suppression (onset 7 days, nadir 10–14 days, recovery 28 days); skin rashes, hyperuricemia, nausea, vomiting, diarrhea, oral ulceration, pulmonary fibrosis, hepatic necrosis, peripheral neuropathy.
Chlorothiazide Diuretic. Generic tablets: 250, 500 mg; suspension: 250 mg/5 mL; powder for injection: 500 mg.	**Treatment of fluid overload states and hypertension (inhibits sodium reabsorption in distal tubule).** *Neonates and infants <6 mo:* oral: 20–40 mg/kg/day divided every 12 hr; IV: 2–8 mg/kg/day divided every 12 hr. *Infants >6 mo and children:* oral: 20 mg/kg/day in 2 divided doses; IV: 4 mg/kg/day. *Adults:* oral: 500 mg–2 g/day in 1–2 doses; IV: 500–1,000 mg/day.	*Adverse events:* Hypkalemia, hypochloremic alkalosis, hyperglycemia, hyperlipidemia, hypercalcemia, hyperuricemia, leukopenia, prerenal azotemia.
Chlorpheniramine Maleate Antihistamine, generic. Capsule: 12 mg; timed-release capsule 6, 8, 12 mg; syrup 2 mg/5 mL; tablet 4, 8, 12 mg; chewable tablet 2 mg; timed-release tablets 8, 12 mg.	**Treat allergic symptoms (compete with histamine for H1-receptor sites).** *Children:* *2–6 yr:* 1 mg every 4–6 hr. *6–12 yr:* 2 mg every 4–6 hr or sustained-release 8 mg at bedtime. *>12 yr and adults:* 4 mg every 4–6 hr or sustained-release 12 mg at bedtime.	*Adverse events:* Drowsiness, excitation or hyperactivity (in children), dry mouth, blurred vision.
Chlorpromazine Phenothiazine. Thorazine. Capsule: 30, 75, 150, 200, 300 mg. Oral concentrate: 30, 100 mg/mL. Suppository: 25, 100 mg. Syrup: 10 mg/5 mL. Tablet: 10, 25, 50, 100, 200 mg. Injection: 25 mg/mL.	**Treatment of psychosis, mania, Tourette syndrome, behavioral problems, nausea and vomiting (blocks postsynaptic mesolimbic dopaminergic receptors in the brain, strong alpha-adrenergic blocking effect).** *Children >6 mo:* Oral: 0.5–1 mg/kg/dose every 4–6 hr; rectal: 1 mg/kg/dose every 6–8 hr; IM or IV: 0.5–1 mg/kg/dose every 6–8 hr. *Adults:* Psychosis: Oral: 30–800 mg/day in 1–4 divided doses (start low and titrate up to effect); IV or IM: 25 mg initial dose and titrate up to effect (max 400 mg/dose every 4–6 hr). Nausea or vomiting: Oral: 10–25 mg every 4–6 hr. IM or IV: 25–50 mg every 4–6 hr. Rectal: 50–100 mg every 6–8 hr.	*Adverse events:* Hypotension, tachycardia, arrhythmias, pseudoparkinsonism, tardive dyskinesia, akathesia, dystonias, constipation, nasal congestion, dry mouth, malignant hyperpyrexia. *Monitoring:* Chlorpromazine concentrations: therapeutic 50–300 ng/mL; toxic >750 ng/mL.

TABLE 728–1 General Medications *Continued*

Drug (Trade Names, Formulations)	Indications (Mechanism of Action) and Dosing	Comments (Cautions, Adverse Events, Monitoring)
Chlorpropamide Sulfonylurea. Diabinese. Tablet: 100, 250 mg.	**Control blood sugar in non-insulin-dependent diabetes diabetes mellitus (type II) (stimulate insulin release from pancreatic islet cells).** *Adults:* initial 250 mg once daily, may increase to response by 125 mg every 3–5 days to response (max 750 mg/day).	*Adverse events:* GI problems, photosensitivity, hepatotoxicity, hyponatremia, SIADH.
Chlorthalidone Thiazide diuretic. Hygroton. Tablets: 20, 25, 100 mg.	**Treatment of fluid overload and mild hypertension (inhibits sodium and chloride reabsorption in the cortical-diluting segment of the ascending loop of Henle).** *Children:* 1–2 mg/kg once daily. *Adults:* 25–100 mg once daily.	*Adverse events:* Photosensitivity, fluid and electrolyte imbalance, hypokalemia.
Chlorzoxazone Skeletal muscle relaxant. Parafon Forte, Paraflex. Tablets: 250, 500 mg.	**Symptomatic relief of muscle spasm and pain (depress polysynaptic reflexes at spinal cord and subcortical levels).** *Children:* 20 mg/kg/day in 3–4 divided doses. *Adults:* 250–500 mg 3–4 times daily.	*Adverse events:* Drowsiness.
Cholestyramine Resin Antilipemic agent. Questran. Powder: 4 g resin/9 g powder.	**Management of elevated cholesterol (forms a nonabsorbable complex with bile salts and LDL-cholesterol).** *Children:* 240 mg/kg/day in 3 divided doses. *Adults:* 4 g/dose 1–6 times daily.	*Adverse events:* Hyperchloremic acidosis, constipation, nausea, vomiting, abdominal pain and distention, malabsorption of fat-soluble vitamins.
Choline magnesium trisalicylate Nonsteroidal antiinflammatory agent (NSAID). Trilisate. Liquid: 500 mg salicylate/5 mL Tablets: 500, 750, 1,000 mg.	**Management of arthritis disorders (inhibit prostaglandin synthesis).** *Children:* 30–60 mg/kg/day in 3–4 divided doses. *Adults:* 500–1,500 mg/dose 1–3 times daily.	*Cautions:* Avoid in patients with suspected influenza or varicella infections due to risk for Reye syndrome; avoid in asthmatics and others at risk for serious hypersensitivity reactions. *Adverse events:* GI intolerance, tinnitus, hepatotoxicity, pulmonary edema. *Monitoring:* Salicylate concentrations: antiinflammatory 150–300 μg/mL; analgesic or antipyretic effect 30–50 μg/mL.
Chorionic gonadotropin Gonadotropin, ovulation stimulator. Chorex, Choron, Pregnyl. Powder for injection 200, 500, 1,000, 2,000 units/mL (10 mL).	**Treatment of hypogonadotropic hypogonadism; cryptorchidism; induce ovulation (stimulate production of gonadal steroid hormones; substitute for leutinizing hormone to stimulate ovulation).** *Children:* *Prepubertal cryptorchidism:* 1,000–2,000 units/m^2/dose 3 times/wk for 3 wk or 500 units 3 times/wk for 4–6 wk. *Hypogonadotropic hypogonadism:* 500–1,000 units/dose 3 times/wk for 3 wk; or 4,000 units 3 times/wk for 6–9 mo then taper to 2,000 units 3 times weekly for 3 mo. *Adults (menotropin dose):* 5,000 units 3 times/wk for 4–6 mo.	*Adverse events:* Mental depression, tiredness, precocious puberty, premature closure of the epiphyses.
Cimetidine Histamine-2 antagonist. Cimetidine. Tablets: 200, 300, 400, 800 mg. Liquid: 300 mg/5 mL. Injection: 150 mg/mL.	**Short-term treatment and long-term prophylaxis of GERD, and gastrointestinal ulcers and hyperacidity (competative inhibition of histamine at H-2 receptors).** *Neonates:* oral, IV, IM: 5–10 mg/kg/day divided every 8–12 hr. *Infants:* oral, IV, IM: 10–20 mg/kg/day divided every 6–12 hr. *Children:* oral IV, IM: 20–40 mg/kg/day divided every 6 hr. *Adults:* 300 mg every 6 hr (prolong dosing interval for creatinine clearance below 40 mL/min).	*Cautions:* Potent enzyme inhibitor thus may cause toxic accumulation of drugs that are metabolized (e.g., antidepressants, anticonvulsants, theophylline, warfarin, cisapride). *Adverse events:* Dizziness, drowsiness, bradycardia. *Monitoring:* Target gastric pH ≥ 5.
Cisapride Prokinetic gastrointestinal agent. Propulsid. Tablet: 10 mg.	**Treatment of gastroesophageal reflux, gastroparesis, and refractory constipation (enhances release of acetylcholine at myenteric plexus).** *Neonates–Children:* 0.15–0.3 mg/kg/dose 3–4 times daily. *Adults:* 10–20 mg 4 times daily. Give doses 15–30 min before meals.	*Cautions:* High doses or combination with enzyme inhibitors (e.g., erythromycin, cimetidine) may cause QT-interval prolongation predisposing to torsades du pointes. *Adverse events:* Tachycardia, prolonged QT interval, headache, anxiety, insomnia, GI cramping, flatulence, diarrhea. *Monitoring:* ECG baseline and early treatment.
Cisplatin Antineoplastic agent, alkylating agent. Platinol. Injection, aqueous: 1 mg/mL. Powder for injection 10, 50 mg.	**Treatment of multiple tumor types (inhibit DNA synthesis).** *Children and adults:* 37–75 mg/m^2 once every 2–3 wk or 50–120 mg/m^2 once every 21–28 days (administer over 4–6 hr). Adjust dose in renal impairment: CrCl 10–50 mL/min = 75% of dose; CrCl <10 mL/min = 50% of dose.	*Adverse events:* Nausea vomiting (lasts up to 1 wk postdose), myelosuppression (onset 10 days, nadir 14–23 days, recovery 21–39 days), acute renal failure, chronic nephropathy (sodium, magnesium, and water wasting; hyperuricemia), peripheral neuropathy (irreversible), ototoxicity (high frequency hearing loss), extravasation injury, elevated liver enzymes, alopecia, optic neuritis, arrhythmias.

Table continued on following page

TABLE 728–1 General Medications *Continued*

Drug (Trade Names, Formulations)	Indications (Mechanism of Action) and Dosing	Comments (Cautions, Adverse Events, Monitoring)
Citrate Solutions Alkalinizing agent. Bicitra (sodium citrate 500 mg and citric acid 334 mg/5 mL = 1 mEq sodium + 1 mEq bicarbonate equivalent per mL). Polycitra (sodium citrate 500 mg and citric acid 334 mg and potassium citrate 550 mg/5 mL = 1 mEq sodium + 1 mEq potassium + 2 mEq bicarbonate equivalent per mL).	**Treatment of chronic metabolic acidosis (citrate salts are oxidized in the body to form bicarbonate).** *Neonates, infants, and children:* 2–3 mEq/kg/day in 3–4 divided doses with water after meals. *Adults:* 15–30 mL with water after meals and at bedtime.	*Adverse events:* Hypernatremia, hyperkalemia, metabolic alkalosis.
Clomipramine Antidepressant. Anafranil. Capsule: 25, 50, 75 mg.	**Treatment of obsessive compulsive disorder and panic attacks (affect serotonin and norepinephrine uptake).** *Children:* start 25 mg/day and gradually increase to response (maximum 200 mg/day). *Adults:* start 25 mg/day and dose to response (max 250 mg/day).	*Adverse events:* Dizziness, drowsiness, dry mouth, constipation, nausea, weight gain, nervousness, anxiety, seizures, hypotension, arrhythmias, parkinsonian syndrome, insomnia.
Clonazepam Benzodiazepine. Klonopin. Tablets: 0.5, 1, 2 mg.	**Prophylaxis of seizure types: absence, Lennox-Gastaut, akinetic, myoclonic (depress nerve transmission in the motor cortex).** *Children:* 0.01–0.03 mg/kg/day in 2–3 divided doses (max 0.05 mg/kg/day). *Adults:* initial dose 0.1 mg twice daily; then 0.2–2.4 mg/day in 2–4 divided doses.	*Adverse events:* Tachycardia, chest pain, drowsiness, fatigue, impaired memory and coordination, depression, blurred vision, nausea, vomiting, dry mouth, hypersalivation, anorexia, bronchial hypersecretion, respiratory depression, physical and psychological dependence. *Monitoring:* Clonazepam concentrations: therapeutic 20–80 ng/mL; toxic >80 ng/mL; loss of efficacy with prolonged use (tachyphylaxis).
Clonidine Alpha-adrenergic agonist. Catapres. Tablet 0.1, 0.2, 0.3 mg. Transdermal patch 0.1, 0.2, 0.3 mg/day.	**Treatment of hypertension; attention deficit disorder; narcotic withdrawal; aid in diagnosis of pheochromocytoma and growth hormone deficiency (stimulates alpha-2 adrenoreceptors in the brain stem).** *Neonates:* Narcotic withdrawal: 1 μg/kg every 6 to 8 hr to start and may titrate to targeted abstinence score (max 2 μg/kg/dose every 4 hr). *Children:* ADD: initial 0.05 mg/day, increase every 3–7 days by 0.05 mg/day given in 3–4 divided doses to response (max 0.4 mg/day). Hypertension: 5–10 μg/kg/day in 2–4 divided doses (max 0.9 mg/day). Clonidine tolerance test for growth hormone release: 4 μg/kg × 1 dose. *Adults:* hypertension oral: 0.2–2.4 mg/day in 2–4 doses titrated to response; transdermal: 0.1–0.3 mg/day titrated to effect.	*Cautions:* Taper doses gradually to avoid sympathetic overactivity symptoms. *Adverse events:* Drowsiness, dizziness, dry mouth, constipation, hypotension.
Clorazepate Benzodiazepine. Tranxene. Tablet 3.75, 7.5, 15 mg.	**Anxiety and panic disorders; adjunct in management of partial seizures (facilitate transmission of the inhibitory neurotransmitter, GABA).** *Children:* *9–12 yr:* 3.75–7.5 mg/dose twice daily (max 60 mg/day). *>12 yr and adults:* 7.5 mg/dose 2–3 times/day (max 90 mg/day). *Adults:* 7.5–15 mg/dose 2–4 times daily.	*Adverse events:* Drowsiness, confusion, depression, blurred vision.
Codeine Narcotic analgesic. Generic, combination products. Injection. Tablet.	**Treatment of mild to moderate pain and cough (inhibition of ascending pain pathways; central action in medulla to suppress cough).** *Children:* Pain: 0.5–1 mg/kg/dose every 4–6 hr (max 60 mg/dose). Cough: 1–1.5 mg/kg/day divided every 4–6 hr. *Adults:* Pain: 15–60 mg/dose every 4–6 hr as needed. Cough: 10–20 mg/dose every 4–6 hr (max 120 mg/day).	*Adverse events:* Drowsiness, constipation, nausea, anorexia, vomiting, sedation, dizziness.
Colchicine Anti-inflammatory/antigout agent. Generic. Injection: 0.5 mg/mL. Tablet: 0.5, 0.6 mg.	**Management of familial Mediterranean fever, acute and chronic gouty arthritis (decrease leukocyte motility and phagocytosis in joints).** *Children:* Prophylaxis of familial Mediterranean fever: *<5 yr:* 0.5 mg/day. *>5 yr:* 1–1.5 mg/day in 2–3 divided doses. *Adults:* gouty arthritis: oral: 0.5–0.6 mg every 2 hr to symptom relief or GI toxicity (max 8 mg/day). IV: 1–3 mg load then 0.5 mg/dose every 6 hr until response (max 4 mg/day).	*Caution:* Reduce dose by 50% if CrCl <10 ml/min. *Adverse events:* Nausea, vomiting, diarrhea, abdominal pain.

TABLE 728–1 General Medications *Continued*

Drug (Trade Names, Formulations)	Indications (Mechanism of Action) and Dosing	Comments (Cautions, Adverse Events, Monitoring)
Colfosceril Palmitate Lung surfactant. Exosurf. Intratracheal suspension, 108 mg/10 mL.	**Neonatal respiratory distress syndrome (replaces deficient surfactant, lowers surface tension at air-fluid interface in alveoli).** *Neonates:* 5 ml/kg/dose as prophylaxis or rescue therapy for RDS (maximum 4 doses although no proven benefit for >2 doses).	*Caution:* Administer via sideport using special ET tube adaptor with ½ dose with head and torso tilted to left and ½ dose head and torso tilted to right; give each half over 1–2 min. *Adverse events:* Pulmonary hemorrhage, overventilation (causing hyperoxia and hypocarbia), PDA.
Corticotropin, ACTH Adrenal corticosteroid. Acthar. Injection, repository: 40, 80 units/mL. Tablet: 5, 10, 25 mg.	**Infantile spasms; diagnostic agent in adrenocortical insufficiency; acute exacerbations of multiple sclerosis; severe muscle weakness in myasthenia gravis (stimulates adrenal cortex to release adrenal steroids, androgenic substances and a small amount of aldosterone).** *Children:* Inflammation or immunosuppression: IV, IM, SC (aqueous): 1.6 units/kg/day or 50 units/m² divided every 6–8 hr; IM (gel): 0.8 units/kg/day divided every 12–24 hr. Infantile spasms: 5–160 units/kg/day has been used for 1 wk–12 mo as IM gel (prednisone 2 mg/kg/day has equal efficacy). *Adults:* Acute exacerbations of MS: 80–120 units/day for 2–3 wk.	*Caution:* May mask signs of infection; do not administer live vaccines; may exacerbate heart failure or hypertension. *Adverse events:* Insomnia, nervousness, increased appetite, indigestion, diabetes mellitus, joint pain, epistaxis, mood swings, pancreatitis, esophagitis, muscle wasting, bone growth suppression, opportunistic infections.
Cortisone Acetate Adrenal corticosteroid. Cortone. Injection: 50 mg/mL. Tablet: 5, 10, 25 mg.	**Management of adrenocortical insufficiency (replacement).** *Children:* oral: 0.5–0.75 mg/kg/day divided every 8 hr. IM: 0.25–0.35 mg/kg once daily. *Adults:* oral, IM: 20–300 mg/day in 1–2 doses.	*Cautions:* Avoid in active fungal infection and most other serious infections except shock or meningitis. *Adverse events:* Insomnia, nervousness, pseudotumor cerebri, headache, increased appetite, peptic ulcer, diabetes mellitus, edema, hypertension, cataracts, glaucoma, hypokalemia. *Comment:* See comparison of corticosteroids under *Hydrocortisone*.
Cosyntropin Adrenal corticosteroid. Cortrosyn. Powder for injection: 0.25 mg.	**Diagnosis of primary versus secondary adrenocortical deficiency (stimulates adrenal cortex to release adrenal steroids).** *Neonates:* 0.015 mg/kg/dose. *Children <2 yr:* 0.125 mg. *Children >2 yr and adult:* 0.25 mg. Give dose in early morning.	*Adverse events:* Flushing, mild fever, pruritis, pancreatitis. *Monitoring:* Measure plasma cortisol before and exactly 30 min after dose. Normal response is serum cortisol increase >7 µg/dL (>193 nmol/L), or peak response increase >18 µg/dL (497 nmol/L).
Cromolyn Sodium Mast cell stabilizer. Intal, Gastrocrom, Nasalcrom Crolom ophthalmic solution. Capsule (oral): 100 mg. Inhalation 20 mg. Metered dose inhaler 800 µg/spray. Nebulizer solution 10 mg/ml (2 ml). Nasal solution 40 mg/mL. Ophthalmic solution 4%.	**Prevention of chronic symptoms of asthma, rhinits, conjunctivitis, systemic mastocytosis, food allergy, and inflammatory bowel disease (prevents mast cell release of histamine and leukotrienes).** *Children and adults:* Asthma: 1–2 puffs (MDI) or 2 ml (nebulizer solution) 3–4 times daily. Rhinitis: 1 spray each nostril 3–4 times daily. Conjunctivitis: 1–2 drops 4–6 times daily. Mastocytosis, food allergy: *Children:* 100 mg/dose 4 times daily (max 40 mg/kg/day). *Adults:* 200 mg/dose 4 times daily (max 400 mg/dose 4 times daily).	*Adverse events:* Hoarseness and coughing (mainly with powder for inhalation), burning and stinging at administration site.
Crotamiton Scabicidal Eurax. Cream: 10%. Lotion: 10%.	**Treatment of scabies (mechanism unknown).** *Infants, children, and adults:* Wash area thoroughly, towel dry, apply a thin layer and massage drug into skin. Repeat application in 24 hr. Take a cleansing bath 48 hr after final application. May repeat in 7 days if needed.	*Adverse events:* Local irritation.
Cyanocabolamin, Vitamin B_{12} Nutritional supplement. Generic. Injection: 100, 1,000 µg/mL. Tablet: 25, 50, 100, 250, 500, 1,000 µg.	**Pernicious anemia, vitamin B12 deficiency (coenzyme for various metabolic functions).** Pernicious anemia: *Children:* 30–50 µg/day to total dose 1,000–5,000 µg, then follow with 100 µg mo. *Adults:* 100 µg/day for 6–7 days, then 100 µg/mo. Vitamin B12 deficiency: *Children:* 100 µg/day for 10–15 days then once or twice wk for several mo. *Adults:* 30 µg/day for 5–10 days then 100–200 µg/mo.	*Monitoring:* Serum B12 levels (normal 150–750 pg/mL). Some reports of neuropsychiatric problems have been reported with levels below 300 pg/mL.

Table continued on following page

TABLE 728–1 General Medications *Continued*

Drug (Trade Names, Formulations)	Indications (Mechanism of Action) and Dosing	Comments (Cautions, Adverse Events, Monitoring)
Cyclizine Antinausea drug. Marezine. Injection: 50 mg/mL. Tablet: 50 mg.	**Prevent and treat motion-related nausea, vomiting, and vertigo; control post-operative nausea and vomiting** (mechanism unknown). *Children 6–12 yr:* oral 25 mg/dose up to 3 times /day as needed. *Adults:* oral 50 mg up to every 4–6 hr (30 min before travel), max 200 mg/day; IM 50 mg every 4–6 hr as needed.	*Adverse events:* Drowsiness, dry mouth, headache, diplopia, urinary retention.
Cyclopentolate Mydriatic. Cyclogyl, AK-Pentolate. Ophthalmic solution: 0.5%, 1%, 2%.	**Diagnostic procedures requiring mydriasis and cycloplegia (prevents the muscles of the ciliary body and iris from responding to cholinergic stimulation).** *Infants:* 1 drop 0.5% into each eye 5–10 min before examination. *Children and adults:* 1 drop 0.5% or 1% in eye 40–50 min before procedure (may repeat 1 drop in 5 min if necessary); may use 2% if heavily pigmented iris.	*Caution:* Avoid in narrow angle glaucoma. *Adverse events:* Tachycardia, CNS stimulation, psychosis, agitation, local burning. *Monitoring:* Cycloplegia and mydriasis begin in 15–60 min and last up to 24 hr (reduce to 3–6 hr with pilocarpine).
Cyclophosphamide Antineoplastic alkylating agent. Cytoxan; Neosar. Powder for injection: 0.1, 0.2, 0.5, 1.0, 2.0 g. Tablet: 25, 50 mg.	**Management of various cancers including Hodgkin disease, malignant lymphomas, leukemias, etc.; nephrotic syndrome; lupus erythematosis; rheumatoid arthritis; and rheumatoid vasculitis (interferes with normal function of DNA by alkylation).** *Children and adults with no hematologic problems:* Induction: IV: 40–50 mg/kg (1.5–1.8 g/m^2) in divided doses over 2–5 days. Oral: 1–5 mg/kg/day. Maintenance: IV: 10–15 mg/kg (350–550 mg/m^2) every 7–10 days or 3–5 mg/kg twice weekly. Oral: *Children:* 2–5 mg/kg twice/wk. *Adults:* 1–5 mg/kg/day. *Children:* SLE: 500–750 mg/m^2 every mo. JRA/vasculitis: IV 10 mg/kg every 2 wk. BMT conditioning: IV 50 mg/kg/day for 3–4 days. Nephrotic syndrome: Oral 2–3 mg/kg/day (when steroids fail, use for up to 12 wk). Adjust doses for: Renal function: CrCl 25–50 mL/min: decrease 50% CrCl <25 mL/min: avoid use. For decreased bone marrow function: reduce does 33–50%.	*Cautions:* Maintain high fluid intake to avoid hemorrhagic cystitis and consider administration of mesna. *Adverse events:* Cardiotoxicity with high doses, pericardial effusion, congestive heart failure, alopecia, nausea, vomiting, taste distortion, stomatitis, anorexia, hemorrhagic cystitis, leukopenia (onset 7 days, nadir 8–15 days, recovery 21 days), thrombocytopenia, hepatotoxicity, jaundice, renal toxicity, secondary malignancy.
Cyclosporine Immunosuppressant. Sandimmune, Neoral. Solution: 100 mg/mL. Injection: 50 mg/mL.	**Immunosuppressant used to prevent graft versus host disease in organ transplantation (inhibit production and release of interleukin II and activation of resting T-lymphocytes by interleukin II).** *Children and adults:* IV: initial 5–6 mg/kg/dose started 4–12 hr prior to organ transplant; maintenance: 2–10 mg/kg/day divided every 8–12 hr. Oral (Neoral preferred): Initial: 14–18 mg/kg/dose started 4–12 hr prior to transplant. Maintenance: 5–15 mg/kg/day divided every 12–24 hr, usually tapered to 3–10 mg/kg/day.	*Cautions:* Drugs inhibiting hepatic metabolism (e.g., erythromycin, ketoconazole, fluconazole, verapamil) may cause toxic accumulation of cyclosporine. Hepatic enzyme inducers may cause cyclosporine levels to become subtherapeutic. *Adverse events:* Hypertension, hirsutism, tremor, nephrotoxicity (especially if combined with other nephrotoxins), gingival hypertrophy, leg cramps, GI discomfort, acne, seizure, headache. *Monitoring:* Trough cyclosporine concentration (12 hr after dose or prior to next dose) should be monitored closely. Reference range depends on organ transplanted and assay method used: Serum RIA 150–300 ng/mL, late post-transplant period 50–150 ng/mL. Whole blood RIA 250–800 ng/mL, late posttransplant period 150–450 ng/mL. Whole blood HPLC 100–500 ng/mL.
Cyproheptadine hydrochloride Antihistamine. Generic, Periactin. Syrup: 2 mg/5 mL. Tablet: 4 mg.	**Treatment of allergic symptoms (H1-receptor and serotonin antagonist).** *Children 2–6 yr:* 2 mg/dose every 8–12 hr. >*7 yr and adults:* 4 mg/dose every 8–12 hr (max 0.5 mg/kg/day).	*Adverse events:* Drowsiness, sedation, thickened bronchial secretions, bronchospasm, appetitie stimulation, photosensitivity.
Cysteine Nutritional supplement. Generic. Injection 50 mg/mL.	**Supplement to crystalline amino acid solutions to meet amino acid nutritional requirements during parenteral nutrition (replace deficiency, also enhances solubility of calcium and phosphate in TPN solutions).** *Neonates and infants:* Add 40 mg cysteine to 1 g of amino acids (typically results in 20–100 mg/kg/day of cysteine).	*Adverse events:* Metabolic acidosis, azotemia, elevated BUN, nausea.

TABLE 728–1 General Medications *Continued*

Drug (Trade Names, Formulations)	Indications (Mechanism of Action) and Dosing	Comments (Cautions, Adverse Events, Monitoring)
Cytarabine HCl, Ara-C Antineoplastic, antimetabolite. Cytosar-U (powder for injection: 0.1, 0.5, 1, 2 g). Tarabine PFS. Injection: 20 mg/mL.	**Used in combination therapy to treat leukemias and lymphomas (inhibits DNA polymerase to inhibit DNA synthesis, works in S-phase of cell division).** *Children and adults:* (doses depend on individual protocols). *Typical dose:* Induction: IV: 100–200 mg/m²/day for 5–10 days or until remission. Maintenance: IV: 70–200 mg/m²/day for 2–5 days at monthly intervals; IM, SC: 1–1.5 mg/kg single dose at 1- to 4-wk intervals. IT: 5–75 mg/m² every 2–7 days until CNS findings normalize (concentration should not exceed 100 mg/mL).	*Adverse events:* fever, rash, oral/anal ulcerations, nausea, vomiting, diarrhea, mucositis, liver dysfunction, bleeding, myelosuppression (onset 4–7 days, nadir 14–18 days, recovery 21–28 days), alopecia, conjunctivitis (administer corticosteroid eye drops around-the-clock before, during, and after high dose Ara-C), dizziness, headache, neuritis (prevent CNS toxicities with pyridoxine administration on days of high-dose Ara-C administration).
Dacarbazine Antineoplastic agent. DTIC-Dome, generic. Injection: 100, 200, 500 mg	**Treatment of various tumors (alkylating agent and possibly some antimetabolite activity).** *Children:* Solid tumors: 200–470 mg/m²/day over 5 days every 21–28 days neuroblastoma: 800–900 mg/m² on day 1 of combination therapy every 3–4 wk. Hodgkin disease: 375 mg/m² on days 1 and 15 of combination treatment; repeat every 28 days. *Adults:* Hodgkin disease: 150 mg/m²/day for 5 days; repeat every 4 wk.	*Adverse events:* Pain and burning at infusion site, nausea and vomiting, leukopenia (onset 7 days, nadir 10–14 days, recovery 21–28 days), weakness, polyneuropathy, paresthesias, elevated liver enzymes, sinus congestion, alopecia, metallic taste.
Dactinomycin, Actinomycin D Antineoplastic agent. Cosmegen. Powder for injection 0.5 mg.	**Treatment of various tumor types (binds to guanine portion of DNA blocking replication and transcription of the DNA template).** *Children >6 mo and adults:* 15 µg/kg/day or 400–600 µg/m²/day for 5 days; may repeat every 3–6 wk.	*Adverse events:* Myelosuppression (onset 7 days, nadir 14–21 days, recovery 21–28 days), fatigue, malais, fever, alopecia, skin eruptions, acne, severe nausea and vomiting, diarrhea, mucositis, stomatitis, hypocalcemia, hyperuricemia.
Dantrolene Sodium Skeletal muscle relaxant. Dantrium. Capsule: 25, 50, 100 mg. Powder for injection: 20 mg.	**Treatment of spasticity associated with upper motor neuron disorders such as spinal cord injury, stroke, cerebral palsy or multiple sclerosis; also used to treat malignant hyperthermia (interferes with release of calcium ion from the sarcoplasmic reticulum).** Spasticity: *Children:* 0.5 mg/kg/dose twice daily; increase frequency every 4–7 days to 3–4 times daily; then increase dose by 0.5 mg/kg to max 3 mg/kg/dose 2–4 times daily. *Adults:* start 25 mg/day and increase dose by 25 mg or frequency every 4–7 days to max of 100 mg 2–4 times daily. Hyperthermia: *Children and adults:* Oral: 4–8 mg/kg/day in 4 divided doses given 1–2 days prior to surgery (prophylaxis), or for 1–3 days postsurgery (postcrisis follow-up). IV: 2.5 mg/kg starting 1.5 hr before surgery and run over 1 hr (prophylaxis) or 1 mg/kg/dose and repeated as needed (crisis); max 10 mg/kg.	*Cautions:* Should not be used where spasticity is used to maintain posture or balance; avoid in patients with active liver disease. *Adverse events:* Drowsiness, fatigue, dizziness, confusion, blurred vision, seizures, diarrhea, stomach cramps, nausea, vomiting, pleural effusion with pericarditis, hepatitis.
Daunorubicin Hydrochloride Antineoplastic. Cerubidine. Powder for injection: 20 mg.	**Treatment of ANLL and myeloblastic leukemia (inhibition of DNA and RNA synthesis).** *Children:* Remission induction for ALL (combination therapy): 25–45 mg/m² on day 1 every wk for 4 cycles (max total 300 mg/m²). *Adults:* 30–60 mg/m²/day for 3–5 days, repeat dose in 3–4 wk; total cumulative dose should not exceed 400–600 mg/m² (lower end if prior cardiotoxic drugs or chest irradiation).	*Caution:* Avoid in patients with heart failure or arrhythmias. Irreversible cardiotoxicity may occur if total dose exposure exceeds: 550 mg/m² in adults, 400 mg/m² if chest irradiation, 300 mg/m² in children >2 yr, 10 mg/kg in children <2 yr. *Adverse events:* Alopecia, red discoloration of urine, nausea, vomiting, diarrhea, GI ulceration, stomatitis, myelosuppression (onset 7 days, nadir 14 days, recovery 21–28 days), extravasation-related tissue ulceration and necrosis, congestive heart failure, hyperuricemia, hepatotoxicity. *Monitoring:* Serum bilirubin and AST (to adjust doses for hepatic impairment): bilirubin 1.2–3 mg/dL or AST 60–180 IU: reduce dose to 75%; bilirubin 3.1–5 mg/dL or AST >180 IU: reduce dose to 50%; bilirubin >5 mg/dL: omit use.

Table continued on following page

TABLE 728–1 General Medications *Continued*

Drug (Trade Names, Formulations)	Indications (Mechanism of Action) and Dosing	Comments (Cautions, Adverse Events, Monitoring)
Deferoxamine Mesylate Chelating agent. Desferal. Powder for injection: 500 mg.	**Treatment of acute iron intoxication or secondary chronic iron overload (forms complex with iron to form ferrioxamine, which is removed by kidneys).** *Children:* Acute iron intoxication: IM: 90 mg/kg/dose every 8 hr. IV: 15 mg/kg/hr (max 6 g/day). Chronic iron overload: IV: 15 mg/kg/hr (max 12 g/day). SC: 20–40 mg/kg/day over 8–12 hr via portable infusion device. *Adults:* Acute iron intoxication: IM: 1 g STAT, then 0.5 g every 4 hr (max 6 g/day). IV: 15 mg/kg/hr (max 6 g/day). Chronic iron overload: IM: 0.5–1 g/day. SC: infuse 1–2 g/day over 8–24 hr.	*Caution:* Contraindicated in patients with primary hemochromatosis. *Adverse events:* Local pain and induration, flushing, hypotension, tachycardia, fever, hearing loss, blurred vision, cataracts. *Monitoring:* Serum ferritin, iron, total iron binding capacity. Audiometry and eye exam with chronic use.
Desipramine Hydrochloride Antidepressant, tricyclic. Norpramin, Pertofrane. Tablet: 10, 25, 50, 75, 100, 150 mg. Capsule: 25, 50 mg.	**Treatment of depression, attention deficit disorder, neuropathic pain (increases synaptic concentrations or serotonin and norepinephrine by inhibiting reuptake).** *Children:* 6–12 yr: 1–3 mg/kg/day (max 5 mg/kg/day). *Adolescents:* initial 25–50 mg/day, gradually increase (max 150 mg/day). *Adults:* initial 75 mg/day, gradually increase (max 300 mg/day).	*Cautions:* Abrupt discontinuation can result in withdrawal symptoms; tablets contain tartrazine (may be problem for asthmatics), contraindicated in narrow angle glaucoma. *Adverse events:* Dizziness, drowsiness, headache, blurred vision, dry mouth, constipation, increased apetite, cardiac arrhythmias, hypotension. *Monitoring:* Desipramine concentrations: therapeutic 100–300 ng/mL, toxic >300 ng/mL; check ECG.
Desmopressin Acetate Vasopressin analog. DDAVP, Stimate. Injection: 4 μg/mL. Nasal solution: 0.1 mg/mL.	**Treatment of diabetes insipidus, control of bleeding in certain types of hemophilia, primary nocturnal enuresis (enhances reabsorption of water in the kidneys, dose-dependent increase in factor VIII and plasminogen activator).** *Children:* Diabetes insipidus: *3 mo–12 yr:* Oral: 0.05 mg initially then titrate to response. IV: 5 μg/day in 1–2 doses. Hemophilia: *>3 mo:* IV: 0.3 μg/kg, may repeat dose if needed, use 30 minutes before procedure. Nocturnal enuresis: *>6 yr:* 20 μg at bedtime. *Children >12 yr and adults:* Diabetes insipidus: Oral: 0.05 mg twice daily then titrate to response. IV, SC: 2–4 μg/day. Intranasal: 5–40 μg/day in 1–3 doses. Hemophilia: IV: 0.3 μg/kg. Intranasal: <50 kg = 150 μg, >50 kg = 300 μg. Enuresis: Oral: 0.2–0.4 mg at bedtime.	*Cautions:* Avoid using in patients with type IIB or platelet-type von Willebrand disease, hemophilia A with factor VII levels <5% or hemophilia B. *Adverse events:* Facial flushing, headache dizziness, increased blood pressure, hyponatremia, water intoxication. *Monitoring:* Serum electrolytes, plasma and urine osmolality, urine output, factor VIII antigen levels, APTT, factor VII activity level.
Dexamethasone Adrenal corticosteroid. Decadron. Aerosol: Oral 84 μg/activation, nasal 84 μg/spray. Cream: 0.1%, 0.04%. Injection: 4, 8, 10, 16, 20, 24 mg/mL. Ophthalmic ointment: 0.05%. Opthalmic suspension: 0.1, 0.5%. Oral solution: 0.5 mg/5 mL. Tablet: 0.25, 0.5, 0.75, 1, 1.5, 2, 4, 6 mg. Elixir: 0.5 mg/5 mL.	**Systemically and locally for acute and chronic inflammation; allergic, neoplastic and autoimmune diseases; cerebral edema, septic shock, *H. influenzae* meningitis, diagnostic agent (decrease inflammation and suppresses normal immune response).** *Neonates:* Airway edema or extubation: IV: 0.25 mg/kg every 12 hr for 3–4 doses (start >4 hr prior to scheduled extubation). Bronchopulmonary dysplasia: IV: Oral: 0.25 mg/kg/dose every 12 hr for 6 doses then taper over 1 to 6 wk (regimens may begin as early as day 1). *Children:* Airway edema or extubation: Oral: IM: IV: 0.5–2 mg/kg/day divided every 6 hr (begin 24 hr prior to extubation and continue for 4–6 doses post extubation). Antiemetic (chemotherapy-induced): IV: 10 mg/m^2 first dose then 5 mg/m^2/dose every 6 hr as needed (start prior to chemotherapy). Anti-inflammatory: oral: IM: IV: 0.08–0.3 mg/kg/day divided every 6–12 hr. Bacterial meningitis: IV: 0.6 mg/kg/day divided every 6 hr for days 1–4 of antibiotics.	*Adverse events:* Insomnia, nervousness, increased apetite, hypertension, hyperglycemia, GI hyperacidity (stress ulcer risk), cataracts, adrenal suppression, poor growth. Comment: See comparison of corticosteroids under *Hydrocortisone*.

TABLE 728–1 General Medications *Continued*

Drug (Trade Names, Formulations)	Indications (Mechanism of Action) and Dosing	Comments (Cautions, Adverse Events, Monitoring)
Dexamethasone *Continued*	Cerebral edema: Oral: IM: IV: loading dose 1–2 mg/kg, then 1–1.5 mg/kg/day divided every 4–6 hr. Inhalation: 2 puffs 3–4 times daily. Nasal spray: 1–2 sprays in each nostril twice daily. Physiologic replacement: Oral: IM: IV: 0.03–0.15 mg/kg/day divided every 6–12 hr. *Adults:* Anti-inflammatory: Oral: IM: IV: 0.5–9 mg/day divided every 6–12 hr. Antiemetic: same as for children. Cerebral edema: IV: 10 mg STAT, then 4 mg every 6 hr. Diagnosis of Cushing syndrome: 1 mg at 11 PM, draw plasma cortisol at 8 AM the following day. Shock: IV: 1–6 mg/kg (max 40 mg) and may repeat every 2–6 hr. *Children and adults:* Ophthalmic: ointment: apply every 3–4 hr to conjunctival sac as thin coating; suspension: instill 2 drops into conjunctival sac every hour during day and every other hour at night. Gradually taper doses when inflammation resolves. Topical: apply 1–4 times daily.	
Dextran Plasma volume expander. Dextran 40 (low molecular weight): Gentran; LMD. Dextran 70 (high molecular weight): Gentran; Macrodex.	**Blood volume expander in shock or impending shock (similar to albumin).** *Children:* Max = 20 mL/kg on day 1, then 10 mL/kg/day for not more than 5 days. *Adults:* 500–1,000 mL at a rate of 20–40 mL/min (max 10 mL/kg/day for 5 days).	*Adverse events:* (Primarily associated with excessive doses)—pulmonary edema, bleeding due to impaired platelet function.
Dextroamphetamine CNS stimulant. Generic, Dexedrine. Tablet: 5, 10 mg. Sustained-release capsule: 5, 10, 15 mg.	**Treatment of attention deficit disorder, narcolepsy, and exogenous obesity (blocks reuptake of dopamine and norepinephrine from the synapse).** *Children 6–12 yr:* Narcolepsy and attention deficit disorder: initial 5 mg/day, may increase by 5 mg/day at weekly intervals to response (max 60 mg/day). *>12 yr and adult:* initial 20 mg/day, may increase at 10 mg increments weekly (max 60 mg/day).	*Caution:* Avoid concurrent use of MAO-inhibitors. *Adverse events:* Hypertension, tachycardia, palpitations, arrhythmias, insomnia, agitation, irritability, nervousness, headache, depression, tremor, exacerbation of tics and movement disorders, mydriasis, physical and psychological dependence, anorexia, nausea, diarrhea, abdominal cramps, growth suppression. *Monitoring:* Blood pressure, growth, CNS activity.
Dextromethorphan Antitussive. Robitussin, generics. Liquid: 7.5 mg/5 mL. Lozenges: 5 mg.	**Symptomatic relief of coughs, best when cough is nonproductive (depress the medullary cough center).** *Children: 2–6 yr:* 2.5–7.5 mg every 4–8 hr or extended-release 15 mg every 12 hr (max 30 mg/day). *Children 6–12 yr:* 10–15 mg every 4–8 hr or extended-release 30 mg twice daily (max 60 mg/day). *Children >12 yr and adults:* 10–30 mg every 4–8 hr or extended-release 60 mg twice daily (max 120 mg/day).	*Adverse events:* (Mainly with overdose)—drowsiness, dizziness, respiratory depression, blurred vision, nausea, GI upset, constipation.
Diazepam Benzodiazepine. Generic, Valium. Tablet: 2, 5, 10 mg. Oral solution: 5 mg/mL. Injection: 5 mg/mL.	**Treatment of anxiety, panic disorders, status epilepticus, alcohol withdrawal, provide sedation and skeletal muscle relaxant (thought to increase neuroinhibitory action of GABA).** *Infants and children:* Status epilepticus: IV: 0.05–0.3 mg/kg/dose given over 2–3 min may repeat every 30 min to max total dose of 5–10 mg. Rectal: 0.5 mg/kg, then 0.25 mg/kg in 10 min if needed. Sedation: Oral: 0.2–0.3 mg/kg (max 10 mg); IM/IV: 0.04–0.3 mg/kg (max 0.6 mg/kg/8 hr). *Adults:* Status epilepticus: IV: 5–10 mg every 30 min (max 30 mg/8 hr). Anxiety, sedation, muscle relaxant: Oral/IM/IV: 2–10 mg 2–4 times daily.	*Adverse events:* Hypotension, bradycardia, cardiac arrest (with IV dose), drowsiness, ataxia, fatigue, confusion, impaired coordination, paradoxical excitement, amnesia, blurred vision, diplopia, sweating, dry mouth, constipation or diarrhea, increased or decreased appetite, hiccups, physical and psychological dependence. *Monitoring:* Desired clinical endpoints and toxic endpoints should be monitored; doses to achieve effects vary considerably between patients.

Table continued on following page

TABLE 728–1 General Medications *Continued*

Drug (Trade Names, Formulations)	Indications (Mechanism of Action) and Dosing	Comments (Cautions, Adverse Events, Monitoring)
Diazoxide Antihypertensive. Hyperstat, injection: 15 mg/mL. Proglycem, oral suspension: 50 mg/mL. Capsule: 50 mg.	**Emergency lowering of blood pressure, treatment of hyperinsulinemic hypoglycemia related to islet cell tumors or nesidioblastosis (smooth muscle relaxation, inhibit insulin release from the pancreas).** Hypertension: *Children and adults:* 1–3 mg/kg, may repeat in 5–15 min, dose every 4–24 hr. Hyperinsulinemic hypoglycemia: *Newborns and infants:* Oral: 8–15 mg/kg/day divided every 8–12 hr (start on low end). *Children and adults:* Oral: 3–8 mg/kg/day divided every 8–12 hr (start on low end).	*Adverse events:* Hypotension, dizziness, weakness, nausea, vomiting.
Dibucaine Local anesthetic. Nupercainal. Cream: 0.5%. Ointment: 1%.	**Temporary relief of pain and itching due to hemorrhoids and minor skin irritation or damage (block initiation and conduction of nerve impulses).** *Children and adults:* Topical: apply gently to affected area (children 7.5 g/day, adults 30 g/day). Rectal: insert with rectal applicator morning, evening, and after each bowel movement.	*Adverse events:* Local irritation, contact dermatitis.
Diclofenac sodium Nonsteroidal anti-inflammatory agent, NSAID. Cataflam, tablets: 50 mg. Voltaren, tablets: 25, 50, 75 mg; ophthalmic solution 0.1%.	**Treatment of mild to moderate acute or chronic pain; postoperative inflammation after cataract extraction (inhibit prostaglandin synthesis)** Oral: *Children:* 2–3 mg/kg/day in 2–4 divided doses. *Adults:* 100–200 mg/day in 2–4 divided doses. Ophthalmic: 1 drop in affected eye 4 times daily for 2 wk, to begin 24 hr after cataract surgery.	*Adverse events:* Dizziness, headache, fluid retention, indigestion, abdominal pain, peptic ulcer, GI bleeding, renal impairment.
Dicyclomine Anticholinergic agent. Antispas, Bentyl, Generic. Capsule: 10, 20 mg. Tablet: 20 mg. Syrup: 10 mg/5 mL. Injection: 10 mg/mL.	**Treatment of functional disturbances of GI motility, e.g., irritable bowel syndrome (block the actions of acetylcholine).** *Infants >6 mo:* Oral: 5 mg/dose 3–4 times daily. *Children:* 10 mg 3–4 times/day. *Adults:* 40 mg 4 times daily (start at 1/2 dose and gradually increase; IM: use 20 mg 4 times/day).	*Cautions:* Avoid in narrow angle glaucoma, GI obstruction, urinary tract obstruction, myasthenia gravis. *Adverse events:* Tachycardia, palpitations, nervousness, irritability, confusion, muscle hypotonia, blurred vision, photophobia, urinary retention, nausea, vomiting, constipation, dry mouth, urticaria, pruritis.
Digoxin Cardiac glycoside. Lanoxin, Generic. Capsule: 50, 100, 200 μg. Elixir: 50 μg/mL. Tablet: 125, 250, 500 μg. Injection: 100, 250 μg/mL.	**Treatment of systolic heart failure and supraventricular tachyarrhythmias (increase intracellular calcium through inhibition of sodium/potassium ATPase pump; suppression of A-V node conduction).** *Neonate:* 10–30 μg/kg IV load, then 5–10 μg/kg/day maintenance dose. *1 mo–2 yr:* 30 μg/kg load, then 10–15 μg/kg/day maintenance dose. *2–10 yr:* 30 μg/kg load, then 5–10 μg/kg/day maintenance dose. *Child >10 yr:* 10 μg/kg load, then 2–5 μg/kg/day maintenance dose. *Adult:* 10–15 μg/kg load, then 0.1 to 0.5 mg/day maintenance dose. Adjust doses for reduced renal function: CrCl 10–50 mL/min: reduce dose to 25–75%; CrCl <10 mL/min: reduce dose to 10–25% of normal.	*Cautions:* Contraindicated in A-V block, idiopathic hypertrophic subaortic stenosis, or constrictive pericarditis. *Adverse events:* Anorexia, nausea, vomiting, diarrhea, feeding intolerance, bradycardia, arrhythmias, lethargy, depression, vertigo, blurred vision, diplopia, photophobia, yellow or green vision. *Monitoring:* Efficacy and toxicity are closely related to serum concentrations and dosing should be guided by measuring serum digoxin concentrations: therapeutic: 0.8–2 ng/mL; toxic: >2–2.5 ng/mL. Digoxin-like immune substances (DLIS) may falsely elevate digoxin levels in neonates and children, so pretreatment digoxin levels can be obtained and subtracted from treatment levels or samples can be run through a free-level filter to remove DLIS before assay. Check post-distribution levels (drawn at least 6–8 hr post dose) at steady-state (2–4 wk) or if ECG or clinical signs of toxicity. Check ECG, serum electrolytes, calcium and magnesium. Check heart rate.
Digoxin Immune Fab Digoxin antidote. Digibind. Powder for injection 38 mg.	**Treatment of digitalis intoxication from digoxin or digitoxin (binds with molecules of unbound digoxin or digitoxin and is renally cleared).** *Infants, children, and adults:* dose is based on amount of digoxin or digitoxin ingested or estimated total body load (TBL) based on post-distributive serum concentration: TBL Digoxin = conc (ng/mL) × 5.6 × weight (kg)/1000. TBL Digoxin = mg ingested × 0.8. TBL Digitoxin = conc (ng/mL) × 0.56 × wt (kg)/1000. TBL Digitoxin = mg ingested. Dose Digoxin Immune Fab (mg) = TBL Digoxin × 76. Dose Digoxin Immune Fab (# vials) = TBL/0.5.	*Adverse events:* Worsening of heart failure or atrial fibrillation, hypokalemia, facial swelling and redness. *Monitoring:* ECG, digoxin serum concentrations will greatly increase with digibind and do not reflect body stores or correlate with clinical toxicity.

TABLE 728–1 General Medications *Continued*

Drug (Trade Names, Formulations)	Indications (Mechanism of Action) and Dosing	Comments (Cautions, Adverse Events, Monitoring)
Dihydrotachysterol Vitamin D analog. Hytakerol, Generic. Capsule: 0.125 mg. Tablet: 0.125 mg. Solution: 0.2 mg/mL, 0.2 mg/5 mL.	**Treatment of hypocalcemia associated with hypoparathyroidism and renal osteodystrophy (stimulates calcium and phosphate intestinal absorption).** *Neonates:* 0.05–0.1 mg/day. *Infants and young children:* 1–5 mg/day for 4 days then 0.5–1.5 mg/day. *Older children and adults:* 0.75–2.5 mg/day for 4 days, then 0.2–1 mg/day (max 1.5 mg/day). Renal osteodystrophy: 0.1–0.6 mg/day.	*Adverse events:* Hypercalcemia, hypercalciuria, elevated serum creatinine.
Diltiazem Calcium channel blocker. Cardizem, Dilacor. Tablet: 30, 60, 90, 120 mg. Capsule (sustained-release): 60, 90, 120, 180, 240, 300 mg. Injection: 5 mg/mL.	**Treatment of hypertension and atrial tachyarrhythmias (inhibit calcium ions from entering the "slow channels" during depolarization),** *Children:* Oral: 1.5–2 mg/kg/day in 3–4 divided doses. *Adolescents and adults:* Oral: 90–480 mg/day in 3–4 divided doses as tablets or 1–2 doses as sustained-release capsules. IV: 0.25 mg/kg load, then 5–15 mg/hr continuous infusion.	*Cautions:* Diltiazem is a hepatic enzyme inhibitor and may cause accumulation and toxicity for concurrently used drugs which are metabolized. *Adverse events:* Hypotension, bradycardia, edema, A-V block, dizziness, nausea, vomiting.
Dimenhydrinate Antihistamine. Dramamine, Generic. Capsule: 50 mg. Injection: 50 mg/mL. Tablet: 50 mg. Liquid: 12.5 mg/4 mL.	**Treatment of nausea, vomiting and vertigo associated with motion sickness (competes with histamine for H1-receptor).** *Children:* *2–5 yr:* 12.5–25 mg every 6–8 hr (max 75 mg/day). *6–12 yr:* 25–50 mg every 6–8 hr (max 150 mg/day). *Adults:* 50–100 mg every 4–6 hr (max 400 mg/day).	*Adverse events:* Drowsiness, dizziness, hypotension, tachycardia.
Dimercaprol BAL. Injection: 100 mg/mL.	**Antidote to gold, arsenic, and mercury poisoning, and adjunct to edetate calcium disodium in lead poisoning (chelates with heavy metals to form nontoxic stable compounds).** *Children and adults:* Mild arsenic and gold poisoning: 2.5 mg/kg/dose IM every 6 hr for 2 days, then every 12 hr on day 3, then every 24 hr for 10 days. Severe arsenic or gold poisoning: 3 mg/kg/dose every 4 hr for 2 days, then every 6 hr on day 3, then every 12 hr for 10 days. Mercury poisoning: 5 mg/kg load, then 2.5 mg/kg/dose 1–2 times/daily for 10 days. Lead poisoning: Mild: 4 mg/kg load, then 3 mg/kg/dose every 4 hr for 2–7 days. Severe: 4 mg/kg/dose every 4 hr for 2–7 days.	*Adverse events:* Hypertension, tachycardia, convulsions, nausea, vomiting, fever, headache, nervousness, blepharospasm, nephrotoxicity. *Monitoring:* Specific heavy metal levels, urine pH should be kept alkaline.
Diphenhydramine Benadryl, Generic. Capsule or tablet: 25, 50 mg. Injection: 10 mg/mL, 50 mg/mL. Syrup or elixir: 12.5 mg/5 mL. Cream or lotion: 1%.	**Antihistamine (competative inhibitor of H-1 receptor).** *Children:* 5 mg/kg/day divided every 6 hr as needed IM, IV, oral (max 300 mg/day). *Adults:* 10–50 mg/dose every 4 hr as needed (max 400 mg/day). *Topical:* apply 3–4 times daily.	*Adverse events:* Hypotension, tachycardia, drowsiness, paradoxical excitement, thickened bronchial secretions, dry mouth.
Diphenoxylate and Atropine Lomotil. Tablet, oral solution.	**Antidiarrheal (diphenoxylate inhibits excessive GI motility, atropine is to prevent abuse).** *Children:* *2–5 yr:* 4 ml (2 mg diphenoxylate) 3 times daily. *5–8 yr:* 4 ml 4 times daily. *8–12 yr:* 4 ml 5 times daily. *Adults:* 15–20 mg/day in 3–4 divided doses.	*Adverse events:* Nervousness, dizziness, drowsiness, headache, dry mouth, urinary retention, blurred vision, paralytic ileus.
Disopyramide Norpace. Capsule: 100, 150 mg.	**Treatment of ventricular arrhythmias and atrial tachyarrhythmias (antiarrhythmic class 1a, decreases myocardial excitability and conduction velocity).** *Children:* *<1 yr:* 10–30 mg/kg/day divided every 6 hr. *1–4 yr:* 10–20 mg/kg/day divided every 6 hr. *4–12 yr:* 10–15 mg/kg/day divided every 6 hr. *12–18 yr:* 6–15 mg/kg/day divided every 6 hr. *Adults:* 100–200 mg every 6 hr.	*Cautions:* Avoid in second or third degree A-V block; will worsen heart failure, urinary retention, glaucoma, and some arrhythmias. *Adverse events:* Urinary retention/hesitancy, dry mouth, fatigue, malaise, constipation, cholestasis, elevated liver enzymes. *Monitoring:* Creatinine clearance (decrease dose to q8h if 30–40 mL/min, q12h if 15–30 mL/min, q24h if <15 mL/min). ECG, blood pressure, signs of heart failure. Blood levels (therapeutic range: atrial arrhythmias 2.8–3.2 μg/mL, ventricular arrhythmias 3.3–7.5 μg/mL).

Table continued on following page

TABLE 728–1 General Medications *Continued*

Drug (Trade Names, Formulations)	Indications (Mechanism of Action) and Dosing	Comments (Cautions, Adverse Events, Monitoring)
Dobutamine Dobutrex. Injection.	**Treatment of hypotension (stimulates beta-1 adrenergic receptors).** *Neonates:* 2–20 μg/kg/min. *Children and adults:* 2.5–40 μg/kg/min constant infusion.	*Cautions:* Avoid in patients with IHSS, atrial fibrillation or flutter, or sulfite sensitivity. *Adverse events:* Tachycardia, ectopic heartbeats, angina, palpitations, tacharrhythmias, tingling sensation, paresthesias, leg cramps.
Docusate Colace, Surfak, Generic. Capsule, liquid, syrup (may be combined with casanthrol).	**Stool softener, laxative (reduces surface tension of oil-water interface of stool).** *<3 yr:* 10–40 mg/day in 1–4 doses. *3–6 yr:* 20–60 mg/day in 1–4 doses. *6–12 yr:* 40–150 mg/day. *>12 yr and adults:* 50–400 mg/day.	*Adverse events:* Diarrhea, abdominal cramping.
Dolasetron Mesylate Anzemet. Tablet: 50, 100 mg. Injection.	**Prevention and treatment of chemotherapy and postoperative nausea and vomiting (5-HT3 receptor antagonist).** *Children >2 yr and adults:* IV, Oral 1.8 mg/kg (max 100 mg) as single dose 30 min before chemotherapy; 0.35 mg/kg (max 12.5 mg) given 15 min before stopping anesthesia for postoperative nausea.	*Adverse events:* Hypotension, headache, tachycardia, dizziness.
Dopamine Intropin. Injection.	**Treatment of hypotension and shock (stimulates dopaminergic receptors and adrenergic receptors).** *Neonates, children, and adults:* 1–20 μg/kg/min IV infusion rate (mL/hr) = 6 × weight (kg) × desired dose (μg/kg/min)/mg drug per 100 mL IV fluid.	*Cautions:* Contains sulfites. *Adverse events:* Tachycardia, ectopic beats, ventricular arrhythmias, tissue necrosis with extravasation, vasoconstriction, gangrene of extremities, excess urine output (doses <5 μg/kg/min), oliguria (doses >10 μg/kg/min).
Dornase Alpha Pulmozyme. Inhalation solution: 1 mg/mL.	**Management of cystic fibrosis to improve pulmonary function (DNA enzyme which reduces mucus viscosity).** *Neonates, children, and adults:* 2.5 mL 1–2 times daily, nebulized with Pulmo-Aide or Pari-Proneb compressor.	*Adverse events:* Pharyngitis, voice alteration, cough, rhinitis, hemoptysis.
Doxacurium Nuromax. Injection: 1 mg/mL.	**Skeletal muscle paralysis (neuromuscular blockade by competing with acetylcholine for neuromuscular receptor).** *Children 2–12 yr:* Initial 30–50 μg/kg, then 5–10 μg/kg/dose every 1–2 hr. *Adults:* Initial 50 μg/kg, then 5–10 μg/kg/dose every 1–2 hr.	*Adverse events:* Skeletal muscle weakness, hypotension. *Monitoring:* Peripheral nerve stimulator.
Doxapram Dopram. Injection: 20 mg/mL.	**Treatment of apnea of prematurity refractory to methylxanthines (respiratory and CNS stimulant).** *Neonates:* Initial 2.5–3 mg/kg followed by infusion of 1 mg/kg/hr (maximum 2.5 mg/kg/hr).	*Caution:* Contains benzyl alcohol (recommended doses deliver 5.4–27 mg/kg/day). *Adverse events:* Hypertension, tachycardia, arrhythmias, CNS stimulation, irritability, seizures, hyperpyrexia, vomiting, increased gastric residuals, hyperglycemia.
Doxepin Adapin, Sinequan. Tricyclic antidepressant. Capsule: 10, 25, 50, 75, 100, 150 mg. Oral concentrate: 10 mg/mL. Cream: 5%.	**Treatment of depression, analgesic for neuropathic pain (increase synaptic concentrations of serotonin and norepinephrine).** *Children:* 1–3 mg/kg/day. *Adolescent:* 25–50 mg/day to start, max 100 mg/day. *Adults:* 30–150 mg/day to start, max 300 mg/day (single dose max 150 mg).	*Caution:* Contraindicated for narrow-angle glaucoma. *Adverse events:* Sedation, drowsiness, dizziness, headache, dry mouth, constipation, increased appetite, weight gain, urinary retention, difficult urination, blurred vision, hypotension, arrhythmias. *Monitoring:* ECG, doxepin concentrations: therapeutic 30–150 ng/mL, toxic >500 ng/mL.
Doxorubicin Hydrochloride Adriamycin, Rubex. Injection: 2 mg/mL. Powder for injection.	**Antineoplastic used for various tumor types (inhibit DNA and RNA synthesis).** *Children:* 35–75 mg/m²/dose repeat every 21 days; or 20–30 mg/m² repeat every wk; or 60–90 mg/m² given as continuous infusion over 96 hr every 3–4 wk. *Adults:* 60–75 mg/m²/dose every 21 days. *Liver disease:* reduce dose: bilirubin 1.2–3 (reduce by 50%), bilirubin >3 (reduce by 75%).	*Caution:* Contraindicated if patient has congestive heart failure, cardiomyopathy, received a total dose of 550 mg/m² (400 mg/m² if prior or concurrent daunorubicin, idarubicin, mitoxantrone, cyclophosphamide, irradiation to cardiac area). *Adverse events:* Cardiotoxicity, alopecia, hyperpigmentation of nail bed, hyperuricemia, stomatitis, esophagitis, mucositis, nausea, vomiting, thrombocytopenia (onset 7 days, nadir 10–14 days, recovery 21–28 days), lacrimation, extravasation tissue necrosis, phlebitis.
Dronabinol, Tetrahydrocannabinol Marinol. Capsule: 2.5, 5, 10 mg.	**Antiemetic for cancer chemotherapy (inhibits the vomiting center).** *Children and adults:* 5 mg/m²/dose every 2–4 hr starting 1–3 hr before chemotherapy (max 15 mg/m²/dose).	*Adverse events:* Drowsiness, difficulty concentrating, mood change, hallucinations. *Monitoring:* Monitor for abuse.

TABLE 728–1 General Medications *Continued*

Drug (Trade Names, Formulations)	Indications (Mechanism of Action) and Dosing	Comments (Cautions, Adverse Events, Monitoring)
Droperidol Inapsine. Injection: 2.5 mg/mL.	**Antiemetic, antipsychotic (alters the action of dopamine in the CNS and has alpha adrenergic blockade).** *Children 2–12 yr:* IV, IM 0.05–0.06 mg/kg/dose every 4–6 hr as needed for nausea. *Adults:* IV, IM 2.5–5 mg/dose every 3–4 hr as needed.	*Adverse events:* Hypotension, tachycardia, extrapyramidal reactions, confusion, memory loss.
D-Xylose. Xylo-pfan. Powder for oral solution.	**Diagnostic agent used to evaluate intestinal disorders due to disease or injury (mechanism not understood).** *Children:* 500 mg/kg as 5–10% solution, max 25 g. *Adults:* 5–25 g as 10% solution followed by 200–400 mL of water.	*Adverse events:* Nausea, vomiting, cramping, intestinal bloating. *Monitoring:* Blood and urinary D-Xylose concentrations.
Edetate Calcium Disodium Calcium Disodium Versenate. Injection: 200 mg/mL.	**Antidote for acute and chronic lead poisoning (chelating agent).** *Children and adults:* 500 mg/m^2/dose once daily.	*Cautions:* Contraindicated in severe renal failure and patients with active tuberculosis or healed calcified tubercular lesions. *Adverse events:* Arrhythmias, hypotension, seizures, headache, chills, skin eruptions, hypomagnesemia, hypokalemia, hypocalcemia, hyperuricemia, vomiting, diarrhea, abdominal cramps, back pain, muscle cramps, paresthesia, tetany, nephrotoxicity, respiratory arrest. *Monitoring:* 24-hr urine collection after first dose for ratio lead excretion/mg calcium EDTA (positive test >0.5–0.6); blood lead level.
Edetate Disodium Chealamide, Disotate, Generic. Injection: 150 mg/mL.	**Emergency treatment of hypercalemia and digitalis-induced ventricular dysrhythmias (chelating agent).** *Children:* 40–70 mg/kg/day slow infusion over 3–4 hr, administer for 5 days then 5 days off drug. *Adults:* 50 mg/kg/dose for 5 days, then 2 days off, then restart for total of 15 doses. *Digitalis arrhythmias (children and adults):* 15 mg/kg/hr continuous infusion (max 60 mg/kg/day).	*Cautions:* Contraindicated in severe renal failure and tuberculosis. *Adverse events:* Arrhythmias, hypotension, seizures, headache, chills, hypokalemia, hypocalcemia, hypomagnesemia, hyperuricemia, vomiting, diarrhea, abdominal cramps, dysuria, back pain, nephrotoxicity.
Edrephonium Chloride Reversol, Tensilon, Enlon. Injection: 10 mg/mL.	**Diagnosis of myesthenia gravis, differentiation of cholinergic crisis from myesthenia crisis, reversal of nondepolarizing neuromuscular blockers, treatment of paroxysmal atrial tachycardia (inhibits destruction of acetylcholine by acetylcholinesterase)** *Infants.* IM 0.5–1 mg, IV 0.1 mg followed by 0.4 mg (if no response). *Children:* diagnosis (initial): IM: <34 kg: 1 mg, >34 kg: 5 mg. IV: 0.04 mg/kg over 1 min followed by 0.16 mg/kg given within 45 sec (if no response), max dose 10 mg total. Titration of oral anticholinesterase therapy: IV 0.04 mg/kg given 1 hr after oral intake of treatment drug; if strength improves increase dose of neostigmine or pyridostigmine. *Adults:* Diagnosis: IM initial 10 mg, if cholinergic reaction occurs given 2 mg in 30 min to rule out false-negative reaction. IV: 2 mg given over 15 sec, 8 mg given 45 sec later (if no response). Titration of oral antichoinesterase therapy: IV 1–2 mg given 1 hr after an oral dose. Increase oral dose if strength improves.	*Adverse events:* Arrhythmias, hypotension, nausea, vomiting, diarrhea, stomach cramps, excess sweating, urinary frequency, lacrimation, diplopia, miosis, laryngospasm, bronchospasm, respiratory paralysis.
Enalapril/Enalaprilat Vasotec. Oral (elanapril): 2.5, 5, 10, 20 mg. Injection (elanaprilat): 1.25 mg/mL. Extemporaneous formulations are available.	**Treatment of hypertension and congestive heart failure (angiotensin-converting enzyme inhibition).** *Neonate:* Oral: 0.1 mg/kg/day in 1–2 doses (may increase to 0.4 mg/kg/day for congestive heart failure or adequate hypertension response). IV: 5–10 μg/kg/dose every 8–24 hr. *Infants and children:* Oral: 0.1–0.5 mg/kg/day in 1–2 doses. IV: 5–10 μg/kg/dose every 8–24 hr. *Adolescent and adults:* Oral: 2.5–5 mg/day and titrate to max 40 mg/day in 2 doses. IV: 0.625–1.25 mg/dose every 6 hr (max 20 mg/day).	*Caution:* Avoid or adjust dose in patients with renal impairment (CrCl 10–50 mL/min, give 75% of dose; CrCl <10 mL/min, give 50% of dose). *Adverse events:* Hypotension, tachycardia, syncope, fatigue, dizzinesss, headache, cough, hyperkalemia, hypoglycemia. *Comments:* Lower doses if concurrent diuretics or reduced renal function, concurrent indomethacin may blunt response.

Table continued on following page

TABLE 728–1 General Medications *Continued*

Drug (Trade Names, Formulations)	Indications (Mechanism of Action) and Dosing	Comments (Cautions, Adverse Events, Monitoring)
Enoxaparin sodium Lovenox. Injection: 30 mg/0.3 mL.	**Prophylaxis and treatment of venous thromboembolism (low molecular weight heparin with activity against factor Xa and IIa).** *Neonates and children:* SC: 1 mg/kg every 8 hr. *Adults:* SC: 30 mg twice daily or 1 mg/kg twice daily (depends on indication).	*Adverse events:* Thrombocytopenia and hemorrhage (less than unfractionated heparin).
Epinephrine Adrenalin. Injection: 0.01 mg/mL, 0.1 mg/mL, 1 mg/mL. Suspension: 5 mg/ml. Aerosol MDI, inhalation solution, ophthalmic solution, topical solution.	**Treatment of cardiac arrest, bronchospasm, anaphylactic reactions, open-angle glaucoma (stimulates alpha, beta-1, and beta-2 receptors).** *Neonates:* IV, intratracheal: 0.01–0.03 mg/kg (0.1–0.3 mL/kg of 1:10,000 solution) every 3–5 min. *Infants and children:* SC: 0.01 mg/kg (0.01 mL/kg/dose of 1:1,000 solution, or 0.005 mL/kg/dose of suspension). IV: 0.01 mg/kg (0.1 mL/kg of 1:10,000 solution) (max 1 mg). Intratracheal: 0.1 mg/kg/dose (0.1 mL/kg of 1:1,000 solution) (max 0.2 mL/kg). Continuous infusion: 0.1–1 μg/kg/min per response. Nebulization: 0.25–0.5 mL of 2.25% racemic epinephrine diluted in 3 mL normal saline. Ophthalmic: instill 1–2 drops in eye(s) 1–2 times daily. *Adults:* IV: 1–5 mg every 3–5 min. Intratracheal: 1 mg initial, max 12.5 mg/dose. IM, SC: 0.1–0.5 mg every 10–15 min. Continuous infusion: 1–10 μg/min. Ophthalmic: instill 1–2 drops in eye(s) 1–2 times daily.	*Adverse events:* Tachycardia, hypertension, nervousness, restlessness, irritability, headache, tremor, weakness, nausea, vomiting, acute urinary retention.
Epoetin Alfa, Erythropoietin, EPO. Epogen, ProCrit. Injection.	**Anemia associated with prematurity, end-stage renal disease, AZT-treated HIV infected patients, cancer patients receiving chemotherapy (induces erythropoiesis).** Administer IV, SC. *Neonates:* 100–500 units/kg/dose every 1–2 days for 10–21 days. *Children and adults:* Cancer patients: 150 units/kg/dose 3 times/wk (may increase to 300 units/kg/dose). Hemodialysis patients: 50–100 units 3 times/wk. Zidovudine-treated patients: 100 units/kg/dose 3 times/wk.	*Caution:* Uncontrolled hypertension, neutropenia in newborns. Must have adequate iron stores and may require oral or intravenous iron supplement. *Adverse events:* Hypertension, edema, headache, fever, rash, arthralgias, hypersensitivity. *Monitoring:* Serum iron, reticulocyte count, hematocrit (reduce dose or stop EPO if hematocrit above 40), blood pressure.
Ergocalciferol Calciferol, Drisdol, Generic. Tablet, capsule: 50,000 units. Liquid: 8,000 units/mL. Injection: 500,000 units/mL (1 μg = 40 units).	**Treatment of refractory ricketts, hypophosphatemia, hypoparathyroidism (vitamin D analog stimulates calcium and phosphate absorption).** Premature infants: 10–20 μg/day. Renal failure: *Children:* 100–1,000 μg/day. *Adults:* 500 μg/day. Hypoparathyroidism: *Children:* 1.25–5 mg/day. *Adults:* 0.625–5 mg/day. Ricketts: *Children:* 75–125 μg/day. *Adults:* 0.25–1.5 mg/day.	*Adverse events:* Hypercalcemia, weakness, lethargy, hypertension, arrhythmias, mild acidosis, hypercholesterolemia, nausea, vomiting, constipation, nephrocalcinosis, photophobia. *Monitoring:* Serum calcium and phosphorus, alkaline phosphatase, bone x-ray.
Ergotamine Cafatine, Cafergot. Tablet: 1 mg/2 mg. Aerosol: 9 mg/mL. Suppository: 2 mg.	**Prevent or abort vascular headaches, e.g., migraine or cluster headache (ergot alkaloid alpha adrenergic blocker).** *Older children and adolescents:* 1 mg SL or oral at onset of attack and every 30 min to relief (max 3 mg per attack). *Adults:* 1–2 mg SL or oral, may repeat every 30 min to max 6 mg (max dose/week is 10 mg).	*Caution:* Reduce dose by 50% if patient is taking chronic methysergide. *Adverse events:* Tachypnea, vasospasm, bradycardia, nausea, vomiting, diarrhea, leg cramps, muscle weakness, paresthesias.
Esmolol Brevibloc. Injection: 10 mg/mL.	**Antiarrhythmic, antihypertensive (beta-blocker, class II antiarrhythmic).** *Children:* 100–500 μg/kg over 1 min then continuous infusion 200–1,000 μg/kg/min. *Adults:* 500 μg/kg over 1 min then 50–200 μg/kg/min.	*Caution:* Contraindicated in sinus bradycardia, heart block, uncompensated heart failure. *Adverse events:* Hypotension, bradycardia, Raynaud phenomenon, dizziness, confusion, lethargy, bronchoconstriction.

TABLE 728–1 General Medications *Continued*

Drug (Trade Names, Formulations)	Indications (Mechanism of Action) and Dosing	Comments (Cautions, Adverse Events, Monitoring)
Ethacrynic Acid Edecrin. Tablet: 25, 50 mg. Injection.	**Diuretic (act at ascending loop of Henle).** *Children:* Oral 1–3 mg/kg/day. IV 0.5–1 mg/kg/dose every 8–24 hr. *Adults:* Oral 25–400 mg/day. IV 0.5–1 mg/kg/dose every 8–24 hr.	*Adverse events:* Hypotension, fluid and electrolyte depletion, hyperuricemia, ototoxicity, tinnitis.
Ethosuximide Zarontin. Capsule: 250 mg. Syrup: 250 mg/5 mL.	**Anticonvulsant for treatment of absence, myoclonic, and akinetic epilepsy (increased seizure threshold).** *Children:* *<6 yr:* start 15 mg/kg/day in 2 doses; increase every 4–7 days to therapeutic level, usually 15–40 mg/kg/day in 2 doses. Max 1.5 g/day. *>6 yr and adults:* start 250 mg twice daily; increase by 250 mg/day every 4–7 days up to therapeutic level or 1.5 g/day.	*Adverse events:* Sedation, lethargy, nausea, vomiting, anorexia, abdominal pain, leukopenia, thrombocytopenia, aplastic anemia. *Monitoring:* Ethosuximide concentrations: therapeutic 40–100 μg/mL; toxic 150 μg/mL.
Etoposide, VP-16 VePesid. Capsule: 50 mg. Injection: 20 mg/mL.	**Antineoplastic for treatment of various cancers (inhibits mitotic activity).** *Children:* IV 150 mg/m²/day for 3 days for 2–3 cycles for AML remission or brain tumor; 160 mg/m²/day for 4 days for BMT conditioning. *Adults:* IV 50–100 mg/m²/day for 3–5 days per course. Oral = IV dose × 2 to nearest 50 mg.	*Adverse events:* Hypotension, tachycardia, fever, headache, chills, alopecia, rash, urticaria, nausea, vomiting, diarrhea, mucositis, myelosuppression, anemia (nadir 7–14 days), thrombocytopenia (nadir 9–16 days), peripheral neuropathy, bronchospasm.
Factor IX Complex (Human) Konyne 80, Proplex, Profilnine. Injection.	**Antihemophilic agent to control bleeding in patients with factor IX deficiency, i.e., hemophilia B or Christmas disease, or with inhibitors to factor VIII, i.e., hemophilia A (replacement of deficient factor).** *Children and adults:* 20–25 units/kg/dose up to every 24 hr; factor VIII-inhibitor patients 75–100 units/kg/dose up to every 6 hr.	*Adverse events:* Flushing, fever, headache, chills, urticaria, thrombosis (with high doses), tingling, tightness of head and neck.
Famotidine Pepcid. Tablet: 20, 40 mg. Injection.	**Treatment of gastric and duodenal ulcer, and control of gastric pH in critically ill patients (blocks histamine-2 receptors).** *Infants and children:* Oral, IV 1–2 mg/kg/day in 1–2 doses; max 40 mg/day. *Adults:* Oral 40 mg/day at bedtime, IV 20 mg every 12 hr.	*Cautions:* Reduce dose for renal function: CrCl 30–50 mL/min give 50% of dose; CrCl <30 mL/min give 25% of dose. *Adverse events:* GI discomfort, thrombocytopenia, increased liver enzymes.
Fat Emulsion Intralipid, Liposyn. Injection: 10%, 20%.	**Source of essential fatty acids and calories (nutritional supplement with parenteral nutrition).** *Premature infants:* start 0.5 g/kg/day and increase by 0.5 g/kg/day as tolerated to 3 g/kg/day. *Infants and children:* start 0.5–1 g/kg/day and increase at 0.5 g/kg/day increments as tolerated to max 3–4 g/kg/day. *Adolescents and adults:* 1 g/kg/day and increase as tolerated to max 2.5 g/kg/day.	*Cautions:* Fat calories should not exceed 60% of total daily calories. Contraindicated in patients with severe egg or soybean allergies. *Adverse events:* Hyperlipidemia, hepatomegaly, dyspnea and hypoxemia may occur if infused too quickly or excessive dose. *Monitoring:* Serum triglycerides.
Felbamate Felbatol. Tablets: 400, 600 mg. Oral suspension: 600 mg/5 mL.	**Adjunctive therapy primarily used for refractory generalized and partial seizures associated with Lennox-Gastaut syndrome (anticonvulsant with unknown mechanism of action).** *Children:* *2–14 yr:* start 15 mg/kg/day in 3–4 doses, increase weekly by 15 mg/kg/day to max of 45 mg/kg/day or 3,600 mg (whichever is less). *>14 yr:* start 1,200 mg/day in 3–4 doses; increase weekly by 1,200 mg/day to max 3600 mg/day.	*Caution:* Over 30 cases each of hepatic failure and aplastic anemia with multiple fatalities have been reported. *Adverse events:* Headache, insomnia, somnolence, fatigue, behavioral changes, depression, ataxia, anorexia, nausea, vomiting, diarrhea, thrombocytopenia, granulocytopenia, leukopenia, agranulocytosis, aplastic anemia, hepatitis, acute liver failure. *Monitoring:* Interacts with phenytoin, carbamazepine, and valproate; monitor drug levels if felbamate added.
Fentanyl citrate Duragesic, Sublimaze. Injection, transdermal, oral lozenge.	**Relief of pain, sedation, preoperative medication, anesthesia adjunct (narcotic analgesic, bind to opioiom receptors).** *Neonates and infants:* IV 1–4 μg/kg/dose, may repeat every 2–4 hr or continuous infusion 0.5–5 μg/kg/hr. *Children 1–12 yr:* Pain: IM, IV 1–3 μg/kg/dose, may repeat every 30–60 min; continuous infusion 1–5 μg/kg/hr; Oralet 5–15 μg/kg. *Children >12 yr and adults:* Pain: IV, IM 0.5–1 μg/kg/dose, may repeat in 30–60 min. Transdermal 25–100 μg/hr system as needed for relief. Oral 5 μg/kg or 400 μg (whichever is less) Anesthesia: IV, IM 2–50 μg/kg.	*Cautions:* Rapid IV infusion may result in skeletal muscle and chest wall rigidity with impaired ventilation and respiratory distress; physical dependence may occur in 3–5 days. *Adverse events:* Hypotension, bradycardia, CNS depression, constipation, biliary tract spasm, nausea, vomiting, urinary tract spasm, respiratory depression.

Table continued on following page

TABLE 728–1 General Medications *Continued*

Drug (Trade Names, Formulations)	Indications (Mechanism of Action) and Dosing	Comments (Cautions, Adverse Events, Monitoring)
Filgastrim, G-CSF Neupogen. Injection: 300 μg/mL.	**Graulocyte colony stimulating factor, reduce duration of neutropenia (stimulate the production, maturation, and activation of neutrophils).** *Neonates:* 5 μg/kg/dose daily for 3–6 doses. *Children and adults:* 5–10 μg/kg/dose daily for up to 14 days, may discontinue if ANC remains >1,000/mm³ for 3 consecutive days.	*Cautions:* Malignancy with myeloid characteristics. *Adverse events:* Hypotension, vasculitis, fever, exacerbation of pre-existing skin disorders, increased uric acid, thrombocytopenia, medullary pain (dose-related and mostly located in lower back, iliac crest, and sternum), hematuria, proteinuria.
Flecainide Tambocor. Tablet: 50, 100, 150 mg. Extemporaneous formulation.	**Treatment of supraventricular tachycardia and ventricular arrhythmias (antiarrhythmic class 1c, slows conduction in cardiac tissue).** *Children:* initial 1–3 mg/kg/day in 3 divided doses, may increase up to 8 mg/kg/day. *Adults:* initial 100 mg every 12 hr; may increase by 100 mg/day every 4 days to max 400 mg/day.	*Caution:* Decrease dose by 25–50% in renal failure; avoid in second- or third-degree heart block. *Adverse events:* Bradycardia, heart block, worsening arrhythmias, congestive heart failure, dizziness, visual disturbances, headache, fatigue, asthenia, nausea, constipation, abdominal pain, elevated liver enzymes, paresthesias, tremor. *Monitoring:* Serum trough concentrations (therapeutic 0.2–1 μg/mL).
Fludarabine, FAMP Fludara. Injection powder.	**Treatment of B-cell chronic lymphocytic leukemia and acute lymphocytic leukemia unresponsive to previous therapy (antineoplastic, antimetabolite).** *Children:* 10 mg/m² over 15 min, followed by 30.5 mg/m²/day by continuous infusion for 5 days. *Adults:* 20–25 mg/m² over 30 minutes for 5 days.	*Adverse events:* Neurotoxicity (primarily progressive demyelinating encephalophapy with mental status deterioration), somnolence, weakness, seizures, metabolic acidosis, hyperuricemia, hyperphosphatemia, hyperkalemia, hypocalcemia, nausea, vomiting, diarrhea, stomatitis, metallic taste, myelosuppression (WBC nadir 8 days, platelet nadir 16 days, recovery 5–7 wk), pneumonitis, dyspnea, nonproductive cough, interstitial pneumonitis, hearing loss, reversible hepatotoxicity.
Fludrocortisone Acetate Florinef. Tablet: 0.1 mg.	**Partial replacement therapy for adrenal insufficiency (mineralocorticoid with glucocorticoid activity).** *Infants and children:* 0.05–0.1 mg/day. *Adults:* 0.05–0.2 mg/day.	*Adverse events:* Hypertension, edema, congestive heart failure, convulsions, headache, acne, rash, bruising, hypokalemia, HPA-axis (adrenal) suppression, peptic ulcer, muscle weakness.
Flumazenil Romazicon. Injection.	**Benzodiazepine antagonist to reverse sedative effects (antagonize benzodiazepine effects on GABA/benzodiazepine receptor complex).** *Children:* 0.005–0.01 mg/kg load, then as continuous infusion 0.005–0.01 mg/kg/hr (max cumulative dose 1 mg).	*Caution:* Avoid if benzodiazepine is used to manage potentially life-threatening conditions, e.g., status epilepticus, increased intracranial pressure. *Adverse events:* Arrhythmias, hypo- or hyper-tension, seizures, acute withdrawal symptoms (if patient dependent on benzodiazepine or tricyclic antidepressant).
Flunisolide AeroBid, Nasalide. Metered dose inhaler 250 μg/puff. Nasal spray 25 μg/actuation.	**Treatment of asthma and rhinitis (inhaled steroid, anti-inflammatory).** *Children and adults:* Oral inhalation: 2–4 puffs twice daily; nasal spray: 1–2 sprays in each nostril 1–3 times daily.	*Adverse events:* Candida infections of nose and throat, dysphonia, sore throat, bitter taste, nasal irritation, headache, dizziness, short-term growth retardation.
Fluocinolone Acetonide Fluonid, Synalar, Generic. Topical cream, ointment, shampoo, solution, oil: 0.01–0.025%.	**Inflammation and corticosteroid-responsive dermatoses (topical adrenocorticosteroid, anti-inflammatory).** *Children and adults:* Apply a thin layer 2–4 times daily.	*Adverse events:* Acne, hypopigmentation, allergic dermatitis, skin atrophy, folliculitis, secondary infection, HPA-axis suppression, growth retardation.
Fluocinonide Fluonex, Lidex, Generic. Cream, gel, ointment, solution: 0.05%.	**Inflammation and corticosteroid-responsive dermatoses (topical adrenocorticosteroid, anti-inflammatory).** *Children and adults:* Apply a thin layer 2–4 times daily.	*Adverse events:* Acne, hypopigmentation, allergic dermatitis, skin atrophy, folliculitis, secondary infection, HPA-axis suppression, growth retardation.
Fluoride Generic. Oral drops, topical gel, lozenge, tablet, topical rinse, oral solution.	**Prevention of dental caries (promotes remineralization, increase resistance to acid dissolution).** Dental rinse or gel: *Children:* 5–10 mL after brushing. *Adults:* 10 mL after brushing.	*Adverse events:* GI upset if swallowed, stannous fluoride may stain teeth.
Fluorometholone Flarex, FML. Ophthalmic ointment 0.1%. Ophthalmic suspension: 0.1, 0.25%.	**Inflammatory conditions of the eye (ophthalmic glucocorticoid, anti-inflammatory).** *Children >2 yr and adults:* Ointment: apply 3 times daily in mild to moderate cases and every 4 hours in severe cases. Drops: instill 1–2 drops into conjunctival sac every hour while awake and every 2 hr at night until response, then every 4–8 hr.	*Adverse events:* Local stinging and burning, increased intraocular pressure.

TABLE 728–1 General Medications *Continued*

Drug (Trade Names, Formulations)	Indications (Mechanism of Action) and Dosing	Comments (Cautions, Adverse Events, Monitoring)
Fluorouracil Adricil, Efudex, Fluoroplex. Injection, topical solution, cream.	**Cancer chemotherapy (antineoplastic antimetabolite that inhibits thymidylate synthase leading to thymidine depletion).** *Children and adults:* IV 12 mg/kg/day (max 800 mg/day) for 4–5 days then 6 mg/kg every other day for 4 doses. Repeat in 4 wk. Cream or solution 5%: apply to entire affected area twice daily.	*Adverse events:* Arrhythmias, hypotension, heart failure, cerebellar ataxia, somnolence, alopecia, skin pigmentation, pruritic maculopapular rash, photosensitivity, erythrodysesthesias of hands and feet, loss of nails, hyperpigmentation of nail beds, nausea, vomiting, diarrhea, GI hemorrhage, esophagitis, stomatitis, hepatotoxicity, conjunctivitis, myelosuppression (WBC and platelets: onset 7–10 days, nadir 9–14 days, recovery 21 days).
Fluoxetine Hydrochloride Prozac. Capsule: 10, 20 mg. Liquid: 20 mg/5 mL.	**Treatment of depression and obsessive-compulsive disorders (antidepressant, inhibits CNS serotonin uptake).** *Children 5–18 yr:* Initial 5–10 mg/day then titrate slowly to effect (max 20 mg/day) *Adults:* initial 20 mg/day then slowly increase daily dose in 20 mg increments to effect (max 80 mg/day).	*Caution:* Avoid in patients on MAO inhibitors. *Adverse events:* Headache, nervousness, insomnia, anxiety, mania, suicidal ideation, tremor, nausea, anorexia, diarrhea, constipation, dry mouth, weight loss. *Monitoring:* Serum concentrations of fluoxetine (therapeutic 100–800 ng/mL), norfluoxetine (therapeutic 100–600 ng/mL).
Fluticasone Flonase, Flovent. Nasal solution: 50 μg/spray. Metered dose inhaler: 44, 110, 220 μg/spray. Rotadisk: 50, 100, 250 μg/dose.	**Treatment of allergic rhinitis and chronic asthma (inhaled corticosteroid).** *Children and adults:* Nasal spray 1–2 sprays in each nostril once daily. MDI 88–880 μg twice daily (depending on asthma severity and need for systemic corticosteroids). Rotadisk 50–1,000 μg twice daily (depending on asthma severity and need for systemic corticosteroids).	*Adverse events:* Dysphonia, oral thrush, adrenal suppression, growth suppression, cataracts.
Folic Acid Generic. Injection. Tablet: 0.4, 0, 8, 1 mg. Extemporaneous formulation.	**Treatment of folate deficiency anemias, i.e., megaloblastic, macrocytic (cofactor for normal erythropoeisis).** *Neonates to 6 mo:* oral 25–35 μg/day. *6 mo–3 yr:* 50 μg/day. *4–6 yr:* 75 μg/day. *7– 10 yr:* 100 μg/day. *11–14 yr:* 150 μg/day. *>15 yr and adults:* 200 μg/day. Folate deficiency: 1 mg/day.	*Caution:* Large folate doses may mask hematologic effects of B_{12} deficiency while allowing the neurologic consequences to progress.
Furosemide Lasix, Generic. Injection. 10 mg/mL. Oral solution: 10 mg/mL, 40 mg/mL. Tablets: 20, 40, 80 mg.	**Diuretic (inhibits sodium and chloride reabsorption at the ascending loop of Henle and distal tubule).** *Premature infants:* 0.5–2 mg/kg IV or 1–4 mg/kg oral every 12–48 hr (dose to response). *Infants and children:* 1–2 mg/kg IV or 1–4 mg/kg oral every 6 to 24 hr or continuous infusion start at 0.05 mg/kg/hr (dose to response). *Adults:* 10–600 mg/day in 1–4 divided doses; or continuous infusion 0.05 mg/kg/hr (adjust dose to effect).	*Adverse events:* Dehydration, electrolyte loss, hyperuricemia, photosensitivity, ischemic hepatitis, hypercalciuria, renal stones, ototoxicity (IV infusion rate >4 mL/min), GI intolerance.
Gabapentin Neurontin. Capsule: 100, 300, 400 mg.	**Adjunct to treatment of partial and secondarily generalized seizures; treatment of neuropathic pain (mechanism not certain).** *Children 2–12 yr:* 5–35 mg/kg/day in 3 divided doses (max 50 mg/kg/day). *Children >12 yr and adults:* start 300 mg daily, then daily increase by 300 mg to 900–3,600 mg/day in 3 divided doses.	*Adverse events:* Somnolence, dizziness, fatigue, depression, hyperactivity, aggression, dyspepsia, constipation, nausea, weight gain, diplopia.
Gamma Globulin	**See Immune Globulin**	
Gentian Violet Generic. Topical solution: 1%, 2%.	**Treatment of cutaneous and mucocutaneous infections (kills *Candida*, staphylococcal species, and some vegetative gram-positive bacteria).** *Infants:* apply 3–4 drops of a 0.5% solution under tongue or on lesion after feedings. *Children and adults:* apply 0.5–2% with cotton to lesion 2–3 times/day for 3 days.	*Caution:* Do not swallow. *Adverse events:* Burning, local irritation or sensitivity reactions.
Glucagon Powder for injection.	**Treatment of hypoglycemia (stimulates hepatic glycolysis and gluconeogenesis).** *Neonates:* 0.3 mg/kg/dose (max 1 mg) IV, IM, SC. *Children:* 0.025–0.1 mg/kg/dose (max 1 mg), may repeat in 20 min. *Adults:* 0.5–1 mg, may repeat in 20 minutes as needed.	*Adverse events:* Nausea, vomiting, hypersensitivity reactions.

Table continued on following page

TABLE 728–1 General Medications *Continued*

Drug (Trade Names, Formulations)	Indications (Mechanism of Action) and Dosing	Comments (Cautions, Adverse Events, Monitoring)
Glycopyrrolate Robinul, Generic. Injection: 0.2 mg/mL. Tablet: 1 mg.	**Inhibits salivation and excessive secretions of the respiratory tract; bronchodilator, adjunct to treatment of peptic ulcer, reversal of muscarinic effects on cholinergic agents (anticholinergic).** *Children:* Control of secretions: Oral 40–100 μg/kg/dose 3–4 times/day. IM, IV 4–10 μg/kg/dose every 3–4 hr. Preoperative IM: 4.4–8.8 μg/kg/dose 30–60 min before procedure.	*Adverse events:* Tachycardia, nervousness, headache, insomnia, drowsiness, dry mouth, constipation, nausea, urinary retention, blurred vision.
Gold Sodium Thiomalate Myochrysine, Generic. Injection: 25 mg/mL.	**Treatment of rheumatoid arthritis (mechanism unknown).** *Children:* Test dose 10 mg IM; followed by 1 mg/kg IM every wk for 20 wk; then 1 mg/kg/dose every 2–4 wk (max 50 mg/dose). *Adults:* Test dose 10 mg IM; then 25–50 mg/wk then 25–50 mg IM every 2–4 wk once response is noted.	*Cautions:* Patient should be sitting or lying for 10 min after the dose; avoid in patients with SLE or blood dyscrasias. *Adverse events:* Headache, flushing, seizures, exfoliative dermatitis, erythema nodosum, hives, alopecia, loss of nails, stomatitis, gingivitis, glossitis, conjunctivitis, eosinophila, leukopenia, thrombocytopenia, hematuria, proteinuria, nephrotic syndrome, pulmonary fibrosis and interstitial penumonitis, hepatotoxicity, peripheral neuropathy. *Monitoring:* Gold serum concentrations (therapeutic 1–3 μg/mL).
Gonadorelin Factrel, Lutrepulse. Injection.	**Evaluate gonadotropin regulation in precocious or delayed puberty, treat primary hypothalamic amenorrhea (stimulate release of leutinizing hormone).** *Children:* IV (HCl salt) 100 μg *Children >12 yr and adults:* IV, SC 100 μg during days 1–7 of menstrual cycle.	*Adverse events:* Flushing, lightheadedness, headache, abdominal discomfort. *Monitoring:* Plasma LH and FSH.
Granisetron Kytril. Injection: 1 mg/mL. Tablet: 1 mg.	**Antiemetic (selective 5-HT3 antagonist).** *Children >2 yr and adults:* IV 10–20 μg/kg 15–30 min prior to chemotherapy, may repeat 2–3 doses in 24 hr. Oral 1 mg twice daily starting 1 hr before chemotherapy.	*Adverse events:* Arrhythmias, bradycardia, transient blood pressure changes, agitation, anxiety, liver enzyme elevations.
Guaifenesin, Glycerol Guaiacolate Generic. ± codeine, dextromethorphan, phenylpropanolamine, or phenylephrine. Syrup, tablet, capsule, liquid.	**Temporary control of cough (expectorant).** *Children <2 yr:* 12 mg/kg/day in 6 divided doses. *2–5 yr:* 50–100 mg every 4 hr (max 600 mg/day). *6–11 yr:* 100–200 mg every 4 hr (max 1,200 mg/day). *>12 yr and adults:* 200–400 mg every 4 hr (max 2.4 g/day).	*Caution:* Monitor doses and toxicities of other drugs in combination products.
Guanethidine Ismelin. Tablet: 10 mg, 25 mg.	**Treatment of moderate to severe hypertension (acts as false neurotransmitter).** *Children:* 0.2 mg/kg/day, may increase by 0.2 mg/kg/day every wk to max 3 mg/kg/day. *Adults:* initial 10 mg/day, increase weekly to max 25–50 mg/day.	*Adverse events:* Palpitations, chest pain, peripheral edema, fatigue, headache drowsiness, confusion, constipation, anorexia, urinary frequency, nocturia, paresthesias, visual disturbances, orthostatic hypotension.
Guanfacine HCl Tenex. Tablet: 1 mg.	**Treatment of hypertension and attention deficit disorder (stimulate alpha-2 receptors in the brain stem)** *Children:* ADD: 1 mg/day. *Adults:* 1 mg/day, may increase every 4 wk to max 3 mg/day.	*Adverse events:* Somnolence, dizziness, dry mouth, constipation, GI upset.
Haloperidol Haldol, Generic. Oral concentrate: 2 mg/mL. Tablet: 0.5, 1, 2, 5, 10, 20 mg. Injection.	**Treatment of severe behavioral problems including psychoses and Tourette's disorder (competative blocker of dopamine receptors).** *Children 3–12 yr:* Oral: start 0.25–0.5 mg/day in 2–3 divided doses, then increase weekly by 0.25–0.5 mg daily based on response to max 0.15 mg/kg/day. *6–12 yr:* IM: 1–3 mg/dose every 4–8 hr (max 0.15 mg/kg/day). *Adults:* Oral: 0.5–5 mg 2–3 times daily. IM: 2–5 mg every 4–8 hr.	*Adverse events:* Drowsiness, restlessness, anxiety, extrapyramidal symptoms, dystonia, akathesia, pseudoparkinsonism, tardive dyskinesia, neuroleptic malignant syndrome, seizures, constipation, weight gain, swelling of breasts, hypotension, tachycardia, arrhythmias, urinary retention, blurred vision, rental pigmentation, cholestatic liver disease, agranulocytosis, leukopenia. *Monitoring:* Plasma concentrations (therapeutic 5–15 ng/mL, toxic >42 ng/mL).

TABLE 728–1 General Medications *Continued*

Drug (Trade Names, Formulations)	Indications (Mechanism of Action) and Dosing	Comments (Cautions, Adverse Events, Monitoring)
Heparin (unfractionated) Generic. Injection.	**Prophylaxis and treatment of thromboembolism (potentiate actions of antithrombin III).** *Neonates, infants, and children:* Thrombosis and ECMO: load 50 units/kg IV bolus, and 15–35 units/kg/hr continuous IV infusion maintenance dose (adjust to target APTT or heparin level). Catheter patency: 0.5–1 unit/mL. *Adults:* load 70–100 units/kg IV push, 15–25 units/kg/hr continuous IV infusion (target APTT or heparin level); SC 5,000 units every 8–12 hr for prophylaxis.	*Caution:* Avoid if severe thrombocytopenia, intracranial hemorrhage, bacterial endocarditis. *Adverse events:* Bleeding from various sites, e.g., urine, gums, nose; bruising, thrombocytopenia, thrombosis. *Monitoring:* APTT (therapeutic, 1.5–2.5 times baseline; toxic >2.5 times baseline); plasma heparin concentration (anti-factor X assay: therapeutic 0.3–0.7 units/mL).
Histrelin Supprelin. Injection.	**Central idiopathic precocious puberty (gonadotropin releasing hormone analog).** *Children:* SC 10 μg/kg once daily. *Adult female:* 100 μg/day for endometriosis.	*Adverse events:* Anxiety, depression, irritability, insomnia, headaches.
Homatropine Hydrobromide Isopto Homatropine, Generic. Ophthalmic solution 2%, 5%.	**Producing cycloplegia and mydriasis for refraction, treatment of uveitis (anticholinergic).** *Children:* For mydriasis: 1 drop of 2% solution before procedure, may repeat every 10 min as needed. Uveitis: 1 drop 2% solution 2–3 times/day. *Adults:* Mydriasis: 1–2 drops of 2% or 5% solution before procedure, may repeat every 10 min. Uveitis: 1–2 drops of 2% or 5% solution 2–3 times daily.	*Adverse events:* Blurred vision, photophobia, local stinging, respiratory congestion.
Human Growth Hormone Humatrope, Nutropin, Protropin. Injection.	**Treatment of growth failure due to inadequate growth hormone secretion (replacement therapy).** *Children:* Humatrope: 0.06 mg/kg (0.15 IU/kg) 3 times/wk. Nutropin: 0.043 mg/kg/day. Protropin: 0.1 mg/kg (0.26 IU/kg) 3 times/wk.	*Adverse events:* Local lipatrophy, hypothyroidism, pain in hip or knee.
Hyaluronidase Wydase. Injection: 150 units/mL.	**Treatment of extravasation, enhance absorption of fluids administered by hypodermoclysis (hydrolysis of hyaluronic acid to modify permeability of connective tissue).** *Neonates, infants, children:* Inject using 25–26 g needle (total 1 mL, 150 U) SC or intradermal at 5 sites (0.2 mL to each) at the leading edge of the extravasation.	*Adverse events:* Tachycardia, hypotension, erythema.
Hydralazine Generic. Injection: 20 mg/mL. Tablet. Extemporaneous formulations.	**Treatment of hypertension, adjunct treatment of congestive heart failure with nitrates (direct vasodilation of arterioles).** *Neonates:* IV 0.1–0.5 mg/kg/dose every 6–8 hr. Oral 0.25–1 mg/kg/dose every 6–8 hr. *Infants and children:* IM, IV start 0.1–0.2 mg/kg/dose every 4–6 hr and titrate to effect (max 3.5 mg/kg/day). Oral 0.75–1 mg/kg/day in 2–4 divided doses (max 7.5 mg/kg/day). *Adults:* IM, IV 10–20 mg/dose every 4–6 hr (max 40 mg/dose). Oral 10–25 mg/dose 4 times daily and titrate to effect (max 300 mg/day).	*Adverse events:* Palpitations, flushing, tachycardia, headache, nausea, vomiting, anorexia, diarrhea, lupus-like syndrome, arthralgias, peripheral neuropathy (related to pyridoxine deficiency).
Hydrochlorothiazide Generic. Oral solution: 50 mg/5 mL. Tablet: 25, 50, 100 mg. Combination products (e.g., spironolactone).	**Treatment of hypertension and fluid overload (edema) states, e.g., BPD, CHF; prevention of recurrent renal calcium stones (diuretic inhibits sodium reabsorption in distal tubule).** *Neonates and infants:* 2–4 mg/kg/day in 2 divided doses. *Infants >6 mo and children:* 2 mg/kg/day in 2 divided doses. *Adults:* 12.5–100 mg/day.	*Adverse events:* Hypokalemia, hypochloremia, hypomagnesemia, hyperglycemia, hyperuricemia, hyperlipidemia, pancreatitis, leukopenia, thrombocytopenia, aplastic anemia, hepatitis, intrahepatic cholestasis, prerenal azotemia.

Table continued on following page

TABLE 728–1 General Medications *Continued*

<table>
<tr><th>Drug
(Trade Names, Formulations)</th><th>Indications
(Mechanism of Action)
and Dosing</th><th>Comments
(Cautions, Adverse Events,
Monitoring)</th></tr>
<tr><td>Hydrocortisone
Generic.
Cream, ointment, gel, lotion, injection, oral suspension, rectal foam.</td><td>Treatment of adrenal insuficiency, congenital adrenal hyperplasia, shock, corticosteroid-responsive dermatoses, adjunctive treatment of ulcerative colitis (anti-inflammatory, glucocorticoid).
Neonates, infants, young children:
Adrenal insufficiency: 1–2 mg/kg IV bolus, then 25–150 mg/day divided every 6 hr.
Congenital adrenal hyperplasia:
IV 0.5–0.7 mg/kg/day start, then 0.3–0.4 mg/kg/day maintenance therapy, give doses as 1/4 in AM, 1/4 at noon, and 1/2 at night.
Shock: IV 35–50 mg/kg, then 50–150 mg/kg/day divided every 6 hr for 48–72 hr.
Infants and older children:
Adrenal insufficiency: 1–2 mg/kg IV bolus, then 150–250 mg/day divided every 6–8 hr.
Anti-inflammatory: IV, IM 1–5 mg/kg/day in 1–2 doses; oral 2.5–10 mg/kg/day divided every 6–8 hr.
Shock: IV 50 mg/kg/dose every 4 hr.
Status asthmaticus: IV 1–2 mg/kg/dose every 6 hr.
Adults:
Anti-inflammatory: IV, IM, Oral 15–240 mg/dose every 12 hr.
Shock: IV 0.5–2 g every 2–6 hr.
Rectal: 1 application 1–2 times/day for 2–3 wk.
Topical: apply 3–4 times/day.</td><td>Caution: Abrupt withdrawal may cause acute adrenal insufficiency.
Adverse events: Hypertension, hyperglycemia, hypokalemia, euphoria, insomnia, headache, Cushing syndrome, peptic ulcer, cataracts, immunosuppression, skin and muscle atrophy, acne, edema.
<table>
<tr><th></th><th colspan="2">Relative Potencies of Corticosteroids</th></tr>
<tr><th>Drug</th><th>Anti-inflammatory Effect (mg)</th><th>Sodium-Retaining Effect (mg)</th></tr>
<tr><td>Hydrocortisone</td><td>100</td><td>100</td></tr>
<tr><td>Cortisone</td><td>80</td><td>80</td></tr>
<tr><td>Prednisolone</td><td>20</td><td>100</td></tr>
<tr><td>Prednisone</td><td>20</td><td>100</td></tr>
<tr><td>Methylprednisolone</td><td>16</td><td>0</td></tr>
<tr><td>Triamcinolone</td><td>16</td><td>0</td></tr>
<tr><td>Dexamethasone</td><td>2</td><td>0</td></tr>
<tr><td>Desoxycorticosterone</td><td>0</td><td>2</td></tr>
</table></td></tr>
<tr><td>Hydromorphone
Dilaudid, Generic.
Injection.
Tablet: 2, 4 mg.
Syrup: 1 mg/5 mL.
Suppository: 3 mg.</td><td>Analgesic, antitusive (narcotic).
Children 6–12 yr:
Cough: Oral 0.5 mg every 3–4 hr as needed.
Pain: Oral 0.03–0.08 mg/kg/dose every 4–6 hr as needed.
IV 0.015 mg/kg/dose every 4–6 hr as needed.
Children >12 yr and adults:
Cough: Oral 1 mg every 3–4 hr as needed.
Pain: Oral, IV, IM, SC 1–4 mg/dose every 4–6 hr as needed.</td><td>Caution: Tablet and syrup contain tartrazine, which may exacerbate asthma; do not discontinue abruptly after continuous use.
Adverse events: Sedation, drowsiness, confusion, restlessness, headache, tachycardia, hypotension, physical and psychological addiction, nausea, vomiting, constipation, stomach cramps, decreased urination, ureteral spasm, respiratory depression, shortness of breath, miosis, antidiuretic hormone release, sensitivity reactions (due to histamine release).
Comment: IV, IM hydromorphone 1.5 mg = morphine 10 mg; oral hydromorphone 7.5 mg = morphine 30 mg (acute) or 60 mg (chronic).</td></tr>
<tr><td>Hydroxocobalamin, Vitamin B_{12}
Codroxomin, Hybalamin, others.
Injection.</td><td>Treatment of pernicious anemia, vitamin B_{12} deficiency, increased vitamin B_{12} requirements (replacement therapy).
Children: 100 μg/day IM to total 1 mg over 2 wk, then 30–50 μg each mo.
Adults: 30 μg/day for 5–10 days, then 100–200 μg/mo.</td><td>Comment: May require coadministration of folate.</td></tr>
<tr><td>Hydroxychloroquine
Plaquenil sulfate.
Tablet: 200 mg.
Extemporaneous formulations.</td><td>Suppression or chemoprophylaxis of malaria; treatment of SLE and rheumatoid arthritis (interferes with digestive vacuole function within sensitive malarial parasites, impairs complement-dependent antigen-antibody reactions).
Children:
Chemoprophylaxis of malaria:
5 mg/kg once wk (begin 1–2 wk before exposure and continue for 4 wk after leaving high-risk area).
Acute malaria attack:
10 mg/kg initial dose followed by 5 mg/kg in 6–8 hr on day 1, 400 mg once on day 2 and day 3.
Adults:
Malaria prophylaxis: 400 mg once wk (timing as above).
Acute malaria attack:
Day 1: 800 mg, then 400 mg in 6–8 hr; day 2: 400 mg once; day 3: 400 mg once.
Rheumatoid arthritis and lupus erythematosus:
400 mg once daily, may increase by 200 mg if inadequate response in 4–12 wk, reduce to 200–400 mg/day once response occurs and long-term maintenance is needed.</td><td>Caution: Avoid in porphyria or psoriasis.
Adverse events: Headache, confusion, agitation, insomnia, nightmares, psychosis, visual field defects, retinitis, blindness, bone marrow suppression, thrombocytopenia, liver failure, anorexia, nausea, vomiting, diarrhea, lichenoid dermatitis, bleaching of hair, itching, ototoxicity.
Monitoring: Ophthalmologic exams for visual field changes.</td></tr>
</table>

TABLE 728–1 General Medications *Continued*

Drug (Trade Names, Formulations)	Indications (Mechanism of Action) and Dosing	Comments (Cautions, Adverse Events, Monitoring)
Hydroxyurea Hydrea, Generic. Capsule: 500 mg.	**Cancer chemotherapy, sickle cell anemia (interfere with DNA synthesis during S-phase of cell division).** *Children:* 1500–3000 mg/m² every 4–6 wk. *Adults:* Cancer chemotherapy: 80 mg/kg every third day, or 20–30 mg/kg/day sickle cell anemia: 10–20 mg/kg/day.	*Adverse events:* Drowsiness, headache, hallucinations, seizures, nausea, vomiting, mucositis, stomatitis, myelosuppression (onset day 7, nadir day 10, recovery day 21), alopecia, maculopapular rash, dry skin, erythema of face and hands, hepatitis, increased BUN and creatinine, hyperuricemia.
Hydroxyzine Generic. Injection, syrup, tablet, capsule.	**Treatment of allergy, itching, anxiety, nausea, and adjunct for chronic pain management (H1-receptor blocker).** Oral, IM: *Children:* 0.6 mg/kg/dose every 6 hr. *Adults:* 10–100 mg/dose 3–4 times daily.	*Caution:* May worsen narrow-angle glaucoma, prostatic hypertrophy, bladder neck obstruction, asthma and COPD. *Adverse events:* Hypotension, drowsiness, dizziness, headache, dry mouth, urinary retention, pain at injection site.
Hyoscyamine (with Atropine, Scopolamine, and Phenobarbital) Donnatal, Generic. Capsule, elixir, tablet.	**Treatment of irritable bowel, spastic colon, spastic bladder, and renal colic (anticholinergic).** *Children:* Donnatal 0.1 mL/kg/dose every 4 hr (max 5 mL). *Adults:* 1–2 tablets (or 5–10 mL) 3–4 times daily.	*Caution:* Contraindicated in narrow-angle glaucoma, myesthenia gravis, GI and GU obstruction. *Adverse events:* Tachycardia, palpitations, headache, drowsiness, nervousness, dry mouth, constipation, dysphagia, paralytic ileus, blurred vision, nasal congestion.
Ibuprofen Generic. Suspension: 100 mg/5 mL. Tablet: 200, 300, 400, 600, 800 mg.	**Treatment of pain, fever, rheumatoid arthritis (nonsteroidal anti-inflammatory, inhibit prostaglandin synthesis).** *Children:* Pain, fever: 5–10 mg/kg/dose every 6–8 hr. Juvenile rheumatoid arthritis: 30–50 mg/kg/day in 4 divided doses. *Adults:* 400–800 mg/dose 3–4 times daily (max 3.2 g/day).	*Adverse events:* Abdominal cramps, heartburn, nausea, GI bleeding, GI perforation, fluid retention, edema, hypertension, tachycardia, acute renal failure.
Idarubicin Idamycin. Injection.	**Combination chemotherapy for AML and ALL (inhibit DNA and RNA synthesis).** *Children:* ALL: 10–12 mg/m² IV once daily for 3 days per treatment course. *Adults:* AML: 8–12 mg/m² IV daily for 3 days per treatment course.	*Adverse events:* Headache, infection, hemorrhage, mucositis, stomatitis, alopecia, rash, urticaria, nausea, vomiting, diarrhea, leukopenia (nadir 8–19 days), thrombocytopenia (nadir 10–15 days), myocardial toxicity (arrhythmias, cardiomyopathy, heart failure, ECG changes). *Monitoring:* Max lifetime dose = 137.5 mg/m². Lower dose by 25% if severe mucositis present or serum creatinine >2 mg/dL; lower dose by 50% if bilirubin >2.5 mg/dL; do not give dose if bilirubin >5 mg/dL.
Ifosfamide Ifex. Injection.	**Cancer chemotherapy (alkylating agent).** *Children:* IV 1,200–1,800 mg/m²/day for 5 days every 21–28 days; or 5 g/m² as single IV infusion. *Adults:* 700–2,000 mg/m²/day for 5 days every 21–28 days; or 5 g/m² as single IV infusion.	*Adverse events:* Alopecia, nausea, vomiting, stomatitis, hemorrhagic cystitis (administer MESNA for uroprotection), hematuria, renal damage, somnolence, confusion, hallucinations, coma, polyneuropathy, depressive psychosis, elevated liver enzymes, myelosuppression (onset day 7, nadir 10–14 days), pulmonary fibrosis, nasal stuffiness, cardiotoxicity.
Imipramine Tofranil, Generic. Injection, capsule, tablet.	**Treatment of depression, enuresis, pain (tricyclic antidepressant, increase synaptic concentrations of norepinephrine and serotonin).** *Children:* Depression: start 1.5 mg/kg/day, may increase by 1 mg/kg/day every 3–4 days (max 5 mg/kg/day) Enuresis: >6 yr, 10–25 mg at bedtime. Cancer pain: 0.2–0.4 mg/kg at bedtime, may increase dose 50% every 3–4 days (max 3 mg/kg). *Adolescents:* Oral: start 25–50 mg/day, may gradually increase to max 200 mg/day. *Adults:* Oral 25 mg 3–4 times daily, may increase dose gradually to max 300 mg/day; IM initial up to 100 mg in divided doses.	*Adverse events:* Arrhythmias, postural hypotension, drowsiness, sedation, confusion, headache, dry mouth, constipation, urinary retention, increased liver enzymes, seizures, urinary retention. *Monitoring:* Imipramine concentrations (therapeutic: imipramine and desipramine 150–250 ng/mL, toxic >1,000 ng/mL).
Immune Globulin, Intravenous (IVIG) Gamimune, Sandoglobulin, Generic. Injection.	**Immunodeficiency syndrome, idiopathic thrombocytopenic purpura, acute bacterial or viral infections in immunocompromised or neutropenic patients, Kawasaki disease, Guillain-Barré syndrome, demyelinating polyneuropathy (replacement therapy or interference with Fc receptors in the reticulo-endothelial system for autoimmune diseases).**	*Caution:* Doses should be based on ideal body weight (not total body weight). *Adverse events:* Flushing, tachycardia, chills, nausea, dyspnea, fever, hypersensitivity reactions, headache, aseptic meningitis.

Table continued on following page

TABLE 728–1 General Medications *Continued*

Drug (Trade Names, Formulations)	Indications (Mechanism of Action) and Dosing	Comments (Cautions, Adverse Events, Monitoring)
Immune Globulin, Intravenous *Continued*	*Neonates:* 500–750 mg/kg once. *Children and adults:* Immunodeficiency syndrome: 100–400 mg/kg/dose every 2–4 wk. Chronic lymphocytic leukemia: 400 mg/kg/dose every 3 wk. Idiopathic thrombocytopenic purpura: 1,000 mg/kg/dose for 2–5 consecutive days then every 3–6 wk. Kawasaki disease: 2 g/kg single dose. CMV infection: 500 mg/kg/dose every other day for 7 doses. Severe systemic infection: 500–1,000 mg/kg once wk. Polyneuropathy: 1 g/kg/day for 2 consecutive days each mo.	
Indomethacin Indocin, Generic (oral forms). Capsule: 25, 50 mg. Suspension: 25 mg/5 mL. Injection.	**Closure of the patent ductus arteriosus (PDA) in neonates, treatment of rheumatoid disorders, acute gouty arthritis, pain (NSAID, prostaglandin inhibition).** *Neonates:* IV 0.10–0.25 mg/kg/dose every 12 hr for 3–6 doses. Inflammatory rheumatoid disorders: *Children:* 1–2 mg/kg/day in 2–4 doses (max 4 mg/kg/day). *Adults:* 25–50 mg/dose 2–3 times/day (max 200 mg/day).	*Caution:* Avoid in premature neonates with necrotizing enterocolitis, poor renal function, or active bleeding, and all patients with active GI bleeding. *Adverse events:* Confusion, dizziness, headache, nausea, vomiting, abdominal pain, GI bleeding, ulcers, GI perforation, bone marrow suppression, impaired platelet aggregation, oliguria, renal failure, hypertension, edema, hyperkalemia. *Monitoring:* Indomethacin (concentrations in PDA closure): therapeutic 1–3 μg/mL.
Insulin ***Rapid-Acting:*** Lispro, Regular, Semilente; ***Intermediate-Acting:*** NPH, Lente; ***Long-Acting:*** Ultralente; ***Combination Products*** (e.g., Novolin 70/30, contains Lente 70 units, Regular 30 units). Humulin, Novolin (human insulin, preferred form); beef insulin, pork insulin. Injection.	**Treatment of insulin dependent diabetes mellitus and non-insulin dependent diabetes not adequately controlled with oral hypoglycemics (replacement therapy).** *Neonates:* Regular insulin 0.01–0.1 units/kg/hr continuous infusion, or SC 0.1–0.2 units/kg every 6–12 hr. *Children and adults:* 0.5–1 unit/kg/day. Adjust doses to blood glucose and hemoglobin A_{1C} results. *Adolescents (during growth spurt):* 0.8–1.2 units/kg/day. Diabetic ketoacidosis: Continuous infusion IV 0.1 units/kg/hr adjusted to serum glucose. Hyperkalemia: Try calcium gluconate and $NaHCO_3$ first, then dextrose 50% 0.5–1 mL/kg and regular insulin 1 unit per 4–5 g dextrose.	*Caution:* Check for drugs that increase or decrease insulin effect, do not change insulin types or brands once patient is regulated since dosing requirements will then change, start new patients on human insulin if possible. *Adverse events:* Hypoglycemia (and associated symptoms of dizziness, weakness, paresthesias, numbness of mouth, fatigue, mental confusion, hunger, nausea, visual problems), hypokalemia. *Monitoring:* Blood glucose (teach patient to monitor at home and make insulin dosing corrections per results), hemoglobin A_{1C}, urine glucose, and acetone.
Interferon Alfa-2a Roferon-A. Injection.	**In children treat hemangiomas of infancy and pulmonary hemangiomas (inhibits cellular growth, alters cellular differentiation).** *Infants and children:* SC 1–3 million units/m² once daily. *Adults:* 3–20 million units/m²/dose daily to 3 times weekly depending on the indication.	*Adverse events:* Tachycardia, arrhythmias, hypotension, edema, CNS depression, confusion, fatigue, dizziness, flu-like symptoms (begin 2–6 hr after dose and last up to 24 hr).
Ipecac Syrup Generic. Syrup: 70 mg/mL.	**Induces vomiting to treat certain toxic ingestions (stimulates medullary chemoreceptor trigger zone).** *Children:* may repeat dose in 20 min one time. *6–12 mo:* 5–10 mL followed by 20 mL/kg of water. *1–12 yr:* 15 mL followed by 20 mL/kg of water. *>12 yr and adults:* 30 mL followed by 300 mL of water.	*Cautions:* Do not use if: patient is unconscious, absent gag reflex, seizures, ingestion of strong bases or acids or volatile oils. Do not confuse with ipecac fluid extract, which is 14 times more potent. *Adverse events:* Lethargy, persistent vomiting, diarrhea.
Ipratropium Atrovent. Nebulization solution: 0.02%. Metered dose inhaler: 18 μg/puff. Nasal spray: 0.3%, 0.6%.	**Bronchodilator, treatment of rhinitis (anticholinergic).** *Neonates:* nebulized 100 μg/dose or MDI 1–2 puffs 3–4 times/day. *Infants and children:* nebulized 125–250 μg or MDI 1–2 puffs 3–6 times/day. *Adults:* nebulized 500 μg or MDI 2 puffs 3–4 times daily. Nasal spray for rhinitis: 1–2 sprays in each nostril 2–3 times daily.	*Adverse events:* Dry mouth, nervousness, dizziness, headache, blurred vision, urinary retention.
Iron Iron dextran complex (injection). Ferrous sulfate, gluconate, etc. (oral).	**Treatment of iron deficiency, hypochromic, microcyticanemia (replacement therapy).** Injection: IM, IV: Give 0.25–0.5 mL test dose 1 hr before starting iron dextran therapy Dose (mL/kg) = Hgb (normal − actual) × 0.0476 + 1 mL/5 kg max: <5kg = 25 mg, 5–10 kg = 50 mg >10kg = 100 mg.	*Adverse events:* (Oral) GI irritation, nausea, constipation, dark stools: (IV, IM) hypotension, flushing, dizziness, fever, headache, metallic taste, arthralgia, anaphylaxis. *Monitoring:* Hemoglobin (normal <15 kg = 12 mg%, >15 kg = 14.8 mg%), reticulocyte count, serum ferritin.

TABLE 728–1 General Medications *Continued*

Drug (Trade Names, Formulations)	Indications (Mechanism of Action) and Dosing	Comments (Cautions, Adverse Events, Monitoring)
Iron *Continued*	Oral (mg iron): *Children:* Prophylaxis: 1–2 mg/kg/day. Deficiency: 3–6 mg/kg/day in 1–3 divided doses. *Adults:* Prophylaxis 60 mg/day. Deficiency: 60 mg 2–4 times/day.	
Isoetharine Generic. Metered dose inhaler, inhalation solution.	**Bronchodilator (beta-agonist stimulation).** *Children:* Nebulize 0.01 mL/kg of 1% solution. *Adults:* Nebulize 0.5–1 mL of 0.5–1% solution; MDI 1–2 puffs every 4 hr as needed.	*Adverse events:* Tachycardia, headache, tremor, excitement, restlessness, nausea.
Isoproterenol Generic. Injection, sublingual tablets, nebulizer solution, metered dose inhaler.	**Asthma or COPD, ventricular arrhythmias due to AV node block, low-output shock states (stimulate beta-1 and beta-2 receptors).** *Neonates, infants, and children:* IV infusion 0.05–2 μg/kg/min. *Children:* MDI 1–2 puffs every 4 hr as needed; nebulize 0.01 mL of 1% solution; SL tablets 5–10 mg every 3–4 hr (max 30 mg/day). *Adults:* MDI 1–2 puffs 4–6 times/day; nebulize 0.25–0.5 mL of 1% solution; SL tablets 10–20 mg every 3–4 hr (max 60 mg/day); IV infusion 2–20 μg/min.	*Adverse events:* Tachycardia, palpitations, chest pain, nervousness, restlessness, anxiety, headache, insomnia, tremor, GI distress, nausea, paradoxical bronchospasm.
Kaolin and Pectin Generic. Oral suspension.	**Treatment of uncomplicated diarrhea (absorbent action).** *Children:* *3–6 yr:* 15–30 mL/dose. *6–12 yr:* 30–60 mL/dose. *>12 yr:* 60–120 mL/dose.	*Cautions:* Some products contain bismuth subsalicylate and may cause bleeding disorders. Avoid in dysentary, toxigenic diarrheas.
Ketamine Ketalar. Injection: 10, 50, 100 mg/mL.	**Anesthesia for short procedures (direct action on cortex and limbic system to produce dissociative anesthesia).** *Children:* Give 30 min prior to procedure. Oral 6–10 mg/kg; IM 3–7 mg/kg; IV 0.5–2 mg/kg. *Adults:* 3–8 mg/kg; IV 1–4.5 mg/kg (supplemental doses are 1/3 of initial dose).	*Adverse events:* Hypertension, tachycardia, hypotension, bradycardia, increased cerebral blood flow and intracranial pressure, hallucinations, delirium, tonic-clonic movements, increased metabolic rate, hypersalivation, nausea, vomiting, respiratory depression, apnea, increased airway resistance, cough, emergence reactions.
Ketorolac Acular. Ophthalmic. Toradol. Tablet, injection.	**Treatment of pain; ocular itching with conjunctivitis (NSAID, inhibits prostaglandin)** *Children 2–16 yr:* IM, IV 0.4–1 mg/kg/dose. Oral 1 mg/kg/dose every 6 hr if needed. *Adults:* IM 60 mg, IV 30 mg up to every 6 hr as needed. Ophthalmic 1 drop in eye 4 times/day for up to 7 days.	*Adverse events:* Edema, somnolence, dizziness, headache, dyspepsia, nausea, diarrhea, GI pain, GI bleeding, peptic ulcer, impaired platelet aggregation, oliguria, acute renal failure, dyspnea, wheezing, pain at injection site.
Labetalol Normodyne, Trandate. Injection: 5 mg/mL. Tablet: 100, 200, 300 mg.	**Treatment of mild to severe hypertension (blocks alpha and beta adrenergic receptors).** *Children:* Oral start 4 mg/kg/day in 2 doses, then gradually increase (max 40 mg/kg/day). IV start 0.2–1 mg/kg/dose (max 20 mg/dose), continuous IV infusion 0.4–1 mg/kg/hr (max 3 mg/kg/hr). *Adults:* Oral 100 mg twice daily, may increase every 2–3 days (max 2.4 g/day). IV start 20 mg, repeat boluses 40 mg every 10 min (max total dose 300 mg), continuous IV infusion 2 mg/min and titrate to response.	*Adverse events:* Orthostatic hypotension, CHF, conduction disturbance, bradycardia, drowsiness, fatigue, headache, dry mouth, nasal congestion, bronchospasm.
Lactulose Generic. Syrup: 10 g/15 mL.	**Treatment of constipation, hepatic encephalopathy (osmotic effect on stool in colon, acidification of stool promotes NH_4^+ elimination).** *Infants:* 2.5–10 mL/day in 3–4 doses. *Children:* 40–90 mL/day in 3–4 doses. *Adults:* 30–45 mL/dose 3–4 times/day.	*Adverse events:* Flatulence, abdominal discomfort, diarrhea, nausea, vomiting. *Monitoring:* Target 2–3 soft stools per day, serum ammonia.

Table continued on following page

TABLE 728–1 General Medications *Continued*

Drug (Trade Names, Formulations)	Indications (Mechanism of Action) and Dosing	Comments (Cautions, Adverse Events, Monitoring)
Lamotrigine Lamictal. Tablet: 25, 50, 100 mg.	**Treatment of partial seizures (blocks sodium channels and inhibit presynaptic release of glutamate and aspartate).** *Children 2–16 yr:* 2 mg/kg/day in 2 doses for 2 wk, then 5 mg/kg/day in 2 doses for 2 wk, then 10 mg/kg/day in 2 doses if needed (usual 5–15 mg/kg/day, max 400 mg/day). *If patient is on Valproate:* 0.2 mg/kg/day in 2 doses for 2 wk, then 0.5 mg/kg/day in 2 doses for 2 wk, then 1 mg/kg/day in 2 doses (max 5 mg/kg/day). *Adults:* Start 50 mg/day for 2 wk, then 100 mg/day, then increase by 100 mg/day at weekly intervals to response (max 500 mg/day). If patient is on *valproate:* 25 mg every other day for 2 wk, then 25 mg/day for 2 wk, then increase by 25 mg/day every wk to response (max 150 mg/day).	*Caution:* Serious skin rashes (potentially fatal) can occur and are particularly common in children and especially if doses are increased too quickly. Slow increases in dosing is especially important for patients on valproic acid. *Adverse events:* Dizziness, sedation, headache, agitation, exacerbation of seizures, rashes (maculopapular or erythematous eruptions), angioedema, photosensitivity, nystagmus, amblyopia, nausea, vomiting.
Lansoprazole Prevacid. Capsule: 15, 30 mg.	**Treatment of gastric or duodenal ulcer (proton pump inhibitor).** *Children:* *Adults:* 15–30 mg/day.	
Leucovorin Wellcovorin, Generic. Tablet: 5, 15 mg. Injection.	**Antidote for folic acid antagonists, e.g., methotrexate, treatment of folate deficient megaloblastic anemias of infancy, nutritional folate deficiency when oral folate can't be used (reduced form of folic acid so conversion is not necessary, replacement therapy).** *Children and adults:* Methotrexate rescue: IV 10 mg/m^2 to start then 10 mg/m^2 orally q6h for 72 hr; increase dose to 100 mg/m^2 every 3 hr if 24 hours after methotrexate dose the serum creatinine is increased by >50%, or methotrexate serum level is $>5 \times 10^{-6}$ M (continue until level $<1 \times 10^{-8}$ M). High-dose methotrexate rescue: IV 100–1000 mg/m^2/dose Intrathecal methotrexate: IV 12 mg/m^2 as single dose Megaloblastic anemia of infancy: IM 3–6 mg/day.	*Adverse events:* Rash, itching erythema. *Monitoring:* Plasma methotrexate levels (a leukovorin dosing nomogram is available based on methotrexate levels at various times after the dose.)
Leuprolide Lupron. Injection.	**Treatment of precocious puberty, prostate cancer (decrease levels of LH and FSH).** *Children:* Precocious puberty: IM depot 0.15–0.3 mg/kg/dose every 28 days (min dose 7.5 mg); SC 20–45 μg/kg/day. *Adults:* Prostate cancer: IM 7.5 mg/dose monthly; SC 1 mg/day.	*Adverse events:* Weight gain, hot flashes, depression, nausea, vomiting, GI bleed, myalgia, bone pain, weakness, blurred vision, estrogenic effects.
Levothyroxine Synthroid, Generic. Injection, tablet.	**Thyroid replacement therapy** Oral: *0–6 mo:* 8–10 μg/kg/day; *6–12 mo:* 6–8 μg/kg/day; *1–5 yr:* 5–6 μg/kg/day; *6–12 yr:* 4–5 μg/kg/day; *>12 yr:* 2–3 μg/kg/day. *Adults:* 12.5–50 μg/day (max 200 μg/day). IV, IM 50–75% of oral dose. Myxedema coma: 200–500 μg for one dose. Thyroid suppression therapy: 2–6 μg/kg/day for 7–10 days.	*Adverse events:* Tachycardia, cardiac arrhythmias, hypertension, nervousness, insomnia, headache, insomnia, hair loss, increased appetite, weight loss, tremor, sweating.
Lidocaine Generic. Injection, Topical (alone or in combination with prilocaine [EMLA]).	**Treatment of ventricular arrhythmias, local anesthetic (class 1B antiarrhythmic, blocks initiation and conduction of impulses).** *Children and adults:* Topical: Apply to affected area (max 3 mg/kg/dose) at least 2 hr apart. Local anesthetic injection: doses per need, max 4.5 mg/kg not closer than 2 hr apart. Arrhythmias: *Children:* load 1 mg/kg (may repeat every 5–10 min to max 3 mg/kg), IV continuous infusion. 20–50 μg/kg/min (1/2 dose if liver disease or poor cardiac output).	*Caution:* Avoid lidocaine with epinephrine preparations for arrhythmias. *Adverse events:* Arrhythmias, heart block, lethargy, coma, seizures, nausea, vomiting, paresthesias, blurred vision, diplopia, local skin irritation or rash. *Monitoring:* Lidocaine serum levels (therapeutic 1–5 μg/mL, toxic >6 μg/mL).

TABLE 728–1 General Medications *Continued*

Drug (Trade Names, Formulations)	Indications (Mechanism of Action) and Dosing	Comments (Cautions, Adverse Events, Monitoring)
Lidocaine *Continued*	*Adults:* load 1–1.5 mg/kg load (may repeat to max 3 mg/kg), IV continuous infusion 2–4 mg/min (1/2 dose for liver disease or heart failure). ET route: 2–2.5 times IV dose. Prehospital post-MI: 300 mg IM.	
Liothyronine Cytomel (oral), Triostat (injection), Generic.	**Replacement therapy in hypothyroidism.** *Neonates, infants, and children <3 yr:* Congenital hypothyroidism (cretinism): Oral 5 μg/day start, then may increase 5 μg every 3 days to max 20 μg/day (50 μg/day for children 1–3 yr). Hypothyroidism: *Children:* 5 μg/day, increase by 5 μg every 1–2 wk (usual 15–20 μg/day). *Adults:* start 5 μg/day, increase by 5 μg/day every 1–2 wk to 25 μg then by 12.5–25 μg every 1–2 wk to max 100 μg/day.	*Adverse events:* Palpitations, tachycardia, hypertension, nervousness, insomnia, headache, hair loss, diarrhea, abdominal cramps, tremor, sweating. *Monitoring:* Thyroid function, T3, TSH.
Lithium Generic. Syrup: 300 mg/5 mL. Tablet: 300 mg. Capsule: 150, 300, 600 mg.	**Management of acute mania, bipolar disorders, and depression (alter cation exchange across cell membranes).** *Children:* 15–60 mg/kg/day in 3–4 doses (start low and increase at weekly intervals). *Adolescents:* 600–1800 mg/day in 3–4 doses at regular intervals. *Adults:* 300 mg 3–4 times/day to start, may gradually increase per blood levels (max 2.4 g/day). **May use twice daily dosing if sustained-release product used.** *Renal impairment:* CrCl 10–50 mL/min 50–75% of normal dose; CrCl <10 mL/min 25–50% of normal dose.	*Adverse events:* Polydipsia, nausea, diarrhea, impaired taste, bloated feeling, weight gain, tremor, muscle twitching, weakness, fatigue, diabetes insipidus, nonspecific nephron atrophy, renal tubular acidosis, leukocytosis, vision problems, hypothyroidism, goiter, skin eruptions, acne. *Monitoring:* Serum lithium concentrations are essential to proper use of lithium, must be drawn 8–12 hr after a dose (therapeutic: acute mania 0.6–1.2 mEq/L, protection against future episodes 0.6–1 mEq/L; toxic >1.5 mEq/L; seizures >2.5 mEq/L. Watch for accumulation during salt loss and dehydration states.
Lomustine, CCNU CeeNu. Capsule 10, 40, 100 mg.	**Treatment of various cancers (alkylating agent, inhibit DNA and RNA synthesis).** *Children:* 75–100 mg/m² as single dose every 6 wk. *Adults:* 100–130 mg/m² as single dose every 6 wk.	*Adverse events:* Nausea, vomiting, myelosuppression (onset 14 days, nadir 4–5 wk, recovery 6 wk), neurotoxicity, stomatitis, diarrhea, anemia, alopecia, hepatotoxicity, renal failure, pulmonary fibrosis (with cumulative doses >600 mg). *Monitoring:* Reduce dose if CrCl <50 mL/min, or platelets and WBC remain low beyond 6 wk.
Loperamide Imodium, Generic. Liquid: 1 mg/5 mL. Tablet: 2 mg. Capsule: 2 mg.	**Treatment of acute and chronic diarrhea (directly inhibit intestinal peristalsis).** *2–5 yr:* 1 mg 3 times/day. *6–8 yr:* 2 mg 2 times/day. *8–12 yr:* 2 mg 3 times/day. *Adults:* 4 mg initially, then 2 mg after each loose stool (max 16 mg/day).	*Adverse events:* Sedation, fatigue, dizziness, nausea, vomiting, constipation.
Loratidine Claritin. Tablet: 10 mg. Syrup: 1 mg/mL.	**Treatment of allergic symptoms (antihistamine, H1 receptor antagonist).** *Children >3 yr:* <30 kg 5 mg/day, >30 kg 10 mg/day. *Adults:* 10 mg/day.	*Caution:* Prolonged Q-T intervals may occur if combined with drugs that inhibit liver enzymes, watch for drug interactions. *Adverse events:* Somnolence, fatigue, anxiety, depression, headache.
Lorazepam Ativan, Generic. Injection. Tablet: 0.5, 1, 2 mg. Oral solution: 2 mg/mL.	**Treatment for anxiety, sedation, and seizures, adjunct to antiemetic therapy (benzodiazepine, increase action of GABA).** Antiemetic therapy: *Children:* IV 0.04–0.08 mg/kg/dose every 6 hr as needed. Anxiety/sedation: *Neonates:* IV 0.1–0.4 mg/kg/dose every 4–6 hr as needed. *Infants and children:* IV 0.05–0.1 mg/kg/dose every 4–8 hr. *Adults:* Oral 1–10 mg/day in 2–3 divided doses. Insomnia: *Adults:* 2–4 mg at bedtime. Status epilepticus: *Neonates:* IV 0.05–0.2 mg/kg/dose over 2–5 min, may repeat in 10–15 min. *Infants and children:* IV 0.1 mg/kg load over 2–5 min, may give additional 0.05 mg/kg bolus in 10–15 min. *Adolescent:* IV 0.07 mg/kg/dose over 2–5 min, may repeat in 10–15 min. *Adults:* IV 4 mg/dose over 2–5 min, may repeat in 10 min.	*Caution:* Do not discontinue abruptly after long-term use to avoid possible abstinence symptoms. *Adverse events:* Several cases of myoclonus have been reported in neonates, tachycardia, drowsiness, depression, confusion, paradoxical excitement, blurred vision, diplopia.

Table continued on following page

TABLE 728–1 General Medications *Continued*

Drug (Trade Names, Formulations)	Indications (Mechanism of Action) and Dosing	Comments (Cautions, Adverse Events, Monitoring)
Magnesium Citrate, Citrate of Magnesia Generic. Solution: 300 mL.	**Evacuation of bowel (osmotic retention of fluid and increased peristalsis).** *Children <6 yr:* 2–4 mL/kg. *Children 6–12 yr:* 100–150 mL. *>12 yr and adult:* 150–300 mL.	*Adverse events:* Hypermagnesemia, hypotension, abdominal cramps, muscle weakness, CNS depression. *Monitoring:* Toxicity related to serum magnesium levels (>3 mg/dL depressed CNA, >5 mg/dL somnolence and depressed deep tendon reflexes, >12 mg/dL respiratory paralysis and heart block.
Magnesium Gluconate Generic. Tablet: 500 mg. **Magnesium Oxide** Generic. Tablet: 400, 420, 500 mg. Capsule: 140 mg.	**Magnesium replacement therapy.** *Children:* 10–20 mg/kg/dose elemental magnesium 4 times daily. *Adults:* 300 mg elemental magnesium 4 times daily.	*Adverse events:* Hypermagnesemia (see Magnesium citrate). *Monitoring:* Serum magnesium concentration (normal: children 1.5–1.9 mg/dL, adults 2.2–2.8 mg/dL).
Magnesium Hydroxide, Milk of Magnesia Generic. Liquid, tablet.	**Short-term treatment of constipation (osmotic retention of fluid promotes peristalsis).** *Children:* *<2 yr:* 0.5 mL/kg/dose. *2–5 yr:* 5–15 mL once daily. *6–12 yr:* 15–30 mL once daily. *>12 yr and adults:* 30–60 mL once daily.	*Adverse events:* (see Magnesium citrate).
Magnesium Sulfate Generic. Granules: 40 mEq/5 g. Injection: 50% solution.	**Treatment of hypomagnesemia, and seizures associated with acute nephritis in children, also used as a cathartic (cofactor for many enzymes in the body, and is important in calcium and potassium hemostasis).** Hypomagnesemia: *Neonates:* IV 25–50 mg/kg/dose every 8 hr for 2–3 doses. *Children:* Oral 100–200 mg/kg/dose 4 times daily; IM, IV 25–50 mg/kg/dose every 6 hr for 3–4 doses. *Adults:* Oral 3 g every 6 hr for 4 doses; IM, IV 1 g every 6 hr for 4 doses. Daily maintenance magnesium: *Neonates, infants, and children:* IV 30–60 mg/kg/day. *Adolescents:* IV 42–54 mg/kg/day. *Adults:* IV 0.5–3 g/day. Infuse IV doses over 2–4 hr (max 125 mg/kg/hr). Management of seizures and hypertension: *Children:* IM, IV 20–100 mg/kg/dose every 4–6 hr as needed. Cathartic: *Children:* Oral 0.25 g/kg/dose. *Adults:* Oral 10–30 g.	*Caution:* Magnesium may accumulate to toxic levels in renal insufficiency. *Adverse events:* (see Magnesium citrate).
Manganese Injection: 0.1 mg/mL.	**Trace element added to parenteral nutrition (cofactor in many enzyme systems).** *Infants:* 2–10 μg/kg/day in TPN solutions. *Adults:* 150–800 μg/day in TPN solutions.	*Monitoring:* Reference manganese plasma level is 4–14 μg/L.
Mannitol Generic. Injection.	**Promotion of diuresis, reduction of increased intracranial pressure.** *Children and adults:* IV 200 mg/kg test dose, initial 0.5–1 g/kg, maintenance 0.25–0.5 g/kg every 4–6 hr.	*Adverse events:* Circulatory overload, congestive heart failure, headache, chills, seizures, fluid and electrolyte imbalance. *Monitoring:* After test dose evaluate urine output of at least 1 mL/kg/hr (children) or 30–50 mL/hr (adults) for 2–3 hr; for increased intracranial pressure maintain serum osmolality 310–320 mOsm/kg.
Mechlorethamine, Nitrogen Mustard Mustargen Hydrochloride. Injection.	**Cancer chemotherapy (alkylating agent, inhibit DNA and RNA synthesis).** *Children:* as part of MOPP regimen, IV 6 mg/m² on days 1 and 8 of 28-day regimen. *Adults:* IV 0.4 mg/kg (12–16 mg/m²) as single monthly dose.	*Caution:* Extravasation should be treated promptly with sterile sodium thiosulfate (1/6 M) and apply cold compress for 6–12 hr. *Adverse events:* Nausea, vomiting, diarrhea, severe myelosuppression (onset 4–7 days, nadir 14 days, recovery 21 days), ototoxicity, precipitation of herpes zoster, alopecia, hyperuricemia.
Meclizine Generic. Tablet, capsule.	**Prevention and treatment of motion sickness, and treatment of vertigo (anticholinergic and CNS depressant effects).** *Children and adults:* Oral 25–50 mg taken 1 hr before travel for motion sickness; 25–100 mg/day in divided doses for vertigo.	*Adverse events:* Drowsiness, headache, fatigue, dry mouth, increased appetite, weight gain.
Medium Chain Triglycerides MCT Oil. Oil: 14 g/15 mL.	**Dietary supplement for those who cannot digest long-chain fats, ketogenic diet for seizure disorders (nutritional supplement).**	*Adverse events:* Nausea, vomiting, abdominal pain, ketosis.

TABLE 728–1 General Medications *Continued*

Drug (Trade Names, Formulations)	Indications (Mechanism of Action) and Dosing	Comments (Cautions, Adverse Events, Monitoring)
Medium Chain Triglycerides *Continued*	*Infants:* 0.5 mL every other feed and may advance by 0.5 mL every 2–3 days as tolerated. *Children:* ketogenic diet for seizures: 50–70% of total calories (usually about 40 mL with each meal); cystic fibrosis: 1 tablespoon 3 times daily. *Adults:* 15 mL 3–4 times daily.	
Medrysone HMS Liquefilm. Opthalmic solution.	**Treatment of conjunctivitis (inhibit inflammatory response).** *Children and adults:* Ophthalmic instill 1 drop in conjunctival sac 2–4 times/day (may use every 1–2 hr for 1–2 days).	*Adverse events:* Local stinging and burning, increased intraocular pressure, cataracts.
Melphalan Alkeran. Injection. Tablet: 2 mg.	**Cancer chemotherapy (alkylating agent, inhibit DNA and RNA synthesis).** *Children:* IV 10–35 mg/m²/dose every 21–28 days; high-dose: 140–220 mg/m² before bone marrow transplantation. Oral 4–20 mg/m²/day for 1–21 days. *Adults:* IV 16 mg/m²/dose every 2 wk for 4 doses monthly. Oral 0.15 mg/kg/day for 7 days or 0.25 mg/kg/day for 4 days, repeat every 4–6 wk.	*Adverse events:* Myelosuppression (onset 7 days, nadir 8–10 days and 27–32 days, recovery 42–50 days), secondary malignancy, alopecia, vesiculation of skin, SIADH, nausea, vomiting, diarrhea, stomatitis, hemorrhagic cystitis, pulmonary fibrosis, interstitial pneumonitis, vasculitis.
Meperidine Generic. Injection, syrup: 50 mg/5 mL. Tablet: 50, 100 mg.	**Narcotic analgesic, adjunct to anesthesia (bind to opiate receptors in CNS).** *Children:* IM, IV, SC 1–1.5 mg/kg/dose every 3–4 hr. *Adults:* IM, IV, SC 50–100 mg/dose every 3–4 hr as needed (equipotent oral dose is 3 times IV dose).	*Caution:* Scheduled use may result in metabolite accumulation in diminished renal function, which may lead to CNS stimulation or seizures. *Adverse events:* Hypotension, weakness, tiredness, headache, anorexia, stomach cramps, hallucination, paradoxical excitation, seizures, physical and psychological dependence. *Comment:* Equianalgesic dose to morphine 10 mg IV is meperidine 100 mg IV, IM or 300 mg oral.
Mephenytoin Mesantoin. Tablet: 100 mg.	**Treatment of tonic-clonic and partial seizures (decrease sodium ion influx across cell membranes)** *Children:* 3–15 mg/kg/day in 3 divided doses. *Adults:* start 50–100 mg/day, then increase weekly by 50–100 mg (max 800 mg/day).	*Adverse events:* Drowsiness, slurred speech, psychiatric changes, confusion, nausea, vomiting, constipation, leukopenia, hepatitis, blurred vision, nystagmus, photophobia, lymphadenopathy. *Monitoring:* Total mephenytoin level (25–40 μg/mL).
Mephobarbital Mebaral. Tablet 32, 50, 100 mg.	**Sedative, treatment of epilepsy (increase seizure threshold).** *Children:* 4–10 mg/kg/day in 2–4 doses. *Adults:* 200–600 mg/day in 2–4 doses.	*Adverse events:* Drowsiness, lethargy, confusion, mental depression, paradoxical excitement, psychological and physical dependence, constipation, nausea, vomiting. *Monitoring:* Phenobarbital concentrations (therapeutic 10–40 μg/mL).
Mercaptopurine Purinethol. Injection, tablet. Extemporaneous formulations.	**Treatment of leukemias and non-Hodgkins lymphoma (antimetabolite, blocks purine synthesis).** *Children:* Oral: induction: 2.5–5 mg/kg once daily; maintenance: 1.5–2.5 mg/kg once daily. IV continuous infusion: 50 mg/m²/hr for 24–48 hr. *Adults:* Oral: induction: 2.5–5 mg/kg once daily; maintenance: 1.5–2.5 mg/kg once daily. *Renal function CrCl <50 mL/min:* dose every 48 hr.	*Adverse events:* Hepatotoxicity (cholestasis and necrosis), nausea, anorexia, vomiting, diarrhea, stomach pain, stomatitis, mucositis, skin rash, hyperpigmentation, myelosuppression (onset 7–10 days, nadir 14 days, recovery 21 days), renal toxicity, hyperuricemia, eosinophilia, drug fever.
Mesna Mesnex. Injection: 100 mg/mL.	**Protect against hemorrhagic cystitis from ifosfamide and cyclophosphamide therapy (binds and detoxifies urotoxic metabolites via active sulfhydryl group).** *Children and adults:* IV 20% W/W of ifosfamide or cyclophosphamide dose started 15 min before alkylating agent dose, and repeat same mesna dose at 3, 6, 9, and 12 hr after alkylating agent dose. Oral 40% W/W of alkylating agent in 3 doses 4 hr apart.	*Adverse events:* Hypotension, headache, nausea, vomiting, bad taste in mouth, limb pain. *Monitoring:* Urinalysis.
Metaproterenol, Orciprenaline Alupent, Metaprel, Generic Metered Dose Inhaler (MDI). Inhalation solution. Tablet: 10, 20 mg. Syrup: 10 mg/5 mL.	**Bronchodilator (stimulate beta-2 receptors).** *Children:* Oral: *<2 yr:* 0.4 mg/kg/dose 3–4 times daily. *2–6 yr:* 1.3–2.6 mg/kg/day divided every 6 hr. *6–9 yr:* 10 mg/dose 4 times daily. *>9 yr and adults:* 20 mg/dose 3–4 times daily.	*Caution:* Some generic nebulizer solutions contain sulfites that may exacerbate asthma. *Adverse events:* Tremor, nervousness, overactivity, tachycardia, hypotension, headache. *Comment:* Dilute nebulizer solution in 2.5 mL normal saline.

Table continued on following page

TABLE 728–1 General Medications *Continued*

Drug (Trade Names, Formulations)	Indications (Mechanism of Action) and Dosing	Comments (Cautions, Adverse Events, Monitoring)
Metaproterenol, Orciprenaline *Continued*	MDI: 2–3 puffs every 4 hr. Nebulizer: *Infants and children:* 0.01–0.02 mL/kg of 5% solution every 4–6 hr. *Adolescents and adults:* 0.3 mL of 5% solution every 4–6 hr.	
Methadone Dolophine, Generic. Injection: 10 mg/mL. Tablet: 5, 10 mg. Oral solution: 5 mg/mL.	**Management of severe pain, narcotic detoxification (binds to opiate receptors in CNS).** *Neonates (abstinence syndrome):* 0.05–0.2 mg/kg/dose every 12 hr then adjust/taper based on abstinence scores. *Children:* analgesia: IV, IM, oral 0.1 mg/kg/dose every 4 hr for 2–3 doses, then every 6–12 hr as needed. Narcotic abstinence: start 0.05–0.1 mg/kg/dose every 6 hr and taper per abstinence scores. *Adults:* IV, IM, SC, oral Analgesia: 2.5–20 mg every 6–8 hr. Detoxification: 15–40 mg/day.	*Adverse events:* Weakness, drowsiness, dizziness, nausea, vomiting, constipation, ileus. *Monitoring:* Methadmonitored accumulates with repeated doses and patients should be monitored for excess CNS depression.
Methimazole Tapazole. Tablets 5, 10 mg.	**Treatment of hyperthyroidism (blocks iodine synthesis in the thyroid gland, inhibits synthesis of thyroid hormone).** *Children:* start 0.4 mg/kg/day, then maintenance 0.2 mg/kg/day. *Adults:* start 5 mg/kg every 8 hr, maintenance dose 5–15 mg/day (max 60 mg/day).	*Adverse events:* Fever, skin rash, leukopenia, agranulocytosis, SLE-like syndrome, nausea, vomiting, stomach pain, loss of taste, cholestatic jaundice, constipation, weight gain. *Monitoring:* Thyroid function tests for hypo- or hyperthyroidism.
Methocarbamol Robaxin, Generic. Injection: 100 mg/mL. Tablet: 500, 750 mg.	**Treatment of muscle spasm (skeletal muscle relaxant through CNS depressive effects)** *Children:* Treatment of tetanus: IV 15 mg/kg/dose every 6 hr for 3 days only. *Adults:* IV 1–2 g every 6 hr. Oral 1.5 g 3–4 times/day for 2–3 days, then decrease to 4–4.5 g/day.	*Adverse events:* Syncope, bradycardia, hypotension, drowsiness, dizziness, headache, nausea, metallic taste.
Methohexital Brevital. Injection.	**Induction and maintenance of general anesthesia (ultra short-acting barbiturate).** *Children:* IM (preoperative) 5–10 mg/kg/dose; IV (induction) 1–2 mg/kg/dose. Rectal 20–35 mg/kg/dose. *Adults:* IV (induction) 50–120 mg, then 20–40 mg every 4–7 min.	*Adverse events:* Apnea, respiratory depression, hiccups, laryngospasm, hypotension, skeletal muscle twitching and rigidity, tremor, seizures, headache, nausea, vomiting.
Methotrexate Generic. Injection. Tablet: 2.5 mg.	**Treatment of neoplasms, psoriasis, rheumatoid arthritis (antimetabolite, inhibition of DNA and purine synthesis).** *Children:* Juvenile rheumatoid arthritis: Oral, IM 5–15 mg/m^2 wk as a single dose. Antineoplastic: Oral, IM 7.5–30 mg/m^2 every 1–2 wk; IV 10–33 g/m^2 bolus dose or infused over 6–42 hr. *Adults:* Rheumatoid arthritis: Oral 7.5 mg once wk. Psoriasis: Oral, IM 10–25 mg/dose once/wk. Antineoplastic: Oral, IM, IV 25–50 mg/m^2/wk. Reduced renal function: CrCl 61–80 mL/min = reduce 25%. CrCl 51–60 mL/min = reduce 33%. CrCl 10–50 mL/min = reduce dose by 50–70%.	*Caution:* Avoid if severe renal or hepatic dysfunction. *Adverse events:* Hepatotoxicity, nephropathy, vasculitis, malaise, fatigue, encephalopathy, headache, seizures, chills, fever, cystitis, stomatitis, enteritis, nausea, vomiting, diarrhea, alopecia, photosensitivity, increase or decrease in skin pigmentation, urticaria, arthralgia, hyperuricemia, myelosuppression (onset 7 days, nadir 10 days, recovery 21 days). *Monitoring:* Methotrexate concentrations (toxic if $>1 \times 10^{-7}$ mol/L for more than 40 hr. Ensure adequate hydration and urinary alkalinization.
Methsuximide Celontin. Capsule: 150, 300 mg.	**Control of absence seizures, and adjunct in partial complex seizure management (increase seizure threshold, suppress nerve transmission).** *Children:* 10–15 mg/kg/day in 3–4 doses, may increase at weekly intervals (max 30 mg/kg/day). *Adults:* start 300 mg/day, may increase by 300 mg/day at weekly intervals (max 1200 mg/day).	*Adverse events:* Dizziness, drowsiness, lethargy, headache, ataxia, aggressiveness, depression, anorexia, nausea, vomiting, hiccups, agranulocytosis, aplastic anemia, leukopenia, thrombocytopenia. *Monitoring:* Methsuximide concentrations (therapeutic 10–40 μg/mL, toxic >4 μg/mL).

TABLE 728–1 General Medications *Continued*

Drug (Trade Names, Formulations)	Indications (Mechanism of Action) and Dosing	Comments (Cautions, Adverse Events, Monitoring)
Methyldopa Aldomet, Generic. Injection: 50 mg/mL. Tablet: 125 mg, 250 mg, 500 mgL. Oral suspension: 250 mg/5 mL.	**Treatment of hypertension (false alpha neurotransmitter metabolite stimulates inhibitory alpha-adrenergic receptors).** *Children:* Oral start 10 mg/kg in 2–4 doses, may increase every 2 days (max 65 mg/kg/day or 3 g/day). IV start 2–4 mg/kg/dose, may increase to 5–10 mg/kg/dose per response (max 65 mg/kg/day). *Adults:* Oral start 250 mg 3 times/day, may increase to max 3 g/day. IV 0.25–1 g every 6 hr (max 4 g/day). Renal dysfunction: extend interval.	*Caution:* Tolerance to effects occurs, so chronic use requires concurrent diuretic. *Adverse events:* Drowsiness, mental depression, headache, dry mouth, fever, chills, vertigo, fluid retention, edema, hepatocellular injury, cholestatic liver disease, cirrhosis, pancreatitis, nausea, vomiting, diarrhea, hemolytic anemia, positive Coombs test, leukopenia, thrombocytopenia, paresthesias, weakness, hypotension, bradycardia. *Monitoring:* Blood pressure, liver enzymes, Coombs test (direct).
Methylene Blue Urolene Blue. Injection: 10 mg/mL. Tablet: 65 mg.	**Antidote for cyanide poisoning and drug-induced methemoglobinemia (promotes conversion of methemoglobin to hemoglobin, combines with cyanide to form cyanmethemoglobin).** *Children and adults:* Methemoglobinemia: IV 1–2 mg/kg, may repeat after 1 hr if needed. NADPH-methemoglobin reductase deficiency: Oral 1–1.5 mg/kg/day (given with 5–8 mg/kg/day of ascorbic acid).	*Caution:* Avoid in G-6-PD deficiency and renal insufficiency. *Adverse events:* Urine and feces turn blue-green, anemia.
Methylphenidate Ritalin, Generic. Tablet: 5, 10, 20 mg. Tablet, sustained release: 20 mg.	**Attention deficit disorder, narcolepsy, adjunct for pain management (CNS stimulant).** *Children >5 yr:* 0.3–0.6 mg/kg/dose (max 2 mg/kg/day). *Adults:* 10 mg 2–3 times/day (max 60 mg/day).	*Cautions:* Avoid in patients with motor tics, Tourette syndrome, or marked agitation or psychosis. May become addictive if used in high doses at frequent intervals. *Adverse events:* Nervousness, insomnia, agitation, anorexia, weight loss, tachycardia, hypertension, movement disorders, tics, growth retardation (controversial and minimal if real), addiction (not a concern with typical ADD dosing).
Methylprednisolone Solu-Medrol (injection) Depo-Medrol (injection, IM) Medrol (tablets), Generic. Topical ointment.	**Anti-inflammatory and immunosuppressant glucocorticoid used in allergic, inflammatory and neoplastic disorders, and acute spinal cord injury.** *Children:* Anti-inflammatory and immunosuppressant: Oral, IM, IV 0.5–2 mg/kg/day divide every 6–12 hr. Lupus nephritis: IV 30 mg/kg every other day for 6 doses. Acute spinal cord injury: 30 mg/kg over 15 min, followed in 45 min by continuous infusion of 5.4 mg/kg/hr for 23 hr. *Adults:* Oral 2–60 mg/day in 1–4 doses. IV 40–250 mg every 4–6 hr. IM 10–80 mg once daily.	*Caution:* Avoid if live virus vaccine given or TB or fungal infection present. *Adverse events:* Hypertension, edema, nervousness, agitation, psychosis, pseudomotor cerebri, headache, mood swing, delirium, euphoria, hyperglycemia, hypokalemia, alkalosis, HPA-axis (adrenal) suppression, Cushing syndrome, skin atrophy, bruising, hyperpigmentation, peptic ulcer disease, muscle weakness, bone loss, joint pain, growth retardation, cataracts, glaucoma, immunosuppression. *Comment:* See comparison of corticosteroids under *Hydrocortisone.*
Metoclopramide Reglan, Generic. Injection: 5 mg/mL. Tablet: 5, 10 mg. Oral solution: 10 mg/mL. Syrup: 5 mg/5 mL.	**Treatment of diabetic gastroparesis, gastroesophageal reflux, and nausea associated with chemotherapy and surgery (blocks dopamine receptors in chemoreceptor trigger zone, enhances GI motility and gastroduodenal sphincter tone).** *Neonates infants, and children:* Gastroesophageal reflux: IV, Oral 0.033–0.1 mg/kg/dose every 8 hr. *Children:* Postoperative antiemetic: IV 0.1–0.2 mg/kg/dose every 6–8 hr as needed. Chemotherapy antiemetic: Oral, IV 1–2 mg/kg/dose every 2–4 hr (pretreat with diphenhydramine to avoid extrapyramidal reactions). *Adults:* Antiemetic: Oral, IV 1–2 mg/kg/dose every 2–4 hr. Gastroesophageal reflux: Oral 10–15 mg 4 times/day. Renal dysfunction: decrease dose.	*Cautions:* May precipitate seizures, acute dystonic reactions, and worsen asthma (if sulfite-containing formulation). In elderly chronic use associated with increased risk and earlier onset Parkinson disease (pediatric studies lacking). *Adverse events:* Weakness, drowsiness, diarrhea, prolactin stimulation, breast tenderness, extrapyramidal reactions, IV administration is associated with an intense feeling of anxiety and restlessness followed by drowsiness. *Comment:* Administer oral doses 30 min before meals and at bedtime. *Monitoring:* Creatinine clearance: CrCl 40–50 mL/min: give 75% of recommended dose; CrCl <40 mL/min: give 50% of recommended dose; CrCl <10 mL/min: give 25% of recommended dose.
Metolazone Zaroxolyn, Mykrox. Tablet.	**Treatment of fluid overload states (diuresis, inhibits sodium reabsorption at distal tubules).** *Children:* 0.2–0.4 mg/kg/day in 1–2 doses. *Adults:* 2.5–20 mg/day.	*Adverse events:* Fluid and electrolyte imbalance, hyperglycemia, hypocalcemia, hypomagnesemia, nausea, vomiting, blood dyscrasias.

Table continued on following page

TABLE 728–1 General Medications *Continued*

Drug (Trade Names, Formulations)	Indications (Mechanism of Action) and Dosing	Comments (Cautions, Adverse Events, Monitoring)
Metoprolol Lopressor. Injection: 1 mg/mL. Tablet: 50, 100 mg.	**Treatment of hypertension, tachyarrhythmias, IHSS, migraine prophylaxis (selective blocker of beta-1 receptors).** *Children:* Oral 1–5 mg/kg/day. *Adults:* Oral 100–450 mg/day in 2–3 doses; IV 5 mg every 2 min for 3 doses.	*Adverse events:* Mental depression, tiredness, weakness, bradycardia, reduced peripheral circulation, worsen diabetes, worsen asthma, insomnia, nightmares.
Mexilitene Mexitil, Generic. Capsule: 150, 200, 250 mg. Extemporaneous formulation.	**Treatment of ventricular arrhythmias, neuropathic pain (class 1B antiarrhythmic).** *Children:* 1.4–5 mg/kg/dose every 8 hr. *Adults:* 200 mg every 8 hr (max 1200 mg/day). Renal dysfunction: CrCl <10 mL/min: give 50% of dose.	*Adverse events:* Atrial and ventricular arrhythmias, bradycardia, hypotension, confusion, dizziness, nervousness, tremor, ataxia, numbness of fingers or toes, weakness, blurred vision, tinnitus, increased liver enzymes, GI discomfort. *Monitoring:* Mexilitene concentrations: therapeutic 0.5–2 μg/mL, toxic >2 μg/mL.
Midazolam Versed. Injection: 1 mg/mL, 5 mg/mL. Extemporaneous formulation.	**Sedation, anticonvulsant (benzodiazepine, increase GABA effect).** *Neonates:* IV continuous infusion 0.15–0.5 μg/kg/min for sedation; IV bolus 0.05–0.15 mg/kg every 2–4 hr. *Infants and children:* Status epilepticus: IV load 0.15 mg/kg followed by continuous infusion 1 μg/kg/min. Sedation: IV 0.05–0.2 mg/kg load, then either same dose every 1–2 hr or continuous infusion 1–2 μg/kg/min. Intranasal: 2.5 mg (0.5 mL) in each naris (total 5 mg) using 5 mg/mL injection. *>12 yr:* 0.5 mg every 3–4 min to effect. *Adults:* 0.5–2 mg every 2 min to effect (usually 2–5 mg).	*Adverse events:* Several cases of myoclonus and prolonged movement disorders have been noted in neonates treated with midazolam, withdrawal reactions may occur if abrupt discontinuation, sedation, amnesia, paradoxical excitation, blurred vision, diplopia, nasal burning, apnea, respiratory depression.
Mitomycin Mutamycin. Injection.	**Cancer chemotherapy (antibiotic type alkylating agent inhibits DNA and RNA synthesis).** *Children and adults:* Depends on protocol; typically IV 3 mg/m²/day for 5 days every 4–6 wk; up to 40–50 mg/m² single dose for BMT.	*Adverse events:* Nausea, vomiting, myelosuppression (onset 21 days, nadir 36 days, recovery 42–56 days), tingling of extremities, paresthesias, alopecia, fingernail discoloration, mouth ulcers, cardiac failure (doses >30 mg), interstitial pneumonitis, pulmonary fibrosis.
Mitoxantrone, DHAD Novantrone. Injection.	**Cancer chemotherapy (Anthracyclin analog inhibits DNA and RNA synthesis throughout entire cell cycle).** ANLL leukemias: *Children <2 yr:* 0.4 mg/kg once daily for 3–5 days. *Children >2 yr and adults:* 8–12 mg/m²/day for 5 days. Solid tumors: *Children:* 18–20 mg/m² every 3–4 wk or 5–8 mg/m² weekly. *Adults:* 12–14 mg/m² every 3–4 wk (max total 80–120 mg/m²).	*Adverse events:* Cardiotoxicity (less than other anthracyclines), seizures, headache, fever, elevated liver enzymes, renal failure, conjunctivitis, myelosuppression (onset 7–10 days, nadir 14 days, recovery 21 days).
Molindone Hydrochloride Moban. Tablet: 5, 10, 25, 50, 100 mg. Oral concentrate: 20 mg/mL.	**Management of psychotic disorder (actions similar to chlorpromazine but more extrapyramidal effects and less sedation).** *Children:* *3–5 yr:* 1–2.5 mg/kg/day in 4 doses. *5–12 yr:* 0.5–1 mg/kg/day in 4 doses. *Adults:* 50–225 mg/day.	*Adverse events:* Extrapyramidal effects, akathesia, dyskinesias, constipation, blurred vision, orthostatic hypotension, seizures, neuroleptic malignant syndrome, dry mouth, weight gain, galactorrhea, urinary retention, agranulocytosis, leukopenia, retinal pigmentation.
Montlukast Singulair. Tablet: 5, 10 mg.	**Prophylaxis and chronic treatment of asthma (leukotriene receptor blocker for LTD4).** *Children: 6–14 yr:* 5 mg once daily in the evening. *>15 yr and adults:* 10 mg once daily in the evening.	*Adverse events:* Headache, dizziness, dyspepsia, fatigue, elevated liver enzymes.
Morphine Generic. Injection, oral solution, suppository. Tablet, sustained-release (SR). Tablet, controlled-release (CR). Tablet.	**Relief of moderate to severe pain (narcotic analgesic).** *Neonates:* IV, IM, SC. Analgesia: 0.05–0.2 mg/kg/dose every 2–4 hr; continuous infusion 0.025–0.05 mg/kg/hr. *Infants and children:* IV, IM, SC 0.1–0.2 mg/kg/dose every 2–4 hr, Oral 0.2–0.5 mg/kg/dose every 4–6 hr. *Adolescents >12 yr:* IV 3–4 mg, may repeat in 5 min if needed. *Adults:* Oral 10–30 mg every 4 hr or CR tablet 15–30 mg every 8–12 hr. IV, IM, SC 2.5–20 mg/dose every 2–6 hr as needed or continuous infusion 0.8–10 mg/hr.	*Cautions:* May develop physical dependence after >5–7 days continuous use; if so, taper dose. Some preparations contain sulfites. *Adverse events:* Hypotension, bradycardia, nausea, vomiting, constipation, sedation, confusion, decreased urination, respiratory depression.
Mupirocin Bactroban. Ointment: 2%.	**Topical treatment of impetigo and other gram-positive skin infections (inhibit bacterial protein and RNA synthesis).**	*Adverse events:* Stinging and irritation at application site.

TABLE 728–1 General Medications *Continued*

Drug (Trade Names, Formulations)	Indications (Mechanism of Action) and Dosing	Comments (Cautions, Adverse Events, Monitoring)
Mupirocin *Continued*	*Children and adults:* Apply to affected area 4–5 times daily. Intranasal (eliminate nasal carriage of *S. aureus*): apply small amount 2–4 times/day for 5–14 days.	
Muromonab-CD3, OKT3 Orthocolone OKT3. Injection: 5 mg/5 mL.	**Treatment of acute allograft rejection in renal transplant patients (coats circulating T lymphocytes facilitating their opsonization by the reticuloendothelial system, and promotes removal of all CD3 molecules from T lymphocyte antigen receptor complex).** *Children <12 yr:* 0.1 mg/kg once daily for 10–14 days, or if <30 kg give 2.5 mg once daily for 10–14 days. *>12 yr and adults:* 5 mg/day for 10–14 days.	*Cautions:* Severe first-dose reactions may occur; recommend methylprednisolone 1 mg/kg IV 2–6 hr prior to first OKT3 dose and hydrocortisone 100 mg IV 30 min after each OKT3 dose and as needed. *Adverse events:* Shortness of breath, pulmonary edema, fever, chills, trembling, nausea, vomiting, diarrhea, headache, stiff neck, photophobia, flu-like symptoms. *Monitoring:* OKT3 serum trough levels (if maintained near 1 μg/mL then CD3 counts remain low).
Mycophenolate Mofetil CellCept. Capsule: 250 mg.	**Prevent rejection of allographic transplants, used in conjunction with other drugs (active metabolite MPA inhibits T- and B-cell proliferation, T-cell generation, and antibody secretion).** *Children:* 600 mg/m²/dose twice daily. *Adults:* 1,000 mg/dose twice daily.	*Adverse events:* Hypertension, insomnia, dizziness, fever, headache, bone marrow suppression, tremor, back pain, myalgia, dyspnea, cough, pharyngitis, hematuria, renal tubular necrosis, lymphoproliferative disease.
Nadolol Corgard. Tablet: 20, 40, 80, 120, 160 mg.	**Antiarrhythmic, antihypertensive, and migraine prophylaxis: (nonselective beta-adrenergic receptor antagonist).** *Child:* 0.1–1 mg/kg PO qd for SVT. *Adult:* 40 mg qd titrate upward to desired effect (usual dose 40–80 mg/day up to 640 mg/day).	*Cautions:* Should not be used in patients with asthma, bronchoconstriction or uncontrolled heart failure. Adjust dose with renal dysfunction (CrCl <50 mL/min). *Adverse effects:* Bradycardia, heart failure, bronchospasm. *Drug interactions:* Other hypotensive drugs, diuretics. Antagonizes beta-sympathomimetic drugs (e.g., albuterol).
Nalbuphine Nubain. IV, IM, SQ: 10 mg/mL.	**Analgesic (opiate agonist with partial opiate antagonistic activity for treatment of moderate to severe pain.)** *Children ≥1 yr:* 0.1–0.2 mg/kg IV, IM, SC, q3–4h. Max single dose 20 mg; max daily dose 160 mg.	*Cautions:* Like most opiate analgesics may stimulate histamine release, cause CNS and respiratory depression. Use with caution in hepatic disease or with other respiratory depressants. Dependence potential. *Adverse effects:* Hypotension, sedation, respiratory depression. Naloxone reverses effects.
Naloxone Narcan, Generic. Injection: 0.4 mg/mL. Injection neonate: 0.02 mg/mL.	**Opiate antagonist: antagonizes all opiate receptors—used in the treatment of opiate excess (overdose, poisoning).** *Neonate/child:* 0.1 mg/kg IV max dose 2 mg. If no response repeat every 2–3 min until desired effect. May give by continuous IV infusion.	*Cautions:* May precipitate acute opiate withdrawal. Duration of effect of many opiates may be longer than naloxone requiring individualized naloxone dosing. Administer via IV push.
Naproxen Aleve, Anaprox, Naprosyn, Generic. Tablet: 220, 250, 275, 375, 550 mg. Suspension: 125 mg/5 mL.	**Nonsteroidal anti-inflammatory drug for the treatment of mild to moderate pain, inflammation, fever (inhibits prostaglandin synthesis).** *Neonates:* Do not use owing to probably negative effects on renal function. *Child:* 5–7 mg/kg PO q8–12 h. *Adult:* 250–375 mg PO q8–12h: max dose 1250 mg/day.	*Cautions:* Gastrointestinal upset/irritation, reversible interference with platelet aggregation. Do not administer to infants <3 mo of age. *Adverse effects:* Dizziness, GI irritation, rash, age-related decreased renal function.
Nedocromil Tilade. Aerosol: 1.75 mg/activation.	**Chronic treatment of asthma/allergic disorders. Mast cell stabilizer (also stabilizes other cells to mediator release—neutrophils, eosinophils, platelets), nonsteroid.** *Child/adult:* 1–2 puffs 2–4 times/day. Dose titrated to clinical response.	*Cautions:* Only effective as chronic therapy. Produces no bronchodilatation. *Adverse effects:* Dysphonia, chest irritation/pain.
Neostigmine Prostigmin, Generic. Tablet: 15 mg (as bromide). Injection: 0.25, 0.5, 1 mg/mL (as methylsulfate).	**Treatment of myasthenia gravis, reversal of nondepolarizing neuromuscular blocking agents (NDNM). Competitively inhibits acetylcholine esterase augmenting effects of endogenous acetylcholine.** *Children:* 0.01–0.04 mg/kg IV, IM, SC q2–4h titrating dose to desired effect. To reverse NDNM 0.025–1 mg/kg/dose (max adult dose 5 mg).	*Cautions:* Patients with asthma/bronchospasm, bradycardia. Does not antagonize succinylcholine. *Adverse effects:* Bradycardia, abdominal cramps, urinary frequency.
Niacin Nicobid, Generic. Tablet: 25, 50, 100, 250, 500 mg. Tablet, timed-release: 150, 250, 500, 750 mg. Capsule, timed-release: 125, 250, 300, 400, 500 mg. Elixir: 50 mg/5 mL. Injection: 100 mg/mL.	**Vitamin supplementation (vitamin B3), hyperlipidemia, vasodilator.** *Children:* IV, IM, SC, PO titrated to desired effect (max 10 mg/kg/day).	*Cautions:* Titrate dose upward and administer IV slowly to avoid/minimize flushing. *Adverse effects:* Flushing, tachycardia, dizziness, hyperuricemia. *Drug interactions:* Augments hypotensive effects of antihypertensives.

Table continued on following page

TABLE 728–1 General Medications *Continued*

Drug (Trade Names, Formulations)	Indications (Mechanism of Action) and Dosing	Comments (Cautions, Adverse Events, Monitoring)
Nifedipine Adalat, Procardia, Generic. Capsule (liquid filled): 10, 20 mg. Tablet, timed-release: 30, 60, 90 mg. Capsule, timed-release: 30, 60, 90 mg.	**Antihypertensive, antiarrhythmic calcium channel antagonist.** *Infant/child:* Hypertensive emergency 0.25–0.5 mg/kg/dose PO/SL q4–6h (max 10 mg). Hypertropic cardiomyopathy: 0.2–0.3 mg/kg PO q8h. *Adult:* 10 mg/dose titrated to effect (max 120–180 mg/day).	*Caution:* Do not crush or break time-release tablet. *Adverse effects:* Profound, acute hypotension, flushing, dizziness. More rapid effect if drug is administered without food. Concurrent grapefruit juice may increase bioavailability and effects. *Drug interactions:* Cimetidine, cyclosporine, phenytoin, possibly digoxin. *Comment:* Preferred route is oral, not SL. Clinical effects due to swallowing. Capsule content approximates 10 mg in 0.34 mL and 20 mg in 0.45 mL.
Nitroprusside Nipride, Generic. Injection: 10 mg/mL, 25 mg/mL.	**Antihypertensive, congestive heart failure: controlled, titratable blood pressure control.** *Children and adults:* 0.3–0.5 μg/kg/min titrating dose to desired effect: rarely requires >6 μg/kg/min; (probable max 8 μg/kg/min).	*Cautions:* Metabolized to thiocyanate/cyanide, which accumulates in renal dysfunction. *Adverse effects:* Profound hypotension, tachycardia, thyroid suppression, acidosis, seizures. Cyanide toxicity—metabolic acidosis, pink skin methemaglobinemia. Administer by continuous IV infusion. Protect solution from direct light. Thiosulfate coadministration prevents toxicity (10 mg thiosulfate for each 1 mg nitroprusside).
Norepinephrine Bitartrate Levophed. Injection: 1 mg/mL base.	**Hypotension/shock. Sympathomimetic/adrenergic agonist.** *Children:* 0.05–0.1 μg/kg/min titrating dose to desired effect (max dose 2 μg/kg/min).	*Cautions:* Extravasation may cause severe tissue necrosis, administer into large vein. Ensure patient fluid status. May cause profound vasoconstriction. *Adverse effects:* Hypertension, cardiac arrhythmias, headache. Administer by continuous IV infusion. Drug dose based on norepinephrine base.
Nortriptyline Aventyl, Pamelor, Generic. Capsule: 10, 25, 50, 75 mg. Solution: 10 mg/5 mL.	**Tricyclic antidepressant, nocturnal enuresis: central synaptic norepinephrine/serotonin reuptake inhibitor.** *Children:* Nocturnal enuresis: 10–20 mg/day titrate upward to max 40 mg/day. Depression: 1–3 mg/kg PO q day (bedtime) titrated to effect. May give in divided doses q6h. Usual max dose 150 mg/day.	*Cautions:* Avoid in patients with cardiac conduction abnormalities, cardiac disease. Slow dose adjustment in patients with hepatic dysfunction. *Adverse effects:* Anticholinergic effects (dry mouth, tachycardia, blurred vision, urinary retention), sedation. *Drug interactions:* Clonidine, MAO inhibitors.
Octrotide Sandostatin. Injection: 0.05, 0.1, 0.2, 0.5, 1 mg/mL.	**Antisecretory somatostatin analog.** *Children:* Secretory diarrhea: 1–10 μg/kg IV, SC q12h titrating dose to effect. May give via continuous IV infusion. *Adults* for treatment of vasoactive intestinal peptide secreting tumors: 100–150 μg IV, SC q12h.	*Cautions:* Continuous long-term use (months) may cause cholelithiasis, hypothyroidism. *Adverse effects:* Flushing, dizziness, hypo/hyper-glycemia. Infuse IV over 20–30 min, IV push over 3 min.
Olsalazine Dipentum. Capsule: 10, 20, 250 mg.	**Inflammatory bowel disease, anti-inflammatory drug, 5-aminosalicylic acid derivative.** *Adults:* 500 mg q12h.	*Cautions:* Administer with food. *Adverse effects:* Headache, cramps, diarrhea, dizziness, rash, cholestasis.
Omeprazole Prilosec. Capsule: 10, 20 mg.	**Gastric acid hypersecretion/ulcer disease. Proton pump inhibitor of parietal cell hydrogen ion secretion.** *Child:* 0.6–0.7 mg/kg PO qd. Dose titrated to desired gastric pH. *Adult:* usual 20–40 mg/day PO qd.	*Caution:* Drug granules in capsule must be swallowed whole; do not chew. *Drug interactions:* May decrease diazepam, phenytoin clearance. May reduce traconazole, digoxin absorption.
Ondansetron Ondansetron. Tablet: 4, 8 mg. Injection: 2 mg/mL.	**Antiemetic. Treatment of nausea/vomiting associated with cancer chemotherapy/surgery other causes (drug toxicity). Selective serotonin-3 receptor antagonist.** *Infant/child:* 0.15 mg/kg IV q8h; may give as continuous IV infusion 0.45 mg/kg/day (max 24–32 mg/day). Child oral dose for mild to moderate nausea/vomiting; 4–8 mg q8–12h).	*Adverse effects:* Headache, chest pain. Does not cause dystonia/sedation. *Comment:* Oral bioavailability ~50%. Doses given ~30 min before starting chemotherapy.
Oxybutynin Ditropan, Generic. Tablet: 5 mg. Syrup: 5 mg/5 mL.	**Urinary antispasmotic. Relaxes smooth muscle by antagonizing acetylcoline.** *Child:* 0.2 mg/kg PO q6–12h (max 5 mg PO q8h). *Adult:* 5 mg per dose up to 4 times daily.	*Cautions:* Patients with renal and/or liver disease. *Adverse effects:* Tachycardia, drowsiness, sedation, dry mouth, blurred vision. *Drug interactions:* Additive anticholinergic effects/CNS depression, e.g., antihistamines.
Oxycodone (Various brands, generic). Tablet: 5 mg.	**Analgesic. Opiate analgesic for the treatment of moderate to severe pain.** *Children:* 0.05–0.15 mg/kg PO q4–6h (max 5 mg). *Adult:* 5 mg per dose PO q4–6h (max 5 mg.)	*Cautions:* Like most opiate analgesics may stimulate histamine release, cause CNS and respiratory depression. Use with caution in hepatic disease or with other respiratory depressants. Dependence potential. *Adverse effects:* Hypotension, sedation, respiratory depression. Naloxone reverses effects.

TABLE 728–1 General Medications *Continued*

Drug (Trade Names, Formulations)	Indications (Mechanism of Action) and Dosing	Comments (Cautions, Adverse Events, Monitoring)
Pamidronate Disodium Aredia. Injection: 30 mg, 60 mg, 90 mg.	**Treatment of hypercalcemia, Paget disease. Bisphosphonate derivative binds to bone inhibiting osteoclast-mediated calcium resorption. Dose based on serum calcium concentration.** *Adult:* Serum calcium 12–13.5 mg/dL: 60–90 mg; Serum calcium >13.5 mg/dL: 90 mg. Wait 7 days to assess full effect of dose before retreatment. Paget disease: 30 mg daily for 3 consecutive days.	*Cautions:* Leukopenia, thrombophlebitis. Drug incompatible with calcium containing IV solutions. *Adverse effects:* Hypertension, syncope, hypocalcemia, hypophosphatemia, hypothyroidism, bone pain.
Pancreatin Various brands. Capsule, tablet, timed-release capsule, powder.	**Pancreatic enzyme replacement. Individual products contain different amounts of lipase, amylase, and protease.** *Children and adults:* Dose titrated to desirable stool frequency and consistency.	*Cautions:* Excessive dosing may lead to impaction; inadequate dosing steratarhea. Exogenous pancreatic enzymes inactivated by gastric acid-use microencapsulated forms when possible. *Drug interactions:* Reduction of gastric acid (e.g., H2 receptor antagonists/omeprazol/antacids) may enhance effectiveness. *Adverse effects:* Rash, abdominal complaints, constipation, hyperuricemia, allergy.
Pancuronium Pavulon, Generic. Injection: 1 mg/mL, 2 mg/mL.	**Anesthetic/skeletal muscle relaxant. Nondepolarizing neuromuscular antagonist.** *Children and adults:* 0.04–0.1 mg/kg IV q20–30 min. Dose titrated to desired effects.	*Cautions:* Ventilation must be supported during neuromuscular blockade. Dose adjustment with renal dysfunction. *Adverse effects:* Tachycardia, hypertension, prolonged muscle weakness. *Drug interactions:* Possible augmented muscle weakness with: aminoglycosides, anesthetics, colistin.
Papaverine Hydrochloride Cerespan, Pavabid, Generic. Capsule: 150 mg. Tablet, time-released. Injection.	**Vasodilator, antimigraine. Generalized smooth muscle relaxant. Common pediatric use for preservation of arterial catheters to prolong function.** *Children:* 30 mg papaverine plus 250 units heparin per 250 mL IV solution (0.45–0.9% NaCl) infused.	*Cautions:* Avoid in neonates as may cause cerebral vasodilitation predisposing to CNS bleed. *Adverse effects:* Flushing, tachycardia, hypotension, dizziness. *Drug interactions:* Additive hypotensive effect.
Paraldehyde Paral, Generic. Liquid: 1 g/mL.	**Anticonvulsant, sedative. Generalized CNS depressant used as adjunct treatment for refractory status epilepticus, alcohol withdrawal.** *Children:* 0.15 mL/kg/dose PO, PR. May repeat once in 4–6 hr. IM formulation not available in USA. *Adults:* 5–10 mL per dose.	*Cautions:* May give IM but inject remote from nerves due to risk of damage. Use glass syringe/ tubing as drug reacts with plastic. Rectal route preferred to IM. Mix rectal solution 2:1 in oil (e.g., olive oil). *Adverse effects:* Sedation, gastric irritation, thrombophlebitis.
Paregoric Generic. Liquid: 2 mg morphine equivalent per 5 mL.	**Antidiarrheal, analgesic. Camphorated tincture of opium.** *Children:* 0.25–0.5 mL/kg PO q6–12h. *Adults:* 5–10 mL PO q6–12h. Neonatal abstinence syndrome: dose titrated to desired effect.	*Comments:* Each 5 mL of paregoric contains 2 mg morphine equivalent, 20 mg camphor, 20 mg benzoic acid. Final alcohol content 45%.
Pegaspargase Oncaspar. Injection.	**Antineoplastic agent used in combination for induction of acute lymphoblastic leukemia. Also called PEG-L-asparaginase.** *Children and adult:* IM, IV 2,500 units/m² every 14 days. Dose usually dictated by specific protocol.	*Cautions:* Hepatotoxic, allergic reactions. Contraindicated in patients with pancreatitis, significantly hemorhagic events associated with L-asparaginase. *Drug interactions:* Possible interactions with methotrexate, vincristine, corticosteroids.
Pemoline Cylert. Tablet: 18.75, 37.5, 75 mg. Tablet, chewable: 37.5 mg.	**Central nervous system stimulant used in the treatment of attention deficit disorder. Structurally unique from methylphenidate.** *Children:* 1 mg/kg/24 hr PO as single dose each morning. Titrate to effect 0.5 mg/kg/24 hours at every 1–2 wk. Usual max dose 3 mg/kg/day (~112.5 mg/day).	*Cautions:* Insomnia, anorexia, weight loss. *Adverse effects:* Central nervous system stimulation, seizures, hypertension, increased liver function studies, hepatitis, movement disorders. *Drug interactions:* Possible with other central nervous system stimulants, sympathomimetics.
Penicillamine Cuprimine, Depen. Capsule: 125 mg, 250 mg. Tablet: 250 mg.	**Metal chelating agent with affinity for copper (Wilson disease) and lead. Also used as an adjunct for the treatment of severe rheumatoid arthritis.** **Wilson disease:** Dose titrated to maintain >1 mg/ day urinary copper excretion. *Infant/child:* 20 mg/kg/day PO q6–12h (max 1 g/ day). *Adult:* 1 g/day PO q6–12h (max 2 g). **Lead intoxication** *Infant/child:* 30–40 mg/kg/day PO q8–12h (max 1.5 g/day). *Adult:* 1–1.5 g/day PO q8–12h. **Rheumatoid arthritis** *Children:* 3 mg/kg/day PO q12 hr, increasing by 3 mg/kg/day every 2–3 mo to max 10 mg/kg/day.	*Cautions:* Cross allergen in patients allergic to penicillin. Do not administer with food or iron/ zinc compounds. *Adverse effects:* Rash, pruritis, nausea, vomiting, anemia, bone marrow suppression, nephrotic syndrome, SLE-like syndrome. *Drug interactions:* Other metals, iron, gold, mercury, antimalarials.

Table continued on following page

TABLE 728–1 General Medications *Continued*

Drug (Trade Names, Formulations)	Indications (Mechanism of Action) and Dosing	Comments (Cautions, Adverse Events, Monitoring)
Pentazocine Talwin. Tablet: 50 mg with 50 mg naloxone (parenteral deterrent). Injection: 30 mg/mL.	**Opiate analgesic of the benzomorphan type for the treatment of moderate to severe pain.** *Children >14 yr of age and adults:* 50 mg PO q3–4h, titrate to effect to 100 mg dose not to exceed 600 mg/day. May give IM or IV reducing oral dose by one third.	*Cautions:* Generalized CNS depressant, possesses weak antagonistic action and may precipitate opiate withdrawal. *Adverse effects:* CNS depression, nausea, vomiting, respiratory depression, histamine release.
Pentobarbital Nembutal, Generic. Capsule 50 mg, 100 mg. Elixer: 18.2 mg/5 mL. Suppository: 30 mg, 60 mg, 120 mg, 200 mg. Injection.	**Short-acting barbiturate used as an anticonvulsant, sedative/hypnotic, anesthetic.** **Sedation** *Children:* 2–6 mg/kg/24 hr PO, IM q6h. May give rectally dosed by body weight: 4.5–10 kg 30 mg; 10–18 kg 30–60 mg; 18–36 kg 60 mg; 36–50 kg 60–120 mg. **Pentobarbital coma** *Children:* Loading dose 10–15 mg/kg IV slowly over 1–2 hr monitoring blood pressure and heart rate. Maintenance infusion 1 mg/kg/hr increasing up to 5 mg/kg/hr to maintain burst suppression on EEG.	*Cautions:* Hypotension in hypovolemic patients; injectables contain propylene glycol. *Adverse effects:* Arrhythmias, bradycardia, hypotension, respiratory depression, laryngospasm, dependence. *Drug interactions:* May increase metabolism of many hepatically cleared drugs; oral contraceptives, griseofulvin, corticosteroids. *Monitoring:* Pentobarbital concentrations: sedation 1–5 μg/mL; coma 20–40 μg/mL.
Pentoxifylline Trental. Tablet, timed-release: 400 mg.	**Used in the treatment of peripheral vascular disease (Raynaud syndrome) and investigationally reducing tumor necrosis factor, neutrophil adhesion and platelet aggregation.** *Children:* Antiplatelet effect in Kawasaki disease: 20 mg/kg/24 hr PO q8h. *Adults:* 400 mg PO three times daily.	*Cautions:* Administer with meals to reduce GI upset. *Adverse effects:* Hypotension, tachycardia, dizziness, nausea, vomiting. *Drug interactions:* Cimetidine, possible augmenting of warfarin, heparin effects.
Phenazopyridine Pyridium, Generic. Tablet: 100 mg, 200 mg.	**Urinary anesthetic for possible symptomatic relief of urinary burning, itching associated with urologic procedures or urinary tract infection.** *Children:* 12 mg/kg/24 hr PO q8h. *Adults:* 100–200 mg PO q6–8h.	*Caution:* Discolors urine to orange or red. *Adverse effects:* Headache, rash, methemoglobinemia. Administer with food to decrease GI side effects.
Phenobarbital Generic. Elixir: 15 mg/5 mL; 20 mg/5 mL. Tablet: 8 mg, 15 mg, 30 mg, 60 mg, 100 mg. Injection: 30 mg/mL, 60 mg/mL, 130 mg/mL.	**Barbiturate central nervous system depressant used as a sedative, hypnotic anticonvulsant, anesthetic.** **Anticonvulsant: loading dose** *Children and adults:* 15–20 mg/kg PO, IV. **Maintenance Dose** *Neonates:* 3–4 mg/kg/24 hr PO, IV, q12–24h. *Children:* 5–6 mg/kg/24 hr PO, IV, q12–24h. *Adult:* 1–3 mg/kg/24 hr PO, IV, q12–24h. **Sedation** *Children:* 2 mg/kg per dose. **Hyperbilirubinemia** *Children:* 3–8 mg/kg/24 hr PO, IV q12–24 h. *Adult:* 90–180 mg/24 hr PO, IV q12–24h.	*Cautions:* Dose titrated to desired effect. Administer IV ≤30 mg/min in infants and children and ≤60 mg/min in adults. *Adverse effects:* Hypotension, drowsiness, respiratory depression, paradoxical hyperactivity. *Drug interactions:* May increase metabolism of many hepatically cleared drugs; oral contraceptives, griseofulvin, corticosteroids. Certain drugs may interfere with phenobarbital metabolism—valproic acid, chloramphenicol, felbamate. *Target serum concentrations:* 15–40 μg/mL; coma (acute) > 60 μg/mL. *Monitoring:* Phenobarbital concentrations: sedation 15–40 μg/mL; coma >60 μg/mL.
Phenoxybenzamine Dibenzyline. Capsule: 10 mg.	**Alpha-adrenergic receptor antagonist used for symptomatic treatment of pheochromocytoma.** *Children:* 0.2–2 mg/kg/24 hr PO qd. Titrate dose to desired effect (e.g., blood pressure). *Adult:* 10 mg per dose PO q12h titrate dose to effect.	*Cautions:* Long-acting alpha-receptor antagonist. *Adverse effects:* Postural hypotension, syncope, dizziness. *Drug interactions:* Sympathomimetics.
Phentolamine Regitine. Injection: 5 mg/mL	**Alpha-adrenergic antagonist used in the diagnosis/treatment of pheochromocytoma and for extravassation of drugs with alpha-adrenergic effects (e.g., dopamine, dobutamine, epinephrine, norepinephrine, phenylephrine).** **Pheochromocytoma** Diagnosis: *Child:* 0.05–0.1 mg/kg/dose; usual max dose 5 mg. *Adult:* 5 mg per dose. Preoperatively: *Children:* 0.05–0.1 mg/kg/dose every 1–2 hr titrating to effect and needed duration. Usual max dose 5 mg. **Extravasation** 5–10 mg in 10 mL 0.95 normal saline—infiltrate area with small volume using 27–30 gauge needle not to exceed total dose of 0.1 mg/kg.	*Cautions:* Short-acting alpha-receptor antagonist. *Adverse effects:* Hypotension, dizziness, gastritis. *Drug interactions:* Sympathomimetics.

TABLE 728–1 General Medications *Continued*

Drug (Trade Names, Formulations)	Indications (Mechanism of Action) and Dosing	Comments (Cautions, Adverse Events, Monitoring)
Phenylephrine Hydrochloride Neo-Synephrine, Generic. Injection: 10 mg/mL. Nasal drops/spray: 0.16–1%. Eye drops.	**Alpha-adrenergic receptor agonist, peripheral vasoconstrictor; used in treatment of hypotension in shock and in many nasal decongestants.** **Nasal decongestant** *Infants:* 1–2 drops per nare q3–4h 0.16% solution. *Children 1–6 yr:* 1–2 drops/spray per nare q3–4h 0.125% solution. *6–12 yr:* 1–2 drops/spray q3–4h 0.25% solution. *>12 yr/adult:* 1–2 drops/spray per nare q3–4h 0.25–0.5% solution. **Hypotension/shock** *Children:* 5–20 µg/kg per dose IV q10–15 min. May give by continuous IV infusion 0.1–0.5 µg/kg/min titrated to desired effects (e.g., blood pressure). *Adults:* 0.1–0.5 mg/dose q10–15 min continuous IV infusion 100–180 µg/min titrating to desired effect. **Paroxysmal supraventricular tachycardia** *Children:* 5–10 µg/kg IV over 20–30 sec. *Adults:* 0.25–0.5 mg IV over 20–30 sec.	*Cautions:* Patients with hypertension. Injection contains sulfites. Rebound nasal stuffiness with prolonged nasal use/abuse. *Adverse effects:* Hypertension, angina, bradycardia, restlessness, necrosis if IV infiltrates. *Drug interactions:* Sympathomimetics, alpha-receptor antagonists, MAO inhibitors.
Phenytoin Dilantin; Generic (use cautiously). Capsule, slow (extended) release: 30 mg, 100 mg. Capsule, prompt release: 30 mg, 100 mg. Suspension: 125 mg/5 mL. Injection: 50 mg/mL.	**Anticonvulsant and antiarrhythmic.** **Status epilepticus: loading dose** *Neonate:* 15–20 mg/kg IV; do not exceed 0.5 mg/kg/min. *Child/adult:* 15–18 mg/kg IV; do not exceed 1–3 mg/kg/min. **Maintenance dose** *Neonate:* 5 mg/kg/24 hr PO, IV q12–24h. *Children: 0.5–6 yr:* 8–10 mg/kg/24 hr *7–9 yr:* 6–8 mg/kg/24 hr PO, IV q12–24h *10–16 yr:* 6–7 mg/kg/24 hr PO, IV q12–24h. *Adult:* 300–600 mg/day q12–24h. **Arrhythmias: loading dose** *Child/adult:* 1.25 mg/kg IV q5 min until desired effect or total dose 15 mg/kg. **Maintenance dose** *Child:* 5–10 mg/kg/24 hr q8–12h. *Adult:* 250 mg per dose q6–8h.	*Cautions:* Infuse slowly IV; variable oral bioavailability; chewable tablet most consistent. Must shake oral suspension very well before use. Follows saturation (Michaelis-Menten) pharmacokinetics. Certain disease states (renal failure, acute head trauma) may lead to imbalance between free and protein-bound drug. *Adverse effects:* Lethargy, dizziness, nystagmus, hypotension, hirsutism, gingival hyperplasia, rash, Stevens-Johnson syndrome, hepatitis, thrombophlebitis. *Drug interactions:* May increase metabolism of certain hepatically cleared drugs; oral contraceptives, griseofulvin, corticosteroids, cyclosporin; highly protein bound and may cause displacement interaction. *Monitoring:* Phenytoin concentrations: therapeutic 8–20 µg/mL. If necessary, measure free drug concentration: therapeutic 1–2 µg/mL.
Physostigmine Antrilirium. Injection, ophthalmic solution, and ointment.	**Competitive antagonist of acetylcholine. Unlike neostigmine, crosses the blood brain barrier with central effects. Used with extreme caution in the reversal of anticholinergic effects.** *Children:* 0.001–0.03 mg/kg/dose IM, IV, SQ, repeated q15–20 min to desired effect (max total dose 2 mg). *Adults:* 0.5–2 mg IM, IV, SQ repeated q15–20 min until desired effect.	*Cautions:* Patients with bradycardia, cardiac dysrhthmias, asthma, ulcer disease. Should be used as an antidote only in life-threatening situations by experienced individuals. *Adverse effects:* Palpitations, restlessness, excessive salivation, secretions, muscle fasciculations, bronchospasm.
Phytonadione AquaMephyton, Mephyton. Tablet: 5 mg. Injection.	**Vitamin K_1 for nutritional supplementation and treatment of hemorrhagic disease of the newborn or from warfarin-like compound anticoagulant toxicity.** *Children:* 1–2 mg/dose IM, IV, SQ dosed to effect; PO dose may increase to 2.5 to 5 mg. *Adults:* 10 mg/24 hr IM, IV, SQ; 5–25 mg/24 hr PO. Higher doses may be required for reversal of warfarin-like anticoagulant toxicity.	*Cautions:* Infuse slowly IV (over 15–30 min) to avoid flushing. Multiple doses may be needed for prolonged period depending upon type of coumarin anticoagulant. *Adverse effects:* Flushing, hypotension.
Piroxicam Feldene. Capsules: 10 mg, 20 mg.	**Nonsteroidal anti-inflammatory agent used as an analgesic and in the treatment of rheumatoid disorders.** *Children:* 0.2–0.3 mg/kg q 24 hr PO (max dose 15 mg/kg/24 hr). *Adults:* 10–20 mg q 24 hr.	*Cautions:* Limited data in infants and children, may require more frequent daily dosing in pediatrics. Administer with food/milk to decrease GI side effects. Do not use in young infants. *Adverse effects:* Dizziness, GI upset, nausea/vomiting, ulcer, hepatitis, decreased renal function.
Polyethylene Glycol-Electrolyte Solution GoLytely, Colovage, Colyte. Powder for reconstitution.	**Bowel lavage solution used prior to bowel radiology or in poisonings.** *Children:* 25–40 mL/kg/hr up to 1.5–2 L/hr until rectal effulent clear; usual max dose 4 L for x-ray may go much higher if used for poisonings (e.g., iron). *Adults:* 2,400 mg q10–20 min until 4 L consumed. May go higher for poisonings.	*Caution:* In patients with bowel disease (colitis) or obstruction. *Adverse effects:* Nausea, cramps, bloating.

Table continued on following page

TABLE 728–1 General Medications *Continued*

Drug (Trade Names, Formulations)	Indications (Mechanism of Action) and Dosing	Comments (Cautions, Adverse Events, Monitoring)
Pralidoxime Protopam (2-PAM). Tablets: 500 mg. Injectable.	**Acetylcholinesterase reactivator used in the treatment of organophosphate poisoning; possible treatment of toxicity from cholinergic drugs.** *Children:* 20–50 mg/kg/dose IM, IV repeated in 1–2 hr if muscle weakness has not been relieved; when desired effect obtained dose q12h. *Adults:* 1–2 g IM, IV q5–6h dose based on clinical response.	*Caution:* As antidote for organophosphate poisoning, use in combination with atropine. Excessive dosing may cause cholinergic effects. Too-rapid IV administration associated with tachycardia, laryngospasm. Infuse IV over 15–30 min. *Adverse effects:* Hypertension, dizziness, nausea, muscle weakness/rigidity.
Prazosin Minipress, Generic. Capsule: 1 mg, 2 mg, 5 mg.	**Competitive antagonist of postsynaptic alpha-adrenergic receptors used in the treatment of hypertension/heart failure.** *Child:* 0.1 mg/kg/24 hr PO q6h titrating dose to desired blood pressure. Usual max dose 0.4 mg/kg/24 hr or 15 mg total dose. Consider additive/synergistic combinations with diuretics. *Adult:* 3 mg/24 hr PO q8–12h titrating dose to desired blood pressure. Usual dose range 3–15 mg/day.	*Caution:* Profound hypotension, may occur after first dose ("first-dose phenomenon") more common in fluid and/or salt depleted patients. *Adverse effects:* Syncope, palpitations, dizziness, fluid retention. *Drug interactions:* Other hypotensive drugs (diuretics, beta-receptor antagonists).
Prednisolone DeltaCortef, Hydeltrasol, Predalone, Generic. Tablet: 5 mg. Suspension. Injection.	**Glucocorticosteroid used in the treatment of inflammatory disorders including allergic, respiratory, rheumatic, endocrine, and neoplastic disorders.** **Asthma** *Children:* 0.5–4 mg/kg/24 hr PO, IV q6–12h. *Adult:* 5–60 mg/24 hr PO, IV. **Anti-inflammatory** *Children:* 0.1–2 mg/kg/24 hr PO, IV q6–q day.	*Cautions:* Dose titrated to desired effect; use shortest treatment course to avoid side effects. May slow growth, increase salt retention. *Adverse effects:* Edema, hypertension, psychosis, Cushing's syndrome. HPA-axis (adrenal) suppression, peptic ulcer. *Drug interactions:* Barbiturate, phenytoin, rifampin. *Comment:* See comparison of corticosteroids under *Hydrocortisone.*
Prednisone Deltasone, Liquid Pred, Generic. Tablet: 1 mg, 2.5 mg, 5 mg, 10 mg, 20 mg, 50 mg. Syrup: 5 mg/5 mL. Injection.	**Glucocorticosteroid used in the treatment of inflammatory disorders including allergic, respiratory, rheumatic, endocrine, and neoplastic disorders.** **Asthma** *Children:* 0.5–4 mg/kg/24 hr PO, IV q6–12h. *Adult:* 5–60 mg/24 hr PO, IV. **Anti-inflammatory** *Children:* 0.1–2 mg/kg/24 hr PO, IV q6–qd.	*Cautions:* Dose titrated to desired effect; use shortest treatment course to avoid side effects. May slow growth, increase salt retention. *Adverse effects:* Edema, hypertension, psychosis, Cushing syndrome. HPA-axis (adrenal) suppression, peptic ulcer. *Drug interactions:* Barbiturate, phenytoin, rifampin. *Comment:* See comparision of corticosteroids under *Hydrocortisone.*
Primidone Mysoline, Generic. Tablet: 50 mg, 250 mg. Suspension: 250 mg/5 mL.	**Anticonvulsant used in the treatment of generalized tonic-clonic, complex partial and focal seizures.** *Neonate:* 12–20 mg/kg/24 hr PO, q8–12h. *Children:* 10–25 mg/kg/24 hr PO q8–12h. *Children >8 yr and adults:* 125–1,500 mg/24 hr PO q8–12h (usual max 2 g/24 hr).	*Caution:* Partially metabolised to phenobarb and PEMA. *Adverse effects:* Sedation, ataxia, rash. *Drug interactions:* Valproate, griseofulvin, phenytoin. *Monitoring:* PEMA concentrations: therapeutic 5–12 μg/mL.
Procainamide Pronestyl, Procan. Tablet and capsule: 250 mg, 375 mg, 500 mg. Tablet, sustained-release: 250 mg, 500 mg, 750 mg, 1,000 mg. Injection.	**Class Ia antiarrhythmic; ventricular tachycardia, PVCs, PAT, atrial fibrillation.** **Loading dose** *Child:* 3–6 mg/kg/dose IV over 5 min not to exceed 100 mg/dose; repeat q5–10 min as needed to max 15 mg/kg total dose. Do not exceed 500 mg in 30 min. **Maintenance dose** *Child:* 15–50 mg/kg/24 hr PO q3–6h; 20–30 mg/kg/24 hr IM, IV; not to exceed 4 g/24 hr; continuous IV infusion 20–80 μg/kg/min, usual max 2 g/24 hr. *Adult:* 250–500 mg/dose q3–6h, max 2–4 g/24 hr.	*Caution:* Causes positive ANA, general cardiodepressant. Metabolized to active NAPA. *Adverse effects:* Hypotension, arrhythmias, A-V block, confusion, agranulocytosis, SLE-like syndrome, fever, rash. *Drug interactions:* Cimetadine, beta-antagonists, anticholinergic agents. *Monitoring:* Procainamide concentrations: therapeutic 4–10 μg/mL. Sum of procainamide and NAPA: therapeutic 10–30 μg/mL.
Procarbazine Capsule: 50 mg.	**Antineoplastic used in the treatment of Hodgkin lymphoma, bronchogenic carcinoma.** **Hodgkin disease** *Child:* 1.5–3 mg/kg/24 hr (50–100 mg/m^2) PO, qd for 10–14 days per 28-day cycle. **BMT preparation** 12.5 mg/kg/dose. **Neuroblastoma/medulloblastoma** *Child:* 100–200 mg/m^2/dose per protocol.	*Caution:* Dose based on disease-based protocol and concurrent drugs. Avoid (alcohol causes disulfiram-like reaction). Possesses some MAO inhibitory activity. *Adverse effects:* CNS depression, confusion, ataxia, marrow suppression, alopecia, flu-like syndrome. *Drug interactions:* Alcohol, tricyclic antidepressants, phenothiazines, tyramine-containing foods sympathomimetics.
Prochlorperazine Compazine, Generic Tablet: 5 mg, 10 mg, 25 mg. Capsule, sustained-release: 10 mg, 15 mg, 30 mg. Injection. Suppository: 2.5 mg, 5 mg, 25 mg. Syrup: 5 mg/5 mL.	**Piperazine-type phenothiazine antiemetic. Use should be avoided in children.** *Child:* 0.4 mg/kg/24 hr PO, rectal, q6–8h; 0.1–0.15 mg/kg/24 hr IM q8–12h. *Adult:* 5–10 mg/dose, PO 3–4 times daily.	*Caution:* Acute dystonic reaction common in children. *Adverse effects:* Sedation, extrapyramidal reactions, photosensitivity, cholestatic jaundice. *Drug interactions:* Additive CNS effects, alpha-receptor antagonists.

TABLE 728–1 General Medications *Continued*

Drug (Trade Names, Formulations)	Indications (Mechanism of Action) and Dosing	Comments (Cautions, Adverse Events, Monitoring)
Prometazine Phenregan; Generic. Tablet: 12.5 mg, 25 mg, 50 mg. Syrup. Suppository. Injection.	**Phenothiazine with primary antihistaminic activity used in the treatment of nausea, vomiting, motion sickness, allergy.** **Motion sickness** *Child:* 0.5 mg/kg PO, 30–60 min before departure; then q8–12h as needed. **Sedation-antiemetic** *Child:* 0.25–1 mg/kg/dose IM, IV, rectal, q4–6h as needed.	*Caution:* Potentiates anticholinergic effects. *Adverse effects:* Sedation, hypotension, extrapyramidal reactions, blurred vision. *Drug interactions:* Additive sedative effects.
Propantheline Bromide ProBanthine, Generic. Tablet: 7.5 mg, 15 mg.	**Synthetic anticholinergic antispasmodic used as adjunctive therapy of GI or bladder spasm, irritable bowel.** *Child:* 1.5–3 mg/kg/24 hr PO, q4–8h. Dose to desired effect.	*Caution:* Avoid in patients with decreased bowel motility. *Adverse effects:* Sedation, tachycardia, dry mouth, blurred vision, mydriasis.
Propofol Diprivan. Injection.	**Nonbarbiturate sedative, hypnotic, general anesthetic.** **Sedation** *Child:* 1.5–3 mg/kg/dose IV over 1–2 min. **Continuous sedation** (mechanical ventilation). *Children:* 5.5 mg/kg for 30 min; increase to 6 mg/kg for 30 min; increase to 8 mg/kg for 1 hr; increase to 10 mg/kg for 1 hr; increase to final infusion rate of 12.5 mg/kg/hr.	*Caution:* Dose titration regimen to permit adequate sedation accomodating drugs complex. Pharmacokinetics. Single-use vials in lipid emulsion. *Adverse effects:* Hypotension, bradycardia, hyperlipidemia, questionable metabolic acidosis.
Propoxyphene Darvon. Capsule. Tablet.	**Analgesic for mild to moderate pain. Binds opiate receptors. Less dependence liability than codeine.** *Child:* 2–3 mg/kg/24 hr PO q4–6h. Titrate dose to desired effect. *Adult:* Hydrochloride 65 mg/dose PO, q4–6h (max dose 390 mg); napsylate salt 100 mg PO, q4–6h (max dose 600 mg).	*Caution:* Weak opiate agonist with limited abuse potential. *Adverse effects:* Sedation, dizziness, nausea, vomiting, constipation, dependence.
Propranolol Inderal, Generic. Tablet: 10 mg, 20 mg, 40 mg, 60 mg, 80 mg. Solution: 4 mg/mL, 8 mg/mL and concentrate 80 mg/mL. Injection: 1 mg/mL. Sustained-release capsule: 60 mg, 80 mg, 120 mg, 160 mg.	**Nonselective beta-adrenergic receptor antagonist (beta-1 and beta-2).** *Neonate:* 0.25 mg/kg/dose PO q6–8h; titrate to desired response, increasing dose slowly; max dose 5 mg/kg/24 hr. IV dose: 0.01 mg/kg over 10–15 min titrate to desired effect; max dose 1 mg/kg/24 hr. **Arrhythmias/hypertension** *Children:* 0.5–1 mg/kg/24 hr PO q6–8h titrated upward to 2–5 (mg/kg/24 hr, over 3 5 days). *IV dose:* 0.01–0.1 mg/kg/dose infused over 10–15 min as needed (max dose 1 mg infants; 3 mg children). *Adult:* 40–80 mg/24 hr, titrating to response; range 40–320 mg/24 hr PO q6–8h. **Thyrotoxicosis** *Neonate:* 2 mg/kg/24 hr PO q6–8h; titrate to response. *Children:* 2–4 mg/kg/24 hr PO q6–8h; titrate to response. **Migraine prophylaxis** *Children:* 0.6–2 mg/kg/24 hr PO q6–8h; usual max 4 mg/kg/24 hr.	*Caution:* Drug undergoes substantial first-pass metabolism explaining huge difference between IV and PO doses. Use cautiously IV and in patients with CHF, asthma, COPD. Monitor heart rate for drug effect. *Adverse effects.* Decreased cardiac contractility, hypotension, bradycardia, hypoglycemia, bronchospasm.
Propylthiouracil (PTU) Generic. Tablet: 50 mg.	**Antithyroid that inhibits thyroid hormone synthesis by interfering with incorporation of iodine.** *Neonate:* 5–10 mg/kg/24 hr PO q8h titrate to effect. *Children:* 5–7 mg/kg/24 hr PO q8h titrate to effect. *Adult:* 300–450 mg/24 hr PO q8h increasing to 600–1,200 mg/24 hr.	*Caution:* Marked drug effect usually requires 24–36 hr. *Adverse effects:* Vertigo, skin rash, blood dyscrasias, hepatitis, arthralgia, interstitial pneumonitis.
Protamine Sulfate Generic. Injection: 10 mg/mL.	**Heparin antidote, neutralizing its anticoagulant effect.** 1 mg protamine neutralizes 90 USP units of lung-derived heparin and 115 USP units of intestinal-derived heparin. Protamine dose calculated on duration of time since last heparin dose using heparin elimination half-life (~1 hr) to determine estimated heparin body stores.	*Caution:* Calculate dose carefully as protamine excess can cause anticoagulation. Monitor PTT with use. *Adverse effects:* Hypotension, dyspnea, hypersensitivity.
Pseudoephedrine Generic. Tablet: 30 mg, 60 mg, time-release 120 mg. Capsule: 60 mg; timed-release: 120 mg. Syrup: 15 mg/mL.	**Indirectly acting sympathomimetic used as a nasal decongestant/symptoms of common cold** *Infant/child:* 4 mg/kg/24 hr PO, q6–12h. *Adult:* 60 mg/dose PO, q6–8h; max 240 mg/24 hr.	*Caution:* In patients with hypertension, heart disease. *Adverse effects:* Tachycardia, headache, nervousness, tremor. *Drug interactions:* MAO inhibitors, propranolol, pressors.

Table continued on following page

TABLE 728–1 General Medications *Continued*

Drug (Trade Names, Formulations)	Indications (Mechanism of Action) and Dosing	Comments (Cautions, Adverse Events, Monitoring)
Pyridostigmine Mestinon. Tablet: 60 mg; sustained-release 180 mg. Syrup: 60 mg/5 mL. Injection: 5 mg/mL.	**Cholinesterase inhibitor used in the treatment of myasthenia gravis; reversal of neuromuscular blocking agents.** **Myasthenia gravis** *Children:* 0.05–0.15 mg/kg/dose IM, IV; max dose 10 mg titrate to desired effect; PO dose 7 mg/kg/day in 5–6 divided doses. *Adult:* 2 mg IM, IV q2–3h; PO dose 60 mg per dose q8h; titrate dose to desired effect. **Reversal of neuromuscular blocking agents** *Children:* 0.1–0.25 mg/kg/dose IM, IV titrate to effect; may need to co-administer atropine/glycopyrrolate. *Adult:* 10–20 mg per dose with atropine/glycopyrrolate.	*Caution:* In patients with asthma, cardiac dysfunction/arrhythmias, peptic ulcer. *Adverse effects:* Bradycardia, A-V block, seizures, headache, diarrhea, abdominal cramping, salivation, urinary frequency, muscle weakness, miosis, lacramation, increased bronchial secretions.
Pyridoxine Nestrex, Generic. Tablets: 25 mg, 50 mg, 100 mg; sustained-release: 100 mg. Injection: 100 mg/mL.	**Vitamin B_6 used for dietary or drug-induced (e.g., INH, hydralazine) deficiency and B_6-dependent seizures.** **Pyridoxine-dependent seizures** *Children:* 50–100 mg PO, IM, IV; maintenance dose 50–100 mg/day. **Dietary deficiency** *Children:* 5–15 mg/day for 3–4 wk then 2.5–5 mg/day. *Adults:* 10–20 mg/day for 3–4 wk. **Drug-induced neuritis.** *Children:* 1 mg/kg/24 hr PO, IM, IV, q day. *Adult:* 100–200 mg/24 hr PO, IM, IV, q day.	*Caution:* May decrease serum phenobarbital and phenytoin concentrations. Large IV doses may precipitate seizures. *Adverse effects:* Nausea, decreased folic acid, increased liver funciton tests, nausea.
Quinidine Quinaglute, Quinidex, Generic. Tablet (sulfate): 200 mg, 300 mg, sustained-release: 300 mg Sustained-release gluconate: 324 mg. Injection, gluconate: 80 mg/mL.	**Myocardial depressent used in the treatment of arrhythmias—supraventricular tachycardia, paroxysmal ventricular tachycardia, premature atrial/ventricular contractions.** *Children:* 2 mg/kg PO, IM, IV test dose to exclude idiosyncrasy: 20–50 mg/kg/24 hr sulfate salt q4h PO; gluconate salt 2–10 mg/kg/dose q3–6h IV. *Adults:* 199–600 mg/dose sulfate salt q4–6h PO; 324–972 mg/dose q8–12h gluconate salt; 200–400 mg/dose sulfate IV titrate to effect.	*Caution:* First-dose syncope; 267 mg quinidine gluconate = 200 mg quinidine sulfate. Infuse IV slowly <10 mg/min. *Adverse effects:* Syncope, hypotension, heart block, fever, abdominal discomfort, bone marrow suppression, thrombocytopenia, ITP, cinchonism. *Drug interactions:* Verapamil, cimetadine, phenytoin, phenobarb, rifampin, digoxin.
Ranitidine Zantac, Generic. Tablet/capsule: 150 mg, 300 mg. Syrup: 15 mg/mL. Injection: 25 mg/mL. Effervescent granules and tablet: 150 mg.	**Histamine-2 (H-2) receptor antagonist competitively inhibits gastric acid secretion in gastric/peptic ulcer disease/stress ulcer prophylaxis, GE reflux disease.** *Neonate:* 1.5–2 mg/kg/24 hr PO, IV q12h; continuous 24 hr IV infusion 0.04 mg/kg/hr max 1 mg/kg/24 hr *Children:* 1–5 mg/kg/24 hr PO, IM, IV q6–8h; continuous 24 hr IV infusion 2–5 mg/kg/24 hr. *Adults:* 150 mg/dose PO q12h or 300 mg PO qhs; 50–100 mg/dose IM, IV q6–8h.	*Caution:* Dose may be titrated to desired gastric pH from gastric aspirate. *Adverse effects:* Headache, mental confusion, pain at injection site. *Comment:* Very few if any clinically important drug–drug interactions.
Riboflavin Generic. Tablet: 25 mg, 50 mg, 100 mg.	**Vitamin used in supplementation and deficiency states.** Deficiency: *Children:* 2.5–10 mg/24 hr PO, q8–12h. *Adults:* 5–30 mg/24 hr PO, q8–12h.	*Adverse effects:* Extremely rare. *Drug interaction:* Probenecid.
Rocuronium Zemuron. Injection: 10 mg/mL.	**Anesthetic/skeletal muscle relaxant—nondepolarizing neuromuscular blocking agent.** *Child/adult:* 0.6–1.2 mg/kg/initial dose: subsequent doses administered as needed 0.2 mg/kg q20–30 min. Continuous IV infusion 10–12 μg/kg/min.	*Cautions:* Ventilation must be supported during neuromuscular blockade. Dose adjustment with hepatic dysfunction. *Adverse effects:* Tachycardia, hypotension, prolonged muscle weakness, bronchospasm. *Drug interactions:* Possible augmented muscle weakness with aminoglycosides, anesthetics, colistin.
Salmeterol Serevent. Aerosol canister.	**Long-acting beta-2 adrenergic agonist (~8–12+ hr), bronchodilator used in the treatment of reversible airways disease. Excellent in patients with nocturnal asthma.** *Child/adult:* 1 (21 μg)-2 puffs, aerosol q12h titrate to desired effect.	*Caution:* Not for use in acute asthma attack. *Adverse effects:* Tachycardia, palpitations, headache, nervousness, muscle tremor, cough, airway irritation.
Sargramostim Leukine, Prokine. Injection: 250 μg, 500 μg.	**Granulocyte-macrophage (Gm-CSF) colony stimulating factor for acceleration of myeloid recovery from chemotherapy/marrow insult.**	*Caution:* Monitor blood count to define duration of therapy. *Adverse effects:* Tachycardia, hypotension, flushing, fluid retention, fever, malaise, bone pain, myalgia, rigors, dyspnea.

TABLE 728–1 General Medications *Continued*

Drug (Trade Names, Formulations)	Indications (Mechanism of Action) and Dosing	Comments (Cautions, Adverse Events, Monitoring)
Scopolamine Transderm Scōp, Generic. Transdermal patch.	**Anticholinergic agent used for control of secretions, postoperative antiemetic and motion sickness.** **Postoperative emesis** *Children:* 6 μg/kg/dose IM, IV, SC q6–8h. *Adult:* 0.3–0.65 mg/dose IM, IV, SC q6–8h. **Motion sickness** *Children and adults:* one patch behind the ear at least 4 hr before movement.	*Caution:* Narrow angle glaucoma, ileus. Use patch cautiously in children under 12 yr. *Adverse effects:* Tachycardia, disorientation, sedation, psychosis, dry mouth, constipation, urinary retention, blurred vision. *Drug interactions:* Other anticholinergic compounds, may interfere with GI absorption of certain drugs.
Senna Senokot, X-Prep, Generic. Syrup: 218 mg/5 mL. Tablet: 187 mg, 217 mg, 600 mg. Granules: 326 mg/teaspoon.	**Stimulant cathartic for short-term treatment of constipation, bowel preparation prior to radiology.** *Child:* 10–20 mg/kg/dose PO, q12–24h.	*Caution:* Avoid prolonged use (>1 wk), dependence. *Adverse effects:* Abdominal cramping, diarrhea, fluid and electrolyte imbalance.
Simethicone Mylicon, Gas-X, Generic. Chewable tablet: 40 mg, 80 mg, 125 mg. Capsule: 125 mg. Drops: 40 mg/0.6 mL.	**Antiflatulent for symptomatic relief of colic, excessive gas.** *Children <2 yr:* 20 mg/dose PO q4–6h. *Children 2–12 yr:* 40 mg/dose q6h. *Children >12 yr and adults:* 40–120 mg PO q6h, dose titrated to effect.	*Comments:* Very safe compound without clinically significant side effects. Dose may be titrated to desired effect by increasing dose or more frequent doses per day. Avoid gas-producing and GI irritant foods.
Sodium Polysterene Sulfonate Kayexalate, Generic. Powder for suspension.	**Ion-exchange resin that removes potassium for sodium for the treatment of hyperkalemia.** *Children:* 4 g/kg/24 hr PO, q4–8h; Rectal: 4–12 g/kg/24 hr PR q2–6h. *Adults:* 15 g/dose PO, q6–12h.	*Cautions:* Follow serum potassium closely. Do not mix with potassium containing liquids (e.g., orange juice). *Adverse effects:* Abdominal cramping, bloating, hypokalemia.
Sodium Thiosulfate Tinver, Generic. Injection: 100 mg/mL, 250 mg/mL.	**Cyanide (nitroprusside) and cisplatin antidote. Provides an extra sulfur to rhodanese enzyme to enhance cyanide detoxification.** **Nitroprusside:** *Children and adults:* 1 g sodium thiosulfate for every 100 mg nitroprusside administered. May infuse in same IV. **Cisplatin:** *Adults:* 12 g IV infused over 6 hr before or concurrent with cisplatin infusion. Alternate: 9 g/m² IV bolus followed by 1.2 g/m²/hr for 6 hr before or during cisplatin infusion.	*Caution:* Rapid IV infusion may cause hypotension. *Adverse effects:* Very unusual. Hypotension, local irritation at infusion site.
Spironolactone Aldactone, Generic. Tablet: 25 mg, 50 mg, 100 mg.	**Competetive aldosterone antagonist used as a mild, potassium-sparing diuretic, antihypertensive, in chronic liver disease.** *Neonates:* 1–3 mg/kg/day PO divided q12–24h. *Children:* 1.5–3.3 mg/kg/day PO divided q8–24h. *Adults:* 25–200 mg per dose PO q12–24h.	*Caution:* Careful monitoring of serum potassium/potassium intake. Suspension may be made with crushed tablets in water/glycerin. *Adverse effects:* Lethargy, hyperkalemia, gynecomastia, nausea, rash.
Streptokinase Streptase. Injection.	**Thrombolytic agent used in the treatment of deep-vein thrombosis, stroke, catheter patency.** Thrombosis: 3,500–4,000 units infused IV over 30 min followed by 1,000–1,500 units IV continuous infusion. Clotted catheter: 10,000–25,000 units in normal saline the volume of the catheter instilled into catheter for ~1 hr then removed (aspirated).	*Caution:* Recent strep infection may reduce efficacy. *Adverse effects:* Bleeding bronchospasm, flushing, rash. *Drug interactions:* Anticoagulants, antiplatelet drugs.
Succimer Chemet. Capsule: 100 mg.	**Metal chelator that forms water-soluble salts with lead, mercury, and arsenic.** *Children/adults:* 10 mg/kg/dose PO q8h for 5 days then, 10 mg/kg/dose PO q12h for 14 days.	*Caution:* Maintain adequate hydration. Capsule may be opened and beads sprinkled onto soft food. *Adverse effects:* Headache, dizzines, nausea, abdominal cramping, flu-like symptoms.
Succinylcholine Anectine. Injection.	**Neuromuscular blocking agent.** *Children:* 1–2 mg IV initial dose; maintenance 0.3–0.6 mg/kg IV q5–10 min dose titrated to level of skeletal muscle relaxation. *Adults:* 0.6 mg/kg up to 150 mg IV initial dose; maintenance 0.04–0.07 mg/kg IV q5–10 min titrated to effect.	*Caution:* In patients with hyperkalemia, severe trauma, increased intraocular or intracranial pressure. *Adverse effects:* Bradycardia, hypotension, malignant hyperthermia, hyperkalemia, bronchospasm. *Drug interactions:* Muscle depressants/relaxants.
Sucralfate Carafate. Tablet: 1 g. Suspension: 1 g/10 mL.	**Aluminum salt of sulfated sucrose in the presence of acid forms a paste-like substance that adheres to damaged mucosa.** *Children:* 40–80 mg/kg/day PO divided q6–8h. Stomatitis 5–10 mL swish/spit or swallow q6h. *Adults:* 1 g per dose PO q4–6h.	*Caution:* May use topically for stomatitis. *Adverse effects:* Headache, constipation, abdominal cramping, rash. *Drug interactions:* Decreases absorption of phenytoin, tetracycline, ketoconazole, theophylline, digoxin, cimetidine.

Table continued on following page

TABLE 728–1 General Medications *Continued*

Drug (Trade Names, Formulations)	Indications (Mechanism of Action) and Dosing	Comments (Cautions, Adverse Events, Monitoring)
Sufentanyl Sufenta. Injection.	**Opioid analgesic used in anesthesia and for pain management.** *Children:* 10–25 μg/kg IV initial dose titrated to desired effect with 25–50 μg/kg. *Adults:* 0.5–8 μg/kg initial dose with maintenance 10–50 μg/kg.	*Caution:* In patients with head trauma, MAO inhibitors adverse effect profiles of all opiates. *Adverse effects:* Bradycardia, vasodilitation, nausea, vomiting, blurred vision, respiratory depression, addiction potential. *Drug interactions:* CNS/respiratory depressants.
Sulfasalazine Azulfidine, Generic. Tablet: 500 mg.	**Anti-inflammatory 5-aminosalicylic acid derivative combined with sulfonamide used in the treatment of inflammatory bowel disease.** *Children:* initial 40–75 mg/kg/day PO divided q4–6h not to exceed 6 g/day; maintenance 30–50 mg/kg/day PO divided q6–8h. *Adults:* 1 g per dose PO q6–8h; max dose 6 g/day.	*Caution:* Hypersensitivity to sulfa drugs. *Adverse effects:* Rash, dizziness, headache, nausea, bone marrow suppression. *Drug interactions:* Decreases folate and digoxin absorption.
Tacrolimus Prograf. Injection. Capsule: 1 mg, 5 mg. Extemporaneous preparation.	**Prevent graft versus host disease in organ transplant (immunosuppressant).** *Children:* Oral 0.15 mg/kg every 12 hr; IV continuous infusion 0.05–0.1 mg/kg/day. *Adults:* Oral 0.075–0.15 mg/kg every 12 hr IV continuous infusion 0.05–0.1 mg/kg/day.	*Adverse events:* Hypertension, headache, insomnia, abdominal and back pain, fever, asthenia, pruritis, hypo/hyperkalemia, hypomagnesemia, hyperglycemia, nausea, vomiting, diarrhea, anemia, leukocytosis, liver damage, nephrotoxicity, dyspnea, pleural effusion, peripheral edema. *Monitoring:* Tacrolimus trough concentrations: therapeutic: 9.8–19.4 ng/mL using whole-blood ELISA assay; 0.5–1.5 ng/mL using serum HPLC assay.
Teniposide, VM-26 Vumon. Injection: 10 mg/mL.	**Treatment of ALL and lung cancer (inhibits cells from entering mitosis).** *Children:* IV start 130 mg/m²/wk, increase at 3 wk to 150 mg/m², and at 6 wk to 180 mg/m². *Adults:* ALL 250 mg/m² wk for 4–8 wk.	*Caution:* Increases intracellular accumulation of methotrexate and thus toxicity. *Adverse events:* Nausea, vomiting, diarrhea, mucositis, myelosuppression, alopecia, rash, fever, hemorrhage, peripheral neuropathy. *Comment:* Down syndrome patients should be started at half the usual dose.
Terbutaline Sulfate Brethine, Generic. Injection. Tablet: 2.5 mg, 5 mg. Metered-dose inhaler (MDI).	**Bronchodilator (beta-2 receptor agonist).** *Children <12 yr:* Oral 0.05 mg/kg/dose (max 5 mg) every 8 hr. SC 0.005–0.01 mg/kg/dose (max 0.4 mg), may repeat in 15–20 min. *Children ≥12 yr and adults:* Oral 2.5–5 mg/dose every 6–8 hr SC 0.25 mg/dose, may repeat in 15 min. *Children and adults:* MDI 1–2 puffs every 6–8 hr as needed.	*Adverse events:* Tachycardia, arrhythmias, flushing, headache, nervousness, tremor, hypokalemia, muscle cramps, paradoxical bronchospasm.
Terfenidine Seldane. Tablet: 60 mg.	**Treatment of allergic symptoms (antihistamine).** *Children:* *3–6 yr:* 15 mg twice daily. *6–12 yr:* 30 mg twice daily. *>12 yr and adults:* 60 mg twice/day.	*Caution:* Q-T interval prolongation and fatal arrhythmias may occur if combined with drugs which inhibit liver enzymes. *Adverse events:* Drowsiness, fatigue. *Drug interactions:* Azole antifungals, macrolides, cimetidine may prolong Qt interval and produce dysrhythmias.
Testosterone Generic. Injection.	**Androgen replacement in male hypogonadism and delayed puberty (replacement therapy).** *Children:* IM **Male hypogonadism:** Initiation of prepubertal growth and delayed puberty: 40–50 mg/m²/dose monthly; terminal growth phase: 100 mg/m²/dose twice mo. *Adults:* Hypogonadism: IM 50–400 mg every 2–4 wk.	*Caution:* May accelerate bone maturation without producing compensating gain in linear growth. *Adverse events:* Acne, bladder irritability, aggressive behavior, depression, sleeplessness, headache, hirsutism, hepatic dysfunction.
Tetanus Antitoxin Injection.	Prevention or treatment of tetanus when tetanus immune globulin unavailable. *Children and adults:* SC, IM Prophylaxis: <30 kg 1500 units; >30 kg 3,000–5,000 units. Treatment: inject 10,000–40,000 units into wound and 40,000–100,000 units IV.	*Adverse events:* Serum sickness, urticaria, skin eruptions, allergic reactions.
Tetanus Immune Globulin Hyper-Tet. Injection.	**Prophylaxis and treatment of tetanus.** Prophylaxis: *Children:* 4 units/kg. *Adults:* 250 units IM. Treatment: *Children:* 500–3,000 units. *Adults:* 3,000–6,000 units (infiltrate some of dose around wound).	*Adverse events:* Allergic reactions.

TABLE 728–1 General Medications *Continued*

Drug (Trade Names, Formulations)	Indications (Mechanism of Action) and Dosing	Comments (Cautions, Adverse Events, Monitoring)
Theophylline Generic. Syrup, solution, elixir, capsule, tablet (sustained-release forms also). (See under *Aminophylline* for intravenous dosing.)	**Treatment of apnea of prematurity, symptoms of reversible airway disease (affect intracellular transport of calcium, phosphodiesterase inhibitor, weak anti-inflammatory).** *Neonates:* Apnea, bronchodilation: loading dose 6–10 mg/kg, maintenance dose 2–4 mg/kg/dose every 12 hr. *Infants and children:* *6 wk–6 mo:* 10 mg/kg/day. *6 mo–1 yr:* 12–18 mg/kg/day. *1–9 yr:* 20–24 mg/kg/day. *9–12 yr:* 16 mg/kg/day. *12–16 yr:* 13 mg/kg/day. *Adults:* 10 mg/kg/day. (Dosing may be increased for smokers and enzyme-inducing drugs; decrease dose if enzyme inhibitors, liver disease, heart failure, or hypothyroid.)	*Cautions:* May cause or worsen arrhythmias, seizures, or gastroesophageal reflux. Theophylline clearance is modified by numerous disease states and drugs requiring dosing adjustments guided by serum theophylline concentrations. Clearance is reduced by viral illnesses, fever >102°F for >24 hr, cor pulmonale, and drugs that inhibit P450 enzymes (cimetidine, verapamil, macrolides, quinolones); reduce dose by 50%. *Adverse events:* Tachycardia, nervousness, hyperactivity, difficulty concentrating, irritability, agitation, headache, nausea, vomiting, abdominal pain, feeding intolerance, frequent urination, seizures and arrhythmias at toxic levels. *Monitoring:* Theophylline concentrations: therapeutic: neonatal apnea: 6–15 μg/mL; prevent intubation or promote extubation 10–20 μg/mL; bronchodilation 5–20 μg/mL; toxic >20 μg/mL.
Thiamine Generic. Injection. Tablet: 50 mg, 100 mg, 250 mg, 500 mg.	**Nutritional supplement, treatment of beriberi and Wernicke encephalopathy (essential coenzyme in carbohydrate metabolism).** Beriberi: *Children:* IM, IV 10–25 mg/day or oral 10–50 mg/day for 2 wk, then 5–10 mg/day for 1 mo. *Adults:* IM, IV 5–30 mg 3 times daily for 2 wk, then oral 5–30 mg/day for 1 mo. Wernicke: IM, IV 100 mg/day until consuming a balanced diet.	*Adverse events:* Cardiovascular collapse with repeated IV doses, angioedema, rash, tingling.
Thioguanine 6-TG. Tablet 40 mg.	**Treatment of leukemias (purine analog inhibits synthesis and utilization of purine nucleotides).** *Children:* <3 yr: acute nonlymphocytic leukemia: oral 3.3 mg/kg/day in 2 doses for 4 days. *Children >3 yr and adults:* Oral 2–3 mg/kg once daily (rounded to nearest 20 mg) until remission.	*Adverse events:* Myelosuppression (onset 7–10 days, nadir 14 days, recovery 21 days), nausea, vomiting, diarrhea, anorexia, stomatitis, hyperuricemia, unsteady gait.
Thiopental Pentothal Sodium. Injection.	**Anesthesia induction and maintenance, intractable seizures, increased intracranial pressure (ultra short-acting barbiturate).** *Neonates:* Anesthesia: 3–4 mg/kg; seizures: 2–3 mg/kg IV, repeat doses 1 mg/kg as needed. *Infants and children:* IV anesthesia: 5–8 mg/kg; seizures: 2–3 mg/kg; increased ICP: 1.5–5 mg/kg repeated as needed. *Adults:* IV 25–250 mg as needed for effect. Sedation: Rectal. *Children:* 5–10 mg/kg/dose. *Adults:* 3–4 g/dose.	*Adverse events:* Cramping, diarrhea, rectal bleeding, hypotension, myocardial depression, prolonged somnolence and recovery, emergence delirium, respiraotry depression, coughing, bronchospasm, laryngospasm, hiccups, sneezing. *Monitoring:* Thiopental concentrations: therapeutic: hypnosis 1–5 μg/mL, anesthesia 7–130 μg/mL, coma 30–100 μg/mL.
Thioridazine Mellaril, Generic. Oral concentrate: 30, 100 mg/mL. Oral suspension: 25, 100 mg/5 mL. Tablet: 10, 15, 25, 50, 100, 150, 200 mg.	**Treatment of psychosis, neurosis, and severe behavior problems in children (phenothiazine, block dopamine receptors in the brain).** *Children:* >2 yr: 0.5–3 mg/kg/day in 2–3 doses. *Children >12 yr and adults:* 25–800 mg/day in 2–4 doses.	*Adverse events:* Pseudoparkinsonism, tardive dyskinesia, akathesia, dystonias, dizziness, neuroleptic malignant syndrome, impaired temperature regulation, orthostatic hypotension, pigmentary retinopathy, cholestatic jaundice, leukopenia, agranulocytosis, urinary retention, constipation, dry mouth, GI upset, hyperpigmentation, photosensitivity.
Thiotepa Thioplex. Injection.	**Cancer chemotherapy (alkylating agent, inhibit DNA, RNA, and protein synthesis).** *Children:* IV (depends on protocol) regular dose: 25–65 mg/m² every 3–4 wk; high dose: 300 mg/m²/day for 3 doses. *Adults:* IV continuous infusion 15–35 mg/m² over 48 hr.	*Adverse events:* Myelosuppression (onset 7–10 days, nadir 14 days, recovery 28 days), dizziness, fever, headache, anorexia, nausea, vomiting, alopecia, rash, pruritis, hyperuricemia, hematuria, hemorrhagic cystitis, stomatitis.
Thiothixene Navane, Generic. Injection. Capsule: 1, 2, 5, 10, 20 mg. Oral concentrate: 5 mg/mL.	**Management of psychosis (phenothiazine, block CNS dopamine receptors).** *Children <12 yr:* 0.25 mg/kg/day in divided doses. *Children >12 yr and adults:* Oral 6–60 mg/day in 3 doses; IM 4 mg 2–4 times/day (max 30 mg/day).	*Adverse events:* Orthostatic hypotension, pseudoparkinsonism, tardive dyskinesia, akathesia, dystonias, constipation, urinary retention, dry mouth, stomach pain, nasal congestion, pigmentary retinopathy, agranulocytosis, leukopenia, neuroleptic malignant syndrome, impaired temperature regulation, finger tremor, cholestatic jaundice.
Thrombin, Topical Thrombinar, Thrombogen, Thrombostat. Powder.	**Hemostasis for minor bleeding from capillaries and venules (catalyze the conversion of fibrinogen to fibrin).** *Children and adults:* apply topically as solution 1,000–2,000 units/mL directly to site.	*Adverse events:* Allergy.

Table continued on following page

TABLE 728–1 General Medications *Continued*

Drug (Trade Names, Formulations)	Indications (Mechanism of Action) and Dosing	Comments (Cautions, Adverse Events, Monitoring)
Timolol Timoptic. Ophthalmic solution, ophthalmic gel, tablet.	**Treat elevated intraocular pressure (block beta-1 and beta-2 receptors, and decrease aqueous humor production).** *Children:* (only ophthalmic use) instill 0.25% solution 1 drop twice daily, may increase to 0.5% solution if response inadequate, may decrease to once daily if controlled. *Adults:* Same ophthalmic dose as children.	*Adverse events:* Bronchospasm, bradycardia, hypotension, visual disturbance, conjunctivitis, keratitis.
Tissue Plasminogen Activator, TPA Alteplase, Retevase. Injection.	**Thrombolytic therapy (enhance conversion of plasminogen to plasmin).** *Neonates:* 0.1–0.5 mg/kg/hr for 3–10 hr. *Children:* 0.1–0.6 mg/kg/hr for 6 hr. *Adults:* 100 mg infused as 60 mg in first hour, 20 mg in 2nd hour, 20 mg in 3rd hour.	*Caution:* Initiate heparin concurrently to avoid tethrombosis and thrombotic emboli. *Adverse events:* Bleeding, arrhythmias (related to post-1st MI reperfusion). *Monitoring:* D-dimer, fibrinogen, bleeding time.
Tolazoline Priscoline. Injection: 25 mg/mL.	**Treatment of persistent pulmonary hypertension (alpha-adrenergic blocker and histamine release).** *Neonates:* IV 1–2 mg/kg load, then 1–2 mg/kg/hr continuous infusion.	*Adverse events:* Hypotension, flushing, tachycardia, increases secretions from respiratory and GI tract, GI bleeding and perforation, oliguria, pulmonary hemorrhage, thrombocytopenia. *Monitoring:* Pre- and post-ductal oxygen saturation, arterial blood gases.
Tolmetin Sodium Tolectin, Generic. Tablet: 200, 600 mg. Capsule: 400 mg.	**Treatment of rheumatoid arthritis including JRA (NSAID, prostaglandin inhibition).** *Children >2 yr:* 15–30 mg/kg/day in 3–4 doses. Analgesia: 5–7 mg/kg/dose. *Adults:* 400–600 mg 3 times/day; max dose 2 g/day.	*Adverse events:* GI upset, peptic ulcer disease, hypertension, edema, dizziness, headache, acute renal failure, tinnitus.
Tranexamic Acid Cyklokapron. Injection: 100 mg/mL. Tablet: 500 mg.	**Use in hemophilia patients during and following tooth extractions to reduce or prevent hemorrhage (competitively inhibits activation of plasminogen).** *Children and adults:* IV 10 mg/kg immediately before surgery, then oral 25 mg/kg/dose 3–4 times/day for 2–8 days.	*Adverse events:* Hypotension, thromboembolic complications (including CNS), thrombocytopenia, nausea, vomiting, diarrhea. *Comment:* Decrease dose in renal impairment (CrCl 50–80 mL/min give 50% of dose; CrCl 10–50 mL/min give 25% of dose; CrCl <10 mL/min give 10% of dose.
Trazodone Desyrel, Generic. Tablet: 50, 100, 150, 300 mg.	**Antidepressant (inhibit serotonin reuptake, alpha-adrenergic blockade).** *Children 6–18 yr:* start 1.5–2 mg/kg/day in 3 doses; may increase every 3–4 days (max 6 mg/kg/day). *Adolescents:* start 25–50 mg/day, may increase gradually (max 150 mg) in 2–3 doses. *Adults:* start 50 mg 3 times/day, may increase by 50 mg every 3 days to effect (max 600 mg/day).	*Adverse events:* Headache, confusion, dizziness, dry mouth, nausea, bad taste in mouth, constipation, blurred vision, muscle tremors, hypotension, tachycardia. *Drug interactions:* Fluoxetine may increase levels. *Monitoring:* Trazodone concentrations (limited correlation with clinical effectiveness): therapeutic 0.5–2.5 μg/mL; toxic >4 μg/mL.
Tretinoin Retin-A. Cream: 0.025%, 0.05%, 0.1%. Topical gel: 0.01%, 0.025%. Topical liquid: 0.05%.	**Treatment of acne vulgaris, photo-damaged skin, and some skin cancers (inhibits microcomedone formation and eliminates lesions).** *Children >12 yr:* apply weaker formulation once daily at bedtime. Increase as needed.	*Adverse events:* Excessive skin dryness, erythema, scaling, and local stinging and burning; photosensitivity (use sun block), initial acne flare-up.
Triamcinolone Generic. Injection (Amcort). Oral (Aristocort). Topical (Aristocort). MDI (Azmacort). Nasal spray (Nasacort).	**Treatment of inflammatory and allergic conditions (corticosteroid).** *Children 6–12 yr:* IM 0.03–0.2 mg/kg every 1–7 days. MDI 2 puffs 2–4 times/day. Intranasal: 1 spray in each nostril 1–2 times/day. Injection: intra-articular, intrabursal, or tendon sheath 2.5–15 mg (repeat as needed). *Children >12 yr and adults:* MDI 2–4 puffs 2–4 times/day; Intranasal: 2 sprays in each nostril once daily (max 4 sprays/day). Intra-articular, intrasynovial; 2.5–40 mg; Oral: 40–100 mg/day in 1–4 doses; Topical: apply thin film 2–3 times daily.	*Adverse events:* Atrophy of tissue at local application site, fatigue, cataracts, osteoporosis, oral candidiasis (with MDI), poor growth. *Comment:* See comparison of corticosteroids under *Hydrocortisone.*
Triamterene Dyrenium. Capsule: 50, 100 mg (combination drugs, e.g., with hydrochlorothiazide).	**Diuretic to treat edema or hypertension (competes with aldosterone for receptor sites in distal renal tubules).** *Children:* Oral 2–4 mg/kg/day in 1–2 doses (max 6 mg/kg/day). *Adults:* 100–300 mg/day in 1–2 doses.	*Caution:* Do not use in patients with renal failure; avoid concurrent potassium supplements to avoid hyperkalemia. *Adverse events:* Constipation, nausea, headache, fatigue, hyperkalemia, hyponatremia, hyperchloremic metabolic acidosis.
Trientine Syprine. Capsule: 250 mg.	**Treatment of Wilson disease in patients intolerant to penicillamine (chelating agent).** *Children <12 yr:* 500–1,500 mg/day in 2–4 doses. *Children >2 yr and adults:* 750–2,000 mg/day in 2–4 doses.	*Comment:* Take 1 hr before or 2 hr after meals. Do not break capsule in any way and take with full glass of water. If capsule breaks wash area of skin where contents touch thoroughly with water. *Adverse events:* Iron-deficiency anemia, malaise, epigastric pain, thickening and fissuring of skin, muscle cramps, SLE.

TABLE 728–1 General Medications *Continued*

Drug (Trade Names, Formulations)	Indications (Mechanism of Action) and Dosing	Comments (Cautions, Adverse Events, Monitoring)
Trifluoperazine Stelazine. Oral concentrate: 10 mg/mL. Tablet: 1, 2, 5, 10 mg. Injection.	**Treatment of psychosis (phenothiazine, block dopamine in the CNS).** *Children 6–12 yr:* Oral 1 mg 1–2 times/day, gradually increase to effect (max 15 mg/day); IM 1 mg twice daily. *>12 yr and adults:* Oral 1–2 mg twice daily; IM 1–2 mg every 4–6 hr as needed (max 10 mg/24 hr).	*Adverse events:* Hypotension, tachycardia, arrhythmias, pseudoparkinsonism, tardive dyskinesia, akathesia, dystonias, constipation, nasal congestion, dry mouth, malignant hypertension.
Trimethaphan Camsylate Arfonad. Injection.	**Treatment of hypertensive emergencies (adrenergic and cholinergic blocker).** *Children:* 50–150 μg/kg/min. *Adults:* 0.5–2 mg/min.	*Adverse events:* Anorexia, nausea, dry mouth, ileus, urinary retention, cycloplegia, itching, urticaria, apnea, hypotension.
Trimethobenzamine Tigan, Generic. Capsule: 100, 250 mg. Rectal suppository: 100, 200 mg. Injection: 100 mg/mL.	**Control of nausea and vomiting (inhibits CNS stimulation of chemoreceptor trigger zone).** *Children:* Oral, rectal 15–20 mg/kg/day in 3–4 doses. *Adults:* Oral 250 mg 3–4 times/day. IM, rectal 200 mg 3–4 times/day.	*Adverse events:* Drowsiness, dizziness, headache, diarrhea, muscle cramps.
Tromethamine Tham. Injection: 0.3 M (1 mEq THAM = 3.3 mL).	**Correction of metabolic acidosis (combines with hydrogen ions to form bicarbonate and buffer).** *Neonates, infants, children, and adults:* Dose (mL of 0.3 M solution) = Weight (kg) × base deficit; or 1–2 mEq/kg/dose.	*Adverse events:* Apnea, hypoglycemia, hyperkalemia, tissue irritation, or necrosis if direct contact.
Tropicamide Mydriacil. Ophthalmic solution 0.5%, 1%.	**Short-acting mydriatic agent (blocks sphincter muscle of iris and ciliary body from responding to cholinergic stimulation).** *Children and adults:* Cycloplegia: instill 1–2 drops of 1% solution, may repeat in 5 min. Mydriasis: instill 1–2 drops of 0.5% solution 15–20 min before exam.	*Adverse events:* Tachycardia, drowsiness, headache, dry mouth, blurred vision, photophobia.
Tubocurarine Injection.	**Neuromuscular blocker used in anesthesia (block acetylcholine receptors).** *Neonates:* start 0.3 mg/kg, maintenance 0.1 mg/kg/dose. *Children:* 0.2–0.5 mg/kg start, then 0.04–0.1 mg/kg/dose maintenance. *Adults:* start 6 9 mg, then 3–4 5 mg maintenance.	*Adverse events:* Hypotension, prolonged respiratory depression.
Urokinase Abbokinase. Injection.	**Thrombolytic agent for treatment of recent onset thrombosis (activates plasminogen conversion to plasmin).** *Neonates, infants, children, and adults:* IV load 4,400 units/kg, maintenance dose 4,000–10,000 units/kg/hr. Occluded IV catheter: fill entire volume of catheter with urokinase 5,000 units/mL and leave in lumen for 1–4 hr.	*Adverse events:* Bleeding, hematoma, allergic reactions, bronchospasm. *Monitoring:* D-dimer, fibrin degradation products, ACT.
Ursodiol, Ursodeoxycholic Acid Actigal. Capsule: 300 mg. Extemporaneous formulations.	**Gallbladder stone dissolution, reversal of TPN-induced cholestasis in neonates (decrease cholesterol content of bile).** *Neonates:* 10–15 mg/kg/day PO qd. *Infants:* 30 mg/kg/day 0.8–12h. *Adults:* 300 mg at bedtime for 6–12 mo.	*Adverse events:* Diarrhea, dyspepsia, biliary pain, rhinitis, pruritus, headache.
Valproic Acid and Derivatives Depakene, Generic, Depakote. Depakote delayed-release tablet, capsule sprinkle: 125, 250, 500 mg. Depakene capsule: 250 mg. Syrup: 250 mg/5 mL. Injection.	**Treatment of simple and complex generalized and partial seizures (block sodium and slow T channels).** *Neonates:* Refractory seizures: load 20 mg/kg orally, then 10 mg/kg/dose every 12 hr. *Children and adults:* Seizures: 10–15 mg/kg/day in 3 doses, then increase weekly by 5–10 mg/kg/day to effect or therapeutic levels.	*Caution:* Hepatic failure with fatalities have been reported, especially if patient <2 yr or receiving other anticonvulsants. If used in neonates, monitor serum ammonia. *Adverse events:* Drowsiness, irritability, confusion, malaise, headache, tremor, sensorineural hearing loss, hyperammonemia, hepatotoxicity, nausea, vomiting, diarrhea, pancreatitis, thrombocytopenia, increased appetite, weight gain. *Monitoring:* Valproate concentrations: therapeutic 50–100 μg/mL; toxic >150 μg/mL.
Vasopressin Pitressin. Injection: 20 pressor units/mL.	**Treatment of diabetes insipidus; prevention and treatment of postoperative abdominal distention; treatment of acute GI hemorrhage (antidiuretic hormone analog).**	*Adverse events:* Increased blood pressure, bradycardia, arrhythmias, fever, flatulence, abdominal cramps, nausea, vomiting, tremor, sweating, circumoral pallor, water intoxication.

Table continued on following page

TABLE 728–1 General Medications *Continued*

Drug (Trade Names, Formulations)	Indications (Mechanism of Action) and Dosing	Comments (Cautions, Adverse Events, Monitoring)
Vasopressin *Continued*	*Children:* Diabetes insipidus: IM, SC 2.5–10 units/dose 2–4 times/day. GI hemorrhage: IV continuous infusion 0.002–0.01 units/kg/min. *Adults:* Diabetes insipidus: IM, SC 5–10 units/dose 2–4 times/day. GI hemorrhage: IV continuous infusion 0.2–0.4 units/min.	
Vecuronium Norcuron. Injection.	**Adjunct to anesthesia, neuromuscular blocker (blocks acetylcholine from binding to motor endplates).** *Neonates:* 0.03–0.15 mg/kg/dose every 1–2 hr as needed. *Infants >7 wk–12 mo:* 0.05–0.1 mg/kg every hour as needed. *Children 1 yr–adults:* 0.05–0.1 mg/kg every hour as needed.	*Adverse events:* Tachycardia, hypotension, flushing, bradycardia, circulatory collapse, hypersensitivity reactions.
Venlafaxine Effexor. Tablet: 25, 37.5, 50, 75, 100 mg.	**Treatment of depression, obsessive-compulsive disorder, attention deficit disorder (serotonin and norepinephrine reuptake inhibitor).** *Children:* 25–200 mg/day, start low and titrate up every 4–7 days. *Adults:* start 75 mg/day, titrate every 4–7 days to effect or max 375 mg/day.	*Caution:* Taper slowly if stopping drug to avoid withdrawal syndrome. *Adverse events:* Headache, somnolence, dizziness, insomnia, nervousness, nausea, dry mouth, constipation, blurred vision.
Verapamil Calan, Isoptin, Generic. Sustained-release capsule: 120 mg, 180 mg, 240 mg, 360 mg. Sustained-release tablet: 120 mg, 180 mg, 240 mg. Tablet: 40 mg, 80 mg, 120 mg. Injection.	**Calcium channel antagonist used in the treatment of hypertension and supraventricular dysrhythmias.** Doses in infants and young children not well established: *Infants:* 0.1–0.2 mg/kg and children 0.1–0.3 mg/kg per dose IV repeated to desired effect. *Children:* 4–8 mg/kg/day PO q6–8h; usual dose 5 mg/kg/day. *Adults:* 240–480 mg/day PO divided q6–8h; q12h with extended-release products. May sprinkle contents of capsule onto soft food without affecting absorption.	*Caution:* Adjust dose in renal disease. Avoid IV use in neonates/young infants, or those with heart failure. *Adverse effects:* Hypotension, bradycardia, heart block, dizziness, seizure, abdominal discomfort. *Drug interactions:* May increase concentrations of caffeine, digoxin, carbamazepine, cyclosporine; decreased concentrations with rifampin, phenobarb.
Vinblastine Sulfate Alkaban-AQ; Velban; Generic. Injection.	**Treatment of several cancers (bind to mitotic spindle to inhibit metaphase).** *Children:* IV Hodgkin disease: 2.5–6 mg/m²/day every 1–2 wk for 3–6 wk (max 12.5 mg/m²/wk). *Adults:* 3.7–18.5 mg/m²/day every 7–10 days.	*Adverse events:* Alopecia, nausea, vomiting, abdominal cramps, constipation, diarrhea, stomatitis, myelosuppression (onset 4–7 days, nadir 4–10 days, recovery 17 days), tachycardia, orthostatic hypotension, dermatitis, photosensitivity, muscle pain, paresthesias, urinary retention, hyperuricemia, peripheral neuropathy (loss of deep tendon reflexes, headache, weakness).
Vincristine Oncovin, Generic. Injection.	**Treatment of various cancers (bind to mitotic spindle to inhibit metaphase).** *Children:* *<10 kg or BSA <1 m²:* 0.05 mg/kg once/wk. *>10 kg or BSA >1 m²:* 1–2 mg/m² once/wk. *Adults:* 0.4–1.4 mg/m² once/wk.	*Adverse events:* Constipation, paralytic ileus, depression, confusion, insomnia, headache, jaw pain, optic atrophy, blindness, loss of deep tendon reflexes in legs, numbness, tingling, pain, stocking and glove paresthesias, foot drop, wrist drop, SIADH, photophobia, hyperuricemia, stomatitis, phlebitis, myelosuppression (onset 7 days, nadir 10 days, recovery 21 days).
Vitamin A Aquasol A, Generic. Injection. Oral drops. Capsule.	**Treatment or prevention of deficiency; supplementation in patients with measles (cofactor for many biochemical processes).** *Children:* Vitamin A deficiency with xerophthalmia: *1–8 yr:* Oral 5000 units/day for 5 days, IM 5000–15,000 units/day for 10 days. *>8 yr and adults:* Oral 500,000 units/day for 3 days, then 50,000 units/day for 14 days, then 20,000 units/day for 2 months. Vitamin A deficiency without corneal changes: *Children:* <1 yr: IM 100,000 units every 4–6 mo. *>1 yr:* IM 200,000 units every 4–6 mo. *>8 yr and adults:* IM 100,000 units/day for 3 days, then 50,000 units/day for 14 days. Prophylaxis of patients at risk and supplementation in measles: Oral dose every 4–6 mo. *Children <1 yr:* 100,000 units. *>1 yr:* 200,000 units.	*Adverse events:* Irritability, vertigo, lethargy, fever, headache, hypercalcemia.

TABLE 728–1 General Medications *Continued*

Drug (Trade Names, Formulations)	Indications (Mechanism of Action) and Dosing	Comments (Cautions, Adverse Events, Monitoring)
Vitamin E Generic. Capsule, oral drops, tablet, cream, ointment.	**Nutritional supplement (antioxidant).** *Neonates, premature infants:* 25–50 units/day. *Children:* 1 unit/kg/day; sickle cell anemia: 450 units/day; cystic fibrosis: 100–400 units/day; beta-thalassemia: 750 units/day. *Adults:* 60–75 units/day.	*Adverse events:* Rare.
Warfarin Coumadin, Generic. Tablet: 1 mg, 2 mg, 2.5 mg, 4 mg, 5 mg, 7.5 mg, 10 mg.	**Anticoagulant that antagonizes hepatic vitamin K synthesis depleting vit K-dependent clotting factors II, VII, IX, and X.** *Children:* initial dose 0.2 mg/kg once PO then usual dose approximates 0.1 mg/kg/day PO. Dose titrated to desired PT and INR targets. Avoid large loading doses as complete anticoagulant effect depends upon elimination half-lives of the target clotting factors. Full effects may not be observed until 2–3 days after a warfarin dose adjustment negating rapid dose changes.	*Caution:* Younger infants require higher doses (typical mean dose 0.3 mg/kg/day). Avoid foods with high vitamin K content (green leafy vegetables). *Adverse effects:* Bleeding, skin necrosis, hemoptysis. *Drug interactions:* Aspirin, barbiturates, carbamazepine, cimetidine, omeprazole, phenytoin, rifampin, vitamin K, ritonavir, delavirdine.
Xylometazoline Otrivin. Nasal solution: 0.05%, 0.1%.	**Symptomatic relief of nasal congestion (stimulate alpha-adrenergic receptors to produce vasoconstriction).** *Children 2–12 yr:* instill 2–3 drops 0.05% solution in each nostril every 8–10 hr. *Children >12 yr and adults:* instill 2–3 drops 0.1% solution in each nostril every 8–10 hr.	*Caution:* Do not use for more than 4 consecutive days or exceed recommended dosage as it may cause rebound congestion, chemical pneumonitis, and create dependence. *Adverse events:* Palpitations, headache, dizzinesss, drowsiness, sweating, blurred vision.
Zafirlukast Accolate. Tablet: 20 mg.	**Leukotriene D4 and E4 antagonist inhibiting the effect of slow-reactive substance(s) of anaphylaxis (SRS-A) on bronchial smooth muscle. Not effective in reversing acute bronchoconstriction, though therapy can be continued in acute attacks.** *Adolescent/adult:* 40 mg/day PO divided q12h. Administration of zafirlucast with food increases bioavailability by as much as 40%.	*Caution:* Based on mechanism of action this drug is effective for prophylaxis and does not reverse bronchoconstriction. *Adverse effects:* Headache, nausea, dyspepsia, elevated liver function tests. *Drug interactions:* Blocks CYP 2C9 and 3A4 hepatic isozymes; macrolides, theophylline, carbamazepine, terfenadine, astemazole.
Zileuton Zyflo. Tablet 600 mg.	**5-lipoxygenase inhibitor inhibiting the formation of leukotrienes LTB1, LTC1, LTD1, and LTE1. Not effective in reversing acute bronchoconstriction, though therapy can be continued in acute attacks.** *Adolescent/adult:* 2400 mg/day PO divided q6h.	*Caution:* Based on mechanism of action this drug is effective for prophylaxis and does not reverse bronchoconstriction. *Adverse effects:* Chest pain, headache, nausea, dyspepsia, elevated liver function tests. *Drug interactions:* Macrolides, theophylline, propranolol, warfarin, terfenadine, astemazole.
Zinc Supplements Generic. Injection, liquid, tablets	**Prevention and treatment of zinc deficiency (replacement therapy).** Zinc deficiency: Oral: *Infants and children:* 0.5–1 mg/kg/day in 1–3 doses. *Adults:* 25–50 mg/dose 3 times/day. TPN supplement: *Preterm infants:* 400 µg/kg/day. *Infants <3 mo:* 250 µg/kg/day. *Infants >3 mo:* 100 µg/kg/day. *Children:* 50 µg/kg/day.	*Adverse events:* Rare, but if excessive doses are used may cause copper deficiency.

TABLE 728–2 Antibacterial Medications (Antibiotics)

Drug (Trade Names, Formulations)	Indications (Mechanism of Action) and Dosing	Comments
Amikacin sulfate Amikin. Injection: 50 mg/mL, 250 mg/mL.	**Aminoglycoside antibiotic effective against gram-negative bacilli, esp. *Pseudomonas, Proteus, E. coli, Klebsiella, Enterobacteria, Serratia.*** *Neonates:* IM, IV (over 30–60 min): *Postnatal age* ≤*7 days: 1,200–2,000 g* 7.5 mg/kg q12–18h; *>2,000 g:* 10 mg/kg q12h; *Postnatal age >7 days: 1,200–2,000 g* 7.5 mg/kg q8–12h; *>2,000 g:* 10 mg/kg q8h. *Children:* 15–25 mg/kg/day divided q8–12h. *Adult:* 15 mg/kg/day divided q8–12h.	*Cautions:* Anaerobes, pneumococci, streptococci are resistant. May cause oto- and nephro-toxicity. Monitor renal function. Drug eliminated renally *Drug interactions:* May potentiate other oto-/nephro-toxins. *Target serum concentrations:* Peak 25–40 mg/L; trough <10 mg/L.
Amoxicillin Amoxil, Polymox. Capsule: 250 mg, 500 mg. Tablet: chewable: 125 mg, 250 mg. Suspension: 125 mg/5 mL, 250 mg/5 mL. Drops: 50 mg/mL.	**Penicillinase-susceptible beta-lactam: gram-positive pathogens except staphylocci; *Salmonella, Shigella, Neiserria, E. coli, P. mirabalis.*** *Children:* 20–50 mg/kg/day PO divided q8–12h. Higher dose 80–90 mg/kg/day for otitis media. *Adult:* 250 mg–500 mg PO q8–12h. Uncomplicated gonorrhea: 3 g + 1 g probenecid.	*Cautions:* Skin rash, diarrhea abdominal cramping. Drug eliminated renally. *Drug interaction:* Probenecid.

Table continued on following page

TABLE 728–2 Antibacterial Medications (Antibiotics) *Continued*

Drug (Trade Names, Formulations)	Indications (Mechanism of Action) and Dosing	Comments
Amoxicillin-Clavulanate Augmentin. Tablet: 250 mg, 500 mg, 875 mg. Tablet, chewable: 125 mg, 200 mg, 250 mg, 400 mg. Suspension: 125 mg/5 mL, 200 mg/5 mL, 250 mg/5 mL, 400 mg/5 mL.	**Beta-lactam (amoxicillin) beta-lactamase inhibitor (clavulanate) enhances amoxicillin activity against penicillinase producing bacteria: *S. aureus, Streptococcus, H. influenzae, M. catarrhalis, E. coli, Klebsiella, B. fragilis.*** *Neonates:* 30 mg/kg/day PO divided q12h. *Children:* 20–45 mg/kg/day PO divided q8–12h. Higher dose 80–90 mg/kg/day for otitis media.	*Caution:* Drug dosed on amoxicillin component. May cause diarrhea, skin rash. Drug eliminated renally. *Drug interaction:* Probenecid. *Comment:* Higher dose may be effective against penicillin tolerant/resistant pneumococci.
Ampicillin Polycillin, Omnipen. Capsule: 250 mg, 500 mg. Suspension: 125 mg/5 mL, 250 mg/5 mL, 500 mg/5 mL. Injection.	**Same spectrum of antibacterial activity as amoxicillin. Available for parenteral administration.** *Neonates:* Postnatal age ≤7 days ≤2,000 g 50 mg/kg/day IM, IV q12h (meningitis 100 mg/kg/day divided q12h); >2,000 g 75 mg/kg/day divided q8h (meningitis 150 mg/kg/day divided q8h). Postnatal age >7 days <1200 g 50 mg/kg/day IM, IV q12h (meningitis 100 mg/kg/day divided q12h); 1,200–2,000 g 75 mg/kg/day divided q8h (meningitis 150 mg/kg/day divided q8h); >2,000 g 100 mg/kg/day divided q6h (meningitis 200 mg/kg/day divided q6h). *Children:* 100–200 mg/kg/day IM, IV divided q6h; meningitis 200–400 mg/kg/day divided q4–6h. *Adults:* 250–500 mg PO, IV, IM q4–8h.	*Cautions:* Less bioavailable than amoxicillin causing greater diarrhea. *Drug interaction:* Probenecid.
Ampicillin-Sulbactam Unasyn. Injection.	**Beta-lactam (ampicillin) beta-lactamase inhibitor (sulbactam) enhances ampicillin activity against penicillinase-producing bacteria: *S. aureus, Streptococcus, H. influenzae, M. catarrhalis, E. coli, Klebsiella, B. fragilis.*** *Children:* 100–200 mg/kg/day IM, IV divided q4–8h. *Adults:* 1–2 g IM, IV q6–8h; max daily dose 8 g.	*Cautions:* Drug dosed on ampicillin component. May cause diarrhea, skin rash. Drug eliminated renally. *Note:* Higher dose may be effective against penicillin tolerant/resistant pneumococci. *Drug interaction:* Probenecid.
Azithromycin Zithromax. Tablets: 250 mg. Suspension: 100 mg/5 mL, 200 mg/5 mL.	**Azilide antibiotic with activity against *S. aureus, Streptococcus, H. influenzae, Mycoplasma, C. trachomatis, Legionella.*** *Children:* 10 mg/kg PO on day 1 (max 500 mg) followed by 5 mg/kg PO qd for 4 days. Suspected strep infection 12 mg/kg/day (max 500 mg) for 5 days. *Adults:* 500 mg PO day 1 followed by 250 mg for 4 days. Uncomplicated chlamydia infection single 1-g dose.	*Note:* Drug with very long t1/2 underscoring single daily dosing. No metabolic-based drug interactions (unlike erythromycin, clarithromycin) and limited GI distress. Newer short-course regimens (e.g., 1–3 days) under investigation.
Aztreonam Azactam. Injection.	**Beta-lactam (monobactam) with activity against gram-negative aerobic bacteria; *P. aeruginosa,* Enterobacteriaceae.** *Neonate:* postnatal age ≤7 days ≤2000 g 60 mg/kg/day IM, IV divided q12h; >2,000 g 90 mg/kg/day divided q8h. Postnatal age >7 days <1,200 g 60 mg/kg/day IM, IV divided q12h; 1,200–2,000 g 90 mg/kg/day divided q8h; >2,000 g 120 mg/kg/day divided q6–8h. *Children:* 90–120 mg/kg/day divided q6–8h. Cystic fibrosis up to 200 mg/kg/day. *Adults:* 1–2 g IM, IV q8–12h (max 8 g/day).	*Cautions:* Rash, thrombophlebitis, eosinophilia. Renally eliminated. *Drug interaction:* Probenecid.
Carbenicillin Geopen Injection. Geocillin oral tablet.	**Extended-spectrum penicillin susceptible to penicillinase destruction active against *Pseudomonas, Enterobacter,* indole-positive *Proteus.*** *Neonate:* postnatal age ≤7 days ≤2,000 g 225 mg/kg/day IM, IV divided q8h; >2000 g 300 mg/kg/day divided q6h; >7 days 300–400 mg/kg/day divided q6h. *Children:* 400–600 mg/kg/day IM, IV divided q4–6h.	*Cautions:* Painful by IM, rash; each gram contains 5.3 mEq sodium. Interferes with platelet aggregation with high doses, increases in liver function tests. Renally eliminated. Oral tablet for treatment of UTI only. *Drug interaction:* Probenecid.
Cefaclor Ceclor. Capsule: 250 mg, 500 mg. Suspension: 125 mg/5 mL, 187 mg/5 mL, 250 mg/5 mL, 375 mg/5 mL.	**Second-generation cephalosporin active against *S. aureus, Streptococcus, pneumococci, H. influenzae, E. coli, Proteus, Klebsiella.*** *Children:* 20–40 mg/kg/day PO divided q8–12h (max dose 2 g). *Adults:* 250 mg–500 mg PO q6–8h.	*Cautions:* Beta-lactam safety profile (rash, eosinophilia) with high incidence of serum sickness reaction. Renally eliminated. *Drug interaction:* Probenecid.
Cefadroxil Duricef, Ultracef. Capsule: 500 mg. Tablet: 1000 mg. Suspension: 125 mg/5 mL, 250 mg/5 mL, 500 mg/5 mL.	**First-generation cephalosporin active against *S. aureus, Streptococcus, E. coli, Proteus, Klebsiella.*** *Children:* 30 mg/kg/day PO divided q12h. *Adults:* 250 mg–500 mg PO q8–12h.	*Cautions:* Beta-lactam safety profile (rash, eosinophilia). Renally eliminated. Long half-life accomodates q12–24h dosing. *Drug interaction:* Probenecid.
Cefazolin Ancef, Kefzol. Injection.	**First-generation cephalosporin active against *S. aureus, Streptococcus, E. coli, Proteus, Klebsiella.*** *Neonates:* Postnatal age ≤7 days 40 mg/kg/day IM, IV divided q12h; >7 days 40–60 mg/kg/day divided q8h. *Children:* 50–100 mg/kg/day IM, IV divided q8h. *Adults:* 0.5–2 g IM, IV q8h (max dose 12 g/day).	*Caution:* Beta-lactam safety profile (rash, eosinophilia). Renally eliminated. Does not adequately penetrate CNS. *Drug interaction:* Probenecid.

TABLE 728–2 Antibacterial Medications (Antibiotics) *Continued*

Drug (Trade Names, Formulations)	Indications (Mechanism of Action) and Dosing	Comments
Cefepime Maxipime. Injection.	**Expanded-spectrum, fourth-generation cephalosporin active against many gram-positive and negative pathogens including many multi-drug-resistant pathogens.** *Children:* 100–150 mg/kg/day IV, IM, q8–12h. *Adults:* 2–4 g/day IV, IM q12h.	*Caution:* Beta-lactam safety profile (rash, eosinophilia). Renally eliminated. *Drug interaction:* Probenecid.
Cefixime Suprax. Tablet: 200 mg, 400 mg. Suspension: 100 mg/5 mL.	**Third-generation cephalosporin active against *Streptococcus, H. influenzae, M. catarrhalis, N. gonorrhoeae, S. marcesens, P. vulgarus.* NO antistaphyloccal or antipseudomonal activity.** *Children:* 8 mg/kg/day PO divided q12–24 h *Adults:* 400 mg/day PO divided q12–24h.	*Caution:* Beta-lactam safety profile (rash, eosinophilia). Renally eliminated. Does not adequately penetrate CNS. *Drug interaction:* Probenecid.
Cefoperazone sodium Cefobid. Injection.	**Third-generation cephalosporin active against gram-positive and negative pathogens.** *Neonates:* 100 mg/kg/day IM, IV divided q12h. *Children:* 100–150 mg/kg/day IM, IV divided q8–12h. *Adults:* 2–4 g/day IM, IV divided q8–12h (max dose 12 g/day).	*Caution:* Highly protein bound cephalosporin with limited potency reflected by weak antipseudomonal activity. Variable gram-positive activity. Primarily eliminated in bile. *Drug interaction:* Disulfiram-like reaction with alcohol.
Cefotaxime sodium Claforan. Injection.	**Third-generation cephalosporin active against gram-positive and negative pathogens. NO antipseudomonal activity.** *Neonates:* ≤7 days 100 mg/kg/day IM, IV divided q12h; >7 days <1,200 g 100 mg/kg/day divided q12h, >12,000 g 150 mg/kg/day divided q8h. *Children:* 150 mg/kg/day IM, IV, divided q6–8h (miningitis 200 mg/kg/day IV divided q6–8h) *Adults:* 1–2 g IM, IV q8–12h (max 12 g/day).	*Caution:* Beta-lactam safety profile (rash, eosinophilia). Renally eliminated. Each gram of drug contains 2.2 mEq sodium. Active metabolite. *Drug interaction:* Probenecid.
Cefotetan disodium Cefotan. Injection.	**Second-generation cephalosporin active against *S. aureus, Streptococcus, H. influenzae, E. coli, Proteus, Klebsiella,* and *Bacteroides* spp. Inactive against *Enterobacter* spp.** *Child:* 40–80 mg/kg/day IM, IV divided q12h. *Adult:* 2–4 g IM, IV/day divided q12h (max 6 g/day).	*Caution:* Highly protein bound cephalsporin, poor CNS penetration; beta-lactam safety profile (rash, eosinophilia), disulfiram-like reaction with alcohol. Renally eliminated (~20% in bile).
Cefoxitin sodium Mefoxin. Injection.	**Second-generation cephalosporin active against *S. aureus, Streptococcus, H. influenzae, E. coli, Proteus, Klebsiella,* and *Bacteroides* spp. Inactive against *Enterobacter* spp.** *Neonate:* 70–100 mg/kg/day IM, IV divided q8–12h. *Children:* 80–160 mg/kg/day IM, IV divided q6–8h. *Adult:* 1–2 g IV, IM q6–8h (max dose 12 g/day).	*Caution:* Poor CNS penetration; beta-lactam safety profile (rash, eosinophilia). Renally eliminated. IM injection painful.
Cefpodoxime proxetil Vantin. Tablet: 100 mg, 200 mg. Suspension: 50 mg/5 mL, 100 mg/5 mL.	**Third-generation cephalosporin active against *S. aureus, Streptococcus, H. influenzae, M. catarrhalis, N. gonorrhoeae, E. coli, Klebsiella,* and *Proteus.* NO antipseudomonal activity.** *Children:* 10 mg/kg/day PO divided q12h *Adults:* 200–800 mg/day PO divided q12h (max dose 800 mg/day). Uncomplicated gonorrhea 200 mg PO single-dose therapy.	*Caution:* Beta-lactam safety profile (rash, eosinophilia). Renally eliminated. Does not adequately penetrate CNS. Increased bioavailability when taken with food. *Drug interaction:* Probenecid.
Cefprozil Cefzil. Tablet: 250 mg, 500 mg. Suspension: 125 mg/5 mL, 250 mg/5 mL.	**Second-generation cephalosporin active against *S. aureus, Streptococcus, H. influenzae, E. coli, M. catarrhalis, Proteus, Klebsiella.*** *Children:* 30 mg/kg/day PO divided q8–12h. *Adults:* 500–1,000 mg/day PO divided q12h (max dose 1.5 g/day).	*Caution:* Beta-lactam safety profile (rash, eosinophilia). Renally eliminated. Good bioavailability; food does not affect bioavailability. *Drug interaction:* Probenecid.
Ceftazidime Fortaz, Ceptaz, Tazicef, Tazidime. Injection.	**Third-generation cephalosporin active against gram-positive and negative pathogens including *Pseudomonas aeruginosa.*** *Neonate:* Postnatal age ≤7 days 100 mg/kg/day IM, IV divided q12h; >7 days <1,200 g 100 mg/kg/day divided q12h, ≥1,200 g 150 mg/kg/day divided q8h. *Children:* 150 mg/kg/day IM, IV, divided q8h (meningitis 150 mg/kg/day IV divided q8h). *Adults:* 1–2 g IM, IV q8–12h (max 8–12 g/day).	*Caution:* Beta-lactam safety profile (rash, eosinophilia). Renally eliminated. Increasing pathogen resistance developing with long-term, widespread use.
Ceftizoxime Ceftizox. Injection.	**Third-generation cephalosporin active against gram-positive and negative pathogens; NO antipseudomonal activity.** *Children:* 150 mg/kg/day IM, IV divided q6–8h. *Adults:* 1–2 g IM, IV q6–8h (max dose 12 g/day).	*Caution:* Beta-lactam safety profile (rash, eosinophilia). Renally eliminated. *Drug interaction:* Probenecid.
Ceftriaxone Sodium Rocephin. Injection.	**Third-generation cephalosporin active against gram-positive and negative pathogens; NO antipseudomonal activity. Very potent and beta-lactamase stable.** *Neonates:* 50–75 mg/kg IM, IV q24h. *Children:* 50–75 mg/kg IM, IV q24h (meningitis 75 mg/kg dose 1 then 80–100 mg/kg/day divided q12–24h). *Adults:* 1–2 g IM, IV q24h (max dose 4 g/day).	*Caution:* Beta-lactam safety profile (rash, eosinophilia). Eliminated via kidney (33–65%) and bile; can cause sludging. Long t1/2 and dose-dependent protein binding favors qd rather than q12h dosing. Can add 1% lidocaine for IM injection.

Table continued on following page

TABLE 728–2 Antibacterial Medications (Antibiotics) *Continued*

Drug (Trade Names, Formulations)	Indications (Mechanism of Action) and Dosing	Comments
Cefuroxime Ceftin, Kefurox, Zinacef. Injection. Suspension: 125 mg/5 mL. Tablet: 125 mg, 250 mg, 500 mg.	**Second-generation cephalosporin active against *S. aureus, Streptococcus, H. influenzae, E. coli, M. catarrhalis, Proteus, Klebsiella.*** *Neonates:* 40–100 mg/kg/day IM, IV divided q12h. *Children:* 200–240 mg/kg/day IM, IV divided q8h; oral administration 20–30 mg/kg/day divided q8h. *Adults:* 750–1,500 mg IM, IV q8h (max dose 6 g/day).	*Caution:* Beta-lactam safety profile (rash, eosinophilia). Renally eliminated. Food increases PO bioavailability. *Drug interaction:* Probenecid.
Cephalexin Keflex, Keftab. Capsule: 250 mg, 500 mg. Tablet: 500 mg, 1 g. Suspension: 125 mg/5 mL, 500 mg/5 mL.	**First-generation cephalosporin active against *S. aureus, Streptococcus, E. coli, Proteus, Klebsiella.*** *Children:* 25–100 mg/kg/day PO divided q6–8h. *Adults:* 250–500 mg PO q6h (max dose 4 g/day).	*Caution:* Beta-lactam safety profile (rash, eosinophilia). Renally eliminated. *Drug interaction:* Probenecid.
Cephradine Velosef.	**First-generation cephalosporin active against *S. aureus, Streptococcus, E. coli, Proteus, Klebsiella.*** *Children:* 50–100 mg/kg/day PO divided q6–12h. *Adults:* 250–500 mg PO q6–12h (max dose 4 g/day).	*Caution:* Beta-lactam safety profile (rash, eosinophilia). Renally eliminated. *Drug interaction:* Probenecid.
Chloramphenicol Chloromycetin. Injection. Capsule: 250 mg. Ophthalmic, otic solutions. Ointment.	**Broad-spectrum protein synthesis inhibitor active against many gram-positive and negative bacteria, *Rickettsia, Chlamydia, Mycoplasma, Salmonella, Bacteroides;* other anerobes, *VRE faecium, Pseudomonas* usually resistant.** *Neonates:* Initial loading dose 20 mg/kg followed 12 h later by: Postnatal age ≤7 days 25 mg/kg/day IV q24h; >7 days ≤2,000 g 25 mg/kg/day IV q24h; >2,000 g 50 mg/kg/day IV divided q12h. *Children:* 50–75 mg/kg/day IV, PO divided q6–8h (meningitis 75–100 mg/kg/day IV divided q6h). *Adults:* 50 mg/kg/day IV, PO divided q6h (max dose 4 g/day).	*Cautions:* Gray baby syndrome—too-high dose in neonate; bone marrow suppression, aplastic anemia (monitor hematocrit, free serum iron). *Drug interactions:* Phenytoin, phenobarbital, rifampin may decrease levels. *Target serum concentrations:* Peak 20–30 mg/L; trough 5–10 mg/L.
Ciprofloxacin HCl Cipro. Tablet: 250 mg, 500 mg, 750 mg. Injection. Ophthalmic solution.	**Quinolone antibiotic active against *P. aeruginosa, Serratia, Enterobacter* spp., *Shigella, Salmonella, Campylobacter, M. catarrhalis, N. gonorrhoea, H. influenzae,* some *S. aureus* and strep spp.** *Children:* 15–30 mg/kg/day PO, IV divided q12h. Cystic fibrosis 20–40 mg/kg/day PO, IV divided q8–12h. *Adults:* 250–750 mg PO q12h; IV 200–400 mg q12h (max dose 1.5 g/day).	*Cautions:* Concerns of joint destruction in juvenile animals not seen in humans; tendonitis, superinfection, dizziness, confusion, crystalluria, some photosensitivity. *Drug interactions:* Theophylline, Mg, Al, Ca containing antacids, sucralfate, probenecid, warfarin, cyclosporine.
Clarithromycin Biaxin. Tablet: 250 mg, 500 mg. Suspension: 125 mg/5 mL, 250 mg/5 mL.	**Newer macroilide (e.g., erythromycin) antibiotic with activity against *S. aureus, Streptococcus, H. influenzae, Mycoplasma, C. trachomatis, Legionella.*** *Children:* 15 mg/kg/day PO divided q12h. *Adults:* 250–500 mg PO q12h (max dose 1 g/day).	*Cautions:* Side effects less than erythromycin; GI upset, dyspepsia, nausea, cramping. *Drug interactions:* Same as erythromycin: astemazole carbamazepine, terfenadine cyclosporine, theophylline, digoxin, tacrolimus.
Clindamycin Cleocin. Capsule: 75 mg, 150 mg, 300 mg. Suspension: 75 mg/5 mL. Injection. Topical solution, lotion, and gel. Vaginal cream.	**Protein synthesis inhibitor active against most gram-positive aerobic and anerobic cocci (not *Enterococcus*).** *Neonates:* Postnatal age ≤7 days ≤200 g 10 mg/kg/day IM, IV divided q12h; >2000 g 15 mg/kg/day divided q8h; >7 days <1,200 g 10 mg/kg/day IM, IV divided q12h; 1,200–2,000 g 15 mg/kg/day divided q8h; >2,000 g 20 mg/kg/day divided 18h. *Children:* 10–40 mg/kg/day IM, IV, PO divided q6–8h. *Adults:* 150–600 mg IM, IV, PO q6–8h (max dose 2 (PO)–5 g (IM, IV) per day).	*Cautions:* Diarrhea, nausea, pseudomembranous colitis, rash. Administer slow IV over 30–60 min. Topically effective as an acne treatment.
Cloxacillin sodium Tegopen. Capsule: 250 mg, 500 mg. Suspension: 125 mg/5 mL.	**Penicillinase-resistant penicillin effective against *S. aureus* and other gram-positive cocci except *Enterococcus* and coagulase-negative staphylococci.** *Children:* 50–100 mg/kg/day PO divided q6h. *Adults:* 250–500 mg PO q6h (max dose 4 g/day).	*Caution:* Beta-lactam safety profile (rash, eosinophilia). Primarily hepatically eliminated, requires dose reduction in renal disease. Food decreases bioavailability. *Drug interaction:* Probenecid.
Co-trimoxazole (trimethoprim-sulfamethoxazole) Bactrim, Cotrim, Septra, Sulfatrim. Tablet: sulfa 400 mg/TMP 80 mg. Tablet DS: sulfa 800 mg TMP 160 mg. Suspension: sulfa 200 mg TMP 40 mg/5 mL. Injection.	**Sequential antagonism of bacterial folate synthesis with broad antibacterial activity: *Shigella, Pneumocystis carinii, Legionella, Nocardia, Chlamydia.*** *Children:* 6–20 mg TMP/kg/day PO, IV divided q12h. *Pneumocystitis:* 15–20 mg TMP/kg/day PO, IV divided q12h. Pneumocystitis prophylaxis 5 mg TMP/kg/day or 3 times/wk. *Adults:* 160 mg TMP PO q12h.	*Cautions:* Drug dosed on TMP (trimethoprim) component. Sulfonamide skin reactions—rash, EM, Stevens-Johnson syndrome, nausea, leukopenia. Renal and hepatic elimination; reduce dose in renal failure. *Drug interactions:* Protein displacement with warfarin, possibly phenytoin, cyclosporine.
Demeclocycline Declomycin. Tablet: 150 mg, 300 mg. Capsule: 150 mg.	**Tetracycline active against most gram-positive cocci (except *Enterococcus*); many gram-negative bacilli, *Mycoplasma, Borrelia burgdorferi* (Lyme disease), *Chlamydia,* anaerobes.** *Children:* 8–12 mg/kg/day PO divided q6–12h. *Adults:* 150 mg PO q6–8h.	*Cautions:* Teeth staining, possibly permanent (<8 yr of age) with prolonged use; photosensitivity, diabetes insipidus, nausea, vomiting, diarrhea, superinfections. *Drug interactions:* Al, Ca, Mg, Zn, Fe containing food, milk, dairy products may decrease absorption.

TABLE 728–2 Antibacterial Medications (Antibiotics) *Continued*

Drug (Trade Names, Formulations)	Indications (Mechanism of Action) and Dosing	Comments
Demeclocycline *Continued*	Syndrome of inappropriate ADH secretion: 900–1,200 mg PO/day or 13–15 mg/kg/day PO divided q6–8h with dose reduction based on response to 600–900 mg/day.	
Dicloxacillin Dynapen, Pethocil. Capsule: 125 mg, 250 mg, 500 mg. Suspension: 62.5 mg/5 mL.	**Penicillinase-resistant penicillin effective against *S. aureus* and other gram-positive cocci except *Enterococcus* and coagulase-negative staphylococci.** *Children:* 12.5–100 mg/kg/day PO divided q6h. *Adults:* 125–500 mg PO q6h.	*Caution:* Beta-lactam safety profile (rash, eosinophilia). Primarily renally (65%) and bile (30%) elimination. Food may decrease bioavailability. *Drug interaction:* Probenecid.
Doxycycline Vibramycin, Doxy. Injection. Capsule: 50 mg, 100 mg. Tablet: 50 mg, 100 mg. Suspension: 25 mg/5 mL. Syrup: 50 mg/5 mL.	**Tetracycline active against most gram-positive cocci (except *Enterococcus*); many gram-negative bacilli, *Mycoplasma, Borrelia burgdorferi* (Lyme disease), *Chlamydia*, anaerobes.** *Children:* 2–5 mg/kg/day PO, IV divided q12–24h (max dose 200 mg/day). *Adults:* 100–200 mg/day).	*Cautions:* Teeth staining, possibly permanent (<8 yr of age) with prolonged use; photosensitivity, diabetes insipidus, nausea, vomiting, diarrhea, superinfections. *Drug interactions:* Al, Ca, Mg, Zn, Fe, kaolin, pectin-containing products, food, milk, dairy products, may decrease absorption. Carbamazepine, rifampin, barbiturates may decrease t1/2.
Erythromycin E-Mycin, Ery-Tab, Ery-C, Ilosone. Estolate 125 mg, 500 mg. Tablet EES: 200 mg. Tablet base: 250 mg, 333 mg, 500 mg. Suspension: estolate 125 mg/5 mL, 250 mg/5 mL, EES 200 mg/5 mL, 400 mg/5 mL. Estolate drops: 100 mg/mL. EES drops: 100 mg/2.5 mL.	**Bacteriostatic macrolide most active against gram-positive organisms, *M. pneumoniae, C. diphtheriae*. Combined with sulfasoxazole (Pediazole), dosed on erythromycin content.** *Neonates: postnatal age ≤7 days:* 20 mg/kg/day PO divided q12; *>7 days <1200 g:* 20 mg/kg/day divided q12h; *≥1200 g:* 30 mg/kg/day PO divided q8h. *Children:* usual max dose 2 g/day: Base: 30–50 mg/kg/day PO divided q6–8h. Estolate: 30–50 mg/kg/day PO divided q8–12h. Stearate: 20–40 mg/kg/day PO divided q6h. Lactobionate: 20–40 mg/kg/day IV divided q6–8h. Gluceptate: 20–50 mg/kg/day IV divided q6h: usual max dose IV 4 g/day. *Adults:* Base 333 mg PO q8h, estolate/stearate/base 250–500 mg PO q6h.	*Cautions:* Motilin agonist leading to marked abdominal cramping, nausea, vomiting, diarrhea. Many different salts with questionable tempering of GI side effects. Rare cardiac toxicity with IV use. Dose of salts differ. Topical formulation to treat acne. *Drug interactions:* Antagonizes hepatic CYP 450 3A3/4 activity: astemazole carbamazepine, terfenadine cyclosporine, theophylline, digoxin, tacrolimus, carbamazepine.
Gentamicin Garamycin. Injection. Ophthalmic solution, ointment, topical cream.	**Aminoglycoside antibiotic effective against gram-negative bacilli, especially *Pseudomonas, Proteus, E. coli, Klebsiella, Enterobacter, Serratia*.** *Neonates:* IM, IV (over 30–60 min): *Postnatal age ≤7 days 1,200–2,000 g:* 2.5 mg/kg q12–18h; *>2,000 g:* 2.5 mg/kg q12h; *postnatal age >7 days 1,200–2,000 g:* 2.5 mg/kg q8–12h; *>2,000 g:* 2.5 mg/kg q8h. *Children:* 2.5 mg/kg/day divided q8–12h. Alternatively may administer 5–7.5 mg/kg/day IV once daily. *Intrathecal:* Preservative-free preparation for intraventricular or intrathecal use: neonate 1 mg/day; child 1–2 mg/day; adult 4–8 mg/day. *Adults:* 3–6 mg/kg/day divided q8h.	*Cautions:* Anaerobes, pneumococci, streptococci are resistant. May cause oto- and nephro-toxicity. Monitor renal function. Drug eliminated renally. *Drug interactions:* May potentiate other oto-/nephro-toxins. *Target serum concentrations:* Peak 6–12 mg/L; trough <2 mg/L.
Imipenem-Cilastatin Primaxin. Injection.	**Carbapenem antibiotic active against broad-spectrum gram-positive cocci and negative bacilli including *P. aeruginosa* (not *Xanthomonas maltophilia*).** *Neonates:* postnatal age ≤7 days <1,200 g 20 mg/kg IM, IV q18–24h; >1,200 g 40 mg/kg divided q12h; postnatal age >7 days 1,200–2,000 g 40 mg/kg q12h; >2,000 g 60 mg/kg q8h. *Children:* 60–100 mg/kg/day divided q6–8h. *Adults:* 2–4 g/day divided q6–8h (max dose 4 g/day).	*Cautions:* Beta-lactam safety profile (rash, eosinophilia), nausea, seizures. Cilastatin possesses no antibacterial activity—reduces renal imipenem metabolism. Primarily renally eliminated. *Drug interaction:* ?Ganciclovir.
Loracarbef Lorabid. Capsule: 200 mg. Suspension: 100 mg/5 mL, 200 mg/5 mL.	**Carbacephem very closely related to cefaclor (second-generation cephalosporin) active against *S. aureus, Streptococcus, H. influenzae, M. catarrhalis, E. coli, Proteus, Klebsiella*.** *Children:* 30 mg/kg/day PO divided q12h (max dose 2 g). *Adults:* 200–400 mg PO q12h (max dose 800 mg/day).	*Caution:* Beta-lactam safety profile (rash, eosinophilia). Renally eliminated.
Meropenem Merrem. Injection.	**Carbapenem antibiotic active against broad-spectrum gram-positive cocci and negative bacilli including *P. aeruginosa* (not *Xanthomonas maltophilia*).** *Children:* 60 mg/kg/day divided q8h. *Meningitis:* 120 mg/kg/day (max 6 g/day) IV q8h. *Adult:* 1.5–3 g IV q8h.	*Cautions:* Beta-lactam safety profile; appears to possess less CNS excitation than imipenem. 80% renal elimination. *Drug interaction:* Probenecid.

Table continued on following page

TABLE 728–2 Antibacterial Medications (Antibiotics) *Continued*

Drug (Trade Names, Formulations)	Indications (Mechanism of Action) and Dosing	Comments
Methicillin sodium Staphcillin. Injection.	**Penicillinase-resistant penicillin effective against *S. aureus* and other gram-positive cocci except *Enterococcus* and coagulase-negative staphylococci.** *Neonates: Postnatal age IM, IV ≤7 days:* 1,200–2,000 g 50 mg/kg/day q12h (meningitis 100 mg/kg/day divided q12h); *>2,000 g:* 75 mg/kg/day divided q8h (meningitis 150 mg/kg/day IV divided q8h); *postnatal age >7 days 1,200–2,000 g:* 75 mg/kg q8h (meningitis 150 mg/kg/day divided q8h); *>2,000 g:* 100 mg/kg IV divided q6–8h (meningitis 200 mg/kg/day IV divided q6h). *Children:* 150–200 mg/kg/day divided q4–6h (mininigitis 200–400 mg/kg/day IV divided q4–6h). *Adults:* 4–12 g/day divided q4–6h (max dose 12 g/day).	*Caution:* Beta-lactam safety profile (rash, eosinophilia); higher incidence of interstitial nephritis. Primarily renally eliminated. *Adverse effects:* Interstitial nephritis, neutropenia.
Metronidazole Flagyl, Metro-IV. Generic. Topical gel, vaginal gel. Injection. Tablet: 250 mg, 500 mg.	**Highly effective in the treatment of infections due to anaerobes.** *Neonate: 0–4 wk <1200 g:* 7.5 mg/kg PO, IV q48h; *postnatal age ≤7 days 1,200–2,000 g:* 7.5 mg/kg/day PO, IV q24h; *2,000 g:* 15 mg/kg/day PO, IV divided q12h. *Postnatal age >7 days:* 1,200–2,000 g 15 mg/kg/day PO, IV divided q12h; *>2,000 g:* 30 mg/kg/day PO, IV divided q12h. *Children:* 30 mg/kg/day PO, IV divided q6–8h. *Adults:* 30 mg/kg/day PO, IV divided q6h. Max dose 4 g/day.	*Cautions:* Dizziness, seizures, metallic taste, nausea, disulfiram-like reaction with alcohol. Administer IV slow over 30–60 min. adjust dose with hepatic impairment. *Drug interactions:* Carbamazepine, rifampin, phenobard may enhance metabolism; may increase levels of warfarin, phenytoin, lithium.
Mezlocillin sodium Mezlin. Injection.	**Extended-spectrum penicillin active against *Enterobacter, Serratia, E. coli, Bacteroides* spp., limited antipseudomonal activity.** *Neonates: postnatal age ≤7 days:* 150 mg/kg/day IV divided q12h; *>7 days:* 225 mg/kg divided q8h. *Children:* 200–300 mg/kg/day divided q4–6h. Cystic fibrosis 300–450 mg/kg/day IV. *Adults:* 2–4 g/dose IV q4–6h (max dose 12 g/day).	*Cautions:* Beta-lactam safety profile (rash, eosinophilia); painful IM; each gram contains 1.8 mEq sodium. Interferes with platelet aggregation with high doses, increases in liver function tests. Renally eliminated. *Drug interaction:* Probenecid.
Mupirocin Bactroban. Ointment.	**Topical antibiotic effective against staphlococci and streptococci.** Topical application: nasal (eliminate nasal carriage) and to the skin 2–4 times per day.	Minimal systemic absorption as drug metabolized within the skin.
Nafcillin sodium Nafcil, Unipen. Injection. Capsule: 500 mg. Tablet: 500 mg.	**Penicillinase-resistant penicillin effective against *S. aureus* and other gram-positive cocci except *Enterococcus* and coagulase-negative staphylococci.** *Neonates: Postnatal age IM, IV ≤7 days:* 1,200–2,000 g 50 mg/kg/day q12h; *>2,000 g:* 75 mg/kg/day divided q8h; *Postnatal age >7 days:* 1,200–2,000 g 75 mg/kg/q8h; *>2,000 g:* 100 mg/kg IV divided q6–8h (meningitis 200 mg/kg/day IV divided q6h). *Children:* 100–200 mg/kg/day divided q4–6h. *Adults:* 4–12 g/day divided q4–6h (max dose 12 g/day).	*Cautions:* Beta-lactam safety profile (rash, eosinophilia), phlebitis; painful IM; oral absorption highly variable and erratic. *Adverse effect:* Neutropenia.
Naldixic Acid NegGram. Tablet: 250 mg, 500 mg, 1,000 mg. Suspension: 250 mg/5 mL.	**First-generation quinolone effective for short-term treatment of lower urinary tract infections caused by *E. coli, Enterobacter, Klebsiella, Proteus.*** *Children:* 50–55 mg/kg/day PO divided q6h; suppressive therapy 25–33 mg/kg/day PO divided q6–8h. *Adults:* 1 g PO q6h; suppressive therapy 500 mg q6h.	*Cautions:* Vertigo, dizziness, rash. Not for use in systemic infections. *Drug interactions:* Liquid antacids.
Neomycin Sulfate Mycifradin, Generics. Tablet: 500 mg. Topical cream/ointment.	**Aminoglycoside antibiotic used for topical application or orally prior to surgery to decrease gastrointestinal flora (nonabsorbable) and hyperammonemia.** *Infants:* 50 mg/kg/day PO divided q6h. *Children:* 50–100 mg/kg/day PO divided q6–8h. *Adults:* 500–2,000 mg per dose PO q6–8h.	*Cautions:* In patients with renal dysfunction as small amount absorbed may accumulate. *Adverse effects:* Primarily related to topical application, abdominal cramps, diarrhea, rash. Aminoglycoside toxicities if absorbed.
Nitrofurantoin Furadantin, Furan, Macrodantin. Capsule: 50 mg, 100 mg. Extended-release capsule: 100 mg. Macrocrystal: 50 mg, 100 mg. Suspension: 25 mg/5 mL.	**Effective in the treatment of lower urinary tract infections caused by gram-positive and negative pathogens.** *Children:* 5–7 mg/kg/day PO divided q6h (max dose 400 mg/day); suppressive therapy 1–2.5 mg/kg/day PO divided q12–24h (max dose 100 mg/day). *Adults:* 50–100 mg PO q6h.	*Cautions:* Vertigo, dizziness, rash, jaundice, interstitial pneumonitis. Do not use with moderate to severe renal dysfunction. *Drug interactions:* Liquid antacids.
Oxacillin Sodium Prostaphlin. Injection. Capsule: 250 mg, 500 mg. Suspension :250 mg/5 mL.	**Penicillinase-resistant penicillin effective against *S. aureus* and other gram-positive cocci except *Enterococcus* and coagulase-negative staphylococci.** *Neonates: postnatal age IM, IV ≤7 days:* 1,200–2,000 g 50 mg/kg/day q12h; *>2,000 g:* 75 mg/kg/day divided q8h; *Postnatal age >7 days ≤1,200 g:* 50 mg/kg/day IV divided q12h; *1,200–2,000 g:* 75 mg/kg/day q8h; *>2,000 g:* 100 mg/kg/day IV divided q6h. *Infants:* 100–200 mg/kg/day divided q4–6h. *Children:* PO 50–100 mg/kg/day divided q4–6h. *Adults:* 2–12 g/day divided q4–6h (max dose 12 g/day).	*Caution:* Beta-lactam safety profile (rash, eosinophilia). Moderate oral bioavailability (35–65%). Primarily renally eliminated. *Drug interaction:* Probenecid. *Adverse effect:* Neutropenia.

TABLE 728–2 Antibacterial Medications (Antibiotics) *Continued*

Drug (Trade Names, Formulations)	Indications (Mechanism of Action) and Dosing	Comments
Penicillin G Injection. Tablets.	**Active against most gram-positive cocci; pneumococci (resistance escalating), group A *S. viridans* and some gram-negative bacteria *(N. gonorrhoeae, N. meningitidis)*.** *Neonates: postnatal age IM, IV ≤7 days:* 1,200–2,000 g 50,000 units/kg/day q12h (meningitis 100,000 units/kg/day divided q12h); *>2,000 g:* 75,000 units/kg/day divided q8h (meningitis 150,000 units/kg/day divided q8h); *postnatal age >7 days ≤1,200 g:* 50,000 units/kg/day IV divided q12h (meningitis 100,000 units/kg/day divided q12h); *1,200–2,000 g:* 75,000 units/kg/day q8h (meningitis 225,000 units/kg/day divided q8h); *>2,000 g:* 100,000 units/kg/day IV divided q6h (meningitis 200,000 units/kg/day IV divided q6h). *Children:* 100,000–250,000 units/kg/day IV, IM, divided q4–6h (up to 400,000 units/kg/day). *Adults:* 2–24 million units/day IM, IV divided q4–6h.	*Caution:* Beta-lactam safety profile (rash, eosinophilia), allergy, seizures with excessive doses particularly in patients with marked renal disease. Substantial pathogen resistance. Primarily renally eliminated. *Drug interaction:* Probenecid.
Penicillin G, Benzathine Bicillin. Injection.	**Long-acting (repository form) penicillin effective in the treatment of infections responsive to persistent, low penicillin concentrations (1–4 wk), e.g., strep pharyngitis, rheumatic fever prophylaxis.** *Neonates:* >1,200 g 50,000 units/kg once IM. *Children:* 300,000–1.2 million units/kg IM once every 3–4 wk, max 1.2–2.4 million units/dose. *Adults:* 1.2 million units IM every 3–4 wk.	*Caution:* Beta-lactam safety profile (rash, eosinophilia), allergy. Administer by IM injection only. Substantial pathogen resistance. Primarily renally eliminated.
Penicillin G, Procaine Crysticillin. Injection.	**Repository form of penicillin providing low penicillin concentrations for ~12 hr.** *Neonates:* >1,200 g 50,000 units/kg, IM, qd. *Children:* 25,000–50,000 units/kg/IM qd for 10 days; max 4.8 million units/dose. Gonorrhea: 100,000 units/kg (max 4.8 million units/day) once with probenecid 25 mg/kg (max dose 1 g). *Adults:* 0.6–4.8 million units IM q12–24h.	*Caution:* Beta-lactam safety profile (rash, eosinophilia), allergy. Administer by IM injection only. Substantial pathogen resistance. Primarily renally eliminated.
Penicillin V PenVK, V-Cillin K. Tablet: 125 mg, 250 mg, 500 mg. Suspension: 125 mg/5 mL, 250 mg/5 mL.	**Preferred oral dosing form of penicillin active against most gram-positive cocci; pneumococci (resistance escalating), other streptococci, and some gram-negative bacteria *(N. gonorrhoeae, N. meningitidis)*.** *Children:* 25–50 mg/kg/day PO divided q4–8h. *Adults:* 125 mg–500 mg PO q6–8h (max dose 3 g/day).	*Caution:* Beta-lactam safety profile (rash, eosinophilia), allergy, seizures with excessive doses particularly in patients with renal disease. Substantial pathogen resistance. Primarily renally eliminated.
Pentamidine Isethionate Pentam. Injection. Aerosol.	**Antiprotozoal agent effective in the prevention and treatment of *Pneumonocystis carinii* infections.** *Children: P. carinii* treatment 4 mg/kg/day IM, IV (preferred) qd for 14 days. Prophylaxis: 4 mg/kg IM, IV every 2–4 wk; aerosol adjusted to minute ventilation (4–8 mg/kg/dose) up to 300 mg/dose. Visceral leishmaniasis: 4 mg/kg/day IM, IV qd for 14 days. *Adults: P. carinii* treatment 4 mg/kg/day IM, IV (preferred) qd for 14 days. *Prophylaxis:* 300 mg/dose every 3–4 wk.	*Cautions:* Hypotension, hypoglycemia, cardiac arrhythmias, pain at injection site, nephrotoxicity; cough/bronchospasm with aerosol. 33–66% renally eliminated. *Drug interactions:* Other nephrotoxins aminoglycosides, amphotericin B, cyclosporine.
Piperacillin-Sodium Pipracil. Injection.	**Extended-spectrum penicillin active against *Enterobacter, Serratia, E. coli, Bacteroides* spp., *P. aeruginosa.*** *Neonates:* postnatal age ≤7 days 150 mg/kg/day IV divided q8–12h; >7 days; 200 mg/kg divided q6–8h. *Children:* 200–300 mg/kg/day divided q4–6h; Cystic fibrosis 350–500 mg/kg/day IV. *Adults:* 2–4 g/dose IV q4–6h (max dose 24 g/day).	*Cautions:* Beta-lactam safety profile (rash, eosinophilia); painful IM; each gram contains 1.9 mEq sodium. Interferes with platelet aggregation/serum sickness-like reaction with high doses; increases in liver function tests. Renally eliminated. *Drug interaction:* Probenecid.
Piperacillin-Tazobactam Zosyn. Injection.	**Extended-spectrum penicillin combined with a beta-lactamase inhibitor (tazobactam) active against *S. aureus, H. influenzae, Enterobacter, Serratia, E. coli, P. aeruginosa. Bacteroides* spp., *Acinetobacter.*** *Children:* 300–400 mg/kg/day IM, IV q6–8h. *Adults:* 3.375 g IM, IV a6–8h.	*Cautions:* Beta-lactam safety profile (rash, eosinophilia); painful IM; each gram contains 1.9 mEq sodium. Interferes with platelet aggregation/serum sickness-like reaction with high doses; increases in liver function tests. Renally eliminated. *Drug interaction:* Probenecid.
Sulfadiazine Tablet: 500 mg.	**Sulfonamide antibiotic primarily indicated for the treatment of lower urinary tract infections due to *E. coli, P. mirabilis, Klebsiella* spp.** **Toxoplasmosis:** *Neonates:* 100 mg/kg/day PO divided q12h with pyrimethamine 1 mg/kg/day PO qd (with folinic acid). *Children:* 120–200 mg/kg/day PO divided q6h with pyrimethamine 2 mg/kg/day PO divided q12h × 3 days then 1 mg/kg/day (max dose 25 mg/day) with folinic acid. **Rheumatic fever prophylaxis:** ≤30 kg 500 mg/day; >30 kg 1 g/day PO qd.	*Cautions:* Rash, Stevens-Johnson syndrome, nausea, leukopenia, crystalluria. Renal and hepatic elimination; avoid use with renal disease. t½ ~10 hr. *Drug interactions:* Protein displacement with warfarin, ?phenytoin, methotrexate.

Table continued on following page

TABLE 728–2 Antibacterial Medications (Antibiotics) *Continued*

Drug (Trade Names, Formulations)	Indications (Mechanism of Action) and Dosing	Comments
Sulfamethoxazole Gantanol. Tablet: 500 mg. Suspension: 500 mg/5 mL.	**Sulfonamide antibiotic used for the treatment of otitis media, chronic bronchitis, and lower urinary tract infections due to susceptible bacteria.** *Children:* 50–60 mg/kg/day PO divided q12h. *Adult:* 1 g/dose PO q12h (max dose 3 g/day).	*Cautions:* Rash, Stevens-Johnson syndrome, nausea, leukopenia, crystalluria. Renal and hepatic elimination; avoid use with renal disease. t½ ~12 hr. Initial dose often a loading dose (doubled). *Drug interactions:* Protein displacement with warfarin, ?phenytoin, methotrexate.
Sulfasoxazole Gantrisin. Tablet: 500 mg. Suspension: 500 mg/5 mL. Ophthalmic solution, ointment.	**Sulfonamide antibiotic used for the treatment of otitis media, chronic bronchitis, and lower urinary tract infections due to susceptible bacteria.** *Children:* 120–150 mg/kg/day PO divided q4–6h (max dose 6 g/day). *Adults:* 4–8 g/day PO q divided q4–6h.	*Cautions:* Rash, Stevens-Johnson syndrome, nausea, leukopenia, crystalluria. Renal and hepatic elimination; avoid use with renal disease. t½ ~7–12 hr. Initial dose often a loading dose (doubled). *Drug interactions:* Protein displacement with warfarin, ?phenytoin, methotrexate.
Ticarcillin Ticar. Injection.	**Extended-spectrum penicillin active against *Enterobacter, Serratia, E. coli, Bacteroides* spp., *P. aeruginosa.*** *Neonates: postnatal age ≤7 days <2,000 g:* 150 mg/kg/day IV divided q8–12h; *>7 days; >2,000 g:* 225 mg/kg/day IV divided q8h; *>7 days <1,200 g:* 150 mg/kg/day IV divided q12h, *1,200–2,000 g:* 225 mg/kg/day divided q8h, *>2,000 g:* 300 mg/kg/day IV divid:ed q6–8h. *Children:* 200–400 mg/kg/day divided q4–6h; Cystic fibrosis 400–600 mg/kg/day IV. *Adults:* 2–4 g/dose IV q4–6h (max dose 24 g/day)	*Cautions:* Beta-lactam safety profile (rash, eosinophilia); painful IM; each gram contains 5–6 mEq sodium. Interferes with platelet aggregation; increases in liver function tests. Renally eliminated. *Drug interaction:* Probenecid.
Ticarcillin-Clavulanate Timentin. Injection.	**Extended-spectrum penicillin combined with a beta-lactamase inhibitor (clavulanate) active against *S. aureus, H. influenzae, Enterobacter, Serratia, E. coli, P. aeruginosa, Bacteroides* spp., *Acinetobacter.*** *Children:* 280–400 mg/kg/day IM, IV q4–8h. *Adults:* 3.1 g IM, IV q4–8h (max dose 18–24 g/day).	*Cautions:* Beta-lactam safety profile (rash, eosinophilia); painful IM; each gram contains 5–6 mEq sodium. Interferes with platelet aggregation; increases in liver function tests. Renally eliminated. *Drug interaction:* Probenecid.
Tobramycin Nebcin, Tobrex. Injection. Ophthalmic solution, ointment.	**Aminoglycoside antibiotic effective against gram-negative bacilli, esp. *Pseudomonas, Proteus, E coli, Klebsiella, Enterobacter,* Serratia.** *Neonates:* IM, IV (over 30–60 min): *postnatal age ≤7 days, 1,200–2,000 g:* 2.5 mg/kg q12–18h; *>2,000 g:* 2.5 mg/kg q12h; *postnatal age >7 days, 1,200–2,000 g:* 2.5 mg/kg q8–12h; *>2,000 g:* 2.5 mg/kg q8h. *Children:* 2.5 mg/kg/day divided q8–12h. Alternatively may administer 5–7.5 mg/kg/day IV qd. Preservative-free preparation for intraventricular or intrathecal use: neonate 1 mg/day; child 1–2 mg/day; adult 4–8 mg/day. *Adults:* 3–6 mg/kg/day divided q8h.	*Cautions:* Anaerobes, pneumococci, streptococci are resistant. May cause oto- and nephro-toxicity. Monitor renal function. Drug eliminated renally *Drug ineractions:* May potentiate other oto-/nephro-toxins. *Target serum concentrations:* Peak 6–12 mg/L; trough <2 mg/L.
Trimethoprim Proloprim, Trimpex. Tablet: 100 mg, 200 mg.	**Folic acid antagonist effective in the prophylaxis and treatment of *E. coli, Klebsiella, Proteus mirabilis,* and *Enterobacter* spp. urinary tract infections; *Pneumocystis carinii* pneumonia.** *Children:* For UTI 4–6 mg/kg/day PO divided q12h *>12 yr and adult:* 100–200 mg PO q12h. *Pneumocystis carinii* pneumonia (with dapsone): 15–20 mg/kg/day PO q6h for 21 days.	*Cautions:* Megaloblastic anemia, bone marrow suppression, nausea, epigastric distress, rash. *Drug interactions:* Possible interactions with phenytoin, cyclosporine, rifampin, warfarin.
Vancomycin Vancocin, Luphocin. Injection. Capsule: 125 mg, 250 mg. Suspension.	**Glycopeptide antibiotic effective against most gram-positive pathogens including staphylococci (methicillin-resistant *S. aureus* and coagulase-negative staphylococci) and enterococci (resistance developing), clostridia, pneumococci including penicillin-resistant strains.** *Neonate: postnatal age ≤7 days, <1200 g:* 15 mg/kg/day IV divided q24h; *1,200–2,000 g:* 15 mg/kg/day IV divided q12–18h; *>2,000 g:* 30 mg/kg/day IV divided q12h; *postnatal age >7 days, <1,200 g:* 15 mg/kg/day IV divided q24h; *1,200–2,000 g:* 15 mg/kg/day IV divided q8–12h; *>2,000 g:* 45 mg/kg/day IV divided q8h. *Children:* 45–60 mg/kg/day IV divided q8–12h; oral dosing for antibiotic-associated enterocolitis; 40–50 mg/kg/day PO divided q6–8h. *Adults:* 0.5–1 g IV q12h.	*Cautions:* Ototoxicity, nephrotoxicity particularly when coadministered with other oto- and nephro-toxins. Infuse IV over 45–60 min. Flushing (red-man syndrome) associated with rapid IV infusions, fever, chills, phlebitis (prefer central line). Renally eliminated. *Target serum concentrations:* Peak (1 hr after 1 hr infusion) 30–40 mg/L; trough 5–10 mg/L.

TABLE 728–3 Antimycobacterial Medications

Drug (Trade Names, Formulations)	Indications (Mechanism of Action) and Dosing	Comments
Cycloserine Seromycin. Capsule: 250 mg.	**Adjunctive antitubercular agent less effective than INH or streptomycin.** *Children:* 10–20 mg/kg/day PO divided q12h. *Adult:* 250–500 mg per dose PO q12h; max daily dose 1,000 mg.	*Cautions:* Headache, dizziness, confusion, psychosis, seizures, photosensitivity, folate vit B_{12} deficiency. Primarily renally eliminated. *Drug interactions:* Phenytoin, additive CNS effects with INH.
Ethambutol HCl Myambutol. Tablet: 100 mg, 400 mg.	**For use in combination with other agents.** *Child:* 15 mg/kg/day PO qd. *Adult:* 15 mg/kg/day PO qd max dose 2.5 g/day.	*Cautions:* Optic neuritis, decreased visual acuity, headache, dizziness, rash, peripheral neuropathy.
Ethionamide Tecator-SC. Tablet: 250 mg.	**For use in combination with other agents. Consider co-administration with vit B_6.** *Child:* 15–20 mg/kg/day PO divided q8–12h (max dose 1,000 mg/day). *Adult:* 500–1,000 mg PO q8–24h.	*Cautions:* GI upset, hepatotoxicity, vit B_6 deficiency, dizziness, headache, metallic taste, optic neuritis.
Isoniazid INH, Nydrazid. Tablet: 50 mg, 100 mg, 300 mg. Syrup: 50 mg/5 mL. Injection.	**For use in combination with other agents.** *Children:* 10–20 mg/kg/day PO divided q12–24h; max dose 300 mg/day; prophylaxis dose 10 mg/kg/day. *Adult:* 5 mg/kg/day PO once daily; usual maximum dose 300 mg/day. Twice weekly therapy (after 3 mo daily therapy): *Children:* 20–40 mg/kg/dose (maxium 900 mg) twice weekly. *Adult:* 15 mg/kg/dose (max 900 mg) twice weekly.	*Cautions:* Dizziness, seizures, rash, pellagra, GI upset, peripheral neuropathy (may give B_6 1–2 mg/kg/day without effect on anti-TB activity), hepatotoxicity. *Drug interactions:* Increase serum concentrations of phenytoin, carbamazepine.
Kanamycin Injection.	**Aminoglycoside antibiotic used in combination with other agents.** *Children:* 15 mg/kg/day IM, IV divided q12h. *Adult:* 1 g/day IM, IV max dose 1 g/day.	*Cautions:* Aminoglycoside side effect profile, oto- and nephro-toxicity.
Pyrazinamide Tablet: 500 mg.	**For use in combination with other agents.** *Children:* 15–40 mg/kg/day PO divided q12–24h (max dose 2 g/day). *Adult:* 15–30 mg/kg/day PO divided q6–24h.	*Cautions:* Photosensitivity, GI upset, hyperuricemia, arthralgia, hepatotoxicity (especially doses >30 mg/kg/day).
Rifabutin Mycobutin. Capsule: 150 mg, 300 mg. Injection. Extemporaneous liquid formulation.	**Treatment (in combination with other antimycobacterial agents) and prevention of infections with *Mycobacterium avium* complex. Inhibits DNA-dependent RNA polymerase.** *Infants and children:* Treatment (preliminary guidelines): 5–7 mg/kg/day PO once daily. Prophylaxis: 5 mg/kg/day PO once daily. *Adults:* 300 mg PO once daily.	*Cautions:* Dosing information in pediatrics is evolving. Fever, headache, confusion, GI upset, increased LFTs, anemia, neutropenia may cause orange-red discoloration of secretions of urine, tears, sweat. *Drug interations:* May enhance metabolism of many drugs: warfarin, corticosteroids, opiates, oral contraceptives.
Rifampin Rifadin, Rimactane. Capsule: 150 mg, 300 mg. Injection. Extemporaneous liquid formulation.	**For use in combination with other agents.** *Children:* 10–20 mg/kg/day PO, IV divided q12–24h. *Adult:* 10 mg/kg/day PO, IV, once daily; max dose 600 mg/day. Twice weekly therapy (after 3 mo daily therapy): *Children:* 10–20 mg/kg/dose (max 600 mg) twice weekly. *Adults:* 10 mg/kg/dose (max 600 mg) twice weekly.	*Cautions:* Hepatotoxicity, influenza-like syndrome, rash, pruritus, leukopenia, arthralgia; may cause orange-red discoloration of urine, tears, sweat. *Drug interactions:* Induces hepatic enzymes decreasing effect/concentrations of opiates, anticoagulants, barbiturates, carbamazepine, phenytoin, azole antifungals, cyclosporine, corticosteroids.
Streptomycin Generic. Injection.	**Aminoglycoside antibiotic used in combination with other agents.** *Neonate:* 10–20 mg/kg/day IM qd. *Children:* 20–40 mg/kg/day IM divided q12h not to exceed 1 g/day. *Adult:* 15 mg/kg/day IM qd, not to exceed 1 g/day.	*Cautions:* Aminoglycoside side effect profile, oto- and nephrotoxicity.

TABLE 728–4 Antifungal Medications

Drug (Trade Names, Formulations)	Indications (Mechanism of Action) and Dosing	Comments
Amphotericin B Fungizone. Injection.	**Polyene effective against a broad spectrum of fungi: *Candida, Aspergillus, Coccidioides, Histoplasma, Torulopsis, Sporotrichum, Blastomyces.* Available as the traditional colloidal suspension and newer lipid-complex/liposomal formulations. Lipid formulations permit higher doses (see below) with increased patient tolerance.** *Children and adults:* 0.1–0.25 mg/kg initial dose. Maintenance dose 0.5–1 mg/kg/day infused IV over 4–6 hr q day. *Bladder irrigation:* 5–15 mg amphotericin B/100 mL.	*Cautions:* Hypotension, fever, chills, flushing; premedicate with meperidine and acetaminophen. Drug augments potassium and magnesium excretion requiring aggressive monitoring and supplementation. Decreases renal function in >80% of patients. Sodium loading prior to or with amphotericin dosing decreases renal toxicity. *Drug interactions:* Concurrent nephrotoxic drugs.

Table continued on following page

TABLE 728–4 Antifungal Medications *Continued*

Drug (Trade Names, Formulations)	Indications (Mechanism of Action) and Dosing	Comments
Amphotericin B Lipid Complexes Abelcet (ABLC); Ambisome (liposome); Amphotec (ABCD). Injection.	**Polyene effective against a broad spectrum of fungi: *Candida, Aspergillus, Coccidioides, Histoplasma, Sporothrix, Blastomyces.* Available as the traditional colloidal suspension and newer lipid-complex/ liposomal formulations. Lipid formulations permit higher doses with increased patient tolerance.** *Children and adults:* 2.5–5 mg/kg IV infused over 1–2 hr q day; may use higher doses of 7.5–10 mg/kg/day if indicated and if tolerated.	*Cautions:* Hypotension, fever, chills, flushing; premedicate with meperidine and acetaminophen. Drug augments potassium and magnesium excretion requiring aggressive monitoring and supplementation. Lipid formulations markedly attenuate renal toxicity. *Drug interactions:* Concurrent nephrotoxic drugs.
Clotrimazole Lotrimin, Gyne-Lotrimin. Troches, topical cream, vaginal tablets, and cream.	**Topical imidazole active against cryptococci, *Aspergillus, Candida,* and *Coccidiodes* for the treatment of oropharyngeal, skin, vaginal infections.** *Children and adults:* 1 troche dissolved 5–6 times daily. Vaginal cream/tablet 100–200 mg qhs. Topical cream: apply twice daily.	*Cautions:* Minimal side effects, nausea, skin irritation. Topical/troche ineffective for systemic infections.
Econazole nitrate Spectazole. Topical cream: 1%.	**Topical agent effective in the treatment of tinea corporis, cruris, pedis, and cutaneous candidiasis.** *Children and adults:* apply over affected areas once daily.	*Cautions:* Minimal side effects—skin irritation.
Fluconazole Diflucan. Tablet: 50 mg, 100 mg, 150 mg, 200 mg. Suspension: 10 mg/mL, 40 mg/mL. Injection.	**Imidazole effective against cryptococci and *Candida* infections of the oropharynx, vagina, meningitis.** *Neonate:* thrush 6 mg/kg, IV, PO qd first day then 3 mg/ kg/day qd for 14–21 days. Systemic infections: postnatal age <14 days 6–12 mg/kg/ day PO, IV q72h; >14 days once daily. *Children:* 6–12 mg/kg/day IV, PO qd; cryptococcal meningitis 12 mg/kg/day first day then 6–12 mg/kg/day IV, PO q day.	*Cautions:* Dizziness, skin rash, nausea, abdominal pain, elevated liver function tests, superinfection with *C. krusei.* Reduce dose with reduced renal function. *Drug interactions:* Warfarin, oral antidiabetic agents, astemizole, cisapride, cyclosporine, phenytoin, rifampin, terfenadine, zidovudine.
Flucytosine Ancobon, 5FC. Capsule: 250 mg, 500 mg.	**5FC used in combination with amphotericin B (resistance develops rapidly) against *Candida, Cryptococcus, Aspergillius,* and *Torulopsis* infections.** *Neonate:* 50–100 mg/kg/day PO divided q12–24 h. *Children and adults:* 100–150 mg/kg/day PO divided q6–8h. Monitor blood levels.	*Cautions:* Confusion, rash, nausea, vomiting, bone marrow suppression with sustained serum concentrations >100 mg/L, elevated liver function tests. *Drug interactions:* Aluminum and magnesium salts delay absorption rate.
Griseofulvin Fulvicin, Grisactin. Microsize capsules: 125 mg, 250 mg. Suspension: 125 mg/5 mL. Tablet: UF 250 mg, 500 mg. Ultra-microsize PG tablet: 125 mg, 165 mg, 250 mg, 330 mg.	**Treatment of tinea infections of the hair, nails, and skin due to *Microsporum, Epidermophyton, Trichophyton.* Ultra-microsize formulation almost complete absorption whereas absorption of microsize is variable (40–80%).** *Children:* microsize 10–20 mg/kg/day PO divided q12–24h; ultra-microsize 5–10 mg/kg/day PO divided q12h. *Adult:* microsize 500–1,000 mg/day PO divided q12–24h; ultra-microsize 330–375 mg/day PO divided q12h.	*Cautions:* Headache, nausea, diarrhea, rash, photosensitivity. Administration with a fatty meal increases oral absorption. *Drug interactions:* Warfarin, phenobarbital, oral contraceptives, ?phenytoin.
Itraconazole Sporanox. Capsule: 100 mg.	**Synthetic triazole active against *Candida, Aspergillus,* cryptococci, *Histoplasma.* Limited dosing data in pediatrics.** *Children:* 3–5 mg/kg/day PO once daily; doses as high as 5–10 mg/kg/day have been used. *Adult:* 200–400 mg/day PO divided q12h; serious infections 600 mg/day q8h for 3–4 days then 200–400 mg/day.	*Cautions:* Hypertension, nausea, headache, dizziness, rash, hepatitis. Food increases bioavailability. *Drug interactions:* Carbamazepine, isoniazid, rifampin, phenytoin, phenobarbital, cyclosporin. Antacids/H_2 antagonists decrease bioavailability.
Miconazole Micatin, Monostat. Topical cream, vaginal tablet, lotion, powder. Injection.	**Imidazole active against cryptococci, *Candida, Coccidioides,* and *Pseudallescheria boydii* for topical or IV use in superficial infections.** *Neonate:* 5–15 mg/kg/day IV divided q8–24h. *Children:* 20–40 mg/kg/day IV divided q8h; vaginal cream/ tablet 100–200 mg qHS; topical cream: apply twice daily. *Adult:* 200 mg stat then 1.2–3.6 g/day IV divided q8h. *Bladder irrigation:* 200 mg in 25 mL saline.	*Cautions:* Dizziness, nausea, hyperlipidemia, tremors, rash, hives. Mostly used for the treatment of topical infections.
Nystatin Mycostatin, Nilstat.	**Polyene effective against many yeasts and molds. IV liposomal formulation for systemic therapy under investigation.** **Oral candidiasis** *Neonate:* 100,000 units 4 times per day. *Infants:* 200,000 units 4 times daily. *Child/adult:* 400,000–600,000 units 4 times daily. Topical: apply 2–4 times daily.	*Cautions:* Minimal side effects with topical application, nausea, skin irritation. Tablet ineffective for systemic infections.

TABLE 728–5 Antiviral Medications

Drug (Trade Names, Formulations)	Indications (Mechanism of Action) and Dosing	Comments
Acyclovir Zovirax. Capsule: 200 mg. Tablet: 400 mg, 800 mg. Suspension: 200 mg/5 mL. Injection. Ointment.	**Herpes simplex (HSV) encephalitis, mucosal, cutaneous, genital infections; herpes zoster, varicella-zoster, cytomegalovirus (CMV) prophylaxis.** *Neonate: HSV encephalitis:* 30–45 mg/kg/day IV divided q8h. *Children and adults:* 15 mg/kg/day IV divided q8–12h. HSV infection in immunocompromised host: *Children and adults:* 15–30 mg/kg/day IV divided q8h. HSV encephalitis/varicella infection/CMV prophylaxis in immunocompromised host: *Children and adults:* 30 mg/kg/day IV divided q8h. Oral dosing for HSV/zoster infection: *Children and adults:* 1,200 mg/day divided q4–8h; maximum pediatric dose 80 mg/kg/day.	*Cautions:* Headache, dizziness, rash, bone marrow suppression. Poor oral bioavailability—best given in frequent daily doses (e.g., q4h). Primarily renally eliminated. 4.2 mEq Na per gram of acyclovir. *Drug interaction:* Probenecid.
Amantadine Symmetrel. Capsule: 100 mg. Syrup: 50 mg/5 mL.	**Prophylaxis and treatment (all ages) of influenza A infections.** Prophylaxis or treatment: *Children: 1–9 yr or <40 kg:* 5 mg/kg/day PO divided q12hr (max 150 mg/day). *Children: >9 yr (and >40 kg) and adults:* 200 mg/day PO divided q12hr.	*Cautions:* Anticholinergic effects, and may potentiate other anticholinergic medications. Drowsiness, dizziness, confusion, hypotension, urinary retention. Renally eliminated; reduce dose with renal impairment. No dosage reduction necessary for hepatic impairment. Not removed by hemodialysis.
Famciclovir Famvir. Tablet: 500 mg.	**Oral prodrug formulation of penciclovir used in the treatment of acute herpes zoster infections. Limited data in pediatrics.** *Adult:* 500 mg PO q8h for 7 days.	*Cautions:* Headache, dizziness, nausea, adjust dose in renal insufficiency (e.g., penciclovir). Rate of absorption, not overall bioavailability, reduced if taken with food.
Foscarnet Foscavir. Injection.	**Treatment of CMV infections, retinitis, and acyclovir-resistant HSV mucocutaneous and herpes zoster infections.** CMV retinitis: IV infusion rate 60 mg/kg per hr. *Children and adults:* induction therapy: 180 mg/kg/day IV divided q8h; maintenance therapy: 90–120 mg/kg/day IV once daily. Acyclovir-resistant HSV infection: *Children and adults:* 120 mg/kg/day divided q8–12h.	*Cautions:* Hypertension, dizziness, seizures, decreased electrolytes (Ca, Mg, K), GU complications, bronchospasm, nephrotoxicity. Adjust dose with renal dysfunction. IV infusion dilution for peripheral administration 12 mg/mL; central administration 24 mg/mL.
Ganciclovir Cytovene. Injection. Capsule: 250 mg.	**Treatment of CMV infections including retinitis.** CMV retinitis: *Children and adults:* Induction therapy: 10 mg/kg/day IV (over 1–2 h) divided q12h for 14–21 days; maintenance therapy: 5–6 mg/kg/day IV once daily. CMV disease and prophylaxis (solid organ transplant): Induction: 10 mg/kg/day IV divided q12h for 7–14 days then 5 6 mg/kg/day IV once daily	*Cautions:* Headache, seizures, hypertension, nausea, marrow suppression, renal/liver toxicity, rash, photophobia. Primarily renally eliminated. *Drug interactions:* Probenecid, immunosuppressants. *Comment:* Oral dose form very poor bioavailability (5–6%).
Idoxuridine (IDU) Herplex. Ophthalmic solution 1%.	**Topical therapy for herpes simplex keratitis.** *Children and adults:* apply ointment 5 times daily and ophthalmic solution (1 drop) to affected eye(s) 7–10 times daily and at bedtime.	*Cautions:* Local irritation, pruritus, ocular edema.
Ribavirin Virazole. Powder for aerosol.	**Aerosol therapy for RSV infections, particularly for patients with underlying conditions, including BPD and/or congenital heart diseases.** *Children and adults:* use SPAG-2 small particle generator at 20 mg/mL concentration for continuous aerosolization 12–18 hr per day. High-dose/short-duration aerosol administration under investigation.	*Cautions:* Rash, irritation, hypotension; drug may precipitate in ventilation tubing; use in well-ventilated areas, minimize staff contact. Best results when initiated early in clinical course.
Rimantadine Flumadine. Tablet: 100 mg. Syrup: 50 mg/5 mL.	**Prophylaxis (all ages) and treatment (>13 yr) of influenza A infections.** Prophylaxis only: *Children 1–9 yr or <40 kg:* 5 mg/kg/day PO divided q12hr (max 150 mg/day). *Children 10–13 yr:* 100 mg PO divided q12hr. Prophylaxis or treatment: *Children >13 yr and adults:* 200 mg/day PO divided q12hr.	*Cautions:* Anticholinergic effects, and may potentiate other anticholinergic medications. Drowsiness, dizziness, confusion, hypotension, urinary retention. Hepatically metabolized; reduce dosage to one-half usual dose for persons with severe liver disease or CrCl ≤10 mL/min.
Trifluridine Viroptic. Ophthalmic solution 1%.	**Treatment of herpes simplex keratitis.** *Children and adults:* instill 1 drop into affected eye(s) q2h while awake and at bedtime for up to 21 days.	*Cautions:* Local irritation, pruritus, ocular edema.
Vidarabine (Ara-A) Vira-A. Injection. Ophthalmic ointment.	**Herpes simplex and varicella zoster infections.** **HSV infections:** *Neonate:* 15–30 mg/kg/day IV infusion over 18–24h. *Children and adults:* 15 mg/kg/day IV once daily over 12h. **Herpes zoster/varicella zoster infections:** *Children and adults:* 10 mg/kg/day IV once daily over 12 hr.	*Cautions:* Bone marrow suppression, disorientation, ataxia, seizures, SIADH. Metabolites primarily renally eliminated. *Drug interactions:* Marrow suppressants.

TABLE 728–6 Antiretroviral-HIV Medications

Drug (Trade Names, Formulations)	Indications (Mechanism of Action) and Dosing	Comments
Didanosine Videx, ddi. Chewable buffered tablet: 25 mg, 50 mg, 100 mg, 150 mg. Buffered powder packet: 100 mg, 167 mg, 250 mg.	**Purine analog—intracellular metabolite inhibits viral RNA-directed DNA polymerase.** *Infants <90 days:* 100 mg/m²/day PO divided q12h. *Children:* 180–300 mg/m²/day PO divided q12h. *Adults (>13 yr):* <60 kg 125 mg PO q12h (buffered oral solution 167 mg PO q12h). >60 kg 200 mg PO q12h (buffered oral solution 250 mg PO q12h). Administer on an empty stomach 1 hr before or 2 hr after a meal to decrease food effect.	*Cautions:* Headache (~30%), diarrhea, pancreatitis, peripheral neuropathy, optic neuritis, liver dysfunction. Renally eliminated. Food decreases bioavailability up to 50%. Tablets dissolved in water stable for 1 hr (4 hr in buffered solution). *Drug interactions:* Antacids/gastric acid antagonists may increase bioavailability; possible decreased absorption of ciprofloxacin, ganciclovir, ketoconazole, itraconazole.
Indinavir Crixivan. Capsule: 200 mg, 400 mg.	**Protease inhibitor for combination use with nucleoside analogs and other protease inhibitors. Evolving experience with neonatal and pediatric dosing.** *Children:* 1,500 mg/m²/day PO divided q8h, max single dose 800 mg. *Adult:* 2,400 mg/day PO divided q8h. Chemoprophylaxis after high-risk exposure given in combination with zidovudine and lamivudine. Administer on an empty stomach 1 hr before or 2 hr after a meal to decrease food effect.	*Cautions:* Nephrolithiasis, nausea, hyperbilirubinemia, headache, diabetes. Reduce dose by ~25% with mild to moderate liver dysfunction. *Drug interactions:* Didanosine decreases absorption; rifampin reduces levels; ketoconazole, ritonavir, and other protease inhibitors decrease indinavir metabolism. Do not co-administer astemizole, cisapride, terfenadine.
Lamivudine Epivir, 3TC. Tablet: 150 mg. Solution: 10 mg/mL.	**Reverse transcriptase inhibitor used in combination with zidovudine and/or other anti-HIV drugs. Evolving experience with neonatal and pediatric dosing.** *Neonates:* 4 mg/kg/day PO divided q12h under study. *Children and adolescents:* 12 mg/kg/day PO divided q12h; max dose 150 mg. *Adult:* 300 mg/day PO divided q12h. Suggested chemoprophylaxis regimen for occupational exposure: 150 mg lamivudine PO q12h with zidovudine 200 mg PO q8h and indinavir 800 mg PO q8h.	*Cautions:* Headache, psychomotor disorders, nausea, feeding problems, abdominal pain, pancreatitis, neutropenia, musculoskeletal pain. Adjust dose in patients with creatinine clearance <30 mL/min. Medication may be administered with or without food. *Drug interactions:* Trimethoprim/sulfamethoxazole may increase 3TC levels.
Nelfinavir Viracept. Tablet: 250 mg. Suspension: 200 mg/5 mL.	**Protease inhibitor as monotherapy or preferably in combination with nucleoside analogs and other protease inhibitors. Evolving experience with neonatal and pediatric dosing.** *Neonates:* 30 mg/kg/day PO divided q8h under study. *Children/adolescents:* 60–90 mg/kg/day PO divided q8h. *Adults:* 750 mg/dose PO q8h. Administer with a meal to optimize absorption; avoid acidic food or drink (e.g., orange juice). Tablet can be dissolved in water to administer as a solution.	*Cautions:* Many adverse effects including hypertension, headaches, dizziness, diarrhea, anemia, leukopenia, hepatitis, iritis, dyspnea, sweating. *Drug interactions:* Rifampin, phenobarb, carbamazepin reduces levels; ketoconazole ritonavir, indinavir, and other protease inhibitors decrease nelfinavir metabolism. Do not co-administer astemizole, cisapride, terfenadine. May interfere with oral contraceptive hormones.
Nevirapine Viramune. Tablet: 200 mg.	**Non-nucleosides reverse transcriptase inhibitor specific for HIV-1 transcriptase (not HIV-2) or human polymerase. Evolving dosing experience with neonatal and pediatric dosing.** *Neonates:* 5 mg/kg PO qd for 14 days, then 240 mg/m²/day PO divided q12h for 14 days, then 400 mg/m²/day divided q12h. *Children:* 240 mg/m²/day PO divided q12h for 14 days; if tolerated increase dose to max dose 400 mg/m²/day PO divided q12h. *Adolescents/adult:* 200 mg PO qd for 14 days if tolerated 200 mg per dose q12h.	*Cautions:* Severe skin rash, Stevens-Johnson syndrome, headache, nausea, diarrhea, increased liver function tests. May give with or without food. *Drug interactions:* Nevirapine induces hepatic CYP450 3A activity and decreases indinavir, saquinavir concentrations; rifampin decreases nevirapine serum levels; cimetidine, macrolides block metabolism.
Ritonavir Novir. Capsule: 100 mg. Solution: 80 mg/mL.	**Protease inhibitor often effective against saquinavir and zidovudine-resistant virus; ritonavir-resistant strains often cross-resistant with other agents.** *Children:* 500 mg/m²/day PO divided q12h, titrate upward in 50 mg/m² per dose increments to 800 mg/m²/day PO q12h. *Adolescents/adults:* 400–600 mg per dose PO q12h. Administer dose with food to enhance bioavailability.	*Cautions:* Headache, nausea, taste aversion, pancreatitis, elevated serum lipids, elevated liver function tests, hypoglycemia, rash *Drug interactions:* Ritonavir is a potent inhibitor of hepatic CYP450 enzyme activity leading to many important drug interactions, e.g., protease inhibitors, antiarrhythmics, antidepressants, cisapride.
Saquinavir Invirase Mesylate capsule: 200 mg. Gelatin capsule: 200 mg.	**Protease inhibitor. Dosing information in neonates, infants, and children is evolving.** *Children:* dose under study; 1,050–2,100 mg/m²/day PO divided q8h. *Adult:* Minimum of 1,800 mg/day—600 to 1,200 mg per dose PO q8h. Administration with a high-fat meal enhances bioavailability. Concurrent grapefruit juice may increase bioavailability.	*Cautions:* Photosensitivity, changes in blood pressure, confusion, ataxia, nausea, elevated liver function tests, rash, marrow suppression, bleeding. *Drug interactions:* Rifampin, phenobarb, carbamazepine decreases serum levels; saquinavir may decrease metabolism of calcium channel antagonists; azoles (e.g., ketoconazole), macrolides, indinavir, ritonavir may increase levels.

TABLE 728–6 Antiretroviral-HIV Medications *Continued*

Drug (Trade Names, Formulations)	Indications (Mechanism of Action) and Dosing	Comments
Stavudine Zerit; d4T. Capsule: 15 mg, 20 mg, 30 mg, 40 mg. Powder for oral suspension.	**Nucleoside analog reverse transcriptase inhibitor. Dosing information in neonates and infants is evolving.** *Children <30 kg:* 2 mg/kg/day PO divided q12h. *Adolescent/adult:* 30–60 kg 30 mg per dose PO q12h; >60 kg 40 mg per dose PO q12h.	*Cautions:* Peripheral neuropathy, headache, nausea, pancreatitis, elevated liver function tests, rash. Primary renal elimination. *Drug interactions:* Other drugs associated with peripheral neuropathy (e.g., cisplatin, gold, INH).
Zalcitabine Hivid; ddc. Tablet: 0.375 mg, 0.75 mg.	**Nucleoside analog reverse transcriptase inhibitor. Dosing information in neonates, infants, and children is evolving.** *Children:* 0.015–0.03 mg/kg/day PO divided q8h. *Adolescents/adult:* 0.75 mg per dose PO q8h.	*Cautions:* Cumulative dose-related peripheral neuropathy, pancreatitis. Cardiac dysfunction, lactic acidosis, marrow suppression, hepatitis, jaundice, rash. Primary renal elimination. *Drug interactions:* Magnesium and aluminum antacids, metoclopramide may decrease absorption; other drugs associated with peripheral neuropathy (e.g., cisplatin, gold, INH).
Zidovudine Retrovir, AZT, ZDV. Capsule: 100 mg. Tablet: 300 mg. Syrup: 50 mg/5 mL. Injection.	**Nucleoside analog reverse transcriptase inhibitor. Dosing information in premature neonates is evolving.** *Neonates:* 8 mg/kg/day PO divided q6h; 6 mg/kg/day IV divided q6h. *Infant/child:* 270–540 mg/m²/day PO divided q6–8h; 480 mg/m²/day IV divided q6h; continuous infusion 20 mg/m²/hr. *Child >12 yr/adult:* 200 mg per dose PO 8 hr or 300 mg per dose PO q12h; 1–2 mg/kg per dose IV q4h.	*Cautions:* Headache, seizure, lactic acidosis, diarrhea, bone marrow suppression, cholestatic hepatitis, rash. Primarily renal elimination. Infuse IV over 1 hr at a final concentration of 4 mg/mL. *Drug interactions:* Rifampin may increase metabolism; cimetidine, fluconazole, valproic acid may decrease metabolism.

TABLE 728–7 Antiparasitic Medications

Drug (Trade Names, Formulations)	Indications (Mechanism of Action) and Dosing	Comments
Atovaquone Mepron. Suspension: 750 mg/5 mL.	**Alternative therapy for mild to moderate *Pneumocystis carinii* pneumonia in patients intolerant of trimethoprim/sulfamethoxazole. Very limited experience with the drug in children.** *Children <40 kg:* 30–40 mg/kg/day PO once daily. *Children >40 kg and adults:* 750 mg/dose PO 3 times daily for 21 days. Administer doses with food.	*Cautions:* Dizziness, fever, rash, elevations in liver enzymes, neutropenia. Drug absorption increased when co-administered with food. *Drug interaction:* Rifampin may decrease levels.
Chloroquine Phosphate Aralen, Generic. Tablets: 250 mg (contains 150 mg base) and 500 mg (contains 300 mg base). Injection.	**Effective in the suppression and treatment of malaria and extraintestinal amebiasis. Dose drug on base equivalent.** **Malaria prophylaxis:** *Child:* 5 mg/kg/wk PO (max dose 300 mg/dose). *Adult:* 300 mg/wk PO. **Acute malaria treatment:** *Child:* 10 mg/kg PO initial dose (max dose 600 mg); 5 mg/kg 6 hr later then 5 mg/kg PO once daily for 2 days. IM 5 mg/kg initial dose, 5 mg/kg 6 hr later (max IM dose 10 mg/kg/24 hr). *Adult:* 600 mg PO initially, 300 mg 6 hr later then 300 mg PO once daily for 2 days. **Extraintestinal amebiasis:** *Child:* 10 mg/kg PO daily for 2–3 wk (max daily dose 300 mg). *Adult:* 600 mg PO once daily for 2 days then 300 mg once daily for 2–3 wk.	*Cautions:* Hypotension, headache, confusion, psychotic episodes, rash, peripheral neuropathy, blood dyscrasias, retinopathy, tinnitus. Administer with meals to decrease GI upset. Liquid may be prepared from tablets using strong flavoring agent (cherry or chocolate) to mask bitter taste.
Furazoladone Furoxone. Tablet: 100 mg. Suspension: 50 mg/15 mL.	**Effective in the treatment of protozoal diarrhea, enteritis.** *Infants >1 mo and children:* 5–9 mg/kg/day PO divided q6h (max daily dose 400 mg). *Adult:* 100 mg per dose PO q6h.	*Cautions:* May cause hemolytic anemia in infants <1 mo of age; caution in G6PD, hypotension, nausea, vomiting, hypoglycemia, hypersensitivity reactions, pulmonary infiltration. *Drug interactions:* MAO inhibitors; disuliram-like alcohol reaction.
Lindane Kwell, Scabene. Lotion: 1%. Shampoo: 1%.	**Topical treatment for scabies, head lice *(Pediculus capitis)*, crab lice *(Pediculus pubis)*.** *Scabies:* Apply thin layer to affected area, remove (shower) in 6–8 hr in children and after 18–24 hr in adults. *Pediculosis:* Shampoo with adequate amount (15–30 mL) and lather for 5 min then rise thoroughly and comb.	*Cautions:* Dermal absorption may cause seizures, dizziness, hepatitis, blood dyscrasias. Do not apply to denuded/inflamed skin; avoid contact to eyes/mucous membranes.
Mebendazole Vermox, Generic. Chewable tablet: 100 mg.	**Treatment of ascariasis (roundworm), hookworm, enterobiasis (pinworm), trichuriasis (whipworm).** *Children and adults:* Pinworm: 100 mg PO once; may repeat in 2 wk. Hookworm/roundworm/whipworm: 100 mg PO q12h for 3 consecutive days; 2nd course, if need, in 3–4 wk. Capillariasis: 200 mg PO q12h for 3 wk.	*Cautions:* Very well tolerated; dizziness, nausea, rash, leukopenia, transient elevation in liver function tests. Enhanced absorption when administered with food. Tablets may be chewed or swallowed whole.

Table continued on following page

TABLE 728–7 Antiparasitic Medications *Continued*

Drug (Trade Names, Formulations)	Indications (Mechanism of Action) and Dosing	Comments
Metronidazole Flagyl, Metro-IV, Generic. Topical gel, vaginal gel. Tablet: 250 mg, 500 mg. Injection.	**Effective in the treatment of anaerobic and protozoal infections particularly, amebiasis, giardiasis, trichomoniasis.** **Amebiasis** *Children:* 35–50 mg/kg/day PO divided q8h. *Adult:* 500–750 mg per dose PO q8h. **Other parasitic infections** *Children:* 15–30 mg/kg/day PO divided q8h. *Adult:* 250 mg per dose PO q8h; alternate dose 2 g single-dose therapy.	*Cautions:* Dizziness, seizures, metallic taste, nausea, disulfiram-like reaction with alcohol. Administer IV slow over 30–60 min. *Drug interactions:* Carbamazepine, rifampin, phenobarb may enhance metabolism; may increase levels of warfarin, phenytoin, lithium.
Niclosamide Niclocide. Chewable tablet: 500 mg.	**Effective in the treatment of tapeworm infections (beef, fish, dog/cat, and dwarf tapeworms). Drug active against intestinal cestodes only.** **Beef and fish tapeworm:** *Child:* 40 mg/kg PO once; max dose 2 g. *Adult:* 2 g PO single dose. May repeat in 7 days. **Dwarf tapeworm:** *Child:* 40 mg/kg PO qd for 7 days (max daily dose 2 g). *Adult:* 2 g PO qd for 7 days.	*Cautions:* Dizziness, headache, rash, alopecia, abdominal pain, nausea. Patients should chew tablets completely. *Drug interactions:* Hepatic enzyme inducers may enhance metabolism (e.g., carbamazepine, rifampin, phenobarb).
Pentamidine Isethionate Pentam, NebuPent. Inhalation, injection.	**For the treatment and prevention of *Pneumocystis carinii* pneumonia usually in patients intolerant of Co-trimox (trimethoprim/sulfamethoxazole).** ***Pneumocystis carinii* pneumonia treatment:** *Infant/child/adult:* 4 mg/kg/day IM or IV for 14–21 days. ***Pneumocystis carinii* prophylaxis:** *Children and adults:* 4 mg/kg/dose IM, IV every 2–4 wk. Aerosol once/mo using Respigard II nebulizer: *Infant:* use dose formula (2.27 mg/kg pentamidine) × [nebulizer output (L/min)] × patient body weight (kg) divided by alveolar ventilation (L/min). *Child >5 yr:* 300 mg per dose every 4 wk. *Adult:* 300 mg every 4 wk.	*Cautions:* Hypotension, tachycardia, dizziness, hypoglycemia, nausea, marrow suppression, pain at injection site, nephrotoxicity, irritation of airway, cough, bronchospasm with aerosol. Adjust dose with renal dysfunction. *Drug interactions:* Other nephrotoxins (aminoglycosides, vancomycin, amphoB, cyclosporine).
Permethrin Elimite, Nix. Cream: 5%. Creme rinse: 1%.	**Topical treatment for scabies, head lice *(Pediculus capitis)*, crab lice *(Pediculis pubis)*.** **Head lice:** *Children and adults:* wash areas, rinse, apply creme rinse liberally, leave on hair for 10-min, rinse and comb. May repeat treatment in 7 days. **Scabies:** *Children and adults:* apply leaving on for 8–16 hr before removing with water.	*Cautions:* Dermal absorption unlikely. Do not apply to denuded/inflamed skin; avoid contact to eyes/mucous membranes. May cause rash.
Piperazine Citrate Vermizine, Generic. Tablet: 250 mg.	**Alternative therapy for pinworm and roundworm.** **Pinworm:** *Children and adults:* 65 mg/kg/day PO once daily for 7 days; may repeat course in 7 days. **Roundworm:** *Children and adults:* 75 mg/kg/day PO once daily for 2 days (max dose 3.5 g/day); may repeat course in 7 days.	*Cautions:* Neurotoxicity, dizziness, seizures, tremor, visual disturbances, allergic reactions.
Praziquantel Biltricide. Tablet: 600 mg.	**Effective in all stages of schistosomiasis and many intestinal tapeworm and trematode infestations.** **Schistosomiasis:** *Children and adults:* 20 mg/kg/dose PO q8h for 1 day. **Trematodes:** *Children and adults:* 75 mg/kg/day PO divided q8h for 1–2 days. **Tapeworm:** *Children and adults:* 5–10 mg/kg as a single dose.	*Cautions:* Central nervous system depression, dizziness, fever, rash, abdominal pain, eosinophilia. *Drug interaction:* Alcohol may increase CNS depression.
Primaquine Phosphate Tablet: 26 mg (15 mg base).	**Effective in the prevention and treatment of malaria. Dose drug on base equivalent.** *Child:* 0.3 mg base/kg/day PO once daily for 14 days (max daily dose 15 mg). *Adult:* 15 mg PO once daily for 14 days.	*Cautions:* Pruritus, abdominal complaints, anemia, methemoglobinemia. Caution in patients with G6PD or NADH methemoglobin reductase deficiency.
Pyrantel Pamoate Antiminth; Pin-Rid. Capsule: 180 mg. Liquid: 50 mg/mL. Suspension: 50 mg/mL.	**Treatment of ascariasis (roundworm) hookworm, enterobiasis (pinworm), and trichostrongyliasis infections.** *Children and adults:* Pinworm, roundworm, trichostrongyliasis: 100 mg PO once; may repeat in 2 wk. Hookworm/roundworm/whipworm: 11 mg/kg PO single dose (max dose 1 g); may repeat in 2 wk for pinworm infestation. Hookworm: 11 mg/kg PO once daily for 3 consecutive days (max dose 1 g/day).	*Cautions:* Rash, elevation in liver function tests, abdominal cramps, dizziness, headache. *Drug interaction:* Possible antagonism of piperazine activity.

TABLE 728–7 Antiparasitic Medications *Continued*

Drug (Trade Names, Formulations)	Indications (Mechanism of Action) and Dosing	Comments
Pyrimethamine Daraprim. Tablet: 25 mg.	**Prophylaxis and in combination with other drugs for the treatment of malaria in combination with sulfa in treatment of toxoplasmosis and in combination with dapsone for prophylaxis against *P. carinii* infection in HIV patients.** **Malaria prophylaxis:** begin drug 2 wk before entering endemic areas. Use for malaria decreasing due to increased resistance and side effects. *Child:* 0.5 mg/kg once wk (max dose 25 mg). Chloroquine-resistant malaria (with quinine and sulfa). **Toxoplasmosis** (with sulfadiazine): *Children:* 2 mg/kg/day PO divided q12h for 2–3 days then 1 mg/kg/day PO qd with sulfadiazine for 6 mo then 1 mg/kg/day PO qd 3 times/wk max daily dose 25 mg/day). *Adult:* 50–75 mg plus 1–4 g sulfadiazine PO 3 times/wk. ***Toxoplasma gondii* prophylaxis:** *Infant >1 mo:* 1 mg/kg/day PO qd plus dapsone. *Adolescents/adult:* 50 mg PO once weekly plus dapsone. ***Pneumocystis carinii* prophylaxis:** *Adolescent/adult:* 50–75 mg PO once wk plus dapsone.	*Cautions:* Administer folinic acid (5–10 mg/kg 3 times wk) to prevent hematologic toxicity; seizures, headache, photosensitivity, rash, folic acid deficiency, marrow suppression, tremor. Tablets may be crushed to prepare an extemporaneous suspension formulation.
Quinine Quinamm, Generic. Capsule: 165 mg, 200 mg, 300 mg, 325 mg. Tablet: 162.5 mg, 260 mg.	**Antimalarial agent with decreasing effectiveness as resistance increasingly develops.** **Chloroquine-resistant malaria:** *Child:* 30 mg/kg/day PO divided q8h for 3–7 days with another antimalarial agent. *Adult:* 650 mg per dose PO q8h for 3–7 days with another antimalarial agent.	*Cautions:* G6PD hemolysis, flushing, tachycardia, fever, headache, rash, nausea, tinnitus, cinchonism. *Drug interactions:* Interferes with digoxin disposition; aluminum-containing antacids decrease absorption.

728.1 Herbal Medicines

Herbal remedies are alternative medications commonly used throughout the world. In addition to various ethnic groups who use folk remedies, most people purchase medicinal herbs from proprietary drug and food supplement stores. As many as 11% of all children in the United States have been treated with these remedies; many of these remedies have no efficacy, whereas others are potentially toxic. Most families do not believe that herbs can be dangerous and are often frustrated about modern prescribed medications that they perceive not to work (e.g., antibiotics for viral upper respiratory tract infections).

Herbs as classified by the 1994 Dietary Supplement and Health Education Act (DSHEA) do not have to be proven effective or safe, nor do they have rigorous quality control. Indeed, bioavailability is not guaranteed; at times there is no active drug or, less often, other pharmacologically active drugs are mixed with the herb (nonsteroidal anti-inflammatory agents, steroids, heavy metals). The herb cannot claim a cure but can claim an effect. The label should state that the FDA has not evaluated the claims. Most herbal plants contain multiple active agents that vary in percent content in the flower, leaf, or root and from preparation to preparation, or in the source of the plant (United States, Europe, Asia). Commonly used over-the-counter herbs for children are cited in Table 728–8. Folk remedies are cited in Table 728–9.

Chan TYK: Monitoring the safety of herbal medicines. Drug Safety 17:209, 1997.
Crone CC, Wise TN: Use of herbal medicines among consultation-liaison populations. Psychosomatics 39:3, 1998.
Kemper K: Seven herbs every pediatrician should know. Contemp Pediatr December 1996, 679.
Shannon M: Herbal, traditional and alternative medicines. *In:* Haddad L, Shannon M, Winchester J (eds): Clinical Management of Poisoning and Drug Overdose, 3rd ed. Philadelphia, WB Saunders, 1998.
Winslow LC, Kroll DJ: Herbs as medicines. Arch Intern Med 158:2192, 1998.

TABLE 728–8 Herbal Remedies

Agent	Proposed Uses	Potential Efficacy	Toxicity
Aloe vera (gel)	Skin wounds, burns, frostbite, sun block, cosmetics, gastric and duodenal ulcers, AIDS, constipation, aphthous stomatitis.	Antibacterial effect on minor wounds. Canker sore healing.	Contact dermatitis. ?May impede healing in severe wounds. Nephritis, diarrhea, nausea, abdominal cramps.
Areca catechu (betel nut)	Similar to nicotine.	No known safe medical use	Cholinergic stimulant, CNS stimulant, high abuse potential, risk of oral/esophageal cancer.
Birch oil	Methyl-salicylate (oils may contain 90% salicylates), antipyretic, analgesic.	None—high toxicity	Salicylate intoxication, contact dermatitis, contraindicated in pregnancy and breast-feeding.
Chamomile AKA manzanilla (tea, tincture)	Antispasmodic (colic), irritable bowel, heartburn, uterine cramps, sedating (insomnia), diaper rash, poison ivy, chickenpox.	Colic, calming effects	Generally safe. Urticaria, angioedema. Excessive fluids may produce water intoxication.

Table continued on following page

TABLE 728–8 Herbal Remedies

Agent	Proposed Uses	Potential Efficacy	Toxicity
Cranberry	Oligosaccharides inhibit *E. coli* fimbriae attachment to bladder.	UTI prophylaxis	Diarrhea if excessive PO, not intended for UTI treatment.
Echinacea (tincture, capsules, tablets)	Immune stimulant (upper respiratory tract infections, HIV), aphthous stomatitis, inflammatory bowel disease, yeast infections, anti-inflammatory effects.	In adults, decreased number of colds (15%); prevents recurrences of genital yeast infections in women if taken with antifungal agent. No proven efficacy in children.	Generally safe. Allergic reactions, tachyphylaxis. Tincture may contain 70% alcohol.
Ephedra AKA ma-huang, herbal ecstasy, Mormon tea	Ephedrine-like. Appetite suppressant (weight loss), decongestant, bronchodilator (asthma), diuretics, uterine contractions. Intoxication—high.	None—traditional medications have better safety record.	Dangerous! Hypertension, tachycardia, anxiety, headache, seizures, coma, psychosis, uterine cramps. Death from overdose.
Feverfew (leaves, capsules)	Migraine prevention, menstrual cramps, arthritis, insect repellent, anti-inflammatory, spasmolytic, antipyretic.	May prevent migraines in adults after 4–6 wk use.	NSAIDS may block its effects. GI upset, tachycardia, rebound headaches if discontinued, allergic reactions, inhibit platelet action.
Ginkgo biloba AKA maidenhair tree	Migraines, depression, heart failure, platelet inhibition, dementia—memory.	Improves or delays defects in Alzheimer patients.	Headache, caution in patients with seizures and bleeding.
Ginseng	Sympathomimetic, aphrodisiac, stimulant (chronic fatigue), athletic performance, digestive aid, oxygen free radical scavenger.	None in children. Lowers fasting blood glucose in adults with diabetes.	Diarrhea, nausea, emesis, anxiety, insomnia, dermatitis, depression, amenorrhea, hypertension, mastalgia. ?Neonatal androgen effect.
Goldenseal (tincture, extract)	Immune stimulation, antimicrobial (common cold, skin infections, eczema, diarrhea, acne, conjunctivitis).	Diarrhea secondary to giardiasis, toxigenic *E. coli*, wound healing.	Hypertension, local irritation, nausea, emesis, displaces bilirubin from albumin, CNS depression.
St. John's wort	Wounds, burns, mild monoamine (MAOI) or serotonin uptake inhibition (SSRI) (anxiety, depression).	Depression in adults.	Photosensitivity; caution with prescribed MAOI or SSRI drugs. Self-diagnosis and treatment of depression—dangerous.
Valerian (tincture)	Anxiolytic, sedative (insomnia), glutamate precursor to GABA.	Mild hypnotic.	Morning drowsiness; avoid with alcohol or barbiturates; hepatotoxic, hallucinogenic.

This table was created with the help of Dr. E. Stremski, Director, Poison Control Center, Children's Hospital of Wisconsin, Milwaukee, WI.

TABLE 728–9 Common Folk Medicines by Cultural Origin

Name	Contents	Potential Toxicity
Hispanic		
Siete jarabes	Almond, castor oil, tolu, wild cherry licorice, cocillana, honey	GI upset, catharsis, electrolyte disturbances
Agua maravilla	Witch hazel, ethanol	Ethanol toxicity
Jarabe maguey	Maguey *(Agave* spp.)	GI upset
Alcanfor	Camphor	Camphor toxicity
Azarcon	Lead	Lead intoxication
Greta	Lead	Lead intoxication
Azogue	Elemental mercury	Mercury intoxication
Ipecacuanha	Ipecac	Vomiting, myopathy
Southeast Asian		
Paylooah	Lead	Lead intoxication
Indian and Ayurvedic		
Surma	Lead	Lead intoxication
Deshi Dawa	Lead	Lead intoxication

Reprinted with permission from Shannon MW: Herbal medicine and miscellaneous agents. In: *Haddad LM, Shannon MW, Winchester JF (eds): Clinical Management of Poisoning and Drug Overdose,* 3rd ed. Philadelphia, WB Saunders, 1998.

INDEX

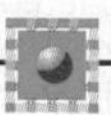

Note: Page numbers in *italics* refer to illustrations; page numbers followed by t refer to tables.

ISBN 0-7216-7767-3